Optum

ICD-10-CM Professional for Hospitals

The complete official code set
Codes valid from October 1, 2024
through September 30, 2025

2025

optumcoding.com

Publisher's Notice

The *ICD-10-CM Professional for Hospitals: The Complete Official Code Set* is designed to be an accurate and authoritative source regarding coding and every reasonable effort has been made to ensure accuracy and completeness of the content. However, Optum makes no guarantee, warranty, or representation that this publication is accurate, complete or without errors. It is understood that Optum is not rendering any legal or other professional services or advice in this publication and that Optum bears no liability for any results or consequences that may arise from the use of this book.

Acknowledgments

Marianne Randall, CPC, *Senior Product Manager*
Anita Schmidt, BS, RHIA, AHIMA-approved ICD-10-CM/PCS Trainer, *Subject Matter Expert*
LaJuana Green, RHIA, CCS, *Subject Matter Expert*
Leanne Patterson, CPC, *Subject Matter Expert*
Jacqueline R. Petersen, MHA, RHIA, CHDA, CPC, *Subject Matter Expert*
Laura M. Anderson, RN, BSN, CCDS, *Subject Matter Expert*
Tara Rose, CPC, CPC-I, CPMA, RHIA, CCS-P, *Subject Matter Expert*
Stacy Perry, *Manager, Desktop Publishing*
Tracy Betzler, *Senior Desktop Publishing Specialist*
Hope M. Dunn, *Senior Desktop Publishing Specialist*
Katie Russell, *Desktop Publishing Specialist*
Kate Holden, *Editor*

Our Commitment to Accuracy

Optum is committed to producing accurate and reliable materials.

To report corrections, please email customerassistance@optum.com. You can also reach customer service by calling 1.800.464.3649, option 1.

Anita Schmidt, BS, RHIA, AHIMA-approved ICD-10-CM/PCS Trainer

Ms. Schmidt has expertise in ICD-10-CM/PCS, DRG, and CPT with more than 20 years' experience in coding in multiple settings, including inpatient, observation, and same-day surgery. Her experience includes analysis of medical record documentation, assignment of ICD-10-CM and PCS codes, and DRG validation. She has collaborated with clinical documentation specialists to identify documentation needs and potential areas for physician education. Most recently she has been developing content for resource and educational products related to ICD-10-CM, ICD-10-PCS, DRG, and CPT. Ms. Schmidt is an AHIMA-approved ICD-10-CM/PCS trainer and is an active member of the American Health Information Management Association (AHIMA) and the Minnesota Health Information Management Association (MHIMA).

Laura M. Anderson, RN, BSN, CCDS

Ms. Anderson is a Registered Nurse and CDI Specialist/Educator with more than 20 years of experience in the healthcare profession. She obtained her BSN at the University of Minnesota and spent most of her bedside nursing career on Medical-Surgical care units. Her clinical documentation experience began in 2007, covering CDI specialist training, education development, and physician engagement. She has served as a CDI Team Lead and consultant, working with senior leadership to incorporate CDI work into documentation compliance and quality metrics. Ms. Anderson also has a BS degree in Biology (Winthrop University), with research experience in liver cancer and radiation-induced leukemia. She has presented at the state and national levels for the Association of Clinical Documentation Integrity Specialists (ACDIS) and has served as a co-lead for the Minnesota state chapter.

2025 ICD-10-CM Official Guidelines for Coding and Reporting

Optum is pleased to provide you with this 2025 ICD-10-CM code book that INCLUDES the 2025 Official Guidelines for Coding and Reporting.

Product Updates

Significant updates to this manual will also be provided on our product updates page at Optumcoding.com, which can be accessed at the following:
https://www.optumcoding.com/ProductUpdates/
Password: HOSPITAL25

Contents

Introduction

ICD-10-CM Professional for Hospitals: The Complete Official Code Set is your definitive coding resource, combining the work of the National Center for Health Statistics (NCHS), Centers for Medicare and Medicaid Services (CMS), American Hospital Association (AHA), and Optum experts to provide the information you need for coding accuracy.

The International Classification of Diseases, 10th Revision, Clinical Modification (ICD-10-CM), is an adaptation of ICD-10, copyrighted by the World Health Organization (WHO). The development and maintenance of this clinical modification (CM) is the responsibility of the NCHS as authorized by WHO. Any new concepts added to ICD-10-CM are based on an established update process through the collaboration of WHO's Update and Revision Committee and the ICD-10-CM Coordination and Maintenance Committee.

In addition to the ICD-10-CM classification, other official government source information has been included in this manual. Depending on the source, updates to information may be annual or quarterly. This manual provides the most current information that was available at the time of publication. For updates to the source documents that may have occurred after this manual was published, please refer to the following:

- **NCHS, International Classification of Diseases, Tenth Revision, Clinical Modification (ICD-10-CM)**

  https://www.cms.gov/medicare/coding-billing/icd-10-codes/2025-icd-10-cm

- **CMS Inpatient Prospective Payment System Proposed Rule and v42 MS-DRG Data Files, FY 2025**

  https://www.cms.gov/medicare/payment/prospective-payment-systems/acute-inpatient-pps/fy-2025-ipps-proposed-rule-home-page

  https://www.cms.gov/medicare/payment/prospective-payment-systems/acute-inpatient-pps/ms-drg-classifications-and-software

- **CMS Risk Adjustment Model, version 28**

  https://www.cms.gov/Medicare/Health-Plans/MedicareAdvtgSpecRateStats/Risk-Adjustors

- **CMS Long-term Care Hospital Prospective Payment System Proposed Rule and Data Files, FY 2025**

  https://www.cms.gov/medicare/payment/prospective-payment-systems/long-term-care-hospital/regulations-notices/cms-1808-p

- **AHA Coding Clinics**

  https://www.codingclinicadvisor.com/

Significant updates to this manual will be provided on our product updates page at Optumcoding.com, which can be accessed at the following:

  https://www.optumcoding.com/ProductUpdates/
  Password: HOSPITAL25

The official NCHS ICD-10-CM classification includes three main sections: the guidelines, the indexes, and the tabular list, all of which make up the bulk of this coding manual. To complement the classification, Optum's coding experts have incorporated Medicare-related coding edits and proprietary features, such as supplementary notations, coding tools, and appendixes, into a comprehensive and easy-to-use reference. This publication is organized as follows:

What's New for 2025

This section provides a high-level overview of the code changes made for FY 2025. The list of codes provided identifies new, revised, and deleted codes. Asterisked codes identify prior midyear changes that were made to the classification, effective April 1, 2024. All changes are based on an official addendum, provided by the NCHS.

Conversion Table

The conversion table was developed by NCHS to help facilitate data retrieval as new codes are added to the ICD-10-CM classification. This table provides a crosswalk from each FY 2025 new code to the equivalent code(s) assigned, prior to October 1, 2024, for that diagnosis or condition. Asterisked codes identify prior midyear additions, effective April 1, 2024. For the full conversion table, refer to the Conversion Table zip file at https://www.cms.gov/medicare/coding-billing/icd-10-codes/2025-icd-10-cm.

10 Steps to Correct Coding

This step-by-step tutorial walks the coder through the process of finding the correct code — from locating the code in the official indexes to verifying the code in the tabular section — while following applicable conventions, guidelines, and instructional notes. Specific examples are provided with detailed explanations of each coding step along with advice for proper sequencing.

Official ICD-10-CM Guidelines for Coding and Reporting

This section provides the full official conventions and guidelines regulating the appropriate assignment and reporting of ICD-10-CM codes. These conventions and guidelines are published by the U.S. Department of Health and Human Services (DHHS) and approved by the cooperating parties (American Health Information Management Association [AHIMA], NCHS, Centers for Disease Control and Prevention [CDC], and the American Hospital Association [AHA]).

Indexes

Index to Diseases and Injuries

The Index to Diseases and Injuries is arranged in alphabetic order by terms specific to a disease, condition, illness, injury, eponym, or abbreviation as well as terms that describe circumstances other than a disease or injury that may require attention from a health care professional.

Neoplasm Table

The Neoplasm Table is arranged in alphabetic order by anatomical site. Codes are then listed in individual columns based upon the histological behavior (malignant, in situ, benign, uncertain, or unspecified) of the neoplasm.

Table of Drugs and Chemicals

The Table of Drugs and Chemicals is arranged in alphabetic order by the specific drug or chemical name. Codes are listed in individual columns based upon the associated intent (poisoning, adverse effect, or underdosing). **Note:** Drugs with an asterisk identify substances added to the table by Optum subject matter experts.

External Causes Index

The External Causes Index is arranged in alphabetic order by main terms that describe the cause, the intent, the place of occurrence, the activity, and the status of the patient at the time the injury occurred or health condition arose.

Index Notations

With

The word "with" or "in" should be interpreted to mean "associated with" or "due to." The classification presumes a causal relationship between the two conditions linked by these terms in the index. These conditions should be coded as related even in the absence of provider documentation explicitly linking them unless the documentation clearly states the conditions are unrelated or when another guideline specifically requires a documented linkage between two conditions (e.g., the sepsis guideline for "acute organ dysfunction that is not clearly associated with the sepsis"). For conditions not specifically linked by these relational terms in the classification or when a guideline requires explicit documentation of a linkage between two conditions, provider documentation must link the conditions to code them as related.

The word "with" in the index is sequenced immediately following the main term, not in alphabetical order.

> **Dermatopolymyositis** M33.9Ø
> with
> myopathy M33.92
> respiratory involvement M33.91
> specified organ involvement NEC M33.99
> amyopathic M33.93

See

When the instruction "see" follows a term in the index, it indicates that another term must be referenced to locate the correct code.

> **Hematoperitoneum** — *see* Hemoperitoneum

See Also

The instructional note "see also" simply provides alternative terms the coder may reference that may be useful in determining the correct code but are not necessary to follow if the main term supplies the appropriate code.

> **Hematinuria** — *see also* Hemaglobinuria
> malarial B5Ø.8

Default Codes

In the index, the default code is the code listed next to the main term and represents the condition most commonly associated with that main term. This code may be assigned when documentation does not support reporting a more specific code. Alternatively, it may provide an unspecified code for the condition.

> **Hemiatrophy** R68.89
> cerebellar G31.9
> face, facial, progressive (Romberg) G51.8
> tongue K14.8

Parentheses

Parentheses in the indexes enclose nonessential modifiers, supplementary words that may be present or absent in the statement of a disease without affecting the code.

> **Pseudomeningocele** (cerebral) (infective) (post-traumatic) G96.198
> postprocedural (spinal) G97.82

Brackets

ICD-10-CM has a coding convention addressing code assignment for manifestations that occur as a result of an underlying condition. This convention requires the underlying condition to be sequenced first, followed by the code or codes for the associated manifestation. In the index, italicized codes in brackets identify manifestation codes.

> **Polyneuropathy** (peripheral) G62.9
> alcoholic G62.1
> amyloid (Portuguese) E85.1 *[G63]*
> transthyretin-related (ATTR) familial E85.1 *[G63]*

Shaded Guides

Exclusive vertical shaded guides in the Index to Diseases and Injuries and External Causes Index help the user easily follow the indent levels for the subentries under a main term. Sequencing rules may apply depending on the level of indent for separate subentries.

> **Hemicrania**
> congenital malformation QØØ.Ø
> continua G44.51
> meaning migraine — *see also* Migraine G43.9Ø9
> paroxysmal G44.Ø39
> chronic G44.Ø49
> intractable G44.Ø41
> not intractable G44.Ø49
> episodic G44.Ø39
> intractable G44.Ø31
> not intractable G44.Ø39
> intractable G44.Ø31
> not intractable G44.Ø39

Following References

The Index to Diseases and Injuries includes "following" references to assist in locating out-of-sequence codes in the tabular list. Out-of-sequence codes contain an alphabetic character (letter) in the third- or fourth-character position. These codes are placed according to the classification rules — according to condition — not according to alphabetic or numeric sequencing rules.

> **Carcinoma** (malignant) — *see also* Neoplasm, by site, malignant
> neuroendocrine — *see also* Tumor, neuroendocrine
> high grade, any site C7A.1 *(following C75)*
> poorly differentiated, any site C7A.1 *(following C75)*

Additional Character Required

The Index to Diseases and Injuries, Neoplasm Table, and External Causes Index provide an icon after certain codes to signify to the user that additional characters are required to make the code valid. The tabular list should be consulted for appropriate character selection.

> **Fall, falling** (accidental) W19 ☑
> building W2Ø.1 ☑

Tabular List of Diseases

ICD-10-CM codes and descriptions are arranged numerically within the tabular list of diseases with 19 separate chapters providing codes associated with a particular body system or nature of injury or disease. There is also a chapter providing codes for external causes of an injury or health conditions, a chapter for codes that address encounters with healthcare facilities for circumstances other than a disease or injury, and finally a chapter for codes that capture special circumstances such as new diseases of uncertain etiology or emergency use codes.

Code and Code Descriptions

ICD-10-CM is an alphanumeric classification system that contains categories, subcategories, and valid codes. The first character is always a letter with any additional characters represented by either a letter or number. A three-character category without further subclassification is equivalent to a valid three-character code. Valid codes may be three, four, five, six, or seven characters in length, with each level of subdivision after a three-character category representing a subcategory. The final level of subdivision is a valid code.

Boldface

Boldface type is used for all codes and descriptions in the tabular list.

Italics

Italicized type is used to identify manifestation codes, those codes that should not be reported as first-listed diagnoses.

Deleted Text

~~Strikethrough~~ on a code and code description indicates a deletion from the classification for the current year.

Key Word

Green font is used throughout the Tabular List of Diseases to differentiate the key words that appear in similar code descriptions in a given category or subcategory. The key word convention is used only in those categories in which there are multiple codes with very similar descriptions with only a few words that differentiate them.

For example, refer to the list of codes below from category H55:

✓4ᵗʰ	**H55**	**Nystagmus and other irregular eye movements**
✓5ᵗʰ	**H55.0**	**Nystagmus**
	H55.00	**Unspecified nystagmus**
	H55.01	**Congenital nystagmus**
	H55.02	**Latent nystagmus**
	H55.03	**Visual deprivation nystagmus**
	H55.04	**Dissociated nystagmus**
	H55.09	**Other forms of nystagmus**

The portion of the code description that appears in **green font** in the tabular list helps the coder quickly identify the key terms and the correct code. This convention is especially useful when the codes describe laterality, such as the following codes from subcategory H40.22:

✓6ᵗʰ	**H40.22**	**Chronic angle-closure glaucoma**
		Chronic primary angle closure glaucoma
✓7ᵗʰ	**H40.221**	**Chronic angle-closure glaucoma, right eye**
✓7ᵗʰ	**H40.222**	**Chronic angle-closure glaucoma, left eye**
✓7ᵗʰ	**H40.223**	**Chronic angle-closure glaucoma, bilateral**
✓7ᵗʰ	**H40.229**	**Chronic angle-closure glaucoma, unspecified eye**

Tabular Notations

Official parenthetical notes as well as Optum's supplementary notations are provided at the chapter, code block, category, subcategory, and individual code level to help the user assign proper codes. The information in the notation can apply to one or more codes depending on where the citation is placed.

Official Notations

Includes Notes

The word INCLUDES appears immediately under certain categories to further define, clarify, or give examples of the content of a code category.

Inclusion Terms

Lists of inclusion terms are included under certain codes. These terms indicate some of the conditions for which that code number may be used. Inclusion terms may be synonyms with the code title, or, in the case of "other specified" codes, the terms may also provide a list of various conditions included within a classification code. The inclusion terms are not exhaustive. The index may provide additional terms that may also be assigned to a given code.

Excludes Notes

ICD-10-CM has two types of excludes notes. Each note has a different definition for use. However, they are similar in that they both indicate that codes excluded from each other are independent of each other.

Excludes 1

An EXCLUDES 1 note is a "pure" excludes. It means "NOT CODED HERE!" An Excludes 1 note indicates mutually exclusive codes: two conditions that cannot be reported together. An Excludes1 note indicates that the code excluded should never be used at the same time as the code above the Excludes1 note. An Excludes1 is used when two conditions cannot occur together, such as a congenital form versus an acquired form of the same condition.

An exception to the Excludes 1 definition is when the two conditions are unrelated to each other. If it is not clear whether the two conditions involving an Excludes 1 note are related or not, query the provider. For example, code F45.8 Other somatoform disorders, has an Excludes 1 note for "sleep related teeth grinding (G47.63)" because "teeth grinding" is an inclusion term under F45.8. Only one of these two codes should be assigned for teeth grinding. However, psychogenic dysmenorrhea is also an inclusion term under F45.8, and a patient could have both this condition and sleep-related teeth grinding. In this case, the two conditions are clearly unrelated to each other, so it would be appropriate to report F45.8 and G47.63 together.

Excludes 2

An EXCLUDES 2 note means "NOT INCLUDED HERE." An Excludes 2 note indicates that although the excluded condition is not part of the condition it is excluded from, a patient may have both conditions at the same time. Therefore, when an Excludes 2 note appears under a code, it may be acceptable to use both the code and the excluded code together if supported by the medical documentation.

Note

The term "NOTE" appears as an icon and precedes the instructional information. These notes function as alerts to highlight coding instructions within the text.

Code First/Use additional code

These instructional notes provide sequencing instruction. They may appear independently of each other or to designate certain etiology/manifestation paired codes. These instructions signal the coder that an additional code should be reported to provide a more complete picture of that diagnosis.

In etiology/manifestation coding, ICD-10-CM requires the underlying condition to be sequenced first, followed by the manifestation. In these situations, codes with "In diseases classified elsewhere" in the code description are never permitted as a first-listed or principal diagnosis code and must be sequenced following the underlying condition code.

Code Also

A "code also" note alerts the coder that more than one code may be required to fully describe the condition. The sequencing depends on the circumstances of the encounter. Factors that may determine sequencing include severity and reason for the encounter.

Revised Text

The revised text ▶◀ "bow ties" alert the user to changes in official notations for the current year. Revised text may include the following:

- A change in a current parenthetical description
- A change in the code(s) associated with a current parenthetical note
- A change in how a current parenthetical note is classified (e.g., an Excludes 1 note that changed to an Excludes 2 note)
- Addition of a new parenthetical note(s) to a code

Deleted Text

~~Strikethrough~~ on official notations indicate a deletion from the classification for the current year.

Optum Notations

AHA Coding Clinic Citations

Coding Clinics are official American Hospital Association (AHA) publications that provide coding advice specific to ICD-10-CM and ICD-10-PCS.

Coding Clinic citations included in this manual are current up to the second quarter of 2024.

These citations identify the year, quarter, and page number of one or more *Coding Clinic* publications that may have coding advice relevant to a particular code or group of codes. With the most current citation listed first, these notations are preceded by the symbol **AHA:** and appear in purple type.

I15.1	**Hypertension secondary to other renal disorders**
	AHA: 2016, 3Q, 22

Definitions

Definitions explain a specific term, condition, or disease process in layman's terms. These notations are preceded by the symbol **DEF:** and appear in purple type.

✓5ᵗʰ **M51.4**	**Schmorl's nodes**
	DEF: Irregular bone defect in the margin of the vertebral body that causes herniation into the end plate of the vertebral body.

Coding Tips

The tips in the tabular list offer coding advice that is not readily available within the ICD-10-CM classification. It may relate official coding guidelines, indexing nuances, or advice from *AHA's Coding Clinic for ICD-10-CM/PCS*. These notations are preceded by the symbol **TIP:** and appear in brown type.

✓5ᵗʰ **M11.2**	**Other chondrocalcinosis**
	Chondrocalcinosis NOS
	AHA: 2018,3Q,20
	TIP: Pseudogout is captured with codes in this subcategory.

Icons

Note: The following icons are placed to the left of the code.

Changes to ICD-10-CM codes since the last published edition of this manual are highlighted in two ways:

The following green icons identify new or revised codes effective April 1, 2024:

- ● **New Code — Midyear**

- ▲ **Revised Code — Midyear**

The following black icons identify new or revised codes effective October 1, 2024:

- ● **New Code**

- ▲ **Revised Code**

- ☑ **Additional Characters Required**

    ✓4ᵗʰ This symbol indicates that the code requires a 4th character.

    ✓5ᵗʰ This symbol indicates that the code requires a 5th character.

    ✓6ᵗʰ This symbol indicates that the code requires a 6th character.

    ✓7ᵗʰ This symbol indicates that the code requires a 7th character.

✓5ᵗʰ **H60.3**	**Other infective otitis externa**	
✓6ᵗʰ **H60.31**	**Diffuse otitis externa**	
	H60.311	Diffuse otitis externa, **right** ear
	H60.312	Diffuse otitis externa, **left** ear
	H60.313	Diffuse otitis externa, **bilateral**
	H60.319	Diffuse otitis externa, unspecified ear

- ✓ₓ7ᵗʰ **Placeholder Alert**

    This symbol indicates that the code requires a 7th character following the placeholder "X". Codes with fewer than six characters that require a 7th character must contain placeholder "X" to fill in the empty character(s).

✓ₓ7ᵗʰ **T16.1**	**Foreign body in right ear**	PE

Most icons in this manual, placed at the end of the code description, include official edits from the following sources:

- Inpatient prospective payment system (IPPS)
- CMS HCC risk-adjustment model

Age Edits

- **N** **Newborn Age: 0**

    These diagnoses are intended for newborns and neonates and the patient's age must be 0 years.

N47.0	**Adherent prepuce, newborn**	N

- **P** **Pediatric Age: 0-17**

    These diagnoses are intended for children and the patient's age must be between 0 and 17 years.

L21.1	**Seborrheic infantile dermatitis**	P

- **M** **Maternity Age: 9-64**

    These diagnoses are intended for childbearing patients between the age of 9 and 64 years.

O02.9	**Abnormal product of conception, unspecified**	M

A **Adult Age: 15-124**

These diagnoses are intended for patients between the age of 15 and 124 years.

R54	Age-related physical debility	**A**
	Frailty	
	Old age	
	Senescence	
	Senile asthenia	
	Senile debility	

EXCLUDES 1 *age-related cognitive decline (R41.81)*
sarcopenia (M62.84)
senile psychosis (F03.-)
senility NOS (R41.81)

Sex Edits

Effective October 1, 2024, the Medicare Code Editor (MCE), a program used to detect and report errors in coding claims data, has deactivated the sex conflict edit. There is no longer a female or male edit restriction for ICD-10-CM codes.

H1 - **H14** **Hospital Acquired Condition (HAC)**

These icons identify codes that are high-cost and/or high-volume (CC or MCC) that when assigned as a secondary diagnosis result in assignment of a case to a higher-paying MS-DRG. The condition or diagnosis represented by these codes is considered reasonably preventable through the application of evidence-based guidelines. If the condition is not present on admission (meaning it developed during the hospital admission), the case will not group to the higher-paying MS-DRG based solely upon the reporting of the HAC code. Many of these HACs are conditional and are based on reporting the specific diagnosis code(s) in combination with certain procedure codes.

Note: Hospital-acquired conditions do not impact MS-LTC-DRG assignment.

N15.1 Renal and perinephric abscess	**MCC** **H6**

CC **CC Condition**

This icon identifies a complication or comorbidity diagnosis that may affect DRG assignment. A complication or comorbidity diagnosis, CC condition, is defined as a significant acute disease, a significant acute manifestation of a chronic disease, an advanced or end-stage chronic disease, or a chronic disease associated with systemic physiological decompensation and debility that have consistently greater impact on hospital resources.

G90.59 Complex regional pain syndrome I of other specified site	**CC**

MCC **MCC Condition**

This icon identifies a major complication or comorbidity diagnosis that may affect DRG assignment. An MCC condition meets the same criteria as a CC condition but is associated with a higher acuity level and hospital resource consumption is expected to be higher than that for a CC condition. There are fewer conditions that meet the criteria as an MCC than those for a CC condition.

J04.11 Acute tracheitis with obstruction	**MCC**

Note: The assignment of an MS-DRG or MS-LTC-DRG often depends on the presence or absence of a secondary diagnosis code that is designated as an MCC or CC. However, in some instances the MCC or CC designation for that secondary diagnosis code is negated due to its relationship with the principal diagnosis; this is referred to as CC exclusion. The ICD-10 MS-DRG Definitions Manual included with the IPPS final rule provides a list of all principal diagnosis codes that would render ineffective the MCC/CC designation for a particular ICD-10-CM code when used as a secondary diagnosis. Optum has provided this CC exclusion list in an easily searchable data file, which can be accessed at the following:

https://www.optumcoding.com/ProductUpdates/
Title: "2025 ICD-10-CM for Hospitals CC Excludes Data File"
Password: HOSPITAL25

UNS **Unspecified Site**

This icon identifies codes that are considered an MCC or CC but lack specificity in regard to their anatomical location. The medical record documentation should be reviewed carefully, to ensure that no other code within the same category or subcategory can be assigned for greater specificity.

G81.00 Flaccid hemiplegia affecting unspecified side	**CC** **UNS** **HCC**

UPD **Unacceptable Principal Diagnosis**

This icon identifies codes that should not be assigned as principal diagnosis for *inpatient* admissions. Codes with an unacceptable principal diagnosis edit are considered supplementary — describing circumstances that influence an individual's health status or an additional code — identifying conditions that are not specific manifestations but may be due to an underlying cause.

✓7ᵗʰ T48.5X5 **Adverse effect** of other anti-common-cold drugs	**UPD** **PE**

HIV **HIV-related Condition**

This icon identifies codes that are considered a major HIV-related diagnosis. When the condition is coded in combination with a diagnosis of human immunodeficiency virus (HIV), code B20, the case will move from MS-DRG/MS-LTC-DRG 977 to MS-DRGs/MS-LTC-DRGs 974-976.

G96.9 Disorder of central nervous system, unspecified	**HIV**

PE **Present on Admission Exempt**

This icon identifies codes that do not require a present on admission (POA) indicator. These codes are considered exempt because they do not represent a current disease or injury or describe conditions that are always present on admission

B90.1 Sequelae of genitourinary tuberculosis	**PE**

HCC **CMS-HCC Condition**

This icon identifies codes that are included in the CMS-HCC risk-adjustment model.

P29.0 Neonatal cardiac failure	**HCC**
Code also associated underlying condition	

Color Bars

Manifestation Code

Codes defined as manifestation codes appear in italic type, with a blue color bar over the code description. A manifestation cannot be reported as a first-listed code; it is sequenced as a secondary diagnosis with the underlying disease code listed first.

G32.89	*Other specified degenerative disorders of nervous system in diseases classified elsewhere*
	Degenerative encephalopathy in diseases classified elsewhere

Questionable Admission Diagnoses

Questionable admission diagnoses will appear with a yellow color bar over the code description. These codes, although not unacceptable as a PDx, may be considered a "questionable admission" when used as PDx in an acute care hospital.

E66.09 Other obesity due to excess calories

Wrong Procedure Performed Edit

An orange color bar over the code title indicates the Wrong Procedure Performed edit. This edit was created to identify cases in which wrong surgeries occurred. Any claim with a code from Y65.51-Y65.53 will be denied and returned to the provider. A surgical or other invasive procedure is considered to be a wrong procedure if one of the following is true:

- The procedure was performed on the wrong site.

- The procedure was performed on the wrong patient.

- The incorrect procedure was performed on a patient.

Y65.51	**Performance of wrong procedure (operation) on correct patient**
	Wrong device implanted into correct surgical site
	EXCLUDES 1 *performance of correct procedure (operation) on wrong side or body part (Y65.53)*

Unspecified Diagnosis

Codes that appear with a gray color bar over the alphanumeric code identify unspecified diagnoses. These codes should be used in limited circumstances, when neither the diagnostic statement nor the documentation provides enough information to assign a more specific diagnosis code. The abbreviation NOS, "not otherwise specified," in the tabular list may be interpreted as "unspecified."

G03.9	**Meningitis, unspecified**	MCC
	Arachnoiditis (spinal) NOS	

Chapter-Level Notations

Chapter-Specific Guidelines with Coding Examples

Each chapter begins with the Official Guidelines for Coding and Reporting specific to that chapter, where provided. Coding examples specific to inpatient care settings have been provided to illustrate the coding and/or sequencing guidance in these guidelines.

Muscle and Tendon Table

ICD-10-CM categorizes certain muscles and tendons in the upper and lower extremities by their action (e.g., extension or flexion) as well as their anatomical location. The Muscle/Tendon table is provided at the beginning of chapter 13 and chapter 19 to help users when code selection depends on the action of the muscle and/or tendon.

Note: This table is not all-inclusive, and proper code assignment should be based on the provider's documentation.

Illustrations

This section includes illustrations of normal anatomy with ICD-10-CM-specific terminology.

Official Updates

A summary of changes to the official ICD-10-CM code set is provided below, identifying changes made for fiscal 2025, effective October 1, 2024, to September 30, 2025. Asterisked codes identify prior midyear changes that were made to the classification, effective April 1, 2024. All code changes were made by the agency charged with maintaining and updating the ICD-10-CM code set, the National Center for Health Statistics (NCHS), a section of the Centers for Disease Control and Prevention (CDC).

252 New Codes

C81.0A	C81.1A	C81.2A	C81.3A	C81.4A
C81.7A	C81.9A	C82.0A	C82.1A	C82.2A
C82.3A	C82.4A	C82.5A	C82.6A	C82.8A
C82.9A	C83.0A	C83.1A	C83.390	C83.398
C83.3A	C83.5A	C83.7A	C83.8A	C83.9A
C84.0A	C84.1A	C84.4A	C84.6A	C84.7B
C84.9A	C84.AA	C84.ZA	C85.1A	C85.2A
C85.8A	C85.9A	C86.00	C86.01	C86.10
C86.11	C86.20	C86.21	C86.30	C86.31
C86.40	C86.41	C86.50	C86.51	C86.60
C86.61	C88.00	C88.01	C88.20	C88.21
C88.30	C88.31	C88.40	C88.41	C88.80
C88.81	C88.90	C88.91	D61.03	E10.A0
E10.A1	E10.A2	E16.A1	E16.A2	E16.A3
E34.00	E34.01	E34.09	E66.811	E66.812
E66.813	E66.89	E74.820	E74.829	E88.82
F50.010	F50.011	F50.012	F50.013	F50.014
F50.019	F50.020	F50.021	F50.022	F50.023
F50.024	F50.029	F50.20	F50.21	F50.22
F50.23	F50.24	F50.25	F50.810	F50.811
F50.812	F50.813	F50.814	F50.819	F50.83
F50.84	G40.841	G40.842	G40.843	G40.844
G90.81	G90.89	G93.45	I26.03	I26.04
I26.95	I26.96	J34.8200	J34.8201	J34.8202
J34.8210	J34.8211	J34.8212	J34.829	K60.30
K60.311	K60.312	K60.313	K60.319	K60.321
K60.322	K60.323	K60.329	K60.40	K60.411
K60.412	K60.413	K60.419	K60.421	K60.422
K60.423	K60.429	K60.50	K60.511	K60.512
K60.513	K60.519	K60.521	K60.522	K60.523
K60.529	L29.81	L29.89	L66.10	L66.11
L66.12	L66.19	L66.81	L66.89	M51.360
M51.361	M51.362	M51.369	M51.370	M51.371
M51.372	M51.379	M62.85	M65.90	M65.911
M65.912	M65.919	M65.921	M65.922	M65.929
M65.931	M65.932	M65.939	M65.941	M65.942
M65.949	M65.951	M65.952	M65.959	M65.961
M65.962	M65.969	M65.971	M65.972	M65.979
M65.98	M65.99	Q23.81	Q23.82	Q23.88
Q87.86	R41.85	T45.AX1A	T45.AX1D	T45.AX1S
T45.AX2A	T45.AX2D	T45.AX2S	T45.AX3A	T45.AX3D
T45.AX3S	T45.AX4A	T45.AX4D	T45.AX4S	T45.AX5A
T45.AX5D	T45.AX5S	T45.AX6A	T45.AX6D	T45.AX6S
T81.320A	T81.320D	T81.320S	T81.321A	T81.321D
T81.321S	T81.328A	T81.328D	T81.328S	T81.329A
T81.329D	T81.329S	Z15.1	Z15.2	Z17.21
Z17.22	Z17.31	Z17.32	Z17.410	Z17.411
Z17.420	Z17.421	Z51.A	Z59.71	Z59.72
Z67.A1	Z67.A2	Z67.A3	Z67.A4	Z68.55
Z68.56	Z83.72	Z86.0100	Z86.0101	Z86.0102
Z86.0109	Z92.26			

13 Revised Codes

Note: Each code is listed with its revised description only.

A77.41	Ehrlichiosis chaffeensis [E. chaffeensis]
F98.21	Rumination disorder of infancy and childhood
G93.42	Megalencephalic leukoencephalopathy with subcortical cysts
H44.2A3	Degenerative myopia with choroidal neovascularization, bilateral
H44.2B3	Degenerative myopia with macular hole, bilateral
H44.2C3	Degenerative myopia with retinal detachment, bilateral
H44.2D3	Degenerative myopia with foveoschisis, bilateral
H44.2E3	Degenerative myopia with other maculopathy, bilateral
I26.93	Single subsegmental thrombotic pulmonary embolism without acute cor pulmonale
I26.94	Multiple subsegmental thrombotic pulmonary emboli without acute cor pulmonale
K58.9	Irritable bowel syndrome, unspecified
Q13.81	Rieger anomaly
Z68.54	Body mass index [BMI] pediatric, 95th percentile for age to less than 120% of the 95th percentile for age

3 Deleted Codes

T81.32XA	Disruption of internal operation (surgical) wound, not elsewhere classified, initial encounter
T81.32XD	Disruption of internal operation (surgical) wound, not elsewhere classified, subsequent encounter
T81.32XS	Disruption of internal operation (surgical) wound, not elsewhere classified, sequela

Proprietary Updates

The following proprietary features have also been added:

- New definitions that describe, in lay terms, a specific condition or disease process

- New coding tips that provide coding advice beyond the code classification

- Updated *AHA Coding Clinic* references through second quarter 2024

Conversion Table of ICD-10-CM Codes

The FY 2025 (October 1, 2024-September 30, 2025) Conversion Table for new ICD-10-CM codes is provided to assist users in data retrieval. For each new code the table shows its previously assigned code equivalent. Asterisks identify new codes added to the classification April 1, 2024.

Code Assignment Beginning 10/1/2024	Previous Code(s) Assignment	Code Assignment Beginning 10/1/2024	Previous Code(s) Assignment	Code Assignment Beginning 10/1/2024	Previous Code(s) Assignment	Code Assignment Beginning 10/1/2024	Previous Code(s) Assignment	Code Assignment Beginning 10/1/2024	Previous Code(s) Assignment
C81.0A	Z85.71	C86.01	Z85.72	E66.89	E66.8	I26.04	I26.09	L29.89	L29.8
C81.1A	Z85.71	C86.10	C86.1	E74.820	E74.89	I26.95	I26.99	L66.10	L66.1
C81.2A	Z85.71	C86.11	Z85.72	E74.829	E74.89	I26.96	I26.99	L66.11	L66.1
C81.3A	Z85.71	C86.20	C86.2	E88.82	E88.89	J34.8200	J34.89	L66.12	L66.1
C81.4A	Z85.71	C86.21	Z85.72	F50.010	F50.01	J34.8201	J34.89	L66.19	L66.1
C81.7A	Z85.71	C86.30	C86.3	F50.011	F50.01	J34.8202	J34.89	L66.81	L66.8
C81.9A	Z85.71	C86.31	Z85.72	F50.012	F50.01	J34.8210	J34.89	L66.89	L66.8
C82.0A	Z85.72	C86.40	C86.4	F50.013	F50.01	J34.8211	J34.89	M51.360	M51.36
C82.1A	Z85.72	C86.41	Z85.72	F50.014	F50.01	J34.8212	J34.89	M51.361	M51.36
C82.2A	Z85.72	C86.50	C86.5	F50.019	F50.01	J34.829	J34.89	M51.362	M51.36
C82.3A	Z85.72	C86.51	Z85.72	F50.020	F50.02	K60.30	K60.3	M51.369	M51.36
C82.4A	Z85.72	C86.60	C86.6	F50.021	F50.02	K60.311	K60.3	M51.370	M51.37
C82.5A	Z85.72	C86.61	Z85.72	F50.022	F50.02	K60.312	K60.3	M51.371	M51.37
C82.6A	Z85.72	C88.00	C88.0	F50.023	F50.02	K60.313	K60.3	M51.372	M51.37
C82.8A	Z85.72	C88.01	Z85.79	F50.024	F50.02	K60.319	K60.3	M51.379	M51.37
C82.9A	Z85.72	C88.20	C88.2	F50.029	F50.02	K60.321	K60.3	M62.85	M62.89
C83.0A	Z85.72	C88.21	Z85.79	F50.20	F50.2	K60.322	K60.3	M65.90	M65.9
C83.1A	Z85.72	C88.30	C88.3	F50.21	F50.2	K60.323	K60.3	M65.911	M65.9
C83.390	Z85.72	C88.31	Z85.79	F50.22	F50.2	K60.329	K60.3	M65.912	M65.9
C83.398	Z85.72	C88.40	C88.4	F50.23	F50.2	K60.40	K60.4	M65.919	M65.9
C83.3A	Z85.72	C88.41	Z85.79	F50.24	F50.2	K60.411	K60.4	M65.921	M65.9
C83.5A	Z85.72	C88.80	C88.8	F50.25	F50.2	K60.412	K60.4	M65.922	M65.9
C83.7A	Z85.72	C88.81	Z85.79	F50.810	F50.81	K60.413	K60.4	M65.929	M65.9
C83.8A	Z85.72	C88.90	C88.9	F50.811	F50.81	K60.419	K60.4	M65.931	M65.9
C83.9A	Z85.72	C88.91	Z85.79	F50.812	F50.81	K60.421	K60.4	M65.932	M65.9
C84.0A	Z85.72	D61.03	D61.09	F50.813	F50.81	K60.422	K60.4	M65.939	M65.9
C84.1A	Z85.72	E10.A0	R73.03	F50.814	F50.81	K60.423	K60.4	M65.941	M65.9
C84.4A	Z85.72	E10.A1	R73.03	F50.819	F50.81	K60.429	K60.4	M65.942	M65.9
C84.6A	Z85.72	E10.A2	R73.03	F50.83	F50.89	K60.50	K60.5	M65.949	M65.9
C84.7B	Z85.72	E16.A1	E16.2	F50.84	F50.89	K60.511	K60.5	M65.951	M65.9
C84.AA	Z85.72	E16.A2	E16.2	G40.841	G40.89	K60.512	K60.5	M65.952	M65.9
C84.ZA	Z85.72	E16.A3	E16.2	G40.842	G40.89	K60.513	K60.5	M65.959	M65.9
C84.9A	Z85.72	E34.00	E34.0	G40.843	G40.89	K60.519	K60.5	M65.961	M65.9
C85.1A	Z85.72	E34.01	E34.0	G40.844	G40.89	K60.521	K60.5	M65.962	M65.9
C85.2A	Z85.72	E34.09	E34.0	G90.81	G90.8	K60.522	K60.5	M65.969	M65.9
C85.8A	Z85.72	E66.811	E66.8	G90.89	G90.8	K60.523	K60.5	M65.971	M65.9
C85.9A	Z85.72	E66.812	E66.8	G93.45	G93.49	K60.529	K60.5	M65.972	M65.9
C86.00	C86.0	E66.813	E66.8	I26.03	I26.09	L29.81	L29.8	M65.979	M65.9

Conversion Table of ICD-10-CM Codes

Code Assignment Beginning 10/1/2024	Previous Code(s) Assignment	Code Assignment Beginning 10/1/2024	Previous Code(s) Assignment	Code Assignment Beginning 10/1/2024	Previous Code(s) Assignment	Code Assignment Beginning 10/1/2024	Previous Code(s) Assignment	Code Assignment Beginning 10/1/2024	Previous Code(s) Assignment
M65.98	M65.9	T45.AX3A	T45.1X3A	T81.320D	T81.32XD	Z17.21	None	Z67.A3	None
M65.99	M65.9	T45.AX3D	T45.1X3D	T81.320S	T81.32XS	Z17.22	None	Z67.A4	None
Q23.81	Q23.8	T45.AX3S	T45.1X3S	T81.321A	T81.32XA	Z17.31	None	Z68.55	Z68.54
Q23.82	Q23.8	T45.AX4A	T45.1X4A	T81.321D	T81.32XD	Z17.32	None	Z68.56	Z68.54
Q23.88	Q23.8	T45.AX4D	T45.1X4D	T81.321S	T81.32XS	Z17.410	None	Z83.72	Z83.718
Q87.86	Q87.89	T45.AX4S	T45.1X4S	T81.328A	T81.32XA	Z17.411	None	Z86.0100	Z86.010
R41.85	R41.89	T45.AX5A	T45.1X5A	T81.328D	T81.32XD	Z17.420	None	Z86.0101	Z86.010
T45.AX1A	T45.1X1A	T45.AX5D	T45.1X5D	T81.328S	T81.32XS	Z17.421	None	Z86.0102	Z86.010
T45.AX1D	T45.1X1D	T45.AX5S	T45.1X5S	T81.329A	T81.32XA	Z51.A	Z51.89	Z86.0109	Z86.010
T45.AX1S	T45.1X1S	T45.AX6A	T45.1X6A	T81.329D	T81.32XD	Z59.71	Z59.7	Z92.26	Z92.29
T45.AX2A	T45.1X2A	T45.AX6D	T45.1X6D	T81.329S	T81.32XS	Z59.72	Z59.7		
T45.AX2D	T45.1X2D	T45.AX6S	T45.1X6S	Z15.1	Z15.89	Z67.A1	None		
T45.AX2S	T45.1X2S	T81.320A	T81.32XA	Z15.2	Z15.89	Z67.A2	None		

10 Steps to Correct Coding

Follow the 10 steps below to correctly code encounters for health care services.

Step 1: Identify the reason for the visit or encounter (i.e., a sign, symptom, diagnosis and/or condition).

The medical record documentation should accurately reflect the patient's condition, using terminology that includes specific diagnoses and symptoms or clearly states the reasons for the encounter.

Choosing the main term that best describes the reason chiefly responsible for the service provided is the most important step in coding. If symptoms are present and documented but a definitive diagnosis has not yet been determined, code the symptoms. *For outpatient cases, do not code conditions that are referred to as "rule out," "suspected," "probable," or "questionable."* Diagnoses often are not established at the time of the initial encounter/visit and may require two or more visits to be established. Code only what is documented in the available outpatient records and only to the highest degree of certainty known at the time of the patient's visit. For inpatient medical records, uncertain diagnoses may be reported if documented at the time of discharge.

Step 2: After selecting the reason for the encounter, consult the alphabetic index.

The most critical rule is to begin code selection in the alphabetic index. Never turn first to the tabular list. The index provides cross-references, essential and nonessential modifiers, and other instructional notations that may not be found in the tabular list.

Step 3: Locate the main term entry.

The alphabetic index lists conditions, which may be expressed as nouns or eponyms, with critical use of adjectives. Some conditions known by several names have multiple main entries. Reasons for encounters may be located under general terms such as admission, encounter, and examination. Other general terms such as history, status (post), or presence (of) can be used to locate other factors influencing health.

Step 4: Scan subterm entries.

Scan the subterm entries, as appropriate, being sure to review continued lines and additional subterms that may appear in the next column or on the next page. Shaded vertical guidelines in the index indicate the indentation level for each subterm in relation to the main terms.

Step 5: Pay close attention to index instructions.

- Parentheses ( ) enclose nonessential modifiers, terms that are supplementary words or explanatory information that may or may not appear in the diagnostic statement and do not affect code selection.

- Brackets [ ] enclose manifestation codes that can be used only as secondary codes to the underlying condition code immediately preceding it. If used, manifestation codes must be reported with the appropriate etiology codes.

- Default codes are listed next to the main term and represent the condition most commonly associated with the main term or the unspecified code for the main term.

- "*See*" cross-references, identified by italicized type and "code by" cross-references indicate that another term *must be referenced* to locate the correct code.

- "*See also*" cross-references, identified by italicized type, provide alternative terms that may be useful to look up but *are not mandatory*.

- "Omit code" cross-references identify instances when a code is not applicable depending on the condition being coded.

- "With" subterms are listed out of alphabetic order and identify a presumed causal relationship between the two conditions they link.

- "Due to" subterms identify a relationship between the two conditions they link.

- "NEC," abbreviation for "not elsewhere classified," follows some main terms or subterms and indicates that there is no specific code for the condition even though the medical documentation may be very specific.

- "NOS," abbreviation for "not otherwise specified," follows some main terms or subterms and is the equivalent of unspecified; NOS signifies that the information in the medical record is insufficient for assigning a more specific code.

- *Following* references help coders locate alphanumeric codes that are out of sequence in the tabular section.

- Check-additional-character symbols flag codes that require additional characters to make the code valid; the characters available to complete the code should be verified in the tabular section.

Step 6: Choose a potential code and locate it in the tabular list.

To prevent coding errors, always use both the alphabetic index (to identify a code) and the tabular list (to verify a code), as the index does not include the important instructional notes found in the tabular list. An added benefit of using the tabular list, which groups like things together, is that while looking at one code in the list, a coder might see a more specific one that would have been missed had the coder relied solely on the alphabetic index. Additionally, many of the codes require a fourth, fifth, sixth, or seventh character to be valid, and many of these characters can be found only in the tabular list.

Step 7: Read all instructional material in the tabular section.

The coder must follow any Includes, Excludes 1 and Excludes 2 notes, and other instructional notes, such as "Code first" and "Use additional code," listed in the tabular list for the chapter, category, subcategory, and subclassification levels of code selection that direct the coder to use a different or additional code. Any codes in the tabular range A00.0–T88.9, Z00–Z99.8, and U00–U85 may be used to identify the diagnostic reason for the encounter. The tabular list encompasses many codes describing disease and injury classifications (e.g., infectious and parasitic diseases, neoplasms, symptoms, nervous and circulatory system, etc.).

Codes that describe symptoms and signs, as opposed to definitive diagnoses, should be reported when an established diagnosis has not been made (confirmed) by the physician. Chapter 18 of the ICD-10-CM code book, "Symptoms, Signs, and Abnormal Clinical and Laboratory Findings, Not Elsewhere Classified" (codes R00–R99), contains many, but not all, codes for symptoms.

ICD-10-CM classifies encounters with health care providers for circumstances other than a disease or injury in chapter 21, "Factors Influencing Health Status and Contact with Health Services" (codes Z00–Z99). Circumstances other than a disease or injury often are recorded as chiefly responsible for the encounter.

A code is invalid if it does not include the full number of characters (greatest level of specificity) required. Codes in ICD-10-CM can contain from three to seven alphanumeric characters. A three-character code is to be used only if the category is not further subdivided into four-, five-, six-, or seven-character codes. Placeholder character X is used as part of an alphanumeric code to allow for future expansion and as a placeholder for empty characters in a code that requires a seventh character but has no fourth, fifth, or sixth character. Note that certain categories require seventh characters that apply to all codes in that category. Always check the category level for applicable seventh characters for that category.

Step 8: Consult the official ICD-10-CM conventions and guidelines.

The *ICD-10-CM Official Guidelines for Coding and Reporting* govern the use of certain codes. These guidelines provide both general and chapter-specific coding guidance.

Step 9: Confirm and assign the code.

Having reviewed all relevant information concerning the possible code choices, assign the code that most completely describes the condition.

Repeat steps 1 through 9 for all additional documented conditions that meet the following criteria:

- They exist at the time of the visit *AND*
- They require or affect patient care, treatment, or management

Step 10: Sequence codes correctly.

Sequencing is the order in which the codes are listed on the claim. List first the ICD-10-CM code for the diagnosis, condition, problem, or other reason for the encounter/visit that is shown in the medical record to be chiefly responsible for the services provided. List additional codes that describe any coexisting conditions. Follow the official coding guidelines (see the guidelines, section II, "Selection of Principal Diagnosis"; section III, "Reporting Additional Diagnoses"; and section IV, "Diagnostic Coding and Reporting Guidelines for Outpatient Services") on proper sequencing of codes.

Coding Examples

Diagnosis: Anorexia

Step 1: The reason for the encounter was the condition, anorexia.

Step 2: Consult the alphabetic index.

Step 3: Locate the main term "Anorexia."

Step 4: Two possible subterms are available, "hysterical" and "nervosa." Neither is documented in this instance, however, so they cannot be used in code selection.

Step 5: The code listed next to the main term is called the default code selection. Because the two subentries (essential modifiers) do not apply in this instance, the default code (R63.0) should be used.

Step 6: Turn to code R63.0 in the tabular list and read all instructional notes.

Step 7: The Excludes 1 note at code R63.0 indicates that anorexia nervosa and loss of appetite determined to be of nonorganic origin should be reported with a code from chapter 5. The diagnostic statement does not describe the condition as anorexia nervosa, however, and does not indicate that the anorexia is of a nonorganic origin. There is no further division of the category past the fourth-character subcategory. Therefore, code R63.0 is at the highest level of specificity.

Step 8: Review of official guideline I.C.18 indicates that a symptom code is appropriate when a more definitive diagnosis is not documented.

Step 9: The default code, R63.0 Anorexia, is the correct code selection.

Repeat steps 1 through 9 for any concomitant diagnoses.

Step 10: Since anorexia is listed as the chief reason for the health care encounter, the first-listed, or principal, diagnosis is R63.0. Note that this is a chapter 18 symptom code but can be assigned for both inpatient and outpatient records since the provider did not establish a more definitive diagnosis, according to sections II.A and IV.D.

Diagnosis: Acute bronchitis

Step 1: The reason for the encounter was the condition, acute bronchitis.

Step 2: Consult the alphabetic index.

Step 3: Locate the main term "Bronchitis."

Step 4: There is a subterm for "acute or subacute." Additional subterms are not included in the diagnostic statement.

Step 5: Nonessential modifiers (with bronchospasm or obstruction) are terms that do not affect code assignment. Since no other subterms indented under "acute" apply here, the code listed next to this subentry—in this case J20.9—should be chosen.

Step 6: Turn to code J20.9 in the tabular list and read all instructional notes.

Step 7: The Includes note under category J20 lists alternative terms for acute bronchitis. Note that the list is not exhaustive but is only a representative selection of diagnoses that are included in the subcategory. The Excludes 1 note refers to category J40 for bronchitis and tracheobronchitis NOS. There are several conditions in the Excludes 2 notes that, if applicable, can be coded in addition to this code.

Note that the codes included in J20 represent acute bronchitis due to various infectious organisms that could be selected if identified in the documentation. In this case, the organism was not identified and there is no further division of the category past the fourth character subcategory. Therefore, code J20.9 is at the highest level of specificity.

Step 8: Review of official guideline I.C.10 provides no additional information affecting the code selected.

Step 9: Assign code J20.9 Acute bronchitis, unspecified.

Repeat steps 1 through 9 for any concomitant diagnoses.

Step 10: In the absence of additional diagnoses that may affect sequencing, code J20.9 should be sequenced as the first-listed, or principal, diagnosis.

Diagnosis: Cerebellar ataxia in myxedema

Step 1: The reason for the encounter was the condition, cerebellar ataxia.

Step 2: Consult the alphabetic index.

Step 3: Locate the main term "Ataxia."

Step 4: Available subterms include "cerebellar (hereditary)," with additional indented subterms for "in" and "myxedema," all essential modifiers that are included in the diagnostic statement. Two codes are provided, E03.9 and G13.2, the latter of which is in brackets.

Step 5: Note the nonessential modifier (in parentheses) after the subterm cerebellar includes the term "hereditary." Because it is in parentheses, this term is not required in the diagnostic statement for this subentry to apply. The brackets around G13.2 identify this code as a manifestation of the condition described by code E03.9 and indicate that the two must be reported together and sequencing rules apply.

Step 6: Locate codes E03.9 and G13.2 in the tabular list, and read all instructional notes.

Step 7: For code E03.9, there are no instructional notes in the tabular list at the category E03 or code level that indicate that this condition should be coded elsewhere in the classification or that additional codes are required. Without further information from the diagnostic statement, myxedema, not otherwise specified (NOS), is appropriately reported with code E03.9 Hypothyroidism, unspecified, according to the inclusion term at this code.

Code G13.2 in the tabular list has an instructional note to "Code first underlying disease," which includes conditions found in category E03.-. Based on this note, codes E03.9 and G13.2 are to be coded together, with G13.2 listed only as a secondary diagnosis. This correlates with what the alphabetic index indicated. As there is no further division of codes in category G13 beyond the fourth character, G13.2 is at the highest level of specificity.

Step 8: Although there are some general conventions, such as how to interpret brackets in the alphabetic index, no chapter-specific guidelines apply to this coding scenario.

Step 9: Assign codes E03.9 Hypothyroidism, unspecified, and G13.2 Systemic atrophy primarily affecting the central nervous system in myxedema.

Repeat steps 1 through 9 for any concomitant diagnoses.

Step 10: Based on the alphabetic index and tabular instructional notations, code E03.9 should be sequenced as the first-listed, or principal, diagnosis followed by G13.2 as a secondary diagnosis.

Diagnosis: Decubitus ulcer of right elbow with skin loss and necrosis of subcutaneous tissue

Step 1: The reason for the encounter was the condition, decubitus ulcer.

Step 2: Consult the alphabetic index.

Step 3: Locate the main term "Ulcer."

Step 4: For the subterm "decubitus," there is no code provided or additional subterms indented, but a cross-reference is listed.

Step 5: The italicized cross-reference instructs the coder to "*see* Ulcer, pressure, by site."

Repeat steps 3 through 5 for the cross-reference:

Step 3: Locate the main term "Ulcer."

Step 4: Review the subentries for the subterm "pressure." The next level of indent lists either the site of the ulcer or the specific stage of the ulcer (stage 1–4, unstageable, and unspecified stages). The diagnostic statement provides the site, right elbow, and the extent of tissue damage (skin loss and necrosis of subcutaneous tissue) but does not specifically state that the ulcer is stage 1, stage 2, etc. Nonessential modifiers (in parentheses) at each stage include a description of the typical extent of damage at each stage. For example, stage 1 describes "pre-ulcer skin changes limited to persistent focal edema." Based on the documentation in the record, the coder can correlate the documentation to the nonessential modifiers and choose the specific stage from the index. The coder can also go directly to the body site, choosing the stage of the ulcer after reviewing the code options and instructional notations in the tabular list.

The diagnostic statement indicates that the extent of the damage to the elbow includes skin loss and necrosis of subcutaneous tissue, coinciding with the nonessential modifier next to the subentry "stage 3." The body site of elbow (L89.0-) is listed as another level of indent with other body sites.

Step 5: Note that code L89.0 is followed by a dash and an additional-character-required icon, which indicate that more characters are needed to complete the code. From here, the tabular listing for L89.0- can be consulted.

Step 6: Locate code L89.0- in the tabular list and read all instructional notes.

Step 7: The tabular listing at category L89 has an Includes note for "decubitus ulcer," which confirms that category L89 is the appropriate category to represent what is documented in the diagnostic statement.

Several Excludes 2 notes are also listed at the category level. Excludes 2 notes represent conditions that can occur concomitantly with the decubitus ulcer and can be coded in addition to code L89, if supported by the documentation.

The subcategory codes under L89.0 indicate that the fifth character describes laterality. Locate the right elbow at subcategory L89.01. See that an additional sixth character to specify the stage of the ulcer is now needed to complete the code. The stage can be determined either by the specific documentation of the stage (e.g., stage 1, stage 2) or, in this case, a description that matches one of the inclusion terms that follow each stage code. For example, the diagnostic description in this case of "skin loss and necrosis of the subcutaneous tissue" matches the inclusion term under L89.013 Pressure ulcer of right elbow, stage 3. No additional characters are required because code L89.013 is at its highest level of specificity.

Step 8: The official guidelines contain quite a bit of information relating to pressure ulcers in chapter-specific guideline I.C.12 as well as

information in general guideline I.B.14. These and any other pertinent guidelines should be reviewed to ensure appropriate code assignment.

Step 9: Assign code L89.013 Pressure ulcer of right elbow, stage 3.

Repeat steps 1 through 9 for any concomitant diagnoses.

Step 10: Since the decubitus ulcer is listed as the chief reason for the health care encounter, the first-listed, or principal, diagnosis is L89.013. However, according to the code first instructional note at the L89 category level, gangrene (I96) would be sequenced before the pressure ulcer if it were documented.

Diagnosis: Emergency department visit for bimalleolar fracture of the right ankle due to trauma

Step 1: The reason for the encounter was the condition, bimalleolar fracture.

Step 2: Consult the alphabetic index.

Step 3: Locate the main term "Fracture." Note that many main terms represent fractures: "Fracture, burst," "Fracture, chronic," "Fracture, insufficiency," "Fracture, nontraumatic NEC," "Fracture, pathological," and "Fracture, traumatic." Since the diagnostic statement specifically states that this fracture was the result of trauma, the main term "Fracture, traumatic" should be used.

Step 4: Subterms that should be referenced are "ankle" and "bimalleolar (displaced)," which lists code S82.84-.

Step 5: A nonessential modifier (in parentheses) next to the term bimalleolar for "displaced" indicates that S82.84- is the default category unless the fracture is specifically identified as "nondisplaced."

Note that code S82.84- is followed by a dash and an additional-character icon, both of which indicate that more characters are required. From here, the tabular list can be consulted.

Step 6: Locate code S82.84- in the tabular list and read all instructional notes.

Step 7: The instructional notes at category S82 indicate that fractures not specified as displaced or nondisplaced default to displaced and that fractures not designated as open or closed default to closed. Additional instructional notes can be found at the category level but none pertain to the current scenario.

Read through the subcategory codes under S82.84, and note that the sixth character specifies displaced or nondisplaced and laterality. Based on the index nonessential modifier (displaced) and the code note at category S82, code selection should identify a displaced fracture of the right side. A displaced bimalleolar fracture of the right lower leg is coded to S82.841.

To complete the code, a seventh character must be assigned to identify the type of encounter (initial, subsequent, or sequela) and whether the fracture is open or closed. Most of the codes in category S82 require a seventh character represented in the list at the category level. However, it is important to note that some subcategories have their own specific set of seventh characters. In this instance, subcategory S82.84- does not have a unique set of seventh characters and the list provided at the category level should be used. Without documentation of the fracture being open, the tabular notation indicates that the default is closed. Character A, representing "initial encounter for closed fracture," listed in the box at the category level is the most appropriate option.

2025 ICD-10-CM Official Guidelines for Coding and Reporting

Narrative changes effective October 1, 2024 appear in **bold** text
Narrative changes effective April 1, 2024 appear in shaded text
Items underlined have been moved within the guidelines since the April 2024, FY 2024 version
Italics are used to indicate revisions to heading changes

The Centers for Medicare and Medicaid Services (CMS) and the National Center for Health Statistics (NCHS), two departments within the U.S. Federal Government's Department of Health and Human Services (DHHS) provide the following guidelines for coding and reporting using the International Classification of Diseases, 10th Revision, Clinical Modification (ICD-10-CM). These guidelines should be used as a companion document to the official version of the ICD-10-CM as published on the NCHS website. The ICD-10-CM is a morbidity classification published by the United States for classifying diagnoses and reason for visits in all health care settings. The ICD-10-CM is based on the ICD-10, the statistical classification of disease published by the World Health Organization (WHO).

These guidelines have been approved by the four organizations that make up the Cooperating Parties for the ICD-10-CM: the American Hospital Association (AHA), the American Health Information Management Association (AHIMA), CMS, and NCHS.

These guidelines are a set of rules that have been developed to accompany and complement the official conventions and instructions provided within the ICD-10-CM itself. The instructions and conventions of the classification take precedence over guidelines. These guidelines are based on the coding and sequencing instructions in the Tabular List and Alphabetic Index of ICD-10-CM, but provide additional instruction. Adherence to these guidelines when assigning ICD-10-CM diagnosis codes is required under the Health Insurance Portability and Accountability Act (HIPAA). The diagnosis codes (Tabular List and Alphabetic Index) have been adopted under HIPAA for all healthcare settings. A joint effort between the healthcare provider and the coder is essential to achieve complete and accurate documentation, code assignment, and reporting of diagnoses and procedures. These guidelines have been developed to assist both the healthcare provider and the coder in identifying those diagnoses that are to be reported. The importance of consistent, complete documentation in the medical record cannot be overemphasized. Without such documentation accurate coding cannot be achieved. The entire record should be reviewed to determine the specific reason for the encounter and the conditions treated.

The term encounter is used for all settings, including hospital admissions. In the context of these guidelines, the term provider is used throughout the guidelines to mean physician or any qualified health care practitioner who is legally accountable for establishing the patient's diagnosis. Only this set of guidelines, approved by the Cooperating Parties, is official.

The guidelines are organized into sections. Section I includes the structure and conventions of the classification and general guidelines that apply to the entire classification, and chapter-specific guidelines that correspond to the chapters as they are arranged in the classification. Section II includes guidelines for selection of principal diagnosis for non-outpatient settings. Section III includes guidelines for reporting additional diagnoses in non-outpatient settings. Section IV is for outpatient coding and reporting. It is necessary to review all sections of the guidelines to fully understand all of the rules and instructions needed to code properly.

Section I. Conventions, general coding guidelines and chapter specific guidelines

The conventions, general guidelines and chapter-specific guidelines are applicable to all health care settings unless otherwise indicated. The conventions and instructions of the classification take precedence over guidelines.

A. Conventions for the ICD-10-CM

The conventions for the ICD-10-CM are the general rules for use of the classification independent of the guidelines. These conventions are incorporated within the Alphabetic Index and Tabular List of the ICD-10-CM as instructional notes.

1. The Alphabetic Index and Tabular List

The ICD-10-CM is divided into the Alphabetic Index, an alphabetical list of terms and their corresponding code, and the Tabular List, a structured list of codes divided into chapters based on body system or condition. The Alphabetic Index consists of the following parts: the Index of Diseases and Injury, the Index of External Causes of Injury, the Table of Neoplasms and the Table of Drugs and Chemicals.

See Section I.C.2. Neoplasms
See Section I.C.19. Adverse effects, poisoning, underdosing and toxic effects

2. Format and Structure:

The ICD-10-CM Tabular List contains categories, subcategories and codes. Characters for categories, subcategories and codes may be either a letter or a number. All categories are 3 characters. A three-character category that has no further subdivision is equivalent to a code. Subcategories are either 4 or 5 characters. Codes may be 3, 4, 5, 6 or 7 characters. That is, each level of subdivision after a category is a subcategory. The final level of subdivision is a code. Codes that have applicable 7th characters are still referred to as codes, not subcategories. A code that has an applicable 7th character is considered invalid without the 7th character.

The ICD-10-CM uses an indented format for ease in reference.

3. Use of codes for reporting purposes

For reporting purposes only codes are permissible, not categories or subcategories, and any applicable 7th character is required.

4. Placeholder character

The ICD-10-CM utilizes a placeholder character "X". The "X" is used as a placeholder at certain codes to allow for future expansion. An example of this is at the poisoning, adverse effect and underdosing codes, categories T36-T50. Where a placeholder exists, the X must be used in order for the code to be considered a valid code.

5. 7th Characters

Certain ICD-10-CM categories have applicable 7th characters. The applicable 7th character is required for all codes within the category, or as the notes in the Tabular List instruct. The 7th character must always be the 7th character in the data field. If a code that requires a 7th character is not 6 characters, a placeholder X must be used to fill in the empty characters.

6. Abbreviations

a. Alphabetic Index abbreviations

NEC "Not elsewhere classifiable"

This abbreviation in the Alphabetic Index represents "other specified." When a specific code is not available for a condition, the Alphabetic Index directs the coder to the "other specified" code in the Tabular List.

NOS "Not otherwise specified"

This abbreviation is the equivalent of unspecified.

b. Tabular List abbreviations

NEC "Not elsewhere classifiable"

This abbreviation in the Tabular List represents "other specified". When a specific code is not available for a condition, the Tabular List includes an NEC entry under a code to identify the code as the "other specified" code.

NOS "Not otherwise specified"

This abbreviation is the equivalent of unspecified.

7. Punctuation

[ ] Brackets are used in the Tabular List to enclose synonyms, alternative wording or explanatory phrases. Brackets are used in the Alphabetic Index to identify manifestation codes.

( ) Parentheses are used in both the Alphabetic Index and Tabular List to enclose supplementary words that may be present or absent in the statement of a disease or procedure without affecting the code number to which it is assigned. The terms within the parentheses are referred to as nonessential modifiers. The nonessential modifiers in the Alphabetic Index to Diseases apply to subterms following a main term except when a nonessential modifier and a subentry are mutually exclusive, the subentry takes precedence. For example, in the ICD-10-CM Alphabetic Index under the main term Enteritis, "acute" is a nonessential modifier and "chronic" is a subentry. In this case, the nonessential modifier "acute" does not apply to the subentry "chronic".

: Colons are used in the Tabular List after an incomplete term which needs one or more of the modifiers following the colon to make it assignable to a given category.

8. Use of "and".

See Section I.A.14. Use of the term "And"

9. Other and Unspecified codes

a. "Other" codes

Codes titled "other" or "other specified" are for use when the information in the medical record provides detail for which a specific code does not exist. Alphabetic Index entries with NEC in the line designate "other" codes in the Tabular List. These Alphabetic Index entries represent specific disease entities for which no specific code exists, so the term is included within an "other" code.

b. "Unspecified" codes

Codes titled "unspecified" are for use when the information in the medical record is insufficient to assign a more specific code. For those categories for which an unspecified code is not provided, the "other specified" code may represent both other and unspecified.

See Section I.B.18. Use of Signs/Symptom/Unspecified Codes

10. Includes Notes

This note appears immediately under a three-character code title to further define, or give examples of, the content of the category.

11. Inclusion terms

List of terms is included under some codes. These terms are the conditions for which that code is to be used. The terms may be synonyms of the code title, or, in the case of "other specified" codes, the terms are a list of the various conditions assigned to that code. The inclusion terms are not necessarily exhaustive. Additional terms found only in the Alphabetic Index may also be assigned to a code.

12. Excludes Notes

The ICD-10-CM has two types of excludes notes. Each type of note has a different definition for use, but they are all similar in that they indicate that codes excluded from each other are independent of each other.

a. Excludes1

A type 1 Excludes note is a pure excludes note. It means "NOT CODED HERE!" An Excludes1 note indicates that the code excluded should never be used at the same time as the code above the Excludes1 note. An Excludes1 is used when two conditions cannot occur together, such as a congenital form versus an acquired form of the same condition.

An exception to the Excludes1 definition is the circumstance when the two conditions are unrelated to each other. If it is not clear whether the two conditions involving an Excludes1 note are related or not, query the provider. For example, code F45.8, Other somatoform disorders, has an Excludes1 note for "sleep related teeth grinding (G47.63)," because "teeth grinding" is an inclusion term under F45.8. Only one of these two codes should be assigned for teeth grinding. However psychogenic dysmenorrhea is also an inclusion term under F45.8, and a patient could have both this condition and sleep related teeth grinding. In this case, the two conditions are clearly unrelated to each other, and so it would be appropriate to report F45.8 and G47.63 together.

b. Excludes2

A type 2 Excludes note represents "Not included here." An excludes2 note indicates that the condition excluded is not part of the condition represented by the code, but a patient may have both conditions at the same time. When an Excludes2 note appears under a code, it is acceptable to use both the code and the excluded code together, when appropriate.

13. Etiology/manifestation convention ("code first", "use additional code" and "in diseases classified elsewhere" notes)

Certain conditions have both an underlying etiology and multiple body system manifestations due to the underlying etiology. For such conditions, the ICD-10-CM has a coding convention that requires the underlying condition be sequenced first, if applicable, followed by the manifestation. Wherever such a combination exists, there is a "use additional code" note at the etiology code, and a "code first" note at the manifestation code. These instructional notes indicate the proper sequencing order of the codes, etiology followed by manifestation.

In most cases the manifestation codes will have in the code title, "in diseases classified elsewhere." Codes with this title are a component of the etiology/ manifestation convention. The code title indicates that it is a manifestation code. "In diseases classified elsewhere" codes are never permitted to be used as first listed or principal diagnosis codes. They must be used in conjunction with an underlying condition code and they must be listed following the underlying condition. See category F02, Dementia in other diseases classified elsewhere, for an example of this convention.

There are manifestation codes that do not have "in diseases classified elsewhere" in the title. For such codes, there is a "use additional code" note at the etiology code and a "code first" note at the manifestation code, and the rules for sequencing apply.

In addition to the notes in the Tabular List, these conditions also have a specific Alphabetic Index entry structure. In the Alphabetic Index both conditions are listed together with the etiology code first followed by the manifestation codes in brackets. The code in brackets is always to be sequenced second.

An example of the etiology/manifestation convention is dementia with Parkinson's disease. In the Alphabetic Index, a code from category G20 is listed first, followed by code F02.80 or F02.81- in brackets. A code from category G20- represents the underlying etiology, Parkinson's disease, and must be sequenced first, whereas codes F02.80 and F02.81- represent the manifestation of dementia in diseases classified elsewhere, with or without behavioral disturbance.

"Code first" and "Use additional code" notes are also used as sequencing rules in the classification for certain codes that are not part of an etiology/ manifestation combination.

See Section I.B.7. Multiple coding for a single condition.

14. "And"

The word "and" should be interpreted to mean either "and" or "or" when it appears in a title.

For example, cases of "tuberculosis of bones", "tuberculosis of joints" and "tuberculosis of bones and joints" are classified to subcategory A18.0, Tuberculosis of bones and joints.

15. "With"

The word "with" or "in" should be interpreted to mean "associated with" or "due to" when it appears in a code title, the Alphabetic Index (either under a main term or subterm), or an instructional note in the Tabular List. The classification presumes a causal relationship between the two conditions linked by these terms in the Alphabetic Index or Tabular List. These conditions should be coded as related even in the absence of provider documentation explicitly linking them, unless the documentation clearly states the conditions are unrelated or when another guideline exists that specifically requires a documented linkage between two conditions (e.g., sepsis guideline for "acute organ dysfunction that is not clearly associated with the sepsis").

For conditions not specifically linked by these relational terms in the classification or when a guideline requires that a linkage between two conditions be explicitly documented, provider documentation must link the conditions in order to code them as related.

The word "with" in the Alphabetic Index is sequenced immediately following the main term or subterm, not in alphabetical order.

16. "See" and "See Also"

The "see" instruction following a main term in the Alphabetic Index indicates that another term should be referenced. It is necessary to go to the main term referenced with the "see" note to locate the correct code.

A "see also" instruction following a main term in the Alphabetic Index instructs that there is another main term that may also be referenced that may provide additional Alphabetic Index entries that may be useful. It is not necessary to follow the "see also" note when the original main term provides the necessary code.

2025 ICD-10-CM Official Guidelines for Coding and Reporting

17. "Code also" note

A "code also" note instructs that two codes may be required to fully describe a condition, but this note does not provide sequencing direction. The sequencing depends on the circumstances of the encounter.

18. Default codes

A code listed next to a main term in the ICD-10-CM Alphabetic Index is referred to as a default code. The default code represents that condition that is most commonly associated with the main term or is the unspecified code for the condition. If a condition is documented in a medical record (for example, appendicitis) without any additional information, such as acute or chronic, the default code should be assigned.

19. Code assignment and Clinical Criteria

The assignment of a diagnosis code is based on the provider's diagnostic statement that the condition exists. The provider's statement that the patient has a particular condition is sufficient. Code assignment is not based on clinical criteria used by the provider to establish the diagnosis. If there is conflicting medical record documentation, query the provider.

B. General Coding Guidelines

1. Locating a code in the ICD-10-CM

To select a code in the classification that corresponds to a diagnosis or reason for visit documented in a medical record, first locate the term in the Alphabetic Index, and then verify the code in the Tabular List. Read and be guided by instructional notations that appear in both the Alphabetic Index and the Tabular List.

It is essential to use both the Alphabetic Index and Tabular List when locating and assigning a code. The Alphabetic Index does not always provide the full code. Selection of the full code, including laterality and any applicable 7th character can only be done in the Tabular List. A dash (-) at the end of an Alphabetic Index entry indicates that additional characters are required. Even if a dash is not included at the Alphabetic Index entry, it is necessary to refer to the Tabular List to verify that no 7th character is required.

2. Level of Detail in Coding

Diagnosis codes are to be used and reported at their highest number of characters available and to the highest level of specificity documented in the medical record.

ICD-10-CM diagnosis codes are composed of codes with 3, 4, 5, 6 or 7 characters. Codes with three characters are included in ICD-10-CM as the heading of a category of codes that may be further subdivided by the use of fourth and/or fifth characters and/or sixth characters, which provide greater detail.

A three-character code is to be used only if it is not further subdivided. A code is invalid if it has not been coded to the full number of characters required for that code, including the 7th character, if applicable.

3. Code or codes from A00.0 through T88.9, Z00-Z99.8, U00-U85

The appropriate code or codes from A00.0 through T88.9, Z00-Z99.8, and U00-U85 must be used to identify diagnoses, symptoms, conditions, problems, complaints or other reason(s) for the encounter/visit.

4. Signs and symptoms

Codes that describe symptoms and signs, as opposed to diagnoses, are acceptable for reporting purposes when a related definitive diagnosis has not been established (confirmed) by the provider. Chapter 18 of ICD-10-CM, Symptoms, Signs, and Abnormal Clinical and Laboratory Findings, Not Elsewhere Classified (codes R00.0-R99) contains many, but not all, codes for symptoms.

See Section I.B.18. Use of Signs/Symptom/Unspecified Codes

5. Conditions that are an integral part of a disease process

Signs and symptoms that are associated routinely with a disease process should not be assigned as additional codes, unless otherwise instructed by the classification.

6. Conditions that are not an integral part of a disease process

Additional signs and symptoms that may not be associated routinely with a disease process should be coded when present.

7. Multiple coding for a single condition

In addition to the etiology/manifestation convention that requires two codes to fully describe a single condition that affects multiple body systems, there are other single conditions that also require more than one code. "Use additional code" notes are found in the Tabular List at codes that are not part of an etiology/manifestation pair where a secondary code is useful to fully describe a condition. The sequencing rule is the same as the etiology/manifestation pair, "use additional code" indicates that a secondary code should be added, if known.

For example, for bacterial infections that are not included in chapter 1, a secondary code from category B95, Streptococcus, Staphylococcus, and Enterococcus, as the cause of diseases classified elsewhere, or B96, Other bacterial agents as the cause of diseases classified elsewhere, may be required to identify the bacterial organism causing the infection. A "use additional code" note will normally be found at the infectious disease code, indicating a need for the organism code to be added as a secondary code.

"Code first" notes are also under certain codes that are not specifically manifestation codes but may be due to an underlying cause. When there is a "code first" note and an underlying condition is present, the underlying condition should be sequenced first, if known.

"Code, if applicable, any causal condition first" notes indicate that this code may be assigned as a principal diagnosis when the causal condition is unknown or not applicable. If a causal condition is known, then the code for that condition should be sequenced as the principal or first-listed diagnosis.

Multiple codes may be needed for sequela, complication codes and obstetric codes to more fully describe a condition. See the specific guidelines for these conditions for further instruction.

8. Acute and Chronic Conditions

If the same condition is described as both acute (subacute) and chronic, and separate subentries exist in the Alphabetic Index at the same indentation level, code both and sequence the acute (subacute) code first.

9. Combination Code

A combination code is a single code used to classify:

> Two diagnoses, or
> A diagnosis with an associated secondary process (manifestation)
> A diagnosis with an associated complication

Combination codes are identified by referring to subterm entries in the Alphabetic Index and by reading the inclusion and exclusion notes in the Tabular List.

Assign only the combination code when that code fully identifies the diagnostic conditions involved or when the Alphabetic Index so directs. Multiple coding should not be used when the classification provides a combination code that clearly identifies all of the elements documented in the diagnosis. When the combination code lacks necessary specificity in describing the manifestation or complication, an additional code should be used as a secondary code.

10. Sequela (Late Effects)

A sequela is the residual effect (condition produced) after the acute phase of an illness or injury has terminated. There is no time limit on when a sequela code can be used. The residual may be apparent early, such as in cerebral infarction, or it may occur months or years later, such as that due to a previous injury. Examples of sequela include: scar formation resulting from a burn, deviated septum due to a nasal fracture, and infertility due to tubal occlusion from old tuberculosis. Coding of sequela generally requires two codes sequenced in the following order: the condition or nature of the sequela is sequenced first. The sequela code is sequenced second.

An exception to the above guidelines are those instances where the code for the sequela is followed by a manifestation code identified in the Tabular List and title, or the sequela code has been expanded (at the fourth, fifth or sixth character levels) to include the manifestation(s). The code for the acute phase of an illness or injury that led to the sequela is never used with a code for the late effect.

See Section I.C.9. Sequelae of cerebrovascular disease
See Section I.C.15. Sequelae of complication of pregnancy, childbirth and the puerperium
See Section I.C.19. Application of 7th characters for Chapter 19

11. Impending or Threatened Condition

Code any condition described at the time of discharge as "impending" or "threatened" as follows:

> If it did occur, code as confirmed diagnosis.
> If it did not occur, reference the Alphabetic Index to determine if the condition has a subentry term for "impending" or "threatened" and also reference main term entries for "Impending" and for "Threatened."
> If the subterms are listed, assign the given code.
> If the subterms are not listed, code the existing underlying condition(s) and not the condition described as impending or threatened.

12. Reporting Same Diagnosis Code More than Once

Each unique ICD-10-CM diagnosis code may be reported only once for an encounter. This applies to bilateral conditions when there are no distinct codes identifying laterality or two different conditions classified to the same ICD-10-CM diagnosis code.

13. Laterality

Some ICD-10-CM codes indicate laterality, specifying whether the condition occurs on the left, right or is bilateral. If no bilateral code is provided and the condition is bilateral, assign separate codes for both the left and right side. If the side is not identified in the medical record, assign the code for the unspecified side.

When a patient has a bilateral condition and each side is treated during separate encounters, assign the "bilateral" code (as the condition still exists on both sides), including for the encounter to treat the first side. For the second encounter for treatment after one side has previously been treated and the condition no longer exists on that side, assign the appropriate unilateral code for the side where the condition still exists (e.g., cataract surgery performed on each eye in separate encounters). The bilateral code would not be assigned for the subsequent encounter, as the patient no longer has the condition in the previously-treated site. If the treatment on the first side did not completely resolve the condition, then the bilateral code would still be appropriate.

When laterality is not documented by the patient's provider, code assignment for the affected side may be based on medical record documentation from other clinicians. If there is conflicting medical record documentation regarding the affected side, the patient's provider should be queried for clarification. Codes for "unspecified" side should rarely be used, such as when the documentation in the record is insufficient to determine the affected side and it is not possible to obtain clarification.

14. Documentation by Clinicians Other than the Patient's Provider

Code assignment is based on the documentation by the patient's provider (i.e., physician or other qualified healthcare practitioner legally accountable for establishing the patient's diagnosis). There are a few exceptions when code assignment may be based on medical record documentation from clinicians who are not the patient's provider (i.e., physician or other qualified healthcare practitioner legally accountable for establishing the patient's diagnosis). In this context, "clinicians" other than the patient's provider refer to healthcare professionals permitted, based on regulatory or accreditation requirements or internal hospital policies, to document in a patient's official medical record. These exceptions include codes for:

- Body Mass Index (BMI)
- Depth of non-pressure chronic ulcers
- Pressure ulcer stage
- Coma scale
- NIH stroke scale (NIHSS)
- Social determinants of health (SDOH) classified to Chapter 21
- Laterality
- Blood alcohol level
- Underimmunization status

This information is typically, or may be, documented by other clinicians involved in the care of the patient (e.g., a dietitian often documents the BMI, a nurse often documents the pressure ulcer stages, and an emergency medical technician often documents the coma scale). However, the associated diagnosis (such as overweight, obesity, acute stroke, pressure ulcer, or a condition classifiable to category F10, Alcohol related disorders) must be documented by the patient's provider. If there is conflicting medical record documentation, either from the same clinician or different clinicians, the patient's provider should be queried for clarification.

The BMI, coma scale, NIHSS, blood alcohol level codes, codes for social determinants of health and underimmunization status should only be reported as secondary diagnoses.

See Section I.C.21.c.17. for additional information regarding coding social determinants of health.

15. Syndromes

Follow the Alphabetic Index guidance when coding syndromes. In the absence of Alphabetic Index guidance, assign codes for the documented manifestations of the syndrome. Additional codes for manifestations that are not an integral part of the disease process may also be assigned when the condition does not have a unique code.

16. Documentation of Complications of Care

Code assignment is based on the provider's documentation of the relationship between the condition and the care or procedure, unless otherwise instructed by the classification. The guideline extends to any complications of care, regardless of the chapter the code is located in. It is important to note that not all conditions that occur during or following medical care or surgery are classified as complications. There must be a cause-and-effect relationship between the care provided and the condition, and the documentation must support that the condition is clinically significant. It is not necessary for the provider to explicitly document the term "complication." For example, if the condition alters the course of the surgery as documented in the operative report, then it would be appropriate to report a complication code. Query the provider for clarification if the documentation is not clear as to the relationship between the condition and the care or procedure.

17. Borderline Diagnosis

If the provider documents a "borderline" diagnosis at the time of discharge, the diagnosis is coded as confirmed, unless the classification provides a specific entry (e.g., borderline diabetes). If a borderline condition has a specific index entry in ICD-10-CM, it should be coded as such. Since borderline conditions are not uncertain diagnoses, no distinction is made between the care setting (inpatient versus outpatient). Whenever the documentation is unclear regarding a borderline condition, coders are encouraged to query for clarification.

18. Use of Sign/Symptom/Unspecified Codes

Sign/symptom and "unspecified" codes have acceptable, even necessary, uses. While specific diagnosis codes should be reported when they are supported by the available medical record documentation and clinical knowledge of the patient's health condition, there are instances when signs/symptoms or unspecified codes are the best choices for accurately reflecting the healthcare encounter. Each healthcare encounter should be coded to the level of certainty known for that encounter.

As stated in the introductory section of these official coding guidelines, a joint effort between the healthcare provider and the coder is essential to achieve complete and accurate documentation, code assignment, and reporting of diagnoses and procedures. The importance of consistent, complete documentation in the medical record cannot be overemphasized. Without such documentation accurate coding cannot be achieved. The entire record should be reviewed to determine the specific reason for the encounter and the conditions treated.

If a definitive diagnosis has not been established by the end of the encounter, it is appropriate to report codes for sign(s) and/or symptom(s) in lieu of a definitive diagnosis. When sufficient clinical information isn't known or available about a particular health condition to assign a more specific code, it is acceptable to report the appropriate "unspecified" code (e.g., a diagnosis of pneumonia has been determined, but not the type). Unspecified codes should be reported when they are the codes that most accurately reflect what is known about the patient's condition at the time of that particular encounter. It would be inappropriate to select a specific code that is not supported by the medical record documentation or conduct medically unnecessary diagnostic testing in order to determine a more specific code.

19. Coding for Healthcare Encounters in Hurricane Aftermath

a. Use of External Cause of Morbidity Codes

An external cause of morbidity code should be assigned to identify the cause of the injury(ies) incurred as a result of the hurricane. The use of external cause of morbidity codes is supplemental to the application of ICD-10-CM codes. External cause of morbidity codes are never to be recorded as a principal diagnosis (first-listed in non-inpatient settings). The appropriate injury code should be sequenced before any external cause codes. The external cause of morbidity codes capture how the injury or health condition happened (cause), the intent (unintentional or accidental; or intentional, such as suicide or assault), the place where the event occurred, the activity of the patient at the time of the event, and the person's status (e.g., civilian, military). They should not be assigned for encounters to treat hurricane victims' medical conditions when no injury, adverse effect or poisoning is involved. External cause of morbidity codes should be assigned for each encounter for care and treatment of the injury. External cause of morbidity codes may be assigned in all health care settings. For the purpose of capturing complete and accurate ICD-10-CM data in the aftermath of the hurricane, a healthcare setting should be considered as any location where medical care is provided by licensed healthcare professionals.

b. Sequencing of External Causes of Morbidity Codes

Codes for cataclysmic events, such as a hurricane, take priority over all other external cause codes except child and adult abuse and terrorism and should be sequenced before other external cause of injury codes. Assign as many external cause of morbidity codes as necessary to fully explain each cause. For example, if an injury occurs as a result of a building collapse during the hurricane, external cause codes for both the hurricane and the building collapse should be assigned, with the external causes code for hurricane being sequenced as the first external cause code. For injuries incurred as a direct result of the hurricane, assign the appropriate code(s) for the injuries, followed by the code X37.0-, Hurricane (with the appropriate 7th character), and any other applicable external cause of injury codes. Code X37.0- also should be assigned when an injury is incurred as a result of flooding caused by a levee breaking related to the hurricane. Code X38.-, Flood (with the appropriate 7th character), should be assigned when an injury is from flooding resulting directly from the storm. Code X36.0-, Collapse of dam or man-made structure, should not be assigned when the cause of the collapse is due to the hurricane. Use of code X36.0- is limited to collapses of man-made structures due to earth surface movements, not due to storm surges directly from a hurricane.

c. Other External Causes of Morbidity Code Issues

For injuries that are not a direct result of the hurricane, such as an evacuee that has incurred an injury as a result of a motor vehicle accident, assign the appropriate external cause of morbidity code(s) to describe the cause of the injury, but do not assign code X37.0-, Hurricane. If it is not clear whether the injury was a direct result of the hurricane, assume the injury is due to the hurricane and assign code X37.0-, Hurricane, as well as any other applicable external cause of morbidity codes. In addition to code X37.0-, Hurricane, other possible applicable external cause of morbidity codes include:

    X30-, Exposure to excessive natural heat
    X31-, Exposure to excessive natural cold
    X38-, Flood

d. Use of Z codes

Z codes (other reasons for healthcare encounters) may be assigned as appropriate to further explain the reasons for presenting for healthcare services, including transfers between healthcare facilities, or provide additional information relevant to a patient encounter. The ICD-10-CM Official Guidelines for Coding and Reporting identify which codes maybe assigned as principal or first-listed diagnosis only, secondary diagnosis only, or principal/first-listed or secondary (depending on the circumstances). Possible applicable Z codes include:

Z59.0-,	Homelessness
Z59.1,	Inadequate housing
Z59.5,	Extreme poverty
Z75.1,	Person awaiting admission to adequate facility elsewhere
Z75.3,	Unavailability and inaccessibility of health-care facilities
Z75.4,	Unavailability and inaccessibility of other helping agencies
Z76.2,	Encounter for health supervision and care of other healthy infant and child
Z99.12,	Encounter for respirator [ventilator] dependence during power failure

The external cause of morbidity codes and the Z codes listed above are not an all-inclusive list. Other codes may be applicable to the encounter based upon the documentation. Assign as many codes as necessary to fully explain each healthcare encounter. Since patient history information may be very limited, use any available documentation to assign the appropriate external cause of morbidity and Z codes.

C. Chapter-Specific Coding Guidelines

In addition to general coding guidelines, there are guidelines for specific diagnoses and/or conditions in the classification. Unless otherwise indicated, these guidelines apply to all health care settings. Please refer to Section II for guidelines on the selection of principal diagnosis.

1. **Chapter 1: Certain Infectious and Parasitic Diseases (A00-B99), U07.1, U09.9**
    a. **Human Immunodeficiency Virus (HIV) Infections**
        1) **Code only confirmed cases**
        Code only confirmed cases of HIV infection/illness. This is an exception to the hospital inpatient guideline Section II, H.
        In this context, "confirmation" does not require documentation of positive serology or culture for HIV; the provider's diagnostic statement that the patient is HIV positive or has an HIV-related illness is sufficient.
        2) **Selection and sequencing of HIV codes**
            (a) **Patient admitted for HIV-related condition**
            If a patient is admitted for an HIV-related condition, the principal diagnosis should be B20, Human immunodeficiency virus [HIV] disease followed by additional diagnosis codes for all reported HIV-related conditions.
            An exception to this guideline is if the reason for admission is hemolytic-uremic syndrome associated with HIV disease. Assign code D59.31, Infection- associated hemolytic-uremic syndrome, followed by code B20, Human immunodeficiency virus [HIV] disease.
            (b) **Patient with HIV disease admitted for unrelated condition**
            If a patient with HIV disease is admitted for an unrelated condition (such as a traumatic injury), the code for the unrelated condition (e.g., the nature of injury code) should be the principal diagnosis. Other diagnoses would be B20 followed by additional diagnosis codes for all reported HIV-related conditions.
            (c) **Whether the patient is newly diagnosed**
            Whether the patient is newly diagnosed or has had previous admissions/encounters for HIV conditions is irrelevant to the sequencing decision.
            (d) **Asymptomatic human immunodeficiency virus**
            Z21, Asymptomatic human immunodeficiency virus [HIV] infection status, is to be applied when the patient without any documentation of symptoms is listed as being "HIV positive," "known HIV," "HIV test positive," or similar terminology. Do not use this code if the term "AIDS" or "HIV disease" is used or if the patient is treated for any HIV-related illness or is described as having any condition(s) resulting from his/her HIV positive status; use B20 in these cases.
            (e) **Patients with inconclusive HIV serology**
            Patients with inconclusive HIV serology, but no definitive diagnosis or manifestations of the illness, may be assigned code R75, Inconclusive laboratory evidence of human immunodeficiency virus [HIV].
            (f) **Previously diagnosed HIV-related illness**
            Patients with any known prior diagnosis of an HIV-related illness should be coded to B20. Once a patient has developed an HIV-related illness, the patient should always be assigned code B20 on every subsequent admission/encounter. Patients previously diagnosed with any HIV illness (B20) should never be assigned to R75 or Z21, Asymptomatic human immunodeficiency virus [HIV] infection status.
            (g) **HIV Infection in Pregnancy, Childbirth and the Puerperium**
            During pregnancy, childbirth or the puerperium, a patient admitted (or presenting for a health care encounter) because of an HIV-related illness should receive a principal diagnosis code of O98.7-, Human immunodeficiency [HIV] disease complicating pregnancy, childbirth and the puerperium, followed by B20 and the code(s) for the HIV-related illness(es). Codes from Chapter 15 always take sequencing priority.
            Patients with asymptomatic HIV infection status admitted (or presenting for a health care encounter) during pregnancy, childbirth, or the puerperium should receive codes of O98.7- and Z21.
            (h) **Encounters for testing for HIV**
            If a patient is being seen to determine his/her HIV status, use code Z11.4, Encounter for screening for human immunodeficiency virus [HIV]. Use additional codes for any associated high-risk behavior, if applicable.
            If a patient with signs or symptoms is being seen for HIV testing, code the signs and symptoms. An additional counseling code Z71.7, Human immunodeficiency virus [HIV] counseling, may be used if counseling is provided during the encounter for the test.
            When a patient returns to be informed of his/her HIV test results and the test result is negative, use code Z71.7, Human immunodeficiency virus [HIV] counseling.
            If the results are positive, see previous guidelines and assign codes as appropriate.
            (i) **HIV managed by antiretroviral medication**
            If a patient with documented HIV disease, HIV-related illness or AIDS is currently managed on antiretroviral medications, assign code B20, Human immunodeficiency virus [HIV] disease. Code Z79.899, Other long term (current) drug therapy, may be assigned as an additional code to identify the long-term (current) use of antiretroviral medications.
            (j) **Encounter for HIV Prophylaxis Measures**
            When a patient is seen for administration of pre-exposure prophylaxis medication for HIV, assign code Z29.81, Encounter for HIV pre-exposure prophylaxis. Pre-exposure prophylaxis (PrEP) is intended to prevent infection in people who are at risk for getting HIV through sex or injection drug use. Any risk factors for HIV should also be coded.
    b. **Infectious agents as the cause of diseases classified to other chapters**
    Certain infections are classified in chapters other than Chapter 1 and no organism is identified as part of the infection code. In these instances, it is necessary to use an additional code from Chapter 1 to identify the organism. A code from category B95, Streptococcus, Staphylococcus, and Enterococcus as the cause of diseases classified to other chapters, B96, Other bacterial agents as the cause of diseases classified to other chapters, or B97, Viral agents as the cause of diseases classified to other chapters, is to be used as an additional code to identify the organism. An instructional note will be found at the infection code advising that an additional organism code is required.
    c. **Infections resistant to antibiotics**
    Many bacterial infections are resistant to current antibiotics. It is necessary to identify all infections documented as antibiotic resistant. Assign a code from category Z16, Resistance to antimicrobial drugs, following the infection code only if the infection code does not identify drug resistance.
    d. **Sepsis, Severe Sepsis, and Septic Shock Infections resistant to antibiotics**
        1) **Coding of Sepsis and Severe Sepsis**
            (a) **Sepsis**
            For a diagnosis of sepsis, assign the appropriate code for the underlying systemic infection. If the type of infection or causal organism is not further specified, assign code A41.9, Sepsis, unspecified organism.
            A code from subcategory R65.2, Severe sepsis, should not be assigned unless severe sepsis or an associated acute organ dysfunction is documented.
                (i) **Negative or inconclusive blood cultures and sepsis**
                Negative or inconclusive blood cultures do not preclude a diagnosis of sepsis in patients with clinical evidence of the condition; however, the provider should be queried.
                (ii) **Urosepsis**
                The term urosepsis is a nonspecific term. It is not to be considered synonymous with sepsis. It has no default code in the Alphabetic Index. Should a provider use this term, he/she must be queried for clarification.
                (iii) **Sepsis with organ dysfunction**
                If a patient has sepsis and associated acute organ dysfunction or multiple organ dysfunction (MOD), follow the instructions for coding severe sepsis.
                (iv) **Acute organ dysfunction that is not clearly associated with the sepsis**
                If a patient has sepsis and an acute organ dysfunction, but the medical record documentation indicates that the acute organ dysfunction is related to a medical condition other than the sepsis, do not assign a code from subcategory R65.2, Severe sepsis. An acute organ dysfunction must be associated with the sepsis in order to assign the severe sepsis code. If the documentation is not clear as to whether an acute organ dysfunction is related to the sepsis or another medical condition, query the provider.
            (b) **Severe sepsis**
            The coding of severe sepsis requires a minimum of 2 codes: first a code for the underlying systemic infection, followed by a code from subcategory R65.2, Severe sepsis. If the causal organism is not documented, assign code A41.9, Sepsis, unspecified organism, for the infection. Additional code(s) for the associated acute organ dysfunction are also required.
            Due to the complex nature of severe sepsis, some cases may require querying the provider prior to assignment of the codes.
        2) **Septic shock**
        Septic shock generally refers to circulatory failure associated with severe sepsis, and therefore, it represents a type of acute organ dysfunction. For cases of septic shock, the code for the systemic infection should be sequenced first, followed by code R65.21, Severe sepsis with septic shock or code T81.12, Postprocedural septic shock.
        Any additional codes for the other acute organ dysfunctions should also be assigned. As noted in the sequencing instructions in the Tabular List, the code for septic shock cannot be assigned as a principal diagnosis.
        3) **Sequencing of severe sepsis**
        If severe sepsis is present on admission, and meets the definition of principal diagnosis, the underlying systemic infection should be assigned as principal diagnosis followed by the appropriate code from subcategory R65.2 as required by the sequencing rules in the Tabular List. A code from subcategory R65.2 can never be assigned as a principal diagnosis.
        When severe sepsis develops during an encounter (it was not present on admission), the underlying systemic infection and the appropriate code from subcategory R65.2 should be assigned as secondary diagnoses.

Severe sepsis may be present on admission, but the diagnosis may not be confirmed until sometime after admission. If the documentation is not clear whether severe sepsis was present on admission, the provider should be queried.

For infection-associated hemolytic-uremic syndrome with severe sepsis, see guideline I.C.1.d.9.

4) **Sepsis or severe sepsis with a localized infection**

If the reason for admission is sepsis or severe sepsis and a localized infection, such as pneumonia or cellulitis, a code(s) for the underlying systemic infection should be assigned first and the code for the localized infection should be assigned as a secondary diagnosis. If the patient has severe sepsis, a code from subcategory R65.2 should also be assigned as a secondary diagnosis. If the patient is admitted with a localized infection, such as pneumonia, and sepsis/severe sepsis doesn't develop until after admission, the localized infection should be assigned first, followed by the appropriate sepsis/severe sepsis codes.

For hemolytic-uremic syndrome associated with sepsis, see guideline I.C.1.d.9.

5) **Sepsis due to a postprocedural infection**

(a) **Documentation of causal relationship**

As with all postprocedural complications, code assignment is based on the provider's documentation of the relationship between the infection and the procedure.

(b) **Sepsis due to a postprocedural infection**

For sepsis following a postprocedural wound (surgical site) infection, a code from T81.41 to T81.43, Infection following a procedure, T81.49, Infection following a procedure, other surgical site, or a code from O86.00 to O86.03, Infection of obstetric surgical wound, or code O86.09, Infection of obstetric surgical wound, other surgical site, that identifies the site of the infection should be sequenced first, if known. Assign an additional code for sepsis following a procedure (T81.44) or sepsis following an obstetrical procedure (O86.04). Use an additional code to identify the infectious agent. If the patient has severe sepsis, the appropriate code from subcategory R65.2 should also be assigned with the additional code(s) for any acute organ dysfunction.

For infections following infusion, transfusion, therapeutic injection, or immunization, a code from subcategory T80.2, Infections following infusion, transfusion, and therapeutic injection, or code T88.0-, Infection following immunization, should be coded first, followed by the code for the specific infection. If the patient has severe sepsis, the appropriate code from subcategory R65.2 should also be assigned, with the additional codes(s) for any acute organ dysfunction.

(c) **Postprocedural infection and postprocedural septic shock**

If a postprocedural infection has resulted in postprocedural septic shock, assign the codes indicated above for sepsis due to a postprocedural infection, followed by code T81.12-, Postprocedural septic shock. Do not assign code R65.21, Severe sepsis with septic shock. Additional code(s) should be assigned for any acute organ dysfunction.

6) **Sepsis and severe sepsis associated with a noninfectious process (condition)**

In some cases, a noninfectious process (condition) such as trauma, may lead to an infection which can result in sepsis or severe sepsis. If sepsis or severe sepsis is documented as associated with a noninfectious condition, such as a burn or serious injury, and this condition meets the definition for principal diagnosis, the code for the noninfectious condition should be sequenced first, followed by the code for the resulting infection. If severe sepsis is present, a code from subcategory R65.2 should also be assigned with any associated organ dysfunction(s) codes. It is not necessary to assign a code from subcategory R65.1, Systemic inflammatory response syndrome (SIRS) of non-infectious origin, for these cases.

If the infection meets the definition of principal diagnosis, it should be sequenced before the non-infectious condition. When both the associated non-infectious condition and the infection meet the definition of principal diagnosis, either may be assigned as principal diagnosis.

Only one code from category R65, Symptoms and signs specifically associated with systemic inflammation and infection, should be assigned. Therefore, when a non-infectious condition leads to an infection resulting in severe sepsis, assign the appropriate code from subcategory R65.2, Severe sepsis. Do not additionally assign a code from subcategory R65.1, Systemic inflammatory response syndrome (SIRS) of non-infectious origin.

See Section I.C.18. SIRS due to non-infectious process

7) **Sepsis and septic shock complicating abortion, pregnancy, childbirth, and the puerperium**

See Section I.C.15. Sepsis and septic shock complicating abortion, pregnancy, childbirth and the puerperium

8) **Newborn sepsis**

See Section I.C.16. f. Bacterial sepsis of Newborn

9) **Hemolytic-uremic syndrome associated with sepsis**

If the reason for admission is hemolytic-uremic syndrome that is associated with sepsis, assign code D59.31, Infection-associated

hemolytic-uremic syndrome, as the principal diagnosis. Codes for the underlying systemic infection and any other conditions (such as severe sepsis) should be assigned as secondary diagnoses.

e. **Methicillin Resistant Staphylococcus aureus (MRSA) Conditions**

1) **Selection and sequencing of MRSA codes**

(a) **Combination codes for MRSA infection**

When a patient is diagnosed with an infection that is due to methicillin resistant *Staphylococcus aureus* (MRSA), and that infection has a combination code that includes the causal organism (e.g., sepsis, pneumonia) assign the appropriate combination code for the condition (e.g., code A41.02, Sepsis due to Methicillin resistant Staphylococcus aureus or code J15.212, Pneumonia due to Methicillin resistant Staphylococcus aureus). Do not assign code B95.62, Methicillin resistant Staphylococcus aureus infection as the cause of diseases classified elsewhere, as an additional code, because the combination code includes the type of infection and the MRSA organism. Do not assign a code from subcategory Z16.11, Resistance to penicillins, as an additional diagnosis.

See Section C.1. for instructions on coding and sequencing of sepsis and severe sepsis.

(b) **Other codes for MRSA infection**

When there is documentation of a current infection (e.g., wound infection, stitch abscess, urinary tract infection) due to MRSA, and that infection does not have a combination code that includes the causal organism, assign the appropriate code to identify the condition along with code B95.62, Methicillin resistant Staphylococcus aureus infection as the cause of diseases classified elsewhere for the MRSA infection. Do not assign a code from subcategory Z16.11, Resistance to penicillins.

(c) **Methicillin susceptible Staphylococcus aureus (MSSA) and MRSA colonization**

The condition or state of being colonized or carrying MSSA or MRSA is called colonization or carriage, while an individual person is described as being colonized or being a carrier.

Colonization means that MSSA or MSRA is present on or in the body without necessarily causing illness. A positive MRSA colonization test might be documented by the provider as "MRSA screen positive" or "MRSA nasal swab positive".

Assign code Z22.322, Carrier or suspected carrier of Methicillin resistant Staphylococcus aureus, for patients documented as having MRSA colonization. Assign code Z22.321, Carrier or suspected carrier of Methicillin susceptible Staphylococcus aureus, for patients documented as having MSSA colonization.

Colonization is not necessarily indicative of a disease process or as the cause of a specific condition the patient may have unless documented as such by the provider.

(d) **MRSA colonization and infection**

If a patient is documented as having both MRSA colonization and infection during a hospital admission, code Z22.322, Carrier or suspected carrier of Methicillin resistant Staphylococcus aureus, and a code for the MRSA infection may both be assigned.

f. **Zika virus infections**

1) **Code only confirmed cases**

Code only a confirmed diagnosis of Zika virus (A92.5, Zika virus disease) as documented by the provider. This is an exception to the hospital inpatient guideline Section II, H. In this context, "confirmation" does not require documentation of the type of test performed; the provider's diagnostic statement that the condition is confirmed is sufficient. This code should be assigned regardless of the stated mode of transmission. If the provider documents "suspected", "possible" or "probable" Zika, do not assign code A92.5. Assign a code(s) explaining the reason for encounter (such as fever, rash, or joint pain) or Z20.821, Contact with and (suspected) exposure to Zika virus.

g. **Coronavirus infections**

1) **COVID-19 infection (infection due to SARS-CoV-2)**

(a) **Code only confirmed cases**

Code only a confirmed diagnosis of the 2019 novel coronavirus disease (COVID-19) as documented by the provider, or documentation of a positive COVID-19 test result. For a confirmed diagnosis, assign code U07.1, COVID-19. This is an exception to the hospital inpatient guideline Section II, H. In this context, "confirmation" does not require documentation of a positive test result for COVID-19; the provider's documentation that the individual has COVID-19 is sufficient.

If the provider documents "suspected," "possible," "probable," or "inconclusive" COVID-19, do not assign code U07.1. Instead, code the signs and symptoms reported. See guideline I.C.1.g.1.g.

(b) **Sequencing of codes**

When COVID-19 meets the definition of principal diagnosis, code U07.1, COVID-19, should be sequenced first, followed by the appropriate codes for associated manifestations, except when another guideline requires that certain codes be sequenced first, such as obstetrics, sepsis, or transplant complications.

For a COVID-19 infection that progresses to sepsis, see Section I.C.1.d. Sepsis, Severe Sepsis, and Septic Shock

See Section I.C.15.s. for COVID-19 infection in pregnancy, childbirth, and the puerperium
See Section I.C.16.h. for COVID-19 infection in newborn
For a COVID-19 infection in a lung transplant patient, see Section I.C.19.g.3.a. Transplant complications other than kidney.

(c) **Acute respiratory manifestations of COVID-19**
When the reason for the encounter/admission is a respiratory manifestation of COVID-19, assign code U07.1, COVID-19, as the principal/first-listed diagnosis and assign code(s) for the respiratory manifestation(s) as additional diagnoses.
The following conditions are examples of common respiratory manifestations of COVID-19.

(i) **Pneumonia**
For a patient with pneumonia confirmed as due to COVID-19, assign codes U07.1, COVID-19, and J12.82, Pneumonia due to coronavirus disease 2019.

(ii) **Acute bronchitis**
For a patient with acute bronchitis confirmed as due to COVID-19, assign codes U07.1, and J20.8, Acute bronchitis due to other specified organisms.
Bronchitis not otherwise specified (NOS) due to COVID-19 should be coded using code U07.1 and J40, Bronchitis, not specified as acute or chronic.

(iii) **Lower respiratory infection**
If the COVID-19 is documented as being associated with a lower respiratory infection, not otherwise specified (NOS), or an acute respiratory infection, NOS, codes U07.1 and J22, Unspecified acute lower respiratory infection, should be assigned.
If the COVID-19 is documented as being associated with a respiratory infection, NOS, codes U07.1 and J98.8, Other specified respiratory disorders, should be assigned.

(iv) **Acute respiratory distress syndrome**
For acute respiratory distress syndrome (ARDS) due to COVID-19, assign codes U07.1, and J80, Acute respiratory distress syndrome.

(v) **Acute respiratory failure**
For acute respiratory failure due to COVID-19, assign code U07.1, and code J96.0-, Acute respiratory failure.

(d) **Non-respiratory manifestations of COVID-19**
When the reason for the encounter/admission is a non-respiratory manifestation (e.g., viral enteritis) of COVID-19, assign code U07.1, COVID-19, as the principal/first-listed diagnosis and assign code(s) for the manifestation(s) as additional diagnoses.

(e) **Exposure to COVID-19**
For asymptomatic individuals with actual or suspected exposure to COVID-19, assign code Z20.822, Contact with and (suspected) exposure to COVID-19.
For symptomatic individuals with actual or suspected exposure to COVID-19 and the infection has been ruled out, or test results are inconclusive or unknown, assign code Z20.822, Contact with and (suspected) exposure to COVID-19. See guideline I.C.21.c.1, Contact/Exposure, for additional guidance regarding the use of category Z20 codes.
If COVID-19 is confirmed, see guideline I.C.1.g.1.a.

(f) **Screening for COVID-19**
For screening for COVID-19, including preoperative testing, assign code Z11.52, Encounter for screening for COVID-19.

(g) **Signs and symptoms without definitive diagnosis of COVID-19**
For patients presenting with any signs/symptoms associated with COVID-19 (such as fever, etc.) but a definitive diagnosis has not been established, assign the appropriate code(s) for each of the presenting signs and symptoms such as:
- R05.1, Acute cough, or R05.9, Cough, unspecified
- R06.02 Shortness of breath
- R50.9 Fever, unspecified

If a patient with signs/symptoms associated with COVID-19 also has an actual or suspected contact with or exposure to COVID-19, assign Z20.822, Contact with and (suspected) exposure to COVID-19, as an additional code.

(h) **Asymptomatic individuals who test positive for COVID-19**
For asymptomatic individuals who test positive for COVID-19, see guideline I.C.1.g.1.a. Although the individual is asymptomatic, the individual has tested positive and is considered to have the COVID-19 infection.

(i) **Personal history of COVID-19**
For patients with a history of COVID-19, assign code Z86.16, Personal history of COVID-19.

(j) **Follow-up visits after COVID-19 infection has resolved**
For individuals who previously had COVID-19, without residual symptom(s) or condition(s), and are being seen for follow-up evaluation, and COVID-19 test results are negative, assign codes Z09, Encounter for follow-up examination after completed treatment for conditions other than malignant neoplasm, and Z86.16, Personal history of COVID-19.

For follow-up visits for individuals with symptom(s) or condition(s) related to a previous COVID-19 infection, see guideline I.C.1.g.1.m.
See Section I.C.21.c.8, Factors influencing health states and contact with health services, Follow-up

(k) **Encounter for antibody testing**
For an encounter for antibody testing that is not being performed to confirm a current COVID-19 infection, nor is a follow-up test after resolution of COVID-19, assign Z01.84, Encounter for antibody response examination.
Follow the applicable guidelines above if the individual is being tested to confirm a current COVID-19 infection.
For follow-up testing after a COVID-19 infection, see guideline I.C.1.g.1.j.

(l) **Multisystem Inflammatory Syndrome**
For individuals with multisystem inflammatory syndrome (MIS) and COVID-19, assign code U07.1, COVID-19, as the principal/first-listed diagnosis and assign code M35.81, Multisystem inflammatory syndrome, as an additional diagnosis.
If an individual with a history of COVID-19 develops MIS, assign codes M35.81, Multisystem inflammatory syndrome, and U09.9, Post COVID-19 condition, unspecified.
If an individual with a known or suspected exposure to COVID-19, and no current COVID-19 infection or history of COVID-19, develops MIS, assign codes M35.81, Multisystem inflammatory syndrome, and Z20.822, Contact with and (suspected) exposure to COVID-19.
Additional codes should be assigned for any associated complications of MIS.

(m) **Post COVID-19 Condition**
For sequela of COVID-19, or associated symptoms or conditions that develop following a previous COVID-19 infection, assign a code(s) for the specific symptom(s) or condition(s) related to the previous COVID-19 infection, if known, and code U09.9, Post COVID-19 condition, unspecified.
Code U09.9 should not be assigned for manifestations of an active (current) COVID-19 infection.
If a patient has a condition(s) associated with a previous COVID-19 infection and develops a new active (current) COVID-19 infection, code U09.9 may be assigned in conjunction with code U07.1, COVID-19, to identify that the patient also has a condition(s) associated with a previous COVID-19 infection. Code(s) for the specific condition(s) associated with the previous COVID-19 infection and code(s) for manifestation(s) of the new active (current) COVID-19 infection should also be assigned.

(n) **Underimmunization for COVID-19 Status**
Code Z28.310, Unvaccinated for COVID-19, may be assigned when the patient has not received a COVID-19 vaccine of any type. Code Z28.311, Partially vaccinated for COVID-19, may be assigned when the patient has been partially vaccinated for COVID-19 as per the recommendations of the Centers for Disease Control and Prevention (CDC) in place at the time of the encounter. For information, visit the CDC's website https://www.cdc.gov/coronavirus/2019-ncov/vaccines/.
See Section I.B.14. for underimmunization documentation by clinicians other than patient's provider.

2. **Chapter 2: Neoplasms (C00-D49)**
General Guidelines
Chapter 2 of the ICD-10-CM contains the codes for most benign and all malignant neoplasms. Certain benign neoplasms, such as prostatic adenomas, may be found in the specific body system chapters. To properly code a neoplasm, it is necessary to determine from the record if the neoplasm is benign, in-situ, malignant, or of uncertain histologic behavior. If malignant, any secondary (metastatic) sites should also be determined.
Primary malignant neoplasms overlapping site boundaries
A primary malignant neoplasm that overlaps two or more contiguous (next to each other) sites should be classified to the subcategory/code .8 ('overlapping lesion'), unless the combination is specifically indexed elsewhere. For multiple neoplasms of the same site that are not contiguous such as tumors in different quadrants of the same breast, codes for each site should be assigned.
Malignant neoplasm of ectopic tissue
Malignant neoplasms of ectopic tissue are to be coded to the site of origin mentioned, e.g., ectopic pancreatic malignant neoplasms involving the stomach are coded to malignant neoplasm of pancreas, unspecified (C25.9).
The neoplasm table in the Alphabetic Index should be referenced first. However, if the histological term is documented, that term should be referenced first, rather than going immediately to the Neoplasm Table, in order to determine which column in the Neoplasm Table is appropriate. For example, if the documentation indicates "adenoma," refer to the term in the Alphabetic Index to review the entries under this term and the instructional note to "see also neoplasm, by site, benign." The table provides the proper code based on the type of neoplasm and the site. It is important to select the proper column in the table that corresponds to the type of neoplasm. The Tabular List should then be referenced to verify that the correct code has been selected from the table and that a more specific site code does not exist.
See Section I.C.21. Factors influencing health status and contact with health services, Status, for information regarding Z15.0, codes for genetic susceptibility to cancer.

a. **Admission/Encounter for treatment of primary site**
If the malignancy is chiefly responsible for occasioning the patient admission/encounter and treatment is directed at the primary site, designate the primary malignancy as the principal/first-listed diagnosis.
The only exception to this guideline is if the administration of chemotherapy, immunotherapy or external beam radiation therapy is chiefly responsible for occasioning the admission/encounter. In that case, assign the appropriate Z51.-- code as the first-listed or principal diagnosis, and the underlying diagnosis or problem for which the service is being performed as a secondary diagnosis.

b. **Admission/Encounter for treatment of secondary site**
When a patient is admitted because of a primary neoplasm with metastasis and treatment is directed toward the secondary site only, the secondary neoplasm is designated as the principal diagnosis even though the primary malignancy is still present.

c. **Coding and sequencing of complications**
Coding and sequencing of complications associated with the malignancies or with the therapy thereof are subject to the following guidelines:

1) **Anemia associated with malignancy**
When admission/encounter is for management of an anemia associated with the malignancy, and the treatment is only for anemia, the appropriate code for the malignancy is sequenced as the principal or first-listed diagnosis followed by the appropriate code for the anemia (such as code D63.0, Anemia in neoplastic disease).

2) **Anemia associated with chemotherapy, immunotherapy and radiation therapy**
When the admission/encounter is for management of an anemia associated with an adverse effect of the administration of chemotherapy or immunotherapy and the only treatment is for the anemia, the anemia code is sequenced first followed by the appropriate codes for the neoplasm and the adverse effect (T45.1X5-, Adverse effect of antineoplastic and immunosuppressive drugs).
When the admission/encounter is for management of an anemia associated with an adverse effect of radiotherapy, the anemia code should be sequenced first, followed by the appropriate neoplasm code and code Y84.2, Radiological procedure and radiotherapy as the cause of abnormal reaction of the patient, or of later complication, without mention of misadventure at the time of the procedure.

3) **Management of dehydration due to the malignancy**
When the admission/encounter is for management of dehydration due to the malignancy and only the dehydration is being treated (intravenous rehydration), the dehydration is sequenced first, followed by the code(s) for the malignancy.

4) **Treatment of a complication resulting from a surgical procedure**
When the admission/encounter is for treatment of a complication resulting from a surgical procedure, designate the complication as the principal or first-listed diagnosis if treatment is directed at resolving the complication.

d. **Primary malignancy previously excised**
When a primary malignancy has been previously excised or eradicated from its site and there is no further treatment directed to that site and there is no evidence of any existing primary malignancy at that site, a code from category Z85, Personal history of malignant neoplasm, should be used to indicate the former site of the malignancy. Any mention of extension, invasion, or metastasis to another site is coded as a secondary malignant neoplasm to that site. The secondary site may be the principal or first-listed diagnosis with the Z85 code used as a secondary code.
See section I.C.2.t. Secondary malignant neoplasm of lymphoid tissue.

e. **Admissions/Encounters involving chemotherapy, immunotherapy and radiation therapy**

1) **Episode of care involves surgical removal of neoplasm**
When an episode of care involves the surgical removal of a neoplasm, primary or secondary site, followed by adjunct chemotherapy or radiation treatment during the same episode of care, the code for the neoplasm should be assigned as principal or first-listed diagnosis.

2) **Patient admission/encounter chiefly for administration of chemotherapy, immunotherapy and radiation therapy**
If a patient admission/encounter is chiefly for the administration of chemotherapy, immunotherapy or external beam radiation therapy assign code Z51.0, Encounter for antineoplastic radiation therapy, or Z51.11, Encounter for antineoplastic chemotherapy, or Z51.12, Encounter for antineoplastic immunotherapy as the first-listed or principal diagnosis. If a patient receives more than one of these therapies during the same admission, more than one of these codes may be assigned, in any sequence.
The malignancy for which the therapy is being administered should be assigned as a secondary diagnosis.
If a patient admission/encounter is for the insertion or implantation of radioactive elements (e.g., brachytherapy) the appropriate code for the malignancy is sequenced as the principal or first-listed diagnosis. Code Z51.0 should not be assigned.

3) **Patient admitted for radiation therapy, chemotherapy or immunotherapy and develops complications**
When a patient is admitted for the purpose of external beam radiotherapy, immunotherapy or chemotherapy and develops complications such as uncontrolled nausea and vomiting or

dehydration, the principal or first-listed diagnosis is Z51.0, Encounter for antineoplastic radiation therapy, or Z51.11, Encounter for antineoplastic chemotherapy, or Z51.12, Encounter for antineoplastic immunotherapy followed by any codes for the complications.
When a patient is admitted for the purpose of insertion or implantation of radioactive elements (e.g., brachytherapy) and develops complications such as uncontrolled nausea and vomiting or dehydration, the principal or first-listed diagnosis is the appropriate code for the malignancy followed by any codes for the complications.

f. **Admission/encounter to determine extent of malignancy**
When the reason for admission/encounter is to determine the extent of the malignancy, or for a procedure such as paracentesis or thoracentesis, the primary malignancy or appropriate metastatic site is designated as the principal or first-listed diagnosis, even though chemotherapy or radiotherapy is administered.

g. **Symptoms, signs, and abnormal findings listed in Chapter 18 associated with neoplasms**
Symptoms, signs, and ill-defined conditions listed in Chapter 18 characteristic of, or associated with, an existing primary or secondary site malignancy cannot be used to replace the malignancy as principal or first-listed diagnosis, regardless of the number of admissions or encounters for treatment and care of the neoplasm.
See section I.C.21. Factors influencing health status and contact with health services, Encounter for prophylactic organ removal.

h. **Admission/encounter for pain control/management**
See Section I.C.6. for information on coding admission/encounter for pain control/management.

i. **Malignancy in two or more noncontiguous sites**
A patient may have more than one malignant tumor in the same organ. These tumors may represent different primaries or metastatic disease, depending on the site. Should the documentation be unclear, the provider should be queried as to the status of each tumor so that the correct codes can be assigned.

j. **Disseminated malignant neoplasm, unspecified**
Code C80.0, Disseminated malignant neoplasm, unspecified, is for use only in those cases where the patient has advanced metastatic disease and no known primary or secondary sites are specified. It should not be used in place of assigning codes for the primary site and all known secondary sites.

k. **Malignant neoplasm without specification of site**
Code C80.1, Malignant (primary) neoplasm, unspecified, equates to Cancer, unspecified. This code should only be used when no determination can be made as to the primary site of a malignancy. This code should rarely be used in the inpatient setting.

l. **Sequencing of neoplasm codes**

1) **Encounter for treatment of primary malignancy**
If the reason for the encounter is for treatment of a primary malignancy, assign the malignancy as the principal/first-listed diagnosis. The primary site is to be sequenced first, followed by any metastatic sites.

2) **Encounter for treatment of secondary malignancy**
When an encounter is for a primary malignancy with metastasis and treatment is directed toward the metastatic (secondary) site(s) only, the metastatic site(s) is designated as the principal/first-listed diagnosis. The primary malignancy is coded as an additional code.

3) **Malignant neoplasm in a pregnant patient**
When a pregnant patient has a malignant neoplasm, a code from subcategory O9A.1-, Malignant neoplasm complicating pregnancy, childbirth, and the puerperium, should be sequenced first, followed by the appropriate code from Chapter 2 to indicate the type of neoplasm.

4) **Encounter for complication associated with a neoplasm**
When an encounter is for management of a complication associated with a neoplasm, such as dehydration, and the treatment is only for the complication, the complication is coded first, followed by the appropriate code(s) for the neoplasm.
The exception to this guideline is anemia. When the admission/encounter is for management of an anemia associated with the malignancy, and the treatment is only for anemia, the appropriate code for the malignancy is sequenced as the principal or first-listed diagnosis followed by code D63.0, Anemia in neoplastic disease.

5) **Complication from surgical procedure for treatment of a neoplasm**
When an encounter is for treatment of a complication resulting from a surgical procedure performed for the treatment of the neoplasm, designate the complication as the principal/first-listed diagnosis. See the guideline regarding the coding of a current malignancy versus personal history to determine if the code for the neoplasm should also be assigned.

6) **Pathologic fracture due to a neoplasm**
When an encounter is for a pathological fracture due to a neoplasm, and the focus of treatment is the fracture, a code from subcategory M84.5, Pathological fracture in neoplastic disease, should be sequenced first, followed by the code for the neoplasm.
If the focus of treatment is the neoplasm with an associated pathological fracture, the neoplasm code should be sequenced first, followed by a code from M84.5 for the pathological fracture.

m. **Current malignancy versus personal history of malignancy**

When a primary malignancy has been excised but further treatment, such as an additional surgery for the malignancy, radiation therapy or chemotherapy is directed to that site, the primary malignancy code should be used until treatment is completed.

When a primary malignancy has been previously excised or eradicated from its site, there is no further treatment (of the malignancy) directed to that site, and there is no evidence of any existing primary malignancy at that site, a code from category Z85, Personal history of malignant neoplasm, should be used to indicate the former site of the malignancy.

Codes from subcategories Z85.0 – Z85.85 should only be assigned for the former site of a primary malignancy, not the site of a secondary malignancy. Code Z85.89 may be assigned for the former site(s) of either a primary or secondary malignancy.

See Section I.C.21. Factors influencing health status and contact with health services, History (of)

n. **Leukemia, Multiple Myeloma, and Malignant Plasma Cell Neoplasms in remission versus personal history**

The categories for leukemia, and category C90, Multiple myeloma and malignant plasma cell neoplasms, have codes indicating whether or not the leukemia has achieved remission. There are also codes Z85.6, Personal history of leukemia, and Z85.79, Personal history of other malignant neoplasms of lymphoid, hematopoietic and related tissues. If the documentation is unclear as to whether the leukemia has achieved remission, the provider should be queried.

See Section I.C.21. Factors influencing health status and contact with health services, History (of)

o. **Aftercare following surgery for neoplasm**

See Section I.C.21. Factors influencing health status and contact with health services, Aftercare

p. **Follow-up care for completed treatment of a malignancy**

See Section I.C.21. Factors influencing health status and contact with health services, Follow-up

q. **Prophylactic organ removal for prevention of malignancy**

See Section I.C. 21, Factors influencing health status and contact with health services, Prophylactic organ removal

r. **Malignant neoplasm associated with transplanted organ**

A malignant neoplasm of a transplanted organ should be coded as a transplant complication. Assign first the appropriate code from category T86.-, Complications of transplanted organs and tissue, followed by code C80.2, Malignant neoplasm associated with transplanted organ. Use an additional code for the specific malignancy.

s. **Breast Implant Associated Anaplastic Large Cell Lymphoma**

Breast implant associated anaplastic large cell lymphoma (BIA-ALCL) is a type of lymphoma that can develop around breast implants. Assign code C84.7A, Anaplastic large cell lymphoma, ALK-negative, breast, for BIA-ALCL **or C84.7B, Anaplastic large cell lymphoma, ALK-negative, in remission, for BIA-ALCL in remission**. Do not assign a complication code from chapter 19.

t. **Secondary malignant neoplasm of lymphoid tissue**

When a malignant neoplasm of lymphoid tissue metastasizes beyond the lymph nodes, a code from categories C81-C85 with a final character identifying "extranodal and solid organ sites" **should be assigned** rather than a code for the secondary neoplasm of the affected solid organ. For example, for metastasis of diffuse large B-cell lymphoma to the lung, brain and left adrenal gland, assign code C83.39**8**, Diffuse large B-cell lymphoma **of other** extranodal and solid organ sites.

3. **Chapter 3: Disease of the blood and blood-forming organs and certain disorders involving the immune mechanism (D50-D89)**

Reserved for future guideline expansion

4. **Chapter 4: Endocrine, Nutritional, and Metabolic Diseases (E00-E89)**

a. **Diabetes mellitus**

The diabetes mellitus codes are combination codes that include the type of diabetes mellitus, the body system affected, and the complications affecting that body system. As many codes within a particular category as are necessary to describe all of the complications of the disease may be used. They should be sequenced based on the reason for a particular encounter. Assign as many codes from categories E08 – E13 as needed to identify all of the associated conditions that the patient has.

1) **Type of diabetes**

The age of a patient is not the sole determining factor, though most type 1 diabetics develop the condition before reaching puberty. For this reason, type 1 diabetes mellitus is also referred to as juvenile diabetes.

(a) **Presymptomatic Type 1 Diabetes Mellitus**

Codes E10.A-, Type 1 diabetes mellitus, presymptomatic, are assigned for early-stage type 1 diabetes that predates the onset of symptoms.

2) **Type of diabetes mellitus not documented**

If the type of diabetes mellitus is not documented in the medical record the default is E11.-, Type 2 diabetes mellitus.

3) **Diabetes mellitus and the use of insulin, oral hypoglycemics, and injectable non-insulin drugs**

If the documentation in a medical record does not indicate the type of diabetes but does indicate that the patient uses insulin, code E11-, Type 2 diabetes mellitus, should be assigned. Additional code(s) should be assigned from category Z79 to identify the long-term (current) use of

insulin, oral hypoglycemic drugs, or injectable non-insulin antidiabetic, as follows:

If the patient is treated with both oral hypoglycemic drugs and insulin, both code Z79.4, Long term (current) use of insulin, and code Z79.84, Long term (current) use of oral hypoglycemic drugs, should be assigned.

If the patient is treated with both insulin and an injectable non-insulin antidiabetic drug, assign codes Z79.4, Long term (current) use of insulin, and Z79.85, Long-term (current) use of injectable non-insulin antidiabetic drugs.

If the patient is treated with both oral hypoglycemic drugs and an injectable non-insulin antidiabetic drug, assign codes Z79.84, Long term (current) use of oral hypoglycemic drugs, and Z79.85, Long-term (current) use of injectable non-insulin antidiabetic drugs.

Code Z79.4 should not be assigned if insulin is given temporarily to bring a type 2 patient's blood sugar under control during an encounter.

4) **Diabetes mellitus in pregnancy and gestational diabetes**

See Section I.C.15. Diabetes mellitus in pregnancy.

See Section I.C.15. Gestational (pregnancy induced) diabetes

5) **Complications due to insulin pump malfunction**

(a) **Underdose of insulin due to insulin pump failure**

An underdose of insulin due to an insulin pump failure should be assigned to a code from subcategory T85.6, Mechanical complication of other specified internal and external prosthetic devices, implants and grafts, that specifies the type of pump malfunction, as the principal or first-listed code, followed by code T38.3X6-, Underdosing of insulin and oral hypoglycemic [antidiabetic] drugs. Additional codes for the type of diabetes mellitus and any associated complications due to the underdosing should also be assigned.

(b) **Overdose of insulin due to insulin pump failure**

The principal or first-listed code for an encounter due to an insulin pump malfunction resulting in an overdose of insulin, should also be T85.6-, Mechanical complication of other specified internal and external prosthetic devices, implants and grafts, followed by code T38.3X1-, Poisoning by insulin and oral hypoglycemic [antidiabetic] drugs, accidental (unintentional).

6) **Secondary diabetes mellitus**

Codes under categories E08, Diabetes mellitus due to underlying condition, E09, Drug or chemical induced diabetes mellitus, and E13, Other specified diabetes mellitus, identify complications/manifestations associated with secondary diabetes mellitus. Secondary diabetes is always caused by another condition or event (e.g., cystic fibrosis, malignant neoplasm of pancreas, pancreatectomy, adverse effect of drug, or poisoning).

(a) **Secondary diabetes mellitus and the use of insulin, oral hypoglycemic drugs, or injectable non-insulin drugs**

For patients with secondary diabetes mellitus who routinely use insulin, oral hypoglycemic drugs, or injectable non-insulin drugs, additional code(s) from category Z79 should be assigned to identify the long-term (current) use of insulin, oral hypoglycemic drugs, or non-injectable non-insulin drugs as follows:

If the patient is treated with both oral hypoglycemic drugs and insulin, both code Z79.4, Long term (current) use of insulin, and code Z79.84, Long term (current) use of oral hypoglycemic drugs, should be assigned.

If the patient is treated with both insulin and an injectable non-insulin antidiabetic drug, assign codes Z79.4, Long-term (current) use of insulin, and Z79.85, Long-term (current) use of injectable non-insulin antidiabetic drugs.

If the patient is treated with both oral hypoglycemic drugs and an injectable non-insulin antidiabetic drug, assign codes Z79.84, Long-term (current) use of oral hypoglycemic drugs, and Z79.85, Long-term (current) use of injectable non-insulin antidiabetic drugs.

Code Z79.4 should not be assigned if insulin is given temporarily to bring a secondary diabetic patient's blood sugar under control during an encounter.

(b) **Assigning and sequencing secondary diabetes codes and its causes**

The sequencing of the secondary diabetes codes in relationship to codes for the cause of the diabetes is based on the Tabular List instructions for categories E08, E09 and E13.

(i) **Secondary diabetes mellitus due to pancreatectomy**

For postpancreatectomy diabetes mellitus (lack of insulin due to the surgical removal of all or part of the pancreas), assign code E89.1, Postprocedural hypoinsulinemia.

Assign a code from category E13 as the principal or first-listed diagnosis and a code from subcategory Z90.41, Acquired absence of pancreas, as an additional code.

(ii) **Secondary diabetes due to drugs**
Secondary diabetes may be caused by an adverse effect of correctly administered medications, poisoning or sequela of poisoning.
See section I.C.19.e. for coding of adverse effects and poisoning, and section I.C.20 for external cause code reporting.

5. **Chapter 5: Mental, Behavioral and Neurodevelopmental disorders (F01-F99)**
   a. **Pain disorders related to psychological factors**
   Assign code F45.41, for pain that is exclusively related to psychological disorders. As indicated by the Excludes 1 note under category G89, a code from category G89 should not be assigned with code F45.41.
   Code F45.42, Pain disorders with related psychological factors, should be used with a code from category G89, Pain, not elsewhere classified, if there is documentation of a psychological component for a patient with acute or chronic pain.
   See Section I.C.6. Pain
   b. **Mental and behavioral disorders due to psychoactive substance use**
   1) **In Remission**
   Selection of codes describing "in remission" for categories F10-F19, Mental and behavioral disorders due to psychoactive substance use (categories F10-F19 with -.11, -.21, -.91) requires the provider's clinical judgment and are assigned only on the basis of provider documentation (as defined in the Official Guidelines for Coding and Reporting), unless otherwise instructed by the classification.
   Mild substance use disorders in early or sustained remission are classified to the appropriate codes for substance abuse in remission, and moderate or severe substance use disorders in early or sustained remission are classified to the appropriate codes for substance dependence in remission.
   2) **Psychoactive Substance Use, Abuse and Dependence**
   When the provider documentation refers to use, abuse and dependence of the same substance (e.g. alcohol, opioid, cannabis, etc.), only one code should be assigned to identify the pattern of use based on the following hierarchy:
   - If both use and abuse are documented, assign only the code for abuse
   - If both abuse and dependence are documented, assign only the code for dependence
   - If use, abuse and dependence are all documented, assign only the code for dependence
   - If both use and dependence are documented, assign only the code for dependence
   3) **Psychoactive Substance Use, Unspecified**
   As with all other unspecified diagnoses, the codes for unspecified psychoactive substance use (F10.9-, F11.9-, F12.9-, F13.9-, F14.9-, F15.9-, F16.9-, F18.9-, F19.9-) should only be assigned based on provider documentation and when they meet the definition of a reportable diagnosis (see Section III, Reporting Additional Diagnoses). These codes are to be used only when the psychoactive substance use is associated with a substance related disorder (chapter 5 disorders such as sexual dysfunction, sleep disorder, or a mental or behavioral disorder) or medical condition, and such a relationship is documented by the provider.
   4) **Medical Conditions Due to Psychoactive Substance Use, Abuse and Dependence**
   Medical conditions due to substance use, abuse, and dependence are not classified as substance-induced disorders. Assign the diagnosis code for the medical condition as directed by the Alphabetical Index along with the appropriate psychoactive substance use, abuse or dependence code. For example, for alcoholic pancreatitis due to alcohol dependence, assign the appropriate code from subcategory K85.2, Alcohol induced acute pancreatitis, and the appropriate code from subcategory F10.2, such as code F10.20, Alcohol dependence, uncomplicated. It would not be appropriate to assign code F10.288, Alcohol dependence with other alcohol-induced disorder.
   5) **Blood Alcohol Level**
   A code from category Y90, Evidence of alcohol involvement determined by blood alcohol level, may be assigned when this information is documented and the patient's provider has documented a condition classifiable to category F10, Alcohol related disorders. The blood alcohol level does not need to be documented by the patient's provider in order for it to be coded.
   See Section I.B.14. for blood alcohol level documentation by clinicians other than patient's provider.
   c. **Factitious Disorder**
   Factitious disorder imposed on self or Munchausen's syndrome is a disorder in which a person falsely reports or causes his or her own physical or psychological signs or symptoms. For patients with documented factitious disorder on self or Munchausen's syndrome, assign the appropriate code from subcategory F68.1-, Factitious disorder imposed on self.
   Munchausen's syndrome by proxy (MSBP) is a disorder in which a caregiver (perpetrator) falsely reports or causes an illness or injury in another person (victim) under his or her care, such as a child, an elderly adult, or a person who has a disability. The condition is also referred to as "factitious disorder imposed on another" or "factitious disorder by proxy." The perpetrator, not the victim, receives this diagnosis. Assign code F68.A, Factitious disorder

imposed on another, to the perpetrator's record. For the victim of a patient suffering from MSBP, assign the appropriate code from categories T74, Adult and child abuse, neglect and other maltreatment, confirmed, or T76, Adult and child abuse, neglect and other maltreatment, suspected.
   See Section I.C.19.f. Adult and child abuse, neglect and other maltreatment
   d. **Dementia**
   The ICD-10-CM classifies dementia (categories F01, F02, and F03) on the basis of the etiology and severity (unspecified, mild, moderate or severe). Selection of the appropriate severity level requires the provider's clinical judgment and codes should be assigned only on the basis of provider documentation (as defined in the *Official Guidelines for Coding and Reporting*), unless otherwise instructed by the classification. If the documentation does not provide information about the severity of the dementia, assign the appropriate code for unspecified severity.
   If a patient is admitted to an inpatient acute care hospital or other inpatient facility setting with dementia at one severity level and it progresses to a higher severity level, assign one code for the highest severity level reported during the stay.

6. **Chapter 6: Diseases of the Nervous System (G00-G99)**
   a. **Dominant/nondominant side**
   Codes from category G81, Hemiplegia and hemiparesis, and subcategories G83.1, Monoplegia of lower limb, G83.2, Monoplegia of upper limb, and G83.3, Monoplegia, unspecified, identify whether the dominant or nondominant side is affected. Should the affected side be documented, but not specified as dominant or nondominant, and the classification system does not indicate a default, code selection is as follows:
   - For ambidextrous patients, the default should be dominant.
   - If the left side is affected, the default is non-dominant.
   - If the right side is affected, the default is dominant.
   b. **Pain - Category G89**
   1) **General coding information**
   Codes in category G89, Pain, not elsewhere classified, may be used in conjunction with codes from other categories and chapters to provide more detail about acute or chronic pain and neoplasm-related pain, unless otherwise indicated below.
   If the pain is not specified as acute or chronic, post-thoracotomy, postprocedural, or neoplasm-related, do not assign codes from category G89.
   A code from category G89 should not be assigned if the underlying (definitive) diagnosis is known, unless the reason for the encounter is pain control/ management and not management of the underlying condition.
   When an admission or encounter is for a procedure aimed at treating the underlying condition (e.g., spinal fusion, kyphoplasty), a code for the underlying condition (e.g., vertebral fracture, spinal stenosis) should be assigned as the principal diagnosis. No code from category G89 should be assigned.
   (a) **Category G89 Codes as Principal or First-Listed Diagnosis**
   Category G89 codes are acceptable as principal diagnosis or the first-listed code:
   - When pain control or pain management is the reason for the admission/encounter (e.g., a patient with displaced intervertebral disc, nerve impingement and severe back pain presents for injection of steroid into the spinal canal). The underlying cause of the pain should be reported as an additional diagnosis, if known.
   - When a patient is admitted for the insertion of a neurostimulator for pain control, assign the appropriate pain code as the principal or first-listed diagnosis. When an admission or encounter is for a procedure aimed at treating the underlying condition and a neurostimulator is inserted for pain control during the same admission/encounter, a code for the underlying condition should be assigned as the principal diagnosis and the appropriate pain code should be assigned as a secondary diagnosis.
   (b) **Use of Category G89 Codes in Conjunction with Site Specific Pain Codes**
   (i) **Assigning Category G89 and Site-Specific Pain Codes**
   Codes from category G89 may be used in conjunction with codes that identify the site of pain (including codes from chapter 18) if the category G89 code provides additional information. For example, if the code describes the site of the pain, but does not fully describe whether the pain is acute or chronic, then both codes should be assigned.
   (ii) **Sequencing of Category G89 Codes with Site-Specific Pain Codes**
   The sequencing of category G89 codes with site-specific pain codes (including chapter 18 codes), is dependent on the circumstances of the encounter/admission as follows:
   - If the encounter is for pain control or pain management, assign the code from category G89 followed by the code identifying the specific site of pain (e.g., encounter for pain management for acute neck pain from trauma is assigned code G89.11, Acute pain due to trauma, followed by code M54.2, Cervicalgia, to identify the site of pain).

- If the encounter is for any other reason except pain control or pain management, and a related definitive diagnosis has not been established (confirmed) by the provider, assign the code for the specific site of pain first, followed by the appropriate code from category G89.

2) Pain due to devices, implants and grafts
See Section I.C.19. Pain due to medical devices

3) Postoperative Pain
The provider's documentation should be used to guide the coding of postoperative pain, as well as *Section III. Reporting Additional Diagnoses* and *Section IV. Diagnostic Coding and Reporting in the Outpatient Setting*. The default for post-thoracotomy and other postoperative pain not specified as acute or chronic is the code for the acute form. Routine or expected postoperative pain immediately after surgery should not be coded.

(a) Postoperative pain not associated with specific postoperative complication
Postoperative pain not associated with a specific postoperative complication is assigned to the appropriate postoperative pain code in category G89.

(b) Postoperative pain associated with specific postoperative complication
Postoperative pain associated with a specific postoperative complication (such as painful wire sutures) is assigned to the appropriate code(s) found in Chapter 19, Injury, poisoning, and certain other consequences of external causes. If appropriate, use additional code(s) from category G89 to identify acute or chronic pain (G89.18 or G89.28).

4) Chronic pain
Chronic pain is classified to subcategory G89.2. There is no time frame defining when pain becomes chronic pain. The provider's documentation should be used to guide use of these codes.

5) Neoplasm Related Pain
Code G89.3 is assigned to pain documented as being related, associated or due to cancer, primary or secondary malignancy, or tumor. This code is assigned regardless of whether the pain is acute or chronic.
This code may be assigned as the principal or first-listed code when the stated reason for the admission/encounter is documented as pain control/pain management. The underlying neoplasm should be reported as an additional diagnosis.
When the reason for the admission/encounter is management of the neoplasm and the pain associated with the neoplasm is also documented, code G89.3 may be assigned as an additional diagnosis. It is not necessary to assign an additional code for the site of the pain.
See Section I.C.2. for instructions on the sequencing of neoplasms for all other stated reasons for the admission/encounter (except for pain control/pain management).

6) Chronic pain syndrome
Central pain syndrome (G89.0) and chronic pain syndrome (G89.4) are different than the term "chronic pain," and therefore codes should only be used when the provider has specifically documented this condition.
See Section I.C.5. Pain disorders related to psychological factors

7. Chapter 7: Diseases of the Eye and Adnexa (H00-H59)
a. Glaucoma
1) Assigning Glaucoma Codes
Assign as many codes from category H40, Glaucoma, as needed to identify the type of glaucoma, the affected eye, and the glaucoma stage.

2) Bilateral glaucoma with same type and stage
When a patient has bilateral glaucoma and both eyes are documented as being the same type and stage, and there is a code for bilateral glaucoma, report only the code for the type of glaucoma, bilateral, with the seventh character for the stage.
When a patient has bilateral glaucoma and both eyes are documented as being the same type and stage, and the classification does not provide a code for bilateral glaucoma (i.e. subcategories H40.10, and H40.20) report only one code for the type of glaucoma with the appropriate seventh character for the stage.

3) Bilateral glaucoma stage with different types or stages
When a patient has bilateral glaucoma and each eye is documented as having a different type or stage, and the classification distinguishes laterality, assign the appropriate code for each eye rather than the code for bilateral glaucoma.
When a patient has bilateral glaucoma and each eye is documented as having a different type, and the classification does not distinguish laterality (i.e., subcategories H40.10, and H40.20), assign one code for each type of glaucoma with the appropriate seventh character for the stage.
When a patient has bilateral glaucoma and each eye is documented as having the same type, but different stage, and the classification does not distinguish laterality (i.e., subcategories H40.10 and H40.20), assign a code for the type of glaucoma for each eye with the seventh character for the specific glaucoma stage documented for each eye.

4) Patient admitted with glaucoma and stage evolves during the admission
If a patient is admitted with glaucoma and the stage progresses during the admission, assign the code for highest stage documented.

5) Indeterminate stage glaucoma
Assignment of the seventh character "4" for "indeterminate stage" should be based on the clinical documentation. The seventh character "4" is used for glaucomas whose stage cannot be clinically determined. This seventh character should not be confused with the seventh character "0", unspecified, which should be assigned when there is no documentation regarding the stage of the glaucoma.

b. Blindness
If "blindness" or "low vision" of both eyes is documented but the visual impairment category is not documented, assign code H54.3, Unqualified visual loss, both eyes. If "blindness" or "low vision" in one eye is documented but the visual impairment category is not documented, assign a code from H54.6-, Unqualified visual loss, one eye. If "blindness" or "visual loss" is documented without any information about whether one or both eyes are affected, assign code H54.7, Unspecified visual loss.

8. Chapter 8: Diseases of the Ear and Mastoid Process (H60-H95)
Reserved for future guideline expansion

9. Chapter 9: Diseases of the Circulatory System (I00-I99)
a. Hypertension
The classification presumes a causal relationship between hypertension and heart involvement and between hypertension and kidney involvement, as the two conditions are linked by the term "with" in the Alphabetic Index. These conditions should be coded as related even in the absence of provider documentation explicitly linking them, unless the documentation clearly states the conditions are unrelated.
For hypertension and conditions not specifically linked by relational terms such as "with," "associated with" or "due to" in the classification, provider documentation must link the conditions in order to code them as related.

1) Hypertension with Heart Disease
Hypertension with heart conditions classified to I50.- or I51.4- I51.7, I51.89, I51.9, are assigned to a code from category I11, Hypertensive heart disease. Use additional code(s) from category I50, Heart failure, to identify the type(s) of heart failure in those patients with heart failure.
The same heart conditions (I50.-, I51.4-I51.7, I51.89, I51.9) with hypertension are coded separately if the provider has documented they are unrelated to the hypertension. Sequence according to the circumstances of the admission/encounter.

2) Hypertensive Chronic Kidney Disease
Assign codes from category I12, Hypertensive chronic kidney disease, when both hypertension and a condition classifiable to category N18, Chronic kidney disease (CKD), are present. CKD should not be coded as hypertensive if the provider indicates the CKD is not related to the hypertension.
The appropriate code from category N18 should be used as a secondary code with a code from category I12 to identify the stage of chronic kidney disease.
See Section I.C.14. Chronic kidney disease.
If a patient has hypertensive chronic kidney disease and acute renal failure, the acute renal failure should also be coded. Sequence according to the circumstances of the admission/encounter.

3) Hypertensive Heart and Chronic Kidney Disease
Assign codes from combination category I13, Hypertensive heart and chronic kidney disease, when there is hypertension with both heart and kidney involvement. If heart failure is present, assign an additional code from category I50 to identify the type of heart failure.
The appropriate code from category N18, Chronic kidney disease, should be used as a secondary code with a code from category I13 to identify the stage of chronic kidney disease.
See Section I.C.14. Chronic kidney disease.
The codes in category I13, Hypertensive heart and chronic kidney disease, are combination codes that include hypertension, heart disease and chronic kidney disease. The Includes note at I13 specifies that the conditions included at I11 and I12 are included together in I13. If a patient has hypertension, heart disease and chronic kidney disease, then a code from I13 should be used, not individual codes for hypertension, heart disease and chronic kidney disease, or codes from I11 or I12.
For patients with both acute renal failure and chronic kidney disease, the acute renal failure should also be coded. Sequence according to circumstances of the admission/encounter.

4) Hypertensive Cerebrovascular Disease
For hypertensive cerebrovascular disease, first assign the appropriate code from categories I60-I69, followed by the appropriate hypertension code.

5) Hypertensive Retinopathy
Subcategory H35.0, Background retinopathy and retinal vascular changes, should be used along with a code from categories I10-I15, in the Hypertensive diseases section, to include the systemic hypertension. The sequencing is based on the reason for the encounter.

6) Hypertension, Secondary
Secondary hypertension is due to an underlying condition. Two codes are required: one to identify the underlying etiology and one from category I15 to identify the hypertension. Sequencing of codes is determined by the reason for admission/encounter.

7) Hypertension, Transient
Assign code R03.0, Elevated blood pressure reading without diagnosis of hypertension, unless patient has an established diagnosis of

hypertension. Assign code O13.-, Gestational [pregnancy-induced] hypertension without significant proteinuria, or O14.-, Pre-eclampsia, for transient hypertension of pregnancy.

8) Hypertension, Controlled
This diagnostic statement usually refers to an existing state of hypertension under control by therapy. Assign the appropriate code from categories I10-I15, Hypertensive diseases.

9) Hypertension, Uncontrolled
Uncontrolled hypertension may refer to untreated hypertension or hypertension not responding to current therapeutic regimen. In either case, assign the appropriate code from categories I10-I15, Hypertensive diseases.

10) Hypertensive Crisis
Assign a code from category I16, Hypertensive crisis, for documented hypertensive urgency, hypertensive emergency or unspecified hypertensive crisis. Code also any identified hypertensive disease (I10-I15). The sequencing is based on the reason for the encounter.

11) Pulmonary Hypertension
Pulmonary hypertension is classified to category I27, Other pulmonary heart diseases. For secondary pulmonary hypertension (I27.1, I27.2-), code also any associated conditions or adverse effects of drugs or toxins. The sequencing is based on the reason for the encounter, except for adverse effects of drugs (See Section I.C.19.e.).

12) Hypertension, Resistant
Resistant hypertension refers to blood pressure of a patient with hypertension that remains above goal in spite of the use of antihypertensive medications. Assign code I1A.0, Resistant hypertension, as an additional code when apparent treatment resistant hypertension, treatment resistant hypertension, or true resistant hypertension is documented by the provider. A code for the specific type of existing hypertension is sequenced first, if known.

b. Atherosclerotic Coronary Artery Disease and Angina
ICD-10-CM has combination codes for atherosclerotic heart disease with angina pectoris. The subcategories for these codes are I25.11, Atherosclerotic heart disease of native coronary artery with angina pectoris and I25.7, Atherosclerosis of coronary artery bypass graft(s) and coronary artery of transplanted heart with angina pectoris.
When using one of these combination codes it is not necessary to use an additional code for angina pectoris. A causal relationship can be assumed in a patient with both atherosclerosis and angina pectoris, unless the documentation indicates the angina is due to something other than the atherosclerosis.
If a patient with coronary artery disease is admitted due to an acute myocardial infarction (AMI), the AMI should be sequenced before the coronary artery disease.
See Section I.C.9. Acute myocardial infarction (AMI)

c. Intraoperative and Postprocedural Cerebrovascular Accident
Medical record documentation should clearly specify the cause- and-effect relationship between the medical intervention and the cerebrovascular accident in order to assign a code for intraoperative or postprocedural cerebrovascular accident.
Proper code assignment depends on whether it was an infarction or hemorrhage and whether it occurred intraoperatively or postoperatively. If it was a cerebral hemorrhage, code assignment depends on the type of procedure performed.

d. Sequelae of Cerebrovascular Disease
1) Category I69, Sequelae of Cerebrovascular disease
Category I69 is used to indicate conditions classifiable to categories I60-I67 as the causes of sequela (neurologic deficits), themselves classified elsewhere. These "late effects" include neurologic deficits that persist after initial onset of conditions classifiable to categories I60-I67. The neurologic deficits caused by cerebrovascular disease may be present from the onset or may arise at any time after the onset of the condition classifiable to categories I60-I67.
Codes from category I69, Sequelae of cerebrovascular disease, that specify hemiplegia, hemiparesis and monoplegia identify whether the dominant or nondominant side is affected. Should the affected side be documented, but not specified as dominant or nondominant, and the classification system does not indicate a default, code selection is as follows:
- For ambidextrous patients, the default should be dominant.
- If the left side is affected, the default is non-dominant.
- If the right side is affected, the default is dominant.

2) Codes from category I69 with codes from I60-I67
Codes from category I69 may be assigned on a health care record with codes from I60-I67, if the patient has a current cerebrovascular disease and deficits from an old cerebrovascular disease.

3) Codes from category I69 and Personal history of transient ischemic attack (TIA) and cerebral infarction (Z86.73)
Codes from category I69 should not be assigned if the patient does not have neurologic deficits.
See Section I.C.21.4. History (of) for use of personal history codes

e. Acute myocardial infarction (AMI)
1) Type 1 ST elevation myocardial infarction (STEMI) and non-ST elevation myocardial infarction (NSTEMI)
The ICD-10-CM codes for type 1 acute myocardial infarction (AMI) identify the site, such as anterolateral wall or true posterior wall. Subcategories I21.0-I21.2 and code I21.3 are used for type 1 ST elevation myocardial infarction (STEMI). Code I21.4, Non-ST elevation (NSTEMI) myocardial infarction, is used for type 1 non-ST elevation myocardial infarction (NSTEMI) and nontransmural MIs.
If a type 1 NSTEMI evolves to STEMI, assign the STEMI code. If a type 1 STEMI converts to NSTEMI due to thrombolytic therapy, it is still coded as STEMI.
For encounters occurring while the myocardial infarction is equal to, or less than, four weeks old, including transfers to another acute setting or a postacute setting, and the myocardial infarction meets the definition for "other diagnoses" (see Section III, Reporting Additional Diagnoses), codes from category I21 may continue to be reported. For encounters after the 4-week time frame and the patient is still receiving care related to the myocardial infarction, the appropriate aftercare code should be assigned, rather than a code from category I21. For old or healed myocardial infarctions not requiring further care, code I25.2, Old myocardial infarction, may be assigned.

2) Acute myocardial infarction, unspecified
Code I21.9, Acute myocardial infarction, unspecified, is the default for unspecified acute myocardial infarction or unspecified type. If only type 1 STEMI or transmural MI without the site is documented, assign code I21.3, ST elevation (STEMI) myocardial infarction of unspecified site.

3) AMI documented as nontransmural or subendocardial but site provided
If an AMI is documented as nontransmural or subendocardial, but the site is provided, it is still coded as a subendocardial AMI.
See Section I.C.21.3. for information on coding status post administration of tPA in a different facility within the last 24 hours.

4) Subsequent acute myocardial infarction
A code from category I22, Subsequent ST elevation (STEMI) and non-ST elevation (NSTEMI) myocardial infarction, is to be used when a patient who has suffered a type 1 or unspecified AMI has a new AMI within the 4 week time frame of the initial AMI. A code from category I22 must be used in conjunction with a code from category I21. The sequencing of the I22 and I21 codes depends on the circumstances of the encounter. Do not assign code I22 for subsequent myocardial infarctions other than type 1 or unspecified. For subsequent type 2 AMI assign only code I21.A1. For subsequent type 4 or type 5 AMI, assign only code I21.A9. If a subsequent myocardial infarction of one type occurs within 4 weeks of a myocardial infarction of a different type, assign the appropriate codes from category I21 to identify each type. Do not assign a code from I22. Codes from category I22 should only be assigned if both the initial and subsequent myocardial infarctions are type 1 or unspecified.

5) Other Types of Myocardial Infarction
The ICD-10-CM provides codes for different types of myocardial infarction. Type 1 myocardial infarctions are assigned to codes I21.0-I21.4.
Type 2 myocardial infarction (myocardial infarction due to demand ischemia or secondary to ischemic imbalance) is assigned to code I21.A1, Myocardial infarction type 2 with the underlying cause coded first, **if applicable**. Do not assign code I24.89, Other forms of acute ischemic heart disease, for the demand ischemia. If a type 2 AMI is described as NSTEMI or STEMI, only assign code I21.A1. Codes I21.01-I21.4 should only be assigned for type 1 AMIs.
Acute myocardial infarctions type 3, 4a, 4b, 4c and 5 are assigned to code I21.A9, Other myocardial infarction type.
The "Code also" and "Code first" notes should be followed related to complications, and for coding of postprocedural myocardial infarctions during or following cardiac surgery.

6) Myocardial Infarction with Coronary Microvascular Dysfunction
Coronary microvascular dysfunction (CMD) is a condition that impacts the microvasculature by restricting microvascular flow and increasing microvascular resistance. Code I21.B, Myocardial infarction with coronary microvascular dysfunction, is assigned for myocardial infarction with coronary microvascular disease, myocardial infarction with coronary microvascular dysfunction, and myocardial infarction with non-obstructive coronary arteries (MINOCA) with microvascular disease.

10. Chapter 10: Diseases of the Respiratory System (J00-J99), U07.0
a. Chronic Obstructive Pulmonary Disease [COPD] and Asthma
1) Acute exacerbation of chronic obstructive bronchitis and asthma
The codes in categories J44 and J45 distinguish between uncomplicated cases and those in acute exacerbation. An acute exacerbation is a worsening or a decompensation of a chronic condition. An acute exacerbation is not equivalent to an infection superimposed on a chronic condition, though an exacerbation may be triggered by an infection.

b. Acute Respiratory Failure
1) Acute respiratory failure as principal diagnosis
A code from subcategory J96.0, Acute respiratory failure, or subcategory J96.2, Acute and chronic respiratory failure, may be assigned as a principal diagnosis when it is the condition established after study to be

chiefly responsible for occasioning the admission to the hospital, and the selection is supported by the Alphabetic Index and Tabular List. However, chapter-specific coding guidelines (such as obstetrics, poisoning, HIV, newborn) that provide sequencing direction take precedence.

2) Acute respiratory failure as secondary diagnosis
Respiratory failure may be listed as a secondary diagnosis if it occurs after admission, or if it is present on admission, but does not meet the definition of principal diagnosis.

3) Sequencing of acute respiratory failure and another acute condition
When a patient is admitted with respiratory failure and another acute condition, (e.g., myocardial infarction, cerebrovascular accident, aspiration pneumonia), the principal diagnosis will not be the same in every situation. This applies whether the other acute condition is a respiratory or nonrespiratory condition. Selection of the principal diagnosis will be dependent on the circumstances of admission. If both the respiratory failure and the other acute condition are equally responsible for occasioning the admission to the hospital, and there are no chapter-specific sequencing rules, the guideline regarding two or more diagnoses that equally meet the definition for principal diagnosis (Section II, C.) may be applied in these situations.
If the documentation is not clear as to whether acute respiratory failure and another condition are equally responsible for occasioning the admission, query the provider for clarification.

c. Influenza due to certain identified influenza viruses
Code only confirmed cases of influenza due to certain identified influenza viruses (category J09), and due to other identified influenza virus (category J10). This is an exception to the hospital inpatient guideline Section II, H. (Uncertain Diagnosis).
In this context, "confirmation" does not require documentation of positive laboratory testing specific for avian or other novel influenza A or other identified influenza virus. However, coding should be based on the provider's diagnostic statement that the patient has avian influenza, or other novel influenza A, for category J09, or has another particular identified strain of influenza, such as H1N1 or H3N2, but not identified as novel or variant, for category J10.
If the provider records "suspected" or "possible" or "probable" avian influenza, or novel influenza, or other identified influenza, then the appropriate influenza code from category J11, Influenza due to unidentified influenza virus, should be assigned. A code from category J09, Influenza due to certain identified influenza viruses, should not be assigned nor should a code from category J10, Influenza due to other identified influenza virus.

d. Ventilator associated Pneumonia
1) Documentation of Ventilator associated Pneumonia
As with all procedural or postprocedural complications, code assignment is based on the provider's documentation of the relationship between the condition and the procedure.
Code J95.851, Ventilator associated pneumonia, should be assigned only when the provider has documented ventilator associated pneumonia (VAP). An additional code to identify the organism (e.g., Pseudomonas aeruginosa, code B96.5) should also be assigned. Do not assign an additional code from categories J12-J18 to identify the type of pneumonia.
Code J95.851 should not be assigned for cases where the patient has pneumonia and is on a mechanical ventilator and the provider has not specifically stated that the pneumonia is ventilator-associated pneumonia. If the documentation is unclear as to whether the patient has a pneumonia that is a complication attributable to the mechanical ventilator, query the provider.
2) Ventilator associated Pneumonia Develops after Admission
A patient may be admitted with one type of pneumonia (e.g., code J13, Pneumonia due to Streptococcus pneumonia) and subsequently develop VAP. In this instance, the principal diagnosis would be the appropriate code from categories J12-J18 for the pneumonia diagnosed at the time of admission. Code J95.851, Ventilator associated pneumonia, would be assigned as an additional diagnosis when the provider has also documented the presence of ventilator associated pneumonia.

e. Vaping-related disorders
For patients presenting with condition(s) related to vaping, assign code U07.0, Vaping-related disorder, as the principal diagnosis. For lung injury due to vaping, assign only code U07.0. Assign additional codes for other manifestations, such as acute respiratory failure (subcategory J96.0-) or pneumonitis (code J68.0).
Associated respiratory signs and symptoms due to vaping, such as cough, shortness of breath, etc., are not coded separately, when a definitive diagnosis has been established. However, it would be appropriate to code separately any gastrointestinal symptoms, such as diarrhea and abdominal pain.
See Section I.C.1.g.1.c.i. for Pneumonia confirmed as due to COVID-19

11. Chapter 11: Diseases of the Digestive System (K00-K95)
Reserved for future guideline expansion

12. Chapter 12: Diseases of the Skin and Subcutaneous Tissue (L00-L99)
a. Pressure ulcer stage codes
1) Pressure ulcer stages
Codes in category L89, Pressure ulcer, identify the site and stage of the pressure ulcer.
The ICD-10-CM classifies pressure ulcer stages based on severity, which is designated by stages 1-4, deep tissue pressure injury, unspecified stage, and unstageable.
Assign as many codes from category L89 as needed to identify all the pressure ulcers the patient has, if applicable.
See Section I.B.14. for pressure ulcer stage documentation by clinicians other than patient's provider.
2) Unstageable pressure ulcers
Assignment of the code for unstageable pressure ulcer (L89.--0) should be based on the clinical documentation. These codes are used for pressure ulcers whose stage cannot be clinically determined (e.g., the ulcer is covered by eschar or has been treated with a skin or muscle graft). This code should not be confused with the codes for unspecified stage (L89.--9). When there is no documentation regarding the stage of the pressure ulcer, assign the appropriate code for unspecified stage (L89.-- 9).
If during an encounter, the stage of an unstageable pressure ulcer is revealed after debridement, assign only the code for the stage revealed following debridement.
3) Documented pressure ulcer stage
Assignment of the pressure ulcer stage code should be guided by clinical documentation of the stage or documentation of the terms found in the Alphabetic Index. For clinical terms describing the stage that are not found in the Alphabetic Index, and there is no documentation of the stage, the provider should be queried.
4) Patients admitted with pressure ulcers documented as healed
No code is assigned if the documentation states that the pressure ulcer is completely healed at the time of admission.
5) Pressure ulcers documented as healing
Pressure ulcers described as healing should be assigned the appropriate pressure ulcer stage code based on the documentation in the medical record. If the documentation does not provide information about the stage of the healing pressure ulcer, assign the appropriate code for unspecified stage.
If the documentation is unclear as to whether the patient has a current (new) pressure ulcer or if the patient is being treated for a healing pressure ulcer, query the provider.
For ulcers that were present on admission but healed at the time of discharge, assign the code for the site and stage of the pressure ulcer at the time of admission.
6) Patient admitted with pressure ulcer evolving into another stage during the admission
If a patient is admitted to an inpatient hospital with a pressure ulcer at one stage and it progresses to a higher stage, two separate codes should be assigned: one code for the site and stage of the ulcer on admission and a second code for the same ulcer site and the highest stage reported during the stay.
7) Pressure-induced deep tissue damage
For pressure-induced deep tissue damage or deep tissue pressure injury, assign only the appropriate code for pressure-induced deep tissue damage (L89.--6).
b. Non-Pressure Chronic Ulcers
1) Patients admitted with non-pressure ulcers documented as healed
No code is assigned if the documentation states that the non-pressure ulcer is completely healed at the time of admission.
2) Non-pressure ulcers documented as healing
Non-pressure ulcers described as healing should be assigned the appropriate non-pressure ulcer code based on the documentation in the medical record. If the documentation does not provide information about the severity of the healing non-pressure ulcer, assign the appropriate code for unspecified severity.
If the documentation is unclear as to whether the patient has a current (new) non-pressure ulcer or if the patient is being treated for a healing non-pressure ulcer, query the provider.
For ulcers that were present on admission but healed at the time of discharge, assign the code for the site and severity of the non-pressure ulcer at the time of admission.
3) Patient admitted with non-pressure ulcer that progresses to another severity level during the admission
If a patient is admitted to an inpatient hospital with a non-pressure ulcer at one severity level and it progresses to a higher severity level, two separate codes should be assigned: one code for the site and severity level of the ulcer on admission and a second code for the same ulcer site and the highest severity level reported during the stay.
See Section I.B.14. for pressure ulcer stage documentation by clinicians other than patient's provider

13. Chapter 13: Diseases of the Musculoskeletal System and Connective Tissue (M00-M99)
a. Site and laterality
Most of the codes within Chapter 13 have site and laterality designations. The site represents the bone, joint or the muscle involved. For some conditions

where more than one bone, joint or muscle is usually involved, such as osteoarthritis, there is a "multiple sites" code available. For categories where no multiple site code is provided and more than one bone, joint or muscle is involved, multiple codes should be used to indicate the different sites involved.

1) Bone versus joint

For certain conditions, the bone may be affected at the upper or lower end, (e.g., avascular necrosis of bone, M87, Osteoporosis, M80, M81). Though the portion of the bone affected may be at the joint, the site designation will be the bone, not the joint.

b. Acute traumatic versus chronic or recurrent musculoskeletal conditions

Many musculoskeletal conditions are a result of previous injury or trauma to a site, or are recurrent conditions. Bone, joint or muscle conditions that are the result of a healed injury are usually found in chapter 13. Recurrent bone, joint or muscle conditions are also usually found in chapter 13. Any current, acute injury should be coded to the appropriate injury code from chapter 19. Chronic or recurrent conditions should generally be coded with a code from chapter 13. If it is difficult to determine from the documentation in the record which code is best to describe a condition, query the provider.

c. Coding of Pathologic Fractures

7th character A is for use as long as the patient is receiving active treatment for the fracture. While the patient may be seen by a new or different provider over the course of treatment for a pathological fracture, assignment of the 7th character is based on whether the patient is undergoing active treatment and not whether the provider is seeing the patient for the first time.

7th character D is to be used for encounters after the patient has completed active treatment for the fracture and is receiving routine care for the fracture during the healing or recovery phase. The other 7th characters, listed under each subcategory in the Tabular List, are to be used for subsequent encounters for treatment of problems associated with the healing, such as malunions, nonunions, and sequelae.

Care for complications of surgical treatment for fracture repairs during the healing or recovery phase should be coded with the appropriate complication codes.

See Section I.C.19. Coding of traumatic fractures.

d. Osteoporosis

Osteoporosis is a systemic condition, meaning that all bones of the musculoskeletal system are affected. Therefore, site is not a component of the codes under category M81, Osteoporosis without current pathological fracture. The site codes under category M80, Osteoporosis with current pathological fracture, identify the site of the fracture, not the osteoporosis.

1) Osteoporosis without pathological fracture

Category M81, Osteoporosis without current pathological fracture, is for use for patients with osteoporosis who do not currently have a pathologic fracture due to the osteoporosis, even if they have had a fracture in the past. For patients with a history of osteoporosis fractures, status code Z87.310, Personal history of (healed) osteoporosis fracture, should follow the code from M81.

2) Osteoporosis with current pathological fracture

Category M80, Osteoporosis with current pathological fracture, is for patients who have a current pathologic fracture at the time of an encounter. The codes under M80 identify the site of the fracture. A code from category M80, not a traumatic fracture code, should be used for any patient with known osteoporosis who suffers a fracture, even if the patient had a minor fall or trauma, if that fall or trauma would not usually break a normal, healthy bone.

e. Multisystem Inflammatory Syndrome

See Section I.C.1.g.1.l. for Multisystem Inflammatory Syndrome

14. Chapter 14: Diseases of Genitourinary System (N00-N99)

a. Chronic kidney disease

1) Stages of chronic kidney disease (CKD)

The ICD-10-CM classifies CKD based on severity. The severity of CKD is designated by stages 1-5. Stage 2, code N18.2, equates to mild CKD; stage 3, codes N18.30-N18.32, equate to moderate CKD; and stage 4, code N18.4, equates to severe CKD. Code N18.6, End stage renal disease (ESRD), is assigned when the provider has documented end-stage renal disease (ESRD).

If both a stage of CKD and ESRD are documented, assign code N18.6 only.

2) Chronic kidney disease and kidney transplant status

Patients who have undergone kidney transplant may still have some form of chronic kidney disease (CKD) because the kidney transplant may not fully restore kidney function. Therefore, the presence of CKD alone does not constitute a transplant complication. Assign the appropriate N18 code for the patient's stage of CKD and code Z94.0, Kidney transplant status. If a transplant complication such as failure or rejection or other transplant complication is documented, see section I.C.19.g for information on coding complications of a kidney transplant. If the documentation is unclear as to whether the patient has a complication of the transplant, query the provider.

3) Chronic kidney disease with other conditions

Patients with CKD may also suffer from other serious conditions, most commonly diabetes mellitus and hypertension. The sequencing of the CKD code in relationship to codes for other contributing conditions is based on the conventions in the Tabular List.

See I.C.9. Hypertensive chronic kidney disease.

See I.C.19. Chronic kidney disease and kidney transplant complications.

15. Chapter 15: Pregnancy, Childbirth, and the Puerperium (O00-O9A)

a. General Rules for Obstetric Cases

1) Codes from chapter 15 and sequencing priority

Obstetric cases require codes from chapter 15, codes in the range O00-O9A, Pregnancy, Childbirth, and the Puerperium. Chapter 15 codes have sequencing priority over codes from other chapters. Additional codes from other chapters may be used in conjunction with chapter 15 codes to further specify conditions. Should the provider document that the pregnancy is incidental to the encounter, then code Z33.1, Pregnant state, incidental, should be used in place of any chapter 15 codes. It is the provider's responsibility to state that the condition being treated is not affecting the pregnancy.

2) Chapter 15 codes used only on the maternal record

Chapter 15 codes are to be used only on the maternal record, never on the record of the newborn.

3) Final character for trimester

The majority of codes in Chapter 15 have a final character indicating the trimester of pregnancy. The timeframes for the trimesters are indicated at the beginning of the chapter. If trimester is not a component of a code, it is because the condition always occurs in a specific trimester, or the concept of trimester of pregnancy is not applicable. Certain codes have characters for only certain trimesters because the condition does not occur in all trimesters, but it may occur in more than just one.

Assignment of the final character for trimester should be based on the provider's documentation of the trimester (or number of weeks) for the current admission/encounter. This applies to the assignment of trimester for pre-existing conditions as well as those that develop during or are due to the pregnancy. The provider's documentation of the number of weeks may be used to assign the appropriate code identifying the trimester.

Whenever delivery occurs during the current admission, and there is an "in childbirth" option for the obstetric complication being coded, the "in childbirth" code should be assigned. When the classification does not provide an obstetric code with an "in childbirth" option, it is appropriate to assign a code describing the current trimester.

4) Selection of trimester for inpatient admissions that encompass more than one trimester

In instances when a patient is admitted to a hospital for complications of pregnancy during one trimester and remains in the hospital into a subsequent trimester, the trimester character for the antepartum complication code should be assigned on the basis of the trimester when the complication developed, not the trimester of the discharge. If the condition developed prior to the current admission/encounter or represents a pre-existing condition, the trimester character for the trimester at the time of the admission/encounter should be assigned.

5) Unspecified trimester

Each category that includes codes for trimester has a code for "unspecified trimester." The "unspecified trimester" code should rarely be used, such as when the documentation in the record is insufficient to determine the trimester and it is not possible to obtain clarification.

6) 7th character for fetus identification

Where applicable, a 7th character is to be assigned for certain categories (O31, O32, O33.3-O33.6, O35, O36, O40, O41, O60.1, O60.2, O64, and O69) to identify the fetus for which the complication code applies. Assign 7th character "0":

- For single gestations
- When the documentation in the record is insufficient to determine the fetus affected and it is not possible to obtain clarification.
- When it is not possible to clinically determine which fetus is affected.

7) Completed weeks of gestation

In ICD-10-CM, "completed" weeks of gestation refers to full weeks. For example, if the provider documents gestation at 39 weeks and 6 days, the code for 39 weeks of gestation should be assigned, as the patient has not yet reached 40 completed weeks.

b. Selection of OB Principal or First-listed Diagnosis

1) Routine outpatient prenatal visits

For routine outpatient prenatal visits when no complications are present, a code from category Z34, Encounter for supervision of normal pregnancy, should be used as the first-listed diagnosis. These codes should not be used in conjunction with chapter 15 codes.

2) Supervision of High-Risk Pregnancy

Codes from category O09, Supervision of high-risk pregnancy, are intended for use only during the prenatal period. For complications during the labor or delivery episode as a result of a high-risk pregnancy, assign the applicable complication codes from Chapter 15. If there are no complications during the labor or delivery episode, assign code O80, Encounter for full-term uncomplicated delivery.

For routine prenatal outpatient visits for patients with high-risk pregnancies, a code from category O09, Supervision of high-risk pregnancy, should be used as the first-listed diagnosis. Secondary chapter 15 codes may be used in conjunction with these codes if appropriate.

3) Episodes when no delivery occurs

In episodes when no delivery occurs, the principal diagnosis should correspond to the principal complication of the pregnancy which necessitated the encounter. Should more than one complication exist, all of which are treated or monitored, any of the complication codes may be sequenced first.

4) **When a delivery occurs**
When an obstetric patient is admitted and delivers during that admission, the condition that prompted the admission should be sequenced as the principal diagnosis. If multiple conditions prompted the admission, sequence the one most related to the delivery as the principal diagnosis. A code for any complication of the delivery should be assigned as an additional diagnosis. In cases of cesarean delivery, if the patient was admitted with a condition that resulted in the performance of a cesarean procedure, that condition should be selected as the principal diagnosis. If the reason for the admission was unrelated to the condition resulting in the cesarean delivery, the condition related to the reason for the admission should be selected as the principal diagnosis.

5) **Outcome of delivery**
A code from category Z37, Outcome of delivery, should be included on every maternal record when a delivery has occurred. These codes are not to be used on subsequent records or on the newborn record.

c. **Pre-existing conditions versus conditions due to the pregnancy**
Certain categories in Chapter 15 distinguish between conditions of the mother that existed prior to pregnancy (pre-existing) and those that are a direct result of pregnancy. When assigning codes from Chapter 15, it is important to assess if a condition was pre-existing prior to pregnancy or developed during or due to the pregnancy in order to assign the correct code.
Categories that do not distinguish between pre-existing and pregnancy-related conditions may be used for either. It is acceptable to use codes specifically for the puerperium with codes complicating pregnancy and childbirth if a condition arises postpartum during the delivery encounter.

d. **Pre-existing hypertension in pregnancy**
Category O10, Pre-existing hypertension complicating pregnancy, childbirth and the puerperium, includes codes for hypertensive heart and hypertensive chronic kidney disease. When assigning one of the O10 codes that includes hypertensive heart disease or hypertensive chronic kidney disease, it is necessary to add a secondary code from the appropriate hypertension category to specify the type of heart failure or chronic kidney disease.
See Section I.C.9. Hypertension.

e. **Fetal Conditions Affecting the Management of the Mother**
1) **Codes from categories O35 and O36**
Codes from categories O35, Maternal care for known or suspected fetal abnormality and damage, and O36, Maternal care for other fetal problems, are assigned only when the fetal condition is actually responsible for modifying the management of the mother, i.e., by requiring diagnostic studies, additional observation, special care, or termination of pregnancy. The fact that the fetal condition exists does not justify assigning a code from this series to the mother's record.

2) **In utero surgery**
In cases when surgery is performed on the fetus, a diagnosis code from category O35, Maternal care for known or suspected fetal abnormality and damage, should be assigned identifying the fetal condition. Assign the appropriate procedure code for the procedure performed.
No code from Chapter 16, the perinatal codes, should be used on the mother's record to identify fetal conditions. Surgery performed in utero on a fetus is still to be coded as an obstetric encounter.

f. **HIV Infection in Pregnancy, Childbirth and the Puerperium**
During pregnancy, childbirth or the puerperium, a patient admitted because of an HIV-related illness should receive a principal diagnosis from subcategory O98.7-, Human immunodeficiency [HIV] disease complicating pregnancy, childbirth and the puerperium, followed by the code(s) for the HIV-related illness(es).
Patients with asymptomatic HIV infection status admitted during pregnancy, childbirth, or the puerperium should receive codes of O98.7- and Z21, Asymptomatic human immunodeficiency virus [HIV] infection status.

g. **Diabetes mellitus in pregnancy**
Diabetes mellitus is a significant complicating factor in pregnancy. Pregnant patients who are diabetic should be assigned a code from category O24, Diabetes mellitus in pregnancy, childbirth, and the puerperium, first, followed by the appropriate diabetes code(s) (E08-E13) from Chapter 4.

h. **Long term use of insulin and oral hypoglycemics**
See section I.C.4.a.3 for information on the long-term use of insulin and oral hypoglycemics.

i. **Gestational (pregnancy induced) diabetes**
Gestational (pregnancy induced) diabetes can occur during the second and third trimester of pregnancy in patients who were not diabetic prior to pregnancy. Gestational diabetes can cause complications in the pregnancy similar to those of pre-existing diabetes mellitus. It also puts the patient at greater risk of developing diabetes after the pregnancy.
Codes for gestational diabetes are in subcategory O24.4, Gestational diabetes mellitus. No other code from category O24, Diabetes mellitus in pregnancy, childbirth, and the puerperium, should be used with a code from O24.4. The codes under subcategory O24.4 include diet controlled, insulin controlled, and controlled by oral hypoglycemic drugs. If a patient with gestational diabetes is treated with both diet and insulin, only the code for insulin-controlled is required. If a patient with gestational diabetes is treated

with both diet and oral hypoglycemic medications, only the code for "controlled by oral hypoglycemic drugs" is required. Codes Z79.4, Long-term (current) use of insulin, Z79.84, Long-term (current) use of oral hypoglycemic drugs, and Z79.85, Long-term (current) use of injectable non-insulin antidiabetic drugs, should not be assigned with codes from subcategory O24.4.
An abnormal glucose tolerance in pregnancy is assigned a code from subcategory O99.81, Abnormal glucose complicating pregnancy, childbirth, and the puerperium.

j. **Sepsis and septic shock complicating abortion, pregnancy, childbirth and the puerperium**
When assigning a chapter 15 code for sepsis complicating abortion, pregnancy, childbirth, and the puerperium, a code for the specific type of infection should be assigned as an additional diagnosis. If severe sepsis is present, a code from subcategory R65.2, Severe sepsis, and code(s) for associated organ dysfunction(s) should also be assigned as additional diagnoses.

k. **Puerperal sepsis**
Code O85, Puerperal sepsis, should be assigned with a secondary code to identify the causal organism (e.g., for a bacterial infection, assign a code from category B95-B96, Bacterial infections in conditions classified elsewhere). A code from category A40, Streptococcal sepsis, or A41, Other sepsis, should not be used for puerperal sepsis. If applicable, use additional codes to identify severe sepsis (R65.2-) and any associated acute organ dysfunction. Code O85 should not be assigned for sepsis following an obstetric procedure (See Section I.C.1.d.5.b., Sepsis due to a postprocedural infection).

l. **Alcohol, tobacco and drug use during pregnancy, childbirth and the puerperium**
1) **Alcohol use during pregnancy, childbirth and the puerperium**
Codes under subcategory O99.31, Alcohol use complicating pregnancy, childbirth, and the puerperium, should be assigned for any pregnancy case when a patient uses alcohol during the pregnancy or postpartum. A secondary code from category F10, Alcohol related disorders, should also be assigned to identify manifestations of the alcohol use.

2) **Tobacco use during pregnancy, childbirth and the puerperium**
Codes under subcategory O99.33, Smoking (tobacco) complicating pregnancy, childbirth, and the puerperium, should be assigned for any pregnancy case when a patient uses any type of tobacco product during the pregnancy or postpartum.
A secondary code from category F17, Nicotine dependence, should also be assigned to identify the type of nicotine dependence.

3) **Drug use during pregnancy, childbirth and the puerperium**
Codes under subcategory O99.32, Drug use complicating pregnancy, childbirth, and the puerperium, should be assigned for any pregnancy case when a patient uses drugs during the pregnancy or postpartum. This can involve illegal drugs, or inappropriate use or abuse of prescription drugs. Secondary code(s) from categories F11-F16 and F18-F19 should also be assigned to identify manifestations of the drug use.

m. **Poisoning, toxic effects, adverse effects and underdosing in a pregnant patient**
A code from subcategory O9A.2, Injury, poisoning and certain other consequences of external causes complicating pregnancy, childbirth, and the puerperium, should be sequenced first, followed by the appropriate injury, poisoning, toxic effect, adverse effect or underdosing code, and then the additional code(s) that specifies the condition caused by the poisoning, toxic effect, adverse effect or underdosing.
See Section I.C.19. Adverse effects, poisoning, underdosing and toxic effects.

n. **Normal Delivery, Code O80**
1) **Encounter for full term uncomplicated delivery**
Code O80 should be assigned when a patient is admitted for a full-term normal delivery and delivers a single, healthy infant without any complications antepartum, during the delivery, or postpartum during the delivery episode. Code O80 is always a principal diagnosis. It is not to be used if any other code from chapter 15 is needed to describe a current complication of the antenatal, delivery, or postnatal period. Additional codes from other chapters may be used with code O80 if they are not related to or are in any way complicating the pregnancy.

2) **Uncomplicated delivery with resolved antepartum complication**
Code O80 may be used if the patient had a complication at some point during the pregnancy, but the complication is not present at the time of the admission for delivery.

3) **Outcome of delivery for O80**
Z37.0, Single live birth, is the only outcome of delivery code appropriate for use with O80.

o. **The Peripartum and Postpartum Periods**
1) **Peripartum and Postpartum periods**
The postpartum period begins immediately after delivery and continues for six weeks following delivery. The peripartum period is defined as the last month of pregnancy to five months postpartum.

2) **Peripartum and postpartum complication**
A postpartum complication is any complication occurring within the six-week period.

3) Pregnancy-related complications after 6-week period

Chapter 15 codes may also be used to describe pregnancy-related complications after the peripartum or postpartum period if the provider documents that a condition is pregnancy related.

4) Admission for routine postpartum care following delivery outside hospital

When the mother delivers outside the hospital prior to admission and is admitted for routine postpartum care and no complications are noted, code Z39.0, Encounter for care and examination of mother immediately after delivery, should be assigned as the principal diagnosis.

5) Pregnancy associated cardiomyopathy

Pregnancy associated cardiomyopathy, code O90.3, is unique in that it may be diagnosed in the third trimester of pregnancy but may continue to progress months after delivery. For this reason, it is referred to as peripartum cardiomyopathy. Code O90.3 is only for use when the cardiomyopathy develops as a result of pregnancy in a patient who did not have pre-existing heart disease.

p. Code O94, Sequelae of complication of pregnancy, childbirth, and the puerperium

1) Code O94

Code O94, Sequelae of complication of pregnancy, childbirth, and the puerperium, is for use in those cases when an initial complication of a pregnancy develops a sequela or sequelae requiring care or treatment at a future date.

2) After the initial postpartum period

This code may be used at any time after the initial postpartum period.

3) Sequencing of Code O94

This code, like all sequela codes, is to be sequenced following the code describing the sequelae of the complication.

q. Termination of Pregnancy and Spontaneous abortions

1) Abortion with Liveborn Fetus

When an attempted termination of pregnancy results in a liveborn fetus, assign code Z33.2, Encounter for elective termination of pregnancy and a code from category Z37, Outcome of Delivery.

2) Retained Products of Conception following an abortion

Subsequent encounters for retained products of conception following a spontaneous abortion or elective termination of pregnancy, without complications are assigned O03.4, Incomplete spontaneous abortion without complication, or code O07.4, Failed attempted termination of pregnancy without complication. This advice is appropriate even when the patient was discharged previously with a discharge diagnosis of complete abortion. If the patient has a specific complication associated with the spontaneous abortion or elective termination of pregnancy in addition to retained products of conception, assign the appropriate complication code (e.g., O03.-, O04.-, O07.-) instead of code O03.4 or O07.4.

3) Complications leading to abortion

Codes from Chapter 15 may be used as additional codes to identify any documented complications of the pregnancy in conjunction with codes in categories in O04, O07 and O08.

4) Hemorrhage following elective abortion

For hemorrhage post elective abortion, assign code O04.6, Delayed or excessive hemorrhage following (induced) termination of pregnancy. Do not assign code O72.1, Other immediate postpartum hemorrhage, as this code should not be assigned for post abortion conditions.

r. Abuse in a pregnant patient

For suspected or confirmed cases of abuse of a pregnant patient, a code(s) from subcategories O9A.3, Physical abuse complicating pregnancy, childbirth, and the puerperium, O9A.4, Sexual abuse complicating pregnancy, childbirth, and the puerperium, and O9A.5, Psychological abuse complicating pregnancy, childbirth, and the puerperium, should be sequenced first, followed by the appropriate codes (if applicable) to identify any associated current injury due to physical abuse, sexual abuse, and the perpetrator of abuse.

See Section I.C.19. Adult and child abuse, neglect and other maltreatment.

s. COVID-19 infection in pregnancy, childbirth, and the puerperium

During pregnancy, childbirth or the puerperium, when COVID-19 is the reason for admission/encounter , code O98.5-, Other viral diseases complicating pregnancy, childbirth and the puerperium, should be sequenced as the principal/first-listed diagnosis, and code U07.1, COVID-19, and the appropriate codes for associated manifestation(s) should be assigned as additional diagnoses. Codes from Chapter 15 always take sequencing priority.

If the reason for admission/encounter is unrelated to COVID-19 but the patient tests positive for COVID-19 during the admission/encounter, the appropriate code for the reason for admission/encounter should be sequenced as the principal/first-listed diagnosis, and codes O98.5- and U07.1, as well as the appropriate codes for associated COVID-19 manifestations, should be assigned as additional diagnoses.

16. Chapter 16: Certain Conditions Originating in the Perinatal Period (P00-P96)

For coding and reporting purposes the perinatal period is defined as before birth through the 28th day following birth. The following guidelines are provided for reporting purposes.

a. General Perinatal Rules

1) Use of Chapter 16 Codes

Codes in this chapter are <u>never</u> for use on the maternal record. Codes from Chapter 15, the obstetric chapter, are never permitted on the newborn record. Chapter 16 codes may be used throughout the life of the patient if the condition is still present.

2) Principal Diagnosis for Birth Record

When coding the birth episode in a newborn record, assign a code from category Z38, Liveborn infants according to place of birth and type of delivery, as the principal diagnosis. A code from category Z38 is assigned only once, to a newborn at the time of birth. If a newborn is transferred to another institution, a code from category Z38 should not be used at the receiving hospital.

A code from category Z38 is used only on the newborn record, not on the mother's record.

3) Use of Codes from other Chapters with Codes from Chapter 16

Codes from other chapters may be used with codes from chapter 16 if the codes from the other chapters provide more specific detail. Codes for signs and symptoms may be assigned when a definitive diagnosis has not been established. If the reason for the encounter is a perinatal condition, the code from chapter 16 should be sequenced first.

4) Use of Chapter 16 Codes after the Perinatal Period

Should a condition originate in the perinatal period, and continue throughout the life of the patient, the perinatal code should continue to be used regardless of the patient's age.

5) Birth process or community acquired conditions

If a newborn has a condition that may be either due to the birth process or community acquired and the documentation does not indicate which it is, the default is due to the birth process and the code from Chapter 16 should be used. If the condition is community-acquired, a code from Chapter 16 should not be assigned.

For COVID-19 infection in a newborn, see guideline I.C.16.h.

6) Code all clinically significant conditions

All clinically significant conditions noted on routine newborn examination should be coded. A condition is clinically significant if it requires:

- clinical evaluation; or
- therapeutic treatment; or
- diagnostic procedures; or
- extended length of hospital stay; or
- increased nursing care and/or monitoring; or
- has implications for future health care needs

Note: The perinatal guidelines listed above are the same as the general coding guidelines for "additional diagnoses," except for the final point regarding implications for future health care needs. Codes should be assigned for conditions that have been specified by the provider as having implications for future health care needs.

b. Observation and Evaluation of Newborns for Suspected Conditions not Found

1) Use of Z05 codes

Assign a code from category Z05, Observation and evaluation of newborn for suspected diseases and conditions ruled out, to identify those instances when a healthy newborn is evaluated for a suspected condition/disease that is determined after study not to be present. Do not use a code from category Z05 when the patient is documented to have signs or symptoms of a suspected problem; in such cases code the sign or symptom.

2) Z05 on other than the birth record

A code from category Z05 may also be assigned as a principal or first-listed code for readmissions or encounters when the code from category Z38 code no longer applies. Codes from category Z05 are for use only for healthy newborns and infants for which no condition after study is found to be present.

3) Z05 on a birth record

A code from category Z05 is to be used as a secondary code after the code from category Z38, Liveborn infants according to place of birth and type of delivery.

c. Coding Additional Perinatal Diagnoses

1) Assigning codes for conditions that require treatment

Assign codes for conditions that require treatment or further investigation, prolong the length of stay, or require resource utilization.

2) Codes for conditions specified as having implications for future health care needs

Assign codes for conditions that have been specified by the provider as having implications for future health care needs.

Note: This guideline should not be used for adult patients.

d. Prematurity and Fetal Growth Retardation

Providers utilize different criteria in determining prematurity. A code for prematurity should not be assigned unless it is documented. Assignment of codes in categories P05, Disorders of newborn related to slow fetal growth and fetal malnutrition, and P07, Disorders of newborn related to short gestation and low birth weight, not elsewhere classified, should be based on the recorded birth weight and estimated gestational age.

When both birth weight and gestational age are available, two codes from category P07 should be assigned, with the code for birth weight sequenced before the code for gestational age.

e. Low birth weight and immaturity status

Codes from category P07, Disorders of newborn related to short gestation and low birth weight, not elsewhere classified, are for use for a child or adult who was premature or had a low birth weight as a newborn and this is affecting the patient's current health status.

See Section I.C.21. Factors influencing health status and contact with health services, Status.

f. Bacterial Sepsis of Newborn

Category P36, Bacterial sepsis of newborn, includes congenital sepsis. If a perinate is documented as having sepsis without documentation of congenital or community acquired, the default is congenital and a code from category P36 should be assigned. If the P36 code includes the causal organism, an additional code from category B95, Streptococcus, Staphylococcus, and Enterococcus as the cause of diseases classified elsewhere, or B96, Other bacterial agents as the cause of diseases classified elsewhere, should not be assigned. If the P36 code does not include the causal organism, assign an additional code from category B96. If applicable, use additional codes to identify severe sepsis (R65.2-) and any associated acute organ dysfunction.

g. Stillbirth

Code P95, Stillbirth, is only for use in institutions that maintain separate records for stillbirths. No other code should be used with P95. Code P95 should not be used on the mother's record.

h. COVID-19 Infection in Newborn

For a newborn that tests positive for COVID-19, assign code U07.1, COVID-19, and the appropriate codes for associated manifestation(s) in neonates/newborns in the absence of documentation indicating a specific type of transmission. For a newborn that tests positive for COVID-19 and the provider documents the condition was contracted in utero or during the birth process, assign codes P35.8, Other congenital viral diseases, and U07.1, COVID-19. When coding the birth episode in a newborn record, the appropriate code from category Z38, Liveborn infants according to place of birth and type of delivery, should be assigned as the principal diagnosis.

17. Chapter 17: Congenital malformations, deformations, and chromosomal abnormalities (Q00-Q99)

Assign an appropriate code(s) from categories Q00-Q99, Congenital malformations, deformations, and chromosomal abnormalities when a malformation/deformation or chromosomal abnormality is documented. A malformation/deformation/or chromosomal abnormality may be the principal/first-listed diagnosis on a record or a secondary diagnosis.

When a malformation/deformation or chromosomal abnormality does not have a unique code assignment, assign additional code(s) for any manifestations that may be present.

When the code assignment specifically identifies the malformation/deformation or chromosomal abnormality, manifestations that are an inherent component of the anomaly should not be coded separately. Additional codes should be assigned for manifestations that are not an inherent component.

Codes from Chapter 17 may be used throughout the life of the patient. If a congenital malformation or deformity has been corrected, a personal history code should be used to identify the history of the malformation or deformity. Although present at birth, a malformation/deformation/or chromosomal abnormality may not be identified until later in life. Whenever the condition is diagnosed by the provider, it is appropriate to assign a code from codes Q00-Q99. For the birth admission, the appropriate code from category Z38, Liveborn infants, according to place of birth and type of delivery, should be sequenced as the principal diagnosis, followed by any congenital anomaly codes, Q00-Q99.

18. Chapter 18: Symptoms, signs, and abnormal clinical and laboratory findings, not elsewhere classified (R00-R99)

Chapter 18 includes symptoms, signs, abnormal results of clinical or other investigative procedures, and ill-defined conditions regarding which no diagnosis classifiable elsewhere is recorded. Signs and symptoms that point to a specific diagnosis have been assigned to a category in other chapters of the classification.

a. Use of symptom codes

Codes that describe symptoms and signs are acceptable for reporting purposes when a related definitive diagnosis has not been established (confirmed) by the provider.

b. Use of a symptom code with a definitive diagnosis code

Codes for signs and symptoms may be reported in addition to a related definitive diagnosis when the sign or symptom is not routinely associated with that diagnosis, such as the various signs and symptoms associated with complex syndromes. The definitive diagnosis code should be sequenced before the symptom code.

Signs or symptoms that are associated routinely with a disease process should not be assigned as additional codes, unless otherwise instructed by the classification.

c. Combination codes that include symptoms

ICD-10-CM contains a number of combination codes that identify both the definitive diagnosis and common symptoms of that diagnosis. When using one of these combination codes, an additional code should not be assigned for the symptom.

d. Repeated falls

Code R29.6, Repeated falls, is for use for encounters when a patient has recently fallen and the reason for the fall is being investigated.

Code Z91.81, History of falling, is for use when a patient has fallen in the past and is at risk for future falls. When appropriate, both codes R29.6 and Z91.81 may be assigned together.

e. Coma

Code R40.20, Unspecified coma, should be assigned when the underlying cause of the coma is not known, or the cause is a traumatic brain injury and the coma scale is not documented in the medical record.

Do not report codes for unspecified coma, individual or total Glasgow coma scale scores for a patient with a medically induced coma or a sedated patient.

1) Coma Scale

The coma scale codes (R40.21- to R40.24-) can be used in conjunction with traumatic brain injury codes. These codes cannot be used with code R40.2A, Nontraumatic coma due to underlying condition. They are primarily for use by trauma registries, but they may be used in any setting where this information is collected. The coma scale codes should be sequenced after the diagnosis code(s).

These codes, one from each subcategory, are needed to complete the scale. The 7th character indicates when the scale was recorded. The 7th character should match for all three codes.

At a minimum, report the initial score documented on presentation at your facility. This may be a score from the emergency medicine technician (EMT) or in the emergency department. If desired, a facility may choose to capture multiple coma scale scores.

Assign code R40.24-, Glasgow coma scale, total score, when only the total score is documented in the medical record and not the individual score(s).

If multiple coma scores are captured within the first 24 hours after hospital admission, assign only the code for the score at the time of admission. ICD-10-CM does not classify coma scores that are reported after admission but less than 24 hours later.

See Section I.B.14. for coma scale documentation by clinicians other than patient's provider

f. Functional quadriplegia

GUIDELINE HAS BEEN DELETED EFFECTIVE OCTOBER 1, 2017

g. SIRS due to Non-Infectious Process

The systemic inflammatory response syndrome (SIRS) can develop as a result of certain non-infectious disease processes, such as trauma, malignant neoplasm, or pancreatitis. When SIRS is documented with a noninfectious condition, and no subsequent infection is documented, the code for the underlying condition, such as an injury, should be assigned, followed by code R65.10, Systemic inflammatory response syndrome (SIRS) of non-infectious origin without acute organ dysfunction, or code R65.11, Systemic inflammatory response syndrome (SIRS) of non-infectious origin with acute organ dysfunction. If an associated acute organ dysfunction is documented, the appropriate code(s) for the specific type of organ dysfunction(s) should be assigned in addition to code R65.11. If acute organ dysfunction is documented, but it cannot be determined if the acute organ dysfunction is associated with SIRS or due to another condition (e.g., directly due to the trauma), the provider should be queried.

h. Death NOS

Code R99, Ill-defined and unknown cause of mortality, is only for use in the very limited circumstance when a patient who has already died is brought into an emergency department or other healthcare facility and is pronounced dead upon arrival. It does not represent the discharge disposition of death.

i. NIHSS Stroke Scale

The NIH stroke scale (NIHSS) codes (R29.7- -) can be used in conjunction with acute stroke codes (I60–I63) to identify the patient's neurological status and the severity of the stroke. The stroke scale codes should be sequenced after the acute stroke diagnosis code(s).

At a minimum, report the initial score documented. If desired, a facility may choose to capture multiple stroke scale scores.

See Section I.B.14. for NIHSS stroke scale documentation by clinicians other than patient's provider

19. Chapter 19: Injury, poisoning, and certain other consequences of external causes (S00-T88)

a. Application of 7th Characters in Chapter 19

Most categories in chapter 19 have a 7th character requirement for each applicable code. Most categories in this chapter have three 7th character values (with the exception of fractures): A, initial encounter, D, subsequent encounter and S, sequela. Categories for traumatic fractures have additional 7th character values. While the patient may be seen by a new or different provider over the course of treatment for an injury, assignment of the 7th character is based on whether the patient is undergoing active treatment and not whether the provider is seeing the patient for the first time.

For complication codes, active treatment refers to treatment for the condition described by the code, even though it may be related to an earlier precipitating problem. For example, code T84.50XA, Infection and inflammatory reaction due to unspecified internal joint prosthesis, initial encounter, is used when active treatment is provided for the infection, even though the condition relates to the prosthetic device, implant or graft that was placed at a previous encounter.

7th character "A", initial encounter is used for each encounter where the patient is receiving active treatment for the condition.

7th character "D" subsequent encounter is used for encounters after the patient has completed active treatment of the condition and is receiving routine care for the condition during the healing or recovery phase.

The aftercare Z codes should not be used for aftercare for conditions such as injuries or poisonings, where 7th characters are provided to identify subsequent care. For example, for aftercare of an injury, assign the acute injury code with the 7th character "D" (subsequent encounter).

7th character "S", sequela, is for use for complications or conditions that arise as a direct result of a condition, such as scar formation after a burn. The scars are sequelae of the burn. When using 7th character "S", it is necessary to use both the injury code that precipitated the sequela and the code for the sequela itself. The "S" is added only to the injury code, not the sequela code. The 7th character "S" identifies the injury responsible for the sequela. The specific type of sequela (e.g. scar) is sequenced first, followed by the injury code.

See Section I.B.10. Sequelae, (Late Effects)

b. Coding of Injuries

When coding injuries, assign separate codes for each injury unless a combination code is provided, in which case the combination code is assigned. Codes from category T07, Unspecified multiple injuries should not be assigned in the inpatient setting unless information for a more specific code is not available. Traumatic injury codes (S00-T14.9) are not to be used for normal, healing surgical wounds or to identify complications of surgical wounds.

The code for the most serious injury, as determined by the provider and the focus of treatment, is sequenced first.

1) Superficial injuries

Superficial injuries such as abrasions or contusions are not coded when associated with more severe injuries of the same site.

2) Primary injury with damage to nerves/blood vessels

When a primary injury results in minor damage to peripheral nerves or blood vessels, the primary injury is sequenced first with additional code(s) for injuries to nerves and spinal cord (such as category S04), and/or injury to blood vessels (such as category S15). When the primary injury is to the blood vessels or nerves, that injury should be sequenced first.

3) Iatrogenic injuries

Injury codes from Chapter 19 should not be assigned for injuries that occur during, or as a result of, a medical intervention. Assign the appropriate complication code(s).

c. Coding of Traumatic Fractures

The principles of multiple coding of injuries should be followed in coding fractures. Fractures of specified sites are coded individually by site in accordance with both the provisions within categories S02, S12, S22, S32, S42, S49, S52, S59, S62, S72, S79, S82, S89, S92 and the level of detail furnished by medical record content.

A fracture not indicated as open or closed should be coded to closed. A fracture not indicated whether displaced or not displaced should be coded to displaced.

More specific guidelines are as follows:

1) Initial vs. subsequent encounter for fractures

Traumatic fractures are coded using the appropriate 7th character for initial encounter (A, B, C) for each encounter where the patient is receiving active treatment for the fracture. The appropriate 7th character for initial encounter should also be assigned for a patient who delayed seeking treatment for the fracture or nonunion.

Fractures are coded using the appropriate 7th character for subsequent care for encounters after the patient has completed active treatment of the fracture and is receiving routine care for the fracture during the healing or recovery phase.

Care for complications of surgical treatment for fracture repairs during the healing or recovery phase should be coded with the appropriate complication codes.

Care of complications of fractures, such as malunion and nonunion, should be reported with the appropriate 7th character for subsequent care with nonunion (K, M, N,) or subsequent care with malunion (P, Q, R). Malunion/nonunion: The appropriate 7th character for initial encounter should also be assigned for a patient who delayed seeking treatment for the fracture or nonunion.

The open fracture designations in the assignment of the 7th character for fractures of the forearm, femur and lower leg, including ankle are based on the Gustilo open fracture classification. When the Gustilo classification type is not specified for an open fracture, the 7th character for open fracture type I or II should be assigned (B, E, H, M, Q).

A code from category M80, not a traumatic fracture code, should be used for any patient with known osteoporosis who suffers a fracture, even if the patient had a minor fall or trauma, if that fall or trauma would not usually break a normal, healthy bone.

See Section I.C.13. Osteoporosis.

The aftercare Z codes should not be used for aftercare for traumatic fractures. For aftercare of a traumatic fracture, assign the acute fracture code with the appropriate 7th character.

2) Multiple fractures sequencing

Multiple fractures are sequenced in accordance with the severity of the fracture.

3) Physeal fractures

For physeal fractures, assign only the code identifying the type of physeal fracture. Do not assign a separate code to identify the specific bone that is fractured.

d. Coding of Burns and Corrosions

The ICD-10-CM makes a distinction between burns and corrosions. The burn codes are for thermal burns, except sunburns, that come from a heat source, such as a fire or hot appliance. The burn codes are also for burns resulting from electricity and radiation. Corrosions are burns due to chemicals. The guidelines are the same for burns and corrosions.

Current burns (T20-T25) are classified by depth, extent and by agent (X code). Burns are classified by depth as first degree (erythema), second degree (blistering), and third degree (full-thickness involvement). Burns of the eye and internal organs (T26-T28) are classified by site, but not by degree.

1) Sequencing of burn and related condition codes

Sequence first the code that reflects the highest degree of burn when more than one burn is present.

a. When the reason for the admission or encounter is for treatment of external multiple burns, sequence first the code that reflects the burn of the highest degree.

b. When a patient has both internal and external burns, the circumstances of admission govern the selection of the principal diagnosis or first-listed diagnosis.

c. When a patient is admitted for burn injuries and other related conditions such as smoke inhalation and/or respiratory failure, the circumstances of admission govern the selection of the principal or first-listed diagnosis.

2) Burns of the same anatomic site

Classify burns of the same anatomic site and on the same side but of different degrees to the subcategory identifying the highest degree recorded in the diagnosis (e.g., for second and third degree burns of right thigh, assign only code T24.311-).

3) Non-healing burns

Non-healing burns are coded as acute burns.

Necrosis of burned skin should be coded as a non-healed burn.

4) Infected burn

For any documented infected burn site, use an additional code for the infection.

5) Assign separate codes for each burn site

When coding burns, assign separate codes for each burn site. Category T30, Burn and corrosion, body region unspecified is extremely vague and should rarely be used.

Codes for burns of "multiple sites" should only be assigned when the medical record documentation does not specify the individual sites.

6) Burns and corrosions classified according to extent of body surface involved

Assign codes from category T31, Burns classified according to extent of body surface involved, or T32, Corrosions classified according to extent of body surface involved, for acute burns or corrosions when the site of the burn or corrosion is not specified or when there is a need for additional data. It is advisable to use category T31 as additional coding when needed to provide data for evaluating burn mortality, such as that needed by burn units. It is also advisable to use category T31 as an additional code for reporting purposes when there is mention of a third-degree burn involving 20 percent or more of the body surface.

Codes from categories T31 and T32 should not be used for sequelae of burns or corrosions.

Categories T31 and T32 are based on the classic "rule of nines" in estimating body surface involved: head and neck are assigned nine percent, each arm nine percent, each leg 18 percent, the anterior trunk 18 percent, posterior trunk 18 percent, and genitalia one percent. Providers may change these percentage assignments where necessary to accommodate infants and children who have proportionately larger heads than adults, and patients who have large buttocks, thighs, or abdomen that involve burns.

7) Encounters for treatment of sequela of burns

Encounters for the treatment of the late effects of burns or corrosions (i.e., scars or joint contractures) should be coded with a burn or corrosion code with the 7th character "S" for sequela.

8) Sequelae with a late effect code and current burn

When appropriate, both a code for a current burn or corrosion with 7th character "A" or "D" and a burn or corrosion code with 7th character "S" may be assigned on the same record (when both a current burn and sequelae of an old burn exist). Burns and corrosions do not heal at the same rate and a current healing wound may still exist with sequela of a healed burn or corrosion.

See Section I.B.10. Sequela (Late Effects)

9) Use of an external cause code with burns and corrosions

An external cause code should be used with burns and corrosions to identify the source and intent of the burn, as well as the place where it occurred.

e. Adverse Effects, Poisoning, Underdosing and Toxic Effects

Codes in categories T36-T65 are combination codes that include the substance that was taken as well as the intent. No additional external cause code is required for poisonings, toxic effects, adverse effects and underdosing codes.

1) Do not code directly from the Table of Drugs

Do not code directly from the Table of Drugs and Chemicals. Always refer back to the Tabular List.

2) **Use as many codes as necessary to describe**
Use as many codes as necessary to describe completely all drugs, medicinal or biological substances.

3) **If the same code would describe the causative agent**
If the same code would describe the causative agent for more than one adverse reaction, poisoning, toxic effect or underdosing, assign the code only once.

4) **If two or more drugs, medicinal or biological substances**
If two or more drugs, medicinal or biological substances are taken, code each individually unless a combination code is listed in the Table of Drugs and Chemicals.
If multiple unspecified drugs, medicinal or biological substances were taken, assign the appropriate code from subcategory T50.91, Poisoning by, adverse effect of and underdosing of multiple unspecified drugs, medicaments and biological substances.

5) **The occurrence of drug toxicity is classified in ICD-10-CM as follows:**

(a) **Adverse Effect**
When coding an adverse effect of a drug that has been correctly prescribed and properly administered, assign the appropriate code for the nature of the adverse effect followed by the appropriate code for the adverse effect of the drug (T36-T50). The code for the drug should have a 5th or 6th character "5" (for example T36.0X5-) Examples of the nature of an adverse effect are tachycardia, delirium, gastrointestinal hemorrhaging, vomiting, hypokalemia, hepatitis, renal failure, or respiratory failure.

(b) **Poisoning**
When coding a poisoning or reaction to the improper use of a medication (e.g., overdose, wrong substance given or taken in error, wrong route of administration), first assign the appropriate code from categories T36-T50. The poisoning codes have an associated intent as their 5th or 6th character (accidental, intentional self-harm, assault and undetermined). If the intent of the poisoning is unknown or unspecified, code the intent as accidental intent. The undetermined intent is only for use if the documentation in the record specifies that the intent cannot be determined. Use additional code(s) for all manifestations of poisonings.
If there is also a diagnosis of abuse or dependence of the substance, the abuse or dependence is assigned as an additional code.
Examples of poisoning include:

(i) Error was made in drug prescription
Errors made in drug prescription or in the administration of the drug by provider, nurse, patient, or other person.

(ii) Overdose of a drug intentionally taken
If an overdose of a drug was intentionally taken or administered and resulted in drug toxicity, it would be coded as a poisoning.

(iii) Nonprescribed drug taken with correctly prescribed and properly administered drug
If a nonprescribed drug or medicinal agent was taken in combination with a correctly prescribed and properly administered drug, any drug toxicity or other reaction resulting from the interaction of the two drugs would be classified as a poisoning.

(iv) Interaction of drug(s) and alcohol
When a reaction results from the interaction of a drug(s) and alcohol, this would be classified as poisoning.

See Section I.C.4. if poisoning is the result of insulin pump malfunctions.
For Sequela (Late Effects) see Section I.B.10.

(c) **Underdosing**
Underdosing refers to taking less of a medication than is prescribed by a provider or a manufacturer's instruction. Discontinuing the use of a prescribed medication on the patient's own initiative (not directed by the patient's provider) is also classified as an underdosing. For underdosing, assign the code from categories T36-T50 (fifth or sixth character "6"). Documentation of a change in the patient's condition is not required in order to assign an underdosing code. Documentation that the patient is taking less of a medication than is prescribed or discontinued the prescribed medication is sufficient for code assignment.
Codes for underdosing should never be assigned as principal or first-listed codes. If a patient has a relapse or exacerbation of the medical condition for which the drug is prescribed because of the reduction in dose, then the medical condition itself should be coded.
Noncompliance (Z91.12-, Z91.13-, Z91.14- and Z91.A4-) or complication of care (Y63.6-Y63.9) codes are to be used with an underdosing code to indicate intent, if known.

(d) **Toxic Effects**
When a harmful substance is ingested or comes in contact with a person, this is classified as a toxic effect. The toxic effect codes are in categories T51-T65. When coding a toxic effect, assign the toxic effect code first, followed by codes for all associated manifestations of the toxic effect.
Toxic effect codes have an associated intent: accidental, intentional self-harm, assault and undetermined.
For Sequela (Late Effects) see Section I.B.10. Sequela

f. **Adult and child abuse, neglect and other maltreatment**
Sequence first the appropriate code from categories T74, Adult and child abuse, neglect and other maltreatment, confirmed, or T76, Adult and child abuse, neglect and other maltreatment, suspected, for abuse, neglect and other maltreatment, followed by any accompanying mental health or injury code(s).
If the documentation in the medical record states abuse or neglect, it is coded as confirmed (T74.-). It is coded as suspected if it is documented as suspected (T76.-).
For cases of confirmed abuse or neglect an external cause code from the assault section (X92-Y09) should be added to identify the cause of any physical injuries. A perpetrator code (Y07) should be added when the perpetrator of the abuse is known. For suspected cases of abuse or neglect, do not report external cause or perpetrator code.
If a suspected case of abuse, neglect or mistreatment is ruled out during an encounter code Z04.71, Encounter for examination and observation following alleged physical adult abuse, ruled out, or code Z04.72, Encounter for examination and observation following alleged child physical abuse, ruled out, should be used, not a code from T76.
If a suspected case of alleged rape or sexual abuse is ruled out during an encounter code Z04.41, Encounter for examination and observation following alleged adult rape or code Z04.42, Encounter for examination and observation following alleged child rape, should be used, not a code from T76.
If a suspected case of forced sexual exploitation or forced labor exploitation is ruled out during an encounter, code Z04.81, Encounter for examination and observation of victim following forced sexual exploitation, or code Z04.82, Encounter for examination and observation of victim following forced labor exploitation, should be used, not a code from T76.
See Section I.C.15. Abuse in a pregnant patient.

g. **Complications of care**

1) **General guidelines for complications of care**

(a) **Documentation of complications of care**
See Section I.B.16. for information on documentation of complications of care.

2) **Pain due to medical devices**
Pain associated with devices, implants or grafts left in a surgical site (for example painful hip prosthesis) is assigned to the appropriate code(s) found in Chapter 19, Injury, poisoning, and certain other consequences of external causes. Specific codes for pain due to medical devices are found in the T code section of the ICD-10-CM. Use additional code(s) from category G89 to identify acute or chronic pain due to presence of the device, implant or graft (G89.18 or G89.28).

3) **Transplant complications**

(a) **Transplant complications other than kidney**
Codes under category T86, Complications of transplanted organs and tissues, are for use for both complications and rejection of transplanted organs. A transplant complication code is only assigned if the complication affects the function of the transplanted organ. Two codes are required to fully describe a transplant complication: the appropriate code from category T86 and a secondary code that identifies the complication.
Pre-existing conditions or conditions that develop after the transplant are not coded as complications unless they affect the function of the transplanted organs.
See I.C.21. for transplant organ removal status
See I.C.2. for malignant neoplasm associated with transplanted organ.
See I.C.1.d.4. for sequencing of sepsis due to infection in transplanted organ

(b) **Kidney transplant complications**
Patients who have undergone kidney transplant may still have some form of chronic kidney disease (CKD) because the kidney transplant may not fully restore kidney function. Code T86.1- should be assigned for documented complications of a kidney transplant, such as transplant failure or rejection or other transplant complication. Code T86.1- should not be assigned for post kidney transplant patients who have chronic kidney (CKD) unless a transplant complication such as transplant failure or rejection is documented. If the documentation is unclear as to whether the patient has a complication of the transplant, query the provider. Conditions that affect the function of the transplanted kidney, other than CKD, should be assigned a code from subcategory T86.1, Complications of transplanted organ, Kidney, and a secondary code that identifies the complication.
For patients with CKD following a kidney transplant, but who do not have a complication such as failure or rejection, *see section I.C.14. Chronic kidney disease and kidney transplant status.*
See I.C.1.d.4. for sequencing of sepsis due to infection in transplanted organ

    4) Complication codes that include the external cause

As with certain other T codes, some of the complications of care codes have the external cause included in the code. The code includes the nature of the complication as well as the type of procedure that caused the complication. No external cause code indicating the type of procedure is necessary for these codes.

    5) Complications of care codes within the body system chapters

Intraoperative and postprocedural complication codes are found within the body system chapters with codes specific to the organs and structures of that body system. These codes should be sequenced first, followed by a code(s) for the specific complication, if applicable. Complication codes from the body system chapters should be assigned for intraoperative and postprocedural complications (e.g., the appropriate complication code from chapter 9 would be assigned for a vascular intraoperative or postprocedural complication) unless the complication is specifically indexed to a T code in chapter 19.

20. Chapter 20: External Causes of Morbidity (V00-Y99)

The external causes of morbidity codes should never be sequenced as the first-listed or principal diagnosis.

External cause codes are intended to provide data for injury research and evaluation of injury prevention strategies. These codes capture how the injury or health condition happened (cause), the intent (unintentional or accidental; or intentional, such as suicide or assault), the place where the event occurred the activity of the patient at the time of the event, and the person's status (e.g., civilian, military).

There is no national requirement for mandatory ICD-10-CM external cause code reporting. Unless a provider is subject to a state-based external cause code reporting mandate or these codes are required by a particular payer, reporting of ICD-10-CM codes in Chapter 20, External Causes of Morbidity, is not required. In the absence of a mandatory reporting requirement, providers are encouraged to voluntarily report external cause codes, as they provide valuable data for injury research and evaluation of injury prevention strategies.

a. General External Cause Guidelines

    1) Used with any code in the range of A00.0-T88.9, Z00-Z99

An external cause code may be used with any code in the range of A00.0-T88.9, Z00-Z99, classification that represents a health condition due to an external cause. Though they are most applicable to injuries, they are also valid for use with such things as infections or diseases due to an external source, and other health conditions, such as a heart attack that occurs during strenuous physical activity.

    2) External cause code used for length of treatment

Assign the external cause code, with the appropriate 7th character (initial encounter, subsequent encounter or sequela) for each encounter for which the injury or condition is being treated.

Most categories in chapter 20 have a 7th character requirement for each applicable code. Most categories in this chapter have three 7th character values: A, initial encounter, D, subsequent encounter and S, sequela. While the patient may be seen by a new or different provider over the course of treatment for an injury or condition, assignment of the 7th character for external cause should match the 7th character of the code assigned for the associated injury or condition for the encounter.

    3) Use the full range of external cause codes

Use the full range of external cause codes to completely describe the cause, the intent, the place of occurrence, and if applicable, the activity of the patient at the time of the event, and the patient's status, for all injuries, and other health conditions due to an external cause.

    4) Assign as many external cause codes as necessary

Assign as many external cause codes as necessary to fully explain each cause. If only one external code can be recorded, assign the code most related to the principal diagnosis.

    5) The selection of the appropriate external cause code

The selection of the appropriate external cause code is guided by the Alphabetic Index of External Causes and by Inclusion and Exclusion notes in the Tabular List.

    6) External cause code can never be a principal diagnosis

An external cause code can never be a principal (first-listed) diagnosis.

    7) Combination external cause codes

Certain of the external cause codes are combination codes that identify sequential events that result in an injury, such as a fall which results in striking against an object. The injury may be due to either event or both. The combination external cause code used should correspond to the sequence of events regardless of which caused the most serious injury.

    8) No external cause code needed in certain circumstances

No external cause code from Chapter 20 is needed if the external cause and intent are included in a code from another chapter (e.g., T36.0X1-, Poisoning by penicillins, accidental (unintentional)).

b. Place of Occurrence Guideline

Codes from category Y92, Place of occurrence of the external cause, are secondary codes for use after other external cause codes to identify the location of the patient at the time of injury or other condition.

Generally, a place of occurrence code is assigned only once, at the initial encounter for treatment. However, in the rare instance that a new injury occurs during hospitalization, an additional place of occurrence code may be assigned. No 7th characters are used for Y92.

Do not use place of occurrence code Y92.9 if the place is not stated or is not applicable.

c. Activity Code

Assign a code from category Y93, Activity code, to describe the activity of the patient at the time the injury or other health condition occurred.

An activity code is used only once, at the initial encounter for treatment. Only one code from Y93 should be recorded on a medical record.

The activity codes are not applicable to poisonings, adverse effects, misadventures or sequela.

Do not assign Y93.9, Unspecified activity, if the activity is not stated.

A code from category Y93 is appropriate for use with external cause and intent codes if identifying the activity provides additional information about the event.

d. Place of Occurrence, Activity, and Status Codes Used with other External Cause Code

When applicable, place of occurrence, activity, and external cause status codes are sequenced after the main external cause code(s). Regardless of the number of external cause codes assigned, generally there should be only one place of occurrence code, one activity code, and one external cause status code assigned to an encounter. However, in the rare instance that a new injury occurs during hospitalization, an additional place of occurrence code may be assigned.

e. If the Reporting Format Limits the Number of External Cause Codes

If the reporting format limits the number of external cause codes that can be used in reporting clinical data, report the code for the cause/intent most related to the principal diagnosis. If the format permits capture of additional external cause codes, the cause/intent, including medical misadventures, of the additional events should be reported rather than the codes for place, activity, or external status.

f. Multiple External Cause Coding Guidelines

More than one external cause code is required to fully describe the external cause of an illness or injury. The assignment of external cause codes should be sequenced in the following priority:

If two or more events cause separate injuries, an external cause code should be assigned for each cause. The first-listed external cause code will be selected in the following order:

External codes for child and adult abuse take priority over all other external cause codes.

See Section I.C.19., Child and Adult abuse guidelines.

External cause codes for terrorism events take priority over all other external cause codes except child and adult abuse.

External cause codes for cataclysmic events take priority over all other external cause codes except child and adult abuse and terrorism.

External cause codes for transport accidents take priority over all other external cause codes except cataclysmic events, child and adult abuse and terrorism.

Activity and external cause status codes are assigned following all causal (intent) external cause codes.

The first-listed external cause code should correspond to the cause of the most serious diagnosis due to an assault, accident, or self-harm, following the order of hierarchy listed above.

g. Child and Adult Abuse Guideline

Adult and child abuse, neglect and maltreatment are classified as assault. Any of the assault codes may be used to indicate the external cause of any injury resulting from the confirmed abuse.

For confirmed cases of abuse, neglect and maltreatment, when the perpetrator is known, a code from Y07, Perpetrator of maltreatment and neglect, should accompany any other assault codes.

See Section I.C.19. Adult and child abuse, neglect and other maltreatment

h. Unknown or Undetermined Intent Guideline

If the intent (accident, self-harm, assault) of the cause of an injury or other condition is unknown or unspecified, code the intent as accidental intent. All transport accident categories assume accidental intent.

    1) Use of undetermined intent

External cause codes for events of undetermined intent are only for use if the documentation in the record specifies that the intent cannot be determined.

i. Sequelae (Late Effects) of External Cause Guidelines

    1) Sequelae external cause codes

Sequela are reported using the external cause code with the 7th character "S" for sequela. These codes should be used with any report of a late effect or sequela resulting from a previous injury.

See Section I.B.10. Sequela (Late Effects)

    2) Sequela external cause code with a related current injury

A sequela external cause code should never be used with a related current nature of injury code.

    3) Use of sequela external cause codes for subsequent visits

Use a late effect external cause code for subsequent visits when a late effect of the initial injury is being treated. Do not use a late effect external cause code for subsequent visits for follow-up care (e.g., to assess healing, to receive rehabilitative therapy) of the injury when no late effect of the injury has been documented.

j. Terrorism Guidelines

    1) Cause of injury identified by the Federal Government (FBI) as terrorism

When the cause of an injury is identified by the Federal Government (FBI) as terrorism, the first-listed external cause code should be a code from category Y38, Terrorism. The definition of terrorism employed by the FBI is found at the inclusion note at the beginning of category Y38. Use additional code for place of occurrence (Y92.-). More than one Y38 code may be assigned if the injury is the result of more than one mechanism of terrorism.

2) **Cause of an injury is suspected to be the result of terrorism**

When the cause of an injury is suspected to be the result of terrorism a code from category Y38 should not be assigned. Suspected cases should be classified as assault.

3) **Code Y38.9, Terrorism, secondary effects**

Assign code Y38.9, Terrorism, secondary effects, for conditions occurring subsequent to the terrorist event. This code should not be assigned for conditions that are due to the initial terrorist act.

It is acceptable to assign code Y38.9 with another code from Y38 if there is an injury due to the initial terrorist event and an injury that is a subsequent result of the terrorist event.

k. External Cause Status

A code from category Y99, External cause status, should be assigned whenever any other external cause code is assigned for an encounter, including an Activity code, except for the events noted below. Assign a code from category Y99, External cause status, to indicate the work status of the person at the time the event occurred. The status code indicates whether the event occurred during military activity, whether a non-military person was at work, whether an individual including a student or volunteer was involved in a non-work activity at the time of the causal event.

A code from Y99, External cause status, should be assigned, when applicable, with other external cause codes, such as transport accidents and falls. The external cause status codes are not applicable to poisonings, adverse effects, misadventures or late effects.

Do not assign a code from category Y99 if no other external cause codes (cause, activity) are applicable for the encounter.

An external cause status code is used only once, at the initial encounter for treatment. Only one code from Y99 should be recorded on a medical record. Do not assign code Y99.9, Unspecified external cause status, if the status is not stated.

21. Chapter 21: Factors influencing health status and contact with health services (Z00-Z99)

Note: The chapter specific guidelines provide additional information about the use of Z codes for specified encounters.

a. Use of Z Codes in Any Healthcare Setting

Z codes are for use in any healthcare setting. Z codes may be used as either a first-listed (principal diagnosis code in the inpatient setting) or secondary code, depending on the circumstances of the encounter. Certain Z codes may only be used as first-listed or principal diagnosis.

b. Z Codes Indicate a Reason for an Encounter or Provide Additional Information about a Patient Encounter

Z codes are not procedure codes. A corresponding procedure code must accompany a Z code to describe any procedure performed.

c. Categories of Z Codes

1) **Contact/Exposure**

Category Z20 indicates contact with, and suspected exposure to, communicable diseases. These codes are for patients who are suspected to have been exposed to a disease by close personal contact with an infected individual or are in an area where a disease is epidemic. Category Z77, Other contact with and (suspected) exposures hazardous to health, indicates contact with and suspected exposures hazardous to health.

Contact/exposure codes may be used as a first-listed code to explain an encounter for testing, or, more commonly, as a secondary code to identify a potential risk.

2) **Inoculations and vaccinations**

Code Z23 is for encounters for inoculations and vaccinations. It indicates that a patient is being seen to receive a prophylactic inoculation against a disease. Procedure codes are required to identify the actual administration of the injection and the type(s) of immunizations given. Code Z23 may be used as a secondary code if the inoculation is given as a routine part of preventive health care, such as a well-baby visit.

3) **Status**

Status codes indicate that a patient is either a carrier of a disease or has the sequelae or residual of a past disease or condition. This includes such things as the presence of prosthetic or mechanical devices resulting from past treatment. A status code is informative, because the status may affect the course of treatment and its outcome. A status code is distinct from a history code. The history code indicates that the patient no longer has the condition.

A status code should not be used with a diagnosis code from one of the body system chapters, if the diagnosis code includes the information provided by the status code. For example, code Z94.1, Heart transplant status, should not be used with a code from subcategory T86.2, Complications of heart transplant. The status code does not provide additional information. The complication code indicates that the patient is a heart transplant patient.

For encounters for weaning from a mechanical ventilator, assign a code from subcategory J96.1, Chronic respiratory failure, followed by code Z99.11, Dependence on respirator [ventilator] status.

The status Z codes/categories are:

Z14	Genetic carrier

Genetic carrier status indicates that a person carries a gene, associated with a particular disease, which may be passed to offspring who may develop that disease. The person does not have the disease and is not at risk of developing the disease.

Z15   Genetic susceptibility to disease

Genetic susceptibility indicates that a person has a gene that increases the risk of that person developing the disease. Codes from category Z15 should not be used as principal or first-listed codes. If the patient has the condition to which he/she is susceptible, and that condition is the reason for the encounter, the code for the current condition should be sequenced first. If the patient is being seen for follow-up after completed treatment for this condition, and the condition no longer exists, a follow-up code should be sequenced first, followed by the appropriate personal history and genetic susceptibility codes. If the purpose of the encounter is genetic counseling associated with procreative management, code Z31.5, Encounter for genetic counseling, should be assigned as the first-listed code, followed by a code from category Z15. Additional codes should be assigned for any applicable family or personal history.

Z16   Resistance to antimicrobial drugs

This code indicates that a patient has a condition that is resistant to antimicrobial drug treatment. Sequence the infection code first.

Z17   Estrogen, **and other hormones and factors** receptor status

Z18   Retained foreign body fragments

Z19   Hormone sensitivity malignancy status

Z21   Asymptomatic HIV infection status

This code indicates that a patient has tested positive for HIV but has manifested no signs or symptoms of the disease.

Z22   Carrier of infectious disease

Carrier status indicates that a person harbors the specific organisms of a disease without manifest symptoms and is capable of transmitting the infection.

Z28.3   Underimmunization status

See Section I.B.14. for underimmunization documentation by clinicians other than the patient's provider.

Z33.1   Pregnant state, incidental

This code is a secondary code only for use when the pregnancy is in no way complicating the reason for visit. Otherwise, a code from the obstetric chapter is required.

Z66   Do not resuscitate

This code may be used when it is documented by the provider that a patient is on do not resuscitate status at any time during the stay.

Z67   Blood type

Z68   Body mass index (BMI)

BMI codes should only be assigned when there is an associated, reportable diagnosis (such as obesity). Do not assign BMI codes during pregnancy.

See Section I.B.14. for BMI documentation by clinicians other than the patient's provider.

Z74.01   Bed confinement status

Z76.82   Awaiting organ transplant status

Z78   Other specified health status

Code Z78.1, Physical restraint status, may be used when it is documented by the provider that a patient has been put in restraints during the current encounter. Please note that this code should not be reported when it is documented by the provider that a patient is temporarily restrained during a procedure.

Z79   Long-term (current) drug therapy

Codes from this category indicate a patient's continuous use of a prescribed drug (including such things as aspirin therapy) for the long-term treatment of a condition or for prophylactic use. It is not for use for patients who have addictions to drugs. This subcategory is not for use of medications for detoxification or maintenance programs to prevent withdrawal symptoms (e.g., methadone maintenance for opiate dependence). Assign the appropriate code for the drug use, abuse, or dependence instead.

Assign a code from Z79 if the patient is receiving a medication for an extended period as a prophylactic measure (such as for the prevention of deep vein thrombosis) or as treatment of a chronic condition (such as arthritis) or a disease requiring a lengthy course of treatment (such as cancer). Do not assign a code from category Z79 for medication being administered for a brief period of time to treat an acute illness or injury (such as a course of antibiotics to treat acute bronchitis).

Z88   Allergy status to drugs, medicaments and biological substances Except: Z88.9, Allergy status to unspecified drugs, medicaments and biological substances status

Z89   Acquired absence of limb

Z90   Acquired absence of organs, not elsewhere classified

Z91.0-   Allergy status, other than to drugs and biological substances

Z92.82   Status post administration of tPA (rtPA) in a different facility within the last 24 hours prior to admission to a current facility

Assign code Z92.82, Status post administration of tPA (rtPA) in a different facility within the last 24 hours prior to admission to current facility, as a secondary diagnosis when a patient is received by transfer into a facility and documentation indicates they were administered tissue plasminogen activator (tPA) within the last 24 hours prior to admission to the current facility. This guideline applies even if the patient is still receiving the tPA at the time they are received into the current facility.

The appropriate code for the condition for which the tPA was administered (such as cerebrovascular disease or myocardial infarction) should be assigned first.

Code Z92.82 is only applicable to the receiving facility record and not to the transferring facility record.

Z93   Artificial opening status

Z94   Transplanted organ and tissue status

Z95   Presence of cardiac and vascular implants and grafts

Z96   Presence of other functional implants

Z97   Presence of other devices

Z98   Other postprocedural states

Assign code Z98.85, Transplanted organ removal status, to indicate that a transplanted organ has been previously removed. This code should not be assigned for the encounter in which the transplanted organ is removed. The complication necessitating removal of the transplant organ should be assigned for that encounter.

See section I.C.19. for information on the coding of organ transplant complications.

Z99   Dependence on enabling machines and devices, not elsewhere classified

Note: Categories Z89-Z90 and Z93-Z99 are for use only if there are no complications or malfunctions of the organ or tissue replaced, the amputation site or the equipment on which the patient is dependent.

4) **History (of)**

There are two types of history Z codes, personal and family. Personal history codes explain a patient's past medical condition that no longer exists and is not receiving any treatment, but that has the potential for recurrence, and therefore may require continued monitoring.

Family history codes are for use when a patient has a family member(s) who has had a particular disease that causes the patient to be at higher risk of also contracting the disease.

Personal history codes may be used in conjunction with follow-up codes and family history codes may be used in conjunction with screening codes to explain the need for a test or procedure. History codes are also acceptable on any medical record regardless of the reason for visit. A history of an illness, even if no longer present, is important information that may alter the type of treatment ordered.

The reason for the encounter (for example, screening or counseling) should be sequenced first and the appropriate personal and/or family history code(s) should be assigned as additional diagnos(es).

The history Z code categories are:

Z80   Family history of primary malignant neoplasm

Z81   Family history of mental and behavioral disorders

Z82   Family history of certain disabilities and chronic diseases (leading to disablement)

Z83   Family history of other specific disorders

Z84   Family history of other conditions

Z85   Personal history of malignant neoplasm

Z86   Personal history of certain other diseases

Z87   Personal history of other diseases and conditions

Z91.4-   Personal history of psychological trauma, not elsewhere classified

Z91.5-   Personal history of self-harm

Z91.81   History of falling

Z91.82   Personal history of military deployment

Z91.85   Personal history of military service

Z92   Personal history of medical treatment

Except: Z92.0, Personal history of contraception

Except: Z92.82, Status post administration of tPA (rtPA) in a different facility within the last 24 hours prior to admission to a current facility

5) **Screening**

Screening is the testing for disease or disease precursors in seemingly well individuals so that early detection and treatment can be provided for those who test positive for the disease (e.g., screening mammogram).

The testing of a person to rule out or confirm a suspected diagnosis because the patient has some sign or symptom is a diagnostic examination, not a screening. In these cases, the sign or symptom is used to explain the reason for the test.

A screening code may be a first-listed code if the reason for the visit is specifically the screening exam. It may also be used as an additional code if the screening is done during an office visit for other health problems. A screening code is not necessary if the screening is inherent to a routine examination, such as a pap smear done during a routine pelvic examination.

Should a condition be discovered during the screening then the code for the condition may be assigned as an additional diagnosis.

The Z code indicates that a screening exam is planned. A procedure code is required to confirm that the screening was performed.

The screening Z codes/categories:

Z11   Encounter for screening for infectious and parasitic diseases

Z12   Encounter for screening for malignant neoplasms

Z13   Encounter for screening for other diseases and disorders Except: Z13.9, Encounter for screening, unspecified

Z36   Encounter for antenatal screening for mother

6) **Observation**

There are three observation Z code categories. They are for use in very limited circumstances when a person is being observed for a suspected condition that is ruled out. The observation codes are not for use if an injury or illness or any signs or symptoms related to the suspected condition are present. In such cases the diagnosis/symptom code is used with the corresponding external cause code.

The observation codes are primarily to be used as a principal/first-listed diagnosis. An observation code may be assigned as a secondary diagnosis code when the patient is being observed for a condition that is ruled out and is unrelated to the principal/first-listed diagnosis. Also, when the principal diagnosis is required to be a code from category Z38, Liveborn infants according to place of birth and type of delivery, then a code from category Z05, Encounter for observation and evaluation of newborn for suspected diseases and conditions ruled out, is sequenced after the Z38 code. Additional codes may be used in addition to the observation code, but only if they are unrelated to the suspected condition being observed.

Codes from subcategory Z03.7, Encounter for suspected maternal and fetal conditions ruled out, may either be used as a first-listed or as an additional code assignment depending on the case. They are for use in very limited circumstances on a maternal record when an encounter is for a suspected maternal or fetal condition that is ruled out during that encounter (for example, a maternal or fetal condition may be suspected due to an abnormal test result). These codes should not be used when the condition is confirmed. In those cases, the confirmed condition should be coded. In addition, these codes are not for use if an illness or any signs or symptoms related to the suspected condition or problem are present. In such cases the diagnosis/symptom code is used.

Additional codes may be used in addition to the code from subcategory Z03.7, but only if they are unrelated to the suspected condition being evaluated.

Codes from subcategory Z03.7 may not be used for encounters for antenatal screening of mother. *See Section I.C.21. Screening.*

For encounters for suspected fetal condition that are inconclusive following testing and evaluation, assign the appropriate code from category O35, O36, O40 or O41.

The observation Z code categories:

Z03   Encounter for medical observation for suspected diseases and conditions ruled out

Z04   Encounter for examination and observation for other reasons Except: Z04.9, Encounter for examination and observation for unspecified reason

Z05   Encounter for observation and evaluation of newborn for suspected diseases and conditions ruled out

7) **Aftercare**

Aftercare visit codes cover situations when the initial treatment of a disease has been performed and the patient requires continued care during the healing or recovery phase, or for the long-term consequences of the disease. The aftercare Z code should not be used if treatment is directed at a current, acute disease. The diagnosis code is to be used in these cases. Exceptions to this rule are codes Z51.0, Encounter for antineoplastic radiation therapy, and codes from subcategory Z51.1, Encounter for antineoplastic chemotherapy and immunotherapy. These codes are to be first listed, followed by the diagnosis code when a patient's encounter is chiefly to receive radiation therapy, chemotherapy, or immunotherapy for the treatment of a neoplasm. If the reason for the encounter is more than one type of antineoplastic therapy, code Z51.0 and a code from subcategory Z51.1 may be assigned together, in which case one of these codes would be reported as a secondary diagnosis.

The aftercare Z codes should also not be used for aftercare for injuries. For aftercare of an injury, assign the acute injury code with the appropriate 7th character (for subsequent encounter).

The aftercare codes are generally first listed to explain the specific reason for the encounter. An aftercare code may be used as an additional code when some type of aftercare is provided in addition to the reason for admission and no diagnosis code is applicable. An example of this would be the closure of a colostomy during an encounter for treatment of another condition.

Aftercare codes should be used in conjunction with other aftercare codes or diagnosis codes to provide better detail on the specifics of an aftercare encounter visit, unless otherwise directed by the classification.

The sequencing of multiple aftercare codes depends on the circumstances of the encounter.

Certain aftercare Z code categories need a secondary diagnosis code to describe the resolving condition or sequelae. For others, the condition is included in the code title.

Additional Z code aftercare category terms include fitting and adjustment, and attention to artificial openings.

Status Z codes may be used with aftercare Z codes to indicate the nature of the aftercare. For example, code Z95.1, Presence of aortocoronary bypass graft, may be used with code Z48.812, Encounter for surgical aftercare following surgery on the circulatory system, to indicate the surgery for which the aftercare is being performed. A status code should not be used when the aftercare code indicates the type of status, such as using Z43.Ø, Encounter for attention to tracheostomy, with Z93.Ø, Tracheostomy status.

The aftercare Z category/codes:

Z42	Encounter for plastic and reconstructive surgery following medical procedure or healed injury
Z43	Encounter for attention to artificial openings
Z44	Encounter for fitting and adjustment of external prosthetic device
Z45	Encounter for adjustment and management of implanted device
Z46	Encounter for fitting and adjustment of other devices
Z47	Orthopedic aftercare
Z48	Encounter for other postprocedural aftercare
Z49	Encounter for care involving renal dialysis
Z51	Encounter for other aftercare and medical care

8) Follow-up

The follow-up codes are used to explain continuing surveillance following completed treatment of a disease, condition, or injury. They imply that the condition has been fully treated and no longer exists. They should not be confused with aftercare codes, or injury codes with a 7th character for subsequent encounter, that explain ongoing care of a healing condition or its sequelae. Follow-up codes may be used in conjunction with history codes to provide the full picture of the healed condition and its treatment. The follow-up code is sequenced first, followed by the history code.

A follow-up code may be used to explain multiple visits. Should a condition be found to have recurred on the follow-up visit, then the diagnosis code for the condition should be assigned in place of the follow-up code.

The follow-up Z codes/categories:

ZØ8	Encounter for follow-up examination after completed treatment for malignant neoplasm
ZØ9	Encounter for follow-up examination after completed treatment for conditions other than malignant neoplasm

Codes ZØ8, Encounter for follow-up examination after completed treatment for malignant neoplasm, and ZØ9, Encounter for follow up examination after completed treatment for conditions other than malignant neoplasm, may be assigned following any type of completed treatment modality (including both medical and surgical treatments).

Z39	Encounter for maternal postpartum care and examination

9) Donor

Codes in category Z52, Donors of organs and tissues, are used for living individuals who are donating blood or other body tissue. These codes are for individuals donating for others, as well as for self-donations. They are not used to identify cadaveric donations.

10) Counseling

Counseling Z codes are used when a patient or family member receives assistance in the aftermath of an illness or injury, or when support is required in coping with family or social problems.

The counseling Z codes/categories:

Z3Ø.Ø-	Encounter for general counseling and advice on contraception
Z31.5	Encounter for procreative genetic counseling
Z31.6-	Encounter for general counseling and advice on procreation
Z32.2	Encounter for childbirth instruction
Z32.3	Encounter for childcare instruction
Z69	Encounter for mental health services for victim and perpetrator of abuse
Z70	Counseling related to sexual attitude, behavior and orientation
Z71	Persons encountering health services for other counseling and medical advice, not elsewhere classified
	Note: Code Z71.84, Encounter for health counseling related to travel, is to be used for health risk and safety counseling for future travel purposes.
	Code Z71.85, Encounter for immunization safety counseling, is to be used for counseling of the patient or caregiver regarding the safety of a vaccine. This code should not be used for the provision of general information regarding risks and potential side effects during routine encounters for the administration of vaccines.
	Code Z71.87, Encounter for pediatric-to-adult transition counseling, should be assigned when pediatric-to-adult transition counseling is the sole reason for the encounter or when this counseling is provided in addition to other services,

such as treatment of a chronic condition. If both transition counseling and treatment of a medical condition are provided during the same encounter, the code(s) for the medical condition(s) treated and code Z71.87 should be assigned, with sequencing depending on the circumstances of the encounter.

Z76.81	Expectant mother prebirth pediatrician visit

11) Encounters for Obstetrical and Reproductive Services

See Section I.C.15. Pregnancy, Childbirth, and the Puerperium, for further instruction on the use of these codes.

Z codes for pregnancy are for use in those circumstances when none of the problems or complications included in the codes from the Obstetrics chapter exist (a routine prenatal visit or postpartum care). Codes in category Z34, Encounter for supervision of normal pregnancy, are always first listed and are not to be used with any other code from the OB chapter.

Codes in category Z3A, Weeks of gestation, may be assigned to provide additional information about the pregnancy. Category Z3A codes should not be assigned for pregnancies with abortive outcomes (categories OØØ-OØ8), elective termination of pregnancy (code Z33.2), nor for postpartum conditions, as category Z3A is not applicable to these conditions. The date of the admission should be used to determine weeks of gestation for inpatient admissions that encompass more than one gestational week.

The outcome of delivery, category Z37, should be included on all maternal delivery records. It is always a secondary code.

Codes in category Z37 should not be used on the newborn record.

Z codes for family planning (contraceptive) or procreative management and counseling should be included on an obstetric record either during the pregnancy or the postpartum stage, if applicable.

Z codes/categories for obstetrical and reproductive services:

Z3Ø	Encounter for contraceptive management
Z31	Encounter for procreative management
Z32.2	Encounter for childbirth instruction
Z32.3	Encounter for childcare instruction
Z33	Pregnant state
Z34	Encounter for supervision of normal pregnancy
Z36	Encounter for antenatal screening of mother
Z3A	Weeks of gestation
Z37	Outcome of delivery
Z39	Encounter for maternal postpartum care and examination
Z76.81	Expectant mother prebirth pediatrician visit

12) Newborns and Infants

See Section I.C.16. Newborn (Perinatal) Guidelines, for further instruction on the use of these codes.

Newborn Z codes/categories:

Z76.1	Encounter for health supervision and care of foundling
ZØØ.1-	Encounter for routine child health examination
Z38	Liveborn infants according to place of birth and type of delivery

13) Routine and Administrative Examinations

The Z codes allow for the description of encounters for routine examinations, such as, a general check-up, or, examinations for administrative purposes, such as, a pre-employment physical. The codes are not to be used if the examination is for diagnosis of a suspected condition or for treatment purposes. In such cases the diagnosis code is used. During a routine exam, should a diagnosis or condition be discovered, it should be coded as an additional code. Pre-existing and chronic conditions and history codes may also be included as additional codes as long as the examination is for administrative purposes and not focused on any particular condition.

Some of the codes for routine health examinations distinguish between "with" and "without" abnormal findings. Code assignment depends on the information that is known at the time the encounter is being coded. For example, if no abnormal findings were found during the examination, but the encounter is being coded before test results are back, it is acceptable to assign the code for "without abnormal findings." When assigning a code for "with abnormal findings," additional code(s) should be assigned to identify the specific abnormal finding(s).

Pre-operative examination and pre-procedural laboratory examination Z codes are for use only in those situations when a patient is being cleared for a procedure or surgery and no treatment is given.

The Z codes/categories for routine and administrative examinations:

ZØØ	Encounter for general examination without complaint, suspected or reported diagnosis
ZØ1	Encounter for other special examination without complaint, suspected or reported diagnosis
ZØ2	Encounter for administrative examination
	Except: ZØ2.9, Encounter for administrative examinations, unspecified
Z32.Ø-	Encounter for pregnancy test

14) Miscellaneous Z Codes

The miscellaneous Z codes capture a number of other health care encounters that do not fall into one of the other categories. Some of these codes identify the reason for the encounter; others are for use as additional codes that provide useful information on circumstances that may affect a patient's care and treatment.

Prophylactic Organ Removal

For encounters specifically for prophylactic removal of an organ (such as prophylactic removal of breasts due to a genetic susceptibility to cancer or a family history of cancer), the principal or first-listed code should be a code from category Z40, Encounter for prophylactic surgery, followed by the appropriate codes to identify the associated risk factor (such as genetic susceptibility or family history).

If the patient has a malignancy of one site and is having prophylactic removal at another site to prevent either a new primary malignancy or metastatic disease, a code for the malignancy should also be assigned in addition to a code from subcategory Z40.0, Encounter for prophylactic surgery for risk factors related to malignant neoplasms. A Z40.0 code should not be assigned if the patient is having organ removal for treatment of a malignancy, such as the removal of the testes for the treatment of prostate cancer.

Miscellaneous Z codes/categories:

Z28	Immunization not carried out
	Except: Z28.3–, Underimmunization status
Z29	Encounter for other prophylactic measures
Z40	Encounter for prophylactic surgery
Z41	Encounter for procedures for purposes other than remedying health state
	Except: Z41.9, Encounter for procedure for purposes other than remedying health state, unspecified
Z53	Persons encountering health services for specific procedures and treatment, not carried out
Z72	Problems related to lifestyle
	Note: These codes should be assigned only when the documentation specifies that the patient has an associated problem
Z73	Problems related to life management difficulty
	Note: These codes should be assigned only when the documentation specifies that the patient has an associated problem.
Z74	Problems related to care provider dependency
	Except: Z74.01, Bed confinement status
Z75	Problems related to medical facilities and other health care
Z76.0	Encounter for issue of repeat prescription
Z76.3	Healthy person accompanying sick person
Z76.4	Other boarder to healthcare facility
Z76.5	Malingerer [conscious simulation]
Z91.1-	Patient's noncompliance with medical treatment and regimen
Z91.A-	Caregiver's noncompliance with patient's medical treatment and regimen
Z91.83	Wandering in diseases classified elsewhere
Z91.84-	Oral health risk factors
Z91.89	Other specified personal risk factors, not elsewhere classified

See Section I.B.14. for Z55-Z65 Persons with potential health hazards related to socioeconomic and psychosocial circumstances, documentation by clinicians other than the patient's provider

15) **Nonspecific Z Codes**

Certain Z codes are so non-specific, or potentially redundant with other codes in the classification, that there can be little justification for their use in the inpatient setting. Their use in the outpatient setting should be limited to those instances when there is no further documentation to permit more precise coding. Otherwise, any sign or symptom or any other reason for visit that is captured in another code should be used.

Nonspecific Z codes/categories:

Z02.9	Encounter for administrative examinations, unspecified
Z04.9	Encounter for examination and observation for unspecified reason
Z13.9	Encounter for screening, unspecified
Z41.9	Encounter for procedure for purposes other than remedying health state, unspecified
Z52.9	Donor of unspecified organ or tissue
Z86.59	Personal history of other mental and behavioral disorders
Z88.9	Allergy status to unspecified drugs, medicaments and biological substances status
Z92.0	Personal history of contraception

16) **Z Codes That May Only be Principal/First-Listed Diagnosis**

The following Z codes/categories may only be reported as the principal/first-listed diagnosis, except when there are multiple encounters on the same day and the medical records for the encounters are combined:

Z00	Encounter for general examination without complaint, suspected or reported diagnosis
	Except: Z00.6
Z01	Encounter for other special examination without complaint, suspected or reported diagnosis
Z02	Encounter for administrative examination
Z04	Encounter for examination and observation for other reasons
Z33.2	Encounter for elective termination of pregnancy
Z31.81	Encounter for male factor infertility in female patient
Z31.83	Encounter for assisted reproductive fertility procedure cycle
Z31.84	Encounter for fertility preservation procedure
Z34	Encounter for supervision of normal pregnancy

Z39	Encounter for maternal postpartum care and examination
Z38	Liveborn infants according to place of birth and type of delivery
Z40	Encounter for prophylactic surgery
Z42	Encounter for plastic and reconstructive surgery following medical procedure or healed injury
Z51.0	Encounter for antineoplastic radiation therapy
Z51.1-	Encounter for antineoplastic chemotherapy and immunotherapy
Z52	Donors of organs and tissues
	Except: Z52.9, Donor of unspecified organ or tissue
Z76.1	Encounter for health supervision and care of foundling
Z76.2	Encounter for health supervision and care of other healthy infant and child
Z99.12	Encounter for respirator [ventilator] dependence during power failure

17) **Social Determinants of Health**

Social determinants of health (SDOH) codes describing social problems, conditions, or risk factors that influence a patient's health should be assigned when this information is documented in the patient's medical record. Assign as many SDOH codes as are necessary to describe all of the social problems, conditions, or risk factors documented during the current episode of care. For example, a patient who lives alone may suffer an acute injury temporarily impacting their ability to perform routine activities of daily living. When documented as such, this would support assignment of code Z60.2, Problems related to living alone. However, merely living alone, without documentation of a risk or unmet need for assistance at home, would not support assignment of code Z60.2. Documentation by a clinician (or patient-reported information that is signed off by a clinician) that the patient expressed concerns with access and availability of food would support assignment of code Z59.41, Food insecurity. Similarly, medical record documentation indicating the patient is homeless would support assignment of a code from subcategory Z59.0-, Homelessness.

For social determinants of health classified to chapter 21, such as information found in categories Z55-Z65, Persons with potential health hazards related to socioeconomic and psychosocial circumstances, code assignment may be based on medical record documentation from clinicians involved in the care of the patient who are not the patient's provider since this information represents social information, rather than medical diagnoses. For example, coding professionals may utilize documentation of social information from social workers, community health workers, case managers, or nurses, if their documentation is included in the official medical record.

Patient self-reported documentation may be used to assign codes for social determinants of health, as long as the patient self-reported information is signed-off by and incorporated into the medical record by either a clinician or provider.

Social determinants of health codes are located primarily in these Z code categories:

Z55	Problems related to education and literacy
Z56	Problems related to employment and unemployment
Z57	Occupational exposure to risk factors
Z58	Problems related to physical environment
Z59	Problems related to housing and economic circumstances
Z60	Problems related to social environment
Z62	Problems related to upbringing
Z63	Other problems related to primary support group, including family circumstances
Z64	Problems related to certain psychosocial circumstances
Z65	Problems related to other psychosocial circumstances

See Section I.B.14. Documentation by Clinicians Other than the Patient's Provider.

22. **Chapter 22: Codes for Special Purposes (U00-U85)**

U07.0	Vaping-related disorder (see Section I.C.10.e., Vaping-related disorders)
U07.1	COVID-19 (see Section I.C.1.g.1., COVID-19 infection)
U09.9	Post COVID-19 condition, unspecified (see Section I.C.1.g.1.m.)

Section II. Selection of Principal Diagnosis

The circumstances of inpatient admission always govern the selection of principal diagnosis. The principal diagnosis is defined in the Uniform Hospital Discharge Data Set (UHDDS) as "that condition established after study to be chiefly responsible for occasioning the admission of the patient to the hospital for care."

The UHDDS definitions are used by hospitals to report inpatient data elements in a standardized manner. These data elements and their definitions can be found in the July 31, 1985, Federal Register (Vol. 50, No, 147), pp. 31038-40.

Since that time, the application of the UHDDS definitions has been expanded to include all non-outpatient settings (acute care, short term, long term care and psychiatric hospitals; home health agencies; rehab facilities; nursing homes, etc.). The UHDDS definitions also apply to hospice services (all levels of care).

In determining principal diagnosis, coding conventions in the ICD-10-CM, the Tabular List and Alphabetic Index take precedence over these official coding guidelines. *(See Section I.A., Conventions for the ICD-10-CM)*

The importance of consistent, complete documentation in the medical record cannot be overemphasized. Without such documentation the application of all coding guidelines is a difficult, if not impossible, task.

A. Codes for symptoms, signs, and ill-defined conditions

Codes for symptoms, signs, and ill-defined conditions from Chapter 18 are not to be used as principal diagnosis when a related definitive diagnosis has been established.

B. Two or more interrelated conditions, each potentially meeting the definition for principal diagnosis.

When there are two or more interrelated conditions (such as diseases in the same ICD-10-CM chapter or manifestations characteristically associated with a certain disease) potentially meeting the definition of principal diagnosis, either condition may be sequenced first, unless the circumstances of the admission, the therapy provided, the Tabular List, or the Alphabetic Index indicate otherwise.

C. Two or more diagnoses that equally meet the definition for principal diagnosis

In the unusual instance when two or more diagnoses equally meet the criteria for principal diagnosis as determined by the circumstances of admission, diagnostic workup and/or therapy provided, and the Alphabetic Index, Tabular List, or another coding guidelines does not provide sequencing direction, any one of the diagnoses may be sequenced first.

D. Two or more comparative or contrasting conditions

In those rare instances when two or more contrasting or comparative diagnoses are documented as "either/or" (or similar terminology), they are coded as if the diagnoses were confirmed and the diagnoses are sequenced according to the circumstances of the admission. If no further determination can be made as to which diagnosis should be principal, either diagnosis may be sequenced first.

E. A symptom(s) followed by contrasting/comparative diagnoses

GUIDELINE HAS BEEN DELETED EFFECTIVE OCTOBER 1, 2014

F. Original treatment plan not carried out

Sequence as the principal diagnosis the condition, which after study occasioned the admission to the hospital, even though treatment may not have been carried out due to unforeseen circumstances.

G. Complications of surgery and other medical care

When the admission is for treatment of a complication resulting from surgery or other medical care, the complication code is sequenced as the principal diagnosis. If the complication is classified to the T80-T88 series and the code lacks the necessary specificity in describing the complication, an additional code for the specific complication should be assigned.

H. Uncertain Diagnosis

If the diagnosis documented at the time of discharge is qualified as "probable," "suspected," "likely," "questionable," "possible," or "still to be ruled out," "compatible with," "consistent with," or other similar terms indicating uncertainty, code the condition as if it existed or was established. The bases for these guidelines are the diagnostic workup, arrangements for further workup or observation, and initial therapeutic approach that correspond most closely with the established diagnosis.

Note: This guideline is applicable only to inpatient admissions to short-term, acute, long-term care and psychiatric hospitals.

I. Admission from Observation Unit

1. Admission Following Medical Observation

When a patient is admitted to an observation unit for a medical condition, which either worsens or does not improve, and is subsequently admitted as an inpatient of the same hospital for this same medical condition, the principal diagnosis would be the medical condition which led to the hospital admission.

2. Admission Following Post-Operative Observation

When a patient is admitted to an observation unit to monitor a condition (or complication) that develops following outpatient surgery, and then is subsequently admitted as an inpatient of the same hospital, hospitals should apply the Uniform Hospital Discharge Data Set (UHDDS) definition of principal diagnosis as "that condition established after study to be chiefly responsible for occasioning the admission of the patient to the hospital for care."

J. Admission from Outpatient Surgery

When a patient receives surgery in the hospital's outpatient surgery department and is subsequently admitted for continuing inpatient care at the same hospital, the following guidelines should be followed in selecting the principal diagnosis for the inpatient admission:

- If the reason for the inpatient admission is a complication, assign the complication as the principal diagnosis.
- If no complication, or other condition, is documented as the reason for the inpatient admission, assign the reason for the outpatient surgery as the principal diagnosis.
- If the reason for the inpatient admission is another condition unrelated to the surgery, assign the unrelated condition as the principal diagnosis.

K. Admissions/Encounters for Rehabilitation

When the purpose for the admission/encounter is rehabilitation, sequence first the code for the condition for which the service is being performed. For example, for an admission/encounter for rehabilitation for right-sided dominant hemiplegia following a cerebrovascular infarction, report code I69.351, Hemiplegia and hemiparesis following cerebral infarction affecting right dominant side, as the first-listed or principal diagnosis.

If the condition for which the rehabilitation service is being provided is no longer present, report the appropriate aftercare code as the first-listed or principal diagnosis, unless the rehabilitation service is being provided following an injury.

For rehabilitation services following active treatment of an injury, assign the injury code with the appropriate seventh character for subsequent encounter as the first-listed or principal diagnosis. For example, if a patient with severe degenerative osteoarthritis of the hip, underwent hip replacement and the current encounter/admission is for rehabilitation, report code Z47.1, Aftercare following joint replacement surgery, as the first-listed or principal diagnosis. If the patient requires rehabilitation post hip replacement for right intertrochanteric femur fracture, report code S72.141D, Displaced intertrochanteric fracture of right femur, subsequent encounter for closed fracture with routine healing, as the first-listed or principal diagnosis.

See Section I.C.21.c.7., Factors influencing health states and contact with health services, Aftercare.

See Section I.C.19.a., for additional information about the use of 7th characters for injury codes.

Section III. Reporting Additional Diagnoses

GENERAL RULES FOR OTHER (ADDITIONAL) DIAGNOSES

For reporting purposes, the definition for "other diagnoses" is interpreted as additional clinically significant conditions that affect patient care in terms of requiring:

    clinical evaluation; or

    therapeutic treatment; or

    diagnostic procedures; or

    extended length of hospital stay; or

    increased nursing care and/or monitoring.

The UHDDS item #11-b defines Other Diagnoses as "all conditions that coexist at the time of admission, that develop subsequently, or that affect the treatment received and/or the length of stay. Diagnoses that relate to an earlier episode which have no bearing on the current hospital stay are to be excluded." UHDDS definitions apply to inpatients in acute care, short-term, long term care and psychiatric hospital setting.

The UHDDS definitions are used by acute care short-term hospitals to report inpatient data elements in a standardized manner. These data elements and their definitions can be found in the July 31, 1985, Federal Register (Vol. 50, No, 147), pp. 31038-40. Since that time, the application of the UHDDS definitions has been expanded to include all non-outpatient settings (acute care, short term, long term care and psychiatric hospitals; home health agencies; rehab facilities; nursing homes, etc.). The UHDDS definitions also apply to hospice services (all levels of care).

The following guidelines are to be applied in designating "other diagnoses" when neither the Alphabetic Index nor the Tabular List in ICD-10-CM provide direction. The listing of the diagnoses in the patient record is the responsibility of the provider.

A. Previous conditions

If the provider has included a diagnosis in the final diagnostic statement, such as the discharge summary or the face sheet, it should ordinarily be coded. Some providers include in the diagnostic statement resolved conditions or diagnoses and status-post procedures from previous admissions that have no bearing on the current stay. Such conditions are not to be reported and are coded only if required by hospital policy.

However, history codes (categories Z80-Z87) may be used as secondary codes if the historical condition or family history has an impact on current care or influences treatment.

B. Abnormal findings

Abnormal findings (laboratory, x-ray, pathologic, and other diagnostic results) are not coded and reported unless the provider indicates their clinical significance. If the findings are outside the normal range and the provider has ordered other tests to evaluate the condition or prescribed treatment, it is appropriate to ask the provider whether the abnormal finding should be added.

Please note: This differs from the coding practices in the outpatient setting for coding encounters for diagnostic tests that have been interpreted by a provider.

C. Uncertain Diagnosis

If the diagnosis documented at the time of discharge is qualified as "probable," "suspected," "likely," "questionable," "possible," or "still to be ruled out," "compatible with," "consistent with," or other similar terms indicating uncertainty, code the condition as if it existed or was established. The bases for these guidelines are the diagnostic workup, arrangements for further workup or observation, and initial therapeutic approach that correspond most closely with the established diagnosis.

Note: This guideline is applicable only to inpatient admissions to short-term, acute, long-term care and psychiatric hospitals.

Section IV. Diagnostic Coding and Reporting Guidelines for Outpatient Services

These coding guidelines for outpatient diagnoses have been approved for use by hospitals/ providers in coding and reporting hospital-based outpatient services and provider-based office visits. Guidelines in Section I, Conventions, general coding guidelines and chapter-specific guidelines, should also be applied for outpatient services and office visits.

Information about the use of certain abbreviations, punctuation, symbols, and other conventions used in the ICD-10-CM Tabular List (code numbers and titles), can be found in Section IA of these guidelines, under "Conventions Used in the Tabular List." Section I.B. contains general guidelines that apply to the entire classification. Section I.C. contains chapter-specific guidelines that correspond to the chapters as they are arranged in the classification. Information about the correct sequence to use in finding a code is also described in Section I.

The terms encounter and visit are often used interchangeably in describing outpatient service contacts and, therefore, appear together in these guidelines without distinguishing one from the other.

Though the conventions and general guidelines apply to all settings, coding guidelines for outpatient and provider reporting of diagnoses will vary in a number of instances from those for inpatient diagnoses, recognizing that:

The Uniform Hospital Discharge Data Set (UHDDS) definition of principal diagnosis does not apply to hospital-based outpatient services and provider-based office visits. Coding guidelines for inconclusive diagnoses (probable, suspected, rule out, etc.) were developed for inpatient reporting and do not apply to outpatients.

A. Selection of first-listed condition

In the outpatient setting, the term first-listed diagnosis is used in lieu of principal diagnosis.

In determining the first-listed diagnosis the coding conventions of ICD-10-CM, as well as the general and disease specific guidelines take precedence over the outpatient guidelines.

Diagnoses often are not established at the time of the initial encounter/visit. It may take two or more visits before the diagnosis is confirmed.

The most critical rule involves beginning the search for the correct code assignment through the Alphabetic Index. Never begin searching initially in the Tabular List as this will lead to coding errors.

1. Outpatient Surgery

When a patient presents for outpatient surgery (same day surgery), code the reason for the surgery as the first-listed diagnosis (reason for the encounter), even if the surgery is not performed due to a contraindication.

2. Observation Stay

When a patient is admitted for observation for a medical condition, assign a code for the medical condition as the first-listed diagnosis.

When a patient presents for outpatient surgery and develops complications requiring admission to observation, code the reason for the surgery as the first reported diagnosis (reason for the encounter), followed by codes for the complications as secondary diagnoses.

B. Codes from A00.0 through T88.9, Z00-Z99, U00-U85

The appropriate code(s) from A00.0 through T88.9, Z00-Z99 and U00-U85 must be used to identify diagnoses, symptoms, conditions, problems, complaints, or other reason(s) for the encounter/visit.

C. Accurate reporting of ICD-10-CM diagnosis codes

For accurate reporting of ICD-10-CM diagnosis codes, the documentation should describe the patient's condition, using terminology which includes specific diagnoses as well as symptoms, problems, or reasons for the encounter. There are ICD-10-CM codes to describe all of these.

D. Codes that describe symptoms and signs

Codes that describe symptoms and signs, as opposed to diagnoses, are acceptable for reporting purposes when a diagnosis has not been established (confirmed) by the provider. Chapter 18 of ICD-10-CM, Symptoms, Signs, and Abnormal Clinical and Laboratory Findings Not Elsewhere Classified (codes R00-R99) contain many, but not all codes for symptoms.

E. Encounters for circumstances other than a disease or injury

ICD-10-CM provides codes to deal with encounters for circumstances other than a disease or injury. The Factors Influencing Health Status and Contact with Health Services codes (Z00-Z99) are provided to deal with occasions when circumstances other than a disease or injury are recorded as diagnosis or problems.

See Section I.C.21. Factors influencing health status and contact with health services.

F. Level of Detail in Coding

1. ICD-10-CM codes with 3, 4, 5, 6 or 7 characters

ICD-10-CM is composed of codes with 3, 4, 5, 6 or 7 characters. Codes with three characters are included in ICD-10-CM as the heading of a category of codes that may be further subdivided by the use of fourth, fifth, sixth or seventh characters to provide greater specificity.

2. Use of full number of characters required for a code

A three-character code is to be used only if it is not further subdivided. A code is invalid if it has not been coded to the full number of characters required for that code, including the 7th character, if applicable.

3. Highest level of specificity

Code to the highest level of specificity when supported by the medical record documentation.

G. ICD-10-CM code for the diagnosis, condition, problem, or other reason for encounter/visit

List first the ICD-10-CM code for the diagnosis, condition, problem, or other reason for encounter/visit shown in the medical record to be chiefly responsible for the services provided. List additional codes that describe any coexisting conditions. In some cases, the first-listed diagnosis may be a symptom when a diagnosis has not been established (confirmed) by the provider.

H. Uncertain diagnosis

Do not code diagnoses documented as "probable", "suspected," "questionable," "rule out," "compatible with," "consistent with," or "working diagnosis" or other similar terms indicating uncertainty. Rather, code the condition(s) to the highest degree of certainty for that encounter/visit, such as symptoms, signs, abnormal test results, or other reason for the visit.

Please note: This differs from the coding practices used by short-term, acute care, long-term care and psychiatric hospitals.

I. Chronic diseases

Chronic diseases treated on an ongoing basis may be coded and reported as many times as the patient receives treatment and care for the condition(s)

J. Code all documented conditions that coexist

Code all documented conditions that coexist at the time of the encounter/visit and that require or affect patient care, treatment or management. Do not code conditions that were previously treated and no longer exist. However, history codes (categories Z80-Z87) may be used as secondary codes if the historical condition or family history has an impact on current care or influences treatment.

K. Patients receiving diagnostic services only

For patients receiving diagnostic services only during an encounter/visit, sequence first the diagnosis, condition, problem, or other reason for encounter/visit shown in the medical record to be chiefly responsible for the outpatient services provided during the encounter/visit. Codes for other diagnoses (e.g., chronic conditions) may be sequenced as additional diagnoses. For encounters for routine laboratory/radiology testing in the absence of any signs, symptoms, or associated diagnosis, assign Z01.89, Encounter for other specified special examinations. If routine testing is performed during the same encounter as a test to evaluate a sign, symptom, or diagnosis, it is appropriate to assign both the Z code and the code describing the reason for the non-routine test.

For outpatient encounters for diagnostic tests that have been interpreted by a physician, and the final report is available at the time of coding, code any confirmed or definitive diagnosis(es) documented in the interpretation. Do not code related signs and symptoms as additional diagnoses.

Please note: This differs from the coding practice in the hospital inpatient setting regarding abnormal findings on test results.

L. Patients receiving therapeutic services only

For patients receiving therapeutic services only during an encounter/visit, sequence first the diagnosis, condition, problem, or other reason for encounter/visit shown in the medical record to be chiefly responsible for the outpatient services provided during the encounter/visit. Codes for other diagnoses (e.g., chronic conditions) may be sequenced as additional diagnoses. The only exception to this rule is that when the primary reason for the admission/encounter is chemotherapy or radiation therapy, the appropriate Z code for the service is listed first, and the diagnosis or problem for which the service is being performed listed second.

M. Patients receiving preoperative evaluations only

For patients receiving preoperative evaluations only, sequence first a code from subcategory Z01.81, Encounter for pre-procedural examinations, to describe the pre-op consultations. Assign a code for the condition to describe the reason for the surgery as an additional diagnosis. Code also any findings related to the pre-op evaluation.

N. Ambulatory surgery

For ambulatory surgery, code the diagnosis for which the surgery was performed. If the postoperative diagnosis is known to be different from the preoperative diagnosis at the time the diagnosis is confirmed, select the postoperative diagnosis for coding, since it is the most definitive.

O. Routine outpatient prenatal visits

See Section I.C.15. Routine outpatient prenatal visits.

P. Encounters for general medical examinations with abnormal findings

The subcategories for encounters for general medical examinations, Z00.0- and encounter for routine child health examination, Z00.12-, provide codes for with and without abnormal findings. Should a general medical examination result in an abnormal finding, the code for general medical examination with abnormal finding should be assigned as the first-listed diagnosis. An examination with abnormal findings refers to a condition/diagnosis that is newly identified or a change in severity of a chronic condition (such as uncontrolled hypertension, or an acute exacerbation of chronic obstructive pulmonary disease) during a routine physical examination. A secondary code for the abnormal finding should also be coded.

Q. Encounters for routine health screenings

See Section I.C.21. Factors influencing health status and contact with health services, Screening

Appendix I. Present on Admission Reporting Guidelines

Introduction

These guidelines are to be used as a supplement to the *ICD-10-CM Official Guidelines for Coding and Reporting* to facilitate the assignment of the Present on Admission (POA) indicator for each diagnosis and external cause of injury code reported on claim forms (UB-04 and 837 Institutional).

These guidelines are not intended to replace any guidelines in the main body of the *ICD-10-CM Official Guidelines for Coding and Reporting*. The POA guidelines are not intended to provide guidance on when a condition should be coded, but rather, how to apply the POA indicator to the final set of diagnosis codes that have been assigned in accordance with Sections I, II, and III of the official coding guidelines. Subsequent to the assignment of the ICD-10-CM codes, the POA indicator should then be assigned to those conditions that have been coded.

As stated in the Introduction to the *ICD-10-CM Official Guidelines for Coding and Reporting*, a joint effort between the healthcare provider and the coder is essential to achieve complete and accurate documentation, code assignment, and reporting of diagnoses and procedures. The importance of consistent, complete documentation in the medical record cannot be overemphasized. Medical record documentation from any provider involved in the care and treatment of the patient may be used to support the determination of whether a condition was present on admission or not. In the context of the official coding guidelines, the term "provider" means a physician or any qualified healthcare practitioner who is legally accountable for establishing the patient's diagnosis.

These guidelines are not a substitute for the provider's clinical judgment as to the determination of whether a condition was/was not present on admission. The provider should be queried regarding issues related to the linking of signs/symptoms, timing of test results, and the timing of findings.

Please see the CDC website for the detailed list of ICD-10-CM codes that do not require the use of a POA indicator **(https://www.cdc.gov/nchs/icd/icd-10-cm/files.html)**. The codes and categories on this exempt list are for circumstances regarding the healthcare encounter or factors influencing health status that do not represent a current disease or injury or that describe conditions that are always present on admission.

General Reporting Requirements

All claims involving inpatient admissions to general acute care hospitals or other facilities that are subject to a law or regulation mandating collection of present on admission information.

Present on admission is defined as present at the time the order for inpatient admission occurs -- conditions that develop during an outpatient encounter, including emergency department, observation, or outpatient surgery, are considered as present on admission.

POA indicator is assigned to principal and secondary diagnoses (as defined in Section II of the Official Guidelines for Coding and Reporting) and the external cause of injury codes.

Issues related to inconsistent, missing, conflicting or unclear documentation must still be resolved by the provider.

If a condition would not be coded and reported based on UHDDS definitions and current official coding guidelines, then the POA indicator would not be reported.

> Reporting Options
> > Y – Yes
> > N – No
> > U – Unknown
> > W – Clinically undetermined
> > Unreported/Not used – (Exempt from POA reporting)
> Reporting Definitions
> > Y = present at the time of inpatient admission
> > N = not present at the time of inpatient admission
> > U = documentation is insufficient to determine if condition is present on admission
> > W = provider is unable to clinically determine whether condition was present on admission or not

Timeframe for POA Identification and Documentation

There is no required timeframe as to when a provider (per the definition of "provider" used in these guidelines) must identify or document a condition to be present on admission. In some clinical situations, it may not be possible for a provider to make a definitive diagnosis (or a condition may not be recognized or reported by the patient) for a period of time after admission. In some cases, it may be several days before the provider arrives at a definitive diagnosis. This does not mean that the condition was not present on admission. Determination of whether the condition was present on admission or not will be based on the applicable POA guideline as identified in this document, or on the provider's best clinical judgment.

If at the time of code assignment the documentation is unclear as to whether a condition was present on admission or not, it is appropriate to query the provider for clarification.

Assigning the POA Indicator

Condition is on the "Exempt from Reporting" list
> Leave the "present on admission" field blank if the condition is on the list of ICD-10-CM codes for which this field is not applicable. This is the only circumstance in which the field may be left blank.

POA Explicitly Documented
> Assign Y for any condition the provider explicitly documents as being present on admission.
> Assign N for any condition the provider explicitly documents as not present at the time of admission.

Conditions diagnosed prior to inpatient admission
> Assign "Y" for conditions that were diagnosed prior to admission (example: hypertension, diabetes mellitus, asthma)

Conditions diagnosed during the admission but clearly present before admission
> Assign "Y" for conditions diagnosed during the admission that were clearly present but not diagnosed until after admission occurred.
> Diagnoses subsequently confirmed after admission are considered present on admission if at the time of admission they are documented as suspected, possible, rule out, differential diagnosis, or constitute an underlying cause of a symptom that is present at the time of admission.

Condition develops during outpatient encounter prior to inpatient admission
> Assign Y for any condition that develops during an outpatient encounter prior to a written order for inpatient admission.

Documentation does not indicate whether condition was present on admission
> Assign "U" when the medical record documentation is unclear as to whether the condition was present on admission. "U" should not be routinely assigned and used only in very limited circumstances. Coders are encouraged to query the providers when the documentation is unclear.

Documentation states that it cannot be determined whether the condition was or was not present on admission

> Assign "W" when the medical record documentation indicates that it cannot be clinically determined whether or not the condition was present on admission.

Chronic condition with acute exacerbation during the admission
> If a single code identifies both the chronic condition and the acute exacerbation, see POA guidelines pertaining to codes that contain multiple clinical concepts.
> If a single code only identifies the chronic condition and not the acute exacerbation (e.g., acute exacerbation of chronic leukemia), assign "Y."

Conditions documented as possible, probable, suspected, or rule out at the time of discharge
> If the final diagnosis contains a possible, probable, suspected, or rule out diagnosis, and this diagnosis was based on signs, symptoms or clinical findings suspected at the time of inpatient admission, assign "Y."
> If the final diagnosis contains a possible, probable, suspected, or rule out diagnosis, and this diagnosis was based on signs, symptoms or clinical findings that were not present on admission, assign "N".

Conditions documented as impending or threatened at the time of discharge
> If the final diagnosis contains an impending or threatened diagnosis, and this diagnosis is based on symptoms or clinical findings that were present on admission, assign "Y".
> If the final diagnosis contains an impending or threatened diagnosis, and this diagnosis is based on symptoms or clinical findings that were not present on admission, assign "N".

Acute and Chronic Conditions
> Assign "Y" for acute conditions that are present at time of admission and N for acute conditions that are not present at time of admission.
> Assign "Y" for chronic conditions, even though the condition may not be diagnosed until after admission.
> If a single code identifies both an acute and chronic condition, see the POA guidelines for codes that contain multiple clinical concepts.

Codes That Contain Multiple Clinical Concepts
> Assign "N" if at least one of the clinical concepts included in the code was not present on admission (e.g., COPD with acute exacerbation, the exacerbation was not present on admission; gastric ulcer that does not start bleeding until after admission; asthma patient develops status asthmaticus after admission).
> Assign "Y" if all of the clinical concepts included in the code were present on admission (e.g., duodenal ulcer that perforates prior to admission).
> For infection codes that include the causal organism, assign "Y" if the infection (or signs of the infection) were present on admission, even though the culture results may not be known until after admission (e.g., patient is admitted with pneumonia and the provider documents Pseudomonas as the causal organism a few days later).

Same Diagnosis Code for Two or More Conditions
> When the same ICD-10-CM diagnosis code applies to two or more conditions during the same encounter (e.g. two separate conditions classified to the same ICD-10-CM diagnosis code):
> Assign "Y" if all conditions represented by the single ICD-10-CM code were present on admission (e.g. bilateral unspecified age-related cataracts).
> Assign "N" if any of the conditions represented by the single ICD-10-CM code was not present on admission (e.g. traumatic secondary and recurrent hemorrhage and seroma is assigned to a single code T79.2, but only one of the conditions was present on admission).

Obstetrical conditions
> Whether or not the patient delivers during the current hospitalization does not affect assignment of the POA indicator. The determining factor for POA assignment is whether the pregnancy complication or obstetrical condition described by the code was present at the time of admission or not.
> If the pregnancy complication or obstetrical condition was present on admission (e.g., patient admitted in preterm labor), assign "Y".
> If the pregnancy complication or obstetrical condition was not present on admission (e.g., 2nd degree laceration during delivery, postpartum hemorrhage that occurred during current hospitalization, fetal distress develops after admission), assign "N".
> If the obstetrical code includes more than one diagnosis and any of the diagnoses identified by the code were not present on admission assign "N". (e.g., Category O11, Pre-existing hypertension with pre-eclampsia)

Perinatal conditions
> Newborns are not considered to be admitted until after birth. Therefore, any condition present at birth or that developed in utero is considered present at admission and should be assigned "Y". This includes conditions that occur during delivery (e.g., injury during delivery, meconium aspiration, exposure to streptococcus B in the vaginal canal).

Congenital conditions and anomalies
> Assign "Y" for congenital conditions and anomalies except for categories Q00-Q99, Congenital anomalies, which are on the exempt list. Congenital conditions are always considered present on admission.

External cause of injury codes
> Assign "Y" for any external cause code representing an external cause of morbidity that occurred prior to inpatient admission (e.g., patient fell out of bed at home, patient fell out of bed in emergency room prior to admission)
> Assign "N" for any external cause code representing an external cause of morbidity that occurred during inpatient hospitalization (e.g., patient fell out of hospital bed during hospital stay, patient experienced an adverse reaction to a medication administered after inpatient admission).

A

Aarskog's syndrome Q87.19
Abandonment — *see* Maltreatment
Abasia (-astasia) (hysterical) F44.4
Abderhalden-Kaufmann-Lignac syndrome (cystinosis) E72.04
Abdomen, abdominal — *see also* condition
  acute R10.0
  angina K55.1
  muscle deficiency syndrome Q79.4
Abdominalgia — *see* Pain, abdominal
Abduction contracture, hip or other joint — *see* Contraction, joint
Aberrant (congenital) — *see also* Malposition, congenital
  adrenal gland Q89.1
  artery (peripheral) Q27.8
    basilar NEC Q28.1
    cerebral Q28.3
    coronary Q24.5
    digestive system Q27.8
    eye Q15.8
    lower limb Q27.8
    precerebral Q28.1
    pulmonary Q25.79
    renal Q27.2
    retina Q14.1
    specified site NEC Q27.8
    subclavian Q27.8
    upper limb Q27.8
    vertebral Q28.1
  breast Q83.8
  endocrine gland NEC Q89.2
  hepatic duct Q44.5
  pancreas Q45.3
  parathyroid gland Q89.2
  pituitary gland Q89.2
  sebaceous glands, mucous membrane, mouth, congenital Q38.6
  spleen Q89.09
  subclavian artery Q27.8
  thymus (gland) Q89.2
  thyroid gland Q89.2
  vein (peripheral) NEC Q27.8
    cerebral Q28.3
    digestive system Q27.8
    lower limb Q27.8
    precerebral Q28.1
    specified site NEC Q27.8
    upper limb Q27.8
Aberration
  distantial — *see* Disturbance, visual
  mental F99
Abetalipoproteinemia E78.6
Abiotrophy R68.89
Ablatio, ablation
  retinae — *see* Detachment, retina
Ablepharia, ablepharon Q10.3
Abnormal, abnormality, abnormalities — *see also* Anomaly
  acid-base balance (mixed) E87.4
  albumin R77.0
  alphafetoprotein R77.2
  alveolar ridge K08.9
  anatomical relationship Q89.9
  apertures, congenital, diaphragm Q79.1
  atrial septal, specified NEC Q21.19
  auditory perception H93.29- ☑
    diplacusis — *see* Diplacusis
    hyperacusis — *see* Hyperacusis
    recruitment — *see* Recruitment, auditory
    threshold shift — *see* Shift, auditory threshold
  autosomes Q99.9
    fragile site Q95.5
  basal metabolic rate R94.8
  biosynthesis, testicular androgen E29.1
  bleeding time R79.1
  blood amino-acid level R79.83
  blood level (of)
    cobalt R79.0
    copper R79.0
    iron R79.0

Abnormal, abnormality, abnormalities — *continued*
  blood level — *continued*
    lithium R78.89
    magnesium R79.0
    mineral NEC R79.0
    zinc R79.0
  blood pressure
    elevated R03.0
    low reading (nonspecific) R03.1
  blood sugar R73.09
  blood-gas level R79.81
  bowel sounds R19.15
    absent R19.11
    hyperactive R19.12
  brain scan R94.02
  breathing R06.9
  caloric test R94.138
  cerebrospinal fluid R83.9
    cytology R83.6
    drug level R83.2
    enzyme level R83.0
    hormones R83.1
    immunology R83.4
    microbiology R83.5
    nonmedicinal level R83.3
    specified type NEC R83.8
  chemistry, blood R79.9
    C-reactive protein R79.82
    drugs — *see* Findings, abnormal, in blood
    gas level R79.81
    minerals R79.0
    pancytopenia D61.818
    PTT R79.1
    specified NEC R79.89
    toxins — *see* Findings, abnormal, in blood
  chest sounds (friction) (rales) R09.89
  chromosome, chromosomal Q99.9
    with more than three X chromosomes, female Q97.1
    analysis result R89.8
      bronchial washings R84.8
      cerebrospinal fluid R83.8
      cervix uteri NEC R87.89
      nasal secretions R84.8
      nipple discharge R89.8
      peritoneal fluid R85.89
      pleural fluid R84.8
      prostatic secretions R86.8
      saliva R85.89
      seminal fluid R86.8
      sputum R84.8
      synovial fluid R89.8
      throat scrapings R84.8
      vagina R87.89
      vulva R87.89
      wound secretions R89.8
    dicentric replacement Q93.2
    ring replacement Q93.2
    sex Q99.8
      female phenotype Q97.9
        specified NEC Q97.8
      male phenotype Q98.9
        specified NEC Q98.8
      structural male Q98.6
    specified NEC Q99.8
  clinical findings NEC R68.89
  coagulation D68.9
    newborn, transient P61.6
    profile R79.1
    time R79.1
  communication — *see* Fistula
  conjunctiva, vascular H11.41- ☑
  coronary artery Q24.5
  cortisol-binding globulin E27.8
  course, eustachian tube Q17.8
  creatinine clearance R94.4
  cytology
    anus R85.619
      atypical squamous cells cannot exclude high grade squamous intraepithelial lesion (ASC-H) R85.611
      atypical squamous cells of undetermined significance (ASC-US) R85.610
      cytologic evidence of malignancy R85.614

Abnormal, abnormality, abnormalities — *continued*
  cytology — *continued*
    anus — *continued*
      high grade squamous intraepithelial lesion (HGSIL) R85.613
      human papillomavirus (HPV) DNA test
        high risk positive R85.81
        low risk postive R85.82
      inadequate smear R85.615
      low grade squamous intraepithelial lesion (LGSIL) R85.612
      satisfactory anal smear but lacking transformation zone R85.616
      specified NEC R85.618
      unsatisfactory smear R85.615
    female genital organs — *see* Abnormal, Papanicolaou (smear)
  dark adaptation curve H53.61
  dentofacial NEC — *see* Anomaly, dentofacial
  development, developmental Q89.9
    central nervous system Q07.9
  diagnostic imaging
    abdomen, abdominal region NEC R93.5
    biliary tract R93.2
    bladder R93.41
    breast R92.8
    central nervous system NEC R90.89
    cerebrovascular NEC R90.89
    coronary circulation R93.1
    digestive tract NEC R93.3
    gastrointestinal (tract) R93.3
    genitourinary organs R93.89
    head R93.0
    heart R93.1
    intrathoracic organ NEC R93.89
    kidney R93.42- ☑
    limbs R93.6
    liver R93.2
    lung (field) R91.8
    musculoskeletal system NEC R93.7
    renal pelvis R93.41
    retroperitoneum R93.5
    site specified NEC R93.89
    skin and subcutaneous tissue R93.89
    skull R93.0
    testis R93.81- ☑
    ureter R93.41
    urinary organs specified NEC R93.49
  direction, teeth, fully erupted M26.30
  ear ossicles, acquired NEC H74.39- ☑
    ankylosis — *see* Ankylosis, ear ossicles
    discontinuity — *see* Discontinuity, ossicles, ear
    partial loss — *see* Loss, ossicles, ear (partial)
  Ebstein Q22.5
  echocardiogram R93.1
  echoencephalogram R90.81
  echogram — *see* Abnormal, diagnostic imaging
  electrocardiogram [ECG] [EKG] R94.31
  electroencephalogram [EEG] R94.01
  electrolyte — *see* Imbalance, electrolyte
  electromyogram [EMG] R94.131
  electro-oculogram [EOG] R94.110
  electrophysiological intracardiac studies R94.39
  electroretinogram [ERG] R94.111
  erythrocytes
    congenital, with perinatal jaundice D58.9
  feces (color) (contents) (mucus) R19.5
  finding — *see* Findings, abnormal, without diagnosis
  fluid
    amniotic — *see* Abnormal, specimen, specified
    cerebrospinal — *see* Abnormal, cerebrospinal fluid
    peritoneal — *see* Abnormal, specimen, digestive organs
    pleural — *see* Abnormal, specimen, respiratory organs
    synovial — *see* Abnormal, specimen, specified
    thorax (bronchial washings) (pleural fluid) — *see* Abnormal, specimen, respiratory organs
    vaginal — *see* Abnormal, specimen, female genital organs
  form
    teeth K00.2
    uterus — *see* Anomaly, uterus

Abnormal, abnormality, abnormalities — *continued*
function studies
auditory R94.120
bladder R94.8
brain R94.09
cardiovascular R94.30
ear R94.128
endocrine NEC R94.7
eye NEC R94.118
kidney R94.4
liver R94.5
nervous system
central NEC R94.09
peripheral NEC R94.138
pancreas R94.8
placenta R94.8
pulmonary R94.2
special senses NEC R94.128
spleen R94.8
thyroid R94.6
vestibular R94.121
gait — *see* Gait
hysterical F44.4
gastrin secretion E16.4
globulin R77.1
cortisol-binding E27.8
thyroid-binding E07.89
glomerular, minor — *see also* N00-N07 with fourth
character .0 N05.0
glucagon secretion E16.3
glucose tolerance (test) (non-fasting) R73.09
gravitational (G) forces or states (effect of) T75.81 ☑
hair (color) (shaft) L67.9
specified NEC L67.8
hard tissue formation in pulp (dental) K04.3
head movement R25.0
heart
rate R00.9
specified NEC R00.8
shadow R93.1
sounds NEC R01.2
hemoglobin (disease) — *see also* Disease, hemoglobin
D58.2
trait — *see* Trait, hemoglobin, abnormal
histology NEC R89.7
immunological findings R89.4
in serum R76.9
specified NEC R76.8
increase in appetite R63.2
involuntary movement — *see* Abnormal, movement,
involuntary
jaw closure M26.51
karyotype R89.8
kidney function test R94.4
knee jerk R29.2
leukocyte (cell) (differential) NEC D72.9
liver function test — *see also* Elevated, liver function, test
R79.89
loss of
height R29.890
weight R63.4
mammogram NEC R92.8
calcification (calculus) R92.1
microcalcification R92.0
Mantoux test R76.11
movement (disorder) — *see also* Disorder, movement
head R25.0
involuntary R25.9
fasciculation R25.3
of head R25.0
spasm R25.2
specified type NEC R25.8
tremor R25.1
myoglobin (Aberdeen) (Annapolis) R89.7
neonatal screening P09.9
for
congenital adrenal hyperplasia P09.2
congenital endocrine disease P09.2
congenital hematologic disorders P09.3
critical congenital heart disease P09.5
cystic fibrosis P09.4
hemoglobinopathy P09.3
hypothyroidism P09.2
inborn errors of metabolism P09.1
neonatal hearing loss P09.6
red cell membrane defects P09.3
sickle cell P09.3
specified NEC P09.8
oculomotor study R94.113

Abnormal, abnormality, abnormalities — *continued*
palmar creases Q82.8
Papanicolaou (smear)
anus R85.619
atypical squamous cells cannot exclude high grade
squamous intraepithelial lesion (ASC-H)
R85.611
atypical squamous cells of undetermined significance (ASC-US) R85.610
cytologic evidence of malignancy R85.614
high grade squamous intraepithelial lesion (HGSIL)
R85.613
human papillomavirus (HPV) DNA test
high risk positive R85.81
low risk postive R85.82
inadequate smear R85.615
low grade squamous intraepithelial lesion (LGSIL)
R85.612
satisfactory anal smear but lacking transformation
zone R85.616
specified NEC R85.618
unsatisfactory smear R85.615
bronchial washings R84.6
cerebrospinal fluid R83.6
cervix R87.619
atypical squamous cells cannot exclude high grade
squamous intraepithelial lesion (ASC-H)
R87.611
atypical squamous cells of undetermined significance (ASC-US) R87.610
cytologic evidence of malignancy R87.614
high grade squamous intraepithelial lesion (HGSIL)
R87.613
inadequate smear R87.615
low grade squamous intraepithelial lesion (LGSIL)
R87.612
non-atypical endometrial cells R87.618
satisfactory cervical smear but lacking transformation zone R87.616
specified NEC R87.618
thin preparaton R87.619
unsatisfactory smear R87.615
nasal secretions R84.6
nipple discharge R89.6
peritoneal fluid R85.69
pleural fluid R84.6
prostatic secretions R86.6
saliva R85.69
seminal fluid R86.6
sites NEC R89.6
sputum R84.6
synovial fluid R89.6
throat scrapings R84.6
vagina R87.629
atypical squamous cells cannot exclude high grade
squamous intraepithelial lesion (ASC-H)
R87.621
atypical squamous cells of undetermined significance (ASC-US) R87.620
cytologic evidence of malignancy R87.624
high grade squamous intraepithelial lesion (HGSIL)
R87.623
inadequate smear R87.625
low grade squamous intraepithelial lesion (LGSIL)
R87.622
specified NEC R87.628
thin preparation R87.629
unsatisfactory smear R87.625
vulva R87.69
wound secretions R89.6
partial thromboplastin time (PTT) R79.1
pelvis (bony) — *see* Deformity, pelvis
percussion, chest (tympany) R09.89
periods (grossly) — *see* Menstruation
phonocardiogram R94.39
plantar reflex R29.2
plasma
protein R77.9
specified NEC R77.8
viscosity R70.1
pleural (folds) Q34.0
posture R29.3
product of conception O02.9
specified type NEC O02.89
prothrombin time (PT) R79.1
pulmonary
artery, congenital Q25.79
function, newborn P28.89
test results R94.2

Abnormal, abnormality, abnormalities — *continued*
pulsations in neck R00.2
pupillary H21.56- ☑
function (reaction) (reflex) — *see* Anomaly, pupil,
function
radiological examination — *see* Abnormal, diagnostic
imaging
red blood cell(s) (morphology) (volume) R71.8
reflex — *see* Reflex
renal function test R94.4
response to nerve stimulation R94.130
retinal correspondence H53.31
retinal function study R94.111
rhythm, heart — *see also* Arrhythmia
saliva — *see* Abnormal, specimen, digestive organs
scan
kidney R94.4
liver R93.2
thyroid R94.6
secretion
gastrin E16.4
glucagon E16.3
semen, seminal fluid — *see* Abnormal, specimen, male
genital organs
serum level (of)
acid phosphatase R74.8
alkaline phosphatase R74.8
amylase R74.8
enzymes R74.9
specified NEC R74.8
lipase R74.8
triacylglycerol lipase R74.8
shape
gravid uterus — *see* Anomaly, uterus
sinus venosus Q21.16
size, tooth, teeth K00.2
spacing, tooth, teeth, fully erupted M26.30
specimen
digestive organs (peritoneal fluid) (saliva) R85.9
cytology R85.69
drug level R85.2
enzyme level R85.0
histology R85.7
hormones R85.1
immunology R85.4
microbiology R85.5
nonmedicinal level R85.3
specified type NEC R85.89
female genital organs (secretions) (smears) R87.9
cytology R87.69
cervix R87.619
human papillomavirus (HPV) DNA test
high risk positive R87.810
low risk positive R87.820
inadequate (unsatisfactory) smear R87.615
non-atypical endometrial cells R87.618
specified NEC R87.618
vagina R87.629
human papillomavirus (HPV) DNA test
high risk positive R87.811
low risk positive R87.821
inadequate (unsatisfactory) smear R87.625
vulva R87.69
drug level R87.2
enzyme level R87.0
histological R87.7
hormones R87.1
immunology R87.4
microbiology R87.5
nonmedicinal level R87.3
specified type NEC R87.89
male genital organs (prostatic secretions) (semen)
R86.9
cytology R86.6
drug level R86.2
enzyme level R86.0
histological R86.7
hormones R86.1
immunology R86.4
microbiology R86.5
nonmedicinal level R86.3
specified type NEC R86.8
nipple discharge — *see* Abnormal, specimen, specified
respiratory organs (bronchial washings) (nasal secretions) (pleural fluid) (sputum) R84.9
cytology R84.6
drug level R84.2
enzyme level R84.0
histology R84.7

☑ **Additional Character Required — Refer to the Tabular List for Character Selection**

Abnormal, abnormality, abnormalities — *continued*
  specimen — *continued*
    respiratory organs — *continued*
      hormones R84.1
      immunology R84.4
      microbiology R84.5
      nonmedicinal level R84.3
      specified type NEC R84.8
    specified organ, system and tissue NOS R89.9
      cytology R89.6
      drug level R89.2
      enzyme level R89.0
      histology R89.7
      hormones R89.1
      immunology R89.4
      microbiology R89.5
      nonmedicinal level R89.3
      specified type NEC R89.8
    synovial fluid — *see* Abnormal, specimen, specified
    thorax (bronchial washings) (pleural fluids) — *see*
        Abnormal, specimen, respiratory organs
    vagina (secretion) (smear) R87.629
    vulva (secretion) (smear) R87.69
    wound secretion — *see* Abnormal, specimen, specified
  spermatozoa — *see* Abnormal, specimen, male genital
      organs
  sputum (amount) (color) (odor) R09.3
  stool (color) (contents) (mucus) R19.5
    bloody K92.1
    guaiac positive R19.5
  synchondrosis Q78.8
  thermography — *see also* Abnormal, diagnostic imaging
      R93.89
  thyroid-binding globulin E07.89
  tooth, teeth (form) (size) K00.2
  toxicology (findings) R78.9
  transport protein E88.09
  tumor marker NEC R97.8
  ultrasound results — *see* Abnormal, diagnostic imaging
  umbilical cord complicating delivery O69.9 ☑
  urination NEC R39.198
  urine (constituents) R82.90
    bile R82.2
    cytological examination R82.89
    drugs R82.5
    fat R82.0
    glucose R81
    heavy metals R82.6
    hemoglobin R82.3
    histological examination R82.89
    ketones R82.4
    microbiological examination (culture) R82.79
    myoglobin R82.1
    positive culture R82.79
    protein — *see* Proteinuria
    specified substance NEC R82.998
      chromoabnormality NEC R82.91
    substances nonmedical R82.6
  uterine hemorrhage — *see* Hemorrhage, uterus
  vectorcardiogram R94.39
  visually evoked potential (VEP) R94.112
  white blood cells D72.9
    specified NEC D72.89
  X-ray examination — *see* Abnormal, diagnostic imaging
Abnormity (any organ or part) — *see* Anomaly
Abocclusion M26.29
  hemolytic disease (newborn) P55.1
  incompatibility reaction ABO — *see* Complication(s),
      transfusion, incompatibility reaction, ABO
Abolition, language R48.8
Aborter, habitual or recurrent — *see* Loss (of), pregnancy,
      recurrent
Abortion (complete) (spontaneous) O03.9
  with
    retained products of conception — *see* Abortion, in-
        complete
  attempted (elective) (failed) O07.4
    complicated by O07.30
      afibrinogenemia O07.1
      cardiac arrest O07.36
      chemical damage of pelvic organ(s) O07.34
      circulatory collapse O07.31
      cystitis O07.38
      defibrination syndrome O07.1
      electrolyte imbalance O07.33
      embolism (air) (amniotic fluid) (blood clot) (fat)
          (pulmonary) (septic) (soap) O07.2
      endometritis O07.0

Abortion — *continued*
  attempted — *continued*
    complicated by — *continued*
      genital tract and pelvic infection O07.0
      hemolysis O07.1
      hemorrhage (delayed) (excessive) O07.1
      infection
          genital tract or pelvic O07.0
          urinary tract tract O07.38
      intravascular coagulation O07.1
      laceration of pelvic organ(s) O07.34
      metabolic disorder O07.33
      oliguria O07.32
      oophoritis O07.0
      parametritis O07.0
      pelvic peritonitis O07.0
      perforation of pelvic organ(s) O07.34
      renal failure or shutdown O07.32
      salpingitis or salpingo-oophoritis O07.0
      sepsis O07.37
      shock O07.31
      specified condition NEC O07.39
      tubular necrosis (renal) O07.32
      uremia O07.32
      urinary tract infection O07.38
      venous complication NEC O07.35
          embolism (air) (amniotic fluid) (blood clot) (fat)
              (pulmonary) (septic) (soap) O07.2
  complicated (by) (following) O03.80
    afibrinogenemia O03.6
    cardiac arrest O03.86
    chemical damage of pelvic organ(s) O03.84
    circulatory collapse O03.81
    cystitis O03.88
    defibrination syndrome O03.6
    electrolyte imbalance O03.83
    embolism (air) (amniotic fluid) (blood clot) (fat) (pul-
        monary) (septic) (soap) O03.7
    endometritis O03.5
    genital tract and pelvic infection O03.5
    hemolysis O03.6
    hemorrhage (delayed) (excessive) O03.6
    infection
        genital tract or pelvic O03.5
        urinary tract O03.88
    intravascular coagulation O03.6
    laceration of pelvic organ(s) O03.84
    metabolic disorder O03.83
    oliguria O03.82
    oophoritis O03.5
    parametritis O03.5
    pelvic peritonitis O03.5
    perforation of pelvic organ(s) O03.84
    renal failure or shutdown O03.82
    salpingitis or salpingo-oophoritis O03.5
    sepsis O03.87
    shock O03.81
    specified condition NEC O03.89
    tubular necrosis (renal) O03.82
    uremia O03.82
    urinary tract infection O03.88
    venous complication NEC O03.85
        embolism (air) (amniotic fluid) (blood clot) (fat)
            (pulmonary) (septic) (soap) O03.7
  failed — *see* Abortion, attempted
  habitual or recurrent N96
    with current abortion — *see* categories O03-O04
    without current pregnancy N96
    care in current pregnancy O26.2- ☑
  incomplete (spontaneous) O03.4
    complicated (by) (following) O03.30
      afibrinogenemia O03.1
      cardiac arrest O03.36
      chemical damage of pelvic organ(s) O03.34
      circulatory collapse O03.31
      cystitis O03.38
      defibrination syndrome O03.1
      electrolyte imbalance O03.33
      embolism (air) (amniotic fluid) (blood clot) (fat)
          (pulmonary) (septic) (soap) O03.2
      endometritis O03.0
      genital tract and pelvic infection O03.0
      hemolysis O03.1
      hemorrhage (delayed) (excessive) O03.1
      infection
          genital tract or pelvic O03.0
          urinary tract O03.38
      intravascular coagulation O03.1
      laceration of pelvic organ(s) O03.34

Abortion — *continued*
  incomplete — *continued*
    complicated — *continued*
      metabolic disorder O03.33
      oliguria O03.32
      oophoritis O03.0
      parametritis O03.0
      pelvic peritonitis O03.0
      perforation of pelvic organ(s) O03.34
      renal failure or shutdown O03.32
      salpingitis or salpingo-oophoritis O03.0
      sepsis O03.37
      shock O03.31
      specified condition NEC O03.39
      tubular necrosis (renal) O03.32
      uremia O03.32
      urinary infection O03.38
      venous complication NEC O03.35
          embolism (air) (amniotic fluid) (blood clot) (fat)
              (pulmonary) (septic) (soap) O03.2
  induced (encounter for) Z33.2
    complicated by O04.80
      afibrinogenemia O04.6
      cardiac arrest O04.86
      chemical damage of pelvic organ(s) O04.84
      circulatory collapse O04.81
      cystitis O04.88
      defibrination syndrome O04.6
      electrolyte imbalance O04.83
      embolism (air) (amniotic fluid) (blood clot) (fat)
          (pulmonary) (septic) (soap) O04.7
      endometritis O04.5
      genital tract and pelvic infection O04.5
      hemolysis O04.6
      hemorrhage (delayed) (excessive) O04.6
      infection
          genital tract or pelvic O04.5
          urinary tract O04.88
      intravascular coagulation O04.6
      laceration of pelvic organ(s) O04.84
      metabolic disorder O04.83
      oliguria O04.82
      oophoritis O04.5
      parametritis O04.5
      pelvic peritonitis O04.5
      perforation of pelvic organ(s) O04.84
      renal failure or shutdown O04.82
      salpingitis or salpingo-oophoritis O04.5
      sepsis O04.87
      shock O04.81
      specified condition NEC O04.89
      tubular necrosis (renal) O04.82
      uremia O04.82
      urinary tract infection O04.88
      venous complication NEC O04.85
          embolism (air) (amniotic fluid) (blood clot) (fat)
              (pulmonary) (septic) (soap) O04.7
  inevitable O03.4
  missed O02.1
  spontaneous — *see* Abortion (complete) (spontaneous)
    threatened O20.0
  threatened (spontaneous) O20.0
  tubal O00.10- ☑
    with intrauterine pregnancy O00.11- ☑
Abortus fever A23.1
Aboulomania F60.7
Abrami's disease D59.8
Abramov-Fiedler myocarditis (acute isolated myocarditis)
      I40.1
Abrasion T14.8 ☑
  abdomen, abdominal (wall) S30.811 ☑
  alveolar process S00.512 ☑
  ankle S90.51- ☑
  antecubital space — *see* Abrasion, elbow
  anus S30.817 ☑
  arm (upper) S40.81- ☑
  auditory canal — *see* Abrasion, ear
  auricle — *see* Abrasion, ear
  axilla — *see* Abrasion, arm
  back, lower S30.810 ☑
  breast S20.11- ☑
  brow S00.81 ☑
  buttock S30.810 ☑
  calf — *see* Abrasion, leg
  canthus — *see* Abrasion, eyelid
  cheek S00.81 ☑
    internal S00.512 ☑
  chest wall — *see* Abrasion, thorax

Index

Abrasion — Abscess

Abrasion — *continued*
  chin S00.81 ☑
  clitoris S30.814 ☑
  cornea S05.0- ☑
  costal region — *see* Abrasion, thorax
  dental K03.1
  digit(s)
    foot — *see* Abrasion, toe
    hand — *see* Abrasion, finger
  ear S00.41- ☑
  elbow S50.31- ☑
  epididymis S30.813 ☑
  epigastric region S30.811 ☑
  epiglottis S10.11 ☑
  esophagus (thoracic) S27.818 ☑
    cervical S10.11 ☑
  eyebrow — *see* Abrasion, eyelid
  eyelid S00.21- ☑
  face S00.81 ☑
  finger(s) S60.41- ☑
    index S60.41- ☑
    little S60.41- ☑
    middle S60.41- ☑
    ring S60.41- ☑
  flank S30.811
  foot (except toe(s) alone) S90.81- ☑
    toe — *see* Abrasion, toe
  forearm S50.81- ☑
    elbow only — *see* Abrasion, elbow
  forehead S00.81 ☑
  genital organs, external
    female S30.816 ☑
    male S30.815 ☑
  groin S30.811 ☑
  gum S00.512 ☑
  hand S60.51- ☑
  head S00.91 ☑
    ear — *see* Abrasion, ear
    eyelid — *see* Abrasion, eyelid
    lip S00.511 ☑
    nose S00.31 ☑
    oral cavity S00.512 ☑
    scalp S00.01 ☑
    specified site NEC S00.81 ☑
  heel — *see* Abrasion, foot
  hip S70.21- ☑
  inguinal region S30.811 ☑
  interscapular region S20.419 ☑
  jaw S00.81 ☑
  knee S80.21- ☑
  labium (majus) (minus) S30.814 ☑
  larynx S10.11 ☑
  leg (lower) S80.81- ☑
    knee — *see* Abrasion, knee
    upper — *see* Abrasion, thigh
  lip S00.511 ☑
  lower back S30.810 ☑
  lumbar region S30.810 ☑
  malar region S00.81 ☑
  mammary — *see* Abrasion, breast
  mastoid region S00.81 ☑
  mouth S00.512 ☑
  nail
    finger — *see* Abrasion, finger
    toe — *see* Abrasion, toe
  nape S10.81 ☑
  nasal S00.31 ☑
  neck S10.91 ☑
    specified site NEC S10.81 ☑
    throat S10.11 ☑
  nose S00.31 ☑
  occipital region S00.01 ☑
  oral cavity S00.512 ☑
  orbital region — *see* Abrasion, eyelid
  palate S00.512 ☑
  palm — *see* Abrasion, hand
  parietal region S00.01 ☑
  pelvis S30.810 ☑
  penis S30.812 ☑
  perineum
    female S30.814 ☑
    male S30.810 ☑
  periocular area — *see* Abrasion, eyelid
  phalanges
    finger — *see* Abrasion, finger
    toe — *see* Abrasion, toe

Abrasion — *continued*
  pharynx S10.11 ☑
  pinna — *see* Abrasion, ear
  popliteal space — *see* Abrasion, knee
  prepuce S30.812 ☑
  pubic region S30.810 ☑
  pudendum
    female S30.816 ☑
    male S30.815 ☑
  sacral region S30.810 ☑
  scalp S00.01 ☑
  scapular region — *see* Abrasion, shoulder
  scrotum S30.813 ☑
  shin — *see* Abrasion, leg
  shoulder S40.21- ☑
  skin NEC T14.8 ☑
  sternal region S20.319 ☑
  submaxillary region S00.81 ☑
  submental region S00.81 ☑
  subungual
    finger(s) — *see* Abrasion, finger
    toe(s) — *see* Abrasion, toe
  supraclavicular fossa S10.81 ☑
  supraorbital S00.81 ☑
  temple S00.81 ☑
  temporal region S00.81 ☑
  testis S30.813 ☑
  thigh S70.31- ☑
  thorax, thoracic (wall) S20.91 ☑
    back S20.41- ☑
    front S20.31- ☑
  throat S10.11 ☑
  thumb S60.31- ☑
  toe(s) (lesser) S90.416 ☑
    great S90.41- ☑
  tongue S00.512 ☑
  tooth, teeth (dentifrice) (habitual) (hard tissues) (occupational) (ritual) (traditional) K03.1
  trachea S10.11 ☑
  tunica vaginalis S30.813 ☑
  tympanum, tympanic membrane — *see* Abrasion, ear
  uvula S00.512 ☑
  vagina S30.814 ☑
  vocal cords S10.11 ☑
  vulva S30.814 ☑
  wrist S60.81- ☑
Abrism — *see* Poisoning, food, noxious, plant
Abruptio placentae O45.9- ☑
  with
    afibrinogenemia O45.01- ☑
    coagulation defect O45.00- ☑
      specified NEC O45.09- ☑
    disseminated intravascular coagulation O45.02- ☑
    hypofibrinogenemia O45.01- ☑
    specified NEC O45.8- ☑
Abruption, placenta — *see* Abruptio placentae
Abscess (connective tissue) (embolic) (fistulous) (infective) (metastatic) (multiple) (pernicious) (pyogenic) (septic) L02.91
  with
    diverticular disease (intestine) K57.80
      with bleeding K57.81
      large intestine K57.20
        with
          bleeding K57.21
          small intestine K57.40
            with bleeding K57.41
      small intestine K57.00
        with
          bleeding K57.01
          large intestine K57.40
            with bleeding K57.41
    lymphangitis — *code by* site under Abscess
  abdomen, abdominal
    cavity K65.1
    wall L02.211
  abdominopelvic K65.1
  accessory sinus — *see* Sinusitis
  adrenal (capsule) (gland) E27.8
  alveolar K04.7
    with sinus K04.6
  amebic A06.4
    brain (and liver or lung abscess) A06.6
    genitourinary tract A06.82
    liver (without mention of brain or lung abscess) A06.4
    lung (and liver) (without mention of brain abscess) A06.5

Abscess — *continued*
  amebic — *continued*
    specified site NEC A06.89
    spleen A06.89
  anerobic A48.0
  ankle — *see* Abscess, lower limb
  anorectal K61.2
  antecubital space — *see* Abscess, upper limb
  antrum (chronic) (Highmore) — *see* Sinusitis, maxillary
  anus K61.0
  apical (tooth) K04.7
    with sinus (alveolar) K04.6
  appendix K35.33
  areola (acute) (chronic) (nonpuerperal) N61.1
    puerperal, postpartum or gestational — *see* Infection, nipple
  arm (any part) — *see* Abscess, upper limb
  artery (wall) I77.89
  atheromatous I77.2
  auricle, ear — *see* Abscess, ear, external
  axilla (region) L02.41- ☑
    lymph gland or node L04.2
  back (any part, except buttock) L02.212
  Bartholin's gland N75.1
    with
      abortion — *see* Abortion, by type complicated by, sepsis
      ectopic or molar pregnancy O08.0
    following ectopic or molar pregnancy O08.0
  Bezold's — *see* Mastoiditis, acute
  bilharziasis B65.1
  bladder (wall) — *see* Cystitis, specified type NEC
  bone (subperiosteal) — *see also* Osteomyelitis, specified type NEC
    accessory sinus (chronic) — *see* Sinusitis
    chronic or old — *see* Osteomyelitis, chronic
    jaw (lower) (upper) M27.2
    mastoid — *see* Mastoiditis, acute, subperiosteal
    petrous — *see* Petrositis
    spinal (tuberculous) A18.01
      nontuberculous — *see* Osteomyelitis, vertebra
  bowel K63.0
  brain (any part) (cystic) (otogenic) G06.0
    amebic (with abscess of any other site) A06.6
    gonococcal A54.82
    pheomycotic (chromomycotic) B43.1
    tuberculous A17.81
  breast (acute) (chronic) (nonpuerperal) N61.1
    newborn P39.0
    puerperal, postpartum, gestational — *see* Mastitis, obstetric, purulent
  broad ligament N73.2
    acute N73.0
    chronic N73.1
  Brodie's (localized) (chronic) M86.8X- ☑
  bronchi J98.09
  buccal cavity K12.2
  bulbourethral gland N34.0
  bursa M71.00
    ankle M71.07- ☑
    elbow M71.02- ☑
    foot M71.07- ☑
    hand M71.04- ☑
    hip M71.05- ☑
    knee M71.06- ☑
    multiple sites M71.09
    pharyngeal J39.1
    shoulder M71.01- ☑
    specified site NEC M71.08
    wrist M71.03- ☑
  buttock L02.31
  canthus — *see* Blepharoconjunctivitis
  cartilage — *see* Disorder, cartilage, specified type NEC
  cecum K35.33
  cerebellum, cerebellar G06.0
    sequelae G09
  cerebral (embolic) G06.0
    sequelae G09
  cervical (meaning neck) L02.11
    lymph gland or node L04.0
  cervix (stump) (uteri) — *see* Cervicitis
  cheek (external) L02.01
    inner K12.2
  chest J86.9
    with fistula J86.0
    wall L02.213
  chin L02.01
  choroid — *see* Inflammation, chorioretinal

☑ **Additional Character Required — Refer to the Tabular List for Character Selection**

Abscess — continued
circumtonsillar J36
cold (lung) (tuberculous) — see also Tuberculosis, abscess, lung
    articular — see Tuberculosis, joint
colon (wall) K63.0
colostomy K94.02
conjunctiva — see Conjunctivitis, acute
cornea H16.31- ☑
corpus
    cavernosum N48.21
    luteum — see Oophoritis
Cowper's gland N34.0
cranium G06.0
cul-de-sac (Douglas') (posterior) — see Peritonitis, pelvic, female
cutaneous — see Abscess, by site
dental K04.7
    with sinus (alveolar) K04.6
dentoalveolar K04.7
    with sinus K04.6
diaphragm, diaphragmatic K65.1
Douglas' cul-de-sac or pouch — see Peritonitis, pelvic, female
Dubois A50.59
ear (middle) — see also Otitis, media, suppurative
    acute — see Otitis, media, suppurative, acute
    external H60.0- ☑
entamebic — see Abscess, amebic
enterostomy K94.12
epididymis N45.4
epidural G06.2
    brain G06.0
    spinal cord G06.1
epiglottis J38.7
epiploon, epiploic K65.1
erysipelatous — see Erysipelas
esophagus K20.80
ethmoid (bone) (chronic) (sinus) J32.2
external auditory canal — see Abscess, ear, external
extradural G06.2
    brain G06.0
        sequelae G09
    spinal cord G06.1
extraperitoneal K68.19
eye — see Endophthalmitis, purulent
eyelid H00.03- ☑
face (any part, except ear, eye and nose) L02.01
fallopian tube — see Salpingitis
fascia M72.8
fauces J39.1
fecal K63.0
femoral (region) — see Abscess, lower limb
filaria, filarial — see Infestation, filarial
finger (any) — see also Abscess, hand
    nail — see Cellulitis, finger
foot L02.61- ☑
forehead L02.01
frontal sinus (chronic) J32.1
gallbladder K81.0
genital organ or tract
    female (external) N76.4
    male N49.9
        multiple sites N49.8
        specified NEC N49.8
gestational mammary O91.11- ☑
gestational subareolar O91.11- ☑
gingival
    aggressive K05.20
        generalized K05.229
            moderate K05.222
            severe K05.223
            slight K05.221
        localized K05.219
            moderate K05.212
            severe K05.213
            slight K05.211
gland, glandular (lymph) (acute) — see Lymphadenitis, acute
gluteal (region) L02.31
gonorrheal — see Gonococcus
groin L02.214
gum
    aggressive K05.20
        generalized K05.229
            moderate K05.222
            severe K05.223
            slight K05.221

Abscess — continued
gum — continued
    aggressive — continued
        localized K05.219
            moderate K05.212
            severe K05.213
            slight K05.211
hand L02.51- ☑
head NEC L02.811
    face (any part, except ear, eye and nose) L02.01
heart — see Carditis
heel — see Abscess, foot
helminthic — see Infestation, helminth
hepatic (cholangitic) (hematogenic) (lymphogenic) (pylephlebitic) K75.0
    amebic A06.4
hip (region) — see Abscess, lower limb
horseshoe K61.31
ileocecal K35.33
ileostomy (bud) K94.12
iliac (region) L02.214
    fossa K35.33
infraclavicular (fossa) — see Abscess, upper limb
inguinal (region) L02.214
    lymph gland or node L04.1
intersphincteric K61.4
intestine, intestinal NEC K63.0
    rectal K61.1
intra-abdominal — see also Abscess, peritoneum K65.1
    following procedure T81.43 ☑
        obstetrical O86.03
    postprocedural T81.43 ☑
        retroperitoneal K68.11
intracranial G06.0
intramammary — see Abscess, breast
intramuscular, following procedure T81.42 ☑
    obstetrical O86.02
intraorbital — see Abscess, orbit
intraperitoneal K65.1
intrasphincteric (anus) K61.4
intraspinal G06.1
intratonsillar J36
ischiorectal (fossa) (specified NEC) K61.39
jaw (bone) (lower) (upper) M27.2
joint — see Arthritis, pyogenic or pyemic
    spine (tuberculous) A18.01
        nontuberculous — see Spondylopathy, infective
kidney N15.1
    with calculus N20.0
        with hydronephrosis N13.6
    puerperal (postpartum) O86.21
knee — see also Abscess, lower limb
    joint M00.9
labium (majus) (minus) N76.4
lacrimal
    caruncle — see Inflammation, lacrimal, passages, acute
    gland — see Dacryoadenitis
    passages (duct) (sac) — see Inflammation, lacrimal, passages, acute
lacunar N34.0
larynx J38.7
lateral (alveolar) K04.7
    with sinus K04.6
leg (any part) — see Abscess, lower limb
lens H27.8
lingual K14.0
    tonsil J36
lip K13.0
Littre's gland N34.0
liver (cholangitic) (hematogenic) (lymphogenic) (pylephlebitic) (pyogenic) K75.0
    amebic (due to Entamoeba histolytica) (dysenteric) (tropical) A06.4
        with
            brain abscess (and liver or lung abscess) A06.6
            lung abscess A06.5
loin (region) L02.211
lower limb L02.41- ☑
lumbar (tuberculous) A18.01
    nontuberculous L02.212
lung (miliary) (putrid) J85.2
    with pneumonia J85.1
        due to specified organism (see Pneumonia, in (due to))
    amebic (with liver abscess) A06.5
        with
            brain abscess A06.6

Abscess — continued
lung — continued
    amebic — continued
        with — continued
            pneumonia A06.5
lymph, lymphatic, gland or node (acute) — see also Lymphadenitis, acute
    mesentery I88.0
malar M27.2
mammary gland — see Abscess, breast
marginal, anus K61.0
mastoid — see Mastoiditis, acute
maxilla, maxillary M27.2
    molar (tooth) K04.7
        with sinus K04.6
    premolar K04.7
    sinus (chronic) J32.0
mediastinum J85.3
meibomian gland — see Hordeolum
meninges G06.2
mesentery, mesenteric K65.1
mesosalpinx — see Salpingitis
mons pubis L02.215
mouth (floor) K12.2
muscle — see Myositis, infective
myocardium I40.0
nabothian (follicle) — see Cervicitis
nasal J32.9
nasopharyngeal J39.1
navel L02.216
    newborn P38.9
        with mild hemorrhage P38.1
        without hemorrhage P38.9
neck (region) L02.11
    lymph gland or node L04.0
nephritic — see Abscess, kidney
nipple N61.1
    associated with
        lactation — see Pregnancy, complicated by
        pregnancy — see Pregnancy, complicated by
nose (external) (fossa) (septum) J34.0
    sinus (chronic) — see Sinusitis
omentum K65.1
operative wound T81.49 ☑
orbit, orbital — see Cellulitis, orbit
otogenic G06.0
ovary, ovarian (corpus luteum) — see Oophoritis
oviduct — see Oophoritis
palate (soft) K12.2
    hard M27.2
palmar (space) — see Abscess, hand
pancreas (duct) — see Pancreatitis, acute
parafrenal N48.21
parametric, parametrium N73.2
    acute N73.0
    chronic N73.1
paranephric N15.1
parapancreatic — see Pancreatitis, acute
parapharyngeal J39.0
pararectal K61.1
parasinus — see Sinusitis
parauterine — see also Disease, pelvis, inflammatory N73.2
paravaginal — see Vaginitis
parietal region (scalp) L02.811
parodontal — see Periodontitis, aggressive, localized
parotid (duct) (gland) K11.3
    region K12.2
pectoral (region) L02.213
pelvis, pelvic
    female — see Disease, pelvis, inflammatory
    male, peritoneal K65.1
penis N48.21
    gonococcal (accessory gland) (periurethral) A54.1
perianal K61.0
periapical K04.7
    with sinus (alveolar) K04.6
periappendicular K35.33
pericardial I30.1
pericecal K35.33
pericemental — see Periodontitis, aggressive, localized
pericholecystic — see Cholecystitis, acute
pericoronal — see Periodontitis, aggressive, localized
peridental — see Periodontitis, aggressive, localized
perimetric — see also Disease, pelvis, inflammatory N73.2
perinephric, perinephritic — see Abscess, kidney
perineum, perineal (superficial) L02.215
    urethra N34.0

Abscess — *continued*
  periodontal (parietal) — *see* Periodontitis, aggressive, localized
    apical K04.7
  periosteum, periosteal — *see also* Osteomyelitis, specified type NEC
    with osteomyelitis — *see also* Osteomyelitis, specified type NEC
      acute — *see* Osteomyelitis, acute
      chronic — *see* Osteomyelitis, chronic
  peripharyngeal J39.0
  peripleuritic J86.9
    with fistula J86.0
  periprostatic N41.2
  perirectal K61.1
  perirenal (tissue) — *see* Abscess, kidney
  perisinuous (nose) — *see* Sinusitis
  peritoneum, peritoneal (perforated) (ruptured) K65.1
    with appendicitis — *see also* Appendicitis K35.33
    pelvic
      female — *see* Peritonitis, pelvic, female
      male K65.1
    postoperative T81.43 ☑
    puerperal, postpartum, childbirth O85
    tuberculous A18.31
  peritonsillar J36
  perityphlic K35.33
  periureteral N28.89
  periurethral N34.0
    gonococcal (accessory gland) (periurethral) A54.1
  periuterine — *see also* Disease, pelvis, inflammatory N73.2
  perivesical — *see* Cystitis, specified type NEC
  petrous bone — *see* Petrositis
  phagedenic NOS L02.91
    chancroid A57
  pharynx, pharyngeal (lateral) J39.1
  pilonidal L05.01
  pituitary (gland) E23.6
  pleura J86.9
    with fistula J86.0
  popliteal — *see* Abscess, lower limb
  postcecal K35.33
  postlaryngeal J38.7
  postnasal J34.0
  postoperative (any site) — *see also* Infection, postoperative wound T81.49 ☑
    retroperitoneal K68.11
  postpharyngeal J39.0
  posttonsillar J36
  post-typhoid A01.09
  pouch of Douglas — *see* Peritonitis, pelvic, female
  premammary — *see* Abscess, breast
  prepatellar — *see* Abscess, lower limb
  presacral K68.19
  prostate N41.2
    gonococcal (acute) (chronic) A54.22
  psoas muscle K68.12
  puerperal — *code by* site under Puerperal, abscess
  pulmonary — *see* Abscess, lung
  pulp, pulpal (dental) K04.01
    irreversible K04.02
    reversible K04.01
  rectovaginal septum K63.0
  rectovesical — *see* Cystitis, specified type NEC
  rectum K61.1
  renal — *see* Abscess, kidney
  retina — *see* Inflammation, chorioretinal
  retrobulbar — *see* Abscess, orbit
  retrocecal K65.1
  retrolaryngeal J38.7
  retromammary — *see* Abscess, breast
  retroperitoneal NEC K68.19
    postprocedural K68.11
  retropharyngeal J39.0
  retrouterine — *see* Peritonitis, pelvic, female
  retrovesical — *see* Cystitis, specified type NEC
  root, tooth K04.7
    with sinus (alveolar) K04.6
  round ligament — *see also* Disease, pelvis, inflammatory N73.2
  rupture (spontaneous) NOS L02.91
  sacrum (tuberculous) A18.01
    nontuberculous M46.28
  salivary (duct) (gland) K11.3
  scalp (any part) L02.811
  scapular — *see* Osteomyelitis, specified type NEC
  sclera — *see* Scleritis
  scrofulous (tuberculous) A18.2

Abscess — *continued*
  scrotum N49.2
  seminal vesicle N49.0
  septal, dental K04.7
    with sinus (alveolar) K04.6
  serous — *see* Periostitis
  shoulder (region) — *see* Abscess, upper limb
  sigmoid K63.0
  sinus (accessory) (chronic) (nasal) — *see also* Sinusitis
    intracranial venous (any) G06.0
  Skene's duct or gland N34.0
  skin — *see* Abscess, by site
  specified site NEC L02.818
  spermatic cord N49.1
  sphenoidal (sinus) (chronic) J32.3
  spinal cord (any part) (staphylococcal) G06.1
    tuberculous A17.81
  spine (column) (tuberculous) A18.01
    epidural G06.1
    nontuberculous — *see* Osteomyelitis, vertebra
  spleen D73.3
    amebic A06.89
  stitch T81.41 ☑
    following an obstetrical procedure O86.01
  subarachnoid G06.2
    brain G06.0
    spinal cord G06.1
  subareolar — *see* Abscess, breast
  subcecal K35.33
  subcutaneous — *see also* Abscess, by site
    following procedure T81.41 ☑
      obstetrical O86.01
    pheomycotic (chromomycotic) B43.2
  subdiaphragmatic K65.1
  subdural G06.2
    brain G06.0
      sequelae G09
    spinal cord G06.1
  sub-fascial, following an obstetrical procedure O86.02
  subgaleal L02.811
  subhepatic K65.1
  sublingual K12.2
    gland K11.3
  submammary — *see* Abscess, breast
  submandibular (region) (space) (triangle) K12.2
    gland K11.3
  submaxillary (region) L02.01
    gland K11.3
  submental L02.01
    gland K11.3
  subperiosteal — *see* Osteomyelitis, specified type NEC
  subphrenic K65.1
    following an obstetrical procedure O86.03
    postoperative T81.43 ☑
  suburethral N34.0
  sudoriparous L75.8
  supraclavicular (fossa) — *see* Abscess, upper limb
  supralevator K61.5
  suprapelvic, acute N73.0
  suprarenal (capsule) (gland) E27.8
  sweat gland L74.8
  tear duct — *see* Inflammation, lacrimal, passages, acute
  temple L02.01
  temporal region L02.01
  temporosphenoidal G06.0
  tendon (sheath) M65.00
    ankle M65.07- ☑
    foot M65.07- ☑
    forearm M65.03- ☑
    hand M65.04- ☑
    lower leg M65.06- ☑
    pelvic region M65.05- ☑
    shoulder region M65.01- ☑
    specified site NEC M65.08
    thigh M65.05- ☑
    upper arm M65.02- ☑
  testis N45.4
  thigh — *see* Abscess, lower limb
  thorax J86.9
    with fistula J86.0
  throat J39.1
  thumb — *see also* Abscess, hand
    nail — *see* Cellulitis, finger
  thymus (gland) E32.1
  thyroid (gland) E06.0
  toe (any) — *see also* Abscess, foot
    nail — *see* Cellulitis, toe
  tongue (staphylococcal) K14.0

Abscess — *continued*
  tonsil(s) (lingual) J36
  tonsillopharyngeal J36
  tooth, teeth (root) K04.7
    with sinus (alveolar) K04.6
    supporting structures NEC — *see* Periodontitis, aggressive, localized
  trachea J39.8
  trunk L02.219
    abdominal wall L02.211
    back L02.212
    chest wall L02.213
    groin L02.214
    perineum L02.215
    umbilicus L02.216
  tubal — *see* Salpingitis
  tuberculous — *see* Tuberculosis, abscess
  tubo-ovarian — *see* Salpingo-oophoritis
  tunica vaginalis N49.1
  umbilicus L02.216
  upper
    limb L02.41- ☑
    respiratory J39.8
  urethral (gland) N34.0
  urinary N34.0
  uterus, uterine (wall) — *see also* Endometritis
    ligament — *see also* Disease, pelvis, inflammatory N73.2
    neck — *see* Cervicitis
  uvula K12.2
  vagina (wall) — *see* Vaginitis
  vaginorectal — *see* Vaginitis
  vas deferens N49.1
  vermiform appendix K35.33
  vertebra (column) (tuberculous) A18.01
    nontuberculous — *see* Osteomyelitis, vertebra
  vesical — *see* Cystitis, specified type NEC
  vesico-uterine pouch — *see* Peritonitis, pelvic, female
  vitreous (humor) — *see* Endophthalmitis, purulent
  vocal cord J38.3
  von Bezold's — *see* Mastoiditis, acute
  vulva N76.4
  vulvovaginal gland N75.1
  web space — *see* Abscess, hand
  wound T81.49 ☑
  wrist — *see* Abscess, upper limb
Absence (of) (organ or part) (complete or partial)
  adrenal (gland) (congenital) Q89.1
    acquired E89.6
  albumin in blood E88.09
  alimentary tract (congenital) Q45.8
    upper Q40.8
  alveolar process (acquired) — *see* Anomaly, alveolar
  ankle (acquired) Z89.44- ☑
  anus (congenital) Q42.3
    with fistula Q42.2
  aorta (congenital) Q25.41
  appendix, congenital Q42.8
  arm (acquired) Z89.20- ☑
    above elbow Z89.22- ☑
      congenital (with hand present) — *see* Agenesis, arm, with hand present
      and hand — *see* Agenesis, forearm, and hand
    below elbow Z89.21- ☑
      congenital (with hand present) — *see* Agenesis, arm, with hand present
      and hand — *see* Agenesis, forearm, and hand
    congenital — *see* Defect, reduction, upper limb
    shoulder (following explanation of shoulder joint prosthesis) (joint) (with or without presence of antibiotic-impregnated cement spacer) Z89.23- ☑
      congenital (with hand present) — *see* Agenesis, arm, with hand present
  artery (congenital) (peripheral) Q27.8
    brain Q28.3
    coronary Q24.5
    pulmonary Q25.79
    specified NEC Q27.8
    umbilical Q27.0
  atrial septum (congenital) Q21.19
  auditory canal (congenital) (external) Q16.1
  auricle (ear), congenital Q16.0
  bile, biliary duct, congenital Q44.5
  bladder (acquired) Z90.6
    congenital Q64.5
  bowel sounds R19.11
  brain Q00.0

☑ **Additional Character Required** — **Refer to the Tabular List for Character Selection**

Absence — *continued*
  brain — *continued*
    part of Q04.3
  breast(s) (and nipple(s)) (acquired) Z90.1- ☑
    congenital Q83.8
  broad ligament Q50.6
  bronchus (congenital) Q32.4
  canaliculus lacrimalis, congenital Q10.4
  cerebellum (vermis) Q04.3
  cervix (acquired) (with uterus) Z90.710
    with remaining uterus Z90.712
    congenital Q51.5
  chin, congenital Q18.8
  cilia (congenital) Q10.3
    acquired — *see* Madarosis
  clitoris (congenital) Q52.6
  coccyx, congenital Q76.49
  cold sense R20.8
  congenital
    lumen — *see* Atresia
    organ or site NEC — *see* Agenesis
    septum — *see* Imperfect, closure
  corpus callosum Q04.0
  cricoid cartilage, congenital Q31.8
  diaphragm (with hernia), congenital Q79.1
  digestive organ(s) or tract, congenital Q45.8
    acquired NEC Z90.49
    upper Q40.8
  ductus arteriosus Q28.8
  duodenum (acquired) Z90.49
    congenital Q41.0
  ear, congenital Q16.9
    acquired H93.8- ☑
    auricle Q16.0
    external Q16.0
    inner Q16.5
    lobe, lobule Q17.8
    middle, except ossicles Q16.4
      ossicles Q16.3
    ossicles Q16.3
  ejaculatory duct (congenital) Q55.4
  endocrine gland (congenital) NEC Q89.2
    acquired E89.89
  epididymis (congenital) Q55.4
    acquired Z90.79
  epiglottis, congenital Q31.8
  esophagus (congenital) Q39.8
    acquired (partial) Z90.49
  eustachian tube (congenital) Q16.2
  extremity (acquired) Z89.9
    congenital Q73.0
    knee (following explantation of knee joint prosthesis) (joint) (with or without presence of antibiotic-impregnated cement spacer) Z89.52- ☑
    lower (above knee) Z89.619
      below knee Z89.51- ☑
    upper — *see* Absence, arm
  eye (acquired) Z90.01
    congenital Q11.1
    muscle (congenital) Q10.3
  eyeball (acquired) Z90.01
  eyelid (fold) (congenital) Q10.3
    acquired Z90.01
  face, specified part NEC Q18.8
  fallopian tube(s) (acquired) Z90.79
    congenital Q50.6
  family member (causing problem in home) NEC — *see also* Disruption, family Z63.32
  femur, congenital — *see* Defect, reduction, lower limb, longitudinal, femur
  fibrinogen (congenital) D68.2
    acquired D65
  finger(s) (acquired) Z89.02- ☑
    congenital — *see* Agenesis, hand
  foot (acquired) Z89.43- ☑
    congenital — *see* Agenesis, foot
  forearm (acquired) — *see* Absence, arm, below elbow
  gallbladder (acquired) Z90.49
    congenital Q44.0
  gamma globulin in blood D80.1
    hereditary D80.0
  genital organs
    acquired (female) (male) Z90.79
    female, congenital Q52.8
      external Q52.71
      internal NEC Q52.8
    male, congenital Q55.8

Absence — *continued*
  genitourinary organs, congenital NEC
    female Q52.8
    male Q55.8
  globe (acquired) Z90.01
    congenital Q11.1
  glottis, congenital Q31.8
  hand and wrist (acquired) Z89.11- ☑
    congenital — *see* Agenesis, hand
  head, part (acquired) NEC Z90.09
  heat sense R20.8
  hip (following explantation of hip joint prosthesis) (joint) (with or without presence of antibiotic-impregnated cement spacer) Z89.62- ☑
  hymen (congenital) Q52.4
  ileum (acquired) Z90.49
    congenital Q41.2
  immunoglobulin, isolated NEC D80.3
    IgA D80.2
    IgG D80.3
    IgM D80.4
  incus (acquired) — *see* Loss, ossicles, ear
    congenital Q16.3
  inner ear, congenital Q16.5
  intestine (acquired) (small) Z90.49
    congenital Q41.9
      specified NEC Q41.8
    large Z90.49
      congenital Q42.9
        specified NEC Q42.8
  iris, congenital Q13.1
  jejunum (acquired) Z90.49
    congenital Q41.1
  joint
    acquired
      hip (following explantation of hip joint prosthesis) (with or without presence of antibiotic-impregnated cement spacer) Z89.62- ☑
      knee (following explantation of knee joint prosthesis) (with or without presence of antibiotic-impregnated cement spacer) Z89.52- ☑
      shoulder (following explantation of shoulder joint prosthesis) (with or without presence of antibiotic-impregnated cement spacer) Z89.23- ☑
    congenital NEC Q74.8
  kidney(s) (acquired) Z90.5
    congenital Q60.2
      bilateral Q60.1
      unilateral Q60.0
  knee (following explantation of knee joint prosthesis) (joint) (with or without presence of antibiotic-impregnated cement spacer) Z89.52- ☑
  labyrinth, membranous Q16.5
  larynx (congenital) Q31.8
    acquired Z90.02
  leg (acquired) (above knee) Z89.61- ☑
    below knee (acquired) Z89.51- ☑
    congenital — *see* Defect, reduction, lower limb
  lens (acquired) — *see also* Aphakia
    congenital Q12.3
    post cataract extraction Z98.4- ☑
  limb (acquired) — *see* Absence, extremity
  lip Q38.6
  liver (congenital) Q44.79
  lung (fissure) (lobe) (bilateral) (unilateral) (congenital) Q33.3
    acquired (any part) Z90.2
  menstruation — *see* Amenorrhea
  muscle (congenital) (pectoral) Q79.8
    ocular Q10.3
  neck, part Q18.8
  neutrophil — *see* Agranulocytosis
  nipple(s) (with breast(s)) (acquired) Z90.1- ☑
    congenital Q83.2
  nose (congenital) Q30.1
    acquired Z90.09
  organ
    of Corti, congenital Q16.5
    or site, congenital NEC Q89.8
      acquired NEC Z90.89
  osseous meatus (ear) Q16.4
  ovary (acquired)
    bilateral Z90.722
    congenital
      bilateral Q50.02
      unilateral Q50.01
    unilateral Z90.721

Absence — *continued*
  oviduct (acquired)
    bilateral Z90.722
    congenital Q50.6
    unilateral Z90.721
  pancreas (congenital) Q45.0
    acquired Z90.410
      complete Z90.410
      partial Z90.411
      total Z90.410
  parathyroid gland (acquired) E89.2
    congenital Q89.2
  patella, congenital Q74.1
  penis (congenital) Q55.5
    acquired Z90.79
  pericardium (congenital) Q24.8
  pituitary gland (congenital) Q89.2
    acquired E89.3
  prostate (acquired) Z90.79
    congenital Q55.4
  pulmonary valve Q22.0
  punctum lacrimale (congenital) Q10.4
  radius, congenital — *see* Defect, reduction, upper limb, longitudinal, radius
  rectum (congenital) Q42.1
    with fistula Q42.0
    acquired Z90.49
  respiratory organ NOS Q34.9
  rib (acquired) Z90.89
    congenital Q76.6
  sacrum, congenital Q76.49
  salivary gland(s), congenital Q38.4
  scrotum, congenital Q55.29
  seminal vesicles (congenital) Q55.4
    acquired Z90.79
  septum
    atrial (congenital) Q21.19
    between aorta and pulmonary artery Q21.4
    ventricular (congenital) Q20.4
  sex chromosome
    female phenotype Q97.8
    male phenotype Q98.8
  skull bone (congenital) Q75.8
    with
      anencephaly Q00.0
      encephalocele — *see* Encephalocele
      hydrocephalus Q03.9
        with spina bifida — *see* Spina bifida, by site, with hydrocephalus
      microcephaly Q02
  spermatic cord, congenital Q55.4
  spine, congenital Q76.49
  spleen (congenital) Q89.01
    acquired Z90.81
  sternum, congenital Q76.7
  stomach (acquired) (partial) Z90.3
    congenital Q40.2
  superior vena cava, congenital Q26.8
  teeth, tooth (congenital) K00.0
    acquired (complete) K08.109
      class I K08.101
      class II K08.102
      class III K08.103
      class IV K08.104
      due to
        caries K08.139
          class I K08.131
          class II K08.132
          class III K08.133
          class IV K08.134
        periodontal disease K08.129
          class I K08.121
          class II K08.122
          class III K08.123
          class IV K08.124
        specified NEC K08.199
          class I K08.191
          class II K08.192
          class III K08.193
          class IV K08.194
        trauma K08.119
          class I K08.111
          class II K08.112
          class III K08.113
          class IV K08.114
      partial K08.409
        class I K08.401
        class II K08.402
        class III K08.403

Absence — *continued*
  teeth, tooth — *continued*
    acquired — *continued*
      partial — *continued*
        class IV K08.404
        due to
          caries K08.439
            class I K08.431
            class II K08.432
            class III K08.433
            class IV K08.434
          periodontal disease K08.429
            class I K08.421
            class II K08.422
            class III K08.423
            class IV K08.424
          specified NEC K08.499
            class I K08.491
            class II K08.492
            class III K08.493
            class IV K08.494
          trauma K08.419
            class I K08.411
            class II K08.412
            class III K08.413
            class IV K08.414
  tendon (congenital) Q79.8
  testis (congenital) Q55.0
    acquired Z90.79
  thumb (acquired) Z89.01- ☑
    congenital — *see* Agenesis, hand
  thymus gland Q89.2
  thyroid (gland) (acquired) E89.0
    cartilage, congenital Q31.8
    congenital E03.1
  toe(s) (acquired) Z89.42- ☑
    with foot — *see* Absence, foot and ankle
    congenital — *see* Agenesis, foot
    great Z89.41- ☑
  tongue, congenital Q38.3
  trachea (cartilage), congenital Q32.1
  transverse aortic arch, congenital Q25.49
  tricuspid valve Q22.4
  umbilical artery, congenital Q27.0
  upper arm and forearm with hand present, congenital — *see* Agenesis, arm, with hand present
  ureter (congenital) Q62.4
    acquired Z90.6
  urethra, congenital Q64.5
  uterus (acquired) Z90.710
    with cervix Z90.710
    with remaining cervical stump Z90.711
    congenital Q51.0
  uvula, congenital Q38.5
  vagina, congenital Q52.0
  vas deferens (congenital) Q55.4
    acquired Z90.79
  vein (peripheral) congenital NEC Q27.8
    cerebral Q28.3
    digestive system Q27.8
    great Q26.8
    lower limb Q27.8
    portal Q26.5
    precerebral Q28.1
    specified site NEC Q27.8
    upper limb Q27.8
  vena cava (inferior) (superior), congenital Q26.8
  ventricular septum Q20.4
  vertebra, congenital Q76.49
  von Willebrand factor, complete (near) — *see also* Disease, von Willebrand D68.03
  vulva, congenital Q52.71
  wrist (acquired) Z89.12- ☑
Absorbent system disease I87.8
Absorption
  carbohydrate, disturbance K90.49
  chemical — *see* Table of Drugs and Chemicals
    through placenta (newborn) P04.9
      environmental substance P04.6
      nutritional substance P04.5
      obstetric anesthetic or analgesic drug P04.0
  drug NEC — *see* Table of Drugs and Chemicals
    addictive
      through placenta (newborn) — *see also* Newborn, affected by, maternal, use of P04.40
        cocaine P04.41
        hallucinogens P04.42
        specified drug NEC P04.49

Absorption — *continued*
  drug — *see* Table of Drugs and Chemicals — *continued*
    medicinal
      through placenta (newborn) P04.19
    through placenta (newborn) P04.19
      obstetric anesthetic or analgesic drug P04.0
  fat, disturbance K90.49
    pancreatic K90.3
  noxious substance — *see* Table of Drugs and Chemicals
  protein, disturbance K90.49
  starch, disturbance K90.49
  toxic substance — *see* Table of Drugs and Chemicals
  uremic — *see* Uremia
Abstinence symptoms, syndrome
  alcohol F10.239
    with delirium F10.231
  cocaine F14.23
  neonatal P96.1
  nicotine — *see* Dependence, drug, nicotine, with, withdrawal
  opioid F11.93
    with dependence F11.23
  psychoactive NEC F19.939
    with
      delirium F19.931
      dependence F19.239
        with
          delirium F19.231
          perceptual disturbance F19.232
        uncomplicated F19.230
      perceptual disturbance F19.932
      uncomplicated F19.930
  sedative F13.939
    with
      delirium F13.931
      dependence F13.239
        with
          delirium F13.231
          perceptual disturbance F13.232
        uncomplicated F13.230
      perceptual disturbance F13.932
      uncomplicated F13.930
  stimulant NEC F15.93
    with dependence F15.23
Abulia R68.89
Abulomania F60.7
Abuse
  adult — *see* Maltreatment, adult
    as reason for
      couple seeking advice (including offender) Z63.0
  alcohol (non-dependent) F10.10
    with
      anxiety disorder F10.180
      intoxication F10.129
        with delirium F10.121
        uncomplicated F10.120
      mood disorder F10.14
      other specified disorder F10.188
      psychosis F10.159
        delusions F10.150
        hallucinations F10.151
      sexual dysfunction F10.181
      sleep disorder F10.182
      unspecified disorder F10.19
      withdrawal F10.139
        with
          perceptual disturbance F10.132
        delirium F10.131
        uncomplicated F10.130
    counseling and surveillance Z71.41
    in remission (early) (sustained) F10.11
  amphetamine (or related substance) — *see also* Abuse, drug, stimulant NEC
    stimulant NEC F15.10
      with
        anxiety disorder F15.180
        intoxication F15.129
          with
            delirium F15.121
            perceptual disturbance F15.122
        withdrawal F15.13
  analgesics (non-prescribed) (over the counter) F55.8
  antacids F55.0
  antidepressants — *see* Abuse, drug, psychoactive NEC
  anxiolytic — *see* Abuse, drug, sedative
  barbiturates — *see* Abuse, drug, sedative
  caffeine — *see* Abuse, drug, stimulant NEC
  cannabis, cannabinoids — *see* Abuse, drug, cannabis

Abuse — *continued*
  child — *see* Maltreatment, child
  cocaine — *see* Abuse, drug, cocaine
  drug NEC (non-dependent) F19.10
    with sleep disorder F19.182
    amphetamine type — *see* Abuse, drug, stimulant NEC
    analgesics (non-prescribed) (over the counter) F55.8
    antacids F55.0
    antidepressants — *see* Abuse, drug, psychoactive NEC
    anxiolytics — *see* Abuse, drug, sedative
    barbiturates — *see* Abuse, drug, sedative
    caffeine — *see* Abuse, drug, stimulant NEC
    cannabis F12.10
      with
        anxiety disorder F12.180
        intoxication F12.129
          with
            delirium F12.121
            perceptual disturbance F12.122
          uncomplicated F12.120
        other specified disorder F12.188
        psychosis F12.159
          delusions F12.150
          hallucinations F12.151
        unspecified disorder F12.19
        withdrawal F12.13
      in remission (early) (sustained) F12.11
    cocaine F14.10
      with
        anxiety disorder F14.180
        intoxication F14.129
          with
            delirium F14.121
            perceptual disturbance F14.122
          uncomplicated F14.120
        mood disorder F14.14
        other specified disorder F14.188
        psychosis F14.159
          delusions F14.150
          hallucinations F14.151
        sexual dysfunction F14.181
        sleep disorder F14.182
        unspecified disorder F14.19
        withdrawal F14.13
      in remission (early) (sustained) F14.11
    counseling and surveillance Z71.51
    hallucinogen F16.10
      with
        anxiety disorder F16.180
        flashbacks F16.183
        intoxication F16.129
          with
            delirium F16.121
            perceptual disturbance F16.122
          uncomplicated F16.120
        mood disorder F16.14
        other specified disorder F16.188
        perception disorder, persisting F16.183
        psychosis F16.159
          delusions F16.150
          hallucinations F16.151
        unspecified disorder F16.19
      in remission (early) (sustained) F16.11
    hashish — *see* Abuse, drug, cannabis
    herbal or folk remedies F55.1
    hormones F55.3
    hypnotics — *see* Abuse, drug, sedative
    in remission (early) (sustained) F19.11
    inhalant F18.10
      with
        anxiety disorder F18.180
        dementia, persisting F18.17
        intoxication F18.129
          with delirium F18.121
          uncomplicated F18.120
        mood disorder F18.14
        other specified disorder F18.188
        psychosis F18.159
          delusions F18.150
          hallucinations F18.151
        unspecified disorder F18.19
      in remission (early) (sustained) F18.11
    laxatives F55.2
    LSD — *see* Abuse, drug, hallucinogen
    marihuana — *see* Abuse, drug, cannabis
    morphine type (opioids) — *see* Abuse, drug, opioid
    opioid F11.10
      with
        intoxication F11.129

☑ **Additional Character Required** — **Refer to the Tabular List for Character Selection**

Abuse — *continued*
  drug — *continued*
    opioid — *continued*
      with — *continued*
        intoxication — *continued*
          with
            delirium F11.121
            perceptual disturbance F11.122
          uncomplicated F11.120
        mood disorder F11.14
        opioid-associated amnestic syndrome F11.188
        other specified disorder F11.188
        psychosis F11.159
          delusions F11.150
          hallucinations F11.151
        sexual dysfunction F11.181
        sleep disorder F11.182
        unspecified disorder F11.19
        withdrawal F11.13
      in remission (early) (sustained) F11.11
    PCP (phencyclidine) (or related substance) — *see* Abuse, drug, hallucinogen
    psychoactive NEC F19.10
      with
        amnestic disorder F19.16
        anxiety disorder F19.180
        dementia F19.17
        intoxication F19.129
          with
            delirium F19.121
            perceptual disturbance F19.122
          uncomplicated F19.120
        mood disorder F19.14
        other specified disorder F19.188
        psychosis F19.159
          delusions F19.150
          hallucinations F19.151
        sexual dysfunction F19.181
        sleep disorder F19.182
        unspecified disorder F19.19
        withdrawal F19.139
          with
            perceptual disturbance F19.132
          delirium F19.131
          uncomplicated F19.130
    sedative, hypnotic or anxiolytic F13.10
      with
        anxiety disorder F13.180
        intoxication F13.129
          with delirium F13.121
          uncomplicated F13.120
        mood disorder F13.14
        other specified disorder F13.188
        psychosis F13.159
          delusions F13.150
          hallucinations F13.151
        sexual dysfunction F13.181
        sleep disorder F13.182
        unspecified disorder F13.19
        withdrawal F13.139
          with
            perceptual disturbance F13.132
          delirium F13.131
          uncomplicated F13.130
      in remission (early) (sustained) F13.11
    solvent — *see* Abuse, drug, inhalant
    steroids F55.3
    stimulant NEC F15.10
      with
        anxiety disorder F15.180
        intoxication F15.129
          with
            delirium F15.121
            perceptual disturbance F15.122
          uncomplicated F15.120
        mood disorder F15.14
        other specified disorder F15.188
        psychosis F15.159
          delusions F15.150
          hallucinations F15.151
        sexual dysfunction F15.181
        sleep disorder F15.182
        unspecified disorder F15.19
        withdrawal F15.13
      in remission (early) (sustained) F15.11
    tranquilizers — *see* Abuse, drug, sedative
    vitamins F55.4
  hallucinogens — *see* Abuse, drug, hallucinogen
  hashish — *see* Abuse, drug, cannabis

Abuse — *continued*
  herbal or folk remedies F55.1
  hormones F55.3
  hypnotic — *see* Abuse, drug, sedative
  inhalant — *see* Abuse, drug, inhalant
  laxatives F55.2
  LSD — *see* Abuse, drug, hallucinogen
  marihuana — *see* Abuse, drug, cannabis
  morphine type (opioids) — *see* Abuse, drug, opioid
  non-psychoactive substance NEC F55.8
    antacids F55.0
    folk remedies F55.1
    herbal remedies F55.1
    hormones F55.3
    laxatives F55.2
    steroids F55.3
    vitamins F55.4
  opioids — *see* Abuse, drug, opioid
  PCP (phencyclidine) (or related substance) — *see* Abuse, drug, hallucinogen
  physical (adult) (child) — *see* Maltreatment
  psychoactive substance — *see* Abuse, drug, psychoactive NEC
  psychological (adult) (child) — *see* Maltreatment
  sedative — *see* Abuse, drug, sedative
  sexual — *see* Maltreatment
  solvent — *see* Abuse, drug, inhalant
  steroids F55.3
  vitamins F55.4
Acalculia R48.8
  developmental F81.2
Acanthamebiasis (with) B60.10
  conjunctiva B60.12
  keratoconjunctivitis B60.13
  meningoencephalitis B60.11
  other specified B60.19
Acanthocephaliasis B83.8
Acanthocheilonemiasis B74.4
Acanthocytosis E78.6
Acantholysis L11.9
Acanthosis (acquired) (nigricans) L83
  benign Q82.8
  congenital Q82.8
  seborrheic L82.1
    inflamed L82.0
  tongue K14.3
Acapnia E87.3
Acarbia E87.29
Acardia, acardius Q89.8
Acardiacus amorphus Q89.8
Acardiotrophia I51.4
Acariasis B88.0
  scabies B86
Acarodermatitis (urticarioides) B88.0
Acarophobia F40.218
Acatalasemia, acatalasia E80.3
Acathisia (drug induced) G25.71
Accelerated atrioventricular conduction I45.6
Accentuation of personality traits (type A) Z73.1
Accessory (congenital)
  adrenal gland Q89.1
  anus Q43.4
  appendix Q43.4
  atrioventricular conduction I45.6
  auditory ossicles Q16.3
  auricle (ear) Q17.0
  biliary duct or passage Q44.5
  bladder Q64.79
  blood vessels NEC Q27.9
    coronary Q24.5
  bone NEC Q79.8
  breast tissue, axilla Q83.1
  carpal bones Q74.0
  cecum Q43.4
  chromosome(s) NEC (nonsex) Q92.9
    with complex rearrangements NEC Q92.5
      seen only at prometaphase Q92.8
    13 — *see* Trisomy, 13
    18 — *see* Trisomy, 18
    21 — *see* Trisomy, 21
    partial Q92.9
    sex
      female phenotype Q97.8
  coronary artery Q24.5
  cusp(s), heart valve NEC Q24.8
    pulmonary Q22.3
  cystic duct Q44.5
  digit(s) Q69.9
  ear (auricle) (lobe) Q17.0

Accessory — *continued*
  endocrine gland NEC Q89.2
  eye muscle Q10.3
  eyelid Q10.3
  face bone(s) Q75.8
  fallopian tube (fimbria) (ostium) Q50.6
  finger(s) Q69.0
  foreskin N47.8
  frontonasal process Q75.8
  gallbladder Q44.1
  genital organ(s)
    female Q52.8
      external Q52.79
      internal NEC Q52.8
    male Q55.8
  genitourinary organs NEC Q89.8
    female Q52.8
    male Q55.8
  hallux Q69.2
  heart Q24.8
    valve NEC Q24.8
      pulmonary Q22.3
  hepatic ducts Q44.5
  hymen Q52.4
  intestine (large) (small) Q43.4
  kidney Q63.0
  lacrimal canal Q10.6
  leaflet, heart valve NEC Q24.8
  ligament, broad Q50.6
  liver Q44.79
    duct Q44.5
  lobule (ear) Q17.0
  lung (lobe) Q33.1
  muscle Q79.8
  navicular of carpus Q74.0
  nervous system, part NEC Q07.8
  nipple Q83.3
  nose Q30.8
  organ or site not listed — *see* Anomaly, by site
  ovary Q50.31
  oviduct Q50.6
  pancreas Q45.3
  parathyroid gland Q89.2
  parotid gland (and duct) Q38.4
  pituitary gland Q89.2
  preauricular appendage Q17.0
  prepuce N47.8
  renal arteries (multiple) Q27.2
  rib Q76.6
    cervical Q76.5
  roots (teeth) K00.2
  salivary gland Q38.4
  sesamoid bones Q74.8
    foot Q74.2
    hand Q74.0
  skin tags Q82.8
  spleen Q89.09
  sternum Q76.7
  submaxillary gland Q38.4
  tarsal bones Q74.2
  teeth, tooth K00.1
  tendon Q79.8
  thumb Q69.1
  thymus gland Q89.2
  thyroid gland Q89.2
  toes Q69.2
  tongue Q38.3
  tooth, teeth K00.1
  tragus Q17.0
  ureter Q62.5
  urethra Q64.79
  urinary organ or tract NEC Q64.8
  uterus Q51.28
  vagina Q52.10
  valve, heart NEC Q24.8
    pulmonary Q22.3
  vertebra Q76.49
  vocal cords Q31.8
  vulva Q52.79
Accident
  birth — *see* Birth, injury
  cardiac — *see* Infarct, myocardium
  cerebrovascular (ischemic) I63.9
    aborted I63.9
    chronic (old) (remote) (imaging) (without sequelae) Z86.73
    with residual defects — *see* Sequelae, disease, cerebrovascular
    embolic I63.- ☑

☑ **Additional Character Required** — Refer to the Tabular List for Character Selection   9

☑ **Additional Character Required** — **Refer to the Tabular List for Character Selection**

Addison's — *continued*
  disease or syndrome — *continued*
    tuberculous A18.7
  keloid L94.0
Addison-Schilder complex E71.528
Additional — *see also* Accessory
  chromosome(s) — *see also* Trisomy Q99.8
    21 — *see* Trisomy, 21
    marker — *see* Extra, marker chromosomes
    sex — *see* Abnormal, chromosome, sex
Adduction contracture, hip or other joint — *see* Contraction, joint
Adenitis — *see also* Lymphadenitis
  acute, unspecified site L04.9
  axillary I88.9
    acute L04.2
    chronic or subacute I88.1
  Bartholin's gland N75.8
  bulbourethral gland — *see* Urethritis
  cervical I88.9
    acute L04.0
    chronic or subacute I88.1
  chancroid (Hemophilus ducreyi) A57
  chronic, unspecified site I88.1
  Cowper's gland — *see* Urethritis
  due to Pasteurella multocida (P. septica) A28.0
  epidemic, acute B27.09
  gangrenous L04.9
  gonorrheal NEC A54.89
  groin I88.9
    acute L04.1
    chronic or subacute I88.1
  infectious (acute) (epidemic) B27.09
  inguinal I88.9
    acute L04.1
    chronic or subacute I88.1
  lymph gland or node, except mesenteric I88.9
    acute — *see* Lymphadenitis, acute
    chronic or subacute I88.1
  mesenteric (acute) (chronic) (nonspecific) (subacute) I88.0
  parotid gland (suppurative) — *see* Sialoadenitis
  salivary gland (any) (suppurative) — *see* Sialoadenitis
  scrofulous (tuberculous) A18.2
  Skene's duct or gland — *see* Urethritis
  strumous, tuberculous A18.2
  subacute, unspecified site I88.1
  sublingual gland (suppurative) — *see* Sialoadenitis
  submandibular gland (suppurative) — *see* Sialoadenitis
  submaxillary gland (suppurative) — *see* Sialoadenitis
  tuberculous — *see* Tuberculosis, lymph gland
  urethral gland — *see* Urethritis
  Wharton's duct (suppurative) — *see* Sialoadenitis
Adenoacanthoma — *see* Neoplasm, malignant, by site
Adenoameloblastoma — *see* Cyst, calcifying odontogenic
Adenocarcinoid (tumor) — *see* Neoplasm, malignant, by site
Adenocarcinoma — *see also* Neoplasm, malignant, by site
  acidophil
    specified site — *see* Neoplasm, malignant, by site
    unspecified site C75.1
  adrenal cortical C74.0- ☑
  alveolar — *see* Neoplasm, lung, malignant
  apocrine
    breast — *see* Neoplasm, breast, malignant
    in situ
      breast D05.8- ☑
      specified site NEC — *see* Neoplasm, skin, in situ
      unspecified site D04.9
    specified site NEC — *see* Neoplasm, skin, malignant
    unspecified site C44.99
  basal cell
    specified site — *see* Neoplasm, skin, malignant
    unspecified site C08.9
  basophil
    specified site — *see* Neoplasm, malignant, by site
    unspecified site C75.1
  bile duct type C22.1
    liver C22.1
    specified site NEC — *see* Neoplasm, malignant, by site
    unspecified site C22.1
  bronchiolar — *see* Neoplasm, lung, malignant
  bronchioloalveolar — *see* Neoplasm, lung, malignant
  ceruminous C44.29- ☑
  cervix, in situ — *see also* Carcinoma, cervix uteri, in situ D06.9
  chromophobe
    specified site — *see* Neoplasm, malignant, by site

Adenocarcinoma — *continued*
  chromophobe — *continued*
    unspecified site C75.1
  diffuse type
    specified site — *see* Neoplasm, malignant, by site
    unspecified site C16.9
  duct
    infiltrating
      with Paget's disease — *see* Neoplasm, breast, malignant
      specified site — *see* Neoplasm, malignant, by site
      unspecified site (female) C50.91- ☑
        male C50.92- ☑
    specified site — *see* Neoplasm, malignant, by site
    unspecified site
      female C56.9
      male C61
  eosinophil
    specified site — *see* Neoplasm, malignant, by site
    unspecified site C75.1
  follicular
    with papillary C73
    moderately differentiated C73
    specified site — *see* Neoplasm, malignant, by site
    trabecular C73
    unspecified site C73
    well differentiated C73
  Hurthle cell C73
  in
    adenomatous
      polyposis coli C18.9
  infiltrating duct
    with Paget's disease — *see* Neoplasm, breast, malignant
    specified site — *see* Neoplasm, by site, malignant
    unspecified site (female) C50.91- ☑
      male C50.92- ☑
  inflammatory
    specified site — *see* Neoplasm, by site, malignant
    unspecified site (female) C50.91- ☑
      male C50.92- ☑
  intestinal type
    specified site — *see* Neoplasm, by site, malignant
    unspecified site C16.9
  intracystic papillary
  intraductal
    breast D05.1- ☑
    noninfiltrating
      breast D05.1- ☑
      papillary
        with invasion
          specified site — *see* Neoplasm, by site, malignant
          unspecified site (female) C50.91- ☑
            male C50.92- ☑
        breast D05.1- ☑
        specified site NEC — *see* Neoplasm, in situ, by site
        unspecified site D05.1- ☑
      specified site NEC — *see* Neoplasm, in situ, by site
      unspecified site D05.1- ☑
    papillary
      with invasion
        specified site — *see* Neoplasm, malignant, by site
        unspecified site (female) C50.91- ☑
          male C50.92- ☑
      breast D05.1- ☑
      specified site — *see* Neoplasm, in situ, by site
      unspecified site D05.1- ☑
    specified site NEC — *see* Neoplasm, in situ, by site
    unspecified site D05.1- ☑
  islet cell
    with exocrine, mixed
      specified site — *see* Neoplasm, malignant, by site
      unspecified site C25.9
    pancreas C25.4
    specified site NEC — *see* Neoplasm, malignant, by site
    unspecified site C25.4
  lobular
    in situ
      breast D05.0- ☑
      specified site NEC — *see* Neoplasm, in situ, by site
      unspecified site D05.0- ☑
    specified site — *see* Neoplasm, malignant, by site
    unspecified site (female) C50.91- ☑
      male C50.92- ☑

Adenocarcinoma — *continued*
  mucoid — *see also* Neoplasm, malignant, by site
    cell
      specified site — *see* Neoplasm, malignant, by site
      unspecified site C75.1
  nonencapsulated sclerosing C73
  papillary
    with follicular C73
    follicular variant C73
    intraductal (noninfiltrating)
      with invasion
        specified site — *see* Neoplasm, malignant, by site
        unspecified site (female) C50.91- ☑
          male C50.92- ☑
      breast D05.1- ☑
      specified site NEC — *see* Neoplasm, in situ, by site
      unspecified site D05.1- ☑
    serous
      specified site — *see* Neoplasm, malignant, by site
      unspecified site C56.9
  papillocystic
    specified site — *see* Neoplasm, malignant, by site
    unspecified site C56.9
  pseudomucinous
    specified site — *see* Neoplasm, malignant, by site
    unspecified site C56.9
  renal cell C64- ☑
  sebaceous — *see* Neoplasm, skin, malignant
  serous — *see also* Neoplasm, malignant, by site
    papillary
      specified site — *see* Neoplasm, malignant, by site
      unspecified site C56.9
  sweat gland — *see* Neoplasm, skin, malignant
  water-clear cell C75.0
Adenocarcinoma-in-situ — *see also* Neoplasm, in situ, by site
  breast D05.9- ☑
Adenofibroma
  clear cell — *see* Neoplasm, benign, by site
  endometrioid D27.9
    borderline malignancy D39.10
    malignant C56- ☑
  mucinous
    specified site — *see* Neoplasm, benign, by site
    unspecified site D27.9
  papillary
    specified site — *see* Neoplasm, benign, by site
    unspecified site D27.9
  prostate — *see* Enlargement, enlarged, prostate
  serous
    specified site — *see* Neoplasm, benign, by site
    unspecified site D27.9
  specified site — *see* Neoplasm, benign, by site
  unspecified site D27.9
Adenofibrosis
  breast — *see* Fibroadenosis, breast
  endometrioid N80.00
Adenoiditis (chronic) J35.02
  with tonsillitis J35.03
  acute J03.90
    recurrent J03.91
    specified organism NEC J03.80
      recurrent J03.81
    staphylococcal J03.80
      recurrent J03.81
    streptococcal J03.00
      recurrent J03.01
Adenoids — *see* condition
Adenolipoma — *see* Neoplasm, benign, by site
Adenolipomatosis, Launois-Bensaude E88.89
Adenolymphoma
  specified site — *see* Neoplasm, benign, by site
  unspecified site D11.9
Adenoma — *see also* Neoplasm, benign, by site
  acidophil
    specified site — *see* Neoplasm, benign, by site
    unspecified site D35.2
  acidophil-basophil, mixed
    specified site — *see* Neoplasm, benign, by site
    unspecified site D35.2
  adrenal (cortical) D35.00
    clear cell D35.00
    compact cell D35.00
    glomerulosa cell D35.00
    heavily pigmented variant D35.00
    mixed cell D35.00

Index

Adenoma — Adhesions, adhesive

Adenoma — continued
alpha-cell
  pancreas D13.7
  specified site NEC — see Neoplasm, benign, by site
  unspecified site D13.7
alveolar D14.30
apocrine
  breast D24- ☑
  specified site NEC — see Neoplasm, skin, benign, by
    site
  unspecified site D23.9
basal cell D11.9
basophil
  specified site — see Neoplasm, benign, by site
  unspecified site D35.2
basophil-acidophil, mixed
  specified site — see Neoplasm, benign, by site
  unspecified site D35.2
beta-cell
  pancreas D13.7
  specified site NEC — see Neoplasm, benign, by site
  unspecified site D13.7
bile duct D13.4
  common D13.5
  extrahepatic D13.5
  intrahepatic D13.4
  specified site NEC — see Neoplasm, benign, by site
  unspecified site D13.4
black D35.00
bronchial D38.1
  cylindroid type — see Neoplasm, lung, malignant
ceruminous D23.2- ☑
chief cell D35.1
chromophobe
  specified site — see Neoplasm, benign, by site
  unspecified site D35.2
colloid
  specified site — see Neoplasm, benign, by site
  unspecified site D34
eccrine, papillary — see Neoplasm, skin, benign
endocrine, multiple
  single specified site — see Neoplasm, uncertain be-
    havior, by site
  two or more specified sites D44- ☑
  unspecified site D44.9
endometrioid — see also Neoplasm, benign
  borderline malignancy — see Neoplasm, uncertain
    behavior, by site
eosinophil
  specified site — see Neoplasm, benign, by site
  unspecified site D35.2
fetal
  specified site — see Neoplasm, benign, by site
  unspecified site D34
follicular
  specified site — see Neoplasm, benign, by site
  unspecified site D34
hepatocellular D13.4
Hurthle cell D34
islet cell
  pancreas D13.7
  specified site NEC — see Neoplasm, benign, by site
  unspecified site D13.7
liver cell D13.4
macrofollicular
  specified site — see Neoplasm, benign, by site
  unspecified site D34
malignant, malignum — see Neoplasm, malignant, by
  site
microcystic
  pancreas D13.6
  specified site NEC — see Neoplasm, benign, by site
  unspecified site D13.6
microfollicular
  specified site — see Neoplasm, benign, by site
  unspecified site D34
mucoid cell
  specified site — see Neoplasm, benign, by site
  unspecified site D35.2
multiple endocrine
  single specified site — see Neoplasm, uncertain be-
    havior, by site
  two or more specified sites D44- ☑
  unspecified site D44.9
nipple D24- ☑
papillary — see also Neoplasm, benign, by site
  eccrine — see Neoplasm, skin, benign, by site

Adenoma — continued
Pick's tubular
  specified site — see Neoplasm, benign, by site
  unspecified site
    female D27.9
    male D29.20
pleomorphic
  carcinoma in — see Neoplasm, salivary gland, malig-
    nant
  specified site — see Neoplasm, malignant, by site
  unspecified site C08.9
polypoid — see also Neoplasm, benign
  adenocarcinoma in — see Neoplasm, malignant, by
    site
  adenocarcinoma in situ — see Neoplasm, in situ, by
    site
prostate — see Neoplasm, prostate, benign
rete cell D29.20
sebaceous — see Neoplasm, skin, benign
Sertoli cell
  specified site — see Neoplasm, benign, by site
  unspecified site
    female D27.9
    male D29.20
skin appendage — see Neoplasm, skin, benign
sudoriferous gland — see Neoplasm, skin, benign
sweat gland — see Neoplasm, skin, benign
testicular
  specified site — see Neoplasm, benign, by site
  unspecified site
    female D27.9
    male D29.20
tubular — see also Neoplasm, benign, by site
  adenocarcinoma in — see Neoplasm, malignant, by
    site
  adenocarcinoma in situ — see Neoplasm, in situ, by
    site
  Pick's
    specified site — see Neoplasm, benign, by site
    unspecified site
      female D27.9
      male D29.20
tubulovillous — see also Neoplasm, benign, by site
  adenocarcinoma in — see Neoplasm, malignant, by
    site
  adenocarcinoma in situ — see Neoplasm, in situ, by
    site
villous — see Neoplasm, uncertain behavior, by site
  adenocarcinoma in — see Neoplasm, malignant, by
    site
  adenocarcinoma in situ — see Neoplasm, in situ, by
    site
water-clear cell D35.1
Adenomatosis
endocrine (multiple) E31.20
  single specified site — see Neoplasm, uncertain be-
    havior, by site
erosive of nipple D24- ☑
pluriendocrine — see Adenomatosis, endocrine
pulmonary D38.1
  malignant — see Neoplasm, lung, malignant
specified site — see Neoplasm, benign, by site
unspecified site D12.6
Adenomatous
goiter (nontoxic) E04.9
  with hyperthyroidism — see Hyperthyroidism, with,
    goiter, nodular
  toxic — see Hyperthyroidism, with, goiter, nodular
Adenomyoma — see also Neoplasm, benign, by site
prostate — see Enlarged, prostate
Adenomyometritis N80.00
Adenomyosis (uterus) N80.03
Adenopathy (lymph gland) R59.9
generalized R59.1
inguinal R59.0
localized R59.0
mediastinal R59.0
mesentery R59.0
syphilitic (secondary) A51.49
tracheobronchial R59.0
  tuberculous A15.4
    primary (progressive) A15.7
tuberculous — see also Tuberculosis, lymph gland
  tracheobronchial A15.4
    primary (progressive) A15.7
Adenosalpingitis — see Salpingitis
Adenosarcoma — see Neoplasm, malignant, by site
Adenosclerosis I88.8
Adenosis (sclerosing) breast — see Fibroadenosis, breast

Adenovirus, as cause of disease classified elsewhere
  B97.0
Adentia (complete) (partial) — see Absence, teeth
Adherent — see also Adhesions
labia (minora) N90.89
pericardium (nonrheumatic) I31.0
  rheumatic I09.2
placenta (with hemorrhage) O72.0
  without hemorrhage O73.0
prepuce, newborn N47.0
scar (skin) L90.5
tendon in scar L90.5
Adhesions, adhesive (postinfective) K66.0
with intestinal obstruction K56.50
  complete K56.52
  incomplete K56.51
  partial K56.51
abdominal (wall) — see Adhesions, peritoneum
appendix K38.8
bile duct (common) (hepatic) K83.8
bladder (sphincter) N32.89
bowel — see Adhesions, peritoneum
cardiac I31.0
  rheumatic I09.2
cecum — see Adhesions, peritoneum
cervicovaginal N88.1
  congenital Q52.8
  postpartal O90.89
    old N88.1
cervix N88.1
ciliary body NEC — see Adhesions, iris
clitoris N90.89
colon — see Adhesions, peritoneum
common duct K83.8
congenital — see also Anomaly, by site
  fingers — see Syndactylism, complex, fingers
  omental, anomalous Q43.3
  peritoneal Q43.3
  tongue (to gum or roof of mouth) Q38.3
conjunctiva (acquired) H11.21- ☑
  congenital Q15.8
cystic duct K82.8
diaphragm — see Adhesions, peritoneum
due to foreign body — see Foreign body
duodenum — see Adhesions, peritoneum
ear
  middle H74.1- ☑
epididymis N50.89
epidural — see Adhesions, meninges
epiglottis J38.7
eyelid H02.59
female pelvis N73.6
gallbladder K82.8
globe H44.89
heart I31.0
  rheumatic I09.2
ileocecal (coil) — see Adhesions, peritoneum
ileum — see Adhesions, peritoneum
intestine — see also Adhesions, peritoneum
  with obstruction K56.50
    complete K56.52
    incomplete K56.51
    partial K56.51
intra-abdominal — see Adhesions, peritoneum
iris H21.50- ☑
  anterior H21.51- ☑
  goniosynechiae H21.52- ☑
  posterior H21.54- ☑
  to corneal graft T85.898 ☑
joint — see Ankylosis
  knee M23.8X
  temporomandibular M26.61- ☑
labium (majus) (minus), congenital Q52.5
liver — see Adhesions, peritoneum
lung J98.4
mediastinum J98.59
meninges (cerebral) (spinal) G96.12
  congenital Q07.8
  tuberculous (cerebral) (spinal) A17.0
mesenteric — see Adhesions, peritoneum
nasal (septum) (to turbinates) J34.89
ocular muscle — see Strabismus, mechanical
omentum — see Adhesions, peritoneum
ovary N73.6
  congenital (to cecum, kidney or omentum) Q50.39
paraovarian N73.6
pelvic (peritoneal)
  female N73.6

☑ Additional Character Required — Refer to the Tabular List for Character Selection

Adhesions, adhesive — *continued*
  pelvic — *continued*
    female — *continued*
      postprocedural N99.4
    male — *see* Adhesions, peritoneum
    postpartal (old) N73.6
    tuberculous A18.17
  penis to scrotum (congenital) Q55.8
  periappendiceal — *see also* Adhesions, peritoneum
  pericardium (nonrheumatic) I31.0
    focal I31.8
    rheumatic I09.2
    tuberculous A18.84
  pericholecystic K82.8
  perigastric — *see* Adhesions, peritoneum
  periovarian N73.6
  periprostatic N42.89
  perirectal — *see* Adhesions, peritoneum
  perirenal N28.89
  peritoneum, peritoneal (postinfective) K66.0
    with obstruction (intestinal) K56.50
      complete K56.52
      incomplete K56.51
      partial K56.51
    congenital Q43.3
    pelvic, female N73.6
      postprocedural N99.4
    postpartal, pelvic N73.6
    postprocedural K66.0
    to uterus N73.6
  peritubal N73.6
  periureteral N28.89
  periuterine N73.6
  perivesical N32.89
  perivesicular (seminal vesicle) N50.89
  pleura, pleuritic J94.8
    tuberculous NEC A15.6
  pleuropericardial J94.8
  postoperative (gastrointestinal tract) K66.0
    with obstruction — *see also* Obstruction, intestine, postoperative K91.30
    due to foreign body accidentally left in wound — *see* Foreign body, accidentally left during a procedure
    pelvic peritoneal N99.4
    urethra — *see* Stricture, urethra, postprocedural
    vagina N99.2
  postpartal, old (vulva or perineum) N90.89
  preputial, prepuce N47.5
  pulmonary J98.4
  pylorus — *see* Adhesions, peritoneum
  sciatic nerve — *see* Lesion, nerve, sciatic
  seminal vesicle N50.89
  shoulder (joint) — *see* Capsulitis, adhesive
  sigmoid flexure — *see* Adhesions, peritoneum
  spermatic cord (acquired) N50.89
    congenital Q55.4
  spinal canal G96.12
  stomach — *see* Adhesions, peritoneum
  subscapular — *see* Capsulitis, adhesive
  temporomandibular M26.61- ☑
  tendinitis (*see also* Tenosynovitis, specified type NEC)
    shoulder — *see* Capsulitis, adhesive
  testis N44.8
  tongue, congenital (to gum or roof of mouth) Q38.3
    acquired K14.8
  trachea J39.8
  tubo-ovarian N73.6
  tunica vaginalis N44.8
  uterus N73.6
    internal N85.6
    to abdominal wall N73.6
  vagina (chronic) N89.5
    postoperative N99.2
  vitreomacular H43.82- ☑
  vitreous H43.89
  vulva N90.89
Adiaspiromycosis B48.8
Adie (-Holmes) **pupil or syndrome** — *see* Anomaly, pupil, function, tonic pupil
Adiponecrosis neonatorum P83.88
Adiposis — *see also* Obesity
  cerebralis E23.6
  dolorosa E88.2
Adiposity — *see also* Obesity
  heart — *see* Degeneration, myocardial
  localized E65
Adiposogenital dystrophy E23.6

Adjustment
  disorder — *see* Disorder, adjustment
  implanted device — *see* Encounter (for), adjustment (of)
  prosthesis, external — *see* Fitting
  reaction — *see* Disorder, adjustment
Administration of tPA (rtPA) in a different facility within the last 24 hours prior to admission to current facility Z92.82
Admission (for) — *see also* Encounter (for)
  adjustment (of)
    artificial
      arm Z44.00- ☑
        complete Z44.01- ☑
        partial Z44.02- ☑
      eye Z44.2 ☑
      leg Z44.10- ☑
        complete Z44.11- ☑
        partial Z44.12- ☑
    brain neuropacemaker Z46.2
      implanted Z45.42
    breast
      implant Z45.81
      prosthesis (external) Z44.3 ☑
    colostomy belt Z46.89
    contact lenses Z46.0
    cystostomy device Z46.6
    dental prosthesis Z46.3
    device NEC
      abdominal Z46.89
      implanted Z45.89
        cardiac Z45.09
          defibrillator (with synchronous cardiac pacemaker) Z45.02
          pacemaker (cardiac resynchronization therapy (CRT-P)) Z45.018
          pulse generator Z45.010
          resynchronization therapy defibrillator (CRT-D) Z45.02
        hearing device Z45.328
          bone conduction Z45.320
          cochlear Z45.321
        infusion pump Z45.1
        nervous system Z45.49
          CSF drainage Z45.41
          hearing device — *see* Admission, adjustment, device, implanted, hearing device
          neuropacemaker Z45.42
          visual substitution Z45.31
        specified NEC Z45.89
        vascular access Z45.2
        visual substitution Z45.31
      nervous system Z46.2
        implanted — *see* Admission, adjustment, device, implanted, nervous system
      orthodontic Z46.4
      prosthetic Z44.9
        arm — *see* Admission, adjustment, artificial, arm
        breast Z44.3 ☑
        dental Z46.3
        eye Z44.2 ☑
        leg — *see* Admission, adjustment, artificial, leg
        specified type NEC Z44.8
      substitution
        auditory Z46.2
          implanted — *see* Admission, adjustment, device, implanted, hearing device
        nervous system Z46.2
          implanted — *see* Admission, adjustment, device, implanted, nervous system
        visual Z46.2
          implanted Z45.31
    urinary Z46.6
    hearing aid Z46.1
      implanted — *see* Admission, adjustment, device, implanted, hearing device
    ileostomy device Z46.89
    intestinal appliance or device NEC Z46.89
    neuropacemaker (brain) (peripheral nerve) (spinal cord) Z46.2
      implanted Z45.42
    orthodontic device Z46.4
    orthopedic (brace) (cast) (device) (shoes) Z46.89
    pacemaker (cardiac resynchronization therapy (CRT-P))
      cardiac Z45.018
        pulse generator Z45.010

Admission — *continued*
  adjustment — *continued*
    pacemaker — *continued*
      nervous system Z46.2
        implanted Z45.42
    portacath (port-a-cath) Z45.2
    prosthesis Z44.9
      arm — *see* Admission, adjustment, artificial, arm
      breast Z44.3 ☑
      dental Z46.3
      eye Z44.2 ☑
      leg — *see* Admission, adjustment, artificial, leg
      specified NEC Z44.8
    spectacles Z46.0
  aftercare — *see also* Aftercare Z51.89
    postpartum
      immediately after delivery Z39.0
      routine follow-up Z39.2
    radiation therapy (antineoplastic) Z51.0
    sepsis Z51.A
  attention to artificial opening (of) Z43.9
    artificial vagina Z43.7
    colostomy Z43.3
    cystostomy Z43.5
    enterostomy Z43.4
    gastrostomy Z43.1
    ileostomy Z43.2
    jejunostomy Z43.4
    nephrostomy Z43.6
    specified site NEC Z43.8
      intestinal tract Z43.4
      urinary tract Z43.6
    tracheostomy Z43.0
    ureterostomy Z43.6
    urethrostomy Z43.6
  breast augmentation or reduction Z41.1
  breast reconstruction following mastectomy Z42.1
  change of
    dressing (nonsurgical) Z48.00
    neuropacemaker device (brain) (peripheral nerve) (spinal cord) Z46.2
      implanted Z45.42
    surgical dressing Z48.01
  circumcision, ritual or routine (in absence of diagnosis) Z41.2
  clinical research investigation (control) (normal comparison) (participant) Z00.6
  contraceptive management Z30.9
  cosmetic surgery NEC Z41.1
  counseling — *see also* Counseling
    dietary Z71.3
    gestational carrier Z31.7
    HIV Z71.7
    human immunodeficiency virus Z71.7
    nonattending third party Z71.0
    procreative management NEC Z31.69
  delivery, full-term, uncomplicated O80
    cesarean, without indication O82
  desensitization to allergens Z51.6
  dietary surveillance and counseling Z71.3
  ear piercing Z41.3
  examination at health care facility (adult) — *see also* Examination Z00.00
    with abnormal findings Z00.01
    clinical research investigation (control) (normal comparison) (participant) Z00.6
    dental Z01.20
      with abnormal findings Z01.21
    donor (potential) Z00.5
    ear Z01.10
      with abnormal findings NEC Z01.118
    eye Z01.00
      with abnormal findings Z01.01
      following failed vision screening Z01.020
        with abnormal findings Z01.021
    general, specified reason NEC Z00.8
    hearing Z01.10
      with abnormal findings NEC Z01.118
      infant or child (over 28 days old) Z00.129
        with abnormal findings Z00.121
    postpartum checkup Z39.2
    psychiatric (general) Z00.8
      requested by authority Z04.6
    vision Z01.00
      with abnormal findings Z01.01
      following failed vision screening Z01.020
        with abnormal findings Z01.021
      infant or child (over 28 days old) Z00.129
        with abnormal findings Z00.121

☑ **Additional Character Required — Refer to the Tabular List for Character Selection**   **13**

Admission — *continued*
  fitting (of)
    artificial
      arm — *see* Admission, adjustment, artificial, arm
      eye Z44.2 ☑
      leg — *see* Admission, adjustment, artificial, leg
    brain neuropacemaker Z46.2
      implanted Z45.42
    breast prosthesis (external) Z44.3 ☑
    colostomy belt Z46.89
    contact lenses Z46.0
    cystostomy device Z46.6
    dental prosthesis Z46.3
    dentures Z46.3
    device NEC
      abdominal Z46.89
      nervous system Z46.2
        implanted — *see* Admission, adjustment, device, implanted, nervous system
      orthodontic Z46.4
      prosthetic Z44.9
        breast Z44.3 ☑
        dental Z46.3
        eye Z44.2 ☑
      substitution
        auditory Z46.2
          implanted — *see* Admission, adjustment, device, implanted, hearing device
        nervous system Z46.2
          implanted — *see* Admission, adjustment, device, implanted, nervous system
        visual Z46.2
          implanted Z45.31
    hearing aid Z46.1
    ileostomy device Z46.89
    intestinal appliance or device NEC Z46.89
    neuropacemaker (brain) (peripheral nerve) (spinal cord) Z46.2
      implanted Z45.42
    orthodontic device Z46.4
    orthopedic device (brace) (cast) (shoes) Z46.89
    prosthesis Z44.9
      arm — *see* Admission, adjustment, artificial, arm
      breast Z44.3 ☑
      dental Z46.3
      eye Z44.2 ☑
      leg — *see* Admission, adjustment, artificial, leg
      specified type NEC Z44.8
    spectacles Z46.0
  follow-up examination Z09
  intrauterine device management Z30.431
    initial prescription Z30.014
  mental health evaluation Z00.8
    requested by authority Z04.6
  observation — *see* Observation
  Papanicolaou smear, cervix Z12.4
    for suspected malignant neoplasm Z12.4
  plastic and reconstructive surgery following medical procedure or healed injury NEC Z42.8
  plastic surgery, cosmetic NEC Z41.1
  postpartum observation
    immediately after delivery Z39.0
    routine follow-up Z39.2
  poststerilization (for restoration) Z31.0
    aftercare Z31.42
  procreative management Z31.9
  prophylactic (measure) — *see also* Encounter, prophylactic measures
    organ removal Z40.00
      breast Z40.01
      fallopian tube(s) Z40.03
        with ovary(s) Z40.02
      ovary(s) Z40.02
      specified organ NEC Z40.09
      testes Z40.09
    vaccination Z23
  psychiatric examination (general) Z00.8
    requested by authority Z04.6
  radiation therapy (antineoplastic) Z51.0
  reconstructive surgery following medical procedure or healed injury NEC Z42.8
  removal of
    cystostomy catheter Z43.5
    drains Z48.03
    dressing (nonsurgical) Z48.00
    implantable subdermal contraceptive Z30.46
    intrauterine contraceptive device Z30.432

Admission — *continued*
  removal of — *continued*
    neuropacemaker (brain) (peripheral nerve) (spinal cord) Z46.2
      implanted Z45.42
    staples Z48.02
    surgical dressing Z48.01
    sutures Z48.02
    ureteral stent Z46.6
  respirator [ventilator] use during power failure Z99.12
  restoration of organ continuity (poststerilization) Z31.0
    aftercare Z31.42
  sensitivity test — *see also* Test, skin
    allergy NEC Z01.82
    Mantoux Z11.1
  tuboplasty following previous sterilization Z31.0
    aftercare Z31.42
  vasoplasty following previous sterilization Z31.0
    aftercare Z31.42
  vision examination Z01.00
    with abnormal findings Z01.01
    following failed vision screening Z01.020
      with abnormal findings Z01.021
    infant or child (over 28 days old) Z00.129
      with abnormal findings Z00.121
  waiting period for admission to other facility Z75.1
Adnexitis (suppurative) — *see* Salpingo-oophoritis
Adolescent X-linked adrenoleukodystrophy E71.521
Adrenal (gland) — *see* condition
Adrenalism, tuberculous A18.7
Adrenalitis, adrenitis E27.8
  autoimmune E27.1
  meningococcal, hemorrhagic A39.1
Adrenarche, premature E27.0
Adrenocortical syndrome — *see* Cushing's, syndrome
Adrenogenital syndrome E25.9
  acquired E25.8
  congenital E25.0
  salt loss E25.0
Adrenogenitalism, congenital E25.0
Adrenoleukodystrophy E71.529
  neonatal E71.511
  X-linked E71.529
    Addison only phenotype E71.528
    Addison-Schilder E71.528
    adolescent E71.521
    adrenomyeloneuropathy E71.522
    childhood cerebral E71.520
    other specified E71.528
Adrenomyeloneuropathy E71.522
Adventitious bursa — *see* Bursopathy, specified type NEC
Adverse effect — *see* Table of Drugs and Chemicals, categories T36-T50, with 6th character 5
Advice — *see* Counseling
Adynamia (episodica) (hereditary) (periodic) G72.3
Aeration lung imperfect, newborn — *see* Atelectasis
Aerobullosis T70.3 ☑
Aerocele — *see* Embolism, air
Aerodermectasia
  subcutaneous (traumatic) T79.7 ☑
Aerodontalgia T70.29 ☑
Aeroembolism T70.3 ☑
Aerogenes capsulatus infection A48.0
Aero-otitis media T70.0 ☑
Aerophagy, aerophagia (psychogenic) F45.8
Aerophobia F40.228
Aerosinusitis T70.1 ☑
Aerotitis T70.0 ☑
Affection — *see* Disease
Afibrinogenemia — *see also* Defect, coagulation D68.8
  acquired D65
  congenital D68.2
  following ectopic or molar pregnancy O08.1
  in abortion — *see* Abortion, by type, complicated by, afibrinogenemia
  puerperal O72.3
African
  sleeping sickness B56.9
  tick fever A68.1
  trypanosomiasis B56.9
    gambian B56.0
    rhodesian B56.1
Aftercare — *see also* Care Z51.89
  following surgery (for) (on)
    amputation Z47.81
    attention to
      drains Z48.03
      dressings (nonsurgical) Z48.00

Aftercare — *continued*
  following surgery — *continued*
    attention to — *continued*
      dressings — *continued*
        surgical Z48.01
        sutures Z48.02
    circulatory system Z48.812
    delayed (planned) wound closure Z48.1
    digestive system Z48.815
    explantation of joint prosthesis (staged procedure)
      hip Z47.32
      knee Z47.33
      shoulder Z47.31
    genitourinary system Z48.816
    joint replacement Z47.1
    neoplasm Z48.3
    nervous system Z48.811
    oral cavity Z48.814
    organ transplant
      bone marrow Z48.290
      heart Z48.21
      heart-lung Z48.280
      kidney Z48.22
      liver Z48.23
      lung Z48.24
      multiple organs NEC Z48.288
      specified NEC Z48.298
    orthopedic NEC Z47.89
    planned wound closure Z48.1
    removal of internal fixation device Z47.2
    respiratory system Z48.813
    scoliosis Z47.82
    sense organs Z48.810
    skin and subcutaneous tissue Z48.817
    specified body system
      circulatory Z48.812
      digestive Z48.815
      genitourinary Z48.816
      nervous Z48.811
      oral cavity Z48.814
      respiratory Z48.813
      sense organs Z48.810
      skin and subcutaneous tissue Z48.817
      teeth Z48.814
    specified NEC Z48.89
    spinal Z47.89
    teeth Z48.814
  fracture — *code to* fracture with seventh character D
  involving
    removal of
      drains Z48.03
      dressings (nonsurgical) Z48.00
      staples Z48.02
      surgical dressings Z48.01
      sutures Z48.02
    neuropacemaker (brain) (peripheral nerve) (spinal cord) Z46.2
      implanted Z45.42
  orthopedic NEC Z47.89
  postprocedural — *see* Aftercare, following surgery
After-cataract — *see* Cataract, secondary
Agalactia (primary) O92.3
  elective, secondary or therapeutic O92.5
Agammaglobulinemia (acquired) (secondary) (nonfamilial) D80.1
  with
    immunoglobulin-bearing B-lymphocytes D80.1
    lymphopenia D81.9
  autosomal recessive (Swiss type) D80.0
  Bruton's X-linked D80.0
  common variable (CVAgamma) D80.1
  congenital sex-linked D80.0
  hereditary D80.0
  lymphopenic D81.9
  Swiss type (autosomal recessive) D80.0
  X-linked (with growth hormone deficiency) (Bruton) D80.0
Aganglionosis (bowel) (colon) Q43.1
Age (old) — *see* Senility
Agenesis
  adrenal (gland) Q89.1
  alimentary tract (complete) (partial) NEC Q45.8
    upper Q40.8
  anus, anal (canal) Q42.3
    with fistula Q42.2
  aorta Q25.41
  appendix Q42.8
  arm (complete) Q71.0- ☑
    with hand present Q71.1- ☑

Agenesis — *continued*
- artery (peripheral) Q27.9
  - brain Q28.3
  - coronary Q24.5
  - pulmonary Q25.79
  - specified NEC Q27.8
  - umbilical Q27.0
- auditory (canal) (external) Q16.1
- auricle (ear) Q16.0
- bile duct or passage Q44.5
- bladder Q64.5
- bone Q79.9
- brain Q00.0
  - part of Q04.3
- breast (with nipple present) Q83.8
  - with absent nipple Q83.0
- bronchus Q32.4
- canaliculus lacrimalis Q10.4
- carpus — *see* Agenesis, hand
- cartilage Q79.9
- cecum Q42.8
- cerebellum Q04.3
- cervix Q51.5
- chin Q18.8
- cilia Q10.3
- circulatory system, part NOS Q28.9
- clavicle Q74.0
- clitoris Q52.6
- coccyx Q76.49
- colon Q42.9
  - specified NEC Q42.8
- corpus callosum Q04.0
- cricoid cartilage Q31.8
- diaphragm (with hernia) Q79.1
- digestive organ(s) or tract (complete) (partial) NEC Q45.8
  - upper Q40.8
- ductus arteriosus Q28.8
- duodenum Q41.0
- ear Q16.9
  - auricle Q16.0
  - lobe Q17.8
- ejaculatory duct Q55.4
- endocrine (gland) NEC Q89.2
- epiglottis Q31.8
- esophagus Q39.8
- eustachian tube Q16.2
- eye Q11.1
  - adnexa Q15.8
- eyelid (fold) Q10.3
- face
  - bones NEC Q75.8
  - specified part NEC Q18.8
- fallopian tube Q50.6
- femur — *see* Defect, reduction, lower limb, longitudinal, femur
- fibula — *see* Defect, reduction, lower limb, longitudinal, fibula
- finger (complete) (partial) — *see* Agenesis, hand
- foot (and toes) (complete) (partial) Q72.3- ☑
- forearm (with hand present) — *see* Agenesis, arm, with hand present
  - and hand Q71.2- ☑
- gallbladder Q44.0
- gastric Q40.2
- genitalia, genital (organ(s))
  - female Q52.8
    - external Q52.71
    - internal NEC Q52.8
  - male Q55.8
- glottis Q31.8
- hair Q84.0
- hand (and fingers) (complete) (partial) Q71.3- ☑
- heart Q24.8
  - valve NEC Q24.8
    - pulmonary Q22.0
- hepatic Q44.79
- humerus — *see* Defect, reduction, upper limb
- hymen Q52.4
- ileum Q41.2
- incus Q16.3
- intestine (small) Q41.9
  - large Q42.9
    - specified NEC Q42.8
- iris (dilator fibers) Q13.1
- jaw M26.09
- jejunum Q41.1
- kidney(s) (partial) Q60.2
  - bilateral Q60.1
  - unilateral Q60.0

Agenesis — *continued*
- labium (majus) (minus) Q52.71
- labyrinth, membranous Q16.5
- lacrimal apparatus Q10.4
- larynx Q31.8
- leg (complete) Q72.0- ☑
  - with foot present Q72.1- ☑
  - lower leg (with foot present) — *see* Agenesis, leg, with foot present
  - and foot Q72.2- ☑
- lens Q12.3
- limb (complete) Q73.0
  - lower — *see* Agenesis, leg
  - upper — *see* Agenesis, arm
- lip Q38.0
- liver Q44.79
- lung (fissure) (lobe) (bilateral) (unilateral) Q33.3
- mandible, maxilla M26.09
- metacarpus — *see* Agenesis, hand
- metatarsus — *see* Agenesis, foot
- muscle Q79.8
  - eyelid Q10.3
  - ocular Q15.8
- musculoskeletal system NEC Q79.8
- nail(s) Q84.3
- neck, part Q18.8
- nerve Q07.8
- nervous system, part NEC Q07.8
- nipple Q83.2
- nose Q30.1
- nuclear Q07.8
- organ
  - of Corti Q16.5
  - or site not listed — *see* Anomaly, by site
- osseous meatus (ear) Q16.1
- ovary
  - bilateral Q50.02
  - unilateral Q50.01
- oviduct Q50.6
- pancreas Q45.0
- parathyroid (gland) Q89.2
- parotid gland(s) Q38.4
- patella Q74.1
- pelvic girdle (complete) (partial) Q74.2
- penis Q55.5
- pericardium Q24.8
- pituitary (gland) Q89.2
- prostate Q55.4
- punctum lacrimale Q10.4
- radioulnar — *see* Defect, reduction, upper limb
- radius — *see* Defect, reduction, upper limb, longitudinal, radius
- rectum Q42.1
  - with fistula Q42.0
- renal Q60.2
  - bilateral Q60.1
  - unilateral Q60.0
- respiratory organ NEC Q34.8
- rib Q76.6
- roof of orbit Q75.8
- round ligament Q52.8
- sacrum Q76.49
- salivary gland Q38.4
- scapula Q74.0
- scrotum Q55.29
- seminal vesicles Q55.4
- septum
  - atrial Q21.19
  - between aorta and pulmonary artery Q21.4
  - ventricular Q20.4
- shoulder girdle (complete) (partial) Q74.0
- skull (bone) Q75.8
  - with
    - anencephaly Q00.0
    - encephalocele — *see* Encephalocele
    - hydrocephalus Q03.9
      - with spina bifida — *see* Spina bifida, by site, with hydrocephalus
    - microcephaly Q02
- spermatic cord Q55.4
- spinal cord Q06.0
- spine Q76.49
- spleen Q89.01
- sternum Q76.7
- stomach Q40.2
- submaxillary gland(s) (congenital) Q38.4
- tarsus — *see* Agenesis, foot
- tendon Q79.8
- testicle Q55.0

Agenesis — *continued*
- thymus (gland) Q89.2
- thyroid (gland) E03.1
  - cartilage Q31.8
- tibia — *see* Defect, reduction, lower limb, longitudinal, tibia
- tibiofibular — *see* Defect, reduction, lower limb, specified type NEC
- toe (and foot) (complete) (partial) — *see* Agenesis, foot
- tongue Q38.3
- trachea (cartilage) Q32.1
- ulna — *see* Defect, reduction, upper limb, longitudinal, ulna
- upper limb — *see* Agenesis, arm
- ureter Q62.4
- urethra Q64.5
- urinary tract NEC Q64.8
- uterus Q51.0
- uvula Q38.5
- vagina Q52.0
- vas deferens Q55.4
- vein(s) (peripheral) Q27.9
  - brain Q28.3
  - great NEC Q26.8
  - portal Q26.5
- vena cava (inferior) (superior) Q26.8
- vermis of cerebellum Q04.3
- vertebra Q76.49
- vulva Q52.71

Ageusia R43.2

Agitated — *see* condition

Agitation R45.1

Aglossia (congenital) Q38.3

Aglossia-adactylia syndrome Q87.0

Aglycogenosis E74.00

Agnosia (body image) (other senses) (tactile) R48.1
- developmental F88
- verbal R48.1
  - auditory R48.1
    - developmental F80.2
  - developmental F80.2
- visual (object) R48.3

Agoraphobia F40.00
- with panic disorder F40.01
- without panic disorder F40.02

Agrammatism R48.8

Agranulocytopenia — *see* Agranulocytosis

Agranulocytosis (chronic) (cyclical) (genetic) (infantile) (periodic) (pernicious) — *see also* Neutropenia D70.9
- congenital D70.0
- cytoreductive cancer chemotherapy sequela D70.1
- drug-induced D70.2
  - due to cytoreductive cancer chemotherapy D70.1
- due to infection D70.3
- secondary D70.4
  - drug-induced D70.2
    - due to cytoreductive cancer chemotherapy D70.1

Agraphia (absolute) R48.8
- with alexia R48.0
- developmental F81.81

Ague (dumb) — *see* Malaria

Agyria Q04.3

Ahumada-del Castillo syndrome E23.0

Aichomophobia F40.298

AIDS (related complex) B20

Ailment heart — *see* Disease, heart

Ailurophobia F40.218

AIN — *see* Neoplasia, intraepithelial, anal

Ainhum (disease) L94.6

AIPHI (acute idiopathic pulmonary hemorrhage in infants (over 28 days old)) R04.81

Air
- anterior mediastinum J98.2
- compressed, disease T70.3 ☑
- conditioner lung or pneumonitis J67.7
- embolism (artery) (cerebral) (any site) T79.0 ☑
  - with ectopic or molar pregnancy O08.2
  - due to implanted device NEC — *see* Complications, by site and type, specified NEC
  - following
    - abortion — *see* Abortion by type, complicated by, embolism
    - ectopic or molar pregnancy O08.2
  - infusion, therapeutic injection or transfusion T80.0 ☑
  - in pregnancy, childbirth or puerperium — *see* Embolism, obstetric
  - traumatic T79.0 ☑
- hunger, psychogenic F45.8

Air — continued
 rarefied, effects of — see Effect, adverse, high altitude
 sickness T75.3 ☑
Airplane sickness T75.3 ☑
Akathisia (drug-induced) (treatment-induced) G25.71
 neuroleptic induced (acute) G25.71
 tardive G25.71
Akinesia R29.898
Akinetic mutism R41.89
Akureyri's disease G93.39
Alactasia, congenital E73.0
Alagille (-Watson) syndrome Q44.71
Alastrim B03
Albers-Schonberg syndrome Q78.2
Albert's syndrome — see Tendinitis, Achilles
Albinism, albino E70.30
 with hematologic abnormality E70.339
 Chediak-Higashi syndrome E70.330
 Hermansky-Pudlak syndrome E70.331
 other specified E70.338
 I E70.320
 II E70.321
 ocular E70.319
 autosomal recessive E70.311
 other specified E70.318
 X-linked E70.310
 oculocutaneous E70.329
 other specified E70.328
 tyrosinase (ty) negative E70.320
 tyrosinase (ty) positive E70.321
 other specified E70.39
Albinismus E70.30
Albright (-McCune)(-Sternberg) **syndrome** Q78.1
Albuminous — see condition
Albuminuria, albuminuric (acute) (chronic) (subacute) —
 see also Proteinuria R80.9
 complicating pregnancy — see Proteinuria, gestational
 with
 gestational hypertension — see Pre-eclampsia
 pre-existing hypertension — see Hypertension,
 complicating pregnancy, pre-existing, with,
 pre-eclampsia
 gestational — see Proteinuria, gestational
 with
 gestational hypertension — see Pre-eclampsia
 pre-existing hypertension — see Hypertension,
 complicating pregnancy, pre-existing, with,
 pre-eclampsia
 orthostatic R80.2
 postural R80.2
 pre-eclamptic — see Pre-eclampsia
 scarlatinal A38.8
Albuminurophobia F40.298
Alcaptonuria E70.29
Alcohol, alcoholic, alcohol-induced
 addiction (without remission) F10.20
 with remission F10.21
 amnestic disorder, persisting F10.96
 with dependence F10.26
 anxiety disorder F10.980
 bipolar and related disorder F10.94
 brain syndrome, chronic F10.97
 with dependence F10.27
 cardiopathy I42.6
 counseling and surveillance Z71.41
 family member Z71.42
 delirium (acute) (tremens) (withdrawal) F10.921
 with intoxication F10.921
 in
 abuse F10.121
 dependence F10.221
 abuse F10.131
 with intoxication F10.121
 dependence (acute) (tremens) (withdrawal) F10.231
 with intoxication F10.221
 use, unspecified F10.931
 with intoxication F10.921
 dementia F10.97
 with dependence F10.27
 depressive disorder F10.94
 deterioration F10.97
 with dependence F10.27
 hallucinosis (acute) F10.951
 in
 abuse F10.151
 dependence F10.251
 insanity F10.959
 intoxication (acute) (without dependence) F10.129

Alcohol, alcoholic, alcohol-induced — continued
 intoxication — continued
 with
 delirium F10.121
 dependence F10.229
 with delirium F10.221
 uncomplicated F10.220
 uncomplicated F10.120
 jealousy F10.988
 Korsakoff's, Korsakov's, Korsakow's F10.26
 liver K70.9
 acute — see Disease, liver, alcoholic, hepatitis
 major neurocognitive disorder, amnestic-confabulatory
 type F10.96
 major neurocognitive disorder, nonamnestic-confabula-
 tory type F10.97
 mania (acute) (chronic) F10.959
 mild neurocognitive disorder F10.988
 paranoia, paranoid (type) psychosis F10.950
 pellagra E52
 poisoning, accidental (acute) NEC — see Table of Drugs
 and Chemicals, alcohol, poisoning
 psychosis — see Psychosis, alcoholic
 psychotic disorder F10.959
 sexual dysfunction F10.981
 sleep disorder F10.982
 withdrawal (without convulsions) F10.239
 with delirium F10.231
Alcoholism (chronic) (without remission) F10.20
 with
 psychosis — see Psychosis, alcoholic
 remission F10.21
 Korsakov's F10.96
 with dependence F10.26
Alder (-Reilly) **anomaly or syndrome** (leukocyte granulation) D72.0
Aldosteronism E26.9
 familial (type I) E26.02
 glucocorticoid-remediable E26.02
 primary (due to (bilateral) adrenal hyperplasia) E26.09
 primary NEC E26.09
 secondary E26.1
 specified NEC E26.89
Aldosteronoma D44.10
Aldrich (-Wiskott) **syndrome** (eczema-thrombocytopenia)
 D82.0
Alektorophobia F40.218
Aleppo boil B55.1
Aleukemic — see condition
Aleukia
 congenital D70.0
 hemorrhagica D61.9
 congenital D61.09
 splenica D73.1
Alexia R48.0
 developmental F81.0
 secondary to organic lesion R48.0
Algoneurodystrophy M89.00
 ankle M89.07- ☑
 foot M89.07- ☑
 forearm M89.03- ☑
 hand M89.04- ☑
 lower leg M89.06- ☑
 multiple sites M89.0- ☑
 shoulder M89.01- ☑
 specified site NEC M89.08
 thigh M89.05- ☑
 upper arm M89.02- ☑
Algophobia F40.298
Alienation, mental — see Psychosis
Alkalemia E87.3
Alkalosis E87.3
 metabolic E87.3
 with respiratory acidosis E87.4
 of newborn P74.41
 respiratory E87.3
Alkaptonuria E70.29
Allen-Masters syndrome N83.8
Allergy, allergic (reaction) (to) T78.40 ☑
 air-borne substance NEC (rhinitis) J30.89
 alveolitis (extrinsic) J67.9
 due to
 Aspergillus clavatus J67.4
 Cryptostroma corticale J67.6
 organisms (fungal, thermophilic actinomycete)
 growing in ventilation (air conditioning)
 systems J67.7
 specified type NEC J67.8

Allergy, allergic — continued
 anaphylactic reaction or shock T78.2 ☑
 angioneurotic edema T78.3 ☑
 animal (dander) (epidermal) (hair) (rhinitis) J30.81
 bee sting (anaphylactic shock) T63.44- ☑
 biological — see Allergy, drug
 colitis — see also Colitis, allergic K52.29
 dander (animal) (rhinitis) J30.81
 dandruff (rhinitis) J30.81
 dental restorative material (existing) K08.55
 dermatitis — see Dermatitis, contact, allergic
 diathesis — see History, allergy
 drug, medicament & biological (any) (external) (internal)
 T78.40 ☑
 correct substance properly administered — see Table
 of Drugs and Chemicals, by drug, adverse effect
 wrong substance given or taken NEC (by accident) —
 see Table of Drugs and Chemicals, by drug,
 poisoning
 due to pollen J30.1
 dust (house) (stock) (rhinitis) J30.89
 with asthma — see Asthma, allergic extrinsic
 eczema — see Dermatitis, contact, allergic
 epidermal (animal) (rhinitis) J30.81
 feathers (rhinitis) J30.89
 food (any) (ingested) NEC T78.1 ☑
 anaphylactic shock — see Shock, anaphylactic, due
 to food
 dermatitis — see Dermatitis, due to, food
 dietary counseling and surveillance Z71.3
 in contact with skin L23.6
 rhinitis J30.5
 status (without reaction) Z91.018
 beef Z91.014
 eggs Z91.012
 lamb Z91.014
 mammalian meats Z91.014
 milk products Z91.011
 peanuts Z91.010
 pork Z91.014
 red meats Z91.014
 seafood Z91.013
 specified NEC Z91.018
 gastrointestinal — see also specific type of allergic reaction
 meaning colitis — see also Colitis, allergic K52.29
 meaning gastroenteritis — see also Gastroenteritis,
 allergic K52.29
 meaning other adverse food reaction not elsewhere
 classified T78.1 ☑
 grain J30.1
 grass (hay fever) (pollen) J30.1
 asthma — see Asthma, allergic extrinsic
 hair (animal) (rhinitis) J30.81
 history (of) — see History, allergy
 horse serum — see Allergy, serum
 inhalant (rhinitis) J30.89
 pollen J30.1
 kapok (rhinitis) J30.89
 medicine — see Allergy, drug
 milk protein — see also Allergy, food Z91.011
 anaphylactic reaction T78.07 ☑
 dermatitis L27.2
 enterocolitis syndrome K52.21
 enteropathy K52.22
 gastroenteritis K52.29
 gastroesophageal reflux — see also Reaction, adverse,
 food K21.9
 with esophagitis (without bleeding) K21.00
 with bleeding K21.01
 proctocolitis K52.29
 nasal, seasonal due to pollen J30.1
 pneumonia J82.89
 pollen (any) (hay fever) J30.1
 asthma — see Asthma, allergic extrinsic
 primrose J30.1
 primula J30.1
 proctocolitis K52.29
 purpura D69.0
 ragweed (hay fever) (pollen) J30.1
 asthma — see Asthma, allergic extrinsic
 rose (pollen) J30.1
 seasonal NEC J30.2
 Senecio jacobae (pollen) J30.1
 serum — see also Reaction, serum T80.69 ☑
 anaphylactic shock T80.59 ☑
 shock (anaphylactic) T78.2 ☑

Allergy, allergic — *continued*
  shock — *continued*
    due to
      administration of blood and blood products
        T80.51 ☑
      adverse effect of correct medicinal substance
        properly administered T88.6 ☑
      immunization T80.52 ☑
      serum NEC T80.59 ☑
      vaccination T80.52 ☑
    specific NEC T78.49 ☑
    tree (any) (hay fever) (pollen) J30.1
      asthma — *see* Asthma, allergic extrinsic
    upper respiratory J30.9
    urticaria L50.0
    vaccine — *see* Allergy, serum
    wheat — *see* Allergy, food
Allescheriasis B48.2
Alligator skin disease Q80.9
Allocheiria, allochiria R20.8
Almeida's disease — *see* Paracoccidioidomycosis
Alopecia (hereditaria) (seborrheica) L65.9
    androgenic L64.9
      drug-induced L64.0
      specified NEC L64.8
    areata L63.9
      ophiasis L63.2
      specified NEC L63.8
      totalis L63.0
      universalis L63.1
    cicatricial L66.9
      central centrifugal L66.81
      specified NEC L66.89
    circumscripta L63.9
    congenital, congenitalis Q84.0
    due to cytotoxic drugs NEC L65.8
    frontal fibrosing L66.12
    mucinosa L65.2
    postinfective NEC L65.8
    postpartum L65.0
    premature L64.8
    specific (syphilitic) A51.32
    specified NEC L65.8
    syphilitic (secondary) A51.32
    totalis (capitis) L63.0
    universalis (entire body) L63.1
    X-ray L58.1
Alpers' disease G31.81
Alpine sickness T70.29 ☑
Alport syndrome Q87.81
ALTE (apparent life threatening event) **in newborn and
    infant** R68.13
Alteration (of), **Altered**
    awareness
      transient R40.4
      unintended under general anesthesia, during proce-
        dure T88.53 ☑
    mental status R41.82
    pattern of family relationships affecting child Z62.898
    sensation
      following
        cerebrovascular disease I69.998
          cerebral infarction I69.398
          intracerebral hemorrhage I69.198
          nontraumatic intracranial hemorrhage NEC
            I69.298
          specified disease NEC I69.898
          subarachnoid hemorrhage I69.098
Alternating — *see* condition
Altitude, high (effects) — *see* Effect, adverse, high altitude
Aluminosis (of lung) J63.0
Alveolitis
    allergic (extrinsic) — *see* Pneumonitis, hypersensitivity
    due to
      Aspergillus clavatus J67.4
      Cryptostroma corticale J67.6
    fibrosing (cryptogenic) (idiopathic) J84.112
    jaw M27.3
    sicca dolorosa M27.3
Alveolus, alveolar — *see* condition
Alymphocytosis D72.810
    thymic (with immunodeficiency) D82.1
Alymphoplasia, thymic D82.1
Alzheimer's disease or sclerosis — *see* Disease,
    Alzheimer's
Amastia (with nipple present) Q83.8
    with absent nipple Q83.0
Amathophobia F40.228

Amaurosis (acquired) (congenital) — *see also* Blindness
    fugax G45.3
    hysterical F44.6
    Leber's congenital H35.50
    uremic — *see* Uremia
Amaurotic idiocy (infantile) (juvenile) (late) E75.4
Amaxophobia F40.248
Ambiguous genitalia Q56.4
Amblyopia (congenital) (ex anopsia) (partial) (suppression)
    H53.00- ☑
    anisometropic — *see* Amblyopia, refractive
    deprivation H53.01- ☑
    hysterical F44.6
    nocturnal — *see also* Blindness, night
      vitamin A deficiency E50.5
    refractive H53.02- ☑
    strabismic H53.03- ☑
    suspect H53.04- ☑
    tobacco H53.8
    toxic NEC H53.8
    uremic — *see* Uremia
Ameba, amebic (histolytica) — *see also* Amebiasis
    abscess (liver) A06.4
Amebiasis A06.9
    with abscess — *see* Abscess, amebic
    acute A06.0
    chronic (intestine) A06.1
      with abscess — *see* Abscess, amebic
    cutaneous A06.7
    cutis A06.7
    cystitis A06.81
    genitourinary tract NEC A06.82
    hepatic — *see* Abscess, liver, amebic
    intestine A06.0
    nondysenteric colitis A06.2
    skin A06.7
    specified site NEC A06.89
Ameboma (of intestine) A06.3
Amelia Q73.0
    lower limb — *see* Agenesis, leg
    upper limb — *see* Agenesis, arm
Ameloblastoma — *see also* Cyst, calcifying odontogenic
    long bones C40.9- ☑
      lower limb C40.2- ☑
      upper limb C40.0- ☑
    malignant C41.1
      jaw (bone) (lower) C41.1
        upper C41.0
    tibial C40.2- ☑
Amelogenesis imperfecta K00.5
    nonhereditaria (segmentalis) K00.4
Amenorrhea N91.2
    hyperhormonal E28.8
    primary N91.0
    secondary N91.1
Amentia — *see* Disability, intellectual
    Meynert's (nonalcoholic) F04
American
    leishmaniasis B55.2
    mountain tick fever A93.2
Ametropia — *see* Disorder, refraction
AMH (asymptomatic microscopic hematuria) R31.21
Amianthosis J61
Amimia R48.8
Amino-acid disorder E72.9
    anemia D53.0
Aminoacidopathy E72.9
Aminoaciduria E72.9
Amnesia R41.3
    anterograde R41.1
    auditory R48.8
    dissociative F44.0
      with dissociative fugue F44.1
    hysterical F44.0
    postictal in epilepsy — *see* Epilepsy
    psychogenic F44.0
    retrograde R41.2
    transient global G45.4
Amnes(t)ic syndrome (post-traumatic) F04
    induced by
      alcohol F10.96
        with dependence F10.26
      psychoactive NEC F19.96
        with
          abuse F19.16
          dependence F19.26
      sedative F13.96
        with dependence F13.26

Amnion, amniotic — *see* condition
Amnionitis — *see* Pregnancy, complicated by
Amok F68.8
Amoral traits F60.89
Amphetamine (or other stimulant) **-induced**
    anxiety disorder F15.980
    bipolar and related disorder F15.94
    delirium F15.921
    depressive disorder F15.94
    obsessive-compulsive and related disorder F15.988
    psychotic disorder F15.959
    sexual dysfunction F15.981
    sleep disorder F15.982
    stimulant withdrawal F15.23
Ampulla
    lower esophagus K22.89
    phrenic K22.89
Amputation — *see also* Absence, by site, acquired
    neuroma (postoperative) (traumatic) — *see* Complica-
      tions, amputation stump, neuroma
    stump (surgical)
      abnormal, painful, or with complication (late) — *see*
        Complications, amputation stump
      healed or old NOS Z89.9
    traumatic (complete) (partial)
      arm (upper) (complete) S48.91- ☑
        at
          elbow S58.01- ☑
            partial S58.02- ☑
          shoulder joint (complete) S48.01- ☑
            partial S48.02- ☑
        between
          elbow and wrist (complete) S58.11- ☑
            partial S58.12- ☑
          shoulder and elbow (complete) S48.11- ☑
            partial S48.12- ☑
        partial S48.92- ☑
      breast (complete) S28.21- ☑
        partial S28.22- ☑
      clitoris (complete) S38.211
        partial S38.212
      ear (complete) S08.11- ☑
        partial S08.12- ☑
      finger (complete) (metacarpophalangeal) S68.11- ☑
        index S68.11- ☑
        little S68.11- ☑
        middle S68.11- ☑
        partial S68.12- ☑
          index S68.12- ☑
          little S68.12- ☑
          middle S68.12- ☑
          ring S68.12- ☑
        ring S68.11- ☑
        thumb — *see* Amputation, traumatic, thumb
        transphalangeal (complete) S68.61- ☑
          index S68.61- ☑
          little S68.61- ☑
          middle S68.61- ☑
          partial S68.62- ☑
            index S68.62- ☑
            little S68.62- ☑
            middle S68.62- ☑
            ring S68.62- ☑
          ring S68.61- ☑
      foot (complete) S98.91- ☑
        at ankle level S98.01- ☑
          partial S98.02- ☑
        midfoot S98.31- ☑
          partial S98.32- ☑
        partial S98.92- ☑
      forearm (complete) S58.91- ☑
        at elbow level (complete) S58.01- ☑
          partial S58.02- ☑
        between elbow and wrist (complete) S58.11- ☑
          partial S58.12- ☑
        partial S58.92- ☑
      genital organ(s) (external)
        female (complete) S38.211 ☑
          partial S38.212 ☑
        male
          penis (complete) S38.221 ☑
            partial S38.222 ☑
          scrotum (complete) S38.231 ☑
            partial S38.232 ☑
          testes (complete) S38.231 ☑
            partial S38.232 ☑

Amputation — *continued*
  traumatic — *continued*
    hand (complete) (wrist level) S68.41- ☑
      finger(s) alone — *see* Amputation, traumatic, finger
      partial S68.42- ☑
      thumb alone — *see* Amputation, traumatic, thumb
      transmetacarpal (complete) S68.71- ☑
        partial S68.72- ☑
    head
      ear — *see* Amputation, traumatic, ear
      nose (partial) S08.812 ☑
        complete S08.811 ☑
      part S08.89 ☑
        scalp S08.0 ☑
    hip (and thigh) (complete) S78.91- ☑
      at hip joint (complete) S78.01- ☑
        partial S78.02- ☑
      between hip and knee (complete) S78.11- ☑
        partial S78.12- ☑
      partial S78.92- ☑
    labium (majus) (minus) (complete) S38.21- ☑
      partial S38.21- ☑
    leg (lower) S88.91- ☑
      at knee level S88.01- ☑
        partial S88.02- ☑
      between knee and ankle S88.11- ☑
        partial S88.12- ☑
      partial S88.92- ☑
    nose (partial) S08.812 ☑
      complete S08.811 ☑
    penis (complete) S38.221 ☑
      partial S38.222 ☑
    scrotum (complete) S38.231 ☑
      partial S38.232 ☑
    shoulder — *see* Amputation, traumatic, arm
      at shoulder joint — *see* Amputation, traumatic, arm, at shoulder joint
    testes (complete) S38.231 ☑
      partial S38.232 ☑
    thigh — *see* Amputation, traumatic, hip
    thorax, part of S28.1 ☑
      breast — *see* Amputation, traumatic, breast
    thumb (complete) (metacarpophalangeal) S68.01- ☑
      partial S68.02- ☑
      transphalangeal (complete) S68.51- ☑
        partial S68.52- ☑
    toe (lesser) S98.13- ☑
      great S98.11- ☑
        partial S98.12- ☑
      more than one S98.21- ☑
        partial S98.22- ☑
      partial S98.14- ☑
    vulva (complete) S38.211 ☑
      partial S38.212 ☑
Amputee (bilateral) (old) Z89.9
Amsterdam dwarfism Q87.19
Amusia R48.8
  developmental F80.89
Amyelencephalus, amyelencephaly Q00.0
Amyelia Q06.0
Amygdalitis — *see* Tonsillitis
Amygdalolith J35.8
Amyloid heart (disease) E85.4 *[I43]*
Amyloidosis (generalized) (primary) E85.9
  with lung involvement E85.4 *[J99]*
  familial E85.2
  genetic E85.2
  heart E85.4 *[I43]*
  hemodialysis-associated E85.3
  light chain (AL) E85.81
  liver E85.4 *[K77]*
  localized E85.4
  neuropathic heredofamilial E85.1
  non-neuropathic heredofamilial E85.0
  organ limited E85.4
  Portuguese E85.1
  pulmonary E85.4 *[J99]*
  secondary systemic E85.3
  senile systemic (SSA) E85.82
  skin (lichen) (macular) E85.4 *[L99]*
  specified NEC E85.89
  subglottic E85.4 *[J99]*
  wild-type transthyretin-related (ATTR) E85.82
Amylopectinosis (brancher enzyme deficiency) E74.03
Amylophagia — *see* Pica
Amyoplasia congenita Q79.8

Amyotonia M62.89
  congenita G70.2
Amyotrophia, amyotrophy, amyotrophic G71.8
  congenita Q79.8
  diabetic — *see* Diabetes, amyotrophy
  lateral sclerosis G12.21
  neuralgic G54.5
  spinal progressive G12.25
Anacidity, gastric K31.83
  psychogenic F45.8
Anaerosis of newborn P28.89
Analbuminemia E88.09
Analgesia — *see* Anesthesia
Analphalipoproteinemia E78.6
Anaphylactic
  purpura D69.0
  shock or reaction — *see* Shock, anaphylactic
Anaphylactoid shock or reaction — *see* Shock, anaphylactic
Anaphylactoid syndrome of pregnancy O88.01- ☑
Anaphylaxis — *see* Shock, anaphylactic
Anaplasia cervix — *see also* Dysplasia, cervix N87.9
Anaplasmosis [A. phagocytophilum] (transfusion transmitted) A79.82
  human A77.49
Anarthria R47.1
Anasarca R60.1
  cardiac — *see* Failure, heart, congestive
  lung J18.2
  newborn P83.2
  nutritional E43
  pulmonary J18.2
  renal N04.9
Anastomosis
  aneurysmal — *see* Aneurysm
  arteriovenous ruptured brain I60.8
    intracerebral I61.8
    intraparenchymal I61.8
    intraventricular I61.5
    subarachnoid I60.8
  intestinal K63.89
    complicated NEC K91.89
      involving urinary tract N99.89
  retinal and choroidal vessels (congenital) Q14.8
Anatomical narrow angle H40.03- ☑
Ancylostoma, ancylostomiasis (braziliense) (caninum) (ceylanicum) (duodenale) B76.0
  Necator americanus B76.1
Andersen's disease (glycogen storage) E74.09
Anderson-Fabry disease E75.21
Andes disease T70.29 ☑
Andrews' disease (bacterid) L08.89
Androblastoma
  benign
    specified site — *see* Neoplasm, benign, by site
    unspecified site
      female D27.9
      male D29.20
  malignant
    specified site — *see* Neoplasm, malignant, by site
    unspecified site
      female C56.9
      male C62.90
  specified site — *see* Neoplasm, uncertain behavior, by site
  tubular
    with lipid storage
      specified site — *see* Neoplasm, benign, by site
      unspecified site
        female D27.9
        male D29.20
    specified site — *see* Neoplasm, benign, by site
    unspecified site
      female D27.9
      male D29.20
  unspecified site
    female D39.10
    male D40.10
Androgen insensitivity syndrome — *see also* Syndrome, androgen insensitivity E34.50
Androgen resistance syndrome — *see also* Syndrome, androgen insensitivity E34.50
Android pelvis Q74.2
  with disproportion (fetopelvic) O33.3 ☑
    causing obstructed labor O65.3
Androphobia F40.290
Anectasis, pulmonary (newborn) — *see* Atelectasis
Anemia (essential) (general) (hemoglobin deficiency) (infantile) (primary) (profound) D64.9

Anemia — *continued*
  with (due to) (in)
    disorder of
      anaerobic glycolysis D55.29
      pentose phosphate pathway D55.1
    koilonychia D50.9
  achlorhydric D50.8
  achrestic D53.1
  Addison (-Biermer) (pernicious) D51.0
  agranulocytic — *see* Agranulocytosis
  amino-acid-deficiency D53.0
  aplastic D61.9
    congenital D61.09
    drug-induced D61.1
    due to
      drugs D61.1
      external agents NEC D61.2
      infection D61.2
      radiation D61.2
    idiopathic D61.3
    red cell (pure) D60.9
      chronic D60.0
      congenital D61.01
      specified type NEC D60.8
      transient D60.1
    specified type NEC D61.89
    toxic D61.2
  aregenerative
    congenital D61.09
  asiderotic D50.9
  atypical (primary) D64.9
  Baghdad spring D55.0
  Balantidium coli A07.0
  Biermer's (pernicious) D51.0
  blood loss (chronic) D50.0
    acute D62
  bothriocephalus B70.0 *[D63.8]*
  brickmaker's B76.9 *[D63.8]*
  cerebral I67.89
  childhood D58.9
  chlorotic D50.8
  chronic
    blood loss D50.0
    hemolytic D58.9
      idiopathic D59.9
    simple D53.9
  chronica congenita aregenerativa D61.09
  combined system disease NEC D51.0 *[G32.0]*
    due to dietary vitamin B12 deficiency D51.3 *[G32.0]*
  complicating pregnancy, childbirth or puerperium — *see* Pregnancy, complicated by (management affected by), anemia
  congenital P61.4
    aplastic D61.09
    due to isoimmunization NOS P55.9
    dyserythropoietic, dyshematopoietic D64.4
    following fetal blood loss P61.3
    Heinz body D58.2
    hereditary hemolytic NOS D58.9
    pernicious D51.0
    spherocytic D58.0
  Cooley's (erythroblastic) D56.1
  cytogenic D51.0
  deficiency D53.9
    2, 3 diphosphoglycurate mutase D55.29
    2, 3 PG D55.29
    6 phosphogluconate dehydrogenase D55.1
    6-PGD D55.1
    amino-acid D53.0
    combined B12 and folate D53.1
    enzyme D55.9
      drug-induced (hemolytic) D59.2
      glucose-6-phosphate dehydrogenase (G6PD) D55.0
      glycolytic D55.29
      nucleotide metabolism D55.3
      related to hexose monophosphate (HMP) shunt pathway NEC D55.1
      specified type NEC D55.8
    erythrocytic glutathione D55.1
    folate D52.9
      dietary D52.0
      drug-induced D52.1
    folic acid D52.9
      dietary D52.0
      drug-induced D52.1
    G SH D55.1
    G6PD D55.0
    GGS-R D55.1

☑ **Additional Character Required** — **Refer to the Tabular List for Character Selection**

Anemia — continued

deficiency — continued
- glucose-6-phosphate dehydrogenase D55.0
- glutathione reductase D55.1
- glyceraldehyde phosphate dehydrogenase D55.29
- hexokinase D55.29
- iron D50.9
  - secondary to blood loss (chronic) D50.0
- nutritional D53.9
  - with
    - poor iron absorption D50.8
    - specified deficiency NEC D53.8
- phosphofructo-aldolase D55.29
- phosphoglycerate kinase D55.29
- PK D55.21
- protein D53.0
- pyruvate kinase D55.21
- transcobalamin II D51.2
- triose-phosphate isomerase D55.29
- vitamin B12 NOS D51.9
  - dietary D51.3
  - due to
    - intrinsic factor deficiency D51.0
    - selective vitamin B12 malabsorption with proteinuria D51.1
  - pernicious D51.0
  - specified type NEC D51.8

Diamond-Blackfan (congenital hypoplastic) D61.01
dibothriocephalus B70.0 [D63.8]
dimorphic D53.1
diphasic D53.1
Diphyllobothrium (Dibothriocephalus) B70.0 [D63.8]
due to (in) (with)
- antineoplastic chemotherapy D64.81
- blood loss (chronic) D50.0
  - acute D62
- chemotherapy, antineoplastic D64.81
- chronic disease classified elsewhere NEC D63.8
- chronic kidney disease D63.1
- deficiency
  - amino-acid D53.0
  - copper D53.8
  - folate (folic acid) D52.9
    - dietary D52.0
    - drug-induced D52.1
  - molybdenum D53.8
  - protein D53.0
  - zinc D53.8
- dietary vitamin B12 deficiency D51.3
- disorder of
  - glutathione metabolism D55.1
  - nucleotide metabolism D55.3
- drug — see Anemia, by type — see also Table of Drugs and Chemicals
- end stage renal disease D63.1
- enzyme disorder D55.9
- fetal blood loss P61.3
- fish tapeworm (D.latum) infestation B70.0 [D63.8]
- hemorrhage (chronic) D50.0
  - acute D62
- impaired absorption D50.9
- loss of blood (chronic) D50.0
  - acute D62
- myxedema E03.9 [D63.8]
- Necator americanus B76.1 [D63.8]
- prematurity P61.2
- selective vitamin B12 malabsorption with proteinuria D51.1
- transcobalamin II deficiency D51.2
Dyke-Young type (secondary) (symptomatic) D59.19
dyserythropoietic (congenital) D64.4
dyshematopoietic (congenital) D64.4
Egyptian B76.9 [D63.8]
elliptocytosis — see Elliptocytosis
enzyme-deficiency, drug-induced D59.2
epidemic — see also Ancylostomiasis B76.9 [D63.8]
erythroblastic
- familial D56.1
- newborn — see also Disease, hemolytic P55.9
- of childhood D56.1
erythrocytic glutathione deficiency D55.1
erythropoietin-resistant anemia (EPO resistant anemia) D63.1
Faber's (achlorhydric anemia) D50.9
factitious (self-induced blood letting) D50.0
familial erythroblastic D56.1
Fanconi ('s) D61.03
favism D55.0
fish tapeworm (D. latum) infestation B70.0 [D63.8]

Anemia — continued

folate (folic acid) deficiency D52.9
glucose-6-phosphate dehydrogenase (G6PD) deficiency D55.0
glutathione-reductase deficiency D55.1
goat's milk D52.0
granulocytic — see Agranulocytosis
Heinz body, congenital D58.2
hemolytic D58.9
- acquired D59.9
  - with hemoglobinuria NEC D59.6
  - autoimmune NEC D59.19
  - infectious D59.4
  - specified type NEC D59.8
  - toxic D59.4
- acute D59.9
  - due to enzyme deficiency specified type NEC D55.8
  - Lederer's D59.19
- autoimmune D59.10
  - cold D59.12
  - drug-induced D59.0
  - mixed D59.13
  - warm D59.11
- chronic D58.9
  - idiopathic D59.9
- cold type (primary) (secondary) (symptomatic) D59.12
- congenital (spherocytic) — see Spherocytosis
- due to
  - cardiac conditions D59.4
  - drugs (nonautoimmune) D59.2
    - autoimmune D59.0
  - enzyme disorder D55.9
    - drug-induced D59.2
  - presence of shunt or other internal prosthetic device D59.4
- familial D58.9
- hereditary D58.9
  - due to enzyme disorder D55.9
    - specified type NEC D55.8
  - specified type NEC D58.8
- idiopathic (chronic) D59.9
- mechanical D59.4
- microangiopathic D59.4
- mixed type (primary) (secondary) (symptomatic) D59.13
- nonautoimmune D59.4
  - drug-induced D59.2
- nonspherocytic
  - congenital or hereditary NEC D55.8
    - glucose-6-phosphate dehydrogenase deficiency D55.0
    - pyruvate kinase deficiency D55.21
    - type
      - I D55.1
      - II D55.29
  - type
    - I D55.1
    - II D55.29
- primary
  - autoimmune
    - cold type D59.12
    - mixed type D59.13
    - warm type D59.11
- secondary D59.4
  - autoimmune
    - cold type D59.12
    - mixed type D59.13
    - warm type D59.11
- specified (hereditary) type NEC D58.8
- Stransky-Regala type — see also Hemoglobinopathy D58.8
- symptomatic D59.4
  - autoimmune
    - cold type D59.12
    - mixed type D59.13
    - warm type D59.11
- toxic D59.4
- warm type (primary) (secondary) (symptomatic) D59.11
hemorrhagic (chronic) D50.0
- acute D62
Herrick's D57.1
hexokinase deficiency D55.29
hookworm B76.9 [D63.8]
hypochromic (idiopathic) (microcytic) (normoblastic) D50.9
- due to blood loss (chronic) D50.0
  - acute D62
- familial sex-linked D64.0

Anemia — continued

hypochromic — continued
- pyridoxine-responsive D64.3
- sideroblastic, sex-linked D64.0
hypoplasia, red blood cells D61.9
- congenital or familial D61.01
hypoplastic (idiopathic) D61.9
- congenital or familial (of childhood) D61.01
hypoproliferative (refractive) D61.9
idiopathic D64.9
- aplastic D61.3
- hemolytic, chronic D59.9
in (due to) (with)
- chronic kidney disease D63.1
- end stage renal disease D63.1
- failure, kidney (renal) D63.1
- neoplastic disease — see also Neoplasm D63.0
intertropical — see also Ancylostomiasis D63.8
iron deficiency D50.9
- secondary to blood loss (chronic) D50.0
  - acute D62
- specified type NEC D50.8
Joseph-Diamond-Blackfan (congenital hypoplastic) D61.01
Lederer's (hemolytic) D59.19
leukoerythroblastic D61.82
macrocytic D53.9
- nutritional D52.0
- tropical D52.8
malarial — see also Malaria B54 [D63.8]
malignant (progressive) D51.0
malnutrition D53.9
marsh — see also Malaria B54 [D63.8]
Mediterranean (with other hemoglobinopathy) D56.9
megaloblastic D53.1
- combined B12 and folate deficiency D53.1
- hereditary D51.1
- nutritional D52.0
- orotic aciduria D53.0
- refractory D53.1
- specified type NEC D53.1
megalocytic D53.1
microcytic (hypochromic) D50.9
- due to blood loss (chronic) D50.0
  - acute D62
- familial D56.8
microdrepanocytosis D57.40
microelliptopoikilocytic (Rietti-Greppi- Micheli) D56.9
miner's B76.9 [D63.8]
myelodysplastic D46.9
myelofibrosis D75.81
myelogenous D64.89
myelopathic D64.89
myelophthisic D61.82
myeloproliferative D47.Z9 (following D47.4)
newborn P61.4
- due to
  - ABO (antibodies, isoimmunization, maternal/fetal incompatibility) P55.1
  - Rh (antibodies, isoimmunization, maternal/fetal incompatibility) P55.0
- following fetal blood loss P61.3
- posthemorrhagic (fetal) P61.3
nonspherocytic hemolytic — see Anemia, hemolytic, nonspherocytic
normocytic (infectional) D64.9
- due to blood loss (chronic) D50.0
  - acute D62
- myelophthisic D61.82
nutritional (deficiency) D53.9
- with
  - poor iron absorption D50.8
  - specified deficiency NEC D53.8
- megaloblastic D52.0
of prematurity P61.2
orotaciduric (congenital) (hereditary) D53.0
osteosclerotic D64.89
ovalocytosis (hereditary) — see Elliptocytosis
paludal — see also Malaria B54 [D63.8]
pernicious (congenital) (malignant) (progressive) D51.0
pleochromic D64.89
- of sprue D52.8
posthemorrhagic (chronic) D50.0
- acute D62
- newborn P61.3
postoperative (postprocedural)
- due to (acute) blood loss D62
  - chronic blood loss D50.0
- specified NEC D64.89

☑ **Additional Character Required — Refer to the Tabular List for Character Selection**

Anemia — continued
  postpartum O9Ø.81
  pressure D64.89
  progressive D64.9
    malignant D51.Ø
    pernicious D51.Ø
  protein-deficiency D53.Ø
  pseudoleukemica infantum D64.89
  pure red cell D6Ø.9
    congenital D61.Ø1
  pyridoxine-responsive D64.3
  pyruvate kinase deficiency D55.21
  refractory D46.4
    with
      excess of blasts D46.2Ø
        1 (RAEB 1) D46.21
        2 (RAEB 2) D46.22
        in transformation (RAEB T) — see Leukemia,
          acute myeloblastic
      hemochromatosis D46.1
      sideroblasts (ring) (RARS) D46.1
    megaloblastic D53.1
    sideroblastic D46.1
    sideropenic D5Ø.9
    without ring sideroblasts, so stated D46.Ø
    without sideroblasts without excess of blasts D46.Ø
  Rietti-Greppi-Micheli D56.9
  scorbutic D53.2
  secondary to
    blood loss (chronic) D5Ø.Ø
      acute D62
    hemorrhage (chronic) D5Ø.Ø
      acute D62
  semiplastic D61.89
  sickle-cell — see Disease, sickle-cell
  sideroblastic D64.3
    hereditary D64.Ø
    hypochromic, sex-linked D64.Ø
    pyridoxine-responsive NEC D64.3
    refractory D46.1
    secondary (due to)
      disease D64.1
      drugs and toxins D64.2
    specified type NEC D64.3
  sideropenic (refractory) D5Ø.9
    due to blood loss (chronic) D5Ø.Ø
      acute D62
  simple chronic D53.9
  specified type NEC D64.89
  spherocytic (hereditary) — see Spherocytosis
  splenic D64.89
  splenomegalic D64.89
  stomatocytosis D58.8
  syphilitic (acquired) (late) A52.79 [D63.8]
  target cell D64.89
  thalassemia D56.9
  thrombocytopenic — see Thrombocytopenia
  toxic D61.2
  tropical B76.9 [D63.8]
    macrocytic D52.8
  tuberculous A18.89 [D63.8]
  vegan D51.3
  vitamin
    B12 deficiency (dietary) pernicious D51.Ø
    B6-responsive D64.3
  von Jaksch's D64.89
  Witts' (achlorhydric anemia) D5Ø.8
Anemophobia F4Ø.228
Anencephalus, anencephaly QØØ.Ø
Anergasia — see Psychosis, organic
Anesthesia, anesthetic R2Ø.Ø
  complication or reaction NEC — see also Complications,
    anesthesia T88.59 ☑
    due to
      correct substance properly administered — see
        Table of Drugs and Chemicals, by drug, ad-
        verse effect
      overdose or wrong substance given — see Table
        of Drugs and Chemicals, by drug, poisoning
    unintended awareness under general anesthesia
      during procedure T88.53 ☑
    personal history of Z92.84
  cornea H18.81- ☑
  dissociative F44.6
  functional (hysterical) F44.6
  hyperesthetic, thalamic G89.Ø
  hysterical F44.6
  local skin lesion R2Ø.Ø
  sexual (psychogenic) F52.1

Anesthesia, anesthetic — continued
  shock (due to) T88.2 ☑
  skin R2Ø.Ø
  testicular N5Ø.Ø
Anetoderma (maculosum) (of) L9Ø.8
  Jadassohn-Pellizzari L9Ø.2
  Schweninger-Buzzi L9Ø.1
Aneurin deficiency E51.9
Aneurysm (anastomotic) (artery) (cirsoid) (diffuse) (false)
    (fusiform) (multiple) (saccular) I72.9
  abdominal (aorta) I71.4Ø
    infrarenal I71.43
      ruptured I71.33
    juxtarenal I71.42
      ruptured I71.32
    pararenal I71.41
      ruptured I71.31
    ruptured I71.3Ø
    syphilitic A52.Ø1
  aorta, aortic (nonsyphilitic) I71.9
    abdominal I71.4Ø
      dissecting — see Dissection, aorta, abdominal
      ruptured I71.3Ø
    arch I71.22
      ruptured I71.12
    arteriosclerotic I71.9
      ruptured I71.8
    ascending I71.21
      ruptured I71.11
    congenital Q25.43
    descending I71.9
      abdominal I71.4Ø
        ruptured I71.3Ø
      ruptured I71.8
      thoracic I71.23
        ruptured I71.13
    dissecting — see Dissection, aorta
    root Q25.43
    ruptured I71.8
    sinus, congenital Q25.43
    syphilitic A52.Ø1
    thoracic I71.2Ø
      ruptured I71.1Ø
    thoracoabdominal I71.6Ø
      paravisceral I71.62
        ruptured I71.52
      supraceliac I71.61
        ruptured I71.51
    thorax, thoracic I71.2Ø
      arch I71.22
        ruptured I71.12
      ascending I71.21
        ruptured I71.11
      descending I71.23
        ruptured I71.13
      ruptured I71.1Ø
        arch I71.12
        ascending I71.11
        descending I71.13
    transverse I71.22
      ruptured I71.12
    valve (heart) — see also Endocarditis, aortic I35.8
  arteriosclerotic I72.9
    cerebral I67.1
      ruptured — see Hemorrhage, intracranial, sub-
        arachnoid
  arteriovenous (congenital) — see also Malformation, ar-
    teriovenous
    acquired I77.Ø
      brain I67.1
        ruptured — see Aneurysm, arteriovenous,
          brain, ruptured
      coronary I25.41
      pulmonary I28.Ø
    brain Q28.2
      ruptured I6Ø.8
        intracerebral I61.8
        intraparenchymal I61.8
        intraventricular I61.5
        subarachnoid I6Ø.8
    peripheral — see Malformation, arteriovenous, periph-
      eral
    precerebral vessels Q28.Ø
    specified site NEC — see also Malformation, arteriove-
      nous
      acquired I77.Ø
  basal — see Aneurysm, brain
  basilar (trunk) I72.5

Aneurysm — continued
  berry (congenital) (nonruptured) I67.1
    ruptured I6Ø.7
  brain I67.1
    arteriosclerotic I67.1
      ruptured — see Hemorrhage, intracranial, sub-
        arachnoid
    arteriovenous (congenital) (nonruptured) Q28.2
      acquired I67.1
        ruptured — see Aneurysm, arteriovenous,
          brain, ruptured
      ruptured — see Aneurysm, arteriovenous, brain,
        ruptured
    berry (congenital) (nonruptured) I67.1
      ruptured — see also Hemorrhage, intracranial,
        subarachnoid I6Ø.7
    congenital Q28.3
      ruptured I6Ø.7
    meninges I67.1
      ruptured I6Ø.8
    miliary (congenital) (nonruptured) I67.1
      ruptured — see also Hemorrhage, intracranial,
        subarachnoid I6Ø.7
    mycotic I67.1
      with endocarditis — see also Endocarditis
      ruptured — see Aneurysm, arteriovenous, brain,
        ruptured I6Ø.8
    syphilitic (hemorrhage) A52.Ø5
  cardiac (false) — see also Aneurysm, heart I25.3
  carotid artery (common) (external) I72.Ø
    internal (intracranial) I67.1
      extracranial portion I72.Ø
    ruptured into brain I6Ø.Ø- ☑
    syphilitic A52.Ø9
      intracranial A52.Ø5
  cavernous sinus I67.1
    arteriovenous (congenital) (nonruptured) Q28.3
      ruptured I6Ø.8
  celiac I72.8
  central nervous system, syphilitic A52.Ø5
  cerebral — see Aneurysm, brain
  chest — see Aneurysm, thorax
  circle of Willis I67.1
    congenital Q28.3
      ruptured I6Ø.6
    ruptured I6Ø.6
  common iliac artery I72.3
  congenital (peripheral) Q27.8
    aorta (root) (sinus) Q25.43
    brain Q28.3
      ruptured I6Ø.7
    coronary Q24.5
    digestive system Q27.8
    lower limb Q27.8
    pulmonary Q25.79
    retina Q14.1
    specified site NEC Q27.8
    upper limb Q27.8
  conjunctiva — see Abnormality, conjunctiva, vascular
  conus arteriosus — see Aneurysm, heart
  coronary (arteriosclerotic) (artery) I25.41
    arteriovenous, congenital Q24.5
    congenital Q24.5
    ruptured — see Infarct, myocardium
    syphilitic A52.Ø6
    vein I25.89
  cylindroid (aorta) I71.9
    ruptured I71.8
    syphilitic A52.Ø1
  ductus arteriosus Q25.Ø
  endocardial, infective (any valve) I33.Ø
  femoral (artery) (ruptured) I72.4
  gastroduodenal I72.8
  gastroepiploic I72.8
  heart (wall) (chronic or with a stated duration of over 4
    weeks) I25.3
    valve — see Endocarditis
  hepatic I72.8
  iliac (common) (artery) (ruptured) I72.3
  infective I72.9
    endocardial (any valve) I33.Ø
  innominate (nonsyphilitic) I72.8
    syphilitic A52.Ø9
  interauricular septum — see Aneurysm, heart
  interventricular septum — see Aneurysm, heart
  intrathoracic (nonsyphilitic) — see also Aneurysm, aorta,
    thorax I71.2Ø
    ruptured — see also Aneurysm, aorta, thorax, ruptured
      I71.1Ø

☑ **Additional Character Required** — Refer to the Tabular List for Character Selection

Aneurysm — *continued*
  intrathoracic — *see also* Aneurysm, aorta, thorax — *continued*
    syphilitic A52.01
  lower limb I72.4
  lung (pulmonary artery) I28.1
  mediastinal (nonsyphilitic) I72.8
    syphilitic A52.09
  miliary (congenital) I67.1
    ruptured — *see* Hemorrhage, intracerebral, subarachnoid, intracranial
  mitral (heart) (valve) I34.89
  mural — *see* Aneurysm, heart
  mycotic I72.9
    endocardial (any valve) I33.0
    ruptured, brain — *see* Hemorrhage, intracerebral, subarachnoid
  myocardium — *see* Aneurysm, heart
  neck I72.0
  pancreaticoduodenal I72.8
  patent ductus arteriosus Q25.0
  peripheral NEC I72.8
    congenital Q27.8
      digestive system Q27.8
      lower limb Q27.8
      specified site NEC Q27.8
      upper limb Q27.8
  popliteal (artery) (ruptured) I72.4
  precerebral
    congenital (nonruptured) Q28.1
    specified site, NEC I72.5
  pulmonary I28.1
    arteriovenous Q25.72
      acquired I28.0
    syphilitic A52.09
    valve (heart) — *see* Endocarditis, pulmonary
  racemose (peripheral) I72.9
    congenital — *see* Aneurysm, congenital
  radial I72.1
  Rasmussen NEC A15.0
  renal (artery) I72.2
  retina — *see also* Disorder, retina, microaneurysms
    congenital Q14.1
    diabetic — *see* E08-E13 with .3-
  sinus of Valsalva Q25.43
  specified NEC I72.8
  spinal (cord) I72.8
    syphilitic (hemorrhage) A52.09
  splenic I72.8
  subclavian (artery) (ruptured) I72.8
    syphilitic A52.09
  superior mesenteric I72.8
  syphilitic (aorta) A52.01
    central nervous system A52.05
    congenital (late) A50.54 *[I79.0]*
    spine, spinal A52.09
  thoracoabdominal (aorta) I71.60
    ruptured I71.50
    syphilitic A52.01
  thorax, thoracic (aorta) (arch) (nonsyphilitic) — *see* Aneurysm, aorta, thorax
    ruptured — *see* Aneurysm, aorta, thorax, ruptured
    syphilitic A52.01
  traumatic (complication) (early), specified site — *see* Injury, blood vessel
  tricuspid (heart) (valve) I07.8
  ulnar I72.1
  upper limb (ruptured) I72.1
  valve, valvular — *see* Endocarditis
  venous — *see also* Varix I86.8
    congenital Q27.8
      digestive system Q27.8
      lower limb Q27.8
      specified site NEC Q27.8
      upper limb Q27.8
  ventricle — *see* Aneurysm, heart
  vertebral artery I72.6
  visceral NEC I72.8
Angelman syndrome Q93.51
Anger R45.4
Angiectasis, angiectopia I99.8
Angiitis I77.6
  allergic granulomatous M30.1
  hypersensitivity M31.0
  necrotizing M31.9
    specified NEC M31.8
  nervous system, granulomatous I67.7
Angina (attack) (cardiac) (chest) (heart) (pectoris) (syndrome) (vasomotor) I20.9

Angina — *continued*
  with
    atherosclerotic heart disease — *see* Arteriosclerosis, coronary (artery),
    coronary microvascular disease I20.81
    coronary microvascular dysfunction I20.81
    documented spasm I20.1
  abdominal K55.1
  accelerated — *see* Angina, unstable
  agranulocytic — *see* Agranulocytosis
  angiospastic — *see* Angina, with documented spasm
  aphthous B08.5
  crescendo — *see* Angina, unstable
  croupous J05.0
  cruris I73.9
  de novo effort — *see* Angina, unstable
  diphtheritic, membranous A36.0
  equivalent I20.89
  exudative, chronic J37.0
  following acute myocardial infarction I23.7
  gangrenous diphtheritic A36.0
  intestinal K55.1
  Ludovici K12.2
  Ludwig's K12.2
  malignant diphtheritic A36.0
  membranous J05.0
    diphtheritic A36.0
    Vincent's A69.1
  mesenteric K55.1
  monocytic — *see* Mononucleosis, infectious
  of effort — *see* Angina, specified NEC
  phlegmonous J36
    diphtheritic A36.0
  post-infarctional I23.7
  pre-infarctional — *see* Angina, unstable
  Prinzmetal — *see* Angina, with documented spasm
  progressive — *see* Angina, unstable
  pseudomembranous A69.1
  pultaceous, diphtheritic A36.0
  refractory I20.2
  spasm-induced — *see* Angina, with documented spasm
  specified NEC I20.89
  stable I20.89
  stenocardia — *see* Angina, specified NEC
  stridulous, diphtheritic A36.2
  tonsil J36
  trachealis J05.0
  unstable I20.0
  variant — *see* Angina, with documented spasm
  Vincent's A69.1
  worsening effort — *see* Angina, unstable
Angioblastoma — *see* Neoplasm, connective tissue, uncertain behavior
Angiocholecystitis — *see* Cholecystitis, acute
Angiocholitis — *see also* Cholecystitis, acute K83.09
Angiodysgenesis spinalis G95.19
Angiodysplasia (cecum) (colon) K55.20
  with bleeding K55.21
  duodenum (and stomach) K31.819
    with bleeding K31.811
  stomach (and duodenum) K31.819
    with bleeding K31.811
Angioedema (allergic) (any site) (with urticaria) T78.3 ☑
  episodic, with eosinophilia D72.118
  hereditary D84.1
Angioendothelioma — *see* Neoplasm, uncertain behavior, by site
  benign D18.00
    intra-abdominal D18.03
    intracranial D18.02
    skin D18.01
    specified site NEC D18.09
  bone — *see* Neoplasm, bone, malignant
  Ewing's — *see* Neoplasm, bone, malignant
Angioendotheliomatosis C85.8- ☑
Angiofibroma — *see also* Neoplasm, benign, by site
  juvenile
    specified site — *see* Neoplasm, benign, by site
    unspecified site D10.6
Angiohemophilia (A) (B) — *see* Disease, von Willebrand
Angioid streaks (choroid) (macula) (retina) H35.33
Angiokeratoma — *see* Neoplasm, skin, benign
  corporis diffusum E75.21
Angioleiomyoma — *see* Neoplasm, connective tissue, benign
Angiolipoma — *see also* Lipoma
  infiltrating — *see* Lipoma
Angioma — *see also* Hemangioma, by site
  capillary I78.1

Angioma — *continued*
  hemorrhagicum hereditaria I78.0
  intra-abdominal D18.03
  intracranial D18.02
  malignant — *see* Neoplasm, connective tissue, malignant
  plexiform D18.00
    intra-abdominal D18.03
    intracranial D18.02
    skin D18.01
    specified site NEC D18.09
  senile I78.1
  serpiginosum L81.7
  skin D18.01
  specified site NEC D18.09
  spider I78.1
  stellate I78.1
  venous Q28.3
Angiomatosis Q82.8
  bacillary A79.89
  encephalotrigeminal Q85.89
  hemorrhagic familial I78.0
  hereditary familial I78.0
  liver K76.4
Angiomyolipoma — *see* Lipoma
Angiomyoliposarcoma — *see* Neoplasm, connective tissue, malignant
Angiomyoma — *see* Neoplasm, connective tissue, benign
Angiomyosarcoma — *see* Neoplasm, connective tissue, malignant
Angiomyxoma — *see* Neoplasm, connective tissue, uncertain behavior
Angioneurosis F45.8
Angioneurotic edema (allergic) (any site) (with urticaria) T78.3 ☑
  hereditary D84.1
Angiopathia, angiopathy I99.9
  cerebral I67.9
    amyloid E85.4 *[I68.0]*
  diabetic (peripheral) — *see* Diabetes, angiopathy
  peripheral I73.9
    diabetic — *see* Diabetes, angiopathy
    specified type NEC I73.89
  retinae syphilitica A52.05
  retinalis (juvenilis)
    diabetic — *see* Diabetes, retinopathy
    proliferative — *see* Retinopathy, proliferative
Angiosarcoma — *see also* Neoplasm, connective tissue, malignant
  liver C22.3
Angiosclerosis — *see* Arteriosclerosis
Angiospasm (peripheral) (traumatic) (vessel) — *see also* Vasospasm I73.9
  brachial plexus G54.0
  cerebral G45.9
  cervical plexus G54.2
  nerve
    arm — *see* Mononeuropathy, upper limb
      axillary G54.0
      median — *see* Lesion, nerve, median
      ulnar — *see* Lesion, nerve, ulnar
    axillary G54.0
    leg — *see* Mononeuropathy, lower limb
    median — *see* Lesion, nerve, median
    plantar — *see* Lesion, nerve, plantar
    ulnar — *see* Lesion, nerve, ulnar
Angiospastic disease or edema I73.9
Angiostrongyliasis
  due to
    Parastrongylus
      cantonensis B83.2
      costaricensis B81.3
  intestinal B81.3
Anguillulosis — *see* Strongyloidiasis
Angulation
  cecum — *see* Obstruction, intestine
  coccyx (acquired) — *see also* subcategory M43.8 ☑
    congenital NEC Q76.49
  femur (acquired) — *see also* Deformity, limb, specified type NEC, thigh
    congenital Q74.2
  intestine (large) (small) — *see* Obstruction, intestine
  sacrum (acquired) — *see also* subcategory M43.8 ☑
    congenital NEC Q76.49
  sigmoid (flexure) — *see* Obstruction, intestine
  spine — *see* Dorsopathy, deforming, specified NEC
  tibia (acquired) — *see also* Deformity, limb, specified type NEC, lower leg
    congenital Q74.2
  ureter N13.5

☑ **Additional Character Required** — Refer to the Tabular List for Character Selection

Angulation — *continued*
 ureter — *continued*
  with infection N13.6
 wrist (acquired) — *see also* Deformity, limb, specified
   type NEC, forearm
  congenital Q74.0
Angulus infectiosus (lips) K13.0
Anhedonia R45.84
 sexual F52.0
Anhidrosis L74.4
Anhydration E86.0
Anhydremia E86.0
Anidrosis L74.4
Aniridia (congenital) Q13.1
Anisakiasis (infection) (infestation) B81.0
Anisakis larvae infestation B81.0
Aniseikonia H52.32
Anisocoria (pupil) H57.02
 congenital Q13.2
Anisocytosis R71.8
Anisometropia (congenital) H52.31
Ankle — *see* condition
Ankyloblepharon (eyelid) (acquired) — *see also* Blepharophimosis
 filiforme (adnatum) (congenital) Q10.3
 total Q10.3
Ankyloglossia Q38.1
Ankylosis (fibrous) (osseous) (joint) M24.60
 ankle M24.67- ☑
 arthrodesis status Z98.1
 cricoarytenoid (cartilage) (joint) (larynx) J38.7
 dental K03.5
 ear ossicles H74.31- ☑
 elbow M24.62- ☑
 foot M24.67- ☑
 hand M24.64- ☑
 hip M24.65- ☑
 incostapedial joint (infectional) — *see* Ankylosis, ear ossicles
 jaw (temporomandibular) M26.61- ☑
 knee M24.66- ☑
 lumbosacral (joint) M43.27
 postoperative (status) Z98.1
 produced by surgical fusion, status Z98.1
 sacro-iliac (joint) M43.28
 shoulder M24.61- ☑
 specified site NEC M24.69
 spine (joint) — *see also* Fusion, spine
  spondylitic — *see* Spondylitis, ankylosing
 surgical Z98.1
 temporomandibular M26.61- ☑
 tooth, teeth (hard tissues) K03.5
 wrist M24.63- ☑
Ankylostoma — *see* Ancylostoma
Ankylostomiasis — *see* Ancylostomiasis
Ankylurethria — *see* Stricture, urethra
Annular — *see also* condition
 detachment, cervix N88.8
 organ or site, congenital NEC — *see* Distortion
 pancreas (congenital) Q45.1
Anoctaminopathy G71.035
Anodontia (complete) (partial) (vera) K00.0
 acquired K08.10 ☑
Anomaly, anomalous (congenital) (unspecified type) Q89.9
 abdominal wall NEC Q79.59
 acoustic nerve Q07.8
 adrenal (gland) Q89.1
 Alder (-Reilly) (leukocyte granulation) D72.0
 alimentary tract Q45.9
  upper Q40.9
 alveolar M26.70
  hyperplasia M26.79
   mandibular M26.72
   maxillary M26.71
  hypoplasia M26.79
   mandibular M26.74
   maxillary M26.73
  ridge (process) M26.79
  specified NEC M26.79
 ankle (joint) Q74.2
 anus Q43.9
 aorta (arch) NEC Q25.40
  coarctation (preductal) (postductal) Q25.1
 aortic cusp or valve Q23.9
 appendix Q43.8
 apple peel syndrome Q41.1
 aqueduct of Sylvius Q03.0

Anomaly, anomalous — *continued*
 aqueduct of Sylvius — *continued*
  with spina bifida — *see* Spina bifida, with hydrocephalus
 arm Q74.0
 arteriovenous NEC
  coronary Q24.5
  gastrointestinal Q27.33
   acquired — *see* Angiodysplasia
 artery (peripheral) Q27.9
  basilar NEC Q28.1
  cerebral Q28.3
  coronary Q24.5
  digestive system Q27.8
  eye Q15.8
  great Q25.9
   specified NEC Q25.8
  lower limb Q27.8
  peripheral Q27.9
   specified NEC Q27.8
  pulmonary NEC Q25.79
  renal Q27.2
  retina Q14.1
  specified site NEC Q27.8
  subclavian Q27.8
   origin Q25.48
  umbilical Q27.0
  upper limb Q27.8
  vertebral NEC Q28.1
 aryteno-epiglottic folds Q31.8
 atrial
  bands or folds Q20.8
  septa Q21.10
 atrioventricular
  excitation I45.6
  septum Q21.0
 auditory canal Q17.8
 auricle
  ear Q17.8
   causing impairment of hearing Q16.9
  heart Q20.8
 Axenfeld's Q15.0
 back Q89.9
 band
  atrial Q20.8
  heart Q24.8
  ventricular Q24.8
 Bartholin's duct Q38.4
 biliary duct or passage Q44.5
 bladder Q64.70
  absence Q64.5
  diverticulum Q64.6
  exstrophy Q64.10
   cloacal Q64.12
   extroversion Q64.19
   specified type NEC Q64.19
   supravesical fissure Q64.11
  neck obstruction Q64.31
  specified type NEC Q64.79
 bone Q79.9
  arm Q74.0
  face Q75.9
  leg Q74.2
  pelvic girdle Q74.2
  shoulder girdle Q74.0
  skull Q75.9
   with
    anencephaly Q00.0
    encephalocele — *see* Encephalocele
    hydrocephalus Q03.9
     with spina bifida — *see* Spina bifida, by
      site, with hydrocephalus
    microcephaly Q02
 brain (multiple) Q04.9
  vessel Q28.3
 breast Q83.9
 broad ligament Q50.6
 bronchus Q32.4
 bulbus cordis Q21.9
 bursa Q79.9
 canal of Nuck Q52.4
 canthus Q10.3
 capillary Q27.9
 cardiac Q24.9
  chambers Q20.9
   specified NEC Q20.8
  septal closure Q21.9
   specified NEC Q21.8
  valve NEC Q24.8

Anomaly, anomalous — *continued*
 cardiac — *continued*
  valve — *continued*
   pulmonary Q22.3
 cardiovascular system Q28.8
 carpus Q74.0
 caruncle, lacrimal Q10.6
 cascade stomach Q40.2
 cauda equina Q06.3
 cecum Q43.9
 cerebral Q04.9
  vessels Q28.3
 cervix Q51.9
 Chediak-Higashi (-Steinbrinck) (congenital gigantism of
  peroxidase granules) E70.330
 cheek Q18.9
 chest wall Q67.8
  bones Q76.9
 chin Q18.9
 chordae tendineae Q24.8
 choroid Q14.3
  plexus Q07.8
 chromosomes, chromosomal Q99.9
  D (1) — *see* condition, chromosome 13
  E (3) — *see* condition, chromosome 18
  G — *see* condition, chromosome 21
  sex
   female phenotype Q97.8
   gonadal dysgenesis (pure) Q99.1
   Klinefelter's Q98.4
   male phenotype Q98.9
   Turner's Q96.9
  specified NEC Q99.8
 cilia Q10.3
 circulatory system Q28.9
 clavicle Q74.0
 clitoris Q52.6
 coccyx Q76.49
 colon Q43.9
 common duct Q44.5
 communication
  coronary artery Q24.5
  left ventricle with right atrium Q21.0
 concha (ear) Q17.3
 connection
  portal vein Q26.5
  pulmonary venous Q26.4
   partial Q26.3
   total Q26.2
  renal artery with kidney Q27.2
 cornea (shape) Q13.4
 coronary artery or vein Q24.5
 cranium — *see* Anomaly, skull
 cricoid cartilage Q31.8
 cystic duct Q44.5
 dental
  alveolar — *see* Anomaly, alveolar
  arch relationship M26.20
   specified NEC M26.29
 dentofacial M26.9
  alveolar — *see* Anomaly, alveolar
  dental arch relationship M26.20
   specified NEC M26.29
  functional M26.50
   specified NEC M26.59
  jaw size M26.00
   macrogenia M26.05
   mandibular
    hyperplasia M26.03
    hypoplasia M26.04
   maxillary
    hyperplasia M26.01
    hypoplasia M26.02
   microgenia M26.06
   specified type NEC M26.09
  jaw-cranial base relationship M26.10
   asymmetry M26.12
    maxillary M26.11
   specified type NEC M26.19
  malocclusion M26.4
   dental arch relationship NEC M26.29
   jaw size — *see* Anomaly, dentofacial, jaw size
   jaw-cranial base relationship — *see* Anomaly,
    dentofacial, jaw-cranial base relationship
  specified type NEC M26.89
  temporomandibular joint M26.60- ☑
   adhesions M26.61- ☑
   ankylosis M26.61- ☑
   arthralgia M26.62- ☑

☑ **Additional Character Required** — **Refer to the Tabular List for Character Selection**

Anomaly, anomalous — *continued*
dentofacial — *continued*
  temporomandibular joint — *continued*
    articular disc M26.63- ☑
    specified type NEC M26.69
  tooth position, fully erupted M26.30
    specified NEC M26.39
dermatoglyphic Q82.8
diaphragm (apertures) NEC Q79.1
digestive organ(s) or tract Q45.9
  lower Q43.9
  upper Q40.9
distance, interarch (excessive) (inadequate) M26.25
distribution, coronary artery Q24.5
ductus
  arteriosus Q25.0
  botalli Q25.0
duodenum Q43.9
dura (brain) Q04.9
  spinal cord Q06.9
ear (external) Q17.9
  causing impairment of hearing Q16.9
  inner Q16.5
  middle (causing impairment of hearing) Q16.4
    ossicles Q16.3
Ebstein's (heart) (tricuspid valve) Q22.5
ectodermal Q82.9
Eisenmenger's (ventricular septal defect) Q21.8
ejaculatory duct Q55.4
elbow Q74.0
endocrine gland NEC Q89.2
epididymis Q55.4
epiglottis Q31.8
esophagus Q39.9
eustachian tube Q17.8
eye Q15.9
  anterior segment Q13.9
    specified NEC Q13.89
  posterior segment Q14.9
    specified NEC Q14.8
  ptosis (eyelid) Q10.0
  specified NEC Q15.8
eyebrow Q18.8
eyelid Q10.3
  ptosis Q10.0
face Q18.9
  bone(s) Q75.9
fallopian tube Q50.6
fascia Q79.9
femur NEC Q74.2
fibula NEC Q74.2
finger Q74.0
fixation, intestine Q43.3
flexion (joint) NOS Q74.9
  hip or thigh Q65.89
foot NEC Q74.2
  varus (congenital) Q66.3- ☑
foramen
  Botalli Q21.12
  ovale Q21.12
forearm Q74.0
forehead Q75.8
form, teeth K00.2
fovea centralis Q14.1
frontal bone — *see* Anomaly, skull
gallbladder (position) (shape) (size) Q44.1
Gartner's duct Q52.4
gastrointestinal tract Q45.9
genitalia, genital organ(s) or system
  female Q52.9
    external Q52.70
    internal NOS Q52.9
  male Q55.9
    hydrocele P83.5
    specified NEC Q55.8
genitourinary NEC
  female Q52.9
  male Q55.9
Gerbode Q21.0
glottis Q31.8
granulation or granulocyte, genetic (constitutional)
  (leukocyte) D72.0
gum Q38.6
gyri Q07.9
hair Q84.2
hand Q74.0
hard tissue formation in pulp K04.3
head — *see* Anomaly, skull
heart Q24.9

Anomaly, anomalous — *continued*
heart — *continued*
  auricle Q20.8
  bands or folds Q24.8
  fibroelastosis cordis I42.4
  obstructive NEC Q22.6
  patent ductus arteriosus (Botalli) Q25.0
  septum Q21.9
    auricular Q21.19
    interatrial Q21.19
    interventricular Q21.0
      with pulmonary stenosis or atresia, dextraposi-
        tion of aorta and hypertrophy of right
        ventricle Q21.3
    specified NEC Q21.8
    ventricular Q21.0
      with pulmonary stenosis or atresia, dextraposi-
        tion of aorta and hypertrophy of right
        ventricle Q21.3
  tetralogy of Fallot Q21.3
  valve NEC Q24.8
    aortic
      bicuspid valve Q23.81
        functional, with stenosis — *see* Stenosis,
          aortic (valve)
      insufficiency Q23.1
      stenosis Q23.0
        subaortic Q24.4
    mitral
      insufficiency Q23.3
      stenosis Q23.2
    pulmonary Q22.3
      atresia Q22.0
      insufficiency Q22.2
      stenosis Q22.1
        infundibular Q24.3
        subvalvular Q24.3
    tricuspid
      atresia Q22.4
      stenosis Q22.4
  ventricle Q20.8
heel NEC Q74.2
Hegglin's D72.0
hemianencephaly Q00.0
hemicephaly Q00.0
hemicrania Q00.0
hepatic duct Q44.5
hip NEC Q74.2
hourglass stomach Q40.2
humerus Q74.0
hydatid of Morgagni
  female Q50.5
  male (epididymal) Q55.4
    testicular Q55.29
hymen Q52.4
hypersegmentation of neutrophils, hereditary D72.0
hypophyseal Q89.2
ileocecal (coil) (valve) Q43.9
ileum Q43.9
ilium NEC Q74.2
integument Q84.9
  specified NEC Q84.8
interarch distance (excessive) (inadequate) M26.25
intervertebral cartilage or disc Q76.49
intestine (large) (small) Q43.9
  with anomalous adhesions, fixation or malrotation
    Q43.3
iris Q13.2
ischium NEC Q74.2
jaw — *see* Anomaly, dentofacial
  alveolar — *see* Anomaly, alveolar
jaw-cranial base relationship — *see* Anomaly, dentofacial,
  jaw-cranial base relationship
jejunum Q43.8
joint Q74.9
  specified NEC Q74.8
Jordan's D72.0
kidney(s) (calyx) (pelvis) Q63.9
  artery Q27.2
  specified NEC Q63.8
Klippel-Feil (brevicollis) Q76.1
knee Q74.1
labium (majus) (minus) Q52.70
labyrinth, membranous Q16.5
lacrimal apparatus or duct Q10.6
larynx, laryngeal (muscle) Q31.9
  web (bed) Q31.0
lens Q12.9
leukocytes, genetic D72.0

Anomaly, anomalous — *continued*
leukocytes, genetic — *continued*
  granulation (constitutional) D72.0
lid (fold) Q10.3
ligament Q79.9
  broad Q50.6
  round Q52.8
limb Q74.9
  lower NEC Q74.2
    reduction deformity — *see* Defect, reduction,
      lower limb
  upper Q74.0
lip Q38.0
liver Q44.70
  duct Q44.5
lower limb NEC Q74.2
lumbosacral (joint) (region) Q76.49
  kyphosis — *see* Kyphosis, congenital
  lordosis — *see* Lordosis, congenital
lung (fissure) (lobe) Q33.9
mandible — *see* Anomaly, dentofacial
maxilla — *see* Anomaly, dentofacial
May (-Hegglin) D72.0
meatus urinarius NEC Q64.79
meningeal bands or folds Q07.9
  constriction of Q07.8
  spinal Q06.9
meninges Q07.9
  cerebral Q04.8
  spinal Q06.9
meningocele Q05.9
mesentery Q45.9
metacarpus Q74.0
metatarsus NEC Q74.2
middle ear Q16.4
  ossicles Q16.3
mitral (leaflets) (valve) Q23.9
  cleft Q23.82
  insufficiency Q23.3
  specified NEC Q23.88
  stenosis Q23.2
mouth Q38.6
Mullerian — *see also* Anomaly, by site
  uterus NEC Q51.818
multiple NEC Q89.7
muscle Q79.9
  eyelid Q10.3
musculoskeletal system, except limbs Q79.9
myocardium Q24.8
nail Q84.6
narrowness, eyelid Q10.3
nasal sinus (wall) Q30.8
neck (any part) Q18.9
nerve Q07.9
  acoustic Q07.8
  optic Q07.8
nervous system (central) Q07.9
nipple Q83.9
nose, nasal (bones) (cartilage) (septum) (sinus) Q30.9
  specified NEC Q30.8
ocular muscle Q15.8
omphalomesenteric duct Q43.0
opening, pulmonary veins Q26.4
optic
  disc Q14.2
  nerve Q07.8
opticociliary vessels Q13.2
orbit (eye) Q10.7
organ Q89.9
  of Corti Q16.5
origin
  artery
    innominate Q25.8
    pulmonary Q25.79
    renal Q27.2
    subclavian Q25.48
osseous meatus (ear) Q16.1
ovary Q50.39
oviduct Q50.6
palate (hard) (soft) NEC Q38.5
pancreas or pancreatic duct Q45.3
papillary muscles Q24.8
parathyroid gland Q89.2
paraurethral ducts Q64.79
parotid (gland) Q38.4
patella Q74.1
Pelger-Huet (hereditary hyposegmentation) D72.0
pelvic girdle NEC Q74.2
pelvis (bony) NEC Q74.2

Anomaly, anomalous — *continued*
- pelvis — *continued*
  - rachitic E64.3
- penis (glans) Q55.69
- pericardium Q24.8
- peripheral vascular system Q27.9
- Peter's Q13.4
- pharynx Q38.8
- pigmentation L81.9
  - congenital Q82.8
- pituitary (gland) Q89.2
- pleural (folds) Q34.0
- portal vein Q26.5
  - connection Q26.5
- position, tooth, teeth, fully erupted M26.30
  - specified NEC M26.39
- precerebral vessel Q28.1
- prepuce Q55.69
- prostate Q55.4
- pulmonary Q33.9
  - artery NEC Q25.79
  - valve Q22.3
    - atresia Q22.0
    - insufficiency Q22.2
    - specified type NEC Q22.3
    - stenosis Q22.1
      - infundibular Q24.3
      - subvalvular Q24.3
  - venous connection Q26.4
    - partial Q26.3
    - total Q26.2
- pupil Q13.2
  - function H57.00
    - anisocoria H57.02
    - Argyll Robertson pupil H57.01
    - miosis H57.03
    - mydriasis H57.04
    - specified type NEC H57.09
    - tonic pupil H57.05- ☑
- pylorus Q40.3
- radius Q74.0
- rectum Q43.9
- reduction (extremity) (limb)
  - femur (longitudinal) — *see* Defect, reduction, lower limb, longitudinal, femur
  - fibula (longitudinal) — *see* Defect, reduction, lower limb, longitudinal, fibula
  - lower limb — *see* Defect, reduction, lower limb
  - radius (longitudinal) — *see* Defect, reduction, upper limb, longitudinal, radius
  - tibia (longitudinal) — *see* Defect, reduction, lower limb, longitudinal, tibia
  - ulna (longitudinal) — *see* Defect, reduction, upper limb, longitudinal, ulna
  - upper limb — *see* Defect, reduction, upper limb
- refraction — *see* Disorder, refraction
- renal Q63.9
  - artery Q27.2
  - pelvis Q63.9
    - specified NEC Q63.8
- respiratory system Q34.9
  - specified NEC Q34.8
- retina Q14.1
- rib Q76.6
  - cervical Q76.5
- Rieger Q13.81
- rotation — *see* Malrotation
  - hip or thigh Q65.89
- round ligament Q52.8
- sacroiliac (joint) NEC Q74.2
- sacrum NEC Q76.49
  - kyphosis — *see* Kyphosis, congenital
  - lordosis — *see* Lordosis, congenital
- saddle nose, syphilitic A50.57
- salivary duct or gland Q38.4
- scapula Q74.0
- scrotum — *see* Malformation, testis and scrotum
- sebaceous gland Q82.9
- seminal vesicles Q55.4
- sense organs NEC Q07.8
- sex chromosomes NEC — *see also* Anomaly, chromosomes
  - female phenotype Q97.8
  - male phenotype Q98.9
- shoulder (girdle) (joint) Q74.0
- sigmoid (flexure) Q43.9
- simian crease Q82.8
- sinus of Valsalva Q25.49
- skeleton generalized Q78.9

Anomaly, anomalous — *continued*
- skin (appendage) Q82.9
- skull Q75.9
  - with
    - anencephaly Q00.0
    - encephalocele — *see* Encephalocele
    - hydrocephalus Q03.9
      - with spina bifida — *see* Spina bifida, by site, with hydrocephalus
    - microcephaly Q02
- specified organ or site NEC Q89.8
- spermatic cord Q55.4
- spine, spinal NEC Q76.49
  - column NEC Q76.49
    - kyphosis — *see* Kyphosis, congenital
    - lordosis — *see* Lordosis, congenital
  - cord Q06.9
  - nerve root Q07.8
- spleen Q89.09
  - agenesis Q89.01
- stenonian duct Q38.4
- sternum NEC Q76.7
- stomach Q40.3
- submaxillary gland Q38.4
- tarsus NEC Q74.2
- tendon Q79.9
- testis — *see* Malformation, testis and scrotum
- thigh NEC Q74.2
- thorax (wall) Q67.8
  - bony Q76.9
- throat Q38.8
- thumb Q74.0
- thymus gland Q89.2
- thyroid (gland) Q89.2
  - cartilage Q31.8
- tibia NEC Q74.2
  - saber A50.56
- toe Q74.2
- tongue Q38.3
- tooth, teeth K00.9
  - eruption K00.6
  - position, fully erupted M26.30
  - spacing, fully erupted M26.30
- trachea (cartilage) Q32.1
- tragus Q17.9
- tricuspid (leaflet) (valve) Q22.9
  - atresia or stenosis Q22.4
  - Ebstein's Q22.5
- Uhl's (hypoplasia of myocardium, right ventricle) Q24.8
- ulna Q74.0
- umbilical artery Q27.0
- union
  - cricoid cartilage and thyroid cartilage Q31.8
  - thyroid cartilage and hyoid bone Q31.8
  - trachea with larynx Q31.8
- upper limb Q74.0
- urachus Q64.4
- ureter Q62.8
  - obstructive NEC Q62.39
    - cecoureterocele Q62.32
    - orthotopic ureterocele Q62.31
- urethra Q64.70
  - absence Q64.5
  - double Q64.74
  - fistula to rectum Q64.73
  - obstructive Q64.39
    - stricture Q64.32
  - prolapse Q64.71
  - specified type NEC Q64.79
- urinary tract Q64.9
- uterus Q51.9
  - with only one functioning horn Q51.4
- uvula Q38.5
- vagina Q52.4
- valleculae Q31.8
- valve (heart) NEC Q24.8
  - coronary sinus Q24.5
  - inferior vena cava Q24.8
  - pulmonary Q22.3
  - sinus coronario Q24.5
  - venae cavae inferioris Q24.8
- vas deferens Q55.4
- vascular Q27.9
  - brain Q28.3
  - ring Q25.45
- vein(s) (peripheral) Q27.9
  - brain Q28.3
  - cerebral Q28.3
  - coronary Q24.5

Anomaly, anomalous — *continued*
- vein(s) — *continued*
  - developmental Q28.3
  - great Q26.9
    - specified NEC Q26.8
- vena cava (inferior) (superior) Q26.9
- venous — *see* Anomaly, vein(s)
- venous return Q26.8
- ventricular
  - bands or folds Q24.8
  - septa Q21.0
- vertebra Q76.49
  - kyphosis — *see* Kyphosis, congenital
  - lordosis — *see* Lordosis, congenital
- vesicourethral orifice Q64.79
- vessel(s) Q27.9
  - optic papilla Q14.2
  - precerebral Q28.1
- vitelline duct Q43.0
- vitreous body or humor Q14.0
- vulva Q52.70
- wrist (joint) Q74.0

Anomia R48.8

Anonychia (congenital) Q84.3
- acquired L60.8

Anophthalmos, anophthalmus (congenital) (globe) Q11.1
- acquired Z90.01

Anopia, anopsia H53.46- ☑
- quadrant H53.46- ☑

Anorchia, anorchism, anorchidism Q55.0

Anorexia R63.0
- hysterical F44.89
- nervosa F50.00
  - atypical F50.9
  - binge-eating type F50.2- ☑
    - with purging F50.02- ☑
  - restricting type F50.01- ☑

Anorgasmy, psychogenic (female) F52.31
- male F52.32

Anosmia R43.0
- hysterical F44.6
- postinfectional J39.8

Anosognosia R41.85

Anosteoplasia Q78.9

Anovulatory cycle N97.0

Anoxemia R09.02
- newborn P84

Anoxia (pathological) R09.02
- altitude T70.29 ☑
- cerebral G93.1
  - complicating
    - anesthesia (general) (local) or other sedation T88.59 ☑
      - in labor and delivery O74.3
      - in pregnancy O29.21- ☑
      - postpartum, puerperal O89.2
    - delivery (cesarean) (instrumental) O75.4
  - during a procedure G97.81
  - newborn P84
  - resulting from a procedure G97.82
- due to
  - drowning T75.1 ☑
  - high altitude T70.29 ☑
- heart — *see* Insufficiency, coronary
- intrauterine P84
- myocardial — *see* Insufficiency, coronary
- newborn P84
- spinal cord G95.11
- systemic (by suffocation) (low content in atmosphere) — *see* Asphyxia, traumatic

Anteflexion — *see* Anteversion

Antenatal
- care (normal pregnancy) Z34.90
- screening (encounter for) of mother — *see also* Encounter, antenatal screening Z36.9

Antepartum — *see* condition

Anterior — *see* condition

Antero-occlusion M26.220

Anteversion
- cervix — *see* Anteversion, uterus
- femur (neck), congenital Q65.89
- uterus, uterine (cervix) (postinfectional) (postpartal, old) N85.4
  - congenital Q51.818
  - in pregnancy or childbirth — *see* Pregnancy, complicated by

Anthophobia F40.228

Anthracosilicosis J60

Anthracosis (lung) (occupational) J60
  lingua K14.3
Anthrax A22.9
  with pneumonia A22.1
  cerebral A22.8
  colitis A22.2
  cutaneous A22.0
  gastrointestinal A22.2
  inhalation A22.1
  intestinal A22.2
  meningitis A22.8
  pulmonary A22.1
  respiratory A22.1
  sepsis A22.7
  specified manifestation NEC A22.8
Anthropoid pelvis Q74.2
  with disproportion (fetopelvic) O33.0
Anthropophobia F40.10
  generalized F40.11
Antibodies, maternal (blood group) — *see* Isoimmunization, affecting management of pregnancy
  anti-D — *see* Isoimmunization, affecting management of pregnancy, Rh
    newborn P55.0
Antibody
  anticardiolipin R76.0
    with
      hemorrhagic disorder D68.312
      hypercoagulable state D68.61
  antiphosphatidylglycerol R76.0
    with
      hemorrhagic disorder D68.312
      hypercoagulable state D68.61
  antiphosphatidylinositol R76.0
    with
      hemorrhagic disorder D68.312
      hypercoagulable state D68.61
  antiphosphatidylserine R76.0
    with
      hemorrhagic disorder D68.312
      hypercoagulable state D68.61
  antiphospholipid R76.0
    with
      hemorrhagic disorder D68.312
      hypercoagulable state D68.61
Anticardiolipin syndrome D68.61
Anticoagulant, circulating (intrinsic) — *see also* Disorder, hemorrhagic D68.318
  drug-induced (extrinsic) — *see also* Disorder, hemorrhagic D68.32
  iatrogenic D68.32
Antidiuretic hormone syndrome E22.2
Antimonial cholera — *see* Poisoning, antimony
Antiphospholipid
  antibody
    with hemorrhagic disorder D68.312
    syndrome D68.61
Antisocial personality F60.2
Antithrombinemia — *see* Circulating anticoagulants
Antithromboplastinemia D68.318
Antithromboplastinogenemia D68.318
Antitoxin complication or reaction — *see* Complications, vaccination
Antlophobia F40.228
Antritis J32.0
  maxilla J32.0
    acute J01.00
      recurrent J01.01
  stomach K29.50
    with bleeding K29.51
Antrum, antral — *see* condition
Anuria R34
  calculus (impacted) (recurrent) — *see also* Calculus, urinary N20.9
  following
    abortion — *see* Abortion by type complicated by, renal failure
    ectopic or molar pregnancy O08.4
  newborn P96.0
  postprocedural N99.0
  postrenal N13.8
  puerperal O90.49
  traumatic (following crushing) T79.5 ☑
Anus, anal — *see* condition
Anusitis K62.89
Anxiety F41.9
  depression F41.8
  episodic paroxysmal F41.0
  generalized F41.1

Anxiety — *continued*
  hysteria F41.8
  neurosis F41.1
  panic type F41.0
  reaction F41.1
  separation, abnormal (of childhood) F93.0
  specified NEC F41.8
  state F41.1
Aorta, aortic — *see* condition
Aortectasia — *see* Ectasia, aorta
  with aneurysm — *see* Aneurysm, aorta
Aortitis (nonsyphilitic) (calcific) I77.6
  arteriosclerotic I70.0
  Doehle-Heller A52.02
  luetic A52.02
  rheumatic — *see* Endocarditis, acute, rheumatic
  specific (syphilitic) A52.02
  syphilitic A52.02
    congenital A50.54 [I79.1]
Apathetic thyroid storm — *see* Thyrotoxicosis
Apathy R45.3
Apeirophobia F40.228
Apepsia K30
  psychogenic F45.8
Aperistalsis, esophagus K22.0
Apertognathia M26.29
Apert's syndrome Q87.0
Aphagia R13.0
  psychogenic F50.9
Aphakia (acquired) (postoperative) H27.0- ☑
  congenital Q12.3
Aphasia (amnestic) (global) (nominal) (semantic) (syntactic) R47.01
  acquired, with epilepsy (Landau-Kleffner syndrome) — *see* Epilepsy, specified NEC
  auditory (developmental) F80.2
  developmental (receptive type) F80.2
    expressive type F80.1
    Wernicke's F80.2
  following
    cerebrovascular disease I69.920
      cerebral infarction I69.320
      intracerebral hemorrhage I69.120
      nontraumatic intracranial hemorrhage NEC I69.220
      specified disease NEC I69.820
      subarachnoid hemorrhage I69.020
  primary progressive — *see also* Dementia, in, diseases specified elsewhere G31.01 [F02.80]
    with behavioral disturbance — *see also* Dementia, in, diseases specified elsewhere G31.01 [F02.81-] ☑
  progressive isolated — *see also* Dementia, in, diseases specified elsewhere G31.01 [F02.80]
    with behavioral disturbance — *see also* Dementia, in, diseases specified elsewhere G31.01 [F02.81-] ☑
  sensory F80.2
  syphilis, tertiary A52.19
  Wernicke's (developmental) F80.2
Aphonia (organic) R49.1
  hysterical F44.4
  psychogenic F44.4
Aphthae, aphthous — *see also* condition
  Bednar's K12.0
  cachectic K14.0
  epizootic B08.8
  fever B08.8
  oral (recurrent) K12.0
  stomatitis (major) (minor) K12.0
  thrush B37.0
  ulcer (oral) (recurrent) K12.0
    genital organ(s) NEC
      female N76.6
      male N50.89
    larynx J38.7
Apical — *see* condition
Apiphobia F40.218
Aplasia — *see also* Agenesis
  abdominal muscle syndrome Q79.4
  alveolar process (acquired) — *see* Anomaly, alveolar
    congenital Q38.6
  aorta (congenital) Q25.41
  axialis extracorticalis (congenita) E75.29
  bone marrow (myeloid) D61.9
    congenital D61.01
  brain Q00.0
    part of Q04.3
  bronchus Q32.4
  cementum K00.4

Aplasia — *continued*
  cerebellum Q04.3
  cervix (congenital) Q51.5
  congenital pure red cell D61.01
  corpus callosum Q04.0
  cutis congenita Q84.8
  erythrocyte congenital D61.01
  extracortical axial E75.29
  eye Q11.1
  fovea centralis (congenital) Q14.1
  gallbladder, congenital Q44.0
  iris Q13.1
  labyrinth, membranous Q16.5
  limb (congenital) Q73.8
    lower — *see* Defect, reduction, lower limb
    upper — *see* Agenesis, arm
  lung, congenital (bilateral) (unilateral) Q33.3
  pancreas Q45.0
  parathyroid-thymic D82.1
  Pelizaeus-Merzbacher E75.27
  penis Q55.5
  prostate Q55.4
  red cell (with thymoma) D60.9
    acquired D60.9
      due to drugs D60.9
    adult D60.9
    chronic D60.0
    congenital D61.01
    constitutional D61.01
    due to drugs D60.9
    hereditary D61.01
    of infants D61.01
    primary D61.01
    pure D61.01
      due to drugs D60.9
    specified type NEC D60.8
    transient D60.1
  round ligament Q52.8
  skin Q84.8
  spermatic cord Q55.4
  spleen Q89.01
  testicle Q55.0
  thymic, with immunodeficiency D82.1
  thyroid (congenital) (with myxedema) E03.1
  uterus Q51.0
  ventral horn cell Q06.1
Apnea, apneic (of) (spells) R06.81
  newborn P28.40
    central P28.41
    mixed P28.43
    obstructive P28.42
    sleep
      primary P28.30
        central P28.31
        mixed P28.33
        obstructive P28.32
        specified NEC P28.39
    specified NEC P28.49
  prematurity P28.49
  sleep G47.30
    central (primary) G47.31
      idiopathic G47.31
      in conditions classified elsewhere G47.37
    obstructive (adult) (pediatric) G47.33
      hypopnea G47.33
    primary central G47.31
    specified NEC G47.39
Apneumatosis, newborn P28.0
Apocrine metaplasia (breast) — *see* Dysplasia, mammary, specified type NEC
Apophysitis (bone) — *see also* Osteochondropathy
  calcaneus M92.6 ☑
  juvenile M92.9
Apoplectiform convulsions (cerebral ischemia) I67.82
Apoplexia, apoplexy, apoplectic
  adrenal A39.1
  heart (auricle) (ventricle) — *see* Infarct, myocardium
  heat T67.01 ☑
  hemorrhagic (stroke) — *see* Hemorrhage, intracranial
  meninges, hemorrhagic — *see* Hemorrhage, intracranial, subarachnoid
  uremic N18.9 [I68.8]
Appearance
  bizarre R46.1
  specified NEC R46.89
  very low level of personal hygiene R46.0
Appendage
  epididymal (organ of Morgagni) Q55.4
  intestine (epiploic) Q43.8

☑ **Additional Character Required** — **Refer to the Tabular List for Character Selection**

Appendage — *continued*
  preauricular Q17.0
  testicular (organ of Morgagni) Q55.29
Appendicitis (pneumococcal) (retrocecal) K37
  with
    gangrene K35.891
      with localized peritonitis K35.31
    perforation NOS K35.32
    peritoneal abscess K35.33
    peritonitis NEC K35.33
      generalized K35.209
        with
          abscess K35.219
            with perforation or rupture K35.211
            following rupture or perforation of appendix NOS K35.211
            without perforation or rupture K35.210
          perforation or rupture K35.201
            following rupture or perforation of appendix NOS K35.201
          without rupture or perforation of appendix K35.200
      localized K35.30
        with
          gangrene K35.31
          perforation K35.32
            and abscess K35.33
      rupture (with localized peritonitis) K35.32
  acute (catarrhal) (fulminating) (obstructive) (retrocecal) (suppurative) K35.80
    with
      gangrene K35.891
      peritoneal abscess K35.33
      peritonitis NEC K35.33
        generalized K35.209
          with
            abscess K35.219
              with perforation or rupture K35.211
              following rupture or perforation of appendix NOS K35.211
              without perforation or rupture K35.210
            perforation or rupture K35.201
              following rupture or perforation of appendix NOS K35.201
            without rupture or perforation of appendix K35.200
        localized K35.30
          with
            gangrene K35.31
            perforation K35.32
              and abscess K35.33
      specified NEC K35.890
        with gangrene K35.891
          with localized peritonitis K35.31
  amebic A06.89
  chronic (recurrent) K36
  exacerbation — *see* Appendicitis, with, gangrene
  gangrenous — *see* Appendicitis, acute
  healed (obliterative) K36
  interval K36
  neurogenic K36
  obstructive K36
  recurrent K36
  relapsing K36
  ruptured NOS (with localized peritonitis) K35.32
  subacute (adhesive) K36
  subsiding K36
  suppurative — *see* Appendicitis, acute
  tuberculous A18.32
Appendicopathia oxyurica B80
Appendix, appendicular — *see also* condition
  epididymis Q55.4
  Morgagni
    female Q50.5
    male (epididymal) Q55.4
      testicular Q55.29
  testis Q55.29
Appetite
  depraved — *see* Pica
  excessive R63.2
  lack or loss — *see also* Anorexia R63.0
    nonorganic origin F50.89
    psychogenic F50.89
  perverted (hysterical) — *see* Pica
Apple peel syndrome Q41.1
Apprehension state F41.1
Apprehensiveness, abnormal F41.9
Approximal wear K03.0

Apraxia (classic) (ideational) (ideokinetic) (ideomotor) (motor) (verbal) R48.2
  following
    cerebrovascular disease I69.990
      cerebral infarction I69.390
      intracerebral hemorrhage I69.190
      nontraumatic intracranial hemorrhage NEC I69.290
      specified disease NEC I69.890
      subarachnoid hemorrhage I69.090
  oculomotor, congenital H51.8
Aptyalism K11.7
Apudoma — *see* Neoplasm, uncertain behavior, by site
Aqueous misdirection H40.83- ☑
Arabicum elephantiasis — *see* Infestation, filarial
Arachnitis — *see* Meningitis
Arachnodactyly — *see* Syndrome, Marfan
Arachnoiditis (acute) (adhesive) (basal) (brain) (cerebrospinal) — *see* Meningitis
Arachnophobia F40.210
Arboencephalitis, Australian A83.4
Arborization block (heart) I45.5
ARC (AIDS-related complex) B20
Arch
  aortic Q25.49
  bovine Q25.49
Arches — *see* condition
Arcuate uterus Q51.810
Arcuatus uterus Q51.810
Arcus (cornea) senilis — *see* Degeneration, cornea, senile
Arc-welder's lung J63.4
Areflexia R29.2
Areola — *see* condition
Argentaffinoma — *see also* Neoplasm, uncertain behavior, by site
  malignant — *see* Neoplasm, malignant, by site
  syndrome E34.09
Argininemia E72.21
Arginosuccinic aciduria E72.22
Argyll Robertson phenomenon, pupil or syndrome (syphilitic) A52.19
  atypical H57.09
  nonsyphilitic H57.09
Argyria, argyriasis
  conjunctival H11.13- ☑
  from drug or medicament — *see* Table of Drugs and Chemicals, by substance
Argyrosis, conjunctival H11.13- ☑
Arhinencephaly Q04.1
Ariboflavinosis E53.0
Arm — *see* condition
Arnold-Chiari disease, obstruction or syndrome (type II) Q07.00
  with
    hydrocephalus Q07.02
      with spina bifida Q07.03
    spina bifida Q07.01
      with hydrocephalus Q07.03
  type III — *see* Encephalocele
  type IV Q04.8
Aromatic amino-acid metabolism disorder E70.9
  specified NEC E70.89
Arousals, confusional G47.51
Arrest, arrested
  cardiac I46.9
    complicating
      abortion — *see* Abortion, by type, complicated by, cardiac arrest
      anesthesia (general) (local) or other sedation — *see* Table of Drugs and Chemicals, by drug
        in labor and delivery O74.2
        in pregnancy O29.11- ☑
        postpartum, puerperal O89.1
      delivery (cesarean) (instrumental) O75.4
    due to
      cardiac condition I46.2
      specified condition NEC I46.8
    intraoperative I97.71- ☑
    newborn P29.81
    personal history, successfully resuscitated Z86.74
    postprocedural I97.12- ☑
      obstetric procedure O75.4
  cardiorespiratory — *see* Arrest, cardiac
  circulatory — *see* Arrest, cardiac
  deep transverse O64.0 ☑
  development or growth
    bone — *see* Disorder, bone, development or growth
    child R62.50
    tracheal rings Q32.1

Arrest, arrested — *continued*
  epiphyseal
    complete
      femur M89.15- ☑
      humerus M89.12- ☑
      tibia M89.16- ☑
      ulna M89.13- ☑
      forearm M89.13- ☑
        specified NEC M89.13- ☑
        ulna — *see* Arrest, epiphyseal, by type, ulna
      lower leg M89.16- ☑
        specified NEC M89.168
        tibia — *see* Arrest, epiphyseal, by type, tibia
    partial
      femur M89.15- ☑
      humerus M89.12- ☑
      tibia M89.16- ☑
      ulna M89.13- ☑
      specified NEC M89.18
  granulopoiesis — *see* Agranulocytosis
  growth plate — *see* Arrest, epiphyseal
  heart — *see* Arrest, cardiac
  legal, anxiety concerning Z65.3
  physeal — *see* Arrest, epiphyseal
  respiratory R09.2
    newborn P28.81
  sinus I45.5
  spermatogenesis (complete) — *see* Azoospermia
    incomplete — *see* Oligospermia
  transverse (deep) O64.0 ☑
Arrhenoblastoma
  benign
    specified site — *see* Neoplasm, benign, by site
    unspecified site
      female D27.9
      male D29.20
  malignant
    specified site — *see* Neoplasm, malignant, by site
    unspecified site
      female C56.9
      male C62.90
  specified site — *see* Neoplasm, uncertain behavior, by site
  unspecified site
    female D39.10
    male D40.10
Arrhythmia (auricle) (cardiac) (juvenile) (nodal) (reflex) (supraventricular) (transitory) (ventricle) I49.9
  block I45.9
  extrasystolic I49.49
  newborn
    bradycardia P29.12
    occurring before birth P03.819
      before onset of labor P03.810
      during labor P03.811
    tachycardia P29.11
  psychogenic F45.8
  sinus I49.8
  specified NEC I49.8
  vagal R55
  ventricular re-entry I47.0
Arrillaga-Ayerza syndrome (pulmonary sclerosis with pulmonary hypertension) I27.0
Arsenical pigmentation L81.8
  from drug or medicament — *see* Table of Drugs and Chemicals
Arsenism — *see* Poisoning, arsenic
Arterial — *see* condition
Arteriofibrosis — *see* Arteriosclerosis
Arteriolar sclerosis — *see* Arteriosclerosis
Arteriolith — *see* Arteriosclerosis
Arteriolitis I77.6
  necrotizing, kidney I77.5
  renal — *see* Hypertension, kidney
Arteriolosclerosis — *see* Arteriosclerosis
Arterionephrosclerosis — *see* Hypertension, kidney
Arteriopathy I77.9
  cerebral autosomal dominant, with subcortical infarcts and leukoencephalopathy (CADASIL) I67.850
Arteriosclerosis, arteriosclerotic (diffuse) (obliterans) (of) (senile) (with calcification) I70.90
  with
    chronic limb-threatening ischemia — *see* Arteriosclerosis, with critical limb ischemia
    critical limb ischemia
      bypass graft I70.329
        autologous vein graft I70.429
          leg I70.429

Arteriosclerosis, arteriosclerotic — *continued*
  with — *continued*
    critical limb ischemia — *continued*
      bypass graft — *continued*
        autologous vein graft — *continued*
          leg — *continued*
            with
              gangrene (and intermittent claudication, rest pain, and ulcer) I70.469
              rest pain (and intermittent claudication) I70.429
            bilateral I70.423
              with
                gangrene (and intermittent claudication, rest pain, and ulcer) I70.463
                rest pain (and intermittent claudication) I70.423
            left I70.422
              with
                gangrene (and intermittent claudication, rest pain, and ulcer) I70.462
                rest pain (and intermittent claudication) I70.422
                ulceration (and intermittent claudication and rest pain) I70.449
                  ankle I70.443
                  calf I70.442
                  foot site NEC I70.445
                  heel I70.444
                  lower leg NEC I70.448
                  mid foot I70.444
                  thigh I70.441
            right I70.421
              with
                gangrene (and intermittent claudication, rest pain, and ulcer) I70.461
                rest pain (and intermittent claudication) I70.421
                ulceration (and intermittent claudication and rest pain) I70.439
                  ankle I70.433
                  calf I70.432
                  foot site NEC I70.435
                  heel I70.434
                  lower leg NEC I70.438
                  midfoot I70.434
                  thigh I70.431
        leg I70.329
          with
            gangrene (and intermittent claudication, rest pain, and ulcer) I70.369
            rest pain (and intermittent claudication) I70.329
          bilateral I70.323
            with
              gangrene (and intermittent claudication, rest pain, and ulcer) I70.363
              rest pain (and intermittent claudication) I70.323
          left I70.322
            with
              gangrene (and intermittent claudication, rest pain, and ulcer) I70.362
              rest pain (and intermittent claudication) I70.322
              ulceration (and intermittent claudication and rest pain) I70.349
                ankle I70.343
                calf I70.342
                foot site NEC I70.345
                heel I70.344
                lower leg NEC I70.348
                midfoot I70.344
                thigh I70.341
          right I70.321
            with
              gangrene (and intermittent claudication, rest pain, and ulcer) I70.361
              rest pain (and intermittent claudication) I70.321

Arteriosclerosis, arteriosclerotic — *continued*
  with — *continued*
    critical limb ischemia — *continued*
      bypass graft — *continued*
        leg — *continued*
          right — *continued*
            with — *continued*
              ulceration (and intermittent claudication and rest pain) I70.339
                ankle I70.333
                calf I70.332
                foot site NEC I70.335
                heel I70.334
                lower leg NEC I70.338
                midfoot I70.334
                thigh I70.331
        nonautologous biological graft I70.529
          leg I70.529
            with
              gangrene (and intermittent claudication, rest pain, and ulcer) I70.569
              rest pain (and intermittent claudication) I70.529
            bilateral I70.523
              with
                gangrene (and intermittent claudication, rest pain, and ulcer) I70.563
                rest pain (and intermittent claudication) I70.523
            left I70.522
              with
                gangrene (and intermittent claudication, rest pain, and ulcer) I70.562
                rest pain (and intermittent claudication) I70.522
                ulceration (and intermittent claudication and rest pain) I70.549
                  ankle I70.543
                  calf I70.542
                  foot site NEC I70.545
                  heel I70.544
                  lower leg NEC I70.548
                  midfoot I70.544
                  thigh I70.541
            right I70.521
              with
                gangrene (and intermittent claudication, rest pain, and ulcer) I70.561
                rest pain (and intermittent claudication) I70.521
                ulceration (and intermittent claudication and rest pain) I70.539
                  ankle I70.533
                  calf I70.532
                  foot site NEC I70.535
                  heel I70.534
                  lower leg NEC I70.538
                  midfoot I70.534
                  thigh I70.531
        nonbiological graft I70.629
          leg I70.629
            with
              gangrene (and intermittent claudication, rest pain, and ulcer) I70.669
              rest pain (and intermittent claudication) I70.629
            bilateral I70.623
              with
                gangrene (and intermittent claudication, rest pain, and ulcer) I70.663
                rest pain (intermittent claudication) I70.623
            left I70.622
              with
                gangrene (and intermittent claudication, rest pain, and ulcer) I70.662
                rest pain (and intermittent claudication) I70.622

Arteriosclerosis, arteriosclerotic — *continued*
  with — *continued*
    critical limb ischemia — *continued*
      bypass graft — *continued*
        nonbiological graft — *continued*
          leg — *continued*
            left — *continued*
              with — *continued*
                ulceration (and intermittent claudication and rest pain) I70.649
                  ankle I70.643
                  calf I70.642
                  foot site NEC I70.645
                  heel I70.644
                  lower leg NEC I70.648
                  midfoot I70.644
                  thigh I70.641
            right I70.621
              with
                gangrene (and intermittent claudication, rest pain, and ulcer) I70.661
                rest pain (and intermittent claudication) I70.621
                ulceration (and intermittent claudication and rest pain) I70.639
                  ankle I70.633
                  calf I70.632
                  foot site NEC I70.635
                  heel I70.634
                  lower leg NEC I70.638
                  midfoot I70.634
                  thigh I70.631
        specified graft NEC I70.729
          leg I70.729
            with
              gangrene (and intermittent claudication, rest pain, and ulcer) I70.769
              rest pain (and intermittent claudication) I70.729
            bilateral I70.723
              with
                gangrene (and intermittent claudication, rest pain, and ulcer) I70.763
                rest pain (and intermittent claudication) I70.723
            left I70.722
              with
                gangrene (and intermittent claudication, rest pain, and ulcer) I70.762
                rest pain (and intermittent claudication) I70.722
                ulceration (and intermittent claudication and rest pain) I70.749
                  ankle I70.743
                  calf I70.742
                  foot site NEC I70.745
                  heel I70.744
                  lower leg NEC I70.748
                  midfoot I70.744
                  thigh I70.741
            right I70.721
              with
                gangrene (and intermittent claudication, rest pain, and ulcer) I70.761
                rest pain (and intermittent claudication) I70.721
                ulceration (and intermittent claudication and rest pain) I70.739
                  ankle I70.733
                  calf I70.732
                  foot site NEC I70.735
                  heel I70.734
                  lower leg NEC I70.738
                  midfoot I70.734
                  thigh I70.731
        leg I70.229
          with
            gangrene (and intermittent claudication, rest pain, and ulcer) I70.269

Arteriosclerosis, arteriosclerotic — *continued*
  with — *continued*
    critical limb ischemia — *continued*
      leg — *continued*
        with — *continued*
          rest pain (and intermittent claudication)
            I70.229
          bilateral I70.223
            with
              gangrene (and intermittent claudica-
                tion, rest pain, and ulcer) I70.263
              rest pain (and intermittent claudication)
                I70.223
          left I70.222
            with
              gangrene (and intermittent claudica-
                tion, rest pain, and ulcer) I70.262
              rest pain (and intermittent claudication)
                I70.222
              ulceration (and intermittent claudica-
                tion and rest pain) I70.249
                ankle I70.243
                calf I70.242
                foot site NEC I70.245
                heel I70.244
                lower leg NEC I70.248
                midfoot I70.244
                thigh I70.241
          right I70.221
            with
              gangrene (and intermittent claudica-
                tion, rest pain, and ulcer) I70.261
              rest pain (and intermittent claudication)
                I70.221
              ulceration (and intermittent claudica-
                tion and rest pain) I70.239
                ankle I70.233
                calf I70.232
                foot site NEC I70.235
                heel I70.234
                lower leg NEC I70.238
                midfoot I70.234
                thigh I70.231
  aorta I70.0
  arteries of extremities — *see* Arteriosclerosis, extremities
    with
      chronic limb-threatening ischemia — *see* Arte-
        riosclerosis, with critical limb ischemia
      critical limb ischemia — *see* Arteriosclerosis, with
        critical limb ischemia
  brain I67.2
    with infarction — *see* Occlusion, artery, brain or
      cerebral, with infarction
  bypass graft
    with
      chronic limb-threatening ischemia — *see* Arte-
        riosclerosis, with critical limb ischemia
      critical limb ischemia — *see* Arteriosclerosis, with
        critical limb ischemia
      coronary — *see* Arteriosclerosis, coronary, bypass
        graft
      extremities — *see* Arteriosclerosis, extremities, bypass
        graft
  cardiac — *see* Disease, heart, ischemic, atherosclerotic
  cardiopathy — *see* Disease, heart, ischemic, atheroscle-
    rotic
  cardiorenal — *see* Hypertension, cardiorenal
  cardiovascular — *see* Disease, heart, ischemic,
    atherosclerotic
  carotid — *see also* Occlusion, artery, carotid I65.2- ☑
  central nervous system I67.2
    with infarction — *see* Occlusion, artery, cerebral or
      precerebral, with infarction
  cerebral I67.2
    with infarction — *see* Occlusion, artery, brain or
      cerebral, with infarction
  cerebrovascular I67.2
    with infarction — *see* Occlusion, artery, brain or
      cerebral, with infarction
  coronary (artery) I25.10
    due to
      calcified coronary lesion (severely) I25.84
      lipid rich plaque I25.83
    bypass graft I25.810
      with
        angina pectoris I25.709
          with documented spasm I25.701
          refractory I25.702
          specified type NEC I25.708

Arteriosclerosis, arteriosclerotic — *continued*
  coronary — *continued*
    bypass graft — *continued*
      with — *continued*
        angina pectoris — *continued*
          unstable I25.700
        ischemic chest pain I25.709
      autologous artery I25.810
        with
          angina pectoris I25.729
            with documented spasm I25.721
            refractory I25.722
            specified type I25.728
            unstable I25.720
          ischemic chest pain I25.729
      autologous vein I25.810
        with
          angina pectoris I25.719
            with documented spasm I25.711
            refractory I25.712
            specified type I25.718
            unstable I25.710
          ischemic chest pain I25.719
      nonautologous biological I25.810
        with
          angina pectoris I25.739
            with documented spasm I25.731
            refractory I25.732
            specified type I25.738
            unstable I25.730
          ischemic chest pain I25.739
      specified type NEC I25.810
        with
          angina pectoris I25.799
            with documented spasm I25.791
            refractory I25.792
            specified type I25.798
            unstable I25.790
          ischemic chest pain I25.799
    native vessel
      with
        angina pectoris I25.119
          with documented spasm I25.111
          refractory I25.112
          specified type NEC I25.118
          unstable I25.110
        ischemic chest pain I25.119
    transplanted heart I25.811
      bypass graft I25.812
        with
          angina pectoris I25.769
            with documented spasm I25.761
            refractory I25.762
            specified type I25.768
            unstable I25.760
          ischemic chest pain I25.769
      native coronary artery I25.811
        with
          angina pectoris I25.759
            with documented spasm I25.751
            refractory I25.752
            specified type I25.758
            unstable I25.750
          ischemic chest pain I25.759
  extremities (native arteries) I70.209
    with
      chronic limb-threatening ischemia — *see* Arte-
        riosclerosis, with critical limb ischemia
      critical limb ischemia — *see* Arteriosclerosis, with
        critical limb ischemia
    bypass graft I70.309
      with
        chronic limb-threatening ischemia — *see* Arte-
          riosclerosis, with critical limb ischemia
        critical limb ischemia — *see* Arteriosclerosis,
          with critical limb ischemia
      autologous vein graft I70.409
        leg I70.409
          with
            gangrene (and intermittent claudica-
              tion, rest pain and ulcer) I70.469
            intermittent claudication I70.419
            rest pain (and intermittent claudication)
              I70.429
          bilateral I70.403
            with
              gangrene (and intermittent claudica-
                tion, rest pain and ulcer)
                I70.463

Arteriosclerosis, arteriosclerotic — *continued*
  extremities — *continued*
    bypass graft — *continued*
      autologous vein graft — *continued*
        leg — *continued*
          bilateral — *continued*
            with — *continued*
              intermittent claudication I70.463
              rest pain (and intermittent claudica-
                tion) I70.423
            specified type NEC I70.493
          left I70.402
            with
              gangrene (and intermittent claudica-
                tion, rest pain and ulcer)
                I70.462
              intermittent claudication I70.412
              rest pain (and intermittent claudica-
                tion) I70.422
              ulceration (and intermittent claudica-
                tion and rest pain) I70.449
                ankle I70.443
                calf I70.442
                foot site NEC I70.445
                heel I70.444
                lower leg NEC I70.448
                midfoot I70.444
                thigh I70.441
            specified type NEC I70.492
          right I70.401
            with
              gangrene (and intermittent claudica-
                tion, rest pain and ulcer)
                I70.461
              intermittent claudication I70.411
              rest pain (and intermittent claudica-
                tion) I70.421
              ulceration (and intermittent claudica-
                tion and rest pain) I70.439
                ankle I70.433
                calf I70.432
                foot site NEC I70.435
                heel I70.434
                lower leg NEC I70.438
                midfoot I70.434
                thigh I70.431
            specified type NEC I70.491
        specified type NEC I70.499
      specified NEC I70.408
        with
          gangrene (and intermittent claudica-
            tion, rest pain and ulcer) I70.468
          intermittent claudication I70.418
          rest pain (and intermittent claudication)
            I70.428
          ulceration (and intermittent claudica-
            tion and rest pain) I70.45
        specified type NEC I70.498
    leg I70.309
      with
        gangrene (and intermittent claudication,
          rest pain and ulcer) I70.369
        intermittent claudication I70.319
        rest pain (and intermittent claudication)
          I70.329
      bilateral I70.303
        with
          gangrene (and intermittent claudica-
            tion, rest pain and ulcer) I70.363
          intermittent claudication I70.313
          rest pain (and intermittent claudication)
            I70.323
        specified type NEC I70.393
      left I70.302
        with
          gangrene (and intermittent claudica-
            tion, rest pain and ulcer) I70.362
          intermittent claudication I70.312
          rest pain (and intermittent claudication)
            I70.322
          ulceration (and intermittent claudica-
            tion and rest pain) I70.349
            ankle I70.343
            calf I70.342
            foot site NEC I70.345
            heel I70.344
            lower leg NEC I70.348
            midfoot I70.344
            thigh I70.341

☑ **Additional Character Required — Refer to the Tabular List for Character Selection**

Arteriosclerosis, arteriosclerotic — *continued*
  extremities — *continued*
    bypass graft — *continued*
      leg — *continued*
        left — *continued*
          specified type NEC I70.392
        right I70.301
          with
            gangrene (and intermittent claudication, rest pain and ulcer) I70.361
            intermittent claudication I70.311
            rest pain (and intermittent claudication) I70.321
            ulceration (and intermittent claudication and rest pain I70.339
              ankle I70.333
              calf I70.332
              foot site NEC I70.335
              heel I70.334
              lower leg NEC I70.338
              midfoot I70.334
              thigh I70.331
          specified type NEC I70.391
        specified type NEC I70.399
      nonautologous biological graft I70.509
        leg I70.509
          with
            gangrene (and intermittent claudication, rest pain and ulcer) I70.569
            intermittent claudication I70.519
            rest pain (and intermittent claudication) I70.529
        bilateral I70.503
          with
            gangrene (and intermittent claudication, rest pain and ulcer) I70.563
            intermittent claudication I70.513
            rest pain (and intermittent claudication) I70.523
          specified type NEC I70.593
        left I70.502
          with
            gangrene (and intermittent claudication, rest pain and ulcer) I70.562
            intermittent claudication I70.512
            rest pain (and intermittent claudication) I70.522
            ulceration (and intermittent claudication and rest pain) I70.549
              ankle I70.543
              calf I70.542
              foot site NEC I70.545
              heel I70.544
              lower leg NEC I70.548
              midfoot I70.544
              thigh I70.541
          specified type NEC I70.592
        right I70.501
          with
            gangrene (and intermittent claudication, rest pain and ulcer) I70.561
            intermittent claudication I70.511
            rest pain (and intermittent claudication) I70.521
            ulceration (and intermittent claudication and rest pain) I70.539
              ankle I70.533
              calf I70.532
              foot site NEC I70.535
              heel I70.534
              lower leg NEC I70.538
              midfoot I70.534
              thigh I70.531
          specified type NEC I70.591
        specified type NEC I70.599
      specified NEC I70.508
        with
          gangrene (and intermittent claudication, rest pain and ulcer) I70.568
          intermittent claudication I70.518
          rest pain (and intermittent claudication) I70.528
          ulceration (and intermittent claudication and rest pain) I70.55
        specified type NEC I70.598
      nonbiological graft I70.609

Arteriosclerosis, arteriosclerotic — *continued*
  extremities — *continued*
    bypass graft — *continued*
      nonbiological graft — *continued*
        leg I70.609
          with
            gangrene (and intermittent claudication, rest pain and ulcer) I70.669
            intermittent claudication I70.619
            rest pain (and intermittent claudication) I70.629
        bilateral I70.603
          with
            gangrene (and intermittent claudication, rest pain and ulcer) I70.663
            intermittent claudication I70.613
            rest pain (and intermittent claudication) I70.623
          specified type NEC I70.693
        left I70.602
          with
            gangrene (and intermittent claudication, rest pain and ulcer) I70.662
            intermittent claudication I70.612
            rest pain (and intermittent claudication) I70.622
            ulceration (and intermittent claudication and rest pain) I70.649
              ankle I70.643
              calf I70.642
              foot site NEC I70.645
              heel I70.644
              lower leg NEC I70.648
              midfoot I70.644
              thigh I70.641
          specified type NEC I70.692
        right I70.601
          with
            gangrene (and intermittent claudication, rest pain and ulcer) I70.661
            intermittent claudication I70.611
            rest pain (and intermittent claudication) I70.621
            ulceration (and intermittent claudication and rest pain) I70.639
              ankle I70.633
              calf I70.632
              foot site NEC I70.635
              heel I70.634
              lower leg NEC I70.638
              midfoot I70.634
              thigh I70.631
          specified type NEC I70.691
        specified type NEC I70.699
      specified NEC I70.608
        with
          gangrene (and intermittent claudication, rest pain and ulcer) I70.668
          intermittent claudication I70.618
          rest pain (and intermittent claudication) I70.628
          ulceration (and intermittent claudication and rest pain) I70.65
        specified type NEC I70.698
      specified graft NEC I70.709
        leg I70.709
          with
            gangrene (and intermittent claudication, rest pain and ulcer) I70.769
            intermittent claudication I70.719
            rest pain (and intermittent claudication) I70.729
        bilateral I70.703
          with
            gangrene (and intermittent claudication, rest pain and ulcer) I70.763
            intermittent claudication I70.713
            rest pain (and intermittent claudication) I70.723
          specified type NEC I70.793
        left I70.702
          with
            gangrene (and intermittent claudication, rest pain and ulcer) I70.762

Arteriosclerosis, arteriosclerotic — *continued*
  extremities — *continued*
    bypass graft — *continued*
      specified graft — *continued*
        leg — *continued*
          left — *continued*
            with — *continued*
              intermittent claudication I70.712
              rest pain (and intermittent claudication) I70.722
              ulceration (and intermittent claudication and rest pain) I70.749
                ankle I70.743
                calf I70.742
                foot site NEC I70.745
                heel I70.744
                lower leg NEC I70.748
                midfoot I70.744
                thigh I70.741
            specified type NEC I70.792
          right I70.701
            with
              gangrene (and intermittent claudication, rest pain and ulcer) I70.761
              intermittent claudication I70.711
              rest pain (and intermittent claudication) I70.721
              ulceration (and intermittent claudication and rest pain) I70.739
                ankle I70.733
                calf I70.732
                foot site NEC I70.735
                heel I70.734
                lower leg NEC I70.738
                midfoot I70.734
                thigh I70.731
            specified type NEC I70.791
          specified type NEC I70.799
        specified NEC I70.708
          with
            gangrene (and intermittent claudication, rest pain and ulcer) I70.768
            intermittent claudication I70.718
            rest pain (and intermittent claudication) I70.728
            ulceration (and intermittent claudication and rest pain) I70.75
          specified type NEC I70.798
      specified NEC I70.308
        with
          gangrene (and intermittent claudication, rest pain and ulcer) I70.368
          intermittent claudication I70.318
          rest pain (and intermittent claudication) I70.328
          ulceration (and intermittent claudication and rest pain) I70.35
        specifiec type NEC I70.398
    leg I70.209
      with
        gangrene (and intermittent claudication, rest pain and ulcer) I70.269
        intermittent claudication I70.219
        rest pain (and intermittent claudication) I70.229
    bilateral I70.203
      with
        gangrene (and intermittent claudication, rest pain and ulcer) I70.263
        intermittent claudication I70.213
        rest pain (and intermittent claudication) I70.223
        specified type NEC I70.293
    left I70.202
      with
        gangrene (and intermittent claudication, rest pain and ulcer) I70.262
        intermittent claudication I70.212
        rest pain (and intermittent claudication) I70.222
        ulceration (and intermittent claudication and rest pain) I70.249
          ankle I70.243
          calf I70.242
          foot site NEC I70.245
          heel I70.244
          lower leg NEC I70.248
          midfoot I70.244
          thigh I70.241

Arteriosclerosis, arteriosclerotic — *continued*
  extremities — *continued*
    leg — *continued*
      left — *continued*
        specified type NEC I70.292
      right I70.201
        with
          gangrene (and intermittent claudication, rest pain and ulcer) I70.261
          intermittent claudication I70.211
          rest pain (and intermittent claudication) I70.221
          ulceration (and intermittent claudication and rest pain) I70.239
            ankle I70.233
            calf I70.232
            foot site NEC I70.235
            heel I70.234
            lower leg NEC I70.238
            midfoot I70.234
            thigh I70.231
        specified type NEC I70.291
      specified type NEC I70.299
    specified site NEC I70.208
      with
        gangrene (and intermittent claudication, rest pain and ulcer) I70.268
        intermittent claudication I70.218
        rest pain (and intermittent claudication) I70.228
        ulceration (and intermittent claudication and rest pain) I70.25
      specified type NEC I70.298
  generalized I70.91
  heart (disease) — *see* Arteriosclerosis, coronary (artery)
  kidney — *see* Hypertension, kidney
  medial — *see* Arteriosclerosis, extremities
  mesenteric (artery) K55.1
  Monckeberg's — *see* Arteriosclerosis, extremities
  myocarditis I51.4
  peripheral (of extremities) — *see* Arteriosclerosis, extremities
  pulmonary (idiopathic) I27.0
  renal (arterioles) — *see also* Hypertension, kidney
    artery I70.1
  retina (vascular) I70.8 *[H35.0-]* ☑
  specified artery NEC I70.8
  spinal (cord) G95.19
  vertebral (artery) I67.2
    with infarction — *see* Occlusion, artery, vertebral, with infarction
Arteriospasm I73.9
Arteriovenous — *see* condition
Arteritis I77.6
  allergic M31.0
  aorta (nonsyphilitic) I77.6
    syphilitic A52.02
  aortic arch M31.4
  brachiocephalic M31.4
  brain I67.7
    syphilitic A52.04
  cerebral I67.7
    in systemic lupus erythematosus M32.19
    listerial A32.89
    syphilitic A52.04
    tuberculous A18.89
  coronary (artery) I25.89
    rheumatic I01.8
      chronic I09.89
    syphilitic A52.06
  cranial (left) (right), giant cell M31.6
  deformans — *see* Arteriosclerosis
  giant cell NEC M31.6
    with polymyalgia rheumatica M31.5
  necrosing or necrotizing M31.9
    specified NEC M31.8
  nodosa M30.0
  obliterans — *see* Arteriosclerosis
  pulmonary I28.8
  rheumatic — *see* Fever, rheumatic
  senile — *see* Arteriosclerosis
  suppurative I77.2
  syphilitic (general) A52.09
    brain A52.04
    coronary A52.06
    spinal A52.09
  temporal, giant cell M31.6
  young female aortic arch syndrome M31.4
Artery, arterial — *see also* condition
  abscess I77.89

Artery, arterial — *continued*
  single umbilical Q27.0
Arthralgia (allergic) — *see also* Pain, joint
  in caisson disease T70.3 ☑
  temporomandibular M26.62- ☑
Arthritis, arthritic (acute) (chronic) (nonpyogenic) (subacute) M19.90
  allergic — *see* Arthritis, specified form NEC
  ankylosing (crippling) (spine) — *see also* Spondylitis, ankylosing
    sites other than spine — *see* Arthritis, specified form NEC
  atrophic — *see* Osteoarthritis
    spine — *see* Spondylitis, ankylosing
  back — *see* Spondylopathy, inflammatory
  blennorrhagic (gonococcal) A54.42
  Charcot's — *see* Arthropathy, neuropathic
    diabetic — *see* Diabetes, arthropathy, neuropathic
    syringomyelic G95.0
  chylous (filarial) — *see also* category M01 B74.9
  climacteric (any site) NEC — *see* Arthritis, specified form NEC
  crystal (-induced) — *see* Arthritis, in, crystals
  deformans — *see* Osteoarthritis
  degenerative — *see* Osteoarthritis
  due to or associated with
    acromegaly E22.0
    brucellosis — *see* Brucellosis
    caisson disease T70.3 ☑
    diabetes — *see* Diabetes, arthropathy
    dracontiasis — *see also* category M01 B72
    enteritis NEC
      regional — *see* Enteritis, regional
    erysipelas — *see also* category M01 A46
    erythema
      epidemic A25.1
      nodosum L52
    filariasis NOS B74.9
    glanders A24.0
    helminthiasis — *see also* category M01 B83.9
    hemophilia D66 *[M36.2]*
    Henoch- (Schonlein) purpura D69.0 *[M36.4]*
    human parvovirus — *see also* category M01 B97.6
    infectious disease NEC M01 ☑
    leprosy (see also category M01) — *see also* Leprosy A30.9
    Lyme disease A69.23
    mycobacteria — *see also* category M01 A31.8
    parasitic disease NEC — *see also* category M01 B89
    paratyphoid fever (see also category M01) — *see also* Fever, paratyphoid A01.4
    rat bite fever — *see also* category M01 A25.1
    regional enteritis — *see* Enteritis, regional
    respiratory disorder NOS J98.9
    serum sickness — *see also* Reaction, serum T80.69 ☑
    syringomyelia G95.0
    typhoid fever A01.04
  epidemic erythema A25.1
  facet joint — *see also* Spondylosis M47.819
  febrile — *see* Fever, rheumatic
  gonococcal A54.42
  gouty (acute) — *see* Gout
  in (due to)
    acromegaly — *see also* subcategory M14.8- E22.0
    amyloidosis — *see also* subcategory M14.8- E85.4
    bacterial disease — *see also* subcategory M01 A49.9
    Behcet's syndrome M35.2
    caisson disease — *see also* subcategory M14.8- T70.3 ☑
    coliform bacilli (Escherichia coli) — *see* Arthritis, in, pyogenic organism NEC
    crystals M11.9
      dicalcium phosphate — *see* Arthritis, in, crystals, specified type NEC
      hydroxyapatite M11.0- ☑
      pyrophosphate — *see* Arthritis, in, crystals, specified type NEC
      specified type NEC M11.80
        ankle M11.87- ☑
        elbow M11.82- ☑
        foot joint M11.87- ☑
        hand joint M11.84- ☑
        hip M11.85- ☑
        knee M11.86- ☑
        multiple sites M11.8- ☑
        shoulder M11.81- ☑
        vertebrae M11.88
        wrist M11.83- ☑

Arthritis, arthritic — *continued*
  in — *continued*
    dermatoarthritis, lipoid E78.81
    dracontiasis (dracunculiasis) — *see also* category M01 B72
    endocrine disorder NEC — *see also* subcategory M14.8- E34.9
    enteritis, infectious NEC — *see also* category M01 A09
      specified organism NEC — *see also* category M01 A08.8
    erythema
      multiforme — *see also* subcategory M14.8- L51.9
      nodosum — *see also* subcategory M14.8- L52
    gout — *see* Gout
    helminthiasis NEC — *see also* category M01 B83.9
    hemochromatosis — *see also* subcategory M14.8- E83.118
    hemoglobinopathy NEC D58.2 *[M36.3]*
    hemophilia NEC D66 *[M36.2]*
    Hemophilus influenzae M00.8- ☑ *[B96.3]*
    Henoch (-Schonlein) purpura D69.0 *[M36.4]*
    hyperparathyroidism NEC — *see also* subcategory M14.8- E21.3
    hypersensitivity reaction NEC T78.49 ☑ *[M36.4]*
    hypogammaglobulinemia — *see also* subcategory M14.8- D80.1
    hypothyroidism NEC — *see also* subcategory M14.8- E03.9
    infection — *see* Arthritis, pyogenic or pyemic
      spine — *see* Spondylopathy, infective
    infectious disease NEC M01
    leprosy — *see also* category M01 A30.9
    leukemia NEC C95.9- ☑ *[M36.1]*
    lipoid dermatoarthritis E78.81
    Lyme disease A69.23
    Mediterranean fever, familial — *see also* subcategory M14.8- M04.1
    Meningococcus A39.83
    metabolic disorder NEC — *see also* subcategory M14.8- E88.9
    multiple myelomatosis C90.0- ☑ *[M36.1]*
    mumps B26.85
    mycosis NEC — *see also* category M01 B49
    myelomatosis (multiple) C90.0- ☑ *[M36.1]*
    neurological disorder NEC G98.0
    ochronosis — *see also* subcategory M14.8- E70.29
    O'nyong-nyong — *see also* category M01 A92.1
    parasitic disease NEC — *see also* category M01 B89
    paratyphoid fever — *see also* category M01 A01.4
    Pseudomonas — *see* Arthritis, pyogenic, bacterial NEC
    psoriasis L40.50
    pyogenic organism NEC — *see* Arthritis, pyogenic, bacterial NEC
    Reiter's disease — *see* Reiter's disease
    respiratory disorder NEC — *see also* subcategory M14.8- J98.9
    reticulosis, malignant — *see also* subcategory M14.8- C86.0- ☑
    rubella B06.82
    Salmonella (arizonae) (cholerae-suis) (enteritidis) (typhimurium) A02.23
    sarcoidosis D86.86
    specified bacteria NEC — *see* Arthritis, pyogenic, bacterial NEC
    sporotrichosis B42.82
    syringomyelia G95.0
    thalassemia NEC D56.9 *[M36.3]*
    tuberculosis — *see* Tuberculosis, arthritis
    typhoid fever A01.04
    urethritis, Reiter's — *see* Reiter's disease
    viral disease NEC — *see also* category M01 B34.9
  infectious or infective — *see also* Arthritis, pyogenic or pyemic
    spine — *see* Spondylopathy, infective
  juvenile M08.90
    with systemic onset — *see* Still's disease
    ankle M08.97- ☑
    elbow M08.92- ☑
    foot joint M08.97- ☑
    hand joint M08.94- ☑
    hip M08.95- ☑
    knee M08.96- ☑
    multiple site M08.99
    pauciarticular M08.40
      ankle M08.47- ☑
      elbow M08.42- ☑
      foot joint M08.47- ☑

Arthritis, arthritic — *continued*
  juvenile — *continued*
    pauciarticular — *continued*
      hand joint M08.44- ☑
      hip M08.45- ☑
      knee M08.46- ☑
      shoulder M08.41- ☑
      specified site NEC M08.4A
      vertebrae M08.48
      wrist M08.43- ☑
    psoriatic L40.54
    rheumatoid — *see* Arthritis, rheumatoid, juvenile
    shoulder M08.91- ☑
    specified site NEC M08.9A
    specified type NEC M08.80
      ankle M08.87- ☑
      elbow M08.82- ☑
      foot joint M08.87- ☑
      hand joint M08.84- ☑
      hip M08.85- ☑
      knee M08.86- ☑
      multiple site M08.89
      shoulder M08.81- ☑
      specified joint NEC M08.88
      vertebrae M08.88
      wrist M08.83- ☑
    wrist M08.93- ☑
  meaning osteoarthritis — *see* Osteoarthritis
  meningococcal A39.83
  menopausal (any site) NEC — *see* Arthritis, specified form NEC
  mutilans (psoriatic) L40.52
  mycotic NEC — *see also* category M01 B49
  neuropathic (Charcot) — *see* Arthropathy, neuropathic
    diabetic — *see* Diabetes, arthropathy, neuropathic
    nonsyphilitic NEC G98.0
    syringomyelic G95.0
  ochronotic — *see also* subcategory M14.8- E70.29
  palindromic (any site) — *see* Rheumatism, palindromic
  pneumococcal M00.10
    ankle M00.17- ☑
    elbow M00.12- ☑
    foot joint — *see* Arthritis, pneumococcal, ankle
    hand joint M00.14- ☑
    hip M00.15- ☑
    knee M00.16- ☑
    multiple site M00.19
    shoulder M00.11- ☑
    vertebra M00.18
    wrist M00.13- ☑
  postdysenteric — *see* Arthropathy, postdysenteric
  postmeningococcal A39.84
  postrheumatic, chronic — *see* Arthropathy, postrheumatic, chronic
  primary progressive — *see also* Arthritis, specified form NEC
    spine — *see* Spondylitis, ankylosing
  psoriatic L40.50
  purulent (any site except spine) — *see* Arthritis, pyogenic or pyemic
    spine — *see* Spondylopathy, infective
  pyogenic or pyemic (any site except spine) M00.9
    bacterial NEC M00.80
      ankle M00.87- ☑
      elbow M00.82- ☑
      foot joint — *see* Arthritis, pyogenic, bacterial NEC, ankle
      hand joint M00.84- ☑
      hip M00.85- ☑
      knee M00.86- ☑
      multiple site M00.89
      shoulder M00.81- ☑
      vertebra M00.88
      wrist M00.83- ☑
    pneumococcal — *see* Arthritis, pneumococcal
    spine — *see* Spondylopathy, infective
    staphylococcal — *see* Arthritis, staphylococcal
    streptococcal — *see* Arthritis, streptococcal NEC
      pneumococcal — *see* Arthritis, pneumococcal
  reactive — *see* Reiter's disease
  rheumatic — *see also* Arthritis, rheumatoid
    acute or subacute — *see* Fever, rheumatic
  rheumatoid M06.9
    with
      carditis — *see* Rheumatoid, carditis
      endocarditis — *see* Rheumatoid, carditis
      heart involvement NEC — *see* Rheumatoid, carditis

Arthritis, arthritic — *continued*
  rheumatoid — *continued*
    with — *continued*
      lung involvement — *see* Rheumatoid, lung
      myocarditis — *see* Rheumatoid, carditis
      myopathy — *see* Rheumatoid, myopathy
      pericarditis — *see* Rheumatoid, carditis
      polyneuropathy — *see* Rheumatoid, polyneuropathy
      rheumatoid factor — *see* Arthritis, rheumatoid, seropositive
      splenoadenomegaly and leukopenia — *see* Felty's syndrome
      vasculitis — *see* Rheumatoid, vasculitis
      visceral involvement NEC — *see* Rheumatoid, arthritis, with involvement of organs NEC
    juvenile (with or without rheumatoid factor) M08.00
      with systemic onset — *see* Still's disease
      ankle M08.07- ☑
      elbow M08.02- ☑
      foot joint M08.07- ☑
      hand joint M08.04- ☑
      hip M08.05- ☑
      knee M08.06- ☑
      multiple site M08.09
      shoulder M08.01- ☑
      specified site NEC M08.0A
      vertebra M08.08
      wrist M08.03- ☑
    seronegative M06.00
      ankle M06.07- ☑
      elbow M06.02- ☑
      foot joint M06.07- ☑
      hand joint M06.04- ☑
      hip M06.05- ☑
      knee M06.06- ☑
      multiple site M06.09
      shoulder M06.01- ☑
      specified site NEC M06.0A
      vertebra M06.08
      wrist M06.03- ☑
    seropositive M05.9
      specified NEC M05.80
        ankle M05.87- ☑
        elbow M05.82- ☑
        foot joint M05.87- ☑
        hand joint M05.84- ☑
        hip M05.85- ☑
        knee M05.86- ☑
        multiple sites M05.89
        shoulder M05.81- ☑
        specified site NEC M05.8A
        vertebra — *see* Spondylitis, ankylosing
        wrist M05.83- ☑
      without organ involvement M05.70
        ankle M05.77- ☑
        elbow M05.72- ☑
        foot joint M05.77- ☑
        hand joint M05.74- ☑
        hip M05.75- ☑
        knee M05.76- ☑
        multiple sites M05.79
        shoulder M05.71- ☑
        specified site NEC M05.7A
        vertebra — *see* Spondylitis, ankylosing
        wrist M05.73- ☑
    specified type NEC M06.80
      ankle M06.87- ☑
      elbow M06.82- ☑
      foot joint M06.87- ☑
      hand joint M06.84- ☑
      hip M06.85- ☑
      knee M06.86- ☑
      multiple site M06.89
      shoulder M06.81- ☑
      specified site NEC M06.8A
      vertebra M06.88
      wrist M06.83- ☑
    spine — *see* Spondylitis, ankylosing
  rubella B06.82
  scorbutic — *see also* subcategory M14.8- E54
  senile or senescent — *see* Osteoarthritis
  septic (any site except spine) — *see* Arthritis, pyogenic or pyemic
    spine — *see* Spondylopathy, infective
  serum (nontherapeutic) (therapeutic) — *see* Arthropathy, postimmunization

Arthritis, arthritic — *continued*
  specified form NEC M13.80
    ankle M13.87- ☑
    elbow M13.82- ☑
    foot joint M13.87- ☑
    hand joint M13.84- ☑
    hip M13.85- ☑
    knee M13.86- ☑
    multiple site M13.89
    shoulder M13.81- ☑
    specified joint NEC M13.88
    wrist M13.83- ☑
  spine — *see also* Spondylosis
    infectious or infective NEC — *see* Spondylopathy, infective
    Marie-Strumpell — *see* Spondylitis, ankylosing
    pyogenic — *see* Spondylopathy, infective
    rheumatoid — *see* Spondylitis, ankylosing
    traumatic (old) — *see* Spondylopathy, traumatic
    tuberculous A18.01
  staphylococcal M00.00
    ankle M00.07- ☑
    elbow M00.02- ☑
    foot joint — *see* Arthritis, staphylococcal, ankle
    hand joint M00.04- ☑
    hip M00.05- ☑
    knee M00.06- ☑
    multiple site M00.09
    shoulder M00.01- ☑
    vertebra M00.08
    wrist M00.03- ☑
  streptococcal NEC M00.20
    ankle M00.27- ☑
    elbow M00.22- ☑
    foot joint — *see* Arthritis, streptococcal, ankle
    hand joint M00.24- ☑
    hip M00.25- ☑
    knee M00.26- ☑
    multiple site M00.29
    shoulder M00.21- ☑
    vertebra M00.28
    wrist M00.23- ☑
  suppurative — *see* Arthritis, pyogenic or pyemic
  syphilitic (late) A52.16
    congenital A50.55 *[M12.80]*
  syphilitica deformans (Charcot) A52.16
  temporomandibular joint M26.64- ☑
  toxic of menopause (any site) — *see* Arthritis, specified form NEC
  transient — *see* Arthropathy, specified form NEC
  traumatic (chronic) — *see* Arthropathy, traumatic
  tuberculous A18.02
    spine A18.01
  uratic — *see* Gout
  urethritica (Reiter's) — *see* Reiter's disease
  vertebral — *see* Spondylopathy, inflammatory
  villous (any site) — *see* Arthropathy, specified form NEC
Arthrocele — *see* Effusion, joint
Arthrodesis status Z98.1
Arthrodynia — *see also* Pain, joint
Arthrodysplasia Q74.9
Arthrofibrosis, joint — *see* Ankylosis
Arthrogryposis (congenital) Q68.8
  multiplex congenita Q74.3
Arthrokatadysis M24.7
Arthropathy — *see also* Arthritis M12.9
  Charcot's — *see* Arthropathy, neuropathic
    diabetic — *see* Diabetes, arthropathy, neuropathic
    syringomyelic G95.0
  cricoarytenoid J38.7
  crystal (-induced) — *see* Arthritis, in, crystals
  diabetic NEC — *see* Diabetes, arthropathy
  distal interphalangeal, psoriatic L40.51
  enteropathic M07.60
    ankle M07.67- ☑
    elbow M07.62- ☑
    foot joint M07.67- ☑
    hand joint M07.64- ☑
    hip M07.65- ☑
    knee M07.66- ☑
    multiple site M07.69
    shoulder M07.61- ☑
    vertebra M07.68
    wrist M07.63- ☑
  facet joint — *see also* Spondylosis M47.819
  following intestinal bypass M02.00
    ankle M02.07- ☑

Arthropathy — *continued*
  following intestinal bypass — *continued*
    elbow M02.02- ✓
    foot joint M02.07- ✓
    hand joint M02.04- ✓
    hip M02.05- ✓
    knee M02.06- ✓
    multiple site M02.09
    shoulder M02.01- ✓
    vertebra M02.08
    wrist M02.03- ✓
  gouty — *see also* Gout
    in (due to)
      Lesch-Nyhan syndrome E79.1 [M14.8-] ✓
      sickle-cell disorders D57- ✓ [M14.8-] ✓
  hemophilic NEC D66 [M36.2]
    in (due to)
      hyperparathyroidism NEC E21.3 [M14.8-] ✓
      metabolic disease NOS E88.9 [M14.8-] ✓
  in (due to)
    acromegaly E22.0 [M14.8-] ✓
    amyloidosis E85.4 [M14.8-] ✓
    blood disorder NOS D75.9 [M36.3]
    diabetes — *see* Diabetes, arthropathy
    endocrine disease NOS E34.9 [M14.8-] ✓
    erythema
      multiforme L51.9 [M14.8-] ✓
      nodosum L52 [M14.8-] ✓
    hemochromatosis E83.118 [M14.8-] ✓
    hemoglobinopathy NEC D58.2 [M36.3]
    hemophilia NEC D66 [M36.2]
    Henoch-Schonlein purpura D69.0 [M36.4]
    hyperthyroidism E05.90 [M14.8-] ✓
    hypothyroidism E03.9 [M14.8-] ✓
    infective endocarditis I33.0 [M12.80]
    leukemia NEC C95.9- ✓ [M36.1]
    malignant histiocytosis C96.A [M36.1]
    metabolic disease NOS E88.9 [M14.8-] ✓
    multiple myeloma C90.0- ✓ [M36.1]
    neoplastic disease NOS (*see also* Neoplasm)
        D49.9 [M36.1]
    nutritional deficiency — *see also* subcategory
        M14.8- E63.9
    psoriasis NOS L40.50
    sarcoidosis D86.86
    syphilis (late) A52.77
      congenital A50.55 [M12.80]
    thyrotoxicosis — *see also* subcategory M14.8- E05.90
    ulcerative colitis K51.90 [M07.60]
    viral hepatitis (postinfectious) NEC B19.9 [M12.80]
    Whipple's disease — *see also* subcategory M14.8-
        K90.81
  Jaccoud — *see* Arthropathy, postrheumatic, chronic
  juvenile — *see* Arthritis, juvenile
    psoriatic L40.54
  mutilans (psoriatic) L40.52
  neuropathic (Charcot) M14.60
    ankle M14.67- ✓
    diabetic — *see* Diabetes, arthropathy, neuropathic
    elbow M14.62- ✓
    foot joint M14.67- ✓
    hand joint M14.64- ✓
    hip M14.65- ✓
    knee M14.66- ✓
    multiple site M14.69
    nonsyphilitic NEC G98.0
    shoulder M14.61- ✓
    syringomyelic G95.0
    vertebra M14.68
    wrist M14.63- ✓
  osteopulmonary — *see* Osteoarthropathy, hypertrophic,
      specified NEC
  postdysenteric M02.10
    ankle M02.17- ✓
    elbow M02.12- ✓
    foot joint M02.17- ✓
    hand joint M02.14- ✓
    hip M02.15- ✓
    knee M02.16- ✓
    multiple site M02.19
    shoulder M02.11- ✓
    vertebra M02.18
    wrist M02.13- ✓
  postimmunization M02.20
    ankle M02.27- ✓
    elbow M02.22- ✓
    foot joint M02.27- ✓

Arthropathy — *continued*
  postimmunization — *continued*
    hand joint M02.24- ✓
    hip M02.25- ✓
    knee M02.26- ✓
    multiple site M02.29
    shoulder M02.21- ✓
    vertebra M02.28
    wrist M02.23- ✓
  postinfectious NEC B99 ✓ [M12.80]
    in (due to)
      enteritis due to Yersinia enterocolitica
          A04.6 [M12.80]
      syphilis A52.77
      viral hepatitis NEC B19.9 [M12.80]
  postrheumatic, chronic (Jaccoud) M12.00
    ankle M12.07- ✓
    elbow M12.02- ✓
    foot joint M12.07- ✓
    hand joint M12.04- ✓
    hip M12.05- ✓
    knee M12.06- ✓
    multiple site M12.09
    shoulder M12.01- ✓
    specified joint NEC M12.08
    vertebrae M12.08
    wrist M12.03- ✓
  psoriatic NEC L40.59
    interphalangeal, distal L40.51
  reactive M02.9
    in (due to)
      infective endocarditis I33.0 [M02.9]
    specified type NEC M02.80
      ankle M02.87- ✓
      elbow M02.82- ✓
      foot joint M02.87- ✓
      hand joint M02.84- ✓
      hip M02.85- ✓
      knee M02.86- ✓
      multiple site M02.89
      shoulder M02.81- ✓
      vertebra M02.88
      wrist M02.83- ✓
  specified form NEC M12.80
    ankle M12.87- ✓
    elbow M12.82- ✓
    foot joint M12.87- ✓
    hand joint M12.84- ✓
    hip M12.85- ✓
    knee M12.86- ✓
    multiple site M12.89
    shoulder M12.81- ✓
    specified joint NEC M12.88
    vertebrae M12.88
    wrist M12.83- ✓
  syringomyelic G95.0
  tabes dorsalis A52.16
  tabetic A52.16
  temporomandibular joint M26.65- ✓
  transient — *see* Arthropathy, specified form NEC
  traumatic M12.50
    ankle M12.57- ✓
    elbow M12.52- ✓
    foot joint M12.57- ✓
    hand joint M12.54- ✓
    hip M12.55- ✓
    knee M12.56- ✓
    multiple site M12.59
    shoulder M12.51- ✓
    specified joint NEC M12.58
    vertebrae M12.58
    wrist M12.53- ✓
Arthropyosis — *see* Arthritis, pyogenic or pyemic
Arthrosis (deformans) (degenerative) (localized) — *see also*
    Osteoarthritis M19.90
  spine — *see* Spondylosis
Arthus' phenomenon or reaction T78.41 ✓
  due to
    drug — *see* Table of Drugs and Chemicals, by drug
Articular — *see* condition
Articulation, reverse (teeth) M26.24
Artificial
  insemination complication — *see* Complications, artifi-
      cial, fertilization
  opening status (functioning) (without complication)
      Z93.9
    anus (colostomy) Z93.3

Artificial — *continued*
  opening status — *continued*
    colostomy Z93.3
    cystostomy Z93.50
      appendico-vesicostomy Z93.52
      cutaneous Z93.51
      specified NEC Z93.59
    enterostomy Z93.4
    gastrostomy Z93.1
    ileostomy (ileal pouch) (Kock pouch) Z93.2
    intestinal tract NEC Z93.4
    jejunostomy Z93.4
    nephrostomy Z93.6
    specified site NEC Z93.8
    tracheostomy Z93.0
    ureterostomy Z93.6
    urethrostomy Z93.6
    urinary tract NEC Z93.6
    vagina Z93.8
  vagina status Z93.8
Arytenoid — *see* condition
Asadollahi-Rauch syndrome Q87.85
Asbestosis (occupational) J61
Ascariasis B77.9
  with
    complications NEC B77.89
    intestinal complications B77.0
    pneumonia, pneumonitis B77.81
Ascaridosis, ascaridiasis — *see* Ascariasis
Ascaris (infection) (infestation) (lumbricoides) — *see* Ascari-
    asis
Ascending — *see* condition
ASC-H (atypical squamous cells cannot exclude high grade
    squamous intraepithelial lesion on cytologic smear)
  anus R85.611
  cervix R87.611
  vagina R87.621
Aschoff's bodies — *see* Myocarditis, rheumatic
Ascites (abdominal) R18.8
  cardiac — *see also* Failure, heart, right I50.810
  chylous (nonfilarial) I89.8
    filarial — *see* Infestation, filarial
  due to
    cirrhosis, alcoholic K70.31
    hepatitis
      alcoholic K70.11
      chronic active K71.51
    S. japonicum B65.2
  heart — *see also* Failure, heart, right I50.810
  malignant R18.0
  pseudochylous R18.8
  syphilitic A52.74
  tuberculous A18.31
ASC-US (atypical squamous cells of undetermined signifi-
    cance on cytologic smear)
  anus R85.610
  cervix R87.610
  vagina R87.620
Aseptic — *see* condition
Asherman's syndrome N85.6
Asialia K11.7
Asiatic cholera — *see* Cholera
Asimultagnosia (simultanagnosia) R48.3
Askin's tumor — *see* Neoplasm, connective tissue, malig-
    nant
Asocial personality F60.2
Asomatognosia R41.4
Aspartylglucosaminuria E77.1
Asperger's disease or syndrome F84.5
Aspergilloma — *see* Aspergillosis
Aspergillosis (with pneumonia) B44.9
  bronchopulmonary, allergic B44.81
  disseminated B44.7
  generalized B44.7
  pulmonary NEC B44.1
    allergic B44.81
    invasive B44.0
  specified NEC B44.89
  tonsillar B44.2
Aspergillus (flavus) (fumigatus) (infection) (terreus) — *see*
    Aspergillosis
Aspermatogenesis — *see* Azoospermia
Aspermia (testis) — *see* Azoospermia
Asphyxia, asphyxiation (by) R09.01
  antenatal P84
  birth P84
  bunny bag — *see* Asphyxia, due to, mechanical threat
      to breathing, trapped in bed clothes
  crushing S28.0 ✓

Asphyxia, asphyxiation — *continued*
  drowning T75.1 ☑
  gas, fumes, or vapor — *see* Table of Drugs and Chemicals
  inhalation — *see* Inhalation
  intrauterine P84
  local I73.00
    with gangrene I73.01
  mucus — *see also* Foreign body, respiratory tract, caus-
    ing, asphyxiation
  newborn P84
  pathological R09.01
  postnatal P84
    mechanical — *see* Asphyxia, due to, mechanical threat
      to breathing
  prenatal P84
  reticularis R23.1
  strangulation — *see* Asphyxia, due to, mechanical threat
    to breathing
  submersion T75.1 ☑
  traumatic T71.9 ☑
    due to
      crushed chest S28.0 ☑
      foreign body (in) — *see* Foreign body, respiratory
        tract, causing asphyxia
      low oxygen content of ambient air T71.20 ☑
        due to
          being trapped in
            low oxygen environment T71.29 ☑
              in car trunk T71.221 ☑
                circumstances undetermined
                  T71.224 ☑
                done with intent to harm by
                  another person T71.223 ☑
                    self T71.222 ☑
              in refrigerator T71.231 ☑
                circumstances undetermined
                  T71.234 ☑
                done with intent to harm by
                  another person T71.233 ☑
                    self T71.232 ☑
            cave-in T71.21 ☑
      mechanical threat to breathing (accidental)
        T71.191 ☑
        circumstances undetermined T71.194 ☑
        done with intent to harm by
          another person T71.193 ☑
            self T71.192 ☑
        hanging T71.161 ☑
          circumstances undetermined T71.164 ☑
          done with intent to harm by
            another person T71.163 ☑
              self T71.162 ☑
        plastic bag T71.121 ☑
          circumstances undetermined T71.124 ☑
          done with intent to harm by
            another person T71.123 ☑
              self T71.122 ☑
        smothering
          in furniture T71.151 ☑
            circumstances undetermined
              T71.154 ☑
            done with intent to harm by
              another person T71.153 ☑
                self T71.152 ☑
          under
            another person's body T71.141 ☑
              circumstances undetermined
                T71.144 ☑
              done with intent to harm T71.143 ☑
            pillow T71.111 ☑
              circumstances undetermined
                T71.114 ☑
              done with intent to harm by
                another person T71.113 ☑
                  self T71.112 ☑
          trapped in bed clothes T71.131 ☑
            circumstances undetermined T71.134 ☑
            done with intent to harm by
              another person T71.133 ☑
                self T71.132 ☑
      vomiting, vomitus — *see* Foreign body, respiratory tract,
        causing asphyxia
Aspiration
  amniotic (clear) fluid (newborn) P24.10
    with
      pneumonia (pneumonitis) P24.11
      respiratory symptoms P24.11

Aspiration — *continued*
  blood
    newborn (without respiratory symptoms) P24.20
      with
        pneumonia (pneumonitis) P24.21
        respiratory symptoms P24.21
      specified age NEC — *see* Foreign body, respiratory
        tract
  bronchitis J69.0
  food or foreign body — *see* Foreign body, by site
  liquor (amnii) (newborn) P24.10
    with
      pneumonia (pneumonitis) P24.11
      respiratory symptoms P24.11
  meconium (newborn) (without respiratory symptoms)
    P24.00
    with
      pneumonitis (pneumonitis) P24.01
      respiratory symptoms P24.01
  milk (newborn) (without respiratory symptoms) P24.30
    with
      pneumonia (pneumonitis) P24.31
      respiratory symptoms P24.31
    specified age NEC — *see* Foreign body, respiratory
      tract
  mucus — *see also* Foreign body, by site, causing asphyxia
    newborn P24.10
      with
        pneumonia (pneumonitis) P24.11
        respiratory symptoms P24.11
  neonatal P24.9
    specific NEC (without respiratory symptoms) P24.80
      with
        pneumonia (pneumonitis) P24.81
        respiratory symptoms P24.81
  newborn P24.9
    specific NEC (without respiratory symptoms) P24.80
      with
        pneumonia (pneumonitis) P24.81
        respiratory symptoms P24.81
  pneumonia J69.0
  pneumonitis J69.0
  syndrome of newborn — *see* Aspiration, by substance,
    with pneumonia
  vernix caseosa (newborn) P24.80
    with
      pneumonia (pneumonitis) P24.81
      respiratory symptoms P24.81
  vomitus — *see also* Foreign body, respiratory tract
    newborn (without respiratory symptoms) P24.30
      with
        pneumonia (pneumonitis) P24.31
        respiratory symptoms P24.31
Asplenia (congenital) Q89.01
  functional D73.0
  postsurgical Z90.81
Assam fever B55.0
Assault, sexual — *see* Maltreatment
Assmann's focus NEC A15.0
Astasia (-abasia) (hysterical) F44.4
Asteatosis cutis L85.3
Astereognosia, astereognosis R48.1
Asterixis R27.8
  in liver disease K71.3
Asteroid hyalitis — *see* Deposit, crystalline
Asthenia, asthenic R53.1
  cardiac — *see also* Failure, heart I50.9
    psychogenic F45.8
  cardiovascular — *see also* Failure, heart I50.9
    psychogenic F45.8
  heart — *see also* Failure, heart I50.9
    psychogenic F45.8
  hysterical F44.4
  myocardial — *see also* Failure, heart I50.9
    psychogenic F45.8
  nervous F48.8
  neurocirculatory F45.8
  neurotic F48.8
  psychogenic F48.8
  psychoneurotic F48.8
  psychophysiologic F48.8
  reaction (psychophysiologic) F48.8
  senile R54
Asthenopia — *see also* Discomfort, visual
  hysterical F44.6
  psychogenic F44.6
Asthenospermia — *see* Abnormal, specimen, male genital
  organs

Asthma, asthmatic (bronchial) (catarrh) (spasmodic)
    J45.909
  with
    chronic obstructive bronchitis J44.89
      with
        acute lower respiratory infection J44.0
        exacerbation (acute) J44.1
    chronic obstructive pulmonary disease J44.89
      with
        acute lower respiratory infection J44.0
        exacerbation (acute) J44.1
    exacerbation (acute) J45.901
    hay fever — *see* Asthma, allergic extrinsic
    rhinitis, allergic — *see* Asthma, allergic extrinsic
    status asthmaticus J45.902
  allergic extrinsic J45.909
    with
      exacerbation (acute) J45.901
      status asthmaticus J45.902
  atopic — *see* Asthma, allergic extrinsic
  cardiac — *see* Failure, ventricular, left
  cardiobronchial I50.1
  childhood J45.909
    with
      exacerbation (acute) J45.901
      status asthmaticus J45.902
  chronic obstructive J44.89
    with
      acute lower respiratory infection J44.0
      exacerbation (acute) J44.1
  collier's J60
  cough variant J45.991
  detergent J69.8
  due to
    detergent J69.8
    inhalation of fumes J68.3
  eosinophilic J82.83
  extrinsic, allergic — *see* Asthma, allergic extrinsic
  grinder's J62.8
  hay — *see* Asthma, allergic extrinsic
  heart I50.1
  idiosyncratic — *see* Asthma, nonallergic
  intermittent (mild) J45.20
    with
      exacerbation (acute) J45.21
      status asthmaticus J45.22
  intrinsic, nonallergic — *see* Asthma, nonallergic
  Kopp's E32.8
  late-onset J45.909
    with
      exacerbation (acute) J45.901
      status asthmaticus J45.902
  mild intermittent J45.20
    with
      exacerbation (acute) J45.21
      status asthmaticus J45.22
  mild persistent J45.30
    with
      exacerbation (acute) J45.31
      status asthmaticus J45.32
  Millar's (laryngismus stridulus) J38.5
  miner's J60
  mixed J45.909
    with
      exacerbation (acute) J45.901
      status asthmaticus J45.902
  moderate persistent J45.40
    with
      exacerbation (acute) J45.41
      status asthmaticus J45.42
  nervous — *see* Asthma, nonallergic
  nonallergic (intrinsic) J45.909
    with
      exacerbation (acute) J45.901
      status asthmaticus J45.902
  persistent
    mild J45.30
      with
        exacerbation (acute) J45.31
        status asthmaticus J45.32
    moderate J45.40
      with
        exacerbation (acute) J45.41
        status asthmaticus J45.42
    severe J45.50
      with
        exacerbation (acute) J45.51
        status asthmaticus J45.52
  platinum J45.998

Asthma, asthmatic — continued
　pneumoconiotic NEC J64
　potter's J62.8
　predominantly allergic J45.909
　psychogenic F54
　pulmonary eosinophilic J82.83
　red cedar J67.8
　Rostan's I50.1
　sandblaster's J62.8
　sequoiosis J67.8
　severe persistent J45.50
　　with
　　　exacerbation (acute) J45.51
　　　status asthmaticus J45.52
　specified NEC J45.998
　stonemason's J62.8
　thymic E32.8
　tuberculous — see Tuberculosis, pulmonary
　Wichmann's (laryngismus stridulus) J38.5
　wood J67.8
Astigmatism (compound) (congenital) H52.20- ☑
　irregular H52.21- ☑
　regular H52.22- ☑
Astraphobia F40.220
Astroblastoma
　specified site — see Neoplasm, malignant, by site
　unspecified site C71.9
Astrocytoma (cystic)
　anaplastic
　　specified site — see Neoplasm, malignant, by site
　　unspecified site C71.9
　fibrillary
　　specified site — see Neoplasm, malignant, by site
　　unspecified site C71.9
　fibrous
　　specified site — see Neoplasm, malignant, by site
　　unspecified site C71.9
　gemistocytic
　　specified site — see Neoplasm, malignant, by site
　　unspecified site C71.9
　juvenile
　　specified site — see Neoplasm, malignant, by site
　　unspecified site C71.9
　pilocytic
　　specified site — see Neoplasm, malignant, by site
　　unspecified site C71.9
　piloid
　　specified site — see Neoplasm, malignant, by site
　　unspecified site C71.9
　protoplasmic
　　specified site — see Neoplasm, malignant, by site
　　unspecified site C71.9
　specified site NEC — see Neoplasm, malignant, by site
　subependymal D43.2
　　giant cell
　　　specified site — see Neoplasm, uncertain behavior, by site
　　　unspecified site D43.2
　　specified site — see Neoplasm, uncertain behavior, by site
　　unspecified site D43.2
　unspecified site C71.9
Astroglioma
　specified site — see Neoplasm, malignant, by site
　unspecified site C71.9
Asymbolia R48.8
Asymmetry — see also Distortion
　between native and reconstructed breast N65.1
　face Q67.0
　jaw (lower) — see Anomaly, dentofacial, jaw-cranial base relationship, asymmetry
Asynergia, asynergy R27.8
　ventricular I51.89
Asystole (heart) — see Arrest, cardiac
At risk
　for
　　dental caries Z91.849
　　　high Z91.843
　　　low Z91.841
　　　moderate Z91.842
　　falling Z91.81
　　feeling loneliness Z65.8
　　social isolation Z91.89
Ataxia, ataxy, ataxic R27.0
　acute R27.8
　autosomal recessive Friedreich G11.11
　brain (hereditary) G11.9
　cerebellar (hereditary) G11.9
　　with defective DNA repair G11.3

Ataxia, ataxy, ataxic — continued
　cerebellar — continued
　　alcoholic G31.2
　　early-onset G11.10
　　with
　　　essential tremor G11.19
　　　myoclonus [Hunt's ataxia] G11.19
　　　retained tendon reflexes G11.19
　　in
　　　alcoholism G31.2
　　　myxedema E03.9 [G13.2]
　　　neoplastic disease — see also Neoplasm D49.9 [G32.81]
　　　specified disease NEC G32.81
　　late-onset (Marie's) G11.2
　cerebral (hereditary) G11.9
　congenital nonprogressive G11.0
　family, familial — see Ataxia, hereditary
　following
　　cerebrovascular disease I69.993
　　　cerebral infarction I69.393
　　　intracerebral hemorrhage I69.193
　　　nontraumatic intracranial hemorrhage NEC I69.293
　　　specified disease NEC I69.893
　　　subarachnoid hemorrhage I69.093
　Friedreich's (heredofamilial) (cerebellar) (spinal) (with retained reflexes) G11.11
　gait R26.0
　　hysterical F44.4
　general R27.8
　gluten M35.9 [G32.81]
　　with celiac disease K90.0 [G32.81]
　hereditary G11.9
　　with neuropathy G60.2
　　cerebellar — see Ataxia, cerebellar
　　spastic G11.4
　　specified NEC G11.8
　　spinal (Friedreich's) G11.11
　heredofamilial — see Ataxia, hereditary
　Hunt's G11.19
　hysterical F44.4
　locomotor (progressive) (syphilitic) (partial) (spastic) A52.11
　　diabetic — see Diabetes, ataxia
　Marie's (cerebellar) (heredofamilial) (late-onset) G11.2
　nonorganic origin F44.4
　nonprogressive, congenital G11.0
　psychogenic F44.4
　Roussy-Levy G60.0
　Sanger-Brown's (hereditary) G11.2
　spastic hereditary G11.4
　spinal
　　hereditary (Friedreich's) G11.11
　　progressive (syphilitic) A52.11
　spinocerebellar, X-linked recessive G11.19
　telangiectasia (Louis-Bar) G11.3
Ataxia-telangiectasia (Louis-Bar) G11.3
Atelocardia Q24.9
Atelomyelia Q06.1
Atheroembolism
　of
　　extremities
　　　lower I75.02- ☑
　　　upper I75.01- ☑
　　kidney I75.81
　　specified NEC I75.89
Atheroma, atheromatous — see also Arteriosclerosis I70.90
　aorta, aortic I70.0
　　valve — see also Endocarditis, aortic I35.8
　aorto-iliac I70.0
　artery — see Arteriosclerosis
　basilar (artery) I67.2
　carotid (artery) (common) (internal) I67.2
　cerebral (arteries) I67.2
　coronary (artery) I25.10
　　with angina pectoris — see Arteriosclerosis, coronary (artery),
　degeneration — see Arteriosclerosis
　heart, cardiac — see Disease, heart, ischemic, atherosclerotic
　mitral (valve) I34.89

Atheroma, atheromatous — continued
　myocardium, myocardial — see Disease, heart, ischemic, atherosclerotic
　pulmonary valve (heart) — see also Endocarditis, pulmonary I37.8
　tricuspid (heart) (valve) I36.8
　valve, valvular — see Endocarditis
　vertebral (artery) I67.2
Atheromatosis — see Arteriosclerosis
Atherosclerosis — see also Arteriosclerosis
　coronary
　　artery I25.10
　　　with angina pectoris — see Arteriosclerosis, coronary (artery),
　　　due to
　　　　calcified coronary lesion (severely) I25.84
　　　　lipid rich plaque I25.83
　　transplanted heart I25.811
　　　bypass graft I25.812
　　　　with angina pectoris — see Arteriosclerosis, coronary (artery),
　　　native coronary artery I25.811
　　　　with angina pectoris — see Arteriosclerosis, coronary (artery),
Athetosis (acquired) R25.8
　bilateral (congenital) G80.3
　congenital (bilateral) (double) G80.3
　double (congenital) G80.3
　unilateral R25.8
Athlete's
　foot B35.3
　heart I51.7
Athrepsia E41
Athyrea (acquired) — see also Hypothyroidism
　congenital E03.1
Atonia, atony, atonic
　bladder (sphincter) (neurogenic) N31.2
　capillary I78.8
　cecum K59.89
　　psychogenic F45.8
　colon — see Atony, intestine
　congenital P94.2
　esophagus K22.89
　intestine K59.89
　　psychogenic F45.8
　stomach K31.89
　　neurotic or psychogenic F45.8
　uterus (during labor) O62.2
　　with hemorrhage (postpartum) O72.1
　　postpartum (with hemorrhage) O72.1
　　　without hemorrhage O75.89
Atopy — see History, allergy
Atransferrinemia, congenital E88.09
Atresia, atretic
　alimentary organ or tract NEC Q45.8
　　upper Q40.8
　ani, anus, anal (canal) Q42.3
　　with fistula Q42.2
　aorta (ring) Q25.29
　aortic (orifice) (valve) Q23.0
　　arch Q25.21
　　congenital with hypoplasia of ascending aorta and defective development of left ventricle (with mitral stenosis) Q23.4
　　in hypoplastic left heart syndrome Q23.4
　aqueduct of Sylvius Q03.0
　　with spina bifida — see Spina bifida, with hydrocephalus
　artery NEC Q27.8
　　cerebral Q28.3
　　coronary Q24.5
　　digestive system Q27.8
　　eye Q15.8
　　lower limb Q27.8
　　pulmonary Q25.5
　　specified site NEC Q27.8
　　umbilical Q27.0
　　upper limb Q27.8
　auditory canal (external) Q16.1
　bile duct (common) (congenital) (hepatic) Q44.2
　　acquired — see Obstruction, bile duct
　bladder (neck) Q64.39
　　obstruction Q64.31
　bronchus Q32.4
　cecum Q42.8
　cervix Q51.828
　　congenital Q51.828
　　in pregnancy or childbirth — see Anomaly, cervix, in pregnancy or childbirth

Atresia, atretic — *continued*
cervix — *continued*
  in pregnancy or childbirth — *see* Anomaly, cervix, in
    pregnancy or childbirth — *continued*
      causing obstructed labor O65.5
choana Q30.0
colon Q42.9
  specified NEC Q42.8
common duct Q44.2
cricoid cartilage Q31.8
cystic duct Q44.2
  acquired K82.8
    with obstruction K82.0
digestive organs NEC Q45.8
duodenum Q41.0
ear canal Q16.1
ejaculatory duct Q55.4
epiglottis Q31.8
esophagus Q39.0
  with tracheoesophageal fistula Q39.1
eustachian tube Q17.8
fallopian tube (congenital) Q50.6
  acquired N97.1
follicular cyst N83.0- ☑
foramen of
  Luschka Q03.1
    with spina bifida — *see* Spina bifida, with hydro-
      cephalus
  Magendie Q03.1
    with spina bifida — *see* Spina bifida, with hydro-
      cephalus
gallbladder Q44.1
genital organ
  external
    female Q52.79
    male Q55.8
  internal
    female Q52.8
    male Q55.8
glottis Q31.8
gullet Q39.0
  with tracheoesophageal fistula Q39.1
heart valve NEC Q24.8
  pulmonary Q22.0
  tricuspid Q22.4
hymen Q52.3
  acquired (postinfective) N89.6
ileum Q41.2
intestine (small) Q41.9
  large Q42.9
    specified NEC Q42.8
iris, filtration angle Q15.0
jejunum Q41.1
lacrimal apparatus Q10.4
larynx Q31.8
meatus urinarius Q64.33
mitral valve Q23.2
  in hypoplastic left heart syndrome Q23.4
nares (anterior) (posterior) Q30.0
nasopharynx Q34.8
nose, nostril Q30.0
  acquired J34.89
organ or site NEC Q89.8
osseous meatus (ear) Q16.1
oviduct (congenital) Q50.6
  acquired N97.1
parotid duct Q38.4
  acquired K11.8
pulmonary (artery) Q25.5
  valve Q22.0
pulmonic Q22.0
pupil Q13.2
rectum Q42.1
  with fistula Q42.0
salivary duct Q38.4
  acquired K11.8
sublingual duct Q38.4
  acquired K11.8
submandibular duct Q38.4
  acquired K11.8
submaxillary duct Q38.4
  acquired K11.8
thyroid cartilage Q31.8
trachea Q32.1
tricuspid valve Q22.4
ureter Q62.10
  pelvic junction Q62.11
  vesical orifice Q62.12
ureteropelvic junction Q62.11

Atresia, atretic — *continued*
ureterovesical orifice Q62.12
urethra (valvular) Q64.39
  stricture Q64.32
urinary tract NEC Q64.8
uterus Q51.818
  acquired N85.8
vagina (congenital) Q52.4
  acquired (postinfectional) (senile) N89.5
vas deferens Q55.3
vascular NEC Q27.8
  cerebral Q28.3
  digestive system Q27.8
  lower limb Q27.8
  specified site NEC Q27.8
  upper limb Q27.8
vein NEC Q27.8
  digestive system Q27.8
  great Q26.8
  lower limb Q27.8
  portal Q26.5
  pulmonary Q26.4
    partial Q26.3
    total Q26.2
  specified site NEC Q27.8
  upper limb Q27.8
vena cava (inferior) (superior) Q26.8
vesicourethral orifice Q64.31
vulva Q52.79
  acquired N90.5
Atrichia, atrichosis — *see* Alopecia
Atrophia — *see also* Atrophy
cutis senilis L90.8
  due to radiation L57.8
gyrata of choroid and retina H31.23
senilis R54
  dermatological L90.8
    due to radiation (nonionizing) (solar) L57.8
unguium L60.3
  congenita Q84.6
Atrophie blanche (en plaque) (de Milian) L95.0
Atrophoderma, atrophodermia (of) L90.9
diffusum (idiopathic) L90.4
maculatum L90.8
  et striatum L90.8
    due to syphilis A52.79
  syphilitic A51.39
neuriticum L90.8
Pasini and Pierini L90.3
pigmentosum Q82.1
reticulatum symmetricum faciei L66.4
senile L90.8
  due to radiation (nonionizing) (solar) L57.8
vermiculata (cheeks) L66.4
Atrophy, atrophic (of)
adrenal (capsule) (gland) E27.49
  primary (autoimmune) E27.1
alveolar process or ridge (edentulous) K08.20
anal sphincter (disuse) N81.84
appendix K38.8
arteriosclerotic — *see* Arteriosclerosis
bile duct (common) (hepatic) K83.8
bladder N32.89
  neurogenic N31.8
blanche (en plaque) (of Milian) L95.0
bone (senile) NEC — *see also* Disorder, bone, specified
    type NEC
  due to
    tabes dorsalis (neurogenic) A52.11
brain (cortex) (progressive) G31.9
  frontotemporal circumscribed — *see also* Dementia,
    in, diseases specified elsewhere G31.01 [F02.80]
    with behavioral disturbance — *see also* Dementia,
      in, diseases specified elsewhere
      G31.01 [F02.81-] ☑
  senile NEC G31.1
breast N64.2
  obstetric — *see* Disorder, breast, specified type NEC
buccal cavity K13.79
cardiac — *see* Degeneration, myocardial
cartilage (infectional) (joint) — *see* Disorder, cartilage,
    specified NEC
cerebellar — *see* Atrophy, brain
cerebral — *see* Atrophy, brain
cervix (mucosa) (senile) (uteri) N88.8
  menopausal N95.8
Charcot-Marie-Tooth G60.0
choroid (central) (macular) (myopic) (retina) H31.10- ☑
  diffuse secondary H31.12- ☑

Atrophy, atrophic — *continued*
choroid — *continued*
  gyrate H31.23
  senile H31.11- ☑
ciliary body — *see* Atrophy, iris
conjunctiva (senile) H11.89
corpus cavernosum N48.89
cortical — *see* Atrophy, brain
cystic duct K82.8
Dejerine-Thomas G23.8
disuse NEC — *see* Atrophy, muscle
Duchenne-Aran G12.21
ear H93.8- ☑
edentulous alveolar ridge K08.20
endometrium (senile) N85.8
  cervix N88.8
enteric K63.89
epididymis N50.89
eyeball — *see* Disorder, globe, degenerated condition,
    atrophy
eyelid (senile) — *see* Disorder, eyelid, degenerative
facial (skin) L90.9
fallopian tube (senile) N83.32- ☑
  with ovary N83.33- ☑
fascioscapulohumeral (Landouzy- Dejerine) G71.02
fatty, thymus (gland) E32.8
gallbladder K82.8
gastric K29.40
  with bleeding K29.41
gastrointestinal K63.89
glandular I89.8
globe H44.52- ☑
gum — *see* Recession, gingival
hair L67.8
heart (brown) — *see* Degeneration, myocardial
hemifacial Q67.4
  Romberg G51.8
infantile E41
  paralysis, acute — *see* Poliomyelitis, paralytic
intestine K63.89
iris (essential) (progressive) H21.26- ☑
  specified NEC H21.29
kidney (senile) (terminal) — *see also* Sclerosis, renal N26.1
  congenital or infantile Q60.5
    bilateral Q60.4
    unilateral Q60.3
  hydronephrotic — *see* Hydronephrosis
lacrimal gland (primary) H04.14- ☑
  secondary H04.15- ☑
Landouzy-Dejerine G71.02
laryngitis, infective J37.0
larynx J38.7
Leber's optic (hereditary) H47.22
lip K13.0
liver (yellow) K72.90
  with coma K72.91
  acute, subacute K72.00
    with coma K72.01
  chronic K72.10
    with coma K72.11
lung (senile) J98.4
macular (dermatological) L90.8
  syphilitic, skin A51.39
    striated A52.79
mandible (edentulous) K08.20
  minimal K08.21
  moderate K08.22
  severe K08.23
maxilla K08.20
  minimal K08.24
  moderate K08.25
  severe K08.26
muscle, muscular (diffuse) (general) (idiopathic) (primary)
    M62.50
  ankle M62.57- ☑
  back M62.5A9
    cervical M62.5A0
    lumbosacral M62.5A2
    thoracic M62.5A1
  Duchenne-Aran G12.21
  foot M62.57- ☑
  forearm M62.53- ☑
  hand M62.54- ☑
  infantile spinal G12.0
  lower leg M62.56- ☑
  multiple sites M62.59
  myelopathic — *see* Atrophy, muscle, spinal
  myotonic G71.11

Atrophy, atrophic — *continued*
  muscle, muscular — *continued*
    neuritic G58.9
    neuropathic (peroneal) (progressive) G60.0
    pelvic (disuse) N81.84
    peroneal G60.0
    progressive (bulbar) G12.21
      adult G12.1
      infantile (spinal) G12.0
      spinal G12.25
        adult G12.1
        infantile G12.0
    pseudohypertrophic G71.02
    shoulder region M62.51- ☑
    specified site NEC M62.58
    spinal G12.9
      adult form G12.1
      Aran-Duchenne G12.21
      childhood form, type II G12.1
      distal G12.1
      hereditary NEC G12.1
      infantile, type I (Werdnig-Hoffmann) G12.0
      juvenile form, type III (Kugelberg- Welander) G12.1
      progressive G12.25
      scapuloperoneal form G12.1
      specified NEC G12.8
    syphilitic A52.78
    thigh M62.55- ☑
    upper arm M62.52- ☑
  myocardium — *see* Degeneration, myocardial
  myometrium (senile) N85.8
    cervix N88.8
  myopathic NEC — *see* Atrophy, muscle
  myotonia G71.11
  nail L60.3
  nasopharynx J31.1
  nerve — *see also* Disorder, nerve
    abducens — *see* Strabismus, paralytic, sixth nerve
    accessory G52.8
    acoustic or auditory H93.3 ☑
    cranial G52.9
      eighth (auditory) H93.3 ☑
      eleventh (accessory) G52.8
      fifth (trigeminal) G50.8
      first (olfactory) G52.0
      fourth (trochlear) — *see* Strabismus, paralytic, fourth nerve
      second (optic) H47.20
      sixth (abducens) — *see* Strabismus, paralytic, sixth nerve
      tenth (pneumogastric) (vagus) G52.2
      third (oculomotor) — *see* Strabismus, paralytic, third nerve
      twelfth (hypoglossal) G52.3
    hypoglossal G52.3
    oculomotor — *see* Strabismus, paralytic, third nerve
    olfactory G52.0
    optic (papillomacular bundle)
      syphilitic (late) A52.15
        congenital A50.44
    pneumogastric G52.2
    trigeminal G50.8
    trochlear — *see* Strabismus, paralytic, fourth nerve
    vagus (pneumogastric) G52.2
  neurogenic, bone, tabetic A52.11
  nutritional E43
    with marasmus E41
  old age R54
  olivopontocerebellar G23.8
  optic (nerve) H47.20
    glaucomatous H47.23- ☑
    hereditary H47.22
    primary H47.21- ☑
    specified type NEC H47.29- ☑
    syphilitic (late) A52.15
      congenital A50.44
  orbit H05.31- ☑
  ovary (senile) N83.31- ☑
    with fallopian tube N83.33- ☑
  oviduct (senile) — *see* Atrophy, fallopian tube
  palsy, diffuse (progressive) G12.22
  pancreas (duct) (senile) K86.89
  parotid gland K11.0
  pelvic muscle N81.84
  penis N48.89
  pharynx J39.2
  pluriglandular E31.8
    autoimmune E31.0

Atrophy, atrophic — *continued*
  polyarthritis M15.9
  prostate N42.89
  pseudohypertrophic (muscle) G71.02
  renal — *see also* Sclerosis, renal N26.1
  retina, retinal (postinfectional) H35.89
  rhinitis J31.0
  salivary gland K11.0
  scar L90.5
  sclerosis, lobar (of brain) — *see also* Dementia, in, diseases specified elsewhere G31.09 *[F02.80]*
    with behavioral disturbance — *see also* Dementia, in, diseases specified elsewhere G31.09 *[F02.81-]* ☑
  scrotum N50.89
  seminal vesicle N50.89
  senile R54
    due to radiation (nonionizing) (solar) L57.8
  skin (patches) (spots) L90.9
    degenerative (senile) L90.8
    due to radiation (nonionizing) (solar) L57.8
    senile L90.8
  spermatic cord N50.89
  spinal (acute) (cord) G95.89
    muscular — *see* Atrophy, muscle, spinal
    paralysis G12.20
      acute — *see* Poliomyelitis, paralytic
      meaning progressive muscular atrophy G12.25
  spine (column) — *see* Spondylopathy, specified NEC
  spleen (senile) D73.0
  stomach K29.40
    with bleeding K29.41
  striate (skin) L90.6
    syphilitic A52.79
  subcutaneous L90.9
  sublingual gland K11.0
  submandibular gland K11.0
  submaxillary gland K11.0
  Sudeck's — *see* Algoneurodystrophy
  suprarenal (capsule) (gland) E27.49
    primary E27.1
  systemic affecting central nervous system
    in
      myxedema E03.9 *[G13.2]*
      neoplastic disease — *see also* Neoplasm D49.9 *[G13.1]*
      specified disease NEC G13.8
  tarso-orbital fascia, congenital Q10.3
  testis N50.0
  thenar, partial — *see* Syndrome, carpal tunnel
  thymus (fatty) E32.8
  thyroid (gland) (acquired) E03.4
    with cretinism E03.1
    congenital (with myxedema) E03.1
  tongue (senile) K14.8
    papillae K14.4
  trachea J39.8
  tunica vaginalis N50.89
  turbinate J34.89
  tympanic membrane (nonflaccid) H73.82- ☑
    flaccid H73.81- ☑
  upper respiratory tract J39.8
  uterus, uterine (senile) N85.8
    cervix N88.8
    due to radiation (intended effect) N85.8
      adverse effect or misadventure N99.89
  vagina (senile) N95.2
  vas deferens N50.89
  vascular I99.8
  vertebra (senile) — *see* Spondylopathy, specified NEC
  vulva (senile) N90.5
  Werdnig-Hoffmann G12.0
  yellow — *see* Failure, hepatic

Attack, attacks
  with alteration of consciousness (with automatisms) — *see* Epilepsy, localization-related, symptomatic, with complex partial seizures
  Adams-Stokes I45.9
  akinetic — *see* Epilepsy, generalized, specified NEC
  angina — *see* Angina
  atonic — *see* Epilepsy, generalized, specified NEC
  benign shuddering G25.83
  cataleptic — *see* Catalepsy
  coronary — *see* Infarct, myocardium
  cyanotic, newborn P28.2
  drop NEC R55
  epileptic — *see* Epilepsy
  heart — *see* infarct, myocardium
  hysterical F44.9

Attack, attacks — *continued*
  jacksonian — *see* Epilepsy, localization-related, symptomatic, with simple partial seizures
  myocardium, myocardial — *see* Infarct, myocardium
  myoclonic — *see* Epilepsy, generalized, specified NEC
  panic F41.0
  psychomotor — *see* Epilepsy, localization-related, symptomatic, with complex partial seizures
  salaam — *see* Epilepsy, spasms
  schizophreniform, brief F23
  shuddering, benign G25.83
  Stokes-Adams I45.9
  syncope R55
  transient ischemic (TIA) G45.9
    specified NEC G45.8
  unconsciousness R55
    hysterical F44.89
  vasomotor R55
  vasovagal (paroxysmal) (idiopathic) R55
  without alteration of consciousness — *see* Epilepsy, localization-related, symptomatic, with simple partial seizures

Attention (to)
  artificial
    opening (of) Z43.9
      digestive tract NEC Z43.4
        colon Z43.3
        ilium Z43.2
        stomach Z43.1
      specified NEC Z43.8
      trachea Z43.0
      urinary tract NEC Z43.6
        cystostomy Z43.5
        nephrostomy Z43.6
        ureterostomy Z43.6
        urethrostomy Z43.6
      vagina Z43.7
  colostomy Z43.3
  cystostomy Z43.5
  deficit disorder or syndrome F98.8
    with hyperactivity — *see* Disorder, attention-deficit hyperactivity
  gastrostomy Z43.1
  ileostomy Z43.2
  jejunostomy Z43.4
  nephrostomy Z43.6
  surgical dressings Z48.01
  sutures Z48.02
  tracheostomy Z43.0
  ureterostomy Z43.6
  urethrostomy Z43.6

Attrition
  gum — *see* Recession, gingival
  tooth, teeth (excessive) (hard tissues) K03.0

Atypical, atypism — *see also* condition
  cells (on cytolgocial smear) (endocervical) (endometrial) (glandular)
    cervix R87.619
    vagina R87.629
  cervical N87.9
  endometrium N85.9
    hyperplasia N85.00
  parenting situation Z62.9

Auditory — *see* condition
Aujeszky's disease B33.8
Aurantiasis, cutis E67.1
Auricle, auricular — *see also* condition
  cervical Q18.2
Auriculotemporal syndrome G50.8
Austin Flint murmur (aortic insufficiency) I35.1
Australian
  Q fever A78
  X disease A83.4
Autism, autistic (childhood) (infantile) F84.0
  atypical F84.9
  spectrum disorder F84.0
Autoantibodies, multiple confirmed islet, with normoglycemia E10.A1
Autodigestion R68.89
Autoerythrocyte sensitization (syndrome) D69.2
Autographism L50.3
Autoimmune
  disease (systemic) M35.9
  inhibitors to clotting factors D68.311
  lymphoproliferative syndrome [ALPS] D89.82
  thyroiditis E06.3
Autoimmunity, confirmed islet, with dysglycemia E10.A2
Autointoxication R68.89
Automatism G93.89

☑ **Additional Character Required — Refer to the Tabular List for Character Selection**

Automatism — *continued*
- with temporal sclerosis G93.81
  - epileptic — *see* Epilepsy, localization-related, symptomatic, with complex partial seizures
  - paroxysmal, idiopathic — *see* Epilepsy, localization-related, symptomatic, with complex partial seizures

Autonomic, autonomous
- bladder (neurogenic) N31.2
- hysteria seizure F44.5

Autosensitivity, erythrocyte D69.2
Autosensitization, cutaneous L30.2
Autosome — *see* condition by chromosome involved
Autotopagnosia R48.1
Autotoxemia R68.89
Autumn — *see* condition
Avellis' syndrome G46.8
Aversion
- oral R63.39
  - newborn P92.- ☑
    - nonorganic origin F98.2 ☑
- sexual F52.1

Aviator's
- disease or sickness — *see* Effect, adverse, high altitude
- ear T70.0 ☑

Avitaminosis (multiple) — *see also* Deficiency, vitamin E56.9
- B E53.9
  - with
    - beriberi E51.11
    - pellagra E52
- B2 E53.0
- B6 E53.1
- B12 E53.8
- D E55.9
  - with rickets E55.0
- G E53.0
- K E56.1
- nicotinic acid E52

AVNRT (atrioventricular nodal re-entrant tachycardia) I47.19
AVRT (atrioventricular nodal re-entrant tachycardia) I47.19
Avulsion (traumatic)
- blood vessel — *see* Injury, blood vessel
- bone — *see* Fracture, by site
- cartilage — *see also* Dislocation, by site
  - symphyseal (inner), complicating delivery O71.6
- external site other than limb — *see* Wound, open, by site
- eye S05.7- ☑
- head (intracranial)
  - external site NEC S08.89 ☑
  - scalp S08.0 ☑
- internal organ or site — *see* Injury, by site
- joint — *see also* Dislocation, by site
  - capsule — *see* Sprain, by site
- kidney S37.06- ☑
- ligament — *see* Sprain, by site
- limb — *see also* Amputation, traumatic, by site
  - skin and subcutaneous tissue — *see* Wound, open, by site
- muscle — *see* Injury, muscle
- nerve (root) — *see* Injury, nerve
- scalp S08.0 ☑
- skin and subcutaneous tissue — *see* Wound, open, by site
- spleen S36.032 ☑
- symphyseal cartilage (inner), complicating delivery O71.6
- tendon — *see* Injury, muscle
- tooth S03.2 ☑

Awareness of heart beat R00.2
Axenfeld's
- anomaly or syndrome Q15.0
- degeneration (calcareous) Q13.4
Axilla, axillary — *see also* condition
- breast Q83.1
Axonotmesis — *see* Injury, nerve
Ayerza's disease or syndrome (pulmonary artery sclerosis with pulmonary hypertension) I27.0
Azoospermia (organic) N46.01
- due to
  - drug therapy N46.021
  - efferent duct obstruction N46.023
  - infection N46.022
  - radiation N46.024
  - specified cause NEC N46.029
  - systemic disease N46.025
Azotemia R79.89
- meaning uremia N19
Aztec ear Q17.3
Azygos
- continuation inferior vena cava Q26.8

Azygos — *continued*
- lobe (lung) Q33.1

B

Baastrup's disease — *see* Kissing spine
Babesiosis B60.00
- due to
  - Babesia
    - divergens B60.03
    - duncani B60.02
    - KO-1 B60.09
    - microti B60.01
    - MO-1 B60.03
    - species
      - unspecified B60.00
    - venatorum B60.09
  - specified NEC B60.09
Babington's disease (familial hemorrhagic telangiectasia) I78.0
Babinski's syndrome A52.79
Baby
- crying constantly R68.11
- floppy (syndrome) P94.2
Bacillary — *see* condition
Bacilluria R82.71
Bacillus — *see also* Infection, bacillus
- abortus infection A23.1
- anthracis infection A22.9
- coli infection — *see also* Escherichia coli B96.20
- Flexner's A03.1
- mallei infection A24.0
- Shiga's A03.0
- suipestifer infection — *see* Infection, salmonella
Back — *see* condition
Backache (postural) M54.9
- sacroiliac M53.3
- specified NEC M54.89
Backflow — *see* Reflux
Backward reading (dyslexia) F81.0
Bacteremia R78.81
- with sepsis — *see* Sepsis
Bactericholia — *see* Cholecystitis, acute
Bacterid, bacteride (pustular) L40.3
Bacterium, bacteria, bacterial
- agent NEC, as cause of disease classified elsewhere B96.89
- in blood — *see* Bacteremia
- in urine — *see* Bacteriuria
Bacteriuria, bacteruria (asymptomatic) R82.71
Bacteroides
- fragilis, as cause of disease classified elsewhere B96.6
Bad
- heart — *see* Disease, heart
- trip
  - due to drug abuse — *see* Abuse, drug, hallucinogen
  - due to drug dependence — *see* Dependence, drug, hallucinogen
Baelz's disease (cheilitis glandularis apostematosa) K13.0
Baerensprung's disease (eczema marginatum) B35.6
Bagasse disease or pneumonitis J67.1
Bagassosis J67.1
Baker's cyst — *see* Cyst, Baker's
Bakwin-Krida syndrome (metaphyseal dysplasia) Q78.5
Balancing side interference M26.56
Balanitis (circinata) (erosiva) (gangrenosa) (phagedenic) (vulgaris) N48.1
- amebic A06.82
- candidal B37.42
- due to Haemophilus ducreyi A57
- gonococcal (acute) (chronic) A54.23
- xerotica obliterans N48.0
Balanoposthitis N47.6
- gonococcal (acute) (chronic) A54.23
- ulcerative (specific) A63.8
Balanorrhagia — *see* Balanitis
Balantidiasis, balantidiosis A07.0
Bald tongue K14.4
Baldness — *see also* Alopecia
- male-pattern — *see* Alopecia, androgenic
Balkan grippe A78
Balloon disease — *see* Effect, adverse, high altitude
Balo's disease (concentric sclerosis) G37.5
Bamberger-Marie disease — *see* Osteoarthropathy, hypertrophic, specified type NEC
Bancroft's filariasis B74.0
Band(s)
- adhesive — *see* Adhesions, peritoneum
- anomalous or congenital — *see also* Anomaly, by site

Band(s) — *continued*
- anomalous or congenital — *see also* Anomaly, by site — *continued*
  - heart (atrial) (ventricular) Q24.8
  - intestine Q43.3
  - omentum Q43.3
- cervix N88.1
- constricting, congenital Q79.8
- gallbladder (congenital) Q44.1
- intestinal (adhesive) — *see* Adhesions, peritoneum
- obstructive
  - intestine K56.50
    - complete K56.52
    - incomplete K56.51
    - partial K56.51
  - peritoneum K56.50
    - complete K56.52
    - incomplete K56.51
    - partial K56.51
- periappendiceal, congenital Q43.3
- peritoneal (adhesive) — *see* Adhesions, peritoneum
- uterus N73.6
  - internal N85.6
- vagina N89.5
Bandemia D72.825
Bandl's ring (contraction), complicating delivery O62.4
Bangkok hemorrhagic fever A91
Bang's disease (brucella abortus) A23.1
Bankruptcy (anxiety concerning) Z59.86
Bannister's disease T78.3 ☑
- hereditary D84.1
Banti's disease or syndrome (with cirrhosis) (with portal hypertension) K76.6
Bar, median, prostate — *see* Enlargement, enlarged, prostate
Barcoo disease or rot — *see* Ulcer, skin
Barlow's disease E54
Barodontalgia T70.29 ☑
Baron Munchausen syndrome — *see* Disorder, factitious
Barosinusitis T70.1 ☑
Barotitis T70.0 ☑
Barotrauma T70.29 ☑
- odontalgia T70.29 ☑
- otitic T70.0 ☑
- sinus T70.1 ☑
Barraquer (-Simons) **disease or syndrome** (progressive lipodystrophy) E88.1
Barre-Guillain disease or syndrome G61.0
Barrel chest M95.4
Barre-Lieou syndrome (posterior cervical sympathetic) M53.0
Barrett's
- disease — *see* Barrett's, esophagus
- esophagus K22.70
  - with dysplasia K22.719
    - high grade K22.711
    - low grade K22.710
  - without dysplasia K22.70
- syndrome — *see* Barrett's, esophagus
- ulcer K22.10
  - with bleeding K22.11
  - without bleeding K22.10
Barsony (-Polgar) (-Teschendorf) **syndrome** (corkscrew esophagus) K22.4
Barth syndrome E78.71
Bartholinitis (suppurating) N75.8
- gonococcal (acute) (chronic) (with abscess) A54.1
Bartonellosis A44.9
- cutaneous A44.1
- mucocutaneous A44.1
- specified NEC A44.8
- systemic A44.0
Barton's fracture S52.56- ☑
Bartter's syndrome E26.81
Basal — *see* condition
Basan's (hidrotic) ectodermal dysplasia Q82.4
Baseball finger — *see* Dislocation, finger
Basedow's disease (exophthalmic goiter) — *see* Hyperthyroidism, with, goiter
Basic — *see* condition
Basilar — *see* condition
Bason's (hidrotic) ectodermal dysplasia Q82.4
Basopenia — *see* Agranulocytosis
Basophilia D72.824
Basophilism (cortico-adrenal) (Cushing's) (pituitary) E24.0
Bassen-Kornzweig disease or syndrome E78.6
Bat ear Q17.5

Bateman's
  disease B08.1
  purpura (senile) D69.2
Bathing cramp T75.1 ☑
Bathophobia F40.248
Batten (-Mayou) **disease** E75.4
  retina E75.4 *[H36.89]*
Batten-Steinert syndrome G71.11
Battered — *see* Maltreatment
Battey Mycobacterium infection A31.0
Battle exhaustion F43.0
Battledore placenta O43.19- ☑
Baumgarten-Cruveilhier cirrhosis, disease or syndrome K74.69
Bauxite fibrosis (of lung) J63.1
Bayle's disease (general paresis) A52.17
Bazin's disease (primary) (tuberculous) A18.4
Beach ear — *see* Swimmer's, ear
Beaded hair (congenital) Q84.1
Beal conjunctivitis or syndrome B30.2
Beard's disease (neurasthenia) F48.8
Beat(s)
  atrial, premature I49.1
  ectopic I49.49
  elbow — *see* Bursitis, elbow
  escaped, heart I49.49
  hand — *see* Bursitis, hand
  knee — *see* Bursitis, knee
  premature I49.40
    atrial I49.1
    auricular I49.1
    supraventricular I49.1
Beau's
  disease or syndrome — *see* Degeneration, myocardial
  lines (transverse furrows on fingernails) L60.4
Bechterev's syndrome — *see* Spondylitis, ankylosing
Becker's
  cardiomyopathy I42.8
  disease
    idiopathic mural endomyocardial disease I42.3
    myotonia congenita, recessive form G71.12
  dystrophy G71.01
  pigmented hairy nevus D22.5
Beck's syndrome (anterior spinal artery occlusion) I65.8
Beckwith-Wiedemann syndrome Q87.3
Bed confinement status Z74.01
Bed sore — *see* Ulcer, pressure, by site
Bedbug bite(s) — *see* Bite(s), by site, superficial, insect
Bedclothes, asphyxiation or suffocation by — *see* Asphyxia, traumatic, due to, mechanical, trapped
Bednar's
  aphthae K12.0
  tumor — *see* Neoplasm, malignant, by site
Bedridden Z74.01
Bed-sharing, infant Z72.823
Bedsore — *see* Ulcer, pressure, by site
Bedwetting — *see* Enuresis
Bee sting (with allergic or anaphylactic shock) T63.44- ☑
Beer drinker's heart (disease) I42.6
Begbie's disease (exophthalmic goiter) — *see* Hyperthyroidism, with, goiter
Behavior
  antisocial
    adult Z72.811
    child or adolescent Z72.810
  disorder, disturbance — *see* Disorder, conduct
  disruptive — *see* Disorder, conduct
  drug seeking Z76.5
  inexplicable R46.2
  marked evasiveness R46.5
  obsessive-compulsive R46.81
  overactivity R46.3
  poor responsiveness R46.4
  self-damaging (life-style) Z72.89
  sleep-incompatible Z72.821
  slowness R46.4
  specified NEC R46.89
  strange (and inexplicable) R46.2
  suspiciousness R46.5
  type A pattern Z73.1
  undue concern or preoccupation with stressful events R46.6
  verbosity and circumstantial detail obscuring reason for contact R46.7
Behcet's disease or syndrome M35.2
Behr's disease — *see* Degeneration, macula
Beigel's disease or morbus (white piedra) B36.2
Bejel A65
Bekhterev's syndrome — *see* Spondylitis, ankylosing

Belching — *see* Eructation
Bell's
  mania F30.8
  palsy, paralysis G51.0
    infant or newborn P11.3
  spasm G51.3- ☑
Bence Jones albuminuria or proteinuria NEC R80.3
Bends T70.3 ☑
Benedikt's paralysis or syndrome G46.3
Benign — *see also* condition
  prostatic hyperplasia — *see* Hyperplasia, prostate
Bennett's fracture (displaced) S62.21- ☑
Benson's disease — *see* Deposit, crystalline
Bent
  back (hysterical) F44.4
  nose M95.0
    congenital Q67.4
Bereavement (uncomplicated) Z63.4
Bergeron's disease (hysterical chorea) F44.4
Berger's disease — *see* Nephropathy, IgA
Beriberi (dry) E51.11
  heart (disease) E51.12
  polyneuropathy E51.11
  wet E51.12
    involving circulatory system E51.11
Berlin's disease or edema (traumatic) S05.8X- ☑
Berlock (berloque) **dermatitis** L56.2
Bernard-Horner syndrome G90.2
Bernard-Soulier disease or thrombopathia D69.1
Bernhardt (-Roth) **disease** — *see* Mononeuropathy, lower limb, meralgia paresthetica
Bernheim's syndrome — *see* Failure, heart, right
Bertielliasis B71.8
Berylliosis (lung) J63.2
Besnier-Boeck (-Schaumann) **disease** — *see* Sarcoidosis
Besnier's
  lupus pernio D86.3
  prurigo L20.0
Bestiality F65.89
Best's disease H35.50
Betalipoproteinemia, broad or floating E78.2
Beta-mercaptolactate-cysteine disulfiduria E72.09
Betting and gambling Z72.6
  pathological (compulsive) F63.0
Bezoar T18.9 ☑
  intestine T18.3 ☑
  stomach T18.2 ☑
Bezold's abscess — *see* Mastoiditis, acute
Bianchi's syndrome R48.8
Bicornate or bicornis uterus Q51.3
  in pregnancy or childbirth O34.00
    causing obstructed labor O65.5
Bicuspid aortic valve (at birth) (congenital) Q23.81
  functional, with stenosis — *see* Stenosis, aortic (valve)
Biedl-Bardet syndrome Q87.83
Bielschowsky (-Jansky) **disease** E75.4
Biermer's (pernicious) **anemia or disease** D51.0
Biett's disease L93.0
Bifid (congenital)
  apex, heart Q24.8
  clitoris Q52.6
  kidney Q63.8
  nose Q30.2
  patella Q74.1
  scrotum Q55.29
  toe NEC Q74.2
  tongue Q38.3
  ureter Q62.8
  uterus Q51.3
  uvula Q35.7
Biforis uterus (suprasimplex) Q51.3
Bifurcation (congenital)
  gallbladder Q44.1
  kidney pelvis Q63.8
  renal pelvis Q63.8
  rib Q76.6
  tongue, congenital Q38.3
  trachea Q32.1
  ureter Q62.8
  urethra Q64.74
  vertebra Q76.49
Big spleen syndrome D73.1
Bigeminal pulse R00.8
Bigorexia F45.22
Bilateral — *see* condition
Bile
  duct — *see* condition
  pigments in urine R82.2

Bilharziasis — *see also* Schistosomiasis
  chyluria B65.0
  cutaneous B65.3
  galacturia B65.0
  hematochyluria B65.0
  intestinal B65.1
  lipemia B65.9
  lipuria B65.0
  oriental B65.2
  piarhemia B65.9
  pulmonary NOS B65.9 *[J99]*
    pneumonia B65.9 *[J17]*
  tropical hematuria B65.0
  vesical B65.0
Biliary — *see* condition
Bilirubin metabolism disorder E80.7
  specified NEC E80.6
Bilirubinemia, familial nonhemolytic E80.4
Bilirubinuria R82.2
Biliuria R82.2
Bilocular stomach K31.2
Binswanger's disease I67.3
Biparta, bipartite
  carpal scaphoid Q74.0
  patella Q74.1
  vagina Q52.10
BI-RADS — *see* Breast, Imaging Reporting and Data System
Bird
  face Q75.8
  fancier's disease or lung J67.2
Birth
  complications in mother — *see* Delivery, complicated
  compression during NOS P15.9
  defect — *see* Anomaly
  immature (less than 37 completed weeks) — *see* Preterm, newborn
    extremely (less than 28 completed weeks) — *see* Immaturity, extreme
  inattention, at or after — *see* Maltreatment, child, neglect
  injury NOS P15.9
    basal ganglia P11.1
    brachial plexus NEC P14.3
    brain (compression) (pressure) P11.2
    central nervous system NOS P11.9
    cerebellum P11.1
    cerebral hemorrhage P10.1
    external genitalia P15.5
    eye P15.3
    face P15.4
    fracture
      bone P13.9
        specified NEC P13.8
      clavicle P13.4
      femur P13.2
      humerus P13.3
      long bone, except femur P13.3
      radius and ulna P13.3
      skull P13.0
      spine P11.5
      tibia and fibula P13.3
    intracranial P11.2
      laceration or hemorrhage P10.9
        specified NEC P10.8
    intraventricular hemorrhage P10.2
    laceration
      brain P10.1
      by scalpel P15.8
      peripheral nerve P14.9
    liver P15.0
    meninges
      brain P11.1
      spinal cord P11.5
    nerve
      brachial plexus P14.3
      cranial NEC (except facial) P11.4
      facial P11.3
      peripheral P14.9
      phrenic (paralysis) P14.2
    paralysis
      facial nerve P11.3
      spinal P11.5
    penis P15.5
    rupture
      spinal cord P11.5
    scalp P12.9
    scalpel wound P15.8
    scrotum P15.5
    skull NEC P13.1
      fracture P13.0

☑ **Additional Character Required — Refer to the Tabular List for Character Selection**

Birth — *continued*
  injury — *continued*
    specified type NEC P15.8
    spinal cord P11.5
    spine P11.5
    spleen P15.1
    sternomastoid (hematoma) P15.2
    subarachnoid hemorrhage P10.3
    subcutaneous fat necrosis P15.6
    subdural hemorrhage P10.0
    tentorial tear P10.4
    testes P15.5
    vulva P15.5
  lack of care, at or after — *see* Maltreatment, child, neglect
  neglect, at or after — *see* Maltreatment, child, neglect
  palsy or paralysis, newborn, NOS (birth injury) P14.9
  premature (infant) — *see* Preterm, newborn
  shock, newborn P96.89
  trauma — *see* Birth, injury
  weight
    low (2499 grams or less) — *see* Low, birthweight
      extremely (999 grams or less) — *see* Low, birth-weight, extreme
    4000 grams to 4499 grams P08.1
    4500 grams or more P08.0
Birthmark Q82.5
Birt-Hogg-Dube syndrome Q87.89
Bisalbuminemia E88.09
Biskra's button B55.1
Bite(s) (animal) (human)
  abdomen, abdominal
    wall S31.159 ☑
      with penetration into peritoneal cavity S31.659 ☑
      epigastric region S31.152 ☑
        with penetration into peritoneal cavity S31.652 ☑
      left
        lower quadrant S31.154 ☑
          with penetration into peritoneal cavity S31.654 ☑
        upper quadrant S31.151 ☑
          with penetration into peritoneal cavity S31.651 ☑
      periumbilic region S31.155 ☑
        with penetration into peritoneal cavity S31.655 ☑
      right
        lower quadrant S31.153 ☑
          with penetration into peritoneal cavity S31.653 ☑
        upper quadrant S31.150 ☑
          with penetration into peritoneal cavity S31.650 ☑
      superficial NEC S30.871 ☑
        insect S30.861 ☑
  alveolar (process) — *see* Bite, oral cavity
  amphibian (venomous) — *see* Venom, bite, amphibian
  animal — *see also* Bite, by site
    venomous — *see* Venom
  ankle S91.05- ☑
    superficial NEC S90.57- ☑
      insect S90.56- ☑
  antecubital space — *see* Bite, elbow
  anus S31.835 ☑
    superficial NEC S30.877 ☑
      insect S30.867 ☑
  arm (upper) S41.15- ☑
    lower — *see* Bite, forearm
    superficial NEC S40.87- ☑
      insect S40.86- ☑
  arthropod NEC — *see* Venom, bite, arthropod
  auditory canal (external) (meatus) — *see* Bite, ear
  auricle, ear — *see* Bite, ear
  axilla — *see* Bite, arm
  back — *see also* Bite, thorax, back
    lower S31.050 ☑
      with penetration into retroperitoneal space S31.051 ☑
      superficial NEC S30.870 ☑
        insect S30.860 ☑
  bedbug — *see* Bite(s), by site, superficial, insect
  breast S21.05- ☑
    superficial NEC S20.17- ☑
      insect S20.16- ☑
  brow — *see* Bite, head, specified site NEC
  buttock S31.805 ☑
    left S31.825 ☑

Bite(s) — *continued*
  buttock — *continued*
    right S31.815 ☑
    superficial NEC S30.870 ☑
      insect S30.860 ☑
  calf — *see* Bite, leg
  canaliculus lacrimalis — *see* Bite, eyelid
  canthus, eye — *see* Bite, eyelid
  centipede — *see* Toxicity, venom, arthropod, centipede
  cheek (external) S01.45- ☑
    internal — *see* Bite, oral cavity
    superficial NEC S00.87 ☑
      insect S00.86 ☑
  chest wall — *see* Bite, thorax
  chigger B88.0
  chin — *see* Bite, head, specified site NEC
  clitoris — *see* Bite, vulva
  costal region — *see* Bite, thorax
  digit(s)
    hand — *see* Bite, finger
    toe — *see* Bite, toe
  ear (canal) (external) S01.35- ☑
    superficial NEC S00.47- ☑
      insect S00.46- ☑
  elbow S51.05- ☑
    superficial NEC S50.37- ☑
      insect S50.36- ☑
  epididymis — *see* Bite, testis
  epigastric region — *see* Bite, abdomen
  epiglottis — *see* Bite, neck, specified site NEC
  esophagus, cervical S11.25 ☑
    superficial NEC S10.17 ☑
      insect S10.16 ☑
  eyebrow — *see* Bite, eyelid
  eyelid S01.15- ☑
    superficial NEC S00.27- ☑
      insect S00.26- ☑
  face NEC — *see* Bite, head, specified site NEC
  finger(s) S61.259 ☑
    with
      damage to nail S61.359 ☑
    index S61.258 ☑
      with
        damage to nail S61.358 ☑
      left S61.251 ☑
        with
          damage to nail S61.351 ☑
      right S61.250 ☑
        with
          damage to nail S61.350 ☑
      superficial NEC S60.478 ☑
        insect S60.46- ☑
    little S61.25- ☑
      with
        damage to nail S61.35- ☑
      superficial NEC S60.47- ☑
        insect S60.46- ☑
    middle S61.25- ☑
      with
        damage to nail S61.35- ☑
      superficial NEC S60.47- ☑
        insect S60.46- ☑
    ring S61.25- ☑
      with
        damage to nail S61.35- ☑
      superficial NEC S60.47- ☑
        insect S60.46- ☑
    superficial NEC S60.479 ☑
      insect S60.469 ☑
    thumb — *see* Bite, thumb
  flank — *see* Bite, abdomen, wall
  flea — *see* Bite, by site, superficial, insect
  foot (except toe(s) alone) S91.35- ☑
    superficial NEC S90.87- ☑
      insect S90.86- ☑
    toe — *see* Bite, toe
  forearm S51.85- ☑
    elbow only — *see* Bite, elbow
    superficial NEC S50.87- ☑
      insect S50.86- ☑
  forehead — *see* Bite, head, specified site NEC
  genital organs, external
    female S31.552 ☑
      superficial NEC S30.876 ☑
        insect S30.866 ☑
      vagina and vulva — *see* Bite, vulva

Bite(s) — *continued*
  genital organs, external — *continued*
    male S31.551 ☑
      penis — *see* Bite, penis
      scrotum — *see* Bite, scrotum
      superficial NEC S30.875 ☑
        insect S30.865 ☑
      testes — *see* Bite, testis
  groin — *see* Bite, abdomen, wall
  gum — *see* Bite, oral cavity
  hand S61.45- ☑
    finger — *see* Bite, finger
    superficial NEC S60.57- ☑
      insect S60.56- ☑
    thumb — *see* Bite, thumb
  head S01.95 ☑
    cheek — *see* Bite, cheek
    ear — *see* Bite, ear
    eyelid — *see* Bite, eyelid
    lip — *see* Bite, lip
    nose — *see* Bite, nose
    oral cavity — *see* Bite, oral cavity
    scalp — *see* Bite, scalp
    specified site NEC S01.85 ☑
      superficial NEC S00.87 ☑
        insect S00.86 ☑
    superficial NEC S00.97 ☑
      insect S00.96 ☑
    temporomandibular area — *see* Bite, cheek
  heel — *see* Bite, foot
  hip S71.05- ☑
    superficial NEC S70.27- ☑
      insect S70.26- ☑
  hymen S31.45 ☑
  hypochondrium — *see* Bite, abdomen, wall
  hypogastric region — *see* Bite, abdomen, wall
  inguinal region — *see* Bite, abdomen, wall
  insect — *see* Bite, by site, superficial, insect
  instep — *see* Bite, foot
  interscapular region — *see* Bite, thorax, back
  jaw — *see* Bite, head, specified site NEC
  knee S81.05- ☑
    superficial NEC S80.27- ☑
      insect S80.26- ☑
  labium (majus) (minus) — *see* Bite, vulva
  lacrimal duct — *see* Bite, eyelid
  larynx S11.015 ☑
    superficial NEC S10.17 ☑
      insect S10.16 ☑
  leg (lower) S81.85- ☑
    ankle — *see* Bite, ankle
    foot — *see* Bite, foot
    knee — *see* Bite, knee
    superficial NEC S80.87- ☑
      insect S80.86- ☑
    toe — *see* Bite, toe
    upper — *see* Bite, thigh
  lip S01.551 ☑
    superficial NEC S00.571 ☑
      insect S00.561 ☑
  lizard (venomous) — *see* Venom, bite, reptile
  loin — *see* Bite, abdomen, wall
  lower back — *see* Bite, back, lower
  lumbar region — *see* Bite, back, lower
  malar region — *see* Bite, head, specified site NEC
  mammary — *see* Bite, breast
  marine animals (venomous) — *see* Toxicity, venom, marine animal
  mastoid region — *see* Bite, head, specified site NEC
  mouth — *see* Bite, oral cavity
  nail
    finger — *see* Bite, finger
    toe — *see* Bite, toe
  nape — *see* Bite, neck, specified site NEC
  nasal (septum) (sinus) — *see* Bite, nose
  nasopharynx — *see* Bite, head, specified site NEC
  neck S11.95 ☑
    involving
      cervical esophagus — *see* Bite, esophagus, cervical
      larynx — *see* Bite, larynx
      pharynx — *see* Bite, pharynx
      thyroid gland S11.15 ☑
      trachea — *see* Bite, trachea
    specified site NEC S11.85 ☑
      superficial NEC S10.87 ☑
        insect S10.86 ☑
    superficial NEC S10.97 ☑

Bite(s) — *continued*
 neck — *continued*
  superficial — *continued*
   insect S10.96 ☑
  throat S11.85 ☑
   superficial NEC S10.17 ☑
    insect S10.16 ☑
 nose (septum) (sinus) S01.25 ☑
  superficial NEC S00.37 ☑
   insect S00.36 ☑
 occipital region — *see* Bite, scalp
 oral cavity S01.552 ☑
  superficial NEC S00.572 ☑
   insect S00.562 ☑
 orbital region — *see* Bite, eyelid
 palate — *see* Bite, oral cavity
 palm — *see* Bite, hand
 parietal region — *see* Bite, scalp
 pelvis S31.050 ☑
  with penetration into retroperitoneal space
   S31.051 ☑
  superficial NEC S30.870 ☑
   insect S30.860 ☑
 penis S31.25 ☑
  superficial NEC S30.872 ☑
   insect S30.862 ☑
 perineum
  female — *see* Bite, vulva
  male — *see* Bite, pelvis
 periocular area (with or without lacrimal passages) —
   see Bite, eyelid
 phalanges
  finger — *see* Bite, finger
  toe — *see* Bite, toe
 pharynx S11.25 ☑
  superficial NEC S10.17 ☑
   insect S10.16 ☑
 pinna — *see* Bite, ear
 poisonous — *see* Venom
 popliteal space — *see* Bite, knee
 prepuce — *see* Bite, penis
 pubic region — *see* Bite, abdomen, wall
 rectovaginal septum — *see* Bite, vulva
 red bug B88.0
 reptile NEC — *see also* Venom, bite, reptile
  nonvenomous — *see* Bite, by site
  snake — *see* Venom, bite, snake
 sacral region — *see* Bite, back, lower
 sacroiliac region — *see* Bite, back, lower
 salivary gland — *see* Bite, oral cavity
 scalp S01.05 ☑
  superficial NEC S00.07 ☑
   insect S00.06 ☑
 scapular region — *see* Bite, shoulder
 scrotum S31.35 ☑
  superficial NEC S30.873 ☑
   insect S30.863 ☑
 sea-snake (venomous) — *see* Toxicity, venom, snake, sea
   snake
 shin — *see* Bite, leg
 shoulder S41.05- ☑
  superficial NEC S40.27- ☑
   insect S40.26- ☑
 snake — *see also* Venom, bite, snake
  nonvenomous — *see* Bite, by site
 spermatic cord — *see* Bite, testis
 spider (venomous) — *see* Toxicity, venom, spider
  nonvenomous — *see* Bite, by site, superficial, insect
 sternal region — *see* Bite, thorax, front
 submaxillary region — *see* Bite, head, specified site NEC
 submental region — *see* Bite, head, specified site NEC
 subungual
  finger(s) — *see* Bite, finger
  toe — *see* Bite, toe
 superficial — *see* Bite, by site, superficial
 supraclavicular fossa S11.85 ☑
 supraorbital — *see* Bite, head, specified site NEC
 temple, temporal region — *see* Bite, head, specified site
   NEC
 temporomandibular area — *see* Bite, cheek
 testis S31.35 ☑
  superficial NEC S30.873 ☑
   insect S30.863 ☑
 thigh S71.15- ☑
  superficial NEC S70.37- ☑
   insect S70.36- ☑
 thorax, thoracic (wall) S21.95 ☑

Bite(s) — *continued*
 thorax, thoracic — *continued*
  back S21.25- ☑
   with penetration into thoracic cavity S21.45- ☑
  breast — *see* Bite, breast
  front S21.15- ☑
   with penetration into thoracic cavity S21.35- ☑
  superficial NEC S20.97 ☑
   back S20.47- ☑
   front S20.37- ☑
   insect S20.96 ☑
    back S20.46- ☑
    front S20.36- ☑
 throat — *see* Bite, neck, throat
 thumb S61.05- ☑
  with
   damage to nail S61.15- ☑
  superficial NEC S60.37- ☑
   insect S60.36- ☑
 thyroid S11.15 ☑
  superficial NEC S10.87 ☑
   insect S10.86 ☑
 toe(s) S91.15- ☑
  with
   damage to nail S91.25- ☑
  great S91.15- ☑
   with
    damage to nail S91.25- ☑
  lesser S91.15- ☑
   with
    damage to nail S91.25- ☑
  superficial NEC S90.47- ☑
   great S90.47- ☑
   insect S90.46- ☑
    great S90.46- ☑
 tongue S01.552 ☑
 trachea S11.025 ☑
  superficial NEC S10.17 ☑
   insect S10.16 ☑
 tunica vaginalis — *see* Bite, testis
 tympanum, tympanic membrane — *see* Bite, ear
 umbilical region S31.155 ☑
 uvula — *see* Bite, oral cavity
 vagina — *see* Bite, vulva
 venomous — *see* Venom
 vocal cords S11.035 ☑
  superficial NEC S10.17 ☑
   insect S10.16 ☑
 vulva S31.45 ☑
  superficial NEC S30.874 ☑
   insect S30.864 ☑
 wrist S61.55- ☑
  superficial NEC S60.87- ☑
   insect S60.86- ☑
Biting, cheek or lip K13.1
Biventricular failure (heart) I50.82
Bjorck (-Thorson) **syndrome** (malignant carcinoid) E34.09
Black
 death A20.9
 eye S00.1- ☑
 hairy tongue K14.3
 heel (foot) S90.3- ☑
 lung (disease) J60
 palm (hand) S60.22- ☑
Blackfan-Diamond anemia or syndrome (congenital hypoplastic anemia) D61.01
Blackhead L70.0
Blackout R55
Bladder — *see* condition
Blast (air) (hydraulic) (immersion) (underwater)
 blindness S05.8X- ☑
 injury
  abdomen or thorax — *see* Injury, by site
  ear (acoustic nerve trauma) — *see* Injury, nerve, acoustic, specified type NEC
  syndrome NEC T70.8 ☑
Blastoma — *see* Neoplasm, malignant, by site
 pulmonary — *see* Neoplasm, lung, malignant
Blastomycosis, blastomycotic B40.9
 Brazilian — *see* Paracoccidioidomycosis
 cutaneous B40.3
 disseminated B40.7
 European — *see* Cryptococcosis
 generalized B40.7
 keloidal B48.0
 North American B40.9
 primary pulmonary B40.0

Blastomycosis, blastomycotic — *continued*
 pulmonary B40.2
  acute B40.0
  chronic B40.1
 skin B40.3
 South American — *see* Paracoccidioidomycosis
 specified NEC B40.89
Bleb(s) R23.8
 emphysematous (lung) (solitary) J43.9
 endophthalmitis H59.43
 filtering (vitreous), after glaucoma surgery Z98.83
 inflamed (infected), postprocedural H59.40
  stage 1 H59.41
  stage 2 H59.42
  stage 3 H59.43
 lung (ruptured) J43.9
  congenital — *see* Atelectasis
  newborn P25.8
 subpleural (emphysematous) J43.9
Blebitis, postprocedural H59.40
 stage 1 H59.41
 stage 2 H59.42
 stage 3 H59.43
Bleeder (familial) (hereditary) — *see* Hemophilia
Bleeding — *see also* Hemorrhage
 anal K62.5
 anovulatory N97.0
 atonic, following delivery O72.1
 capillary I78.8
  puerperal O72.2
 contact (postcoital) N93.0
 due to uterine subinvolution N85.3
 ear — *see* Otorrhagia
 excessive, associated with menopausal onset N92.4
 familial — *see* Defect, coagulation
 following intercourse N93.0
 gastrointestinal K92.2
 hemorrhoids — *see* Hemorrhoids
 intermenstrual (regular) N92.3
  irregular N92.1
 intraoperative — *see* Complication, intraoperative, hemorrhage
 irregular N92.6
 menopausal N92.4
 newborn, intraventricular — *see* Newborn, affected by, hemorrhage, intraventricular
 nipple N64.59
 nose R04.0
 ovulation N92.3
 perimenopausal N92.4
 postclimacteric N95.0
 postcoital N93.0
 postmenopausal N95.0
 postoperative — *see* Complication, postprocedural, hemorrhage
 preclimacteric N92.4
 pre-pubertal vaginal N93.1
 puberty (excessive, with onset of menstrual periods) N92.2
 rectum, rectal K62.5
  newborn P54.2
 tendencies — *see* Defect, coagulation
 throat R04.1
 tooth socket (post-extraction) K91.840
 umbilical stump P51.9
 uterus, uterine NEC N93.9
  climacteric N92.4
  dysfunctional or functional N93.8
  menopausal N92.4
  preclimacteric or premenopausal N92.4
  unrelated to menstrual cycle N93.9
 vagina, vaginal (abnormal) N93.9
  dysfunctional or functional N93.8
  newborn P54.6
  pre-pubertal N93.1
 vicarious N94.89
Blennorrhagia, blennorrhagic — *see* Gonorrhea
Blennorrhea (acute) (chronic) — *see* Gonorrhea
 inclusion (neonatal) (newborn) P39.1
 lower genitourinary tract (gonococcal) A54.00
 neonatorum (gonococcal ophthalmia) A54.31
Blepharelosis — *see* Entropion
Blepharitis (angularis) (ciliaris) (eyelid) (marginal) (nonulcerative) H01.009
 herpes zoster B02.39
 left H01.006
  lower H01.005
  upper H01.004
  upper and lower H01.00B

Blepharitis — *continued*
  right H01.003
    lower H01.002
    upper H01.001
    upper and lower H01.00A
  squamous H01.029
    left H01.026
      lower H01.025
      upper H01.024
      upper and lower H01.02B
    right H01.023
      lower H01.022
      upper H01.021
      upper and lower H01.02A
  ulcerative H01.019
    left H01.016
      lower H01.015
      upper H01.014
      upper and lower H01.01B
    right H01.013
      lower H01.012
      upper H01.011
      upper and lower H01.01A
Blepharochalasis H02.30
  congenital Q10.0
  left H02.36
    lower H02.35
    upper H02.34
  right H02.33
    lower H02.32
    upper H02.31
Blepharoclonus H02.59
Blepharoconjunctivitis H10.50- ☑
  angular H10.52- ☑
  contact H10.53- ☑
  ligneous H10.51- ☑
Blepharophimosis (eyelid) H02.529
  congenital Q10.3
  left H02.526
    lower H02.525
    upper H02.524
  right H02.523
    lower H02.522
    upper H02.521
Blepharoptosis H02.40- ☑
  congenital Q10.0
  mechanical H02.41- ☑
  myogenic H02.42- ☑
  neurogenic H02.43- ☑
  paralytic H02.43- ☑
Blepharopyorrhea, gonococcal A54.39
Blepharospasm G24.5
  drug induced G24.01
Blighted ovum O02.0
Blind — *see also* Blindness
  bronchus (congenital) Q32.4
  loop syndrome K90.2
    congenital Q43.8
  sac, fallopian tube (congenital) Q50.6
  spot, enlarged — *see* Defect, visual field, localized, scotoma, blind spot area
  tract or tube, congenital NEC — *see* Atresia, by site
Blindness (acquired) (congenital) (both eyes) H54.0X- ☑
  blast S05.8X- ☑
  color — *see* Deficiency, color vision
  concussion S05.8X- ☑
  cortical H47.619
    left brain H47.612
    right brain H47.611
  day H53.11
  due to injury (current episode) S05.9- ☑
    sequelae — *code to* injury with seventh character S
  eclipse (total) — *see* Retinopathy, solar
  emotional (hysterical) F44.6
  face H53.16
  hysterical F44.6
  legal (both eyes) (USA definition) H54.8
  mind R48.8
  night H53.60
    abnormal dark adaptation curve H53.61
    acquired H53.62
    congenital H53.63
    specified type NEC H53.69
    vitamin A deficiency E50.5
  one eye (other eye normal) H54.40
    left (normal vision on right) H54.42- ☑
      low vision on right H54.12- ☑
    low vision, other eye H54.10

Blindness — *continued*
  one eye — *continued*
    right (normal vision on left) H54.41- ☑
      low vision on left H54.11- ☑
  psychic R48.8
  river B73.01
  snow — *see* Photokeratitis
  sun, solar — *see* Retinopathy, solar
  transient — *see* Disturbance, vision, subjective, loss, transient
  traumatic (current episode) S05.9- ☑
  word (developmental) F81.0
    acquired R48.0
    secondary to organic lesion R48.0
Blister (nonthermal)
  abdominal wall S30.821 ☑
  alveolar process S00.522 ☑
  ankle S90.52- ☑
  antecubital space — *see* Blister, elbow
  anus S30.827 ☑
  arm (upper) S40.82- ☑
  auditory canal — *see* Blister, ear
  auricle — *see* Blister, ear
  axilla — *see* Blister, arm
  back, lower S30.820 ☑
  beetle dermatitis L24.89
  breast S20.12- ☑
  brow S00.82 ☑
  calf — *see* Blister, leg
  canthus — *see* Blister, eyelid
  cheek S00.82 ☑
    internal S00.522 ☑
  chest wall — *see* Blister, thorax
  chin S00.82 ☑
  costal region — *see* Blister, thorax
  digit(s)
    foot — *see* Blister, toe
    hand — *see* Blister, finger
  due to burn — *see* Burn, by site, second degree
  ear S00.42- ☑
  elbow S50.32- ☑
  epiglottis S10.12 ☑
  esophagus, cervical S10.12 ☑
  eyebrow — *see* Blister, eyelid
  eyelid S00.22- ☑
  face S00.82 ☑
  fever B00.1
  finger(s) S60.429 ☑
    index S60.42- ☑
    little S60.42- ☑
    middle S60.42- ☑
    ring S60.42- ☑
  foot (except toe(s) alone) S90.82- ☑
    toe — *see* Blister, toe
  forearm S50.82- ☑
    elbow only — *see* Blister, elbow
  forehead S00.82 ☑
  fracture — *omit code*
  genital organ
    female S30.826 ☑
    male S30.825 ☑
  gum S00.522 ☑
  hand S60.52- ☑
  head S00.92 ☑
    ear — *see* Blister, ear
    eyelid — *see* Blister, eyelid
    lip S00.521 ☑
    nose S00.32 ☑
    oral cavity S00.522 ☑
    scalp S00.02 ☑
    specified site NEC S00.82 ☑
  heel — *see* Blister, foot
  hip S70.22- ☑
  interscapular region S20.429 ☑
  jaw S00.82 ☑
  knee S80.22- ☑
  larynx S10.12 ☑
  leg (lower) S80.82- ☑
    knee — *see* Blister, knee
    upper — *see* Blister, thigh
  lip S00.521 ☑
  malar region S00.82 ☑
  mammary — *see* Blister, breast
  mastoid region S00.82 ☑
  mouth S00.522 ☑
  multiple, skin, nontraumatic R23.8

Blister — *continued*
  nail
    finger — *see* Blister, finger
    toe — *see* Blister, toe
  nasal S00.32 ☑
  neck S10.92 ☑
    specified site NEC S10.82 ☑
    throat S10.12 ☑
  nose S00.32 ☑
  occipital region S00.02 ☑
  oral cavity S00.522 ☑
  orbital region — *see* Blister, eyelid
  palate S00.522 ☑
  palm — *see* Blister, hand
  parietal region S00.02 ☑
  pelvis S30.820 ☑
  penis S30.822 ☑
  periocular area — *see* Blister, eyelid
  phalanges
    finger — *see* Blister, finger
    toe — *see* Blister, toe
  pharynx S10.12 ☑
  pinna — *see* Blister, ear
  popliteal space — *see* Blister, knee
  scalp S00.02 ☑
  scapular region — *see* Blister, shoulder
  scrotum S30.823 ☑
  shin — *see* Blister, leg
  shoulder S40.22- ☑
  sternal region S20.329 ☑
  submaxillary region S00.82 ☑
  submental region S00.82 ☑
  subungual
    finger(s) — *see* Blister, finger
    toe(s) — *see* Blister, toe
  supraclavicular fossa S10.82 ☑
  supraorbital S00.82 ☑
  temple S00.82 ☑
  temporal region S00.82 ☑
  testis S30.823 ☑
  thermal — *see* Burn, by site, second degree
  thigh S70.32- ☑
  thorax, thoracic (wall) S20.92 ☑
    back S20.42- ☑
    front S20.32- ☑
  throat S10.12 ☑
  thumb S60.32- ☑
  toe(s) S90.42- ☑
    great S90.42- ☑
  tongue S00.522 ☑
  trachea S10.12 ☑
  tympanum, tympanic membrane — *see* Blister, ear
  upper arm — *see* Blister, arm (upper)
  uvula S00.522 ☑
  vagina S30.824 ☑
  vocal cords S10.12 ☑
  vulva S30.824 ☑
  wrist S60.82- ☑
Bloating R14.0
Bloch-Sulzberger disease or syndrome Q82.3
Block, blocked
  alveolocapillary J84.10
  arborization (heart) I45.5
  arrhythmic I45.9
  atrioventricular (incomplete) (partial) I44.30
    with atrioventricular dissociation I44.2
    complete I44.2
      congenital Q24.6
    congenital Q24.6
    first degree I44.0
    second degree (types I and II) I44.1
    specified NEC I44.39
    third degree I44.2
    types I and II I44.1
  auriculoventricular — *see* Block, atrioventricular
  bifascicular (cardiac) I45.2
  bundle-branch (complete) (false) (incomplete) I45.4
    bilateral I45.2
    left I44.7
      with right bundle branch block I45.2
      hemiblock I44.60
        anterior I44.4
        posterior I44.5
      incomplete I44.7
        with right bundle branch block I45.2
    right I45.10

Block, blocked — *continued*
- bundle-branch — *continued*
  - right — *continued*
    - with
      - left bundle branch block I45.2
      - left fascicular block I45.2
    - specified NEC I45.19
  - Wilson's type I45.19
- cardiac I45.9
- conduction I45.9
  - complete I44.2
- fascicular (left) I44.60
  - anterior I44.4
  - posterior I44.5
  - right I45.0
  - specified NEC I44.69
- foramen Magendie (acquired) G91.1
  - congenital Q03.1
    - with spina bifida — *see* Spina bifida, by site, with hydrocephalus
- heart I45.9
  - bundle branch I45.4
    - bilateral I45.2
  - complete (atrioventricular) I44.2
  - congenital Q24.6
  - first degree (atrioventricular) I44.0
  - second degree (atrioventricular) I44.1
  - specified type NEC I45.5
  - third degree (atrioventricular) I44.2
- hepatic vein I82.0
- intraventricular (nonspecific) I45.4
  - bundle branch
    - bilateral I45.2
- kidney N28.9
  - postcystoscopic or postprocedural N99.0
- Mobitz (types I and II) I44.1
- myocardial — *see* Block, heart
- nodal I45.5
- organ or site, congenital NEC — *see* Atresia, by site
- portal (vein) I81
- second degree (types I and II) I44.1
- sinoatrial I45.5
- sinoauricular I45.5
- third degree I44.2
- trifascicular I45.3
- tubal N97.1
- vein NOS I82.90
- Wenckebach (types I and II) I44.1

Blockage — *see* Obstruction
Blocq's disease F44.4
Blood
- constituents, abnormal R78.9
- disease D75.9
- donor — *see* Donor, blood
- dyscrasia D75.9
  - with
    - abortion — *see* Abortion, by type, complicated by, hemorrhage
    - ectopic pregnancy O08.1
    - molar pregnancy O08.1
  - following ectopic or molar pregnancy O08.1
  - newborn P61.9
  - puerperal, postpartum O72.3
- flukes NEC — *see* Schistosomiasis
- in
  - feces K92.1
    - occult R19.5
  - urine — *see* Hematuria
- mole O02.0
- occult in feces R19.5
- pressure
  - decreased, due to shock following injury T79.4 ☑
  - examination only Z01.30
  - fluctuating I99.8
  - high — *see* Hypertension
    - borderline R03.0
    - incidental reading, without diagnosis of hypertension R03.0
  - low — *see also* Hypotension
    - incidental reading, without diagnosis of hypotension R03.1
- spitting — *see* Hemoptysis
- staining cornea — *see* Pigmentation, cornea, stromal
- transfusion
  - reaction or complication — *see* Complications, transfusion
- type
  - A (Rh positive) Z67.10
    - Rh negative Z67.11

Blood — *continued*
- type — *continued*
  - AB (Rh positive) Z67.30
    - Rh negative Z67.31
  - B (Rh positive) Z67.20
    - Rh negative Z67.21
  - O (Rh positive) Z67.40
    - Rh negative Z67.41
  - Rh (positive) Z67.90
    - negative Z67.91
- vessel rupture — *see* Hemorrhage
- vomiting — *see* Hematemesis

Blood-forming organs, disease D75.9
Bloodgood's disease — *see* Mastopathy, cystic
Bloom (-Machacek)(-Torre) **syndrome** Q82.8
Blount disease or osteochondrosis M92.51- ☑
Blue
- baby Q24.9
- diaper syndrome E72.09
- dome cyst (breast) — *see* Cyst, breast
- dot cataract Q12.0
- nevus D22.9
- sclera Q13.5
  - with fragility of bone and deafness Q78.0
- toe syndrome I75.02- ☑

Blueness — *see* Cyanosis
Blues, postpartal O90.6
- baby O90.6
Blurring, visual H53.8
Blushing (abnormal) (excessive) R23.2
BMI — *see* Body, mass index
Boarder, hospital NEC Z76.4
- accompanying sick person Z76.3
- healthy infant or child Z76.2
  - foundling Z76.1
Bockhart's impetigo L01.02
Bodechtel-Guttman disease (subacute sclerosing panencephalitis) A81.1
Boder-Sedgwick syndrome (ataxia-telangiectasia) G11.3
Body, bodies
- Aschoff's — *see* Myocarditis, rheumatic
- asteroid, vitreous — *see* Deposit, crystalline
- cytoid (retina) — *see* Occlusion, artery, retina
- drusen (degenerative) (macula) (retinal) — *see also* Degeneration, macula, drusen
  - optic disc — *see* Drusen, optic disc
- foreign — *see* Foreign body
- loose
  - joint, except knee — *see* Loose, body, joint
    - knee M23.4- ☑
  - sheath, tendon — *see* Disorder, tendon, specified type NEC
- mass index (BMI)
  - adult
    - 19.9 or less Z68.1
    - 20.0-20.9 Z68.20
    - 21.0-21.9 Z68.21
    - 22.0-22.9 Z68.22
    - 23.0-23.9 Z68.23
    - 24.0-24.9 Z68.24
    - 25.0-25.9 Z68.25
    - 26.0-26.9 Z68.26
    - 27.0-27.9 Z68.27
    - 28.0-28.9 Z68.28
    - 29.0-29.9 Z68.29
    - 30.0-30.9 Z68.30
    - 31.0-31.9 Z68.31
    - 32.0-32.9 Z68.32
    - 33.0-33.9 Z68.33
    - 34.0-34.9 Z68.34
    - 35.0-35.9 Z68.35
    - 36.0-36.9 Z68.36
    - 37.0-37.9 Z68.37
    - 38.0-38.9 Z68.38
    - 39.0-39.9 Z68.39
    - 40.0-44.9 Z68.41
    - 45.0-49.9 Z68.42
    - 50.0-59.9 Z68.43
    - 60.0-69.9 Z68.44
    - 70 and over Z68.45
  - pediatric
    - 5th percentile to less than 85th percentile for age Z68.52
    - 85th percentile to less than 95th percentile for age Z68.53
    - 95th percentile for age to less than 120% of the 95th percentile for age Z68.54
    - 120% of the 95th percentile for age to less than 140% of the 95th percentile for age Z68.55

Body, bodies — *continued*
- mass index — *continued*
  - pediatric — *continued*
    - greater than or equal to 140% of the 95th percentile for age Z68.56
    - less than fifth percentile for age Z68.51
  - Mooser's A75.2
  - rice — *see also* Loose, body, joint
    - knee M23.4- ☑
  - rocking F98.4
Boeck's
- disease or sarcoid — *see* Sarcoidosis
- lupoid (miliary) D86.3
Boerhaave's syndrome (spontaneous esophageal rupture) K22.3
Boggy
- cervix N88.8
- uterus N85.8
Boil — *see also* Furuncle, by site
- Aleppo B55.1
- Baghdad B55.1
- Delhi B55.1
- lacrimal
  - gland — *see* Dacryoadenitis
  - passages (duct) (sac) — *see* Inflammation, lacrimal, passages, acute
- Natal B55.1
- orbit, orbital — *see* Abscess, orbit
- tropical B55.1
Bold hives — *see* Urticaria
Bombé, iris — *see* Membrane, pupillary
Bone — *see* condition
Bonnevie-Ullrich syndrome — *see also* Turner's syndrome Q87.19
Bonnier's syndrome H81.8 ☑
Bonvale dam fever T73.3 ☑
Bony block of joint — *see* Ankylosis
BOOP (bronchiolitis obliterans organized pneumonia) J84.89
Borderline
- diabetes mellitus R73.03
- hypertension R03.0
- osteopenia M85.8- ☑
- pelvis, with obstruction during labor O65.1
- personality F60.3
Borna disease A83.9
Bornholm disease B33.0
Boston exanthem A88.0
Botalli, ductus (patent) (persistent) Q25.0
Bothriocephalus latus infestation B70.0
Botulism (foodborne intoxication) A05.1
- infant A48.51
- non-foodborne A48.52
- wound A48.52
Bouba — *see* Yaws
Bouchard's nodes (with arthropathy) M15.2
Bouffée délirante F23
Bouillaud's disease or syndrome (rheumatic heart disease) I01.9
Bourneville's disease Q85.1
Boutonniere deformity (finger) —- *see* Deformity, finger, boutonniere
Bouveret (-Hoffmann) **syndrome** (paroxysmal tachycardia) I47.9
Bovine heart — *see* Hypertrophy, cardiac
Bowel — *see* condition
Bowen's
- dermatosis (precancerous) — *see* Neoplasm, skin, in situ
- disease — *see* Neoplasm, skin, in situ
- epithelioma — *see* Neoplasm, skin, in situ
- type
  - epidermoid carcinoma-in-situ — *see* Neoplasm, skin, in situ
  - intraepidermal squamous cell carcinoma — *see* Neoplasm, skin, in situ
Bowing
- femur — *see also* Deformity, limb, specified type NEC, thigh
  - congenital Q68.3
- fibula — *see also* Deformity, limb, specified type NEC, lower leg
  - congenital Q68.4
- forearm — *see* Deformity, limb, specified type NEC, forearm
- leg(s), long bones, congenital Q68.5
- radius — *see* Deformity, limb, specified type NEC, forearm
- tibia — *see also* Deformity, limb, specified type NEC, lower leg
  - congenital Q68.4

☑ **Additional Character Required** — **Refer to the Tabular List for Character Selection**

Bowleg(s) (acquired) M21.16- ☑
  congenital Q68.5
  rachitic E64.3
Boyd's dysentery A03.2
Brachial — *see* condition
Brachycardia R00.1
Brachycephaly, non-deformational Q75.022
Bradley's disease A08.19
Bradyarrhythmia, cardiac I49.8
Bradycardia (sinoatrial) (sinus) (vagal) R00.1
  neonatal P29.12
  reflex G90.09
  tachycardia syndrome I49.5
Bradykinesia R25.8
Bradypnea R06.89
Bradytachycardia I49.5
Brailsford's disease or osteochondrosis — *see* Osteochondrosis, juvenile, radius
Brain — *see also* condition
  death G93.82
  syndrome — *see* Syndrome, brain
Branched-chain amino-acid disorder E71.2
Branchial — *see* condition
  cartilage, congenital Q18.2
Branchiogenic remnant (in neck) Q18.0
Brandt's syndrome (acrodermatitis enteropathica) E83.2
Brash (water) R12
Bravais-jacksonian epilepsy — *see* Epilepsy, localization-related, symptomatic, with simple partial seizures
Braxton Hicks contractions — *see* False, labor
Brazilian leishmaniasis B55.2
BRBPR K62.5
Break, retina (without detachment) H33.30- ☑
  with retinal detachment — *see* Detachment, retina
  horseshoe tear H33.31- ☑
  multiple H33.33- ☑
  round hole H33.32- ☑
Breakdown
  device, graft or implant — *see also* Complications, by site and type, mechanical T85.618 ☑
    arterial graft NEC — *see* Complication, cardiovascular device, mechanical, vascular
    breast (implant) T85.41 ☑
    catheter NEC T85.618 ☑
      cystostomy T83.010 ☑
      dialysis (renal) T82.41 ☑
        intraperitoneal T85.611 ☑
      Hopkins T83.018 ☑
      ileostomy T83.018 ☑
      infusion NEC T82.514 ☑
        cranial T85.610- ☑
        epidural T85.610 ☑
        intrathecal T85.610 ☑
        spinal T85.610 ☑
        subarachnoid T85.610 ☑
        subdural T85.610 ☑
      nephrostomy T83.012 ☑
      urethral indwelling T83.011 ☑
      urinary NEC T83.018 ☑
      urostomy T83.018 ☑
    electronic (electrode) (pulse generator) (stimulator)
      bone T84.310 ☑
      cardiac T82.119 ☑
        electrode T82.110 ☑
        pulse generator T82.111 ☑
        specified type NEC T82.118 ☑
      nervous system — *see* Complication, prosthetic device, mechanical, electronic nervous system stimulator
      urinary — *see* Complication, genitourinary, device, urinary, mechanical
    fixation, internal (orthopedic) NEC — *see* Complication, fixation device, mechanical
    gastrointestinal — *see* Complications, prosthetic device, mechanical, gastrointestinal device
    genital NEC T83.418 ☑
      intrauterine contraceptive device T83.31 ☑
      penile prosthesis (cylinder) (implanted) (pump) (reservoir) T83.410 ☑
      testicular prosthesis T83.411 ☑
    heart NEC — *see* Complication, cardiovascular device, mechanical
    intrathecal infusion pump T85.615 ☑
    joint prosthesis — *see* Complications, joint prosthesis, internal, mechanical, by site
    nervous system, specified device NEC T85.615 ☑

Breakdown — *continued*
  device, graft or implant — *see also* Complications, by site and type, mechanical — *continued*
    ocular NEC — *see* Complications, prosthetic device, mechanical, ocular device
    orthopedic NEC — *see* Complication, orthopedic, device, mechanical
    specified NEC T85.618 ☑
    subcutaneous device pocket
      nervous system prosthetic device, implant, or graft T85.890 ☑
      other internal prosthetic device, implant, or graft T85.898 ☑
    sutures, permanent T85.612 ☑
      used in bone repair — *see* Complications, fixation device, internal (orthopedic), mechanical
    urinary NEC T83.118 ☑
      graft T83.21 ☑
      sphincter, implanted T83.111 ☑
      stent (ileal conduit) (nephroureteral) T83.113 ☑
        ureteral indwelling T83.112 ☑
    vascular NEC — *see* Complication, cardiovascular device, mechanical
    ventricular intracranial shunt T85.01 ☑
  nervous F48.8
  perineum O90.1
  respirator J95.850
    specified NEC J95.859
  ventilator J95.850
    specified NEC J95.859
Breast — *see also* condition
  buds E30.1
    in newborn P96.89
  dense R92.3- ☑
  Imaging Reporting and Data System (BI-RADS) : A R92.31- ☑
  Imaging Reporting and Data System (BI-RADS) : B R92.32- ☑
  Imaging Reporting and Data System (BI-RADS) : C R92.33- ☑
  Imaging Reporting and Data System (BI-RADS) : D R92.34- ☑
  Imaging Reporting and Data System (BI-RADS) : 1 R92.31- ☑
  Imaging Reporting and Data System (BI-RADS) : 2 R92.32- ☑
  Imaging Reporting and Data System (BI-RADS) : 3 R92.33- ☑
  Imaging Reporting and Data System (BI-RADS) : 4 R92.34- ☑
  nodule — *see also* Lump, breast N63.0
Breath
  foul R19.6
  holder, child R06.89
  holding spell R06.89
  shortness R06.02
Breathing
  labored — *see* Hyperventilation
  mouth R06.5
    causing malocclusion M26.5 ☑
  periodic R06.3
    high altitude G47.32
Breathlessness R06.81
Breda's disease — *see* Yaws
Breech presentation (mother) O32.1 ☑
  causing obstructed labor O64.1 ☑
  footling O32.8 ☑
    causing obstructed labor O64.8 ☑
  incomplete O32.8 ☑
    causing obstructed labor O64.8 ☑
Breisky's disease N90.4
Brennemann's syndrome I88.0
Brenner
  tumor (benign) D27.9
    borderline malignancy D39.1- ☑
    malignant C56 ☑
    proliferating D39.1- ☑
Bretonneau's disease or angina A36.0
Breus' mole O02.0
Brevicollis Q76.49
Brickmakers' anemia B76.9 *[D63.8]*
Bridge, myocardial Q24.5
Bright red blood per rectum (BRBPR) K62.5
Bright's disease — *see also* Nephritis
  arteriosclerotic — *see* Hypertension, kidney
Brill (-Zinsser) **disease** (recrudescent typhus) A75.1
Brill-Symmers' disease C82.90

Brion-Kayser disease — *see* Fever, paratyphoid
Briquet's disorder or syndrome F45.0
Brissaud's
  infantilism or dwarfism E23.0
  motor-verbal tic F95.2
Brittle
  bones disease Q78.0
  nails L60.3
    congenital Q84.6
Broad — *see also* condition
  beta disease E78.2
  ligament laceration syndrome N83.8
Broad- or floating-betalipoproteinemia E78.2
Brock's syndrome (atelectasis due to enlarged lymph nodes) J98.19
Brocq-Duhring disease (dermatitis herpetiformis) L13.0
Brodie's abscess or disease M86.8X- ☑
Broken
  arches — *see also* Deformity, limb, flat foot
  arm (meaning upper limb) — *see* Fracture, arm
  back — *see* Fracture, vertebra
  bone — *see* Fracture
  implant or internal device — *see* Complications, by site and type, mechanical
  leg (meaning lower limb) — *see* Fracture, leg
  nose S02.2 ☑
  tooth, teeth — *see* Fracture, tooth
Bromhidrosis, bromidrosis L75.0
Bromidism, bromism G92.8
  due to
    correct substance properly administered — *see* Table of Drugs and Chemicals, by drug, adverse effect
    overdose or wrong substance given or taken — *see* Table of Drugs and Chemicals, by drug, poisoning
  chronic (dependence) F13.20
Bromidrosiphobia F40.298
Bronchi, bronchial — *see* condition
Bronchiectasis (cylindrical) (diffuse) (fusiform) (localized) (saccular) J47.9
  with
    acute
      bronchitis J47.0
      lower respiratory infection J47.0
    exacerbation (acute) J47.1
  congenital Q33.4
  tuberculous NEC — *see* Tuberculosis, pulmonary
Bronchiolectasis — *see* Bronchiectasis
Bronchiolitis (acute) (infective) (subacute) J21.9
  with
    bronchospasm or obstruction J21.9
    influenza, flu or grippe — *see* Influenza, with, respiratory manifestations NEC
  chemical (chronic) J68.4
    acute J68.0
  chronic (fibrosing) J44.89
    obliterative J44.81
  due to
    external agent — *see* Bronchitis, acute, due to
    human metapneumovirus J21.1
    respiratory syncytial virus (RSV) J21.0
    specified organism NEC J21.8
  fibrosa obliterans J44.81
  influenzal — *see* Influenza, with, respiratory manifestations NEC
  obliterans — *see also* Bronchiolitis, obliterative J44.81
    with organizing pneumonia (BOOP) J84.89
    syndrome J44.81
  obliterative (chronic) (subacute) — *see also* Bronchiolitis, obliterans J44.81
    due to chemicals, gases, fumes or vapors (inhalation) — *see also* Disease, respiratory, chronic, due to chemicals, gases, fumes or vapors J44.81
    due to fumes or vapors — *see also* Disease, respiratory, chronic, due to chemicals, gases, fumes or vapors J44.81
  respiratory, interstitial lung disease J84.115
Bronchitis (diffuse) (fibrinous) (hypostatic) (infective) (membranous) J40
  with
    influenza, flu or grippe — *see* Influenza, with, respiratory manifestations NEC
    obstruction (airway) (lung) J44.89
    tracheitis (15 years of age and above) J40
      acute or subacute J20.9
      chronic J42
      under 15 years of age J20.9
  acute or subacute (with bronchospasm or obstruction) J20.9

Bronchitis — *continued*
  acute or subacute — *continued*
    with
      bronchiectasis J47.Ø
      chronic obstructive pulmonary disease J44.Ø
    chemical (due to gases, fumes or vapors) J68.Ø
    due to
      fumes or vapors J68.Ø
      Haemophilus influenzae J2Ø.1
      Mycoplasma pneumoniae J2Ø.Ø
      radiation J7Ø.Ø
      specified organism NEC J2Ø.8
      Streptococcus J2Ø.2
      virus
        coxsackie J2Ø.3
        echovirus J2Ø.7
        parainfluenzae J2Ø.4
        respiratory syncytial (RSV) J2Ø.5
        rhinovirus J2Ø.6
      viral NEC J2Ø.8
  allergic (acute) J45.9Ø9
    with
      exacerbation (acute) J45.9Ø1
      status asthmaticus J45.9Ø2
  arachidic T17.528 ☑
  aspiration (due to food and vomit) J69.Ø
  asthmatic J45.9 ☑
    chronic J44.89
      with
        acute lower respiratory infection J44.Ø
        exacerbation (acute) J44.1
  capillary — *see* Pneumonia, broncho
  caseous (tuberculous) A15.5
  Castellani's A69.8
  catarrhal (l5 years of age and above) J4Ø
    acute — *see* Bronchitis, acute
    chronic J41.Ø
    under l5 years of age J2Ø.9
  chemical (acute) (subacute) J68.Ø
    chronic — *see also* Disease, respiratory, chronic, due to chemicals, gases, fumes or vapors J42
    due to fumes or vapors — *see also* Disease, respiratory, chronic, due to chemicals, gases, fumes or vapors J42
      chronic J68.4
  chronic J42
    with
      airways obstruction J44.89
      tracheitis (chronic) J42
    asthmatic (obstructive) J44.89
    catarrhal J41.Ø
    chemical (due to fumes or vapors) — *see also* Disease, respiratory, chronic, due to chemicals, gases, fumes or vapors J42
    due to
      chemicals, gases, fumes or vapors (inhalation) — *see also* Disease, respiratory, chronic, due to chemicals, gases, fumes or vapors J42
      radiation J7Ø.1
      tobacco smoking J41.Ø
    emphysematous J44.89
    mucopurulent J41.1
    non-obstructive J41.Ø
    obliterans — *see* Bronchiolitis, obliterans
    obstructive J44.89
    purulent J41.1
    simple J41.Ø
  croupous — *see* Bronchitis, acute
  due to gases, fumes or vapors (chemical) J68.Ø
  emphysematous (obstructive) J44.89
  exudative — *see* Bronchitis, acute
  fetid J41.1
  grippal — *see* Influenza, with, respiratory manifestations NEC
  in those under l5 years age — *see* Bronchitis, acute
    chronic — *see* Bronchitis, chronic
  influenzal — *see* Influenza, with, respiratory manifestations NEC
  mixed simple and mucopurulent J41.8
  moulder's J62.8
  mucopurulent (chronic) (recurrent) J41.1
    acute or subacute J2Ø.9
    simple (mixed) J41.8
  obliterans (chronic) — *see* Bronchiolitis, obliterans
  obstructive (chronic) (diffuse) J44.89
  pituitous J41.1
  pneumococcal, acute or subacute J2Ø.2
  pseudomembranous, acute or subacute — *see* Bronchitis, acute

Bronchitis — *continued*
  purulent (chronic) (recurrent) J41.1
    acute or subacute — *see* Bronchitis, acute
  putrid J41.1
  senile (chronic) J42
  simple and mucopurulent (mixed) J41.8
  smokers' J41.Ø
  spirochetal NEC A69.8
  subacute — *see* Bronchitis, acute
  suppurative (chronic) J41.1
    acute or subacute — *see* Bronchitis, acute
  tuberculous A15.5
  under l5 years of age — *see* Bronchitis, acute
    chronic — *see* Bronchitis, chronic
  viral NEC, acute or subacute — *see also* Bronchitis, acute J2Ø.8
Bronchoalveolitis J18.Ø
Bronchoaspergillosis B44.1
Bronchocele meaning goiter E04.Ø
Broncholithiasis J98.Ø9
  tuberculous NEC A15.5
Bronchomalacia J98.Ø9
  congenital Q32.2
Bronchomycosis NOS B49 *[J99]*
  candidal B37.1
Bronchopleuropneumonia — *see* Pneumonia, broncho
Bronchopneumonia — *see* Pneumonia, broncho
Bronchopneumonitis — *see* Pneumonia, broncho
Bronchopulmonary — *see* condition
Bronchopulmonitis — *see* Pneumonia, broncho
Bronchorrhagia (see Hemoptysis)
Bronchorrhea J98.Ø9
  acute J2Ø.9
  chronic (infective) (purulent) J42
Bronchospasm (acute) J98.Ø1
  with
    bronchiolitis, acute J21.9
    bronchitis, acute (conditions in J2Ø) — *see* Bronchitis, acute
  due to external agent — *see* condition, respiratory, acute, due to
  exercise induced J45.99Ø
Bronchospirochetosis A69.8
  Castellani A69.8
Bronchostenosis J98.Ø9
Bronchus — *see* condition
Brontophobia F4Ø.22Ø
Bronze baby syndrome P83.88
Brooke's tumor — *see* Neoplasm, skin, benign
Brown enamel of teeth (hereditary) KØØ.5
Brown's sheath syndrome H5Ø.61- ☑
Brown-Sequard disease, paralysis or syndrome G83.81
Bruce sepsis A23.Ø
Brucellosis (infection) A23.9
  abortus A23.1
  canis A23.3
  dermatitis A23.9
  melitensis A23.Ø
  mixed A23.8
  sepsis A23.9
    melitensis A23.Ø
    specified NEC A23.8
  suis A23.2
Bruck-de Lange disease Q87.19
Bruck's disease — *see* Deformity, limb
BRUE (brief resolved unexplained event) R68.13
Brugsch's syndrome Q82.8
Bruise (skin surface intact) — *see also* Contusion
  with
    open wound — *see* Wound, open
  internal organ — *see* Injury, by site
  newborn P54.5
  scalp, due to birth injury, newborn P12.3
  umbilical cord O69.5 ☑
Bruit (arterial) RØ9.89
  cardiac RØ1.1
Brush burn — *see* Abrasion, by site
Bruton's X-linked agammaglobulinemia D8Ø.Ø
Bruxism
  psychogenic F45.8
  sleep related G47.63
Bubbly lung syndrome P27.Ø
Bubo I88.8
  blennorrhagic (gonococcal) A54.89
  chancroidal A57
  climatic A55
  due to Haemophilus ducreyi A57
  gonococcal A54.89
  indolent (nonspecific) I88.8

Bubo — *continued*
  inguinal (nonspecific) I88.8
    chancroidal A57
    climatic A57
    due to H. ducreyi A57
    infective I88.8
  scrofulous (tuberculous) A18.2
  soft chancre A57
  suppurating — *see* Lymphadenitis, acute
  syphilitic (primary) A51.Ø
    congenital A5Ø.Ø7
  tropical A55
  virulent (chancroidal) A57
Bubonic plague A2Ø.Ø
Bubonocele — *see* Hernia, inguinal
Buccal — *see* condition
Buchanan's disease or osteochondrosis M91.Ø
Buchem's syndrome (hyperostosis corticalis) M85.2
Bucket-handle fracture or tear (semilunar cartilage) — *see* Tear, meniscus
Budd-Chiari syndrome (hepatic vein thrombosis) I82.Ø
Budgerigar fancier's disease or lung J67.2
Buds
  breast E3Ø.1
    in newborn P96.89
Buerger's disease (thromboangiitis obliterans) I73.1
Bulbar — *see* condition
Bulbus cordis (left ventricle) (persistent) Q21.8
Bulimia (nervosa) F5Ø.2- ☑
  atypical F5Ø.9
  normal weight F5Ø.9
Bulky
  stools R19.5
  uterus N85.2
Bulla (e) R23.8
  lung (emphysematous) (solitary) J43.9
    newborn P25.8
Bullet wound — *see also* Puncture
  fracture — *code as* Fracture, by site
  internal organ — *see* Injury, by site
Bundle
  branch block (complete) (false) (incomplete) — *see* Block, bundle-branch
  of His — *see* condition
Bunion M21.61- ☑
  tailor's M21.62- ☑
Bunionette M21.62- ☑
Buphthalmia, buphthalmos (congenital) Q15.Ø
Burdwan fever B55.Ø
Burger-Grutz disease or syndrome E78.3
Buried
  penis (congenital) Q55.64
    acquired N48.83
  roots KØ8.3
Burke's syndrome K86.89
Burkholderia
  cepacia A49.8
  mallei A24.Ø
  pseudomallei — *see* Melioidosis
Burkitt
  cell leukemia C91.Ø- ☑
  lymphoma (malignant) C83.7- ☑
    small noncleaved, diffuse C83.7- ☑
    spleen C83.77
    undifferentiated C83.7- ☑
  tumor C83.7- ☑
  type
    acute lymphoblastic leukemia C91.Ø- ☑
    undifferentiated C83.7- ☑
Burn (electricity) (flame) (hot gas, liquid or hot object) (radiation) (steam) (thermal) T3Ø.Ø
  abdomen, abdominal (muscle) (wall) T21.Ø2 ☑
    first degree T21.12 ☑
    second degree T21.22 ☑
    third degree T21.32 ☑
  above elbow T22.Ø39 ☑
    first degree T22.139 ☑
    left T22.Ø32 ☑
      first degree T22.132 ☑
      second degree T22.232 ☑
      third degree T22.332 ☑
    right T22.Ø31 ☑
      first degree T22.131 ☑
      second degree T22.231 ☑
      third degree T22.331 ☑
    second degree T22.239 ☑
    third degree T22.339 ☑

Burn — *continued*
- acid (caustic) (external) (internal) — *see* Corrosion, by site
- alimentary tract NEC T28.2 ☑
  - esophagus T28.1 ☑
  - mouth T28.0 ☑
  - pharynx T28.0 ☑
- alkaline (caustic) (external) (internal) — *see* Corrosion, by site
- ankle T25.019 ☑
  - first degree T25.119 ☑
  - left T25.012 ☑
    - first degree T25.112 ☑
    - second degree T25.212 ☑
    - third degree T25.312 ☑
  - multiple with foot — *see* Burn, lower, limb, multiple, ankle and foot
  - right T25.011 ☑
    - first degree T25.111 ☑
    - second degree T25.211 ☑
    - third degree T25.311 ☑
  - second degree T25.219 ☑
  - third degree T25.319 ☑
- anus — *see* Burn, buttock
- arm (lower) (upper) — *see* Burn, upper, limb
- axilla T22.049 ☑
  - first degree T22.149 ☑
  - left T22.042 ☑
    - first degree T22.142 ☑
    - second degree T22.242 ☑
    - third degree T22.342 ☑
  - right T22.041 ☑
    - first degree T22.141 ☑
    - second degree T22.241 ☑
    - third degree T22.341 ☑
  - second degree T22.249 ☑
  - third degree T22.349 ☑
- back (lower) T21.04 ☑
  - first degree T21.14 ☑
  - second degree T21.24 ☑
  - third degree T21.34 ☑
  - upper T21.03 ☑
    - first degree T21.13 ☑
    - second degree T21.23 ☑
    - third degree T21.33 ☑
- blisters — *code as* Burn, second degree, by site
- breast(s) — *see* Burn, chest wall
- buttock(s) T21.05 ☑
  - first degree T21.15 ☑
  - second degree T21.25 ☑
  - third degree T21.35 ☑
- calf T24.039 ☑
  - first degree T24.139 ☑
  - left T24.032 ☑
    - first degree T24.132 ☑
    - second degree T24.232 ☑
    - third degree T24.332 ☑
  - right T24.031 ☑
    - first degree T24.131 ☑
    - second degree T24.231 ☑
    - third degree T24.331 ☑
  - second degree T24.239 ☑
  - third degree T24.339 ☑
- canthus (eye) — *see* Burn, eyelid
- caustic acid or alkaline — *see* Corrosion, by site
- cervix T28.3 ☑
- cheek T20.06 ☑
  - first degree T20.16 ☑
  - second degree T20.26 ☑
  - third degree T20.36 ☑
- chemical (acids) (alkalines) (caustics) (external) (internal) — *see* Corrosion, by site
- chest wall T21.01 ☑
  - first degree T21.11 ☑
  - second degree T21.21 ☑
  - third degree T21.31 ☑
- chin T20.03 ☑
  - first degree T20.13 ☑
  - second degree T20.23 ☑
  - third degree T20.33 ☑
- colon T28.2 ☑
- conjunctiva (and cornea) — *see* Burn, cornea
- cornea (and conjunctiva) T26.1- ☑
  - chemical — *see* Corrosion, cornea
- corrosion (external) (internal) — *see* Corrosion, by site

Burn — *continued*
- deep necrosis of underlying tissue — *code as* Burn, third degree, by site
- dorsum of hand T23.069 ☑
  - first degree T23.169 ☑
  - left T23.062 ☑
    - first degree T23.162 ☑
    - second degree T23.262 ☑
    - third degree T23.362 ☑
  - right T23.061 ☑
    - first degree T23.161 ☑
    - second degree T23.261 ☑
    - third degree T23.361 ☑
  - second degree T23.269 ☑
  - third degree T23.369 ☑
- due to ingested chemical agent — *see* Corrosion, by site
- ear (auricle) (external) (canal) T20.01 ☑
  - first degree T20.11 ☑
  - second degree T20.21 ☑
  - third degree T20.31 ☑
- elbow T22.029 ☑
  - first degree T22.129 ☑
  - left T22.022 ☑
    - first degree T22.122 ☑
    - second degree T22.222 ☑
    - third degree T22.322 ☑
  - right T22.021 ☑
    - first degree T22.121 ☑
    - second degree T22.221 ☑
    - third degree T22.321 ☑
  - second degree T22.229 ☑
  - third degree T22.329 ☑
- epidermal loss — *code as* Burn, second degree, by site
- erythema, erythematous — *code as* Burn, first degree, by site
- esophagus T28.1 ☑
- extent (percentage of body surface)
  - less than 10 percent T31.0
  - 10-19 percent T31.10
    - with 0-9 percent third degree burns T31.10
    - with 10-19 percent third degree burns T31.11
  - 20-29 percent T31.20
    - with 0-9 percent third degree burns T31.20
    - with 10-19 percent third degree burns T31.21
    - with 20-29 percent third degree burns T31.22
  - 30-39 percent T31.30
    - with 0-9 percent third degree burns T31.30
    - with 10-19 percent third degree burns T31.31
    - with 20-29 percent third degree burns T31.32
    - with 30-39 percent third degree burns T31.33
  - 40-49 percent T31.40
    - with 0-9 percent third degree burns T31.40
    - with 10-19 percent third degree burns T31.41
    - with 20-29 percent third degree burns T31.42
    - with 30-39 percent third degree burns T31.43
    - with 40-49 percent third degree burns T31.44
  - 50-59 percent T31.50
    - with 0-9 percent third degree burns T31.50
    - with 10-19 percent third degree burns T31.51
    - with 20-29 percent third degree burns T31.52
    - with 30-39 percent third degree burns T31.53
    - with 40-49 percent third degree burns T31.54
    - with 50-59 percent third degree burns T31.55
  - 60-69 percent T31.60
    - with 0-9 percent third degree burns T31.60
    - with 10-19 percent third degree burns T31.61
    - with 20-29 percent third degree burns T31.62
    - with 30-39 percent third degree burns T31.63
    - with 40-49 percent third degree burns T31.64
    - with 50-59 percent third degree burns T31.65
    - with 60-69 percent third degree burns T31.66
  - 70-79 percent T31.70
    - with 0-9 percent third degree burns T31.70
    - with 10-19 percent third degree burns T31.71
    - with 20-29 percent third degree burns T31.72
    - with 30-39 percent third degree burns T31.73
    - with 40-49 percent third degree burns T31.74
    - with 50-59 percent third degree burns T31.75
    - with 60-69 percent third degree burns T31.76
    - with 70-79 percent third degree burns T31.77
  - 80-89 percent T31.80
    - with 0-9 percent third degree burns T31.80
    - with 10-19 percent third degree burns T31.81
    - with 20-29 percent third degree burns T31.82
    - with 30-39 percent third degree burns T31.83
    - with 40-49 percent third degree burns T31.84
    - with 50-59 percent third degree burns T31.85

Burn — *continued*
- extent — *continued*
  - 80-89 percent — *continued*
    - with 60-69 percent third degree burns T31.86
    - with 70-79 percent third degree burns T31.87
    - with 80-89 percent third degree burns T31.88
  - 90 percent or more T31.90
    - with 0-9 percent third degree burns T31.90
    - with 10-19 percent third degree burns T31.91
    - with 20-29 percent third degree burns T31.92
    - with 30-39 percent third degree burns T31.93
    - with 40-49 percent third degree burns T31.94
    - with 50-59 percent third degree burns T31.95
    - with 60-69 percent third degree burns T31.96
    - with 70-79 percent third degree burns T31.97
    - with 80-89 percent third degree burns T31.98
    - with 90 percent or more third degree burns T31.99
- extremity — *see* Burn, limb
- eye(s) and adnexa T26.4- ☑
  - with resulting rupture and destruction of eyeball T26.2-
  - conjunctival sac — *see* Burn, cornea
  - cornea — *see* Burn, cornea
  - lid — *see* Burn, eyelid
  - periocular area — *see* Burn, eyelid
  - specified site NEC T26.3- ☑
- eyeball — *see* Burn, eye
- eyelid(s) T26.0- ☑
  - chemical — *see* Corrosion, eyelid
- face — *see* Burn, head
- finger T23.029 ☑
  - first degree T23.129 ☑
  - left T23.022 ☑
    - first degree T23.122 ☑
    - second degree T23.222 ☑
    - third degree T23.322 ☑
  - multiple sites (without thumb) T23.039 ☑
    - with thumb T23.049 ☑
      - first degree T23.149 ☑
      - left T23.042 ☑
        - first degree T23.142 ☑
        - second degree T23.242 ☑
        - third degree T23.342 ☑
      - right T23.041 ☑
        - first degree T23.141 ☑
        - second degree T23.241 ☑
        - third degree T23.341 ☑
      - second degree T23.249 ☑
      - third degree T23.349 ☑
    - first degree T23.139 ☑
    - left T23.032 ☑
      - first degree T23.132 ☑
      - second degree T23.232 ☑
      - third degree T23.332 ☑
    - right T23.031 ☑
      - first degree T23.131 ☑
      - second degree T23.231 ☑
      - third degree T23.331 ☑
    - second degree T23.239 ☑
    - third degree T23.339 ☑
  - right T23.021 ☑
    - first degree T23.121 ☑
    - second degree T23.221 ☑
    - third degree T23.321 ☑
  - second degree T23.229 ☑
  - third degree T23.329 ☑
- flank — *see* Burn, abdominal wall
- foot T25.029 ☑
  - first degree T25.129 ☑
  - left T25.022 ☑
    - first degree T25.122 ☑
    - second degree T25.222 ☑
    - third degree T25.322 ☑
  - multiple with ankle — *see* Burn, lower, limb, multiple, ankle and foot
  - right T25.021 ☑
    - first degree T25.121 ☑
    - second degree T25.221 ☑
    - third degree T25.321 ☑
  - second degree T25.229 ☑
  - third degree T25.329 ☑
- forearm T22.019 ☑
  - first degree T22.119 ☑
  - left T22.012 ☑
    - first degree T22.112 ☑
    - second degree T22.212 ☑

Burn — *continued*
 forearm — *continued*
  left — *continued*
   third degree T22.312 ☑
  right T22.011 ☑
   first degree T22.111 ☑
   second degree T22.211 ☑
   third degree T22.311 ☑
  second degree T22.219 ☑
  third degree T22.319 ☑
 forehead T20.06 ☑
  first degree T20.16 ☑
  second degree T20.26 ☑
  third degree T20.36 ☑
 fourth degree — *code as* Burn, third degree, by site
 friction — *see* Burn, by site
 from swallowing caustic or corrosive substance NEC — *see* Corrosion, by site
 full thickness skin loss — *code as* Burn, third degree, by site
 gastrointestinal tract NEC T28.2 ☑
  from swallowing caustic or corrosive substance T28.7 ☑
 genital organs
  external
   female T21.07 ☑
    first degree T21.17 ☑
    second degree T21.27 ☑
    third degree T21.37 ☑
   male T21.06 ☑
    first degree T21.16 ☑
    second degree T21.26 ☑
    third degree T21.36 ☑
  internal T28.3 ☑
   from caustic or corrosive substance T28.8 ☑
 groin — *see* Burn, abdominal wall
 hand(s) T23.009 ☑
  back — *see* Burn, dorsum of hand
  finger — *see* Burn, finger
  first degree T23.109 ☑
  left T23.002 ☑
   first degree T23.102 ☑
   second degree T23.202 ☑
   third degree T23.302 ☑
  multiple sites with wrist T23.099 ☑
   first degree T23.199 ☑
   left T23.092 ☑
    first degree T23.192 ☑
    second degree T23.292 ☑
    third degree T23.392 ☑
   right T23.091 ☑
    first degree T23.191 ☑
    second degree T23.291 ☑
    third degree T23.391 ☑
   second degree T23.299 ☑
   third degree T23.399 ☑
  palm — *see* Burn, palm
  right T23.001 ☑
   first degree T23.101 ☑
   second degree T23.201 ☑
   third degree T23.301 ☑
  second degree T23.209 ☑
  third degree T23.309 ☑
  thumb — *see* Burn, thumb
 head (and face) (and neck) T20.00 ☑
  cheek — *see* Burn, cheek
  chin — *see* Burn, chin
  ear — *see* Burn, ear
  eye(s) only — *see* Burn, eye
  first degree T20.10 ☑
  forehead — *see* Burn, forehead
  lip — *see* Burn, lip
  multiple sites T20.09 ☑
   first degree T20.19 ☑
   second degree T20.29 ☑
   third degree T20.39 ☑
  neck — *see* Burn, neck
  nose — *see* Burn, nose
  scalp — *see* Burn, scalp
  second degree T20.20 ☑
  third degree T20.30 ☑
 hip(s) — *see* Burn, thigh
 inhalation — *see* Burn, respiratory tract
  caustic or corrosive substance (fumes) — *see* Corrosion, respiratory tract
 internal organ(s) T28.40 ☑

Burn — *continued*
 internal organ(s) — *continued*
  alimentary tract T28.2 ☑
   esophagus T28.1 ☑
  eardrum T28.41 ☑
  esophagus T28.1 ☑
  from caustic or corrosive substance (swallowing) NEC — *see* Corrosion, by site
  genitourinary T28.3 ☑
  mouth T28.0 ☑
  pharynx T28.0 ☑
  respiratory tract — *see* Burn, respiratory tract
  specified organ NEC T28.49 ☑
 interscapular region — *see* Burn, back, upper
 intestine (large) (small) T28.2 ☑
 knee T24.029 ☑
  first degree T24.129 ☑
  left T24.022 ☑
   first degree T24.122 ☑
   second degree T24.222 ☑
   third degree T24.322 ☑
  right T24.021 ☑
   first degree T24.121 ☑
   second degree T24.221 ☑
   third degree T24.321 ☑
  second degree T24.229 ☑
  third degree T24.329 ☑
 labium (majus) (minus) — *see* Burn, genital organs, external, female
 lacrimal apparatus, duct, gland or sac — *see* Burn, eye, specified site NEC
 larynx T27.0 ☑
  with lung T27.1 ☑
 leg(s) (lower) (upper) — *see* Burn, lower, limb
 lightning — *see* Burn, by site
 limb(s)
  lower (except ankle or foot alone) — *see* Burn, lower, limb
  upper — *see* Burn, upper limb
 lip(s) T20.02 ☑
  first degree T20.12 ☑
  second degree T20.22 ☑
  third degree T20.32 ☑
 lower
  back — *see* Burn, back
  limb T24.009 ☑
   ankle — *see* Burn, ankle
   calf — *see* Burn, calf
   first degree T24.109 ☑
   foot — *see* Burn, foot
   hip — *see* Burn, thigh
   knee — *see* Burn, knee
   left T24.002 ☑
    first degree T24.102 ☑
    second degree T24.202 ☑
    third degree T24.302 ☑
   multiple sites, except ankle and foot T24.099 ☑
    ankle and foot T25.099 ☑
     first degree T25.199 ☑
     left T25.092 ☑
      first degree T25.192 ☑
      second degree T25.292 ☑
      third degree T25.392 ☑
     right T25.091 ☑
      first degree T25.191 ☑
      second degree T25.291 ☑
      third degree T25.391 ☑
     second degree T25.299 ☑
     third degree T25.399 ☑
    first degree T24.199 ☑
    left T24.092 ☑
     first degree T24.192 ☑
     second degree T24.292 ☑
     third degree T24.392 ☑
    right T24.091 ☑
     first degree T24.191 ☑
     second degree T24.291 ☑
     third degree T24.391 ☑
    second degree T24.299 ☑
    third degree T24.399 ☑
   right T24.001 ☑
    first degree T24.101 ☑
    second degree T24.201 ☑
    third degree T24.301 ☑
   second degree T24.209 ☑
   thigh — *see* Burn, thigh

Burn — *continued*
 lower — *continued*
  limb — *continued*
   third degree T24.309 ☑
   toe — *see* Burn, toe
 lung (with larynx and trachea) T27.1 ☑
 mouth T28.0 ☑
 neck T20.07 ☑
  first degree T20.17 ☑
  second degree T20.27 ☑
  third degree T20.37 ☑
 nose (septum) T20.04 ☑
  first degree T20.14 ☑
  second degree T20.24 ☑
  third degree T20.34 ☑
 ocular adnexa — *see* Burn, eye
 orbit region — *see* Burn, eyelid
 palm T23.059 ☑
  first degree T23.159 ☑
  left T23.052 ☑
   first degree T23.152 ☑
   second degree T23.252 ☑
   third degree T23.352 ☑
  right T23.051 ☑
   first degree T23.151 ☑
   second degree T23.251 ☑
   third degree T23.351 ☑
  second degree T23.259 ☑
  third degree T23.359 ☑
 partial thickness — *code as* Burn, by site, second degree
 pelvis — *see* Burn, trunk
 penis — *see* Burn, genital organs, external, male
 perineum
  female — *see* Burn, genital organs, external, female
  male — *see* Burn, genital organs, external, male
 periocular area — *see* Burn, eyelid
 pharynx T28.0 ☑
 rectum T28.2 ☑
 respiratory tract T27.3 ☑
  larynx — *see* Burn, larynx
  specified part NEC T27.2 ☑
  trachea — *see* Burn, trachea
 sac, lacrimal — *see* Burn, eye, specified site NEC
 scalp T20.05 ☑
  first degree T20.15 ☑
  second degree T20.25 ☑
  third degree T20.35 ☑
 scapular region T22.069 ☑
  first degree T22.169 ☑
  left T22.062 ☑
   first degree T22.162 ☑
   second degree T22.262 ☑
   third degree T22.362 ☑
  right T22.061 ☑
   first degree T22.161 ☑
   second degree T22.261 ☑
   third degree T22.361 ☑
  second degree T22.269 ☑
  third degree T22.369 ☑
 sclera — *see* Burn, eye, specified site NEC
 scrotum — *see* Burn, genital organs, external, male
 shoulder T22.059 ☑
  first degree T22.159 ☑
  left T22.052 ☑
   first degree T22.152 ☑
   second degree T22.252 ☑
   third degree T22.352 ☑
  right T22.051 ☑
   first degree T22.151 ☑
   second degree T22.251 ☑
   third degree T22.351 ☑
  second degree T22.259 ☑
  third degree T22.359 ☑
 stomach T28.2 ☑
 temple — *see* Burn, head
 testis — *see* Burn, genital organs, external, male
 thigh T24.019 ☑
  first degree T24.119 ☑
  left T24.012 ☑
   first degree T24.112 ☑
   second degree T24.212 ☑
   third degree T24.312 ☑
  right T24.011 ☑
   first degree T24.111 ☑
   second degree T24.211 ☑
   third degree T24.311 ☑

Burn — *continued*
thigh — *continued*
  second degree T24.219 ☑
  third degree T24.319 ☑
thorax (external) — *see* Burn, trunk
throat (meaning pharynx) T28.0 ☑
thumb(s) T23.019 ☑
  first degree T23.119 ☑
  left T23.012 ☑
    first degree T23.112 ☑
    second degree T23.212 ☑
    third degree T23.312 ☑
  multiple sites with fingers T23.049 ☑
    first degree T23.149 ☑
    left T23.042 ☑
      first degree T23.142 ☑
      second degree T23.242 ☑
      third degree T23.342 ☑
    right T23.041 ☑
      first degree T23.141 ☑
      second degree T23.241 ☑
      third degree T23.341 ☑
    second degree T23.249 ☑
    third degree T23.349 ☑
  right T23.011 ☑
    first degree T23.111 ☑
    second degree T23.211 ☑
    third degree T23.311 ☑
  second degree T23.219 ☑
  third degree T23.319 ☑
toe T25.039 ☑
  first degree T25.139 ☑
  left T25.032 ☑
    first degree T25.132 ☑
    second degree T25.232 ☑
    third degree T25.332 ☑
  right T25.031 ☑
    first degree T25.131 ☑
    second degree T25.231 ☑
    third degree T25.331 ☑
  second degree T25.239 ☑
  third degree T25.339 ☑
tongue T28.0 ☑
tonsil(s) T28.0 ☑
trachea T27.0 ☑
  with lung T27.1 ☑
trunk T21.00 ☑
  abdominal wall — *see* Burn, abdominal wall
  anus — *see* Burn, buttock
  axilla — *see* Burn, upper limb
  back — *see* Burn, back
  breast — *see* Burn, chest wall
  buttock — *see* Burn, buttock
  chest wall — *see* Burn, chest wall
  first degree T21.10 ☑
  flank — *see* Burn, abdominal wall
  genital
    female — *see* Burn, genital organs, external, female
    male — *see* Burn, genital organs, external, male
  groin — *see* Burn, abdominal wall
  interscapular region — *see* Burn, back, upper
  labia — *see* Burn, genital organs, external, female
  lower back — *see* Burn, back
  penis — *see* Burn, genital organs, external, male
  perineum
    female — *see* Burn, genital organs, external, female
    male — *see* Burn, genital organs, external, male
  scapula region — *see* Burn, scapular region
  scrotum — *see* Burn, genital organs, external, male
  second degree T21.20 ☑
  specified site NEC T21.09 ☑
    first degree T21.19 ☑
    second degree T21.29 ☑
    third degree T21.39 ☑
  testes — *see* Burn, genital organs, external, male
  third degree T21.30 ☑
  upper back — *see* Burn, back, upper
  vulva — *see* Burn, genital organs, external, female
unspecified site with extent of body surface involved specified
  less than 10 percent T31.0
  10-19 percent (0-9 percent third degree) T31.10
    with 10-19 percent third degree T31.11
  20-29 percent (0-9 percent third degree) T31.20

Burn — *continued*
unspecified site with extent of body surface involved specified — *continued*
  20-29 percent — *continued*
    with
      10-19 percent third degree T31.21
      20-29 percent third degree T31.22
  30-39 percent (0-9 percent third degree) T31.30
    with
      10-19 percent third degree T31.31
      20-29 percent third degree T31.32
      30-39 percent third degree T31.33
  40-49 percent (0-9 percent third degree) T31.40
    with
      10-19 percent third degree T31.41
      20-29 percent third degree T31.42
      30-39 percent third degree T31.43
      40-49 percent third degree T31.44
  50-59 percent (0-9 percent third degree) T31.50
    with
      10-19 percent third degree T31.51
      20-29 percent third degree T31.52
      30-39 percent third degree T31.53
      40-49 percent third degree T31.54
      50-59 percent third degree T31.55
  60-69 percent (0-9 percent third degree) T31.60
    with
      10-19 percent third degree T31.61
      20-29 percent third degree T31.62
      30-39 percent third degree T31.63
      40-49 percent third degree T31.64
      50-59 percent third degree T31.65
      60-69 percent third degree T31.66
  70-79 percent (0-9 percent third degree) T31.70
    with
      10-19 percent third degree T31.71
      20-29 percent third degree T31.72
      30-39 percent third degree T31.73
      40-49 percent third degree T31.74
      50-59 percent third degree T31.75
      60-69 percent third degree T31.76
      70-79 percent third degree T31.77
  80-89 percent (0-9 percent third degree) T31.80
    with
      10-19 percent third degree T31.81
      20-29 percent third degree T31.82
      30-39 percent third degree T31.83
      40-49 percent third degree T31.84
      50-59 percent third degree T31.85
      60-69 percent third degree T31.86
      70-79 percent third degree T31.87
      80-89 percent third degree T31.88
  90 percent or more (0-9 percent third degree) T31.90
    with
      10-19 percent third degree T31.91
      20-29 percent third degree T31.92
      30-39 percent third degree T31.93
      40-49 percent third degree T31.94
      50-59 percent third degree T31.95
      60-69 percent third degree T31.96
      70-79 percent third degree T31.97
      80-89 percent third degree T31.98
      90-99 percent third degree T31.99
upper limb T22.00 ☑
  above elbow — *see* Burn, above elbow
  axilla — *see* Burn, axilla
  elbow — *see* Burn, elbow
  first degree T22.10 ☑
  forearm — *see* Burn, forearm
  hand — *see* Burn, hand
  interscapular region — *see* Burn, back, upper
  multiple sites T22.099 ☑
    first degree T22.199 ☑
    left T22.092 ☑
      first degree T22.192 ☑
      second degree T22.292 ☑
      third degree T22.392 ☑
    right T22.091 ☑
      first degree T22.191 ☑
      second degree T22.291 ☑
      third degree T22.391 ☑
    second degree T22.299 ☑
    third degree T22.399 ☑
  scapular region — *see* Burn, scapular region
  second degree T22.20 ☑
  shoulder — *see* Burn, shoulder
  third degree T22.30 ☑
  wrist — *see* Burn, wrist

Burn — *continued*
uterus T28.3 ☑
vagina T28.3 ☑
vulva — *see* Burn, genital organs, external, female
wrist T23.079 ☑
  first degree T23.179 ☑
  left T23.072 ☑
    first degree T23.172 ☑
    second degree T23.272 ☑
    third degree T23.372 ☑
  multiple sites with hand T23.099 ☑
    first degree T23.199 ☑
    left T23.092 ☑
      first degree T23.192 ☑
      second degree T23.292 ☑
      third degree T23.392 ☑
    right T23.091 ☑
      first degree T23.191 ☑
      second degree T23.291 ☑
      third degree T23.391 ☑
    second degree T23.299 ☑
    third degree T23.399 ☑
  right T23.071 ☑
    first degree T23.171 ☑
    second degree T23.271 ☑
    third degree T23.371 ☑
  second degree T23.279 ☑
  third degree T23.379 ☑
Burnett's syndrome E83.52
Burning
  feet syndrome E53.9
  sensation R20.8
  tongue K14.6
Burn-out (state) Z73.0
Burns' disease or osteochondrosis — *see* Osteochondrosis, juvenile, ulna
Bursa — *see* condition
Bursitis M71.9
  Achilles — *see* Tendinitis, Achilles
  adhesive — *see* Bursitis, specified NEC
  ankle — *see* Enthesopathy, ankle and tarsus
  calcaneal — *see* Enthesopathy, foot, specified type NEC
  collateral ligament, tibial — *see* Bursitis, tibial collateral
  due to use, overuse, pressure — *see also* Disorder, soft tissue, due to use, specified type NEC
    specified NEC — *see* Disorder, soft tissue, due to use, specified NEC
  Duplay's M75.0 ☑
  elbow NEC M70.3- ☑
    olecranon M70.2- ☑
  finger — *see* Disorder, soft tissue, due to use, specified type NEC, hand
  foot — *see* Enthesopathy, foot, specified type NEC
  gonococcal A54.49
  gouty — *see* Gout
  hand M70.1- ☑
  hip NEC M70.7- ☑
    trochanteric M70.6- ☑
  infective NEC M71.10
    abscess — *see* Abscess, bursa
    ankle M71.17- ☑
    elbow M71.12- ☑
    foot M71.17- ☑
    hand M71.14- ☑
    hip M71.15- ☑
    knee M71.16- ☑
    multiple sites M71.19
    shoulder M71.11- ☑
    specified site NEC M71.18
    wrist M71.13- ☑
  ischial — *see* Bursitis, hip
  knee NEC M70.5- ☑
    prepatellar M70.4- ☑
  occupational NEC — *see also* Disorder, soft tissue, due to, use
  olecranon — *see* Bursitis, elbow, olecranon
  pharyngeal J39.1
  popliteal — *see* Bursitis, knee
  prepatellar M70.4- ☑
  radiohumeral M70.3- ☑
  rheumatoid M06.20
    ankle M06.27- ☑
    elbow M06.22- ☑
    foot joint M06.27- ☑
    hand joint M06.24- ☑
    hip M06.25- ☑

Bursitis — *continued*
  rheumatoid — *continued*
    knee M06.26- ☑
    multiple site M06.29
    shoulder M06.21- ☑
    vertebra M06.28
    wrist M06.23- ☑
  scapulohumeral — *see* Bursitis, shoulder
  semimembranous muscle (knee) — *see* Bursitis, knee
  shoulder M75.5- ☑
    adhesive — *see* Capsulitis, adhesive
  specified NEC M71.50
    ankle M71.57- ☑
    due to use, overuse or pressure — *see* Disorder, soft
      tissue, due to, use
    elbow M71.52- ☑
    foot M71.57- ☑
    hand M71.54- ☑
    hip M71.55- ☑
    knee M71.56- ☑
    shoulder — *see* Bursitis, shoulder
    specified site NEC M71.58
    tibial collateral M76.4- ☑
    wrist M71.53- ☑
  subacromial — *see* Bursitis, shoulder
  subcoracoid — *see* Bursitis, shoulder
  subdeltoid — *see* Bursitis, shoulder
  syphilitic A52.78
  Thornwaldt, Tornwaldt J39.2
  tibial collateral M76.4- ☑
  toe — *see* Enthesopathy, foot, specified type NEC
  trochanteric (area) — *see* Bursitis, hip, trochanteric
  wrist — *see* Bursitis, hand
Bursopathy M71.9
  specified type NEC M71.80
    ankle M71.87- ☑
    elbow M71.82- ☑
    foot M71.87- ☑
    hand M71.84- ☑
    hip M71.85- ☑
    knee M71.86- ☑
    multiple sites M71.89
    shoulder M71.81- ☑
    specified site NEC M71.88
    wrist M71.83- ☑
Burst stitches or sutures (complication of surgery)
  T81.31 ☑
  external operation wound T81.31 ☑
  internal operation wound — *see also* Dehiscence, closure
    T81.328 ☑
    abdominal wall muscle or fascia T81.321 ☑
    specified NEC T81.328 ☑
Buruli ulcer A31.1
Bury's disease L95.1
Buschke's
  disease — *see* Cryptococcosis by site
  scleredema — *see* Sclerosis, systemic
Busse-Buschke disease — *see* Cryptococcosis by site
Buttock — *see* condition
Button
  Biskra B55.1
  Delhi B55.1
  oriental B55.1
Buttonhole deformity (finger) — *see* Deformity, finger,
  boutonniere
Bwamba fever A92.8
Byssinosis J66.0
Bywaters' syndrome T79.5 ☑

C

Cachexia R64
  cancerous R64
  cardiac — *see* Disease, heart
  dehydration E86.0
  due to
    malnutrition — *see also* Malnutrition, severe E88.A
    underlying condition E88.A
  exophthalmic — *see* Hyperthyroidism
  heart — *see* Disease, heart
  hypophyseal E23.0
  hypopituitary E23.0
  lead — *see* Poisoning, lead
  malignant R64
  marsh — *see* Malaria
  nervous F48.8
  old age R54

Cachexia — *continued*
  paludal — *see* Malaria
  pituitary E23.0
  pulmonary R64
  renal N28.9
  saturnine — *see* Poisoning, lead
  senile R54
  Simmonds' E23.0
  splenica D73.0
  strumipriva E03.4
  tuberculous NEC — *see* Tuberculosis
CADASIL (cerebral autosomal dominant arteriopathy with
  subcortical infarcts and leukoencephalopathy) I67.850
Cafe, au lait spots L81.3
Caffeine-induced
  anxiety disorder F15.980
  sleep disorder F15.982
Caffey's syndrome Q78.8
Caisson disease T70.3 ☑
Cake kidney Q63.1
Caked breast (puerperal, postpartum) O92.79
Calabar swelling B74.3
Calcaneal spur — *see* Spur, bone, calcaneal
Calcaneo-apophysitis M92.6 ☑
Calcareous — *see* condition
Calcicosis J62.8
Calciferol (vitamin D) **deficiency** E55.9
  with rickets E55.0
Calcification
  adrenal (capsule) (gland) E27.49
    tuberculous B90.8 *[E35]*
  aorta I70.0
  artery (annular) — *see* Arteriosclerosis
  auricle (ear) — *see* Disorder, pinna, specified type NEC
  basal ganglia G23.8
  bladder N32.89
    due to Schistosoma hematobium B65.0
  brain (cortex) — *see* Calcification, cerebral
  bronchus J98.09
  bursa M71.40
    ankle M71.47- ☑
    elbow M71.42- ☑
    foot M71.47- ☑
    hand M71.44- ☑
    hip M71.45- ☑
    knee M71.46- ☑
    multiple sites M71.49
    shoulder M75.3- ☑
    specified site NEC M71.48
    wrist M71.43- ☑
  cardiac — *see* Degeneration, myocardial
  cerebral (cortex) G93.89
    artery I67.2
  cervix (uteri) N88.8
  choroid plexus G93.89
  conjunctiva — *see* Concretion, conjunctiva
  corpora cavernosa (penis) N48.89
  cortex (brain) — *see* Calcification, cerebral
  dental pulp (nodular) K04.2
  dentinal papilla K00.4
  fallopian tube N83.8
  falx cerebri G96.198
  gallbladder K82.8
  general E83.59
  heart — *see also* Degeneration, myocardial
    valve — *see also* Endocarditis
      mitral — *see* Calcification, mitral
  idiopathic infantile arterial (IIAC) Q28.8
  intervertebral cartilage or disc (postinfective) — *see*
    Disorder, disc, specified NEC
  intracranial — *see* Calcification, cerebral
  joint — *see* Disorder, joint, specified type NEC
  kidney N28.89
    tuberculous N29 *[B90.1]*
  larynx (senile) J38.7
  lens — *see* Cataract, specified NEC
  lung (active) (postinfectional) J98.4
    tuberculous B90.9
  lymph gland or node (postinfectional) I89.8
    tuberculous — *see also* Tuberculosis, lymph gland
      B90.8
  mammographic R92.1
  massive (paraplegic) — *see* Myositis, ossificans, in,
    quadriplegia
  medial — *see* Arteriosclerosis, extremities
  meninges (cerebral) (spinal) G96.198
  metastatic E83.59

Calcification — *continued*
  mitral (valve)
    annular I34.81
      nonrheumatic I34.81
      rheumatic I05.8
    annulus I34.81
      nonrheumatic I34.81
      rheumatic I05.8
  Monckeberg's — *see* Arteriosclerosis, extremities
  muscle M61.9
    due to burns — *see* Myositis, ossificans, in, burns
    paralytic — *see* Myositis, ossificans, in, quadriplegia
    specified type NEC M61.40
      ankle M61.47- ☑
      foot M61.47- ☑
      forearm M61.43- ☑
      hand M61.44- ☑
      lower leg M61.46- ☑
      multiple sites M61.49
      pelvic region M61.45- ☑
      shoulder region M61.41- ☑
      specified site NEC M61.48
      thigh M61.45- ☑
      upper arm M61.42- ☑
  myocardium, myocardial — *see* Degeneration, myocar-
    dial
  ovary N83.8
  pancreas K86.89
  penis N48.89
  periarticular — *see* Disorder, joint, specified type NEC
  pericardium — *see also* Pericarditis I31.1
  pineal gland E34.8
  pleura J94.8
    postinfectional J94.8
    tuberculous NEC B90.9
  pulpal (dental) (nodular) K04.2
  sclera H15.89
  spleen D73.89
  subcutaneous L94.2
  suprarenal (capsule) (gland) E27.49
  tendon (sheath) — *see also* Tenosynovitis, specified type
    NEC
    with bursitis, synovitis or tenosynovitis — *see* Tendini-
      tis, calcific
  trachea J39.8
  ureter N28.89
  uterus N85.8
  vitreous — *see* Deposit, crystalline
Calcified — *see* Calcification
Calcinosis (interstitial) (tumoral) (universalis) E83.59
  with Raynaud's phenomenon, esophageal dysfunction,
    sclerodactyly, telangiectasia (CREST syndrome)
    M34.1
  circumscripta (skin) L94.2
  cutis L94.2
Calciphylaxis — *see also* Calcification, by site E83.59
Calcium
  deposits — *see* Calcification, by site
  metabolism disorder E83.50
  salts or soaps in vitreous — *see* Deposit, crystalline
Calciuria R82.994
Calculi — *see* Calculus
Calculosis, intrahepatic — *see* Calculus, bile duct
Calculus, calculi, calculous
  ampulla of Vater — *see* Calculus, bile duct
  anuria (impacted) (recurrent) — *see also* Calculus, urinary
    N20.9
  appendix K38.1
  bile duct (common) (hepatic) K80.50
    with
      calculus of gallbladder — *see* Calculus, gallbladder
        and bile duct
      cholangitis K80.30
        with
          cholecystitis — *see* Calculus, bile duct, with
            cholecystitis
          obstruction K80.31
        acute K80.32
          with
            chronic cholangitis K80.36
              with obstruction K80.37
            obstruction K80.33
        chronic K80.34
          with
            acute cholangitis K80.36
              with obstruction K80.37
            obstruction K80.35
      cholecystitis (with cholangitis) K80.40

Calculus, calculi, calculous — *continued*
  bile duct — *continued*
    with — *continued*
      cholecystitis — *continued*
        with obstruction K80.41
        acute K80.42
          with
            chronic cholecystitis K80.46
              with obstruction K80.47
            obstruction K80.43
        chronic K80.44
          with
            acute cholecystitis K80.46
              with obstruction K80.47
            obstruction K80.45
  biliary — *see also* Calculus, gallbladder
    with bile duct involvement — *see also* Calculus, bile duct
    specified NEC K80.80
      with obstruction K80.81
  bilirubin, multiple — *see* Calculus, gallbladder
  bladder (encysted) (impacted) (urinary) (diverticulum) N21.0
  bronchus J98.09
  calyx (kidney) (renal) — *see* Calculus, kidney
  cholesterol (pure) (solitary) — *see* Calculus, gallbladder
  common duct (bile) — *see* Calculus, bile duct
  conjunctiva — *see* Concretion, conjunctiva
  cystic N21.0
    duct — *see* Calculus, gallbladder
  dental (subgingival) (supragingival) K03.6
  diverticulum
    bladder N21.0
    kidney N20.0
  epididymis N50.89
  gallbladder K80.20
    with
      bile duct calculus — *see* Calculus, gallbladder and bile duct
      cholecystitis K80.10
        with obstruction K80.11
        acute K80.00
          with
            chronic cholecystitis K80.12
              with obstruction K80.13
            obstruction K80.01
        chronic K80.10
          with
            acute cholecystitis K80.12
              with obstruction K80.13
            obstruction K80.11
      specified NEC K80.18
        with obstruction K80.19
      obstruction K80.21
  gallbladder and bile duct K80.70
    with
      cholecystitis K80.60
        with obstruction K80.61
        acute K80.62
          with
            chronic cholecystitis K80.66
              with obstruction K80.67
            obstruction K80.63
        chronic K80.64
          with
            acute cholecystitis K80.66
              with obstruction K80.67
            obstruction K80.65
      obstruction K80.71
  hepatic (duct) — *see* Calculus, bile duct
  ileal conduit N21.8
  intestinal (impaction) (obstruction) K56.49
  kidney (impacted) (multiple) (pelvis) (recurrent) (staghorn) N20.0
    with calculus, ureter N20.2
      with hydronephrosis N13.2
        with infection N13.6
    congenital Q63.8
      with hydronephrosis N13.2
        with infection N13.6
  lacrimal passages — *see* Dacryolith
  liver (impacted) — *see* Calculus, bile duct
  lung J98.4
  mammographic R92.1
  nephritic (impacted) (recurrent) — *see* Calculus, kidney
  nose J34.89
  pancreas (duct) K86.89
  parotid duct or gland K11.5
  pelvis, encysted — *see* Calculus, kidney

Calculus, calculi, calculous — *continued*
  prostate N42.0
  pulmonary J98.4
  pyelitis (impacted) (recurrent) N20.0
    with hydronephrosis N13.6
  pyelonephritis (impacted) (recurrent) — *see* category N20 ☑
    with hydronephrosis N13.6
  renal (impacted) (recurrent) — *see* Calculus, kidney
  salivary (duct) (gland) K11.5
  seminal vesicle N50.89
  staghorn — *see* Calculus, kidney
  Stensen's duct K11.5
  stomach K31.89
  sublingual duct or gland K11.5
    congenital Q38.4
  submandibular duct, gland or region K11.5
  submaxillary duct, gland or region K11.5
  suburethral N21.8
  tonsil J35.8
  tooth, teeth (subgingival) (supragingival) K03.6
  tunica vaginalis N50.89
  ureter (impacted) (recurrent) N20.1
    with calculus, kidney N20.2
      with hydronephrosis N13.2
        with infection N13.6
    with hydronephrosis N13.2
      with infection N13.6
  ureteropelvic junction N20.1
  urethra (impacted) N21.1
  urinary (duct) (impacted) (passage) (tract) N20.9
    with hydronephrosis N13.2
      with infection N13.6
    in (due to)
    lower N21.9
      specified NEC N21.8
  vagina N89.8
  vesical (impacted) N21.0
  Wharton's duct K11.5
  xanthine E79.82 *[N22]*

Calicectasis N28.89
Caliectasis N28.89
California
  disease B38.9
  encephalitis A83.5
Caligo cornea — *see* Opacity, cornea, central
Callositas, callosity (infected) L84
Callus (infected) L84
  bone — *see* Osteophyte
    excessive, following fracture — *code as* Sequelae of fracture
CALME (childhood asymmetric labium majus enlargement) N90.61
Calorie deficiency or malnutrition — *see also* Malnutrition E46
Calpainopathy (primary) G71.032
  autosomal dominant G71.031
  autosomal recessive G71.032
Calve-Perthes disease — *see* Legg-Calve-Perthes disease
Calve's disease — *see* Osteochondrosis, juvenile, spine
Calvities — *see* Alopecia, androgenic
Cameroon fever — *see* Malaria
Camptocormia (hysterical) F44.4
Camurati-Engelmann syndrome Q78.3
Canal — *see also* condition
  atrioventricular Q21.20
    common Q21.23
    incomplete Q21.21
    intermediate Q21.22
    partial Q21.21
    transitional Q21.22
Canaliculitis (lacrimal) (acute) (subacute) H04.33- ☑
  Actinomyces A42.89
  chronic H04.42- ☑
Canavan disease E75.28
Canceled procedure (surgical) Z53.9
  because of
    contraindication Z53.09
      smoking Z53.01
    left against medical advice (AMA) Z53.29
    patient's decision Z53.20
      for reasons of belief or group pressure Z53.1
      specified reason NEC Z53.29
    specified reason NEC Z53.8
Cancer — *see also* Neoplasm, by site, malignant
  bile duct type liver C22.1
  blood — *see* Leukemia
  breast — *see also* Neoplasm, breast, malignant C50.91- ☑

Cancer — *continued*
  hepatocellular C22.0
  lung — *see also* Neoplasm, lung, malignant C34.90
  ovarian — *see also* Neoplasm ovary, malignant C56.9
  unspecified site (primary) C80.1
Cancer (o) **phobia** F45.29
Cancerous — *see* Neoplasm, malignant, by site
Cancrum oris A69.0
Candidiasis, candidal B37.9
  balanitis B37.42
  bronchitis B37.1
  cheilitis B37.83
  congenital P37.5
  cystitis B37.41
  disseminated B37.7
  endocarditis B37.6
  enteritis B37.82
  esophagitis B37.81
  intertrigo B37.2
  lung B37.1
  meningitis B37.5
  mouth B37.0
  nails B37.2
  neonatal P37.5
  onychia B37.2
  oral B37.0
  osteomyelitis B37.89
  otitis externa B37.84
  paronychia B37.2
  perionyxis B37.2
  pneumonia B37.1
  proctitis B37.82
  pulmonary B37.1
  pyelonephritis B37.49
  sepsis B37.7
  skin B37.2
  specified site NEC B37.89
  stomatitis B37.0
  systemic B37.7
  urethritis B37.41
  urogenital site NEC B37.49
  vagina (acute) B37.31
    chronic (recurrent) B37.32
  vulva (acute) B37.31
    chronic (recurrent) B37.32
  vulvovaginitis (acute) B37.31
    chronic (recurrent) B37.32
Candidid L30.2
Candidosis — *see* Candidiasis
Candiru infection or infestation B88.8
Canities (premature) L67.1
  congenital Q84.2
Canker (mouth) (sore) K12.0
  rash A38.9
Cannabinosis J66.2
Cannabis induced
  anxiety disorder F12.980
  psychotic disorder F12.959
  sleep disorder F12.988
Canton fever A75.9
Cantrell's syndrome Q87.89
Capillariasis (intestinal) B81.1
  hepatic B83.8
Capillary — *see* condition
Caplan's syndrome — *see* Rheumatoid, lung
Capsule — *see* condition
Capsulitis (joint) — *see also* Enthesopathy
  adhesive (shoulder) M75.0- ☑
  hepatic K65.8
  labyrinthine — *see* Otosclerosis, specified NEC
  thyroid E06.9
Caput
  crepitus Q75.8
  medusae I86.8
  succedaneum P12.81
Car sickness T75.3 ☑
Carapata (disease) A68.0
Carate — *see* Pinta
Carbon lung J60
Carbuncle L02.93
  abdominal wall L02.231
  anus K61.0
  auditory canal, external — *see* Abscess, ear, external
  auricle ear — *see* Abscess, ear, external
  axilla L02.43- ☑
  back (any part) L02.232
  breast N61.1
  buttock L02.33
  cheek (external) L02.03

Carbuncle — *continued*
chest wall L02.233
chin L02.03
corpus cavernosum N48.21
ear (any part) (external) (middle) — *see* Abscess, ear, external
external auditory canal — *see* Abscess, ear, external
eyelid — *see* Abscess, eyelid
face NEC L02.03
femoral (region) — *see* Carbuncle, lower limb
finger — *see* Carbuncle, hand
flank L02.231
foot L02.63- ☑
forehead L02.03
genital — *see* Abscess, genital
gluteal (region) L02.33
groin L02.234
hand L02.53- ☑
head NEC L02.831
heel — *see* Carbuncle, foot
hip — *see* Carbuncle, lower limb
kidney — *see* Abscess, kidney
knee — *see* Carbuncle, lower limb
labium (majus) (minus) N76.4
lacrimal
   gland — *see* Dacryoadenitis
   passages (duct) (sac) — *see* Inflammation, lacrimal, passages, acute
leg — *see* Carbuncle, lower limb
lower limb L02.43- ☑
malignant A22.0
navel L02.236
neck L02.13
nose (external) (septum) J34.0
orbit, orbital — *see* Abscess, orbit
palmar (space) — *see* Carbuncle, hand
partes posteriores L02.33
pectoral region L02.233
penis N48.21
perineum L02.235
pinna — *see* Abscess, ear, external
popliteal — *see* Carbuncle, lower limb
scalp L02.831
seminal vesicle N49.0
shoulder — *see* Carbuncle, upper limb
specified site NEC L02.838
temple (region) L02.03
thumb — *see* Carbuncle, hand
toe — *see* Carbuncle, foot
trunk L02.239
   abdominal wall L02.231
   back L02.232
   chest wall L02.233
   groin L02.234
   perineum L02.235
   umbilicus L02.236
umbilicus L02.236
upper limb L02.43- ☑
urethra N34.0
vulva N76.4
Carbunculus — *see* Carbuncle
Carcinoid (tumor) — *see* Tumor, carcinoid
Carcinoidosis E34.00
heart E34.01
Carcinoma (malignant) — *see also* Neoplasm, by site, malignant
acidophil
   specified site — *see* Neoplasm, malignant, by site
   unspecified site C75.1
acidophil-basophil, mixed
   specified site — *see* Neoplasm, malignant, by site
   unspecified site C75.1
adnexal (skin) — *see* Neoplasm, skin, malignant
adrenal cortical C74.0- ☑
alveolar — *see* Neoplasm, lung, malignant
   cell — *see* Neoplasm, lung, malignant
ameloblastic C41.1
   upper jaw (bone) C41.0
apocrine
   breast — *see* Neoplasm, breast, malignant
   specified site NEC — *see* Neoplasm, skin, malignant
   unspecified site C44.99
basal cell (pigmented) (*see also* Neoplasm, skin, malignant) C44.91
   fibro-epithelial — *see* Neoplasm, skin, malignant
   morphea — *see* Neoplasm, skin, malignant
   multicentric — *see* Neoplasm, skin, malignant

Carcinoma — *continued*
basaloid
basal-squamous cell, mixed — *see* Neoplasm, skin, malignant
basophil
   specified site — *see* Neoplasm, malignant, by site
   unspecified site C75.1
basophil-acidophil, mixed
   specified site — *see* Neoplasm, malignant, by site
   unspecified site C75.1
basosquamous — *see* Neoplasm, skin, malignant
bile duct
   with hepatocellular, mixed C22.0
   liver C22.1
   specified site NEC — *see* Neoplasm, malignant, by site
   unspecified site C22.1
branchial or branchiogenic C10.4
bronchial or bronchogenic — *see* Neoplasm, lung, malignant
bronchiolar — *see* Neoplasm, lung, malignant
bronchioloalveolar — *see* Neoplasm, lung, malignant
C cell
   specified site — *see* Neoplasm, malignant, by site
   unspecified site C73
ceruminous C44.29- ☑
cervix uteri
   in situ D06.9
      endocervix D06.0
      exocervix D06.1
      specified site NEC D06.7
chorionic
   specified site — *see* Neoplasm, malignant, by site
   unspecified site
      female C58
      male C62.90
chromophobe
   specified site — *see* Neoplasm, malignant, by site
   unspecified site C75.1
cloacogenic
   specified site — *see* Neoplasm, malignant, by site
   unspecified site C21.2
diffuse type
   specified site — *see* Neoplasm, malignant, by site
   unspecified site C16.9
duct (cell)
   with Paget's disease — *see* Neoplasm, breast, malignant
   infiltrating
      with lobular carcinoma (in situ)
         specified site — *see* Neoplasm, malignant, by site
         unspecified site (female) C50.91- ☑
            male C50.92- ☑
      specified site — *see* Neoplasm, malignant, by site
      unspecified site (female) C50.91- ☑
         male C50.92- ☑
ductal
   with lobular
      specified site — *see* Neoplasm, malignant, by site
      unspecified site (female) C50.91- ☑
         male C50.92- ☑
ductular, infiltrating
   specified site — *see* Neoplasm, malignant, by site
   unspecified site (female) C50.91- ☑
      male C50.92- ☑
embryonal
   liver C22.7
endometrioid
   specified site — *see* Neoplasm, malignant, by site
   unspecified site
      female C56.9
      male C61
eosinophil
   specified site — *see* Neoplasm, malignant, by site
   unspecified site C75.1
epidermoid — *see also* Neoplasm, skin, malignant
   in situ, Bowen's type — *see* Neoplasm, skin, in situ
fibroepithelial, basal cell — *see* Neoplasm, skin, malignant
follicular
   with papillary (mixed) C73
   moderately differentiated C73
   pure follicle C73
   specified site — *see* Neoplasm, malignant, by site
   trabecular C73
   unspecified site C73
   well differentiated C73

Carcinoma — *continued*
generalized, with unspecified primary site C80.0
glycogen-rich — *see* Neoplasm, breast, malignant
granulosa cell C56- ☑
hepatic cell C22.0
hepatocellular C22.0
   with bile duct, mixed C22.0
   fibrolamellar C22.0
hepatocholangiolitic C22.0
Hurthle cell C73
in
   adenomatous
      polyposis coli C18.9
   pleomorphic adenoma — *see* Neoplasm, salivary gland or duct, malignant
   situ — *see* Carcinoma-in-situ
infiltrating
   duct
      with lobular
         specified site — *see* Neoplasm, malignant, by site
         unspecified site (female) C50.91- ☑
            male C50.92- ☑
      with Paget's disease — *see* Neoplasm, breast, malignant
      specified site — *see* Neoplasm, malignant
      unspecified site (female) C50.91- ☑
         male C50.92- ☑
   ductular
      specified site — *see* Neoplasm, malignant
      unspecified site (female) C50.91- ☑
         male C50.92- ☑
   lobular
      specified site — *see* Neoplasm, malignant
      unspecified site (female) C50.91- ☑
         male C50.92- ☑
inflammatory
   specified site — *see* Neoplasm, malignant
   unspecified site (female) C50.91- ☑
      male C50.92- ☑
intestinal type
   specified site — *see* Neoplasm, malignant, by site
   unspecified site C16.9
intracystic
   noninfiltrating — *see* Neoplasm, in situ, by site
intraductal (noninfiltrating)
   with Paget's disease — *see* Neoplasm, breast, malignant
   breast D05.1- ☑
   papillary
      with invasion
         specified site — *see* Neoplasm, malignant, by site
         unspecified site (female) C50.91- ☑
            male C50.92- ☑
      breast D05.1- ☑
      specified site NEC — *see* Neoplasm, in situ, by site
      unspecified site (female) D05.1- ☑
   specified site NEC — *see* Neoplasm, in situ, by site
   unspecified site (female) D05.1- ☑
intraepidermal — *see* Neoplasm, in situ
   squamous cell, Bowen's type — *see* Neoplasm, skin, in situ
intraepithelial — *see* Neoplasm, in situ, by site
   squamous cell — *see* Neoplasm, in situ, by site
intraosseous C41.1
   upper jaw (bone) C41.0
islet cell
   with exocrine, mixed
      specified site — *see* Neoplasm, malignant, by site
      unspecified site C25.9
   pancreas C25.4
   specified site NEC — *see* Neoplasm, malignant, by site
   unspecified site C25.4
juvenile, breast — *see* Neoplasm, breast, malignant
large cell
   small cell
      specified site — *see* Neoplasm, malignant, by site
      unspecified site C34.90
Leydig cell (testis)
   specified site — *see* Neoplasm, malignant, by site
   unspecified site
      female C56.9
      male C62.90
lipid-rich (female) C50.91- ☑
   male C50.92- ☑
liver cell C22.0

Carcinoma — *continued*
  liver NEC C22.7
  lobular (infiltrating)
    with intraductal
      specified site — *see* Neoplasm, malignant, by site
      unspecified site (female) C50.91- ☑
        male C50.92- ☑
    noninfiltrating
      breast D05.0- ☑
      specified site NEC — *see* Neoplasm, in situ, by site
      unspecified site D05.0- ☑
    specified site — *see* Neoplasm, malignant, by site
    unspecified site (female) C50.91- ☑
      male C50.92- ☑
  medullary
    with
      amyloid stroma
        specified site — *see* Neoplasm, malignant, by site
        unspecified site C73
      lymphoid stroma
        specified site — *see* Neoplasm, malignant, by site
        unspecified site (female) C50.91- ☑
          male C50.92- ☑
  Merkel cell C4A.9 *(following* C43)
    anal margin C4A.51 *(following* C43)
    anal skin C4A.51 *(following* C43)
    canthus C4A.1- ☑ *(following* C43)
    ear and external auricular canal C4A.2- ☑ *(following* C43)
    external auricular canal C4A.2- ☑ *(following* C43)
    eyelid, including canthus C4A.1- ☑ *(following* C43)
    face C4A.30 *(following* C43)
      specified NEC C4A.39 *(following* C43)
    hip C4A.7- ☑ *(following* C43)
    lip C4A.0 *(following* C43)
    lower limb, including hip C4A.7- ☑ *(following* C43)
    neck C4A.4 *(following* C43)
    nodal presentation C7B.1 *(following* C75)
    nose C4A.31 *(following* C43)
    overlapping sites C4A.8 *(following* C43)
    perianal skin C4A.51 *(following* C43)
    scalp C4A.4 *(following* C43)
    secondary C7B.1 *(following* C75)
    shoulder C4A.6- ☑ *(following* C43)
    skin of breast C4A.52 *(following* C43)
    trunk NEC C4A.59 *(following* C43)
    upper limb, including shoulder C4A.6- ☑ *(following* C43)
    visceral metastatic C7B.1 *(following* C75)
  metastatic — *see* Neoplasm, secondary, by site
  metatypical — *see* Neoplasm, skin, malignant
  morphea, basal cell — *see* Neoplasm, skin, malignant
  mucoid
    cell
      specified site — *see* Neoplasm, malignant, by site
      unspecified site C75.1
  neuroendocrine — *see also* Tumor, neuroendocrine
    high grade, any site C7A.1 *(following* C75)
    poorly differentiated, any site C7A.1 *(following* C75)
  nonencapsulated sclerosing C73
  noninfiltrating
    intracystic — *see* Neoplasm, in situ, by site
    intraductal
      breast D05.1- ☑
      papillary
        breast D05.1- ☑
        specified site NEC — *see* Neoplasm, in situ, by site
        unspecified site D05.1- ☑
      specified site — *see* Neoplasm, in situ, by site
      unspecified site D05.1- ☑
    lobular
      breast D05.0- ☑
      specified site NEC — *see* Neoplasm, in situ, by site
      unspecified site (female) D05.0- ☑
  oat cell
    specified site — *see* Neoplasm, malignant, by site
    unspecified site C34.90
  odontogenic C41.1
    upper jaw (bone) C41.0
  papillary
    with follicular (mixed) C73
      follicular variant C73

Carcinoma — *continued*
  papillary — *continued*
    intraductal (noninfiltrating)
      with invasion
        specified site — *see* Neoplasm, malignant, by site
        unspecified site (female) C50.91- ☑
          male C50.92- ☑
      breast D05.1- ☑
      specified site NEC — *see* Neoplasm, in situ, by site
      unspecified site D05.1- ☑
    serous
      specified site — *see* Neoplasm, malignant, by site
      surface
        specified site — *see* Neoplasm, malignant, by site
        unspecified site C56.9
      unspecified site C56.9
  papillocystic
    specified site — *see* Neoplasm, malignant, by site
    unspecified site C56.9
  parafollicular cell
    specified site — *see* Neoplasm, malignant, by site
    unspecified site C73
  pilomatrix — *see* Neoplasm, skin, malignant
  pseudomucinous
    specified site — *see* Neoplasm, malignant, by site
    unspecified site C56.9
  renal cell C64- ☑
  Schmincke — *see* Neoplasm, nasopharynx, malignant
  Schneiderian
    specified site — *see* Neoplasm, malignant, by site
    unspecified site C30.0
  sebaceous — *see* Neoplasm, skin, malignant
  secondary — *see also* Neoplasm, secondary, by site
    Merkel cell C7B.1 *(following* C75)
  secretory, breast — *see* Neoplasm, breast, malignant
  serous
    papillary
      specified site — *see* Neoplasm, malignant, by site
      unspecified site C56.9
    surface, papillary
      specified site — *see* Neoplasm, malignant, by site
      unspecified site C56.9
  Sertoli cell
    specified site — *see* Neoplasm, malignant, by site
    unspecified site C62.90
      female C56.9
      male C62.90
  skin appendage — *see* Neoplasm, skin, malignant
  small cell
    fusiform cell
      specified site — *see* Neoplasm, malignant, by site
      unspecified site C34.90
    intermediate cell
      specified site — *see* Neoplasm, malignant, by site
      unspecified site C34.90
    large cell
      specified site — *see* Neoplasm, malignant, by site
      unspecified site C34.90
  solid
    with amyloid stroma
      specified site — *see* Neoplasm, malignant, by site
      unspecified site C73
    microinvasive
      specified site — *see* Neoplasm, malignant, by site
      unspecified site C53.9
  sweat gland — *see* Neoplasm, skin, malignant
  theca cell C56.- ☑
  thymic C37
  unspecified site (primary) C80.1
  water-clear cell C75.0
Carcinoma-in-situ — *see also* Neoplasm, in situ, by site
  breast NOS D05.9- ☑
    specified type NEC D05.8- ☑
  epidermoid — *see also* Neoplasm, in situ, by site
    with questionable stromal invasion
      cervix D06.9
      specified site NEC — *see* Neoplasm, in situ, by site
      unspecified site D06.9
    Bowen's type — *see* Neoplasm, skin, in situ
  intraductal
    breast D05.1- ☑
    specified site NEC — *see* Neoplasm, in situ, by site
    unspecified site D05.1- ☑

Carcinoma-in-situ — *continued*
  lobular
    with
      infiltrating duct
        breast (female) C50.91- ☑
          male C50.92- ☑
        specified site NEC — *see* Neoplasm, malignant
        unspecified site (female) C50.91- ☑
          male C50.92- ☑
      intraductal
        breast D05.8- ☑
        specified site NEC — *see* Neoplasm, in situ, by site
        unspecified site (female) D05.8- ☑
    breast D05.0- ☑
    specified site NEC — *see* Neoplasm, in situ, by site
    unspecified site D05.0- ☑
  squamous cell — *see also* Neoplasm, in situ, by site
    with questionable stromal invasion
      cervix D06.9
      specified site NEC — *see* Neoplasm, in situ, by site
      unspecified site D06.9
Carcinomaphobia F45.29
Carcinomatosis C80.0
  peritonei C78.6
  unspecified site (primary) (secondary) C80.0
Carcinosarcoma — *see* Neoplasm, malignant, by site
  embryonal — *see* Neoplasm, malignant, by site
Cardia, cardial — *see* condition
Cardiac — *see also* condition
  death, sudden — *see* Arrest, cardiac
  pacemaker
    in situ Z95.0
    management or adjustment Z45.018
  tamponade I31.4
Cardialgia — *see* Pain, precordial
Cardiectasis — *see* Hypertrophy, cardiac
Cardiochalasia K21.9
Cardiomalacia I51.5
Cardiomegalia glycogenica diffusa E74.02 *[I43]*
Cardiomegaly — *see also* Hypertrophy, cardiac
  congenital Q24.8
  glycogen E74.02 *[I43]*
  idiopathic I51.7
Cardiomyoliposis I51.5
Cardiomyopathy (familial) (idiopathic) I42.9
  alcoholic I42.6
  amyloid E85.4 *[I43]*
    transthyretin-related (ATTR) familial E85.4 *[I43]*
  arteriosclerotic — *see* Disease, heart, ischemic, atherosclerotic
  beriberi E51.12
  cobalt-beer I42.6
  congenital I42.4
  congestive I42.0
  constrictive NOS I42.5
  dilated I42.0
  due to
    alcohol I42.6
    beriberi E51.12
    cardiac glycogenosis E74.02 *[I43]*
    drugs I42.7
    external agents NEC I42.7
    Friedreich's ataxia G11.11
    myotonia atrophica G71.11 *[I43]*
    progressive muscular dystrophy — *see also* Dystrophy, muscular, by type G71.09 *[I43]*
  glycogen storage E74.02 *[I43]*
  hypertensive — *see* Hypertension, heart
  hypertrophic (nonobstructive) I42.2
    obstructive I42.1
      congenital Q24.8
  in
    Chagas' disease (chronic) B57.2
      acute B57.0
    sarcoidosis D86.85
  ischemic I25.5
  metabolic E88.9 *[I43]*
    thyrotoxic E05.90 *[I43]*
      with thyroid storm E05.91 *[I43]*
  newborn I42.8
    congenital I42.4
  non-ischemic — *see also* by cause I42.8
  nutritional E63.9 *[I43]*
    beriberi E51.12
  obscure of Africa I42.8
  peripartum O90.3
  postpartum O90.3

Cardiomyopathy — *continued*
  restrictive NEC I42.5
  rheumatic I09.0
  secondary I42.9
  specified NEC I42.8
  stress induced I51.81
  takotsubo I51.81
  thyrotoxic E05.90 *[I43]*
    with thyroid storm E05.91 *[I43]*
  toxic NEC I42.7
  transthyretin-related (ATTR) familial amyloid E85.4
  tuberculous A18.84
  viral B33.24
Cardionephritis — *see* Hypertension, cardiorenal
Cardionephropathy — *see* Hypertension, cardiorenal
Cardionephrosis — *see* Hypertension, cardiorenal
Cardiopathia nigra I27.0
Cardiopathy — *see also* Disease, heart I51.9
  idiopathic I42.9
  mucopolysaccharidosis E76.3 *[I52]*
Cardiopericarditis — *see* Pericarditis
Cardiophobia F45.29
Cardiorenal — *see* condition
Cardiorrhexis — *see* Infarct, myocardium
Cardiosclerosis — *see* Disease, heart, ischemic,
  atherosclerotic
Cardiosis — *see* Disease, heart
Cardiospasm (esophagus) (reflex) (stomach) K22.0
  congenital Q39.5
    with megaesophagus Q39.5
Cardiostenosis — *see* Disease, heart
Cardiosymphysis I31.0
Cardiovascular — *see* condition
Carditis (acute) (bacterial) (chronic) (subacute) I51.89
  meningococcal A39.50
  rheumatic — *see* Disease, heart, rheumatic
  rheumatoid — *see* Rheumatoid, carditis
  viral B33.20
Care (of) (for) (following)
  child (routine) Z76.2
  family member (handicapped) (sick)
    creating problem for family Z63.6
    provided away from home for holiday relief Z75.5
    unavailable, due to
      absence (person rendering care) (sufferer) Z74.2
      inability (any reason) of person rendering care
        Z74.2
  foundling Z76.1
  holiday relief Z75.5
  improper — *see* Maltreatment
  lack of (at or after birth) (infant) — *see* Maltreatment,
    child, neglect
  lactating mother Z39.1
  palliative Z51.5
  postpartum
    immediately after delivery Z39.0
    routine follow-up Z39.2
  respite Z75.5
  unavailable, due to
    absence of person rendering care Z74.2
    inability (any reason) of person rendering care Z74.2
  well-baby Z76.2
Caries
  bone NEC A18.03
  dental (dentino enamel junction) (early childhood) (of
    dentine) (pre-eruptive) (recurrent) (to the pulp)
    K02.9
    arrested (coronal) (root) K02.3
    chewing surface
      limited to enamel K02.51
      penetrating into dentin K02.52
      penetrating into pulp K02.53
    coronal surface
      chewing surface
        limited to enamel K02.51
        penetrating into dentin K02.52
        penetrating into pulp K02.53
      pit and fissure surface
        limited to enamel K02.51
        penetrating into dentin K02.52
        penetrating into pulp K02.53
      smooth surface
        limited to enamel K02.61
        penetrating into dentin K02.62
        penetrating into pulp K02.63
    pit and fissure surface
      limited to enamel K02.51
      penetrating into dentin K02.52
      penetrating into pulp K02.53

Caries — *continued*
  dental — *continued*
    primary, cervical origin K02.52
    root K02.7
    smooth surface
      limited to enamel K02.61
      penetrating into dentin K02.62
      penetrating into pulp K02.63
  external meatus — *see* Disorder, ear, external, specified
    type NEC
  hip (tuberculous) A18.02
  initial (tooth)
    chewing surface K02.51
    pit and fissure surface K02.51
    smooth surface K02.61
  knee (tuberculous) A18.02
  labyrinth H83.8 ☑
  limb NEC (tuberculous) A18.03
  mastoid process (chronic) — *see* Mastoiditis, chronic
    tuberculous A18.03
  middle ear H74.8 ☑
  nose (tuberculous) A18.03
  orbit (tuberculous) A18.03
  ossicles, ear — *see* Abnormal, ear ossicles
  petrous bone — *see* Petrositis
  root (dental) (tooth) K02.7
  sacrum (tuberculous) A18.01
  spine, spinal (column) (tuberculous) A18.01
  syphilitic A52.77
    congenital (early) A50.02 *[M90.80]*
  tooth, teeth — *see* Caries, dental
  tuberculous A18.03
  vertebra (column) (tuberculous) A18.01
Carious teeth — *see* Caries, dental
Carneous mole O02.0
Carnitine insufficiency E71.40
Carotenemia (dietary) E67.1
Carotenosis (cutis) (skin) E67.1
Carotid body or sinus syndrome G90.01
Carotidynia G90.01
Carpal tunnel syndrome — *see* Syndrome, carpal tunnel
Carpenter's syndrome Q87.0
Carpopedal spasm — *see* Tetany
Carr-Barr-Plunkett syndrome Q97.1
Carrier (suspected) of
  Acinetobacter baumannii Z22.349
    carbapenem-resistant Z22.340
    carbapenem-sensitive Z22.341
  amebiasis Z22.1
  bacterial disease NEC Z22.39
    diphtheria Z22.2
    intestinal infectious NEC Z22.1
      typhoid Z22.0
    meningococcal Z22.31
    sexually transmitted Z22.4
    specified NEC Z22.39
    staphylococcal (Methicillin susceptible) Z22.321
      Methicillin resistant Z22.322
    streptococcal Z22.338
      group B Z22.330
        complicating pregnancy or delivery O99.82- ☑
    typhoid Z22.0
  cholera Z22.1
  diphtheria Z22.2
  E. coli (Escherichia coli) Z22.35- ☑
  Enterobacterales Z22.359
    carbapenem-resistant Z22.350
    carbapenem-sensitive Z22.358
    Enterobacterales, specified type NEC Z22.358
    ESBL-producing Z22.358
    extended-spectrum beta-lactamase producing
      Z22.358
  gastrointestinal pathogens NEC Z22.1
  genetic Z14.8
    cystic fibrosis Z14.1
    hemophilia A (asymptomatic) Z14.01
      symptomatic Z14.02
  gestational, pregnant Z33.1
  gonorrhea Z22.4
  HAA (hepatitis Australian-antigen) B18.8
  HB (c)(s)-AG B18.1
  hepatitis (viral) B18.9
    Australia-antigen (HAA) B18.8
    B surface antigen (HBsAg) B18.1
      with acute delta- (super)infection B17.0
    C B18.2
    specified NEC B18.8
  human T-cell lymphotropic virus type-1 (HTLV-1) infec-
    tion Z22.6

Carrier of — *continued*
  infectious organism Z22.9
    specified NEC Z22.8
  K. pneumoniae (Klebsiella pneumoniae) Z22.35- ☑
  meningococci Z22.31
  Salmonella typhosa Z22.0
  serum hepatitis — *see* Carrier, hepatitis
  staphylococci (Methicillin susceptible) Z22.321
    Methicillin resistant Z22.322
  streptococci Z22.338
    group B Z22.330
      complicating pregnancy or delivery O99.82- ☑
  syphilis Z22.4
  typhoid Z22.0
  venereal disease NEC Z22.4
Carrion's disease A44.0
Carter's relapsing fever (Asiatic) A68.1
Cartilage — *see* condition
Caruncle (inflamed)
  conjunctiva (acute) — *see* Conjunctivitis, acute
  labium (majus) (minus) N90.89
  lacrimal — *see* Inflammation, lacrimal, passages
  myrtiform N89.8
  urethral (benign) N36.2
Cascade stomach K31.2
Caseation lymphatic gland (tuberculous) A18.2
Cassidy (-Scholte) **syndrome** (malignant carcinoid) E34.09
Castellani's disease A69.8
Castration, traumatic, male S38.231 ☑
Casts in urine R82.998
Cat
  cry syndrome Q93.4
  ear Q17.3
  eye syndrome Q92.8
Catabolism, senile R54
Catalepsy (hysterical) F44.2
  schizophrenic F20.2
Cataplexy (idiopathic) — *see* Narcolepsy
Cataract (cortical) (immature) (incipient) H26.9
  with
    neovascularization — *see* Cataract, complicated
  age-related — *see* Cataract, senile
  anterior
    and posterior axial embryonal Q12.0
    pyramidal Q12.0
  associated with
    galactosemia E74.21 *[H28]*
    myotonic disorders G71.19 *[H28]*
  blue Q12.0
  central Q12.0
  cerulean Q12.0
  complicated H26.20
    with
      neovascularization H26.21- ☑
      ocular disorder H26.22- ☑
      glaucomatous flecks H26.23- ☑
  congenital Q12.0
  coraliform Q12.0
  coronary Q12.0
  crystalline Q12.0
  diabetic — *see* Diabetes, cataract
  drug-induced H26.3- ☑
  due to
    ocular disorder — *see* Cataract, complicated
    radiation H26.8
  electric H26.8
  extraction status Z98.4- ☑
  glass-blower's H26.8
  heat ray H26.8
  heterochromic — *see* Cataract, complicated
  hypermature — *see* Cataract, senile, morgagnian type
  in (due to)
    chronic iridocyclitis — *see* Cataract, complicated
    diabetes — *see* Diabetes, cataract
    endocrine disease E34.9 *[H28]*
    eye disease — *see* Cataract, complicated
    hypoparathyroidism E20.9 *[H28]*
    malnutrition-dehydration E46 *[H28]*
    metabolic disease E88.9 *[H28]*
    myotonic disorders G71.19 *[H28]*
    nutritional disease E63.9 *[H28]*
  infantile — *see* Cataract, presenile
  irradiational — *see* Cataract, specified NEC
  juvenile — *see* Cataract, presenile
  malnutrition-dehydration E46 *[H28]*
  morgagnian — *see* Cataract, senile, morgagnian type
  myotonic G71.19 *[H28]*
  myxedema E03.9 *[H28]*

Cataract — continued
- nuclear
  - embryonal Q12.0
  - sclerosis — see Cataract, senile, nuclear
- presenile H26.00- ☑
  - combined forms H26.06- ☑
  - cortical H26.01- ☑
  - lamellar — see Cataract, presenile, cortical
  - nuclear H26.03- ☑
  - specified NEC H26.09
  - subcapsular polar (anterior) H26.04- ☑
    - posterior H26.05- ☑
  - zonular — see Cataract, presenile, cortical
- secondary H26.40
  - Soemmering's ring H26.41- ☑
  - specified NEC H26.49- ☑
  - to eye disease — see Cataract, complicated
- senile H25.9
  - brunescens — see Cataract, senile, nuclear
  - combined forms H25.81- ☑
  - coronary — see Cataract, senile, incipient
  - cortical H25.01- ☑
  - hypermature — see Cataract, senile, morgagnian type
  - incipient (mature) (total) H25.09- ☑
    - cortical — see Cataract, senile, cortical
    - subcapsular — see Cataract, senile, subcapsular
  - morgagnian type (hypermature) H25.2- ☑
  - nuclear (sclerosis) H25.1- ☑
  - polar subcapsular (anterior) (posterior) — see Cataract, senile, incipient
  - punctate — see Cataract, senile, incipient
  - specified NEC H25.89
  - subcapsular polar (anterior) H25.03- ☑
    - posterior H25.04- ☑
- snowflake — see Diabetes, cataract
- specified NEC H26.8
- toxic — see Cataract, drug-induced
- traumatic H26.10- ☑
  - localized H26.11- ☑
  - partially resolved H26.12- ☑
  - total H26.13- ☑
- zonular (perinuclear) Q12.0

Cataracta — see also Cataract
- brunescens — see Cataract, senile, nuclear
- centralis pulverulenta Q12.0
- cerulea Q12.0
- complicata — see Cataract, complicated
- congenita Q12.0
- coralliformis Q12.0
- coronaria Q12.0
- diabetic — see Diabetes, cataract
- membranacea
  - accreta — see Cataract, secondary
  - congenita Q12.0
- nigra — see Cataract, senile, nuclear
- sunflower — see Cataract, complicated

Catarrh, catarrhal (acute) (febrile) (infectious) (inflammation) — see also condition J00
- bronchial — see Bronchitis
- chest — see Bronchitis
- chronic J31.0
- due to congenital syphilis A50.03
- enteric — see Enteritis
- eustachian H68.009
- fauces — see Pharyngitis
- gastrointestinal — see Enteritis
- gingivitis K05.00
  - nonplaque induced K05.01
  - plaque induced K05.00
- hay — see Fever, hay
- intestinal — see Enteritis
- larynx, chronic J37.0
- liver B15.9
  - with hepatic coma B15.0
- lung — see Bronchitis
- middle ear, chronic — see Otitis, media, nonsuppurative, chronic, serous
- mouth K12.1
- nasal (chronic) — see Rhinitis
- nasobronchial J31.1
- nasopharyngeal (chronic) J31.1
  - acute J00
- pulmonary — see Bronchitis
- spring (eye) (vernal) — see Conjunctivitis, acute, atopic
- summer (hay) — see Fever, hay
- throat J31.2
- tubotympanal — see also Otitis, media, nonsuppurative

Catarrh, catarrhal — continued
- tubotympanal — see also Otitis, media, nonsuppurative — continued
  - chronic — see Otitis, media, nonsuppurative, chronic, serous

Catatonia (schizophrenic) F20.2

Catatonic
- disorder due to known physiologic condition F06.1
- schizophrenia F20.2
- stupor R40.1

Cat-scratch — see also Abrasion
- disease or fever A28.1

Cauda equina — see condition

Cauliflower ear M95.1-

Causalgia (upper limb) G56.4- ☑
- lower limb G57.7- ☑

Cause
- external, general effects T75.89 ☑

Caustic burn — see Corrosion, by site

Cavare's disease (familial periodic paralysis) G72.3

Cave-in, injury
- crushing (severe) — see Crush
- suffocation — see Asphyxia, traumatic, due to low oxygen, due to cave-in

Cavernitis (penis) N48.29

Cavernositis N48.29

Cavernous — see condition

Cavitation of lung — see also Tuberculosis, pulmonary
- nontuberculous J98.4

Cavities, dental — see Caries, dental

Cavity
- lung — see Cavitation of lung
- optic papilla Q14.2
- pulmonary — see Cavitation of lung

Cavovarus foot, congenital Q66.1- ☑

Cavus foot (congenital) Q66.7- ☑
- acquired — see Deformity, limb, foot, specified NEC

Cazenave's disease L10.2

CCCA (central centrifugal cicatricial alopecia) L66.81

CDKL5 (Cyclin-Dependent Kinase-Like 5 Deficiency Disorder) G40.42

Cecitis K52.9
- with perforation, peritonitis, or rupture K65.8

Cecoureterocele Q62.32

Cecum — see condition

Celiac
- artery compression syndrome I77.4
- disease (with steatorrhea) K90.0
- infantilism K90.0

Cell(s), **cellular** — see also condition
- in urine R82.998

Cellulitis (diffuse) (phlegmonous) (septic) (suppurative) L03.90
- abdominal wall L03.311
- anaerobic A48.0
- ankle — see Cellulitis, lower limb
- anus K61.0
- arm — see Cellulitis, upper limb
- auricle (ear) — see Cellulitis, ear
- axilla L03.11- ☑
- back (any part) L03.312
- breast (acute) (nonpuerperal) (subacute) N61.0
  - nipple N61.0
- broad ligament
  - acute N73.0
- buttock L03.317
- cervical (meaning neck) L03.221
- cervix (uteri) — see Cervicitis
- cheek (external) L03.211
  - internal K12.2
- chest wall L03.313
- chronic L03.90
- clostridial A48.0
- corpus cavernosum N48.22
- digit
  - finger — see Cellulitis, finger
  - toe — see Cellulitis, toe
- Douglas' cul-de-sac or pouch
  - acute N73.0
- drainage site (following operation) T81.49 ☑
- ear (external) H60.1- ☑
- eosinophilic (granulomatous) L98.3
- erysipelatous — see Erysipelas
- external auditory canal — see Cellulitis, ear
- eyelid — see Abscess, eyelid
- face NEC L03.211
- finger (intrathecal) (periosteal) (subcutaneous) (subcuticular) L03.01- ☑

Cellulitis — continued
- foot — see Cellulitis, lower limb
- gangrenous — see Gangrene
- genital organ NEC
  - female (external) N76.4
  - male N49.9
    - multiple sites N49.8
    - specified NEC N49.8
- gluteal (region) L03.317
- gonococcal A54.89
- groin L03.314
- hand — see Cellulitis, upper limb
- head NEC L03.811
  - face (any part, except ear, eye and nose) L03.211
- heel — see Cellulitis, lower limb
- hip — see Cellulitis, lower limb
- jaw (region) L03.211
- knee — see Cellulitis, lower limb
- labium (majus) (minus) — see Vulvitis
- lacrimal passages — see Inflammation, lacrimal, passages
- larynx J38.7
- leg — see Cellulitis, lower limb
- lip K13.0
- lower limb L03.11- ☑
  - toe — see Cellulitis, toe
- mouth (floor) K12.2
- multiple sites, so stated L03.90
- nasopharynx J39.1
- navel L03.316
  - newborn P38.9
    - with mild hemorrhage P38.1
    - without hemorrhage P38.9
- neck (region) L03.221
- nipple (acute) (nonpuerperal) (subacute) N61.0
- nose (septum) (external) J34.0
- orbit, orbital H05.01- ☑
- palate (soft) K12.2
- pectoral (region) L03.313
- pelvis, pelvic (chronic)
  - female — see also Disease, pelvis, inflammatory N73.2
    - acute N73.0
  - following ectopic or molar pregnancy O08.0
  - male K65.0
- penis N48.22
- perineal, perineum L03.315
- periorbital L03.213
- perirectal K61.1
- peritonsillar J36
- periurethral N34.0
- periuterine — see also Disease, pelvis, inflammatory N73.2
  - acute N73.0
- pharynx J39.1
- preseptal L03.213
- rectum K61.1
- retroperitoneal K68.9
- round ligament
  - acute N73.0
- scalp (any part) L03.811
- scrotum N49.2
- seminal vesicle N49.0
- shoulder — see Cellulitis, upper limb
- specified site NEC L03.818
- submandibular (region) (space) (triangle) K12.2
  - gland K11.3
- submaxillary (region) K12.2
  - gland K11.3
- thigh — see Cellulitis, lower limb
- thumb (intrathecal) (periosteal) (subcutaneous) (subcuticular) — see Cellulitis, finger
- toe (intrathecal) (periosteal) (subcutaneous) (subcuticular) L03.03- ☑
- tonsil J36
- trunk L03.319
  - abdominal wall L03.311
  - back (any part) L03.312
  - buttock L03.317
  - chest wall L03.313
  - groin L03.314
  - perineal, perineum L03.315
  - umbilicus L03.316
- tuberculous (primary) A18.4
- umbilicus L03.316
- upper limb L03.11- ☑
  - axilla — see Cellulitis, axilla
  - finger — see Cellulitis, finger
  - thumb — see Cellulitis, finger
- vaccinal T88.0 ☑

Cellulitis — *continued*
  vocal cord J38.3
  vulva — *see* Vulvitis
  wrist — *see* Cellulitis, upper limb
Cementoblastoma, benign — *see* Cyst, calcifying odontogenic
Cementoma — *see* Cyst, calcifying odontogenic
Cementoperiostitis — *see* Periodontitis
Cementosis K03.4
Central auditory processing disorder H93.25
Central pain syndrome G89.0
Cephalematocele, cephal (o)hematocele
  newborn P52.8
    birth injury P10.8
  traumatic — *see* Hematoma, brain
Cephalematoma, cephalhematoma (calcified)
  newborn (birth injury) P12.0
  traumatic — *see* Hematoma, brain
Cephalgia, cephalalgia — *see also* Headache
  histamine G44.009
    intractable G44.001
    not intractable G44.009
  trigeminal autonomic (TAC) NEC G44.099
    intractable G44.091
    not intractable G44.099
Cephalic — *see* condition
Cephalitis — *see* Encephalitis
Cephalocele — *see* Encephalocele
Cephalomenia N94.89
Cephalopelvic — *see* condition
Cerclage (with cervical incompetence) in pregnancy — *see* Incompetence, cervix, in pregnancy
Cerebellitis — *see* Encephalitis
Cerebellum, cerebellar — *see* condition
Cerebral — *see* condition
Cerebritis — *see* Encephalitis
Cerebro-hepato-renal syndrome Q87.89
Cerebromalacia — *see* Softening, brain
  sequelae of cerebrovascular disease I69.398
Cerebroside lipidosis E75.22
Cerebrospasticity (congenital) G80.1
Cerebrospinal — *see* condition
Cerebrum — *see* condition
Ceroid-lipofuscinosis, neuronal E75.4
Cerumen (accumulation) (impacted) H61.2- ☑
Cervical — *see also* condition
  auricle Q18.2
  dysplasia in pregnancy — *see* Abnormal, cervix, in pregnancy or childbirth
  erosion in pregnancy — *see* Abnormal, cervix, in pregnancy or childbirth
  fibrosis in pregnancy — *see* Abnormal, cervix, in pregnancy or childbirth
  fusion syndrome Q76.1
  rib Q76.5
  shortening (complicating pregnancy) O26.87- ☑
Cervicalgia M54.2
Cervicitis (acute) (atrophic) (chronic) (nonvenereal) (senile) (subacute) (with ulceration) N72
  with
    abortion — *see* Abortion, by type complicated by genital tract and pelvic infection
    ectopic pregnancy O08.0
    molar pregnancy O08.0
  chlamydial A56.09
  gonococcal A54.03
  herpesviral A60.03
  puerperal (postpartum) O86.11
  syphilitic A52.76
  trichomonal A59.09
  tuberculous A18.16
Cervicocolpitis (emphysematosa) — *see also* Cervicitis N72
Cervix — *see* condition
Cesarean delivery, previous, affecting management of pregnancy O34.219
  classical (vertical) scar O34.212
  isthmocele (non-pregnant state) N85.A
    maternal care for O34.22
  low transverse scar O34.211
  mid-transverse T incision O34.218
  scar
    defect (non-pregnant state) N85.A
      maternal care for O34.22
    specified type NEC O34.218
Cestan (-Chenais) **paralysis or syndrome** G46.3
Cestan-Raymond syndrome I65.8
Cestode infestation B71.9
  specified type NEC B71.8
Cestodiasis B71.9

Chabert's disease A22.9
Chacaleh E53.8
Chafing L30.4
Chagas' (-Mazza) disease (chronic) B57.2
  with
    cardiovascular involvement NEC B57.2
    digestive system involvement B57.30
      megacolon B57.32
      megaesophagus B57.31
      other specified B57.39
    megacolon B57.32
    megaesophagus B57.31
    myocarditis B57.2
    nervous system involvement B57.40
      meningitis B57.41
      meningoencephalitis B57.42
      other specified B57.49
    specified organ involvement NEC B57.5
  acute (with) B57.1
    cardiovascular NEC B57.0
    myocarditis B57.0
Chagres fever B50.9
Chairridden Z74.09
Chalasia (cardiac sphincter) K21.9
Chalazion H00.19
  left H00.16
    lower H00.15
    upper H00.14
  right H00.13
    lower H00.12
    upper H00.11
Chalcosis — *see also* Disorder, globe, degenerative, chalcosis
  cornea — *see* Deposit, cornea
  crystalline lens — *see* Cataract, complicated
  retina H35.89
Chalicosis (pulmonum) J62.8
Chancre (any genital site) (hard) (hunterian) (mixed) (primary) (seronegative) (seropositive) (syphilitic) A51.0
  congenital A50.07
  conjunctiva NEC A51.2
  ducreyi A57
  Ducrey's A57
  extragenital A51.2
  eyelid A51.2
  lip A51.2
  nipple A51.2
  Nisbet's A57
  of
    carate A67.0
    pinta A67.0
    yaws A66.0
  palate, soft A51.2
  phagedenic A57
  simple A57
  soft A57
    bubo A57
    palate A51.2
  urethra A51.0
  yaws A66.0
Chancroid (anus) (genital) (penis) (perineum) (rectum) (urethra) (vulva) A57
Chandler's disease (osteochondritis dissecans, hip) — *see* Osteochondritis, dissecans, hip
Change(s) (in) (of) — *see also* Removal
  arteriosclerotic — *see* Arteriosclerosis
  bone — *see also* Disorder, bone
    diabetic — *see* Diabetes, bone change
  bowel habit R19.4
  cardiorenal (vascular) — *see* Hypertension, cardiorenal
  cardiovascular — *see* Disease, cardiovascular
  circulatory I99.9
  cognitive (mild) (organic) R41.89
  color, tooth, teeth
    during formation K00.8
    posteruptive K03.7
  contraceptive device Z30.433
  corneal membrane H18.30
    Bowman's membrane fold or rupture H18.31- ☑
    Descemet's membrane
      fold H18.32- ☑
      rupture H18.33- ☑
  coronary — *see* Disease, heart, ischemic
  degenerative, spine or vertebra — *see* Spondylosis
  dental pulp, regressive K04.2
  dressing (nonsurgical) Z48.00
    surgical Z48.01
  heart — *see* Disease, heart
  hip joint — *see* Derangement, joint, hip

Change(s) — *continued*
  hyperplastic larynx J38.7
  hypertrophic
    nasal sinus J34.89
    turbinate, nasal J34.3
    upper respiratory tract J39.8
  indwelling catheter Z46.6
  inflammatory — *see also* Inflammation
    sacroiliac M46.1
  job, anxiety concerning Z56.1
  joint — *see* Derangement, joint
  life — *see* Menopause
  mental status R41.82
  minimal (glomerular) — *see also* N00-N07 with fourth character .0 N05.0
  myocardium, myocardial — *see* Degeneration, myocardial
  of life — *see* Menopause
  pacemaker Z45.018
    pulse generator Z45.010
  personality (enduring) F68.8
    due to (secondary to)
      general medical condition F07.0
    secondary (nonspecific) F60.89
  regressive, dental pulp K04.2
  renal — *see* Disease, renal
  retina H35.9
    myopic — *see also* Myopia, degenerative H44.2- ☑
  sacroiliac joint M53.3
  senile — *see also* condition R54
  sensory R20.8
  skin R23.9
    acute, due to ultraviolet radiation L56.9
      specified NEC L56.8
    chronic, due to nonionizing radiation L57.9
      specified NEC L57.8
    cyanosis R23.0
    flushing R23.2
    pallor R23.1
    petechiae R23.3
    specified change NEC R23.8
    swelling — *see* Mass, localized
    texture R23.4
  trophic
    arm — *see* Mononeuropathy, upper limb
    leg — *see* Mononeuropathy, lower limb
  vascular I99.9
  vasomotor I73.9
  voice R49.9
    psychogenic F44.4
    specified NEC R49.8
Changing sleep-work schedule, affecting sleep G47.26
Changuinola fever A93.1
Chapping skin T69.8 ☑
Charcot-Marie-Tooth disease, paralysis or syndrome G60.0
Charcot's
  arthropathy — *see* Arthropathy, neuropathic
  cirrhosis K74.3
  disease (tabetic arthropathy) A52.16
  joint (disease) (tabetic) A52.16
    diabetic — *see* Diabetes, with, arthropathy
    syringomyelic G95.0
  syndrome (intermittent claudication) I73.9
CHARGE association Q89.8
Charley-horse (quadriceps) M62.831
  traumatic (quadriceps) S76.11- ☑
Charlouis' disease — *see* Yaws
Cheadle's disease E54
Checking (of)
  cardiac pacemaker (battery) (electrode(s)) Z45.018
    pulse generator Z45.010
  implantable subdermal contraceptive Z30.46
  intrauterine contraceptive device Z30.431
  wound Z48.0- ☑
    due to injury — code to Injury, by site, using appropriate seventh character for subsequent encounter
    postoperative — *see* Aftercare
Check-up — *see* Examination
Chediak-Higashi (-Steinbrinck) **syndrome** (congenital gigantism of peroxidase granules) E70.330
Cheek — *see* condition
Cheese itch B88.0
Cheese-washer's lung J67.8
Cheese-worker's lung J67.8
Cheilitis (acute) (angular) (catarrhal) (chronic) (exfoliative) (gangrenous) (glandular) (infectional) (suppurative) (ulcerative) (vesicular) K13.0

Cheilitis — *continued*
  actinic (due to sun) L56.8
    other than from sun L59.8
  candidal B37.83
Cheilodynia K13.0
Cheiloschisis — *see* Cleft, lip
Cheilosis (angular) K13.0
  with pellagra E52
  due to
    vitamin B2 (riboflavin) deficiency E53.0
Cheiromegaly M79.89
Cheiropompholyx L30.1
Cheloid — *see* Keloid
Chemical burn — *see* Corrosion, by site
Chemodectoma — *see* Paraganglioma, nonchromaffin
Chemosis, conjunctiva — *see* Edema, conjunctiva
Chemotherapy (session) (for)
  cancer Z51.11
  neoplasm Z51.11
Cherubism M27.8
Chest — *see* condition
Cheyne-Stokes breathing (respiration) R06.3
Chiari's
  disease or syndrome (hepatic vein thrombosis) I82.0
  malformation
    type I G93.5
    type II — *see* Spina bifida
  net Q24.8
Chicago disease B40.9
Chickenpox — *see* Varicella
Chiclero ulcer or sore B55.1
Chigger (infestation) B88.0
Chignon (disease) B36.8
  newborn (from vacuum extraction) (birth injury) P12.1
Chilaiditi's syndrome (subphrenic displacement, colon) Q43.3
Chilblain(s) (lupus) T69.1 ☑
Child — *see also* Problem, child
  custody dispute Z65.3
Childbirth — *see* Delivery
Childhood
  cerebral X-linked adrenoleukodystrophy E71.520
  period of rapid growth Z00.2
Chill(s) R68.83
  with fever R50.9
  congestive in malarial regions B54
  without fever R68.83
Chilomastigiasis A07.8
Chimera 46,XX/46,XY Q99.0
Chin — *see* condition
Chinese dysentery A03.9
Chionophobia F40.228
Chitral fever A93.1
Chlamydia, chlamydial A74.9
  cervicitis A56.09
  conjunctivitis A74.0
  cystitis A56.01
  endometritis A56.11
  epididymitis A56.19
  female
    pelvic inflammatory disease A56.11
    pelviperitonitis A56.11
  orchitis A56.19
  peritonitis A74.81
  pharyngitis A56.4
  proctitis A56.3
  psittaci (infection) A70
  salpingitis A56.11
  sexually-transmitted infection NEC A56.8
  specified NEC A74.89
  urethritis A56.01
  vulvovaginitis A56.02
Chlamydiosis — *see* Chlamydia
Chloasma (skin) (idiopathic) (symptomatic) L81.1
  eyelid H02.719
    hyperthyroid E05.90 *[H02.719]*
      with thyroid storm E05.91 *[H02.719]*
    left H02.716
      lower H02.715
      upper H02.714
    right H02.713
      lower H02.712
      upper H02.711
Chloroma C92.3- ☑
Chlorosis D50.9
  Egyptian B76.9 *[D63.8]*
  miner's B76.9 *[D63.8]*
Chlorotic anemia D50.8
Chocolate cyst (ovary) N80.10- ☑

Choked
  disc or disk — *see* Papilledema
  on food, phlegm, or vomitus NOS — *see* Foreign body, by site
  while vomiting NOS — *see* Foreign body, by site
Chokes (resulting from bends) T70.3 ☑
Choking sensation R09.89
Cholangiectasis K83.8
Cholangiocarcinoma
  with hepatocellular carcinoma, combined C22.0
  liver C22.1
  specified site NEC — *see* Neoplasm, malignant, by site
  unspecified site C22.1
Cholangiohepatitis K83.8
  due to fluke infestation B66.1
Cholangiohepatoma C22.0
Cholangiolitis (acute) (chronic) (extrahepatic) (gangrenous) (intrahepatic) K83.09
  paratyphoidal — *see* Fever, paratyphoid
  typhoidal A01.09
Cholangioma D13.4
  malignant — *see* Cholangiocarcinoma
Cholangitis (ascending) (recurrent) (secondary) (stenosing) (suppurative) K83.09
  with calculus, bile duct — *see* Calculus, bile duct, with cholangitis
  chronic nonsuppurative destructive K74.3
  primary K83.09
    sclerosing K83.01
  sclerosing K83.09
Cholecystectasia K82.8
Cholecystitis K81.9
  with
    calculus, stones in
      bile duct (common) (hepatic) — *see* Calculus, bile duct, with cholecystitis
      cystic duct — *see* Calculus, gallbladder, with cholecystitis
      gallbladder — *see* Calculus, gallbladder, with cholecystitis
    choledocholithiasis — *see* Calculus, bile duct, with cholecystitis
    cholelithiasis — *see* Calculus, gallbladder, with cholecystitis
    gangrene of gallbladder K82.A1
    perforation of gallbladder K82.A2
  acute (emphysematous) (gangrenous) (suppurative) K81.0
    with
      calculus, stones in
        cystic duct — *see* Calculus, gallbladder, with cholecystitis, acute
        gallbladder — *see* Calculus, gallbladder, with cholecystitis, acute
      choledocholithiasis — *see* Calculus, bile duct, with cholecystitis, acute
      cholelithiasis — *see* Calculus, gallbladder, with cholecystitis, acute
      chronic cholecystitis K81.2
        with gallbladder calculus K80.12
          with obstruction K80.13
  chronic K81.1
    with acute cholecystitis K81.2
      with gallbladder calculus K80.12
        with obstruction K80.13
  emphysematous (acute) — *see* Cholecystitis, acute
  gangrenous — *see* Cholecystitis, acute
  paratyphoidal, current A01.4
  suppurative — *see* Cholecystitis, acute
  typhoidal A01.09
Cholecystolithiasis — *see* Calculus, gallbladder
Choledochitis (suppurative) K83.09
Choledocholith — *see* Calculus, bile duct
Choledocholithiasis (common duct) (hepatic duct) — *see* Calculus, bile duct
  cystic — *see* Calculus, gallbladder
  typhoidal A01.09
Cholelithiasis (cystic duct) (gallbladder) (impacted) (multiple) — *see* Calculus, gallbladder
  bile duct (common) (hepatic) — *see* Calculus, bile duct
  hepatic duct — *see* Calculus, bile duct
  specified NEC K80.80
    with obstruction K80.81
Cholemia — *see also* Jaundice
  familial (simple) (congenital) E80.4
  Gilbert's E80.4
Choleperitoneum, choleperitonitis K65.3
Cholera (Asiatic) (epidemic) (malignant) A00.9
  antimonial — *see* Poisoning, antimony

Cholera — *continued*
  classical A00.0
  due to Vibrio cholerae 01 A00.9
    biovar cholerae A00.0
    biovar eltor A00.1
    el tor A00.1
  el tor A00.1
Cholerine — *see* Cholera
Cholestasis NEC K83.1
  with hepatocyte injury K71.0
  due to total parenteral nutrition (TPN) K76.89
  pure K71.0
Cholesteatoma (ear) (middle) (with reaction) H71.9- ☑
  attic H71.0- ☑
  external ear (canal) H60.4- ☑
  mastoid H71.2- ☑
  postmastoidectomy cavity (recurrent) — *see* Complications, postmastoidectomy, recurrent cholesteatoma
  recurrent (postmastoidectomy) — *see* Complications, postmastoidectomy, recurrent cholesteatoma
  tympanum H71.1- ☑
Cholesteatosis, diffuse H71.3- ☑
Cholesteremia E78.00
Cholesterin in vitreous — *see* Deposit, crystalline
Cholesterol
  deposit
    retina H35.89
    vitreous — *see* Deposit, crystalline
  elevated (high) E78.00
    with elevated (high) triglycerides E78.2
    screening for Z13.220
  imbibition of gallbladder K82.4
Cholesterolemia (essential) (pure) E78.00
  familial E78.01
  hereditary E78.01
Cholesterolosis, cholesterosis (gallbladder) K82.4
  cerebrotendinous E75.5
Cholocolic fistula K82.3
Choluria R82.2
Chondritis M94.8X9
  aurical H61.03- ☑
  costal (Tietze's) M94.0
  external ear H61.03- ☑
  patella, posttraumatic — *see* Chondromalacia, patella
  pinna H61.03- ☑
  purulent M94.8X- ☑
  tuberculous NEC A18.02
    intervertebral A18.01
Chondroblastoma — *see also* Neoplasm, bone, benign
  malignant — *see* Neoplasm, bone, malignant
Chondrocalcinosis M11.20
  ankle M11.27- ☑
  elbow M11.22- ☑
  familial M11.10
    ankle M11.17- ☑
    elbow M11.12- ☑
    foot joint M11.17- ☑
    hand joint M11.14- ☑
    hip M11.15- ☑
    knee M11.16- ☑
    multiple site M11.19
    shoulder M11.11- ☑
    vertebrae M11.18
    wrist M11.13- ☑
  foot joint M11.27- ☑
  hand joint M11.24- ☑
  hip M11.25- ☑
  knee M11.26- ☑
  multiple site M11.29
  shoulder M11.21- ☑
  specified type NEC M11.20
    ankle M11.27- ☑
    elbow M11.22- ☑
    foot joint M11.27- ☑
    hand joint M11.24- ☑
    hip M11.25- ☑
    knee M11.26- ☑
    multiple site M11.29
    shoulder M11.21- ☑
    vertebrae M11.28
    wrist M11.23- ☑
  vertebrae M11.28
  wrist M11.23- ☑
Chondrodermatitis nodularis helicis or anthelicis — *see* Perichondritis, ear
Chondrodysplasia Q78.9

Chondrodysplasia — *continued*
with hemangioma Q78.4
calcificans congenita Q77.3
fetalis Q77.4
metaphyseal (Jansen's) (McKusick's) (Schmid's) Q78.8
punctata Q77.3
Chondrodystrophy, chondrodystrophia (familial) (fetalis) (hypoplastic) Q78.9
calcificans congenita Q77.3
myotonic (congenital) G71.13
punctata Q77.3
Chondroectodermal dysplasia Q77.6
Chondrogenesis imperfecta Q77.4
Chondrolysis M94.35- ☑
Chondroma — *see also* Neoplasm, cartilage, benign
juxtacortical — *see* Neoplasm, bone, benign
periosteal — *see* Neoplasm, bone, benign
Chondromalacia (systemic) M94.20
acromioclavicular joint M94.21- ☑
ankle M94.27- ☑
elbow M94.22- ☑
foot joint M94.27- ☑
glenohumeral joint M94.21- ☑
hand joint M94.24- ☑
hip M94.25- ☑
knee M94.26- ☑
patella M22.4- ☑
multiple sites M94.29
patella M22.4- ☑
rib M94.28
sacroiliac joint M94.259
shoulder M94.21- ☑
sternoclavicular joint M94.21- ☑
vertebral joint M94.28
wrist M94.23- ☑
Chondromatosis — *see also* Neoplasm, cartilage, uncertain behavior
internal Q78.4
Chondromyxosarcoma — *see* Neoplasm, cartilage, malignant
Chondro-osteodysplasia (Morquio-Brailsford type) E76.219
Chondro-osteodystrophy E76.29
Chondro-osteoma — *see* Neoplasm, bone, benign
Chondropathia tuberosa M94.0
Chondrosarcoma — *see* Neoplasm, cartilage, malignant
juxtacortical — *see* Neoplasm, bone, malignant
mesenchymal — *see* Neoplasm, connective tissue, malignant
myxoid — *see* Neoplasm, cartilage, malignant
Chordee (nonvenereal) N48.89
congenital Q54.4
gonococcal A54.09
Chorditis (fibrinous) (nodosa) (tuberosa) J38.2
Chordoma — *see* Neoplasm, vertebral (column), malignant
Chorea (chronic) (gravis) (posthemiplegic) (senile) (spasmodic) G25.5
with
heart involvement I02.0
active or acute (conditions in I01-) I02.0
rheumatic I02.9
with valvular disorder I02.0
rheumatic heart disease (chronic) (inactive) (quiescent) — *code to* rheumatic heart condition involved
drug-induced G25.4
habit F95.8
hereditary G10
Huntington's G10
hysterical F44.4
minor I02.9
with heart involvement I02.0
progressive G25.5
hereditary G10
rheumatic (chronic) I02.9
with heart involvement I02.0
Sydenham's I02.9
with heart involvement — *see* Chorea, with rheumatic heart disease
nonrheumatic G25.5
Choreoathetosis (paroxysmal) G25.5
Chorioadenoma (destruens) D39.2
Chorioamnionitis O41.12- ☑
Chorioangioma D26.7
Choriocarcinoma — *see* Neoplasm, malignant, by site
combined with
embryonal carcinoma — *see* Neoplasm, malignant, by site

Choriocarcinoma — *continued*
combined with — *continued*
other germ cell elements — *see* Neoplasm, malignant, by site
teratoma — *see* Neoplasm, malignant, by site
specified site — *see* Neoplasm, malignant, by site
unspecified site
female C58
male C62.90
Chorioencephalitis (acute) (lymphocytic) (serous) A87.2
Chorioepithelioma — *see* Choriocarcinoma
Choriomeningitis (acute) (lymphocytic) (serous) A87.2
Chorionepithelioma — *see* Choriocarcinoma
Chorioretinitis — *see also* Inflammation, chorioretinal
disseminated — *see also* Inflammation, chorioretinal, disseminated
in neurosyphilis A52.19
Egyptian B76.9 *[D63.8]*
focal — *see also* Inflammation, chorioretinal, focal
histoplasmic B39.9 *[H32]*
in (due to)
histoplasmosis B39.9 *[H32]*
syphilis (secondary) A51.43
late A52.71
toxoplasmosis (acquired) B58.01
congenital (active) P37.1 *[H32]*
tuberculosis A18.53
juxtapapillary, juxtapapillaris — *see* Inflammation, chorioretinal, focal, juxtapapillary
leprous A30.9 *[H32]*
miner's B76.9 *[D63.8]*
progressive myopia (degeneration) — *see also* Myopia, degenerative H44.2- ☑
syphilitic (secondary) A51.43
congenital (early) A50.01 *[H32]*
late A50.32
late A52.71
tuberculous A18.53
Chorioretinopathy, central serous H35.71- ☑
Choroid — *see* condition
Choroideremia H31.21
Choroiditis — *see* Chorioretinitis
Choroidopathy — *see* Disorder, choroid
Choroidoretinitis — *see* Chorioretinitis
Choroidoretinopathy, central serous — *see* Chorioretinopathy, central serous
Christian-Weber disease M35.6
Christmas disease D67
Chromaffinoma — *see also* Neoplasm, benign, by site
malignant — *see* Neoplasm, malignant, by site
Chromatopsia — *see* Deficiency, color vision
Chromhidrosis, chromidrosis L75.1
Chromoblastomycosis — *see* Chromomycosis
Chromoconversion R82.91
Chromomycosis B43.9
brain abscess B43.1
cerebral B43.1
cutaneous B43.0
skin B43.0
specified NEC B43.8
subcutaneous abscess or cyst B43.2
Chromophytosis B36.0
Chromosome — *see* Anomaly, by chromosome involved
D (1) — *see* Anomaly, chromosome 13
E (3) — *see* Anomaly, chromosome 18
G — *see* Anomaly, chromosome 21
Chromotrichomycosis B36.8
Chronic — *see* condition
fracture — *see* Fracture, pathological
Churg-Strauss syndrome M30.1
Chyle cyst, mesentery I89.8
Chylocele (nonfilarial) I89.8
filarial — *see also* Infestation, filarial B74.9 *[N51]*
tunica vaginalis N50.89
filarial — *see also* Infestation, filarial B74.9 *[N51]*
Chylomicronemia (fasting) (with hyperprebetalipoproteinemia) E78.3
Chylopericardium I31.39
acute I30.9
Chylothorax (nonfilarial) J94.0
filarial — *see also* Infestation, filarial B74.9 *[J91.8]*
Chylous — *see* condition
Chyluria (nonfilarial) R82.0
due to
bilharziasis B65.0
Brugia (malayi) B74.1
timori B74.2
schistosomiasis (bilharziasis) B65.0
Wuchereria (bancrofti) B74.0

Chyluria — *continued*
filarial — *see* Infestation, filarial
Cicatricial (deformity) — *see* Cicatrix
Cicatrix (adherent) (contracted) (painful) (vicious) — *see also* Scar L90.5
adenoid (and tonsil) J35.8
alveolar process M26.79
anus K62.89
auricle — *see* Disorder, pinna, specified type NEC
bile duct (common) (hepatic) K83.8
bladder N32.89
bone — *see* Disorder, bone, specified type NEC
brain G93.89
cervix (postoperative) (postpartal) N88.1
common duct K83.8
cornea H17.9
tuberculous A18.59
duodenum (bulb), obstructive K31.5
esophagus K22.2
eyelid — *see* Disorder, eyelid function
hypopharynx J39.2
lacrimal passages — *see* Obstruction, lacrimal
larynx J38.7
lung J98.4
middle ear H74.8 ☑
mouth K13.79
muscle M62.89
with contracture — *see* Contraction, muscle NEC
nasopharynx J39.2
palate (soft) K13.79
penis N48.89
pharynx J39.2
prostate N42.89
rectum K62.89
retina — *see* Scar, chorioretinal
semilunar cartilage — *see* Derangement, meniscus
seminal vesicle N50.89
skin L90.5
infected L08.89
postinfective L90.5
tuberculous B90.8
specified site NEC L90.5
throat J39.2
tongue K14.8
tonsil (and adenoid) J35.8
trachea J39.8
tuberculous NEC B90.9
urethra N36.8
uterus N85.8
vagina N89.8
postoperative N99.2
vocal cord J38.3
wrist, constricting (annular) L90.5
CIDP (chronic inflammatory demyelinating polyneuropathy) G61.81
CIN — *see* Neoplasia, intraepithelial, cervix
CINCA (chronic infantile neurological, cutaneous and articular syndrome) M04.2
Cinchonism — *see* Deafness, ototoxic
correct substance properly administered — *see* Table of Drugs and Chemicals, by drug, adverse effect
overdose or wrong substance given or taken — *see* Table of Drugs and Chemicals, by drug, poisoning
Circle of Willis — *see* condition
Circular — *see* condition
Circulating anticoagulants — *see also* Disorder, hemorrhagic D68.318
due to drugs — *see also* Disorder, hemorrhagic D68.32
following childbirth O72.3
Circulation
collateral, any site I99.8
defective (lower extremity) I99.9
congenital Q28.9
embryonic Q28.9
failure (peripheral) R57.9
newborn P29.89
fetal, persistent P29.38
heart, incomplete Q28.9
Circulatory system — *see* condition
Circulus senilis (cornea) — *see* Degeneration, cornea, senile
Circumcision (in absence of medical indication) (ritual) (routine) Z41.2
Circumscribed — *see* condition
Circumvallate placenta O43.11- ☑
Cirrhosis, cirrhotic (hepatic) (liver) K74.60
alcoholic K70.30
with ascites K70.31
atrophic — *see* Cirrhosis, liver
Baumgarten-Cruveilhier K74.69

☑ **Additional Character Required — Refer to the Tabular List for Character Selection**

Cirrhosis, cirrhotic — continued
  biliary (cholangiolitic) (cholangitic) (hypertrophic) (obstructive) (pericholangiolitic) K74.5
    due to
      Clonorchiasis B66.1
      flukes B66.3
    primary K74.3
    secondary K74.4
  cardiac (of liver) K76.1
  Charcot's K74.3
  cholangiolitic, cholangitic, cholostatic (primary) K74.3
  congestive K76.1
  Cruveilhier-Baumgarten K74.69
  cryptogenic (liver) K74.69
  due to
    hepatolenticular degeneration E83.01
    Wilson's disease E83.01
    xanthomatosis E78.2
  fatty K76.0
    alcoholic K70.0
  Hanot's (hypertrophic) K74.3
  hepatic — see Cirrhosis, liver
  hypertrophic K74.3
  Indian childhood K74.69
  kidney — see Sclerosis, renal
  Laennec's K70.30
    with ascites K70.31
    alcoholic K70.30
      with ascites K70.31
    nonalcoholic K74.69
  liver K74.60
    alcoholic K70.30
      with ascites K70.31
      fatty K70.0
    congenital P78.81
    syphilitic A52.74
  lung (chronic) J84.10
  macronodular K74.69
    alcoholic K70.30
      with ascites K70.31
  micronodular K74.69
    alcoholic K70.30
      with ascites K70.31
  mixed type K74.69
  monolobular K74.3
  nephritis — see Sclerosis, renal
  nutritional K74.69
    alcoholic K70.30
      with ascites K70.31
  obstructive — see Cirrhosis, biliary
  ovarian N83.8
  pancreas (duct) K86.89
  pigmentary E83.110
  portal K74.69
    alcoholic K70.30
      with ascites K70.31
  postnecrotic K74.69
    alcoholic K70.30
      with ascites K70.31
  pulmonary J84.10
  renal — see Sclerosis, renal
  spleen D73.2
  stasis K76.1
  Todd's K74.3
  unilobar K74.3
  xanthomatous (biliary) K74.5
    due to xanthomatosis (familial) (metabolic) (primary) E78.2
Cistern, subarachnoid R93.0
Citrullinemia E72.23
Citrullinuria E72.23
Civatte's disease or poikiloderma L57.3
CLAD — see Dysfunction, chronic, lung allograft
Clam digger's itch B65.3
Clammy skin R23.1
Clap — see Gonorrhea
Clarke-Hadfield syndrome (pancreatic infantilism) K86.89
Clark's paralysis G80.9
Clastothrix L67.8
Claude Bernard-Horner syndrome G90.2
  traumatic — see Injury, nerve, cervical sympathetic
Claude's disease or syndrome G46.3
Claudicatio venosa intermittens I87.8
Claudication (intermittent) I73.9
  cerebral (artery) G45.9
  spinal cord (arteriosclerotic) G95.19
    syphilitic A52.09
  venous (axillary) I87.8
Claustrophobia F40.240

Clavus (infected) L84
Clawfoot (congenital) Q66.89
  acquired — see Deformity, limb, clawfoot
Clawhand (acquired) — see also Deformity, limb, clawhand
  congenital Q68.1
Clawtoe (congenital) Q66.89
  acquired — see Deformity, toe, specified NEC
Clay eating — see Pica
Cleansing of artificial opening — see Attention to, artificial, opening
Cleft (congenital) — see also Imperfect, closure
  alveolar process M26.79
  branchial (persistent) Q18.2
    cyst Q18.0
      fistula Q18.0
      sinus Q18.0
  cricoid cartilage, posterior Q31.8
  cyst Q18.0
    fistula Q18.0
    sinus Q18.0
  foot Q72.7 ☑
  hand Q71.6 ☑
  lip (unilateral) Q36.9
    with cleft palate Q37.9
      hard Q37.1
        with soft Q37.5
      soft Q37.3
        with hard Q37.5
    bilateral Q36.0
      with cleft palate Q37.8
        hard Q37.0
          with soft Q37.4
        soft Q37.2
          with hard Q37.4
    median Q36.1
  mitral valve leaflet (at birth) (congenital) Q23.82
  nose Q30.2
  palate Q35.9
    with cleft lip (unilateral) Q37.9
      bilateral Q37.8
    hard Q35.1
      with
        cleft lip (unilateral) Q37.1
          bilateral Q37.0
        soft Q35.5
          with cleft lip (unilateral) Q37.5
            bilateral Q37.4
    medial Q35.5
    soft Q35.3
      with
        cleft lip (unilateral) Q37.3
          bilateral Q37.2
        hard Q35.5
          with cleft lip (unilateral) Q37.5
            bilateral Q37.4
  penis Q55.69
  scrotum Q55.29
  thyroid cartilage Q31.8
  uvula Q35.7
Cleidocranial dysostosis Q74.0
Cleptomania F63.2
Clicking hip (newborn) R29.4
Climacteric (female) — see also Menopause
  arthritis (any site) NEC — see Arthritis, specified form NEC
  depression (single episode) F32.89
    recurrent episode F33.8
  male (symptoms) (syndrome) NEC N50.89
  melancholia (single episode) F32.89
    recurrent episode F33.8
  paranoid state F22
  polyarthritis NEC — see Arthritis, specified form NEC
  symptoms (female) N95.1
Clinical research investigation (clinical trial) (control subject) (normal comparison) (participant) Z00.6
Clitoris — see condition
Cloaca (persistent) Q43.7
Clonorchiasis, clonorchis infection (liver) B66.1
Clonus R25.8
Closed bite M26.29
Clostridium (C.) **perfringens, as cause of disease classified elsewhere** B96.7
Closure
  congenital, nose Q30.0
  cranial sutures, premature Q75.009
  defective or imperfect NEC — see Imperfect, closure
  fistula, delayed — see Fistula
  foramen ovale, imperfect Q21.12
  hymen N89.6

Closure — continued
  interauricular septum, defective Q21.19
  interventricular septum, defective Q21.0
  lacrimal duct — see also Stenosis, lacrimal, duct
    congenital Q10.5
  nose (congenital) Q30.0
    acquired M95.0
  of artificial opening — see Attention to, artificial, opening
  vagina N89.5
  valve — see Endocarditis
  vulva N90.5
Clot (blood) — see also Embolism
  artery (obstruction) (occlusion) — see Embolism
  bladder N32.89
  brain (intradural or extradural) — see Occlusion, artery, cerebral
  circulation I74.9
  heart — see also Infarct, myocardium
    not resulting in infarction I51.3
  vein — see Thrombosis
Clouded state R40.1
  epileptic — see Epilepsy, specified NEC
  paroxysmal — see Epilepsy, specified NEC
Cloudy antrum, antra J32.0
Clouston's (hidrotic) **ectodermal dysplasia** Q82.4
Cloverleaf skull Q75.051
Clubbed nail pachydermoperiostosis M89.40 [L62]
Clubbing of finger(s) (nails) R68.3
Clubfinger R68.3
  congenital Q68.1
Clubfoot (congenital) Q66.89
  acquired — see Deformity, limb, clubfoot
  equinovarus Q66.0- ☑
  paralytic — see Deformity, limb, clubfoot
Clubhand (congenital) (radial) Q71.4- ☑
  acquired — see Deformity, limb, clubhand
Clubnail R68.3
  congenital Q84.6
Clump, kidney Q63.1
Clumsiness, clumsy child syndrome F82
Cluttering F80.81
Clutton's joints A50.51 [M12.80]
Coagulation, intravascular (diffuse) (disseminated) — see also Defibrination syndrome
  complicating abortion — see Abortion, by type, complicated by, intravascular coagulation
  COVID-19 associated — see also COVID-19 D65
  following ectopic or molar pregnancy O08.1
Coagulopathy — see also Defect, coagulation
  consumption D65
  intravascular D65
    newborn P60
Coalition
  calcaneo-scaphoid Q66.89
  tarsal Q66.89
Coalminer's
  elbow — see Bursitis, elbow, olecranon
  lung or pneumoconiosis J60
Coalworker's lung or pneumoconiosis J60
Coarctation
  aorta (preductal) (postductal) Q25.1
  pulmonary artery Q25.71
Coated tongue K14.3
Coats' disease (exudative retinopathy) — see Retinopathy, exudative
Cocaine-induced
  anxiety disorder F14.980
  bipolar and related disorder F14.94
  depressive disorder F14.94
  obsessive-compulsive and related disorder F14.988
  psychotic disorder F14.959
  sexual dysfunction F14.981
  sleep disorder F14.982
Cocainism — see Disorder, cocaine use
Coccidioidomycosis B38.9
  cutaneous B38.3
  disseminated B38.7
  generalized B38.7
  meninges B38.4
  prostate B38.81
  pulmonary B38.2
    acute B38.0
    chronic B38.1
  skin B38.3
  specified NEC B38.89
Coccidioidosis — see Coccidioidomycosis
Coccidiosis (intestinal) A07.3
Coccydynia, coccygodynia M53.3
Coccyx — see condition

Cochin-China diarrhea K90.1
Cockayne's syndrome Q87.19
Cocked up toe — *see* Deformity, toe, specified NEC
Cock's peculiar tumor L72.3
Codman's tumor — *see* Neoplasm, bone, benign
Coenurosis B71.8
Coffee-worker's lung J67.8
Cogan's syndrome H16.32- ☑
　oculomotor apraxia H51.8
Coitus, painful (female) N94.10
　male N53.12
　psychogenic F52.6
Cold J00
　with influenza, flu, or grippe — *see* Influenza, with, res-
　　piratory manifestations NEC
　agglutinin disease or hemoglobinuria (chronic) D59.12
　bronchial — *see* Bronchitis
　chest — *see* Bronchitis
　common (head) J00
　effects of T69.9 ☑
　　specified effect NEC T69.8 ☑
　excessive, effects of T69.9 ☑
　　specified effect NEC T69.8 ☑
　exhaustion from T69.8 ☑
　exposure to T69.9 ☑
　　specified effect NEC T69.8 ☑
　head J00
　injury syndrome (newborn) P80.0
　on lung — *see* Bronchitis
　rose J30.1
　sensitivity, auto-immune D59.12
　symptoms J00
　virus J00
Coldsore B00.1
Colibacillosis A49.8
　as the cause of other disease — *see also* Escherichia coli
　　B96.20
　generalized — *see also* Sepsis, Escherichia coli A41.51
Colic (bilious) (infantile) (intestinal) (recurrent) (spasmodic)
　　R10.83
　abdomen R10.83
　　psychogenic F45.8
　appendix, appendicular K38.8
　bile duct — *see* Calculus, bile duct
　biliary — *see* Calculus, bile duct
　common duct — *see* Calculus, bile duct
　cystic duct — *see* Calculus, gallbladder
　Devonshire NEC — *see* Poisoning, lead
　gallbladder — *see* Calculus, gallbladder
　gallstone — *see* Calculus, gallbladder
　　gallbladder or cystic duct — *see* Calculus, gallbladder
　hepatic (duct) — *see* Calculus, bile duct
　hysterical F45.8
　kidney N23
　lead NEC — *see* Poisoning, lead
　mucous K58.9
　　with diarrhea K58.0
　　psychogenic F54
　nephritic N23
　painter's NEC — *see* Poisoning, lead
　pancreas K86.89
　psychogenic F45.8
　renal N23
　saturnine NEC — *see* Poisoning, lead
　ureter N23
　urethral N36.8
　　due to calculus N21.1
　uterus NEC N94.89
　　menstrual — *see* Dysmenorrhea
　worm NOS B83.9
Colicystitis — *see* Cystitis
Colitis (acute) (catarrhal) (chronic) (noninfective) (hemor-
　　rhagic) — *see also* Enteritis K52.9
　allergic K52.29
　　with
　　　food protein-induced enterocolitis syndrome
　　　　K52.21
　　　proctocolitis K52.29
　amebic (acute) — *see also* Amebiasis A06.0
　　nondysenteric A06.2
　anthrax A22.2
　bacillary — *see* Infection, Shigella
　balantidial A07.0
　Clostridioides difficile
　　not specified as recurrent A04.72
　　recurrent A04.71
　Clostridium difficile
　　not specified as recurrent A04.72

Colitis — *continued*
　Clostridium difficile — *continued*
　　recurrent A04.71
　coccidial A07.3
　collagenous K52.831
　cystica superficialis K52.89
　dietary counseling and surveillance (for) Z71.3
　dietetic — *see also* Colitis, allergic K52.29
　drug-induced K52.1
　due to radiation K52.0
　eosinophilic K52.82
　food hypersensitivity — *see also* Colitis, allergic K52.29
　giardial A07.1
　granulomatous — *see* Enteritis, regional, large intestine
　indeterminate, so stated K52.3
　infectious — *see* Enteritis, infectious
　ischemic K55.9
　　acute (subacute) — *see also* Ischemia, intestine, acute
　　　K55.039
　　chronic K55.1
　　due to mesenteric artery insufficiency K55.1
　　fulminant (acute) — *see also* Ischemia, intestine, acute
　　　K55.039
　left sided K51.50
　　with
　　　abscess K51.514
　　　complication K51.519
　　　　specified NEC K51.518
　　　fistula K51.513
　　　obstruction K51.512
　　　rectal bleeding K51.511
　lymphocytic K52.832
　membranous
　　psychogenic F54
　microscopic K52.839
　　specified NEC K52.838
　mucous — *see* Syndrome, irritable, bowel
　　psychogenic F54
　noninfective K52.9
　　specified NEC K52.89
　polyposa — *see* Polyp, colon, inflammatory
　protozoal A07.9
　pseudomembranous
　　not specified as recurrent A04.72
　　recurrent A04.71
　pseudomucinous — *see* Syndrome, irritable, bowel
　regional — *see* Enteritis, regional, large intestine
　　infectious A09
　segmental — *see* Enteritis, regional, large intestine
　septic — *see* Enteritis, infectious
　spastic K58.9
　　with diarrhea K58.0
　　psychogenic F54
　staphylococcal A04.8
　　foodborne A05.0
　subacute ischemic — *see also* Ischemia, intestine, acute
　　K55.039
　thromboulcerative — *see also* Ischemia, intestine, acute
　　K55.039
　toxic NEC K52.1
　　due to
　　　Clostridioides difficile
　　　　not specified as recurrent A04.72
　　　　recurrent A04.71
　　　Clostridium difficile
　　　　not specified as recurrent A04.72
　　　　recurrent A04.71
　transmural — *see* Enteritis, regional, large intestine
　trichomonal A07.8
　tuberculous (ulcerative) A18.32
　ulcerative (chronic) K51.90
　　with
　　　complication K51.919
　　　　abscess K51.914
　　　　fistula K51.913
　　　　obstruction K51.912
　　　　rectal bleeding K51.911
　　　　specified complication NEC K51.918
　　enterocolitis — *see* Enterocolitis, ulcerative
　　ileocolitis — *see* Ileocolitis, ulcerative
　　mucosal proctocolitis — *see* Proctocolitis, mucosal
　　proctitis — *see* Proctitis, ulcerative
　　pseudopolyposis — *see* Polyp, colon, inflammatory
　　psychogenic F54
　　rectosigmoiditis — *see* Rectosigmoiditis, ulcerative
　　specified type NEC K51.80
　　　with
　　　　complication K51.819
　　　　　abscess K51.814

Colitis — *continued*
　ulcerative — *continued*
　　specified type — *continued*
　　　with — *continued*
　　　　complication — *continued*
　　　　　fistula K51.813
　　　　　obstruction K51.812
　　　　　rectal bleeding K51.811
　　　　　specified complication NEC K51.818
Collagenosis, collagen disease (nonvascular) (vascular)
　　M35.9
　cardiovascular I42.8
　reactive perforating L87.1
　specified NEC M35.89
Collapse R55
　adrenal E27.2
　cardiorespiratory R57.0
　cardiovascular R57.0
　　newborn P29.89
　circulatory (peripheral) R57.9
　　during or after labor and delivery O75.1
　　following ectopic or molar pregnancy O08.3
　　newborn P29.89
　during or
　　after labor and delivery O75.1
　　resulting from a procedure, not elsewhere classified
　　　T81.10 ☑
　external ear canal — *see* Stenosis, external ear canal
　general R55
　heart — *see* Disease, heart
　heat T67.1 ☑
　hysterical F44.89
　labyrinth, membranous (congenital) Q16.5
　lung (massive) — *see also* Atelectasis J98.19
　　pressure due to anesthesia (general) (local) or other
　　　sedation T88.2 ☑
　　during labor and delivery O74.1
　　in pregnancy O29.02- ☑
　　postpartum, puerperal O89.09
　myocardial — *see* Disease, heart
　nasal valve J34.829
　　external J34.8210
　　　dynamic J34.8212
　　　static J34.8211
　　internal J34.8200
　　　dynamic J34.8202
　　　static J34.8201
　nervous F48.8
　neurocirculatory F45.8
　nose M95.0
　　lower sidewall or nostril, on inspiration J34.8212
　　upper, middle sidewall, on inspiration J34.8202
　postoperative T81.10 ☑
　pulmonary — *see also* Atelectasis J98.19
　　newborn — *see* Atelectasis
　trachea J39.8
　tracheobronchial J98.09
　valvular — *see* Endocarditis
　vascular (peripheral) R57.9
　　during or after labor and delivery O75.1
　　following ectopic or molar pregnancy O08.3
　　newborn P29.89
　vertebra M48.50- ☑
　　cervical region M48.52- ☑
　　cervicothoracic region M48.53- ☑
　　in (due to)
　　　neoplasm (metastasis) M84.58- ☑
　　　osteoporosis — *see also* Osteoporosis M80.88 ☑
　　　　cervical region M80.88 ☑
　　　　cervicothoracic region M80.88 ☑
　　　　lumbar region M80.88 ☑
　　　　lumbosacral region M80.88 ☑
　　　　multiple sites M80.88 ☑
　　　　occipito-atlanto-axial region M80.88 ☑
　　　　sacrococcygeal region M80.88 ☑
　　　　thoracic region M80.88 ☑
　　　　thoracolumbar region M80.88 ☑
　　　specified disease NEC M48.50- ☑
　　　　cervical region M48.52- ☑
　　　　cervicothoracic region M48.53- ☑
　　　　lumbar region M48.56- ☑
　　　　lumbosacral region M48.57- ☑
　　　　occipito-atlanto-axial region M48.51- ☑
　　　　sacrococcygeal region M48.58- ☑
　　　　thoracic region M48.54- ☑
　　　　thoracolumbar region M48.55- ☑
　　lumbar region M48.56- ☑

☑ **Additional Character Required — Refer to the Tabular List for Character Selection**

Collapse — *continued*
  vertebra — *continued*
    lumbosacral region M48.57- ☑
    occipito-atlanto-axial region M48.51- ☑
    sacrococcygeal region M48.58- ☑
    thoracic region M48.54- ☑
    thoracolumbar region M48.55- ☑
Collateral — *see also* condition
  circulation (venous) I87.8
  dilation, veins I87.8
Colles' fracture S52.53- ☑
Collet (-Sicard) **syndrome** G52.7
Collier's asthma or lung J60
Collodion baby Q80.2
Colloid nodule (of thyroid) (cystic) E04.1
Coloboma (iris) Q13.0
  eyelid Q10.3
  fundus Q14.8
  lens Q12.2
  optic disc (congenital) Q14.2
    acquired H47.31- ☑
Coloenteritis — *see* Enteritis
Colon — *see* condition
Colonization
  MRSA (Methicillin resistant Staphylococcus aureus)
    Z22.322
  MSSA (Methicillin susceptible Staphylococcus aureus)
    Z22.321
  status — *see* Carrier (suspected) of
Coloptosis K63.4
Color blindness — *see* Deficiency, color vision
Colostomy
  attention to Z43.3
  fitting or adjustment Z46.89
  malfunctioning K94.03
  status Z93.3
Colpitis (acute) — *see* Vaginitis
Colpocele N81.5
Colpocystitis — *see* Vaginitis
Colpospasm N94.2
Column, spinal, vertebral — *see* condition
Coma R40.20
  with
    motor response (none) R40.231 ☑
      abnormal extensor posturing to pain or noxious
        stimuli (< 2 years of age) R40.232 ☑
      abnormal flexure posturing to pain or noxious
        stimuli (0-5 years of age) R40.233 ☑
      extensor posturing to pain or noxious stimuli (2-5
        years of age) R40.232 ☑
      flexion/decorticate posturing (< 2 years of age)
        R40.233 ☑
      localizes pain (2-5 years of age) R40.235 ☑
      normal or spontaneous movement (< 2 years of
        age) R40.236 ☑
      obeys commands (2-5 years of age) R40.236 ☑
      score of
        1 R40.231 ☑
        2 R40.232 ☑
        3 R40.233 ☑
        4 R40.234 ☑
        5 R40.235 ☑
        6 R40.236 ☑
      withdraws from pain or noxious stimuli (0-5 years
        of age) R40.234 ☑
      withdraws to touch (< 2 years of age) R40.235 ☑
    opening of eyes (never) R40.211 ☑
      in response to
        pain R40.212 ☑
        sound R40.213 ☑
      score of
        1 R40.211 ☑
        2 R40.212 ☑
        3 R40.213 ☑
        4 R40.214 ☑
      spontaneous R40.214 ☑
    verbal response (none) R40.221 ☑
      confused conversation R40.224 ☑
      cooing or babbling or crying appropriately (<2
        years of age) R40.225 ☑
      inappropriate crying or screaming (< 2 years of
        age) R40.223 ☑
      inappropriate words (2-5 years of age) R40.224 ☑
      inappropriate words R40.223 ☑
      incomprehensible sounds (2-5 years of age)
        R40.222 ☑
      incomprehensible words R40.222 ☑

Coma — *continued*
  with — *continued*
    verbal response — *continued*
      irritable cries (< 2 years of age) R40.224 ☑
      moans/grunts to pain; restless (< 2 years old)
        R40.222 ☑
      oriented R40.225 ☑
      score of
        1 R40.221 ☑
        2 R40.222 ☑
        3 R40.223 ☑
        4 R40.224 ☑
        5 R40.225 ☑
      screaming (2-5 years of age) R40.223 ☑
      uses appropriate words (2-5 years of age)
        R40.225 ☑
  eclamptic — *see* Eclampsia
  epileptic — *see* Epilepsy
  Glasgow, scale score — *see* Glasgow coma scale
  hepatic — *see* Failure, hepatic, by type, with coma
  hyperglycemic (diabetic) — *see* Diabetes, by type, with
    hyperosmolarity, with coma
  hyperosmolar (diabetic) — *see* Diabetes, by type, with
    hyperosmolarity, with coma
  hypoglycemic (diabetic) — *see* Diabetes, by type, with
    hypoglycemia, with coma
    nondiabetic E15
  in diabetes — *see* Diabetes, coma
  insulin-induced — *see* Coma, hypoglycemic
  ketoacidotic (diabetic) — *see* Diabetes, by type, with
    ketoacidosis, with coma
  myxedematous E03.5
  newborn P91.5
  nontraumatic, due to underlying condition R40.2A
  persistent vegetative state R40.3
  secondary R40.2A
  specified NEC, without documented Glasgow coma scale
    score, or with partial Glasgow coma scale score
    reported R40.244 ☑
Comatose — *see* Coma
Combat fatigue F43.0
Combined — *see* condition
Comedo, comedones (giant) L70.0
Comedocarcinoma — *see also* Neoplasm, breast, malignant
  noninfiltrating
    breast D05.8- ☑
    specified site — *see* Neoplasm, in situ, by site
    unspecified site D05.8- ☑
Comedomastitis — *see* Ectasia, mammary duct
Comminuted fracture — *code as* Fracture, closed
Common
  arterial trunk Q20.0
  atrioventricular canal Q21.23
  atrium Q21.19
  cold (head) J00
  truncus (arteriosus) Q20.0
  variable immunodeficiency — *see* Immunodeficiency,
    common variable
  ventricle Q20.4
Commotio, commotion (current)
  brain — *see* Injury, intracranial, concussion
  cerebri — *see* Injury, intracranial, concussion
  retinae S05.8X- ☑
  spinal cord — *see* Injury, spinal cord, by region
  spinalis — *see* Injury, spinal cord, by region
Communication
  between
    base of aorta and pulmonary artery Q21.4
    left ventricle and right atrium Q20.5
    pericardial sac and pleural sac Q34.8
    pulmonary artery and pulmonary vein, congenital
      Q25.72
  congenital between uterus and digestive or urinary tract
    Q51.7
Compartment syndrome (deep) (posterior) (traumatic)
  T79.A0 ☑ (*following* T79.7)
  abdomen T79.A3 ☑ (*following* T79.7)
  lower extremity (hip, buttock, thigh, leg, foot, toes)
    T79.A2 ☑ (*following* T79.7)
  nontraumatic
    abdomen M79.A3 (*following* M79.7)
    lower extremity (hip, buttock, thigh, leg, foot, toes)
      M79.A2- ☑ (*following* M79.7)
    specified site NEC M79.A9 (*following* M79.7)
    upper extremity (shoulder, arm, forearm, wrist, hand,
      fingers) M79.A1- ☑ (*following* M79.7)
  specified site NEC T79.A9 ☑ (*following* T79.7)

Compartment syndrome — *continued*
  upper extremity (shoulder, arm, forearm, wrist, hand,
    fingers) T79.A1- ☑ (*following* T79.7)
Compensation
  failure — *see* Disease, heart
  neurosis, psychoneurosis — *see* Disorder, factitious
Complaint — *see also* Disease
  bowel, functional K59.9
    psychogenic F45.8
  intestine, functional K59.9
    psychogenic F45.8
  kidney — *see* Disease, renal
  miners' J60
Complete — *see* condition
Complex
  Addison-Schilder E71.528
  cardiorenal — *see* Hypertension, cardiorenal
  Costen's M26.69
  disseminated mycobacterium avium- intracellulare
    (DMAC) A31.2
  Eisenmenger's (ventricular septal defect) I27.83
  hypersexual F52.8
  jumped process, spine — *see* Dislocation, vertebra
  primary, tuberculous A15.7
  Schilder-Addison E71.528
  subluxation (vertebral) M99.19
    abdomen M99.19
    acromioclavicular M99.17
    cervical region M99.11
    cervicothoracic M99.11
    costochondral M99.18
    costovertebral M99.18
    head region M99.10
    hip M99.15
    lower extremity M99.16
    lumbar region M99.13
    lumbosacral M99.13
    occipitocervical M99.10
    pelvic region M99.15
    pubic M99.15
    rib cage M99.18
    sacral region M99.14
    sacrococcygeal M99.14
    sacroiliac M99.14
    specified NEC M99.19
    sternochondral M99.18
    sternoclavicular M99.17
    thoracic region M99.12
    thoracolumbar M99.12
    upper extremity M99.17
  Taussig-Bing (transposition, aorta and overriding pul-
    monary artery) Q20.1
Complication(s) (from) (of)
  accidental puncture or laceration during a procedure (of)
    — *see* Complications, intraoperative (intraproce-
    dural), puncture or laceration
  amputation stump (surgical) (late) NEC T87.9
    dehiscence T87.81
    infection or inflammation T87.40
      lower limb T87.4- ☑
      upper limb T87.4- ☑
    necrosis T87.50
      lower limb T87.5- ☑
      upper limb T87.5- ☑
    neuroma T87.30
      lower limb T87.3- ☑
      upper limb T87.3- ☑
    specified type NEC T87.89
  anastomosis (and bypass) — *see also* Complications,
    prosthetic device or implant
    intestinal (internal) NEC K91.89
      involving urinary tract N99.89
    urinary tract (involving intestinal tract) N99.89
    vascular — *see* Complications, cardiovascular device
      or implant
  anesthesia, anesthetic — *see also* Anesthesia, complica-
    tion T88.59 ☑
    brain, postpartum, puerperal O89.2
    cardiac
      in
        labor and delivery O74.2
        pregnancy O29.19- ☑
      postpartum, puerperal O89.1
    central nervous system
      in
        labor and delivery O74.3
        pregnancy O29.29- ☑
      postpartum, puerperal O89.2

Complication(s) — *continued*
anesthesia, anesthetic — *see also* Anesthesia, complication — *continued*
difficult or failed intubation T88.4 ☑
in pregnancy O29.6- ☑
failed sedation (conscious) (moderate) during procedure T88.52 ☑
general, unintended awareness during procedure
T88.53 ☑
hyperthermia, malignant T88.3 ☑
hypothermia T88.51 ☑
intubation failure T88.4 ☑
malignant hyperthermia T88.3 ☑
pulmonary
in
labor and delivery O74.1
pregnancy NEC O29.09- ☑
postpartum, puerperal O89.09
shock T88.2 ☑
spinal and epidural
in
labor and delivery NEC O74.6
headache O74.5
pregnancy NEC O29.5X- ☑
postpartum, puerperal NEC O89.5
headache O89.4
unintended awareness under general anesthesia
during procedure T88.53 ☑
anti-reflux device — *see* Complications, esophageal anti-
reflux device
aortic (bifurcation) graft — *see* Complications, graft,
vascular
aortocoronary (bypass) graft — *see* Complications,
coronary artery (bypass) graft
aortofemoral (bypass) graft — *see* Complications, extremity artery (bypass) graft
arteriovenous
fistula, surgically created T82.9 ☑
embolism T82.818 ☑
fibrosis T82.828 ☑
hemorrhage T82.838 ☑
infection or inflammation T82.7 ☑
mechanical
breakdown T82.510 ☑
displacement T82.520 ☑
leakage T82.530 ☑
malposition T82.520 ☑
obstruction T82.590 ☑
perforation T82.590 ☑
protrusion T82.590 ☑
pain T82.848 ☑
specified type NEC T82.898 ☑
stenosis T82.858 ☑
thrombosis T82.868 ☑
shunt, surgically created T82.9 ☑
embolism T82.818 ☑
fibrosis T82.828 ☑
hemorrhage T82.838 ☑
infection or inflammation T82.7 ☑
mechanical
breakdown T82.511 ☑
displacement T82.521 ☑
leakage T82.531 ☑
malposition T82.521 ☑
obstruction T82.591 ☑
perforation T82.591 ☑
protrusion T82.591 ☑
pain T82.848 ☑
specified type NEC T82.898 ☑
stenosis T82.858 ☑
thrombosis T82.868 ☑
arthroplasty — *see* Complications, joint prosthesis
artificial
fertilization or insemination N98.9
attempted introduction (of)
embryo in embryo transfer N98.3
ovum following in vitro fertilization N98.2
hyperstimulation of ovaries N98.1
infection N98.0
specified NEC N98.8
heart T82.9 ☑
embolism T82.817 ☑
fibrosis T82.827 ☑
hemorrhage T82.837 ☑
infection or inflammation T82.7 ☑

Complication(s) — *continued*
artificial — *continued*
heart — *continued*
mechanical
breakdown T82.512 ☑
displacement T82.522 ☑
leakage T82.532 ☑
malposition T82.522 ☑
obstruction T82.592 ☑
perforation T82.592 ☑
protrusion T82.592 ☑
pain T82.847 ☑
specified type NEC T82.897 ☑
stenosis T82.857 ☑
thrombosis T82.867 ☑
opening
cecostomy — *see* Complications, colostomy
colostomy — *see* Complications, colostomy
cystostomy — *see* Complications, cystostomy
enterostomy — *see* Complications, enterostomy
gastrostomy — *see* Complications, gastrostomy
ileostomy — *see* Complications, enterostomy
jejunostomy — *see* Complications, enterostomy
nephrostomy — *see* Complications, stoma, urinary
tract
tracheostomy — *see* Complications, tracheostomy
ureterostomy — *see* Complications, stoma, urinary
tract
urethrostomy — *see* Complications, stoma, urinary
tract
balloon implant or device
gastrointestinal T85.9 ☑
embolism T85.818 ☑
fibrosis T85.828 ☑
hemorrhage T85.838 ☑
infection and inflammation T85.79 ☑
pain T85.848 ☑
specified type NEC T85.898 ☑
stenosis T85.858 ☑
thrombosis T85.868 ☑
vascular (counterpulsation) T82.9 ☑
embolism T82.818 ☑
fibrosis T82.828 ☑
hemorrhage T82.838 ☑
infection or inflammation T82.7 ☑
mechanical
breakdown T82.513 ☑
displacement T82.523 ☑
leakage T82.533 ☑
malposition T82.523 ☑
obstruction T82.593 ☑
perforation T82.593 ☑
protrusion T82.593 ☑
pain T82.848 ☑
specified type NEC T82.898 ☑
stenosis T82.858 ☑
thrombosis T82.868 ☑
bariatric procedure
gastric band procedure K95.09
infection K95.01
specified procedure NEC K95.89
infection K95.81
bile duct implant (prosthetic) T85.9 ☑
embolism T85.818 ☑
fibrosis T85.828 ☑
hemorrhage T85.838 ☑
infection and inflammation T85.79 ☑
mechanical
breakdown T85.510 ☑
displacement T85.520 ☑
malfunction T85.510 ☑
malposition T85.520 ☑
obstruction T85.590 ☑
perforation T85.590 ☑
protrusion T85.590 ☑
specified NEC T85.590 ☑
pain T85.848 ☑
specified type NEC T85.898 ☑
stenosis T85.858 ☑
thrombosis T85.868 ☑
bladder device (auxiliary) — *see* Complications, genitourinary, device or implant, urinary system
bleeding (postoperative) — *see* Complication, postoperative, hemorrhage
intraoperative — *see* Complication, intraoperative,
hemorrhage

Complication(s) — *continued*
blood vessel graft — *see* Complications, graft, vascular
bone
device NEC T84.9 ☑
embolism T84.81 ☑
fibrosis T84.82 ☑
hemorrhage T84.83 ☑
infection or inflammation T84.7 ☑
mechanical
breakdown T84.318 ☑
displacement T84.328 ☑
malposition T84.328 ☑
obstruction T84.398 ☑
perforation T84.398 ☑
protrusion T84.398 ☑
pain T84.84 ☑
specified type NEC T84.89 ☑
stenosis T84.85 ☑
thrombosis T84.86 ☑
graft — *see* Complications, graft, bone
growth stimulator (electrode) — *see* Complications,
electronic stimulator device, bone
marrow transplant — *see* Complications, transplant,
bone, marrow
brain neurostimulator (electrode) — *see* Complications,
electronic stimulator device, brain
breast implant (prosthetic) T85.9 ☑
capsular contracture T85.44 ☑
embolism T85.818 ☑
fibrosis T85.828 ☑
hemorrhage T85.838 ☑
infection and inflammation T85.79 ☑
mechanical
breakdown T85.41 ☑
displacement T85.42 ☑
leakage T85.43 ☑
malposition T85.42 ☑
obstruction T85.49 ☑
perforation T85.49 ☑
protrusion T85.49 ☑
specified NEC T85.49 ☑
pain T85.848 ☑
specified type NEC T85.898 ☑
stenosis T85.858 ☑
thrombosis T85.868 ☑
bypass — *see also* Complications, prosthetic device or
implant
aortocoronary — *see* Complications, coronary artery
(bypass) graft
arterial — *see also* Complications, graft, vascular
extremity — *see* Complications, extremity artery
(bypass) graft
cardiac — *see also* Disease, heart
device, implant or graft T82.9 ☑
embolism T82.817 ☑
fibrosis T82.827 ☑
hemorrhage T82.837 ☑
infection or inflammation T82.7 ☑
valve prosthesis T82.6 ☑
mechanical
breakdown T82.519 ☑
specified device NEC T82.518 ☑
displacement T82.529 ☑
specified device NEC T82.528 ☑
leakage T82.539 ☑
specified device NEC T82.538 ☑
malposition T82.529 ☑
specified device NEC T82.528 ☑
obstruction T82.599 ☑
specified device NEC T82.598 ☑
perforation T82.599 ☑
specified device NEC T82.598 ☑
protrusion T82.599 ☑
specified device NEC T82.598 ☑
pain T82.847 ☑
specified type NEC T82.897 ☑
stenosis T82.857 ☑
thrombosis T82.867 ☑
cardiovascular device, graft or implant T82.9 ☑
aortic graft — *see* Complications, graft, vascular
arteriovenous
fistula, artificial — *see* Complication, arteriovenous,
fistula, surgically created
shunt — *see* Complication, arteriovenous, shunt,
surgically created
artificial heart — *see* Complication, artificial, heart

Index

Complication — Complication

Complication(s) — *continued*
  cardiovascular device, graft or implant — *continued*
    balloon (counterpulsation) device — *see* Complication, balloon implant, vascular
    carotid artery graft — *see* Complications, graft, vascular
    coronary bypass graft — *see* Complication, coronary artery (bypass) graft
    dialysis catheter (vascular) — *see* Complication, catheter, dialysis
    electronic T82.9
      electrode T82.9 ☑
        embolism T82.817 ☑
        fibrosis T82.827 ☑
        hemorrhage T82.837 ☑
        infection T82.7 ☑
        mechanical
          breakdown T82.110 ☑
          displacement T82.120 ☑
          leakage T82.190 ☑
          obstruction T82.190 ☑
          perforation T82.190 ☑
          protrusion T82.190 ☑
          specified type NEC T82.190 ☑
        pain T82.847 ☑
        specified NEC T82.897 ☑
        stenosis T82.857 ☑
        thrombosis T82.867 ☑
      embolism T82.817 ☑
      fibrosis T82.827 ☑
      hemorrhage T82.837 ☑
      infection T82.7 ☑
      mechanical
        breakdown T82.119 ☑
        displacement T82.129 ☑
        leakage T82.199 ☑
        obstruction T82.199 ☑
        perforation T82.199 ☑
        protrusion T82.199 ☑
        specified type NEC T82.199 ☑
      pain T82.847 ☑
      pulse generator T82.9 ☑
        embolism T82.817 ☑
        fibrosis T82.827 ☑
        hemorrhage T82.837 ☑
        infection T82.7 ☑
        mechanical
          breakdown T82.111 ☑
          displacement T82.121 ☑
          leakage T82.191 ☑
          obstruction T82.191 ☑
          perforation T82.191 ☑
          protrusion T82.191 ☑
          specified type NEC T82.191 ☑
        pain T82.847 ☑
        specified NEC T82.897 ☑
        stenosis T82.857 ☑
        thrombosis T82.867 ☑
      specified condition NEC T82.897 ☑
      specified device NEC T82.9 ☑
        embolism T82.817 ☑
        fibrosis T82.827 ☑
        hemorrhage T82.837 ☑
        infection T82.7 ☑
        mechanical
          breakdown T82.118 ☑
          displacement T82.128 ☑
          leakage T82.198 ☑
          obstruction T82.198 ☑
          perforation T82.198 ☑
          protrusion T82.198 ☑
          specified type NEC T82.198 ☑
        pain T82.847 ☑
        specified NEC T82.897 ☑
        stenosis T82.857 ☑
        thrombosis T82.867 ☑
      stenosis T82.857 ☑
      thrombosis T82.867 ☑
    extremity artery graft — *see* Complication, extremity artery (bypass) graft
    femoral artery graft — *see* Complication, extremity artery (bypass) graft
    heart
      transplant — *see* Complication, transplant, heart
      valve — *see* Complication, prosthetic device, heart valve

Complication(s) — *continued*
  cardiovascular device, graft or implant — *continued*
    heart — *continued*
      valve — *see* Complication, prosthetic device, heart valve — *continued*
        graft — *see* Complication, heart, valve, graft
      heart-lung transplant — *see* Complication, transplant, heart, with lung
      infection or inflammation T82.7 ☑
      umbrella device — *see* Complication, umbrella device, vascular
      vascular graft (or anastomosis) — *see* Complication, graft, vascular
    carotid artery (bypass) graft — *see* Complications, graft, vascular
    catheter (device) NEC — *see also* Complications, prosthetic device or implant
      cranial infusion
        infection and inflammation T85.735 ☑
        mechanical
          breakdown T85.610 ☑
          displacement T85.620 ☑
          leakage T85.630 ☑
          malfunction T85.690 ☑
          malposition T85.620 ☑
          obstruction T85.690 ☑
          perforation T85.690 ☑
          protrusion T85.690 ☑
          specified NEC T85.690 ☑
      cystostomy T83.9 ☑
        embolism T83.81 ☑
        fibrosis T83.82 ☑
        hemorrhage T83.83 ☑
        infection and inflammation T83.510 ☑
        mechanical
          breakdown T83.010 ☑
          displacement T83.020 ☑
          leakage T83.030 ☑
          malposition T83.020 ☑
          obstruction T83.090 ☑
          perforation T83.090 ☑
          protrusion T83.090 ☑
          specified NEC T83.090 ☑
        pain T83.84 ☑
        specified type NEC T83.89 ☑
        stenosis T83.85 ☑
        thrombosis T83.86 ☑
      dialysis (vascular) T82.9 ☑
        embolism T82.818 ☑
        fibrosis T82.828 ☑
        hemorrhage T82.838 ☑
        infection and inflammation T82.7 ☑
        intraperitoneal — *see* Complications, catheter, intraperitoneal dialysis
        mechanical
          breakdown T82.41 ☑
          displacement T82.42 ☑
          leakage T82.43 ☑
          malposition T82.42 ☑
          obstruction T82.49 ☑
          perforation T82.49 ☑
          protrusion T82.49 ☑
        pain T82.848 ☑
        specified type NEC T82.898 ☑
        stenosis T82.858 ☑
        thrombosis T82.868 ☑
      epidural infusion T85.9 ☑
        embolism T85.810 ☑
        fibrosis T85.820 ☑
        hemorrhage T85.830 ☑
        infection and inflammation T85.735 ☑
        mechanical
          breakdown T85.610 ☑
          displacement T85.620 ☑
          leakage T85.630 ☑
          malfunction T85.690 ☑
          malposition T85.620 ☑
          obstruction T85.690 ☑
          perforation T85.690 ☑
          protrusion T85.690 ☑
          specified NEC T85.690 ☑
        pain T85.840 ☑
        specified type NEC T85.890 ☑
        stenosis T85.850 ☑
        thrombosis T85.860 ☑
      intraperitoneal dialysis T85.9 ☑

Complication(s) — *continued*
  catheter — *see also* Complications, prosthetic device or implant — *continued*
    intraperitoneal dialysis — *continued*
      embolism T85.818 ☑
      fibrosis T85.828 ☑
      hemorrhage T85.838 ☑
      infection and inflammation T85.71 ☑
      mechanical
        breakdown T85.611 ☑
        displacement T85.621 ☑
        leakage T85.631 ☑
        malfunction T85.611 ☑
        malposition T85.621 ☑
        obstruction T85.691 ☑
        perforation T85.691 ☑
        protrusion T85.691 ☑
        specified NEC T85.691 ☑
      pain T85.848 ☑
      specified type NEC T85.898 ☑
      stenosis T85.858 ☑
      thrombosis T85.868 ☑
    intrathecal infusion
      infection and inflammation T85.735 ☑
      mechanical
        breakdown T85.610 ☑
        displacement T85.620 ☑
        leakage T85.630 ☑
        malfunction T85.690 ☑
        malposition T85.620 ☑
        obstruction T85.690 ☑
        perforation T85.690 ☑
        protrusion T85.690 ☑
        specified NEC T85.690 ☑
    intravenous infusion T82.9 ☑
      embolism T82.818 ☑
      fibrosis T82.828 ☑
      hemorrhage T82.838 ☑
      infection or inflammation T82.7 ☑
      mechanical
        breakdown T82.514 ☑
        displacement T82.524 ☑
        leakage T82.534 ☑
        malposition T82.524 ☑
        obstruction T82.594 ☑
        perforation T82.594 ☑
        protrusion T82.594 ☑
      pain T82.848 ☑
      specified type NEC T82.898 ☑
      stenosis T82.858 ☑
      thrombosis T82.868 ☑
    spinal infusion
      infection and inflammation T85.735 ☑
      mechanical
        breakdown T85.610 ☑
        displacement T85.620 ☑
        leakage T85.630 ☑
        malfunction T85.690 ☑
        malposition T85.620 ☑
        obstruction T85.690 ☑
        perforation T85.690 ☑
        protrusion T85.690 ☑
        specified NEC T85.690 ☑
    subarachnoid infusion
      infection and inflammation T85.735 ☑
      mechanical
        breakdown T85.610 ☑
        displacement T85.620 ☑
        leakage T85.630 ☑
        malfunction T85.690 ☑
        malposition T85.620 ☑
        obstruction T85.690 ☑
        perforation T85.690 ☑
        protrusion T85.690 ☑
        specified NEC T85.690 ☑
    subdural infusion T85.9 ☑
      embolism T85.810 ☑
      fibrosis T85.820 ☑
      hemorrhage T85.830 ☑
      infection and inflammation T85.735 ☑
      mechanical
        breakdown T85.610 ☑
        displacement T85.620 ☑
        leakage T85.630 ☑
        malfunction T85.690 ☑

Complication(s) — *continued*
  catheter — *see also* Complications, prosthetic device or implant — *continued*
    subdural infusion — *continued*
      mechanical — *continued*
        malposition T85.620 ☑
        obstruction T85.690 ☑
        perforation T85.690 ☑
        protrusion T85.690 ☑
        specified NEC T85.690 ☑
      pain T85.840 ☑
      specified type NEC T85.890 ☑
      stenosis T85.850 ☑
      thrombosis T85.860 ☑
    urethral T83.9 ☑
      displacement T83.028 ☑
      embolism T83.81 ☑
      fibrosis T83.82 ☑
      hemorrhage T83.83 ☑
      indwelling
        breakdown T83.011 ☑
        displacement T83.021 ☑
        infection and inflammation T83.511 ☑
        leakage T83.031 ☑
        specified complication NEC T83.091 ☑
      infection and inflammation T83.511 ☑
      leakage T83.038 ☑
      malposition T83.028 ☑
      mechanical
        breakdown T83.011 ☑
      obstruction (mechanical) T83.091 ☑
      pain T83.84 ☑
      perforation T83.091 ☑
      protrusion T83.091 ☑
      specified type NEC T83.091 ☑
      stenosis T83.85 ☑
      thrombosis T83.86 ☑
    urinary NEC
      breakdown T83.018 ☑
      displacement T83.028 ☑
      infection and inflammation T83.518 ☑
      leakage T83.038 ☑
      specified complication NEC T83.098 ☑
  cecostomy (stoma) — *see* Complications, colostomy
  cesarean delivery wound NEC O90.89
    disruption O90.0
    hematoma O90.2
    infection (following delivery) O86.00
  chemotherapy (antineoplastic) NEC T88.7
  chimeric antigen receptor (CAR-T) cell therapy T80.82 ☑
  chin implant (prosthetic) — *see* Complication, prosthetic device or implant, specified NEC
  circulatory system I99.8
    intraoperative I97.88
    postprocedural I97.89
      following cardiac surgery — *see also* Infarct, myocardium, associated with revascularization procedure I97.19- ☑
        postcardiotomy syndrome I97.0
      hypertension I97.3
      lymphedema after mastectomy I97.2
      postcardiotomy syndrome I97.0
      specified NEC I97.89
  colostomy (stoma) K94.00
    hemorrhage K94.01
    infection K94.02
    malfunction K94.03
    mechanical K94.03
    specified complication NEC K94.09
  contraceptive device, intrauterine — *see* Complications, intrauterine, contraceptive device
  cord (umbilical) — *see* Complications, umbilical cord
  corneal graft — *see* Complications, graft, cornea
  coronary artery (bypass) graft T82.9
    atherosclerosis — *see* Arteriosclerosis, coronary (artery)
    embolism T82.817 ☑
    fibrosis T82.827 ☑
    hemorrhage T82.837 ☑
    infection and inflammation T82.7 ☑
    mechanical
      breakdown T82.211 ☑
      displacement T82.212 ☑
      leakage T82.213 ☑
      malposition T82.212 ☑
      obstruction T82.218 ☑

Complication(s) — *continued*
  coronary artery graft — *continued*
    mechanical — *continued*
      perforation T82.218 ☑
      protrusion T82.218 ☑
      specified NEC T82.218 ☑
    pain T82.847 ☑
    specified type NEC T82.898 ☑
    stenosis T82.857 ☑
    thrombosis T82.867 ☑
  counterpulsation device (balloon), intra-aortic — *see* Complications, balloon implant, vascular
  cystostomy (stoma) N99.518
    catheter — *see* Complications, catheter, cystostomy
    hemorrhage N99.510
    infection N99.511
    malfunction N99.512
    specified type NEC N99.518
  delivery — *see also* Complications, obstetric O75.9
    procedure (instrumental) (manual) (surgical) O75.4
    specified NEC O75.89
  dialysis (peritoneal) (renal) — *see also* Complications, infusion
    catheter (vascular) — *see* Complication, catheter, dialysis
    peritoneal, intraperitoneal — *see* Complications, catheter, intraperitoneal
  dorsal column (spinal) neurostimulator — *see* Complications, electronic stimulator device, spinal cord
  drug NEC T88.7 ☑
  ear procedure — *see also* Disorder, ear
    intraoperative H95.88
      hematoma — *see* Complications, intraoperative, hemorrhage (hematoma) (of), ear
      hemorrhage — *see* Complications, intraoperative, hemorrhage (hematoma) (of), ear
      laceration — *see* Complications, intraoperative, puncture or laceration, ear
      specified NEC H95.88
    postoperative H95.89
      external ear canal stenosis H95.81- ☑
      hematoma — *see* Complications, postprocedural, hematoma (of), ear
      hemorrhage — *see* Complications, postprocedural, hemorrhage (of), ear
      postmastoidectomy — *see* Complications, postmastoidectomy
      seroma — *see* Complications, postprocedural, seroma (of), mastoid process
      specified NEC H95.89
  ectopic pregnancy O08.9
    damage to pelvic organs O08.6
    embolism O08.2
    genital infection O08.0
    hemorrhage (delayed) (excessive) O08.1
    metabolic disorder O08.5
    renal failure O08.4
    shock O08.3
    specified type NEC O08.0
    venous complication NEC O08.7
  electronic stimulator device
    bladder (urinary) — *see* Complications, electronic stimulator device, urinary
    bone T84.9 ☑
      breakdown T84.310 ☑
      displacement T84.320 ☑
      embolism T84.81 ☑
      fibrosis T84.82 ☑
      hemorrhage T84.83 ☑
      infection or inflammation T84.7 ☑
      malfunction T84.310 ☑
      malposition T84.320 ☑
      mechanical NEC T84.390 ☑
      obstruction T84.390 ☑
      pain T84.84 ☑
      perforation T84.390 ☑
      protrusion T84.390 ☑
      specified type NEC T84.89 ☑
      stenosis T84.85 ☑
      thrombosis T84.86 ☑
    brain T85.9 ☑
      embolism T85.810 ☑
      fibrosis T85.820 ☑
      hemorrhage T85.830 ☑
      infection and inflammation T85.731 ☑
      mechanical
        breakdown T85.110 ☑

Complication(s) — *continued*
  electronic stimulator device — *continued*
    brain — *continued*
      mechanical — *continued*
        displacement T85.120 ☑
        leakage T85.190 ☑
        malposition T85.120 ☑
        obstruction T85.190 ☑
        perforation T85.190 ☑
        protrusion T85.190 ☑
        specified NEC T85.190 ☑
      pain T85.840 ☑
      specified type NEC T85.890 ☑
      stenosis T85.850 ☑
      thrombosis T85.860 ☑
    cardiac (defibrillator) (pacemaker) — *see* Complications, cardiovascular device or implant, electronic
    generator (brain) (gastric) (peripheral) (sacral) (spinal)
      breakdown T85.113 ☑
      displacement T85.123 ☑
      leakage T85.193 ☑
      malposition T85.123 ☑
      obstruction T85.193 ☑
      perforation T85.193 ☑
      protrusion T85.193 ☑
      specified type NEC T85.193 ☑
    muscle T84.9 ☑
      breakdown T84.418 ☑
      displacement T84.428 ☑
      embolism T84.81 ☑
      fibrosis T84.82 ☑
      hemorrhage T84.83 ☑
      infection or inflammation T84.7 ☑
      mechanical NEC T84.498 ☑
      pain T84.84 ☑
      specified type NEC T84.89 ☑
      stenosis T84.85 ☑
      thrombosis T84.86 ☑
    nervous system T85.9 ☑
      brain — *see* Complications, electronic stimulator device, brain
      cranial nerve — *see* Complications, electronic stimulator device, peripheral nerve
      embolism T85.810 ☑
      fibrosis T85.820 ☑
      gastric nerve — *see* Complications, electronic stimulator device, peripheral nerve
      hemorrhage T85.830 ☑
      infection and inflammation T85.738 ☑
      mechanical
        breakdown T85.118 ☑
        displacement T85.128 ☑
        leakage T85.199 ☑
        malposition T85.128 ☑
        obstruction T85.199 ☑
        perforation T85.199 ☑
        protrusion T85.199 ☑
        specified NEC T85.199 ☑
      pain T85.840 ☑
      peripheral nerve — *see* Complications, electronic stimulator device, peripheral nerve
      sacral nerve — *see* Complications, electronic stimulator device, peripheral nerve
      specified type NEC T85.890 ☑
      spinal cord — *see* Complications, electronic stimulator device, spinal cord
      stenosis T85.850 ☑
      thrombosis T85.860 ☑
      vagal nerve — *see* Complications, electronic stimulator device, peripheral nerve
    peripheral nerve T85.9 ☑
      embolism T85.810 ☑
      fibrosis T85.820 ☑
      hemorrhage T85.830 ☑
      infection and inflammation T85.732 ☑
      mechanical
        breakdown T85.111 ☑
        displacement T85.121 ☑
        leakage T85.191 ☑
        malposition T85.121 ☑
        obstruction T85.191 ☑
        perforation T85.191 ☑
        protrusion T85.191 ☑
        specified NEC T85.191 ☑
      pain T85.840 ☑

Complication(s) — *continued*
  electronic stimulator device — *continued*
    peripheral nerve — *continued*
      specified type NEC T85.890 ☑
      stenosis T85.850 ☑
      thrombosis T85.860 ☑
    spinal cord T85.9 ☑
      embolism T85.810 ☑
      fibrosis T85.820 ☑
      hemorrhage T85.830 ☑
      infection and inflammation T85.733 ☑
      mechanical
        breakdown T85.112 ☑
        displacement T85.122 ☑
        leakage T85.192 ☑
        malposition T85.122 ☑
        obstruction T85.192 ☑
        perforation T85.192 ☑
        protrusion T85.192 ☑
        specified NEC T85.192 ☑
      pain T85.840 ☑
      specified type NEC T85.890 ☑
      stenosis T85.850 ☑
      thrombosis T85.860 ☑
    urinary T83.9 ☑
      embolism T83.81 ☑
      fibrosis T83.82 ☑
      hemorrhage T83.83 ☑
      infection and inflammation T83.598 ☑
      mechanical
        breakdown T83.110 ☑
        displacement T83.120 ☑
        malposition T83.120 ☑
        perforation T83.190 ☑
        protrusion T83.190 ☑
        specified NEC T83.190 ☑
      pain T83.84 ☑
      specified type NEC T83.89 ☑
      stenosis T83.85 ☑
      thrombosis T83.86 ☑
  electroshock therapy T88.9 ☑
    specified NEC T88.8 ☑
  endocrine E34.9
    postprocedural
      adrenal hypofunction E89.6
      hypoinsulinemia E89.1
      hypoparathyroidism E89.2
      hypopituitarism E89.3
      hypothyroidism E89.0
      ovarian failure E89.40
        asymptomatic E89.40
        symptomatic E89.41
      specified NEC E89.89
      testicular hypofunction E89.5
  endodontic treatment NEC M27.59
  enterostomy (stoma) K94.10
    hemorrhage K94.11
    infection K94.12
    malfunction K94.13
    mechanical K94.13
    specified complication NEC K94.19
  episiotomy, disruption O90.1
  esophageal anti-reflux device T85.9 ☑
    embolism T85.818 ☑
    fibrosis T85.828 ☑
    hemorrhage T85.838 ☑
    infection and inflammation T85.79 ☑
    mechanical
      breakdown T85.511 ☑
      displacement T85.521 ☑
      malfunction T85.511 ☑
      malposition T85.521 ☑
      obstruction T85.591 ☑
      perforation T85.591 ☑
      protrusion T85.591 ☑
      specified NEC T85.591 ☑
    pain T85.848 ☑
    specified type NEC T85.898 ☑
    stenosis T85.858 ☑
    thrombosis T85.868 ☑
  esophagostomy K94.30
    hemorrhage K94.31
    infection K94.32
    malfunction K94.33
    mechanical K94.33
    specified complication NEC K94.39

Complication(s) — *continued*
  extracorporeal circulation T80.90 ☑
  extremity artery (bypass) graft T82.9 ☑
    arteriosclerosis — *see* Arteriosclerosis, extremities,
        bypass graft
    embolism T82.818 ☑
    fibrosis T82.828 ☑
    hemorrhage T82.838 ☑
    infection and inflammation T82.7 ☑
    mechanical
      breakdown T82.318 ☑
        femoral artery T82.312 ☑
      displacement T82.328 ☑
        femoral artery T82.322 ☑
      leakage T82.338 ☑
        femoral artery T82.332 ☑
      malposition T82.328 ☑
        femoral artery T82.322 ☑
      obstruction T82.398 ☑
        femoral artery T82.392 ☑
      perforation T82.398 ☑
        femoral artery T82.392 ☑
      protrusion T82.398 ☑
        femoral artery T82.392 ☑
    pain T82.848 ☑
    specified type NEC T82.898 ☑
    stenosis T82.858 ☑
    thrombosis T82.868 ☑
  eye H57.9
    corneal graft — *see* Complications, graft, cornea
    implant (prosthetic) T85.9 ☑
      embolism T85.818 ☑
      fibrosis T85.828 ☑
      hemorrhage T85.838 ☑
      infection and inflammation T85.79 ☑
      mechanical
        breakdown T85.318 ☑
        displacement T85.328 ☑
        leakage T85.398 ☑
        malposition T85.328 ☑
        obstruction T85.398 ☑
        perforation T85.398 ☑
        protrusion T85.398 ☑
        specified NEC T85.398 ☑
      pain T85.848 ☑
      specified type NEC T85.898 ☑
      stenosis T85.858 ☑
      thrombosis T85.868 ☑
    intraocular lens — *see* Complications, intraocular lens
    orbital prosthesis — *see* Complications, orbital pros-
        thesis
  female genital N94.9
    device, implant or graft NEC — *see* Complications,
        genitourinary, device or implant, genital tract
  femoral artery (bypass) graft — *see* Complication, extrem-
      ity artery (bypass) graft
  fixation device, internal (orthopedic) T84.9 ☑
    infection and inflammation T84.60 ☑
      arm T84.61- ☑
        humerus T84.61- ☑
        radius T84.61- ☑
        ulna T84.61- ☑
      leg T84.629 ☑
        femur T84.62- ☑
        fibula T84.62- ☑
        tibia T84.62- ☑
      specified site NEC T84.89 ☑
      spine T84.63 ☑
    mechanical
      breakdown
        limb T84.119 ☑
          carpal T84.210 ☑
          femur T84.11- ☑
          fibula T84.11- ☑
          humerus T84.11- ☑
          metacarpal T84.210 ☑
          metatarsal T84.213 ☑
          phalanx
            foot T84.213 ☑
            hand T84.210 ☑
          radius T84.11- ☑
          tarsal T84.213 ☑
          tibia T84.11- ☑
          ulna T84.11- ☑
        specified bone NEC T84.218 ☑
        spine T84.216 ☑

Complication(s) — *continued*
  fixation device, internal — *continued*
    mechanical — *continued*
      displacement
        limb T84.129 ☑
          carpal T84.220 ☑
          femur T84.12- ☑
          fibula T84.12- ☑
          humerus T84.12- ☑
          metacarpal T84.220 ☑
          metatarsal T84.223 ☑
          phalanx
            foot T84.223 ☑
            hand T84.220 ☑
          radius T84.12- ☑
          tarsal T84.223 ☑
          tibia T84.12- ☑
          ulna T84.12- ☑
        specified bone NEC T84.228 ☑
        spine T84.226 ☑
      malposition — *see* Complications, fixation device,
          internal, mechanical, displacement
      obstruction — *see* Complications, fixation device,
          internal, mechanical, specified type NEC
      perforation — *see* Complications, fixation device,
          internal, mechanical, specified type NEC
      protrusion — *see* Complications, fixation device,
          internal, mechanical, specified type NEC
      specified type NEC
        limb T84.199 ☑
          carpal T84.290 ☑
          femur T84.19- ☑
          fibula T84.19- ☑
          humerus T84.19- ☑
          metacarpal T84.290 ☑
          metatarsal T84.293 ☑
          phalanx
            foot T84.293 ☑
            hand T84.290 ☑
          radius T84.19- ☑
          tarsal T84.293 ☑
          tibia T84.19- ☑
          ulna T84.19- ☑
        specified bone NEC T84.298 ☑
        vertebra T84.296 ☑
    specified type NEC T84.89 ☑
      embolism T84.81 ☑
      fibrosis T84.82 ☑
      hemorrhage T84.83 ☑
      pain T84.84 ☑
      specified complication NEC T84.89 ☑
      stenosis T84.85 ☑
      thrombosis T84.86 ☑
  following
    acute myocardial infarction NEC I23.8
      aneurysm (false) (of cardiac wall) (of heart wall)
          (ruptured) I23.3
      angina I23.7
      atrial
        septal defect I23.1
        thrombosis I23.6
      cardiac wall rupture I23.3
      chordae tendinae rupture I23.4
      defect
        septal
          atrial (heart) I23.1
          ventricular (heart) I23.2
      hemopericardium I23.0
      papillary muscle rupture I23.5
      rupture
        cardiac wall I23.3
          with hemopericardium I23.0
        chordae tendineae I23.4
        papillary muscle I23.5
      specified NEC I23.8
      thrombosis
        atrium I23.6
        auricular appendage I23.6
        ventricle (heart) I23.6
      ventricular
        septal defect I23.2
        thrombosis I23.6
    ectopic or molar pregnancy O08.9
      cardiac arrest O08.81
      sepsis O08.82
      specified type NEC O08.89
      urinary tract infection O08.83

☑ **Additional Character Required — Refer to the Tabular List for Character Selection**

Complication(s) — *continued*
following — *continued*
termination of pregnancy — *see* Abortion
gastrointestinal K92.9
bile duct prosthesis — *see* Complications, bile duct implant
esophageal anti-reflux device — *see* Complications, esophageal anti-reflux device
postoperative
colostomy — *see* Complications, colostomy
dumping syndrome K91.1
enterostomy — *see* Complications, enterostomy
gastrostomy — *see* Complications, gastrostomy
malabsorption NEC K91.2
obstruction — *see also* Obstruction, intestine, postoperative K91.30
postcholecystectomy syndrome K91.5
specified NEC K91.89
vomiting after GI surgery K91.0
prosthetic device or implant
bile duct prosthesis — *see* Complications, bile duct implant
esophageal anti-reflux device — *see* Complications, esophageal anti-reflux device
specified type NEC
embolism T85.818 ☑
fibrosis T85.828 ☑
hemorrhage T85.838 ☑
mechanical
breakdown T85.518 ☑
displacement T85.528 ☑
malfunction T85.518 ☑
malposition T85.528 ☑
obstruction T85.598 ☑
perforation T85.598 ☑
protrusion T85.598 ☑
specified NEC T85.598 ☑
pain T85.848 ☑
specified complication NEC T85.898 ☑
stenosis T85.858 ☑
thrombosis T85.868 ☑
gastrostomy (stoma) K94.20
hemorrhage K94.21
infection K94.22
malfunction K94.23
mechanical K94.23
specified complication NEC K94.29
genitourinary
device or implant T83.9 ☑
genital tract T83.9 ☑
infection or inflammation T83.69 ☑
intrauterine contraceptive device — *see* Complications, intrauterine, contraceptive device
mechanical — *see* Complications, by device, mechanical
mesh — *see* Complications, prosthetic device or implant, mesh
penile prosthesis — *see* Complications, prosthetic device, penile
specified type NEC T83.89 ☑
embolism T83.81 ☑
fibrosis T83.82 ☑
hemorrhage T83.83 ☑
pain T83.84 ☑
specified complication NEC T83.89 ☑
stenosis T83.85 ☑
thrombosis T83.86 ☑
vaginal mesh — *see* Complications, prosthetic device or implant, mesh
urinary system T83.9 ☑
cystostomy catheter — *see* Complication, catheter, cystostomy
electronic stimulator — *see* Complications, electronic stimulator device, urinary
indwelling urethral catheter — *see* Complications, catheter, urethral, indwelling
infection or inflammation T83.598 ☑
indwelling urethral catheter T83.511 ☑
kidney transplant — *see* Complication, transplant, kidney
organ graft — *see* Complication, graft, urinary organ
specified type NEC T83.89 ☑
embolism T83.81 ☑
fibrosis T83.82 ☑
hemorrhage T83.83 ☑

Complication(s) — *continued*
genitourinary — *continued*
device or implant — *continued*
urinary system — *continued*
specified type — *continued*
mechanical T83.198 ☑
breakdown T83.118 ☑
displacement T83.128 ☑
malfunction T83.118 ☑
malposition T83.128 ☑
obstruction T83.198 ☑
perforation T83.198 ☑
protrusion T83.198 ☑
specified NEC T83.198 ☑
sphincter implant — *see* Complications, implant, urinary sphincter
sphincter, implanted T83.191 ☑
stent (ileal conduit) (nephroureteral) T83.193 ☑
pain T83.84 ☑
specified complication NEC T83.89 ☑
stenosis T83.85 ☑
thrombosis T83.86 ☑
ureteral indwelling T83.192 ☑
postprocedural
pelvic peritoneal adhesions N99.4
renal failure N99.0
specified NEC N99.89
stoma — *see* Complications, stoma, urinary tract
urethral stricture — *see* Stricture, urethra, postprocedural
vaginal
adhesions N99.2
vault prolapse N99.3
graft (bypass) (patch) — *see also* Complications, prosthetic device or implant
aorta — *see* Complications, graft, vascular
arterial — *see* Complication, graft, vascular
bone T86.839
failure T86.831
infection T86.832
mechanical T84.318 ☑
breakdown T84.318 ☑
displacement T84.328 ☑
protrusion T84.398 ☑
specified type NEC T84.398 ☑
rejection T86.830
specified type NEC T86.838
carotid artery — *see* Complications, graft, vascular
cornea T86.849-
failure T86.841-
infection T86.842-
mechanical T85.398 ☑
breakdown T85.318 ☑
displacement T85.328 ☑
protrusion T85.398 ☑
specified type NEC T85.398 ☑
rejection T86.840-
retroprosthetic membrane T85.398 ☑
specified type NEC T86.848-
femoral artery (bypass) — *see* Complication, extremity artery (bypass) graft
genital organ or tract — *see* Complications, genitourinary, device or implant, genital tract
muscle T84.9 ☑
breakdown T84.410 ☑
displacement T84.420 ☑
embolism T84.81 ☑
fibrosis T84.82 ☑
hemorrhage T84.83 ☑
infection and inflammation T84.7 ☑
mechanical NEC T84.490 ☑
pain T84.84 ☑
specified type NEC T84.89 ☑
stenosis T84.85 ☑
thrombosis T84.86 ☑
nerve — *see* Complication, prosthetic device or implant, specified NEC
skin — *see* Complications, prosthetic device or implant, skin graft
tendon T84.9 ☑
breakdown T84.410 ☑
displacement T84.420 ☑
embolism T84.81 ☑
fibrosis T84.82 ☑
hemorrhage T84.83 ☑

Complication(s) — *continued*
graft — *see also* Complications, prosthetic device or implant — *continued*
tendon — *continued*
infection and inflammation T84.7 ☑
mechanical NEC T84.490 ☑
pain T84.84 ☑
specified type NEC T84.89 ☑
stenosis T84.85 ☑
thrombosis T84.86 ☑
urinary organ T83.9 ☑
embolism T83.81 ☑
fibrosis T83.82 ☑
hemorrhage T83.83 ☑
infection and inflammation T83.598 ☑
indwelling urethral catheter T83.511 ☑
mechanical
breakdown T83.21 ☑
displacement T83.22 ☑
erosion T83.24 ☑
exposure T83.25 ☑
leakage T83.23 ☑
malposition T83.22 ☑
obstruction T83.29 ☑
perforation T83.29 ☑
protrusion T83.29 ☑
specified NEC T83.29 ☑
pain T83.84 ☑
specified type NEC T83.89 ☑
stenosis T83.85 ☑
thrombosis T83.86 ☑
vascular T82.9 ☑
embolism T82.818 ☑
femoral artery — *see* Complication, extremity artery (bypass) graft
fibrosis T82.828 ☑
hemorrhage T82.838 ☑
mechanical
breakdown T82.319 ☑
aorta (bifurcation) T82.310 ☑
carotid artery T82.311 ☑
specified vessel NEC T82.318 ☑
displacement T82.329 ☑
aorta (bifurcation) T82.320 ☑
carotid artery T82.321 ☑
specified vessel NEC T82.328 ☑
leakage T82.339 ☑
aorta (bifurcation) T82.330 ☑
carotid artery T82.331 ☑
specified vessel NEC T82.338 ☑
malposition T82.329 ☑
aorta (bifurcation) T82.320 ☑
carotid artery T82.321 ☑
specified vessel NEC T82.328 ☑
obstruction T82.399 ☑
aorta (bifurcation) T82.390 ☑
carotid artery T82.391 ☑
specified vessel NEC T82.398 ☑
perforation T82.399 ☑
aorta (bifurcation) T82.390 ☑
carotid artery T82.391 ☑
specified vessel NEC T82.398 ☑
protrusion T82.399 ☑
aorta (bifurcation) T82.390 ☑
carotid artery T82.391 ☑
specified vessel NEC T82.398 ☑
pain T82.848 ☑
specified complication NEC T82.898 ☑
stenosis T82.858 ☑
thrombosis T82.868 ☑
heart I51.9
assist device
infection and inflammation T82.7 ☑
following acute myocardial infarction — *see* Complications, following, acute myocardial infarction
postoperative — *see* Complications, circulatory system
transplant — *see* Complication, transplant, heart
and lung(s) — *see* Complications, transplant, heart, with lung
valve
graft (biological) T82.9 ☑
embolism T82.817 ☑
fibrosis T82.827 ☑
hemorrhage T82.837 ☑
infection and inflammation T82.7 ☑

Complication(s) — *continued*
　heart — *continued*
　　valve — *continued*
　　　graft — *continued*
　　　　mechanical T82.228 ☑
　　　　　breakdown T82.221 ☑
　　　　　displacement T82.222 ☑
　　　　　leakage T82.223 ☑
　　　　　malposition T82.222 ☑
　　　　　obstruction T82.228 ☑
　　　　　perforation T82.228 ☑
　　　　　protrusion T82.228 ☑
　　　　pain T82.847 ☑
　　　　specified type NEC T82.897 ☑
　　　　stenosis T82.857 ☑
　　　　thrombosis T82.867 ☑
　　　prosthesis T82.9 ☑
　　　　embolism T82.817 ☑
　　　　fibrosis T82.827 ☑
　　　　hemorrhage T82.837 ☑
　　　　infection or inflammation T82.6 ☑
　　　　mechanical T82.09 ☑
　　　　　breakdown T82.01 ☑
　　　　　displacement T82.02 ☑
　　　　　leakage T82.03 ☑
　　　　　malposition T82.02 ☑
　　　　　obstruction T82.09 ☑
　　　　　perforation T82.09 ☑
　　　　　protrusion T82.09 ☑
　　　　pain T82.847 ☑
　　　　specified type NEC T82.897 ☑
　　　　　mechanical T82.09 ☑
　　　　stenosis T82.857 ☑
　　　　thrombosis T82.867 ☑
　hematoma
　　intraoperative — *see* Complication, intraoperative, hemorrhage
　　postprocedural — *see* Complication, postprocedural, hematoma
　hemodialysis — *see* Complications, dialysis
　hemorrhage
　　intraoperative — *see* Complication, intraoperative, hemorrhage
　　postprocedural — *see* Complication, postprocedural, hemorrhage
　IEC (immune effector cellular) therapy T80.82 ☑
　ileostomy (stoma) — *see* Complications, enterostomy
　immune effector cellular (IEC) therapy T80.82 ☑
　immunization (procedure) — *see* Complications, vaccination
　implant — *see also* Complications, by site and type
　　urinary sphincter T83.9 ☑
　　　embolism T83.81 ☑
　　　fibrosis T83.82 ☑
　　　hemorrhage T83.83 ☑
　　　infection and inflammation T83.591 ☑
　　　mechanical
　　　　breakdown T83.111 ☑
　　　　displacement T83.121 ☑
　　　　leakage T83.191 ☑
　　　　malposition T83.121 ☑
　　　　obstruction T83.191 ☑
　　　　perforation T83.191 ☑
　　　　protrusion T83.191 ☑
　　　　specified NEC T83.191 ☑
　　　pain T83.84 ☑
　　　specified type NEC T83.89 ☑
　　　stenosis T83.85 ☑
　　　thrombosis T83.86 ☑
　infusion (procedure) T80.90 ☑
　　air embolism T80.0 ☑
　　blood — *see* Complications, transfusion
　　catheter — *see* Complications, catheter
　　infection T80.29 ☑
　　pump — *see* Complications, cardiovascular, device or implant
　　sepsis T80.29 ☑
　　serum reaction — *see also* Reaction, serum T80.69 ☑
　　　anaphylactic shock — *see also* Shock, anaphylactic T80.59 ☑
　　specified type NEC T80.89 ☑
　inhalation therapy NEC T81.81 ☑
　injection (procedure) T80.90 ☑
　　drug reaction — *see* Reaction, drug
　　infection T80.29 ☑
　　sepsis T80.29 ☑

Complication(s) — *continued*
　injection — *continued*
　　serum (prophylactic) (therapeutic) — *see* Complications, vaccination
　　specified type NEC T80.89 ☑
　　vaccine (any) — *see* Complications, vaccination
　inoculation (any) — *see* Complications, vaccination
　insulin pump
　　infection and inflammation T85.72 ☑
　　mechanical
　　　breakdown T85.614 ☑
　　　displacement T85.624 ☑
　　　leakage T85.633 ☑
　　　malposition T85.624 ☑
　　　obstruction T85.694 ☑
　　　perforation T85.694 ☑
　　　protrusion T85.694 ☑
　　　specified NEC T85.694 ☑
　intestinal pouch NEC K91.858
　intraocular lens (prosthetic) T85.9 ☑
　　embolism T85.818 ☑
　　fibrosis T85.828 ☑
　　hemorrhage T85.838 ☑
　　infection and inflammation T85.79 ☑
　　mechanical
　　　breakdown T85.21 ☑
　　　displacement T85.22 ☑
　　　malposition T85.22 ☑
　　　obstruction T85.29 ☑
　　　perforation T85.29 ☑
　　　protrusion T85.29 ☑
　　　specified NEC T85.29 ☑
　　pain T85.848 ☑
　　specified type NEC T85.898 ☑
　　stenosis T85.858 ☑
　　thrombosis T85.868 ☑
　intraoperative (intraprocedural)
　　cardiac arrest — *see also* Infarct, myocardium, associated with revascularization procedure
　　　during cardiac surgery I97.710
　　　during other surgery I97.711
　　cardiac functional disturbance NEC — *see also* Infarct, myocardium, associated with revascularization procedure
　　　during cardiac surgery I97.790
　　　during other surgery I97.791
　　hemorrhage (hematoma) (of)
　　　circulatory system organ or structure
　　　　during cardiac bypass I97.411
　　　　during cardiac catheterization I97.410
　　　　during other circulatory system procedure I97.418
　　　　during other procedure I97.42
　　　digestive system organ
　　　　during procedure on digestive system K91.61
　　　　during procedure on other organ K91.62
　　　ear
　　　　during procedure on ear and mastoid process H95.21
　　　　during procedure on other organ H95.22
　　　endocrine system organ or structure
　　　　during procedure on endocrine system organ or structure E36.01
　　　　during procedure on other organ E36.02
　　　eye and adnexa
　　　　during ophthalmic procedure H59.11- ☑
　　　　during other procedure H59.12- ☑
　　　genitourinary organ or structure
　　　　during procedure on genitourinary organ or structure N99.61
　　　　during procedure on other organ N99.62
　　　mastoid process
　　　　during procedure on ear and mastoid process H95.21
　　　　during procedure on other organ H95.22
　　　musculoskeletal structure
　　　　during musculoskeletal surgery M96.810
　　　　during non-orthopedic surgery M96.811
　　　　during orthopedic surgery M96.810
　　　nervous system
　　　　during a nervous system procedure G97.31
　　　　during other procedure G97.32
　　　respiratory system
　　　　during other procedure J95.62
　　　　during procedure on respiratory system organ or structure J95.61

Complication(s) — *continued*
　intraoperative — *continued*
　　hemorrhage — *continued*
　　　skin and subcutaneous tissue
　　　　during a dermatologic procedure L76.01
　　　　during a procedure on other organ L76.02
　　　spleen
　　　　during a procedure on other organ D78.02
　　　　during a procedure on the spleen D78.01
　　puncture or laceration (accidental) (unintentional) (of)
　　　brain
　　　　during a nervous system procedure G97.48
　　　　during other procedure G97.49
　　　circulatory system organ or structure
　　　　during circulatory system procedure I97.51
　　　　during other procedure I97.52
　　　digestive system
　　　　during procedure on digestive system K91.71
　　　　during procedure on other organ K91.72
　　　ear
　　　　during procedure on ear and mastoid process H95.31
　　　　during procedure on other organ H95.32
　　　endocrine system organ or structure
　　　　during procedure on endocrine system organ or structure E36.11
　　　　during procedure on other organ E36.12
　　　eye and adnexa
　　　　during ophthalmic procedure H59.21- ☑
　　　　during other procedure H59.22- ☑
　　　genitourinary organ or structure
　　　　during procedure on genitourinary organ or structure N99.71
　　　　during procedure on other organ N99.72
　　　mastoid process
　　　　during procedure on ear and mastoid process H95.31
　　　　during procedure on other organ H95.32
　　　musculoskeletal structure
　　　　during musculoskeletal surgery M96.820
　　　　during non-orthopedic surgery M96.821
　　　　during orthopedic surgery M96.820
　　　nervous system
　　　　during a nervous system procedure G97.48
　　　　during other procedure G97.49
　　　respiratory system
　　　　during other procedure J95.72
　　　　during procedure on respiratory system organ or structure J95.71
　　　skin and subcutaneous tissue
　　　　during a dermatologic procedure L76.11
　　　　during a procedure on other organ L76.12
　　　spleen
　　　　during a procedure on other organ D78.12
　　　　during a procedure on the spleen D78.11
　　specified NEC
　　　circulatory system I97.88
　　　digestive system K91.81
　　　ear H95.88
　　　endocrine system E36.8
　　　eye and adnexa H59.88
　　　genitourinary system N99.81
　　　mastoid process H95.88
　　　musculoskeletal structure M96.89
　　　nervous system G97.81
　　　respiratory system J95.88
　　　skin and subcutaneous tissue L76.81
　　　spleen D78.81
　intraperitoneal catheter (dialysis) (infusion) — *see* Complication(s), catheter, intraperitoneal dialysis
　intrathecal infusion pump
　　infection and inflammation T85.738 ☑
　　mechanical
　　　breakdown T85.615 ☑
　　　displacement T85.625 ☑
　　　leakage T85.635 ☑
　　　malfunction T85.695 ☑
　　　malposition T85.625 ☑
　　　obstruction T85.695 ☑
　　　perforation T85.695 ☑
　　　protrusion T85.695 ☑
　　　specified NEC T85.695 ☑
　intrauterine
　　contraceptive device
　　　embolism T83.81 ☑
　　　fibrosis T83.82 ☑
　　　hemorrhage T83.83 ☑

Complication(s) — *continued*
  intrauterine — *continued*
    contraceptive device — *continued*
      infection and inflammation T83.69 ☑
      mechanical
        breakdown T83.31 ☑
        displacement T83.32 ☑
        malposition T83.32 ☑
        obstruction T83.39 ☑
        perforation T83.39 ☑
        protrusion T83.39 ☑
        specified NEC T83.39 ☑
      pain T83.84 ☑
      specified type NEC T83.89 ☑
      stenosis T83.85 ☑
      thrombosis T83.86 ☑
    procedure (fetal), to newborn P96.5
  jejunostomy (stoma) — *see* Complications, enterostomy
  joint prosthesis, internal T84.9 ☑
    breakage (fracture) T84.01- ☑
    dislocation T84.02- ☑
    fracture T84.01- ☑
    infection or inflammation T84.50 ☑
      hip T84.5- ☑
      knee T84.5- ☑
      specified joint NEC T84.59 ☑
    instability T84.02- ☑
    malposition — *see* Complications, joint prosthesis, mechanical, displacement
    mechanical
      breakage, broken T84.01- ☑
      dislocation T84.02- ☑
      displacement T84.02- ☑
      fracture T84.01- ☑
      instability T84.02- ☑
      leakage — *see* Complications, joint prosthesis, mechanical, specified NEC
      loosening T84.039 ☑
        hip T84.03- ☑
        knee T84.03- ☑
        specified joint NEC T84.038 ☑
      obstruction — *see* Complications, joint prosthesis, mechanical, specified NEC
      osteolysis T84.059 ☑
        hip T84.05- ☑
        knee T84.05- ☑
      perforation — *see* Complications, joint prosthesis, mechanical, specified NEC
        osteolysis T84.059 ☑
          other specified joint T84.058 ☑
      periprosthetic osteolysis, by site T84.05- ☑
      protrusion — *see* Complications, joint prosthesis, mechanical, specified NEC
      specified complication NEC T84.099 ☑
        hip T84.09- ☑
        knee T84.09- ☑
        other specified joint T84.098 ☑
      subluxation T84.02- ☑
      wear of articular bearing surface T84.069 ☑
        hip T84.06- ☑
        knee T84.06- ☑
        other specified joint T84.068 ☑
    specified joint NEC T84.89 ☑
      embolism T84.81 ☑
      fibrosis T84.82 ☑
      hemorrhage T84.83 ☑
      pain T84.84 ☑
      specified complication NEC T84.89 ☑
      stenosis T84.85 ☑
      thrombosis T84.86 ☑
    subluxation T84.02- ☑
  kidney transplant — *see* Complications, transplant, kidney
  labor O75.9
    specified NEC O75.89
  liver transplant (immune or nonimmune) — *see* Complications, transplant, liver
  lumbar puncture G97.1
    cerebrospinal fluid leak G97.0
    headache or reaction G97.1
  lung transplant — *see* Complications, transplant, lung
    and heart — *see* Complications, transplant, lung, with heart
  male genital N50.9
    device, implant or graft — *see* Complications, genitourinary, device or implant, genital tract

Complication(s) — *continued*
  male genital — *continued*
    postprocedural or postoperative — *see* Complications, genitourinary, postprocedural
    specified NEC N99.89
  mastoid (process) procedure
    intraoperative H95.88
      hematoma — *see* Complications, intraoperative, hemorrhage (hematoma) (of), mastoid process
      hemorrhage — *see* Complications, intraoperative, hemorrhage (hematoma) (of), mastoid process
      laceration — *see* Complications, intraoperative, puncture or laceration, mastoid process
      specified NEC H95.88
    postmastoidectomy — *see* Complications, postmastoidectomy
    postoperative H95.89
      external ear canal stenosis H95.81 ☑
      hematoma — *see* Complications, postprocedural, hematoma (of), mastoid process
      hemorrhage — *see* Complications, postprocedural, hemorrhage (of), mastoid process
      postmastoidectomy — *see* Complications, postmastoidectomy
      seroma — *see* Complications, postprocedural, seroma (of), mastoid process
      specified NEC H95.89
  mastoidectomy cavity — *see* Complications, postmastoidectomy
  mechanical — *see* Complications, by site and type, mechanical
  medical procedures — *see also* Complication(s), intraoperative T88.9 ☑
  metabolic E88.9
    postoperative E89.89
      specified NEC E89.89
  molar pregnancy NOS O08.9
    damage to pelvic organs O08.6
    embolism O08.2
    genital infection O08.0
    hemorrhage (delayed) (excessive) O08.1
    metabolic disorder O08.5
    renal failure O08.4
    shock O08.3
    specified type NEC O08.0
    venous complication NEC O08.7
  musculoskeletal system — *see also* Complication, intraoperative (intraprocedural), by site
    device, implant or graft NEC — *see* Complications, orthopedic, device or implant
    internal fixation (nail) (plate) (rod) — *see* Complications, fixation device, internal
    joint prosthesis — *see* Complications, joint prosthesis
    post radiation M96.89
      kyphosis M96.2
      scoliosis M96.5
      specified complication NEC M96.89
    postoperative (postprocedural) M96.89
      with osteoporosis — *see* Osteoporosis
      fracture following insertion of device — *see* Fracture, following insertion of orthopedic implant, joint prosthesis or bone plate
      joint instability after prosthesis removal M96.89
      lordosis M96.4
      postlaminectomy syndrome NEC M96.1
        kyphosis M96.3
      pseudarthrosis M96.0
      specified complication NEC M96.89
  nephrostomy (stoma) — *see* Complications, stoma, urinary tract, external NEC
  nervous system G98.8
    central G96.9
    device, implant or graft — *see also* Complication, prosthetic device or implant, specified NEC
    electronic stimulator (electrode(s)) — *see* Complications, electronic stimulator device
    specified NEC
      infection and inflammation T85.738 ☑
      mechanical T85.695 ☑
        breakdown T85.615 ☑
        displacement T85.625 ☑
        leakage T85.635 ☑
        malfunction T85.695 ☑
        malposition T85.625 ☑
        obstruction T85.695 ☑
        perforation T85.695 ☑

Complication(s) — *continued*
  nervous system — *continued*
    device, implant or graft — *see also* Complication, prosthetic device or implant, specified — *continued*
      specified — *continued*
        mechanical — *continued*
          protrusion T85.695 ☑
          specified NEC T85.695 ☑
      ventricular shunt — *see* Complications, ventricular shunt
    electronic stimulator (electrode(s)) — *see* Complications, electronic stimulator device
    postprocedural G97.82
      intracranial hypotension G97.2
      specified NEC G97.82
      spinal fluid leak G97.0
  newborn, due to intrauterine (fetal) procedure P96.5
  nonabsorbable (permanent) sutures — *see* Complication, sutures, permanent
  obstetric O75.9
    procedure (instrumental) (manual) (surgical) specified NEC O75.4
    specified NEC O75.89
    surgical wound NEC O90.89
      hematoma O90.2
      infection O86.00
  ocular lens implant — *see* Complications, intraocular lens
  ophthalmologic
    postprocedural bleb — *see* Blebitis
  orbital prosthesis T85.9 ☑
    embolism T85.818 ☑
    fibrosis T85.828 ☑
    hemorrhage T85.838 ☑
    infection and inflammation T85.79 ☑
    mechanical
      breakdown T85.31- ☑
      displacement T85.32- ☑
      malposition T85.32- ☑
      obstruction T85.39- ☑
      perforation T85.39- ☑
      protrusion T85.39- ☑
      specified NEC T85.39- ☑
    pain T85.848 ☑
    specified type NEC T85.898 ☑
    stenosis T85.858 ☑
    thrombosis T85.868 ☑
  organ or tissue transplant (partial) (total) — *see* Complications, transplant
  orthopedic — *see also* Disorder, soft tissue
    device or implant T84.9 ☑
      bone
        device or implant — *see* Complication, bone, device NEC
        graft — *see* Complication, graft, bone
      breakdown T84.418 ☑
      displacement T84.428 ☑
      electronic bone stimulator — *see* Complications, electronic stimulator device, bone
      embolism T84.81 ☑
      fibrosis T84.82 ☑
      fixation device — *see* Complication, fixation device, internal
      hemorrhage T84.83 ☑
      infection or inflammation T84.7 ☑
      joint prosthesis — *see* Complication, joint prosthesis, internal
      malfunction T84.418 ☑
      malposition T84.428 ☑
      mechanical NEC T84.498 ☑
      muscle graft — *see* Complications, graft, muscle
      obstruction T84.498 ☑
      pain T84.84 ☑
      perforation T84.498 ☑
      protrusion T84.498 ☑
      specified complication NEC T84.89 ☑
      stenosis T84.85 ☑
      tendon graft — *see* Complications, graft, tendon
      thrombosis T84.86 ☑
    fracture (following insertion of device) — *see* Fracture, following insertion of orthopedic implant, joint prosthesis or bone plate
    postprocedural M96.89
      fracture — *see* Fracture, following insertion of orthopedic implant, joint prosthesis or bone plate

☑ **Additional Character Required — Refer to the Tabular List for Character Selection**

Complication(s) — *continued*
  orthopedic — *see also* Disorder, soft tissue — *continued*
    postprocedural — *continued*
      postlaminectomy syndrome NEC M96.1
        kyphosis M96.3
        lordosis M96.4
      postradiation
        kyphosis M96.2
        scoliosis M96.5
      pseudarthrosis post-fusion M96.0
      specified type NEC M96.89
  pacemaker (cardiac) — *see* Complications, cardiovascular device or implant, electronic
  pancreas transplant — *see* Complications, transplant, pancreas
  penile prosthesis (implant) — *see* Complications, prosthetic device, penile
  perfusion NEC T80.90 ☑
  perineal repair (obstetrical) NEC O90.89
    disruption O90.1
    hematoma O90.2
    infection (following delivery) O86.09
  phototherapy T88.9 ☑
    specified NEC T88.8 ☑
  postmastoidectomy NEC H95.19- ☑
    cyst, mucosal H95.13- ☑
    granulation H95.12- ☑
    inflammation, chronic H95.11- ☑
    recurrent cholesteatoma H95.0- ☑
  postoperative — *see* Complications, postprocedural
    circulatory — *see* Complications, circulatory system
    ear — *see* Complications, ear
    endocrine — *see* Complications, endocrine
    eye — *see* Complications, eye
    lumbar puncture G97.1
      cerebrospinal fluid leak G97.0
    nervous system (central) (peripheral) — *see* Complications, nervous system
    respiratory system — *see* Complications, respiratory system
  postprocedural — *see also* Complications, surgical procedure
    cardiac arrest — *see also* Infarct, myocardium, associated with revascularization procedure
      following cardiac surgery I97.120
      following other surgery I97.121
    cardiac functional disturbance NEC — *see also* Infarct, myocardium, associated with revascularization procedure
      following cardiac surgery I97.190
      following other surgery I97.191
    cardiac insufficiency
      following cardiac surgery I97.110
      following other surgery I97.111
    chorioretinal scars following retinal surgery H59.81- ☑
    following cataract surgery
      cataract (lens) fragments H59.02- ☑
      cystoid macular edema H59.03- ☑
      specified NEC H59.09- ☑
      vitreous (touch) syndrome H59.01- ☑
    heart failure
      following cardiac surgery I97.130
      following other surgery I97.131
    hematoma (of)
      circulatory system organ or structure
        following cardiac bypass I97.631
        following cardiac catheterization I97.630
        following other circulatory system procedure I97.638
        following other procedure I97.621
      digestive system
        following procedure on digestive system K91.870
        following procedure on other organ K91.871
      ear
        following other procedure H95.52
        following procedure on ear and mastoid process H95.51
      endocrine system
        following endocrine system procedure E89.820
        following other procedure E89.821
      eye and adnexa
        following ophthalmic procedure H59.33- ☑
        following other procedure H59.34- ☑

Complication(s) — *continued*
  postprocedural — *see also* Complications, surgical procedure — *continued*
    hematoma — *continued*
      genitourinary organ or structure
        following procedure on genitourinary organ or structure N99.840
        following procedure on other organ N99.841
      mastoid process
        following other procedure H95.52
        following procedure on ear and mastoid process H95.51
      musculoskeletal structure
        following musculoskeletal surgery M96.840
        following non-orthopedic surgery M96.841
        following orthopedic surgery M96.840
      nervous system
        following nervous system procedure G97.61
        following other procedure G97.62
      respiratory system
        following other procedure J95.861
        following procedure on respiratory system organ or structure J95.860
      skin and subcutaneous tissue
        following dermatologic procedure L76.31
        following procedure on other organ L76.32
      spleen
        following procedure on other organ D78.32
        following procedure on the spleen D78.31
    hemorrhage (of)
      circulatory system organ or structure
        following cardiac bypass I97.611
        following cardiac catheterization I97.610
        following other circulatory system procedure I97.618
        following other procedure I97.620
      digestive system
        following procedure on digestive system K91.840
        following procedure on other organ K91.841
      ear
        following other procedure H95.42
        following procedure on ear and mastoid process H95.41
      endocrine system
        following endocrine system procedure E89.810
        following other procedure E89.811
      eye and adnexa
        following ophthalmic procedure H59.31- ☑
        following other procedure H59.32- ☑
      genitourinary organ or structure
        following procedure on genitourinary organ or structure N99.820
        following procedure on other organ N99.821
      mastoid process
        following other procedure H95.42
        following procedure on ear and mastoid process H95.41
      musculoskeletal structure
        following musculoskeletal surgery M96.830
        following non-orthopedic surgery M96.831
        following orthopedic surgery M96.830
      nervous system
        following nervous system procedure G97.51
        following other procedure G97.52
      respiratory system
        following a respiratory system procedure J95.830
        following other procedure J95.831
      skin and subcutaneous tissue
        following a procedure on other organ L76.22
        following dermatologic procedure L76.21
      spleen
        following procedure on other organ D78.22
        following procedure on the spleen D78.21
    seroma (of)
      circulatory system organ or structure
        following cardiac bypass I97.641
        following cardiac catheterization I97.640
        following other circulatory system procedure I97.648
        following other procedure I97.622
      digestive system
        following procedure on digestive system K91.872
        following procedure on other organ K91.873
      ear
        following other procedure H95.54

Complication(s) — *continued*
  postprocedural — *see also* Complications, surgical procedure — *continued*
    seroma — *continued*
      ear — *continued*
        following procedure on ear and mastoid process H95.53
      endocrine system
        following endocrine system procedure E89.822
        following other procedure E89.823
      eye and adnexa
        following ophthalmic procedure H59.35- ☑
        following other procedure H59.36- ☑
      genitourinary organ or structure
        following procedure on genitourinary organ or structure N99.842
        following procedure on other organ N99.843
      mastoid process
        following other procedure H95.54
        following procedure on ear and mastoid process H95.53
      musculoskeletal structure
        following musculoskeletal surgery M96.842
        following non-orthopedic surgery M96.843
        following orthopedic surgery M96.842
      nervous system
        following nervous system procedure G97.63
        following other procedure G97.64
      respiratory system
        following other procedure J95.863
        following procedure on respiratory system organ or structure J95.862
      skin and subcutaneous tissue
        following dermatologic procedure L76.33
        following procedure on other organ L76.34
      spleen
        following procedure on other organ D78.34
        following procedure on the spleen D78.33
    specified NEC
      circulatory system I97.89
      digestive K91.89
      ear H95.89
      endocrine E89.89
      eye and adnexa H59.89
      genitourinary N99.89
      mastoid process H95.89
      metabolic E89.89
      musculoskeletal structure M96.89
      nervous system G97.82
      respiratory system J95.89
      skin and subcutaneous tissue L76.82
      spleen D78.89
  pregnancy NEC — *see* Pregnancy, complicated by
  prosthetic device or implant T85.9 ☑
    bile duct — *see* Complications, bile duct implant
    breast — *see* Complications, breast implant
    bulking agent
      ureteral
        erosion T83.714 ☑
        exposure T83.724 ☑
      urethral
        erosion T83.713 ☑
        exposure T83.723 ☑
    cardiac and vascular NEC — *see* Complications, cardiovascular device or implant
    corneal transplant — *see* Complications, graft, cornea
    electronic nervous system stimulator — *see* Complications, electronic stimulator device
    epidural infusion catheter — *see* Complications, catheter, epidural
    esophageal anti-reflux device — *see* Complications, esophageal anti-reflux device
    genital organ or tract — *see* Complications, genitourinary, device or implant, genital tract
      specified NEC T83.79- ☑
    heart valve — *see* Complications, heart, valve, prosthesis
    infection or inflammation T85.79 ☑
      intestine transplant T86.852
      liver transplant T86.43
      lung transplant T86.812
      pancreas transplant T86.892
      skin graft T86.822
    intraocular lens — *see* Complications, intraocular lens
    intraperitoneal (dialysis) catheter — *see* Complication(s), catheter, intraperitoneal dialysis
    joint — *see* Complications, joint prosthesis, internal
    mechanical NEC T85.698 ☑

☑ Additional Character Required — Refer to the Tabular List for Character Selection

Complication(s) — *continued*
prosthetic device or implant — *continued*
    mechanical — *continued*
        dialysis catheter (vascular) — *see also* Complication, catheter, dialysis, mechanical
            peritoneal — *see* Complication(s), catheter, intraperitoneal dialysis
        gastrointestinal device T85.598 ☑
        ocular device T85.398 ☑
        subdural (infusion) catheter T85.690 ☑
        suture, permanent T85.692 ☑
            that for bone repair — *see* Complications, fixation device, internal (orthopedic), mechanical
        ventricular shunt
            breakdown T85.01 ☑
            displacement T85.02 ☑
            leakage T85.03 ☑
            malposition T85.02 ☑
            obstruction T85.09 ☑
            perforation T85.09 ☑
            protrusion T85.09 ☑
            specified NEC T85.09 ☑
    mesh
        erosion (to surrounding organ or tissue) T83.718 ☑
            urethral (into pelvic floor muscles) T83.712 ☑
            vaginal (into pelvic floor muscles) T83.711 ☑
        exposure (into surrounding organ or tissue) T83.728 ☑
            urethral (through urethral wall) T83.722 ☑
            vaginal (into vagina) (through vaginal wall) T83.721 ☑
    orbital — *see* Complications, orbital prosthesis
    penile T83.9 ☑
        embolism T83.81 ☑
        fibrosis T83.82 ☑
        hemorrhage T83.83 ☑
        infection and inflammation T83.61 ☑
        mechanical
            breakdown T83.410 ☑
            displacement T83.420 ☑
            leakage T83.490 ☑
            malposition T83.420 ☑
            obstruction T83.490 ☑
            perforation T83.490 ☑
            protrusion T83.490 ☑
            specified NEC T83.490 ☑
        pain T83.84 ☑
        specified type NEC T83.89 ☑
        stenosis T83.85 ☑
        thrombosis T83.86 ☑
    prosthetic materials NEC
        erosion (to surrounding organ or tissue) T83.718 ☑
        exposure (into surrounding organ or tissue) T83.728 ☑
    skin graft T86.829
        artificial skin or decellularized allodermis
            embolism T85.818 ☑
            fibrosis T85.828 ☑
            hemorrhage T85.838 ☑
            infection and inflammation T85.79 ☑
            mechanical
                breakdown T85.613 ☑
                displacement T85.623 ☑
                malfunction T85.613 ☑
                malposition T85.623 ☑
                obstruction T85.693 ☑
                perforation T85.693 ☑
                protrusion T85.693 ☑
                specified NEC T85.693 ☑
            pain T85.848 ☑
            specified type NEC T85.898 ☑
            stenosis T85.858 ☑
            thrombosis T85.868 ☑
        failure T86.821
        infection T86.822
        rejection T86.820
        specified NEC T86.828
    sling
        urethral (female) (male)
            erosion T83.712 ☑
            exposure T83.722 ☑
    specified NEC T85.9 ☑
        embolism T85.818 ☑

Complication(s) — *continued*
prosthetic device or implant — *continued*
    specified — *continued*
        fibrosis T85.828 ☑
        hemorrhage T85.838 ☑
        infection and inflammation T85.79 ☑
        mechanical
            breakdown T85.618 ☑
            displacement T85.628 ☑
            leakage T85.638 ☑
            malfunction T85.618 ☑
            malposition T85.628 ☑
            obstruction T85.698 ☑
            perforation T85.698 ☑
            protrusion T85.698 ☑
            specified NEC T85.698 ☑
        pain T85.848 ☑
        specified type NEC T85.898 ☑
        stenosis T85.858 ☑
        thrombosis T85.868 ☑
    subdural infusion catheter — *see* Complications, catheter, subdural
    sutures — *see* Complications, sutures
    urinary organ or tract NEC — *see* Complications, genitourinary, device or implant, urinary system
    vascular — *see* Complications, cardiovascular device, graft or implant
    ventricular shunt — *see* Complications, ventricular shunt (device)
puerperium — *see* Puerperal
puncture, spinal G97.1
    cerebrospinal fluid leak G97.0
    headache or reaction G97.1
pyelogram N99.89
radiation
    kyphosis M96.2
    scoliosis M96.5
reattached
    extremity (infection) (rejection)
        lower T87.1X-
        upper T87.0X-
    specified body part NEC T87.2
reconstructed breast
    asymmetry between native and reconstructed breast N65.1
    deformity N65.0
    disproportion between native and reconstructed breast N65.1
    excess tissue N65.0
    misshappen N65.0
reimplant NEC — *see also* Complications, prosthetic device or implant
    limb (infection) (rejection) — *see* Complications, reattached, extremity
    organ (partial) (total) — *see* Complications, transplant
    prosthetic device NEC — *see* Complications, prosthetic device
renal N28.9
    allograft — *see* Complications, transplant, kidney
    dialysis — *see* Complications, dialysis
respirator
    mechanical J95.850
        specified NEC J95.859
respiratory system J98.9
    device, implant or graft — *see* Complication, prosthetic device or implant, specified NEC
    lung transplant — *see* Complications, prosthetic device or implant, lung transplant
    postoperative J95.89
        air leak J95.812
        Mendelson's syndrome (chemical pneumonitis) J95.4
        pneumothorax J95.811
        pulmonary insufficiency (acute) (after nonthoracic surgery) J95.2
            chronic J95.3
            following thoracic surgery J95.1
        respiratory failure (acute) J95.821
            acute and chronic J95.822
        specified NEC J95.89
        subglottic stenosis J95.5
        tracheostomy complication — *see* Complications, tracheostomy
    therapy T81.89 ☑
sedation during labor and delivery O74.9
    cardiac O74.2
    central nervous system O74.3
    pulmonary NEC O74.1

Complication(s) — *continued*
shunt — *see also* Complications, prosthetic device or implant
    arteriovenous — *see* Complications, arteriovenous, shunt
    ventricular (communicating) — *see* Complications, ventricular shunt
skin
    graft T86.829
        failure T86.821
        infection T86.822
        rejection T86.820
        specified type NEC T86.828
spinal
    anesthesia — *see* Complications, anesthesia, spinal
    catheter (epidural) (subdural) — *see* Complications, catheter
    puncture or tap G97.1
        cerebrospinal fluid leak G97.0
        headache or reaction G97.1
stent
    bile duct — *see* Complications, bile duct prosthesis
    ureteral indwelling
        breakdown T83.112 ☑
        displacement T83.122 ☑
        leakage T83.192 ☑
        malposition T83.122 ☑
        obstruction T83.192 ☑
        perforation T83.192 ☑
        protrusion T83.192 ☑
        specified NEC T83.192 ☑
    urinary NEC (ileal conduit) (nephroureteral) T83.193 ☑
        embolism T83.81 ☑
        fibrosis T83.82 ☑
        hemorrhage T83.83 ☑
        infection and inflammation T83.593 ☑
        mechanical
            breakdown T83.113 ☑
            displacement T83.123 ☑
            leakage T83.193 ☑
            malposition T83.123 ☑
            obstruction T83.193 ☑
            perforation T83.193 ☑
            protrusion T83.193 ☑
            specified NEC T83.193 ☑
        pain T83.84 ☑
        specified type NEC T83.89 ☑
        stenosis T83.85 ☑
        thrombosis T83.86 ☑
    vascular
        end stent stenosis — *see* Restenosis, stent
        in stent stenosis — *see* Restenosis, stent
stoma
    digestive tract
        colostomy — *see* Complications, colostomy
        enterostomy — *see* Complications, enterostomy
        esophagostomy — *see* Complications, esophagostomy
        gastrostomy — *see* Complications, gastrostomy
    urinary tract N99.528
        continent N99.538
            hemorrhage N99.530
            herniation N99.533
            infection N99.531
            malfunction N99.532
            specified type NEC N99.538
            stenosis N99.534
        cystostomy — *see* Complications, cystostomy
        external NOS N99.528
        hemorrhage N99.520
        herniation N99.523
        incontinent N99.528
            hemorrhage N99.520
            herniation N99.523
            infection N99.521
            malfunction N99.522
            specified type NEC N99.528
            stenosis N99.524
        infection N99.521
        malfunction N99.522
        specified type NEC N99.528
        stenosis N99.524
stomach banding — *see* Complication(s), bariatric procedure
stomach stapling — *see* Complication(s), bariatric procedure

☑ **Additional Character Required** — **Refer to the Tabular List for Character Selection**

Complication(s) — *continued*

surgical material, nonabsorbable — *see* Complication, suture, permanent
surgical procedure (on) T81.9 ☑
  amputation stump (late) — *see* Complications, amputation stump
  cardiac — *see* Complications, circulatory system
  cholesteatoma, recurrent — *see* Complications, postmastoidectomy, recurrent cholesteatoma
  circulatory (early) — *see* Complications, circulatory system
  digestive system — *see* Complications, gastrointestinal
  dumping syndrome (postgastrectomy) K91.1
  ear — *see* Complications, ear
  elephantiasis or lymphedema I97.89
    postmastectomy I97.2
  emphysema (surgical) T81.82 ☑
  endocrine — *see* Complications, endocrine
  eye — *see* Complications, eye
  fistula (persistent postoperative) T81.83 ☑
  foreign body inadvertently left in wound (sponge) (suture) (swab) — *see* Foreign body, accidentally left during a procedure
  gastrointestinal — *see* Complications, gastrointestinal
  genitourinary NEC N99.89
  hematoma
    intraoperative — *see* Complication, intraoperative, hemorrhage
    postprocedural — *see* Complication, postprocedural, hematoma
  hemorrhage
    intraoperative — *see* Complication, intraoperative, hemorrhage
    postprocedural — *see* Complication, postprocedural, hemorrhage
  hepatic failure K91.82
  hyperglycemia (postpancreatectomy) E89.1
  hypoinsulinemia (postpancreatectomy) E89.1
  hypoparathyroidism (postparathyroidectomy) E89.2
  hypopituitarism (posthypophysectomy) E89.3
  hypothyroidism (post-thyroidectomy) E89.0
  intestinal obstruction — *see also* Obstruction, intestine, postoperative K91.30
  intracranial hypotension following ventricular shunting (ventriculostomy) G97.2
  lymphedema I97.89
    postmastectomy I97.2
  malabsorption (postsurgical) NEC K91.2
    osteoporosis — *see* Osteoporosis, postsurgical malabsorption
  mastoidectomy cavity NEC — *see* Complications, postmastoidectomy
  metabolic E89.89
    specified NEC E89.89
  musculoskeletal — *see* Complications, musculoskeletal system
  nervous system (central) (peripheral) — *see* Complications, nervous system
  ovarian failure E89.40
    asymptomatic E89.40
    symptomatic E89.41
  peripheral vascular — *see* Complications, surgical procedure, vascular
  postcardiotomy syndrome I97.0
  postcholecystectomy syndrome K91.5
  postcommissurotomy syndrome I97.0
  postgastrectomy dumping syndrome K91.1
  postlaminectomy syndrome NEC M96.1
    kyphosis M96.3
  postmastectomy lymphedema syndrome I97.2
  postmastoidectomy cholesteatoma — *see* Complications, postmastoidectomy, recurrent cholesteatoma
  postvagotomy syndrome K91.1
  postvalvulotomy syndrome I97.0
  pulmonary insufficiency (acute) J95.2
    chronic J95.3
    following thoracic surgery J95.1
  reattached body part — *see* Complications, reattached
  respiratory — *see* Complications, respiratory system
  shock (hypovolemic) T81.19 ☑
  spleen (postoperative) D78.89
    intraoperative D78.81
  stitch abscess T81.41 ☑
  subglottic stenosis (postsurgical) J95.5
  testicular hypofunction E89.5

Complication(s) — *continued*

surgical procedure — *continued*
  transplant — *see* Complications, organ or tissue transplant
  urinary NEC N99.89
  vaginal vault prolapse (posthysterectomy) N99.3
  vascular (peripheral)
    artery T81.719 ☑
      mesenteric T81.710 ☑
      renal T81.711 ☑
      specified NEC T81.718 ☑
    vein T81.72 ☑
  wound infection T81.49 ☑
suture, permanent (wire) NEC T85.9 ☑
  with repair of bone — *see* Complications, fixation device, internal
  embolism T85.818 ☑
  fibrosis T85.828 ☑
  hemorrhage T85.838 ☑
  infection and inflammation T85.79 ☑
  mechanical
    breakdown T85.612 ☑
    displacement T85.622 ☑
    malfunction T85.612 ☑
    malposition T85.622 ☑
    obstruction T85.692 ☑
    perforation T85.692 ☑
    protrusion T85.692 ☑
    specified NEC T85.692 ☑
  pain T85.843 ☑
  specified type NEC T85.898 ☑
  stenosis T85.858 ☑
  thrombosis T85.868 ☑
tracheostomy J95.00
  granuloma J95.09
  hemorrhage J95.01
  infection J95.02
  malfunction J95.03
  mechanical J95.03
  obstruction J95.03
  specified type NEC J95.09
  tracheo-esophageal fistula J95.04
transfusion (blood) (lymphocytes) (plasma) T80.92 ☑
  air embolism T80.0 ☑
  circulatory overload E87.71
  febrile nonhemolytic transfusion reaction R50.84
  hemochromatosis E83.111
  hemolysis T80.89 ☑
  hemolytic reaction (antigen unspecified) T80.919 ☑
  incompatibility reaction (antigen unspecified) T80.919 ☑
    ABO T80.30 ☑
      delayed serologic (DSTR) T80.39 ☑
      hemolytic transfusion reaction (HTR) (unspecified time after transfusion) T80.319 ☑
      acute (AHTR) (less than 24 hours after transfusion) T80.310 ☑
      delayed (DHTR) (24 hours or more after transfusion) T80.311 ☑
      specified NEC T80.39 ☑
    acute (antigen unspecified) T80.910 ☑
    delayed (antigen unspecified) T80.911 ☑
    delayed serologic (DSTR) T80.89 ☑
    non-ABO (minor antigens (Duffy) (K) (Kell) (Kidd) (Lewis) (M) (N) (P) (S)) T80.A0 ☑ (*following* T80.4)
      delayed serologic (DSTR) T80.A9 ☑ (*following* T80.4)
      hemolytic transfusion reaction (HTR) (unspecified time after transfusion) T80.A19 ☑ (*following* T80.4)
      acute (AHTR) (less than 24 hours after transfusion) T80.A10 ☑ (*following* T80.4)
      delayed (DHTR) (24 hours or more after transfusion) T80.A11 ☑ (*following* T80.4)
      specified NEC T80.A9 ☑ (*following* T80.4)
    Rh (antigens (C) (c) (D) (E) (e)) (factor) T80.40 ☑
      delayed serologic (DSTR) T80.49 ☑
      hemolytic transfusion reaction (HTR) (unspecified time after transfusion) T80.419 ☑
      acute (AHTR) (less than 24 hours after transfusion) T80.410 ☑
      delayed (DHTR) (24 hours or more after transfusion) T80.411 ☑

Complication(s) — *continued*

transfusion — *continued*
  incompatibility reaction — *continued*
    Rh — *continued*
      specified NEC T80.49 ☑
  infection T80.29 ☑
    acute T80.22- ☑
  reaction NEC T80.89 ☑
  sepsis T80.29 ☑
  shock T80.89 ☑
transplant T86.90
  bone T86.839
    failure T86.831
    infection T86.832
    rejection T86.830
    specified type NEC T86.838
  bone marrow T86.00
    failure T86.02
    infection T86.03
    rejection T86.01
    specified type NEC T86.09
  cornea T86.849- ☑
    failure T86.841- ☑
    infection T86.842- ☑
    rejection T86.840- ☑
    specified type NEC T86.848- ☑
  failure T86.92
  heart T86.20
    with lung T86.30
    cardiac allograft vasculopathy T86.290
      failure T86.32
      infection T86.33
      rejection T86.31
      specified type NEC T86.39
    failure T86.22
    infection T86.23
    rejection T86.21
    specified type NEC T86.298
  infection T86.93
  intestine T86.859
    failure T86.851
    infection T86.852
    rejection T86.850
    specified type NEC T86.858
  kidney T86.10
    failure T86.12
    infection T86.13
    rejection T86.11
    specified type NEC T86.19
  liver T86.40
    failure T86.42
    infection T86.43
    rejection T86.41
    specified type NEC T86.49
  lung T86.819
    with heart T86.30
      failure T86.32
      infection T86.33
      rejection T86.31
      specified type NEC T86.39
    failure T86.811
    infection T86.812
    rejection T86.810
    specified type NEC T86.818
  malignant neoplasm C80.2
  pancreas T86.899
    failure T86.891
    infection T86.892
    rejection T86.890
    specified type NEC T86.898
  peripheral blood stem cells T86.5
  post-transplant lymphoproliferative disorder (PTLD) D47.Z1 (*following* D47.4)
  rejection T86.91
  skin T86.829
    failure T86.821
    infection T86.822
    rejection T86.820
    specified type NEC T86.828
  specified
    tissue T86.899
      failure T86.891
      infection T86.892
      rejection T86.890
      specified type NEC T86.898
    type NEC T86.99
  stem cell (from peripheral blood) (from umbilical cord) T86.5

Complication(s) — *continued*
  transplant — *continued*
    umbilical cord stem cells T86.5
  trauma (early) T79.9 ☑
    specified NEC T79.8 ☑
  ultrasound therapy NEC T88.9 ☑
  umbilical cord NEC
    complicating delivery O69.9 ☑
      specified NEC O69.89 ☑
  umbrella device, vascular T82.9 ☑
    embolism T82.818 ☑
    fibrosis T82.828 ☑
    hemorrhage T82.838 ☑
    infection or inflammation T82.7 ☑
    mechanical
      breakdown T82.515 ☑
      displacement T82.525 ☑
      leakage T82.535 ☑
      malposition T82.525 ☑
      obstruction T82.595 ☑
      perforation T82.595 ☑
      protrusion T82.595 ☑
    pain T82.848 ☑
    specified type NEC T82.898 ☑
    stenosis T82.858 ☑
    thrombosis T82.868 ☑
  urethral catheter — *see* Complications, catheter, urethral,
      indwelling
  vaccination T88.1 ☑
    anaphylaxis NEC T80.52 ☑
    arthropathy — *see* Arthropathy, postimmunization
    cellulitis T88.0 ☑
    encephalitis or encephalomyelitis G04.02
    infection (general) (local) NEC T88.0 ☑
    meningitis G03.8
    myelitis G04.02
    protein sickness T80.62 ☑
    rash T88.1 ☑
    reaction (allergic) T88.1 ☑
      serum T80.62 ☑
    sepsis T88.0 ☑
    serum intoxication, sickness, rash, or other serum re-
        action NEC T80.62 ☑
    anaphylactic shock T80.52 ☑
    shock (allergic) (anaphylactic) T80.52 ☑
    vaccinia (generalized) (localized) T88.1 ☑
  vas deferens device or implant — *see* Complications,
      genitourinary, device or implant, genital tract
  vascular I99.9
    device or implant T82.9 ☑
      embolism T82.818 ☑
      fibrosis T82.828 ☑
      hemorrhage T82.838 ☑
      infection or inflammation T82.7 ☑
      mechanical
        breakdown T82.519 ☑
          specified device NEC T82.518 ☑
        displacement T82.529 ☑
          specified device NEC T82.528 ☑
        leakage T82.539 ☑
          specified device NEC T82.538 ☑
        malposition T82.529 ☑
          specified device NEC T82.528 ☑
        obstruction T82.599 ☑
          specified device NEC T82.598 ☑
        perforation T82.599 ☑
          specified device NEC T82.598 ☑
        protrusion T82.599 ☑
          specified device NEC T82.598 ☑
      pain T82.848 ☑
      specified type NEC T82.898 ☑
      stenosis T82.858 ☑
      thrombosis T82.868 ☑
    dialysis catheter — *see* Complication, catheter, dialysis
    following infusion, therapeutic injection or transfusion
        T80.1 ☑
    graft T82.9 ☑
      embolism T82.818 ☑
      fibrosis T82.828 ☑
      hemorrhage T82.838 ☑
      mechanical
        breakdown T82.319 ☑
          aorta (bifurcation) T82.310 ☑
          carotid artery T82.311 ☑
          specified vessel NEC T82.318 ☑
        displacement T82.329 ☑

Complication(s) — *continued*
  vascular — *continued*
    graft — *continued*
      mechanical — *continued*
        displacement — *continued*
          aorta (bifurcation) T82.320 ☑
          carotid artery T82.321 ☑
          specified vessel NEC T82.328 ☑
        leakage T82.339 ☑
          aorta (bifurcation) T82.330 ☑
          carotid artery T82.331 ☑
          femoral artery T82.332 ☑
          specified vessel NEC T82.338 ☑
        malposition T82.329 ☑
          aorta (bifurcation) T82.320 ☑
          carotid artery T82.321 ☑
          specified vessel NEC T82.328 ☑
        obstruction T82.399 ☑
          aorta (bifurcation) T82.390 ☑
          carotid artery T82.391 ☑
          specified vessel NEC T82.398 ☑
        perforation T82.399 ☑
          aorta (bifurcation) T82.390 ☑
          carotid artery T82.391 ☑
          specified vessel NEC T82.398 ☑
        protrusion T82.399 ☑
          aorta (bifurcation) T82.390 ☑
          carotid artery T82.391 ☑
          specified vessel NEC T82.398 ☑
      pain T82.848 ☑
      specified complication NEC T82.898 ☑
      stenosis T82.858 ☑
      thrombosis T82.868 ☑
    postoperative — *see* Complications, postoperative,
        circulatory
  vena cava device (filter) (sieve) (umbrella) — *see* Compli-
      cations, umbrella device, vascular
  ventilation therapy NEC T81.81 ☑
  ventilator
    mechanical J95.850
      specified NEC J95.859
  ventricular (communicating) shunt (device) T85.9 ☑
    embolism T85.810 ☑
    fibrosis T85.820 ☑
    hemorrhage T85.830 ☑
    infection and inflammation T85.730 ☑
    mechanical
      breakdown T85.01 ☑
      displacement T85.02 ☑
      leakage T85.03 ☑
      malposition T85.02 ☑
      obstruction T85.09 ☑
      perforation T85.09 ☑
      protrusion T85.09 ☑
      specified NEC T85.09 ☑
    pain T85.840 ☑
    specified type NEC T85.890 ☑
    stenosis T85.850 ☑
    thrombosis T85.860 ☑
  wire suture, permanent (implanted) — *see* Complica-
      tions, suture, permanent
Compressed air disease T70.3 ☑
Compression
  with injury — *code by* Nature of injury
  artery I77.1
    celiac, syndrome I77.4
  brachial plexus G54.0
  brain (stem) G93.5
    due to
      contusion (diffuse) — *see also* Injury, intracranial,
          diffuse S06.A0 ☑
        with herniation S06.A1 ☑
        focal — *see also* Injury, intracranial, focal
            S06.A0 ☑
          with herniation S06.A1 ☑
      injury NEC — *see also* Injury, intracranial, diffuse
          S06.A0 ☑
    nontraumatic G93.5
    traumatic — *see also* Injury, intracranial, diffuse
        S06.A0 ☑
      with herniation S06.A1 ☑
  bronchus J98.09
  cauda equina G83.4
  celiac (artery) (axis) I77.4
  cerebral — *see* Compression, brain
  cervical plexus G54.2

Compression — *continued*
  cord
    spinal — *see* Compression, spinal
    umbilical — *see* Compression, umbilical cord
  cranial nerve G52.9
    eighth H93.3
    eleventh G52.8
    fifth G50.8
    first G52.0
    fourth — *see* Strabismus, paralytic, fourth nerve
    ninth G52.1
    second — *see* Disorder, nerve, optic
    seventh G51.8
    sixth — *see* Strabismus, paralytic, sixth nerve
    tenth G52.2
    third — *see* Strabismus, paralytic, third nerve
    twelfth G52.3
  diver's squeeze T70.3 ☑
  during birth (newborn) P15.9
  esophagus K22.2
  eustachian tube — *see* Obstruction, eustachian tube,
      cartilagenous
  facies Q67.1
  fracture
    nontraumatic NOS — *see* Collapse, vertebra
    pathological — *see* Fracture, pathological
    traumatic — *see* Fracture, traumatic
  heart — *see* Disease, heart
  intestine — *see* Obstruction, intestine
  laryngeal nerve, recurrent G52.2
    with paralysis of vocal cords and larynx J38.00
      bilateral J38.02
      unilateral J38.01
  lumbosacral plexus G54.1
  lung J98.4
  lymphatic vessel I89.0
  medulla — *see* Compression, brain
  nerve — *see also* Disorder, nerve G58.9
    arm NEC — *see* Mononeuropathy, upper limb
    axillary G54.0
    cranial — *see* Compression, cranial nerve
    leg NEC — *see* Mononeuropathy, lower limb
    median (in carpal tunnel) — *see* Syndrome, carpal
        tunnel
    optic — *see* Disorder, nerve, optic
    plantar — *see* Lesion, nerve, plantar
    posterior tibial (in tarsal tunnel) — *see* Syndrome,
        tarsal tunnel
    root or plexus NOS (in) G54.9
      intervertebral disc disorder NEC — *see* Disorder,
          disc, with, radiculopathy
        with myelopathy — *see* Disorder, disc, with,
            myelopathy
      neoplastic disease — *see also* Neoplasm
          D49.9 *[G55]*
      spondylosis — *see* Spondylosis, with radiculopathy
    sciatic (acute) — *see* Lesion, nerve, sciatic
    sympathetic G90.89
    traumatic — *see* Injury, nerve
    ulnar — *see* Lesion, nerve, ulnar
    upper extremity NEC — *see* Mononeuropathy, upper
        limb
  spinal (cord) G95.20
    by displacement of intervertebral disc NEC — *see also*
        Disorder, disc, with, myelopathy
    nerve root NOS G54.9
      due to displacement of intervertebral disc NEC —
          see Disorder, disc, with, radiculopathy
        with myelopathy — *see* Disorder, disc, with,
            myelopathy
    specified NEC G95.29
    spondylogenic (cervical) (lumbar, lumbosacral) (tho-
        racic) — *see* Spondylosis, with myelopathy NEC
      anterior — *see* Syndrome, anterior, spinal artery,
          compression
    traumatic — *see* Injury, spinal cord, by region
  subcostal nerve (syndrome) — *see* Mononeuropathy,
      upper limb, specified NEC
  sympathetic nerve NEC G90.89
  syndrome T79.5 ☑
  trachea J39.8
  ulnar nerve (by scar tissue) — *see* Lesion, nerve, ulnar
  umbilical cord
    complicating delivery O69.2 ☑
      cord around neck O69.1 ☑
      prolapse O69.0 ☑
      specified NEC O69.2 ☑
  ureter N13.5

Compression — continued
vein I87.1
vena cava (inferior) (superior) I87.1
Compulsion, compulsive
gambling F63.0
neurosis F42.8
personality F60.5
states F42.8
swearing F42.8
in Gilles de la Tourette's syndrome F95.2
tics and spasms F95.9
Concato's disease (pericardial polyserositis) A19.9
nontubercular I31.1
pleural — see Pleurisy, with effusion
Concavity chest wall M95.4
Concealed penis Q55.64
Concern (normal) **about sick person in family** Z63.6
Concrescence (teeth) K00.2
Concretio cordis I31.1
rheumatic I09.2
Concretion — see also Calculus
appendicular K38.1
canaliculus — see Dacryolith
clitoris N90.89
conjunctiva H11.12- ☑
eyelid — see Disorder, eyelid, specified type NEC
lacrimal passages — see Dacryolith
prepuce (male) N47.8
salivary gland (any) K11.5
seminal vesicle N50.89
tonsil J35.8
Concussion (brain) (cerebral) (current) S06.0X9 ☑
with
loss of consciousness
30 minutes or less S06.0X1 ☑
brief S06.0X1 ☑
status unknown S06.0XA ☑
unspecified duration S06.0X9 ☑
no loss of consciousness S06.0X0 ☑
blast (air) (hydraulic) (immersion) (underwater)
abdomen or thorax — see Injury, blast, by site
ear with acoustic nerve injury — see Injury, nerve,
acoustic, specified type NEC
cauda equina S34.3 ☑
conus medullaris S34.02 ☑
ocular S05.8X- ☑
spinal (cord)
cervical S14.0 ☑
lumbar S34.01 ☑
sacral S34.02 ☑
thoracic S24.0 ☑
syndrome F07.81
without loss of consciousness S06.0X0 ☑
Condition — see also Disease
post COVID-19 U09.9
Conditions arising in the perinatal period — see Newborn, affected by
Conduct disorder — see Disorder, conduct
Condyloma A63.0
acuminatum A63.0
gonorrheal A54.09
latum A51.31
syphilitic A51.31
congenital A50.07
venereal, syphilitic A51.31
Conflagration — see also Burn
asphyxia (by inhalation of gases, fumes or vapors) — see
also Table of Drugs and Chemicals T59.9- ☑
Conflict (with) — see also Discord
family Z73.9
grandparent-child Z62.831
group home staff-child Z62.833
kinship-care child Z62.831
marital Z63.0
involving divorce or estrangement Z63.5
non-parental relative legal guardian-child Z62.831
non-parental relative-child Z62.831
non-relative guardian-child Z62.832
other relative-child Z62.831
parent-child Z62.820
parent-adopted child Z62.821
parent-biological child Z62.820
parent-foster child Z62.822
parent-step child Z62.823
social role NEC Z73.5
Confluent — see condition
Confusion, confused R41.0
epileptic F05

Confusion, confused — continued
mental state (psychogenic) F44.89
psychogenic F44.89
reactive (from emotional stress, psychological trauma)
F44.89
Confusional arousals G47.51
Congelation T69.9 ☑
Congenital — see also condition
aortic septum Q25.49
intrinsic factor deficiency D51.0
malformation — see Anomaly
Congestion, congestive
bladder N32.89
bowel K63.89
brain G93.89
breast N64.59
bronchial J98.09
catarrhal J31.0
chest R09.89
chill, malarial — see Malaria
circulatory NEC I99.8̷
duodenum K31.89
eye — see Hyperemia, conjunctiva
facial, due to birth injury P15.4
general R68.89
glottis J37.0
heart — see Failure, heart, congestive
hepatic K76.1
hypostatic (lung) — see Edema, lung
intestine K63.89
kidney N28.89
labyrinth H83.8 ☑
larynx J37.0
liver K76.1
lung R09.89
active or acute — see Pneumonia
malaria, malarial — see Malaria
nasal R09.81
nose R09.81
orbit, orbital — see also Exophthalmos
inflammatory (chronic) — see Inflammation, orbit
ovary N83.8
pancreas K86.89
pelvic, female N94.89
pleural J94.8
prostate (active) N42.1
pulmonary — see Congestion, lung
renal N28.89
retina H35.81
seminal vesicle N50.1
spinal cord G95.19
spleen (chronic) D73.2
stomach K31.89
trachea — see Tracheitis
urethra N36.8
uterus N85.8
with subinvolution N85.3
venous (passive) I87.8
viscera R68.89
Congestive — see Congestion
Conical
cervix (hypertrophic elongation) N88.4
cornea — see Keratoconus
teeth K00.2
Conjoined twins Q89.4
Conjugal maladjustment Z63.0
involving divorce or estrangement Z63.5
Conjunctiva — see condition
Conjunctivitis (staphylococcal) (streptococcal) NOS H10.9
Acanthamoeba B60.12
acute H10.3- ☑
atopic H10.1- ☑
chemical — see also Corrosion, cornea H10.21- ☑
mucopurulent H10.02- ☑
follicular H10.01- ☑
pseudomembranous H10.22- ☑
serous except viral H10.23- ☑
viral — see Conjunctivitis, viral
toxic H10.21- ☑
adenoviral (acute) (follicular) B30.1
allergic (acute) — see Conjunctivitis, acute, atopic
chronic H10.45
vernal H10.44
anaphylactic — see Conjunctivitis, acute, atopic
Apollo B30.3
atopic (acute) — see Conjunctivitis, acute, atopic
Beal's B30.2
blennorrhagic (gonococcal) (neonatorum) A54.31

Conjunctivitis — continued
chemical (acute) — see also Corrosion, cornea H10.21- ☑
chlamydial A74.0
due to trachoma A71.1
neonatal P39.1
chronic (nodosa) (petrificans) (phlyctenular) H10.40- ☑
allergic H10.45
vernal H10.44
follicular H10.43- ☑
giant papillary H10.41- ☑
simple H10.42- ☑
vernal H10.44
coxsackievirus 24 B30.3
diphtheritic A36.86
due to
dust — see Conjunctivitis, acute, atopic
filariasis B74.9
mucocutaneous leishmaniasis B55.2
enterovirus type 70 (hemorrhagic) B30.3
epidemic (viral) B30.9
hemorrhagic B30.3
gonococcal (neonatorum) A54.31
granular (trachomatous) A71.1
sequelae (late effect) B94.0
hemorrhagic (acute) (epidemic) B30.3
herpes zoster B02.31
in (due to)
Acanthamoeba B60.12
adenovirus (acute) (follicular) B30.1
Chlamydia A74.0
coxsackievirus 24 B30.3
diphtheria A36.86
enterovirus type 70 (hemorrhagic) B30.3
filariasis B74.9
gonococci A54.31
herpes (simplex) virus B00.53
zoster B02.31
infectious disease NEC B99 ☑
meningococci A39.89
mucocutaneous leishmaniasis B55.2
rosacea H10.82- ☑
syphilis (late) A52.71
zoster B02.31
inclusion A74.0
infantile P39.1
gonococcal A54.31
Koch-Weeks' — see Conjunctivitis, acute, mucopurulent
light — see Conjunctivitis, acute, atopic
ligneous — see Blepharoconjunctivitis, ligneous
meningococcal A39.89
mucopurulent — see Conjunctivitis, acute, mucopurulent
neonatal P39.1
gonococcal A54.31
Newcastle B30.8
of Beal B30.2
parasitic
filariasis B74.9
mucocutaneous leishmaniasis B55.2
Parinaud's H10.89
petrificans H10.89
rosacea H10.82- ☑
specified NEC H10.89
swimming-pool B30.1
trachomatous A71.1
acute A71.0
sequelae (late effect) B94.0
traumatic NEC H10.89
tuberculous A18.59
tularemic A21.1
tularensis A21.1
viral B30.9
due to
adenovirus B30.1
enterovirus B30.3
specified NEC B30.8
Conjunctivochalasis H11.82- ☑
Connective tissue — see condition
Conn's syndrome E26.01
Conradi (-Hunermann) **disease** Q77.3
Consanguinity Z84.3
counseling Z71.89
Conscious simulation (of illness) Z76.5
Consecutive — see condition
Consolidation lung (base) — see Pneumonia, lobar
Constipation (atonic) (neurogenic) (simple) (spastic) K59.00
chronic K59.09
idiopathic K59.04
drug-induced K59.03

Constipation — *continued*
 functional K59.04
 outlet dysfunction K59.02
 psychogenic F45.8
 slow transit K59.01
 specified NEC K59.09
Constitutional — *see also* condition
 substandard F60.7
Constitutionally substandard F60.7
Constriction — *see also* Stricture
 auditory canal — *see* Stenosis, external ear canal
 bronchial J98.09
 duodenum K31.5
 esophagus K22.2
 external
  abdomen, abdominal (wall) S30.841 ☑
  alveolar process S00.542 ☑
  ankle S90.54-
  antecubital space — *see* Constriction, external, forearm
  arm (upper) S40.84- ☑
  auricle — *see* Constriction, external, ear
  axilla — *see* Constriction, external, arm
  back, lower S30.840 ☑
  breast S20.14- ☑
  brow S00.84 ☑
  buttock S30.840 ☑
  calf — *see* Constriction, external, leg
  canthus — *see* Constriction, external, eyelid
  cheek S00.84 ☑
   internal S00.542 ☑
  chest wall — *see* Constriction, external, thorax
  chin S00.84 ☑
  clitoris S30.844 ☑
  costal region — *see* Constriction, external, thorax
  digit(s)
   foot — *see* Constriction, external, toe
   hand — *see* Constriction, external, finger
  ear S00.44- ☑
  elbow S50.34- ☑
  epididymis S30.843 ☑
  epigastric region S30.841 ☑
  esophagus, cervical S10.14 ☑
  eyebrow — *see* Constriction, external, eyelid
  eyelid S00.24- ☑
  face S00.84 ☑
  finger(s) S60.44- ☑
   index S60.44- ☑
   little S60.44- ☑
   middle S60.44- ☑
   ring S60.44- ☑
  flank S30.841 ☑
  foot (except toe(s) alone) S90.84- ☑
   toe — *see* Constriction, external, toe
  forearm S50.84- ☑
   elbow only — *see* Constriction, external, elbow
  forehead S00.84 ☑
  genital organs, external
   female S30.846 ☑
   male S30.845 ☑
  groin S30.841 ☑
  gum S00.542 ☑
  hand S60.54- ☑
  head S00.94 ☑
   ear — *see* Constriction, external, ear
   eyelid — *see* Constriction, external, eyelid
   lip S00.541 ☑
   nose S00.34 ☑
   oral cavity S00.542 ☑
   scalp S00.04 ☑
   specified site NEC S00.84 ☑
  heel — *see* Constriction, external, foot
  hip S70.24- ☑
  inguinal region S30.841 ☑
  interscapular region S20.449 ☑
  jaw S00.84 ☑
  knee S80.24- ☑
  labium (majus) (minus) S30.844 ☑
  larynx S10.14 ☑
  leg (lower) S80.84- ☑
   knee — *see* Constriction, external, knee
   upper — *see* Constriction, external, thigh
  lip S00.541 ☑
  lower back S30.840 ☑
  lumbar region S30.840 ☑
  malar region S00.84 ☑

Constriction — *continued*
 external — *continued*
  mammary — *see* Constriction, external, breast
  mastoid region S00.84 ☑
  mouth S00.542 ☑
  nail
   finger — *see* Constriction, external, finger
   toe — *see* Constriction, external, toe
  nasal S00.34 ☑
  neck S10.94 ☑
   specified site NEC S10.84 ☑
   throat S10.14 ☑
  nose S00.34 ☑
  occipital region S00.04 ☑
  oral cavity S00.542 ☑
  orbital region — *see* Constriction, external, eyelid
  palate S00.542 ☑
  palm — *see* Constriction, external, hand
  parietal region S00.04 ☑
  pelvis S30.840 ☑
  penis S30.842 ☑
  perineum
   female S30.844 ☑
   male S30.840 ☑
  periocular area — *see* Constriction, external, eyelid
  phalanges
   finger — *see* Constriction, external, finger
   toe — *see* Constriction, external, toe
  pharynx S10.14 ☑
  pinna — *see* Constriction, external, ear
  popliteal space — *see* Constriction, external, knee
  prepuce S30.842 ☑
  pubic region S30.840 ☑
  pudendum
   female S30.846 ☑
   male S30.845 ☑
  sacral region S30.840 ☑
  scalp S00.04 ☑
  scapular region — *see* Constriction, external, shoulder
  scrotum S30.843 ☑
  shin — *see* Constriction, external, leg
  shoulder S40.24- ☑
  sternal region S20.349 ☑
  submaxillary region S00.84 ☑
  submental region S00.84 ☑
  subungual
   finger(s) — *see* Constriction, external, finger
   toe(s) — *see* Constriction, external, toe
  supraclavicular fossa S10.84 ☑
  supraorbital S00.84 ☑
  temple S00.84 ☑
  temporal region S00.84 ☑
  testis S30.843 ☑
  thigh S70.34- ☑
  thorax, thoracic (wall) S20.94 ☑
   back S20.44- ☑
   front S20.34- ☑
  throat S10.14 ☑
  thumb S60.34- ☑
  toe(s) (lesser) S90.44- ☑
   great S90.44- ☑
  tongue S00.542 ☑
  trachea S10.14 ☑
  tunica vaginalis S30.843 ☑
  uvula S00.542 ☑
  vagina S30.844 ☑
  vulva S30.844 ☑
  wrist S60.84- ☑
 gallbladder — *see* Obstruction, gallbladder
 intestine — *see* Obstruction, intestine
 larynx J38.6
  congenital Q31.8
   specified NEC Q31.8
   subglottic Q31.1
 organ or site, congenital NEC — *see* Atresia, by site
 prepuce (acquired) (congenital) N47.1
 pylorus (adult hypertrophic) K31.1
  congenital or infantile Q40.0
  newborn Q40.0
 ring dystocia (uterus) O62.4
 spastic — *see also* Spasm
  ureter N13.5
 ureter N13.5
  with infection N13.6
 urethra — *see* Stricture, urethra
 visual field (peripheral) (functional) — *see* Defect, visual field

Constrictive — *see* condition
Consultation
 medical — *see* Counseling, medical
 religious Z71.81
 specified reason NEC Z71.89
 spiritual Z71.81
 without complaint or sickness Z71.9
  feared complaint unfounded Z71.1
  specified reason NEC Z71.89
Consumption — *see* Tuberculosis
Contact (with) — *see also* Exposure (to)
 acariasis Z20.7
 AIDS virus Z20.6
 air pollution Z77.110
 algae and algae toxins Z77.121
 algae bloom Z77.121
 anthrax Z20.810
 aromatic amines Z77.020
 aromatic (hazardous) compounds NEC Z77.028
 aromatic dyes NOS Z77.028
 arsenic Z77.010
 asbestos Z77.090
 bacterial disease NEC Z20.818
 benzene Z77.021
 blue-green algae bloom Z77.121
 body fluids (potentially hazardous) Z77.21
 brown tide Z77.121
 chemicals (chiefly nonmedicinal) (hazardous) NEC Z77.098
 cholera Z20.09
 chromium compounds Z77.018
 communicable disease Z20.9
  bacterial NEC Z20.818
  specified NEC Z20.89
  viral NEC Z20.828
  Zika virus Z20.821
 coronavirus (disease) (novel) 2019 Z20.822
 COVID-19 Z20.822
 cyanobacteria bloom Z77.121
 dyes Z77.098
 Escherichia coli (E. coli) Z20.01
 fiberglass — *see* Table of Drugs and Chemicals, fiberglass
 German measles Z20.4
 gonorrhea Z20.2
 hazardous metals NEC Z77.018
 hazardous substances NEC Z77.29
 hazards in the physical environment NEC Z77.128
 hazards to health NEC Z77.9
 HIV Z20.6
 HTLV-III/LAV Z20.6
 human immunodeficiency virus (HIV) Z20.6
 infection Z20.9
  specified NEC Z20.89
 infestation (parasitic) NEC Z20.7
 intestinal infectious disease NEC Z20.09
  Escherichia coli (E. coli) Z20.01
 lead Z77.011
 meningococcus Z20.811
 mold (toxic) Z77.120
 nickel dust Z77.018
 noise Z77.122
 parasitic disease Z20.7
 pediculosis Z20.7
 pfiesteria piscicida Z77.121
 poliomyelitis Z20.89
 pollution
  air Z77.110
  environmental NEC Z77.118
  soil Z77.112
  water Z77.111
 polycyclic aromatic hydrocarbons Z77.028
 positive maternal group B streptococcus P00.82
 rabies Z20.3
 radiation, naturally occurring NEC Z77.123
 radon Z77.123
 red tide (Florida) Z77.121
 rubella Z20.4
 SARS-CoV-2 Z20.822
 sexually-transmitted disease Z20.2
 smallpox (laboratory) Z20.89
 syphilis Z20.2
 tuberculosis Z20.1
 uranium Z77.012
 varicella Z20.820
 venereal disease Z20.2
 viral disease NEC Z20.828
 viral hepatitis Z20.5
 water pollution Z77.111
 Zika virus Z20.821

☑ **Additional Character Required** — Refer to the Tabular List for Character Selection

Contamination, food — *see* Intoxication, foodborne
Contraception, contraceptive
  advice Z30.09
  counseling Z30.09
  device (intrauterine) (in situ) Z97.5
    causing menorrhagia T83.83 ☑
    checking Z30.431
    complications — *see* Complications, intrauterine, contraceptive device
    in place Z97.5
    initial prescription Z30.014
    reinsertion Z30.433
    removal Z30.432
    replacement Z30.433
  emergency (postcoital) Z30.012
  initial prescription Z30.019
    barrier Z30.018
    diaphragm Z30.018
    injectable Z30.013
    intrauterine device Z30.014
    pills Z30.011
    postcoital (emergency) Z30.012
    specified type NEC Z30.018
    subdermal implantable Z30.017
    transdermal patch hormonal Z30.016
    vaginal ring hormonal Z30.015
  maintenance Z30.40
    barrier Z30.49
    diaphragm Z30.49
    examination Z30.8
    injectable Z30.42
    intrauterine device Z30.431
    pills Z30.41
    specified type NEC Z30.49
    subdermal implantable Z30.46
    transdermal patch hormonal Z30.45
    vaginal ring hormonal Z30.44
  management Z30.9
    specified NEC Z30.8
  postcoital (emergency) Z30.012
  prescription Z30.019
    repeat Z30.40
  sterilization Z30.2
  surveillance (drug) — *see* Contraception, maintenance
Contraction(s), contracture, contracted
  Achilles tendon — *see also* Short, tendon, Achilles
    congenital Q66.89
  amputation stump (surgical) (flexion) (late) (next proximal joint) T87.89
  anus K59.89
  bile duct (common) (hepatic) K83.8
  bladder N32.89
    neck or sphincter N32.0
  bowel, cecum, colon or intestine, any part — *see* Obstruction, intestine
  Braxton Hicks — *see* False, labor
  breast implant, capsular T85.44 ☑
  bronchial J98.09
  burn (old) — *see* Cicatrix
  cervix — *see* Stricture, cervix
  cicatricial — *see* Cicatrix
  conjunctiva, trachomatous, active A71.1
    sequelae (late effect) B94.0
  Dupuytren's M72.0
  eyelid — *see* Disorder, eyelid function
  fascia (lata) (postural) M72.8
    Dupuytren's M72.0
    palmar M72.0
    plantar M72.2
  finger NEC — *see also* Deformity, finger
    congenital Q68.1
    joint — *see* Contraction, joint, hand
  flaccid — *see* Contraction, paralytic
  gallbladder K82.0
  heart valve — *see* Endocarditis
  hip — *see* Contraction, joint, hip
  hourglass
    bladder N32.89
      congenital Q64.79
    gallbladder K82.0
      congenital Q44.1
    stomach K31.89
      congenital Q40.2
      psychogenic F45.8
    uterus (complicating delivery) O62.4
  hysterical F44.4
  internal os — *see* Stricture, cervix
  joint (abduction) (acquired) (adduction) (flexion) (rotation) M24.50

Contraction(s), contracture, contracted — *continued*
  joint — *continued*
    ankle M24.57- ☑
    congenital NEC Q68.8
      hip Q65.89
    elbow M24.52- ☑
    foot joint M24.57- ☑
    hand joint M24.54- ☑
    hip M24.55- ☑
      congenital Q65.89
    hysterical F44.4
    knee M24.56- ☑
    shoulder M24.51- ☑
    specified site NEC M24.59
    wrist M24.53- ☑
  kidney (granular) (secondary) N26.9
    congenital Q63.8
    hydronephritic — *see* Hydronephrosis Page N26.2
    pyelonephritic — *see* Pyelitis, chronic
    tuberculous A18.11
  ligament — *see also* Disorder, ligament
    congenital Q79.8
  muscle (postinfective) (postural) NEC M62.40
    with contracture of joint — *see* Contraction, joint
    ankle M62.47- ☑
    congenital Q79.8
      sternocleidomastoid Q68.0
    extraocular — *see* Strabismus
    eye (extrinsic) — *see* Strabismus
    foot M62.47- ☑
    forearm M62.43- ☑
    hand M62.44- ☑
    hysterical F44.4
    ischemic (Volkmann's) T79.6 ☑
    lower leg M62.46- ☑
    multiple sites M62.49
    pelvic region M62.45- ☑
    posttraumatic — *see* Strabismus, paralytic
    psychogenic F45.8
      conversion reaction F44.4
    shoulder region M62.41- ☑
    specified site NEC M62.48
    thigh M62.45- ☑
    upper arm M62.42- ☑
  neck — *see* Torticollis
  ocular muscle — *see* Strabismus
  organ or site, congenital NEC — *see* Atresia, by site
  outlet (pelvis) — *see* Contraction, pelvis
  palmar fascia M72.0
  paralytic
    joint — *see* Contraction, joint
    muscle — *see also* Contraction, muscle NEC
      ocular — *see* Strabismus, paralytic
  pelvis (acquired) (general) M95.5
    with disproportion (fetopelvic) O33.1
      causing obstructed labor O65.1
    inlet O33.2
    mid-cavity O33.3 ☑
    outlet O33.3 ☑
  plantar fascia M72.2
  premature
    atrium I49.1
    auriculoventricular I49.49
    heart I49.49
    junctional I49.2
    supraventricular I49.1
    ventricular I49.3
  prostate N42.89
  pylorus NEC — *see also* Pylorospasm
    psychogenic F45.8
  rectum, rectal (sphincter) K59.89
  ring (Bandl's) (complicating delivery) O62.4
  scar — *see* Cicatrix
  spine — *see* Dorsopathy, deforming
  sternocleidomastoid (muscle), congenital Q68.0
  stomach K31.89
    hourglass K31.89
      congenital Q40.2
      psychogenic F45.8
    psychogenic F45.8
  tendon (sheath) M62.40
    with contracture of joint — *see* Contraction, joint
    Achilles — *see* Short, tendon, Achilles
    ankle M62.47- ☑
      Achilles — *see* Short, tendon, Achilles
    foot M62.47- ☑
    forearm M62.43- ☑

Contraction(s), contracture, contracted — *continued*
  tendon — *continued*
    hand M62.44- ☑
    lower leg M62.46- ☑
    multiple sites M62.49
    neck M62.48
    pelvic region M62.45- ☑
    shoulder region M62.41- ☑
    specified site NEC M62.48
    thigh M62.45- ☑
    thorax M62.48
    trunk M62.48
    upper arm M62.42- ☑
  toe — *see* Deformity, toe, specified NEC
  ureterovesical orifice (postinfectional) N13.5
    with infection N13.6
  urethra — *see also* Stricture, urethra
    orifice N32.0
  uterus N85.8
    abnormal NEC O62.9
    clonic (complicating delivery) O62.4
    dyscoordinate (complicating delivery) O62.4
    hourglass (complicating delivery) O62.4
    hypertonic O62.4
    hypotonic NEC O62.2
    inadequate
      primary O62.0
      secondary O62.1
    incoordinate (complicating delivery) O62.4
    poor O62.2
    tetanic (complicating delivery) O62.4
  vagina (outlet) N89.5
  vesical N32.89
    neck or urethral orifice N32.0
  visual field — *see* Defect, visual field, generalized
  Volkmann's (ischemic) T79.6 ☑
Contusion (skin surface intact) T14.8
  abdomen, abdominal (muscle) (wall) S30.1 ☑
  adnexa, eye NEC S05.8X- ☑
  adrenal gland S37.812 ☑
  alveolar process S00.532 ☑
  ankle S90.0- ☑
  antecubital space — *see* Contusion, forearm
  anus S30.3 ☑
  arm (upper) S40.02- ☑
    lower (with elbow) — *see* Contusion, forearm
  auditory canal — *see* Contusion, ear
  auricle — *see* Contusion, ear
  axilla — *see* Contusion, arm, upper
  back — *see also* Contusion, thorax, back
    lower S30.0 ☑
  bile duct S36.13 ☑
  bladder S37.22 ☑
  bone NEC T14.8 ☑
  brain (diffuse) — *see* Injury, intracranial, diffuse
    focal — *see* Injury, intracranial, focal
  brainstem S06.38- ☑
  breast S20.0- ☑
  broad ligament S37.892 ☑
  brow S00.83 ☑
  buttock S30.0 ☑
  canthus, eye S00.1- ☑
  cauda equina S34.3 ☑
  cerebellar, traumatic S06.37- ☑
  cerebral S06.33- ☑
    left side S06.32- ☑
    right side S06.31- ☑
  cheek S00.83 ☑
    internal S00.532 ☑
  chest (wall) — *see* Contusion, thorax
  chin S00.83 ☑
  clitoris S30.23 ☑
  colon — *see* Injury, intestine, large, contusion
  common bile duct S36.13 ☑
  conjunctiva S05.1- ☑
    with foreign body (in conjunctival sac) — *see* Foreign body, conjunctival sac
  conus medullaris (spine) S34.139 ☑
  cornea — *see* Contusion, eyeball
    with foreign body — *see* Foreign body, cornea
  corpus cavernosum S30.21 ☑
  cortex (brain) (cerebral) — *see* Injury, intracranial, diffuse
    focal — *see* Injury, intracranial, focal
  costal region — *see* Contusion, thorax
  cystic duct S36.13 ☑
  diaphragm S27.802 ☑
  duodenum S36.420 ☑

Contusion — *continued*
- ear S00.43- ☑
- elbow S50.0- ☑
  - with forearm — *see* Contusion, forearm
- epididymis S30.22 ☑
- epigastric region S30.1 ☑
- epiglottis S10.0 ☑
- esophagus (thoracic) S27.812 ☑
  - cervical S10.0 ☑
- eyeball S05.1- ☑
- eyebrow S00.1- ☑
- eyelid (and periocular area) S00.1- ☑
- face NEC S00.83 ☑
- fallopian tube S37.529 ☑
  - bilateral S37.522 ☑
  - unilateral S37.521 ☑
- femoral triangle S30.1 ☑
- finger(s) S60.00 ☑
  - with damage to nail (matrix) S60.10 ☑
  - index S60.02- ☑
    - with damage to nail S60.12- ☑
  - little S60.05- ☑
    - with damage to nail S60.15- ☑
  - middle S60.03- ☑
    - with damage to nail S60.13- ☑
  - ring S60.04- ☑
    - with damage to nail S60.14- ☑
  - thumb — *see* Contusion, thumb
- flank S30.1 ☑
- foot (except toe(s) alone) S90.3- ☑
  - toe — *see* Contusion, toe
- forearm S50.1- ☑
  - elbow only — *see* Contusion, elbow
- forehead S00.83 ☑
- gallbladder S36.122 ☑
- genital organs, external
  - female S30.202 ☑
  - male S30.201 ☑
- globe (eye) — *see* Contusion, eyeball
- groin S30.1 ☑
- gum S00.532 ☑
- hand S60.22- ☑
  - finger(s) — *see* Contusion, finger
  - wrist — *see* Contusion, wrist
- head S00.93 ☑
  - ear — *see* Contusion, ear
  - eyelid — *see* Contusion, eyelid
  - lip S00.531 ☑
  - nose S00.33 ☑
  - oral cavity S00.532 ☑
  - scalp S00.03 ☑
  - specified part NEC S00.83 ☑
- heart — *see also* Injury, heart S26.91 ☑
- heel — *see* Contusion, foot
- hepatic duct S36.13 ☑
- hip S70.0- ☑
- ileum S36.428 ☑
- iliac region S30.1 ☑
- inguinal region S30.1 ☑
- interscapular region S20.229 ☑
- intra-abdominal organ S36.92 ☑
  - colon — *see* Injury, intestine, large, contusion
  - liver S36.112 ☑
  - pancreas — *see* Contusion, pancreas
  - rectum S36.62 ☑
  - small intestine — *see* Injury, intestine, small, contusion
  - specified organ NEC S36.892 ☑
  - spleen — *see* Contusion, spleen
  - stomach S36.32 ☑
- iris (eye) — *see* Contusion, eyeball
- jaw S00.83 ☑
- jejunum S36.428 ☑
- kidney S37.01- ☑
  - major (greater than 2 cm) S37.02- ☑
  - minor (less than 2 cm) S37.01- ☑
- knee S80.0- ☑
- labium (majus) (minus) S30.23 ☑
- lacrimal apparatus, gland or sac S05.8X- ☑
- larynx S10.0 ☑
- leg (lower) S80.1- ☑
  - knee — *see* Contusion, knee
- lens — *see* Contusion, eyeball
- lip S00.531 ☑
- liver S36.112 ☑
- lower back S30.0 ☑

Contusion — *continued*
- lumbar region S30.0 ☑
- lung S27.329 ☑
  - bilateral S27.322 ☑
  - unilateral S27.321 ☑
- malar region S00.83 ☑
- mastoid region S00.83 ☑
- membrane, brain — *see* Injury, intracranial, diffuse
  - focal — *see* Injury, intracranial, focal
- mesentery S36.892 ☑
- mesosalpinx S37.892 ☑
- mouth S00.532 ☑
- muscle — *see* Contusion, by site
- nail
  - finger — *see* Contusion, finger, with damage to nail
  - toe — *see* Contusion, toe, with damage to nail
- nasal S00.33 ☑
- neck S10.93 ☑
  - specified site NEC S10.83 ☑
  - throat S10.0 ☑
- nerve — *see* Injury, nerve
- newborn P54.5
- nose S00.33 ☑
- occipital
  - lobe (brain) — *see* Injury, intracranial, diffuse
    - focal — *see* Injury, intracranial, focal
  - region (scalp) S00.03 ☑
- orbit (region) (tissues) S05.1- ☑
- ovary S37.429 ☑
  - bilateral S37.422 ☑
  - unilateral S37.421 ☑
- palate S00.532 ☑
- pancreas S36.229 ☑
  - body S36.221 ☑
  - head S36.220 ☑
  - tail S36.222 ☑
- parietal
  - lobe (brain) — *see* Injury, intracranial, diffuse
    - focal — *see* Injury, intracranial, focal
  - region (scalp) S00.03 ☑
- pelvic organ S37.92 ☑
  - adrenal gland S37.812 ☑
  - bladder S37.22 ☑
  - fallopian tube — *see* Contusion, fallopian tube
  - kidney — *see* Contusion, kidney
  - ovary — *see* Contusion, ovary
  - prostate S37.822 ☑
  - specified organ NEC S37.892 ☑
  - ureter S37.12 ☑
  - urethra S37.32 ☑
  - uterus S37.62 ☑
- pelvis S30.0 ☑
- penis S30.21 ☑
- perineum
  - female S30.23 ☑
  - male S30.0 ☑
- periocular area S00.1- ☑
- peritoneum S36.81 ☑
- periurethral tissue — *see* Contusion, urethra
- pharynx S10.0 ☑
- pinna — *see* Contusion, ear
- popliteal space — *see* Contusion, knee
- prepuce S30.21 ☑
- prostate S37.822 ☑
- pubic region S30.1 ☑
- pudendum
  - female S30.202 ☑
  - male S30.201 ☑
- quadriceps femoris — *see* Contusion, thigh
- rectum S36.62 ☑
- retroperitoneum S36.892 ☑
- round ligament S37.892 ☑
- sacral region S30.0 ☑
- scalp S00.03 ☑
  - due to birth injury P12.3
- scapular region — *see* Contusion, shoulder
- sclera — *see* Contusion, eyeball
- scrotum S30.22 ☑
- seminal vesicle S37.892 ☑
- shoulder S40.01- ☑
- skin NEC T14.8 ☑
- small intestine — *see* Injury, intestine, small, contusion
- spermatic cord S30.22 ☑
- spinal cord — *see* Injury, spinal cord, by region
  - cauda equina S34.3 ☑
  - conus medullaris S34.139 ☑

Contusion — *continued*
- spleen S36.029 ☑
  - major S36.021 ☑
  - minor S36.020 ☑
- sternal region S20.219 ☑
- stomach S36.32 ☑
- subconjunctival S05.1- ☑
- subcutaneous NEC T14.8 ☑
- submaxillary region S00.83 ☑
- submental region S00.83 ☑
- subperiosteal NEC T14.8 ☑
- subungual
  - finger — *see* Contusion, finger, with damage to nail
  - toe — *see* Contusion, toe, with damage to nail
- supraclavicular fossa S10.83 ☑
- supraorbital S00.83 ☑
- suprarenal gland S37.812 ☑
- temple (region) S00.83 ☑
- temporal
  - lobe (brain) — *see* Injury, intracranial, diffuse
    - focal — *see* Injury, intracranial, focal
  - region S00.83 ☑
- testis S30.22 ☑
- thigh S70.1- ☑
- thorax (wall) S20.20 ☑
  - back S20.22- ☑
  - front S20.21- ☑
- throat S10.0 ☑
- thumb S60.01- ☑
  - with damage to nail S60.11- ☑
- toe(s) (lesser) S90.12- ☑
  - with damage to nail S90.22- ☑
  - great S90.11- ☑
    - with damage to nail S90.21- ☑
- tongue S00.532 ☑
- trachea (cervical) S10.0 ☑
  - thoracic S27.52 ☑
- tunica vaginalis S30.22 ☑
- tympanum, tympanic membrane — *see* Contusion, ear
- ureter S37.12 ☑
- urethra S37.32 ☑
- urinary organ NEC S37.892 ☑
- uterus S37.62 ☑
- uvula S00.532 ☑
- vagina S30.23 ☑
- vas deferens S37.892 ☑
- vesical S37.22 ☑
- vocal cord(s) S10.0 ☑
- vulva S30.23 ☑
- wrist S60.21- ☑

Conus (congenital) (any type) Q14.8
- cornea — *see* Keratoconus
- medullaris syndrome G95.81

Conversion hysteria, neurosis or reaction F44.9

Converter, tuberculosis (test reaction) R76.11

Conviction (legal), **anxiety concerning** Z65.0
- with imprisonment Z65.1

Convulsions (idiopathic) — *see also* Seizure(s) R56.9
- apoplectiform (cerebral ischemia) I67.82
- dissociative F44.5
- epileptic — *see* Epilepsy
- epileptiform, epileptoid — *see* Epilepsy
- ether (anesthetic) — *see* Table of Drugs and Chemicals, by drug
- febrile R56.00
  - with status epilepticus G40.901
  - complex R56.01
    - with status epilepticus G40.901
  - simple R56.00
- hysterical F44.5
- infantile P90
  - epilepsy — *see* Epilepsy
- jacksonian — *see* Epilepsy, localization-related, symptomatic, with simple partial seizures
- myoclonic G25.3
- newborn P90
- obstetrical (nephritic) (uremic) — *see* Eclampsia
- paretic A52.17
- post traumatic R56.1
- psychomotor — *see* Epilepsy, localization-related, symptomatic, with complex partial seizures
- recurrent R56.9
- reflex R25.8
- scarlatinal A38.8
- tetanus, tetanic — *see* Tetanus
- thymic E32.8

Convulsive — *see also* Convulsions

☑ **Additional Character Required** — **Refer to the Tabular List for Character Selection**

Cooley's anemia D56.1
Coolie itch B76.9
Cooper's
  disease — *see* Mastopathy, cystic
  hernia — *see* Hernia, abdomen, specified site NEC
Copra itch B88.0
Coprophagy F50.89
Coprophobia F40.298
Coproporphyria, hereditary E80.29
Cor
  biloculare Q20.8
  bovis, bovinum — *see* Hypertrophy, cardiac
  pulmonale I27.81
    acute I26.09
      without pulmonary embolism I27.81
    chronic I27.81
      with chronic pulmonary embolism I27.82
  triatriatum, triatrium Q24.2
  triloculare Q20.8
    biatrium Q20.4
    biventriculare Q21.19
Corbus' disease (gangrenous balanitis) N48.1
Cord — *see also* condition
  around neck
    complicating delivery O69.81 ☑
      with compression O69.1 ☑
  bladder G95.89
    tabetic A52.19
Cordis ectopia Q24.8
Corditis (spermatic) N49.1
Corectopia Q13.2
Cori's disease (glycogen storage) E74.03
Corkhandler's disease or lung J67.3
Corkscrew esophagus K22.4
Corkworker's disease or lung J67.3
Corn (infected) L84
Cornea — *see also* condition
  donor Z52.5
  plana Q13.4
Cornelia de Lange syndrome Q87.19
Cornu cutaneum L85.8
Cornual gestation or pregnancy O00.80
  with intrauterine pregnancy O00.81
Coronary (artery) — *see* condition
Coronavirus (infection)
  2019 — *see also* COVID-19 U07.1
  as cause of diseases classified elsewhere B97.29
  coronavirus-19 — *see also* COVID-19 U07.1
  COVID-19 — *see also* COVID-19 U07.1
  SARS-associated B97.21
Corpora — *see also* condition
  amylacea, prostate N42.89
  cavernosa — *see* condition
Corpulence — *see* Obesity
Corpus — *see* condition
Corrected transposition Q20.5
Corrosion (injury) (acid) (caustic) (chemical) (lime) (external)
    (internal) T30.4
  abdomen, abdominal (muscle) (wall) T21.42 ☑
    first degree T21.52 ☑
    second degree T21.62 ☑
    third degree T21.72 ☑
  above elbow T22.439 ☑
    first degree T22.539 ☑
    left T22.432 ☑
      first degree T22.532 ☑
      second degree T22.632 ☑
      third degree T22.732 ☑
    right T22.431 ☑
      first degree T22.531 ☑
      second degree T22.631 ☑
      third degree T22.731 ☑
    second degree T22.639 ☑
    third degree T22.739 ☑
  alimentary tract NEC T28.7 ☑
  ankle T25.419 ☑
    first degree T25.519 ☑
    left T25.412 ☑
      first degree T25.512 ☑
      second degree T25.612 ☑
      third degree T25.712 ☑
    multiple with foot — *see* Corrosion, lower, limb,
        multiple, ankle and foot
    right T25.411 ☑
      first degree T25.511 ☑
      second degree T25.611 ☑
      third degree T25.711 ☑

Corrosion — *continued*
  ankle — *continued*
    second degree T25.619 ☑
    third degree T25.719 ☑
  anus — *see* Corrosion, buttock
  arm(s) (meaning upper limb(s)) — *see* Corrosion, upper
      limb
  axilla T22.449 ☑
    first degree T22.549 ☑
    left T22.442 ☑
      first degree T22.542 ☑
      second degree T22.642 ☑
      third degree T22.742 ☑
    right T22.441 ☑
      first degree T22.541 ☑
      second degree T22.641 ☑
      third degree T22.741 ☑
    second degree T22.649 ☑
    third degree T22.749 ☑
  back (lower) T21.44 ☑
    first degree T21.54 ☑
    second degree T21.64 ☑
    third degree T21.74 ☑
    upper T21.43 ☑
      first degree T21.53 ☑
      second degree T21.63 ☑
      third degree T21.73 ☑
  blisters — *code as* Corrosion, second degree, by site
  breast(s) — *see* Corrosion, chest wall
  buttock(s) T21.45 ☑
    first degree T21.55 ☑
    second degree T21.65 ☑
    third degree T21.75 ☑
  calf T24.439 ☑
    first degree T24.539 ☑
    left T24.432 ☑
      first degree T24.532 ☑
      second degree T24.632 ☑
      third degree T24.732 ☑
    right T24.431 ☑
      first degree T24.531 ☑
      second degree T24.631 ☑
      third degree T24.731 ☑
    second degree T24.639 ☑
    third degree T24.739 ☑
  canthus (eye) — *see* Corrosion, eyelid
  cervix T28.8 ☑
  cheek T20.46 ☑
    first degree T20.56 ☑
    second degree T20.66 ☑
    third degree T20.76 ☑
  chest wall T21.41 ☑
    first degree T21.51 ☑
    second degree T21.61 ☑
    third degree T21.71 ☑
  chin T20.43 ☑
    first degree T20.53 ☑
    second degree T20.63 ☑
    third degree T20.73 ☑
  colon T28.7 ☑
  conjunctiva (and cornea) — *see* Corrosion, cornea
  cornea (and conjunctiva) T26.6- ☑
  deep necrosis of underlying tissue — *code as* Corrosion,
      third degree, by site
  dorsum of hand T23.469 ☑
    first degree T23.569 ☑
    left T23.462 ☑
      first degree T23.562 ☑
      second degree T23.662 ☑
      third degree T23.762 ☑
    right T23.461 ☑
      first degree T23.561 ☑
      second degree T23.661 ☑
      third degree T23.761 ☑
    second degree T23.669 ☑
    third degree T23.769 ☑
  ear (auricle) (external) (canal) T20.41 ☑
    drum T28.91 ☑
    first degree T20.51 ☑
    second degree T20.61 ☑
    third degree T20.71 ☑
  elbow T22.429 ☑
    first degree T22.529 ☑
    left T22.422 ☑
      first degree T22.522 ☑

Corrosion — *continued*
  elbow — *continued*
    left — *continued*
      second degree T22.622 ☑
      third degree T22.722 ☑
    right T22.421 ☑
      first degree T22.521 ☑
      second degree T22.621 ☑
      third degree T22.721 ☑
    second degree T22.629 ☑
    third degree T22.729 ☑
  entire body — *see* Corrosion, multiple body regions
  epidermal loss — *code as* Corrosion, second degree, by
      site
  epiglottis T27.4 ☑
  erythema, erythematous — *code as* Corrosion, first de-
      gree, by site
  esophagus T28.6 ☑
  extent (percentage of body surface)
    less than 10 percent T32.0
    10-19 percent (0-9 percent third degree) T32.10
      with 10-19 percent third degree T32.11
    20-29 percent (0-9 percent third degree) T32.20
      with
        10-19 percent third degree T32.21
        20-29 percent third degree T32.22
    30-39 percent (0-9 percent third degree) T32.30
      with
        10-19 percent third degree T32.31
        20-29 percent third degree T32.32
        30-39 percent third degree T32.33
    40-49 percent (0-9 percent third degree) T32.40
      with
        10-19 percent third degree T32.41
        20-29 percent third degree T32.42
        30-39 percent third degree T32.43
        40-49 percent third degree T32.44
    50-59 percent (0-9 percent third degree) T32.50
      with
        10-19 percent third degree T32.51
        20-29 percent third degree T32.52
        30-39 percent third degree T32.53
        40-49 percent third degree T32.54
        50-59 percent third degree T32.55
    60-69 percent (0-9 percent third degree) T32.60
      with
        10-19 percent third degree T32.61
        20-29 percent third degree T32.62
        30-39 percent third degree T32.63
        40-49 percent third degree T32.64
        50-59 percent third degree T32.65
        60-69 percent third degree T32.66
    70-79 percent (0-9 percent third degree) T32.70
      with
        10-19 percent third degree T32.71
        20-29 percent third degree T32.72
        30-39 percent third degree T32.73
        40-49 percent third degree T32.74
        50-59 percent third degree T32.75
        60-69 percent third degree T32.76
        70-79 percent third degree T32.77
    80-89 percent (0-9 percent third degree) T32.80
      with
        10-19 percent third degree T32.81
        20-29 percent third degree T32.82
        30-39 percent third degree T32.83
        40-49 percent third degree T32.84
        50-59 percent third degree T32.85
        60-69 percent third degree T32.86
        70-79 percent third degree T32.87
        80-89 percent third degree T32.88
    90 percent or more (0-9 percent third degree) T32.90
      with
        10-19 percent third degree T32.91
        20-29 percent third degree T32.92
        30-39 percent third degree T32.93
        40-49 percent third degree T32.94
        50-59 percent third degree T32.95
        60-69 percent third degree T32.96
        70-79 percent third degree T32.97
        80-89 percent third degree T32.98
        90-99 percent third degree T32.99
  extremity — *see* Corrosion, limb
  eye(s) and adnexa T26.9- ☑
    with resulting rupture and destruction of eyeball
        T26.7- ☑
    conjunctival sac — *see* Corrosion, cornea
    cornea — *see* Corrosion, cornea

Corrosion — *continued*
  eye(s) and adnexa — *continued*
    lid — *see* Corrosion, eyelid
    periocular area — *see* Corrosion eyelid
    specified site NEC T26.8- ☑
  eyeball — *see* Corrosion, eye
  eyelid(s) T26.5- ☑
  face — *see* Corrosion, head
  finger T23.429 ☑
    first degree T23.529 ☑
    left T23.422 ☑
      first degree T23.522 ☑
      second degree T23.622 ☑
      third degree T23.722 ☑
    multiple sites (without thumb) T23.439 ☑
      with thumb T23.449 ☑
        first degree T23.549 ☑
        left T23.442 ☑
          first degree T23.542 ☑
          second degree T23.642 ☑
          third degree T23.742 ☑
        right T23.441 ☑
          first degree T23.541 ☑
          second degree T23.641 ☑
          third degree T23.741 ☑
      second degree T23.649 ☑
      third degree T23.749 ☑
    first degree T23.539 ☑
    left T23.432 ☑
      first degree T23.532 ☑
      second degree T23.632 ☑
      third degree T23.732 ☑
    right T23.431 ☑
      first degree T23.531 ☑
      second degree T23.631 ☑
      third degree T23.731 ☑
    second degree T23.639 ☑
    third degree T23.739 ☑
    right T23.421 ☑
      first degree T23.521 ☑
      second degree T23.621 ☑
      third degree T23.721 ☑
    second degree T23.629 ☑
    third degree T23.729 ☑
  flank — *see* Corrosion, abdomen
  foot T25.429 ☑
    first degree T25.529 ☑
    left T25.422 ☑
      first degree T25.522 ☑
      second degree T25.622 ☑
      third degree T25.722 ☑
    multiple with ankle — *see* Corrosion, lower, limb,
        multiple, ankle and foot
    right T25.421 ☑
      first degree T25.521 ☑
      second degree T25.621 ☑
      third degree T25.721 ☑
    second degree T25.629 ☑
    third degree T25.729 ☑
  forearm T22.419 ☑
    first degree T22.519 ☑
    left T22.412 ☑
      first degree T22.512 ☑
      second degree T22.612 ☑
      third degree T22.712 ☑
    right T22.411 ☑
      first degree T22.511 ☑
      second degree T22.611 ☑
      third degree T22.711 ☑
    second degree T22.619 ☑
    third degree T22.719 ☑
  forehead T20.46 ☑
    first degree T20.56 ☑
    second degree T20.66 ☑
    third degree T20.76 ☑
  fourth degree — *code as* Corrosion, third degree, by site
  full thickness skin loss — *code as* Corrosion, third degree,
      by site
  gastrointestinal tract NEC T28.7 ☑
  genital organs
    external
      female T21.47 ☑
        first degree T21.57 ☑
        second degree T21.67 ☑
        third degree T21.77 ☑

Corrosion — *continued*
  genital organs — *continued*
    external — *continued*
      male T21.46 ☑
        first degree T21.56 ☑
        second degree T21.66 ☑
        third degree T21.76 ☑
    internal T28.8 ☑
  groin — *see* Corrosion, abdominal wall
  hand(s) T23.409 ☑
    back — *see* Corrosion, dorsum of hand
    finger — *see* Corrosion, finger
    first degree T23.509 ☑
    left T23.402 ☑
      first degree T23.502 ☑
      second degree T23.602 ☑
      third degree T23.702 ☑
    multiple sites with wrist T23.499 ☑
      first degree T23.599 ☑
      left T23.492 ☑
        first degree T23.592 ☑
        second degree T23.692 ☑
        third degree T23.792 ☑
      right T23.491 ☑
        first degree T23.591 ☑
        second degree T23.691 ☑
        third degree T23.791 ☑
      second degree T23.699 ☑
      third degree T23.799 ☑
    palm — *see* Corrosion, palm
    right T23.401 ☑
      first degree T23.501 ☑
      second degree T23.601 ☑
      third degree T23.701 ☑
    second degree T23.609 ☑
    third degree T23.709 ☑
    thumb — *see* Corrosion, thumb
  head (and face) (and neck) T20.40 ☑
    cheek — *see* Corrosion, cheek
    chin — *see* Corrosion, chin
    ear — *see* Corrosion, ear
    eye(s) only — *see* Corrosion, eye
    first degree T20.50 ☑
    forehead — *see* Corrosion, forehead
    lip — *see* Corrosion, lip
    multiple sites T20.49 ☑
      first degree T20.59 ☑
      second degree T20.69 ☑
      third degree T20.79 ☑
    neck — *see* Corrosion, neck
    nose — *see* Corrosion, nose
    scalp — *see* Corrosion, scalp
    second degree T20.60 ☑
    third degree T20.70 ☑
  hip(s) — *see* Corrosion, lower, limb
  inhalation — *see* Corrosion, respiratory tract
  internal organ(s) — *see also* Corrosion, by site T28.90 ☑
    alimentary tract T28.7 ☑
      esophagus T28.6 ☑
    esophagus T28.6 ☑
    genitourinary T28.8 ☑
    mouth T28.5 ☑
    pharynx T28.5 ☑
    specified organ NEC T28.99 ☑
  interscapular region — *see* Corrosion, back, upper
  intestine (large) (small) T28.7 ☑
  knee T24.429 ☑
    first degree T24.529 ☑
    left T24.422 ☑
      first degree T24.522 ☑
      second degree T24.622 ☑
      third degree T24.722 ☑
    right T24.421 ☑
      first degree T24.521 ☑
      second degree T24.621 ☑
      third degree T24.721 ☑
    second degree T24.629 ☑
    third degree T24.729 ☑
  labium (majus) (minus) — *see* Corrosion, genital organs,
      external, female
  lacrimal apparatus, duct, gland or sac — *see* Corrosion,
      eye, specified site NEC
  larynx T27.4 ☑
    with lung T27.5 ☑
  leg(s) (meaning lower limb(s)) — *see* Corrosion, lower
      limb

Corrosion — *continued*
  limb(s)
    lower — *see* Corrosion, lower, limb
    upper — *see* Corrosion, upper limb
  lip(s) T20.42 ☑
    first degree T20.52 ☑
    second degree T20.62 ☑
    third degree T20.72 ☑
  lower
    back — *see* Corrosion, back
    limb T24.409 ☑
      ankle — *see* Corrosion, ankle
      calf — *see* Corrosion, calf
      first degree T24.509 ☑
      foot — *see* Corrosion, foot
      knee — *see* Corrosion, knee
      left T24.402 ☑
        first degree T24.502 ☑
        second degree T24.602 ☑
        third degree T24.702 ☑
      multiple sites, except ankle and foot T24.499 ☑
        ankle and foot T25.499 ☑
          first degree T25.599 ☑
          left T25.492 ☑
            first degree T25.592 ☑
            second degree T25.692 ☑
            third degree T25.792 ☑
          right T25.491 ☑
            first degree T25.591 ☑
            second degree T25.691 ☑
            third degree T25.791 ☑
          second degree T25.699 ☑
          third degree T25.799 ☑
        first degree T24.599 ☑
        left T24.492 ☑
          first degree T24.592 ☑
          second degree T24.692 ☑
          third degree T24.792 ☑
        right T24.491 ☑
          first degree T24.591 ☑
          second degree T24.691 ☑
          third degree T24.791 ☑
        second degree T24.699 ☑
        third degree T24.799 ☑
      right T24.401 ☑
        first degree T24.501 ☑
        second degree T24.601 ☑
        third degree T24.701 ☑
      second degree T24.609 ☑
      thigh — *see* Corrosion, thigh
      third degree T24.709 ☑
  lung (with larynx and trachea) T27.5 ☑
  mouth T28.5 ☑
  neck T20.47 ☑
    first degree T20.57 ☑
    second degree T20.67 ☑
    third degree T20.77 ☑
  nose (septum) T20.44 ☑
    first degree T20.54 ☑
    second degree T20.64 ☑
    third degree T20.74 ☑
  ocular adnexa — *see* Corrosion, eye
  orbit region — *see* Corrosion, eyelid
  palm T23.459 ☑
    first degree T23.559 ☑
    left T23.452 ☑
      first degree T23.552 ☑
      second degree T23.652 ☑
      third degree T23.752 ☑
    right T23.451 ☑
      first degree T23.551 ☑
      second degree T23.651 ☑
      third degree T23.751 ☑
    second degree T23.659 ☑
    third degree T23.759 ☑
  partial thickness — *code as* Corrosion, unspecified de-
      gree, by site
  pelvis — *see* Corrosion, trunk
  penis — *see* Corrosion, genital organs, external, male
  perineum
    female — *see* Corrosion, genital organs, external, fe-
        male
    male — *see* Corrosion, genital organs, external, male
  periocular area — *see* Corrosion, eyelid
  pharynx T28.5 ☑
  rectum T28.7 ☑

Corrosion — *continued*
- respiratory tract T27.7 ☑
  - larynx — *see* Corrosion, larynx
  - specified part NEC T27.6 ☑
  - trachea — *see* Corrosion, larynx
- sac, lacrimal — *see* Corrosion, eye, specified site NEC
- scalp T20.45 ☑
  - first degree T20.55 ☑
  - second degree T20.65 ☑
  - third degree T20.75 ☑
- scapular region T22.469 ☑
  - first degree T22.569 ☑
  - left T22.462 ☑
    - first degree T22.562 ☑
    - second degree T22.662 ☑
    - third degree T22.762 ☑
  - right T22.461 ☑
    - first degree T22.561 ☑
    - second degree T22.661 ☑
    - third degree T22.761 ☑
  - second degree T22.669 ☑
  - third degree T22.769 ☑
- sclera — *see* Corrosion, eye, specified site NEC
- scrotum — *see* Corrosion, genital organs, external, male
- shoulder T22.459 ☑
  - first degree T22.559 ☑
  - left T22.452 ☑
    - first degree T22.552 ☑
    - second degree T22.652 ☑
    - third degree T22.752 ☑
  - right T22.451 ☑
    - first degree T22.551 ☑
    - second degree T22.651 ☑
    - third degree T22.751 ☑
  - second degree T22.659 ☑
  - third degree T22.759 ☑
- stomach T28.7 ☑
- temple — *see* Corrosion, head
- testis — *see* Corrosion, genital organs, external, male
- thigh T24.419 ☑
  - first degree T24.519 ☑
  - left T24.412 ☑
    - first degree T24.512 ☑
    - second degree T24.612 ☑
    - third degree T24.712 ☑
  - right T24.411 ☑
    - first degree T24.511 ☑
    - second degree T24.611 ☑
    - third degree T24.711 ☑
  - second degree T24.619 ☑
  - third degree T24.719 ☑
- thorax (external) — *see* Corrosion, trunk
- throat (meaning pharynx) T28.5 ☑
- thumb(s) T23.419 ☑
  - first degree T23.519 ☑
  - left T23.412 ☑
    - first degree T23.512 ☑
    - second degree T23.612 ☑
    - third degree T23.712 ☑
  - multiple sites with fingers T23.449 ☑
    - first degree T23.549 ☑
    - left T23.442 ☑
      - first degree T23.542 ☑
      - second degree T23.642 ☑
      - third degree T23.742 ☑
    - right T23.441 ☑
      - first degree T23.541 ☑
      - second degree T23.641 ☑
      - third degree T23.741 ☑
    - second degree T23.649 ☑
    - third degree T23.749 ☑
  - right T23.411 ☑
    - first degree T23.511 ☑
    - second degree T23.611 ☑
    - third degree T23.711 ☑
  - second degree T23.619 ☑
  - third degree T23.719 ☑
- toe T25.439 ☑
  - first degree T25.539 ☑
  - left T25.432 ☑
    - first degree T25.532 ☑
    - second degree T25.632 ☑
    - third degree T25.732 ☑
  - right T25.431 ☑
    - first degree T25.531 ☑

Corrosion — *continued*
- toe — *continued*
  - right — *continued*
    - second degree T25.631 ☑
    - third degree T25.731 ☑
  - second degree T25.639 ☑
  - third degree T25.739 ☑
- tongue T28.5 ☑
- tonsil(s) T28.5 ☑
- total body — *see* Corrosion, multiple body regions
- trachea T27.4 ☑
  - with lung T27.5 ☑
- trunk T21.40 ☑
  - abdominal wall — *see* Corrosion, abdominal wall
  - anus — *see* Corrosion, buttock
  - axilla — *see* Corrosion, upper limb
  - back — *see* Corrosion, back
  - breast — *see* Corrosion, chest wall
  - buttock — *see* Corrosion, buttock
  - chest wall — *see* Corrosion, chest wall
  - first degree T21.50 ☑
  - flank — *see* Corrosion, abdominal wall
  - genital
    - female — *see* Corrosion, genital organs, external, female
    - male — *see* Corrosion, genital organs, external, male
  - groin — *see* Corrosion, abdominal wall
  - interscapular region — *see* Corrosion, back, upper
  - labia — *see* Corrosion, genital organs, external, female
  - lower back — *see* Corrosion, back
  - penis — *see* Corrosion, genital organs, external, male
  - perineum
    - female — *see* Corrosion, genital organs, external, female
    - male — *see* Corrosion, genital organs, external, male
  - scapular region — *see* Corrosion, upper limb
  - scrotum — *see* Corrosion, genital organs, external, male
  - second degree T21.60 ☑
  - shoulder — *see* Corrosion, upper limb
  - specified site NEC T21.49 ☑
    - first degree T21.59 ☑
    - second degree T21.69 ☑
    - third degree T21.79 ☑
  - testes — *see* Corrosion, genital organs, external, male
  - third degree T21.70 ☑
  - upper back — *see* Corrosion, back, upper
  - vagina T28.8 ☑
  - vulva — *see* Corrosion, genital organs, external, female
- unspecified site with extent of body surface involved specified
  - less than 10 percent T32.0
  - 10-19 percent (0-9 percent third degree) T32.10
    - with 10-19 percent third degree T32.11
  - 20-29 percent (0-9 percent third degree) T32.20
    - with
      - 10-19 percent third degree T32.21
      - 20-29 percent third degree T32.22
  - 30-39 percent (0-9 percent third degree) T32.30
    - with
      - 10-19 percent third degree T32.31
      - 20-29 percent third degree T32.32
      - 30-39 percent third degree T32.33
  - 40-49 percent (0-9 percent third degree) T32.40
    - with
      - 10-19 percent third degree T32.41
      - 20-29 percent third degree T32.42
      - 30-39 percent third degree T32.43
      - 40-49 percent third degree T32.44
  - 50-59 percent (0-9 percent third degree) T32.50
    - with
      - 10-19 percent third degree T32.51
      - 20-29 percent third degree T32.52
      - 30-39 percent third degree T32.53
      - 40-49 percent third degree T32.54
      - 50-59 percent third degree T32.55
  - 60-69 percent (0-9 percent third degree) T32.60
    - with
      - 10-19 percent third degree T32.61
      - 20-29 percent third degree T32.62
      - 30-39 percent third degree T32.63
      - 40-49 percent third degree T32.64
      - 50-59 percent third degree T32.65
      - 60-69 percent third degree T32.66
  - 70-79 percent (0-9 percent third degree) T32.70

Corrosion — *continued*
- unspecified site with extent of body surface involved specified — *continued*
  - 70-79 percent — *continued*
    - with
      - 10-19 percent third degree T32.71
      - 20-29 percent third degree T32.72
      - 30-39 percent third degree T32.73
      - 40-49 percent third degree T32.74
      - 50-59 percent third degree T32.75
      - 60-69 percent third degree T32.76
      - 70-79 percent third degree T32.77
  - 80-89 percent (0-9 percent third degree) T32.80
    - with
      - 10-19 percent third degree T32.81
      - 20-29 percent third degree T32.82
      - 30-39 percent third degree T32.83
      - 40-49 percent third degree T32.84
      - 50-59 percent third degree T32.85
      - 60-69 percent third degree T32.86
      - 70-79 percent third degree T32.87
      - 80-89 percent third degree T32.88
  - 90 percent or more (0-9 percent third degree) T32.90
    - with
      - 10-19 percent third degree T32.91
      - 20-29 percent third degree T32.92
      - 30-39 percent third degree T32.93
      - 40-49 percent third degree T32.94
      - 50-59 percent third degree T32.95
      - 60-69 percent third degree T32.96
      - 70-79 percent third degree T32.97
      - 80-89 percent third degree T32.98
      - 90-99 percent third degree T32.99
- upper limb (axilla) (scapular region) T22.40 ☑
  - above elbow — *see* Corrosion, above elbow
  - axilla — *see* Corrosion, axilla
  - elbow — *see* Corrosion, elbow
  - first degree T22.50 ☑
  - forearm — *see* Corrosion, forearm
  - hand — *see* Corrosion, hand
  - interscapular region — *see* Corrosion, back, upper
  - multiple sites T22.499 ☑
    - first degree T22.599 ☑
    - left T22.492 ☑
      - first degree T22.592 ☑
      - second degree T22.692 ☑
      - third degree T22.792 ☑
    - right T22.491 ☑
      - first degree T22.591 ☑
      - second degree T22.691 ☑
      - third degree T22.791 ☑
    - second degree T22.699 ☑
    - third degree T22.799 ☑
  - scapular region — *see* Corrosion, scapular region
  - second degree T22.60 ☑
  - shoulder — *see* Corrosion, shoulder
  - third degree T22.70 ☑
  - wrist — *see* Corrosion, hand
- uterus T28.8 ☑
- vagina T28.8 ☑
- vulva — *see* Corrosion, genital organs, external, female
- wrist T23.479 ☑
  - first degree T23.579 ☑
  - left T23.472 ☑
    - first degree T23.572 ☑
    - second degree T23.672 ☑
    - third degree T23.772 ☑
  - multiple sites with hand T23.499 ☑
    - first degree T23.599 ☑
    - left T23.492 ☑
      - first degree T23.592 ☑
      - second degree T23.692 ☑
      - third degree T23.792 ☑
    - right T23.491 ☑
      - first degree T23.591 ☑
      - second degree T23.691 ☑
      - third degree T23.791 ☑
    - second degree T23.699 ☑
    - third degree T23.799 ☑
  - right T23.471 ☑
    - first degree T23.571 ☑
    - second degree T23.671 ☑
    - third degree T23.771 ☑
  - second degree T23.679 ☑
  - third degree T23.779 ☑

Corrosive burn — *see* Corrosion

Corsican fever — *see* Malaria

☑ **Additional Character Required — Refer to the Tabular List for Character Selection**

Cortical — *see* condition
Cortico-adrenal — *see* condition
Coryza (acute) J00
  with grippe or influenza — *see* Influenza, with, respiratory manifestations NEC
  syphilitic
    congenital (chronic) A50.05
Co-sleeping, child-caregiver Z72.823
Costen's syndrome or complex M26.69
Costiveness — *see* Constipation
Costochondritis M94.0
Cot death R99
Cotard's syndrome F22
Cotia virus B08.8
Cotton wool spots (retinal) H35.81
Cotugno disease — *see* Sciatica
Cough (affected) (epidemic) (nervous) R05.9
  with hemorrhage — *see* Hemoptysis
  acute R05.1
  bronchial R05.8
    with grippe or influenza — *see* Influenza, with, respiratory manifestations NEC
  chronic R05.3
  functional F45.8
  hysterical F45.8
  laryngeal, spasmodic R05.8
  paroxysmal, due to Bordetella pertussis (without pneumonia) A37.00
    with pneumonia A37.01
  persistent R05.3
  psychogenic F45.8
  refractory R05.3
  smokers' J41.0
  specified NEC R05.8
  subacute R05.2
  syncope R05.4
  tea taster's B49
  unexplained R05.3
Counseling (for) Z71.9
  abuse NEC
    perpetrator Z69.82
    victim Z69.81
  alcohol abuser Z71.41
    family Z71.42
  child abuse
    nonparental
      perpetrator Z69.021
      victim Z69.020
    parental
      perpetrator Z69.011
      victim Z69.010
  consanguinity Z71.89
  contraceptive Z30.09
  dietary Z71.3
  drug abuser Z71.51
    family member Z71.52
  exercise Z71.82
  family Z71.89
  fertility preservation (prior to cancer therapy) (prior to removal of gonads) Z31.62
  for non-attending third party Z71.0
    related to sexual behavior or orientation Z70.2
  genetic
    nonprocreative Z71.83
    procreative NEC Z31.5
  gestational carrier Z31.7
  health (advice) (education) (instruction) — *see* Counseling, medical
    risk for travel (international) Z71.84
  human immunodeficiency virus (HIV) Z71.7
  immunization safety Z71.85
  impotence Z70.1
  insulin pump use Z46.81
  medical (for) Z71.9
    boarding school resident Z59.3
    consanguinity Z71.89
    feared complaint and no disease found Z71.1
    human immunodeficiency virus (HIV) Z71.7
    institutional resident Z59.3
    on behalf of another Z71.0
      related to sexual behavior or orientation Z70.2
    person living alone — *see also* Consultation, specified reason NEC Z60.2
    specified reason NEC Z71.89
  natural family planning
    procreative Z31.61
    to avoid pregnancy Z30.02
  pediatric-to-adult transition Z71.87

Counseling — *continued*
  perpetrator (of)
    abuse NEC Z69.82
    child abuse
      non-parental Z69.021
      parental Z69.011
    rape NEC Z69.82
    spousal abuse Z69.12
  procreative NEC Z31.69
    fertility preservation (prior to cancer therapy) (prior to removal of gonads) Z31.62
    using natural family planning Z31.61
  promiscuity Z70.1
  rape victim Z69.81
  religious Z71.81
  safety for travel (international) Z71.84
  sex, sexual (related to) Z70.9
    attitude(s) Z70.0
    behavior or orientation Z70.1
    combined concerns Z70.3
    non-responsiveness Z70.1
    on behalf of third party Z70.2
    specified reason NEC Z70.8
  socioeconomic factors Z71.88
  specified reason NEC Z71.89
  spiritual Z71.81
  spousal abuse (perpetrator) Z69.12
    victim Z69.11
  substance abuse Z71.89
    alcohol Z71.41
    drug Z71.51
    tobacco Z71.6
  tobacco use Z71.6
  travel (international) Z71.84
  use (of)
    insulin pump Z46.81
  vaccine product safety Z71.85
  victim (of)
    abuse Z69.81
    child abuse
      by parent Z69.010
      non-parental Z69.020
    rape NEC Z69.81
Coupled rhythm R00.8
Couvelaire syndrome or uterus (complicating delivery) O45.8X- ☑
COVID-19 U07.1
  condition post U09.9
  contact (with) Z20.822
  exposure (to) Z20.822
  history of (personal) Z86.16
  long (haul) U09.9
  partially vaccinated (for) Z28.311
  pneumonia J12.82
  screening Z11.52
  sequelae (post acute) U09.9
  unvaccinated (for) Z28.310
Cowperitis — *see* Urethritis
Cowper's gland — *see* condition
Cowpox B08.010
  due to vaccination T88.1 ☑
Coxa
  magna M91.4- ☑
  plana M91.2- ☑
  valga (acquired) — *see also* Deformity, limb, specified type NEC, thigh
    congenital Q65.81
    sequelae (late effect) of rickets E64.3
  vara (acquired) — *see also* Deformity, limb, specified type NEC, thigh
    congenital Q65.82
    sequelae (late effect) of rickets E64.3
Coxalgia, coxalgic (nontuberculous) — *see also* Pain, joint, hip
  tuberculous A18.02
Coxitis — *see* Monoarthritis, hip
Coxsackie (virus) (infection) B34.1
  as cause of disease classified elsewhere B97.11
  carditis B33.20
  central nervous system NEC A88.8
  endocarditis B33.21
  enteritis A08.39
  meningitis (aseptic) A87.0
  myocarditis B33.22
  pericarditis B33.23
  pharyngitis B08.5
  pleurodynia B33.0
  specific disease NEC B33.8
Crabs, meaning pubic lice B85.3

Crack baby P04.41
Cracked nipple N64.0
  associated with
    lactation O92.13
    pregnancy O92.11- ☑
    puerperium O92.12
Cracked tooth K03.81
Cradle cap L21.0
Craft neurosis F48.8
Cramp(s) R25.2
  abdominal — *see* Pain, abdominal
  bathing T75.1 ☑
  colic R10.83
    psychogenic F45.8
  due to immersion T75.1 ☑
  fireman T67.2 ☑
  heat T67.2 ☑
  immersion T75.1 ☑
  intestinal — *see* Pain, abdominal
    psychogenic F45.8
  leg, sleep related G47.62
  limb (lower) (upper) NEC R25.2
    sleep related G47.62
  linotypist's F48.8
    organic G25.89
  muscle (limb) (general) R25.2
    due to immersion T75.1 ☑
    psychogenic F45.8
  occupational (hand) F48.8
    organic G25.89
  salt-depletion E87.1
  sleep related, leg G47.62
  stoker's T67.2 ☑
  swimmer's T75.1 ☑
  telegrapher's F48.8
    organic G25.89
  typist's F48.8
    organic G25.89
  uterus N94.89
    menstrual — *see* Dysmenorrhea
  writer's F48.8
    organic G25.89
Cranial — *see* condition
Craniocleidodysostosis Q74.0
Craniofenestria (skull) Q75.8
Craniolacunia (skull) Q75.8
Craniopagus Q89.4
Craniopathy, metabolic M85.2
Craniopharyngeal — *see* condition
Craniopharyngioma D44.4
Craniorachischisis (totalis) Q00.1
Cranioschisis Q75.8
Craniostenosis Q75.009
Craniosynostosis Q75.009
  bilateral Q75.002
  coronal Q75.029
    bilateral Q75.022
    unilateral Q75.021
  lambdoid Q75.049
    bilateral Q75.042
    unilateral Q75.041
  metopic Q75.03
  multi-suture, specified NEC Q75.058
  sagittal Q75.01
  single-suture, specified NEC Q75.08
  unilateral Q75.001
Craniotabes (cause unknown) M83.8
  neonatal P96.3
  rachitic E64.3
  syphilitic A50.56
Cranium — *see* condition
Craw-craw — *see* Onchocerciasis
Creaking joint — *see* Derangement, joint, specified type NEC
Creeping
  eruption B76.9
  palsy or paralysis G12.22
Crenated tongue K14.8
Creotoxism A05.9
Crepitus
  caput Q75.8
  joint — *see* Derangement, joint, specified type NEC
Crescent or conus choroid, congenital Q14.3
CREST syndrome M34.1
Cretin, cretinism (congenital) (endemic) (nongoitrous) (sporadic) E00.9
  pelvis
    with disproportion (fetopelvic) O33.0

☑ **Additional Character Required** — **Refer to the Tabular List for Character Selection**

Cretin, cretinism — continued
  pelvis — continued
    with disproportion — continued
      causing obstructed labor O65.0
    type
      hypothyroid E00.1
      mixed E00.2
      myxedematous E00.1
      neurological E00.0
Creutzfeldt-Jakob disease or syndrome (with dementia)
      A81.00
  familial A81.09
  iatrogenic A81.09
  specified NEC A81.09
  sporadic A81.09
  variant (vCJD) A81.01
Crib death R99
Cribriform hymen Q52.3
Cri-du-chat syndrome Q93.4
Crigler-Najjar disease or syndrome E80.5
Crime, victim of Z65.4
Crimean hemorrhagic fever A98.0
Criminalism F60.2
Crisis
  abdomen R10.0
  acute reaction F43.0
  addisonian E27.2
  adrenal (cortical) E27.2
  celiac K90.0
  Dietl's N13.8
  emotional — see also Disorder, adjustment
    acute reaction to stress F43.0
    specific to childhood and adolescence F93.8
  glaucomatocyclitic — see Glaucoma, secondary, inflam-
      mation
  heart — see Failure, heart
  nitritoid I95.2
    correct substance properly administered — see Table
        of Drugs and Chemicals, by drug, adverse effect
    overdose or wrong substance given or taken — see
        Table of Drugs and Chemicals, by drug, poison-
        ing
  oculogyric H51.8
    psychogenic F45.8
  Pel's (tabetic) A52.11
  psychosexual identity F64.2
  renal N28.0
  sickle-cell — see also Disease, sickle-cell, by type, with
      crisis D57.00
    with
      acute chest syndrome D57.01
      cerebral vascular involvement D57.03
      complication specified NEC D57.09
      pain (vaso-occlusive) D57.00
      splenic sequestration D57.02
  state (acute reaction) F43.0
  tabetic A52.11
  thyroid — see Thyrotoxicosis with thyroid storm
  thyrotoxic — see Thyrotoxicosis with thyroid storm
Crocq's disease (acrocyanosis) I73.89
Crohn's disease — see Enteritis, regional
Crooked septum, nasal J34.2
Cross syndrome E70.328
Crossbite (anterior) (posterior) M26.24
Cross-eye — see Strabismus, convergent concomitant
Croup, croupous (catarrhal) (infectious) (inflammatory)
      (nondiphtheritic) J05.0
  bronchial J20.9
  diphtheritic A36.2
  false J38.5
  spasmodic J38.5
    diphtheritic A36.2
  stridulous J38.5
    diphtheritic A36.2
Crouzon's disease Q75.1
Crowding, tooth, teeth, fully erupted M26.31
CRST syndrome M34.1
Cruchet's disease A85.8
Cruelty in children — see also Disorder, conduct
Crural ulcer — see Ulcer, lower limb
Crush, crushed, crushing T14.8 ☑
  abdomen S38.1 ☑
  ankle S97.0- ☑
  arm (upper) (and shoulder) S47.- ☑
  axilla — see Crush, arm
  back, lower S38.1 ☑
  buttock S38.1 ☑
  cheek S07.0 ☑

Crush, crushed, crushing — continued
  chest S28.0 ☑
  cranium S07.1 ☑
  ear S07.0 ☑
  elbow S57.0- ☑
  extremity
    lower
      ankle — see Crush, ankle
      below knee — see Crush, leg
      foot — see Crush, foot
      hip — see Crush, hip
      knee — see Crush, knee
      thigh — see Crush, thigh
      toe — see Crush, toe
    upper
      below elbow S67.9- ☑
      elbow — see Crush, elbow
      finger — see Crush, finger
      forearm — see Crush, forearm
      hand — see Crush, hand
      thumb — see Crush, thumb
      upper arm — see Crush, arm
      wrist — see Crush, wrist
  face S07.0 ☑
  finger(s) S67.1- ☑
    with hand (and wrist) — see Crush, hand, specified
        site NEC
    index S67.19- ☑
    little S67.19- ☑
    middle S67.19- ☑
    ring S67.19- ☑
    thumb — see Crush, thumb
  foot S97.8- ☑
    toe — see Crush, toe
  forearm S57.8- ☑
  genitalia, external
    female S38.002 ☑
      vagina S38.03 ☑
      vulva S38.03 ☑
    male S38.001 ☑
      penis S38.01 ☑
      scrotum S38.02 ☑
      testis S38.02 ☑
  hand (except fingers alone) S67.2- ☑
    with wrist S67.4- ☑
  head S07.9 ☑
    specified NEC S07.8 ☑
  heel — see Crush, foot
  hip S77.0- ☑
    with thigh S77.2- ☑
  internal organ (abdomen, chest, or pelvis) NEC T14.8 ☑
  knee S87.0- ☑
  labium (majus) (minus) S38.03 ☑
  larynx S17.0 ☑
  leg (lower) S87.8- ☑
    knee — see Crush, knee
  lip S07.0 ☑
  lower
    back S38.1 ☑
    leg — see Crush, leg
  neck S17.9 ☑
  nerve — see Injury, nerve
  nose S07.0 ☑
  pelvis S38.1 ☑
  penis S38.01 ☑
  scalp S07.8 ☑
  scapular region — see Crush, arm
  scrotum S38.02 ☑
  severe, unspecified site T14.8 ☑
  shoulder (and upper arm) — see Crush, arm
  skull S07.1 ☑
  syndrome (complication of trauma) T79.5 ☑
  testis S38.02 ☑
  thigh S77.1- ☑
    with hip S77.2- ☑
  throat S17.8 ☑
  thumb S67.0- ☑
    with hand (and wrist) — see Crush, hand, specified
        site NEC
  toe(s) S97.10- ☑
    great S97.11- ☑
    lesser S97.12- ☑
  trachea S17.0 ☑
  vagina S38.03 ☑
  vulva S38.03 ☑
  wrist S67.3- ☑

Crush, crushed, crushing — continued
  wrist — continued
    with hand S67.4- ☑
Crusta lactea L21.0
Crusts R23.4
Crutch paralysis — see Injury, brachial plexus
Cruveilhier-Baumgarten cirrhosis, disease or syndrome
      K74.69
Cruveilhier's atrophy or disease G12.8
Crying (constant) (continuous) (excessive)
  child, adolescent, or adult R45.83
  infant (baby) (newborn) R68.11
Cryofibrinogenemia D89.2
Cryoglobulinemia (essential) (idiopathic) (mixed) (primary)
      (purpura) (secondary) (vasculitis) D89.1
  with lung involvement D89.1 [J99]
Cryptitis (anal) (rectal) K62.89
Cryptococcosis, cryptococcus (infection) (neoformans)
      B45.9
  bone B45.3
  cerebral B45.1
  cutaneous B45.2
  disseminated B45.7
  generalized B45.7
  meningitis B45.1
  meningocerebralis B45.1
  osseous B45.3
  pulmonary B45.0
  skin B45.2
  specified NEC B45.8
Cryptopapillitis (anus) K62.89
Cryptophthalmos Q11.2
  syndrome Q87.0
Cryptorchid, cryptorchism, cryptorchidism Q53.9
  bilateral Q53.20
    abdominal Q53.211
    perineal Q53.22
  unilateral Q53.10
    abdominal Q53.111
    perineal Q53.12
Cryptosporidiosis A07.2
  hepatobiliary B88.8
  respiratory B88.8
Cryptostromosis J67.6
Crystalluria R82.998
Cubitus
  congenital Q68.8
  valgus (acquired) M21.0- ☑
    congenital Q68.8
    sequelae (late effect) of rickets E64.3
  varus (acquired) M21.1- ☑
    congenital Q68.8
    sequelae (late effect) of rickets E64.3
Cultural deprivation or shock Z60.3
Curling esophagus K22.4
Curling's ulcer — see Ulcer, peptic, acute
Curschmann (-Batten) (-Steinert) **disease or syndrome**
      G71.11
Curse, Ondine's — see Apnea, sleep
Curvature
  organ or site, congenital NEC — see Distortion
  penis (lateral) Q55.61
  Pott's (spinal) A18.01
  radius, idiopathic, progressive (congenital) Q74.0
  spine (acquired) (angular) (idiopathic) (incorrect) (postu-
      ral) — see Dorsopathy, deforming
    congenital Q67.5
    due to or associated with
      Charcot-Marie-Tooth disease — see also subcate-
          gory M49.8 G60.0
      osteitis
        deformans M88.88
        fibrosa cystica — see also subcategory M49.8
            E21.0
      tuberculosis (Pott's curvature) A18.01
    sequelae (late effect) of rickets E64.3
    tuberculous A18.01
Cushingoid due to steroid therapy E24.2
  correct substance properly administered — see Table of
      Drugs and Chemicals, by drug, adverse effect
  overdose or wrong substance given or taken — see Table
      of Drugs and Chemicals, by drug, poisoning
Cushing's
  syndrome or disease E24.9
    drug-induced E24.2
    iatrogenic E24.2
    pituitary-dependent E24.0
    specified NEC E24.8
  ulcer — see Ulcer, peptic, acute

☑ **Additional Character Required** — **Refer to the Tabular List for Character Selection**

Cusp, Carabelli — omit code
Cut (external) — see also Laceration
  muscle — see Injury, muscle
Cutaneous — see also condition
  hemorrhage R23.3
  larva migrans B76.9
Cutis — see also condition
  hyperelastica Q82.8
    acquired L57.4
  laxa (hyperelastica) — see Dermatolysis
  marmorata R23.8
  osteosis L94.2
  pendula — see Dermatolysis
  rhomboidalis nuchae L57.2
  verticis gyrata Q82.8
    acquired L91.8
Cyanosis R23.0
  due to
    patent foramen botalli Q21.12
    persistent foramen ovale Q21.12
  enterogenous D74.8
  paroxysmal digital — see Raynaud's disease
    with gangrene I73.01
  retina, retinal H35.89
Cyanotic heart disease I24.9
  congenital Q24.9
Cycle
  anovulatory N97.0
  menstrual, irregular N92.6
Cyclencephaly Q04.9
Cyclical vomiting, in migraine — see also Vomiting,
  cyclical G43.A0 (following G43.7)
  psychogenic F50.89
Cyclitis — see also Iridocyclitis H20.9
  chronic — see Iridocyclitis, chronic
  Fuchs' heterochromic H20.81- ☑
  granulomatous — see Iridocyclitis, chronic
  lens-induced — see Iridocyclitis, lens-induced
  posterior H30.2- ☑
Cycloid personality F34.0
Cyclophoria H50.54
Cyclopia, cyclops Q87.0
Cyclopism Q87.0
Cyclosporiasis A07.4
Cyclothymia F34.0
Cyclothymic personality F34.0
Cyclotropia H50.41- ☑
Cylindroma — see also Neoplasm, malignant, by site
  eccrine dermal — see Neoplasm, skin, benign
  skin — see Neoplasm, skin, benign
Cylindruria R82.998
Cynanche
  diphtheritic A36.2
  tonsillaris J36
Cynophobia F40.218
Cynorexia R63.2
Cyphosis — see Kyphosis
Cyprus fever — see Brucellosis
Cyst (colloid) (mucous) (simple) (retention)
  adenoid (infected) J35.8
  adrenal gland E27.8
    congenital Q89.1
  air, lung J98.4
  allantoic Q64.4
  alveolar process (jaw bone) M27.40
  amnion, amniotic O41.8X- ☑
  aneurysmal M27.49
  anterior
    chamber (eye) — see Cyst, iris
    nasopalatine K09.1
  antrum J34.1
  anus K62.89
  apical (tooth) (periodontal) K04.8
  appendix K38.8
  arachnoid, brain (acquired) G93.0
    congenital Q04.6
  arytenoid J38.7
  Baker's M71.2- ☑
    ruptured M66.0
    tuberculous A18.02
  Bartholin's gland N75.0
  bile duct (common) (hepatic) K83.5
  bladder (multiple) (trigone) N32.89
  blue dome (breast) — see Cyst, breast
  bone (local) NEC M85.60
    aneurysmal M85.50
      ankle M85.57- ☑
      foot M85.57- ☑

Cyst — continued
  bone — continued
    aneurysmal — continued
      forearm M85.53- ☑
      hand M85.54- ☑
      jaw M27.49
      lower leg M85.56- ☑
      multiple site M85.59
      neck M85.58
      rib M85.58
      shoulder M85.51- ☑
      skull M85.58
      specified site NEC M85.58
      thigh M85.55- ☑
      toe M85.57- ☑
      upper arm M85.52- ☑
      vertebra M85.58
    solitary M85.40
      ankle M85.47- ☑
      fibula M85.46- ☑
      foot M85.47- ☑
      hand M85.44- ☑
      humerus M85.42- ☑
      jaw M27.49
      neck M85.48
      pelvis M85.45- ☑
      radius M85.43- ☑
      rib M85.48
      shoulder M85.41- ☑
      skull M85.48
      specified site NEC M85.48
      tibia M85.46- ☑
      toe M85.47- ☑
      ulna M85.43- ☑
      vertebra M85.48
    specified type NEC M85.60
      ankle M85.67- ☑
      foot M85.67- ☑
      forearm M85.63- ☑
      hand M85.64- ☑
      jaw M27.40
        developmental (nonodontogenic) K09.1
          odontogenic K09.0
        latent M27.0
      lower leg M85.66- ☑
      multiple site M85.69
      neck M85.68
      rib M85.68
      shoulder M85.61- ☑
      skull M85.68
      specified site NEC M85.68
      thigh M85.65- ☑
      toe M85.67- ☑
      upper arm M85.62- ☑
      vertebra M85.68
  brain (acquired) G93.0
    congenital Q04.6
    hydatid B67.99 [G94]
    third ventricle (colloid), congenital Q04.6
  branchial (cleft) Q18.0
  branchiogenic Q18.0
  breast (benign) (blue dome) (pedunculated) (solitary)
    N60.0- ☑
    involution — see Dysplasia, mammary, specified type
      NEC
    sebaceous — see Dysplasia, mammary, specified type
      NEC
  broad ligament (benign) N83.8
  bronchogenic (mediastinal) (sequestration) J98.4
    congenital Q33.0
  buccal K09.8
  bulbourethral gland N36.8
  bursa, bursal NEC M71.30
    with rupture — see Rupture, synovium
    ankle M71.37- ☑
    elbow M71.32- ☑
    foot M71.37- ☑
    hand M71.34- ☑
    hip M71.35- ☑
    multiple sites M71.39
    pharyngeal J39.2
    popliteal space — see Cyst, Baker's
    shoulder M71.31- ☑
    specified site NEC M71.38
    wrist M71.33- ☑
  calcifying odontogenic D16.5
    upper jaw (bone) (maxilla) D16.4

Cyst — continued
  canal of Nuck (female) N94.89
    congenital Q52.4
  canthus — see Cyst, conjunctiva
  carcinomatous — see Neoplasm, malignant, by site
  cauda equina G95.89
  cavum septi pellucidi — see Cyst, brain
  celomic (pericardium) Q24.8
  cerebellopontine (angle) — see Cyst, brain
  cerebellum — see Cyst, brain
  cerebral — see Cyst, brain
  cervical lateral Q18.0
  cervix NEC N88.8
    embryonic Q51.6
    nabothian N88.8
  chiasmal optic NEC — see Disorder, optic, chiasm
  chocolate (ovary) N80.10- ☑
  choledochus, congenital Q44.4
  chorion O41.8X- ☑
  choroid plexus G93.0
    congenital Q04.6
  ciliary body — see Cyst, iris
  clitoris N90.7
  colon K63.89
  common (bile) duct K83.5
  congenital NEC Q89.8
    adrenal gland Q89.1
    epiglottis Q31.8
    esophagus Q39.8
    fallopian tube Q50.4
    kidney Q61.00
      more than one (multiple) Q61.02
        specified as polycystic Q61.3
          adult type Q61.2
          infantile type NEC Q61.19
            collecting duct dilation Q61.11
      solitary Q61.01
    larynx Q31.8
    liver Q44.6
    lung Q33.0
    mediastinum Q34.1
    ovary Q50.1
    oviduct Q50.4
    periurethral (tissue) Q64.79
    prepuce Q55.69
    salivary gland (any) Q38.4
    sublingual Q38.6
    submaxillary gland Q38.6
    thymus (gland) Q89.2
    tongue Q38.3
    ureterovesical orifice Q62.8
    vulva Q52.79
  conjunctiva H11.44- ☑
  cornea H18.89- ☑
  corpora quadrigemina G93.0
  corpus
    albicans N83.29- ☑
    luteum (hemorrhagic) (ruptured) N83.1- ☑
  Cowper's gland (benign) (infected) N36.8
  cranial meninges G93.0
  craniobuccal pouch E23.6
  craniopharyngeal pouch E23.6
  cystic duct K82.8
  Cysticercus — see Cysticercosis
  Dandy-Walker Q03.1
    with spina bifida — see Spina bifida
  dental (root) K04.8
    developmental K09.0
    eruption K09.0
    primordial K09.0
  dentigerous (mandible) (maxilla) K09.0
  dermoid — see Neoplasm, benign, by site
    with malignant transformation C56.- ☑
    implantation
      external area or site (skin) NEC L72.0
      iris — see Cyst, iris, implantation
      vagina N89.8
      vulva N90.7
    mouth K09.8
    oral soft tissue K09.8
    sacrococcygeal — see Cyst, pilonidal
  developmental K09.1
    odontogenic K09.0
    oral region (nonodontogenic) K09.1
    ovary, ovarian Q50.1
  dura (cerebral) G93.0
    spinal G96.198
  ear (external) Q18.1

Cyst — *continued*
- echinococcal — *see* Echinococcus
- embryonic
  - cervix uteri Q51.6
  - fallopian tube Q50.4
  - vagina Q52.4
- endometrium, endometrial (uterus) N85.8
  - ectopic — *see* Endometriosis
- enterogenous Q43.8
- epidermal, epidermoid (inclusion) (*see also* Cyst, skin) L72.0
  - mouth K09.8
  - oral soft tissue K09.8
- epididymis N50.3
- epiglottis J38.7
- epiphysis cerebri E34.8
- epithelial (inclusion) L72.0
- epoophoron Q50.5
- eruption K09.0
- esophagus K22.89
- ethmoid sinus J34.1
- external female genital organs NEC N90.7
- eyelid (sebaceous) H02.829
  - infected — *see* Hordeolum
  - left H02.826
    - lower H02.825
    - upper H02.824
  - right H02.823
    - lower H02.822
    - upper H02.821
- eye NEC H57.89
  - congenital Q15.8
- fallopian tube N83.8
  - congenital Q50.4
- fimbrial (twisted) Q50.4
- fissural (oral region) K09.1
- follicle (graafian) (hemorrhagic) N83.0- ☑
  - nabothian N88.8
- follicular (atretic) (hemorrhagic) (ovarian) N83.0- ☑
  - dentigerous K09.0
  - odontogenic K09.0
  - skin L72.9
    - specified NEC L72.8
- frontal sinus J34.1
- gallbladder K82.8
- ganglion — *see* Ganglion
- Gartner's duct Q52.4
- gingiva K09.0
- gland of Moll — *see* Cyst, eyelid
- globulomaxillary K09.1
- graafian follicle (hemorrhagic) N83.0- ☑
- granulosal lutein (hemorrhagic) N83.1- ☑
- hemangiomatous D18.00
  - intra-abdominal D18.03
  - intracranial D18.02
  - skin D18.01
  - specified site NEC D18.09
- hemorrhagic M27.49
- hydatid — *see also* Echinococcus B67.90
  - brain B67.99 *[G94]*
  - liver — *see also* Cyst, liver, hydatid B67.8
  - lung NEC B67.99 *[J99]*
  - Morgagni
    - female Q50.5
    - male (epididymal) Q55.4
      - testicular Q55.29
  - specified site NEC B67.99
- hymen N89.8
  - embryonic Q52.4
- hypopharynx J39.2
- hypophysis, hypophyseal (duct) (recurrent) E23.6
  - cerebri E23.6
- implantation (dermoid)
  - external area or site (skin) NEC L72.0
  - iris — *see* Cyst, iris, implantation
  - vagina N89.8
  - vulva N90.7
- incisive canal K09.1
- inclusion (epidermal) (epithelial) (epidermoid) (squamous) L72.0
  - not of skin — *code under* Cyst, by site
- intestine (large) (small) K63.89
- intracranial — *see* Cyst, brain
- intraligamentous — *see also* Disorder, ligament
  - knee — *see* Derangement, knee
- intrasellar E23.6
- iris H21.309
  - exudative H21.31- ☑

Cyst — *continued*
- iris — *continued*
  - idiopathic H21.30- ☑
  - implantation H21.32- ☑
  - parasitic H21.33- ☑
  - pars plana (primary) H21.34- ☑
    - exudative H21.35- ☑
- jaw (bone) M27.40
  - aneurysmal M27.49
  - developmental (odontogenic) K09.0
  - fissural K09.1
  - hemorrhagic M27.49
  - traumatic M27.49
- joint NEC — *see* Disorder, joint, specified type NEC
- kidney N28.1
  - acquired N28.1
  - calyceal — *see* Hydronephrosis
  - congenital Q61.00
    - more than one (multiple) Q61.02
      - specified as polycystic Q61.3
        - adult type (autosomal dominant) Q61.2
        - infantile type (autosomal recessive) NEC Q61.19
          - collecting duct dilation Q61.11
  - pyelogenic — *see* Hydronephrosis
  - simple N28.1
  - solitary (single) N28.1
    - acquired N28.1
    - congenital Q61.01
- labium (majus) (minus) N90.7
  - sebaceous N90.7
- lacrimal — *see also* Disorder, lacrimal system, specified NEC
  - gland H04.13- ☑
  - passages or sac — *see* Disorder, lacrimal system, specified NEC
- larynx J38.7
- lateral periodontal K09.0
- lens H27.8
  - congenital Q12.8
- lip (gland) K13.0
- liver (idiopathic) (simple) K76.89
  - congenital Q44.6
  - hydatid B67.8
    - granulosus B67.0
    - multilocularis B67.5
- lung J98.4
  - congenital Q33.0
  - giant bullous J43.9
- lutein N83.1- ☑
- lymphangiomatous D18.1
- lymphoepithelial, oral soft tissue K09.8
- macula — *see* Degeneration, macula, hole
- malignant — *see* Neoplasm, malignant, by site
- mammary gland — *see* Cyst, breast
- mandible M27.40
  - dentigerous K09.0
  - radicular K04.8
- maxilla M27.40
  - dentigerous K09.0
  - radicular K04.8
- medial, face and neck Q18.8
- median
  - anterior maxillary K09.1
  - palatal K09.1
- mediastinum, congenital Q34.1
- meibomian (gland) — *see* Chalazion
  - infected — *see* Hordeolum
- membrane, brain G93.0
- meninges (cerebral) G93.0
  - spinal G96.198
- meniscus, knee — *see* Derangement, knee, meniscus, cystic
- mesentery, mesenteric K66.8
  - chyle I89.8
- mesonephric duct
  - female Q50.5
  - male Q55.4
- milk N64.89
- Morgagni (hydatid)
  - female Q50.5
  - male (epididymal) Q55.4
    - testicular Q55.29
- mouth K09.8
- Mullerian duct Q50.4
  - appendix testis Q55.29
  - cervix Q51.6
  - fallopian tube Q50.4
  - female Q50.4

Cyst — *continued*
- Mullerian duct — *continued*
  - male Q55.29
  - prostatic utricle Q55.4
  - vagina (embryonal) Q52.4
- multilocular (ovary) D39.10
  - benign — *see* Neoplasm, benign, by site
- myometrium N85.8
- nabothian (follicle) (ruptured) N88.8
- nasoalveolar K09.1
- nasolabial K09.1
- nasopalatine (anterior) (duct) K09.1
- nasopharynx J39.2
- neoplastic — *see* Neoplasm, uncertain behavior, by site
  - benign — *see* Neoplasm, benign, by site
- nerve root
  - cervical G96.191
  - lumbar G96.191
  - sacral G96.191
  - thoracic G96.191
- nervous system NEC G96.89
- neuroenteric (congenital) Q06.8
- nipple — *see* Cyst, breast
- nose (turbinates) J34.1
  - sinus J34.1
- odontogenic, developmental K09.0
- omentum (lesser) K66.8
  - congenital Q45.8
- ora serrata — *see* Cyst, retina, ora serrata
- oral
  - region K09.9
    - developmental (nonodontogenic) K09.1
      - specified NEC K09.8
  - soft tissue K09.9
    - specified NEC K09.8
- orbit H05.81- ☑
- ovary, ovarian (twisted) N83.20- ☑
  - adherent N83.20- ☑
  - chocolate N80.10- ☑
  - corpus
    - albicans N83.29- ☑
    - luteum (hemorrhagic) N83.1- ☑
  - dermoid D27.9
  - developmental Q50.1
  - due to failure of involution NEC N83.20- ☑
  - endometrial N80.10- ☑
  - follicular (graafian) (hemorrhagic) N83.0- ☑
  - hemorrhagic N83.20- ☑
  - in pregnancy or childbirth O34.8- ☑
    - with obstructed labor O65.5
  - multilocular D39.10
  - pseudomucinous D27.9
  - retention N83.29- ☑
  - serous N83.20- ☑
  - specified NEC N83.29- ☑
  - theca lutein (hemorrhagic) N83.1- ☑
  - tuberculous A18.18
- oviduct N83.8
- palate (median) (fissural) K09.1
- palatine papilla (jaw) K09.1
- pancreas, pancreatic (hemorrhagic) (true) K86.2
  - congenital Q45.2
  - false K86.3
- paralabral
  - hip M24.85- ☑
  - shoulder S43.43- ☑
- paramesonephric duct Q50.4
  - female Q50.4
  - male Q55.29
- paranephric N28.1
- paraphysis, cerebri, congenital Q04.6
- parasitic B89
- parathyroid (gland) E21.4
- paratubal N83.8
- paraurethral duct N36.8
- paroophoron Q50.5
- parotid gland K11.6
- parovarian Q50.5
- pelvis, female N94.89
  - in pregnancy or childbirth O34.8- ☑
    - causing obstructed labor O65.5
- penis (sebaceous) N48.89
- periapical K04.8
- pericardial (congenital) Q24.8
  - acquired (secondary) I31.8
- pericoronal K09.0
- perineural G96.191
- periodontal K04.8

Cyst — *continued*
  periodontal — *continued*
    lateral K09.0
  peripelvic (lymphatic) N28.1
  peritoneum K66.8
    chylous I89.8
  periventricular, acquired, newborn P91.1
  pharynx (wall) J39.2
  pilar L72.11
  pilonidal (infected) (rectum) L05.91
    with abscess L05.01
    malignant C44.59- ☑
  pituitary (duct) (gland) E23.6
  placenta O43.19- ☑
  pleura J94.8
  popliteal — *see* Cyst, Baker's
  porencephalic Q04.6
    acquired G93.0
  postanal (infected) — *see* Cyst, pilonidal
  postmastoidectomy cavity (mucosal) — *see* Complications, postmastoidectomy, cyst
  preauricular Q18.1
  prepuce N47.4
    congenital Q55.69
  primordial (jaw) K09.0
  prostate N42.83
  pseudomucinous (ovary) D27.9
  pupillary, miotic H21.27- ☑
  radicular (residual) K04.8
  radiculodental K04.8
  ranular K11.8
  Rathke's pouch E23.6
  rectum (epithelium) (mucous) K62.89
  renal — *see* Cyst, kidney
  residual (radicular) K04.8
  retention (ovary) N83.29- ☑
    salivary gland K11.6
  retina H33.19- ☑
    ora serrata H33.11- ☑
    parasitic H33.12- ☑
  retroperitoneal K68.9
  sacrococcygeal (dermoid) — *see* Cyst, pilonidal
  salivary gland or duct (mucous extravasation or retention) K11.6
  Sampson's N80.10- ☑
  sclera H15.89
  scrotum L72.9
    sebaceous L72.3
  sebaceous (duct) (gland) L72.3
    breast — *see* Dysplasia, mammary, specified type NEC
    eyelid — *see* Cyst, eyelid
    genital organ NEC
      female N94.89
      male N50.89
    scrotum L72.3
  semilunar cartilage (knee) (multiple) — *see* Derangement, knee, meniscus, cystic
  seminal vesicle N50.89
  serous (ovary) N83.20- ☑
  sinus (accessory) (nasal) J34.1
  Skene's gland N36.8
  skin L72.9
    breast — *see* Dysplasia, mammary, specified type NEC
    epidermal, epidermoid L72.0
    epithelial L72.0
    eyelid — *see* Cyst, eyelid
    genital organ NEC
      female N90.7
      male N50.89
    inclusion L72.0
    scrotum L72.9
    sebaceous L72.3
    sweat gland or duct L74.8
  solitary
    bone — *see* Cyst, bone, solitary
    jaw M27.40
    kidney N28.1
  spermatic cord N50.89
  sphenoid sinus J34.1
  spinal meninges G96.198
  spleen NEC D73.4
    congenital Q89.09
    hydatid — *see also* Echinococcus B67.99 [D77]
  Stafne's M27.0
  subarachnoid intrasellar R93.0
  subcutaneous, pheomycotic (chromomycotic) B43.2
  subdural (cerebral) G93.0
    spinal cord G96.198

Cyst — *continued*
  sublingual gland K11.6
  submandibular gland K11.6
  submaxillary gland K11.6
  suburethral N36.8
  suprarenal gland E27.8
  suprasellar — *see* Cyst, brain
  sweat gland or duct L74.8
  synovial — *see also* Cyst, bursa
    ruptured — *see* Rupture, synovium
  Tarlov G96.191
  tarsal — *see* Chalazion
  tendon (sheath) — *see* Disorder, tendon, specified type NEC
  testis N44.2
    tunica albuginea N44.1
  theca lutein (ovary) N83.1- ☑
  Thornwaldt's J39.2
  thymus (gland) E32.8
  thyroglossal duct (infected) (persistent) Q89.2
  thyroid (gland) E04.1
  thyrolingual duct (infected) (persistent) Q89.2
  tongue K14.8
  tonsil J35.8
  tooth — *see* Cyst, dental
  Tornwaldt's J39.2
  trichilemmal (proliferating) L72.12
  trichodermal L72.12
  tubal (fallopian) N83.8
    inflammatory — *see* Salpingitis, chronic
  tubo-ovarian N83.8
    inflammatory N70.13
  tunica
    albuginea testis N44.1
    vaginalis N50.89
  turbinate (nose) J34.1
  Tyson's gland N48.89
  urachus, congenital Q64.4
  ureter N28.89
  ureterovesical orifice N28.89
  urethra, urethral (gland) N36.8
  uterine ligament N83.8
  uterus (body) (corpus) (recurrent) N85.8
    embryonic Q51.818
      cervix Q51.6
  vagina, vaginal (implantation) (inclusion) (squamous cell) (wall) N89.8
    embryonic Q52.4
  vallecula, vallecular (epiglottis) J38.7
  vesical (orifice) N32.89
  vitreous body H43.89
  vulva (implantation) (inclusion) N90.7
    congenital Q52.79
    sebaceous gland N90.7
  vulvovaginal gland N90.7
  wolffian
    female Q50.5
    male Q55.4
Cystadenocarcinoma — *see* Neoplasm, malignant, by site
  bile duct C22.1
  endometrioid — *see* Neoplasm, malignant, by site
    specified site — *see* Neoplasm, malignant, by site
    unspecified site
      female C56.9
      male C61
  mucinous
    papillary
      specified site — *see* Neoplasm, malignant, by site
      unspecified site C56.9
    specified site — *see* Neoplasm, malignant, by site
    unspecified site C56.9
  papillary
    mucinous
      specified site — *see* Neoplasm, malignant, by site
      unspecified site C56.9
    pseudomucinous
      specified site — *see* Neoplasm, malignant, by site
      unspecified site C56.9
    serous
      specified site — *see* Neoplasm, malignant, by site
      unspecified site C56.9
    specified site — *see* Neoplasm, malignant, by site
    unspecified site C56.9
  pseudomucinous
    papillary
      specified site — *see* Neoplasm, malignant, by site
      unspecified site C56.9
    specified site — *see* Neoplasm, malignant, by site
    unspecified site C56.9

Cystadenocarcinoma — *continued*
  serous
    papillary
      specified site — *see* Neoplasm, malignant, by site
      unspecified site C56.9
    specified site — *see* Neoplasm, malignant, by site
    unspecified site C56.9
Cystadenofibroma
  clear cell — *see* Neoplasm, benign, by site
  endometrioid D27.9
    borderline malignancy D39.1- ☑
    malignant C56.- ☑
  mucinous
    specified site — *see* Neoplasm, benign, by site
    unspecified site D27.9
  serous
    specified site — *see* Neoplasm, benign, by site
    unspecified site D27.9
  specified site — *see* Neoplasm, benign, by site
  unspecified site D27.9
Cystadenoma — *see also* Neoplasm, benign, by site
  bile duct D13.4
  endometrioid — *see* Neoplasm, benign, by site
    borderline malignancy — *see* Neoplasm, uncertain behavior, by site
  malignant — *see* Neoplasm, malignant, by site
  mucinous
    borderline malignancy
      ovary C56.- ☑
      specified site NEC — *see* Neoplasm, uncertain behavior, by site
      unspecified site C56.9
    papillary
      borderline malignancy
        ovary C56.- ☑
        specified site NEC — *see* Neoplasm, uncertain behavior, by site
        unspecified site C56.9
      specified site — *see* Neoplasm, benign, by site
      unspecified site D27.9
    specified site — *see* Neoplasm, benign, by site
    unspecified site D27.9
  papillary
    borderline malignancy
      ovary C56.- ☑
      specified site NEC — *see* Neoplasm, uncertain behavior, by site
      unspecified site C56.9
    lymphomatosum
      specified site — *see* Neoplasm, benign, by site
      unspecified site D11.9
    mucinous
      borderline malignancy
        ovary C56.- ☑
        specified site NEC — *see* Neoplasm, uncertain behavior, by site
        unspecified site C56.9
      specified site — *see* Neoplasm, benign, by site
      unspecified site D27.9
    pseudomucinous
      borderline malignancy
        ovary C56.- ☑
        specified site NEC — *see* Neoplasm, uncertain behavior, by site
        unspecified site C56.9
      specified site — *see* Neoplasm, benign, by site
      unspecified site D27.9
    serous
      borderline malignancy
        ovary C56.- ☑
        specified site NEC — *see* Neoplasm, uncertain behavior, by site
        unspecified site C56.9
      specified site — *see* Neoplasm, benign, by site
      unspecified site D27.9
    specified site — *see* Neoplasm, benign, by site
    unspecified site D27.9
  pseudomucinous
    borderline malignancy
      ovary C56.- ☑
      specified site NEC — *see* Neoplasm, uncertain behavior, by site
      unspecified site C56.9
    papillary
      borderline malignancy
        ovary C56.- ☑
        specified site NEC — *see* Neoplasm, uncertain behavior, by site

Cystadenoma — *continued*
  pseudomucinous — *continued*
    papillary — *continued*
      borderline malignancy — *continued*
        unspecified site C56.9
      specified site — *see* Neoplasm, benign, by site
      unspecified site D27.9
    specified site — *see* Neoplasm, benign, by site
    unspecified site D27.9
  serous
    borderline malignancy
      ovary C56.- ☑
      specified site NEC — *see* Neoplasm, uncertain behavior, by site
      unspecified site C56.9
    papillary
      borderline malignancy
        ovary C56.- ☑
        specified site NEC — *see* Neoplasm, uncertain behavior, by site
        unspecified site C56.9
      specified site — *see* Neoplasm, benign, by site
      unspecified site D27.9
    specified site — *see* Neoplasm, benign, by site
    unspecified site D27.9
Cystathionine synthase deficiency E72.11
Cystathioninemia E72.19
Cystathioninuria E72.19
Cystic — *see also* condition
  breast (chronic) — *see* Mastopathy, cystic
  corpora lutea (hemorrhagic) N83.1- ☑
  duct — *see* condition
  eyeball (congenital) Q11.0
  fibrosis — *see* Fibrosis, cystic
  kidney (congenital) Q61.9
    adult type Q61.2
    infantile type NEC Q61.19
      collecting duct dilatation Q61.11
    medullary Q61.5
  liver, congenital Q44.6
  lung disease J98.4
    congenital Q33.0
  mastitis, chronic — *see* Mastopathy, cystic
  medullary, kidney Q61.5
  meniscus — *see* Derangement, knee, meniscus, cystic
  ovary N83.20- ☑
Cysticercosis, cysticerciasis B69.9
  with
    epileptiform fits B69.0
    myositis B69.81
  brain B69.0
  central nervous system B69.0
  cerebral B69.0
  ocular B69.1
  specified NEC B69.89
Cysticercus cellulose infestation — *see* Cysticercosis
Cystinosis (malignant) E72.04

Cystinuria E72.01
Cystitis (exudative) (hemorrhagic) (septic) (suppurative) N30.90
  with
    fibrosis — *see* Cystitis, chronic, interstitial
    hematuria N30.91
    leukoplakia — *see* Cystitis, chronic, interstitial
    malakoplakia — *see* Cystitis, chronic, interstitial
    metaplasia — *see* Cystitis, chronic, interstitial
    prostatitis N41.3
  acute N30.00
    with hematuria N30.01
    of trigone N30.30
      with hematuria N30.31
  allergic — *see* Cystitis, specified type NEC
  amebic A06.81
  bilharzial B65.9 *[N33]*
  blennorrhagic (gonococcal) A54.01
  bullous — *see* Cystitis, specified type NEC
  calculous N21.0
  chlamydial A56.01
  chronic N30.20
    with hematuria N30.21
    interstitial N30.10
      with hematuria N30.11
    of trigone N30.30
      with hematuria N30.31
    specified NEC N30.20
      with hematuria N30.21
  cystic (a) — *see* Cystitis, specified type NEC
  diphtheritic A36.85
  echinococcal
    granulosus B67.39
    multilocularis B67.69
  emphysematous — *see* Cystitis, specified type NEC
  encysted — *see* Cystitis, specified type NEC
  eosinophilic — *see* Cystitis, specified type NEC
  follicular — *see* Cystitis, of trigone
  gangrenous — *see* Cystitis, specified type NEC
  glandularis — *see* Cystitis, specified type NEC
  gonococcal A54.01
  incrusted — *see* Cystitis, specified type NEC
  interstitial (chronic) — *see* Cystitis, chronic, interstitial
  irradiation N30.40
    with hematuria N30.41
  irritation — *see* Cystitis, specified type NEC
  malignant — *see* Cystitis, specified type NEC
  of trigone N30.30
    with hematuria N30.31
  panmural — *see* Cystitis, chronic, interstitial
  polyposa — *see* Cystitis, specified type NEC
  prostatic N41.3
  puerperal (postpartum) O86.22
  radiation — *see* Cystitis, irradiation
  specified type NEC N30.80
    with hematuria N30.81
  subacute — *see* Cystitis, chronic
  submucous — *see* Cystitis, chronic, interstitial

Cystitis — *continued*
  syphilitic (late) A52.76
  trichomonal A59.03
  tuberculous A18.12
  ulcerative — *see* Cystitis, chronic, interstitial
Cystocele (-urethrocele)
  female N81.10
    with prolapse of uterus — *see* Prolapse, uterus
    lateral N81.12
    midline N81.11
    paravaginal N81.12
  in pregnancy or childbirth O34.8- ☑
    causing obstructed labor O65.5
  male N32.89
Cystolithiasis N21.0
Cystoma — *see also* Neoplasm, benign, by site
  endometrial, ovary N80.10- ☑
  mucinous
    specified site — *see* Neoplasm, benign, by site
    unspecified site D27.9
  serous
    specified site — *see* Neoplasm, benign, by site
    unspecified site D27.9
  simple (ovary) N83.29- ☑
Cystoplegia N31.2
Cystoptosis N32.89
Cystopyelitis — *see* Pyelonephritis
Cystorrhagia N32.89
Cystosarcoma phyllodes D48.6- ☑
  benign D24- ☑
  malignant — *see* Neoplasm, breast, malignant
Cystostomy
  attention to Z43.5
  complication — *see* Complications, cystostomy
  status Z93.50
    appendico-vesicostomy Z93.52
    cutaneous Z93.51
    specified NEC Z93.59
Cystourethritis — *see* Urethritis
Cystourethrocele — *see also* Cystocele
  female N81.10
    with uterine prolapse — *see* Prolapse, uterus
    lateral N81.12
    midline N81.11
    paravaginal N81.12
  male N32.89
Cytomegalic inclusion disease
  congenital P35.1
Cytomegalovirus infection B25.9
Cytomycosis (reticuloendothelial) B39.4
Cytopenia D75.9
  refractory
    with multilineage dysplasia D46.A (*following* D46.2)
      and ring sideroblasts (RCMD RS) D46.B (*following* D46.2)
Czerny's disease (periodic hydrarthrosis of the knee) — *see* Effusion, joint, knee

D

Da Costa's syndrome F45.8
Daae (-Finsen) **disease** (epidemic pleurodynia) B33.0
Dabney's grip B33.0
Dacryoadenitis, dacryadenitis H04.00- ☑
  acute H04.01- ☑
  chronic H04.02- ☑
Dacryocystitis H04.30- ☑
  acute H04.32- ☑
  chronic H04.41- ☑
  neonatal P39.1
  phlegmonous H04.31- ☑
  syphilitic A52.71
    congenital (early) A50.01
  trachomatous, active A71.1
    sequelae (late effect) B94.0
Dacryocystoblennorrhea — *see* Inflammation, lacrimal, passages, chronic
Dacryocystocele — *see* Disorder, lacrimal system, changes
Dacryolith, dacryolithiasis H04.51- ☑
Dacryoma — *see* Disorder, lacrimal system, changes
Dacryopericystitis — *see* Dacryocystitis
Dacryops H04.11- ☑
Dacryostenosis — *see also* Stenosis, lacrimal
  congenital Q10.5
Dactylitis
  bone — *see* Osteomyelitis
  sickle-cell D57.00
    Hb C D57.219
    Hb SS D57.00
    specified NEC D57.819
  skin L08.9
  syphilitic A52.77
  tuberculous A18.03
Dactylolysis spontanea (ainhum) L94.6
Dactylosymphysis Q70.9
  fingers — *see* Syndactylism, complex, fingers
  toes — *see* Syndactylism, complex, toes
Damage
  arteriosclerotic — *see* Arteriosclerosis
  brain (nontraumatic) G93.9
    anoxic, hypoxic G93.1
      resulting from a procedure G97.82
    child NEC G80.9
    due to birth injury P11.2
  cardiorenal (vascular) — *see* Hypertension, cardiorenal
  cerebral NEC — *see* Damage, brain
  coccyx, complicating delivery O71.6
  coronary — *see* Disease, heart, ischemic
  deep tissue, pressure-induced — *see also* L89 with final character .6
  eye, birth injury P15.3
  liver (nontraumatic) K76.9
    alcoholic K70.9
    due to drugs — *see* Disease, liver, toxic
    toxic — *see* Disease, liver, toxic
  lung
    dabbing (related) U07.0
    electronic cigarette (related) U07.0
    vaping (associated) (device) (product) (use) U07.0
  medication T88.7 ☑
  organ
    dabbing (related) U07.0
    electronic cigarette (related) U07.0
    vaping (associated) (device) (product) (use) U07.0
  pelvic
    joint or ligament, during delivery O71.6
    organ NEC
      during delivery O71.5
      following ectopic or molar pregnancy O08.6
  renal — *see* Disease, renal
  subendocardium, subendocardial — *see* Degeneration, myocardial
  vascular I99.9
Dana-Putnam syndrome (subacute combined sclerosis with pernicious anemia) — *see* Degeneration, combined
Danbolt (-Cross) **syndrome** (acrodermatitis enteropathica) E83.2
Dandruff L21.0
Dandy-Walker syndrome Q03.1
  with spina bifida — *see* Spina bifida
Danlos' syndrome — *see also* Syndrome, Ehlers-Danlos Q79.60
Darier (-White) **disease** (congenital) Q82.8
  meaning erythema annulare centrifugum L53.1

Darier-Roussy sarcoid D86.3
Darling's disease or histoplasmosis B39.4
Darwin's tubercle Q17.8
Dawson's (inclusion body) **encephalitis** A81.1
De Beurmann (-Gougerot) **disease** B42.1
De la Tourette's syndrome F95.2
De Lange's syndrome Q87.19
De Morgan's spots (senile angiomas) I78.1
De Quervain's
  disease (tendon sheath) M65.4
  syndrome E34.51
  thyroiditis (subacute granulomatous thyroiditis) E06.1
De Toni-Fanconi (-Debre) **syndrome** E72.09
  with cystinosis E72.04
Dead
  fetus, retained (mother) O36.4 ☑
    early pregnancy O02.1
  labyrinth H83.2 ☑
  ovum, retained O02.0
Deaf nonspeaking NEC H91.3
Deafmutism (acquired) (congenital) NEC H91.3
  hysterical F44.6
  syphilitic, congenital — *see also* subcategory H94.8 A50.09
Deafness (acquired) (complete) (hereditary) (partial) H91.9- ☑
  with blue sclera and fragility of bone Q78.0
  auditory fatigue — *see* Deafness, specified type NEC
  aviation T70.0 ☑
    nerve injury — *see* Injury, nerve, acoustic, specified type NEC
  boilermaker's H83.3 ☑
  central — *see* Deafness, sensorineural
  conductive H90.2
    and sensorineural
      mixed H90.8
        bilateral H90.6
    bilateral H90.0
    unilateral H90.1- ☑
      with restricted hearing on the contralateral side H90.A- ☑
  congenital H90.5
    with blue sclera and fragility of bone Q78.0
  due to toxic agents — *see* Deafness, ototoxic
  emotional (hysterical) F44.6
  functional (hysterical) F44.6
  high frequency H91.9- ☑
  hysterical F44.6
  low frequency H91.9- ☑
  mental R48.8
  mixed conductive and sensorineural H90.8
    bilateral H90.6
    unilateral H90.7- ☑
  nerve — *see* Deafness, sensorineural
  neural — *see* Deafness, sensorineural
  noise-induced — *see also* subcategory H83.3 ☑
    nerve injury — *see* Injury, nerve, acoustic, specified type NEC
  nonspeaking H91.3
  ototoxic H91.0 ☑
  perceptive — *see* Deafness, sensorineural
  psychogenic (hysterical) F44.6
  sensorineural H90.5
    and conductive
      bilateral H90.6
      mixed H90.8
        bilateral H90.6
    bilateral H90.3
    unilateral H90.4- ☑
      with restricted hearing on the contralateral side H90.A- ☑
  sensory — *see* Deafness, sensorineural
  specified type NEC H91.8 ☑
  sudden (idiopathic) H91.2- ☑
  syphilitic A52.15
  transient ischemic H93.01- ☑
  traumatic — *see* Injury, nerve, acoustic, specified type NEC
  word (developmental) H93.25
Death (cause unknown) (of) (unexplained) (unspecified cause) R99
  brain G93.82
  cardiac (sudden) (with successful resuscitation) — *see* Arrest, cardiac
    family history of Z82.41
    personal history of Z86.74
  family member (assumed) Z63.4
Debility (chronic) (general) (nervous) R53.81

Debility — *continued*
  congenital or neonatal NOS P96.9
  nervous R53.81
  old age R54
  senile R54
Debove's disease (splenomegaly) R16.1
Debt, burdensome Z59.86
Decalcification
  bone — *see* Osteoporosis
  teeth K03.89
Decapsulation, kidney N28.89
Decay
  dental — *see* Caries, dental
  senile R54
  tooth, teeth — *see* Caries, dental
Deciduitis (acute)
  following ectopic or molar pregnancy O08.0
Decline (general) — *see* Debility
  cognitive, age-associated R41.81
Decompensation
  cardiac (acute) (chronic) — *see* Disease, heart
  cardiovascular — *see* Disease, cardiovascular
  heart — *see* Disease, heart
  hepatic — *see* Failure, hepatic
  myocardial (acute) (chronic) — *see* Disease, heart
  respiratory J98.8
Decompression sickness T70.3 ☑
Decrease (d)
  absolute neutrophile count — *see* Neutropenia
  blood
    glucose
      level 1 E16.A1
      level 2 E16.A2
      level 3 E16.A3
    platelets — *see* Thrombocytopenia
    pressure R03.1
      due to shock following
        injury T79.4 ☑
        operation T81.19 ☑
  estrogen E28.39
    postablative E89.40
      asymptomatic E89.40
      symptomatic E89.41
  fragility of erythrocytes D58.8
  function
    lipase (pancreatic) K90.3
    ovary in hypopituitarism E23.0
    parenchyma of pancreas K86.89
    pituitary (gland) (anterior) (lobe) E23.0
      posterior (lobe) E23.0
  functional activity R68.89
  glucose R73.09
  hematocrit R71.0
  hemoglobin R71.0
  leukocytes D72.819
    specified NEC D72.818
  libido R68.82
  lymphocytes D72.810
  platelets D69.6
  respiration, due to shock following injury T79.4 ☑ ☑
  sexual desire R68.82
  tear secretion NEC — *see* Syndrome, dry eye
  tolerance
    fat K90.49
    glucose R73.09
    pancreatic K90.3
    salt and water E87.8
  vision NEC H54.7
  white blood cell count D72.819
    specified NEC D72.818
Decubitus (ulcer) — *see* Ulcer, pressure, by site
  cervix N86
Deepening acetabulum — *see* Derangement, joint, specified type NEC, hip
Defect, defective Q89.9
  3-beta-hydroxysteroid dehydrogenase E25.0
  11-hydroxylase E25.0
  21-hydroxylase E25.0
  abdominal wall, congenital Q79.59
  antibody immunodeficiency D80.9
  aorticopulmonary septum Q21.4
  atrial septal Q21.10
    coronary sinus Q21.13
    following acute myocardial infarction (current complication) I23.1
    ostium primum type (type I) Q21.20
    with
      common atrioventricular valves and moderate or larger inlet VSD Q21.23

Defect, defective — *continued*
  atrial septal — *continued*
    ostium primum type — *continued*
      with — *continued*
        separate atrioventricular valves Q21.21
          and small or restrictive inlet VSD Q21.22
      ostium secundum type (patent persistent) (type II) Q21.11
      sinus venosus Q21.16
        inferior Q21.15
        superior Q21.14
      specified NEC Q21.19
      vena cava type
        inferior Q21.15
        superior Q21.14
  atrioventricular
    canal Q21.20
    septal
      common Q21.23
      complete Q21.23
      incomplete Q21.21
      intermediate Q21.22
      partial Q21.21
      transitional Q21.22
      unspecified as to partial or complete Q21.20
    septum Q21.20
  auricular septal Q21.10
  bilirubin excretion NEC E80.6
  biosynthesis, androgen (testicular) E29.1
  bulbar septum Q21.0
  catalase E80.3
  cell membrane receptor complex (CR3) D71
  circulation I99.9
    congenital Q28.9
    newborn Q28.9
  coagulation (factor) — *see also* Deficiency, factor D68.9
    with
      COVID-19 associated coagulopathy D68.8
      ectopic pregnancy O08.1
      molar pregnancy O08.1
    acquired D68.4
    antepartum with hemorrhage — *see* Hemorrhage, antepartum, with coagulation defect
    due to
      liver disease D68.4
      vitamin K deficiency D68.4
    hereditary NEC D68.2
    intrapartum O67.0
    newborn, transient P61.6
    postpartum O99.13
      with hemorrhage O72.3
    specified type NEC D68.8
  complement system D84.1
  conduction (heart) I45.9
    bone — *see* Deafness, conductive
  congenital, organ or site not listed — *see* Anomaly, by site
  coronary sinus Q21.13
  cushion, endocardial Q21.20
    common Q21.23
    incomplete Q21.21
    intermediate Q21.22
    transitional Q21.22
  degradation, glycoprotein E77.1
  dental bridge, crown, fillings — *see* Defect, dental restoration
  dental restoration K08.50
    specified NEC K08.59
  dentin (hereditary) K00.5
  Descemet's membrane, congenital Q13.89
  developmental — *see also* Anomaly
    cauda equina Q06.3
  diaphragm
    with elevation, eventration or hernia — *see* Hernia, diaphragm
    congenital Q79.1
      with hernia Q79.0
      gross (with hernia) Q79.0
  ectodermal, congenital Q82.9
  Eisenmenger's Q21.8
  enzyme
    catalase E80.3
    peroxidase E80.3
  esophagus, congenital Q39.9
  extensor retinaculum M62.89
  fibrin polymerization D68.2
  filling
    bladder R93.41
    kidney R93.42- ☑

Defect, defective — *continued*
  filling — *continued*
    renal pelvis R93.41
    stomach R93.3
    ureter R93.41
    urinary organs, specified NEC R93.49
  GABA (gamma aminobutyric acid) metabolic E72.81
  Gerbode Q21.0
  glucose transport, blood-brain barrier E74.810
  glycoprotein degradation E77.1
  Hageman (factor) D68.2
  hearing — *see* Deafness
  high grade F70
  home, technical, preventing adequate care Z59.19
  interatrial septal Q21.19
  interauricular septal Q21.19
  interventricular septal Q21.0
    with dextroposition of aorta, pulmonary stenosis and hypertrophy of right ventricle Q21.3
    in tetralogy of Fallot Q21.3
  intervertebral annular fibrosis — *see also* Disease, intervertebral disc, by site M51.9
    lumbar M51.A0
      large M51.A2
      small M51.A1
    lumbosacral M51.A3
      large M51.A5
      small M51.A4
  learning (specific) — *see* Disorder, learning
  lymphocyte function antigen-1 (LFA-1) D84.0
  lysosomal enzyme, post-translational modification E77.0
  major osseous M89.70
    ankle M89.77- ☑
    carpus M89.74- ☑
    clavicle M89.71- ☑
    femur M89.75- ☑
    fibula M89.76- ☑
    fingers M89.74- ☑
    foot M89.77- ☑
    forearm M89.73- ☑
    hand M89.74- ☑
    humerus M89.72- ☑
    lower leg M89.76- ☑
    metacarpus M89.74- ☑
    metatarsus M89.77- ☑
    multiple sites M89.79
    pelvic region M89.75- ☑
    pelvis M89.75- ☑
    radius M89.73- ☑
    scapula M89.71- ☑
    shoulder region M89.71- ☑
    specified NEC M89.78
    tarsus M89.77- ☑
    thigh M89.75- ☑
    tibia M89.76- ☑
    toes M89.77- ☑
    ulna M89.73- ☑
  mental — *see* Disability, intellectual
  modification, lysosomal enzymes, post-translational E77.0
  obstructive, congenital
    renal pelvis Q62.39
    ureter Q62.39
      atresia — *see* Atresia, ureter
      cecoureterocele Q62.32
      megaureter Q62.2
      orthotopic ureterocele Q62.31
  osseous, major M89.70
    ankle M89.77- ☑
    carpus M89.74- ☑
    clavicle M89.71- ☑
    femur M89.75- ☑
    fibula M89.76- ☑
    fingers M89.74- ☑
    foot M89.77- ☑
    forearm M89.73- ☑
    hand M89.74- ☑
    humerus M89.72- ☑
    lower leg M89.76- ☑
    metacarpus M89.74- ☑
    metatarsus M89.77- ☑
    multiple sites M89.9
    pelvic region M89.75- ☑
    pelvis M89.75- ☑
    radius M89.73- ☑
    scapula M89.71- ☑
    shoulder region M89.71- ☑
    specified NEC M89.78

Defect, defective — *continued*
  osseous, major — *continued*
    tarsus M89.77- ☑
    thigh M89.75- ☑
    tibia M89.76- ☑
    toes M89.77- ☑
    ulna M89.73- ☑
  osteochondral NEC — *see also* Deformity M95.8
  ostium
    primum Q21.20
    secundum Q21.11
  peroxidase E80.3
  placental blood supply — *see* Insufficiency, placental
  platelets, qualitative D69.1
    constitutional — *see* Disease, von Willebrand
  postural NEC, spine — *see* Dorsopathy, deforming
  qualitative, of von Willebrand factor
    with
      decreased platelet adhesion and selective deficiency of high-molecular-weight multimers — *see* Disease, von Willebrand D68.020
      defective platelet adhesion with a normal size distribution of von Willebrand factor multimers — *see also* Disease, von Willebrand D68.022
      defective von Willebrand factor to factor VIII binding — *see also* Disease, von Willebrand D68.023
      high-molecular-weight von Willebrand factor loss — *see also* Disease, von Willebrand D68.021
      hyper-adhesive forms — *see also* Disease, von Willebrand D68.021
      increased affinity for platelet glycoprotein Ib — *see also* Disease, von Willebrand D68.021
      markedly decreased affinity for factor VIII — *see also* Disease, von Willebrand D68.023
    in von Willebrand factor function, with no further subtyping — *see also* Disease, von Willebrand D68.029
  reduction
    limb Q73.8
      lower Q72.9- ☑
        absence — *see* Agenesis, leg
        foot — *see* Agenesis, foot
        longitudinal
          femur Q72.4- ☑
          fibula Q72.6- ☑
          tibia Q72.5- ☑
        specified type NEC Q72.89- ☑
        split foot Q72.7- ☑
      specified type NEC Q73.8
      upper Q71.9- ☑
        absence — *see* Agenesis, arm
        forearm — *see* Agenesis, forearm
        hand — *see* Agenesis, hand
        lobster-claw hand Q71.6- ☑
        longitudinal
          radius Q71.4- ☑
          ulna Q71.5- ☑
        specified type NEC Q71.89- ☑
  renal pelvis Q63.8
    obstructive Q62.39
  respiratory system, congenital Q34.9
  restoration, dental K08.50
    specified NEC K08.59
  retinal nerve bundle fibers H35.89
  septal (heart) NOS Q21.9
    acquired (atrial) (auricular) (ventricular) (old) I51.0
    atrial — *see also* Defect, atrial septal Q21.10
      concurrent with acute myocardial infarction — *see* Infarct, myocardium
      following acute myocardial infarction (current complication) I23.1
      ventricular — *see also* Defect, ventricular septal Q21.0
  sinus venosus — *see also* Defect, atrial septal, sinus venosus Q21.16
  speech — *see* Disorder, speech
    developmental F80.9
    specified NEC R47.89
  Taussig-Bing (aortic transposition and overriding pulmonary artery) Q20.1
  teeth, wedge K03.1
  vascular (local) I99.9
    congenital Q27.9
  ventricular septal Q21.0
    concurrent with acute myocardial infarction — *see* Infarct, myocardium

Defect, defective — *continued*
  ventricular septal — *continued*
    following acute myocardial infarction (current complication) I23.2
    in tetralogy of Fallot Q21.3
  vision NEC H54.7
  visual field H53.40
    bilateral
      heteronymous H53.47
      homonymous H53.46- ☑
    generalized contraction H53.48- ☑
    localized
      arcuate H53.43- ☑
      scotoma (central area) H53.41- ☑
        blind spot area H53.42- ☑
      sector H53.43- ☑
      specified type NEC H53.45- ☑
  voice R49.9
    specified NEC R49.8
  wedge, tooth, teeth (abrasion) K03.1
Deferentitis N49.1
  gonorrheal (acute) (chronic) A54.23
Defibrination (syndrome) D65
  antepartum — *see* Hemorrhage, antepartum, with coagulation defect, disseminated intravascular coagulation
  following ectopic or molar pregnancy O08.1
  intrapartum O67.0
  newborn P60
  postpartum O72.3
Deficiency, deficient
  3-beta hydroxysteroid dehydrogenase E25.0
  5-alpha reductase (with male pseudohermaphroditism) E29.1
  11-hydroxylase E25.0
  21-hydroxylase E25.0
  AADC (aromatic L-amino acid decarboxylase) E70.81
  abdominal muscle syndrome Q79.4
  AC globulin (congenital) (hereditary) D68.2
    acquired D68.4
  accelerator globulin (Ac G) (blood) D68.2
  acid phosphatase E83.39
  acid sphingomyelinase (ASMD) E75.249
    type
      A E75.240
      A/B E75.244
      B E75.241
  activating factor (blood) D68.2
  ADA2 (adenosine deaminase 2) D81.32
  adenosine deaminase (ADA) D81.30
    with severe combined immunodeficiency (SCID) D81.31
    partial (type 1) D81.39
    specified NEC D81.39
    type 1 (without SCID) (without severe combined immunodeficiency) D81.39
    type 2 D81.32
  aldolase (hereditary) E74.19
  alpha-1-antitrypsin E88.01
  amino-acids E72.9
  anemia — *see* Anemia
  aneurin E51.9
  antibody with
    hyperimmunoglobulinemia D80.6
    near-normal immunoglobins D80.6
  antidiuretic hormone E23.2
  anti-hemophilic
    factor (A) D66
      B D67
      C D68.1
    globulin (AHG) NEC D66
  antithrombin (antithrombin III) D68.59
  aromatic L-amino acid decarboxylase (AADC) E70.81
  ascorbic acid E54
  attention (disorder) (syndrome) F98.8
    with hyperactivity — *see* Disorder, attention-deficit hyperactivity
  autoprothrombin
    I D68.2
    II D67
    C D68.2
  beta-glucuronidase E76.29
  biotin E53.8
  biotin-dependent carboxylase D81.819
  biotinidase D81.810
  brancher enzyme (amylopectinosis) E74.03
  C1 esterase inhibitor (C1-INH) D84.1
  calciferol E55.9

Deficiency, deficient — *continued*
  calciferol — *continued*
    with
      adult osteomalacia M83.8
      rickets — *see* Rickets
  calcium (dietary) E58
  calorie, severe E43
    with marasmus E41
      and kwashiorkor E42
  cardiac — *see* Insufficiency, myocardial
  carnitine E71.40
    due to
      hemodialysis E71.43
      inborn errors of metabolism E71.42
      Valproic acid therapy E71.43
    iatrogenic E71.43
    muscle palmityltransferase E71.314
    primary E71.41
    secondary E71.448
  carotene E50.9
  central nervous system G96.89
  ceruloplasmin (Wilson) E83.01
  choline E53.8
  Christmas factor D67
  chromium E61.4
  chronic neurovisceral acid sphingomyelinase E75.244
  chronic visceral acid sphingomyelinase E75.241
  clotting (blood) — *see also* Deficiency, coagulation factor D68.9
  clotting factor NEC (hereditary) — *see also* Deficiency, factor D68.2
  coagulation NOS D68.9
    with
      ectopic pregnancy O08.1
      molar pregnancy O08.1
    acquired (any) D68.4
    antepartum hemorrhage — *see* Hemorrhage, antepartum, with coagulation defect
    clotting factor NEC — *see also* Deficiency, factor D68.2
    due to
      hyperprothrombinemia D68.4
      liver disease D68.4
      vitamin K deficiency D68.4
    newborn, transient P61.6
    postpartum O72.3
    specified NEC D68.8
  cognitive F09
  color vision H53.50
    achromatopsia H53.51
    acquired H53.52
    deuteranomaly H53.53
    protanomaly H53.54
    specified type NEC H53.59
    tritanomaly H53.55
  combined glucocorticoid and mineralocorticoid E27.49
  contact factor D68.2
  copper (nutritional) E61.0
  corticoadrenal E27.40
    primary E27.1
  craniofacial axis Q75.009
  cyanocobalamin E53.8
  debrancher enzyme (limit dextrinosis) E74.03
  dehydrogenase
    long chain/very long chain acyl CoA E71.310
    medium chain acyl CoA E71.311
    short chain acyl CoA E71.312
  diet E63.9
  dihydropyrimidine dehydrogenase (DPD) E88.89
  disaccharidase E73.9
  edema — *see* Malnutrition, severe
  endocrine E34.9
  energy-supply — *see* Malnutrition
  enzymes, circulating NEC E88.09
  ergosterol E55.9
    with
      adult osteomalacia M83.8
      rickets — *see* Rickets
  essential fatty acid (EFA) E63.0
  eye movements
    saccadic H55.81
    smooth pursuit H55.82
  factor — *see also* Deficiency, coagulation
    Hageman D68.2
    I (congenital) (hereditary) D68.2
    II (congenital) (hereditary) D68.2
    IX (congenital) (functional) (hereditary) (with functional defect) D67
    multiple (congenital) D68.8
      acquired D68.4

Deficiency, deficient — *continued*
  factor — *see also* Deficiency, coagulation — *continued*
    V (congenital) (hereditary) D68.2
    VII (congenital) (hereditary) D68.2
    VIII (congenital) (functional) (hereditary) (with functional defect) D66
      with vascular defect — *see* Disease, von Willebrand
    X (congenital) (hereditary) D68.2
    XI (congenital) (hereditary) D68.1
    XII (congenital) (hereditary) D68.2
    XIII (congenital) (hereditary) D68.2
  femoral, proximal focal (congenital) — *see* Defect, reduction, lower limb, longitudinal, femur
  fibrinase D68.2
  fibrinogen (congenital) (hereditary) D68.2
    acquired D65
  fibrin-stabilizing factor (congenital) (hereditary) D68.2
    acquired D68.4
  folate E53.8
  folic acid E53.8
  foreskin N47.3
  fructokinase E74.11
  fructose 1,6-diphosphatase E74.19
  fructose-1-phosphate aldolase E74.19
  GABA (gamma aminobutyric acid) transaminase E72.81
  GABA-T (gamma aminobutyric acid transaminase) E72.81
  galactokinase E74.29
  galactose-1-phosphate uridyl transferase E74.29
  gammaglobulin in blood D80.1
    hereditary D80.0
  glass factor D68.2
  glucocorticoid E27.49
    mineralocorticoid E27.49
  glucose transporter protein type 1 E74.810
  glucose-6-phosphatase E74.01
  glucose-6-phosphate dehydrogenase
    anemia D55.0
    without anemia D75.A
  glucuronyl transferase E80.5
  Glut1 E74.810
  glycogen synthetase E74.09
  gonadotropin (isolated) E23.0
  growth hormone (idiopathic) (isolated) E23.0
  Hageman factor D68.2
  hemoglobin D64.9
  hepatophosphorylase E74.09
  homogentisate 1,2-dioxygenase E70.29
  hormone
    anterior pituitary (partial) NEC E23.0
      growth E23.0
    growth (isolated) E23.0
    pituitary E23.0
    testicular E29.1
  hypoxanthine- (guanine)-phosphoribosyltransferase (HG- PRT) (total H-PRT) E79.1
  immunity D84.9
    cell-mediated D84.89
      with thrombocytopenia and eczema D82.0
    combined D81.9
    humoral D80.9
    IgA (secretory) D80.2
    IgG D80.3
    IgM D80.4
  immuno — *see* Immunodeficiency
  immunoglobulin, selective
    A (IgA) D80.2
    G (IgG) (subclasses) D80.3
    M (IgM) D80.4
  infantile neurovisceral acid sphingomyelinase E75.240
  inositol (B complex) E53.8
  intrinsic
    factor (congenital) D51.0
    sphincter N36.42
      with urethral hypermobility N36.43
  iodine E61.8
    congenital syndrome — *see* Syndrome, iodine-deficiency, congenital
  iron E61.1
    anemia D50.9
  kalium E87.6
  kappa-light chain D80.8
  labile factor (congenital) (hereditary) D68.2
    acquired D68.4
  lacrimal fluid (acquired) — *see also* Syndrome, dry eye
    congenital Q10.6
  lactase
    congenital E73.0
    secondary E73.1

☑ **Additional Character Required** — **Refer to the Tabular List for Character Selection**

Deficiency, deficient — continued
  Laki-Lorand factor D68.2
  LCAD (long chain acyl CoA dehydrogenase deficiency) E71.31Ø
  lecithin cholesterol acyltransferase E78.6
  lipocaic K86.89
  lipoprotein (familial) (high density) E78.6
  liver phosphorylase E74.Ø9
  lysosomal alpha-1, 4 glucosidase E74.Ø2
  lysosome-associated membrane protein 2 [LAMP2] E74.Ø5
  magnesium E61.2
  major histocompatibility complex
    class I D81.6
    class II D81.7
  manganese E61.3
  MCAD (medium chain acyl CoA dehydrogenase deficiency) E71.311
  menadione (vitamin K) E56.1
    newborn P53
  mental (familial) (hereditary) — see Disability, intellectual
  methylenetetrahydrofolate reductase (MTHFR) E72.12
  mevalonate kinase MØ4.1
  mineralocorticoid E27.49
    with glucocorticoid E27.49
  mineral NEC E61.8
  molybdenum (nutritional) E61.5
  moral F6Ø.2
  multiple nutrient elements E61.7
  multiple sulfatase (MSD) E75.26
  muscle
    carnitine (palmityltransferase) E71.314
    phosphofructokinase E74.Ø9
  myoadenylate deaminase E79.2
  myocardial — see Insufficiency, myocardial
  myophosphorylase E74.Ø4
  NADH diaphorase or reductase (congenital) D74.Ø
  NADH-methemoglobin reductase (congenital) D74.Ø
  natrium E87.1
  niacin (amide) (-tryptophan) E52
  nicotinamide E52
  nicotinic acid E52
  number of teeth — see Anodontia
  nutrient element E61.9
    multiple E61.7
    specified NEC E61.8
  nutrition, nutritional — see also Nutrition deficient E63.9
    sequelae — see Sequelae, nutritional deficiency
    specified NEC E63.8
  of interleukin 1 receptor antagonist [DIRA] MØ4.8
  ornithine transcarbamylase E72.4
  ovarian E28.39
  oxygen — see Anoxia
  pantothenic acid E53.8
  parathyroid (gland) E2Ø.9
  perineum (female) N81.89
  phenylalanine hydroxylase E7Ø.1
  phosphoenolpyruvate carboxykinase E74.4
  phosphofructokinase E74.19
  phosphomannomutase E74.818
  phosphomannose isomerase E74.818
  phosphomannosyl mutase E74.818
  phosphorylase kinase, liver E74.Ø9
  pituitary hormone (isolated) E23.Ø
  plasma thromboplastin
    antecedent (PTA) D68.1
    component (PTC) D67
  plasminogen (type 1) (type 2) E88.Ø2
  platelet NEC D69.1
    constitutional — see Disease, von Willebrand
  polyglandular E31.8
    autoimmune E31.Ø
  potassium (K) E87.6
  prepuce N47.3
  proaccelerin (congenital) (hereditary) D68.2
    acquired D68.4
  proconvertin factor (congenital) (hereditary) D68.2
    acquired D68.4
  protein — see also Malnutrition E46
    anemia D53.Ø
    C D68.59
    S D68.59
  prothrombin (congenital) (hereditary) D68.2
    acquired D68.4
  Prower factor D68.2
  pseudocholinesterase E88.Ø9
  PTA (plasma thromboplastin antecedent) D68.1
  PTC (plasma thromboplastin component) D67
  purine nucleoside phosphorylase (PNP) D81.5

Deficiency, deficient — continued
  pyracin (alpha) (beta) E53.1
  pyridoxal E53.1
  pyridoxamine E53.1
  pyridoxine (derivatives) E53.1
  pyruvate
    carboxylase E74.4
    dehydrogenase E74.4
  riboflavin (vitamin B2) E53.Ø
  salt E87.1
  SCAD (short chain acyl CoA dehydrogenase deficiency) E71.312
  secretion
    ovary E28.39
    salivary gland (any) K11.7
    urine R34
  selenium (dietary) E59
  serum antitrypsin, familial E88.Ø1
  short stature homeobox gene (SHOX)
    with
      dyschondrosteosis Q78.8
      short stature (idiopathic) E34.328
      Turner's syndrome Q96.9
  sodium (Na) E87.1
  SPCA (factor VII) D68.2
  sphincter, intrinsic N36.42
    with urethral hypermobility N36.43
  stable factor (congenital) (hereditary) D68.2
    acquired D68.4
  Stuart-Prower (factor X) D68.2
  succinic semialdehyde dehydrogenase E72.81
  sucrase E74.39
  sulfatase E75.26
  sulfite oxidase E72.19
  thiamin, thiaminic (chloride) E51.9
    beriberi (dry) E51.11
      wet E51.12
  thrombokinase D68.2
    newborn P53
  thyroid (gland) — see Hypothyroidism
  tocopherol E56.Ø
  tooth bud KØØ.Ø
  transcobalamine II (anemia) D51.2
  vanadium E61.6
  vascular I99.9
  vasopressin E23.2
  vertical ridge KØ6.8
  viosterol — see Deficiency, calciferol
  vitamin (multiple) NOS E56.9
    A E5Ø.9
      with
        Bitot's spot (corneal) E5Ø.1
        follicular keratosis E5Ø.8
        keratomalacia E5Ø.4
        manifestations NEC E5Ø.8
        night blindness E5Ø.5
        scar of cornea, xerophthalmic E5Ø.6
        xeroderma E5Ø.8
        xerophthalmia E5Ø.7
        xerosis
          conjunctival E5Ø.Ø
            and Bitot's spot E5Ø.1
          cornea E5Ø.2
            and ulceration E5Ø.3
      sequelae E64.1
    B (complex) NOS E53.9
      with
        beriberi (dry) E51.11
          wet E51.12
        pellagra E52
    B1 NOS E51.9
      beriberi (dry) E51.11
        with circulatory system manifestations E51.11
        wet E51.12
    B12 E53.8
    B2 (riboflavin) E53.Ø
    B6 E53.1
    C E54
      sequelae E64.2
    D E55.9
      with
        adult osteomalacia M83.8
        rickets — see Rickets
      25-hydroxylase E83.32
    E E56.Ø
    folic acid E53.8
    G E53.Ø
    group B E53.9
      specified NEC E53.8

Deficiency, deficient — continued
  vitamin — continued
    H (biotin) E53.8
    K E56.1
      of newborn P53
    nicotinic E52
    P E56.8
    PP (pellagra-preventing) E52
    specified NEC E56.8
    thiamin E51.9
      beriberi — see Beriberi
  VLCAD (very long chain acyl CoA dehydrogenase deficiency) E71.31Ø
  von Willebrand factor
    partial quantitative — see also Disease, von Willebrand D68.Ø1
    total quantitative — see also Disease, von Willebrand D68.Ø3
  zinc, dietary E6Ø
Deficit — see also Deficiency
  attention and concentration R41.84Ø
    disorder — see Attention, deficit
    following
      cerebral infarction I69.31Ø
      cerebrovascular disease I69.91Ø
        specified disease NEC I69.81Ø
      nontraumatic
        intracerebral hemorrhage I69.11Ø
        specified intracranial hemorrhage NEC I69.21Ø
        subarachnoid hemorrhage I69.Ø1Ø
  cognitive
    communication R41.841
    emotional
      following
        cerebral infarction I69.315
        cerebrovascular disease I69.915
          specified disease NEC I69.815
        nontraumatic
          intracerebral hemorrhage I69.115
          specified intracranial hemorrhage NEC I69.215
          subarachnoid hemorrhage I69.Ø15
    following
      cerebral infarction I69.319
      cerebrovascular disease I69.919
        specified disease NEC I69.819
      nontraumatic
        intracerebral hemorrhage I69.119
        specified intracranial hemorrhage NEC I69.219
        subarachnoid hemorrhage I69.Ø19
    social
      following
        cerebral infarction I69.315
        cerebrovascular disease I69.915
          specified disease NEC I69.815
        nontraumatic
          intracerebral hemorrhage I69.115
          specified intracranial hemorrhage NEC I69.215
          subarachnoid hemorrhage I69.Ø15
  cognitive NEC R41.89
    following
      cerebral infarction I69.318
      cerebrovascular disease I69.918
        specified disease NEC I69.818
      nontraumatic
        intracerebral hemorrhage I69.118
        specified intracranial hemorrhage NEC I69.218
        subarachnoid hemorrhage I69.Ø18
  concentration R41.84Ø
  executive function R41.844
    following
      cerebral infarction I69.314
      cerebrovascular disease I69.914
        specified disease NEC I69.814
      nontraumatic
        intracerebral hemorrhage I69.114
        specified intracranial hemorrhage NEC I69.214
        subarachnoid hemorrhage I69.Ø14
  frontal lobe R41.844
    following
      cerebral infarction I69.314
      cerebrovascular disease I69.914
        specified disease NEC I69.814
      nontraumatic
        intracerebral hemorrhage I69.114
        specified intracranial hemorrhage NEC I69.214
        subarachnoid hemorrhage I69.Ø14

Deficit — *continued*
  memory
    following
      cerebral infarction I69.311
      cerebrovascular disease I69.911
        specified disease NEC I69.811
      nontraumatic
        intracerebral hemorrhage I69.111
        specified intracranial hemorrhage NEC I69.211
        subarachnoid hemorrhage I69.011
  neurologic NEC R29.818
    ischemic
      reversible (RIND) I63.9
        prolonged (PRIND) I63.9
  oxygen R09.02
  prolonged reversible ischemic neurologic (PRIND) I63.9
  psychomotor R41.843
    following
      cerebral infarction I69.313
      cerebrovascular disease I69.913
        specified disease NEC I69.813
      nontraumatic
        intracerebral hemorrhage I69.113
        specified intracranial hemorrhage NEC I69.213
        subarachnoid hemorrhage I69.013
  visuospatial R41.842
    following
      cerebral infarction I69.312
      cerebrovascular disease I69.912
        specified disease NEC I69.812
      nontraumatic
        intracerebral hemorrhage I69.112
        specified intracranial hemorrhage NEC I69.212
        subarachnoid hemorrhage I69.012

Deflection
  radius — *see* Deformity, limb, specified type NEC, forearm
  septum (acquired) (nasal) (nose) J34.2
  spine — *see* Curvature, spine
  turbinate (nose) J34.2

Defluvium
  capillorum — *see* Alopecia
  ciliorum — *see* Madarosis
  unguium L60.8

Deformity Q89.9
  abdomen, congenital Q89.9
  abdominal wall
    acquired M95.8
    congenital Q79.59
  acquired (unspecified site) M95.9
  adrenal gland Q89.1
  alimentary tract, congenital Q45.9
    upper Q40.9
  ankle (joint) (acquired) — *see also* Deformity, limb, lower leg
    abduction — *see* Contraction, joint, ankle
    congenital Q68.8
    contraction — *see* Contraction, joint, ankle
    specified type NEC — *see* Deformity, limb, foot, specified NEC
  anus (acquired) K62.89
    congenital Q43.9
  aorta (arch) (congenital) Q25.40
    acquired I77.89
  aortic
    arch, acquired I77.89
    cusp or valve (congenital) Q23.88
      acquired — *see also* Endocarditis, aortic I35.8
  arm (acquired) (upper) — *see also* Deformity, limb, upper arm
    congenital Q68.8
    forearm — *see* Deformity, limb, forearm
  artery (congenital) (peripheral) NOS Q27.9
    acquired I77.89
    coronary (acquired) I25.9
      congenital Q24.5
    umbilical Q27.0
  atrial septal — *see also* Defect, atrial septal Q21.10
  auditory canal (external) (congenital) — *see also* Malformation, ear, external
    acquired — *see* Disorder, ear, external, specified type NEC
  auricle
    ear (congenital) — *see also* Malformation, ear, external
      acquired — *see* Disorder, pinna, deformity
  back — *see* Dorsopathy, deforming
  bile duct (common) (congenital) (hepatic) Q44.5
    acquired K83.8
  biliary duct or passage (congenital) Q44.5
    acquired K83.8

Deformity — *continued*
  bladder (neck) (trigone) (sphincter) (acquired) N32.89
    congenital Q64.79
  bone (acquired) NOS M95.9
    congenital Q79.9
    turbinate M95.0
  brain (congenital) Q04.9
    acquired G93.89
    reduction Q04.3
  breast (acquired) N64.89
    congenital Q83.9
    reconstructed N65.0
  bronchus (congenital) Q32.4
    acquired NEC J98.09
  bursa, congenital Q79.9
  canaliculi (lacrimalis) (acquired) — *see also* Disorder, lacrimal system, changes
    congenital Q10.6
  canthus, acquired — *see* Disorder, eyelid, specified type NEC
  capillary (acquired) I78.8
  cardiovascular system, congenital Q28.9
  caruncle, lacrimal (acquired) — *see also* Disorder, lacrimal system, changes
    congenital Q10.6
  cascade, stomach K31.2
  cecum (congenital) Q43.9
    acquired K63.89
  cerebral, acquired G93.89
    congenital Q04.9
  cervix (uterus) (acquired) NEC N88.8
    congenital Q51.9
  cheek (acquired) M95.2
    congenital Q18.9
  chest (acquired) (wall) M95.4
    congenital Q67.8
    sequelae (late effect) of rickets E64.3
  chin (acquired) M95.2
    congenital Q18.9
  choroid (congenital) Q14.3
    acquired H31.8
    plexus Q07.8
      acquired G96.198
  cicatricial — *see* Cicatrix
  cilia, acquired — *see* Disorder, eyelid, specified type NEC
  clavicle (acquired) M95.8
    congenital Q68.8
  clitoris (congenital) Q52.6
    acquired N90.89
  clubfoot — *see* Clubfoot
  coccyx (acquired) — *see* subcategory M43.8 ☑
  colon (congenital) Q43.9
    acquired K63.89
  concha (ear), congenital — *see also* Malformation, ear, external
    acquired — *see* Disorder, pinna, deformity
  cornea (acquired) H18.70
    congenital Q13.4
    descemetocele — *see* Descemetocele
    ectasia — *see* Ectasia, cornea
    specified NEC H18.79- ☑
    staphyloma — *see* Staphyloma, cornea
  coronary artery (acquired) I25.9
    congenital Q24.5
  cranium (acquired) — *see* Deformity, skull
  cricoid cartilage (congenital) Q31.8
    acquired J38.7
  cystic duct (congenital) Q44.5
    acquired K82.8
  Dandy-Walker Q03.1
    with spina bifida — *see* Spina bifida
  diaphragm (congenital) Q79.1
    acquired J98.6
  digestive organ NOS Q45.9
  ductus arteriosus Q25.0
  duodenal bulb K31.89
  duodenum (congenital) Q43.9
    acquired K31.89
  dura — *see* Deformity, meninges
  ear (acquired) — *see also* Disorder, pinna, deformity
    congenital (external) Q17.9
      internal Q16.5
      middle Q16.4
        ossicles Q16.3
      ossicles Q16.3
  ectodermal (congenital) NEC Q84.9
  ejaculatory duct (congenital) Q55.4
    acquired N50.89

Deformity — *continued*
  elbow (joint) (acquired) — *see also* Deformity, limb, upper arm
    congenital Q68.8
    contraction — *see* Contraction, joint, elbow
  endocrine gland NEC Q89.2
  epididymis (congenital) Q55.4
    acquired N50.89
  epiglottis (congenital) Q31.8
    acquired J38.7
  esophagus (congenital) Q39.9
    acquired K22.89
  eustachian tube (congenital) NEC Q17.8
  eye, congenital Q15.9
  eyebrow (congenital) Q18.8
  eyelid (acquired) — *see also* Disorder, eyelid, specified type NEC
    congenital Q10.3
  face (acquired) M95.2
    congenital Q18.9
  fallopian tube, acquired N83.8
  femur (acquired) — *see* Deformity, limb, specified type NEC, thigh
  fetal
    with fetopelvic disproportion O33.7 ☑
    causing obstructed labor O66.3
  finger (acquired) M20.00- ☑
    boutonniere M20.02- ☑
    congenital Q68.1
    flexion contracture — *see* Contraction, joint, hand
    mallet finger M20.01- ☑
    specified NEC M20.09- ☑
    swan-neck M20.03- ☑
  flexion (joint) (acquired) — *see also* Deformity, limb, flexion M21.20
    congenital NOS Q74.9
    hip Q65.89
  foot (acquired) — *see also* Deformity, limb, lower leg
    cavovarus (congenital) Q66.1- ☑
    congenital NOS Q66.9- ☑
      specified type NEC Q66.89
    specified type NEC — *see* Deformity, limb, foot, specified NEC
    valgus (congenital) Q66.6
      acquired — *see* Deformity, valgus, ankle
    varus (congenital) NEC Q66.3- ☑
      acquired — *see* Deformity, varus, ankle
  forearm (acquired) — *see also* Deformity, limb, forearm
    congenital Q68.8
  forehead (acquired) M95.2
    congenital Q75.8
  frontal bone (acquired) M95.2
    congenital Q75.8
  gallbladder (congenital) Q44.1
    acquired K82.8
  gastrointestinal tract (congenital) NOS Q45.9
    acquired K63.89
  genitalia, genital organ(s) or system NEC
    female (congenital) Q52.9
      acquired N94.89
      external Q52.70
    male (congenital) Q55.9
      acquired N50.89
  globe (eye) (congenital) Q15.8
    acquired H44.89
  gum, acquired NEC K06.8
  hand (acquired) — *see* Deformity, limb, hand
    congenital Q68.1
  head (acquired) M95.2
    congenital Q75.8
  heart (congenital) Q24.9
    septum Q21.9
      auricular — *see also* Defect, atrial septal Q21.10
      ventricular Q21.0
    valve (congenital) NEC Q24.8
      acquired — *see* Endocarditis
  heel (acquired) — *see* Deformity, foot
  hepatic duct (congenital) Q44.5
    acquired K83.8
  hip (joint) (acquired) (*see also* Deformity, limb, thigh)
    congenital Q65.9
    due to (previous) juvenile osteochondrosis — *see* Coxa, plana
    flexion — *see* Contraction, joint, hip
  hourglass — *see* Contraction, hourglass
  humerus (acquired) M21.82- ☑
    congenital Q74.0
  hypophyseal (congenital) Q89.2

Deformity — *continued*
 ileocecal (coil) (valve) (acquired) K63.89
  congenital Q43.9
 ileum (congenital) Q43.9
  acquired K63.89
 ilium (acquired) M95.5
  congenital Q74.2
 integument (congenital) Q84.9
 intervertebral cartilage or disc (acquired) — *see* Disorder,
   disc, specified NEC
 intestine (large) (small) (congenital) NOS Q43.9
  acquired K63.89
 intrinsic minus or plus (hand) — *see* Deformity, limb,
   specified type NEC, forearm
 iris (acquired) H21.89
  congenital Q13.2
 ischium (acquired) M95.5
  congenital Q74.2
 jaw (acquired) (congenital) M26.9
 joint (acquired) NEC M21.90
  congenital Q68.8
  elbow M21.92- ☑
  hand M21.94- ☑
  hip M21.95- ☑
  knee M21.96- ☑
  shoulder M21.92- ☑
  wrist M21.93- ☑
 kidney(s) (calyx) (pelvis) (congenital) Q63.9
  acquired N28.89
  artery (congenital) Q27.2
   acquired I77.89
 Klippel-Feil (brevicollis) Q76.1
 knee (acquired) NEC — *see also* Deformity, limb, lower
   leg
  congenital Q68.2
 labium (majus) (minus) (congenital) Q52.79
  acquired N90.89
 lacrimal passages or duct (congenital) NEC Q10.6
  acquired — *see* Disorder, lacrimal system, changes
 larynx (muscle) (congenital) Q31.8
  acquired J38.7
  web (glottic) Q31.0
 leg (upper) (acquired) NEC — *see also* Deformity, limb,
   thigh
  congenital Q68.8
  lower leg — *see* Deformity, limb, lower leg
 lens (acquired) H27.8
  congenital Q12.9
 lid (fold) (acquired) — *see also* Disorder, eyelid, specified
   type NEC
  congenital Q10.3
 ligament (acquired) — *see* Disorder, ligament
  congenital Q79.9
 limb (acquired) M21.90
  clawfoot M21.53- ☑
  clawhand M21.51- ☑
   congenital Q68.1
  clubfoot M21.54- ☑
  clubhand M21.52- ☑
  congenital, except reduction deformity Q74.9
  flat foot M21.4- ☑
  flexion M21.20
   ankle M21.27- ☑
   elbow M21.22- ☑
   finger M21.24- ☑
   hip M21.25- ☑
   knee M21.26- ☑
   shoulder M21.21- ☑
   toe M21.27- ☑
   wrist M21.23- ☑
  foot
   claw — *see* Deformity, limb, clawfoot
   club — *see* Deformity, limb, clubfoot
   drop M21.37- ☑
   flat — *see* Deformity, limb, flat foot
   specified NEC M21.6X- ☑
  forearm M21.93- ☑
  hand M21.94- ☑
  lower leg M21.96- ☑
  specified type NEC M21.80
   forearm M21.83- ☑
   lower leg M21.86- ☑
   thigh M21.85- ☑
   upper arm M21.82- ☑
  thigh M21.95- ☑
  unequal length M21.70

Deformity — *continued*
 limb — *continued*
  unequal length — *continued*
   short site is
    femur M21.75- ☑
    fibula M21.76- ☑
    humerus M21.72- ☑
    radius M21.73- ☑
    tibia M21.76- ☑
    ulna M21.73- ☑
   upper arm M21.92- ☑
  valgus — *see* Deformity, valgus
  varus — *see* Deformity, varus
  wrist drop M21.33- ☑
 lip (acquired) NEC K13.0
  congenital Q38.0
 liver (congenital) Q44.70
  acquired K76.89
 lumbosacral (congenital) (joint) (region) Q76.49
  acquired — *see* subcategory M43.8
  kyphosis — *see* Kyphosis, congenital
  lordosis — *see* Lordosis, congenital
 lung (congenital) Q33.9
  acquired J98.4
 lymphatic system, congenital Q89.9
 Madelung's (radius) Q74.0
 mandible (acquired) (congenital) M26.9
 maxilla (acquired) (congenital) M26.9
 meninges or membrane (congenital) Q07.9
  cerebral Q04.8
   acquired G96.198
  spinal cord (congenital) Q06.- ☑
   acquired G96.198
 metacarpus (acquired) — *see* Deformity, limb, forearm
  congenital Q74.0
 metatarsus (acquired) — *see* Deformity, foot
  congenital Q66.9- ☑
 middle ear (congenital) Q16.4
  ossicles Q16.3
 mitral (leaflets) (valve) I05.8
  parachute Q23.2
  stenosis, congenital Q23.2
 mouth (acquired) K13.79
  congenital Q38.6
 multiple, congenital NEC Q89.7
 muscle (acquired) M62.89
  congenital Q79.9
   sternocleidomastoid Q68.0
 musculoskeletal system (acquired) M95.9
  congenital Q79.9
  specified NEC M95.8
 nail (acquired) L60.8
  congenital Q84.6
 nasal — *see* Deformity, nose
 neck (acquired) M95.3
  congenital Q18.9
   sternocleidomastoid Q68.0
 nervous system (congenital) Q07.9
 nipple (congenital) Q83.9
  acquired N64.89
 nose (acquired) (cartilage) M95.0
  bone (turbinate) M95.0
  congenital Q30.9
   bent or squashed Q67.4
  saddle M95.0
   syphilitic A50.57
  septum (acquired) J34.2
   congenital Q30.8
  sinus (wall) (congenital) Q30.8
   acquired M95.0
  syphilitic (congenital) A50.57
   late A52.73
 ocular muscle (congenital) Q10.3
  acquired — *see* Strabismus, mechanical
 opticociliary vessels (congenital) Q13.2
 orbit (eye) (acquired) H05.30
  atrophy — *see* Atrophy, orbit
  congenital Q10.7
  due to
   bone disease NEC H05.32- ☑
   trauma or surgery H05.33- ☑
  enlargement — *see* Enlargement, orbit
  exostosis — *see* Exostosis, orbit
 organ of Corti (congenital) Q16.5
 ovary (congenital) Q50.39
  acquired N83.8
 oviduct, acquired N83.8
 palate (congenital) Q38.5

Deformity — *continued*
 palate — *continued*
  acquired M27.8
  cleft (congenital) — *see* Cleft, palate
 pancreas (congenital) Q45.3
  acquired K86.89
 parathyroid (gland) Q89.2
 parotid (gland) (congenital) Q38.4
  acquired K11.8
 patella (acquired) — *see* Disorder, patella, specified NEC
 pelvis, pelvic (acquired) (bony) M95.5
  with disproportion (fetopelvic) O33.0
   causing obstructed labor O65.0
  congenital Q74.2
  rachitic sequelae (late effect) E64.3
 penis (glans) (congenital) Q55.69
  acquired N48.89
 pericardium (congenital) Q24.8
  acquired — *see* Pericarditis
 pharynx (congenital) Q38.8
  acquired J39.2
 pinna, acquired — *see also* Disorder, pinna, deformity
  congenital Q17.9
 pituitary (congenital) Q89.2
 posture — *see* Dorsopathy, deforming
 prepuce (congenital) Q55.69
  acquired N47.8
 prostate (congenital) Q55.4
  acquired N42.89
 pupil (congenital) Q13.2
  acquired — *see* Abnormality, pupillary
 pylorus (congenital) Q40.3
  acquired K31.89
 rachitic (acquired), old or healed E64.3
 radius (acquired) — *see also* Deformity, limb, forearm
  congenital Q68.8
 rectum (congenital) Q43.9
  acquired K62.89
 reduction (extremity) (limb), congenital — *see also* condition and site Q73.8
  brain Q04.3
  lower — *see* Defect, reduction, lower limb
  upper — *see* Defect, reduction, upper limb
 renal — *see* Deformity, kidney
 respiratory system (congenital) Q34.9
 rib (acquired) M95.4
  congenital Q76.6
  cervical Q76.5
 rotation (joint) (acquired) — *see* Deformity, limb, specified site NEC
  congenital Q74.9
  hip — *see* Deformity, limb, specified type NEC, thigh
   congenital Q65.89
 sacroiliac joint (congenital) — *see* subcategory Q74.2
  acquired — *see* subcategory M43.8 ☑
 sacrum (acquired) — *see* subcategory M43.8 ☑
 saddle
  back — *see* Lordosis
  nose M95.0
   syphilitic A50.57
 salivary gland or duct (congenital) Q38.4
  acquired K11.8
 scapula (acquired) M95.8
  congenital Q68.8
 scrotum (congenital) — *see also* Malformation, testis and
   scrotum
  acquired N50.89
 seminal vesicles (congenital) Q55.4
  acquired N50.89
 septum, nasal (acquired) J34.2
 shoulder (joint) (acquired) — *see* Deformity, limb, upper
   arm
  congenital Q74.0
  contraction — *see* Contraction, joint, shoulder
 sigmoid (flexure) (congenital) Q43.9
  acquired K63.89
 skin (congenital) Q82.9
 skull (acquired) M95.2
  congenital Q75.8
   with
    anencephaly Q00.0
    encephalocele — *see* Encephalocele
    hydrocephalus Q03.9
     with spina bifida — *see* Spina bifida, by
       site, with hydrocephalus
    microcephaly Q02
 soft parts, organs or tissues (of pelvis)
  in pregnancy or childbirth NEC O34.8- ☑
   causing obstructed labor O65.5

Deformity — *continued*
spermatic cord (congenital) Q55.4
  acquired N50.89
    torsion — *see* Torsion, spermatic cord
spinal — *see* Dorsopathy, deforming
  column (acquired) — *see* Dorsopathy, deforming
  congenital Q67.5
  cord (congenital) Q06.9
    acquired G95.89
  nerve root (congenital) Q07.9
spine (acquired) — *see also* Dorsopathy, deforming
  congenital Q67.5
  rachitic E64.3
  specified NEC — *see* Dorsopathy, deforming, specified NEC
spleen
  acquired D73.89
  congenital Q89.09
Sprengel's (congenital) Q74.0
sternocleidomastoid (muscle), congenital Q68.0
sternum (acquired) M95.4
  congenital NEC Q76.7
stomach (congenital) Q40.3
  acquired K31.89
submandibular gland (congenital) Q38.4
submaxillary gland (congenital) Q38.4
  acquired K11.8
talipes — *see* Talipes
testis (congenital) — *see also* Malformation, testis and scrotum
  acquired N44.8
    torsion — *see* Torsion, testis
thigh (acquired) — *see also* Deformity, limb, thigh
  congenital NEC Q68.8
thorax (acquired) (wall) M95.4
  congenital Q67.8
  sequelae of rickets E64.3
thumb (acquired) — *see also* Deformity, finger
  congenital NEC Q68.1
thymus (tissue) (congenital) Q89.2
thyroid (gland) (congenital) Q89.2
  cartilage Q31.8
    acquired J38.7
tibia (acquired) — *see also* Deformity, limb, specified type NEC, lower leg
  congenital NEC Q68.8
  saber (syphilitic) A50.56
toe (acquired) M20.6- ☑
  congenital Q66.9- ☑
  hallux rigidus M20.2- ☑
  hallux valgus M20.1- ☑
  hallux varus M20.3- ☑
  hammer toe M20.4- ☑
  specified NEC M20.5X- ☑
tongue (congenital) Q38.3
  acquired K14.8
tooth, teeth K00.2
trachea (rings) (congenital) Q32.1
  acquired J39.8
transverse aortic arch (congenital) Q25.49
tricuspid (leaflets) (valve) I07.8
  atresia or stenosis Q22.4
  Ebstein's Q22.5
trunk (acquired) M95.8
  congenital Q89.9
ulna (acquired) — *see also* Deformity, limb, forearm
  congenital NEC Q68.8
urachus, congenital Q64.4
ureter (opening) (congenital) Q62.8
  acquired N28.89
urethra (congenital) Q64.79
  acquired N36.8
urinary tract (congenital) Q64.9
  urachus Q64.4
uterus (congenital) Q51.9
  acquired N85.8
uvula (congenital) Q38.5
vagina (acquired) N89.8
  congenital Q52.4
valgus NEC M21.00
  ankle M21.07- ☑
  elbow M21.02- ☑
  hip M21.05- ☑
  knee M21.06- ☑
valve, valvular (congenital) (heart) Q24.8
  acquired — *see* Endocarditis
varus NEC M21.10
  ankle M21.17- ☑

Deformity — *continued*
varus — *continued*
  elbow M21.12- ☑
  hip M21.15 ☑
  knee M21.16- ☑
  tibia — *see* Osteochondrosis, juvenile, tibia
vas deferens (congenital) Q55.4
  acquired N50.89
vein (congenital) Q27.9
  great Q26.9
vertebra — *see* Dorsopathy, deforming
vertical talus (congenital) Q66.80
  left foot Q66.82
  right foot Q66.81
vesicourethral orifice (acquired) N32.89
  congenital NEC Q64.79
vessels of optic papilla (congenital) Q14.2
visual field (contraction) — *see* Defect, visual field
vitreous body, acquired H43.89
vulva (congenital) Q52.79
  acquired N90.89
wrist (joint) (acquired) — *see also* Deformity, limb, forearm
  congenital Q68.8
  contraction — *see* Contraction, joint, wrist

Degeneration, degenerative
adrenal (capsule) (fatty) (gland) (hyaline) (infectional) E27.8
amyloid — *see also* Amyloidosis E85.9
anterior cornua, spinal cord G12.29
anterior labral S43.49- ☑
aorta, aortic I70.0
  fatty I77.89
aortic valve (heart) — *see* Endocarditis, aortic
arteriovascular — *see* Arteriosclerosis
artery, arterial (atheromatous) (calcareous) — *see also* Arteriosclerosis
  cerebral, amyloid E85.4 [I68.0]
  medial — *see* Arteriosclerosis, extremities
articular cartilage NEC — *see* Derangement, joint, articular cartilage, by site
atheromatous — *see* Arteriosclerosis
basal nuclei or ganglia G23.9
  specified NEC G23.8
bone NEC — *see* Disorder, bone, specified type NEC
brachial plexus G54.0
brain (cortical) (progressive) G31.9
  alcoholic G31.2
  arteriosclerotic I67.2
  childhood G31.9
    specified NEC G31.89
  cystic G31.89
    congenital Q04.6
  in
    alcoholism G31.2
    beriberi E51.2
    cerebrovascular disease I67.9
    congenital hydrocephalus Q03.9
      with spina bifida — *see also* Spina bifida
    Fabry-Anderson disease E75.21
    Gaucher's disease E75.22
    Hunter's syndrome E76.1
    lipidosis
      cerebral E75.4
      generalized E75.6
    mucopolysaccharidosis — *see* Mucopolysaccharidosis
    myxedema E03.9 [G32.89]
    neoplastic disease — *see also* Neoplasm D49.6 [G32.89]
    Niemann-Pick disease E75.249 [G32.89]
    sphingolipidosis E75.3 [G32.89]
    vitamin B12 deficiency E53.8 [G32.89]
  senile NEC G31.1
breast N64.89
Bruch's membrane — *see* Degeneration, choroid
capillaries (fatty) I78.8
  amyloid E85.89 [I79.8]
cardiac — *see also* Degeneration, myocardial
  valve, valvular — *see* Endocarditis
cardiorenal — *see* Hypertension, cardiorenal
cardiovascular — *see also* Disease, cardiovascular
  renal — *see* Hypertension, cardiorenal
cerebellar NOS G31.9
  alcoholic G31.2
  primary (hereditary) (sporadic) G11.9
cerebral — *see* Degeneration, brain
cerebrovascular I67.9
  due to hypertension I67.4

Degeneration, degenerative — *continued*
cervical plexus G54.2
cervix N88.8
  due to radiation (intended effect) N88.8
    adverse effect or misadventure N99.89
chamber angle H21.21- ☑
changes, spine or vertebra — *see* Spondylosis
chorioretinal — *see also* Degeneration, choroid
  hereditary H31.20
choroid (colloid) (drusen) H31.10- ☑
  atrophy — *see* Atrophy, choroidal
  hereditary — *see* Dystrophy, choroidal, hereditary
ciliary body H21.22- ☑
cochlear — *see* subcategory H83.8 ☑
combined (spinal cord) (subacute) E53.8 [G32.0]
  with anemia (pernicious) D51.0 [G32.0]
    due to dietary vitamin B12 deficiency D51.3 [G32.0]
  in (due to)
    vitamin B12 deficiency E53.8 [G32.0]
      anemia D51.9 [G32.0]
conjunctiva H11.10
  concretions — *see* Concretion, conjunctiva
  deposits — *see* Deposit, conjunctiva
  pigmentations — *see* Pigmentation, conjunctiva
  pinguecula — *see* Pinguecula
  xerosis — *see* Xerosis, conjunctiva
cornea H18.40
  calcerous H18.43
    band keratopathy H18.42- ☑
  familial, hereditary — *see* Dystrophy, cornea
  hyaline (of old scars) H18.49
  keratomalacia — *see* Keratomalacia
  nodular H18.45- ☑
  peripheral H18.46- ☑
  senile H18.41- ☑
  specified type NEC H18.49
cortical (cerebellar) (parenchymatous) G31.89
  alcoholic G31.2
  diffuse, due to arteriopathy I67.2
corticobasal G31.85
cutis L98.8
  amyloid E85.4 [L99]
dental pulp K04.2
disc disease — *see* Degeneration, intervertebral disc, by site
dorsolateral (spinal cord) — *see* Degeneration, combined
extrapyramidal G25.9
eye, macular — *see also* Degeneration, macula
  congenital or hereditary — *see* Dystrophy, retina
facet joints — *see* Spondylosis
fatty
  liver NEC K76.0
    alcoholic K70.0
grey matter (brain) (Alpers') G31.81
heart — *see also* Degeneration, myocardial
  amyloid E85.4 [I43]
  atheromatous — *see* Disease, heart, ischemic, atherosclerotic
  ischemic — *see* Disease, heart, ischemic
hepatolenticular (Wilson's) E83.01
hepatorenal K76.7
hyaline (diffuse) (generalized)
  localized — *see* Degeneration, by site
infrapatellar fat pad M79.4
intervertebral disc
  with
    myelopathy — *see* Disorder, disc, with, myelopathy
    radiculitis or radiculopathy — *see* Disorder, disc, with, radiculopathy
  cervical, cervicothoracic — *see* Disorder, disc, cervical, degeneration
    with
      myelopathy — *see* Disorder, disc, cervical, with myelopathy
      neuritis, radiculitis or radiculopathy — *see* Disorder, disc, cervical, with neuritis
  lumbar region M51.36- ☑
    with
      myelopathy M51.06
      neuritis, radiculitis, radiculopathy or sciatica M51.16
  lumbosacral region M51.37- ☑
    with
      neuritis, radiculitis, radiculopathy or sciatica M51.17
  sacrococcygeal region M53.3
  thoracic region M51.34

Degeneration, degenerative — continued
  intervertebral disc — continued
    thoracic region — continued
      with
        myelopathy M51.04
        neuritis, radiculitis, radiculopathy M51.14
    thoracolumbar region M51.35
      with
        myelopathy M51.05
        neuritis, radiculitis, radiculopathy M51.15
  intestine, amyloid E85.4
  iris (pigmentary) H21.23- ✓
  ischemic — see Ischemia
  joint disease — see Osteoarthritis
  kidney N28.89
    amyloid E85.4 [N29]
    cystic, congenital Q61.9
    fatty N28.89
    polycystic Q61.3
      adult type (autosomal dominant) Q61.2
      infantile type (autosomal recessive) NEC Q61.19
        collecting duct dilatation Q61.11
  Kuhnt-Junius — see also Degeneration, macula
    H35.32- ✓
  lens — see Cataract
  lenticular (familial) (progressive) (Wilson's) (with cirrhosis of liver) E83.01
  liver (diffuse) NEC K76.89
    amyloid E85.4 [K77]
    cystic K76.89
      congenital Q44.6
    fatty NEC K76.0
      alcoholic K70.0
    hypertrophic K76.89
    parenchymatous, acute or subacute K72.00
      with coma K72.01
    pigmentary K76.89
    toxic (acute) K71.9
  lung J98.4
  lymph gland I89.8
    hyaline I89.8
  macula, macular (acquired) (age-related) (senile) H35.30
    angioid streaks H35.33
    atrophic age-related H35.31- ✓
    congenital or hereditary — see Dystrophy, retina
    cystoid H35.35- ✓
    drusen H35.36- ✓
    dry age-related H35.31- ✓
    exudative H35.32- ✓
    hole H35.34- ✓
    nonexudative H35.31- ✓
    puckering H35.37- ✓
    toxic H35.38- ✓
    wet age-related H35.32- ✓
  membranous labyrinth, congenital (causing impairment of hearing) Q16.5
  meniscus — see Derangement, meniscus
  mitral — see Insufficiency, mitral
  Monckeberg's — see Arteriosclerosis, extremities
  motor centers, senile G31.1
  multi-system G90.3
  mural — see Degeneration, myocardial
  muscle (fatty) (fibrous) (hyaline) (progressive) M62.89
    heart — see Degeneration, myocardial
  myelin, central nervous system G37.9
  myocardial, myocardium (fatty) (hyaline) (senile) I51.5
    with rheumatic fever (conditions in I00) I09.0
      active, acute or subacute I01.2
        with chorea I02.0
      inactive or quiescent (with chorea) I09.0
    hypertensive — see Hypertension, heart
    rheumatic — see Degeneration, myocardial, with rheumatic fever
    syphilitic A52.06
  nasal sinus (mucosa) J32.9
    frontal J32.1
    maxillary J32.0
  nerve — see Disorder, nerve
  nervous system G31.9
    alcoholic G31.2
    amyloid E85.4 [G99.8]
    autonomic G90.9
    fatty G31.89
    specified NEC G31.89
  nipple N64.89
  olivopontocerebellar (hereditary) (familial) G23.8
  osseous labyrinth — see subcategory H83.8 ✓
  ovary N83.8

Degeneration, degenerative — continued
  ovary — continued
    cystic N83.20- ✓
      microcystic N83.20- ✓
  pallidal pigmentary (progressive) G23.0
  pancreas K86.89
    tuberculous A18.83
  penis N48.89
  pigmentary (diffuse) (general)
    localized — see Degeneration, by site
    pallidal (progressive) G23.0
  pineal gland E34.8
  pituitary (gland) E23.6
  popliteal fat pad M79.4
  posterolateral (spinal cord) — see Degeneration, combined
  pulmonary valve (heart) I37.8
  pulp (tooth) K04.2
  pupillary margin H21.24- ✓
  renal — see Degeneration, kidney
  retina H35.9
    hereditary (cerebroretinal) (congenital) (juvenile) (macula) (peripheral) (pigmentary) — see Dystrophy, retina
    Kuhnt-Junius — see also Degeneration, macula H35.32- ✓
    macula (cystic) (exudative) (hole) (nonexudative) (pseudohole) (senile) (toxic) — see Degeneration, macula
    peripheral H35.40
      lattice H35.41- ✓
      microcystoid H35.42- ✓
      paving stone H35.43- ✓
      secondary
        pigmentary H35.45- ✓
        vitreoretinal H35.46- ✓
      senile reticular H35.44- ✓
    pigmentary (primary) — see also Dystrophy, retina
      secondary — see Degeneration, retina, peripheral, secondary
    posterior pole — see Degeneration, macula
  saccule, congenital (causing impairment of hearing) Q16.5
  senile R54
    brain G31.1
    cardiac, heart or myocardium — see Degeneration, myocardial
    motor centers G31.1
    vascular — see Arteriosclerosis
  sinus (cystic) — see also Sinusitis
    polypoid J33.1
  skin L98.8
    amyloid E85.4 [L99]
    colloid L98.8
  spinal (cord) G31.89
    amyloid E85.4 [G32.89]
    combined (subacute) — see Degeneration, combined
    dorsolateral — see Degeneration, combined
    familial NEC G31.89
    fatty G31.89
    funicular — see Degeneration, combined
    posterolateral — see Degeneration, combined
    subacute combined — see Degeneration, combined
    tuberculous A17.81
  spleen D73.0
    amyloid E85.4 [D77]
  stomach K31.89
  striatonigral G23.2
  suprarenal (capsule) (gland) E27.8
  synovial membrane (pulpy) — see Disorder, synovium, specified type NEC
  tapetoretinal — see Dystrophy, retina
  thymus (gland) E32.8
    fatty E32.8
  thyroid (gland) E07.89
  tricuspid (heart) (valve) I07.9
  tuberculous NEC — see Tuberculosis
  turbinate J34.89
  uterus (cystic) N85.8
  vascular (senile) — see Arteriosclerosis
    hypertensive — see Hypertension
  vitreoretinal, secondary — see Degeneration, retina, peripheral, secondary, vitreoretinal
  vitreous (body) H43.81- ✓
  Wallerian — see Disorder, nerve
  Wilson's hepatolenticular E83.01
Deglutition
  paralysis R13.0

Deglutition — continued
  paralysis — continued
    hysterical F44.4
    pneumonia J69.0
Degos' disease I77.89
Dehiscence (of)
  amputation stump T87.81
  cesarean wound O90.0
  closure of
    abdominal wall muscle or fascia T81.321 ✓
    cornea T81.31 ✓
    craniotomy T81.328 ✓
    fascia (muscular) (superficial) T81.328 ✓
    gastrointestinal tract anastomosis, repair, or closure T81.320 ✓
    internal organ or tissue T81.328 ✓
    laceration (external) (internal) T81.33 ✓
    ligament T81.328 ✓
    mucosa T81.31 ✓
    muscle or muscle flap T81.328 ✓
    ribs or rib cage T81.328 ✓
    skin and subcutaneous tissue (full-thickness) (superficial) T81.31 ✓
    skull T81.328 ✓
    sternum (sternotomy) T81.328 ✓
    tendon T81.328 ✓
    traumatic laceration (external) (internal) T81.33 ✓
  episiotomy O90.1
  operation wound NEC T81.31 ✓
    deep T81.329 ✓
    external operation wound (superficial) T81.31 ✓
    internal operation wound (deep) T81.329 ✓
      abdominal wall muscle or fascia T81.321 ✓
      specified NEC T81.328 ✓
  perineal wound (postpartum) O90.1
  traumatic injury wound repair T81.33 ✓
  wound T81.30 ✓
    traumatic repair T81.33 ✓
Dehydration E86.0
  newborn P74.1
Dejerine-Roussy syndrome G89.0
Dejerine-Sottas disease or neuropathy (hypertrophic) G60.0
Dejerine-Thomas atrophy G23.8
Delay, delayed
  any plane in pelvis
    complicating delivery O66.9
  birth or delivery NOS O63.9
  closure, ductus arteriosus (Botalli) P29.38
  coagulation — see Defect, coagulation
  conduction (cardiac) (ventricular) I45.9
  delivery, second twin, triplet, etc O63.2
  development R62.50
    global F88
    intellectual (specific) F81.9
    language F80.9
      due to hearing loss F80.4
    learning F81.9
    milestone R62.0
    pervasive F84.9
    physiological R62.50
      specified stage NEC R62.0
    reading F81.0
    sexual E30.0
    speech F80.9
      due to hearing loss F80.4
    spelling F81.81
  ejaculation F52.32
  gastric emptying K30
  menarche E30.0
  menstruation (cause unknown) N91.0
  milestone R62.0
  passage of meconium (newborn) P76.0
  primary respiration P28.9
  puberty (constitutional) E30.0
  separation of umbilical cord P96.82
  sexual maturation, female E30.0
  sleep phase syndrome G47.21
  union, fracture — see Fracture, by site
  vaccination Z28.9
Deletion(s)
  autosome Q93.9
    identified by fluorescence in situ hybridization (FISH) Q93.89
    identified by in situ hybridization (ISH) Q93.89
  chromosome
    with complex rearrangements NEC Q93.7
    part of NEC Q93.59

Deletion(s) — *continued*
  chromosome — *continued*
    seen only at prometaphase Q93.89
    short arm
      22q11.2 Q93.81
      4 Q93.3
      5p Q93.4
    specified NEC Q93.89
    long arm chromosome 18 or 21 Q93.89
      with complex rearrangements NEC Q93.7
    microdeletions NEC Q93.88
Delhi boil or button B55.1
Delinquency (juvenile) (neurotic) F91.8
  group Z72.810
Delinquent immunization status Z28.39
  COVID-19 Z28.31- ☑
Delirium, delirious (acute or subacute) (not alcohol- or drug-induced) R41.0
  with
    dementia — *see also* Dementia F05
  alcoholic (acute) (tremens) (withdrawal) F10.921
    with intoxication F10.921
      in
        abuse F10.121
        dependence F10.221
  due to (secondary to)
    alcohol
      intoxication F10.921
        in
          abuse F10.121
          dependence F10.221
      withdrawal F10.231
    amphetamine intoxication F15.921
      in
        abuse F15.121
        dependence F15.221
    anxiolytic
      intoxication F13.921
        in
          abuse F13.121
          dependence F13.221
      withdrawal F13.231
    cannabis intoxication (acute) F12.921
      in
        abuse F12.121
        dependence F12.221
    cocaine intoxication (acute) F14.921
      in
        abuse F14.121
        dependence F14.221
    general medical condition F05
    hallucinogen intoxication F16.921
      in
        abuse F16.121
        dependence F16.221
    hypnotic
      intoxication F13.921
        in
          abuse F13.121
          dependence F13.221
      withdrawal F13.231
    inhalant intoxication (acute) F18.921
      in
        abuse F18.121
        dependence F18.221
    multiple etiologies F05
    opioid intoxication (acute) F11.921
      in
        abuse F11.121
        dependence F11.221
    other (or unknown) substance F19.921
    phencyclidine intoxication (acute) F16.921
      in
        abuse F16.121
        dependence F16.221
    psychoactive substance NEC intoxication (acute) F19.921
      in
        abuse F19.121
        dependence F19.221
    sedative
      intoxication F13.921
        in
          abuse F13.121
          dependence F13.221
      withdrawal F13.231
    unknown etiology R41.0
  exhaustion F43.0
  hysterical F44.89

Delirium, delirious — *continued*
  postprocedural (postoperative) F05
  puerperal F05
  thyroid — *see* Thyrotoxicosis with thyroid storm
  traumatic — *see* Injury, intracranial
  tremens (alcohol-induced) F10.231
    sedative-induced F13.231
Delivery (childbirth) (labor)
  arrested active phase O62.1
  cesarean (for)
    abnormal
      pelvis (bony) (deformity) (major) NEC with dispro-portion (fetopelvic) O33.0
        with obstructed labor O65.0
      presentation or position O32.9 ☑
    abruptio placentae — *see also* Abruptio placentae O45.9- ☑
    acromion presentation O32.2 ☑
    atony, uterus O62.2
    breech presentation O32.1 ☑
      incomplete O32.8 ☑
    brow presentation O32.3 ☑
    cephalopelvic disproportion O33.9
    cerclage O34.3- ☑
    chin presentation O32.3 ☑
    cicatrix of cervix O34.4- ☑
    contracted pelvis (general)
      inlet O33.2
      outlet O33.3 ☑
    cord presentation or prolapse O69.0 ☑
    cystocele O34.8- ☑
    deformity (acquired) (congenital)
      pelvic organs or tissues NEC O34.8- ☑
      pelvis (bony) NEC O33.0
    disproportion NOS O33.9
    eclampsia — *see* Eclampsia
    face presentation O32.3 ☑
    failed
      forceps O66.5
      induction of labor O61.9
        instrumental O61.1
        mechanical O61.1
        medical O61.0
        specified NEC O61.8
        surgical O61.1
      trial of labor NOS O66.40
        following previous cesarean delivery O66.41
      vacuum extraction O66.5
      ventouse O66.5
    fetal-maternal hemorrhage O43.01- ☑
    hemorrhage (intrapartum) O67.9
      with coagulation defect O67.0
      specified cause NEC O67.8
    high head at term O32.4 ☑
    hydrocephalic fetus O33.6 ☑
    incarceration of uterus O34.51- ☑
    incoordinate uterine action O62.4
    increased size, fetus O33.5 ☑
    inertia, uterus O62.2
      primary O62.0
      secondary O62.1
    isthmocele O34.22
    lateroversion, uterus O34.59- ☑
    mal lie O32.9 ☑
    malposition
      fetus O32.9 ☑
      pelvic organs or tissues NEC O34.8- ☑
      uterus NEC O34.59- ☑
    malpresentation NOS O32.9 ☑
    oblique presentation O32.2 ☑
    occurring after 37 completed weeks of gestation but before 39 completed weeks gestation due to (spontaneous) onset of labor O75.82
    oversize fetus O33.5 ☑
    pelvic tumor NEC O34.8- ☑
    placenta previa O44.0- ☑
      complete O44.0- ☑
        with hemorrhage O44.1- ☑
    placental insufficiency O36.51- ☑
    planned, occurring after 37 completed weeks of gesta-tion but before 39 completed weeks gesta-tion due to (spontaneous) onset of labor O75.82
    polyp, cervix O34.4- ☑
      causing obstructed labor O65.5
    poor dilatation, cervix O62.0
    pre-eclampsia O14.94
      mild O14.04

Delivery — *continued*
  cesarean — *continued*
    pre-eclampsia — *continued*
      moderate O14.04
      severe O14.14
        with hemolysis, elevated liver enzymes and low platelet count (HELLP) O14.24
    previous
      cesarean delivery O34.219
        classical (vertical) scar O34.212
        isthmocele O34.22
        low transverse scar O34.211
        mid-transverse T incision O34.218
        scar
          defect (isthmocele) O34.22
          specified type NEC O34.218
      surgery (to)
        cervix O34.4- ☑
        gynecological NEC O34.8- ☑
        rectum O34.7- ☑
        uterus O34.29
        vagina O34.6- ☑
    prolapse
      arm or hand O32.2 ☑
      uterus O34.52- ☑
    prolonged labor NOS O63.9
    rectocele O34.8- ☑
    retroversion
      uterus O34.53- ☑
    rigid
      cervix O34.4- ☑
      pelvic floor O34.8- ☑
      perineum O34.7- ☑
      vagina O34.6- ☑
      vulva O34.7- ☑
    sacculation, pregnant uterus O34.59- ☑
    scar(s)
      cervix O34.4- ☑
      cesarean delivery O34.219
        classical (vertical) O34.212
        isthmocele O34.22
        low transverse O34.211
        mid-transverse T incision O34.218
        scar
          defect (isthmocele) O34.22
          specified type NEC O34.218
      defect (isthmocele) O34.22
      transmural uterine O34.29
      uterus O34.29
    Shirodkar suture in situ O34.3- ☑
    shoulder presentation O32.2 ☑
    stenosis or stricture, cervix O34.4- ☑
    streptococcus group B (GBS) carrier state O99.824
    transmural uterine scar O34.29
    transverse presentation or lie O32.2 ☑
    tumor, pelvic organs or tissues NEC O34.8- ☑
      cervix O34.4- ☑
    umbilical cord presentation or prolapse O69.0 ☑
    without indication O82
  completely normal case O80
  complicated O75.9
    by
      abnormal, abnormality (of)
        forces of labor O62.9
          specified type NEC O62.8
        glucose O99.814
        uterine contractions NOS O62.9
      abruptio placentae — *see also* Abruptio placentae O45.9- ☑
      abuse
        physical O9A.32 (*following* O99)
        psychological O9A.52 (*following* O99)
        sexual O9A.42 (*following* O99)
      adherent placenta O72.0
        without hemorrhage O73.0
      alcohol use O99.314
      anemia (pre-existing) O99.02
      anesthetic death O74.8
      annular detachment of cervix O71.3
      atony, uterus O62.2
      attempted vacuum extraction and forceps O66.5
      Bandl's ring O62.4
      bariatric surgery status O99.844
      biliary tract disorder O26.62
      bleeding — *see* Delivery, complicated by, hemor-rhage
      blood disorder NEC O99.12
      cervical dystocia (hypotonic) O62.2

Delivery — *continued*
  complicated — *continued*
    by — *continued*
      cervical dystocia — *continued*
        primary O62.0
        secondary O62.1
      circulatory system disorder O99.42
      compression of cord (umbilical) NEC O69.2 ☑
      condition NEC O99.892
      contraction, contracted ring O62.4
      cord (umbilical)
        around neck
          with compression O69.1 ☑
          without compression O69.81 ☑
        bruising O69.5 ☑
        complication O69.9 ☑
          specified NEC O69.89 ☑
        compression NEC O69.2 ☑
        entanglement O69.2 ☑
          without compression O69.82 ☑
        hematoma O69.5 ☑
        presentation O69.0 ☑
        prolapse O69.0 ☑
        short O69.3 ☑
        thrombosis (vessels) O69.5 ☑
        vascular lesion O69.5 ☑
      Couvelaire uterus O45.8X- ☑
      damage to (injury to) NEC
        perineum O71.82
        periurethral tissue O71.82
        vulva O71.82
      delay following rupture of membranes (sponta-
        neous) — *see* Pregnancy, complicated by,
        premature rupture of membranes
      depressed fetal heart tones O76
      diabetes O24.92
        gestational O24.429
          diet controlled O24.420
          insulin controlled O24.424
          oral drug controlled (antidiabetic) (hypo-
            glycemic) O24.425
        pre-existing O24.32
          specified NEC O24.82
          type 1 O24.02
          type 2 O24.12
      diastasis recti (abdominis) O71.89
      dilatation
        bladder O66.8
        cervix incomplete, poor or slow O62.0
      disease NEC O99.892
      disruptio uteri — *see* Delivery, complicated by,
        rupture, uterus
      drug use O99.324
      dysfunction, uterus NOS O62.9
        hypertonic O62.4
        hypotonic O62.2
          primary O62.0
          secondary O62.1
        incoordinate O62.4
      eclampsia O15.1
      embolism (pulmonary) — *see* Embolism, obstetric
      endocrine, nutritional or metabolic disease NEC
        O99.284
      failed
        attempted vaginal birth after previous cesarean
          delivery O66.41
        induction of labor O61.9
          instrumental O61.1
          mechanical O61.1
          medical O61.0
          specified NEC O61.8
          surgical O61.1
        trial of labor O66.40
      female genital mutilation O65.5
      fetal
        abnormal acid-base balance O68
        acidemia O68
        acidosis O68
        alkalosis O68
        death, early O02.1
        deformity O66.3
        heart rate or rhythm (abnormal) (non-reassur-
          ing) O76
        hypoxia O77.8
        stress O77.9
          due to drug administration O77.1
          electrocardiographic evidence of O77.8
          specified NEC O77.8

Delivery — *continued*
  complicated — *continued*
    by — *continued*
      fetal — *continued*
        stress — *continued*
          ultrasound evidence of O77.8
      fever during labor O75.2
      gastric banding status O99.844
      gastric bypass status O99.844
      gastrointestinal disease NEC O99.62
      gestational
        diabetes O24.429
          diet controlled O24.420
          insulin (and diet) controlled O24.424
          oral drug controlled (antidiabetic) (hypo-
            glycemic) O24.425
        edema O12.04
          with proteinuria O12.24
        proteinuria O12.14
      gonorrhea O98.22
      hematoma O71.7
        ischial spine O71.7
        pelvic O71.7
        vagina O71.7
        vulva or perineum O71.7
      hemorrhage (uterine) O67.9
        associated with
          afibrinogenemia O67.0
          coagulation defect O67.0
          hyperfibrinolysis O67.0
          hypofibrinogenemia O67.0
        due to
          low implantation of placenta O44.5- ☑
          low-lying placenta O44.5- ☑
          placenta previa O44.1- ☑
            marginal O44.3- ☑
            partial O44.3- ☑
          premature separation of placenta (normal-
            ly implanted) — *see also* Abruptio
            placentae O45.9- ☑
          retained placenta O72.0
          uterine leiomyoma O67.8
        placenta NEC O67.8
        postpartum NEC (atonic) (immediate) O72.1
          with retained or trapped placenta O72.0
          delayed O72.2
          secondary O72.2
          third stage O72.0
      hourglass contraction, uterus O62.4
      hypertension, hypertensive (pre-existing) — *see*
        Hypertension, complicated by, childbirth
        (labor)
      hypotension O26.5- ☑
      incomplete dilatation (cervix) O62.0
      incoordinate uterus contractions O62.4
      inertia, uterus O62.2
        during latent phase of labor O62.0
        primary O62.0
        secondary O62.1
      infection (maternal) O98.92
        carrier state NEC O99.834
        gonorrhea O98.22
        human immunodeficiency virus (HIV) O98.72
        sexually transmitted NEC O98.32
        specified NEC O98.82
        syphilis O98.12
        tuberculosis O98.02
        viral hepatitis O98.42
        viral NEC O98.52
      injury (to mother) — *see also* Delivery, complicat-
        ed, by, damage to O71.9
        nonobstetric O9A.22 (*following* O99)
          caused by abuse — *see* Delivery, compli-
            cated by, abuse
      intrauterine fetal death, early O02.1
      inversion, uterus O71.2
      laceration (perineal) O70.9
        anus (sphincter) O70.4
          with third degree laceration — *see also*
            Delivery, complicated, by, laceration,
            perineum, third degree O70.20
            with mucosa O70.3
          without third degree laceration O70.2 ☑
        bladder (urinary) O71.5
        bowel O71.5
        cervix (uteri) O71.3
        fourchette O70.0
        hymen O70.0

Delivery — *continued*
  complicated — *continued*
    by — *continued*
      laceration — *continued*
        labia O70.0
        pelvic
          floor O70.1
          organ NEC O71.5
        perineum, perineal O70.9
          first degree O70.0
          fourth degree O70.3
          muscles O70.1
          second degree O70.1
          skin O70.0
          slight O70.0
          third degree O70.20
            with
              both external anal sphincter (EAS)
                and internal anal sphincter
                (IAS) torn (IIIc) O70.23
              less than 50% of external anal
                sphincter (EAS) thickness torn
                (IIIa) O70.21
              more than 50% external anal sphinc-
                ter (EAS) thickness torn (IIIb)
                O70.22
            IIIa O70.21
            IIIb O70.22
            IIIc O70.23
        peritoneum (pelvic) O71.5
        rectovaginal (septum) (without perineal lacer-
          ation) O71.4
          with perineum — *see also* Delivery, compli-
            cated, by, laceration, perineum, third
            degree O70.20
          with anal or rectal mucosa O70.3
        specified NEC O71.89
        sphincter ani — *see* Delivery, complicated, by,
          laceration, anus (sphincter)
        urethra O71.5
        uterus O71.81
          before labor O71.81
        vagina, vaginal (deep) (high) (without perineal
          laceration) O71.4
          with perineum O70.0
          muscles, with perineum O70.1
        vulva O70.0
      liver disorder O26.62
      malignancy O9A.12 (*following* O99)
      malnutrition O25.2
      malposition, malpresentation
        uterus or cervix O65.5
        placenta O44.0- ☑
          with hemorrhage O44.1- ☑
        without obstruction — *see also* Delivery, com-
          plicated by, obstruction O32.9 ☑
          breech O32.1 ☑
          compound O32.6 ☑
          face (brow) (chin) O32.3 ☑
          footling O32.8 ☑
          high head O32.4 ☑
          oblique O32.2 ☑
          specified NEC O32.8 ☑
          transverse O32.2 ☑
          unstable lie O32.0 ☑
      meconium in amniotic fluid O77.0
      mental disorder NEC O99.344
      metrorrhexis — *see* Delivery, complicated by,
        rupture, uterus
      nervous system disorder O99.354
      obesity (pre-existing) O99.214
      obesity surgery status O99.844
      obstetric trauma O71.9
        specified NEC O71.89
      obstructed labor
        due to
          breech (complete) (frank) presentation
            O64.1 ☑
            incomplete O64.8 ☑
          brow presentation O64.3 ☑
          buttock presentation O64.1 ☑
          chin presentation O64.2 ☑
          compound presentation O64.5 ☑
          contracted pelvis O65.1
          deep transverse arrest O64.0 ☑
          deformed pelvis O65.0
          dystocia (fetal) O66.9

Delivery — *continued*
 complicated — *continued*
  by — *continued*
   obstructed labor — *continued*
    due to — *continued*
     dystocia — *continued*
      due to
       conjoined twins O66.3
       fetal
        abnormality NEC O66.3
        ascites O66.3
        hydrops O66.3
        meningomyelocele O66.3
        sacral teratoma O66.3
        tumor O66.3
       hydrocephalic fetus O66.3
       shoulder O66.0
     face presentation O64.2 ☑
     fetopelvic disproportion O65.4
     footling presentation O64.8 ☑
     impacted shoulders O66.0
     incomplete rotation of fetal head O64.0 ☑
     large fetus O66.2
     locked twins O66.1
     malposition O64.9 ☑
      specified NEC O64.8 ☑
     malpresentation O64.9 ☑
      specified NEC O64.8 ☑
     multiple fetuses NEC O66.6
     pelvic
      abnormality (maternal) O65.9
       organ O65.5
       specified NEC O65.8
      contraction
       inlet O65.2
       mid-cavity O65.3
       outlet O65.3
     persistent (position)
      occipitoiliac O64.0 ☑
      occipitoposterior O64.0 ☑
      occipitosacral O64.0 ☑
      occipitotransverse O64.0 ☑
     prolapsed arm O64.4 ☑
     shoulder presentation O64.4 ☑
    specified NEC O66.8
   pathological retraction ring, uterus O62.4
   penetration, pregnant uterus by instrument O71.1
   perforation — *see* Delivery, complicated by, laceration
   placenta, placental
    ablatio — *see also* Abruptio placentae
     O45.9- ☑
    abnormality O43.9- ☑
     specified NEC O43.89- ☑
    abruptio — *see also* Abruptio placentae
     O45.9- ☑
    accreta O43.21- ☑
    adherent (with hemorrhage) O72.0
     without hemorrhage O73.0
    detachment (premature) — *see also* Abruptio
     placentae O45.9- ☑
    disorder O43.9- ☑
     specified NEC O43.89- ☑
    hemorrhage NEC O67.8
    increta O43.22- ☑
    low (implantation) (lying) O44.4- ☑
     with hemorrhage O44.5- ☑
    malformation O43.10- ☑
    malposition O44.0- ☑
     without hemorrhage O44.1- ☑
    percreta O43.23- ☑
    previa (central) (complete) (lateral) (total)
     O44.0- ☑
     with hemorrhage O44.1- ☑
     marginal O44.2- ☑
      with hemorrhage O44.3- ☑
     partial O44.2- ☑
      with hemorrhage O44.3- ☑
    retained (with hemorrhage) O72.0
     without hemorrhage O73.0
    separation (premature) O45.9- ☑
     specified NEC O45.8X- ☑
    vicious insertion O44.1- ☑
   precipitate labor O62.3
   premature rupture, membranes — *see also* Pregnancy, complicated by, premature rupture of membranes O42.90

Delivery — *continued*
 complicated — *continued*
  by — *continued*
   prolapse
    arm or hand O32.2 ☑
    cord (umbilical) O69.0 ☑
    foot or leg O32.8 ☑
    uterus O34.52- ☑
   prolonged labor O63.9
    first stage O63.0
    second stage O63.1
   protozoal disease (maternal) O98.62
   respiratory disease NEC O99.52
   retained membranes or portions of placenta O72.2
    without hemorrhage O73.1
   retarded birth O63.9
   retention of secundines (with hemorrhage) O72.0
    without hemorrhage O73.0
    partial O72.2
     without hemorrhage O73.1
   rupture
    bladder (urinary) O71.5
    cervix O71.3
    pelvic organ NEC O71.5
    urethra O71.5
    uterus (during or after labor) O71.1
     before labor O71.0- ☑
   separation, pubic bone (symphysis pubis) O71.6
   shock O75.1
   shoulder presentation O64.4 ☑
   skin disorder NEC O99.72
   spasm, cervix O62.4
   stenosis or stricture, cervix O65.5
   streptococcus group B (GBS) carrier state O99.824
   subluxation of symphysis (pubis) O26.72
   syphilis (maternal) O98.12
   tear — *see* Delivery, complicated by, laceration
   tetanic uterus O62.4
   trauma (obstetrical) — *see also* Delivery, complicated, by, damage to O71.9
    non-obstetric O9A.22 (*following* O99)
    periurethral O71.82
    specified NEC O71.89
   tuberculosis (maternal) O98.02
   tumor, pelvic organs or tissues NEC O65.5
   umbilical cord around neck
    with compression O69.1 ☑
    without compression O69.81 ☑
   uterine inertia O62.2
    during latent phase of labor O62.0
    primary O62.0
    secondary O62.1
   vasa previa O69.4 ☑
   velamentous insertion of cord O43.12- ☑
  specified complication NEC O75.89
  delayed NOS O63.9
   following rupture of membranes
    artificial O75.5
   second twin, triplet, etc. O63.2
  forceps, low following failed vacuum extraction O66.5
  missed (at or near term) O36.4 ☑
  normal O80
  obstructed — *see* Delivery, complicated by, obstructed labor
  precipitate O62.3
  preterm — *see also* Pregnancy, complicated by, preterm labor O60.10 ☑
  spontaneous O80
  term pregnancy NOS O80
  uncomplicated O80
  vaginal, following previous cesarean delivery O34.219
   classical (vertical) scar O34.212
   low transverse scar O34.211
   mid-transverse T incision O34.218
   scar
    defect (isthmocele) O34.22
    specified type NEC O34.218
Delusions (paranoid) — *see* Disorder, delusional
Dementia (degenerative (primary)) (persisting) (unspecified severity) (without behavioral disturbance, psychotic disturbance, mood disturbance, and anxiety) F03.90
 with
  aberrant motor behavior (exit-seeking) (pacing) (restlessness) (rocking) F03.911
  acute confusional state F05
  agitation F03.911
  anxiety F03.94

Dementia — *continued*
 with — *continued*
  behavioral disturbances (sexual disinhibition) (sleep disturbance) (social disinhibition) F03.918
   specified NEC F03.918
  Lewy bodies — *see also* Dementia, in, diseases specified elsewhere G31.83 *[F02.80]*
   with behavioral disturbance — *see also* Dementia, in, diseases specified elsewhere G31.83 *[F02.81-]* ☑
  mood disturbance (anhedonia) (apathy) (depression) F03.93
  Parkinsonism — *see also* Dementia, in, diseases specified elsewhere G20.C *[F02.80]*
   with behavioral disturbance –– *see also* Dementia, in, diseases specified elsewhere G20.C *[F02.81-]* ☑
  Parkinson's disease — *see also* Dementia, in, diseases specified elsewhere G20.A1 *[F02.80]*
   with behavioral disturbance –– *see also* Dementia, in, diseases specified elsewhere G20.A1 *[F02.81-]* ☑
  psychotic disturbance (delusional state) (hallucinations) (paranoia) (suspiciousness) F03.92
  verbal or physical behaviors (anger) (aggression) (combativeness) (profanity) (shouting) (threatening) (violence) F03.911
 alcoholic F10.97
  with dependence F10.27
 Alzheimer's type — *see* Disease, Alzheimer's
 arteriosclerotic — *see* Dementia, vascular
 atypical, Alzheimer's type — *see* Disease, Alzheimer's, specified NEC
 congenital — *see* Disability, intellectual
 frontal (lobe) — *see also* Dementia, in, diseases specified elsewhere G31.09 *[F02.80]*
  with behavioral disturbance — *see also* Dementia, in, diseases specified elsewhere G31.09 *[F02.81-]* ☑
 frontotemporal G31.09 *[F02.80]*
  with behavioral disturbance G31.09 *[F02.81]* ☑
  specified NEC — *see also* Dementia, in, diseases specified elsewhere G31.09 *[F02.80]*
   with behavioral disturbance — *see also* Dementia, in, diseases specified elsewhere G31.09 *[F02.81-]* ☑
 in (due to)
  alcohol F10.97
   with dependence F10.27
  Alzheimer's disease — *see* Disease, Alzheimer's
  arteriosclerotic brain disease — *see* Dementia, vascular
  cerebral lipidoses — *see also* Dementia, in, diseases specified elsewhere E75.- ☑ *[F02.80]*
   with behavioral disturbance — *see also* Dementia, in, diseases specified elsewhere E75.- ☑ *[F02.81-]* ☑
  Creutzfeldt-Jakob disease — *see also* Creutzfeldt-Jakob disease or syndrome (with dementia) A81.00
  diseases specified elsewhere (unspecified severity) (without behavioral disturbance, psychotic disturbance, mood disturbance, and anxiety) F02.80
   with
    aberrant motor behavior (exit-seeking) (pacing) (restlessness) (rocking) F02.811
    agitation F02.811
    anxiety F02.84
    behavioral disturbances (sexual disinhibition) (sleep disturbance) (social disinhibition) F02.818
     specified NEC F02.818
    mood disturbance (anhedonia) (apathy) (depression) F02.83
    psychotic disturbance (delusional state) (hallucinations) (paranoia) (suspiciousness) F02.82
    verbal or physical behaviors (anger) (aggression) (combativeness) (profanity) (shouting) (threatening) (violence) F02.811
   mild F02.A0
    with
     aberrant motor behavior (exit-seeking) (pacing) (restlessness) (rocking) F02.A11
     agitation F02.A11

☑ **Additional Character Required** — **Refer to the Tabular List for Character Selection**

Dementia — *continued*
  in — *continued*
    diseases specified elsewhere — *continued*
      mild — *continued*
        with — *continued*
          anxiety F02.A4
          behavioral disturbances (sexual disinhibition) (sleep disturbance) (social disinhibition) F02.A18
            specified NEC F02.A18
          mood disturbance (anhedonia) (apathy) (depression) F02.A3
          psychotic disturbance (delusional state) (hallucinations) (paranoia) (suspiciousness) F02.A2
          verbal or physical behaviors (anger) (aggression) (combativeness) (profanity) (shouting) (threatening) (violence) F02.A11
      moderate F02.B0
        with
          aberrant motor behavior (exit-seeking) (pacing) (restlessness) (rocking) F02.B11
          agitation F02.B11
          anxiety F02.B4
          behavioral disturbances (sexual disinhibition) (sleep disturbance) (social disinhibition) F02.B18
            specified NEC F02.B18
          mood disturbance (anhedonia) (apathy) (depression) F02.B3
          psychotic disturbance (delusional state) (hallucinations) (paranoia) (suspiciousness) F02.B2
          verbal or physical behaviors (anger) (aggression) (combativeness) (profanity) (shouting) (threatening) (violence) F02.B11
      severe F02.C0
        with
          aberrant motor behavior (exit-seeking) (pacing) (restlessness) (rocking) F02.C11
          agitation F02.C11
          anxiety F02.C4
          behavioral disturbances (sexual disinhibition) (sleep disturbance) (social disinhibition) F02.C18
            specified NEC F02.C18
          mood disturbance (anhedonia) (apathy) (depression) F02.C3
          psychotic disturbance (delusional state) (hallucinations) (paranoia) (suspiciousness) F02.C2
          verbal or physical behaviors (anger) (aggression) (combativeness) (profanity) (shouting) (threatening) (violence) F02.C11
    epilepsy — *see also* Dementia, in, diseases specified elsewhere G40.- ☑ *[F02.80]*
      with behavioral disturbance — *see also* Dementia, in, diseases specified elsewhere G40.- ☑ *[F02.81-]* ☑
    hepatolenticular degeneration — *see also* Dementia, in, diseases specified elsewhere E83.01 *[F02.80]*
      with behavioral disturbance — *see also* Dementia, in, diseases specified elsewhere E83.01 *[F02.81-]* ☑
    human immunodeficiency virus (HIV) disease — *see also* Dementia, in, diseases specified elsewhere B20 *[F02.80]*
      with behavioral disturbance — *see also* Dementia, in, diseases specified elsewhere B20 *[F02.81-]* ☑
    Huntington's disease or chorea — *see also* Dementia, in, diseases specified elsewhere G10 *[F02.80]*
      with behavioral disturbance — *see also* Dementia, in, diseases specified elsewhere G10 *[F02.81-]* ☑
    hypercalcemia — *see also* Dementia, in, diseases specified elsewhere E83.52 *[F02.80]*
      with behavioral disturbance — *see also* Dementia, in, diseases specified elsewhere E83.52 *[F02.81-]* ☑
    hypothyroidism, acquired — *see also* Dementia, in, diseases specified elsewhere E03.9 *[F02.80]*

Dementia — *continued*
  in — *continued*
    hypothyroidism, acquired — *see also* Dementia, in, diseases specified elsewhere — *continued*
      with behavioral disturbance — *see also* Dementia, in, diseases specified elsewhere E03.9 *[F02.81-]* ☑
      due to iodine deficiency — *see also* Dementia, in, diseases specified elsewhere E01.8 *[F02.80]*
        with behavioral disturbance — *see also* Dementia, in, diseases specified elsewhere E01.8 *[F02.81-]* ☑
    inhalants F18.97
      with dependence F18.27
    multiple
      etiologies F03 ☑
      sclerosis — *see also* Dementia, in, diseases specified elsewhere G35 *[F02.80]*
        with behavioral disturbance — *see also* Dementia, in, diseases specified elsewhere G35 *[F02.81-]* ☑
    neurosyphilis — *see also* Dementia, in, diseases specified elsewhere A52.17 *[F02.80]*
      with behavioral disturbance — *see also* Dementia, in, diseases specified elsewhere A52.17 *[F02.81-]* ☑
      juvenile — *see also* Dementia, in, diseases specified elsewhere A50.49 *[F02.80]*
        with behavioral disturbance — *see also* Dementia, in, diseases specified elsewhere A50.49 *[F02.81-]* ☑
    niacin deficiency — *see also* Dementia, in, diseases specified elsewhere E52 *[F02.80]*
      with behavioral disturbance — *see also* Dementia, in, diseases specified elsewhere E52 *[F02.81-]* ☑
    paralysis agitans — *see also* Dementia, in, diseases specified elsewhere G20.C *[F02.80]*
      with behavioral disturbance — *see also* Dementia, in, diseases specified elsewhere G20.C *[F02.81-]* ☑
    Parkinson's disease — *see also* Dementia, in, diseases specified elsewhere G20.A1 *[F02.80]*
    pellagra — *see also* Dementia, in, diseases specified elsewhere E52 *[F02.80]*
      with behavioral disturbance — *see also* Dementia, in, diseases specified elsewhere E52 *[F02.81-]* ☑
    Pick's — *see also* Dementia, in, diseases specified elsewhere G31.01 *[F02.80]*
      with behavioral disturbance — *see also* Dementia, in, diseases specified elsewhere G31.01 *[F02.81-]* ☑
    polyarteritis nodosa — *see also* Dementia, in, diseases specified elsewhere M30.0 *[F02.80]*
      with behavioral disturbance — *see also* Dementia, in, diseases specified elsewhere M30.0 *[F02.81-]* ☑
    psychoactive drug F19.97
      with dependence F19.27
      inhalants F18.97
        with dependence F18.27
      sedatives, hypnotics or anxiolytics F13.97
        with dependence F13.27
    sedatives, hypnotics or anxiolytics F13.97
      with dependence F13.27
    systemic lupus erythematosus — *see also* Dementia, in, diseases specified elsewhere M32.- ☑ *[F02.80]*
      with behavioral disturbance — *see also* Dementia, in, diseases specified elsewhere M32.- ☑ *[F02.81-]* ☑
    trypanosomiasis
      African — *see also* Dementia, in, diseases specified elsewhere B56.9 *[F02.80]*
        with behavioral disturbance — *see also* Dementia, in, diseases specified elsewhere B56.9 *[F02.81-]* ☑
    unknown etiology F03.- ☑
    vitamin B12 deficiency — *see also* Dementia, in, diseases specified elsewhere E53.8 *[F02.80]*
      with behavioral disturbance — *see also* Dementia, in, diseases specified elsewhere E53.8 *[F02.81-]* ☑
    volatile solvents F18.97
      with dependence F18.27
  infantile, infantilis F84.3

Dementia — *continued*
  Lewy body — *see also* Dementia, in, diseases specified elsewhere G31.83 *[F02.80]*
    with behavioral disturbance — *see also* Dementia, in, diseases specified elsewhere G31.83 *[F02.81-]* ☑
    mild F03.A0
      with
        aberrant motor behavior (exit-seeking) (pacing) (restlessness) (rocking) F03.A11
        agitation F03.A11
        anxiety F03.A4
        behavioral disturbances (sexual disinhibition) (sleep disturbance) (social disinhibition) F03.A18
          specified NEC F03.A18
        mood disturbance (anhedonia) (apathy) (depression) F03.A3
        psychotic disturbance (delusional state) (hallucinations) (paranoia) (suspiciousness) F03.A2
        verbal or physical behaviors (anger) (aggression) (combativeness) (profanity) (shouting) (threatening) (violence) F03.A11
    moderate F03.B0
      with
        aberrant motor behavior (exit-seeking) (pacing) (restlessness) (rocking) F03.B11
        agitation F03.B11
        anxiety F03.B4
        behavioral disturbances (sexual disinhibition) (sleep disturbance) (social disinhibition) F03.B18
          specified NEC F03.B18
        mood disturbance (anhedonia) (apathy) (depression) F03.B3
        psychotic disturbance (delusional state) (hallucinations) (paranoia) (suspiciousness) F03.B2
        verbal or physical behaviors (anger) (aggression) (combativeness) (profanity) (shouting) (threatening) (violence) F03.B11
  multi-infarct — *see* Dementia, vascular
  old age (senile) F03 ☑
    Alzheimer's type — *see* Disease, Alzheimer's, late onset
  paralytica, paralytic (syphilitic) — *see also* Dementia, in, diseases specified elsewhere A52.17 *[F02.80]*
    with behavioral disturbance — *see also* Dementia, in, diseases specified elsewhere A52.17 *[F02.81-]* ☑
    juvenilis A50.45
  paretic A52.17
  praecox — *see* Schizophrenia
  presenile F03 ☑
    Alzheimer's type — *see* Disease, Alzheimer's, early onset
  primary degenerative F03 ☑
  progressive, syphilitic A52.17
  senile F03 ☑
    Alzheimer's type — *see* Disease, Alzheimer's, late onset
    depressed or paranoid type F03 ☑
  severe F03.C0
    with
      aberrant motor behavior (exit-seeking) (pacing) (restlessness) (rocking) F03.C11
      agitation F03.C11
      anxiety F03.C4
      behavioral disturbances (sexual disinhibition) (sleep disturbance) (social disinhibition) F03.C18
        specified NEC F03.C18
      mood disturbance (anhedonia) (apathy) (depression) F03.C3
      psychotic disturbance (delusional state) (hallucinations) (paranoia) (suspiciousness) F03.C2
      verbal or physical behaviors (anger) (aggression) (combativeness) (profanity) (shouting) (threatening) (violence) F03.C11
  vascular (acute onset) (mixed) (multi-infarct) (subcortical) (unspecified severity) (without behavioral disturbance, psychotic disturbance, mood disturbance, and anxiety) F01.50
    with
      aberrant motor behavior (exit-seeking) (pacing) (restlessness) (rocking) F01.511
      agitation F01.511
      anxiety F01.54

☑ **Additional Character Required** — **Refer to the Tabular List for Character Selection**

Dementia — *continued*
- vascular — *continued*
  - with — *continued*
    - behavioral disturbances (sleep disturbance) (sexual disinhibition) (social disinhibition) F01.518
      - specified NEC F01.518
    - mood disturbance (anhedonia) (apathy) (depression) F01.53
    - psychotic disturbance (delusional state) (hallucinations) (paranoia) (suspiciousness) F01.52
    - verbal or physical behaviors (anger) (aggression) (combativeness) (profanity) (shouting) (threatening) (violence) F01.511
  - mild F01.A0
    - with
      - aberrant motor behavior (exit-seeking) (pacing) (restlessness) (rocking) F01.A11
      - agitation F01.A11
      - anxiety F01.A4
      - behavioral disturbances (sleep disturbance) (sexual disinhibition) (social disinhibition) F01.A18
        - specified NEC F01.A18
      - mood disturbance (anhedonia) (apathy) (depression) F01.A3
      - psychotic disturbance (delusional state) (hallucinations) (paranoia) (suspiciousness) F01.A2
      - verbal or physical behaviors (anger) (aggression) (combativeness) (profanity) (shouting) (threatening) (violence) F01.A11
  - moderate F01.B0
    - with
      - aberrant motor behavior (exit-seeking) (pacing) (restlessness) (rocking) F01.B11
      - agitation F01.B11
      - anxiety F01.B4
      - behavioral disturbances (sleep disturbance) (sexual disinhibition) (social disinhibition) F01.B18
        - specified NEC F01.B18
      - mood disturbance (anhedonia) (apathy) (depression) F01.B3
      - psychotic disturbance (delusional state) (hallucinations) (paranoia) (suspiciousness) F01.B2
      - verbal or physical behaviors (anger) (aggression) (combativeness) (profanity) (shouting) (threatening) (violence) F01.B11
  - severe F01.C0
    - with
      - aberrant motor behavior (exit-seeking) (pacing) (restlessness) (rocking) F01.C11
      - agitation F01.C11
      - anxiety F01.C4
      - behavioral disturbances (sleep disturbance) (sexual disinhibition) (social disinhibition) F01.C18
        - specified NEC F01.C18
      - mood disturbance (anhedonia) (apathy) (depression) F01.C3
      - psychotic disturbance (delusional state) (hallucinations) (paranoia) (suspiciousness) F01.C2
      - verbal or physical behaviors (anger) (aggression) (combativeness) (profanity) (shouting) (threatening) (violence) F01.C11

Demineralization, bone — *see* Osteoporosis
Demodex folliculorum (infestation) B88.0
Demophobia F40.248
Demoralization R45.3
Demyelination, demyelinization
- central nervous system G37.9
  - specified NEC G37.89
- corpus callosum (central) G37.1
- disseminated, acute G36.9
  - specified NEC G36.8
- global G35
- in optic neuritis G36.0

Dengue (classical) (fever) A90
- hemorrhagic A91
- sandfly A93.1

Dennie-Marfan syphilitic syndrome A50.45
Dens evaginatus, in dente or invaginatus K00.2
Dense breasts — *see also* Density, breast R92.30

Density R92.30
- breast R92.30
  - mammographic
    - extreme R92.34- ☑
    - fatty tissue R92.31- ☑
    - fibroglandular R92.32- ☑
    - heterogeneous R92.33- ☑
- increased, bone (disseminated) (generalized) (spotted) — *see* Disorder, bone, density and structure, specified type NEC
- low R92.30
- lung (nodular) J98.4

Dental — *see also* condition
- examination Z01.20
  - with abnormal findings Z01.21
- restoration
  - aesthetically inadequate or displeasing K08.56
  - defective K08.50
    - specified NEC K08.59
  - failure of marginal integrity K08.51
  - failure of periodontal anatomical integrity K08.54

Dentia praecox K00.6
Denticles (pulp) K04.2
Dentigerous cyst K09.0
Dentin
- irregular (in pulp) K04.3
- opalescent K00.5
- secondary (in pulp) K04.3
- sensitive K03.89

Dentinogenesis imperfecta K00.5
Dentinoma — *see* Cyst, calcifying odontogenic
Dentition (syndrome) K00.7
- delayed K00.6
- difficult K00.7
- precocious K00.6
- premature K00.6
- retarded K00.6

Dependence (on) (syndrome) F19.20
- with remission F19.21
- alcohol (ethyl) (methyl) (without remission) F10.20
  - with
    - amnestic disorder, persisting F10.26
    - anxiety disorder F10.280
    - dementia, persisting F10.27
    - intoxication F10.229
      - with delirium F10.221
      - uncomplicated F10.220
    - mood disorder F10.24
    - psychotic disorder F10.259
      - with
        - delusions F10.250
        - hallucinations F10.251
    - remission F10.21
    - sexual dysfunction F10.281
    - sleep disorder F10.282
    - specified disorder NEC F10.288
    - withdrawal F10.239
      - with
        - delirium F10.231
        - perceptual disturbance F10.232
      - uncomplicated F10.230
  - counseling and surveillance Z71.41
  - in remission F10.21
- amobarbital — *see* Dependence, drug, sedative
- amphetamine(s) (type) — *see* Dependence, drug, stimulant NEC
- amytal (sodium) — *see* Dependence, drug, sedative
- analgesic NEC F55.8
- anesthetic (agent) (gas) (general) (local) NEC — *see* Dependence, drug, psychoactive NEC
- anxiolytic NEC — *see* Dependence, drug, sedative
- barbital(s) — *see* Dependence, drug, sedative
- barbiturate(s) (compounds) (drugs classifiable to T42) — *see* Dependence, drug, sedative
- benzedrine — *see* Dependence, drug, stimulant NEC
- bhang — *see* Dependence, drug, cannabis
- bromide(s) NEC — *see* Dependence, drug, sedative
- caffeine — *see* Dependence, drug, stimulant NEC
- cannabis (sativa) (indica) (resin) (derivatives) (type) — *see* Dependence, drug, cannabis
- chloral (betaine) (hydrate) — *see* Dependence, drug, sedative
- chlordiazepoxide — *see* Dependence, drug, sedative
- coca (leaf) (derivatives) — *see* Dependence, drug, cocaine
- cocaine — *see* Dependence, drug, cocaine
- codeine — *see* Dependence, drug, opioid
- combinations of drugs F19.20
- dagga — *see* Dependence, drug, cannabis
- demerol — *see* Dependence, drug, opioid

Dependence — *continued*
- dexamphetamine — *see* Dependence, drug, stimulant NEC
- dexedrine — *see* Dependence, drug, stimulant NEC
- dextromethorphan — *see* Dependence, drug, opioid
- dextromoramide — *see* Dependence, drug, opioid
- dextro-nor-pseudo-ephedrine — *see* Dependence, drug, stimulant NEC
- dextrorphan — *see* Dependence, drug, opioid
- diazepam — *see* Dependence, drug, sedative
- dilaudid — *see* Dependence, drug, opioid
- D-lysergic acid diethylamide — *see* Dependence, drug, hallucinogen
- drug NEC F19.20
  - with sleep disorder F19.282
  - cannabis F12.20
    - with
      - anxiety disorder F12.280
      - intoxication F12.229
        - with
          - delirium F12.221
          - perceptual disturbance F12.222
        - uncomplicated F12.220
      - other specified disorder F12.288
      - psychosis F12.259
        - delusions F12.250
        - hallucinations F12.251
      - unspecified disorder F12.29
      - withdrawal F12.23
    - in remission F12.21
  - cocaine F14.20
    - with
      - anxiety disorder F14.280
      - intoxication F14.229
        - with
          - delirium F14.221
          - perceptual disturbance F14.222
        - uncomplicated F14.220
      - mood disorder F14.24
      - other specified disorder F14.288
      - psychosis F14.259
        - delusions F14.250
        - hallucinations F14.251
      - sexual dysfunction F14.281
      - sleep disorder F14.282
      - unspecified disorder F14.29
      - withdrawal F14.23
    - in remission F14.21
    - withdrawal symptoms in newborn P96.1
  - counseling and surveillance Z71.51
  - hallucinogen F16.20
    - with
      - anxiety disorder F16.280
      - flashbacks F16.283
      - intoxication F16.229
        - with delirium F16.221
        - uncomplicated F16.220
      - mood disorder F16.24
      - other specified disorder F16.288
      - perception disorder, persisting F16.283
      - psychosis F16.259
        - delusions F16.250
        - hallucinations F16.251
      - unspecified disorder F16.29
    - in remission F16.21
  - in remission F19.21
  - inhalant F18.20
    - with
      - anxiety disorder F18.280
      - dementia, persisting F18.27
      - intoxication F18.229
        - with delirium F18.221
        - uncomplicated F18.220
      - mood disorder F18.24
      - other specified disorder F18.288
      - psychosis F18.259
        - delusions F18.250
        - hallucinations F18.251
      - unspecified disorder F18.29
    - in remission F18.21
  - nicotine F17.200
    - with disorder F17.209
      - in remission F17.201
      - specified disorder NEC F17.208
      - withdrawal F17.203
    - chewing tobacco F17.220
      - with disorder F17.229
        - in remission F17.221
        - specified disorder NEC F17.228

☑ **Additional Character Required — Refer to the Tabular List for Character Selection**

Dependence — *continued*
  drug — *continued*
    nicotine — *continued*
      chewing tobacco — *continued*
        with disorder — *continued*
          withdrawal F17.223
      cigarettes F17.210
        with disorder F17.219
          in remission F17.211
          specified disorder NEC F17.218
          withdrawal F17.213
      specified product NEC F17.290
        with disorder F17.299
          remission F17.291
          specified disorder NEC F17.298
          withdrawal F17.293
    opioid F11.20
      with
        intoxication F11.229
          with
            delirium F11.221
            perceptual disturbance F11.222
          uncomplicated F11.220
        mood disorder F11.24
        opioid-associated amnestic syndrome F11.288
        other specified disorder F11.288
        psychosis F11.259
          delusions F11.250
          hallucinations F11.251
        sexual dysfunction F11.281
        sleep disorder F11.282
        unspecified disorder F11.29
        withdrawal F11.23
      in remission F11.21
    psychoactive NEC F19.20
      with
        amnestic disorder F19.26
        anxiety disorder F19.280
        dementia F19.27
        intoxication F19.229
          with
            delirium F19.221
            perceptual disturbance F19.222
          uncomplicated F19.220
        mood disorder F19.24
        other specified disorder F19.288
        psychosis F19.259
          delusions F19.250
          hallucinations F19.251
        sexual dysfunction F19.281
        sleep disorder F19.282
        unspecified disorder F19.29
        withdrawal F19.239
          with
            delirium F19.231
            perceptual disturbance F19.232
          uncomplicated F19.230
      in remission F19.21
    sedative, hypnotic or anxiolytic F13.20
      with
        amnestic disorder F13.26
        anxiety disorder F13.280
        dementia, persisting F13.27
        intoxication F13.229
          with delirium F13.221
          uncomplicated F13.220
        mood disorder F13.24
        other specified disorder F13.288
        psychosis F13.259
          delusions F13.250
          hallucinations F13.251
        sexual dysfunction F13.281
        sleep disorder F13.282
        unspecified disorder F13.29
        withdrawal F13.239
          with
            delirium F13.231
            perceptual disturbance F13.232
          uncomplicated F13.230
      in remission F13.21
    stimulant NEC F15.20
      with
        anxiety disorder F15.280
        intoxication F15.229
          with
            delirium F15.221
            perceptual disturbance F15.222
          uncomplicated F15.220
        mood disorder F15.24

Dependence — *continued*
  drug — *continued*
    stimulant — *continued*
      with — *continued*
        other specified disorder F15.288
        psychosis F15.259
          delusions F15.250
          hallucinations F15.251
        sexual dysfunction F15.281
        sleep disorder F15.282
        unspecified disorder F15.29
        withdrawal F15.23
      in remission F15.21
    ethyl
      alcohol (without remission) F10.20
        with remission F10.21
      bromide — *see* Dependence, drug, sedative
      carbamate F19.20
      chloride F19.20
      morphine — *see* Dependence, drug, opioid
    ganja — *see* Dependence, drug, cannabis
    glue (airplane) (sniffing) — *see* Dependence, drug, inhalant
    glutethimide — *see* Dependence, drug, sedative
    hallucinogenics — *see* Dependence, drug, hallucinogen
    hashish — *see* Dependence, drug, cannabis
    hemp — *see* Dependence, drug, cannabis
    heroin (salt) (any) — *see* Dependence, drug, opioid
    hypnotic NEC — *see* Dependence, drug, sedative
    Indian hemp — *see* Dependence, drug, cannabis
    inhalants — *see* Dependence, drug, inhalant
    khat — *see* Dependence, drug, stimulant NEC
    laudanum — *see* Dependence, drug, opioid
    LSD (-25) (derivatives) — *see* Dependence, drug, hallucinogen
    luminal — *see* Dependence, drug, sedative
    lysergic acid — *see* Dependence, drug, hallucinogen
    maconha — *see* Dependence, drug, cannabis
    marihuana — *see* Dependence, drug, cannabis
    meprobamate — *see* Dependence, drug, sedative
    mescaline — *see* Dependence, drug, hallucinogen
    methadone — *see* Dependence, drug, opioid
    methamphetamine(s) — *see* Dependence, drug, stimulant NEC
    methaqualone — *see* Dependence, drug, sedative
    methyl
      alcohol (without remission) F10.20
        with remission F10.21
      bromide — *see* Dependence, drug, sedative
      morphine — *see* Dependence, drug, opioid
      phenidate — *see* Dependence, drug, stimulant NEC
      sulfonal — *see* Dependence, drug, sedative
    morphine (sulfate) (sulfite) (type) — *see* Dependence, drug, opioid
    narcotic (drug) NEC — *see* Dependence, drug, opioid
    nembutal — *see* Dependence, drug, sedative
    neraval — *see* Dependence, drug, sedative
    neravan — *see* Dependence, drug, sedative
    neurobarb — *see* Dependence, drug, sedative
    nicotine — *see* Dependence, drug, nicotine
    nitrous oxide F19.20
    nonbarbiturate sedatives and tranquilizers with similar effect — *see* Dependence, drug, sedative
  on
    artificial heart (fully implantable) (mechanical) Z95.812
    aspirator Z99.0
    care provider (because of) Z74.9
      impaired mobility Z74.09
      need for
        assistance with personal care Z74.1
        continuous supervision Z74.3
      no other household member able to render care Z74.2
      specified reason NEC Z74.8
    machine Z99.89
      enabling NEC Z99.89
      specified type NEC Z99.89
    renal dialysis (hemodialysis) (peritoneal) Z99.2
    respirator Z99.11
    ventilator Z99.11
    wheelchair Z99.3
  opiate — *see* Dependence, drug, opioid
  opioids — *see* Dependence, drug, opioid
  opium (alkaloids) (derivatives) (tincture) — *see* Dependence, drug, opioid
  oxygen (long-term) (supplemental) Z99.81
  paraldehyde — *see* Dependence, drug, sedative
  paregoric — *see* Dependence, drug, opioid

Dependence — *continued*
  PCP (phencyclidine) (or related substance) — *see* Dependence, drug, hallucinogen
  pentobarbital — *see* Dependence, drug, sedative
  pentobarbitone (sodium) — *see* Dependence, drug, sedative
  pentothal — *see* Dependence, drug, sedative
  peyote — *see* Dependence, drug, hallucinogen
  phencyclidine (PCP) (or related substance) — *see* Dependence, drug, hallucinogen
  phenmetrazine — *see* Dependence, drug, stimulant NEC
  phenobarbital — *see* Dependence, drug, sedative
  polysubstance F19.20
  psilocibin, psilocin, psilocyn, psilocyline — *see* Dependence, drug, hallucinogen
  psychostimulant NEC — *see* Dependence, drug, stimulant NEC
  secobarbital — *see* Dependence, drug, sedative
  seconal — *see* Dependence, drug, sedative
  sedative NEC — *see* Dependence, drug, sedative
  specified drug NEC — *see* Dependence, drug
  stimulant NEC — *see* Dependence, drug, stimulant NEC
  substance NEC — *see* Dependence, drug
  supplemental oxygen Z99.81
  tobacco — *see* Dependence, drug, nicotine
    counseling and surveillance Z71.6
  tranquilizer NEC — *see* Dependence, drug, sedative
  vitamin B6 E53.1
  volatile solvents — *see* Dependence, drug, inhalant

Dependency
  care-provider Z74.9
  passive F60.7
  reactions (persistent) F60.7

Depersonalization (in neurotic state) (neurotic) (syndrome) F48.1

Depletion
  extracellular fluid E86.9
  plasma E86.1
  potassium E87.6
    nephropathy N25.89
  salt or sodium E87.1
    causing heat exhaustion or prostration T67.4 ☑
    nephropathy N28.9
  volume NOS E86.9

Deployment (current) (military) status Z56.82
  in theater or in support of military war, peacekeeping and humanitarian operations Z56.82
  personal history of Z91.82
    military war, peacekeeping and humanitarian deployment (current or past conflict) Z91.82
  returned from Z91.82

Depolarization, premature I49.40
  atrial I49.1
  junctional I49.2
  specified NEC I49.49
  ventricular I49.3

Deposit
  bone in Boeck's sarcoid D86.89
  calcareous, calcium — *see* Calcification
  cholesterol
    retina H35.89
    vitreous (body) (humor) — *see* Deposit, crystalline
  conjunctiva H11.11- ☑
  cornea H18.00- ☑
    argentous H18.02- ☑
    due to metabolic disorder H18.03- ☑
    Kayser-Fleischer ring H18.04- ☑
    pigmentation — *see* Pigmentation, cornea
  crystalline, vitreous (body) (humor) H43.2- ☑
  hemosiderin in old scars of cornea — *see* Pigmentation, cornea, stromal
  metallic in lens — *see* Cataract, specified NEC
  skin R23.8
  tooth, teeth (betel) (black) (green) (materia alba) (orange) (tobacco) K03.6
  urate, kidney — *see* Calculus, kidney

Depraved appetite — *see* Pica

Depressed
  HDL cholesterol E78.6

Depression (acute) (mental) F32.A
  agitated (single episode) F32.2
  anaclitic — *see* Disorder, adjustment
  anxiety F41.8
    persistent F34.1
  arches — *see also* Deformity, limb, flat foot
  atypical (single episode) F32.89
    recurrent episode F33.9
  basal metabolic rate R94.8

Depression — *continued*
bone marrow D75.89
central nervous system G98.8
cerebral R29.818
newborn P91.4
cerebrovascular I67.9
chest wall M95.4
climacteric (single episode) F32.89
recurrent episode F33.8
endogenous (without psychotic symptoms) F33.2
with psychotic symptoms F33.3
functional activity R68.89
hysterical F44.89
involutional (single episode) F32.89
recurrent episode F33.8
major F32.9
with psychotic symptoms F32.3
recurrent — *see* Disorder, depressive, recurrent
manic-depressive — *see* Disorder, depressive, recurrent
masked (single episode) F32.89
medullary G93.89
menopausal (single episode) F32.89
recurrent episode F33.8
metatarsus — *see* Depression, arches
monopolar F33.9
nervous F34.1
neurotic F34.1
nose M95.0
postnatal (NOS) F53.0
postpartum (NOS) F53.0
post-psychotic of schizophrenia F32.89
post-schizophrenic F32.89
psychogenic (reactive) (single episode) F32.9
psychoneurotic F34.1
psychotic (single episode) F32.3
recurrent F33.3
reactive (psychogenic) (single episode) F32.9
psychotic (single episode) F32.3
recurrent — *see* Disorder, depressive, recurrent
respiratory center G93.89
seasonal — *see* Disorder, depressive, recurrent
senile F03 ☑
severe, single episode F32.2
situational F43.21
skull Q67.4
specified NEC (single episode) F32.89
sternum M95.4
visual field — *see* Defect, visual field
vital (recurrent) (without psychotic symptoms) F33.2
with psychotic symptoms F33.3
single episode F32.2
Deprivation
cultural Z60.3
effects NOS T73.9 ☑
specified NEC T73.8 ☑
emotional NEC Z65.8
affecting infant or child — *see* Maltreatment, child, psychological
food T73.0 ☑
material due to limited financial resources, specified NEC Z59.87
protein — *see* Malnutrition
sleep Z72.820
social Z60.4
affecting infant or child — *see* Maltreatment, child, psychological
specified NEC T73.8 ☑
vitamins — *see* Deficiency, vitamin
water T73.1 ☑
Derangement
ankle (internal) — *see* Derangement, joint, articular cartilage, ankle
cartilage (articular) NEC — *see* Derangement, joint, articular cartilage, by site
recurrent — *see* Dislocation, recurrent
cruciate ligament, anterior, current injury — *see* Sprain, knee, cruciate, anterior
elbow (internal) — *see* Derangement, joint, articular cartilage, elbow
hip (joint) (internal) (old) — *see* Derangement, joint, articular cartilage, hip
joint (internal) M24.9
ankylosis — *see* Ankylosis
articular cartilage M24.10
ankle M24.17- ☑
elbow M24.12- ☑
foot M24.17- ☑
hand M24.14- ☑

Derangement — *continued*
joint — *continued*
articular cartilage — *continued*
hip M24.15- ☑
knee NEC M23.9- ☑
loose body — *see* Loose, body
shoulder M24.11- ☑
specified site NEC M24.19
wrist M24.13- ☑
contracture — *see* Contraction, joint
current injury — *see also* Dislocation
knee, meniscus or cartilage — *see* Tear, meniscus
dislocation
pathological — *see* Dislocation, pathological
recurrent — *see* Dislocation, recurrent
knee — *see* Derangement, knee
ligament — *see* Disorder, ligament
loose body — *see* Loose, body
recurrent — *see* Dislocation, recurrent
specified type NEC M24.80
ankle M24.87- ☑
elbow M24.82- ☑
foot joint M24.87- ☑
hand joint M24.84- ☑
hip M24.85- ☑
shoulder M24.81- ☑
specified site NEC M24.89
wrist M24.83- ☑
temporomandibular M26.69
knee (recurrent) M23.9- ☑
ligament disruption, spontaneous M23.60- ☑
anterior cruciate M23.61- ☑
capsular M23.67- ☑
instability, chronic M23.5- ☑
lateral collateral M23.64- ☑
medial collateral M23.63- ☑
posterior cruciate M23.62- ☑
loose body M23.4- ☑
meniscus M23.30- ☑
cystic M23.00- ☑
lateral M23.002
anterior horn M23.04- ☑
posterior horn M23.05- ☑
specified NEC M23.06- ☑
medial M23.005
anterior horn M23.01- ☑
posterior horn M23.02- ☑
specified NEC M23.03- ☑
degenerate — *see* Derangement, knee, meniscus, specified NEC
detached — *see* Derangement, knee, meniscus, specified NEC
due to old tear or injury M23.20- ☑
lateral M23.20- ☑
anterior horn M23.24- ☑
posterior horn M23.25- ☑
specified NEC M23.26- ☑
medial M23.20- ☑
anterior horn M23.21- ☑
posterior horn M23.22- ☑
specified NEC M23.23- ☑
retained — *see* Derangement, knee, meniscus, specified NEC
specified NEC M23.30- ☑
lateral M23.30- ☑
anterior horn M23.34- ☑
posterior horn M23.35- ☑
specified NEC M23.36- ☑
medial M23.30- ☑
anterior horn M23.31- ☑
posterior horn M23.32- ☑
specified NEC M23.33- ☑
old M23.8X- ☑
specified NEC — *see* subcategory M23.8 ☑
low back NEC — *see* Dorsopathy, specified NEC
meniscus — *see* Derangement, knee, meniscus
mental — *see* Psychosis
patella, specified NEC — *see* Disorder, patella, derangement NEC
semilunar cartilage (knee) — *see* Derangement, knee, meniscus, specified NEC
shoulder (internal) — *see* Derangement, joint, shoulder
Dercum's disease E88.2
Derealization (neurotic) F48.1
Dermal — *see* condition
Dermaphytid — *see* Dermatophytosis

Dermatitis (eczematous) L30.9
ab igne L59.0
acarine B88.0
actinic (due to sun) L57.8
other than from sun L59.8
allergic — *see* Dermatitis, contact, allergic
ambustionis, due to burn or scald — *see* Burn
amebic A06.7
ammonia L22
arsenical (ingested) L27.8
artefacta L98.1
psychogenic F54
atopic L20.9
psychogenic F54
specified NEC L20.89
autoimmune progesterone L30.8
berlock, berloque L56.2
blastomycotic B40.3
blister beetle L24.89
bullous, bullosa L13.9
mucosynechial, atrophic L12.1
seasonal L30.8
specified NEC L13.8
calorica L59.0
due to burn or scald — *see* Burn
caterpillar L24.89
cercarial B65.3
combustionis L59.0
due to burn or scald — *see* Burn
congelationis T69.1 ☑
contact (occupational) L25.9
allergic L23.9
due to
adhesives L23.1
cement L23.5
chemical products NEC L23.5
chromium L23.0
cosmetics L23.2
dander (cat) (dog) L23.81
drugs in contact with skin L23.3
dyes L23.4
food in contact with skin L23.6
hair (cat) (dog) L23.81
insecticide L23.5
metals L23.0
nickel L23.0
plants, non-food L23.7
plastic L23.5
rubber L23.5
specified agent NEC L23.89
due to
cement L25.3
chemical products NEC L25.3
cosmetics L25.0
dander (cat) (dog) L23.81
drugs in contact with skin L25.1
dyes L25.2
food in contact with skin L25.4
hair (cat) (dog) L23.81
plants, non-food L25.5
specified agent NEC L25.8
irritant L24.9
due to
body fluids L24.A0
feces L24.A2
incontinence (dual) (fecal) (urinary) L24.A2
saliva L24.A1
specified NEC L24.A9
urine L24.A2
wound exudate L24.A9
cement L24.5
chemical products NEC L24.5
cosmetics L24.3
detergents L24.0
drugs in contact with skin L24.4
exudate L24.A9
food in contact with skin L24.6
friction L24.A0
oils and greases L24.1
plants, non-food L24.7
solvents L24.2
specified agent NEC L24.89
related to
colostomy L24.B3
endotracheal tube L24.A9
enterocutaneous fistula L24.B3
gastrostomy L24.B1
ileostomy L24.B3
jejunostomy L24.B1

Dermatitis — *continued*
 contact — *continued*
  irritant — *continued*
   related to — *continued*
    saliva or spit fistula L24.B1
    stoma or fistula L24.B0
     digestive L24.B1
     fecal or urinary L24.B3
     respiratory L24.B2
     tracheostomy L24.B2
 contusiformis L52
 desquamative L30.8
 diabetic — *see* E08-E13 with .620
 diaper L22
 diphtheritica A36.3
 dry skin L85.3
 due to
  acetone (contact) (irritant) L24.2
  acids (contact) (irritant) L24.5
  adhesive(s) (allergic) (contact) (plaster) L23.1
   irritant L24.5
  alcohol (irritant) (skin contact) (substances in category T51) L24.2
   taken internally L27.8
  alkalis (contact) (irritant) L24.5
  arsenic (ingested) L27.8
  carbon disulfide (contact) (irritant) L24.2
  caustics (contact) (irritant) L24.5
  cement (contact) L25.3
  cereal (ingested) L27.2
  chemical(s) NEC L25.3
   taken internally L27.8
  chlorocompounds L24.2
  chromium (contact) (irritant) L24.81
  coffee (ingested) L27.2
  cold weather L30.8
  cosmetics (contact) L25.0
   allergic L23.2
   irritant L24.3
  cyclohexanes L24.2
  dander (cat) (dog) L23.81
  Demodex species B88.0
  Dermanyssus gallinae B88.0
  detergents (contact) (irritant) L24.0
  dichromate L24.81
  drugs and medicaments (generalized) (internal use) L27.0
   external — *see* Dermatitis, due to, drugs, in contact with skin
   in contact with skin L25.1
    allergic L23.3
    irritant L24.4
   localized skin eruption L27.1
   specified substance — *see* Table of Drugs and Chemicals
  dyes (contact) L25.2
   allergic L23.4
   irritant L24.89
  epidermophytosis — *see* Dermatophytosis
  esters L24.2
  external irritant NEC L24.9
  exudate (wound fluids) L24.A9
  fish (ingested) L27.2
  flour (ingested) L27.2
  food (ingested) L27.2
   in contact with skin L25.4
  fruit (ingested) L27.2
  furs (allergic) (contact) L23.81
  glues — *see* Dermatitis, due to, adhesives
  glycols L24.2
  greases NEC (contact) (irritant) L24.1
  hair (cat) (dog) L23.81
  hot
   objects and materials — *see* Burn
   weather or places L59.0
  hydrocarbons L24.2
  infrared rays L59.8
  ingestion, ingested substance L27.9
   chemical NEC L27.8
   drugs and medicaments — *see* Dermatitis, due to, drugs
   food L27.2
   specified NEC L27.8
  insecticide in contact with skin L24.5
  internal agent L27.9
   drugs and medicaments (generalized) — *see* Dermatitis, due to, drugs
   food L27.2

Dermatitis — *continued*
 due to — *continued*
  irradiation — *see* Dermatitis, due to, radioactive substance
  ketones L24.2
  lacquer tree (allergic) (contact) L23.7
  light (sun) NEC L57.8
   acute L56.8
   other L59.8
  Liponyssoides sanguineus B88.0
  low temperature L30.8
  meat (ingested) L27.2
  metals, metal salts (contact) (irritant) L24.81
  milk (ingested) L27.2
  nickel (contact) (irritant) L24.81
  nylon (contact) (irritant) L24.5
  oils NEC (contact) (irritant) L24.1
  paint solvent (contact) (irritant) L24.2
  petroleum products (contact) (irritant) (substances in T52.0) L24.2
  plants NEC (contact) L25.5
   allergic L23.7
   irritant L24.7
  plasters (adhesive) (any) (allergic) (contact) L23.1
   irritant L24.5
  plastic (contact) L25.3
  preservatives (contact) — *see* Dermatitis, due to, chemical, in contact with skin
  primrose (allergic) (contact) L23.7
  primula (allergic) (contact) L23.7
  radiation L59.8
   nonionizing (chronic exposure) L57.8
   sun NEC L57.8
    acute L56.8
  radioactive substance L58.9
   acute L58.0
   chronic L58.1
  radium L58.9
   acute L58.0
   chronic L58.1
  ragweed (allergic) (contact) L23.7
  Rhus (allergic) (contact) (diversiloba) (radicans) (toxicodendron) (venenata) (verniciflua) L23.7
  rubber (contact) L24.5
  Senecio jacobaea (allergic) (contact) L23.7
  solvents (contact) (irritant) (substances in category T52) L24.2
  specified agent NEC (contact) L25.8
   allergic L23.89
   irritant L24.89
  sunshine NEC L57.8
   acute L56.8
  tetrachlorethylene (contact) (irritant) L24.2
  toluene (contact) (irritant) L24.2
  turpentine (contact) L24.2
  ultraviolet rays (sun NEC) (chronic exposure) L57.8
   acute L56.8
  vaccine or vaccination L27.0
   specified substance — *see* Table of Drugs and Chemicals
  varicose veins — *see* Varix, leg, with, inflammation
  X-rays L58.9
   acute L58.0
   chronic L58.1
 dyshydrotic L30.1
 dysmenorrheica N94.6
 escharotica — *see* Burn
 exfoliative, exfoliativa (generalized) L26
  neonatorum L00
 eyelid — *see also* Dermatosis, eyelid H01.9
  allergic H01.119
   left H01.116
    lower H01.115
    upper H01.114
   right H01.113
    lower H01.112
    upper H01.111
  contact — *see* Dermatitis, eyelid, allergic
  due to
   Demodex species B88.0
   herpes (zoster) B02.39
    simplex B00.59
  eczematous H01.139
   left H01.136
    lower H01.135
    upper H01.134
   right H01.133
    lower H01.132
    upper H01.131

Dermatitis — *continued*
 eyelid — *see also* Dermatosis, eyelid — *continued*
  specified NEC H01.8
 facta, factitia, factitial L98.1
  psychogenic F54
 flexural NEC L20.82
 friction L30.4
 fungus B36.9
  specified type NEC B36.8
 gangrenosa, gangrenous infantum L08.0
 harvest mite B88.0
 heat L59.0
 herpesviral, vesicular (ear) (lip) B00.1
 herpetiformis (bullous) (erythematous) (pustular) (vesicular) L13.0
  juvenile L12.2
  senile L12.0
 hiemalis L30.8
 hypostatic, hypostatica — *see* Varix, leg, with, inflammation
 infectious eczematoid L30.3
 infective L30.3
 irritant — *see* Dermatitis, contact, irritant
 Jacquet's (diaper dermatitis) L22
 Leptus B88.0
 lichenified NEC L28.0
 medicamentosa (generalized) (internal use) — *see* Dermatitis, due to drugs
 mite B88.0
 multiformis L13.0
  juvenile L12.2
 napkin L22
 neurotica L13.0
 nummular L30.0
 papillaris capillitii L73.0
 pellagrous E52
 perioral L71.0
 photocontact L56.2
 polymorpha dolorosa L13.0
 pruriginosa L13.0
 pruritic NEC L30.8
 psychogenic F54
 purulent L08.0
 pustular
  contagious B08.02
  subcorneal L13.1
 pyococcal L08.0
 pyogenica L08.0
 repens L40.2
 Ritter's (exfoliativa) L00
 Schamberg's L81.7
 schistosome B65.3
 seasonal bullous L30.8
 seborrheic L21.9
  infantile L21.1
  specified NEC L21.8
 sensitization NOS L23.9
 septic L08.0
 solare L57.8
 specified NEC L30.8
 stasis I87.2
  with
   varicose ulcer — *see* Varix, leg, with ulcer, with inflammation
   varicose veins — *see* Varix, leg, with, inflammation
  due to postthrombotic syndrome — *see* Syndrome, postthrombotic
 suppurative L08.0
 traumatic NEC L30.4
 trophoneurotica L13.0
 ultraviolet (sun) (chronic exposure) L57.8
  acute L56.8
 varicose — *see* Varix, leg, with, inflammation
 vegetans L10.1
 vegetous B43.0
 verrucosa B43.0
 vesicular, herpesviral B00.1
Dermatoarthritis, lipoid E78.81
Dermatochalasis, eyelid H02.839
 left H02.836
  lower H02.835
  upper H02.834
 right H02.833
  lower H02.832
  upper H02.831
Dermatofibroma (lenticulare) — *see* Neoplasm, skin, benign
 protuberans — *see* Neoplasm, skin, uncertain behavior
Dermatofibrosarcoma (pigmented) (protuberans) — *see* Neoplasm, skin, malignant

Dermatographia L50.3
Dermatolysis (exfoliativa) (congenital) Q82.8
  acquired L57.4
  eyelids — see Blepharochalasis
  palpebrarum — see Blepharochalasis
  senile L57.4
Dermatomegaly NEC Q82.8
Dermatomucosomyositis — see also Dermatomyositis
  M33.10
  with
    myopathy M33.12
    respiratory involvement M33.11
    specified organ involvement NEC M33.19
Dermatomycosis B36.9
  furfuracea B36.0
  specified type NEC B36.8
Dermatomyositis (acute) (chronic) — see also Dermatopolymyositis
  adult — see also Dermatomyositis, specified NEC M33.10
  in (due to) neoplastic disease — see also Neoplasm
    D49.9 [M36.0]
  juvenile M33.00
    with
      myopathy M33.02
      respiratory involvement M33.01
      specified organ involvement NEC M33.09
    amyopathic M33.03
    without myopathy M33.03
  specified NEC M33.10
    with
      myopathy M33.12
      respiratory involvement M33.11
      specified organ involvement NEC M33.19
    amyopathic M33.13
    without myopathy M33.13
Dermatoneuritis of children — see Poisoning, mercury
Dermatophilosis A48.8
Dermatophytid L30.2
Dermatophytide — see Dermatophytosis
Dermatophytosis (epidermophyton) (infection) (Microsporum) (tinea) (Trichophyton) B35.9
  beard B35.0
  body B35.4
  capitis B35.0
  corporis B35.4
  deep-seated B35.8
  disseminated B35.8
  foot B35.3
  granulomatous B35.8
  groin B35.6
  hand B35.2
  nail B35.1
  perianal (area) B35.6
  scalp B35.0
  specified NEC B35.8
Dermatopolymyositis M33.90
  with
    myopathy M33.92
    respiratory involvement M33.91
    specified organ involvement NEC M33.99
  amyopathic M33.93
  in neoplastic disease — see also Neoplasm D49.9 [M36.0]
  juvenile M33.00
    with
      myopathy M33.02
      respiratory involvement M33.01
      specified organ involvement NEC M33.09
    amyopathic M33.03
    without myopathy M33.03
  specified NEC M33.10
    amyopathic M33.13
    myopathy M33.12
    respiratory involvement M33.11
    specified organ involvement NEC M33.19
    without myopathy M33.13
  without myopathy M33.93
Dermatopolyneuritis — see Poisoning, mercury
Dermatorrhexis — see also Syndrome, Ehlers-Danlos
  Q79.60
  acquired L57.4
Dermatosclerosis — see also Scleroderma
  localized L94.0
Dermatosis L98.9
  Andrews' L08.89
  Bowen's — see Neoplasm, skin, in situ
  bullous L13.9
    specified NEC L13.8
  exfoliativa L26
  eyelid (noninfectious) — see also Dermatitis, eyelid H01.9

Dermatosis — continued
  eyelid — see also Dermatitis, eyelid — continued
    discoid lupus erythematosus — see Lupus, erythematosus, eyelid
    xeroderma — see Xeroderma, acquired, eyelid
  factitial L98.1
  febrile neutrophilic L98.2
  gonococcal A54.89
  herpetiformis L13.0
    juvenile L12.2
  linear IgA L13.8
  menstrual NEC L98.8
  neutrophilic, febrile L98.2
  occupational — see Dermatitis, contact
  papulosa nigra L82.1
  pigmentary L81.9
    progressive L81.7
    Schamberg's L81.7
  psychogenic F54
  purpuric, pigmented L81.7
  pustular, subcorneal L13.1
  transient acantholytic L11.1
Dermographia, dermographism L50.3
Dermoid (cyst) — see also Neoplasm, benign, by site
  with malignant transformation C56- ☑
  due to radiation (nonionizing) L57.8
Dermopathy
  infiltrative with thyrotoxicosis — see Thyrotoxicosis
  nephrogenic fibrosing L90.8
Dermophytosis — see Dermatophytosis
Descemetocele H18.73- ☑
Descemet's membrane — see condition
Descending — see condition
Descensus uteri — see Prolapse, uterus
Desert
  rheumatism B38.0
  sore — see Ulcer, skin
Desertion (newborn) — see Maltreatment
Desmoid (extra-abdominal) (tumor) — see Neoplasm, connective tissue, uncertain behavior
  abdominal wall D48.113
  back D48.117
  buttock D48.116
  chest wall D48.111
  extremity
    lower D48.116
    upper D48.115
  head and neck D48.110
  intraabdominal D48.114
  intrathoracic D48.112
  pelvic cavity D48.114
  pelvic girdle D48.116
  peritoneal D48.114
  retroperitoneal D48.114
  shoulder girdle D48.115
  site unspecified D48.119
  specified site NEC D48.118
Despondency F32.A
Desquamation, skin R23.4
Destruction, destructive — see also Damage
  articular facet — see also Derangement, joint, specified type NEC
    knee M23.8X- ☑
    vertebra — see Spondylosis
  bone — see also Disorder, bone, specified type NEC
    syphilitic A52.77
  joint — see also Derangement, joint, specified type NEC
    sacroiliac M53.3
  rectal sphincter K62.89
  septum (nasal) J34.89
  tuberculous NEC — see Tuberculosis
  tympanum, tympanic membrane (nontraumatic) — see Disorder, tympanic membrane, specified NEC
  vertebral disc — see Degeneration, intervertebral disc
Destructiveness — see also Disorder, conduct
  adjustment reaction — see Disorder, adjustment
Desultory labor O62.2
Detachment
  cartilage — see Sprain
  cervix, annular N88.8
    complicating delivery O71.3
  choroid (old) (postinfectional) (simple) (spontaneous)
    H31.40- ☑
    hemorrhagic H31.41- ☑
    serous H31.42- ☑
  ligament — see Sprain
  meniscus (knee) — see also Derangement, knee, meniscus, specified NEC

Detachment — continued
  meniscus — see also Derangement, knee, meniscus, specified — continued
    current injury — see Tear, meniscus
    due to old tear or injury — see Derangement, knee, meniscus, due to old tear
  retina (without retinal break) (serous) H33.2- ☑
    with retinal:
      break H33.00- ☑
        giant H33.03- ☑
        multiple H33.02- ☑
        single H33.01- ☑
      dialysis H33.04- ☑
    pigment epithelium — see Degeneration, retina, separation of layers, pigment epithelium detachment
    rhegmatogenous — see Detachment, retina, with retinal, break
    specified NEC H33.8
    total H33.05- ☑
    traction H33.4- ☑
  vitreous (body) H43.81 ☑
Detergent asthma J69.8
Deterioration
  epileptic F06.8
  general physical R53.81
  heart, cardiac — see Degeneration, myocardial
  mental — see Psychosis
  myocardial, myocardium — see Degeneration, myocardial
  senile (simple) R54
Deuteranomaly (anomalous trichromat) H53.53
Deuteranopia (complete) (incomplete) H53.53
Development
  abnormal, bone Q79.9
  arrested R62.50
    bone — see Arrest, development or growth, bone
    child R62.50
    due to malnutrition E45
  defective, congenital — see also Anomaly, by site
    cauda equina Q06.3
    left ventricle Q24.8
      in hypoplastic left heart syndrome Q23.4
    valve Q24.8
      pulmonary Q22.3
  delayed — see also Delay, development R62.50
    arithmetical skills F81.2
    language (skills) (expressive) F80.1
    learning skill F81.9
    mixed skills F88
    motor coordination F82
    reading F81.0
    specified learning skill NEC F81.89
    speech F80.9
    spelling F81.81
    written expression F81.81
  imperfect, congenital — see also Anomaly, by site
    heart Q24.9
    lungs Q33.6
  incomplete
    bronchial tree Q32.4
    organ or site not listed — see Hypoplasia, by site
    respiratory system Q34.9
    sexual, precocious NEC E30.1
  tardy, mental — see also Disability, intellectual F79
Developmental — see condition
  testing, infant or child — see Examination, child
Devergie's disease (pityriasis rubra pilaris) L44.0
Deviation (in)
  conjugate palsy (eye) (spastic) H51.0
  esophagus (acquired) K22.89
  eye, skew H51.8
  midline (jaw) (teeth) (dental arch) M26.29
    specified site NEC — see Malposition
  nasal septum J34.2
    congenital Q67.4
  opening and closing of the mandible M26.53
  organ or site, congenital NEC — see Malposition, congenital
  septum (nasal) (acquired) J34.2
    congenital Q67.4
  sexual F65.9
    bestiality F65.89
    erotomania F52.8
    exhibitionism F65.2
    fetishism, fetishistic F65.0
      transvestism F65.1
    frotteurism F65.81

☑ Additional Character Required — Refer to the Tabular List for Character Selection

Deviation — continued
  sexual — continued
    masochism F65.51
    multiple F65.89
    necrophilia F65.89
    nymphomania F52.8
    pederosis F65.4
    pedophilia F65.4
    sadism, sadomasochism F65.52
    satyriasis F52.8
    specified type NEC F65.89
    transvestism F64.1
    voyeurism F65.3
  teeth, midline M26.29
  trachea J39.8
  ureter, congenital Q62.61
Device
  cerebral ventricle (communicating) in situ Z98.2
  contraceptive — see Contraceptive, device
  drainage, cerebrospinal fluid, in situ Z98.2
Devic's disease G36.0
Devil's
  grip B33.0
  pinches (purpura simplex) D69.2
Devitalized tooth K04.99
Devonshire colic — see Poisoning, lead
Dextraposition, aorta Q20.3
  in tetralogy of Fallot Q21.3
Dextrinosis, limit (debrancher enzyme deficiency) E74.03
Dextrocardia (true) Q24.0
  with
    complete transposition of viscera Q89.3
    situs inversus Q89.3
Dextrotransposition, aorta Q20.3
d-glycericacidemia E72.59
Dhat syndrome F48.8
Dhobi itch B35.6
Di George's syndrome D82.1
Di Guglielmo's disease C94.0- ☑
Diabetes, diabetic (mellitus) (sugar) E11.9
  with
    amyotrophy E11.44
    arthropathy NEC E11.618
    autonomic (poly)neuropathy E11.43
    cataract E11.36
    Charcot's joints E11.610
    chronic kidney disease E11.22
    circulatory complication NEC E11.59
    coma due to
      hyperosmolarity E11.01
      hypoglycemia E11.641
      ketoacidosis E11.11
    complication E11.8
      specified NEC E11.69
    dermatitis E11.620
    foot ulcer E11.621
    gangrene E11.52
    gastroparalysis E11.43
    gastroparesis E11.43
    glomerulonephrosis, intracapillary E11.21
    glomerulosclerosis, intercapillary E11.21
    hyperglycemia E11.65
    hyperosmolarity E11.00
      with coma E11.01
    hypoglycemia E11.649
      with coma E11.641
    ketoacidosis E11.10
      with coma E11.11
    kidney complications NEC E11.29
    Kimmelstiel-Wilson disease E11.21
    loss of protective sensation (LOPS) — see Diabetes, by type, with neuropathy
    mononeuropathy E11.41
    myasthenia E11.44
    necrobiosis lipoidica E11.620
    nephropathy E11.21
    neuralgia E11.42
    neurologic complication NEC E11.49
    neuropathic arthropathy E11.610
    neuropathy E11.40
    ophthalmic complication NEC E11.39
    oral complication NEC E11.638
    osteomyelitis E11.69
    periodontal disease E11.630
    peripheral angiopathy E11.51
      with gangrene E11.52
    polyneuropathy E11.42
    renal complication NEC E11.29
    renal tubular degeneration E11.29

Diabetes, diabetic — continued
  with — continued
    retinopathy E11.319
      with macular edema E11.311
      resolved following treatment E11.37- ☑
      nonproliferative E11.329 ☑
        with macular edema E11.321 ☑
        mild E11.329 ☑
          with macular edema E11.321 ☑
        moderate E11.339 ☑
          with macular edema E11.331 ☑
        severe E11.349 ☑
          with macular edema E11.341 ☑
      proliferative E11.359 ☑
        with
          combined traction retinal detachment and rhegmatogenous retinal detachment E11.354 ☑
          macular edema E11.351 ☑
          stable proliferative diabetic retinopathy E11.355 ☑
          traction retinal detachment involving the macula E11.352 ☑
          traction retinal detachment not involving the macula E11.353 ☑
    skin complication NEC E11.628
    skin ulcer NEC E11.622
  brittle — see Diabetes, type 1
  bronzed E83.110
  complicating pregnancy — see Pregnancy, complicated by, diabetes
  dietary counseling and surveillance Z71.3
  due to
    autoimmune process — see Diabetes, type 1
    immune mediated pancreatic islet beta-cell destruction — see Diabetes, type 1
    pancreatectomy — see Diabetes, specified type NEC
  due to drug or chemical E09.9
    with
      amyotrophy E09.44
      arthropathy NEC E09.618
      autonomic (poly)neuropathy E09.43
      cataract E09.36
      Charcot's joints E09.610
      chronic kidney disease E09.22
      circulatory complication NEC E09.59
      complication E09.8
        specified NEC E09.69
      dermatitis E09.620
      foot ulcer E09.621
      gangrene E09.52
      gastroparalysis E09.43
      gastroparesis E09.43
      glomerulonephrosis, intracapillary E09.21
      glomerulosclerosis, intercapillary E09.21
      hyperglycemia E09.65
      hyperosmolarity E09.00
        with coma E09.01
      hypoglycemia E09.649
        with coma E09.641
      ketoacidosis E09.10
        with coma E09.11
      kidney complications NEC E09.29
      Kimmelstiel-Wilson disease E09.21
      mononeuropathy E09.41
      myasthenia E09.44
      necrobiosis lipoidica E09.620
      nephropathy E09.21
      neuralgia E09.42
      neurologic complication NEC E09.49
      neuropathic arthropathy E09.610
      neuropathy E09.40
      ophthalmic complication NEC E09.39
      oral complication NEC E09.638
      periodontal disease E09.630
      peripheral angiopathy E09.51
        with gangrene E09.52
      polyneuropathy E09.42
      renal complication NEC E09.29
      renal tubular degeneration E09.29
      retinopathy E09.319
        with macular edema E09.311
        resolved following treatment E09.37 ☑
        nonproliferative E09.329 ☑
          with macular edema E09.321 ☑
          mild E09.329 ☑
            with macular edema E09.321 ☑
          moderate E09.339 ☑

Diabetes, diabetic — continued
  due to drug or chemical — continued
    with — continued
      retinopathy — continued
        nonproliferative — continued
          moderate — continued
            with macular edema E09.331 ☑
          severe E09.349 ☑
            with macular edema E09.341 ☑
        proliferative E09.359 ☑
          with
            combined traction retinal detachment and rhegmatogenous retinal detachment E09.354 ☑
            macular edema E09.351 ☑
            stable proliferative diabetic retinopathy E09.355 ☑
            traction retinal detachment involving the macula E09.352 ☑
            traction retinal detachment not involving the macula E09.353 ☑
    skin complication NEC E09.628
    skin ulcer NEC E09.622
  due to underlying condition E08.9
    with
      amyotrophy E08.44
      arthropathy NEC E08.618
      autonomic (poly)neuropathy E08.43
      cataract E08.36
      Charcot's joints E08.610
      chronic kidney disease E08.22
      circulatory complication NEC E08.59
      complication E08.8
        specified NEC E08.69
      dermatitis E08.620
      foot ulcer E08.621
      gangrene E08.52
      gastroparalysis E08.43
      gastroparesis E08.43
      glomerulonephrosis, intracapillary E08.21
      glomerulosclerosis, intercapillary E08.21
      hyperglycemia E08.65
      hyperosmolarity E08.00
        with coma E08.01
      hypoglycemia E08.649
        with coma E08.641
      ketoacidosis E08.10
        with coma E08.11
      kidney complications NEC E08.29
      Kimmelstiel-WIlson disease E08.21
      mononeuropathy E08.41
      myasthenia E08.44
      necrobiosis lipoidica E08.620
      nephropathy E08.21
      neuralgia E08.42
      neurologic complication NEC E08.49
      neuropathic arthropathy E08.610
      neuropathy E08.40
      ophthalmic complication NEC E08.39
      oral complication NEC E08.638
      periodontal disease E08.630
      peripheral angiopathy E08.51
        with gangrene E08.52
      polyneuropathy E08.42
      renal complication NEC E08.29
      renal tubular degeneration E08.29
      retinopathy E08.319
        with macular edema E08.311
        resolved following treatment E08.37 ☑
        nonproliferative E08.329 ☑
          with macular edema E08.321 ☑
          mild E08.329 ☑
            with macular edema E08.321 ☑
          moderate E08.339 ☑
            with macular edema E08.331 ☑
          severe E08.349 ☑
            with macular edema E08.341 ☑
        proliferative E08.359 ☑
          with
            combined traction retinal detachment and rhegmatogenous retinal detachment E08.354 ☑
            macular edema E08.351 ☑
            stable proliferative diabetic retinopathy E08.355 ☑
            traction retinal detachment involving the macula E08.352 ☑

Diabetes, diabetic — *continued*
  due to underlying condition — *continued*
    with — *continued*
      retinopathy — *continued*
        proliferative — *continued*
          with — *continued*
            traction retinal detachment not involving the macula E08.353 ☑
      skin complication NEC E08.628
      skin ulcer NEC E08.622
  gestational (in pregnancy) O24.419
    affecting newborn P70.0
    diet controlled O24.410
    in childbirth O24.429
      diet controlled O24.420
      insulin (and diet) controlled O24.424
      oral drug controlled (antidiabetic) (hypoglycemic) O24.425
    insulin (and diet) controlled O24.414
    oral drug controlled (antidiabetic) (hypoglycemic) O24.415
    puerperal O24.439
      diet controlled O24.430
      insulin (and diet) controlled O24.434
      oral drug controlled (antidiabetic) (hypoglycemic) O24.435
  hepatogenous E13.9
  idiopathic — *see* Diabetes, type 1
  inadequately controlled — *see* Diabetes, by type, with hyperglycemia
  insipidus E23.2
    nephrogenic N25.1
    pituitary E23.2
    vasopressin resistant N25.1
  insulin dependent — *code to* type of diabetes
  juvenile-onset — *see* Diabetes, type 1
  ketosis-prone — *see* Diabetes, type 1
  latent R73.03
  neonatal (transient) P70.2
  non-insulin dependent — *code to* type of diabetes
  out of control — *see* Diabetes, by type, with hyperglycemia
  phosphate E83.39
  poorly controlled — *see* Diabetes, by type, with hyperglycemia
  postpancreatectomy — *see* Diabetes, specified type NEC
  postprocedural — *see* Diabetes, specified type NEC
  retina, hemorrhage E13.39
  secondary diabetes mellitus NEC — *see* Diabetes, specified type NEC
  specified type NEC E13.9
    with
      amyotrophy E13.44
      arthropathy NEC E13.618
      autonomic (poly)neuropathy E13.43
      cataract E13.36
      Charcot's joints E13.610
      chronic kidney disease E13.22
      circulatory complication NEC E13.59
      complication E13.8
        specified NEC E13.69
      dermatitis E13.620
      foot ulcer E13.621
      gangrene E13.52
      gastroparalysis E13.43
      gastroparesis E13.43
      glomerulonephrosis, intracapillary E13.21
      glomerulosclerosis, intercapillary E13.21
      hyperglycemia E13.65
      hyperosmolarity E13.00
        with coma E13.01
      hypoglycemia E13.649
        with coma E13.641
      ketoacidosis E13.10
        with coma E13.11
      kidney complications NEC E13.29
      Kimmelstiel-Wilson disease E13.21
      mononeuropathy E13.41
      myasthenia E13.44
      necrobiosis lipoidica E13.620
      nephropathy E13.21
      neuralgia E13.42
      neurologic complication NEC E13.49
      neuropathic arthropathy E13.610
      neuropathy E13.40
      ophthalmic complication NEC E13.39
      oral complication NEC E13.638
      periodontal disease E13.630
      peripheral angiopathy E13.51

Diabetes, diabetic — *continued*
  specified type — *continued*
    with — *continued*
      peripheral angiopathy — *continued*
        with gangrene E13.52
      polyneuropathy E13.42
      renal complication NEC E13.29
      renal tubular degeneration E13.29
      retinopathy E13.319
        with macular edema E13.311
        resolved following treatment E13.37 ☑
        nonproliferative E13.329 ☑
          with macular edema E13.321 ☑
          mild E13.329 ☑
            with macular edema E13.321 ☑
          moderate E13.339 ☑
            with macular edema E13.331 ☑
          severe E13.349 ☑
            with macular edema E13.341 ☑
        proliferative E13.359 ☑
          with
            combined traction retinal detachment and rhegmatogenous retinal detachment E13.354 ☑
            macular edema E13.351 ☑
            stable proliferative diabetic retinopathy E13.355 ☑
            traction retinal detachment involving the macula E13.352 ☑
            traction retinal detachment not involving the macula E13.353 ☑
      skin complication NEC E13.628
      skin ulcer NEC E13.622
  steroid-induced — *see* Diabetes, due to, drug or chemical
  type 1 E10.9
    with
      amyotrophy E10.44
      arthropathy NEC E10.618
      autonomic (poly)neuropathy E10.43
      cataract E10.36
      Charcot's joints E10.610
      chronic kidney disease E10.22
      circulatory complication NEC E10.59
      coma due to
        hypoglycemia E10.641
        ketoacidosis E10.11
      complication E10.8
        specified NEC E10.69
      dermatitis E10.620
      foot ulcer E10.621
      gangrene E10.52
      gastroparalysis E10.43
      gastroparesis E10.43
      glomerulonephrosis, intracapillary E10.21
      glomerulosclerosis, intercapillary E10.21
      hyperglycemia E10.65
      hypoglycemia E10.649
        with coma E10.641
      ketoacidosis E10.10
        with coma E10.11
      kidney complications NEC E10.29
      Kimmelstiel-Wilson disease E10.21
      mononeuropathy E10.41
      myasthenia E10.44
      necrobiosis lipoidica E10.620
      nephropathy E10.21
      neuralgia E10.42
      neurologic complication NEC E10.49
      neuropathic arthropathy E10.610
      neuropathy E10.40
      ophthalmic complication NEC E10.39
      oral complication NEC E10.638
      osteomyelitis E10.69
      periodontal disease E10.630
      peripheral angiopathy E10.51
        with gangrene E10.52
      polyneuropathy E10.42
      renal complication NEC E10.29
      renal tubular degeneration E10.29
      retinopathy E10.319
        with macular edema E10.311
        resolved following treatment E10.37 ☑
        nonproliferative E10.329 ☑
          with macular edema E10.321 ☑
          mild E10.329 ☑
            with macular edema E10.321 ☑
          moderate E10.339 ☑
            with macular edema E10.331 ☑

Diabetes, diabetic — *continued*
  type 1 — *continued*
    with — *continued*
      retinopathy — *continued*
        nonproliferative — *continued*
          severe E10.349 ☑
            with macular edema E10.341 ☑
        proliferative E10.359 ☑
          with
            combined traction retinal detachment and rhegmatogenous retinal detachment E10.354 ☑
            macular edema E10.351 ☑
            stable proliferative diabetic retinopathy E10.355 ☑
            traction retinal detachment involving the macula E10.352 ☑
            traction retinal detachment not involving the macula E10.353 ☑
      skin complication NEC E10.628
      skin ulcer NEC E10.622
    early-stage E10.A- ☑
    presymptomatic E10.A0
    Stage 1 E10.A1
    Stage 2 E10.A2
  type 2 E11.9
    with
      amyotrophy E11.44
      arthropathy NEC E11.618
      autonomic (poly)neuropathy E11.43
      cataract E11.36
      Charcot's joints E11.610
      chronic kidney disease E11.22
      circulatory complication NEC E11.59
      coma due to
        hyperosmolarity E11.01
        hypoglycemia E11.641
        ketoacidosis E11.1- ☑
      complication E11.8
        specified NEC E11.69
      dermatitis E11.620
      foot ulcer E11.621
      gangrene E11.52
      gastroparalysis E11.43
      gastroparesis E11.43
      glomerulonephrosis, intracapillary E11.21
      glomerulosclerosis, intercapillary E11.21
      hyperglycemia E11.65
      hyperosmolarity E11.00
        with coma E11.01
      hypoglycemia E11.649
        with coma E11.641
      ketoacidosis E11.10
        with coma E11.11
      kidney complications NEC E11.29
      Kimmelstiel-Wilson disease E11.21
      mononeuropathy E11.41
      myasthenia E11.44
      necrobiosis lipoidica E11.620
      nephropathy E11.21
      neuralgia E11.42
      neurologic complication NEC E11.49
      neuropathic arthropathy E11.610
      neuropathy E11.40
      ophthalmic complication NEC E11.39
      oral complication NEC E11.638
      osteomyelitis E11.69
      periodontal disease E11.630
      peripheral angiopathy E11.51
        with gangrene E11.52
      polyneuropathy E11.42
      renal complication NEC E11.29
      renal tubular degeneration E11.29
      retinopathy E11.319
        with macular edema E11.311
        resolved following treatment E11.37 ☑
        nonproliferative E11.329 ☑
          with macular edema E11.321 ☑
          mild E11.329 ☑
            with macular edema E11.321 ☑
          moderate E11.339 ☑
            with macular edema E11.331 ☑
          severe E11.349 ☑
            with macular edema E11.341 ☑
        proliferative E11.359 ☑

Diabetes, diabetic — *continued*
  type 2 — *continued*
    with — *continued*
      retinopathy — *continued*
        proliferative — *continued*
          with
            combined traction retinal detachment
              and rhegmatogenous retinal de-
              tachment E11.354 ☑
            macular edema E11.351 ☑
            stable proliferative diabetic retinopathy
              E11.355 ☑
            traction retinal detachment involving
              the macula E11.352 ☑
            traction retinal detachment not involv-
              ing the macula E11.353 ☑
      skin complication NEC E11.628
      skin ulcer NEC E11.622
  uncontrolled
    meaning
      hyperglycemia — *see* Diabetes, by type, with, hy-
        perglycemia
      hypoglycemia — *see* Diabetes, by type, with, hy-
        poglycemia
Diacyclothrombopathia D69.1
Diagnosis deferred R69
Dialysis (intermittent) (treatment)
  noncompliance (with) Z91.158
    due to financial hardship Z91.151
  renal (hemodialysis) (peritoneal), status Z99.2
  retina, retinal — *see* Detachment, retina, with retinal,
    dialysis
Diamond-Blackfan anemia (congenital hypoplastic) D61.01
Diamond-Gardener syndrome (autoerythrocyte sensitiza-
  tion) D69.2
Diaper rash L22
Diaphoresis (excessive) R61
Diaphragm — *see* condition
Diaphragmalgia R07.1
Diaphragmatitis, diaphragmitis J98.6
Diaphysial aclasis Q78.6
Diaphysitis — *see* Osteomyelitis, specified type NEC
Diarrhea, diarrheal (disease) (infantile) (inflammatory)
  R19.7
  achlorhydric K31.83
  allergic K52.29
    due to
      colitis — *see* Colitis, allergic
      enteritis — *see* Enteritis, allergic
  amebic — *see also* Amebiasis A06.0
    with abscess — *see* Abscess, amebic
    acute A06.0
    chronic A06.1
    nondysenteric A06.2
  bacillary — *see* Dysentery, bacillary
  balantidial A07.0
  cachectic NEC K52.89
  Chilomastix A07.8
  choleriformis A00.1
  chronic (noninfectious) K52.9
  coccidial A07.3
  Cochin-China K90.1
    strongyloidiasis B78.0
  Dientamoeba A07.8
  dietetic — *see also* Diarrhea, allergic K52.29
  drug-induced K52.1
  due to
    bacteria A04.9
      specified NEC A04.8
    Campylobacter A04.5
    Capillaria philippinensis B81.1
    Clostridium difficile
      not specified as recurrent A04.72
      recurrent A04.71
    Clostridium perfringens (C) (F) A04.8
    Cryptosporidium A07.2
    drugs K52.1
    Escherichia coli A04.4
      enteroaggregative A04.4
      enterohemorrhagic A04.3
      enteroinvasive A04.2
      enteropathogenic A04.0
      enterotoxigenic A04.1
      specified NEC A04.4
    food hypersensitivity — *see also* Diarrhea, allergic
      K52.29
    Necator americanus B76.1
    S. japonicum B65.2

Diarrhea, diarrheal — *continued*
  due to — *continued*
    specified organism NEC A08.8
      bacterial A04.8
      viral A08.39
    Staphylococcus A04.8
    Trichuris trichiuria B79
    virus — *see* Enteritis, viral
    Yersinia enterocolitica A04.6
  dysenteric A09
  endemic A09
  epidemic A09
  flagellate A07.9
  Flexner's (ulcerative) A03.1
  functional K59.1
    following gastrointestinal surgery K91.89
    psychogenic F45.8
  Giardia lamblia A07.1
  giardial A07.1
  hill K90.1
  infectious A09
  malarial — *see* Malaria
  mite B88.0
  mycotic NEC B49
  neonatal (noninfectious) P78.3
  nervous F45.8
  neurogenic K59.1
  noninfectious K52.9
  postgastrectomy K91.1
  postvagotomy K91.1
  protozoal A07.9
    specified NEC A07.8
  psychogenic F45.8
  specified
    bacterium NEC A04.8
    virus NEC A08.39
  strongyloidiasis B78.0
  toxic K52.1
  trichomonal A07.8
  tropical K90.1
  tuberculous A18.32
  viral — *see* Enteritis, viral
Diastasis
  cranial bones M84.88
    congenital NEC Q75.8
  joint (traumatic) — *see* Dislocation
  muscle M62.00
    ankle M62.07- ☑
    congenital Q79.8
    foot M62.07- ☑
    forearm M62.03- ☑
    hand M62.04- ☑
    lower leg M62.06- ☑
    pelvic region M62.05- ☑
    shoulder region M62.01- ☑
    specified site NEC M62.08
    thigh M62.05- ☑
    upper arm M62.02- ☑
  recti (abdomen)
    complicating delivery O71.89
    congenital Q79.59
Diastema, tooth, teeth, fully erupted M26.32
Diastematomyelia Q06.2
Diataxia, cerebral G80.4
Diathesis
  allergic — *see* History, allergy
  bleeding (familial) D69.9
  cystine (familial) E72.00
  gouty — *see* Gout
  hemorrhagic (familial) D69.9
    newborn NEC P53
  spasmophilic R29.0
Diaz's disease or osteochondrosis (juvenile) (talus) — *see*
  Osteochondrosis, juvenile, tarsus
Dibothriocephalus, dibothriocephaliasis (latus) (infec-
  tion) (infestation) B70.0
  larval B70.1
Dicephalus, dicephaly Q89.4
Dichotomy, teeth K00.2
Dichromat, dichromatopsia (congenital) — *see* Deficiency,
  color vision
Dichuchwa A65
Dicroceliasis B66.2
Didelphia, didelphys — *see* Double uterus
Didymytis N45.1
  with orchitis N45.3
Dietary
  inadequacy or deficiency E63.9

Dietary — *continued*
  surveillance and counseling Z71.3
Dietl's crisis N13.8
Dieulafoy lesion (hemorrhagic)
  duodenum K31.82
  esophagus K22.89
  intestine (colon) K63.81
  stomach K31.82
Difficult, difficulty (in)
  acculturation Z60.3
  feeding R63.30
    elderly R63.39
    infant NOS R63.39
    newborn P92.9
      breast P92.5
      specified NEC P92.8
    nonorganic (infant or child) F98.29
    specified NEC R63.39
  intubation, in anesthesia T88.4 ☑
  mechanical, gastroduodenal stoma K91.89
    causing obstruction — *see also* Obstruction, intestine,
      postoperative K91.30
  micturition
    need to immediately re-void R39.191
    position dependent R39.192
    specified NEC R39.198
  reading (developmental) F81.0
    secondary to emotional disorders F93.9
  spelling (specific) F81.81
    with reading disorder F81.89
    due to inadequate teaching Z55.8
  swallowing — *see* Dysphagia
  understanding
    health related information Z55.6
    medication instructions Z55.6
  walking R26.2
  work
    conditions NEC Z56.5
    schedule Z56.3
Diffuse — *see* condition
Digestive — *see* condition
Dihydropyrimidine dehydrogenase disease (DPD) E88.89
Diktyoma — *see* Neoplasm, malignant, by site
Dilaceration, tooth K00.4
Dilatation
  anus K59.89
    venule — *see* Hemorrhoids
  aorta (focal) (general) — *see* Ectasia, aorta
    with aneurysm — *see* Aneurysm, aorta
    congenital Q25.44
  artery — *see* Aneurysm
  bladder (sphincter) N32.89
    congenital Q64.79
  blood vessel I99.8
  bronchial J47.9
    with
      exacerbation (acute) J47.1
      lower respiratory infection J47.0
  calyx N28.89
    due to obstruction — *see* Hydronephrosis
  capillaries I78.8
  cardiac (acute) (chronic) — *see also* Hypertrophy, cardiac
    congenital Q24.8
      valve NEC Q24.8
        pulmonary Q22.3
    valve — *see* Endocarditis
  cavum septi pellucidi Q06.8
  cervix (uteri) — *see also* Incompetency, cervix
    incomplete, poor, slow complicating delivery O62.0
  colon K59.39
    congenital Q43.1
    psychogenic F45.8
    toxic K59.31
  common duct (acquired) K83.8
    congenital Q44.5
  cystic duct (acquired) K82.8
    congenital Q44.5
  duct, mammary — *see* Ectasia, mammary duct
  duodenum K59.89
  esophagus K22.89
    congenital Q39.5
    due to achalasia K22.0
  eustachian tube, congenital Q17.8
  gallbladder K82.8
  gastric — *see* Dilatation, stomach
  heart (acute) (chronic) — *see also* Hypertrophy, cardiac
    congenital Q24.8
    valve — *see* Endocarditis
  ileum K59.89

Dilatation — continued
ileum — continued
psychogenic F45.8
jejunum K59.89
psychogenic F45.8
kidney (calyx) (collecting structures) (cystic) (parenchyma) (pelvis) (idiopathic) N28.89
due to obstruction — see Hydronephrosis
lacrimal passages or duct — see Disorder, lacrimal system, changes
lymphatic vessel I89.0
mammary duct — see Ectasia, mammary duct
Meckel's diverticulum (congenital) Q43.0
malignant — see Table of Neoplasms, small intestine, malignant
myocardium (acute) (chronic) — see Hypertrophy, cardiac
organ or site, congenital NEC — see Distortion
pancreatic duct K86.89
pericardium — see Pericarditis
pharynx J39.2
prostate N42.89
pulmonary
artery (idiopathic) I28.8
valve, congenital Q22.3
pupil H57.04
rectum K59.39
saccule, congenital Q16.5
salivary gland (duct) K11.8
sphincter ani K62.89
stomach K31.89
acute K31.0
psychogenic F45.8
submaxillary duct K11.8
trachea, congenital Q32.1
ureter (idiopathic) N28.82
congenital Q62.2
due to obstruction N13.4
urethra (acquired) N36.8
vasomotor I73.9
vein I86.8
ventricular, ventricle (acute) (chronic) — see also Hypertrophy, cardiac
cerebral, congenital Q04.8
venule NEC I86.8
vesical orifice N32.89
Dilated, dilation — see Dilatation
Diminished, diminution
hearing (acuity) — see Deafness
sense or sensation (cold) (heat) (tactile) (vibratory) R20.8
vision NEC H54.7
vital capacity R94.2
Diminuta taenia B71.0
Dimitri-Sturge-Weber disease Q85.89
Dimple
congenital sacral Q82.6
parasacral Q82.6
pilonidal or postanal — see Cyst, pilonidal
Dioctophyme renalis (infection) (infestation) B83.8
Dipetalonemiasis B74.4
Diphallus Q55.69
Diphtheria, diphtheritic (gangrenous) (hemorrhagic) A36.9
carrier (suspected) Z22.2
cutaneous A36.3
faucial A36.0
infection of wound A36.3
laryngeal A36.2
myocarditis A36.81
nasal, anterior A36.89
nasopharyngeal A36.1
neurological complication A36.89
pharyngeal A36.0
specified site NEC A36.89
tonsillar A36.0
Diphyllobothriasis (intestine) B70.0
larval B70.1
Diplacusis H93.22- ☑
Diplegia (upper limbs) G83.0
congenital (cerebral) G80.8
facial G51.0
lower limbs G82.20
spastic G80.1
Diplococcus, diplococcal — see condition
Diplopia H53.2
Dipsomania F10.20
with
psychosis — see Psychosis, alcoholic
remission F10.21
Dipylidiasis B71.1
DIRA (deficiency of interleukin 1 receptor antagonist) M04.8

Direction, teeth, abnormal, fully erupted M26.30
Dirofilariasis B74.8
Dirt-eating child F98.3
Disability, disabilities
heart — see Disease, heart
intellectual F79
with
autistic features F84.9
pathogenic CHAMP1 (genetic) (variant) F78.A9
pathogenic HNRNPH2 (genetic) (variant) F78.A9
pathogenic SATB2 (genetic) (variant) F78.A9
pathogenic SETBP1 (genetic) (variant) F78.A9
pathogenic STXBP1 (genetic) (variant) F78.A9
pathogenic SYNGAP1 (genetic) (variant) F78.A1
autosomal dominant F78.A9
autosomal recessive F78.A9
genetic related F78.A9
with
pathogenic CHAMP1 (variant) F78.A9
pathogenic HNRNPH2 (variant) F78.A9
pathogenic SATB2 (variant) F78.A9
pathogenic SETBP1 (variant) F78.A9
pathogenic STXBP1 (variant) F78.A9
pathogenic SYNGAP1 (variant) F78.A1
specified NEC F78.A9
SYNGAP1-related F78.A1
in
autosomal dominant mental retardation F78.A9
autosomal recessive mental retardation F78.A9
SATB2-associated syndrome F78.A9
SETBP1 disorder F78.A9
STXBP1 encephalopathy with epilepsy — see also Encephalopathy; and — see also Epilepsy
X-linked mental retardation (syndromic) (Bain type) F78.A9
mild (I.Q. 50-69) F70
moderate (I.Q. 35-49) F71
profound (I.Q. under 20) F73
severe (I.Q. 20-34) F72
specified level NEC F78.A9
SYNGAP1-related F78.A1
X-linked (syndromic) (Bain type) F78.A9
knowledge acquisition F81.9
learning F81.9
limiting activities Z73.6
spelling, specific F81.81
Disappearance of family member Z63.4
Disarticulation — see Amputation
meaning traumatic amputation — see Amputation, traumatic
Discharge (from)
abnormal finding in — see Abnormal, specimen
breast (female) (male) N64.52
diencephalic autonomic idiopathic — see Epilepsy, specified NEC
ear — see also Otorrhea
blood — see Otorrhagia
excessive urine R35.89
nipple N64.52
penile R36.9
postnasal R09.82
prison, anxiety concerning Z65.2
urethral R36.9
without blood R36.0
hematospermia R36.1
vaginal N89.8
Discitis, diskitis M46.40
cervical region M46.42
cervicothoracic region M46.43
lumbar region M46.46
lumbosacral region M46.47
multiple sites M46.49
occipito-atlanto-axial region M46.41
pyogenic — see Infection, intervertebral disc, pyogenic
sacrococcygeal region M46.48
thoracic region M46.44
thoracolumbar region M46.45
Discoid
meniscus (congenital) Q68.6
semilunar cartilage (congenital) — see Derangement, knee, meniscus, specified NEC
Discoloration
nails L60.8
teeth (posteruptive) K03.7
during formation K00.8
Discomfort
chest R07.89
visual H53.14- ☑
Discontinuity, ossicles, ear H74.2- ☑

Discord (with)
boss Z56.4
classmates Z55.4
counselor Z64.4
employer Z56.4
family Z63.8
fellow employees Z56.4
in-laws Z63.1
landlord Z59.2
lodgers Z59.2
neighbors Z59.2
probation officer Z64.4
social worker Z64.4
teachers Z55.4
workmates Z56.4
Discordant connection
atrioventricular (congenital) Q20.5
ventriculoarterial Q20.3
Discrepancy
centric occlusion maximum intercuspation M26.55
leg length (acquired) — see Deformity, limb, unequal length
congenital — see Defect, reduction, lower limb
uterine size date O26.84- ☑
Discrimination
ethnic Z60.5
political Z60.5
racial Z60.5
religious Z60.5
sex Z60.5
Disease, diseased — see also Syndrome
absorbent system I87.8
acid-peptic K30
Acosta's T70.29 ☑
Adams-Stokes (-Morgagni) (syncope with heart block) I45.9
Addison's anemia (pernicious) D51.0
adenoids (and tonsils) J35.9
adrenal (capsule) (cortex) (gland) (medullary) E27.9
hyperfunction E27.0
specified NEC E27.8
ainhum L94.6
airway
obstructive, chronic J44.9
due to
cotton dust J66.0
specific organic dusts NEC J66.8
reactive — see Asthma
akamushi (scrub typhus) A75.3
Albers-Schonberg (marble bones) Q78.2
Albert's — see Tendinitis, Achilles
Alexander G31.86
alimentary canal K63.9
alligator-skin Q80.9
acquired L85.0
alpha heavy chain C88.3- ☑
alpine T70.29 ☑
altitude T70.20 ☑
alveolar ridge
edentulous K06.9
specified NEC K06.8
alveoli, teeth K08.9
Alzheimer's — see also Dementia, in, diseases specified elsewhere G30.9 [F02.80]
with behavioral disturbance — see also Dementia, in, diseases specified elsewhere G30.9 [F02.81-] ☑
early onset — see also Dementia, in, diseases specified elsewhere G30.0 [F02.80]
with behavioral disturbance — see also Dementia, in, diseases specified elsewhere G30.0 [F02.81-] ☑
late onset — see also Dementia, in, diseases specified elsewhere G30.1 [F02.80]
with behavioral disturbance — see also Dementia, in, diseases specified elsewhere G30.1 [F02.81-] ☑
specified NEC — see also Dementia, in, diseases specified elsewhere G30.8 [F02.80]
with behavioral disturbance — see also Dementia, in, diseases specified elsewhere G30.8 [F02.81] ☑
amyloid — see Amyloidosis
Andersen's (glycogenosis IV) E74.09
Andes T70.29 ☑
Andrews' (bacterid) L08.89
angiospastic I73.9
cerebral G45.9
vein I87.8

☑ **Additional Character Required** — Refer to the Tabular List for Character Selection

Disease, diseased — *continued*

anterior
chamber H21.9
horn cell G12.29
antiglomerular basement membrane (anti- GBM) antibody M31.0
tubulo-interstitial nephritis N12
Antopol E74.05
antral — *see* Sinusitis, maxillary
anus K62.9
specified NEC K62.89
aorta (nonsyphilitic) I77.9
syphilitic NEC A52.02
aortic (heart) (valve) I35.9
rheumatic I06.9
Apollo B30.3
aponeuroses — *see* Enthesopathy
appendix K38.9
specified NEC K38.8
aqueous (chamber) H21.9
Arnold-Chiari — *see* Arnold-Chiari disease
arterial — *see also* Disease, artery I77.9
occlusive — *see also* Occlusion, by site
due to stricture or stenosis I77.1
peripheral I73.9
arteriocardiorenal — *see* Hypertension, cardiorenal
arteriolar (generalized) (obliterative) I77.9
arteriorenal — *see* Hypertension, kidney
arteriosclerotic — *see also* Arteriosclerosis
cardiovascular — *see* Disease, heart, ischemic,
atherosclerotic
coronary (artery) — *see* Disease, heart, ischemic,
atherosclerotic
heart — *see* Disease, heart, ischemic, atherosclerotic
artery — *see also* Disease, arterial I77.9
cerebral I67.9
coronary I25.10
with angina pectoris — *see* Arteriosclerosis, coronary (artery)
peripheral I73.9
arthropod-borne NOS (viral) A94
specified type NEC A93.8
atticoantral, chronic H66.20
left H66.22
with right H66.23
right H66.21
with left H66.23
auditory canal — *see* Disorder, ear, external
auricle, ear NEC — *see* Disorder, pinna
Australian X A83.4
autoimmune (systemic) NOS M35.9
hemolytic D59.10
cold type (primary) (secondary) (symptomatic)
D59.12
drug-induced D59.0
mixed type (primary) (secondary) (symptomatic)
D59.13
warm type (primary) (secondary) (symptomatic)
D59.11
thyroid E06.3
autoinflammatory M04.9
NOD2-associated M04.8
specified type NEC M04.8
aviator's — *see* Effect, adverse, high altitude
Ayerza's (pulmonary artery sclerosis with pulmonary
hypertension) I27.0
Babington's (familial hemorrhagic telangiectasia) I78.0
bacterial A49.9
specified NEC A48.8
zoonotic A28.9
specified type NEC A28.8
Baelz's (cheilitis glandularis apostematosa) K13.0
bagasse J67.1
balloon — *see* Effect, adverse, high altitude
Bang's (brucella abortus) A23.1
Bannister's T78.3 ☑
barometer makers' — *see* Poisoning, mercury
Barraquer (-Simons') (progressive lipodystrophy) E88.1
Barrett's — *see* Barrett's, esophagus
Bartholin's gland N75.9
basal ganglia G25.9
degenerative G23.9
specified NEC G23.8
specified NEC G25.89
Basedow's (exophthalmic goiter) — *see* Hyperthyroidism,
with, goiter (diffuse)
Bateman's B08.1
Batten-Steinert G71.11
Battey A31.0

Disease, diseased — *continued*

Beard's (neurasthenia) F48.8
Becker
idiopathic mural endomyocardial I42.3
myotonia congenita G71.12
Begbie's (exophthalmic goiter) — *see* Hyperthyroidism,
with, goiter (diffuse)
behavioral, organic F07.9
Beigel's (white piedra) B36.2
Benson's — *see* Deposit, crystalline
Bernard-Soulier (thrombopathy) D69.1
Bernhardt (-Roth) — *see* Mononeuropathy, lower limb,
meralgia paresthetica
Biermer's (pernicious anemia) D51.0
bile duct (common) (hepatic) K83.9
with calculus, stones — *see* Calculus, bile duct
specified NEC K83.8
biliary (tract) K83.9
specified NEC K83.8
Billroth's — *see* Spina bifida
bird fancier's J67.2
black lung J60
bladder N32.9
in (due to)
schistosomiasis (bilharziasis) B65.0 *[N33]*
specified NEC N32.89
bleeder's D66
blood D75.9
forming organs D75.9
vessel I99.9
Bloodgood's — *see* Mastopathy, cystic
Blount M92.51- ☑
Bodechtel-Guttmann (subacute sclerosing panencephalitis) A81.1
bone — *see also* Disorder, bone
aluminum M83.4
fibrocystic NEC
jaw M27.49
bone-marrow D75.9
Borna A83.9
Bornholm (epidemic pleurodynia) B33.0
Bouchard's (myopathic dilatation of the stomach) K31.0
Bouillaud's (rheumatic heart disease) I01.9
Bourneville (-Brissaud) (tuberous sclerosis) Q85.1
Bouveret (-Hoffmann) (paroxysmal tachycardia) I47.9
bowel K63.9
functional K59.9
psychogenic F45.8
brain — *see also* Dementia, in, diseases specified elsewhere G93.9
arterial, artery I67.9
arteriosclerotic I67.2
congenital Q04.9
degenerative — *see* Degeneration, brain
inflammatory — *see* Encephalitis
organic G93.9
arteriosclerotic I67.2
parasitic NEC B71.9 *[G94]*
senile NEC G31.1
specified NEC G93.89
breast — *see also* Disorder, breast N64.9
cystic (chronic) — *see* Mastopathy, cystic
fibrocystic — *see* Mastopathy, cystic
Paget's
female, unspecified side C50.91- ☑
male, unspecified side C50.92- ☑
specified NEC N64.89
Breda's — *see* Yaws
Bretonneau's (diphtheritic malignant angina) A36.0
Bright's — *see* Nephritis
arteriosclerotic — *see* Hypertension, kidney
Brill's (recrudescent typhus) A75.1
Brill-Zinsser (recrudescent typhus) A75.1
Brion-Kayser — *see* Fever, paratyphoid
broad
beta E78.2
ligament (noninflammatory) N83.9
inflammatory — *see* Disease, pelvis, inflammatory
specified NEC N83.8
Brocq-Duhring (dermatitis herpetiformis) L13.0
Brocq's
meaning
dermatitis herpetiformis L13.0
prurigo L28.2
bronchopulmonary J98.4
bronchus NEC J98.09
bronze Addison's E27.1
tuberculous A18.7
budgerigar fancier's J67.2

Disease, diseased — *continued*

Buerger's (thromboangiitis obliterans) I73.1
bullous L13.9
chronic of childhood L12.2
specified NEC L13.8
Burger-Grutz (essential familial hyperlipemia) E78.3
bursa — *see* Bursopathy
caisson T70.3 ☑
California — *see* Coccidioidomycosis
Canavan E75.28
capillaries I78.9
specified NEC I78.8
Carapata A68.0
carcinoid E34.00
heart E34.01
specified NEC E34.09
cardiac — *see* Disease, heart
cardiopulmonary, chronic I27.9
cardiorenal (hepatic) (hypertensive) (vascular) — *see*
Hypertension, cardiorenal
cardiovascular (atherosclerotic) I25.10
with angina pectoris — *see* Arteriosclerosis, coronary
(artery),
congenital Q28.9
hypertensive — *see* Hypertension, heart
newborn P29.9
specified NEC P29.89
renal (hypertensive) — *see* Hypertension, cardiorenal
syphilitic (asymptomatic) A52.00
cartilage — *see* Disorder, cartilage
Castellani's A69.8
Castleman (unicentric) (multicentric) D47.Z2
HHV-8-associated — *see also* Herpesvirus, human, 8
D47.Z2
cat-scratch A28.1
Cavare's (familial periodic paralysis) G72.3
cecum K63.9
celiac (adult) (infantile) (with steatorrhea) K90.0
cellular tissue L98.9
central core G71.29
cerebellar, cerebellum — *see* Disease, brain
cerebral — *see also* Disease, brain
degenerative — *see* Degeneration, brain
cerebrospinal G96.9
cerebrovascular I67.9
acute I67.89
embolic I63.4- ☑
thrombotic I63.3- ☑
arteriosclerotic I67.2
hereditary NEC I67.858
specified NEC I67.89
cervix (uteri) (noninflammatory) N88.9
inflammatory — *see* Cervicitis
specified NEC N88.8
Chabert's A22.9
Chandler's (osteochondritis dissecans, hip) — *see* Osteochondritis, dissecans, hip
Charlouis — *see* Yaws
Chediak-Steinbrinck (-Higashi) (congenital gigantism of
peroxidase granules) E70.330
chest J98.9
Chiari's (hepatic vein thrombosis) I82.0
Chicago B40.9
Chignon B36.8
chigo, chigoe B88.1
childhood granulomatous D71
Chinese liver fluke B66.1
chlamydial A74.9
specified NEC A74.89
cholecystic K82.9
choroid H31.9
specified NEC H31.8
Christmas D67
chronic bullous of childhood L12.2
chylomicron retention E78.3
ciliary body H21.9
specified NEC H21.89
circulatory (system) NEC I99.8
newborn P29.9
syphilitic A52.00
congenital A50.54
coagulation factor deficiency (congenital) — *see* Defect,
coagulation
coccidioidal — *see* Coccidioidomycosis
cold
agglutinin or hemoglobinuria D59.12
paroxysmal D59.6
hemagglutinin (chronic) D59.12
collagen NOS (nonvascular) (vascular) M35.9

Disease, diseased — *continued*
  collagen — *continued*
    specified NEC M35.89
  colon K63.9
    functional K59.9
      congenital Q43.2
    ischemic — *see also* Ischemia, intestine, acute K55.039
  colonic inflammatory bowel, unclassified (IBDU) K52.3
  combined system — *see* Degeneration, combined
  compressed air T70.3 ☑
  Concato's (pericardial polyserositis) A19.9
    nontubercular I31.1
    pleural — *see* Pleurisy, with effusion
  conjunctiva H11.9
    chlamydial A74.0
    specified NEC H11.89
    viral B30.9
      specified NEC B30.8
  connective tissue, systemic (diffuse) M35.9
    in (due to)
      hypogammaglobulinemia D80.1 *[M36.8]*
      ochronosis E70.29 *[M36.8]*
    specified NEC M35.89
  Conor and Bruch's (boutonneuse fever) A77.1
  Cooper's — *see* Mastopathy, cystic
  Cori's (glycogenosis III) E74.03
  corkhandler's or corkworker's J67.3
  cornea H18.9
    specified NEC H18.89- ☑
  coronary (artery) — *see* Disease, heart, ischemic, atherosclerotic
    congenital Q24.5
    microvascular
      with
        angina pectoris I20.81
        myocardial infarction I21.B
      acute I24.81
      chronic I25.85
    ostial, syphilitic (aortic) (mitral) (pulmonary) A52.03
  corpus cavernosum N48.9
    specified NEC N48.89
  Cotugno — *see* Sciatica
  COVID-19 U07.1
  coxsackie (virus) NEC B34.1
  cranial nerve NOS G52.9
  Creutzfeldt-Jakob — *see* Creutzfeldt-Jakob disease or syndrome
  Crocq's (acrocyanosis) I73.89
  Crohn's — *see* Enteritis, regional
  Curschmann G71.11
  cystic
    breast (chronic) — *see* Mastopathy, cystic
    kidney, congenital Q61.9
    liver, congenital Q44.6
    lung J98.4
      congenital Q33.0
  cytomegalic inclusion (generalized) B25.9
    with pneumonia B25.0
    congenital P35.1
  cytomegaloviral B25.9
    specified NEC B25.8
  Czerny's (periodic hydrarthrosis of the knee) — *see* Effusion, joint, knee
  Daae (-Finsen) (epidemic pleurodynia) B33.0
  Danon E74.05
  Darling's — *see* Histoplasmosis capsulati
  de Quervain's (tendon sheath) M65.4
    thyroid (subacute granulomatous thyroiditis) E06.1
  Debove's (splenomegaly) R16.1
  deer fly — *see* Tularemia
  Degos' I77.89
  demyelinating, demyelinizating (nervous system) G37.9
    multiple sclerosis G35
    specified NEC G37.89
  dense deposit — *see also* N00-N07 with fourth character .6 N05.6
  deposition, hydroxyapatite — *see* Disease, hydroxyapatite deposition
  Devergie's (pityriasis rubra pilaris) L44.0
  Devic's G36.0
  diaphorase deficiency D74.0
  diaphragm J98.6
  diarrheal, infectious NEC A09
  digestive system K92.9
    specified NEC K92.89
  disc, degenerative — *see* Degeneration, intervertebral disc
  discogenic — *see also* Displacement, intervertebral disc NEC

Disease, diseased — *continued*
  discogenic — *see also* Displacement, intervertebral disc — *continued*
    with myelopathy — *see* Disorder, disc, with, myelopathy
  diverticular — *see* Diverticula
  Dubois (thymus) A50.59 *[E35]*
  Duchenne-Griesinger G71.01
  Duchenne's
    muscular dystrophy G71.01
    pseudohypertrophy, muscles G71.01
  ductless glands E34.9
  Duhring's (dermatitis herpetiformis) L13.0
  duodenum K31.9
    specified NEC K31.89
  Dupre's (meningism) R29.1
  Dupuytren's (muscle contracture) M72.0
  Durand-Nicholas-Favre (climatic bubo) A55
  Duroziez's (congenital mitral stenosis) Q23.2
  ear — *see* Disorder, ear
  Eberth's — *see* Fever, typhoid
  Ebola (virus) A98.4
  Ebstein's heart Q22.5
  Echinococcus — *see* Echinococcus
  echovirus NEC B34.1
  Eddowes' (brittle bones and blue sclera) Q78.0
  edentulous (alveolar) ridge K06.9
    specified NEC K06.8
  Edsall's T67.2 ☑
  Eichstedt's (pityriasis versicolor) B36.0
  Eisenmenger's (irreversible) I27.83
  Ellis-van Creveld (chondroectodermal dysplasia) Q77.6
  end stage renal (ESRD) N18.6
    due to hypertension I12.0
  endocrine glands or system NEC E34.9
  endomyocardial (eosinophilic) I42.3
  English (rickets) E55.0
  enteroviral, enterovirus NEC B34.1
    central nervous system NEC A88.8
  epidemic B99.9
    specified NEC B99.8
  epididymis N50.9
  Erb (-Landouzy) G71.02
  Erdheim-Chester (ECD) E88.89
  esophagus K22.9
    functional K22.4
    psychogenic F45.8
    specified NEC K22.89
  Eulenburg's (congenital paramyotonia) G71.19
  eustachian tube — *see* Disorder, eustachian tube
  external
    auditory canal — *see* Disorder, ear, external
    ear — *see* Disorder, ear, external
  extrapyramidal G25.9
    specified NEC G25.89
  eye H57.9
    anterior chamber H21.9
    inflammatory NEC H57.89
    muscle (external) — *see* Strabismus
    specified NEC H57.89
    syphilitic — *see* Oculopathy, syphilitic
  eyeball H44.9
    specified NEC H44.89
  eyelid — *see* Disorder, eyelid
    specified NEC — *see* Disorder, eyelid, specified type NEC
  eyeworm of Africa B74.3
  facial nerve (seventh) G51.9
    newborn (birth injury) P11.3
  Fahr (of brain) G23.8
  Fahr Volhard (of kidney) I12.- ☑
  fallopian tube (noninflammatory) N83.9
    inflammatory — *see* Salpingo-oophoritis
    specified NEC N83.8
  familial periodic paralysis G72.3
  Fanconi ('s) D61.03
  fascia NEC — *see also* Disorder, muscle
    inflammatory — *see* Myositis
    specified NEC M62.89
  Fauchard's (periodontitis) — *see* Periodontitis
  Favre-Durand-Nicolas (climatic bubo) A55
  Fede's K14.0
  Feer's — *see* Poisoning, mercury
  female pelvic inflammatory — *see also* Disease, pelvis, inflammatory N73.9
    syphilitic (secondary) A51.42
    tuberculous A18.17
  Fernels' (aortic aneurysm) I71.9
  fibrocaseous of lung — *see* Tuberculosis, pulmonary

Disease, diseased — *continued*
  fibrocystic — *see* Fibrocystic disease
  Fiedler's (leptospiral jaundice) A27.0
  fifth B08.3
  file-cutter's — *see* Poisoning, lead
  fish-skin Q80.9
    acquired L85.0
  Flajani (-Basedow) (exophthalmic goiter) — *see* Hyperthyroidism, with, goiter (diffuse)
  flax-dresser's J66.1
  fluke — *see* Infestation, fluke
  foot and mouth B08.8
  foot process N04.9
  Forbes' (glycogenosis III) E74.03
  Fordyce-Fox (apocrine miliaria) L75.2
  Fordyce's (ectopic sebaceous glands) (mouth) Q38.6
  Forestier's (rhizomelic pseudopolyarthritis) M35.3
    meaning ankylosing hyperostosis — *see* Hyperostosis, ankylosing
  Fothergill's
    neuralgia — *see* Neuralgia, trigeminal
    scarlatina anginosa A38.9
  Fournier (gangrene) N49.3
    female N76.82
    vagina and vulva N76.82
  fourth B08.8
  Fox (-Fordyce) (apocrine miliaria) L75.2
  Francis' — *see* Tularemia
  Franklin C88.2- ☑
  Frei's (climatic bubo) A55
  Friedreich's
    combined systemic or ataxia G11.11
    myoclonia G25.3
  frontal sinus — *see* Sinusitis, frontal
  fungus NEC B49
  Gaisböck's (polycythemia hypertonica) D75.1
  gallbladder K82.9
    calculus — *see* Calculus, gallbladder
    cholecystitis — *see* Cholecystitis
    cholesterolosis K82.4
    fistula — *see* Fistula, gallbladder
    hydrops K82.1
    obstruction — *see* Obstruction, gallbladder
    perforation K82.2
    specified NEC K82.8
  gamma heavy chain C88.2- ☑
  Gamna's (siderotic splenomegaly) D73.2
  Gamstorp's (adynamia episodica hereditaria) G72.3
  Gandy-Nanta (siderotic splenomegaly) D73.2
  ganister J62.8
  gastric — *see* Disease, stomach
  gastroesophageal reflux (GERD) K21.9
    with esophagitis (without bleeding) K21.00
      with bleeding K21.01
  gastrointestinal (tract) K92.9
    amyloid E85.4
    functional K59.9
      psychogenic F45.8
    specified NEC K92.89
  Gee (-Herter) (-Heubner) (-Thaysen) (nontropical sprue) K90.0
  genital organs
    female N94.9
    male N50.9
  Gerhardt's (erythromelalgia) I73.81
  Gibert's (pityriasis rosea) L42
  Gierke's (glycogenosis I) E74.01
  Gilles de la Tourette's (motor-verbal tic) F95.2
  gingiva K06.9
    plaque induced K05.00
    specified NEC K06.8
  gland (lymph) I89.9
  Glanzmann's (hereditary hemorrhagic thrombasthenia) D69.1
  glass-blower's (cataract) — *see* Cataract, specified NEC
    salivary gland hypertrophy K11.1
  Glisson's — *see* Rickets
  globe H44.9
    specified NEC H44.89
  glomerular — *see also* Glomerulonephritis
    with edema — *see* Nephrosis
    acute — *see* Nephritis, acute
    chronic — *see* Nephritis, chronic
    minimal change N05.0
    rapidly progressive N01.9
  glycogen storage E74.00
    Andersen's E74.09
    Cori's E74.03
    Forbes' E74.03

Disease, diseased — *continued*
glycogen storage — *continued*
generalized E74.00
glucose-6-phosphatase deficiency E74.01
heart E74.02 *[I43]*
hepatorenal E74.09
Hers' E74.09
liver and kidney E74.09
lysosomal E74.02
with acid maltase deficiency E74.02
without acid maltase deficiency E74.05
McArdle's E74.04
muscle phosphofructokinase E74.09
myocardium E74.02 *[I43]*
Pompe's E74.02
Tauri's E74.09
type 0 E74.09
type I E74.01
type II E74.02
type IIB E74.05
type III E74.03
type IV E74.09
type V E74.04
type VI-XI E74.09
Von Gierke's E74.01
Goldstein's (familial hemorrhagic telangiectasia) I78.0
gonococcal NOS A54.9
graft-versus-host (GVH) D89.813
acute D89.810
acute on chronic D89.812
chronic D89.811
grainhandler's J67.8
granulomatous (childhood) (chronic) D71
Graves' (exophthalmic goiter) — *see* Hyperthyroidism, with, goiter (diffuse)
Griesinger's — *see* Ancylostomiasis
Grisel's M43.6
Gruby's (tinea tonsurans) B35.0
Guillain-Barre G61.0
Guinon's (motor-verbal tic) F95.2
gum K06.9
gynecological N94.9
H (Hartnup's) E72.02
Haff — *see* Poisoning, mercury
Hageman (congenital factor XII deficiency) D68.2
hair (color) (shaft) L67.9
follicles L73.9
specified NEC L73.8
Hamman's (spontaneous mediastinal emphysema) J98.2
hand, foot and mouth B08.4
Hansen's — *see* Leprosy
Hantavirus, with pulmonary manifestations B33.4
with renal manifestations A98.5
Harada's H30.81- ☑
Hartnup (pellagra-cerebellar ataxia-renal aminoaciduria) E72.02
Hart's (pellagra-cerebellar ataxia-renal aminoaciduria) E72.02
Hashimoto's (struma lymphomatosa) E06.3
Hb — *see* Disease, hemoglobin
heart (organic) I51.9
with
pulmonary edema (acute) — *see also* Failure, ventricular, left I50.1
rheumatic fever (conditions in I00)
active I01.9
with chorea I02.0
specified NEC I01.8
inactive or quiescent (with chorea) I09.9
specified NEC I09.89
amyloid E85.4 *[I43]*
aortic (valve) I35.9
arteriosclerotic or sclerotic (senile) — *see* Disease, heart, ischemic, atherosclerotic
artery, arterial — *see* Disease, heart, ischemic, atherosclerotic
beer drinkers' I42.6
beriberi (wet) E51.12
black I27.0
congenital Q24.9
cyanotic Q24.9
specified NEC Q24.8
coronary — *see* Disease, heart, ischemic
cryptogenic I51.9
fibroid — *see* Myocarditis
functional I51.89
psychogenic F45.8
glycogen storage E74.02 *[I43]*
gonococcal A54.83

Disease, diseased — *continued*
heart — *continued*
hypertensive — *see* Hypertension, heart
hyperthyroid — *see also* Hyperthyroidism E05.90 *[I43]*
with thyroid storm E05.91 *[I43]*
ischemic (chronic or with a stated duration of over 4 weeks) I25.9
atherosclerotic (of) I25.10
with angina pectoris — *see* Arteriosclerosis, coronary (artery)
coronary artery bypass graft — *see* Arteriosclerosis, coronary (artery),
cardiomyopathy I25.5
diagnosed on ECG or other special investigation, but currently presenting no symptoms I25.6
silent I25.6
specified form NEC
acute I24.89
chronic I25.89
kyphoscoliotic I27.1
meningococcal A39.50
endocarditis A39.51
myocarditis A39.52
pericarditis A39.53
mitral I05.9
specified NEC I05.8
muscular — *see* Degeneration, myocardial
psychogenic (functional) F45.8
pulmonary (chronic) I27.9
in schistosomiasis B65.9 *[I52]*
specified NEC I27.89
rheumatic (chronic) (inactive) (old) (quiescent) (with chorea) I09.9
active or acute I01.9
with chorea (acute) (rheumatic) (Sydenham's) I02.0
specified NEC I09.89
senile — *see* Myocarditis
syphilitic A52.06
aortic A52.03
aneurysm A52.01
congenital A50.54 *[I52]*
thyrotoxic — *see also* Thyrotoxicosis E05.90 *[I43]*
with thyroid storm E05.91 *[I43]*
valve, valvular (obstructive) (regurgitant) — *see also* Endocarditis
congenital NEC Q24.8
pulmonary Q22.3
vascular — *see* Disease, cardiovascular
heavy chain NEC C88.2- ☑
alpha C88.3- ☑
gamma C88.2- ☑
mu C88.2- ☑
Hebra's
pityriasis
maculata et circinata L42
rubra pilaris L44.0
prurigo L28.2
hematopoietic organs D75.9
hemoglobin or Hb
abnormal (mixed) NEC D58.2
with thalassemia D56.9
AS genotype D57.3
Bart's D56.0
C (Hb-C) D58.2
with other abnormal hemoglobin NEC D58.2
elliptocytosis D58.1
Hb-S D57.2- ☑
sickle-cell D57.2- ☑
thalassemia D56.8
Constant Spring D58.2
D (Hb-D) D58.2
E (Hb-E) D58.2
E-beta thalassemia D56.5
elliptocytosis D58.1
H (Hb-H) (thalassemia) D56.0
with other abnormal hemoglobin NEC D56.9
Constant Spring D56.0
I thalassemia D56.9
M D74.0
S or SS D57.1
with
acute chest syndrome D57.01
cerebral vascular involvement D57.03
crisis (painful) D57.00
with complication specified NEC D57.09
pain (vaso-occlusive) D57.00
splenic sequestration D57.02

Disease, diseased — *continued*
hemoglobin or Hb — *continued*
S or SS — *continued*
beta plus D57.44
with
acute chest syndrome D57.451
cerebral vascular involvement D57.453
crisis D57.459
with specified complication NEC D57.458
pain (vaso-occlusive) D57.459
splenic sequestration D57.452
without crisis D57.44
beta zero D57.42
with
acute chest syndrome D57.431
cerebral vascular involvement D57.433
crisis D57.439
with specified complication NEC D57.438
pain (vaso-occlusive) D57.439
splenic sequestration D57.432
without crisis D57.42
SC D57.2- ☑
SD D57.8- ☑
SE D57.8- ☑
spherocytosis D58.0
unstable, hemolytic D58.2
hemolytic (newborn) P55.9
autoimmune D59.10
cold type (primary) (secondary) (symptomatic) D59.12
mixed type (primary) (secondary) (symptomatic) D59.13
warm type (primary) (secondary) (symptomatic) D59.11
drug-induced D59.0
due to or with
incompatibility
ABO (blood group) P55.1
blood (group) (Duffy) (K) (Kell) (Kidd) (Lewis) (M) (S) NEC P55.8
Rh (blood group) (factor) P55.0
Rh negative mother P55.0
specified type NEC P55.8
unstable hemoglobin D58.2
hemorrhagic D69.9
newborn P53
Henoch (-Schonlein) (purpura nervosa) D69.0
hepatic — *see* Disease, liver
hepatolenticular E83.01
heredodegenerative NEC
spinal cord G95.89
herpesviral, disseminated B00.7
Hers' (glycogenosis VI) E74.09
Herter (-Gee) (-Heubner) (nontropical sprue) K90.0
Heubner-Herter (nontropical sprue) K90.0
high fetal gene or hemoglobin thalassemia D56.9
Hildenbrand's — *see* Typhus
hip (joint) M25.9
congenital Q65.89
suppurative M00.9
tuberculous A18.02
His (-Werner) (trench fever) A79.0
Hodgson's — *see also* Aneurysm, aorta, thorax I71.20
ruptured — *see also* Aneurysm, aorta, thorax, ruptured I71.10
Holla — *see* Spherocytosis
hookworm B76.9
specified NEC B76.8
host-versus-graft D89.813
acute D89.810
acute on chronic D89.812
chronic D89.811
human immunodeficiency virus (HIV) B20
Huntington's G10
with dementia — *see also* Dementia, in, diseases specified elsewhere G10 *[F02.80]*
Hunt's (herpetic geniculate ganglionitis) (neuralgia) B02.21
dyssynergia cerebellaris myoclonica G11.19
Hutchinson's (cheiropompholyx) — *see* Hutchinson's disease
hyaline (diffuse) (generalized)
membrane (lung) (newborn) P22.0
adult J80
hydatid — *see* Echinococcus
hydroxyapatite deposition M11.00
ankle M11.07- ☑

☑ **Additional Character Required** — **Refer to the Tabular List for Character Selection**

Disease, diseased — *continued*
hydroxyapatite deposition — *continued*
  elbow M11.02- ☑
  foot joint M11.07- ☑
  hand joint M11.04- ☑
  hip M11.05- ☑
  knee M11.06- ☑
  multiple site M11.09
  shoulder M11.01- ☑
  vertebra M11.08
  wrist M11.03- ☑
hyperkinetic — *see* Hyperkinesia
hypertensive — *see* Hypertension
hypophysis E23.7
Iceland G93.39
I-cell E77.0
IgG4-related D89.84
immune D89.9
immunoglobulin G4-related D89.84
immunoproliferative (malignant) C88.9- ☑
  small intestinal C88.3- ☑
  specified NEC C88.8- ☑
inclusion B25.9
  salivary gland B25.9
infectious, infective B99.9
  congenital P37.9
    specified NEC P37.8
    viral P35.9
      specified type NEC P35.8
  specified NEC B99.8
inflammatory
  penis N48.29
    abscess N48.21
    cellulitis N48.22
  prepuce N47.7
    balanoposthitis N47.6
  tubo-ovarian — *see* Salpingo-oophoritis
intervertebral disc — *see also* Disorder, disc
  with myelopathy — *see* Disorder, disc, with, myelopathy
  cervical, cervicothoracic — *see* Disorder, disc, cervical
    with
      myelopathy — *see* Disorder, disc, cervical, with myelopathy
      neuritis, radiculitis or radiculopathy — *see* Disorder, disc, cervical, with neuritis
      specified NEC — *see* Disorder, disc, cervical, specified type NEC
  lumbar (with)
    myelopathy M51.06
    neuritis, radiculitis, radiculopathy or sciatica M51.16
    specified NEC M51.86
  lumbosacral (with)
    neuritis, radiculitis, radiculopathy or sciatica M51.17
    specified NEC M51.87
  specified NEC — *see* Disorder, disc, specified NEC
  thoracic (with)
    myelopathy M51.04
    neuritis, radiculitis or radiculopathy M51.14
    specified NEC M51.84
  thoracolumbar (with)
    myelopathy M51.05
    neuritis, radiculitis or radiculopathy M51.15
    specified NEC M51.85
intestine K63.9
  functional K59.9
    psychogenic F45.8
    specified NEC K59.89
  organic K63.9
  protozoal A07.9
  specified NEC K63.89
iris H21.9
  specified NEC H21.89
iron metabolism or storage E83.10
island (scrub typhus) A75.3
itai-itai — *see* Poisoning, cadmium
Jakob-Creutzfeldt — *see* Creutzfeldt-Jakob disease or syndrome
jaw M27.9
  fibrocystic M27.49
  specified NEC M27.8
jigger B88.1
joint — *see also* Disorder, joint
  Charcot's — *see* Arthropathy, neuropathic (Charcot)
  degenerative — *see* Osteoarthritis
    multiple M15.9

Disease, diseased — *continued*
joint — *see also* Disorder, joint — *continued*
  degenerative — *see* Osteoarthritis — *continued*
    spine — *see* Spondylosis
  facet joint — *see also* Spondylosis M47.819
  hypertrophic — *see* Osteoarthritis
  sacroiliac M53.3
  specified NEC — *see* Disorder, joint, specified type NEC
  spine NEC — *see* Dorsopathy
  suppurative — *see* Arthritis, pyogenic or pyemic
Jourdain's (acute gingivitis) K05.00
  nonplaque induced K05.01
  plaque induced K05.00
Kaschin-Beck (endemic polyarthritis) M12.10
  ankle M12.17- ☑
  elbow M12.12- ☑
  foot joint M12.17- ☑
  hand joint M12.14- ☑
  hip M12.15- ☑
  knee M12.16- ☑
  multiple site M12.19
  shoulder M12.11- ☑
  vertebra M12.18
  wrist M12.13- ☑
Katayama B65.2
Kedani (scrub typhus) A75.3
Keshan E59
kidney (functional) (pelvis) N28.9
  chronic N18.9
    hypertensive — *see* Hypertension, kidney
    stage 1 N18.1
    stage 2 (mild) N18.2
    stage 3 (moderate) N18.30
    stage 3a N18.31
    stage 3b N18.32
    stage 4 (severe) N18.4
    stage 5 N18.5
  complicating pregnancy — *see* Pregnancy, complicated by, renal disease
  cystic (congenital) Q61.9
  fibrocystic (congenital) Q61.8
  hypertensive — *see* Hypertension, kidney
  in (due to)
    schistosomiasis (bilharziasis) B65.9 *[N29]*
  multicystic Q61.4
  polycystic Q61.3
    adult type Q61.2
    childhood type NEC Q61.19
      collecting duct dilatation Q61.11
Kimmelstiel (-Wilson) (intercapillary polycystic (congenital) glomerulosclerosis) — *see* E08-E13 with .21
Kinnier Wilson's (hepatolenticular degeneration) E83.01
kissing — *see* Mononucleosis, infectious
Klebs' — *see also* Glomerulonephritis N05- ☑
Klippel-Feil (brevicollis) Q76.1
Kohler-Pellegrini-Stieda (calcification, knee joint) — *see* Bursitis, tibial collateral
Kok Q89.8
Konig's (osteochondritis dissecans) — *see* Osteochondritis, dissecans
Korsakoff's (nonalcoholic) F04
  alcoholic F10.96
    with dependence F10.26
Kostmann's (infantile genetic agranulocytosis) D70.0
kuru A81.81
Kyasanur Forest A98.2
labyrinth, ear — *see* Disorder, ear, inner
lacrimal system — *see* Disorder, lacrimal system
Lafora body — *see also* Epilepsy, progressive, Lafora G40.C09
Lancereaux-Mathieu (leptospiral jaundice) A27.0
Landry's G61.0
Larrey-Weil (leptospiral jaundice) A27.0
larynx J38.7
legionnaires' A48.1
  nonpneumonic A48.2
Lenegre's I44.2
lens H27.9
  specified NEC H27.8
Lev's (acquired complete heart block) I44.2
Lewy body (dementia) — *see also* Dementia, in, diseases specified elsewhere G31.83 *[F02.80]*
  with behavioral disturbance — *see also* Dementia, in, diseases specified elsewhere G31.83 *[F02.81-]* ☑
Lichtheim's (subacute combined sclerosis with pernicious anemia) D51.0

Disease, diseased — *continued*
Lightwood's (renal tubular acidosis) N25.89
Lignac's (cystinosis) E72.04
lip K13.0
lipid-storage E75.6
  specified NEC E75.5
Lipschutz's N76.6
liver (chronic) (organic) K76.9
  alcoholic (chronic) K70.9
    acute — *see* Disease, liver, alcoholic, hepatitis
    cirrhosis K70.30
      with ascites K70.31
    failure K70.40
      with coma K70.41
    fatty liver K70.0
    fibrosis K70.2
    hepatitis K70.10
      with ascites K70.11
    sclerosis K70.2
  cystic, congenital Q44.6
  drug-induced (idiosyncratic) (toxic) (predictable) (unpredictable) — *see* Disease, liver, toxic
  end stage K72.1- ☑
    due to hepatitis — *see* Hepatitis
    with coma K72.11
  fatty, nonalcoholic (NAFLD) K76.0
    alcoholic K70.0
  fibrocystic (congenital) Q44.6
  fluke
    Chinese B66.1
    oriental B66.1
    sheep B66.3
  gestational alloimmune (GALD) P78.84
  glycogen storage E74.09 *[K77]*
  in (due to)
    schistosomiasis (bilharziasis) B65.9 *[K77]*
  inflammatory K75.9
    alcoholic K70.1 ☑
    specified NEC K75.89
  polycystic (congenital) Q44.6
  toxic K71.9
    with
      cholestasis K71.0
      cirrhosis (liver) K71.7
      fibrosis (liver) K71.7
      focal nodular hyperplasia K71.8
      hepatic granuloma K71.8
      hepatic necrosis K71.10
        with coma K71.11
      hepatitis NEC K71.6
        acute K71.2
        chronic
          active K71.50
            with ascites K71.51
          lobular K71.4
          persistent K71.3
        lupoid K71.50
          with ascites K71.51
      peliosis hepatis K71.8
      veno-occlusive disease (VOD) of liver K71.8
    veno-occlusive K76.5
Lobo's (keloid blastomycosis) B48.0
Lobstein's (brittle bones and blue sclera) Q78.0
Ludwig's (submaxillary cellulitis) K12.2
lumbosacral region M53.87
lung J98.4
  black J60
  congenital Q33.9
  cystic J98.4
    congenital Q33.0
  dabbing (related) U07.0
  electronic cigarette (related) U07.0
  fibroid (chronic) — *see* Fibrosis, lung
  fluke B66.4
    oriental B66.4
  in
    amyloidosis E85.4 *[J99]*
    sarcoidosis D86.0
    Sjogren's syndrome M35.02
    systemic
      lupus erythematosus M32.13
      sclerosis M34.81
  interstitial J84.9
    with progressive fibrotic phenotype, in diseases classified elsewhere J84.170
    drug-induced — *see* Disorder, lung, interstitial, drug-induced
    of childhood, specified NEC J84.848

☑ **Additional Character Required — Refer to the Tabular List for Character Selection**

Disease, diseased — *continued*
- lung — *continued*
  - interstitial — *continued*
    - of childhood, specified — *continued*
      - drug-induced — *see* Disorder, lung, interstitial, drug-induced
      - respiratory bronchiolitis J84.115
      - specified NEC J84.89
    - obstructive (chronic) J44.9
      - with
        - acute
          - bronchitis J44.0
            - exacerbation NEC J44.1
            - lower respiratory infection J44.0
        - alveolitis, allergic J67.9
        - asthma J44.89
        - bronchiectasis J47.9
          - with
            - exacerbation (acute) J47.1
            - lower respiratory infection J47.0
        - bronchitis J44.89
          - with
            - exacerbation (acute) J44.1
            - lower respiratory infection J44.0
        - emphysema J43.9
        - hypersensitivity pneumonitis J67.9
      - decompensated J44.1
        - with
          - exacerbation (acute) J44.1
    - polycystic J98.4
      - congenital Q33.0
    - rheumatoid (diffuse) (interstitial) — *see* Rheumatoid, lung
    - vaping (associated) (device) (product) (use) U07.0
- Lutembacher's (atrial septal defect with mitral stenosis) Q21.19
- Lyme A69.20
- lymphatic (gland) (system) (channel) (vessel) I89.9
- lymphoproliferative D47.9
  - specified NEC D47.Z9 (*following* D47.4)
  - T-gamma D47.Z9 (*following* D47.4)
  - X-linked D82.3
- Magitot's M27.2
- malarial — *see* Malaria
- malignant — *see also* Neoplasm, malignant, by site
- Manson's B65.1
- maple bark J67.6
- maple-syrup-urine E71.0
- Marburg (virus) A98.3
- Marion's (bladder neck obstruction) N32.0
- Marsh's (exophthalmic goiter) — *see* Hyperthyroidism, with, goiter (diffuse)
- mastoid (process) — *see* Disorder, ear, middle
- Mathieu's (leptospiral jaundice) A27.0
- Maxcy's A75.2
- McArdle (-Schmid-Pearson) (glycogenosis V) E74.04
- mediastinum J98.59
- medullary center (idiopathic) (respiratory) G93.89
- Meige's (chronic hereditary edema) Q82.0
- meningococcal — *see* Infection, meningococcal
- mental F99
  - organic F09
- mesenchymal M35.9
- mesenteric embolic — *see also* Ischemia, intestine, acute K55.039
- metabolic, metabolism E88.9
  - bilirubin E80.7
- metal-polisher's J62.8
- metastatic — *see also* Neoplasm, secondary, by site C79.9
- microvascular - code to condition
- microvillus
  - atrophy Q43.8
  - inclusion (MVD) Q43.8
- middle ear — *see* Disorder, ear, middle
- Mikulicz' (dryness of mouth, absent or decreased lacrimation) K11.8
- Milroy's (chronic hereditary edema) Q82.0
- Minamata — *see* Poisoning, mercury
- minicore G71.29
- Minor's G95.19
- Minot's (hemorrhagic disease, newborn) P53
- Minot-von Willebrand-Jurgens (angiohemophilia) — *see* Disease, von Willebrand
- Mitchell's (erythromelalgia) I73.81
- mitral (valve) I05.9
  - nonrheumatic I34.9
- mixed connective tissue M35.1
- MOG antibody G37.81
- moldy hay J67.0

Disease, diseased — *continued*
- Monge's T70.29 ☑
- Morgagni-Adams-Stokes (syncope with heart block) I45.9
- Morgagni's (syndrome) (hyperostosis frontalis interna) M85.2
- Morton's (with metatarsalgia) — *see* Lesion, nerve, plantar
- Morvan's G60.8
- motor neuron (bulbar) (mixed type) (spinal) G12.20
  - amyotrophic lateral sclerosis G12.21
  - familial G12.24
  - progressive bulbar palsy G12.22
  - specified NEC G12.29
- moyamoya I67.5
- mu heavy chain disease C88.2- ☑
- multicore G71.29
- multiminicore G71.29
- muscle — *see also* Disorder, muscle
  - inflammatory — *see* Myositis
  - ocular (external) — *see* Strabismus
- musculoskeletal system, soft tissue — *see also* Disorder, soft tissue
  - specified NEC — *see* Disorder, soft tissue, specified type NEC
- mushroom workers' J67.5
- mycotic B49
- myelin oligodendrocyte glycoprotein antibody G37.81
- myelodysplastic — *see also* Syndrome, myelodysplastic C94.6
- myelodysplastic/myeloproliferative neoplasm, unclassifiable C94.6
- myeloproliferative D47.1
  - chronic D47.1
  - not classified C94.6
  - specified NEC C94.6
  - unclassifiable C94.6
- myocardium, myocardial — *see also* Degeneration, myocardial I51.5
  - primary (idiopathic) I42.9
- myoneural G70.9
- Naegeli's D69.1
- nails L60.9
  - specified NEC L60.8
- Nairobi (sheep virus) A93.8
- nasal J34.9
- nemaline body G71.21
- nerve — *see* Disorder, nerve
- nervous system G98.8
  - autonomic G90.9
  - central G96.9
    - specified NEC G96.89
  - congenital Q07.9
  - parasympathetic G90.9
  - specified NEC G98.8
  - sympathetic G90.9
  - vegetative G90.9
- neuromuscular system G70.9
- Newcastle B30.8
- Nicolas (-Durand)-Favre (climatic bubo) A55
- nipple N64.9
  - Paget's C50.01- ☑
    - female C50.01- ☑
    - male C50.02- ☑
- Nishimoto (-Takeuchi) I67.5
- nonarthropod-borne NOS (viral) B34.9
  - enterovirus NEC B34.1
- nonautoimmune hemolytic D59.4
  - drug-induced D59.2
- Nonne-Milroy-Meige (chronic hereditary edema) Q82.0
- nose J34.9
- nucleus pulposus — *see* Disorder, disc
- nutritional E63.9
- oast-house-urine E72.19
  - ocular
    - herpesviral B00.50
    - zoster B02.30
- obliterative vascular I77.1
- Ohara's — *see* Tularemia
- Opitz's (congestive splenomegaly) D73.2
- Oppenheim-Urbach (necrobiosis lipoidica diabeticorum) — *see* E08-E13 with .620
- optic nerve NEC — *see* Disorder, nerve, optic
- orbit — *see* Disorder, orbit
- organ
  - dabbing (related) U07.0
  - electronic cigarette (related) U07.0
  - vaping (associated) (device) (product) (use) U07.0
- Oriental liver fluke B66.1

Disease, diseased — *continued*
- Oriental lung fluke B66.4
- Ormond's N13.5
- Oropouche virus A93.0
- Osler-Rendu (familial hemorrhagic telangiectasia) I78.0
- osteofibrocystic E21.0
- Otto's M24.7
- outer ear — *see* Disorder, ear, external
- ovary (noninflammatory) N83.9
  - cystic N83.20- ☑
  - inflammatory — *see* Salpingo-oophoritis
  - polycystic E28.2
  - specified NEC N83.8
- Owren's (congenital) — *see* Defect, coagulation
- p110d-activating mutation causing senescent T cells, lymphadenopathy, and immunodeficiency [PASLI] D81.82
- pancreas K86.9
  - cystic K86.2
  - fibrocystic E84.9
  - specified NEC K86.89
- panvalvular I08.9
  - specified NEC I08.8
- parametrium (noninflammatory) N83.9
- parasitic B89
  - cerebral NEC B71.9 *[G94]*
  - intestinal NOS B82.9
  - mouth B37.0
  - skin NOS B88.9
  - specified type — *see* Infestation
  - tongue B37.0
- parathyroid (gland) E21.5
  - specified NEC E21.4
- Parkinson's G20.A1
  - with dyskinesia
    - with
      - fluctuations G20.B2
      - OFF episodes G20.B2
    - without mention of
      - fluctuations G20.B1
      - OFF episodes G20.B1
  - without dyskinesia
    - with
      - fluctuations G20.A2
      - OFF episodes G20.A2
    - without mention of
      - fluctuations G20.A1
      - OFF episodes G20.A1
- parodontal K05.6
- Parrot's (syphilitic osteochondritis) A50.02
- Parry's (exophthalmic goiter) — *see* Hyperthyroidism, with, goiter (diffuse)
- Parson's (exophthalmic goiter) — *see* Hyperthyroidism, with, goiter (diffuse)
- Paxton's (white piedra) B36.2
- pearl-worker's — *see* Osteomyelitis, specified type NEC
- Pellegrini-Stieda (calcification, knee joint) — *see* Bursitis, tibial collateral
- pelvis, pelvic
  - female NOS N94.9
    - specified NEC N94.89
  - gonococcal (acute) (chronic) A54.24
  - inflammatory (female) N73.9
    - acute N73.0
    - chlamydial A56.11
    - chronic N73.1
    - specified NEC N73.8
    - syphilitic (secondary) A51.42
      - late A52.76
    - tuberculous A18.17
  - organ, female N94.9
  - peritoneum, female NEC N94.89
- penis N48.9
  - inflammatory N48.29
    - abscess N48.21
    - cellulitis N48.22
  - specified NEC N48.89
- periapical tissues NOS K04.90
- periodontal K05.6
  - specified NEC K05.5
- periosteum — *see* Disorder, bone, specified type NEC
- peripheral
  - arterial I73.9
  - autonomic nervous system G90.9
  - nerves — *see* Polyneuropathy
  - vascular NOS I73.9
    - in diabetes mellitus — *see* Diabetes, by type, with peripheral angiopathy
- peritoneum K66.9

Disease, diseased — *continued*

peritoneum — *continued*
  pelvic, female NEC N94.89
  specified NEC K66.8
persistent mucosal (middle ear) H66.20
  left H66.22
    with right H66.23
  right H66.21
    with left H66.23
Petit's — *see* Hernia, abdomen, specified site NEC
pharynx J39.2
  specified NEC J39.2
Phocas' — *see* Mastopathy, cystic
photochromogenic (acid-fast bacilli) (pulmonary) A31.0
  nonpulmonary A31.9
Pick's — *see also* Dementia, in, diseases specified elsewhere G31.01 *[F02.80]*
  with behavioral disturbance — *see also* Dementia, in,
    diseases specified elsewhere
    G31.01 *[F02.81-]* ✓
  brain G31.01 *[F02.80]*
    with behavioral disturbance — *see also* Dementia,
     in, diseases specified elsewhere
     G31.01 *[F02.81-]* ✓
  of pericardium (pericardial pseudocirrhosis of liver)
    I31.1
pigeon fancier's J67.2
pineal gland E34.8
pink — *see* Poisoning, mercury
Pinkus' (lichen nitidus) L44.1
pinworm B80
Piry virus A93.8
pituitary (gland) E23.7
pituitary-snuff-taker's J67.8
pleura (cavity) J94.9
  specified NEC J94.8
pneumatic drill (hammer) T75.21 ✓
Pollitzer's (hidradenitis suppurativa) L73.2
polycystic
  kidney or renal Q61.3
    adult type Q61.2
    childhood type NEC Q61.19
      collecting duct dilatation Q61.11
  liver or hepatic Q44.6
  lung or pulmonary J98.4
    congenital Q33.0
  ovary, ovaries E28.2
  spleen Q89.09
polyethylene T84.05- ✓
Pompe's (glycogenosis II) E74.02
Posadas-Wernicke B38.9
Potain's (pulmonary edema) — *see* Edema, lung
prepuce N47.8
  inflammatory N47.7
    balanoposthitis N47.6
Pringle's (tuberous sclerosis) Q85.1
prion, central nervous system A81.9
  specified NEC A81.89
prostate N42.9
  specified NEC N42.89
protozoal B64
  acanthamebiasis — *see* Acanthamebiasis
  African trypanosomiasis — *see* African trypanosomi-
    asis
  babesiosis — *see also* Babesiosis B60.00
  Chagas disease — *see* Chagas disease
  intestine, intestinal A07.9
  leishmaniasis — *see* Leishmaniasis
  malaria — *see* Malaria
  naegleriasis B60.2
  pneumocystosis B59
  specified organism NEC B60.8
  toxoplasmosis — *see* Toxoplasmosis
pseudo-Hurler's E77.0
psychiatric F99
psychotic — *see* Psychosis
Puente's (simple glandular cheilitis) K13.0
puerperal — *see also* Puerperal O90.89
pulmonary — *see also* Disease, lung
  artery I28.9
  chronic obstructive J44.9
    with
      acute bronchitis J44.0
      exacerbation (acute) J44.1
      lower respiratory infection (acute) J44.0
    decompensated J44.1
      with
        exacerbation (acute) J44.1
  heart I27.9

Disease, diseased — *continued*

pulmonary — *see also* Disease, lung — *continued*
  heart — *continued*
    specified NEC I27.89
    hypertensive (vascular) — *see also* Hypertension,
     pulmonary I27.20
     NEC I27.2 ✓
     primary (idiopathic) I27.0
  valve I37.9
    rheumatic I09.89
pulp (dental) NOS K04.90
pulseless M31.4
Putnam's (subacute combined sclerosis with pernicious
  anemia) D51.0
Pyle (-Cohn) (metaphyseal dysplasia) Q78.5
ragpicker's or ragsorter's A22.1
Raynaud's — *see* Raynaud's disease
reactive airway — *see* Asthma
Reclus' (cystic) — *see* Mastopathy, cystic
rectum K62.9
  specified NEC K62.89
Refsum's (heredopathia atactica polyneuritiformis) G60.1
renal (functional) (pelvis) — *see also* Disease, kidney
  N28.9
  with
    edema — *see* Nephrosis
    glomerular lesion — *see* Glomerulonephritis
     with edema — *see* Nephrosis
    interstitial nephritis N12
  acute N28.9
  chronic — *see also* Disease, kidney, chronic N18.9
  cystic, congenital Q61.9
  diabetic — *see* E08-E13 with .22
  end-stage (failure) N18.6
    due to hypertension I12.0
  fibrocystic (congenital) Q61.8
  hypertensive — *see* Hypertension, kidney
  lupus M32.14
  phosphate-losing (tubular) N25.0
  polycystic (congenital) Q61.3
    adult type Q61.2
    childhood type NEC Q61.19
      collecting duct dilatation Q61.11
  rapidly progressive N01.9
  subacute N01.9
Rendu-Osler-Weber (familial hemorrhagic telangiectasia)
  I78.0
renovascular (arteriosclerotic) — *see* Hypertension, kidney
respiratory (tract) J98.9
  acute or subacute NOS J06.9
    due to
      chemicals, gases, fumes or vapors (inhalation)
        J68.3
      external agent J70.9
        specified NEC J70.8
      radiation J70.0
      smoke inhalation J70.5
    noninfectious J39.8
  chronic NOS J98.9
    due to
      chemicals, gases, fumes or vapors J68.4
      external agent J70.9
        specified NEC J70.8
      radiation J70.1
  newborn P27.9
    specified NEC P27.8
  due to
    chemicals, gases, fumes or vapors J68.9
      acute or subacute NEC J68.3
      chronic J68.4
    external agent J70.9
      specified NEC J70.8
  newborn P28.9
    specified type NEC P28.89
  upper J39.9
    acute or subacute J06.9
    noninfectious NEC J39.8
    specified NEC J39.8
    streptococcal J06.9
retina, retinal H35.9
  Batten's or Batten-Mayou E75.4 *[H36.89]*
  specified NEC H35.89
rheumatoid — *see* Arthritis, rheumatoid
rickettsial NOS A79.9
  specified type NEC A79.89
Riga (-Fede) (cachectic aphthae) K14.0
Riggs' (compound periodontitis) — *see* Periodontitis
Ritter's L00

Disease, diseased — *continued*

Rivalta's (cervicofacial actinomycosis) A42.2
Robles' (onchocerciasis) B73.01
rod body G71.21
Roger's (congenital interventricular septal defect) Q21.0
Rosenthal's (factor XI deficiency) D68.1
Ross River B33.1
Rossbach's (hyperchlorhydria) K31.89
  psychogenic F45.8
Rotes Querol — *see* Hyperostosis, ankylosing
Roth (-Bernhardt) — *see* Mononeuropathy, lower limb,
  meralgia paresthetica
Runeberg's (progressive pernicious anemia) D51.0
sacroiliac NEC M53.3
salivary gland or duct K11.9
  inclusion B25.9
  specified NEC K11.8
  virus B25.9
sandworm B76.9
Schimmelbusch's — *see* Mastopathy, cystic
Schmorl's — *see* Schmorl's disease or nodes
Schonlein (-Henoch) (purpura rheumatica) D69.0
Schottmuller's — *see* Fever, paratyphoid
Schultz's (agranulocytosis) — *see* Agranulocytosis
Schwalbe-Ziehen-Oppenheim G24.1
Schwartz-Jampel G71.13
sclera H15.9
  specified NEC H15.89
scrofulous (tuberculous) A18.2
scrotum N50.9
sebaceous glands L73.9
semilunar cartilage, cystic — *see also* Derangement, knee,
  meniscus, cystic
seminal vesicle N50.9
serum NEC — *see also* Reaction, serum T80.69 ✓
sexually transmitted A64
  anogenital
    herpesviral infection — *see* Herpes, anogenital
    warts A63.0
  chancroid A57
  chlamydial infection — *see* Chlamydia
  gonorrhea — *see* Gonorrhea
  granuloma inguinale A58
  specified organism NEC A63.8
  syphilis — *see* Syphilis
  trichomoniasis — *see* Trichomoniasis
Sezary C84.1- ✓
shimamushi (scrub typhus) A75.3
shipyard B30.0
sickle-cell D57.1
  with
    acute chest syndrome D57.01
    cerebral vascular involvement D57.03
    crisis (painful) D57.00
      with
        complication specified NEC D57.09
        dactylitis D57.04
    dactylitis D57.04
    pain (vaso-occlusive) D57.00
    priapism D57.09
    splenic sequestration D57.02
  elliptocytosis D57.8- ✓
  Hb-C D57.20
    with
      acute chest syndrome D57.211
      cerebral vascular involvement D57.213
      crisis D57.219
        with
          dactylitis D57.214
          specified complication NEC D57.218
      dactylitis D57.214
      pain (vaso-occlusive) D57.219
      priapism D57.218
      splenic sequestration D57.212
    without crisis D57.20
  Hb-SD D57.80
    with
      acute chest syndrome D57.811
      cerebral vascular involvement D57.813
      crisis D57.819
        with
          complication specified NEC D57.818
          dactylitis D57.814
      dactylitis D57.814
      pain (vaso-occlusive) D57.819
      splenic sequestration D57.812
    without crisis D57.80
  Hb-SE D57.80

Disease, diseased — *continued*
  sickle-cell — *continued*
    Hb-SE — *continued*
      with
        acute chest syndrome D57.811
        cerebral vascular involvement D57.813
        crisis D57.819
          with
            complication specified NEC D57.818
            dactylitis D57.814
        dactylitis D57.814
        pain (vaso-occlusive) D57.819
        splenic sequestration D57.812
      without crisis D57.80
    specified NEC D57.80
      with
        acute chest syndrome D57.811
        cerebral vascular involvement D57.813
        crisis D57.819
          with
            complication specified NEC D57.818
            dactylitis D57.814
        dactylitis D57.814
        pain (vaso-occlusive) D57.819
        splenic sequestration D57.812
      without crisis D57.80
    spherocytosis D57.80
      with
        acute chest syndrome D57.811
        cerebral vascular involvement D57.813
        crisis D57.819
          with complication specified NEC D57.818
        pain (vaso-occlusive) D57.819
        splenic sequestration D57.812
      without crisis D57.80
    thalassemia D57.40
      with
        acute chest syndrome D57.411
          with dactylitis D57.414
          with specified complication NEC D57.418
        cerebral vascular involvement D57.413
        crisis (painful) D57.419
          with specified complication NEC D57.418
        dactylitis D57.414
        pain (vaso-occlusive) D57.419
        splenic sequestration D57.412
      beta plus D57.44
        with
          acute chest syndrome D57.451
            with dactylitis D57.454
          cerebral vascular involvement D57.453
          crisis D57.459
            with specified complication NEC D57.458
          dactylitis D57.454
          pain (vaso-occlusive) D57.459
          splenic sequestration D57.452
        without crisis D57.44
      beta zero D57.42
        with
          acute chest syndrome D57.431
            with dactylitis D57.434
          cerebral vascular involvement D57.433
          crisis D57.439
            with specified complication NEC D57.438
          dactylitis D57.434
          pain (vaso-occlusive) D57.439
          splenic sequestration D57.432
        without crisis D57.42
  silo-filler's J68.8
    bronchitis J68.0
    pneumonitis J68.0
    pulmonary edema J68.1
  simian B B00.4
  Simons' (progressive lipodystrophy) E88.1
  sin nombre virus B33.4
  sinus — *see* Sinusitis
  Sirkari's B55.0
  sixth B08.20
    due to human herpesvirus 6 B08.21
    due to human herpesvirus 7 B08.22
  skin L98.9
    due to metabolic disorder NEC E88.9 *[L99]*
    specified NEC L98.8
  slim (HIV) B20
  small vessel I73.9
  Sneddon-Wilkinson (subcorneal pustular dermatosis)
    L13.1

Disease, diseased — *continued*
  South African creeping B88.0
  spinal (cord) G95.9
    congenital Q06.9
    specified NEC G95.89
  spine — *see also* Spondylopathy
    joint — *see* Dorsopathy
    tuberculous A18.01
  spinocerebellar (hereditary) G11.9
    specified NEC G11.8
  spleen D73.9
    amyloid E85.4 *[D77]*
    organic D73.9
    polycystic Q89.09
    postinfectional D73.89
  sponge-diver's — *see* Toxicity, venom, marine animal,
    sea anemone
  Startle Q89.8
  Steinert's G71.11
  Sticker's (erythema infectiosum) B08.3
  Stieda's (calcification, knee joint) — *see* Bursitis, tibial
    collateral
  Stokes' (exophthalmic goiter) — *see* Hyperthyroidism,
    with, goiter (diffuse)
  Stokes-Adams (syncope with heart block) I45.9
  stomach K31.9
    functional, psychogenic F45.8
    specified NEC K31.89
  stonemason's J62.8
  storage
    glycogen — *see* Disease, glycogen storage
    mucopolysaccharide — *see* Mucopolysaccharidosis
  striatopallidal system NEC G25.89
  Stuart-Prower (congenital factor X deficiency) D68.2
  Stuart's (congenital factor X deficiency) D68.2
  subcutaneous tissue — *see* Disease, skin
  supporting structures of teeth K08.9
    specified NEC K08.89
  suprarenal (capsule) (gland) E27.9
    hyperfunction E27.0
    specified NEC E27.8
  sweat glands L74.9
    specified NEC L74.8
  Sweeley-Klionsky E75.21
  Swift (-Feer) — *see* Poisoning, mercury
  swimming-pool granuloma A31.1
  Sylvest's (epidemic pleurodynia) B33.0
  sympathetic nervous system G90.9
  synovium — *see* Disorder, synovium
  syphilitic — *see* Syphilis
  systemic tissue mast cell D47.02
  tanapox (virus) B08.71
  Tangier E78.6
  Tarral-Besnier (pityriasis rubra pilaris) L44.0
  Tauri's E74.09
  tear duct — *see* Disorder, lacrimal system
  tendon, tendinous — *see also* Disorder, tendon
    nodular — *see* Trigger finger
  terminal vessel I73.9
  testis N50.9
  thalassemia Hb-S — *see* Disease, sickle-cell, thalassemia
  Thaysen-Gee (nontropical sprue) K90.0
  Thomsen G71.12
  throat J39.2
    septic J02.0
  thromboembolic — *see* Embolism
  thymus (gland) E32.9
    specified NEC E32.8
  thyroid (gland) E07.9
    heart — *see also* Hyperthyroidism E05.90 *[I43]*
      with thyroid storm E05.91 *[I43]*
    specified NEC E07.89
  Tietze's M94.0
  tongue K14.9
    specified NEC K14.8
  tonsils, tonsillar (and adenoids) J35.9
  tooth, teeth K08.9
    hard tissues K03.9
      specified NEC K03.89
    pulp NEC K04.99
    specified NEC K08.89
  Tourette's F95.2
  trachea NEC J39.8
  tricuspid I07.9
    nonrheumatic I36.9
  triglyceride-storage E75.5
  trophoblast c — *see* Mole, hydatidiform
  tsutsugamushi A75.3
  tube (fallopian) (noninflammatory) N83.9

Disease, diseased — *continued*
  tube — *continued*
    inflammatory — *see* Salpingitis
    specified NEC N83.8
  tuberculous NEC — *see* Tuberculosis
  tubo-ovarian (noninflammatory) N83.9
    inflammatory — *see* Salpingo-oophoritis
    specified NEC N83.8
  tubotympanic, chronic — *see* Otitis, media, suppurative,
    chronic, tubotympanic
  tubulo-interstitial N15.9
    specified NEC N15.8
  tympanum — *see* Disorder, tympanic membrane
  Uhl's Q24.8
  Underwood's (sclerema neonatorum) P83.0
  Unverricht (-Lundborg) — *see* Epilepsy, generalized, id-
    iopathic
  Urbach-Oppenheim (necrobiosis lipoidica diabeticorum)
    — *see* E08-E13 with .620
  ureter N28.9
    in (due to)
      schistosomiasis (bilharziasis) B65.0 *[N29]*
  urethra N36.9
    specified NEC N36.8
  urinary (tract) N39.9
    bladder N32.9
      specified NEC N32.89
    specified NEC N39.8
  uterus (noninflammatory) N85.9
    infective — *see* Endometritis
    inflammatory — *see* Endometritis
    specified NEC N85.8
  uveal tract (anterior) H21.9
    posterior H31.9
  vagabond's B85.1
  vagina, vaginal (noninflammatory) N89.9
    inflammatory NEC N76.89
    specified NEC N89.8
  valve, valvular I38
    multiple I08.9
      specified NEC I08.8
  van Creveld-von Gierke (glycogenosis I) E74.01
  vas deferens N50.9
  vascular I99.9
    arteriosclerotic — *see* Arteriosclerosis
    ciliary body NEC — *see* Disorder, iris, vascular
    hypertensive — *see* Hypertension
    iris NEC — *see* Disorder, iris, vascular
    obliterative I77.1
      peripheral I73.9
    occlusive I99.8
    peripheral (occlusive) I73.9
      in diabetes mellitus — *see* E08-E13 with .51
  vasomotor I73.9
  vasospastic I73.9
  vein I87.9
  venereal — *see also* Disease, sexually transmitted A64
    chlamydial NEC A56.8
      anus A56.3
      genitourinary NOS A56.2
      pharynx A56.4
      rectum A56.3
    fifth A55
    sixth A55
    specified nature or type NEC A63.8
  vertebra, vertebral — *see also* Spondylopathy
    disc — *see* Disorder, disc
  vibration — *see* Vibration, adverse effects
  viral, virus — *see also* Disease, by type of virus B34.9
    arbovirus NOS A94
    arthropod-borne NOS A94
    congenital P35.9
      specified NEC P35.8
    Hanta (with renal manifestations) (Dobrava) (Pu-
      umala) (Seoul) A98.5
      with pulmonary manifestations (Andes) (Bayou)
        (Bermejo) (Black Creek Canal) (Choclo)
        (Juquitiba) (Laguna negra) (Lechiguanas)
        (New York) (Oran) (Sin nombre) B33.4
    Hantaan (Korean hemorrhagic fever) A98.5
    human immunodeficiency (HIV) B20
    Kunjin A83.4
    nonarthropod-borne NOS B34.9
    Powassan A84.81
    Rocio (encephalitis) A83.6
    Sin nombre (Hantavirus) (cardio)-pulmonary syn-
      drome) B33.4
    Tahyna B33.8
    vesicular stomatitis A93.8

☑ **Additional Character Required** — **Refer to the Tabular List for Character Selection**

Index

Disease, diseased — Dislocation

Disease, diseased — *continued*
- vitreous H43.9
  - specified NEC H43.89
- vocal cord J38.3
- Volkmann's, acquired T79.6 ☑
- von Eulenburg's (congenital paramyotonia) G71.19
- von Gierke's (glycogenosis I) E74.01
- von Graefe's — *see* Strabismus, paralytic, ophthalmoplegia, progressive
- von Willebrand (-Jurgens) (angiohemophilia) D68.00
  - acquired D68.04
  - platelet-type D68.09
  - pseudo D68.09
  - specified NEC D68.09
  - type 1 D68.01
  - type 1C D68.01
  - type 2 D68.029
    - type 2A D68.020
    - type 2B D68.021
    - type 2M D68.022
    - type 2N D68.023
  - type 3 D68.03
- Vrolik's (osteogenesis imperfecta) Q78.0
- vulva (noninflammatory) N90.9
  - inflammatory NEC N76.89
  - specified NEC N90.89
- Wallgren's (obstruction of splenic vein with collateral circulation) I87.8
- Wassilieff's (leptospiral jaundice) A27.0
- wasting NEC E88.A
  - due to
    - malnutrition E43
      - with marasmus E41
    - underlying condition E88.A
      - with marasmus E41
- Waterhouse-Friderichsen A39.1
- Wegner's (syphilitic osteochondritis) A50.02
- Weil's (leptospiral jaundice of lung) A27.0
- Weir Mitchell's (erythromelalgia) I73.81
- Werdnig-Hoffmann G12.0
- Wermer's E31.21
- Werner-His (trench fever) A79.0
- Werner-Schultz (neutropenic splenomegaly) D73.81
- Wernicke-Posadas B38.9
- whipworm B79
- white blood cells D72.9
  - specified NEC D72.89
- white matter R90.82
- white-spot, meaning lichen sclerosus et atrophicus L90.0
  - penis N48.0
  - vulva N90.4
- Wilkie's K55.1
- Wilkinson-Sneddon (subcorneal pustular dermatosis) L13.1
- Willis' — *see* Diabetes
- Wilson's (hepatolenticular degeneration) E83.01
- woolsorter's A22.1
- yaba monkey tumor B08.72
- yaba pox (virus) B08.72
- Zika virus A92.5
  - congenital P35.4
- zoonotic, bacterial A28.9
  - specified type NEC A28.8

Disfigurement (due to scar) L90.5
Disgerminoma — *see* Dysgerminoma
DISH (diffuse idiopathic skeletal hyperostosis) — *see* Hyperostosis, ankylosing
Disinsertion, retina — *see* Detachment, retina
Dislocatable hip, congenital Q65.6
Dislocation (articular)
- with fracture — *see* Fracture
- acromioclavicular (joint) S43.10- ☑
  - with displacement
    - 100%-200% S43.12- ☑
    - more than 200% S43.13- ☑
  - inferior S43.14- ☑
  - posterior S43.15- ☑
- ankle S93.0- ☑
- astragalus — *see* Dislocation, ankle
- atlantoaxial S13.121 ☑
- atlantooccipital S13.111 ☑
- atloidooccipital S13.111 ☑
- breast bone S23.29 ☑
- capsule, joint — *code by* site under Dislocation
- carpal (bone) — *see* Dislocation, wrist
- carpometacarpal (joint) NEC S63.05- ☑
  - thumb S63.04- ☑

Dislocation — *continued*
- cartilage (joint) — *code by* site under Dislocation
- cervical spine (vertebra) — *see* Dislocation, vertebra, cervical
- chronic — *see* Dislocation, recurrent
- clavicle — *see* Dislocation, acromioclavicular joint
- coccyx S33.2 ☑
- congenital NEC Q68.8
- coracoid — *see* Dislocation, shoulder
- costal cartilage S23.29 ☑
- costochondral S23.29 ☑
- cricoarytenoid articulation S13.29 ☑
- cricothyroid articulation S13.29 ☑
- dorsal vertebra — *see* Dislocation, vertebra, thoracic
- ear ossicle — *see* Discontinuity, ossicles, ear
- elbow S53.10- ☑
  - congenital Q68.8
  - pathological — *see* Dislocation, pathological NEC, elbow
  - radial head alone — *see* Dislocation, radial head
  - recurrent — *see* Dislocation, recurrent, elbow
  - traumatic S53.10- ☑
    - anterior S53.11- ☑
    - lateral S53.14- ☑
    - medial S53.13- ☑
    - posterior S53.12- ☑
    - specified type NEC S53.19- ☑
- eye, nontraumatic — *see* Luxation, globe
- eyeball, nontraumatic — *see* Luxation, globe
- femur
  - distal end — *see* Dislocation, knee
  - proximal end — *see* Dislocation, hip
- fibula
  - distal end — *see* Dislocation, ankle
  - proximal end — *see* Dislocation, knee
- finger S63.25- ☑
  - index S63.25- ☑
  - interphalangeal S63.27- ☑
    - distal S63.29- ☑
      - index S63.29- ☑
      - little S63.29- ☑
      - middle S63.29- ☑
      - ring S63.29- ☑
    - index S63.27- ☑
    - little S63.27- ☑
    - middle S63.27- ☑
    - proximal S63.28- ☑
      - index S63.28- ☑
      - little S63.28- ☑
      - middle S63.28- ☑
      - ring S63.28- ☑
    - ring S63.27- ☑
  - little S63.25- ☑
  - metacarpophalangeal S63.26- ☑
    - index S63.26- ☑
    - little S63.26- ☑
    - middle S63.26- ☑
    - ring S63.26- ☑
  - middle S63.25- ☑
  - recurrent — *see* Dislocation, recurrent, finger
  - ring S63.25- ☑
  - thumb — *see* Dislocation, thumb
- foot S93.30- ☑
  - recurrent — *see* Dislocation, recurrent, foot
  - specified site NEC S93.33- ☑
  - tarsal joint S93.31- ☑
  - tarsometatarsal joint S93.32- ☑
  - toe — *see* Dislocation, toe
- fracture — *see* Fracture
- glenohumeral (joint) — *see* Dislocation, shoulder
- glenoid — *see* Dislocation, shoulder
- habitual — *see* Dislocation, recurrent
- hip S73.00- ☑
  - anterior S73.03- ☑
    - obturator S73.02- ☑
  - central S73.04- ☑
  - congenital (total) Q65.2
    - bilateral Q65.1
    - partial Q65.5
      - bilateral Q65.4
      - unilateral Q65.3- ☑
    - unilateral Q65.0- ☑
  - developmental M24.85- ☑
  - pathological — *see* Dislocation, pathological NEC, hip
  - posterior S73.01- ☑
  - recurrent — *see* Dislocation, recurrent, hip

Dislocation — *continued*
- humerus, proximal end — *see* Dislocation, shoulder
- incomplete — *see* Subluxation, by site
- incus — *see* Discontinuity, ossicles, ear
- infracoracoid — *see* Dislocation, shoulder
- innominate (pubic junction) (sacral junction) S33.39 ☑
  - acetabulum — *see* Dislocation, hip
- interphalangeal (joint(s))
  - finger S63.279 ☑
    - distal S63.29- ☑
      - index S63.29- ☑
      - little S63.29- ☑
      - middle S63.29- ☑
      - ring S63.29- ☑
    - index S63.27- ☑
    - little S63.27- ☑
    - middle S63.27- ☑
    - proximal S63.28- ☑
      - index S63.28- ☑
      - little S63.28- ☑
      - middle S63.28- ☑
      - ring S63.28- ☑
    - ring S63.27- ☑
  - foot or toe — *see* Dislocation, toe
  - thumb S63.12- ☑
- jaw (cartilage) (meniscus) S03.0- ☑
- joint prosthesis — *see* Complications, joint prosthesis, mechanical, displacement, by site
- knee S83.106 ☑
  - cap — *see* Dislocation, patella
  - congenital Q68.2
  - old M23.8X- ☑
  - patella — *see* Dislocation, patella
  - pathological — *see* Dislocation, pathological NEC, knee
  - proximal tibia
    - anteriorly S83.11- ☑
    - laterally S83.14- ☑
    - medially S83.13- ☑
    - posteriorly S83.12- ☑
  - recurrent — *see also* Derangement, knee, specified NEC
  - specified type NEC S83.19- ☑
- lacrimal gland H04.16- ☑
- lens (complete) H27.10
  - anterior H27.12- ☑
  - congenital Q12.1
  - ocular implant — *see* Complications, intraocular lens
  - partial H27.11- ☑
  - posterior H27.13- ☑
  - traumatic S05.8X- ☑
- ligament — *code by* site under Dislocation
- lumbar (vertebra) — *see* Dislocation, vertebra, lumbar
- lumbosacral (vertebra) — *see also* Dislocation, vertebra, lumbar
  - congenital Q76.49
- mandible S03.0- ☑
- meniscus (knee) — *see* Tear, meniscus
  - other sites - code by site under Dislocation
- metacarpal (bone)
  - distal end — *see* Dislocation, finger
  - proximal end S63.06- ☑
- metacarpophalangeal (joint)
  - finger S63.26- ☑
    - index S63.26- ☑
    - little S63.26- ☑
    - middle S63.26- ☑
    - ring S63.26- ☑
  - thumb S63.11- ☑
- metatarsal (bone) — *see* Dislocation, foot
- metatarsophalangeal (joint(s)) — *see* Dislocation, toe
- midcarpal (joint) S63.03- ☑
- midtarsal (joint) — *see* Dislocation, foot
- neck S13.20 ☑
  - specified site NEC S13.29 ☑
  - vertebra — *see* Dislocation, vertebra, cervical
- nose (septal cartilage) S03.1 ☑
- occipitoatloid S13.111 ☑
- old — *see* Derangement, joint, specified type NEC
- ossicles, ear — *see* Discontinuity, ossicles, ear
- partial — *see* Subluxation, by site
- patella S83.006 ☑
  - congenital Q74.1
  - lateral S83.01- ☑
  - recurrent (nontraumatic) M22.0- ☑
    - incomplete M22.1- ☑

☑ Additional Character Required — Refer to the Tabular List for Character Selection

Dislocation — *continued*
  patella — *continued*
    specified type NEC S83.09- ☑
    pathological NEC M24.30
      ankle M24.37- ☑
      elbow M24.32- ☑
      foot joint M24.37- ☑
      hand joint M24.34- ☑
      hip M24.35- ☑
      knee M24.36- ☑
      lumbosacral joint — *see* subcategory M53.2
      pelvic region — *see* Dislocation, pathological, hip
      sacroiliac — *see* subcategory M53.2
      shoulder M24.31- ☑
      specified site NEC M24.39
      wrist M24.33- ☑
    pelvis NEC S33.30 ☑
      specified NEC S33.39 ☑
  phalanx
    finger or hand — *see* Dislocation, finger
    foot or toe — *see* Dislocation, toe
  prosthesis, internal — *see* Complications, prosthetic device, by site, mechanical
  radial head S53.006 ☑
    anterior S53.01- ☑
    posterior S53.02- ☑
    specified type NEC S53.09- ☑
  radiocarpal (joint) S63.02- ☑
  radiohumeral (joint) — *see* Dislocation, radial head
  radioulnar (joint)
    distal S63.01- ☑
    proximal — *see* Dislocation, elbow
  radius
    distal end — *see* Dislocation, wrist
    proximal end — *see* Dislocation, radial head
  recurrent M24.40
    ankle M24.47- ☑
    elbow M24.42- ☑
    finger M24.44- ☑
    foot joint M24.47- ☑
    hand joint M24.44- ☑
    hip M24.45- ☑
    knee M24.46- ☑
      patella — *see* Dislocation, patella, recurrent
    patella — *see* Dislocation, patella, recurrent
    sacroiliac — *see* subcategory M53.2 ☑
    shoulder M24.41- ☑
    specified site NEC M24.49
    toe M24.47- ☑
    vertebra — *see also* subcategory M43.5 ☑
      atlantoaxial M43.4
        with myelopathy M43.3
    wrist M24.43- ☑
  rib (cartilage) S23.29 ☑
  sacrococcygeal S33.2 ☑
  sacroiliac (joint) (ligament) S33.2 ☑
    congenital Q74.2
    recurrent — *see* subcategory M53.2 ☑
  sacrum S33.2 ☑
  scaphoid (bone) (hand) (wrist) — *see* Dislocation, wrist
    foot — *see* Dislocation, foot
  scapula — *see* Dislocation, shoulder, girdle, scapula
  semilunar cartilage, knee — *see* Tear, meniscus
  septal cartilage (nose) S03.1 ☑
  septum (nasal) (old) J34.2
  sesamoid bone — *code by* site under Dislocation
  shoulder (blade) (ligament) (joint) (traumatic) S43.006 ☑
    acromioclavicular — *see* Dislocation, acromioclavicular
    chronic — *see* Dislocation, recurrent, shoulder
    congenital Q68.8
    girdle S43.30- ☑
      scapula S43.31- ☑
      specified site NEC S43.39- ☑
    humerus S43.00- ☑
      anterior S43.01- ☑
      inferior S43.03- ☑
      posterior S43.02- ☑
    pathological — *see* Dislocation, pathological NEC, shoulder
    recurrent — *see* Dislocation, recurrent, shoulder
    specified type NEC S43.08- ☑
  spine
    cervical — *see* Dislocation, vertebra, cervical
    congenital Q76.49
    due to birth trauma P11.5
    lumbar — *see* Dislocation, vertebra, lumbar

Dislocation — *continued*
  spine — *continued*
    thoracic — *see* Dislocation, vertebra, thoracic
  spontaneous — *see* Dislocation, pathological
  sternoclavicular (joint) S43.206 ☑
    anterior S43.21- ☑
    posterior S43.22- ☑
  sternum S23.29 ☑
  subglenoid — *see* Dislocation, shoulder
  symphysis pubis S33.4 ☑
  talus — *see* Dislocation, ankle
  tarsal (bone(s)) (joint(s)) — *see* Dislocation, foot
  tarsometatarsal (joint(s)) — *see* Dislocation, foot
  temporomandibular (joint) S03.0- ☑
  thigh, proximal end — *see* Dislocation, hip
  thorax S23.20 ☑
    specified site NEC S23.29 ☑
    vertebra — *see* Dislocation, vertebra
  thumb S63.10- ☑
    interphalangeal joint — *see* Dislocation, interphalangeal (joint), thumb
    metacarpophalangeal joint — *see* Dislocation, metacarpophalangeal (joint), thumb
  thyroid cartilage S13.29 ☑
  tibia
    distal end — *see* Dislocation, ankle
    proximal end — *see* Dislocation, knee
  tibiofibular (joint)
    distal — *see* Dislocation, ankle
    superior — *see* Dislocation, knee
  toe(s) S93.106 ☑
    great S93.10- ☑
      interphalangeal joint S93.11- ☑
      metatarsophalangeal joint S93.12- ☑
      interphalangeal joint S93.119 ☑
    lesser S93.106 ☑
      interphalangeal joint S93.11- ☑
      metatarsophalangeal joint S93.12- ☑
      metatarsophalangeal joint S93.12- ☑
  tooth S03.2 ☑
  trachea S23.29 ☑
  ulna
    distal end S63.07- ☑
    proximal end — *see* Dislocation, elbow
  ulnohumeral (joint) — *see* Dislocation, elbow
  vertebra (articular process) (body) (traumatic)
    cervical S13.101 ☑
      atlantoaxial joint S13.121 ☑
      atlantoccipital joint S13.111 ☑
      atloidoccipital joint S13.111 ☑
      joint between
        C0 and C1 S13.111 ☑
        C1 and C2 S13.121 ☑
        C2 and C3 S13.131 ☑
        C3 and C4 S13.141 ☑
        C4 and C5 S13.151 ☑
        C5 and C6 S13.161 ☑
        C6 and C7 S13.171 ☑
        C7 and T1 S13.181 ☑
      occipitcatloid joint S13.111 ☑
    congenital Q76.49
    lumbar S33.101 ☑
      joint between
        L1 and L2 S33.111 ☑
        L2 and L3 S33.121 ☑
        L3 and L4 S33.131 ☑
        L4 and L5 S33.141 ☑
    nontraumatic — *see* Displacement, intervertebral disc
    partial — *see* Subluxation, by site
    recurrent NEC — *see* subcategory M43.5 ☑
    thoracic S23.101 ☑
      joint between
        T1 and T2 S23.111 ☑
        T2 and T3 S23.121 ☑
        T3 and T4 S23.123 ☑
        T4 and T5 S23.131 ☑
        T5 and T6 S23.133 ☑
        T6 and T7 S23.141 ☑
        T7 and T8 S23.143 ☑
        T8 and T9 S23.151 ☑
        T9 and T10 S23.153 ☑
        T10 and T11 S23.161 ☑
        T11 and T12 S23.163 ☑
        T12 and L1 S23.171 ☑
  wrist (carpal bone) S63.006 ☑

Dislocation — *continued*
  wrist — *continued*
    carpometacarpal joint — *see* Dislocation, carpometacarpal (joint)
    distal radioulnar joint — *see* Dislocation, radioulnar (joint), distal
    metacarpal bone, proximal — *see* Dislocation, metacarpal (bone), proximal end
    midcarpal — *see* Dislocation, midcarpal (joint)
    radiocarpal joint — *see* Dislocation, radiocarpal (joint)
    recurrent — *see* Dislocation, recurrent, wrist
    specified site NEC S63.09- ☑
    ulna — *see* Dislocation, ulna, distal end
  xiphoid cartilage S23.29 ☑
Disorder (of) — *see also* Disease
  acantholytic L11.9
    specified NEC L11.8
  acute
    psychotic — *see* Psychosis, acute
    stress F43.0
  adjustment (grief) F43.20
    with
      anxiety F43.22
        with depressed mood F43.23
      conduct disturbance F43.24
        with emotional disturbance F43.25
      depressed mood F43.21
        with anxiety F43.23
      other specified symptom F43.29
  adrenal (capsule) (gland) (medullary) E27.9
    specified NEC E27.8
  adrenogenital — *see also* Adrenogenital syndrome E25.9
    drug-induced E25.8
    iatrogenic E25.8
    idiopathic E25.8
  adult personality (and behavior) F69
    specified NEC F68.8
  affective (mood) — *see* Disorder, mood
  aggressive, unsocialized F91.1
  alcohol use
    mild F10.10
      with
        alcohol intoxication F10.129
          delirium F10.121
        alcohol-induced
          anxiety disorder F10.180
          bipolar and related disorder F10.14
          depressive disorder F10.14
          psychotic disorder F10.159
          sexual dysfunction F10.181
          sleep disorder F10.182
      in remission (early) (sustained) F10.11
    moderate or severe F10.20
      with
        alcohol intoxication F10.229
          delirium F10.221
        alcohol-induced
          anxiety disorder F10.280
          bipolar and related disorder F10.24
          depressive disorder F10.24
          major neurocognitive disorder, amnestic-confabulatory type F10.26
          major neurocognitive disorder, nonamnestic-confabulatory type F10.27
          mild neurocognitive disorder F10.288
          psychotic disorder F10.259
          sexual dysfunction F10.281
          sleep disorder F10.282
      in remission (early) (sustained) F10.21
  alcohol-related F10.99
    with
      amnestic disorder, persisting F10.96
      anxiety disorder F10.980
      dementia, persisting F10.97
      intoxication F10.929
        with delirium F10.921
        uncomplicated F10.920
      mood disorder F10.94
      other specified F10.988
      psychotic disorder F10.959
        with
          delusions F10.950
          hallucinations F10.951
      sexual dysfunction F10.981
      sleep disorder F10.982
  allergic — *see* Allergy
  alveolar NEC J84.09
  amino-acid
    cystathioninuria E72.19

Disorder — continued
amino-acid — continued
cystinosis E72.04
cystinuria E72.01
glycinuria E72.09
homocystinuria E72.11
metabolism — see Disturbance, metabolism, amino-
acid
specified NEC E72.89
neonatal, transitory P74.8
renal transport NEC E72.09
transport NEC E72.09
amnesic, amnestic
alcohol-induced F10.96
with dependence F10.26
due to (secondary to) general medical condition F04
psychoactive NEC-induced F19.96
with
abuse F19.16
dependence F19.26
sedative, hypnotic or anxiolytic-induced F13.96
with dependence F13.26
amphetamine (or other stimulant) use
mild
with
amphetamine, cocaine, or other stimulant intoxication
with perceptual disturbances F15.122
without perceptual disturbances F15.129
amphetamine (or other stimulant) -induced
anxiety disorder F15.180
bipolar and related disorder F15.14
depressive disorder F15.14
obsessive-compulsive and related disorder
F15.188
psychotic disorder F15.159
sexual dysfunction F15.181
intoxication delirium F15.121
moderate or severe
with
amphetamine, cocaine, or other stimulant intoxication
with perceptual disturbances F15.222
without perceptual disturbances F15.229
amphetamine (or other stimulant) -induced
anxiety disorder F15.280
bipolar and related disorder F15.24
depressive disorder F15.24
obsessive-compulsive and related disorder
F15.288
psychotic disorder F15.259
sexual dysfunction F15.281
intoxication delirium F15.221
amphetamine-type substance use
mild F15.10
in remission (early) (sustained) F15.11
moderate F15.20
in remission (early) (sustained) F15.21
severe F15.20
in remission (early) (sustained) F15.21
anaerobic glycolysis with anemia D55.29
anxiety F41.9
due to (secondary to)
alcohol F10.980
in
abuse F10.180
dependence F10.280
amphetamine F15.980
in
abuse F15.180
dependence F15.280
anxiolytic F13.980
in
abuse F13.180
dependence F13.280
caffeine F15.980
in
abuse F15.180
dependence F15.280
cannabis F12.980
in
abuse F12.180
dependence F12.280
cocaine F14.980
in
abuse F14.180
dependence F14.180
general medical condition F06.4
hallucinogen F16.980

Disorder — continued
anxiety — continued
due to — continued
hallucinogen — continued
in
abuse F16.180
dependence F16.280
hypnotic F13.980
in
abuse F13.180
dependence F13.280
inhalant F18.980
in
abuse F18.180
dependence F18.280
phencyclidine F16.980
in
abuse F16.180
dependence F16.280
psychoactive substance NEC F19.980
in
abuse F19.180
dependence F19.280
sedative F13.980
in
abuse F13.180
dependence F13.280
volatile solvents F18.980
in
abuse F18.180
dependence F18.280
generalized F41.1
illness F45.21
mixed
with depression (mild) F41.8
specified NEC F41.3
organic F06.4
phobic F40.9
of childhood F40.8
specified NEC F41.8
aortic valve — see Endocarditis, aortic
aromatic amino-acid metabolism E70.9
specified NEC E70.89
arteriole NEC I77.89
artery NEC I77.89
articulation — see Disorder, joint
attachment (childhood)
disinhibited F94.2
reactive F94.1
attention-deficit hyperactivity (adolescent) (adult) (child)
F90.9
combined
presentation F90.2
type F90.2
hyperactive
impulsive presentation F90.1
type F90.1
inattentive
presentation F90.0
type F90.0
specified type NEC F90.8
attention-deficit without hyperactivity (adolescent)
(adult) (child) F98.8
auditory processing (central) H93.25
autism spectrum F84.0
autistic F84.0
autoimmune D89.89
autonomic nervous system G90.9
specified NEC G90.89
avoidant
child or adolescent F40.10
restrictive food intake F50.82
balance
acid-base E87.8
mixed E87.4
electrolyte E87.8
fluid NEC E87.8
behavioral (disruptive) — see Disorder, conduct
bereavement, persistent complex F43.81
beta-amino-acid metabolism E72.89
bile acid and cholesterol metabolism E78.70
Barth syndrome E78.71
other specified E78.79
Smith-Lemli-Opitz syndrome E78.72
bilirubin excretion E80.6
binge eating F50.81- ☑
binocular
movement H51.9

Disorder — continued
binocular — continued
movement — continued
convergence
excess H51.12
insufficiency H51.11
internuclear ophthalmoplegia — see Ophthalmoplegia, internuclear
palsy of conjugate gaze H51.0
specified type NEC H51.8
vision NEC — see Disorder, vision, binocular
bipolar (I) (seasonal) (type I) F31.9
and related due to a known physiological condition
with
manic features F06.33
manic- or hypomanic-like episodes F06.33
mixed features F06.34
current (or most recent) episode
depressed F31.9
with psychotic features F31.5
without psychotic features F31.30
mild F31.31
moderate F31.32
severe (without psychotic features) F31.4
with psychotic features F31.5
hypomanic F31.0
manic F31.9
with psychotic features F31.2
without psychotic features F31.10
mild F31.11
moderate F31.12
severe (without psychotic features) F31.13
with psychotic features F31.2
mixed F31.60
mild F31.61
moderate F31.62
severe (without psychotic features) F31.63
with psychotic features F31.64
severe depression (without psychotic features)
F31.4
with psychotic features F31.5
II (type 2) F31.81
in remission (currently) F31.70
in full remission
most recent episode
depressed F31.76
hypomanic F31.72
manic F31.74
mixed F31.78
in partial remission
most recent episode
depressed F31.75
hypomanic F31.71
manic F31.73
mixed F31.77
organic F06.30
single manic episode F30.9
mild F30.11
moderate F30.12
severe (without psychotic symptoms) F30.13
with psychotic symptoms F30.2
specified NEC F31.89
bladder N32.9
functional NEC N31.9
in schistosomiasis B65.0 [N33]
specified NEC N32.89
bleeding D68.9
blood D75.9
in congenital early syphilis A50.09 [D77]
body dysmorphic F45.22
bone M89.9
continuity M84.9
specified type NEC M84.80
ankle M84.87- ☑
fibula M84.86- ☑
foot M84.87- ☑
hand M84.84- ☑
humerus M84.82- ☑
neck M84.88
pelvis M84.859
radius M84.83- ☑
rib M84.88
shoulder M84.81- ☑
skull M84.88
thigh M84.85- ☑
tibia M84.86- ☑
ulna M84.83- ☑
vertebra M84.88

Disorder — *continued*
  bone — *continued*
    density and structure M85.9
      cyst — *see also* Cyst, bone, specified type NEC
        aneurysmal — *see* Cyst, bone, aneurysmal
        solitary — *see* Cyst, bone, solitary
      diffuse idiopathic skeletal hyperostosis — *see* Hyperostosis, ankylosing
      fibrous dysplasia (monostotic) — *see* Dysplasia, fibrous, bone
      fluorosis — *see* Fluorosis, skeletal
      hyperostosis of skull M85.2
      osteitis condensans — *see* Osteitis, condensans
      specified type NEC M85.8- ☑
        ankle M85.87- ☑
        foot M85.87- ☑
        forearm M85.83- ☑
        hand M85.84- ☑
        lower leg M85.86- ☑
        multiple sites M85.89
        neck M85.88
        rib M85.88
        shoulder M85.81- ☑
        skull M85.88
        thigh M85.85- ☑
        upper arm M85.82- ☑
        vertebra M85.88
    development and growth NEC M89.20
      carpus M89.24- ☑
      clavicle M89.21- ☑
      femur M89.25- ☑
      fibula M89.26- ☑
      finger M89.24- ☑
      humerus M89.22- ☑
      ilium M89.28
      ischium M89.28
      metacarpus M89.24- ☑
      metatarsus M89.27- ☑
      multiple sites M89.29
      neck M89.28
      radius M89.23- ☑
      rib M89.28
      scapula M89.21- ☑
      skull M89.28
      tarsus M89.27- ☑
      tibia M89.26- ☑
      toe M89.27- ☑
      ulna M89.23- ☑
      vertebra M89.28
    specified type NEC M89.8X- ☑
  brachial plexus G54.0
  branched-chain amino-acid metabolism E71.2
    specified NEC E71.19
  breast N64.9
    agalactia — *see* Agalactia
    associated with
      lactation O92.70
        specified NEC O92.79
      pregnancy O92.20
        specified NEC O92.29
      puerperium O92.20
        specified NEC O92.29
    cracked nipple — *see* Cracked nipple
    galactorrhea — *see* Galactorrhea
    hypogalactia O92.4
    lactation disorder NEC O92.79
    mastitis — *see* Mastitis
    nipple infection — *see* Infection, nipple
    retracted nipple — *see* Retraction, nipple
    specified type NEC N64.89
  Briquet's F45.0
  bullous, in diseases classified elsewhere L14
  caffeine use
    mild
      with
        caffeine-induced
          anxiety disorder F15.180
          sleep disorder F15.182
    moderate or severe
      with
        caffeine-induced
          anxiety disorder F15.280
          sleep disorder F15.282
  cannabis use
    mild F12.10
      with
        cannabis intoxication delirium F12.121
          with perceptual disturbances F12.122

Disorder — *continued*
  cannabis use — *continued*
    mild — *continued*
      with — *continued*
        cannabis intoxication delirium — *continued*
          without perceptual disturbances F12.129
        cannabis-induced
          anxiety disorder F12.180
          psychotic disorder F12.159
          sleep disorder F12.188
      in remission (early) (sustained) F12.11
    moderate or severe F12.20
      with
        cannabis intoxication
          with perceptual disturbances F12.222
          without perceptual disturbances F12.229
        cannabis-induced
          anxiety disorder F12.280
          psychotic disorder F12.259
          sleep disorder F12.288
        delirium F12.221
      in remission (early) (sustained) F12.21
  carbohydrate
    absorption, intestinal NEC E74.39
    metabolism (congenital) E74.9
      specified NEC E74.89
  cardiac, functional I51.39
  carnitine metabolism E71.40
  cartilage M94.9
    articular NEC — *see* Derangement, joint, articular cartilage
    chondrocalcinosis — *see* Chondrocalcinosis
    specified type NEC M94.8X- ☑
      articular — *see* Derangement, joint, articular cartilage
      multiple sites M94.8X0
  catatonia (due to known physiological condition) (with another mental disorder) F06.1
  catatonic NOS F06.1
    due to (secondary to) known physiological condition F06.1
    organic NOS F06.1
  central auditory processing H93.25
  cervical
    region NEC M53.82
    root (nerve) NEC G54.2
  character NOS F60.9
  childhood disintegrative NEC F84.3
  cholesterol and bile acid metabolism E78.70
    Barth syndrome E78.71
    other specified E78.79
    Smith-Lemli-Opitz syndrome E78.72
  choroid H31.9
    atrophy — *see* Atrophy, choroid
    degeneration — *see* Degeneration, choroid
    detachment — *see* Detachment, choroid
    dystrophy — *see* Dystrophy, choroid
    hemorrhage — *see* Hemorrhage, choroid
    rupture — *see* Rupture, choroid
    scar — *see* Scar, chorioretinal
    solar retinopathy — *see* Retinopathy, solar
    specified type NEC H31.8
  ciliary body — *see* Disorder, iris
    degeneration — *see* Degeneration, ciliary body
  citrate metabolism NEC E74.829
  citrate transporter, SLC13A5 E74.820
  coagulation (factor) — *see also* Defect, coagulation D68.9
    newborn, transient P61.6
  cocaine use
    mild F14.10
      with
        amphetamine, cocaine, or other stimulant intoxication
          with perceptual disturbances F14.122
          without perceptual disturbances F14.129
        cocaine intoxication delirium F14.121
        cocaine-induced
          anxiety disorder F14.180
          bipolar and related disorder F14.14
          depressive disorder F14.14
          obsessive-compulsive and related disorder F14.188
          psychotic disorder F14.159
          sexual dysfunction F14.181
          sleep disorder F14.182
      in remission (early) (sustained) F14.11
    moderate or severe F14.20

Disorder — *continued*
  cocaine use — *continued*
    moderate or severe — *continued*
      with
        amphetamine, cocaine, or other stimulant intoxication
          with perceptual disturbances F14.222
          without perceptual disturbances F14.229
        cocaine intoxication delirium F14.221
        cocaine-induced
          anxiety disorder F14.280
          bipolar and related disorder F14.24
          depressive disorder F14.24
          obsessive-compulsive and related disorder F14.288
          psychotic disorder F14.259
          sexual dysfunction F14.281
          sleep disorder F14.282
      in remission (early) (sustained) F14.21
  coccyx NEC M53.3
  cognitive F09
    due to (secondary to) general medical condition F09
    persisting R41.89
      due to
        alcohol F10.97
          with dependence F10.27
        anxiolytics F13.97
          with dependence F13.27
        hypnotics F13.97
          with dependence F13.27
        sedatives F13.97
          with dependence F13.27
        specified substance NEC F19.97
          with
            abuse F19.17
            dependence F19.27
  communication F80.9
    social pragmatic F80.82
  conduct (childhood) F91.9
    adjustment reaction — *see* Disorder, adjustment
    adolescent onset type F91.2
    childhood onset type F91.1
    compulsive F63.9
    confined to family context F91.0
    depressive F91.8
    group type F91.2
    hyperkinetic — *see* Disorder, attention-deficit hyperactivity
    oppositional defiance F91.3
    socialized F91.2
    solitary aggressive type F91.1
    specified NEC F91.8
    unsocialized (aggressive) F91.1
  conduction, heart I45.9
  congenital glycosylation (CDG) E74.89
  conjunctiva H11.9
    infection — *see* Conjunctivitis
  connective tissue, localized L94.9
    specified NEC L94.8
  conversion (functional neurological symptom disorder)
    with
      abnormal movement F44.4
      anesthesia or sensory loss F44.6
      attacks or seizures F44.5
      mixed symptoms F44.7
      special sensory symptoms F44.6
      speech symptoms F44.4
      swallowing symptoms F44.4
      weakness or paralysis F44.4
  convulsive (secondary) — *see* Convulsions
  cornea H18.9
    deformity — *see* Deformity, cornea
    degeneration — *see* Degeneration, cornea
    deposits — *see* Deposit, cornea
    due to contact lens H18.82- ☑
      specified as edema — *see* Edema, cornea
    edema — *see* Edema, cornea
    keratitis — *see* Keratitis
    keratoconjunctivitis — *see* Keratoconjunctivitis
    membrane change — *see* Change, corneal membrane
    neovascularization — *see* Neovascularization, cornea
    scar — *see* Opacity, cornea
    specified type NEC H18.89- ☑
    ulcer — *see* Ulcer, cornea
  corpus cavernosum N48.9
  cranial nerve — *see* Disorder, nerve, cranial
  Cyclin-Dependent Kinase-Like 5 Deficiency (CDKL5) G40.42
  cyclothymic F34.0

☑ **Additional Character Required — Refer to the Tabular List for Character Selection**

Disorder — *continued*
defiant oppositional F91.3
delusional (persistent) (systematized) F22
   induced F24
depersonalization F48.1
depressive F32.A
   due to known physiological condition
      with
         depressive features F06.31
         major depressive-like episode F06.32
         mixed features F06.34
   major F32.9
      with psychotic symptoms F32.3
      in remission (full) F32.5
         partial F32.4
      recurrent F33.9
         with psychotic features F33.3
      single episode F32.9
         mild F32.0
         moderate F32.1
         severe (without psychotic symptoms) F32.2
            with psychotic symptoms F32.3
   organic F06.31
   persistent F34.1
   recurrent F33.9
      current episode
         mild F33.0
         moderate F33.1
         severe (without psychotic symptoms) F33.2
            with psychotic symptoms F33.3
      in remission F33.40
         full F33.42
         partial F33.41
      specified NEC F33.8
   single episode — *see* Episode, depressive
   specified NEC F32.89
developmental F89
   arithmetical skills F81.2
   coordination (motor) F82
   expressive writing F81.81
   language F80.9
      expressive F80.1
      mixed receptive and expressive F80.2
      receptive type F80.2
      specified NEC F80.89
   learning F81.9
      arithmetical F81.2
      reading F81.0
   mixed F88
   motor coordination or function F82
   pervasive F84.9
      specified NEC F84.8
   phonological F80.0
   reading F81.0
   scholastic skills — *see also* Disorder, learning
      mixed F81.89
   specified NEC F88
   speech F80.9
      articulation F80.0
      specified NEC F80.89
   written expression F81.81
diaphragm J98.6
digestive (system) K92.9
   newborn P78.9
      specified NEC P78.89
   postprocedural — *see* Complication, gastrointestinal
   psychogenic F45.8
disc (intervertebral) M51.9
   with
      myelopathy
         cervical region M50.00
         cervicothoracic region M50.03
         high cervical region M50.01
         lumbar region M51.06
         mid-cervical region M50.020
         sacrococcygeal region M53.3
         thoracic region M51.04
         thoracolumbar region M51.05
      radiculopathy
         cervical region M50.10
         cervicothoracic region M50.13
         high cervical region M50.11
         lumbar region M51.16
         lumbosacral region M51.17
         mid-cervical region M50.120
         sacrococcygeal region M53.3
         thoracic region M51.14
         thoracolumbar region M51.15
   cervical M50.90

Disorder — *continued*
disc — *continued*
   cervical — *continued*
      with
         myelopathy M50.00
            C2-C3 M50.01
            C3-C4 M50.01
            C4-C5 M50.021
            C5-C6 M50.022
            C6-C7 M50.023
            C7-T1 M50.03
            cervicothoracic region M50.03
            high cervical region M50.01
            mid-cervical region M50.020
         neuritis, radiculitis or radiculopathy M50.10
            C2-C3 M50.11
            C3-C4 M50.11
            C4-C5 M50.121
            C5-C6 M50.122
            C6-C7 M50.123
            C7-T1 M50.13
            cervicothoracic region M50.13
            high cervical region M50.11
            mid-cervical region M50.120
      C2-C3 M50.91
      C3-C4 M50.91
      C4-C5 M50.921
      C5-C6 M50.922
      C6-C7 M50.923
      C7-T1 M50.93
      cervicothoracic region M50.93
      degeneration M50.30
         C2-C3 M50.31
         C3-C4 M50.31
         C4-C5 M50.321
         C5-C6 M50.322
         C6-C7 M50.323
         C7-T1 M50.33
         cervicothoracic region M50.33
         high cervical region M50.31
         mid-cervical region M50.320
      displacement M50.20
         C2-C3 M50.21
         C3-C4 M50.21
         C4-C5 M50.221
         C5-C6 M50.222
         C6-C7 M50.223
         C7-T1 M50.23
         cervicothoracic region M50.23
         high cervical region M50.21
         mid-cervical region M50.220
      high cervical region M50.91
      mid-cervical region M50.920
      specified type NEC M50.80
         C2-C3 M50.81
         C3-C4 M50.81
         C4-C5 M50.821
         C5-C6 M50.822
         C6-C7 M50.823
         C7-T1 M50.83
         cervicothoracic region M50.83
         high cervical region M50.81
         mid-cervical region M50.820
   specified NEC
      lumbar region M51.86
      lumbosacral region M51.87
      sacrococcygeal region M53.3
      thoracic region M51.84
      thoracolumbar region M51.85
disinhibited attachment (childhood) F94.2
disintegrative, childhood NEC F84.3
disruptive F91.9
   mood dysregulation F34.81
   specified NEC F91.8
disruptive behavior — *see* Disorder, conduct
dissocial personality F60.2
dissociative F44.9
   affecting
      motor function F44.4
         and sensation F44.7
      sensation F44.6
         and motor function F44.7
   brief reactive F43.0
   due to (secondary to) general medical condition F06.8
   mixed F44.7
   organic F06.8
   other specified NEC F44.89
double heterozygous sickling — *see* Disease, sickle-cell
dream anxiety F51.5

Disorder — *continued*
drug induced hemorrhagic D68.32
drug related F19.99
   abuse — *see* Abuse, drug
   dependence — *see* Dependence, drug
dysmorphic body F45.22
dysthymic F34.1
ear H93.9- ☑
   bleeding — *see* Otorrhagia
   deafness — *see* Deafness
   degenerative H93.09- ☑
   discharge — *see* Otorrhea
   external H61.9- ☑
      auditory canal stenosis — *see* Stenosis, external ear canal
      exostosis — *see* Exostosis, external ear canal
      impacted cerumen — *see* Impaction, cerumen
      otitis — *see* Otitis, externa
      perichondritis — *see* Perichondritis, ear
      pinna — *see* Disorder, pinna
      specified type NEC H61.89- ☑
   inner H83.9- ☑
      vestibular dysfunction — *see* Disorder, vestibular function
   middle H74.9- ☑
      adhesive H74.1- ☑
      ossicle — *see* Abnormal, ear ossicles
      polyp — *see* Polyp, ear (middle)
      specified NEC, in diseases classified elsewhere H75.8- ☑
   postprocedural — *see* Complications, ear, procedure
   specified NEC, in diseases classified elsewhere H94.8- ☑
eating (adult) (psychogenic) F50.9
   anorexia — *see* Anorexia
   binge F50.81- ☑
   bulimia F50.2- ☑
   child F98.29
      pica (in remission) F98.3
      rumination disorder (in remission) F98.21
   pica F50.89
      adult (in remission) F50.83
      childhood (in remission) F98.3
   rumination — *see also* Rumination R11.10
      adult (in remission) F50.84
      infancy or childhood (in remission) F98.21
   specified NEC F50.89
electrolyte (balance) NEC E87.8
   with
      abortion — *see* Abortion by type complicated by specified condition NEC
      ectopic pregnancy O08.5
      molar pregnancy O08.5
   acidosis (lactic) (metabolic) E87.20
      acute E87.21
      chronic E87.22
      respiratory E87.29
      specified NEC E87.29
   alkalosis (metabolic) (respiratory) E87.3
elimination, transepidermal L87.9
   specified NEC L87.8
emotional (persistent) F34.9
   of childhood F93.9
      specified NEC F93.8
endocrine E34.9
   postprocedural E89.89
      specified NEC E89.89
erectile (male) (organic) — *see also* Dysfunction, sexual, male, erectile N52.9
   nonorganic F52.21
erythematous — *see* Erythema
esophagus K22.9
   functional K22.4
   psychogenic F45.8
eustachian tube H69.9- ☑
   infection — *see* Salpingitis, eustachian
   obstruction — *see* Obstruction, eustachian tube
   patulous — *see* Patulous, eustachian tube
   specified NEC H69.8- ☑
exhibitionistic F65.2
extrapyramidal G25.9
   in deseases classified elsewhere — *see* category G26
   specified type NEC G25.89
eye H57.9
   postprocedural — *see* Complication, postprocedural, eye
eyelid H02.9
   cyst — *see* Cyst, eyelid

Disorder — *continued*
eyelid — *continued*
  degenerative H02.70
    chloasma — *see* Chloasma, eyelid
    madarosis — *see* Madarosis
    specified type NEC H02.79
    vitiligo — *see* Vitiligo, eyelid
    xanthelasma — *see* Xanthelasma
  dermatochalasis — *see* Dermatochalasis
  edema — *see* Edema, eyelid
  elephantiasis — *see* Elephantiasis, eyelid
  foreign body, retained — *see* Foreign body, retained,
    eyelid
  function H02.59
    abnormal innervation syndrome — *see* Syndrome,
      abnormal innervation
    blepharochalasis — *see* Blepharochalasis
    blepharoclonus — *see* Blepharoclonus
    blepharophimosis — *see* Blepharophimosis
    blepharoptosis — *see* Blepharoptosis
    lagophthalmos — *see* Lagophthalmos
    lid retraction — *see* Retraction, lid
  hypertrichosis — *see* Hypertrichosis, eyelid
  specified type NEC H02.89
  vascular H02.879
    left H02.876
      lower H02.875
      upper H02.874
    right H02.873
      lower H02.872
      upper H02.871
factitious
  by proxy F68.A
  imposed on another F68.A
  imposed on self F68.10
    with predominantly
      psychological symptoms F68.11
        with physical symptoms F68.13
      physical symptoms F68.12
        with psychological symptoms F68.13
factor, coagulation — *see* Defect, coagulation
fatty acid
  metabolism E71.30
    specified NEC E71.39
  oxidation
    LCAD E71.310
    MCAD E71.311
    SCAD E71.312
    specified deficiency NEC E71.318
feeding (infant or child) — *see also* Disorder, eating
  R63.30
  or eating disorder F50.9
  pediatric
    acute R63.31
    chronic R63.32
  specified NEC F50.9
feigned (with obvious motivation) Z76.5
  without obvious motivation — *see* Disorder, factitious
female
  hypoactive sexual desire F52.0
  orgasmic F52.31
  sexual interest/arousal F52.22
fetishistic F65.0
fibroblastic M72.9
  specified NEC M72.8
fluency
  adult onset F98.5
  childhood onset F80.81
  following
    cerebral infarction I69.323
    cerebrovascular disease I69.923
      specified disease NEC I69.823
    intracerebral hemorrhage I69.123
    nontraumatic intracranial hemorrhage NEC I69.223
    subarachnoid hemorrhage I69.023
  in conditions classified elsewhere R47.82
fluid balance E87.8
follicular (skin) L73.9
  specified NEC L73.8
frotteuristic F65.81
fructose metabolism E74.10
  essential fructosuria E74.11
  fructokinase deficiency E74.11
  fructose-1, 6-diphosphatase deficiency E74.19
  hereditary fructose intolerance E74.12
  other specified E74.19
functional polymorphonuclear neutrophils D71
gallbladder, biliary tract and pancreas in diseases classified elsewhere K87

Disorder — *continued*
gambling F63.0
gamma aminobutyric acid (GABA) metabolism E72.81
gamma-glutamyl cycle E72.89
gastric (functional) K31.9
  motility K30
  psychogenic F45.8
  secretion K30
gastrointestinal (functional) NOS K92.9
  newborn P78.9
  psychogenic F45.8
gender incongruence F64.9
  in adolescents and adults F64.0
  of childhood F64.2
gender-identity or -role F64.9
  childhood F64.2
  effect on relationship F66
  of adolescence or adulthood F64.0
    nontranssexual F64.8
  specified NEC F64.8
  uncertainty F66
genito-pelvic pain penetration F52.6
genitourinary system
  female N94.9
  male N50.9
  psychogenic F45.8
globe H44.9
  degenerated condition H44.50
    absolute glaucoma H44.51- ☑
    atrophy H44.52- ☑
    leucocoria H44.53- ☑
  degenerative H44.30
    chalcosis H44.31- ☑
    myopia — *see also* Myopia, degenerative H44.2- ☑
    siderosis H44.32- ☑
    specified type NEC H44.39- ☑
  endophthalmitis — *see* Endophthalmitis
  foreign body, retained — *see* Foreign body, intraocu-
    lar, old, retained
  hemophthalmos — *see* Hemophthalmos
  hypotony H44.40
    due to
      ocular fistula H44.42- ☑
      specified disorder NEC H44.43- ☑
    flat anterior chamber H44.41- ☑
    primary H44.44- ☑
  luxation — *see* Luxation, globe
  specified type NEC H44.89
glomerular (in) N05.9
  amyloidosis E85.4 *[N08]*
  cryoglobulinemia D89.1 *[N08]*
  disseminated intravascular coagulation D65 *[N08]*
  Fabry's disease E75.21 *[N08]*
  familial lecithin cholesterol acyltransferase deficiency
    E78.6 *[N08]*
  Goodpasture's syndrome M31.0
  hemolytic-uremic syndrome — *see* Syndrome,
    hemolytic-uremic
  Henoch (-Schonlein) purpura D69.0 *[N08]*
  malariae malaria B52.0
  microscopic polyangiitis M31.7 *[N08]*
  multiple myeloma C90.0- ☑ *[N08]*
  mumps B26.83
  schistosomiasis B65.9 *[N08]*
  sepsis NEC A41.- ☑ *[N08]*
    streptococcal A40.- ☑ *[N08]*
  sickle-cell disorders D57.- ☑ *[N08]*
  strongyloidiasis B78.9 *[N08]*
  subacute bacterial endocarditis I33.0 *[N08]*
  syphilis A52.75
  systemic lupus erythematosus M32.14
  thrombotic thrombocytopenic purpura M31.19 *[N08]*
  Waldenstrom macroglobulinemia C88.0- ☑ *[N08]*
  Wegener's granulomatosis M31.31
gluconeogenesis E74.4
glucosaminoglycan metabolism — *see* Disorder,
  metabolism, glucosaminoglycan
glucose transport E74.819
  specified NEC E74.818
glycine metabolism E72.50
  d-glycericacidemia E72.59
  hyperhydroxyprolinemia E72.59
  hyperoxaluria R82.992
    primary E72.53
  hyperprolinemia E72.59
  non-ketotic hyperglycinemia E72.51
  oxalosis E72.53
  oxaluria E72.53

Disorder — *continued*
glycine metabolism — *continued*
  sarcosinemia E72.59
  trimethylaminuria E72.52
glycoprotein metabolism E77.9
  specified NEC E77.8
grief
  complicated F43.81
  prolonged F43.81
habit (and impulse) F63.9
  involving sexual behavior NEC F65.9
  specified NEC F63.89
hallucinogen use
  mild F16.10
    with
      hallucinogen intoxication delirium F16.121
      hallucinogen-induced
        anxiety disorder F16.180
        bipolar and related disorder F16.14
        depressive disorder F16.14
        psychotic disorder F16.159
      other hallucinogen intoxication F16.129
    in remission (early) (sustained) F16.11
  moderate or severe F16.20
    with
      hallucinogen intoxication delirium F16.221
      hallucinogen-induced
        anxiety disorder F16.280
        bipolar and related disorder F16.24
        depressive disorder F16.24
        psychotic disorder F16.259
      other hallucinogen intoxication F16.229
    in remission (early) (sustained) F16.21
heart action I49.9
hematological D75.9
  newborn (transient) P61.9
    specified NEC P61.8
hematopoietic organs D75.9
hemorrhagic NEC D69.9
  drug-induced D68.32
  due to
    extrinsic circulating anticoagulants D68.32
    increase in
      anti-IIa D68.32
      anti-Xa D68.32
    intrinsic
      circulating anticoagulants D68.318
      increase in
        anti-IXa D68.318
        antithrombin D68.318
        anti-VIIIa D68.318
        anti-XIa D68.318
  following childbirth O72.3
hemostasis — *see* Defect, coagulation
histidine metabolism E70.40
  histidinemia E70.41
  other specified E70.49
hoarding F42.3
hyperkinetic — *see* Disorder, attention-deficit hyperactivity
hyperleucine-isoleucinemia E71.19
hypervalinemia E71.19
hypoactive sexual desire F52.0
hypochondriacal F45.20
  body dysmorphic F45.22
  neurosis F45.21
  other specified F45.29
identity
  dissociative F44.81
  illness anxiety F45.21
  of childhood F93.8
immune mechanism (immunity) D89.9
  specified type NEC D89.89
impaired renal tubular function N25.9
  specified NEC N25.89
impulse (control) F63.9
inflammatory
  pelvic, in diseases classified elsewhere — *see* category
    N74
  penis N48.29
    abscess N48.21
    cellulitis N48.22
inhalant use
  mild F18.10
    with
      inhalant intoxication F18.129
      inhalant intoxication delirium F18.121
      inhalant-induced
        anxiety disorder F18.180

Disorder — continued
  inhalant use — continued
    mild — continued
      with — continued
        inhalant-induced — continued
          depressive disorder F18.14
          major neurocognitive disorder F18.17
          mild neurocognitive disorder F18.188
          psychotic disorder F18.159
        in remission (early) (sustained) F18.11
      moderate or severe F18.20
        with
          inhalant intoxication F18.229
          inhalant intoxication delirium F18.221
          inhalant-induced
            anxiety disorder F18.280
            depressive disorder F18.24
            major neurocognitive disorder F18.27
            mild neurocognitive disorder F18.288
            psychotic disorder F18.259
        in remission (early) (sustained) F18.21
  integument, newborn P83.9
    specified NEC P83.88
  intermittent explosive F63.81
  internal secretion pancreas — see Increased, secretion, pancreas, endocrine
  intestine, intestinal
    carbohydrate absorption NEC E74.39
      postoperative K91.2
    functional NEC K59.9
      postoperative K91.89
    psychogenic F45.8
    vascular K55.9
      chronic K55.1
      specified NEC K55.8
  intraoperative (intraprocedural) — see Complications, intraoperative
  involuntary emotional expression (IEED) F07.89
  iris H21.9
    adhesions — see Adhesions, iris
    atrophy — see Atrophy, iris
    chamber angle recession — see Recession, chamber angle
    cyst — see Cyst, iris
    degeneration — see Degeneration, iris
    in diseases classified elsewhere H22
    iridodialysis — see Iridodialysis
    iridoschisis — see Iridoschisis
    miotic pupillary cyst — see Cyst, pupillary
    pupillary
      abnormality — see Abnormality, pupillary
      membrane — see Membrane, pupillary
    specified type NEC H21.89
    vascular NEC H21.1X- ☑
  iron metabolism E83.10
    specified NEC E83.19
  isovaleric acidemia E71.110
  jaw, developmental M27.0
    temporomandibular — see also Anomaly, dentofacial, temporomandibular joint M26.60- ☑
  joint M25.9
    derangement — see Derangement, joint
    effusion — see Effusion, joint
    fistula — see Fistula, joint
    hemarthrosis — see Hemarthrosis
    instability — see Instability, joint
    osteophyte — see Osteophyte
    pain — see Pain, joint
    psychogenic F45.8
    specified type NEC M25.80
      ankle M25.87- ☑
      elbow M25.82- ☑
      foot joint M25.87- ☑
      hand joint M25.84- ☑
      hip M25.85- ☑
      knee M25.86- ☑
      shoulder M25.81- ☑
      wrist M25.83- ☑
    stiffness — see Stiffness, joint
  ketone metabolism E71.32
  kidney N28.9
    functional (tubular) N25.9
    in
      schistosomiasis B65.9 [N29]
    tubular function N25.9
      specified NEC N25.89
  lacrimal system H04.9
    changes H04.69

Disorder — continued
  lacrimal system — continued
    changes — continued
      fistula — see Fistula, lacrimal
      gland H04.19
        atrophy — see Atrophy, lacrimal gland
        cyst — see Cyst, lacrimal, gland
        dacryops — see Dacryops
        dislocation — see Dislocation, lacrimal gland
        dry eye syndrome — see Syndrome, dry eye
        infection — see Dacryoadenitis
      granuloma — see Granuloma, lacrimal
      inflammation — see Inflammation, lacrimal
      obstruction — see Obstruction, lacrimal
      specified NEC H04.89
  lactation NEC O92.79
  language (developmental) F80.9
    expressive F80.1
    mixed receptive and expressive F80.2
    receptive F80.2
  late luteal phase dysphoric N94.89
  learning (specific) F81.9
    acalculia R48.8
    alexia R48.0
    mathematics F81.2
    reading F81.0
    specified
      with impairment in
        mathematics F81.2
        reading F81.0
        written expression F81.81
    specified NEC F81.89
    spelling F81.81
    written expression F81.81
  lens H27.9
    aphakia — see Aphakia
    cataract — see Cataract
    dislocation — see Dislocation, lens
    specified type NEC H27.8
  ligament M24.20
    ankle M24.27- ☑
    attachment, spine — see Enthesopathy, spinal
    elbow M24.22- ☑
    foot joint M24.27- ☑
    hand joint M24.24- ☑
    hip M24.25- ☑
    knee — see Derangement, knee, specified NEC
    shoulder M24.21- ☑
    specified site NEC M24.29
    vertebra M24.28
    wrist M24.23- ☑
  ligamentous attachments — see also Enthesopathy
    spine — see Enthesopathy, spinal
  lipid
    metabolism, congenital E78.9
    storage E75.6
      specified NEC E75.5
  lipoprotein
    deficiency (familial) E78.6
    metabolism E78.9
      specified NEC E78.89
  liver K76.9
    malarial B54 [K77]
  low back — see also Dorsopathy, specified NEC
  lumbosacral
    plexus G54.1
    root (nerve) NEC G54.4
  lung, interstitial, drug-induced J70.4
    acute J70.2
    chronic J70.3
    dabbing (related) U07.0
    e-cigarette (related) U07.0
    electronic cigarette (related) U07.0
    vaping (associated) (device) (product) (related) (use) U07.0
  lymphoproliferative, post-transplant (PTLD) D47.Z1 (following D47.4)
  lysine and hydroxylysine metabolism E72.3
  major neurocognitive — see also Dementia, in (due to) F03- ☑
  male
    erectile (organic) — see also Dysfunction, sexual, male, erectile N52.9
      nonorganic F52.21
    hypoactive sexual desire F52.0
    orgasmic F52.32
  manic F30.9
    organic F06.33

Disorder — continued
  mast cell activation — see Activation, mast cell
  mastoid — see also Disorder, ear, middle
    postprocedural — see Complications, ear, procedure
  meninges, specified type NEC G96.198
  meniscus — see Derangement, knee, meniscus
  menopausal N95.9
    specified NEC N95.8
  menstrual N92.6
    psychogenic F45.8
    specified NEC N92.5
  mental (or behavioral) (nonpsychotic) F99
    due to (secondary to)
      amphetamine
        due to drug abuse — see Abuse, drug, stimulant
        due to drug dependence — see Dependence, drug, stimulant
      brain disease, damage and dysfunction F09
      caffeine use
        due to drug abuse — see Abuse, drug, stimulant
        due to drug dependence — see Dependence, drug, stimulant
      cannabis use
        due to drug abuse — see Abuse, drug, cannabis
        due to drug dependence — see Dependence, drug, cannabis
      general medical condition F09
      sedative or hypnotic use
        due to drug abuse — see Abuse, drug, sedative
        due to drug dependence — see Dependence, drug, sedative
      tobacco (nicotine) use — see Dependence, drug, nicotine
    following organic brain damage F07.9
      frontal lobe syndrome F07.0
      personality change F07.0
      postconcussional syndrome F07.81
      specified NEC F07.89
    infancy, childhood or adolescence F98.9
    neurotic — see Neurosis
    organic or symptomatic F09
    presenile, psychotic F03 ☑
    problem NEC
    psychoneurotic — see Neurosis
    psychotic — see Psychosis
    puerperal F53.0
    senile, psychotic NEC F03 ☑
  metabolic, amino acid, transitory, newborn P74.8
  metabolism NOS E88.9
    amino-acid E72.9
      aromatic E70.9
        albinism — see Albinism
        histidine E70.40
          histidinemia E70.41
          other specified E70.49
        hyperphenylalaninemia E70.1
          classical phenylketonuria E70.0
        other specified E70.89
        tryptophan E70.5
        tyrosine E70.20
          hypertyrosinemia E70.21
          other specified E70.29
      branched chain E71.2
        3-methylglutaconic aciduria E71.111
        hyperleucine-isoleucinemia E71.19
        hypervalinemia E71.19
        isovaleric acidemia E71.110
        maple syrup urine disease E71.0
        methylmalonic acidemia E71.120
        organic aciduria NEC E71.118
        other specified E71.19
        propionate NEC E71.128
        propionic acidemia E71.121
      glycine E72.50
        d-glycericacidemia E72.59
        hyperhydroxyprolinemia E72.59
        hyperoxaluria R82.992
          primary E72.53
        hyperprolinemia E72.59
        non-ketotic hyperglycinemia E72.51
        other specified E72.59
        sarcosinemia E72.59
        trimethylaminuria E72.52
      hydroxylysine E72.3
      lysine E72.3
      ornithine E72.4
      other specified E72.89

Disorder — *continued*
  metabolism — *continued*
    amino-acid — *continued*
      other specified — *continued*
        beta-amino acid E72.89
        gamma-glutamyl cycle E72.89
      straight-chain E72.89
      sulfur-bearing E72.10
        homocystinuria E72.11
        methylenetetrahydrofolate reductase deficiency E72.12
        other specified E72.19
    bile acid and cholesterol metabolism E78.70
    bilirubin E80.7
      specified NEC E80.6
    calcium E83.50
      hypercalcemia E83.52
      hypocalcemia E83.51
      other specified E83.59
    carbohydrate E74.9
      specified NEC E74.89
    cholesterol and bile acid metabolism E78.70
    citrate NEC E74.829
    congenital E88.9
    copper E83.00
      specified type NEC E83.09
      Wilson's disease E83.01
    cystinuria E72.01
    fructose E74.10
    galactose E74.20
    glucosaminoglycan E76.9
      mucopolysaccharidosis — *see* Mucopolysaccharidosis
      specified NEC E76.8
    glutamine E72.89
    glycine E72.50
    glycogen storage (hepatorenal) E74.09
    glycoprotein E77.9
      specified NEC E77.8
    glycosaminoglycan E76.9
      specified NEC E76.8
    in labor and delivery O75.89
    iron E83.10
    isoleucine E71.19
    leucine E71.19
    lipoid E78.9
    lipoprotein E78.9
      specified NEC E78.89
    magnesium E83.40
      hypermagnesemia E83.41
      hypomagnesemia E83.42
      other specified E83.49
    mineral E83.9
      specified NEC E83.89
    mitochondrial E88.40
      MELAS syndrome E88.41
      MERRF syndrome (myoclonic epilepsy associated with ragged-red fibers) E88.42
      other specified E88.49
      tRNA synthetases E88.43
    ornithine E72.4
    phosphatases E83.30
    phosphorus E83.30
      acid phosphatase deficiency E83.39
      hypophosphatasia E83.39
      hypophosphatemia E83.39
        familial E83.31
      other specified E83.39
      pseudovitamin D deficiency E83.32
    plasma protein NEC E88.09
    porphyrin — *see* Porphyria
    postprocedural E89.89
      specified NEC E89.89
    purine E79.9
      specified NEC E79.89
    pyrimidine E79.9
      specified NEC E79.89
    pyruvate E74.4
    serine E72.89
    sodium E87.8
    specified NEC E88.89
    threonine E72.89
    valine E71.19
    zinc E83.2
  methylmalonic acidemia E71.120
  micturition NEC — *see also* Difficulty, micturition R39.198
    feeling of incomplete emptying R39.14
    hesitancy R39.11
    poor stream R39.12

Disorder — *continued*
  micturition — *see also* Difficulty, micturition — *continued*
    psychogenic F45.8
    split stream R39.13
    straining R39.16
    urgency R39.15
  mild neurocognitive G31.84
    due to known physiological condition (without behavioral disturbance) F06.70
      with behavioral disturbance F06.71
  mitochondrial metabolism E88.40
  mitral (valve) — *see* Endocarditis, mitral
  mixed
    anxiety and depressive F41.8
    of scholastic skills (developmental) F81.89
    receptive expressive language F80.2
  mood F39
    bipolar — *see* Disorder, bipolar
    depressive — *see* Disorder, depressive
    due to (secondary to)
      alcohol F10.94
      amphetamine F15.94
        in
          abuse F15.14
          dependence F15.24
      anxiolytic F13.94
        in
          abuse F13.14
          dependence F13.24
      cocaine F14.94
        in
          abuse F14.14
          dependence F14.24
      general medical condition F06.30
      hallucinogen F16.94
        in
          abuse F16.14
          dependence F16.24
      hypnotic F13.94
        in
          abuse F13.14
          dependence F13.24
      inhalant F18.94
        in
          abuse F18.14
          dependence F18.24
      opioid F11.94
        in
          abuse F11.14
          dependence F11.24
      phencyclidine (PCP) F16.94
        in
          abuse F16.14
          dependence F16.24
      physiological condition F06.30
        with
          depressive features F06.31
          major depressive-like episode F06.32
          manic features F06.33
          mixed features F06.34
      psychoactive substance NEC F19.94
        in
          abuse F19.14
          dependence F19.24
      sedative F13.94
        in
          abuse F13.14
          dependence F13.24
      volatile solvents F18.94
        in
          abuse F18.14
          dependence F18.24
    manic episode F30.9
      with psychotic symptoms F30.2
      in remission (full) F30.4
        partial F30.3
      specified type NEC F30.8
      without psychotic symptoms F30.10
        mild F30.11
        moderate F30.12
        severe F30.13
    organic F06.30
      right hemisphere F07.89
    persistent F34.9
      cyclothymia F34.0
      dysthymia F34.1
      specified type NEC F34.89
    recurrent F39

Disorder — *continued*
  mood — *continued*
    right hemisphere organic F07.89
  movement G25.9
    drug-induced G25.70
      akathisia G25.71
      specified NEC G25.79
    hysterical F44.4
    in diseases classified elsewhere — *see* category G26
    periodic limb G47.61
      sleep related G47.61
    sleep related NEC G47.69
    specified NEC G25.89
    stereotyped F98.4
    treatment-induced G25.9
  multiple personality F44.81
  muscle M62.9
    attachment, spine — *see* Enthesopathy, spinal
    in trichinellosis — *see* Trichinellosis, with muscle disorder
    psychogenic F45.8
    specified type NEC M62.89
    tone, newborn P94.9
      specified NEC P94.8
  muscular
    attachments — *see also* Enthesopathy
      spine — *see* Enthesopathy, spinal
    urethra N36.44
  musculoskeletal system, soft tissue — *see* Disorder, soft tissue
    postprocedural M96.89
    psychogenic F45.8
  myoneural G70.9
    due to lead G70.1
    specified NEC G70.89
    toxic G70.1
  myotonic NEC G71.19
  nail, in diseases classified elsewhere L62
  neck region NEC — *see* Dorsopathy, specified NEC
  neonatal onset multisystemic inflammatory (NOMID) M04.2
  nerve G58.9
    abducent NEC — *see* Strabismus, paralytic, sixth nerve
    accessory G52.8
    acoustic — *see* subcategory H93.3 ☑
    auditory — *see* subcategory H93.3 ☑
    auriculotemporal G50.8
    axillary G54.0
    cerebral — *see* Disorder, nerve, cranial
    cranial G52.9
      eighth — *see* subcategory H93.3 ☑
      eleventh G52.8
      fifth G50.9
      first G52.0
      fourth NEC — *see* Strabismus, paralytic, fourth nerve
      multiple G52.7
      ninth G52.1
      second NEC — *see* Disorder, nerve, optic
      seventh NEC G51.8
      sixth NEC — *see* Strabismus, paralytic, sixth nerve
      specified NEC G52.8
      tenth G52.2
      third NEC — *see* Strabismus, paralytic, third nerve
      twelfth G52.3
    entrapment — *see* Neuropathy, entrapment
    facial G51.9
      specified NEC G51.8
    femoral — *see* Lesion, nerve, femoral
    glossopharyngeal NEC G52.1
    hypoglossal G52.3
    intercostal G58.0
    lateral
      cutaneous of thigh — *see* Mononeuropathy, lower limb, meralgia paresthetica
      popliteal — *see* Lesion, nerve, popliteal
    lower limb — *see* Mononeuropathy, lower limb
    medial popliteal — *see* Lesion, nerve, popliteal, medial
    median NEC — *see* Lesion, nerve, median
    multiple G58.7
    oculomotor NEC — *see* Strabismus, paralytic, third nerve
    olfactory G52.0
    optic NEC H47.09- ☑
      hemorrhage into sheath — *see* Hemorrhage, optic nerve
      ischemic H47.01- ☑
    peroneal — *see* Lesion, nerve, popliteal

☑ **Additional Character Required — Refer to the Tabular List for Character Selection**

Disorder — *continued*
  nerve — *continued*
    phrenic G58.8
    plantar — *see* Lesion, nerve, plantar
    pneumogastric G52.2
    posterior tibial — *see* Syndrome, tarsal tunnel
    radial — *see* Lesion, nerve, radial
    recurrent laryngeal G52.2
    root G54.9
      cervical G54.2
      lumbosacral G54.1
      specified NEC G54.8
      thoracic G54.3
    sciatic NEC — *see* Lesion, nerve, sciatic
    specified NEC G58.8
      lower limb — *see* Mononeuropathy, lower limb, specified NEC
      upper limb — *see* Mononeuropathy, upper limb, specified NEC
    sympathetic G90.9
    tibial — *see* Lesion, nerve, popliteal, medial
    trigeminal G50.9
      specified NEC G50.8
    trochlear NEC — *see* Strabismus, paralytic, fourth nerve
    ulnar — *see* Lesion, nerve, ulnar
    upper limb — *see* Mononeuropathy, upper limb
    vagus G52.2
  nervous system G98.8
    autonomic (peripheral) G90.9
      specified NEC G90.89
    central G96.9
      specified NEC G96.89
    parasympathetic G90.9
    specified NEC G98.8
    sympathetic G90.9
    vegetative G90.9
  neurocognitive R41.9
    with Lewy bodies — *see also* Dementia, in, diseases specified elsewhere G31.83 *[F02.-]* ☑
    frontotemporal, specified NEC — *see also* Dementia, in, diseases specified elsewhere G31.09 *[F02.-]* ☑
    major — *see also* Dementia F03.- ☑
      due to vascular disease — *see* Dementia, vascular
        mild — *see* Dementia, vascular, mild
        moderate — *see* Dementia, vascular, moderate
        severe — *see* Dementia, vascular, severe
      in (due to) (other diseases classified elsewhere) — *see also* Dementia, in (due to) F02.80
        with
          aggressive behavior — *see also* Dementia, in (due to) F02.81- ☑
          combative behavior — *see also* Dementia, in (due to) F02.81- ☑
          violent behavior — *see also* Dementia, in (due to) F02.81- ☑
    mild (of uncertain or unknown etiology) — *see also* Disorder, mild neurocognitive G31.84
  neurodevelopmental F89
    specified NEC F88
  neurohypophysis NEC E23.3
  neurological NEC R29.818
  neuromuscular G70.9
    hereditary NEC G71.9
    specified NEC G70.89
    toxic G70.1
  neurotic F48.9
    specified NEC F48.8
  neutrophil, polymorphonuclear D71
  nicotine use — *see* Dependence, drug, nicotine
  nightmare F51.5
  non-rapid eye movement sleep arousal
    sleep terror type F51.4
    sleepwalking type F51.3
  nose J34.9
    specified NEC J34.89
  obsessive-compulsive F42.9
    and related disorder due to a known physiological condition F06.8
  odontogenesis NOS K00.9
  opioid use
    with
      opioid-induced psychotic disorder F11.959
        with
          delusions F11.950
          hallucinations F11.951
    due to drug abuse — *see* Abuse, drug, opioid

Disorder — *continued*
  opioid use — *continued*
    due to drug dependence — *see* Dependence, drug, opioid
    mild F11.10
      with
        opioid-induced
          anxiety disorder F11.188
          depressive disorder F11.14
          sexual dysfunction F11.181
        opioid intoxication
          with perceptual disturbances F11.122
          delirium F11.121
          without perceptual disturbances F11.129
      in remission (early) (sustained) F11.11
    moderate or severe F11.20
      with
        opioid-induced
          anxiety disorder F11.288
          anxiety disorder F11.988
          depressive disorder F11.24
          depressive disorder F11.94
          sexual dysfunction F11.281
          sexual dysfunction F11.981
        opioid intoxication
          with perceptual disturbances F11.222
          delirium F11.221
          without perceptual disturbances F11.229
      in remission (early) (sustained) F11.21
  oppositional defiant F91.3
  optic
    chiasm H47.49
      due to
        inflammatory disorder H47.41
        neoplasm H47.42
        vascular disorder H47.43
    disc H47.39- ☑
      coloboma — *see* Coloboma, optic disc
      drusen — *see* Drusen, optic disc
      pseudopapilledema — *see* Pseudopapilledema
    radiations — *see* Disorder, visual, pathway
    tracts — *see* Disorder, visual, pathway
  orbit H05.9
    cyst — *see* Cyst, orbit
    deformity — *see* Deformity, orbit
    edema — *see* Edema, orbit
    enophthalmos — *see* Enophthalmos
    exophthalmos — *see* Exophthalmos
    hemorrhage — *see* Hemorrhage, orbit
    inflammation — *see* Inflammation, orbit
    myopathy — *see* Myopathy, extraocular muscles
    retained foreign body — *see* Foreign body, orbit, old
    specified type NEC H05.89
  organic
    anxiety F06.4
    catatonic NOS F06.1
    delusional F06.2
    dissociative F06.8
    emotionally labile (asthenic) F06.8
    mood (affective) F06.30
    schizophrenia-like F06.2
  orgasmic (female) F52.31
    male F52.32
  ornithine metabolism E72.4
  overanxious F41.1
    of childhood F93.8
  pain
    with related psychological factors F45.42
    exclusively related to psychological factors F45.41
    genito-pelvic penetration disorder F52.6
  pancreatic internal secretion E16.9
    specified NEC E16.8
  panic F41.0
    with agoraphobia F40.01
  papulosquamous L44.9
    in diseases classified elsewhere L45
    specified NEC L44.8
  paranoid F22
    induced F24
    shared F24
  paraphilic F65.9
    specified NEC F65.89
  parathyroid (gland) E21.5
    specified NEC E21.4
  parietoalveolar NEC J84.09
  paroxysmal, mixed R56.9
  patella M22.9- ☑
    chondromalacia — *see* Chondromalacia, patella
    derangement NEC M22.3X- ☑

Disorder — *continued*
  patella — *continued*
    recurrent
      dislocation — *see* Dislocation, patella, recurrent
      subluxation — *see* Dislocation, patella, recurrent, incomplete
    specified NEC M22.8X- ☑
  patellofemoral M22.2X- ☑
  pedophilic F65.4
  pentose phosphate pathway with anemia D55.1
  perception, due to hallucinogens F16.983
    in
      abuse F16.183
      dependence F16.283
  peripheral nervous system NEC G64
  peroxisomal E71.50
    biogenesis
      neonatal adrenoleukodystrophy E71.511
      specified disorder NEC E71.518
      Zellweger syndrome E71.510
    rhizomelic chondrodysplasia punctata E71.540
    specified form NEC E71.548
      group 1 E71.518
      group 2 E71.53
      group 3 E71.542
    X-linked adrenoleukodystrophy E71.529
      adolescent E71.521
      adrenomyeloneuropathy E71.522
      childhood E71.520
      specified form NEC E71.528
    Zellweger-like syndrome E71.541
  persistent
    (somatoform) pain F45.41
    affective (mood) F34.9
  personality — *see also* Personality F60.9
    affective F34.0
    aggressive F60.3
    amoral F60.2
    anankastic F60.5
    antisocial F60.2
    anxious F60.6
    asocial F60.2
    asthenic F60.7
    avoidant F60.6
    borderline F60.3
    change (secondary) due to general medical condition F07.0
    compulsive F60.5
    cyclothymic F34.0
    dependent (passive) F60.7
    depressive F34.1
    dissocial F60.2
    emotional instability F60.3
    expansive paranoid F60.0
    explosive F60.3
    following organic brain damage F07.9
    histrionic F60.4
    hyperthymic F34.0
    hypothymic F34.1
    hysterical F60.4
    immature F60.89
    inadequate F60.7
    labile F60.3
    mixed (nonspecific) F60.89
    moral deficiency F60.2
    narcissistic F60.81
    negativistic F60.89
    obsessional F60.5
    obsessive (-compulsive) F60.5
    organic F07.9
    overconscientious F60.5
    paranoid F60.0
    passive (-dependent) F60.7
    passive-aggressive F60.89
    pathological NEC F60.9
    pseudosocial F60.2
    psychopathic F60.2
    schizoid F60.1
    schizotypal F21
    self-defeating F60.7
    specified NEC F60.89
    type A F60.5
    unstable (emotional) F60.3
  pervasive, developmental F84.9
  phencyclidine use
    mild F16.10
      with
        phencyclidine intoxication F16.129
        phencyclidine intoxication delirium F16.121

☑ **Additional Character Required** — **Refer to the Tabular List for Character Selection**

Disorder — *continued*
  phencyclidine use — *continued*
    mild — *continued*
      with — *continued*
        phencyclidine-induced
          anxiety disorder F16.18Ø
          bipolar and related disorder F16.14
          depressive disorder F16.14
          psychotic disorder F16.159
        in remission (early) (sustained) F16.11
    moderate or severe F16.2Ø
      with
        phencyclidine intoxication F16.229
        phencyclidine intoxication delirium F16.221
        phencyclidine-induced
          anxiety disorder F16.28Ø
          bipolar and related disorder F16.14
          depressive disorder F16.24
          psychotic disorder F16.259
        in remission (early) (sustained) F16.21
  phobic anxiety, childhood F40.8
  phosphate-losing tubular N25.Ø
  pigmentation L81.9
    choroid, congenital Q14.3
    diminished melanin formation L81.6
    iron L81.8
    specified NEC L81.8
  pinna (noninfective) H61.1Ø- ☑
    deformity, acquired H61.11- ☑
    hematoma H61.12- ☑
    perichondritis — *see* Perichondritis, ear
    specified type NEC H61.19- ☑
  pituitary gland E23.7
    iatrogenic (postprocedural) E89.3
    specified NEC E23.6
  platelet-activating anti-PF4, specified NEC D75.84
  platelets D69.1
  plexus G54.9
    specified NEC G54.8
  polymorphonuclear neutrophils D71
  porphyrin metabolism — *see* Porphyria
  postconcussional FØ7.81
  posthallucinogen perception F16.983
    in
      abuse F16.183
      dependence F16.283
  postmenopausal N95.9
    specified NEC N95.8
  postprocedural (postoperative) — *see* Complications, postprocedural
  post-transplant lymphoproliferative D47.Z1 (*following* D47.4)
  post-traumatic stress (PTSD) F43.1Ø
    acute F43.11
    chronic F43.12
  premenstrual dysphoric (PMDD) F32.81
  prepuce N47.8
  propionic acidemia E71.121
  prostate N42.9
    specified NEC N42.89
  psychogenic NOS — *see also* condition F45.9
    anxiety F41.8
    appetite F5Ø.9
    asthenic F48.8
    cardiovascular (system) F45.8
    compulsive F42.8
    cutaneous F54
    depressive F32.9
    digestive (system) F45.8
    dysmenorrheic F45.8
    dyspneic F45.8
    endocrine (system) F54
    eye NEC F45.8
    feeding — *see* Disorder, eating
    functional NEC F45.8
    gastric F45.8
    gastrointestinal (system) F45.8
    genitourinary (system) F45.8
    heart (function) (rhythm) F45.8
    hyperventilatory F45.8
    hypochondriacal — *see* Disorder, hypochondriacal
    intestinal F45.8
    joint F45.8
    learning F81.9
    limb F45.8
    lymphatic (system) F45.8
    menstrual F45.8
    micturition F45.8
    monoplegic NEC F44.4

Disorder — *continued*
  psychogenic — *see also* condition — *continued*
    motor F44.4
    muscle F45.8
    musculoskeletal F45.8
    neurocirculatory F45.8
    obsessive F42.8
    occupational F48.8
    organ or part of body NEC F45.8
    paralytic NEC F44.4
    phobic F4Ø.9
    physical NEC F45.8
    rectal F45.8
    respiratory (system) F45.8
    rheumatic F45.8
    sexual (function) F52.9
    skin (allergic) (eczematous) F54
    sleep F51.9
    specified part of body NEC F45.8
    stomach F45.8
  psychological F99
    associated with
      disease classified elsewhere F54
      sexual
        development F66
        relationship F66
      uncertainty about gender identity F64.9
  psychomotor NEC F44.4
    hysterical F44.4
  psychoneurotic — *see also* Neurosis
    mixed NEC F48.8
  psychophysiologic — *see* Disorder, somatoform
  psychosexual F65.9
    development F66
    identity of childhood F64.2
  psychosomatic NOS — *see* Disorder, somatoform
    multiple F45.Ø
    undifferentiated F45.1
  psychotic — *see* Psychosis
    transient (acute) F23
  puberty E3Ø.9
    specified NEC E3Ø.8
  pulmonary (valve) — *see* Endocarditis, pulmonary
  purine metabolism E79.9
  pyrimidine metabolism E79.9
  pyruvate metabolism E74.4
  reactive attachment (childhood) F94.1
  reading R48.Ø
    developmental (specific) F81.Ø
  receptive language F8Ø.2
  receptor, hormonal, peripheral — *see also* Syndrome, androgen insensitivity E34.5Ø
  recurrent brief depressive F33.8
  reflex R29.2
  refraction H52.7
    aniseikonia H52.32
    anisometropia H52.31
    astigmatism — *see* Astigmatism
    hypermetropia — *see* Hypermetropia
    myopia — *see* Myopia
    presbyopia H52.4
    specified NEC H52.6
  relationship F68.8
    due to sexual orientation F66
  REM sleep behavior G47.52
  renal function, impaired (tubular) N25.9
  resonance R49.9
    specified NEC R49.8
  respiratory function, impaired — *see also* Failure, respiration
    postprocedural — *see* Complication, postoperative, respiratory system
    psychogenic F45.8
  retina H35.9
    angioid streaks H35.33
    changes in vascular appearance H35.Ø1- ☑
    degeneration — *see* Degeneration, retina
    dystrophy (hereditary) — *see* Dystrophy, retina
    edema H35.81
    hemorrhage — *see* Hemorrhage, retina
    ischemia H35.82
    macular degeneration — *see* Degeneration, macula
    microaneurysms H35.Ø4- ☑
    microvascular abnormality NEC H35.Ø9
    neovascularization — *see* Neovascularization, retina
    retinopathy — *see* Retinopathy
    separation of layers H35.7Ø
      central serous chorioretinopathy H35.71- ☑

Disorder — *continued*
  retina — *continued*
    separation of layers — *continued*
      pigment epithelium detachment (serous) H35.72- ☑
        hemorrhagic H35.73- ☑
      specified type NEC H35.89
    telangiectasis — *see* Telangiectasis, retina
    vasculitis — *see* Vasculitis, retina
  retroperitoneal K68.9
  right hemisphere organic affective FØ7.89
  rumination (infant or child) (in remission) F98.21
    adult (in remission) F5Ø.84
  sacrum, sacrococcygeal NEC M53.3
  schizoaffective F25.9
    bipolar type F25.Ø
    depressive type F25.1
    manic type F25.Ø
    mixed type F25.Ø
    specified NEC F25.8
  schizoid of childhood F84.5
  schizophrenia spectrum and other psychotic disorder F29
    specified NEC F28
  schizophreniform F2Ø.81
    brief F23
  schizotypal (personality) F21
  seasonal affective, recurrent episodes F33.- ☑
  secretion, thyrocalcitonin EØ7.Ø
  sedative, hypnotic, or anxiolytic use
    mild F13.1Ø
      with
        sedative, hypnotic, or anxiolytic intoxication F13.129
        sedative, hypnotic, or anxiolytic intoxication delirium F13.121
        sedative, hypnotic, or anxiolytic-induced
          anxiety disorder F13.18Ø
          bipolar and related disorder F13.14
          depressive disorder F13.14
          psychotic disorder F13.159
          sexual dysfunction F13.181
        in remission (early) (sustained) F13.11
    moderate or severe F13.2Ø
      with
        sedative, hypnotic, or anxiolytic intoxication F13.229
        sedative, hypnotic, or anxiolytic intoxication delirium F13.221
        sedative, hypnotic, or anxiolytic-induced
          anxiety disorder F13.28Ø
          bipolar and related disorder F13.24
          depressive disorder F13.24
          major neurocognitive disorder F13.27
          mild neurocognitive disorder F13.288
          psychotic disorder F13.259
          sexual dysfunction F13.281
        in remission (early) (sustained) F13.21
  seizure — *see also* Epilepsy G4Ø.9Ø9
    intractable G4Ø.919
      with status epilepticus G4Ø.911
  semantic pragmatic F8Ø.89
    with autism F84.Ø
  sense of smell R43.1
    psychogenic F45.8
  separation anxiety, of childhood F93.Ø
  sexual
    aversion F52.1
    function, psychogenic F52.9
    interest/arousal, female F52.22
    masochism F65.51
    maturation F66
    nonorganic F52.9
    preference — *see also* Deviation, sexual F65.9
      fetishistic transvestism F65.1
    relationship F66
    sadism F65.52
  shyness, of childhood and adolescence F4Ø.1Ø
  sibling rivalry F93.8
  sickle-cell (sickling) (homozygous) — *see* Disease, sickle-cell
    heterozygous D57.3
    specified type NEC D57.8- ☑
    trait D57.3
  sinus (nasal) J34.9
    specified NEC J34.89
  skin L98.9
    atrophic L9Ø.9
      specified NEC L9Ø.8

☑ **Additional Character Required — Refer to the Tabular List for Character Selection**

☑ **Additional Character Required — Refer to the Tabular List for Character Selection**

Disorder — *continued*
   temporomandibular joint M26.60- ☑
   tendon M67.90
      acromioclavicular M67.91- ☑
      ankle M67.97- ☑
      contracture — *see* Contracture, tendon
      elbow M67.92- ☑
      foot M67.97- ☑
      forearm M67.93- ☑
      hand M67.94- ☑
      hip M67.95- ☑
      knee M67.96- ☑
      multiple sites M67.99
      rupture — *see* Rupture, tendon
      shoulder M67.91- ☑
      specified type NEC M67.80
         acromioclavicular M67.81- ☑
         ankle M67.87- ☑
         elbow M67.82- ☑
         foot M67.87- ☑
         hand M67.84- ☑
         hip M67.85- ☑
         knee M67.86- ☑
         multiple sites M67.89
         trunk M67.88
         wrist M67.83- ☑
      synovitis — *see* Synovitis
      tendinitis — *see* Tendinitis
      tenosynovitis — *see* Tenosynovitis
      trunk M67.98
      upper arm M67.92- ☑
      wrist M67.93- ☑
   thoracic root (nerve) NEC G54.3
   thyrocalcitonin hypersecretion E07.0
   thyroid (gland) E07.9
      function NEC, neonatal, transitory P72.2
      iodine-deficiency related E01.8
      specified NEC E07.89
   tic — *see* Tic
   tobacco use
      chewing tobacco (mild) (moderate) (severe)
         in remission (early) (sustained) F17.221
      cigarettes (mild) (moderate) (severe)
         in remission (early) (sustained) F17.211
      mild F17.200
         in remission (early) (sustained) F17.201
      moderate F17.200
         in remission (early) (sustained) F17.201
      severe F17.200
         in remission (early) (sustained) F17.201
      specified product NEC (mild) (moderate) (severe)
         in remission (early) (sustained) F17.291
   tooth K08.9
      development K00.9
         specified NEC K00.8
      eruption K00.6
   Tourette's F95.2
   trance and possession F44.89
   transvestic F65.1
   trauma and stressor-related NOS F43.9
      other specified F43.89
      unspecified F43.9
   tricuspid (valve) — *see* Endocarditis, tricuspid
   tryptophan metabolism E70.5
   tubular, phosphate-losing N25.0
   tubulo-interstitial (in)
      brucellosis A23.9 *[N16]*
      cystinosis E72.04
      diphtheria A36.84
      glycogen storage disease E74.00 *[N16]*
      leukemia NEC C95.9- ☑ *[N16]*
      lymphoma NEC C85.9- ☑ *[N16]*
      mixed cryoglobulinemia D89.1 *[N16]*
      multiple myeloma C90.0- ☑ *[N16]*
      Salmonella infection A02.25
      sarcoidosis D86.84
      sepsis A41.9 *[N16]*
         streptococcal A40.9 *[N16]*
      systemic lupus erythematosus M32.15
      toxoplasmosis B58.83
      transplant rejection T86.91 *[N16]*
      Wilson's disease E83.01 *[N16]*
   tubulo-renal function, impaired N25.9
      specified NEC N25.89
   tympanic membrane H73.9- ☑
      atrophy — *see* Atrophy, tympanic membrane
      infection — *see* Myringitis
      perforation — *see* Perforation, tympanum

Disorder — *continued*
   tympanic membrane — *continued*
      specified NEC H73.89- ☑
   unsocialized aggressive F91.1
   urea cycle metabolism E72.20
      argininemia E72.21
      arginosuccinic aciduria E72.22
      citrullinemia E72.23
      ornithine transcarbamylase deficiency E72.4
      other specified E72.29
   ureter (in) N28.9
      schistosomiasis B65.0 *[N29]*
      tuberculosis A18.11
   urethra N36.9
      specified NEC N36.8
   urinary system N39.9
      specified NEC N39.8
   valve, heart
      aortic — *see* Endocarditis, aortic
      mitral — *see* Endocarditis, mitral
      pulmonary — *see* Endocarditis, pulmonary
      rheumatic
         aortic — *see* Endocarditis, aortic, rheumatic
         mitral — *see* Endocarditis, mitral
         pulmonary — *see* Endocarditis, pulmonary, rheumatic
         tricuspid — *see* Endocarditis, tricuspid
      tricuspid — *see* Endocarditis, tricuspid
   vestibular function H81.9- ☑
      specified NEC — *see* subcategory H81.8 ☑
         in diseases classified elsewhere H82.- ☑
      vertigo — *see* Vertigo
   vision, binocular H53.30
      abnormal retinal correspondence H53.31
      diplopia H53.2
      fusion with defective stereopsis H53.32
      simultaneous perception H53.33
      suppression H53.34
   visual
      cortex
         blindness H47.619
            left brain H47.612
            right brain H47.611
         due to
            inflammatory disorder H47.629
               left brain H47.622
               right brain H47.621
            neoplasm H47.639
               left brain H47.632
               right brain H47.631
            vascular disorder H47.649
               left brain H47.642
               right brain H47.641
      pathway H47.9
         due to
            inflammatory disorder H47.51- ☑
            neoplasm H47.52- ☑
            vascular disorder H47.53- ☑
      optic chiasm — *see* Disorder, optic, chiasm
   vitreous body H43.9
      crystalline deposits — *see* Deposit, crystalline
      degeneration — *see* Degeneration, vitreous
      hemorrhage — *see* Hemorrhage, vitreous
      opacities — *see* Opacity, vitreous
      prolapse — *see* Prolapse, vitreous
      specified type NEC H43.89
   voice R49.9
      specified type NEC R49.8
   volatile solvent use
      due to drug abuse — *see* Abuse, drug, inhalant
      due to drug dependence — *see* Dependence, drug, inhalant
   voyeuristic F65.3
   white blood cells D72.9
      specified NEC D72.89
   withdrawing, child or adolescent F40.10
Disorientation R41.0
Displacement, displaced
   acquired traumatic of bone, cartilage, joint, tendon NEC — *see* Dislocation
   adrenal gland (congenital) Q89.1
   appendix, retrocecal (congenital) Q43.8
   auricle (congenital) Q17.4
   bladder (acquired) N32.89
      congenital Q64.19
   brachial plexus (congenital) Q07.8
   brain stem, caudal (congenital) Q04.8
   canaliculus (lacrimalis), congenital Q10.6

Displacement, displaced — *continued*
   cardia through esophageal hiatus (congenital) Q40.1
   cerebellum, caudal (congenital) Q04.8
   cervix — *see* Malposition, uterus
   colon (congenital) Q43.3
   device, implant or graft — *see also* Complications, by site and type, mechanical T85.628 ☑
      arterial graft NEC — *see* Complication, cardiovascular device, mechanical, vascular
      breast (implant) T85.42 ☑
      catheter NEC T85.628 ☑
         dialysis (renal) T82.42 ☑
            intraperitoneal T85.621 ☑
         infusion NEC T82.524 ☑
            spinal (epidural) (subdural) T85.620 ☑
         urinary
            cystostomy T83.020 ☑
            Hopkins T83.028 ☑
            ileostomy T83.028 ☑
            indwelling T83.021 ☑
            nephrostomy T83.022 ☑
            specified NEC T83.028 ☑
            urostomy T83.028 ☑
      electronic (electrode) (pulse generator) (stimulator) — *see* Complication, electronic stimulator
      fixation, internal (orthopedic) NEC — *see* Complication, fixation device, mechanical
      gastrointestinal — *see* Complications, prosthetic device, mechanical, gastrointestinal device
      genital NEC T83.428 ☑
         intrauterine contraceptive device (string) T83.32 ☑
         penile prosthesis (cylinder) (implanted) (pump) (reservoir) T83.420 ☑
         testicular prosthesis T83.421 ☑
      heart NEC — *see* Complication, cardiovascular device, mechanical
      joint prosthesis — *see* Complications, joint prosthesis, mechanical
      ocular — *see* Complications, prosthetic device, mechanical, ocular device
      orthopedic NEC — *see* Complication, orthopedic, device or graft, mechanical
      specified NEC T85.628 ☑
      urinary NEC T83.128 ☑
         graft T83.22 ☑
         sphincter, implanted T83.121 ☑
         stent (ileal conduit) (nephroureteral) T83.123 ☑
            ureteral indwelling T83.122 ☑
      vascular NEC — *see* Complication, cardiovascular device, mechanical
      ventricular intracranial shunt T85.02 ☑
   electronic stimulator
      bone T84.320 ☑
      cardiac — *see* Complications, cardiac device, electronic
      nervous system — *see* Complication, prosthetic device, mechanical, electronic nervous system stimulator
      urinary — *see* Complications, electronic stimulator, urinary
   esophageal mucosa into cardia of stomach, congenital Q39.8
   esophagus (acquired) K22.89
      congenital Q39.8
   eyeball (acquired) (lateral) (old) — *see* Displacement, globe
      congenital Q15.8
      current — *see* Avulsion, eye
   fallopian tube (acquired) N83.4- ☑
      congenital Q50.6
      opening (congenital) Q50.6
   gallbladder (congenital) Q44.1
   gastric mucosa (congenital) Q40.2
   globe (acquired) (old) (lateral) H05.21- ☑
      current — *see* Avulsion, eye
   heart (congenital) Q24.8
      acquired I51.89
   hymen (upward) (congenital) Q52.4
   intervertebral disc NEC
      with myelopathy — *see* Disorder, disc, with, myelopathy
      cervical, cervicothoracic (with) M50.20
         myelopathy — *see* Disorder, disc, cervical, with myelopathy
         neuritis, radiculitis or radiculopathy — *see* Disorder, disc, cervical, with neuritis

Displacement, displaced — *continued*
  intervertebral disc — *continued*
    due to trauma — *see* Dislocation, vertebra
    lumbar region M51.26
      with
        myelopathy M51.06
        neuritis, radiculitis, radiculopathy or sciatica M51.16
    lumbosacral region M51.27
      with
        neuritis, radiculitis, radiculopathy or sciatica M51.17
    sacrococcygeal region M53.3
    thoracic region M51.24
      with
        myelopathy M51.04
        neuritis, radiculitis, radiculopathy M51.14
    thoracolumbar region M51.25
      with
        myelopathy M51.05
        neuritis, radiculitis, radiculopathy M51.15
  intrauterine device (string) T83.32 ☑
  kidney (acquired) N28.83
    congenital Q63.2
  lachrymal, lacrimal apparatus or duct (congenital) Q10.6
  lens, congenital Q12.1
  macula (congenital) Q14.1
  Meckel's diverticulum Q43.0
    malignant — *see* Table of Neoplasms, small intestine, malignant
  nail (congenital) Q84.6
    acquired L60.8
  opening of Wharton's duct in mouth Q38.4
  organ or site, congenital NEC — *see* Malposition, congenital
  ovary (acquired) N83.4- ☑
    congenital Q50.39
    free in peritoneal cavity (congenital) Q50.39
    into hernial sac N83.4- ☑
  oviduct (acquired) N83.4- ☑
    congenital Q50.6
  parathyroid (gland) E21.4
  parotid gland (congenital) Q38.4
  punctum lacrimale (congenital) Q10.6
  sacro-iliac (joint) (congenital) Q74.2
    current injury S33.2 ☑
    old — *see* subcategory M53.2 ☑
  salivary gland (any) (congenital) Q38.4
  spleen (congenital) Q89.09
  stomach, congenital Q40.2
  sublingual duct Q38.4
  tongue (downward) (congenital) Q38.3
  tooth, teeth, fully erupted M26.30
    horizontal M26.33
    vertical M26.34
  trachea (congenital) Q32.1
  ureter or ureteric opening or orifice (congenital) Q62.62
  uterine opening of oviducts or fallopian tubes Q50.6
  uterus, uterine — *see* Malposition, uterus
  ventricular septum Q21.0
    with rudimentary ventricle Q20.4

Disproportion
  between native and reconstructed breast N65.1
  fiber-type G71.20
    congenital G71.29

Disruptio uteri — *see* Rupture, uterus

Disruption (of)
  ciliary body NEC H21.89
  closure of
    abdominal wall muscle or fascia T81.321 ☑
    cornea T81.31 ☑
    craniotomy T81.328 ☑
    fascia (muscular) (superficial) T81.328 ☑
    gastrointestinal tract anastomosis, repair, or closure T81.320 ☑
    internal organ or tissue T81.328 ☑
    laceration (external) (internal) T81.33 ☑
    ligament T81.328 ☑
    mucosa T81.31 ☑
    muscle or muscle flap T81.328 ☑
    ribs or rib cage T81.328 ☑
    skin and subcutaneous tissue (full-thickness) (superficial) T81.31 ☑
    skull T81.328 ☑
    sternum (sternotomy) T81.328 ☑
    tendon T81.328 ☑
    traumatic laceration (external) (internal) T81.33 ☑
  family Z63.8

Disruption — *continued*
  family — *continued*
    due to
      absence of family member due to military deployment Z63.31
      absence of family member NEC Z63.32
      alcoholism and drug addiction in family Z63.72
      bereavement Z63.4
      death (assumed) or disappearance of family member Z63.4
      divorce or separation Z63.5
      drug addiction in family Z63.72
      return of family member from military deployment (current or past conflict) Z63.71
      stressful life events NEC Z63.79
  iris NEC H21.89
  ligament(s) — *see also* Sprain
    knee
      current injury — *see* Dislocation, knee
      old (chronic) — *see* Derangement, knee, instability
      spontaneous NEC — *see* Derangement, knee, disruption ligament
  ossicular chain — *see* Discontinuity, ossicles, ear
  pelvic ring (stable) S32.810 ☑
    unstable S32.811 ☑
  traumatic injury wound repair T81.33 ☑
  wound T81.30 ☑
    episiotomy O90.1
    operation T81.31 ☑
      cesarean O90.0
      deep T81.329 ☑
      external operation wound (superficial) T81.31 ☑
      internal operation wound (deep) T81.329 ☑
        abdominal wall muscle or fascia T81.321 ☑
        specified NEC T81.328 ☑
    perineal (obstetric) O90.1
    traumatic injury repair T81.33 ☑

Dissatisfaction with
  employment Z56.9
  school environment Z55.4

Dissecting — *see* condition

Dissection
  aorta I71.00
    abdominal I71.02
    thoracic I71.019
      aortic arch I71.011
      ascending aorta I71.010
      descending thoracic aorta I71.012
    thoracoabdominal I71.03
  artery I77.70
    basilar (trunk) I77.75
    carotid I77.71
    cerebral (nonruptured) I67.0
      ruptured — *see* Hemorrhage, intracranial, subarachnoid
    coronary I25.42
    extremity
      lower I77.77
      upper I77.76
    iliac I77.72
    precerebral
      congenital (nonruptured) Q28.1
      specified site NEC I77.75
    renal I77.73
    specified NEC I77.79
    vertebral I77.74
  precerebral artery, congenital (nonruptured) Q28.1
    Heartland A93.8
  traumatic — *see* Wound, open, by site
  vascular I99.8
  wound — *see* Wound, open

Disseminated — *see* condition

Dissociation
  auriculoventricular or atrioventricular (AV) (any degree) (isorhythmic) I45.89
    with heart block I44.2
  interference I45.89

Dissociative reaction, state F44.9

Dissolution, vertebra — *see* Osteoporosis

Distension, distention
  abdomen R14.0
  bladder N32.89
  cecum K63.89
  colon K63.89
  gallbladder K82.8
  intestine K63.89
  kidney N28.89
  liver K76.89

Distension, distention — *continued*
  seminal vesicle N50.89
  stomach K31.89
    acute K31.0
    psychogenic F45.8
  ureter — *see* Dilatation, ureter
  uterus N85.8

Distoma hepaticum infestation B66.3

Distomiasis B66.9
  bile passages B66.3
  hemic B65.9
  hepatic B66.3
    due to Clonorchis sinensis B66.1
  intestinal B66.5
  liver B66.3
    due to Clonorchis sinensis B66.1
  lung B66.4
  pulmonary B66.4

Distomolar (fourth molar) K00.1

Disto-occlusion (Division I) (Division II) M26.212

Distortion(s) (congenital)
  adrenal (gland) Q89.1
  arm NEC Q68.8
  bile duct or passage Q44.5
  bladder Q64.79
  brain Q04.9
  cervix (uteri) Q51.9
  chest (wall) Q67.8
    bones Q76.8
  clavicle Q74.0
  clitoris Q52.6
  coccyx Q76.49
  common duct Q44.5
  coronary Q24.5
  cystic duct Q44.5
  ear (auricle) (external) Q17.3
    inner Q16.5
    middle Q16.4
      ossicles Q16.3
  endocrine NEC Q89.2
  eustachian tube Q17.8
  eye (adnexa) Q15.8
  face bone(s) NEC Q75.8
  fallopian tube Q50.6
  femur NEC Q68.8
  fibula NEC Q68.8
  finger(s) Q68.1
  foot Q66.9- ☑
  genitalia, genital organ(s)
    female Q52.8
      external Q52.79
      internal NEC Q52.8
  gyri Q04.8
  hand bone(s) Q68.1
  heart (auricle) (ventricle) Q24.8
    valve (cusp) Q24.8
  hepatic duct Q44.5
  humerus NEC Q68.8
  hymen Q52.4
  intrafamilial communications Z63.8
  jaw NEC M26.89
  labium (majus) (minus) Q52.79
  leg NEC Q68.8
  lens Q12.8
  liver Q44.79
  lumbar spine Q76.49
    with disproportion O33.8
      causing obstructed labor O65.0
  lumbosacral (joint) (region) Q76.49
    kyphosis — *see* Kyphosis, congenital
    lordosis — *see* Lordosis, congenital
  nerve Q07.8
  nose Q30.8
  organ
    of Corti Q16.5
    or site not listed — *see* Anomaly, by site
  ossicles, ear Q16.3
  oviduct Q50.6
  pancreas Q45.3
  parathyroid (gland) Q89.2
  pituitary (gland) Q89.2
  radius NEC Q68.8
  sacroiliac joint Q74.2
  sacrum Q76.49
  scapula Q74.0
  shoulder girdle Q74.0
  skull bone(s) NEC Q75.8
    with
      anencephalus Q00.0

Distortion(s) — *continued*
  skull bone(s) — *continued*
    with — *continued*
      encephalocele — *see* Encephalocele
      hydrocephalus Q03.9
        with spina bifida — *see* Spina bifida, with hydrocephalus
      microcephaly Q02
  spinal cord Q06.8
  spine Q76.49
    kyphosis — *see* Kyphosis, congenital
    lordosis — *see* Lordosis, congenital
  spleen Q89.09
  sternum NEC Q76.7
  thorax (wall) Q67.8
    bony Q76.8
  thymus (gland) Q89.2
  thyroid (gland) Q89.2
  tibia NEC Q68.8
  toe(s) Q66.9- ☑
  tongue Q38.3
  trachea (cartilage) Q32.1
  ulna NEC Q68.8
  ureter Q62.8
  urethra Q64.79
    causing obstruction Q64.39
  uterus Q51.9
  vagina Q52.4
  vertebra Q76.49
    kyphosis — *see* Kyphosis, congenital
    lordosis — *see* Lordosis, congenital
  visual — *see also* Disturbance, vision
    shape and size H53.15
  vulva Q52.79
  wrist (bones) (joint) Q68.8

Distress
  abdomen — *see* Pain, abdominal
  acute respiratory R06.03
    syndrome (adult) (child) J80
  epigastric R10.13
  fetal P84
    complicating pregnancy — *see* Stress, fetal
  gastrointestinal (functional) K30
    psychogenic F45.8
  intestinal (functional) NOS K59.9
    psychogenic F45.8
  maternal, during labor and delivery O75.0
  relationship, with spouse or intimate partner Z63.0
  respiratory (adult) (child) R06.03
    newborn P22.9
      specified NEC P22.8
    orthopnea R06.01
    psychogenic F45.8
    shortness of breath R06.02
    specified type NEC R06.09

Distribution vessel, atypical Q27.9
  coronary artery Q24.5
  precerebral Q28.1

Districhiasis L68.8

Disturbance(s) — *see also* Disease
  absorption K90.9
    calcium E58
    carbohydrate K90.49
    fat K90.49
      pancreatic K90.3
    protein K90.49
    starch K90.49
    vitamin — *see* Deficiency, vitamin
  acid-base equilibrium E87.8
    mixed E87.4
  activity and attention (with hyperkinesis) — *see* Disorder, attention-deficit hyperactivity
  amino acid transport E72.00
  assimilation, food K90.9
  auditory nerve, except deafness — *see* subcategory H93.3 ☑
  behavior — *see* Disorder, conduct
  blood clotting (mechanism) — *see also* Defect, coagulation D68.9
  cerebral
    nerve — *see* Disorder, nerve, cranial
    status, newborn P91.9
      specified NEC P91.88
  circulatory I99.9
  conduct — *see also* Disorder, conduct F91.9
    adjustment reaction — *see* Disorder, adjustment
    compulsive F63.9
    disruptive F91.9

Disturbance(s) — *continued*
  conduct — *see also* Disorder, conduct — *continued*
    hyperkinetic — *see* Disorder, attention-deficit hyperactivity
    socialized F91.2
    specified NEC F91.8
    unsocialized F91.1
  coordination R27.8
  cranial nerve — *see* Disorder, nerve, cranial
  deep sensibility — *see* Disturbance, sensation
  digestive K30
    psychogenic F45.8
  electrolyte — *see also* Imbalance, electrolyte
    newborn, transitory P74.49
      hyperammonemia P74.6
      hyperchloremia P74.421
      hyperchloremic metabolic acidosis P74.421
      hypochloremia P74.422
      potassium balance
        hyperkalemia P74.31
        hypokalemia P74.32
      sodium balance
        hypernatremia P74.21
        hyponatremia P74.22
      specified type NEC P74.49
  emotions specific to childhood and adolescence F93.9
    with
      anxiety and fearfulness NEC F93.8
      elective mutism F94.0
      oppositional disorder F91.3
      sensitivity (withdrawal) F40.10
      shyness F40.10
      social withdrawal F40.10
    involving relationship problems F93.8
    mixed F93.8
    specified NEC F93.8
  endocrine (gland) E34.9
    neonatal, transitory P72.9
      specified NEC P72.8
  equilibrium R42
  fructose metabolism E74.10
  gait — *see* Gait
    hysterical F44.4
    psychogenic F44.4
  gastrointestinal (functional) K30
    psychogenic F45.8
  habit, child F98.9
  hearing, except deafness and tinnitus — *see* Abnormal, auditory perception
  heart, functional (conditions in I44-I50)
    due to presence of (cardiac) prosthesis I97.19- ☑
    postoperative I97.89
      cardiac surgery — *see also* Infarct, myocardium, associated with revascularization procedure I97.19- ☑
  hormones E34.9
  innervation uterus (parasympathetic) (sympathetic) N85.8
  keratinization NEC
    gingiva K05.10
      nonplaque induced K05.11
      plaque induced K05.10
    lip K13.0
    oral (mucosa) (soft tissue) K13.29
    tongue K13.29
  learning (specific) — *see* Disorder, learning
  memory — *see* Amnesia
    mild, following organic brain damage F06.8
  mental F99
    associated with diseases classified elsewhere F54
  metabolism E88.9
    with
      abortion — *see* Abortion, by type with other specified complication
      ectopic pregnancy O08.5
      molar pregnancy O08.5
    amino-acid E72.9
      aromatic E70.9
      branched-chain E71.2
      straight-chain E72.89
      sulfur-bearing E72.10
    ammonia E72.20
    arginine E72.21
    arginosuccinic acid E72.22
    carbohydrate E74.9
    cholesterol E78.9
    citrulline E72.23
    cystathionine E72.19
    general E88.9

Disturbance(s) — *continued*
  metabolism — *continued*
    glutamine E72.89
    histidine E70.40
    homocystine E72.19
    hydroxylysine E72.3
    in labor or delivery O75.89
    iron E83.10
    lipoid E78.9
    lysine E72.3
    methionine E72.19
    neonatal, transitory P74.9
      calcium and magnesium P71.9
        specified type NEC P71.8
      carbohydrate metabolism P70.9
        specified type NEC P70.8
      specified NEC P74.8
    ornithine E72.4
    phosphate E83.39
    sodium NEC E87.8
    threonine E72.89
    tryptophan E70.5
    tyrosine E70.20
    urea cycle E72.20
  motor R29.2
  nervous, functional R45.0
  neuromuscular mechanism (eye), due to syphilis A52.15
  nutritional E63.9
    nail L60.3
  ocular motion H51.9
    psychogenic F45.8
  oculogyric H51.8
    psychogenic F45.8
  oculomotor H51.9
    psychogenic F45.8
  olfactory nerve R43.1
  optic nerve NEC — *see* Disorder, nerve, optic
  oral epithelium, including tongue NEC K13.29
  perceptual due to
    alcohol withdrawal F10.232
    amphetamine intoxication F15.922
      in
        abuse F15.122
        dependence F15.222
    anxiolytic withdrawal F13.232
    cannabis intoxication (acute) F12.922
      in
        abuse F12.122
        dependence F12.222
    cocaine intoxication (acute) F14.922
      in
        abuse F14.122
        dependence F14.222
    hypnotic withdrawal F13.232
    opioid intoxication (acute) F11.922
      in
        abuse F11.122
        dependence F11.222
    phencyclidine intoxication (acute) F16.122
    sedative withdrawal F13.232
  personality (pattern) (trait) — *see also* Disorder, personality F60.9
    following organic brain damage F07.9
  polyglandular E31.9
    specified NEC E31.8
  potassium balance, newborn
    hyperkalemia P74.31
    hypokalemia P74.32
  psychogenic F45.9
  psychomotor F44.4
  psychophysical visual H53.16
  pupillary — *see* Anomaly, pupil, function
  reflex R29.2
  rhythm, heart I49.9
  salivary secretion K11.7
  sensation (cold) (heat) (localization) (tactile discrimination) (texture) (vibratory) NEC R20.9
    hysterical F44.6
    skin R20.9
      anesthesia R20.0
      hyperesthesia R20.3
      hypoesthesia R20.1
      paresthesia R20.2
      specified type NEC R20.8
    smell R43.9
      and taste (mixed) R43.8
      anosmia R43.0
      parosmia R43.1
      specified NEC R43.8

Disturbance(s) — continued
  sensation — continued
    taste R43.9
      and smell (mixed) R43.8
      parageusia R43.2
      specified NEC R43.8
    sensory — see Disturbance, sensation
    situational (transient) — see also Disorder, adjustment
      acute F43.0
    sleep G47.9
      nonorganic origin F51.9
    smell — see Disturbance, sensation, smell
  sociopathic F60.2
  sodium balance, newborn
    hypernatremia P74.21
    hyponatremia P74.22
  speech R47.9
    developmental F80.9
    specified NEC R47.89
  stomach (functional) K31.9
  sympathetic (nerve) G90.9
  taste — see Disturbance, sensation, taste
  temperature
    regulation, newborn P81.9
      specified NEC P81.8
    sense R20.8
      hysterical F44.6
  tooth
    eruption K00.6
    formation K00.4
    structure, hereditary NEC K00.5
  touch — see Disturbance, sensation
  vascular I99.9
    arteriosclerotic — see Arteriosclerosis
  vasomotor I73.9
  vasospastic I73.9
  vision, visual H53.9
    following
      cerebral infarction I69.398
      cerebrovascular disease I69.998
        specified NEC I69.898
      intracerebral hemorrhage I69.198
      nontraumatic intracranial hemorrhage NEC I69.298
      specified disease NEC I69.898
      subarachnoid hemorrhage I69.098
    psychophysical H53.16
    specified NEC H53.8
    subjective H53.10
      day blindness H53.11
      discomfort H53.14- ☑
      distortions of shape and size H53.15
      loss
        sudden H53.13- ☑
        transient H53.12- ☑
      specified type NEC H53.19
  voice R49.9
    psychogenic F44.4
    specified NEC R49.8
Diuresis R35.89
Diver's palsy, paralysis or squeeze T70.3 ☑
Diverticulitis (acute) K57.92
  bladder — see Cystitis
  ileum — see Diverticulitis, intestine, small
  intestine K57.92
    with
      abscess, perforation K57.80
        with bleeding K57.81
      bleeding K57.93
    congenital Q43.8
    large K57.32
      with
        abscess, perforation K57.20
          with bleeding K57.21
        bleeding K57.33
        small intestine K57.52
          with
            abscess, perforation K57.40
              with bleeding K57.41
            bleeding K57.53
    small K57.12
      with
        abscess, perforation K57.00
          with bleeding K57.01
        bleeding K57.13
        large intestine K57.52
          with
            abscess, perforation K57.40
              with bleeding K57.41
            bleeding K57.53

Diverticulosis K57.90
  with bleeding K57.91
  large intestine K57.30
    with
      bleeding K57.31
      small intestine K57.50
        with bleeding K57.51
  small intestine K57.10
    with
      bleeding K57.11
      large intestine K57.50
        with bleeding K57.51
Diverticulum, diverticula (multiple) K57.90
  appendix (noninflammatory) K38.2
  bladder (sphincter) N32.3
    congenital Q64.6
  bronchus (congenital) Q32.4
    acquired J98.09
  calyx, calyceal (kidney) N28.89
  cardia (stomach) K31.4
  cecum — see Diverticulosis, intestine, large
    congenital Q43.8
  colon — see Diverticulosis, intestine, large
    congenital Q43.8
  duodenum — see Diverticulosis, intestine, small
    congenital Q43.8
  epiphrenic (esophagus) K22.5
  esophagus (congenital) Q39.6
    acquired (epiphrenic) (pulsion) (traction) K22.5
  eustachian tube — see Disorder, eustachian tube, speci-
    fied NEC
  fallopian tube N83.8
  gastric K31.4
  heart (congenital) Q24.8
  ileum — see Diverticulosis, intestine, small
  jejunum — see Diverticulosis, intestine, small
  kidney (pelvis) (calyces) N28.89
    with calculus — see Calculus, kidney
  Meckel's (displaced) (hypertrophic) Q43.0
    malignant — see Table of Neoplasms, small intestine,
      malignant
  midthoracic K22.5
  organ or site, congenital NEC — see Distortion
  pericardium (congenital) (cyst) Q24.8
    acquired I31.8
  pharyngoesophageal (congenital) Q39.6
    acquired K22.5
  pharynx (congenital) Q38.7
  rectosigmoid — see Diverticulosis, intestine, large
    congenital Q43.8
  rectum — see Diverticulosis, intestine, large
  Rokitansky's K22.5
  seminal vesicle N50.89
  sigmoid — see Diverticulosis, intestine, large
    congenital Q43.8
  stomach (acquired) K31.4
    congenital Q40.2
  trachea (acquired) J39.8
  ureter (acquired) N28.89
    congenital Q62.8
  ureterovesical orifice N28.89
  urethra (acquired) N36.1
    congenital Q64.79
  ventricle, left (congenital) Q24.8
  vesical N32.3
    congenital Q64.6
  Zenker's (esophagus) K22.5
Division
  cervix uteri (acquired) N88.8
  glans penis Q55.69
  labia minora (congenital) Q52.79
  ligament (partial or complete) (current) — see also Sprain
    with open wound — see Wound, open
  muscle (partial or complete) (current) — see also Injury,
    muscle
    with open wound — see Wound, open
  nerve (traumatic) — see Injury, nerve
  spinal cord — see Injury, spinal cord, by region
  vein I87.8
Divorce, causing family disruption Z63.5
Dix-Hallpike neurolabyrinthitis — see Neuronitis,
    vestibular
Dizziness R42
  hysterical F44.89
  psychogenic F45.8
DMAC (disseminated mycobacterium avium- intracellulare
    complex) A31.2
DNR (do not resuscitate) Z66

Doan-Wiseman syndrome (primary splenic neutropenia)
    — see Agranulocytosis
Doehle-Heller aortitis A52.02
Dog bite — see Bite
Dohle body panmyelopathic syndrome D72.0
Dolichocephaly Q67.2
  non-deformational Q75.01
Dolichocolon Q43.8
Dolichostenomelia — see Syndrome, Marfan
Donohue's syndrome E34.8
Donor (organ or tissue) Z52.9
  blood (whole) Z52.000
    autologous Z52.010
    specified component (lymphocytes) (platelets) NEC
      Z52.008
      autologous Z52.018
      specified donor NEC Z52.098
    specified donor NEC Z52.090
    stem cells Z52.001
      autologous Z52.011
      specified donor NEC Z52.091
  bone Z52.20
    autologous Z52.21
    marrow Z52.3
    specified type NEC Z52.29
  cornea Z52.5
  egg (Oocyte) Z52.819
    age 35 and over Z52.812
      anonymous recipient Z52.812
      designated recipient Z52.813
    under age 35 Z52.810
      anonymous recipient Z52.810
      designated recipient Z52.811
  kidney Z52.4
  liver Z52.6
  lung Z52.89
  lymphocyte — see Donor, blood, specified components
    NEC
  Oocyte — see Donor, egg
  platelets Z52.008
  potential, examination of Z00.5
  semen Z52.89
  skin Z52.10
    autologous Z52.11
    specified type NEC Z52.19
  specified organ or tissue NEC Z52.89
  sperm Z52.89
Donovanosis A58
Dorsalgia M54.9
  psychogenic F45.41
  specified NEC M54.89
Dorsopathy M53.9
  deforming M43.9
    specified NEC — see subcategory M43.8 ☑
  specified NEC M53.80
    cervical region M53.82
    cervicothoracic region M53.83
    lumbar region M53.86
    lumbosacral region M53.87
    occipito-atlanto-axial region M53.81
    sacrococcygeal region M53.88
    thoracic region M53.84
    thoracolumbar region M53.85
Double
  albumin E88.09
  aortic arch Q25.45
  auditory canal Q17.8
  auricle (heart) Q20.8
  bladder Q64.79
  cervix Q51.820
    with doubling of uterus (and vagina) Q51.10
      with obstruction Q51.11
  inlet ventricle Q20.4
  kidney with double pelvis (renal) Q63.0
  meatus urinarius Q64.75
  monster Q89.4
  outlet
    left ventricle Q20.2
    right ventricle Q20.1
  pelvis (renal) with double ureter Q62.5
  tongue Q38.3
  ureter (one or both sides) Q62.5
    with double pelvis (renal) Q62.5
  urethra Q64.74
  urinary meatus Q64.75
  uterus Q51.28
    with
      doubling of cervix (and vagina) Q51.10
        with obstruction Q51.11

☑ **Additional Character Required — Refer to the Tabular List for Character Selection**

Double — *continued*
  uterus — *continued*
    complete Q51.21
    in pregnancy or childbirth O34.0- ☑
      causing obstructed labor O65.5
    partial Q51.22
    specified NEC Q51.28
  vagina Q52.10
    with doubling of uterus (and cervix) Q51.10
      with obstruction Q51.11
  vision H53.2
  vulva Q52.79
Doubled up Z59.01
Douglas' pouch, cul-de-sac — *see* condition
Down syndrome Q90.9
  meiotic nondisjunction Q90.0
  mitotic nondisjunction Q90.1
  mosaicism Q90.1
  translocation Q90.2
DPD (dihydropyrimidine dehydrogenase deficiency) E88.89
Dracontiasis B72
Dracunculiasis, dracunculosis B72
Dream state, hysterical F44.89
Drepanocytic anemia — *see* Disease, sickle-cell
Dresbach's syndrome (elliptocytosis) D58.1
Dreschlera (hawaiiensis) (infection) B43.8
Dressler's syndrome I24.1
Drift, ulnar — *see* Deformity, limb, specified type NEC, forearm
Drinking (alcohol)
  excessive, to excess NEC (without dependence) F10.10
    habitual (continual) (without remission) F10.20
      with remission F10.21
Drip, postnasal (chronic) R09.82
  due to
    allergic rhinitis — *see* Rhinitis, allergic
    common cold J00
    gastroesophageal reflux — *see* Reflux, gastroe-sophageal
    nasopharyngitis — *see* Nasopharyngitis
    other known condition — *code to* condition
    sinusitis — *see* Sinusitis
Droop
  facial R29.810
    cerebrovascular disease I69.992
      cerebral infarction I69.392
      intracerebral hemorrhage I69.192
      nontraumatic intracranial hemorrhage NEC I69.292
      specified disease NEC I69.892
      subarachnoid hemorrhage I69.092
Drop (in)
  attack NEC R55
  finger — *see* Deformity, finger
  foot — *see* Deformity, limb, foot, drop
  hematocrit (precipitous) R71.0
  hemoglobin R71.0
  toe — *see* Deformity, toe, specified NEC
  wrist — *see* Deformity, limb, wrist drop
Dropped heart beats I45.9
Dropsy, dropsical — *see also* Hydrops
  abdomen R18.8
  brain — *see* Hydrocephalus
  cardiac, heart — *see* Failure, heart, congestive
  gangrenous — *see* Gangrene
  heart — *see* Failure, heart, congestive
  kidney — *see* Nephrosis
  lung — *see* Edema, lung
  newborn due to isoimmunization P56.0
  pericardium — *see* Pericarditis
Drowned, drowning (near) T75.1 ☑
Drowsiness R40.0
Drug
  abuse counseling and surveillance Z71.51
  addiction — *see* Dependence
  dependence — *see* Dependence
  habit — *see* Dependence
  harmful use — *see* Abuse, drug
  induced fever R50.2
  overdose — *see* Table of Drugs and Chemicals, by drug, poisoning
  poisoning — *see* Table of Drugs and Chemicals, by drug, poisoning
  resistant organism infection — *see also* Resistant, organism, to, drug Z16.30
  therapy
    long term (current) (prophylactic) — *see* Therapy, drug long-term (current) (prophylactic)

Drug — *continued*
  therapy — *continued*
    short term — *omit code*
    wrong substance given or taken in error — *see* Table of Drugs and Chemicals, by drug, poisoning
Drunkenness (without dependence) F10.129
  acute in alcoholism F10.229
  chronic (without remission) F10.20
    with remission F10.21
  pathological (without dependence) F10.129
    with dependence F10.229
  sleep F51.9
Drusen
  macula (degenerative) (retina) — *see* Degeneration, macula, drusen
  optic disc H47.32- ☑
Dry, dryness — *see also* condition
  larynx J38.7
  mouth R68.2
    due to dehydration E86.0
  nose J34.89
  socket (teeth) M27.3
  throat J39.2
DSAP L56.5
Duane's syndrome H50.81- ☑
Dubin-Johnson disease or syndrome E80.6
Dubois' disease (thymus gland) A50.59 *[E35]*
Dubowitz' syndrome Q87.19
Duchenne-Aran muscular atrophy G12.21
Duchenne-Griesinger disease G71.01
Duchenne's
  disease or syndrome
    motor neuron disease G12.22
    muscular dystrophy G71.01
  locomotor ataxia (syphilitic) A52.11
  paralysis
    birth injury P14.0
    due to or associated with
      motor neuron disease G12.22
      muscular dystrophy G71.01
Ducreyi chancre A57
Ducrey's chancre A57
Duct, ductus — *see* condition
Duffy phenotype — *see* Phenotype, Duffy
Duhring's disease (dermatitis herpetiformis) L13.0
Dullness, cardiac (decreased) (increased) R01.2
Dumb ague — *see* Malaria
Dumbness — *see* Aphasia
Dumdum fever B55.0
Dumping syndrome (postgastrectomy) K91.1
Duodenitis (nonspecific) (peptic) K29.80
  with bleeding K29.81
  erosive — *see* Ulcer, duodenum
Duodenocholangitis — *see* Cholangitis
Duodenum, duodenal — *see* condition
Duplay's bursitis or periarthritis M75.0 ☑
Duplication, duplex — *see also* Accessory
  alimentary tract Q45.8
  anus Q43.4
  appendix (and cecum) Q43.4
  biliary duct (any) Q44.5
  bladder Q64.79
  cecum (and appendix) Q43.4
  cervix Q51.820
  chromosome NEC — *see also* Trisomy
    with complex rearrangements NEC Q92.5
    seen only at prometaphase Q92.8
  cystic duct Q44.5
  digestive organs Q45.8
  esophagus Q39.8
  frontonasal process Q75.8
  intestine (large) (small) Q43.4
  kidney Q63.0
  liver Q44.79
  pancreas Q45.3
  penis Q55.69
  respiratory organs NEC Q34.8
  salivary duct Q38.4
  spinal cord (incomplete) Q06.2
  stomach Q40.2
Dupre's disease (meningism) R29.1
Dupuytren's contraction or disease M72.0
Durand-Nicolas-Favre disease A55
Durotomy (inadvertent) (incidental) G97.41
Duroziez's disease (congenital mitral stenosis) Q23.2
Dutton's relapsing fever (West African) A68.1
Dwarfism — *see also* Short, stature E34.328
  achondroplastic Q77.4
  congenital — *see also* Short, stature E34.328

Dwarfism — *continued*
  constitutional E34.31
  hypochondroplastic Q77.4
  hypophyseal E23.0
  infantile — *see also* Short, stature E34.328
  Laron-type — *see also* Short, stature E34.321
  Lorain (-Levi) type E23.0
  metatropic Q77.8
  nephrotic-glycosuric (with hypophosphatemic rickets) E72.09
  nutritional E45
  pancreatic K86.89
  pituitary E23.0
  renal N25.0
  thanatophoric Q77.1
Dyke-Young anemia (secondary) (symptomatic) D59.19
Dysacusis — *see* Abnormal, auditory perception
Dysadrenocortism E27.9
  hyperfunction E27.0
Dysarthria R47.1
  following
    cerebral infarction I69.322
    cerebrovascular disease I69.922
      specified disease NEC I69.822
    intracerebral hemorrhage I69.122
    nontraumatic intracranial hemorrhage NEC I69.222
    subarachnoid hemorrhage I69.022
Dysautonomia (familial) G90.1
Dysbarism T70.3 ☑
Dysbasia R26.2
  angiosclerotica intermittens I73.9
  hysterical F44.4
  lordotica (progressiva) G24.1
  nonorganic origin F44.4
  psychogenic F44.4
Dysbetalipoproteinemia (familial) E78.2
Dyscalculia R48.8
  developmental F81.2
Dyschezia K59.00
Dyschondroplasia (with hemangiomata) Q78.4
Dyschromia (skin) L81.9
Dyscollagenosis M35.9
Dyscranio-pygo-phalangy Q87.0
Dyscrasia
  blood (with) D75.9
    antepartum hemorrhage — *see* Hemorrhage, antepartum, with coagulation defect
    intrapartum hemorrhage O67.0
    newborn P61.9
      specified type NEC P61.8
    puerperal, postpartum O72.3
  polyglandular, pluriglandular E31.9
Dysendocrinism E34.9
Dysentery, dysenteric (catarrhal) (diarrhea) (epidemic) (hemorrhagic) (infectious) (sporadic) (tropical) A09
  abscess, liver A06.4
  amebic — *see also* Amebiasis A06.0
    with abscess — *see* Abscess, amebic
    acute A06.0
    chronic A06.1
  arthritis — *see also* category M01 A09
    bacillary (*see also* category M01) A03.9
  bacillary A03.9
    arthritis — *see also* category M01 A03.9
    Boyd A03.2
    Flexner A03.1
    Schmitz (-Stutzer) A03.0
    Shiga (-Kruse) A03.0
    Shigella A03.9
      boydii A03.2
      dysenteriae A03.0
      flexneri A03.1
      group A A03.0
      group B A03.1
      group C A03.2
      group D A03.3
      sonnei A03.3
      specified type NEC A03.8
    Sonne A03.3
    specified type NEC A03.8
  balantidial A07.0
  Balantidium coli A07.0
  Boyd's A03.2
  candidal B37.82
  Chilomastix A07.8
  Chinese A03.9
  coccidial A07.3
  Dientamoeba (fragilis) A07.8
  Embadomonas A07.8

Dysentery, dysenteric — *continued*
  Entamoeba, entambic — *see* Dysentery, amebic
  Flexner-Boyd A03.2
  Flexner's A03.1
  Giardia lamblia A07.1
  Hiss-Russell A03.1
  Lamblia A07.1
  leishmanial B55.0
  malarial — *see* Malaria
  metazoal B82.0
  monilial B37.82
  protozoal A07.9
  Salmonella A02.0
  schistosomal B65.1
  Schmitz (-Stutzer) A03.0
  Shiga (-Kruse) A03.0
  Shigella NOS — *see* Dysentery, bacillary
  Sonne A03.3
  strongyloidiasis B78.0
  trichomonal A07.8
  viral — *see also* Enteritis, viral A08.4
Dysequilibrium R42
Dysesthesia R20.8
  hysterical F44.6
Dysferlinopathy G71.033
Dysfibrinogenemia (congenital) D68.2
Dysfunction
  adrenal E27.9
    hyperfunction E27.0
  autonomic
    due to alcohol G31.2
    somatoform F45.8
  bladder N31.9
    neurogenic NOS — *see* Dysfunction, bladder, neuro-
      muscular
    neuromuscular NOS N31.9
      atonic (motor) (sensory) N31.2
      autonomous N31.2
      flaccid N31.2
      nonreflex N31.2
      reflex N31.1
      specified NEC N31.8
      uninhibited N31.0
  bleeding, uterus N93.8
  cerebral G93.89
  chronic
    coronary microvascular I25.85
    lung allograft J4A.9
      mixed J4A.0
      specified NEC J4A.8
  colon K59.9
    psychogenic F45.8
  colostomy K94.03
  coronary microvascular I25.85
    with
      angina pectoris I20.81
      myocardial infarction I21.B
    acute I24.81
    chronic I25.85
  cystic duct K82.8
  cystostomy (stoma) — *see* Complications, cystostomy
  ejaculatory N53.19
    anejaculatory orgasm N53.13
    painful N53.12
    premature F52.4
    retarded N53.11
  endocrine NOS E34.9
  endometrium N85.8
  enterostomy K94.13
  erectile — *see* Dysfunction, sexual, male, erectile
  feeding, pediatric
    acute R63.31
    chronic R63.32
  gallbladder K82.8
  gastrostomy (stoma) K94.23
  gland, glandular NOS E34.9
    meibomian, of eyelid — *see* Dysfunction, meibomian
      gland
  heart I51.89
  hemoglobin D75.89
  hepatic K76.89
  hypophysis E23.7
  hypothalamic NEC E23.3
  ileostomy (stoma) K94.13
  jejunostomy (stoma) K94.13
  kidney — *see* Disease, renal
  labyrinthine — *see* subcategory H83.2 ☑
  left ventricular, following sudden emotional stress I51.81
  liver K76.89

Dysfunction — *continued*
  male — *see* Dysfunction, sexual, male
  meibomian gland, of eyelid H02.889
    left H02.886
      lower H02.885
      upper H02.884
      upper and lower eyelids H02.88B
    right H02.883
      lower H02.882
      upper H02.881
      upper and lower eyelids H02.88A
  multifidus muscles, lumbar region M62.85
  orgasmic (female) F52.31
    male F52.32
  ovary E28.9
    specified NEC E28.8
  papillary muscle I51.89
  parathyroid E21.4
  physiological NEC R68.89
    psychogenic F59
  pineal gland E34.8
  pituitary (gland) E23.3
  platelets D69.1
  polyglandular E31.9
    specified NEC E31.8
  psychophysiologic F59
  psychosexual F52.9
    with
      dyspareunia F52.6
      premature ejaculation F52.4
      vaginismus F52.5
  pylorus K31.9
  rectum K59.9
    psychogenic F45.8
  reflex (sympathetic) — *see* Syndrome, pain, complex re-
    gional I
  segmental — *see* Dysfunction, somatic
  senile R54
  sexual (due to) R37
    alcohol F10.981
    amphetamine F15.981
      in
        abuse F15.181
        dependence F15.281
    anxiolytic F13.981
      in
        abuse F13.181
        dependence F13.281
    cocaine F14.981
      in
        abuse F14.181
        dependence F14.281
    excessive sexual drive F52.8
    failure of genital response (male) F52.21
      female F52.22
    female N94.9
      aversion F52.1
      dyspareunia N94.10
        psychogenic F52.6
      frigidity F52.22
      nymphomania F52.8
      orgasmic F52.31
      psychogenic F52.9
        aversion F52.1
        dyspareunia F52.6
        frigidity F52.22
        nymphomania F52.8
        orgasmic F52.31
        vaginismus F52.5
      vaginismus N94.2
        psychogenic F52.5
    hypnotic F13.981
      in
        abuse F13.181
        dependence F13.281
    inhibited orgasm (female) F52.31
      male F52.32
    lack
      of sexual enjoyment F52.1
      or loss of sexual desire F52.0
    male N53.9
      anejaculatory orgasm N53.13
      ejaculatory N53.19
        painful N53.12
        premature F52.4
        retarded N53.11
      erectile N52.9
        drug induced N52.2

Dysfunction — *continued*
  sexual — *continued*
    male — *continued*
      erectile — *continued*
        due to
          disease classified elsewhere N52.1
          drug N52.2
        postoperative (postprocedural) N52.39
          following
            cryotherapy N52.37
            interstitial seed therapy N52.36
            prostate ablative therapy N52.37
            prostatectomy N52.34
              radical N52.31
            radiation therapy N52.35
            radical cystectomy N52.32
            ultrasound ablative therapy N52.37
            urethral surgery N52.33
        psychogenic F52.21
        specified cause NEC N52.8
        vasculogenic
          arterial insufficiency N52.01
            with corporo-venous occlusive N52.03
          corporo-venous occlusive N52.02
            with arterial insufficiency N52.03
      impotence — *see* Dysfunction, sexual, male, erec-
        tile
      psychogenic F52.9
        aversion F52.1
        erectile F52.21
        orgasmic F52.32
        premature ejaculation F52.4
        satyriasis F52.8
        specified type NEC F52.8
      specified type NEC N53.8
    nonorganic F52.9
      specified NEC F52.8
    opioid F11.981
      in
        abuse F11.181
        dependence F11.281
    orgasmic dysfunction (female) F52.31
      male F52.32
    premature ejaculation F52.4
    psychoactive substances NEC F19.981
      in
        abuse F19.181
        dependence F19.281
    psychogenic F52.9
    sedative F13.981
      in
        abuse F13.181
        dependence F13.281
    sexual aversion F52.1
    vaginismus (nonorganic) (psychogenic) F52.5
  sinoatrial node I49.5
  somatic M99.09
    abdomen M99.09
    acromioclavicular M99.07
    cervical region M99.01
    cervicothoracic M99.01
    costochondral M99.08
    costovertebral M99.08
    head region M99.00
    hip M99.05
    lower extremity M99.06
    lumbar region M99.03
    lumbosacral M99.03
    occipitocervical M99.00
    pelvic region M99.05
    pubic M99.05
    rib cage M99.08
    sacral region M99.04
    sacrococcygeal M99.04
    sacroiliac M99.04
    specified NEC M99.09
    sternochondral M99.08
    sternoclavicular M99.07
    thoracic region M99.02
    thoracolumbar M99.02
    upper extremity M99.07
  somatoform autonomic F45.8
  stomach K31.89
    psychogenic F45.8
  suprarenal E27.9
    hyperfunction E27.0
  symbolic R48.9
    specified type NEC R48.8
  temporomandibular (joint) M26.69

☑ **Additional Character Required — Refer to the Tabular List for Character Selection**

Dysfunction — *continued*
  temporomandibular — *continued*
    joint-pain syndrome M26.62- ☑
  testicular (endocrine) E29.9
    specified NEC E29.8
  thymus E32.9
  thyroid E07.9
  ureterostomy (stoma) — *see* Complications, stoma, urinary tract
  urethrostomy (stoma) — *see* Complications, stoma, urinary tract
  uterus, complicating delivery O62.9
    hypertonic O62.4
    hypotonic O62.2
      primary O62.0
      secondary O62.1
  ventricular I51.9
    with congestive heart failure — *see also* Failure, heart I50.9
    left, reversible, following sudden emotional stress I51.81
Dysgenesis
  gonadal (due to chromosomal anomaly) Q96.9
    pure Q99.1
  renal Q60.5
    bilateral Q60.4
    unilateral Q60.3
  reticular D72.0
  tidal platelet D69.3
Dysgerminoma
  specified site — *see* Neoplasm, malignant, by site
  unspecified site
    female C56.9
    male C62.90
Dysgeusia R43.2
Dysgraphia R27.8
Dyshidrosis, dysidrosis L30.1
Dyskaryotic cervical smear R87.619
Dyskeratosis L85.8
  cervix — *see* Dysplasia, cervix
  congenital Q82.8
  uterus NEC N85.8
Dyskinesia G24.9
  biliary (cystic duct or gallbladder) K82.8
  drug induced
    orofacial G24.01
  esophagus K22.4
  hysterical F44.4
  intestinal K59.89
  nonorganic origin F44.4
  orofacial (idiopathic) G24.4
    drug induced G24.01
  psychogenic F44.4
  subacute, drug induced G24.01
  tardive G24.01
    neuroleptic induced G24.01
  trachea J39.8
  tracheobronchial J98.09
Dyslalia (developmental) F80.0
Dyslexia R48.0
  developmental F81.0
Dyslipidemia E78.5
  depressed HDL cholesterol E78.6
  elevated fasting triglycerides E78.1
Dysmaturity — *see also* Light for dates
  pulmonary (newborn) (Wilson-Mikity) P27.0
Dysmenorrhea (essential) (exfoliative) N94.6
  congestive (syndrome) N94.6
  primary N94.4
  psychogenic F45.8
  secondary N94.5
Dysmetabolic syndrome X E88.810
Dysmetria R27.8
Dysmorphia
  muscle F45.22
Dysmorphism (due to)
  alcohol Q86.0
  exogenous cause NEC Q86.8
  hydantoin Q86.1
  warfarin Q86.2
Dysmorphophobia (nondelusional) F45.22
  delusional F22
Dysnomia R47.01
Dysorexia R63.0
  psychogenic F50.89
Dysostosis
  cleidocranial, cleidocranialis Q74.0
  craniofacial Q75.1

Dysostosis — *continued*
  Fairbank's (idiopathic familial generalized osteophytosis) Q78.9
  mandibulofacial (incomplete) Q75.4
  multiplex E76.01
  oculomandibular Q75.5
Dyspareunia (female) N94.10
  deep N94.12
  male N53.12
  nonorganic F52.6
  psychogenic F52.6
  secondary N94.19
  specified NEC N94.19
  superficial (introital) N94.11
Dyspepsia R10.13
  atonic K30
  functional (allergic) (congenital) (gastrointestinal) (occupational) (reflex) K30
  intestinal K59.89
  nervous F45.8
  neurotic F45.8
  psychogenic F45.8
Dysphagia R13.10
  cervical R13.19
  following
    cerebral infarction I69.391
    cerebrovascular disease I69.991
      specified NEC I69.891
    intracerebral hemorrhage I69.191
    nontraumatic intracranial hemorrhage NEC I69.291
    specified disease NEC I69.891
    subarachnoid hemorrhage I69.091
  functional (hysterical) F45.8
  hysterical F45.8
  nervous (hysterical) F45.8
  neurogenic R13.19
  oral phase R13.11
  oropharyngeal phase R13.12
  pharyngeal phase R13.13
  pharyngoesophageal phase R13.14
  psychogenic F45.8
  sideropenic D50.1
  spastica K22.4
  specified NEC R13.19
Dysphagocytosis, congenital D71
Dysphasia R47.02
  developmental
    expressive type F80.1
    receptive type F80.2
  following
    cerebrovascular disease I69.921
      cerebral infarction I69.321
      intracerebral hemorrhage I69.121
      nontraumatic intracranial hemorrhage NEC I69.221
      specified disease NEC I69.821
      subarachnoid hemorrhage I69.021
Dysphonia R49.0
  functional F44.4
  hysterical F44.4
  psychogenic F44.4
  spastica J38.3
Dysphoria
  gender F64.9
    in
      adolescence and adulthood F64.0
      children F64.2
    specified NEC F64.8
  postpartal O90.6
Dyspituitarism E23.3
Dysplasia — *see also* Anomaly
  acetabular, congenital Q65.89
  alveolar capillary, with vein misalignment J84.843
  anus (histologically confirmed) (mild) (moderate) K62.82
    severe D01.3
  arrhythmogenic right ventricular I42.8
  arterial, fibromuscular I77.3
  asphyxiating thoracic (congenital) Q77.2
  brain Q07.9
  bronchopulmonary, perinatal P27.1
  cervix (uteri) N87.9
    mild N87.0
    moderate N87.1
    severe D06.9
  chondroectodermal Q77.6
  colon D12.6
  craniometaphyseal Q78.8
  dentinal K00.5
  diaphyseal, progressive Q78.3
  dystrophic Q77.5

Dysplasia — *continued*
  ectodermal (anhidrotic) (congenital) (hereditary) Q82.4
    hydrotic Q82.8
  epithelial, uterine cervix — *see* Dysplasia, cervix
  eye (congenital) Q11.2
  fibrous
    bone NEC (monostotic) M85.00
      ankle M85.07- ☑
      foot M85.07- ☑
      forearm M85.03- ☑
      hand M85.04- ☑
      lower leg M85.06- ☑
      multiple site M85.09
      neck M85.08
      rib M85.08
      shoulder M85.01- ☑
      skull M85.08
      specified site NEC M85.08
      thigh M85.05- ☑
      toe M85.07- ☑
      upper arm M85.02- ☑
      vertebra M85.08
    diaphyseal, progressive Q78.3
    jaw M27.8
    polyostotic Q78.1
  florid osseous — *see also* Cyst, calcifying odontogenic
  high grade, focal D12.6
  hip, congenital Q65.89
  joint, congenital Q74.8
  kidney Q61.4
    multicystic Q61.4
  leg Q74.2
  lung, congenital (not associated with short gestation) Q33.6
  mammary (gland) (benign) N60.9- ☑
    cyst (solitary) — *see* Cyst, breast
    cystic — *see* Mastopathy, cystic
    duct ectasia — *see* Ectasia, mammary duct
    fibroadenosis — *see* Fibroadenosis, breast
    fibrosclerosis — *see* Fibrosclerosis, breast
    specified type NEC N60.8- ☑
  metaphyseal Q78.5
  muscle Q79.8
  oculodentodigital Q87.0
  periapical (cemental) (cemento-osseous) — *see* Cyst, calcifying odontogenic
  periosteum — *see* Disorder, bone, specified type NEC
  polyostotic fibrous Q78.1
  prostate — *see also* Neoplasia, intraepithelial, prostate N42.30
    severe D07.5
    specified NEC N42.39
  renal Q61.4
    multicystic Q61.4
  retinal, congenital Q14.1
  right ventricular, arrhythmogenic I42.8
  septo-optic Q04.4
  skin L98.8
  spinal cord Q06.1
  spondyloepiphyseal Q77.7
  thymic, with immunodeficiency D82.1
  vagina N89.3
    mild N89.0
    moderate N89.1
    severe NEC D07.2
  vulva N90.3
    mild N90.0
    moderate N90.1
    severe NEC D07.1
Dysplasminogenemia E88.02
Dyspnea (nocturnal) (paroxysmal) R06.00
  asthmatic (bronchial) J45.909
    with
      bronchitis J45.909
        with
          exacerbation (acute) J45.901
          status asthmaticus J45.902
        chronic J44.89
      exacerbation (acute) J45.901
      status asthmaticus J45.902
  cardiac — *see* Failure, ventricular, left
  cardiac — *see* Failure, ventricular, left
  functional F45.8
  hyperventilation R06.4
  hysterical F45.8
  newborn P28.89
  orthopnea R06.01
  psychogenic F45.8

Dyspnea — *continued*
  shortness of breath R06.02
  specified type NEC R06.09
  transfusion-associated [TAD] J95.87
Dyspraxia R27.8
  developmental (syndrome) F82
Dysproteinemia E88.09
Dysreflexia, autonomic G90.4
Dysrhythmia
  cardiac I49.9
    newborn
      bradycardia P29.12
        occurring before birth P03.819
          before onset of labor P03.810
          during labor P03.811
      tachycardia P29.11
    postoperative I97.89
  cerebral or cortical — *see* Epilepsy
Dyssomnia — *see* Disorder, sleep
Dyssynergia
  biliary K83.8
  bladder sphincter N36.44
  cerebellaris myoclonica (Hunt's ataxia) G11.19
Dysthymia F34.1
Dysthyroidism E07.9
Dystocia O66.9
  affecting newborn P03.1
  cervical (hypotonic) O62.2
    affecting newborn P03.6
    primary O62.0
    secondary O62.1
  contraction ring O62.4
  fetal O66.9
    abnormality NEC O66.3
    conjoined twins O66.3
    oversize O66.2
  maternal O66.9
  positional O64.9 ☑
  shoulder (girdle) O66.0
    causing obstructed labor O66.0
  uterine NEC O62.4
Dystonia G24.9
  cervical G24.3
  deformans progressiva G24.1
  drug induced NEC G24.09
    acute G24.02
    specified NEC G24.09
  familial G24.1
  idiopathic G24.1
    familial G24.1
    nonfamilial G24.2
    orofacial G24.4
  lenticularis G24.8
  musculorum deformans G24.1
  neuroleptic induced (acute) G24.02
  orofacial (idiopathic) G24.4
  oromandibular G24.4
    due to drug G24.01
  specified NEC G24.8
  torsion (familial) (idiopathic) G24.1
    acquired G24.8
    genetic G24.1
    symptomatic (nonfamilial) G24.2
Dystonic movements R25.8
Dystrophy, dystrophia
  adiposogenital E23.6
  autosomal recessive, childhood type, muscular dystrophy resembling Duchenne or Becker G71.01
  Becker's type G71.01
  cervical sympathetic G90.2
  choroid (hereditary) H31.20
    central areolar H31.22
    choroideremia H31.21
    gyrate atrophy H31.23
    specified type NEC H31.29
  cornea (hereditary) H18.50- ☑
    endothelial H18.51- ☑
    epithelial H18.52- ☑
    granular H18.53- ☑
    lattice H18.54- ☑
    macular H18.55- ☑
    specified type NEC H18.59- ☑
  Duchenne's type G71.01
  due to malnutrition E45
  Erb's G71.02
  Fuchs' H18.51- ☑
  Gower's muscular G71.01
  hair L67.8

Dystrophy, dystrophia — *continued*
  infantile neuraxonal G31.89
  Landouzy-Dejerine G71.02
  Leyden-Mobius — *see also* Dystrophy, muscular, limb-girdle, by type G71.039
    meaning Limb girdle muscular dystrophy NOS G71.039
    meaning Limb girdle muscular dystrophy, other specified type — *see* by type
    meaning Limb girdle muscular dystrophy, specified type NEC G71.038
    meaning Limb girdle muscular dystrophy type 2A (autosomal recessive) G71.032
  muscular G71.00
    autosomal recessive, childhood type, muscular dystrophy resembling Duchenne or Becker G71.01
    benign (Becker type) G71.01
      scapuloperoneal with early contractures [Emery-Dreifuss] G71.09
    congenital (hereditary) (progressive) (with specific morphological abnormalities of the muscle fiber) G71.09
      myotonic G71.11
    distal G71.09
    Duchenne type G71.01
    Emery-Dreifuss G71.09
    Erb type G71.02
    facioscapulohumeral G71.02
    Gower's G71.01
    hereditary (progressive) — *see also* Dystrophy, muscular, by type G71.09
    Landouzy-Dejerine type G71.02
    limb-girdle G71.039
      alpha-sarcoglycan-relate G71.0341
      anoctamin-5-related autosomal recessive (R12) G71.035
      autosomal recessive NEC G71.038
      beta-sarcoglycan-related G71.0342
      calpain-3-related G71.032
        autosomal dominant G71.031
        autosomal recessive G71.032
      collagen VI related
        autosomal dominant G71.031
        autosomal recessive G71.038
      D1 (autosomal dominant) G71.031
      D2 (autosomal dominant) G71.031
      D3 (autosomal dominant) G71.031
      D4 (autosomal dominant) G71.031
      D5 (autosomal dominant) G71.031
      delta-sarcoglycan-related G71.0349
      due to
        alpha sarcoglycan dysfunction G71.0341
        anoctamin-5 dysfunction G71.035
        beta sarcoglycan dysfunction G71.0342
        fukutin related protein dysfunction G71.038
        sarcoglycan dysfunction, specified NEC G71.0349
      FKRP-related autosomal recessive G71.038
      gamma-sarcoglycan-related G71.0349
      R1 (autosomal recessive) G71.032
      R2 (autosomal recessive) G71.033
      R3 (autosomal recessive) G71.0341
      R4 (autosomal recessive) G71.0342
      R5 (autosomal recessive) G71.0349
      R6 (autosomal recessive) G71.0349
      R7 (autosomal recessive) G71.038
      R8 (autosomal recessive) G71.038
      R9 (autosomal recessive) G71.038
      R10 (autosomal recessive) G71.038
      R11 (autosomal recessive) G71.038
      R12 (autosomal recessive) G71.035
      R13 (autosomal recessive) G71.038
      R14 (autosomal recessive) G71.038
      R15 (autosomal recessive) G71.038
      R16 (autosomal recessive) G71.038
      R17 (autosomal recessive) G71.038
      R18 (autosomal recessive) G71.038
      R19 (autosomal recessive) G71.038
      R20 (autosomal recessive) G71.038
      R21 (autosomal recessive) G71.038
      R22 (autosomal recessive) G71.038
      R23 (autosomal recessive) G71.038
      R24 (autosomal recessive) G71.038
      type 1 (autosomal dominant) G71.031
      type 1A (autosomal dominant) G71.031
      type 1B (autosomal dominant) G71.031
      type 1C (autosomal dominant) G71.031
      type 1E (autosomal dominant) G71.031
      type 1H (autosomal dominant) G71.031

Dystrophy, dystrophia — *continued*
  muscular — *continued*
    limb-girdle — *continued*
      type 1I (autosomal dominant) G71.031
      type 2 (autosomal recessive) G71.038
        specified NEC G71.038
      type 2A (autosomal recessive) G71.032
      type 2B (autosomal recessive) G71.033
      type 2C (autosomal recessive) G71.0349
      type 2D (autosomal recessive) G71.0341
      type 2E (autosomal recessive) G71.0342
      type 2F (autosomal recessive) G71.0349
      type 2I (autosomal recessive) G71.038
      type 2L (autosomal recessive) G71.035
    myotonic G71.11
    progressive (hereditary) — *see also* Dystrophy, muscular, by type G71.09
      Charcot-Marie (-Tooth) type G60.0
    pseudohypertrophic (infantile) G71.01
    scapulohumeral G71.02
    scapuloperoneal G71.09
    severe (Duchenne type) G71.01
    specified type NEC G71.09
  myocardium, myocardial — *see* Degeneration, myocardial
  nail L60.3
    congenital Q84.6
  nutritional E45
  ocular G71.09
  oculocerebrorenal E72.03
  oculopharyngeal G71.09
  ovarian N83.8
  polyglandular E31.8
  reflex (neuromuscular) (sympathetic) — *see* Syndrome, pain, complex regional I
  retinal (hereditary) H35.50
    in
      lipid storage disorders E75.6 [H36.89]
      systemic lipidoses E75.6 [H36.89]
    involving
      pigment epithelium H35.54
      sensory area H35.53
    pigmentary H35.52
    vitreoretinal H35.51
  Salzmann's nodular — *see* Degeneration, cornea, nodular
  scapuloperoneal G71.09
  skin NEC L98.8
  sympathetic (reflex) — *see* Syndrome, pain, complex regional I
    cervical G90.2
  tapetoretinal H35.54
  thoracic, asphyxiating Q77.2
  unguium L60.3
    congenital Q84.6
  vitreoretinal H35.51
  vulva N90.4
  yellow (liver) — *see* Failure, hepatic
Dysuria R30.0
  psychogenic F45.8

E

Eales' disease H35.06- ☑
Ear — *see also* condition
  piercing Z41.3
  tropical NEC B36.9 [H62.40]
    in
      aspergillosis B44.89
      candidiasis B37.84
      moniliasis B37.84
  wax (impacted) H61.20
    left H61.22
      with right H61.23
    right H61.21
      with left H61.23
Earache — *see* subcategory H92.0 ☑
Early satiety R68.81
Eaton-Lambert syndrome — *see* Syndrome, Lambert-Eaton
Eberth's disease (typhoid fever) A01.00
Ebola virus disease A98.4
Ebstein's anomaly or syndrome (heart) Q22.5
Eccentro-osteochondrodysplasia E76.29
Ecchondroma — *see* Neoplasm, bone, benign
Ecchondrosis D48.0
Ecchymosis R58
  conjunctiva — *see* Hemorrhage, conjunctiva
  eye (traumatic) — *see* Contusion, eyeball

Ecchymosis — *continued*
  eyelid (traumatic) — *see* Contusion, eyelid
  newborn P54.5
  spontaneous R23.3
  traumatic — *see* Contusion
Echinococciasis — *see* Echinococcus
Echinococcosis — *see* Echinococcus
Echinococcus (infection) B67.90
  granulosus B67.4
    bone B67.2
    liver B67.0
    lung B67.1
    multiple sites B67.32
    specified site NEC B67.39
    thyroid B67.31
  liver NOS B67.8
    granulosus B67.0
    multilocularis B67.5
  lung NEC B67.99
    granulosus B67.1
    multilocularis B67.69
  multilocularis B67.7
    liver B67.5
    multiple sites B67.61
    specified site NEC B67.69
  specified site NEC B67.99
    granulosus B67.39
    multilocularis B67.69
  thyroid NEC B67.99
    granulosus B67.31
    multilocularis B67.69 [E35]
Echinorhynchiasis B83.8
Echinostomiasis B66.8
Echolalia R48.8
Echovirus, as cause of disease classified elsewhere B97.12
Eclampsia, eclamptic (coma) (convulsions) (delirium) (with hypertension) NEC O15.9
  complicating
    labor and delivery O15.1
    postpartum O15.2
    pregnancy O15.0- ☑
    puerperium O15.2
Economic circumstances affecting care Z59.9
Economo's disease A85.8
Ectasia, ectasis
  annuloaortic I35.8
  aorta I77.819
    with aneurysm — *see* Aneurysm, aorta
    abdominal I77.811
    thoracic I77.810
    thoracoabdominal I77.812
  breast — *see* Ectasia, mammary duct
  capillary I78.8
  cornea H18.71- ☑
  gastric antral vascular (GAVE) K31.819
    with hemorrhage K31.811
    without hemorrhage K31.819
  mammary duct N60.4- ☑
  salivary gland (duct) K11.8
  sclera — *see* Sclerectasia
Ecthyma L08.0
  contagiosum B08.02
  gangrenosum L08.0
  infectiosum B08.02
Ectocardia Q24.8
Ectodermal dysplasia (anhidrotic) Q82.4
Ectodermosis erosiva pluriorificialis L51.1
Ectopic, ectopia (congenital)
  abdominal viscera Q45.8
    due to defect in anterior abdominal wall Q79.59
  ACTH syndrome E24.3
  adrenal gland Q89.1
  anus Q43.5
  atrial beats I49.1
  beats I49.49
    atrial I49.1
    ventricular I49.3
  bladder Q64.10
  bone and cartilage in lung Q33.5
  brain Q04.8
  breast tissue Q83.8
  cardiac Q24.8
  cerebral Q04.8
  cordis Q24.8
  endometrium — *see* Endometriosis
  gastric mucosa Q40.2
  gestation — *see* Pregnancy, by site
  heart Q24.8

Ectopic, ectopia — *continued*
  hormone secretion NEC E34.2
  kidney (crossed) (pelvis) Q63.2
  lens, lentis Q12.1
  mole — *see* Pregnancy, by site
  organ or site NEC — *see* Malposition, congenital
  pancreas Q45.3
  pregnancy — *see* Pregnancy, ectopic
  pupil — *see* Abnormality, pupillary
  renal Q63.2
  sebaceous glands of mouth Q38.6
  spleen Q89.09
  testis Q53.00
    bilateral Q53.02
    unilateral Q53.01
  thyroid Q89.2
  tissue in lung Q33.5
  ureter Q62.63
  ventricular beats I49.3
  vesicae Q64.10
Ectromelia Q73.8
  lower limb — *see* Defect, reduction, limb, lower, specified type NEC
  upper limb — *see* Defect, reduction, limb, upper, specified type NEC
Ectropion H02.109
  cervix N86
    with cervicitis N72
  congenital Q10.1
  eyelid H02.109
    cicatricial H02.119
      left H02.116
        lower H02.115
        upper H02.114
      right H02.113
        lower H02.112
        upper H02.111
    congenital Q10.1
    left H02.106
      lower H02.105
      upper H02.104
    mechanical H02.129
      left H02.126
        lower H02.125
        upper H02.124
      right H02.123
        lower H02.122
        upper H02.121
    paralytic H02.159
      left H02.156
        lower H02.155
        upper H02.154
      right H02.153
        lower H02.152
        upper H02.151
    right H02.103
      lower H02.102
      upper H02.101
    senile H02.139
      left H02.136
        lower H02.135
        upper H02.134
      right H02.133
        lower H02.132
        upper H02.131
    spastic H02.149
      left H02.146
        lower H02.145
        upper H02.144
      right H02.143
        lower H02.142
        upper H02.141
  iris H21.89
  lip (acquired) K13.0
    congenital Q38.0
  urethra N36.8
  uvea H21.89
Eczema (acute) (chronic) (erythematous) (fissum) (rubrum) (squamous) — *see also* Dermatitis L30.9
  contact — *see* Dermatitis, contact
  dyshydrotic L30.1
  external ear — *see* Otitis, externa, acute, eczematoid
  flexural L20.82
  herpeticum B00.0
  hypertrophicum L28.0
  hypostatic — *see* Varix, leg, with, inflammation
  impetiginous L01.1
  infantile (due to any substance) L20.83
    intertriginous L21.1

Eczema — *continued*
  infantile — *continued*
    seborrheic L21.1
  intertriginous NEC L30.4
    infantile L21.1
  intrinsic (allergic) L20.84
  lichenified NEC L28.0
  marginatum (hebrae) B35.6
  pustular L30.3
  stasis I87.2
    with varicose veins — *see* Varix, leg, with, inflammation
  vaccination, vaccinatum T88.1 ☑
  varicose — *see* Varix, leg, with, inflammation
Eczematid L30.2
Eddowes (-Spurway) **syndrome** Q78.0
Edema, edematous (infectious) (pitting) (toxic) R60.9
  with nephritis — *see* Nephrosis
  allergic T78.3 ☑
  amputation stump (surgical) (sequelae (late effect)) T87.89
  angioneurotic (allergic) (any site) (with urticaria) T78.3 ☑
    hereditary D84.1
  angiospastic I73.9
  Berlin's (traumatic) S05.8X- ☑
  brain (cytotoxic) (vasogenic) G93.6
    due to birth injury P11.0
    newborn (anoxia or hypoxia) P52.4
      birth injury P11.0
    traumatic — *see* Injury, intracranial, cerebral edema
  cardiac — *see* Failure, heart, congestive
  cardiovascular — *see* Failure, heart, congestive
  cerebral — *see* Edema, brain
  cerebrospinal — *see* Edema, brain
  cervix (uteri) (acute) N88.8
    puerperal, postpartum O90.89
  chronic hereditary Q82.0
  circumscribed, acute T78.3 ☑
    hereditary D84.1
  conjunctiva H11.42- ☑
  cornea H18.2- ☑
    idiopathic H18.22- ☑
    secondary H18.23- ☑
      due to contact lens H18.21- ☑
  due to
    lymphatic obstruction I89.0
    salt retention E87.0
  epiglottis — *see* Edema, glottis
  essential, acute T78.3 ☑
    hereditary D84.1
  extremities, lower — *see* Edema, legs
  eyelid NEC H02.849
    left H02.846
      lower H02.845
      upper H02.844
    right H02.843
      lower H02.842
      upper H02.841
  familial, hereditary Q82.0
  famine — *see* Malnutrition, severe
  generalized R60.1
  glottis, glottic, glottidis (obstructive) (passive) J38.4
    allergic T78.3 ☑
      hereditary D84.1
  heart — *see* Failure, heart, congestive
  heat T67.7 ☑
  hereditary Q82.0
  inanition — *see* Malnutrition, severe
  intracranial G93.6
  iris H21.89
  joint — *see* Effusion, joint
  larynx — *see* Edema, glottis
  legs R60.0
    due to venous obstruction I87.1
    hereditary Q82.0
  localized R60.0
    due to venous obstruction I87.1
  lower limbs — *see* Edema, legs
  lung J81.1
    with heart condition or failure — *see* Failure, ventricular, left
    newborn P29.0
    acute J81.0
    chemical (acute) J68.1
      chronic J68.1
    chronic J81.1

Edema, edematous — *continued*
  lung — *continued*
    chronic — *continued*
      due to
        chemicals, gases, fumes or vapors (inhalation) J68.1
        external agent J70.9
          specified NEC J70.8
        radiation J70.1
      due to
        chemicals, fumes or vapors (inhalation) J68.1
        external agent J70.9
          specified NEC J70.8
        high altitude T70.29 ☑
        near drowning T75.1 ☑
        radiation J70.0
      meaning failure, left ventricle I50.1
  lymphatic I89.0
    due to mastectomy I97.2
  macula H35.81
    cystoid, following cataract surgery — *see* Complications, postprocedural, following cataract surgery
    diabetic — *see* Diabetes, by type, with, retinopathy, with macular edema
  malignant — *see* Gangrene, gas
  Milroy's Q82.0
  nasopharynx J39.2
  newborn P83.30
    hydrops fetalis — *see* Hydrops, fetalis
    specified NEC P83.39
  nutritional — *see also* Malnutrition, severe
    with dyspigmentation, skin and hair E40
  optic disc or nerve — *see* Papilledema
  orbit H05.22- ☑
  pancreas K86.89
  papilla, optic — *see* Papilledema
  penis N48.89
  periodic T78.3 ☑
    hereditary D84.1
  pharynx J39.2
  pulmonary — *see* Edema, lung
  Quincke's T78.3 ☑
    hereditary D84.1
  renal — *see* Nephrosis
  retina H35.81
    diabetic — *see* Diabetes, by type, with, retinopathy, with macular edema
  salt E87.0
  scrotum N50.89
  seminal vesicle N50.89
  spermatic cord N50.89
  spinal (cord) (vascular) (nontraumatic) G95.19
  starvation — *see* Malnutrition, severe
  stasis — *see* Hypertension, venous, (chronic)
  subglottic — *see* Edema, glottis
  supraglottic — *see* Edema, glottis
  testis N44.8
  tunica vaginalis N50.89
  vas deferens N50.89
  vulva (acute) N90.89
Edentulism — *see* Absence, teeth, acquired
Edsall's disease T67.2 ☑
Educational handicap Z55.9
  less than a high school diploma Z55.5
  no general equivalence degree (GED) Z55.5
  specified NEC Z55.8
Edward's syndrome — *see* Trisomy, 18
Effect(s) (of) (from) — *see* Effect, adverse NEC
Effect, adverse
  abnormal gravitational (G) forces or states T75.81 ☑
  abuse — *see* Maltreatment
  air pressure T70.9 ☑
    specified NEC T70.8 ☑
  altitude (high) — *see* Effect, adverse, high altitude
  anesthesia — *see also* Anesthesia T88.59 ☑
    in labor and delivery O74.9
    local, toxic
      in labor and delivery O74.4
      in pregnancy NEC O29.3- ☑
      postpartum, puerperal O89.3
    postpartum, puerperal O89.9
    specified NEC T88.59 ☑
      in labor and delivery O74.8
      postpartum, puerperal O89.8
    spinal and epidural T88.59 ☑
      headache T88.59 ☑
        in labor and delivery O74.5

Effect, adverse — *continued*
  anesthesia — *see also* Anesthesia — *continued*
    spinal and epidural — *continued*
      headache — *continued*
        postpartum, puerperal O89.4
      specified NEC
        in labor and delivery O74.6
        postpartum, puerperal O89.5
  antitoxin — *see* Complications, vaccination
  atmospheric pressure T70.9 ☑
    due to explosion T70.8 ☑
    high T70.3 ☑
    low — *see* Effect, adverse, high altitude
    specified effect NEC T70.8 ☑
  biological, correct substance properly administered — *see* Effect, adverse, drug
  blood (derivatives) (serum) (transfusion) — *see* Complications, transfusion
  chemical substance — *see* Table of Drugs and Chemicals
  cold (temperature) (weather) T69.9 ☑
    chilblains T69.1 ☑
    frostbite — *see* Frostbite
    specified effect NEC T69.8 ☑
  drugs and medicaments T88.7 ☑
    specified drug — *see* Table of Drugs and Chemicals, by drug, adverse effect
    specified effect — *code to* condition
  electric current, electricity (shock) T75.4 ☑
    burn — *see* Burn
  exertion (excessive) T73.3 ☑
  exposure — *see* Exposure
  external cause NEC T75.89 ☑
  foodstuffs T78.1 ☑
    allergic reaction — *see* Allergy, food
      causing anaphylaxis — *see* Shock, anaphylactic, due to food
    noxious — *see* Poisoning, food, noxious
  gases, fumes, or vapors T59.9- ☑
    specified agent — *see* Table of Drugs and Chemicals
  glue (airplane) sniffing
    due to drug abuse — *see* Abuse, drug, inhalant
    due to drug dependence — *see* Dependence, drug, inhalant
  heat — *see* Heat
  high altitude NEC T70.29 ☑
    anoxia T70.29 ☑
    on
      ears T70.0 ☑
      sinuses T70.1 ☑
    polycythemia D75.1
  high pressure fluids T70.4 ☑
  hot weather — *see* Heat
  hunger T73.0 ☑
  immersion, foot — *see* Immersion
  immunization — *see* Complications, vaccination
  immunological agents — *see* Complications, vaccination
  infrared (radiation) (rays) NOS T66 ☑
    dermatitis or eczema L59.8
  infusion — *see* Complications, infusion
  lack of care of infants — *see* Maltreatment, child
  lightning — *see* Lightning
  medical care T88.9 ☑
    specified NEC T88.8 ☑
  medicinal substance, correct, properly administered — *see* Effect, adverse, drug
  motion T75.3 ☑
  noise, on inner ear — *see* subcategory H83.3 ☑
  overheated places — *see* Heat
  psychosocial, of work environment Z56.5
  radiation (diagnostic) (infrared) (natural source) (therapeutic) (ultraviolet) (X-ray) NOS T66 ☑
    dermatitis or eczema — *see* Dermatitis, due to, radiation
    fibrosis of lung J70.1
    pneumonitis J70.0
    pulmonary manifestations
      acute J70.0
      chronic J70.1
    skin L59.9
  radioactive substance NOS
    dermatitis or eczema — *see* Radiodermatitis
  reduced temperature T69.9 ☑
    immersion foot or hand — *see* Immersion
    specified effect NEC T69.8 ☑
  serum NEC — *see also* Reaction, serum T80.69 ☑
  specified NEC T78.8 ☑
    external cause NEC T75.89 ☑

Effect, adverse — *continued*
  strangulation — *see* Asphyxia, traumatic
  submersion T75.1 ☑
  thirst T73.1 ☑
  toxic — *see* Toxicity
  transfusion — *see* Complications, transfusion
  ultraviolet (radiation) (rays) NOS T66 ☑
    burn — *see* Burn
    dermatitis or eczema — *see* Dermatitis, due to, ultraviolet rays
      acute L56.8
  vaccine (any) — *see* Complications, vaccination
  vibration — *see* Vibration, adverse effects
  water pressure NEC T70.9 ☑
    specified NEC T70.8 ☑
  weightlessness T75.82 ☑
  whole blood — *see* Complications, transfusion
  work environment Z56.5
Effects, late — *see* Sequelae
Effluvium
  anagen L65.1
  telogen L65.0
Effort syndrome (psychogenic) F45.8
Effusion
  amniotic fluid — *see* Pregnancy, complicated by, premature rupture of membranes
  brain (serous) G93.6
  bronchial — *see* Bronchitis
  cerebral G93.6
  cerebrospinal — *see also* Meningitis
    vessel G93.6
  chest — *see* Effusion, pleura
  chylous, chyliform (pleura) J94.0
  intracranial G93.6
  joint M25.40
    ankle M25.47- ☑
    elbow M25.42- ☑
    foot joint M25.47- ☑
    hand joint M25.44- ☑
    hip M25.45- ☑
    knee M25.46- ☑
    shoulder M25.41- ☑
    specified joint NEC M25.48
    wrist M25.43- ☑
  malignant pleural J91.0
  meninges — *see* Meningitis
  pericardium, pericardial (noninflammatory) I31.39
    acute — *see* Pericarditis, acute
    malignant, in disease classified elsewhere I31.31
    specified type, NEC I31.39
  peritoneal (chronic) R18.8
  pleura, pleurisy, pleuritic, pleuropericardial J90
    chylous, chyliform J94.0
    due to systemic lupus erythematosis M32.13
    in conditions classified elsewhere J91.8
    influenzal — *see* Influenza, with, respiratory manifestations NEC
    malignant J91.0
    newborn P28.89
    tuberculous NEC A15.6
      primary (progressive) A15.7
  spinal — *see* Meningitis
  thorax, thoracic — *see* Effusion, pleura
Egg shell nails L60.3
  congenital Q84.6
EGPA (eosinophilic granulomatosis with polyangiitis) M30.1
Egyptian splenomegaly B65.1
Ehlers-Danlos syndrome — *see also* Syndrome, Ehlers-Danlos Q79.60
Ehrlichiosis A77.40
  due to
    E. chaffeensis A77.41
    E. ewingii A77.49
    E. muris euclairensis A77.49
    E. sennetsu A79.81
    specified organism NEC A77.49
Eichstedt's disease B36.0
Eisenmenger's
  complex or syndrome I27.83
  defect Q21.8
Ejaculation
  delayed F52.32
  painful N53.12
  premature F52.4
  retarded N53.11
  retrograde N53.14
  semen, painful N53.12
    psychogenic F52.6

☑ **Additional Character Required — Refer to the Tabular List for Character Selection**

Ekbom's syndrome (restless legs) G25.81
Ekman's syndrome (brittle bones and blue sclera) Q78.0
Elastic skin Q82.8
   acquired L57.4
Elastofibroma — *see* Neoplasm, connective tissue, benign
Elastoma (juvenile) Q82.8
   Miescher's L87.2
Elastomyofibrosis I42.4
Elastosis
   actinic, solar L57.8
   atrophicans (senile) L57.4
   perforans serpiginosa L87.2
   senilis L57.4
Elbow — *see* condition
Electric current, electricity, effects (concussion) (fatal)
   (nonfatal) (shock) T75.4 ☑
   burn — *see* Burn
Electric feet syndrome E53.8
Electrocution T75.4 ☑
   from electroshock gun (taser) T75.4 ☑
Electrolyte imbalance E87.8
   with
      abortion — *see* Abortion by type, complicated by,
         electrolyte imbalance
      ectopic pregnancy O08.5
      molar pregnancy O08.5
Elephantiasis (nonfilarial) I89.0
   arabicum — *see* Infestation, filarial
   bancroftian B74.0
   congenital (any site) (hereditary) Q82.0
   due to
      Brugia (malayi) B74.1
         timori B74.2
      mastectomy I97.2
      Wuchereria (bancrofti) B74.0
   eyelid H02.859
      left H02.856
         lower H02.855
         upper H02.854
      right H02.853
         lower H02.852
         upper H02.851
   filarial, filariensis — *see* Infestation, filarial
   glandular I89.0
   graecorum A30.9
   lymphangiectatic I89.0
   lymphatic vessel I89.0
      due to mastectomy I97.2
   scrotum (nonfilarial) I89.0
   streptococcal I89.0
   surgical I97.89
      postmastectomy I97.2
   telangiectodes I89.0
   vulva (nonfilarial) N90.89
Elevated, elevation
   alanine transaminase (ALT) R74.01
   ALT (alanine transaminase) R74.01
   antibody titer R76.0
   aspartate transaminase (AST) R74.01
   AST (aspartate transaminase) R74.01
   basal metabolic rate R94.8
   blood pressure — *see also* Hypertension
      reading (incidental) (isolated) (nonspecific), no diag-
         nosis of hypertension R03.0
   blood sugar R73.9
   body temperature (of unknown origin) R50.9
   cancer antigen 125 [CA 125] R97.1
   carcinoembryonic antigen [CEA] R97.0
   cholesterol E78.00
      with high triglycerides E78.2
   conjugate, eye H51.0
   C-reactive protein (CRP) R79.82
   diaphragm, congenital Q79.1
   erythrocyte sedimentation rate R70.0
   fasting glucose R73.01
   fasting triglycerides E78.1
   finding on laboratory examination — *see* Findings, ab-
      normal, inconclusive, without diagnosis, by type
      of exam
   GFR (glomerular filtration rate) — *see* Findings, abnormal,
      inconclusive, without diagnosis, by type of exam
   glucose tolerance (oral) R73.02
   immunoglobulin level R76.8
   indoleacetic acid R82.5
   lactic acid dehydrogenase (LDH) level R74.02
   leukocytes D72.829
   lipoprotein a (Lp(a)) level E78.41
   liver function
      study R94.5

Elevated, elevation — *continued*
   liver function — *continued*
      test R79.89
         alkaline phosphatase R74.8
         aminotransferase R74.01
         bilirubin R17
         hepatic enzyme R74.8
         lactate dehydrogenase R74.02
   Lp(a) (lipoprotein(a)) E78.41
   lymphocytes D72.820
   prostate specific antigen [PSA] R97.20
   Rh titer — *see* Complication(s), transfusion, incompatibil-
      ity reaction, Rh (factor)
   scapula, congenital Q74.0
   sedimentation rate R70.0
   SGOT R74.01
   SGPT R74.01
   transaminase level R74.01
   triglycerides E78.1
      with high cholesterol E78.2
   troponin R79.89
   tumor associated antigens [TAA] NEC R97.8
   tumor specific antigens [TSA] NEC R97.8
   urine level of
      17-ketosteroids R82.5
      catecholamine R82.5
      indoleacetic acid R82.5
      steroids R82.5
      vanillylmandelic acid (VMA) R82.5
   venous pressure I87.8
   white blood cell count D72.829
      specified NEC D72.828
Elliptocytosis (congenital) (hereditary) D58.1
   Hb C (disease) D58.1
   hemoglobin disease D58.1
   sickle-cell (disease) D57.8- ☑
      trait D57.3
Ellison-Zollinger syndrome E16.4
Ellis-van Creveld syndrome (chondroectodermal dysplasia)
   Q77.6
Elongated, elongation (congenital) — *see also* Distortion
   bone Q79.9
   cervix (uteri) Q51.828
      acquired N88.4
      hypertrophic N88.4
   colon Q43.8
   common bile duct Q44.5
   cystic duct Q44.5
   frenulum, penis Q55.69
   labia minora (acquired) N90.69
   ligamentum patellae Q74.1
   petiolus (epiglottidis) Q31.8
   tooth, teeth K00.2
   uvula Q38.6
Eltor cholera A00.1
Emaciation R64
   due to malnutrition E43
Embadomoniasis A07.8
Embedded tooth, teeth K01.0
   root only K08.3
Embolic — *see* condition
Embolism (multiple) (paradoxical) I74.9
   air (any site) (traumatic) T79.0 ☑
      following
         abortion — *see* Abortion by type complicated by
            embolism
         ectopic pregnancy O08.2
         infusion, therapeutic injection or transfusion
            T80.0 ☑
         molar pregnancy O08.2
         procedure NEC
            artery T81.719 ☑
               mesenteric T81.710 ☑
               renal T81.711 ☑
               specified NEC T81.718 ☑
            vein T81.72 ☑
      in pregnancy, childbirth or puerperium — *see* Em-
         bolism, obstetric
   amniotic fluid (pulmonary) — *see also* Embolism, obstet-
      ric
      following
         abortion — *see* Abortion by type complicated by
            embolism
         ectopic pregnancy O08.2
         molar pregnancy O08.2
   aorta, aortic I74.10
      abdominal I74.09
      saddle I74.01

Embolism — *continued*
   aorta, aortic — *continued*
      bifurcation I74.09
      saddle I74.01
      thoracic I74.11
   artery I74.9
      auditory, internal I65.8
      basilar — *see* Occlusion, artery, basilar
      carotid (common) (internal) — *see* Occlusion, artery,
         carotid
      cerebellar (anterior inferior) (posterior inferior) (supe-
         rior) I66.3
      cerebral — *see* Occlusion, artery, cerebral
      choroidal (anterior) I65.8
      communicating posterior I65.8
      coronary — *see also* Infarct, myocardium
         not resulting in infarction I24.0
      extremity I74.4
         lower I74.3
         upper I74.2
      hypophyseal I65.8
      iliac I74.5
      limb I74.4
         lower I74.3
         upper I74.2
      mesenteric (with gangrene) — *see also* Ischemia, in-
         testine, acute K55.059
      ophthalmic — *see* Occlusion, artery, retina
      peripheral I74.4
      pontine I65.8
      precerebral — *see* Occlusion, artery, precerebral
      pulmonary — *see* Embolism, pulmonary
      renal N28.0
      retinal — *see* Occlusion, artery, retina
      septic I76
      specified NEC I74.8
      vertebral — *see* Occlusion, artery, vertebral
   basilar (artery) I65.1
   blood clot
      following
         abortion — *see* Abortion by type complicated by
            embolism
         ectopic or molar pregnancy O08.2
      in pregnancy, childbirth or puerperium — *see* Em-
         bolism, obstetric
   brain — *see also* Occlusion, artery, cerebral
      following
         abortion — *see* Abortion by type complicated by
            embolism
         ectopic or molar pregnancy O08.2
      puerperal, postpartum, childbirth — *see* Embolism,
         obstetric
   capillary I78.8
   cardiac — *see also* Infarct, myocardium
      not resulting in infarction I51.3
   carotid (artery) (common) (internal) — *see* Occlusion,
      artery, carotid
   cavernous sinus (venous) — *see* Embolism, intracranial,
      venous sinus
   cement
      pulmonary artery I26.95
         with acute cor pulmonale I26.03
   cerebral — *see* Occlusion, artery, cerebral
   cholesterol — *see* Atheroembolism
   coronary (artery or vein) (systemic) — *see* Occlusion,
      coronary
   due to device, implant or graft — *see also* Complications,
      by site and type, specified NEC
      arterial graft NEC T82.818 ☑
      breast (implant) T85.818 ☑
      catheter NEC T85.818 ☑
         dialysis (renal) T82.818 ☑
            intraperitoneal T85.818 ☑
         infusion NEC T82.818 ☑
            spinal (epidural) (subdural) T85.810 ☑
         urinary (indwelling) T83.81 ☑
      electronic (electrode) (pulse generator) (stimulator)
         bone T84.81 ☑
         cardiac T82.817 ☑
         nervous system (brain) (peripheral nerve) (spinal)
            T85.810 ☑
         urinary T83.81 ☑
      fixation, internal (orthopedic) NEC T84.81 ☑
      gastrointestinal (bile duct) (esophagus) T85.818 ☑
      genital NEC T83.81 ☑
      heart (graft) (valve) T82.817 ☑
      joint prosthesis T84.81 ☑
      ocular (corneal graft) (orbital implant) T85.818 ☑

Embolism — *continued*
due to device, implant or graft — *see also* Complications, by site and type, specified — *continued*
    orthopedic (bone graft) NEC T86.838
    specified NEC T85.818 ☑
    urinary (graft) NEC T83.81 ☑
    vascular NEC T82.818 ☑
    ventricular intracranial shunt T85.810 ☑
extremities
  lower — *see* Embolism, vein, lower extremity
    arterial I74.3
  upper I74.2
eye H34.9
fat (cerebral) (pulmonary) (systemic) T79.1 ☑
  complicating delivery — *see* Embolism, obstetric
  following
    abortion — *see* Abortion by type complicated by embolism
    ectopic or molar pregnancy O08.2
  pulmonary artery I26.96
    with acute cor pulmonale I26.04
following
  abortion — *see* Abortion by type complicated by embolism
  ectopic or molar pregnancy O08.2
  infusion, therapeutic injection or transfusion
    air T80.0 ☑
heart (fatty) — *see also* Infarct, myocardium
  not resulting in infarction I51.3
hepatic (vein) I82.0
in pregnancy, childbirth or puerperium — *see* Embolism, obstetric
intestine (artery) (vein) (with gangrene) — *see also* Ischemia, intestine, acute K55.039
intracranial — *see also* Occlusion, artery, cerebral
  venous sinus (any) G08
    nonpyogenic I67.6
intraspinal venous sinuses or veins G08
  nonpyogenic G95.19
kidney (artery) N28.0
lateral sinus (venous) — *see* Embolism, intracranial, venous sinus
leg — *see* Embolism, vein, lower extremity
  arterial I74.3
longitudinal sinus (venous) — *see* Embolism, intracranial, venous sinus
lung (massive) — *see* Embolism, pulmonary
meninges I66.8
mesenteric (artery) (vein) (with gangrene) — *see also* Ischemia, intestine, acute K55.059
obstetric (in) (pulmonary)
  childbirth O88.22
    air O88.02
    amniotic fluid O88.12
    blood clot O88.22
    fat O88.82
    pyemic O88.32
    septic O88.32
    specified type NEC O88.82
  pregnancy O88.21- ☑
    air O88.01- ☑
    amniotic fluid O88.11- ☑
    blood clot O88.21- ☑
    fat O88.81- ☑
    pyemic O88.31- ☑
    septic O88.31- ☑
    specified type NEC O88.81- ☑
  puerperal O88.23
    air O88.03
    amniotic fluid O88.13
    blood clot O88.23
    fat O88.83
    pyemic O88.33
    septic O88.33
    specified type NEC O88.83
ophthalmic — *see* Occlusion, artery, retina
penis N48.81
peripheral artery NOS I74.4
pituitary E23.6
popliteal (artery) I74.3
portal (vein) I81
postoperative, postprocedural
  artery T81.719 ☑
    mesenteric T81.710 ☑
    renal T81.711 ☑
    specified NEC T81.718 ☑
  vein T81.72 ☑
precerebral artery — *see* Occlusion, artery, precerebral

Embolism — *continued*
puerperal — *see* Embolism, obstetric
pulmonary (acute) (artery) (vein) I26.99
  with acute cor pulmonale I26.09
  cement I26.95
    with acute cor pulmonale I26.03
  chronic I27.82
  fat I26.96
    with acute cor pulmonale I26.04
  following
    abortion — *see* Abortion by type complicated by embolism
    ectopic or molar pregnancy O08.2
  healed or old Z86.711
  in pregnancy, childbirth or puerperium — *see* Embolism, obstetric
  multiple subsegmental without acute cor pulmonale I26.94
  personal history of Z86.711
  saddle I26.92
    with acute cor pulmonale I26.02
  septic I26.90
    with acute cor pulmonale I26.01
  single subsegmental without acute cor pulmonale I26.93
  subsegmental NOS I26.93
pyemic (multiple) I76
  following
    abortion — *see* Abortion by type complicated by embolism
    ectopic or molar pregnancy O08.2
  Hemophilus influenzae A41.3
  pneumococcal A40.3
    with pneumonia J13
  puerperal, postpartum, childbirth (any organism) — *see* Embolism, obstetric
  specified organism NEC A41.89
  staphylococcal A41.2
  streptococcal A40.9
renal (artery) N28.0
  vein I82.3
retina, retinal — *see* Occlusion, artery, retina
saddle
  abdominal aorta I74.01
  pulmonary artery I26.92
    with acute cor pulmonale I26.02
septic (arterial) I76
  complicating abortion — *see* Abortion, by type, complicated by, embolism
sinus — *see* Embolism, intracranial, venous sinus
soap complicating abortion — *see* Abortion, by type, complicated by, embolism
spinal cord G95.19
  pyogenic origin G06.1
spleen, splenic (artery) I74.8
thrombotic
  specified NEC I26.99
    with acute cor pulmonale I26.09
upper extremity I74.2
vein (acute) I82.90
  antecubital I82.61- ☑
    chronic I82.71- ☑
  axillary I82.A1- ☑ (*following* I82.7)
    chronic I82.A2- ☑ (*following* I82.7)
  basilic I82.61- ☑
    chronic I82.71- ☑
  brachial I82.62- ☑
    chronic I82.72- ☑
  brachiocephalic (innominate) I82.290
    chronic I82.291
  calf, muscle I82.46- ☑
    chronic I82.56- ☑
  cephalic I82.61- ☑
    chronic I82.71- ☑
  chronic I82.91
  deep (DVT) I82.40- ☑
    calf I82.4Z- ☑
      chronic I82.5Z- ☑
    lower leg I82.4Z- ☑
      chronic I82.5Z- ☑
    thigh I82.4Y- ☑
      chronic I82.5Y- ☑
    upper leg I82.4Y ☑
      chronic I82.5Y-
  femoral I82.41- ☑
    chronic I82.51- ☑
  gastrocnemial I82.46- ☑
    chronic I82.56- ☑

Embolism — *continued*
vein — *continued*
  iliac (iliofemoral) I82.42- ☑
    chronic I82.52- ☑
  innominate I82.290
    chronic I82.291
  internal jugular I82.C1- ☑ (*following* I82.7)
    chronic I82.C2- ☑ (*following* I82.7)
  lower extremity
    deep I82.40- ☑
      chronic I82.50- ☑
      specified NEC I82.49- ☑
        chronic NEC I82.59- ☑
    distal
      deep I82.4Z- ☑
    proximal
      deep I82.4Y- ☑
        chronic I82.5Y- ☑
    superficial I82.81- ☑
  peroneal I82.45- ☑
    chronic I82.55- ☑
  popliteal I82.43- ☑
    chronic I82.53- ☑
  radial I82.62- ☑
    chronic I82.72- ☑
  renal I82.3
  saphenous (greater) (lesser) I82.81- ☑
  soleal I82.46- ☑
    chronic I82.56- ☑
  specified NEC I82.890
    chronic NEC I82.891
  subclavian I82.B1- ☑ (*following* I82.7)
    chronic I82.B2- ☑ (*following* I82.7)
  thoracic NEC I82.290
    chronic I82.291
  tibial I82.44- ☑
    chronic I82.54- ☑
  ulnar I82.62- ☑
    chronic I82.72- ☑
  upper extremity I82.60- ☑
    chronic I82.70- ☑
    deep I82.62- ☑
      chronic I82.72- ☑
    superficial I82.61- ☑
      chronic I82.71- ☑
  vena cava
    inferior (acute) I82.220
      chronic I82.221
    superior (acute) I82.210
      chronic I82.211
  venous sinus G08
  vessels of brain — *see* Occlusion, artery, cerebral
Embolus — *see* Embolism
Embryoma — *see also* Neoplasm, uncertain behavior, by site
  benign — *see* Neoplasm, benign, by site
  kidney C64.- ☑
  liver C22.0
  malignant — *see also* Neoplasm, malignant, by site
    kidney C64.- ☑
    liver C22.0
    testis C62.9- ☑
      descended (scrotal) C62.1- ☑
      undescended C62.0- ☑
  testis C62.9- ☑
    descended (scrotal) C62.1- ☑
    undescended C62.0- ☑
Embryonic
  circulation Q28.9
  heart Q28.9
  vas deferens Q55.4
Embryopathia NOS Q89.9
Embryotoxon Q13.4
Emesis — *see* Vomiting
Emotional lability R45.86
Emotionality, pathological F60.3
Emotogenic disease — *see* Disorder, psychogenic
Emphysema (atrophic) (bullous) (chronic) (interlobular) (lung) (obstructive) (pulmonary) (senile) (vesicular) J43.9
  cellular tissue (traumatic) T79.7 ☑
    surgical T81.82 ☑
  centrilobular J43.2
  compensatory J98.3
  congenital (interstitial) P25.0
  conjunctiva H11.89
  connective tissue (traumatic) T79.7 ☑

Emphysema — *continued*
  connective tissue — *continued*
    surgical T81.82 ☑
  due to chemicals, gases, fumes or vapors — *see also*
      Disease, respiratory, chronic, due to chemicals,
      gases, fumes or vapors J43- ☑
  eyelid(s) — *see* Disorder, eyelid, specified type NEC
    surgical T81.82 ☑
    traumatic T79.7 ☑
  interstitial J98.2
    congenital P25.0
    perinatal period P25.0
  laminated tissue T79.7 ☑
    surgical T81.82 ☑
  mediastinal J98.2
    newborn P25.2
  orbit, orbital — *see* Disorder, orbit, specified type NEC
  panacinar J43.1
  panlobular J43.1
  specified NEC J43.8
  subcutaneous (traumatic) T79.7 ☑
    nontraumatic J98.2
    postprocedural T81.82 ☑
    surgical T81.82 ☑
  surgical T81.82 ☑
  thymus (gland) (congenital) E32.8
  traumatic (subcutaneous) T79.7 ☑
  unilateral J43.0
Empty nest syndrome Z60.0
Empyema (acute) (chest) (double) (pleura) (supradiaphragmatic) (thorax) J86.9
  with fistula J86.0
  accessory sinus (chronic) — *see* Sinusitis
  antrum (chronic) — *see* Sinusitis, maxillary
  brain (any part) — *see* Abscess, brain
  ethmoidal (chronic) (sinus) — *see* Sinusitis, ethmoidal
  extradural — *see* Abscess, extradural
  frontal (chronic) (sinus) — *see* Sinusitis, frontal
  gallbladder K81.0
  mastoid (process) (acute) — *see* Mastoiditis, acute
  maxilla, maxillary M27.2
    sinus (chronic) — *see* Sinusitis, maxillary
  nasal sinus (chronic) — *see* Sinusitis
  sinus (accessory) (chronic) (nasal) — *see* Sinusitis
  sphenoidal (sinus) (chronic) — *see* Sinusitis, sphenoidal
  subarachnoid — *see* Abscess, extradural
  subdural — *see* Abscess, subdural
  tuberculous A15.6
  ureter — *see* Ureteritis
  ventricular — *see* Abscess, brain
En coup de sabre lesion L94.1
Enamel pearls K00.2
Enameloma K00.2
Enanthema, viral B09
Encephalitis (chronic) (hemorrhagic) (idiopathic) (nonepidemic) (spurious) (subacute) G04.90
  acute — *see also* Encephalitis, viral A86
    disseminated G04.00
      infectious G04.01
      noninfectious G04.81
      postimmunization (postvaccination) G04.02
      postinfectious G04.01
    inclusion body A85.8
    necrotizing hemorrhagic G04.30
      postimmunization G04.32
      postinfectious G04.31
      specified NEC G04.39
  arboviral, arbovirus NEC A85.2
  arthropod-borne NEC (viral) A85.2
  Australian A83.4
  California (virus) A83.5
  Central European (tick-borne) A84.1
  Czechoslovakian A84.1
  Dawson's (inclusion body) A81.1
  diffuse sclerosing A81.1
  disseminated, acute G04.00
  due to
    cat scratch disease A28.1
    human immunodeficiency virus (HIV) disease B20 *[G05.3]*
    malaria — *see* Malaria
    rickettsiosis — *see* Rickettsiosis
    smallpox inoculation G04.02
    typhus — *see* Typhus
  Eastern equine A83.2
  endemic (viral) A86
  epidemic NEC (viral) A86
  equine (acute) (infectious) (viral) A83.9

Encephalitis — *continued*
  equine — *continued*
    Eastern A83.2
    Venezuelan A92.2
    Western A83.1
  Far Eastern (tick-borne) A84.0
  following vaccination or other immunization procedure G04.02
  herpes zoster B02.0
  herpesviral B00.4
    due to herpesvirus 6 B10.01
    due to herpesvirus 7 B10.09
    specified NEC B10.09
  Ilheus (virus) A83.8
  in (due to)
    actinomycosis A42.82
    adenovirus A85.1
    African trypanosomiasis B56.9 *[G05.3]*
    Chagas' disease (chronic) B57.42
    cytomegalovirus B25.8
    enterovirus A85.0
    herpes (simplex) virus B00.4
      due to herpesvirus 6 B10.01
      due to herpesvirus 7 B10.09
      specified NEC B10.09
    infectious disease NEC B99 ☑ *[G05.3]*
    influenza — *see* Influenza, with, encephalopathy
    listeriosis A32.12
    measles B05.0
    mumps B26.2
    naegleriasis B60.2
    parasitic disease NEC B89 *[G05.3]*
    poliovirus A80.9 *[G05.3]*
    rubella B06.01
    syphilis
      congenital A50.42
      late A52.14
    systemic lupus erythematosus M32.19 *[G05.3]*
    toxoplasmosis (acquired) B58.2
      congenital P37.1
    tuberculosis A17.82
    zoster B02.0
  inclusion body A81.1
  infectious (acute) (virus) NEC A86
  Japanese (B type) A83.0
  La Crosse A83.5
  lead — *see* Poisoning, lead
  lethargica (acute) (infectious) A85.8
  louping ill A84.89
  lupus erythematosus, systemic M32.19 *[G05.3]*
  lymphatica A87.2
  Mengo A85.8
  meningococcal A39.81
  Murray Valley A83.4
  otitic NEC H66.40 *[G05.3]*
  parasitic NOS B71.9
  periaxial G37.0
  periaxialis (concentrica) (diffuse) G37.5
  postchickenpox B01.11
  postexanthematous NEC B09
  postimmunization G04.02
  postinfectious NEC G04.01
  postmeasles B05.0
  postvaccinal G04.02
  postvaricella B01.11
  postviral NEC A86
  Powassan A84.81
  Rasmussen G04.81
  Rio Bravo A85.8
  Russian
    autumnal A83.0
    spring-summer (taiga) A84.0
  saturnine — *see* Poisoning, lead
  specified NEC G04.81
  St. Louis A83.3
  subacute sclerosing A81.1
  summer A83.0
  suppurative G04.81
  tick-borne A84.9
  Torula, torular (cryptococcal) B45.1
  toxic NEC G92.8
  trichinosis B75 *[G05.3]*
  type
    B A83.0
    C A83.3
  van Bogaert's A81.1
  Venezuelan equine A92.2
  Vienna A85.8
  viral, virus A86

Encephalitis — *continued*
  viral, virus — *continued*
    arthropod-borne NEC A85.2
      mosquito-borne A83.9
        Australian X disease A83.4
        California virus A83.5
        Eastern equine A83.2
        Japanese (B type) A83.0
        Murray Valley A83.4
        specified NEC A83.8
        St. Louis A83.3
        type B A83.0
        type C A83.3
        Western equine A83.1
      tick-borne A84.9
        biundulant A84.1
        central European A84.1
        Czechoslovakian A84.1
        diphasic meningoencephalitis A84.1
        Far Eastern A84.0
        Russian spring-summer (taiga) A84.0
        specified NEC A84.89
      specified type NEC A85.8
      tick-borne, specified NEC A84.89
  Western equine A83.1
Encephalocele Q01.9
  frontal Q01.0
  nasofrontal Q01.1
  occipital Q01.2
  specified NEC Q01.8
Encephalocystocele — *see* Encephalocele
Encephaloduroarteriomyosynangiosis (EDAMS) I67.5
Encephalomalacia (brain) (cerebellar) (cerebral) — *see*
      Softening, brain
Encephalomeningitis — *see* Meningoencephalitis
Encephalomeningocele — *see* Encephalocele
Encephalomeningomyelitis — *see* Meningoencephalitis
Encephalomyelitis — *see also* Encephalitis G04.90
  acute disseminated G04.00
    infectious G04.01
    noninfectious G04.81
    postimmunization G04.02
    postinfectious G04.01
  acute necrotizing hemorrhagic G04.30
    postimmunization G04.32
    postinfectious G04.31
    specified NEC G04.39
  equine A83.9
    Eastern A83.2
    Venezuelan A92.2
    Western A83.1
  in diseases classified elsewhere G05.3
  myalgic G93.32
    chronic fatigue syndrome [ME/CFS] G93.32
  postchickenpox B01.11
  postinfectious NEC G04.01
  postmeasles B05.0
  postvaccinal G04.02
  postvaricella B01.11
  rubella B06.01
  specified NEC G04.81
  Venezuelan equine A92.2
Encephalomyelocele — *see* Encephalocele
Encephalomyelomeningitis — *see* Meningoencephalitis
Encephalomyelopathy G96.9
Encephalomyeloradiculitis (acute) G61.0
Encephalomyeloradiculoneuritis (acute) (Guillain-Barre) G61.0
Encephalomyeloradiculopathy G96.9
Encephalopathia hyperbilirubinemica, newborn P57.9
  due to isoimmunization (conditions in P55) P57.0
Encephalopathy (acute) G93.40
  acute necrotizing hemorrhagic G04.30
    postimmunization G04.32
    postinfectious G04.31
    specified NEC G04.39
  alcoholic G31.2
  anoxic — *see* Damage, brain, anoxic
  arteriosclerotic I67.2
  centrolobar progressive (Schilder) G37.0
  congenital Q07.9
  degenerative, in specified disease NEC G32.89
  demyelinating callosal G37.1
  developmental and epileptic G93.45
  due to
    drugs — *see also* Table of Drugs and Chemicals G92.8
  early infantile epileptic G93.45
  hepatic (without coma) K76.82
  hyperbilirubinemic, newborn P57.9

Encephalopathy — *continued*
hyperbilirubinemic, newborn — *continued*
  due to isoimmunization (conditions in P55) P57.0
hypertensive I67.4
hypoglycemic E16.2
hypoxic — *see* Damage, brain, anoxic
hypoxic ischemic P91.60
  mild P91.61
  moderate P91.62
  severe P91.63
in (due to) (with)
  birth injury P11.1
  hyperinsulinism E16.1 *[G94]*
  influenza — *see* Influenza, with, encephalopathy
  lack of vitamin — *see also* Deficiency, vitamin
    E56.9 *[G32.89]*
  neoplastic disease — *see also* Neoplasm D49.9 *[G13.1]*
  serum — *see also* Reaction, serum T80.69 ☑
  syphilis A52.17
  trauma (postconcussional) F07.81
    current injury — *see* Injury, intracranial
  vaccination G04.02
lead — *see* Poisoning, lead
metabolic G93.41
  drug induced G92.8
  toxic G92.8
myoclonic, early, symptomatic — *see* Epilepsy, generalized, specified NEC
necrotizing, subacute (Leigh) G31.82
neonatal P91.819
  in diseases classified elsewhere P91.811
pellagrous E52 *[G32.89]*
portal-systemic K76.82
postcontusional F07.81
  current injury — *see* Injury, intracranial, diffuse
posthypoglycemic (coma) E16.1 *[G94]*
postradiation G93.89
saturnine — *see* Poisoning, lead
septic G93.41
specified NEC G93.49
spongiform, subacute (viral) A81.09
toxic G92.9
  metabolic G92.8
traumatic (postconcussional) F07.81
  current injury — *see* Injury, intracranial
vitamin B deficiency NEC E53.9 *[G32.89]*
  vitamin B1 E51.2
  Wernicke's E51.2
Encephalorrhagia — *see* Hemorrhage, intracranial, intracerebral
Encephalosis, posttraumatic F07.81
Enchondroma — *see also* Neoplasm, bone, benign
Enchondromatosis (cartilaginous) (multiple) Q78.4
Encopresis R15.9
functional F98.1
nonorganic origin F98.1
psychogenic F98.1
Encounter (with health service) (for) Z76.89
adjustment and management (of)
  breast implant Z45.81 ☑
  implanted device NEC Z45.89
  myringotomy device (stent) (tube) Z45.82
  neurostimulator (brain) (gastric) (peripheral nerve)
    (sacral nerve) (spinal cord) (vagus nerve) Z45.42
administrative purpose only Z02.9
  examination for
    adoption Z02.82
    armed forces Z02.3
    child welfare Z02.84
    disability determination Z02.71
    driving license Z02.4
    employment Z02.1
    insurance Z02.6
    medical certificate NEC Z02.79
    paternity testing Z02.81
    residential institution admission Z02.2
    school admission Z02.0
    sports Z02.5
  specified reason NEC Z02.89
aftercare — *see* Aftercare
antenatal screening Z36.9
  cervical length Z36.86
  chromosomal anomalies Z36.0
  congenital cardiac abnormalities Z36.83
  elevated maternal serum alphafetoprotein Z36.1
  fetal growth retardation Z36.4
  fetal lung maturity Z36.84
  fetal macrosomia Z36.88
  hydrops fetalis Z36.81

Encounter — *continued*
antenatal screening — *continued*
  intrauterine growth restriction (IUGR) /small-for-dates
    Z36.4
  isoimmunization Z36.5
  large-for-dates Z36.88
  malformations Z36.3
  non-visualized anatomy on a previous scan Z36.2
  nuchal translucency Z36.82
  raised alphafetoprotein level Z36.1
  risk of pre-term labor Z36.86
  specified follow-up NEC Z36.2
  specified genetic defects NEC Z36.8A
  specified type NEC Z36.89
  Streptococcus B Z36.85
  suspected anomaly Z36.3
  uncertain dates Z36.87
assisted reproductive fertility procedure cycle Z31.83
blood typing Z01.83
  Rh typing Z01.83
breast augmentation or reduction Z41.1
breast implant exchange (different material) (different
  size) Z45.81 ☑
breast reconstruction following mastectomy Z42.1
check-up — *see* Examination
chemotherapy for neoplasm Z51.11
child welfare screening exam Z02.84
colonoscopy, screening Z12.11
counseling — *see* Counseling
delivery, full-term, uncomplicated O80
  cesarean, without indication O82
desensitization to allergens Z51.6
ear piercing Z41.3
examination — *see* Examination
expectant parent(s) (adoptive) pre-birth pediatrician
  visit Z76.81
fertility preservation procedure (prior to cancer therapy)
  (prior to removal of gonads) Z31.84
fitting (of) — *see* Fitting (and adjustment) (of)
genetic
  counseling
    nonprocreative Z71.83
    procreative Z31.5
  testing — *see* Test, genetic
hearing conservation and treatment Z01.12
HIV
  pre-exposure prophylaxis Z29.81
  PrEP Z29.81
immunotherapy for neoplasm Z51.12
in vitro fertilization cycle Z31.83
instruction (in)
  child care (postpartal) (prenatal) Z32.3
  childbirth Z32.2
  natural family planning
    procreative Z31.61
    to avoid pregnancy Z30.02
insulin pump titration Z46.81
joint prosthesis insertion following prior explantation of
  joint prosthesis (staged procedure)
    hip Z47.32
    knee Z47.33
    shoulder Z47.31
laboratory (as part of a general medical examination)
  Z00.00
  with abnormal findings Z00.01
mental health services (for)
  abuse NEC
    perpetrator Z69.82
    victim Z69.81
  child abuse
    nonparental
      perpetrator Z69.021
      victim Z69.020
    parental
      perpetrator Z69.011
      victim Z69.010
  child neglect
    nonparental
      perpetrator Z69.021
      victim Z69.020
    parental
      perpetrator Z69.011
      victim Z69.010
  child psychological abuse
    nonparental
      perpetrator Z69.021
      victim Z69.020
    parental
      perpetrator Z69.011

Encounter — *continued*
mental health services — *continued*
  child psychological abuse — *continued*
    parental — *continued*
      victim Z69.010
  child sexual abuse
    nonparental
      perpetrator Z69.021
      victim Z69.020
    parental
      perpetrator Z69.011
      victim Z69.010
  non-spousal adult abuse
    perpetrator Z69.82
    victim Z69.81
  spousal or partner
    abuse
      perpetrator Z69.12
      victim Z69.11
    neglect
      perpetrator Z69.12
      victim Z69.11
    psychological abuse
      perpetrator Z69.12
      victim Z69.11
    violence
      perpetrator (physical) (sexual) Z69.12
      victim (physical) Z69.11
      sexual Z69.81
observation (for) (ruled out)
  alarm, without findings
    apnea Z03.83
    bradycardia Z03.83
    oximeter Z03.83
  condition suspected related to home physiologic
    monitoring device Z03.83
    newborn Z05.81
      apnea alarm Z05.81
      bradycardia alarm Z05.81
      malfunction of home cardiorespiratory monitor
        Z05.81
      non-specific findings home physiologic monitoring device Z05.81
      pulse oximeter alarm without findings Z05.81
  exposure to (suspected)
    anthrax Z03.810
    biological agent NEC Z03.818
  malfunction of home cardiorespiratory monitor Z03.83
  non-specific findings home physiologic monitoring
    device Z03.83
palliative care Z51.5
pediatrician visit, by expectant parent(s) (adoptive)
  Z76.81
placental sample (taken vaginally) — *see also* Encounter,
  antenatal screening Z36.9
plastic and reconstructive surgery following medical
  procedure or healed injury NEC Z42.8
postoperative — *see* Aftercare
pregnancy
  supervision of — *see* Pregnancy, supervision of
  test Z32.00
    result negative Z32.02
    result positive Z32.01
procreative management and counseling for gestational
  carrier Z31.7
prophylactic measures Z29.9
  antivenin Z29.12
  fluoride administration Z29.3
  HIV pre-exposure Z29.81
  immunotherapy for respiratory syncytial virus (RSV)
    Z29.11
  rabies immune globin Z29.14
  Rho (D) immune globulin Z29.13
  specified NEC Z29.89
radiation therapy (antineoplastic) Z51.0
radiological (as part of a general medical examination)
  Z00.00
  with abnormal findings Z00.01
reconstructive surgery following medical procedure or
  healed injury NEC Z42.8
removal (of) — *see also* Removal
  artificial
    arm Z44.00- ☑
      complete Z44.01- ☑
      partial Z44.02- ☑
    eye Z44.2- ☑
    leg Z44.10- ☑
      complete Z44.11- ☑

☑ **Additional Character Required — Refer to the Tabular List for Character Selection**

Encounter — *continued*
  removal — *see also* Removal — *continued*
    artificial — *continued*
      leg — *continued*
        partial Z44.12- ☑
      breast implant Z45.81 ☑
        tissue expander (with or without synchronous insertion of permanent implant) Z45.81 ☑
    device Z46.9
      specified NEC Z46.89
    external
      fixation device — *code to* fracture with seventh character D
    prosthesis, prosthetic device Z44.9
      breast Z44.3- ☑
      specified NEC Z44.8
    implanted device NEC Z45.89
    insulin pump Z46.81
    internal fixation device Z47.2
    myringotomy device (stent) (tube) Z45.82
    nervous system device NEC Z46.2
      brain neuropacemaker Z46.2
      visual substitution device Z46.2
        implanted Z45.31
    non-vascular catheter Z46.82
    orthodontic device Z46.4
    stent
      ureteral Z46.6
    urinary device Z46.6
  repeat cervical smear to confirm findings of recent normal smear following initial abnormal smear Z01.42
  respirator [ventilator] use during power failure Z99.12
  Rh typing Z01.83
  screening — *see* Screening
  specified NEC Z76.89
  sterilization Z30.2
  suspected condition, ruled out
    amniotic cavity and membrane Z03.71
    cervical shortening Z03.75
    fetal anomaly Z03.73
    fetal growth Z03.74
    maternal and fetal conditions NEC Z03.79
    oligohydramnios Z03.71
    placental problem Z03.72
    polyhydramnios Z03.71
  suspected exposure (to), ruled out
    anthrax Z03.810
    biological agents NEC Z03.818
  termination of pregnancy, elective Z33.2
  testing — *see* Test
  therapeutic drug level monitoring Z51.81
  titration, insulin pump Z46.81
  to determine fetal viability of pregnancy O36.80 ☑
  training
    insulin pump Z46.81
  X-ray of chest (as part of a general medical examination) Z00.00
    with abnormal findings Z00.01
Encystment — *see* Cyst
Endarteritis (bacterial, subacute) (infective) I77.6
  brain I67.7
  cerebral or cerebrospinal I67.7
  deformans — *see* Arteriosclerosis
  embolic — *see* Embolism
  obliterans — *see also* Arteriosclerosis
    pulmonary I28.8
  pulmonary I28.8
  retina — *see* Vasculitis, retina
  senile — *see* Arteriosclerosis
  syphilitic A52.09
    brain or cerebral A52.04
    congenital A50.54 [I79.8]
  tuberculous A18.89
Endemic — *see* condition
Endocarditis (chronic) (marantic) (nonbacterial) (thrombotic) (valvular) I38
  with rheumatic fever (conditions in I00)
    active — *see* Endocarditis, acute, rheumatic
    inactive or quiescent (with chorea) I09.1
  acute or subacute I33.9
    infective I33.0
    rheumatic (aortic) (mitral) (pulmonary) (tricuspid) I01.1
      with chorea (acute) (rheumatic) (Sydenham's) I02.0
  aortic (heart) (nonrheumatic) (valve) I35.8
    with
      mitral disease I08.0
        with tricuspid (valve) disease I08.3

Endocarditis — *continued*
  aortic — *continued*
    with — *continued*
      mitral disease — *continued*
        active or acute I01.1
          with chorea (acute) (rheumatic) (Sydenham's) I02.0
      rheumatic fever (conditions in I00)
        active — *see* Endocarditis, acute, rheumatic
        inactive or quiescent (with chorea) I06.9
      tricuspid (valve) disease I08.2
        with mitral (valve) disease I08.3
    acute or subacute I33.9
    arteriosclerotic I35.8
    rheumatic I06.9
      with mitral disease I08.0
        with tricuspid (valve) disease I08.3
        active or acute I01.1
          with chorea (acute) (rheumatic) (Sydenham's) I02.0
      active or acute I01.1
        with chorea (acute) (rheumatic) (Sydenham's) I02.0
      specified NEC I06.8
    specified cause NEC I35.8
    syphilitic A52.03
  arteriosclerotic I38
  atypical verrucous (Libman-Sacks) M32.11
  bacterial (acute) (any valve) (subacute) I33.0
  candidal B37.6
  congenital Q24.8
  constrictive I33.0
  Coxiella burnetii A78 [I39]
  Coxsackie B33.21
  due to
    prosthetic cardiac valve T82.6 ☑
    Q fever A78 [I39]
    Serratia marcescens I33.0
    typhoid (fever) A01.02
  gonococcal A54.83
  infectious or infective (acute) (any valve) (subacute) I33.0
  lenta (acute) (any valve) (subacute) I33.0
  Libman-Sacks M32.11
  listerial A32.82
  Loffler's I42.3
  malignant (acute) (any valve) (subacute) I33.0
  meningococcal A39.51
  mitral (chronic) (double) (fibroid) (heart) (inactive) (valve) (with chorea) I05.9
    with
      aortic (valve) disease I08.0
        with tricuspid (valve) disease I08.3
        active or acute I01.1
          with chorea (acute) (rheumatic) (Sydenham's) I02.0
      rheumatic fever (conditions in I00)
        active — *see* Endocarditis, acute, rheumatic
        inactive or quiescent (with chorea) I05.9
      tricuspid (valve) disease I08.1
        with aortic (valve) disease I08.3
    active or acute I01.1
      with chorea (acute) (rheumatic) (Sydenham's) I02.0
    bacterial I33.0
    arteriosclerotic I34.89
    nonrheumatic I34.89
      acute or subacute I33.9
    specified NEC I05.8
  monilial B37.6
  multiple valves I08.9
    specified disorders I08.8
  mycotic (acute) (any valve) (subacute) I33.0
  pneumococcal (acute) (any valve) (subacute) I33.0
  pulmonary (chronic) (heart) (valve) I37.8
    with rheumatic fever (conditions in I00)
      active — *see* Endocarditis, acute, rheumatic
      inactive or quiescent (with chorea) I09.89
        with aortic, mitral or tricuspid disease I08.8
    acute or subacute I33.9
      rheumatic I01.1
        with chorea (acute) (rheumatic) (Sydenham's) I02.0
    arteriosclerotic I37.8
    congenital Q22.2
    rheumatic (chronic) (inactive) (with chorea) I09.89
      active or acute I01.1
        with chorea (acute) (rheumatic) (Sydenham's) I02.0
    syphilitic A52.03
  purulent (acute) (any valve) (subacute) I33.0

Endocarditis — *continued*
  Q fever A78 [I39]
  rheumatic (chronic) (inactive) (with chorea) I09.1
    active or acute (aortic) (mitral) (pulmonary) (tricuspid) I01.1
      with chorea (acute) (rheumatic) (Sydenham's) I02.0
  rheumatoid — *see* Rheumatoid, carditis
  septic (acute) (any valve) (subacute) I33.0
  streptococcal (acute) (any valve) (subacute) I33.0
  subacute — *see* Endocarditis, acute
  suppurative (acute) (any valve) (subacute) I33.0
  syphilitic A52.03
  toxic I33.9
  tricuspid (chronic) (heart) (inactive) (rheumatic) (valve) (with chorea) I07.9
    with
      aortic (valve) disease I08.2
        mitral (valve) disease I08.3
      mitral (valve) disease I08.1
        aortic (valve) disease I08.3
      rheumatic fever (conditions in I00)
        active — *see* Endocarditis, acute, rheumatic
        inactive or quiescent (with chorea) I07.8
    active or acute I01.1
      with chorea (acute) (rheumatic) (Sydenham's) I02.0
    arteriosclerotic I36.8
    nonrheumatic I36.8
      acute or subacute I33.9
    specified cause, except rheumatic I36.8
  tuberculous — *see* Tuberculosis, endocarditis
  typhoid A01.02
  ulcerative (acute) (any valve) (subacute) I33.0
  vegetative (acute) (any valve) (subacute) I33.0
  verrucous (atypical) (nonbacterial) (nonrheumatic) M32.11
Endocardium, endocardial — *see also* condition
  cushion defect Q21.20
Endocervicitis — *see also* Cervicitis
  due to intrauterine (contraceptive) device T83.69 ☑
  hyperplastic N72
Endocrine — *see* condition
Endocrinopathy, pluriglandular E31.9
Endodontic
  overfill M27.52
  underfill M27.53
Endodontitis K04.01
  irreversible K04.02
  reversible K04.01
Endomastoiditis — *see* Mastoiditis
Endometrioma N80.12- ☑
Endometriosis N80.9
  abdomen, abdominal N80.C0
    specified site, NEC N80.C9
    wall N80.C19
      fascia and muscular layers N80.C11
      subcutaneous tissue N80.C10
      unspecified depth N80.C19
  appendix N80.549
    deep N80.542
    superficial N80.541
  bladder (unspecified depth) N80.A0
    deep N80.A2
    superficial N80.A1
  bowel N80.50
  broad ligament N80.3C ☑
  cardiothoracic space N80.B6
  cecum N80.539
    deep N80.532
    superficial N80.531
  cervix N80.0- ☑
  colon N80.559
    descending N80.559
      deep N80.552
      superficial N80.551
    sigmoid N80.529
      deep N80.522
      superficial N80.521
    transverse N80.559
      deep N80.552
      superficial N80.551
  cul-de-sac (Douglas')
    anterior (unspecified depth) N80.319
      deep N80.312
      superficial N80.311
    posterior (unspecified depth) N80.329
      deep N80.322
      superficial N80.321

Endometriosis — *continued*
  deep
    involving muscular wall of fallopian tube N80.22 ☑
    retrocervical N80.02
  diaphragm N80.B39
    deep N80.B32
    superficial N80.B31
    unspecified depth N80.B39
  exocervix N80.01
  extra-pelvic abdominal peritoneum N80.C4
  fallopian tube (unspecified depth) N80.20- ☑
    deep N80.22- ☑
    superficial N80.21- ☑
  female genital organ NEC N80.8
  gallbladder N80.8
  in scar of skin N80.6
  inguinal canal N80.C3
  internal N80.02
  intestine N80.50
    small N80.569
      deep (multifocal) N80.562
      superficial N80.561
  lung N80.B2
  mediastinal space N80.B5
  myometrium N80.03
  nerve
    femoral N80.D6
    obturator N80.D3
    pelvic N80.D0
      splanchnic N80.D1
    pudendal N80.D5
    retroperitoneum, NEC N80.D9
    sacral splanchnic N80.D1
    sciatic N80.D4
    specified, NEC N80.D9
  ovary (unspecified depth) N80.10- ☑
    deep N80.12- ☑
    superficial N80.11- ☑
  parametrium N80.399
  pelvic
    brim N80.38- ☑
      deep N80.37- ☑
      superficial N80.36- ☑
    peritoneum N80.30
      specified sites, NEC N80.399
        deep N80.392
        superficial N80.391
    sidewall N80.35- ☑
      deep N80.34- ☑
      superficial N80.33- ☑
  pericardial space N80.B4
  peritoneal (pelvic) N80.30
  pleura N80.B1
  rectovaginal septum N80.40
    with involvement of vagina N80.42
    without involvement of vagina N80.41
  rectum N80.519
    deep (multifocal) N80.512
    superficial N80.511
  retroperitoneum N80.30
  round ligament N80.3C9
  sacral nerve roots N80.D2
  skin (scar) N80.6
  specified site NEC N80.8
  stromal D39.0
  thorax N80.B- ☑
  umbilicus N80.C2
  ureter N80.A69
    deep N80.A5- ☑
    extrinsic N80.A4- ☑
    intrinsic N80.A5- ☑
    superficial N80.A4- ☑
    unspecified depth N80.A6- ☑
  uterosacral ligament(s) N80.3C- ☑
    deep N80.3B- ☑
    superficial N80.3A- ☑
  uterus N80.00
    deep N80.02
    internal N80.02
    superficial N80.01
  vagina N80.42
  vulva N80.8
Endometritis (decidual) (nonspecific) (purulent) (senile) (atrophic) (suppurative) N71.9
  with ectopic pregnancy O08.0
  acute N71.0
  blennorrhagic (gonococcal) (acute) (chronic) A54.24

Endometritis — *continued*
  cervix, cervical (with erosion or ectropion) — *see also* Cervicitis
    hyperplastic N72
  chlamydial A56.11
  chronic N71.1
  following
    abortion — *see* Abortion by type complicated by genital infection
    ectopic or molar pregnancy O08.0
  gonococcal, gonorrheal (acute) (chronic) A54.24
  hyperplastic — *see also* Hyperplasia, endometrial N85.00
    cervix N72
  puerperal, postpartum, childbirth O86.12
  subacute N71.9
  tuberculous A18.17
Endometrium — *see* condition
Endomyocardiopathy, South African I42.3
Endomyocarditis — *see* Endocarditis
Endomyofibrosis I42.3
Endomyometritis — *see* Endometritis
Endopericarditis — *see* Endocarditis
Endoperineuritis — *see* Disorder, nerve
Endophlebitis — *see* Phlebitis
Endophthalmia — *see* Endophthalmitis, purulent
Endophthalmitis (acute) (infective) (metastatic) (subacute) H44.009
  bleb associated — *see also* Bleb, inflamed (infected), postprocedural H59.4 ☑
  gonorrheal A54.39
  in (due to)
    cysticercosis B69.1
    onchocerciasis B73.01
    toxocariasis B83.0
  panuveitis — *see* Panuveitis
  parasitic H44.12- ☑
  purulent H44.00- ☑
    panophthalmitis — *see* Panophthalmitis
    vitreous abscess H44.02- ☑
  specified NEC H44.19
  sympathetic — *see* Uveitis, sympathetic
Endosalpingioma D28.2
Endosalpingiosis N94.89
Endosteitis — *see* Osteomyelitis
Endothelioma, bone — *see* Neoplasm, bone, malignant
Endotheliosis (hemorrhagic infectional) D69.8
Endotoxemia — code to condition
Endotrachelitis — *see* Cervicitis
Engelmann (-Camurati) **syndrome** Q78.3
English disease — *see* Rickets
Engman's disease L30.3
Engorgement
  breast N64.59
    newborn P83.4
    puerperal, postpartum O92.79
  lung (passive) — *see* Edema, lung
  pulmonary (passive) — *see* Edema, lung
  stomach K31.89
  venous, retina — *see* Occlusion, retina, vein, engorgement
Enlargement, enlarged — *see also* Hypertrophy
  adenoids J35.2
    with tonsils J35.3
  alveolar ridge K08.89
    congenital — *see* Anomaly, alveolar
  apertures of diaphragm (congenital) Q79.1
  gingival K06.1
  heart, cardiac — *see* Hypertrophy, cardiac
  labium majus, childhood asymmetric (CALME) N90.61
  lacrimal gland, chronic H04.03- ☑
  liver — *see* Hypertrophy, liver
  lymph gland or node R59.9
    generalized R59.1
    localized R59.0
  orbit H05.34- ☑
  organ or site, congenital NEC — *see* Anomaly, by site
  parathyroid (gland) E21.0
  pituitary fossa R93.0
  prostate N40.0
    with lower urinary tract symptoms (LUTS) N40.1
      nodular N40.3
    nodular N40.2
      with lower urinary tract symptoms (LUTS) N40.3
    without lower urinary tract symptoms (LUTS) N40.0
      nodular N40.2
  sella turcica R93.0
  spleen — *see* Splenomegaly
  thymus (gland) (congenital) E32.0

Enlargement, enlarged — *continued*
  thyroid (gland) — *see* Goiter
  tongue K14.8
  tonsils J35.1
    with adenoids J35.3
  uterus N85.2
  vestibular aqueduct Q16.5
Enophthalmos H05.40- ☑
  due to
    orbital tissue atrophy H05.41- ☑
    trauma or surgery H05.42- ☑
Enostosis M27.8
Entamebic, entamebiasis — *see* Amebiasis
Entanglement
  umbilical cord(s) O69.82 ☑
    with compression O69.2 ☑
    around neck
      with compression O69.1 ☑
      without compression O69.81 ☑
    of twins in monoamniotic sac O69.2 ☑
    other, with compression O69.2 ☑
    other, without compression O69.82 ☑
    without compression O69.82 ☑
Enteralgia — *see* Pain, abdominal
Enteric — *see* condition
Enteritis (acute) (diarrheal) (hemorrhagic) (noninfective) K52.9
  adenovirus A08.2
  aertrycke infection A02.0
  allergic K52.29
    with
      eosinophilic gastritis or gastroenteritis K52.81
      food protein-induced enterocolitis syndrome K52.21
      food protein-induced enteropathy K52.22
      FPIES K52.21
  amebic (acute) A06.0
    with abscess — *see* Abscess, amebic
    chronic A06.1
      with abscess — *see* Abscess, amebic
      nondysenteric A06.2
    nondysenteric A06.2
  astrovirus A08.32
  bacillary NOS A03.9
  bacterial A04.9
    specified NEC A04.8
  calicivirus A08.31
  candidal B37.82
  Chilomastix A07.8
  choleriformis A00.1
  chronic (noninfectious) K52.9
    ulcerative — *see* Colitis, ulcerative
  cicatrizing (chronic) — *see* Enteritis, regional, small intestine
  Clostridioides difficile
    not specified as recurrent A04.72
    recurrent A04.71
  Clostridium
    botulinum (food poisoning) A05.1
    difficile
      not specified as recurrent A04.72
      recurrent A04.71
  coccidial A07.3
  coxsackie virus A08.39
  dietetic — *see also* Enteritis, allergic K52.29
  drug-induced K52.1
  due to
    astrovirus A08.32
    calicivirus A08.31
    coxsackie virus A08.39
    drugs K52.1
    echovirus A08.39
    enterovirus NEC A08.39
    food hypersensitivity — *see also* Enteritis, allergic K52.29
    infectious organism (bacterial) (viral) — *see* Enteritis, infectious
    torovirus A08.39
    Yersinia enterocolitica A04.6
  echovirus A08.39
  eltor A00.1
  enterovirus NEC A08.39
  eosinophilic K52.81
  epidemic (infectious) A09
  fulminant — *see also* Ischemia, intestine, acute K55.019
  gangrenous — *see* Enteritis, infectious
  giardial A07.1
  infectious NOS A09

Enteritis — *continued*
  infectious — *continued*
    due to
      adenovirus A08.2
      Aerobacter aerogenes A04.8
      Arizona (bacillus) A02.0
      bacteria NOS A04.9
        specified NEC A04.8
      Campylobacter A04.5
      Clostridioides difficile
        not specified as recurrent A04.72
        recurrent A04.71
      Clostridium difficile
        not specified as recurrent A04.72
        recurrent A04.71
      Clostridium perfringens A04.8
      Enterobacter aerogenes A04.8
      enterovirus A08.39
      Escherichia coli A04.4
        enteroaggregative A04.4
        enterohemorrhagic A04.3
        enteroinvasive A04.2
        enteropathogenic A04.0
        enterotoxigenic A04.1
        specified NEC A04.4
      specified
        bacteria NEC A04.8
        virus NEC A08.39
      Staphylococcus A04.8
      virus NEC A08.4
        specified type NEC A08.39
      Yersinia enterocolitica A04.6
    specified organism NEC A08.8
  influenzal — *see* Influenza, with, digestive manifestations
  ischemic K55.9
    acute — *see also* Ischemia, intestine, acute K55.019
    chronic K55.1
  microsporidial A07.8
  mucomembranous, myxomembranous — *see* Syndrome, irritable bowel
  mucous — *see* Syndrome, irritable bowel
  necroticans A05.2
  necrotizing of newborn — *see* Enterocolitis, necrotizing, in newborn
  neurogenic — *see* Syndrome, irritable bowel
  newborn necrotizing — *see* Enterocolitis, necrotizing, in newborn
  noninfectious K52.9
  norovirus A08.11
  parasitic NEC B82.9
  paratyphoid (fever) — *see* Fever, paratyphoid
  protozoal A07.9
    specified NEC A07.8
  radiation K52.0
  regional (of) K50.90
    with
      complication K50.919
        abscess K50.914
        fistula K50.913
        intestinal obstruction K50.912
        rectal bleeding K50.911
        specified complication NEC K50.918
    colon — *see* Enteritis, regional, large intestine
    duodenum — *see* Enteritis, regional, small intestine
    ileum — *see* Enteritis, regional, small intestine
    jejunum — *see* Enteritis, regional, small intestine
    large bowel — *see* Enteritis, regional, large intestine
    large intestine (colon) (rectum) K50.10
      with
        complication K50.119
          abscess K50.114
          fistula K50.113
          intestinal obstruction K50.112
          rectal bleeding K50.111
          small intestine (duodenum) (ileum) (jejunum) involvement K50.80
            with
              complication K50.819
                abscess K50.814
                fistula K50.813
                intestinal obstruction K50.812
                rectal bleeding K50.811
                specified complication NEC K50.818
        specified complication NEC K50.118
    rectum — *see* Enteritis, regional, large intestine
    small intestine (duodenum) (ileum) (jejunum) K50.00
      with
        complication K50.019

Enteritis — *continued*
  regional — *continued*
    small intestine — *continued*
      with — *continued*
        complication — *continued*
          abscess K50.014
          fistula K50.013
          intestinal obstruction K50.012
          large intestine (colon) (rectum) involvement K50.80
            with
              complication K50.819
                abscess K50.814
                fistula K50.813
                intestinal obstruction K50.812
                rectal bleeding K50.811
                specified complication NEC K50.818
          rectal bleeding K50.011
          specified complication NEC K50.018
  rotaviral A08.0
  Salmonella, salmonellosis (arizonae) (cholerae-suis) (enteritidis) (typhimurium) A02.0
  segmental — *see* Enteritis, regional
  septic A09
  Shigella — *see* Infection, Shigella
  small round structured NEC A08.19
  spasmodic, spastic — *see* Syndrome, irritable bowel
  staphylococcal A04.8
    due to food A05.0
  torovirus A08.39
  toxic NEC K52.1
    due to
      Clostridioides difficile
        not specified as recurrent A04.72
        recurrent A04.71
      Clostridium difficile
        not specified as recurrent A04.72
        recurrent A04.71
  trichomonal A07.8
  tuberculous A18.32
  typhosa A01.00
  ulcerative (chronic) — *see* Colitis, ulcerative
  viral A08.4
    adenovirus A08.2
    enterovirus A08.39
    Rotavirus A08.0
    small round structured NEC A08.19
    specified NEC A08.39
    virus specified NEC A08.39
Enterobiasis B80
Enterobius vermicularis (infection) (infestation) B80
Enterocele — *see also* Hernia, abdomen
  pelvic, pelvis (acquired) (congenital) N81.5
  vagina, vaginal (acquired) (congenital) NEC N81.5
Enterocolitis — *see also* Enteritis K52.9
  due to
    Clostridioides difficile
      not specified as recurrent A04.72
      recurrent A04.71
    Clostridium difficile
      not specified as recurrent A04.72
      recurrent A04.71
  fulminant ischemic — *see also* Ischemia, intestine, acute K55.059
  granulomatous — *see* Enteritis, regional
  hemorrhagic (acute) — *see also* Ischemia, intestine, acute K55.059
    chronic K55.1
  infectious NEC A09
  ischemic K55.9
  necrotizing K55.30
    with
      perforation K55.33
      pneumatosis K55.32
        and perforation K55.33
    due to
      Clostridioides difficile
        not specified as recurrent A04.72
        recurrent A04.71
      Clostridium difficile
        not specified as recurrent A04.72
        recurrent A04.71
    in non-newborn K55.30
      stage 1 (without pneumatosis, without perforation) K55.31
      stage 2 (with pneumatosis, without perforation) K55.32

Enterocolitis — *continued*
  necrotizing — *continued*
    in non-newborn — *continued*
      stage 3 (with pneumatosis, with perforation) K55.33
    in newborn P77.9
      stage 1 (without pneumatosis, without perforation) P77.1
      stage 2 (with pneumatosis, without perforation) P77.2
      stage 3 (with pneumatosis, with perforation) P77.3
    without pneumatosis or perforation K55.31
  noninfectious K52.9
    newborn — *see* Enterocolitis, necrotizing, in newborn
  pseudomembranous (newborn)
    not specified as recurrent A04.72
    recurrent A04.71
  radiation K52.0
    newborn — *see* Enterocolitis, necrotizing, in newborn
  ulcerative (chronic) — *see* Pancolitis, ulcerative (chronic)
Enterogastritis — *see* Enteritis
Enteropathy K63.9
  celiac-gluten-sensitive K90.0
    non-celiac K90.41
  food protein-induced K52.22
  hemorrhagic, terminal — *see also* Ischemia, intestine, acute K55.059
  protein-losing K90.49
Enteroperitonitis — *see* Peritonitis
Enteroptosis K63.4
Enterorrhagia K92.2
Enterospasm — *see also* Syndrome, irritable, bowel
  psychogenic F45.8
Enterostenosis — *see also* Obstruction, intestine, specified NEC K56.699
Enterostomy
  complication — *see* Complication, enterostomy
  status Z93.4
Enterovirus, as cause of disease classified elsewhere B97.10
  coxsackievirus B97.11
  echovirus B97.12
  other specified B97.19
Enthesopathy (peripheral) M77.9
  Achilles tendinitis — *see* Tendinitis, Achilles
  ankle and tarsus M77.5- ☑
    specified type NEC — *see* Enthesopathy, foot, specified type NEC
  anterior tibial syndrome M76.81- ☑
  calcaneal spur — *see* Spur, bone, calcaneal
  elbow region M77.8
    lateral epicondylitis — *see* Epicondylitis, lateral
    medial epicondylitis — *see* Epicondylitis, medial
  foot NEC M77.8
    metatarsalgia — *see* Metatarsalgia
    specified type NEC M77.5- ☑
  forearm M77.8
  gluteal tendinitis — *see* Tendinitis, gluteal
  hand M77.8
  hip — *see* Enthesopathy, lower limb, specified type NEC
  iliac crest spur — *see* Spur, bone, iliac crest
  iliotibial band syndrome — *see* Syndrome, iliotibial band
  knee — *see* Enthesopathy, lower limb, lower leg, specified type NEC
  lateral epicondylitis — *see* Epicondylitis, lateral
  lower limb (excluding foot) M76.9
    Achilles tendinitis — *see* Tendinitis, Achilles
    ankle and tarsus M77.5- ☑
      specified type NEC — *see* Enthesopathy, foot, specified type NEC
    anterior tibial syndrome M76.81- ☑
    gluteal tendinitis — *see* Tendinitis, gluteal
    iliac crest spur — *see* Spur, bone, iliac crest
    iliotibial band syndrome — *see* Syndrome, iliotibial band
    patellar tendinitis — *see* Tendinitis, patellar
    pelvic region — *see* Enthesopathy, lower limb, specified type NEC
    peroneal tendinitis — *see* Tendinitis, peroneal
    posterior tibial syndrome M76.82- ☑
    psoas tendinitis — *see* Tendinitis, psoas
    specified type NEC M76.89- ☑
    tibial collateral bursitis — *see* Bursitis, tibial collateral
  medial epicondylitis — *see* Epicondylitis, medial
  metatarsalgia — *see* Metatarsalgia
  multiple sites M77.8
  patellar tendinitis — *see* Tendinitis, patellar
  pelvis M77.8

Enthesopathy — *continued*
 periarthritis of wrist — *see* Periarthritis, wrist
 peroneal tendinitis — *see* Tendinitis, peroneal
 posterior tibial syndrome M76.82- ☑
 psoas tendinitis — *see* Tendinitis, psoas
 shoulder M77.8
 shoulder region — *see* Lesion, shoulder
 specified type NEC M77.8
 spinal M46.00
  cervical region M46.02
  cervicothoracic region M46.03
  lumbar region M46.06
  lumbosacral region M46.07
  multiple sites M46.09
  occipito-atlanto-axial region M46.01
  sacrococcygeal region M46.08
  thoracic region M46.04
  thoracolumbar region M46.05
 tibial collateral bursitis — *see* Bursitis, tibial collateral
 upper arm M77.8
 wrist and carpus NEC M77.8
  calcaneal spur — *see* Spur, bone, calcaneal
  periarthritis of wrist — *see* Periarthritis, wrist
Entomophobia F40.218
Entomophthoromycosis B46.8
Entrance, air into vein — *see* Embolism, air
Entrapment
 muscle
  eye
   extraocular H50.68- ☑
   oblique
    inferior H50.62- ☑
    superior H50.66- ☑
   rectus
    inferior H50.63- ☑
    lateral H50.64- ☑
    medial H50.65- ☑
    superior H50.67- ☑
 nerve — *see* Neuropathy, entrapment
Entropion (eyelid) (paralytic) H02.009
 cicatricial H02.019
  left H02.016
   lower H02.015
   upper H02.014
  right H02.013
   lower H02.012
   upper H02.011
 congenital Q10.2
 left H02.006
  lower H02.005
  upper H02.004
 mechanical H02.029
  left H02.026
   lower H02.025
   upper H02.024
  right H02.023
   lower H02.022
   upper H02.021
 right H02.003
  lower H02.002
  upper H02.001
 senile H02.039
  left H02.036
   lower H02.035
   upper H02.034
  right H02.033
   lower H02.032
   upper H02.031
 spastic H02.049
  left H02.046
   lower H02.045
   upper H02.044
  right H02.043
   lower H02.042
   upper H02.041
Enucleated eye (traumatic, current) S05.7- ☑
Enuresis R32
 functional F98.0
 habit disturbance F98.0
 nocturnal N39.44
  psychogenic F98.0
 nonorganic origin F98.0
 psychogenic F98.0
Eosinopenia — *see* Agranulocytosis
Eosinophilia (allergic) (idiopathic) (secondary) D72.10
 with
  angiolymphoid hyperplasia (ALHE) D18.01
 familial D72.19

Eosinophilia — *continued*
 hereditary D72.19
 in disease classified elsewhere D72.18
 infiltrative — *see* Eosinophilia, pulmonary
 Loffler's J82.89
 peritoneal — *see* Peritonitis, eosinophilic
 pulmonary NEC J82.89
  acute J82.82
  asthmatic J82.83
  chronic J82.81
 specified NEC D72.19
 tropical (pulmonary) J82.89
Eosinophilia-myalgia syndrome M35.89
Ependymitis (acute) (cerebral) (chronic) (granular) — *see* Encephalomyelitis
Ependymoblastoma
 specified site — *see* Neoplasm, malignant, by site
 unspecified site C71.9
Ependymoma (epithelial) (malignant)
 anaplastic
  specified site — *see* Neoplasm, malignant, by site
  unspecified site C71.9
 benign
  specified site — *see* Neoplasm, benign, by site
  unspecified site D33.2
 myxopapillary D43.2
  specified site — *see* Neoplasm, uncertain behavior, by site
  unspecified site D43.2
 papillary D43.2
  specified site — *see* Neoplasm, uncertain behavior, by site
  unspecified site D43.2
 specified site — *see* Neoplasm, malignant, by site
 unspecified site C71.9
Ependymopathy G93.89
Ephelis, ephelides L81.2
Epiblepharon (congenital) Q10.3
Epicanthus, epicanthic fold (eyelid) (congenital) Q10.3
Epicondylitis (elbow)
 lateral M77.1- ☑
 medial M77.0- ☑
Epicystitis — *see* Cystitis
Epidemic — *see* condition
Epidermidalization, cervix — *see* Dysplasia, cervix
Epidermis, epidermal — *see* condition
Epidermodysplasia verruciformis B07.8
Epidermolysis
 bullosa (congenital) Q81.9
  acquired L12.30
   drug-induced L12.31
   specified cause NEC L12.35
  dystrophica Q81.2
  letalis Q81.1
  simplex Q81.0
  specified NEC Q81.8
 necroticans combustiformis L51.2
  due to drug — *see* Table of Drugs and Chemicals, by drug
Epidermophytid — *see* Dermatophytosis
Epidermophytosis (infected) — *see* Dermatophytosis
Epididymis — *see* condition
Epididymitis (acute) (nonvenereal) (recurrent) (residual) N45.1
 with orchitis N45.3
 blennorrhagic (gonococcal) A54.23
 caseous (tuberculous) A18.15
 chlamydial A56.19
 filarial — *see also* Infestation, filarial B74.9 *[N51]*
 gonococcal A54.23
 syphilitic A52.76
 tuberculous A18.15
Epididymo-orchitis — *see also* Epididymitis N45.3
Epidural — *see* condition
Epigastrium, epigastric — *see* condition
Epigastrocele — *see* Hernia, ventral
Epiglottis — *see* condition
Epiglottitis, epiglottiditis (acute) J05.10
 with obstruction J05.11
 chronic J37.0
Epignathus Q89.4
Epilepsia partialis continua — *see also* Kozhevnikof's epilepsy G40.1- ☑

Epilepsy, epileptic, epilepsia (attack) (cerebral) (convulsion) (fit) (seizure) G40.909

> *Note: the following terms are to be considered equivalent to intractable: pharmacoresistant (pharmacologically resistant), treatment resistant, refractory (medically) and poorly controlled*

 with
  complex partial seizures — *see* Epilepsy, localization-related, symptomatic, with complex partial seizures
  grand mal seizures on awakening — *see* Epilepsy, generalized, specified NEC
  myoclonic absences — *see* Epilepsy, generalized, specified NEC
  myoclonic-astatic seizures — *see* Epilepsy, generalized, specified NEC
  simple partial seizures — *see* Epilepsy, localization-related, symptomatic, with simple partial seizures
 akinetic — *see* Epilepsy, generalized, specified NEC
 benign childhood with centrotemporal EEG spikes — *see* Epilepsy, localization-related, idiopathic
 benign myoclonic in infancy G40.80- ☑
 Bravais-jacksonian — *see* Epilepsy, localization-related, symptomatic, with simple partial seizures
 childhood
  with occipital EEG paroxysms — *see* Epilepsy, localization-related, idiopathic
  absence G40.A09 (*following* G40.3)
   intractable G40.A19 (*following* G40.3)
    with status epilepticus G40.A11 (*following* G40.3)
    without status epilepticus G40.A19 (*following* G40.3)
   not intractable G40.A09 (*following* G40.3)
    with status epilepticus G40.A01 (*following* G40.3)
    without status epilepticus G40.A09 (*following* G40.3)
 climacteric — *see* Epilepsy, specified NEC
 cysticercosis B69.0
 deterioration (mental) F06.8
 due to syphilis A52.19
 focal — *see* Epilepsy, localization-related, symptomatic, with simple partial seizures
 generalized
  idiopathic G40.309
   intractable G40.319
    with status epilepticus G40.311
    without status epilepticus G40.319
   not intractable G40.309
    with status epilepticus G40.301
    without status epilepticus G40.309
  specified NEC G40.409
   intractable G40.419
    with status epilepticus G40.411
    without status epilepticus G40.419
   not intractable G40.409
    with status epilepticus G40.401
    without status epilepticus G40.409
 impulsive petit mal — *see* Epilepsy, juvenile myoclonic
 intractable G40.919
  with status epilepticus G40.911
  without status epilepticus G40.919
 juvenile absence G40.A09 (*following* G40.3)
  intractable G40.A19 (*following* G40.3)
   with status epilepticus G40.A11 (*following* G40.3)
   without status epilepticus G40.A19 (*following* G40.3)
  not intractable G40.A09 (*following* G40.3)
   with status epilepticus G40.A01 (*following* G40.3)
   without status epilepticus G40.A09 (*following* G40.3)
 juvenile myoclonic G40.B09 (*following* G40.3)
  intractable G40.B19 (*following* G40.3)
   with status epilepticus G40.B11 (*following* G40.3)
   without status epilepticus G40.B19 (*following* G40.3)
  not intractable G40.B09 (*following* G40.3)
   with status epilepticus G40.B01 (*following* G40.3)
   without status epilepticus G40.B09 (*following* G40.3)
 KCNQ2-related G40.842
  intractable G40.844
   with status epilepticus G40.843
   without status epilepticus G40.844
  not intractable G40.842
   with status epilepticus G40.841

Epilepsy, epileptic, epilepsia — *continued*
  KCNQ2-related — *continued*
    not intractable — *continued*
      without status epilepticus G40.842
  Lafora progressive myoclonus — *see also* Epilepsy, progressive, Lafora G40.C09
  localization-related (focal) (partial)
    idiopathic G40.009
      with seizures of localized onset G40.009
        intractable G40.019
          with status epilepticus G40.011
          without status epilepticus G40.019
        not intractable G40.009
          with status epilepticus G40.001
          without status epilepticus G40.009
    symptomatic
      with complex partial seizures G40.209
        intractable G40.219
          with status epilepticus G40.211
          without status epilepticus G40.219
        not intractable G40.209
          with status epilepticus G40.201
          without status epilepticus G40.209
      with simple partial seizures G40.109
        intractable G40.119
          with status epilepticus G40.111
          without status epilepticus G40.119
        not intractable G40.109
          with status epilepticus G40.101
          without status epilepticus G40.109
  myoclonus, myoclonic — *see also* Epilepsy, generalized, specified NEC
    progressive — *see also* Epilepsy, generalized, idiopathic
    Lafora G40.C09
      intractable G40.C19
        with status epilepticus G40.C11
        without status epilepticus G40.C19
      not intractable G40.C09
        with status epilepticus G40.C01
        without status epilepticus G40.C09
    type 1 — *see* Epilepsy, generalized, idiopathic
    type 2 — *see* Epilepsy, myoclonus, progressive, Lafora
  severe, in infancy (SMEI) G40.83- ☑
  not intractable G40.909
    with status epilepticus G40.901
    without status epilepticus G40.909
  on awakening — *see* Epilepsy, generalized, specified NEC
  parasitic NOS B71.9 *[G94]*
  partial — *see* Epilepsy, localization-related, symptomatic, with simple partial seizures
  partialis continua — *see also* Kozhevnikof's epilepsy G40.1- ☑
  peripheral — *see* Epilepsy, specified NEC
  polymorphic, in infancy (PMEI) G40.83- ☑
  procursiva — *see* Epilepsy, localization-related, symptomatic, with simple partial seizures
  progressive (familial) myoclonic — *see* Epilepsy, myoclonus, progressive
    Lafora — *see also* Epilepsy, progressive, Lafora G40.C09
  reflex — *see* Epilepsy, specified NEC
  related to
    alcohol G40.509
      not intractable G40.509
        with status epilepticus G40.501
        without status epliepticus G40.509
    drugs G40.509
      not intractable G40.509
        with status epilepticus G40.501
        without status epliepticus G40.509
    external causes G40.509
      not intractable G40.509
        with status epilepticus G40.501
        without status epliepticus G40.509
    hormonal changes G40.509
      not intractable G40.509
        with status epilepticus G40.501
        without status epliepticus G40.509
    sleep deprivation G40.509
      not intractable G40.509
        with status epilepticus G40.501
        without status epliepticus G40.509
    stress G40.509
      not intractable G40.509
        with status epilepticus G40.501
        without status epliepticus G40.509

Epilepsy, epileptic, epilepsia — *continued*
  somatomotor — *see* Epilepsy, localization-related, symptomatic, with simple partial seizures
  somatosensory — *see* Epilepsy, localization-related, symptomatic, with simple partial seizures
  spasms G40.822
    intractable G40.824
      with status epilepticus G40.823
      without status epilepticus G40.824
    not intractable G40.822
      with status epilepticus G40.821
      without status epilepticus G40.822
  specified NEC G40.802
    intractable G40.804
      with status epilepticus G40.803
      without status epilepticus G40.804
    not intractable G40.802
      with status epilepticus G40.801
      without status epilepticus G40.802
  syndromes
    generalized
      idiopathic G40.309
        intractable G40.319
          with status epilepticus G40.311
          without status epilepticus G40.319
        not intractable G40.309
          with status epilepticus G40.301
          without status epilepticus G40.309
      specified NEC G40.409
        intractable G40.419
          with status epilepticus G40.411
          without status epilepticus G40.419
        not intractable G40.409
          with status epilepticus G40.401
          without status epilepticus G40.409
    localization-related (focal) (partial)
      idiopathic G40.009
        with seizures of localized onset G40.009
          intractable G40.019
            with status epilepticus G40.011
            without status epilepticus G40.019
          not intractable G40.009
            with status epilepticus G40.001
            without status epilepticus G40.009
      symptomatic
        with complex partial seizures G40.209
          intractable G40.219
            with status epilepticus G40.211
            without status epilepticus G40.219
          not intractable G40.209
            with status epilepticus G40.201
            without status epilepticus G40.209
        with simple partial seizures G40.109
          intractable G40.119
            with status epilepticus G40.111
            without status epilepticus G40.119
          not intractable G40.109
            with status epilepticus G40.101
            without status epilepticus G40.109
    specified NEC G40.802
      intractable G40.804
        with status epilepticus G40.803
        without status epilepticus G40.804
      not intractable G40.802
        with status epilepticus G40.801
        without status epilepticus G40.802
  tonic (-clonic) — *see* Epilepsy, generalized, specified NEC
  twilight F05
  uncinate (gyrus) — *see* Epilepsy, localization-related, symptomatic, with complex partial seizures
  Unverricht (-Lundborg) (familial myoclonic) — *see* Epilepsy, generalized, idiopathic
  visceral — *see* Epilepsy, specified NEC
  visual — *see* Epilepsy, specified NEC
Epiloia Q85.1
Epimenorrhea N92.0
Epipharyngitis — *see* Nasopharyngitis
Epiphora H04.20- ☑
  due to
    excess lacrimation H04.21- ☑
    insufficient drainage H04.22- ☑
Epiphyseal arrest — *see* Arrest, epiphyseal
Epiphyseolysis, epiphysiolysis — *see* Osteochondropathy
Epiphysitis — *see also* Osteochondropathy
  juvenile M92.9
  syphilitic (congenital) A50.02
Epiplocele — *see* Hernia, abdomen
Epiploitis — *see* Peritonitis
Epiplosarcomphalocele — *see* Hernia, umbilicus

Episcleritis (suppurative) H15.10- ☑
  in (due to)
    syphilis A52.71
    tuberculosis A18.51
  nodular H15.12- ☑
  periodica fugax H15.11- ☑
    angioneurotic — *see* Edema, angioneurotic
  syphilitic (late) A52.71
  tuberculous A18.51
Episode
  affective, mixed F39
  depersonalization (in neurotic state) F48.1
  depressive F32.A
    major F32.9
      mild F32.0
      moderate F32.1
      severe (without psychotic symptoms) F32.2
        with psychotic symptoms F32.3
    recurrent F33.9
      brief F33.8
    specified NEC F32.89
  hypomanic F30.8
  manic F30.9
    with
      psychotic symptoms F30.2
      remission (full) F30.4
        partial F30.3
    other specified F30.8
    recurrent F31.89
    without psychotic symptoms F30.10
      mild F30.11
      moderate F30.12
      severe (without psychotic symptoms) F30.13
        with psychotic symptoms F30.2
  psychotic F23
    organic F06.8
  schizophrenic (acute) NEC, brief F23
Epispadias (female) (male) Q64.0
Episplenitis D73.89
Epistaxis (multiple) R04.0
  hereditary I78.0
  vicarious menstruation N94.89
Epithelioma (malignant) — *see also* Neoplasm, malignant, by site
  adenoides cysticum — *see* Neoplasm, skin, benign
  basal cell — *see* Neoplasm, skin, malignant
  benign — *see* Neoplasm, benign, by site
  Bowen's — *see* Neoplasm, skin, in situ
  calcifying, of Malherbe — *see* Neoplasm, skin, benign
  external site — *see* Neoplasm, skin, malignant
  intraepidermal, Jadassohn — *see* Neoplasm, skin, benign
  squamous cell — *see* Neoplasm, malignant, by site
Epitheliomatosis pigmented Q82.1
Epitheliopathy, multifocal placoid pigment H30.14- ☑
Epithelium, epithelial — *see* condition
Epituberculosis (with atelectasis) (allergic) A15.7
Eponychia Q84.6
Epstein's
  nephrosis or syndrome — *see* Nephrosis
  pearl K09.8
Epulis (gingiva) (fibrous) (giant cell) K06.8
Equinia A24.0
Equinovarus (congenital) (talipes) Q66.0- ☑
  acquired — *see* Deformity, limb, clubfoot
Equivalent
  convulsive (abdominal) — *see* Epilepsy, specified NEC
  epileptic (psychic) — *see* Epilepsy, localization-related, symptomatic, with complex partial seizures
Erb (-Duchenne) **paralysis** (birth injury) (newborn) P14.0
Erb-Goldflam disease or syndrome G70.00
  with exacerbation (acute) G70.01
  in crisis G70.01
Erb's
  disease G71.02
  palsy, paralysis (brachial) (birth) (newborn) P14.0
    spinal (spastic) syphilitic A52.17
  pseudohypertrophic muscular dystrophy G71.02
Erdheim's syndrome (acromegalic macrospondylitis) E22.0
Erection, painful (persistent) — *see* Priapism
Ergosterol deficiency (vitamin D) E55.9
  with
    adult osteomalacia M83.8
    rickets — *see* Rickets
Ergotism — *see also* Poisoning, food, noxious, plant
  from ergot used as drug (migraine therapy) — *see* Table of Drugs and Chemicals
Erosio interdigitalis blastomycetica B37.2

Erosion
- artery I77.2
  - without rupture I77.89
- bone — *see* Disorder, bone, density and structure, specified NEC
- bronchus J98.09
- cameron — *see* Ulcer, stomach
- cartilage (joint) — *see* Disorder, cartilage, specified type NEC
- cervix (uteri) (acquired) (chronic) (congenital) N86
  - with cervicitis N72
- cornea (nontraumatic) — *see* Ulcer, cornea
  - recurrent H18.83- ☑
  - traumatic — *see* Abrasion, cornea
- dental (idiopathic) (occupational) (due to diet, drugs or vomiting) K03.2
- duodenum, postpyloric — *see* Ulcer, duodenum
- esophagus K22.10
  - with bleeding K22.11
- gastric — *see* Ulcer, stomach
- gastrojejunal — *see* Ulcer, gastrojejunal
- implanted mesh — *see* Complications, prosthetic device or implant, mesh
- intestine K63.3
- lymphatic vessel I89.8
- pylorus, pyloric (ulcer) — *see* Ulcer, stomach
- spine, aneurysmal A52.09
- stomach — *see* Ulcer, stomach
- subcutaneous device pocket
  - nervous system prosthetic device, implant, or graft T85.890 ☑
  - other internal prosthetic device, implant, or graft T85.898 ☑
- teeth (idiopathic) (occupational) (due to diet, drugs or vomiting) K03.2
- urethra N36.8
- uterus N85.8
Erotomania F52.8
Error
- metabolism, inborn — *see* Disorder, metabolism
- refractive — *see* Disorder, refraction
Eructation R14.2
- nervous or psychogenic F45.8
Eruption
- creeping B76.9
- drug (generalized) (taken internally) L27.0
  - fixed L27.1
  - in contact with skin — *see* Dermatitis, due to drugs
  - localized L27.1
- Hutchinson, summer L56.4
- Kaposi's varicelliform B00.0
- napkin L22
- polymorphous light (sun) L56.4
- recalcitrant pustular L13.8
- ringed R23.8
- skin (nonspecific) R21
  - creeping (meaning hookworm) B76.9
  - due to inoculation/vaccination (generalized) — *see also* Dermatitis, due to, vaccine L27.0
    - localized L27.1
  - erysipeloid A26.0
  - feigned L98.1
  - Kaposi's varicelliform B00.0
  - lichenoid L28.0
  - meaning dermatitis — *see* Dermatitis
  - toxic NEC L53.0
- tooth, teeth, abnormal (incomplete) (late) (premature) (sequence) K00.6
- vesicular R23.8
Erysipelas (gangrenous) (infantile) (newborn) (phlegmonous) (suppurative) A46
- external ear A46 *[H62.40]*
- puerperal, postpartum O86.89
Erysipeloid A26.9
- cutaneous (Rosenbach's) A26.0
- disseminated A26.8
- sepsis A26.7
- specified NEC A26.8
Erythema, erythematous (infectional) (inflammation) L53.9
- ab igne L59.0
- annulare (centrifugum) (rheumaticum) L53.1
- arthriticum epidemicum A25.1
- brucellum — *see* Brucellosis
- chronic figurate NEC L53.3
- chronicum migrans (Borrelia burgdorferi) A69.20
- diaper L22
- due to
  - chemical NEC L53.0
    - in contact with skin L24.5

Erythema, erythematous — *continued*
- due to — *continued*
  - drug (internal use) — *see* Dermatitis, due to, drugs
- elevatum diutinum L95.1
- endemic E52
- epidemic, arthritic A25.1
- figuratum perstans L53.3
- gluteal L22
- heat — *code by site under* Burn, first degree
- ichthyosiforme congenitum bullous Q80.3
- in diseases classified elsewhere L54
- induratum (nontuberculous) L52
  - tuberculous A18.4
- infectiosum B08.3
- intertrigo L30.4
- iris L51.9
- marginatum L53.2
  - in (due to) acute rheumatic fever I00
- medicamentosum — *see* Dermatitis, due to, drugs
- migrans A26.0
  - chronicum A69.20
  - tongue K14.1
- multiforme (major) (minor) L51.9
  - bullous, bullosum L51.1
  - conjunctiva L51.1
  - nonbullous L51.0
  - pemphigoides L12.0
  - specified NEC L51.8
- napkin L22
- neonatorum P83.88
  - toxic P83.1
- nodosum L52
  - tuberculous A18.4
- palmar L53.8
- pernio T69.1 ☑
- rash, newborn P83.88
- scarlatiniform (recurrent) (exfoliative) L53.8
- solare L55.0
- specified NEC L53.8
- toxic, toxicum NEC L53.0
  - newborn P83.1
- tuberculous (primary) A18.4
Erythematous, erythematosus — *see* condition
Erythermalgia (primary) I73.81
Erythralgia I73.81
Erythrasma L08.1
Erythredema (polyneuropathy) — *see* Poisoning, mercury
Erythremia (acute) C94.0- ☑
- chronic D45
- secondary D75.1
Erythroblastopenia — *see also* Aplasia, red cell D60.9
- congenital D61.01
Erythroblastophthisis D61.09
Erythroblastosis (fetalis) (newborn) P55.9
- due to
  - ABO (antibodies) (incompatibility) (isoimmunization) P55.1
  - Rh (antibodies) (incompatibility) (isoimmunization) P55.0
Erythrocyanosis (crurum) I73.89
Erythrocythemia — *see* Erythremia
Erythrocytosis (megalosplenic) (secondary) D75.1
- familial D75.0
- oval, hereditary — *see* Elliptocytosis
- secondary D75.1
- stress D75.1
Erythroderma (secondary) — *see also* Erythema L53.9
- bullous ichthyosiform, congenital Q80.3
- desquamativum L21.1
- ichthyosiform, congenital (bullous) Q80.3
- neonatorum P83.88
- psoriaticum L40.8
Erythrodysesthesia, palmar plantar (PPE) L27.1
Erythrogenesis imperfecta D61.09
Erythroleukemia C94.0- ☑
Erythromelalgia I73.81
Erythrophagocytosis D75.89
Erythrophobia F40.298
Erythroplakia, oral epithelium, and tongue K13.29
Erythroplasia (Queyrat) D07.4
- specified site — *see* Neoplasm, skin, in situ
- unspecified site D07.4
Escherichia coli (E. coli), **as cause of disease classified elsewhere** B96.89
- non-O157 Shiga toxin-producing (with known O group) B96.22
- non-Shiga toxin-producing B96.29
- O157 B96.21

Escherichia coli (E. coli), **as cause of disease classified elsewhere** — *continued*
- O157 with confirmation of Shiga toxin when H antigen is unknown, or is not H7 B96.21
- O157:H- (nonmotile) with confirmation of Shiga toxin B96.21
- O157:H7 with or without confirmation of Shiga toxin-production B96.21
  - specified NEC B96.22
- Shiga toxin-producing (with unspecified O group) (STEC) B96.23
- specified NEC B96.29
Esophagismus K22.4
Esophagitis (acute) (alkaline) (chemical) (chronic) (infectional) (necrotic) (peptic) (postoperative) (without bleeding) K20.90
- with bleeding K20.91
- candidal B37.81
- due to gastrointestinal reflux disease (without bleeding) K21.00
  - with bleeding K21.01
- eosinophilic K20.0
- reflux K21.00
  - with bleeding K21.01
- specified NEC (without bleeding) K20.80
  - with bleeding K20.81
- tuberculous A18.83
- ulcerative K22.10
  - with bleeding K22.11
Esophagocele K22.5
Esophagomalacia K22.89
Esophagospasm K22.4
Esophagostenosis K22.2
Esophagostomiasis B81.8
Esophagotracheal — *see* condition
Esophagus — *see* condition
Esophoria H50.51
- convergence, excess H51.12
- divergence, insufficiency H51.8
Esotropia — *see* Strabismus, convergent concomitant
Espundia B55.2
Essential — *see* condition
Esthesioneuroblastoma C30.0
Esthesioneurocytoma C30.0
Esthesioneuroepithelioma C30.0
Esthiomene A55
Estivo-autumnal malaria (fever) B50.9
Estrangement (marital) Z63.5
- parent-child NEC Z62.890
Estriasis — *see* Myiasis
Ethanolism — *see* Alcoholism
Etherism — *see* Dependence, drug, inhalant
Ethmoid, ethmoidal — *see* condition
Ethmoiditis (chronic) (nonpurulent) (purulent) — *see also* Sinusitis, ethmoidal
- influenzal — *see* Influenza, with, respiratory manifestations NEC
- Woakes' J33.1
Ethylism — *see* Alcoholism
Eulenburg's disease (congenital paramyotonia) G71.19
Eumycetoma B47.0
Eunuchoidism E29.1
- hypogonadotropic E23.0
European blastomycosis — *see* Cryptococcosis
Eustachian — *see* condition
Evaluation (for) (of)
- development state
  - adolescent Z00.3
  - period of
    - delayed growth in childhood Z00.70
      - with abnormal findings Z00.71
    - rapid growth in childhood Z00.2
  - puberty Z00.3
- growth and developmental state (period of rapid growth) Z00.2
- delayed growth Z00.70
  - with abnormal findings Z00.71
- mental health (status) Z00.8
  - requested by authority Z04.6
- period of
  - delayed growth in childhood Z00.70
    - with abnormal findings Z00.71
  - rapid growth in childhood Z00.2
- suspected condition — *see* Observation
Evans syndrome D69.41
Event
- apparent life threatening in newborn and infant (ALTE) R68.13
- brief resolved unexplained event (BRUE) R68.13

☑ **Additional Character Required — Refer to the Tabular List for Character Selection**

Eventration — see also Hernia, ventral
  colon into chest — see Hernia, diaphragm
  diaphragm (congenital) Q79.1
Eversion
  bladder N32.89
  cervix (uteri) N86
    with cervicitis N72
  foot NEC — see also Deformity, valgus, ankle
    congenital Q66.6
  punctum lacrimale (postinfectional) (senile) H04.52- ☑
  ureter (meatus) N28.89
  urethra (meatus) N36.8
  uterus N81.4
Evidence
  cytologic
    of malignancy on anal smear R85.614
    of malignancy on cervical smear R87.614
    of malignancy on vaginal smear R87.624
Evisceration
  birth injury P15.8
  traumatic NEC
    eye — see Enucleated eye
Evulsion — see Avulsion
Ewing's sarcoma or tumor — see Neoplasm, bone, malignant
Examination (for) (following) (general) (of) (routine) Z00.00
  with abnormal findings Z00.01
  abuse, physical (alleged), ruled out
    adult Z04.71
    child Z04.72
  adolescent (development state) Z00.3
  alleged rape or sexual assault (victim), ruled out
    adult Z04.41
    child Z04.42
  allergy Z01.82
  annual (adult) (periodic) (physical) Z00.00
    with abnormal findings Z00.01
    gynecological Z01.419
      with abnormal findings Z01.411
  antibody response Z01.84
  blood — see Examination, laboratory
  blood pressure Z01.30
    with abnormal findings Z01.31
  cancer staging — see Neoplasm, malignant, by site
  cervical Papanicolaou smear Z12.4
    as part of routine gynecological examination Z01.419
      with abnormal findings Z01.411
  child (over 28 days old) Z00.129
    with abnormal findings Z00.121
    under 28 days old — see Newborn, examination
  clinical research control or normal comparison (control) (participant) Z00.6
  contraceptive (drug) maintenance (routine) Z30.8
    device (intrauterine) Z30.431
  dental Z01.20
    with abnormal findings Z01.21
  developmental — see Examination, child
  donor (potential) Z00.5
  ear Z01.10
    with abnormal findings NEC Z01.118
  eye Z01.00
    with abnormal findings Z01.01
    following failed vision screening Z01.020
      with abnormal findings Z01.021
  follow-up (routine) (following) Z09
    chemotherapy NEC Z09
      malignant neoplasm Z08
    fracture Z09
    malignant neoplasm Z08
    postpartum Z39.2
    psychotherapy Z09
    radiotherapy NEC Z09
      malignant neoplasm Z08
    surgery NEC Z09
      malignant neoplasm Z08
  following
    accident NEC Z04.3
      transport Z04.1
      work Z04.2
    assault, alleged, ruled out
      adult Z04.71
      child Z04.72
    motor vehicle accident Z04.1
    treatment (for) Z09
      combined NEC Z09
        fracture Z09
          malignant neoplasm Z08
        malignant neoplasm Z08
        mental disorder Z09

Examination — continued
  following — continued
    treatment — continued
      specified condition NEC Z09
  forced sexual exploitation Z04.81
  forced labor exploitation Z04.82
  gynecological Z01.419
    with abnormal findings Z01.411
    for contraceptive maintenance Z30.8
  health — see Examination, medical
  hearing Z01.10
    with abnormal findings NEC Z01.118
    following failed hearing screening Z01.110
    infant or child (over 28 days old) Z00.129
      with abnormal findings Z00.121
  immunity status testing Z01.84
  laboratory (as part of a general medical examination) Z00.00
    with abnormal findings Z00.01
    preprocedural Z01.812
  lactating mother Z39.1
  medical (adult) (for) (of) Z00.00
    with abnormal findings Z00.01
    administrative purpose only Z02.9
      specified NEC Z02.89
    admission to
      armed forces Z02.3
      old age home Z02.2
      prison Z02.89
      residential institution Z02.2
      school Z02.0
        following illness or medical treatment Z02.0
      summer camp Z02.89
    adoption Z02.82
    blood alcohol or drug level Z02.83
    camp (summer) Z02.89
    clinical research, normal subject (control) (participant) Z00.6
    control subject in clinical research (normal comparison) (participant) Z00.6
    donor (potential) Z00.5
    driving license Z02.4
    general (adult) Z00.00
      with abnormal findings Z00.01
    immigration Z02.89
    insurance purposes Z02.6
    marriage Z02.89
    medicolegal reasons NEC Z04.89
    naturalization Z02.89
    participation in sport Z02.5
    paternity testing Z02.81
    population survey Z00.8
    pre-employment Z02.1
    pre-operative — see Examination, pre-procedural
    pre-procedural
      cardiovascular Z01.810
      respiratory Z01.811
      specified NEC Z01.818
    preschool children
      for admission to school Z02.0
    prisoners
      for entrance into prison Z02.89
    recruitment for armed forces Z02.3
    specified NEC Z00.8
    sport competition Z02.5
  medicolegal reason NEC Z04.89
    following
      forced sexual exploitation Z04.81
      forced labor exploitation Z04.82
  newborn — see Newborn, examination
  pelvic (annual) (periodic) Z01.419
    with abnormal findings Z01.411
  period of rapid growth in childhood Z00.2
  periodic (adult) (annual) (routine) Z00.00
    with abnormal findings Z00.01
  physical (adult) — see also Examination, medical Z00.00
    sports Z02.5
  postpartum
    immediately after delivery Z39.0
    routine follow-up Z39.2
  pre-chemotherapy (antineoplastic) Z01.818
  prenatal (normal pregnancy) — see also Pregnancy, normal Z34.9- ☑
  pre-procedural (pre-operative)
    cardiovascular Z01.810
    laboratory Z01.812
    respiratory Z01.811
    specified NEC Z01.818
  prior to chemotherapy (antineoplastic) Z01.818

Examination — continued
  psychiatric NEC Z00.8
    follow-up not needing further care Z09
    requested by authority Z04.6
  radiological (as part of a general medical examination) Z00.00
    with abnormal findings Z00.01
  repeat cervical smear to confirm findings of recent normal smear following initial abnormal smear Z01.42
  skin (hypersensitivity) Z01.82
  special — see also Examination, by type Z01.89
    specified type NEC Z01.89
  specified type or reason NEC Z04.89
  teeth Z01.20
    with abnormal findings Z01.21
  urine — see Examination, laboratory
  vision Z01.00
    with abnormal findings Z01.01
    following failed vision screening Z01.020
      with abnormal findings Z01.021
    infant or child (over 28 days old) Z00.129
      with abnormal findings Z00.121
Exanthem, exanthema — see also Rash
  with enteroviral vesicular stomatitis B08.4
  Boston A88.0
  epidemic with meningitis A88.0 [G02]
  subitum B08.20
    due to human herpesvirus 6 B08.21
    due to human herpesvirus 7 B08.22
  viral, virus B09
    specified type NEC B08.8
Excess, excessive, excessively
  alcohol level in blood R78.0
  androgen (ovarian) E28.1
  attrition, tooth, teeth K03.0
  carotene, carotin (dietary) E67.1
  cold, effects of T69.9 ☑
    specified effect NEC T69.8 ☑
  convergence H51.12
  crying
    in child, adolescent, or adult R45.83
    in infant R68.11
  development, breast N62
  divergence H51.8
  drinking (alcohol) NEC (without dependence) F10.10
    habitual (continual) (without remission) F10.20
  eating R63.2
  estrogen E28.0
  fat — see also Obesity
    in heart — see Degeneration, myocardial
    localized E65
  foreskin N47.8
  gas R14.0
  glucagon E16.3
  heat — see Heat
  intermaxillary vertical dimension of fully erupted teeth M26.37
  interocclusal distance of fully erupted teeth M26.37
  kalium E87.5
  large
    colon K59.39
      congenital Q43.8
    infant P08.0
    organ or site, congenital NEC — see Anomaly, by site
  long
    organ or site, congenital NEC — see Anomaly, by site
  menstruation (with regular cycle) N92.0
    with irregular cycle N92.1
  napping Z72.821
  natrium E87.0
  number of teeth K00.1
  nutrient (dietary) NEC R63.2
  potassium (K) E87.5
  salivation K11.7
  secretion — see also Hypersecretion
    milk O92.6
    sputum R09.3
    sweat R61
  sexual drive F52.8
  short
    organ or site, congenital NEC — see Anomaly, by site
    umbilical cord in labor or delivery O69.3 ☑
  skin L98.7
    and subcutaneous tissue L98.7
    eyelid (acquired) — see Blepharochalasis
      congenital Q10.3
  sodium (Na) E87.0
  spacing of fully erupted teeth M26.32
  sputum R09.3

Excess, excessive, excessively — *continued*
  sweating R61
  thirst R63.1
    due to deprivation of water T73.1 ☑
  transportation time Z59.82
  tuberosity of jaw M26.07
  vitamin
    A (dietary) E67.0
      administered as drug (prolonged intake) — *see*
        Table of Drugs and Chemicals, vitamins,
        adverse effect
      overdose or wrong substance given or taken —
        see Table of Drugs and Chemicals, vitamins,
        poisoning
    D (dietary) E67.3
      administered as drug (prolonged intake) — *see*
        Table of Drugs and Chemicals, vitamins,
        adverse effect
      overdose or wrong substance given or taken —
        see Table of Drugs and Chemicals, vitamins,
        poisoning
  weight
    gain R63.5
    loss R63.4
Excitability, abnormal, under minor stress (personality
    disorder) F60.3
Excitation
  anomalous atrioventricular I45.6
  psychogenic F30.8
  reactive (from emotional stress, psychological trauma)
    F30.8
Excitement
  hypomanic F30.8
  manic F30.9
  mental, reactive (from emotional stress, psychological
    trauma) F30.8
  state, reactive (from emotional stress, psychological
    trauma) F30.8
Excoriation (traumatic) — *see also* Abrasion
  neurotic L98.1
  skin picking disorder F42.4
Exfoliation
  due to erythematous conditions according to extent of
    body surface involved L49.0
    10-19 percent of body surface L49.1
    20-29 percent of body surface L49.2
    30-39 percent of body surface L49.3
    40-49 percent of body surface L49.4
    50-59 percent of body surface L49.5
    60-69 percent of body surface L49.6
    70-79 percent of body surface L49.7
    80-89 percent of body surface L49.8
    90-99 percent of body surface L49.9
    less than 10 percent of body surface L49.0
  teeth, due to systemic causes K08.0
Exfoliative — *see* condition
Exhaustion, exhaustive (physical NEC) R53.83
  battle F43.0
  cardiac — *see* Failure, heart
  delirium F43.0
  due to
    cold T69.8 ☑
    excessive exertion T73.3 ☑
    exposure T73.2 ☑
    neurasthenia F48.8
  heart — *see* Failure, heart
  heat — *see also* Heat, exhaustion T67.5 ☑
    due to
      salt depletion T67.4 ☑
      water depletion T67.3 ☑
  maternal, complicating delivery O75.81
  mental F48.8
  myocardium, myocardial — *see* Failure, heart
  nervous F48.8
  old age R54
  psychogenic F48.8
  psychosis F43.0
  senile R54
  vital NEC Z73.0
Exhibitionism F65.2
Exocervicitis — *see* Cervicitis
Exomphalos Q79.2
  meaning hernia — *see* Hernia, umbilicus
Exophoria H50.52
  convergence, insufficiency H51.11
  divergence, excess H51.8
Exophthalmos H05.2- ☑
  congenital Q15.8

Exophthalmos — *continued*
  constant NEC H05.24- ☑
  displacement, globe — *see* Displacement, globe
  due to thyrotoxicosis (hyperthyroidism) — *see* Hyperthy-
    roidism, with, goiter (diffuse)
  dysthyroid — *see* Hyperthyroidism, with, goiter (diffuse)
  goiter — *see* Hyperthyroidism, with, goiter (diffuse)
  intermittent NEC H05.25- ☑
  malignant — *see* Hyperthyroidism, with, goiter (diffuse)
  orbital
    edema — *see* Edema, orbit
    hemorrhage — *see* Hemorrhage, orbit
  pulsating NEC H05.26- ☑
  thyrotoxic, thyrotropic — *see* Hyperthyroidism, with,
    goiter (diffuse)
Exostosis — *see also* Disorder, bone
  cartilaginous — *see* Neoplasm, bone, benign
  congenital (multiple) Q78.6
  external ear canal H61.81- ☑
  gonococcal A54.49
  jaw (bone) M27.8
  multiple, congenital Q78.6
  orbit H05.35- ☑
  osteocartilaginous — *see* Neoplasm, bone, benign
  syphilitic A52.77
Exotropia — *see* Strabismus, divergent concomitant
Explanation of
  investigation finding Z71.2
  medication Z71.89
Exploitation
  labor
    confirmed
      adult forced T74.61 ☑
      child forced T74.62 ☑
    suspected
      adult forced T76.61 ☑
      child forced T76.62 ☑
  sexual
    confirmed
      adult forced T74.51 ☑
      child T74.52 ☑
    suspected
      adult forced T76.51 ☑
      child T76.52 ☑
Exposure (to) — *see also* Contact, with T75.89 ☑
  acariasis Z20.7
  AIDS virus Z20.6
  air pollution Z77.110
  algae and algae toxins Z77.121
  algae bloom Z77.121
  anthrax Z20.810
  aromatic amines Z77.020
  aromatic (hazardous) compounds NEC Z77.028
  aromatic dyes NOS Z77.028
  arsenic Z77.010
  asbestos Z77.090
  bacterial disease NEC Z20.818
  benzene Z77.021
  blue-green algae bloom Z77.121
  body fluids (potentially hazardous) Z77.21
  brown tide Z77.121
  chemicals (chiefly nonmedicinal) (hazardous) NEC
    Z77.098
  cholera Z20.09
  chromium compounds Z77.018
  cold, effects of T69.9 ☑
    specified effect NEC T69.8 ☑
  communicable disease Z20.9
    bacterial NEC Z20.818
    specified NEC Z20.89
    viral NEC Z20.828
    Zika virus Z20.821
  coronavirus (disease) (novel) 2019 Z20.822
  COVID-19 Z20.822
  cyanobacteria bloom Z77.121
  disaster Z65.5
  discrimination Z60.5
  dyes Z77.098
  effects of T73.9 ☑
  environmental tobacco smoke (acute) (chronic) Z77.22
  Escherichia coli (E. coli) Z20.01
  exhaustion due to T73.2 ☑
  fiberglass — *see* Table of Drugs and Chemicals, fiberglass
  German measles Z20.4
  gonorrhea Z20.2
  hazardous metals NEC Z77.018
  hazardous substances NEC Z77.29
  hazards in the physical environment NEC Z77.128

Exposure — *continued*
  hazards to health NEC Z77.9
  human immunodeficiency virus (HIV) Z20.6
  human T-lymphotropic virus type-1 (HTLV-1) Z20.89
  implanted
    mesh — *see* Complications, prosthetic device or im-
      plant, mesh
    prosthetic materials NEC — *see* Complications, pros-
      thetic materials NEC
  infestation (parasitic) NEC Z20.7
  intestinal infectious disease NEC Z20.09
    Escherichia coli (E. coli) Z20.01
  lead Z77.011
  meningococcus Z20.811
  mold (toxic) Z77.120
  nickel dust Z77.018
  noise Z77.122
  occupational
    air contaminants NEC Z57.39
    dust Z57.2
    environmental tobacco smoke Z57.31
    extreme temperature Z57.6
    noise Z57.0
    radiation Z57.1
    risk factors Z57.9
      specified NEC Z57.8
    toxic agents (gases) (liquids) (solids) (vapors) in agri-
      culture Z57.4
    toxic agents (gases) (liquids) (solids) (vapors) in indus-
      try NEC Z57.5
    vibration Z57.7
  parasitic disease NEC Z20.7
  pediculosis Z20.7
  persecution Z60.5
  pfiesteria piscicida Z77.121
  poliomyelitis Z20.89
  pollution
    air Z77.110
    environmental NEC Z77.118
    soil Z77.112
    water Z77.111
  polycyclic aromatic hydrocarbons Z77.028
  prenatal (drugs) (toxic chemicals) — *see* Newborn, affect-
    ed by, noxious substances transmitted via placenta
    or breast milk
  rabies Z20.3
  radiation, naturally occurring NEC Z77.123
  radon Z77.123
  red tide (Florida) Z77.121
  rubella Z20.4
  SARS-CoV-2 Z20.822
  second hand tobacco smoke (acute) (chronic) Z77.22
    in the perinatal period P96.81
  sexually-transmitted disease Z20.2
  smallpox (laboratory) Z20.89
  syphilis Z20.2
  terrorism Z65.4
  torture Z65.4
  tuberculosis Z20.1
  uranium Z77.012
  varicella Z20.820
  venereal disease Z20.2
  viral disease NEC Z20.828
  war Z65.5
  water pollution Z77.111
  Zika virus Z20.821
Exsanguination — *see* Hemorrhage
Exstrophy
  abdominal contents Q45.8
  bladder Q64.10
    cloacal Q64.12
    specified type NEC Q64.19
    supravesical fissure Q64.11
Extensive — *see* condition
Extra — *see also* Accessory
  marker chromosomes (normal individual) Q92.61
    in abnormal individual Q92.62
  rib Q76.6
    cervical Q76.5
Extrasystoles (supraventricular) I49.49
  atrial I49.1
  auricular I49.1
  junctional I49.2
  ventricular I49.3
Extrauterine gestation or pregnancy — *see* Pregnancy,
    by site
Extravasation
  blood R58
  chyle into mesentery I89.8

☑ **Additional Character Required — Refer to the Tabular List for Character Selection**

Extravasation — *continued*
  pelvicalyceal N13.8
  pyelosinus N13.8
  urine (from ureter) R39.0
  vesicant agent
    antineoplastic chemotherapy T80.810 ☑
    other agent NEC T80.818 ☑
Extremity — *see* condition, limb
Extrophy — *see* Exstrophy
Extroversion
  bladder Q64.19
  uterus N81.4
    complicating delivery O71.2
    postpartal (old) N81.4
Extruded tooth (teeth) M26.34
Extrusion
  breast implant (prosthetic) T85.42 ☑
  eye implant (globe) (ball) T85.328 ☑
  intervertebral disc — *see* Displacement, intervertebral disc
  ocular lens implant (prosthetic) — *see* Complications, intraocular lens
  vitreous — *see* Prolapse, vitreous
Exudate
  causing irritant dermatitis L24.A9
  pleural — *see* Effusion, pleura
  retina H35.89
  wound fluids causing irritant dermatitis L24.A9
Exudative — *see* condition
Eye, eyeball, eyelid — *see* condition
Eyestrain — *see* Disturbance, vision, subjective
Eyeworm disease of Africa B74.3

F

Faber's syndrome (achlorhydric anemia) D50.9
Fabry (-Anderson) disease E75.21
Facet syndrome M47.89- ☑
Faciocephalalgia, autonomic — *see also* Neuropathy, peripheral, autonomic G90.09
Factor(s)
  psychic, associated with diseases classified elsewhere F54
  psychological
    affecting physical conditions F54
    or behavioral
      affecting general medical condition F54
      associated with disorders or diseases classified elsewhere F54
Fahr disease (of brain) G23.8
Fahr Volhard disease (of kidney) I12.- ☑
Failure, failed
  abortion — *see* Abortion, attempted
  aortic (valve) I35.8
    rheumatic I06.8
  attempted abortion — *see* Abortion, attempted
  biventricular I50.82
    due to left heart failure I50.814
  bone marrow — *see* Anemia, aplastic
  cardiac — *see* Failure, heart
  cardiorenal (chronic) — *see also* Failure, renal, and Failure, heart I50.9
    hypertensive I13.2
  cardiorespiratory — *see also* Failure, heart R09.2
  cardiovascular (chronic) — *see* Failure, heart
  cerebrovascular I67.9
  cervical dilatation in labor O62.0
  circulation, circulatory (peripheral) R57.9
    newborn P29.89
  compensation — *see* Disease, heart
  compliance with medical treatment or regimen — *see* Noncompliance
  congestive — *see* Failure, heart, congestive
  dental implant (endosseous) M27.69
    due to
      failure of dental prosthesis M27.63
      lack of attached gingiva M27.62
      occlusal trauma (poor prosthetic design) M27.62
      parafunctional habits M27.62
      periodontal infection (peri-implantitis) M27.62
      poor oral hygiene M27.62
    osseointegration M27.61
      due to
        complications of systemic disease M27.61
        poor bone quality M27.61
      iatrogenic M27.61
    post-osseointegration
      biological M27.62

Failure, failed — *continued*
  dental implant — *continued*
    post-osseointegration — *continued*
      due to complications of systemic disease M27.62
      iatrogenic M27.62
      mechanical M27.63
    pre-integration M27.61
    pre-osseointegration M27.61
    specified NEC M27.69
  descent of head (at term) of pregnancy (mother) O32.4 ☑
  endosseous dental implant — *see* Failure, dental implant
  engagement of head (term of pregnancy) (mother) O32.4 ☑
  erection (penile) — *see also* Dysfunction, sexual, male, erectile N52.9
    nonorganic F52.21
  examination(s), anxiety concerning Z55.2
  expansion terminal respiratory units (newborn) (primary) P28.0
  forceps NOS (with subsequent cesarean delivery) O66.5
  gain weight (child over 28 days old) R62.51
    adult R62.7
    newborn P92.6
  genital response (male) F52.21
    female F52.22
  heart (acute) (senile) (sudden) I50.9
    with
      acute pulmonary edema — *see* Failure, ventricular, left
      decompensation I50.9
        with
          normal ejection fraction I50.33
          preserved ejection fraction I50.33
          reduced ejection fraction I50.23
            with diastolic dysfunction I50.43
          combined systolic and diastolic I50.43
          diastolic I50.33
          right I50.813
          systolic I50.23
      dilatation — *see* Disease, heart
      hypertension — *see* Hypertension, heart
      normal ejection fraction — *see* Failure, heart, diastolic
      preserved ejection fraction — *see* Failure, heart, diastolic
      reduced ejection fraction — *see* Failure, heart, systolic
    arteriosclerotic I70.90
    biventricular I50.82
      due to left heart failure I50.814
    combined left-right sided I50.82
      due to left heart failure I50.814
    compensated — *see also* Failure, heart, by type as diastolic or systolic, chronic I50.9
    complicating
      anesthesia (general) (local) or other sedation
        in labor and delivery O74.2
        in pregnancy O29.12- ☑
        postpartum, puerperal O89.1
      delivery (cesarean) (instrumental) O75.4
    congestive I50.9
      with rheumatic fever (conditions in I00)
        active I01.8
        inactive or quiescent (with chorea) I09.81
      newborn P29.0
      rheumatic (chronic) (inactive) (with chorea) I09.81
        active or acute I01.8
          with chorea I02.0
    decompensated — *see also* Failure, heart, by type as diastolic or systolic, acute and chronic I50.9
    degenerative — *see* Degeneration, myocardial
    diastolic (congestive) (left ventricular) I50.30
      acute (congestive) I50.31
        and (on) chronic (congestive) I50.33
      chronic (congestive) I50.32
        and (on) acute (congestive) I50.33
      combined with systolic (congestive) I50.40
        acute (congestive) I50.41
          and (on) chronic (congestive) I50.43
        chronic (congestive) I50.42
          and (on) acute (congestive) I50.43
    due to presence of cardiac prosthesis I97.13- ☑
    end stage — *see also* Failure, heart, by type as diastolic or systolic, chronic I50.84
    following cardiac surgery I97.13- ☑
    high output NOS I50.83
    hypertensive — *see* Hypertension, heart

Failure, failed — *continued*
  heart — *continued*
    left (ventricular) — *see also* Failure, ventricular, left
      combined diastolic and systolic — *see* Failure, heart, diastolic, combined with systolic
      diastolic — *see* Failure, heart, diastolic
      systolic — *see* Failure, heart, systolic
    low output (syndrome) NOS I50.9
    newborn P29.0
    organic — *see* Disease, heart
    peripartum O90.3
    postprocedural I97.13- ☑
    rheumatic (chronic) (inactive) I09.9
    right (isolated) (ventricular) I50.810
      acute I50.811
        and (on) chronic I50.813
      chronic I50.812
        and acute I50.813
      secondary to left heart failure I50.814
    specified NEC I50.89

> Note: heart failure stages A, B, C, and D are based on the American College of Cardiology and American Heart Association stages of heart failure, which complement and should not be confused with the New York Heart Association Classification of Heart Failure, into Class I, Class II, Class III, and Class IV

    stage A Z91.89
    stage B — *see also* Failure, heart, by type as diastolic or systolic I50.9
    stage C — *see also* Failure, heart, by type as diastolic or systolic I50.9
    stage D — *see also* Failure, heart, by type as diastolic or systolic, chronic I50.84
    systolic (congestive) (left ventricular) I50.20
      acute (congestive) I50.21
        and (on) chronic (congestive) I50.23
      chronic (congestive) I50.22
        and (on) acute (congestive) I50.23
      combined with diastolic (congestive) I50.40
        acute (congestive) I50.41
          and (on) chronic (congestive) I50.43
        chronic (congestive) I50.42
          and (on) acute (congestive) I50.43
    thyrotoxic — *see also* Thyrotoxicosis E05.90 *[I43]*
      with
        high output — *see also* Thyrotoxicosis I50.83
        thyroid storm E05.91 *[I43]*
          high output — *see also* Thyrotoxicosis I50.83
    valvular — *see* Endocarditis
  hepatic K72.90
    with coma K72.91
    acute or subacute K72.00
      with coma K72.01
      due to drugs K71.10
        with coma K71.11
    alcoholic (acute) (chronic) (subacute) K70.40
      with coma K70.41
    chronic K72.10
      with coma K72.11
      due to drugs (acute) (subacute) (chronic) K71.10
        with coma K71.11
    due to drugs (acute) (subacute) (chronic) K71.10
      with coma K71.11
    end stage K72.10
      with coma K72.11
    postprocedural K91.82
  hepatorenal K76.7
  induction (of labor) O61.9
    abortion — *see* Abortion, attempted
    by
      oxytocic drugs O61.0
      prostaglandins O61.0
    instrumental O61.1
    mechanical O61.1
    medical O61.0
    specified NEC O61.8
    surgical O61.1
  intestinal failure K90.83
  intubation during anesthesia T88.4 ☑
    in pregnancy O29.6- ☑
    labor and delivery O74.7
    postpartum, puerperal O89.6
  involution, thymus (gland) E32.0
  kidney — *see also* Disease, kidney, chronic N19
    acute — *see also* Failure, renal, acute N17.9
  lactation (complete) O92.3
    partial O92.4

Failure, failed — *continued*
- Leydig's cell, adult E29.1
- liver — *see* Failure, hepatic
- menstruation at puberty N91.0
- mitral I05.8
- myocardial, myocardium — *see also* Failure, heart I50.9
  - chronic — *see also* Failure, heart, congestive I50.9
  - congestive — *see also* Failure, heart, congestive I50.9
- newborn screening — *see* Abnormal, neonatal screening
  - neonatal congenital heart disease P09.5
- orgasm (female) (psychogenic) F52.31
  - male F52.32
- ovarian (primary) E28.39
  - iatrogenic E89.40
    - asymptomatic E89.40
    - symptomatic E89.41
  - postprocedural (postablative) (postirradiation) (postsurgical) E89.40
    - asymptomatic E89.40
    - symptomatic E89.41
- ovulation causing infertility N97.0
- polyglandular, autoimmune E31.0
- prosthetic joint implant — *see* Complications, joint prosthesis, mechanical, breakdown, by site
- renal N19
  - with
    - tubular necrosis (acute) N17.0
  - acute N17.9
    - with
      - cortical necrosis N17.1
      - medullary necrosis N17.2
      - tubular necrosis N17.0
    - specified NEC N17.8
  - chronic N18.9
    - hypertensive — *see* Hypertension, kidney
  - congenital P96.0
  - end stage (chronic) N18.6
    - due to hypertension I12.0
  - following
    - abortion — *see* Abortion by type complicated by specified condition NEC
    - crushing T79.5 ☑
    - ectopic or molar pregnancy O08.4
    - labor and delivery (acute) O90.49
  - hypertensive — *see* Hypertension, kidney
  - postprocedural N99.0
- respiration, respiratory J96.90
  - with
    - hypercapnia J96.92
    - hypercarbia J96.92
    - hypoxia J96.91
  - acute J96.00
    - with
      - hypercapnia J96.02
      - hypercarbia J96.02
      - hypoxia J96.01
  - center G93.89
  - acute and (on) chronic J96.20
    - with
      - hypercapnia J96.22
      - hypercarbia J96.22
      - hypoxia J96.21
  - chronic J96.10
    - with
      - hypercapnia J96.12
      - hypercarbia J96.12
      - hypoxia J96.11
  - newborn P28.5
  - postprocedural (acute) J95.821
    - acute and chronic J95.822
- rotation
  - cecum Q43.3
  - colon Q43.3
  - intestine Q43.3
  - kidney Q63.2
- sedation (conscious) (moderate) during procedure T88.52 ☑
  - history of Z92.83
- segmentation — *see also* Fusion
  - fingers — *see* Syndactylism, complex, fingers
  - vertebra Q76.49
    - with scoliosis Q76.3
- seminiferous tubule, adult E29.1
- senile (general) R54
- sexual arousal (male) F52.21
  - female F52.22
- testicular endocrine function E29.1
- to thrive (child over 28 days old) R62.51
  - adult R62.7

Failure, failed — *continued*
- to thrive — *continued*
  - newborn P92.6
- transplant T86.92
  - bone T86.831
    - marrow T86.02
  - cornea T86.841- ☑
  - heart T86.22
    - with lung(s) T86.32
  - intestine T86.851
  - kidney T86.12
  - liver T86.42
  - lung(s) T86.811
    - with heart T86.32
  - pancreas T86.891
  - skin (allograft) (autograft) T86.821
  - specified organ or tissue NEC T86.891
  - stem cell (peripheral blood) (umbilical cord) T86.5
- trial of labor (with subsequent cesarean delivery) O66.40
  - following previous cesarean delivery O66.41
- tubal ligation N99.89
- urinary — *see* Disease, kidney, chronic
- vacuum extraction NOS (with subsequent cesarean delivery) O66.5
- vasectomy N99.89
- ventouse NOS (with subsequent cesarean delivery) O66.5
- ventricular — *see also* Failure, heart I50.9
  - left — *see also* Failure, heart, left I50.1
    - with rheumatic fever (conditions in I00)
      - active I01.8
        - with chorea I02.0
      - inactive or quiescent (with chorea) I09.81
      - rheumatic (chronic) (inactive) (with chorea) I09.81
        - active or acute I01.8
          - with chorea I02.0
  - right — *see* Failure, heart, right
- vital centers, newborn P91.88

Fainting (fit) R55
Fallen arches — *see* Deformity, limb, flat foot
Falling, falls (repeated) R29.6
- any organ or part — *see* Prolapse
Fallopian
- insufflation Z31.41
- tube — *see* condition
Fallot's
- pentalogy Q21.8
- tetrad or tetralogy Q21.3
- triad or trilogy Q22.3
False — *see also* condition
- croup J38.5
- joint — *see* Nonunion, fracture
- labor (pains) O47.9
  - at or after 37 completed weeks of gestation O47.1
  - before 37 completed weeks of gestation O47.0- ☑
- passage, urethra (prostatic) N36.5
- pregnancy F45.8
Family, familial — *see also* condition
- disruption Z63.8
  - involving divorce or separation Z63.5
- Li-Fraumeni (syndrome) Z15.01
- planning advice Z30.09
- problem Z63.9
  - specified NEC Z63.8
- retinoblastoma C69.2- ☑
Famine (effects of) T73.0 ☑
- edema — *see* Malnutrition, severe
Fanconi ('s) **anemia** D61.03
Fanconi hypoplastic anemia D61.03
Fanconi panmyelopathy D61.03
Fanconi (-de Toni)(-Debre) **syndrome** E72.09
- with cystinosis E72.04
Farber's disease or syndrome E75.29
Farcy A24.0
Farmer's
- lung J67.0
- skin L57.8
Farsightedness — *see* Hypermetropia
Fascia — *see* condition
Fasciculation R25.3
Fasciitis M72.9
- diffuse (eosinophilic) M35.4
- infective M72.8
  - necrotizing M72.6
- necrotizing M72.6
- nodular M72.4
- perirenal (with ureteral obstruction) N13.5
  - with infection N13.6
- plantar M72.2
- specified NEC M72.8

Fasciitis — *continued*
- traumatic (old) M72.8
  - current — *code by* site under Sprain
Fascioliasis B66.3
Fasciolopsis, fasciolopsiasis (intestinal) B66.5
Fascioscapulohumeral myopathy G71.02
Fast pulse R00.0
Fat
- embolism — *see* Embolism, fat
- excessive — *see also* Obesity
  - in heart — *see* Degeneration, myocardial
- in stool R19.5
- localized (pad) E65
  - heart — *see* Degeneration, myocardial
  - knee M79.4
  - retropatellar M79.4
- necrosis
  - breast N64.1
  - mesentery K65.4
  - omentum K65.4
- pad E65
  - knee M79.4
Fatigue R53.83
- auditory deafness — *see* Deafness
- chronic R53.82
- combat F43.0
- general R53.83
  - psychogenic F48.8
- heat (transient) T67.6 ☑
- muscle M62.89
- myocardium — *see* Failure, heart
- neoplasm-related R53.0
- nervous, neurosis F48.8
- operational F48.8
- psychogenic (general) F48.8
- senile R54
- voice R49.8
Fatness — *see* Obesity
Fatty — *see also* condition
- apron E65
- degeneration — *see* Degeneration, fatty
- heart (enlarged) — *see* Degeneration, myocardial
- liver NEC K76.0
  - alcoholic K70.0
  - nonalcoholic K76.0
- necrosis — *see* Degeneration, fatty
Fauces — *see* condition
Fauchard's disease (periodontitis) — *see* Periodontitis
Faucitis J02.9
Favism (anemia) D55.0
Favus — *see* Dermatophytosis
Fazio-Londe disease or syndrome G12.1
Fear complex or reaction F40.9
Fear of — *see* Phobia
Feared complaint unfounded Z71.1
Febris, febrile — *see also* Fever
- flava — *see also* Fever, yellow A95.9
- melitensis A23.0
- pestis — *see* Plague
- recurrens — *see* Fever, relapsing
- rubra A38.9
Fecal
- incontinence R15.9
- smearing R15.1
- soiling R15.1
- urgency R15.2
Fecalith (impaction) K56.41
- appendix K38.1
- congenital P76.8
Fede's disease K14.0
Feeble rapid pulse due to shock following injury T79.4 ☑
Feeble-minded F70
Feeding
- difficulties R63.30
- problem (elderly) (infant) R63.39
  - newborn P92.9
    - specified NEC P92.8
  - nonorganic (adult) — *see* Disorder, eating
Feeling (of)
- foreign body in throat R09.A2
Feer's disease — *see* Poisoning, mercury
Feet — *see* condition
Feigned illness Z76.5
Feil-Klippel syndrome (brevicollis) Q76.1
Feinmesser's (hidrotic) **ectodermal dysplasia** Q82.4
Felinophobia F40.218
Felon — *see also* Cellulitis, digit
- with lymphangitis — *see* Lymphangitis, acute, digit
Felty's syndrome M05.00

☑ **Additional Character Required** — Refer to the Tabular List for Character Selection

Felty's syndrome — *continued*
ankle MØ5.Ø7- ☑
elbow MØ5.Ø2- ☑
foot joint MØ5.Ø7- ☑
hand joint MØ5.Ø4- ☑
hip MØ5.Ø5- ☑
knee MØ5.Ø6- ☑
multiple site MØ5.Ø9
shoulder MØ5.Ø1- ☑
vertebra — *see* Spondylitis, ankylosing
wrist MØ5.Ø3- ☑
Female genital cutting status — *see* Female genital mutilation status (FGM)
Female genital mutilation status (FGM) N9Ø.81Ø
specified NEC N9Ø.818
type I (clitorectomy status) N9Ø.811
type II (clitorectomy with excision of labia minora status) N9Ø.812
type III (infibulation status) N9Ø.813
type IV N9Ø.818
Femur, femoral — *see* condition
Fenestration, fenestrated — *see also* Imperfect, closure
aortico-pulmonary Q21.4
atrial septum Q21.11
cusps, heart valve NEC Q24.8
pulmonary Q22.3
pulmonic cusps Q22.3
Fernell's disease (aortic aneurysm) I71.9
Fertile eunuch syndrome E23.Ø
Fetid
breath R19.6
sweat L75.Ø
Fetishism F65.Ø
transvestic F65.1
Fetus, fetal — *see also* condition
alcohol syndrome (dysmorphic) Q86.Ø
compressus O31.Ø- ☑
hydantoin syndrome Q86.1
lung tissue P28.Ø
papyraceous O31.Ø- ☑
Fever (inanition) (of unknown origin) (persistent) (with chills) (with rigor) R5Ø.9
abortus A23.1
Aden (dengue) A9Ø
African tick bite A77.8
African tick-borne A68.1
American
mountain (tick) A93.2
spotted A77.Ø
aphthous BØ8.8
arbovirus, arboviral A94
hemorrhagic A94
specified NEC A93.8
Argentinian hemorrhagic A96.Ø
Assam B55.Ø
Australian Q A78
Bangkok hemorrhagic A91
Barmah forest A92.8
Bartonella A44.Ø
bilious, hemoglobinuric B5Ø.8
blackwater B5Ø.8
blister BØØ.1
Bolivian hemorrhagic A96.1
Bonvale dam T73.3 ☑
boutonneuse A77.1
brain — *see* Encephalitis
Brazilian purpuric A48.4
breakbone A9Ø
Bullis A77.Ø
Bunyamwera A92.8
Burdwan B55.Ø
Bwamba A92.8
Cameroon — *see* Malaria
Canton A75.9
catarrhal (acute) JØØ
chronic J31.Ø
cat-scratch A28.1
Central Asian hemorrhagic A98.Ø
cerebral — *see* Encephalitis
cerebrospinal meningococcal A39.Ø
Chagres B5Ø.9
Chandipura A92.8
Changuinola A93.1
Charcot's (biliary) (hepatic) (intermittent) — *see* Calculus, bile duct
Chikungunya (viral) (hemorrhagic) A92.Ø
Chitral A93.1
Colombo — *see* Fever, paratyphoid

Fever — *continued*
Colorado tick (virus) A93.2
congestive (remittent) — *see* Malaria
Congo virus A98.Ø
continued malarial B5Ø.9
Corsican — *see* Malaria
Crimean-Congo hemorrhagic A98.Ø
Cyprus — *see* Brucellosis
dandy A9Ø
deer fly — *see* Tularemia
dengue (virus) A9Ø
hemorrhagic A91
sandfly A93.1
desert B38.Ø
drug induced R5Ø.2
due to
conditions classified elsewhere R5Ø.81
heat T67.Ø1 ☑
enteric AØ1.ØØ
enteroviral exanthematous (Boston exanthem) A88.Ø
ephemeral (of unknown origin) R5Ø.9
epidemic hemorrhagic A98.5
erysipelatous — *see* Erysipelas
estivo-autumnal (malarial) B5Ø.9
famine A75.Ø
five day A79.Ø
following delivery O86.4
Fort Bragg A27.89
gastroenteric AØ1.ØØ
gastromalarial — *see* Malaria
Gibraltar — *see* Brucellosis
glandular — *see* Mononucleosis, infectious
Guama (viral) A92.8
Haverhill A25.1
hay (allergic) J3Ø.1
with asthma (bronchial) J45.9Ø9
with
exacerbation (acute) J45.9Ø1
status asthmaticus J45.9Ø2
due to
allergen other than pollen J3Ø.89
pollen, any plant or tree J3Ø.1
heat (effects) T67.Ø1 ☑
hematuric, bilious B5Ø.8
hemoglobinuric (malarial) (bilious) B5Ø.8
hemorrhagic (arthropod-borne) NOS A94
with renal syndrome A98.5
arenaviral A96.9
specified NEC A96.8
Argentinian A96.Ø
Bangkok A91
Bolivian A96.1
Central Asian A98.Ø
Chikungunya A92.Ø
Crimean-Congo A98.Ø
dengue (virus) A91
epidemic A98.5
Junin (virus) A96.Ø
Korean A98.5
Kyasanur forest A98.2
Machupo (virus) A96.1
mite-borne A93.8
mosquito-borne A92.8
Omsk A98.1
Philippine A91
Russian A98.5
Singapore A91
Southeast Asia A91
Thailand A91
tick-borne NEC A93.8
viral A99
specified NEC A98.8
hepatic — *see* Cholecystitis
herpetic — *see* Herpes
icterohemorrhagic A27.Ø
Indiana A93.8
infective B99.9
specified NEC B99.8
intermittent (bilious) — *see also* Malaria
of unknown origin R5Ø.9
pernicious B5Ø.9
iodide R5Ø.2
Japanese river A75.3
jungle — *see also* Malaria
yellow A95.Ø
Junin (virus) hemorrhagic A96.Ø
Katayama B65.2
kedani A75.3
Kenya (tick) A77.1

Fever — *continued*
Kew Garden A79.1
Korean hemorrhagic A98.5
Lassa A96.2
Lone Star A77.Ø
Machupo (virus) hemorrhagic A96.1
malaria, malarial — *see* Malaria
Malta A23.9
Marseilles A77.1
marsh — *see* Malaria
Mayaro (viral) A92.8
Mediterranean — *see also* Brucellosis A23.9
familial MØ4.1
tick A77.1
meningeal — *see* Meningitis
Meuse A79.Ø
Mexican A75.2
mianeh A68.1
miasmatic — *see* Malaria
mosquito-borne (viral) A92.9
hemorrhagic A92.8
mountain — *see also* Brucellosis
meaning Rocky Mountain spotted fever A77.Ø
tick (American) (Colorado) (viral) A93.2
Mucambo (viral) A92.8
mud A27.9
Neapolitan — *see* Brucellosis
neutropenic D7Ø.9
newborn P81.9
environmental P81.Ø
Nine-Mile A78
non-exanthematous tick A93.2
North Asian tick-borne A77.2
Omsk hemorrhagic A98.1
O'nyong-nyong (viral) A92.1
Oropouche (viral) A93.Ø
Oroya A44.Ø
pacific coast tick A77.8
paludal — *see* Malaria
Panama (malarial) B5Ø.9
Pappataci A93.1
paratyphoid AØ1.4
A AØ1.1
B AØ1.2
C AØ1.3
parrot A7Ø
periodic (Mediterranean) MØ4.1
persistent (of unknown origin) R5Ø.9
petechial A39.Ø
pharyngoconjunctival B3Ø.2
Philippine hemorrhagic A91
phlebotomus A93.1
Piry (virus) A93.8
Pixuna (viral) A92.8
Plasmodium ovale B53.Ø
poliovirial (nonparalytic) A8Ø.4
Pontiac A48.2
postimmunization R5Ø.83
postoperative R5Ø.82
due to infection T81.4Ø ☑
posttransfusion R5Ø.84
postvaccination R5Ø.83
presenting with conditions classified elsewhere R5Ø.81
pretibial A27.89
puerperal O86.4
Q A78
quadrilateral A78
quartan (malaria) B52.9
Queensland (coastal) (tick) A77.3
quintan A79.Ø
rabbit — *see* Tularemia
rat-bite A25.9
due to
Spirillum A25.Ø
Streptobacillus moniliformis A25.1
recurrent — *see* Fever, relapsing
relapsing (Borrelia) A68.9
Carter's (Asiatic) A68.1
Dutton's (West African) A68.1
Koch's A68.9
louse-borne A68.Ø
Novy's
louse-borne A68.Ø
tick-borne A68.1
Obermeyer's (European) A68.Ø
tick-borne A68.1
remittent (bilious) (congestive) (gastric) — *see* Malaria
rheumatic (active) (acute) (chronic) (subacute) IØØ
with central nervous system involvement IØ2.9

☑ Additional Character Required — Refer to the Tabular List for Character Selection

Fever — continued
  rheumatic — continued
    active with heart involvement — see category I01 ✓
    inactive or quiescent with
      cardiac hypertrophy I09.89
      carditis I09.9
      endocarditis I09.1
        aortic (valve) I06.9
          with mitral (valve) disease I08.0
        mitral (valve) I05.9
          with aortic (valve) disease I08.0
        pulmonary (valve) I09.89
        tricuspid (valve) I07.8
      heart disease NEC I09.89
      heart failure (congestive) (conditions in category I50.) I09.81
      left ventricular failure (conditions in I50.1-I50.4-) I09.81
      myocarditis, myocardial degeneration (conditions in I51.4) I09.0
      pancarditis I09.9
      pericarditis I09.2
  Rift Valley (viral) A92.4
  Rocky Mountain spotted A77.0
  rose J30.1
  Ross River B33.1
  Russian hemorrhagic A98.5
  San Joaquin (Valley) B38.0
  sandfly A93.1
  Sao Paulo A77.0
  scarlet A38.9
  seven day (leptospirosis) (autumnal) (Japanese) A27.89
    dengue A90
  shin-bone A79.0
  Singapore hemorrhagic A91
  solar A90
  Songo A98.5
  sore B00.1
  South African tick-bite A68.1
  Southeast Asia hemorrhagic A91
  spinal — see Meningitis
  spirillary A25.0
  splenic — see Anthrax
  spotted A77.9
    American A77.0
    Brazilian A77.0
    cerebrospinal meningitis A39.0
    Colombian A77.0
    due to Rickettsia
      africae (African tick bite fever) A77.8
      australis A77.3
      conorii A77.1
      parkeri A77.8
      rickettsii A77.0
      sibirica A77.2
      specified type NEC A77.8
    Ehrlichiosis A77.40
      due to
        E. chaffeensis A77.41
        specified organism NEC A77.49
    Rocky Mountain A77.0
  steroid R50.2
  streptobacillary A25.1
  subtertian B50.9
  Sumatran mite A75.3
  sun A90
  swamp A27.9
  swine A02.8
  sylvatic, yellow A95.0
  Tahyna B33.8
  tertian — see Malaria, tertian
  Thailand hemorrhagic A91
  thermic T67.01 ✓
  three-day A93.1
  tick
    American mountain A93.2
    Colorado A93.2
    Kemerovo A93.8
    Mediterranean A77.1
    mountain A93.2
    nonexanthematous A93.2
    Quaranfil A93.8
  tick-bite NEC A93.8
  tick-borne (hemorrhagic) NEC A93.8
  trench A79.0
  tsutsugamushi A75.3
  typhogastric A01.00
  typhoid (abortive) (hemorrhagic) (intermittent) (malignant) A01.00

Fever — continued
  typhoid — continued
    complicated by
      arthritis A01.04
      heart involvement A01.02
      meningitis A01.01
      osteomyelitis A01.05
      pneumonia A01.03
      specified NEC A01.09
  typhomalarial — see Malaria
  typhus — see Typhus (fever)
  undulant — see Brucellosis
  unknown origin R50.9
  uveoparotid D86.89
  valley B38.0
  Venezuelan equine A92.2
  vesicular stomatitis A93.8
  viral hemorrhagic — see Fever, hemorrhagic, by type of virus
  Volhynian A79.0
  Wesselsbron (viral) A92.8
  West
    African B50.8
    Nile (viral) A92.30
      with
        complications NEC A92.39
        cranial nerve disorders A92.32
        encephalitis A92.31
        encephalomyelitis A92.31
        neurologic manifestation NEC A92.32
        optic neuritis A92.32
        polyradiculitis A92.32
  Whitmore's — see Melioidosis
  Wolhynian A79.0
  worm B83.9
  yellow A95.9
    jungle A95.0
    sylvatic A95.0
    urban A95.1
  Zika virus A92.5
FFA (frontal fibrosing alopecia) L66.12
Fibrillation
  atrial or auricular (established) I48.91
    chronic I48.20
      persistent I48.19
    paroxysmal I48.0
    permanent I48.21
    persistent (chronic) (NOS) (other) I48.19
      longstanding I48.11
  cardiac I49.8
  heart I49.8
  muscular M62.89
  ventricular I49.01
Fibrin
  ball or bodies, pleural (sac) J94.1
  chamber, anterior (eye) (gelatinous exudate) — see Iridocyclitis, acute
Fibrinogenolysis — see Fibrinolysis
Fibrinogenopenia D68.8
  acquired D65
  congenital D68.2
Fibrinolysis (hemorrhagic) (acquired) D65
  antepartum hemorrhage — see Hemorrhage, antepartum, with coagulation defect
  following
    abortion — see Abortion by type complicated by hemorrhage
    ectopic or molar pregnancy O08.1
  intrapartum O67.0
  newborn, transient P60
  postpartum O72.3
Fibrinopenia (hereditary) D68.2
  acquired D68.4
Fibrinopurulent — see condition
Fibrinous — see condition
Fibroadenoma
  cellular intracanalicular D24- ✓
  giant D24- ✓
  intracanalicular
    cellular D24- ✓
    giant D24- ✓
    specified site — see Neoplasm, benign, by site
    unspecified site D24- ✓
  juvenile D24- ✓
  pericanalicular
    specified site — see Neoplasm, benign, by site
    unspecified site D24- ✓
  phyllodes D24- ✓

Fibroadenoma — continued
  prostate D29.1
  specified site NEC — see Neoplasm, benign, by site
  unspecified site D24- ✓
Fibroadenosis, breast (chronic) (cystic) (diffuse) (periodic) (segmental) N60.2- ✓
Fibroangioma — see also Neoplasm, benign, by site
  juvenile
    specified site — see Neoplasm, benign, by site
    unspecified site D10.6
Fibrochondrosarcoma — see Neoplasm, cartilage, malignant
Fibrocystic
  disease — see also Fibrosis, cystic
    breast — see Mastopathy, cystic
    jaw M27.49
    kidney (congenital) Q61.8
    liver Q44.6
    pancreas E84.9
  kidney (congenital) Q61.8
Fibrodysplasia ossificans progressiva — see Myositis, ossificans, progressiva
Fibroelastosis (cordis) (endocardial) (endomyocardial) I42.4
Fibroid (tumor) — see also Neoplasm, connective tissue, benign
  disease, lung (chronic) — see Fibrosis, lung
  heart (disease) — see Myocarditis
  in pregnancy or childbirth O34.1- ✓
    causing obstructed labor O65.5
  induration, lung (chronic) — see Fibrosis, lung
  lung — see Fibrosis, lung
  pneumonia (chronic) — see Fibrosis, lung
  uterus — see also Leiomyoma, uterus D25.9
Fibrolipoma — see Lipoma
Fibroliposarcoma — see Neoplasm, connective tissue, malignant
Fibroma — see also Neoplasm, connective tissue, benign
  ameloblastic — see Cyst, calcifying odontogenic
  bone (nonossifying) — see Disorder, bone, specified type NEC
    ossifying — see Neoplasm, bone, benign
  cementifying — see Neoplasm, bone, benign
  chondromyxoid — see Neoplasm, bone, benign
  desmoplastic — see Neoplasm, connective tissue, uncertain behavior
  durum — see Neoplasm, connective tissue, benign
  fascial — see Neoplasm, connective tissue, benign
  invasive — see Neoplasm, connective tissue, uncertain behavior
  molle — see Lipoma
  myxoid — see Neoplasm, connective tissue, benign
  nasopharynx, nasopharyngeal (juvenile) D10.6
  nonosteogenic (nonossifying) — see Dysplasia, fibrous
  odontogenic (central) — see Cyst, calcifying odontogenic
  ossifying — see Neoplasm, bone, benign
  periosteal — see Neoplasm, bone, benign
  soft — see Lipoma
Fibromatosis M72.9
  abdominal — see Neoplasm, connective tissue, uncertain behavior
  aggressive — see Neoplasm, connective tissue, uncertain behavior
  congenital generalized — see Neoplasm, connective tissue, uncertain behavior
  Dupuytren's M72.0
  gingival K06.1
  palmar (fascial) M72.0
  plantar (fascial) M72.2
  pseudosarcomatous (proliferative) (subcutaneous) M72.4
  retroperitoneal D48.3
  specified NEC M72.8
Fibromyalgia M79.7
Fibromyoma — see also Neoplasm, connective tissue, benign
  uterus (corpus) — see also Leiomyoma, uterus
    in pregnancy or childbirth — see Fibroid, in pregnancy or childbirth
      causing obstructed labor O65.5
Fibromyositis M79.7
Fibromyxolipoma D17.9
Fibromyxoma — see Neoplasm, connective tissue, benign
Fibromyxosarcoma — see Neoplasm, connective tissue, malignant
Fibro-odontoma, ameloblastic — see Cyst, calcifying odontogenic
Fibro-osteoma — see Neoplasm, bone, benign
Fibroplasia, retrolental H35.17- ✓
Fibropurulent — see condition

✓ **Additional Character Required — Refer to the Tabular List for Character Selection**

Fibrosarcoma — *see also* Neoplasm, connective tissue, malignant
  ameloblastic C41.1
    upper jaw (bone) C41.0
  congenital — *see* Neoplasm, connective tissue, malignant
  fascial — *see* Neoplasm, connective tissue, malignant
  infantile — *see* Neoplasm, connective tissue, malignant
  odontogenic C41.1
    upper jaw (bone) C41.0
  periosteal — *see* Neoplasm, bone, malignant
Fibrosclerosis
  breast N60.3- ☑
  multifocal M35.5
  penis (corpora cavernosa) N48.6
Fibrosis, fibrotic
  adrenal (gland) E27.8
  amnion O41.8X- ☑
  anal papillae K62.89
  arteriocapillary — *see* Arteriosclerosis
  bladder N32.89
    interstitial — *see* Cystitis, chronic, interstitial
    localized submucosal — *see* Cystitis, chronic, interstitial
    panmural — *see* Cystitis, chronic, interstitial
  breast — *see* Fibrosclerosis, breast
  capillary — *see also* Arteriosclerosis I70.90
    lung (chronic) — *see* Fibrosis, lung
  cardiac — *see* Myocarditis
  cervix N88.8
  chorion O41.8X- ☑
  corpus cavernosum (sclerosing) N48.6
  cystic (of pancreas) E84.9
    with
      distal intestinal obstruction syndrome E84.19
      fecal impaction E84.19
      intestinal manifestations NEC E84.19
      pulmonary manifestations E84.0
      specified manifestations NEC E84.8
  due to device, implant or graft — *see also* Complications, by site and type, specified NEC T85.828 ☑
    arterial graft NEC T82.828 ☑
    breast (implant) T85.828 ☑
    catheter NEC T85.828 ☑
      dialysis (renal) T82.828 ☑
        intraperitoneal T85.828 ☑
      infusion NEC T82.828 ☑
        spinal (epidural) (subdural) T85.820 ☑
      urinary (indwelling) T83.82 ☑
    electronic (electrode) (pulse generator) (stimulator)
      bone T84.82 ☑
      cardiac T82.827 ☑
      nervous system (brain) (peripheral nerve) (spinal) T85.820 ☑
      urinary T83.82 ☑
    fixation, internal (orthopedic) NEC T84.82 ☑
    gastrointestinal (bile duct) (esophagus) T85.828 ☑
    genital NEC T83.82 ☑
    heart NEC T82.827 ☑
    joint prosthesis T84.82 ☑
    ocular (corneal graft) (orbital implant) NEC T85.828 ☑
    orthopedic NEC T84.82 ☑
    specified NEC T85.828 ☑
    urinary NEC T83.82 ☑
    vascular NEC T82.828 ☑
    ventricular intracranial shunt T85.820 ☑
  ejaculatory duct N50.89
  endocardium — *see* Endocarditis
  endomyocardial (tropical) I42.3
  epididymis N50.89
  eye muscle — *see* Strabismus, mechanical
  heart — *see* Myocarditis
  hepatic — *see* Fibrosis, liver
  hepatolienal (portal hypertension) K76.6
  hepatosplenic (portal hypertension) K76.6
  infrapatellar fat pad M79.4
  intrascrotal N50.89
  kidney N26.9
  liver K74.00
    with sclerosis K74.2
      advanced K74.02
      alcoholic K70.2
      early K74.01
    stage
      F1 or F2 K74.01
      F3 K74.02
  lung (atrophic) (chronic) (confluent) (massive) (perialveolar) (peribronchial) J84.10

Fibrosis, fibrotic — *continued*
  lung — *continued*
    with
      anthracosilicosis J60
      anthracosis J60
      asbestosis J61
      bagassosis J67.1
      bauxite J63.1
      berylliosis J63.2
      byssinosis J66.0
      calcicosis J62.8
      chalicosis J62.8
      dust reticulation J64
      farmer's lung J67.0
      ganister disease J62.8
      graphite J63.3
      pneumoconiosis NOS J64
      siderosis J63.4
      silicosis J62.8
    capillary J84.10
    congenital P27.8
    diffuse (idiopathic) J84.10
      chemicals, gases, fumes or vapors (inhalation) — *see also* Disease, respiratory, chronic, due to chemicals, gases, fumes or vapors J84.10
    interstitial J84.10
      acute J84.114
    talc J62.0
    following radiation J70.1
    idiopathic J84.112
    postinflammatory J84.10
    silicotic J62.8
    tuberculous — *see* Tuberculosis, pulmonary
  lymphatic gland I89.8
  median bar — *see* Hyperplasia, prostate
  mediastinum (idiopathic) J98.59
  meninges G96.198
  myocardium, myocardial — *see* Myocarditis
  ovary N83.8
  oviduct N83.8
  pancreas K86.89
  penis NEC N48.6
  pericardium I31.0
  perineum, in pregnancy or childbirth O34.7- ☑
    causing obstructed labor O65.5
  pleura J94.1
  popliteal fat pad M79.4
  prostate (chronic) — *see* Hyperplasia, prostate
  pulmonary — *see also* Fibrosis, lung J84.10
    congenital P27.8
    idiopathic J84.112
  rectal sphincter K62.89
  retroperitoneal K68.2
    with infection N13.6
    idiopathic (with ureteral obstruction) N13.5
  sclerosing mesenteric (idiopathic) K65.4
  scrotum N50.89
  seminal vesicle N50.89
  senile R54
  skin L90.5
  spermatic cord N50.89
  spleen D73.89
    in schistosomiasis (bilharziasis) B65.9 *[D77]*
  subepidermal nodular — *see* Neoplasm, skin, benign
  submucous (oral) (tongue) K13.5
  testis N44.8
    chronic, due to syphilis A52.76
  thymus (gland) E32.8
  tongue, submucous K13.5
  tunica vaginalis N50.89
  uterus (non-neoplastic) N85.8
  vagina N89.8
  valve, heart — *see* Endocarditis
  vas deferens N50.89
  vein I87.8
Fibrositis (periarticular) M79.7
  nodular, chronic (Jaccoud's) (rheumatoid) — *see* Arthropathy, postrheumatic, chronic
Fibrothorax J94.1
Fibrotic — *see* Fibrosis
Fibrous — *see* condition
Fibroxanthoma — *see also* Neoplasm, connective tissue, benign
  atypical — *see* Neoplasm, connective tissue, uncertain behavior
  malignant — *see* Neoplasm, connective tissue, malignant
Fibroxanthosarcoma — *see* Neoplasm, connective tissue, malignant

Fiedler's
  disease (icterohemorrhagic leptospirosis) A27.0
  myocarditis (acute) I40.1
Fifth disease B08.3
  venereal A55
Filaria, filarial, filariasis — *see* Infestation, filarial
Filatov's disease — *see* Mononucleosis, infectious
File-cutter's disease — *see* Poisoning, lead
Filling defect
  biliary tract R93.2
  bladder R93.41
  duodenum R93.3
  gallbladder R93.2
  gastrointestinal tract R93.3
  intestine R93.3
  kidney R93.42- ☑
  stomach R93.3
  ureter R93.41
  urinary organs, specified NEC R93.49
Fimbrial cyst Q50.4
Financial problem affecting care NOS Z59.9
  bankruptcy Z59.89
  foreclosure on loan Z59.89
    home loan Z59.81- ☑
  strain Z59.86
Findings, abnormal, inconclusive, without diagnosis — *see also* Abnormal
  17-ketosteroids, elevated R82.5
  acetonuria R82.4
  alcohol in blood R78.0
  anisocytosis R71.8
  antenatal screening of mother O28.9
    biochemical O28.1
    chromosomal O28.5
    cytological O28.2
    genetic O28.5
    hematological O28.0
    radiological O28.4
    specified NEC O28.8
    ultrasonic O28.3
  antibody titer, elevated R76.0
  anticardiolipin antibody R76.0
  antiphosphatidylglycerol antibody R76.0
  antiphosphatidylinositol antibody R76.0
  antiphosphatidylserine antibody R76.0
  antiphospholipid antibody R76.0
  bacteriuria R82.71
  bicarbonate E87.8
  bile in urine R82.2
  blood sugar R73.09
    high R73.9
    low (transient) E16.2
  body fluid or substance, specified NEC R88.8
  casts, urine R82.998
  catecholamines R82.5
  cells, urine R82.998
  chloride E87.8
  cholesterol E78.9
    high E78.00
      with high triglycerides E78.2
  chyluria R82.0
  cloudy
    dialysis effluent R88.0
    urine R82.90
  creatinine clearance R94.4
  crystals, urine R82.998
  culture
    blood R78.81
    positive — *see* Positive, culture
  echocardiogram R93.1
  electrolyte level, urinary R82.998
  function study NEC R94.8
    bladder R94.8
    endocrine NEC R94.7
      thyroid R94.6
    kidney R94.4
    liver R94.5
    pancreas R94.8
    placenta R94.8
    pulmonary R94.2
    spleen R94.8
  gallbladder, nonvisualization R93.2
  glucose (tolerance test) (non-fasting) R73.09
  glycosuria R81
  heart
    shadow R93.1
    sounds R01.2
  hematinuria R82.3
  hematocrit drop (precipitous) R71.0

Fistula — *continued*
  cervical, lateral Q18.1
  cervicoaural Q18.1
  cervicosigmoidal N82.4
  cervicovesical N82.1
  cervix N82.8
  chest (wall) J86.0
  cholecystenteric — *see* Fistula, gallbladder
  cholecystocolic — *see* Fistula, gallbladder
  cholecystocolonic — *see* Fistula, gallbladder
  cholecystoduodenal — *see* Fistula, gallbladder
  cholecystogastric — *see* Fistula, gallbladder
  cholecystointestinal — *see* Fistula, gallbladder
  choledochoduodenal — *see* Fistula, bile duct
  cholocolic K82.3
  coccyx — *see* Sinus, pilonidal
  colon K63.2
  colostomy K94.09
  colovesical N32.1
  common duct — *see* Fistula, bile duct
  congenital, site not listed — *see* Anomaly, by site
  coronary, arteriovenous I25.41
    congenital Q24.5
  costal region J86.0
  cul-de-sac, Douglas' N82.8
  cystic duct — *see also* Fistula, gallbladder
    congenital Q44.5
  dental K04.6
  diaphragm J86.0
  duodenum K31.6
  ear (external) (canal) — *see* Disorder, ear, external,
    specified type NEC
  enterocolic K63.2
  enterocutaneous K63.2
  enterouterine N82.4
    congenital Q51.7
  enterovaginal N82.4
    congenital Q52.2
    large intestine N82.3
    small intestine N82.2
  enterovesical N32.1
  epididymis N50.89
    tuberculous A18.15
  esophagobronchial J86.0
    congenital Q39.2
      with atresia of esophagus Q39.1
  esophagocutaneous K22.89
  esophagopleural-cutaneous J86.0
  esophagotracheal J86.0
    congenital Q39.2
      with atresia of esophagus Q39.1
  esophagus K22.89
    congenital Q39.2
      with atresia of esophagus Q39.1
  ethmoid — *see* Sinusitis, ethmoidal
  eyeball (cornea) (sclera) — *see* Disorder, globe, hypotony
  eyelid H01.8
  fallopian tube, external N82.5
  fecal K63.2
    congenital Q43.6
  from periapical abscess K04.6
  frontal sinus — *see* Sinusitis, frontal
  gallbladder K82.3
    with calculus, cholelithiasis, stones — *see* Calculus,
      gallbladder
  gastric K31.6
  gastrocolic K31.6
    congenital Q40.2
    tuberculous A18.32
  gastroenterocolic K31.6
  gastroesophageal K31.6
  gastrojejunal K31.6
  gastrojejunocolic K31.6
  genital tract (female) N82.9
    specified NEC N82.8
    to intestine NEC N82.4
    to skin N82.5
  hepatic artery-portal vein, congenital Q26.6
  hepatopleural J86.0
  hepatopulmonary J86.0
  ileorectal or ileosigmoidal K63.2
  ileovaginal N82.2
  ileovesical N32.1
  ileum K63.2
  in ano K60.30
    tuberculous A18.32
  inner ear (labyrinth) — *see* subcategory H83.1 ☑
  intestine NEC K63.2
  intestinocolonic (abdominal) K63.2

Fistula — *continued*
  intestinoureteral N28.89
  intestinouterine N82.4
  intestinovaginal N82.4
    large intestine N82.3
    small intestine N82.2
  intestinovesical N32.1
  ischiorectal (fossa) K61.39
  jejunum K63.2
  joint M25.10
    ankle M25.17- ☑
    elbow M25.12- ☑
    foot joint M25.17- ☑
    hand joint M25.14- ☑
    hip M25.15- ☑
    knee M25.16- ☑
    shoulder M25.11- ☑
    specified joint NEC M25.18
    tuberculous — *see* Tuberculosis, joint
    vertebrae M25.18
    wrist M25.13- ☑
  kidney N28.89
  labium (majus) (minus) N82.8
  labyrinth — *see* subcategory H83.1 ☑
  lacrimal (gland) (sac) H04.61- ☑
  lacrimonasal duct — *see* Fistula, lacrimal
  laryngotracheal, congenital Q34.8
  larynx J38.7
  lip K13.0
    congenital Q38.0
  lumbar, tuberculous A18.01
  lung J86.0
  lymphatic I89.8
  mammary (gland) N61.0
  mastoid (process) (region) — *see* Mastoiditis, chronic
  maxillary J32.0
  medial, face and neck Q18.8
  mediastinal J86.0
  mediastinobronchial J86.0
  mediastinocutaneous J86.0
  middle ear — *see* subcategory H74.8 ☑
  mouth K12.2
  nasal J34.89
    sinus — *see* Sinusitis
  nasopharynx J39.2
  nipple N64.0
  nose J34.89
  oral (cutaneous) K12.2
    maxillary J32.0
    nasal (with cleft palate) — *see* Cleft, palate
  orbit, orbital — *see* Disorder, orbit, specified type NEC
  oroantral J32.0
  oviduct, external N82.5
  palate (hard) M27.8
  pancreatic K86.89
  pancreaticoduodenal K86.89
  parotid (gland) K11.4
    region K12.2
  penis N48.89
  perianal K60.30
  pericardium (pleura) (sac) — *see* Pericarditis
  pericecal K63.2
  perineorectal K60.40
  perineosigmoidal K63.2
  perineum, perineal (with urethral involvement) NEC
    N36.0
    tuberculous A18.13
    ureter N28.89
  perirectal K60.40
    tuberculous A18.32
  peritoneum K65.9
  pharyngoesophageal J39.2
  pharynx J39.2
    branchial cleft (congenital) Q18.0
  pilonidal (infected) (rectum) — *see* Sinus, pilonidal
  pleura, pleural, pleurocutaneous, pleuroperitoneal J86.0
    tuberculous NEC A15.6
  pleuropericardial I31.8
  portal vein-hepatic artery, congenital Q26.6
  postauricular H70.81- ☑
  postoperative, persistent T81.83 ☑
    specified site — *see* Fistula, by site
  preauricular (congenital) Q18.1
  prostate N42.89
  pulmonary J86.0
    arteriovenous I28.0
      congenital Q25.72
    tuberculous — *see* Tuberculosis, pulmonary

Fistula — *continued*
  pulmonoperitoneal J86.0
  rectal (infectional) K60.40
    complex K60.429
      chronic K60.422
      initial K60.421
      new K60.421
      occurring following complete healing K60.423
      persistent K60.422
      recurrent K60.423
    extrasphincteric K60.42- ☑
    high intersphincteric K60.42- ☑
    low intersphincteric K60.41- ☑
    simple K60.419
      chronic K60.412
      initial K60.411
      new K60.411
      occurring following complete healing K60.413
      persistent K60.412
      recurrent K60.413
    superficial K60.41- ☑
    suprasphincteric K60.42- ☑
    transsphincteric K60.42- ☑
  rectolabial N82.4
  rectosigmoid (intercommunicating) K63.2
  rectoureteral N28.89
  rectourethral N36.0
    congenital Q64.73
  rectouterine N82.4
    congenital Q51.7
  rectovaginal N82.3
    congenital Q52.2
    tuberculous A18.18
  rectovesical N32.1
    congenital Q64.79
  rectovesicovaginal N82.3
  rectovulval N82.4
    congenital Q52.79
  rectum (to skin) K60.40
    congenital Q43.6
      with absence, atresia and stenosis Q42.0
    tuberculous A18.32
  renal N28.89
  retroauricular — *see* Fistula, postauricular
  salivary duct or gland (any) K11.4
    congenital Q38.4
  scrotum (urinary) N50.89
    tuberculous A18.15
  semicircular canals — *see* subcategory H83.1 ☑
  sigmoid K63.2
    to bladder N32.1
  sinus — *see* Sinusitis
  skin L98.8
    to genital tract (female) N82.5
  splenocolic D73.89
  stercoral K63.2
  stomach K31.6
  sublingual gland K11.4
  submandibular gland K11.4
  submaxillary (gland) K11.4
    region K12.2
  thoracic J86.0
    duct I89.8
  thoracoabdominal J86.0
  thoracogastric J86.0
  thoracointestinal J86.0
  thorax J86.0
  thyroglossal duct Q89.2
  thyroid E07.89
  trachea, congenital (external) (internal) Q32.1
  tracheoesophageal J86.0
    congenital Q39.2
      with atresia of esophagus Q39.1
    following tracheostomy J95.04
  traumatic arteriovenous — *see* Injury, blood vessel, by
    site
  tuberculous — *code by* site under Tuberculosis
  typhoid A01.09
  umbilicourinary Q64.8
  urachus, congenital Q64.4
  ureter (persistent) N28.89
  ureteroabdominal N28.89
  ureterorectal N28.89
  ureterosigmoido-abdominal N28.89
  ureterovaginal N82.1
  ureterovesical N32.2
  urethra N36.0
    congenital Q64.79

☑ **Additional Character Required** — **Refer to the Tabular List for Character Selection**

Fistula — *continued*
- urethra — *continued*
  - tuberculous A18.13
- urethroperineal N36.0
- urethroperineovesical N32.2
- urethrorectal N36.0
  - congenital Q64.73
- urethroscrotal N50.89
- urethrovaginal N82.1
- urethrovesical N32.2
- urinary (tract) (persistent) (recurrent) N36.0
- uteroabdominal N82.5
  - congenital Q51.7
- uteroenteric, uterointestinal N82.4
  - congenital Q51.7
- uterorectal N82.4
  - congenital Q51.7
- uteroureteric N82.1
- uteroourethral Q51.7
- uterovaginal N82.8
- uterovesical N82.1
  - congenital Q51.7
- uterus N82.8
- vagina (postpartal) (wall) N82.8
- vaginocutaneous (postpartal) N82.5
- vaginointestinal NEC N82.4
  - large intestine N82.3
  - small intestine N82.2
- vaginoperineal N82.5
- vasocutaneous, congenital Q55.7
- vesical NEC N32.2
- vesicoabdominal N32.2
- vesicocervicovaginal N82.1
- vesicocolic N32.1
- vesicocutaneous N32.2
- vesicoenteric N32.1
- vesicointestinal N32.1
- vesicometrorectal N82.4
- vesicoperineal N32.2
- vesicorectal N32.1
  - congenital Q64.79
- vesicosigmoidal N32.1
- vesicosigmoidovaginal N82.3
- vesicoureteral N32.2
- vesicoureterovaginal N82.1
- vesicourethral N32.2
- vesicourethrorectal N32.1
- vesicouterine N82.1
  - congenital Q51.7
- vesicovaginal N82.0
- vulvorectal N82.4
  - congenital Q52.79

Fit R56.9
- epileptic — *see* Epilepsy
- fainting R55
- hysterical F44.5
- newborn P90

Fitting (and adjustment) (of)
- artificial
  - arm — *see* Admission, adjustment, artificial, arm
  - breast Z44.3 ☑
  - eye Z44.2 ☑
  - leg — *see* Admission, adjustment, artificial, leg
- automatic implantable cardiac defibrillator (with synchronous cardiac pacemaker) Z45.02
- brain neuropacemaker Z46.2
  - implanted Z45.42
- cardiac defibrillator — *see* Fitting (and adjustment) (of), automatic implantable cardiac defibrillator
- catheter, non-vascular Z46.82
- colostomy belt Z46.89
- contact lenses Z46.0
- CRT-D (resynchronization therapy defibrillator) Z45.02
- CRT-P (cardiac resynchronization therapy pacemaker) Z45.018
  - pulse generator Z45.010
- cystostomy device Z46.6
- defibrillator, cardiac — *see* Fitting (and adjustment) (of), automatic implantable cardiac defibrillator
- dentures Z46.3
- device NOS Z46.9
  - abdominal Z46.89
  - gastrointestinal NEC Z46.59
  - implanted NEC Z45.89
  - nervous system Z46.2
    - implanted — *see* Admission, adjustment, device, implanted, nervous system
  - orthodontic Z46.4
  - orthoptic Z46.0

Fitting — *continued*
- device — *continued*
  - orthotic Z46.89
  - prosthetic (external) Z44.9
    - breast Z44.3 ☑
    - dental Z46.3
    - eye Z44.2 ☑
    - specified NEC Z44.8
  - specified NEC Z46.89
  - substitution
    - auditory Z46.2
      - implanted — *see* Admission, adjustment, device, implanted, hearing device
    - nervous system Z46.2
      - implanted — *see* Admission, adjustment, device, implanted, nervous system
    - visual Z46.2
      - implanted Z45.31
    - urinary Z46.6
  - gastric lap band Z46.51
  - gastrointestinal appliance NEC Z46.59
  - glasses (reading) Z46.0
  - hearing aid Z46.1
  - ileostomy device Z46.89
  - insulin pump Z46.81
  - intestinal appliance NEC Z46.89
  - myringotomy device (stent) (tube) Z45.82
  - neuropacemaker Z46.2
    - implanted Z45.42
  - non-vascular catheter Z46.82
  - orthodontic device Z46.4
  - orthopedic device (brace) (cast) (corset) (shoes) Z46.89
  - pacemaker (cardiac) (cardiac resynchronization therapy (CRT-P)) Z45.018
    - nervous system (brain) (peripheral nerve) (spinal cord) Z46.2
      - implanted Z45.42
    - pulse generator Z45.010
  - portacath (port-a-cath) Z45.2
  - prosthesis (external) Z44.9
    - arm — *see* Admission, adjustment, artificial, arm
    - breast Z44.3 ☑
    - dental Z46.3
    - eye Z44.2 ☑
    - leg — *see* Admission, adjustment, artificial, leg
    - specified NEC Z44.8
  - spectacles Z46.0
  - wheelchair Z46.89

Fitzhugh-Curtis syndrome
- due to
  - Chlamydia trachomatis A74.81
  - Neisseria gonorrhea (gonococcal peritonitis) A54.85

Fitz's syndrome (acute hemorrhagic pancreatitis) — *see also* Pancreatitis, acute K85.80

Fixation
- joint — *see* Ankylosis
- larynx J38.7
- stapes — *see* Ankylosis, ear ossicles
  - deafness — *see* Deafness, conductive
- uterus (acquired) — *see* Malposition, uterus
- vocal cord J38.3

Flabby ridge K06.8

Flaccid — *see also* condition
- palate, congenital Q38.5

Flail
- chest S22.5 ☑
  - associated with chest compression and cardiopulmonary resuscitation M96.A4
  - newborn (birth injury) P13.8
- joint (paralytic) M25.20
  - ankle M25.27- ☑
  - elbow M25.22- ☑
  - foot joint M25.27- ☑
  - hand joint M25.24- ☑
  - hip M25.25- ☑
  - knee M25.26- ☑
  - shoulder M25.21- ☑
  - specified joint NEC M25.28
  - wrist M25.23- ☑

Flajani's disease — *see* Hyperthyroidism, with, goiter (diffuse)

Flap, liver K71.3

Flashbacks (residual to hallucinogen use) F16.283

Flat
- affect R45.89
- chamber (eye) — *see* Disorder, globe, hypotony, flat anterior chamber
- chest, congenital Q67.8

Flat — *continued*
- foot (acquired) (fixed type) (painful) (postural) — *see also* Deformity, limb, flat foot
  - congenital (rigid) (spastic (everted)) Q66.5- ☑
  - rachitic sequelae (late effect) E64.3
- organ or site, congenital NEC — *see* Anomaly, by site
- pelvis M95.5
  - with disproportion (fetopelvic) O33.0
    - causing obstructed labor O65.0
  - congenital Q74.2

Flatau-Schilder disease G37.0

Flatback syndrome M40.30
- lumbar region M40.36
- lumbosacral region M40.37
- thoracolumbar region M40.35

Flattening
- head, femur M89.8X5
- hip — *see* Coxa, plana
- lip (congenital) Q18.8
- nose (congenital) Q67.4
  - acquired M95.0

Flatulence R14.3
- psychogenic F45.8

Flatus R14.3
- vaginalis N89.8

Flax-dresser's disease J66.1

Flea bite — *see* Injury, bite, by site, superficial, insect

Flecks, glaucomatous (subcapsular) — *see* Cataract, complicated

Fleischer (-Kayser) **ring** (cornea) H18.04- ☑

Fleshy mole O02.0

Flexibilitas cerea — *see* Catalepsy

Flexion
- amputation stump (surgical) T87.89
- cervix — *see* Malposition, uterus
- contracture, joint — *see* Contraction, joint
- deformity, joint — *see also* Deformity, limb, flexion M21.20
  - hip, congenital Q65.89
- uterus — *see also* Malposition, uterus
  - lateral — *see* Lateroversion, uterus

Flexner-Boyd dysentery A03.2

Flexner's dysentery A03.1

Flexure — *see* Flexion

Flint murmur (aortic insufficiency) I35.1

Floater, vitreous — *see* Opacity, vitreous

Floating
- cartilage (joint) — *see also* Loose, body, joint
  - knee — *see* Derangement, knee, loose body
- gallbladder, congenital Q44.1
- kidney N28.89
  - congenital Q63.8
- spleen D73.89

Flooding N92.0

Floor — *see* condition

Floppy
- baby syndrome (nonspecific) P94.2
- iris syndrome (intraoperative) (IFIS) H21.81
- nonrheumatic mitral valve syndrome I34.1

Flu — *see also* Influenza
- avian — *see also* Influenza, due to, identified novel influenza A virus J09.X2
- bird — *see also* Influenza, due to, identified novel influenza A virus J09.X2
- intestinal NEC A08.4
- swine (viruses that normally cause infections in pigs) — *see also* Influenza, due to, identified novel influenza A virus J09.X2

Fluctuating blood pressure I99.8

Fluid
- abdomen R18.8
- chest J94.8
- heart — *see* Failure, heart, congestive
- joint — *see* Effusion, joint
- loss (acute) E86.9
- lung — *see* Edema, lung
- overload E87.70
  - specified NEC E87.79
- peritoneal cavity R18.8
- pleural cavity J94.8
- retention R60.9

Flukes NEC — *see also* Infestation, fluke
- blood NEC — *see* Schistosomiasis
- liver B66.3

Fluor (vaginalis) N89.8
- trichomonal or due to Trichomonas (vaginalis) A59.00

Fluorosis
- dental K00.3
- skeletal M85.10

Fluorosis — *continued*
  skeletal — *continued*
    ankle M85.17- ☑
    foot M85.17- ☑
    forearm M85.13- ☑
    hand M85.14- ☑
    lower leg M85.16- ☑
    multiple site M85.19
    neck M85.18
    rib M85.18
    shoulder M85.11- ☑
    skull M85.18
    specified site NEC M85.18
    thigh M85.15- ☑
    toe M85.17- ☑
    upper arm M85.12- ☑
    vertebra M85.18
Flush syndrome E34.09
Flushing R23.2
  menopausal N95.1
Flutter
  atrial or auricular I48.92
    atypical I48.4
    type I I48.3
    type II I48.4
    typical I48.3
  heart I49.8
    atrial or auricular I48.92
      atypical I48.4
      type I I48.3
      type II I48.4
      typical I48.3
    ventricular I49.02
  ventricular I49.02
FNHTR (febrile nonhemolytic transfusion reaction) R50.84
Fochier's abscess — *code by* site under Abscess
Focus, Assmann's — *see* Tuberculosis, pulmonary
Fogo selvagem L10.3
Foix-Alajouanine syndrome G95.19
Fold, folds (anomalous) — *see also* Anomaly, by site
  Descemet's membrane — *see* Change, corneal membrane, Descemet's, fold
  epicanthic Q10.3
  heart Q24.8
Folie a deux F24
Follicle
  cervix (nabothian) (ruptured) N88.8
  graafian, ruptured, with hemorrhage N83.0- ☑
  nabothian N88.8
Follicular — *see* condition
Folliculitis (superficial) L73.9
  abscedens et suffodiens L66.3
  cyst N83.0- ☑
  decalvans L66.2
  deep — *see* Furuncle, by site
  gonococcal (acute) (chronic) A54.01
  keloid, keloidalis L73.0
  pustular L01.02
  ulerythematosa reticulata L66.4
Folliculome lipidique
  specified site — *see* Neoplasm, benign, by site
  unspecified site
    female D27.9
    male D29.20
Følling's disease E70.0
Follow-up — *see* Examination, follow-up
Fong's syndrome (hereditary osteo-onychodysplasia) Q87.2
Food
  allergy L27.2
  asphyxia (from aspiration or inhalation) — *see* Foreign body, by site
  choked on — *see* Foreign body, by site
  deprivation T73.0 ☑
    specified kind of food NEC E63.8
  insecurity Z59.41
  intoxication — *see* Poisoning, food
  lack of T73.0 ☑
  poisoning — *see* Poisoning, food
  rejection NEC — *see* Disorder, eating
  strangulation or suffocation — *see* Foreign body, by site
  toxemia — *see* Poisoning, food
Foot — *see* condition
Foramen ovale (nonclosure) (patent) (persistent) Q21.12
Forbes' glycogen storage disease E74.03
Fordyce-Fox disease L75.2
Fordyce's disease (mouth) Q38.6
Forearm — *see* condition
Foreclosure on loan Z59.89

Foreign body
  with
    laceration — *see* Laceration, by site, with foreign body
    puncture wound — *see* Puncture, by site, with foreign body
  accidentally left following a procedure T81.509 ☑
    aspiration T81.506 ☑
      resulting in
        adhesions T81.516 ☑
        obstruction T81.526 ☑
        perforation T81.536 ☑
        specified complication NEC T81.596 ☑
    cardiac catheterization T81.505 ☑
      resulting in
        acute reaction T81.60 ☑
          aseptic peritonitis T81.61 ☑
          specified NEC T81.69 ☑
        adhesions T81.515 ☑
        obstruction T81.525 ☑
        perforation T81.535 ☑
        specified complication NEC T81.595 ☑
      causing
        acute reaction T81.60 ☑
          aseptic peritonitis T81.61 ☑
          specified complication NEC T81.69 ☑
        adhesions T81.519 ☑
        aseptic peritonitis T81.61 ☑
        obstruction T81.529 ☑
        perforation T81.539 ☑
        specified complication NEC T81.599 ☑
    endoscopy T81.504 ☑
      resulting in
        adhesions T81.514 ☑
        obstruction T81.524 ☑
        perforation T81.534 ☑
        specified complication NEC T81.594 ☑
    immunization T81.503 ☑
      resulting in
        adhesions T81.513 ☑
        obstruction T81.523 ☑
        perforation T81.533 ☑
        specified complication NEC T81.593 ☑
    infusion T81.501 ☑
      resulting in
        adhesions T81.511 ☑
        obstruction T81.521 ☑
        perforation T81.531 ☑
        specified complication NEC T81.591 ☑
    injection T81.503 ☑
      resulting in
        adhesions T81.513 ☑
        obstruction T81.523 ☑
        perforation T81.533 ☑
        specified complication NEC T81.593 ☑
    kidney dialysis T81.502 ☑
      resulting in
        adhesions T81.512 ☑
        obstruction T81.522 ☑
        perforation T81.532 ☑
        specified complication NEC T81.592 ☑
    packing removal T81.507 ☑
      resulting in
        acute reaction T81.60 ☑
          aseptic peritonitis T81.61 ☑
          specified NEC T81.69 ☑
        adhesions T81.517 ☑
        obstruction T81.527 ☑
        perforation T81.537 ☑
        specified complication NEC T81.597 ☑
    puncture T81.506 ☑
      resulting in
        adhesions T81.516 ☑
        obstruction T81.526 ☑
        perforation T81.536 ☑
        specified complication NEC T81.596 ☑
    specified procedure NEC T81.508 ☑
      resulting in
        acute reaction T81.60 ☑
          aseptic peritonitis T81.61 ☑
          specified NEC T81.69 ☑
        adhesions T81.518 ☑
        obstruction T81.528 ☑
        perforation T81.538 ☑
        specified complication NEC T81.598 ☑
    surgical operation T81.500 ☑

Foreign body — *continued*
  accidentally left following a procedure — *continued*
    surgical operation — *continued*
      resulting in
        acute reaction T81.60 ☑
          aseptic peritonitis T81.61 ☑
          specified NEC T81.69 ☑
        adhesions T81.510 ☑
        obstruction T81.520 ☑
        perforation T81.530 ☑
        specified complication NEC T81.590 ☑
    transfusion T81.501 ☑
      resulting in
        adhesions T81.511 ☑
        obstruction T81.521 ☑
        perforation T81.531 ☑
        specified complication NEC T81.591 ☑
  alimentary tract T18.9 ☑
    anus T18.5 ☑
    colon T18.4 ☑
    esophagus — *see* Foreign body, esophagus
    mouth T18.0 ☑
    multiple sites T18.8 ☑
    rectosigmoid (junction) T18.5 ☑
    rectum T18.5 ☑
    small intestine T18.3 ☑
    specified site NEC T18.8 ☑
    stomach T18.2 ☑
  anterior chamber (eye) S05.5- ☑
  auditory canal — *see* Foreign body, entering through orifice, ear
  bronchus T17.508 ☑
    causing
      asphyxiation T17.500 ☑
        food (bone) (seed) T17.520 ☑
        gastric contents (vomitus) T17.510 ☑
        specified NEC T17.590 ☑
      injury NEC T17.508 ☑
        food (bone) (seed) T17.528 ☑
        gastric contents (vomitus) T17.518 ☑
        specified type NEC T17.598 ☑
  canthus — *see* Foreign body, conjunctival sac
  ciliary body (eye) S05.5- ☑
  conjunctival sac T15.1- ☑
  cornea T15.0- ☑
  entering through orifice
    accessory sinus T17.0 ☑
    alimentary canal T18.9 ☑
      multiple parts T18.8 ☑
      specified part NEC T18.8 ☑
    alveolar process T18.0 ☑
    antrum (Highmore's) T17.0 ☑
    anus T18.5 ☑
    appendix T18.4 ☑
    auditory canal — *see* Foreign body, entering through orifice, ear
    auricle — *see* Foreign body, entering through orifice, ear
    bladder T19.1 ☑
    bronchioles — *see* Foreign body, respiratory tract, specified site NEC
    bronchus (main) — *see* Foreign body, bronchus
    buccal cavity T18.0 ☑
    canthus (inner) — *see* Foreign body, conjunctival sac
    cecum T18.4 ☑
    cervix (canal) (uteri) T19.3 ☑
    colon T18.4 ☑
    conjunctival sac — *see* Foreign body, conjunctival sac
    cornea — *see* Foreign body, cornea
    digestive organ or tract NOS T18.9 ☑
      multiple parts T18.8 ☑
      specified part NEC T18.8 ☑
    duodenum T18.3 ☑
    ear (external) T16.- ☑
    esophagus — *see* Foreign body, esophagus
    eye (external) NOS T15.9- ☑
      conjunctival sac — *see* Foreign body, conjunctival sac
      cornea — *see* Foreign body, cornea
      specified part NEC T15.8- ☑
    eyeball — *see also* Foreign body, entering through orifice, eye, specified part NEC
      with penetrating wound — *see* Puncture, eyeball
    eyelid — *see also* Foreign body, conjunctival sac

☑ **Additional Character Required** — **Refer to the Tabular List for Character Selection**

Fracture, pathological — *continued*
  due to — *continued*
    specified disease — *continued*
      tibia M84.66- ☑
      toe M84.67- ☑
      ulna M84.63- ☑
      vertebra M84.68 ☑
    femur M84.45- ☑
    fibula M84.46- ☑
    finger M84.44- ☑
    hip M84.459 ☑
    humerus M84.42- ☑
    ilium M84.454 ☑
    ischium M84.454 ☑
    joint prosthesis — *see* Complications, joint prosthesis, mechanical, breakdown, by site
      periprosthetic — *see* Fracture, pathological, periprosthetic
    metacarpus M84.44- ☑
    metatarsus M84.47- ☑
    neck M84.48 ☑
    pelvis M84.454 ☑
    periprosthetic M97.9 ☑
      ankle M97.2- ☑
      elbow M97.4- ☑
      finger M97.8 ☑
      hip M97.0- ☑
      knee M97.1- ☑
      other specified joint M97.8 ☑
      shoulder M97.3- ☑
      spinal joint M97.8 ☑
      toe joint M97.8 ☑
      wrist joint M97.8 ☑
    radius M84.43- ☑
    restorative material (dental) K08.539
      with loss of material K08.531
      without loss of material K08.530
    rib M84.48 ☑
    scapula M84.41- ☑
    skull M84.48 ☑
    tarsus M84.47- ☑
    tibia M84.46- ☑
    toe M84.47- ☑
    ulna M84.43- ☑
    vertebra M84.48 ☑

Fracture, traumatic (abduction) (adduction) (separation)
  — *see also* Fracture, pathological T14.8 ☑
  acetabulum S32.40- ☑
    column
      anterior (displaced) (iliopubic) S32.43- ☑
        nondisplaced S32.436
      posterior (displaced) (ilioischial) S32.443 ☑
        nondisplaced S32.44- ☑
    dome (displaced) S32.48- ☑
      nondisplaced S32.48 ☑
    specified NEC S32.49- ☑
    transverse (displaced) S32.45- ☑
      with associated posterior wall fracture (displaced) S32.46- ☑
        nondisplaced S32.46- ☑
      nondisplaced S32.45- ☑
    wall
      anterior (displaced) S32.41- ☑
        nondisplaced S32.41- ☑
      medial (displaced) S32.47- ☑
        nondisplaced S32.47- ☑
      posterior (displaced) S32.42- ☑
        with associated transverse fracture (displaced) S32.46- ☑
          nondisplaced S32.46- ☑
        nondisplaced S32.42- ☑
  acromion — *see* Fracture, scapula, acromial process
  ankle S82.899 ☑
    bimalleolar (displaced) S82.84- ☑
      nondisplaced S82.84- ☑
    lateral malleolus only (displaced) S82.6- ☑
      nondisplaced S82.6- ☑
    medial malleolus (displaced) S82.5- ☑
      associated with Maisonneuve's fracture — *see* Fracture, Maisonneuve's
      nondisplaced S82.5- ☑
    talus — *see* Fracture, tarsal, talus
    trimalleolar (displaced) S82.85- ☑
      nondisplaced S82.85- ☑
  arm (upper) — *see also* Fracture, humerus, shaft
    humerus — *see* Fracture, humerus

Fracture, traumatic — *continued*
  arm — *see also* Fracture, humerus, shaft — *continued*
    radius — *see* Fracture, radius
    ulna — *see* Fracture, ulna
  associated with chest compression and cardiopulmonary resuscitation M96.A9
  astragalus — *see* Fracture, tarsal, talus
  atlas — *see* Fracture, neck, cervical vertebra, first
  axis — *see* Fracture, neck, cervical vertebra, second
  back — *see* Fracture, vertebra
  Barton's — *see* Barton's fracture
  base of skull — *see* Fracture, skull, base
  basicervical (basal) (femoral) S72.0 ☑
  Bennett's — *see* Bennett's fracture
  bimalleolar — *see* Fracture, ankle, bimalleolar
  blow-out S02.3- ☑
  bone NEC T14.8 ☑
    birth injury P13.9
    following insertion of orthopedic implant, joint prosthesis or bone plate — *see* Fracture, following insertion of orthopedic implant, joint prosthesis or bone plate
    in (due to) neoplastic disease NEC — *see* Fracture, pathological, due to, neoplastic disease
    pathological (cause unknown) — *see* Fracture, pathological
  breast bone — *see* Fracture, sternum
  bucket handle (semilunar cartilage) — *see* Tear, meniscus
  buckle — *see* Fracture, by site, torus
  burst — *see* Fracture, traumatic, by site
  calcaneus — *see* Fracture, tarsal, calcaneus
  carpal bone(s) S62.10- ☑
    capitate (displaced) S62.13- ☑
      nondisplaced S62.13- ☑
    cuneiform — *see* Fracture, carpal bone, triquetrum
    hamate (body) (displaced) S62.143 ☑
      hook process (displaced) S62.15- ☑
        nondisplaced S62.15- ☑
      nondisplaced S62.14- ☑
    larger multangular — *see* Fracture, carpal bones, trapezium
    lunate (displaced) S62.12- ☑
      nondisplaced S62.12- ☑
    navicular S62.00- ☑
      distal pole (displaced) S62.01- ☑
        nondisplaced S62.01- ☑
      middle third (displaced) S62.02- ☑
        nondisplaced S62.02- ☑
      proximal third (displaced) S62.03- ☑
        nondisplaced S62.03- ☑
      volar tuberosity — *see* Fracture, carpal bones, navicular, distal pole
    os magnum — *see* Fracture, carpal bones, capitate
    pisiform (displaced) S62.16- ☑
      nondisplaced S62.16- ☑
    semilunar — *see* Fracture, carpal bones, lunate
    smaller multangular — *see* Fracture, carpal bones, trapezoid
    trapezium (displaced) S62.17- ☑
      nondisplaced S62.17- ☑
    trapezoid (displaced) S62.18- ☑
      nondisplaced S62.18- ☑
    triquetrum (displaced) S62.11- ☑
      nondisplaced S62.11- ☑
    unciform — *see* Fracture, carpal bones, hamate
  cervical — *see* Fracture, vertebra, cervical
  clavicle S42.00- ☑
    acromial end (displaced) S42.03- ☑
      nondisplaced S42.03- ☑
    birth injury P13.4
    lateral end — *see* Fracture, clavicle, acromial end
    shaft (displaced) S42.02- ☑
      nondisplaced S42.02- ☑
    sternal end (anterior) (displaced) S42.01- ☑
      nondisplaced S42.01- ☑
      posterior S42.01- ☑
  coccyx S32.2
  collapsed — *see* Collapse, vertebra
  collar bone — *see* Fracture, clavicle
  Colles' — *see* Colles' fracture
  coronoid process — *see* Fracture, ulna, upper end, coronoid process
  corpus cavernosum penis S39.840 ☑
  costochondral cartilage S23.41
  costochondral, costosternal junction — *see* Fracture, rib
  cranium — *see* Fracture, skull
  cricoid cartilage S12.8 ☑

Fracture, traumatic — *continued*
  cuboid (ankle) — *see* Fracture, tarsal, cuboid
  cuneiform
    foot — *see* Fracture, tarsal, cuneiform
    wrist — *see* Fracture, carpal, triquetrum
  delayed union — *see* Delay, union, fracture
  dental restorative material K08.539
    with loss of material K08.531
    without loss of material K08.530
  due to
    birth injury — *see* Birth, injury, fracture
    osteoporosis — *see* Osteoporosis, with fracture
  Dupuytren's — *see* Fracture, ankle, lateral malleolus
  elbow S42.40- ☑
  ethmoid (bone) (sinus) — *see* Fracture, skull, base
  face bone S02.92 ☑
  fatigue — *see also* Fracture, stress
    vertebra M48.40 ☑
      cervical region M48.42 ☑
      cervicothoracic region M48.43 ☑
      lumbar region M48.46 ☑
      lumbosacral region M48.47 ☑
      occipito-atlanto-axial region M48.41 ☑
      sacrococcygeal region M48.48 ☑
      thoracic region M48.44 ☑
      thoracolumbar region M48.45 ☑
  femur, femoral S72.9- ☑
    basicervical (basal) S72.0 ☑
    birth injury P13.2
    capital epiphyseal S79.01- ☑
    condyles, epicondyles — *see* Fracture, femur, lower end
    distal end — *see* Fracture, femur, lower end
    epiphysis
      head — *see* Fracture, femur, upper end, epiphysis
      lower — *see* Fracture, femur, lower end, epiphysis
      upper — *see* Fracture, femur, upper end, epiphysis
    following insertion of implant, prosthesis or plate M96.66- ☑
    head — *see* Fracture, femur, upper end, head
    intertrochanteric — *see* Fracture, femur, trochanteric
    intratrochanteric — *see* Fracture, femur, trochanteric
    lower end S72.40- ☑
      condyle (displaced) S72.41- ☑
        lateral (displaced) S72.42- ☑
          nondisplaced S72.42- ☑
        medial (displaced) S72.43- ☑
          nondisplaced S72.43- ☑
        nondisplaced S72.41- ☑
      epiphysis (displaced) S72.44- ☑
        nondisplaced S72.44- ☑
      physeal S79.10- ☑
        Salter-Harris
          Type I S79.11- ☑
          Type II S79.12- ☑
          Type III S79.13- ☑
          Type IV S79.14- ☑
        specified NEC S79.19- ☑
      specified NEC S72.49- ☑
      supracondylar (displaced) S72.45- ☑
        with intracondylar extension (displaced) S72.46- ☑
          nondisplaced S72.46- ☑
        nondisplaced S72.45- ☑
      torus S72.47- ☑
    neck — *see* Fracture, femur, upper end, neck
    pertrochanteric — *see* Fracture, femur, trochanteric
    shaft (lower third) (middle third) (upper third) S72.30- ☑
      comminuted (displaced) S72.35- ☑
        nondisplaced S72.35- ☑
      oblique (displaced) S72.33- ☑
        nondisplaced S72.33- ☑
      segmental (displaced) S72.36- ☑
        nondisplaced S72.36- ☑
      specified NEC S72.39- ☑
      spiral (displaced) S72.34- ☑
        nondisplaced S72.34- ☑
      transverse (displaced) S72.32- ☑
        nondisplaced S72.32- ☑
    specified site NEC — *see* subcategory S72.8 ☑
    subcapital S72.01- ☑
    subtrochanteric (region) (section) (displaced) S72.2- ☑
      nondisplaced S72.2- ☑
    transcervical — *see* Fracture, femur, midcervical

Fracture, traumatic — *continued*
  femur, femoral — *continued*
    transtrochanteric — *see* Fracture, femur, trochanteric
    trochanteric S72.10- ✓
      apophyseal (displaced) S72.13- ✓
        nondisplaced S72.13- ✓
      greater trochanter (displaced) S72.11- ✓
        nondisplaced S72.11- ✓
      intertrochanteric (displaced) S72.14- ✓
        nondisplaced S72.14- ✓
      lesser trochanter (displaced) S72.12- ✓
        nondisplaced S72.12- ✓
    upper end S72.00- ✓
      apophyseal (displaced) S72.13- ✓
        nondisplaced S72.13- ✓
      cervicotrochanteric — *see* Fracture, femur, upper end, neck, base
      epiphysis (displaced) S72.02- ✓
        nondisplaced S72.02- ✓
      head S72.05- ✓
        articular (displaced) S72.06- ✓
          nondisplaced S72.06- ✓
        specified NEC S72.09- ✓
      intertrochanteric (displaced) S72.14- ✓
        nondisplaced S72.14- ✓
      intracapsular S72.01- ✓
      midcervical (displaced) S72.03- ✓
        nondisplaced S72.03- ✓
      neck S72.00- ✓
        base (displaced) S72.04- ✓
          nondisplaced S72.04- ✓
        specified NEC S72.09- ✓
      pertrochanteric — *see* Fracture, femur, upper end, trochanteric
      physeal S79.00- ✓
        Salter-Harris type I S79.01- ✓
        specified NEC S79.09- ✓
      subcapital (displaced) S72.01- ✓
      subtrochanteric (displaced) S72.2- ✓
        nondisplaced S72.2- ✓
      transcervical — *see* Fracture, femur, upper end, midcervical
      trochanteric S72.10- ✓
        greater (displaced) S72.11- ✓
          nondisplaced S72.11- ✓
        lesser (displaced) S72.12- ✓
          nondisplaced S72.12- ✓
  fibula (shaft) (styloid) S82.40- ✓
    comminuted (displaced) S82.45- ✓
      nondisplaced S82.45- ✓
    following insertion of implant, prosthesis or plate M96.67- ✓
    involving ankle or malleolus — *see* Fracture, fibula, lateral malleolus
    lateral malleolus (displaced) S82.6- ✓
      nondisplaced S82.6- ✓
    lower end
      physeal S89.30- ✓
        Salter-Harris
          Type I S89.31- ✓
          Type II S89.32- ✓
        specified NEC S89.39- ✓
      specified NEC S82.83- ✓
      torus S82.82- ✓
    oblique (displaced) S82.43- ✓
      nondisplaced S82.43- ✓
    segmental (displaced) S82.46- ✓
      nondisplaced S82.46- ✓
    specified NEC S82.49- ✓
    spiral (displaced) S82.44- ✓
      nondisplaced S82.44- ✓
    transverse (displaced) S82.42- ✓
      nondisplaced S82.42- ✓
    upper end
      physeal S89.20- ✓
        Salter-Harris
          Type I S89.21- ✓
          Type II S89.22- ✓
        specified NEC S89.29- ✓
      specified NEC S82.83- ✓
      torus S82.81- ✓
  finger (except thumb) S62.60- ✓
    distal phalanx (displaced) S62.63- ✓
      nondisplaced S62.66- ✓
    index S62.60- ✓

Fracture, traumatic — *continued*
  finger — *continued*
    index — *continued*
      distal phalanx (displaced) S62.63- ✓
        nondisplaced S62.66- ✓
      middle phalanx (displaced) S62.62- ✓
        nondisplaced S62.65- ✓
      proximal phalanx (displaced) S62.61- ✓
        nondisplaced S62.64- ✓
    little S62.60- ✓
      distal phalanx (displaced) S62.63- ✓
        nondisplaced S62.66- ✓
      middle phalanx (displaced) S62.62- ✓
        nondisplaced S62.65- ✓
      proximal phalanx (displaced) S62.61- ✓
        nondisplaced S62.64- ✓
    middle S62.60- ✓
      distal phalanx (displaced) S62.63- ✓
        nondisplaced S62.66- ✓
      middle phalanx (displaced) S62.62- ✓
        nondisplaced S62.65- ✓
      proximal phalanx (displaced) S62.61- ✓
        nondisplaced S62.64- ✓
    middle phalanx (displaced) S62.62- ✓
      nondisplaced S62.65- ✓
    proximal phalanx (displaced) S62.61- ✓
      nondisplaced S62.64- ✓
    ring S62.60- ✓
      distal phalanx (displaced) S62.63- ✓
        nondisplaced S62.66- ✓
      middle phalanx (displaced) S62.62- ✓
        nondisplaced S62.65- ✓
      proximal phalanx (displaced) S62.61- ✓
        nondisplaced S62.64- ✓
    thumb — *see* Fracture, thumb
  following insertion (intraoperative) (postoperative) of orthopedic implant, joint prosthesis or bone plate M96.69
    femur M96.66- ✓
    fibula M96.67- ✓
    humerus M96.62- ✓
    pelvis M96.65
    radius M96.63- ✓
    specified bone NEC M96.69
    tibia M96.67- ✓
    ulna M96.63- ✓
  foot S92.90- ✓
    astragalus — *see* Fracture, tarsal, talus
    calcaneus — *see* Fracture, tarsal, calcaneus
    cuboid — *see* Fracture, tarsal, cuboid
    cuneiform — *see* Fracture, tarsal, cuneiform
    metatarsal — *see* Fracture, metatarsal
    navicular — *see* Fracture, tarsal, navicular
    sesamoid S92.81- ✓
    specified NEC S92.81- ✓
    talus — *see* Fracture, tarsal, talus
    tarsal — *see* Fracture, tarsal
    toe — *see* Fracture, toe
  forearm S52.9- ✓
    radius — *see* Fracture, radius
    ulna — *see* Fracture, ulna
  fossa (anterior) (middle) (posterior) S02.19 ✓
  fragility — *see* Fracture, pathological, due to osteoporosis
  frontal (bone) (skull) S02.0 ✓
    sinus S02.19 ✓
  glenoid (cavity) (scapula) — *see* Fracture, scapula, glenoid cavity
  greenstick — *see* Fracture, by site
  hallux — *see* Fracture, toe, great
  hand S62.9- ✓
    carpal — *see* Fracture, carpal bone
    finger (except thumb) — *see* Fracture, finger
    metacarpal — *see* Fracture, metacarpal
    navicular (scaphoid) (hand) — *see* Fracture, carpal bone, navicular
    thumb — *see* Fracture, thumb
  healed or old
    with complications — *code by* Nature of the complication
  heel bone — *see* Fracture, tarsal, calcaneus
  Hill-Sachs S42.29- ✓
  hip — *see* Fracture, femur, neck
  humerus S42.30- ✓
    anatomical neck — *see* Fracture, humerus, upper end
    articular process — *see* Fracture, humerus, lower end
    capitellum — *see* Fracture, humerus, lower end, condyle, lateral

Fracture, traumatic — *continued*
  humerus — *continued*
    distal end — *see* Fracture, humerus, lower end
    epiphysis
      lower — *see* Fracture, humerus, lower end, physeal
      upper — *see* Fracture, humerus, upper end, physeal
    external condyle — *see* Fracture, humerus, lower end, condyle, lateral
    following insertion of implant, prosthesis or plate M96.62- ✓
    great tuberosity — *see* Fracture, humerus, upper end, greater tuberosity
    intercondylar — *see* Fracture, humerus, lower end
    internal epicondyle — *see* Fracture, humerus, lower end, epicondyle, medial
    lesser tuberosity — *see* Fracture, humerus, upper end, lesser tuberosity
    lower end S42.40- ✓
      condyle
        lateral (displaced) S42.45- ✓
          nondisplaced S42.45- ✓
        medial (displaced) S42.46- ✓
          nondisplaced S42.46- ✓
      epicondyle
        lateral (displaced) S42.43- ✓
          nondisplaced S42.43- ✓
        medial (displaced) S42.44- ✓
          incarcerated S42.44- ✓
          nondisplaced S42.44- ✓
      physeal S49.10- ✓
        Salter-Harris
          Type I S49.11- ✓
          Type II S49.12- ✓
          Type III S49.13- ✓
          Type IV S49.14- ✓
        specified NEC S49.19- ✓
      specified NEC (displaced) S42.49- ✓
        nondisplaced S42.49- ✓
      supracondylar (simple) (displaced) S42.41- ✓
        with intercondylar fracture — *see* Fracture, humerus, lower end
        comminuted (displaced) S42.42- ✓
          nondisplaced S42.42- ✓
        nondisplaced S42.41- ✓
      torus S42.48- ✓
      transcondylar (displaced) S42.47- ✓
        nondisplaced S42.47- ✓
    proximal end — *see* Fracture, humerus, upper end
    shaft S42.30- ✓
      comminuted (displaced) S42.35- ✓
        nondisplaced S42.35- ✓
      greenstick S42.31- ✓
      oblique (displaced) S42.33- ✓
        nondisplaced S42.33- ✓
      segmental (displaced) S42.36- ✓
        nondisplaced S42.36- ✓
      specified NEC S42.39- ✓
      spiral (displaced) S42.34- ✓
        nondisplaced S42.34- ✓
      transverse (displaced) S42.32- ✓
        nondisplaced S42.32- ✓
    supracondylar — *see* Fracture, humerus, lower end
    surgical neck — *see* Fracture, humerus, upper end, surgical neck
    trochlea — *see* Fracture, humerus, lower end, condyle, medial
    tuberosity — *see* Fracture, humerus, upper end
    upper end S42.20- ✓
      anatomical neck — *see* Fracture, humerus, upper end, specified NEC
      articular head — *see* Fracture, humerus, upper end, specified NEC
      epiphysis — *see* Fracture, humerus, upper end, physeal
      greater tuberosity (displaced) S42.25- ✓
        nondisplaced S42.25- ✓
      lesser tuberosity (displaced) S42.26- ✓
        nondisplaced S42.26- ✓
      physeal S49.00- ✓
        Salter-Harris
          Type I S49.01- ✓
          Type II S49.02- ✓
          Type III S49.03- ✓
          Type IV S49.04- ✓
        specified NEC S49.09- ✓

Fracture, traumatic — *continued*
  humerus — *continued*
    upper end — *continued*
      specified NEC (displaced) S42.29- ☑
        nondisplaced S42.29- ☑
      surgical neck (displaced) S42.21- ☑
        four-part S42.24- ☑
        nondisplaced S42.21- ☑
        three-part S42.23- ☑
        two-part (displaced) S42.22- ☑
          nondisplaced S42.22- ☑
      torus S42.27- ☑
      transepiphyseal — *see* Fracture, humerus, upper
        end, physeal
  hyoid bone S12.8 ☑
  ilium S32.30- ☑
    with disruption of pelvic ring — *see* Disruption, pelvic
      ring
    avulsion (displaced) S32.31- ☑
      nondisplaced S32.31- ☑
    specified NEC S32.39- ☑
  impaction, impacted — *code as* Fracture, by site
  innominate bone — *see* Fracture, ilium
  instep — *see* Fracture, foot
  ischium S32.60- ☑
    with disruption of pelvic ring — *see* Disruption, pelvic
      ring
    avulsion (displaced) S32.61- ☑
      nondisplaced S32.61- ☑
    specified NEC S32.69- ☑
  jaw (bone) (lower) — *see* Fracture, mandible
    upper — *see* Fracture, maxilla
  joint prosthesis — *see* Complications, joint prosthesis,
    mechanical, breakdown, by site
    periprosthetic — *see* Fracture, traumatic, periprosthet-
      ic
  knee cap — *see* Fracture, patella
  larynx S12.8 ☑
  late effects — *see* Sequelae, fracture
  leg (lower) S82.9- ☑
    ankle — *see* Fracture, ankle
    femur — *see* Fracture, femur
    fibula — *see* Fracture, fibula
    malleolus — *see* Fracture, ankle
    patella — *see* Fracture, patella
    specified site NEC S82.89- ☑
    tibia — *see* Fracture, tibia
  lumbar spine — *see* Fracture, vertebra, lumbar
  lumbosacral spine S32.9 ☑
  Maisonneuve's (displaced) S82.86- ☑
    nondisplaced S82.86- ☑
  malar bone — *see also* Fracture, maxilla S02.400 ☑
    left side S02.40B ☑
    right side S02.40A ☑
  malleolus — *see* Fracture, ankle
  malunion — *see* Fracture, by site
  mandible (lower jaw (bone)) S02.609 ☑
    alveolus S02.67- ☑
    angle (of jaw) S02.65- ☑
    body, unspecified S02.600 ☑
      left side S02.602 ☑
      right side S02.601 ☑
    condylar process S02.61- ☑
    coronoid process S02.62- ☑
    ramus, unspecified S02.64- ☑
    specified site NEC S02.69 ☑
    subcondylar process S02.62- ☑
    symphysis S02.66 ☑
  manubrium (sterni) S22.21 ☑
    dissociation from sternum S22.23 ☑
  march — *see* Fracture, traumatic, stress, by site
  maxilla, maxillary (bone) (sinus) (superior) (upper jaw)
    S02.401 ☑
    alveolus S02.42 ☑
    inferior — *see* Fracture, mandible
    LeFort I S02.411 ☑
    LeFort II S02.412 ☑
    LeFort III S02.413 ☑
    left side S02.40D ☑
    right side S02.40C ☑
  metacarpal S62.309 ☑
    base (displaced) S62.319 ☑
      nondisplaced S62.349 ☑
    fifth S62.30- ☑
      base (displaced) S62.31- ☑
        nondisplaced S62.34- ☑

Fracture, traumatic — *continued*
  metacarpal — *continued*
    fifth — *continued*
      neck (displaced) S62.33- ☑
        nondisplaced S62.36- ☑
      shaft (displaced) S62.32- ☑
        nondisplaced S62.35- ☑
      specified NEC S62.398 ☑
    first S62.20- ☑
      base NEC (displaced) S62.23- ☑
      Bennett's — *see* Bennett's fracture
      neck (displaced) S62.25- ☑
        nondisplaced S62.25- ☑
      shaft (displaced) S62.24- ☑
        nondisplaced S62.24- ☑
      specified NEC S62.29- ☑
    fourth S62.30- ☑
      base (displaced) S62.31- ☑
        nondisplaced S62.34- ☑
      neck (displaced) S62.33- ☑
        nondisplaced S62.36- ☑
      shaft (displaced) S62.32- ☑
        nondisplaced S62.35- ☑
      specified NEC S62.39- ☑
    neck (displaced) S62.33- ☑
      nondisplaced S62.36- ☑
    Rolando's — *see* Rolando's fracture
    second S62.30- ☑
      base (displaced) S62.31- ☑
        nondisplaced S62.34- ☑
      neck (displaced) S62.33- ☑
        nondisplaced S62.36- ☑
      shaft (displaced) S62.32- ☑
        nondisplaced S62.35- ☑
      specified NEC S62.39- ☑
    shaft (displaced) S62.32- ☑
      nondisplaced S62.35- ☑
    specified NEC S62.399 ☑
    third S62.30- ☑
      base (displaced) S62.31- ☑
        nondisplaced S62.34- ☑
      neck (displaced) S62.33- ☑
        nondisplaced S62.36- ☑
      shaft (displaced) S62.32- ☑
        nondisplaced S62.35- ☑
      specified NEC S62.39- ☑
  metaphyseal — *see* Fracture, traumatic, by site, shaft
  metastatic — *see* Fracture, pathological, due to, neoplas-
    tic disease — *see also* Neoplasm
  metatarsal bone S92.30- ☑
    fifth (displaced) S92.35- ☑
      nondisplaced S92.35- ☑
    first (displaced) S92.31- ☑
      nondisplaced S92.31- ☑
    fourth (displaced) S92.34- ☑
      nondisplaced S92.34- ☑
    physeal S99.10- ☑
      Salter-Harris
        Type I S99.11- ☑
        Type II S99.12- ☑
        Type III S99.13- ☑
        Type IV S99.14- ☑
      specified NEC S99.19- ☑
    second (displaced) S92.32- ☑
      nondisplaced S92.32- ☑
    third (displaced) S92.33- ☑
      nondisplaced S92.33- ☑
  Monteggia's — *see* Monteggia's fracture
  multiple
    hand (and wrist) NEC — *see* Fracture, by site
    ribs — *see* Fracture, rib, multiple
  nasal (bone(s)) S02.2 ☑
  navicular (scaphoid) (foot) — *see also* Fracture, tarsal,
    navicular
    hand — *see* Fracture, carpal, navicular
  neck S12.9 ☑
    cervical vertebra S12.9 ☑
      fifth (displaced) S12.400 ☑
        nondisplaced S12.401 ☑
        specified type NEC (displaced) S12.490 ☑
          nondisplaced S12.491 ☑
      first (displaced) S12.000 ☑
        burst (stable) S12.01 ☑
        unstable S12.02 ☑

Fracture, traumatic — *continued*
  neck — *continued*
    cervical vertebra — *continued*
      first — *continued*
        lateral mass (displaced) S12.040 ☑
          nondisplaced S12.041 ☑
        nondisplaced S12.001 ☑
        posterior arch (displaced) S12.030 ☑
          nondisplaced S12.031 ☑
        specified type NEC (displaced) S12.090 ☑
          nondisplaced S12.091 ☑
      fourth (displaced) S12.300 ☑
        nondisplaced S12.301 ☑
        specified type NEC (displaced) S12.390 ☑
          nondisplaced S12.391 ☑
      second (displaced) S12.100 ☑
        dens (anterior) (displaced) (type II) S12.110 ☑
          nondisplaced S12.112 ☑
          posterior S12.111 ☑
          specified type NEC (displaced) S12.120 ☑
            nondisplaced S12.121 ☑
        nondisplaced S12.101 ☑
        specified type NEC (displaced) S12.190 ☑
          nondisplaced S12.191 ☑
      seventh (displaced) S12.600 ☑
        nondisplaced S12.601 ☑
        specified type NEC (displaced) S12.690 ☑
          nondisplaced S12.691 ☑
      sixth (displaced) S12.500 ☑
        nondisplaced S12.501 ☑
        specified type NEC (displaced) S12.590 ☑
          nondisplaced S12.591 ☑
      third (displaced) S12.200 ☑
        nondisplaced S12.201 ☑
        specified type NEC (displaced) S12.290 ☑
          nondisplaced S12.291 ☑
    hyoid bone S12.8 ☑
    larynx S12.8 ☑
    specified site NEC S12.8 ☑
    thyroid cartilage S12.8 ☑
    trachea S12.8 ☑
  neoplastic NEC — *see* Fracture, pathological, due to,
    neoplastic disease
  neural arch — *see* Fracture, vertebra
  newborn — *see* Birth, injury, fracture
  nontraumatic — *see* Fracture, pathological
  nonunion — *see* Nonunion, fracture
  nose, nasal (bone) (septum) S02.2 ☑
  occiput — *see* Fracture, skull, base, occiput
  odontoid process — *see* Fracture, neck, cervical vertebra,
    second
  olecranon (process) (ulna) — *see* Fracture, ulna, upper
    end, olecranon process
  orbit, orbital (bone) (region) S02.85 ☑
    floor (blow-out) S02.3- ☑
    roof S02.12- ☑
    wall S02.85 ☑
      lateral S02.84- ☑
      medial S02.83- ☑
  os
    calcis — *see* Fracture, tarsal, calcaneus
    magnum — *see* Fracture, carpal, capitate
    pubis — *see* Fracture, pubis
  palate S02.8- ☑
  parietal bone (skull) S02.0 ☑
  patella S82.00- ☑
    comminuted (displaced) S82.04- ☑
      nondisplaced S82.04- ☑
    longitudinal (displaced) S82.02- ☑
      nondisplaced S82.02- ☑
    osteochondral (displaced) S82.01- ☑
      nondisplaced S82.01- ☑
    specified NEC S82.09- ☑
    transverse (displaced) S82.03- ☑
      nondisplaced S82.03- ☑
  pedicle (of vertebral arch) — *see* Fracture, vertebra
  pelvis, pelvic (bone) S32.9 ☑
    acetabulum — *see* Fracture, acetabulum
    circle — *see* Disruption, pelvic ring
    following insertion of implant, prosthesis or plate
      M96.65
    ilium — *see* Fracture, ilium
    ischium — *see* Fracture, ischium
    multiple
      with disruption of pelvic ring (circle) — *see* Disrup-
        tion, pelvic ring

Fracture, traumatic — *continued*
- pelvis, pelvic — *continued*
  - multiple — *continued*
    - without disruption of pelvic ring (circle) S32.82 ☑
  - pubis — *see* Fracture, pubis
  - sacrum — *see* Fracture, sacrum
  - specified site NEC S32.89 ☑
- periprosthetic, around internal prosthetic joint M97.9 ☑
  - ankle M97.2- ☑
  - elbow M97.4- ☑
  - finger M97.8 ☑
  - hip M97.0- ☑
  - knee M97.1- ☑
  - shoulder M97.3- ☑
  - specified joint NEC M97.8 ☑
  - spine M97.8 ☑
  - toe M97.8 ☑
  - wrist M97.8 ☑
- phalanx
  - foot — *see* Fracture, toe
  - hand — *see* Fracture, finger
- pisiform — *see* Fracture, carpal, pisiform
- pond — *see* Fracture, skull
- prosthetic device, internal — *see* Complications, prosthetic device, by site, mechanical
- pubis S32.50- ☑
  - with disruption of pelvic ring — *see* Disruption, pelvic ring
  - specified site NEC S32.59- ☑
  - superior rim S32.51- ☑
- radius S52.9- ☑
  - distal end — *see* Fracture, radius, lower end
  - following insertion of implant, prosthesis or plate M96.63- ☑
  - head — *see* Fracture, radius, upper end, head
  - lower end S52.50- ☑
    - Barton's — *see* Barton's fracture
    - Colles' — *see* Colles' fracture
    - extraarticular NEC S52.55- ☑
    - intraarticular NEC S52.57- ☑
    - physeal S59.20- ☑
      - Salter-Harris
        - Type I S59.21- ☑
        - Type II S59.22- ☑
        - Type III S59.23- ☑
        - Type IV S59.24- ☑
      - specified NEC S59.29- ☑
    - Smith's — *see* Smith's fracture
    - specified NEC S52.59- ☑
    - styloid process (displaced) S52.51- ☑
      - nondisplaced S52.51- ☑
    - torus S52.52- ☑
  - neck — *see* Fracture, radius, upper end
  - proximal end — *see* Fracture, radius, upper end
  - shaft S52.30- ☑
    - bent bone S52.38- ☑
    - comminuted (displaced) S52.35- ☑
      - nondisplaced S52.35- ☑
    - Galeazzi's — *see* Galeazzi's fracture
    - greenstick S52.31- ☑
    - oblique (displaced) S52.33- ☑
      - nondisplaced S52.33- ☑
    - segmental (displaced) S52.36- ☑
      - nondisplaced S52.36- ☑
    - specified NEC S52.39- ☑
    - spiral (displaced) S52.34- ☑
      - nondisplaced S52.34- ☑
    - transverse (displaced) S52.32- ☑
      - nondisplaced S52.32- ☑
  - upper end S52.10- ☑
    - head (displaced) S52.12- ☑
      - nondisplaced S52.12- ☑
    - neck (displaced) S52.13- ☑
      - nondisplaced S52.13- ☑
    - physeal S59.10- ☑
      - Salter-Harris
        - Type I S59.11- ☑
        - Type II S59.12- ☑
        - Type III S59.13- ☑
        - Type IV S59.14- ☑
      - specified NEC S59.19- ☑
    - specified NEC S52.18- ☑
    - torus S52.11- ☑
- ramus
  - inferior or superior, pubis — *see* Fracture, pubis
  - mandible — *see* Fracture, mandible

Fracture, traumatic — *continued*
- restorative material (dental) K08.539
  - with loss of material K08.531
  - without loss of material K08.530
- rib S22.3-
  - with flail chest — *see* Flail, chest
  - associated with chest compression and cardiopulmonary resuscitation M96.A2
  - multiple S22.4-
    - with flail chest — *see* Flail, chest
    - associated with chest compression and cardiopulmonary resuscitation M96.A3
- root, tooth — *see* Fracture, tooth
- sacrum S32.10 ☑
  - specified NEC S32.19 ☑
  - Type
    - 1 S32.14 ☑
    - 2 S32.15 ☑
    - 3 S32.16 ☑
    - 4 S32.17 ☑
  - Zone
    - I S32.119 ☑
      - displaced (minimally) S32.111 ☑
        - severely S32.112 ☑
      - nondisplaced S32.110 ☑
    - II S32.129 ☑
      - displaced (minimally) S32.121 ☑
        - severely S32.122 ☑
      - nondisplaced S32.120 ☑
    - III S32.139 ☑
      - displaced (minimally) S32.131 ☑
        - severely S32.132 ☑
      - nondisplaced S32.130 ☑
- scaphoid (hand) — *see also* Fracture, carpal, navicular
  - foot — *see* Fracture, tarsal, navicular
- scapula S42.10- ☑
  - acromial process (displaced) S42.12- ☑
    - nondisplaced S42.12- ☑
  - body (displaced) S42.11- ☑
    - nondisplaced S42.11- ☑
  - coracoid process (displaced) S42.13- ☑
    - nondisplaced S42.13- ☑
  - glenoid cavity (displaced) S42.14- ☑
    - nondisplaced S42.14- ☑
  - neck (displaced) S42.15- ☑
    - nondisplaced S42.15- ☑
  - specified NEC S42.19- ☑
- semilunar bone, wrist — *see* Fracture, carpal, lunate
- sequelae — *see* Sequelae, fracture
- sesamoid bone
  - foot S92.81- ☑
  - hand — *see* Fracture, carpal
  - other — *see* Fracture, traumatic, by site
- shepherd's — *see* Fracture, tarsal, talus
- shoulder (girdle) S42.9- ☑
  - blade — *see* Fracture, scapula
- sinus (ethmoid) (frontal) S02.19 ☑
- skull S02.91 ☑
  - base S02.10- ☑
    - occiput S02.119 ☑
      - condyle S02.113 ☑
      - specified NEC S02.118 ☑
        - left side S02.11H ☑
        - right side S02.11G ☑
      - type I S02.110 ☑
        - left side S02.11B ☑
        - right side S02.11A ☑
      - type II S02.111 ☑
        - left side S02.11D ☑
        - right side S02.11C ☑
      - type III S02.112 ☑
        - left side S02.11F ☑
        - right side S02.11E ☑
    - specified NEC S02.19 ☑
  - birth injury P13.0
  - frontal bone S02.0 ☑
  - parietal bone S02.0 ☑
  - specified site NEC S02.8- ☑
  - temporal bone S02.19 ☑
  - vault S02.0 ☑
- Smith's — *see* Smith's fracture
- sphenoid (bone) (sinus) S02.19 ☑
- spine — *see* Fracture, vertebra
- spinous process — *see* Fracture, vertebra
- spontaneous (cause unknown) — *see* Fracture, pathological

Fracture, traumatic — *continued*
- stave (of thumb) — *see* Fracture, metacarpal, first
- sternum S22.20 ☑
  - with flail chest — *see* Flail, chest
  - associated with chest compression and cardiopulmonary resuscitation M96.A1
  - body S22.22 ☑
  - manubrium S22.21 ☑
  - xiphoid (process) S22.24 ☑
    - associated with chest compression and cardiopulmonary resuscitation M96.A1
- stress M84.30 ☑
  - ankle M84.37- ☑
  - carpus M84.34- ☑
  - clavicle M84.31- ☑
  - femoral neck M84.359 ☑
  - femur M84.35- ☑
  - fibula M84.36- ☑
  - finger M84.34- ☑
  - hip M84.35- ☑
  - humerus M84.32- ☑
  - ilium M84.350 ☑
  - ischium M84.350 ☑
  - metacarpus M84.34- ☑
  - metatarsus M84.37- ☑
  - neck — *see* Fracture, fatigue, vertebra
  - pelvis M84.350 ☑
  - radius M84.33- ☑
  - rib M84.38 ☑
  - scapula M84.31- ☑
  - skull M84.38 ☑
  - tarsus M84.37- ☑
  - tibia M84.36- ☑
  - toe M84.37- ☑
  - ulna M84.33- ☑
  - vertebra — *see* Fracture, fatigue, vertebra
- supracondylar, elbow — *see* Fracture, humerus, lower end, supracondylar
- symphysis pubis — *see* Fracture, pubis
- talus (ankle bone) — *see* Fracture, tarsal, talus
- tarsal bone(s) S92.20- ☑
  - astragalus — *see* Fracture, tarsal, talus
  - calcaneus S92.00- ☑
    - anterior process (displaced) S92.02- ☑
      - nondisplaced S92.02- ☑
    - body (displaced) S92.01- ☑
      - nondisplaced S92.01- ☑
    - extraarticular NEC (displaced) S92.05- ☑
      - nondisplaced S92.05- ☑
    - intraarticular (displaced) S92.06- ☑
      - nondisplaced S92.06- ☑
    - physeal S99.00- ☑
      - Salter-Harris
        - Type I S99.01- ☑
        - Type II S99.02- ☑
        - Type III S99.03- ☑
        - Type IV S99.04- ☑
      - specified NEC S99.09- ☑
    - tuberosity (displaced) S92.04- ☑
      - avulsion (displaced) S92.03- ☑
        - nondisplaced S92.03- ☑
      - nondisplaced S92.04- ☑
  - cuboid (displaced) S92.21- ☑
    - nondisplaced S92.21- ☑
  - cuneiform
    - intermediate (displaced) S92.23- ☑
      - nondisplaced S92.23- ☑
    - lateral (displaced) S92.22- ☑
      - nondisplaced S92.22- ☑
    - medial (displaced) S92.24- ☑
      - nondisplaced S92.24- ☑
  - navicular (displaced) S92.25- ☑
    - nondisplaced S92.25- ☑
  - scaphoid — *see* Fracture, tarsal, navicular
  - talus S92.10- ☑
    - avulsion (displaced) S92.15- ☑
      - nondisplaced S92.15- ☑
    - body (displaced) S92.12- ☑
      - nondisplaced S92.12- ☑
    - dome (displaced) S92.14- ☑
      - nondisplaced S92.14- ☑
    - head (displaced) S92.12- ☑
      - nondisplaced S92.12- ☑
    - lateral process (displaced) S92.14- ☑
      - nondisplaced S92.14- ☑

☑ **Additional Character Required** — **Refer to the Tabular List for Character Selection**

Fracture, traumatic — *continued*
  vertebra, vertebral — *continued*
    lumbar — *continued*
      burst (stable) S32.001 ☑
        unstable S32.002 ☑
      fifth S32.059 ☑
        burst (stable) S32.051 ☑
          unstable S32.052 ☑
        specified type NEC S32.058 ☑
        wedge compression S32.050 ☑
      first S32.019 ☑
        burst (stable) S32.011 ☑
          unstable S32.012 ☑
        specified type NEC S32.018 ☑
        wedge compression S32.010 ☑
      fourth S32.049 ☑
        burst (stable) S32.041 ☑
          unstable S32.042 ☑
        specified type NEC S32.048 ☑
        wedge compression S32.040 ☑
      second S32.029 ☑
        burst (stable) S32.021 ☑
          unstable S32.022 ☑
        specified type NEC S32.028 ☑
        wedge compression S32.020 ☑
      specified type NEC S32.008 ☑
      third S32.039 ☑
        burst (stable) S32.031 ☑
          unstable S32.032 ☑
        specified type NEC S32.038 ☑
        wedge compression S32.030 ☑
      wedge compression S32.000 ☑
    metastatic — *see* Collapse, vertebra, in, specified disease NEC — *see also* Neoplasm
  newborn (birth injury) P11.5
  sacrum S32.10 ☑
    specified NEC S32.19 ☑
    Type
      1 S32.14 ☑
      2 S32.15 ☑
      3 S32.16 ☑
      4 S32.17 ☑
    Zone
      I S32.119 ☑
        displaced (minimally) S32.111 ☑
          severely S32.112 ☑
        nondisplaced S32.110 ☑
      II S32.129 ☑
        displaced (minimally) S32.121 ☑
          severely S32.122 ☑
        nondisplaced S32.120 ☑
      III S32.139 ☑
        displaced (minimally) S32.131 ☑
          severely S32.132 ☑
        nondisplaced S32.130 ☑
    thoracic — *see* Fracture, thorax, vertebra
  vertex S02.0 ☑
  vomer (bone) S02.2 ☑
  wrist S62.10- ☑
    carpal — *see* Fracture, carpal bone
    navicular (scaphoid) (hand) — *see* Fracture, carpal, navicular
  xiphisternum, xiphoid (process) S22.24 ☑
    associated with chest compression and cardiopulmonary resuscitation M96.A1
  zygoma S02.402 ☑
    left side S02.40F ☑
    right side S02.40E ☑

Fragile, fragility
  autosomal site Q95.5
  bone, congenital (with blue sclera) Q78.0
  capillary (hereditary) D69.8
  hair L67.8
  nails L60.3
  non-sex chromosome site Q95.5
  X chromosome Q99.2

Fragilitas
  crinium L67.8
  ossium (with blue sclerae) (hereditary) Q78.0
  unguium L60.3
    congenital Q84.6

Fragments, cataract (lens), **following cataract surgery** H59.02- ☑
  retained foreign body — *see* Retained, foreign body fragments (type of)

Frailty (frail) R54

Frailty — *continued*
  mental R41.81

Frambesia, frambesial (tropica) — *see also* Yaws
  initial lesion or ulcer A66.0
  primary A66.0

Frambeside
  gummatous A66.4
  of early yaws A66.2

Frambesioma A66.1

Franceschetti-Klein (-Wildervanck) **disease or syndrome** Q75.4

Francis' disease — *see* Tularemia

Franklin disease C88.2- ☑

Frank's essential thrombocytopenia D69.3

Fraser's syndrome Q87.0

Freckle(s) L81.2
  malignant melanoma in — *see* Melanoma
  melanotic (Hutchinson's) — *see* Melanoma, in situ
  retinal D49.81

Frederickson's hyperlipoproteinemia, type
  I and V E78.3
  IIA E78.00
  IIB and III E78.2
  IV E78.1

Freeman Sheldon syndrome Q87.0

Freezing — *see also* Effect, adverse, cold T69.9 ☑

Freiberg's disease (infraction of metatarsal head or osteochondrosis) — *see* Osteochondrosis, juvenile, metatarsus

Frei's disease A55

Fremitus, friction, cardiac R01.2

Frenum, frenulum
  external os Q51.828
  tongue (shortening) (congenital) Q38.1

Frequency micturition (nocturnal) R35.0
  psychogenic F45.8

Frey's syndrome
  auriculotemporal G50.8
  hyperhidrosis L74.52

Friction
  burn — *see* Burn, by site
  fremitus, cardiac R01.2
  precordial R01.2
  sounds, chest R09.89

Friderichsen-Waterhouse syndrome or disease A39.1

Friedlander's B (bacillus) **NEC** — *see also* condition A49.8

Friedreich's
  ataxia G11.11
  combined systemic disease G11.11
  facial hemihypertrophy Q67.4
  sclerosis (cerebellum) (spinal cord) G11.11

Frigidity F52.22

Frohlich's syndrome E23.6

Frontal — *see also* condition
  lobe syndrome F07.0

Frostbite (superficial) T33.90 ☑
  with
    partial thickness skin loss — *see* Frostbite (superficial), by site
    tissue necrosis T34.90 ☑
  abdominal wall T33.3
    with tissue necrosis T34.3
  ankle T33.81- ☑
    with tissue necrosis T34.81- ☑
  arm T33.4- ☑
    with tissue necrosis T34.4- ☑
    finger(s) — *see* Frostbite, finger
    hand — *see* Frostbite, hand
    wrist — *see* Frostbite, wrist
  ear T33.01- ☑
    with tissue necrosis T34.01- ☑
  face T33.09 ☑
    with tissue necrosis T34.09 ☑
  finger T33.53- ☑
    with tissue necrosis T34.53- ☑
  foot T33.82- ☑
    with tissue necrosis T34.82- ☑
  hand T33.52- ☑
    with tissue necrosis T34.52- ☑
  head T33.09 ☑
    with tissue necrosis T34.09 ☑
    ear — *see* Frostbite, ear
    nose — *see* Frostbite, nose
  hip (and thigh) T33.6- ☑
    with tissue necrosis T34.6- ☑
  knee T33.7- ☑
    with tissue necrosis T34.7- ☑

Frostbite — *continued*
  leg T33.9- ☑
    with tissue necrosis T34.9- ☑
    ankle — *see* Frostbite, ankle
    foot — *see* Frostbite, foot
    knee — *see* Frostbite, knee
    lower T33.7- ☑
      with tissue necrosis T34.7- ☑
    thigh — *see* Frostbite, hip
    toe — *see* Frostbite, toe
  limb
    lower T33.99 ☑
      with tissue necrosis T34.99 ☑
    upper — *see* Frostbite, arm
  neck T33.1 ☑
    with tissue necrosis T34.1 ☑
  nose T33.02 ☑
    with tissue necrosis T34.02 ☑
  pelvis T33.3 ☑
    with tissue necrosis T34.3 ☑
  specified site NEC T33.99 ☑
    with tissue necrosis T34.99 ☑
  thigh — *see* Frostbite, hip
  thorax T33.2 ☑
    with tissue necrosis T34.2 ☑
  toes T33.83- ☑
    with tissue necrosis T34.83- ☑
  trunk T33.99 ☑
    with tissue necrosis T34.99 ☑
  wrist T33.51- ☑
    with tissue necrosis T34.51- ☑

Frotteurism F65.81

Frozen — *see also* Effect, adverse, cold T69.9 ☑
  pelvis (female) N94.89
    male K66.8
  shoulder — *see* Capsulitis, adhesive

Fructokinase deficiency E74.11

Fructose 1,6 diphosphatase deficiency E74.19

Fructosemia (benign) (essential) E74.12

Fructosuria (benign) (essential) E74.11

Fuchs'
  black spot (myopic) — *see also* Myopia, degenerative H44.2- ☑
  dystrophy (corneal endothelium) H18.51- ☑
  heterochromic cyclitis — *see* Cyclitis, Fuchs' heterochromic

Fucosidosis E77.1

Fugue R68.89
  dissociative F44.1
  hysterical (dissociative) F44.1
  postictal in epilepsy — *see* Epilepsy
  reaction to exceptional stress (transient) F43.0

Fulminant, fulminating — *see* condition

Functional — *see also* condition
  bleeding (uterus) N93.8

Functioning, intellectual, borderline R41.83

Fundus — *see* condition

Fungemia NOS B49

Fungus, fungous
  cerebral G93.89
  disease NOS B49
  infection — *see* Infection, fungus

Funiculitis (acute) (chronic) (endemic) N49.1
  gonococcal (acute) (chronic) A54.23
  tuberculous A18.15

Funnel
  breast (acquired) M95.4
    congenital Q67.6
    sequelae (late effect) of rickets E64.3
  chest (acquired) M95.4
    congenital Q67.6
    sequelae (late effect) of rickets E64.3
  pelvis (acquired) M95.5
    with disproportion (fetopelvic) O33.3 ☑
      causing obstructed labor O65.3
    congenital Q74.2

FUO (fever of unknown origin) R50.9

Furfur L21.0
  microsporon B36.0

Furrier's lung J67.8

Furrowed K14.5
  nail(s) (transverse) L60.4
    congenital Q84.6
  tongue K14.5
    congenital Q38.3

Furuncle L02.92
  abdominal wall L02.221
  ankle — *see* Furuncle, lower limb

☑ **Additional Character Required** — **Refer to the Tabular List for Character Selection**

Furuncle — continued
- antecubital space — see Furuncle, upper limb
- anus K61.0
- arm — see Furuncle, upper limb
- auditory canal, external — see Abscess, ear, external
- auricle (ear) — see Abscess, ear, external
- axilla (region) L02.42- ☑
- back (any part) L02.222
- breast N61.1
- buttock L02.32
- cheek (external) L02.02
- chest wall L02.223
- chin L02.02
- corpus cavernosum N48.21
- ear, external — see Abscess, ear, external
- external auditory canal — see Abscess, ear, external
- eyelid — see Abscess, eyelid
- face L02.02
- femoral (region) — see Furuncle, lower limb
- finger — see Furuncle, hand
- flank L02.221
- foot L02.62- ☑
- forehead L02.02
- gluteal (region) L02.32
- groin L02.224
- hand L02.52- ☑
- head L02.821
  - face L02.02
- hip — see Furuncle, lower limb
- kidney — see Abscess, kidney
- knee — see Furuncle, lower limb
- labium (majus) (minus) N76.4
- lacrimal
  - gland — see Dacryoadenitis
  - passages (duct) (sac) — see Inflammation, lacrimal, passages, acute
- leg (any part) — see Furuncle, lower limb
- lower limb L02.42- ☑
- malignant A22.0
- mouth K12.2
- navel L02.226
- neck L02.12
- nose J34.0
- orbit, orbital — see Abscess, orbit
- palmar (space) — see Furuncle, hand
- partes posteriores L02.32
- pectoral region L02.223

Furuncle — continued
- penis N48.21
- perineum L02.225
- pinna — see Abscess, ear, external
- popliteal — see Furuncle, lower limb
- prepatellar — see Furuncle, lower limb
- scalp L02.821
- seminal vesicle N49.0
- shoulder — see Furuncle, upper limb
- specified site NEC L02.828
- submandibular K12.2
- temple (region) L02.02
- thumb — see Furuncle, hand
- toe — see Furuncle, foot
- trunk L02.229
  - abdominal wall L02.221
  - back L02.222
  - chest wall L02.223
  - groin L02.224
  - perineum L02.225
  - umbilicus L02.226
- umbilicus L02.226
- upper limb L02.42- ☑
- vulva N76.4

Furunculosis — see Furuncle

Fused — see Fusion, fused

Fusion, fused (congenital)
- astragaloscaphoid Q74.2
- atria Q21.19
- auditory canal Q16.1
- auricles, heart Q21.19
- binocular with defective stereopsis H53.32
- bone Q79.8
- cervical spine M43.22
- choanal Q30.0
- commissure, mitral valve Q23.2
- cusps, heart valve NEC Q24.8
  - mitral Q23.2
  - pulmonary Q22.1
  - tricuspid Q22.4
- ear ossicles Q16.3
- fingers Q70.0 ☑
- hymen Q52.3
- joint (acquired) — see also Ankylosis
  - congenital Q74.8
- kidneys (incomplete) Q63.1
- labium (majus) (minus) Q52.5

Fusion, fused — continued
- larynx and trachea Q34.8
- limb, congenital Q74.8
  - lower Q74.2
  - upper Q74.0
- lobes, lung Q33.8
- lumbosacral (acquired) M43.27
  - arthrodesis status Z98.1
  - congenital Q76.49
  - postprocedural status Z98.1
- nares, nose, nasal, nostril(s) Q30.0
- organ or site not listed — see Anomaly, by site
- ossicles Q79.9
  - auditory Q16.3
- pulmonic cusps Q22.1
- ribs Q76.6
- sacroiliac (joint) (acquired) M43.28
  - arthrodesis status Z98.1
  - congenital Q74.2
  - postprocedural status Z98.1
- spine (acquired) NEC M43.20
  - arthrodesis status Z98.1
  - cervical region M43.22
  - cervicothoracic region M43.23
  - congenital Q76.49
  - lumbar M43.26
  - lumbosacral region M43.27
  - occipito-atlanto-axial region M43.21
  - postoperative status Z98.1
  - sacrococcygeal region M43.28
  - thoracic region M43.24
  - thoracolumbar region M43.25
- sublingual duct with submaxillary duct at opening in mouth Q38.4
- testes Q55.1
- toes Q70.2- ☑
- tooth, teeth K00.2
- trachea and esophagus Q39.8
- twins Q89.4
- vagina Q52.4
- ventricles, heart Q21.0
- vertebra (arch) — see Fusion, spine
- vulva Q52.5

Fusospirillosis (mouth) (tongue) (tonsil) A69.1

Fussy baby R68.12

G

Gain in weight (abnormal) (excessive) — *see also* Weight, gain
Gaisbock's disease (polycythemia hypertonica) D75.1
Gait abnormality R26.9
  ataxic R26.0
  falling R29.6
  hysterical (ataxic) (staggering) F44.4
  paralytic R26.1
  spastic R26.1
  specified type NEC R26.89
  staggering R26.0
  unsteadiness R26.81
  walking difficulty NEC R26.2
Galactocele (breast) N64.89
  puerperal, postpartum O92.79
Galactokinase deficiency E74.29
Galactophoritis N61.0
  gestational, puerperal, postpartum O91.2- ☑
Galactorrhea O92.6
  not associated with childbirth N64.3
Galactosemia (classic) (congenital) E74.21
Galactosuria E74.29
Galacturia R82.0
  schistosomiasis (bilharziasis) B65.0
GALD (gestational alloimmune liver disease) P78.84
Galeazzi's fracture S52.37- ☑
Galen's vein — *see* condition
Galeophobia F40.218
Gall duct — *see* condition
Gallbladder — *see also* condition
  acute K81.0
Gallop rhythm R00.8
Gallstone (colic) (cystic duct) (gallbladder) (impacted)
   (multiple) — *see also* Calculus, gallbladder
  with
    cholecystitis — *see* Calculus, gallbladder, with chole-
     cystitis
  bile duct (common) (hepatic) — *see* Calculus, bile duct
  causing intestinal obstruction K56.3
  specified NEC K80.80
    with obstruction K80.81
Gambling Z72.6
  pathological (compulsive) F63.0
Gammopathy (of undetermined significance [MGUS]) D47.2
  associated with lymphoplasmacytic dyscrasia D47.2
  monoclonal D47.2
  polyclonal D89.0
Gamna's disease (siderotic splenomegaly) D73.1
Gamophobia F40.298
Gampsodactylia (congenital) Q66.7- ☑
Gamstorp's disease (adynamia episodica hereditaria) G72.3
Gandy-Nanta disease (siderotic splenomegaly) D73.1
Gang
  membership offenses Z72.810
Gangliocytoma D36.10
Ganglioglioma — *see* Neoplasm, uncertain behavior, by
  site
Ganglion (compound) (diffuse) (joint) (tendon (sheath))
   M67.40
  ankle M67.47- ☑
  foot M67.47- ☑
  forearm M67.43- ☑
  hand M67.44- ☑
  lower leg M67.46- ☑
  multiple sites M67.49
  of yaws (early) (late) A66.6
  pelvic region M67.45- ☑
  periosteal — *see* Periostitis
  shoulder region M67.41- ☑
  specified site NEC M67.48
  thigh region M67.45- ☑
  tuberculous A18.09
  upper arm M67.42- ☑
  wrist M67.43- ☑
Ganglioneuroblastoma — *see* Neoplasm, nerve, malignant
Ganglioneuroma D36.10
  malignant — *see* Neoplasm, nerve, malignant
Ganglioneuromatosis D36.10
Ganglionitis
  fifth nerve — *see* Neuralgia, trigeminal
  gasserian (postherpetic) (postzoster) B02.21
  geniculate G51.1
    newborn (birth injury) P11.3
    postherpetic, postzoster B02.21
  herpes zoster B02.21

Ganglionitis — *continued*
  postherpetic geniculate B02.21
Gangliosidosis E75.10
  GM1 E75.19
  GM2 E75.00
    other specified E75.09
    Sandhoff disease E75.01
    Tay-Sachs disease E75.02
  GM3 E75.19
  mucolipidosis IV E75.11
Gangosa A66.5
Gangrene, gangrenous (connective tissue) (dropsical) (dry)
   (moist) (skin) (ulcer) — *see also* Necrosis I96
  with diabetes (mellitus) — *see* Diabetes, with, gangrene
  abdomen (wall) I96
  alveolar M27.3
  appendix K35.80
    with
     peritonitis, localized — *see also* Appendicitis
      K35.31
  arteriosclerotic (general) (senile) — *see* Arteriosclerosis,
    extremities, with, gangrene
  auricle I96
  Bacillus welchii A48.0
  bladder (infectious) — *see* Cystitis, specified type NEC
  bowel, cecum, or colon — *see* Gangrene, intestine
  Clostridium perfringens or welchii A48.0
  cornea H18.89- ☑
  corpora cavernosa N48.29
    noninfective N48.89
  cutaneous, spreading I96
  decubital — *see* Ulcer, pressure, by site
  diabetic (any site) — *see* Diabetes, with, gangrene
  emphysematous — *see* Gangrene, gas
  epidemic — *see* Poisoning, food, noxious, plant
  epididymis (infectional) N45.1
  erysipelas — *see* Erysipelas
  extremity (lower) (upper) I96
  Fournier N49.3
    female N76.82
    vagina and vulva N76.82
  fusospirochetal A69.0
  gallbladder — *see* Cholecystitis, acute
  gas (bacillus) A48.0
    following
     abortion — *see* Abortion by type complicated by
      infection
     ectopic or molar pregnancy O08.0
  glossitis K14.0
  hernia — *see* Hernia, by site, with gangrene
  intestine, intestinal (hemorrhagic) (massive) — *see also*
    Infarct, intestine K55.069
    with
     mesenteric embolism — *see also* Infarct, intestine
      K55.069
     obstruction — *see* Obstruction, intestine
  laryngitis J04.0
  limb (lower) (upper) I96
  lung J85.0
    spirochetal A69.8
  lymphangitis I89.1
  Meleney's (synergistic) — *see* Ulcer, skin
  mesentery — *see also* Infarct, intestine K55.069
    with
     embolism — *see also* Infarct, intestine K55.069
     intestinal obstruction — *see* Obstruction, intestine
  mouth A69.0
  ovary — *see* Oophoritis
  pancreas — *see* Pancreatitis, acute
  penis N48.29
    noninfective N48.89
  perineum I96
  pharynx — *see also* Pharyngitis
    Vincent's A69.1
  presenile I73.1
  progressive synergistic — *see* Ulcer, skin
  pulmonary J85.0
  pulpal (dental) K04.1
  quinsy J36
  Raynaud's (symmetric gangrene) I73.01
  retropharyngeal J39.2
  scrotum N49.3
    noninfective N50.89
  senile (atherosclerotic) — *see* Arteriosclerosis, extremi-
    ties, with, gangrene
  spermatic cord N49.1
    noninfective N50.89
  spine I96
  spirochetal NEC A69.8

Gangrene, gangrenous — *continued*
  spreading cutaneous I96
  stomatitis A69.0
  symmetrical I73.01
  testis (infectional) N45.2
    noninfective N44.8
  throat — *see also* Pharyngitis
    diphtheritic A36.0
    Vincent's A69.1
  thyroid (gland) E07.89
  tooth (pulp) K04.1
  tuberculous NEC — *see* Tuberculosis
  tunica vaginalis N49.1
    noninfective N50.89
  umbilicus I96
  uterus — *see* Endometritis
  uvulitis K12.2
  vas deferens N49.1
    noninfective N50.89
  vulva N76.82
Ganister disease J62.8
Ganser's syndrome (hysterical) F44.89
Gardner-Diamond syndrome (autoerythrocyte sensitization) D69.2
Gargoylism E76.01
Garre's disease, osteitis (sclerosing), osteomyelitis — *see*
  Osteomyelitis, specified type NEC
Garrod's pad, knuckle M72.1
Gartner's duct
  cyst Q52.4
  persistent Q50.6
Gas R14.3
  asphyxiation, inhalation, poisoning, suffocation NEC —
    see Table of Drugs and Chemicals
  excessive R14.0
  gangrene A48.0
    following
     abortion — *see* Abortion by type complicated by
      infection
     ectopic or molar pregnancy O08.0
  on stomach R14.0
  pains R14.1
Gastralgia — *see also* Pain, abdominal
Gastrectasis K31.0
  psychogenic F45.8
Gastric — *see* condition
Gastrinoma
  malignant
    pancreas C25.4
    specified site NEC — *see* Neoplasm, malignant, by
     site
    unspecified site C25.4
  specified site — *see* Neoplasm, uncertain behavior
  unspecified site D37.9
Gastritis (simple) K29.70
  with bleeding K29.71
  acute (erosive) K29.00
    with bleeding K29.01
  alcoholic K29.20
    with bleeding K29.21
  allergic K29.60
    with bleeding K29.61
  atrophic (chronic) K29.40
    with bleeding K29.41
  chronic (antral) (fundal) K29.50
    with bleeding K29.51
    atrophic K29.40
     with bleeding K29.41
    superficial K29.30
     with bleeding K29.31
  dietary counseling and surveillance Z71.3
  due to diet deficiency E63.9
  eosinophilic K52.81
  giant hypertrophic K29.60
    with bleeding K29.61
  granulomatous K29.60
    with bleeding K29.61
  hypertrophic (mucosa) K29.60
    with bleeding K29.61
  nervous F54
  spastic K29.60
    with bleeding K29.61
  specified NEC K29.60
    with bleeding K29.61
  superficial chronic K29.30
    with bleeding K29.31
  tuberculous A18.83
  viral NEC A08.4
Gastrocarcinoma — *see* Neoplasm, malignant, stomach

Gastrocolic — see condition
Gastrodisciasis, gastrodiscoidiasis B66.8
Gastroduodenitis K29.90
  with bleeding K29.91
  virus, viral A08.4
    specified type NEC A08.39
Gastrodynia — see Pain, abdominal
Gastroenteritis (acute) (chronic) (noninfectious) — see also
  Enteritis K52.9
  allergic K52.29
    with
      eosinophilic gastritis or gastroenteritis K52.81
      food protein-induced enterocolitis syndrome
        K52.21
      food protein-induced enteropathy K52.22
  dietetic — see also Gastroenteritis, allergic K52.29
  drug-induced K52.1
  due to
    Cryptosporidium A07.2
    drugs K52.1
    food poisoning — see Intoxication, foodborne
    radiation K52.0
  eosinophilic K52.81
  epidemic (infectious) A09
  food hypersensitivity — see also Gastroenteritis, allergic
    K52.29
  infectious — see Enteritis, infectious
  influenzal — see Influenza, with gastroenteritis
  noninfectious K52.9
    specified NEC K52.89
  rotaviral A08.0
  Salmonella A02.0
  toxic K52.1
  viral NEC A08.4
    acute infectious A08.39
      type Norwalk A08.11
    infantile (acute) A08.39
    Norwalk agent A08.11
    rotaviral A08.0
    severe of infants A08.39
    specified type NEC A08.39
Gastroenteropathy — see also Gastroenteritis K52.9
  acute, due to Norovirus A08.11
  acute, due to Norwalk agent A08.11
  infectious A09
Gastroenteroptosis K63.4
Gastroesophageal laceration- hemorrhage syndrome
  K22.6
Gastrointestinal — see condition
Gastrojejunal — see condition
Gastrojejunitis — see also Enteritis K52.9
Gastrojejunocolic — see condition
Gastroliths K31.89
Gastromalacia K31.89
Gastroparalysis K31.84
  diabetic — see Diabetes, gastroparalysis
Gastroparesis K31.84
  diabetic — see Diabetes, by type, with gastroparesis
Gastropathy K31.9
  congestive portal — see also Hypertension, portal K31.89
  erythematous K29.70
  exudative K90.89
  portal hypertensive — see also Hypertension, portal
    K31.89
  specified NEC K31.89
Gastroptosis K31.89
Gastrorrhagia K92.2
  psychogenic F45.8
Gastroschisis (congenital) Q79.3
Gastrospasm (neurogenic) (reflex) K31.89
  neurotic F45.8
  psychogenic F45.8
Gastrostaxis — see Gastritis, with bleeding
Gastrostenosis K31.89
Gastrostomy
  attention to Z43.1
  status Z93.1
Gastrosuccorrhea (continuous) (intermittent) K31.89
  neurotic F45.8
  psychogenic F45.8
Gatophobia F40.218
Gaucher's disease or splenomegaly (adult) (infantile)
  E75.22
Gee (-Herter)(-Thaysen) **disease** (nontropical sprue) K90.0
Gelineau's syndrome G47.419
  with cataplexy G47.411
Gemination, tooth, teeth K00.2
Gemistocytoma
  specified site — see Neoplasm, malignant, by site

Gemistocytoma — continued
  unspecified site C71.9
General, generalized — see condition
Genetic
  carrier (status)
    cystic fibrosis Z14.1
    hemophilia A (asymptomatic) Z14.01
      symptomatic Z14.02
    specified NEC Z14.8
  susceptibility to disease NEC Z15.89
    epilepsy Z15.1
    malignant neoplasm Z15.09
      breast Z15.01
      endometrium Z15.04
      ovary Z15.02
      prostate Z15.03
      specified NEC Z15.09
    multiple endocrine neoplasia Z15.81
    neurodevelopmental disorders Z15.1
    obesity Z15.2
Genital — see condition
Genito-anorectal syndrome A55
Genitourinary system — see condition
Genu
  congenital Q74.1
  extrorsum (acquired) — see also Deformity, varus, knee
    congenital Q74.1
    sequelae (late effect) of rickets E64.3
  introrsum (acquired) — see also Deformity, valgus, knee
    congenital Q74.1
    sequelae (late effect) of rickets E64.3
  rachitic (old) E64.3
  recurvatum (acquired) — see also Deformity, limb,
    specified type NEC, lower leg
    congenital Q68.2
    sequelae (late effect) of rickets E64.3
  valgum (acquired) (knock-knee) M21.06- ☑
    congenital Q74.1
    sequelae (late effect) of rickets E64.3
  varum (acquired) (bowleg) M21.16- ☑
    congenital Q74.1
    sequelae (late effect) of rickets E64.3
Geographic tongue K14.1
Geophagia — see Pica
Geotrichosis B48.3
  stomatitis B48.3
Gephyrophobia F40.242
Gerbode defect Q21.0
GERD (gastroesophageal reflux disease) K21.9
Gerhardt's
  disease (erythromelalgia) I73.81
  syndrome (vocal cord paralysis) J38.00
    bilateral J38.02
    unilateral J38.01
German measles — see also Rubella
  exposure to Z20.4
Germinoblastoma (diffuse) C85.9- ☑
  follicular C82.9- ☑
Germinoma — see Neoplasm, malignant, by site
Gerontoxon — see Degeneration, cornea, senile
Gerstmann's syndrome R48.8
  developmental F81.2
Gerstmann-Straussler-Scheinker syndrome (GSS) A81.82
Gestation (period) — see also Pregnancy
  ectopic — see Pregnancy, by site
  multiple O30.9- ☑
    greater than quadruplets — see Pregnancy, multiple
      (gestation), specified NEC
    specified NEC — see Pregnancy, multiple (gestation),
      specified NEC
Gestational
  mammary abscess O91.11- ☑
  purulent mastitis O91.11- ☑
  subareolar abscess O91.11- ☑
Ghon tubercle, primary infection A15.7
Ghost
  teeth K00.4
  vessels (cornea) H16.41- ☑
Ghoul hand A66.3
Gianotti-Crosti disease L44.4
Giant
  cell
    epulis K06.8
    peripheral granuloma K06.8
  esophagus, congenital Q39.5
  kidney, congenital Q63.3
  urticaria T78.3 ☑
    hereditary D84.1

Giardiasis A07.1
Gibert's disease or pityriasis L42
Giddiness R42
  hysterical F44.89
  psychogenic F45.8
Gierke's disease (glycogenosis I) E74.01
Gigantism (cerebral) (hypophyseal) (pituitary) E22.0
  constitutional E34.4
Gilbert's disease or syndrome E80.4
Gilchrist's disease B40.9
Gilford-Hutchinson disease E34.8
Gilles de la Tourette's disease or syndrome (motor-verbal
  tic) F95.2
Gingivitis K05.10
  acute (catarrhal) K05.00
    necrotizing A69.1
    nonplaque induced K05.01
    plaque induced K05.00
  chronic (desquamative) (hyperplastic) (simple marginal)
    (pregnancy associated) (ulcerative) K05.10
    nonplaque induced K05.11
    plaque induced K05.10
  expulsiva — see Periodontitis
  necrotizing ulcerative (acute) A69.1
  pellagrous E52
    acute necrotizing A69.1
  Vincent's A69.1
Gingivoglossitis K14.0
Gingivopericementitis — see Periodontitis
Gingivosis — see Gingivitis, chronic
Gingivostomatitis K05.10
  herpesviral B00.2
  necrotizing ulcerative (acute) A69.1
Gland, glandular — see condition
Glanders A24.0
Glanzmann (-Naegeli) **disease or thrombasthenia** D69.1
Glasgow coma scale
  total score
    3-8 R40.243 ☑
    9-12 R40.242 ☑
    13-15 R40.241 ☑
Glass-blower's disease (cataract) — see Cataract, specified
  NEC
Glaucoma H40.9
  with
    increased episcleral venous pressure H40.81- ☑
    pseudoexfoliation of lens — see Glaucoma, open an-
      gle, primary, capsular
  absolute H44.51- ☑
  angle-closure (primary) H40.20- ☑
    acute (attack) (crisis) H40.21- ☑
    chronic H40.22- ☑
    intermittent H40.23- ☑
    residual stage H40.24- ☑
  borderline H40.00- ☑
  capsular (with pseudoexfoliation of lens) — see Glauco-
    ma, open angle, primary, capsular
  childhood Q15.0
  closed angle — see Glaucoma, angle-closure
  congenital Q15.0
  corticosteroid-induced — see Glaucoma, secondary,
    drugs
  hypersecretion H40.82- ☑
  in (due to)
    amyloidosis E85.4 [H42]
    aniridia Q13.1 [H42]
    concussion of globe — see Glaucoma, secondary,
      trauma
    dislocation of lens — see Glaucoma, secondary
    disorder of lens NEC — see Glaucoma, secondary
    drugs — see Glaucoma, secondary, drugs
    endocrine disease NOS E34.9 [H42]
    eye
      inflammation — see Glaucoma, secondary, inflam-
        mation
      trauma — see Glaucoma, secondary, trauma
    hypermature cataract — see Glaucoma, secondary
    iridocyclitis — see Glaucoma, secondary, inflammation
    lens disorder — see Glaucoma, secondary
    Lowe's syndrome E72.03 [H42]
    metabolic disease NOS E88.9 [H42]
    ocular disorders NEC — see Glaucoma, secondary
    onchocerciasis B73.02
    pupillary block — see Glaucoma, secondary
    retinal vein occlusion — see Glaucoma, secondary
    Rieger anomaly Q13.81 [H42]
    rubeosis of iris — see Glaucoma, secondary
    tumor of globe — see Glaucoma, secondary

Glaucoma — *continued*
  infantile Q15.0
  low tension — *see* Glaucoma, open angle, primary, low-tension
  malignant H40.83- ☑
  narrow angle — *see* Glaucoma, angle-closure
  newborn Q15.0
  noncongestive (chronic) — *see* Glaucoma, open angle
  nonobstructive — *see* Glaucoma, open angle
  obstructive — *see also* Glaucoma, angle-closure
    due to lens changes — *see* Glaucoma, secondary
  open angle H40.10- ☑
    primary H40.11- ☑
      capsular (with pseudoexfoliation of lens) H40.14- ☑
      low-tension H40.12- ☑
      pigmentary H40.13- ☑
      residual stage H40.15- ☑
  phacolytic — *see* Glaucoma, secondary
  pigmentary — *see* Glaucoma, open angle, primary, pigmentary
  postinfectious — *see* Glaucoma, secondary, inflammation
  secondary (to) H40.5- ☑
    drugs H40.6- ☑
    inflammation H40.4- ☑
    trauma H40.3- ☑
  simple (chronic) H40.11- ☑
  simplex H40.11- ☑
  specified type NEC H40.89
  suspect H40.00- ☑
  syphilitic A52.71
  traumatic — *see also* Glaucoma, secondary, trauma
    newborn (birth injury) P15.3
  tuberculous A18.59
Glaucomatous flecks (subcapsular) — *see* Cataract, complicated
Glazed tongue K14.4
Gleet (gonococcal) A54.01
Glenard's disease K63.4
Glioblastoma (multiforme)
  with sarcomatous component
    specified site — *see* Neoplasm, malignant, by site
    unspecified site C71.9
  giant cell
    specified site — *see* Neoplasm, malignant, by site
    unspecified site C71.9
  specified site — *see* Neoplasm, malignant, by site
  unspecified site C71.9
Glioma (malignant)
  astrocytic
    specified site — *see* Neoplasm, malignant, by site
    unspecified site C71.9
  mixed
    specified site — *see* Neoplasm, malignant, by site
    unspecified site C71.9
  nose Q30.8
  specified site NEC — *see* Neoplasm, malignant, by site
  subependymal D43.2
    specified site — *see* Neoplasm, uncertain behavior, by site
    unspecified site D43.2
  unspecified site C71.9
Gliomatosis cerebri C71.0
Glioneuroma — *see* Neoplasm, uncertain behavior, by site
Gliosarcoma
  specified site — *see* Neoplasm, malignant, by site
  unspecified site C71.9
Gliosis (cerebral) G93.89
  spinal G95.89
Glisson's disease — *see* Rickets
Globinuria R82.3
Globus (hystericus) F45.8
Glomangioma D18.00
  intra-abdominal D18.03
  intracranial D18.02
  skin D18.01
  specified site NEC D18.09
Glomangiomyoma D18.00
  intra-abdominal D18.03
  intracranial D18.02
  skin D18.01
  specified site NEC D18.09
Glomangiosarcoma — *see* Neoplasm, connective tissue, malignant
Glomerular
  disease in syphilis A52.75
  nephritis — *see* Glomerulonephritis
Glomerulitis — *see* Glomerulonephritis

Glomerulonephritis — *see also* Nephritis N05.9
  with
    C3
      glomerulonephritis N05.A
      glomerulopathy N05.A
        with dense deposit disease N05.6
    edema — *see* Nephrosis
    minimal change N05.0
    minor glomerular abnormality N05.0
  acute N00.9
  chronic N03.9
  crescentic (diffuse) NEC — *see also* N00-N07 with fourth character .7 N05.7
  dense deposit — *see also* N00-N07 with fourth character .6 N05.6
  diffuse
    crescentic — *see also* N00-N07 with fourth character .7 N05.7
    endocapillary proliferative — *see also* N00-N07 with fourth character .4 N05.4
    membranous — *see also* N00-N07 with fourth character .2 N05.2
    mesangial proliferative — *see also* N00-N07 with fourth character .3 N05.3
    mesangiocapillary — *see also* N00-N07 with fourth character .5 N05.5
    sclerosing N18.9
  endocapillary proliferative (diffuse) NEC — *see also* N00-N07 with fourth character .4 N05.4
  extracapillary NEC — *see also* N00-N07 with fourth character .7 N05.7
  focal (and segmental) — *see also* N00-N07 with fourth character .1 N05.1
  hypocomplementemic — *see* Glomerulonephritis, membranoproliferative
  IgA — *see* Nephropathy, IgA
  immune complex (circulating) NEC N05.8
  in (due to)
    amyloidosis E85.4 *[N08]*
    bilharziasis B65.9 *[N08]*
    cryoglobulinemia D89.1 *[N08]*
    defibrination syndrome D65 *[N08]*
    diabetes mellitus — *see* Diabetes, glomerulosclerosis
    disseminated intravascular coagulation D65 *[N08]*
    Fabry (-Anderson) disease E75.21 *[N08]*
    Goodpasture's syndrome M31.0
    hemolytic-uremic syndrome — *see* Syndrome, hemolytic-uremic
    Henoch (-Schonlein) purpura D69.0 *[N08]*
    lecithin cholesterol acyltransferase deficiency E78.6 *[N08]*
    microscopic polyangiitis M31.7 *[N08]*
    multiple myeloma C90.0- ☑ *[N08]*
    Plasmodium malariae B52.0
    schistosomiasis B65.9 *[N08]*
    sepsis A41.9 *[N08]*
      streptococcal A40- ☑ *[N08]*
    sickle-cell disorders D57.- ☑ *[N08]*
    strongyloidiasis B78.9 *[N08]*
    subacute bacterial endocarditis I33.0 *[N08]*
    syphilis (late) congenital A50.59 *[N08]*
    systemic lupus erythematosus M32.14
    thrombotic thrombocytopenic purpura M31.19 *[N08]*
    typhoid fever A01.09
    Waldenstrom macroglobulinemia C88.0- ☑ *[N08]*
    Wegener's granulomatosis M31.31
  latent or quiescent N03.9
  lobular, lobulonodular — *see* Glomerulonephritis, membranoproliferative
  membranoproliferative (diffuse)(type 1 or 3) — *see also* N00-N07 with fourth character .5 N05.5
    dense deposit (type 2) NEC — *see also* N00-N07 with fourth character .6 N05.6
  membranous (diffuse) NEC — *see also* N00-N07 with fourth character .2 N05.2
  mesangial
    IgA/IgG — *see* Nephropathy, IgA
    proliferative (diffuse) NEC — *see also* N00-N07 with fourth character .3 N05.3
  mesangiocapillary (diffuse) NEC — *see also* N00-N07 with fourth character .5 N05.5
  necrotic, necrotizing NEC — *see also* N00-N07 with fourth character .8 N05.8
  nodular — *see* Glomerulonephritis, membranoproliferative
  poststreptococcal NEC N05.9
    acute N00.9
    chronic N03.9
    rapidly progressive N01.9

Glomerulonephritis — *continued*
  proliferative NEC — *see also* N00-N07 with fourth character .8 N05.8
    diffuse (lupus) M32.14
  rapidly progressive N01.9
  sclerosing, diffuse N18.9
  specified pathology NEC — *see also* N00-N07 with fourth character .8 N05.8
  subacute N01.9
Glomerulopathy — *see* Glomerulonephritis
Glomerulosclerosis — *see also* Sclerosis, renal
  intercapillary (nodular) (with diabetes) — *see* Diabetes, glomerulosclerosis
  intracapillary — *see* Diabetes, glomerulosclerosis
Glossagra K14.6
Glossalgia K14.6
Glossitis (chronic superficial) (gangrenous) (Moeller's) K14.0
  areata exfoliativa K14.1
  atrophic K14.4
  benign migratory K14.1
  cortical superficial, sclerotic K14.0
  Hunter's D51.0
  interstitial, sclerous K14.0
  median rhomboid K14.2
  pellagrous E52
  superficial, chronic K14.0
Glossocele K14.8
Glossodynia K14.6
  exfoliativa K14.4
Glossoncus K14.8
Glossopathy K14.9
Glossophytia K14.3
Glossoplegia K14.8
Glossoptosis K14.8
Glossopyrosis K14.6
Glossotrichia K14.3
Glossy skin L90.8
Glottis — *see* condition
Glottitis — *see also* Laryngitis J04.0
Glucagonoma
  pancreas
    benign D13.7
    malignant C25.4
    uncertain behavior D37.8
  specified site NEC
    benign — *see* Neoplasm, benign, by site
    malignant — *see* Neoplasm, malignant, by site
    uncertain behavior — *see* Neoplasm, uncertain behavior, by site
  unspecified site
    benign D13.7
    malignant C25.4
    uncertain behavior D37.8
Glucoglycinuria E72.51
Glucose-galactose malabsorption E74.39
Glue
  ear — *see* Otitis, media, nonsuppurative, chronic, mucoid
  sniffing (airplane) — *see* Abuse, drug, inhalant
  dependence — *see* Dependence, drug, inhalant
GLUT1 deficiency syndrome 1, infantile onset E74.810
GLUT1 deficiency syndrome 2, childhood onset E74.810
Glutaric aciduria E72.3
Glycinemia E72.51
Glycinuria (renal) (with ketosis) E72.09
Glycogen
  infiltration — *see* Disease, glycogen storage
  storage disease — *see* Disease, glycogen storage
Glycogenosis (diffuse) (generalized) — *see also* Disease, glycogen storage
  cardiac E74.02 *[I43]*
  diabetic, secondary — *see* Diabetes, glycogenosis, secondary
  pulmonary interstitial J84.842
Glycopenia E16.2
Glycosuria R81
  renal E74.818
Gnathostoma spinigerum (infection) (infestation), **gnathostomiasis** (wandering swelling) B83.1
Goiter (plunging) (substernal) E04.9
  with
    hyperthyroidism (recurrent) — *see* Hyperthyroidism, with, goiter
    thyrotoxicosis — *see* Hyperthyroidism, with, goiter
  adenomatous — *see* Goiter, nodular
  cancerous C73
  congenital (nontoxic) E03.0
    diffuse E03.0
    parenchymatous E03.0
    transitory, with normal functioning P72.0

Goiter — *continued*
  cystic E04.2
    due to iodine-deficiency E01.1
  due to
    enzyme defect in synthesis of thyroid hormone E07.1
    iodine-deficiency (endemic) E01.2
  dyshormonogenetic (familial) E07.1
  endemic (iodine-deficiency) E01.2
    diffuse E01.0
    multinodular E01.1
  exophthalmic — *see* Hyperthyroidism, with, goiter
  iodine-deficiency (endemic) E01.2
    diffuse E01.0
    multinodular E01.1
    nodular E01.1
  lingual Q89.2
  lymphadenoid E06.3
  malignant C73
  multinodular (cystic) (nontoxic) E04.2
    toxic or with hyperthyroidism E05.20
      with thyroid storm E05.21
  neonatal NEC P72.0
  nodular (nontoxic) (due to) E04.9
    with
      hyperthyroidism E05.20
        with thyroid storm E05.21
      thyrotoxicosis E05.20
        with thyroid storm E05.21
    endemic E01.1
    iodine-deficiency E01.1
    sporadic E04.9
    toxic E05.20
      with thyroid storm E05.21
  nontoxic E04.9
    diffuse (colloid) E04.0
    multinodular E04.2
    simple E04.0
    specified NEC E04.8
    uninodular E04.1
  simple E04.0
  toxic — *see* Hyperthyroidism, with, goiter
  uninodular (nontoxic) E04.1
    toxic or with hyperthyroidism E05.10
      with thyroid storm E05.11
Goiter-deafness syndrome E07.1
Goldberg syndrome Q89.8
Goldberg-Maxwell syndrome E34.51
Goldblatt's hypertension or kidney I70.1
Goldenhar (-Gorlin) **syndrome** Q87.0
Goldflam-Erb disease or syndrome G70.00
  with exacerbation (acute) G70.01
  in crisis G70.01
Goldscheider's disease Q81.8
Goldstein's disease (familial hemorrhagic telangiectasia) I78.0
Golfer's elbow — *see* Epicondylitis, medial
Gonadoblastoma
  specified site — *see* Neoplasm, uncertain behavior, by site
  unspecified site
    female D39.10
    male D40.10
Gonecystitis — *see* Vesiculitis
Gongylonemiasis B83.8
Goniosynechiae — *see* Adhesions, iris, goniosynechiae
Gonococcemia A54.86
Gonococcus, gonococcal (disease) (infection) — *see also* condition A54.9
  anus A54.6
  bursa, bursitis A54.49
  conjunctiva, conjunctivitis (neonatorum) A54.31
  endocardium A54.83
  eye A54.30
    conjunctivitis A54.31
    iridocyclitis A54.32
    keratitis A54.33
    newborn A54.31
    other specified A54.39
  fallopian tubes (acute) (chronic) A54.24
  genitourinary (organ) (system) (tract) (acute)
    lower A54.00
      with abscess (accessory gland) (periurethral) A54.1
    upper — *see also* condition A54.29
  heart A54.83
  iridocyclitis A54.32
  joint A54.42
  lymphatic (gland) (node) A54.89
  meninges, meningitis A54.81
  musculoskeletal A54.40

Gonococcus, gonococcal — *continued*
  musculoskeletal — *continued*
    arthritis A54.42
    osteomyelitis A54.43
    other specified A54.49
    spondylopathy A54.41
  pelviperitonitis A54.24
  pelvis (acute) (chronic) A54.24
  pharynx A54.5
  proctitis A54.6
  pyosalpinx (acute) (chronic) A54.24
  rectum A54.6
  skin A54.89
  specified site NEC A54.89
  tendon sheath A54.49
  throat A54.5
  urethra (acute) (chronic) A54.01
    with abscess (accessory gland) (periurethral) A54.1
  vulva (acute) (chronic) A54.02
Gonocytoma
  specified site — *see* Neoplasm, uncertain behavior, by site
  unspecified site
    female D39.10
    male D40.10
Gonorrhea (acute) (chronic) A54.9
  Bartholin's gland (acute) (chronic) (purulent) A54.02
    with abscess (accessory gland) (periurethral) A54.1
  bladder A54.01
  cervix A54.03
  conjunctiva, conjunctivitis (neonatorum) A54.31
  contact Z20.2
  Cowper's gland (with abscess) A54.1
  exposure to Z20.2
  fallopian tube (acute) (chronic) A54.24
  kidney (acute) (chronic) A54.21
  lower genitourinary tract A54.00
    with abscess (accessory gland) (periurethral) A54.1
  ovary (acute) (chronic) A54.24
  pelvis (acute) (chronic) A54.24
    female pelvic inflammatory disease A54.24
  penis A54.09
  prostate (acute) (chronic) A54.22
  seminal vesicle (acute) (chronic) A54.23
  specified site not listed — *see also* Gonococcus A54.89
  spermatic cord (acute) (chronic) A54.23
  urethra A54.01
    with abscess (accessory gland) (periurethral) A54.1
  vagina A54.02
  vas deferens (acute) (chronic) A54.23
  vulva A54.02
Goodall's disease A08.19
Goodpasture's syndrome M31.0
Gopalan's syndrome (burning feet) E53.0
Gorlin-Chaudry-Moss syndrome Q87.0
Gottron's papules L94.4
Gougerot-Blum syndrome (pigmented purpuric lichenoid dermatitis) L81.7
Gougerot-Carteaud disease or syndrome (confluent reticulate papillomatosis) L83
Gougerot's syndrome (trisymptomatic) L81.7
Gouley's syndrome (constrictive pericarditis) I31.1
Goundou A66.6
Gout, chronic — *see also* Gout, gouty M1A.9 ☑ (*following* M08)
  drug-induced M1A.20 ☑ (*following* M08)
    ankle M1A.27- ☑ (*following* M08)
    elbow M1A.22- ☑ (*following* M08)
    foot joint M1A.27- ☑ (*following* M08)
    hand joint M1A.24- ☑ (*following* M08)
    hip M1A.25- ☑ (*following* M08)
    knee M1A.26- ☑ (*following* M08)
    multiple site M1A.29- ☑ (*following* M08)
    shoulder M1A.21- ☑ (*following* M08)
    vertebrae M1A.28 ☑ (*following* M08)
    wrist M1A.23- ☑ (*following* M08)
  idiopathic M1A.00 ☑ (*following* M08)
    ankle M1A.07- ☑ (*following* M08)
    elbow M1A.02- ☑ (*following* M08)
    foot joint M1A.07- ☑ (*following* M08)
    hand joint M1A.04- ☑ (*following* M08)
    hip M1A.05- ☑ (*following* M08)
    knee M1A.06- ☑ (*following* M08)
    multiple site M1A.09 ☑ (*following* M08)
    shoulder M1A.01- ☑ (*following* M08)
    vertebrae M1A.08 ☑ (*following* M08)
    wrist M1A.03- ☑ (*following* M08)
  in (due to) renal impairment M1A.30 ☑ (*following* M08)

Gout, chronic — *continued*
  in renal impairment — *continued*
    ankle M1A.37- ☑ (*following* M08)
    elbow M1A.32- ☑ (*following* M08)
    foot joint M1A.37- ☑ (*following* M08)
    hand joint M1A.34- ☑ (*following* M08)
    hip M1A.35- ☑ (*following* M08)
    knee M1A.36- ☑ (*following* M08)
    multiple site M1A.39 ☑ (*following* M08)
    shoulder M1A.31- ☑ (*following* M08)
    vertebrae M1A.38 ☑ (*following* M08)
    wrist M1A.33- ☑ (*following* M08)
  lead-induced M1A.10 ☑ (*following* M08)
    ankle M1A.17- ☑ (*following* M08)
    elbow M1A.12- ☑ (*following* M08)
    foot joint M1A.17- ☑ (*following* M08)
    hand joint M1A.14- ☑ (*following* M08)
    hip M1A.15- ☑ (*following* M08)
    knee M1A.16- ☑ (*following* M08)
    multiple site M1A.19 ☑ (*following* M08)
    shoulder M1A.11- ☑ (*following* M08)
    vertebrae M1A.18 ☑ (*following* M08)
    wrist M1A.13- ☑ (*following* M08)
  primary — *see* Gout, chronic, idiopathic
  saturnine — *see* Gout, chronic, lead-induced
  secondary NEC M1A.40 ☑ (*following* M08)
    ankle M1A.47- ☑ (*following* M08)
    elbow M1A.42- ☑ (*following* M08)
    foot joint M1A.47- ☑ (*following* M08)
    hand joint M1A.44- ☑ (*following* M08)
    hip M1A.45- ☑ (*following* M08)
    knee M1A.46- ☑ (*following* M08)
    multiple site M1A.49 ☑ (*following* M08)
    shoulder M1A.41- ☑ (*following* M08)
    vertebrae M1A.48 ☑ (*following* M08)
    wrist M1A.43- ☑ (*following* M08)
  syphilitic — *see also* subcategory M14.8- A52.77
  tophi M1A.9 ☑ (*following* M08)
Gout, gouty (acute) (attack) (flare) — *see also* Gout, chronic M10.9
  drug-induced M10.20
    ankle M10.27- ☑
    elbow M10.22- ☑
    foot joint M10.27- ☑
    hand joint M10.24- ☑
    hip M10.25- ☑
    knee M10.26- ☑
    multiple site M10.29
    shoulder M10.21- ☑
    vertebrae M10.28
    wrist M10.23- ☑
  idiopathic M10.00
    ankle M10.07- ☑
    elbow M10.02- ☑
    foot joint M10.07- ☑
    hand joint M10.04- ☑
    hip M10.05- ☑
    knee M10.06- ☑
    multiple site M10.09
    shoulder M10.01- ☑
    vertebrae M10.08
    wrist M10.03- ☑
  in (due to) renal impairment M10.30
    ankle M10.37- ☑
    elbow M10.32- ☑
    foot joint M10.37- ☑
    hand joint M10.34- ☑
    hip M10.35- ☑
    knee M10.36- ☑
    multiple site M10.39
    shoulder M10.31- ☑
    vertebrae M10.38
    wrist M10.33- ☑
  lead-induced M10.10
    ankle M10.17- ☑
    elbow M10.12- ☑
    foot joint M10.17- ☑
    hand joint M10.14- ☑
    hip M10.15- ☑
    knee M10.16- ☑
    multiple site M10.19
    shoulder M10.11- ☑
    vertebrae M10.18
    wrist M10.13- ☑
  primary — *see* Gout, idiopathic
  saturnine — *see* Gout, lead-induced

☑ **Additional Character Required** — **Refer to the Tabular List for Character Selection**

Gout, gouty — continued
  secondary NEC M10.40
    ankle M10.47- ☑
    elbow M10.42- ☑
    foot joint M10.47- ☑
    hand joint M10.44- ☑
    hip M10.45- ☑
    knee M10.46- ☑
    multiple site M10.49
    shoulder M10.41- ☑
    vertebrae M10.48
    wrist M10.43- ☑
  syphilitic — see also subcategory M14.8- A52.77
  tophi — see Gout, chronic
Gower's
  muscular dystrophy G71.01
  syndrome (vasovagal attack) R55
Gradenigo's syndrome — see Otitis, media, suppurative, acute
Graefe's disease — see Strabismus, paralytic, ophthalmoplegia, progressive
Graft-versus-host disease D89.813
  acute D89.810
  acute on chronic D89.812
  chronic D89.811
Grain mite (itch) B88.0
Grainhandler's disease or lung J67.8
Grand mal — see Epilepsy, generalized, specified NEC
Grand multipara status only (not pregnant) Z64.1
  pregnant — see Pregnancy, complicated by, grand multiparity
Granite worker's lung J62.8
Granular — see also condition
  inflammation, pharynx J31.2
  kidney (contracting) — see Sclerosis, renal
  liver K74.69
Granulation tissue (abnormal) (excessive) L92.9
  postmastoidectomy cavity — see Complications, postmastoidectomy, granulation
Granulocytopenia (primary) (malignant) — see Agranulocytosis
Granuloma L92.9
  abdomen K66.8
    from residual foreign body L92.3
    pyogenicum L98.0
  actinic L57.5
  annulare (perforating) L92.0
  apical K04.5
  aural — see Otitis, externa, specified NEC
  beryllium (skin) L92.3
  bone
    eosinophilic C96.6
    from residual foreign body — see Osteomyelitis, specified type NEC
    lung C96.6
  brain (any site) G06.0
    schistosomiasis B65.9 [G07]
  canaliculus lacrimalis — see Granuloma, lacrimal
  candidal (cutaneous) B37.2
  cerebral (any site) G06.0
  coccidioidal (primary) (progressive) B38.7
    lung B38.1
    meninges B38.4
  colon K63.89
  conjunctiva H11.22- ☑
  dental K04.5
  ear, middle — see Cholesteatoma
  eosinophilic C96.6
    bone C96.6
    lung C96.6
    oral mucosa K13.4
    skin L92.2
  eyelid H01.8
  facial (e) L92.2
  foreign body (in soft tissue) NEC M60.20
    ankle M60.27- ☑
    foot M60.27- ☑
    forearm M60.23- ☑
    hand M60.24- ☑
    in operation wound — see Foreign body, accidentally left during a procedure
    lower leg M60.26- ☑
    pelvic region M60.25- ☑
    shoulder region M60.21- ☑
    skin L92.3
    specified site NEC M60.28
    subcutaneous tissue L92.3
    thigh M60.25- ☑

Granuloma — continued
  foreign body — continued
    upper arm M60.22- ☑
  gangraenescens M31.2
  genito-inguinale A58
  giant cell (central) (reparative) (jaw) M27.1
    gingiva (peripheral) K06.8
  gland (lymph) I88.8
  hepatic NEC K75.3
    in (due to)
      berylliosis J63.2 [K77]
      sarcoidosis D86.89
  Hodgkin C81.9- ☑
  ileum K63.89
  infectious B99.9
    specified NEC B99.8
  inguinale (Donovan) (venereal) A58
  intestine NEC K63.89
  intracranial (any site) G06.0
  intraspinal (any part) G06.1
  iridocyclitis — see Iridocyclitis, chronic
  jaw (bone) (central) M27.1
    reparative giant cell M27.1
  kidney — see also Infection, kidney N15.8
  lacrimal H04.81- ☑
  larynx J38.7
  lethal midline (faciale(e)) M31.2
  liver NEC — see Granuloma, hepatic
  lung (infectious) — see also Fibrosis, lung
    coccidioidal B38.1
    eosinophilic C96.6
  Majocchi's B35.8
  malignant (facial(e)) M31.2
  mandible (central) M27.1
  midline (lethal) M31.2
  monilial (cutaneous) B37.2
  nasal sinus — see Sinusitis
  operation wound T81.89 ☑
    foreign body — see Foreign body, accidentally left during a procedure
    stitch T81.89 ☑
    talc — see Foreign body, accidentally left during a procedure
  oral mucosa K13.4
  orbit, orbital H05.11- ☑
  paracoccidioidal B41.8
  penis, venereal A58
  periapical K04.5
  peritoneum K66.8
    due to ova of helminths NOS — see also Helminthiasis B83.9 [K67]
  postmastoidectomy cavity — see Complications, postmastoidectomy, recurrent cholesteatoma
  prostate N42.89
  pudendi (ulcerating) A58
  pulp, internal (tooth) K03.3
  pyogenic, pyogenicum (of) (skin) L98.0
    gingiva K06.8
    maxillary alveolar ridge K04.5
    oral mucosa K13.4
  rectum K62.89
  reticulohistiocytic D76.3
  rubrum nasi L74.8
  Schistosoma — see Schistosomiasis
  septic (skin) L98.0
  silica (skin) L92.3
  sinus (accessory) (infective) (nasal) — see Sinusitis
  skin L92.9
    from residual foreign body L92.3
    pyogenicum L98.0
  spine
    syphilitic (epidural) A52.19
    tuberculous A18.01
  stitch (postoperative) T81.89 ☑
  suppurative (skin) L98.0
  swimming pool A31.1
  talc — see also Granuloma, foreign body
    in operation wound — see Foreign body, accidentally left during a procedure
  telangiectaticum (skin) L98.0
  tracheostomy J95.09
  trichophyticum B35.8
  tropicum A66.4
  umbilical P83.81
  umbilicus P83.81
  urethra N36.8
  uveitis — see Iridocyclitis, chronic
  vagina A58

Granuloma — continued
  venereum A58
  vocal cord J38.3
Granulomatosis L92.9
  with polyangiitis M31.3- ☑
  eosinophilic, with polyangiitis [EGPA] M30.1
  lymphoid C83.8- ☑
  miliary (listerial) A32.89
  necrotizing, respiratory M31.30
  progressive septic D71
  specified NEC L92.8
  Wegener's M31.30
    with renal involvement M31.31
Granulomatous tissue (abnormal) (excessive) L92.9
Granulosis rubra nasi L74.8
Graphite fibrosis (of lung) J63.3
Graphospasm F48.8
  organic G25.89
Grating scapula M89.8X1
Gravel (urinary) — see Calculus, urinary
Graves' disease — see Hyperthyroidism, with, goiter
Gravis — see condition
Grawitz tumor C64.- ☑
Gray syndrome (newborn) P93.0
Grayness, hair (premature) L67.1
  congenital Q84.2
Green sickness D50.8
Greenfield's disease
  meaning
    concentric sclerosis (encephalitis periaxialis concentrica) G37.5
    metachromatic leukodystrophy E75.25
Greenstick fracture — code as Fracture, by site
Grey syndrome (newborn) P93.0
Grief F43.21
  complicated F43.81
  prolonged F43.81
  reaction — see also Disorder, adjustment F43.20
Griesinger's disease B76.0
Grinder's lung or pneumoconiosis J62.8
Grinding, teeth
  psychogenic F45.8
  sleep related G47.63
Grip
  Dabney's B33.0
  devil's B33.0
Grippe, grippal — see also Influenza
  Balkan A78
  summer, of Italy A93.1
Grisel's disease M43.6
Groin — see condition
Grooved tongue K14.5
Ground itch B76.9
Grover's disease or syndrome L11.1
Growing pains, children R29.898
Growth (fungoid) (neoplastic) (new) — see also Neoplasm
  adenoid (vegetative) J35.8
  benign — see Neoplasm, benign, by site
  malignant — see Neoplasm, malignant, by site
  rapid, childhood Z00.2
  secondary — see Neoplasm, secondary, by site
Gruby's disease B35.0
Guardianship by non-parental relative Z62.23
Gubler-Millard paralysis or syndrome G46.3
Guerin-Stern syndrome Q74.3
Guidance, insufficient anterior (occlusal) M26.54
Guillain-Barre disease or syndrome G61.0
  sequelae G65.0
Guinea worms (infection) (infestation) B72
Guinon's disease (motor-verbal tic) F95.2
Gull's disease E03.4
Gum — see condition
Gumboil K04.7
  with sinus K04.6
Gumma (syphilitic) A52.79
  artery A52.09
    cerebral A52.04
  bone A52.77
    of yaws (late) A66.6
  brain A52.19
  cauda equina A52.19
  central nervous system A52.3
  ciliary body A52.71
  congenital A50.59
  eyelid A52.71
  heart A52.06
  intracranial A52.19
  iris A52.71
  kidney A52.75

Gumma — *continued*
  larynx A52.73
  leptomeninges A52.19
  liver A52.74
  meninges A52.19
  myocardium A52.06
  nasopharynx A52.73
  neurosyphilitic A52.3
  nose A52.73
  orbit A52.71
  palate (soft) A52.79
  penis A52.76
  pericardium A52.06
  pharynx A52.73
  pituitary A52.79
  scrofulous (tuberculous) A18.4
  skin A52.79
  specified site NEC A52.79
  spinal cord A52.19
  tongue A52.79
  tonsil A52.73
  trachea A52.73
  tuberculous A18.4
  ulcerative due to yaws A66.4
  ureter A52.75
  yaws A66.4
    bone A66.6
Gunn's syndrome Q07.8
Gunshot wound — *see also* Puncture, open
  fracture — *code as* Fracture, by site
  internal organs — *see* Injury, by site
Gynandrism Q56.0
Gynandroblastoma
  specified site — *see* Neoplasm, uncertain behavior, by site
  unspecified site
    female D39.10
    male D40.10
Gynecological examination (periodic) (routine) Z01.419
  with abnormal findings Z01.411
Gynecomastia N62
Gynephobia F40.291
Gyrate scalp Q82.8

H

H (Hartnup's) **disease** E72.02
Haas' disease or osteochondrosis (juvenile) (head of humerus) — *see* Osteochondrosis, juvenile, humerus
H-ABC (hypomyelination with atrophy of the basal ganglia and cerebellum) G23.3
Habit, habituation
  bad sleep Z72.821
  chorea F95.8
  disturbance, child F98.9
  drug — *see* Dependence, drug
  irregular sleep Z72.821
  laxative F55.2
  spasm — *see* Tic
  tic — *see* Tic
Haemophilus (H.) **influenzae, as cause of disease classified elsewhere** B96.3
Haff disease — *see* Poisoning, mercury
Hageman's factor defect, deficiency or disease D68.2
Haglund's disease or osteochondrosis (juvenile) (os tibiale externum) — *see* Osteochondrosis, juvenile, tarsus
Hailey-Hailey disease Q82.8
Hair — *see also* condition
  plucking F63.3
    in stereotyped movement disorder F98.4
  tourniquet syndrome — *see also* Constriction, external, by site
    finger S60.44- ☑
    penis S30.842 ☑
    thumb S60.34- ☑
    toe S90.44- ☑
Hairball in stomach T18.2 ☑
Hair-pulling, pathological (compulsive) F63.3
Hairy black tongue K14.3
Half vertebra Q76.49
Halitosis R19.6
Hallerman-Streiff syndrome Q87.0
Hallervorden-Spatz disease G23.0
Hallopeau's acrodermatitis or disease L40.2
Hallucination R44.3
  auditory R44.0
  gustatory R44.2
  olfactory R44.2

Hallucination — *continued*
  specified NEC R44.2
  tactile R44.2
  visual R44.1
Hallucinosis (chronic) F28
  alcoholic (acute) F10.951
    in
      abuse F10.151
      dependence F10.251
  drug-induced F19.951
    cannabis F12.951
    cocaine F14.951
    hallucinogen F16.151
    in
      abuse F19.151
        cannabis F12.151
        cocaine F14.151
        hallucinogen F16.151
        inhalant F18.151
        opioid F11.151
        sedative, anxiolytic or hypnotic F13.151
        stimulant NEC F15.151
      dependence F19.251
        cannabis F12.251
        cocaine F14.251
        hallucinogen F16.251
        inhalant F18.251
        opioid F11.251
        sedative, anxiolytic or hypnotic F13.251
        stimulant NEC F15.251
    inhalant F18.951
    opioid F11.951
    sedative, anxiolytic or hypnotic F13.951
    stimulant NEC F15.951
  organic F06.0
Hallux
  deformity (acquired) NEC M20.5X- ☑
  limitus M20.5X- ☑
  malleus (acquired) NEC M20.3- ☑
  rigidus (acquired) M20.2- ☑
    congenital Q74.2
    sequelae (late effect) of rickets E64.3
  valgus (acquired) M20.1- ☑
    congenital Q66.6
  varus (acquired) M20.3- ☑
    congenital Q66.3- ☑
Halo, visual H53.19
Hamartoma, hamartoblastoma Q85.9
  epithelial (gingival), odontogenic, central or peripheral — *see* Cyst, calcifying odontogenic
Hamartosis Q85.9
Hamman-Rich syndrome J84.114
Hammer toe (acquired) NEC — *see also* Deformity, toe, hammer toe
  congenital Q66.89
  sequelae (late effect) of rickets E64.3
Hand — *see* condition
Hand-foot syndrome L27.1
Handicap, handicapped
  educational Z55.9
    specified NEC Z55.8
Hand-Schuller-Christian disease or syndrome C96.5
Hanging (asphyxia) (strangulation) (suffocation) — *see* Asphyxia, traumatic, due to mechanical threat
Hangnail — *see also* Cellulitis, digit
  with lymphangitis — *see* Lymphangitis, acute, digit
Hangover (alcohol) F10.129
Hanhart's syndrome Q87.0
Hanot-Chauffard (-Troisier) **syndrome** E83.19
Hanot's cirrhosis or disease K74.3
Hansen's disease — *see* Leprosy
Hantaan virus disease (Korean hemorrhagic fever) A98.5
Hantavirus disease (with renal manifestations) (Dobrava) (Puumala) (Seoul) A98.5
  with pulmonary manifestations (Andes) (Bayou) (Bermejo) (Black Creek Canal) (Choclo) (Juquitiba) (Laguna negra) (Lechiguanas) (New York) (Oran) (Sin nombre) B33.4
Happy puppet syndrome Q93.51
Harada's disease or syndrome H30.81- ☑
Hardening
  artery — *see* Arteriosclerosis
  brain G93.89
Hardship, material, due to limited financial resources, specified NEC Z59.87
Harelip (complete) (incomplete) — *see* Cleft, lip
Harlequin (newborn) Q80.4
Harley's disease D59.6

Harmful use (of)
  alcohol F10.10
  anxiolytics — *see* Abuse, drug, sedative
  cannabinoids — *see* Abuse, drug, cannabis
  cocaine — *see* Abuse, drug, cocaine
  drug — *see* Abuse, drug
  hallucinogens — *see* Abuse, drug, hallucinogen
  hypnotics — *see* Abuse, drug, sedative
  opioids — *see* Abuse, drug, opioid
  PCP (phencyclidine) — *see* Abuse, drug, hallucinogen
  sedatives — *see* Abuse, drug, sedative
  stimulants NEC — *see* Abuse, drug, stimulant
Harris' lines — *see* Arrest, epiphyseal
Hartnup's disease E72.02
Harvester's lung J67.0
Harvesting ovum for in vitro fertilization Z31.83
Hashimoto's disease or thyroiditis E06.3
Hashitoxicosis (transient) E06.3
Hassal-Henle bodies or warts (cornea) H18.49
Haut mal — *see* Epilepsy, generalized, specified NEC
Haverhill fever A25.1
Hay fever — *see also* Fever, hay J30.1
Hayem-Widal syndrome D59.8
Haygarth's nodes M15.8
Haymaker's lung J67.0
Hb (abnormal)
  Bart's disease D56.0
  disease — *see* Disease, hemoglobin
  trait — *see* Trait
Head — *see* condition
Headache R51.9
  with
    orthostatic component NEC R51.0
    positional component NEC R51.0
  allergic NEC G44.89
  associated with sexual activity G44.82
  cervicogenic G44.86
  chronic daily R51.9
  cluster G44.009
    chronic G44.029
      intractable G44.021
      not intractable G44.029
    episodic G44.019
      intractable G44.011
      not intractable G44.019
    intractable G44.001
    not intractable G44.009
  cough (primary) G44.83
  daily chronic R51.9
  drug-induced NEC G44.40
    intractable G44.41
    not intractable G44.40
  exertional (primary) G44.84
  histamine G44.009
    intractable G44.001
    not intractable G44.009
  hypnic G44.81
  lumbar puncture G97.1
  medication overuse G44.40
    intractable G44.41
    not intractable G44.40
  menstrual — *see* Migraine, menstrual
  migraine (type) — *see also* Migraine G43.909
  nasal septum R51.9
  neuralgiform, short lasting unilateral, with conjunctival injection and tearing (SUNCT) G44.059
    intractable G44.051
    not intractable G44.059
  new daily persistent (NDPH) G44.52
  orgasmic G44.82
  periodic syndromes in adults and children G43.C0 (*following* G43.7)
    with refractory migraine G43.C1 (*following* G43.7)
    intractable G43.C1 (*following* G43.7)
    not intractable G43.C0 (*following* G43.7)
    without refractory migraine G43.C0 (*following* G43.7)
  postspinal puncture G97.1
  post-traumatic G44.309
    acute G44.319
      intractable G44.311
      not intractable G44.319
    chronic G44.329
      intractable G44.321
      not intractable G44.329
    intractable G44.301
    not intractable G44.309
  pre-menstrual — *see* Migraine, menstrual
  preorgasmic G44.82

Headache — *continued*
  primary
    cough G44.83
    exertional G44.84
    stabbing G44.85
    thunderclap G44.53
  rebound G44.40
    intractable G44.41
    not intractable G44.40
  short lasting unilateral neuralgiform, with conjunctival
    injection and tearing (SUNCT) G44.059
    intractable G44.051
    not intractable G44.059
  specified syndrome NEC G44.89
  spinal and epidural anesthesia - induced T88.59 ☑
    in labor and delivery O74.5
    in pregnancy O29.4- ☑
    postpartum, puerperal O89.4
  spinal fluid loss (from puncture) G97.1
  stabbing (primary) G44.85
  tension (-type) G44.209
    chronic G44.229
      intractable G44.221
      not intractable G44.229
    episodic G44.219
      intractable G44.211
      not intractable G44.219
    intractable G44.201
    not intractable G44.209
  thunderclap (primary) G44.53
  vascular NEC G44.1
Healthy
  infant
    accompanying sick mother Z76.3
    receiving care Z76.2
  person accompanying sick person Z76.3
Hearing examination Z01.10
  with abnormal findings NEC Z01.118
  following failed hearing screening Z01.110
  for hearing conservation and treatment Z01.12
  infant or child (over 28 days old) Z00.129
    with abnormal findings Z00.121
Heart — *see* condition
  carcinoid — *see* Syndrome, carcinoid, heart
Heart beat
  abnormality R00.9
    specified NEC R00.8
  awareness R00.2
  rapid R00.0
  slow R00.1
Heartburn R12
  psychogenic F45.8
Heartland virus disease A93.8
Heat (effects) T67.9 ☑
  apoplexy T67.01 ☑
  burn — *see also* Burn L55.9
  collapse T67.1 ☑
  cramps T67.2 ☑
  dermatitis or eczema L59.0
  edema T67.7 ☑
  erythema — *code by site under* Burn, first degree
  excessive T67.9 ☑
    specified effect NEC T67.8 ☑
  exhaustion T67.5 ☑
    anhydrotic T67.3 ☑
    due to
      salt (and water) depletion T67.4 ☑
      water depletion T67.3 ☑
        with salt depletion T67.4 ☑
  fatigue (transient) T67.6 ☑
  fever T67.01 ☑
  hyperpyrexia T67.01 ☑
  prickly L74.0
  prostration — *see* Heat, exhaustion
  pyrexia T67.01 ☑
  rash L74.0
  specified effect NEC T67.8 ☑
  stroke T67.01 ☑
    exertional T67.02 ☑
    specified NEC T67.09 ☑
  sunburn — *see* Sunburn
  syncope T67.1 ☑
Heavy-for-dates NEC (infant) (4000g to 4499g) P08.1
  exceptionally (4500g or more) P08.0
Hebephrenia, hebephrenic (schizophrenia) F20.1
Heberden's disease or nodes (with arthropathy) M15.1
Hebra's
  pityriasis L26

Hebra's — *continued*
  prurigo L28.2
Heel — *see* condition
Heerfordt's disease D86.89
Hegglin's anomaly or syndrome D72.0
Heilmeyer-Schoner disease D45
Heine-Medin disease A80.9
Heinz body anemia, congenital D58.2
Heliophobia F40.228
Heller's disease or syndrome F84.3
HELLP syndrome (hemolysis, elevated liver enzymes and
  low platelet count) O14.2- ☑
  complicating
    childbirth O14.24
    puerperium O14.25
Helminthiasis — *see also* Infestation, helminth
  Ancylostoma B76.0
  intestinal B82.0
    mixed types (types classifiable to more than one of
      the titles B65.0-B81.3 and B81.8) B81.4
    specified type NEC B81.8
  mixed types (intestinal) (types classifiable to more than
    one of the titles B65.0-B81.3 and B81.8) B81.4
  Necator (americanus) B76.1
  specified type NEC B83.8
Heloma L84
Hemangioblastoma — *see* Neoplasm, connective tissue,
  uncertain behavior
  malignant — *see* Neoplasm, connective tissue, malignant
Hemangioendothelioma — *see also* Neoplasm, uncertain
  behavior, by site
  benign D18.00
    intra-abdominal D18.03
    intracranial D18.02
    skin D18.01
    specified site NEC D18.09
  bone (diffuse) — *see* Neoplasm, bone, malignant
  epithelioid — *see also* Neoplasm, uncertain behavior, by
    site
    malignant — *see* Neoplasm, malignant, by site
  malignant — *see* Neoplasm, connective tissue, malignant
Hemangiofibroma — *see* Neoplasm, benign, by site
Hemangiolipoma — *see* Lipoma
Hemangioma D18.00
  arteriovenous D18.00
    intra-abdominal D18.03
    intracranial D18.02
    skin D18.01
    specified site NEC D18.09
  capillary I78.1
    intra-abdominal D18.03
    intracranial D18.02
    skin D18.01
    specified site NEC D18.09
  cavernous D18.00
    intra-abdominal D18.03
    intracranial D18.02
    skin D18.01
    specified site NEC D18.09
  epithelioid D18.00
    intra-abdominal D18.03
    intracranial D18.02
    skin D18.01
    specified site NEC D18.09
  histiocytoid D18.00
    intra-abdominal D18.03
    intracranial D18.02
    skin D18.01
    specified site NEC D18.09
  infantile D18.00
    intra-abdominal D18.03
    intracranial D18.02
    skin D18.01
    specified site NEC D18.09
  intra-abdominal D18.03
  intracranial D18.02
  intramuscular D18.00
    intra-abdominal D18.03
    intracranial D18.02
    skin D18.01
    specified site NEC D18.09
  intrathoracic structures D18.09
  juvenile D18.00
  malignant — *see* Neoplasm, connective tissue, malignant
  plexiform D18.00
    intra-abdominal D18.03
    intracranial D18.02
    skin D18.01
    specified site NEC D18.09

Hemangioma — *continued*
  racemose D18.00
    intra-abdominal D18.03
    intracranial D18.02
    skin D18.01
    specified site NEC D18.09
  sclerosing — *see* Neoplasm, skin, benign
  simplex D18.00
    intra-abdominal D18.03
    intracranial D18.02
    skin D18.01
    specified site NEC D18.09
  skin D18.01
  specified site NEC D18.09
  venous D18.00
    intra-abdominal D18.03
    intracranial D18.02
    skin D18.01
    specified site NEC D18.09
  verrucous keratotic D18.00
    intra-abdominal D18.03
    intracranial D18.02
    skin D18.01
    specified site NEC D18.09
Hemangiomatosis (systemic) I78.8
  involving single site — *see* Hemangioma
Hemangiopericytoma — *see also* Neoplasm, connective
  tissue, uncertain behavior
  benign — *see* Neoplasm, connective tissue, benign
  malignant — *see* Neoplasm, connective tissue, malignant
Hemangiosarcoma — *see* Neoplasm, connective tissue,
  malignant
Hemarthrosis (nontraumatic) M25.00
  ankle M25.07- ☑
  elbow M25.02- ☑
  foot joint M25.07- ☑
  hand joint M25.04- ☑
  hip M25.05- ☑
  in hemophilic arthropathy — *see* Arthropathy,
    hemophilic
  knee M25.06- ☑
  shoulder M25.01- ☑
  specified joint NEC M25.08
  traumatic — *see* Sprain, by site
  vertebrae M25.08
  wrist M25.03- ☑
Hematemesis K92.0
  with ulcer — *code by site under* Ulcer, with hemorrhage
    K27.4
  newborn, neonatal P54.0
    due to swallowed maternal blood P78.2
Hematidrosis L74.8
Hematinuria — *see also* Hemoglobinuria
  malarial B50.8
Hematobilia K83.8
Hematocele
  female NEC N94.89
    with ectopic pregnancy O00.90
      with intrauterine pregnancy O00.91
    ovary N83.8
  male N50.1
Hematochezia — *see also* Melena K92.1
Hematochyluria — *see also* Infestation, filarial
  schistosomiasis (bilharziasis) B65.0
Hematocolpos (with hematometra or hematosalpinx) N89.7
Hematocornea — *see* Pigmentation, cornea, stromal
Hematogenous — *see* condition
Hematoma (traumatic) (skin surface intact) — *see also*
  Contusion
  with
    injury of internal organs — *see* Injury, by site
    open wound — *see* Wound, open
  amputation stump (surgical) (late) T87.89
  aorta, dissecting I71.00
    abdominal I71.02
    thoracic — *see also* Dissection, aorta, thoracic I71.019
    thoracoabdominal I71.03
  aortic intramural — *see* Dissection, aorta
  arterial (complicating trauma) — *see* Injury, blood vessel,
    by site
  auricle — *see* Contusion, ear
    nontraumatic — *see* Disorder, pinna, hematoma
  birth injury NEC P15.8
  brain (traumatic)
    with
      cerebral laceration or contusion (diffuse) — *see*
        Injury, intracranial, diffuse
        focal — *see* Injury, intracranial, focal

Hematoma — continued
- brain — continued
  - cerebellar, traumatic S06.37- ☑
  - intracerebral, traumatic — see Injury, intracranial, intracerebral hemorrhage
  - newborn NEC P52.4
    - birth injury P10.1
  - nontraumatic — see Hemorrhage, intracranial
  - subarachnoid, arachnoid, traumatic — see Injury, intracranial, subarachnoid hemorrhage
  - subdural, traumatic — see Injury, intracranial, subdural hemorrhage
- breast (nontraumatic) N64.89
- broad ligament (nontraumatic) N83.7
  - traumatic S37.892 ☑
- cerebellar, traumatic S06.37- ☑
- cerebral — see Hematoma, brain
- cerebrum S06.36- ☑
  - left S06.35- ☑
  - right S06.34- ☑
- cesarean delivery wound O90.2
- complicating delivery (perineal) (pelvic) (vagina) (vulva) O71.7
- corpus cavernosum (nontraumatic) N48.89
- epididymis (nontraumatic) N50.1
- epidural (traumatic) — see Injury, intracranial, epidural hemorrhage
  - spinal — see Injury, spinal cord, by region
- episiotomy O90.2
- face, birth injury P15.4
- genital organ NEC (nontraumatic)
  - female (nonobstetric) N94.89
    - traumatic S30.202 ☑
  - male N50.1
    - traumatic S30.201 ☑
- internal organs — see Injury, by site
- intracerebral, traumatic — see Injury, intracranial, intracerebral hemorrhage
- intraoperative — see Complications, intraoperative, hemorrhage
- labia (nontraumatic) (nonobstetric) N90.89
- liver (subcapsular) (nontraumatic) K76.89
  - birth injury P15.0
- mediastinum — see Injury, intrathoracic
- mesosalpinx (nontraumatic) N83.7
  - traumatic S37.898 ☑
- muscle — code by site under Contusion
- nontraumatic
  - muscle M79.81
  - soft tissue M79.81
- obstetrical surgical wound O90.2
- orbit, orbital (nontraumatic) — see also Hemorrhage, orbit
  - traumatic — see Contusion, orbit
- pelvis (female) (nontraumatic) (nonobstetric) N94.89
  - obstetric O71.7
  - traumatic — see Injury, by site
- penis (nontraumatic) N48.89
  - birth injury P15.5
- perianal (nontraumatic) K64.5
- perineal S30.23 ☑
  - complicating delivery O71.7
- perirenal — see Injury, kidney
- peritoneal K66.1
- pinna — see Contusion, ear
  - nontraumatic — see Disorder, pinna, hematoma
- placenta O43.89- ☑
- postoperative (postprocedural) — see Complication, postprocedural, hematoma
- retroperitoneal (nontraumatic) K68.3
  - traumatic S36.892 ☑
- scrotum, superficial S30.22 ☑
  - birth injury P15.5
- seminal vesicle (nontraumatic) N50.1
  - traumatic S37.892 ☑
- spermatic cord (traumatic) S37.892 ☑
  - nontraumatic N50.1
- spinal (cord) (meninges) — see also Injury, spinal cord, by region
  - newborn (birth injury) P11.5
- spleen D73.5
  - intraoperative — see Complications, intraoperative, hemorrhage, spleen
  - postprocedural (postoperative) — see Complications, postprocedural, hemorrhage, spleen
- sternocleidomastoid, birth injury P15.2
- sternomastoid, birth injury P15.2

Hematoma — continued
- subarachnoid (traumatic) — see Injury, intracranial, subarachnoid hemorrhage
  - newborn (nontraumatic) P52.5
    - due to birth injury P10.3
  - nontraumatic — see Hemorrhage, intracranial, subarachnoid
- subdural (traumatic) — see Injury, intracranial, subdural hemorrhage
  - newborn (localized) P52.8
    - birth injury P10.0
  - nontraumatic — see Hemorrhage, intracranial, subdural
- superficial, newborn P54.5
- testis (nontraumatic) N50.1
  - birth injury P15.5
- tunica vaginalis (nontraumatic) N50.1
- umbilical cord, complicating delivery O69.5 ☑
- uterine ligament (broad) (nontraumatic) N83.7
  - traumatic S37.892 ☑
- vagina (ruptured) (nontraumatic) N89.8
  - complicating delivery O71.7
- vas deferens (nontraumatic) N50.1
  - traumatic S37.892 ☑
- vitreous — see Hemorrhage, vitreous
- vulva (nontraumatic) (nonobstetric) N90.89
  - complicating delivery O71.7
  - newborn (birth injury) P15.5

Hematometra N85.7
- with hematocolpos N89.7

Hematomyelia (central) G95.19
- newborn (birth injury) P11.5
- traumatic T14.8 ☑

Hematomyelitis G04.90

Hematoperitoneum — see Hemoperitoneum

Hematopneumothorax (see Hemothorax)

Hematophobia F40.230

Hematopoiesis, cyclic D70.4

Hematoporphyria — see Porphyria

Hematorachis, hematorrhachis G95.19
- newborn (birth injury) P11.5

Hematosalpinx N83.6
- with
  - hematocolpos N89.7
  - hematometra N85.7
    - with hematocolpos N89.7
- infectional — see Salpingitis

Hematospermia R36.1

Hematothorax (see Hemothorax)

Hematuria R31.9
- benign (familial) (of childhood) — see also Hematuria, idiopathic
  - essential microscopic R31.1
- due to sulphonamide, sulfonamide — see Table of Drugs and Chemicals, by drug
- endemic — see also Schistosomiasis B65.0
- gross R31.0
- idiopathic N02.9
  - with glomerular lesion
    - C3
      - glomerulonephritis N02.A
      - glomerulopathy N02.A
        - with dense deposit disease N02.6
    - crescentic (diffuse) glomerulonephritis N02.7
    - dense deposit disease N02.6
    - endocapillary proliferative glomerulonephritis N02.4
    - focal and segmental hyalinosis or sclerosis N02.1
    - membranoproliferative (diffuse) N02.5
    - membranous (diffuse) N02.2
    - mesangial proliferative (diffuse) N02.3
    - mesangiocapillary (diffuse) N02.5
    - minor abnormality N02.0
    - proliferative NEC N02.8
    - specified pathology NEC N02.8
- intermittent — see Hematuria, idiopathic
- malarial B50.8
- microscopic NEC (with symptoms) R31.29
  - asymptomatic R31.21
  - benign essential R31.1
- paroxysmal — see also Hematuria, idiopathic
  - nocturnal D59.5
- persistent — see Hematuria, idiopathic
- recurrent — see Hematuria, idiopathic
- tropical — see also Schistosomiasis B65.0
- tuberculous A18.13

Hemeralopia (day blindness) H53.11
- vitamin A deficiency E50.5

Hemi-akinesia R41.4

Hemianalgesia R20.0

Hemianencephaly Q00.0

Hemianesthesia R20.0

Hemianopia, hemianopsia (heteronymous) H53.47
- homonymous H53.46- ☑
- syphilitic A52.71

Hemiathetosis R25.8

Hemiatrophy R68.89
- cerebellar G31.9
- face, facial, progressive (Romberg) G51.8
- tongue K14.8

Hemiballism (us) G25.5

Hemicardia Q24.8

Hemicephalus, hemicephaly Q00.0

Hemichorea G25.5

Hemicolitis, left — see Colitis, left sided

Hemicrania
- congenital malformation Q00.0
- continua G44.51
- meaning migraine — see also Migraine G43.909
- paroxysmal G44.039
  - chronic G44.049
    - intractable G44.041
    - not intractable G44.049
  - episodic G44.039
    - intractable G44.031
    - not intractable G44.039
  - intractable G44.031
  - not intractable G44.039

Hemidystrophy — see Hemiatrophy

Hemiectromelia Q73.8

Hemihypalgesia R20.8

Hemihypesthesia R20.1

Hemi-inattention R41.4

Hemimegalencephaly Q04.5

Hemimelia Q73.8
- lower limb — see Defect, reduction, lower limb, specified type NEC
- upper limb — see Defect, reduction, upper limb, specified type NEC

Hemiparalysis — see Hemiplegia

Hemiparesis — see Hemiplegia

Hemiparesthesia R20.2

Hemiparkinsonism G20.C

Hemiplegia G81.9- ☑
- alternans facialis G83.89
- ascending NEC G81.90
  - spinal G95.89
- congenital (cerebral) G80.8
  - spastic G80.2
- embolic (current episode) I63.4- ☑
- flaccid G81.0- ☑
- following
  - cerebrovascular disease I69.959
    - cerebral infarction I69.35- ☑
    - intracerebral hemorrhage I69.15- ☑
    - nontraumatic intracranial hemorrhage NEC I69.25- ☑
    - specified disease NEC I69.85- ☑
    - stroke NOS I69.35- ☑
    - subarachnoid hemorrhage I69.05- ☑
- hysterical F44.4
- newborn NEC P91.88
  - birth injury P11.9
- spastic G81.1- ☑
  - congenital G80.2
- thrombotic (current episode) I63.3- ☑

Hemisection, spinal cord — see Injury, spinal cord, by region

Hemispasm (facial) R25.2

Hemisporosis B48.8

Hemitremor R25.1

Hemivertebra Q76.49
- failure of segmentation with scoliosis Q76.3
- fusion with scoliosis Q76.3

Hemochromatosis E83.119
- with refractory anemia D46.1
- due to repeated red blood cell transfusion E83.111
- hereditary (primary) E83.110
- neonatal P78.84
- primary E83.110
- specified NEC E83.118

Hemoglobin — see also condition
- abnormal (disease) — see Disease, hemoglobin
- AS genotype D57.3
- Constant Spring D58.2
- E-beta thalassemia D56.5
- fetal, hereditary persistence (HPFH) D56.4

Hemoglobin — *continued*
  H Constant Spring D56.0
  low NOS D64.9
  S (Hb S), heterozygous D57.3
Hemoglobinemia D59.9
  due to blood transfusion T80.89 ☑
  paroxysmal D59.6
    nocturnal D59.5
Hemoglobinopathy (mixed) D58.2
  with thalassemia D56.8
  sickle-cell D57.1
    with thalassemia D57.40
      with
        acute chest syndrome D57.411
        cerebral vascular involvement D57.413
        crisis (painful) D57.419
          with specified complication NEC D57.418
        pain (vaso-occlusive) D57.419
        splenic sequestration D57.412
      without crisis D57.40
Hemoglobinuria R82.3
  with anemia, hemolytic, acquired (chronic) NEC D59.6
  cold (paroxysmal) (with Raynaud's syndrome) D59.6
    agglutinin D59.12
  due to exertion or hemolysis NEC D59.6
  intermittent D59.6
  malarial B50.8
  march D59.6
  nocturnal (paroxysmal) D59.5
  paroxysmal (cold) D59.6
    nocturnal D59.5
Hemolymphangioma D18.1
Hemolysis
  intravascular
    with
      abortion — *see* Abortion, by type, complicated by, hemorrhage
      ectopic or molar pregnancy O08.1
      hemorrhage
        antepartum — *see* Hemorrhage, antepartum, with coagulation defect
        intrapartum — *see also* Hemorrhage, complicating, delivery O67.0
    postpartum O72.3
  neonatal (excessive) P58.9
    specified NEC P58.8
Hemolytic — *see* condition
Hemopericardium I31.2
  following acute myocardial infarction (current complication) I23.0
  newborn P54.8
  traumatic — *see* Injury, heart, with hemopericardium
Hemoperitoneum K66.1
  infectional K65.9
  traumatic S36.899 ☑
    with open wound — *see* Wound, open, abdominal, wall, by site if known, with penetration into peritoneal cavity
Hemophilia (classical) (familial) (hereditary) D66
  A D66
  acquired D68.311
  autoimmune D68.311
  B D67
  C D68.1
  calcipriva — *see also* Defect, coagulation D68.4
  nonfamilial — *see also* Defect, coagulation D68.4
  secondary D68.311
  vascular — *see* Disease, von Willebrand
Hemophthalmos H44.81- ☑
Hemopneumothorax — *see also* Hemothorax
  traumatic S27.2 ☑
Hemoptysis R04.2
  newborn P26.9
  tuberculous — *see* Tuberculosis, pulmonary
Hemorrhage, hemorrhagic (concealed) R58
  abdomen R58
  accidental antepartum — *see* Hemorrhage, antepartum
  acute idiopathic pulmonary, in infants R04.81
  adenoid J35.8
  adrenal (capsule) (gland) E27.49
    medulla E27.8
    newborn P54.4
  after delivery — *see* Hemorrhage, postpartum
  alveolar
    lung, newborn P26.8
    process K08.89
  alveolus K08.89
  amputation stump (surgical) T87.89
  anemia (chronic) D50.0

Hemorrhage, hemorrhagic — *continued*
  anemia — *continued*
    acute D62
  antepartum (with) O46.90
    with coagulation defect O46.00- ☑
      afibrinogenemia O46.01- ☑
      disseminated intravascular coagulation O46.02- ☑
      hypofibrinogenemia O46.01- ☑
      specified defect NEC O46.09- ☑
    before 20 weeks gestation O20.9
      specified type NEC O20.8
      threatened abortion O20.0
    due to
      abruptio placenta — *see also* Abruptio placentae O45.9-
      leiomyoma, uterus — *see* Hemorrhage, antepartum, specified cause NEC
      placenta previa O44.1- ☑
      specified cause NEC — *see* subcategory O46.8X- ☑
  anus (sphincter) K62.5
  apoplexy (stroke) — *see* Hemorrhage, intracranial, intracerebral
  arachnoid — *see* Hemorrhage, intracranial, subarachnoid
  artery R58
    brain — *see* Hemorrhage, intracranial, intracerebral
  basilar (ganglion) I61.0
  bladder N32.89
  bowel K92.2
    newborn P54.3
  brain (miliary) (nontraumatic) — *see* Hemorrhage, intracranial, intracerebral
    due to
      birth injury P10.1
      syphilis A52.05
    epidural or extradural (traumatic) — *see* Injury, intracranial, epidural hemorrhage
    newborn P52.4
      birth injury P10.1
    subarachnoid — *see* Hemorrhage, intracranial, subarachnoid
    subdural — *see* Hemorrhage, intracranial, subdural
  brainstem (nontraumatic) I61.3
    traumatic S06.38- ☑
  breast N64.59
  bronchial tube — *see* Hemorrhage, lung
  bronchopulmonary — *see* Hemorrhage, lung
  bronchus — *see* Hemorrhage, lung
  bulbar I61.5
  capillary I78.8
    primary D69.8
  cecum K92.2
  cerebellar, cerebellum (nontraumatic) I61.4
    newborn P52.6
    traumatic S06.37- ☑
  cerebral, cerebrum — *see also* Hemorrhage, intracranial, intracerebral
    lobe I61.1
    newborn (anoxic) P52.4
      birth injury P10.1
  cerebromeningeal I61.8
  cerebrospinal — *see* Hemorrhage, intracranial, intracerebral
  cervix (uteri) (stump) NEC N88.8
  chamber, anterior (eye) — *see* Hyphema
  childbirth — *see* Hemorrhage, complicating, delivery
  choroid H31.30- ☑
    expulsive H31.31- ☑
  ciliary body — *see* Hyphema
  cochlea — *see* subcategory H83.8 ☑
  colon K92.2
  complicating
    abortion — *see* Abortion, by type, complicated by, hemorrhage
    delivery O67.9
      associated with coagulation defect (afibrinogenemia) (DIC) (hyperfibrinolysis) O67.0
      specified cause NEC O67.8
    surgical procedure — *see* Hemorrhage, intraoperative
  conjunctiva H11.3- ☑
    newborn P54.8
  cord, newborn (stump) P51.9
  corpus luteum (ruptured) cyst N83.1- ☑
  cortical (brain) I61.1
  cranial — *see* Hemorrhage, intracranial
  cutaneous R23.3
    due to autosensitivity, erythrocyte D69.2
    newborn P54.5

Hemorrhage, hemorrhagic — *continued*
  delayed
    following ectopic or molar pregnancy O08.1
    postpartum O72.2
  diathesis (familial) D69.9
  disease D69.9
    newborn P53
    specified type NEC D69.8
  due to or associated with
    afibrinogenemia or other coagulation defect (conditions in categories D65- D69)
      antepartum — *see* Hemorrhage, antepartum, with coagulation defect
      intrapartum O67.0
    dental implant M27.61
    device, implant or graft — *see also* Complications, by site and type, specified NEC T85.838 ☑
      arterial graft NEC T82.838 ☑
      breast T85.838 ☑
      catheter NEC T85.838 ☑
        dialysis (renal) T82.838 ☑
          intraperitoneal T85.838 ☑
        infusion NEC T82.838 ☑
          spinal (epidural) (subdural) T85.830 ☑
        urinary (indwelling) T83.83 ☑
      electronic (electrode) (pulse generator) (stimulator)
        bone T84.83 ☑
        cardiac T82.837 ☑
        nervous system (brain) (peripheral nerve) (spinal) T85.830 ☑
        urinary T83.83 ☑
      fixation, internal (orthopedic) NEC T84.83 ☑
      gastrointestinal (bile duct) (esophagus) T85.838 ☑
      genital NEC T83.83 ☑
      heart NEC T82.837 ☑
      joint prosthesis T84.83 ☑
      ocular (corneal graft) (orbital implant) NEC T85.838 ☑
      orthopedic NEC T84.83 ☑
        bone graft T86.838 ☑
      specified NEC T85.838 ☑
      urinary NEC T83.83 ☑
      vascular NEC T82.838 ☑
      ventricular intracranial shunt T85.830 ☑
  duodenum, duodenal K92.2
    ulcer — *see* Ulcer, duodenum, with hemorrhage
  dura mater — *see* Hemorrhage, intracranial, subdural
  endotracheal — *see* Hemorrhage, lung
  epicranial subaponeurotic (massive), birth injury P12.2
  epidural (traumatic) — *see also* Injury, intracranial, epidural hemorrhage
    nontraumatic I62.1
  esophagus K22.89
    varix I85.01
      secondary I85.11
  excessive, following ectopic gestation (subsequent episode) O08.1
  extradural (traumatic) — *see* Injury, intracranial, epidural hemorrhage
    birth injury P10.8
    newborn (anoxic) (nontraumatic) P52.8
    nontraumatic I62.1
  eye NEC H57.89
    fundus — *see* Hemorrhage, retina
    lid — *see* Disorder, eyelid, specified type NEC
  fallopian tube N83.6
  fibrinogenolysis — *see* Fibrinolysis
  fibrinolytic (acquired) — *see* Fibrinolysis
  from
    ear (nontraumatic) — *see* Otorrhagia
    tracheostomy stoma J95.01
  fundus, eye — *see* Hemorrhage, retina
  funis — *see* Hemorrhage, umbilicus, cord
  gastric — *see* Hemorrhage, stomach
  gastroenteric K92.2
    newborn P54.3
  gastrointestinal (tract) K92.2
    newborn P54.3
  genital organ, male N50.1
  genitourinary (tract) NOS R31.9
  gingiva K06.8
  globe (eye) — *see* Hemophthalmos
  graafian follicle cyst (ruptured) N83.0- ☑
  gum K06.8
  heart I51.89
  hypopharyngeal (throat) R04.1
  intermenstrual (regular) N92.3

Hemorrhage, hemorrhagic — *continued*
  intermenstrual — *continued*
    irregular N92.1
  internal (organs) NEC R58
    capsule I61.0
    ear — *see* subcategory H83.8 ☑
    newborn P54.8
  intestine K92.2
    newborn P54.3
  intra-abdominal R58
  intra-alveolar (lung), newborn P26.8
  intracerebral (nontraumatic) — *see* Hemorrhage, intracranial, intracerebral
  intracranial (nontraumatic) I62.9
    birth injury P10.9
    epidural, nontraumatic I62.1
    extradural, nontraumatic I62.1
    intracerebral (nontraumatic) (in) I61.9
      brain stem I61.3
      cerebellum I61.4
      hemisphere I61.2
        cortical (superficial) I61.1
        subcortical (deep) I61.0
      intraoperative
        during a nervous system procedure G97.31
        during other procedure G97.32
      intraventricular I61.5
      multiple localized I61.6
      newborn P52.4
        birth injury P10.1
      postprocedural
        following a nervous system procedure G97.51
        following other procedure G97.52
      specified NEC I61.8
      superficial I61.1
      traumatic — *see* Injury, intracranial, intracerebral hemorrhage, traumatic
    newborn P52.9
      specified NEC P52.8
    subarachnoid (nontraumatic) (from) I60.9
      intracranial (cerebral) artery I60.7
        anterior communicating I60.2
        basilar I60.4
        carotid siphon and bifurcation I60.0- ☑
        communicating I60.7
          anterior I60.2
          posterior I60.3- ☑
        middle cerebral I60.1- ☑
        posterior communicating I60.3- ☑
        specified artery NEC I60.6
        vertebral I60.5- ☑
      newborn P52.5
        birth injury P10.3
      specified NEC I60.8
      traumatic S06.6X- ☑
    subdural (nontraumatic) I62.00
      acute I62.01
      birth injury P10.0
      chronic I62.03
      newborn (anoxic) (hypoxic) P52.8
        birth injury P10.0
      spinal G95.19
      subacute I62.02
      traumatic — *see* Injury, intracranial, subdural hemorrhage
    traumatic — *see* Injury, intracranial, focal brain injury
  intramedullary NEC G95.19
  intraocular — *see* Hemophthalmos
  intraoperative, intraprocedural — *see* Complication, hemorrhage (hematoma), intraoperative (intraprocedural), by site
  intrapartum — *see* Hemorrhage, complicating, delivery
  intrapelvic
    female N94.89
    male K66.1
  intraperitoneal K66.1
  intrapontine I61.3
  intraprocedural — *see* Complication, hemorrhage (hematoma), intraoperative (intraprocedural), by site
  intrauterine N85.7
    complicating delivery — *see also* Hemorrhage, complicating, delivery O67.9
    postpartum — *see* Hemorrhage, postpartum
  intraventricular I61.5
    newborn (nontraumatic) — *see also* Newborn, affected by, hemorrhage P52.3
      due to birth injury P10.2

Hemorrhage, hemorrhagic — *continued*
  intraventricular — *continued*
    newborn — *see also* Newborn, affected by, hemorrhage — *continued*
      grade
        1 P52.0
        2 P52.1
        3 P52.21
        4 P52.22
  intravesical N32.89
  iris (postinfectional) (postinflammatory) (toxic) — *see* Hyphema
  joint (nontraumatic) — *see* Hemarthrosis
  kidney N28.89
  knee (joint) (nontraumatic) — *see* Hemarthrosis, knee
  labyrinth — *see* subcategory H83.8 ☑
  lenticular striate artery I61.0
  ligature, vessel — *see* Hemorrhage, postoperative
  liver K76.89
  lung R04.89
    newborn P26.9
      massive P26.1
      specified NEC P26.8
    tuberculous — *see* Tuberculosis, pulmonary
  massive umbilical, newborn P51.0
  mediastinum — *see* Hemorrhage, lung
  medulla I61.3
  membrane (brain) I60.8
    spinal cord — *see* Hemorrhage, spinal cord
  meninges, meningeal (brain) (middle) I60.8
    spinal cord — *see* Hemorrhage, spinal cord
  mesentery K66.1
  metritis — *see* Endometritis
  mouth K13.79
  mucous membrane NEC R58
    newborn P54.8
  muscle M62.89
  nail (subungual) L60.8
  nasal turbinate R04.0
    newborn P54.8
  navel, newborn P51.9
  newborn P54.9
    specified NEC P54.8
  nipple N64.59
  nose R04.0
    newborn P54.8
  omentum K66.1
  optic nerve (sheath) H47.02- ☑
  orbit, orbital H05.23- ☑
  ovary NEC N83.8
  oviduct N83.6
  pancreas K86.89
  parathyroid (gland) (spontaneous) E21.4
  parturition — *see* Hemorrhage, complicating, delivery
  penis N48.89
  pericardium, pericarditis I31.2
  peritoneum, peritoneal K66.1
  peritonsillar tissue J35.8
    due to infection J36
  petechial R23.3
    due to autosensitivity, erythrocyte D69.2
  pituitary (gland) E23.6
  pleura — *see* Hemorrhage, lung
  polioencephalitis, superior E51.2
  polymyositis — *see* Polymyositis
  pons, pontine I61.3
  posterior fossa (nontraumatic) I61.8
    newborn P52.6
  postmenopausal N95.0
  postnasal R04.0
  postoperative — *see* Complications, postprocedural, hemorrhage, by site
  postpartum NEC (following delivery of placenta) O72.1
    delayed or secondary O72.2
    retained placenta O72.0
    third stage O72.0
  pregnancy — *see* Hemorrhage, antepartum
  preretinal — *see* Hemorrhage, retina
  prostate N42.1
  puerperal — *see* Hemorrhage, postpartum
    delayed or secondary O72.2
  pulmonary R04.89
    newborn P26.9
      massive P26.1
      specified NEC P26.8
    tuberculous — *see* Tuberculosis, pulmonary
  purpura (primary) D69.3
  rectum (sphincter) K62.5
    newborn P54.2

Hemorrhage, hemorrhagic — *continued*
  recurring, following initial hemorrhage at time of injury T79.2 ☑
  renal N28.89
  respiratory passage or tract R04.9
    specified NEC R04.89
  retina, retinal (vessels) H35.6- ☑
    diabetic — *see* Microaneurysm, retinal, diabetic
  retroperitoneal K68.3
  scalp R58
  scrotum N50.1
  secondary (nontraumatic) R58
    following initial hemorrhage at time of injury T79.2 ☑
  seminal vesicle N50.1
  skin R23.3
    newborn P54.5
  slipped umbilical ligature P51.8
  spermatic cord N50.1
  spinal (cord) G95.19
    newborn (birth injury) P11.5
  spleen D73.5
    intraoperative — *see* Complications, intraoperative, hemorrhage, spleen
    postprocedural — *see* Complications, postprocedural, hemorrhage, spleen
  stomach K92.2
    newborn P54.3
    ulcer — *see* Ulcer, stomach, with hemorrhage
  subarachnoid (nontraumatic) — *see* Hemorrhage, intracranial, subarachnoid
  subconjunctival — *see also* Hemorrhage, conjunctiva
    birth injury P15.3
  subcortical (brain) I61.0
  subcutaneous R23.3
  subdiaphragmatic R58
  subdural (acute) (nontraumatic) — *see* Hemorrhage, intracranial, subdural
  subependymal
    newborn P52.0
      with intraventricular extension P52.1
        and intracerebral extension P52.22
  subgaleal P12.2
  subhyaloid — *see* Hemorrhage, retina
  subperiosteal — *see* Disorder, bone, specified type NEC
  subretinal — *see* Hemorrhage, retina
  subtentorial — *see* Hemorrhage, intracranial, subdural
  subungual L60.8
  suprarenal (capsule) (gland) E27.49
    newborn P54.4
  tentorium (traumatic) NEC — *see* Hemorrhage, brain
    newborn (birth injury) P10.4
  testis N50.1
  third stage (postpartum) O72.0
  thorax — *see* Hemorrhage, lung
  throat R04.1
  thymus (gland) E32.8
  thyroid (cyst) (gland) E07.89
  tongue K14.8
  tonsil J35.8
  trachea — *see* Hemorrhage, lung
  tracheobronchial R04.89
    newborn P26.0
  traumatic — *code to* specific injury
    cerebellar — *see* Hemorrhage, brain
    intracranial — *see* Hemorrhage, brain
    recurring or secondary (following initial hemorrhage at time of injury) T79.2 ☑
  tuberculous NEC — *see also* Tuberculosis, pulmonary A15.0
  tunica vaginalis N50.1
  ulcer — *code by* site under Ulcer, with hemorrhage K27.4
  umbilicus, umbilical
    cord
      after birth, newborn P51.9
      complicating delivery O69.5 ☑
    newborn P51.9
      massive P51.0
      slipped ligature P51.8
    stump P51.9
  urethra (idiopathic) N36.8
  uterus, uterine (abnormal) N93.9
    climacteric N92.4
    complicating delivery — *see* Hemorrhage, complicating, delivery
    dysfunctional or functional N93.8
    intermenstrual (regular) N92.3
      irregular N92.1
    postmenopausal N95.0

☑ **Additional Character Required** — **Refer to the Tabular List for Character Selection**

Hemorrhage, hemorrhagic — continued
 uterus, uterine — continued
  postpartum — see Hemorrhage, postpartum
  preclimacteric or premenopausal N92.4
  prepubertal N93.8
  pubertal N92.2
 vagina (abnormal) N93.9
  newborn P54.6
 vas deferens N50.1
 vasa previa O69.4 ☑
 ventricular I61.5
 vesical N32.89
 viscera NEC R58
  newborn P54.8
 vitreous (humor) (intraocular) H43.1- ☑
 vulva N90.89
Hemorrhoids (bleeding) (without mention of degree) K64.9
 1st degree (grade/stage I) (without prolapse outside of anal canal) K64.0
 2nd degree (grade/stage II) (that prolapse with straining but retract spontaneously) K64.1
 3rd degree (grade/stage III) (that prolapse with straining and require manual replacement back inside anal canal) K64.2
 4th degree (grade/stage IV) (with prolapsed tissue that cannot be manually replaced) K64.3
 complicating
  pregnancy O22.4 ☑
  puerperium O87.2
 external K64.4
  with
   thrombosis K64.5
 internal (without mention of degree) K64.8
 prolapsed K64.8
 skin tags
  anus K64.4
  residual K64.4
 specified NEC K64.8
 strangulated — see also Hemorrhoids, by degree K64.8
 thrombosed — see also Hemorrhoids, by degree K64.5
 ulcerated — see also Hemorrhoids, by degree K64.8
Hemosalpinx N83.6
 with
  hematocolpos N89.7
  hematometra N85.7
   with hematocolpos N89.7
Hemosiderosis (dietary) E83.19
 pulmonary, idiopathic E83.1- ☑ [J84.03]
 transfusion T80.89 ☑
Hemothorax (bacterial) (nontuberculous) J94.2
 newborn P54.8
 traumatic S27.1 ☑
  with pneumothorax S27.2 ☑
 tuberculous NEC A15.6
Henoch (-Schonlein) **disease or syndrome** (purpura) D69.0
Henpue, henpuye A66.6
Hepar lobatum (syphilitic) A52.74
Hepatalgia K76.89
Hepatitis K75.9
 A — see Hepatitis, viral, type, A
 acute B17.9
  with coma K72.01
  with hepatic failure — see Failure, hepatic
  alcoholic — see Hepatitis, alcoholic
  infectious B17.9
  non-viral K72.0 ☑
  viral — see also, Hepatitis, viral B17.9
 alcoholic (acute) (chronic) K70.10
  with ascites K70.11
 amebic — see Abscess, liver, amebic
 anicteric, (viral) — see Hepatitis, viral
 antigen-associated (HAA) — see Hepatitis, B
 Australia-antigen (positive) — see Hepatitis, B
 autoimmune K75.4
 B B19.10
  with B19.11
   delta (agent) — see Hepatitis, D
   hepatic coma B19.11
  acute B16.9
   with
    delta-agent (coinfection) (without hepatic coma) B16.1
     with hepatic coma B16.0
    hepatic coma (without delta-agent coinfection) B16.2
  chronic B18.1
   with delta-agent B18.0
 bacterial NEC K75.89

Hepatitis — continued
 C (viral) B19.20
  with hepatic coma B19.21
  acute B17.10
   with hepatic coma B17.11
  chronic B18.2
 catarrhal (acute) B15.9
  with hepatic coma B15.0
 cholangiolitic K75.89
 cholestatic K75.89
 chronic K73.9
  active NEC K73.2
   toxic — see Disease, liver, toxic, with, hepatitis, chronic, active
  lobular NEC K73.1
  persistent NEC K73.0
  specified NEC K73.8
  toxic — see Disease, liver, toxic, with, hepatitis, chronic
  viral — see Hepatitis, viral, chronic
 cytomegaloviral B25.1
 D B16.1
  acute B16.1
   with hepatic coma B16.0
   in hepatitis B carrier B17.0
  chronic B18.0
 delta (agent) — see Hepatitis, D
 due to ethanol (acute) (chronic) — see Hepatitis, alcoholic
 epidemic B15.9
  with hepatic coma B15.0
 fulminant NEC (viral) — see Hepatitis, viral
 granulomatous NEC K75.3
 herpesviral B00.81
 history of
  B Z86.19
  C Z86.19
 homologous serum — see Hepatitis, viral, type B
 in (due to)
  mumps B26.81
  toxoplasmosis (acquired) B58.1
   congenital (active) P37.1 [K77]
 infectious, infective B15.9
  acute (subacute) B17.9
  chronic B18.9
 inoculation — see Hepatitis, viral, type B
 interstitial (chronic) K74.69
 ischemia, ischemic K72.00
 lupoid NEC K75.4
 malignant NEC (with hepatic failure) K72.90
  with coma K72.91
 neonatal (idiopathic) (toxic) P59.29
 neonatal giant cell P59.29
  newborn P59.29
 non-viral K72.0 ☑
 postimmunization — see Hepatitis, viral, type B
 post-transfusion — see Hepatitis, viral, type B
 reactive, nonspecific K75.2
 serum — see Hepatitis, viral, type B
 shock K72.00
 specified type NEC
  with hepatic failure — see Failure, hepatic
 syphilitic (late) A52.74
  congenital (early) A50.08 [K77]
   late A50.59 [K77]
  secondary A51.45
 toxic — see also Disease, liver, toxic K71.6
 tuberculous A18.83
 viral, virus B19.9
  with hepatic coma B19.0
  acute B17.9
  chronic B18.9
   specified NEC B18.8
   type
    B B18.1
     with delta-agent B18.0
    C B18.2
    D B18.0
  congenital P35.3
  coxsackie B33.8 [K77]
  cytomegalic inclusion B25.1
  in remission, any type — code to Hepatitis, chronic, by type
  non-A, non-B B17.8
  specified type NEC (with or without coma) B17.8
  type
   A B15.9
    with hepatic coma B15.0
   B B19.10
    with hepatic coma B19.11

Hepatitis — continued
 viral, virus — continued
  type — continued
   B — continued
    acute B16.9
     with
      delta-agent (coinfection) (without hepatic coma) B16.1
       with hepatic coma B16.0
      hepatic coma (without delta-agent coinfection) B16.2
    chronic B18.1
     with delta-agent B18.0
   C B19.20
    with hepatic coma B19.21
    acute B17.10
     with hepatic coma B17.11
    chronic B18.2
   D B16.1
    acute B16.1
     with hepatic coma B16.0
     in hepatitis B carrier B17.0
    chronic B18.0
   delta (agent) — see Hepatitis, viral, type, D
   E B17.2
   non-A, non-B B17.8
Hepatization lung (acute) — see Pneumonia, lobar
Hepatoblastoma C22.2
Hepatocarcinoma C22.0
Hepatocholangiocarcinoma C22.0
Hepatocholangioma, benign D13.4
Hepatocholangitis K75.89
Hepatolenticular degeneration E83.01
Hepatoma (malignant) C22.0
 benign D13.4
 embryonal C22.0
Hepatomegaly — see also Hypertrophy, liver
 with splenomegaly R16.2
 congenital Q44.79
 in mononucleosis
  gammaherpesviral B27.09
  infectious specified NEC B27.89
Hepatoptosis K76.89
Hepatorenal syndrome following labor and delivery O90.41
Hepatosis K76.89
Hepatosplenomegaly R16.2
 hyperlipemic (Burger-Grutz type) E78.3 [K77]
Hereditary — see condition
Hereditary alpha tryptasemia (syndrome) D89.44
Heredodegeneration, macular — see Dystrophy, retina
Heredopathia atactica polyneuritiformis G60.1
Heredosyphilis — see Syphilis, congenital
Herlitz' syndrome Q81.1
Hermansky-Pudlak syndrome E70.331
Hermaphrodite, hermaphroditism (true) Q56.0
 46,XX with streak gonads Q99.1
 46,XX/46,XY Q99.0
 46,XY with streak gonads Q99.1
 chimera 46,XX/46,XY Q99.0
Hernia, hernial (acquired) (recurrent) K46.9
 with
  gangrene — see Hernia, by site, with, gangrene
  incarceration — see Hernia, by site, with, obstruction
  irreducible — see Hernia, by site, with, obstruction
  obstruction — see Hernia, by site, with, obstruction
  strangulation — see Hernia, by site, with, obstruction
 abdomen, abdominal K46.9
  with
   gangrene (and obstruction) K46.1
   obstruction K46.0
  femoral — see Hernia, femoral
  incisional — see Hernia, incisional
  inguinal — see Hernia, inguinal
  specified site NEC K45.8
   with
    gangrene (and obstruction) K45.1
    obstruction K45.0
  umbilical — see Hernia, umbilical
  wall — see Hernia, ventral
 appendix — see Hernia, abdomen
 bladder (mucosa) (sphincter)
  congenital (female) (male) Q79.51
  female — see Cystocele
  male N32.89
 brain, congenital — see Encephalocele
 cartilage, vertebra — see Displacement, intervertebral disc
 cerebral, congenital — see also Encephalocele

Hernia, hernial — *continued*
- cerebral, congenital — *see also* Encephalocele — *continued*
  - endaural Q01.8
- ciliary body (traumatic) S05.2- ☑
- colon — *see* Hernia, abdomen
- Cooper's — *see* Hernia, abdomen, specified site NEC
- crural — *see* Hernia, femoral
- diaphragm, diaphragmatic K44.9
  - with
    - gangrene (and obstruction) K44.1
    - obstruction K44.0
  - congenital Q79.0
- direct (inguinal) — *see* Hernia, inguinal
- diverticulum, intestine — *see* Hernia, abdomen
- double (inguinal) — *see* Hernia, inguinal, bilateral
- due to adhesions (with obstruction) K56.50
- epigastric — *see also* Hernia, ventral K43.9
- esophageal hiatus — *see* Hernia, hiatal
- external (inguinal) — *see* Hernia, inguinal
- fallopian tube N83.4- ☑
- fascia M62.89
- femoral K41.90
  - with
    - gangrene (and obstruction) K41.40
      - not specified as recurrent K41.40
      - recurrent K41.41
    - obstruction K41.30
      - not specified as recurrent K41.30
      - recurrent K41.31
  - not specified as recurrent K41.90
  - recurrent K41.91
  - bilateral K41.20
    - with
      - gangrene (and obstruction) K41.10
        - not specified as recurrent K41.10
        - recurrent K41.11
      - obstruction K41.00
        - not specified as recurrent K41.00
        - recurrent K41.01
    - not specified as recurrent K41.20
    - recurrent K41.21
  - unilateral K41.90
    - with
      - gangrene (and obstruction) K41.40
        - not specified as recurrent K41.40
        - recurrent K41.41
      - obstruction K41.30
        - not specified as recurrent K41.30
        - recurrent K41.31
    - not specified as recurrent K41.90
    - recurrent K41.91
- foramen magnum G93.5
  - congenital Q01.8
- funicular (umbilical) — *see also* Hernia, umbilicus
  - spermatic (cord) — *see* Hernia, inguinal
- gastrointestinal tract — *see* Hernia, abdomen
- Hesselbach's — *see* Hernia, femoral, specified site NEC
- hiatal (esophageal) (sliding) K44.9
  - with
    - gangrene (and obstruction) K44.1
    - obstruction K44.0
  - congenital Q40.1
- hypogastric — *see* Hernia, ventral
- incarcerated — *see also* Hernia, by site, with obstruction
  - with gangrene — *see* Hernia, by site, with gangrene
- incisional K43.2
  - with
    - gangrene (and obstruction) K43.1
    - obstruction K43.0
- indirect (inguinal) — *see* Hernia, inguinal
- inguinal (direct) (external) (funicular) (indirect) (internal) (oblique) (scrotal) (sliding) K40.90
  - with
    - gangrene (and obstruction) K40.40
      - not specified as recurrent K40.40
      - recurrent K40.41
    - obstruction K40.30
      - not specified as recurrent K40.30
      - recurrent K40.31
  - not specified as recurrent K40.90
  - recurrent K40.91
  - bilateral K40.20
    - with
      - gangrene (and obstruction) K40.10
        - not specified as recurrent K40.10
        - recurrent K40.11
      - obstruction K40.00
        - not specified as recurrent K40.00

Hernia, hernial — *continued*
- inguinal — *continued*
  - bilateral — *continued*
    - with — *continued*
      - obstruction — *continued*
        - recurrent K40.01
      - not specified as recurrent K40.20
      - recurrent K40.21
    - unilateral K40.90
      - with
        - gangrene (and obstruction) K40.40
          - not specified as recurrent K40.40
          - recurrent K40.41
        - obstruction K40.30
          - not specified as recurrent K40.30
          - recurrent K40.31
      - not specified as recurrent K40.90
      - recurrent K40.91
- internal — *see also* Hernia, abdomen
  - inguinal — *see* Hernia, inguinal
- interstitial — *see* Hernia, abdomen
- intervertebral cartilage or disc — *see* Displacement, intervertebral disc
- intestine, intestinal — *see* Hernia, by site
- intra-abdominal — *see* Hernia, abdomen
- iris (traumatic) S05.2- ☑
- irreducible — *see also* Hernia, by site, with obstruction
  - with gangrene — *see* Hernia, by site, with gangrene
- ischiatic — *see* Hernia, abdomen, specified site NEC
- ischiorectal — *see* Hernia, abdomen, specified site NEC
- lens (traumatic) S05.2- ☑
- linea (alba) (semilunaris) — *see* Hernia, ventral
- Littre's — *see* Hernia, abdomen
- lumbar — *see* Hernia, abdomen, specified site NEC
- lung (subcutaneous) J98.4
- mediastinum J98.59
- mesenteric (internal) — *see* Hernia, abdomen
- midline — *see* Hernia, ventral
- muscle (sheath) M62.89
- nucleus pulposus — *see* Displacement, intervertebral disc
- oblique (inguinal) — *see* Hernia, inguinal
- obstructive — *see also* Hernia, by site, with obstruction
  - with gangrene — *see* Hernia, by site, with gangrene
- obturator — *see* Hernia, abdomen, specified site NEC
- omental — *see* Hernia, abdomen
- ovary N83.4- ☑
- oviduct N83.4- ☑
- paraesophageal — *see also* Hernia, diaphragm
  - congenital Q40.1
- parastomal K43.5
  - with
    - gangrene (and obstruction) K43.4
    - obstruction K43.3
- paraumbilical — *see* Hernia, umbilicus
- perineal — *see* Hernia, abdomen, specified site NEC
- Petit's — *see* Hernia, abdomen, specified site NEC
- postoperative — *see* Hernia, incisional
- pregnant uterus — *see* Abnormal, uterus in pregnancy or childbirth
- prevesical N32.89
- properitoneal — *see* Hernia, abdomen, specified site NEC
- pudendal — *see* Hernia, abdomen, specified site NEC
- rectovaginal N81.6
- retroperitoneal — *see* Hernia, abdomen, specified site NEC
- Richter's — *see* Hernia, abdomen, with obstruction
- Rieux's, Riex's — *see* Hernia, abdomen, specified site NEC
- sac condition (adhesion) (dropsy) (inflammation) (laceration) (suppuration) — *code by site under* Hernia
- sciatic — *see* Hernia, abdomen, specified site NEC
- scrotum, scrotal — *see* Hernia, inguinal
- sliding (inguinal) — *see also* Hernia, inguinal
  - hiatus — *see* Hernia, hiatal
- spigelian — *see* Hernia, ventral
- spinal — *see* Spina bifida
- strangulated — *see also* Hernia, by site, with obstruction
  - with gangrene — *see* Hernia, by site, with gangrene
- subxiphoid — *see* Hernia, ventral
- supra-umbilicus — *see* Hernia, ventral
- tendon — *see* Disorder, tendon, specified type NEC
- Treitz's (fossa) — *see* Hernia, abdomen, specified site NEC
- tunica vaginalis Q55.29
- umbilicus, umbilical K42.9
  - with
    - gangrene (and obstruction) K42.1
    - obstruction K42.0
- ureter N28.89

Hernia, hernial — *continued*
- urethra, congenital Q64.79
- urinary meatus, congenital Q64.79
- uterus N81.4
  - pregnant — *see* Abnormal, uterus in pregnancy or childbirth
- vaginal (anterior) (wall) — *see* Cystocele
- Velpeau's — *see* Hernia, femoral
- ventral K43.9
  - with
    - gangrene (and obstruction) K43.7
    - obstruction K43.6
  - incisional K43.2
    - with
      - gangrene (and obstruction) K43.1
      - obstruction K43.0
  - recurrent — *see* Hernia, incisional
  - specified NEC K43.9
    - with
      - gangrene (and obstruction) K43.7
      - obstruction K43.6
- vesical
  - congenital (female) (male) Q79.51
  - female — *see* Cystocele
  - male N32.89
- vitreous (into wound) S05.2- ☑
  - into anterior chamber — *see* Prolapse, vitreous

Herniation — *see also* Hernia
- brain (stem) G93.5
  - nontraumatic G93.5
  - traumatic S06.A1 ☑
    - cerebellar S06.A1 ☑
    - subfalcine (cingulate) S06.A1 ☑
    - tonsillar S06.A1 ☑
    - transtentorial (central) (upward cerebellar) S06.A1 ☑
    - uncal S06.A1 ☑
- cerebral G93.5
  - nontraumatic G93.5
  - traumatic S06.A1 ☑
- mediastinum J98.59
- nucleus pulposus — *see* Displacement, intervertebral disc

Herpangina B08.5

Herpes, herpesvirus, herpetic B00.9
- anogenital A60.9
  - perianal skin A60.1
  - rectum A60.1
  - urogenital tract A60.00
    - cervix A60.03
    - male genital organ NEC A60.02
    - penis A60.01
    - specified site NEC A60.09
    - vagina A60.04
    - vulva A60.04
- blepharitis (zoster) B02.39
  - simplex B00.59
- circinatus B35.4
  - bullosus L12.0
- conjunctivitis (simplex) B00.53
  - zoster B02.31
- cornea B02.33
- encephalitis B00.4
  - due to herpesvirus 6 B10.01
  - due to herpesvirus 7 B10.09
  - specified NEC B10.09
- eye (zoster) B02.30
  - simplex B00.50
- eyelid (zoster) B02.39
  - simplex B00.59
- facialis B00.1
- febrilis B00.1
- geniculate ganglionitis B02.21
- genital, genitalis A60.00
  - female A60.09
  - male A60.02
- gestational, gestationis O26.4- ☑
- gingivostomatitis B00.2
- human B00.9
  - 1 — *see* Herpes, simplex
  - 2 — *see* Herpes, simplex
  - 3 — *see* Varicella
  - 4 — *see* Mononucleosis, Epstein-Barr (virus)
  - 5 — *see* Disease, cytomegalic inclusion (generalized)
  - 6
    - encephalitis B10.01
    - specified NEC B10.81

Herpes, herpesvirus, herpetic — *continued*
  human — *continued*
    7
      encephalitis B10.09
      specified NEC B10.82
    8 B10.89
    infection NEC B10.89
      Kaposi's sarcoma associated B10.89
    iridocyclitis (simplex) B00.51
      zoster B02.32
    iris (vesicular erythema multiforme) L51.9
    iritis (simplex) B00.51
    Kaposi's sarcoma associated B10.89
    keratitis (simplex) (dendritic) (disciform) (interstitial) B00.52
      zoster (interstitial) B02.33
    keratoconjunctivitis (simplex) B00.52
      zoster B02.33
    labialis B00.1
    lip B00.1
    meningitis (simplex) B00.3
      zoster B02.1
    ophthalmicus (zoster) NEC B02.30
      simplex B00.50
    penis A60.01
    perianal skin A60.1
    pharyngitis, pharyngotonsillitis B00.2
    rectum A60.1
    scrotum A60.02
    sepsis B00.7
    simplex B00.9
      complicated NEC B00.89
      congenital P35.2
      conjunctivitis B00.53
      external ear B00.1
      eyelid B00.59
      hepatitis B00.81
      keratitis (interstitial) B00.52
      myelitis B00.82
      specified complication NEC B00.89
      visceral B00.89
    stomatitis B00.2
    tonsurans B35.0
    visceral B00.89
    vulva A60.04
    whitlow B00.89
    zoster — *see also* condition B02.9
      auricularis B02.21
      complicated NEC B02.8
      conjunctivitis B02.31
      disseminated B02.7
      encephalitis B02.0
      eye (lid) B02.39
      geniculate ganglionitis B02.21
      keratitis (interstitial) B02.33
      meningitis B02.1
      myelitis B02.24
      neuritis, neuralgia B02.29
      ophthalmicus NEC B02.30
      oticus B02.21
      polyneuropathy B02.23
      specified complication NEC B02.8
      trigeminal neuralgia B02.22
Herpesvirus (human) — *see* Herpes
Herpetophobia F40.218
Herrick's anemia — *see* Disease, sickle-cell
Hers' disease E74.09
Herter-Gee syndrome K90.0
Herxheimer's reaction R68.89
Hesitancy
  of micturition R39.11
  urinary R39.11
Hesselbach's hernia — *see* Hernia, femoral, specified site NEC
Heterochromia (congenital) Q13.2
  cataract — *see* Cataract, complicated
  cyclitis (Fuchs) — *see* Cyclitis, Fuchs' heterochromic
  hair L67.1
  iritis — *see* Cyclitis, Fuchs' heterochromic
  retained metallic foreign body (nonmagnetic) — *see* Foreign body, intraocular, old, retained
    magnetic — *see* Foreign body, intraocular, old, re-tained, magnetic
  uveitis — *see* Cyclitis, Fuchs' heterochromic
Heterophoria — *see* Strabismus, heterophoria
Heterophyes, heterophyiasis (small intestine) B66.8
Heterotopia, heterotopic — *see also* Malposition, congenital
  cerebralis Q04.8

Heterotropia — *see* Strabismus
Heubner-Herter disease K90.0
Hexadactylism Q69.9
HGSIL (cytology finding) (high grade squamous intraepithelial lesion on cytologic smear) (Pap smear finding)
  anus R85.613
  cervix R87.613
    biopsy (histology) finding — *see* Neoplasia, intraep-ithelial, cervix, grade II or grade III
  vagina R87.623
    biopsy (histology) finding — *see* Neoplasia, intraep-ithelial, cervix, grade II or grade III
Hibernoma — *see* Lipoma
Hiccup, hiccough R06.6
  epidemic B33.0
  psychogenic F45.8
Hidden penis (congenital) Q55.64
  acquired N48.83
Hidradenitis (axillaris) (suppurative) L73.2
Hidradenoma (nodular) — *see also* Neoplasm, skin, benign
  clear cell — *see* Neoplasm, skin, benign
  papillary — *see* Neoplasm, skin, benign
Hidrocystoma — *see* Neoplasm, skin, benign
High
  altitude effects T70.20 ☑
    anoxia T70.29 ☑
    on
      ears T70.0 ☑
      sinuses T70.1 ☑
    polycythemia D75.1
  arch
    foot Q66.7- ☑
    palate, congenital Q38.5
  arterial tension — *see* Hypertension
  basal metabolic rate R94.8
  blood pressure — *see also* Hypertension
    borderline R03.0
    reading (incidental) (isolated) (nonspecific), without diagnosis of hypertension R03.0
  cholesterol E78.00
    with high triglycerides E78.2
  diaphragm (congenital) Q79.1
  expressed emotional level within family Z63.8
  head at term O32.4 ☑
  palate, congenital Q38.5
  risk
    infant NEC Z76.2
    sexual behavior (heterosexual) Z72.51
      bisexual Z72.53
      homosexual Z72.52
  scrotal testis, testes
    bilateral Q53.23
    unilateral Q53.13
  temperature (of unknown origin) R50.9
  thoracic rib Q76.6
  triglycerides E78.1
    with high cholesterol E78.2
Hildenbrand's disease A75.0
Hilum — *see* condition
Hip — *see* condition
Hippel's disease Q85.83
Hippophobia F40.218
Hippus H57.09
Hirschsprung's disease or megacolon Q43.1
Hirsutism, hirsuties L68.0
Hirudiniasis
  external B88.3
  internal B83.4
Hiss-Russell dysentery A03.1
Histidinemia, histidinuria E70.41
Histiocytoma — *see also* Neoplasm, skin, benign
  fibrous — *see also* Neoplasm, skin, benign
    atypical — *see* Neoplasm, connective tissue, uncertain behavior
    malignant — *see* Neoplasm, connective tissue, malig-nant
Histiocytosis D76.3
  acute differentiated progressive C96.0
  Langerhans' cell NEC C96.6
    multifocal X
      multisystemic (disseminated) C96.0
      unisystemic C96.5
    pulmonary, adult (adult PLCH) J84.82
    unifocal (X) C96.6
  lipid, lipoid D76.3
    essential E75.29
  malignant C96.A (*following* C96.6)
  mononuclear phagocytes NEC D76.1

Histiocytosis — *continued*
  mononuclear phagocytes — *continued*
    Langerhans' cells C96.6
  non-Langerhans cell D76.3
  polyostotic sclerosing D76.3
  sinus, with massive lymphadenopathy D76.3
  syndrome NEC D76.3
  X NEC C96.6
    acute (progressive) C96.0
    chronic C96.6
    multifocal C96.5
    multisystemic C96.0
    unifocal C96.6
Histoplasmosis B39.9
  with pneumonia NEC B39.2
  African B39.5
  American — *see* Histoplasmosis, capsulati
  capsulati B39.4
    disseminated B39.3
    generalized B39.3
    pulmonary B39.2
      acute B39.0
      chronic B39.1
  Darling's B39.4
  duboisii B39.5
  lung NEC B39.2
History
  family (of) — *see also* History, personal (of)
    adenomatous polyposis Z83.72
    alcohol abuse Z81.1
    allergy NEC Z84.89
    anemia Z83.2
    arthritis Z82.61
    asthma Z82.5
    blindness Z82.1
    cardiac death (sudden) Z82.41
    carrier of genetic disease Z84.81
    chromosomal anomaly Z82.79
    chronic
      disabling disease NEC Z82.8
      lower respiratory disease Z82.5
    colonic polyps Z83.719
      adenomatous and serrated Z83.710
      hyperplastic Z83.711
      inflammatory Z83.718
      specified, NEC Z83.718
      tubular adenoma Z83.710
      tubulovillous adenoma Z83.710
      villous adenoma Z83.710
    congenital malformations and deformations Z82.79
      polycystic kidney Z82.71
    consanguinity Z84.3
    deafness Z82.2
    diabetes mellitus Z83.3
    disability NEC Z82.8
    disease or disorder (of)
      allergic NEC Z84.89
      behavioral NEC Z81.8
      blood and blood-forming organs Z83.2
      cardiovascular NEC Z82.49
      chronic disabling NEC Z82.8
      digestive Z83.79
      ear NEC Z83.52
      elevated lipoprotein (a) (Lp(a)) Z83.430
      endocrine NEC Z83.49
      eye NEC Z83.518
        glaucoma Z83.511
      familial hypercholesterolemia Z83.42
      genitourinary NEC Z84.2
      glaucoma Z83.511
      hematological Z83.2
      immune mechanism Z83.2
      infectious NEC Z83.1
      ischemic heart Z82.49
      kidney Z84.1
      lipoprotein metabolism Z83.438
      mental NEC Z81.8
      metabolic Z83.49
      musculoskeletal NEC Z82.69
      neurological NEC Z82.0
      nutritional Z83.49
      parasitic NEC Z83.1
      psychiatric NEC Z81.8
      respiratory NEC Z83.6
      skin and subcutaneous tissue NEC Z84.0
      specified NEC Z84.89
    drug abuse NEC Z81.3
    elevated lipoprotein (a) (Lp(a)) Z83.430
    epilepsy Z82.0

History — *continued*
    family — *see also* History, personal — *continued*
        familial hypercholesterolemia Z83.42
        genetic disease carrier Z84.81
        glaucoma Z83.511
        hearing loss Z82.2
        human immunodeficiency virus (HIV) infection Z83.0
        Huntington's chorea Z82.0
        hyperlipidemia, familial combined Z83.438
        intellectual disability Z81.0
        leukemia Z80.6
        lipidemia NEC Z83.438
        malignant neoplasm (of) NOS Z80.9
            bladder Z80.52
            breast Z80.3
            bronchus Z80.1
            digestive organ Z80.0
            gastrointestinal tract Z80.0
            genital organ Z80.49
                ovary Z80.41
                prostate Z80.42
                specified organ NEC Z80.49
                testis Z80.43
            hematopoietic NEC Z80.7
            intrathoracic organ NEC Z80.2
            kidney Z80.51
            lung Z80.1
            lymphatic NEC Z80.7
            ovary Z80.41
            prostate Z80.42
            respiratory organ NEC Z80.2
            specified site NEC Z80.8
            testis Z80.43
            trachea Z80.1
            urinary organ or tract Z80.59
                bladder Z80.52
                kidney Z80.51
        mental
            disorder NEC Z81.8
        multiple endocrine neoplasia (MEN) syndrome Z83.41
        osteoporosis Z82.62
        polycystic kidney Z82.71
        polyposis, adenomatous Z83.72
        polyps (colon) — *see also* History, family, colonic
            polyps Z83.719
        psychiatric disorder Z81.8
        psychoactive substance abuse NEC Z81.3
        respiratory condition NEC Z83.6
            asthma and other lower respiratory conditions
                Z82.5
        self-harmful behavior Z81.8
        SIDS (sudden infant death syndrome) Z84.82
        skin condition Z84.0
        specified condition NEC Z84.89
        stroke (cerebrovascular) Z82.3
        substance abuse NEC Z81.4
            alcohol Z81.1
            drug NEC Z81.3
            psychoactive NEC Z81.3
            tobacco Z81.2
        sudden
            cardiac death Z82.41
            infant death syndrome (SIDS) Z84.82
        tobacco abuse Z81.2
        violence, violent behavior Z81.8
        visual loss Z82.1
    personal (of) — *see also* History, family (of)
        abuse
            adult Z91.419
                financial Z91.413
                forced labor or sexual exploitation Z91.42
                intimate partner Z91.414
                physical and sexual Z91.410
                psychological Z91.411
            childhood Z62.819
                financial Z62.814
                forced labor or sexual exploitation in childhood
                    Z62.813
                intimate partner Z62.815
                physical Z62.810
                psychological Z62.811
                sexual Z62.810
            in adolescence — *see* History, personal, abuse,
                childhood
        alcohol dependence F10.21
        allergy (to) Z88.9
            analgesic agent NEC Z88.6
            anesthetic Z88.4
            antibiotic agent NEC Z88.1

History — *continued*
    personal — *see also* History, family — *continued*
        allergy — *continued*
            anti-infective agent NEC Z88.3
            contrast media Z91.041
            drugs, medicaments and biological substances
                Z88.9
                specified NEC Z88.8
            food Z91.018
                additives Z91.02
                beef Z91.014
                eggs Z91.012
                lamb Z91.014
                mammalian meats Z91.014
                milk products Z91.011
                peanuts Z91.010
                pork Z91.014
                red meats Z91.014
                seafood Z91.013
                specified food NEC Z91.018
            insect Z91.038
                bee Z91.030
            latex Z91.040
            medicinal agents Z88.9
                specified NEC Z88.8
            narcotic agent NEC Z88.5
            nonmedicinal agents Z91.048
            penicillin Z88.0
            serum Z88.7
            specified NEC Z91.09
            sulfonamides Z88.2
            vaccine Z88.7
        anaphylactic shock Z87.892
        anaphylaxis Z87.892
        behavioral disorders Z86.59
        benign carcinoid tumor Z86.012
        benign neoplasm Z86.018
            brain Z86.011
            carcinoid Z86.012
            colonic polyps — *see* History, personal, neoplasm,
                benign, colon polyp
        brain injury (traumatic) Z87.820
        breast implant removal Z98.86
        calculi, renal Z87.442
        cancer — *see* History, personal (of), malignant neo-
            plasm (of)
        cardiac arrest (death), successfully resuscitated Z86.74
        CAR-T (Chimeric Antigen Receptor T-cell) therapy
            Z92.850
        cellular therapy Z92.859
            specified NEC Z92.858
        cerebral infarction without residual deficit Z86.73
        certain (corrected) conditions arising in the perinatal
            period, specified NEC Z87.68
        cervical dysplasia Z87.410
        chemotherapy for neoplastic condition Z92.21
        childhood abuse — *see* History, personal (of), abuse
        Chimeric Antigen Receptor T-cell (CAR-T) therapy
            Z92.850
        cleft lip (corrected) Z87.730
        cleft palate (corrected) Z87.730
        cloaca, persistent Z87.732
        cloacal malformations Z87.732
        collapsed vertebra (healed) Z87.311
            due to osteoporosis Z87.310
        combat and operational stress reaction Z86.51
        congenital malformation (corrected) Z87.798
            circulatory system (corrected) Z87.74
            diaphragmatic hernia Z87.760
            digestive system (corrected) NEC Z87.738
            ear (corrected) Z87.721
            eye (corrected) Z87.720
            face and neck (corrected) Z87.790
            gastroschisis Z87.761
            genitourinary system (corrected) NEC Z87.718
            heart (corrected) Z87.74
            integument (corrected) Z87.768
            limb(s) (corrected) Z87.768
            malformations
                abdominal wall Z87.763
                diaphragm NEC Z87.760
                integument Z87.768
                limbs Z87.768
                musculoskeletal system Z87.768
                prune belly Z87.762
            musculoskeletal system (corrected) Z87.768
            neck (corrected) Z87.790
            nervous system (corrected) NEC Z87.728
            respiratory system (corrected) Z87.75

History — *continued*
    personal — *see also* History, family — *continued*
        congenital malformation — *continued*
            sense organs (corrected) NEC Z87.728
            specified NEC Z87.798
        contraception Z92.0
        coronavirus (disease) (novel) 2019 Z86.16
        COVID-19 Z86.16
        deployment (military) Z91.82
        diabetic foot ulcer Z86.31
        disease or disorder (of) Z87.898
            anaphylaxis Z87.892
            blood and blood-forming organs Z86.2
            circulatory system Z86.79
                specified condition NEC Z86.79
            connective tissue Z87.39
            digestive system Z87.19
                colonic polyp — *see* History, personal, neo-
                    plasm, benign, colon polyp
                peptic ulcer disease Z87.11
                specified condition NEC Z87.19
            ear Z86.69
            endocrine Z86.39
                diabetic foot ulcer Z86.31
                gestational diabetes Z86.32
                specified type NEC Z86.39
            eye Z86.69
            genital (track) system NEC
                female Z87.42
                male Z87.438
            hematological Z86.2
            Hodgkin Z85.71
            immune mechanism Z86.2
            infectious Z86.19
                coronavirus (disease) (novel) 2019 Z86.16
                COVID-19 Z86.16
                malaria Z86.13
                Methicillin resistant Staphylococcus aureus
                    (MRSA) Z86.14
                poliomyelitis Z86.12
                SARS-CoV-2 Z86.16
                specified NEC Z86.19
                tuberculosis Z86.11
            mental NEC Z86.59
            metabolic Z86.39
                diabetic foot ulcer Z86.31
                gestational diabetes Z86.32
                specified type NEC Z86.39
            musculoskeletal NEC Z87.39
            nervous system Z86.69
            nutritional Z86.39
            parasitic Z86.19
            respiratory system NEC Z87.09
            sense organs Z86.69
            skin Z87.2
            specified site or type NEC Z87.898
            subcutaneous tissue Z87.2
            trophoblastic Z87.59
            urinary system NEC Z87.448
        drug dependence — *see* Dependence, drug, by type,
            in remission
        drug therapy
            antineoplastic chemotherapy Z92.21
            estrogen Z92.23
            ICI (immune checkpoint inhibitor) drug therapy
                Z92.26
            immunosuppression Z92.25
            inhaled steroids Z92.240
            monoclonal drug Z92.22
            specified NEC Z92.29
            steroid Z92.241
            systemic steroids Z92.241
        dysplasia
            cervical (mild) (moderate) Z87.410
                severe (grade III) Z86.001
            prostatic Z87.430
            vaginal (mild) (moderate) Z87.411
                severe (grade III) Z86.002
            vulvar (mild) (moderate) Z87.412
                severe (grade III) Z86.002
        embolism (venous) Z86.718
            pulmonary Z86.711
        encephalitis Z86.61
        estrogen therapy Z92.23
        extracorporeal membrane oxygenation (ECMO)
            Z92.81
        failed conscious sedation Z92.83
        failed moderate sedation Z92.83
        fall, falling Z91.81

☑ **Additional Character Required** — Refer to the Tabular List for Character Selection

History — continued
  personal — see also History, family — continued
    forced labor or sexual exploitation Z91.42
      in childhood Z62.813
    fracture (healed)
      fatigue Z87.312
      fragility Z87.310
      osteoporosis Z87.310
      pathological NEC Z87.311
      stress Z87.312
      traumatic Z87.81
    gene therapy Z92.86
    gestational diabetes Z86.32
    hepatitis
      B Z86.19
      C Z86.19
    Hodgkin disease Z85.71
    hyperthermia, malignant Z88.4
    hypospadias (corrected) Z87.710
    hysterectomy Z90.710
    ICI (immune checkpoint inhibitor) drug therapy Z92.26
    immune checkpoint inhibitor (ICI) therapy Z92.26
    immunosuppression therapy Z92.25
    in situ neoplasm
      breast Z86.000
      cervix uteri Z86.001
      digestive organs, specified NEC Z86.004
      esophagus Z86.003
      genital organs, specified NEC Z86.002
      melanoma Z86.006
      middle ear Z86.005
      oral cavity Z86.003
      respiratory system Z86.005
      skin Z86.007
      specified NEC Z86.008
      stomach Z86.003
    in utero procedure during pregnancy Z98.870
    in utero procedure while a fetus Z98.871
    infection NEC Z86.19
      central nervous system Z86.61
      coronavirus (disease) (novel) 2019 Z86.16
      COVID-19 Z86.16
      latent tuberculosis Z86.15
      Methicillin resistant Staphylococcus aureus (MRSA) Z86.14
      SARS-CoV-2 Z86.16
      urinary (recurrent) (tract) Z87.440
    injury NEC Z87.828
    irradiation Z92.3
    kidney stones Z87.442
    latent tuberculosis infection Z86.15
    leukemia Z85.6
    lymphoma (non-Hodgkin) Z85.72
    malignant melanoma (skin) Z85.820
    malignant neoplasm (of) Z85.9
      accessory sinuses Z85.22
      anus NEC Z85.048
        carcinoid Z85.040
      bladder Z85.51
      bone Z85.830
      brain Z85.841
      breast Z85.3
      bronchus NEC Z85.118
        carcinoid Z85.110
      carcinoid — see History, personal (of), malignant neoplasm, by site, carcinoid
      cervix Z85.41
      colon NEC Z85.038
        carcinoid Z85.030
      digestive organ Z85.00
        specified NEC Z85.09
      endocrine gland NEC Z85.858
      epididymis Z85.48
      esophagus Z85.01
      eye Z85.840
      gastrointestinal tract — see History, malignant neoplasm, digestive organ
      genital organ
        female Z85.40
          specified NEC Z85.44
        male Z85.45
          specified NEC Z85.49
      hematopoietic NEC Z85.79
      intrathoracic organ Z85.20
      kidney NEC Z85.528
        carcinoid Z85.520
      large intestine NEC Z85.038
        carcinoid Z85.030
      larynx Z85.21

History — continued
  personal — see also History, family — continued
    malignant neoplasm — continued
      liver Z85.05
      lung NEC Z85.118
        carcinoid Z85.110
      mediastinum Z85.29
      Merkel cell Z85.821
      middle ear Z85.22
      nasal cavities Z85.22
      nervous system NEC Z85.848
      oral cavity Z85.819
        specified site NEC Z85.818
      ovary Z85.43
      pancreas Z85.07
      pelvis Z85.53
      pharynx Z85.819
        specified site NEC Z85.818
      pleura Z85.29
      prostate Z85.46
      rectosigmoid junction NEC Z85.048
        carcinoid Z85.040
      rectum NEC Z85.048
        carcinoid Z85.040
      respiratory organ Z85.20
      sinuses, accessory Z85.22
      skin NEC Z85.828
        melanoma Z85.820
        Merkel cell Z85.821
      small intestine NEC Z85.068
        carcinoid Z85.060
      soft tissue Z85.831
      specified site NEC Z85.89
      stomach NEC Z85.028
        carcinoid Z85.020
      testis Z85.47
      thymus NEC Z85.238
        carcinoid Z85.230
      thyroid Z85.850
      tongue Z85.810
      trachea Z85.12
      urinary organ or tract Z85.50
        specified NEC Z85.59
      uterus Z85.42
    maltreatment Z91.89
    medical treatment NEC Z92.89
    melanoma Z85.820
      in situ Z86.006
      malignant (skin) Z85.820
    meningitis Z86.61
    mental disorder Z86.59
    Merkel cell carcinoma (skin) Z85.821
    Methicillin resistant Staphylococcus aureus (MRSA) Z86.14
    military deployment Z91.82
    military service Z91.85
    military war, peacekeeping and humanitarian deployment (current or past conflict) Z91.82
    myocardial infarction (old) I25.2
    necrotizing enterocolitis of newborn (corrected) Z87.61
    neglect (in)
      adult Z91.412
      childhood Z62.812
    neoplasia
      anal intraepithelial, III [AIN III] Z86.004
      high-grade prostatic intraepithelial, III [HGPIN III] Z86.002
      vaginal intraepithelial, III [VAIN III] Z86.002
      vulvar intraepithelial, III [VIN III] Z86.002
    neoplasm
      benign Z86.018
        brain Z86.011
        colon polyp Z86.0100
          adenomatous (sessile) Z86.0101
          hyperplastic Z86.0102
          serrated (sessile) Z86.0101
          specified NEC Z86.0109
          traditional serrated adenoma Z86.0101
          tubular adenoma Z86.0101
          tubulovillous adenoma Z86.0101
          villous adenoma Z86.0101
      in situ
        breast Z86.000
        cervix uteri Z86.001
        digestive organs, specified NEC Z86.004
        esophagus Z86.003
        genital organs, specified NEC Z86.002
        melanoma Z86.006

History — continued
  personal — see also History, family — continued
    neoplasm — continued
      in situ — continued
        middle ear Z86.005
        oral cavity Z86.003
        respiratory system Z86.005
        skin Z86.007
        specified NEC Z86.008
        stomach Z86.003
      malignant — see History of, malignant neoplasm
      uncertain behavior Z86.03
    nephrotic syndrome Z87.441
    nicotine dependence Z87.891
    noncompliance with medical treatment or regimen — see Noncompliance
    nutritional deficiency Z86.39
    obstetric complications Z87.59
      childbirth Z87.59
      pregnancy Z87.59
      pre-term labor Z87.51
      puerperium Z87.59
    osteoporosis fractures Z87.31 ☑
    parasuicide (attempt) Z91.51
    physical trauma NEC Z87.828
      self-harm or suicide attempt Z91.51
    pneumonia (recurrent) Z87.01
    poisoning NEC Z91.89
      self-harm or suicide attempt Z91.51
    poor personal hygiene Z91.89
    preterm labor Z87.51
    procedure during pregnancy Z98.870
    procedure while a fetus Z98.871
    prolonged reversible ischemic neurologic deficit (PRIND) Z86.73
    prostatic dysplasia Z87.430
    psychological
      abuse
        adult Z91.411
        child Z62.811
      trauma, specified NEC Z91.49
    radiation therapy Z92.3
    removal
      implant
        breast Z98.86
    renal calculi Z87.442
    respiratory condition NEC Z87.09
    retained foreign body fully removed Z87.821
    risk factors NEC Z91.89
    SARS-CoV-2 infection Z86.16
    self-harm
      nonsuicidal Z91.52
      suicidal Z91.51
    self-inflicted injury without suicidal intent Z91.52
    self-injury
      nonsuicidal Z91.52
    self-mutilation Z91.52
    self-poisoning attempt Z91.51
    sex reassignment Z87.890
    sleep-wake cycle problem Z72.821
    specified NEC Z87.898
    steroid therapy (systemic) Z92.241
      inhaled Z92.240
    stroke without residual deficits Z86.73
    substance abuse NEC F10-F19
    sudden cardiac arrest Z86.74
    sudden cardiac death successfully resuscitated Z86.74
    suicidal behavior Z91.51
    suicide attempt Z91.51
    surgery NEC Z98.890
      with uterine scar Z98.891
      sex reassignment Z87.890
      transplant — see Transplant
    thrombophlebitis Z86.72
    thrombosis (venous) Z86.718
      pulmonary Z86.711
    tobacco dependence Z87.891
    tracheoesophageal
      atresia Z87.731
      fistula Z87.731
    transient ischemic attack (TIA) without residual deficits Z86.73
    trauma (physical) NEC Z87.828
      psychological NEC Z91.49
      self-harm Z91.51
    traumatic brain injury Z87.820
    tuberculosis, latent infection Z86.15
    unhealthy sleep-wake cycle Z72.821

History — *continued*
  personal — *see also* History, family — *continued*
    unintended awareness under general anesthesia Z92.84
    urinary calculi Z87.442
    urinary (recurrent) (tract) infection(s) Z87.440
    uterine scar from previous surgery Z98.891
    vaginal dysplasia Z87.411
    venous thrombosis or embolism Z86.718
      pulmonary Z86.711
    vulvar dysplasia Z87.412
His-Werner disease A79.0
HIV — *see also* Human, immunodeficiency virus B20
  laboratory evidence (nonconclusive) R75
  nonconclusive test (in infants) R75
  positive, seropositive Z21
Hives (bold) — *see* Urticaria
Hoarseness R49.0
Hobo Z59.00
Hodgkin disease — *see* Lymphoma, Hodgkin
Hodgson's — *see also* Aneurysm, aorta, thorax I71.20
  ruptured — *see also* Aneurysm, aorta, thorax, ruptured I71.10
Hoffa-Kastert disease E88.89
Hoffa's disease E88.89
Hoffmann-Bouveret syndrome I47.9
Hoffmann's syndrome E03.9 *[G73.7]*
Hole (round)
  macula H35.34- ☑
  retina (without detachment) — *see* Break, retina, round hole
    with detachment — *see* Detachment, retina, with retinal, break
Holiday relief care Z75.5
Hollenhorst's plaque — *see* Occlusion, artery, retina
Hollow foot (congenital) Q66.7- ☑
  acquired — *see* Deformity, limb, foot, specified NEC
Holoprosencephaly Q04.2
Holt-Oram syndrome Q87.2
Homelessness Z59.00
  sheltered Z59.01
  unsheltered Z59.02
Homesickness — *see* Disorder, adjustment
Homocysteinemia R79.83
Homocystinemia R79.83
Homocystinuria E72.11
Homogentisate 1,2-dioxygenase deficiency E70.29
Homologous serum hepatitis (prophylactic) (therapeutic) — *see* Hepatitis, viral, type B
Honeycomb lung J98.4
  congenital Q33.0
Hooded
  clitoris Q52.6
  penis Q55.69
Hookworm (disease) (infection) (infestation) B76.9
  with anemia B76.9 *[D63.8]*
  specified NEC B76.8
Hordeolum (eyelid) (externum) (recurrent) H00.019
  internum H00.029
    left H00.026
      lower H00.025
      upper H00.024
    right H00.023
      lower H00.022
      upper H00.021
  left H00.016
    lower H00.015
    upper H00.014
  right H00.013
    lower H00.012
    upper H00.011
Horn
  cutaneous L85.8
  nail L60.2
    congenital Q84.6
Horner (-Claude Bernard) **syndrome** G90.2
  traumatic — *see* Injury, nerve, cervical sympathetic
Horseshoe kidney (congenital) Q63.1
Horton's headache or neuralgia G44.099
  intractable G44.091
  not intractable G44.099
Hospital hopper syndrome — *see* Disorder, factitious
Hospitalism in children — *see* Disorder, adjustment
Hostility R45.5
  towards child Z62.3
Hot flashes
  menopausal N95.1
Hourglass (contracture) — *see also* Contraction, hourglass
  stomach K31.89

Hourglass — *continued*
  stomach — *continued*
    congenital Q40.2
    stricture K31.2
Household, housing circumstance affecting care Z59.9
  specified NEC Z59.89
Housemaid's knee — *see* Bursitis, prepatellar
HSCT-TMA (hematopoietic stem cell transplantation-associated thrombotic microangiopathy) M31.11
Hudson (-Stahli) **line** (cornea) — *see* Pigmentation, cornea, anterior
Human
  bite (open wound) — *see also* Bite
    intact skin surface — *see* Bite, superficial
  herpesvirus — *see* Herpes
  immunodeficiency virus (HIV) disease (infection) B20
    asymptomatic status Z21
    contact Z20.6
    counseling Z71.7
    dementia — *see also* Dementia, in, diseases specified elsewhere B20 *[F02.80]*
      with behavioral disturbance — *see also* Dementia, in, diseases specified elsewhere B20 *[F02.81-]* ☑
    exposure to Z20.6
    laboratory evidence R75
    type-2 (HIV 2) as cause of disease classified elsewhere B97.35
  papillomavirus (HPV)
    DNA test positive
      high risk
        cervix R87.810
        vagina R87.811
      low risk
        cervix R87.820
        vagina R87.821
    screening for Z11.51
  T-cell lymphotropic virus
    type-1 (HTLV-I) infection B33.3
      as cause of disease classified elsewhere B97.33
      carrier Z22.6
    type-2 (HTLV-II) as cause of disease classified elsewhere B97.34
Humidifier lung or pneumonitis J67.7
Humiliation (experience) **in childhood** Z62.898
Humpback (acquired) — *see* Kyphosis
Hunchback (acquired) — *see* Kyphosis
Hunger T73.0 ☑
  air, psychogenic F45.8
Hungry bone syndrome E83.81
Hunner's ulcer — *see* Cystitis, chronic, interstitial
Hunter's
  glossitis D51.0
  syndrome E76.1
Huntington's disease or chorea G10
  with dementia — *see also* Dementia, in, diseases specified elsewhere G10 *[F02.80]*
    with behavioral disturbance — *see also* Dementia, in, diseases specified elsewhere G10 *[F02.81-]* ☑
Hunt's
  disease or syndrome (herpetic geniculate ganglionitis) B02.21
    dyssynergia cerebellaris myoclonica G11.19
  neuralgia B02.21
Hurler (-Scheie) **disease or syndrome** E76.02
Hurst's disease G36.1
Hurthle cell
  adenocarcinoma C73
  adenoma D34
  carcinoma C73
  tumor D34
Hutchinson-Boeck disease or syndrome — *see* Sarcoidosis
Hutchinson-Gilford disease or syndrome E34.8
Hutchinson's
  disease, meaning
    angioma serpiginosum L81.7
    pompholyx (cheiropompholyx) L30.1
    prurigo estivalis L56.4
    summer eruption or summer prurigo L56.4
  melanotic freckle — *see* Melanoma, in situ
    malignant melanoma in — *see* Melanoma
  teeth or incisors (congenital syphilis) A50.52
  triad (congenital syphilis) A50.53
Hyalin plaque, sclera, senile H15.89
Hyaline membrane (disease) (lung) (pulmonary) (newborn) P22.0
Hyalinosis
  cutis (et mucosae) E78.89

Hyalinosis — *continued*
  focal and segmental (glomerular) — *see also* N00-N07
    with fourth character .1 N05.1
Hyalitis, hyalosis, asteroid — *see* Deposit, crystalline
  syphilitic (late) A52.71
Hydatid
  cyst or tumor — *see* Echinococcus
  mole — *see* Hydatidiform mole
  Morgagni
    female Q50.5
    male (epididymal) Q55.4
    testicular Q55.29
Hydatidiform mole (benign) (complicating pregnancy) (delivered) (undelivered) O01.9
  classical O01.0
  complete O01.0
  incomplete O01.1
  invasive D39.2
  malignant D39.2
  partial O01.1
Hydatidosis — *see* Echinococcus
Hydradenitis (axillaris) (suppurative) L73.2
Hydradenoma — *see* Hidradenoma
Hydramnios O40.- ☑
Hydrancephaly, hydranencephaly Q04.3
  with spina bifida — *see* Spina bifida, with hydrocephalus
Hydrargyrism NEC — *see* Poisoning, mercury
Hydrarthrosis — *see also* Effusion, joint
  gonococcal A54.42
  intermittent M12.40
    ankle M12.47- ☑
    elbow M12.42- ☑
    foot joint M12.47- ☑
    hand joint M12.44- ☑
    hip M12.45- ☑
    knee M12.46- ☑
    multiple site M12.49
    shoulder M12.41- ☑
    specified joint NEC M12.48
    wrist M12.43- ☑
  of yaws (early) (late) — *see also* subcategory M14.8- A66.6
  syphilitic (late) A52.77
    congenital A50.55 *[M12.80]*
Hydremia D64.89
Hydrencephalocele (congenital) — *see* Encephalocele
Hydrencephalomeningocele (congenital) — *see* Encephalocele
Hydroa R23.8
  aestivale L56.4
  vacciniforme L56.4
Hydroadenitis (axillaris) (suppurative) L73.2
Hydrocalycosis — *see* Hydronephrosis
Hydrocele (spermatic cord) (testis) (tunica vaginalis) N43.3
  canal of Nuck N94.89
  communicating N43.2
    congenital P83.5
  congenital P83.5
  encysted N43.0
  female NEC N94.89
  infected N43.1
  newborn P83.5
  round ligament N94.89
  specified NEC N43.2
  spinalis — *see* Spina bifida
  vulva N90.89
Hydrocephalus (acquired) (external) (internal) (malignant) (recurrent) G91.9
  aqueduct Sylvius stricture Q03.0
  causing disproportion O33.6 ☑
    with obstructed labor O66.3
  communicating G91.0
  congenital (external) (internal) Q03.9
    with spina bifida Q05.4
      cervical Q05.0
      dorsal Q05.1
      lumbar Q05.2
      lumbosacral Q05.2
      sacral Q05.3
      thoracic Q05.1
      thoracolumbar Q05.1
    specified NEC Q03.8
  due to toxoplasmosis (congenital) P37.1
  foramen Magendie block (acquired) G91.1
    congenital — *see also* Hydrocephalus, congenital Q03.1
  in (due to)
    infectious disease NEC B89 *[G91.4]*
    neoplastic disease NEC — *see also* Neoplasm G91.4

☑ **Additional Character Required** — **Refer to the Tabular List for Character Selection**

Hydrocephalus — continued
 in — continued
  parasitic disease B89 [G91.4]
 newborn Q03.9
  with spina bifida — see Spina bifida, with hydrocephalus
 noncommunicating G91.1
 normal pressure G91.2
  secondary G91.0
 obstructive G91.1
 otitic G93.2
 post-traumatic NEC G91.3
 secondary G91.4
  post-traumatic G91.3
 specified NEC G91.8
 syphilitic, congenital A50.49
Hydrocolpos (congenital) N89.8
Hydrocystoma — see Neoplasm, skin, benign
Hydroencephalocele (congenital) — see Encephalocele
Hydroencephalomeningocele (congenital) — see Encephalocele
Hydrohematopneumothorax — see Hemothorax
Hydromeningitis — see Meningitis
Hydromeningocele (spinal) — see also Spina bifida
 cranial — see Encephalocele
Hydrometra N85.8
Hydrometrocolpos N89.8
Hydromicrocephaly Q02
Hydromphalos (since birth) Q45.8
Hydromyelia Q06.4
Hydromyelocele — see Spina bifida
Hydronephrosis (atrophic) (early) (functionless) (intermittent) (primary) (secondary) NEC N13.30
 with
  infection N13.6
  obstruction (by) (of)
   renal calculus N13.2
    with infection N13.6
   ureteral NEC N13.1
    with infection N13.6
    calculus N13.2
     with infection N13.6
   ureteropelvic junction (congenital) Q62.11
    acquired N13.0
     with infection N13.6
   ureteral stricture NEC N13.1
    with infection N13.6
 congenital Q62.0
  due to acquired occlusion of ureteropelvic junction
   N13.0
 specified type NEC N13.39
 tuberculous A18.11
Hydropericarditis — see Pericarditis
Hydropericardium — see Pericarditis
Hydroperitoneum R18.8
Hydrophobia — see Rabies
Hydrophthalmos Q15.0
Hydropneumohemothorax — see Hemothorax
Hydropneumopericarditis — see Pericarditis
Hydropneumopericardium — see Pericarditis
Hydropneumothorax J94.8
 traumatic — see Injury, intrathoracic, lung
 tuberculous NEC A15.6
Hydrops R60.9
 abdominis R18.8
 articulorum intermittens — see Hydrarthrosis, intermittent
 cardiac — see Failure, heart, congestive
 causing obstructed labor (mother) O66.3
 endolymphatic H81.0- ☑
 fetal — see Pregnancy, complicated by, hydrops, fetalis
 fetalis P83.2
  due to
   ABO isoimmunization P56.0
   alpha thalassemia D56.0
   hemolytic disease P56.90
    specified NEC P56.99
   isoimmunization (ABO) (Rh) P56.0
   other specified nonhemolytic disease NEC P83.2
   Rh incompatibility P56.0
  during pregnancy — see Pregnancy, complicated by,
   hydrops, fetalis
 gallbladder K82.1
 joint — see Effusion, joint
 labyrinth H81.0- ☑
 newborn (idiopathic) P83.2
  due to
   ABO isoimmunization P56.0
   alpha thalassemia D56.0

Hydrops — continued
 newborn — continued
  due to — continued
   hemolytic disease P56.90
    specified NEC P56.99
   isoimmunization (ABO) (Rh) P56.0
   Rh incompatibility P56.0
 nutritional — see Malnutrition, severe
 pericardium — see Pericarditis
 pleura — see Hydrothorax
 spermatic cord — see Hydrocele
Hydropyonephrosis N13.6
Hydrorachis Q06.4
Hydrorrhea (nasal) J34.89
 pregnancy — see Rupture, membranes, premature
Hydrosadenitis (axillaris) (suppurative) L73.2
Hydrosalpinx (fallopian tube) (follicularis) N70.11
Hydrothorax (double) (pleura) J94.8
 chylous (nonfilarial) I89.8
  filarial — see also Infestation, filarial B74.9 [J91.8]
 traumatic — see Injury, intrathoracic
 tuberculous NEC (non primary) A15.6
Hydroureter — see also Hydronephrosis N13.4
 with infection N13.6
 congenital Q62.39
Hydroureteronephrosis — see Hydronephrosis
Hydrourethra N36.8
Hydroxykynureninuria E70.89
Hydroxylysinemia E72.3
Hydroxyprolinemia E72.59
Hygiene, sleep
 abuse Z72.821
 inadequate Z72.821
 poor Z72.821
Hygroma (congenital) (cystic) D18.1
 praepatellare, prepatellar — see Bursitis, prepatellar
 subdural — see Leak, cerebrospinal fluid
Hymen — see condition
Hymenolepis, hymenolepiasis (diminuta) (infection) (infestation) (nana) B71.0
Hypalgesia R20.8
Hyperacidity (gastric) K31.89
 psychogenic F45.8
Hyperactive, hyperactivity F90.9
 basal cell, uterine cervix — see Dysplasia, cervix
 bowel sounds R19.12
 cervix epithelial (basal) — see Dysplasia, cervix
 child F90.9
  attention deficit — see Disorder, attention-deficit
   hyperactivity
 detrusor muscle N32.81
 gastrointestinal K31.89
  psychogenic F45.8
 nasal mucous membrane J34.3
 stomach K31.89
 thyroid (gland) — see Hyperthyroidism
Hyperacusis H93.23- ☑
Hyperadrenalism E27.5
Hyperadrenocorticism E24.9
 congenital E25.0
 iatrogenic E24.2
  correct substance properly administered — see Table
   of Drugs and Chemicals, by drug, adverse effect
  overdose or wrong substance given or taken — see
   Table of Drugs and Chemicals, by drug, poisoning
 not associated with Cushing's syndrome E27.0
 pituitary-dependent E24.0
Hyperaldosteronism E26.9
 familial (type I) E26.02
 glucocorticoid-remediable E26.02
 primary (due to (bilateral) adrenal hyperplasia) E26.09
 primary NEC E26.09
 secondary E26.1
 specified NEC E26.89
Hyperalgesia R20.8
Hyperalimentation R63.2
 carotene, carotin E67.1
 specified NEC E67.8
 vitamin
  A E67.0
  D E67.3
Hyperaminoaciduria
 arginine E72.21
 cystine E72.01
 lysine E72.3
 ornithine E72.4
Hyperammonemia (congenital) E72.20
Hyperazotemia — see Uremia

Hyperbetalipoproteinemia (familial) E78.00
 with prebetalipoproteinemia E78.2
Hyperbicarbonatemia P74.41
Hyperbilirubinemia
 constitutional E80.6
 familial conjugated E80.6
 neonatal (transient) — see Jaundice, newborn
Hypercalcemia, hypocalciuric, familial E83.52
Hypercalciuria, idiopathic R82.994
Hypercapnia R06.89
 newborn P84
Hypercarotenemia (dietary) E67.1
Hypercementosis K03.4
Hyperchloremia E87.8
Hyperchlorhydria K31.89
 neurotic F45.8
 psychogenic F45.8
Hypercholesterinemia — see Hypercholesterolemia
Hypercholesterolemia (essential) (primary) (pure) E78.00
 with hyperglyceridemia, endogenous E78.2
 dietary counseling and surveillance Z71.3
 familial E78.01
 hereditary E78.01
Hyperchylia gastrica, psychogenic F45.8
Hyperchylomicronemia (familial) (primary) E78.3
 with hyperbetalipoproteinemia E78.3
Hypercoagulable (state) D68.59
 activated protein C resistance D68.51
 antithrombin (III) deficiency D68.59
 factor V Leiden mutation D68.51
 primary NEC D68.59
 protein C deficiency D68.59
 protein S deficiency D68.59
 prothrombin gene mutation D68.52
 secondary D68.69
 specified NEC D68.69
Hypercoagulation (state) D68.59
Hypercorticalism, pituitary-dependent E24.0
Hypercorticosolism — see Cushing's, syndrome
Hypercorticosteronism E24.2
 correct substance properly administered — see Table of
  Drugs and Chemicals, by drug, adverse effect
 overdose or wrong substance given or taken — see Table
  of Drugs and Chemicals, by drug, poisoning
Hypercortisonism E24.2
 correct substance properly administered — see Table of
  Drugs and Chemicals, by drug, adverse effect
 overdose or wrong substance given or taken — see Table
  of Drugs and Chemicals, by drug, poisoning
Hyperekplexia Q89.8
Hyperelectrolytemia E87.8
Hyperemesis R11.10
 with nausea R11.2
 gravidarum (mild) O21.0
  with
   carbohydrate depletion O21.1
   dehydration O21.1
   electrolyte imbalance O21.1
   metabolic disturbance O21.1
  severe (with metabolic disturbance) O21.1
 projectile R11.12
 psychogenic F45.8
Hyperemia (acute) (passive) R68.89
 anal mucosa K62.89
 bladder N32.89
 cerebral I67.89
 conjunctiva H11.43- ☑
 ear internal, acute — see subcategory H83.0 ☑
 enteric K59.89
 eye — see Hyperemia, conjunctiva
 eyelid (active) (passive) — see Disorder, eyelid, specified
  type NEC
 intestine K59.89
 iris — see Disorder, iris, vascular
 kidney N28.89
 labyrinth — see subcategory H83.0 ☑
 liver (active) K76.89
 lung (passive) — see Edema, lung
 pulmonary (passive) — see Edema, lung
 renal N28.89
 retina H35.89
 stomach K31.89
Hyperesthesia (body surface) R20.3
 larynx (reflex) J38.7
  hysterical F44.89
 pharynx (reflex) J39.2
  hysterical F44.89
Hyperestrogenism (drug-induced) (iatrogenic) E28.0
Hyperexplexia Q89.8

Hyperfibrinolysis — *see* Fibrinolysis
Hyperfructosemia E74.19
Hyperfunction
　adrenal cortex, not associated with Cushing's syndrome
　　E27.0
　　medulla E27.5
　　　adrenomedullary E27.5
　　virilism E25.9
　　　congenital E25.0
　ovarian E28.8
　pancreas K86.89
　parathyroid (gland) E21.3
　pituitary (gland) (anterior) E22.9
　　specified NEC E22.8
　polyglandular E31.1
　testicular E29.0
Hypergammaglobulinemia D89.2
　polyclonal D89.0
　Waldenstrom D89.0
Hypergastrinemia E16.4
Hyperglobulinemia R77.1
Hyperglycemia, hyperglycemic (transient) R73.9
　coma — *see* Diabetes, by type, with coma
　postpancreatectomy E89.1
Hyperglyceridemia (endogenous) (essential) (familial)
　(hereditary) (pure) E78.1
　mixed E78.3
Hyperglycinemia (non-ketotic) E72.51
Hypergonadism
　ovarian E28.8
　testicular (primary) (infantile) E29.0
Hyperheparinemia D68.32
Hyperhidrosis, hyperidrosis R61
　focal
　　primary L74.519
　　　axilla L74.510
　　　face L74.511
　　　palms L74.512
　　　soles L74.513
　　secondary L74.52
　generalized R61
　localized
　　primary L74.519
　　　axilla L74.510
　　　face L74.511
　　　palms L74.512
　　　soles L74.513
　　secondary L74.52
　psychogenic F45.8
　secondary R61
　　focal L74.52
Hyperhistidinemia E70.41
Hyperhomocysteinemia E72.11
Hyperhydroxyprolinemia E72.59
Hyperinsulinism (functional) E16.1
　with
　　coma (hypoglycemic) E15
　　encephalopathy E16.1 [G94]
　ectopic E16.1
　therapeutic misadventure (from administration of insulin)
　　— *see* subcategory T38.3 ☑
Hyperkalemia E87.5
Hyperkeratosis — *see also* Keratosis L85.9
　cervix N88.0
　due to yaws (early) (late) (palmar or plantar) A66.3
　follicularis Q82.8
　　penetrans (in cutem) L87.0
　palmoplantaris climacterica L85.1
　pinta A67.1
　senile (with pruritus) L57.0
　universalis congenita Q80.8
　vocal cord J38.3
　vulva N90.4
Hyperkinesia, hyperkinetic (disease) (reaction) (syndrome)
　(childhood) (adolescence) — *see also* Disorder, atten-
　tion-deficit hyperactivity
　heart I51.89
Hyperleucine-isoleucinemia E71.19
Hyperlipemia, hyperlipidemia E78.5
　combined E78.2
　　familial E78.49
　group
　　A E78.00
　　B E78.1
　　C E78.2
　　D E78.3
　mixed E78.2
　specified NEC E78.49
Hyperlipidosis E75.6

Hyperlipidosis — *continued*
　hereditary NEC E75.5
Hyperlipoproteinemia E78.5
　Fredrickson's type
　　I E78.3
　　IIa E78.00
　　IIb E78.2
　　III E78.2
　　IV E78.1
　　V E78.3
　low-density-lipoprotein-type (LDL) E78.00
　very-low-density-lipoprotein-type (VLDL) E78.1
Hyperlucent lung, unilateral J43.0
Hyperlysinemia E72.3
Hypermagnesemia E83.41
　neonatal P71.8
Hypermenorrhea N92.0
Hypermethioninemia E72.19
Hypermetropia (congenital) H52.0- ☑
Hypermobility, hypermotility
　cecum — *see* Syndrome, irritable bowel
　coccyx — *see* subcategory M53.2
　colon — *see* Syndrome, irritable bowel
　　psychogenic F45.8
　ileum K58.9
　intestine — *see also* Syndrome, irritable bowel K58.9
　　psychogenic F45.8
　meniscus (knee) — *see* Derangement, knee, meniscus
　scapula — *see* Instability, joint, shoulder
　stomach K31.89
　　psychogenic F45.8
　syndrome M35.7
　urethra N36.41
　　with intrinsic sphincter deficiency N36.43
Hypernasality R49.21
Hypernatremia E87.0
Hypernephroma C64.- ☑
Hyperopia — *see* Hypermetropia
Hyperorexia nervosa F50.2- ☑
Hyperornithinemia E72.4
Hyperosmia R43.1
Hyperosmolality — *see also* Diabetes, by type, with hyper-
　osmolarity E87.0
Hyperostosis (monomelic) — *see also* Disorder, bone,
　density and structure, specified NEC
　ankylosing (spine) M48.10
　　cervical region M48.12
　　cervicothoracic region M48.13
　　lumbar region M48.16
　　lumbosacral region M48.17
　　multiple sites M48.19
　　occipito-atlanto-axial region M48.11
　　sacrococcygeal region M48.18
　　thoracic region M48.14
　　thoracolumbar region M48.15
　cortical (skull) M85.2
　　infantile M89.8X- ☑
　frontal, internal of skull M85.2
　interna frontalis M85.2
　skeletal, diffuse idiopathic — *see* Hyperostosis, ankylos-
　　ing
　skull M85.2
　　congenital Q75.8
　vertebral, ankylosing — *see* Hyperostosis, ankylosing
Hyperovarism E28.8
Hyperoxaluria R82.992
　primary E72.53
Hyperparathyroidism E21.3
　primary E21.0
　secondary (renal) N25.81
　　non-renal E21.1
　specified NEC E21.2
　tertiary E21.2
Hyperpathia R20.8
Hyperperistalsis R19.2
　psychogenic F45.8
Hyperpermeability, capillary I78.8
Hyperphagia R63.2
Hyperphenylalaninemia NEC E70.1
Hyperphoria (alternating) H50.53
Hyperphosphatemia E83.39
Hyperpiesis, hyperpiesia — *see* Hypertension
Hyperpigmentation — *see also* Pigmentation
　melanin NEC L81.4
　postinflammatory L81.0
Hyperpinealism E34.8
Hyperpituitarism E22.9

Hyperplasia, hyperplastic
　adenoids J35.2
　adrenal (capsule) (cortex) (gland) E27.8
　　with
　　　sexual precocity (male) E25.9
　　　　congenital E25.0
　　　virilism, adrenal E25.9
　　　　congenital E25.0
　　　virilization (female) E25.9
　　　　congenital E25.0
　　congenital E25.0
　　　salt-losing E25.0
　adrenomedullary E27.5
　angiolymphoid, eosinophilia (ALHE) D18.01
　appendix (lymphoid) K38.0
　artery, fibromuscular I77.3
　bone — *see also* Hypertrophy, bone
　　marrow D75.89
　breast — *see also* Hypertrophy, breast
　　atypical, atypia N60.9- ☑
　　　ductal N60.9- ☑
　　　lobular N60.9- ☑
　C-cell, thyroid E07.0
　cementation (tooth) (teeth) K03.4
　cervical gland R59.0
　cervix (uteri) (basal cell) (endometrium) (polypoid) —
　　see also Dysplasia, cervix
　　congenital Q51.828
　clitoris, congenital Q52.6
　denture K06.2
　endocervicitis N72
　endometrium, endometrial (adenomatous) (cystic)
　　(glandular) (glandular-cystic) (polypoid) N85.00
　　with atypia N85.02
　　benign N85.01
　　cervix — *see* Dysplasia, cervix
　　complex (without atypia) N85.01
　　simple (without atypia) N85.01
　epithelial L85.9
　　focal, oral, including tongue K13.29
　　nipple N62
　　skin L85.9
　　tongue K13.29
　　vaginal wall N89.3
　erythroid D75.89
　fibromuscular of artery (carotid) (renal) I77.3
　genital
　　female NEC N94.89
　　male N50.89
　gingiva K06.1
　glandularis cystica uteri (interstitialis) — *see also* Hyper-
　　plasia, endometrial N85.00
　gum K06.1
　hymen, congenital Q52.4
　irritative, edentulous (alveolar) K06.2
　jaw M26.09
　　alveolar M26.79
　　　lower M26.03
　　　　alveolar M26.72
　　　upper M26.01
　　　　alveolar M26.71
　kidney (congenital) Q63.3
　labia N90.69
　　epithelial N90.3
　liver (congenital) Q44.79
　　nodular, focal K76.89
　lymph gland or node R59.9
　mandible, mandibular M26.03
　　alveolar M26.72
　　unilateral condylar M27.8
　maxilla, maxillary M26.01
　　alveolar M26.71
　myometrium, myometrial N85.2
　neuroendocrine cell, of infancy J84.841
　nose
　　lymphoid J34.89
　　polypoid J33.9
　oral mucosa (irritative) K13.6
　organ or site, congenital NEC — *see* Anomaly, by site
　ovary N83.8
　palate, papillary (irritative) K13.6
　pancreatic islet cells E16.9
　　alpha E16.8
　　　with excess
　　　　gastrin E16.4
　　　　glucagon E16.3
　　beta E16.1
　parathyroid (gland) E21.0
　pharynx (lymphoid) J39.2

☑ **Additional Character Required** — **Refer to the Tabular List for Character Selection**

Hyperplasia, hyperplastic — *continued*
  prostate (adenofibromatous) N40.0
    with lower urinary tract symptoms (LUTS) N40.1
      nodular N40.3
    nodular N40.2
      with lower urinary tract symptoms (LUTS) N40.3
      without lower urinary tract symptoms (LUTS) N40.0
        nodular N40.2
  renal artery I77.89
  reticulo-endothelial (cell) D75.89
  salivary gland (any) K11.1
  Schimmelbusch's — *see* Mastopathy, cystic
  suprarenal capsule (gland) E27.8
  thymus (gland) (persistent) E32.0
  thyroid (gland) — *see* Goiter
  tonsils (faucial) (infective) (lingual) (lymphoid) J35.1
    with adenoids J35.3
  unilateral condylar M27.8
  uterus, uterine N85.2
    endometrium (glandular) — *see also* Hyperplasia,
      endometrial N85.00
  vulva N90.69
    epithelial N90.3
Hyperpnea — *see* Hyperventilation
Hyperpotassemia E87.5
Hyperprebetalipoproteinemia (familial) E78.1
Hyperprolactinemia E22.1
Hyperprolinemia (type I) (type II) E72.59
Hyperproteinemia E88.09
Hyperprothrombinemia, causing coagulation factor
  deficiency D68.4
Hyperpyrexia R50.9
  heat (effects) T67.01 ☑
  malignant, due to anesthetic T88.3 ☑
  rheumatic — *see* Fever, rheumatic
  unknown origin R50.9
Hyper-reflexia R29.2
Hypersalivation K11.7
Hypersecretion
  ACTH (not associated with Cushing's syndrome) E27.0
    pituitary E24.0
  adrenaline E27.5
  adrenomedullary E27.5
  androgen (testicular) E29.0
    ovarian (drug-induced) (iatrogenic) E28.1
  calcitonin E07.0
  catecholamine E27.5
  corticoadrenal E24.9
  cortisol E24.9
  epinephrine E27.5
  estrogen E28.0
  gastric K31.89
    psychogenic F45.8
  gastrin E16.4
  glucagon E16.3
  hormone(s)
    ACTH (not associated with Cushing's syndrome) E27.0
      pituitary E24.0
    antidiuretic E22.2
    growth E22.0
    intestinal NEC E34.1
    ovarian androgen E28.1
    pituitary E22.9
    testicular E29.0
    thyroid stimulating E05.80
      with thyroid storm E05.81
  insulin — *see* Hyperinsulinism
  lacrimal glands — *see* Epiphora
  medulloadrenal E27.5
  milk O92.6
  ovarian androgens E28.1
  salivary gland (any) K11.7
  thyrocalcitonin E07.0
  upper respiratory J39.8
Hypersegmentation, leukocytic, hereditary D72.0
Hypersensitive, hypersensitiveness, hypersensitivity
  — *see also* Allergy
  carotid sinus G90.01
  colon — *see* Irritable, colon
  drug T88.7 ☑
  gastrointestinal K52.29
    immediate K52.29
    psychogenic F45.8
  labyrinth — *see* subcategory H83.2 ☑
  pain R20.8
  pneumonitis — *see* Pneumonitis, allergic
  reaction T78.40 ☑
    upper respiratory tract NEC J39.3

Hypersomnia (organic) G47.10
  due to
    alcohol
      abuse F10.182
      dependence F10.282
      use F10.982
    amphetamines
      abuse F15.182
      dependence F15.282
      use F15.982
    caffeine
      abuse F15.182
      dependence F15.282
      use F15.982
    cocaine
      abuse F14.182
      dependence F14.282
      use F14.982
    drug NEC
      abuse F19.182
      dependence F19.282
      use F19.982
    medical condition G47.14
    mental disorder F51.13
    opioid
      abuse F11.182
      dependence F11.282
      use F11.982
    psychoactive substance NEC
      abuse F19.182
      dependence F19.282
      use F19.982
    sedative, hypnotic, or anxiolytic
      abuse F13.182
      dependence F13.282
      use F13.982
    stimulant NEC
      abuse F15.182
      dependence F15.282
      use F15.982
  idiopathic G47.11
    with long sleep time G47.11
    without long sleep time G47.12
  menstrual related G47.13
  nonorganic origin F51.11
    specified NEC F51.19
  not due to a substance or known physiological condition
    F51.11
    specified NEC F51.19
  primary F51.11
  recurrent G47.13
  specified NEC G47.19
Hypersplenia, hypersplenism D73.1
Hyperstimulation, ovaries (associated with induced ovulation) N98.1
Hypersusceptibility — *see* Allergy
Hypertelorism (ocular) (orbital) Q75.2
Hypertension, hypertensive (accelerated) (benign) (essential) (idiopathic) (malignant) (systemic) I10
  with
    heart failure (congestive) I11.0
    heart involvement (conditions in I50.- or I51.4-I51.7,
      I51.89, I51.9, due to hypertension) — *see* Hypertension, heart
    kidney involvement — *see* Hypertension, kidney
  benign, intracranial G93.2
  borderline R03.0
  cardiorenal (disease) I13.10
    with heart failure I13.0
      with stage 1 through stage 4 chronic kidney disease I13.0
      with stage 5 or end stage renal disease I13.2
    without heart failure I13.10
      with stage 1 through stage 4 chronic kidney disease I13.10
      with stage 5 or end stage renal disease I13.11
  cardiovascular
    disease (arteriosclerotic) (sclerotic) — *see* Hypertension, heart
    renal (disease) — *see* Hypertension, cardiorenal
  chronic venous — *see* Hypertension, venous (chronic)
  complicating
    childbirth (labor) O16.4
      pre-existing O10.92
        with
          heart disease O10.12
            with renal disease O10.32
          pre-eclampsia O11.4
          renal disease O10.22

Hypertension, hypertensive — *continued*
  complicating — *continued*
    childbirth — *continued*
      pre-existing — *continued*
        with — *continued*
          renal disease — *continued*
            with heart disease O10.32
          essential O10.02
        secondary O10.42
    pregnancy O16.- ☑
      with edema — *see also* Pre-eclampsia O14.9- ☑
      gestational (pregnancy induced) (without proteinuria) O13.- ☑
        with proteinuria O14.9- ☑
          mild pre-eclampsia O14.0- ☑
          moderate pre-eclampsia O14.0- ☑
          severe pre-eclampsia O14.1- ☑
            with hemolysis, elevated liver enzymes
              and low platelet count (HELLP)
              O14.2- ☑
      pre-existing O10.91- ☑
        with
          heart disease O10.11- ☑
            with renal disease O10.31- ☑
          pre-eclampsia — *see* category O11
          renal disease O10.21- ☑
            with heart disease O10.31- ☑
        essential O10.01- ☑
        secondary O10.41- ☑
      transient O13- ☑
    puerperium, pre-existing O16.5
      pre-existing
        with
          heart disease O10.13
            with renal disease O10.33
          pre-eclampsia O11.5
          renal disease O10.23
            with heart disease O10.33
        essential O10.03
      pregnancy-induced O13.9
      secondary O10.43
  crisis I16.9
  due to
    endocrine disorders I15.2
    pheochromocytoma — *see also* Pheochromocytoma,
      by type I15.2
    renal disorders NEC I15.1
      arterial I15.0
    renovascular disorders I15.0
    specified disease NEC I15.8
  emergency I16.1
  encephalopathy I67.4
  gestational (without significant proteinuria) (pregnancy-
    induced) (transient) O13.- ☑
    with significant proteinuria — *see* Pre-eclampsia
    complicating
      delivery O13.4
      puerperium O13.5
  Goldblatt's I70.1
  heart (disease) (conditions in I51.4-I51.9 due to hypertension) I11.9
    with
      heart failure (congestive) I11.0
      kidney disease (chronic) — *see* Hypertension, cardiorenal
  intracranial, benign G93.2
  kidney I12.9
    with
      heart disease — *see* Hypertension, cardiorenal
      stage 1 through stage 4 chronic kidney disease I12.9
      stage 5 chronic kidney disease (CKD) or end stage
        renal disease (ESRD) I12.0
  lesser circulation I27.0
  maternal O16- ☑
  newborn P29.2
    pulmonary (persistent) P29.30
  ocular H40.05- ☑
  pancreatic duct — *code to* underlying condition
    with chronic pancreatitis K86.1
  portal (due to chronic liver disease) (idiopathic) K76.6
    gastropathy K31.89
    in (due to) schistosomiasis (bilharziasis) B65.9 [K77]
  postoperative I97.3
  psychogenic F45.8
  pulmonary I27.20
    with
      cor pulmonale (chronic) I27.29

Hypertension, hypertensive — *continued*
pulmonary — *continued*
  with — *continued*
    cor pulmonale — *continued*
      acute I26.09
    right heart ventricular strain/failure I27.29
      acute I26.09
    right to left shunt related to congenital heart disease I27.83
    unclear multifactorial mechanisms I27.29
  arterial (associated) (drug-induced) (toxin-induced) I27.21
  chronic thromboembolic I27.24
  due to
    hematologic disorders I27.29
    kyphoscoliotic heart disease I27.1
    left heart disease I27.22
    lung diseases and hypoxia I27.23
    metabolic disorders I27.29
    specified systemic disorders I27.29
  group 1 (associated) (drug-induced) (toxin-induced) I27.21
  group 2 I27.22
  group 3 I27.23
  group 4 I27.24
  group 5 I27.29
  of newborn (persistent) P29.30
  primary (idiopathic) I27.0
  secondary
    arterial I27.21
    specified NEC I27.29
renal — *see* Hypertension, kidney
renovascular I15.0
resistant (apparent treatment) (treatment) (true) I1A.0
secondary NEC I15.9
  due to
    endocrine disorders I15.2
    pheochromocytoma — *see also* Pheochromocytoma, by type I15.2
    renal disorders NEC I15.1
      arterial I15.0
    renovascular disorders I15.0
  specified NEC I15.8
transient R03.0
  of pregnancy O13.- ☑
urgency I16.0
venous (chronic)
  due to
    deep vein thrombosis — *see* Syndrome, postthrombotic
  idiopathic I87.309
    with
      inflammation I87.32- ☑
        with ulcer I87.33- ☑
      specified complication NEC I87.39- ☑
      ulcer I87.31- ☑
        with inflammation I87.33- ☑
    asymptomatic I87.30- ☑
Hypertensive urgency — *see* Hypertension
Hyperthecosis ovary E28.8
Hyperthermia (of unknown origin) — *see also* Hyperpyrexia
malignant, due to anesthesia T88.3 ☑
newborn P81.9
  environmental P81.0
Hyperthyroid (recurrent) — *see* Hyperthyroidism
Hyperthyroidism (latent) (pre-adult) (recurrent) E05.90
with
  goiter (diffuse) E05.00
    with thyroid storm E05.01
    nodular (multinodular) E05.20
      with thyroid storm E05.21
      uninodular E05.10
        with thyroid storm E05.11
  storm E05.91
due to ectopic thyroid tissue E05.30
  with thyroid storm E05.31
neonatal, transitory P72.1
specified NEC E05.80
  with thyroid storm E05.81
Hypertony, hypertonia, hypertonicity
bladder N31.8
congenital P94.1
stomach K31.89
  psychogenic F45.8
uterus, uterine (contractions) (complicating delivery) O62.4
Hypertrichosis L68.9
congenital Q84.2

Hypertrichosis — *continued*
eyelid H02.869
  left H02.866
    lower H02.865
    upper H02.864
  right H02.863
    lower H02.862
    upper H02.861
lanuginosa Q84.2
  acquired L68.1
localized L68.2
specified NEC L68.8
Hypertriglyceridemia, essential E78.1
Hypertrophy, hypertrophic
adenofibromatous, prostate — *see* Enlargement, enlarged, prostate
adenoids (infective) J35.2
  with tonsils J35.3
adrenal cortex E27.8
alveolar process or ridge — *see* Anomaly, alveolar
anal papillae K62.89
artery I77.89
  congenital NEC Q27.8
    digestive system Q27.8
    lower limb Q27.8
    specified site NEC Q27.8
    upper limb Q27.8
auricular — *see* Hypertrophy, cardiac
Bartholin's gland N75.8
bile duct (common) (hepatic) K83.8
bladder (sphincter) (trigone) N32.89
bone M89.30
  carpus M89.34- ☑
  clavicle M89.31- ☑
  femur M89.35- ☑
  fibula M89.36- ☑
  finger M89.34- ☑
  humerus M89.32- ☑
  ilium M89.38
  ischium M89.38
  metacarpus M89.34- ☑
  metatarsus M89.37- ☑
  multiple sites M89.39
  neck M89.38
  pubic ramus M89.38
  radius M89.33- ☑
  rib M89.38
  scapula M89.31- ☑
  skull M89.38
  tarsus M89.37- ☑
  tibia M89.36- ☑
  toe M89.37- ☑
  ulna M89.33- ☑
  vertebra M89.38
brain G93.89
breast N62
  cystic — *see* Mastopathy, cystic
  newborn P83.4
  pubertal, massive N62
  puerperal, postpartum — *see* Disorder, breast, specified type NEC
  senile (parenchymatous) N62
cardiac (chronic) (idiopathic) I51.7
  with rheumatic fever (conditions in I00)
    active I01.8
    inactive or quiescent (with chorea) I09.89
  congenital NEC Q24.8
  fatty — *see* Degeneration, myocardial
  hypertensive — *see* Hypertension, heart
  rheumatic (with chorea) I09.89
    active or acute I01.8
      with chorea I02.0
  valve — *see* Endocarditis
cartilage — *see* Disorder, cartilage, specified type NEC
cecum — *see* Megacolon
cervix (uteri) N88.8
  congenital Q51.828
  elongation N88.4
clitoris (cirrhotic) N90.89
  congenital Q52.6
colon — *see also* Megacolon
  congenital Q43.2
conjunctiva, lymphoid H11.89
corpora cavernosa N48.89
cystic duct K82.8
duodenum K31.89
endometrium (glandular) — *see also* Hyperplasia, endometrial N85.00

Hypertrophy, hypertrophic — *continued*
endometrium — *see also* Hyperplasia, endometrial — *continued*
  cervix N88.8
epididymis N50.89
esophageal hiatus (congenital) Q79.1
  with hernia — *see* Hernia, hiatal
eyelid — *see* Disorder, eyelid, specified type NEC
facet joint — *see also* Spondylosis M47.819
fat pad E65
  knee (infrapatellar) (popliteal) (prepatellar) (retropatellar) M79.4
foot (congenital) Q74.2
frenulum, frenum (tongue) K14.8
  lip K13.0
gallbladder K82.8
gastric mucosa K29.60
  with bleeding K29.61
gland, glandular R59.9
  generalized R59.1
  localized R59.0
gum (mucous membrane) K06.1
heart (idiopathic) — *see also* Hypertrophy, cardiac
  valve — *see also* Endocarditis I38
hemifacial Q67.4
hepatic — *see* Hypertrophy, liver
hiatus (esophageal) Q79.1
hilus gland R59.0
hymen, congenital Q52.4
ileum K63.89
intestine NEC K63.89
jejunum K63.89
kidney (compensatory) N28.81
  congenital Q63.3
labium (majus) (minus) N90.60
ligament — *see* Disorder, ligament
lingual tonsil (infective) J35.1
  with adenoids J35.3
lip K13.0
  congenital Q18.6
liver R16.0
  acute K76.89
  cirrhotic — *see* Cirrhosis, liver
  congenital Q44.79
  fatty — *see* Fatty, liver
lymph, lymphatic gland R59.9
  generalized R59.1
  localized R59.0
  tuberculous — *see* Tuberculosis, lymph gland
mammary gland — *see* Hypertrophy, breast
Meckel's diverticulum (congenital) Q43.0
  malignant — *see* Table of Neoplasms, small intestine, malignant
median bar — *see* Hyperplasia, prostate
meibomian gland — *see* Chalazion
meniscus, knee, congenital Q74.1
metatarsal head — *see* Hypertrophy, bone, metatarsus
metatarsus — *see* Hypertrophy, bone, metatarsus
mucous membrane
  alveolar ridge K06.2
  gum K06.1
  nose (turbinate) J34.3
muscle M62.89
muscular coat, artery I77.89
myocardium — *see also* Hypertrophy, cardiac
  idiopathic I42.2
myometrium N85.2
nail L60.2
  congenital Q84.5
nasal J34.89
  alae J34.89
  bone J34.89
  cartilage J34.89
  mucous membrane (septum) J34.3
  sinus J34.89
  turbinate J34.3
nasopharynx, lymphoid (infectional) (tissue) (wall) J35.2
nipple N62
organ or site, congenital NEC — *see* Anomaly, by site
ovary N83.8
palate (hard) M27.8
  soft K13.79
pancreas, congenital Q45.3
parathyroid (gland) E21.0
parotid gland K11.1
penis N48.89
pharyngeal tonsil J35.2
pharynx J39.2
  lymphoid (infectional) (tissue) (wall) J35.2

☑ **Additional Character Required** — Refer to the Tabular List for Character Selection

Hypertrophy, hypertrophic — *continued*
- pituitary (anterior) (fossa) (gland) E23.6
- prepuce (congenital) N47.8
  - female N90.89
- prostate — *see* Enlargement, enlarged, prostate
  - congenital Q55.4
- pseudomuscular — *see also* Dystrophy, muscular, by type, if applicable G71.09
- pylorus (adult) (muscle) (sphincter) K31.1
  - congenital or infantile Q40.0
- rectal, rectum (sphincter) K62.89
- rhinitis (turbinate) J31.0
- salivary gland (any) K11.1
  - congenital Q38.4
- scaphoid (tarsal) — *see* Hypertrophy, bone, tarsus
- scar L91.0
- scrotum N50.89
- seminal vesicle N50.89
- sigmoid — *see* Megacolon
- skin L91.9
  - specified NEC L91.8
- spermatic cord N50.89
- spleen — *see* Splenomegaly
- spondylitis — *see* Spondylosis
- stomach K31.89
- sublingual gland K11.1
- submandibular gland K11.1
- suprarenal cortex (gland) E27.8
- synovial NEC M67.20
  - acromioclavicular M67.21- ☑
  - ankle M67.27- ☑
  - elbow M67.22- ☑
  - foot M67.27- ☑
  - hand M67.24- ☑
  - hip M67.25- ☑
  - knee M67.26- ☑
  - multiple sites M67.29
  - specified site NEC M67.28
  - wrist M67.23- ☑
- tendon — *see* Disorder, tendon, specified type NEC
- testis N44.8
  - congenital Q55.29
- thymic, thymus (gland) (congenital) E32.0
- thyroid (gland) — *see* Goiter
- toe (congenital) Q74.2
  - acquired — *see also* Deformity, toe, specified NEC
- tongue K14.8
  - congenital Q38.2
  - papillae (foliate) K14.3
- tonsils (faucial) (infective) (lingual) (lymphoid) J35.1
  - with adenoids J35.3
- tunica vaginalis N50.89
- ureter N28.89
- urethra N36.8
- uterus N85.2
  - neck (with elongation) N88.4
  - puerperal O90.89
- uvula K13.79
- vagina N89.8
- vas deferens N50.89
- vein I87.8
- ventricle, ventricular (heart) — *see also* Hypertrophy, cardiac
  - congenital Q24.8
  - in tetralogy of Fallot Q21.3
- verumontanum N36.8
- vocal cord J38.3
- vulva N90.60
  - stasis (nonfilarial) N90.69

Hypertropia H50.2- ☑
Hypertyrosinemia E70.21
Hyperuricemia (asymptomatic) E79.0
Hyperuricosuria R82.993
Hypervalinemia E71.19
Hyperventilation (tetany) R06.4
- hysterical F45.8
- psychogenic F45.8
- syndrome F45.8

Hypervitaminosis (dietary) NEC E67.8
- A E67.0
  - administered as drug (prolonged intake) — *see* Table of Drugs and Chemicals, vitamins, adverse effect
  - overdose or wrong substance given or taken — *see* Table of Drugs and Chemicals, vitamins, poisoning
- B6 E67.2
- D E67.3

Hypervitaminosis — *continued*
- D — *continued*
  - administered as drug (prolonged intake) — *see* Table of Drugs and Chemicals, vitamins, adverse effect
  - overdose or wrong substance given or taken — *see* Table of Drugs and Chemicals, vitamins, poisoning
- K E67.8
  - administered as drug (prolonged intake) — *see* Table of Drugs and Chemicals, vitamins, adverse effect
  - overdose or wrong substance given or taken — *see* Table of Drugs and Chemicals, vitamins, poisoning

Hypervolemia E87.70
- specified NEC E87.79

Hypesthesia R20.1
- cornea — *see* Anesthesia, cornea

Hyphema H21.0- ☑
- traumatic S05.1- ☑

Hypoacidity, gastric K31.89
- psychogenic F45.8

Hypoadrenalism, hypoadrenia E27.40
- primary E27.1
- tuberculous A18.7

Hypoadrenocorticism E27.40
- pituitary E23.0
- primary E27.1

Hypoalbuminemia E88.09
Hypoaldosteronism E27.40
Hypoalphalipoproteinemia E78.6
Hypobarism T70.29 ☑
Hypobaropathy T70.29 ☑
Hypobetalipoproteinemia (familial) E78.6
Hypocalcemia E83.51
- autosomal dominant E20.810
  - type 1 (ADH1) E20.810
  - type 2 (ADH2) E20.810
- dietary E58
- neonatal P71.1
  - due to cow's milk P71.0
- phosphate-loading (newborn) P71.1

Hypochloremia E87.8
Hypochlorhydria K31.89
- neurotic F45.8
- psychogenic F45.8

Hypochondria, hypochondriac, hypochondriasis (reaction) F45.21
- sleep F51.03

Hypochondrogenesis Q77.0
Hypochondroplasia Q77.4
Hypochromasia, blood cells D50.8
Hypocitraturia R82.991
Hypodontia — *see* Anodontia
Hypoeosinophilia D72.89
Hypoesthesia R20.1
Hypofibrinogenemia D68.8
- acquired D65
- congenital (hereditary) D68.2

Hypofunction
- adrenocortical E27.40
  - drug-induced E27.3
  - postprocedural E89.6
  - primary E27.1
- adrenomedullary, postprocedural E89.6
- cerebral R29.818
- corticoadrenal NEC E27.40
- intestinal K59.89
- labyrinth — *see* subcategory H83.2 ☑
- ovary E28.39
- pituitary (gland) (anterior) E23.0
- testicular E29.1
  - postprocedural (postsurgical) (postirradiation) (iatrogenic) E89.5

Hypogalactia O92.4
Hypogammaglobulinemia — *see also* Agammaglobulinemia D80.1
- hereditary D80.0
- nonfamilial D80.1
- transient, of infancy D80.7

Hypogenitalism (congenital) — *see* Hypogonadism
Hypoglossia Q38.3
Hypoglycemia (spontaneous) E16.2
- coma E15
  - diabetic — *see* Diabetes, by type, with hypoglycemia, with coma
- diabetic — *see* Diabetes, hypoglycemia

Hypoglycemia — *continued*
- dietary counseling and surveillance Z71.3
- drug-induced E16.0
  - with coma (nondiabetic) E15
- due to insulin E16.0
  - with coma (nondiabetic) E15
  - therapeutic misadventure — *see* subcategory T38.3 ☑
- functional, nonhyperinsulinemic E16.1
- iatrogenic E16.0
  - with coma (nondiabetic) E15
- in infant of diabetic mother P70.1
  - gestational diabetes P70.0
- infantile E16.1
- leucine-induced E71.19
- level
  - 1 E16.A1
  - 2 E16.A2
  - 3 E16.A3
- neonatal (transitory) P70.4
  - iatrogenic P70.3
- reactive (not drug-induced) E16.1
- transitory neonatal P70.4

Hypogonadism
- female E28.39
- hypogonadotropic E23.0
- male E29.1
- ovarian (primary) E28.39
- pituitary E23.0
- testicular (primary) E29.1

Hypohidrosis, hypoidrosis L74.4
Hypoinsulinemia, postprocedural E89.1
Hypokalemia E87.6
Hypoleukocytosis — *see* Agranulocytosis
Hypolipoproteinemia (alpha) (beta) E78.6
Hypomagnesemia E83.42
- neonatal P71.2

Hypomania, hypomanic reaction F30.8
Hypomenorrhea — *see* Oligomenorrhea
Hypometabolism R63.8
Hypomotility
- gastrointestinal (tract) K31.89
  - psychogenic F45.8
- intestine K59.89
  - psychogenic F45.8
- stomach K31.89
  - psychogenic F45.8

Hypomyelination - hypogonadotropic hypogonadism - hypodontia G11.5
Hypomyelination with atrophy of the basal ganglia and cerebellum (H-ABC) G23.3
Hyponasality R49.22
Hyponatremia E87.1
Hypo-osmolality E87.1
Hypo-ovarianism, hypo-ovarism E28.39
Hypoparathyroidism E20.9
- autoimmune E20.812
- due to impaired parathyroid hormone secretion, unspecified E20.819
- familial E20.89
  - isolated E20.818
- idiopathic E20.0
- neonatal, transitory P71.4
- postprocedural E89.2
- secondary, in diseases classified elsewhere E20.811
- specified NEC E20.89
  - due to impaired parathyroid hormone secretion E20.818

Hypoperfusion (in)
- newborn P96.89

Hypopharyngitis — *see* Laryngopharyngitis
Hypophoria H50.53
Hypophosphatemia, hypophosphatasia (acquired) (congenital) (renal) E83.39
- familial E83.31

Hypophyseal, hypophysis — *see also* condition
- dwarfism E23.0
- gigantism E22.0

Hypopiesis — *see* Hypotension
Hypopinealism E34.8
Hypopituitarism (juvenile) E23.0
- drug-induced E23.1
- due to
  - hypophysectomy E89.3
  - radiotherapy E89.3
- iatrogenic NEC E23.1
- postirradiation E89.3
- postpartum O99.285
- postprocedural E89.3

☑ **Additional Character Required** — **Refer to the Tabular List for Character Selection**

Hypoplasia, hypoplastic
adrenal (gland), congenital Q89.1
alimentary tract, congenital Q45.8
  upper Q40.8
anus, anal (canal) Q42.3
  with fistula Q42.2
aorta, aortic Q25.42
  ascending, in hypoplastic left heart syndrome Q23.4
  valve Q23.1
    in hypoplastic left heart syndrome Q23.4
areola, congenital Q83.8
arm (congenital) — see Defect, reduction, upper limb
artery (peripheral) Q27.8
  brain (congenital) Q28.3
  coronary Q24.5
  digestive system Q27.8
  lower limb Q27.8
  pulmonary Q25.79
    functional, unilateral J43.0
  retinal (congenital) Q14.1
  specified site NEC Q27.8
  umbilical Q27.0
  upper limb Q27.8
auditory canal Q17.8
  causing impairment of hearing Q16.9
biliary duct or passage Q44.5
bone NOS Q79.9
  face Q75.8
  marrow D61.9
    megakaryocytic D69.49
  skull — see Hypoplasia, skull
brain Q02
  gyri Q04.3
  part of Q04.3
breast (areola) N64.82
bronchus Q32.4
cardiac Q24.8
carpus — see Defect, reduction, upper limb, specified
  type NEC
cartilage hair Q78.8
cecum Q42.8
cementum K00.4
cephalic Q02
cerebellum Q04.3
cervix (uteri), congenital Q51.821
clavicle (congenital) Q74.0
coccyx Q76.49
colon Q42.9
  specified NEC Q42.8
corpus callosum Q04.0
cricoid cartilage Q31.2
digestive organ(s) or tract NEC Q45.8
  upper (congenital) Q40.8
ear (auricle) (lobe) Q17.2
  middle Q16.4
enamel of teeth (neonatal) (postnatal) (prenatal) K00.4
endocrine (gland) NEC Q89.2
endometrium N85.8
epididymis (congenital) Q55.4
epiglottis Q31.2
erythroid, congenital D61.01
esophagus (congenital) Q39.8
eustachian tube Q17.8
eye Q11.2
eyelid (congenital) Q10.3
face Q18.8
  bone(s) Q75.8
femur (congenital) — see Defect, reduction, lower limb,
  specified type NEC
fibula (congenital) — see Defect, reduction, lower limb,
  specified type NEC
finger (congenital) — see Defect, reduction, upper limb,
  specified type NEC
focal dermal Q82.8
foot — see Defect, reduction, lower limb, specified type
  NEC
gallbladder Q44.0
genitalia, genital organ(s)
  female, congenital Q52.8
    external Q52.79
    internal NEC Q52.8
  in adiposogenital dystrophy E23.6
glottis Q31.2
hair Q84.2
hand (congenital) — see Defect, reduction, upper limb,
  specified type NEC
heart Q24.8
humerus (congenital) — see Defect, reduction, upper
  limb, specified type NEC

Hypoplasia, hypoplastic — continued
intestine (small) Q41.9
  large Q42.9
    specified NEC Q42.8
jaw M26.09
  alveolar M26.79
  lower M26.04
    alveolar M26.74
  upper M26.02
    alveolar M26.73
kidney(s) Q60.5
  bilateral Q60.4
  unilateral Q60.3
labium (majus) (minus), congenital Q52.79
larynx Q31.2
left heart syndrome Q23.4
leg (congenital) — see Defect, reduction, lower limb
limb Q73.8
  lower (congenital) — see Defect, reduction, lower
    limb
  upper (congenital) — see Defect, reduction, upper
    limb
liver Q44.79
lung (lobe) (not associated with short gestation) Q33.6
  associated with immaturity, low birth weight, prema-
    turity, or short gestation P28.0
mammary (areola), congenital Q83.8
mandible, mandibular M26.04
  alveolar M26.74
  unilateral condylar M27.8
maxillary M26.02
  alveolar M26.73
medullary D61.9
megakaryocytic D69.49
metacarpus — see Defect, reduction, upper limb, specified type NEC
metatarsus — see Defect, reduction, lower limb, specified
  type NEC
muscle Q79.8
nail(s) Q84.6
nose, nasal Q30.1
optic nerve H47.03- ☑
osseous meatus (ear) Q17.8
ovary, congenital Q50.39
pancreas Q45.0
parathyroid (gland) Q89.2
parotid gland Q38.4
patella Q74.1
pelvis, pelvic girdle Q74.2
penis (congenital) Q55.62
peripheral vascular system Q27.8
  digestive system Q27.8
  lower limb Q27.8
  specified site NEC Q27.8
  upper limb Q27.8
pituitary (gland) (congenital) Q89.2
pulmonary (not associated with short gestation) Q33.6
  artery, functional J43.0
  associated with short gestation P28.0
radioulnar — see Defect, reduction, upper limb, specified
  type NEC
radius — see Defect, reduction, upper limb
rectum Q42.1
  with fistula Q42.0
respiratory system NEC Q34.8
rib Q76.6
right heart syndrome Q22.6
sacrum Q76.49
scapula Q74.0
scrotum Q55.1
shoulder girdle Q74.0
skin Q82.8
skull (bone) Q75.8
  with
    anencephaly Q00.0
    encephalocele — see Encephalocele
    hydrocephalus Q03.9
      with spina bifida — see Spina bifida, by site,
        with hydrocephalus
    microcephaly Q02
spinal (cord) (ventral horn cell) Q06.1
spine Q76.49
sternum Q76.7
tarsus — see Defect, reduction, lower limb, specified type
  NEC
testis Q55.1
thymic, with immunodeficiency D82.1
thymus (gland) Q89.2
  with immunodeficiency D82.1

Hypoplasia, hypoplastic — continued
thyroid (gland) E03.1
  cartilage Q31.2
tibiofibular (congenital) — see Defect, reduction, lower
  limb, specified type NEC
toe — see Defect, reduction, lower limb, specified type
  NEC
tongue Q38.3
Turner's K00.4
ulna (congenital) — see Defect, reduction, upper limb
umbilical artery Q27.0
unilateral condylar M27.8
ureter Q62.8
uterus, congenital Q51.811
vagina Q52.4
vascular NEC peripheral Q27.8
  brain Q28.3
  digestive system Q27.8
  lower limb Q27.8
  specified site NEC Q27.8
  upper limb Q27.8
vein(s) (peripheral) Q27.8
  brain Q28.3
  digestive system Q27.8
  great Q26.8
  lower limb Q27.8
  specified site NEC Q27.8
  upper limb Q27.8
vena cava (inferior) (superior) Q26.8
vertebra Q76.49
vulva, congenital Q52.79
zonule (ciliary) Q12.8
Hypoplasminogenemia E88.02
Hypopnea, obstructive sleep apnea G47.33
Hypopotassemia E87.6
Hypoproconvertinemia, congenital (hereditary) D68.2
Hypoproteinemia E77.8
Hypoprothrombinemia (congenital) (hereditary) (idiopathic) D68.2
  acquired D68.4
  newborn, transient P61.6
Hypoptyalism K11.7
Hypopyon (eye) (anterior chamber) — see Iridocyclitis,
  acute, hypopyon
Hypopyrexia R68.0
Hyporeflexia R29.2
Hyposecretion
  ACTH E23.0
  antidiuretic hormone E23.2
  ovary E28.39
  salivary gland (any) K11.7
  vasopressin E23.2
Hyposegmentation, leukocytic, hereditary D72.0
Hyposiderinemia D50.9
Hypospadias Q54.9
  balanic Q54.0
  coronal Q54.0
  glandular Q54.0
  penile Q54.1
  penoscrotal Q54.2
  perineal Q54.3
  specified NEC Q54.8
Hypospermatogenesis — see Oligospermia
Hyposplenism D73.0
Hypostasis pulmonary, passive — see Edema, lung
Hypostatic — see condition
Hyposthenuria N28.89
Hypotension (arterial) (constitutional) I95.9
  chronic I95.89
  due to (of) hemodialysis I95.3
  drug-induced I95.2
  iatrogenic I95.89
  idiopathic (permanent) I95.0
  intracranial G96.810
    following
      lumbar cerebrospinal fluid shunting G97.83
      specified procedure NEC G97.84
      ventricular shunting (ventriculostomy) G97.2
    specified NEC G96.819
    spontaneous G96.811
  intra-dialytic I95.3
  maternal, syndrome (following labor and delivery)
    O26.5- ☑
  neurogenic, orthostatic G90.3
  orthostatic (chronic) I95.1
    due to drugs I95.2
    neurogenic G90.3
  postoperative I95.81
  postural I95.1

☑ **Additional Character Required — Refer to the Tabular List for Character Selection**

Hypotension — continued
  specified NEC I95.89
Hypothermia (accidental) T68 ☑
  due to anesthesia, anesthetic T88.51 ☑
  low environmental temperature T68 ☑
  neonatal P80.9
    environmental (mild) NEC P80.8
    mild P80.8
    severe (chronic) (cold injury syndrome) P80.0
    specified NEC P80.8
  not associated with low environmental temperature
    R68.0
Hypothyroidism (acquired) E03.9
  autoimmune — see Thyroiditis, autoimmune
  congenital (without goiter) E03.1
    with goiter (diffuse) E03.0
  due to
    exogenous substance NEC E03.2
    iodine-deficiency, acquired E01.8
      subclinical E02
    irradiation therapy E89.0
    medicament NEC E03.2
    P-aminosalicylic acid (PAS) E03.2
    phenylbutazone E03.2
    resorcinol E03.2
    sulfonamide E03.2
    surgery E89.0
    thiourea group drugs E03.2
  iatrogenic NEC E03.2
  iodine-deficiency (acquired) E01.8
    congenital — see Syndrome, iodine- deficiency, con-
      genital
    subclinical E02
  neonatal, transitory P72.2
  postinfectious E03.3
  postirradiation E89.0
  postprocedural E89.0
  postsurgical E89.0
  specified NEC E03.8
  subclinical, iodine-deficiency related E02
Hypotonia, hypotonicity, hypotony
  bladder N31.2
  congenital (benign) P94.2
  eye — see Disorder, globe, hypotony
Hypotrichosis — see Alopecia
Hypotropia H50.2- ☑
Hypoventilation R06.89
  congenital central alveolar G47.35
  sleep related
    idiopathic nonobstructive alveolar G47.34
    in conditions classified elsewhere G47.36
Hypovitaminosis — see Deficiency, vitamin
Hypovolemia E86.1
  surgical shock T81.19 ☑
  traumatic (shock) T79.4 ☑
Hypoxemia R09.02
  newborn P84
  sleep related, in conditions classified elsewhere G47.36
Hypoxia — see also Anoxia R09.02
  cerebral, during a procedure NEC G97.81
    postprocedural NEC G97.82
  intrauterine P84
  myocardial — see Insufficiency, coronary
  newborn P84
  sleep-related G47.34
Hypsarrhythmia — see Epilepsy, generalized, specified
  NEC
Hysteralgia, pregnant uterus O26.89- ☑
Hysteria, hysterical (conversion) (dissociative state) F44.9
  anxiety F41.8
  convulsions F44.5
  psychosis, acute F44.9
Hysteroepilepsy F44.5

I

IBDU (colonic inflammatory bowel dissease unclassified)
  K52.3
ICANS (immune effector cell-associated neurotoxicity syndrome) — see Syndrome, immune effector cell-associated neurotoxicity
Ichthyoparasitism due to Vandellia cirrhosa B88.8
Ichthyosis (congenital) Q80.9
  acquired L85.0
  fetalis Q80.4
  hystrix Q80.8
  lamellar Q80.2
  lingual K13.29

Ichthyosis — continued
  palmaris and plantaris Q82.8
  simplex Q80.0
  vera Q80.8
  vulgaris Q80.0
  X-linked Q80.1
Ichthyotoxism — see Poisoning, fish
  bacterial — see Intoxication, foodborne
Icteroanemia, hemolytic (acquired) D59.9
  congenital — see Spherocytosis
Icterus — see also Jaundice
  conjunctiva R17
  gravis, newborn P55.0
  hematogenous (acquired) D59.9
  hemolytic (acquired) D59.9
    congenital — see Spherocytosis
  hemorrhagic (acute) (leptospiral) (spirochetal) A27.0
    newborn P53
  infectious B15.9
    with hepatic coma B15.0
    leptospiral A27.0
    spirochetal A27.0
  neonatorum — see Jaundice, newborn
  newborn P59.9
  spirochetal A27.0
Ictus solaris, solis T67.01 ☑
Id reaction (due to bacteria) L30.2
Ideation
  homicidal R45.850
  suicidal R45.851
Identity disorder (child) F64.9
  gender role F64.2
  psychosexual F64.2
Idioglossia F80.0
Idiopathic — see condition
Idiot, idiocy (congenital) F73
  amaurotic (Bielschowsky(-Jansky)) (family) (infantile
    (late)) (juvenile (late)) (Vogt-Spielmeyer) E75.4
  microcephalic Q02
IgE asthma J45.909
IIAC (idiopathic infantile arterial calcification) Q28.8
Ileitis (chronic) (noninfectious) — see also Enteritis K52.9
  backwash — see Pancolitis, ulcerative (chronic)
  infectious A09
  regional (ulcerative) — see Enteritis, regional, small intes-
    tine
  segmental — see Enteritis, regional
  terminal (ulcerative) — see Enteritis, regional, small in-
    testine
Ileocolitis — see also Enteritis K52.9
  infectious A09
  regional — see Enteritis, regional
  ulcerative K51.0- ☑
Ileostomy
  attention to Z43.2
  malfunctioning K94.13
  status (ileal pouch) (Kock pouch) Z93.2
    with complication — see Complications, enterostomy
Ileotyphus — see Typhoid
Ileum — see condition
Ileus (bowel) (colon) (inhibitory) (intestine) K56.7
  adynamic K56.0
  due to gallstone (in intestine) K56.3
  duodenal (chronic) K31.5
  gallstone K56.3
  mechanical NEC — see also Obstruction, intestine, spec-
    ified NEC K56.699
  meconium P76.0
    in cystic fibrosis E84.11
    meaning meconium plug (without cystic fibrosis)
      P76.0
  myxedema K59.89
  neurogenic K56.0
    Hirschsprung's disease or megacolon Q43.1
  newborn
    due to meconium P76.0
      in cystic fibrosis E84.11
      meaning meconium plug (without cystic fibrosis)
        P76.0
    transitory P76.1
  obstructive — see also Obstruction, intestine, specified
    NEC K56.699
  paralytic K56.0
  postoperative K91.89
Iliac — see condition
Iliotibial band syndrome M76.3- ☑
Illiteracy Z55.0
  health Z55.6
Illness — see also Disease R69

Illness — continued
  manic-depressive — see Disorder, bipolar
Imbalance R26.89
  autonomic G90.89
  constituents of food intake E63.1
  electrolyte E87.8
    with
      abortion — see Abortion by type, complicated by,
        electrolyte imbalance
      molar pregnancy O08.5
    due to hyperemesis gravidarum O21.1
    following ectopic or molar pregnancy O08.5
    neonatal, transitory NEC P74.49
      potassium
        hyperkalemia P74.31
        hypokalemia P74.32
      sodium
        hypernatremia P74.21
        hyponatremia P74.22
  endocrine E34.9
  eye muscle NOS H50.9
  hormone E34.9
  hysterical F44.4
  labyrinth — see subcategory H83.2 ☑
  posture R29.3
  protein-energy — see Malnutrition
  sympathetic G90.89
Imbecile, imbecility (I.Q. 35-49) F71
Imbedding, intrauterine device T83.39 ☑
Imbibition, cholesterol (gallbladder) K82.4
Imbrication, teeth,, fully erupted M26.30
Imerslund (-Gräsbeck) **syndrome** D51.1
Immature — see also Immaturity
  birth (less than 37 completed weeks) — see Preterm,
    newborn
    extremely (less than 28 completed weeks) — see Im-
      maturity, extreme
  personality F60.89
Immaturity (less than 37 completed weeks) — see also
  Preterm, newborn
  extreme of newborn (less than 28 completed weeks of
    gestation) (less than 196 completed days of gesta-
    tion) (unspecified weeks of gestation) P07.20
    gestational age
      23 completed weeks (23 weeks, 0 days through
        23 weeks, 6 days) P07.22
      24 completed weeks (24 weeks, 0 days through
        24 weeks, 6 days) P07.23
      25 completed weeks (25 weeks, 0 days through
        25 weeks, 6 days) P07.24
      26 completed weeks (26 weeks, 0 days through
        26 weeks, 6 days) P07.25
      27 completed weeks (27 weeks, 0 days through
        27 weeks, 6 days) P07.26
      less than 23 completed weeks P07.21
  fetus or infant light-for-dates — see Light-for-dates
  lung, newborn P28.0
  organ or site NEC — see Hypoplasia
  pulmonary, newborn P28.0
  reaction F60.89
  sexual (female) (male), after puberty E30.0
Immersion T75.1 ☑
  foot T69.02- ☑
  hand T69.01- ☑
Immobile, immobility
  complete, due to severe physical disability or frailty R53.2
  intestine K59.89
  syndrome (paraplegic) M62.3
Immune reconstitution (inflammatory) syndrome [IRIS]
  D89.3
Immunization — see also Vaccination
  ABO — see Incompatibility, ABO
    in newborn P55.1
  appropriate for age
    child (over 28 days old) Z00.129
      with abnormal findings Z00.121
  complication — see Complications, vaccination
  encounter for Z23
  not done (not carried out) — see also Underimmunization
    status Z28.9
    because (of)
      acute illness of patient Z28.01
      allergy to vaccine (or component) Z28.04
      caregiver refusal Z28.82
      chronic illness of patient Z28.02
      contraindication NEC Z28.09
      delay in delivery of vaccine Z28.83
      group pressure Z28.1

Immunization — *continued*
  not done — *see also* Underimmunization status — *continued*
    because — *continued*
      guardian refusal Z28.82
      immune compromised state of patient Z28.03
      lack of availability of vaccine Z28.83
      manufacturer delay of vaccine Z28.83
      parent refusal Z28.82
      patient had disease being vaccinated against Z28.81
      patient refusal Z28.21
      patient's belief Z28.1
      religious beliefs of patient Z28.1
      specified reason NEC Z28.89
        of patient Z28.29
      unavailability of vaccine Z28.83
      unspecified patient reason Z28.20
  partial — *see also* Underimmunization status
    for COVID-19 Z28.311
  Rh factor
    affecting management of pregnancy NEC O36.09- ☑
    anti-D antibody O36.01- ☑
    from transfusion — *see* Complication(s), transfusion, incompatibility reaction, Rh (factor)
Immunocompromised NOS D84.9
Immunocytoma C83.0- ☑
Immunodeficiency D84.9
  with
    adenosine-deaminase deficiency — *see also* Deficiency, adenosine deaminase D81.30
    antibody defects D80.9
      specified type NEC D80.8
    hyperimmunoglobulinemia D80.6
    increased immunoglobulin M (IgM) D80.5
    major defect D82.9
      specified type NEC D82.8
    partial albinism D82.8
    short-limbed stature D82.2
    thrombocytopenia and eczema D82.0
  antibody with
    hyperimmunoglobulinemia D80.6
    near-normal immunoglobulins D80.6
  autosomal recessive, Swiss type D80.0
  combined D81.9
    biotin-dependent carboxylase D81.819
      biotinidase D81.810
      holocarboxylase synthetase D81.818
      specified type NEC D81.818
    severe (SCID) D81.9
      with
        low or normal B-cell numbers D81.2
        low T- and B-cell numbers D81.1
        reticular dysgenesis D81.0
    specified type NEC D81.89
  common variable D83.9
    with
      abnormalities of B-cell numbers and function D83.0
      autoantibodies to B- or T-cells D83.2
      immunoregulatory T-cell disorders D83.1
    specified type NEC D83.8
  due to
    conditions classified elsewhere D84.81
    drugs D84.821
    external causes D84.822
    medication (current or past) D84.821
  following hereditary defective response to Epstein-Barr virus (EBV) D82.3
  selective, immunoglobulin
    A (IgA) D80.2
    G (IgG) (subclasses) D80.3
    M (IgM) D80.4
  severe combined (SCID) D81.9
    due to adenosine deaminase deficiency D81.31
  specified type NEC D84.89
  X-linked, with increased IgM D80.5
Immunodeficient NOS D84.9
Immunosuppressed NOS D84.9
Immunotherapy (encounter for)
  antineoplastic Z51.12
Impaction, impacted
  bowel, colon, rectum — *see also* Impaction, fecal K56.49
    by gallstone K56.3
  calculus — *see* Calculus
  cerumen (ear) (external) H61.2- ☑
  cuspid — *see* Impaction, tooth
  dental (same or adjacent tooth) K01.1
  fecal, feces K56.41

Impaction, impacted — *continued*
  fracture — *see* Fracture, by site
  gallbladder — *see* Calculus, gallbladder
  gallstone(s) — *see* Calculus, gallbladder
    bile duct (common) (hepatic) — *see* Calculus, bile duct
    cystic duct — *see* Calculus, gallbladder
    in intestine, with obstruction (any part) K56.3
  intestine (calculous) NEC — *see also* Impaction, fecal K56.49
    gallstone, with ileus K56.3
  intrauterine device (IUD) T83.39 ☑
  molar — *see* Impaction, tooth
  shoulder, causing obstructed labor O66.0
  tooth, teeth K01.1
  turbinate J34.89
Impaired, impairment (function)
  auditory discrimination — *see* Abnormal, auditory perception
  cognitive, mild, of uncertain or unknown etiology G31.84
  dual sensory Z73.82
  fasting glucose R73.01
  glucose tolerance (oral) R73.02
  hearing — *see* Deafness
  heart — *see* Disease, heart
  kidney N28.9
    disorder resulting from N25.9
      specified NEC N25.89
  liver K72.90
    with coma K72.91
  mastication K08.89
  mild cognitive G31.84
    of uncertain or unknown etiology G31.84
  mild neurocognitive
    due to known physiological condition (without behavioral disturbance) F06.70
      with behavioral disturbance F06.71
  mobility
    ear ossicles — *see* Ankylosis, ear ossicles
    requiring care provider Z74.09
  myocardium, myocardial — *see* Insufficiency, myocardial
  rectal sphincter R19.8
  renal (acute) (chronic) N28.9
    disorder resulting from N25.9
      specified NEC N25.89
  vision NEC H54.7
    both eyes H54.3
Impediment, speech — *see also* Disorder, speech R47.9
  psychogenic (childhood) F98.8
  slurring R47.81
  specified NEC R47.89
Impending
  coronary syndrome I20.0
  delirium tremens F10.239
  myocardial infarction I20.0
Imperception auditory (acquired) — *see also* Deafness
  congenital H93.25
Imperfect
  aeration, lung (newborn) NEC — *see* Atelectasis
  closure (congenital)
    alimentary tract NEC Q45.8
      lower Q43.8
      upper Q40.8
    atrioventricular ostium Q21.20
    atrium (secundum) Q21.11
    branchial cleft NOS Q18.2
      cyst Q18.0
      fistula Q18.0
      sinus Q18.0
    choroid Q14.3
    cricoid cartilage Q31.8
    cusps, heart valve NEC Q24.8
      pulmonary Q22.3
    ductus
      arteriosus Q25.0
      Botalli Q25.0
    ear drum (causing impairment of hearing) Q16.4
    esophagus with communication to bronchus or trachea Q39.1
    eyelid Q10.3
    foramen
      botalli Q21.12
      ovale Q21.12
    genitalia, genital organ(s) or system
      female Q52.8
        external Q52.79
        internal NEC Q52.8
      male Q55.8
    glottis Q31.8

Imperfect — *continued*
  closure — *continued*
    interatrial ostium or septum Q21.19
    interauricular ostium or septum Q21.19
    interventricular ostium or septum Q21.0
    larynx Q31.8
    lip — *see* Cleft, lip
    nasal septum Q30.3
    nose Q30.2
    omphalomesenteric duct Q43.0
    optic nerve entry Q14.2
    organ or site not listed — *see* Anomaly, by site
    ostium
      interatrial Q21.19
      interauricular Q21.19
      interventricular Q21.0
    palate — *see* Cleft, palate
    preauricular sinus Q18.1
    retina Q14.1
    roof of orbit Q75.8
    sclera Q13.5
    septum
      aorticopulmonary Q21.4
      atrial (secundum) Q21.19
      between aorta and pulmonary artery Q21.4
      heart Q21.9
      interatrial (secundum) Q21.19
      interauricular (secundum) Q21.19
      interventricular Q21.0
        in tetralogy of Fallot Q21.3
      nasal Q30.3
      ventricular Q21.0
        with pulmonary stenosis or atresia, dextraposition of aorta, and hypertrophy of right ventricle Q21.3
        in tetralogy of Fallot Q21.3
    skull Q75.009
      with
        anencephaly Q00.0
        encephalocele — *see* Encephalocele
        hydrocephalus Q03.9
          with spina bifida — *see* Spina bifida, by site, with hydrocephalus
        microcephaly Q02
    spine (with meningocele) — *see* Spina bifida
    trachea Q32.1
    tympanic membrane (causing impairment of hearing) Q16.4
    uterus Q51.818
    vitelline duct Q43.0
  erection — *see* Dysfunction, sexual, male, erectile
  fusion — *see* Imperfect, closure
  inflation, lung (newborn) — *see* Atelectasis
  posture R29.3
  rotation, intestine Q43.3
  septum, ventricular Q21.0
Imperfectly descended testis — *see* Cryptorchid
Imperforate (congenital) — *see also* Atresia
  anus Q42.3
    with fistula Q42.2
  cervix (uteri) Q51.828
  esophagus Q39.0
    with tracheoesophageal fistula Q39.1
  hymen Q52.3
  jejunum Q41.1
  pharynx Q38.8
  rectum Q42.1
    with fistula Q42.0
  urethra Q64.39
  vagina Q52.4
Impervious (congenital) — *see also* Atresia
  anus Q42.3
    with fistula Q42.2
  bile duct Q44.2
  esophagus Q39.0
    with tracheoesophageal fistula Q39.1
  intestine (small) Q41.9
    large Q42.9
      specified NEC Q42.8
  rectum Q42.1
    with fistula Q42.0
  ureter — *see* Atresia, ureter
  urethra Q64.39
Impetiginization of dermatoses L01.1
Impetigo (any organism) (any site) (circinate) (contagiosa) (simplex) (vulgaris) L01.00
  Bockhart's L01.02
  bullous, bullosa L01.03
  external ear L01.00 [H62.40]

Impetigo — continued
  follicularis L01.02
  furfuracea L30.5
  herpetiformis L40.1
    nonobstetrical L40.1
  neonatorum L01.03
  nonbullous L01.01
  specified type NEC L01.09
  ulcerative L01.09
Impingement (on teeth)
  joint — see Disorder, joint, specified type NEC
  soft tissue
    anterior M26.81
    posterior M26.82
Implant, endometrial N80.9
Implantation
  anomalous — see Anomaly, by site
    ureter Q62.63
  cyst
    external area or site (skin) NEC L72.0
    iris — see Cyst, iris, implantation
    vagina N89.8
    vulva N90.7
  dermoid (cyst) — see Implantation, cyst
Impotence (sexual) N52.9
  counseling Z70.1
  organic origin — see also Dysfunction, sexual, male,
      erectile N52.9
  psychogenic F52.21
Impression, basilar Q75.8
Imprisonment, anxiety concerning Z65.1
Improper care (child) (newborn) — see Maltreatment
Improperly tied umbilical cord (causing hemorrhage)
    P51.8
Impulsiveness (impulsive) R45.87
Inability to
  comply with dietary regimen Z91.118
  swallow — see Aphagia
Inaccessible, inaccessibility
  health care NEC Z75.3
    due to
      waiting period Z75.2
        for admission to facility elsewhere Z75.1
  other helping agencies Z75.4
  transportation Z59.82
Inactive — see condition
Inadequate, inadequacy
  aesthetics of dental restoration K08.56
  biologic, constitutional, functional, or social F60.7
  development
    child R62.50
    genitalia
      after puberty NEC E30.0
      congenital
        female Q52.8
          external Q52.79
          internal Q52.8
        male Q55.8
    lungs Q33.6
      associated with short gestation P28.0
    organ or site not listed — see Anomaly, by site
  diet (causing nutritional deficiency) E63.9
  drinking-water supply Z58.6
  eating habits Z72.4
  environment, household Z59.11
  family support Z63.8
  food (supply) NEC Z59.48
    hunger effects T73.0 ☑
  functional F60.7
  household care, due to
    family member
      handicapped or ill Z74.2
      on vacation Z75.5
      temporarily away from home Z74.2
    technical defects in home Z59.19
    temporary absence from home of person rendering
        care Z74.2
  housing Z59.10
    environmental temperature Z59.11
    heating Z59.11
    space Z59.19
    specified NEC Z59.19
    utilities Z59.12
  income (financial) Z59.6
  intrafamilial communication Z63.8
  material resources due to limited financial resources,
      specified NEC Z59.87
  mental — see Disability, intellectual
  parental supervision or control of child Z62.0

Inadequate, inadequacy — continued
  personality F60.7
  pulmonary
    function R06.89
      newborn P28.5
    ventilation, newborn P28.5
  sample of cytologic smear
    anus R85.615
    cervix R87.615
    vagina R87.625
  social F60.7
    insurance Z59.71
    skills NEC Z73.4
    social support Z60.8
  supervision of child by parent Z62.0
  teaching affecting education Z55.8
  transportation Z59.82
  welfare support Z59.72
Inanition R64
  with edema — see Malnutrition, severe
  due to
    deprivation of food T73.0 ☑
    malnutrition — see Malnutrition
  fever R50.9
Inappropriate
  change in quantitative human chorionic gonadotropin
      (hCG) in early pregnancy O02.81
  diet or eating habits Z72.4
  level of quantitative human chorionic gonadotropin
      (hCG) for gestational age in early pregnancy
      O02.81
  secretion
    antidiuretic hormone (ADH) (excessive) E22.2
      deficiency E23.2
    pituitary (posterior) E22.2
  sinus tachycardia, so stated (IST) I47.11
Inattention at or after birth — see Neglect
Incarceration, incarcerated
  enterocele K46.0
    gangrenous K46.1
  epiplocele K46.0
    gangrenous K46.1
  exomphalos K42.0
    gangrenous K42.1
  hernia — see also Hernia, by site, with obstruction
    with gangrene — see Hernia, by site, with gangrene
  iris, in wound — see Injury, eye, laceration, with prolapse
  lens, in wound — see Injury, eye, laceration, with prolapse
  omphalocele K42.0
  prison, anxiety concerning Z65.1
  rupture — see Hernia, by site
  sarcoepiplocele K46.0
    gangrenous K46.1
  sarcoepiplomphalocele K42.0
    with gangrene K42.1
  uterus N85.8
    gravid O34.51- ☑
      causing obstructed labor O65.5
Incised wound
  external — see Laceration
  internal organs — see Injury, by site
Incision, incisional
  hernia K43.2
    with
      gangrene (and obstruction) K43.1
      obstruction K43.0
  surgical, complication — see Complications, surgical
      procedure
  traumatic
    external — see Laceration
    internal organs — see Injury, by site
Inclusion
  azurophilic leukocytic D72.0
  blennorrhea (neonatal) (newborn) P39.1
  gallbladder in liver (congenital) Q44.1
Incompatibility
  ABO
    affecting management of pregnancy O36.11- ☑
      anti-A sensitization O36.11- ☑
      anti-B sensitization O36.19- ☑
      specified NEC O36.19- ☑
    infusion or transfusion reaction — see Complication(s), transfusion, incompatibility reaction, ABO
    newborn P55.1
  blood (group) (Duffy) (K) (Kell) (Kidd) (Lewis) (M) (S) NEC
    affecting management of pregnancy O36.11- ☑

Incompatibility — continued
  blood (S) — continued
    affecting management of pregnancy — continued
      anti-A sensitization O36.11- ☑
      anti-B sensitization O36.19- ☑
    infusion or transfusion reaction T80.89 ☑
    newborn P55.8
  divorce or estrangement Z63.5
  Rh (blood group) (factor) Z31.82
    affecting management of pregnancy NEC O36.09- ☑
      anti-D antibody O36.01- ☑
    infusion or transfusion reaction — see Complication(s), transfusion, incompatibility reaction, Rh (factor)
    newborn P55.0
  rhesus — see Incompatibility, Rh
Incompetency, incompetent, incompetence
  annular
    aortic (valve) — see Insufficiency, aortic
    mitral (valve) I34.0
    pulmonary valve (heart) I37.1
  aortic (valve) — see Insufficiency, aortic
  cardiac valve — see Endocarditis
  cervix, cervical (os) N88.3
    in pregnancy O34.3- ☑
  chronotropic I45.89
    with
      autonomic dysfunction G90.89
      ischemic heart disease I25.89
      left ventricular dysfunction I51.89
      sinus node dysfunction I49.8
  esophagogastric (junction) (sphincter) K22.0
  mitral (valve) — see Insufficiency, mitral
  pelvic fundus N81.89
  pubocervical tissue N81.82
  pulmonary valve (heart) I37.1
    congenital Q22.3
  rectovaginal tissue N81.83
  tricuspid (annular) (valve) — see Insufficiency, tricuspid
  valvular — see Endocarditis
    congenital Q24.8
  vein, venous (saphenous) (varicose) — see Varix, leg
Incomplete — see also condition
  atrioventricular
    canal Q21.21
    septal defect Q21.21
  bladder, emptying R33.9
  defecation R15.0
  endocardial cushion defect Q21.21
  expansion lungs (newborn) NEC — see Atelectasis
  rotation, intestine Q43.3
Inconclusive
  diagnostic imaging due to excess body fat of patient
      R93.9
  findings on diagnostic imaging of breast NEC R92.8
  mammogram R92.2
Incontinence R32
  anal sphincter R15.9
  coital N39.491
  feces R15.9
    nonorganic origin F98.1
  insensible (urinary) N39.42
  overflow N39.490
  postural (urinary) N39.492
  psychogenic F45.8
  rectal R15.9
  reflex N39.498
  stress (female) (male) N39.3
    and urge N39.46
  urethral sphincter R32
  urge N39.41
    and stress (female) (male) N39.46
  urine (urinary) R32
    continuous N39.45
    due to cognitive impairment, or severe physical disability or immobility R39.81
    functional R39.81
    insensible N39.42
    mixed (stress and urge) N39.46
    nocturnal N39.44
    nonorganic origin F98.0
    overflow N39.490
    post dribbling N39.43
    postural N39.492
    reflex N39.498
    specified NEC N39.498
    stress (female) (male) N39.3
      and urge N39.46

Incontinence — *continued*
  urine — *continued*
    total N39.498
    unaware N39.42
    urge N39.41
      and stress (female) (male) N39.46
Incontinentia pigmenti Q82.3
Incoordinate, incoordination
  esophageal-pharyngeal (newborn) — *see* Dysphagia
  muscular R27.8
  uterus (action) (contractions) (complicating delivery)
    O62.4
Increase, increased
  abnormal, in development R63.8
  androgens (ovarian) E28.1
  anticoagulants (antithrombin) (anti-VIIIa) (anti-IXa) (anti-
    Xa) (anti-XIa) — *see* Circulating anticoagulants
  cold sense R20.8
  estrogen E28.0
  function
    adrenal
      cortex — *see* Cushing's, syndrome
      medulla E27.5
    pituitary (gland) (anterior) (lobe) E22.9
      posterior E22.2
  heat sense R20.8
  intracranial pressure (benign) G93.2
  permeability, capillaries I78.8
  pressure, intracranial G93.2
  secretion
    gastrin E16.4
    glucagon E16.3
    pancreas, endocrine E16.9
      growth hormone-releasing hormone E16.8
      pancreatic polypeptide E16.8
      somatostatin E16.8
      vasoactive-intestinal polypeptide E16.8
  sphericity, lens Q12.4
  splenic activity D73.1
  venous pressure I87.8
    portal K76.6
Increta placenta O43.22- ☑
Incrustation, cornea, foreign body (lead)(zinc) — *see*
  Foreign body, cornea
Incyclophoria H50.54
Incyclotropia — *see* Cyclotropia
Indeterminate sex Q56.4
India rubber skin Q82.8
Indigestion (acid) (bilious) (functional) K30
  catarrhal K31.89
  due to decomposed food NOS A05.9
  nervous F45.8
  psychogenic F45.8
Indirect — *see* condition
Induratio penis plastica N48.6
Induration, indurated
  brain G93.89
  breast (fibrous) N64.51
    puerperal, postpartum O92.29
  broad ligament N83.8
  chancre
    anus A51.1
    congenital A50.07
    extragenital NEC A51.2
  corpora cavernosa (penis) (plastic) N48.6
  liver (chronic) K76.89
  lung (black) (chronic) (fibroid) — *see also* Fibrosis, lung
    J84.10
    essential brown J84.03
  penile (plastic) N48.6
  phlebitic — *see* Phlebitis
  skin R23.4
Inebriety (without dependence) — *see* Alcohol, intoxication
Inefficiency, kidney N28.9
Inelasticity, skin R23.4
Inequality, leg (length) (acquired) — *see also* Deformity,
  limb, unequal length
  congenital — *see* Defect, reduction, lower limb
  lower leg — *see* Deformity, limb, unequal length
Inertia
  bladder (neurogenic) N31.2
  stomach K31.89
    psychogenic F45.8
  uterus, uterine during labor O62.2
    during latent phase of labor O62.0
    primary O62.0
    secondary O62.1
  vesical (neurogenic) N31.2
Infancy, infantile, infantilism — *see also* condition

Infancy, infantile, infantilism — *continued*
  celiac K90.0
  genitalia, genitals (after puberty) E30.0
  Herter's (nontropical sprue) K90.0
  intestinal K90.0
  Lorain E23.0
  pancreatic K86.89
  pelvis M95.5
    with disproportion (fetopelvic) O33.1
      causing obstructed labor O65.1
  pituitary E23.0
  renal N25.0
  uterus — *see* Infantile, genitalia
Infant(s) — *see also* Infancy
  excessive crying R68.11
  irritable child R68.12
  lack of care — *see* Neglect
  liveborn (singleton) Z38.2
    born in hospital Z38.00
      by cesarean Z38.01
    born outside hospital Z38.1
    multiple NEC Z38.8
      born in hospital Z38.68
        by cesarean Z38.69
      born outside hospital Z38.7
    quadruplet Z38.8
      born in hospital Z38.63
        by cesarean Z38.64
      born outside hospital Z38.7
    quintuplet Z38.8
      born in hospital Z38.65
        by cesarean Z38.66
      born outside hospital Z38.7
    triplet Z38.8
      born in hospital Z38.61
        by cesarean Z38.62
      born outside hospital Z38.7
    twin Z38.5
      born in hospital Z38.30
        by cesarean Z38.31
      born outside hospital Z38.4
  of diabetic mother (syndrome of) P70.1
    gestational diabetes P70.0
Infantile — *see also* condition
  genitalia, genitals E30.0
  os, uterine E30.0
  penis E30.0
  testis E29.1
  uterus E30.0
Infantilism — *see* Infancy
Infarct, infarction
  adrenal (capsule) (gland) E27.49
  appendices epiploicae — *see also* Infarct, intestine
    K55.069
  bowel — *see also* Infarct, intestine K55.069
  brain (stem) — *see* Infarct, cerebral
  breast N64.89
  brewer's (kidney) N28.0
  cardiac — *see* Infarct, myocardium
  cerebellar — *see* Infarct, cerebral
  cerebral (acute) — *see also* Occlusion, artery cerebral or
    precerebral, with infarction I63.9-
    aborted I63.9
    chronic (imaging) (old) (remote) (without sequelae)
      Z86.73
      with residual defects — *see* Sequelae, disease,
        cerebrovascular
    cortical I63.9
    due to
      cerebral venous thrombosis, nonpyogenic I63.6
      embolism
        cerebral arteries I63.4- ☑
        precerebral arteries I63.1- ☑
      occlusion NEC
        cerebral arteries I63.5- ☑
        precerebral arteries I63.2- ☑
        small artery I63.81
      stenosis NEC
        cerebral arteries I63.5- ☑
        precerebral arteries I63.2- ☑
        small artery I63.81
      thrombosis
        cerebral artery I63.3- ☑
        precerebral artery I63.0- ☑
    intraoperative
      during cardiac surgery I97.810
      during other surgery I97.811
    neonatal P91.82- ☑

Infarct, infarction — *continued*
  cerebral — *see also* Occlusion, artery cerebral or precere-
    bral, with infarction — *continued*
    perinatal (arterial ischemic) P91.82- ☑
    postprocedural
      following cardiac surgery I97.820
      following other surgery I97.821
    specified NEC I63.89
  colon (acute) (agnogenic) (embolic) (hemorrhagic)
    (nonocclusive) (nonthrombotic) (occlusive) (seg-
    mental) (thrombotic) (with gangrene) — *see also*
    Infarct, intestine K55.049
  coronary artery — *see* Infarct, myocardium
  embolic — *see* Embolism
  fallopian tube N83.8
  gallbladder K82.8
  heart — *see* Infarct, myocardium
  hepatic K76.3
  hypophysis (anterior lobe) E23.6
  impending (myocardium) I20.0
  intestine (acute) (agnogenic) (embolic) (hemorrhagic)
    (nonocclusive) (nonthrombotic) (occlusive)
    (thrombotic) (with gangrene) K55.069
    diffuse K55.062
    focal K55.061
    large K55.049
      diffuse K55.042
      focal K55.041
    small K55.029
      diffuse K55.022
      focal K55.021
  kidney N28.0
  lacunar I63.81
  liver K76.3
  lung (embolic) (thrombotic) — *see* Embolism, pulmonary
  lymph node I89.8
  mesentery, mesenteric (embolic) (thrombotic) (with
    gangrene) — *see also* Infarct, intestine K55.069
  muscle (ischemic) M62.20
    ankle M62.27- ☑
    foot M62.27- ☑
    forearm M62.23- ☑
    hand M62.24- ☑
    lower leg M62.26- ☑
    pelvic region M62.25- ☑
    shoulder region M62.21- ☑
    specified site NEC M62.28
    thigh M62.25- ☑
    upper arm M62.22- ☑
  myocardium, myocardial (acute) (with stated duration
    of 4 weeks or less) I21.9
    with
      coronary microvascular disease I21.B
      coronary microvascular dysfunction I21.B
      nonobstructive coronary arteries [MINOCA] with
        microvascular disease I21.B
    associated with revascularization procedure I21.A9
    diagnosed on ECG, but presenting no symptoms I25.2
    due to
      demand ischemia I21.A1
      ischemic imbalance I21.A1
    healed or old I25.2
    intraoperative — *see also* Infarct, myocardium, asso-
      ciated with revascularization procedure
      during cardiac surgery I97.790
      during other surgery I97.791
    non-Q wave I21.4
    non-ST elevation (NSTEMI) I21.4
      subsequent I22.2
    nontransmural I21.4
    past (diagnosed on ECG or other investigation, but
      currently presenting no symptoms) I25.2
    postprocedural — *see also* Infarct, myocardium, asso-
      ciated with revascularization procedure
      following cardiac surgery — *see also* Infarct, my-
        ocardium, type 4 or type 5 I97.190
      following other surgery I97.191
    Q wave — *see also* Infarct, myocardium, ST elevation,
      by site I21.3
    secondary to
      demand ischemia I21.A1
      ischemic imbalance I21.A1
    ST elevation (STEMI) I21.3
      anterior (anteroapical) (anterolateral) (anterosep-
        tal) (Q wave) (wall) I21.09
        subsequent I22.0
      inferior (diaphragmatic) (inferolateral) (inferopos-
        terior) (wall) NEC I21.19

Infarct, infarction — *continued*
  myocardium, myocardial — *continued*
    ST elevation — *continued*
      inferior — *continued*
        subsequent I22.1
      inferoposterior transmural (Q wave) I21.11
      involving
        coronary artery of anterior wall NEC I21.09
        coronary artery of inferior wall NEC I21.19
        diagonal coronary artery I21.02
        left anterior descending coronary artery I21.02
        left circumflex coronary artery I21.21
        left main coronary artery I21.01
        oblique marginal coronary artery I21.21
        right coronary artery I21.11
      lateral (apical-lateral) (basal-lateral) (high) I21.29
        subsequent I22.8
      posterior (posterobasal) (posterolateral) (posteroseptal) (true) I21.29
        subsequent I22.8
      septal I21.29
        subsequent I22.8
      specified NEC I21.29
        subsequent I22.8
      subsequent I22.9
    subsequent (recurrent) (reinfarction) I22.9
      anterior (anteroapical) (anterolateral) (anteroseptal) (wall) I22.0
      diaphragmatic (wall) I22.1
      inferior (diaphragmatic) (inferolateral) (inferoposterior) (wall) I22.1
      lateral (apical-lateral) (basal-lateral) (high) I22.8
      non-ST elevation (NSTEMI) I22.2
      posterior (posterobasal) (posterolateral) (posteroseptal) (true) I22.8
      septal I22.8
      specified NEC I22.8
      ST elevation I22.9
        anterior (anteroapical) (anterolateral) (anteroseptal) (wall) I22.0
        inferior (diaphragmatic) (inferolateral) (inferoposterior) (wall) I22.1
        specified NEC I22.8
      subendocardial I22.2
      transmural I22.9
        anterior (anteroapical) (anterolateral) (anteroseptal) (wall) I22.0
        diaphragmatic (wall) I22.1
        inferior (diaphragmatic) (inferolateral) (inferoposterior) (wall) I22.1
        lateral (apical-lateral) (basal-lateral) (high) I22.8
        posterior (posterobasal) (posterolateral) (posteroseptal) (true) I22.8
        specified NEC I22.8
    type 1 — *see also* Infarction, myocardial, subsequent, by site, or by ST elevation or non-ST elevation I22.9
    type 2 I21.A1
    type 3 I21.A9
    type 4 I21.A9
    type 5 I21.A9
  syphilitic A52.06
  transmural — *see also*, Infarct, myocardium, ST elevation, by site I21.3
    anterior (anteroapical) (anterolateral) (anteroseptal) (Q wave) (wall) NEC I21.09
    inferior (diaphragmatic) (inferolateral) (inferoposterior) (Q wave) (wall) NEC I21.19
    inferoposterior (Q wave) I21.11
    lateral (apical-lateral) (basal-lateral) (high) NEC I21.29
    posterior (posterobasal) (posterolateral) (posteroseptal) (true) NEC I21.29
    septal NEC I21.29
    specified NEC I21.29
  type 1 — *see also* Infarction, myocardial, by site, or by ST elevation or non-ST elevation I21.9
  type 2 I21.A1
  type 3 I21.A9
  type 4 (a) (b) (c) I21.A9
  type 5 I21.A9
  nontransmural I21.4
  omentum — *see also* Infarct, intestine K55.069
  ovary N83.8
  pancreas K86.89
  papillary muscle — *see* Infarct, myocardium
  parathyroid gland E21.4
  pituitary (gland) E23.6
  placenta O43.81- ☑

Infarct, infarction — *continued*
  prostate N42.89
  pulmonary (artery) (vein) (hemorrhagic) — *see* Embolism, pulmonary
  renal (embolic) (thrombotic) N28.0
  retina, retinal (artery) — *see* Occlusion, artery, retina
  spinal (cord) (acute) (embolic) (nonembolic) G95.11
  spleen D73.5
    embolic or thrombotic I74.8
  subendocardial (acute) (nontransmural) I21.4
  suprarenal (capsule) (gland) E27.49
  testis N50.1
  thrombotic — *see also* Thrombosis
    artery, arterial — *see* Embolism
  thyroid (gland) E07.89
  ventricle (heart) — *see* Infarct, myocardium
Infecting — *see* condition
Infection, infected, infective (opportunistic) B99.9
  with
    drug resistant organism — *see* Resistance (to), drug
      — *see also* specific organism
    lymphangitis — *see* Lymphangitis
    organ dysfunction (acute) R65.20
      with septic shock R65.21
  abscess (skin) — *code by* site under Abscess
  Absidia — *see* Mucormycosis
  Acanthamoeba — *see* Acanthamebiasis
  Acanthocheilonema (perstans) (streptocerca) B74.4
  accessory sinus (chronic) — *see* Sinusitis
  achorion — *see* Dermatophytosis
  Acinetobacter baumannii, as cause of disease classified elsewhere B96.83
  Acremonium falciforme B47.0
  acromioclavicular M00.9
  Actinobacillus (actinomycetem-comitans) A28.8
    mallei A24.0
    muris A25.1
  Actinomadura B47.1
  Actinomyces (israelii) — *see also* Actinomycosis A42.9
  Actinomycetales — *see* Actinomycosis
  actinomycotic NOS — *see* Actinomycosis
  adenoid (and tonsil) J03.90
    chronic J35.02
  adenovirus NEC
    as cause of disease classified elsewhere B97.0
    unspecified nature or site B34.0
  aerogenes capsulatus A48.0
  aertrycke — *see* Infection, salmonella
  alimentary canal NOS — *see* Enteritis, infectious
  Allescheria boydii B48.2
  Alternaria B48.8
  alveolus, alveolar (process) K04.7
  Ameba, amebic (histolytica) — *see* Amebiasis
  amniotic fluid, sac or cavity O41.10- ☑
    chorioamnionitis O41.12- ☑
    placentitis O41.14- ☑
  amputation stump (surgical) — *see* Complication, amputation stump, infection
  Ancylostoma (duodenalis) B76.0
  Anisakiasis, Anisakis larvae B81.0
  anthrax — *see* Anthrax
  antrum (chronic) — *see* Sinusitis, maxillary
  anus, anal (papillae) (sphincter) K62.89
  arbovirus (arbor virus) A94
    specified type NEC A93.8
  artificial insemination N98.0
  Ascaris lumbricoides — *see* Ascariasis
  Ascomycetes B47.0
  Aspergillus (flavus) (fumigatus) (terreus) — *see* Aspergillosis
  atypical
    acid-fast (bacilli) — *see* Mycobacterium, atypical
    mycobacteria — *see* Mycobacterium, atypical
    virus A81.9
      specified type NEC A81.89
  auditory meatus (external) — *see* Otitis, externa, infective
  auricle (ear) — *see* Otitis, externa, infective
  axillary gland (lymph) L04.2
  Bacillus A49.9
    abortus A23.1
    anthracis — *see* Anthrax
    ducreyi (any location) A57
    Flexner's A03.1
    Friedlander's NEC A49.8
    gas (gangrene) A48.0
    mallei A24.0
    melitensis A23.0
    paratyphoid, paratyphosus A01.4
      A A01.1

Infection, infected, infective — *continued*
  Bacillus — *continued*
    paratyphoid, paratyphosus — *continued*
      B A01.2
      C A01.3
    Shiga (-Kruse) A03.0
    suipestifer — *see* Infection, salmonella
    swimming pool A31.1
    typhosa A01.00
    welchii — *see* Gangrene, gas
  bacterial NOS A49.9
    as cause of disease classified elsewhere B96.89
      Acinetobacter baumannii B96.83
      Bacteroides fragilis [B. fragilis] B96.6
      Clostridium perfringens [C. perfringens] B96.7
      Cronobacter (sakazakii) B96.89
      Enterobacter sakazakii B96.89
      Enterococcus B95.2
      Escherichia coli [E. coli] — *see also* Escherichia coli B96.20
      Helicobacter pylori [H.pylori] B96.81
      Hemophilus influenzae [H. influenzae] B96.3
      Klebsiella pneumoniae [K. pneumoniae] B96.1
      Mycoplasma pneumoniae [M. pneumoniae] B96.0
      Proteus (mirabilis) (morganii) B96.4
      Pseudomonas (aeruginosa) (mallei) (pseudomallei) B96.5
      Staphylococcus B95.8
        aureus (methicillin susceptible) (MSSA) B95.61
        methicillin resistant (MRSA) B95.62
        specified NEC B95.7
      Streptococcus B95.5
        group A B95.0
        group B B95.1
        pneumoniae B95.3
        specified NEC B95.4
      Vibrio vulnificus B96.82
    specified NEC A48.8
  Bacterium
    paratyphosum A01.4
      A A01.1
      B A01.2
      C A01.3
    typhosum A01.00
  Bacteroides NEC A49.8
    fragilis, as cause of disease classified elsewhere B96.6
  Balantidium coli A07.0
  Bartholin's gland N75.8
  Basidiobolus B46.8
  bile duct (common) (hepatic) — *see* Cholangitis
  bladder — *see* Cystitis
  Blastomyces, blastomycotic — *see also* Blastomycosis
    brasiliensis — *see* Paracoccidioidomycosis
    dermatitidis — *see* Blastomycosis
    European — *see* Cryptococcosis
    Loboi B48.0
    North American B40.9
    South American — *see* Paracoccidioidomycosis
  bleb, postprocedure — *see* Blebitis
  bone — *see* Osteomyelitis
  Bordetella — *see* Whooping cough
  Borrelia bergdorfi A69.20
  brain — *see also* Encephalitis G04.90
    membranes — *see* Meningitis
    septic G06.0
      meninges — *see* Meningitis, bacterial
  branchial cyst Q18.0
  breast — *see* Mastitis
  bronchus — *see* Bronchitis
  Brucella A23.9
    abortus A23.1
    canis A23.3
    melitensis A23.0
    mixed A23.8
    specified NEC A23.8
    suis A23.2
  Brugia (malayi) B74.1
    timori B74.2
  bursa — *see* Bursitis, infective
  buttocks (skin) L08.9
  Campylobacter, intestinal A04.5
    as cause of disease classified elsewhere B96.81
  Candida (albicans) (tropicalis) — *see* Candidiasis
  candiru B88.8
  Capillaria (intestinal) B81.1
    hepatica B83.8
    philippinensis B81.1
  cartilage — *see* Disorder, cartilage, specified type NEC
  cat liver fluke B66.0

☑ **Additional Character Required — Refer to the Tabular List for Character Selection**

Infection, infected, infective — *continued*
- catheter-related bloodstream (CRBSI) T80.211 ☑
- cellulitis — *code by* site under Cellulitis
- central line-associated T80.219 ☑
  - bloodstream (CLABSI) T80.211 ☑
  - specified NEC T80.218 ☑
- Cephalosporium falciforme B47.0
- cerebrospinal — *see* Meningitis
- cervical gland (lymph) L04.0
- cervix — *see* Cervicitis
- cesarean delivery wound (puerperal) O86.00
- cestodes — *see* Infestation, cestodes
- chest J22
- Chilomastix (intestinal) A07.8
- Chlamydia, chlamydial A74.9
  - anus A56.3
  - genitourinary tract A56.2
    - lower A56.00
    - specified NEC A56.19
  - lymphogranuloma A55
  - pharynx A56.4
  - psittaci A70
  - rectum A56.3
  - sexually transmitted NEC A56.8
- cholera — *see* Cholera
- Cladosporium
  - bantianum (brain abscess) B43.1
  - carrionii B43.0
  - castellanii B36.1
  - trichoides (brain abscess) B43.1
  - werneckii B36.1
- Clonorchis (sinensis) (liver) B66.1
- Clostridioides
  - difficile
    - as cause of disease classified elsewhere B96.89
    - foodborne (disease)
      - not specified as recurrent A04.72
      - recurrent A04.71
    - gas gangrene A48.0
    - necrotizing enterocolitis
      - not specified as recurrent A04.72
      - recurrent A04.71
    - sepsis A41.4
- Clostridium NEC
  - bifermentans A48.0
  - botulinum (food poisoning) A05.1
    - infant A48.51
    - wound A48.52
  - difficile
    - as cause of disease classified elsewhere B96.89
    - foodborne (disease)
      - not specified as recurrent A04.72
      - recurrent A04.71
    - gas gangrene A48.0
    - necrotizing enterocolitis
      - not specified as recurrent A04.72
      - recurrent A04.71
    - sepsis A41.4
  - gas-forming NEC A48.0
  - histolyticum A48.0
  - novyi, causing gas gangrene A48.0
  - oedematiens A48.0
  - perfringens
    - as cause of disease classified elsewhere B96.7
    - due to food A05.2
    - foodborne (disease) A05.2
    - gas gangrene A48.0
    - sepsis A41.4
  - septicum, causing gas gangrene A48.0
  - sordellii, causing gas gangrene A48.0
  - welchii
    - as cause of disease classified elsewhere B96.7
    - foodborne (disease) A05.2
    - gas gangrene A48.0
    - necrotizing enteritis A05.2
    - sepsis A41.4
- Coccidioides (immitis) — *see* Coccidioidomycosis
- colon — *see* Enteritis, infectious
- colostomy K94.02
- common duct — *see* Cholangitis
- congenital P39.9
  - Candida (albicans) P37.5
  - cytomegalovirus P35.1
  - hepatitis, viral P35.3
  - herpes simplex P35.2
  - infectious or parasitic disease P37.9
    - specified NEC P37.8
  - listeriosis (disseminated) P37.2
  - malaria NEC P37.4

Infection, infected, infective — *continued*
- congenital — *continued*
  - malaria — *continued*
    - falciparum P37.3
  - Plasmodium falciparum P37.3
  - poliomyelitis P35.8
  - rubella P35.0
  - skin P39.4
  - toxoplasmosis (acute) (subacute) (chronic) P37.1
  - tuberculosis P37.0
  - urinary (tract) P39.3
  - vaccinia P35.8
  - virus P35.9
    - specified type NEC P35.8
- Conidiobolus B46.8
- coronavirus-2019 U07.1
- coronavirus NEC B34.2
  - as cause of disease classified elsewhere B97.29
  - severe acute respiratory syndrome (SARS associated) B97.21
- corpus luteum — *see* Salpingo-oophoritis
- Corynebacterium diphtheriae — *see* Diphtheria
- cotia virus B08.8
- COVID-19 — *see also* COVID-19 U07.1
- Coxiella burnetii A78
- coxsackie — *see* Coxsackie
- Cronobacter (sakazakii) B96.89
  - as cause of disease classified elsewhere B96.89
  - generalized A41.59
- Cryptococcus neoformans — *see* Cryptococcosis
- Cryptosporidium A07.2
- Cunninghamella — *see* Mucormycosis
- cyst — *see* Cyst
- cystic duct — *see also* Cholecystitis K81.9
- Cysticercus cellulosae — *see* Cysticercosis
- cytomegalovirus, cytomegaloviral B25.9
  - congenital P35.1
  - maternal, maternal care for (suspected) damage to fetus O35.3
  - mononucleosis B27.10
    - with
      - complication NEC B27.19
      - meningitis B27.12
      - polyneuropathy B27.11
- delta-agent (acute), in hepatitis B carrier B17.0
- dental (pulpal origin) K04.7
- Deuteromycetes B47.0
- Dicrocoelium dendriticum B66.2
- Dipetalonema (perstans) (streptocerca) B74.4
- diphtherial — *see* Diphtheria
- Diphyllobothrium (adult) (latum) (pacificum) B70.0
  - larval B70.1
- Diplogonoporus (grandis) B71.8
- Dipylidium caninum B67.4
- Dirofilaria B74.8
- Dracunculus medinensis B72
- Drechslera (hawaiiensis) B43.8
- ducreyi Haemophilus (any location) A57
- due to or resulting from
  - artificial insemination N98.0
  - Babesia
    - divergens (-like) strain B60.03
    - duncani (-type) species B60.02
    - microti B60.01
    - species
      - specified NEC B60.09
  - central venous catheter T80.219 ☑
    - bloodstream T80.211 ☑
    - exit or insertion site T80.212 ☑
    - localized T80.212 ☑
    - port or reservoir T80.212 ☑
    - specified NEC T80.218 ☑
    - tunnel T80.212 ☑
  - device, implant or graft — *see also* Complications, by site and type, infection or inflammation T85.79 ☑
    - arterial graft NEC T82.7 ☑
    - breast (implant) T85.79 ☑
    - catheter NEC T85.79 ☑
      - dialysis (renal) T82.7 ☑
        - central line T80.211 ☑
        - intraperitoneal T85.71 ☑
      - infusion NEC T82.7 ☑
        - cranial T85.735 ☑
        - intrathecal T85.735 ☑
        - spinal (epidural) (subdural) T85.735 ☑
        - subarachnoid T85.735 ☑
      - urinary T83.518 ☑

Infection, infected, infective — *continued*
- due to or resulting from — *continued*
  - device, implant or graft — *see also* Complications, by site and type, infection or inflammation — *continued*
    - catheter — *continued*
      - urinary — *continued*
        - cystostomy T83.510 ☑
        - Hopkins T83.518 ☑
        - ileostomy T83.518 ☑
        - nephrostomy T83.512 ☑
        - specified NEC T83.518 ☑
        - urethral indwelling T83.511 ☑
        - urostomy T83.518 ☑
    - electronic (electrode) (pulse generator) (stimulator)
      - bone T84.7 ☑
      - cardiac T82.7 ☑
      - nervous system T85.738 ☑
        - brain T85.731 ☑
        - cranial nerve T85.732 ☑
        - gastric nerve T85.732 ☑
        - generator pocket T85.734 ☑
        - neurostimulator generator T85.734 ☑
        - peripheral nerve T85.732 ☑
        - sacral nerve T85.732 ☑
        - spinal cord T85.733 ☑
        - vagal nerve T85.732 ☑
      - urinary (indwelling) T83.51 ☑
    - fixation, internal (orthopedic) NEC — *see* Complication, fixation device, infection
    - gastrointestinal (bile duct) (esophagus) T85.79 ☑
      - neurostimulator electrode (lead) T85.732 ☑
    - genital NEC T83.69 ☑
    - heart NEC T82.7 ☑
      - valve (prosthesis) T82.6 ☑
      - graft T82.7 ☑
    - joint prosthesis — *see* Complication, joint prosthesis, infection
    - ocular (corneal graft) (orbital implant) NEC T85.79 ☑
    - orthopedic NEC T84.7 ☑
    - penile (cylinder) (pump) (reservoir) T83.61 ☑
    - specified NEC T85.79 ☑
    - testicular T83.62 ☑
    - urinary NEC T83.598 ☑
      - ileal conduit stent T83.593 ☑
      - implanted neurostimulation T83.590 ☑
      - implanted sphincter T83.591 ☑
      - indwelling ureteral stent T83.592 ☑
      - nephroureteral stent T83.593 ☑
      - specified stent NEC T83.593 ☑
    - vascular NEC T82.7 ☑
    - ventricular intracranial (communicating) shunt T85.730 ☑
  - Hickman catheter T80.219 ☑
    - bloodstream T80.211 ☑
    - localized T80.212 ☑
    - specified NEC T80.218 ☑
  - immunization or vaccination T88.0 ☑
  - infusion, injection or transfusion NEC T80.29 ☑
  - injury NEC — *code by* site under Wound, open
  - peripherally inserted central catheter (PICC) T80.219 ☑
    - bloodstream T80.211 ☑
    - localized T80.212 ☑
    - specified NEC T80.218 ☑
  - portacath (port-a-cath) T80.219 ☑
    - bloodstream T80.211 ☑
    - localized T80.212 ☑
    - specified NEC T80.218 ☑
  - protozoa of the order Piroplasmida NEC B60.09
  - pulmonary artery catheter — *see* Infection, due to or resulting from, central venous catheter
  - surgery T81.40 ☑
  - Swan Ganz catheter — *see* Infection, due to or resulting from, central venous catheter
  - triple lumen catheter T80.219 ☑
    - bloodstream T80.211 ☑
    - localized T80.212 ☑
    - specified NEC T80.218 ☑
  - umbilical venous catheter T80.219 ☑
    - bloodstream T80.211 ☑
    - localized T80.212 ☑
    - specified NEC T80.218 ☑
- during labor NEC O75.3

☑ **Additional Character Required — Refer to the Tabular List for Character Selection**

Infection, infected, infective — *continued*
- ear (middle) — *see also* Otitis media
  - external — *see* Otitis, externa, infective
  - inner — *see* subcategory H83.0 ☑
- Eberthella typhosa A01.00
- Echinococcus — *see* Echinococcus
- echovirus
  - as cause of disease classified elsewhere B97.12
  - unspecified nature or site B34.1
- endocardium I33.0
- endocervix — *see* Cervicitis
- Entamoeba — *see* Amebiasis
- enteric — *see* Enteritis, infectious
- Enterobacter sakazakii B96.89
- Enterobius vermicularis B80
- enterostomy K94.12
- enterovirus B34.1
  - as cause of disease classified elsewhere B97.10
    - coxsackievirus B97.11
    - echovirus B97.12
    - specified NEC B97.19
- Entomophthora B46.8
- Epidermophyton — *see* Dermatophytosis
- epididymis — *see* Epididymitis
- episiotomy (puerperal) O86.09
- Erysipelothrix (insidiosa) (rhusiopathiae) — *see* Erysipeloid
- erythema infectiosum B08.3
- Escherichia (E.) coli NEC A49.8
  - as cause of disease classified elsewhere — *see also* Escherichia coli B96.20
  - congenital P39.8
    - sepsis P36.4
  - generalized A41.51
  - intestinal — *see* Enteritis, infectious, due to, Escherichia coli
- ethmoidal (chronic) (sinus) — *see* Sinusitis, ethmoidal
- eustachian tube (ear) — *see* Salpingitis, eustachian
- external auditory canal (meatus) NEC — *see* Otitis, externa, infective
- eye (purulent) — *see* Endophthalmitis, purulent
- eyelid — *see* Inflammation, eyelid
- fallopian tube — *see* Salpingo-oophoritis
- Fasciola (gigantica) (hepatica) (indica) B66.3
- Fasciolopsis (buski) B66.5
- filarial — *see* Infestation, filarial
- finger (skin) L08.9
  - nail L03.01- ☑
    - fungus B35.1
- fish tapeworm B70.0
  - larval B70.1
- flagellate, intestinal A07.9
- fluke — *see* Infestation, fluke
- focal
  - teeth (pulpal origin) K04.7
  - tonsils J35.01
- Fonsecaea (compactum) (pedrosoi) B43.0
- food — *see* Intoxication, foodborne
- foot (skin) L08.9
  - dermatophytic fungus B35.3
- Francisella tularensis — *see* Tularemia
- frontal (sinus) (chronic) — *see* Sinusitis, frontal
- fungus NOS B49
  - beard B35.0
  - dermatophytic — *see* Dermatophytosis
  - foot B35.3
  - groin B35.6
  - hand B35.2
  - nail B35.1
  - pathogenic to compromised host only B48.8
  - perianal (area) B35.6
  - scalp B35.0
  - skin B36.9
    - foot B35.3
    - hand B35.2
    - toenails B35.1
- Fusarium B48.8
- gallbladder — *see* Cholecystitis
- gas bacillus — *see* Gangrene, gas
- gastrointestinal — *see* Enteritis, infectious
- generalized NEC — *see* Sepsis
- generator pocket, implanted electronic neurostimulator T85.734 ☑
- genital organ or tract
  - female — *see* Disease, pelvis, inflammatory
  - male N49.9
    - multiple sites N49.8
    - specified NEC N49.8
- Ghon tubercle, primary A15.7

Infection, infected, infective — *continued*
- Giardia lamblia A07.1
- gingiva (chronic) K05.10
  - acute K05.00
    - nonplaque induced K05.01
    - plaque induced K05.00
  - nonplaque induced K05.11
  - plaque induced K05.10
- glanders A24.0
- glenosporopsis B48.0
- Gnathostoma (spinigerum) B83.1
- Gongylonema B83.8
- gonococcal — *see* Gonococcus
- gram-negative bacilli NOS A49.9
- guinea worm B72
- gum (chronic) K05.10
  - acute K05.00
    - nonplaque induced K05.01
    - plaque induced K05.00
  - nonplaque induced K05.11
  - plaque induced K05.10
- Haemophilus — *see* Infection, Hemophilus
- heart — *see* Carditis
- Helicobacter pylori A04.8
  - as cause of disease classified elsewhere B96.81
- helminths B83.9
  - intestinal B82.0
    - mixed (types classifiable to more than one of the titles B65.0-B81.3 and B81.8) B81.4
    - specified type NEC B81.8
  - specified type NEC B83.8
- Hemophilus
  - aegyptius, systemic A48.4
  - ducreyi (any location) A57
  - generalized A41.3
  - influenzae NEC A49.2
    - as cause of disease classified elsewhere B96.3
- herpes (simplex) — *see also* Herpes
  - congenital P35.2
  - disseminated B00.7
  - zoster B02.9
- herpesvirus, herpesviral — *see* Herpes
- Heterophyes (heterophyes) B66.8
- hip (joint) NEC M00.9
  - due to internal joint prosthesis
    - left T84.52 ☑
    - right T84.51 ☑
  - skin NEC L08.9
- Histoplasma — *see* Histoplasmosis
  - American B39.4
  - capsulatum B39.4
- hookworm B76.9
- human
  - papilloma virus A63.0
  - T-cell lymphotropic virus type-1 (HTLV-1) B33.3
- hydrocele N43.0
- Hymenolepis B71.0
- hypopharynx — *see* Pharyngitis
- inguinal (lymph) glands L04.1
  - due to soft chancre A57
- intervertebral disc, pyogenic M46.30
  - cervical region M46.32
  - cervicothoracic region M46.33
  - lumbar region M46.36
  - lumbosacral region M46.37
  - multiple sites M46.39
  - occipito-atlanto-axial region M46.31
  - sacrococcygeal region M46.38
  - thoracic region M46.34
  - thoracolumbar region M46.35
- intestine, intestinal — *see* Enteritis, infectious
  - specified NEC A08.8
- intra-amniotic affecting newborn NEC P39.2
- intrauterine inflammation O41.12- ☑
- Isospora belli or hominis A07.3
- Japanese B encephalitis A83.0
- jaw (bone) (lower) (upper) M27.2
- joint NEC M00.9
  - due to internal joint prosthesis T84.50 ☑
- kidney (cortex) (hematogenous) N15.9
  - with calculus N20.0
    - with hydronephrosis N13.6
  - following ectopic gestation O08.83
  - pelvis and ureter (cystic) N28.85
  - puerperal (postpartum) O86.21
  - specified NEC N15.8
- Klebsiella (K.) pneumoniae NEC A49.8
  - as cause of disease classified elsewhere B96.1
- knee (joint) NEC M00.9

Infection, infected, infective — *continued*
- knee — *continued*
  - joint M00.9
  - due to internal joint prosthesis
    - left T84.54 ☑
    - right T84.53 ☑
  - skin L08.9
- Koch's — *see* Tuberculosis
- labia (majora) (minora) (acute) — *see* Vulvitis
- lacrimal
  - gland — *see* Dacryoadenitis
  - passages (duct) (sac) — *see* Inflammation, lacrimal, passages
- lancet fluke B66.2
- larynx NEC J38.7
- leg (skin) NOS L08.9
- Legionella pneumophila A48.1
  - nonpneumonic A48.2
- Leishmania — *see also* Leishmaniasis
  - aethiopica B55.1
  - braziliensis B55.2
  - chagasi B55.0
  - donovani B55.0
  - infantum B55.0
  - major B55.1
  - mexicana B55.1
  - tropica B55.1
- lentivirus, as cause of disease classified elsewhere B97.31
- Leptosphaeria senegalensis B47.0
- Leptospira interrogans A27.9
  - autumnalis A27.89
  - canicola A27.89
  - hebdomadis A27.89
  - icterohaemorrhagiae A27.0
  - pomona A27.89
  - specified type NEC A27.89
- leptospirochetal NEC — *see* Leptospirosis
- Listeria monocytogenes — *see also* Listeriosis
  - congenital P37.2
- Loa loa B74.3
  - with conjunctival infestation B74.3
  - eyelid B74.3
- Loboa loboi B48.0
- local, skin (staphylococcal) (streptococcal) L08.9
  - abscess — *code by* site under Abscess
  - cellulitis — *code by* site under Cellulitis
  - specified NEC L08.89
  - ulcer — *see* Ulcer, skin
- Loefflerella mallei A24.0
- lung — *see also* Pneumonia J18.9
  - atypical Mycobacterium A31.0
  - spirochetal A69.8
  - tuberculous — *see* Tuberculosis, pulmonary
  - virus — *see* Pneumonia, viral
- lymph gland — *see also* Lymphadenitis, acute
  - mesenteric I88.0
- lymphoid tissue, base of tongue or posterior pharynx, NEC (chronic) J35.03
- Madurella (grisea) (mycetomii) B47.0
- major
  - following ectopic or molar pregnancy O08.0
  - puerperal, postpartum, childbirth O85
- Malassezia furfur B36.0
- Malleomyces
  - mallei A24.0
  - pseudomallei (whitmori) — *see* Melioidosis
- mammary gland N61.0
- Mansonella (ozzardi) (perstans) (streptocerca) B74.4
- mastoid — *see* Mastoiditis
- maxilla, maxillary M27.2
  - sinus (chronic) — *see* Sinusitis, maxillary
- mediastinum J98.51
- Medina (worm) B72
- meibomian cyst or gland — *see* Hordeolum
- meninges — *see* Meningitis, bacterial
- meningococcal — *see also* condition A39.9
  - adrenals A39.1
  - brain A39.81
  - cerebrospinal A39.0
  - conjunctiva A39.89
  - endocardium A39.51
  - heart A39.50
    - endocardium A39.51
    - myocardium A39.52
    - pericardium A39.53
  - joint A39.83
  - meninges A39.0
  - meningococcemia A39.4
    - acute A39.2

☑ **Additional Character Required** — **Refer to the Tabular List for Character Selection**

Infection, infected, infective — *continued*
  meningococcal — *see also* condition — *continued*
    meningococcemia — *continued*
      chronic A39.3
     myocardium A39.52
     pericardium A39.53
     retrobulbar neuritis A39.82
     specified site NEC A39.89
  mesenteric lymph nodes or glands NEC I88.0
  Metagonimus B66.8
  metatarsophalangeal M00.9
  methicillin
    resistant Staphylococcus aureus (MRSA) A49.02
    susceptible Staphylococcus aureus (MSSA) A49.01
  Microsporum, microsporic — *see* Dermatophytosis
  mixed flora (bacterial) NEC A49.8
  Monilia — *see* Candidiasis
  Monosporium apiospermum B48.2
  mouth, parasitic B37.0
  Mucor — *see* Mucormycosis
  muscle NEC — *see* Myositis, infective
  mycelium NOS B49
  mycetoma B47.9
    actinomycotic NEC B47.1
    mycotic NEC B47.0
  Mycobacterium, mycobacterial — *see* Mycobacterium
  Mycoplasma NEC A49.3
    pneumoniae, as cause of disease classified elsewhere B96.0
  mycotic NOS B49
    pathogenic to compromised host only B48.8
    skin NOS B36.9
  myocardium NEC I40.0
  nail (chronic)
    with lymphangitis — *see* Lymphangitis, acute, digit
    finger L03.01- ☑
      fungus B35.1
    ingrowing L60.0
    toe L03.03- ☑
      fungus B35.1
  nasal sinus (chronic) — *see* Sinusitis
  nasopharynx — *see* Nasopharyngitis
  navel L08.82
  Necator americanus B76.1
  Neisseria — *see* Gonococcus
  Neotestudina rosatii B47.0
  newborn P39.9
    intra-amniotic NEC P39.2
    skin P39.4
    specified type NEC P39.8
  nipple N61.0
    associated with
      lactation O91.03
      pregnancy O91.01- ☑
      puerperium O91.02
  Nocardia — *see* Nocardiosis
  obstetrical surgical wound (puerperal) O86.00
    incisional site
      deep O86.02
      superficial O86.01
    organ and space site O86.03
    surgical site specified NEC O86.09
  Oesophagostomum (apiostomum) B81.8
  Oestrus ovis — *see* Myiasis
  Oidium albicans B37.9
  Onchocerca (volvulus) — *see* Onchocerciasis
  oncovirus, as cause of disease classified elsewhere B97.32
  operation wound T81.49 ☑
  Opisthorchis (felineus) (viverrini) B66.0
  orbit, orbital — *see* Inflammation, orbit
  orthopoxvirus NEC B08.09
  ovary — *see* Salpingo-oophoritis
  Oxyuris vermicularis B80
  pancreas (acute) — *see* Pancreatitis, acute
    abscess — *see* Pancreatitis, acute
    specified NEC — *see also* Pancreatitis, acute K85.80
  papillomavirus, as cause of disease classified elsewhere B97.7
  papovavirus NEC B34.4
  Paracoccidioides brasiliensis — *see* Paracoccidioidomy-cosis
  Paragonimus (westermani) B66.4
  parainfluenza virus B34.8
  parameningococcus NOS A39.9
  parapoxvirus B08.60
    specified NEC B08.69
  parasitic B89
  Parastrongylus
    cantonensis B83.2

Infection, infected, infective — *continued*
  Parastrongylus — *continued*
    costaricensis B81.3
  paratyphoid A01.4
    Type A A01.1
    Type B A01.2
    Type C A01.3
  paraurethral ducts N34.2
  parotid gland — *see* Sialoadenitis
  parvovirus NEC B34.3
    as cause of disease classified elsewhere B97.6
  Pasteurella NEC A28.0
    multocida A28.0
    pestis — *see* Plague
    pseudotuberculosis A28.0
    septica (cat bite) (dog bite) A28.0
    tularensis — *see* Tularemia
  pelvic, female — *see* Disease, pelvis, inflammatory
  Penicillium (marneffei) B48.4
  penis (glans) (retention) NEC N48.29
  periapical K04.5
  peridental, periodontal K05.20
    generalized — *see* Periodontitis, aggressive, generalized
    localized — *see* Periodontitis, aggressive, localized
  perinatal period P39.9
    specified type NEC P39.8
  perineal repair (puerperal) O86.09
  periorbital — *see* Inflammation, orbit
  perirectal K62.89
  perirenal — *see* Infection, kidney
  peritoneal — *see* Peritonitis
  periureteral N28.89
  Petriellidium boydii B48.2
  pharynx — *see also* Pharyngitis
    coxsackievirus B08.5
    posterior, lymphoid (chronic) J35.03
  Phialophora
    gougerotii (subcutaneous abscess or cyst) B43.2
    jeanselmei (subcutaneous abscess or cyst) B43.2
    verrucosa (skin) B43.0
  Piedraia hortae B36.3
  pinta A67.9
    intermediate A67.1
    late A67.2
    mixed A67.3
    primary A67.0
  pinworm B80
  pityrosporum furfur B36.0
  pleuro-pneumonia-like organism (PPLO) NEC A49.3
    as cause of disease classified elsewhere B96.0
  pneumococcus, pneumococcal NEC A49.1
    as cause of disease classified elsewhere B95.3
    generalized (purulent) A40.3
      with pneumonia J13
  Pneumocystis carinii (pneumonia) B59
  Pneumocystis jiroveci (pneumonia) B59
  port or reservoir T80.212 ☑
  postoperative T81.40 ☑
  postoperative wound T81.49 ☑
    surgical site
      deep incisional T81.42 ☑
      organ and space T81.43 ☑
      specified NEC T81.49 ☑
      superficial incisional T81.41 ☑
  postprocedural T81.40 ☑
  postvaccinal T88.0 ☑
  prepuce NEC N47.7
    with penile inflammation N47.6
  prion — *see* Disease, prion, central nervous system
  prostate (capsule) — *see* Prostatitis
  Proteus (mirabilis) (morganii) (vulgaris) NEC A49.8
    as cause of disease classified elsewhere B96.4
  protozoal NEC B64
    intestinal A07.9
      specified NEC A07.8
    specified NEC B60.8
  Pseudoallescheria boydii B48.2
  Pseudomonas NEC A49.8
    as cause of disease classified elsewhere B96.5
    generalized A41.52
    mallei A24.0
    pneumonia J15.1
    pseudomallei — *see* Melioidosis
  puerperal O86.4
    genitourinary tract NEC O86.89
    major or generalized O85
    minor O86.4

Infection, infected, infective — *continued*
  puerperal — *continued*
    specified NEC O86.89
  pulmonary — *see* Infection, lung
  purulent — *see* Abscess
  Pyrenochaeta romeroi B47.0
  Q fever A78
  rectum (sphincter) K62.89
  renal — *see also* Infection, kidney
    pelvis and ureter (cystic) N28.85
  reovirus, as cause of disease classified elsewhere B97.5
  respiratory (tract) NEC J98.8
    acute J22
    chronic J98.8
    influenzal (upper) (acute) — *see* Influenza, with, respiratory manifestations NEC
    lower (acute) J22
      chronic — *see* Bronchitis, chronic
    rhinovirus J00
    syncytial virus (RSV) — *see* Infection, virus, respiratory syncytial (RSV)
    upper (acute) NOS J06.9
      chronic J39.8
      streptococcal J06.9
      viral NOS J06.9
        due to respiratory syncytial virus (RSV) J06.9 [B97.4]
  resulting from
    presence of internal prosthesis, implant, graft — *see* Complications, by site and type, infection
  retortamoniasis A07.8
  retroperitoneal NEC K68.9
  retrovirus B33.3
    as cause of disease classified elsewhere B97.30
      human
        immunodeficiency, type 2 (HIV 2) B97.35
        T-cell lymphotropic
          type I (HTLV-I) B97.33
          type II (HTLV-II) B97.34
      lentivirus B97.31
      oncovirus B97.32
      specified NEC B97.39
  Rhinosporidium (seeberi) B48.1
  rhinovirus
    as cause of disease classified elsewhere B97.89
    unspecified nature or site B34.8
  Rhizopus — *see* Mucormycosis
  rickettsial NOS A79.9
  roundworm (large) NEC B82.0
    Ascariasis — *see also* Ascariasis B77.9
  rubella — *see* Rubella
  Saccharomyces — *see* Candidiasis
  salivary duct or gland (any) — *see* Sialoadenitis
  Salmonella (aertrycke) (arizonae) (cholerae-suis) (enteritidis) (gallinarum) (suipestifer) (typhimurium) A02.9
    with
      (gastro)enteritis A02.0
      sepsis A02.1
      specified manifestation NEC A02.8
    due to food (poisoning) A02.9
    hirschfeldii A01.3
    localized A02.20
      arthritis A02.23
      meningitis A02.21
      osteomyelitis A02.24
      pneumonia A02.22
      pyelonephritis A02.25
      specified NEC A02.29
    paratyphi A01.4
      A A01.1
      B A01.2
      C A01.3
    schottmuelleri A01.2
    typhi, typhosa — *see* Typhoid
  Sarcocystis A07.8
  SARS-CoV-2 — *see* Infection, COVID-19
  scabies B86
  Schistosoma — *see* Infestation, Schistosoma
  scrotum (acute) NEC N49.2
  seminal vesicle — *see* Vesiculitis
  septic
    localized, skin — *see* Abscess
  Serratia NEC A49.8
    as cause of disease classified elsewhere B96.89
    generalized A41.53
  sheep liver fluke B66.3
  Shigella A03.9
    boydii A03.2

☑ Additional Character Required — Refer to the Tabular List for Character Selection

Infection, infected, infective — *continued*
Shigella — *continued*
dysenteriae A03.0
flexneri A03.1
group
A A03.0
B A03.1
C A03.2
D A03.3
Schmitz (-Stutzer) A03.0
schmitzii A03.0
shigae A03.0
sonnei A03.3
specified NEC A03.8
shoulder (joint) NEC M00.9
due to internal joint prosthesis T84.59 ☑
skin NEC L08.9
sinus (accessory) (chronic) (nasal) — *see also* Sinusitis
pilonidal — *see* Sinus, pilonidal
skin NEC L08.89
Skene's duct or gland — *see* Urethritis
skin (local) (staphylococcal) (streptococcal) L08.9
abscess — *code by* site under Abscess
cellulitis — *code by* site under Cellulitis
due to fungus B36.9
specified type NEC B36.8
mycotic B36.9
specified type NEC B36.8
newborn P39.4
ulcer — *see* Ulcer, skin
slow virus A81.9
specified NEC A81.89
Sparganum (mansoni) (proliferum) (baxteri) B70.1
specific — *see also* Syphilis
to perinatal period — *see* Infection, congenital
specified NEC B99.8
spermatic cord NEC N49.1
sphenoidal (sinus) — *see* Sinusitis, sphenoidal
spinal cord NOS — *see also* Myelitis G04.91
abscess G06.1
meninges — *see* Meningitis
streptococcal G04.89
Spirillum A25.0
spirochetal NOS A69.9
lung A69.8
specified NEC A69.8
Spirometra larvae B70.1
spleen D73.89
Sporotrichum, Sporothrix (schenckii) — *see* Sporotrichosis
staphylococcal, unspecified site
as cause of disease classified elsewhere B95.8
aureus (methicillin susceptible) (MSSA) B95.61
methicillin resistant (MRSA) B95.62
specified NEC B95.7
aureus (methicillin susceptible) (MSSA) A49.01
methicillin resistant (MRSA) A49.02
food poisoning A05.0
generalized (purulent) A41.2
pneumonia — *see* Pneumonia, staphylococcal
Stellantchasmus falcatus B66.8
streptobacillus moniliformis A25.1
streptococcal NEC A49.1
as cause of disease classified elsewhere B95.5
B genitourinary complicating
childbirth O98.82
pregnancy O98.81- ☑
puerperium O98.83
congenital
sepsis P36.10
group B P36.0
specified NEC P36.19
generalized (purulent) A40.9
Streptomyces B47.1
Strongyloides (stercoralis) — *see* Strongyloidiasis
stump (amputation) (surgical) — *see* Complication, amputation stump, infection
subcutaneous tissue, local L08.9
suipestifer — *see* Infection, salmonella
swimming pool bacillus A31.1
Taenia — *see* Infestation, Taenia
Taeniarhynchus saginatus B68.1
tapeworm — *see* Infestation, tapeworm
tendon (sheath) — *see* Tenosynovitis, infective NEC
Ternidens diminutus B81.8
testis — *see* Orchitis
threadworm B80
throat — *see* Pharyngitis
thyroglossal duct K14.8

Infection, infected, infective — *continued*
toe (skin) L08.9
cellulitis L03.03- ☑
fungus B35.1
nail L03.03- ☑
fungus B35.1
tongue NEC K14.0
parasitic B37.0
tonsil (and adenoid) (faucial) (lingual) (pharyngeal) —
see Tonsillitis
tooth, teeth K04.7
periapical K04.7
peridental, periodontal K05.20
generalized — *see* Periodontitis, aggressive, generalized
localized — *see* Periodontitis, aggressive, localized
pulp K04.01
irreversible K04.02
reversible K04.01
socket M27.3
TORCH — *see* Infection, congenital
without active infection P00.2
Torula histolytica — *see* Cryptococcosis
Toxocara (canis) (cati) (felis) B83.0
Toxoplasma gondii — *see* Toxoplasma
trachea, chronic J42
trematode NEC — *see* Infestation, fluke
trench fever A79.0
Treponema pallidum — *see* Syphilis
Trichinella (spiralis) B75
Trichomonas A59.9
cervix A59.09
intestine A07.8
prostate A59.02
specified site NEC A59.8
urethra A59.03
urogenitalis A59.00
vagina A59.01
vulva A59.01
Trichophyton, trichophytic — *see* Dermatophytosis
Trichosporon (beigelii) cutaneum B36.2
Trichostrongylus B81.2
Trichuris (trichiura) B79
Trombicula (irritans) B88.0
Trypanosoma
brucei
gambiense B56.0
rhodesiense B56.1
cruzi — *see* Chagas' disease
tubal — *see* Salpingo-oophoritis
tuberculous
latent (LTBI) Z22.7
NEC — *see* Tuberculosis
tubo-ovarian — *see* Salpingo-oophoritis
tunica vaginalis N49.1
tunnel T80.212 ☑
tympanic membrane NEC — *see* Myringitis
typhoid (abortive) (ambulant) (bacillus) — *see* Typhoid
typhus A75.9
flea-borne A75.2
mite-borne A75.3
recrudescent A75.1
tick-borne A77.9
African A77.1
North Asian A77.2
umbilicus L08.82
ureter — *see* Ureteritis
urethra — *see* Urethritis
urinary (tract) N39.0
bladder — *see* Cystitis
complicating
pregnancy O23.4- ☑
specified type NEC O23.3- ☑
kidney — *see* Infection, kidney
newborn P39.3
puerperal (postpartum) O86.20
tuberculous A18.13
urethra — *see* Urethritis
uterus, uterine — *see* Endometritis
vaccination T88.0 ☑
vaccinia not from vaccination B08.011
vagina (acute) — *see* Vaginitis
varicella B01.9
varicose veins — *see* Varix
vas deferens NEC N49.1
vesical — *see* Cystitis
Vibrio
cholerae A00.0

Infection, infected, infective — *continued*
Vibrio — *continued*
cholerae — *continued*
El Tor A00.1
parahaemolyticus (food poisoning) A05.3
vulnificus
as cause of disease classified elsewhere B96.82
foodborne intoxication A05.5
Vincent's (gum) (mouth) (tonsil) A69.1
virus, viral NOS B34.9
adenovirus
as cause of disease classified elsewhere B97.0
unspecified nature or site B34.0
arbovirus, arbovirus arthropod-borne A94
as cause of disease classified elsewhere B97.89
adenovirus B97.0
coronavirus B97.29
SARS-associated B97.21
coxsackievirus B97.11
echovirus B97.12
enterovirus B97.10
coxsackievirus B97.11
echovirus B97.12
specified NEC B97.19
human
immunodeficiency, type 2 (HIV 2) B97.35
metapneumovirus B97.81
T-cell lymphotropic,
type I (HTLV-I) B97.33
type II (HTLV-II) B97.34
papillomavirus B97.7
parvovirus B97.6
reovirus B97.5
respiratory syncytial (RSV) — *see* Infection, virus,
respiratory syncytial (RSV)
retrovirus B97.30
human
immunodeficiency, type 2 (HIV 2) B97.35
T-cell lymphotropic,
type I (HTLV-I) B97.33
type II (HTLV-II) B97.34
lentivirus B97.31
oncovirus B97.32
specified NEC B97.39
specified NEC B97.89
central nervous system A89
atypical A81.9
specified NEC A81.89
enterovirus NEC A88.8
meningitis A87.0
slow virus A81.9
specified NEC A81.89
specified NEC A88.8
chest J98.8
cotia B08.8
COVID-19 U07.1
coxsackie — *see also* Infection, coxsackie B34.1
as cause of disease classified elsewhere B97.11
ECHO
as cause of disease classified elsewhere B97.12
unspecified nature or site B34.1
encephalitis, tick-borne A84.9
enterovirus, as cause of disease classified elsewhere
B97.10
coxsackievirus B97.11
echovirus B97.12
specified NEC B97.19
exanthem NOS B09
human metapneumovirus as cause of disease classified elsewhere B97.81
human papilloma as cause of disease classified elsewhere B97.7
intestine — *see* Enteritis, viral
respiratory syncytial (RSV)
as cause of disease classified elsewhere B97.4
bronchiolitis J21.0
bronchitis J20.5
bronchopneumonia J12.1
otitis media H65- ☑ [B97.4]
pneumonia J12.1
upper respiratory infection J06.9 [B97.4]
rhinovirus
as cause of disease classified elsewhere B97.89
unspecified nature or site B34.8
slow A81.9
specified NEC A81.89
specified type NEC B33.8
as cause of disease classified elsewhere B97.89
unspecified nature or site B34.8

Infection, infected, infective — *continued*
  virus, viral — *continued*
    unspecified nature or site B34.9
    West Nile — *see* Virus, West Nile
    vulva (acute) — *see* Vulvitis
  West Nile — *see* Virus, West Nile
  whipworm B79
  worms B83.9
    specified type NEC B83.8
  Wuchereria (bancrofti) B74.0
    malayi B74.1
  yatapoxvirus B08.70
    specified NEC B08.79
  yeast — *see also* Candidiasis B37.9
  yellow fever — *see* Fever, yellow
  Yersinia
    enterocolitica (intestinal) A04.6
    pestis — *see* Plague
    pseudotuberculosis A28.2
  Zeis' gland — *see* Hordeolum
  Zika virus A92.5
    congenital P35.4
  zoonotic bacterial NOS A28.9
  Zopfia senegalensis B47.0
Infective, infectious — *see* condition
Infertility
  female N97.9
    age-related N97.8
    associated with
      anovulation N97.0
      cervical (mucus) disease or anomaly N88.3
      congenital anomaly
        cervix N88.3
        fallopian tube N97.1
        uterus N97.2
        vagina N97.8
      dysmucorrhea N88.3
      fallopian tube disease or anomaly N97.1
      pituitary-hypothalamic origin E23.0
      specified origin NEC N97.8
      Stein-Leventhal syndrome E28.2
      uterine disease or anomaly N97.2
      vaginal disease or anomaly N97.8
    due to
      cervical anomaly N88.3
      fallopian tube anomaly N97.1
      ovarian failure E28.39
      Stein-Leventhal syndrome E28.2
      uterine anomaly N97.2
      vaginal anomaly N97.8
    nonimplantation N97.2
    origin
      cervical N88.3
      tubal (block) (occlusion) (stenosis) N97.1
      uterine N97.2
      vaginal N97.8
  male N46.9
    azoospermia N46.01
      extratesticular cause N46.029
        drug therapy N46.021
        efferent duct obstruction N46.023
        infection N46.022
        radiation N46.024
        specified cause NEC N46.029
        systemic disease N46.025
    oligospermia N46.11
      extratesticular cause N46.129
        drug therapy N46.121
        efferent duct obstruction N46.123
        infection N46.122
        radiation N46.124
        specified cause NEC N46.129
        systemic disease N46.125
    specified type NEC N46.8
Infestation B88.9
  Acanthocheilonema (perstans) (streptocerca) B74.4
  Acariasis B88.0
    demodex folliculorum B88.0
    sarcoptes scabiei B86
    trombiculae B88.0
  Agamofilaria streptocerca B74.4
  Ancylostoma, ankylostoma (braziliense) (caninum) (ceylanicum) (duodenale) B76.0
    americanum B76.1
    new world B76.1
  Anisakis larvae, anisakiasis B81.0
  arthropod NEC B88.2
  Ascaris lumbricoides — *see* Ascariasis
  Balantidium coli A07.0

Infestation — *continued*
  beef tapeworm B68.1
  Bothriocephalus (latus) B70.0
    larval B70.1
  broad tapeworm B70.0
    larval B70.1
  Brugia (malayi) B74.1
    timori B74.2
  candiru B88.8
  Capillaria
    hepatica B83.8
    philippinensis B81.1
  cat liver fluke B66.0
  cestodes B71.9
    diphyllobothrium — *see* Infestation, diphyllobothrium
    dipylidiasis B71.1
    hymenolepiasis B71.0
    specified type NEC B71.8
  chigger B88.0
  chigo, chigoe B88.1
  Clonorchis (sinensis) (liver) B66.1
  coccidial A07.3
  crab-lice B85.3
  Cysticercus cellulosae — *see* Cysticercosis
  Demodex (folliculorum) B88.0
  Dermanyssus gallinae B88.0
  Dermatobia (hominis) — *see* Myiasis
  Dibothriocephalus (latus) B70.0
    larval B70.1
  Dicrocoelium dendriticum B66.2
  Diphyllobothrium (adult) (latum) (intestinal) (pacificum) B70.0
    larval B70.1
  Diplogonoporus (grandis) B71.8
  Dipylidium caninum B67.4
  Distoma hepaticum B66.3
  dog tapeworm B67.4
  Dracunculus medinensis B72
  dragon worm B72
  dwarf tapeworm B71.0
  Echinococcus — *see* Echinococcus
  Echinostomum ilocanum B66.8
  Entamoeba (histolytica) — *see* Infection, Ameba
  Enterobius vermicularis B80
  eyelid
    in (due to)
      leishmaniasis B55.1
      loiasis B74.3
      onchocerciasis B73.09
      phthiriasis B85.3
      parasitic NOS B89
  eyeworm B74.3
  Fasciola (gigantica) (hepatica) (indica) B66.3
  Fasciolopsis (buski) (intestine) B66.5
  filarial B74.9
    bancroftian B74.0
    conjunctiva B74.9
    due to
      Acanthocheilonema (perstans) (streptocerca) B74.4
      Brugia (malayi) B74.1
        timori B74.2
      Dracunculus medinensis B72
      guinea worm B72
      loa loa B74.3
      Mansonella (ozzardi) (perstans) (streptocerca) B74.4
      Onchocerca volvulus B73.00
        eye B73.00
        eyelid B73.09
      Wuchereria (bancrofti) B74.0
    Malayan B74.1
    ozzardi B74.4
    specified type NEC B74.8
  fish tapeworm B70.0
    larval B70.1
  fluke B66.9
    blood NOS — *see* Schistosomiasis
    cat liver B66.0
    intestinal B66.5
    lancet B66.2
    liver (sheep) B66.3
      cat B66.0
      Chinese B66.1
      due to clonorchiasis B66.1
      oriental B66.1
    lung (oriental) B66.4
    sheep liver B66.3
    specified type NEC B66.8
  fly larvae — *see* Myiasis

Infestation — *continued*
  Gasterophilus (intestinalis) — *see* Myiasis
  Gastrodiscoides hominis B66.8
  Giardia lamblia A07.1
  Gnathostoma (spinigerum) B83.1
  Gongylonema B83.8
  guinea worm B72
  helminth B83.9
    angiostrongyliasis B83.2
      intestinal B81.3
    gnathostomiasis B83.1
    hirudiniasis, internal B83.4
    intestinal B82.0
      angiostrongyliasis B81.3
      anisakiasis B81.0
      ascariasis — *see* Ascariasis
      capillariasis B81.1
      cysticercosis — *see* Cysticercosis
      diphyllobothriasis — *see* Infestation, diphyllobothriasis
      dracunculiasis B72
      echinococcus — *see* Echinococcosis
      enterobiasis B80
      filariasis — *see* Infestation, filarial
      fluke — *see* Infestation, fluke
      hookworm — *see* Infestation, hookworm
      mixed (types classifiable to more than one of the titles B65.0-B81.3 and B81.8) B81.4
      onchocerciasis — *see* Onchocerciasis
      schistosomiasis — *see* Infestation, schistosoma
      specified
        cestode NEC — *see* Infestation, cestode
        type NEC B81.8
      strongyloidiasis — *see* Strongyloidiasis
      taenia — *see* Infestation, taenia
      trichinellosis B75
      trichostrongyliasis B81.2
      trichuriasis B79
    specified type NEC B83.8
    syngamiasis B83.3
    visceral larva migrans B83.0
  Heterophyes (heterophyes) B66.8
  hookworm B76.9
    ancylostomiasis B76.0
    necatoriasis B76.1
    specified type NEC B76.8
  Hymenolepis (diminuta) (nana) B71.0
  intestinal NEC B82.9
  leeches (aquatic) (land) — *see* Hirudiniasis
  Leishmania — *see* Leishmaniasis
  lice, louse — *see* Infestation, Pediculus
  Linguatula B88.8
  Liponyssoides sanguineus B88.0
  Loa loa B74.3
    conjunctival B74.3
    eyelid B74.3
  louse — *see* Infestation, Pediculus
  maggots — *see* Myiasis
  Mansonella (ozzardi) (perstans) (streptocerca) B74.4
  Medina (worm) B72
  Metagonimus (yokogawai) B66.8
  microfilaria streptocerca — *see* Onchocerciasis
    eye B73.00
    eyelid B73.09
  mites B88.9
    scabic B86
  Monilia (albicans) — *see* Candidiasis
  mouth B37.0
  Necator americanus B76.1
  nematode NEC (intestinal) B82.0
    Ancylostoma B76.0
    conjunctiva NEC B83.9
    Enterobius vermicularis B80
    Gnathostoma spinigerum B83.1
    physaloptera B80
    specified NEC B81.8
    trichostrongylus B81.2
    trichuris (trichuria) B79
  Oesophagostomum (apiostomum) B81.8
  Oestrus ovis — *see also* Myiasis B87.9
  Onchocerca (volvulus) — *see* Onchocerciasis
  Opisthorchis (felineus) (viverrini) B66.0
  orbit, parasitic NOS B89
  Oxyuris vermicularis B80
  Paragonimus (westermani) B66.4
  parasite, parasitic B89
    eyelid B89
    intestinal NOS B82.9
    mouth B37.0

Infestation — *continued*
  parasite, parasitic — *continued*
    skin B88.9
    tongue B37.0
  Parastrongylus
    cantonensis B83.2
    costaricensis B81.3
  Pediculus B85.2
    body B85.1
    capitis (humanus) (any site) B85.0
    corporis (humanus) (any site) B85.1
    head B85.0
    mixed (classifiable to more than one of the titles B85.0 - B85.3) B85.4
    pubis (any site) B85.3
  Pentastoma B88.8
  pest Z59.19
  Phthirus (pubis) (any site) B85.3
    with any infestation classifiable to B85.0 - B85.2 B85.4
  pinworm B80
  pork tapeworm (adult) B68.0
  protozoal NEC B64
    intestinal A07.9
      specified NEC A07.8
    specified NEC B60.8
  pubic, louse B85.3
  rat tapeworm B71.0
  red bug B88.0
  roundworm (large) NEC B82.0
    Ascariasis — *see also* Ascariasis B77.9
  sandflea B88.1
  Sarcoptes scabiei B86
  scabies B86
  Schistosoma B65.9
    bovis B65.8
    cercariae B65.3
    haematobium B65.0
    intercalatum B65.8
    japonicum B65.2
    mansoni B65.1
    mattheei B65.8
    mekongi B65.8
    specified type NEC B65.8
    spindale B65.8
  screw worms — *see* Myiasis
  skin NOS B88.9
  Sparganum (mansoni) (proliferum) (baxteri) B70.1
    larval B70.1
  specified type NEC B88.8
  Spirometra larvae B70.1
  Stellantchasmus falcatus B66.8
  Strongyloides stercoralis — *see* Strongyloidiasis
  Taenia B68.9
    diminuta B71.0
    echinococcus — *see* Echinococcus
    mediocanellata B68.1
    nana B71.0
    saginata B68.1
    solium (intestinal form) B68.0
      larval form — *see* Cysticercosis
  Taeniarhynchus saginatus B68.1
  tapeworm B71.9
    beef B68.1
    broad B70.0
      larval B70.1
    dog B67.4
    dwarf B71.0
    fish B70.0
      larval B70.1
    pork B68.0
    rat B71.0
  Ternidens diminutus B81.8
  Tetranychus molestissimus B88.0
  threadworm B80
  tongue B37.0
  Toxocara (canis) (cati) (felis) B83.0
  trematode(s) NEC — *see* Infestation, fluke
  Trichinella (spiralis) B75
  Trichocephalus B79
  Trichomonas — *see* Trichomoniasis
  Trichostrongylus B81.2
  Trichuris (trichiura) B79
  Trombicula (irritans) B88.0
  Tunga penetrans B88.1
  Uncinaria americana B76.1
  Vandellia cirrhosa B88.8
  whipworm B79
  worms B83.9
    intestinal B82.0

Infestation — *continued*
  Wuchereria (bancrofti) B74.0
Infiltrate, infiltration
  amyloid (generalized) (localized) — *see* Amyloidosis
  calcareous NEC R89.7
    localized — *see* Degeneration, by site
  calcium salt R89.7
  cardiac
    fatty — *see* Degeneration, myocardial
    glycogenic E74.02 *[43]*
  corneal — *see* Edema, cornea
  eyelid — *see* Inflammation, eyelid
  glycogen, glycogenic — *see* Disease, glycogen storage
  heart, cardiac
    fatty — *see* Degeneration, myocardial
    glycogenic E74.02 *[43]*
  inflammatory in vitreous H43.89
  kidney N28.89
  leukemic — *see* Leukemia
  liver K76.89
    fatty — *see* Fatty, liver NEC
    glycogen — *see also* Disease, glycogen storage E74.03 *[K77]*
  lung R91.8
    eosinophilic — *see* Eosinophilia, pulmonary
  lymphatic — *see also* Leukemia, lymphatic C91.9- ☑
    gland I88.9
  muscle, fatty M62.89
  myocardium, myocardial
    fatty — *see* Degeneration, myocardial
    glycogenic E74.02 *[43]*
  on chest x-ray R91.8
  pulmonary R91.8
    with eosinophilia — *see* Eosinophilia, pulmonary
  skin (lymphocytic) L98.6
  thymus (gland) (fatty) E32.8
  urine R39.0
  vesicant agent
    antineoplastic chemotherapy T80.810 ☑
    other agent NEC T80.818 ☑
  vitreous body H43.89
Infirmity R68.89
  senile R54
Inflammation, inflamed, inflammatory (with exudation)
  abducent (nerve) — *see* Strabismus, paralytic, sixth nerve
  accessory sinus (chronic) — *see* Sinusitis
  adrenal (gland) E27.8
  alveoli, teeth M27.3
    scorbutic E54
  anal canal, anus K62.89
  antrum (chronic) — *see* Sinusitis, maxillary
  appendix — *see* Appendicitis
  arachnoid — *see* Meningitis
  areola N61.0
    puerperal, postpartum or gestational — *see* Infection, nipple
  areolar tissue NOS L08.9
  artery — *see* Arteritis
  auditory meatus (external) — *see* Otitis, externa
  Bartholin's gland N75.8
  bile duct (common) (hepatic) or passage — *see* Cholangitis
  bladder — *see* Cystitis
  bone — *see* Osteomyelitis
  brain — *see also* Encephalitis
    membrane — *see* Meningitis
  breast N61.0
    puerperal, postpartum, gestational — *see* Mastitis, obstetric
  broad ligament — *see* Disease, pelvis, inflammatory
  bronchi — *see* Bronchitis
  catarrhal J00
  cecum — *see* Appendicitis
  cerebral — *see also* Encephalitis
    membrane — *see* Meningitis
  cerebrospinal
    meningococcal A39.0
  cervix (uteri) — *see* Cervicitis
  chest J98.8
  chorioretinal H30.9- ☑
    cyclitis — *see* Cyclitis
    disseminated H30.10- ☑
      generalized H30.13- ☑
      peripheral H30.12- ☑
      posterior pole H30.11- ☑
    epitheliopathy — *see* Epitheliopathy
    focal H30.00- ☑
      juxtapapillary H30.01- ☑

Inflammation, inflamed, inflammatory — *continued*
  chorioretinal — *continued*
    focal — *continued*
      macular H30.04- ☑
      paramacular — *see* Inflammation, chorioretinal, focal, macular
      peripheral H30.03- ☑
      posterior pole H30.02- ☑
    specified type NEC H30.89- ☑
  choroid — *see* Inflammation, chorioretinal
  chronic, postmastoidectomy cavity — *see* Complications, postmastoidectomy, inflammation
  colon — *see* Enteritis
  connective tissue (diffuse) NEC — *see* Disorder, soft tissue, specified type NEC
  cornea — *see* Keratitis
  corpora cavernosa N48.29
  cranial nerve — *see* Disorder, nerve, cranial
  Douglas' cul-de-sac or pouch (chronic) N73.0
  due to device, implant or graft — *see also* Complications, by site and type, infection or inflammation
    arterial graft T82.7 ☑
    breast (implant) T85.79 ☑
    catheter T85.79 ☑
      dialysis (renal) T82.7 ☑
        intraperitoneal T85.71 ☑
      infusion T82.7 ☑
        cranial T85.735 ☑
        intrathecal T85.735 ☑
        spinal (epidural) (subdural) T85.735 ☑
        subarachnoid T85.735 ☑
      urinary T83.518 ☑
        cystostomy T83.510 ☑
        Hopkins T83.518 ☑
        ileostomy T83.518 ☑
        nephrostomy T83.512 ☑
        specified NEC T83.518 ☑
        urethral indwelling T83.511 ☑
        urostomy T83.518 ☑
    electronic (electrode) (pulse generator) (stimulator)
      bone T84.7 ☑
      cardiac T82.7 ☑
      nervous system T85.738 ☑
        brain T85.731 ☑
        cranial nerve T85.732 ☑
        gastric nerve T85.732 ☑
        neurostimulator generator T85.734 ☑
        peripheral nerve T85.732 ☑
        sacral nerve T85.732 ☑
        spinal cord T85.733 ☑
        vagal nerve T85.732 ☑
      urinary T83.590 ☑
    fixation, internal (orthopedic) NEC — *see* Complication, fixation device, infection
    gastrointestinal (bile duct) (esophagus) T85.79 ☑
      neurostimulator electrode (lead) T85.732 ☑
    genital NEC T83.69 ☑
    heart NEC T82.7 ☑
      valve (prosthesis) T82.6 ☑
        graft T82.7 ☑
    joint prosthesis — *see* Complication, joint prosthesis, infection
    ocular (corneal graft) (orbital implant) NEC T85.79 ☑
    orthopedic NEC T84.7 ☑
    penile (cylinder) (pump) (reservoir) T83.61 ☑
    specified NEC T85.79 ☑
    testicular T83.62 ☑
    urinary NEC T83.598 ☑
      ileal conduit stent T83.593 ☑
      implanted neurostimulation T83.590 ☑
      implanted sphincter T83.591 ☑
      indwelling ureteral stent T83.592 ☑
      nephroureteral stent T83.593 ☑
      specified stent NEC T83.593 ☑
    vascular NEC T82.7 ☑
    ventricular intracranial (communicating) shunt T85.730 ☑
  duodenum K29.80
    with bleeding K29.81
  dura mater — *see* Meningitis
  ear (middle) — *see also* Otitis, media
    external — *see* Otitis, externa
    inner — *see* subcategory H83.0 ☑
  epididymis — *see* Epididymitis
  esophagus — *see* Esophagitis
  ethmoidal (sinus) (chronic) — *see* Sinusitis, ethmoidal

Inflammation, inflamed, inflammatory — *continued*
- eustachian tube (catarrhal) — *see* Salpingitis, eustachian
- eyelid H01.9
  - abscess — *see* Abscess, eyelid
  - blepharitis — *see* Blepharitis
  - chalazion — *see* Chalazion
  - dermatosis (noninfectious) — *see* Dermatosis, eyelid
  - hordeolum — *see* Hordeolum
  - specified NEC H01.8
- fallopian tube — *see* Salpingo-oophoritis
- fascia — *see* Myositis
- follicular, pharynx J31.2
- frontal (sinus) (chronic) — *see* Sinusitis, frontal
- gallbladder — *see* Cholecystitis
- gastric — *see* Gastritis
- gastrointestinal — *see* Enteritis
- genital organ (internal) (diffuse)
  - female — *see* Disease, pelvis, inflammatory
  - male N49.9
    - multiple sites N49.8
    - specified NEC N49.8
- gland (lymph) — *see* Lymphadenitis
- glottis — *see* Laryngitis
- granular, pharynx J31.2
- gum K05.10
  - nonplaque induced K05.11
  - plaque induced K05.10
- heart — *see* Carditis
- hepatic duct — *see* Cholangitis
- ileoanal (internal) pouch K91.850
- ileum — *see also* Enteritis
  - regional or terminal — *see* Enteritis, regional
- intestinal pouch K91.850
- intestine (any part) — *see* Enteritis
- jaw (acute) (bone) (chronic) (lower) (suppurative) (upper) M27.2
- joint NEC — *see* Arthritis
  - sacroiliac M46.1
- kidney — *see* Nephritis
- knee (joint) M13.169
  - tuberculous A18.02
- labium (majus) (minus) — *see* Vulvitis
- lacrimal
  - gland — *see* Dacryoadenitis
  - passages (duct) (sac) — *see also* Dacryocystitis
    - canaliculitis — *see* Canaliculitis, lacrimal
- larynx — *see* Laryngitis
- leg NOS L08.9
- lip K13.0
- liver (capsule) — *see also* Hepatitis
  - chronic K73.9
  - suppurative K75.0
- lung (acute) — *see also* Pneumonia
  - chronic J98.4
- lymph gland or node — *see* Lymphadenitis
- lymphatic vessel — *see* Lymphangitis
- maxilla, maxillary M27.2
  - sinus (chronic) — *see* Sinusitis, maxillary
- membranes of brain or spinal cord — *see* Meningitis
- meninges — *see* Meningitis
- mouth K12.1
- muscle — *see* Myositis
- myocardium — *see* Myocarditis
- nasal sinus (chronic) — *see* Sinusitis
- nasopharynx — *see* Nasopharyngitis
- navel L08.82
- nerve NEC — *see* Neuritis
- nipple N61.0
  - puerperal, postpartum or gestational — *see* Infection, nipple
- nose — *see* Rhinitis
- oculomotor (nerve) — *see* Strabismus, paralytic, third nerve
- optic nerve — *see* Neuritis, optic
- orbit (chronic) H05.10
  - acute H05.00
    - abscess — *see* Abscess, orbit
    - cellulitis — *see* Cellulitis, orbit
    - osteomyelitis — *see* Osteomyelitis, orbit
    - periostitis — *see* Periostitis, orbital
    - tenonitis — *see* Tenonitis, eye
  - granuloma — *see* Granuloma, orbit
  - myositis — *see* Myositis, orbital
- ovary — *see* Salpingo-oophoritis
- oviduct — *see* Salpingo-oophoritis
- pancreas (acute) — *see* Pancreatitis
- parametrium N73.0
- parotid region L08.9
- pelvis, female — *see* Disease, pelvis, inflammatory

Inflammation, inflamed, inflammatory — *continued*
- penis (corpora cavernosa) N48.29
- perianal K62.89
- pericardium — *see* Pericarditis
- perineum (female) (male) L08.9
- perirectal K62.89
- peritoneum — *see* Peritonitis
- periuterine — *see* Disease, pelvis, inflammatory
- perivesical — *see* Cystitis
- petrous bone (acute) (chronic) — *see* Petrositis
- pharynx (acute) — *see* Pharyngitis
- pia mater — *see* Meningitis
- pleura — *see* Pleurisy
- polyp, colon — *see also* Polyp, colon, inflammatory K51.40
- prostate — *see also* Prostatitis
  - specified type NEC N41.8
- rectosigmoid — *see* Rectosigmoiditis
- rectum — *see also* Proctitis K62.89
- respiratory, upper — *see also* Infection, respiratory, upper J06.9
  - acute, due to radiation J70.0
  - chronic, due to external agent — *see* condition, respiratory, chronic, due to
  - due to
    - chemicals, gases, fumes or vapors (inhalation) J68.2
    - radiation J70.1
- retina — *see* Chorioretinitis
- retrocecal — *see* Appendicitis
- retroperitoneal — *see* Peritonitis
- salivary duct or gland (any) (suppurative) — *see* Sialoadenitis
- scorbutic, alveoli, teeth E54
- scrotum N49.2
- seminal vesicle — *see* Vesiculitis
- sigmoid — *see* Enteritis
- sinus — *see* Sinusitis
- Skene's duct or gland — *see* Urethritis
- skin L08.9
- spermatic cord N49.1
- sphenoidal (sinus) — *see* Sinusitis, sphenoidal
- spinal
  - cord — *see* Encephalitis
  - membrane — *see* Meningitis
  - nerve — *see* Disorder, nerve
- spine — *see* Spondylopathy, inflammatory
- spleen (capsule) D73.89
- stomach — *see* Gastritis
- subcutaneous tissue L08.9
- suprarenal (gland) E27.8
- synovial — *see* Tenosynovitis
- tendon (sheath) NEC — *see* Tenosynovitis
- testis — *see* Orchitis
- throat (acute) — *see* Pharyngitis
- thymus (gland) E32.8
- thyroid (gland) — *see* Thyroiditis
- tongue K14.0
- tonsil — *see* Tonsillitis
- trachea — *see* Tracheitis
- trochlear (nerve) — *see* Strabismus, paralytic, fourth nerve
- tubal — *see* Salpingo-oophoritis
- tuberculous NEC — *see* Tuberculosis
- tubo-ovarian — *see* Salpingo-oophoritis
- tunica vaginalis N49.1
- tympanic membrane — *see* Tympanitis
- umbilicus, umbilical L08.82
- uterine ligament — *see* Disease, pelvis, inflammatory
- uterus (catarrhal) — *see* Endometritis
- uveal tract (anterior) NOS — *see also* Iridocyclitis
  - posterior — *see* Chorioretinitis
- vagina — *see* Vaginitis
- vas deferens N49.1
- vein — *see also* Phlebitis
  - intracranial or intraspinal (septic) G08
  - thrombotic I80.9
    - leg — *see* Phlebitis, leg
    - lower extremity — *see* Phlebitis, leg
- vocal cord J38.3
- vulva — *see* Vulvitis
- Wharton's duct (suppurative) — *see* Sialoadenitis

Inflation, lung, imperfect (newborn) — *see* Atelectasis
Influenza (bronchial) (epidemic) (respiratory (upper)) (unidentified influenza virus) J11.1
- with
  - digestive manifestations J11.2
  - encephalopathy J11.81
  - enteritis J11.2

Influenza — *continued*
- with — *continued*
  - gastroenteritis J11.2
  - gastrointestinal manifestations J11.2
  - laryngitis J11.1
  - myocarditis J11.82
  - otitis media J11.83
  - pharyngitis J11.1
  - pneumonia J11.00
    - specified type J11.08
  - respiratory manifestations NEC J11.1
  - specified manifestation NEC J11.89
- A (non-novel) J10- ☑
- A/H5N1 — *see also* Influenza, due to, identified novel influenza A virus J09.X2
- avian — *see also* Influenza, due to, identified novel influenza A virus J09.X2
- B J10- ☑
- bird — *see also* Influenza, due to, identified novel influenza A virus J09.X2
- C J10- ☑
- due to
  - avian — *see also* Influenza, due to, identified novel influenza A virus J09.X2
  - identified influenza virus NEC J10.1
    - with
      - digestive manifestations J10.2
      - encephalopathy J10.81
      - enteritis J10.2
      - gastroenteritis J10.2
      - gastrointestinal manifestations J10.2
      - laryngitis J10.1
      - myocarditis J10.82
      - otitis media J10.83
      - pharyngitis J10.1
      - pneumonia (unspecified type) J10.00
        - with same identified influenza virus J10.01
        - specified type NEC J10.08
      - respiratory manifestations NEC J10.1
      - specified manifestation NEC J10.89
  - identified novel influenza A virus J09.X2
    - with
      - digestive manifestations J09.X3
      - encephalopathy J09.X9
      - enteritis J09.X3
      - gastroenteritis J09.X3
      - gastrointestinal manifestations J09.X3
      - laryngitis J09.X2
      - myocarditis J09.X9
      - otitis media J09.X9
      - pharyngitis J09.X2
      - pneumonia J09.X1
      - respiratory manifestations NEC J09.X2
      - specified manifestation NEC J09.X9
      - upper respiratory symptoms J09.X2
  - novel (2009) H1N1 influenza — *see also* Influenza, due to, identified influenza virus NEC J10.1
  - novel influenza A/H1N1 — *see also* Influenza, due to, identified influenza virus NEC J10.1
  - of other animal origin, not bird or swine — *see also* Influenza, due to, identified novel influenza A virus J09.X2
  - swine (viruses that normally cause infections in pigs) — *see also* Influenza, due to, identified novel influenza A virus J09.X2
Influenzal — *see* Influenza
Influenza-like disease — *see* Influenza
Infraction, Freiberg's (metatarsal head) — *see* Osteochondrosis, juvenile, metatarsus
Infraeruption of tooth (teeth) M26.34
Infusion complication, misadventure, or reaction — *see* Complications, infusion
Ingestion
- chemical — *see* Table of Drugs and Chemicals, by substance, poisoning
- drug or medicament
  - correct substance properly administered — *see* Table of Drugs and Chemicals, by drug, adverse effect
  - overdose or wrong substance given or taken — *see* Table of Drugs and Chemicals, by drug, poisoning
- foreign body — *see* Foreign body, alimentary tract
- multiple drug — *see* Table of Drugs and Chemicals, multiple
- tularemia A21.3
Ingrowing
- hair (beard) L73.1
- nail (finger) (toe) L60.0
Inguinal — *see also* condition

☑ **Additional Character Required** — Refer to the Tabular List for Character Selection

Inguinal — *continued*
  testicle Q53.9
    bilateral Q53.212
    unilateral Q53.112
Inhalant-induced
  anxiety disorder F18.980
  depressive disorder F18.94
  major neurocognitive disorder F18.97
  mild neurocognitive disorder F18.988
  psychotic disorder F18.959
Inhalation
  anthrax A22.1
  flame T27.3
  food or foreign body — *see* Foreign body, by site
  gases, fumes, or vapors T59.9- ☑
    specified agent NEC — *see* Table of Drugs and Chemicals, by substance T59.89- ☑
  liquid or vomitus — *see* Asphyxia
  meconium (newborn) P24.00
    with
      with respiratory symptoms P24.01
      pneumonia (pneumonitis) P24.01
  mucus — *see* Asphyxia, mucus
  oil or gasoline (causing suffocation) — *see* Foreign body, by site
  smoke T59.81- ☑
    with respiratory conditions J70.5
      due to chemicals, gases, fumes and vapors J68.9
  steam — *see also* Burn, respiratory tract T59.9- ☑
  stomach contents or secretions — *see* Foreign body, by site
    due to anesthesia (general) (local) or other sedation T88.59 ☑
      in labor and delivery O74.0
      in pregnancy O29.01- ☑
      postpartum, puerperal O89.01
Inhibition, orgasm
  female F52.31
  male F52.32
Inhibitor, systemic lupus erythematosus (presence of) D68.62
Iniencephalus, iniencephaly Q00.2
Injection, traumatic jet (air) (industrial) (water) (paint or dye) T70.4 ☑
Injury — *see also* specified injury type T14.90 ☑
  abdomen, abdominal S39.91 ☑
    blood vessel — *see* Injury, blood vessel, abdomen
    cavity — *see* Injury, intra-abdominal
    contusion S30.1 ☑
    internal — *see* Injury, intra-abdominal
    intra-abdominal organ — *see* Injury, intra-abdominal
    nerve — *see* Injury, nerve, abdomen
    open — *see* Wound, open, abdomen
    specified NEC S39.81 ☑
    superficial — *see* Injury, superficial, abdomen
  Achilles tendon S86.00- ☑
    laceration S86.02- ☑
    specified type NEC S86.09- ☑
    strain S86.01- ☑
  acoustic, resulting in deafness — *see* Injury, nerve, acoustic
  adrenal (gland) S37.819 ☑
    contusion S37.812 ☑
    laceration S37.813 ☑
    specified type NEC S37.818 ☑
  alveolar (process) S09.93 ☑
  ankle S99.91- ☑
    contusion — *see* Contusion, ankle
    dislocation — *see* Dislocation, ankle
    fracture — *see* Fracture, ankle
    nerve — *see* Injury, nerve, ankle
    open — *see* Wound, open, ankle
    specified type NEC S99.81- ☑
    sprain — *see* Sprain, ankle
    superficial — *see* Injury, superficial, ankle
  anterior chamber, eye — *see* Injury, eye, specified site NEC
  anus — *see* Injury, abdomen
  aorta (thoracic) S25.00 ☑
    abdominal S35.00 ☑
      laceration (minor) (superficial) S35.01 ☑
        major S35.02 ☑
      specified type NEC S35.09 ☑
    laceration (minor) (superficial) S25.01 ☑
      major S25.02 ☑
    specified type NEC S25.09 ☑
  arm (upper) S49.9- ☑

Injury — *continued*
  arm — *continued*
    blood vessel — *see* Injury, blood vessel, arm
    contusion — *see* Contusion, arm, upper
    fracture — *see* Fracture, humerus
    lower — *see* Injury, forearm
    muscle — *see* Injury, muscle, shoulder
    nerve — *see* Injury, nerve, arm
    open — *see* Wound, open, arm
    specified type NEC S49.8- ☑
    superficial — *see* Injury, superficial, arm
  artery (complicating trauma) — *see also* Injury, blood vessel, by site
    cerebral or meningeal — *see* Injury, intracranial
  auditory canal (external) (meatus) S09.91 ☑
  auricle, auris, ear S09.91 ☑
  axilla — *see* Injury, shoulder
  back — *see* Injury, back, lower
  bile duct S36.13 ☑
  birth — *see also* Birth, injury P15.9
  bladder (sphincter) S37.20 ☑
    at delivery O71.5
    contusion S37.22 ☑
    laceration S37.23 ☑
    obstetrical trauma O71.5
    specified type NEC S37.29 ☑
  blast (air) (hydraulic) (immersion) (underwater) NEC T14.8 ☑
    acoustic nerve trauma — *see* Injury, nerve, acoustic
    bladder — *see* Injury, bladder
    brain — *see* Concussion
      primary, specified NEC S06.8A- ☑
    colon — *see* Injury, intestine, large
    ear (primary) S09.31- ☑
      secondary S09.39- ☑
    generalized T70.8 ☑
    lung — *see* Injury, intrathoracic, lung
    multiple body organs T70.8 ☑
    peritoneum S36.81 ☑
    rectum S36.61 ☑
    retroperitoneum S36.898 ☑
    small intestine S36.419 ☑
      duodenum S36.410 ☑
      specified site NEC S36.418 ☑
    specified
      intra-abdominal organ NEC S36.898 ☑
      pelvic organ NEC S37.899 ☑
  blood vessel NEC T14.8 ☑
    abdomen S35.9 ☑
      aorta — *see* Injury, aorta, abdominal
      celiac artery — *see* Injury, blood vessel, celiac artery
      iliac vessel — *see* Injury, blood vessel, iliac
      laceration S35.91 ☑
      mesenteric vessel — *see* Injury, mesenteric
      portal vein — *see* Injury, blood vessel, portal vein
      renal vessel — *see* Injury, blood vessel, renal
      specified vessel NEC S35.8X- ☑
      splenic vessel — *see* Injury, blood vessel, splenic
      vena cava — *see* Injury, vena cava, inferior
    ankle — *see* Injury, blood vessel, foot
    aorta (abdominal) (thoracic) — *see* Injury, aorta
    arm (upper) NEC S45.90- ☑
      forearm — *see* Injury, blood vessel, forearm
      laceration S45.91- ☑
      specified
        site NEC S45.80- ☑
          laceration S45.81- ☑
          specified type NEC S45.89- ☑
        type NEC S45.99- ☑
      superficial vein S45.30- ☑
        laceration S45.31- ☑
        specified type NEC S45.39- ☑
    axillary
      artery S45.00- ☑
        laceration S45.01- ☑
        specified type NEC S45.09- ☑
      vein S45.20- ☑
        laceration S45.21- ☑
        specified type NEC S45.29- ☑
    azygos vein — *see* Injury, blood vessel, thoracic, specified site NEC
    brachial
      artery S45.10- ☑
        laceration S45.11- ☑
        specified type NEC S45.19- ☑
      vein S45.20- ☑

Injury — *continued*
  blood vessel — *continued*
    brachial — *continued*
      vein — *continued*
        laceration S45.219 ☑
        specified type NEC S45.29- ☑
    carotid artery (common) (external) (internal, extracranial) S15.00- ☑
      internal, intracranial S06.8- ☑
      laceration (minor) (superficial) S15.01- ☑
        major S15.02- ☑
      specified type NEC S15.09- ☑
    celiac artery S35.219 ☑
      branch S35.299 ☑
        laceration (minor) (superficial) S35.291 ☑
          major S35.292 ☑
        specified NEC S35.298 ☑
      laceration (minor) (superficial) S35.211 ☑
        major S35.212 ☑
      specified type NEC S35.218 ☑
    cerebral — *see* Injury, intracranial
    deep plantar — *see* Injury, blood vessel, plantar artery
    digital (hand) — *see* Injury, blood vessel, finger
    dorsal
      artery (foot) S95.00- ☑
        laceration S95.01- ☑
        specified type NEC S95.09- ☑
      vein (foot) S95.20- ☑
        laceration S95.21- ☑
        specified type NEC S95.29- ☑
    due to accidental laceration during procedure — *see* Laceration, accidental complicating surgery
    extremity — *see* Injury, blood vessel, limb
    femoral
      artery (common) (superficial) S75.00- ☑
        laceration (minor) (superficial) S75.01- ☑
          major S75.02- ☑
        specified type NEC S75.09- ☑
      vein (hip level) (thigh level) S75.10- ☑
        laceration (minor) (superficial) S75.11- ☑
          major S75.12- ☑
        specified type NEC S75.19- ☑
    finger S65.50- ☑
      index S65.50- ☑
        laceration S65.51- ☑
        specified type NEC S65.59- ☑
      laceration S65.51- ☑
      little S65.50- ☑
        laceration S65.51- ☑
        specified type NEC S65.59- ☑
      middle S65.50- ☑
        laceration S65.51- ☑
        specified type NEC S65.59- ☑
      specified type NEC S65.59- ☑
      thumb — *see* Injury, blood vessel, thumb
    foot S95.90- ☑
      dorsal
        artery — *see* Injury, blood vessel, dorsal, artery
        vein — *see* Injury, blood vessel, dorsal, vein
      laceration S95.91- ☑
      plantar artery — *see* Injury, blood vessel, plantar artery
      specified
        site NEC S95.80- ☑
          laceration S95.81- ☑
          specified type NEC S95.89- ☑
        specified type NEC S95.99- ☑
    forearm S55.90- ☑
      laceration S55.91- ☑
      radial artery — *see* Injury, blood vessel, radial artery
      specified
        site NEC S55.80- ☑
          laceration S55.81- ☑
          specified type NEC S55.89- ☑
        type NEC S55.99- ☑
      ulnar artery — *see* Injury, blood vessel, ulnar artery
      vein S55.20- ☑
        laceration S55.21- ☑
        specified type NEC S55.29- ☑
    gastric
      artery — *see* Injury, mesenteric, artery, branch
      vein — *see* Injury, blood vessel, abdomen
    gastroduodenal artery — *see* Injury, mesenteric, artery, branch
    greater saphenous vein (lower leg level) S85.30- ☑

Injury — *continued*
  blood vessel — *continued*
    greater saphenous vein — *continued*
      hip (and thigh) level S75.20- ☑
        laceration (minor) (superficial) S75.21- ☑
          major S75.22- ☑
        specified type NEC S75.29- ☑
      laceration S85.31- ☑
      specified type NEC S85.39- ☑
    hand (level) S65.90- ☑
      finger — *see* Injury, blood vessel, finger
      laceration S65.91- ☑
      palmar arch — *see* Injury, blood vessel, palmar arch
      radial artery — *see* Injury, blood vessel, radial artery, hand
      specified
        site NEC S65.80- ☑
          laceration S65.81- ☑
          specified type NEC S65.89- ☑
        type NEC S65.99- ☑
      thumb — *see* Injury, blood vessel, thumb
      ulnar artery — *see* Injury, blood vessel, ulnar artery, hand
    head S09.0 ☑
      intracranial — *see* Injury, intracranial
      multiple S09.0 ☑
    hepatic
      artery — *see* Injury, mesenteric, artery
      vein — *see* Injury, vena cava, inferior
    hip S75.90- ☑
      femoral artery — *see* Injury, blood vessel, femoral, artery
      femoral vein — *see* Injury, blood vessel, femoral, vein
      greater saphenous vein — *see* Injury, blood vessel, greater saphenous, hip level
      laceration S75.91- ☑
      specified
        site NEC S75.80- ☑
          laceration S75.81- ☑
          specified type NEC S75.89- ☑
        type NEC S75.99- ☑
    hypogastric (artery) (vein) — *see* Injury, blood vessel, iliac
    iliac S35.5- ☑
      artery S35.51- ☑
      specified vessel NEC S35.5- ☑
      uterine vessel — *see* Injury, blood vessel, uterine
      vein S35.51- ☑
    innominate — *see* Injury, blood vessel, thoracic, innominate
    intercostal (artery) (vein) — *see* Injury, blood vessel, thoracic, intercostal
    jugular vein (external) S15.20- ☑
      internal S15.30- ☑
        laceration (minor) (superficial) S15.31- ☑
          major S15.32- ☑
        specified type NEC S15.39- ☑
      laceration (minor) (superficial) S15.21- ☑
        major S15.22- ☑
      specified type NEC S15.29- ☑
    leg (level) (lower) S85.90- ☑
      greater saphenous — *see* Injury, blood vessel, greater saphenous
      laceration S85.91- ☑
      lesser saphenous — *see* Injury, blood vessel, lesser saphenous
      peroneal artery — *see* Injury, blood vessel, peroneal artery
      popliteal
        artery — *see* Injury, blood vessel, popliteal, artery
        vein — *see* Injury, blood vessel, popliteal, vein
      specified
        site NEC S85.80- ☑
          laceration S85.81- ☑
          specified type NEC S85.89- ☑
        type NEC S85.99- ☑
      thigh — *see* Injury, blood vessel, hip
      tibial artery — *see* Injury, blood vessel, tibial artery
    lesser saphenous vein (lower leg level) S85.40- ☑
      laceration S85.41- ☑
      specified type NEC S85.49- ☑
    limb
      lower — *see* Injury, blood vessel, leg
      upper — *see* Injury, blood vessel, arm

Injury — *continued*
  blood vessel — *continued*
    lower back — *see* Injury, blood vessel, abdomen
      specified NEC — *see* Injury, blood vessel, abdomen, specified, site NEC
    mammary (artery) (vein) — *see* Injury, blood vessel, thoracic, specified site NEC
    mesenteric (inferior) (superior)
      artery — *see* Injury, mesenteric, artery
      vein — *see* Injury, blood vessel, mesenteric, vein
    neck S15.9 ☑
      specified site NEC S15.8 ☑
    ovarian (artery) (vein) — *see* subcategory S35.8 ☑
    palmar arch (superficial) S65.20- ☑
      deep S65.30- ☑
        laceration S65.31- ☑
        specified type NEC S65.39- ☑
      laceration S65.21- ☑
      specified type NEC S65.29- ☑
    pelvis — *see* Injury, blood vessel, abdomen
      specified NEC — *see* Injury, blood vessel, abdomen, specified, site NEC
    peroneal artery S85.20- ☑
      laceration S85.21- ☑
      specified type NEC S85.29- ☑
    plantar artery (deep) (foot) S95.10- ☑
      laceration S95.11- ☑
      specified type NEC S95.19- ☑
    popliteal
      artery S85.00- ☑
        laceration S85.01- ☑
        specified type NEC S85.09- ☑
      vein S85.50- ☑
        laceration S85.51- ☑
        specified type NEC S85.59- ☑
    portal vein S35.319 ☑
      laceration S35.311 ☑
      specified type NEC S35.318 ☑
    precerebral — *see* Injury, blood vessel, neck
    pulmonary (artery) (vein) — *see* Injury, blood vessel, thoracic, pulmonary
    radial artery (forearm level) S55.10- ☑
      hand and wrist (level) S65.10- ☑
        laceration S65.11- ☑
        specified type NEC S65.19- ☑
      laceration S55.11- ☑
      specified type NEC S55.19- ☑
    renal
      artery S35.40- ☑
        laceration S35.41- ☑
        specified NEC S35.49- ☑
      vein S35.40- ☑
        laceration S35.41- ☑
        specified NEC S35.49- ☑
    saphenous vein (greater) (lower leg level) — *see* Injury, blood vessel, greater saphenous
      hip and thigh level — *see* Injury, blood vessel, greater saphenous, hip level
      lesser — *see* Injury, blood vessel, lesser saphenous
    shoulder
      specified NEC — *see* Injury, blood vessel, arm, specified site NEC
      superficial vein — *see* Injury, blood vessel, arm, superficial vein
    specified NEC T14.8 ☑
    splenic
      artery — *see* Injury, blood vessel, celiac artery, branch
      vein S35.329 ☑
        laceration S35.321 ☑
        specified NEC S35.328 ☑
    subclavian — *see* Injury, blood vessel, thoracic, innominate
    thigh — *see* Injury, blood vessel, hip
    thoracic S25.90 ☑
      aorta S25.00 ☑
        laceration (minor) (superficial) S25.01 ☑
          major S25.02 ☑
        specified type NEC S25.09 ☑
      azygos vein — *see* Injury, blood vessel, thoracic, specified, site NEC
      innominate
        artery S25.10- ☑
          laceration (minor) (superficial) S25.11- ☑
            major S25.12- ☑
          specified type NEC S25.19- ☑

Injury — *continued*
  blood vessel — *continued*
    thoracic — *continued*
      innominate — *continued*
        vein S25.30- ☑
          laceration (minor) (superficial) S25.31- ☑
            major S25.32- ☑
          specified type NEC S25.39- ☑
      intercostal S25.50- ☑
        laceration S25.51- ☑
        specified type NEC S25.59- ☑
      laceration S25.91 ☑
      mammary vessel — *see* Injury, blood vessel, thoracic, specified, site NEC
      pulmonary S25.40- ☑
        laceration (minor) (superficial) S25.41- ☑
          major S25.42- ☑
        specified type NEC S25.49- ☑
      specified
        site NEC S25.80- ☑
          laceration S25.81 ☑
          specified type NEC S25.89 ☑
        type NEC S25.99 ☑
      subclavian — *see* Injury, blood vessel, thoracic, innominate
      vena cava (superior) S25.20 ☑
        laceration (minor) (superficial) S25.21 ☑
          major S25.22 ☑
        specified type NEC S25.29 ☑
    thumb S65.40- ☑
      laceration S65.41- ☑
      specified type NEC S65.49- ☑
    tibial artery S85.10- ☑
      anterior S85.13- ☑
        laceration S85.14- ☑
        specified injury NEC S85.15- ☑
      laceration S85.11- ☑
      posterior S85.16- ☑
        laceration S85.17- ☑
        specified injury NEC S85.18- ☑
      specified injury NEC S85.12- ☑
    ulnar artery (forearm level) S55.00- ☑
      hand and wrist (level) S65.00- ☑
        laceration S65.01- ☑
        specified type NEC S65.09- ☑
      laceration S55.01- ☑
      specified type NEC S55.09- ☑
    upper arm (level) — *see* Injury, blood vessel, arm
      superficial vein — *see* Injury, blood vessel, arm, superficial vein
    uterine S35.5- ☑
      artery S35.53- ☑
      vein S35.53- ☑
    vena cava — *see* Injury, vena cava
    vertebral artery S15.10- ☑
      laceration (minor) (superficial) S15.11- ☑
        major S15.12- ☑
      specified type NEC S15.19- ☑
    wrist (level) — *see* Injury, blood vessel, hand
  brachial plexus S14.3 ☑
    newborn P14.3
  brain (traumatic) S06.9- ☑
    diffuse (axonal) S06.2X- ☑
    focal S06.30- ☑
  brainstem S06.38- ☑
  breast NOS S29.9 ☑
  broad ligament — *see* Injury, pelvic organ, specified site NEC
  bronchus, bronchi — *see* Injury, intrathoracic, bronchus
  brow S09.90 ☑
  buttock S39.92 ☑
  canthus, eye S05.90 ☑
  cardiac plexus — *see* Injury, nerve, thorax, sympathetic
  cauda equina S34.3 ☑
  cavernous sinus — *see* Injury, intracranial
  cecum — *see* Injury, colon
  celiac ganglion or plexus — *see* Injury, nerve, lumbosacral, sympathetic
  cerebellum — *see* Injury, intracranial
  cerebral — *see* Injury, intracranial
  cervix (uteri) — *see* Injury, uterus
  cheek (wall) S09.93 ☑
  chest — *see* Injury, thorax
  childbirth (newborn) — *see also* Birth, injury
    maternal NEC O71.9
  chin S09.93 ☑

☑ **Additional Character Required** — **Refer to the Tabular List for Character Selection**

Injury — *continued*
 choroid (eye) — *see* Injury, eye, specified site NEC
 clitoris S39.94 ☑
 coccyx — *see also* Injury, back, lower
  complicating delivery O71.6
 colon — *see* Injury, intestine, large
 common bile duct — *see* Injury, liver
 conjunctiva (superficial) — *see* Injury, eye, conjunctiva
 conus medullaris — *see* Injury, spinal, sacral
 cord
  spermatic (pelvic region) S37.898 ☑
   scrotal region S39.848 ☑
  spinal — *see* Injury, spinal cord, by region
 cornea — *see* Injury, eye, specified site NEC
  abrasion — *see* Injury, eye, cornea, abrasion
 cortex (cerebral) — *see also* Injury, intracranial
  visual — *see* Injury, nerve, optic
 costal region NEC S29.9 ☑
 costochondral NEC S29.9 ☑
 cranial
  cavity — *see* Injury, intracranial
  nerve — *see* Injury, nerve, cranial
 crushing — *see* Crush
 cutaneous sensory nerve
 cystic duct — *see* Injury, liver
 deep tissue — *see* Contusion, by site
  meaning pressure ulcer — *see* Ulcer, pressure L89
   with final character .6
 delivery (newborn) P15.9
  maternal NEC O71.9
 Descemet's membrane — *see* Injury, eyeball, penetrating
 diaphragm — *see* Injury, intrathoracic, diaphragm
 duodenum — *see* Injury, intestine, small, duodenum
 ear (auricle) (external) (canal) S09.91 ☑
  abrasion — *see* Abrasion, ear
  bite — *see* Bite, ear
  blister — *see* Blister, ear
  bruise — *see* Contusion, ear
  contusion — *see* Contusion, ear
  external constriction — *see* Constriction, external, ear
  hematoma — *see* Hematoma, ear
  inner — *see* Injury, ear, middle
  laceration — *see* Laceration, ear
  middle S09.30- ☑
   blast — *see* Injury, blast, ear
   specified NEC S09.39- ☑
  puncture — *see* Puncture, ear
  superficial — *see* Injury, superficial, ear
 eighth cranial nerve (acoustic or auditory) — *see* Injury, nerve, acoustic
 elbow S59.90- ☑
  contusion — *see* Contusion, elbow
  dislocation — *see* Dislocation, elbow
  fracture — *see* Fracture, ulna, upper end
  open — *see* Wound, open, elbow
  specified NEC S59.80- ☑
  sprain — *see* Sprain, elbow
  superficial — *see* Injury, superficial, elbow
 eleventh cranial nerve (accessory) — *see* Injury, nerve, accessory
 epididymis S39.94 ☑
 epigastric region S39.91 ☑
 epiglottis NEC S19.89 ☑
 esophageal plexus — *see* Injury, nerve, thorax, sympathetic
 esophagus (thoracic part) — *see also* Injury, intrathoracic, esophagus
  cervical NEC S19.85 ☑
 eustachian tube S09.30 ☑
 eye S05.9- ☑
  avulsion S05.7- ☑
  ball — *see* Injury, eyeball
  conjunctiva S05.0- ☑
  cornea
   abrasion S05.0- ☑
  laceration S05.3- ☑
   with prolapse S05.2- ☑
  lacrimal apparatus S05.8X- ☑
  orbit penetration S05.4- ☑
  specified site NEC S05.8X- ☑
 eyeball S05.8X- ☑
  contusion S05.1- ☑
  penetrating S05.6- ☑
   with
    foreign body S05.5- ☑
    prolapse or loss of intraocular tissue S05.2- ☑

Injury — *continued*
 eyeball — *continued*
  penetrating — *continued*
   without prolapse or loss of intraocular tissue S05.3- ☑
  specified type NEC S05.8- ☑
 eyebrow S09.93 ☑
 eyelid S09.93 ☑
  abrasion — *see* Abrasion, eyelid
  contusion — *see* Contusion, eyelid
  open — *see* Wound, open, eyelid
 face S09.93 ☑
 fallopian tube S37.509 ☑
  bilateral S37.502 ☑
   blast injury S37.512 ☑
   contusion S37.522 ☑
   laceration S37.532 ☑
   specified type NEC S37.592 ☑
  blast injury (primary) S37.519 ☑
   bilateral S37.512 ☑
   secondary — *see* Injury, fallopian tube, specified type NEC
   unilateral S37.511 ☑
  contusion S37.529 ☑
   bilateral S37.522 ☑
   unilateral S37.521 ☑
  laceration S37.539 ☑
   bilateral S37.532 ☑
   unilateral S37.531 ☑
  specified type NEC S37.599 ☑
   bilateral S37.592 ☑
   unilateral S37.591 ☑
  unilateral S37.501 ☑
   blast injury S37.511 ☑
   contusion S37.521 ☑
   laceration S37.531 ☑
   specified type NEC S37.591 ☑
 fascia — *see* Injury, muscle
 fifth cranial nerve (trigeminal) — *see* Injury, nerve, trigeminal
 finger (nail) S69.9- ☑
  blood vessel — *see* Injury, blood vessel, finger
  contusion — *see* Contusion, finger
  dislocation — *see* Dislocation, finger
  fracture — *see* Fracture, finger
  muscle — *see* Injury, muscle, finger
  nerve — *see* Injury, nerve, digital, finger
  open — *see* Wound, open, finger
  specified NEC S69.8- ☑
  sprain — *see* Sprain, finger
  superficial — *see* Injury, superficial, finger
 first cranial nerve (olfactory) — *see* Injury, nerve, olfactory
 flank — *see* Injury, abdomen
 foot S99.92- ☑
  blood vessel — *see* Injury, blood vessel, foot
  contusion — *see* Contusion, foot
  dislocation — *see* Dislocation, foot
  fracture — *see* Fracture, foot
  muscle — *see* Injury, muscle, foot
  open — *see* Wound, open, foot
  specified type NEC S99.82- ☑
  sprain — *see* Sprain, foot
  superficial — *see* Injury, superficial, foot
 forceps NOS P15.9
 forearm S59.91- ☑
  blood vessel — *see* Injury, blood vessel, forearm
  contusion — *see* Contusion, forearm
  fracture — *see* Fracture, forearm
  muscle — *see* Injury, muscle, forearm
  nerve — *see* Injury, nerve, forearm
  open — *see* Wound, open, forearm
  specified NEC S59.81- ☑
  superficial — *see* Injury, superficial, forearm
 forehead S09.90 ☑
 fourth cranial nerve (trochlear) — *see* Injury, nerve, trochlear
 gallbladder S36.129 ☑
  contusion S36.122 ☑
  laceration S36.123 ☑
  specified NEC S36.128 ☑
 ganglion
  celiac, coeliac — *see* Injury, nerve, lumbosacral, sympathetic
  gasserian — *see* Injury, nerve, trigeminal
  stellate — *see* Injury, nerve, thorax, sympathetic
  thoracic sympathetic — *see* Injury, nerve, thorax, sympathetic

Injury — *continued*
 gasserian ganglion — *see* Injury, nerve, trigeminal
 gastric artery — *see* Injury, blood vessel, celiac artery, branch
 gastroduodenal artery — *see* Injury, blood vessel, celiac artery, branch
 gastrointestinal tract — *see* Injury, intra-abdominal
  with open wound into abdominal cavity — *see* Wound, open, with penetration into peritoneal cavity
  colon — *see* Injury, intestine, large
  rectum — *see* Injury, intestine, large, rectum
   with open wound into abdominal cavity S36.61 ☑
  small intestine — *see* Injury, intestine, small
  specified site NEC — *see* Injury, intra-abdominal, specified, site NEC
  stomach — *see* Injury, stomach
 genital organ(s)
  external S39.94 ☑
   specified NEC S39.848 ☑
  internal S37.90 ☑
   fallopian tube — *see* Injury, fallopian tube
   ovary — *see* Injury, ovary
   prostate — *see* Injury, prostate
   seminal vesicle — *see* Injury, pelvis, organ, specified site NEC
   uterus — *see* Injury, uterus
   vas deferens — *see* Injury, pelvis, organ, specified site NEC
  obstetrical trauma O71.9
 gland
  lacrimal laceration — *see* Injury, eye, specified site NEC
  salivary S09.93 ☑
  thyroid NEC S19.84 ☑
 globe (eye) S05.90 ☑
  specified NEC S05.8X- ☑
 groin — *see* Injury, abdomen
 gum S09.90 ☑
 hand S69.9- ☑
  blood vessel — *see* Injury, blood vessel, hand
  contusion — *see* Contusion, hand
  fracture — *see* Fracture, hand
  muscle — *see* Injury, muscle, hand
  nerve — *see* Injury, nerve, hand
  open — *see* Wound, open, hand
  specified NEC S69.8- ☑
  sprain — *see* Sprain, hand
  superficial — *see* Injury, superficial, hand
 head S09.90 ☑
  with loss of consciousness S06.9- ☑
  specified NEC S09.8 ☑
 heart (traumatic) S26.90 ☑
  with hemopericardium S26.00 ☑
   contusion S26.01 ☑
   laceration (mild) S26.020 ☑
    major S26.022 ☑
    moderate S26.021 ☑
   specified type NEC S26.09 ☑
  contusion S26.91 ☑
  laceration S26.92 ☑
  non-traumatic (acute) (chronic) (non-ischemic) I5A
  specified type NEC S26.99 ☑
  without hemopericardium S26.10 ☑
   contusion S26.11 ☑
   laceration S26.12 ☑
   specified type NEC S26.19 ☑
 heel — *see* Injury, foot
 hepatic
  artery — *see* Injury, blood vessel, celiac artery, branch
  duct — *see* Injury, liver
  vein — *see* Injury, vena cava, inferior
 hip S79.91- ☑
  blood vessel — *see* Injury, blood vessel, hip
  contusion — *see* Contusion, hip
  dislocation — *see* Dislocation, hip
  fracture — *see* Fracture, femur, neck
  muscle — *see* Injury, muscle, hip
  nerve — *see* Injury, nerve, hip
  open — *see* Wound, open, hip
  specified NEC S79.81- ☑
  sprain — *see* Sprain, hip
  superficial — *see* Injury, superficial, hip
 hymen S39.94 ☑
 hypogastric
  blood vessel — *see* Injury, blood vessel, iliac
  plexus — *see* Injury, nerve, lumbosacral, sympathetic

Injury — *continued*
  ileum — *see* Injury, intestine, small
  iliac region S39.91 ☑
  instrumental (during surgery) — *see* Laceration, accidental complicating surgery
    birth injury — *see* Birth, injury
    nonsurgical — *see* Injury, by site
    obstetrical O71.9
      bladder O71.5
      cervix O71.3
      high vaginal O71.4
      perineal NOS O70.9
      urethra O71.5
      uterus O71.5
        with rupture or perforation O71.1
  internal T14.8 ☑
    aorta — *see* Injury, aorta
    bladder (sphincter) — *see* Injury, bladder
      with
        ectopic or molar pregnancy O08.6
      following ectopic or molar pregnancy O08.6
      obstetrical trauma O71.5
    bronchus, bronchi — *see* Injury, intrathoracic, bronchus
    cecum — *see* Injury, intestine, large
    cervix (uteri) — *see also* Injury, uterus
      with ectopic or molar pregnancy O08.6
      following ectopic or molar pregnancy O08.6
      obstetrical trauma O71.3
    chest — *see* Injury, intrathoracic
    gastrointestinal tract — *see* Injury, intra-abdominal
    heart — *see* Injury, heart
    intestine NEC — *see* Injury, intestine
    intrauterine — *see* Injury, uterus
    mesentery — *see* Injury, intra-abdominal, specified, site NEC
    pelvis, pelvic (organ) S37.90 ☑
      following ectopic or molar pregnancy (subsequent episode) O08.6
      obstetrical trauma NEC O71.5
        rupture or perforation O71.1
      specified NEC S39.83 ☑
    rectum — *see* Injury, intestine, large, rectum
    stomach — *see* Injury, stomach
    ureter — *see* Injury, ureter
    urethra (sphincter) following ectopic or molar pregnancy O08.6
    uterus — *see* Injury, uterus
  interscapular area — *see* Injury, thorax
  intestine
    large S36.509 ☑
      ascending (right) S36.500 ☑
        blast injury (primary) S36.510 ☑
          secondary S36.590 ☑
        contusion S36.520 ☑
        laceration S36.530 ☑
        specified type NEC S36.590 ☑
      blast injury (primary) S36.519 ☑
        ascending (right) S36.510 ☑
        descending (left) S36.512 ☑
        rectum S36.61 ☑
        sigmoid S36.513 ☑
        specified site NEC S36.518 ☑
        transverse S36.511 ☑
      contusion S36.529 ☑
        ascending (right) S36.520 ☑
        descending (left) S36.522 ☑
        rectum S36.62 ☑
        sigmoid S36.523 ☑
        specified site NEC S36.528 ☑
        transverse S36.521 ☑
      descending (left) S36.502 ☑
        blast injury (primary) S36.512 ☑
          secondary S36.592 ☑
        contusion S36.522 ☑
        laceration S36.532 ☑
        specified type NEC S36.592 ☑
      laceration S36.539 ☑
        ascending (right) S36.530 ☑
        descending (left) S36.532 ☑
        rectum S36.63 ☑
        sigmoid S36.533 ☑
        specified site NEC S36.538 ☑
        transverse S36.531 ☑
      rectum S36.60 ☑
        blast injury (primary) S36.61 ☑
          secondary S36.69 ☑

Injury — *continued*
  intestine — *continued*
    large — *continued*
      rectum — *continued*
        contusion S36.62 ☑
        laceration S36.63 ☑
        specified type NEC S36.69 ☑
      sigmoid S36.503 ☑
        blast injury (primary) S36.513 ☑
          secondary S36.593 ☑
        contusion S36.523 ☑
        laceration S36.533 ☑
        specified type NEC S36.593 ☑
      specified
        site NEC S36.508 ☑
          blast injury (primary) S36.518 ☑
            secondary S36.598 ☑
          contusion S36.528 ☑
          laceration S36.538 ☑
          specified type NEC S36.598 ☑
        type NEC S36.599 ☑
          ascending (right) S36.590 ☑
          descending (left) S36.592 ☑
          rectum S36.69 ☑
          sigmoid S36.593 ☑
          specified site NEC S36.598 ☑
          transverse S36.591 ☑
      transverse S36.501 ☑
        blast injury (primary) S36.511 ☑
          secondary S36.591 ☑
        contusion S36.521 ☑
        laceration S36.531 ☑
        specified type NEC S36.591 ☑
    small S36.409 ☑
      blast injury (primary) S36.419 ☑
        duodenum S36.410 ☑
        secondary S36.499 ☑
          duodenum S36.490 ☑
          specified site NEC S36.498 ☑
        specified site NEC S36.418 ☑
      contusion S36.429 ☑
        duodenum S36.420 ☑
        specified site NEC S36.428 ☑
      duodenum S36.400 ☑
        blast injury (primary) S36.410 ☑
          secondary S36.490 ☑
        contusion S36.420 ☑
        laceration S36.430 ☑
        specified NEC S36.490 ☑
      laceration S36.439 ☑
        duodenum S36.430 ☑
        specified site NEC S36.438 ☑
      specified
        site NEC S36.408 ☑
        type NEC S36.499 ☑
          duodenum S36.490 ☑
          specified site NEC S36.498 ☑
    intra-abdominal S36.90 ☑
      adrenal gland — *see* Injury, adrenal gland
      bladder — *see* Injury, bladder
      colon — *see* Injury, intestine, large
      contusion S36.92 ☑
      fallopian tube — *see* Injury, fallopian tube
      gallbladder — *see* Injury, gallbladder
      intestine — *see* Injury, intestine
      kidney — *see* Injury, kidney
      laceration S36.93 ☑
      liver — *see* Injury, liver
      ovary — *see* Injury, ovary
      pancreas — *see* Injury, pancreas
      pelvic NOS S37.90 ☑
      peritoneum — *see* Injury, intra-abdominal, specified, site NEC
      prostate — *see* Injury, prostate
      rectum — *see* Injury, intestine, large, rectum
      retroperitoneum — *see* Injury, intra-abdominal, specified, site NEC
      seminal vesicle — *see* Injury, pelvis, organ, specified site NEC
      small intestine — *see* Injury, intestine, small
      specified
        pelvic S37.90 ☑
        specified
          site NEC S37.899 ☑
            specified type NEC S37.898 ☑
          type NEC S37.99 ☑

Injury — *continued*
  intra-abdominal — *continued*
    specified — *continued*
      site NEC S36.899 ☑
        contusion S36.892 ☑
        laceration S36.893 ☑
        specified type NEC S36.898 ☑
      type NEC S36.99 ☑
    spleen — *see* Injury, spleen
    stomach — *see* Injury, stomach
    ureter — *see* Injury, ureter
    urethra — *see* Injury, urethra
    uterus — *see* Injury, uterus
    vas deferens — *see* Injury, pelvis, organ, specified site NEC
  intracranial (traumatic) — *see also* if applicable, Compression, brain, traumatic S06.9- ☑
    cerebellar hemorrhage, traumatic — *see* Injury, intracranial, focal
    cerebral edema, traumatic S06.1X- ☑
      diffuse S06.1X- ☑
      focal S06.1X- ☑
    diffuse (axonal) S06.2X- ☑
    epidural hemorrhage (traumatic) S06.4X- ☑
    focal brain injury S06.30- ☑
      contusion — *see* Contusion, cerebral
      laceration — *see* Laceration, cerebral
      intracerebral hemorrhage, traumatic S06.36- ☑
        left side S06.35- ☑
        right side S06.34- ☑
      specified NEC S06.89- ☑
    subarachnoid hemorrhage, traumatic S06.6X- ☑
    subdural hemorrhage, traumatic S06.5X- ☑
  intraocular — *see* Injury, eyeball, penetrating
  intrathoracic S27.9 ☑
    bronchus S27.409 ☑
      bilateral S27.402 ☑
      blast injury (primary) S27.419 ☑
        bilateral S27.412 ☑
        secondary — *see* Injury, intrathoracic, bronchus, specified type NEC
        unilateral S27.411 ☑
      contusion S27.429 ☑
        bilateral S27.422 ☑
        unilateral S27.421 ☑
      laceration S27.439 ☑
        bilateral S27.432 ☑
        unilateral S27.431 ☑
      specified type NEC S27.499 ☑
        bilateral S27.492 ☑
        unilateral S27.491 ☑
      unilateral S27.401 ☑
    diaphragm S27.809 ☑
      contusion S27.802 ☑
      laceration S27.803 ☑
      specified type NEC S27.808 ☑
    esophagus (thoracic) S27.819 ☑
      contusion S27.812 ☑
      laceration S27.813 ☑
      specified type NEC S27.818 ☑
    heart — *see* Injury, heart
    hemopneumothorax S27.2 ☑
    hemothorax S27.1 ☑
    lung S27.309 ☑
      aspiration J69.0
      bilateral S27.302 ☑
      blast injury (primary) S27.319 ☑
        bilateral S27.312 ☑
        secondary — *see* Injury, intrathoracic, lung, specified type NEC
        unilateral S27.311 ☑
      contusion S27.329 ☑
        bilateral S27.322 ☑
        unilateral S27.321 ☑
      laceration S27.339 ☑
        bilateral S27.332 ☑
        unilateral S27.331 ☑
      specified type NEC S27.399 ☑
        bilateral S27.392 ☑
        unilateral S27.391 ☑
      unilateral S27.301 ☑
    pleura S27.60 ☑
      laceration S27.63 ☑
      specified type NEC S27.69 ☑
    pneumothorax S27.0 ☑
    specified organ NEC S27.899 ☑

Injury — *continued*
 intrathoracic — *continued*
  specified organ — *continued*
   contusion S27.892 ☑
   laceration S27.893 ☑
   specified type NEC S27.898 ☑
  thoracic duct — *see* Injury, intrathoracic, specified organ NEC
  thymus gland — *see* Injury, intrathoracic, specified organ NEC
  trachea, thoracic S27.50 ☑
   blast (primary) S27.51 ☑
   contusion S27.52 ☑
   laceration S27.53 ☑
   specified type NEC S27.59 ☑
 iris — *see* Injury, eye, specified site NEC
  penetrating — *see* Injury, eyeball, penetrating
 jaw S09.93 ☑
 jejunum — *see* Injury, intestine, small
 joint NOS T14.8 ☑
  old or residual — *see* Disorder, joint, specified type NEC
 kidney S37.00- ☑
  acute (nontraumatic) N17.9
  contusion — *see* Contusion, kidney
  laceration — *see* Laceration, kidney
  specified NEC S37.09- ☑
 knee S89.9- ☑
  contusion — *see* Contusion, knee
  dislocation — *see* Dislocation, knee
  meniscus (lateral) (medial) — *see* Sprain, knee, specified site NEC
   old injury or tear — *see* Derangement, knee, meniscus, due to old injury
  open — *see* Wound, open, knee
  specified NEC S89.8- ☑
  sprain — *see* Sprain, knee
  superficial — *see* Injury, superficial, knee
 labium (majus) (minus) S39.94 ☑
 labyrinth, ear S09.30- ☑
 lacrimal apparatus, duct, gland, or sac — *see* Injury, eye, specified site NEC
 larynx NEC S19.81 ☑
 leg (lower) S89.9- ☑
  blood vessel — *see* Injury, blood vessel, leg
  contusion — *see* Contusion, leg
  fracture — *see* Fracture, leg
  muscle — *see* Injury, muscle, leg
  nerve — *see* Injury, nerve, leg
  open — *see* Wound, open, leg
  specified NEC S89.8- ☑
  superficial — *see* Injury, superficial, leg
 lens, eye — *see* Injury, eye, specified site NEC
  penetrating — *see* Injury, eyeball, penetrating
 limb NEC T14.8 ☑
 lip S09.93 ☑
 liver S36.119 ☑
  contusion S36.112 ☑
  laceration S36.113 ☑
   major (stellate) S36.116 ☑
   minor S36.114 ☑
   moderate S36.115 ☑
  specified NEC S36.118 ☑
 lower back S39.92 ☑
  specified NEC S39.82 ☑
 lumbar, lumbosacral (region) S39.92 ☑
  plexus — *see* Injury, lumbosacral plexus
 lumbosacral plexus S34.4 ☑
 lung — *see also* Injury, intrathoracic, lung
  aspiration J69.0
  dabbing (related) U07.0
  electronic cigarette (related) U07.0
  EVALI - [e-cigarette, or vaping, product use associated] U07.0
  transfusion-related (TRALI) J95.84
  vaping (associated) (device) (product) (use) U07.0
 lymphatic thoracic duct — *see* Injury, intrathoracic, specified organ NEC
 malar region S09.93 ☑
 mastoid region S09.90 ☑
 maxilla S09.93 ☑
 mediastinum — *see* Injury, intrathoracic, specified organ NEC
 membrane, brain — *see* Injury, intracranial
 meningeal artery — *see* Injury, intracranial, subdural hemorrhage
 meninges (cerebral) — *see* Injury, intracranial

Injury — *continued*
 mesenteric
  artery
   branch S35.299 ☑
    laceration (minor) (superficial) S35.291 ☑
     major S35.292 ☑
    specified NEC S35.298 ☑
   inferior S35.239 ☑
    laceration (minor) (superficial) S35.231 ☑
     major S35.232 ☑
    specified NEC S35.238 ☑
   superior S35.229 ☑
    laceration (minor) (superficial) S35.221 ☑
     major S35.222 ☑
    specified NEC S35.228 ☑
   plexus (inferior) (superior) — *see* Injury, nerve, lumbosacral, sympathetic
  vein
   inferior S35.349 ☑
    laceration S35.341 ☑
    specified NEC S35.348 ☑
   superior S35.339 ☑
    laceration S35.331 ☑
    specified NEC S35.338 ☑
 mesentery — *see* Injury, intra-abdominal, specified site NEC
 mesosalpinx — *see* Injury, pelvic organ, specified site NEC
 middle ear S09.30- ☑
 midthoracic region NOS S29.9 ☑
 mouth S09.93 ☑
 multiple NOS T07 ☑
 muscle (and fascia) (and tendon)
  abdomen S39.001 ☑
   laceration S39.021 ☑
   specified type NEC S39.091 ☑
   strain S39.011 ☑
  abductor
   thumb, forearm level — *see* Injury, muscle, thumb, abductor
  adductor
   thigh S76.20- ☑
    laceration S76.22- ☑
    specified type NEC S76.29- ☑
    strain S76.21- ☑
  ankle — *see* Injury, muscle, foot
  anterior muscle group, at leg level (lower) S86.20- ☑
   laceration S86.22- ☑
   specified type NEC S86.29- ☑
   strain S86.21- ☑
  arm (upper) — *see* Injury, muscle, shoulder
  biceps (parts NEC) S46.20- ☑
   laceration S46.22- ☑
   long head S46.10- ☑
    laceration S46.12- ☑
    specified type NEC S46.19- ☑
    strain S46.11- ☑
   specified type NEC S46.29- ☑
   strain S46.21- ☑
  extensor
   finger(s) (other than thumb) — *see* Injury, muscle, finger by site, extensor
   forearm level, specified NEC — *see* Injury, muscle, forearm, extensor
   thumb — *see* Injury, muscle, thumb, extensor
   toe (large) (ankle level) (foot level) — *see* Injury, muscle, toe, extensor
  finger
   extensor (forearm level) S56.40- ☑
    hand level S66.309 ☑
     laceration S66.329 ☑
     specified type NEC S66.399 ☑
     strain S66.319 ☑
    laceration S56.429 ☑
    specified type NEC S56.499 ☑
    strain S56.419 ☑
   flexor (forearm level) S56.10- ☑
    hand level S66.109 ☑
     laceration S66.129 ☑
     specified type NEC S66.199 ☑
     strain S66.119 ☑
    laceration S56.129 ☑
    specified type NEC S56.199 ☑
    strain S56.119 ☑

Injury — *continued*
 muscle — *continued*
  finger — *continued*
   index
    extensor (forearm level)
     hand level S66.308 ☑
      laceration S66.32- ☑
      specified type NEC S66.39- ☑
      strain S66.31- ☑
     specified type NEC S56.492- ☑
    flexor (forearm level)
     hand level S66.108 ☑
      laceration S66.12- ☑
      specified type NEC S66.19- ☑
      strain S66.11- ☑
     specified type NEC S56.19- ☑
     strain S56.11- ☑
    intrinsic S66.50- ☑
     laceration S66.52- ☑
     specified type NEC S66.59- ☑
     strain S66.51- ☑
   intrinsic S66.509 ☑
    laceration S66.529 ☑
    specified type NEC S66.599 ☑
    strain S66.519 ☑
   little
    extensor (forearm level)
     hand level S66.30- ☑
      laceration S66.32- ☑
      specified type NEC S66.39- ☑
      strain S66.31- ☑
     laceration S56.42- ☑
     specified type NEC S56.49- ☑
     strain S56.41- ☑
    flexor (forearm level)
     hand level S66.10- ☑
      laceration S66.12- ☑
      specified type NEC S66.19- ☑
      strain S66.11- ☑
     laceration S56.12- ☑
     specified type NEC S56.19- ☑
     strain S56.11- ☑
    intrinsic S66.50- ☑
     laceration S66.52- ☑
     specified type NEC S66.59- ☑
     strain S66.51- ☑
   middle
    extensor (forearm level)
     hand level S66.30- ☑
      laceration S66.32- ☑
      specified type NEC S66.39- ☑
      strain S66.31- ☑
     laceration S56.42- ☑
     specified type NEC S56.49- ☑
     strain S56.41- ☑
    flexor (forearm level)
     hand level S66.10- ☑
      laceration S66.12- ☑
      specified type NEC S66.19- ☑
      strain S66.11- ☑
     laceration S56.12- ☑
     specified type NEC S56.19- ☑
     strain S56.11- ☑
    intrinsic S66.50- ☑
     laceration S66.52- ☑
     specified type NEC S66.59- ☑
     strain S66.51- ☑
   ring
    extensor (forearm level)
     hand level S66.30- ☑
      laceration S66.32- ☑
      specified type NEC S66.39- ☑
      strain S66.31- ☑
     laceration S56.42- ☑
     specified type NEC S56.49- ☑
     strain S56.41- ☑
    flexor (forearm level)
     hand level S66.10- ☑
      laceration S66.12- ☑
      specified type NEC S66.19- ☑
      strain S66.11- ☑
     laceration S56.12- ☑
     specified type NEC S56.19- ☑
     strain S56.11- ☑
    intrinsic S66.50- ☑

Injury — *continued*
  muscle — *continued*
    finger — *continued*
      ring — *continued*
        intrinsic — *continued*
          laceration S66.52- ☑
          specified type NEC S66.59- ☑
          strain S66.51- ☑
      flexor
        finger(s) (other than thumb) — *see* Injury, muscle, finger
        forearm level, specified NEC — *see* Injury, muscle, forearm, flexor
        thumb — *see* Injury, muscle, thumb, flexor
        toe (long) (ankle level) (foot level) — *see* Injury, muscle, toe, flexor
      foot S96.90- ☑
        intrinsic S96.20- ☑
          laceration S96.22- ☑
          specified type NEC S96.29- ☑
          strain S96.21- ☑
        laceration S96.92- ☑
        long extensor, toe — *see* Injury, muscle, toe, extensor
        long flexor, toe — *see* Injury, muscle, toe, flexor
        specified
          site NEC S96.80- ☑
            laceration S96.82- ☑
            specified type NEC S96.89- ☑
            strain S96.81- ☑
          type S96.99- ☑
        strain S96.91- ☑
      forearm (level) S56.90- ☑
        extensor S56.50- ☑
          laceration S56.52- ☑
          specified type NEC S56.59- ☑
          strain S56.51- ☑
        flexor S56.20- ☑
          laceration S56.22- ☑
          specified type NEC S56.29- ☑
          strain S56.21- ☑
        laceration S56.92- ☑
        specified S56.99- ☑
          site NEC S56.80- ☑
            laceration S56.82- ☑
            strain S56.81- ☑
            type NEC S56.89- ☑
        strain S56.91- ☑
      hand (level) S66.90- ☑
        laceration S66.92- ☑
        specified
          site NEC S66.80- ☑
            laceration S66.82- ☑
            specified type NEC S66.89- ☑
            strain S66.81- ☑
            type NEC S66.99- ☑
        strain S66.91- ☑
      head S09.10 ☑
        laceration S09.12 ☑
        specified type NEC S09.19 ☑
        strain S09.11 ☑
      hip NEC S76.00- ☑
        laceration S76.02- ☑
        specified type NEC S76.09- ☑
        strain S76.01- ☑
      intrinsic
        ankle and foot level — *see* Injury, muscle, foot, intrinsic
        finger (other than thumb) — *see* Injury, muscle, finger by site, intrinsic
        foot (level) — *see* Injury, muscle, foot, intrinsic
        thumb — *see* Injury, muscle, thumb, intrinsic
      leg (level) (lower) S86.90- ☑
        Achilles tendon — *see* Injury, Achilles tendon
        anterior muscle group — *see* Injury, muscle, anterior muscle group
        laceration S86.92- ☑
        peroneal muscle group — *see* Injury, muscle, peroneal muscle group
        posterior muscle group — *see* Injury, muscle, posterior muscle group, leg level
        specified
          site NEC S86.80- ☑
            laceration S86.82- ☑
            specified type NEC S86.89- ☑
            strain S86.81- ☑

Injury — *continued*
  muscle — *continued*
    leg — *continued*
      specified — *continued*
        type NEC S86.99- ☑
      strain S86.91- ☑
    long
      extensor toe, at ankle and foot level — *see* Injury, muscle, toe, extensor
      flexor, toe, at ankle and foot level — *see* Injury, muscle, toe, flexor
      head, biceps — *see* Injury, muscle, biceps, long head
    lower back S39.002 ☑
      laceration S39.022 ☑
      specified type NEC S39.092 ☑
      strain S39.012 ☑
    neck (level) S16.9 ☑
      laceration S16.2 ☑
      specified type NEC S16.8 ☑
      strain S16.1 ☑
    pelvis S39.003 ☑
      laceration S39.023 ☑
      specified type NEC S39.093 ☑
      strain S39.013 ☑
    peroneal muscle group, at leg level (lower) S86.30- ☑
      laceration S86.32- ☑
      specified type NEC S86.39- ☑
      strain S86.31- ☑
    posterior muscle (group)
      leg level (lower) S86.10- ☑
        laceration S86.12- ☑
        specified type NEC S86.19- ☑
        strain S86.11- ☑
      thigh level S76.30- ☑
        laceration S76.32- ☑
        specified type NEC S76.39- ☑
        strain S76.31- ☑
    quadriceps (thigh) S76.10- ☑
      laceration S76.12- ☑
      specified type NEC S76.19- ☑
      strain S76.11- ☑
    shoulder S46.90- ☑
      laceration S46.92- ☑
      rotator cuff — *see* Injury, rotator cuff
      specified site NEC S46.80- ☑
        laceration S46.82- ☑
        specified type NEC S46.89- ☑
        strain S46.81- ☑
      specified type NEC S46.99- ☑
      strain S46.91- ☑
    thigh NEC (level) S76.90- ☑
      adductor — *see* Injury, muscle, adductor, thigh
      laceration S76.92- ☑
      posterior muscle (group) — *see* Injury, muscle, posterior muscle, thigh level
      quadriceps — *see* Injury, muscle, quadriceps
      specified
        site NEC S76.80- ☑
          laceration S76.82- ☑
          specified type NEC S76.89- ☑
          strain S76.81- ☑
        type NEC S76.99- ☑
      strain S76.91- ☑
    thorax (level) S29.009 ☑
      back wall S29.002 ☑
      front wall S29.001 ☑
      laceration S29.029 ☑
        back wall S29.022 ☑
        front wall S29.021 ☑
      specified type NEC S29.099 ☑
        back wall S29.092 ☑
        front wall S29.091 ☑
      strain S29.019 ☑
        back wall S29.012 ☑
        front wall S29.011 ☑
    thumb
      abductor (forearm level) S56.30- ☑
        laceration S56.32- ☑
        specified type NEC S56.39- ☑
        strain S56.31- ☑
      extensor (forearm level) S56.30- ☑
        hand level S66.20- ☑
          laceration S66.22- ☑
          specified type NEC S66.29- ☑
          strain S66.21- ☑

Injury — *continued*
  muscle — *continued*
    thumb — *continued*
      extensor — *continued*
        laceration S56.32- ☑
        specified type NEC S56.39- ☑
        strain S56.31- ☑
      flexor (forearm level) S56.00- ☑
        hand level S66.00- ☑
          laceration S66.02- ☑
          specified type NEC S66.09- ☑
          strain S66.01- ☑
        laceration S56.02- ☑
        specified type NEC S56.09- ☑
        strain S56.01- ☑
        wrist level — *see* Injury, muscle, thumb, flexor, hand level
      intrinsic S66.40- ☑
        laceration S66.42- ☑
        specified type NEC S66.49- ☑
        strain S66.41- ☑
    toe — *see also* Injury, muscle, foot
      extensor, long S96.10- ☑
        laceration S96.12- ☑
        specified type NEC S96.19- ☑
        strain S96.11- ☑
      flexor, long S96.00- ☑
        laceration S96.02- ☑
        specified type NEC S96.09- ☑
        strain S96.01- ☑
    triceps S46.30- ☑
      laceration S46.32- ☑
      specified type NEC S46.39- ☑
      strain S46.31- ☑
    wrist (and hand) level — *see* Injury, muscle, hand
  musculocutaneous nerve — *see* Injury, nerve, musculocutaneous
  myocardial (acute) (chronic) (non-ischemic) (non-traumatic) I5A
    traumatic — *see* Injury, heart
  myocardium — *see also* Injury, heart
    non-traumatic — *see* Injury, myocardial
  nape — *see* Injury, neck
  nasal (septum) (sinus) S09.92 ☑
  nasopharynx S09.92 ☑
  neck S19.9 ☑
    specified NEC S19.80 ☑
      specified site NEC S19.89 ☑
  nerve NEC T14.8 ☑
    abdomen S34.9 ☑
      peripheral S34.6 ☑
      specified site NEC S34.8 ☑
    abducens S04.4- ☑
      contusion S04.4- ☑
      laceration S04.4- ☑
      specified type NEC S04.4- ☑
    abducent — *see* Injury, nerve, abducens
    accessory S04.7- ☑
      contusion S04.7- ☑
      laceration S04.7- ☑
      specified type NEC S04.7- ☑
    acoustic S04.6- ☑
      contusion S04.6- ☑
      laceration S04.6- ☑
      specified type NEC S04.6- ☑
    ankle S94.9- ☑
      cutaneous sensory S94.3- ☑
      specified site NEC — *see* subcategory S94.8 ☑
    anterior crural, femoral — *see* Injury, nerve, femoral
    arm (upper) S44.9- ☑
      axillary — *see* Injury, nerve, axillary
      cutaneous — *see* Injury, nerve, cutaneous, arm
      median — *see* Injury, nerve, median, upper arm
      musculocutaneous — *see* Injury, nerve, musculocutaneous
      radial — *see* Injury, nerve, radial, upper arm
      specified site NEC — *see* subcategory S44.8 ☑
      ulnar — *see* Injury, nerve, ulnar, arm
    auditory — *see* Injury, nerve, acoustic
    axillary S44.3- ☑
    brachial plexus — *see* Injury, brachial plexus
    cervical sympathetic S14.5 ☑
    cranial S04.9 ☑
      contusion S04.9 ☑
      eighth (acoustic or auditory) — *see* Injury, nerve, acoustic

Injury — *continued*
  nerve — *continued*
    cranial — *continued*
      eleventh (accessory) — *see* Injury, nerve, accessory
      fifth (trigeminal) — *see* Injury, nerve, trigeminal
      first (olfactory) — *see* Injury, nerve, olfactory
      fourth (trochlear) — *see* Injury, nerve, trochlear
      laceration S04.9 ☑
      ninth (glossopharyngeal) — *see* Injury, nerve, glossopharyngeal
      second (optic) — *see* Injury, nerve, optic
      seventh (facial) — *see* Injury, nerve, facial
      sixth (abducent) — *see* Injury, nerve, abducens
      specified
        nerve NEC S04.89- ☑
          contusion S04.89- ☑
          laceration S04.89- ☑
          specified type NEC S04.89- ☑
        type NEC S04.9 ☑
      tenth (pneumogastric or vagus) — *see* Injury, nerve, vagus
      third (oculomotor) — *see* Injury, nerve, oculomotor
      twelfth (hypoglossal) — *see* Injury, nerve, hypoglossal
    cutaneous sensory
      ankle (level) S94.3- ☑
      arm (upper) (level) S44.5- ☑
      foot (level) — *see* Injury, nerve, cutaneous sensory, ankle
      forearm (level) S54.3- ☑
      hip (level) S74.2- ☑
      leg (lower level) S84.2- ☑
      shoulder (level) — *see* Injury, nerve, cutaneous sensory, arm
      thigh (level) — *see* Injury, nerve, cutaneous sensory, hip
    deep peroneal — *see* Injury, nerve, peroneal, foot
    digital
      finger S64.4- ☑
        index S64.49- ☑
        little S64.49- ☑
        middle S64.49- ☑
        ring S64.49- ☑
      thumb S64.3- ☑
      toe — *see* Injury, nerve, ankle, specified site NEC
    eighth cranial (acoustic or auditory) — *see* Injury, nerve, acoustic
    eleventh cranial (accessory) — *see* Injury, nerve, accessory
    facial S04.5- ☑
      contusion S04.5- ☑
      laceration S04.5- ☑
      newborn P11.3
      specified type NEC S04.5- ☑
    femoral (hip level) (thigh level) S74.1- ☑
    fifth cranial (trigeminal) — *see* Injury, nerve, trigeminal
    finger (digital) — *see* Injury, nerve, digital, finger
    first cranial (olfactory) — *see* Injury, nerve, olfactory
    foot S94.9- ☑
      cutaneous sensory S94.3- ☑
      deep peroneal S94.2- ☑
      lateral plantar S94.0- ☑
      medial plantar S94.1- ☑
      specified site NEC — *see* subcategory S94.8 ☑
    forearm (level) S54.9- ☑
      cutaneous sensory — *see* Injury, nerve, cutaneous sensory, forearm
      median — *see* Injury, nerve, median
      radial — *see* Injury, nerve, radial
      specified site NEC — *see* subcategory S54.8 ☑
      ulnar — *see* Injury, nerve, ulnar
    fourth cranial (trochlear) — *see* Injury, nerve, trochlear
    glossopharyngeal S04.89- ☑
      specified type NEC S04.89- ☑
    hand S64.9- ☑
      median — *see* Injury, nerve, median, hand
      radial — *see* Injury, nerve, radial, hand
      specified NEC — *see* subcategory S64.8 ☑
      ulnar — *see* Injury, nerve, ulnar, hand
    hip (level) S74.9- ☑
      cutaneous sensory — *see* Injury, nerve, cutaneous sensory, hip
      femoral — *see* Injury, nerve, femoral
      sciatic — *see* Injury, nerve, sciatic
      specified site NEC — *see* subcategory S74.8 ☑
    hypoglossal S04.89- ☑

Injury — *continued*
  nerve — *continued*
    hypoglossal — *continued*
      specified type NEC S04.89- ☑
    lateral plantar S94.0- ☑
    leg (lower) S84.9- ☑
      cutaneous sensory — *see* Injury, nerve, cutaneous sensory, leg
      peroneal — *see* Injury, nerve, peroneal
      specified site NEC — *see* subcategory S84.8 ☑
      tibial — *see* Injury, nerve, tibial
      upper — *see* Injury, nerve, thigh
    lower
      back — *see* Injury, nerve, abdomen, specified site NEC
        peripheral — *see* Injury, nerve, abdomen, peripheral
      limb — *see* Injury, nerve, leg
    lumbar plexus — *see* Injury, nerve, lumbosacral, sympathetic
    lumbar spinal — *see* Injury, spinal, lumbar
      peripheral S34.6 ☑
      root S34.21
      sympathetic S34.5 ☑
    lumbosacral
      plexus — *see* Injury, nerve, lumbosacral, sympathetic
      sympathetic S34.5 ☑
    medial plantar S94.1- ☑
    median (forearm level) S54.1- ☑
      hand S64.1- ☑
      upper arm (level) S44.1- ☑
      wrist (level) — *see* Injury, nerve, median, hand
    musculocutaneous S44.4- ☑
    musculospiral (upper arm level) — *see* Injury, nerve, radial, upper arm
    neck S14.9 ☑
      peripheral S14.4 ☑
      specified site NEC S14.8 ☑
      sympathetic S14.5 ☑
    ninth cranial (glossopharyngeal) — *see* Injury, nerve, glossopharyngeal
    oculomotor S04.1- ☑
      contusion S04.1- ☑
      laceration S04.1- ☑
      specified type NEC S04.1- ☑
    olfactory S04.81- ☑
      specified type NEC S04.81- ☑
    optic S04.01- ☑
      contusion S04.01- ☑
      laceration S04.01- ☑
      specified type NEC S04.01- ☑
    pelvic girdle — *see* Injury, nerve, hip
    pelvis — *see* Injury, nerve, abdomen, specified site NEC
      peripheral — *see* Injury, nerve, abdomen, peripheral
    peripheral NEC T14.8 ☑
      abdomen — *see* Injury, nerve, abdomen, peripheral
      lower back — *see* Injury, nerve, abdomen, peripheral
      neck — *see* Injury, nerve, neck, peripheral
      pelvis — *see* Injury, nerve, abdomen, peripheral
      specified NEC T14.8 ☑
    peroneal (lower leg level) S84.1- ☑
      foot S94.2- ☑
    plexus
      brachial — *see* Injury, brachial plexus
      celiac, coeliac — *see* Injury, nerve, lumbosacral, sympathetic
      mesenteric, inferior — *see* Injury, nerve, lumbosacral, sympathetic
      sacral — *see* Injury, lumbosacral plexus
      spinal
        brachial — *see* Injury, brachial plexus
        lumbosacral — *see* Injury, lumbosacral plexus
    pneumogastric — *see* Injury, nerve, vagus
    radial (forearm level) S54.2- ☑
      hand (level) S64.2- ☑
      upper arm (level) S44.2- ☑
      wrist (level) — *see* Injury, nerve, radial, hand
    root — *see* Injury, nerve, spinal, root
    sacral plexus — *see* Injury, lumbosacral plexus
    sacral spinal — *see* Injury, spinal, sacral
      peripheral S34.6 ☑
      root S34.22 ☑

Injury — *continued*
  nerve — *continued*
    sacral spinal — *see* Injury, spinal, sacral — *continued*
      sympathetic S34.5 ☑
    sciatic (hip level) (thigh level) S74.0- ☑
    second cranial (optic) — *see* Injury, nerve, optic
    seventh cranial (facial) — *see* Injury, nerve, facial
    shoulder — *see* Injury, nerve, arm
    sixth cranial (abducent) — *see* Injury, nerve, abducens
    spinal
      plexus — *see* Injury, nerve, plexus, spinal
      root
        cervical S14.2 ☑
        dorsal S24.2 ☑
        lumbar S34.21 ☑
        sacral S34.22 ☑
        thoracic — *see* Injury, nerve, spinal, root, dorsal
    splanchnic — *see* Injury, nerve, lumbosacral, sympathetic
    sympathetic NEC — *see* Injury, nerve, lumbosacral, sympathetic
      cervical — *see* Injury, nerve, cervical sympathetic
    tenth cranial (pneumogastric or vagus) — *see* Injury, nerve, vagus
    thigh (level) — *see* Injury, nerve, hip
      cutaneous sensory — *see* Injury, nerve, cutaneous sensory, hip
      femoral — *see* Injury, nerve, femoral
      sciatic — *see* Injury, nerve, sciatic
      specified NEC — *see* Injury, nerve, hip
    third cranial (oculomotor) — *see* Injury, nerve, oculomotor
    thorax S24.9 ☑
      peripheral S24.3 ☑
      specified site NEC S24.8 ☑
      sympathetic S24.4 ☑
    thumb, digital — *see* Injury, nerve, digital, thumb
    tibial (lower leg level) (posterior) S84.0- ☑
    toe — *see* Injury, nerve, ankle
    trigeminal S04.3- ☑
      contusion S04.3- ☑
      laceration S04.3- ☑
      specified type NEC S04.3- ☑
    trochlear S04.2- ☑
      contusion S04.2- ☑
      laceration S04.2- ☑
      specified type NEC S04.2- ☑
    twelfth cranial (hypoglossal) — *see* Injury, nerve, hypoglossal
    ulnar (forearm level) S54.0- ☑
      arm (upper) (level) S44.0- ☑
      hand (level) S64.0- ☑
      wrist (level) — *see* Injury, nerve, ulnar, hand
    vagus S04.89- ☑
      specified type NEC S04.89- ☑
    wrist (level) — *see* Injury, nerve, hand
  ninth cranial nerve (glossopharyngeal) — *see* Injury, nerve, glossopharyngeal
  nose (septum) S09.92 ☑
  obstetrical O71.9
    specified NEC O71.89
  occipital (region) (scalp) S09.90 ☑
    lobe — *see* Injury, intracranial
  optic chiasm S04.02 ☑
  optic radiation S04.03- ☑
  optic tract and pathways S04.03- ☑
  orbit, orbital (region) — *see* Injury, eye
    penetrating (with foreign body) — *see* Injury, eye, orbit, penetrating
    specified NEC — *see* Injury, eye, specified site NEC
  ovary, ovarian S37.409 ☑
    bilateral S37.402 ☑
      contusion S37.422 ☑
      laceration S37.432 ☑
      specified type NEC S37.492 ☑
    blood vessel — *see* Injury, blood vessel, ovarian
    contusion S37.429 ☑
      bilateral S37.422 ☑
      unilateral S37.421 ☑
    laceration S37.439 ☑
      bilateral S37.432 ☑
      unilateral S37.431 ☑
    specified type NEC S37.499 ☑
      bilateral S37.492 ☑
      unilateral S37.491 ☑
    unilateral S37.401 ☑

Injury — *continued*
- ovary, ovarian — *continued*
  - unilateral — *continued*
    - contusion S37.421 ☑
    - laceration S37.431 ☑
    - specified type NEC S37.491 ☑
- palate (hard) (soft) S09.93 ☑
- pancreas S36.209 ☑
  - body S36.201 ☑
    - contusion S36.221 ☑
    - laceration S36.231 ☑
      - major S36.261 ☑
      - minor S36.241 ☑
      - moderate S36.251 ☑
    - specified type NEC S36.291 ☑
  - contusion S36.229 ☑
  - head S36.200 ☑
    - contusion S36.220 ☑
    - laceration S36.230 ☑
      - major S36.260 ☑
      - minor S36.240 ☑
      - moderate S36.250 ☑
    - specified type NEC S36.290 ☑
  - laceration S36.239 ☑
    - major S36.269 ☑
    - minor S36.249 ☑
    - moderate S36.259 ☑
  - specified type NEC S36.299 ☑
  - tail S36.202 ☑
    - contusion S36.222 ☑
    - laceration S36.232 ☑
      - major S36.262 ☑
      - minor S36.242 ☑
      - moderate S36.252 ☑
    - specified type NEC S36.292 ☑
- parietal (region) (scalp) S09.90 ☑
  - lobe — *see* Injury, intracranial
- patellar ligament (tendon) S76.10- ☑
  - laceration S76.12- ☑
  - specified NEC S76.19- ☑
  - strain S76.11- ☑
- pelvis, pelvic (floor) S39.93 ☑
  - complicating delivery O70.1
  - joint or ligament, complicating delivery O71.6
  - organ S37.90 ☑
    - with ectopic or molar pregnancy O08.6
    - complication of abortion — *see* Abortion
    - contusion S37.92 ☑
    - following ectopic or molar pregnancy O08.6
    - laceration S37.93 ☑
    - obstetrical trauma NEC O71.5
    - specified
      - site NEC S37.899 ☑
        - contusion S37.892 ☑
        - laceration S37.893 ☑
        - specified type NEC S37.898 ☑
      - type NEC S37.99 ☑
  - specified NEC S39.83 ☑
- penis S39.94 ☑
- perineum S39.94 ☑
- peritoneum S36.81 ☑
  - laceration S36.893 ☑
- periurethral tissue — *see* Injury, urethra
  - complicating delivery O71.82
- phalanges
  - foot — *see* Injury, foot
  - hand — *see* Injury, hand
- pharynx NEC S19.85 ☑
- pleura — *see* Injury, intrathoracic, pleura
- plexus
  - brachial — *see* Injury, brachial plexus
  - cardiac — *see* Injury, nerve, thorax, sympathetic
  - celiac, coeliac — *see* Injury, nerve, lumbosacral, sympathetic
  - esophageal — *see* Injury, nerve, thorax, sympathetic
  - hypogastric — *see* Injury, nerve, lumbosacral, sympathetic
  - lumbar, lumbosacral — *see* Injury, lumbosacral plexus
  - mesenteric — *see* Injury, nerve, lumbosacral, sympathetic
  - pulmonary — *see* Injury, nerve, thorax, sympathetic
- postcardiac surgery (syndrome) I97.0
- prepuce S39.94 ☑
- pressure
  - injury — *see* Ulcer, pressure, by site
- prostate S37.829 ☑

Injury — *continued*
- prostate — *continued*
  - contusion S37.822 ☑
  - laceration S37.823 ☑
  - specified type NEC S37.828 ☑
- pubic region S39.94 ☑
- pudendum S39.94 ☑
- pulmonary plexus — *see* Injury, nerve, thorax, sympathetic
- rectovaginal septum NEC S39.83 ☑
- rectum — *see* Injury, intestine, large, rectum
- retina — *see* Injury, eye, specified site NEC
  - penetrating — *see* Injury, eyeball, penetrating
- retroperitoneal — *see* Injury, intra-abdominal, specified site NEC
- rotator cuff (muscle(s)) (tendon(s)) S46.00- ☑
  - laceration S46.02- ☑
  - specified type NEC S46.09- ☑
  - strain S46.01- ☑
- round ligament — *see* Injury, pelvic organ, specified site NEC
- sacral plexus — *see* Injury, lumbosacral plexus
- salivary duct or gland S09.93 ☑
- scalp S09.90 ☑
  - newborn (birth injury) P12.9
    - due to monitoring (electrode) (sampling incision) P12.4
    - specified NEC P12.89
      - caput succedaneum P12.81
- scapular region — *see* Injury, shoulder
- sclera — *see* Injury, eye, specified site NEC
  - penetrating — *see* Injury, eyeball, penetrating
- scrotum S39.94 ☑
- second cranial nerve (optic) — *see* Injury, nerve, optic
- self-inflicted, without suicidal intent R45.88
- seminal vesicle — *see* Injury, pelvic organ, specified site NEC
- seventh cranial nerve (facial) — *see* Injury, nerve, facial
- shoulder S49.9- ☑
  - blood vessel — *see* Injury, blood vessel, arm
  - contusion — *see* Contusion, shoulder
  - dislocation — *see* Dislocation, shoulder
  - fracture — *see* Fracture, shoulder
  - muscle — *see* Injury, muscle, shoulder
  - nerve — *see* Injury, nerve, shoulder
  - open — *see* Wound, open, shoulder
  - specified type NEC S49.8- ☑
  - sprain — *see* Sprain, shoulder girdle
  - superficial — *see* Injury, superficial, shoulder
- sinus
  - cavernous — *see* Injury, intracranial
  - nasal S09.92 ☑
- sixth cranial nerve (abducent) — *see* Injury, nerve, abducens
- skeleton, birth injury P13.9
  - specified part NEC P13.8
- skin NEC T14.8 ☑
  - surface intact — *see* Injury, superficial
- skull NEC S09.90 ☑
- specified NEC T14.8 ☑
- spermatic cord (pelvic region) S37.898 ☑
  - scrotal region S39.848 ☑
- spinal (cord)
  - cervical (neck) S14.109 ☑
    - anterior cord syndrome S14.139 ☑
      - C1 level S14.131 ☑
      - C2 level S14.132 ☑
      - C3 level S14.133 ☑
      - C4 level S14.134 ☑
      - C5 level S14.135 ☑
      - C6 level S14.136 ☑
      - C7 level S14.137 ☑
      - C8 level S14.138 ☑
    - Brown-Sequard syndrome S14.149 ☑
      - C1 level S14.141 ☑
      - C2 level S14.142 ☑
      - C3 level S14.143 ☑
      - C4 level S14.144 ☑
      - C5 level S14.145 ☑
      - C6 level S14.146 ☑
      - C7 level S14.147 ☑
      - C8 level S14.148 ☑
    - C1 level S14.101 ☑
    - C2 level S14.102 ☑
    - C3 level S14.103 ☑
    - C4 level S14.104 ☑
    - C5 level S14.105 ☑

Injury — *continued*
- spinal — *continued*
  - cervical — *continued*
    - C6 level S14.106 ☑
    - C7 level S14.107 ☑
    - C8 level S14.108 ☑
    - central cord syndrome S14.129 ☑
      - C1 level S14.121 ☑
      - C2 level S14.122 ☑
      - C3 level S14.123 ☑
      - C4 level S14.124 ☑
      - C5 level S14.125 ☑
      - C6 level S14.126 ☑
      - C7 level S14.127 ☑
      - C8 level S14.128 ☑
    - complete lesion S14.119 ☑
      - C1 level S14.111 ☑
      - C2 level S14.112 ☑
      - C3 level S14.113 ☑
      - C4 level S14.114 ☑
      - C5 level S14.115 ☑
      - C6 level S14.116 ☑
      - C7 level S14.117 ☑
      - C8 level S14.118 ☑
    - concussion S14.0 ☑
    - edema S14.0 ☑
    - incomplete lesion specified NEC S14.159 ☑
      - C1 level S14.151 ☑
      - C2 level S14.152 ☑
      - C3 level S14.153 ☑
      - C4 level S14.154 ☑
      - C5 level S14.155 ☑
      - C6 level S14.156 ☑
      - C7 level S14.157 ☑
      - C8 level S14.158 ☑
    - posterior cord syndrome S14.159 ☑
      - C1 level S14.151 ☑
      - C2 level S14.152 ☑
      - C3 level S14.153 ☑
      - C4 level S14.154 ☑
      - C5 level S14.155 ☑
      - C6 level S14.156 ☑
      - C7 level S14.157 ☑
      - C8 level S14.158 ☑
  - dorsal — *see* Injury, spinal, thoracic
  - lumbar S34.109 ☑
    - complete lesion S34.119 ☑
      - L1 level S34.111 ☑
      - L2 level S34.112 ☑
      - L3 level S34.113 ☑
      - L4 level S34.114 ☑
      - L5 level S34.115 ☑
    - concussion S34.01 ☑
    - edema S34.01 ☑
    - incomplete lesion S34.129 ☑
      - L1 level S34.121 ☑
      - L2 level S34.122 ☑
      - L3 level S34.123 ☑
      - L4 level S34.124 ☑
      - L5 level S34.125 ☑
    - L1 level S34.101 ☑
    - L2 level S34.102 ☑
    - L3 level S34.103 ☑
    - L4 level S34.104 ☑
    - L5 level S34.105 ☑
  - nerve root NEC
    - cervical — *see* Injury, nerve, spinal, root, cervical
    - dorsal — *see* Injury, nerve, spinal, root, dorsal
    - lumbar S34.21 ☑
    - sacral S34.22 ☑
    - thoracic — *see* Injury, nerve, spinal, root, dorsal
  - plexus
    - brachial — *see* Injury, brachial plexus
    - lumbosacral — *see* Injury, lumbosacral plexus
  - sacral S34.139 ☑
    - complete lesion S34.131 ☑
    - incomplete lesion S34.132 ☑
  - thoracic S24.109 ☑
    - anterior cord syndrome S24.139 ☑
      - T1 level S24.131 ☑
      - T2-T6 level S24.132 ☑
      - T7-T10 level S24.133 ☑
      - T11-T12 level S24.134 ☑
    - Brown-Sequard syndrome S24.149 ☑
      - T1 level S24.141 ☑

☑ Additional Character Required — Refer to the Tabular List for Character Selection

Injury — *continued*
  spinal — *continued*
    thoracic — *continued*
      Brown-Sequard syndrome — *continued*
        T2-T6 level S24.142 ☑
        T7-T10 level S24.143 ☑
        T11-T12 level S24.144 ☑
      complete lesion S24.119 ☑
        T1 level S24.111 ☑
        T2-T6 level S24.112 ☑
        T7-T10 level S24.113 ☑
        T11-T12 level S24.114 ☑
      concussion S24.0 ☑
      edema S24.0 ☑
      incomplete lesion specified NEC S24.159 ☑
        T1 level S24.151 ☑
        T2-T6 level S24.152 ☑
        T7-T10 level S24.153 ☑
        T11-T12 level S24.154 ☑
      posterior cord syndrome S24.159 ☑
        T1 level S24.151 ☑
        T2-T6 level S24.152 ☑
        T7-T10 level S24.153 ☑
        T11-T12 level S24.154 ☑
      T1 level S24.101 ☑
      T2-T6 level S24.102 ☑
      T7-T10 level S24.103 ☑
      T11-T12 level S24.104 ☑
  splanchnic nerve — *see* Injury, nerve, lumbosacral, sympathetic
  spleen S36.00 ☑
    contusion S36.029 ☑
      major S36.021 ☑
      minor S36.020 ☑
    laceration S36.039 ☑
      major (massive) (stellate) S36.032 ☑
      moderate S36.031 ☑
      superficial (capsular) (minor) S36.030 ☑
    specified type NEC S36.09 ☑
  splenic artery — *see* Injury, blood vessel, celiac artery, branch
  stellate ganglion — *see* Injury, nerve, thorax, sympathetic
  sternal region S29.9 ☑
  stomach S36.30 ☑
    contusion S36.32 ☑
    laceration S36.33 ☑
    specified type NEC S36.39 ☑
  subconjunctival — *see* Injury, eye, conjunctiva
  subcutaneous NEC T14.8 ☑
  submaxillary region S09.93 ☑
  submental region S09.93 ☑
  subungual
    fingers — *see* Injury, hand
    toes — *see* Injury, foot
  superficial NEC T14.8 ☑
    abdomen, abdominal (wall) S30.92 ☑
      abrasion S30.811 ☑
      bite S30.871 ☑
        insect S30.861 ☑
      contusion S30.1 ☑
      external constriction S30.841 ☑
      foreign body S30.851 ☑
    abrasion — *see* Abrasion, by site
    adnexa, eye NEC — *see* Injury, eye, specified site NEC
    alveolar process — *see* Injury, superficial, oral cavity
    ankle S90.91- ☑
      abrasion — *see* Abrasion, ankle
      bite — *see* Bite, ankle
      blister — *see* Blister, ankle
      contusion — *see* Contusion, ankle
      external constriction — *see* Constriction, external, ankle
      foreign body — *see* Foreign body, superficial, ankle
    anus S30.98 ☑
    arm (upper) S40.92- ☑
      abrasion — *see* Abrasion, arm
      bite — *see* Bite, superficial, arm
      blister — *see* Blister, arm (upper)
      contusion — *see* Contusion, arm
      external constriction — *see* Constriction, external, arm
      foreign body — *see* Foreign body, superficial, arm
    auditory canal (external) (meatus) — *see* Injury, superficial, ear
    auricle — *see* Injury, superficial, ear
    axilla — *see* Injury, superficial, arm

Injury — *continued*
  superficial — *continued*
    back — *see also* Injury, superficial, thorax, back
      lower S30.91 ☑
        abrasion S30.810 ☑
        contusion S30.0 ☑
        external constriction S30.840 ☑
        superficial
          bite NEC S30.870 ☑
            insect S30.860 ☑
          foreign body S30.850 ☑
    bite NEC — *see* Bite, superficial NEC, by site
    blister — *see* Blister, by site
    breast S20.10- ☑
      abrasion — *see* Abrasion, breast
      bite — *see* Bite, superficial, breast
      contusion — *see* Contusion, breast
      external constriction — *see* Constriction, external, breast
      foreign body — *see* Foreign body, superficial, breast
    brow — *see* Injury, superficial, head, specified NEC
    buttock S30.91 ☑
    calf — *see* Injury, superficial, leg
    canthus, eye — *see* Injury, superficial, periocular area
    cheek (external) — *see* Injury, superficial, head, specified NEC
      internal — *see* Injury, superficial, oral cavity
    chest wall — *see* Injury, superficial, thorax
    chin — *see* Injury, superficial, head NEC
    clitoris S30.95 ☑
    conjunctiva — *see* Injury, eye, conjunctiva
      with foreign body (in conjunctival sac) — *see* Foreign body, conjunctival sac
    contusion — *see* Contusion, by site
    costal region — *see* Injury, superficial, thorax
    digit(s)
      hand — *see* Injury, superficial, finger
    ear (auricle) (canal) (external) S00.40- ☑
      abrasion — *see* Abrasion, ear
      bite — *see* Bite, superficial, ear
      contusion — *see* Contusion, ear
      external constriction — *see* Constriction, external, ear
      foreign body — *see* Foreign body, superficial, ear
    elbow S50.90- ☑
      abrasion — *see* Abrasion, elbow
      bite — *see* Bite, superficial, elbow
      blister — *see* Blister, elbow
      contusion — *see* Contusion, elbow
      external constriction — *see* Constriction, external, elbow
      foreign body — *see* Foreign body, superficial, elbow
    epididymis S30.94 ☑
    epigastric region S30.92 ☑
    epiglottis — *see* Injury, superficial, throat
    esophagus
      cervical — *see* Injury, superficial, throat
    external constriction — *see* Constriction, external, by site
    extremity NEC T14.8 ☑
    eyeball NEC — *see* Injury, eye, specified site NEC
    eyebrow — *see* Injury, superficial, periocular area
    eyelid S00.20- ☑
      abrasion — *see* Abrasion, eyelid
      bite — *see* Bite, superficial, eyelid
      contusion — *see* Contusion, eyelid
      external constriction — *see* Constriction, external, eyelid
      foreign body — *see* Foreign body, superficial, eyelid
    face NEC — *see* Injury, superficial, head, specified NEC
    finger(s) S60.949 ☑
      abrasion — *see* Abrasion, finger
      bite — *see* Bite, superficial, finger
      blister — *see* Blister, finger
      contusion — *see* Contusion, finger
      external constriction — *see* Constriction, external, finger
      foreign body — *see* Foreign body, superficial, finger
      index S60.94- ☑
      insect bite — *see* Bite, by site, superficial, insect
      little S60.94- ☑
      middle S60.94- ☑
      ring S60.94- ☑
    flank S30.92 ☑

Injury — *continued*
  superficial — *continued*
    foot S90.92- ☑
      abrasion — *see* Abrasion, foot
      bite — *see* Bite, foot
      blister — *see* Blister, foot
      contusion — *see* Contusion, foot
      external constriction — *see* Constriction, external, foot
      foreign body — *see* Foreign body, superficial, foot
    forearm S50.91- ☑
      abrasion — *see* Abrasion, forearm
      bite — *see* Bite, forearm, superficial
      blister — *see* Blister, forearm
      contusion — *see* Contusion, forearm
      elbow only — *see* Injury, superficial, elbow
      external constriction — *see* Constriction, external, forearm
      foreign body — *see* Foreign body, superficial, forearm
    forehead — *see* Injury, superficial, head NEC
    foreign body — *see* Foreign body, superficial
    genital organs, external
      female S30.97 ☑
      male S30.96 ☑
    globe (eye) — *see* Injury, eye, specified site NEC
    groin S30.92 ☑
    gum — *see* Injury, superficial, oral cavity
    hand S60.92- ☑
      abrasion — *see* Abrasion, hand
      bite — *see* Bite, superficial, hand
      contusion — *see* Contusion, hand
      external constriction — *see* Constriction, external, hand
      foreign body — *see* Foreign body, superficial, hand
    head S00.90 ☑
      ear — *see* Injury, superficial, ear
      eyelid — *see* Injury, superficial, eyelid
      nose S00.30 ☑
      oral cavity S00.502 ☑
      scalp S00.00 ☑
      specified site NEC S00.80 ☑
    heel — *see* Injury, superficial, foot
    hip S70.91- ☑
      abrasion — *see* Abrasion, hip
      bite — *see* Bite, superficial, hip
      blister — *see* Blister, hip
      contusion — *see* Contusion, hip
      external constriction — *see* Constriction, external, hip
      foreign body — *see* Foreign body, superficial, hip
    iliac region — *see* Injury, superficial, abdomen
    inguinal region — *see* Injury, superficial, abdomen
    insect bite — *see* Bite, by site, superficial, insect
    interscapular region — *see* Injury, superficial, thorax, back
    jaw — *see* Injury, superficial, head, specified NEC
    knee S80.91- ☑
      abrasion — *see* Abrasion, knee
      bite — *see* Bite, superficial, knee
      blister — *see* Blister, knee
      contusion — *see* Contusion, knee
      external constriction — *see* Constriction, external, knee
      foreign body — *see* Foreign body, superficial, knee
    labium (majus) (minus) S30.95 ☑
    lacrimal (apparatus) (gland) (sac) — *see* Injury, eye, specified site NEC
    larynx — *see* Injury, superficial, throat
    leg (lower) S80.92- ☑
      abrasion — *see* Abrasion, leg
      bite — *see* Bite, superficial, leg
      contusion — *see* Contusion, leg
      external constriction — *see* Constriction, external, leg
      foreign body — *see* Foreign body, superficial, leg
      knee — *see* Injury, superficial, knee
    limb NEC T14.8 ☑
    lip S00.501 ☑
    lower back S30.91 ☑
    lumbar region S30.91 ☑
    malar region — *see* Injury, superficial, head, specified NEC
    mammary — *see* Injury, superficial, breast
    mastoid region — *see* Injury, superficial, head, specified NEC
    mouth — *see* Injury, superficial, oral cavity
    muscle NEC T14.8 ☑

Injury — *continued*
  superficial — *continued*
    nail NEC T14.8
      finger — *see* Injury, superficial, finger
      toe — *see* Injury, superficial, toe
    nasal (septum) — *see* Injury, superficial, nose
    neck S10.90 ☑
      specified site NEC S10.80 ☑
    nose (septum) S00.30 ☑
    occipital region — *see* Injury, superficial, scalp
    oral cavity S00.502 ☑
    orbital region — *see* Injury, superficial, periocular area
    palate — *see* Injury, superficial, oral cavity
    palm — *see* Injury, superficial, hand
    parietal region — *see* Injury, superficial, scalp
    pelvis S30.91 ☑
      girdle — *see* Injury, superficial, hip
    penis S30.93 ☑
    perineum
      female S30.95 ☑
      male S30.91 ☑
    periocular area S00.20- ☑
      abrasion — *see* Abrasion, eyelid
      bite — *see* Bite, superficial, eyelid
      contusion — *see* Contusion, eyelid
      external constriction — *see* Constriction, external, eyelid
      foreign body — *see* Foreign body, superficial, eyelid
    phalanges
      finger — *see* Injury, superficial, finger
      toe — *see* Injury, superficial, toe
    pharynx — *see* Injury, superficial, throat
    pinna — *see* Injury, superficial, ear
    popliteal space — *see* Injury, superficial, knee
    prepuce S30.93 ☑
    pubic region S30.91 ☑
    pudendum
      female S30.97 ☑
      male S30.96 ☑
    sacral region S30.91 ☑
    scalp S00.00 ☑
    scapular region — *see* Injury, superficial, shoulder
    sclera — *see* Injury, eye, specified site NEC
    scrotum S30.94 ☑
    shin — *see* Injury, superficial, leg
    shoulder S40.91- ☑
      abrasion — *see* Abrasion, shoulder
      bite — *see* Bite, superficial, shoulder
      blister — *see* Blister, shoulder
      contusion — *see* Contusion, shoulder
      external constriction — *see* Constriction, external, shoulder
      foreign body — *see* Foreign body, superficial, shoulder
    skin NEC T14.8 ☑
    sternal region — *see* Injury, superficial, thorax, front
    subconjunctival — *see* Injury, eye, specified site NEC
    subcutaneous NEC T14.8 ☑
    submaxillary region — *see* Injury, superficial, head, specified NEC
    submental region — *see* Injury, superficial, head, specified NEC
    subungual
      finger(s) — *see* Injury, superficial, finger
      toe(s) — *see* Injury, superficial, toe
    supraclavicular fossa — *see* Injury, superficial, neck
    supraorbital — *see* Injury, superficial, head, specified NEC
    temple — *see* Injury, superficial, head, specified NEC
    temporal region — *see* Injury, superficial, head, specified NEC
    testis S30.94 ☑
    thigh S70.92- ☑
      abrasion — *see* Abrasion, thigh
      bite — *see* Bite, superficial, thigh
      blister — *see* Blister, thigh
      contusion — *see* Contusion, thigh
      external constriction — *see* Constriction, external, thigh
      foreign body — *see* Foreign body, superficial, thigh
    thorax, thoracic (wall) S20.90 ☑
      abrasion — *see* Abrasion, thorax
      back S20.40- ☑
      bite — *see* Bite, thorax, superficial
      blister — *see* Blister, thorax
      contusion — *see* Contusion, thorax

Injury — *continued*
  superficial — *continued*
    thorax, thoracic — *continued*
      external constriction — *see* Constriction, external, thorax
      foreign body — *see* Foreign body, superficial, thorax
      front S20.30- ☑
    throat S10.10 ☑
      abrasion S10.11 ☑
      bite S10.17 ☑
        insect S10.16 ☑
      blister S10.12 ☑
      contusion S10.0 ☑
      external constriction S10.14 ☑
      foreign body S10.15 ☑
    thumb S60.93- ☑
      abrasion — *see* Abrasion, thumb
      bite — *see* Bite, superficial, thumb
      blister — *see* Blister, thumb
      contusion — *see* Contusion, thumb
      external constriction — *see* Constriction, external, thumb
      foreign body — *see* Foreign body, superficial, thumb
      insect bite — *see* Bite, by site, superficial, insect
      specified type NEC S60.39 ☑
    toe(s) S90.93- ☑
      abrasion — *see* Abrasion, toe
      bite — *see* Bite, toe
      blister — *see* Blister, toe
      contusion — *see* Contusion, toe
      external constriction — *see* Constriction, external, toe
      foreign body — *see* Foreign body, superficial, toe
      great S90.93- ☑
    tongue — *see* Injury, superficial, oral cavity
    tooth, teeth — *see* Injury, superficial, oral cavity
    trachea S10.10 ☑
    tunica vaginalis S30.94 ☑
    tympanum, tympanic membrane — *see* Injury, superficial, ear
    uvula — *see* Injury, superficial, oral cavity
    vagina S30.95 ☑
    vocal cords — *see* Injury, superficial, throat
    vulva S30.95 ☑
    wrist S60.91- ☑
  supraclavicular region — *see* Injury, neck
  supraorbital S09.93 ☑
  suprarenal gland (multiple) — *see* Injury, adrenal
  surgical complication (external or internal site) — *see* Laceration, accidental complicating surgery
  temple S09.90 ☑
  temporal region S09.90 ☑
  tendon — *see also* Injury, muscle, by site
    abdomen — *see* Injury, muscle, abdomen
    Achilles — *see* Injury, Achilles tendon
    lower back — *see* Injury, muscle, lower back
    pelvic organs — *see* Injury, muscle, pelvis
  tenth cranial nerve (pneumogastric or vagus) — *see* Injury, nerve, vagus
  testis S39.94 ☑
  thigh S79.92- ☑
    blood vessel — *see* Injury, blood vessel, hip
    contusion — *see* Contusion, thigh
    fracture — *see* Fracture, femur
    muscle — *see* Injury, muscle, thigh
    nerve — *see* Injury, nerve, thigh
    open — *see* Wound, open, thigh
    specified NEC S79.82- ☑
    superficial — *see* Injury, superficial, thigh
  third cranial nerve (oculomotor) — *see* Injury, nerve, oculomotor
  thorax, thoracic S29.9 ☑
    blood vessel — *see* Injury, blood vessel, thorax
    cavity — *see* Injury, intrathoracic
    dislocation — *see* Dislocation, thorax
    external (wall) S29.9 ☑
      contusion — *see* Contusion, thorax
      nerve — *see* Injury, nerve, thorax
      open — *see* Wound, open, thorax
      specified NEC S29.8 ☑
      sprain — *see* Sprain, thorax
      superficial — *see* Injury, superficial, thorax
    fracture — *see* Fracture, thorax
    internal — *see* Injury, intrathoracic
    intrathoracic organ — *see* Injury, intrathoracic

Injury — *continued*
  thorax, thoracic — *continued*
    sympathetic ganglion — *see* Injury, nerve, thorax, sympathetic
  throat — *see also* Injury, neck S19.9 ☑
  thumb S69.9- ☑
    blood vessel — *see* Injury, blood vessel, thumb
    contusion — *see* Contusion, thumb
    dislocation — *see* Dislocation, thumb
    fracture — *see* Fracture, thumb
    muscle — *see* Injury, muscle, thumb
    nerve — *see* Injury, nerve, digital, thumb
    open — *see* Wound, open, thumb
    specified NEC S69.8- ☑
    sprain — *see* Sprain, thumb
    superficial — *see* Injury, superficial, thumb
  thymus (gland) — *see* Injury, intrathoracic, specified organ NEC
  thyroid (gland) NEC S19.84 ☑
  toe S99.92- ☑
    contusion — *see* Contusion, toe
    dislocation — *see* Dislocation, toe
    fracture — *see* Fracture, toe
    muscle — *see* Injury, muscle, toe
    open — *see* Wound, open, toe
    specified type NEC S99.82- ☑
    sprain — *see* Sprain, toe
    superficial — *see* Injury, superficial, toe
  tongue S09.93 ☑
  tonsil S09.93 ☑
  tooth S09.93 ☑
  trachea (cervical) NEC S19.82 ☑
    thoracic — *see* Injury, intrathoracic, trachea, thoracic
  transfusion-related acute lung (TRALI) J95.84
  tunica vaginalis S39.94 ☑
  twelfth cranial nerve (hypoglossal) — *see* Injury, nerve, hypoglossal
  ureter S37.10 ☑
    contusion S37.12 ☑
    laceration S37.13 ☑
    specified type NEC S37.19 ☑
  urethra (sphincter) S37.30 ☑
    at delivery O71.5
    contusion S37.32 ☑
    laceration S37.33 ☑
    specified type NEC S37.39 ☑
  urinary organ S37.90 ☑
    contusion S37.92 ☑
    laceration S37.93 ☑
    specified
      site NEC S37.899 ☑
        contusion S37.892 ☑
        laceration S37.893 ☑
        specified type NEC S37.898 ☑
      type NEC S37.99 ☑
  uterus, uterine S37.60 ☑
    with ectopic or molar pregnancy O08.6
    blood vessel — *see* Injury, blood vessel, iliac
    contusion S37.62 ☑
    laceration S37.63 ☑
      cervix at delivery O71.3
    rupture associated with obstetrics — *see* Rupture, uterus
    specified type NEC S37.69 ☑
  uvula S09.93 ☑
  vagina S39.93 ☑
    abrasion S30.814 ☑
    bite S31.45 ☑
      insect S30.864 ☑
      superficial NEC S30.874 ☑
    contusion S30.23 ☑
    crush S38.03 ☑
    during delivery — *see* Laceration, vagina, during delivery
    external constriction S30.844 ☑
    insect bite S30.864 ☑
    laceration S31.41 ☑
      with foreign body S31.42 ☑
    open wound S31.40 ☑
    puncture S31.43 ☑
      with foreign body S31.44 ☑
    superficial S30.95 ☑
      foreign body S30.854 ☑
  vas deferens — *see* Injury, pelvic organ, specified site NEC
  vascular NEC T14.8 ☑

☑ **Additional Character Required** — **Refer to the Tabular List for Character Selection**

Injury — *continued*
   vein — *see* Injury, blood vessel
   vena cava (superior) S25.20 ☑
      inferior S35.10 ☑
         laceration (minor) (superficial) S35.11 ☑
            major S35.12 ☑
         specified type NEC S35.19 ☑
      laceration (minor) (superficial) S25.21 ☑
         major S25.22 ☑
      specified type NEC S25.29 ☑
   vesical (sphincter) — *see* Injury, bladder
   visual cortex S04.04-
   vitreous (humor) S05.90 ☑
      specified NEC S05.8X- ☑
   vocal cord NEC S19.83 ☑
   vulva S39.94 ☑
      abrasion S30.814 ☑
      bite S31.45 ☑
         insect S30.864 ☑
         superficial NEC S30.874 ☑
      contusion S30.23 ☑
      crush S38.03 ☑
      during delivery — *see* Laceration, perineum, female, during delivery
      external constriction S30.844 ☑
      insect bite S30.864 ☑
      laceration S31.41 ☑
         with foreign body S31.42 ☑
      open wound S31.40 ☑
      puncture S31.43 ☑
         with foreign body S31.44 ☑
      superficial S30.95 ☑
         foreign body S30.854 ☑
   whiplash (cervical spine) S13.4 ☑
   wrist S69.9- ☑
      blood vessel — *see* Injury, blood vessel, hand
      contusion — *see* Contusion, wrist
      dislocation — *see* Dislocation, wrist
      fracture — *see* Fracture, wrist
      muscle — *see* Injury, muscle, hand
      nerve — *see* Injury, nerve, hand
      open — *see* Wound, open, wrist
      specified NEC S69.8- ☑
      sprain — *see* Sprain, wrist
      superficial — *see* Injury, superficial, wrist
Inoculation — *see also* Vaccination
   complication or reaction — *see* Complications, vaccination
Insanity, insane — *see also* Psychosis
   adolescent — *see* Schizophrenia
   confusional F28
      acute or subacute F05
   delusional F22
   senile F03 ☑
Insect
   bite — *see* Bite, by site, superficial, insect
   venomous, poisoning NEC (by) — *see* Venom, arthropod
Insecurity
   financial Z59.86
   food Z59.41
   transportation Z59.82
Insensitivity
   adrenocorticotropin hormone (ACTH) E27.49
   androgen E34.50
      complete E34.51
      partial E34.52
Insertion
   cord (umbilical) lateral or velamentous O43.12- ☑
   intrauterine contraceptive device (encounter for) — *see* Intrauterine contraceptive device
Insolation (sunstroke) T67.01 ☑
Insomnia (organic) G47.00
   adjustment F51.02
   adjustment disorder F51.02
   behavioral, of childhood Z73.819
      combined type Z73.812
      limit setting type Z73.811
      sleep-onset association type Z73.810
   childhood Z73.819
   chronic F51.04
      somatized tension F51.04
   conditioned F51.04
   due to
      alcohol
         abuse F10.182
         dependence F10.282
         use F10.982

Insomnia — *continued*
   due to — *continued*
      amphetamines
         abuse F15.182
         dependence F15.282
         use F15.982
      anxiety disorder F51.05
      caffeine
         abuse F15.182
         dependence F15.282
         use F15.982
      cocaine
         abuse F14.182
         dependence F14.282
         use F14.982
      depression F51.05
      drug NEC
         abuse F19.182
         dependence F19.282
         use F19.982
      medical condition G47.01
      mental disorder NEC F51.05
      opioid
         abuse F11.182
         dependence F11.282
         use F11.982
      psychoactive substance NEC
         abuse F19.182
         dependence F19.182
         use F19.982
      sedative, hypnotic, or anxiolytic
         abuse F13.182
         dependence F13.282
         use F13.982
      stimulant NEC
         abuse F15.182
         dependence F15.282
         use F15.982
   fatal familial (FFI) A81.83
   idiopathic F51.01
   learned F51.3
   nonorganic origin F51.01
   not due to a substance or known physiological condition F51.01
      specified NEC F51.09
   paradoxical F51.03
   primary F51.01
   psychiatric F51.05
   psychophysiologic F51.04
   related to psychopathology F51.05
   short-term F51.02
   specified NEC G47.09
   stress-related F51.02
   transient F51.02
   without objective findings F51.02
Inspiration
   food or foreign body — *see* Foreign body, by site
   mucus — *see* Asphyxia, mucus
Inspissated bile syndrome (newborn) P59.1
Instability
   emotional (excessive) F60.3
   housing
      housed Z59.819
         with risk of homelessness Z59.811
         homelessness in past 12 months Z59.812
   joint (post-traumatic) M25.30
      ankle M25.37- ☑
      due to old ligament injury — *see* Disorder, ligament
      elbow M25.32- ☑
      flail — *see* Flail, joint
      foot M25.37- ☑
      hand M25.34- ☑
      hip M25.35- ☑
      knee M25.36- ☑
      lumbosacral — *see* subcategory M53.2 ☑
      prosthesis — *see* Complications, joint prosthesis, mechanical, displacement, by site
      sacroiliac — *see* subcategory M53.2 ☑
      secondary to
         old ligament injury — *see* Disorder, ligament
         removal of joint prosthesis M96.89
      shoulder (region) M25.31- ☑
      specified site NEC M25.39
      spine — *see* subcategory M53.2 ☑
      wrist M25.33- ☑
   knee (chronic) M23.5- ☑
   lumbosacral — *see* subcategory M53.2 ☑
   nervous F48.8

Instability — *continued*
   personality (emotional) F60.3
   spine — *see* Instability, joint, spine
   vasomotor R55
Institutional syndrome (childhood) F94.2
Institutionalization, affecting child Z62.22
   disinhibited attachment F94.2
Insufficiency, insufficient
   accommodation, old age H52.4
   adrenal (gland) E27.40
      primary E27.1
   adrenocortical E27.40
      drug-induced E27.3
      iatrogenic E27.3
      primary E27.1
   anatomic crown height K08.89
   anterior (occlusal) guidance M26.54
   anus K62.89
   aortic (valve) I35.1
      with
         mitral (valve) disease I08.0
            with tricuspid (valve) disease I08.3
         stenosis I35.2
         tricuspid (valve) disease I08.2
            with mitral (valve) disease I08.3
      congenital Q23.1
      rheumatic I06.1
         with
            mitral (valve) disease I08.0
               with tricuspid (valve) disease I08.3
            stenosis I06.2
               with mitral (valve) disease I08.0
                  with tricuspid (valve) disease I08.3
            tricuspid (valve) disease I08.2
               with mitral (valve) disease I08.3
      specified cause NEC I35.1
      syphilitic A52.03
   arterial I77.1
      basilar G45.0
      carotid (hemispheric) G45.1
      cerebral I67.81
      coronary (acute or subacute) I24.89
      mesenteric K55.1
      peripheral I73.9
      precerebral (multiple) (bilateral) G45.2
      vertebral G45.0
   arteriovenous I99.8
   biliary K83.8
   cardiac — *see also* Insufficiency, myocardial
      due to presence of (cardiac) prosthesis I97.11- ☑
      postprocedural I97.11- ☑
   cardiorenal, hypertensive I13.2
   cardiovascular — *see* Disease, cardiovascular
   cerebrovascular (acute) I67.81
      with transient focal neurological signs and symptoms G45.8
   circulatory NEC I99.8
      newborn P29.89
   clinical crown length K08.89
   convergence H51.11
   coronary (acute or subacute) I24.89
      chronic or with a stated duration of over 4 weeks I25.89
   corticoadrenal E27.40
      primary E27.1
   dietary E63.9
   divergence H51.8
   food T73.0 ☑
   gastroesophageal K22.89
   gonadal
      ovary E28.39
      testis E29.1
   health insurance coverage Z59.71
   heart — *see also* Insufficiency, myocardial
      newborn P29.0
      valve — *see* Endocarditis
   hepatic — *see* Failure, hepatic
   idiopathic autonomic G90.09
   interocclusal distance of fully erupted teeth (ridge) M26.36
   kidney N28.9
      acute N28.9
      chronic N18.9
   lacrimal (secretion) H04.12- ☑
      passages — *see* Stenosis, lacrimal
   liver — *see* Failure, hepatic
   lung — *see* Insufficiency, pulmonary
   mental (congenital) — *see* Disability, intellectual
   mesenteric K55.1

Index

Injury — Insufficiency, insufficient

Insufficiency, insufficient — continued
- mitral (valve) I34.0
  - with
    - aortic valve disease I08.0
      - with tricuspid (valve) disease I08.3
    - obstruction or stenosis I05.2
      - with aortic valve disease I08.0
    - tricuspid (valve) disease I08.1
      - with aortic (valve) disease I08.3
  - congenital Q23.3
  - rheumatic I05.1
    - with
      - aortic valve disease I08.0
        - with tricuspid (valve) disease I08.3
      - obstruction or stenosis I05.2
        - with aortic valve disease I08.0
          - with tricuspid (valve) disease I08.3
      - tricuspid (valve) disease I08.1
        - with aortic (valve) disease I08.3
    - active or acute I01.1
      - with chorea, rheumatic (Sydenham's) I02.0
  - specified cause, except rheumatic I34.0
- muscle — see also Disease, muscle
  - heart — see Insufficiency, myocardial
- ocular NEC H50.9
- myocardial, myocardium (with arteriosclerosis) — see also Failure, heart I50.9
  - with
    - rheumatic fever (conditions in I00) I09.0
      - active, acute or subacute I01.2
        - with chorea I02.0
      - inactive or quiescent (with chorea) I09.0
  - congenital Q24.8
  - hypertensive — see Hypertension, heart
  - newborn P29.0
  - rheumatic I09.0
    - active, acute, or subacute I01.2
  - syphilitic A52.06
- nourishment — see also Nutrition deficient T73.0 ☑
- pancreatic K86.89
  - exocrine K86.81
- parathyroid (gland) E20.9
- peripheral vascular (arterial) I73.9
- pituitary E23.0
- placental (mother) O36.51- ☑
- platelets D69.6
- prenatal care affecting management of pregnancy O09.3- ☑
- progressive pluriglandular E31.0
- pulmonary J98.4
  - acute, following surgery (nonthoracic) J95.2
    - thoracic J95.1
  - chronic, following surgery J95.3
  - following
    - shock J98.4
    - trauma J98.4
  - newborn P28.89
  - valve I37.1
    - with stenosis I37.2
    - congenital Q22.2
    - rheumatic I09.89
      - with aortic, mitral or tricuspid (valve) disease I08.8
- pyloric K31.89
- renal (acute) N28.9
  - chronic N18.9
- respiratory R06.89
  - newborn P28.5
- rotation — see Malrotation
- sleep syndrome F51.12
- social insurance Z59.71
- suprarenal E27.40
  - primary E27.1
- tarso-orbital fascia, congenital Q10.3
- testis E29.1
- thyroid (gland) (acquired) E03.9
  - congenital E03.1
- tricuspid (valve) (rheumatic) I07.1
  - with
    - aortic (valve) disease I08.2
      - with mitral (valve) disease I08.3
    - mitral (valve) disease I08.1
      - with aortic (valve) disease I08.3
    - obstruction or stenosis I07.2
      - with aortic (valve) disease I08.2
        - with mitral (valve) disease I08.3
  - congenital Q22.8
  - nonrheumatic I36.1
    - with stenosis I36.2

Insufficiency, insufficient — continued
- urethral sphincter R32
- valve, valvular (heart) I38
  - aortic — see Insufficiency, aortic (valve)
  - congenital Q24.8
  - mitral — see Insufficiency, mitral (valve)
  - pulmonary — see Insufficiency, pulmonary, valve
  - tricuspid — see Insufficiency, tricuspid (valve)
- vascular I99.8
  - intestine K55.9
    - acute — see also Ischemia, intestine, acute K55.059
  - mesenteric K55.1
  - peripheral I73.9
  - renal — see Hypertension, kidney
- velopharyngeal
  - acquired K13.79
  - congenital Q38.8
- venous (chronic) (peripheral) I87.2
- ventricular — see Insufficiency, myocardial
- welfare support Z59.72

Insufflation, fallopian Z31.41

Insular — see condition

Insulinoma
- pancreas
  - benign D13.7
  - malignant C25.4
  - uncertain behavior D37.8
- specified site
  - benign — see Neoplasm, by site, benign
  - malignant — see Neoplasm, by site, malignant
  - uncertain behavior — see Neoplasm, by site, uncertain behavior
- unspecified site
  - benign D13.7
  - malignant C25.4
  - uncertain behavior D37.8

Insuloma — see Insulinoma

Interference
- balancing side M26.56
- non-working side M26.56

Intermenstrual — see condition

Intermittent — see condition

Internal — see condition

Interrogation
- cardiac defibrillator (automatic) (implantable) Z45.02
- cardiac pacemaker Z45.018
- cardiac (event) (loop) recorder Z45.09
- infusion pump (implanted) (intrathecal) Z45.1
- neurostimulator Z46.2

Interruption
- aortic arch Q25.21
- bundle of His I44.30
- phase-shift, sleep cycle — see Disorder, sleep, circadian rhythm
- sleep phase-shift, or 24 hour sleep-wake cycle — see Disorder, sleep, circadian rhythm

Interstitial — see condition

Intertrigo L30.4
- labialis K13.0

Intervertebral disc — see condition

Intestine, intestinal — see condition

Intolerance
- carbohydrate K90.49
- disaccharide, hereditary E73.0
- fat NEC K90.49
  - pancreatic K90.3
- food K90.49
  - dietary counseling and surveillance Z71.3
- fructose E74.10
  - hereditary E74.12
- glucose (-galactose) E74.39
- gluten K90.41
- lactose E73.9
  - specified NEC E73.8
- lysine E72.3
- milk NEC K90.49
  - lactose E73.9
- orthostatic, chronic G90.A
- protein K90.49
- starch NEC K90.49
- sucrose (-isomaltose) E74.31

Intoxicated NEC (without dependence) — see Alcohol, intoxication

Intoxication
- acid — see also Acidosis E87.29
- alcoholic (acute) (without dependence) — see Alcohol, intoxication
- alimentary canal K52.1

Intoxication — continued
- amphetamine (without dependence) — see also Abuse, drug, stimulant, with intoxication
  - with dependence — see Dependence, drug, stimulant, with intoxication
  - stimulant NEC F15.10
    - with
      - anxiety disorder F15.180
      - intoxication F15.129
        - with
          - delirium F15.121
          - perceptual disturbance F15.122
- anxiolytic (acute) (without dependence) — see Abuse, drug, sedative, with intoxication
  - with dependence — see Dependence, drug, sedative, with intoxication
- caffeine F15.929
  - with dependence — see Dependence, drug, stimulant, with intoxication
- cannabinoids (acute) (without dependence) — see Use, cannabis, with intoxication
  - with
    - abuse — see Abuse, drug, cannabis, with intoxication
    - dependence — see Dependence, drug, cannabis, with intoxication
- chemical — see Table of Drugs and Chemicals
  - via placenta or breast milk — see - Absorption, chemical, through placenta
- cocaine (acute) (without dependence) — see Abuse, drug, cocaine, with intoxication
  - with dependence — see Dependence, drug, cocaine, with intoxication
- drug
  - acute (without dependence) — see Abuse, drug, by type with intoxication
    - with dependence — see Dependence, drug, by type with intoxication
  - addictive
    - via placenta or breast milk — see Absorption, drug, addictive, through placenta
  - newborn P93.8
    - gray baby syndrome P93.0
  - overdose or wrong substance given or taken — see Table of Drugs and Chemicals, by drug, poisoning
- enteric K52.1
- foodborne A05.9
  - bacterial A05.9
  - classical (Clostridium botulinum) A05.1
  - due to
    - Bacillus cereus A05.4
    - bacterium A05.9
      - specified NEC A05.8
    - Clostridium
      - botulinum A05.1
      - perfringens A05.2
      - welchii A05.2
    - Salmonella A02.9
      - with
        - (gastro)enteritis A02.0
        - localized infection(s) A02.20
          - arthritis A02.23
          - meningitis A02.21
          - osteomyelitis A02.24
          - pneumonia A02.22
          - pyelonephritis A02.25
          - specified NEC A02.29
        - sepsis A02.1
        - specified manifestation NEC A02.8
    - Staphylococcus A05.0
    - Vibrio
      - parahaemolyticus A05.3
      - vulnificus A05.5
  - enterotoxin, staphylococcal A05.0
  - noxious — see Poisoning, food, noxious
- gastrointestinal K52.1
- hallucinogenic (without dependence) — see Abuse, drug, hallucinogen, with intoxication
  - with dependence — see Dependence, drug, hallucinogen, with intoxication
- hepatocerebral K76.82
- hypnotic (acute) (without dependence) — see Abuse, drug, sedative, with intoxication
  - with dependence — see Dependence, drug, sedative, with intoxication
- inhalant (acute) (without dependence) — see Abuse, drug, inhalant, with intoxication

Intoxication — continued
- inhalant — see Abuse, drug, inhalant, with intoxication — continued
  - with dependence — see Dependence, drug, inhalant, with intoxication
- meaning
  - inebriation — see category F10 ☑
  - poisoning — see Table of Drugs and Chemicals
- methyl alcohol (acute) (without dependence) — see Alcohol, intoxication
- opioid (acute) (without dependence) — see Abuse, drug, opioid, with intoxication
  - with dependence — see Dependence, drug, opioid, with intoxication
- pathologic NEC (without dependence) — see Alcohol, intoxication
- phencyclidine (without dependence) — see Abuse, drug, hallucinogen, with intoxication
  - with dependence — see Dependence, drug, hallucinogen, with intoxication
- potassium (K) E87.5
- psychoactive substance NEC (without dependence) — see Abuse, drug, psychoactive NEC, with intoxication
  - with dependence — see Dependence, drug, psychoactive NEC, with intoxication
- sedative (acute) (without dependence) — see Abuse, drug, sedative, with intoxication
  - with dependence — see Dependence, drug, sedative, with intoxication
- serum — see also Reaction, serum T80.69 ☑
- uremic — see Uremia
- volatile solvents (acute) (without dependence) — see Abuse, drug, inhalant, with intoxication
  - with dependence — see Dependence, drug, inhalant, with intoxication
- water E87.79

Intraabdominal testis, testes
- bilateral Q53.211
- unilateral Q53.111

Intracranial — see condition
Intrahepatic gallbladder Q44.1
Intraligamentous — see condition
Intrathoracic — see also condition
- kidney Q63.2

Intrauterine contraceptive device
- checking Z30.431
- in situ Z97.5
- insertion Z30.430
  - immediately following removal Z30.433
- management Z30.431
- reinsertion Z30.433
- removal Z30.432
- replacement Z30.433
- retention in pregnancy O26.3- ☑

Intraventricular — see condition
Intrinsic deformity — see Deformity
Intubation, difficult or failed T88.4 ☑
Intumescence, lens (eye) (cataract) — see Cataract
Intussusception (bowel) (colon) (enteric) (ileocecal) (ileocolic) (intestine) (rectum) K56.1
- appendix K38.8
- congenital Q43.8
- ureter (with obstruction) N13.5
Invagination (bowel, colon, intestine or rectum) K56.1
Inversion
- albumin-globulin (A-G) ratio E88.09
- bladder N32.89
- cecum — see Intussusception
- cervix N88.8
- chromosome in normal individual Q95.1
- circadian rhythm — see Disorder, sleep, circadian rhythm
- nipple N64.59
  - congenital Q83.8
  - gestational — see Retraction, nipple
  - puerperal, postpartum — see Retraction, nipple
- nyctohemeral rhythm — see Disorder, sleep, circadian rhythm
- optic papilla Q14.2
- organ or site, congenital NEC — see Anomaly, by site
- sleep rhythm — see Disorder, sleep, circadian rhythm
- testis (congenital) Q55.29
- uterus (chronic) (postinfectional) (postpartal, old) N85.5
  - postpartum O71.2
- vagina (posthysterectomy) N99.3
- ventricular Q20.5
Investigation — see also Examination Z04.9
- clinical research subject (control) (normal comparison) (participant) Z00.6

Involuntary movement, abnormal R25.9
Involution, involutional — see also condition
- breast, cystic — see Dysplasia, mammary, specified type NEC
- depression (single episode) F32.89
  - recurrent episode F33.9
- melancholia (single episode) F32.89
  - recurrent episode F33.8
- ovary, senile — see Atrophy, ovary
- thymus failure E32.8

I.Q.
- 20-34 F72
- 35-49 F71
- 50-69 F70
- under 20 F73
IRDS (type I) P22.0
- type II P22.1
Irideremia Q13.1
Iridis rubeosis — see Disorder, iris, vascular
Iridochoroiditis (panuveitis) — see Panuveitis
Iridocyclitis H20.9
- acute H20.0- ☑
  - hypopyon H20.05- ☑
  - primary H20.01- ☑
  - recurrent H20.02- ☑
  - secondary (noninfectious) H20.04- ☑
    - infectious H20.03- ☑
- chronic H20.1- ☑
- due to allergy — see Iridocyclitis, acute, secondary
- endogenous — see Iridocyclitis, acute, primary
- Fuchs' — see Cyclitis, Fuchs' heterochromic
- gonococcal A54.32
- granulomatous — see Iridocyclitis, chronic
- herpes, herpetic (simplex) B00.51
  - zoster B02.32
- hypopyon — see Iridocyclitis, acute, hypopyon
- in (due to)
  - ankylosing spondylitis M45.9
  - gonococcal infection A54.32
  - herpes (simplex) virus B00.51
    - zoster B02.32
  - infectious disease NOS B99 ☑
  - parasitic disease NOS B89 [H22]
  - sarcoidosis D86.83
  - syphilis A51.43
  - tuberculosis A18.54
  - zoster B02.32
- lens-induced H20.2- ☑
- nongranulomatous — see Iridocyclitis, acute
- recurrent — see Iridocyclitis, acute, recurrent
- rheumatic — see Iridocyclitis, chronic
- subacute — see Iridocyclitis, acute
- sympathetic — see Uveitis, sympathetic
- syphilitic (secondary) A51.43
- tuberculous (chronic) A18.54
- Vogt-Koyanagi H20.82- ☑
Iridocyclochoroiditis (panuveitis) — see Panuveitis
Iridodialysis H21.53- ☑
Iridodonesis H21.89
Iridoplegia (complete) (partial) (reflex) H57.09
Iridoschisis H21.25- ☑
Iris — see also condition
- bombé — see Membrane, pupillary
Iritis — see also Iridocyclitis
- chronic — see Iridocyclitis, chronic
- diabetic — see E08-E13 with .39
- due to
  - herpes simplex B00.51
  - leprosy A30.9 [H22]
- gonococcal A54.32
- gouty — see also Gout, by type M10.9 [H22]
- granulomatous — see Iridocyclitis, chronic
- lens induced — see Iridocyclitis, lens-induced
- papulosa (syphilitic) A52.71
- rheumatic — see Iridocyclitis, chronic
- syphilitic (secondary) A51.43
  - congenital (early) A50.01
  - late A52.71
- tuberculous A18.54
Iron — see condition
Iron-miner's lung J63.4
Irradiated enamel (tooth, teeth) K03.89
Irradiation effects, adverse T66 ☑
Irreducible, irreducibility — see condition
Irregular, irregularity
- action, heart I49.9
- alveolar process K08.89
- bleeding N92.6

Irregular, irregularity — continued
- breathing R06.89
- contour of cornea (acquired) — see Deformity, cornea
  - congenital Q13.4
- contour, reconstructed breast N65.0
- dentin (in pulp) K04.3
- eye movements H55.89
  - deficient
    - saccadic H55.81
    - smooth H55.82
  - nystagmus — see Nystagmus
- labor O62.2
- menstruation (cause unknown) N92.6
- periods N92.6
- prostate N42.9
- pupil — see Abnormality, pupillary
- reconstructed breast N65.0
- respiratory R06.89
- septum (nasal) J34.2
- shape, organ or site, congenital NEC — see Distortion
- sleep-wake pattern (rhythm) G47.23
Irritable, irritability R45.4
- bladder N32.89
- bowel (syndrome) K58.9
  - with
    - constipation K58.1
    - diarrhea K58.0
  - mixed K58.2
  - psychogenic F45.8
  - specified NEC K58.8
- bronchial — see Bronchitis
- cerebral, in newborn P91.3
- colon — see also Irritable, bowel K58.9
  - with diarrhea K58.0
  - psychogenic F45.8
- duodenum K59.89
- heart (psychogenic) F45.8
- hip — see Derangement, joint, specified type NEC, hip
- ileum K59.89
- infant R68.12
- jejunum K59.89
- rectum K59.89
- stomach K31.89
  - psychogenic F45.8
- sympathetic G90.89
- urethra N36.8
- without diarrhea K58.9
Irritation
- anus K62.89
- axillary nerve G54.0
- bladder N32.89
- brachial plexus G54.0
- bronchial — see Bronchitis
- cervical plexus G54.2
- cervix — see Cervicitis
- choroid, sympathetic — see Endophthalmitis
- cranial nerve — see Disorder, nerve, cranial
- gastric K31.89
  - psychogenic F45.8
- globe, sympathetic — see Uveitis, sympathetic
- labyrinth — see subcategory H83.2 ☑
- lumbosacral plexus G54.1
- meninges (traumatic) — see Injury, intracranial
  - nontraumatic — see Meningismus
- nerve — see Disorder, nerve
- nervous R45.0
- penis N48.89
- perineum NEC L29.3
- peripheral autonomic nervous system G90.89
- peritoneum — see Peritonitis
- pharynx J39.2
- plantar nerve — see Lesion, nerve, plantar
- spinal (cord) (traumatic) — see also Injury, spinal cord, by region
  - nerve G58.9
    - root NEC — see Radiculopathy
  - nontraumatic — see Myelopathy
- stomach K31.89
  - psychogenic F45.8
- sympathetic nerve NEC G90.89
- ulnar nerve — see Lesion, nerve, ulnar
- vagina N89.8
Ischemia, ischemic I99.8
- bowel (transient)
  - acute — see also Ischemia, intestine, acute K55.059
  - chronic K55.1
  - due to mesenteric artery insufficiency K55.1
- brain — see Ischemia, cerebral
- cardiac — see Disease, heart, ischemic

Ischemia, ischemic — *continued*
cardiomyopathy I25.5
cerebral (chronic) (generalized) I67.82
arteriosclerotic I67.2
intermittent G45.9
newborn P91.0
recurrent focal G45.8
transient G45.9
colon chronic (due to mesenteric artery insufficiency) K55.1
coronary — *see* Disease, heart, ischemic
demand (coronary) — *see also* Angina I24.89
with myocardial infarction I21.A1
resulting in myocardial infarction I21.A1
heart (chronic or with a stated duration of over 4 weeks) I25.9
acute or with a stated duration of 4 weeks or less I24.9
subacute I24.9
infarction, muscle — *see* Infarct, muscle
intestine (large) (small) (transient) K55.9
acute K55.059
diffuse K55.052
focal K55.051
large K55.039
diffuse K55.032
focal K55.031
small K55.019
diffuse K55.012
focal K55.011
chronic K55.1
due to mesenteric artery insufficiency K55.1
kidney N28.0
limb, critical — *see* Arteriosclerosis, with critical limb ischemia
limb-threatening, chronic — *see* Arteriosclerosis, with critical limb ischemia
mesenteric, acute — *see also* Ischemia, intestine, acute K55.059
muscle, traumatic T79.6 ☑
myocardium, myocardial (chronic or with a stated duration of over 4 weeks) I25.9
acute, without myocardial infarction I51.3
silent (asymptomatic) I25.6
transient of newborn P29.4
renal N28.0
retina, retinal — *see* Occlusion, artery, retina
small bowel
acute K55.019
diffuse K55.012
focal K55.011
chronic K55.1
due to mesenteric artery insufficiency K55.1
spinal cord G95.11
subendocardial — *see* Insufficiency, coronary
supply (coronary) — *see also* Angina I25.9
due to vasospasm I20.1
Ischial spine — *see* condition
Ischialgia — *see* Sciatica
Ischiopagus Q89.4
Ischium, ischial — *see* condition
Ischuria R34
Iselin's disease or osteochondrosis — *see* Osteochondrosis, juvenile, metatarsus
Islands of
parotid tissue in
lymph nodes Q38.6
neck structures Q38.6
submaxillary glands in
fascia Q38.6
lymph nodes Q38.6
neck muscles Q38.6
Islet cell tumor, pancreas D13.7
Isoimmunization NEC — *see also* Incompatibility
affecting management of pregnancy (ABO) (with hydrops fetalis) O36.11- ☑
anti-A sensitization O36.11- ☑
anti-B sensitization O36.19- ☑
anti-c sensitization O36.09- ☑
anti-C sensitization O36.09- ☑
anti-e sensitization O36.09- ☑
anti-E sensitization O36.09- ☑
Rh NEC O36.09- ☑
anti-D antibody O36.01- ☑
specified NEC O36.19- ☑
newborn P55.9
with
hydrops fetalis P56.0
kernicterus P57.0

Isoimmunization — *continued*
newborn — *continued*
ABO (blood groups) P55.1
Rhesus (Rh) factor P55.0
specified type NEC P55.8
Isolation, isolated
dwelling Z59.89
family Z63.79
social Z60.4
Isoleucinosis E71.19
Isomerism atrial appendages (with asplenia or polysplenia) Q20.6
Isosporiasis, isosporosis A07.3
Isovaleric acidemia E71.110
Issue of
medical certificate Z02.79
for disability determination Z02.71
repeat prescription (appliance) (glasses) (medicinal substance, medicament, medicine) Z76.0
contraception — *see* Contraception
IST (inappropriate sinus tachycardia, so stated) I47.11
Itch, itching — *see also* Pruritus
baker's L23.6
barber's B35.0
bricklayer's L24.5
cheese B88.0
clam digger's B65.3
coolie B76.9
copra B88.0
dew B76.9
dhobi B35.6
filarial — *see* Infestation, filarial
grain B88.0
grocer's B88.0
ground B76.9
harvest B88.0
jock B35.6
Malabar B35.5
beard B35.0
foot B35.3
scalp B35.0
meaning scabies B86
Norwegian B86
perianal L29.0
poultrymen's B88.0
sarcoptic B86
scabies B86
scrub B88.0
straw B88.0
swimmer's B65.3
water B76.9
winter L29.89
Ivemark's syndrome (asplenia with congenital heart disease) Q89.01
Ivory bones Q78.2
Ixodiasis NEC B88.8

J

Jaccoud's syndrome — *see* Arthropathy, postrheumatic, chronic
Jackson's
membrane Q43.3
paralysis or syndrome G83.89
veil Q43.3
Jacquet's dermatitis (diaper dermatitis) L22
Jadassohn-Pellizari's disease or anetoderma L90.2
Jadassohn's
blue nevus — *see* Nevus
intraepidermal epithelioma — *see* Neoplasm, skin, benign
Jaffe-Lichtenstein (-Uehlinger) **syndrome** — *see* Dysplasia, fibrous, bone NEC
Jakob-Creutzfeldt disease or syndrome — *see* Creutzfeldt-Jakob disease or syndrome
Jaksch-Luzet disease D64.89
Jamaican
neuropathy G92.8
paraplegic tropical ataxic-spastic syndrome G92.8
Janet's disease F48.8
Janiceps Q89.4
Jansky-Bielschowsky amaurotic idiocy E75.4
Japanese
B-type encephalitis A83.0
river fever A75.3
Jaundice (yellow) R17
acholuric (familial) (splenomegalic) — *see also* Spherocytosis
acquired D59.8

Jaundice — *continued*
breast-milk (inhibitor) P59.3
catarrhal (acute) B15.9
with hepatic coma B15.0
cholestatic (benign) R17
due to or associated with
delayed conjugation P59.8
associated with (due to) preterm delivery P59.0
preterm delivery P59.0
epidemic (catarrhal) B15.9
with hepatic coma B15.0
leptospiral A27.0
spirochetal A27.0
familial nonhemolytic (congenital) (Gilbert) E80.4
Crigler-Najjar E80.5
febrile (acute) B15.9
with hepatic coma B15.0
leptospiral A27.0
spirochetal A27.0
hematogenous D59.9
hemolytic (acquired) D59.9
congenital — *see* Spherocytosis
hemorrhagic (acute) (leptospiral) (spirochetal) A27.0
infectious (acute) (subacute) B15.9
with hepatic coma B15.0
leptospiral A27.0
spirochetal A27.0
leptospiral (hemorrhagic) A27.0
malignant (without coma) K72.90
with coma K72.91
neonatal — *see* Jaundice, newborn
newborn P59.9
due to or associated with
ABO
antibodies P55.1
incompatibility, maternal/fetal P55.1
isoimmunization P55.1
absence or deficiency of enzyme system for bilirubin conjugation (congenital) P59.8
bleeding P58.1
breast milk inhibitors to conjugation P59.3
associated with preterm delivery P59.0
bruising P58.0
Crigler-Najjar syndrome E80.5
delayed conjugation P59.8
associated with preterm delivery P59.0
drugs or toxins
given to newborn P58.42
transmitted from mother P58.41
excessive hemolysis P58.9
due to
bleeding P58.1
bruising P58.0
drugs or toxins
given to newborn P58.42
transmitted from mother P58.41
infection P58.2
polycythemia P58.3
swallowed maternal blood P58.5
specified type NEC P58.8
galactosemia E74.21
Gilbert syndrome E80.4
hemolytic disease P55.9
ABO isoimmunization P55.1
Rh isoimmunization P55.0
specified NEC P55.8
hepatocellular damage P59.20
specified NEC P59.29
hereditary hemolytic anemia P58.8
hypothyroidism, congenital E03.1
incompatibility, maternal/fetal NOS P55.9
infection P58.2
inspissated bile syndrome P59.1
isoimmunization NOS P55.9
mucoviscidosis E84.9
polycythemia P58.3
preterm delivery P59.0
Rh
antibodies P55.0
incompatibility, maternal/fetal P55.0
isoimmunization P55.0
specified cause NEC P59.8
swallowed maternal blood P58.5
spherocytosis (congenital) D58.0
nonhemolytic congenital familial (Gilbert) E80.4
nuclear, newborn — *see also* Kernicterus of newborn P57.9
obstructive — *see also* Obstruction, bile duct K83.1
post-immunization — *see* Hepatitis, viral, type, B

☑ **Additional Character Required — Refer to the Tabular List for Character Selection**

Jaundice — *continued*
  post-transfusion — *see* Hepatitis, viral, type, B
  regurgitation — *see also* Obstruction, bile duct K83.1
  serum (homologous) (prophylactic) (therapeutic) — *see* Hepatitis, viral, type, B
  spirochetal (hemorrhagic) A27.Ø
  symptomatic R17
    newborn P59.9
Jaw — *see* condition
Jaw-winking phenomenon or syndrome QØ7.8
Jealousy
  alcoholic F1Ø.988
  childhood F93.8
  sibling F93.8
Jejunitis — *see* Enteritis
Jejunostomy status Z93.4
Jejunum, jejunal — *see* condition
Jensen's disease — *see* Inflammation, chorioretinal, focal, juxtapapillary
Jerks, myoclonic G25.3
Jervell-Lange-Nielsen syndrome I45.81
Jeune's disease Q77.2
Jigger disease B88.1
Job's syndrome (chronic granulomatous disease) D71
Joint — *see also* condition
  mice — *see* Loose, body, joint
    knee M23.4- ☑
Jordan's anomaly or syndrome D72.Ø
Joseph-Diamond-Blackfan anemia (congenital hypoplastic) D61.Ø1
Jungle yellow fever A95.Ø
Jüngling's disease — *see* Sarcoidosis
Juvenile — *see* condition

K

Kahler's disease C9Ø.Ø- ☑
Kakke E51.11
Kala-azar B55.Ø
Kallmann's syndrome E23.Ø
Kanner's syndrome (autism) — *see* Psychosis, childhood
Kaposi's
  dermatosis (xeroderma pigmentosum) Q82.1
  lichen ruber L44.Ø
    acuminatus L44.Ø
  sarcoma
    colon C46.4
    connective tissue C46.1
    gastrointestinal organ C46.4
    lung C46.5- ☑
    lymph node (multiple) C46.3
    palate (hard) (soft) C46.2
    rectum C46.4
    skin (multiple sites) C46.Ø
    specified site NEC C46.7
    stomach C46.4
    unspecified site C46.9
  varicelliform eruption BØØ.Ø
    vaccinia T88.1 ☑
Kartagener's syndrome or triad (sinusitis, bronchiectasis, situs inversus) Q89.3
Karyotype
  with abnormality except iso (Xq) Q96.2
  45,X Q96.Ø
  46,X
    iso (Xq) Q96.1
  46,XX Q98.3
    with streak gonads Q5Ø.32
    hermaphrodite (true) Q99.1
    male Q98.3
  46,XY
    with streak gonads Q56.1
    female Q97.3
    hermaphrodite (true) Q99.1
  47,XXX Q97.Ø
  47,XXY Q98.Ø
  47,XYY Q98.5
Kaschin-Beck disease — *see* Disease, Kaschin-Beck
Katayama's disease or fever B65.2
Kawasaki's syndrome M3Ø.3
Kayser-Fleischer ring (cornea) (pseudosclerosis) H18.Ø4- ☑
Kaznelson's syndrome (congenital hypoplastic anemia) D61.Ø1
Kearns-Sayre syndrome H49.81- ☑
Kedani fever A75.3
Kelis L91.Ø
Kelly (-Patterson) **syndrome** (sideropenic dysphagia) D5Ø.1
Keloid, cheloid L91.Ø

Keloid, cheloid — *continued*
  acne L73.Ø
  Addison's L94.Ø
  cornea — *see* Opacity, cornea
  Hawkin's L91.Ø
  scar L91.Ø
Keloma L91.Ø
Kenya fever A77.1
Keratectasia — *see also* Ectasia, cornea
  congenital Q13.4
Keratinization of alveolar ridge mucosa
  excessive K13.23
  minimal K13.22
Keratinized residual ridge mucosa
  excessive K13.23
  minimal K13.22
Keratitis (nodular) (nonulcerative) (simple) (zonular) H16.9
  with ulceration (central) (marginal) (perforated) (ring) — *see* Ulcer, cornea
  actinic — *see* Photokeratitis
  arborescens (herpes simplex) BØØ.52
  areolar H16.11- ☑
  bullosa H16.8
  deep H16.3Ø9
    specified type NEC H16.399
  dendritic (a) (herpes simplex) BØØ.52
  disciform (is) (herpes simplex) BØØ.52
    varicella BØ1.81
  filamentary H16.12- ☑
  gonococcal (congenital or prenatal) A54.33
  herpes, herpetic (simplex) BØØ.52
    zoster BØ2.33
  in (due to)
    acanthamebiasis B6Ø.13
    adenovirus B3Ø.Ø
    exanthema — *see also* Exanthem BØ9
    herpes (simplex) virus BØØ.52
    measles BØ5.81
    syphilis A5Ø.31
    tuberculosis A18.52
    zoster BØ2.33
  interstitial (nonsyphilitic) H16.3Ø- ☑
    diffuse H16.32- ☑
    herpes, herpetic (simplex) BØØ.52
      zoster BØ2.33
    sclerosing H16.33- ☑
    specified type NEC H16.39- ☑
    syphilitic (congenital) (late) A5Ø.31
    tuberculous A18.52
  macular H16.11- ☑
  nummular H16.11- ☑
  oyster shuckers' H16.8
  parenchymatous — *see* Keratitis, interstitial
  petrificans H16.8
  postmeasles BØ5.81
  punctata
    leprosa A3Ø.9 *[H16.14-]* ☑
    syphilitic (profunda) A5Ø.31
  punctate H16.14- ☑
  purulent H16.8
  rosacea L71.8
  sclerosing H16.33- ☑
  specified type NEC H16.8
  stellate H16.11- ☑
  striate H16.11- ☑
  superficial H16.1Ø- ☑
    with conjunctivitis — *see* Keratoconjunctivitis
    due to light — *see* Photokeratitis
  suppurative H16.8
  syphilitic (congenital) (prenatal) A5Ø.31
  trachomatous A71.1
    sequelae B94.Ø
  tuberculous A18.52
  vesicular H16.8
  xerotic — *see also* Keratomalacia H16.8
    vitamin A deficiency E5Ø.4
Keratoacanthoma L85.8
Keratocele — *see* Descemetocele
Keratoconjunctivitis H16.2Ø- ☑
  Acanthamoeba B6Ø.13
  adenoviral B3Ø.Ø
  epidemic B3Ø.Ø
  exposure H16.21- ☑
  herpes, herpetic (simplex) BØØ.52
    zoster BØ2.33
  in exanthema — *see also* Exanthem BØ9
  infectious B3Ø.Ø

Keratoconjunctivitis — *continued*
  lagophthalmic — *see* Keratoconjunctivitis, specified type NEC
  neurotrophic H16.23- ☑
  phlyctenular H16.25- ☑
  postmeasles BØ5.81
  shipyard B3Ø.Ø
  sicca (Sjogren's) M35.Ø- ☑
    not Sjogren's H16.22- ☑
  specified type NEC H16.29- ☑
  tuberculous (phlyctenular) A18.52
  vernal H16.26- ☑
Keratoconus H18.6Ø- ☑
  congenital Q13.4
  stable H18.61- ☑
  unstable H18.62- ☑
Keratocyst (dental) (odontogenic) — *see* Cyst, calcifying odontogenic
Keratoderma, keratodermia (congenital) (palmaris et plantaris) (symmetrical) Q82.8
  acquired L85.1
    in diseases classified elsewhere L86
  climactericum L85.1
  gonococcal A54.89
  gonorrheal A54.89
  punctata L85.2
  Reiter's — *see* Reiter's disease
Keratodermatocele — *see* Descemetocele
Keratoglobus H18.79 ☑
  congenital Q15.8
    with glaucoma Q15.Ø
Keratohemia — *see* Pigmentation, cornea, stromal
Keratoiritis — *see also* Iridocyclitis
  syphilitic A5Ø.39
  tuberculous A18.54
Keratoma L57.Ø
  palmaris and plantaris hereditarium Q82.8
  senile L57.Ø
Keratomalacia H18.44- ☑
  vitamin A deficiency E5Ø.4
Keratomegaly Q13.4
Keratomycosis B49
  nigrans, nigricans (palmaris) B36.1
Keratopathy H18.9
  band H18.42- ☑
  bullous (aphakic), following cataract surgery H59.Ø1- ☑
  bullous H18.1- ☑
Keratoscleritis, tuberculous A18.52
Keratosis L57.Ø
  actinic L57.Ø
  arsenical L85.8
  congenital, specified NEC Q8Ø.8
  female genital NEC N94.89
  follicularis Q82.8
    acquired L11.Ø
    congenita Q82.8
    et parafollicularis in cutem penetrans L87.Ø
    spinulosa (decalvans) Q82.8
    vitamin A deficiency E5Ø.8
  gonococcal A54.89
  lichenoid L82.Ø
  male genital (external) N5Ø.89
  nigricans L83
  obturans, external ear (canal) — *see* Cholesteatoma, external ear
  palmaris et plantaris (inherited) (symmetrical) Q82.8
    acquired L85.1
  penile N48.89
  pharynx J39.2
  pilaris, acquired L85.8
  punctata (palmaris et plantaris) L85.2
  scrotal N5Ø.89
  seborrheic L82.1
    inflamed L82.Ø
  senile L57.Ø
  solar L57.Ø
  tonsillaris J35.8
  vagina N89.4
  vegetans Q82.8
  vitamin A deficiency E5Ø.8
  vocal cord J38.3
Kerato-uveitis — *see* Iridocyclitis
Keraunoparalysis T75.Ø9 ☑
Kerion (celsi) B35.Ø
Kernicterus of newborn (not due to isoimmunization) P57.9
  due to isoimmunization (conditions in P55.Ø-P55.9) P57.Ø
  specified type NEC P57.8

Keshan disease E59
Ketoacidosis E87.29
  diabetic — *see* Diabetes, by type, with ketoacidosis
Ketonuria R82.4
Ketosis NEC E88.89
  diabetic — *see* Diabetes, by type, with ketoacidosis
Kew Garden fever A79.1
Kidney — *see* condition
Kienbock's disease — *see also* Osteochondrosis, juvenile, hand, carpal lunate
  adult M93.1
Kimmelstiel (-Wilson) disease — *see* Diabetes, Kimmelstiel (-Wilson) disease
Kink, kinking
  artery I77.1
  hair (acquired) L67.8
  ileum or intestine — *see* Obstruction, intestine
  Lane's — *see* Obstruction, intestine
  organ or site, congenital NEC — *see* Anomaly, by site
  ureter (pelvic junction) N13.5
    with
      hydronephrosis N13.1
        with infection N13.6
      pyelonephritis (chronic) N11.1
    congenital Q62.39
  vein(s) I87.8
    caval I87.1
    peripheral I87.1
Kinnier Wilson's disease (hepatolenticular degeneration) E83.01
Kissing spine M48.20
  cervical region M48.22
  cervicothoracic region M48.23
  lumbar region M48.26
  lumbosacral region M48.27
  occipito-atlanto-axial region M48.21
  thoracic region M48.24
  thoracolumbar region M48.25
Klatskin's tumor C22.1
Klauder's disease A26.8
Klebs' disease — *see also* Glomerulonephritis N05- ☑
Klebsiella (K.) pneumoniae, as cause of disease classified elsewhere B96.1
Kleeblattschaedel skull Q75.051
Klein (e)-Levin syndrome G47.13
Kleptomania F63.2
Klinefelter's syndrome Q98.4
  karyotype 47,XXY Q98.0
  male with more than two X chromosomes Q98.1
Klippel-Feil deficiency, disease, or syndrome (brevicollis) Q76.1
Klippel's disease I67.2
Klippel-Trenaunay (-Weber) syndrome Q87.2
Klumpke (-Dejerine) palsy, paralysis (birth) (newborn) P14.1
Knee — *see* condition
Knock knee (acquired) M21.06- ☑
  congenital Q74.1
Knot(s)
  intestinal, syndrome (volvulus) K56.2
  surfer S89.8- ☑
  umbilical cord (true) O69.2 ☑
Knotting (of)
  hair L67.8
  intestine K56.2
Knuckle pad (Garrod's) M72.1
Koch's
  infection — *see* Tuberculosis
  relapsing fever A68.9
Koch-Weeks' conjunctivitis — *see* Conjunctivitis, acute, mucopurulent
Koebner's syndrome Q81.8
Koenig's disease (osteochondritis dissecans) — *see* Osteochondritis, dissecans
Kohler-Pellegrini-Stieda disease or syndrome (calcification, knee joint) — *see* Bursitis, tibial collateral
Kohler's disease
  patellar — *see* Osteochondrosis, juvenile, patella
  tarsal navicular — *see* Osteochondrosis, juvenile, tarsus
Koilonychia L60.3
  congenital Q84.6
Kojevnikov's, epilepsy — *see* Kozhevnikof's epilepsy
Koplik's spots B05.9
Kopp's asthma E32.8
Korsakoff's (Wernicke) disease, psychosis or syndrome (alcoholic) F10.96
  with dependence F10.26

Korsakoff's (Wernicke) disease, psychosis or syndrome — *continued*
  drug-induced
    due to drug abuse — *see* Abuse, drug, by type, with amnestic disorder
    due to drug dependence — *see* Dependence, drug, by type, with amnestic disorder
  nonalcoholic F04
Korsakov's disease, psychosis or syndrome — *see* Korsakoff's disease
Korsakow's disease, psychosis or syndrome — *see* Korsakoff's disease
Kostmann's disease or syndrome (infantile genetic agranulocytosis) — *see* Agranulocytosis
Kozhevnikof's epilepsy G40.109
  intractable G40.119
    with status epilepticus G40.111
    without status epilepticus G40.119
  not intractable G40.109
    with status epilepticus G40.101
    without status epilepticus G40.109
Krabbe's
  disease E75.23
  syndrome, congenital muscle hypoplasia Q79.8
Kraepelin-Morel disease — *see* Schizophrenia
Kraft-Weber-Dimitri disease Q85.89
Kraurosis
  ani K62.89
  penis N48.0
  vagina N89.8
  vulva N90.4
Kreotoxism A05.9
Krukenberg's
  spindle — *see* Pigmentation, cornea, posterior
  tumor C79.6- ☑
Kufs' disease E75.4
Kugelberg-Welander disease G12.1
Kuhnt-Junius degeneration — *see also* Degeneration, macula H35.32- ☑
Kummell's disease or spondylitis — *see* Spondylopathy, traumatic
Kupffer cell sarcoma C22.3
Kuru A81.81
Kussmaul's
  disease M30.0
  respiration E87.29
    in diabetic acidosis — *see* Diabetes, by type, with ketoacidosis
Kwashiorkor E40
  marasmic, marasmus type E42
Kyasanur Forest disease A98.2
Kyphoscoliosis, kyphoscoliotic (acquired) — *see also* Scoliosis M41.9
  congenital Q67.5
  heart (disease) I27.1
  sequelae of rickets E64.3
  tuberculous A18.01
Kyphosis, kyphotic (acquired) M40.209
  cervical region M40.202
  cervicothoracic region M40.203
  congenital Q76.419
    cervical region Q76.412
    cervicothoracic region Q76.413
    occipito-atlanto-axial region Q76.411
    thoracic region Q76.414
    thoracolumbar region Q76.415
  Morquio-Brailsford type (spinal) — *see also* subcategory M49.8 E76.219
  postlaminectomy M96.3
  postradiation therapy M96.2
  postural (adolescent) M40.00
    cervicothoracic region M40.03
    thoracic region M40.04
    thoracolumbar region M40.05
  secondary NEC M40.10
    cervical region M40.12
    cervicothoracic region M40.13
    thoracic region M40.14
    thoracolumbar region M40.15
  sequelae of rickets E64.3
  specified type NEC M40.299
    cervical region M40.292
    cervicothoracic region M40.293
    thoracic region M40.294
    thoracolumbar region M40.295
  syphilitic, congenital A50.56
  thoracic region M40.204
  thoracolumbar region M40.205
  tuberculous A18.01

Kyrle disease L87.0

L

Labia, labium — *see* condition
Labile
  blood pressure R09.89
  vasomotor system I73.9
Labioglossal paralysis G12.29
Labium leporinum — *see* Cleft, lip
Labor — *see* Delivery
Labored breathing — *see* Hyperventilation
Labyrinthitis (circumscribed) (destructive) (diffuse) (inner ear) (latent) (purulent) (suppurative) — *see also* subcategory H83.0 ☑
  syphilitic A52.79
Laceration
  with abortion — *see* Abortion, by type, complicated by laceration of pelvic organs
  abdomen, abdominal
    wall S31.119 ☑
      with
        foreign body S31.129 ☑
        penetration into peritoneal cavity S31.619 ☑
          with foreign body S31.629 ☑
      epigastric region S31.112 ☑
        with
          foreign body S31.122 ☑
          penetration into peritoneal cavity S31.612 ☑
            with foreign body S31.622 ☑
      left
        lower quadrant S31.114 ☑
          with
            foreign body S31.124 ☑
            penetration into peritoneal cavity S31.614 ☑
              with foreign body S31.624 ☑
        upper quadrant S31.111 ☑
          with
            foreign body S31.121 ☑
            penetration into peritoneal cavity S31.611 ☑
              with foreign body S31.621 ☑
      periumbilic region S31.115 ☑
        with
          foreign body S31.125 ☑
          penetration into peritoneal cavity S31.615 ☑
            with foreign body S31.625 ☑
      right
        lower quadrant S31.113 ☑
          with
            foreign body S31.123 ☑
            penetration into peritoneal cavity S31.613 ☑
              with foreign body S31.623 ☑
        upper quadrant S31.110 ☑
          with
            foreign body S31.120 ☑
            penetration into peritoneal cavity S31.610 ☑
              with foreign body S31.620 ☑
  accidental, complicating surgery — *see* Complications, surgical, accidental puncture or laceration
  Achilles tendon S86.02- ☑
  adrenal gland S37.813 ☑
  alveolar (process) — *see* Laceration, oral cavity
  ankle S91.01- ☑
    with
      foreign body S91.02- ☑
  antecubital space — *see* Laceration, elbow
  anus (sphincter) S31.831 ☑
    with
      ectopic or molar pregnancy O08.6
      foreign body S31.832 ☑
    complicating delivery — *see* Delivery, complicated, by, laceration, anus (sphincter)
    following ectopic or molar pregnancy O08.6
    nontraumatic, nonpuerperal — *see* Fissure, anus
  arm (upper) S41.11- ☑
    with foreign body S41.12- ☑
    lower — *see* Laceration, forearm
  auditory canal (external) (meatus) — *see* Laceration, ear
  auricle, ear — *see* Laceration, ear
  axilla — *see* Laceration, arm
  back — *see also* Laceration, thorax, back

☑ **Additional Character Required** — Refer to the Tabular List for Character Selection

Laceration — *continued*
- back — *see also* Laceration, thorax, back — *continued*
  - lower S31.010 ☑
    - with
      - foreign body S31.020 ☑
        - with penetration into retroperitoneal space S31.021 ☑
        - penetration into retroperitoneal space S31.011 ☑
- bile duct S36.13 ☑
- bladder S37.23 ☑
  - with ectopic or molar pregnancy O08.6
  - following ectopic or molar pregnancy O08.6
  - obstetrical trauma O71.5
- blood vessel — *see* Injury, blood vessel
- bowel — *see also* Laceration, intestine
  - with ectopic or molar pregnancy O08.6
  - complicating abortion — *see* Abortion, by type, complicated by, specified condition NEC
  - following ectopic or molar pregnancy O08.6
  - obstetrical trauma O71.5
- brain (any part) (cortex) (diffuse) (membrane) — *see also* Injury, intracranial, diffuse
  - during birth P10.8
    - with hemorrhage P10.1
  - focal — *see* Injury, intracranial, focal brain injury
- brainstem S06.38- ☑
- breast S21.01- ☑
  - with foreign body S21.02- ☑
- broad ligament S37.893 ☑
  - with ectopic or molar pregnancy O08.6
  - following ectopic or molar pregnancy O08.6
  - laceration syndrome N83.8
  - obstetrical trauma O71.6
  - syndrome (laceration) N83.8
- buttock S31.801 ☑
  - with foreign body S31.802 ☑
  - left S31.821 ☑
    - with foreign body S31.822 ☑
  - right S31.811 ☑
    - with foreign body S31.812 ☑
- calf — *see* Laceration, leg
- canaliculus lacrimalis — *see* Laceration, eyelid
- canthus, eye — *see* Laceration, eyelid
- capsule, joint — *see* Sprain
- causing eversion of cervix uteri (old) N86
- central (perineal), complicating delivery O70.9
- cerebellum, traumatic S06.37- ☑
- cerebral S06.33- ☑
  - during birth P10.8
    - with hemorrhage P10.1
  - left side S06.32- ☑
  - right side S06.31- ☑
- cervix (uteri)
  - with ectopic or molar pregnancy O08.6
  - following ectopic or molar pregnancy O08.6
  - nonpuerperal, nontraumatic N88.1
  - obstetrical trauma (current) O71.3
  - old (postpartal) N88.1
  - traumatic S37.63 ☑
- cheek (external) S01.41- ☑
  - with foreign body S01.42- ☑
  - internal — *see* Laceration, oral cavity
- chest wall — *see* Laceration, thorax
- chin — *see* Laceration, head, specified site NEC
- chordae tendinae NEC I51.1
  - concurrent with acute myocardial infarction — *see* Infarct, myocardium
  - following acute myocardial infarction (current complication) I23.4
- clitoris — *see* Laceration, vulva
- colon — *see* Laceration, intestine, large, colon
- common bile duct S36.13 ☑
- cortex (cerebral) — *see* Injury, intracranial, diffuse
- costal region — *see* Laceration, thorax
- cystic duct S36.13 ☑
- diaphragm S27.803 ☑
- digit(s)
  - foot — *see* Laceration, toe
  - hand — *see* Laceration, finger
- duodenum S36.430 ☑
- ear (canal) (external) S01.31- ☑
  - with foreign body S01.32- ☑
  - drum S09.2- ☑
- elbow S51.01- ☑
  - with
    - foreign body S51.02- ☑

Laceration — *continued*
- epididymis — *see* Laceration, testis
- epigastric region — *see* Laceration, abdomen, wall, epigastric region
- esophagus K22.89
  - traumatic
    - cervical S11.21 ☑
      - with foreign body S11.22 ☑
    - thoracic S27.813 ☑
- eye (ball) S05.3- ☑
  - with prolapse or loss of intraocular tissue S05.2- ☑
  - penetrating S05.6- ☑
- eyebrow — *see* Laceration, eyelid
- eyelid S01.11- ☑
  - with foreign body S01.12- ☑
- face NEC — *see* Laceration, head, specified site NEC
- fallopian tube S37.539 ☑
  - bilateral S37.532 ☑
  - unilateral S37.531 ☑
- finger(s) S61.219 ☑
  - with
    - damage to nail S61.319 ☑
      - with
        - foreign body S61.329 ☑
    - foreign body S61.229 ☑
  - index S61.218 ☑
    - with
      - damage to nail S61.318 ☑
        - with
          - foreign body S61.328 ☑
      - foreign body S61.228 ☑
    - left S61.211 ☑
      - with
        - damage to nail S61.311 ☑
          - with
            - foreign body S61.321 ☑
        - foreign body S61.221 ☑
    - right S61.210 ☑
      - with
        - damage to nail S61.310 ☑
          - with
            - foreign body S61.320 ☑
        - foreign body S61.220 ☑
  - little S61.218 ☑
    - with
      - damage to nail S61.318 ☑
        - with
          - foreign body S61.328 ☑
      - foreign body S61.228 ☑
    - left S61.217 ☑
      - with
        - damage to nail S61.317 ☑
          - with
            - foreign body S61.327 ☑
        - foreign body S61.227 ☑
    - right S61.216 ☑
      - with
        - damage to nail S61.316 ☑
          - with
            - foreign body S61.326 ☑
        - foreign body S61.226 ☑
  - middle S61.218 ☑
    - with
      - damage to nail S61.318 ☑
        - with
          - foreign body S61.328 ☑
      - foreign body S61.228 ☑
    - left S61.213 ☑
      - with
        - damage to nail S61.313 ☑
          - with
            - foreign body S61.323 ☑
        - foreign body S61.223 ☑
    - right S61.212 ☑
      - with
        - damage to nail S61.312 ☑
          - with
            - foreign body S61.322 ☑
        - foreign body S61.222 ☑
  - ring S61.218 ☑
    - with
      - damage to nail S61.318 ☑
        - with
          - foreign body S61.328 ☑
      - foreign body S61.228 ☑
    - left S61.215 ☑

Laceration — *continued*
- finger(s) — *continued*
  - ring — *continued*
    - left — *continued*
      - with
        - damage to nail S61.315 ☑
          - with
            - foreign body S61.325 ☑
        - foreign body S61.225 ☑
    - right S61.214 ☑
      - with
        - damage to nail S61.314 ☑
          - with
            - foreign body S61.324 ☑
        - foreign body S61.224 ☑
- flank S31.119 ☑
  - with foreign body S31.129 ☑
- foot (except toe(s) alone) S91.319 ☑
  - with foreign body S91.329 ☑
  - left S91.312 ☑
    - with foreign body S91.322 ☑
  - right S91.311 ☑
    - with foreign body S91.321 ☑
  - toe — *see* Laceration, toe
- forearm S51.819 ☑
  - with
    - foreign body S51.829 ☑
  - elbow only — *see* Laceration, elbow
  - left S51.812 ☑
    - with
      - foreign body S51.822 ☑
  - right S51.811 ☑
    - with
      - foreign body S51.821 ☑
- forehead S01.81 ☑
  - with foreign body S01.82 ☑
- fourchette O70.0
  - with ectopic or molar pregnancy O08.6
  - complicating delivery O70.0
  - following ectopic or molar pregnancy O08.6
- gallbladder S36.123 ☑
- genital organs, external
  - female S31.512 ☑
    - with foreign body S31.522 ☑
    - vagina — *see* Laceration, vagina
    - vulva — *see* Laceration, vulva
  - male S31.511 ☑
    - with foreign body S31.521 ☑
    - penis — *see* Laceration, penis
    - scrotum — *see* Laceration, scrotum
    - testis — *see* Laceration, testis
- groin — *see* Laceration, abdomen, wall
- gum — *see* Laceration, oral cavity
- hand S61.419 ☑
  - with
    - foreign body S61.429 ☑
  - finger — *see* Laceration, finger
  - left S61.412 ☑
    - with
      - foreign body S61.422 ☑
  - right S61.411 ☑
    - with
      - foreign body S61.421 ☑
  - thumb — *see* Laceration, thumb
- head S01.91 ☑
  - with foreign body S01.92 ☑
  - cheek — *see* Laceration, cheek
  - ear — *see* Laceration, ear
  - eyelid — *see* Laceration, eyelid
  - lip — *see* Laceration, lip
  - nose — *see* Laceration, nose
  - oral cavity — *see* Laceration, oral cavity
  - scalp S01.01 ☑
    - with foreign body S01.02 ☑
  - specified site NEC S01.81 ☑
    - with foreign body S01.82 ☑
  - temporomandibular area — *see* Laceration, cheek
- heart — *see* Injury, heart, laceration
- heel — *see* Laceration, foot
- hepatic duct S36.13 ☑
- hip S71.019 ☑
  - with foreign body S71.029 ☑
  - left S71.012 ☑
    - with foreign body S71.022 ☑
  - right S71.011 ☑
    - with foreign body S71.021 ☑
- hymen — *see* Laceration, vagina

Index

Laceration — Laceration

Laceration — *continued*
  hypochondrium — *see* Laceration, abdomen, wall
  hypogastric region — *see* Laceration, abdomen, wall
  ileum S36.438 ☑
  inguinal region — *see* Laceration, abdomen, wall
  instep — *see* Laceration, foot
  internal organ — *see* Injury, by site
  interscapular region — *see* Laceration, thorax, back
  intestine
    large
      colon S36.539 ☑
        ascending S36.530 ☑
        descending S36.532 ☑
        sigmoid S36.533 ☑
        specified site NEC S36.538 ☑
      rectum S36.63 ☑
      transverse S36.531 ☑
    small S36.439 ☑
      duodenum S36.430 ☑
      specified site NEC S36.438 ☑
  intra-abdominal organ S36.93 ☑
    intestine — *see* Laceration, intestine
    liver — *see* Laceration, liver
    pancreas — *see* Laceration, pancreas
    peritoneum S36.81
    specified site NEC S36.893 ☑
    spleen — *see* Laceration, spleen
    stomach — *see* Laceration, stomach
  intracranial NEC — *see also* Injury, intracranial, diffuse
    birth injury P10.9
  jaw — *see* Laceration, head, specified site NEC
  jejunum S36.438 ☑
  joint capsule — *see* Sprain, by site
  kidney S37.03-
    major (greater than 3 cm) (massive) (stellate)
      S37.06-
    minor (less than 1 cm) S37.04- ☑
    moderate (1 to 3 cm) S37.05- ☑
      multiple S37.06- ☑
  knee S81.01- ☑
    with foreign body S81.02- ☑
  labium (majus) (minus) — *see* Laceration, vulva
  lacrimal duct — *see* Laceration, eyelid
  large intestine — *see* Laceration, intestine, large
  larynx S11.011 ☑
    with foreign body S11.012 ☑
  leg (lower) S81.819 ☑
    with foreign body S81.829 ☑
    foot — *see* Laceration, foot
    knee — *see* Laceration, knee
    left S81.812 ☑
      with foreign body S81.822 ☑
    right S81.811 ☑
      with foreign body S81.821 ☑
    upper — *see* Laceration, thigh
  ligament — *see* Sprain
  lip S01.511 ☑
    with foreign body S01.521 ☑
  liver S36.113 ☑
    major (stellate) S36.116 ☑
    minor S36.114 ☑
    moderate S36.115 ☑
  loin — *see* Laceration, abdomen, wall
  lower back — *see* Laceration, back, lower
  lumbar region — *see* Laceration, back, lower
  lung S27.339 ☑
    bilateral S27.332 ☑
    unilateral S27.331 ☑
  malar region — *see* Laceration, head, specified site NEC
  mammary — *see* Laceration, breast
  mastoid region — *see* Laceration, head, specified site
      NEC
  meninges — *see* Injury, intracranial, diffuse
  meniscus — *see* Tear, meniscus
  mesentery S36.893 ☑
  mesosalpinx S37.893 ☑
  mouth — *see* Laceration, oral cavity
  muscle — *see* Injury, muscle, by site, laceration
  nail
    finger — *see* Laceration, finger, with damage to nail
    toe — *see* Laceration, toe, with damage to nail
  nasal (septum) (sinus) — *see* Laceration, nose
  nasopharynx — *see* Laceration, head, specified site NEC
  neck S11.91 ☑
    with foreign body S11.92 ☑
    involving
      cervical esophagus S11.21 ☑

Laceration — *continued*
  neck — *continued*
    involving — *continued*
      cervical esophagus — *continued*
        with foreign body S11.22 ☑
      larynx — *see* Laceration, larynx
      pharynx — *see* Laceration, pharynx
      thyroid gland — *see* Laceration, thyroid gland
      trachea — *see* Laceration, trachea
    specified site NEC S11.81 ☑
      with foreign body S11.82 ☑
  nerve — *see* Injury, nerve
  nose (septum) (sinus) S01.21 ☑
    with foreign body S01.22 ☑
  ocular NOS S05.3- ☑
    adnexa NOS S01.11- ☑
  oral cavity S01.512 ☑
    with foreign body S01.522 ☑
  orbit (eye) — *see* Wound, open, ocular, orbit
  ovary S37.439 ☑
    bilateral S37.432 ☑
    unilateral S37.431 ☑
  palate — *see* Laceration, oral cavity
  palm — *see* Laceration, hand
  pancreas S36.239 ☑
  pelvic S31.010 ☑
    with
      foreign body S31.020 ☑
        penetration into retroperitoneal cavity
          S31.021 ☑
      penetration into retroperitoneal cavity S31.011 ☑
    floor — *see also* Laceration, back, lower
      with ectopic or molar pregnancy O08.6
      complicating delivery O70.1
      following ectopic or molar pregnancy O08.6
      old (postpartal) N81.89
    organ S37.93 ☑
  penis S31.21 ☑
    with foreign body S31.22 ☑
  perineum
    female S31.41 ☑
      with
        ectopic or molar pregnancy O08.6
        foreign body S31.42 ☑
      during delivery O70.9
        first degree O70.0
        fourth degree O70.3
        second degree O70.1
        third degree — *see also* Delivery, complicated,
          by, laceration, perineum, third degree
          O70.20
      old (postpartal) N81.89
      postpartal N81.89
      secondary (postpartal) O90.1
    male S31.119 ☑
      with foreign body S31.129 ☑
  periocular area (with or without lacrimal passages) —
      see Laceration, eyelid
  peritoneum S36.893 ☑
  periumbilic region — *see* Laceration, abdomen, wall,
      periumbilic
  periurethral tissue — *see* Laceration, urethra
  phalanges
    finger — *see* Laceration, finger
    toe — *see* Laceration, toe
  pharynx S11.21 ☑
    with foreign body S11.22 ☑
  pinna — *see* Laceration, ear
  popliteal space — *see* Laceration, knee
  prepuce — *see* Laceration, penis
  prostate S37.823 ☑
  pubic region S31.119 ☑
    with foreign body S31.129 ☑
  pudendum — *see* Laceration, genital organs, external
  rectovaginal septum — *see* Laceration, vagina
  rectum S36.63 ☑
  retroperitoneum S36.893 ☑
  round ligament S37.893 ☑
  sacral region — *see* Laceration, back, lower
  sacroiliac region — *see* Laceration, back, lower
  salivary gland — *see* Laceration, oral cavity
  scalp S01.01 ☑
    with foreign body S01.02 ☑
  scapular region — *see* Laceration, shoulder
  scrotum S31.31 ☑
    with foreign body S31.32 ☑
  seminal vesicle S37.893 ☑

Laceration — *continued*
  shin — *see* Laceration, leg
  shoulder S41.019 ☑
    with foreign body S41.029 ☑
    left S41.012 ☑
      with foreign body S41.022 ☑
    right S41.011 ☑
      with foreign body S41.021 ☑
  small intestine — *see* Laceration, intestine, small
  spermatic cord — *see* Laceration, testis
  spinal cord (meninges) — *see also* Injury, spinal cord, by
      region
    due to injury at birth P11.5
    newborn (birth injury) P11.5
  spleen S36.039 ☑
    major (massive) (stellate) S36.032 ☑
    moderate S36.031 ☑
    superficial (minor) S36.030 ☑
  sternal region — *see* Laceration, thorax, front
  stomach S36.33 ☑
  submaxillary region — *see* Laceration, head, specified
      site NEC
  submental region — *see* Laceration, head, specified site
      NEC
  subungual
    finger(s) — *see* Laceration, finger, with damage to
      nail
    toe(s) — *see* Laceration, toe, with damage to nail
  suprarenal gland — *see* Laceration, adrenal gland
  temple, temporal region — *see* Laceration, head, speci-
      fied site NEC
  temporomandibular area — *see* Laceration, cheek
  tendon — *see* Injury, muscle, by site, laceration
    Achilles S86.02- ☑
  tentorium cerebelli — *see* Injury, intracranial, diffuse
  testis S31.31 ☑
    with foreign body S31.32 ☑
  thigh S71.11- ☑
    with foreign body S71.12- ☑
  thorax, thoracic (wall) S21.91 ☑
    with foreign body S21.92 ☑
      back S21.22- ☑
        with penetration into thoracic cavity S21.42- ☑
      front S21.12- ☑
        with penetration into thoracic cavity S21.32- ☑
    back S21.21- ☑
      with
        foreign body S21.22- ☑
          with penetration into thoracic cavity
            S21.42- ☑
        penetration into thoracic cavity S21.41- ☑
    breast — *see* Laceration, breast
    front S21.11- ☑
      with
        foreign body S21.12- ☑
          with penetration into thoracic cavity
            S21.32- ☑
        penetration into thoracic cavity S21.31- ☑
  thumb S61.019 ☑
    with
      damage to nail S61.119 ☑
        with
          foreign body S61.129 ☑
      foreign body S61.029 ☑
    left S61.012 ☑
      with
        damage to nail S61.112 ☑
          with
            foreign body S61.122 ☑
        foreign body S61.022 ☑
    right S61.011 ☑
      with
        damage to nail S61.111 ☑
          with
            foreign body S61.121 ☑
        foreign body S61.021 ☑
  thyroid gland S11.11 ☑
    with foreign body S11.12 ☑
  toe(s) S91.119 ☑
    with
      damage to nail S91.219 ☑
        with
          foreign body S91.229 ☑
      foreign body S91.129 ☑
    great S91.113 ☑

☑ **Additional Character Required — Refer to the Tabular List for Character Selection**

Laceration — *continued*
  toe(s) — *continued*
    great — *continued*
      with
        damage to nail S91.213 ☑
          with
            foreign body S91.223 ☑
        foreign body S91.123 ☑
      left S91.112 ☑
        with
          damage to nail S91.212 ☑
            with
              foreign body S91.222 ☑
          foreign body S91.122 ☑
      right S91.111 ☑
        with
          damage to nail S91.211 ☑
            with
              foreign body S91.221 ☑
          foreign body S91.121 ☑
    lesser S91.116 ☑
      with
        damage to nail S91.216 ☑
          with
            foreign body S91.226 ☑
        foreign body S91.126 ☑
      left S91.115 ☑
        with
          damage to nail S91.215 ☑
            with
              foreign body S91.225 ☑
          foreign body S91.125 ☑
      right S91.114 ☑
        with
          damage to nail S91.214 ☑
            with
              foreign body S91.224 ☑
          foreign body S91.124 ☑
  tongue — *see* Laceration, oral cavity
  trachea S11.021 ☑
    with foreign body S11.022 ☑
  tunica vaginalis — *see* Laceration, testis
  tympanum, tympanic membrane — *see* Laceration, ear, drum
  umbilical region S31.115 ☑
    with foreign body S31.125 ☑
  ureter S37.13 ☑
  urethra S37.33 ☑
    with or following ectopic or molar pregnancy O08.6
    obstetrical trauma O71.5
  urinary organ NEC S37.893 ☑
  uterus S37.63 ☑
    with ectopic or molar pregnancy O08.6
    following ectopic or molar pregnancy O08.6
    nonpuerperal, nontraumatic N85.8
    obstetrical trauma NEC O71.81
    old (postpartal) N85.8
  uvula — *see* Laceration, oral cavity
  vagina S31.41 ☑
    with
      ectopic or molar pregnancy O08.6
      foreign body S31.42 ☑
    during delivery O71.4
      with perineal laceration — *see* Laceration, perineum, female, during delivery
    following ectopic or molar pregnancy O08.6
    nonpuerperal, nontraumatic N89.8
    old (postpartal) N89.8
  vas deferens S37.893 ☑
  vesical — *see* Laceration, bladder
  vocal cords S11.031 ☑
    with foreign body S11.032 ☑
  vulva S31.41 ☑
    with
      ectopic or molar pregnancy O08.6
      foreign body S31.42 ☑
    complicating delivery O70.0
    following ectopic or molar pregnancy O08.6
    nonpuerperal, nontraumatic N90.89
    old (postpartal) N90.89
  wrist S61.519 ☑
    with
      foreign body S61.529 ☑
    left S61.512 ☑
      with
        foreign body S61.522 ☑
    right S61.511 ☑

Laceration — *continued*
  wrist — *continued*
    right — *continued*
      with
        foreign body S61.521 ☑
Lack of
  achievement in school Z55.3
  adequate
    food Z59.48
    intermaxillary vertical dimension of fully erupted teeth M26.36
    sleep Z72.820
  air conditioning Z59.11
  appetite (see Anorexia) R63.0
  awareness R41.9
  basic services in physical environment Z58.81
  care
    in home Z74.2
    of infant (at or after birth) T76.02 ☑
      confirmed T74.02 ☑
  cognitive functions R41.9
  coordination R27.9
    ataxia R27.0
    specified type NEC R27.8
  development (physiological) R62.50
    failure to thrive (child over 28 days old) R62.51
      adult R62.7
      newborn P92.6
    short stature R62.52
    specified type NEC R62.59
  electricity services Z59.12
  emotional support Z60.8
  energy R53.83
  financial resources Z59.6
  food Z59.48
  gas services Z59.12
  growth R62.52
  heating Z59.11
  housing (permanent) (temporary) Z59.00
    adequate Z59.10
  learning experiences in childhood Z62.898
  leisure time (affecting life-style) Z73.2
  material resources due to limited financial resources, specified NEC Z59.87
  memory — *see also* Amnesia
    mild, following organic brain damage F06.8
  oil services Z59.12
  ovulation N97.0
  parental supervision or control of child Z62.0
  person able to render necessary care Z74.2
  physical exercise Z72.3
  play experience in childhood Z62.898
  posterior occlusal support M26.57
  relaxation (affecting life-style) Z73.2
  safe drinking water Z58.6
  sexual
    desire F52.0
    enjoyment F52.1
  shelter Z59.02
  sleep (adequate) Z72.820
  supervision of child by parent Z62.0
  support, posterior occlusal M26.57
  transportation Z59.82
  water T73.1 ☑
    safe drinking Z58.6
    services Z59.12
Lacrimal — *see* condition
Lacrimation, abnormal — *see* Epiphora
Lacrimonasal duct — *see* condition
Lactate, elevated — *see* Acidosis, lactic
Lactation, lactating (breast) (puerperal, postpartum)
  associated
    cracked nipple O92.13
    retracted nipple O92.03
  defective O92.4
  disorder NEC O92.79
  excessive O92.6
  failed (complete) O92.3
    partial O92.4
  mastitis NEC — *see* Mastitis, obstetric
  mother (care and/or examination) Z39.1
  nonpuerperal N64.3
Lacticemia, excessive — *see also* Acidosis E87.20
Lacunar skull Q75.8
Laennec's cirrhosis K70.30
  with ascites K70.31
  nonalcoholic K74.69
Lafora disease — *see also* Epilepsy, progressive, Lafora G40.C09

Lag, lid (nervous) — *see* Retraction, lid
Lagophthalmos (eyelid) (nervous) H02.209
  bilateral, upper and lower eyelids H02.20C
  cicatricial H02.219
    bilateral, upper and lower eyelids H02.21C
    left H02.216
      lower H02.215
      upper H02.214
      upper and lower eyelids H02.21B
    right H02.213
      lower H02.212
      upper H02.211
      upper and lower eyelids H02.21A
  keratoconjunctivitis — *see* Keratoconjunctivitis
  left H02.206
    lower H02.205
    upper H02.204
    upper and lower eyelids H02.20B
  mechanical H02.229
    bilateral, upper and lower eyelids H02.22C
    left H02.226
      lower H02.225
      upper H02.224
      upper and lower eyelids H02.22B
    right H02.223
      lower H02.222
      upper H02.221
      upper and lower eyelids H02.22A
  paralytic H02.239
    bilateral, upper and lower eyelids H02.23C
    left H02.236
      lower H02.235
      upper H02.234
      upper and lower eyelids H02.23B
    right H02.233
      lower H02.232
      upper H02.231
      upper and lower eyelids H02.23A
  right H02.203
    lower H02.202
    upper H02.201
    upper and lower eyelids H02.20A
Laki-Lorand factor deficiency — *see* Defect, coagulation, specified type NEC
Lalling F80.0
Lambert-Eaton syndrome — *see* Syndrome, Lambert-Eaton
Lambliasis, lambliosis A07.1
Landau-Kleffner syndrome — *see* Epilepsy, specified NEC
Landouzy-Dejerine dystrophy or facioscapulohumeral atrophy G71.02
Landouzy's disease (icterohemorrhagic leptospirosis) A27.0
Landry-Guillain-Barre, syndrome or paralysis G61.0
Landry's disease or paralysis G61.0
Lane's
  band Q43.3
  kink — *see* Obstruction, intestine
  syndrome K90.2
Langdon Down syndrome — *see* Trisomy, 21
Lapsed immunization schedule status Z28.39
Large
  baby (regardless of gestational age) (4000g to 4499g) P08.1
  ear, congenital Q17.1
  physiological cup Q14.2
  stature R68.89
Large-for-dates NEC (infant) (4000g to 4499g) P08.1
  affecting management of pregnancy O36.6- ☑
  exceptionally (4500g or more) P08.0
Larsen-Johansson disease or osteochondrosis — *see* Osteochondrosis, juvenile, patella
Larsen's syndrome (flattened facies and multiple congenital dislocations) Q74.8
Larva migrans
  cutaneous B76.9
    Ancylostoma B76.0
  visceral B83.0
Laryngeal — *see* condition
Laryngismus (stridulus) J38.5
  congenital P28.89
  diphtheritic A36.2
Laryngitis (acute) (edematous) (fibrinous) (infective) (infiltrative) (malignant) (membranous) (phlegmonous) (pneumococcal) (pseudomembranous) (septic) (subglottic) (suppurative) (ulcerative) J04.0
  with
    influenza, flu, or grippe — *see* Influenza, with, laryngitis
    tracheitis (acute) — *see* Laryngotracheitis

Laryngitis — *continued*
 atrophic J37.0
 catarrhal J37.0
 chronic J37.0
  with tracheitis (chronic) J37.1
 diphtheritic A36.2
 due to external agent — *see* Inflammation, respiratory, upper, due to
 H. influenzae J04.0
 Hemophilus influenzae J04.0
 hypertrophic J37.0
 influenzal — *see* Influenza, with, respiratory manifestations NEC
 obstructive J05.0
 sicca J37.0
 spasmodic J05.0
  acute J04.0
 streptococcal J04.0
 stridulous J05.0
 syphilitic (late) A52.73
  congenital A50.59 *[J99]*
   early A50.03 *[J99]*
 tuberculous A15.5
 Vincent's A69.1
Laryngocele (congenital) (ventricular) Q31.3
Laryngofissure J38.7
 congenital Q31.8
Laryngomalacia (congenital) Q31.5
Laryngopharyngitis (acute) J06.0
 chronic J37.0
 due to external agent — *see* Inflammation, respiratory, upper, due to
Laryngoplegia J38.00
 bilateral J38.02
 unilateral J38.01
Laryngoptosis J38.7
Laryngospasm J38.5
Laryngostenosis J38.6
Laryngotracheitis (acute) (Infectional) (infective) (viral) J04.2
 atrophic J37.1
 catarrhal J37.1
 chronic J37.1
 diphtheritic A36.2
 due to external agent — *see* Inflammation, respiratory, upper, due to
 Hemophilus influenzae J04.2
 hypertrophic J37.1
 influenzal — *see* Influenza, with, respiratory manifestations NEC
 pachydermic J38.7
 sicca J37.1
 spasmodic J38.5
  acute J05.0
 streptococcal J04.2
 stridulous J38.5
 syphilitic (late) A52.73
  congenital A50.59 *[J99]*
   early A50.03 *[J99]*
 tuberculous A15.5
 Vincent's A69.1
Laryngotracheobronchitis — *see* Bronchitis
Larynx, laryngeal — *see* condition
Lassa fever A96.2
Lassitude — *see* Weakness
Late
 talker R62.0
 walker R62.0
Late effect(s) — *see* Sequelae
Latent — *see* condition
Laterocession — *see* Lateroversion
Lateroflexion — *see* Lateroversion
Lateroversion
 cervix — *see* Lateroversion, uterus
 uterus, uterine (cervix) (postinfectional) (postpartal, old) N85.4
  congenital Q51.818
  in pregnancy or childbirth O34.59- ☑
Lathyrism — *see* Poisoning, food, noxious, plant
Launois' syndrome (pituitary gigantism) E22.0
Launois-Bensaude adenolipomatosis E88.89
Laurence-Moon syndrome Q87.84
Lax, laxity — *see also* Relaxation
 ligament (ous) — *see also* Disorder, ligament
  familial M35.7
  knee — *see* Derangement, knee
 skin (acquired) L57.4
  congenital Q82.8
Laxative habit F55.2

Lazy leukocyte syndrome D70.8
Lead miner's lung J63.6
Leak, leakage
 air NEC J93.82
  postprocedural J95.812
 amniotic fluid — *see* Rupture, membranes, premature
 blood (microscopic), fetal, into maternal circulation affecting management of pregnancy — *see* Pregnancy, complicated by
 cerebrospinal fluid G96.00
  cranial
   postoperative G96.08
   specified NEC G96.08
   spontaneous G96.01
   traumatic G96.08
  from spinal (lumbar) puncture G97.0
  spinal
   postoperative G96.09
   post-traumatic G96.09
   specified NEC G96.09
   spontaneous G96.02
  spontaneous
   from
    skull base G96.01
    spine G96.02
 CSF — *see* Leak, cerebrospinal fluid
 device, implant or graft — *see also* Complications, by site and type, mechanical
  arterial graft NEC — *see* Complication, vascular, graft, mechanical, leakage T82.838 ☑
  breast (implant) T85.43 ☑
  catheter NEC T85.638 ☑
   dialysis (renal) T82.43 ☑
    intraperitoneal T85.631 ☑
   infusion NEC T82.534 ☑
    spinal (epidural) (subdural) T85.630 ☑
   urinary T83.038 ☑
    cystostomy T83.030 ☑
    Hopkins T83.038 ☑
    ileostomy T83.038 ☑
    indwelling T83.031 ☑
    nephrostomy T83.032 ☑
    specified T83.038 ☑
    urostomy T83.038 ☑
  gastrointestinal — *see* Complications, prosthetic device, mechanical, gastrointestinal device
  genital NEC T83.498 ☑
   penile prosthesis (cylinder) (implanted) (pump) (reservoir) T83.490 ☑
   testicular prosthesis T83.491 ☑
  heart NEC — *see* Complication, cardiovascular device, mechanical
  joint prosthesis — *see* Complications, joint prosthesis, mechanical, specified NEC, by site
  ocular NEC — *see* Complications, prosthetic device, mechanical, ocular device
  orthopedic NEC — *see* Complication, orthopedic, device, mechanical
  persistent air J93.82
  specified NEC T85.638 ☑
  urinary NEC — *see also* Complication, genitourinary, device, urinary, mechanical
   graft T83.23 ☑
  vascular NEC — *see* Complication, cardiovascular device, mechanical
  ventricular intracranial shunt T85.03 ☑
 urine — *see* Incontinence
Leaky heart — *see* Endocarditis
Learning defect (specific) F81.9
Leather bottle stomach C16.9
Leber's
 congenital amaurosis H35.50
 optic atrophy (hereditary) H47.22
Lederer's anemia D59.19
Leeches (external) — *see* Hirudiniasis
Leg — *see* condition
Legg (-Calve)-**Perthes disease, syndrome or osteochondrosis** M91.1- ☑
Legionellosis A48.1
 nonpneumonic A48.2
Legionnaires'
 disease A48.1
  nonpneumonic A48.2
 pneumonia A48.1
Leigh's disease G31.82
Leiner's disease L21.1
Leiofibromyoma — *see* Leiomyoma

Leiomyoblastoma — *see* Neoplasm, connective tissue, benign
Leiomyofibroma — *see also* Neoplasm, connective tissue, benign
 uterus (cervix) (corpus) D25.9
Leiomyoma — *see also* Neoplasm, connective tissue, benign
 bizarre — *see* Neoplasm, connective tissue, benign
 cellular — *see* Neoplasm, connective tissue, benign
 epithelioid — *see* Neoplasm, connective tissue, benign
 uterus (cervix) (corpus) D25.9
  intramural D25.1
  submucous D25.0
  subserosal D25.2
 vascular — *see* Neoplasm, connective tissue, benign
Leiomyoma, leiomyomatosis (intravascular) — *see* Neoplasm, connective tissue, uncertain behavior
Leiomyosarcoma — *see also* Neoplasm, connective tissue, malignant
 epithelioid — *see* Neoplasm, connective tissue, malignant
 myxoid — *see* Neoplasm, connective tissue, malignant
Leishmaniasis B55.9
 American (mucocutaneous) B55.2
  cutaneous B55.1
 Asian Desert B55.1
 Brazilian B55.2
 cutaneous (any type) B55.1
 dermal — *see also* Leishmaniasis, cutaneous
  post-kala-azar B55.0
 eyelid B55.1
 infantile B55.0
 Mediterranean B55.0
 mucocutaneous (American) (New World) B55.2
 naso-oral B55.2
 nasopharyngeal B55.2
 old world B55.1
 tegumentaria diffusa B55.1
 visceral B55.0
Leishmanoid, dermal — *see also* Leishmaniasis, cutaneous post-kala-azar B55.0
Lenegre's disease I44.2
Lengthening, leg — *see* Deformity, limb, unequal length
Lennert's lymphoma — *see* Lymphoma, Lennert's
Lennox-Gastaut syndrome G40.812
 intractable G40.814
  with status epilepticus G40.813
  without status epilepticus G40.814
 not intractable G40.812
  with status epilepticus G40.811
  without status epilepticus G40.812
Lens — *see* condition
Lenticonus (anterior) (posterior) (congenital) Q12.8
Lenticular degeneration, progressive E83.01
Lentiglobus (posterior) (congenital) Q12.8
Lentigo (congenital) L81.4
 maligna — *see also* Melanoma, in situ
 melanoma — *see* Melanoma
Lentivirus, as cause of disease classified elsewhere B97.31
Leontiasis
 ossium M85.2
 syphilitic (late) A52.78
  congenital A50.59
Lepothrix A48.8
Lepra — *see* Leprosy
Leprechaunism E34.8
Leprosy A30.- ☑
 with muscle disorder A30.9 *[M63.80]*
  ankle A30.9 *[M63.87-]* ☑
  foot A30.9 *[M63.87-]* ☑
  forearm A30.9 *[M63.83-]* ☑
  hand A30.9 *[M63.84-]* ☑
  lower leg A30.9 *[M63.86-]* ☑
  multiple sites A30.9 *[M63.89]*
  pelvic region A30.9 *[M63.85-]* ☑
  shoulder region A30.9 *[M63.81-]* ☑
  specified site NEC A30.9 *[M63.88]*
  thigh A30.9 *[M63.85-]* ☑
  upper arm A30.9 *[M63.82-]* ☑
 anesthetic A30.9
 BB A30.3
 BL A30.4
 borderline (infiltrated) (neuritic) A30.3
  lepromatous A30.4
  tuberculoid A30.2
 BT A30.2
 dimorphous (infiltrated) (neuritic) A30.3
 I A30.0

☑ **Additional Character Required** — **Refer to the Tabular List for Character Selection**

Leprosy — *continued*
  indeterminate (macular) (neuritic) A30.0
  lepromatous (diffuse) (infiltrated) (macular) (neuritic) (nodular) A30.5
  LL A30.5
  macular (early) (neuritic) (simple) A30.9
  maculoanesthetic A30.9
  mixed A30.3
  neural A30.9
  nodular A30.5
  primary neuritic A30.3
  specified type NEC A30.8
  TT A30.1
  tuberculoid (major) (minor) A30.1
Leptocytosis, hereditary D56.9
Leptomeningitis (chronic) (circumscribed) (hemorrhagic) (nonsuppurative) — *see* Meningitis
Leptomeningopathy G96.198
Leptospiral — *see* condition
Leptospirochetal — *see* condition
Leptospirosis A27.9
  canicola A27.89
  due to Leptospira interrogans serovar icterohaemorrhagiae A27.0
  icterohemorrhagica A27.0
  pomona A27.89
  Weil's disease A27.0
Leptus dermatitis B88.0
Leriche's syndrome (aortic bifurcation occlusion) I74.09
Leri's pleonosteosis Q78.8
Leri-Weill syndrome Q77.8
Lermoyez' syndrome — *see* Vertigo, peripheral NEC
Lesch-Nyhan syndrome E79.1
Leser-Trélat disease L82.1
  inflamed L82.0
Lesion(s) (nontraumatic)
  abducens nerve — *see* Strabismus, paralytic, sixth nerve
  alveolar process K08.9
  angiocentric immunoproliferative D47.Z9 (*following* D47.4)
  anorectal K62.9
  aortic (valve) I35.9
  auditory nerve — *see* subcategory H93.3 ☑
  basal ganglion G25.9
  bile duct — *see* Disease, bile duct
  biomechanical M99.9
    specified type NEC M99.89
      abdomen M99.89
      acromioclavicular M99.87
      cervical region M99.81
      cervicothoracic M99.81
      costochondral M99.88
      costovertebral M99.88
      head region M99.80
      hip M99.85
      lower extremity M99.86
      lumbar region M99.83
      lumbosacral M99.83
      occipitocervical M99.80
      pelvic region M99.85
      pubic M99.85
      rib cage M99.88
      sacral region M99.84
      sacrococcygeal M99.84
      sacroiliac M99.84
      specified NEC M99.89
      sternochondral M99.88
      sternoclavicular M99.87
      thoracic region M99.82
      thoracolumbar M99.82
      upper extremity M99.87
  bladder N32.9
  bone — *see* Disorder, bone
  brachial plexus G54.0
  brain G93.9
    congenital Q04.9
    vascular I67.9
      degenerative I67.9
      hypertensive I67.4
  buccal cavity K13.79
  calcified — *see* Calcification
  cameron — *see* Ulcer, stomach
  canthus — *see* Disorder, eyelid
  carate — *see* Pinta, lesions
  cardia K31.9
  cardiac — *see also* Disease, heart I51.9
    congenital Q24.9
    valvular — *see* Endocarditis
  cauda equina G83.4

Lesion(s) — *continued*
  cecum K63.9
  cerebral — *see* Lesion, brain
  cerebrovascular I67.9
    degenerative I67.9
    hypertensive I67.4
  cervical (nerve) root NEC G54.2
  chiasmal — *see* Disorder, optic, chiasm
  chorda tympani G51.8
  coin, lung R91.1
  colon K63.9
  combined periodontic - endodontic K05.5
  congenital — *see* Anomaly, by site
  conjunctiva H11.9
  conus medullaris — *see* Injury, conus medullaris
  coronary artery — *see* Ischemia, heart
  cranial nerve G52.9
    eighth — *see* Disorder, ear
    eleventh G52.9
    fifth G50.9
    first G52.0
    fourth — *see* Strabismus, paralytic, fourth nerve
    seventh G51.9
    sixth — *see* Strabismus, paralytic, sixth nerve
    tenth G52.2
    twelfth G52.3
  cystic — *see* Cyst
  degenerative — *see* Degeneration
  duodenum K31.9
  edentulous (alveolar) ridge, associated with trauma, due to traumatic occlusion K06.2
  en coup de sabre L94.1
  eyelid — *see* Disorder, eyelid
  gasserian ganglion G50.8
  gastric K31.9
  gastroduodenal K31.9
  gastrointestinal K63.9
  gingiva, associated with trauma K06.2
  glomerular
    focal and segmental — *see also* N00-N07 with fourth character .1 N05.1
    minimal change — *see also* N00-N07 with fourth character .0 N05.0
  heart (organic) — *see* Disease, heart
  hyperchromic, due to pinta (carate) A67.1
  hyperkeratotic — *see* Hyperkeratosis
  hypothalamic E23.7
  ileocecal K63.9
  ileum K63.9
  iliohypogastric nerve G57.8- ☑
  inflammatory — *see* Inflammation
  intestine K63.9
  intracerebral — *see* Lesion, brain
  intrachiasmal (optic) — *see* Disorder, optic, chiasm
  intracranial, space-occupying R90.0
  joint — *see* Disorder, joint
    sacroiliac (old) M53.3
  keratotic — *see* Keratosis
  kidney — *see* Disease, renal
  laryngeal nerve (recurrent) G52.2
  lip K13.0
  liver K76.9
  lumbosacral
    plexus G54.1
    root (nerve) NEC G54.4
  lung (coin) R91.1
  maxillary sinus J32.0
  mitral I05.9
  Morel-Lavallée — *see* Hematoma, by site
  motor cortex NEC G93.89
  mouth K13.79
  nerve G58.9
    femoral G57.2- ☑
    median G56.1- ☑
      carpal tunnel syndrome — *see* Syndrome, carpal tunnel
    plantar G57.6- ☑
    popliteal (lateral) G57.3- ☑
      medial G57.4- ☑
    radial G56.3- ☑
    sciatic G57.0- ☑
    spinal — *see* Injury, nerve, spinal
    ulnar G56.2- ☑
  nervous system, congenital Q07.9
  nonallopathic — *see* Lesion, biomechanical
  nose (internal) J34.89
  obstructive — *see* Obstruction
  obturator nerve G57.8- ☑

Lesion(s) — *continued*
  oral mucosa K13.70
  organ or site NEC — *see* Disease, by site
  osteolytic — *see* Osteolysis
  peptic K27.9
  periodontal, due to traumatic occlusion K05.5
  pharynx J39.2
  pigment, pigmented (skin) L81.9
  pinta — *see* Pinta, lesions
  polypoid — *see* Polyp
  prechiasmal (optic) — *see* Disorder, optic, chiasm
  primary — *see also* Syphilis, primary A51.0
    carate A67.0
    pinta A67.0
    yaws A66.0
  pulmonary J98.4
    valve I37.9
  pylorus K31.9
  rectosigmoid K63.9
  retina, retinal H35.9
  sacroiliac (joint) (old) M53.3
  salivary gland K11.9
    benign lymphoepithelial K11.8
  saphenous nerve G57.8- ☑
  sciatic nerve G57.0- ☑
  secondary — *see* Syphilis, secondary
  shoulder (region) M75.9- ☑
    specified NEC M75.8- ☑
  sigmoid K63.9
  sinus (accessory) (nasal) J34.89
  skin L98.9
    suppurative L08.0
  SLAP S43.43- ☑
  spinal cord G95.9
    congenital Q06.9
  spleen D73.89
  stomach K31.9
  superior glenoid labrum S43.43- ☑
  syphilitic — *see* Syphilis
  tertiary — *see* Syphilis, tertiary
  thoracic root (nerve) NEC G54.3
  tonsillar fossa J35.9
  tooth, teeth K08.9
    white spot
      chewing surface K02.51
      pit and fissure surface K02.51
      smooth surface K02.61
  traumatic — *see* specific type of injury by site
  tricuspid (valve) I07.9
    nonrheumatic I36.9
  trigeminal nerve G50.9
  ulcerated or ulcerative — *see* Ulcer, skin
  uterus N85.9
  vagina N89.8
  vagus nerve G52.2
  valvular — *see* Endocarditis
  vascular I99.9
    affecting central nervous system I67.9
    following trauma NEC T14.8 ☑
    umbilical cord, complicating delivery O69.5 ☑
  vulva N90.89
  warty — *see* Verruca
  white spot (tooth)
    chewing surface K02.51
    pit and fissure surface K02.51
    smooth surface K02.61
Less than a high school diploma Z55.5
Lethargic — *see* condition
Lethargy R53.83
Letterer-Siwe's disease C96.0
Leukemia, leukemic C95.9- ☑
  acute basophilic C94.8- ☑
  acute bilineal C95.0- ☑
  acute erythroid C94.0- ☑
  acute lymphoblastic C91.0- ☑
  acute megakaryoblastic C94.2- ☑
  acute megakaryocytic C94.2- ☑
  acute mixed lineage C95.0- ☑
  acute monoblastic (monoblastic/monocytic) C93.0- ☑
  acute monocytic (monoblastic/monocytic) C93.0- ☑
  acute myeloblastic (minimal differentiation) (with maturation) C92.0- ☑
  acute myeloid, NOS C92.0- ☑
    with
      11q23-abnormality C92.6- ☑
      dysplasia of remaining hematopoesis and/or myelodysplastic disease in its history C92.A- ☑ (*following* C92.6)

Leukemia, leukemic — *continued*
  acute myeloid, — *continued*
    with — *continued*
      multilineage dysplasia C92.A- ☑ (*following* C92.6)
      variation of MLL-gene C92.6- ☑
    M6 (a)(b) C94.0- ☑
    M7 C94.2- ☑
  acute myelomonocytic C92.5- ☑
  acute promyelocytic C92.4- ☑
  adult T-cell (HTLV-1-associated) (acute variant) (chronic variant) (lymphomatoid variant) (smouldering variant) C91.5- ☑
  aggressive NK-cell C94.8- ☑
  AML (1/ETO) (MØ) (M1) (M2) (without a FAB classification) C92.0- ☑
  AML M3 C92.4- ☑
  AML M4 (Eo with inv(16) or t(16;16)) C92.5- ☑
  AML M5 C93.0- ☑
  AML M5a C93.0- ☑
  AML M5b C93.0- ☑
  AML Me with t (15;17) and variants C92.4- ☑
  atypical chronic myeloid, BCR/ABL-negative C92.2- ☑
  biphenotypic acute C95.0- ☑
  blast cell C95.0- ☑
  Burkitt-type, mature B-cell C91.A- ☑ (*following* C91.6)
  chronic eosinophilic — *see also* Syndrome, hypereosinophilic, myeloid C94.8- ☑
  chronic lymphocytic, of B-cell type C91.1- ☑
  chronic monocytic C93.1- ☑
  chronic myelogenous (Philadelphia chromosome (Ph1) positive) (t(9;22)) (q34;q11) (with crisis of blast cells) C92.1- ☑
  chronic myeloid, BCR/ABL-positive C92.1- ☑
    atypical, BCR/ABL-negative C92.2- ☑
  chronic myelomonocytic C93.1- ☑
  chronic neutrophilic D47.1
  CMML (-1) (-2) (with eosinophilia) C93.1- ☑
  granulocytic — *see also* Category C92 C92.9- ☑
  hairy cell C91.4- ☑
  juvenile myelomonocytic C93.3- ☑
  lymphoid C91.9- ☑
    specified NEC C91.Z- ☑ (*following* C91.6)
  mast cell C94.3- ☑
  mature B-cell, Burkitt-type C91.A- ☑ (*following* C91.6)
  monocytic (subacute) C93.9- ☑
    specified NEC C93.Z- ☑ (*following* C93.3)
  myelogenous — *see also* Category C92 C92.9- ☑
  myeloid C92.9- ☑
    specified NEC C92.Z- ☑ (*following* C92.6)
  plasma cell C90.1- ☑
  plasmacytic C90.1- ☑
  prolymphocytic
    of B-cell type C91.3- ☑
    of T-cell type C91.6- ☑
  specified NEC C94.8- ☑
  stem cell, of unclear lineage C95.0- ☑
  subacute lymphocytic C91.9- ☑
  T-cell large granular lymphocytic C91.Z- ☑ (*following* C91.6)
  unspecified cell type C95.9- ☑
    acute C95.0- ☑
    chronic C95.1- ☑
Leukemoid reaction — *see also* Reaction, leukemoid D72.823
Leukoaraiosis (hypertensive) I67.81
Leukoariosis — *see* Leukoaraiosis
Leukocoria — *see* Disorder, globe, degenerated condition, leucocoria
Leukocytopenia D72.819
Leukocytosis D72.829
  eosinophilic D72.19
Leukoderma, leukodermia NEC L81.5
  syphilitic A51.39
    late A52.79
Leukodystrophy G31.80
  with vanishing white matter disease G11.6
  LMNB1-related autosomal dominant G90.B
  metachromatic E75.25
  pol III-related G11.5
Leukoedema, oral epithelium K13.29
Leukoencephalitis G04.81
  acute (subacute) hemorrhagic G36.1
    postimmunization or postvaccinal G04.02
  postinfectious G04.01
  subacute sclerosing A81.1
  van Bogaert's (sclerosing) A81.1

Leukoencephalopathy — *see also* Encephalopathy G93.49
  with calcifications and cysts G93.43
  adult-onset, with axonal spheroids (and pigmented glia) G93.44
  Binswanger's I67.3
  heroin vapor G92.8
  megalencephalic, with subcortical cysts G93.42
  metachromatic E75.25
  multifocal (progressive) A81.2
  postimmunization and postvaccinal G04.02
  progressive multifocal A81.2
  reversible, posterior G93.6
  van Bogaert's (sclerosing) A81.1
  vascular, progressive I67.3
Leukoerythroblastosis D75.9
Leukokeratosis — *see also* Leukoplakia
  mouth K13.21
  nicotina palati K13.24
  oral mucosa K13.21
  tongue K13.21
  vocal cord J38.3
Leukokraurosis vulva (e) N90.4
Leukoma (cornea) — *see also* Opacity, cornea
  adherent H17.0- ☑
  interfering with central vision — *see* Opacity, cornea, central
Leukomalacia, cerebral, newborn P91.2
  periventricular P91.2
Leukomelanopathy, hereditary D72.0
Leukonychia (punctata) (striata) L60.8
  congenital Q84.4
Leukopathia unguium L60.8
  congenital Q84.4
Leukopenia D72.819
  basophilic D72.818
  chemotherapy (cancer) induced D70.1
  congenital D70.0
  cyclic D70.0
  drug induced NEC D70.2
    due to cytoreductive cancer chemotherapy D70.1
  eosinophilic D72.818
  familial D70.0
  infantile genetic D70.0
  malignant D70.9
  periodic D70.0
  transitory neonatal P61.5
Leukopenic — *see* condition
Leukoplakia
  anus K62.89
  bladder (postinfectional) N32.89
  buccal K13.21
  cervix (uteri) N88.0
  esophagus K22.89
  gingiva K13.21
  hairy (oral mucosa) (tongue) K13.3
  kidney (pelvis) N28.89
  larynx J38.7
  lip K13.21
  mouth K13.21
  oral epithelium, including tongue (mucosa) K13.21
  palate K13.21
  pelvis (kidney) N28.89
  penis (infectional) N48.0
  rectum K62.89
  syphilitic (late) A52.79
  tongue K13.21
  ureter (postinfectional) N28.89
  urethra (postinfectional) N36.8
  uterus N85.8
  vagina N89.4
  vocal cord J38.3
  vulva N90.4
Leukorrhea N89.8
  due to Trichomonas (vaginalis) A59.00
  trichomonal A59.00
Leukosarcoma C85.9- ☑
Levocardia (isolated) Q24.1
  with situs inversus Q89.3
Levotransposition Q20.5
Lev's disease or syndrome (acquired complete heart block) I44.2
Levulosuria — *see* Fructosuria
Levurid L30.2
Lewy body (ies) (disease) G31.83
Leyden-Mobius dystrophy — *see* Dystrophy, Leyden-Mobius
Leydig cell
  carcinoma
    specified site — *see* Neoplasm, malignant, by site

Leydig cell — *continued*
  carcinoma — *continued*
    unspecified site
      female C56.9
      male C62.9- ☑
  tumor
    benign
      specified site — *see* Neoplasm, benign, by site
      unspecified site
        female D27.- ☑
        male D29.2- ☑
    malignant
      specified site — *see* Neoplasm, malignant, by site
      unspecified site
        female C56.- ☑
        male C62.9- ☑
    specified site — *see* Neoplasm, uncertain behavior, by site
    unspecified site
      female D39.1- ☑
      male D40.1- ☑
Leydig-Sertoli cell tumor
  specified site — *see* Neoplasm, benign, by site
  unspecified site
    female D27.- ☑
    male D29.2- ☑
LGMD — *see* Dystrophy, muscular, limb-girdle
LGSIL (Low grade squamous intraepithelial lesion on cytologic smear of)
  anus R85.612
  cervix R87.612
  vagina R87.622
Liar, pathologic F60.2
Libido
  decreased R68.82
Libman-Sacks disease M32.11
Lice (infestation) B85.2
  body (Pediculus corporis) B85.1
  crab B85.3
  head (Pediculus capitis) B85.0
  mixed (classifiable to more than one of the titles B85.0-B85.3) B85.4
  pubic (Phthirus pubis) B85.3
Lichen L28.0
  albus L90.0
    penis N48.0
    vulva N90.4
  amyloidosis E85.4 [L99]
  atrophicus L90.0
    penis N48.0
    vulva N90.4
  congenital Q82.8
  myxedematosus L98.5
  nitidus L44.1
  pilaris Q82.8
    acquired L85.8
  planopilaris L66.10
    classic L66.11
    follicular L66.11
    specified NEC L66.19
  planus (chronicus) L43.9
    annularis L43.8
    bullous L43.1
    follicular L66.11
    hypertrophic L43.0
    moniliformis L44.3
    of Wilson L43.9
    specified NEC L43.8
    subacute (active) L43.3
    tropicus L43.3
  ruber
    acuminatus L44.0
    moniliformis L44.3
    planus L43.9
  sclerosus (et atrophicus) L90.0
    penis N48.0
    vulva N90.4
  scrofulosus (primary) (tuberculous) A18.4
  simplex (chronicus) (circumscriptus) L28.0
  striatus L44.2
  urticatus L28.2
Lichenification L28.0
Lichenoid keratosis — *see* Keratosis, lichenoid
Lichenoides tuberculosis (primary) A18.4
Lichtheim's disease or syndrome D51.0
Lien migrans D73.89
Ligament — *see* condition

Light

for gestational age — *see* Light for dates
headedness R42
Light-for-dates (infant) P05.00
with weight of
499 grams or less P05.01
500-749 grams P05.02
750-999 grams P05.03
1000-1249 grams P05.04
1250-1499 grams P05.05
1500-1749 grams P05.06
1750-1999 grams P05.07
2000-2499 grams P05.08
2500 grams and over P05.09
affecting management of pregnancy O36.59- ☑
and small-for-dates — *see* Small for dates
specified NEC P05.09
Lightning (effects) (stroke) (struck by) T75.00 ☑
burn — *see* Burn
foot E53.8
shock T75.01 ☑
specified effect NEC T75.09 ☑
Lightwood-Albright syndrome N25.89
Lightwood's disease or syndrome (renal tubular acidosis)
N25.89
Lignac (-de Toni) (-Fanconi) (-Debre) **disease or syndrome**
E72.09
with cystinosis E72.04
Ligneous thyroiditis E06.5
Likoff's syndrome I20.89
Limb — *see* condition
Limbic epilepsy personality syndrome F07.0
Limitation, limited
activities due to disability Z73.6
cardiac reserve — *see* Disease, heart
eye muscle duction, traumatic — *see* Strabismus, mechanical
mandibular range of motion M26.52
Lindau (-von Hippel) **disease** Q85.83
Line(s)
Beau's L60.4
Harris' — *see* Arrest, epiphyseal
Hudson's (cornea) — *see* Pigmentation, cornea, anterior
Stahli's (cornea) — *see* Pigmentation, cornea, anterior
Linea corneae senilis — *see* Change, cornea, senile
Lingua
geographica K14.1
nigra (villosa) K14.3
plicata K14.5
tylosis K13.29
Lingual — *see* condition
Linguatulosis B88.8
Linitis (gastric) **plastica** C16.9
Lip — *see* condition
Lipedema — *see* Edema
Lipemia — *see also* Hyperlipidemia
retina, retinalis E78.3
Lipidosis E75.6
cerebral (infantile) (juvenile) (late) E75.4
cerebroretinal E75.4
cerebroside E75.22
cholesterol (cerebral) E75.5
glycolipid E75.21
hepatosplenomegalic E78.3
sphingomyelin — *see* Niemann-Pick disease or syndrome
sulfatide E75.29
Lipoadenoma — *see* Neoplasm, benign, by site
Lipoblastoma — *see* Lipoma
Lipoblastomatosis — *see* Lipoma
Lipochondrodystrophy E76.01
Lipochrome histiocytosis (familial) D71
Lipodermatosclerosis — *see also* Insufficiency, venous
M79.3
with
varicose veins — *see* Varix, leg, with, inflammation
ulcerated — *see* Varix, leg, with, ulcer, with inflammation by site
ulcerated — *see* Ulcer, by site
Lipodystrophia progressiva E88.1
Lipodystrophy (progressive) E88.1
insulin E88.1
intestinal K90.81
mesenteric K65.4
Lipofibroma — *see* Lipoma
Lipofuscinosis, neuronal (with ceroidosis) E75.4
Lipogranuloma, sclerosing L92.8
Lipogranulomatosis E78.89
Lipoid — *see also* condition
histiocytosis D76.3

Lipoid — *continued*
histiocytosis — *continued*
essential E75.29
nephrosis N04.9
proteinosis of Urbach E78.89
Lipoidemia — *see* Hyperlipidemia
Lipoidosis — *see* Lipidosis
Lipoma D17.9
fetal D17.9
fat cell D17.9
infiltrating D17.9
intramuscular D17.9
pleomorphic D17.9
site classification
arms (skin) (subcutaneous) D17.2- ☑
connective tissue D17.30
intra-abdominal D17.5
intrathoracic D17.4
peritoneum D17.79
retroperitoneum D17.79
specified site NEC D17.39
spermatic cord D17.6
face (skin) (subcutaneous) D17.0
genitourinary organ NEC D17.72
head (skin) (subcutaneous) D17.0
intra-abdominal D17.5
intrathoracic D17.4
kidney D17.71
legs (skin) (subcutaneous) D17.2- ☑
neck (skin) (subcutaneous) D17.0
peritoneum D17.79
retroperitoneum D17.79
skin D17.30
specified site NEC D17.39
specified site NEC D17.79
spermatic cord D17.6
subcutaneous D17.30
specified site NEC D17.39
trunk (skin) (subcutaneous) D17.1
unspecified D17.9
spindle cell D17.9
Lipomatosis E88.2
dolorosa (Dercum) E88.2
fetal — *see* Lipoma
Launois-Bensaude E88.89
Lipomyoma — *see* Lipoma
Lipomyxoma — *see* Lipoma
Lipomyxosarcoma — *see* Neoplasm, connective tissue, malignant
Lipoprotein metabolism disorder E78.9
Lipoproteinemia E78.5
broad-beta E78.2
floating-beta E78.2
hyper-pre-beta E78.1
Liposarcoma — *see also* Neoplasm, connective tissue, malignant
dedifferentiated — *see* Neoplasm, connective tissue, malignant
differentiated type — *see* Neoplasm, connective tissue, malignant
embryonal — *see* Neoplasm, connective tissue, malignant
mixed type — *see* Neoplasm, connective tissue, malignant
myxoid — *see* Neoplasm, connective tissue, malignant
pleomorphic — *see* Neoplasm, connective tissue, malignant
round cell — *see* Neoplasm, connective tissue, malignant
well differentiated type — *see* Neoplasm, connective tissue, malignant
Liposynovitis prepatellaris E88.89
Lipping, cervix N86
Lipschütz disease or ulcer N76.6
Lipuria R82.0
schistosomiasis (bilharziasis) B65.0
Lisping F80.0
Lissauer's paralysis A52.17
Lissencephalia, lissencephaly Q04.3
Listeriosis, listerellosis A32.9
congenital (disseminated) P37.2
cutaneous A32.0
neonatal, newborn (disseminated) P37.2
oculoglandular A32.81
specified NEC A32.89
Lithemia E79.0
Lithiasis — *see* Calculus
Lithosis J62.8
Lithuria R82.998
Litigation, anxiety concerning Z65.3

Little leaguer's elbow — *see* Epicondylitis, medial
Little's disease G80.9
Littre's
gland — *see* condition
hernia — *see* Hernia, abdomen
Littritis — *see* Urethritis
Livedo (annularis) (racemosa) (reticularis) R23.1
Liver — *see* condition
Living alone (problems with) Z60.2
with handicapped person Z74.2
Living in a shelter (motel) (scattered site housing) (temporary or transitional living situation) Z59.01
Lloyd's syndrome — *see* Adenomatosis, endocrine
Loa loa (loiasis) B74.3
Lobar — *see* condition
Lobomycosis B48.0
Lobo's disease B48.0
Lobotomy syndrome F07.0
Lobstein (-Ekman) **disease or syndrome** Q78.0
Lobster-claw hand Q71.6- ☑
Lobulation (congenital) — *see also* Anomaly, by site
kidney, Q63.1
liver, abnormal Q44.79
spleen Q89.09
Lobule, lobular — *see* condition
Local, localized — *see* condition
Locked twins causing obstructed labor O66.1
Locked-in state G83.5
Locking
joint — *see* Derangement, joint, specified type NEC
knee — *see* Derangement, knee
Lockjaw — *see* Tetanus
Loffler's
endocarditis I42.3
eosinophilia J82.89
pneumonia J82.89
syndrome (eosinophilic pneumonitis) J82.89
Loiasis (with conjunctival infestation) (eyelid) B74.3
Lone Star fever A77.0
Loneliness R45.89
Long
COVID (-19) — *see also* COVID-19 U09.9
labor O63.9
first stage O63.0
second stage O63.1
QT syndrome I45.81
Longitudinal stripes or grooves, nails L60.8
congenital Q84.6
Long-term (current) (prophylactic) **drug therapy** (use of)
5-fluorouracil Z79.631
6-mercaptopurine Z79.631
adalimumab Z79.620
agents affecting estrogen receptors and estrogen levels
NEC Z79.818
alkylating agent Z79.630
anastrozole (Arimidex) Z79.811
antibiotics Z79.2
short-term use — *omit code*
anticoagulants Z79.01
antidiabetic drugs, injectable, non-insulin Z79.85
anti-inflammatory, non-steroidal (NSAID) Z79.1
antimetabolite agent Z79.631
antiplatelet Z79.02
antithrombotics Z79.02
antitumor antibiotic Z79.632
apremilast Z79.61
aromatase inhibitors Z79.811
aspirin Z79.82
azathioprine Z79.624
birth control pill or patch Z79.3
bisphosphonates Z79.83
bleomycin Z79.632
calcineurin inhibitor Z79.621
chlorambucil Z79.630
cisplatin Z79.630
contraceptive, oral Z79.3
cyclophosphamide Z79.630
cyclosporine Z79.621
cytarabine Z79.631
doxorubicin Z79.632
drug, specified NEC Z79.899
estrogen receptor downregulators Z79.818
etanercept Z79.620
etoposide Z79.634
Evista Z79.810
exemestane (Aromasin) Z79.811
Fareston Z79.810
fulvestrant (Faslodex) Z79.818
gonadotropin-releasing hormone (GnRH) agonist Z79.818

☑ **Additional Character Required** — Refer to the Tabular List for Character Selection

Long-term (current) (prophylactic) **drug therapy** — *continued*
- goserelin acetate (Zoladex) Z79.818
- hormone replacement Z79.890
- hydroxyurea Z79.64
- immunomodulators, unspecified Z79.60
  - specified NEC Z79.69
- immunomodulatory imide drug Z79.61
- immunosuppressants, unspecified Z79.60
  - specified NEC Z79.69
- immunosuppressive biologic Z79.620
- infliximab Z79.620
- inhibitors of nucleotide synthesis Z79.624
- insulin Z79.4
- irinotecan Z79.634
- Janus kinase inhibitor Z79.622
- lenalidomide Z79.61
- letrozole (Femara) Z79.811
- leuprolide acetate (leuprorelin) (Lupron) Z79.818
- mammalian target of rapamycin (mTOR) inhibitor Z79.623
- megestrol acetate (Megace) Z79.818
- methadone for pain management Z79.891
- mitomycin C Z79.632
- mitotic inhibitor Z79.633
- monoclonal antibodies Z79.620
- mycophenolate Z79.624
- myelosuppressive agent Z79.64
- Nolvadex Z79.810
- non-insulin antidiabetic drug, injectable Z79.85
- non-steroidal anti-inflammatories (NSAID) Z79.1
- opiate analgesic Z79.891
- oral
  - antidiabetic Z79.84
  - contraceptive Z79.3
  - hypoglycemic Z79.84
- paclitaxel Z79.633
- plant alkaloids Z79.633
- pomalidomide Z79.61
- purine synthesis (IMDH) inhibitors Z79.624
- raloxifene (Evista) Z79.810
- selective estrogen receptor modulators (SERMs) Z79.810
- sirolimus Z79.623
- steroids
  - inhaled Z79.51
  - systemic Z79.52
- tacrolimus Z79.621
- tamoxifen (Nolvadex) Z79.810
- tofacitinib Z79.622
- topoisomerase inhibitor Z79.634
- topotecan Z79.634
- toremifene (Fareston) Z79.810
- vinblastine Z79.633
- vincristine Z79.633

Loop
- intestine — *see* Volvulus
- vascular on papilla (optic) Q14.2

Loose — *see also* condition
- body
  - joint M24.00
    - ankle M24.07- ☑
    - elbow M24.02- ☑
    - hand M24.04- ☑
    - hip M24.05- ☑
    - knee M23.4-
    - shoulder (region) M24.01- ☑
    - specified site NEC M24.08
    - temporomandibular M24.08
    - toe M24.07- ☑
    - vertebra M24.08
    - wrist M24.03- ☑
  - knee M23.4- ☑
  - sheath, tendon — *see* Disorder, tendon, specified type NEC
- cartilage — *see* Loose, body, joint
- skin and subcutaneous tissue (following bariatric surgery weight loss) (following dietary weight loss) L98.7
- tooth, teeth K08.89

Loosening
- aseptic
  - joint prosthesis — *see* Complications, joint prosthesis, mechanical, loosening, by site
- epiphysis — *see* Osteochondropathy
- mechanical
  - joint prosthesis — *see* Complications, joint prosthesis, mechanical, loosening, by site

Looser-Milkman (-Debray) **syndrome** M83.8
Lop ear (deformity) Q17.3

Lorain (-Levi) **short stature syndrome** E23.0
Lordosis M40.50
- acquired — *see* Lordosis, specified type NEC
- congenital Q76.429
  - lumbar region Q76.426
  - lumbosacral region Q76.427
  - sacral region Q76.428
  - sacrococcygeal region Q76.428
  - thoracolumbar region Q76.425
- lumbar region M40.56
- lumbosacral region M40.57
- postsurgical M96.4
- postural — *see* Lordosis, specified type NEC
- rachitic (late effect) (sequelae) E64.3
- sequelae of rickets E64.3
- specified type NEC M40.40
  - lumbar region M40.46
  - lumbosacral region M40.47
  - thoracolumbar region M40.45
- thoracolumbar region M40.55
- tuberculous A18.01

Loss (of)
- appetite — *see also* Anorexia R63.0
  - hysterical F50.89
  - nonorganic origin F50.89
  - psychogenic F50.89
- blood — *see* Hemorrhage
- bone —*see* Loss, substance of, bone
- consciousness, transient R55
  - traumatic — *see* Injury, intracranial
- control, sphincter, rectum R15.9
  - nonorganic origin F98.1
- elasticity, skin R23.4
- family (member) in childhood Z62.898
- fluid (acute) E86.9
- function of labyrinth — *see* subcategory H83.2 ☑
- hair, nonscarring — *see* Alopecia
- hearing — *see also* Deafness
  - central NOS H90.5
  - conductive H90.2
    - bilateral H90.0
    - unilateral
      - with
        - restricted hearing on the contralateral side H90.A1- ☑
        - unrestricted hearing on the contralateral side H90.1- ☑
  - mixed conductive and sensorineural hearing loss H90.8
    - bilateral H90.6
    - unilateral
      - with
        - restricted hearing on the contralateral side H90.A3- ☑
        - unrestricted hearing on the contralateral side H90.7- ☑
  - neural NOS H90.5
  - perceptive NOS H90.5
  - sensorineural NOS H90.5
    - bilateral H90.3
    - unilateral
      - with
        - restricted hearing onthe contralateral side H90.A2- ☑
        - unrestricted hearing on the contralateral side H90.4- ☑
  - sensory NOS H90.5
- height R29.890
- limb or member, traumatic, current — *see* Amputation, traumatic
- love relationship in childhood Z62.898
- memory — *see also* Amnesia
  - mild, following organic brain damage F06.8
- mind — *see* Psychosis
- occlusal vertical dimension of fully erupted teeth M26.37
- organ or part — *see* Absence, by site, acquired
- ossicles, ear (partial) H74.32- ☑
- parent in childhood Z63.4
- pregnancy, recurrent N96
  - care in current pregnancy O26.2- ☑
  - without current pregnancy N96
- recurrent pregnancy — *see* Loss, pregnancy, recurrent
- self-esteem, in childhood Z62.898
- sense of
  - smell — *see* Disturbance, sensation, smell
  - taste — *see* Disturbance, sensation, taste
  - touch R20.8
- sensory R44.9

Loss — *continued*
- sensory — *continued*
  - dissociative F44.6
- sexual desire F52.0
- sight (acquired) (complete) (congenital) — *see* Blindness
- substance of
  - bone — *see* Disorder, bone, density and structure, specified NEC
    - horizontal alveolar K06.3
  - cartilage — *see* Disorder, cartilage, specified type NEC
    - auricle (ear) — *see* Disorder, pinna, specified type NEC
  - vitreous (humor) H15.89
- tooth, teeth — *see* Absence, teeth, acquired
- vision, visual H54.7
  - both eyes H54.3
  - one eye H54.60
    - left (normal vision on right) H54.62
    - right (normal vision on left) H54.61
  - specified as blindness — *see* Blindness
  - subjective
    - sudden H53.13- ☑
    - transient H53.12- ☑
- vitreous — *see* Prolapse, vitreous
- voice — *see* Aphonia
- weight (abnormal) (cause unknown) R63.4

Louis-Bar syndrome (ataxia-telangiectasia) G11.3
Louping ill (encephalitis) A84.89
Louse, lousiness — *see* Lice
Low
- achiever, school Z55.3
- back syndrome M54.50
- basal metabolic rate R94.8
- birthweight (2499 grams or less) P07.10
  - with weight of
    - 1000-1249 grams P07.14
    - 1250-1499 grams P07.15
    - 1500-1749 grams P07.16
    - 1750-1999 grams P07.17
    - 2000-2499 grams P07.18
  - extreme (999 grams or less) P07.00
    - with weight of
      - 499 grams or less P07.01
      - 500-749 grams P07.02
      - 750-999 grams P07.03
  - for gestational age — *see* Light for dates
- blood pressure — *see also* Hypotension
  - reading (incidental) (isolated) (nonspecific) R03.1
- cardiac reserve — *see* Disease, heart
- function — *see also* Hypofunction
  - kidney N28.9
- hematocrit D64.9
- hemoglobin D64.9
- income Z59.6
- level of literacy Z55.0
- lying
  - kidney N28.89
  - organ or site, congenital — *see* Malposition, congenital
- output syndrome (cardiac) — *see* Failure, heart
- platelets (blood) — *see* Thrombocytopenia
- reserve, kidney N28.89
- salt syndrome E87.1
- self esteem R45.81
- set ears Q17.4
- vision H54.2X- ☑
  - one eye (other eye normal) H54.50
    - left (normal vision on right)
      - category 1 H54.52A1
      - category 2 H54.52A2
    - other eye blind — *see* Blindness
    - right (normal vision on left)
      - category 1 H54.511A
      - category 2 H54.512A
- von Willebrand factor R79.1

Low-density-lipoprotein-type (LDL) **hyperlipoproteine-mia** E78.00
Lowe's syndrome E72.03
Lown-Ganong-Levine syndrome I45.6
LSD reaction (acute) (without dependence) F16.90
- with dependence F16.20

L-shaped kidney Q63.8
LTBI (latent tuberculosis infection) Z22.7
Ludwig's angina or disease K12.2
Lues (venerea), **luetic** — *see* Syphilis
Luetscher's syndrome (dehydration) E86.0
Lumbago, lumbalgia M54.50
- with sciatica M54.4- ☑
  - due to intervertebral disc disorder M51.17

Lumbago, lumbalgia — *continued*
  due to displacement, intervertebral disc M51.27
    with sciatica M51.17
Lumbar — *see* condition
Lumbarization, vertebra, congenital Q76.49
Lumbermen's itch B88.0
Lump — *see also* Mass
  breast N63.0
    axillary tail
      left N63.32
      right N63.31
    left
      lower inner quadrant N63.24
      lower outer quadrant N63.23
      overlapping quadrants N63.25
      unspecified quadrant N63.20
      upper inner quadrant N63.22
      upper outer quadrant N63.21
    right
      lower inner quadrant N63.14
      lower outer quadrant N63.13
      overlapping quadrants N63.15
      unspecified quadrant N63.10
      upper inner quadrant N63.12
      upper outer quadrant N63.11
    subareolar
      left N63.42
      right N63.41
Lunacy — *see* Psychosis
Lung — *see* condition
Lupoid (miliary) **of Boeck** D86.3
Lupus
  anticoagulant D68.62
    with
      hemorrhagic disorder D68.312
      hypercoagulable state D68.62
    finding without diagnosis R76.0
  discoid (local) L93.0
  erythematosus (discoid) (local) L93.0
    disseminated — *see* Lupus, erythematosus, systemic
    eyelid H01.129
      left H01.126
        lower H01.125
        upper H01.124
      right H01.123
        lower H01.122
        upper H01.121
    profundus L93.2
    specified NEC L93.2
    subacute cutaneous L93.1
    systemic M32.9
      with organ or system involvement M32.10
        endocarditis M32.11
        lung M32.13
        pericarditis M32.12
        renal (glomerular) M32.14
          tubulo-interstitial M32.15
        specified organ or system NEC M32.19
      drug-induced M32.0
      inhibitor (presence of) D68.62
        with
          hemorrhagic disorder D68.312
          hypercoagulable state D68.62
        finding without diagnosis R76.0
      specified NEC M32.8
  exedens A18.4
  hydralazine M32.0
    correct substance properly administered — *see* Table of Drugs and Chemicals, by drug, adverse effect
    overdose or wrong substance given or taken — *see* Table of Drugs and Chemicals, by drug, poisoning
  nephritis (chronic) M32.14
  nontuberculous, not disseminated L93.0
  panniculitis L93.2
  pernio (Besnier) D86.3
  systemic — *see* Lupus, erythematosus, systemic
  tuberculous A18.4
    eyelid A18.4
  vulgaris A18.4
    eyelid A18.4
Luteinoma D27.- ☑
Lutembacher's disease or syndrome (atrial septal defect with mitral stenosis) Q21.19
Luteoma D27.- ☑
Lutz (-Splendore-de Almeida) **disease** — *see* Paracoccidioidomycosis
Luxation — *see also* Dislocation
  eyeball (nontraumatic) — *see* Luxation, globe

Luxation — *continued*
  eyeball — *see* Luxation, globe — *continued*
    birth injury P15.3
    globe, nontraumatic H44.82- ☑
    lacrimal gland — *see* Dislocation, lacrimal gland
    lens (old) (partial) (spontaneous)
      congenital Q12.1
      syphilitic A50.39
Lycanthropy F22
Lyell's syndrome L51.2
  due to drug L51.2
    correct substance properly administered — *see* Table of Drugs and Chemicals, by drug, adverse effect
    overdose or wrong substance given or taken — *see* Table of Drugs and Chemicals, by drug, poisoning
Lyme disease A69.20
Lymph
  gland or node — *see* condition
  scrotum — *see* Infestation, filarial
Lymphadenitis I88.9
  with ectopic or molar pregnancy O08.0
  acute L04.9
    axilla L04.2
    face L04.0
    head L04.0
    hip L04.3
    limb
      lower L04.3
      upper L04.2
    neck L04.0
    shoulder L04.2
    specified site NEC L04.8
    trunk L04.1
  anthracosis (occupational) J60
  any site, except mesenteric I88.9
    chronic I88.1
    subacute I88.1
  breast
    gestational — *see* Mastitis, obstetric
    puerperal, postpartum (nonpurulent) O91.22
  chancroidal (congenital) A57
  chronic I88.1
    mesenteric I88.0
  due to
    Brugia (malayi) B74.1
      timori B74.2
    chlamydial lymphogranuloma A55
    diphtheria (toxin) A36.89
    lymphogranuloma venereum A55
    Wuchereria bancrofti B74.0
  following ectopic or molar pregnancy O08.0
  gonorrheal A54.89
  infective — *see* Lymphadenitis, acute
  mesenteric (acute) (chronic) (nonspecific) (subacute) I88.0
    due to Salmonella typhi A01.09
    tuberculous A18.39
  mycobacterial A31.8
  purulent — *see* Lymphadenitis, acute
  pyogenic — *see* Lymphadenitis, acute
  regional, nonbacterial I88.8
  septic — *see* Lymphadenitis, acute
  subacute, unspecified site I88.1
  suppurative — *see* Lymphadenitis, acute
  syphilitic (early) (secondary) A51.49
    late A52.79
  tuberculous — *see* Tuberculosis, lymph gland
  venereal (chlamydial) A55
Lymphadenoid goiter E06.3
Lymphadenopathy (generalized) R59.1
  angioimmunoblastic, with dysproteinemia (AILD) C86.5- ☑
  due to toxoplasmosis (acquired) B58.89
    congenital (acute) (subacute) (chronic) P37.1
  localized R59.0
  syphilitic (early) (secondary) A51.49
Lymphadenosis R59.1
Lymphangiectasis I89.0
  conjunctiva H11.89
  postinfectional I89.0
  scrotum I89.0
Lymphangiectatic elephantiasis, nonfilarial I89.0
Lymphangioendothelioma
  malignant — *see* Neoplasm, connective tissue, malignant
Lymphangioleiomyomatosis J84.81
Lymphangioma D18.1
  capillary D18.1
  cavernous D18.1

Lymphangioma — *continued*
  cystic D18.1
  malignant — *see* Neoplasm, connective tissue, malignant
Lymphangiomyoma D18.1
Lymphangiomyomatosis J84.81
Lymphangiosarcoma — *see* Neoplasm, connective tissue, malignant
Lymphangitis I89.1
  with
    abscess — *code by* site under Abscess
    cellulitis — *code by* site under Cellulitis
    ectopic or molar pregnancy O08.0
  acute L03.91
    abdominal wall L03.321
    ankle — *see* Lymphangitis, acute, lower limb
    arm — *see* Lymphangitis, acute, upper limb
    auricle (ear) — *see* Lymphangitis, acute, ear
    axilla L03.12- ☑
    back (any part) L03.322
    buttock L03.327
    cervical (meaning neck) L03.222
    cheek (external) L03.212
    chest wall L03.323
    digit
      finger — *see* Lymphangitis, acute, finger
      toe — *see* Lymphangitis, acute, toe
    ear (external) H60.1- ☑
    external auditory canal — *see* Lymphangitis, acute, ear
    eyelid — *see* Abscess, eyelid
    face NEC L03.212
    finger (intrathecal) (periosteal) (subcutaneous) (subcuticular) L03.02- ☑
    foot — *see* Lymphangitis, acute, lower limb
    gluteal (region) L03.327
    groin L03.324
    hand — *see* Lymphangitis, acute, upper limb
    head NEC L03.891
      face (any part, except ear, eye and nose) L03.212
    heel — *see* Lymphangitis, acute, lower limb
    hip — *see* Lymphangitis, acute, lower limb
    jaw (region) L03.212
    knee — *see* Lymphangitis, acute, lower limb
    leg — *see* Lymphangitis, acute, lower limb
    lower limb L03.12- ☑
      toe — *see* Lymphangitis, acute, toe
    navel L03.326
    neck (region) L03.222
    orbit, orbital — *see* Cellulitis, orbit
    pectoral (region) L03.323
    perineal, perineum L03.325
    scalp (any part) L03.891
    shoulder — *see* Lymphangitis, acute, upper limb
    specified site NEC L03.898
    thigh — *see* Lymphangitis, acute, lower limb
    thumb (intrathecal) (periosteal) (subcutaneous) (subcuticular) — *see* Lymphangitis, acute, finger
    toe (intrathecal) (periosteal) (subcutaneous) (subcuticular) L03.04- ☑
    trunk L03.329
      abdominal wall L03.321
      back (any part) L03.322
      buttock L03.327
      chest wall L03.323
      groin L03.324
      perineal, perineum L03.325
      umbilicus L03.326
    umbilicus L03.326
    upper limb L03.12- ☑
      axilla — *see* Lymphangitis, acute, axilla
      finger — *see* Lymphangitis, acute, finger
      thumb — *see* Lymphangitis, acute, finger
      wrist — *see* Lymphangitis, acute, upper limb
  breast
    gestational — *see* Mastitis, obstetric
  chancroidal A57
  chronic (any site) I89.1
  due to
    Brugia (malayi) B74.1
      timori B74.2
    Wuchereria bancrofti B74.0
  following ectopic or molar pregnancy O08.89
  penis
    acute N48.29
    gonococcal (acute) (chronic) A54.09
  puerperal, postpartum, childbirth O86.89
  strumous, tuberculous A18.2

Lymphangitis — continued
  subacute (any site) I89.1
  tuberculous — see Tuberculosis, lymph gland
Lymphatic (vessel) — see condition
Lymphatism E32.8
Lymphectasia I89.0
Lymphedema (acquired) — see also Elephantiasis
  congenital Q82.0
  hereditary (chronic) (idiopathic) Q82.0
  postmastectomy I97.2
  praecox I89.0
  secondary I89.0
  surgical NEC I97.89
    postmastectomy (syndrome) I97.2
Lymphoblastic — see condition
Lymphoblastoma (diffuse) — see Lymphoma, lymphoblastic (diffuse)
  giant follicular — see Lymphoma, lymphoblastic (diffuse)
  macrofollicular — see Lymphoma, lymphoblastic (diffuse)
Lymphocele I89.8
Lymphocytic
  chorioencephalitis (acute) (serous) A87.2
  choriomeningitis (acute) (serous) A87.2
  meningoencephalitis A87.2
Lymphocytoma, benign cutis L98.8
Lymphocytopenia D72.810
Lymphocytosis (symptomatic) D72.820
  infectious (acute) B33.8
Lymphoepithelioma — see Neoplasm, malignant, by site
Lymphogranuloma (malignant) — see also Lymphoma, Hodgkin
  chlamydial A55
  inguinale A55
  venereum (any site) (chlamydial) (with stricture of rectum) A55
Lymphogranulomatosis (malignant) — see also Lymphoma, Hodgkin
  benign (Boeck's sarcoid) (Schaumann's) D86.1
Lymphohistiocytosis, hemophagocytic (familial) D76.1
Lymphoid — see condition
Lymphoma (of) (malignant) C85.90
  adult T-cell (HTLV-1-associated) (acute variant) (chronic variant) (lymphomatoid variant) (smouldering variant) C91.5- ☑
  anaplastic large cell
    ALK-negative C84.7- ☑
    ALK-positive C84.6- ☑
    breast implant associated (BIA-ALCL) C84.7A
    CD30-positive C84.6- ☑
    primary cutaneous C86.6- ☑
  angioimmunoblastic T-cell C86.5- ☑
  BALT C88.4- ☑
  B-cell C85.1- ☑
  blastic NK-cell C86.4- ☑
  blastic plasmacytoid dendritic cell neoplasm (BPDCN) C86.4- ☑
  B-precursor C83.5- ☑
  brain, primary — see Lymphoma, primary central nervous system
  bronchial-associated lymphoid tissue [BALT-lymphoma] C88.4- ☑
  Burkitt (atypical) C83.7- ☑
  Burkitt-like C83.7- ☑
  central nervous system, primary — see Lymphoma, primary central nervous system
  centrocytic C83.1- ☑
  cutaneous follicle center C82.6- ☑
  cutaneous T-cell C84.A- ☑ (following C84.7)
  diffuse follicle center C82.5- ☑
  diffuse large cell C83.3- ☑
    anaplastic C83.3- ☑
    B-cell C83.3- ☑
    CD30-positive C83.3- ☑
    centroblastic C83.3- ☑
    extranodal and solid organ sites NEC C83.398
    immunoblastic C83.3- ☑
    plasmablastic C83.3- ☑
    primary central nervous system (brain) (meninges) (PCNSL) (spinal cord) C83.390
    subtype not specified C83.3- ☑
    T-cell rich C83.3- ☑
  enteropathy-type (associated) (intestinal) T-cell C86.2- ☑
  extranodal marginal zone B-cell lymphoma of mucosa-associated lymphoid tissue [MALT-lymphoma] C88.4- ☑
  extranodal NK/T-cell, nasal type C86.0- ☑
  follicular C82.9- ☑

Lymphoma — continued
  follicular — continued
    grade
      I C82.0- ☑
      II C82.1- ☑
      III C82.2- ☑
      IIIa C82.3- ☑
      IIIb C82.4- ☑
      specified NEC C82.8- ☑
    hepatosplenic T-cell (alpha-beta) (gamma-delta) C86.1- ☑
    histiocytic C85.9- ☑
      true C96.A (following C96.6)
    Hodgkin C81.9- ☑
      lymphocyte depleted (classical) C81.3- ☑
      lymphocyte-rich (classical) C81.4- ☑
      mixed cellularity (classical) C81.2- ☑
      nodular
        lymphocyte predominant C81.0- ☑
        sclerosis (classical) C81.1- ☑
      nodular sclerosis (classical) C81.1- ☑
      specified NEC (classical) C81.7- ☑
    intravascular large B-cell C83.8- ☑
    Lennert's C84.4- ☑
    lymphoblastic (diffuse) C83.5- ☑
    lymphoblastic B-cell C83.5- ☑
    lymphoblastic T-cell C83.5- ☑
    lymphoepithelioid C84.4- ☑
    lymphoplasmacytic C83.0- ☑
      with IgM-production C88.0- ☑
    MALT C88.4- ☑
    mantle cell C83.1- ☑
    mature T-cell NEC C84.4- ☑
    mature T/NK-cell C84.9- ☑
      specified NEC C84.Z- ☑ (following C84.7)
    mediastinal (thymic) large B-cell C85.2- ☑
    Mediterranean C88.3- ☑
    meninges, primary — see Lymphoma, primary central nervous system
    mucosa-associated lymphoid tissue [MALT-lymphoma] C88.4- ☑
    NK/T cell C84.9- ☑
    nodal marginal zone C83.0- ☑
    non-follicular (diffuse) C83.9- ☑
      specified NEC C83.8- ☑
    non-Hodgkin — see also Lymphoma, by type C85.9- ☑
      specified NEC C85.8- ☑
    non-leukemic variant of B-CLL C83.0- ☑
    peripheral T-cell NEC C84.4- ☑
    primary central nervous system (brain) (meninges) (PCNSL) (spinal cord) C83.390
      Burkitt C83.79
      diffuse large B-cell C83.390
      lymphoblastic C83.59
      peripheral T-cell C84.49
    primary cutaneous
      anaplastic large cell C86.6- ☑
      CD30-positive large T-cell C86.6- ☑
    primary effusion B-cell C83.8- ☑
    SALT C88.4- ☑
    skin-associated lymphoid tissue [SALT-lymphoma] C88.4- ☑
    small cell B-cell C83.0- ☑
    spinal cord, primary — see Lymphoma, primary central nervous system
    splenic marginal zone C83.0- ☑
    subcutaneous panniculitis-like T-cell C86.3- ☑
    T-precursor C83.5- ☑
    true histiocytic C96.A (following C96.6)
Lymphomatosis — see Lymphoma
Lymphopathia venereum, veneris A55
Lymphopenia D72.810
Lymphoplasmacytic leukemia — see Leukemia, chronic lymphocytic, B-cell type
Lymphoproliferation, X-linked disease D82.3
Lymphoreticulosis, benign (of inoculation) A28.1
Lymphorrhea I89.8
Lymphosarcoma (diffuse) — see also Lymphoma C85.9- ☑
Lymphostasis I89.8
Lypemania — see Melancholia
Lysine and hydroxylysine metabolism disorder E72.3
Lyssa — see Rabies

M

Macacus ear Q17.3

Maceration, wet feet, tropical (syndrome) T69.02- ☑
MacLeod's syndrome J43.0
Macrocephalia, macrocephaly Q75.3
Macrocheilia, macrochilia (congenital) Q18.6
Macrocolon — see also Megacolon Q43.1
Macrocornea Q15.8
  with glaucoma Q15.0
Macrocytic — see condition
Macrocytosis D75.89
Macrodactylia, macrodactylism (fingers) (thumbs) Q74.0
  toes Q74.2
Macrodontia K00.2
Macrogenia M26.05
Macrogenitosomia (adrenal) (male) (praecox) E25.9
  congenital E25.0
Macroglobulinemia (idiopathic) (primary) C88.0- ☑
  monoclonal (essential) D47.2
  Waldenstrom C88.0- ☑
Macroglossia (congenital) Q38.2
  acquired K14.8
Macrognathia, macrognathism (congenital) (mandibular) (maxillary) M26.09
Macrogyria (congenital) Q04.8
Macrohydrocephalus — see Hydrocephalus
Macromastia — see Hypertrophy, breast
Macrophthalmos Q11.3
  in congenital glaucoma Q15.0
Macropsia H53.15
Macrosigmoid K59.39
  congenital Q43.2
Macrospondylitis , acromegalic E22.0
Macrostomia (congenital) Q18.4
Macrotia (external ear) (congenital) Q17.1
Macula
  cornea, corneal — see Opacity, cornea
  degeneration (atrophic) (exudative) (senile) — see also Degeneration, macula
  hereditary — see Dystrophy, retina
Maculae ceruleae B85.1
Maculopathy, toxic — see Degeneration, macula, toxic
Madarosis (eyelid) H02.729
  left H02.726
    lower H02.725
    upper H02.724
  right H02.723
    lower H02.722
    upper H02.721
Madelung's
  deformity (radius) Q74.0
  disease
    radial deformity Q74.0
    symmetrical lipomas, neck E88.89
Madness — see Psychosis
Madura
  foot B47.9
    actinomycotic B47.1
    mycotic B47.0
Maduromycosis B47.0
Maffucci's syndrome Q78.4
Magnesium metabolism disorder — see Disorder, metabolism, magnesium
Main en griffe (acquired) — see also Deformity, limb, clawhand
  congenital Q68.1
Maintenance (encounter for)
  antineoplastic chemotherapy Z51.11
  antineoplastic radiation therapy Z51.0
  methadone F11.20
Majocchi's
  disease L81.7
  granuloma B35.8
Major — see condition
Mal de los pintos — see Pinta
Mal de mer T75.3 ☑
Malabar itch (any site) B35.5
Malabsorption K90.9
  calcium K90.89
  carbohydrate K90.49
  disaccharide E73.9
  fat K90.49
  galactose E74.20
  glucose (-galactose) E74.39
  intestinal K90.9
    specified NEC K90.89
  isomaltose E74.31
  lactose E73.9
  methionine E72.19
  monosaccharide E74.39
  postgastrectomy K91.2

☑ **Additional Character Required — Refer to the Tabular List for Character Selection**

Malabsorption — *continued*
  postsurgical K91.2
  protein K90.49
  starch K90.49
  sucrose E74.39
  syndrome K90.9
    postsurgical K91.2
Malacia, bone (adult) M83.9
  juvenile — *see* Rickets
Malacoplakia
  bladder N32.89
  pelvis (kidney) N28.89
  ureter N28.89
  urethra N36.8
Malacosteon, juvenile — *see* Rickets
Maladaptation — *see* Maladjustment
Maladie de Roger Q21.0
Maladjustment
  conjugal Z63.0
    involving divorce or estrangement Z63.5
  educational Z55.4
  family Z63.9
  marital Z63.0
    involving divorce or estrangement Z63.5
  occupational NEC Z56.89
  simple, adult — *see* Disorder, adjustment
  situational — *see* Disorder, adjustment
  social Z60.9
    due to
      acculturation difficulty Z60.3
      discrimination and persecution (perceived) Z60.5
      exclusion and isolation Z60.4
      life-cycle (phase of life) transition Z60.0
      rejection Z60.4
      specified reason NEC Z60.8
Malaise R53.81
Malakoplakia — *see* Malacoplakia
Malaria, malarial (fever) B54
  with
    blackwater fever B50.8
      hemoglobinuric (bilious) B50.8
    hemoglobinuria B50.8
  accidentally induced (therapeutically) — *code by* type
    under Malaria
  algid B50.9
  cerebral B50.0 *[G94]*
  clinically diagnosed (without parasitological confirma-
    tion) B54
  congenital NEC P37.4
    falciparum P37.3
  congestion, congestive B54
  continued (fever) B50.9
  estivo-autumnal B50.9
  falciparum B50.9
    with complications NEC B50.8
      cerebral B50.0 *[G94]*
    severe B50.8
  hemorrhagic B54
  malariae B52.9
    with
      complications NEC B52.8
      glomerular disorder B52.0
  malignant (tertian) — *see* Malaria, falciparum
  mixed infections — *code to* first listed type in B50-B53
  ovale B53.0
  parasitologically confirmed NEC B53.8
  pernicious, acute — *see* Malaria, falciparum
  Plasmodium (P.)
    falciparum NEC — *see* Malaria, falciparum
    malariae NEC B52.9
      with Plasmodium
        falciparum (and or vivax) — *see* Malaria, falci-
          parum
        vivax — *see also* Malaria, vivax
          and falciparum — *see* Malaria, falciparum
    ovale B53.0
      with Plasmodium malariae — *see also* Malaria,
        malariae
        and vivax — *see also* Malaria, vivax
          and falciparum — *see* Malaria, falciparum
    simian B53.1
      with Plasmodium malariae — *see also* Malaria,
        malariae
        and vivax — *see also* Malaria, vivax
          and falciparum — *see* Malaria, falciparum
    vivax NEC B51.9
      with Plasmodium falciparum — *see* Malaria, falci-
        parum
  quartan — *see* Malaria, malariae

Malaria, malarial — *continued*
  quotidian — *see* Malaria, falciparum
  recurrent B54
  remittent B54
  specified type NEC (parasitologically confirmed) B53.8
  spleen B54
  subtertian (fever) — *see* Malaria, falciparum
  tertian (benign) — *see also* Malaria, vivax
    malignant B50.9
  tropical B50.9
  typhoid B54
  vivax B51.9
    with
      complications NEC B51.8
      ruptured spleen B51.0
Malassez's disease (cystic) N50.89
Malassimilation K90.9
Maldescent, testis Q53.9
  bilateral Q53.20
    abdominal Q53.211
    perineal Q53.22
  unilateral Q53.10
    abdominal Q53.111
    perineal Q53.12
Maldevelopment — *see also* Anomaly
  brain Q07.9
  colon Q43.9
  hip Q74.2
    congenital dislocation Q65.2
      bilateral Q65.1
      unilateral Q65.0- ☑
  mastoid process Q75.8
  middle ear Q16.4
    except ossicles Q16.4
    ossicles Q16.3
  ossicles Q16.3
  spine Q76.49
  toe Q74.2
Male type pelvis Q74.2
  with disproportion (fetopelvic) O33.3 ☑
    causing obstructed labor O65.3
Malformation (congenital) — *see also* Anomaly
  adrenal gland Q89.1
  affecting multiple systems with skeletal changes NEC
    Q87.5
  alimentary tract Q45.9
    specified type NEC Q45.8
    upper Q40.9
      specified type NEC Q40.8
  aorta Q25.40
    absence Q25.41
    aneurysm, congenital Q25.43
    aplasia Q25.41
    atresia Q25.29
      aortic arch Q25.21
    coarctation (preductal) (postductal) Q25.1
    dilatation, congenital Q25.44
    hypoplasia Q25.42
    patent ductus arteriosus Q25.0
    specified type NEC Q25.49
    stenosis Q25.1
      supravalvular Q25.3
  aortic valve Q23.9
    specified NEC Q23.88
  arteriovenous, aneurysmatic (congenital) Q27.30
    brain Q28.2
      ruptured I60.8
        intracerebral I61.8
        intraparenchymal I61.8
        intraventricular I61.5
        subarachnoid I60.8
    cerebral — *see also* Malformation, arteriovenous,
      brain Q28.2
    peripheral Q27.30
      digestive system — *see* Angiodysplasia
      congenital Q27.33
      lower limb Q27.32
      other specified site Q27.39
      renal vessel Q27.34
      upper limb Q27.31
    precerebral vessels (nonruptured) Q28.0
  auricle
    ear (congenital) Q17.3
      acquired H61.119
        left H61.112
          with right H61.113
        right H61.111
          with left H61.113
  bile duct Q44.5

Malformation — *continued*
  bladder Q64.79
    aplasia Q64.5
    diverticulum Q64.6
    exstrophy — *see* Exstrophy, bladder
    neck obstruction Q64.31
  bone Q79.9
    face Q75.9
      specified type NEC Q75.8
    skull Q75.9
      specified type NEC Q75.8
  brain (multiple) Q04.9
    arteriovenous Q28.2
    specified type NEC Q04.8
  branchial cleft Q18.2
  breast Q83.9
    specified type NEC Q83.8
  broad ligament Q50.6
  bronchus Q32.4
  bursa Q79.9
  cardiac
    chambers Q20.9
      specified type NEC Q20.8
    septum Q21.9
      specified type NEC Q21.8
  cerebral Q04.9
    vessels Q28.3
  cervix uteri Q51.9
    specified type NEC Q51.828
  Chiari
    Type I G93.5
    Type II Q07.01
  choroid (congenital) Q14.3
    plexus Q07.8
  circulatory system Q28.9
  cochlea Q16.5
  cornea Q13.4
  coronary vessels Q24.5
  corpus callosum (congenital) Q04.0
  diaphragm Q79.1
  digestive system NEC, specified type NEC Q45.8
  dura Q07.9
    brain Q04.9
    spinal Q06.9
  ear Q17.9
    causing impairment of hearing Q16.9
    external Q17.9
      accessory auricle Q17.0
      causing impairment of hearing Q16.9
        absence of
          auditory canal Q16.1
          auricle Q16.0
      macrotia Q17.1
      microtia Q17.2
      misplacement Q17.4
      misshapen NEC Q17.3
      prominence Q17.5
      specified type NEC Q17.8
    inner Q16.5
    middle Q16.4
      absence of eustachian tube Q16.2
      ossicles (fusion) Q16.3
    ossicles Q16.3
    specified type NEC Q17.8
  epididymis Q55.4
  esophagus Q39.9
    specified type NEC Q39.8
  eye Q15.9
    lid Q10.3
    specified NEC Q15.8
  fallopian tube Q50.6
  genital organ — *see* Anomaly, genitalia
  great
    artery Q25.9
      aorta — *see* Malformation, aorta
      pulmonary artery — *see* Malformation, pulmonary,
        artery
      specified type NEC Q25.8
    vein Q26.9
      anomalous
        portal venous connection Q26.5
        pulmonary venous connection Q26.4
          partial Q26.3
          total Q26.2
      persistent left superior vena cava Q26.1
      portal vein-hepatic artery fistula Q26.6
      specified type NEC Q26.8
      vena cava stenosis, congenital Q26.0
  gum Q38.6

Malformation — continued
  hair Q84.2
  heart Q24.9
    specified type NEC Q24.8
  integument Q84.9
    specified type NEC Q84.8
  internal ear Q16.5
  intestine Q43.9
    specified type NEC Q43.8
  iris Q13.2
  joint Q74.9
    ankle Q74.2
    lumbosacral Q76.49
    sacroiliac Q74.2
    specified type NEC Q74.8
  kidney Q63.9
    accessory Q63.0
    giant Q63.3
    horseshoe Q63.1
    hydronephrosis Q62.0
    malposition Q63.2
    specified type NEC Q63.8
  lacrimal apparatus Q10.6
  lingual Q38.3
  lip Q38.0
  liver Q44.70
  lung Q33.9
  meninges or membrane (congenital) Q07.9
    cerebral Q04.8
    spinal (cord) Q06.9
  middle ear Q16.4
    ossicles Q16.3
  mitral valve Q23.9
    specified NEC Q23.88
  Mondini's (congenital) (malformation, cochlea) Q16.5
  mouth (congenital) Q38.6
  multiple types NEC Q89.7
  musculoskeletal system Q79.9
  myocardium Q24.8
  nail Q84.6
  nervous system (central) Q07.9
  nose Q30.9
    specified type NEC Q30.8
  optic disc Q14.2
  orbit Q10.7
  ovary Q50.39
  palate Q38.5
  parathyroid gland Q89.2
  pelvic organs or tissues NEC
    in pregnancy or childbirth O34.8- ☑
      causing obstructed labor O65.5
  penis Q55.69
    aplasia Q55.5
    curvature (lateral) Q55.61
    hypoplasia Q55.62
  pericardium Q24.8
  peripheral vascular system Q27.9
    specified type NEC Q27.8
  pharynx Q38.8
  precerebral vessels Q28.1
  prostate Q55.4
  pulmonary
    arteriovenous Q25.72
    artery Q25.9
      atresia Q25.5
      specified type NEC Q25.79
      stenosis Q25.6
    valve Q22.3
  renal artery Q27.2
  respiratory system Q34.9
  retina Q14.1
  scrotum — see Malformation, testis and scrotum
  seminal vesicles Q55.4
  sense organs NEC Q07.9
  skin Q82.9
  specified NEC Q89.8
  spinal
    cord Q06.9
    nerve root Q07.8
  spine Q76.49
    kyphosis — see Kyphosis, congenital
    lordosis — see Lordosis, congenital
  spleen Q89.09
  stomach Q40.3
    specified type NEC Q40.2
  teeth, tooth K00.9
  tendon Q79.9
  testis and scrotum Q55.20
    aplasia Q55.0

Malformation — continued
  testis and scrotum — continued
    hypoplasia Q55.1
    polyorchism Q55.21
    retractile testis Q55.22
    scrotal transposition Q55.23
    specified NEC Q55.29
  thorax, bony Q76.9
  throat Q38.8
  thyroid gland Q89.2
  tongue (congenital) Q38.3
    hypertrophy Q38.2
    tie Q38.1
  trachea Q32.1
  tricuspid valve Q22.9
    specified type NEC Q22.8
  umbilical cord NEC (complicating delivery) O69.89 ☑
  umbilicus Q89.9
  ureter Q62.8
    agenesis Q62.4
    duplication Q62.5
    malposition — see Malposition, congenital, ureter
    obstructive defect — see Defect, obstructive, ureter
    vesico-uretero-renal reflux Q62.7
  urethra Q64.79
    aplasia Q64.5
    duplication Q64.74
    posterior valves Q64.2
    prolapse Q64.71
    stricture Q64.32
  urinary system Q64.9
  uterus Q51.9
    specified type NEC Q51.818
  vagina Q52.4
  vas deferens Q55.4
    atresia Q55.3
  vascular system, peripheral Q27.9
  venous — see Anomaly, vein(s)
  vulva Q52.70

Malfunction — see also Dysfunction
  cardiac electronic device T82.119 ☑
    electrode T82.110 ☑
    pulse generator T82.111 ☑
    specified type NEC T82.118 ☑
  catheter device NEC T85.618 ☑
    cystostomy T83.010 ☑
    dialysis (renal) (vascular) T82.41 ☑
      intraperitoneal T85.611 ☑
    infusion NEC T82.514 ☑
      cranial — see also Complication(s), catheter, cranial infusion, mechanical T85.690 ☑
      epidural — see also Complication(s), catheter, cranial infusion, mechanical T85.690 ☑
      intrathecal — see also Complication(s), catheter, cranial infusion, mechanical T85.690 ☑
      spinal — see also Complication(s), catheter, cranial infusion, mechanical T85.690 ☑
      subarachnoid — see also Complication(s), catheter, cranial infusion, mechanical T85.690 ☑
      subdural — see also Complication(s), catheter, cranial infusion, mechanical T85.690 ☑
    urinary — see also Breakdown, device, catheter T83.018 ☑
  colostomy K94.03
    valve K94.03
  cystostomy (stoma) N99.512
    catheter T83.010 ☑
  enteric stoma K94.13
  enterostomy K94.13
  esophagostomy K94.33
  gastroenteric K31.89
  gastrostomy K94.23
  ileostomy K94.13
    valve K94.13
  intrathecal infusion pump T85.615 ☑
  jejunostomy K94.13
  nervous system device, implant or graft, specified NEC T85.615 ☑
  pacemaker — see Malfunction, cardiac electronic device
  prosthetic device, internal — see Complications, prosthetic device, by site, mechanical
  tracheostomy J95.03
  urinary device NEC — see Complication, genitourinary, device, urinary, mechanical
  valve
    colostomy K94.03
    heart T82.09 ☑
    ileostomy K94.13

Malfunction — continued
  vascular graft or shunt NEC — see Complication, cardio-vascular device, mechanical, vascular
  ventricular (communicating shunt) T85.01 ☑
Malherbe's tumor — see Neoplasm, skin, benign
Malibu disease L98.8
Malignancy — see also Neoplasm, malignant, by site
  unspecified site (primary) C80.1
Malignant — see condition
Malingerer, malingering Z76.5
Mallet finger (acquired) — see Deformity, finger, mallet
  finger
  congenital Q74.0
  sequelae of rickets E64.3
Malleus A24.0
Mallory's bodies R89.7
Mallory-Weiss syndrome K22.6
Malnutrition E46
  degree
    first E44.1
      mild (protein) E44.1
      moderate (protein) E44.0
    second E44.0
    severe (protein-energy) E43
      with
        kwashiorkor E40
        marasmus E41
        intermediate form E42
          with
            kwashiorkor E42
    third E43
  following gastrointestinal surgery K91.2
  intrauterine
    light-for-dates — see Light for dates
    small-for-dates — see Small for dates
  lack of care, or neglect (child) (infant) T76.02 ☑
    confirmed T74.02 ☑
  malignant E40
  protein E46
    calorie E46
      mild E44.1
      moderate E44.0
      severe E43
        with
          kwashiorkor E40
          marasmus E41
          intermediate form E42
            with
              kwashiorkor (and marasmus) E42
    energy E46
      mild E44.1
      moderate E44.0
      severe E43
        with
          kwashiorkor E40
          marasmus E41
          intermediate form E42
            with
              kwashiorkor (and marasmus) E42
    severe (protein-energy) E43
      with
        kwashiorkor E40
          with marasmus E42
        intermediate form E42
          with
            kwashiorkor (and marasmus) E42
        marasmus E41
Malocclusion (teeth) M26.4
  Angle's M26.219
    class I M26.211
    class II M26.212
    class III M26.213
  due to
    abnormal swallowing M26.59
    mouth breathing M26.59
    tongue, lip or finger habits M26.59
  temporomandibular (joint) M26.69
Malposition
  cervix — see Malposition, uterus
  congenital
    adrenal (gland) Q89.1
    alimentary tract Q45.8
      lower Q43.8
      upper Q40.8
    aorta Q25.49
    appendix Q43.8
    arterial trunk Q20.0
    artery (peripheral) Q27.8
      coronary Q24.5

Malposition — *continued*
  congenital — *continued*
    artery — *continued*
      digestive system Q27.8
      lower limb Q27.8
      pulmonary Q25.79
      specified site NEC Q27.8
      upper limb Q27.8
    auditory canal Q17.8
      causing impairment of hearing Q16.9
    auricle (ear) Q17.4
      causing impairment of hearing Q16.9
      cervical Q18.2
    biliary duct or passage Q44.5
    bladder (mucosa) — *see* Exstrophy, bladder
    brachial plexus Q07.8
    brain tissue Q04.8
    breast Q83.8
    bronchus Q32.4
    cecum Q43.8
    clavicle Q74.0
    colon Q43.8
    digestive organ or tract NEC Q45.8
      lower Q43.8
      upper Q40.8
    ear (auricle) (external) Q17.4
      ossicles Q16.3
    endocrine (gland) NEC Q89.2
    epiglottis Q31.8
    eustachian tube Q17.8
    eye Q15.8
    facial features Q18.8
    fallopian tube Q50.6
    finger(s) Q68.1
      supernumerary Q69.0
    foot Q66.9- ☑
    gallbladder Q44.1
    gastrointestinal tract Q45.8
    genitalia, genital organ(s) or tract
      female Q52.8
        external Q52.79
        internal NEC Q52.8
      male Q55.8
    glottis Q31.8
    hand Q68.1
    heart Q24.8
      dextrocardia Q24.0
        with complete transposition of viscera Q89.3
    hepatic duct Q44.5
    hip (joint) Q65.89
    intestine (large) (small) Q43.8
      with anomalous adhesions, fixation or malrotation Q43.3
    joint NEC Q68.8
    kidney Q63.2
    larynx Q31.8
    limb Q68.8
      lower Q68.8
      upper Q68.8
    liver Q44.79
    lung (lobe) Q33.8
    nail(s) Q84.6
    nerve Q07.8
    nervous system NEC Q07.8
    nose, nasal (septum) Q30.8
    organ or site not listed — *see* Anomaly, by site
    ovary Q50.39
    pancreas Q45.3
    parathyroid (gland) Q89.2
    patella Q74.1
    peripheral vascular system Q27.8
    pituitary (gland) Q89.2
    respiratory organ or system NEC Q34.8
    rib (cage) Q76.6
      supernumerary in cervical region Q76.5
    scapula Q74.0
    shoulder Q74.0
    spinal cord Q06.8
    spleen Q89.09
    sternum NEC Q76.7
    stomach Q40.2
    symphysis pubis Q74.2
    thymus (gland) Q89.2
    thyroid (gland) (tissue) Q89.2
      cartilage Q31.8
    toe(s) Q66.9- ☑
      supernumerary Q69.2
    tongue Q38.3
    trachea Q32.1

Malposition — *continued*
  congenital — *continued*
    ureter Q62.60
      deviation Q62.61
      displacement Q62.62
      ectopia Q62.63
      specified type NEC Q62.69
    uterus Q51.818
    vein(s) (peripheral) Q27.8
      great Q26.8
    vena cava (inferior) (superior) Q26.8
  device, implant or graft — *see also* Complications, by site and type, mechanical T85.628 ☑
    arterial graft NEC — *see* Complication, cardiovascular device, mechanical, vascular
    breast (implant) T85.42 ☑
    catheter NEC T85.628 ☑
      cystostomy T83.020 ☑
      dialysis (renal) T82.42 ☑
        intraperitoneal T85.621 ☑
      infusion NEC T82.524 ☑
        spinal (epidural) (subdural) T85.620 ☑
      urinary — *see also* Displacement, device, catheter, urinary T83.028 ☑
    electronic (electrode) (pulse generator) (stimulator)
      bone T84.320 ☑
      cardiac T82.129 ☑
        electrode T82.120 ☑
        pulse generator T82.121 ☑
        specified type NEC T82.128 ☑
      nervous system — *see* Complication, prosthetic device, mechanical, electronic nervous system stimulator
      urinary — *see* Complication, genitourinary, device, urinary, mechanical
    fixation, internal (orthopedic) NEC — *see* Complication, fixation device, mechanical
    gastrointestinal — *see* Complications, prosthetic device, mechanical, gastrointestinal device
    genital NEC T83.428 ☑
      intrauterine contraceptive device (string) T83.32 ☑
      penile prosthesis (cylinder) (implanted) (pump) (reservoir) T83.420 ☑
      testicular prosthesis T83.421 ☑
    heart NEC — *see* Complication, cardiovascular device, mechanical
    joint prosthesis — *see* Complication, joint prosthesis, mechanical
    ocular NEC — *see* Complications, prosthetic device, mechanical, ocular device
    orthopedic NEC — *see* Complication, orthopedic, device, mechanical
    specified NEC T85.628 ☑
    urinary NEC — *see also* Complication, genitourinary, device, urinary, mechanical
      graft T83.22 ☑
    vascular NEC — *see* Complication, cardiovascular device, mechanical
    ventricular intracranial shunt T85.02 ☑
  fetus — *see* Pregnancy, complicated by (management affected by), presentation, fetal
  gallbladder K82.8
  gastrointestinal tract, congenital Q45.8
  heart, congenital NEC Q24.8
  joint prosthesis — *see* Complications, joint prosthesis, mechanical, displacement, by site
  stomach K31.89
    congenital Q40.2
  tooth, teeth, fully erupted M26.30
  uterus (acute) (acquired) (adherent) (asymptomatic) (postinfectional) (postpartal, old) N85.4
    anteflexion or anteversion N85.4
      congenital Q51.818
    flexion N85.4
      lateral — *see* Lateroversion, uterus
    inversion N85.5
    lateral (flexion) (version) — *see* Lateroversion, uterus
      in pregnancy or childbirth — *see* subcategory O34.5
    retroflexion or retroversion — *see* Retroversion, uterus
Malposture R29.3
Malrotation
  cecum Q43.3
  colon Q43.3
  intestine Q43.3
  kidney Q63.2
Malta fever — *see* Brucellosis

Maltreatment
  adult
    abandonment
      confirmed T74.01 ☑
      suspected T76.01 ☑
    bullying
      confirmed T74.31 ☑
      suspected T76.31 ☑
    confirmed T74.91 ☑
    financial
      confirmed T74.A1 ☑
      suspected T76.A1 ☑
    history of Z91.419
    intimidation (through social media)
      confirmed T74.31 ☑
      suspected T76.31 ☑
    neglect
      confirmed T74.01 ☑
      suspected T76.01 ☑
    physical abuse
      confirmed T74.11 ☑
      suspected T76.11 ☑
    psychological abuse
      confirmed T74.31 ☑
      history of Z91.411
      suspected T76.31 ☑
    sexual abuse
      confirmed T74.21 ☑
      suspected T76.21 ☑
    suspected T76.91 ☑
    threatened abuse (harm) (physical violence) (sexual abuse)
      confirmed T74.31 ☑
      suspected T76.31 ☑
  child
    abandonment
      confirmed T74.02 ☑
      suspected T76.02 ☑
    bullying
      confirmed T74.32 ☑
      suspected T76.32 ☑
    confirmed T74.92 ☑
    financial
      confirmed T74.A2 ☑
      suspected T76.A2 ☑
    history of — *see* History, personal (of), abuse
    intimidation (through social media)
      confirmed T74.32 ☑
      suspected T76.32 ☑
    neglect
      confirmed T74.02 ☑
      history of — *see* History, personal (of), abuse
      suspected T76.02 ☑
    physical abuse
      confirmed T74.12 ☑
      history of — *see* History, personal (of), abuse
      suspected T76.12 ☑
    psychological abuse
      confirmed T74.32 ☑
      history of — *see* History, personal (of), abuse
      suspected T76.32 ☑
    sexual abuse
      confirmed T74.22 ☑
      history of — *see* History, personal (of), abuse
      suspected T76.22 ☑
    suspected T76.92 ☑
    threatened abuse (harm) (physical violence) (sexual abuse)
      confirmed T74.32 ☑
      suspected T76.32 ☑
  personal history of Z91.89
Maltworker's lung J67.4
Malunion, fracture — *see* Fracture, by site
Mammillitis N61.0
  puerperal, postpartum O91.02
Mammitis — *see* Mastitis
Mammogram (examination) Z12.39
  routine Z12.31
Mammoplasia N62
Management (of)
  bone conduction hearing device (implanted) Z45.320
  cardiac pacemaker NEC Z45.018
  cerebrospinal fluid drainage device Z45.41
  cochlear device (implanted) Z45.321
  contraceptive Z30.9
    specified NEC Z30.8
  implanted device Z45.9

Management — *continued*
  implanted device — *continued*
    specified NEC Z45.89
  infusion pump Z45.1
  procreative Z31.9
    male factor infertility in female Z31.81
    specified NEC Z31.89
  prosthesis (external) — *see also* Fitting Z44.9
    implanted Z45.9
      specified NEC Z45.89
  renal dialysis catheter Z49.01
  vascular access device Z45.2
Mangled — *see* specified injury by site
Mania (monopolar) — *see also* Disorder, mood, manic
    episode
  with psychotic symptoms F30.2
  without psychotic symptoms F30.10
    mild F30.11
    moderate F30.12
    severe F30.13
  Bell's F30.8
  chronic (recurrent) F31.89
  hysterical F44.89
  puerperal F30.8
  recurrent F31.89
Manic depression F31.9
Manic-depressive insanity, psychosis, or syndrome —
    see Disorder, bipolar
Mannosidosis E77.1
Mansonelliasis, mansonellosis B74.4
Manson's
  disease B65.1
  schistosomiasis B65.1
Manual — *see* condition
Maple-bark-stripper's lung (disease) J67.6
Maple-syrup-urine disease E71.0
Marable's syndrome (celiac artery compression) I77.4
Marasmus E41
  due to malnutrition E41
  intestinal E41
  nutritional E41
  senile R54
  tuberculous NEC — *see* Tuberculosis
Marble
  bones Q78.2
  skin R23.8
Marburg virus disease A98.3
March
  fracture — *see* Fracture, traumatic, stress, by site
  hemoglobinuria D59.6
Marchesani (-Weill) **syndrome** Q87.0
Marchiafava (-Bignami) **syndrome or disease** G37.1
Marchiafava-Micheli syndrome D59.5
Marcus Gunn's syndrome Q07.8
Marfan syndrome — *see* Syndrome, Marfan
Marie-Bamberger disease — *see* Osteoarthropathy, hyper-
    trophic, specified NEC
Marie-Charcot-Tooth neuropathic muscular atrophy
    G60.0
Marie's
  cerebellar ataxia (late-onset) G11.2
  disease or syndrome (acromegaly) E22.0
Marie-Strumpell arthritis, disease or spondylitis — *see*
    Spondylitis, ankylosing
Marion's disease (bladder neck obstruction) N32.0
Marital conflict Z63.0
Mark
  port wine Q82.5
  raspberry Q82.5
  strawberry Q82.5
  stretch L90.6
  tattoo L81.8
Marker heterochromatin — *see* Extra, marker chromo-
    somes
Maroteaux-Lamy syndrome (mild) (severe) E76.29
Marrow (bone)
  arrest D61.9
  poor function D75.89
Marseilles fever A77.1
Marsh fever — *see* Malaria
Marshall's (hidrotic) **ectodermal dysplasia** Q82.4
Marsh's disease (exophthalmic goiter) E05.00
  with storm E05.01
Masculinization (female) **with adrenal hyperplasia** E25.9
  congenital E25.0
Masculinovoblastoma D27.- ☑
Masochism (sexual) F65.51
Mason's lung J62.8

Mass
  abdominal R19.00
    epigastric R19.06
    generalized R19.07
    left lower quadrant R19.04
    left upper quadrant R19.02
    periumbilic R19.05
    right lower quadrant R19.03
    right upper quadrant R19.01
    specified site NEC R19.09
  breast — *see also* Lump, breast N63.0
  chest R22.2
  cystic — *see* Cyst
  ear H93.8- ☑
  head R22.0
  intra-abdominal (diffuse) (generalized) — *see* Mass, ab-
    dominal
  kidney N28.89
  liver R16.0
  localized (skin) R22.9
    chest R22.2
    head R22.0
    limb
      lower R22.4- ☑
      upper R22.3- ☑
    neck R22.1
    trunk R22.2
  lung R91.8
  malignant — *see* Neoplasm, malignant, by site
  neck R22.1
  pelvic (diffuse) (generalized) — *see* Mass, abdominal
  specified organ NEC — *see* Disease, by site
  splenic R16.1
  substernal thyroid — *see* Goiter
  superficial (localized) R22.9
  umbilical (diffuse) (generalized) R19.09
Massive — *see* condition
Mast cell
  disease, systemic tissue D47.02
  leukemia C94.3- ☑
  neoplasm
    malignant C96.20
      specified type NEC C96.29
    of uncertain behavior NEC D47.09
  sarcoma C96.22
  tumor D47.09
Mastalgia N64.4
Masters-Allen syndrome N83.8
Mastitis (acute) (diffuse) (nonpuerperal) (subacute) N61.0
  with abscess N61.1
  chronic (cystic) — *see* Mastopathy, cystic
  cystic (Schimmelbusch's type) — *see* Mastopathy, cystic
  fibrocystic — *see* Mastopathy, cystic
  granulomatous N61.2- ☑
  infective N61.0
    newborn P39.0
  interstitial, gestational or puerperal — *see* Mastitis, ob-
    stetric
  neonatal (noninfective) P83.4
    infective P39.0
  obstetric (interstitial) (nonpurulent)
    associated with
      lactation O91.23
      pregnancy O91.21- ☑
      puerperium O91.22
    purulent
      associated with
        lactation O91.13
        pregnancy O91.11- ☑
        puerperium O91.12
  periductal — *see* Ectasia, mammary duct
  phlegmonous — *see* Mastopathy, cystic
  plasma cell — *see* Ectasia, mammary duct
  without abscess N61.0
Mastocytoma (extracutaneous) D47.09
  malignant C96.29
  solitary D47.01
Mastocytosis D47.09
  aggressive systemic C96.21
  cutaneous (diffuse) (maculopapular) D47.01
    congenital Q82.2
    of neonatal onset Q82.2
    of newborn onset Q82.2
  indolent systemic D47.02
  isolated bone marrow D47.02
  malignant C96.29

Mastocytosis — *continued*
  systemic (indolent) (smoldering)
    with an associated hematological non-mast cell lin-
      eage disease (SM-AHNMD) D47.02
Mastodynia N64.4
Mastoid — *see* condition
Mastoidalgia — *see* subcategory H92.0 ☑
Mastoiditis (coalescent) (hemorrhagic) (suppurative)
  H70.9- ☑
  acute, subacute H70.00- ☑
    complicated NEC H70.09- ☑
    subperiosteal H70.01- ☑
  chronic (necrotic) (recurrent) H70.1- ☑
  in (due to)
    infectious disease NEC B99 *[H75.0-]* ☑
    parasitic disease NEC B89 *[H75.0-]* ☑
    tuberculosis A18.03
  petrositis — *see* Petrositis
  postauricular fistula — *see* Fistula, postauricular
  specified NEC H70.89- ☑
  tuberculous A18.03
Mastopathy, mastopathia N64.9
  chronica cystica — *see* Mastopathy, cystic
  cystic (chronic) (diffuse) N60.1- ☑
    with epithelial proliferation N60.3- ☑
  diffuse cystic — *see* Mastopathy, cystic
  estrogenic, oestrogenica, oestrogenic N64.89
  ovarian origin N64.89
Mastoplasia, mastoplastia N62
Masturbation (excessive) F98.8
Maternal care (for) — *see* Pregnancy (complicated by)
  (management affected by)
Mathieu's disease (leptospiral jaundice) A27.0
Mauclaire's disease or osteochondrosis — *see* Osteochon-
  drosis, juvenile, hand, metacarpal
Maxcy's disease A75.2
Maxilla, maxillary — *see* condition
May (-Hegglin) **anomaly or syndrome** D72.0
McArdle (-Schmid)(-Pearson) **disease** (glycogen storage)
  E74.04
McCune-Albright syndrome Q78.1
McQuarrie's syndrome (idiopathic familial hypoglycemia)
  E16.2
Meadow's syndrome Q86.1
Measles (black) (hemorrhagic) (suppressed) B05.9
  with
    complications NEC B05.89
    encephalitis B05.0
    intestinal complications B05.4
    keratitis (keratoconjunctivitis) B05.81
    meningitis B05.1
    otitis media B05.3
    pneumonia B05.2
  French — *see* Rubella
  German — *see* Rubella
  Liberty — *see* Rubella
Meatitis, urethral — *see* Urethritis
Meatus, meatal — *see* condition
Meat-wrappers' asthma J68.9
ME/CFS (myalgic encephalomyelitis/chronic fatigue syn-
  drome) G93.32
Meckel-Gruber syndrome Q61.9
Meckel's diverticulitis, diverticulum (displaced) (hyper-
  trophic) Q43.0
  malignant — *see* Table of Neoplasms, small intestine,
    malignant
Meconium
  ileus, newborn P76.0
    in cystic fibrosis E84.11
    meaning meconium plug (without cystic fibrosis)
      P76.0
  obstruction, newborn P76.0
    due to fecaliths P76.0
    in mucoviscidosis E84.11
  peritonitis P78.0
  plug syndrome (newborn) NEC P76.0
MED13L (mediator complex subunit 13L) **syndrome** Q87.85
Median — *see also* condition
  arcuate ligament syndrome I77.4
  bar (prostate) (vesical orifice) — *see* Hyperplasia, prostate
  rhomboid glossitis K14.2
Mediastinal shift R93.89
Mediastinitis (acute) (chronic) J98.51
  syphilitic A52.73
  tuberculous A15.8
Mediastinopericarditis — *see also* Pericarditis
  acute I30.9
  adhesive I31.0

Mediastinopericarditis — *continued*
  chronic I31.8
    rheumatic I09.2
Mediastinum, mediastinal — *see* condition
Mediator complex subunit 13L (MED13L) **syndrome** Q87.85
Medicine poisoning — *see* Table of Drugs and Chemicals, by drug, poisoning
Mediterranean
  fever — *see* Brucellosis
    familial M04.1
      tick A77.1
  kala-azar B55.0
  leishmaniasis B55.0
  tick fever A77.1
Medulla — *see* condition
Medullary cystic kidney Q61.5
Medullated fibers
  optic (nerve) Q14.8
  retina Q14.1
Medulloblastoma
  desmoplastic C71.6
  specified site — *see* Neoplasm, malignant, by site
  unspecified site C71.6
Medulloepithelioma — *see also* Neoplasm, malignant, by site
  teratoid — *see* Neoplasm, malignant, by site
Medullomyoblastoma
  specified site — *see* Neoplasm, malignant, by site
  unspecified site C71.6
Meekeren-Ehlers-Danlos syndrome — *see also* Syndrome, Ehlers-Danlos Q79.69
Megacolon (acquired) (functional) (not Hirschsprung's disease) (in) K59.39
  Chagas' disease B57.32
  congenital, congenitum (aganglionic) Q43.1
  Hirschsprung's (disease) Q43.1
  toxic NEC K59.31
    due to
      Clostridioides difficile
        not specified as recurrent A04.72
        recurrent A04.71
      Clostridium difficile
        not specified as recurrent A04.72
        recurrent A04.71
Megaesophagus (functional) K22.0
  congenital Q39.5
  in (due to) Chagas' disease B57.31
Megalencephaly Q04.5
Megalerythema (epidemic) B08.3
Megaloappendix Q43.8
Megalocephalus, megalocephaly NEC Q75.3
Megalocornea Q15.8
  with glaucoma Q15.0
Megalocytic anemia D53.1
Megalodactylia (fingers) (thumbs) (congenital) Q74.0
  toes Q74.2
Megaloduodenum Q43.8
Megaloesophagus (functional) K22.0
  congenital Q39.5
Megalogastria (acquired) K31.89
  congenital Q40.2
Megalophthalmos Q11.3
Megalopsia H53.15
Megalosplenia — *see* Splenomegaly
Megaloureter N28.82
  congenital Q62.2
Megarectum K62.89
Megasigmoid K59.39
  congenital Q43.2
Megaureter N28.82
  congenital Q62.2
Megavitamin-B6 syndrome E67.2
Megrim — *see* Migraine
Meibomian
  cyst, infected — *see* Hordeolum
  gland — *see* condition
  sty, stye — *see* Hordeolum
Meibomitis — *see* Hordeolum
Meige-Milroy disease (chronic hereditary edema) Q82.0
Meige's syndrome Q82.0
Melalgia, nutritional E53.8
Melancholia F32.A
  climacteric (single episode) F32.89
    recurrent episode F33.8
  hypochondriac F45.29
  intermittent (single episode) F32.89
    recurrent episode F33.8
  involutional (single episode) F32.89

Melancholia — *continued*
  involutional — *continued*
    recurrent episode F33.8
  menopausal (single episode) F32.89
    recurrent episode F33.8
  puerperal F32.89
  reactive (emotional stress or trauma) F32.3
  recurrent F33.9
  senile F03 ☑
  stuporous (single episode) F32.89
    recurrent episode F33.8
Melanemia R79.89
Melanoameloblastoma — *see* Neoplasm, bone, benign
Melanoblastoma — *see* Melanoma
Melanocarcinoma — *see* Melanoma
Melanocytoma, eyeball D31.9- ☑
Melanocytosis, neurocutaneous Q82.8
Melanoderma, melanodermia L81.4
Melanodontia, infantile K03.89
Melanodontoclasia K03.89
Melanoepithelioma — *see* Melanoma
Melanoma (malignant) C43.9
  acral lentiginous, malignant — *see* Melanoma, skin, by site
  amelanotic — *see* Melanoma, skin, by site
  balloon cell — *see* Melanoma, skin, by site
  benign — *see* Nevus
  desmoplastic, malignant — *see* Melanoma, skin, by site
  epithelioid cell — *see* Melanoma, skin, by site
    with spindle cell, mixed — *see* Melanoma, skin, by site
  in
    giant pigmented nevus — *see* Melanoma, skin, by site
    Hutchinson's melanotic freckle — *see* Melanoma, skin, by site
    junctional nevus — *see* Melanoma, skin, by site
    precancerous melanosis — *see* Melanoma, skin, by site
  in situ D03.9
    abdominal wall D03.59
    ala nasi D03.39
    ankle D03.7- ☑
    anus, anal (margin) (skin) D03.51
    arm D03.6- ☑
    auditory canal D03.2- ☑
    auricle (ear) D03.2- ☑
    auricular canal (external) D03.2- ☑
    axilla, axillary fold D03.59
    back D03.59
    breast D03.52
    brow D03.39
    buttock D03.59
    canthus (eye) D03.1- ☑
    cheek (external) D03.39
    chest wall D03.59
    chin D03.39
    choroid D03.8
    conjunctiva D03.8
    ear (external) D03.2- ☑
    external meatus (ear) D03.2- ☑
    eye D03.8
    eyebrow D03.39
    eyelid (lower) (upper) D03.1- ☑
    face D03.30
      specified NEC D03.39
    female genital organ (external) NEC D03.8
    finger D03.6- ☑
    flank D03.59
    foot D03.7- ☑
    forearm D03.6- ☑
    forehead D03.39
    foreskin D03.8
    gluteal region D03.59
    groin D03.59
    hand D03.6- ☑
    heel D03.7- ☑
    helix D03.2- ☑
    hip D03.7- ☑
    interscapular region D03.59
    iris D03.8
    jaw D03.39
    knee D03.7- ☑
    labium (majus) (minus) D03.8
    lacrimal gland D03.8
    leg D03.7- ☑
    lip (lower) (upper) D03.0
    lower limb NEC D03.7- ☑

Melanoma — *continued*
  in situ — *continued*
    male genital organ (external) NEC D03.8
    nail D03.9
      finger D03.6- ☑
      toe D03.7- ☑
    neck D03.4
    nose (external) D03.39
    orbit D03.8
    penis D03.8
    perianal skin D03.51
    perineum D03.51
    pinna D03.2- ☑
    popliteal fossa or space D03.7- ☑
    prepuce D03.8
    pudendum D03.8
    retina D03.8
    retrobulbar D03.8
    scalp D03.4
    scrotum D03.8
    shoulder D03.6- ☑
    specified site NEC D03.8
    submammary fold D03.52
    temple D03.39
    thigh D03.7- ☑
    toe D03.7- ☑
    trunk NEC D03.59
    umbilicus D03.59
    upper limb NEC D03.6- ☑
    vulva D03.8
  juvenile — *see* Nevus
  malignant, of soft parts except skin — *see* Neoplasm, connective tissue, malignant
  metastatic
    breast C79.81
    genital organ C79.82
    specified site NEC C79.89
  neurotropic, malignant — *see* Melanoma, skin, by site
  nodular — *see* Melanoma, skin, by site
  regressing, malignant — *see* Melanoma, skin, by site
  skin C43.9
    abdominal wall C43.59
    ala nasi C43.31
    ankle C43.7- ☑
    anus, anal (skin) C43.51
    arm C43.6- ☑
    auditory canal (external) C43.2- ☑
    auricle (ear) C43.2- ☑
    auricular canal (external) C43.2- ☑
    axilla, axillary fold C43.59
    back C43.59
    breast (female) (male) C43.52
    brow C43.39
    buttock C43.59
    canthus (eye) C43.1- ☑
    cheek (external) C43.39
    chest wall C43.59
    chin C43.39
    ear (external) C43.2- ☑
    elbow C43.6- ☑
    external meatus (ear) C43.2- ☑
    eyebrow C43.39
    eyelid (lower) (upper) C43.1- ☑
    face C43.30
      specified NEC C43.39
    female genital organ (external) NEC C51.9
    finger C43.6- ☑
    flank C43.59
    foot C43.7- ☑
    forearm C43.6- ☑
    forehead C43.39
    foreskin C60.0
    glabella C43.39
    gluteal region C43.59
    groin C43.59
    hand C43.6- ☑
    heel C43.7- ☑
    helix C43.2- ☑
    hip C43.7- ☑
    interscapular region C43.59
    jaw (external) C43.39
    knee C43.7- ☑
    labium C51.9
      majus C51.0
      minus C51.1
    leg C43.7- ☑
    lip (lower) (upper) C43.0

Melanoma — continued
  skin — continued
    lower limb NEC C43.7- ☑
    male genital organ (external) NEC C63.9
    nail
      finger C43.6- ☑
      toe C43.7- ☑
    nasolabial groove C43.39
    nates C43.59
    neck C43.4
    nose (external) C43.31
    overlapping site C43.8
    palpebra C43.1- ☑
    penis C60.9
    perianal skin C43.51
    perineum C43.51
    pinna C43.2- ☑
    popliteal fossa or space C43.7- ☑
    prepuce C60.0
    pudendum C51.9
    scalp C43.4
    scrotum C63.2
    shoulder C43.6- ☑
    skin NEC C43.9
    submammary fold C43.52
    temple C43.39
    thigh C43.7- ☑
    toe C43.7- ☑
    trunk NEC C43.59
    umbilicus C43.59
    upper limb NEC C43.6- ☑
    vulva C51.9
      overlapping sites C51.8
  spindle cell
    with epithelioid, mixed — see Melanoma, skin, by site
    type A C69.4- ☑
    type B C69.4- ☑
  superficial spreading — see Melanoma, skin, by site
Melanosarcoma — see also Melanoma
  epithelioid cell — see Melanoma
Melanosis L81.4
  addisonian E27.1
    tuberculous A18.7
  adrenal E27.1
  colon K63.89
  conjunctiva — see Pigmentation, conjunctiva
    congenital Q13.89
  cornea (presenile) (senile) — see also Pigmentation, cornea
    congenital Q13.4
  eye NEC H57.89
    congenital Q15.8
  lenticularis progressiva Q82.1
  liver K76.89
  precancerous — see also Melanoma, in situ
    malignant melanoma in — see Melanoma
  Riehl's L81.4
  sclera H15.89
    congenital Q13.89
  suprarenal E27.1
  tar L81.4
  toxic L81.4
Melanuria R82.998
MELAS syndrome E88.41
Melasma L81.1
  adrenal (gland) E27.1
  suprarenal (gland) E27.1
Melena K92.1
  with ulcer — code by site under Ulcer, with hemorrhage K27.4
  due to swallowed maternal blood P78.2
  newborn, neonatal P54.1
    due to swallowed maternal blood P78.2
Meleney's
  gangrene (cutaneous) — see Ulcer, skin
  ulcer (chronic undermining) — see Ulcer, skin
Melioidosis A24.9
  acute A24.1
  chronic A24.2
  fulminating A24.1
  pneumonia A24.1
  pulmonary (chronic) A24.2
    acute A24.1
    subacute A24.2
  sepsis A24.1
  specified NEC A24.3
  subacute A24.2
Melitensis, febris A23.0

Melkersson (-Rosenthal) **syndrome** G51.2
Mellitus, diabetes — see Diabetes
Melorheostosis (bone) — see Disorder, bone, density and structure, specified NEC
Meloschisis Q18.4
Melotia Q17.4
Membrana
  capsularis lentis posterior Q13.89
  epipapillaris Q14.2
Membranacea placenta O43.19- ☑
Membranaceous uterus N85.8
Membrane(s), membranous — see also condition
  cyclitic — see Membrane, pupillary
  folds, congenital — see Web
  Jackson's Q43.3
  over face of newborn P28.9
  premature rupture — see Rupture, membranes, premature
  pupillary H21.4- ☑
    persistent Q13.89
  retained (with hemorrhage) (complicating delivery) O72.2
    without hemorrhage O73.1
  secondary cataract — see Cataract, secondary
  unruptured (causing asphyxia) — see Asphyxia, newborn
  vitreous — see Opacity, vitreous, membranes and strands
Membranitis — see Chorioamnionitis
Memory disturbance, lack or loss — see also Amnesia
  mild, following organic brain damage F06.8
Menadione deficiency E56.1
Menarche
  delayed E30.0
  precocious E30.1
Mendacity, pathologic F60.2
Mendelson's syndrome (due to anesthesia) J95.4
  in labor and delivery O74.0
  in pregnancy O29.01- ☑
  obstetric O74.0
  postpartum, puerperal O89.01
Menetrier's disease or syndrome K29.60
  with bleeding K29.61
Meniere's disease, syndrome or vertigo H81.0- ☑
Meninges, meningeal — see condition
Meningioma — see also Neoplasm, meninges, benign
  angioblastic — see Neoplasm, meninges, benign
  angiomatous — see Neoplasm, meninges, benign
  atypical — see Neoplasm, meninges, uncertain behavior
  endotheliomatous — see Neoplasm, meninges, benign
  fibroblastic — see Neoplasm, meninges, benign
  fibrous — see Neoplasm, meninges, benign
  hemangioblastic — see Neoplasm, meninges, benign
  hemangiopericytic — see Neoplasm, meninges, benign
  malignant — see Neoplasm, meninges, malignant
  meningiothelial — see Neoplasm, meninges, benign
  meningotheliomatous — see Neoplasm, meninges, benign
  mixed — see Neoplasm, meninges, benign
  multiple — see Neoplasm, meninges, uncertain behavior
  papillary — see Neoplasm, meninges, uncertain behavior
  psammomatous — see Neoplasm, meninges, benign
  syncytial — see Neoplasm, meninges, benign
  transitional — see Neoplasm, meninges, benign
Meningiomatosis (diffuse) — see Neoplasm, meninges, uncertain behavior
Meningism — see Meningismus
Meningismus (infectional) (pneumococcal) R29.1
  due to serum or vaccine R29.1
  influenzal — see Influenza, with, manifestations NEC
Meningitis (basal) (basic) (brain) (cerebral) (cervical) (congestive) (diffuse) (hemorrhagic) (infantile) (membranous) (metastatic) (nonspecific) (pontine) (progressive) (simple) (spinal) (subacute) (sympathetic) (toxic) G03.9
  abacterial G03.0
  actinomycotic A42.81
  adenoviral A87.1
  arbovirus A87.8
  aseptic (acute) G03.0
  bacterial G00.9
    Escherichia coli (E. coli) G00.8
    Friedlander (bacillus) G00.8
    gram-negative G00.9
    H. influenzae G00.0
    Klebsiella G00.8
    pneumococcal G00.1
    specified organism NEC G00.8
    staphylococcal G00.3
    streptococcal (acute) G00.2
  benign recurrent (Mollaret) G03.2
  candidal B37.5

Meningitis — continued
  caseous (tuberculous) A17.0
  cerebrospinal A39.0
  chronic NEC G03.1
  clear cerebrospinal fluid NEC G03.0
  coxsackievirus A87.0
  cryptococcal B45.1
  diplococcal (gram positive) A39.0
  echovirus A87.0
  enteroviral A87.0
  eosinophilic B83.2
  epidemic NEC A39.0
  Escherichia coli (E. coli) G00.8
  fibrinopurulent G00.9
    specified organism NEC G00.8
  Friedlander (bacillus) G00.8
  gonococcal A54.81
  gram-negative cocci G00.9
  gram-positive cocci G00.9
  H. influenzae G00.0
  Haemophilus (influenzae) G00.0
  in (due to)
    adenovirus A87.1
    African trypanosomiasis B56.9 [G02]
    anthrax A22.8
    bacterial disease NEC A48.8 [G01]
    Chagas' disease (chronic) B57.41
    chickenpox B01.0
    coccidioidomycosis B38.4
    Diplococcus pneumoniae G00.1
    enterovirus A87.0
    herpes (simplex) virus B00.3
      zoster B02.1
    infectious mononucleosis B27.92
    leptospirosis A27.81
    Listeria monocytogenes A32.11
    Lyme disease A69.21
    measles B05.1
    mumps (virus) B26.1
    neurosyphilis (late) A52.13
    parasitic disease NEC B89 [G02]
    poliovirus A80.9 [G02]
    preventive immunization, inoculation or vaccination G03.8
    rubella B06.02
    Salmonella infection A02.21
    specified cause NEC G03.8
    Streptococcal pneumoniae G00.1
    typhoid fever A01.01
    varicella B01.0
    viral disease NEC A87.8
    whooping cough A37.90
    zoster B02.1
  infectious G00.9
  influenzal (H. influenzae) G00.0
  Klebsiella G00.8
  leptospiral (aseptic) A27.81
  lymphocytic (acute) (benign) (serous) A87.2
  meningococcal A39.0
  Mima polymorpha G00.8
  Mollaret (benign recurrent) G03.2
  monilial B37.5
  mycotic NEC B49 [G02]
  Neisseria A39.0
  nonbacterial G03.0
  nonpyogenic NEC G03.0
  ossificans G96.198
  pneumococcal streptococcus pneumoniae G00.1
  poliovirus A80.9 [G02]
  postmeasles B05.1
  purulent G00.9
    specified organism NEC G00.8
  pyogenic G00.9
    specified organism NEC G00.8
  Salmonella (arizonae) (Cholerae-Suis) (enteritidis) (typhimurium) A02.21
  septic G00.9
    specified organism NEC G00.8
  serosa circumscripta NEC G03.0
  serous NEC G93.2
  specified organism NEC G00.8
  sporotrichosis B42.81
  staphylococcal G00.3
  sterile G03.0
  Streptococcal (acute) G00.2
    pneumoniae G00.1
  suppurative G00.9
    specified organism NEC G00.8
  syphilitic (late) (tertiary) A52.13

☑ **Additional Character Required** — Refer to the Tabular List for Character Selection

Meningitis — *continued*
　syphilitic — *continued*
　　acute A51.41
　　congenital A50.41
　　secondary A51.41
　Torula histolytica (cryptococcal) B45.1
　traumatic (complication of injury) T79.8 ☑
　tuberculous A17.0
　typhoid A01.01
　viral NEC A87.9
　Yersinia pestis A20.3
Meningocele (spinal) — *see also* Spina bifida
　with hydrocephalus — *see* Spina bifida, by site, with hydrocephalus
　acquired (traumatic) G96.198
　cerebral — *see* Encephalocele
Meningocerebritis — *see* Meningoencephalitis
Meningococcemia A39.4
　acute A39.2
　chronic A39.3
Meningococcus, meningococcal — *see also* condition A39.9
　adrenalitis, hemorrhagic A39.1
　carrier (suspected) of Z22.31
　meningitis (cerebrospinal) A39.0
Meningoencephalitis — *see also* Encephalitis G04.90
　acute NEC — *see also* Encephalitis, viral A86
　bacterial NEC G04.2
　California A83.5
　diphasic A84.1
　eosinophilic B83.2
　epidemic A39.81
　herpesviral, herpetic B00.4
　　due to herpesvirus 6 B10.01
　　due to herpesvirus 7 B10.09
　　specified NEC B10.09
　in (due to)
　　blastomycosis NEC B40.81
　　diseases classified elsewhere G05.3
　　free-living amebae B60.2
　　H. influenzae G00.0
　　Hemophilus influenzae (H .influenzae) G00.0
　　herpes B00.4
　　　due to herpesvirus 6 B10.01
　　　due to herpesvirus 7 B10.09
　　　specified NEC B10.09
　　Lyme disease A69.22
　　mercury — *see* subcategory T56.1 ☑
　　mumps B26.2
　　Naegleria (amebae) (organisms) (fowleri) B60.2
　　Parastrongylus cantonensis B83.2
　　toxoplasmosis (acquired) B58.2
　　　congenital P37.1
　infectious (acute) (viral) A86
　influenzal (H. influenzae) G00.0
　Listeria monocytogenes A32.12
　lymphocytic (serous) A87.2
　mumps B26.2
　parasitic NEC B89 [G05.3]
　pneumococcal G04.2
　primary amebic B60.2
　specific (syphilitic) A52.14
　specified organism NEC G04.81
　staphylococcal G04.2
　streptococcal G04.2
　syphilitic A52.14
　toxic NEC G92.8
　　due to mercury — *see* subcategory T56.1 ☑
　tuberculous A17.82
　virus NEC A86
Meningoencephalocele — *see also* Encephalocele
　syphilitic A52.19
　　congenital A50.49
Meningoencephalomyelitis — *see also* Meningoencephalitis
　acute NEC (viral) A86
　　disseminated G04.00
　　　postimmunization or postvaccination G04.02
　　　postinfectious G04.01
　　due to
　　　actinomycosis A42.82
　　　Torula B45.1
　　　Toxoplasma or toxoplasmosis (acquired) B58.2
　　　　congenital P37.1
　　postimmunization or postvaccination G04.02
Meningoencephalomyelopathy G96.9
Meningoencephalopathy G96.9
Meningomyelitis — *see also* Meningoencephalitis
　bacterial NEC G04.2

Meningomyelitis — *continued*
　blastomycotic NEC B40.81
　cryptococcal B45.1
　in diseases classified elsewhere G05.4
　meningococcal A39.81
　syphilitic A52.14
　tuberculous A17.82
Meningomyelocele — *see also* Spina bifida
　syphilitic A52.19
Meningomyeloneuritis — *see* Meningoencephalitis
Meningoradiculitis — *see* Meningitis
Meningovascular — *see* condition
Menkes' disease or syndrome E83.09
　meaning maple-syrup-urine disease E71.0
Menometrorrhagia N92.1
Menopause, menopausal (asymptomatic) (state) Z78.0
　arthritis (any site) NEC — *see* Arthritis, specified form NEC
　bleeding N92.4
　depression (single episode) F32.89
　　agitated (single episode) F32.2
　　　recurrent episode F33.9
　　psychotic (single episode) F32.89
　　　recurrent episode F33.9
　　recurrent episode F33.8
　melancholia (single episode) F32.89
　　recurrent episode F33.8
　paranoid state F22
　postirradiation (postprocedural)
　　asymptomatic E89.40
　　symptomatic E89.41
　premature E28.319
　　asymptomatic E28.319
　　　postirradiation E89.40
　　　postsurgical E89.40
　　symptomatic E28.310
　　　postirradiation E89.41
　　　postsurgical E89.41
　psychosis NEC F28
　symptomatic N95.1
　toxic polyarthritis NEC — *see* Arthritis, specified form NEC
Menorrhagia (primary) N92.0
　climacteric N92.4
　　menopausal N92.4
　menopausal N92.4
　perimenopausal N92.4
　postclimacteric N95.0
　postmenopausal N95.0
　preclimacteric or premenopausal N92.4
　pubertal (menses retained) N92.2
Menostaxis N92.0
Menses, retention N94.89
Menstrual — *see* Menstruation
Menstruation
　absent — *see* Amenorrhea
　anovulatory N97.0
　cycle, irregular N92.6
　delayed N91.0
　disorder N93.9
　　psychogenic F45.8
　during pregnancy O20.8
　excessive (with regular cycle) N92.0
　　with irregular cycle N92.1
　　at puberty N92.2
　frequent N92.0
　infrequent — *see* Oligomenorrhea
　irregular N92.6
　　specified NEC N92.5
　latent N92.5
　membranous N92.5
　painful — *see also* Dysmenorrhea N94.6
　　primary N94.4
　　psychogenic F45.8
　　secondary N94.5
　passage of clots N92.0
　precocious E30.1
　protracted N92.5
　rare — *see* Oligomenorrhea
　retained N94.89
　retrograde N92.5
　scanty — *see* Oligomenorrhea
　suppression N94.89
　vicarious (nasal) N94.89
Mental — *see also* condition
　deficiency — *see* Disability, intellectual
　deterioration — *see* Psychosis
　disorder — *see* Disorder, mental
　exhaustion F48.8

Mental — *continued*
　insufficiency (congenital) — *see* Disability, intellectual
　observation without need for further medical care Z03.89
　retardation — *see* Disability, intellectual
　subnormality — *see* Disability, intellectuall
　upset — *see* Disorder, mental
Meralgia paresthetica G57.1- ☑
Mercurial — *see* condition
Mercurialism — *see* subcategory T56.1 ☑
Merkel cell tumor — *see* Carcinoma, Merkel cell
Merocele — *see* Hernia, femoral
Meromelia
　lower limb — *see* Defect, reduction, lower limb
　　intercalary
　　　femur — *see* Defect, reduction, lower limb, specified type NEC
　　　　tibiofibular (complete) (incomplete) — *see* Defect, reduction, lower limb
　upper limb — *see* Defect, reduction, upper limb
　　intercalary, humeral, radioulnar — *see* Agenesis, arm, with hand present
MERRF syndrome (myoclonic epilepsy associated with ragged-red fiber) E88.42
Merzbacher-Pelizaeus disease E75.27
Mesaortitis — *see* Aortitis
Mesarteritis — *see* Arteritis
Mesencephalitis — *see* Encephalitis
Mesenchymoma — *see also* Neoplasm, connective tissue, uncertain behavior
　benign — *see* Neoplasm, connective tissue, benign
　malignant — *see* Neoplasm, connective tissue, malignant
Mesenteritis
　retractile K65.4
　sclerosing K65.4
Mesentery, mesenteric — *see* condition
Mesiodens, mesiodentes K00.1
Mesio-occlusion M26.213
Mesocolon — *see* condition
Mesonephroma (malignant) — *see* Neoplasm, malignant, by site
　benign — *see* Neoplasm, benign, by site
Mesophlebitis — *see* Phlebitis
Mesostromal dysgenesis Q13.89
Mesothelioma (malignant) C45.9
　benign
　　mesentery D19.1
　　mesocolon D19.1
　　omentum D19.1
　　peritoneum D19.1
　　pleura D19.0
　　specified site NEC D19.7
　　unspecified site D19.9
　biphasic C45.9
　　benign
　　　mesentery D19.1
　　　mesocolon D19.1
　　　omentum D19.1
　　　peritoneum D19.1
　　　pleura D19.0
　　　specified site NEC D19.7
　　　unspecified site D19.9
　cystic D48.4
　epithelioid C45.9
　　benign
　　　mesentery D19.1
　　　mesocolon D19.1
　　　omentum D19.1
　　　peritoneum D19.1
　　　pleura D19.0
　　　specified site NEC D19.7
　　　unspecified site D19.9
　fibrous C45.9
　　benign
　　　mesentery D19.1
　　　mesocolon D19.1
　　　omentum D19.1
　　　peritoneum D19.1
　　　pleura D19.0
　　　specified site NEC D19.7
　　　unspecified site D19.9
　site classification
　　liver C45.7
　　lung C45.7
　　mediastinum C45.7
　　mesentery C45.1
　　mesocolon C45.1
　　omentum C45.1
　　pericardium C45.2
　　peritoneum C45.1

Mesothelioma — *continued*
  site classification — *continued*
    pleura C45.0
      parietal C45.0
    retroperitoneum C45.7
    specified site NEC C45.7
    unspecified C45.9
Metabolic syndrome E88.810
Metagonimiasis B66.8
Metagonimus infestation (intestine) B66.8
Metal
  pigmentation L81.8
  polisher's disease J62.8
Metamorphopsia H53.15
Metaplasia
  apocrine (breast) — *see* Dysplasia, mammary, specified
    type NEC
  cervix (squamous) — *see* Dysplasia, cervix
  endometrium (squamous) (uterus) N85.8
  esophagus K22.7- ☑
  gastric intestinal K31.A0
    with dysplasia K31.A29
      high grade K31.A22
      low grade K31.A21
    indefinite for dysplasia K31.A0
    without dysplasia K31.A19
      involving
        antrum K31.A11
        body (corpus) K31.A12
        cardia K31.A14
        fundus K31.A13
        multiple sites K31.A15
  kidney (pelvis) (squamous) N28.89
  myelogenous D73.1
  myeloid (agnogenic) (megakaryocytic) D73.1
  spleen D73.1
  squamous cell, bladder N32.89
Metastasis, metastatic
  abscess — *see* Abscess
  calcification E83.59
  cancer
    from specified site — *see* Neoplasm, malignant, by
      site
    to specified site — *see* Neoplasm, secondary, by site
  deposits (in) — *see* Neoplasm, secondary, by site
  disease — *see also* Neoplasm, secondary, by site C79.9
  spread (to) — *see* Neoplasm, secondary, by site
Metastrongyliasis B83.8
Metatarsalgia M77.4- ☑
  anterior G57.6- ☑
  Morton's G57.6- ☑
Metatarsus, metatarsal — *see also* condition
  adductus, congenital Q66.22- ☑
  valgus (abductus), congenital Q66.6
  varus (congenital) Q66.22- ☑
    primus Q66.21- ☑
Methadone use — *see* Use, opioid
Methemoglobinemia D74.9
  acquired (with sulfhemoglobinemia) D74.8
  congenital D74.0
  enzymatic (congenital) D74.0
  Hb M disease D74.0
  hereditary D74.0
  toxic D74.8
Methemoglobinuria — *see* Hemoglobinuria
Methioninemia E72.19
Methylmalonic acidemia E71.120
Metritis (catarrhal) (hemorrhagic) (septic) (suppurative) —
  see also Endometritis
  cervical — *see* Cervicitis
Metropathia hemorrhagica N93.8
Metroperitonitis — *see* Peritonitis, pelvic, female
Metrorrhagia N92.1
  climacteric N92.4
  menopausal N92.4
  perimenopausal N92.4
  postpartum NEC (atonic) (following delivery of placenta)
    O72.1
    delayed or secondary O72.2
  preclimacteric or premenopausal N92.4
  psychogenic F45.8
Metrorrhexis — *see* Rupture, uterus
Metrosalpingitis N70.91
Metrostaxis N93.8
Metrovaginitis — *see* Endometritis
Meyer-Schwickerath and Weyers syndrome Q87.0
Meynert's amentia (nonalcoholic) F04
  alcoholic F10.96

Meynert's amentia — *continued*
  alcoholic — *continued*
    with dependence F10.26
Mibelli's disease (porokeratosis) Q82.8
Mice, joint — *see* Loose, body, joint
  knee M23.4- ☑
Micrencephalon, micrencephaly Q02
Microalbuminuria R80.9
Microaneurysm, retinal — *see also* Disorder, retina, microa-
  neurysms
  diabetic — *see* E08-E13 with .31
Microangiopathy (peripheral) I73.9
  thrombotic M31.10
    hematopoietic stem cell transplantation-associated
      [HSCT-TMA] M31.11
Microcalcifications, breast R92.0
Microcephalus, microcephalic, microcephaly Q02
  due to toxoplasmosis (congenital) P37.1
Microcheilia Q18.7
Microcolon (congenital) Q43.8
Microcornea (congenital) Q13.4
Microcytic — *see* condition
Microdeletions NEC Q93.88
Microdontia K00.2
Microdrepanocytosis D57.40
  with
    acute chest syndrome D57.411
    cerebral vascular involvement D57.413
    crisis (painful) D57.419
      with specified complication NEC D57.418
    pain (vaso-occlusive) D57.419
    splenic sequestration D57.412
Microembolism
  atherothrombotic — *see* Atheroembolism
  retinal — *see* Occlusion, artery, retina
Microencephalon Q02
Microfilaria streptocerca infestation — *see* Onchocercia-
  sis
Microgastria (congenital) Q40.2
Microgenia M26.06
Microgenitalia, congenital
  female Q52.8
  male Q55.8
Microglioma — *see* Lymphoma, non-Hodgkin, specified
  NEC
Microglossia (congenital) Q38.3
Micrognathia, micrognathism (congenital) (mandibular)
  (maxillary) M26.09
Microgyria (congenital) Q04.3
Microinfarct of heart — *see* Insufficiency, coronary
Microlentia (congenital) Q12.8
Microlithiasis, alveolar, pulmonary J84.02
Micromastia N64.82
Micromyelia (congenital) Q06.8
Micropenis Q55.62
Microphakia (congenital) Q12.8
Microphthalmos, microphthalmia (congenital) Q11.2
  due to toxoplasmosis P37.1
Micropsia H53.15
Microscopic polyangiitis (polyarteritis) M31.7
Microsporidiosis B60.8
  intestinal A07.8
Microsporon furfur infestation B36.0
Microsporosis — *see also* Dermatophytosis
  nigra B36.1
Microstomia (congenital) Q18.5
Microtia (congenital) (external ear) Q17.2
Microtropia H50.40
Microvillus inclusion disease (MVD) (MVID) Q43.8
Micturition
  disorder NEC — *see also* Difficulty, micturition R39.198
    psychogenic F45.8
  frequency R35.0
    psychogenic F45.8
  hesitancy R39.11
  incomplete emptying R39.14
  nocturnal R35.1
  painful R30.9
    dysuria R30.0
    psychogenic F45.8
    tenesmus R30.1
  poor stream R39.12
  position dependent R39.192
  split stream R39.13
  straining R39.16
  urgency R39.15
Mid plane — *see* condition
Middle
  ear — *see* condition

Middle — *continued*
  lobe (right) syndrome J98.19
Miescher's elastoma L87.2
Mietens' syndrome Q87.2
Migraine (idiopathic) G43.909
  with refractory migraine G43.919
    with status migrainosus G43.911
    without status migrainosus G43.919
  with aura (acute-onset) (prolonged) (typical) (without
    headache) G43.109
    with refractory migraine G43.119
      with status migrainosus G43.111
      without status migrainosus G43.119
    chronic G43.E09
      with refractory migraine G43.E19
        with status migrainosus G43.E11
        without status migrainosus G43.E19
      intractable
        with status migrainosus G43.E11
        without status migrainosus G43.E19
      not intractable
        with status migrainosus G43.E01
        without status migrainosus G43.E09
      without refractory migraine G43.E09
        with status migrainosus G43.E01
        without status migrainosus G43.E09
    intractable G43.119
      with status migrainosus G43.111
      without status migrainosus G43.119
    not intractable G43.109
      with status migrainosus G43.101
      without status migrainosus G43.109
    persistent G43.509
      with cerebral infarction G43.609
        with refractory migraine G43.619
          with status migrainosus G43.611
          without status migrainosus G43.619
        intractable G43.619
          with status migrainosus G43.611
          without status migrainosus G43.619
        not intractable G43.609
          with status migrainosus G43.601
          without status migrainosus G43.609
        without refractory migraine G43.609
          with status migrainosus G43.601
          without status migrainosus G43.609
      without cerebral infarction G43.509
        with refractory migraine G43.519
          with status migrainosus G43.511
          without status migrainosus G43.519
        intractable G43.519
          with status migrainosus G43.511
          without status migrainosus G43.519
        not intractable G43.509
          with status migrainosus G43.501
          without status migrainosus G43.509
        without refractory migraine G43.509
          with status migrainosus G43.501
          without status migrainosus G43.509
    without mention of refractory migraine G43.109
      with status migrainosus G43.101
      without status migrainosus G43.109
  abdominal G43.D0 (*following* G43.7)
    with refractory migraine G43.D1 (*following* G43.7)
    intractable G43.D1 (*following* G43.7)
    not intractable G43.D0 (*following* G43.7)
    without refractory migraine G43.D0 (*following* G43.7)
  basilar — *see* Migraine, with aura
  classical — *see* Migraine, with aura
  common — *see* Migraine, without aura
  complicated G43.109
  equivalents — *see* Migraine, with aura
  familiar — *see* Migraine, hemiplegic
  hemiplegic G43.409
    with refractory migraine G43.419
      with status migrainosus G43.411
      without status migrainosus G43.419
    intractable G43.419
      with status migrainosus G43.411
      without status migrainosus G43.419
    not intractable G43.409
      with status migrainosus G43.401
      without status migrainosus G43.409
    without refractory migraine G43.409
      with status migrainosus G43.401
      without status migrainosus G43.409
  intractable G43.919
    with status migrainosus G43.911
    without status migrainosus G43.919

☑ **Additional Character Required** — Refer to the Tabular List for Character Selection

Migraine — *continued*
  menstrual G43.829
    with refractory migraine G43.839
      with status migrainosus G43.831
      without status migrainosus G43.839
    intractable G43.839
      with status migrainosus G43.831
      without status migrainosus G43.839
    not intractable G43.829
      with status migrainosus G43.821
      without status migrainosus G43.829
    without refractory migraine G43.829
      with status migrainosus G43.821
      without status migrainosus G43.829
  menstrually related — *see* Migraine, menstrual
  not intractable G43.909
    with status migrainosus G43.901
    without status migrainosus G43.909
  ophthalmoplegic G43.B0 (*following* G43.7)
    with refractory migraine G43.B1 (*following* G43.7)
    intractable G43.B1 (*following* G43.7)
    not intractable G43.B0 (*following* G43.7)
    without refractory migraine G43.B0 (*following* G43.7)
  persistent aura (with, without) cerebral infarction — *see* Migraine, with aura, persistent
  preceded or accompanied by transient focal neurological phenomena — *see* Migraine, with aura
  pre-menstrual — *see* Migraine, menstrual
  pure menstrual — *see* Migraine, menstrual
  retinal — *see* Migraine, with aura
  specified NEC G43.809
    intractable G43.819
      with status migrainosus G43.811
      without status migrainosus G43.819
    not intractable G43.809
      with status migrainosus G43.801
      without status migrainosus G43.809
  sporadic — *see* Migraine, hemiplegic
  transformed — *see* Migraine, without aura, chronic
  triggered seizures — *see* Migraine, with aura
  without aura G43.009
    with refractory migraine G43.019
      with status migrainosus G43.011
      without status migrainosus G43.019
    chronic G43.709
      with refractory migraine G43.719
        with status migrainosus G43.711
        without status migrainosus G43.719
      intractable
        with status migrainosus G43.711
        without status migrainosus G43.719
      not intractable
        with status migrainosus G43.701
        without status migrainosus G43.709
      without refractory migraine G43.709
        with status migrainosus G43.701
        without status migrainosus G43.709
    intractable
      with status migrainosus G43.011
      without status migrainosus G43.019
    not intractable
      with status migrainosus G43.001
      without status migrainosus G43.009
    without mention of refractory migraine G43.009
      with status migrainosus G43.001
      without status migrainosus G43.009
    without refractory migraine G43.909
      with status migrainosus G43.901
      without status migrainosus G43.909
Migrant, social Z59.00
Migration, anxiety concerning Z60.3
Migratory, migrating — *see also* condition
  person Z59.00
  testis Q55.29
Mikity-Wilson disease or syndrome P27.0
Mikulicz' disease or syndrome K11.8
Miliaria L74.3
  alba L74.1
  apocrine L75.2
  crystallina L74.1
  profunda L74.2
  rubra L74.0
  tropicalis L74.2
Miliary — *see* condition
Milium L72.0
  colloid L57.8
Milk
  crust L21.0
  excessive secretion O92.6

Milk — *continued*
  poisoning — *see* Poisoning, food, noxious
  retention O92.79
  sickness — *see* Poisoning, food, noxious
  spots I31.0
Milk-alkali disease or syndrome E83.52
Milk-leg (deep vessels) (nonpuerperal) — *see* Embolism, vein, lower extremity
  complicating pregnancy O22.3- ☑
  puerperal, postpartum, childbirth O87.1
Milkman's disease or syndrome M83.8
Milky urine — *see* Chyluria
Millard-Gubler (-Foville) **paralysis or syndrome** G46.3
Millar's asthma J38.5
Miller Fisher syndrome G61.0
Mills' disease — *see* Hemiplegia
Millstone maker's pneumoconiosis J62.8
Milroy's disease (chronic hereditary edema) Q82.0
Minamata disease T56.1 ☑
Miners' asthma or lung J60
Minkowski-Chauffard syndrome — *see* Spherocytosis
Minor — *see* condition
Minor's disease (hematomyelia) G95.19
Minot's disease (hemorrhagic disease), newborn P53
Minot-von Willebrand-Jurgens disease or syndrome (angiohemophilia) — *see* Disease, von Willebrand
Minus (and plus) **hand** (intrinsic) — *see* Deformity, limb, specified type NEC, forearm
Miosis (pupil) H57.03
Mirizzi's syndrome (hepatic duct stenosis) K83.1
Mirror writing F81.0
MIS-A M35.81
Misadventure (of) (prophylactic) (therapeutic) — *see also* Complications T88.9 ☑
  administration of insulin (by accident) — *see* subcategory T38.3 ☑
  infusion — *see* Complications, infusion
  local applications (of fomentations, plasters, etc.) T88.9 ☑
    burn or scald — *see* Burn
    specified NEC T88.8 ☑
  medical care (early) (late) T88.9 ☑
    adverse effect of drugs or chemicals — *see* Table of Drugs and Chemicals
    burn or scald — *see* Burn
    specified NEC T88.8 ☑
  specified NEC T88.8 ☑
  surgical procedure (early) (late) — *see* Complications, surgical procedure
  transfusion — *see* Complications, transfusion
  vaccination or other immunological procedure — *see* Complications, vaccination
MIS-C M35.81
Miscarriage O03.9
Misdirection, aqueous H40.83- ☑
Misperception, sleep state F51.02
Misplaced, misplacement
  ear Q17.4
  kidney (acquired) N28.89
    congenital Q63.2
  organ or site, congenital NEC — *see* Malposition, congenital
Missed
  abortion O02.1
  delivery O36.4 ☑
Missing — *see also* Absence
  string of intrauterine contraceptive device T83.32- ☑
Misuse of drugs F19.99
Mitchell's disease (erythromelalgia) I73.81
Mite(s) (infestation) B88.9
  diarrhea B88.0
  grain (itch) B88.0
  hair follicle (itch) B88.0
  in sputum B88.0
Mitral — *see* condition
Mittelschmerz N94.0
Mixed — *see* condition
MMN (multifocal motor neuropathy) G61.82
MNGIE (Mitochondrial Neurogastrointestinal Encephalopathy) **syndrome** E88.49
Mobile, mobility
  cecum Q43.3
  excessive — *see* Hypermobility
  gallbladder, congenital Q44.1
  kidney N28.89
  organ or site, congenital NEC — *see* Malposition, congenital
Mobitz heart block (atrioventricular) I44.1

Moebius, Möbius
  disease (ophthalmoplegic migraine) — *see* Migraine, ophthalmoplegic
  syndrome Q87.0
    congenital oculofacial paralysis (with other anomalies) Q87.0
    ophthalmoplegic migraine — *see* Migraine, ophthalmoplegic
Moeller's glossitis K14.0
MOGAD (myelin oligodendrocyte glycoprotein antibody disease) G37.81
Mohr's syndrome (Types I and II) Q87.0
Mola destruens D39.2
Molar pregnancy O02.0
Molarization of premolars K00.2
Molding, head (during birth) — *omit code*
Mole (pigmented) — *see also* Nevus
  blood O02.0
  Breus' O02.0
  cancerous — *see* Melanoma
  carneous O02.0
  destructive D39.2
  fleshy O02.0
  hydatid, hydatidiform (benign) (complicating pregnancy) (delivered) (undelivered) O01.9
    classical O01.0
    complete O01.0
    incomplete O01.1
    invasive D39.2
    malignant D39.2
    partial O01.1
  intrauterine O02.0
  invasive (hydatidiform) D39.2
  malignant
    meaning
      malignant hydatidiform mole D39.2
      melanoma — *see* Melanoma
  nonhydatidiform O02.0
  nonpigmented — *see* Nevus
  pregnancy NEC O02.0
  skin — *see* Nevus
  tubal O00.10- ☑
    with intrauterine pregnancy O00.11- ☑
  vesicular — *see* Mole, hydatidiform
Molimen, molimina (menstrual) N94.3
Molluscum contagiosum (epitheliale) B08.1
Monckeberg's arteriosclerosis, disease, or sclerosis — *see* Arteriosclerosis, extremities
Mondini's malformation (cochlea) Q16.5
Mondor's disease I80.8
Monge's disease T70.29 ☑
Monilethrix (congenital) Q84.1
Moniliasis — *see also* Candidiasis B37.9
  neonatal P37.5
Monitoring (encounter for)
  therapeutic drug level Z51.81
Monkey malaria B53.1
Monkeypox B04
Monoarthritis M13.10
  ankle M13.17- ☑
  elbow M13.12- ☑
  foot joint M13.17- ☑
  hand joint M13.14- ☑
  hip M13.15- ☑
  knee M13.16- ☑
  shoulder M13.11- ☑
  wrist M13.13- ☑
Monoblastic — *see* condition
Monochromat (ism), monochromatopsia (acquired) (congenital) H53.51
Monocytic — *see* condition
Monocytopenia D72.818
Monocytosis (symptomatic) D72.821
Monomania — *see* Psychosis
Mononeuritis G58.9
  cranial nerve — *see* Disorder, nerve, cranial
  femoral nerve G57.2- ☑
  lateral
    cutaneous nerve of thigh G57.1- ☑
    popliteal nerve G57.3- ☑
  lower limb G57.9- ☑
    specified nerve NEC G57.8- ☑
  medial popliteal nerve G57.4- ☑
  median nerve G56.1- ☑
  multiplex G58.7
  plantar nerve G57.6- ☑
  posterior tibial nerve G57.5- ☑
  radial nerve G56.3- ☑

Mononeuritis — *continued*
  sciatic nerve G57.0- ☑
  specified NEC G58.8
  tibial nerve G57.4- ☑
  ulnar nerve G56.2- ☑
  upper limb G56.9- ☑
    specified nerve NEC G56.8- ☑
  vestibular — *see* subcategory H93.3 ☑
Mononeuropathy G58.9
  carpal tunnel syndrome — *see* Syndrome, carpal tunnel
  diabetic NEC — *see* E08-E13 with .41
  femoral nerve — *see* Lesion, nerve, femoral
  ilioinguinal nerve G57.8- ☑
  in diseases classified elsewhere — *see* category G59
  intercostal G58.0
  lower limb G57.9- ☑
    causalgia — *see* Causalgia, lower limb
    femoral nerve — *see* Lesion, nerve, femoral
    meralgia paresthetica G57.1- ☑
    plantar nerve — *see* Lesion, nerve, plantar
    popliteal nerve — *see* Lesion, nerve, popliteal
    sciatic nerve — *see* Lesion, nerve, sciatic
    specified NEC G57.8- ☑
    tarsal tunnel syndrome — *see* Syndrome, tarsal tunnel
  median nerve — *see* Lesion, nerve, median
  multiplex G58.7
  obturator nerve G57.8- ☑
  popliteal nerve — *see* Lesion, nerve, popliteal
  radial nerve — *see* Lesion, nerve, radial
  saphenous nerve G57.8- ☑
  specified NEC G58.8
  tarsal tunnel syndrome — *see* Syndrome, tarsal tunnel
  tuberculous A17.83
  ulnar nerve — *see* Lesion, nerve, ulnar
  upper limb G56.9- ☑
    carpal tunnel syndrome — *see* Syndrome, carpal tunnel
    causalgia — *see* Causalgia
    median nerve — *see* Lesion, nerve, median
    radial nerve — *see* Lesion, nerve, radial
    specified site NEC G56.8- ☑
    ulnar nerve — *see* Lesion, nerve, ulnar
Mononucleosis, infectious B27.90
  with
    complication NEC B27.99
    meningitis B27.92
    polyneuropathy B27.91
  cytomegaloviral B27.10
    with
      complication NEC B27.19
      meningitis B27.12
      polyneuropathy B27.11
  Epstein-Barr (virus) B27.00
    with
      complication NEC B27.09
      meningitis B27.02
      polyneuropathy B27.01
  gammaherpesviral B27.00
    with
      complication NEC B27.09
      meningitis B27.02
      polyneuropathy B27.01
  specified NEC B27.80
    with
      complication NEC B27.89
      meningitis B27.82
      polyneuropathy B27.81
Monoparesis — *see* Monoplegia
Monoplegia G83.3- ☑
  congenital (cerebral) G80.8
    spastic G80.1
  embolic (current episode) I63.4- ☑
  following
    cerebrovascular disease
      cerebral infarction
        lower limb I69.34- ☑
        upper limb I69.33- ☑
      intracerebral hemorrhage
        lower limb I69.14- ☑
        upper limb I69.13- ☑
      lower limb I69.94- ☑
      nontraumatic intracranial hemorrhage NEC
        lower limb I69.24- ☑
        upper limb I69.23- ☑
      specified disease NEC
        lower limb I69.84- ☑
        upper limb I69.83- ☑

Monoplegia — *continued*
  following — *continued*
    cerebrovascular disease — *continued*
      stroke NOS
        lower limb I69.34- ☑
        upper limb I69.33- ☑
      subarachnoid hemorrhage
        lower limb I69.04- ☑
        upper limb I69.03- ☑
      upper limb I69.93- ☑
  hysterical (transient) F44.4
  lower limb G83.1-
  psychogenic (conversion reaction) F44.4
  thrombotic (current episode) I63.3- ☑
  transient R29.818
  upper limb G83.2- ☑
Monorchism, monorchidism Q55.0
Monosomy — *see also* Deletion, chromosome Q93.9
  specified NEC Q93.89
  whole chromosome
    meiotic nondisjunction Q93.0
    mitotic nondisjunction Q93.1
    mosaicism Q93.1
  X Q96.9
Monster, monstrosity (single) Q89.7
  acephalic Q00.0
  twin Q89.4
Monteggia's fracture (-dislocation) S52.27- ☑
Mooren's ulcer (cornea) — *see* Ulcer, cornea, Mooren's
Moore's syndrome — *see* Epilepsy, specified NEC
Mooser-Neill reaction A75.2
Mooser's bodies A75.2
Morbidity not stated or unknown R69
Morbilli — *see* Measles
Morbus — *see also* Disease
  angelicus, anglorum E55.0
  Beigel B36.2
  caducus — *see* Epilepsy
  celiacus K90.0
  comitialis — *see* Epilepsy
  cordis — *see also* Disease, heart I51.9
    valvulorum — *see* Endocarditis
  coxae senilis M16.9
    tuberculous A18.02
  hemorrhagicus neonatorum P53
  maculosus neonatorum P54.5
Morel (-Stewart)(-Morgagni) **syndrome** M85.2
Morel-Kraepelin disease — *see* Schizophrenia
Morel-Moore syndrome M85.2
Morgagni's
  cyst, organ, hydatid, or appendage
    female Q50.5
    male (epididymal) Q55.4
      testicular Q55.29
  syndrome M85.2
Morgagni-Stewart-Morel syndrome M85.2
Morgagni-Stokes-Adams syndrome I45.9
Morgagni-Turner (-Albright) **syndrome** Q96.9
Moria F07.0
Moron (I.Q. 50-69) F70
Morphea L94.0
Morphinism (without remission) F11.20
  with remission F11.21
Morphinomania (without remission) F11.20
  with remission F11.21
Morquio (-Ullrich)(-Brailsford) **disease or syndrome** — *see* Mucopolysaccharidosis
Mortification (dry) (moist) — *see* Gangrene
Morton's metatarsalgia (neuralgia) (neuroma) (syndrome) G57.6- ☑
Morvan's disease or syndrome G60.8
Mosaicism, mosaic (autosomal) (chromosomal)
  45,X/46,XX Q96.3
  45,X/other cell lines NEC with abnormal sex chromosome Q96.4
  sex chromosome
    female Q97.8
    lines with various numbers of X chromosomes Q97.2
    male Q98.7
  XY Q96.3
Moschowitz' disease M31.19
Mother yaw A66.0
Motion sickness (from travel, any vehicle) (from round-abouts or swings) T75.3 ☑
Mottled, mottling, teeth (enamel) (endemic) (nonendemic) K00.3
Mounier-Kuhn syndrome Q32.4
  with bronchiectasis J47.9

Mounier-Kuhn syndrome — *continued*
  with bronchiectasis — *continued*
    exacerbation (acute) J47.1
    lower respiratory infection J47.0
  acquired J98.09
    with bronchiectasis J47.9
      with
        exacerbation (acute) J47.1
        lower respiratory infection J47.0
Mountain
  sickness T70.29 ☑
    with polycythemia , acquired (acute) D75.1
  tick fever A93.2
Mouse, joint — *see* Loose, body, joint
  knee M23.4- ☑
Mouth — *see* condition
Movable
  coccyx — *see* subcategory M53.2 ☑
  kidney N28.89
    congenital Q63.8
  spleen D73.89
Movements, dystonic R25.8
Moyamoya disease I67.5
Mpox B04
MRSA (Methicillin resistant Staphylococcus aureus)
  infection A49.02
    as the cause of diseases classified elsewhere B95.62
  sepsis A41.02
MSD (multiple sulfatase deficiency) E75.26
MSSA (Methicillin susceptible Staphylococcus aureus)
  infection A49.01
    as the cause of diseases classified elsewhere B95.61
  sepsis A41.01
Mucha-Habermann disease L41.0
Mucinosis (cutaneous) (focal) (papular) (skin) L98.5
  oral K13.79
Mucocele
  appendix K38.8
  buccal cavity K13.79
  gallbladder K82.1
  lacrimal sac, chronic H04.43- ☑
  nasal sinus J34.1
  nose J34.1
  salivary gland (any) K11.6
  sinus (accessory) (nasal) J34.1
  turbinate (bone) (middle) (nasal) J34.1
  uterus N85.8
Mucolipidosis
  I E77.1
  II, III E77.0
  IV E75.11
Mucopolysaccharidosis E76.3
  beta-gluduronidase deficiency E76.29
  cardiopathy E76.3 *[I52]*
  Hunter's syndrome E76.1
  Hurler's syndrome E76.01
  Hurler-Scheie syndrome E76.02
  Maroteaux-Lamy syndrome E76.29
  Morquio syndrome E76.219
    A E76.210
    B E76.211
    classic E76.210
  Sanfilippo syndrome E76.22
  Scheie's syndrome E76.03
  specified NEC E76.29
  type
    I
      Hurler's syndrome E76.01
      Hurler-Scheie syndrome E76.02
      Scheie's syndrome E76.03
    II E76.1
    III E76.22
    IV E76.219
    IVA E76.210
    IVB E76.211
    VI E76.29
    VII E76.29
Mucormycosis B46.5
  cutaneous B46.3
  disseminated B46.4
  gastrointestinal B46.2
  generalized B46.4
  pulmonary B46.0
  rhinocerebral B46.1
  skin B46.3
  subcutaneous B46.3
Mucositis (ulcerative) K12.30
  due to drugs NEC K12.32
  gastrointestinal K92.81

Mucositis — *continued*
- mouth (oral) (oropharyngeal) K12.30
  - due to antineoplastic therapy K12.31
  - due to drugs NEC K12.32
  - due to radiation K12.33
  - specified NEC K12.39
  - viral K12.39
- nasal J34.81
- oral cavity — *see* Mucositis, mouth
- oral soft tissues — *see* Mucositis, mouth
- vagina and vulva N76.81

Mucositis necroticans agranulocytica — *see* Agranulocytosis

Mucous — *see also* condition
- patches (syphilitic) A51.39
  - congenital A50.07

Mucoviscidosis E84.9
- with meconium obstruction E84.11

Mucus
- asphyxia or suffocation — *see* Asphyxia, mucus
- in stool R19.5
- plug — *see* Asphyxia, mucus

Muguet B37.0

Mulberry molars (congenital syphilis) A50.52

Mullerian mixed tumor
- specified site — *see* Neoplasm, malignant, by site
- unspecified site C54.9

Multicystic kidney (development) Q61.4

Multiparity (grand) Z64.1
- affecting management of pregnancy, labor and delivery (supervision only) O09.4- ☑
- requiring contraceptive management — *see* Contraception

Multipartita placenta O43.19- ☑

Multiple, multiplex — *see also* condition
- digits (congenital) Q69.9
- endocrine neoplasia — *see* Neoplasia, endocrine, multiple (MEN)
- personality F44.81

Multisystem inflammatory syndrome (in adult) (in children) M35.81

Mumps B26.9
- arthritis B26.85
- complication NEC B26.89
- encephalitis B26.2
- hepatitis B26.81
- meningitis (aseptic) B26.1
- meningoencephalitis B26.2
- myocarditis B26.82
- oophoritis B26.89
- orchitis B26.0
- pancreatitis B26.3
- polyneuropathy B26.84

Mumu — *see also* Infestation, filarial B74.9 *[N51]*

Munchhausen's syndrome — *see* Disorder, factitious

Munchmeyer's syndrome — *see* Myositis, ossificans, progressiva

Mural — *see* condition

Murmur (cardiac) (heart) (organic) R01.1
- abdominal R19.15
- aortic (valve) — *see* Endocarditis, aortic
- benign R01.0
- diastolic — *see* Endocarditis
- Flint I35.1
- functional R01.0
- Graham Steell I37.1
- innocent R01.0
- mitral (valve) — *see* Insufficiency, mitral
- nonorganic R01.0
- presystolic, mitral — *see* Insufficiency, mitral
- pulmonic (valve) I37.8
- systolic R01.1
- tricuspid (valve) I07.9
- valvular — *see* Endocarditis

Murri's disease (intermittent hemoglobinuria) D59.6

Muscle, muscular — *see also* condition
- carnitine (palmityltransferase) deficiency E71.314

Musculoneuralgia — *see* Neuralgia

Mushrooming hip — *see* Derangement, joint, specified NEC, hip

Mushroom-workers' (pickers') **disease or lung** J67.5

Mutation(s)
- factor V Leiden D68.51
- prothrombin gene D68.52
- surfactant, of lung J84.83

Mutism — *see also* Aphasia
- deaf (acquired) (congenital) NEC H91.3
- elective (adjustment reaction) (childhood) F94.0
- hysterical F44.4

Mutism — *continued*
- selective (childhood) F94.0

MVD (microvillus inclusion disease) Q43.8

MVID (microvillus inclusion disease) Q43.8

Myalgia M79.10
- auxiliary muscles, head and neck M79.12
- epidemic (cervical) B33.0
- mastication muscle M79.11
- site specified NEC M79.18
- traumatic NEC T14.8 ☑

Myasthenia G70.9
- congenital G70.2
- cordis — *see* Failure, heart
- developmental G70.2
- gravis G70.00
  - with exacerbation (acute) G70.01
  - in crisis G70.01
  - neonatal, transient P94.0
  - pseudoparalytica G70.00
    - with exacerbation (acute) G70.01
    - in crisis G70.01
- stomach, psychogenic F45.8
- syndrome
  - in
    - diabetes mellitus — *see* E08-E13 with .44
    - neoplastic disease — *see also* Neoplasm D49.9 *[G73.3]*
    - pernicious anemia D51.0 *[G73.3]*
    - thyrotoxicosis E05.90 *[G73.3]*
      - with thyroid storm E05.91 *[G73.3]*

Myasthenic M62.81

Mycelium infection B49

Mycetismus — *see* Poisoning, food, noxious, mushroom

Mycetoma B47.9
- actinomycotic B47.1
- bone (mycotic) B47.9 *[M90.80]*
- eumycotic B47.0
- foot B47.9
  - actinomycotic B47.1
  - mycotic B47.0
- madurae NEC B47.9
  - mycotic B47.0
- maduromycotic B47.0
- mycotic B47.0
- nocardial B47.1

Mycobacteriosis — *see* Mycobacterium

Mycobacterium, mycobacterial (infection) A31.9
- anonymous A31.9
- atypical A31.9
  - cutaneous A31.1
  - pulmonary A31.0
    - tuberculous — *see* Tuberculosis, pulmonary
  - specified site NEC A31.8
- avium (intracellulare complex) A31.0
- balnei A31.1
- Battey A31.0
- chelonei A31.8
- cutaneous A31.1
- extrapulmonary systemic A31.8
- fortuitum A31.8
- intracellulare (Battey bacillus) A31.0
- kakaferifu A31.8
- kansasii (yellow bacillus) A31.0
- kasongo A31.8
- leprae — *see also* Leprosy A30.9
- luciflavum A31.1
- marinum (M. balnei) A31.1
- nonspecific — *see* Mycobacterium, atypical
- pulmonary (atypical) A31.0
  - tuberculous — *see* Tuberculosis, pulmonary
- scrofulaceum A31.8
- simiae A31.8
- systemic, extrapulmonary A31.8
- szulgai A31.8
- terrae A31.8
- triviale A31.8
- tuberculosis (human, bovine) — *see* Tuberculosis
- ulcerans A31.1
- xenopi A31.8

Mycoplasma (M.) **pneumoniae, as cause of disease classified elsewhere** B96.0

Mycosis, mycotic B49
- cutaneous NEC B36.9
- ear B36.9
  - in
    - aspergillosis E44.89
    - candidiasis B37.84
    - moniliasis B37.84
- fungoides (extranodal) (solid organ) C84.0- ☑

Mycosis, mycotic — *continued*
- mouth B37.0
- nails B35.1
- opportunistic B48.8
- skin NEC B36.9
- specified NEC B48.8
- stomatitis B37.0
- vagina, vaginitis (candidal) (acute) B37.31
  - chronic (recurrent) B37.32

Mydriasis (pupil) H57.04

Myelatelia Q06.1

Myelinolysis, pontine, central G37.2

Myelitis (acute) (ascending) (childhood) (chronic) (descending) (diffuse) (disseminated) (idiopathic) (pressure) (progressive) (spinal cord) (subacute) — *see also* Encephalitis G04.91
- flaccid G04.82
- herpes simplex B00.82
- herpes zoster B02.24
- in diseases classified elsewhere G05.4
- necrotizing, subacute G37.4
- optic neuritis in G36.0
- postchickenpox B01.12
- postherpetic B02.24
- postimmunization G04.02
- postinfectious NEC G04.89
- postvaccinal G04.02
- specified NEC G04.89
- syphilitic (transverse) A52.14
- toxic G92.9
- transverse (in demyelinating diseases of central nervous system) G37.3
- tuberculous A17.82
- varicella B01.12

Myeloblastic — *see* condition

Myeloblastoma
- granular cell — *see also* Neoplasm, connective tissue
  - malignant — *see* Neoplasm, connective tissue, malignant
  - tongue D10.1

Myelocele — *see* Spina bifida

Myelocystocele — *see* Spina bifida

Myelocytic — *see* condition

Myelodysplasia D46.9
- specified NEC D46.Z (*following* D46.4)
- spinal cord (congenital) Q06.1

Myelodysplastic syndrome — *see also* Syndrome, myelodysplastic D46.9
- with
  - 5q deletion D46.C (*following* D46.2)
  - isolated del (5q) chromosomal abnormality D46.C (*following* D46.2)
  - pancytopenia, acquired — *see* Syndrome, myelodysplastic, pancytopenia
- specified NEC D46.Z (*following* D46.4)

Myeloencephalitis — *see* Encephalitis

Myelofibrosis D75.81
- with myeloid metaplasia D47.4
- acute C94.4- ☑
- idiopathic (chronic) D47.4
- primary D47.1
- secondary D75.81
  - in myeloproliferative disease D47.4

Myelogenous — *see* condition

Myeloid — *see* condition

Myelokathexis D70.9

Myeloleukodystrophy E75.29

Myelolipoma — *see* Lipoma

Myeloma (multiple) C90.0- ☑
- monostotic C90.3 ☑
  - plasma cell C90.0- ☑
- plasma cell C90.0- ☑
- solitary — *see also* Plasmacytoma, solitary C90.3- ☑

Myelomalacia G95.89

Myelomatosis C90.0- ☑

Myelomeningitis — *see* Meningoencephalitis

Myelomeningocele (spinal cord) — *see* Spina bifida

Myelo-osteo-musculodysplasia hereditaria Q79.8

Myelopathic
- anemia D64.89
- muscle atrophy — *see* Atrophy, muscle, spinal
- pain syndrome G89.0

Myelopathy (spinal cord) G95.9
- drug-induced G95.89
- in (due to)
  - degeneration or displacement, intervertebral disc NEC — *see* Disorder, disc, with, myelopathy
  - disease classified elsewhere G99.2

Myelopathy — continued
  in — continued
    infection — see Encephalitis
    intervertebral disc disorder — see also Disorder, disc, with, myelopathy
    mercury — see subcategory T56.1 ☑
    neoplastic disease — see also Neoplasm D49.9 [G99.2]
    pernicious anemia D51.0 [G99.2]
    spondylosis — see Spondylosis, with myelopathy NEC
  necrotic (subacute) (vascular) G95.19
  radiation-induced G95.89
  spondylogenic NEC — see Spondylosis, with myelopathy NEC
  toxic G95.89
  transverse, acute G37.3
  vascular G95.19
  vitamin B12 E53.8 [G32.0]
Myelophthisis D61.82
Myeloradiculitis G04.91
Myeloradiculodysplasia (spinal) Q06.1
Myelosarcoma C92.3- ☑
Myelosclerosis D75.89
  with myeloid metaplasia D47.4
  disseminated, of nervous system G35
  megakaryocytic D47.4
    with myeloid metaplasia D47.4
Myelosis
  acute C92.0- ☑
  aleukemic C92.9- ☑
  chronic D47.1
  erythremic (acute) C94.0- ☑
  megakaryocytic C94.2- ☑
  nonleukemic D72.828
  subacute C92.9- ☑
Myiasis (cavernous) B87.9
  aural B87.4
  creeping B87.0
  cutaneous B87.0
  dermal B87.0
  ear (externa) (middle) B87.4
  eye B87.2
  genitourinary B87.81
  intestinal B87.82
  laryngeal B87.3
  nasopharyngeal B87.3
  ocular B87.2
  orbit B87.2
  skin B87.0
  specified site NEC B87.89
  traumatic B87.1
  wound B87.1
Myoadenoma prostate — see Hyperplasia, prostate
Myoblastoma
  granular cell — see also Neoplasm, connective tissue, benign
    malignant — see Neoplasm, connective tissue, malignant
  tongue D10.1
Myocardial — see condition
Myocardiopathy (congestive) (constrictive) (familial) (hypertrophic nonobstructive) (idiopathic) (infiltrative) (obstructive) (primary) (restrictive) (sporadic) — see also Cardiomyopathy I42.9
  alcoholic I42.6
  cobalt-beer I42.6
  glycogen storage E74.02 [I43]
  hypertrophic obstructive I42.1
  in (due to)
    beriberi E51.12
    cardiac glycogenosis E74.02 [I43]
    Friedreich's ataxia G11.11 [I43]
    myotonia atrophica G71.11 [I43]
    progressive muscular dystrophy — see also Dystrophy, muscular, by type G71.09 [I43]
  obscure (African) I42.8
  secondary I42.9
  thyrotoxic E05.90 [I43]
    with storm E05.91 [I43]
  toxic NEC I42.7
Myocarditis (with arteriosclerosis) (chronic) (fibroid) (interstitial) (old) (progressive) (senile) I51.4
  with
    rheumatic fever (conditions in I00) I09.0
      active — see Myocarditis, acute, rheumatic
      inactive or quiescent (with chorea) I09.0
    active I40.9
      rheumatic I01.2
        with chorea (acute) (rheumatic) (Sydenham's) I02.0

Myocarditis — continued
  acute or subacute (interstitial) I40.9
    due to
      streptococcus (beta-hemolytic) I01.2
    idiopathic I40.1
    rheumatic I01.2
      with chorea (acute) (rheumatic) (Sydenham's) I02.0
    specified NEC I40.8
  aseptic of newborn B33.22
  bacterial (acute) I40.0
  Coxsackie (virus) B33.22
  diphtheritic A36.81
  eosinophilic I40.1
  epidemic of newborn (Coxsackie) B33.22
  Fiedler's (acute) (isolated) I40.1
  giant cell (acute) (subacute) I40.1
  gonococcal A54.83
  granulomatous (idiopathic) (isolated) (nonspecific) I40.1
  hypertensive — see Hypertension, heart
  idiopathic (granulomatous) I40.1
  in (due to)
    diphtheria A36.81
    epidemic louse-borne typhus A75.0 [I41]
    Lyme disease A69.29
    sarcoidosis D86.85
    scarlet fever A38.1
    toxoplasmosis (acquired) B58.81
    typhoid A01.02
    typhus NEC A75.9 [I41]
  infective I40.0
  influenzal — see Influenza, with, myocarditis
  isolated (acute) I40.1
  meningococcal A39.52
  mumps B26.82
  nonrheumatic, active I40.9
  parenchymatous I40.9
  pneumococcal I40.0
  rheumatic (chronic) (inactive) (with chorea) I09.0
    active or acute I01.2
      with chorea (acute) (rheumatic) (Sydenham's) I02.0
  rheumatoid — see Rheumatoid, carditis
  septic I40.0
  staphylococcal I40.0
  suppurative I40.0
  syphilitic (chronic) A52.06
  toxic I40.8
    rheumatic — see Myocarditis, acute, rheumatic
  tuberculous A18.84
  typhoid A01.02
  valvular — see Endocarditis
  virus, viral I40.0
    of newborn (Coxsackie) B33.22
Myocardium, myocardial — see condition
Myocardosis — see Cardiomyopathy
Myoclonus, myoclonic, myoclonia (familial) (essential) (multifocal) (simplex) G25.3
  drug-induced G25.3
  epilepsy — see also Epilepsy, generalized, specified NEC G40.4- ☑
    familial (progressive) — see Epilepsy, myoclonus Lafora — see Epilepsy, myoclonus, progressive, Lafora
  epileptica — see also Epilepsy, myoclonus G40.409
    with status epilepticus G40.401
  facial G51.3- ☑
  familial progressive G25.3
    epilepsy — see Epilepsy, myoclonus, progressive
  Friedreich's G25.3
  jerks G25.3
  massive G25.3
  palatal G25.3
  pharyngeal G25.3
Myocytolysis I51.5
Myodiastasis — see Diastasis, muscle
Myoendocarditis — see Endocarditis
Myoepithelioma — see Neoplasm, benign, by site
Myofasciitis (acute) — see Myositis
Myofibroma — see also Neoplasm, connective tissue, benign
  uterus (cervix) (corpus) — see Leiomyoma
Myofibromatosis D48.19
  infantile Q89.8
Myofibrosis M62.89
  heart — see Myocarditis
  scapulohumeral — see Lesion, shoulder, specified NEC
Myofibrositis M79.7
  scapulohumeral — see Lesion, shoulder, specified NEC
Myoglobulinuria, myoglobinuria (primary) R82.1
Myokymia, facial G51.4
Myolipoma — see Lipoma

Myoma — see also Neoplasm, connective tissue, benign
  malignant — see Neoplasm, connective tissue, malignant
  prostate D29.1
  uterus (cervix) (corpus) — see Leiomyoma
Myomalacia M62.89
Myometritis — see Endometritis
Myometrium — see condition
Myonecrosis, clostridial A48.0
Myopathy G72.9
  acute
    necrotizing G72.81
    quadriplegic G72.81
  alcoholic G72.1
  benign congenital G71.20
  central core G71.29
  centronuclear G71.228
    autosomal (dominant) (recessive) G71.228
    other specified NEC G71.228
  congenital (benign) G71.20
  critical illness G72.81
  distal G71.09
  drug-induced G72.0
  endocrine NEC E34.9 [G73.7]
  extraocular muscles H05.82- ☑
  facioscapulohumeral G71.02
  hereditary G71.9
    specified NEC G71.8
  hyaline body G71.29
  immune NEC G72.49
  in (due to)
    Addison's disease E27.1 [G73.7]
    alcohol G72.1
    amyloidosis E85.0 [G73.7]
    cretinism E00.9 [G73.7]
    Cushing's syndrome E24.9 [G73.7]
    drugs G72.0
    endocrine disease NEC E34.9 [G73.7]
    giant cell arteritis M31.6 [G73.7]
    glycogen storage disease E74.00 [G73.7]
    hyperadrenocorticism E24.9 [G73.7]
    hyperparathyroidism NEC E21.3 [G73.7]
    hypoparathyroidism E20.9 [G73.7]
    hypopituitarism E23.0 [G73.7]
    hypothyroidism E03.9 [G73.7]
    infectious disease NEC B99 ☑ [G73.7]
    lipid storage disease E75.6 [G73.7]
    metabolic disease NEC E88.9 [G73.7]
    myxedema E03.9 [G73.7]
    parasitic disease NEC B89 [G73.7]
    polyarteritis nodosa M30.0 [G73.7]
    rheumatoid arthritis — see Rheumatoid, myopathy
    sarcoidosis D86.87
    scleroderma M34.82
    sicca syndrome M35.03
    Sjogren's syndrome M35.03
    systemic lupus erythematosus M32.19
    thyrotoxicosis (hyperthyroidism) E05.90 [G73.7]
      with thyroid storm E05.91 [G73.7]
    toxic agent NEC G72.2
  inflammatory NEC G72.49
  intensive care (ICU) G72.81
  limb-girdle — see Dystrophy, muscular, limb-girdle
  mitochondrial NEC G71.3
  Miyoshi, type 3 G71.035
  myosin storage G71.29
  myotubular (centronuclear) G71.220
    X-linked G71.220
  myotonic, proximal (PROMM) G71.11
  nemaline G71.21
  ocular G71.09
  oculopharyngeal G71.09
  of critical illness G72.81
  primary G71.9
    specified NEC G71.8
  progressive NEC G72.89
  proximal myotonic (PROMM) G71.11
  rod (body) G71.21
  scapulohumeral G71.02
  specified NEC G72.89
  toxic G72.2
Myopericarditis — see also Pericarditis
  chronic rheumatic I09.2
Myopia (axial) (congenital) H52.1- ☑
  degenerative (malignant) H44.20
    with
      choroidal neovascularization H44.2A- ☑
      foveoschisis H44.2D- ☑
      macular hole H44.2B- ☑

Myopia — *continued*
  degenerative — *continued*
    with — *continued*
      retinal detachment H44.2C- ☑
      specified maculopathy NEC H44.2E- ☑
    bilateral H44.23
    left eye H44.22
    right eye H44.21
  malignant — *see also* Myopia, degenerative H44.2- ☑
  pernicious — *see also* Myopia, degenerative H44.2- ☑
  progressive high (degenerative) — *see also* Myopia, degenerative H44.2- ☑
Myosarcoma — *see* Neoplasm, connective tissue, malignant
Myosis (pupil) H57.03
  stromal (endolymphatic) D39.0
Myositis M60.9
  clostridial A48.0
  due to posture — *see* Myositis, specified type NEC
  epidemic B33.0
  fibrosa or fibrous (chronic), Volkmann's T79.6 ☑
  foreign body granuloma — *see* Granuloma, foreign body
  in (due to)
    bilharziasis B65.9 *[M63.8-]* ☑
    cysticercosis B69.81
    leprosy A30.9 *[M63.8-]* ☑
    mycosis B49 *[M63.8-]* ☑
    sarcoidosis D86.87
    schistosomiasis B65.9 *[M63.8-]* ☑
    syphilis
      late A52.78
      secondary A51.49
    toxoplasmosis (acquired) B58.82
    trichinellosis B75 *[M63.8-]* ☑
    tuberculosis A18.09
  inclusion body [IBM] G72.41
  infective M60.009
    arm M60.002
      left M60.001
      right M60.000
    leg M60.005
      left M60.004
      right M60.003
    lower limb M60.005
      ankle M60.07- ☑
      foot M60.07- ☑
      lower leg M60.06- ☑
      thigh M60.05- ☑
      toe M60.07- ☑
    multiple sites M60.09
    specified site NEC M60.08
    upper limb M60.002
      finger M60.04- ☑
      forearm M60.03- ☑
      hand M60.04- ☑
      shoulder region M60.01- ☑
      upper arm M60.02- ☑
  interstitial M60.10
    ankle M60.17- ☑
    foot M60.17- ☑
    forearm M60.13- ☑
    hand M60.14- ☑
    lower leg M60.16- ☑
    multiple sites M60.19
    shoulder region M60.11- ☑

Myositis — *continued*
  interstitial — *continued*
    specified site NEC M60.18
    thigh M60.15- ☑
    upper arm M60.12- ☑
  mycotic B49 *[M63.8-]* ☑
  orbital, chronic H05.12- ☑
  ossificans or ossifying (circumscripta) — *see also* Ossification, muscle, specified NEC
  in (due to)
    burns M61.30
      ankle M61.37- ☑
      foot M61.37- ☑
      forearm M61.33- ☑
      hand M61.34- ☑
      lower leg M61.36- ☑
      multiple sites M61.39
      pelvic region M61.35- ☑
      shoulder region M61.31- ☑
      specified site NEC M61.38
      thigh M61.35- ☑
      upper arm M61.32- ☑
    quadriplegia or paraplegia M61.20
      ankle M61.27- ☑
      foot M61.27- ☑
      forearm M61.23- ☑
      hand M61.24- ☑
      lower leg M61.26- ☑
      multiple sites M61.29
      pelvic region M61.25- ☑
      shoulder region M61.21- ☑
      specified site NEC M61.28
      thigh M61.25- ☑
      upper arm M61.22- ☑
    progressiva M61.10
      ankle M61.17- ☑
      finger M61.14- ☑
      foot M61.17- ☑
      forearm M61.13- ☑
      hand M61.14- ☑
      lower leg M61.16- ☑
      multiple sites M61.19
      pelvic region M61.15- ☑
      shoulder region M61.11- ☑
      specified site NEC M61.18
      thigh M61.15- ☑
      toe M61.17- ☑
      upper arm M61.12- ☑
    traumatica M61.00
      ankle M61.07- ☑
      foot M61.07- ☑
      forearm M61.03- ☑
      hand M61.04- ☑
      lower leg M61.06- ☑
      multiple sites M61.09
      pelvic region M61.05- ☑
      shoulder region M61.01- ☑
      specified site NEC M61.08
      thigh M61.05- ☑
      upper arm M61.02- ☑
  purulent — *see* Myositis, infective
  specified type NEC M60.80
    ankle M60.87- ☑

Myositis — *continued*
  specified type — *continued*
    foot M60.87- ☑
    forearm M60.83- ☑
    hand M60.84- ☑
    lower leg M60.86- ☑
    multiple sites M60.89
    pelvic region M60.85- ☑
    shoulder region M60.81- ☑
    specified site NEC M60.88
    thigh M60.85- ☑
    upper arm M60.82- ☑
  suppurative — *see* Myositis, infective
  traumatic (old) — *see* Myositis, specified type NEC
Myospasia impulsiva F95.2
Myotonia (acquisita) (intermittens) M62.89
  atrophica G71.11
  chondrodystrophic G71.13
  congenita (acetazolamide responsive) (dominant) (recessive) G71.12
  drug-induced G71.14
  dystrophica G71.11
  fluctuans G71.19
  levior G71.12
  permanens G71.19
  symptomatic G71.19
Myotonic pupil — *see* Anomaly, pupil, function, tonic pupil
Myriapodiasis B88.2
Myringitis H73.2- ☑
  with otitis media — *see* Otitis, media
  acute H73.00- ☑
    bullous H73.01- ☑
    specified NEC H73.09- ☑
  bullous — *see* Myringitis, acute, bullous
  chronic H73.1- ☑
Mysophobia F40.228
Mytilotoxism — *see* Poisoning, fish
Myxadenitis labialis K13.0
Myxedema (adult) (idiocy) (infantile) (juvenile) — *see also* Hypothyroidism E03.9
  circumscribed E05.90
    with storm E05.91
  coma E03.5
  congenital E00.1
  cutis L98.5
  localized (pretibial) E05.90
    with storm E05.91
  papular L98.5
Myxochondrosarcoma — *see* Neoplasm, cartilage, malignant
Myxofibroma — *see* Neoplasm, connective tissue, benign
  odontogenic — *see* Cyst, calcifying odontogenic
Myxofibrosarcoma — *see* Neoplasm, connective tissue, malignant
Myxolipoma D17.9
Myxoliposarcoma — *see* Neoplasm, connective tissue, malignant
Myxoma — *see also* Neoplasm, connective tissue, benign
  nerve sheath — *see* Neoplasm, nerve, benign
  odontogenic — *see* Cyst, calcifying odontogenic
Myxosarcoma — *see* Neoplasm, connective tissue, malignant

N

Naegeli's
  disease Q82.8
  leukemia, monocytic C93.1- ☑
Naegleriasis (with meningoencephalitis) B60.2
Naffziger's syndrome G54.0
Naga sore — *see* Ulcer, skin
Nägele's pelvis M95.5
  with disproportion (fetopelvic) O33.0
    causing obstructed labor O65.0
Nail — *see also* condition
  biting F98.8
  patella syndrome Q87.2
Nanism, nanosomia — *see* Dwarfism
Nanophyetiasis B66.8
Nanukayami A27.89
Napkin rash L22
Narcolepsy G47.419
  with cataplexy G47.411
  in conditions classified elsewhere G47.429
    with cataplexy G47.421
Narcosis R06.89
Narcotism — *see* Dependence
NARP (Neuropathy, Ataxia and Retinitis pigmentosa) syndrome E88.49
Narrow
  anterior chamber angle H40.03- ☑
  gingival width (of periodontal soft tissue) K05.5
  pelvis — *see* Contraction, pelvis
Narrowing — *see also* Stenosis
  artery I77.1
    auditory, internal I65.8
    basilar — *see* Occlusion, artery, basilar
    carotid — *see* Occlusion, artery, carotid
    cerebellar — *see* Occlusion, artery, cerebellar
    cerebral — *see* Occlusion artery, cerebral
    choroidal — *see* Occlusion, artery, precerebral, specified NEC
    communicating posterior — *see* Occlusion, artery, precerebral, specified NEC
    coronary — *see also* Disease, heart, ischemic, atherosclerotic
      congenital Q24.5
      syphilitic A50.54 *[I52]*
      due to syphilis NEC A52.06
    hypophyseal — *see* Occlusion, artery, precerebral, specified NEC
    pontine — *see* Occlusion, artery, precerebral, specified NEC
    precerebral — *see* Occlusion, artery, precerebral
    vertebral — *see* Occlusion, artery, vertebral
  auditory canal (external) — *see* Stenosis, external ear canal
  caudal septum, fixed, lower lateral cartilage, alar rim and nasal sill J34.8211
  eustachian tube — *see* Obstruction, eustachian tube
  eyelid — *see* Disorder, eyelid function
  larynx J38.6
  mesenteric artery — *see also* Ischemia, intestine, acute K55.059
  nasal septum, head of the inferior turbinate and the upper lateral cartilage J34.8201
  palate M26.89
  palpebral fissure — *see* Disorder, eyelid function
  ureter N13.5
    with infection N13.6
  urethra — *see* Stricture, urethra
Narrowness, abnormal, eyelid Q10.3
Nasal — *see* condition
Nasolachrymal, nasolacrimal — *see* condition
Nasopharyngeal — *see also* condition
  pituitary gland Q89.2
  torticollis M43.6
Nasopharyngitis (acute) (infective) (streptococcal) (subacute) J00
  chronic (suppurative) (ulcerative) J31.1
Nasopharynx, nasopharyngeal — *see* condition
Natal tooth, teeth K00.6
Nausea (without vomiting) R11.0
  with vomiting R11.2
  gravidarum — *see* Hyperemesis, gravidarum
  marina T75.3 ☑
  navalis T75.3 ☑
Navel — *see* condition
Neapolitan fever — *see* Brucellosis
Near drowning T75.1 ☑

Nearsightedness — *see* Myopia
Near-syncope R55
Nebula, cornea — *see* Opacity, cornea
Necator americanus infestation B76.1
Necatoriasis B76.1
Neck — *see* condition
Necrobiosis R68.89
  lipoidica NEC L92.1
    with diabetes — *see* E08-E13 with .620
Necrolysis, toxic epidermal L51.2
  due to drug
    correct substance properly administered — *see* Table of Drugs and Chemicals, by drug, adverse effect
    overdose or wrong substance given or taken — *see* Table of Drugs and Chemicals, by drug, poisoning
Necrophilia F65.89
Necrosis, necrotic (ischemic) — *see also* Gangrene
  adrenal (capsule) (gland) E27.49
  amputation stump (surgical) (late) T87.50
    arm T87.5- ☑
    leg T87.5- ☑
  antrum J32.0
  aorta (hyaline) — *see also* Aneurysm, aorta
    cystic medial — *see* Dissection, aorta
  artery I77.5
  bladder (aseptic) (sphincter) N32.89
  bone — *see also* Osteonecrosis M87.9
    aseptic or avascular — *see* Osteonecrosis
      idiopathic M87.00
    ethmoid J32.2
    jaw M27.2
    tuberculous — *see* Tuberculosis, bone
  brain I67.89
  breast (aseptic) (fat) (segmental) N64.1
  bronchus J98.09
  central nervous system NEC I67.89
  cerebellar I67.89
  cerebral I67.89
  colon — *see also* Infarct, intestine K55.049
  cornea H18.89- ☑
  cortical (acute) (renal) N17.1
  cystic medial (aorta) — *see* Dissection, aorta
  dental pulp K04.1
  esophagus K22.89
  ethmoid (bone) J32.2
  eyelid — *see* Disorder, eyelid, degenerative
  fat, fatty (generalized) — *see also* Disorder, soft tissue, specified type NEC
    abdominal wall K65.4
    breast (aseptic) (segmental) N64.1
    localized — *see* Degeneration, by site, fatty
    mesentery K65.4
    omentum K65.4
    pancreas K86.89
    peritoneum K65.4
    skin (subcutaneous), newborn P83.0
    subcutaneous, due to birth injury P15.6
  gallbladder — *see* Cholecystitis, acute
  heart — *see* Infarct, myocardium
  hip, aseptic or avascular — *see* Osteonecrosis, by type, femur
  intestine (acute) (hemorrhagic) (massive) — *see also* Infarct, intestine K55.069
  jaw M27.2
  kidney (bilateral) N28.0
    acute N17.9
    cortical (acute) (bilateral) N17.1
      with ectopic or molar pregnancy O08.4
    medullary (bilateral) (in acute renal failure) (papillary) N17.2
    papillary (bilateral) (in acute renal failure) N17.2
    tubular N17.0
      with ectopic or molar pregnancy O08.4
      complicating
        abortion — *see* Abortion, by type, complicated by, tubular necrosis
        ectopic or molar pregnancy O08.4
        pregnancy — *see* Pregnancy, complicated by, diseases of, specified type or system NEC
      following ectopic or molar pregnancy O08.4
      traumatic T79.5 ☑
  larynx J38.7
  liver (with hepatic failure) (cell) — *see* Failure, hepatic hemorrhagic, central K76.2
  lung J85.0
  lymphatic gland — *see* Lymphadenitis, acute
  mammary gland (fat) (segmental) N64.1
  mastoid (chronic) — *see* Mastoiditis, chronic

Necrosis, necrotic — *continued*
  medullary (acute) (renal) N17.2
  mesentery — *see also* Infarct, intestine K55.069
    fat K65.4
  mitral valve — *see* Insufficiency, mitral
  myocardium, myocardial — *see* Infarct, myocardium
  nose J34.0
  omentum (with mesenteric infarction) — *see also* Infarct, intestine K55.069
    fat K65.4
  orbit, orbital — *see* Osteomyelitis, orbit
  ossicles, ear — *see* Abnormal, ear ossicles
  ovary N70.92
  pancreas (aseptic) (duct) (fat) K86.89
    acute (infective) — *see* Pancreatitis, acute
    infective — *see* Pancreatitis, acute
  papillary (acute) (renal) N17.2
  perineum N90.89
  peritoneum (with mesenteric infarction) — *see also* Infarct, intestine K55.069
    fat K65.4
  pharynx J02.9
    in granulocytopenia — *see* Neutropenia
    Vincent's A69.1
  phosphorus — *see* subcategory T54.2 ☑
  pituitary (gland) E23.0
    postpartum O99.285
    Sheehan O99.285
  pressure — *see* Ulcer, pressure, by site
  pulmonary J85.0
  pulp (dental) K04.1
  radiation — *see* Necrosis, by site
  radium — *see* Necrosis, by site
  renal — *see* Necrosis, kidney
  sclera H15.89
  scrotum N50.89
  skin or subcutaneous tissue NEC I96
  spine, spinal (column) — *see also* Osteonecrosis, by type, vertebra
    cord G95.19
  spleen D73.5
  stomach K31.89
  stomatitis (ulcerative) A69.0
  subcutaneous fat, newborn P83.88
  subendocardial (acute) I21.4
    chronic I25.89
  suprarenal (capsule) (gland) E27.49
  testis N50.89
  thymus (gland) E32.8
  tonsil J35.8
  trachea J39.8
  tuberculous NEC — *see* Tuberculosis
  tubular (acute) (anoxic) (renal) (toxic) N17.0
    postprocedural N99.0
  vagina N89.8
  vertebra — *see also* Osteonecrosis, by type, vertebra
    tuberculous A18.01
  vulva N90.89
  X-ray — *see* Necrosis, by site
Necrospermia — *see* Infertility, male
Need (for)
  care provider because (of)
    assistance with personal care Z74.1
    continuous supervision required Z74.3
    impaired mobility Z74.09
    no other household member able to render care Z74.2
    specified reason NEC Z74.8
  immunization — *see* Vaccination
  vaccination — *see* Vaccination
Neglect
  adult
    confirmed T74.01 ☑
    history of Z91.412
    suspected T76.01 ☑
  child (childhood)
    confirmed T74.02 ☑
    history of Z62.812
    suspected T76.02 ☑
  emotional, in childhood Z62.898
  hemispatial R41.4
  left-sided R41.4
  sensory R41.4
  visuospatial R41.4
Neisserian infection NEC — *see* Gonococcus
Nelaton's syndrome G60.8
Nelson's syndrome E24.1
Nematodiasis (intestinal) B82.0
  Ancylostoma B76.0

Neonatal — *see also* Newborn
  acne L70.4
  bradycardia P29.12
  screening, abnormal findings on — *see* Abnormal,
    neonatal screening
  tachycardia P29.11
  tooth, teeth K00.6
Neonatorum — *see* condition
Neoplasia
  endocrine, multiple (MEN) E31.20
    type I E31.21
    type IIA E31.22
    type IIB E31.23
  intraepithelial (histologically confirmed)
    anal (AIN) (histologically confirmed) K62.82
      grade I K62.82
      grade II K62.82
      severe D01.3
    cervical glandular (histologically confirmed) D06.9
    cervix (uteri) (CIN) (histologically confirmed) N87.9
      glandular D06.9
      grade I N87.0
      grade II N87.1
      grade III (severe dysplasia) — *see also* Carcinoma,
        cervix uteri, in situ D06.9
    prostate (histologically confirmed) (PIN) N42.31
      grade I N42.31
      grade II N42.31
      grade III (severe dysplasia) D07.5
    vagina (histologically confirmed) (VAIN) N89.3
      grade I N89.0
      grade II N89.1
      grade III (severe dysplasia) D07.2
    vulva (histologically confirmed) (VIN) N90.3
      grade I N90.0
      grade II N90.1
      grade III (severe dysplasia) D07.1
Neoplasm, neoplastic — *see also* Table of Neoplasms
  lipomatous, benign — *see* Lipoma
  malignant mast cell C96.20
    specified type NEC C96.29
  mast cell, of uncertain behavior NEC D47.09
  myelodysplastic/myeloproliferative, unclassifiable C94.6
Neovascularization
  ciliary body — *see* Disorder, iris, vascular
  cornea H16.40- ☑
    deep H16.44- ☑
    ghost vessels — *see* Ghost, vessels
    localized H16.43- ☑
    pannus — *see* Pannus
  iris — *see* Disorder, iris, vascular
  retina H35.05- ☑
Nephralgia N23
Nephritis, nephritic (albuminuric) (azotemic) (congenital)
    (disseminated) (epithelial) (familial) (focal) (granulo-
    matous) (hemorrhagic) (infantile) (nonsuppurative,
    excretory) (uremic) N05.9
  with
    C3
      glomerulonephritis N05.A
      glomerulopathy N05.A
        with dense deposit disease N05.6
      dense deposit disease N05.6
      diffuse
        crescentic glomerulonephritis N05.7
        endocapillary proliferative glomerulonephritis
          N05.4
        membranous glomerulonephritis N05.2
        mesangial proliferative glomerulonephritis N05.3
        mesangiocapillary glomerulonephritis N05.5
      edema — *see* Nephrosis
      focal and segmental glomerular lesions N05.1
      foot process disease N04.9
      glomerular lesion
        diffuse sclerosing N05.8
        hypocomplementemic — *see* Nephritis, membra-
          noproliferative
        IgA — *see* Nephropathy, IgA
        lobular, lobulonodular — *see* Nephritis, membra-
          noproliferative
        nodular — *see* Nephritis, membranoproliferative
      lesion of
        glomerulonephritis, proliferative N05.8
        renal necrosis N05.9
      minor glomerular abnormality N05.0
      specified morphological changes NEC N05.8
  acute N00.9

Nephritis, nephritic — *continued*
  acute — *continued*
    with
      C3
        glomerulonephritis N00.A
        glomerulopathy N00.A
          with dense deposit disease N00.6
        dense deposit disease N00.6
        diffuse
          crescentic glomerulonephritis N00.7
          endocapillary proliferative glomerulonephritis
            N00.4
          membranous glomerulonephritis N00.2
          mesangial proliferative glomerulonephritis
            N00.3
          mesangiocapillary glomerulonephritis N00.5
        focal and segmental glomerular lesions N00.1
        minor glomerular abnormality N00.0
        specified morphological changes NEC N00.8
    amyloid E85.4 *[N08]*
    antiglomerular basement membrane (anti-GBM) anti-
      body NEC
      in Goodpasture's syndrome M31.0
    antitubular basement membrane (tubulo-interstitial)
      NEC N12
      toxic — *see* Nephropathy, toxic
    arteriolar — *see* Hypertension, kidney
    arteriosclerotic — *see* Hypertension, kidney
    ascending — *see* Nephritis, tubulo-interstitial
    atrophic N03.9
    Balkan (endemic) N15.0
    calculous, calculus — *see* Calculus, kidney
    cardiac — *see* Hypertension, kidney
    cardiovascular — *see* Hypertension, kidney
    chronic N03.9
      with
        C3
          glomerulonephritis N03.A
          glomerulopathy N03.A
            with dense deposit disease N03.6
          dense deposit disease N03.6
          diffuse
            crescentic glomerulonephritis N03.7
            endocapillary proliferative glomerulonephritis
              N03.4
            membranous glomerulonephritis N03.2
            mesangial proliferative glomerulonephritis
              N03.3
            mesangiocapillary glomerulonephritis N03.5
          focal and segmental glomerular lesions N03.1
          minor glomerular abnormality N03.0
          specified morphological changes NEC N03.8
    arteriosclerotic — *see* Hypertension, kidney
    cirrhotic N26.9
    complicating pregnancy O26.83- ☑
    croupous N00.9
    degenerative — *see* Nephrosis
    diffuse sclerosing N05.8
    due to
      diabetes mellitus — *see* E08-E13 with .21
      subacute bacterial endocarditis I33.0
      systemic lupus erythematosus (chronic) M32.14
      typhoid fever A01.09
    gonococcal (acute) (chronic) A54.21
    hypocomplementemic — *see* Nephritis, membranopro-
      liferative
    IgA — *see* Nephropathy, IgA
    immune complex (circulating) NEC N05.8
    infective — *see* Nephritis, tubulo-interstitial
    interstitial — *see* Nephritis, tubulo-interstitial
    lead N14.3
    membranoproliferative (diffuse) (type 1 or 3) — *see also*
      N00-N07 with fourth character .5 N05.5
      type 2 — *see also* N00-N07 with fourth character .6
        N05.6
    minimal change N05.0
    necrotic, necrotizing NEC — *see also* N00-N07 with fourth
      character .8 N05.8
    nephrotic — *see* Nephrosis
    nodular — *see* Nephritis, membranoproliferative
    polycystic Q61.3
      adult type Q61.2
      autosomal
        dominant Q61.2
        recessive NEC Q61.19
          childhood type NEC Q61.19
          infantile type NEC Q61.19
    poststreptococcal N05.9
      acute N00.9

Nephritis, nephritic — *continued*
  poststreptococcal — *continued*
    chronic N03.9
    rapidly progressive N01.9
  proliferative NEC — *see also* N00-N07 with fourth charac-
    ter .8 N05.8
  purulent — *see* Nephritis, tubulo-interstitial
  rapidly progressive N01.9
    with
      C3
        glomerulonephritis N01.A
        glomerulopathy N01.A
          with dense deposit disease N01.6
        dense deposit disease N01.6
        diffuse
          crescentic glomerulonephritis N01.7
          endocapillary proliferative glomerulonephritis
            N01.4
          membranous glomerulonephritis N01.2
          mesangial proliferative glomerulonephritis
            N01.3
          mesangiocapillary glomerulonephritis N01.5
        focal and segmental glomerular lesions N01.1
        minor glomerular abnormality N01.0
        specified morphological changes NEC N01.8
  salt losing or wasting NEC N28.89
  saturnine N14.3
  sclerosing, diffuse N05.8
  septic — *see* Nephritis, tubulo-interstitial
  specified pathology NEC — *see also* N00-N07 with fourth
    character .8 N05.8
  subacute N01.9
  suppurative — *see* Nephritis, tubulo-interstitial
  syphilitic (late) A52.75
    congenital A50.59 *[N08]*
    early (secondary) A51.44
  toxic — *see* Nephropathy, toxic
  tubal, tubular — *see* Nephritis, tubulo-interstitial
  tuberculous A18.11
  tubulo-interstitial (in) N12
    acute (infectious) N10
    chronic (infectious) N11.9
      nonobstructive N11.8
        reflux-associated N11.0
      obstructive N11.1
      specified NEC N11.8
    due to
      brucellosis A23.9 *[N16]*
      cryoglobulinemia D89.1 *[N16]*
      glycogen storage disease E74.00 *[N16]*
      Sjogren's syndrome M35.04
  vascular — *see* Hypertension, kidney
  war N00.9
Nephroblastoma (epithelial) (mesenchymal) C64- ☑
Nephrocalcinosis E83.59 *[N29]*
Nephrocystitis, pustular — *see* Nephritis, tubulo-interstitial
Nephrolithiasis (congenital) (pelvis) (recurrent) — *see also*
    Calculus, kidney
Nephroma C64- ☑
  mesoblastic D41.0- ☑
Nephronephritis — *see* Nephrosis
Nephronophthisis Q61.5
Nephropathia epidemica A98.5
Nephropathy — *see also* Nephritis N28.9
  with
    edema — *see* Nephrosis
    glomerular lesion — *see* Glomerulonephritis
  amyloid, hereditary E85.0
  analgesic N14.0
    with medullary necrosis, acute N17.2
  Balkan (endemic) N15.0
  chemical — *see* Nephropathy, toxic
  contrast medium, radiography N14.11
  contrast-induced N14.11
  diabetic — *see* E08-E13 with .21
  drug-induced N14.2
    contrast-induced N14.11
    specified NEC N14.19
  focal and segmental hyalinosis or sclerosis N02.1
  heavy metal-induced N14.3
  hereditary NEC N07.9
    with
      C3
        glomerulonephritis N07.A
        glomerulopathy N07.A
          with dense deposit disease N07.6
        dense deposit disease N07.6
        diffuse
          crescentic glomerulonephritis N07.7

Nephropathy — *continued*
  hereditary — *continued*
    with — *continued*
      diffuse — *continued*
        endocapillary proliferative glomerulonephritis N07.4
        membranous glomerulonephritis N07.2
        mesangial proliferative glomerulonephritis N07.3
        mesangiocapillary glomerulonephritis N07.5
      focal and segmental glomerular lesions N07.1
      minor glomerular abnormality N07.0
      specified morphological changes NEC N07.8
  hypercalcemic N25.89
  hypertensive — *see* Hypertension, kidney
  hypokalemic (vacuolar) N25.89
  IgA N02.B- ☑
    with glomerular lesion N02.B1
      focal and segmental hyalinosis or sclerosis N02.B2
      membranoproliferative (diffuse) N02.B3
      membranous (diffuse) N02.B4
      mesangial proliferative (diffuse) N02.B5
      mesangiocapillary (diffuse) N02.B6
      proliferative NEC N02.B9
      specified pathology NEC N02.B9
  lead N14.3
  membranoproliferative (diffuse) N02.5
  membranous (diffuse) N06.20
    with
      nephrotic syndrome N04.20
        primary N04.21
        secondary N04.22
      idiopathic, with nephrotic syndrome N04.21
      primary N06.21
        with nephrotic syndrome N04.21
      secondary N06.22
        with nephrotic syndrome N04.22
  mesangial (IgA/IgG) — *see* Nephropathy, IgA
    proliferative (diffuse) N02.3
  mesangiocapillary (diffuse) N02.5
  obstructive N13.8
  phenacetin N17.2
  phosphate-losing N25.0
  potassium depletion N25.89
  pregnancy-related O26.83- ☑
  proliferative NEC — *see also* N00-N07 with fourth character .8 N05.8
  protein-losing N25.89
  saturnine N14.3
  sickle-cell D57.- ☑ *[N08]*
  toxic NEC N14.4
    due to
      drugs N14.2
        analgesic N14.0
        specified NEC N14.19
      heavy metals N14.3
  vasomotor N17.0
  water-losing N25.89
Nephroptosis N28.83
Nephropyosis — *see* Abscess, kidney
Nephrorrhagia N28.89
Nephrosclerosis (arteriolar) (arteriosclerotic) (chronic) (hyaline) — *see also* Hypertension, kidney
  hyperplastic — *see* Hypertension, kidney
  senile N26.9
Nephrosis, nephrotic (Epstein's) (syndrome) (congenital) N04.9
  with
    foot process disease N04.9
    glomerular lesion N04.1
    hypocomplementemic N04.5
  acute N04.9
  anoxic — *see* Nephrosis, tubular
  chemical — *see* Nephrosis, tubular
  cholemic K76.7
  diabetic — *see* E08-E13 with .21
  Finnish type (congenital) Q89.8
  hemoglobin N10
  hemoglobinuric — *see* Nephrosis, tubular
  in
    amyloidosis E85.4 *[N08]*
    diabetes mellitus — *see* E08-E13 with .21
    epidemic hemorrhagic fever A98.5
    malaria (malariae) B52.0
  ischemic — *see* Nephrosis, tubular
  lipoid N04.9
  lower nephron — *see* Nephrosis, tubular
  malarial (malariae) B52.0
  minimal change N04.0

Nephrosis, nephrotic — *continued*
  myoglobin N10
  necrotizing — *see* Nephrosis, tubular
  osmotic (sucrose) N25.89
  radiation N04.9
  syphilitic (late) A52.75
  toxic — *see* Nephrosis, tubular
  tubular (acute) N17.0
    postprocedural N99.0
    radiation N04.9
Nephrosonephritis, hemorrhagic (endemic) A98.5
Nephrostomy
  attention to Z43.6
  status Z93.6
Nerve — *see also* condition
  injury — *see* Injury, nerve, by body site
Nerves R45.0
Nervous — *see also* condition R45.0
  heart F45.8
  stomach F45.8
  tension R45.0
Nervousness R45.0
Nesidioblastoma
  pancreas D13.7
  specified site NEC — *see* Neoplasm, benign, by site
  unspecified site D13.7
Nettleship's syndrome — *see* Urticaria pigmentosa
Neumann's disease or syndrome L10.1
Neuralgia, neuralgic (acute) M79.2
  accessory (nerve) G52.8
  acoustic (nerve) — *see* subcategory H93.3 ☑
  auditory (nerve) — *see* subcategory H93.3 ☑
  ciliary G44.009
    intractable G44.001
    not intractable G44.009
  cranial
    nerve — *see also* Disorder, nerve, cranial
      fifth or trigeminal — *see* Neuralgia, trigeminal
    postherpetic, postzoster B02.29
  ear — *see* subcategory H92.0 ☑
  facialis vera G51.1
  Fothergill's — *see* Neuralgia, trigeminal
  glossopharyngeal (nerve) G52.1
  Horton's G44.099
    intractable G44.091
    not intractable G44.099
  Hunt's B02.21
  hypoglossal (nerve) G52.3
  infraorbital — *see* Neuralgia, trigeminal
  malarial — *see* Malaria
  migrainous G44.009
    intractable G44.001
    not intractable G44.009
  Morton's G57.6- ☑
  nerve, cranial — *see* Disorder, nerve, cranial
  nose G52.0
  occipital M54.81
  olfactory G52.0
  penis N48.9
  perineum R10.2
  postherpetic NEC B02.29
    trigeminal B02.22
  pubic region R10.2
  scrotum R10.2
  Sluder's G44.89
  specified nerve NEC G58.8
  spermatic cord R10.2
  sphenopalatine (ganglion) G90.09
  trifacial — *see* Neuralgia, trigeminal
  trigeminal G50.0
    postherpetic, postzoster B02.22
  vagus (nerve) G52.2
  writer's F48.8
    organic G25.89
Neurapraxia — *see* Injury, nerve
Neurasthenia F48.8
  cardiac F45.8
  gastric F45.8
  heart F45.8
Neurilemmoma — *see also* Neoplasm, nerve, benign
  acoustic (nerve) D33.3
  malignant — *see also* Neoplasm, nerve, malignant
    acoustic (nerve) C72.4- ☑
Neurilemmosarcoma — *see* Neoplasm, nerve, malignant
Neurinoma — *see* Neoplasm, nerve, benign
Neurinomatosis — *see* Neoplasm, nerve, uncertain behavior
Neuritis (rheumatoid) M79.2

Neuritis — *continued*
  abducens (nerve) — *see* Strabismus, paralytic, sixth nerve
  accessory (nerve) G52.8
  acoustic (nerve) — *see also* subcategory H93.3 ☑
    in (due to)
      infectious disease NEC B99 ☑ *[H94.0-]* ☑
      parasitic disease NEC B89 *[H94.0-]* ☑
    syphilitic A52.15
  alcoholic G62.1
    with psychosis — *see* Psychosis, alcoholic
  amyloid, any site E85.4 *[G63]*
  auditory (nerve) — *see* subcategory H93.3 ☑
  brachial — *see* Radiculopathy
    due to displacement, intervertebral disc — *see* Disorder, disc, cervical, with neuritis
  cranial nerve
    due to Lyme disease A69.22
    eighth or acoustic or auditory — *see* subcategory H93.3 ☑
    eleventh or accessory G52.8
    fifth or trigeminal G50.- ☑
    first or olfactory G52.0
    fourth or trochlear — *see* Strabismus, paralytic, fourth nerve
    second or optic — *see* Neuritis, optic
    seventh or facial G51.8
      newborn (birth injury) P11.3
    sixth or abducent — *see* Strabismus, paralytic, sixth nerve
    tenth or vagus G52.2
    third or oculomotor — *see* Strabismus, paralytic, third nerve
    twelfth or hypoglossal G52.3
  Dejerine-Sottas G60.0
  diabetic (mononeuropathy) — *see* E08-E13 with .41
    polyneuropathy — *see* E08-E13 with .42
  due to
    beriberi E51.11
    displacement, prolapse or rupture, intervertebral disc — *see* Disorder, disc, with, radiculopathy
    herniation, nucleus pulposus M51.9 *[G55]*
  endemic E51.11
  facial G51.8
    newborn (birth injury) P11.3
  general — *see* Polyneuropathy
  geniculate ganglion G51.1
    due to herpes (zoster) B02.21
  gouty — *see also* Gout, by type M10.9 *[G63]*
  hypoglossal (nerve) G52.3
  ilioinguinal (nerve) G57.9- ☑
  infectious (multiple) NEC G61.0
  interstitial hypertrophic progressive G60.0
  lumbar M54.16
  lumbosacral M54.17
  multiple — *see also* Polyneuropathy
    endemic E51.11
    infective, acute G61.0
  multiplex endemica E51.11
  nerve root — *see* Radiculopathy
  oculomotor (nerve) — *see* Strabismus, paralytic, third nerve
  olfactory nerve G52.0
  optic (nerve) (hereditary) (sympathetic) H46.9
    with demyelination G36.0
    in myelitis G36.0
    nutritional H46.2
    papillitis — *see* Papillitis, optic
    retrobulbar H46.1- ☑
    specified type NEC H46.8
    toxic H46.3
  peripheral (nerve) G62.9
    multiple — *see* Polyneuropathy
    single — *see* Mononeuritis
  pneumogastric (nerve) G52.2
  postherpetic, postzoster B02.29
  progressive hypertrophic interstitial G60.0
  retrobulbar — *see also* Neuritis, optic, retrobulbar
    in (due to)
      late syphilis A52.15
      meningococcal infection A39.82
    meningococcal A39.82
    syphilitic A52.15
  sciatic (nerve) — *see also* Sciatica
    due to displacement of intervertebral disc — *see* Disorder, disc, with, radiculopathy
  serum — *see also* Reaction, serum T80.69 ☑
  shoulder-girdle G54.5
  specified nerve NEC G58.8

☑ **Additional Character Required** — **Refer to the Tabular List for Character Selection**

Neuritis — *continued*
  spinal (nerve) root — *see* Radiculopathy
  syphilitic A52.15
  thenar (median) G56.1- ☑
  thoracic M54.14
  toxic NEC G62.2
  trochlear (nerve) — *see* Strabismus, paralytic, fourth nerve
  vagus (nerve) G52.2
Neuroastrocytoma — *see* Neoplasm, uncertain behavior, by site
Neuroavitaminosis E56.9 *[G99.8]*
Neuroblastoma
  olfactory C30.0
  specified site — *see* Neoplasm, malignant, by site
  unspecified site C74.90
Neurochorioretinitis — *see* Chorioretinitis
Neurocirculatory asthenia F45.8
Neurocysticercosis B69.0
Neurocytoma — *see* Neoplasm, benign, by site
Neurodermatitis (circumscribed) (circumscripta) (local) L28.0
  atopic L20.81
  diffuse (Brocq) L20.81
  disseminated L20.81
Neuroencephalomyelopathy, optic G36.0
Neuroepithelioma — *see also* Neoplasm, malignant, by site
  olfactory C30.0
Neurofibroma — *see also* Neoplasm, nerve, benign
  melanotic — *see* Neoplasm, nerve, benign
  multiple — *see* Neurofibromatosis
  plexiform — *see* Neoplasm, nerve, benign
Neurofibromatosis (multiple) (nonmalignant) Q85.00
  acoustic Q85.02
  malignant — *see* Neoplasm, nerve, malignant
  specified NEC Q85.09
  type 1 (von Recklinghausen) Q85.01
  type 2 Q85.02
Neurofibrosarcoma — *see* Neoplasm, nerve, malignant
Neurogenic — *see also* condition
  bladder — *see also* Dysfunction, bladder, neuromuscular N31.9
    cauda equina syndrome G83.4
  bowel NEC K59.2
  heart F45.8
Neuroglioma — *see* Neoplasm, uncertain behavior, by site
Neurolabyrinthitis (of Dix and Hallpike) — *see* Neuronitis, vestibular
Neurolathyrism — *see* Poisoning, food, noxious, plant
Neuroleprosy A30.9
Neuroma — *see also* Neoplasm, nerve, benign
  acoustic (nerve) D33.3
  amputation (stump) (traumatic) (surgical complication) (late) T87.3- ☑
    arm T87.3- ☑
    leg T87.3- ☑
  digital (toe) G57.6- ☑
  interdigital G58.8
    lower limb (toe) G57.8- ☑
    upper limb G56.8- ☑
  intermetatarsal G57.8- ☑
  Morton's G57.6- ☑
  nonneoplastic
    arm G56.9- ☑
    leg G57.9- ☑
    lower extremity G57.9- ☑
    upper extremity G56.9- ☑
  optic (nerve) D33.3
  plantar G57.6- ☑
  plexiform — *see* Neoplasm, nerve, benign
  surgical (nonneoplastic)
    arm G56.9- ☑
    leg G57.9- ☑
    lower extremity G57.9- ☑
    upper extremity G56.9- ☑
Neuromyalgia — *see* Neuralgia
Neuromyasthenia (epidemic) (postinfectious) G93.39
Neuromyelitis G36.9
  ascending G61.0
  optica G36.0
Neuromyopathy G70.9
  paraneoplastic — *see also*, Neoplasm, by site, if known D49.9 *[G13.0]*
Neuromyotonia (Isaacs) G71.19
Neuronevus — *see* Nevus
Neuronitis G58.9
  ascending (acute) G57.2- ☑

Neuronitis — *continued*
  vestibular H81.2- ☑
Neuroparalytic — *see* condition
Neuropathy, neuropathic G62.9
  acute motor G62.81
  alcoholic G62.1
    with psychosis — *see* Psychosis, alcoholic
  arm G56.9- ☑
  autonomic, peripheral — *see* Neuropathy, peripheral, autonomic
  axillary G56.9- ☑
  bladder N31.9
    atonic (motor) (sensory) N31.2
    autonomous N31.2
    flaccid N31.2
    nonreflex N31.2
    reflex N31.1
    uninhibited N31.0
  brachial plexus G54.0
  cervical plexus G54.2
  chronic
    progressive segmentally demyelinating G62.89
    relapsing demyelinating G62.89
  Dejerine-Sottas G60.0
  diabetic — *see* E08-E13 with .40
    mononeuropathy — *see* E08-E13 with .41
    polyneuropathy — *see* E08-E13 with .42
  entrapment G58.9
    iliohypogastric nerve G57.8- ☑
    ilioinguinal nerve G57.8- ☑
    lateral cutaneous nerve of thigh G57.1- ☑
    median nerve G56.0- ☑
    obturator nerve G57.8- ☑
    peroneal nerve G57.3- ☑
    posterior tibial nerve G57.5- ☑
    saphenous nerve G57.8- ☑
    ulnar nerve G56.2- ☑
  facial nerve G51.9
  hereditary G60.9
    motor and sensory (types I-IV) G60.0
    sensory G60.8
    specified NEC G60.8
  hypertrophic G60.0
    Charcot-Marie-Tooth G60.0
    Dejerine-Sottas G60.0
    interstitial progressive G60.0
    of infancy G60.0
    Refsum G60.1
  idiopathic G60.9
    progressive G60.3
    specified NEC G60.8
  in association with hereditary ataxia G60.2
  intercostal G58.0
  ischemic — *see* Disorder, nerve
  Jamaica (ginger) G62.2
  leg NEC G57.9- ☑
  lower extremity G57.9- ☑
  lumbar plexus G54.1
  median nerve G56.1- ☑
  motor and sensory — *see also* Polyneuropathy
    hereditary (types I-IV) G60.0
  multifocal motor (MMN) G61.82
  multiple (acute) (chronic) — *see* Polyneuropathy
  optic (nerve) — *see also* Neuritis, optic
    ischemic H47.01- ☑
  paraneoplastic (sensorial) (Denny Brown) — *see also*, Neoplasm, by site, if known D49.9 *[G13.0]*
  peripheral (nerve) — *see also* Polyneuropathy G62.9
    autonomic G90.9
      idiopathic G90.09
      in (due to)
        amyloidosis E85.4 *[G99.0]*
        diabetes mellitus — *see* E08-E13 with .43
        endocrine disease NEC E34.9 *[G99.0]*
        gout M10.00 *[G99.0]*
        hyperthyroidism E05.90 *[G99.0]*
          with thyroid storm E05.91 *[G99.0]*
        metabolic disease NEC E88.9 *[G99.0]*
    idiopathic G60.9
      progressive G60.3
    in (due to)
      antitetanus serum G62.0
      arsenic G62.2
      drugs NEC G62.0
      lead G62.2
      organophosphate compounds G62.2
      toxic agent NEC G62.2
  plantar nerves G57.6- ☑

Neuropathy, neuropathic — *continued*
  progressive
    hypertrophic interstitial G60.0
    inflammatory G62.81
  radicular NEC — *see* Radiculopathy
  sacral plexus G54.1
  sciatic G57.0- ☑
  serum G61.1
  toxic NEC G62.2
  trigeminal sensory G50.8
  ulnar nerve G56.2- ☑
  uremic N18.9 *[G63]*
  vitamin B12 E53.8 *[G63]*
    with anemia (pernicious) D51.0 *[G63]*
      due to dietary deficiency D51.3 *[G63]*
Neurophthisis — *see also* Disorder, nerve
  peripheral, diabetic — *see* E08-E13 with .42
Neuroretinitis — *see* Chorioretinitis
Neuroretinopathy, hereditary optic H47.22
Neurosarcoma — *see* Neoplasm, nerve, malignant
Neurosclerosis — *see* Disorder, nerve
Neurosis, neurotic F48.9
  anankastic F42.8
  anxiety (state) F41.1
    panic type F41.0
  asthenic F48.8
  bladder F45.8
  cardiac (reflex) F45.8
  cardiovascular F45.8
  character F60.9
  colon F45.8
  compensation F68.10
  compulsive, compulsion F42.8
  conversion F44.9
  craft F48.8
  cutaneous F45.8
  depersonalization F48.1
  depressive (reaction) (type) F34.1
  environmental F48.8
  excoriation L98.1
  fatigue F48.8
  functional — *see* Disorder, somatoform
  gastric F45.8
  gastrointestinal F45.8
  heart F45.8
  hypochondriacal F45.21
  hysterical F44.9
  incoordination F45.8
    larynx F45.8
    vocal cord F45.8
  intestine F45.8
  larynx (sensory) F45.8
    hysterical F44.4
  mixed NEC F48.8
  musculoskeletal F45.8
  obsessional F42.8
  obsessive-compulsive F42.8
  occupational F48.8
  ocular NEC F45.8
  organ — *see* Disorder, somatoform
  pharynx F45.8
  phobic F40.9
  posttraumatic (situational) F43.10
    acute F43.11
    chronic F43.12
  psychasthenic (type) F48.8
  railroad F48.8
  rectum F45.8
  respiratory F45.8
  rumination F45.8
  sexual F65.9
  situational F48.8
  social F40.10
    generalized F40.11
  specified type NEC F48.8
  state F48.9
    with depersonalization episode F48.1
  stomach F45.8
  traumatic F43.10
    acute F43.11
    chronic F43.12
  vasomotor F45.8
  visceral F45.8
  war F48.8
Neurospongioblastosis diffusa Q85.1
Neurosyphilis (arrested) (early) (gumma) (late) (latent) (recurrent) (relapse) A52.3
  with ataxia (cerebellar) (locomotor) (spastic) (spinal) A52.19

☑ **Additional Character Required** — Refer to the Tabular List for Character Selection

Neurosyphilis — *continued*
- aneurysm (cerebral) A52.05
- arachnoid (adhesive) A52.13
- arteritis (any artery) (cerebral) A52.04
- asymptomatic A52.2
- congenital A50.40
- dura (mater) A52.13
- general paresis A52.17
- hemorrhagic A52.05
- juvenile (asymptomatic) (meningeal) A50.40
- leptomeninges (aseptic) A52.13
- meningeal, meninges (adhesive) A52.13
- meningitis A52.13
- meningovascular (diffuse) A52.13
- optic atrophy A52.15
- parenchymatous (degenerative) A52.19
- paresis, paretic A52.17
  - juvenile A50.45
- remission in (sustained) A52.3
- serological without symptoms A52.2
- specified nature or site NEC A52.19
- tabes, tabetic (dorsalis) A52.11
  - juvenile A50.45
- taboparesis (taboparetic) A52.17
  - juvenile A50.45
- thrombosis (cerebral) A52.05
- vascular (cerebral) NEC A52.05

Neurothekeoma — *see* Neoplasm, nerve, benign
Neurotic — *see* Neurosis
Neurotoxemia — *see* Toxemia
Neuroclusion M26.211
Neutropenia, neutropenic (chronic) (genetic) (idiopathic) (immune) (infantile) (malignant) (pernicious) (splenic) D70.9
- benign ethnic — *see* Phenotype, Duffy, null
- congenital (primary) D70.0
- cyclic D70.4
- cytoreductive cancer chemotherapy sequela D70.1
- drug-induced D70.2
  - due to cytoreductive cancer chemotherapy D70.1
- due to infection D70.3
- fever D70.9
- neonatal, transitory (isoimmune) (maternal transfer) P61.5
- periodic D70.4
- secondary (cyclic) (periodic) (splenic) D70.4
  - drug-induced D70.2
    - due to cytoreductive cancer chemotherapy D70.1
- specified NEC D70.8
- toxic D70.8

Neutrophilia, hereditary giant D72.0
Nevocarcinoma — *see* Melanoma
Nevus D22.9
- achromic — *see* Neoplasm, skin, benign
- amelanotic — *see* Neoplasm, skin, benign
- angiomatous D18.00
  - intra-abdominal D18.03
  - intracranial D18.02
  - skin D18.01
  - specified site NEC D18.09
- araneus I78.1
- balloon cell — *see* Neoplasm, skin, benign
- bathing trunk D48.5
- blue — *see* Neoplasm, skin, benign
  - cellular — *see* Neoplasm, skin, benign
  - giant — *see* Neoplasm, skin, benign
  - Jadassohn's — *see* Neoplasm, skin, benign
  - malignant — *see* Melanoma
- capillary D18.00
  - intra-abdominal D18.03
  - intracranial D18.02
  - skin D18.01
  - specified site NEC D18.09
- cavernous D18.00
  - intra-abdominal D18.03
  - intracranial D18.02
  - skin D18.01
  - specified site NEC D18.09
- cellular — *see* Neoplasm, skin, benign
  - blue — *see* Neoplasm, skin, benign
- choroid D31.3- ☑
- comedonicus Q82.5
- conjunctiva D31.0- ☑
- dermal — *see* Neoplasm, skin, benign
  - with epidermal nevus — *see* Neoplasm, skin, benign
- dysplastic — *see* Neoplasm, skin, benign
- eye D31.9- ☑
- flammeus Q82.5
- hemangiomatous D18.00

Nevus — *continued*
- hemangiomatous — *continued*
  - intra-abdominal D18.03
  - intracranial D18.02
  - skin D18.01
  - specified site NEC D18.09
- iris D31.4- ☑
- lacrimal gland D31.5- ☑
- lymphatic D18.1
- magnocellular
  - specified site — *see* Neoplasm, benign, by site
  - unspecified site D31.40
- malignant — *see* Melanoma
- meaning hemangioma D18.00
  - intra-abdominal D18.03
  - intracranial D18.02
  - skin D18.01
  - specified site NEC D18.09
- mouth (mucosa) D10.30
  - specified site NEC D10.39
  - white sponge Q38.6
- multiplex Q85.1
- non-neoplastic I78.1
- oral mucosa D10.30
  - specified site NEC D10.39
  - white sponge Q38.6
- orbit D31.6- ☑
- pigmented
  - giant — *see also* Neoplasm, skin, uncertain behavior D48.5
    - malignant melanoma in — *see* Melanoma
- portwine Q82.5
- retina D31.2- ☑
- retrobulbar D31.6- ☑
- sanguineous Q82.5
- senile I78.1
- skin D22.9
  - abdominal wall D22.5
  - ala nasi D22.39
  - ankle D22.7- ☑
  - anus, anal D22.5
  - arm D22.6- ☑
  - auditory canal (external) D22.2- ☑
  - auricle (ear) D22.2- ☑
  - auricular canal (external) D22.2- ☑
  - axilla, axillary fold D22.5
  - back D22.5
  - breast D22.5
  - brow D22.39
  - buttock D22.5
  - canthus (eye) D22.1- ☑
  - cheek (external) D22.39
  - chest wall D22.5
  - chin D22.39
  - ear (external) D22.2- ☑
  - external meatus (ear) D22.2- ☑
  - eyebrow D22.39
  - eyelid (lower) (upper) D22.1- ☑
  - face D22.30
    - specified NEC D22.39
  - female genital organ (external) NEC D28.0
  - finger D22.6- ☑
  - flank D22.5
  - foot D22.7- ☑
  - forearm D22.6- ☑
  - forehead D22.39
  - foreskin D29.0
  - genital organ (external) NEC
    - female D28.0
    - male D29.9
  - gluteal region D22.5
  - groin D22.5
  - hand D22.6- ☑
  - heel D22.7- ☑
  - helix D22.2- ☑
  - hip D22.7- ☑
  - interscapular region D22.5
  - jaw D22.39
  - knee D22.7- ☑
  - labium (majus) (minus) D28.0
  - leg D22.7- ☑
  - lip (lower) (upper) D22.0
  - lower limb D22.7- ☑
  - male genital organ (external) D29.9
  - nail D22.9
    - finger D22.6- ☑
    - toe D22.7- ☑
  - nasolabial groove D22.39

Nevus — *continued*
- skin — *continued*
  - nates D22.5
  - neck D22.4
  - nose (external) D22.39
  - palpebra D22.1- ☑
  - penis D29.0
  - perianal skin D22.5
  - perineum D22.5
  - pinna D22.2- ☑
  - popliteal fossa or space D22.7- ☑
  - prepuce D29.0
  - pudendum D28.0
  - scalp D22.4
  - scrotum D29.4
  - shoulder D22.6- ☑
  - submammary fold D22.5
  - temple D22.39
  - thigh D22.7- ☑
  - toe D22.7- ☑
  - trunk NEC D22.5
  - umbilicus D22.5
  - upper limb D22.6- ☑
  - vulva D28.0
- specified site NEC — *see* Neoplasm, by site, benign
- spider I78.1
- stellar I78.1
- strawberry Q82.5
- Sutton's benign D22.9
- unius lateris Q82.5
- Unna's Q82.5
- vascular Q82.5
- verrucous Q82.5

Newborn (infant) (liveborn) (singleton) Z38.2
- abstinence syndrome P96.1
- acne L70.4
- affected by
  - abnormalities of membranes P02.9
    - specified NEC P02.8
  - abruptio placenta P02.1
  - amino-acid metabolic disorder, transitory P74.8
  - amniocentesis (while in utero) P00.6
  - amnionitis P02.78
  - apparent life threatening event (ALTE) R68.13
  - bleeding (into)
    - cerebral cortex P52.22
    - germinal matrix P52.0
    - ventricles P52.1
  - breech delivery P03.0
  - cardiac arrest P29.81
  - cardiomyopathy I42.8
    - congenital I42.4
  - cerebral ischemia P91.0
  - Cesarean delivery P03.4
  - chemotherapy agents P04.11
  - chorioamnionitis P02.78
  - cocaine (crack) P04.41
  - complications of labor and delivery P03.9
    - specified NEC P03.89
  - compression of umbilical cord NEC P02.5
  - contracted pelvis P03.1
  - cyanosis P28.2
  - delivery P03.9
    - Cesarean P03.4
    - forceps P03.2
    - vacuum extractor P03.3
  - drugs of addiction P04.40
    - cocaine P04.41
    - hallucinogens P04.42
    - specified drug NEC P04.49
  - entanglement (knot) in umbilical cord P02.5
  - environmental chemicals P04.6
  - fetal (intrauterine)
    - growth retardation P05.9
    - inflammatory response syndrome (FIRS) P02.70
    - malnutrition not light or small for gestational age P05.2
  - FIRS (fetal inflammatory response syndrome) P02.70
  - forceps delivery P03.2
  - heart rate abnormalities
    - bradycardia P29.12
    - intrauterine P03.819
      - before onset of labor P03.810
      - during labor P03.811
    - tachycardia P29.11
  - hemorrhage (antepartum) P02.1
    - cerebellar (nontraumatic) P52.6
    - intracerebral (nontraumatic) P52.4

☑ **Additional Character Required — Refer to the Tabular List for Character Selection**

Newborn — continued
  affected by — continued
    hemorrhage — continued
      intracranial (nontraumatic) P52.9
        specified NEC P52.8
      intraventricular (nontraumatic) P52.3
        grade 1 P52.0
        grade 2 P52.1
        grade 3 P52.21
        grade 4 P52.22
      posterior fossa (nontraumatic) P52.6
      subarachnoid (nontraumatic) P52.5
      subependymal P52.0
        with intracerebral extension P52.22
        with intraventricular extension P52.1
          with enlargment of ventricles P52.21
        without intraventricular extension P52.0
    hypoxic ischemic encephalopathy [HIE] P91.60
      mild P91.61
      moderate P91.62
      severe P91.63
    induction of labor P03.89
    intestinal perforation P78.0
    intrauterine (fetal) blood loss P50.9
      due to (from)
        cut end of co-twin cord P50.5
        hemorrhage into
          co-twin P50.3
            maternal circulation P50.4
        placenta P50.2
        ruptured cord blood P50.1
        vasa previa P50.0
      specified NEC P50.8
    intrauterine (fetal) hemorrhage P50.9
    intrauterine (in utero) procedure P96.5
    malpresentation (malposition) NEC P03.1
    maternal (complication) (use of)
      alcohol P04.3
      amphetamines P04.16
      analgesia (maternal) P04.0
      anesthesia (maternal) P04.0
      anticonvulsants P04.13
      antidepressants P04.15
      antineoplastic chemotherapy P04.11
      anxiolytics P04.1A
      blood loss P02.1
      cannabis P04.81
      circulatory disease P00.3
      condition P00.9
        specified NEC P00.89
      cytotoxic drugs P04.12
      delivery P03.9
        Cesarean P03.4
        forceps P03.2
        vacuum extractor P03.3
      diabetes mellitus (pre-existing) P70.1
      disorder P00.9
        specified NEC P00.89
      drugs (addictive) (illegal) NEC P04.49
      ectopic pregnancy P01.4
      gestational diabetes P70.0
      group B streptococcus (GBS) colonization (positive) P00.82
      hemorrhage P02.1
      hypertensive disorder P00.0
      incompetent cervix P01.0
      infectious disease P00.2
      injury P00.5
      labor and delivery P03.9
      malpresentation before labor P01.7
      maternal death P01.6
      medical procedure P00.7
      medication P04.19
        specified type NEC P04.18
      multiple pregnancy P01.5
      nutritional disorder P00.4
      oligohydramnios P01.2
      opiates P04.14
        administered for procedures during pregnancy or labor and delivery P04.0
      parasitic disease P00.2
      periodontal disease P00.81
      placenta previa P02.0
      polyhydramnios P01.3
      precipitate delivery P03.5
      pregnancy P01.9
        specified P01.8
      premature rupture of membranes P01.1
      renal disease P00.1

Newborn — continued
  affected by — continued
    maternal — continued
      respiratory disease P00.3
      sedative-hypnotics P04.17
      surgical procedure P00.6
      tranquilizers administered for procedures during pregnancy or labor and delivery P04.0
      urinary tract disease P00.1
      uterine contraction (abnormal) P03.6
    meconium peritonitis P78.0
    medication (legal) (maternal use) (prescribed) P04.19
    membrane abnormalities P02.9
      specified NEC P02.8
    membranitis P02.78
    methamphetamine(s) P04.49
    mixed metabolic and respiratory acidosis P84
    neonatal abstinence syndrome P96.1
    noxious substances transmitted via placenta or breast milk P04.9
      cannabis P04.81
      specified NEC P04.89
    nutritional supplements P04.5
    placenta previa P02.0
    placental
      abnormality (functional) (morphological) P02.20
        specified NEC P02.29
      dysfunction P02.29
      infarction P02.29
      insufficiency P02.29
      separation NEC P02.1
      transfusion syndromes P02.3
    placentitis P02.78
    precipitate delivery P03.5
    prolapsed cord P02.4
    respiratory arrest P28.81
    slow intrauterine growth P05.9
    tobacco P04.2
    twin to twin transplacental transfusion P02.3
    umbilical cord (tightly) around neck P02.5
    umbilical cord condition P02.60
      short cord P02.69
      specified NEC P02.69
    uterine contractions (abnormal) P03.6
    vasa previa P02.69
      from intrauterine blood loss P50.0
  apnea — see also Apnea, newborn P28.40
    obstructive P28.42
    primary — see also Apnea, newborn, sleep, primary P28.30
    sleep (central) (obstructive) (primary) — see also Apnea, newborn, sleep, primary P28.30
  born in hospital Z38.00
    by cesarean Z38.01
  born outside hospital Z38.1
  breast buds P96.89
  breast engorgement P83.4
  check-up — see Newborn, examination
  convulsion P90
  dehydration P74.1
  examination
    8 to 28 days old Z00.111
    under 8 days old Z00.110
  fever P81.9
    environmentally-induced P81.0
  hyperbilirubinemia P59.9
    of prematurity P59.0
  hypernatremia P74.21
  hyponatremia P74.22
  infection P39.9
    candidal P37.5
    specified NEC P39.8
    urinary tract P39.3
  jaundice P59.9
    due to
      breast milk inhibitor P59.3
      hepatocellular damage P59.20
        specified NEC P59.29
      preterm delivery P59.0
    of prematurity P59.0
    specified NEC P59.8
  late metabolic acidosis P74.0
  mastitis P39.0
    infective P39.0
    noninfective P83.4
  multiple born NEC Z38.8
    born in hospital Z38.68
      by cesarean Z38.69
    born outside hospital Z38.7

Newborn — continued
  omphalitis P38.9
    with mild hemorrhage P38.1
    without hemorrhage P38.9
  post-term P08.21
  prolonged gestation (over 42 completed weeks) P08.22
  quadruplet Z38.8
    born in hospital Z38.63
      by cesarean Z38.64
    born outside hospital Z38.7
  quintuplet Z38.8
    born in hospital Z38.65
      by cesarean Z38.66
    born outside hospital Z38.7
  seizure P90
  sepsis (congenital) P36.9
    due to
      anaerobes NEC P36.5
      Escherichia coli P36.4
      Staphylococcus P36.30
        aureus P36.2
        specified NEC P36.39
      Streptococcus P36.10
        group B P36.0
        specified NEC P36.19
      specified NEC P36.8
  triplet Z38.8
    born in hospital Z38.61
      by cesarean Z38.62
    born outside hospital Z38.7
  twin Z38.5
    born in hospital Z38.30
      by cesarean Z38.31
    born outside hospital Z38.4
  vomiting P92.09
    bilious P92.01
  weight check Z00.111
Newcastle conjunctivitis or disease B30.8
Nezelof's syndrome (pure alymphocytosis) D81.4
Niacin (amide) **deficiency** E52
Nicolas (-Durand)-**Favre disease** A55
Nicotine — see Tobacco
Nicotinic acid deficiency E52
Niemann-Pick disease or syndrome E75.249
  specified NEC E75.248
  type
    A E75.240
    A/B E75.244
    B E75.241
    C E75.242
    D E75.243
Night
  blindness — see Blindness, night
  sweats R61
  terrors (child) F51.4
Nightmares (REM sleep type) F51.5
NIHSS (National Institutes of Health Stroke Scale) **score** R29.7- ☑
Nipple — see condition
Nisbet's chancre A57
Nishimoto (-Takeuchi) **disease** I67.5
Nitritoid crisis or reaction — see Crisis, nitritoid
Nitrosohemoglobinemia D74.8
Njovera A65
No
  general equivalence degree (GED) Z55.5
  health insurance coverage Z59.71
Nocardiosis, nocardiasis A43.9
  cutaneous A43.1
  lung A43.0
  pneumonia A43.0
  pulmonary A43.0
  specified site NEC A43.8
Nocturia R35.1
  psychogenic F45.8
Nocturnal — see condition
Nodal rhythm I49.8
Node(s) — see also Nodule
  Bouchard's (with arthropathy) M15.2
  Haygarth's M15.8
  Heberden's (with arthropathy) M15.1
  larynx J38.7
  lymph — see condition
  milker's B08.03
  Osler's I33.0
  Schmorl's — see Schmorl's disease
  singer's J38.2
  teacher's J38.2
  tuberculous — see Tuberculosis, lymph gland

Node(s) — *continued*
vocal cord J38.2
Nodule(s), **nodular**
actinomycotic — *see* Actinomycosis
breast NEC — *see also* Lump, breast N63.0
colloid (cystic), thyroid E04.1
cutaneous — *see* Swelling, localized
endometrial (stromal) D26.1
Haygarth's M15.8
inflammatory — *see* Inflammation
juxta-articular
syphilitic A52.77
yaws A66.7
larynx J38.7
lung, solitary (subsegmental branch of the bronchial tree)
R91.1
multiple R91.8
milker's B08.03
prostate N40.2
with lower urinary tract symptoms (LUTS) N40.3
without lower urinary tract symptoms (LUTS) N40.2
pulmonary, solitary (subsegmental branch of the
bronchial tree) R91.1
retrocardiac R09.89
rheumatoid M06.30
ankle M06.37- ☑
elbow M06.32- ☑
foot joint M06.37- ☑
hand joint M06.34- ☑
hip M06.35- ☑
knee M06.36- ☑
multiple site M06.39
shoulder M06.31- ☑
vertebra M06.38
wrist M06.33- ☑
scrotum (inflammatory) N49.2
singer's J38.2
solitary, lung (subsegmental branch of the bronchial tree)
R91.1
multiple R91.8
subcutaneous — *see* Swelling, localized
teacher's J38.2
thyroid (cold) (gland) (nontoxic) E04.1
with thyrotoxicosis E05.20
with thyroid storm E05.21
toxic or with hyperthyroidism E05.20
with thyroid storm E05.21
vocal cord J38.2
Noma (gangrenous) (hospital) (infective) A69.0
auricle I96
mouth A69.0
pudendi N76.89
vulvae N76.89
Nomad, nomadism Z59.00
NOMID (neonatal onset multisystemic inflammatory disorder) M04.2
Non-accidental trauma — *see* Abuse, physical
Nonadherence to medical treatment, specified NEC
Z91.199
due to
financial hardship Z91.190
specified reason NEC Z91.198
Nonautoimmune hemolytic anemia D59.4
drug-induced D59.2
Nonclosure — *see also* Imperfect, closure
ductus arteriosus (Botallo's) Q25.0
foramen
botalli Q21.12
ovale Q21.12
Noncompliance Z91.199
with
dialysis Z91.158
due to financial hardship Z91.151
dietary regimen Z91.119
due to
financial hardship Z91.110
specified reason NEC Z91.118
medical treatment, specified NEC Z91.199
due to
financial hardship Z91.190
specified reason NEC Z91.198
medication regimen NEC Z91.148
due to financial hardship Z91.141
underdosing — *see also* Table of Drugs and
Chemicals, categories T36-T50, with final
character 6 Z91.148
intentional NEC Z91.128

Noncompliance — *continued*
with — *continued*
medication regimen — *continued*
underdosing — *see also* Table of Drugs and
Chemicals, categories T36-T50, with final
character 6 — *continued*
intentional — *continued*
by caregiver
due to
financial hardship Z91.A20
specified reason NEC Z91.A28
due to financial hardship of patient
Z91.120
unintentional NEC Z91.138
by caregiver Z91.A3
due to patient's age related debility
Z91.130
renal dialysis Z91.158
due to financial hardship Z91.151
caregiver
with patient's
dietary regimen
due to
financial hardship Z91.A10
specified reason NEC Z91.A18
medical treatment and regimen
due to financial hardship Z91.A91
specified reason NEC Z91.A98
medication regimen
due to financial hardship Z91.A41
specified reason NEC Z91.A48
renal dialysis
due to financial hardship Z91.A51
specified reason NEC Z91.A58
Nondescent (congenital) — *see also* Malposition, congenital
cecum Q43.3
colon Q43.3
testicle Q53.9
bilateral Q53.20
abdominal Q53.211
perineal Q53.22
unilateral Q53.10
abdominal Q53.111
perineal Q53.12
Nondevelopment
brain Q02
part of Q04.3
heart Q24.8
organ or site, congenital NEC — *see* Hypoplasia
Nonengagement
head NEC O32.4 ☑
in labor, causing obstructed labor O64.8 ☑
Nonexanthematous tick fever A93.2
Nonexpansion, lung (newborn) P28.0
Nonfunctioning
cystic duct — *see also* Disease, gallbladder K82.8
gallbladder — *see also* Disease, gallbladder K82.8
kidney N28.9
labyrinth — *see* subcategory H83.2 ☑
Non-Hodgkin lymphoma NEC — *see* Lymphoma, non-
Hodgkin
Nonimplantation, ovum N97.2
Noninsufflation, fallopian tube N97.1
Non-ketotic hyperglycinemia E72.51
Nonne-Milroy syndrome Q82.0
Nonovulation N97.0
Non-palpable testicle(s)
bilateral R39.84
unilateral R39.83
Nonpatent fallopian tube N97.1
Nonpneumatization, lung NEC P28.0
Nonrotation — *see* Malrotation
Nonsecretion, urine — *see* Anuria
Nonunion
fracture — *see* Fracture, by site
joint, following fusion or arthrodesis M96.0
organ or site, congenital NEC — *see* Imperfect, closure
symphysis pubis, congenital Q74.2
Nonvisualization, gallbladder R93.2
Nonvital, nonvitalized tooth K04.99
Non-working side interference M26.56
Noonan's syndrome Q87.19
Normocytic anemia (infectional) due to blood loss
(chronic) D50.0
acute D62
Norrie's disease (congenital) Q15.8
North American blastomycosis B40.9
Norwegian itch B86
Nose, nasal — *see* condition

Nosebleed R04.0
Nose-picking F98.8
Nosomania F45.21
Nosophobia F45.22
Nostalgia F43.20
Notch of iris Q13.2
Notching nose, congenital (tip) Q30.2
Nothnagel's
syndrome — *see* Strabismus, paralytic, third nerve
vasomotor acroparesthesia I73.89
Novy's relapsing fever A68.9
louse-borne A68.0
tick-borne A68.1
Noxious
foodstuffs, poisoning by — *see* Poisoning, food, noxious,
plant
substances transmitted through placenta or breast milk
P04.9
Nucleus pulposus — *see* condition
Numbness R20.0
Nuns' knee — *see* Bursitis, prepatellar
Nursemaid's elbow S53.03-
Nutcracker esophagus K22.4
Nutmeg liver K76.1
Nutrient element deficiency E61.9
specified NEC E61.8
Nutrition deficient or insufficient — *see also* Malnutrition
E63.9
due to
insufficient food T73.0 ☑
lack of
care (child) T76.02 ☑
adult T76.01 ☑
food T73.0 ☑
specific element deficiency — *see* Nutrient element
deficiency, or by element
sequelae — *see* Sequelae, nutritional deficiency
specified NEC E63.8
Nutritional stunting E45
Nyctalopia (night blindness) — *see* Blindness, night
Nycturia R35.1
psychogenic F45.8
Nymphomania F52.8
Nystagmus H55.00
benign paroxysmal — *see* Vertigo, benign paroxysmal
central positional H81.4
congenital H55.01
dissociated H55.04
latent H55.02
miners' H55.09
positional
benign paroxysmal H81.4
central H81.4
specified form NEC H55.09
visual deprivation H55.03

O

Obermeyer's relapsing fever (European) A68.0
Obesity E66.9
with alveolar hypoventilation E66.2
adrenal E27.8
class
1 E66.811
2 E66.812
3 E66.813
complicating
childbirth O99.214
pregnancy O99.21- ☑
puerperium O99.215
constitutional E66.89
dietary counseling and surveillance Z71.3
drug-induced E66.1
due to
disruption of MC4R pathway E88.82
drug E66.1
excess calories E66.09
morbid E66.01
severe E66.01
gene mutation
leptin (LEP) E88.82
leptin receptor (LEPR) E88.82
melanocortin 4 Receptor (MC4R) E88.82
nuclear receptor coactivator 1 (NCOA1) E88.82
proopiomelanocortin (POMC) E88.82
proprotein convertase subtilisin/kexin type 1 (PC-
SK1) E88.82

☑ **Additional Character Required** — **Refer to the Tabular List for Character Selection**

Obesity — *continued*
due to — *continued*
gene mutation — *continued*
src homology 2B adaptor signaling protein (SH2B1) E88.82
endocrine E66.89
endogenous E66.89
exogenous E66.09
familial E66.89
glandular E66.89
hypothyroid — *see* Hypothyroidism
hypoventilation syndrome (OHS) E66.2
morbid E66.01
with
alveolar hypoventilation E66.2
obesity hypoventilation syndrome (OHS) E66.2
due to excess calories E66.01
nutritional E66.09
pituitary E23.6
severe E66.01
specified type NEC E66.89
Oblique — *see* condition
Obliteration
appendix (lumen) K38.8
artery I77.1
bile duct (noncalculous) K83.1
common duct (noncalculous) K83.1
cystic duct — *see* Obstruction, gallbladder
disease, arteriolar I77.1
endometrium N85.8
eye, anterior chamber — *see* Disorder, globe, hypotony
fallopian tube N97.1
lymphatic vessel I89.0
due to mastectomy I97.2
organ or site, congenital NEC — *see* Atresia, by site
ureter N13.5
with infection N13.6
urethra — *see* Stricture, urethra
vein I87.8
vestibule (oral) K08.89
Observation (following) (for) (without need for further medical care) Z04.9
accident NEC Z04.3
at work Z04.2
transport Z04.1
adverse effect of drug Z03.6
alleged rape or sexual assault (victim), ruled out
adult Z04.41
child Z04.42
criminal assault Z04.89
development state
adolescent Z00.3
period of rapid growth in childhood Z00.2
puberty Z00.3
disease, specified NEC Z03.89
following work accident Z04.2
forced sexual exploitation Z04.81
forced labor exploitation Z04.82
growth and development state — *see* Observation, development state
injuries (accidental) NEC — *see also* Observation, accident
newborn (for)
suspected condition, related to exposure from the mother or birth process — *see* Newborn, affected by, maternal
ruled out Z05.9
cardiac Z05.0
connective tissue Z05.73
gastrointestinal Z05.5
genetic Z05.41
genitourinary Z05.6
immunologic Z05.43
infectious Z05.1
metabolic Z05.42
musculoskeletal Z05.72
neurological Z05.2
respiratory Z05.3
skin and subcutaneous tissue Z05.71
specified condition NEC Z05.89
postpartum
immediately after delivery Z39.0
routine follow-up Z39.2
pregnancy (normal) (without complication) Z34.9- ☑
high risk O09.9- ☑
suicide attempt, alleged NEC Z03.89
self-poisoning Z03.6
suspected, ruled out — *see also* Suspected condition, ruled out

Observation — *continued*
suspected, ruled out — *see also* Suspected condition, ruled out — *continued*
abuse, physical
adult Z04.71
child Z04.72
accident at work Z04.2
adult battering victim Z04.71
child battering victim Z04.72
condition NEC Z03.89
newborn — *see also* Observation, newborn (for), suspected condition, ruled out Z05.9
drug poisoning or adverse effect Z03.6
exposure (to)
anthrax Z03.810
biological agent NEC Z03.818
foreign body
aspirated (inhaled) Z03.822
ingested Z03.821
inserted (injected), in (eye) (orifice) (skin) Z03.823
inflicted injury NEC Z04.89
suicide attempt, alleged Z03.89
self-poisoning Z03.6
toxic effects from ingested substance (drug) (poison) Z03.6
toxic effects from ingested substance (drug) (poison) Z03.6
Obsession, obsessional state F42.8
mixed thoughts and acts F42.2
Obsessive-compulsive neurosis or reaction F42.8
Obstetric embolism, septic — *see* Embolism, obstetric, septic
Obstetrical trauma (complicating delivery) O71.9
with or following ectopic or molar pregnancy O08.6
specified type NEC O71.89
Obstipation — *see* Constipation
Obstruction, obstructed, obstructive
airway J98.8
with
allergic alveclitis J67.9
asthma J45.909
with
exacerbation (acute) J45.901
status asthmaticus J45.902
bronchiectasis J47.9
with
exacerbation (acute) J47.1
lower respiratory infection J47.0
bronchitis (chronic) J44.89
emphysema J43.9
chronic J44.9
with
allergic alveolitis — *see* Pneumonitis, hypersensitivity
bronchiectasis J47.9
with
exacerbation (acute) J47.1
lower respiratory infection J47.0
due to
foreign body — *see* Foreign body, by site, causing asphyxia
inhalation of fumes or vapors J68.9
laryngospasm J38.5
ampulla of Vater K83.1
aortic (heart) (valve) — *see* Stenosis, aortic
aortoiliac I74.09
aqueduct of Sylvius G91.1
congenital Q03.0
with spina bifida — *see* Spina bifida, by site, with hydrocephalus
Arnold-Chiari — *see* Arnold-Chiari disease
artery — *see also* Atherosclerosis, artery I70.9 ☑
basilar (complete) (partial) — *see* Occlusion, artery, basilar
carotid (complete) (partial) — *see* Occlusion, artery, carotid
cerebellar — *see* Occlusion, artery, cerebellar
cerebral (anterior) (middle) (posterior) — *see* Occlusion, artery, cerebral
precerebral — *see* Occlusion, artery, precerebral
renal N28.0
retinal NEC — *see* Occlusion, artery, retina
stent — *see* Restenosis, stent
vertebral (complete) (partial) — *see* Occlusion, artery, vertebral
band (intestinal) — *see also* Obstruction, intestine, specified NEC K56.699
bile duct or passage (common) (hepatic) (noncalculous) K83.1

Obstruction, obstructed, obstructive — *continued*
bile duct or passage — *continued*
with calculus K80.51
congenital (causing jaundice) Q44.3
biliary (duct) (tract) K83.1
gallbladder K82.0
bladder-neck (acquired) N32.0
congenital Q64.31
due to hyperplasia (hypertrophy) of prostate — *see* Hyperplasia, prostate
bowel — *see* Obstruction, intestine
bronchus J98.09
canal, ear — *see* Stenosis, external ear canal
cardia K22.2
caval veins (inferior) (superior) I87.1
cecum — *see* Obstruction, intestine
circulatory I99.8
colon — *see* Obstruction, intestine
common duct (noncalculous) K83.1
coronary (artery) — *see* Occlusion, coronary
cystic duct — *see also* Obstruction, gallbladder
with calculus K80.21
device, implant or graft — *see also* Complications, by site and type, mechanical T85.698 ☑
arterial graft NEC — *see* Complication, cardiovascular device, mechanical, vascular
catheter NEC T85.628 ☑
cystostomy T83.090 ☑
dialysis (renal) T82.49 ☑
intraperitoneal T85.691 ☑
Hopkins T83.098 ☑
ileostomy T83.098 ☑
infusion NEC T82.594 ☑
spinal (epidural) (subdural) T85.690 ☑
nephrostomy T83.092 ☑
urethral indwelling T83.091 ☑
urinary T83.098 ☑
urostomy T83.098 ☑
due to infection T85.79 ☑
gastrointestinal — *see* Complications, prosthetic device, mechanical, gastrointestinal device
genital NEC T83.498 ☑
intrauterine contraceptive device T83.39 ☑
penile prosthesis (cylinder) (implanted) (pump) (reservoir) T83.490 ☑
testicular prosthesis T83.491 ☑
heart NEC — *see* Complication, cardiovascular device, mechanical
joint prosthesis — *see* Complications, joint prosthesis, mechanical, specified NEC, by site
orthopedic NEC — *see* Complication, orthopedic, device, mechanical
specified NEC T85.628 ☑
urinary NEC — *see also* Complication, genitourinary, device, urinary, mechanical
graft T83.29 ☑
vascular NEC — *see* Complication, cardiovascular device, mechanical
ventricular intracranial shunt T85.09 ☑
due to foreign body accidentally left in operative wound T81.529 ☑
duodenum K31.5
ejaculatory duct N50.89
esophagus K22.2
eustachian tube (complete) (partial) H68.10- ☑
cartilagenous (extrinsic) H68.13- ☑
intrinsic H68.12- ☑
osseous H68.11- ☑
fallopian tube (bilateral) N97.1
fecal K56.41
with hernia — *see* Hernia, by site, with obstruction
foramen of Monro (congenital) Q03.8
with spina bifida — *see* Spina bifida, by site, with hydrocephalus
foreign body — *see* Foreign body
gallbladder K82.0
with calculus, stones K80.21
congenital Q44.1
gastric outlet K31.1
gastrointestinal — *see* Obstruction, intestine
hepatic K76.89
duct (noncalculous) K83.1
ileum — *see* Obstruction, intestine
iliofemoral (artery) I74.5
intestine K56.609
with
adhesions (intestinal) (peritoneal) K56.50
complete K56.52

Obstruction, obstructed, obstructive — *continued*
- intestine — *continued*
  - with — *continued*
    - adhesions — *continued*
      - incomplete K56.51
      - partial K56.51
    - adynamic K56.0
    - by gallstone K56.3
    - complete K56.601
    - congenital (small) Q41.9
      - large Q42.9
        - specified part NEC Q42.8
    - incomplete K56.600
    - neurogenic K56.0
      - Hirschsprung's disease or megacolon Q43.1
    - newborn P76.9
      - due to
        - fecaliths P76.8
        - inspissated milk P76.2
        - meconium (plug) P76.0
          - in mucoviscidosis E84.11
      - specified NEC P76.8
    - partial K56.600
    - postoperative K91.30
      - complete K91.32
      - incomplete K91.31
      - partial K91.31
    - reflex K56.0
    - specified NEC K56.699
      - complete K56.691
      - incomplete K56.690
      - partial K56.690
    - volvulus K56.2
- intracardiac ball valve prosthesis T82.09 ☑
- jejunum — *see* Obstruction, intestine
- joint prosthesis — *see* Complications, joint prosthesis, mechanical, specified NEC, by site
- kidney (calices) — *see also* Hydronephrosis N28.89
- labor — *see* Delivery
- lacrimal (passages) (duct)
  - by
    - dacryolith — *see* Dacryolith
    - stenosis — *see* Stenosis, lacrimal
  - congenital Q10.5
  - neonatal H04.53- ☑
- lacrimonasal duct — *see* Obstruction, lacrimal
- lacteal, with steatorrhea K90.2
- laryngitis — *see* Laryngitis
- larynx NEC J38.6
  - congenital Q31.8
- lung J98.4
  - disease, chronic J44.9
- lymphatic I89.0
- meconium (plug)
  - newborn P76.0
    - due to fecaliths P76.0
    - in mucoviscidosis E84.11
- mitral — *see* Stenosis, mitral
- nasal J34.89
- nasolacrimal duct — *see also* Obstruction, lacrimal
  - congenital Q10.5
- nasopharynx J39.2
- nose J34.89
- organ or site, congenital NEC — *see* Atresia, by site
- pancreatic duct K86.89
- parotid duct or gland K11.8
- pelviureteral junction N13.5
  - with hydronephrosis N13.0
  - congenital Q62.39
- pharynx J39.2
- portal (circulation) (vein) I81
- prostate — *see also* Hyperplasia, prostate
  - valve (urinary) N32.0
- pulmonary valve (heart) I37.0
- pyelonephritis (chronic) N11.1
- pylorus
  - adult K31.1
  - congenital or infantile Q40.0
- rectosigmoid — *see* Obstruction, intestine
- rectum K62.4
- renal — *see also* Hydronephrosis N28.89
  - outflow N13.8
  - pelvis, congenital Q62.39
- respiratory J98.8
  - chronic J44.9
- retinal (vessels) H34.9
- salivary duct (any) K11.8
  - with calculus K11.5
- sigmoid — *see* Obstruction, intestine

Obstruction, obstructed, obstructive — *continued*
- sinus (accessory) (nasal) J34.89
- Stensen's duct K11.8
- stomach NEC K31.89
  - acute K31.0
  - congenital Q40.2
  - due to pylorospasm K31.3
- submandibular duct K11.8
- submaxillary gland K11.8
  - with calculus K11.5
- thoracic duct I89.0
- thrombotic — *see* Thrombosis
- trachea J39.8
- tracheostomy airway J95.03
- tricuspid (valve) — *see* Stenosis, tricuspid
- upper respiratory, congenital Q34.8
- ureter (functional) (pelvic junction) NEC N13.5
  - with
    - hydronephrosis N13.1
      - with infection N13.6
      - congenital Q62.39
    - pyelonephritis (chronic) N11.1
  - congenital Q62.39
  - due to calculus — *see* Calculus, ureter
- urethra NEC N36.8
  - congenital Q64.39
- urinary (moderate) N13.9
  - due to hyperplasia (hypertrophy) of prostate — *see* Hyperplasia, prostate
  - organ or tract (lower) N13.9
  - prostatic valve N32.0
  - specified NEC N13.8
- uropathy N13.9
- uterus N85.8
- vagina N89.5
- valvular — *see* Endocarditis
- vein, venous I87.1
  - caval (inferior) (superior) I87.1
  - thrombotic — *see* Thrombosis
- vena cava (inferior) (superior) I87.1
- vesical NEC N32.0
- vesicourethral orifice N32.0
  - congenital Q64.31
- vessel NEC I99.8
  - stent — *see* Restenosis, stent

Obturator — *see* condition
Occlusal wear, teeth K03.0
Occlusio pupillae — *see* Membrane, pupillary
Occlusion, occluded
- anus K62.4
  - congenital Q42.3
    - with fistula Q42.2
- aortoiliac (chronic) I74.09
- aqueduct of Sylvius G91.1
  - congenital Q03.0
    - with spina bifida — *see* Spina bifida, by site, with hydrocephalus
- artery — *see also* Atherosclerosis, artery I70.9 ☑
  - auditory, internal I65.8
  - basilar I65.1
    - with
      - infarction I63.22
        - due to
          - embolism I63.12
          - thrombosis I63.02
  - brain or cerebral I66.9
    - with infarction (due to) I63.5- ☑
      - embolism I63.4- ☑
      - thrombosis I63.3- ☑
  - carotid I65.2- ☑
    - with
      - infarction I63.23- ☑
        - due to
          - embolism I63.13- ☑
          - thrombosis I63.03- ☑
  - cerebellar (anterior inferior) (posterior inferior) (superior) I66.3
    - with infarction I63.54- ☑
      - due to
        - embolism I63.44- ☑
        - thrombosis I63.34- ☑
  - cerebral I66.9
    - with infarction I63.50
      - due to
        - embolism I63.40
          - specified NEC I63.49
        - thrombosis I63.30
          - specified NEC I63.39

Occlusion, occluded — *continued*
- artery — *see also* Atherosclerosis, artery — *continued*
  - cerebral — *continued*
    - anterior I66.1- ☑
      - with infarction I63.52- ☑
        - due to
          - embolism I63.42- ☑
          - thrombosis I63.32- ☑
    - middle I66.0- ☑
      - with infarction I63.51- ☑
        - due to
          - embolism I63.41- ☑
          - thrombosis I63.31- ☑
    - posterior I66.2- ☑
      - with infarction I63.53- ☑
        - due to
          - embolism I63.43- ☑
          - thrombosis I63.33- ☑
    - specified NEC I66.8
      - with infarction I63.59
        - due to
          - embolism I63.4- ☑
          - thrombosis I63.3- ☑
  - choroidal (anterior) — *see* Occlusion, artery, precerebral, specified NEC
  - communicating posterior — *see* Occlusion, artery, precerebral, specified NEC
  - complete
    - coronary I25.82
    - extremities I70.92
  - coronary (acute) (thrombotic) (without myocardial infarction) I24.0
    - with myocardial infarction — *see* Infarction, myocardium
    - chronic total I25.82
    - complete I25.82
    - healed or old I25.2
    - total (chronic) I25.82
  - hypophyseal — *see* Occlusion, artery, precerebral, specified NEC
  - iliac I74.5
  - lower extremities due to stenosis or stricture I77.1
  - mesenteric (embolic) (thrombotic) — *see also* Infarct, intestine K55.069
  - perforating — *see* Occlusion, artery, cerebral, specified NEC
  - peripheral I77.9
    - thrombotic or embolic I74.4
  - pontine — *see* Occlusion, artery, precerebral, specified NEC
  - precerebral I65.9
    - with infarction I63.20
      - specified NEC I63.29
      - due to
        - embolism I63.10
          - specified NEC I63.19
        - thrombosis I63.00
          - specified NEC I63.09
    - basilar — *see* Occlusion, artery, basilar
    - carotid — *see* Occlusion, artery, carotid
    - puerperal O88.23
    - specified NEC I65.8
      - with infarction I63.29
        - due to
          - embolism I63.19
          - thrombosis I63.09
    - vertebral — *see* Occlusion, artery, vertebral
  - renal N28.0
  - retinal
    - branch H34.23- ☑
    - central H34.1- ☑
    - partial H34.21- ☑
    - transient H34.0- ☑
  - spinal — *see* Occlusion, artery, precerebral, vertebral
  - total (chronic)
    - coronary I25.82
    - extremities I70.92
  - vertebral I65.0- ☑
    - with
      - infarction I63.21- ☑
        - due to
          - embolism I63.11- ☑
          - thrombosis I63.01- ☑
- basilar artery — *see* Occlusion, artery, basilar
- bile duct (common) (hepatic) (noncalculous) K83.1
- bowel — *see* Obstruction, intestine
- carotid (artery) (common) (internal) — *see* Occlusion, artery, carotid

☑ **Additional Character Required** — **Refer to the Tabular List for Character Selection**

Occlusion, occluded — *continued*
  centric (of teeth) M26.59
    maximum intercuspation discrepancy M26.55
  cerebellar (artery) — *see* Occlusion, artery, cerebellar
  cerebral (artery) — *see* Occlusion, artery, cerebral
  cerebrovascular — *see also* Occlusion, artery, cerebral
    with infarction I63.5- ☑
  cervical canal — *see* Stricture, cervix
  cervix (uteri) — *see* Stricture, cervix
  choanal Q30.0
  choroidal (artery) — *see* Occlusion, artery, precerebral, specified NEC
  colon — *see* Obstruction, intestine
  communicating posterior artery — *see* Occlusion, artery, precerebral, specified NEC
  coronary (artery) (vein) (thrombotic) — *see also* Infarct, myocardium
    chronic total I25.82
    healed or old I25.2
    not resulting in infarction I24.0
    total (chronic) I25.82
  cystic duct — *see* Obstruction, gallbladder
  embolic — *see* Embolism
  fallopian tube N97.1
    congenital Q50.6
  gallbladder — *see also* Obstruction, gallbladder
    congenital (causing jaundice) Q44.1
  gingiva, traumatic K06.2
  hymen N89.6
    congenital Q52.3
  hypophyseal (artery) — *see* Occlusion, artery, precerebral, specified NEC
  iliac artery I74.5
  intestine — *see* Obstruction, intestine
  lacrimal passages — *see* Obstruction, lacrimal
  lung J98.4
  lymph or lymphatic channel I89.0
  mammary duct N64.89
  mesenteric artery (embolic) (thrombotic) — *see also* Infarct, intestine K55.069
  nose J34.89
    congenital Q30.0
  organ or site, congenital NEC — *see* Atresia, by site
  oviduct N97.1
    congenital Q50.6
  peripheral arteries
    due to stricture or stenosis I77.1
    upper extremity I74.2
  pontine (artery) — *see* Occlusion, artery, precerebral, specified NEC
  posterior lingual, of mandibular teeth M26.29
  precerebral artery — *see* Occlusion, artery, precerebral
  punctum lacrimale — *see* Obstruction, lacrimal
  pupil — *see* Membrane, pupillary
  pylorus, adult — *see also* Stricture, pylorus K31.1
  renal artery N28.0
  retina, retinal
    artery — *see* Occlusion, artery, retinal
    vein (central) H34.81- ☑
      engorgement H34.82- ☑
      tributary H34.83- ☑
    vessels H34.9
  spinal artery — *see* Occlusion, artery, precerebral, vertebral
  teeth (mandibular) (posterior lingual) M26.29
  thoracic duct I89.0
  thrombotic — *see* Thrombosis, artery
  traumatic
    edentulous (alveolar) ridge K06.2
    gingiva K06.2
    periodontal K05.5
  tubal N97.1
  ureter (complete) (partial) N13.5
    congenital Q62.10
  ureteropelvic junction N13.5
    congenital Q62.11
  ureterovesical orifice N13.5
    congenital Q62.12
  urethra — *see* Stricture, urethra
  uterus N85.8
  vagina N89.5
  vascular NEC I99.8
  vein — *see* Thrombosis
    retinal — *see* Occlusion, retinal, vein
  vena cava (inferior) (superior) — *see* Embolism, vena cava
  ventricle (brain) NEC G91.1
  vertebral (artery) — *see* Occlusion, artery, vertebral
  vessel (blood) I99.8

Occlusion, occluded — *continued*
  vulva N90.5
Occult
  blood in feces (stools) R19.5
Occupational
  problems NEC Z56.89
Ochlophobia — *see* Agoraphobia
Ochronosis (endogenous) E70.29
Ocular muscle — *see* condition
Oculogyric crisis or disturbance H51.8
  psychogenic F45.8
Oculomotor syndrome H51.9
Oculopathy
  syphilitic NEC A52.71
    congenital
      early A50.01
      late A50.30
    early (secondary) A51.43
    late A52.71
Oddi's sphincter spasm K83.4
Odontalgia K08.89
Odontoameloblastoma — *see* Cyst, calcifying odontogenic
Odontoclasia K03.89
Odontodysplasia, regional K00.4
Odontogenesis imperfecta K00.5
Odontoma (ameloblastic) (complex) (compound) (fibroameloblastic) — *see* Cyst, calcifying odontogenic
Odontomyelitis (closed) (open) K04.01
  irreversible K04.02
  reversible K04.01
Odontorrhagia K08.89
Odontosarcoma, ameloblastic C41.1
  upper jaw (bone) C41.0
Oestriasis — *see* Myiasis
Oguchi's disease H53.63
Ohara's disease — *see* Tularemia
OHS (obesity hypoventilation syndrome) E66.2
Oidiomycosis — *see* Candidiasis
Oidium albicans infection — *see* Candidiasis
Old age (without mention of debility) R54
  dementia F03 ☑
Old (previous) **myocardial infarction** I25.2
Olfactory — *see* condition
Oligemia — *see* Anemia
Oligoastrocytoma
  specified site — *see* Neoplasm, malignant, by site
  unspecified site C71.9
Oligocythemia D64.9
Oligodendroblastoma
  specified site — *see* Neoplasm, malignant
  unspecified site C71.9
Oligodendroglioma
  anaplastic type
    specified site — *see* Neoplasm, malignant, by site
    unspecified site C71.9
  specified site — *see* Neoplasm, malignant, by site
  unspecified site C71.9
Oligodontia — *see* Anodontia
Oligoencephalon Q02
Oligohidrosis L74.4
Oligohydramnios O41.0- ☑
Oligohydrosis L74.4
Oligomenorrhea N91.5
  primary N91.3
  secondary N91.4
Oligophrenia — *see also* Disability, intellectual
  phenylpyruvic E70.0
Oligospermia N46.11
  due to
    drug therapy N46.121
    efferent duct obstruction N46.123
    infection N46.122
    radiation N46.124
    specified cause NEC N46.129
    systemic disease N46.125
Oligotrichia — *see* Alopecia
Oliguria R34
  with, complicating or following ectopic or molar pregnancy O08.4
  postprocedural N99.0
  puerperal O90.49
Ollier's disease Q78.4
Omentitis — *see* Peritonitis
Omentocele — *see* Hernia, abdomen, specified site NEC
Omentum, omental — *see* condition
Omphalitis (congenital) (newborn) P38.9
  with mild hemorrhage P38.1
  without hemorrhage P38.9
  not of newborn L08.82

Omphalitis — *continued*
  tetanus A33
Omphalocele Q79.2
Omphalomesenteric duct, persistent Q43.0
Omphalorrhagia, newborn P51.9
Omsk hemorrhagic fever A98.1
Onanism (excessive) F98.8
Onchocerciasis, onchocercosis B73.1
  with
    eye disease B73.00
      endophthalmitis B73.01
      eyelid B73.09
      glaucoma B73.02
      specified NEC B73.09
    eyelid B73.09
    eye NEC B73.00
Oncocytoma — *see* Neoplasm, benign, by site
Oncovirus, as cause of disease classified elsewhere B97.32
Ondine's curse — *see* Apnea, sleep
Oneirophrenia F23
Onychauxis L60.2
  congenital Q84.5
Onychia — *see also* Cellulitis, digit
  with lymphangitis — *see* Lymphangitis, acute, digit
  candidal B37.2
  dermatophytic B35.1
Onychitis — *see also* Cellulitis, digit
  with lymphangitis — *see* Lymphangitis, acute, digit
Onychocryptosis L60.0
Onychodystrophy L60.3
  congenital Q84.6
Onychogryphosis, onychogryposis L60.2
Onycholysis L60.1
Onychomadesis L60.8
Onychomalacia L60.3
Onychomycosis (finger) (toe) B35.1
Onycho-osteodysplasia Q87.2
Onychophagia F98.8
Onychophosis L60.8
Onychoptosis L60.8
Onychorrhexis L60.3
  congenital Q84.6
Onychoschizia L60.3
Onyxis (finger) (toe) L60.0
Onyxitis — *see also* Cellulitis, digit
  with lymphangitis — *see* Lymphangitis, acute, digit
Oophoritis (cystic) (infectional) (interstitial) N70.92
  with salpingitis N70.93
  acute N70.02
    with salpingitis N70.03
  chronic N70.12
    with salpingitis N70.13
  complicating abortion — *see* Abortion, by type, complicated by, oophoritis
Oophorocele N83.4- ☑
Opacity, opacities
  cornea H17.- ☑
    central H17.1- ☑
    congenital Q13.3
    degenerative — *see* Degeneration, cornea
    hereditary — *see* Dystrophy, cornea
    inflammatory — *see* Keratitis
    minor H17.81- ☑
    peripheral H17.82- ☑
    sequelae of trachoma (healed) B94.0
    specified NEC H17.89
  enamel (teeth) (fluoride) (nonfluoride) K00.3
  lens — *see* Cataract
  snowball — *see* Deposit, crystalline
  vitreous (humor) NEC H43.39- ☑
    congenital Q14.0
    membranes and strands H43.31- ☑
Opalescent dentin (hereditary) K00.5
Open, opening
  abnormal, organ or site, congenital — *see* Imperfect, closure
  angle with
    borderline
      findings
        high risk H40.02- ☑
        low risk H40.01- ☑
      intraocular pressure H40.00- ☑
    cupping of discs H40.01- ☑
    glaucoma (primary) — *see* Glaucoma, open angle
  bite
    anterior M26.220
    posterior M26.221

☑ **Additional Character Required — Refer to the Tabular List for Character Selection**

Open, opening — *continued*
  false — *see* Imperfect, closure
  margin on tooth restoration K08.51
  restoration margins of tooth K08.51
  wound — *see* Wound, open
Operational fatigue F48.8
Operative — *see* condition
Operculitis — *see* Periodontitis
Operculum — *see* Break, retina
Ophiasis L63.2
Ophthalmia — *see also* Conjunctivitis H10.9
  actinic rays — *see* Photokeratitis
  allergic (acute) — *see* Conjunctivitis, acute, atopic
  blennorrhagic (gonococcal) (neonatorum) A54.31
  diphtheritic A36.86
  Egyptian A71.1
  electrica — *see* Photokeratitis
  gonococcal (neonatorum) A54.31
  metastatic — *see* Endophthalmitis, purulent
  migraine — *see* Migraine, ophthalmoplegic
  neonatorum, newborn P39.1
    gonococcal A54.31
  nodosa H16.24- ☑
  purulent — *see* Conjunctivitis, acute, mucopurulent
  spring — *see* Conjunctivitis, acute, atopic
  sympathetic — *see* Uveitis, sympathetic
Ophthalmitis — *see* Ophthalmia
Ophthalmocele (congenital) Q15.8
Ophthalmoneuromyelitis G36.0
Ophthalmoplegia — *see also* Strabismus, paralytic
  anterior internuclear — *see* Ophthalmoplegia, internu-clear
  ataxia-areflexia G61.0
  diabetic — *see* E08-E13 with .39
  exophthalmic E05.00
    with thyroid storm E05.01
  external H49.88- ☑
    progressive H49.4- ☑
      with pigmentary retinopathy — *see* Kearns-Sayre syndrome
    total H49.3- ☑
  internal (complete) (total) H52.51- ☑
  internuclear H51.2- ☑
  migraine — *see* Migraine, ophthalmoplegic
  Parinaud's H49.88- ☑
  progressive external — *see* Ophthalmoplegia, external, progressive
  supranuclear, progressive G23.1
  total (external) — *see* Ophthalmoplegia, external, total
Opioid(s)
  abuse — *see* Abuse, drug, opioids
  dependence — *see* Dependence, drug, opioids
  induced, without use disorder
    anxiety disorder F11.988
    delirium F11.921
    depressive disorder F11.94
    sexual dysfunction F11.981
    sleep disorder F11.982
Opisthognathism M26.09
Opisthorchiasis (felineus) (viverrini) B66.0
Opitz' disease D73.2
Opiumism — *see* Dependence, drug, opioid
Oppenheim's disease G70.2
Oppenheim-Urbach disease (necrobiosis lipoidica diabeti-corum) — *see* E08-E13 with .620
Optic nerve — *see* condition
Orbit — *see* condition
Orchioblastoma C62.9- ☑
Orchitis (gangrenous) (nonspecific) (septic) (suppurative) N45.2
  blennorrhagic (gonococcal) (acute) (chronic) A54.23
  chlamydial A56.19
  filarial — *see also* Infestation, filarial B74.9 *[N51]*
  gonococcal (acute) (chronic) A54.23
  mumps B26.0
  syphilitic A52.76
  tuberculous A18.15
Orf (virus disease) B08.02
Organic — *see also* condition
  brain syndrome F09
  heart — *see* Disease, heart
  mental disorder F09
  psychosis F09
Orgasm
  anejaculatory N53.13
Oriental
  bilharziasis B65.2
  schistosomiasis B65.2

Orifice — *see* condition
Origin of both great vessels from right ventricle Q20.1
Ormond's disease (with ureteral obstruction) N13.5
  with infection N13.6
Ornithine metabolism disorder E72.4
Ornithinemia (Type I) (Type II) E72.4
Ornithosis A70
Orotaciduria, oroticaciduria (congenital) (hereditary) (pyrimidine deficiency) E79.89
  anemia D53.0
Orthodontics
  adjustment Z46.4
  fitting Z46.4
Orthopnea R06.01
Orthopoxvirus B08.09
Os, uterus — *see* condition
Osgood-Schlatter disease or osteochondrosis M92.52- ☑
Osler (-Weber)-**Rendu disease** I78.0
Osler's nodes I33.0
Osmidrosis L75.0
Osseous — *see* condition
Ossification
  artery — *see* Arteriosclerosis
  auricle (ear) — *see* Disorder, pinna, specified type NEC
  bronchial J98.09
  cardiac — *see* Degeneration, myocardial
  cartilage (senile) — *see* Disorder, cartilage, specified type NEC
  coronary (artery) — *see* Disease, heart, ischemic, atherosclerotic
  diaphragm J98.6
  ear, middle — *see* Otosclerosis
  falx cerebri G96.198
  fontanel, premature Q75.009
  heart — *see also* Degeneration, myocardial
    valve — *see* Endocarditis
  larynx J38.7
  ligament — *see* Disorder, tendon, specified type NEC
    posterior longitudinal — *see* Spondylopathy, specified NEC
  meninges (cerebral) (spinal) G96.198
  multiple, eccentric centers — *see* Disorder, bone, devel-opment or growth
  muscle — *see also* Calcification, muscle
    due to burns — *see* Myositis, ossificans, in, burns
    paralytic — *see* Myositis, ossificans, in, quadriplegia
    progressive — *see* Myositis, ossificans, progressiva
    specified NEC M61.50
      ankle M61.57- ☑
      foot M61.57- ☑
      forearm M61.53- ☑
      hand M61.54- ☑
      lower leg M61.56- ☑
      multiple sites M61.59
      pelvic region M61.55- ☑
      shoulder region M61.51- ☑
      specified site NEC M61.58
      thigh M61.55- ☑
      upper arm M61.52- ☑
    traumatic — *see* Myositis, ossificans, traumatica
  myocardium, myocardial — *see* Degeneration, myocar-dial
  penis N48.89
  periarticular — *see* Disorder, joint, specified type NEC
  pinna — *see* Disorder, pinna, specified type NEC
  rider's bone — *see* Ossification, muscle, specified NEC
  sclera H15.89
  subperiosteal, post-traumatic M89.8X- ☑
  tendon — *see* Disorder, tendon, specified type NEC
  trachea J39.8
  tympanic membrane — *see* Disorder, tympanic mem-brane, specified NEC
  vitreous (humor) — *see* Deposit, crystalline
Osteitis — *see also* Osteomyelitis
  alveolar M27.3
  condensans M85.30
    ankle M85.37- ☑
    foot M85.37- ☑
    forearm M85.33- ☑
    hand M85.34- ☑
    lower leg M85.36- ☑
    multiple site M85.39
    neck M85.38
    rib M85.38
    shoulder M85.31- ☑
    skull M85.38
    specified site NEC M85.38
    thigh M85.35- ☑

Osteitis — *continued*
  condensans — *continued*
    toe M85.37- ☑
    upper arm M85.32- ☑
    vertebra M85.38
  deformans — *see also* Paget's disease, bone M88.9
    in (due to)
      malignant neoplasm of bone — *see also* Neoplasm, malignant, by site C41.9 *[M90.60]*
      neoplastic disease — *see also* Neoplasm, by type and site D49.9 *[M90.60]*
      carpus D49.2 *[M90.64-]* ☑
      clavicle D49.2 *[M90.61-]* ☑
      femur D49.2 *[M90.65-]* ☑
      fibula D49.2 *[M90.66-]* ☑
      finger D49.2 *[M90.64-]* ☑
      humerus D49.2 *[M90.62-]* ☑
      ilium D49.2 *[M90.68]*
      ischium D49.2 *[M90.68]*
      metacarpus D49.2 *[M90.64-]* ☑
      metatarsus D49.2 *[M90.67-]* ☑
      multiple sites D49.89 *[M90.69]*
      neck D49.2 *[M90.68]*
      pubic ramus D49.2 *[M90.68]*
      radius D49.2 *[M90.63-]* ☑
      rib D49.2 *[M90.68]*
      scapula D49.2 *[M90.61-]* ☑
      skull D49.2 *[M90.68]*
      tarsus D49.2 *[M90.67-]* ☑
      tibia D49.2 *[M90.66-]* ☑
      toe D49.2 *[M90.67-]* ☑
      ulna D49.2 *[M90.63-]* ☑
      vertebra D49.2 *[M90.68]*
    skull M88.0
    specified NEC — *see* Paget's disease, bone, by site
    vertebra M88.1
  due to yaws A66.6
  fibrosa NEC — *see* Cyst, bone, by site
    circumscripta — *see* Dysplasia, fibrous, bone NEC
    cystica (generalisata) E21.0
    disseminata Q78.1
    osteoplastica E21.0
  fragilitans Q78.0
  Garr's (sclerosing) — *see* Osteomyelitis, specified type NEC
  jaw (acute) (chronic) (lower) (suppurative) (upper) M27.2
  parathyroid E21.0
  petrous bone (acute) (chronic) — *see* Petrositis
  sclerotic, nonsuppurative — *see* Osteomyelitis, specified type NEC
  tuberculosa A18.09
    cystica D86.89
    multiplex cystoides D86.89
Osteoarthritis M19.90
  ankle M19.07- ☑
    post-traumatic M19.17- ☑
    primary M19.07- ☑
    secondary M19.27- ☑
  elbow M19.02- ☑
    post-traumatic M19.12- ☑
    primary M19.02- ☑
    secondary M19.22- ☑
  foot joint M19.07- ☑
    post-traumatic M19.17- ☑
    primary M19.07- ☑
    secondary M19.27- ☑
  generalized (multiple joints) M15.9
    erosive M15.4
    primary M15.0
    specified NEC M15.8
  hand joint M19.04- ☑
    first carpometacarpal joint M18.9
      post-traumatic — *see* Osteoarthritis, post-traumat-ic NEC, hand joint, first carpometacarpal joint
      primary — *see* Osteoarthritis, primary, hand joint, first carpometacarpal joint
      secondary — *see* Osteoarthritis, secondary, hand joint, first carpometacarpal joint
    post-traumatic M19.14- ☑
    primary M19.04- ☑
    secondary M19.24- ☑
  hip M16.9
    bilateral M16.0
      due to hip dysplasia M16.2
      post-traumatic M16.4
      secondary M16.6

☑ **Additional Character Required — Refer to the Tabular List for Character Selection**

Osteoarthritis — *continued*
- hip — *continued*
  - due to hip dysplasia (unilateral) M16.3- ☑
    - bilateral M16.2
  - post-traumatic — *see* Osteoarthritis, post-traumatic, hip
  - primary M16.1- ☑
  - secondary — *see* Osteoarthritis, secondary, hip
  - unilateral M16.1- ☑
    - due to hip dysplasia M16.3- ☑
    - post-traumatic M16.5- ☑
    - primary M16.1- ☑
    - secondary NEC M16.7
- interphalangeal
  - distal (Heberden) M15.1
  - proximal (Bouchard) M15.2
- knee M17.9
  - bilateral M17.0
    - post-traumatic M17.2
    - secondary M17.4
  - post-traumatic — *see* Osteoarthritis, post-traumatic, knee
  - primary M17.1- ☑
    - bilateral M17.0
  - secondary — *see* Osteoarthritis, secondary, knee
  - unilateral M17.1- ☑
    - post-traumatic M17.3- ☑
    - primary M17.1- ☑
    - secondary NEC M17.5
- post-traumatic NEC M19.92
  - ankle M19.17- ☑
  - elbow M19.12- ☑
  - foot joint M19.17- ☑
  - hand joint M19.14- ☑
    - first carpometacarpal joint M18.3- ☑
      - bilateral M18.2
  - hip M16.5- ☑
    - bilateral M16.4
  - knee M17.3- ☑
    - bilateral M17.2
  - shoulder M19.11- ☑
  - specified site NEC M19.19
  - wrist M19.13- ☑
- primary M19.91
  - ankle M19.07- ☑
  - elbow M19.02- ☑
  - foot joint M19.07- ☑
  - hand joint M19.04- ☑
    - first carpometacarpal joint M18.1- ☑
      - bilateral M18.0
  - hip M16.1- ☑
    - bilateral M16.0
  - knee M17.1- ☑
    - bilateral M17.0
  - multiple sites M15.9
  - shoulder M19.01- ☑
  - specified site NEC M19.09
  - spine — *see* Spondylosis
  - wrist M19.03- ☑
- secondary M19.93
  - ankle M19.27- ☑
  - elbow M19.22- ☑
  - foot joint M19.27- ☑
  - hand joint M19.24- ☑
    - first carpometacarpal joint M18.5- ☑
      - bilateral M18.4
  - hip M16.7-
    - bilateral M16.6
  - knee M17.5-
    - bilateral M17.4
  - multiple M15.3
  - shoulder M19.21- ☑
  - specified site NEC M19.29
  - spine — *see* Spondylosis
  - wrist M19.23- ☑
- shoulder M19.01- ☑
  - post-traumatic M19.11- ☑
  - primary M19.01- ☑
  - secondary M19.21- ☑
- specified site NEC M19.09
- spine — *see* Spondylosis
- wrist M19.03- ☑
  - first carpometacarpal joint — *see* Osteoarthritis, hand joint, first carpometacarpal joint
  - post-traumatic M19.13- ☑
  - primary M19.03- ☑
  - secondary M19.23 ☑

Osteoarthropathy (hypertrophic) M19.90
- ankle — *see* Osteoarthritis, primary, ankle
- elbow — *see* Osteoarthritis, primary, elbow
- foot joint — *see* Osteoarthritis, primary, foot
- hand joint — *see* Osteoarthritis, primary, hand joint
- knee joint — *see* Osteoarthritis, primary, knee
- multiple site — *see* Osteoarthritis, primary, multiple joint
- pulmonary — *see also* Osteoarthropathy, specified type NEC
  - hypertrophic — *see* Osteoarthropathy, hypertrophic, specified type NEC
- secondary — *see* Osteoarthropathy, specified type NEC
- secondary hypertrophic — *see* Osteoarthropathy, specified type NEC
- shoulder — *see* Osteoarthritis, primary, shoulder
- specified joint NEC — *see* Osteoarthritis, primary, specified joint NEC
- specified type NEC M89.40
  - carpus M89.44- ☑
  - clavicle M89.41- ☑
  - femur M89.45- ☑
  - fibula M89.46- ☑
  - finger M89.44- ☑
  - humerus M89.42- ☑
  - ilium M89.48
  - ischium M89.48
  - metacarpus M89.44- ☑
  - metatarsus M89.47- ☑
  - multiple sites M89.49
  - neck M89.48
  - pubic ramus M89.48
  - radius M89.43- ☑
  - rib M89.48
  - scapula M89.41- ☑
  - skull M89.48
  - tarsus M89.47- ☑
  - tibia M89.46- ☑
  - toe M89.47- ☑
  - ulna M89.43- ☑
  - vertebra M89.48
- spine — *see* Spondylosis
- wrist — *see* Osteoarthritis, primary, wrist

Osteoarthrosis (degenerative) (hypertrophic) (joint) — *see also* Osteoarthritis
- deformans alkaptonurica E70.29 *[M36.8]*
- erosive M15.4
- generalized M15.9
  - primary M15.0
- polyarticular M15.9
- spine — *see* Spondylosis

Osteoblastoma — *see* Neoplasm, bone, benign
- aggressive — *see* Neoplasm, bone, uncertain behavior

Osteochondritis — *see also* Osteochondropathy, by site
- Brailsford's — *see* Osteochondrosis, juvenile, radius
- dissecans M93.20
  - ankle M93.27- ☑
  - elbow M93.22- ☑
  - foot M93.27- ☑
  - hand M93.24- ☑
  - hip M93.25- ☑
  - knee M93.26- ☑
  - multiple sites M93.29
  - shoulder joint M93.21- ☑
  - specified site NEC M93.28
  - wrist M93.23- ☑
- juvenile M92.9
  - patellar — *see* Osteochondrosis, juvenile, patella
- syphilitic (congenital) (early) A50.02 *[M90.80]*
  - ankle A50.02 *[M90.87-]* ☑
  - elbow A50.02 *[M90.82-]* ☑
  - foot A50.02 *[M90.87-]* ☑
  - forearm A50.02 *[M90.83-]* ☑
  - hand A50.02 *[M90.84-]* ☑
  - hip A50.02 *[M90.85-]* ☑
  - knee A50.02 *[M90.86-]* ☑
  - multiple sites A50.02 *[M90.89]*
  - shoulder joint A50.02 *[M90.81-]* ☑
  - specified site NEC A50.02 *[M90.88]*

Osteochondroarthrosis deformans endemica — *see* Disease, Kaschin-Beck

Osteochondrodysplasia Q78.9
- with defects of growth of tubular bones and spine Q77.9
  - specified NEC Q77.8
- specified NEC Q78.8

Osteochondrodystrophy E78.9

Osteochondrolysis — *see* Osteochondritis, dissecans

Osteochondroma — *see* Neoplasm, bone, benign

Osteochondromatosis D16.9
- syndrome Q78.4

Osteochondromyxosarcoma — *see* Neoplasm, bone, malignant

Osteochondropathy M93.90
- ankle M93.97- ☑
- elbow M93.92- ☑
- foot M93.97- ☑
- hand M93.94- ☑
- hip M93.95- ☑
- Kienbock's disease of adults M93.1
- knee M93.96- ☑
- multiple joints M93.99
- osteochondritis dissecans — *see* Osteochondritis, dissecans
- osteochondrosis — *see* Osteochondrosis
- shoulder region M93.91- ☑
- slipped upper femoral epiphysis — *see* Slipped, epiphysis, upper femoral
- specified joint NEC M93.98
- specified type NEC M93.80
  - ankle M93.87- ☑
  - elbow M93.82- ☑
  - foot M93.87- ☑
  - hand M93.84- ☑
  - hip M93.85- ☑
  - knee M93.86- ☑
  - multiple joints M93.89
  - shoulder region M93.81- ☑
  - specified joint NEC M93.88
  - wrist M93.83- ☑
- syphilitic, congenital
  - early A50.02 *[M90.80]*
  - late A50.56 *[M90.80]*
- wrist M93.93- ☑

Osteochondrosarcoma — *see* Neoplasm, bone, malignant

Osteochondrosis — *see also* Osteochondropathy, by site
- acetabulum (juvenile) M91.0
- adult — *see* Osteochondropathy, specified type NEC, by site
- astragalus (juvenile) — *see* Osteochondrosis, juvenile, tarsus
- Blount's M92.51- ☑
- Buchanan's M91.0
- Burns' — *see* Osteochondrosis, juvenile, ulna
- calcaneus (juvenile) — *see* Osteochondrosis, juvenile, tarsus
- capitular epiphysis (femur) (juvenile) — *see* Legg-Calve-Perthes disease
- carpal (juvenile) (lunate) (scaphoid) — *see* Osteochondrosis, juvenile, hand, carpal lunate
  - adult M93.1
- coxae juvenilis — *see* Legg-Calve-Perthes disease
- deformans juvenilis, coxae — *see* Legg-Calve-Perthes disease
- Diaz's — *see* Osteochondrosis, juvenile, tarsus
- dissecans (knee) (shoulder) — *see* Osteochondritis, dissecans
- femoral capital epiphysis (juvenile) — *see* Legg-Calve-Perthes disease
- femur (head), juvenile — *see* Legg-Calve-Perthes disease
- fibula (juvenile) — *see* Osteochondrosis, juvenile, fibula
- foot NEC (juvenile) M92.8
- Freiberg's — *see* Osteochondrosis, juvenile, metatarsus
- Haas' (juvenile) — *see* Osteochondrosis, juvenile, humerus
- Haglund's — *see* Osteochondrosis, juvenile, tarsus
- hip (juvenile) — *see* Legg-Calve-Perthes disease
- humerus (capitulum) (head) (juvenile) — *see* Osteochondrosis, juvenile, humerus
- ilium, iliac crest (juvenile) M91.0
- ischiopubic synchondrosis M91.0
- Iselin's — *see* Osteochondrosis, juvenile, metatarsus
- juvenile, juvenilis M92.9
  - after congenital dislocation of hip reduction — *see* Osteochondrosis, juvenile, hip, specified NEC
  - arm — *see* Osteochondrosis, juvenile, upper limb NEC
  - capitular epiphysis (femur) — *see* Legg-Calve-Perthes disease
  - clavicle, sternal epiphysis — *see* Osteochondrosis, juvenile, upper limb NEC
  - coxae — *see* Legg-Calve-Perthes disease
  - deformans M92.9
  - fibula M92.50- ☑
  - foot NEC M92.8
  - hand M92.20- ☑
    - carpal lunate M92.21- ☑
    - metacarpal head M92.22- ☑

Osteochondrosis — *continued*
  juvenile, juvenilis — *continued*
    hand — *continued*
      specified site NEC M92.29- ☑
    head of femur — *see* Legg-Calve-Perthes disease
    hip and pelvis M91.9- ☑
      coxa plana — *see* Coxa, plana
      femoral head — *see* Legg-Calve-Perthes disease
      pelvis M91.0
      pseudocoxalgia — *see* Pseudocoxalgia
      specified NEC M91.8- ☑
    humerus M92.0- ☑
    limb
      lower NEC M92.8
      upper NEC — *see* Osteochondrosis, juvenile, upper limb NEC
    medial cuneiform bone — *see* Osteochondrosis, juvenile, tarsus
    metatarsus M92.7- ☑
    patella M92.4- ☑
    radius M92.1- ☑
    specified
      site NEC M92.8
      type NEC M92.8
        tibia and fibula M92.59- ☑
    spine M42.00
      cervical region M42.02
      cervicothoracic region M42.03
      lumbar region M42.06
      lumbosacral region M42.07
      multiple sites M42.09
      occipito-atlanto-axial region M42.01
      sacrococcygeal region M42.08
      thoracic region M42.04
      thoracolumbar region M42.05
    tarsus M92.6- ☑
    tibia M92.50- ☑
      proximal M92.51- ☑
      tubercle M92.52- ☑
    ulna M92.1- ☑
    upper limb NEC M92.3- ☑
    vertebra (body) (epiphyseal plates) (Calve's) (Scheuermann's) — *see* Osteochondrosis, juvenile, spine
  Kienbock's — *see* Osteochondrosis, juvenile, hand, carpal lunate
    adult M93.1
  Kohler's
    patellar — *see* Osteochondrosis, juvenile, patella
    tarsal navicular — *see* Osteochondrosis, juvenile, tarsus
  Legg-Perthes (-Calve) (-Waldenstrom) — *see* Legg-Calve-Perthes disease
  limb
    lower NEC (juvenile) M92.8
      tibia and fibula M92.59- ☑
    upper NEC (juvenile) — *see* Osteochondrosis, juvenile, upper limb NEC
  lunate bone (carpal) (juvenile) — *see also* Osteochondrosis, juvenile, hand, carpal lunate
    adult M93.1
  Mauclaire's — *see* Osteochondrosis, juvenile, hand, metacarpal
  metacarpal (head) (juvenile) — *see* Osteochondrosis, juvenile, hand, metacarpal
  metatarsus (fifth) (head) (juvenile) (second) — *see* Osteochondrosis, juvenile, metatarsus
  navicular (juvenile) — *see* Osteochondrosis, juvenile, tarsus
  os
    calcis (juvenile) — *see* Osteochondrosis, juvenile, tarsus
    tibiale externum (juvenile) — *see* Osteochondrosis, juvenile, tarsus
  Osgood-Schlatter M92.52- ☑
  Panner's — *see* Osteochondrosis, juvenile, humerus
  patellar center (juvenile) (primary) (secondary) — *see* Osteochondrosis, juvenile, patella
  pelvis (juvenile) M91.0
  Pierson's M91.0
  radius (head) (juvenile) — *see* Osteochondrosis, juvenile, radius
  Scheuermann's — *see* Osteochondrosis, juvenile, spine
  Sever's — *see* Osteochondrosis, juvenile, tarsus
  Sinding-Larsen — *see* Osteochondrosis, juvenile, patella
  spine M42.9
    adult M42.10
      cervical region M42.12

Osteochondrosis — *continued*
  spine — *continued*
    adult — *continued*
      cervicothoracic region M42.13
      lumbar region M42.16
      lumbosacral region M42.17
      multiple sites M42.19
      occipito-atlanto-axial region M42.11
      sacrococcygeal region M42.18
      thoracic region M42.14
      thoracolumbar region M42.15
    juvenile — *see* Osteochondrosis, juvenile, spine
  symphysis pubis (juvenile) M91.0
  syphilitic (congenital) A50.02
  talus (juvenile) — *see* Osteochondrosis, juvenile, tarsus
  tarsus (navicular) (juvenile) — *see* Osteochondrosis, juvenile, tarsus
  tibia (proximal) (tubercle) (juvenile) — *see* Osteochondrosis, juvenile, tibia
  tuberculous — *see* Tuberculosis, bone
  ulna (lower) (juvenile) — *see* Osteochondrosis, juvenile, ulna
  van Neck's M91.0
  vertebral — *see* Osteochondrosis, spine
Osteoclastoma D48.0
  malignant — *see* Neoplasm, bone, malignant
Osteodynia — *see* Disorder, bone, specified type NEC
Osteodystrophy Q78.9
  azotemic N25.0
  congenital Q78.9
  parathyroid, secondary E21.1
  renal N25.0
Osteofibroma — *see* Neoplasm, bone, benign
Osteofibrosarcoma — *see* Neoplasm, bone, malignant
Osteogenesis imperfecta Q78.0
Osteogenic — *see* condition
Osteolysis M89.50
  carpus M89.54- ☑
  clavicle M89.51- ☑
  femur M89.55- ☑
  fibula M89.56- ☑
  finger M89.54- ☑
  humerus M89.52- ☑
  ilium M89.58
  ischium M89.58
  joint prosthesis (periprosthetic) — *see* Complications, joint prosthesis, mechanical, periprosthetic, osteolysis, by site
  metacarpus M89.54- ☑
  metatarsus M89.57- ☑
  multiple sites M89.59
  neck M89.58
  periprosthetic — *see* Complications, joint prosthesis, mechanical, periprosthetic, osteolysis, by site
  pubic ramus M89.58
  radius M89.53- ☑
  rib M89.58
  scapula M89.51- ☑
  skull M89.58
  tarsus M89.57- ☑
  tibia M89.56- ☑
  toe M89.57- ☑
  ulna M89.53- ☑
  vertebra M89.58
Osteoma — *see also* Neoplasm, bone, benign
  osteoid — *see also* Neoplasm, bone, benign
    giant — *see* Neoplasm, bone, benign
Osteomalacia M83.9
  adult M83.9
    drug-induced NEC M83.5
    due to
      malabsorption (postsurgical) M83.2
      malnutrition M83.3
    specified NEC M83.8
  aluminium-induced M83.4
  infantile — *see* Rickets
  juvenile — *see* Rickets
  oncogenic E83.89
  pelvis M83.8
  puerperal M83.0
  senile M83.1
  vitamin-D-resistant in adults E83.31 *[M90.8-]* ☑
    carpus E83.31 *[M90.84-]* ☑
    clavicle E83.31 *[M90.81-]* ☑
    femur E83.31 *[M90.85-]* ☑
    fibula E83.31 *[M90.86-]* ☑
    finger E83.31 *[M90.84-]* ☑
    humerus E83.31 *[M90.82-]* ☑

Osteomalacia — *continued*
  vitamin-D-resistant in adults — *continued*
    ilium E83.31 *[M90.88]*
    ischium E83.31 *[M90.88]*
    metacarpus E83.31 *[M90.84-]* ☑
    metatarsus E83.31 *[M90.87-]* ☑
    multiple sites E83.31 *[M90.89]*
    neck E83.31 *[M90.88]*
    pubic ramus E83.31 *[M90.88]*
    radius E83.31 *[M90.83-]* ☑
    rib E83.31 *[M90.88]*
    scapula E83.31 *[M90.819]*
    skull E83.31 *[M90.88]*
    tarsus E83.31 *[M90.879]*
    tibia E83.31 *[M90.869]*
    toe E83.31 *[M90.879]*
    ulna E83.31 *[M90.839]*
    vertebra E83.31 *[M90.88]*
Osteomyelitis (general) (infective) (localized) (neonatal) (purulent) (septic) (staphylococcal) (streptococcal) (suppurative) (with periostitis) M86.9
  acute M86.10
    carpus M86.14- ☑
    clavicle M86.11- ☑
    femur M86.15- ☑
    fibula M86.16- ☑
    finger M86.14- ☑
    hematogenous M86.00
      carpus M86.04- ☑
      clavicle M86.01- ☑
      femur M86.05- ☑
      fibula M86.06- ☑
      finger M86.04- ☑
      humerus M86.02- ☑
      ilium M86.08
      ischium M86.08
      mandible M27.2
      metacarpus M86.04- ☑
      metatarsus M86.07- ☑
      multiple sites M86.09
      neck M86.08
      orbit H05.02- ☑
      petrous bone — *see* Petrositis
      radius M86.03- ☑
      rib M86.08
      scapula M86.01- ☑
      skull M86.08
      tarsus M86.07- ☑
      tibia M86.06- ☑
      toe M86.07- ☑
      ulna M86.03- ☑
      vertebra — *see* Osteomyelitis, vertebra
    humerus M86.12- ☑
    ilium M86.18
    ischium M86.18
    mandible M27.2
    metacarpus M86.14- ☑
    metatarsus M86.17- ☑
    multiple sites M86.19
    neck M86.18
    orbit H05.02- ☑
    petrous bone — *see* Petrositis
    radius M86.13- ☑
    rib M86.18
    scapula M86.11- ☑
    skull M86.18
    tarsus M86.17- ☑
    tibia M86.16- ☑
    toe M86.17- ☑
    ulna M86.13- ☑
    vertebra — *see* Osteomyelitis, vertebra
  chronic (or old) M86.60
    with draining sinus M86.40
      carpus M86.44- ☑
      clavicle M86.41- ☑
      femur M86.45- ☑
      fibula M86.46- ☑
      finger M86.44- ☑
      humerus M86.42- ☑
      ilium M86.48
      ischium M86.48
      mandible M27.2
      metacarpus M86.44- ☑
      metatarsus M86.47- ☑
      multiple sites M86.49
      neck M86.48
      orbit H05.02- ☑

Osteomyelitis — continued
  chronic — continued
    with draining sinus — continued
      petrous bone — see Petrositis
      pubic ramus M86.48
      radius M86.43- ☑
      rib M86.48
      scapula M86.41- ☑
      skull M86.48
      tarsus M86.47- ☑
      tibia M86.46- ☑
      toe M86.47- ☑
      ulna M86.43- ☑
      vertebra — see Osteomyelitis, vertebra
    carpus M86.64- ☑
    clavicle M86.61- ☑
    femur M86.65- ☑
    fibula M86.66- ☑
    finger M86.64- ☑
    hematogenous NEC M86.50
      carpus M86.54- ☑
      clavicle M86.51- ☑
      femur M86.55- ☑
      fibula M86.56- ☑
      finger M86.54- ☑
      humerus M86.52- ☑
      ilium M86.58
      ischium M86.58
      mandible M27.2
      metacarpus M86.54- ☑
      metatarsus M86.57- ☑
      multifocal M86.30
        carpus M86.34- ☑
        clavicle M86.31- ☑
        femur M86.35- ☑
        fibula M86.36- ☑
        finger M86.34- ☑
        humerus M86.32- ☑
        ilium M86.38
        ischium M86.38
        metacarpus M86.34- ☑
        metatarsus M86.37- ☑
        multiple sites M86.39
        neck M86.38
        pubic ramus M86.38
        radius M86.33- ☑
        rib M86.38
        scapula M86.31- ☑
        skull M86.38
        tarsus M86.37- ☑
        tibia M86.36- ☑
        toe M86.37- ☑
        ulna M86.33- ☑
        vertebra — see Osteomyelitis, vertebra
      multiple sites M86.59
      neck M86.58
      orbit H05.02- ☑
      petrous bone — see Petrositis
      pubic ramus M86.58
      radius M86.53- ☑
      rib M86.58
      scapula M86.51- ☑
      skull M86.58
      tarsus M86.57- ☑
      tibia M86.56- ☑
      toe M86.57- ☑
      ulna M86.53- ☑
      vertebra — see Osteomyelitis, vertebra
    humerus M86.62- ☑
    ilium M86.659
    ischium M86.659
    mandible M27.2
    metacarpus M86.64- ☑
    metatarsus M86.67- ☑
    multifocal — see Osteomyelitis, chronic, hematogenous, multifocal
    multiple sites M86.69
    neck M86.68
    orbit H05.02- ☑
    petrous bone — see Petrositis
    radius M86.63- ☑
    rib M86.68
    scapula M86.61- ☑
    skull M86.68
    tarsus M86.67- ☑
    tibia M86.66- ☑

Osteomyelitis — continued
  chronic — continued
    toe M86.67- ☑
    ulna M86.63- ☑
    vertebra — see Osteomyelitis, vertebra
  echinococcal B67.2
  Garr's — see Osteomyelitis, specified type NEC
  in diabetes mellitus — see E08-E13 with .69
  jaw (acute) (chronic) (lower) (neonatal) (suppurative) (upper) M27.2
  nonsuppurating — see Osteomyelitis, specified type NEC
  orbit H05.02- ☑
  petrous bone — see Petrositis
  Salmonella (arizonae) (cholerae-suis) (enteritidis) (typhimurium) A02.24
  sclerosing, nonsuppurative — see Osteomyelitis, specified type NEC
  specified type NEC — see also subcategory M86.8X- ☑
    mandible M27.2
    orbit H05.02- ☑
    petrous bone — see Petrositis
    vertebra — see Osteomyelitis, vertebra
  subacute M86.20
    carpus M86.24- ☑
    clavicle M86.21- ☑
    femur M86.25- ☑
    fibula M86.26- ☑
    finger M86.24- ☑
    humerus M86.22- ☑
    mandible M27.2
    metacarpus M86.24- ☑
    metatarsus M86.27- ☑
    multiple sites M86.29
    neck M86.28
    orbit H05.02- ☑
    petrous bone — see Petrositis
    radius M86.23- ☑
    rib M86.28
    scapula M86.21- ☑
    skull M86.28
    tarsus M86.27- ☑
    tibia M86.26- ☑
    toe M86.27- ☑
    ulna M86.23- ☑
    vertebra — see Osteomyelitis, vertebra
  syphilitic A52.77
    congenital (early) A50.02 [M90.80]
  tuberculous — see Tuberculosis, bone
  typhoid A01.05
  vertebra M46.20
    cervical region M46.22
    cervicothoracic region M46.23
    lumbar region M46.26
    lumbosacral region M46.27
    occipito-atlanto-axial region M46.21
    sacrococcygeal region M46.28
    thoracic region M46.24
    thoracolumbar region M46.25
Osteomyelofibrosis D47.4
Osteomyelosclerosis D75.89
Osteonecrosis M87.9
  due to
    drugs — see Osteonecrosis, secondary, due to, drugs
    trauma — see Osteonecrosis, secondary, due to, trauma
  idiopathic aseptic M87.00
    ankle M87.07- ☑
    carpus M87.03- ☑
    clavicle M87.01- ☑
    femur M87.05- ☑
    fibula M87.06- ☑
    finger M87.04- ☑
    humerus M87.02- ☑
    ilium M87.050
    ischium M87.050
    metacarpus M87.04- ☑
    metatarsus M87.07- ☑
    multiple sites M87.09
    neck M87.08
    pelvis M87.050
    pubic ramus M87.050
    radius M87.03- ☑
    rib M87.08
    scapula M87.01- ☑
    skull M87.08
    tarsus M87.07- ☑
    tibia M87.06- ☑

Osteonecrosis — continued
  idiopathic aseptic — continued
    toe M87.07- ☑
    ulna M87.03- ☑
    vertebra M87.08
  secondary NEC M87.30
    carpus M87.33- ☑
    clavicle M87.31- ☑
    due to
      drugs M87.10
        carpus M87.13- ☑
        clavicle M87.11- ☑
        femur M87.15- ☑
        fibula M87.16- ☑
        finger M87.14- ☑
        humerus M87.12- ☑
        ilium M87.150
        ischium M87.150
        jaw M87.180
        metacarpus M87.14- ☑
        metatarsus M87.17- ☑
        multiple sites M87.19
        neck M87.18
        pubic ramus M87.150
        radius M87.13- ☑
        rib M87.18 ☑
        scapula M87.11- ☑
        skull M87.18
        tarsus M87.17- ☑
        tibia M87.16- ☑
        toe M87.17- ☑
        ulna M87.13- ☑
        vertebra M87.18
      hemoglobinopathy NEC D58.2 [M90.50]
        carpus D58.2 [M90.54-] ☑
        clavicle D58.2 [M90.51-] ☑
        femur D58.2 [M90.55-] ☑
        fibula D58.2 [M90.56-] ☑
        finger D58.2 [M90.54-] ☑
        humerus D58.2 [M90.52-] ☑
        ilium D58.2 [M90.58]
        ischium D58.2 [M90.58]
        metacarpus D58.2 [M90.54-] ☑
        metatarsus D58.2 [M90.57-] ☑
        multiple sites D58.2 [M90.59]
        neck D58.2 [M90.58]
        pubic ramus D58.2 [M90.58]
        radius D58.2 [M90.53-] ☑
        rib D58.2 [M90.58]
        scapula D58.2 [M90.51-] ☑
        skull D58.2 [M90.58]
        specified NEC D58.2 [M90.58]
        tarsus D58.2 [M90.57-] ☑
        tibia D58.2 [M90.56-] ☑
        toe D58.2 [M90.57-] ☑
        ulna D58.2 [M90.53-] ☑
        vertebra D58.2 [M90.58]
      trauma (previous) M87.20
        carpus M87.23- ☑
        clavicle M87.21- ☑
        femur M87.25- ☑
        fibula M87.26- ☑
        finger M87.24- ☑
        humerus M87.22- ☑
        ilium M87.250
        ischium M87.250
        metacarpus M87.24- ☑
        metatarsus M87.27- ☑
        multiple sites M87.29
        neck M87.28
        pubic ramus M87.250
        radius M87.23- ☑
        rib M87.28
        scapula M87.21- ☑
        skull M87.28
        tarsus M87.27- ☑
        tibia M87.26- ☑
        toe M87.27- ☑
        ulna M87.23- ☑
        vertebra M87.28
    femur M87.35- ☑
    fibula M87.36- ☑
    finger M87.34- ☑
    humerus M87.32- ☑
    ilium M87.350

Osteonecrosis — *continued*
  secondary — *continued*
    in
      caisson disease T70.3 ✓ *[M90.50]*
        carpus T70.3 ✓ *[M90.54-]* ✓
        clavicle T70.3 ✓ *[M90.51-]* ✓
        femur T70.3 ✓ *[M90.55-]* ✓
        fibula T70.3 ✓ *[M90.56-]* ✓
        finger T70.3 ✓ *[M90.54-]* ✓
        humerus T70.3 ✓ *[M90.52-]* ✓
        ilium T70.3 ✓ *[M90.58]*
        ischium T70.3 ✓ *[M90.58]*
        metacarpus T70.3 ✓ *[M90.54-]* ✓
        metatarsus T70.3 ✓ *[M90.57-]* ✓
        multiple sites T70.3 ✓ *[M90.59]*
        neck T70.3 ✓ *[M90.58]*
        pubic ramus T70.3 ✓ *[M90.58]*
        radius T70.3 ✓ *[M90.53-]* ✓
        rib T70.3 ✓ *[M90.58]*
        scapula T70.3 ✓ *[M90.51-]* ✓
        skull T70.3 ✓ *[M90.58]*
        tarsus T70.3 ✓ *[M90.57-]* ✓
        tibia T70.3 ✓ *[M90.56-]* ✓
        toe T70.3 ✓ *[M90.57-]* ✓
        ulna T70.3 ✓ *[M90.53-]* ✓
        vertebra T70.3 ✓ *[M90.58]*
      ischium M87.350
      metacarpus M87.34- ✓
      metatarsus M87.37- ✓
      multiple site M87.39
      neck M87.38
      pubic ramus M87.350
      radius M87.33- ✓
      rib M87.38
      scapula M87.319
      skull M87.38
      tarsus M87.379
      tibia M87.366
      toe M87.379
      ulna M87.33- ✓
      vertebra M87.38
    specified type NEC M87.80
      carpus M87.83- ✓
      clavicle M87.81- ✓
      femur M87.85- ✓
      fibula M87.86- ✓
      finger M87.84- ✓
      humerus M87.82- ✓
      ilium M87.850
      ischium M87.850
      metacarpus M87.84- ✓
      metatarsus M87.87- ✓
      multiple sites M87.89
      neck M87.88
      pubic ramus M87.850
      radius M87.83- ✓
      rib M87.88
      scapula M87.81- ✓
      skull M87.88
      tarsus M87.87- ✓
      tibia M87.86- ✓
      toe M87.87- ✓
      ulna M87.83- ✓
      vertebra M87.88
Osteo-onycho-arthro-dysplasia Q87.2
Osteo-onychodysplasia, hereditary Q87.2
Osteopathia condensans disseminata Q78.8
Osteopathy — *see also* Osteomyelitis, Osteonecrosis, Osteoporosis
  after poliomyelitis M89.60
    carpus M89.64- ✓
    clavicle M89.61- ✓
    femur M89.65- ✓
    fibula M89.66- ✓
    finger M89.64- ✓
    humerus M89.62- ✓
    ilium M89.68
    ischium M89.68
    metacarpus M89.64- ✓
    metatarsus M89.67- ✓
    multiple sites M89.69
    neck M89.68
    pubic ramus M89.68
    radius M89.63- ✓
    rib M89.68
    scapula M89.61- ✓

Osteopathy — *continued*
  after poliomyelitis — *continued*
    skull M89.68
    tarsus M89.67- ✓
    tibia M89.66- ✓
    toe M89.67- ✓
    ulna M89.63- ✓
    vertebra M89.68
  in (due to)
    renal osteodystrophy N25.0
    specified diseases classified elsewhere — *see* subcategory M90.8 ✓
Osteopenia M85.8- ✓
  borderline M85.8- ✓
Osteoperiostitis — *see* Osteomyelitis, specified type NEC
Osteopetrosis (familial) Q78.2
Osteophyte M25.70
  ankle M25.77- ✓
  elbow M25.72- ✓
  foot joint M25.77- ✓
  hand joint M25.74- ✓
  hip M25.75- ✓
  knee M25.76- ✓
  shoulder M25.71- ✓
  spine M25.78
  vertebrae M25.78
  wrist M25.73- ✓
Osteopoikilosis Q78.8
Osteoporosis (female) (male) M81.0
  with current pathological fracture M80.00 ✓
  age-related M81.0
    with current pathologic fracture M80.00 ✓
      carpus M80.04- ✓
      clavicle M80.01- ✓
      femur M80.05- ✓
      fibula M80.06- ✓
      finger M80.04- ✓
      hip M80.05- ✓
      humerus M80.02- ✓
      ilium M80.0A ✓
      ischium M80.0A ✓
      metacarpus M80.04- ✓
      metatarsus M80.07- ✓
      pelvis M80.0B- ✓
      pubis ramus M80.0A ✓
      radius M80.03- ✓
      rib(s) M80.0A ✓
      scapula M80.01- ✓
      site specified NEC M80.0A ✓
      specified site NEC M80.0A ✓
      tarsus M80.07- ✓
      tibia M80.06- ✓
      toe M80.07- ✓
      ulna M80.03- ✓
      vertebra M80.08 ✓
  disuse M81.8
    with current pathological fracture M80.80 ✓
      carpus M80.84- ✓
      clavicle M80.81- ✓
      femur M80.85- ✓
      fibula M80.86- ✓
      finger M80.84- ✓
      hip M80.85- ✓
      humerus M80.82- ✓
      ilium M80.8A ✓
      ischium M80.8A ✓
      metacarpus M80.84- ✓
      metatarsus M80.87- ✓
      pelvis M80.8B- ✓
      pubis ramus M80.8A ✓
      radius M80.83- ✓
      scapula M80.81- ✓
      site specified NEC M80.8A ✓
      tarsus M80.87- ✓
      tibia M80.86- ✓
      toe M80.87- ✓
      ulna M80.83- ✓
      vertebra M80.88 ✓
  drug-induced — *see* Osteoporosis, specified type NEC
  idiopathic — *see* Osteoporosis, specified type NEC
  involutional — *see* Osteoporosis, age-related
  Lequesne M81.6
  localized M81.6
  postmenopausal M81.0
    with pathological fracture M80.00 ✓
      carpus M80.04- ✓

Osteoporosis — *continued*
  postmenopausal — *continued*
    with pathological fracture — *continued*
      clavicle M80.01- ✓
      femur M80.05- ✓
      fibula M80.06- ✓
      finger M80.04- ✓
      hip M80.05- ✓
      humerus M80.02- ✓
      ilium M80.0A ✓
      ischium M80.0A ✓
      metacarpus M80.04- ✓
      metatarsus M80.07- ✓
      pelvis M80.0B- ✓
      pubis ramus M80.0A ✓
      radius M80.03- ✓
      scapula M80.01- ✓
      site specified NEC M80.0A ✓
      tarsus M80.07- ✓
      tibia M80.06- ✓
      toe M80.07- ✓
      ulna M80.03- ✓
      vertebra M80.08 ✓
  postoophorectomy — *see* Osteoporosis, specified type NEC
  postsurgical malabsorption — *see* Osteoporosis, specified type NEC
  post-traumatic — *see* Osteoporosis, specified type NEC
  senile — *see* Osteoporosis, age-related
  specified type NEC M81.8
    with pathological fracture M80.80 ✓
      carpus M80.84- ✓
      clavicle M80.81- ✓
      femur M80.85- ✓
      fibula M80.86- ✓
      finger M80.84- ✓
      hip M80.85- ✓
      humerus M80.82- ✓
      ilium M80.8A ✓
      ischium M80.8A ✓
      metacarpus M80.84- ✓
      metatarsus M80.87- ✓
      pelvis M80.8B- ✓
      pubis ramus M80.8A ✓
      radius M80.83- ✓
      scapula M80.81- ✓
      site specified NEC M80.8A ✓
      tarsus M80.87- ✓
      tibia M80.86- ✓
      toe M80.87- ✓
      ulna M80.83- ✓
      vertebra M80.88 ✓
Osteopsathyrosis (idiopathica) Q78.0
Osteoradionecrosis, jaw (acute) (chronic) (lower) (suppurative) (upper) M27.2
Osteosarcoma (any form) — *see* Neoplasm, bone, malignant
Osteosclerosis Q78.2
  acquired M85.8- ✓
  congenita Q77.4
  fragilitas (generalisata) Q78.2
  myelofibrosis D75.81
Osteosclerotic anemia D64.89
Osteosis
  cutis L94.2
  renal fibrocystic N25.0
Österreicher-Turner syndrome Q87.2
Ostium
  atrioventriculare commune Q21.23
  primum (arteriosum) (defect) (persistent) Q21.20
  secundum (arteriosum) (defect) (patent) (persistent) Q21.11
Ostrum-Furst syndrome Q75.8
Otalgia H92.0
Otitis (acute) H66.90
  with effusion — *see also* Otitis, media, nonsuppurative
    purulent — *see* Otitis, media, suppurative
  adhesive — *see* subcategory H74.1 ✓
  chronic — *see also* Otitis, media
    with effusion — *see also* Otitis, media, nonsuppurative, chronic
  externa H60.9- ✓
    abscess — *see* Abscess, ear, external
    acute (noninfective) H60.50- ✓
      actinic H60.51- ✓
      chemical H60.52- ✓

Otitis — *continued*
  externa — *continued*
    acute — *continued*
      contact H60.53- ☑
      eczematoid H60.54- ☑
      infective — *see* Otitis, externa, infective
      reactive H60.55- ☑
      specified NEC H60.59- ☑
    cellulitis — *see* Cellulitis, ear
    chronic H60.6- ☑
    diffuse — *see* Otitis, externa, infective, diffuse
    hemorrhagic — *see* Otitis, externa, infective, hemorrhagic
    in (due to)
      aspergillosis B44.89
      candidiasis B37.84
      erysipelas A46 *[H62.40]*
      herpes (simplex) virus infection B00.1
        zoster B02.8
      impetigo L01.00 *[H62.40]*
      infectious disease NEC B99 *[H62.4-]* ☑
      mycosis NEC B36.9 *[H62.40]*
      parasitic disease NEC B89 *[H62.40]*
      viral disease NEC B34.9 *[H62.40]*
      zoster B02.8
    infective NEC H60.39- ☑
      abscess — *see* Abscess, ear, external
      cellulitis — *see* Cellulitis, ear
      diffuse H60.31- ☑
      hemorrhagic H60.32- ☑
      swimmer's ear — *see* Swimmer's, ear
    malignant H60.2- ☑
    mycotic NEC B36.9 *[H62.40]*
      in
        aspergillosis B44.89
        candidiasis B37.84
        moniliasis B37.84
    necrotizing — *see* Otitis, externa, malignant
    Pseudomonas aeruginosa — *see* Otitis, externa, malignant
    reactive — *see* Otitis, externa, acute, reactive
    specified NEC — *see* subcategory H60.8 ☑
    tropical NEC B36.9 *[H62.40]*
      in
        aspergillosis B44.89
        candidiasis B37.84
        moniliasis B37.84
  insidiosa — *see* Otosclerosis
  interna H83.0 ☑
  media (hemorrhagic) (staphylococcal) (streptococcal) H66.9-
    with effusion (nonpurulent) — *see* Otitis, media, nonsuppurative
    acute, subacute H66.90
      allergic — *see* Otitis, media, nonsuppurative, acute, allergic
      exudative — *see* Otitis, media, suppurative, acute
      mucoid — *see* Otitis, media, nonsuppurative, acute
      necrotizing — *see also* Otitis, media, suppurative, acute
        in
          measles B05.3
          scarlet fever A38.0
      nonsuppurative NEC — *see* Otitis, media, nonsuppurative, acute
      purulent — *see* Otitis, media, suppurative, acute
      sanguinous — *see* Otitis, media, nonsuppurative, acute
      secretory — *see* Otitis, media, nonsuppurative, acute, serous
      seromucinous — *see* Otitis, media, nonsuppurative, acute
      serous — *see* Otitis, media, nonsuppurative, acute, serous
      suppurative — *see* Otitis, media, suppurative, acute
    allergic — *see* Otitis, media, nonsuppurative
    catarrhal — *see* Otitis, media, nonsuppurative
    chronic H66.90
      with effusion (nonpurulent) — *see* Otitis, media, nonsuppurative, chronic
      allergic — *see* Otitis, media, nonsuppurative, chronic, allergic
      benign suppurative — *see* Otitis, media, suppurative, chronic, tubotympanic
      catarrhal — *see* Otitis, media, nonsuppurative, chronic, serous

Otitis — *continued*
  media — *continued*
    chronic — *continued*
      exudative — *see* Otitis, media, nonsuppurative, chronic
      mucinous — *see* Otitis, media, nonsuppurative, chronic, mucoid
      mucoid — *see* Otitis, media, nonsuppurative, chronic, mucoid
      nonsuppurative NEC — *see* Otitis, media, nonsuppurative, chronic
      purulent — *see* Otitis, media, suppurative, chronic
      secretory — *see* Otitis, media, nonsuppurative, chronic, mucoid
      seromucinous — *see* Otitis, media, nonsuppurative, chronic
      serous — *see* Otitis, media, nonsuppurative, chronic, serous
      suppurative — *see* Otitis, media, suppurative, chronic
      transudative — *see* Otitis, media, nonsuppurative, chronic, mucoid
    exudative — *see* Otitis, media, suppurative
    in (due to) (with)
      influenza — *see* Influenza, with, otitis media
      measles B05.3
      scarlet fever A38.0
      tuberculosis A18.6
      viral disease NEC B34.- ☑ *[H67.-]* ☑
    mucoid — *see* Otitis, media, nonsuppurative
    nonsuppurative H65.9- ☑
      acute or subacute NEC H65.19- ☑
        allergic H65.11- ☑
          recurrent H65.11- ☑
        recurrent H65.19- ☑
        secretory — *see* Otitis, media, nonsuppurative, serous
        serous H65.0- ☑
          recurrent H65.0- ☑
      chronic H65.49- ☑
        allergic H65.41- ☑
        mucoid H65.3- ☑
        serous H65.2- ☑
    postmeasles B05.3
    purulent — *see* Otitis, media, suppurative
    secretory — *see* Otitis, media, nonsuppurative
    seromucinous — *see* Otitis, media, nonsuppurative
    serous — *see* Otitis, media, nonsuppurative
    suppurative H66.4- ☑
      acute H66.00- ☑
        with rupture of ear drum H66.01- ☑
        recurrent H66.00- ☑
          with rupture of ear drum H66.01- ☑
      chronic — *see also* subcategory H66.3 ☑
        atticoantral H66.2- ☑
        benign — *see* Otitis, media, suppurative, chronic, tubotympanic
        tubotympanic H66.1- ☑
    transudative — *see* Otitis, media, nonsuppurative
    tuberculous A18.6
Otocephaly Q18.2
Otolith syndrome — *see* subcategory H81.8 ☑
Otomycosis (diffuse) NEC B36.9 *[H62.40]*
  in
    aspergillosis B44.89
    candidiasis B37.84
    moniliasis B37.84
Otoporosis — *see* Otosclerosis
Otorrhagia (nontraumatic) H92.2- ☑
  traumatic — *code by* Type of injury
Otorrhea H92.1- ☑
  cerebrospinal (fluid) G96.01
    postoperative G96.08
    specified NEC G96.08
    spontaneous G96.01
    traumatic G96.08
Otosclerosis (general) H80.9- ☑
  cochlear (endosteal) H80.2- ☑
  involving
    otic capsule — *see* Otosclerosis, cochlear
    oval window
      nonobliterative H80.0- ☑
      obliterative H80.1- ☑
    round window — *see* Otosclerosis, cochlear
  nonobliterative — *see* Otosclerosis, involving, oval window, nonobliterative

Otosclerosis — *continued*
  obliterative — *see* Otosclerosis, involving, oval window, obliterative
  specified NEC H80.8- ☑
Otospongiosis — *see* Otosclerosis
Otto's disease or pelvis M24.7
Outcome of delivery Z37.9
  multiple births Z37.9
    all liveborn Z37.50
      quadruplets Z37.52
      quintuplets Z37.53
      sextuplets Z37.54
      specified number NEC Z37.59
      triplets Z37.51
    all stillborn Z37.7
    some liveborn Z37.60
      quadruplets Z37.62
      quintuplets Z37.63
      sextuplets Z37.64
      specified number NEC Z37.69
      triplets Z37.61
  single NEC Z37.9
    liveborn Z37.0
    stillborn Z37.1
  twins NEC Z37.9
    both liveborn Z37.2
    both stillborn Z37.4
    one liveborn, one stillborn Z37.3
Outlet — *see* condition
Ovalocytosis (congenital) (hereditary) — *see* Elliptocytosis
Ovarian — *see* Condition
Ovariocele N83.4- ☑
Ovaritis (cystic) — *see* Oophoritis
Ovary, ovarian — *see also* condition
  resistant syndrome E28.39
  vein syndrome N13.8
Overactive — *see also* Hyperfunction
  adrenal cortex NEC E27.0
  bladder N32.81
  hypothalamus E23.3
  thyroid — *see* Hyperthyroidism
Overactivity R46.3
  child — *see* Disorder, attention-deficit hyperactivity
Overbite (deep) (excessive) (horizontal) (vertical) M26.29
Overbreathing — *see* Hyperventilation
Overconscientious personality F60.5
Overdevelopment — *see* Hypertrophy
Overdistension — *see* Distension
Overdose, overdosage (drug) — *see* Table of Drugs and Chemicals, by drug, poisoning
Overeating R63.2
  nonorganic origin F50.89
  psychogenic F50.89
Overexertion (effects) (exhaustion) T73.3 ☑
Overexposure (effects) T73.9 ☑
  exhaustion T73.2 ☑
Overfeeding — *see* Overeating
  newborn P92.4
Overfill, endodontic M27.52
Overgrowth
  bacterial
    small intestinal K63.8219
      fungal K63.822
      hydrogen-subtype K63.8211
      hydrogen sulfide-subtype K63.8212
  bone — *see* Hypertrophy, bone
  intestinal methanogen K63.829
Overhanging of dental restorative material (unrepairable) K08.52
Overheated (places) (effects) — *see* Heat
Overjet (excessive horizontal) M26.23
Overlaid, overlying (suffocation) — *see* Asphyxia, traumatic, due to mechanical threat
Overlap, excessive horizontal (teeth) M26.23
Overlapping toe (acquired) — *see also* Deformity, toe, specified NEC
  congenital (fifth toe) Q66.89
Overload
  circulatory, due to transfusion (blood) (blood components) (TACO) E87.71
  fluid E87.70
    due to transfusion (blood) (blood components) E87.71
    specified NEC E87.79
  iron, due to repeated red blood cell transfusions E83.111
  potassium (K) E87.5
  sodium (Na) E87.0
Overnutrition — *see* Hyperalimentation
Overproduction — *see also* Hypersecretion

Index

Otitis — Overproduction

Index

Overproduction — *continued*
ACTH E27.0
catecholamine E27.5
growth hormone E22.0
Overprotection, child by parent Z62.1
Overriding
aorta Q25.49
finger (acquired) — *see* Deformity, finger
congenital Q68.1
toe (acquired) — *see also* Deformity, toe, specified NEC
congenital Q66.89
Overstrained F53.83
heart — *see* Hypertrophy, cardiac
Overuse, muscle NEC M70.8- ☑
Overweight E66.3
Overworked F53.83
Oviduct — *see* condition
Ovotestis Q56.0
Ovulation (cycle)
failure or lack of N97.0
pain N94.0
Ovum — *see* condition
Owren's disease or syndrome (parahemophilia) D68.2
Ox heart — *see* Hypertrophy, cardiac
Oxalosis E72.53
Oxaluria E72.53
Oxycephaly, oxycephalic Q75.009
syphilitic, congenital A50.02
Oxyuriasis B80
Oxyuris vermicularis (infestation) B80
Ozena J31.0

P

Pachyderma, pachydermia L85.9
larynx (verrucosa) J38.7
Pachydermatocele (congenital) Q82.8
Pachydermoperiostosis — *see also* Osteoarthropathy, hypertrophic, specified type NEC
clubbed nail M89.40 *[L62]*
Pachygyria Q04.3
Pachymeningitis (adhesive) (basal) (brain) (cervical) (chronic) (circumscribed) (external) (fibrous) (hemorrhagic) (hypertrophic) (internal) (purulent) (spinal) (suppurative) — *see* Meningitis
Pachyonychia (congenital) Q84.5
Pacinian tumor — *see* Neoplasm, skin, benign
Pad, knuckle or Garrod's M72.1
Paget's disease
with infiltrating duct carcinoma — *see* Neoplasm, breast, malignant
bone M88.9
carpus M88.84- ☑
clavicle M88.81- ☑
femur M88.85- ☑
fibula M88.86- ☑
finger M88.84- ☑
humerus M88.82- ☑
ilium M88.88
in neoplastic disease — *see* Osteitis, deformans, in neoplastic disease
ischium M88.88
metacarpus M88.84- ☑
metatarsus M88.87- ☑
multiple sites M88.89
neck M88.88
pubic ramus M88.88
radius M88.83- ☑
rib M88.88
scapula M88.81- ☑
skull M88.0
specified NEC M88.88
tarsus M88.87- ☑
tibia M88.86- ☑
toe M88.87- ☑
ulna M88.83- ☑
vertebra M88.1
breast (female) C50.01- ☑
male C50.02- ☑
extramammary — *see also* Neoplasm, skin, malignant
anus C21.0
margin C44.590
skin C44.590
intraductal carcinoma — *see* Neoplasm, breast, malignant
malignant — *see* Neoplasm, skin, malignant
breast (female) C50.01- ☑
male C50.02- ☑

Paget's disease — *continued*
malignant — *see* Neoplasm, skin, malignant — *continued*
unspecified site (female) C50.01- ☑
male C50.02- ☑
mammary — *see* Paget's disease, breast
nipple — *see* Paget's disease, breast
osteitis deformans — *see* Paget's disease, bone
Paget-Schroetter syndrome I82.890
Pain(s) — *see also* Painful R52
abdominal R10.9
colic R10.83
generalized R10.84
with acute abdomen R10.0
lower R10.30
left quadrant R10.32
pelvic or perineal R10.2
periumbilical R10.33
right quadrant R10.31
rebound — *see* Tenderness, abdominal, rebound
severe with abdominal rigidity R10.0
tenderness — *see* Tenderness, abdominal
upper R10.10
epigastric R10.13
left quadrant R10.12
right quadrant R10.11
acute R52
due to trauma G89.11
neoplasm related G89.3
postprocedural NEC G89.18
post-thoracotomy G89.12
specified by site — *code to* Pain, by site
adnexa (uteri) R10.2
anginoid — *see* Pain, precordial
anus K62.89
arm — *see* Pain, limb, upper
axillary (axilla) M79.62- ☑
back (postural) M54.9
bladder R39.89
associated with micturition — *see* Micturition, painful
chronic R39.82
bone — *see* Disorder, bone, specified type NEC
breast N64.4
broad ligament R10.2
cancer associated (acute) (chronic) G89.3
cecum — *see* Pain, abdominal
cervicobrachial M53.1
chest (central) R07.9
anterior wall R07.89
atypical R07.89
ischemic I20.9
musculoskeletal R07.89
non-cardiac R07.89
on breathing R07.1
pleurodynia R07.81
precordial R07.2
wall (anterior) R07.89
chronic G89.29
associated with significant psychosocial dysfunction G89.4
due to trauma G89.21
neoplasm related G89.3
postoperative NEC G89.28
postprocedural NEC G89.28
post-thoracotomy G89.22
specified NEC G89.29
coccyx M53.3
colon — *see* Pain, abdominal
coronary — *see* Angina
costochondral R07.1
diaphragm R07.1
due to cancer G89.3
due to device, implant or graft — *see also* Complications, by site and type, specified NEC T85.848 ☑
arterial graft NEC T82.848 ☑
breast (implant) T85.848 ☑
catheter NEC T85.848 ☑
dialysis (renal) T82.848 ☑
intraperitoneal T85.848 ☑
infusion NEC T82.848 ☑
spinal (epidural) (subdural) T85.840 ☑
urinary (indwelling) T83.84 ☑
electronic (electrode) (pulse generator) (stimulator)
bone T85.840 ☑
cardiac T82.847 ☑
nervous system (brain) (peripheral nerve) (spinal) T85.84 ☑
urinary T83.84 ☑

Pain(s) — *continued*
due to device, implant or graft — *see also* Complications, by site and type, specified — *continued*
fixation, internal (orthopedic) NEC T84.84 ☑
gastrointestinal (bile duct) (esophagus) T85.848 ☑
genital NEC T83.84 ☑
heart NEC T82.847 ☑
infusion NEC T85.848 ☑
joint prosthesis T84.84 ☑
ocular (corneal graft) (orbital implant) NEC T85.848 ☑
orthopedic NEC T84.84 ☑
specified NEC T85.848 ☑
urinary NEC T83.84 ☑
vascular NEC T82.848 ☑
ventricular intracranial shunt T85.840 ☑
due to malignancy (primary) (secondary) G89.3
ear — *see* subcategory H92.0 ☑
epigastric, epigastrium R10.13
eye — *see* Pain, ocular
face, facial R51.9
atypical G50.1
female genital organs NEC N94.89
finger — *see* Pain, limb, upper
flank — *see* Pain, abdominal
foot — *see* Pain, limb, lower
gallbladder K82.9
gas (intestinal) R14.1
gastric — *see* Pain, abdominal
generalized NOS R52
genital organ
female N94.89
male N50.89
groin — *see* Pain, abdominal, lower
hand — *see* Pain, limb, upper
head — *see* Headache
heart — *see* Pain, precordial
infra-orbital — *see* Neuralgia, trigeminal
intercostal R07.82
intermenstrual N94.0
jaw R68.84
joint M25.50
ankle M25.57- ☑
elbow M25.52- ☑
finger M25.54- ☑
foot M25.57- ☑
hand M25.54- ☑
hip M25.55- ☑
knee M25.56- ☑
shoulder M25.51- ☑
specified site NEC M25.59
toe M25.57- ☑
wrist M25.53- ☑
kidney N23
laryngeal R07.0
leg — *see* Pain, limb, lower
limb M79.609
lower M79.60- ☑
foot M79.67- ☑
lower leg M79.66- ☑
thigh M79.65- ☑
toe M79.67- ☑
upper M79.60- ☑
axilla M79.62- ☑
finger M79.64- ☑
forearm M79.63- ☑
hand M79.64- ☑
upper arm M79.62- ☑
loin M54.50
low back M54.50
specified NEC M54.59
vertebral end plate M54.51
vertebrogenic M54.51
lumbar region M54.50
vertebral end plate M54.51
vertebrogenic M54.51
mandibular R68.84
mastoid — *see* subcategory H92.0 ☑
maxilla R68.84
menstrual — *see also* Dysmenorrhea N94.6
metacarpophalangeal (joint) — *see* Pain, joint, hand
metatarsophalangeal (joint) — *see* Pain, joint, foot
mouth K13.79
muscle — *see* Myalgia
musculoskeletal — *see also* Pain, by site M79.18
myofascial M79.18
nasal J34.89
nasopharynx J39.2

Overproduction — Pain

Pain(s) — *continued*
neck NEC M54.2
nerve NEC — *see* Neuralgia
neuromuscular — *see* Neuralgia
nose J34.89 ☑
ocular H57.1- ☑
ophthalmic — *see* Pain, ocular
orbital region — *see* Pain, ocular
ovary N94.89
over heart — *see* Pain, precordial
ovulation N94.0
pelvic (female) R10.2
penis N48.89
pericardial — *see* Pain, precordial
perineal, perineum R10.2
pharynx J39.2
pleura, pleural, pleuritic R07.81
postoperative NOS G89.18
postprocedural NOS G89.18
post-thoracotomy G89.12
precordial (region) R07.2
premenstrual N94.3
psychogenic (persistent) (any site) F45.41
radicular (spinal) — *see* Radiculopathy
rectum K62.89
respiration R07.1
retrosternal R07.2
rheumatoid, muscular — *see* Myalgia
rib R07.81
root (spinal) — *see* Radiculopathy
round ligament (stretch) R10.2
sacroiliac M53.3
sciatic — *see* Sciatica
scrotum N50.82
seminal vesicle N50.89
shoulder M25.51- ☑
spermatic cord N50.89
spinal root — *see* Radiculopathy
spine M54.9
cervical M54.2
low back M54.50
with sciatica M54.4- ☑
thoracic M54.6
stomach — *see* Pain, abdominal
substernal R07.2
temporomandibular (joint) M26.62- ☑
testis N50.81- ☑
thoracic spine M54.6
with radicular and visceral pain M54.14
throat R07.0
tibia — *see* Pain, limb, lower
toe — *see* Pain, limb, lower
tongue K14.6
tooth K08.89
trigeminal — *see* Neuralgia, trigeminal
tumor associated G89.3
ureter N23
urinary (organ) (system) N23
uterus NEC N94.89
vagina R10.2
vertebral end plate — *see* Pain, vertebrogenic
vertebrogenic M54.89
low back M54.51
lumbar M54.51
syndrome M54.89
vesical R39.89
associated with micturition — *see* Micturition, painful
vulva R10.2
Painful — *see also* Pain
coitus
female N94.10
male N53.12
psychogenic F52.6
ejaculation (semen) N53.12
psychogenic F52.6
erection — *see* Priapism
feet syndrome E53.8
joint replacement (hip) (knee) T84.84 ☑
menstruation — *see* Dysmenorrhea
psychogenic F45.8
micturition — *see* Micturition, painful
respiration R07.1
scar NEC L90.5
wire sutures T81.89 ☑
Painter's colic — *see* subcategory T56.0 ☑
Palate — *see* condition
Palatoplegia K13.79
Palatoschisis — *see* Cleft, palate

Palilalia R48.8
Palliative care Z51.5
Pallor R23.1
optic disc, temporal — *see* Atrophy, optic
Palmar — *see also* condition
fascia — *see* condition
Palpable
cecum K63.89
kidney N28.89
ovary N83.8
prostate N42.9
spleen — *see* Splenomegaly
Palpitations (heart) R00.2
psychogenic F45.8
Palsy — *see also* Paralysis G83.9
atrophic diffuse (progressive) G12.22
Bell's — *see also* Palsy, facial
newborn P11.3
brachial plexus NEC G54.0
newborn (birth injury) P14.3
brain — *see* Palsy, cerebral
bulbar (progressive) (chronic) G12.22
of childhood (Fazio-Londe) G12.1
pseudo NEC G12.29
supranuclear (progressive) G23.1
cerebral (congenital) G80.9
ataxic G80.4
athetoid G80.3
choreathetoid G80.3
diplegic G80.8
spastic G80.1
dyskinetic G80.3
athetoid G80.3
choreathetoid G80.3
distonic G80.3
dystonic G80.3
hemiplegic G80.8
spastic G80.2
mixed G80.8
monoplegic G80.8
spastic G80.1
paraplegic G80.8
spastic G80.1
quadriplegic G80.8
spastic G80.0
spastic G80.1
diplegic G80.1
hemiplegic G80.2
monoplegic G80.1
quadriplegic G80.0
specified NEC G80.1
tetrapelgic G80.0
specified NEC G80.8
syphilitic A52.12
congenital A50.49
tetraplegic G80.8
spastic G80.0
cranial nerve — *see also* Disorder, nerve, cranial
multiple G52.7
in
infectious disease B99 ☑ *[G53]*
neoplastic disease — *see also* Neoplasm
D49.9 *[G53]*
parasitic disease B89 *[G53]*
sarcoidosis D86.82
creeping G12.22
diver's T70.3 ☑
Erb's P14.0
facial G51.0
newborn (birth injury) P11.3
glossopharyngeal G52.1
Klumpke (-Dejerine) P14.1
lead — *see* subcategory T56.0 ☑
median nerve (tardy) G56.1- ☑
nerve G58.9
specified NEC G58.8
peroneal nerve (acute) (tardy) G57.3- ☑
progressive supranuclear G23.1
pseudobulbar NEC G12.29
radial nerve (acute) G56.3- ☑
seventh nerve — *see also* Palsy, facial
newborn P11.3
shaking — *see* Parkinsonism
spastic (cerebral) (spinal) G80.1
ulnar nerve (tardy) G56.2- ☑
wasting G12.29
Paludism — *see* Malaria
Panangiitis M30.0

Panaris, panaritium — *see also* Cellulitis, digit
with lymphangitis — *see* Lymphangitis, acute, digit
Panarteritis nodosa M30.0
brain or cerebral I67.7
Pancake heart R93.1
with cor pulmonale (chronic) I27.81
Pancarditis (acute) (chronic) I51.89
rheumatic I09.89
active or acute I01.8
Pancoast's syndrome or tumor C34.1- ☑
Pancolitis — *see also* Colitis
ulcerative (chronic) K51.00
with
abscess K51.014
complication K51.019
fistula K51.013
obstruction K51.012
rectal bleeding K51.011
specified complication NEC K51.018
Pancreas, pancreatic — *see* condition
Pancreatitis (annular) (apoplectic) (calcareous) (edematous)
(hemorrhagic) (malignant) (subacute) (suppurative)
K85.90
with necrosis (uninfected) K85.91
infected K85.92
acute (without necrosis or infection) K85.90
with necrosis (uninfected) K85.91
infected K85.92
alcohol induced (without necrosis or infection) K85.20
with necrosis (uninfected) K85.21
infected K85.22
biliary (without necrosis or infection) K85.10
with necrosis (uninfected) K85.11
infected K85.12
drug induced (without necrosis or infection) K85.30
with necrosis (uninfected) K85.31
infected K85.32
gallstone (without necrosis or infection) K85.10
with necrosis (uninfected) K85.11
infected K85.12
idiopathic (without necrosis or infection) K85.00
with necrosis (uninfected) K85.01
infected K85.02
specified NEC (without necrosis or infection) K85.80
with necrosis (uninfected) K85.81
infected K85.82
chronic (infectious) K86.1
alcohol-induced K86.0
recurrent K86.1
relapsing K86.1
cystic (chronic) K86.1
cytomegaloviral B25.2
fibrous (chronic) K86.1
gallstone (without necrosis or infection) K85.10
with necrosis (uninfected) K85.11
infected K85.12
gangrenous — *see* Pancreatitis, acute
interstitial (chronic) K86.1
acute — *see also* Pancreatitis, acute K85.80
mumps B26.3
recurrent
acute — *see* Pancreatitis, acute by type
chronic K86.1
relapsing, chronic K86.1
syphilitic A52.74
Pancreatoblastoma — *see* Neoplasm, pancreas, malignant
Pancreolithiasis K86.89
Pancytolysis D75.89
Pancytopenia (acquired) D61.818
with
malformations D61.09
myelodysplastic syndrome — *see* Syndrome,
myelodysplastic, pancytopenia (acquired)
antineoplastic chemotherapy induced D61.810
congenital D61.09
drug-induced NEC D61.811
Fanconi D61.03
PANDAS (pediatric autoimmune neuropsychiatric disorders
associated with streptococcal infections syndrome)
D89.89
Panencephalitis, subacute, sclerosing A81.1
Panhematopenia D61.9
congenital D61.09
constitutional D61.09
splenic, primary D73.1
Panhemocytopenia D61.9
congenital D61.09
constitutional D61.09
Panhypogonadism E29.1

Panhypopituitarism E23.0
  prepubertal E23.0
Panic (attack) (state) F41.0
  reaction to exceptional stress (transient) F43.0
Panmyelopathy, familial, constitutional D61.09
Panmyelophthisis D61.82
  congenital D61.09
Panmyelosis (acute) (with myelofibrosis) C94.4- ☑
Panner's disease — *see* Osteochondrosis, juvenile, humerus
Panneuritis endemica E51.11
Panniculitis (nodular) (nonsuppurative) M79.3
  back M54.00
    cervical region M54.02
    cervicothoracic region M54.03
    lumbar region M54.06
    lumbosacral region M54.07
    multiple sites M54.09
    occipito-atlanto-axial region M54.01
    sacrococcygeal region M54.08
    thoracic region M54.04
    thoracolumbar region M54.05
  lupus L93.2
  mesenteric K65.4
  neck M54.02
    cervicothoracic region M54.03
    occipito-atlanto-axial region M54.01
  relapsing M35.6
Panniculus adiposus (abdominal) E65
Pannus (allergic) (cornea) (degenerativus) (keratic)
    H16.42- ☑
  abdominal (symptomatic) E65
  trachomatosus, trachomatous (active) A71.1
Panophthalmitis H44.01- ☑
Pansinusitis (chronic) (hyperplastic) (nonpurulent) (purulent) J32.4
  acute J01.40
    recurrent J01.41
  tuberculous A15.8
Pansynostosis Q75.052
Panuveitis (sympathetic) H44.11- ☑
Panvalvular disease I08.9
  specified NEC I08.8
PAPA (pyogenic arthritis, pyoderma gangrenosum, and acne syndrome) M04.8
Papanicolaou smear, cervix Z12.4
  as part of routine gynecological examination Z01.419
    with abnormal findings Z01.411
  for suspected neoplasm Z12.4
  nonspecific abnormal finding R87.619
  routine Z01.419
    with abnormal findings Z01.411
Papilledema (choked disc) H47.10
  associated with
    decreased ocular pressure H47.12
    increased intracranial pressure H47.11
    retinal disorder H47.13
  Foster-Kennedy syndrome H47.14- ☑
Papillitis H46.00
  anus K62.89
  chronic lingual K14.4
  necrotizing, kidney N17.2
  optic H46.0- ☑
  rectum K62.89
  renal, necrotizing N17.2
  tongue K14.0
Papilloma — *see also* Neoplasm, benign, by site
  acuminatum (female) (male) (anogenital) A63.0
  basal cell L82.1
    inflamed L82.0
  benign pinta (primary) A67.0
  bladder (urinary) (transitional cell) D41.4
  choroid plexus (lateral ventricle) (third ventricle) D33.0
    anaplastic C71.5
    fourth ventricle D33.1
    malignant C71.5
  renal pelvis (transitional cell) D41.1- ☑
    benign D30.1- ☑
  Schneiderian
    specified site — *see* Neoplasm, benign, by site
    unspecified site D14.0
  serous surface
    borderline malignancy
      specified site — *see* Neoplasm, uncertain behavior, by site
      unspecified site D39.10
    specified site — *see* Neoplasm, benign, by site
    unspecified site D27.9

Papilloma — *continued*
  transitional (cell)
    bladder (urinary) D41.4
    inverted type — *see* Neoplasm, uncertain behavior, by site
    renal pelvis D41.1- ☑
    ureter D41.2- ☑
  ureter (transitional cell) D41.2- ☑
    benign D30.2- ☑
  urothelial — *see* Neoplasm, uncertain behavior, by site
  villous — *see* Neoplasm, uncertain behavior, by site
    adenocarcinoma in — *see* Neoplasm, malignant, by site
    in situ — *see* Neoplasm, in situ
  yaws, plantar or palmar A66.1
Papillomata, multiple, of yaws A66.1
Papillomatosis — *see also* Neoplasm, benign, by site
  confluent and reticulated L83
  cystic, breast — *see* Mastopathy, cystic
  ductal, breast — *see* Mastopathy, cystic
  intraductal (diffuse) — *see* Neoplasm, benign, by site
  subareolar duct D24- ☑
Papillomavirus, as cause of disease classified elsewhere B97.7
Papillon-Léage and Psaume syndrome Q87.0
Papule(s) R23.8
  carate (primary) A67.0
  fibrous, of nose D22.39
  Gottron's L94.4
  pinta (primary) A67.0
Papulosis
  lymphomatoid C86.6- ☑
  malignant I77.89
Papyraceous fetus O31.0- ☑
Para-albuminemia E88.09
Paracephalus Q89.7
Parachute mitral valve Q23.2
Paracoccidioidomycosis B41.9
  disseminated B41.7
  generalized B41.7
  mucocutaneous-lymphangitic B41.8
  pulmonary B41.0
  specified NEC B41.8
  visceral B41.8
Paradentosis K05.4
Paraffinoma T88.8 ☑
Paraganglioma D44.7
  adrenal D35.0- ☑
    malignant C74.1- ☑
  aortic body D44.7
    malignant C75.5
  carotid body D44.6
    malignant C75.4
  chromaffin — *see also* Neoplasm, benign, by site
    malignant — *see* Neoplasm, malignant, by site
  extra-adrenal D44.7
    malignant C75.5
      specified site — *see* Neoplasm, malignant, by site
      unspecified site C75.5
    specified site — *see* Neoplasm, uncertain behavior, by site
    unspecified site D44.7
  gangliocytic D13.2
    specified site — *see* Neoplasm, benign, by site
    unspecified site D13.2
  glomus jugulare D44.7
    malignant C75.5
  jugular D44.7
  malignant C75.5
    specified site — *see* Neoplasm, malignant, by site
    unspecified site C75.5
  nonchromaffin D44.7
    malignant C75.5
      specified site — *see* Neoplasm, malignant, by site
      unspecified site C75.5
    specified site — *see* Neoplasm, uncertain behavior, by site
    unspecified site D44.7
  parasympathetic D44.7
    specified site — *see* Neoplasm, uncertain behavior, by site
    unspecified site D44.7
  specified site — *see* Neoplasm, uncertain behavior, by site
  sympathetic D44.7
    specified site — *see* Neoplasm, uncertain behavior, by site
    unspecified site D44.7

Paraganglioma — *continued*
  unspecified site D44.7
Parageusia R43.2
  psychogenic F45.8
Paragonimiasis B66.4
Paragranuloma, Hodgkin — *see* Lymphoma, Hodgkin, specified NEC
Parahemophilia — *see also* Defect, coagulation D68.2
Parakeratosis R23.4
  variegata L41.0
Paralysis, paralytic (complete) (incomplete) G83.9
  with
    syphilis A52.17
  abducens, abducent (nerve) — *see* Strabismus, paralytic, sixth nerve
  abductor, lower extremity G57.9- ☑
  accessory nerve G52.8
  accommodation — *see also* Paresis, of accommodation
    hysterical F44.89
  acoustic nerve (except Deafness) H93.3 ☑
  agitans — *see also* Parkinsonism G20.C
    arteriosclerotic G21.4
  alternating (oculomotor) G83.89
  amyotrophic G12.21
  ankle G57.9- ☑
  anus (sphincter) K62.89
  arm — *see* Monoplegia, upper limb
  ascending (spinal), acute G61.0
  association G12.29
  asthenic bulbar G70.00
    with exacerbation (acute) G70.01
    in crisis G70.01
  ataxic (hereditary) G11.9
    general (syphilitic) A52.17
  atrophic G58.9
    infantile, acute — *see* Poliomyelitis, paralytic
    progressive G12.22
    spinal (acute) — *see* Poliomyelitis, paralytic
  axillary G54.0
  Babinski-Nageotte's G83.89
  Bell's G51.0
    newborn P11.3
  Benedikt's G46.3
  birth injury P14.9
    spinal cord P11.5
  bladder (neurogenic) (sphincter) N31.2
  bowel, colon or intestine K56.0
  brachial plexus G54.0
    birth injury P14.3
    newborn (birth injury) P14.3
  brain G83.9
    diplegia G83.0
    triplegia G83.89
  bronchial J98.09
  Brown-Séquard G83.81
  bulbar (chronic) (progressive) G12.22
    infantile — *see* Poliomyelitis, paralytic
    poliomyelitic — *see* Poliomyelitis, paralytic
    pseudo G12.29
  bulbospinal G70.00
    with exacerbation (acute) G70.01
    in crisis G70.01
  cardiac — *see also* Failure, heart I50.9
  cerebrocerebellar, diplegic G80.1
  cervical
    plexus G54.2
    sympathetic G90.09
  Céstan-Chenais G46.3
  Charcot-Marie-Tooth type G60.0
  Clark's G80.9
  colon K56.0
  compressed air T70.3 ☑
  compression
    arm G56.9- ☑
    leg G57.9- ☑
    lower extremity G57.9- ☑
    upper extremity G56.9- ☑
  congenital (cerebral) — *see* Palsy, cerebral
  conjugate movement (gaze) (of eye) H51.0
    cortical (nuclear) (supranuclear) H51.0
  cordis — *see* Failure, heart
  cranial or cerebral nerve G52.9
  creeping G12.22
  crossed leg G83.89
  crutch — *see* Injury, brachial plexus
  deglutition R13.0
    hysterical F44.4
  dementia A52.17

Paralysis, paralytic — *continued*

descending (spinal) NEC G12.29
diaphragm (flaccid) J98.6
  due to accidental dissection of phrenic nerve during procedure — *see* Puncture, accidental complicating surgery
digestive organs NEC K59.89
diplegic — *see* Diplegia
divergence (nuclear) H51.8
diver's T70.3 ☑
Duchenne's
  birth injury P14.0
  due to or associated with
    motor neuron disease G12.22
    muscular dystrophy G71.01
due to intracranial or spinal birth injury — *see* Palsy, cerebral
embolic (current episode) I63.4- ☑
Erb (-Duchenne) (birth) (newborn) P14.0
Erb's syphilitic spastic spinal A52.17
esophagus K22.89
eye muscle (extrinsic) H49.9
  intrinsic — *see also* Paresis, of accommodation
facial (nerve) G51.0
  birth injury P11.3
  congenital P11.3
  following operation NEC — *see* Puncture, accidental complicating surgery
  newborn (birth injury) P11.3
familial (recurrent) (periodic) G72.3
  spastic G11.4
fauces J39.2
finger G56.9- ☑
gait R26.1
gastric nerve (nondiabetic) G52.2
gaze, conjugate H51.0
general (progressive) (syphilitic) A52.17
  juvenile A50.45
glottis J38.00
  bilateral J38.02
  unilateral J38.01
gluteal G54.1
Gubler (-Millard) G46.3
hand — *see* Monoplegia, upper limb
heart — *see* Arrest, cardiac
hemiplegic — *see* Hemiplegia
hyperkalemic periodic (familial) G72.3
hypoglossal (nerve) G52.3
hypokalemic periodic G72.3
hysterical F44.4
ileus K56.0
infantile — *see also* Poliomyelitis, paralytic A80.30
  bulbar — *see* Poliomyelitis, paralytic
  cerebral — *see* Palsy, cerebral
  spastic — *see* Palsy, cerebral, spastic
infective — *see* Poliomyelitis, paralytic
inferior nuclear G83.9
internuclear — *see* Ophthalmoplegia, internuclear
intestine K56.0
iris H57.09
  due to diphtheria (toxin) A36.89
ischemic, Volkmann's (complicating trauma) T79.6 ☑
Jackson's G83.89
jake — *see* Poisoning, food, noxious, plant
Jamaica ginger (jake) G62.2
juvenile general A50.45
Klumpke (-Dejerine) (birth) (newborn) P14.1
labioglossal (laryngeal) (pharyngeal) G12.29
Landry's G61.0
laryngeal nerve (recurrent) (superior) (unilateral) J38.00
  bilateral J38.02
  unilateral J38.01
larynx J38.00
  bilateral J38.02
  due to diphtheria (toxin) A36.2
  unilateral J38.01
lateral G12.23
lead T56.0 ☑
left side — *see* Hemiplegia
leg G83.1- ☑
  both — *see* Paraplegia
  crossed G83.89
  hysterical F44.4
  psychogenic F44.4
  transient or transitory R29.818
    traumatic NEC — *see* Injury, nerve, leg
levator palpebrae superioris — *see* Blepharoptosis, paralytic

Paralysis, paralytic — *continued*

limb — *see* Monoplegia
lip K13.0
Lissauer's A52.17
lower limb — *see* Monoplegia, lower limb
  both — *see* Paraplegia
lung J98.4
median nerve G56.1- ☑
medullary (tegmental) G83.89
mesencephalic NEC G83.89
  tegmental G83.89
middle alternating G83.89
Millard-Gubler-Foville G46.3
monoplegic — *see* Monoplegia
motor G83.9
muscle, muscular NEC G72.89
  due to nerve lesion G58.9
  eye (extrinsic) H49.9
    intrinsic — *see* Paresis, of accommodation
    oblique — *see* Strabismus, paralytic, fourth nerve
  iris sphincter H21.9
  ischemic (Volkmann's) (complicating trauma) T79.6 ☑
  progressive G12.21
  progressive, spinal G12.25
  pseudohypertrophic G71.02
  spinal progressive G12.25
musculocutaneous nerve G56.9- ☑
musculospiral G56.9- ☑
nerve — *see also* Disorder, nerve
  abducent — *see* Strabismus, paralytic, sixth nerve
  accessory G52.8
  auditory (except Deafness) H93.3 ☑
  birth injury P14.9
  cranial or cerebral G52.9
  facial G51.0
    birth injury P11.3
    congenital P11.3
    newborn (birth injury) P11.3
  fourth or trochlear — *see* Strabismus, paralytic, fourth nerve
  newborn (birth injury) P14.9
  oculomotor — *see* Strabismus, paralytic, third nerve
  phrenic (birth injury) P14.2
  radial G56.3- ☑
  seventh or facial G51.0
    newborn (birth injury) P11.3
  sixth or abducent — *see* Strabismus, paralytic, sixth nerve
  syphilitic A52.15
  third or oculomotor — *see* Strabismus, paralytic, third nerve
  trigeminal G50.9
  trochlear — *see* Strabismus, paralytic, fourth nerve
  ulnar G56.2- ☑
normokalemic periodic G72.3
ocular H49.9
  alternating G83.89
oculofacial, congenital (Moebius) Q87.0
oculomotor (external bilateral) (nerve) — *see* Strabismus, paralytic, third nerve
palate (soft) K13.79
paratrigeminal G50.9
periodic (familial) (hyperkalemic) (hypokalemic) (myotonic) (normokalemic) (potassium sensitive) (secondary) G72.3
peripheral autonomic nervous system — *see* Neuropathy, peripheral, autonomic
peroneal (nerve) G57.3- ☑
pharynx J39.2
phrenic nerve G56.8- ☑
plantar nerve(s) G57.6- ☑
pneumogastric nerve G52.2
poliomyelitis (current) — *see* Poliomyelitis, paralytic
popliteal nerve G57.3- ☑
postepileptic transitory G83.84
progressive (atrophic) (bulbar) (spinal) G12.22
  general A52.17
  infantile acute — *see* Poliomyelitis, paralytic
  supranuclear G23.1
pseudobulbar G12.29
pseudohypertrophic (muscle) — *see also* Dystrophy, muscular, by type, if applicable G71.09
psychogenic F44.4
quadriceps G57.9- ☑
quadriplegic — *see* Tetraplegia
radial nerve G56.3- ☑
rectus muscle (eye) H49.9
recurrent isolated sleep G47.53

Paralysis, paralytic — *continued*

respiratory (muscle) (system) (tract) R06.81
  center NEC G93.89
  congenital P28.89
  newborn P28.89
right side — *see* Hemiplegia
saturnine T56.0 ☑
sciatic nerve G57.0- ☑
senile G83.9
shaking — *see* Parkinsonism
shoulder G56.9- ☑
sleep, recurrent isolated G47.53
spastic G83.9
  cerebral — *see* Palsy, cerebral, spastic
  congenital (cerebral) — *see* Palsy, cerebral, spastic
  familial G11.4
  hereditary G11.4
  quadriplegic G80.0
  syphilitic (spinal) A52.17
sphincter, bladder — *see* Paralysis, bladder
spinal (cord) G83.9
  accessory nerve G52.8
  acute — *see* Poliomyelitis, paralytic
  ascending acute G61.0
  atrophic (acute) — *see also* Poliomyelitis, paralytic
    spastic, syphilitic A52.17
  congenital NEC — *see* Palsy, cerebral
  hereditary G95.89
  infantile — *see* Poliomyelitis, paralytic
  progressive G12.21
  muscle G12.25
  sequelae NEC G83.89
sternomastoid G52.8
stomach K31.84
  diabetic — *see* Diabetes, by type, with gastroparesis
  nerve G52.2
    diabetic — *see* Diabetes, by type, with gastroparesis
stroke — *see* Infarct, brain
subscapularis G56.8- ☑
supranuclear (progressive) G23.1
sympathetic G90.89
  cervical G90.09
  nervous system — *see* Neuropathy, peripheral, autonomic
syndrome G83.9
  specified NEC G83.89
syphilitic spastic spinal (Erb's) A52.17
thigh G57.9- ☑
throat J39.2
  diphtheritic A36.0
  muscle J39.2
thrombotic (current episode) I63.3- ☑
thumb G56.9- ☑
tick — *see* Toxicity, venom, arthropod, specified NEC
Todd's (postepileptic transitory paralysis) G83.84
toe G57.6- ☑
tongue K14.8
transient R29.5
  arm or leg NEC R29.818
  traumatic NEC — *see* Injury, nerve
trapezius G52.8
traumatic, transient NEC — *see* Injury, nerve
trembling — *see* Parkinsonism
triceps brachii G56.9- ☑
trigeminal nerve G50.9
trochlear (nerve) — *see* Strabismus, paralytic, fourth nerve
ulnar nerve G56.2- ☑
upper limb — *see* Monoplegia, upper limb
uremic N18.9 [G99.8]
uveoparotitic D86.89
uvula K13.79
  postdiphtheritic A36.0
vagus nerve G52.2
vasomotor NEC G90.89
velum palati K13.79
vesical — *see* Paralysis, bladder
vestibular nerve (except Vertigo) H93.3 ☑
vocal cords J38.00
  bilateral J38.02
  unilateral J38.01
Volkmann's (complicating trauma) T79.6 ☑
wasting G12.29
Weber's G46.3
wrist G56.9- ☑
Paramedial urethrovesical orifice Q64.79
Paramenia N92.6

Parametritis — *see also* Disease, pelvis, inflammatory N73.2
  acute N73.0
  complicating abortion — *see* Abortion, by type, complicated by, parametritis
Parametrium, parametric — *see* condition
Paramnesia — *see* Amnesia
Paramolar K00.1
Paramyloidosis E85.89
Paramyoclonus multiplex G25.3
Paramyotonia (congenita) G71.19
Parangi — *see* Yaws
Paranoia (querulans) F22
  senile F03 ☑
Paranoid
  dementia (senile) F03 ☑
    praecox — *see* Schizophrenia
  personality F60.0
  psychosis (climacteric) (involutional) (menopausal) F22
    psychogenic (acute) F23
    senile F03 ☑
  reaction (acute) F23
    chronic F22
  schizophrenia F20.0
  state (climacteric) (involutional) (menopausal) (simple) F22
    senile F03 ☑
  tendencies F60.0
  traits F60.0
  trends F60.0
  type, psychopathic personality F60.0
Paraparesis — *see* Paraplegia
Paraphasia R47.02
Paraphilia F65.9
Paraphimosis (congenital) N47.2
  chancroidal A57
Paraphrenia, paraphrenic (late) F22
  schizophrenia F20.0
Paraplegia (lower) G82.20
  ataxic — *see* Degeneration, combined, spinal cord
  complete G82.21
  congenital (cerebral) G80.8
    spastic G80.1
  familial spastic G11.4
  functional (hysterical) F44.4
  hereditary, spastic G11.4
  hysterical F44.4
  incomplete G82.22
  Pott's A18.01
  psychogenic F44.4
  spastic
    Erb's spinal, syphilitic A52.17
    hereditary G11.4
    tropical G04.1
  syphilitic (spastic) A52.17
  traumatic
    current injury — code to injury with seventh character A
    sequela of previous injury — code to injury with seventh character S
  tropical spastic G04.1
Parapoxvirus B08.60
  specified NEC B08.69
Paraproteinemia D89.2
  benign (familial) D89.2
  monoclonal D47.2
  secondary to malignant disease D47.2
Parapsoriasis L41.9
  en plaques L41.4
  guttata L41.1
  large plaque L41.4
  retiform, retiformis L41.5
  small plaque L41.3
  specified NEC L41.8
  varioliformis (acuta) L41.0
Parasitic — *see also* condition
  disease NEC B89
  stomatitis B37.0
  sycosis (beard) (scalp) B35.0
  twin Q89.4
Parasitism B89
  intestinal B82.9
  skin B88.9
  specified — *see* Infestation
Parasitophobia F40.218
Parasomnia G47.50
  due to
    alcohol
      abuse F10.182
      dependence F10.282

Parasomnia — *continued*
  due to — *continued*
    alcohol — *continued*
      use F10.982
    amphetamines
      abuse F15.182
      dependence F15.282
      use F15.982
    caffeine
      abuse F15.182
      dependence F15.282
      use F15.982
    cocaine
      abuse F14.182
      dependence F14.282
      use F14.982
    drug NEC
      abuse F19.182
      dependence F19.282
      use F19.982
    opioid
      abuse F11.182
      dependence F11.282
      use F11.982
    psychoactive substance NEC
      abuse F19.182
      dependence F19.282
      use F19.982
    sedative, hypnotic, or anxiolytic
      abuse F13.182
      dependence F13.282
      use F13.982
    stimulant NEC
      abuse F15.182
      dependence F15.282
      use F15.982
  in conditions classified elsewhere G47.54
  nonorganic origin F51.8
  organic G47.50
  specified NEC G47.59
Paraspadias Q54.9
Paraspasmus facialis G51.8
Parasuicide (attempt)
  history of (personal) Z91.51
    in family Z81.8
Parathyroid gland — *see* condition
Parathyroid tetany E20.9
Paratrachoma A74.0
Paratyphilitis — *see* Appendicitis
Paratyphoid (fever) — *see* Fever, paratyphoid
Paratyphus — *see* Fever, paratyphoid
Paraurethral duct Q64.79
Paraurethritis — *see also* Urethritis
  gonococcal (acute) (chronic) (with abscess) A54.1
Paravaccinia NEC B08.04
Paravaginitis — *see* Vaginitis
Parencephalitis — *see also* Encephalitis
  sequelae G09
Parent-child conflict — *see* Conflict, parent-child
  estrangement NEC Z62.890
Paresis — *see also* Paralysis
  accommodation — *see* Paresis, of accommodation
  Bernhardt's G57.1- ☑
  bladder (sphincter) — *see also* Paralysis, bladder
    tabetic A52.17
  bowel, colon or intestine K56.0
  extrinsic muscle, eye H49.9
  general (progressive) (syphilitic) A52.17
    juvenile A50.45
  heart — *see* Failure, heart
  insane (syphilitic) A52.17
  juvenile (general) A50.45
  of accommodation H52.52- ☑
  peripheral progressive (idiopathic) G60.3
  pseudohypertrophic — *see also* Dystrophy, muscular, by type, if applicable G71.09
  senile G83.9
  syphilitic (general) A52.17
    congenital A50.45
  vesical NEC N31.2
Paresthesia — *see also* Disturbance, sensation, skin R20.2
  Bernhardt G57.1- ☑
Paretic — *see* condition
Parinaud's
  conjunctivitis H10.89
  oculoglandular syndrome H10.89
  ophthalmoplegia H49.88- ☑
Parkinsonism (idiopathic) (primary) G20.C

Parkinsonism — *continued*
  with neurogenic orthostatic hypotension (symptomatic) G90.3
  arteriosclerotic G21.4
  dementia — *see also* Dementia, in, diseases specified elsewhere G20.C [F02.80]
    with behavioral disturbance — *see also* Dementia, in, diseases specified elsewhere G20.C [F02.81-] ☑
  due to
    drugs NEC G21.19
      neuroleptic G21.11
  medication-induced NEC G21.19
  neuroleptic induced G21.11
  postencephalitic G21.3
  secondary G21.9
    due to
      arteriosclerosis G21.4
      drugs NEC G21.19
        neuroleptic G21.11
      encephalitis G21.3
      external agents NEC G21.2
      syphilis A52.19
    specified NEC G21.8
  syphilitic A52.19
  treatment-induced NEC G21.19
  vascular G21.4
Parkinson's disease, syndrome or tremor — *see* Parkinsonism
Parodontitis — *see* Periodontitis
Parodontosis K05.4
Paronychia — *see also* Cellulitis, digit
  with lymphangitis — *see* Lymphangitis, acute, digit
  candidal (chronic) B37.2
  tuberculous (primary) A18.4
Parorexia (psychogenic) F50.89
Parosmia R43.1
  psychogenic F45.8
Parotid gland — *see* condition
Parotitis, parotiditis (allergic) (nonspecific toxic) (purulent) (septic) (suppurative) — *see also* Sialoadenitis
  epidemic — *see* Mumps
  infectious — *see* Mumps
  postoperative K91.89
  surgical K91.89
Parrot fever A70
Parrot's disease (early congenital syphilitic pseudoparalysis) A50.02
Parry-Romberg syndrome G51.8
Parry's disease or syndrome E05.00
  with thyroid storm E05.01
Pars planitis — *see* Cyclitis
Parsonage (-Aldren)-**Turner syndrome** G54.5
Parson's disease (exophthalmic goiter) E05.00
  with thyroid storm E05.01
Particolored infant Q82.8
Parturition — *see* Delivery
Parulis K04.7
  with sinus K04.6
Parvovirus, as cause of disease classified elsewhere B97.6
Pasini and Pierini's atrophoderma L90.3
Passage
  false, urethra N36.5
  meconium (newborn) during delivery P03.82
  of sounds or bougies — *see* Attention to, artificial, opening
Passive — *see* condition
  smoking Z77.22
Past due on rent or mortgage Z59.81- ☑
Pasteurella septica A28.0
Pasteurellosis — *see* Infection, Pasteurella
PAT (paroxysmal atrial tachycardia) I47.19
Patau's syndrome — *see* Trisomy, 13
Patches
  mucous (syphilitic) A51.39
    congenital A50.07
  smokers' (mouth) K13.24
Patellar — *see* condition
Patent — *see also* Imperfect, closure
  canal of Nuck Q52.4
  cervix N88.3
  ductus arteriosus or Botallo's Q25.0
  foramen
    botalli Q21.12
    ovale Q21.12
  interauricular septum Q21.19
  interventricular septum Q21.0
  omphalomesenteric duct Q43.0
  os (uteri) — *see* Patent, cervix

☑ **Additional Character Required — Refer to the Tabular List for Character Selection**

Patent — *continued*
ostium secundum (type II) Q21.11
urachus Q64.4
vitelline duct Q43.0
Paterson (-Brown) (-Kelly) **syndrome or web** D50.1
Pathologic, pathological — *see also* condition
asphyxia R09.01
fire-setting F63.1
gambling F63.0
ovum O02.0
resorption, tooth K03.3
stealing F63.2
Pathology (of) — *see* Disease
periradicular, associated with previous endodontic
treatment NEC M27.59
Pattern, sleep-wake, irregular G47.23
Patulous — *see also* Imperfect, closure (congenital)
alimentary tract Q45.8
lower Q43.8
upper Q40.8
eustachian tube H69.0- ☑
Pause, sinoatrial I49.5
Paxton's disease B36.2
Pearl(s)
enamel K00.2
Epstein's K09.8
Pearl-worker's disease — *see* Osteomyelitis, specified type
NEC
Pectenosis K62.4
Pectoral — *see* condition
Pectus
carinatum (congenital) Q67.7
acquired M95.4
rachitic sequelae (late effect) E64.3
excavatum (congenital) Q67.6
acquired M95.4
rachitic sequelae (late effect) E64.3
recurvatum (congenital) Q67.6
Pedatrophia E41
Pederosis F65.4
Pediatric inflammatory multisystem syndrome M35.81
Pediculosis (infestation) B85.2
capitis (head-louse) (any site) B85.0
corporis (body-louse) (any site) B85.1
eyelid B85.0
mixed (classifiable to more than one of the titles B85.0-
B85.3) B85.4
pubis (pubic louse) (any site) B85.3
vestimenti B85.1
vulvae B85.3
Pediculus (infestation) — *see* Pediculosis
Pedophilia F65.4
Peg-shaped teeth K00.2
Pelade — *see* Alopecia, areata
Pelger-Huet anomaly or syndrome D72.0
Peliosis (rheumatica) D69.0
hepatis K76.4
with toxic liver disease K71.8
Pelizaeus-Merzbacher disease E75.27
Pellagra (alcoholic) E52
with
polyneuropathy E52 *[G63]*
**Pellagra-cerebellar-ataxia-renal aminoaciduria syn-
drome** E72.02
Pellegrini (-Stieda) **disease or syndrome** — *see* Bursitis,
tibial collateral
Pellizzi's syndrome E34.8
Pel's crisis A52.11
Pelvic — *see also* condition
examination (periodic) (routine) Z01.419
with abnormal findings Z01.411
kidney, congenital Q63.2
Pelviolithiasis — *see* Calculus, kidney
Pelviperitonitis — *see also* Peritonitis, pelvic
gonococcal A54.24
puerperal O85
Pelvis — *see* condition or type
Pemphigoid L12.9
benign, mucous membrane L12.1
bullous L12.0
cicatricial L12.1
juvenile L12.2
ocular L12.1
specified NEC L12.8
Pemphigus L10.9
benign familial (chronic) Q82.8
Brazilian L10.3
circinatus L13.0
conjunctiva L12.1

Pemphigus — *continued*
drug-induced L10.5
erythematosus L10.4
foliaceous L10.2
gangrenous — *see* Gangrene
neonatorum L01.03
ocular L12.1
paraneoplastic L10.81
specified NEC L10.89
syphilitic (congenital) A50.06
vegetans L10.1
vulgaris L10.0
wildfire L10.3
Pendred's syndrome E07.1
Pendulous
abdomen, in pregnancy — *see* Pregnancy, complicated
by, abnormal, pelvic organs or tissues NEC
breast N64.89
Penetrating wound — *see also* Puncture
with internal injury — *see* Injury, by site
eyeball — *see* Puncture, eyeball
orbit (with or without foreign body) — *see* Puncture,
orbit
uterus by instrument with or following ectopic or molar
pregnancy O08.6
Penicillosis B48.4
Penis — *see* condition
Penitis N48.29
Pentalogy of Fallot Q21.8
Pentasomy X syndrome Q97.1
Pentosuria (essential) E74.89
Percreta placenta - O43.23 ☑
Peregrinating patient — *see* Disorder, factitious
Perforation, perforated (nontraumatic) (of)
accidental during procedure (blood vessel) (nerve) (organ) — *see* Complication, accidental puncture or
laceration
antrum — *see* Sinusitis, maxillary
appendix K35.32
with localized peritonitis K35.32
atrial septum, multiple Q21.19
attic, ear — *see* Perforation, tympanum, attic
bile duct (common) (hepatic) K83.2
cystic K82.2
bladder (urinary)
with or following ectopic or molar pregnancy O08.6
obstetrical trauma O71.5
traumatic S37.29 ☑
at delivery O71.5
bowel K63.1
with or following ectopic or molar pregnancy O08.6
newborn P78.0
obstetrical trauma O71.5
traumatic — *see* Laceration, intestine
broad ligament N83.8
with or following ectopic or molar pregnancy O08.6
obstetrical trauma O71.6
by
device, implant or graft — *see also* Complications, by
site and type, mechanical T85.628 ☑
arterial graft NEC — *see* Complication, cardiovascular device, mechanical, vascular
breast (implant) T85.49 ☑
catheter NEC T85.698 ☑
cystostomy T83.090 ☑
dialysis (renal) T82.49 ☑
intraperitoneal T85.691 ☑
infusion NEC T82.594 ☑
spinal (epidural) (subdural) T85.690 ☑
urinary — *see also* Complications, catheter,
urinary T83.098 ☑
electronic (electrode) (pulse generator) (stimulator)
bone T84.390 ☑
cardiac T82.199 ☑
electrode T82.190 ☑
pulse generator T82.191 ☑
specified type NEC T82.198 ☑
nervous system — *see* Complication, prosthetic
device, mechanical, electronic nervous
system stimulator
urinary — *see* Complication, genitourinary,
device, urinary, mechanical
fixation, internal (orthopedic) NEC — *see* Complication, fixation device, mechanical
gastrointestinal — *see* Complications, prosthetic
device, mechanical, gastrointestinal device
genital NEC T83.498 ☑

Perforation, perforated — *continued*
by — *continued*
device, implant or graft — *see also* Complications, by
site and type, mechanical — *continued*
genital — *continued*
intrauterine contraceptive device T83.39 ☑
penile prosthesis T83.490 ☑
heart NEC — *see* Complication, cardiovascular
device, mechanical
joint prosthesis — *see* Complications, joint prosthesis, mechanical, specified NEC, by site
ocular NEC — *see* Complications, prosthetic device,
mechanical, ocular device
orthopedic NEC — *see* Complication, orthopedic,
device, mechanical
specified NEC T85.628 ☑
urinary NEC — *see also* Complication, genitourinary, device, urinary, mechanical
graft T83.29 ☑
vascular NEC — *see* Complication, cardiovascular
device, mechanical
ventricular intracranial shunt T85.09 ☑
foreign body left accidentally in operative wound
T81.539 ☑
instrument (any) during a procedure, accidental —
see Puncture, accidental complicating surgery
cecum K35.32
with localized peritonitis K35.32
cervix (uteri) N88.8
with or following ectopic or molar pregnancy O08.6
obstetrical trauma O71.3
colon K63.1
newborn P78.0
obstetrical trauma O71.5
traumatic — *see* Laceration, intestine, large
common duct (bile) K83.2
cornea (due to ulceration) — *see* Ulcer, cornea, perforated
cystic duct K82.2
diverticulum (intestine) K57.80
with bleeding K57.81
large intestine K57.20
with
bleeding K57.21
small intestine K57.40
with bleeding K57.41
small intestine K57.00
with
bleeding K57.01
large intestine K57.40
with bleeding K57.41
ear drum — *see* Perforation, tympanum
esophagus K22.3
ethmoidal sinus — *see* Sinusitis, ethmoidal
frontal sinus — *see* Sinusitis, frontal
gallbladder K82.2
heart valve — *see* Endocarditis
ileum K63.1
newborn P78.0
obstetrical trauma O71.5
traumatic — *see* Laceration, intestine, small
instrumental, surgical (accidental) (blood vessel) (nerve)
(organ) — *see* Puncture, accidental complicating
surgery
intestine NEC K63.1
with ectopic or molar pregnancy O08.6
newborn P78.0
obstetrical trauma O71.5
traumatic — *see* Laceration, intestine
ulcerative NEC K63.1
newborn P78.0
jejunum, jejunal K63.1
obstetrical trauma O71.5
traumatic — *see* Laceration, intestine, small
ulcer — *see* Ulcer, gastrojejunal, with perforation
joint prosthesis — *see* Complications, joint prosthesis,
mechanical, specified NEC, by site
mastoid (antrum) (cell) — *see* Disorder, mastoid, specified
NEC
maxillary sinus — *see* Sinusitis, maxillary
membrana tympani — *see* Perforation, tympanum
nasal
septum J34.89
congenital Q30.3
syphilitic A52.73
sinus J34.89
congenital Q30.8
due to sinusitis — *see* Sinusitis

Perforation, perforated — *continued*
palate — *see also* Cleft, palate Q35.9
  syphilitic A52.79
palatine vault — *see also* Cleft, palate, hard Q35.1
  syphilitic A52.79
    congenital A50.59
pars flaccida (ear drum) — *see* Perforation, tympanum, attic
pelvic
  floor S31.030 ☑
    with
      ectopic or molar pregnancy O08.6
      penetration into retroperitoneal space S31.031 ☑
      retained foreign body S31.040 ☑
        with penetration into retroperitoneal space S31.041 ☑
    following ectopic or molar pregnancy O08.6
    obstetrical trauma O70.1
  organ S37.99 ☑
    adrenal gland S37.818 ☑
    bladder — *see* Perforation, bladder
    fallopian tube S37.599 ☑
      bilateral S37.592 ☑
      unilateral S37.591 ☑
    kidney S37.09- ☑
    obstetrical trauma O71.5
    ovary S37.499 ☑
      bilateral S37.492 ☑
      unilateral S37.491 ☑
    prostate S37.828 ☑
    specified organ NEC S37.898 ☑
    ureter — *see* Perforation, ureter
    urethra — *see* Perforation, urethra
    uterus — *see* Perforation, uterus
perineum — *see* Laceration, perineum
pharynx J39.2
rectum K63.1
  newborn P78.0
  obstetrical trauma O71.5
  traumatic S36.63 ☑
root canal space due to endodontic treatment M27.51
sigmoid K63.1
  newborn P78.0
  obstetrical trauma O71.5
  traumatic S36.533 ☑
sinus (accessory) (chronic) (nasal) J34.89
sphenoidal sinus — *see* Sinusitis, sphenoidal
surgical (accidental) (by instrument) (blood vessel) (nerve) (organ) — *see* Puncture, accidental complicating surgery
traumatic
  external — *see* Puncture
  eye — *see* Puncture, eyeball
  internal organ — *see* Injury, by site
tympanum, tympanic (membrane) (persistent posttraumatic) (postinflammatory) H72.9- ☑
  attic H72.1- ☑
    multiple — *see* Perforation, tympanum, multiple
    total — *see* Perforation, tympanum, total
  central H72.0- ☑
    multiple — *see* Perforation, tympanum, multiple
    total — *see* Perforation, tympanum, total
  marginal NEC — *see* subcategory H72.2 ☑
  multiple H72.81- ☑
  pars flaccida — *see* Perforation, tympanum, attic
  total H72.82- ☑
traumatic, current episode S09.2- ☑
typhoid, gastrointestinal — *see* Typhoid
ulcer — *see* Ulcer, by site, with perforation
ureter N28.89
  traumatic S37.19 ☑
urethra N36.8
  with ectopic or molar pregnancy O08.6
  following ectopic or molar pregnancy O08.6
  obstetrical trauma O71.5
  traumatic S37.39 ☑
    at delivery O71.5
uterus
  with ectopic or molar pregnancy O08.6
  by intrauterine contraceptive device T83.39 ☑
  following ectopic or molar pregnancy O08.6
  obstetrical trauma O71.1
  traumatic S37.69 ☑
    obstetric O71.1
uvula K13.79
  syphilitic A52.79

Perforation, perforated — *continued*
vagina O71.4
  obstetrical trauma O71.4
  other trauma — *see* Puncture, vagina
Periadenitis mucosa necrotica recurrens K12.0
Periappendicitis (acute) — *see* Appendicitis
Periarteritis nodosa (disseminated) (infectious) (necrotizing) M30.0
Periarthritis (joint) — *see also* Enthesopathy
  Duplay's M75.0- ☑
  gonococcal A54.42
  humeroscapularis — *see* Capsulitis, adhesive
  scapulohumeral — *see* Capsulitis, adhesive
  shoulder — *see* Capsulitis, adhesive
  wrist M77.2- ☑
Periarthrosis (angioneural) — *see* Enthesopathy
Pericapsulitis, adhesive (shoulder) — *see* Capsulitis, adhesive
Pericarditis (with decompensation) (with effusion) I31.9
  with rheumatic fever (conditions in I00)
    active — *see* Pericarditis, rheumatic
    inactive or quiescent I09.2
  acute (hemorrhagic) (nonrheumatic) (Sicca) I30.9
    with chorea (acute) (rheumatic) (Sydenham's) I02.0
    benign I30.8
    nonspecific I30.0
    rheumatic I01.0
      with chorea (acute) (Sydenham's) I02.0
  adhesive or adherent (chronic) (external) (internal) I31.0
    acute — *see* Pericarditis, acute
    rheumatic I09.2
  bacterial (acute) (subacute) (with serous or seropurulent effusion) I30.1
  calcareous I31.1
  cholesterol (chronic) I31.8
    acute I30.9
  chronic (nonrheumatic) I31.9
    rheumatic I09.2
  constrictive (chronic) I31.1
  coxsackie B33.23
  fibrinocaseous (tuberculous) A18.84
  fibrinopurulent I30.1
  fibrinous I30.8
  fibrous I31.0
  gonococcal A54.83
  idiopathic I30.0
  in systemic lupus erythematosus M32.12
  infective I30.1
  meningococcal A39.53
  neoplastic (chronic) I31.8
    acute I30.9
  obliterans, obliterating I31.0
  plastic I31.0
  pneumococcal I30.1
  postinfarction I24.1
  purulent I30.1
  rheumatic (active) (acute) (with effusion) (with pneumonia) I01.0
    with chorea (acute) (rheumatic) (Sydenham's) I02.0
    chronic or inactive (with chorea) I09.2
  rheumatoid — *see* Rheumatoid, carditis
  septic I30.1
  serofibrinous I30.8
  staphylococcal I30.1
  streptococcal I30.1
  suppurative I30.1
  syphilitic A52.06
  tuberculous A18.84
  uremic N18.9 [I32]
  viral I30.1
Pericardium, pericardial — *see* condition
Pericellulitis — *see* Cellulitis
Pericementitis (chronic) (suppurative) — *see also* Periodontitis
  acute K05.20
    generalized — *see* Periodontitis, aggressive, generalized
    localized — *see* Periodontitis, aggressive, localized
Perichondritis
  auricle — *see* Perichondritis, ear
  bronchus J98.09
  ear (external) H61.00- ☑
    acute H61.01- ☑
    chronic H61.02- ☑
  external auditory canal — *see* Perichondritis, ear
  larynx J38.7
    syphilitic A52.73
    typhoid A01.09

Perichondritis — *continued*
  nose J34.89
  pinna — *see* Perichondritis, ear
  trachea J39.8
Periclasia K05.4
Pericoronitis — *see* Periodontitis
Pericystitis N30.90
  with hematuria N30.91
Peridiverticulitis (intestine) K57.92
  cecum — *see* Diverticulitis, intestine, large
  colon — *see* Diverticulitis, intestine, large
  duodenum — *see* Diverticulitis, intestine, small
  intestine — *see* Diverticulitis, intestine
  jejunum — *see* Diverticulitis, intestine, small
  rectosigmoid — *see* Diverticulitis, intestine, large
  rectum — *see* Diverticulitis, intestine, large
  sigmoid — *see* Diverticulitis, intestine, large
Periendocarditis — *see* Endocarditis
Periepididymitis N45.1
Perifolliculitis L01.02
  abscedens, caput, scalp L66.3
  capitis, abscedens (et suffodiens) L66.3
  superficial pustular L01.02
Perihepatitis K65.8
Perilabyrinthitis (acute) — *see* subcategory H83.0 ☑
Perimeningitis — *see* Meningitis
Perimetritis — *see* Endometritis
Perimetrosalpingitis — *see* Salpingo-oophoritis
Perineocele N81.81
Perinephric, perinephritic — *see* condition
Perinephritis — *see also* Infection, kidney
  purulent — *see* Abscess, kidney
Perineum, perineal — *see* condition
Perineuritis NEC — *see* Neuralgia
Periodic — *see* condition
Periodontitis (chronic) (complex) (compound) (local) (simplex) K05.30
  acute K05.20
    generalized K05.229
      moderate K05.222
      severe K05.223
      slight K05.221
    localized K05.219
      moderate K05.212
      severe K05.213
      slight K05.211
  aggressive K05.20
    generalized K05.229
      moderate K05.222
      severe K05.223
      slight K05.221
    localized K05.219
      moderate K05.212
      severe K05.213
      slight K05.211
  apical K04.5
    acute (pulpal origin) K04.4
  generalized K05.329
    moderate K05.322
    severe K05.323
    slight K05.321
  localized K05.319
    moderate K05.312
    severe K05.313
    slight K05.311
Periodontoclasia K05.4
Periodontosis (juvenile) K05.4
Periods — *see also* Menstruation
  heavy N92.0
  irregular N92.6
  shortened intervals (irregular) N92.1
Perionychia — *see also* Cellulitis, digit
  with lymphangitis — *see* Lymphangitis, acute, digit
Perioophoritis — *see* Salpingo-oophoritis
Periorchitis N45.2
Periosteum, periosteal — *see* condition
Periostitis (albuminosa) (circumscribed) (diffuse) (infective) (monomelic) — *see also* Osteomyelitis
  alveolar M27.3
  alveolodental M27.3
  dental M27.3
  gonorrheal A54.43
  jaw (lower) (upper) M27.2
  orbit H05.03- ☑
  syphilitic A52.77
    congenital (early) A50.02 [M90.80]
    secondary A51.46
  tuberculous — *see* Tuberculosis, bone
  yaws (hypertrophic) (early) (late) A66.6 [M90.80]

☑ **Additional Character Required** — **Refer to the Tabular List for Character Selection**

Periostosis (hyperplastic) — *see also* Disorder, bone, specified type NEC
  with osteomyelitis — *see* Osteomyelitis, specified type NEC
Peripartum
  cardiomyopathy O90.3
Periphlebitis — *see* Phlebitis
Periproctitis K62.89
Periprostatitis — *see* Prostatitis
Perirectal — *see* condition
Perirenal — *see* condition
Perisalpingitis — *see* Salpingo-oophoritis
Perisplenitis (infectional) D73.89
Peristalsis, visible or reversed R19.2
Peritendinitis — *see* Enthesopathy
Peritoneum, peritoneal — *see* condition
Peritonitis (adhesive) (bacterial) (fibrinous) (hemorrhagic) (idiopathic) (localized) (perforative) (primary) (with adhesions) (with effusion) K65.9
  with or following
    abscess K65.1
    appendicitis
      with perforation or rupture K35.32
      generalized — *see also* Appendicitis K35.209
      localized — *see also* Appendicitis K35.30
    diverticular disease (intestine) K57.80
      with bleeding K57.81
      ectopic or molar pregnancy O08.0
      large intestine K57.20
        with
          bleeding K57.21
          small intestine K57.40
            with bleeding K57.41
      small intestine K57.00
        with
          bleeding K57.01
          large intestine K57.40
            with bleeding K57.41
  acute (generalized) K65.0
  aseptic T81.61 ☑
  bile, biliary K65.3
  chemical T81.61 ☑
  chlamydial A74.81
  chronic proliferative K65.8
  complicating abortion — *see* Abortion, by type, complicated by, pelvic peritonitis
  congenital P78.1
  diaphragmatic K65.0
  diffuse K65.0
  diphtheritic A36.89
  disseminated K65.0
  due to
    bile K65.3
    foreign
      body or object accidentally left during a procedure (instrument) (sponge) (swab) T81.599 ☑
      substance accidentally left during a procedure (chemical) (powder) (talc) T81.61 ☑
    talc T81.61 ☑
    urine K65.8
  eosinophilic K65.8
    acute K65.0
  fibrocaseous (tuberculous) A18.31
  fibropurulent K65.0
  following ectopic or molar pregnancy O08.0
  general (ized) K65.0
  gonococcal A54.85
  meconium (newborn) P78.0
  neonatal P78.1
    meconium P78.0
  pancreatic K65.0
  paroxysmal, familial E85.0
    benign E85.0
  pelvic
    female N73.5
      acute N73.3
      chronic N73.4
        with adhesions N73.6
    male K65.0
  periodic, familial E85.0
  proliferative, chronic K65.8
  puerperal, postpartum, childbirth O85
  purulent K65.0
  septic K65.0
  specified NEC K65.8
  spontaneous bacterial K65.2
  subdiaphragmatic K65.0
  subphrenic K65.0

Peritonitis — *continued*
  suppurative K65.0
  syphilitic A52.74
    congenital (early) A50.08 *[K67]*
  talc T81.61 ☑
  tuberculous A18.31
  urine K65.8
Peritonsillar — *see* condition
Peritonsillitis J36
Perityphlitis — *see also* Cecitis K37
Periureteritis N28.89
Periurethral — *see* condition
Periurethritis (gangrenous) — *see* Urethritis
Periuterine — *see* condition
Perivaginitis — *see* Vaginitis
Perivasculitis, retinal H35.06- ☑
Perivasitis (chronic) N49.1
Perivesiculitis (seminal) — *see* Vesiculitis
Perlèche NEC K13.0
  due to
    candidiasis B37.83
    moniliasis B37.83
    riboflavin deficiency E53.0
    vitamin B2 (riboflavin) deficiency E53.0
Pernicious — *see* condition
Pernio, perniosis T69.1 ☑
Perpetrator (of abuse) — *see* Index to External Causes of Injury, Perpetrator
Persecution
  delusion F22
  social Z60.5
Perseveration (tonic) R48.8
Persistence, persistent (congenital)
  anal membrane Q42.3
    with fistula Q42.2
  arteria stapedia Q16.3
  atrioventricular canal Q21.20
  branchial cleft NOS Q18.2
    cyst Q18.0
    fistula Q18.0
    sinus Q18.0
  bulbus cordis in left ventricle Q21.8
  canal of Cloquet Q14.0
  capsule (opaque) Q12.8
  cilioretinal artery or vein Q14.8
  cloaca Q43.7
  communication — *see* Fistula, congenital
  convolutions
    aortic arch Q25.46
    fallopian tube Q50.6
    oviduct Q50.6
    uterine tube Q50.6
  double aortic arch Q25.45
  ductus arteriosus (Botalli) Q25.0
  fetal
    circulation P29.38
    form of cervix (uteri) Q51.828
    hemoglobin, hereditary (HPFH) D56.4
  foramen
    Botalli Q21.12
    ovale Q21.12
  Gartner's duct Q52.4
  hemoglobin, fetal (hereditary) (HPFH) D56.4
  hyaloid
    artery (generally incomplete) Q14.0
    system Q14.8
  hymen, in pregnancy or childbirth — *see* Pregnancy, complicated by, abnormal, vulva
  lanugo Q84.2
  left
    posterior cardinal vein Q26.8
    root with right arch of aorta Q25.49
    superior vena cava Q26.1
  Meckel's diverticulum Q43.0
    malignant — *see* Table of Neoplasms, small intestine, malignant
  mucosal disease (middle ear) — *see* Otitis, media, suppurative, chronic, tubotympanic
  nail(s), anomalous Q84.6
  omphalomesenteric duct Q43.0
  organ or site not listed — *see* Anomaly, by site
  ostium
    atrioventriculare commune Q21.23
    primum Q21.20
    secundum Q21.11
  ovarian rests in fallopian tube Q50.6
  pancreatic tissue in intestinal tract Q43.8
  primary (deciduous)
    teeth K00.6

Persistence, persistent — *continued*
  primary — *continued*
    vitreous hyperplasia Q14.0
  pupillary membrane Q13.89
  rhesus (Rh) titer — *see* Complication(s), transfusion, incompatibility reaction, Rh (factor)
  right aortic arch Q25.47
  sinus
    urogenitalis
      female Q52.8
      male Q55.8
    venosus with imperfect incorporation in right auricle Q26.8
  thymus (gland) (hyperplasia) E32.0
  thyroglossal duct Q89.2
  thyrolingual duct Q89.2
  truncus arteriosus or communis Q20.0
  tunica vasculosa lentis Q12.2
  umbilical sinus Q64.4
  urachus Q64.4
  vitelline duct Q43.0
Person (with)
  admitted for clinical research, as a control subject (normal comparison) (participant) Z00.6
  awaiting admission to adequate facility elsewhere Z75.1
  concern (normal) about sick person in family Z63.6
  consulting on behalf of another Z71.0
  feigning illness Z76.5
  living (in)
    alone Z60.2
    boarding school Z59.3
    residential institution Z59.3
    without
      adequate housing Z59.10
        air conditioning Z59.11
        environmental temperature Z59.11
        heating Z59.11
        space Z59.19
      housing (permanent) (temporary) Z59.00
      person able to render necessary care Z74.2
      shelter Z59.02
  on waiting list Z75.1
  sick or handicapped in family Z63.6
Personality (disorder) F60.9
  accentuation of traits (type A pattern) Z73.1
  affective F34.0
  aggressive F60.3
  amoral F60.2
  anacastic, anankastic F60.5
  antisocial F60.2
  anxious F60.6
  asocial F60.2
  asthenic F60.7
  avoidant F60.6
  borderline F60.3
  change due to organic condition (enduring) F07.0
  compulsive F60.5
  cycloid F34.0
  cyclothymic F34.0
  dependent F60.7
  depressive F34.1
  dissocial F60.2
  dual F44.81
  eccentric F60.89
  emotionally unstable F60.3
  expansive paranoid F60.0
  explosive F60.3
  fanatic F60.0
  haltose type F60.89
  histrionic F60.4
  hyperthymic F34.0
  hypothymic F34.1
  hysterical F60.4
  immature F60.89
  inadequate F60.7
  labile (emotional) F60.3
  mixed (nonspecific) F60.89
  morally defective F60.2
  multiple F44.81
  narcissistic F60.81
  obsessional F60.5
  obsessive (-compulsive) F60.5
  organic F07.0
  overconscientious F60.5
  paranoid F60.0
  passive (-dependent) F60.7
  passive-aggressive F60.89
  pathologic F60.9
  pattern defect or disturbance F60.9

Personality — *continued*
 pseudopsychopathic (organic) F07.0
 pseudoretarded (organic) F07.0
 psychoinfantile F60.4
 psychoneurotic NEC F60.89
 psychopathic F60.2
 querulant F60.0
 sadistic F60.89
 schizoid F60.1
 self-defeating F60.89
 sensitive paranoid F60.0
 sociopathic (amoral) (antisocial) (asocial) (dissocial) F60.2
 specified NEC F60.89
 type A Z73.1
 unstable (emotional) F60.3
Perthes' disease — *see* Legg-Calve-Perthes disease
Pertussis — *see also* Whooping cough A37.90
Perversion, perverted
 appetite F50.89
  psychogenic F50.89
 function
  pituitary gland E23.2
   posterior lobe E22.2
 sense of smell and taste R43.8
  psychogenic F45.8
 sexual — *see* Deviation, sexual
Pervious, congenital — *see also* Imperfect, closure
 ductus arteriosus Q25.0
Pes (congenital) — *see also* Talipes
 acquired — *see also* Deformity, limb, foot, specified NEC
  planus — *see* Deformity, limb, flat foot
 adductus Q66.89
 cavus Q66.7- ☑
 deformity NEC, acquired — *see* Deformity, limb, foot, specified NEC
 planus (acquired) (any degree) — *see also* Deformity, limb, flat foot
  rachitic sequelae (late effect) E64.3
 valgus Q66.6
Pest, pestis — *see* Plague
Petechia, petechiae R23.3
 newborn P54.5
Petechial typhus A75.9
Peter's anomaly Q13.4
Petit mal seizure — *see* Epilepsy, childhood, absence
Petit's hernia — *see* Hernia, abdomen, specified site NEC
Petrellidosis B48.2
Petrositis H70.20- ☑
 acute H70.21- ☑
 chronic H70.22- ☑
Peutz-Jeghers disease or syndrome Q85.89
Peyronie's disease N48.6
PFAPA (periodic fever, aphthous stomatitis, pharyngitis, and adenopathy syndrome) M04.8
Pfeiffer's disease — *see* Mononucleosis, infectious
Phagedena (dry) (moist) (sloughing) — *see also* Gangrene
 geometric L88
 penis N48.29
 tropical — *see* Ulcer, skin
 vulva N76.6
Phagedenic — *see* condition
Phakoma H35.89
Phakomatosis — *see also* specific eponymous syndromes Q85.9
 Bourneville's Q85.1
 specified NEC Q85.89
Phantom limb syndrome (without pain) G54.7
 with pain G54.6
Pharyngeal pouch syndrome D82.1
Pharyngitis (acute) (catarrhal) (gangrenous) (infective) (malignant) (membranous) (phlegmonous) (pseudomembranous) (simple) (subacute) (suppurative) (ulcerative) (viral) J02.9
 with influenza, flu, or grippe — *see* Influenza, with, pharyngitis
 aphthous E08.5
 atrophic J31.2
 chlamydial A56.4
 chronic (atrophic) (granular) (hypertrophic) J31.2
 coxsackievirus B08.5
 diphtheritic A36.0
 enteroviral vesicular B08.5
 follicular (chronic) J31.2
 fusospirochetal A69.1
 gonococca A54.5
 granular (chronic) J31.2
 herpesviral B00.2
 hypertrophic J31.2
 infectional, chronic J31.2

Pharyngitis — *continued*
 influenzal — *see* Influenza, with, respiratory manifestations NEC
 lymphonodular, acute (enteroviral) B08.8
 pneumococcal J02.8
 purulent J02.9
 putrid J02.9
 septic J02.0
 sicca J31.2
 specified organism NEC J02.8
 staphylococcal J02.8
 streptococcal J02.0
 syphilitic, congenital (early) A50.03
 tuberculous A15.8
 vesicular, enteroviral B08.5
 viral NEC J02.8
Pharyngoconjunctivitis, viral B30.2
Pharyngolaryngitis (acute) J06.0
 chronic J37.0
Pharyngoplegia J39.2
Pharyngotonsillitis, herpesviral B00.2
Pharyngotracheitis, chronic J42
Pharynx, pharyngeal — *see* condition
Phelan-McDermid syndrome Q93.52
Phencyclidine-induced
 anxiety disorder F16.980
 bipolar and related disorder F16.94
 depressive disorder F16.94
 psychotic disorder F16.959
Phenomenon
 Arthus' — *see* Arthus' phenomenon
 jaw-winking Q07.8
 lupus erythematosus (LE) cell M32.9
 Raynaud's (secondary) I73.00
  with gangrene I73.01
 vasomotor R55
 vasospastic I73.9
 vasovagal R55
 Wenckebach's I44.1
Phenotype
 Duffy
  a positive Z67.A2
  a and b positive Z67.A4
  b positive Z67.A3
  Fy (a+b-) Z67.A2
  Fy (a-b-) Z67.A1
  Fy (a-b+) Z67.A3
  Fy (a+b+) Z67.A4
  null Z67.A1
Phenylketonuria E70.1
 classical E70.0
 maternal E70.1
Pheochromoblastoma
 specified site — *see* Neoplasm, malignant, by site
 unspecified site C74.10
Pheochromocytoma
 malignant
  specified site — *see* Neoplasm, malignant, by site
  unspecified site C74.10
 specified site — *see* Neoplasm, benign, by site
 unspecified site D35.00
Pheohyphomycosis — *see* Chromomycosis
Pheomycosis — *see* Chromomycosis
Phimosis (congenital) (due to infection) N47.1
 chancroidal A57
Phlebectasia — *see also* Varix
 congenital Q27.4
Phlebitis (infective) (pyemic) (septic) (suppurative) I80.9
 antepartum — *see* Thrombophlebitis, antepartum
 blue — *see* Phlebitis, leg, deep
 breast, superficial I80.8
 calf muscular vein (NOS) I80.25- ☑
 cavernous (venous) sinus — *see* Phlebitis, intracranial (venous) sinus
 cerebral (venous) sinus — *see* Phlebitis, intracranial (venous) sinus
 chest wall, superficial I80.8
 cranial (venous) sinus — *see* Phlebitis, intracranial (venous) sinus
 deep (vessels) — *see* Phlebitis, leg, deep
 due to implanted device — *see* Complications, by site and type, specified NEC
 during or resulting from a procedure T81.72 ☑
 femoral vein (superficial) I80.1- ☑
 femoropopliteal vein I80.0- ☑
 gastrocnemial vein I80.25- ☑
 gestational — *see* Phlebopathy, gestational
 hepatic veins I80.8

Phlebitis — *continued*
 iliac vein (common) (external) (internal) I80.21- ☑
 iliofemoral — *see* Phlebitis, femoral vein
 intracranial (venous) sinus (any) G08
  nonpyogenic I67.6
 intraspinal venous sinuses and veins G08
  nonpyogenic G95.19
 lateral (venous) sinus — *see* Phlebitis, intracranial (venous) sinus
 leg I80.3
  antepartum — *see* Thrombophlebitis, antepartum
  deep (vessels) NEC I80.20- ☑
   iliac I80.21- ☑
   popliteal vein I80.22- ☑
   specified vessel NEC I80.29- ☑
   tibial vein (anterior) (posterior) I80.23- ☑
  femoral vein (superficial) I80.1- ☑
  superficial (vessels) I80.0- ☑
 longitudinal sinus — *see* Phlebitis, intracranial (venous) sinus
 lower limb — *see* Phlebitis, leg
 migrans, migrating (superficial) I82.1
 pelvic
  with ectopic or molar pregnancy O08.0
  following ectopic or molar pregnancy O08.0
  puerperal, postpartum O87.1
 peroneal vein I80.24- ☑
 popliteal vein — *see* Phlebitis, leg, deep, popliteal
 portal (vein) K75.1
 postoperative T81.72 ☑
 pregnancy — *see* Thrombophlebitis, antepartum
 puerperal, postpartum, childbirth O87.0
  deep O87.1
  pelvic O87.1
  superficial O87.0
 retina — *see* Vasculitis, retina
 saphenous (accessory) (great) (long) (small) — *see* Phlebitis, leg, superficial
 sinus (meninges) — *see* Phlebitis, intracranial (venous) sinus
 soleal vein I80.25- ☑
 specified site NEC I80.8
 syphilitic A52.09
 tibial vein — *see* Phlebitis, leg, deep, tibial
 ulcerative I80.9
  leg — *see* Phlebitis, leg
 umbilicus I80.8
 uterus (septic) — *see* Endometritis
 varicose (leg) (lower limb) — *see* Varix, leg, with, inflammation
Phlebofibrosis I87.8
Phleboliths I87.8
Phlebopathy,
 gestational O22.9- ☑
 puerperal O87.9
Phlebosclerosis I87.8
Phlebothrombosis — *see also* Thrombosis
 antepartum — *see* Thrombophlebitis, antepartum
 pregnancy — *see* Thrombophlebitis, antepartum
 puerperal — *see* Thrombophlebitis, puerperal
Phlebotomus fever A93.1
Phlegmasia
 alba dolens O87.1
  nonpuerperal — *see* Phlebitis, femoral vein
 cerulea dolens — *see* Phlebitis, leg, deep
Phlegmon — *see* Abscess
Phlegmonous — *see* condition
Phlyctenulosis (allergic) (keratoconjunctivitis) (nontuberculous) — *see also* Keratoconjunctivitis
 cornea — *see* Keratoconjunctivitis
 tuberculous A18.52
Phobia, phobic F40.9
 animal F40.218
  spiders F40.210
 examination F40.298
 reaction F40.9
 simple F40.298
 social F40.10
  generalized F40.11
 specific (isolated) F40.298
  animal F40.218
   spiders F40.210
  blood F40.230
  injection F40.231
  injury F40.233
  men F40.290
  natural environment F40.228
   thunderstorms F40.220

☑ **Additional Character Required** — **Refer to the Tabular List for Character Selection**

Phobia, phobic — *continued*
  specific — *continued*
    situational F40.248
      bridges F40.242
      closed in spaces F40.240
      flying F40.243
      heights F40.241
    specified focus NEC F40.298
    transfusion F40.231
    women F40.291
  specified NEC F40.8
    medical care NEC F40.232
  state F40.9
Phocas' disease — *see* Mastopathy, cystic
Phocomelia Q73.1
  lower limb — *see* Agenesis, leg, with foot present
  upper limb — *see* Agenesis, arm, with hand present
Phoria H50.50
Phosphate-losing tubular disorder N25.0
Phosphatemia E83.39
Phosphaturia E83.39
Photodermatitis (sun) L56.8
  chronic L57.8
  due to drug L56.8
  light other than sun L59.8
Photokeratitis H16.13- ☑
Photophobia H53.14- ☑
Photophthalmia — *see* Photokeratitis
Photopsia H53.19
Photoretinitis — *see* Retinopathy, solar
Photosensitivity, photosensitization (sun) skin L56.8
  light other than sun L59.8
Phrenitis — *see* Encephalitis
Phrynoderma (vitamin A deficiency) E50.8
Phthiriasis (pubis) B85.3
  with any infestation classifiable to B85.0-B85.2 B85.4
Phthirus infestation — *see* Phthiriasis
Phthisis — *see also* Tuberculosis
  bulbi (infectional) — *see* Disorder, globe, degenerated condition, atrophy
  eyeball (due to infection) — *see* Disorder, globe, degenerated condition, atrophy
PHTS Q85.81
Phycomycosis — *see* Zygomycosis
Physalopteriasis B81.8
Physical restraint status Z78.1
Phytobezoar T18.9 ☑
  intestine T18.3 ☑
  stomach T18.2 ☑
Pian — *see* Yaws
Pianoma A66.1
Pica F50.89
  in adults (in remission) F50.83
  infant or child (in remission) F98.3
Picking, nose F98.8
Pick-Niemann disease — *see* Niemann-Pick disease or syndrome
Pick's
  cerebral atrophy — *see also* Dementia, in, diseases specified elsewhere G31.01 *[F02.80]*
    with behavioral disturbance — *see also* Dementia, in, diseases specified elsewhere G31.01 *[F02.81-]* ☑
  disease or syndrome (brain) — *see also* Dementia, in, diseases specified elsewhere G31.01 *[F02.80]*
    with behavioral disturbance — *see also* Dementia, in, diseases specified elsewhere G31.01 *[F02.81-]* ☑
    brain — *see also* Dementia, in, diseases specified elsewhere G31.01 *[F02.80]*
      with behavioral disturbance — *see also* Dementia, in, diseases specified elsewhere G31.01 *[F02.81-]* ☑
  pericardium (pericardial pseudocirrhosis of liver) I31.1
  syndrome
    brain — *see also* Dementia, in, diseases specified elsewhere G31.01 *[F02.80]*
      with behavioral disturbance — *see also* Dementia, in, diseases specified elsewhere G31.01 *[F02.81-]* ☑
    of heart (pericardial pseudocirrhosis of liver) I31.1
Pickwickian syndrome E66.2
Piebaldism E70.39
Piedra (beard) (scalp) B36.8
  black B36.3
  white B36.2
Pierre Robin deformity or syndrome Q87.0
Pierson's disease or osteochondrosis M91.0

Pig-bel A05.2
Pigeon
  breast or chest (acquired) M95.4
    congenital Q67.7
      rachitic sequelae (late effect) E64.3
  breeder's disease or lung J67.2
  fancier's disease or lung J67.2
  toe — *see* Deformity, toe, specified NEC
Pigmentation (abnormal) (anomaly) L81.9
  conjunctiva H11.13- ☑
  cornea (anterior) H18.01- ☑
    posterior H18.05- ☑
    stromal H18.06- ☑
  diminished melanin formation NEC L81.6
  iron L81.8
  lids, congenital Q82.8
  limbus corneae — *see* Pigmentation, cornea
  metals L81.8
  optic papilla, congenital Q14.2
  retina, congenital (grouped) (nevoid) Q14.1
  scrotum, congenital Q82.8
  tattoo L81.8
Piles — *see also* Hemorrhoids K64.9
Pili
  annulati or torti (congenital) Q84.1
  incarnati L73.1
Pill roller hand (intrinsic) — *see* Parkinsonism
Pilomatrixoma — *see* Neoplasm, skin, benign
  malignant — *see* Neoplasm, skin, malignant
Pilonidal — *see* condition
Pimple R23.8
PIMS M35.81
PIN — *see* Neoplasia, intraepithelial, prostate
Pinched nerve — *see* Neuropathy, entrapment
Pindborg tumor — *see* Cyst, calcifying odontogenic
Pineal body or gland — *see* condition
Pinealoblastoma C75.3
Pinealoma D44.5
  malignant C75.3
Pineoblastoma C75.3
Pineocytoma D44.5
Pinguecula H11.15- ☑
Pingueculitis H10.81- ☑
Pinhole meatus — *see also* Stricture, urethra N35.919
Pink
  disease — *see* subcategory T56.1 ☑
  eye — *see* Conjunctivitis, acute, mucopurulent
Pinkus' disease (lichen nitidus) L44.1
Pinpoint
  meatus — *see* Stricture, urethra
  os (uteri) — *see* Stricture, cervix
Pins and needles R20.2
Pinta A67.9
  cardiovascular lesions A67.2
  chancre (primary) A67.0
  erythematous plaques A67.1
  hyperchromic lesions A67.1
  hyperkeratosis A67.1
  lesions A67.9
    cardiovascular A67.2
    hyperchromic A67.1
    intermediate A67.1
    late A67.2
    mixed A67.3
    primary A67.0
    skin (achromic) (cicatricial) (dyschromic) A67.2
      hyperchromic A67.1
      mixed (achromic and hyperchromic) A67.3
  papule (primary) A67.0
  skin lesions (achromic) (cicatricial) (dyschromic) A67.2
    hyperchromic A67.1
    mixed (achromic and hyperchromic) A67.3
  vitiligo A67.2
Pintids A67.1
Pinworm (disease) (infection) (infestation) B80
Piroplasmosis — *see also* Babesiosis B60.00
  specified NEC B60.09
Pistol wound — *see* Gunshot wound
Pitchers' elbow — *see* Derangement, joint, specified type NEC, elbow
Pithecoid pelvis Q74.2
  with disproportion (fetopelvic) O33.0
    causing obstructed labor O65.0
Pithiatism F48.8
Pitted — *see* Pitting
Pitting — *see also* Edema R60.9
  lip R60.0
  nail L60.8

Pitting — *continued*
  teeth K00.4
Pituitary gland — *see* condition
Pituitary-snuff-taker's disease J67.8
Pityriasis (capitis) L21.0
  alba L30.5
  circinata (et maculata) L42
  furfuracea L21.0
  Hebra's L26
  lichenoides L41.0
    chronica L41.1
    et varioliformis (acuta) L41.0
  maculata (et circinata) L30.5
  nigra B36.1
  pilaris, Hebra's L44.0
  rosea L42
  rotunda L44.8
  rubra (Hebra) pilaris L44.0
  simplex L30.5
  specified type NEC L30.5
  streptogenes L30.5
  versicolor (scrotal) B36.0
Placenta, placental — *see* Pregnancy, complicated by (care of) (management affected by), specified condition
Placentitis O41.14- ☑
Plagiocephaly Q67.3
  non-deformational
    anterior Q75.021
    posterior Q75.04- ☑
Plague A20.9
  abortive A20.8
  ambulatory A20.8
  asymptomatic A20.8
  bubonic A20.0
  cellulocutaneous A20.1
  cutaneobubonic A20.1
  lymphatic gland A20.0
  meningitis A20.3
  pharyngeal A20.8
  pneumonic (primary) (secondary) A20.2
  pulmonary, pulmonic A20.2
  septicemic A20.7
  tonsillar A20.8
    septicemic A20.7
Planning, family
  contraception Z30.9
  procreation Z31.69
Plaque(s)
  artery, arterial — *see* Arteriosclerosis
  calcareous — *see* Calcification
  coronary, lipid rich I25.83
  epicardial I31.8
  erythematous, of pinta A67.1
  Hollenhorst's — *see* Occlusion, artery, retina
  lipid rich, coronary I25.83
  pleural (without asbestos) J92.9
    with asbestos J92.0
  tongue K13.29
Plasmacytoma C90.3- ☑
  extramedullary C90.2- ☑
  medullary C90.0- ☑
  solitary C90.3- ☑
Plasmacytopenia D72.818
Plasmacytosis D72.822
Plaster ulcer — *see* Ulcer, pressure, by site
Plateau iris syndrome (post-iridectomy) (postprocedural) (without glaucoma) H21.82
  with glaucoma H40.22- ☑
Platybasia Q75.8
Platyonychia (congenital) Q84.6
  acquired L60.8
Platypelloid pelvis M95.5
  with disproportion (fetopelvic) O33.0
    causing obstructed labor O65.0
  congenital Q74.2
Platyspondylisis Q76.49
Plaut (-Vincent) **disease** — *see also* Vincent's A69.1
Plethora R23.2
  newborn P61.1
Pleura, pleural — *see* condition
Pleuralgia R07.81
Pleurisy (acute) (adhesive) (chronic) (costal) (diaphragmatic) (double) (dry) (fibrinous) (fibrous) (interlobar) (latent) (plastic) (primary) (residual) (sicca) (sterile) (subacute) (unresolved) R09.1
  with
    adherent pleura J86.0
    effusion J90

Pleurisy — *continued*
  with — *continued*
    effusion — *continued*
      chylous, chyliform J94.0
      tuberculous (non primary) A15.6
        primary (progressive) A15.7
    tuberculosis — *see* Pleurisy, tuberculous (non primary)
    encysted — *see* Pleurisy, with effusion
    exudative — *see* Pleurisy, with effusion
    fibrinopurulent, fibropurulent — *see* Pyothorax
    hemorrhagic — *see* Hemothorax
    pneumococcal J90
    purulent — *see* Pyothorax
    septic — *see* Pyothorax
    serofibrinous — *see* Pleurisy, with effusion
    seropurulent — *see* Pyothorax
    serous — *see* Pleurisy, with effusion
    staphylococcal J86.9
    streptococcal J90
    suppurative — *see* Pyothorax
    traumatic (post) (current) — *see* Injury, intrathoracic, pleura
    tuberculous (with effusion) (non primary) A15.6
      primary (progressive) A15.7
Pleuritis sicca — *see* Pleurisy
Pleurobronchopneumonia — *see* Pneumonia, broncho-
Pleurodynia R07.81
  epidemic B33.0
  viral B33.0
Pleuropericarditis — *see also* Pericarditis
  acute I30.9
Pleuropneumonia (acute) (bilateral) (double) (septic) — *see also* Pneumonia J18.8
  chronic — *see* Fibrosis, lung
Pleuro-pneumonia-like-organism (PPLO), as cause of disease classified elsewhere B96.0
Pleurorrhea — *see* Pleurisy, with effusion
Plexitis, brachial G54.0
Plica
  polonica B85.0
  syndrome, knee M67.5- ☑
  tonsil J35.8
Plicated tongue K14.5
Plug
  bronchus NEC J98.09
  meconium (newborn) NEC syndrome P76.0
  mucus — *see* Asphyxia, mucus
Plumbism — *see* subcategory T56.0 ☑
Plummer's disease E05.20
  with thyroid storm E05.21
Plummer-Vinson syndrome D50.1
Pluricarential syndrome of infancy E40
Plus (and minus) **hand** (intrinsic) — *see* Deformity, limb, specified type NEC, forearm
PMEI (polymorphic epilepsy in infancy) G40.83- ☑
Pneumathemia — *see* Air, embolism
Pneumatic hammer (drill) syndrome T75.21 ☑
Pneumatocele (lung) J98.4
  intracranial G93.89
  tension J98.8
Pneumatosis
  cystoides intestinalis K63.89
  intestinalis K63.89
  peritonei K66.8
Pneumaturia R39.89
Pneumoblastoma — *see* Neoplasm, lung, malignant
Pneumocephalus G93.89
Pneumococcemia A40.3
Pneumococcus, pneumococcal — *see* condition
Pneumoconiosis (due to) (inhalation of) J64
  with tuberculosis (any type in A15) J65
  aluminum J63.0
  asbestos J61
  bagasse, bagassosis J67.1
  bauxite J63.1
  beryllium J63.2
  coal miners' (simple) J60
  coalworkers' (simple) J60
  collier's J60
  cotton dust J66.0
  diatomite (diatomaceous earth) J62.8
  dust
    inorganic NEC J63.6
    lime J62.8
    marble J62.8
    organic NEC J66.8
  fumes or vapors (from silo) J68.9
  graphite J63.3
  grinder's J62.8

Pneumoconiosis — *continued*
  kaolin J62.8
  mica J62.8
  millstone maker's J62.8
  mineral fibers NEC J61
  miner's J60
  moldy hay J67.0
  potter's J62.8
  rheumatoid — *see* Rheumatoid, lung
  sandblaster's J62.8
  silica, silicate NEC J62.8
    with carbon J60
  stonemason's J62.8
  talc (dust) J62.0
Pneumocystis carinii pneumonia B59
Pneumocystis jiroveci (pneumonia) B59
Pneumocystosis (with pneumonia) B59
Pneumohemopericardium I31.2
Pneumohemothorax J94.2
  traumatic S27.2 ☑
Pneumohydropericardium — *see* Pericarditis
Pneumohydrothorax — *see* Hydrothorax
Pneumomediastinum J98.2
  congenital or perinatal P25.2
Pneumomycosis B49 [J99]
Pneumonia (acute) (double) (migratory) (purulent) (septic) (unresolved) J18.9
  with
    influenza — *see* Influenza, with, pneumonia
    lung abscess J85.1
      due to specified organism — *see* Pneumonia, in (due to)
  2019 (novel) coronavirus J12.82
  adenoviral J12.0
  adynamic J18.2
  alba A50.04
  allergic — *see also* Pneumonitis, hypersensitivity J82.89
  alveolar — *see* Pneumonia, lobar
  anaerobes J15.8
  anthrax A22.1
  apex, apical — *see* Pneumonia, lobar
  Ascaris B77.81
  aspiration J69.0
    due to
      aspiration of microorganisms
        bacterial J15.9
        viral J12.9
      food (regurgitated) J69.0
      gastric secretions J69.0
      milk (regurgitated) J69.0
      oils, essences J69.1
      solids, liquids NEC J69.8
      vomitus J69.0
    newborn P24.81
      amniotic fluid (clear) P24.11
      blood P24.21
      food (regurgitated) P24.31
      liquor (amnii) P24.11
      meconium P24.01
      milk P24.31
      mucus P24.11
      specified NEC P24.81
      stomach contents P24.31
    postprocedural J95.4
  atypical NEC J18.9
  bacillus J15.9
    specified NEC J15.8
  bacterial J15.9
    specified NEC J15.8
  Bacteroides (fragilis) (oralis) (melaninogenicus) J15.8
  basal, basic, basilar — *see* Pneumonia, by type
  bronchiolitis obliterans organized (BOOP) J84.89
  broncho-, bronchial (confluent) (croupous) (diffuse) (disseminated) (hemorrhagic) (involving lobes) (lobar) (terminal) J18.0
    allergic — *see also* Pneumonitis, hypersensitivity J82.89
    aspiration — *see* Pneumonia, aspiration
    bacterial J15.9
      specified NEC J15.8
    chronic — *see* Fibrosis, lung
    diplococcal J13
    Eaton's agent J15.7
    Escherichia coli (E. coli) J15.5
    Friedlander's bacillus J15.0
    Hemophilus influenzae J14
    hypostatic J18.2
    inhalation — *see also* Pneumonia, aspiration
      due to fumes or vapors (chemical) J68.0

Pneumonia — *continued*
  broncho-, bronchial — *continued*
    inhalation — *see also* Pneumonia, aspiration — *continued*
      of oils or essences J69.1
    Klebsiella (pneumoniae) J15.0
    lipid, lipoid J69.1
      endogenous J84.89
    Mycoplasma (pneumoniae) J15.7
    pleuro-pneumonia-like-organisms (PPLO) J15.7
    pneumococcal J13
    Proteus J15.69
    Pseudomonas J15.1
    Serratia marcescens J15.69
    specified organism NEC J16.8
    staphylococcal — *see* Pneumonia, staphylococcal
    streptococcal NEC J15.4
      group B J15.3
      pneumoniae J13
    viral, virus — *see* Pneumonia, viral
  Butyrivibrio (fibriosolvens) J15.8
  Candida B37.1
  caseous — *see* Tuberculosis, pulmonary
  catarrhal — *see* Pneumonia, broncho
  chlamydial J16.0
    congenital P23.1
  cholesterol J84.89
  cirrhotic (chronic) — *see* Fibrosis, lung
  Clostridium (haemolyticum) (novyi) J15.8
  confluent — *see* Pneumonia, broncho
  congenital (infective) P23.9
    due to
      bacterium NEC P23.6
      Chlamydia P23.1
      Escherichia coli P23.4
      Haemophilus influenzae P23.6
      infective organism NEC P23.8
      Klebsiella pneumoniae P23.6
      Mycoplasma P23.6
      Pseudomonas P23.5
      Staphylococcus P23.2
      Streptococcus (except group B) P23.6
        group B P23.3
      viral agent P23.0
    specified NEC P23.8
  coronavirus (novel) (disease) 2019 J12.82
  COVID-19 J12.82
  croupous — *see* Pneumonia, lobar
  cryptogenic organizing J84.116
  cytomegalic inclusion B25.0
  cytomegaloviral B25.0
  deglutition — *see* Pneumonia, aspiration
  desquamative interstitial J84.117
  diffuse — *see* Pneumonia, broncho
  diplococcal, diplococcus (broncho-) (lobar) J13
  disseminated (focal) — *see* Pneumonia, broncho
  Eaton's agent J15.7
  embolic, embolism — *see* Embolism, pulmonary
  Enterobacter J15.69
  eosinophilic J82.81
    acute J82.82
    chronic J82.81
  Escherichia coli (E. coli) J15.5
  Eubacterium J15.8
  fibrinous — *see* Pneumonia, lobar
  fibroid, fibrous (chronic) — *see* Fibrosis, lung
  Friedlander's bacillus J15.0
  Fusobacterium (nucleatum) J15.8
  gangrenous J85.0
  giant cell (measles) B05.2
  gonococcal A54.84
  gram-negative bacteria NEC J15.69
    anaerobic J15.8
  Hemophilus influenzae (broncho) (lobar) J14
  human metapneumovirus J12.3
  hypostatic (broncho) (lobar) J18.2
  in (due to)
    Acinetobacter baumannii J15.61
    actinomycosis A42.0
    adenovirus J12.0
    anthrax A22.1
    ascariasis B77.81
    aspergillosis B44.9
    Bacillus anthracis A22.1
    Bacterium anitratum J15.69
    candidiasis B37.1
    chickenpox B01.2
    Chlamydia J16.0
      neonatal P23.1

☑ **Additional Character Required** — **Refer to the Tabular List for Character Selection**

Pneumonia — *continued*
  in — *continued*
    coccidioidomycosis B38.2
      acute B38.0
      chronic B38.1
    cytomegalovirus disease B25.0
    Diplococcus (pneumoniae) J13
    Eaton's agent J15.7
    Enterobacter J15.69
    Escherichia coli (E. coli) J15.5
    Friedlander's bacillus J15.0
    fumes and vapors (chemical) (inhalation) J68.0
    gonorrhea A54.84
    Hemophilus influenzae (H. influenzae) J14
    Herellea J15.69
    histoplasmosis B39.2
      acute B39.0
      chronic B39.1
    human metapneumovirus J12.3
    Klebsiella (pneumoniae) J15.0
    measles B05.2
    Mycoplasma (pneumoniae) J15.7
    nocardiosis, nocardiasis A43.0
    ornithosis A70
    parainfluenza virus J12.2
    pleuro-pneumonia-like-organism (PPLO) J15.7
    pneumococcus J13
    pneumocystosis (Pneumocystis carinii) (Pneumocystis jiroveci) B59
    Proteus J15.69
    Pseudomonas NEC J15.1
      pseudomallei A24.1
    psittacosis A70
    Q fever A78
    respiratory syncytial virus (RSV) J12.1
    rheumatic fever I00 *[J17]*
    rubella B06.81
    Salmonella (infection) A02.22
      typhi A01.03
    schistosomiasis B65.9 *[J17]*
    Serratia marcescens J15.69
    specified
      bacterium NEC J15.8
      organism NEC J16.8
    spirochetal NEC A69.8
    Staphylococcus J15.20
      aureus (methicillin susceptible) (MSSA) J15.211
        methicillin resistant (MRSA) J15.212
      specified NEC J15.29
    Streptococcus J15.4
      group B J15.3
      pneumoniae J13
      specified NEC J15.4
    toxoplasmosis B58.3
    tularemia A21.2
    typhoid (fever) A01.03
    varicella B01.2
    virus — *see* Pneumonia, viral
    whooping cough A37.91
      due to
        Bordetella parapertussis A37.11
        Bordetella pertussis A37.01
        specified NEC A37.81
    Yersinia pestis A20.2
  inhalation of food or vomit — *see* Pneumonia, aspiration
  interstitial J84.9
    chronic J84.111
    desquamative J84.117
    due to
      collagen vascular disease J84.178
      known underlying cause J84.178
    idiopathic NOS J84.111
    in disease classified elsewhere J84.178
    lymphocytic (due to collagen vascular disease) (in diseases classified elsewhere) J84.178
    lymphoid J84.2
    non-specific J84.89
      due to
        collagen vascular disease J84.178
        known underlying cause J84.178
      idiopathic J84.113
      in diseases classified elsewhere J84.178
    plasma cell B59
    pseudomonas J15.1
    usual J84.112
      due to collagen vascular disease J84.178
      idiopathic J84.112
      in diseases classified elsewhere J84.178
  Klebsiella (pneumoniae) J15.0

Pneumonia — *continued*
  lipid, lipoid (exogenous) J69.1
    endogenous J84.89
  lobar (disseminated) (double) (interstitial) J18.1
    bacterial J15.9
      specified NEC J15.8
    chronic — *see* Fibrosis, lung
    Escherichia coli (E. coli) J15.5
    Friedlander's bacillus J15.0
    Hemophilus influenzae J14
    hypostatic J18.2
    Klebsiella (pneumoniae) J15.0
    pneumococcal J13
    Proteus J15.69
    Pseudomonas J15.1
    specified organism NEC J16.8
    staphylococcal — *see* Pneumonia, staphylococcal
    streptococcal NEC J15.4
    Streptococcus pneumoniae J13
    viral, virus — *see* Pneumonia, viral
  lobular — *see* Pneumonia, broncho
  Loffler's J82.89
  lymphoid interstitial J84.2
  massive — *see* Pneumonia, lobar
  meconium P24.01
  MRSA (methicillin resistant Staphylococcus aureus) J15.212
  MSSA (methicillin susceptible Staphylococcus aureus) J15.211
  multilobar — *see* Pneumonia, by type
  Mycoplasma (pneumoniae) J15.7
  necrotic J85.0
  neonatal P23.9
    aspiration — *see* Aspiration, by substance, with pneumonia
  nitrogen dioxide J68.0
  organizing J84.89
    due to
      collagen vascular disease J84.178
      known underlying cause J84.178
    in diseases classified elsewhere J84.178
  orthostatic J18.2
  parainfluenza virus J12.2
  parenchymatous — *see* Fibrosis, lung
  passive J18.2
  patchy — *see* Pneumonia, broncho
  Peptococcus J15.8
  Peptostreptococcus J15.8
  plasma cell (of infants) B59
  pleurolobar — *see* Pneumonia, lobar
  pleuro-pneumonia-like organism (PPLO) J15.7
  pneumococcal (broncho) (lobar) J13
  Pneumocystis (carinii) (jiroveci) B59
  postinfectional NEC B99 ☑ *[J17]*
  postmeasles B05.2
  Proteus J15.69
  Pseudomonas J15.1
  psittacosis A70
  radiation J70.0
  respiratory syncytial virus (RSV) J12.1
  resulting from a procedure J95.89
  rheumatic I00 *[J17]*
  Salmonella (arizonae) (cholerae-suis) (enteritidis) (typhimurium) A02.22
    typhi A01.03
    typhoid fever A01.03
  SARS-associated coronavirus J12.81
  SARS-CoV-2 J12.82
  segmented, segmental — *see* Pneumonia, broncho-
  Serratia marcescens J15.69
  specified NEC J18.8
    bacterium NEC J15.8
    organism NEC J16.8
    virus NEC J12.89
  spirochetal NEC A69.8
  staphylococcal (broncho) (lobar) J15.20
    aureus (methicillin susceptible) (MSSA) J15.211
      methicillin resistant (MRSA) J15.212
    specified NEC J15.29
  static, stasis J18.2
  streptococcal NEC (broncho) (lobar) J15.4
    group
      A J15.4
      B J15.3
      specified NEC J15.4
  Streptococcus pneumoniae J13
  syphilitic, congenital (early) A50.04
  traumatic (complication) (early) (secondary) T79.8 ☑
  tuberculous (any) — *see* Tuberculosis, pulmonary

Pneumonia — *continued*
  tularemic A21.2
  varicella B01.2
  Veillonella J15.8
  ventilator associated J95.851
  viral, virus (broncho) (interstitial) (lobar) J12.9
    adenoviral J12.0
    congenital P23.0
    human metapneumovirus J12.3
    parainfluenza J12.2
    respiratory syncytial (RSV) J12.1
    SARS-associated coronavirus J12.81
    specified NEC J12.89
  white (congenital) A50.04
Pneumonic — *see* condition
Pneumonitis (acute) (primary) — *see also* Pneumonia J98.4
  air-conditioner J67.7
  allergic (due to) J67.9
    organic dust NEC J67.8
    red cedar dust J67.8
    sequoiosis J67.8
    wood dust J67.8
  aspiration J69.0
    due to
      anesthesia J95.4
        during
          labor and delivery O74.0
          pregnancy O29.01- ☑
          puerperium O89.01
      fumes or gases J68.0
    obstetric O74.0
  chemical (due to gases, fumes or vapors) (inhalation) J68.0
    due to anesthesia J95.4
  cholesterol J84.89
  chronic — *see* Fibrosis, lung
  congenital rubella P35.0
  crack (cocaine) J68.0
  due to
    beryllium J68.0
    cadmium J68.0
    crack (cocaine) J68.0
    detergent J69.8
    fluorocarbon-polymer J68.0
    food, vomit (aspiration) J69.0
    fumes or vapors J68.0
    gases, fumes or vapors (inhalation) J68.0
    inhalation
      blood J69.8
      essences J69.1
      food (regurgitated), milk, vomit J69.0
      oils, essences J69.1
      saliva J69.0
      solids, liquids NEC J69.8
    manganese J68.0
    nitrogen dioxide J68.0
    oils, essences J69.1
    solids, liquids NEC J69.8
    toxoplasmosis (acquired) B58.3
      congenital P37.1
    vanadium J68.0
    ventilator J95.851
  eosinophilic J82.81
    acute J82.82
    chronic J82.81
  hypersensitivity J67.9
    air conditioner lung J67.7
    bagassosis J67.1
    bird fancier's lung J67.2
    farmer's lung J67.0
    maltworker's lung J67.4
    maple bark-stripper's lung J67.6
    mushroom worker's lung J67.5
    specified organic dust NEC J67.8
    suberosis J67.3
  interstitial (chronic) J84.89
    acute J84.114
    lymphoid J84.2
    non-specific J84.89
      idiopathic J84.113
  lymphoid, interstitial J84.2
  meconium P24.01
  noninfectious J98.4
  postanesthetic J95.4
    correct substance properly administered — *see* Table of Drugs and Chemicals, by drug, adverse effect
    in labor and delivery O74.0
    in pregnancy O29.01- ☑
    obstetric O74.0

Pneumonitis — continued
  postanesthetic — continued
    overdose or wrong substance given or taken (by accident) — see Table of Drugs and Chemicals, by drug, poisoning
  postpartum, puerperal O89.01
  postoperative J95.4
    obstetric O74.0
  radiation J70.0
  rubella, congenital P35.0
  specified NEC J98.4
  ventilation (air-conditioning) J67.7
  ventilator associated J95.851
  wood-dust J67.8
Pneumoconiosis — see Pneumoconiosis
Pneumoparotid K11.8
Pneumopathy NEC J98.4
  alveolar J84.09
  due to organic dust NEC J66.8
  parietoalveolar J84.09
Pneumopericarditis — see also Pericarditis
  acute I30.9
Pneumopericardium — see also Pericarditis
  congenital P25.3
  newborn P25.3
  traumatic (post) — see Injury, heart
Pneumophagia (psychogenic) F45.8
Pneumopleurisy, pneumopleuritis — see also Pneumonia J18.8
Pneumopyopericardium I30.1
Pneumopyothorax — see Pyopneumothorax
  with fistula J86.0
Pneumorrhagia — see also Hemorrhage, lung
  tuberculous — see Tuberculosis, pulmonary
Pneumothorax NOS J93.9
  acute J93.83
  chronic J93.81
  congenital P25.1
  perinatal period P25.1
  postprocedural J95.811
  specified NEC J93.83
  spontaneous NOS J93.83
    newborn P25.1
    primary J93.11
    secondary J93.12
    tension J93.0
  tense valvular, infectional J93.0
  tension (spontaneous) J93.0
  traumatic S27.0 ☑
    with hemothorax S27.2 ☑
  tuberculous — see Tuberculosis, pulmonary
Podagra — see also Gout M10.9
Podencephalus Q01.9
Poikilocytosis R71.8
Poikiloderma L81.6
  Civatte's L57.3
  congenital Q82.8
  vasculare atrophicans L94.5
Poikilodermatomyositis M33.10
  with
    myopathy M33.12
    respiratory involvement M33.11
    specified organ involvement NEC M33.19
  amyopathic M33.13
  without myopathy M33.13
Pointed ear (congenital) Q17.3
Poison ivy, oak, sumac or other plant dermatitis (allergic) (contact) L23.7
Poisoning (acute) — see also Table of Drugs and Chemicals
  algae and toxins T65.82- ☑
  Bacillus B (aertrycke) (cholerae (suis)) (paratyphosus) (suipestifer) A02.9
    botulinus A05.1
  bacterial toxins A05.9
  berries, noxious — see Poisoning, food, noxious, berries
  botulism A05.1
  ciguatera fish T61.0- ☑
  Clostridium botulinum A05.1
  death-cap (Amanita phalloides) (Amanita verna) — see Poisoning, food, noxious, mushrooms
  drug — see Table of Drugs and Chemicals, by drug, poisoning
  epidemic, fish (noxious) — see Poisoning, seafood
    bacterial A05.9
  fava bean D55.0
  fish (noxious) T61.9- ☑
    bacterial — see Intoxication, foodborne, by agent
    ciguatera fish — see Poisoning, ciguatera fish

Poisoning — continued
  fish — continued
    scombroid fish — see Poisoning, scombroid fish
    specified type NEC T61.77- ☑
  food NEC A05.9
    bacterial — see Intoxication, foodborne, by agent
    due to
      Bacillus (aertrycke) (choleraesuis) (paratyphosus) (suipestifer) A02.9
        botulinus A05.1
      Clostridium (perfringens) (Welchii) A05.2
      salmonella (aertrycke) (choleraesuis) (enteritidis) (gallinarum) (paratyphi) (suipestifer) A02.9
        with
          gastroenteritis A02.0
          sepsis A02.1
      staphylococcus A05.0
      Vibrio
        parahaemolyticus A05.3
        vulnificus A05.5
    noxious or naturally toxic T62.9- ☑
      berries — see subcategory T62.1 ☑
      fish — see Poisoning, seafood
      mushrooms — see subcategory T62.0X ☑
      plants NEC — see subcategory T62.2X ☑
      seafood — see Poisoning, seafood
      specified NEC — see subcategory T62.8X ☑
  ichthyotoxism — see Poisoning, seafood
  kreotoxism, food A05.9
  latex T65.81- ☑
  lead T56.0- ☑
  mushroom — see Poisoning, food, noxious, mushroom
  mussels — see also Poisoning, shellfish
    bacterial — see Intoxication, foodborne, by agent
  nicotine (tobacco) T65.2- ☑
  noxious foodstuffs — see Poisoning, food, noxious
  plants, noxious — see Poisoning, food, noxious, plants NEC
  ptomaine — see Poisoning, food
  radiation J70.0
  Salmonella (arizonae) (cholerae-suis) (enteritidis) (typhimurium) A02.9
  scombroid fish T61.1- ☑
  seafood (noxious) T61.9- ☑
    bacterial — see Intoxication, foodborne, by agent
    fish — see Poisoning, fish
    shellfish — see Poisoning, shellfish
    specified NEC — see subcategory T61.8X ☑
  shellfish (amnesic) (azaspiracid) (diarrheic) (neurotoxic) (noxious) (paralytic) T61.78- ☑
    bacterial — see Intoxication, foodborne, by agent
    ciguatera mollusk — see Poisoning, ciguatera fish
  specified substance NEC T65.891 ☑
  Staphylococcus, food A05.0
  tobacco (nicotine) T65.2- ☑
  water E87.79
Poker spine — see Spondylitis, ankylosing
Poland syndrome Q79.8
Polioencephalitis (acute) (bulbar) A80.9
  inferior G12.22
  influenzal — see Influenza, with, encephalopathy
  superior hemorrhagic (acute) (Wernicke's) E51.2
  Wernicke's E51.2
Polioencephalomyelitis (acute) (anterior) A80.9
  with beriberi E51.2
Polioencephalopathy, superior hemorrhagic E51.2
  with
    beriberi E51.11
    pellagra E52
Poliomeningoencephalitis — see Meningoencephalitis
Poliomyelitis (acute) (anterior) (epidemic) A80.9
  with paralysis (bulbar) — see Poliomyelitis, paralytic
  abortive A80.4
  ascending (progressive) — see Poliomyelitis, paralytic
  bulbar (paralytic) — see Poliomyelitis, paralytic
  congenital P35.8
  nonepidemic A80.9
  nonparalytic A80.4
  paralytic A80.30
    specified NEC A80.39
    vaccine-associated A80.0
    wild virus
      imported A80.1
      indigenous A80.2
  spinal, acute A80.9
Poliosis (eyebrow) (eyelashes) L67.1
  circumscripta, acquired L67.1
Pollakiuria R35.0

Pollakiuria — continued
  psychogenic F45.8
Pollinosis J30.1
Pollitzer's disease L73.2
Polyadenitis — see also Lymphadenitis
  malignant A20.0
Polyalgia M79.89
Polyangiitis M30.0
  microscopic M31.7
  overlap syndrome M30.8
Polyarteritis
  microscopic M31.7
  nodosa M30.0
    with lung involvement M30.1
    juvenile M30.2
    related condition NEC M30.8
Polyarthralgia — see Pain, joint
Polyarthritis, polyarthropathy — see also Arthritis M13.0
  due to or associated with other specified conditions — see Arthritis
  epidemic (Australian) (with exanthema) B33.1
  infective — see Arthritis, pyogenic or pyemic
  inflammatory M06.4
  juvenile (chronic) (seronegative) M08.3
  migratory M13.8- ☑
  rheumatic, acute — see Fever, rheumatic
Polyarthrosis M15.9
  post-traumatic M15.3
  primary M15.0
  specified NEC M15.8
Polycarential syndrome of infancy E40
Polychondritis (atrophic) (chronic) — see also Disorder, cartilage, specified type NEC
  relapsing M94.1
Polycoria Q13.2
Polycystic (disease)
  degeneration, kidney Q61.3
    autosomal dominant (adult type) Q61.2
    autosomal recessive (infantile type) NEC Q61.19
  kidney Q61.3
    autosomal
      dominant Q61.2
      recessive NEC Q61.19
    autosomal dominant (adult type) Q61.2
    autosomal recessive (childhood type) NEC Q61.19
    infantile type NEC Q61.19
  liver Q44.6
  lung J98.4
    congenital Q33.0
  ovary, ovaries E28.2
  spleen Q89.09
Polycythemia (secondary) D75.1
  acquired D75.1
  benign (familial) D75.0
  due to
    donor twin P61.1
    erythropoietin D75.1
    fall in plasma volume D75.1
    high altitude D75.1
    maternal-fetal transfusion P61.1
    stress D75.1
  emotional D75.1
  erythropoietin D75.1
  familial (benign) D75.0
  Gaisbock's (hypertonica) D75.1
  high altitude D75.1
  hypertonica D75.1
  hypoxemic D75.1
  neonatorum P61.1
  nephrogenous D75.1
  relative D75.1
  secondary D75.1
  spurious D75.1
  stress D75.1
  vera D45
Polycytosis cryptogenica D75.1
Polydactylism, polydactyly Q69.9
  toes Q69.2
Polydipsia R63.1
Polydystrophy, pseudo-Hurler E77.0
Polyembryoma — see Neoplasm, malignant, by site
Polyglandular
  deficiency E31.0
  dyscrasia E31.9
  dysfunction E31.9
  syndrome E31.8
Polyhydramnios O40.- ☑
Polymastia Q83.1
Polymenorrhea N92.0

Polymyalgia M35.3
  arteritica, giant cell M31.5
  rheumatica M35.3
    with giant cell arteritis M31.5
Polymyositis (acute) (chronic) (hemorrhagic) M33.20
  with
    myopathy M33.22
    respiratory involvement M33.21
    skin involvement — see Dermatopolymyositis
    specified organ involvement NEC M33.29
  ossificans (generalisata) (progressiva) — see Myositis,
    ossificans, progressiva
Polyneuritis, polyneuritic — see also Polyneuropathy
  acute (post-)infective G61.0
  alcoholic G62.1
  cranialis G52.7
  demyelinating, chronic inflammatory (CIDP) G61.81
  diabetic — see Diabetes, polyneuropathy
  diphtheritic A36.83
  due to lack of vitamin NEC E56.9 [G63]
  endemic E51.11
  erythredema — see subcategory T56.1 ☑
  febrile, acute G61.0
  hereditary ataxic G60.1
  idiopathic, acute G61.0
  infective (acute) G61.0
  inflammatory, chronic demyelinating (CIDP) G61.81
  nutritional E63.9 [G63]
  postinfective (acute) G61.0
  specified NEC G62.89
Polyneuropathy (peripheral) G62.9
  alcoholic G62.1
  amyloid (Portuguese) E85.1 [G63]
    transthyretin-related (ATTR) familial E85.1 [G63]
  arsenical G62.2
  critical illness G62.81
  demyelinating, chronic inflammatory (CIDP) G61.81
  diabetic — see Diabetes, polyneuropathy
  drug-induced G62.0
  hereditary G60.9
    specified NEC G60.8
  idiopathic G60.9
    progressive G60.3
  in (due to)
    alcohol G62.1
      sequelae G65.2
    amyloidosis, familial (Portuguese) E85.1 [G63]
    antitetanus serum G61.1
    arsenic G62.2
      sequelae G65.2
    avitaminosis NEC E56.9 [G63]
    beriberi E51.11
    collagen vascular disease NEC M35.9 [G63]
    deficiency (of)
      B (-complex) vitamins E53.9 [G63]
      vitamin B6 E53.1 [G63]
    diabetes — see Diabetes, polyneuropathy
    diphtheria A36.83
    drug or medicament G62.0
      correct substance properly administered — see
        Table of Drugs and Chemicals, by drug, ad-
        verse effect
      overdose or wrong substance given or taken —
        see Table of Drugs and Chemicals, by drug,
        poisoning
    endocrine disease NEC E34.9 [G63]
    herpes zoster B02.23
    hypoglycemia E16.2 [G63]
    infectious
      disease NEC B99 ☑ [G63]
      mononucleosis B27.91
    lack of vitamin NEC E56.9 [G63]
    lead G62.2
      sequelae G65.2
    leprosy A30.9 [G63]
    Lyme disease A69.22
    metabolic disease NEC E88.9 [G63]
    microscopic polyangiitis M31.7 [G63]
    mumps B26.84
    neoplastic disease — see also Neoplasm D49.9 [G63]
    nutritional deficiency NEC E63.9 [G63]
    organophosphate compounds G62.2
      sequelae G65.2
    parasitic disease NEC B89 [G63]
    pellagra E52 [G63]
    polyarteritis nodosa M30.0
    porphyria E80.20 [G63]
    radiation G62.82

Polyneuropathy — continued
  in — continued
    rheumatoid arthritis — see Rheumatoid, polyneuropa-
      thy
    sarcoidosis D86.89
    serum G61.1
    syphilis (late) A52.15
      congenital A50.43
    systemic
      connective tissue disorder M35.9 [G63]
      lupus erythematosus M32.19
    toxic agent NEC G62.2
      sequelae G65.2
    transthyretin-related (ATTR) familial amyloid E85.1
    triorthocresyl phosphate G62.2
      sequelae G65.2
    tuberculosis A17.89
    uremia N18.9 [G63]
    vitamin B12 deficiency E53.8 [G63]
      with anemia (pernicious) D51.0 [G63]
        due to dietary deficiency D51.3, G63
    zoster B02.23
  inflammatory G61.9
    chronic demyelinating (CIDP) G61.81
    sequelae G65.1
    specified NEC G61.89
  lead G62.2
    sequelae G65.2
  nutritional NEC E63.9 [G63]
  postherpetic (zoster) B02.23
  progressive G60.3
  radiation-induced G62.82
  sensory (hereditary) (idiopathic) G60.8
  specified NEC G62.89
  syphilitic (late) A52.15
    congenital A50.43
Polyopia H53.8
Polyorchism, polyorchidism Q55.21
Polyosteoarthritis — see also Osteoarthritis, generalized
    M15.9
  post-traumatic M15.3
  specified NEC M15.8
Polyostotic fibrous dysplasia Q78.1
Polyotia Q17.0
Polyp, polypus
  accessory sinus J33.8
  adenocarcinoma in — see Neoplasm, malignant, by site
  adenocarcinoma in situ in — see Neoplasm, in situ, by
    site
  adenoid tissue J33.0
  adenomatous — see also Neoplasm, benign, by site
    adenocarcinoma in — see Neoplasm, malignant, by
      site
    adenocarcinoma in situ in — see Neoplasm, in situ,
      by site
    carcinoma in — see Neoplasm, malignant, by site
    carcinoma in situ in — see Neoplasm, in situ, by site
    multiple — see Neoplasm, benign
      adenocarcinoma in — see Neoplasm, malignant,
        by site
      adenocarcinoma in situ in — see Neoplasm, in situ,
        by site
  antrum J33.8
  anus, anal (canal) K62.0
  Bartholin's gland N84.3
  bladder D41.4
  carcinoma in — see Neoplasm, malignant, by site
  carcinoma in situ in — see Neoplasm, in situ, by site
  cecum D12.0
  cervix (uteri) N84.1
    in pregnancy or childbirth — see Pregnancy, compli-
      cated by, abnormal, cervix
    mucous N84.1
    nonneoplastic N84.1
  choanal J33.0
  cholesterol K82.4
  clitoris N84.3
  colon K63.5
    adenomatous D12.6
      ascending D12.2
      cecum D12.0
      descending D12.4
      sigmoid D12.5
      transverse D12.3
    ascending K63.5
    cecum K63.5
    descending K63.5
    hyperplastic, (any site) K63.5
    inflammatory K51.40

Polyp, polypus — continued
  colon — continued
    inflammatory — continued
      with
        abscess K51.414
        complication K51.419
          specified NEC K51.418
        fistula K51.413
        intestinal obstruction K51.412
        rectal bleeding K51.411
    sigmoid K63.5
    transverse K63.5
  corpus uteri N84.0
  dental K04.01
    irreversible K04.02
    reversible K04.01
  duodenum K31.7
  ear (middle) H74.4- ☑
  endometrium N84.0
  esophageal K22.81
  esophagogastric junction K22.82
  ethmoidal (sinus) J33.8
  fallopian tube N84.8
  female genital tract N84.9
    specified NEC N84.8
  frontal (sinus) J33.8
  gallbladder K82.4
  gingiva, gum K06.8
  labia, labium (majus) (minus) N84.3
  larynx (mucous) J38.1
    adenomatous D14.1
  malignant — see Neoplasm, malignant, by site
  maxillary (sinus) J33.8
  middle ear — see Polyp, ear (middle)
  myometrium N84.0
  nares
    anterior J33.9
    posterior J33.0
  nasal (mucous) J33.9
    cavity J33.0
    septum J33.0
  nasopharyngeal J33.0
  nose (mucous) J33.9
  oviduct N84.8
  pharynx J39.2
  placenta O90.89
  prostate — see Enlargement, enlarged, prostate
  pudenda, pudendum N84.3
  pulpal (dental) K04.01
    irreversible K04.02
    reversible K04.01
  rectum (nonadenomatous) K62.1
    adenomatous — see Polyp, adenomatous
  septum (nasal) J33.0
  sinus (accessory) (ethmoidal) (frontal) (maxillary) (sphe-
    noidal) J33.8
  sphenoidal (sinus) J33.8
  stomach K31.7
    adenomatous D13.1
  tube, fallopian N84.8
  turbinate, mucous membrane J33.8
  umbilical, newborn P83.6
  ureter N28.89
  urethra N36.2
  uterus (body) (corpus) (mucous) N84.0
    cervix N84.1
    in pregnancy or childbirth — see Pregnancy, compli-
      cated by, tumor, uterus
  vagina N84.2
  vocal cord (mucous) J38.1
  vulva N84.3
Polyphagia R63.2
Polyploidy Q92.7
Polypoid — see condition
Polyposis — see also Polyp
  adenomatous D13.91
  coli (adenomatous) D12.6
    adenocarcinoma in C18.9
    adenocarcinoma in situ in — see Neoplasm, in situ,
      by site
    carcinoma in C18.9
  colon (adenomatous) D12.6
  familial D12.6
    adenocarcinoma in situ in — see Neoplasm, in situ,
      by site
    adenomatous D13.91
  intestinal D12.6
    adenomatous D13.91
  malignant lymphomatous C83.1- ☑

☑ **Additional Character Required — Refer to the Tabular List for Character Selection**

Polyposis — continued
multiple, adenomatous — see also Neoplasm, benign D36.9
Polyradiculitis — see Polyneuropathy
Polyradiculoneuropathy (acute) (postinfective) (segmentally demyelinating) G61.0
Polyserositis
due to pericarditis I31.1
pericardial I31.1
periodic, familial E85.0
tuberculous A19.9
acute A19.1
chronic A19.8
Polysplenia syndrome Q89.09
Polysyndactyly — see also Syndactylism, syndactyly Q70.4
Polytrichia L68.3
Polyunguia Q84.6
Polyuria R35.89
nocturnal R35.81
psychogenic F45.8
specified NEC R35.89
Pompe's disease (glycogen storage) E74.02
Pompholyx L30.1
Poncet's disease (tuberculous rheumatism) A18.09
Pond fracture — see Fracture, skull
Ponos B55.0
Pons, pontine — see condition
Poor
aesthetic of existing restoration of tooth K08.56
contractions, labor O62.2
gingival margin to tooth restoration K08.51
personal hygiene R46.0
prenatal care, affecting management of pregnancy — see Pregnancy, complicated by, insufficient, prenatal care
sucking reflex (newborn) R29.2
urinary stream R39.12
vision NEC H54.7
Poradenitis, nostras inguinalis or venerea A55
Porencephaly (congenital) (developmental) (true) Q04.6
acquired G93.0
nondevelopmental G93.0
traumatic (post) F07.89
Porocephaliasis B88.8
Porokeratosis Q82.8
Poroma, eccrine — see Neoplasm, skin, benign
Porphyria (South African) E80.20
acquired E80.20
acute intermittent (hepatic) (Swedish) E80.21
cutanea tarda (hereditary) (symptomatic) E80.1
due to drugs E80.20
correct substance properly administered — see Table of Drugs and Chemicals, by drug, adverse effect
overdose or wrong substance given or taken — see Table of Drugs and Chemicals, by drug, poisoning
erythropoietic (congenital) (hereditary) E80.0
hepatocutaneous type E80.1
secondary E80.20
toxic NEC E80.20
variegata E80.20
Porphyrinuria — see Porphyria
Porphyruria — see Porphyria
Port wine nevus, mark, or stain Q82.5
Portal — see condition
Posadas-Wernicke disease B38.9
Positive
culture (nonspecific)
blood R78.81
bronchial washings R84.5
cerebrospinal fluid R83.5
cervix uteri R87.5
nasal secretions R84.5
nipple discharge R89.5
nose R84.5
staphylococcus (Methicillin susceptible) Z22.321
Methicillin resistant Z22.322
peritoneal fluid R85.5
pleural fluid R84.5
prostatic secretions R86.5
saliva R85.5
seminal fluid R86.5
sputum R84.5
synovial fluid R89.5
throat scrapings R84.5
urine R82.79
vagina R87.5
vulva R87.5
wound secretions R89.5

Positive — continued
PPD (skin test) R76.11
serology for syphilis A53.0
false R76.8
with signs or symptoms — code as Syphilis, by site and stage
skin test, tuberculin (without active tuberculosis) R76.11
test, human immunodeficiency virus (HIV) R75
VDRL A53.0
with signs or symptoms — code by site and stage under Syphilis A53.9
Wassermann reaction A53.0
Post COVID-19 condition, unspecified U09.9
Postcardiotomy syndrome I97.0
Postcaval ureter Q62.62
Postcholecystectomy syndrome K91.5
Postclimacteric bleeding N95.0
Postcommissurotomy syndrome I97.0
Postconcussion syndrome F07.81
Postcontusional syndrome F07.81
Postcricoid region — see condition
Post-dates (40-42 weeks) (pregnancy) (mother) O48.0
more than 42 weeks gestation O48.1
Postencephalitic syndrome F07.89
Posterior — see condition
Posterolateral sclerosis (spinal cord) — see Degeneration, combined
Postexanthematous — see condition
Postfebrile — see condition
Postgastrectomy dumping syndrome K91.1
Posthemiplegic chorea — see Monoplegia
Posthemorrhagic anemia (chronic) D50.0
acute D62
newborn P61.3
Postherpetic neuralgia (zoster) B02.29
trigeminal B02.22
Posthitis N47.7
Postimmunization complication or reaction — see Complications, vaccination
Postinfectious — see condition
Postlaminectomy syndrome NEC M96.1
Postleukotomy syndrome F07.0
Postmastectomy lymphedema (syndrome) I97.2
Postmaturity, postmature (over 42 weeks)
maternal (over 42 weeks gestation) O48.1
newborn P08.22
Postmeasles complication NEC — see also condition B05.89
Postmenopausal
endometrium (atrophic) N95.8
suppurative — see also Endometritis N71.9
osteoporosis — see Osteoporosis, postmenopausal
Postnasal drip R09.82
due to
allergic rhinitis — see Rhinitis, allergic
common cold J00
gastroesophageal reflux — see Reflux, gastroesophageal
nasopharyngitis — see Nasopharyngitis
other known condition — code to condition
sinusitis — see Sinusitis
Postnatal — see condition
Postoperative (postprocedural) — see also Complication, postoperative
pneumothorax, therapeutic Z98.3
state NEC Z98.890
visit — see Aftercare
wound check — see Aftercare
Postpancreatectomy hyperglycemia E89.1
Postpartum — see Puerperal
Postphlebitic syndrome — see Syndrome, postthrombotic
Postpolio (myelitic) **syndrome** G14
Postpoliomyelitic — see also condition
osteopathy — see Osteopathy, after poliomyelitis
Postprocedural — see also Postoperative
hypoinsulinemia E89.1
Postschizophrenic depression F32.89
Postsurgery status — see also Status (post)
pneumothorax, therapeutic Z98.3
Post-term (40-42 weeks) (pregnancy) (mother) O48.0
infant P08.21
more than 42 weeks gestation (mother) O48.1
Post-traumatic brain syndrome, nonpsychotic F07.81
Post-typhoid abscess A01.09
Postures, hysterical F44.2
Postvaccinal reaction or complication — see Complications, vaccination
Postvalvulotomy syndrome I97.0

Potain's
disease (pulmonary edema) — see Edema, lung
syndrome (gastrectasis with dyspepsia) K31.0
POTS (postural orthostatic tachycardia syndrome) G90.A
Potter's
asthma J62.8
facies Q60.6
lung J62.8
syndrome (with renal agenesis) Q60.6
Pott's
curvature (spinal) A18.01
disease or paraplegia A18.01
spinal curvature A18.01
tumor, puffy — see Osteomyelitis, specified type NEC
Pouch
bronchus Q32.4
Douglas' — see condition
esophagus, esophageal, congenital Q39.6
acquired K22.5
gastric K31.4
Hartmann's K82.8
pharynx, pharyngeal (congenital) Q38.7
Pouchitis K91.850
Poultrymen's itch B88.0
Poverty NEC Z59.6
extreme Z59.5
Poxvirus NEC B08.8
Prader-Willi syndrome Q87.11
Prader-Willi-like syndrome Q87.19
Preauricular appendage or tag Q17.0
Prebetalipoproteinemia (acquired) (essential) (familial) (hereditary) (primary) (secondary) E78.1
with chylomicronemia E78.3
Precipitate labor or delivery O62.3
Preclimacteric bleeding (menorrhagia) N92.4
Precocious
adrenarche E30.1
menarche E30.1
menstruation E30.1
pubarche E30.1
puberty E30.1
central E22.8
sexual development NEC E30.1
thelarche E30.1
Precocity, sexual (constitutional) (cryptogenic) (female) (idiopathic) (male) E30.1
with adrenal hyperplasia E25.9
congenital E25.0
Precordial pain R07.2
Predeciduous teeth K00.2
Prediabetes, prediabetic R73.03
complicating
pregnancy — see Pregnancy, complicated by, diseases of, specified type or system NEC
puerperium O99.893
Predislocation status of hip at birth Q65.6
Pre-eclampsia O14.9- ☑
with pre-existing hypertension — see Hypertension, complicating pregnancy, pre-existing, with, pre-eclampsia
complicating
childbirth O14.94
puerperium O14.95
mild O14.0- ☑
complicating
childbirth O14.04
puerperium O14.05
moderate O14.0- ☑
complicating
childbirth O14.04
puerperium O14.05
severe O14.1- ☑
with hemolysis, elevated liver enzymes and low platelet count (HELLP) O14.2- ☑
complicating
childbirth O14.24
puerperium O14.25
complicating
childbirth O14.14
puerperium O14.15
Pre-eruptive color change, teeth, tooth K00.8
Pre-excitation atrioventricular conduction I45.6
Preglaucoma H40.00- ☑

☑ **Additional Character Required** — Refer to the Tabular List for Character Selection

Pregnancy (single) (uterine) — *see also* Delivery and Puerperal Z33.1

> *Note: The Tabular must be reviewed for assignment of appropriate seventh character for multiple gestation codes in Chapter 15*

> *Note: The Tabular must be reviewed for assignment of the appropriate character indicating the trimester of the pregnancy*

abdominal (ectopic) O00.00
  with intrauterine pregnancy O00.01
  with viable fetus O36.7- ☑
ampullar O00.10- ☑
  with intrauterine pregnancy O00.11- ☑
biochemical O02.81
broad ligament O00.80
  with intrauterine pregnancy O00.81
cervical O00.8
  with intrauterine pregnancy O00.81
chemical O02.81
complicated by (care of) (management affected by)
  abnormal, abnormality
    cervix O34.4- ☑
      causing obstructed labor O65.5
    cord (umbilical) O69.9 ☑
    fetal heart rate or rhythm O36.83- ☑
    findings on antenatal screening of mother O28.9
      biochemical O28.1
      chromosomal O28.5
      cytological O28.2
      genetic O28.5
      hematological O28.0
      radiological O28.4
      specified NEC O28.8
      ultrasonic O28.3
    glucose (tolerance) NEC O99.810
    pelvic organs O34.9- ☑
      specified NEC O34.8- ☑
        causing obstructed labor O65.5
    pelvis (bony) (major) NEC O33.0
    perineum O34.7- ☑
    position
      placenta O44.0- ☑
        with hemorrhage O44.1- ☑
      uterus O34.59- ☑
    uterus O34.59- ☑
      causing obstructed labor O65.5
      congenital O34.0- ☑
    vagina O34.6- ☑
      causing obstructed labor O65.5
    vulva O34.7- ☑
      causing obstructed labor O65.5
  abruptio placentae — *see* Abruptio placentae
  abscess or cellulitis
    bladder O23.1- ☑
    breast O91.11- ☑
    genital organ or tract O23.9- ☑
  abuse
    physical O9A.31 ☑ (*following* O99)
    psychological O9A.51 ☑ (*following* O99)
    sexual O9A.41 ☑ (*following* O99)
  adverse effect anesthesia O29.9- ☑
    aspiration pneumonitis O29.01- ☑
    cardiac arrest O29.11- ☑
    cardiac complication NEC O29.19- ☑
    cardiac failure O29.12- ☑
    central nervous system complication NEC O29.29- ☑
    cerebral anoxia O29.21- ☑
    failed or difficult intubation O29.6- ☑
    inhalation of stomach contents or secretions NOS O29.01- ☑
    local, toxic reaction O29.3X- ☑
    Mendelson's syndrome O29.01- ☑
    pressure collapse of lung O29.02- ☑
    pulmonary complications NEC O29.09- ☑
    specified NEC O29.8X- ☑
    spinal and epidural type NEC O29.5X ☑
      induced headache O29.4- ☑
  albuminuria — *see also* Proteinuria, gestational O12.1- ☑
  alcohol use O99.31- ☑
  amnionitis O41.12- ☑
  anaphylactoid syndrome of pregnancy O88.01- ☑
  anemia (conditions in D50-D64) (pre-existing) O99.01- ☑

Pregnancy — *continued*
  complicated by — *continued*
    anemia — *continued*
      complicating childbirth O99.02
      complicating the puerperium O99.03
    antepartum hemorrhage O46.9- ☑
      with coagulation defect — *see* Hemorrhage, antepartum, with coagulation defect
      specified NEC O46.8X- ☑
    appendicitis O99.61- ☑
    atrophy (yellow) (acute) liver (subacute) O26.61- ☑
    bariatric surgery status O99.84- ☑
    bicornis or bicornuate uterus O34.0- ☑
    biliary tract problems O26.61- ☑
    breech presentation O32.1 ☑
    cardiovascular diseases (conditions in I00-I09, I20-I52, I70-I99) O99.41- ☑
    cerebrovascular disorders (conditions in I60-I69) O99.41- ☑
    cervical shortening O26.87- ☑
    cervicitis O23.51- ☑
    cesarean scar defect (isthmocele) O34.22
    chloasma (gravidarum) O26.89- ☑
    cholecystitis O99.61- ☑
    cholestasis (intrahepatic) O26.64- ☑
    chorioamnionitis O41.12- ☑
    circulatory system disorder (conditions in I00-I09, I20-I99, O99.41-)
    compound presentation O32.6 ☑
    conjoined twins O30.02- ☑
    connective system disorders (conditions in M00-M99) O99.891
    contracted pelvis (general) O33.1
      inlet O33.2
      outlet O33.3
    convulsions (eclamptic) (uremic) — *see also* Eclampsia O15.9
    cracked nipple O92.11- ☑
    cystitis O23.1- ☑
    cystocele O34.8- ☑
    death of fetus (near term) O36.4 ☑
      early pregnancy O02.1
      of one fetus or more in multiple gestation O31.2- ☑
    deciduitis O41.14- ☑
    decreased fetal movement O36.81- ☑
    dental problems O99.61- ☑
    diabetes (mellitus) O24.91- ☑
      gestational (pregnancy induced) — *see* Diabetes, gestational
      pre-existing O24.31- ☑
        specified NEC O24.81- ☑
        type 1 O24.01- ☑
        type 2 O24.11- ☑
    digestive system disorders (conditions in K00-K93) O99.61- ☑
    diseases of — *see* Pregnancy, complicated by, specified body system disease
      biliary tract O26.61- ☑
      blood NEC (conditions in D65-D77) O99.11- ☑
      liver O26.61- ☑
      specified NEC O99.891
    disorders of — *see* Pregnancy, complicated by, specified body system disorder
      amniotic fluid and membranes O41.9- ☑
        specified NEC O41.8X- ☑
      biliary tract O26.61- ☑
      ear and mastoid process (conditions in H60-H95) O99.891
      eye and adnexa (conditions in H00-H59) O99.891
      liver O26.61- ☑
      skin (conditions in L00-L99) O99.71- ☑
      specified NEC O99.891
    displacement, uterus NEC O34.59- ☑
      causing obstructed labor O65.5
    disproportion (due to) O33.9
      fetal (ascites) (hydrops) (meningomyelocele) (sacral teratoma) (tumor) deformities NEC O33.7
      generally contracted pelvis O33.1
      hydrocephalic fetus O33.6
      inlet contraction of pelvis O33.2
      mixed maternal and fetal origin O33.4
      specified NEC O33.8
    double uterus O34.0- ☑
      causing obstructed labor O65.5
    drug use (conditions in F11-F19) O99.32- ☑

Pregnancy — *continued*
  complicated by — *continued*
    eclampsia, eclamptic (coma) (convulsions) (delirium) (nephritis) (uremia) — *see also* Eclampsia O15.- ☑
    ectopic pregnancy — *see* Pregnancy, ectopic
    edema O12.0- ☑
      with
        gestational hypertension, mild — *see also* Pre-eclampsia O14.0- ☑
        proteinuria O12.2- ☑
    effusion, amniotic fluid — *see* Pregnancy, complicated by, premature rupture of membranes
    elderly
      multigravida O09.52- ☑
      primigravida O09.51- ☑
    embolism — *see also* Embolism, obstetric, pregnancy O88.- ☑
    endocrine diseases NEC O99.28- ☑
    endometritis O86.12
    excessive weight gain O26.0- ☑
    exhaustion O26.81- ☑
      during labor and delivery O75.81
    face presentation O32.3 ☑
    failed induction of labor O61.9
      instrumental O61.1
      mechanical O61.1
      medical O61.0
      specified NEC O61.8
      surgical O61.1
    failed or difficult intubation for anesthesia O29.6- ☑
    false labor (pains) O47.9
      at or after 37 completed weeks of pregnancy O47.1
      before 37 completed weeks of pregnancy O47.0- ☑
    fatigue O26.81- ☑
      during labor and delivery O75.81
    fatty metamorphosis of liver O26.61- ☑
    female genital mutilation O34.8- ☑ *[N90.81-]* ☑
    fetal (maternal care for)
      abnormality or damage O35.9 ☑
        acid-base balance O68
        specified type NEC O35.8 ☑
      acidemia O68
      acidosis O68
      agenesis of corpus callosum O35.01 ☑
      alkalosis O68
      anemia and thrombocytopenia O36.82- ☑
      anencephaly O35.02 ☑
      bradycardia O36.83- ☑
      cardiac anomalies O35.B
      central nervous system malformation or damage O35.00 ☑
        specified type NEC O35.09 ☑
      choroid plexus cysts O35.03 ☑
      chromosomal abnormality (conditions in Q90-Q99) O35.10 ☑
        sex chromosome O35.15 ☑
        specified NEC O35.19 ☑
        Trisomy 13 O35.11 ☑
        Trisomy 18 O35.12 ☑
        Trisomy 21 O35.13 ☑
        Turner Syndrome O35.14 ☑
      conjoined twins O30.02- ☑
      damage from
        amniocentesis O35.7 ☑
        biopsy procedures O35.7 ☑
        drug addiction O35.5 ☑
        hematological investigation O35.7 ☑
        intrauterine contraceptive device O35.7 ☑
        maternal
          alcohol addiction O35.4 ☑
          cytomegalovirus infection O35.3 ☑
          disease NEC O35.8 ☑
          drug addiction O35.5 ☑
          listeriosis O35.8 ☑
          rubella O35.3 ☑
          toxoplasmosis O35.8 ☑
          viral infection O35.3 ☑
        medical procedure NEC O35.7 ☑
        radiation O35.6 ☑
      death (near term) O36.4 ☑
        early pregnancy O02.1
      decreased movement O36.81- ☑
      depressed heart rate tones O36.83- ☑
      disproportion due to deformity (fetal) O33.7

Pregnancy — *continued*
  complicated by — *continued*
    fetal — *continued*
      encephalocele O35.04 ☑
      excessive growth (large for dates) O36.6- ☑
      facial anomalies O35.A ☑
      gastrointestinal anomalies O35.D ☑
      genitourinary anomalies O35.E ☑
      growth retardation O36.59- ☑
        light for dates O36.59- ☑
        small for dates O36.59- ☑
      heart rate irregularity (abnormal variability) (bradycardia) (decelerations) (tachycardia) O36.83- ☑
      hereditary disease O35.2 ☑
      holoprosencephaly O35.05 ☑
      hydrocephalus O35.06 ☑
      hydrocephaly O35.06 ☑
      intrauterine death O36.4 ☑
      microcephaly O35.07 ☑
      musculoskeletal anomalies
        lower extremities O35.H ☑
        trunk O35.F ☑
        upper extremities O35.G ☑
      non-reassuring heart rate or rhythm O36.83- ☑
      poor growth O36.59- ☑
        light for dates O36.59- ☑
        small for dates O36.59- ☑
      problem O36.9- ☑
        specified NEC O36.89- ☑
      pulmonary anomalies O35.C ☑
      reduction (elective) O31.3- ☑
      selective termination O31.3- ☑
      spina bifida O35.08 ☑
      thrombocytopenia O36.82- ☑
    fibroid (tumor) (uterus) O34.1- ☑
    fissure of nipple O92.11- ☑
    gallstones O99.61- ☑
    gastric banding status O99.84- ☑
    gastric bypass status O99.84- ☑
    genital herpes (asymptomatic) (history of) (inactive) O98.3- ☑
    genital tract infection O23.9- ☑
    glomerular diseases (conditions in N00-N07) O26.83- ☑
      with hypertension, pre-existing — *see* Hypertension, complicating, pregnancy, pre-existing, with, renal disease
    gonorrhea O98.21- ☑
    grand multiparity O09.4 ☑
    habitual aborter — *see* Pregnancy, complicated by, recurrent pregnancy loss
    HELLP syndrome (hemolysis, elevated liver enzymes and low platelet count) O14.2- ☑
    hemorrhage
      antepartum — *see* Hemorrhage, antepartum
      before 20 completed weeks gestation O20.9
        specified NEC O20.8
      due to premature separation, placenta — *see also* Abruptio placentae O45.9- ☑
      early O20.9
        specified NEC O20.8
      threatened abortion O20.0
    hemorrhoids O22.4- ☑
    hepatitis (viral) O98.41- ☑
    herniation of uterus O34.59- ☑
    high
      head at term O32.4 ☑
      risk — *see* Supervision (of) (for), high-risk
    history of in utero procedure during previous pregnancy O09.82- ☑
    HIV O98.71- ☑
    human immunodeficiency virus (HIV) disease O98.71- ☑
    hydatidiform mole — *see also* Mole, hydatidiform O01.9
    hydramnios O40.- ☑
    hydrocephalic fetus (disproportion) O33.6 ☑
    hydrops
      amnii O40.- ☑
      fetalis O36.2- ☑
        associated with isoimmunization — *see also* Pregnancy, complicated by, isoimmunization O36.11- ☑
    hydrorrhea O42.90

Pregnancy — *continued*
  complicated by — *continued*
    hyperemesis (gravidarum) (mild) — *see also* Hyperemesis, gravidarum O21.0
    hypertension — *see* Hypertension, complicating pregnancy
    hypertensive
      heart and renal disease, pre-existing — *see* Hypertension, complicating, pregnancy, pre-existing, with, heart disease, with renal disease
      heart disease, pre-existing — *see* Hypertension, complicating, pregnancy, pre-existing, with, heart disease
      renal disease, pre-existing — *see* Hypertension, complicating, pregnancy, pre-existing, with, renal disease
    hypotension O26.5- ☑
    immune disorders NEC (conditions in D80-D89) O99.11- ☑
    incarceration, uterus O34.51- ☑
    incompetent cervix O34.3- ☑
    inconclusive fetal viability O36.80 ☑
    infection(s) O98.91- ☑
      amniotic fluid or sac O41.10- ☑
      bladder O23.1- ☑
      carrier state NEC O99.830
        streptococcus B O99.820
      genital organ or tract O23.9- ☑
        specified NEC O23.59- ☑
      genitourinary tract O23.9- ☑
      gonorrhea O98.21- ☑
      hepatitis (viral) O98.41- ☑
      HIV O98.71- ☑
      human immunodeficiency virus (HIV) O98.71- ☑
      intrauterine O41.12 ☑
      kidney O23.0- ☑
      nipple O91.01- ☑
      parasitic disease O98.91- ☑
        specified NEC O98.81- ☑
      protozoal disease O98.61- ☑
      sexually transmitted NEC O98.31- ☑
      specified type NEC O98.81- ☑
      syphilis O98.11- ☑
      tuberculosis O98.01- ☑
      urethra O23.2- ☑
      urinary (tract) O23.4- ☑
        specified NEC O23.3- ☑
      viral disease O98.51- ☑
    inflammation
      intrauterine O41.12 ☑
    injury or poisoning (conditions in S00-T88) O9A.21- ☑ (*following* O99)
      due to abuse
        physical O9A.31- ☑ (*following* O99)
        psychological O9A.51- ☑ (*following* O99)
        sexual O9A.41- ☑ (*following* O99)
    insufficient
      prenatal care O09.3- ☑
      weight gain O26.1- ☑
    insulin resistance O26.89 ☑
    intrauterine fetal death (near term) O36.4 ☑
      early pregnancy O02.1
      multiple gestation (one fetus or more) O31.2- ☑
    isoimmunization O36.11- ☑
      anti-A sensitization O36.11- ☑
      anti-B sensitization O36.19- ☑
      Rh O36.09- ☑
        anti-D antibody O36.01- ☑
      specified NEC O36.19- ☑
    laceration of uterus NEC O71.81
    malformation
      central nervous system O35.00 ☑
        specified type NEC O35.09 ☑
      placenta, placental (vessel) O43.10- ☑
        specified NEC O43.19- ☑
      uterus (congenital) O34.0- ☑
    malnutrition (conditions in E40-E46) O25.1- ☑
    maternal hypotension syndrome O26.5- ☑
    mental disorders (conditions in F01-F09, F20-F52 and F54-F99) O99.34- ☑
      alcohol use O99.31- ☑
      drug use O99.32- ☑
      smoking O99.33- ☑
    mentum presentation O32.3 ☑
    metabolic disorders O99.28- ☑

Pregnancy — *continued*
  complicated by — *continued*
    missed
      abortion O02.1
      delivery O36.4 ☑
    multiple gestations O30.9- ☑
      conjoined twins O30.02- ☑
      quadruplet — *see* Pregnancy, quadruplet
      specified complication NEC O31.8X- ☑
      specified number of multiples NEC — *see* Pregnancy, multiple (gestation), specified NEC
      triplet — *see* Pregnancy, triplet
      twin — *see* Pregnancy, twin
    musculoskeletal condition (conditions is M00-M99) O99.891
    necrosis, liver (conditions in K72) O26.61- ☑
    neoplasm
      benign
        cervix O34.4- ☑
        corpus uteri O34.1- ☑
        uterus O34.1- ☑
      malignant O9A.11- ☑ (*following* O99)
    nephropathy NEC O26.83- ☑
    nervous system condition (conditions in G00-G99) O99.35- ☑
    nutritional diseases NEC O99.28- ☑
    obesity (pre-existing) O99.21- ☑
    obesity surgery status O99.84- ☑
    oblique lie or presentation O32.2 ☑
    older mother — *see* Pregnancy, complicated by, elderly
    oligohydramnios O41.0- ☑
      with premature rupture of membranes — *see also* Pregnancy, complicated by, premature rupture of membranes O42.- ☑
    onset (spontaneous) of labor after 37 completed weeks of gestation but before 39 completed weeks gestation, with delivery by (planned) cesarean section O75.82
    oophoritis O23.52- ☑
    overdose, drug — *see also* Table of Drugs and Chemicals, by drug, poisoning O9A.21- ☑ (*following* O99)
    oversize fetus O33.5 ☑
    papyraceous fetus O31.0- ☑
    pelvic inflammatory disease O99.891
    periodontal disease O99.61- ☑
    peripheral neuritis O26.82- ☑
    peritoneal (pelvic) adhesions O99.891
    phlebitis O22.9- ☑
    phlebopathy O22.9- ☑
    phlebothrombosis (superficial) O22.2- ☑
      deep O22.3- ☑
    placenta accreta O43.21- ☑
    placenta increta O43.22- ☑
    placenta percreta O43.23- ☑
    placenta previa O44.0- ☑
      complete O44.0- ☑
        with hemorrhage O44.1- ☑
      marginal O44.2- ☑
        with hemorrhage O44.3- ☑
      partial O44.2- ☑
        with hemorrhage O44.3- ☑
    placental disorder O43.9- ☑
      specified NEC O43.89- ☑
    placental dysfunction O43.89- ☑
    placental infarction O43.81- ☑
    placental insufficiency O36.51- ☑
    placental transfusion syndromes
      fetomaternal O43.01- ☑
      fetus to fetus O43.02- ☑
      maternofetal O43.01- ☑
    placentitis O41.14- ☑
    pneumonia O99.51- ☑
    poisoning — *see also* Table of Drugs and Chemicals O9A.21 ☑ (*following* O99)
    polyhydramnios O40- ☑
    polymorphic eruption of pregnancy O26.86
    poor obstetric history NEC O09.29- ☑
    postmaturity (post-term) (40 to 42 weeks) O48.0
      more than 42 completed weeks gestation (prolonged) O48.1
    pre-eclampsia O14.9- ☑
      mild O14.0- ☑
      moderate O14.0- ☑
      severe O14.1- ☑

Index

Pregnancy — *continued*
  complicated by — *continued*
    pre-eclampsia — *continued*
      severe — *continued*
        with hemolysis, elevated liver enzymes and low platelet count (HELLP) O14.2- ☑
    premature labor — *see* Pregnancy, complicated by, preterm labor
    premature rupture of membranes O42.90
      with onset of labor
        within 24 hours O42.00
          at or after 37 weeks gestation, onset of labor within 24 hours of rupture O42.02
          pre-term (before 37 completed weeks of gestation) O42.01- ☑
        after 24 hours O42.10
          at or after 37 weeks gestation, onset of labor more than 24 hours following rupture O42.12
          pre-term (before 37 completed weeks of gestation) O42.11- ☑
      at or after 37 weeks gestation, unspecified as to length of time between rupture and onset of labor O42.92
      full-term, unspecified as to length of time between rupture and onset of labor O42.92
      pre-term (before 37 completed weeks of gestation) O42.91- ☑
    premature separation of placenta — *see also* Abruptio placentae O45.9- ☑
    presentation, fetal — *see* Delivery, complicated by, malposition
    preterm delivery O60.10 ☑
    preterm labor
      with delivery O60.10 ☑
        preterm O60.10 ☑
        term O60.20 ☑
      second trimester
        with term delivery O60.22 ☑
        without delivery O60.02
        with preterm delivery
          second trimester O60.12 ☑
          third trimester O60.13 ☑
      third trimester
        with term delivery O60.23 ☑
        without delivery O60.03
        with third trimester preterm delivery O60.14 ☑
      without delivery O60.00
        second trimester O60.02
        third trimester O60.03
    previous history of — *see* Pregnancy, supervision of, high-risk
    prolapse, uterus O34.52- ☑
    proteinuria (gestational) — *see also* Proteinuria, gestational O12.1- ☑
      with edema O12.2- ☑
    pruritic urticarial papules and plaques of pregnancy (PUPPP) O26.86
    pruritus (neurogenic) O26.89- ☑
    psychosis or psychoneurosis (puerperal) F53.1
    ptyalism O26.89- ☑
    PUPPP (pruritic urticarial papules and plaques of pregnancy) O26.86
    pyelitis O23.0- ☑
    recurrent pregnancy loss O26.2- ☑
    renal disease or failure NEC O26.83- ☑
      with secondary hypertension, pre-existing — *see* Hypertension, complicating, pregnancy, pre-existing, secondary
      hypertensive, pre-existing — *see* Hypertension, complicating, pregnancy, pre-existing, with, renal disease
    respiratory condition (conditions in J00-J99) O99.51- ☑
    retained, retention
      dead ovum O02.0
      intrauterine contraceptive device O26.3- ☑
    retroversion, uterus O34.53- ☑
    Rh immunization, incompatibility or sensitization NEC O36.09- ☑
      anti-D antibody O36.01- ☑
    rupture
      amnion (premature) — *see also* Pregnancy, complicated by, premature rupture of membranes O42- ☑

      membranes (premature) — *see also* Pregnancy, complicated by, premature rupture of membranes O42- ☑
      uterus (during labor) O71.1
        before onset of labor O71.0- ☑
    salivation (excessive) O26.89- ☑
    salpingitis O23.52- ☑
    salpingo-oophoritis O23.52- ☑
    sepsis (conditions in A40, A41) O98.81- ☑
    size date discrepancy (uterine) O26.84- ☑
    skin condition (conditions in L00-L99) O99.71- ☑
    smoking (tobacco) O99.33- ☑
    social problem O09.7- ☑
    specified condition NEC O26.89- ☑
    spotting O26.35- ☑
    streptococcus group B (GBS) carrier state O99.820
    subluxation of symphysis (pubis) O26.71- ☑
    syphilis (conditions in A50-A53) O98.11- ☑
    threatened
      abortion O20.0
      labor O47.9
        at or after 37 completed weeks of gestation O47.1
        before 37 completed weeks of gestation O47.0- ☑
    thrombophlebitis (superficial) O22.2- ☑
    thrombosis O22.9- ☑
      cerebral venous O22.5- ☑
      cerebrovenous sinus O22.5- ☑
      deep O22.3- ☑
    tobacco use disorder (smoking) O99.33- ☑
    torsion of uterus O34.59- ☑
    toxemia O14.9- ☑
    transverse lie or presentation O32.2 ☑
    tuberculosis (conditions in A15-A19) O98.01- ☑
    tumor (benign)
      cervix O34.4- ☑
      malignant O9A.11- ☑ (*following* O99)
      uterus O34.1- ☑
    unstable lie O32.0 ☑
    upper respiratory infection O99.51- ☑
    urethritis O23.2- ☑
    uterine size date discrepancy O26.84- ☑
    vaginitis or vulvitis O23.59- ☑
    varicose veins (lower extremities) O22.0- ☑
      genitals O22.1- ☑
      legs O22.0- ☑
      perineal O22.1- ☑
      vaginal or vulval O22.1- ☑
    venereal disease NEC (conditions in A63.8) O98.31- ☑
    venous disorders O22.9- ☑
      specified NEC O22.8X- ☑
    very young mother — *see* Pregnancy, complicated by, young mother
    viral diseases (conditions in A80-B09, B25-B34) O98.51- ☑
    vomiting O21.9
      due to diseases classified elsewhere O21.8
      hyperemesis gravidarum (mild) — *see also* Hyperemesis, gravidarum O21.0
      late (occurring after 20 weeks of gestation) O21.2
    young mother
      multigravida O09.62- ☑
      primigravida O09.61- ☑
  complicated NOS O26.9- ☑
  concealed O09.3- ☑
  continuing following
    elective fetal reduction of one or more fetus O31.3- ☑
    intrauterine death of one or more fetus O31.2- ☑
    spontaneous abortion of one or more fetus O31.1- ☑
  cornual O00.80
    with intrauterine pregnancy O00.81
  ectopic (ruptured) O00.90
    with intrauterine pregnancy O00.91
    abdominal O00.00
      with
        intrauterine pregnancy O00.01
        viable fetus O36.7- ☑
    cervical O00.80
      with intrauterine pregnancy O00.81
    complicated (by) O08.9
      afibrinogenemia O08.1
      cardiac arrest O08.81

Pregnancy — *continued*
  ectopic — *continued*
    complicated — *continued*
      chemical damage of pelvic organ(s) O08.6
      circulatory collapse O08.3
      defibrination syndrome O08.1
      electrolyte imbalance O08.5
      embolism (amniotic fluid) (blood clot) (pulmonary) (septic) O08.2
      endometritis O08.0
      genital tract and pelvic infection O08.0
      hemorrhage (delayed) (excessive) O08.1
      infection
        genital tract or pelvic O08.0
        kidney O08.83
        urinary tract O08.83
      intravascular coagulation O08.1
      laceration of pelvic organ(s) O08.6
      metabolic disorder O08.5
      oliguria O08.4
      oophoritis O08.0
      parametritis O08.0
      pelvic peritonitis O08.0
      perforation of pelvic organ(s) O08.6
      renal failure or shutdown O08.4
      salpingitis or salpingo-oophoritis O08.0
      sepsis O08.82
      shock O08.83
        septic O08.82
      specified condition NEC O08.89
      tubular necrosis (renal) O08.4
      uremia O08.4
      urinary infection O08.83
      venous complication NEC O08.7
        embolism O08.2
    cornual O00.80
      with intrauterine pregnancy O00.81
    intraligamentous O00.80
      with intrauterine pregnancy O00.81
    mural O00.80
      with intrauterine pregnancy O00.81
    ovarian O00.20-
      with intrauterine pregnancy O00.21- ☑
    specified site NEC O00.80
      with intrauterine pregnancy O00.81
    tubal (ruptured) O00.10-
      with intrauterine pregnancy O00.11- ☑
  examination (normal) Z34.9- ☑
    first Z34.0- ☑
    high-risk — *see* Pregnancy, supervision of, high-risk
    specified Z34.8- ☑
  extrauterine — *see* Pregnancy, ectopic
  fallopian O00.10- ☑
    with intrauterine pregnancy O00.11- ☑
  false F45.8
  gestational carrier Z33.3
  heptachorionic, hepta-amniotic (septuplets) O30.83- ☑
  hexachorionic, hexa-amniotic (sextuplets) O30.83- ☑
  hidden O09.3- ☑
  high-risk — *see* Pregnancy, supervision of, high-risk
  incidental finding Z33.1
  interstitial O00.80
    with intrauterine pregnancy O00.81
  intraligamentous O00.80
    with intrauterine pregnancy O00.81
  intramural O00.80
    with intrauterine pregnancy O00.81
  intraperitoneal O00.00
    with intrauterine pregnancy O00.01
  isthmian O00.10- ☑
    with intrauterine pregnancy O00.11- ☑
  mesometric (mural) O00.80
    with intrauterine pregnancy O00.81
  molar NEC O02.0
    complicated (by) O08.9
      afibrinogenemia O08.1
      cardiac arrest O08.81
      chemical damage of pelvic organ(s) O08.6
      circulatory collapse O08.3
      defibrination syndrome O08.1
      electrolyte imbalance O08.5
      embolism (amniotic fluid) (blood clot) (pulmonary) (septic) O08.2
      endometritis O08.0
      genital tract and pelvic infection O08.0
      hemorrhage (delayed) (excessive) O08.1
      infection
        genital tract or pelvic O08.0

Pregnancy — Pregnancy

☑ **Additional Character Required** — **Refer to the Tabular List for Character Selection**

Index

Pregnancy — Prescription of contraceptives

Pregnancy — *continued*
  molar — *continued*
    complicated — *continued*
      infection — *continued*
        kidney O08.83
        urinary tract O08.83
      intravascular coagulation O08.1
      laceration of pelvic organ(s) O08.6
      metabolic disorder O08.5
      oliguria O08.4
      oophoritis O08.0
      parametritis O08.0
      pelvic peritonitis O08.0
      perforation of pelvic organ(s) O08.6
      renal failure or shutdown O08.4
      salpingitis or salpingo-oophoritis O08.0
      sepsis O08.82
      shock O08.3
        septic O08.82
      specified condition NEC O08.89
      tubular necrosis (renal) O08.4
      uremia O08.4
      urinary infection O08.83
      venous complication NEC O08.7
        embolism O08.2
    hydatidiform — *see also* Mole, hydatidiform O01.9
  multiple (gestation) O30.9- ☑
    greater than quadruplets — *see* Pregnancy, multiple (gestation), specified NEC
    specified NEC O30.80- ☑
      with
        two or more monoamniotic fetuses O30.82- ☑
        two or more monochorionic fetuses O30.81- ☑
        number of chorions and amnions are both equal to the number of fetuses O30.83- ☑
        two or more monoamniotic fetuses O30.82- ☑
        two or more monochorionic fetuses O30.81- ☑
        unable to determine number of placenta and number of amniotic sacs O30.89- ☑
        unspecified number of placenta and unspecified number of amniotic sacs O30.80- ☑
  mural O00.80
    with intrauterine pregnancy O00.81
  normal (supervision of) Z34.9- ☑
    first Z34.0- ☑
    high-risk — *see* Pregnancy, supervision of, high-risk
    specified Z34.8- ☑
  ovarian O00.20- ☑
    with intrauterine pregnancy O00.21- ☑
  pentachorionic, penta-amniotic (quintuplets) O30.83- ☑
  postmature (40 to 42 weeks) O48.0
    more than 42 weeks gestation O48.1
  post-term (40 to 42 weeks) O48.0
  prenatal care only Z34.9- ☑
    first Z34.0- ☑
    high-risk — *see* Pregnancy, supervision of, high-risk
    specified Z34.8- ☑
  prolonged (more than 42 weeks gestation) O48.1
  quadruplet O30.20- ☑
    with
      two or more monoamniotic fetuses O30.22- ☑
      two or more monochorionic fetuses O30.21- ☑
      quadrachorionic/quadra-amniotic O30.23- ☑
      two or more monoamniotic fetuses O30.22- ☑
      two or more monochorionic fetuses O30.21- ☑
      unable to determine number of placenta and number of amniotic sacs O30.29- ☑
      unspecified number of placenta and unspecified number of amniotic sacs O30.20- ☑
  quintuplet — *see* Pregnancy, multiple (gestation), specified NEC
  sextuplet — *see* Pregnancy, multiple (gestation), specified NEC
  supervision of
    concealed pregnancy O09.3- ☑
    elderly mother
      multigravida O09.52- ☑
      primigravida O09.51- ☑
    hidden pregnancy O09.3- ☑
    high-risk O09.9- ☑
      due to (history of)
        ectopic pregnancy O09.1- ☑
        elderly — *see* Pregnancy, supervision, elderly mother
        grand multiparity O09.4 ☑
        in utero procedure during previous pregnancy O09.82- ☑

Pregnancy — *continued*
  supervision of — *continued*
    high-risk — *continued*
      due to — *continued*
        in vitro fertilization O09.81- ☑
        infertility O09.0- ☑
        insufficient prenatal care O09.3- ☑
        molar pregnancy O09.A- ☑
        multiple previous pregnancies O09.4- ☑
        older mother — *see* Pregnancy, supervision of, elderly mother
        poor reproductive or obstetric history NEC O09.29- ☑
        pre-term labor O09.21- ☑
        previous
          neonatal death O09.29- ☑
        social problems O09.7- ☑
        specified NEC O09.89- ☑
        very young mother — *see* Pregnancy, supervision, young mother
      resulting from in vitro fertilization O09.81- ☑
    normal Z34.9- ☑
      first Z34.0- ☑
      specified NEC Z34.8- ☑
    young mother
      multigravida O09.62- ☑
      primigravida O09.61- ☑
  triplet O30.10- ☑
    with
      two or more monoamniotic fetuses O30.12- ☑
      two or more monochorionic fetuses O30.11- ☑
      trichorionic/triamniotic O30.13- ☑
      two or more monoamniotic fetuses O30.12- ☑
      two or more monochorionic fetuses O30.11- ☑
      unable to determine number of placenta and number of amniotic sacs O30.19- ☑
      unspecified number of placenta and unspecified number of amniotic sacs O30.10- ☑
  tubal (with abortion) (with rupture) O00.10- ☑
    with intrauterine pregnancy O00.11- ☑
  twin O30.00- ☑
    conjoined O30.02- ☑
    dichorionic/diamniotic (two placenta, two amniotic sacs) O30.04- ☑
    monochorionic/diamniotic (one placenta, two amniotic sacs) O30.03- ☑
    monochorionic/monoamniotic (one placenta, one amniotic sac) O30.01- ☑
    unable to determine number of placenta and number of amniotic sacs O30.09- ☑
    unspecified number of placenta and unspecified number of amniotic sacs O30.00- ☑
  unwanted Z64.0
  weeks of gestation
    8 weeks Z3A.08 (*following* Z36)
    9 weeks Z3A.09 (*following* Z36)
    10 weeks Z3A.10 (*following* Z36)
    11 weeks Z3A.11 (*following* Z36)
    12 weeks Z3A.12 (*following* Z36)
    13 weeks Z3A.13 (*following* Z36)
    14 weeks Z3A.14 (*following* Z36)
    15 weeks Z3A.15 (*following* Z36)
    16 weeks Z3A.16 (*following* Z36)
    17 weeks Z3A.17 (*following* Z36)
    18 weeks Z3A.18 (*following* Z36)
    19 weeks Z3A.19 (*following* Z36)
    20 weeks Z3A.20 (*following* Z36)
    21 weeks Z3A.21 (*following* Z36)
    22 weeks Z3A.22 (*following* Z36)
    23 weeks Z3A.23 (*following* Z36)
    24 weeks Z3A.24 (*following* Z36)
    25 weeks Z3A.25 (*following* Z36)
    26 weeks Z3A.26 (*following* Z36)
    27 weeks Z3A.27 (*following* Z36)
    28 weeks Z3A.28 (*following* Z36)
    29 weeks Z3A.29 (*following* Z36)
    30 weeks Z3A.30 (*following* Z36)
    31 weeks Z3A.31 (*following* Z36)
    32 weeks Z3A.32 (*following* Z36)
    33 weeks Z3A.33 (*following* Z36)
    34 weeks Z3A.34 (*following* Z36)
    35 weeks Z3A.35 (*following* Z36)
    36 weeks Z3A.36 (*following* Z36)
    37 weeks Z3A.37 (*following* Z36)
    38 weeks Z3A.38 (*following* Z36)
    39 weeks Z3A.39 (*following* Z36)
    40 weeks Z3A.40 (*following* Z36)

Pregnancy — *continued*
  weeks of gestation — *continued*
    41 weeks Z3A.41 (*following* Z36)
    42 weeks Z3A.42 (*following* Z36)
    greater than 42 weeks Z3A.49 (*following* Z36)
    less than 8 weeks Z3A.01 (*following* Z36)
    not specified Z3A.00 (*following* Z36)
Preiser's disease — *see* Osteonecrosis, secondary, due to, trauma, metacarpus
Pre-kwashiorkor — *see* Malnutrition, severe
Preleukemia (syndrome) D46.9
Preluxation, hip, congenital Q65.6
Premature — *see also* condition
  adrenarche E27.0
  aging E34.8
  beats I49.40
    atrial I49.1
    auricular I49.1
    supraventricular I49.1
  birth NEC — *see* Preterm, newborn
  closure, foramen ovale Q21.8
  contraction
    atrial I49.1
    atrioventricular I49.2
    auricular I49.1
    auriculoventricular I49.49
    heart (extrasystole) I49.49
    junctional I49.2
    ventricular I49.3
  delivery — *see also* Pregnancy, complicated by, preterm labor O60.10 ☑
  ejaculation F52.4
  infant NEC — *see* Preterm, newborn
    light-for-dates — *see* Light for dates
  labor — *see* Pregnancy, complicated by, preterm labor
  lungs P28.0
  menopause E28.319
    asymptomatic E28.319
    symptomatic E28.310
  newborn
    extreme (less than 28 completed weeks) — *see* Immaturity, extreme
    less than 37 completed weeks — *see* Preterm, newborn
  puberty E30.1
  rupture membranes or amnion — *see* Pregnancy, complicated by, premature rupture of membranes
  senility E34.8
  thelarche E30.8
  ventricular systole I49.3
Prematurity NEC (less than 37 completed weeks) — *see* Preterm, newborn
  extreme (less than 28 completed weeks) — *see* Immaturity, extreme
Premenstrual
  dysphoric disorder (PMDD) F32.81
  tension (syndrome) N94.3
Premolarization, cuspids K00.2
Prenatal
  care, normal pregnancy — *see* Pregnancy, normal
  screening of mother — *see also* Encounter, antenatal screening Z36.9
  teeth K00.6
Preparatory care for subsequent treatment NEC
  for dialysis Z49.01
    peritoneal Z49.02
Prepartum — *see* condition
Preponderance, left or right ventricular I51.7
Prepuce — *see* condition
PRES (posterior reversible encephalopathy syndrome) I67.83
Presbycardia R54
Presbycusis, presbyacusia H91.1- ☑
Presbyesophagus K22.89
Presbyophrenia F03 ☑
Presbyopia H52.4
Prescription of contraceptives (initial) Z30.019
  barrier Z30.018
  diaphragm Z30.018
  emergency (postcoital) Z30.012
  implantable subdermal Z30.017
  injectable Z30.013
  intrauterine contraceptive device Z30.014
  pills Z30.011
  postcoital (emergency) Z30.012
  repeat Z30.40
    barrier Z30.49
    diaphragm Z30.49
    implantable subdermal Z30.46
    injectable Z30.42

☑ **Additional Character Required** — **Refer to the Tabular List for Character Selection**

Prescription of contraceptives — *continued*
  repeat — *continued*
    pills Z30.41
    specified type NEC Z30.49
    transdermal patch hormonal Z30.45
    vaginal ring hormonal Z30.44
  specified type NEC Z30.018
    transdermal patch hormonal Z30.016
    vaginal ring hormonal Z30.015
Presence (of)
  ankle-joint implant (functional) (prosthesis) Z96.66- ☑
  aortocoronary (bypass) graft Z95.1
  arterial-venous shunt (dialysis) Z99.2
  artificial
    eye (globe) Z97.0
    heart (fully implantable) (mechanical) Z95.812
      valve Z95.2
    larynx Z96.3
    lens (intraocular) Z96.1
    limb (complete) (partial) Z97.1- ☑
      arm Z97.1- ☑
        bilateral Z97.15
      leg Z97.1- ☑
        bilateral Z97.16
  audiological implant (functional) Z96.29
  bladder implant (functional) Z96.0
  bone
    conduction hearing device Z96.29
    implant (functional) NEC Z96.7
    joint (prosthesis) — *see* Presence, joint implant
  cardiac
    defibrillator (functional) (with synchronous cardiac
      pacemaker) Z95.810
    implant or graft Z95.9
      specified type NEC Z95.818
    pacemaker Z95.0
    resynchronization therapy
      defibrillator Z95.810
      pacemaker Z95.0
  cardioverter-defibrillator (ICD) Z95.810
  cerebrospinal fluid drainage device Z98.2
  cochlear implant (functional) Z96.21
  contact lens (es) Z97.3
  coronary artery graft or prosthesis Z95.5
  CRT-D (cardiac resynchronization therapy defibrillator)
    Z95.810
  CRT-P (cardiac resynchronization therapy pacemaker)
    Z95.0
  CSF shunt Z98.2
  dental prosthesis device Z97.2
  dentures Z97.2
  device (external) NEC Z97.8
    cardiac NEC Z95.818
    heart assist Z95.811
    implanted (functional) Z96.9
      specified NEC Z96.89
    prosthetic Z97.8
  ear implant Z96.20
    cochlear implant Z96.21
    myringotomy tube Z96.22
    specified type NEC Z96.29
  elbow-joint implant (functional) (prosthesis) Z96.62- ☑
  endocrine implant (functional) NEC Z96.49
  eustachian tube stent or device (functional) Z96.29
  external hearing-aid or device Z97.4
  finger-joint implant (functional) (prosthetic) Z96.69- ☑
  functional implant Z96.9
    specified NEC Z96.89
  graft
    cardiac NEC Z95.818
    vascular NEC Z95.828
  hearing-aid or device (external) Z97.4
    implant (bone) (cochlear) (functional) Z96.21
  heart assist device Z95.811
  heart valve implant (functional) Z95.2
    prosthetic Z95.2
    specified type NEC Z95.4
    xenogenic Z95.3
  hip-joint implant (functional) (prosthesis) Z96.64- ☑
  ICD (cardioverter-defibrillator) Z95.810
  implanted device (artificial) (functional) (prosthetic) Z96.9
    automatic cardiac defibrillator (with synchronous
      cardiac pacemaker) Z95.810
    cardiac pacemaker Z95.0
    cochlear Z96.21
    dental Z96.5
    heart Z95.812
    heart valve Z95.2

Presence — *continued*
  implanted device — *continued*
    heart valve — *continued*
      prosthetic Z95.2
      specified NEC Z95.4
      xenogenic Z95.3
    insulin pump Z96.41
    intraocular lens Z96.1
    joint Z96.60
      ankle Z96.66- ☑
      elbow Z96.62- ☑
      finger Z96.69- ☑
      hip Z96.64- ☑
      knee Z96.65- ☑
      shoulder Z96.61- ☑
      specified NEC Z96.698
      wrist Z96.63- ☑
    larynx Z96.3
    myringotomy tube Z96.22
    otological Z96.20
      cochlear Z96.21
      eustachian stent Z96.29
      myringotomy Z96.22
      specified NEC Z96.29
      stapes Z96.29
    skin Z96.81
    skull plate Z96.7
    specified NEC Z96.89
    urogenital Z96.0
  insulin pump (functional) Z96.41
  intestinal bypass or anastomosis Z98.0
  intraocular lens (functional) Z96.1
  intrauterine contraceptive device (IUD) Z97.5
  intravascular implant (functional) (prosthetic) NEC Z95.9
    coronary artery Z95.5
    defibrillator (with synchronous cardiac pacemaker)
      Z95.810
    peripheral vessel (with angioplasty) Z95.820
  joint implant (prosthetic) (any) Z96.60
    ankle — *see* Presence, ankle joint implant
    elbow — *see* Presence, elbow joint implant
    finger — *see* Presence, finger joint implant
    hip — *see* Presence, hip joint implant
    knee — *see* Presence, knee joint implant
    shoulder — *see* Presence, shoulder joint implant
    specified joint NEC Z96.698
    wrist — *see* Presence, wrist joint implant
  knee-joint implant (functional) (prosthesis) Z96.65- ☑
  laryngeal implant (functional) Z96.3
  mandibular implant (dental) Z96.5
  myringotomy tube(s) Z96.22
  neurostimulator (brain) (gastric) (peripheral nerve) (sacral
    nerve) (spinal cord) (vagus nerve) Z96.82
  orthopedic-joint implant (prosthetic) (any) — *see* Pres-
    ence, joint implant
  otological implant (functional) Z96.29
  shoulder-joint implant (functional) (prosthesis)
    Z96.61- ☑
  skull-plate implant Z96.7
  spectacles Z97.3
  stapes implant (functional) Z96.29
  systemic lupus erythematosus [SLE] inhibitor D68.62
  tendon implant (functional) (graft) Z96.7
  tooth root(s) implant Z96.5
  ureteral stent Z96.0
  urethral stent Z96.0
  urogenital implant (functional) Z96.0
  vascular implant or device Z95.9
    access port device Z95.828
    specified type NEC Z95.828
  wrist-joint implant (functional) (prosthesis) Z96.63- ☑
Presenile — *see also* condition
  dementia F03 ☑
  premature aging E34.8
Presentation, fetal — *see* Delivery, complicated by, malposition
Prespondylolisthesis (congenital) Q76.2
Pressure
  area, skin — *see* Ulcer, pressure, by site
  brachial plexus G54.0
  brain G93.5
    injury at birth NEC P11.1
  cerebral — *see* Pressure, brain
  chest R07.89
  cone, tentorial G93.5
  hyposystolic — *see also* Hypotension
    incidental reading, without diagnosis of hypotension
      R03.1

Pressure — *continued*
  increased
    intracranial benign G93.2
      injury at birth P11.0
    intraocular H40.05- ☑
  injury — *see* Ulcer, pressure, by site
  lumbosacral plexus G54.1
  mediastinum J98.59
  necrosis (chronic) — *see* Ulcer, pressure, by site
  parental, inappropriate (excessive) Z62.6
  sore (chronic) — *see* Ulcer, pressure, by site
  spinal cord G95.20
  ulcer (chronic) — *see* Ulcer, pressure, by site
  venous, increased I87.8
Pre-syncope R55
Preterm
  delivery — *see also* Pregnancy, complicated by, preterm
    labor O60.10 ☑
  labor — *see* Pregnancy, complicated by, preterm labor
  newborn (infant) P07.30
    gestational age
      28 completed weeks (28 weeks, 0 days through
        28 weeks, 6 days) P07.31
      29 completed weeks (29 weeks, 0 days through
        29 weeks, 6 days) P07.32
      30 completed weeks (30 weeks, 0 days through
        30 weeks, 6 days) P07.33
      31 completed weeks (31 weeks, 0 days through
        31 weeks, 6 days) P07.34
      32 completed weeks (32 weeks, 0 days through
        32 weeks, 6 days) P07.35
      33 completed weeks (33 weeks, 0 days through
        33 weeks, 6 days) P07.36
      34 completed weeks (34 weeks, 0 days through
        34 weeks, 6 days) P07.37
      35 completed weeks (35 weeks, 0 days through
        35 weeks, 6 days) P07.38
      36 completed weeks (36 weeks, 0 days through
        36 weeks, 6 days) P07.39
Previa
  placenta (total) (without hemorrhage) O44.0- ☑
    with hemorrhage O44.1- ☑
    complete O44.0- ☑
      with hemorrhage O44.1- ☑
    low — *see also* Delivery, complicated, by, placenta,
      low O44.4- ☑
      with hemorrhage O44.5- ☑
    marginal O44.2- ☑
      with hemorrhage O44.3- ☑
    partial O44.2- ☑
      with hemorrhage O44.3- ☑
  vasa O69.4 ☑
Priapism N48.30
  due to
    disease classified elsewhere N48.32
    drug N48.33
    specified cause NEC N48.39
    trauma N48.31
Prickling sensation (skin) R20.2
Prickly heat L74.0
Primary — *see* condition
Primigravida
  elderly, affecting management of pregnancy, labor and
    delivery (supervision only) — *see* Pregnancy,
    complicated by, elderly, primigravida
  older, affecting management of pregnancy, labor and
    delivery (supervision only) — *see* Pregnancy,
    complicated by, elderly, primigravida
  very young, affecting management of pregnancy, labor
    and delivery (supervision only) — *see* Pregnancy,
    complicated by, young mother, primigravida
Primipara
  elderly, affecting management of pregnancy, labor and
    delivery (supervision only) — *see* Pregnancy,
    complicated by, elderly, primigravida
  older, affecting management of pregnancy, labor and
    delivery (supervision only) — *see* Pregnancy,
    complicated by, elderly, primigravida
  very young, affecting management of pregnancy, labor
    and delivery (supervision only) — *see* Pregnancy,
    complicated by, young mother, primigravida
Primus varus Q66.21- ☑
PRIND (Prolonged reversible ischemic neurologic deficit)
  I63.9
Pringle's disease (tuberous sclerosis) Q85.1
Prinzmetal angina I20.1
Prizefighter ear — *see* Cauliflower ear

Problem (with) (related to)
academic Z55.8
acculturation Z60.3
adjustment (to)
  change of job Z56.1
  life-cycle transition Z60.0
  pension Z60.0
  retirement Z60.0
adopted child Z62.821
alcoholism in family Z63.72
atypical parenting situation Z62.9
bankruptcy Z59.89
behavioral (adult) F69
  drug seeking Z76.5
birth of sibling affecting child Z62.898
care (of)
  provider dependency Z74.9
    specified NEC Z74.8
  sick or handicapped person in family or household
    Z63.6
child
  abuse (affecting the child) — see Maltreatment, child
  custody or support proceedings Z65.3
  in
    care of non-parental family member Z62.23
    custody of
      grandparent Z62.23
      non-parental relative Z62.23
      non-relative guardian Z62.24
    foster care Z62.21
    kinship care Z62.23
    welfare
      custody Z62.21
      guardianship Z62.21
  leaving living situation without permission Z62.892
  living in
    group home Z62.22
    orphanage Z62.22
child-rearing Z62.9
  specified NEC Z62.898
communication (developmental) F80.9
completing medical forms Z55.6
conflict or discord (with)
  boss Z56.4
  classmates Z55.4
  counselor Z64.4
  employer Z56.4
  family Z63.9
    specified NEC Z63.8
  probation officer Z64.4
  social worker Z64.4
  teachers Z55.4
  workmates Z56.4
conviction in legal proceedings Z65.0
  with imprisonment Z65.1
counselor Z64.4
creditors Z59.89
digestive K92.9
drug addict in family Z63.72
ear — see Disorder, ear
economic Z59.9
  affecting care Z59.9
  specified NEC Z59.89
  strain Z59.86
education Z55.9
  specified NEC Z55.8
employment Z56.9
  change of job Z56.1
  discord Z56.4
  environment Z56.5
  sexual harassment Z56.81
  specified NEC Z56.89
  stressful schedule Z56.3
  stress NEC Z56.6
  threat of job loss Z56.2
  unemployment Z56.0
enuresis, child F98.0
eye H57.9
failed examinations (school) Z55.2
falling Z91.81
family — see also Disruption, family Z63.9
  specified NEC Z63.8
feeding (elderly) (infant) NOS R63.39
  newborn P92.9
    breast P92.5
    overfeeding P92.4
    slow P92.2
    specified NEC P92.8
    underfeeding P92.3

Problem — continued
feeding — continued
  nonorganic F50.89
finance Z59.9
  specified NEC Z59.89
foreclosure on loan Z59.89
foster child Z62.822
frightening experience(s) in childhood Z62.898
genital NEC
  female N94.9
  male N50.9
health care Z75.9
  specified NEC Z75.8
health literacy Z55.6
hearing — see Deafness
homelessness Z59.00
housing Z59.9
  inadequate Z59.10
  isolated Z59.89
  specified NEC Z59.89
identity (of childhood) F93.8
illegitimate pregnancy (unwanted) Z64.0
illiteracy Z55.0
impaired mobility Z74.09
imprisonment or incarceration Z65.1
inadequate teaching affecting education Z55.8
inappropriate (excessive) parental pressure Z62.6
influencing health status NEC Z78.9
in-law Z63.1
institutionalization, affecting child Z62.22
intrafamilial communication Z63.8
jealousy, child F93.8
landlord Z59.2
language (developmental) F80.9
learning (developmental) F81.9
legal Z65.3
  conviction without imprisonment Z65.0
  imprisonment Z65.1
  release from prison Z65.2
life-management Z73.9
  specified NEC Z73.89
life-style Z72.9
  gambling Z72.6
  high-risk sexual behavior (heterosexual) Z72.51
    bisexual Z72.53
    homosexual Z72.52
  inappropriate eating habits Z72.4
  self-damaging behavior NEC Z72.89
  specified NEC Z72.89
  tobacco use Z72.0
literacy Z55.9
  low level Z55.0
  specified NEC Z55.8
living alone Z60.2
lodgers Z59.2
loss of love relationship in childhood Z62.898
marital Z63.0
  involving
    divorce Z63.5
    estrangement Z63.5
    gender identity F66
mastication K08.89
medical
  care, within family Z63.6
  facilities Z75.9
    specified NEC Z75.8
mental F48.9
money Z59.86
multiparity Z64.1
negative life events in childhood Z62.9
  altered pattern of family relationships Z62.898
  frightening experience Z62.898
  loss of
    love relationship Z62.898
    self-esteem Z62.898
  physical abuse (alleged) — see Maltreatment, child
  removal from home Z62.29
  specified event NEC Z62.898
neighbor Z59.2
neurological NEC R29.818
new step-parent affecting child Z62.898
none (feared complaint unfounded) Z71.1
occupational NEC Z56.89
parent-child — see Conflict, parent-child
personal hygiene Z91.89
personality F69
phase-of-life transition, adjustment Z60.0
presence of sick or disabled person in family or household
  Z63.79

Problem — continued
presence of sick or disabled person in family or household
  — continued
  needing care Z63.6
primary support group (family) Z63.9
  specified NEC Z63.8
probation officer Z64.4
psychiatric F99
psychosexual (development) F66
psychosocial Z65.9
  religious or spiritual Z65.8
  specified NEC Z65.8
related to physical environment, specified NEC Z58.89
relationship Z63.9
  childhood F93.8
release from prison Z65.2
  religious or spiritual Z65.8
removal from home affecting child Z62.29
seeking and accepting known hazardous and harmful
  behavioral or psychological interventions Z65.8
  chemical, nutritional or physical interventions Z65.8
sexual function (nonorganic) F52.9
sight H54.7
sleep disorder, child F51.9
smell — see Disturbance, sensation, smell
social
  environment Z60.9
    specified NEC Z60.8
  exclusion and rejection Z60.4
  worker Z64.4
speech R47.9
  developmental F80.9
  specified NEC R47.89
swallowing — see Dysphagia
taste — see Disturbance, sensation, taste
tic, child F95.0
underachievement in school Z55.3
unemployment Z56.0
  threatened Z56.2
unwanted pregnancy Z64.0
upbringing Z62.9
  specified NEC Z62.898
urinary N39.9
voice production R47.89
work schedule (stressful) Z56.3
Procedure (surgical)
converted
  arthroscopic to open Z53.33
  laparoscopic to open Z53.31
  specified procedure NEC to open Z53.39
  thoracoscopic to open Z53.32
for purpose other than remedying health state Z41.9
  specified NEC Z41.8
not done Z53.9
  because of
    administrative reasons Z53.8
    contraindication Z53.09
      smoking Z53.01
    patient's decision Z53.20
      for reasons of belief or group pressure Z53.1
      left against medical advice (AMA) Z53.29
      left without being seen Z53.21
      specified reason NEC Z53.29
    specified reason NEC Z53.8
Procidentia (uteri) N81.3
Proctalgia K62.89
  fugax K59.4
  spasmodic K59.4
Proctitis K62.89
  amebic (acute) A06.0
  chlamydia A56.3
  gonococcal A54.6
  granulomatous — see Enteritis, regional, large intestine
  herpetic A60.1
  radiation K62.7
  tuberculous A18.32
  ulcerative (chronic) K51.20
    with
      complication K51.219
        abscess K51.214
        fistula K51.213
        obstruction K51.212
        rectal bleeding K51.211
        specified NEC K51.218
Proctocele
  female (without uterine prolapse) N81.6
    with uterine prolapse N81.2
      complete N81.3
  male K62.3

☑ **Additional Character Required — Refer to the Tabular List for Character Selection**

Proctocolitis
  allergic K52.29
  food protein-induced K52.29
  food-induced eosinophilic K52.29
  milk protein-induced K52.29
  mucosal — see Rectosigmoiditis, ulcerative
Proctoptosis K62.3
Proctorrhagia K62.5
Proctosigmoiditis K63.89
  ulcerative (chronic) — see Rectosigmoiditis, ulcerative
Proctospasm K59.4
  psychogenic F45.8
Profichet's disease — see Disorder, soft tissue, specified
    type NEC
Progeria E34.8
Prognathism (mandibular) (maxillary) M26.19
Progonoma (melanotic) — see Neoplasm, benign, by site
Progressive — see condition
Prolactinoma
  specified site — see Neoplasm, benign, by site
  unspecified site D35.2
Prolapse, prolapsed
  anus, anal (canal) (sphincter) K62.2
  arm or hand O32.2 ☑
    causing obstructed labor O64.4 ☑
  bladder (mucosa) (sphincter) (acquired)
    congenital Q79.4
    female — see Cystocele
    male N32.89
  breast implant (prosthetic) T85.49 ☑
  cecostomy K94.09
  cecum K63.4
  cervix, cervical (hypertrophied) N81.2
    anterior lip, obstructing labor O65.5
    congenital Q51.828
    postpartal, old N81.2
    stump N81.85
  ciliary body (traumatic) — see Laceration, eye(ball), with
      prolapse or loss of interocular tissue
  colon (pedunculated) K63.4
  colostomy K94.09
  disc (intervertebral) — see Displacement, intervertebral
      disc
  eye implant (orbital) T85.398 ☑
    lens (ocular) — see Complications, intraocular lens
  fallopian tube N83.4- ☑
  gastric (mucosa) K31.89
  genital, female N81.9
    specified NEC N81.89
  globe, nontraumatic — see Luxation, globe
  ileostomy bud K94.19
  intervertebral disc — see Displacement, intervertebral
      disc
  intestine (small) K63.4
  iris (traumatic) — see Laceration, eye(ball), with prolapse
      or loss of interocular tissue
    nontraumatic H21.89
  kidney N28.83
    congenital Q63.2
  laryngeal muscles or ventricle J38.7
  liver K76.89
  meatus urinarius N36.8
  mitral (valve) I34.1
  ocular lens implant — see Complications, intraocular
      lens
  organ or site, congenital NEC — see Malposition, congen-
      ital
  ovary N83.4- ☑
  pelvic floor, female N81.89
  perineum, female N81.89
  rectum (mucosa) (sphincter) K62.3
    due to trichuris trichuria B79
  spleen D73.89
  stomach K31.89
  umbilical cord
    complicating delivery O69.0 ☑
  urachus, congenital Q64.4
  ureter N28.89
    with obstruction N13.5
      with infection N13.6
  ureterovesical orifice N28.89
  urethra (acquired) (infected) (mucosa) N36.8
    congenital Q64.71
  urinary meatus N36.8
    congenital Q64.72
  uterovaginal N81.4
    complete N81.3
    incomplete N81.2

Prolapse, prolapsed — continued
  uterus (with prolapse of vagina) N81.4
    complete N81.3
    congenital Q51.818
    first degree N81.2
    in pregnancy or childbirth — see Pregnancy, compli-
        cated by, abnormal, uterus
    incomplete N81.2
    postpartal (old) N81.4
    second degree N81.2
    third degree N81.3
  uveal (traumatic) — see Laceration, eye(ball), with pro-
      lapse or loss of interocular tissue
  vagina (anterior) (wall) — see Cystocele
    with prolapse of uterus N81.4
      complete N81.3
      incomplete N81.2
    posterior wall N81.6
    posthysterectomy N99.3
  vitreous (humor) H43.0- ☑
    in wound — see Laceration, eye(ball), with prolapse
        or loss of interocular tissue
  womb — see Prolapse, uterus
Prolapsus, female N81.9
  specified NEC N81.89
Proliferation(s)
  primary cutaneous CD30-positive large T-cell C86.6- ☑
  prostate, atypical small acinar N42.32
Proliferative — see condition
Prolonged, prolongation (of)
  bleeding (time) (idiopathic) R79.1
  coagulation (time) R79.1
  gestation (over 42 completed weeks)
    mother O48.1
    newborn P08.22
  interval I44.0
  labor O63.9
    first stage O63.0
    second stage O63.1
  partial thromboplastin time (PTT) R79.1
  pregnancy (more than 42 weeks gestation) O48.1
  prothrombin time R79.1
  QT interval R94.31
  uterine contractions in labor O62.4
Prominence, prominent
  auricle (congenital) (ear) Q17.5
  ischial spine or sacral promontory with disproportion
      (fetopelvic) O33.0
    causing obstructed labor O65.0
  nose (congenital) acquired M95.0
Promiscuity — see High, risk, sexual behavior
Pronation
  ankle — see Deformity, limb, foot, specified NEC
  foot — see also Deformity, limb, foot, specified NEC
    congenital Q74.2
Prophylactic
  administration of
    antibiotics, long-term Z79.2
      short-term use — omit code
    drug — see also Long-term (current) drug therapy
        (use of) Z79.899
  medication Z79.899
  organ removal (for neoplasia management) Z40.00
    breast Z40.01
    fallopian tube(s) Z40.03
      with ovary(s) Z40.02
    ovary(s) Z40.02
    specified site NEC Z40.09
  surgery Z40.9
    for risk factors related to malignant neoplasm — see
        Prophylactic, organ removal
    specified NEC Z40.8
  vaccination Z23
Propionic acidemia E71.121
Proptosis (ocular) — see also Exophthalmos
  thyroid — see Hyperthyroidism, with goiter
Prosecution, anxiety concerning Z65.3
Prosopagnosia R48.3
Prostadynia N42.81
Prostate, prostatic — see condition
Prostatism — see Hyperplasia, prostate
Prostatitis (congestive) (suppurative) (with cystitis) N41.9
  acute N41.0
  cavitary N41.8
  chronic N41.1
  diverticular N41.8
  due to Trichomonas (vaginalis) A59.02
  fibrous N41.1
  gonococcal (acute) (chronic) A54.22

Prostatitis — continued
  granulomatous N41.4
  hypertrophic N41.1
  subacute N41.1
  trichomonal A59.02
  tuberculous A18.14
Prostatocystitis N41.3
Prostatorrhea N42.89
Prostatosis N42.82
Prostration R53.83
  heat — see also Heat, exhaustion
    anhydrotic T67.3 ☑
    due to
      salt (and water) depletion T67.4 ☑
      water depletion T67.3 ☑
  nervous F48.8
  senile R54
Protanomaly (anomalous trichromat) H53.54
Protanopia (complete) (incomplete) H53.54
Protection (against) (from) — see Prophylactic
Protein
  deficiency NEC — see Malnutrition
  malnutrition — see Malnutrition
  sickness — see also Reaction, serum T80.69 ☑
Proteinemia R77.9
Proteinosis
  alveolar (pulmonary) J84.01
  lipid or lipoid (of Urbach) E78.89
Proteinuria R80.9
  Bence Jones R80.3
  complicating pregnancy — see Proteinuria, gestational
  gestational
    complicating
      childbirth O12.14
      pregnancy O12.1- ☑
        with edema O12.2- ☑
      puerperium O12.15
  idiopathic R80.0
  isolated R80.0
    with glomerular lesion N06.9
      C3
        glomerulonephritis N06.A
        glomerulopathy N06.A
          with dense deposit disease N06.6
      dense deposit disease N06.6
      diffuse
        crescentic glomerulonephritis N06.7
        endocapillary proliferative glomerulonephritis
            N06.4
        mesangiocapillary glomerulonephritis N06.5
      focal and segmental hyalinosis or sclerosis N06.1
      membranous (diffuse) — see also Nephropathy,
          membranous N06.20
        with diffuse membranous glomerulonephritis
            N06.29
      mesangial proliferative (diffuse) N06.3
      minimal change N06.0
      specified pathology NEC N06.8
  orthostatic R80.2
    with glomerular lesion — see Proteinuria, isolated,
        with glomerular lesion
  persistent R80.1
    with glomerular lesion — see Proteinuria, isolated,
        with glomerular lesion
  postural R80.2
    with glomerular lesion — see Proteinuria, isolated,
        with glomerular lesion
  pre-eclamptic — see Pre-eclampsia
  puerperal O12.15
  specified type NEC R80.8
Proteolysis, pathologic D65
Proteus (mirabilis) (morganii), **as cause of disease classi-
    fied elsewhere** B96.4
Prothrombin gene mutation D68.52
Protoporphyria, erythropoietic E80.0
Protozoal — see also condition
  disease B64
  specified NEC B60.8
Protrusion, protrusio
  acetabuli M24.7
  acetabulum (into pelvis) M24.7
  device, implant or graft — see also Complications, by site
      and type, mechanical T85.698 ☑
    arterial graft NEC — see Complication, cardiovascular
        device, mechanical, vascular
    breast (implant) T85.49 ☑
    catheter NEC T85.698 ☑
      cystostomy T83.090 ☑

Protrusion, protrusio — continued
device, implant or graft — see also Complications, by site and type, mechanical — continued
catheter — continued
dialysis (renal) T82.49 ☑
intraperitoneal T85.691 ☑
infusion NEC T82.594 ☑
spinal (epidural) (subdural) T85.690 ☑
urinary — see also Complications, catheter, urinary T83.098 ☑
electronic (electrode) (pulse generator) (stimulator) bone T84.390 ☑
nervous system — see Complication, prosthetic device, mechanical, electronic nervous system stimulator
fixation, internal (orthopedic) NEC — see Complication, fixation device, mechanical
gastrointestinal — see Complications, prosthetic device, mechanical, gastrointestinal device
genital NEC T83.498 ☑
intrauterine contraceptive device T83.39 ☑
penile prosthesis (cylinder) (implanted) (pump) (reservoir) T83.490 ☑
testicular prosthesis T83.491 ☑
heart NEC — see Complication, cardiovascular device, mechanical
joint prosthesis — see Complications, joint prosthesis, mechanical, specified NEC, by site
ocular NEC — see Complications, prosthetic device, mechanical, ocular device
orthopedic NEC — see Complication, orthopedic, device, mechanical
specified NEC T85.628 ☑
urinary NEC — see also Complication, genitourinary, device, urinary, mechanical
graft T83.29 ☑
vascular NEC — see Complication, cardiovascular device, mechanical
ventricular intracranial shunt T85.09 ☑
intervertebral disc — see Displacement, intervertebral disc
joint prosthesis — see Complications, joint prosthesis, mechanical, specified NEC, by site
nucleus pulposus — see Displacement, intervertebral disc
Prune belly (syndrome) Q79.4
Prurigo (ferox) (gravis) (Hebrae) (Hebra's) (mitis) (simplex) L28.2
Besnier's L20.0
estivalis L56.4
nodularis L28.1
psychogenic F45.8
Pruritus, pruritic (essential) L29.9
ani, anus L29.0
psychogenic F45.8
anogenital L29.3
psychogenic F45.8
cholestatic L29.81
due to onchocerca volvulus B73.1
gravidarum — see Pregnancy, complicated by, specified pregnancy-related condition NEC
hiemalis L29.89
neurogenic (any site) F45.8
perianal L29.0
psychogenic (any site) F45.8
scroti, scrotum L29.1
psychogenic F45.8
senile, senilis L29.89
specified NEC L29.89
psychogenic F45.8
Trichomonas A59.9
vulva, vulvae L29.2
psychogenic F45.8
Pseudarthrosis, pseudoarthrosis (bone) — see Nonunion, fracture
clavicle, congenital Q74.0
joint, following fusion or arthrodesis M96.0
Pseudoaneurysm — see Aneurysm
Pseudoangina (pectoris) — see Angina
Pseudoangioma I81
Pseudoarteriosus Q28.8
Pseudoarthrosis — see Pseudarthrosis
Pseudobulbar affect (PBA) F48.2
Pseudochromhidrosis L67.8
Pseudocirrhosis, liver, pericardial I31.1
Pseudocowpox B08.03
Pseudocoxalgia M91.3- ☑
Pseudocroup J38.5

Pseudo-Cushing's syndrome, alcohol-induced E24.4
Pseudocyesis F45.8
Pseudocyst
lung J98.4
pancreas K86.3
retina — see Cyst, retina
Pseudoelephantiasis neuroarthritica Q82.0
Pseudoexfoliation, capsule (lens) — see Cataract, specified NEC
Pseudofolliculitis barbae L73.1
Pseudoglioma H44.89
Pseudohemophilia (Bernuth's) (hereditary) (type B) — see Disease, von Willebrand
Type A D69.8
vascular D69.8
Pseudohermaphroditism Q56.3
adrenal E25.8
female — see also Disorder, adrenogenital Q56.2
with adrenocortical disorder E25.8
without adrenocortical disorder Q56.2
adrenal (congenital) E25.0
male — see also Disorder, adrenogenital Q56.1
with
5-alpha-reductase deficiency E29.1
adrenocortical disorder E25.8
androgen resistance E34.51
cleft scrotum Q56.1
feminizing testis E34.51
without gonadal disorder Q56.1
adrenal E25.8
Pseudo-Hurler's polydystrophy E77.0
Pseudohydrocephalus G93.2
Pseudohypertrophic muscular dystrophy (Erb's) G71.02
Pseudohypertrophy, muscle — see also Dystrophy, muscular, by type, if applicable G71.09
Pseudohypoparathyroidism E20.1
Pseudoinsomnia F51.03
Pseudoleukemia, infantile D64.89
Pseudomembranous — see condition
Pseudomeningocele (cerebral) (infective) (post-traumatic) G96.198
postprocedural (spinal) G97.82
Pseudomenses (newborn) P54.6
Pseudomenstruation (newborn) P54.6
Pseudomonas
aeruginosa, as cause of disease classified elsewhere B96.5
mallei infection A24.0
as cause of disease classified elsewhere B96.5
pseudomallei, as cause of disease classified elsewhere B96.5
Pseudomyotonia G71.19
Pseudomyxoma peritonei C78.6
Pseudoneuritis, optic (nerve) (disc) (papilla), **congenital** Q14.2
Pseudo-obstruction intestine (acute) (chronic) (idiopathic) (intermittent secondary) (primary) K59.89
colonic K59.81
Pseudopapilledema H47.33- ☑
congenital Q14.2
Pseudoparalysis
arm or leg R29.818
atonic, congenital P94.2
Pseudopelade L66.0
Pseudophakia Z96.1
Pseudopolyarthritis, rhizomelic M35.3
Pseudopolycythemia D75.1
Pseudopseudohypoparathyroidism E20.1
Pseudopterygium H11.81- ☑
Pseudoptosis (eyelid) — see Blepharochalasis
Pseudopuberty, precocious
female heterosexual E25.8
male isosexual E25.8
Pseudorickets (renal) N25.0
Pseudorubella B08.20
Pseudosclerema, newborn P83.88
Pseudosclerosis (brain)
Jakob's — see Creutzfeldt-Jakob disease or syndrome of Westphal (Strumpell) E83.01
spastic — see Creutzfeldt-Jakob disease or syndrome
Pseudotetanus — see Convulsions
Pseudotetany R29.0
hysterical F44.5
Pseudotruncus arteriosus Q25.49
Pseudotuberculosis A28.2
enterocolitis A04.8
pasteurella (infection) A28.0
Pseudotumor G93.2
cerebri G93.2
orbital H05.11 ☑

Pseudoxanthoma elasticum Q82.8
Psilosis (sprue) (tropical) K90.1
nontropical K90.0
Psittacosis A70
Psoitis M60.88
Psoriasis L40.9
arthropathic L40.50
arthritis mutilans L40.52
distal interphalangeal L40.51
juvenile L40.54
other specified L40.59
spondylitis L40.53
buccal K13.29
flexural L40.8
guttate L40.4
mouth K13.29
nummular L40.0
plaque L40.0
psychogenic F54
pustular (generalized) L40.1
palmaris et plantaris L40.3
specified NEC L40.8
vulgaris L40.0
Psychasthenia F48.8
Psychiatric disorder or problem F99
Psychogenic — see also condition
factors associated with physical conditions F54
Psychological and behavioral factors affecting medical condition F59
Psychoneurosis, psychoneurotic — see also Neurosis
anxiety (state) F41.1
depersonalization F48.1
hypochondriacal F45.21
hysteria F44.9
neurasthenic F48.8
personality NEC F60.89
Psychopathy, psychopathic
affectionless F94.2
autistic F84.5
constitution, post-traumatic F07.81
personality — see Disorder, personality
sexual — see Deviation, sexual
state F60.2
Psychosexual identity disorder of childhood F64.2
Psychosis, psychotic F29
acute (transient) F23
hysterical F44.9
affective — see Disorder, mood
alcoholic F10.959
with
abuse F10.159
anxiety disorder F10.980
with
abuse F10.180
dependence F10.280
delirium tremens F10.231
delusions F10.950
with
abuse F10.150
dependence F10.250
dementia F10.97
with dependence F10.27
dependence F10.259
hallucinosis F10.951
with
abuse F10.151
dependence F10.251
mood disorder F10.94
with
abuse F10.14
dependence F10.24
paranoia F10.950
with
abuse F10.150
dependence F10.250
persisting amnesia F10.96
with dependence F10.26
amnestic confabulatory F10.96
with dependence F10.26
delirium tremens F10.231
Korsakoff's, Korsakov's, Korsakow's F10.26
paranoid type F10.950
with
abuse F10.150
dependence F10.250
anergastic — see Psychosis, organic
arteriosclerotic (simple type) (uncomplicated) — see also Dementia, vascular F01.50
with behavioral disturbance — see Dementia, vascular

Psychosis, psychotic — *continued*
- childhood F84.0
  - atypical F84.8
- climacteric — *see* Psychosis, involutional
- confusional F29
  - acute or subacute F05
  - reactive F23
- cycloid F23
- depressive — *see* Disorder, depressive
- disintegrative (childhood) F84.3
- drug-induced — *see* F11-F19 with .X59
  - paranoid and hallucinatory states — *see* F11-F19 with .X50 or .X51
- due to or associated with
  - addiction, drug — *see* F11-F19 with .X59
  - dependence
    - alcohol F10.259
    - drug — *see* F11-F19 with .X59
  - epilepsy F06.8
  - Huntington's chorea F06.8
  - ischemia, cerebrovascular (generalized) F06.8
  - multiple sclerosis F06.8
  - physical disease F06.8
  - presenile dementia F03 ☑
  - senile dementia F03 ☑
  - vascular disease (arteriosclerotic) (cerebral) — *see also* Dementia, vascular F01.50
    - with behavioral disturbance — *see* Dementia, vascular
- epileptic F06.8
- episode F23
  - due to or associated with physical condition F06.8
- exhaustive F43.0
- hallucinatory, chronic F28
- hypomanic F30.8
- hysterical (acute) F44.9
- induced F24
- infantile F84.0
  - atypical F84.8
- infective (acute) (subacute) F05
- involutional F28
  - depressive — *see* Disorder, depressive
  - melancholic — *see* Disorder, depressive
  - paranoid (state) F22
- Korsakoff's, Korsakov's, Korsakow's (nonalcoholic) F04
  - alcoholic F10.96
    - in dependence F10.26
  - induced by other psychoactive substance — *see* categories F11-F19 with .X5X
- mania, manic (single episode) F30.2
  - recurrent type F31.89
- manic-depressive — *see* Disorder, bipolar
- menopausal — *see* Psychosis, involutional
- mixed schizophrenic and affective F25.8
- multi-infarct (cerebrovascular) — *see also* Dementia, vascular F01.50
  - with behavioral disturbance — *see* Dementia, vascular
- nonorganic F29
  - specified NEC F28
- organic F09
  - due to or associated with
    - arteriosclerosis (cerebral) — *see* Psychosis, arteriosclerotic
    - cerebrovascular disease, arteriosclerotic — *see* Psychosis, arteriosclerotic
    - childbirth — *see* Psychosis, puerperal
    - Creutzfeldt-Jakob disease or syndrome — *see* Creutzfeldt-Jakob disease or syndrome
    - dependence, alcohol F10.259
    - disease
      - alcoholic liver F10.259
      - brain, arteriosclerotic — *see* Psychosis, arteriosclerotic
      - cerebrovascular — *see also* Dementia, vascular F01.50
        - with behavioral disturbance — *see* Dementia, vascular
      - Creutzfeldt-Jakob — *see* Creutzfeldt-Jakob disease or syndrome
      - endocrine or metabolic F06.8
        - acute or subacute F05
      - liver, alcoholic F10.259
    - epilepsy transient (acute) F05
    - infection
      - brain (intracranial) F06.8
        - acute or subacute F05
    - intoxication
      - alcoholic (acute) F10.259

Psychosis, psychotic — *continued*
- organic — *continued*
  - due to or associated with — *continued*
    - intoxication — *continued*
      - drug F11-F19 with .x59
      - ischemia, cerebrovascular (generalized) — *see* Psychosis, arteriosclerotic
    - puerperium — *see* Psychosis, puerperal
    - trauma, brain (birth) (from electric current) (surgical) F06.8
      - acute or subacute F05
  - infective F06.8
    - acute or subacute F05
  - post-traumatic F06.8
    - acute or subacute F05
- paranoiac F22
- paranoid (climacteric) (involutional) (menopausal) F22
  - psychogenic (acute) F23
  - schizophrenic F20.0
  - senile F03 ☑
- postpartum (NOS) F53.1
- presbyophrenic (type) F03 ☑
- presenile F03 ☑
- psychogenic (paranoid) F23
  - depressive F32.3
- puerperal (NOS) F53.1
  - specified type — *see* Psychosis, by type
- reactive (brief) (transient) (emotional stress) (psychological trauma) F23
  - depressive F32.3
    - recurrent F33.3
  - excitative type F30.8
- schizoaffective F25.9
  - depressive type F25.1
  - manic type F25.0
- schizophrenia, schizophrenic — *see* Schizophrenia
- schizophrenia-like, in epilepsy F06.2
- schizophreniform F20.81
  - affective type F25.9
  - brief F23
  - confusional type F23
  - mixed type F25.0
- senile NEC F03 ☑
  - depressed or paranoid type F03 ☑
  - simple deterioration F03 ☑
  - specified type — *code to* condition
- shared F24
- situational (reactive) F23
- symbiotic (childhood) F84.3
- symptomatic F09

Psychosomatic — *see* Disorder, psychosomatic
Psychosyndrome, organic F07.9
Psychotic episode due to or associated with physical condition F06.8
Pterygium (eye) H11.00- ☑
- amyloid H11.01- ☑
- central H11.02- ☑
- colli Q18.3
- double H11.03- ☑
- peripheral
  - progressive H11.05- ☑
  - stationary H11.04- ☑
- recurrent H11.06- ☑
Ptilosis (eyelid) — *see* Madarosis
Ptomaine (poisoning) — *see* Poisoning, food
Ptosis — *see also* Blepharoptosis
- adiposa (false) — *see* Blepharoptosis
- breast N64.81-
- brow H57.81- ☑
- cecum K63.4
- colon K63.4
- congenital (eyelid) Q10.0
  - specified site NEC — *see* Anomaly, by site
- eyebrow H57.81- ☑
- eyelid — *see* Blepharoptosis
  - congenital Q10.0
- gastric K31.89
- intestine K63.4
- kidney N28.83
- liver K76.89
- renal N28.83
- splanchnic K63.4
- spleen D73.89
- stomach K31.89
- viscera K63.4
PTP D69.51
Ptyalism (periodic) K11.7
- hysterical F45.8

Ptyalism — *continued*
- pregnancy — *see* Pregnancy, complicated by, specified pregnancy-related condition NEC
- psychogenic F45.8
Ptyalolithiasis K11.5
Pubarche, precocious E30.1
Pubertas praecox E30.1
Puberty (development state) Z00.3
- bleeding (excessive) N92.2
- delayed E30.0
- precocious (constitutional) (cryptogenic) (idiopathic) E30.1
  - central E22.8
  - due to
    - ovarian hyperfunction E28.1
      - estrogen E28.0
    - testicular hyperfunction E29.0
- premature E30.1
  - due to
    - adrenal cortical hyperfunction E25.8
    - pineal tumor E34.8
    - pituitary (anterior) hyperfunction E22.8
Puckering, macula — *see* Degeneration, macula, puckering
Pudenda, pudendum — *see* condition
Puente's disease (simple glandular cheilitis) K13.0
Puerperal, puerperium (complicated by, complications)
- abnormal glucose (tolerance test) O99.815
- abscess
  - areola O91.02
    - associated with lactation O91.03
  - Bartholin's gland O86.19
  - breast O91.12
    - associated with lactation O91.13
  - cervix (uteri) O86.11
  - genital organ NEC O86.19
  - kidney O86.21
  - mammary O91.12
    - associated with lactation O91.13
  - nipple O91.02
    - associated with lactation O91.03
  - peritoneum O85
  - subareolar O91.12
    - associated with lactation O91.13
  - urinary tract — *see* Puerperal, infection, urinary
  - uterus O86.12
  - vagina (wall) O86.13
  - vaginorectal O86.13
  - vulvovaginal gland O86.13
- adnexitis O86.19
- afibrinogenemia, or other coagulation defect O72.3
- albuminuria (acute) (subacute) — *see* Proteinuria, gestational
- alcohol use O99.315
- anemia O90.81
  - pre-existing (pre-pregnancy) O99.03
- anesthetic death O89.8
- apoplexy O99.43
- bariatric surgery status O99.845
- blood disorder NEC O99.13
- blood dyscrasia O72.3
- cardiomyopathy O90.3
- cerebrovascular disorder (conditions in I60-I69) O99.43
- cervicitis O86.11
- circulatory system disorder O99.43
- coagulopathy (any) O99.13
  - with hemorrhage O72.3
- complications O90.9
  - specified NEC O90.89
- convulsions — *see* Eclampsia
- cystitis O86.22
- cystopyelitis O86.29
- delirium NEC F05
- diabetes O24.93
  - gestational — *see* Puerperal, gestational diabetes
  - pre-existing O24.33
    - specified NEC O24.83
    - type 1 O24.03
    - type 2 O24.13
- digestive system disorder O99.63
- disease O90.9
  - breast NEC O92.29
  - cerebrovascular (acute) O99.43
  - nonobstetric NEC O99.893
  - tubo-ovarian O86.19
  - Valsuani's O99.03
- disorder O90.9
  - biliary tract O26.63
  - lactation O92.70
  - liver O26.63

Puerperal, puerperium — *continued*
    disorder — *continued*
        nonobstetric NEC O99.893
    disruption
        cesarean wound O90.0
        episiotomy wound O90.1
        perineal laceration wound O90.1
    drug use O99.325
    eclampsia (with pre-existing hypertension) O15.2
    embolism (pulmonary) (blood clot) — *see* Embolism, obstetric, puerperal
    endocrine, nutritional or metabolic disease NEC O99.285
    endophlebitis — *see* Puerperal, phlebitis
    endotrachelitis O86.11
    failure
        lactation (complete) O92.3
            partial O92.4
        renal, acute O90.49
    fever (of unknown origin) O86.4
        septic O85
    fissure, nipple O92.12
        associated with lactation O92.13
    fistula
        breast (due to mastitis) O91.12
            associated with lactation O91.13
        nipple O91.02
            associated with lactation O91.03
    galactophoritis O91.22
        associated with lactation O91.23
    galactorrhea O92.6
    gastric banding status O99.845
    gastric bypass status O99.845
    gastrointestinal disease NEC O99.63
    gestational
        diabetes O24.439
            diet controlled O24.430
            insulin (and diet) controlled O24.434
            oral drug controlled (antidiabetic) (hypoglycemic) O24.435
        edema O12.05
            with proteinuria O12.25
        proteinuria O12.15
    gonorrhea O98.23
    hematoma, subdural O99.43
    hemiplegia, cerebral O99.355
        due to cerbrovascular disorder O99.43
    hemorrhage O72.1
        brain O99.43
        bulbar O99.43
        cerebellar O99.43
        cerebral O99.43
        cortical O99.43
        delayed or secondary O72.2
        extradural O99.43
        internal capsule O99.43
        intracranial O99.43
        intrapontine O99.43
        meningeal O99.43
        pontine O99.43
        retained placenta O72.0
        subarachnoid O99.43
        subcortical O99.43
        subdural O99.43
        third stage O72.0
        uterine, delayed O72.2
        ventricular O99.43
    hemorrhoids O87.2
    hepatorenal syndrome O90.41
    hypertension — *see* Hypertension, complicating, puerperium
    hypertrophy, breast O92.29
    induration breast (fibrous) O92.29
    infection O86.4
        cervix O86.11
        generalized O85
        genital tract NEC O86.19
            obstetric surgical wound O86.09
        kidney (bacillus coli) O86.21
        maternal O98.93
            carrier state NEC O99.835
            gonorrhea O98.23
            human immunodeficiency virus (HIV) O98.73
            protozoal O98.63
            sexually transmitted NEC O98.33
            specified NEC O98.83
            streptococcus group B (GBS) carrier state O99.825
            syphilis O98.13
            tuberculosis O98.03
            viral hepatitis O98.43

Puerperal, puerperium — *continued*
    infection — *continued*
        maternal — *continued*
            viral NEC O98.53
        nipple O91.02
            associated with lactation O91.03
        peritoneum O85
        renal O86.21
        specified NEC O86.89
        urinary (asymptomatic) (tract) NEC O86.20
            bladder O86.22
            kidney O86.21
            specified site NEC O86.29
            urethra O86.22
        vagina O86.13
        vein — *see* Puerperal, phlebitis
    ischemia, cerebral O99.43
    lymphangitis O86.89
        breast O91.22
            associated with lactation O91.23
    malignancy O9A.13 (*following* O99)
    malnutrition O25.3
    mammillitis O91.02
        associated with lactation O91.03
    mammitis O91.22
        associated with lactation O91.23
    mania F30.8
    mastitis O91.22
        associated with lactation O91.23
        purulent O91.12
            associated with lactation O91.13
    melancholia — *see* Disorder, depressive
    mental disorder NEC O99.345
    metroperitonitis O85
    metrorrhagia — *see* Hemorrhage, postpartum
    metrosalpingitis O86.19
    metrovaginitis O86.13
    milk leg O87.1
    monoplegia, cerebral O99.43
    mood disturbance O90.6
    necrosis, liver (acute) (subacute) (conditions in subcategory K72.0) O26.63
        with renal failure O90.49
    nervous system disorder O99.355
    neuritis O90.89
    obesity (pre-existing prior to pregnancy) O99.215
    obesity surgery status O99.845
    occlusion, precerebral artery O99.43
    paralysis
        bladder (sphincter) O90.89
        cerebral O99.43
    paralytic stroke O99.43
    parametritis O85
    paravaginitis O86.13
    pelviperitonitis O85
    perimetritis O86.12
    perimetrosalpingitis O86.19
    perinephritis O86.21
    periphlebitis — *see* Puerperal phlebitis
    peritoneal infection O85
    peritonitis (pelvic) O85
    perivaginitis O86.13
    phlebitis O87.0
        deep O87.1
        pelvic O87.1
        superficial O87.0
    phlebothrombosis, deep O87.1
    phlegmasia alba dolens O87.1
    placental polyp O90.89
    pneumonia, embolic — *see* Embolism, obstetric, puerperal
    pre-eclampsia — *see* Pre-eclampsia
    psychosis (NOS) F53.1
    pyelitis O86.21
    pyelocystitis O86.29
    pyelonephritis O86.21
    pyelonephrosis O86.21
    pyemia O85
    pyocystitis O86.29
    pyohemia O85
    pyometra O86.12
    pyonephritis O86.21
    pyosalpingitis O86.19
    pyrexia (of unknown origin) O86.4
    renal
        disease NEC O90.89
        failure O90.49
    respiratory disease NEC O99.53

Puerperal, puerperium — *continued*
    retention
        decidua — *see* Retention, decidua
        placenta O72.0
        secundines — *see* Retention, secundines
    retrated nipple O92.02
    salpingo-ovaritis O86.19
    salpingoperitonitis O85
    secondary perineal tear O90.1
    sepsis (pelvic) O85
    septic thrombophlebitis O86.81
    skin disorder NEC O99.73
    specified condition NEC O99.893
    stroke O99.43
    subinvolution (uterus) O90.89
    subluxation of symphysis (pubis) O26.73
    suppuration — *see* Puerperal, abscess
    tetanus A34
    thelitis O91.02
        associated with lactation O91.03
    thrombocytopenia O72.3
    thrombophlebitis (superficial) O87.0
        deep O87.1
        pelvic O87.1
        septic O86.81
    thrombosis (venous) — *see* Thrombosis, puerperal
    thyroiditis O90.5
    toxemia (eclamptic) (pre-eclamptic) (with convulsions) O15.2
    trauma, non-obstetric O9A.23 (*following* O99)
        caused by abuse (physical) (suspected) O9A.33 (*following* O99)
            confirmed O9A.33 (*following* O99)
            psychological (suspected) O9A.53 (*following* O99)
                confirmed O9A.53 (*following* O99)
            sexual (suspected) O9A.43 (*following* O99)
                confirmed O9A.43 (*following* O99)
    uremia (due to renal failure) O90.49
    urethritis O86.22
    vaginitis O86.13
    varicose veins (legs) O87.4
        vulva or perineum O87.8
    venous O87.9
    vulvitis O86.19
    vulvovaginitis O86.13
    white leg O87.1
Puerperium — *see* Puerperal
Pulmolithiasis J98.4
Pulmonary — *see* condition
Pulpitis (acute) (anachoretic) (chronic) (hyperplastic) (putrescent) (suppurative) (ulcerative) K04.01
    irreversible K04.02
    reversible K04.01
Pulpless tooth K04.99
Pulse
    alternating R00.8
    bigeminal R00.8
    fast R00.0
    feeble, rapid due to shock following injury T79.4 ☑
    rapid R00.0
    weak R09.89
Pulsus alternans or trigeminus R00.8
Punch drunk F07.81
Punctum lacrimale occlusion — *see* Obstruction, lacrimal
Puncture
    abdomen, abdominal
        wall S31.139 ☑
            with
                foreign body S31.149 ☑
                penetration into peritoneal cavity S31.639 ☑
                    with foreign body S31.649 ☑
            epigastric region S31.132 ☑
                with
                    foreign body S31.142 ☑
                    penetration into peritoneal cavity S31.632 ☑
                        with foreign body S31.642 ☑
            left
                lower quadrant S31.134 ☑
                    with
                        foreign body S31.144 ☑
                        penetration into peritoneal cavity S31.634 ☑
                            with foreign body S31.644 ☑
                upper quadrant S31.131 ☑
                    with
                        foreign body S31.141 ☑

Puncture — *continued*
  abdomen, abdominal — *continued*
    wall — *continued*
      left — *continued*
        upper quadrant — *continued*
          with — *continued*
            penetration into peritoneal cavity S31.631 ✓
              with foreign body S31.641 ✓
      periumbilic region S31.135 ✓
        with
          foreign body S31.145 ✓
          penetration into peritoneal cavity S31.635 ✓
            with foreign body S31.645 ✓
      right
        lower quadrant S31.133 ✓
          with
            foreign body S31.143 ✓
            penetration into peritoneal cavity S31.633 ✓
              with foreign body S31.643 ✓
        upper quadrant S31.130 ✓
          with
            foreign body S31.140 ✓
            penetration into peritoneal cavity S31.630 ✓
              with foreign body S31.640 ✓
  accidental, complicating surgery — *see* Complication, accidental puncture or laceration
  alveolar (process) — *see* Puncture, oral cavity
  ankle S91.039 ✓
    with
      foreign body S91.049 ✓
    left S91.032 ✓
      with
        foreign body S91.042 ✓
    right S91.031 ✓
      with
        foreign body S91.041 ✓
  anus S31.833 ✓
    with foreign body S31.834 ✓
  arm (upper) S41.139 ✓
    with foreign body S41.149 ✓
    left S41.132 ✓
      with foreign body S41.142 ✓
    lower — *see* Puncture, forearm
    right S41.131 ✓
      with foreign body S41.141 ✓
  auditory canal (external) (meatus) — *see* Puncture, ear
  auricle, ear — *see* Puncture, ear
  axilla — *see* Puncture, arm
  back — *see also* Puncture, thorax, back
    lower S31.030 ✓
      with
        foreign body S31.040 ✓
          with penetration into retroperitoneal space S31.041 ✓
        penetration into retroperitoneal space S31.031 ✓
  bladder (traumatic) S37.29 ✓
    nontraumatic N32.89
  breast S21.039 ✓
    with foreign body S21.049 ✓
    left S21.032 ✓
      with foreign body S21.042 ✓
    right S21.031 ✓
      with foreign body S21.041 ✓
  buttock S31.803 ✓
    with foreign body S31.804 ✓
    left S31.823 ✓
      with foreign body S31.824 ✓
    right S31.813 ✓
      with foreign body S31.814 ✓
  by
    device, implant or graft — *see* Complications, by site and type, mechanical
    foreign body left accidentally in operative wound T81.539 ✓
    instrument (any) during a procedure, accidental — *see* Puncture, accidental complicating surgery
  calf — *see* Puncture, leg
  canaliculus lacrimalis — *see* Puncture, eyelid
  canthus, eye — *see* Puncture, eyelid
  cervical esophagus S11.23 ✓
    with foreign body S11.24 ✓

Puncture — *continued*
  cheek (external) S01.439 ✓
    with foreign body S01.449 ✓
    internal — *see* Puncture, oral cavity
    left S01.432 ✓
      with foreign body S01.442 ✓
    right S01.431 ✓
      with foreign body S01.441 ✓
  chest wall — *see* Puncture, thorax
  chin — *see* Puncture, head, specified site NEC
  clitoris — *see* Puncture, vulva
  costal region — *see* Puncture, thorax
  digit(s)
    foot — *see* Puncture, toe
    hand — *see* Puncture, finger
  ear (canal) (external) S01.339 ✓
    with foreign body S01.349 ✓
    drum S09.2- ✓
    left S01.332 ✓
      with foreign body S01.342 ✓
    right S01.331 ✓
      with foreign body S01.341 ✓
  elbow S51.039 ✓
    with
      foreign body S51.049 ✓
    left S51.032 ✓
      with
        foreign body S51.042 ✓
    right S51.031 ✓
      with
        foreign body S51.041 ✓
  epididymis — *see* Puncture, testis
  epigastric region — *see* Puncture, abdomen, wall, epigastric
  epiglottis S11.83 ✓
    with foreign body S11.84 ✓
  esophagus
    cervical S11.23 ✓
      with foreign body S11.24 ✓
    thoracic S27.818 ✓
  eyeball S05.6- ✓
    with foreign body S05.5- ✓
  eyebrow — *see* Puncture, eyelid
  eyelid S01.13- ✓
    with foreign body S01.14- ✓
    left S01.132 ✓
      with foreign body S01.142 ✓
    right S01.131 ✓
      with foreign body S01.141 ✓
  face NEC — *see* Puncture, head, specified site NEC
  finger(s) S61.239 ✓
    with
      damage to nail S61.339 ✓
        with
          foreign body S61.349 ✓
      foreign body S61.249 ✓
    index S61.238 ✓
      with
        damage to nail S51.338 ✓
          with
            foreign body S61.348 ✓
        foreign body S61.248 ✓
      left S61.231 ✓
        with
          damage to nail S61.331 ✓
            with
              foreign body S61.341 ✓
          foreign body S61.241 ✓
      right S61.230 ✓
        with
          damage to nail S61.330 ✓
            with
              foreign body S61.340 ✓
          foreign body S61.240 ✓
    little S61.238 ✓
      with
        damage to nail S61.338 ✓
          with
            foreign body S61.348 ✓
        foreign body S61.248 ✓
      left S61.237 ✓
        with
          damage to nail S61.337 ✓
            with
              foreign body S61.347 ✓
          foreign body S61.247 ✓

Puncture — *continued*
  finger(s) — *continued*
    little — *continued*
      right S61.236 ✓
        with
          damage to nail S61.336 ✓
            with
              foreign body S61.346 ✓
          foreign body S61.246 ✓
    middle S61.238 ✓
      with
        damage to nail S61.338 ✓
          with
            foreign body S61.348 ✓
        foreign body S61.248 ✓
      left S61.233 ✓
        with
          damage to nail S61.333 ✓
            with
              foreign body S61.343 ✓
          foreign body S61.243 ✓
      right S61.232 ✓
        with
          damage to nail S61.332 ✓
            with
              foreign body S61.342 ✓
          foreign body S61.242 ✓
    ring S61.238 ✓
      with
        damage to nail S61.338 ✓
          with
            foreign body S61.348 ✓
        foreign body S61.248 ✓
      left S61.235 ✓
        with
          damage to nail S61.335 ✓
            with
              foreign body S61.345 ✓
          foreign body S61.245 ✓
      right S61.234 ✓
        with
          damage to nail S61.334 ✓
            with
              foreign body S61.344 ✓
          foreign body S61.244 ✓
  flank S31.139 ✓
    with foreign body S31.149 ✓
  foot (except toe(s) alone) S91.339 ✓
    with foreign body S91.349 ✓
    left S91.332 ✓
      with foreign body S91.342 ✓
    right S91.331 ✓
      with foreign body S91.341 ✓
    toe — *see* Puncture, toe
  forearm S51.839 ✓
    with
      foreign body S51.849 ✓
    elbow only — *see* Puncture, elbow
    left S51.832 ✓
      with
        foreign body S51.842 ✓
    right S51.831 ✓
      with
        foreign body S51.841 ✓
  forehead — *see* Puncture, head, specified site NEC
  genital organs, external
    female S31.532 ✓
      with foreign body S31.542 ✓
      vagina — *see* Puncture, vagina
      vulva — *see* Puncture, vulva
    male S31.531 ✓
      with foreign body S31.541 ✓
      penis — *see* Puncture, penis
      scrotum — *see* Puncture, scrotum
      testis — *see* Puncture, testis
  groin — *see* Puncture, abdomen, wall
  gum — *see* Puncture, oral cavity
  hand S61.439 ✓
    with
      foreign body S61.449 ✓
    finger — *see* Puncture, finger
    left S61.432 ✓
      with
        foreign body S61.442 ✓
    right S61.431 ✓

Puncture — *continued*
  hand — *continued*
    right — *continued*
      with
        foreign body S61.441 ☑
      thumb — *see* Puncture, thumb
  head S01.93 ☑
    with foreign body S01.94 ☑
    cheek — *see* Puncture, cheek
    ear — *see* Puncture, ear
    eyelid — *see* Puncture, eyelid
    lip — *see* Puncture, oral cavity
    nose — *see* Puncture, nose
    oral cavity — *see* Puncture, oral cavity
    scalp S01.03 ☑
      with foreign body S01.04 ☑
    specified site NEC S01.83 ☑
      with foreign body S01.84 ☑
    temporomandibular area — *see* Puncture, cheek
  heart S26.99 ☑
    with hemopericardium S26.09 ☑
    without hemopericardium S26.19 ☑
  heel — *see* Puncture, foot
  hip S71.039 ☑
    with foreign body S71.049 ☑
    left S71.032 ☑
      with foreign body S71.042 ☑
    right S71.031 ☑
      with foreign body S71.041 ☑
  hymen — *see* Puncture, vagina
  hypochondrium — *see* Puncture, abdomen, wall
  hypogastric region — *see* Puncture, abdomen, wall
  inguinal region — *see* Puncture, abdomen, wall
  instep — *see* Puncture, foot
  internal organs — *see* Injury, by site
  interscapular region — *see* Puncture, thorax, back
  intestine
    large
      colon S36.599 ☑
        ascending S36.590 ☑
        descending S36.592 ☑
        sigmoid S36.593 ☑
        specified site NEC S36.598 ☑
        transverse S36.591 ☑
      rectum S36.69 ☑
    small S36.499 ☑
      duodenum S36.490 ☑
      specified site NEC S36.498 ☑
  intra-abdominal organ S36.99 ☑
    gallbladder S36.128 ☑
    intestine — *see* Puncture, intestine
    liver S36.118 ☑
    pancreas — *see* Puncture, pancreas
    peritoneum S36.81 ☑
    specified site NEC S36.898 ☑
    spleen S36.09 ☑
    stomach S36.39 ☑
  jaw — *see* Puncture, head, specified site NEC
  knee S81.039 ☑
    with foreign body S81.049 ☑
    left S81.032 ☑
      with foreign body S81.042 ☑
    right S81.031 ☑
      with foreign body S81.041 ☑
  labium (majus) (minus) — *see* Puncture, vulva
  lacrimal duct — *see* Puncture, eyelid
  larynx S11.013 ☑
    with foreign body S11.014 ☑
  leg (lower) S81.839 ☑
    with foreign body S81.849 ☑
    foot — *see* Puncture, foot
    knee — *see* Puncture, knee
    left S81.832 ☑
      with foreign body S81.842 ☑
    right S81.831 ☑
      with foreign body S81.841 ☑
    upper — *see* Puncture, thigh
  lip S01.531 ☑
    with foreign body S01.541 ☑
  loin — *see* Puncture, abdomen, wall
  lower back — *see* Puncture, back, lower
  lumbar region — *see* Puncture, back, lower
  malar region — *see* Puncture, head, specified site NEC
  mammary — *see* Puncture, breast
  mastoid region — *see* Puncture, head, specified site NEC
  mouth — *see* Puncture, oral cavity

Puncture — *continued*
  nail
    finger — *see* Puncture, finger, with damage to nail
    toe — *see* Puncture, toe, with damage to nail
  nasal (septum) (sinus) — *see* Puncture, nose
  nasopharynx — *see* Puncture, head, specified site NEC
  neck S11.93 ☑
    with foreign body S11.94 ☑
    involving
      cervical esophagus — *see* Puncture, cervical esophagus
      larynx — *see* Puncture, larynx
      pharynx — *see* Puncture, pharynx
      thyroid gland — *see* Puncture, thyroid gland
      trachea — *see* Puncture, trachea
    specified site NEC S11.83 ☑
      with foreign body S11.84 ☑
  nose (septum) (sinus) S01.23 ☑
    with foreign body S01.24 ☑
  ocular — *see* Puncture, eyeball
  oral cavity S01.532 ☑
    with foreign body S01.542 ☑
  orbit S05.4-
  palate — *see* Puncture, oral cavity
  palm — *see* Puncture, hand
  pancreas S36.299 ☑
    body S36.291 ☑
    head S36.290 ☑
    tail S36.292 ☑
  pelvis — *see* Puncture, back, lower
  penis S31.23 ☑
    with foreign body S31.24 ☑
  perineum
    female S31.43 ☑
      with foreign body S31.44 ☑
    male S31.139 ☑
      with foreign body S31.149 ☑
  periocular area (with or without lacrimal passages) — *see* Puncture, eyelid
  phalanges
    finger — *see* Puncture, finger
    toe — *see* Puncture, toe
  pharynx S11.23 ☑
    with foreign body S11.24 ☑
  pinna — *see* Puncture, ear
  popliteal space — *see* Puncture, knee
  prepuce — *see* Puncture, penis
  pubic region S31.139 ☑
    with foreign body S31.149 ☑
  pudendum — *see* Puncture, genital organs, external
  rectovaginal septum — *see* Puncture, vagina
  sacral region — *see* Puncture, back, lower
  sacroiliac region — *see* Puncture, back, lower
  salivary gland — *see* Puncture, oral cavity
  scalp S01.03 ☑
    with foreign body S01.04 ☑
  scapular region — *see* Puncture, shoulder
  scrotum S31.33 ☑
    with foreign body S31.34 ☑
  shin — *see* Puncture, leg
  shoulder S41.039 ☑
    with foreign body S41.049 ☑
    left S41.032 ☑
      with foreign body S41.042 ☑
    right S41.031 ☑
      with foreign body S41.041 ☑
  spermatic cord — *see* Puncture, testis
  sternal region — *see* Puncture, thorax, front
  submaxillary region — *see* Puncture, head, specified site NEC
  submental region — *see* Puncture, head, specified site NEC
  subungual
    finger(s) — *see* Puncture, finger, with damage to nail
    toe — *see* Puncture, toe, with damage to nail
  supraclavicular fossa — *see* Puncture, neck, specified site NEC
  temple, temporal region — *see* Puncture, head, specified site NEC
  temporomandibular area — *see* Puncture, cheek
  testis S31.33 ☑
    with foreign body S31.34 ☑
  thigh S71.139 ☑
    with foreign body S71.149 ☑
    left S71.132 ☑
      with foreign body S71.142 ☑
    right S71.131 ☑

Puncture — *continued*
  thigh — *continued*
    right — *continued*
      with foreign body S71.141 ☑
  thorax, thoracic (wall) S21.93 ☑
    with foreign body S21.94 ☑
    back S21.23- ☑
      with
        foreign body S21.24- ☑
          with penetration S21.44 ☑
        penetration S21.43 ☑
    breast — *see* Puncture, breast
    front S21.13- ☑
      with
        foreign body S21.14- ☑
          with penetration S21.34 ☑
        penetration S21.33 ☑
  throat — *see* Puncture, neck
  thumb S61.039 ☑
    with
      damage to nail S61.139 ☑
        with
          foreign body S61.149 ☑
      foreign body S61.049 ☑
    left S61.032 ☑
      with
        damage to nail S61.132 ☑
          with
            foreign body S61.142 ☑
        foreign body S61.042 ☑
    right S61.031 ☑
      with
        damage to nail S61.131 ☑
          with
            foreign body S61.141 ☑
        foreign body S61.041 ☑
  thyroid gland S11.13 ☑
    with foreign body S11.14 ☑
  toe(s) S91.139 ☑
    with
      damage to nail S91.239 ☑
        with
          foreign body S91.249 ☑
      foreign body S91.149 ☑
    great S91.133 ☑
      with
        damage to nail S91.233 ☑
          with
            foreign body S91.243 ☑
        foreign body S91.143 ☑
      left S91.132 ☑
        with
          damage to nail S91.232 ☑
            with
              foreign body S91.242 ☑
          foreign body S91.142 ☑
      right S91.131 ☑
        with
          damage to nail S91.231 ☑
            with
              foreign body S91.241 ☑
          foreign body S91.141 ☑
    lesser S91.136 ☑
      with
        damage to nail S91.236 ☑
          with
            foreign body S91.246 ☑
        foreign body S91.146 ☑
      left S91.135 ☑
        with
          damage to nail S91.235 ☑
            with
              foreign body S91.245 ☑
          foreign body S91.145 ☑
      right S91.134 ☑
        with
          damage to nail S91.234 ☑
            with
              foreign body S91.244 ☑
          foreign body S91.144 ☑
  tongue — *see* Puncture, oral cavity
  trachea S11.023 ☑
    with foreign body S11.024 ☑
  tunica vaginalis — *see* Puncture, testis
  tympanum, tympanic membrane S09.2- ☑
  umbilical region S31.135 ☑

Puncture — *continued*
umbilical region — *continued*
  with foreign body S31.145 ☑
uvula — *see* Puncture, oral cavity
vagina S31.43 ☑
  with foreign body S31.44 ☑
vocal cords S11.033 ☑
  with foreign body S11.034 ☑
vulva S31.43 ☑
  with foreign body S31.44 ☑
wrist S61.539 ☑
  with
    foreign body S61.549 ☑
  left S61.532 ☑
    with
      foreign body S61.542 ☑
  right S61.531 ☑
    with
      foreign body S61.541 ☑
PUO (pyrexia of unknown origin) R50.9
Pupillary membrane (persistent) Q13.89
Pupillotonia — *see* Anomaly, pupil, function, tonic pupil
Purpura D69.2
abdominal D69.0
allergic D69.0
anaphylactoid D69.0
annularis telangiectodes L81.7
arthritic D69.0
autoerythrocyte sensitization D69.2
autoimmune D69.0
bacterial D69.0
Bateman's (senile) D69.2
capillary fragility (hereditary) (idiopathic) D69.8
cryoglobulinemic D89.1
Devil's pinches D69.2
fibrinolytic — *see* Fibrinolysis
fulminans, fulminous D65
gangrenous D65
hemorrhagic, hemorrhagica D69.3
  not due to thrombocytopenia D69.0
Henoch (-Schonlein) (allergic) D69.0
hypergammaglobulinemic (benign) (Waldenstrom) D89.0
idiopathic (thrombocytopenic) D69.3
  nonthrombocytopenic D69.0
immune thrombocytopenic D69.3
infectious D69.0
malignant D69.0
neonatorum P54.5
nervosa D69.0
newborn P54.5
nonthrombocytopenic D69.2
  hemorrhagic D69.0
  idiopathic D69.0
nonthrombopenic D69.2
peliosis rheumatica D69.0
posttransfusion (post-transfusion) (from (fresh) whole blood or blood products) D69.51
primary D69.49
red cell membrane sensitivity D69.2
rheumatica D69.0
Schonlein (-Henoch) (allergic) D69.0
scorbutic E54 [D77]
senile D69.2
simplex D69.2
symptomatica D69.0
telangiectasia annularis L81.7
thrombocytopenic D69.49
  congenital D69.42
  hemorrhagic D69.3
  hereditary D69.42
  idiopathic D69.3
  immune D69.3
  neonatal, transitory P61.0
  thrombotic M31.19
thrombohemolytic — *see* Fibrinolysis
thrombolytic — *see* Fibrinolysis
thrombopenic D69.49
thrombotic, thrombocytopenic M31.19
toxic D69.0
vascular D69.0
visceral symptoms D69.0
Purpuric spots R23.3
Purulent — *see* condition
Pus
in
  stool R19.5
  urine N39.0
tube (rupture) — *see* Salpingo-oophoritis

Pustular rash L08.0
Pustule (nonmalignant) L08.9
malignant A22.0
Pustulosis palmaris et plantaris L40.3
Putnam (-Dana) **disease or syndrome** — *see* Degeneration, combined
Putrescent pulp (dental) K04.1
Pyarthritis, pyarthrosis — *see* Arthritis, pyogenic or pyemic
tuberculous — *see* Tuberculosis, joint
Pyelectasis — *see* Hydronephrosis
Pyelitis (congenital) (uremic) — *see also* Pyelonephritis
with
  calculus — *see* category N20 ☑
    with hydronephrosis N13.6
  contracted kidney N11.9
acute N10
chronic N11.9
  with calculus — *see* category N20 ☑
    with hydronephrosis N13.6
cystica N28.84
puerperal (postpartum) O86.21
tuberculous A18.11
Pyelocystitis — *see* Pyelonephritis
Pyelonephritis — *see also* Nephritis, tubulo-interstitial
with
  calculus — *see* category N20 ☑
    with hydronephrosis N13.6
  contracted kidney N11.9
acute N10
calculus — *see* category N20 ☑
  with hydronephrosis N13.6
chronic N11.9
  with calculus — *see* category N20 ☑
    with hydronephrosis N13.6
  associated with ureteral obstruction or stricture N11.1
  nonobstructive N11.8
    with reflux (vesicoureteral) N11.0
  obstructive N11.1
  specified NEC N11.8
in (due to)
  brucellosis A23.9 *[N16]*
  cryoglobulinemia (mixed) D89.1 *[N16]*
  cystinosis E72.04
  diphtheria A36.84
  glycogen storage disease E74.09 *[N16]*
  leukemia NEC C95.9- ☑ *[N16]*
  lymphoma NEC C85.90 *[N16]*
  multiple myeloma C90.0- ☑ *[N16]*
  obstruction N11.1
  Salmonella infection A02.25
  sarcoidosis D86.84
  sepsis A41.9 *[N16]*
  Sjogren's disease M35.04
  toxoplasmosis B58.83
  transplant rejection T86.91 *[N16]*
  Wilson's disease E83.01 *[N16]*
nonobstructive N12
  with reflux (vesicoureteral) N11.0
  chronic N11.8
syphilitic A52.75
Pyelonephrosis (obstructive) N11.1
chronic N11.9
Pyelophlebitis I80.8
Pyeloureteritis cystica N28.85
Pyemia, pyemic (fever) (infection) (purulent) — *see also* Sepsis
joint — *see* Arthritis, pyogenic or pyemic
liver K75.1
pneumococcal A40.3
portal K75.1
postvaccinal T88.0 ☑
puerperal, postpartum, childbirth O85
specified organism NEC A41.89
tuberculous — *see* Tuberculosis, miliary
Pygopagus Q89.4
Pyknoepilepsy (idiopathic) — *see* Pyknolepsy
Pyknolepsy G40.A09 (*following* G40.3)
intractable G40.A19 (*following* G40.3)
  with status epilepticus G40.A11 (*following* G40.3)
  without status epilepticus G40.A19 (*following* G40.3)
not intractable G40.A09 (*following* G40.3)
  with status epilepticus G40.A01 (*following* G40.3)
  without status epilepticus G40.A09 (*following* G40.3)
Pylephlebitis K75.1
Pyle's syndrome Q78.5
Pylethrombophlebitis K75.1
Pylethrombosis K75.1
Pyloritis K29.90

Pyloritis — *continued*
with bleeding K29.91
Pylorospasm (reflex) **NEC** K31.3
congenital or infantile Q40.0
neurotic F45.8
newborn Q40.0
psychogenic F45.8
Pylorus, pyloric — *see* condition
Pyoarthrosis — *see* Arthritis, pyogenic or pyemic
Pyocele
mastoid — *see* Mastoiditis, acute
sinus (accessory) — *see* Sinusitis
turbinate (bone) J32.9
urethra — *see also* Urethritis N34.0
Pyocolpos — *see* Vaginitis
Pyocystitis N30.80
with hematuria N30.81
Pyoderma, pyodermia L08.0
gangrenosum L88
newborn P39.4
phagedenic L88
vegetans L08.81
Pyodermatitis L08.0
vegetans L08.81
Pyogenic — *see* condition
Pyohydronephrosis N13.6
Pyometra, pyometrium, pyometritis — *see* Endometritis
Pyomyositis (tropical) — *see* Myositis, infective
Pyonephritis N12
Pyonephrosis N13.6
tuberculous A18.11
Pyo-oophoritis — *see* Salpingo-oophoritis
Pyo-ovarium — *see* Salpingo-oophoritis
Pyopericarditis, pyopericardium I30.1
Pyophlebitis — *see* Phlebitis
Pyopneumopericardium I30.1
Pyopneumothorax (infective) J86.9
with fistula J86.0
tuberculous NEC A15.6
Pyosalpinx, pyosalpingitis — *see also* Salpingo-oophoritis
Pyothorax J86.9
with fistula J86.0
tuberculous NEC A15.6
Pyoureter N28.89
tuberculous A18.11
Pyramidopallidonigral syndrome G20.C
Pyrexia (of unknown origin) R50.9
atmospheric T67.01 ☑
during labor NEC O75.2
heat T67.01 ☑
newborn P81.9
  environmentally-induced P81.0
persistent R50.9
puerperal O86.4
Pyroglobulinemia NEC E88.09
Pyromania F63.1
Pyrosis R12
Pyuria (bacterial) (sterile) R82.81

Q

Q fever A78
with pneumonia A78
Quadricuspid aortic valve Q23.88
Quadrilateral fever A78
Quadriparesis — *see* Quadriplegia
meaning muscle weakness M62.81
Quadriplegia G82.50
complete
  C1-C4 level G82.51
  C5-C7 level G82.53
congenital (cerebral) (spinal) G80.8
  spastic G80.0
embolic (current episode) I63.4- ☑
functional R53.2
incomplete
  C1-C4 level G82.52
  C5-C7 level G82.54
thrombotic (current episode) I63.3- ☑
traumatic — *code to* injury with seventh character S
  current episode — *see* Injury, spinal (cord), cervical
Quadruplet, pregnancy — *see* Pregnancy, quadruplet
Quarrelsomeness F60.3
Queensland fever A77.3
Quervain's disease M65.4
thyroid E06.1
Queyrat's erythroplasia D07.4
penis D07.4

Queyrat's erythroplasia — *continued*
  specified site — *see* Neoplasm, skin, in situ
  unspecified site D07.4
Quincke's disease or edema T78.3 ☑
  hereditary D84.1
Quinsy (gangrenous) J36
Quintan fever A79.0
Quintuplet, pregnancy — *see* Pregnancy, quintuplet

R

Rabbit fever — *see* Tularemia
Rabies A82.9
  contact Z20.3
  exposure to Z20.3
  inoculation reaction — *see* Complications, vaccination
  sylvatic A82.0
  urban A82.1
Rachischisis — *see* Spina bifida
Rachitic — *see also* condition
  deformities of spine (late effect) (sequelae) E64.3
  pelvis (late effect) (sequelae) E64.3
    with disproportion (fetopelvic) O33.0
      causing obstructed labor O65.0
Rachitis, rachitism (acute) (tarda) — *see also* Rickets
  renalis N25.0
  sequelae E64.3
Radial nerve — *see* condition
Radiation
  burn — *see* Burn
  effects NOS T66 ☑
  sickness NOS T66 ☑
  therapy, encounter for Z51.0
Radiculitis (pressure) (vertebrogenic) — *see* Radiculopathy
Radiculomyelitis — *see also* Encephalitis
  toxic, due to
    Clostridium tetani A35
    Corynebacterium diphtheriae A36.82
Radiculopathy M54.10
  cervical region M54.12
  cervicothoracic region M54.13
  due to
    disc disorder
      C3 M50.11
      C4 M50.11
      C5 M50.121
      C6 M50.122
      C7 M50.123
    displacement of intervertebral disc — *see* Disorder, disc, with, radiculopathy
  leg M54.1-
  lumbar region M54.16
  lumbosacral region M54.17
  occipito-atlanto-axial region M54.11
  postherpetic B02.29
  sacrococcygeal region M54.18
  syphilitic A52.11
  thoracic region (with visceral pain) M54.14
  thoracolumbar region M54.15
Radiodermal burns (acute, chronic, or occupational) — *see* Burn
Radiodermatitis L58.9
  acute L58.0
  chronic L58.1
Radiotherapy session Z51.0
RAEB (refractory anemia with excess blasts) D46.2- ☑
Rage, meaning rabies — *see* Rabies
Ragpicker's disease A22.1
Ragsorter's disease A22.1
Raillietiniasis B71.8
Railroad neurosis F48.8
Railway spine F48.8
Raised — *see also* Elevated
  antibody titer R76.0
Rake teeth, tooth M26.39
Rales R09.89
Ramifying renal pelvis Q63.8
Ramsay-Hunt disease or syndrome — *see also* Hunt's, disease B02.21
  meaning dyssynergia cerebellaris myoclonica G11.19
Ranula K11.6
  congenital Q38.4
Rape
  adult
    confirmed T74.21 ☑
    suspected T76.21 ☑
  alleged, observation or examination, ruled out — adult Z04.41

Rape — *continued*
  alleged, observation or examination, ruled out — *continued*
    child Z04.42
  child
    confirmed T74.22 ☑
    suspected T76.22 ☑
Rapid
  feeble pulse, due to shock, following injury T79.4 ☑
  heart (beat) R00.0
    psychogenic F45.8
  second stage (delivery) O62.3
  time-zone change syndrome G47.25
Rarefaction, bone — *see* Disorder, bone, density and structure, specified NEC
Rash (toxic) R21
  canker A38.9
  diaper L22
  drug (internal use) L27.0
    contact — *see also* Dermatitis, due to, drugs, external L25.1
  following immunization T88.1 ☑
  food — *see* Dermatitis, due to, food
  heat L74.0
  napkin (psoriasiform) L22
  nettle — *see* Urticaria
  pustular L08.0
  rose R21
    epidemic B06.9
  scarlet A38.9
  serum — *see also* Reaction, serum T80.69 ☑
  wandering tongue K14.1
Rasmussen aneurysm — *see* Tuberculosis, pulmonary
Rasmussen encephalitis G04.81
Rat-bite fever A25.9
  due to Streptobacillus moniliformis A25.1
  spirochetal (morsus muris) A25.0
Rathke's pouch tumor D44.3
Raymond (-Cestan) **syndrome** I65.8
Raynaud's disease, phenomenon or syndrome (secondary) I73.00
  with gangrene (symmetric) I73.01
RDS (newborn) (type I) P22.0
  type II P22.1
Reaction — *see also* Disorder
  withdrawing, child or adolescent F93.8
  adaptation — *see* Disorder, adjustment
  adjustment (anxiety) (conduct disorder) (depressiveness) (distress) — *see* Disorder, adjustment
    with
      mutism, elective (child) (adolescent) F94.0
  adverse
    food (any) (ingested) NEC T78.1 ☑
      anaphylactic — *see* Shock, anaphylactic, due to, food
  affective — *see* Disorder, mood
  allergic — *see* Allergy
  anaphylactic — *see* Shock, anaphylactic
  anaphylactoid — *see* Shock, anaphylactic
  anesthesia — *see* Anesthesia, complication
  antitoxin (prophylactic) (therapeutic) — *see* Complications, vaccination
  anxiety F41.1
  Arthus — *see* Arthus' phenomenon
  asthenic F48.8
  combat and operational stress F43.0
  compulsive F42.8
  conversion F44.9
  crisis, acute F43.0
  deoxyribonuclease (DNA) (DNase) hypersensitivity D69.2
  depressive (single episode) F32.9
    affective (single episode) F31.4
      recurrent episode F33.9
    neurotic F34.1
    psychoneurotic F34.1
    psychotic F32.3
    recurrent — *see* Disorder, depressive, recurrent
  dissociative F44.9
  drug NEC T88.7 ☑
    addictive — *see* Dependence, drug
      transmitted via placenta or breast milk — *see* Absorption, drug, addictive, through placenta
    allergic — *see* Allergy, drug
    lichenoid L43.2
    newborn P93.8
      gray baby syndrome P93.0
    overdose or poisoning (by accident) — *see* Table of Drugs and Chemicals, by drug, poisoning

Reaction — *continued*
  drug — *continued*
    photoallergic L56.1
    phototoxic L56.0
    withdrawal — *see* Dependence, by drug, with, withdrawal
      infant of dependent mother P96.1
      newborn P96.1
    wrong substance given or taken (by accident) — *see* Table of Drugs and Chemicals, by drug, poisoning
  fear F40.9
    child (abnormal) F93.8
  febrile nonhemolytic transfusion (FNHTR) R50.84
  fluid loss, cerebrospinal G97.1
  foreign
    body NEC — *see* Granuloma, foreign body
      in operative wound (inadvertently left) — *see* Foreign body, accidentally left during a procedure
    substance accidentally left during a procedure (chemical) (powder) (talc) T81.60 ☑
      aseptic peritonitis T81.61 ☑
      body or object (instrument) (sponge) (swab) — *see* Foreign body, accidentally left during a procedure
      specified reaction NEC T81.69 ☑
  grief — *see* Disorder, adjustment
  Herxheimer's R68.89
  hyperkinetic — *see* Hyperkinesia
  hypochondriacal F45.20
  hypoglycemic, due to insulin E16.0
    with coma (diabetic) — *see* Diabetes, coma
      nondiabetic E15
    therapeutic misadventure — *see* subcategory T38.3 ☑
  hypomanic F30.8
  hysterical F44.9
  immunization — *see* Complications, vaccination
  incompatibility
    ABO blood group (infusion) (transfusion) — *see* Complication(s), transfusion, incompatibility reaction, ABO
    delayed serologic T80.39 ☑
    minor blood group (Duffy) (E) (K) (Kell) (Kidd) (Lewis) (M) (N) (P) (S) T80.89 ☑
    Rh (factor) (infusion) (transfusion) — *see* Complication(s), transfusion, incompatibility reaction, Rh (factor)
  inflammatory — *see* Infection
  infusion — *see* Complications, infusion
  inoculation (immune serum) — *see* Complications, vaccination
  insulin T38.3- ☑
  involutional psychotic — *see* Disorder, depressive
  leukemoid D72.823
    basophilic D72.823
    lymphocytic D72.823
    monocytic D72.823
    myelocytic D72.823
    neutrophilic D72.823
  LSD (acute)
    due to drug abuse — *see* Abuse, drug, hallucinogen
    due to drug dependence — *see* Dependence, drug, hallucinogen
  lumbar puncture G97.1
  manic-depressive — *see* Disorder, bipolar
  neurasthenic F48.8
  neurogenic — *see* Neurosis
  neurotic F48.9
  neurotic-depressive F34.1
  nitritoid — *see* Crisis, nitritoid
  nonspecific
    to
      cell mediated immunity measurement of gamma interferon antigen response without active tuberculosis R76.12
      QuantiFERON-TB test (QFT) without active tuberculosis R76.12
      tuberculin test — *see also* Reaction, tuberculin skin test R76.11
  obsessive-compulsive F42.8
  organic, acute or subacute — *see* Delirium
  paranoid (acute) F23
    chronic F22
    senile F03 ☑
  passive dependency F60.7
  phobic F40.9

Reaction — *continued*
  post-traumatic stress, uncomplicated Z73.3
  psychogenic F99
  psychoneurotic — *see also* Neurosis
    compulsive F42.8
    depersonalization F48.1
    depressive F34.1
    hypochondriacal F45.20
    neurasthenic F48.8
    obsessive F42.8
  psychophysiologic — *see* Disorder, somatoform
  psychosomatic — *see* Disorder, somatoform
  psychotic — *see* Psychosis
  scarlet fever toxin — *see* Complications, vaccination
  schizophrenic F23
    acute (brief) (undifferentiated) F23
    latent F21
    undifferentiated (acute) (brief) F23
  serological for syphilis — *see* Serology for syphilis
  serum T80.69 ☑
    anaphylactic (immediate) — *see also* Shock, anaphylactic T80.59 ☑
    specified reaction NEC
      due to
        administration of blood and blood products T80.61 ☑
        immunization T80.62 ☑
        serum specified NEC T80.69 ☑
        vaccination T80.62 ☑
  situational — *see* Disorder, adjustment
  somatization — *see* Disorder, somatoform
  spinal puncture G97.1
    dural G97.1
  stress (severe) F43.9
    acute (agitation) ("daze") (disorientation) (disturbance of consciousness) (flight reaction) (fugue) F43.0
    specified NEC F43.89
  surgical procedure — *see* Complications, surgical procedure
  tetanus antitoxin — *see* Complications, vaccination
  toxic, to local anesthesia T88.59 ☑
    in labor and delivery O74.4
    in pregnancy O29.3X- ☑
    postpartum, puerperal O89.3
  toxin-antitoxin — *see* Complications, vaccination
  transfusion (blood) (bone marrow) (lymphocytes) (allergic) — *see* Complications, transfusion
  tuberculin skin test, abnormal R76.11
  vaccination (any) — *see* Complications, vaccination
Reactive airway disease — *see* Asthma
Reactive depression — *see* Reaction, depressive
Rearrangement
  chromosomal
    balanced (in) Q95.9
      abnormal individual (autosomal) Q95.2
        non-sex (autosomal) chromosomes Q95.2
        sex/non-sex chromosomes Q95.3
      specified NEC Q95.8
Recalcitrant patient — *see* Noncompliance
Recanalization, thrombus — *see* Thrombosis
Recession, receding
  chamber angle (eye) H21.55- ☑
  chin M26.09
  gingival (postinfective) (postoperative)
    generalized K06.020
      minimal K06.021
      moderate K06.022
      severe K06.023
    localized K06.010
      minimal K06.011
      moderate K06.012
      severe K06.013
Recklinghausen disease Q85.01
  bones E21.0
Reclus' disease (cystic) — *see* Mastopathy, cystic
Recrudescence
  deficit
    cerebral infarction — *see* Sequelae, infarction, cerebral
    stroke — *see* Sequelae, infarction, cerebral
  sequelae
    cerebral infarction — *see* Sequelae, infarction, cerebral
    stroke — *see* Sequelae, infarction, cerebral
Recrudescent typhus (fever) A75.1
Recruitment, auditory H93.21- ☑
Rectalgia K62.89
Rectitis K62.89
Rectocele
  female (without uterine prolapse) N81.6

Rectocele — *continued*
  female — *continued*
    with uterine prolapse N81.4
      complete N81.3
      incomplete N81.2
    in pregnancy — *see* Pregnancy, complicated by, abnormal, pelvic organs or tissues NEC
    male K62.3
Rectosigmoid junction — *see* condition
Rectosigmoiditis K63.89
  ulcerative (chronic) K51.30
    with
      complication K51.319
        abscess K51.314
        fistula K51.313
        obstruction K51.312
        rectal bleeding K51.311
        specified NEC K51.318
Rectourethral — *see* condition
Rectovaginal — *see* condition
Rectovesical — *see* condition
Rectum, rectal — *see* condition
Recurrent — *see* condition
  pregnancy loss — *see* Loss (of), pregnancy, recurrent
Red bugs B88.0
Red tide — *see also* Table of Drugs and Chemicals T65.82- ☑
Red-cedar lung or pneumonitis J67.8
Reduced
  mobility Z74.09
  ventilatory or vital capacity R94.2
Redundant, redundancy
  anus (congenital) Q43.8
  clitoris N90.89
  colon (congenital) Q43.8
  foreskin (congenital) N47.8
  intestine (congenital) Q43.8
  labia N90.69
  organ or site, congenital NEC — *see* Accessory
  panniculus (abdominal) E65
  prepuce (congenital) N47.8
  pylorus K31.89
  rectum (congenital) Q43.8
  scrotum N50.89
  sigmoid (congenital) Q43.8
  skin L98.7
    and subcutaneous tissue L98.7
    of face L57.4
      eyelids — *see* Blepharochalasis
  stomach K31.89
Reduplication — *see* Duplication
Reflex R29.2
  hyperactive gag J39.2
  pupillary, abnormal — *see* Anomaly, pupil, function
  vasoconstriction I73.9
  vasovagal R55
Reflux K21.9
  acid K21.9
  esophageal K21.9
    with esophagitis (without bleeding) K21.00
      with bleeding K21.01
    newborn P78.83
  gastroesophageal K21.9
    with esophagitis (without bleeding) K21.00
      with bleeding K21.01
  mitral — *see* Insufficiency, mitral
  ureteral — *see* Reflux, vesicoureteral
  vesicoureteral (with scarring) N13.70
    with
      nephropathy N13.729
        with hydroureter N13.739
          bilateral N13.732
          unilateral N13.731
        bilateral N13.722
        unilateral N13.721
        without hydroureter N13.729
          bilateral N13.722
          unilateral N13.721
      pyelonephritis (chronic) N11.0
    congenital Q62.7
    without nephropathy N13.71
Reforming, artificial openings — *see* Attention to, artificial, opening
Refractive error — *see* Disorder, refraction
Refsum's disease or syndrome G60.1
Refusal of
  food, psychogenic F50.89
  treatment (because of) Z53.20
    left against medical advice (AMA) Z53.29

Refusal of — *continued*
  treatment — *continued*
    left without being seen Z53.21
    patient's decision NEC Z53.29
    reasons of belief or group pressure Z53.1
Regional — *see* condition
Regurgitation R11.10
  aortic (valve) — *see* Insufficiency, aortic
  food — *see also* Vomiting
    with reswallowing — *see* Rumination
    newborn P92.1
  gastric contents — *see* Vomiting
  heart — *see* Endocarditis
  mitral (valve) — *see* Insufficiency, mitral
    congenital Q23.3
  myocardial — *see* Endocarditis
  pulmonary (valve) (heart) I37.1
    congenital Q22.2
    syphilitic A52.03
  tricuspid — *see* Insufficiency, tricuspid
  valve, valvular — *see* Endocarditis
    congenital Q24.8
  vesicoureteral — *see* Reflux, vesicoureteral
Reichmann's disease or syndrome K31.89
Reifenstein syndrome E34.52
Reinsertion
  implantable subdermal contraceptive Z30.46
  intrauterine contraceptive device Z30.433
Reiter's disease, syndrome, or urethritis M02.30
  ankle M02.37- ☑
  elbow M02.32- ☑
  foot joint M02.37- ☑
  hand joint M02.34- ☑
  hip M02.35- ☑
  knee M02.36- ☑
  multiple site M02.39
  shoulder M02.31- ☑
  vertebra M02.38
  wrist M02.33- ☑
Rejection
  food, psychogenic F50.89
  transplant T86.91
    bone T86.830
      marrow T86.01
    cornea T86.840- ☑
    heart T86.21
      with lung(s) T86.31
    intestine T86.850
    kidney T86.11
    liver T86.41
    lung(s) T86.810
      with heart T86.31
    organ (immune or nonimmune cause) T86.91
    pancreas T86.890
    skin (allograft) (autograft) T86.820
    specified NEC T86.890
    stem cell (peripheral blood) (umbilical cord) T86.5
Relapsing fever A68.9
  Carter's (Asiatic) A68.1
  Dutton's (West African) A68.1
  Koch's A68.9
  louse-borne (epidemic) A68.0
  Novy's (American) A68.1
  Obermeyers's (European) A68.0
  Spirillum A68.9
  tick-borne (endemic) A68.1
Relationship
  occlusal
    open anterior M26.220
    open posterior M26.221
Relaxation
  anus (sphincter) K62.89
    psychogenic F45.8
  arch (foot) — *see also* Deformity, limb, flat foot
  back ligaments — *see* Instability, joint, spine
  bladder (sphincter) N31.2
  cardioesophageal K21.9
  cervix — *see* Incompetency, cervix
  diaphragm J98.6
  joint (capsule) (ligament) (paralytic) — *see* Flail, joint
    congenital NEC Q74.8
  lumbosacral (joint) — *see* subcategory M53.2 ☑
  pelvic floor N81.89
  perineum N81.89
  posture R29.3
  rectum (sphincter) K62.89
  sacroiliac (joint) — *see* subcategory M53.2 ☑
  scrotum N50.89

Relaxation — *continued*
  urethra (sphincter) N36.44
  vesical N31.2
Release from prison, anxiety concerning Z65.2
Remains
  canal of Cloquet Q14.0
  capsule (opaque) Q14.8
Remittent fever (malarial) B54
Remnant
  canal of Cloquet Q14.0
  capsule (opaque) Q14.8
  cervix, cervical stump (acquired) (postoperative) N88.8
  cystic duct, postcholecystectomy K91.5
  fingernail L60.8
    congenital Q84.6
  meniscus, knee — *see* Derangement, knee, meniscus,
    specified NEC
  thyroglossal duct Q89.2
  tonsil J35.8
    infected (chronic) J35.01
  urachus Q64.4
Removal (from) (of)
  artificial
    arm Z44.00- ☑
      complete Z44.01- ☑
      partial Z44.02- ☑
    eye Z44.2- ☑
    leg Z44.10- ☑
      complete Z44.11- ☑
      partial Z44.12- ☑
  breast implant Z45.81
  cardiac pulse generator (battery) (end-of-life) Z45.010
  catheter (urinary) (indwelling) Z46.6
    from artificial opening — *see* Attention to, artificial,
      opening
    non-vascular Z46.82
    vascular NEC Z45.2
  device Z46.9
    contraceptive Z30.432
      implantable subdermal Z30.46
    implanted NEC Z45.89
    specified NEC Z46.89
  drains Z48.03
  dressing (nonsurgical) Z48.00
    surgical Z48.01
  external
    fixation device — *code to* fracture with seventh char-
      acter D
    prosthesis, prosthetic device Z44.9
      breast Z44.3- ☑
      specified NEC Z44.8
  home in childhood (to foster home or institution) Z62.29
  ileostomy Z43.2
  insulin pump Z46.81
  myringotomy device (stent) (tube) Z45.82
  nervous system device NEC Z46.2
    brain neuropacemaker Z46.2
    visual substitution device Z46.2
      implanted Z45.31
  non-vascular catheter Z46.82
  organ, prophylactic (for neoplasia management) — *see*
    Prophylactic, organ removal
  orthodontic device Z46.4
  staples Z48.02
  stent
    ureteral Z46.6
  suture Z48.02
  urinary device Z46.6
  vascular access device or catheter Z45.2
Ren
  arcuatus Q63.1
  mobile, mobilis N28.89
    congenital Q63.8
  unguliformis Q63.1
Renal — *see* condition
Rendu-Osler-Weber disease or syndrome I78.0
Reninoma D41.0- ☑
Renon-Delille syndrome E23.3
Reovirus, as cause of disease classified elsewhere B97.5
Repeated falls NEC R29.6
Replaced chromosome by dicentric ring Q93.2
Replacement by artificial or mechanical device or
    prosthesis of
  bladder Z96.0
  blood vessel NEC Z95.828
  bone NEC Z96.7
  cochlea Z96.21
  coronary artery Z95.5

Replacement by artificial or mechanical device or
    prosthesis of — *continued*
  eustachian tube Z96.29
  eye globe Z97.0
  heart Z95.812
    valve Z95.2
      prosthetic Z95.2
      specified NEC Z95.4
      xenogenic Z95.3
  intestine Z96.89
  joint Z96.60
    hip — *see* Presence, hip joint implant
    knee — *see* Presence, knee joint implant
    specified site NEC Z96.698
  larynx Z96.3
  lens Z96.1
  limb(s) — *see* Presence, artificial, limb
  mandible NEC (for tooth root implant(s)) Z96.5
  organ NEC Z96.89
  peripheral vessel NEC Z95.828
  stapes Z96.29
  teeth Z97.2
  tendon Z96.7
  tissue NEC Z96.89
  tooth root(s) Z96.5
  vessel NEC Z95.828
    coronary (artery) Z95.5
Request for expert evidence Z04.89
Reserve, decreased or low
  cardiac — *see* Disease, heart
  kidney N28.89
Residing
  in place not meant for human habitation (abandoned
    building) (car) (park) (sidewalk) Z59.02
  on the street Z59.02
Residual — *see also* condition
  ovary syndrome N99.83
  state, schizophrenic F20.5
  urine R39.198
Resistance, resistant (to)
  activated protein C D68.51
  insulin E88.819
    complicating pregnancy O26.89- ☑
    specified type NEC E88.818
  organism(s)
    to
      drug Z16.30
        aminoglycosides Z16.29
        amoxicillin Z16.11
        ampicillin Z16.11
        antibiotic(s) Z16.20
          multiple Z16.24
          specified NEC Z16.29
        antifungal Z16.32
        antimicrobial (single) Z16.30
          multiple Z16.35
          specified NEC Z16.39
        antimycobacterial (single) Z16.341
          multiple Z16.342
        antiparasitic Z16.31
        antiviral Z16.33
        beta lactam antibiotics Z16.10
          specified NEC Z16.19
        carbapenem Z16.13
        cephalosporins Z16.19
        extended beta lactamase (ESBL) Z16.12
        fluoroquinolones Z16.23
        macrolides Z16.29
        methicillin — *see* MRSA
        multiple drugs (MDRO)
          antibiotics Z16.24
          antimicrobial Z16.35
          antimycobacterials Z16.342
        penicillins Z16.11
        quinine (and related compounds) Z16.31
        quinolones Z16.23
        sulfonamides Z16.29
        tetracyclines Z16.29
        tuberculostatics (single) Z16.341
          multiple Z16.342
        vancomycin Z16.21
          related antibiotics Z16.22
  thyroid hormone E07.89
Resorption
  dental (roots) K03.3
    alveoli M26.79
  teeth (external) (internal) (pathological) (roots) K03.3
Respiration
  Cheyne-Stokes R06.3

Respiration — *continued*
  decreased due to shock, following injury T79.4 ☑
  disorder of, psychogenic F45.8
  insufficient, or poor R06.89
    newborn P28.5
  painful R07.1
  sighing, psychogenic F45.8
Respiratory — *see also* condition
  distress syndrome (newborn) (type I) P22.0
    type II P22.1
  syncytial virus, as cause of disease classified elsewhere
    — *see also* Virus, respiratory syncytial (RSV) B97.4
Respite care Z75.5
Response (drug)
  photoallergic L56.1
  phototoxic L56.0
Restenosis
  stent
    vascular
      end stent
        adjacent to stent — *see* Arteriosclerosis
        within the stent
          coronary T82.855 ☑
          peripheral T82.856 ☑
      in stent
        coronary vessel T82.855 ☑
        peripheral vessel T82.856 ☑
Restless legs (syndrome) G25.81
Restlessness R45.1
Restoration (of)
  dental
    aesthetically inadequate or displeasing K08.56
    defective K08.50
      specified NEC K08.59
    failure of marginal integrity K08.51
    failure of periodontal anatomical intergrity K08.54
  organ continuity from previous sterilization (tuboplasty)
    (vasoplasty) Z31.0
    aftercare Z31.42
  tooth (existing)
    contours biologically incompatible with oral health
      K08.54
    open margins K08.51
    overhanging K08.52
    poor aesthetic K08.56
    poor gingival margins K08.51
    unsatisfactory, of tooth K08.50
      specified NEC K08.59
Restorative material (dental)
  allergy to K08.55
  fractured K08.539
    with loss of material K08.531
    without loss of material K08.530
  unrepairable overhanging of K08.52
Restriction of housing space Z59.19
Rests, ovarian, in fallopian tube Q50.6
Restzustand (schizophrenic) F20.5
Retained — *see also* Retention
  cholelithiasis following cholecystectomy K91.86
  foreign body fragments (type of) Z18.9
    acrylics Z18.2
    animal quill(s) or spines Z18.31
    cement Z18.83
    concrete Z18.83
    crystalline Z18.83
    depleted isotope Z18.09
    depleted uranium Z18.01
    diethylhexyl phthalates Z18.2
    glass Z18.81
    isocyanate Z18.2
    magnetic metal Z18.11
    metal Z18.10
    nonmagnectic metal Z18.12
    nontherapeutic radioactive Z18.09
    organic NEC Z18.39
    plastic Z18.2
    quill(s) (animal) Z18.31
    radioactive (nontherapeutic) NEC Z18.09
    specified NEC Z18.89
    spine(s) (animal) Z18.31
    stone Z18.83
    tooth (teeth) Z18.32
    wood Z18.33
  fragments (type of) Z18.9
    acrylics Z18.2
    animal quill(s) or spines Z18.31
    cement Z18.83
    concrete Z18.83

☑ **Additional Character Required** — **Refer to the Tabular List for Character Selection**

Retained — *continued*
  fragments — *continued*
    crystalline Z18.83
    depleted isotope Z18.09
    depleted uranium Z18.01
    diethylhexyl phthalates Z18.2
    glass Z18.81
    isocyanate Z18.2
    magnetic metal Z18.11
    metal Z18.10
    nonmagnectic metal Z18.12
    nontherapeutic radioactive Z18.09
    organic NEC Z18.39
    plastic Z18.2
    quill(s) (animal) Z18.31
    radioactive (nontherapeutic) NEC Z18.09
    specified NEC Z18.89
    spine(s) (animal) Z18.31
    stone Z18.83
    tooth (teeth) Z18.32
    wood Z18.33
  gallstones, following cholecystectomy K91.86
Retardation
  development, developmental, specific — *see* Disorder, developmental
  endochondral bone growth — *see* Disorder, bone, development or growth
  growth R62.50
    due to malnutrition E45
  mental — *see* Disability, intellectual
  motor function, specific F82
  physical (child) R62.52
    due to malnutrition E45
  reading (specific) F81.0
  spelling (specific) (without reading disorder) F81.81
Retching — *see* Vomiting
Retention — *see also* Retained
  bladder — *see* Retention, urine
  carbon dioxide E87.29
  cholelithiasis following cholecystectomy K91.86
  cyst — *see* Cyst
  dead
    fetus (at or near term) (mother) O36.4 ☑
      early fetal death O02.1
    ovum O02.0
  decidua (fragments) (following delivery) (with hemorrhage) O72.2
    without hemorrhage O73.1
  deciduous tooth K00.6
  dental root K08.3
  fecal — *see* Constipation
  fetus
    dead O36.4 ☑
      early O02.1
  fluid R60.9
  foreign body — *see also* Foreign body, retained
    current trauma — *code as* Foreign body, by site or type
  gallstones, following cholecystectomy K91.86
  gastric K31.89
  intrauterine contraceptive device, in pregnancy — *see* Pregnancy, complicated by, retention, intrauterine device
  membranes (complicating delivery) (with hemorrhage) O72.2
    with abortion — *see* Abortion, by type
    without hemorrhage O73.1
  meniscus — *see* Derangement, meniscus
  menses N94.89
  milk (puerperal, postpartum) O92.79
  nitrogen, extrarenal R39.2
  ovary syndrome N99.83
  placenta (total) (with hemorrhage) O72.0
    without hemorrhage O73.0
    portions or fragments (with hemorrhage) O72.2
      without hemorrhage O73.1
  products of conception
    early pregnancy (dead fetus) O02.1
    following
      delivery (with hemorrhage) O72.2
        without hemorrhage O73.1
  secundines (following delivery) (with hemorrhage) O72.0
    without hemorrhage O73.0
    complicating puerperium (delayed hemorrhage) O72.2
    partial O72.2
      without hemorrhage O73.1
  smegma, clitoris N90.89
  urine R33.9

Retention — *continued*
  urine — *continued*
    due to hyperplasia (hypertrophy) of prostate — *see* Hyperplasia, prostate
    drug-induced R33.0
    organic R33.8
      drug-induced R33.0
    psychogenic F45.8
    specified NEC R33.8
  water (in tissues) — *see* Edema
Reticulation, dust — *see* Pneumoconiosis
Reticulocytosis R70.1
Reticuloendotheliosis
  acute infantile C96.0
  leukemic C91.4- ☑
  nonlipid C96.0
Reticulohistiocytoma (giant-cell) D76.3
Reticuloid, actinic L57.1
Reticulosis (skin)
  acute of infancy C96.0
  hemophagocytic, familial D76.1
  histiocytic medullary C96.A (*following* C96.6)
  lipomelanotic I89.8
  malignant (midline) C86.0- ☑
  polymorphic C86.0- ☑
  Sezary — *see* Sezary disease
Retina, retinal — *see also* condition
  dark area D49.81
Retinitis — *see also* Inflammation, chorioretinal
  albuminurica N18.9 *[H32]*
  diabetic — *see* Diabetes, retinitis
  disciformis — *see* Degeneration, macula
  focal — *see* Inflammation, chorioretinal, focal
  gravidarum — *see* Pregnancy, complicated by, specified pregnancy-related condition NEC
  juxtapapillaris — *see* Inflammation, chorioretinal, focal, juxtapapillary
  luetic — *see* Retinitis, syphilitic
  pigmentosa H35.52
  proliferans — *see* Disorder, globe, degenerative, specified type NEC
  proliferating — *see* Disorder, globe, degenerative, specified type NEC
  renal N18.9 *[H32]*
  syphilitic (early) (secondary) A51.43
    central, recurrent A52.71
    congenital (early) A50.01 *[H32]*
    late A52.71
  tuberculous A18.53
Retinoblastoma C69.2- ☑
  differentiated C69.2- ☑
  undifferentiated C69.2- ☑
Retinochoroiditis — *see also* Inflammation, chorioretinal
  disseminated — *see* Inflammation, chorioretinal, disseminated
    syphilitic A52.71
  focal — *see* Inflammation, chorioretinal
  juxtapapillaris — *see* Inflammation, chorioretinal, focal, juxtapapillary
Retinopathy (background) H35.00
  arteriosclerotic I70.8 *[H35.0-]* ☑
  atherosclerotic I70.8 *[H35.0-]* ☑
  central serous — *see* Chorioretinopathy, central serous
  Coats H35.02- ☑
  diabetic — *see* Diabetes, retinopathy
  exudative H35.02- ☑
  hypertensive H35.03- ☑
  in (due to)
    diabetes — *see* Diabetes, retinopathy
    sickle-cell disorders
      nonproliferative D57.- *[H36.81-]* ☑
      proliferative D57.- *[H36.82-]* ☑
  of prematurity H35.10- ☑
    stage 0 H35.11- ☑
    stage 1 H35.12- ☑
    stage 2 H35.13- ☑
    stage 3 H35.14- ☑
    stage 4 H35.15- ☑
    stage 5 H35.16- ☑
  pigmentary, congenital — *see* Dystrophy, retina
  proliferative NEC H35.2- ☑
    diabetic — *see* Diabetes, retinopathy, proliferative
    sickle-cell D57.- *[H36.82-]* ☑
    thalassemia H35.2 ☑
  solar H31.02- ☑
Retinoschisis H33.10- ☑
  congenital Q14.1
  specified type NEC H33.19- ☑

Retortamoniasis A07.8
Retractile testis Q55.22
Retraction
  cervix — *see* Retroversion, uterus
  drum (membrane) — *see* Disorder, tympanic membrane, specified NEC
  finger — *see* Deformity, finger
  lid H02.539
    left H02.536
      lower H02.535
      upper H02.534
    right H02.533
      lower H02.532
      upper H02.531
  lung J98.4
  mediastinum J98.59
  nipple N64.53
    associated with
      lactation O92.03
      pregnancy O92.01- ☑
      puerperium O92.02
    congenital Q83.8
  palmar fascia M72.0
  pleura — *see* Pleurisy
  ring, uterus (Bandl's) (pathological) O62.4
  sternum (congenital) Q76.7
    acquired M95.4
  uterus — *see* Retroversion, uterus
  valve (heart) — *see* Endocarditis
Retrobulbar — *see* condition
Retrocecal — *see* condition
Retrocession — *see* Retroversion
Retrodisplacement — *see* Retroversion
Retroflection, retroflexion — *see* Retroversion
Retrognathia, retrognathism (mandibular) (maxillary) M26.19
Retrograde menstruation N92.5
Retroperineal — *see* condition
Retroperitoneal — *see* condition
Retroperitonitis K68.9
Retropharyngeal — *see* condition
Retroplacental — *see* condition
Retroposition — *see* Retroversion
Retroprosthetic membrane T85.398 ☑
Retrosternal thyroid (congenital) Q89.2
Retroversion, retroverted
  cervix — *see* Retroversion, uterus
  female NEC — *see* Retroversion, uterus
  iris H21.89
  testis (congenital) Q55.29
  uterus (acquired) (acute) (any degree) (asymptomatic) (cervix) (postinfectional) (postpartal, old) N85.4
    congenital Q51.818
    in pregnancy O34.53- ☑
Retrovirus, as cause of disease classified elsewhere B97.30
  human
    immunodeficiency, type 2 (HIV 2) B97.35
    T-cell lymphotropic
      type I (HTLV-I) B97.33
      type II (HTLV-II) B97.34
  lentivirus B97.31
  oncovirus B97.32
  specified NEC B97.39
Retrusion, premaxilla (developmental) M26.09
Rett's disease or syndrome F84.2
Reverse peristalsis R19.2
Reye's syndrome G93.7
Rh (factor)
  hemolytic disease (newborn) P55.0
  incompatibility, immunization or sensitization
    affecting management of pregnancy NEC O36.09- ☑
      anti-D antibody O36.01- ☑
    newborn P55.0
    transfusion reaction — *see* Complication(s), transfusion, incompatibility reaction, Rh (factor)
  negative mother affecting newborn P55.0
  titer elevated — *see* Complication(s), transfusion, incompatibility reaction, Rh (factor)
  transfusion reaction — *see* Complication(s), transfusion, incompatibility reaction, Rh (factor)
Rhabdomyolysis (idiopathic) NEC M62.82
  traumatic T79.6
Rhabdomyoma — *see also* Neoplasm, connective tissue, benign
  adult — *see* Neoplasm, connective tissue, benign
  fetal — *see* Neoplasm, connective tissue, benign
  glycogenic — *see* Neoplasm, connective tissue, benign

Rhabdomyosarcoma (any type) — *see* Neoplasm, connective tissue, malignant
Rhabdosarcoma — *see* Rhabdomyosarcoma
Rhesus (factor) **incompatibility** — *see* Rh, incompatibility
Rheumatic (acute) (subacute)
  adherent pericardium I09.2
  chronic I09.89
  coronary arteritis I01.8
  degeneration, myocardium I09.0
  fever (acute) — *see* Fever, rheumatic
  heart — *see* Disease, heart, rheumatic
  myocardial degeneration — *see* Degeneration, myocardium
  myocarditis (chronic) (inactive) (with chorea) I09.0
    active or acute I01.2
      with chorea (acute) (rheumatic) (Sydenham's) I02.0
  pancarditis, acute I01.8
    with chorea (acute (rheumatic) Sydenham's) I02.0
  pericarditis (active) (acute) (with effusion) (with pneumonia) I01.0
    with chorea (acute) (rheumatic) (Sydenham's) I02.0
    chronic or inactive I09.2
  pneumonia I00 [J17]
  torticollis M43.6
  typhoid fever A01.09
Rheumatism (articular) (neuralgic) (nonarticular) M79.0
  gout — *see* Arthritis, rheumatoid
  intercostal, meaning Tietze's disease M94.0
  palindromic (any site) M12.30
    ankle M12.37- ☑
    elbow M12.32- ☑
    foot joint M12.37- ☑
    hand joint M12.34- ☑
    hip M12.35- ☑
    knee M12.36- ☑
    multiple site M12.39
    shoulder M12.31- ☑
    specified joint NEC M12.38
    vertebrae M12.38
    wrist M12.33- ☑
  sciatic M54.4- ☑
Rheumatoid — *see also* condition
  arthritis — *see also* Arthritis, rheumatoid
    with involvement of organs NEC M05.60
      ankle M05.67- ☑
      elbow M05.62- ☑
      foot joint M05.67- ☑
      hand joint M05.64- ☑
      hip M05.65- ☑
      knee M05.66- ☑
      multiple site M05.69
      shoulder M05.61- ☑
      vertebra — *see* Spondylitis, ankylosing
      wrist M05.63- ☑
    seronegative — *see* Arthritis, rheumatoid, seronegative
    seropositive — *see* Arthritis, rheumatoid, seropositive
  carditis M05.30
    ankle M05.37- ☑
    elbow M05.32- ☑
    foot joint M05.37- ☑
    hand joint M05.34- ☑
    hip M05.35- ☑
    knee M05.36- ☑
    multiple site M05.39
    shoulder M05.31- ☑
    vertebra — *see* Spondylitis, ankylosing
    wrist M05.33- ☑
  endocarditis — *see* Rheumatoid, carditis
  lung (disease) M05.10
    ankle M05.17- ☑
    elbow M05.12- ☑
    foot joint M05.17- ☑
    hand joint M05.14- ☑
    hip M05.15- ☑
    knee M05.16- ☑
    multiple site M05.19
    shoulder M05.11- ☑
    vertebra — *see* Spondylitis, ankylosing
    wrist M05.13- ☑
  myocarditis — *see* Rheumatoid, carditis
  myopathy M05.40
    ankle M05.47- ☑
    elbow M05.42- ☑
    foot joint M05.47- ☑
    hand joint M05.44- ☑
    hip M05.45- ☑

Rheumatoid — *continued*
  myopathy — *continued*
    knee M05.46- ☑
    multiple site M05.49
    shoulder M05.41- ☑
    vertebra — *see* Spondylitis, ankylosing
    wrist M05.43- ☑
  pericarditis — *see* Rheumatoid, carditis
  polyarthritis — *see* Arthritis, rheumatoid
  polyneuropathy M05.50
    ankle M05.57- ☑
    elbow M05.52- ☑
    foot joint M05.57- ☑
    hand joint M05.54- ☑
    hip M05.55- ☑
    knee M05.56- ☑
    multiple site M05.59
    shoulder M05.51- ☑
    vertebra — *see* Spondylitis, ankylosing
    wrist M05.53- ☑
  vasculitis M05.20
    ankle M05.27- ☑
    elbow M05.22- ☑
    foot joint M05.27- ☑
    hand joint M05.24- ☑
    hip M05.25- ☑
    knee M05.26- ☑
    multiple site M05.29
    shoulder M05.21- ☑
    vertebra — *see* Spondylitis, ankylosing
    wrist M05.23- ☑
Rhinitis (atrophic) (catarrhal) (chronic) (croupous) (fibrinous) (granulomatous) (hyperplastic) (hypertrophic) (membranous) (obstructive) (purulent) (suppurative) (ulcerative) J31.0
  with
    sore throat — *see* Nasopharyngitis
  acute J00
  allergic J30.9
    with asthma J45.909
      with
        exacerbation (acute) J45.901
        status asthmaticus J45.902
    due to
      food J30.5
      pollen J30.1
    nonseasonal J30.89
    perennial J30.89
    seasonal NEC J30.2
    specified NEC J30.89
  infective J00
  pneumococcal J00
  syphilitic A52.73
    congenital A50.05 [J99]
  tuberculous A15.8
  vasomotor J30.0
Rhinoantritis (chronic) — *see* Sinusitis, maxillary
Rhinodacryolith — *see* Dacryolith
Rhinolith (nasal sinus) J34.89
Rhinomegaly J34.89
Rhinopharyngitis (acute) (subacute) — *see also* Nasopharyngitis
  chronic J31.1
  destructive ulcerating A66.5
  mutilans A66.5
Rhinophyma L71.1
Rhinorrhea J34.89
  cerebrospinal (fluid) G96.01
    postoperative G96.08
    specified NEC G96.08
    spontaneous G96.01
    traumatic G96.08
  paroxysmal — *see* Rhinitis, allergic
  spasmodic — *see* Rhinitis, allergic
Rhinosalpingitis — *see* Salpingitis, eustachian
Rhinoscleroma A48.8
Rhinosinusitis — *see* Sinusitis
Rhinosporidiosis B48.1
Rhinovirus infection NEC B34.8
Rhizomelic chondrodysplasia punctata E71.540
Rhythm
  atrioventricular nodal I49.8
  disorder I49.9
    coronary sinus I49.8
    ectopic I49.8
    nodal I49.8
  escape I49.9
  heart, abnormal I49.9

Rhythm — *continued*
  idioventricular I44.2
  nodal I49.8
  sleep, inversion G47.2- ☑
    nonorganic origin — *see* Disorder, sleep, circadian rhythm, psychogenic
Rhytidosis facialis L98.8
Rib — *see also* condition
  cervical Q76.5
Riboflavin deficiency E53.0
Rice bodies — *see also* Loose, body, joint
  knee M23.4- ☑
Richter syndrome — *see* Leukemia, chronic lymphocytic, B-cell type
Richter's hernia — *see* Hernia, abdomen, with obstruction
Ricinism — *see* Poisoning, food, noxious, plant
Rickets (active) (acute) (adolescent) (chest wall) (congenital) (current) (infantile) (intestinal) E55.0
  adult — *see* Osteomalacia
  celiac K90.0
  hypophosphatemic with nephrotic-glycosuric dwarfism E72.09
  inactive E64.3
  kidney N25.0
  renal N25.0
  sequelae, any E64.3
  vitamin-D-resistant E83.31 [M90.80]
Rickettsia 364D/R. philipii (Pacific Coast tick fever) A77.8
Rickettsial disease A79.9
  specified type NEC A79.89
Rickettsialpox (Rickettsia akari) A79.1
Rickettsiosis A79.9
  due to
    Ehrlichia sennetsu A79.81
    Neorickettsia sennetsu A79.81
    Rickettsia akari (rickettsialpox) A79.1
  specified type NEC A79.89
  tick-borne A77.9
  vesicular A79.1
Rider's bone — *see* Ossification, muscle, specified NEC
Ridge, alveolus — *see also* condition
  flabby K06.8
Ridged ear, congenital Q17.3
Riedel's
  lobe, liver Q44.79
  struma, thyroiditis or disease E06.5
Rieger anomaly or syndrome Q13.81
Riehl's melanosis L81.4
Rietti-Greppi-Micheli anemia D56.9
Rieux's hernia — *see* Hernia, abdomen, specified site NEC
Riga (-Fede) **disease** K14.0
Riggs' disease — *see* Periodontitis
Right aortic arch Q25.47
Right middle lobe syndrome J98.11
Rigid, rigidity — *see also* condition
  abdominal R19.30
    with severe abdominal pain R10.0
    epigastric R19.36
    generalized R19.37
    left lower quadrant R19.34
    left upper quadrant R19.32
    periumbilic R19.35
    right lower quadrant R19.33
    right upper quadrant R19.31
  articular, multiple, congenital Q68.8
  cervix (uteri) in pregnancy — *see* Pregnancy, complicated by, abnormal, cervix
  hymen (acquired) (congenital) N89.6
  nuchal R29.1
  pelvic floor in pregnancy — *see* Pregnancy, complicated by, abnormal, pelvic organs or tissues NEC
  perineum or vulva in pregnancy — *see* Pregnancy, complicated by, abnormal, vulva
  spine — *see* Dorsopathy, specified NEC
  vagina in pregnancy — *see* Pregnancy, complicated by, abnormal, vagina
Rigors R68.89
  with fever R50.9
Riley-Day syndrome G90.1
RIND (reversible ischemic neurologic deficit) I63.9
Ring(s)
  aorta (vascular) Q25.45
  Bandl's O62.3
  contraction, complicating delivery O62.4
  esophageal, lower (muscular) K22.2
  Fleischer's (cornea) H18.04- ☑
  hymenal, tight (acquired) (congenital) N89.6
  Kayser-Fleischer (cornea) H18.04- ☑
  retraction, uterus, pathological O62.4

Ring(s) — *continued*
Schatzki's (esophagus) (lower) K22.2
congenital Q39.3
Soemmerring's — *see* Cataract, secondary
vascular (congenital) Q25.8
aorta Q25.45
Ringed hair (congenital) Q84.1
Ringworm B35.9
beard B35.0
black dot B35.0
body B35.4
Burmese B35.5
corporeal B35.4
foot B35.3
groin B35.6
hand B35.2
honeycomb B35.0
nails B35.1
perianal (area) B35.6
scalp B35.0
specified NEC B35.8
Tokelau B35.5
Rise, venous pressure I87.8
Rising, PSA following treatment for malignant neoplasm of prostate R97.21
Risk
for
dental caries Z91.849
high Z91.843
low Z91.841
moderate Z91.842
homelessness, imminent Z59.811
suffocation (smothering) under another while sleeping Z72.823
suicidal
meaning personal history of attempted suicide Z91.51
meaning suicidal ideation — *see* Ideation, suicidal
Ritter's disease L00
Rivalry, sibling Z62.891
Rivalta's disease A42.2
River blindness B73.01
Robert's pelvis Q74.2
with disproportion (fetopelvic) O33.0
causing obstructed labor O65.0
Robin (-Pierre) **syndrome** Q87.0
Robinow-Silverman-Smith syndrome Q87.19
Robinson's (hidrotic) **ectodermal dysplasia or syndrome** Q82.4
Robles' disease B73.01
Rocky Mountain (spotted) **fever** A77.0
Roetheln — *see* Rubella
Roger's disease Q21.0
Rokitansky-Aschoff sinuses (gallbladder) K82.8
Rolando's fracture (displaced) S62.22- ☑
nondisplaced S62.22- ☑
Romano-Ward (prolonged QT interval) **syndrome** I45.81
Romberg's disease or syndrome G51.8
Roof, mouth — *see* condition
Rosacea L71.9
acne L71.9
keratitis L71.8
specified NEC L71.8
Rosary, rachitic E55.0
Rose
cold J30.1
fever J30.1
rash R21
epidemic B06.9
Rosenbach's erysipeloid A26.0
Rosenthal's disease or syndrome D68.1
Roseola B09
infantum B08.20
due to human herpesvirus 6 B08.21
due to human herpesvirus 7 B08.22
Ross River disease or fever B33.1
Rossbach's disease K31.89
psychogenic F45.8
Rostan's asthma (cardiac) — *see* Failure, ventricular, left
Rotation
anomalous, incomplete or insufficient, intestine Q43.3
cecum (congenital) Q43.3
colon (congenital) Q43.3
spine, incomplete or insufficient — *see* Dorsopathy, deforming, specified NEC
tooth, teeth, fully erupted M26.35
vertebra, incomplete or insufficient — *see* Dorsopathy, deforming, specified NEC
Rotes Querol disease or syndrome — *see* Hyperostosis, ankylosing

Roth (-Bernhardt) **disease or syndrome** — *see* Meralgia paraesthetica
Rothmund (-Thomson) **syndrome** Q82.8
Rotor's disease or syndrome E80.6
Round
back (with wedging of vertebrae) — *see* Kyphosis
sequelae (late effect) of rickets E64.3
worms (large) (infestation) NEC B82.0
Ascariasis — *see also* Ascariasis B77.9
Roussy-Levy syndrome G60.0
Rubella (German measles) B06.9
complication NEC B06.09
neurological B06.00
congenital P35.0
contact Z20.4
exposure to Z20.4
maternal
care for (suspected) damage to fetus O35.3 ☑
manifest rubella in infant P35.0
suspected damage to fetus affecting management of pregnancy O35.3 ☑
specified complications NEC B06.89
Rubeola (meaning measles) — *see* Measles
meaning rubella — *see* Rubella
Rubeosis, iris — *see* Disorder, iris, vascular
Rubinstein-Taybi syndrome Q87.2
Rudimentary (congenital) — *see also* Agenesis
arm — *see* Defect, reduction, upper limb
bone Q79.9
cervix uteri Q51.828
eye Q11.2
lobule of ear Q17.3
patella Q74.1
respiratory organs in thoracopagus Q89.4
tracheal bronchus Q32.4
uterus Q51.818
in male Q56.1
vagina Q52.0
Ruled out condition — *see* Observation, suspected
Rumination R11.10
with nausea R11.2
disorder of infancy or childhood (in remission) F98.21
in adults (in remission) F50.84
neurotic F42.8
newborn P92.1
obsessional F42.8
psychogenic F42.8
Runaway [from current living environment] Z62.892
Runeberg's disease D51.0
Running out of money Z59.86
Runny nose R09.89
Rupia (syphilitic) A51.39
congenital A50.06
tertiary A52.79

Rupture, ruptured
abscess (spontaneous) — *code by* site under Abscess
aneurysm — *see* Aneurysm
anus (sphincter) — *see* Laceration, anus
aorta, aortic I71.8
abdominal I71.30
infrarenal I71.33
juxtarenal I71.32
pararenal I71.31
arch I71.12
ascending I71.11
descending I71.8
abdominal I71.30
thoracic I71.13
syphilitic A52.01
thoracoabdominal I71.50
paravisceral I71.52
supraceliac I71.51
thorax, thoracic I71.10
transverse I71.12
traumatic — *see* Injury, aorta, laceration, major
valve or cusp — *see also* Endocarditis, aortic I35.8
appendix (with peritonitis) — *see also* Appendicitis K35.32
with localized peritonitis — *see also* Appendicitis K35.32
arteriovenous fistula, brain — *see* Fistula, arteriovenous, brain, ruptured
artery I77.2
brain — *see* Hemorrhage, intracranial, intracerebral
coronary — *see* Infarct, myocardium
heart — *see* Infarct, myocardium
pulmonary I28.8
traumatic (complication) — *see* Injury, blood vessel
bile duct (common) (hepatic) K83.2

Rupture, ruptured — *continued*
bile duct — *continued*
cystic K82.2
bladder (sphincter) (nontraumatic) (spontaneous) N32.89
following ectopic or molar pregnancy O08.6
obstetrical trauma O71.5
traumatic S37.29 ☑
blood vessel — *see also* Hemorrhage
brain — *see* Hemorrhage, intracranial, intracerebral
heart — *see* Infarct, myocardium
traumatic (complication) — *see* Injury, blood vessel, laceration, major, by site
bone — *see* Fracture
bowel (nontraumatic) K63.1
brain
aneurysm (congenital) — *see also* Hemorrhage, intracranial, subarachnoid
syphilitic A52.05
hemorrhagic — *see* Hemorrhage, intracranial, intracerebral
capillaries I78.8
cardiac (auricle) (ventricle) (wall) I23.3
with hemopericardium I23.0
infectional I40.9
traumatic — *see* Injury, heart
cartilage (articular) (current) — *see also* Sprain
knee S83.3- ☑
semilunar — *see* Tear, meniscus
cecum (with peritonitis) K65.0
with peritoneal abscess K35.33
traumatic S36.598 ☑
celiac artery, traumatic — *see* Injury, blood vessel, celiac artery, laceration, major
cerebral aneurysm (congenital) (see Hemorrhage, intracranial, subarachnoid)
cervix (uteri)
with ectopic or molar pregnancy O08.6
following ectopic or molar pregnancy O08.6
obstetrical trauma O71.3
traumatic S37.69 ☑
chordae tendineae NEC I51.1
concurrent with acute myocardial infarction — *see* Infarct, myocardium
following acute myocardial infarction (current complication) I23.4
choroid (direct) (indirect) (traumatic) H31.32- ☑
circle of Willis I60.6
colon (nontraumatic) K63.1
traumatic — *see* Injury, intestine, large
cornea (traumatic) — *see* Injury, eye, laceration
coronary (artery) (thrombotic) — *see* Infarct, myocardium
corpus luteum (infected) (ovary) N83.1- ☑
cyst — *see* Cyst
cystic duct K82.2
Descemet's membrane — *see* Change, corneal membrane, Descemet's, rupture
traumatic — *see* Injury, eye, laceration
diaphragm, traumatic — *see* Injury, intrathoracic, diaphragm
disc — *see* Rupture, intervertebral disc
diverticulum (intestine) K57.80
with bleeding K57.81
bladder N32.3
large intestine K57.20
with
bleeding K57.21
small intestine K57.40
with bleeding K57.41
small intestine K57.00
with
bleeding K57.01
large intestine K57.40
with bleeding K57.41
duodenal stump K31.89
ear drum (nontraumatic) — *see also* Perforation, tympanum
traumatic S09.2- ☑
due to blast injury — *see* Injury, blast, ear
esophagus K22.3
eye (without prolapse or loss of intraocular tissue) — *see* Injury, eye, laceration
fallopian tube NEC (nonobstetric) (nontraumatic) N83.8
due to pregnancy O00.10- ☑
with intrauterine pregnancy O00.11- ☑
fontanel P13.1
gallbladder K82.2
traumatic S36.128 ☑
gastric — *see also* Rupture, stomach

Rupture, ruptured — *continued*

gastric — *see also* Rupture, stomach — *continued*
  vessel K92.2
globe (eye) (traumatic) — *see* Injury, eye, laceration
  nontraumatic — *see also* Disorder, globe H44.89
graafian follicle (hematoma) N83.0- ☑
heart — *see* Rupture, cardiac
hymen (nontraumatic) (nonintentional) N89.8
internal organ, traumatic — *see* Injury, by site
intervertebral disc — *see* Displacement, intervertebral
    disc
  traumatic — *see* Rupture, traumatic, intervertebral
      disc
intestine NEC (nontraumatic) K63.1
  traumatic — *see* Injury, intestine
iris — *see also* Abnormality, pupillary
  traumatic — *see* Injury, eye, laceration
joint capsule, traumatic — *see* Sprain
kidney (traumatic) S37.06- ☑
  birth injury P15.8
  nontraumatic N28.89
lacrimal duct (traumatic) — *see* Injury, eye, specified site
    NEC
lens (cataract) (traumatic) — *see* Cataract, traumatic
ligament, traumatic — *see* Rupture, traumatic, ligament,
    by site
liver S36.116 ☑
  birth injury P15.0
lymphatic vessel I89.8
marginal sinus (placental) (with hemorrhage) — *see*
    Hemorrhage, antepartum, specified cause NEC
membrana tympani (nontraumatic) — *see* Perforation,
    tympanum
membranes (spontaneous)
  artificial
    delayed delivery following O75.5
  delayed delivery following — *see* Pregnancy, compli-
      cated by, premature rupture of membranes
meningeal artery I60.8
meniscus (knee) — *see also* Tear, meniscus
  old — *see* Derangement, meniscus
  site other than knee — *code as* Sprain
mesenteric artery, traumatic — *see* Injury, mesenteric,
    artery, laceration, major
mesentery (nontraumatic) K66.8
  traumatic — *see* Injury, intra-abdominal, specified,
      site NEC
mitral (valve) I34.89
muscle (traumatic) — *see also* Strain
  diastasis — *see* Diastasis, muscle
  nontraumatic M62.10
    ankle M62.17- ☑
    foot M62.17- ☑
    forearm M62.13- ☑
    hand M62.14- ☑
    lower leg M62.16- ☑
    pelvic region M62.15- ☑
    shoulder region M62.11- ☑
    specified site NEC M62.18
    thigh M62.15- ☑
    upper arm M62.12- ☑
  traumatic — *see* Strain, by site
musculotendinous junction NEC, nontraumatic — *see*
    Rupture, tendon, spontaneous
mycotic aneurysm causing cerebral hemorrhage — *see*
    Hemorrhage, intracranial, subarachnoid
myocardium, myocardial — *see* Rupture, cardiac
  traumatic — *see* Injury, heart
nontraumatic, meaning hernia — *see* Hernia
obstructed — *see* Hernia, by site, obstructed
operation wound — *see* Disruption, wound, operation
ovary, ovarian N83.8
  corpus luteum cyst N83.1- ☑
  follicle (graafian) N83.0- ☑
oviduct (nonobstetric) (nontraumatic) N83.8
  due to pregnancy O00.10- ☑
    with intrauterine pregnancy O00.11- ☑
pancreas (nontraumatic) K86.89
  traumatic S36.299 ☑
papillary muscle NEC I51.2
  following acute myocardial infarction (current compli-
      cation) I23.5
pelvic
  floor, complicating delivery O70.1
  organ NEC, obstetrical trauma O71.5
perineum (nonobstetric) (nontraumatic) N90.89
  complicating delivery — *see* Delivery, complicated,
      by, laceration, anus (sphincter)

Rupture, ruptured — *continued*

postoperative wound — *see* Disruption, wound, opera-
    tion
prostate (traumatic) S37.828 ☑
pulmonary
  artery I28.8
    valve (heart) I37.8
  vein I28.8
  vessel I28.8
pus tube — *see* Salpingitis
pyosalpinx — *see* Salpingitis
rectum (nontraumatic) K63.1
  traumatic S36.69 ☑
retina, retinal (traumatic) (without detachment) — *see*
    also Break, retina
  with detachment — *see* Detachment, retina, with
      retinal, break
rotator cuff (nontraumatic) M75.10- ☑
  complete M75.12- ☑
  incomplete M75.11- ☑
sclera — *see* Injury, eye, laceration
sigmoid (nontraumatic) K63.1
  traumatic S36.593 ☑
spinal cord — *see also* Injury, spinal cord, by region
  due to injury at birth P11.5
  newborn (birth injury) P11.5
spleen (traumatic) S36.09 ☑
  birth injury P15.1
  congenital (birth injury) P15.1
  due to P. vivax malaria B51.0
  nontraumatic D73.5
  spontaneous D73.5
splenic vein R58
  traumatic — *see* Injury, blood vessel, splenic vein
stomach (nontraumatic) (spontaneous) K31.89
  traumatic S36.39 ☑
supraspinatus (complete) (incomplete) (nontraumatic)
    — *see* Tear, rotator cuff
symphysis pubis
  obstetric O71.6
  traumatic S33.4 ☑
synovium (cyst) M66.10
  ankle M66.17- ☑
  elbow M66.12- ☑
  finger M66.14- ☑
  foot M66.17- ☑
  forearm M66.13- ☑
  hand M66.14- ☑
  pelvic region M66.15- ☑
  shoulder region M66.11- ☑
  specified site NEC M66.18
  thigh M66.15- ☑
  toe M66.17- ☑
  upper arm M66.12- ☑
  wrist M66.13- ☑
tendon (traumatic) — *see* Strain
  nontraumatic (spontaneous) M66.9
    ankle M66.87- ☑
    extensor M66.20
      ankle M66.27- ☑
      foot M66.27- ☑
      forearm M66.23- ☑
      hand M66.24- ☑
      lower leg M66.26- ☑
      multiple sites M66.29
      pelvic region M66.25- ☑
      shoulder region M66.21- ☑
      specified site NEC M66.28
      thigh M66.25- ☑
      upper arm M66.22- ☑
    flexor M66.30
      ankle M66.37- ☑
      foot M66.37- ☑
      forearm M66.33- ☑
      hand M66.34- ☑
      lower leg M66.36- ☑
      multiple sites M66.39
      pelvic region M66.35- ☑
      shoulder region M66.31- ☑
      specified site NEC M66.38
      thigh M66.35- ☑
      upper arm M66.32- ☑
    foot M66.87- ☑
    forearm M66.83- ☑
    hand M66.84- ☑
    lower leg M66.86- ☑
    multiple sites M66.89

Rupture, ruptured — *continued*

tendon — *see* Strain — *continued*
  nontraumatic — *continued*
    pelvic region M66.85- ☑
    shoulder region M66.81- ☑
    specified
      site NEC M66.88
      tendon M66.80
    thigh M66.85- ☑
    upper arm M66.82- ☑
thoracic duct I89.8
tonsil J35.8
traumatic
  aorta — *see* Injury, aorta, laceration, major
  diaphragm — *see* Injury, intrathoracic, diaphragm
  external site — *see* Wound, open, by site
  eye — *see* Injury, eye, laceration
  internal organ — *see* Injury, by site
  intervertebral disc
    cervical S13.0
    lumbar S33.0 ☑
    thoracic S23.0 ☑
  kidney S37.06- ☑
  ligament — *see also* Sprain
    ankle — *see* Sprain, ankle
    carpus — *see* Rupture, traumatic, ligament, wrist
    collateral (hand) — *see* Rupture, traumatic, liga-
        ment, finger, collateral
    finger (metacarpophalangeal) (interphalangeal)
        S63.40- ☑
      collateral S63.41- ☑
        index S63.41- ☑
        little S63.41- ☑
        middle S63.41- ☑
        ring S63.41- ☑
      index S63.40- ☑
      little S63.40- ☑
      middle S63.40- ☑
      palmar S63.42- ☑
        index S63.42- ☑
        little S63.42- ☑
        middle S63.42- ☑
        ring S63.42- ☑
      ring S63.40- ☑
      specified site NEC S63.499 ☑
        index S63.49- ☑
        little S63.49- ☑
        middle S63.49- ☑
        ring S63.49- ☑
      volar plate S63.43- ☑
        index S63.43- ☑
        little S63.43- ☑
        middle S63.43- ☑
        ring S63.43- ☑
    foot — *see* Sprain, foot
    radial collateral S53.2- ☑
    radiocarpal — *see* Rupture, traumatic, ligament,
        wrist, radiocarpal
    ulnar collateral S53.3- ☑
    ulnocarpal — *see* Rupture, traumatic, ligament,
        wrist, ulnocarpal
    wrist S63.30- ☑
      collateral S63.31- ☑
      radiocarpal S63.32- ☑
      specified site NEC S63.39- ☑
      ulnocarpal (palmar) S63.33- ☑
  liver S36.116 ☑
  membrana tympani — *see* Rupture, ear drum, trau-
      matic
  muscle or tendon — *see* Strain
  myocardium — *see* Injury, heart
  pancreas S36.299 ☑
  rectum S36.69 ☑
  sigmoid S36.593 ☑
  spleen S36.09 ☑
  stomach S36.39 ☑
  symphysis pubis S33.4 ☑
  tympanum, tympanic (membrane) — *see* Rupture,
      ear drum, traumatic
  ureter S37.19 ☑
  uterus S37.69 ☑
  vagina — *see* Injury, vagina
  vena cava — *see* Injury, vena cava, laceration, major
tricuspid (heart) (valve) I07.8
tube, tubal (nonobstetric) (nontraumatic) N83.8
  abscess — *see* Salpingitis

☑ **Additional Character Required** — Refer to the Tabular List for Character Selection

Sarcoma — continued
osteogenic — see also Neoplasm, bone, malignant
  juxtacortical — see Neoplasm, bone, malignant
  periosteal — see Neoplasm, bone, malignant
periosteal — see also Neoplasm, bone, malignant
  osteogenic — see Neoplasm, bone, malignant
pleomorphic cell — see Neoplasm, connective tissue, malignant
reticulum cell (diffuse) — see Lymphoma, diffuse large cell
  nodular — see Lymphoma, follicular
  pleomorphic cell type — see Lymphoma, diffuse large cell
rhabdoid — see Neoplasm, malignant, by site
round cell — see Neoplasm, connective tissue, malignant
small cell — see Neoplasm, connective tissue, malignant
soft tissue — see Neoplasm, connective tissue, malignant
spindle cell — see Neoplasm, connective tissue, malignant
stromal (endometrial) C54.1
  isthmus C54.0
synovial — see also Neoplasm, connective tissue, malignant
  biphasic — see Neoplasm, connective tissue, malignant
  epithelioid cell — see Neoplasm, connective tissue, malignant
  spindle cell — see Neoplasm, connective tissue, malignant

Sarcomatosis
meningeal — see Neoplasm, meninges, malignant
specified site NEC — see Neoplasm, connective tissue, malignant
unspecified site C80.1

Sarcopenia (age-related) M62.84
Sarcosinemia E72.59
Sarcosporidiosis (intestinal) A07.8
SARS-CoV-2 — see also COVID-19
  sequelae (post acute) U09.9
Satiety, early R68.81
Saturnine — see condition
Saturnism
  overdose or wrong substance given or taken — see Table of Drugs and Chemicals, by drug, poisoning
Satyriasis F52.8
Sauriasis — see Ichthyosis
SBE (subacute bacterial endocarditis) I33.0
Scabies (any site) B86
Scabs R23.4
Scaglietti-Dagnini syndrome E22.0
Scald — see Burn
Scalenus anticus (anterior) **syndrome** G54.0
Scales R23.4
Scaling, skin R23.4
Scalp — see condition
Scapegoating affecting child Z62.3
Scaphocephaly, non-deformational Q75.01
Scapulalgia M89.8X1
Scapulohumeral myopathy G71.02
Scar, scarring — see also Cicatrix L90.5
  adherent L90.5
  atrophic L90.5
  cervix
    in pregnancy or childbirth — see Pregnancy, complicated by, abnormal cervix
  cheloid L91.0
  chorioretinal H31.00- ☑
    posterior pole macula H31.01- ☑
    postsurgical H59.81- ☑
    solar retinopathy H31.02- ☑
    specified type NEC H31.09- ☑
  choroid — see Scar, chorioretinal
  conjunctiva H11.24- ☑
  cornea H17.9
    xerophthalmic — see also Opacity, cornea
      vitamin A deficiency E50.6
  defect (isthmocele) O34.22
  duodenum, obstructive K31.5
  hypertrophic L91.0
  keloid L91.0
  labia N90.89
  lung (base) J98.4
  macula — see Scar, chorioretinal, posterior pole
  muscle M62.89
  myocardium, myocardial I25.2
  painful L90.5
  posterior pole (eye) — see Scar, chorioretinal, posterior pole

Scar, scarring — continued
retina — see Scar, chorioretinal
trachea J39.8
transmural uterine, in pregnancy O34.29
uterus N85.8
  in pregnancy O34.29
vagina N89.8
  postoperative N99.2
vulva N90.89
Scarabiasis B88.2
Scarlatina (anginosa) (maligna) A38.9
  myocarditis (acute) A38.1
    old — see Myocarditis
  otitis media A38.0
  ulcerosa A38.8
Scarlet fever (albuminuria) (angina) A38.9
Schamberg's disease (progressive pigmentary dermatosis) L81.7
Schatzki's ring (acquired) (esophagus) (lower) K22.2
  congenital Q39.3
Schaufenster krankheit I20.89
Schaumann's
  benign lymphogranulomatosis D86.1
  disease or syndrome — see Sarcoidosis
Scheie's syndrome E76.03
Schenck's disease B42.1
Scheuermann's disease or osteochondrosis — see Osteochondrosis, juvenile, spine
Schilder (-Flatau) **disease** G37.0
Schilling-type monocytic leukemia C93.0- ☑
Schimmelbusch's disease, cystic mastitis, or hyperplasia — see Mastopathy, cystic
Schistosoma infestation — see Infestation, Schistosoma
Schistosomiasis B65.9
  with muscle disorder B65.9 [M63.80]
    ankle B65.9 [M63.87-] ☑
    foot B65.9 [M63.87-] ☑
    forearm B65.9 [M63.83-] ☑
    hand B65.9 [M63.84-] ☑
    lower leg B65.9 [M63.86-] ☑
    multiple sites B65.9 [M63.89]
    pelvic region B65.9 [M63.85-] ☑
    shoulder region B65.9 [M63.81-] ☑
    specified site NEC B65.9 [M63.88]
    thigh B65.9 [M63.85-] ☑
    upper arm B65.9 [M63.82-] ☑
  Asiatic B65.2
  bladder B65.0
  chestermani B65.8
  colon B65.1
  cutaneous B65.3
  due to
    S. haematobium B65.0
    S. japonicum B65.2
    S. mansoni B65.1
    S. mattheii B65.8
  Eastern B65.2
  genitourinary tract B65.0
  intestinal B65.1
  lung NEC B65.9 [J99]
    pneumonia B65.9 [J17]
  Manson's (intestinal) B65.1
  oriental B65.2
  pulmonary NEC B65.9 [J99]
    pneumonia B65.9
  Schistosoma
    haematobium B65.0
    japonicum B65.2
    mansoni B65.1
  specified site NEC B65.8
  urinary B65.0
  vesical B65.0
Schizencephaly Q04.6
Schizoaffective psychosis F25.9
Schizodontia K00.2
Schizoid personality F60.1
Schizophrenia, schizophrenic F20.9
  acute (brief) (undifferentiated) F23
  atypical (form) F20.3
  borderline F21
  catalepsy F20.2
  catatonic (type) (excited) (withdrawn) F20.2
  cenesthopathic, cenesthesiopathic F20.89
  childhood type F20.9
  chronic undifferentiated F20.9
  cyclic F25.0
  disorganized (type) F20.1
  flexibilitas cerea F20.2

Schizophrenia, schizophrenic — continued
hebephrenic (type) F20.1
incipient F21
latent F21
negative type F20.5
paranoid (type) F20.0
paraphrenic F20.0
post-psychotic depression F32.89
prepsychotic F21
prodromal F21
pseudoneurotic F21
pseudopsychopathic F21
reaction F23
residual (state) (type) F20.5
restzustand F20.5
schizoaffective (type) — see Psychosis, schizoaffective
simple (type) F20.89
simplex F20.89
specified type NEC F20.89
spectrum and other psychotic disorder F29
  specified NEC F28
stupor F20.2
syndrome of childhood F84.5
undifferentiated (type) F20.3
  chronic F20.5
Schizothymia (persistent) F60.1
Schlatter-Osgood disease or osteochondrosis M92.52- ☑
Schlatter's tibia — see Osteochondrosis, juvenile, tibia
Schmidt's syndrome (polyglandular, autoimmune) E31.0
Schmincke's carcinoma or tumor — see Neoplasm, nasopharynx, malignant
Schmitz (-Stutzer) **dysentery** A03.0
Schmorl's disease or nodes
  lumbar region M51.46
  lumbosacral region M51.47
  sacrococcygeal region M53.3
  thoracic region M51.44
  thoracolumbar region M51.45
Schneiderian
  papilloma — see Neoplasm, nasopharynx, benign
    specified site — see Neoplasm, benign, by site
    unspecified site D14.0
  specified site — see Neoplasm, malignant, by site
    unspecified site C30.0
Scholte's syndrome (malignant carcinoid) E34.09
Scholz (-Bielchowsky-Henneberg) **disease or syndrome** E75.25
Schonlein (-Henoch) disease or purpura (primary) (rheumatic) D69.0
Schottmuller's disease A01.4
Schroeder's syndrome (endocrine hypertensive) E27.0
Schuller-Christian disease or syndrome C96.5
Schultze's type acroparesthesia, simple I73.89
Schultz's disease or syndrome — see Agranulocytosis
Schwalbe-Ziehen-Oppenheim disease G24.1
Schwannoma — see also Neoplasm, nerve, benign
  malignant — see also Neoplasm, nerve, malignant
    with rhabdomyoblastic differentiation — see Neoplasm, nerve, malignant
  melanocytic — see Neoplasm, nerve, benign
  pigmented — see Neoplasm, nerve, benign
Schwannomatosis Q85.03
Schwartz (-Jampel) **syndrome** G71.13
Schwartz-Bartter syndrome E22.2
Schweninger-Buzzi anetoderma L90.1
Sciatic — see condition
Sciatica (infective) M54.3- ☑
  with lumbago M54.4- ☑
  due to intervertebral disc disorder — see Disorder, disc, with, radiculopathy
  due to displacement of intervertebral disc (with lumbago) — see Disorder, disc, with, radiculopathy
  wallet M54.3- ☑
Scimitar syndrome Q26.8
Sclera — see condition
Sclerectasia H15.84- ☑
Scleredema
  adultorum — see Sclerosis, systemic
  Buschke's — see Sclerosis, systemic
  newborn P83.0
Sclerema (adiposum) (edematosum) (neonatorum) (newborn) P83.0
  adultorum — see Sclerosis, systemic
Scleriasis — see Scleroderma
Scleritis H15.00- ☑
  with corneal involvement H15.04- ☑
  anterior H15.01- ☑
  brawny H15.02- ☑

☑ Additional Character Required — Refer to the Tabular List for Character Selection

Scleritis — *continued*
  in (due to) zoster B02.34
  posterior H15.03-
  specified type NEC H15.09- ☑
  syphilitic A52.71
  tuberculous (nodular) A18.51
Sclerochoroiditis H31.8
Scleroconjunctivitis — *see* Scleritis
Sclerocystic ovary syndrome E28.2
Sclerodactyly, sclerodactylia L94.3
Scleroderma, sclerodermia (acrosclerotic) (diffuse) (generalized) (progressive) (pulmonary) — *see also* Sclerosis, systemic M34.9
  circumscribed L94.0
  linear L94.1
  localized L94.0
  newborn P83.88
  systemic M34.9
Sclerokeratitis H16.8
  tuberculous A18.52
Scleroma nasi A48.8
Scleromalacia (perforans) H15.05- ☑
Scleromyxedema L98.5
Sclerose en plaques G35
Sclerosis, sclerotic
  adrenal (gland) E27.8
  Alzheimer's — *see* Disease, Alzheimer's
  amyotrophic (lateral) G12.21
  aorta, aortic I70.0
    valve — *see* Endocarditis, aortic
  artery, arterial, arteriolar, arteriovascular — *see* Arteriosclerosis
  ascending multiple G35
  brain (generalized) (lobular) G37.9
    artery, arterial I67.2
    diffuse G37.0
    disseminated G35
    insular G35
    Krabbe's E75.23
    miliary G35
    multiple G35
    presenile (Alzheimer's) — *see* Disease, Alzheimer's, early onset
    senile (arteriosclerotic) I67.2
    stem, multiple G35
    tuberous Q85.1
  bulbar, multiple G35
  bundle of His I44.39
  cardiac — *see* Disease, heart, ischemic, atherosclerotic
  cardiorenal — *see* Hypertension, cardiorenal
  cardiovascular — *see also* Disease, cardiovascular
    renal — *see* Hypertension, cardiorenal
  cerebellar — *see* Sclerosis, brain
  cerebral — *see* Sclerosis, brain
  cerebrospinal (disseminated) (multiple) G35
  cerebrovascular I67.2
  choroid — *see* Degeneration, choroid
  combined (spinal cord) — *see also* Degeneration, combined
    multiple G35
  concentric (Balo) G37.5
  cornea — *see* Opacity, cornea
  coronary (artery) I25.10
    with angina pectoris — *see* Arteriosclerosis, coronary (artery),
  corpus cavernosum
    female N90.89
    male N48.6
  diffuse (brain) (spinal cord) G37.0
  disseminated G35
  dorsal G35
  dorsolateral (spinal cord) — *see* Degeneration, combined
  endometrium N85.5
  extrapyramidal G25.9
  eye, nuclear (senile) — *see* Cataract, senile, nuclear
  focal and segmental (glomerular) — *see also* N00-N07
    with fourth character .1 N05.1
  Friedreich's (spinal cord) G11.11
  funicular (spermatic cord) N50.89
  general (vascular) — *see* Arteriosclerosis
  gland (lymphatic) I89.8
  hepatic K74.1
    alcoholic K70.2
  hereditary
    cerebellar G11.9
    spinal (Friedreich's ataxia) G11.11
  hippocampal G93.81
  insular G35
  kidney — *see* Sclerosis, renal

Sclerosis, sclerotic — *continued*
  larynx J38.7
  lateral (amyotrophic) (descending) (spinal) G12.21
    primary G12.23
  lens, senile nuclear — *see* Cataract, senile, nuclear
  liver K74.1
    with fibrosis K74.2
      alcoholic K70.2
    alcoholic K70.2
    cardiac K76.1
  lung — *see* Fibrosis, lung
  mastoid — *see* Mastoiditis, chronic
  mesial temporal G93.81
  mitral I05.8
  Monckeberg's (medial) — *see* Arteriosclerosis, extremities
  multiple (brain stem) (cerebral) (generalized) (spinal cord) G35
  myocardium, myocardial — *see* Disease, heart, ischemic, atherosclerotic
  nuclear (senile), eye — *see* Cataract, senile, nuclear
  ovary N83.8
  pancreas K86.89
  penis N48.6
  peripheral arteries — *see* Arteriosclerosis, extremities
  plaques G35
  pluriglandular E31.8
  polyglandular E31.8
  posterolateral (spinal cord) — *see* Degeneration, combined
  presenile (Alzheimer's) — *see* Disease, Alzheimer's, early onset
  primary, lateral G12.23
  progressive, systemic M34.0
  pulmonary — *see* Fibrosis, lung
    artery I27.0
    valve (heart) — *see* Endocarditis, pulmonary
  renal N26.9
    with
      cystine storage disease E72.09
      hypertensive heart disease (conditions in I11) — *see* Hypertension, cardiorenal
      arteriolar (hyaline) (hyperplastic) — *see* Hypertension, kidney
  retina (senile) (vascular) H35.00
  senile (vascular) — *see* Arteriosclerosis
  spinal (cord) (progressive) G95.89
    ascending G61.0
    combined — *see also* Degeneration, combined
      multiple G35
      syphilitic A52.11
    disseminated G35
    dorsolateral — *see* Degeneration, combined
    hereditary (Friedreich's) (mixed form) G11.11
    lateral (amyotrophic) G12.21
      progressive G12.23
    multiple G35
    posterior (syphilitic) A52.11
  stomach K31.89
  subendocardial, congenital I42.4
  systemic M34.9
    with
      lung involvement M34.81
      myopathy M34.82
      polyneuropathy M34.83
    drug-induced M34.2
    due to chemicals NEC M34.2
    progressive M34.0
    specified NEC M34.89
  temporal (mesial) G93.81
  tricuspid (heart) (valve) I07.8
  tuberous (brain) Q85.1
  tympanic membrane — *see* Disorder, tympanic membrane, specified NEC
  valve, valvular (heart) — *see* Endocarditis
  vascular — *see* Arteriosclerosis
  vein I87.8
Scoliosis (acquired) (postural) M41.9
  adolescent (idiopathic) — *see* Scoliosis, idiopathic, adolescent
  congenital Q67.5
    due to bony malformation Q76.3
    failure of segmentation (hemivertebra) Q76.3
    hemivertebra fusion Q76.3
    postural Q67.5
  degenerative M41.5- ☑
  idiopathic M41.20
    adolescent M41.129
      cervical region M41.122
      cervicothoracic region M41.123

Scoliosis — *continued*
  idiopathic — *continued*
    adolescent — *continued*
      lumbar region M41.126
      lumbosacral region M41.127
      thoracic region M41.124
      thoracolumbar region M41.125
    cervical region M41.22
    cervicothoracic region M41.23
    infantile M41.00
      cervical region M41.02
      cervicothoracic region M41.03
      lumbar region M41.06
      lumbosacral region M41.07
      sacrococcygeal M41.08
      thoracic region M41.04
      thoracolumbar region M41.05
    juvenile M41.119
      cervical region M41.112
      cervicothoracic region M41.113
      lumbar region M41.116
      lumbosacral region M41.117
      thoracic region M41.114
      thoracolumbar region M41.115
    lumbar region M41.26
    lumbosacral region M41.27
    thoracic region M41.24
    thoracolumbar region M41.25
  infantile — *see* Scoliosis, idiopathic, infantile
  neuromuscular M41.40
    cervical region M41.42
    cervicothoracic region M41.43
    lumbar region M41.46
    lumbosacral region M41.47
    occipito-atlanto-axial region M41.41
    thoracic region M41.44
    thoracolumbar region M41.45
  paralytic — *see* Scoliosis, neuromuscular
  postprocedural M96.89
  postradiation therapy M96.5
  rachitic (late effect or sequelae) E64.3 *[M49.80]*
    cervical region E64.3 *[M49.82]*
    cervicothoracic region E64.3 *[M49.83]*
    lumbar region E64.3 *[M49.86]*
    lumbosacral region E64.3 *[M49.87]*
    multiple sites E64.3 *[M49.89]*
    occipito-atlanto-axial region E64.3 *[M49.81]*
    sacrococcygeal region E64.3 *[M49.88]*
    thoracic region E64.3 *[M49.84]*
    thoracolumbar region E64.3 *[M49.85]*
  sciatic M54.4- ☑
  secondary (to) NEC M41.50
    cerebral palsy, Friedreich's ataxia, poliomyelitis, neuromuscular disorders — *see* Scoliosis, neuromuscular
    cervical region M41.52
    cervicothoracic region M41.53
    lumbar region M41.56
    lumbosacral region M41.57
    thoracic region M41.54
    thoracolumbar region M41.55
  specified form NEC M41.80
    cervical region M41.82
    cervicothoracic region M41.83
    lumbar region M41.86
    lumbosacral region M41.87
    thoracic region M41.84
    thoracolumbar region M41.85
  thoracogenic M41.30
    thoracic region M41.34
    thoracolumbar region M41.35
  tuberculous A18.01
Scoliotic pelvis
  with disproportion (fetopelvic) O33.0
    causing obstructed labor O65.0
Scorbutus, scorbutic — *see also* Scurvy
  anemia D53.2
Score, NIHSS (National Institutes of Health Stroke Scale) R29.7- ☑
Scotoma (arcuate) (Bjerrum) (central) (ring) — *see also* Defect, visual field, localized, scotoma
  scintillating H53.12- ☑
Scratch — *see* Abrasion
Scratchy throat R09.89
Screening (for) Z13.9
  alcoholism Z13.39
  anemia Z13.0
  anomaly, congenital Z13.89

Screening — *continued*
- antenatal, of mother — *see also* Encounter, antenatal
  - screening Z36.9
- arterial hypertension Z13.6
- arthropod-borne viral disease NEC Z11.59
- autism Z13.41
- bacteriuria, asymptomatic Z13.89
- behavioral disorder Z13.30
  - specified NEC Z13.39
- brain injury, traumatic Z13.850
- bronchitis, chronic Z13.83
- brucellosis Z11.2
- cardiovascular disorder Z13.6
- cataract Z13.5
- chlamydial diseases Z11.8
- cholera Z11.0
- chromosomal abnormalities (nonprocreative) NEC Z13.79
- colonoscopy Z12.11
- congenital
  - dislocation of hip Z13.89
  - eye disorder Z13.5
  - malformation or deformation Z13.89
- contamination NEC Z13.88
- coronavirus (disease) (novel) 2019 Z11.52
- COVID-19 Z11.52
- cystic fibrosis Z13.228
- dengue fever Z11.59
- dental disorder Z13.84
- depression (adult) (adolescent) (child) Z13.31
  - maternal Z13.32
  - perinatal Z13.32
- developmental
  - delays Z13.40
    - global (milestones) Z13.42
    - specified NEC Z13.49
  - handicap Z13.42
    - in early childhood Z13.42
- diabetes mellitus Z13.1
- diphtheria Z11.2
- disability, intellectual Z13.39
- disease or disorder Z13.9
  - bacterial NEC Z11.2
    - intestinal infectious Z11.0
    - respiratory tuberculosis Z11.1
  - behavioral Z13.30
    - specified NEC Z13.39
  - blood or blood-forming organ Z13.0
  - cardiovascular Z13.6
  - Chagas' Z11.6
  - chlamydial Z11.8
  - coronavirus (novel) 2019 Z11.52
  - COVID-19 Z11.52
  - dental Z13.89
  - developmental delays Z13.40
    - global (milestones) Z13.42
    - specified NEC Z13.49
  - digestive tract NEC Z13.818
    - lower GI Z13.811
    - upper GI Z13.810
  - ear Z13.5
  - endocrine Z13.29
  - eye Z13.5
  - genitourinary Z13.89
  - heart Z13.6
  - human immunodeficiency virus (HIV) infection Z11.4
  - immunity Z13.0
  - infection
    - intestinal Z11.0
      - specified NEC Z11.6
  - infectious Z11.9
  - mental health and behavioral Z13.30
    - specified NEC Z13.39
  - metabolic Z13.228
  - neurological Z13.89
  - nutritional Z13.21
    - metabolic Z13.228
      - lipoid disorders Z13.220
  - protozoal Z11.6
    - intestinal Z11.0
  - respiratory Z13.83
  - rheumatic Z13.828
  - rickettsial Z11.8
  - sexually-transmitted NEC Z11.3
    - human immunodeficiency virus (HIV) Z11.4
  - sickle-cell (trait) Z13.0
  - skin Z13.89
  - specified NEC Z13.89
  - spirochetal Z11.8
  - thyroid Z13.29

Screening — *continued*
- disease or disorder — *continued*
  - vascular Z13.6
  - venereal Z11.3
  - viral NEC Z11.59
    - coronavirus (novel) 2019 Z11.52
    - COVID-19 Z11.52
    - human immunodeficiency virus (HIV) Z11.4
    - intestinal Z11.0
    - SARS-CoV-2 Z11.52
- elevated titer Z13.89
- emphysema Z13.83
- encephalitis, viral (mosquito- or tick-borne) Z11.59
- exposure to contaminants (toxic) Z13.88
- fever
  - dengue Z11.59
  - hemorrhagic Z11.59
  - yellow Z11.59
- filariasis Z11.6
- galactosemia Z13.228
- gastrointestinal condition Z13.818
- genetic (nonprocreative) - for procreative management
  - — *see* Testing, genetic, for procreative management
  - disease carrier status (nonprocreative) Z13.71
  - specified NEC (nonprocreative) Z13.79
- genitourinary condition Z13.89
- glaucoma Z13.5
- gonorrhea Z11.3
- gout Z13.89
- helminthiasis (intestinal) Z11.6
- hematopoietic malignancy Z12.89
- hemoglobinopathies NEC Z13.0
- hemorrhagic fever Z11.59
- Hodgkin disease Z12.89
- human immunodeficiency virus (HIV) Z11.4
- human papillomavirus Z11.51
- hypertension Z13.6
- immunity disorders Z13.0
- infant or child (over 28 days old) Z00.129
  - with abnormal findings Z00.121
- infection
  - mycotic Z11.8
  - parasitic Z11.8
- ingestion of radioactive substance Z13.88
- intellectual disability Z13.39
- intestinal
  - helminthiasis Z11.6
  - infectious disease Z11.0
- leishmaniasis Z11.6
- leprosy Z11.2
- leptospirosis Z11.8
- leukemia Z12.89
- lymphoma Z12.89
- malaria Z11.6
- malnutrition Z13.29
  - metabolic Z13.228
  - nutritional Z13.21
- measles Z11.59
- mental health disorder Z13.30
  - specified NEC Z13.39
- metabolic errors, inborn Z13.228
- multiphasic Z13.89
- musculoskeletal disorder Z13.828
  - osteoporosis Z13.820
- mycoses Z11.8
- myocardial infarction (acute) Z13.6
- neoplasm (malignant) (of) Z12.9
  - bladder Z12.6
  - blood Z12.89
  - breast Z12.39
    - routine mammogram Z12.31
  - cervix Z12.4
  - colon Z12.11
  - genitourinary organs NEC Z12.79
    - bladder Z12.6
    - cervix Z12.4
    - ovary Z12.73
    - prostate Z12.5
    - testis Z12.71
    - vagina Z12.72
  - hematopoietic system Z12.89
  - intestinal tract Z12.10
    - colon Z12.11
    - rectum Z12.12
    - small intestine Z12.13
  - lung Z12.2
  - lymph (glands) Z12.89
  - nervous system Z12.82

Screening — *continued*
- neoplasm — *continued*
  - oral cavity Z12.81
  - prostate Z12.5
  - rectum Z12.12
  - respiratory organs Z12.2
  - skin Z12.83
  - small intestine Z12.13
  - specified site NEC Z12.89
  - stomach Z12.0
- nephropathy Z13.89
- nervous system disorders NEC Z13.858
- neurological condition Z13.89
- osteoporosis Z13.820
- parasitic infestation Z11.9
  - specified NEC Z11.8
- phenylketonuria Z13.228
- plague Z11.2
- poisoning (chemical) (heavy metal) Z13.88
- poliomyelitis Z11.59
- postnatal, chromosomal abnormalities Z13.89
- prenatal, of mother — *see also* Encounter, antenatal
  - screening Z36.9
- protozoal disease Z11.6
  - intestinal Z11.0
- pulmonary tuberculosis Z11.1
- radiation exposure Z13.88
- respiratory condition Z13.83
- respiratory tuberculosis Z11.1
- rheumatoid arthritis Z13.828
- rubella Z11.59
- SARS-CoV-2 Z11.52
- schistosomiasis Z11.6
- sexually-transmitted disease NEC Z11.3
  - human immunodeficiency virus (HIV) Z11.4
- sickle-cell disease or trait Z13.0
- skin condition Z13.89
- sleeping sickness Z11.6
- special Z13.9
  - specified NEC Z13.89
- syphilis Z11.3
- tetanus Z11.2
- trachoma Z11.8
- traumatic brain injury Z13.850
- trypanosomiasis Z11.6
- tuberculosis, respiratory Z11.1
  - active Z11.1
  - latent Z11.7
- venereal disease Z11.3
- viral encephalitis (mosquito- or tick-borne) Z11.59
- whooping cough Z11.2
- worms, intestinal Z11.6
- yaws Z11.8
- yellow fever Z11.59

Scrofula, scrofulosis (tuberculosis of cervical lymph glands) A18.2
Scrofulide (primary) (tuberculous) A18.4
Scrofuloderma, scrofulodermia (any site) (primary) A18.4
Scrofulosus lichen (primary) (tuberculous) A18.4
Scrofulous — *see* condition
Scrotal tongue K14.5
Scrotum — *see* condition
Scurvy, scorbutic E54
- anemia D53.2
- gum E54
- infantile E54
- rickets E55.0 *[M90.80]*
Sealpox B08.62
Seasickness T75.3 ☑
Seatworm (infection) (infestation) B80
Sebaceous — *see also* condition
- cyst — *see* Cyst, sebaceous
Seborrhea, seborrheic L21.9
- capillitii R23.8
- capitis L21.0
- dermatitis L21.9
  - infantile L21.1
- eczema L21.9
  - infantile L21.1
- sicca L21.0
Seckel's syndrome Q87.19
Seclusion, pupil — *see* Membrane, pupillary
Second hand tobacco smoke exposure (acute) (chronic) Z77.22
- in the perinatal period P96.81
Secondary
- dentin (in pulp) K04.3
- neoplasm, secondaries — *see* Table of Neoplasms, secondary

Secretion
- antidiuretic hormone, inappropriate E22.2
- catecholamine, by pheochromocytoma — *see also* Pheochromocytoma, by type E27.5
- hormone
  - antidiuretic, inappropriate (syndrome) E22.2
  - by
    - carcinoid tumor — *see also* Tumor, carcinoid E34.09
    - pheochromocytoma — *see also* Pheochromocytoma, by type E27.5
  - ectopic NEC E34.2
- urinary
  - excessive R35.89
  - suppression R34

Section
- nerve, traumatic — *see* Injury, nerve

Sedative, hypnotic, or anxiolytic-induced
- anxiety disorder F13.980
- bipolar and related disorder F13.94
- delirium F13.921
- depressive disorder F13.94
- major neurocognitive disorder F13.97
- mild neurocognitive disorder F13.988
- psychotic disorder F13.959
- sexual dysfunction F13.981
- sleep disorder F13.982

Segmentation, incomplete (congenital) — *see also* Fusion
- bone NEC Q78.8
- lumbosacral (joint) (vertebra) Q76.49

SEID (systemic exertion intolerance disease) G93.32

Seitelberger's syndrome (infantile neuraxonal dystrophy) G31.89

Seizure(s) — *see also* Convulsions R56.9
- absence G40.A- ☑ (*following* G40.3)
- akinetic — *see* Epilepsy, generalized, specified NEC
- atonic — *see* Epilepsy, generalized, specified NEC
- autonomic (hysterical) F44.5
- convulsive — *see* Convulsions
- cortical (focal) (motor) — *see* Epilepsy, localization-related, symptomatic, with simple partial seizures
- disorder — *see also* Epilepsy G40.909
- due to stroke — *see* Sequelae (of), disease, cerebrovascular, by type, specified NEC
- epileptic — *see* Epilepsy
- febrile (simple) R56.00
  - with status epilepticus G40.901
  - complex (atypical) (complicated) R56.01
    - with status epilepticus G40.901
- grand mal G40.409
  - intractable G40.419
    - with status epilepticus G40.411
    - without status epilepticus G40.419
  - not intractable G40.409
    - with status epilepticus G40.401
    - without status epilepticus G40.409
- heart — *see* Disease, heart
- hysterical F44.5
- intractable G40.919
  - with status epilepticus G40.911
- Jacksonian (focal) (motor type) (sensory type) — *see* Epilepsy, localization-related, symptomatic, with simple partial seizures
- newborn P90
- nonspecific epileptic
  - atonic — *see* Epilepsy, generalized, specified NEC
  - clonic — *see* Epilepsy, generalized, specified NEC
  - myoclonic — *see* Epilepsy, generalized, specified NEC
  - tonic — *see* Epilepsy, generalized, specified NEC
  - tonic-clonic — *see* Epilepsy, generalized, specified NEC
- partial, developing into secondarily generalized seizures
  - complex — *see* Epilepsy, localization-related, symptomatic, with complex partial seizures
  - simple — *see* Epilepsy, localization-related, symptomatic, with simple partial seizures
- petit mal G40.A- ☑ (*following* G40.3)
  - intractable G40.A1- ☑ (*following* G40.3)
    - with status epilepticus G40.A11 (*following* G40.3)
    - without status epilepticus G40.A19 (*following* G40.3)
  - not intractable G40.A0- ☑ (*following* G40.3)
    - with status epilepticus G40.A01 (*following* G40.3)
    - without status epilepticus G40.A09 (*following* G40.3)
- post traumatic R56.1
- recurrent G40.909
- specified NEC G40.89

Seizure(s) — *continued*
- uncinate — *see* Epilepsy, localization-related, symptomatic, with complex partial seizures

Selenium deficiency, dietary E59

Self-damaging behavior (life-style) Z72.89

Self-harm (attempted)
- history (personal)
  - in family Z81.8
  - nonsuicidal Z91.52
  - suicidal Z91.51
- nonsuicidal R45.88

Self-injury, nonsuicidal R45.88
- personal history Z91.52

Self-mutilation (attempted)
- history (personal)
  - in family Z81.8
  - nonsuicidal Z91.52
  - suicidal Z91.51
- nonsuicidal R45.88

Self-poisoning
- history (personal) Z91.51
  - in family Z81.8
- observation following (alleged) attempt Z03.6

Semicoma R40.1

Seminal vesiculitis N49.0

Seminoma C62.9- ☑
- specified site — *see* Neoplasm, malignant, by site

Senear-Usher disease or syndrome L10.4

Senectus R54

Senescence (without mention of psychosis) R54

Senile, senility — *see also* condition R41.81
- with
  - acute confusional state F05
  - mental changes NOS F03 ☑
  - psychosis NEC — *see* Psychosis, senile
- asthenia R54
- cervix (atrophic) N88.8
- debility R54
- endometrium (atrophic) N85.8
- fallopian tube (atrophic) — *see* Atrophy, fallopian tube
- heart (failure) R54
- ovary (atrophic) — *see* Atrophy, ovary
- premature E34.8
- vagina, vaginitis (atrophic) N95.2
- wart L82.1

Sensation
- burning (skin) R20.8
  - tongue K14.6
- foreign body R09.A0
  - eye H57.8A- ☑
  - globus R09.A2
  - nose R09.A1
  - specified site NEC R09.A9
  - throat R09.A2
- loss of R20.8
- prickling (skin) R20.2
- tingling (skin) R20.2

Sense loss
- smell — *see* Disturbance, sensation, smell
- taste — *see* Disturbance, sensation, taste
- touch R20.8

Sensibility disturbance (cortical) (deep) (vibratory) R20.9

Sensitive, sensitivity — *see also* Allergy
- carotid sinus G90.01
- child (excessive) F93.8
- cold, autoimmune D59.12
- dentin K03.89
- gluten (non-celiac) K90.41
- latex Z91.040
- methemoglobin D74.8
- tuberculin, without clinical or radiological symptoms R76.11
- visual
  - glare H53.71
  - impaired contrast H53.72

Sensitiver Beziehungswahn F22

Sensitization, auto-erythrocytic D69.2

Separation
- anxiety, abnormal (of childhood) F93.0
- apophysis, traumatic — *code as* Fracture, by site
- choroid — *see* Detachment, choroid
- epiphysis, epiphyseal
  - nontraumatic — *see also* Osteochondropathy, specified type NEC
    - upper femoral — *see* Slipped, epiphysis, upper femoral
  - traumatic — *code as* Fracture, by site
- fracture — *see* Fracture

Separation — *continued*
- infundibulum cardiac from right ventricle by a partition Q24.3
- joint (traumatic) (current) — *code by* site under Dislocation
- muscle (nontraumatic) — *see* Diastasis, muscle
- pubic bone, obstetrical trauma O71.6
- retina, retinal — *see* Detachment, retina
- symphysis pubis, obstetrical trauma O71.6
- tracheal ring, incomplete, congenital Q32.1

Sepsis (generalized) (unspecified organism) A41.9
- with
  - organ dysfunction (acute) (multiple) R65.20
    - with septic shock R65.21
- Acinetobacter baumannii A41.54
- actinomycotic A42.7
- adrenal hemorrhage syndrome (meningococcal) A39.1
- anaerobic A41.4
- Bacillus anthracis A22.7
- Brucella — *see also* Brucellosis A23.9
- candidal B37.7
- Cronobacter A41.59
- cryptogenic A41.9
- due to device, implant or graft T85.79 ☑
  - arterial graft NEC T82.7 ☑
  - breast (implant) T85.79 ☑
  - catheter NEC T85.79 ☑
    - dialysis (renal) T82.7 ☑
      - intraperitoneal T85.71 ☑
    - infusion NEC T82.7 ☑
      - spinal (cranial) (epidural) (intrathecal) (spinal) (subarachnoid) (subdural) T85.735 ☑
    - urethral indwelling T83.511 ☑
    - urinary T83.518 ☑
  - ectopic or molar pregnancy O08.82
  - electronic (electrode) (pulse generator) (stimulator)
    - bone T84.7 ☑
    - cardiac T82.7 ☑
    - nervous system T85.738 ☑
      - brain T85.731 ☑
      - neurostimulator generator T85.734 ☑
      - peripheral nerve T85.732 ☑
      - spinal cord T85.733 ☑
    - urinary T83.590 ☑
  - fixation, internal (orthopedic) — *see* Complication, fixation device, infection
  - gastrointestinal (bile duct) (esophagus) T85.79 ☑
    - neurostimulator electrode (lead) T85.732 ☑
  - genital T83.69 ☑
  - heart NEC T82.7 ☑
    - valve (prosthesis) T82.6 ☑
      - graft T82.7 ☑
  - joint prosthesis — *see* Complication, joint prosthesis, infection
  - ocular (corneal graft) (orbital implant) T85.79 ☑
  - orthopedic NEC T84.7 ☑
    - fixation device, internal — *see* Complication, fixation device, infection
  - specified NEC T85.79 ☑
  - vascular T82.7 ☑
  - ventricular intracranial (communicating) shunt T85.730 ☑
- during labor O75.3
- Enterococcus A41.81
- Erysipelothrix (rhusiopathiae) (erysipeloid) A26.7
- Escherichia coli (E. coli) A41.51
- extraintestinal yersiniosis A28.2
- following
  - abortion (subsequent episode) O08.0
    - current episode — *see* Abortion
  - ectopic or molar pregnancy O08.82
  - immunization T88.0 ☑
  - infusion, therapeutic injection or transfusion NEC T80.29 ☑
  - obstetrical procedure O86.04
- gangrenous A41.9
- gonococcal A54.86
- Gram-negative (organism) A41.50
  - anaerobic A41.4
- Haemophilus influenzae A41.3
- herpesviral B00.7
- intra-abdominal K65.1
- intraocular — *see* Endophthalmitis, purulent
- Listeria monocytogenes A32.7
- localized — *code to* specific localized infection
  - in operation wound T81.49 ☑
  - skin — *see* Abscess

Sepsis — *continued*
  malleus A24.0
  melioidosis A24.1
  meningeal — *see* Meningitis
  meningococcal A39.4
    acute A39.2
    chronic A39.3
  MRSA (Methicillin resistant Staphylococcus aureus) A41.02
  MSSA (Methicillin susceptible Staphylococcus aureus) A41.01
  newborn P36.9
    due to
      anaerobes NEC P36.5
      Escherichia coli P36.4
      Staphylococcus P36.30
        aureus P36.2
        specified NEC P36.39
      Streptococcus P36.10
        group B P36.0
        specified NEC P36.19
    specified NEC P36.8
  other gram-negative A41.59
  Pasteurella multocida A28.0
  pelvic, puerperal, postpartum, childbirth O85
  pneumococcal A40.3
  postprocedural T81.44 ☑
  Pseudomonas (pseudomonas aeruginosa) A41.52
  puerperal, postpartum, childbirth (pelvic) O85
  Salmonella (arizonae) (cholerae-suis) (enteritidis) (typhimurium) A02.1
  Serratia A41.53
  severe R65.20
    with septic shock R65.21
  Shigella — *see also* Dysentery, bacillary A03.9
  skin, localized — *see* Abscess
  specified organism NEC A41.89
  Staphylococcus, staphylococcal A41.2
    aureus (methicillin susceptible) (MSSA) A41.01
      methicillin resistant (MRSA) A41.02
    coagulase-negative A41.1
    specified NEC A41.1
  Streptococcus, streptococcal A40.9
    agalactiae A40.1
    group
      A A40.0
      B A40.1
      D A41.81
    neonatal P36.10
      group B P36.0
      specified NEC P36.19
    pneumoniae A40.3
    pyogenes A40.0
    specified NEC A40.8
  tracheostomy stoma J95.02
  tularemic A21.7
  umbilical, umbilical cord (newborn) — *see* Sepsis, newborn
  Yersinia pestis A20.7
Septate — *see* Septum
Septic — *see* condition
  arm — *see* Cellulitis, upper limb
    with lymphangitis — *see* Lymphangitis, acute, upper limb
  embolus — *see* Embolism
  finger — *see* Cellulitis, digit
    with lymphangitis — *see* Lymphangitis, acute, digit
  foot — *see* Cellulitis, lower limb
    with lymphangitis — *see* Lymphangitis, acute, lower limb
  gallbladder (acute) K81.0
  hand — *see* Cellulitis, upper limb
    with lymphangitis — *see* Lymphangitis, acute, upper limb
  joint — *see* Arthritis, pyogenic or pyemic
  leg — *see* Cellulitis, lower limb
    with lymphangitis — *see* Lymphangitis, acute, lower limb
  nail — *see also* Cellulitis, digit
    with lymphangitis — *see* Lymphangitis, acute, digit
  sore — *see also* Abscess
    throat J02.0
      streptococcal J02.0
  spleen (acute) D73.89
  teeth, tooth (pulpal origin) K04.4
  throat — *see* Pharyngitis
  thrombus — *see* Thrombosis
  toe — *see* Cellulitis, digit
    with lymphangitis — *see* Lymphangitis, acute, digit

Septic — *continued*
  tonsils, chronic J35.01
    with adenoiditis J35.03
  uterus — *see* Endometritis
Septicemia A41.9
  meaning sepsis — *see* Sepsis
Septum, septate (congenital) — *see also* Anomaly, by site
  anal Q42.3
    with fistula Q42.2
  aqueduct of Sylvius Q03.0
    with spina bifida — *see* Spina bifida, by site, with hydrocephalus
  uterus Q51.28
    complete Q51.21
    partial Q51.22
    specified NEC Q51.28
  vagina Q52.10
    in pregnancy — *see* Pregnancy, complicated by, abnormal vagina
      causing obstructed labor O65.5
    longitudinal Q52.129
      microperforate
        left side Q52.124
        right side Q52.123
      nonobstruction Q52.120
      obstructing Q52.129
        left side Q52.122
        right side Q52.121
    transverse Q52.11
Sequelae (of) — *see also* condition
  abscess, intracranial or intraspinal (conditions in G06) G09
  amputation — *code to* injury with seventh character S
  burn and corrosion — *code to* injury with seventh character S
  calcium deficiency E64.8
  cerebrovascular disease — *see* Sequelae, disease, cerebrovascular
  childbirth O94
  contusion — *code to* injury with seventh character S
  corrosion — *see* Sequelae, burn and corrosion
  COVID-19 (post acute) U09.9
  crushing injury — *code to* injury with seventh character S
  disease
    cerebrovascular I69.90
      alteration of sensation I69.998
      aphasia I69.920
      apraxia I69.990
      ataxia I69.993
      cognitive deficits I69.91 ☑
      disturbance of vision I69.998
      dysarthria I69.922
      dysphagia I69.991
      dysphasia I69.921
      facial droop I69.992
      facial weakness I69.992
      fluency disorder I69.923
      hemiplegia I69.95- ☑
      hemorrhage
        intracerebral — *see* Sequelae, hemorrhage, intracerebral
        intracranial, nontraumatic NEC — *see* Sequelae, hemorrhage, intracranial, nontraumatic
        subarachnoid — *see* Sequelae, hemorrhage, subarachnoid
      language deficit I69.928
      monoplegia
        lower limb I69.94- ☑
        upper limb I69.93- ☑
      paralytic syndrome I69.96- ☑
      specified effect NEC I69.998
      specified type NEC I69.80
        alteration of sensation I69.898
        aphasia I69.820
        apraxia I69.890
        ataxia I69.893
        cognitive deficits I69.81 ☑
        disturbance of vision I69.898
        dysarthria I69.822
        dysphagia I69.891
        dysphasia I69.821
        facial droop I69.892
        facial weakness I69.892
        fluency disorder I69.823
        hemiplegia I69.85- ☑
        language deficit I69.828

Sequelae — *continued*
  disease — *continued*
    cerebrovascular — *continued*
      specified type — *continued*
        monoplegia
          lower limb I69.84- ☑
          upper limb I69.83- ☑
        paralytic syndrome I69.86- ☑
        specified effect NEC I69.898
      speech deficit I69.928
      speech deficit I69.828
      stroke NOS — *see* Sequelae, stroke NOS
  dislocation — *code to* injury with seventh character S
  encephalitis or encephalomyelitis (conditions in G04) G09
    in infectious disease NEC B94.8
    viral B94.1
  external cause — *code to* injury with seventh character S
  foreign body entering natural orifice — *code to* injury with seventh character S
  fracture — *code to* injury with seventh character S
  frostbite — *code to* injury with seventh character S
  Hansen's disease B92
  hemorrhage
    intracerebral I69.10
      alteration of sensation I69.198
      aphasia I69.120
      apraxia I69.190
      ataxia I69.193
      cognitive deficits I69.11 ☑
      disturbance of vision I69.198
      dysarthria I69.122
      dysphagia I69.191
      dysphasia I69.121
      facial droop I69.192
      facial weakness I69.192
      fluency disorder I69.123
      hemiplegia I69.15- ☑
      language deficit NEC I69.128
      monoplegia
        lower limb I69.14- ☑
        upper limb I69.13- ☑
      paralytic syndrome I69.16- ☑
      specified effect NEC I69.198
      speech deficit NEC I69.128
    intracranial, nontraumatic NEC I69.20
      alteration of sensation I69.298
      aphasia I69.220
      apraxia I69.290
      ataxia I69.293
      cognitive deficits I69.21 ☑
      disturbance of vision I69.298
      dysarthria I69.222
      dysphagia I69.291
      dysphasia I69.221
      facial droop I69.292
      facial weakness I69.292
      fluency disorder I69.223
      hemiplegia I69.25- ☑
      language deficit NEC I69.228
      monoplegia
        lower limb I69.24- ☑
        upper limb I69.23- ☑
      paralytic syndrome I69.26- ☑
      specified effect NEC I69.298
      speech deficit NEC I69.228
    subarachnoid I69.00
      alteration of sensation I69.098
      aphasia I69.020
      apraxia I69.090
      ataxia I69.093
      cognitive deficits — *see* subcategory I69.01- ☑
      disturbance of vision I69.098
      dysarthria I69.022
      dysphagia I69.091
      dysphasia I69.021
      facial droop I69.092
      facial weakness I69.092
      fluency disorder I69.023
      hemiplegia I69.05- ☑
      language deficit NEC I69.028
      monoplegia
        lower limb I69.04- ☑
        upper limb I69.03- ☑
      paralytic syndrome I69.06- ☑
      specified effect NEC I69.098
      speech deficit NEC I69.028

Sequelae — *continued*
  hepatitis, viral B94.2
  hyperalimentation E68
  infarction
    cerebral I69.30
      alteration of sensation I69.398
      aphasia I69.320
      apraxia I69.390
      ataxia I69.393
      cognitive deficits I69.31 ☑
      disturbance of vision I69.398
      dysarthria I69.322
      dysphagia I69.391
      dysphasia I69.321
      facial droop I69.392
      facial weakness I69.392
      fluency disorder I69.323
      hemiplegia I69.35- ☑
      language deficit NEC I69.328
      monoplegia
        lower limb I69.34- ☑
        upper limb I69.33- ☑
      paralytic syndrome I69.36- ☑
      specified effect NEC I69.398
      speech deficit NEC I69.328
  infection, pyogenic, intracranial or intraspinal G09
  infectious disease B94.9
    specified NEC B94.8
  injury — *code to* injury with seventh character S
  leprosy B92
  meningitis
    bacterial (conditions in G00) G09
    other or unspecified cause (conditions in G03) G09
  muscle (and tendon) injury — *code to* injury with seventh character S
  myelitis — *see* Sequelae, encephalitis
  niacin deficiency E64.8
  nutritional deficiency E64.9
    specified NEC E64.8
  obstetrical condition O94
  parasitic disease B94.9
  phlebitis or thrombophlebitis of intracranial or intraspinal venous sinuses and veins (conditions in G08) G09
  poisoning — *code to* poisoning with seventh character S
    nonmedicinal substance — *see* Sequelae, toxic effect, nonmedicinal substance
  poliomyelitis (acute) B91
  pregnancy O94
  protein-energy malnutrition E64.0
  puerperium O94
  rickets E64.3
  SARS-CoV-2 (post acute) U09.9
  selenium deficiency E64.8
  sprain and strain — *code to* injury with seventh character S
  stroke NOS I69.30
    alteration in sensation I69.398
    aphasia I69.320
    apraxia I69.390
    ataxia I69.393
    cognitive deficits I69.31 ☑
    disturbance of vision I69.398
    dysarthria I69.322
    dysphagia I69.391
    dysphasia I69.321
    facial droop I69.392
    facial weakness I69.392
    hemiplegia I69.35- ☑
    language deficit NEC I69.328
    monoplegia
      lower limb I69.34- ☑
      upper limb I69.33- ☑
    paralytic syndrome I69.36- ☑
    specified effect NEC I69.398
    speech deficit NEC I69.328
  tendon and muscle injury — *code to* injury with seventh character S
  thiamine deficiency E64.8
  trachoma B94.0
  tuberculosis B90.9
    bones and joints B90.2
    central nervous system B90.0
    genitourinary B90.1
    pulmonary (respiratory) B90.9
    specified organs NEC B90.8
  viral
    encephalitis B94.1

Sequelae — *continued*
  viral — *continued*
    hepatitis B94.2
  vitamin deficiency NEC E64.8
    A E64.1
    B E64.8
    C E64.2
  wound, open — *code to* injury with seventh character S
Sequestration — *see also* Sequestrum
  disc — *see* Displacement, intervertebral disc
  lung, congenital Q33.2
Sequestrum
  bone — *see* Osteomyelitis, chronic
  dental M27.2
  jaw bone M27.2
  orbit — *see* Osteomyelitis, orbit
  sinus (accessory) (nasal) — *see* Sinusitis
Sequoiosis lung or pneumonitis J67.8
Serology for syphilis
  doubtful
    with signs or symptoms — *code by* site and stage under Syphilis
    follow-up of latent syphilis — *see* Syphilis, latent
  negative, with signs or symptoms — *code by* site and stage under Syphilis
  positive A53.0
    with signs or symptoms — *code by* site and stage under Syphilis
  reactivated A53.0
Seroma — *see also* Hematoma
  postprocedural — *see* Complication, postprocedural, seroma
  traumatic, secondary and recurrent T79.2 ☑
Seropurulent — *see* condition
Serositis, multiple K65.8
  pericardial I31.1
  peritoneal K65.8
Serous — *see* condition
Sertoli cell
  adenoma
    specified site — *see* Neoplasm, benign, by site
    unspecified site
      female D27.9
      male D29.20
  carcinoma
    specified site — *see* Neoplasm, malignant, by site
    unspecified site (male) C62.9- ☑
      female C56.9
  tumor
    with lipid storage
      specified site — *see* Neoplasm, benign, by site
      unspecified site
        female D27.9
        male D29.20
    specified site — *see* Neoplasm, benign, by site
    unspecified site
      female D27.9
      male D29.20
Sertoli-Leydig cell tumor — *see* Neoplasm, benign, by site
  specified site — *see* Neoplasm, benign, by site
  unspecified site
    female D27.9
    male D29.20
Serum
  allergy, allergic reaction — *see also* Reaction, serum T80.69 ☑
    shock — *see also* Shock, anaphylactic T80.59 ☑
  arthritis — *see also* Reaction, serum T80.69 ☑
  complication or reaction NEC — *see also* Reaction, serum T80.69 ☑
  disease NEC — *see also* Reaction, serum T80.69 ☑
  hepatitis — *see also* Hepatitis, viral, type B
    carrier (suspected) of B18.1
  intoxication — *see also* Reaction, serum T80.69 ☑
  neuritis — *see also* Reaction, serum T80.69 ☑
  neuropathy G61.1
  poisoning NEC — *see also* Reaction, serum T80.69 ☑
  rash NEC — *see also* Reaction, serum T80.69 ☑
  reaction NEC — *see also* Reaction, serum T80.69 ☑
  sickness NEC — *see also* Reaction, serum T80.69 ☑
  urticaria — *see also* Reaction, serum T80.69 ☑
Sesamoiditis M25.8- ☑
Severe sepsis R65.20
  with septic shock R65.21
Sever's disease or osteochondrosis — *see* Osteochondrosis, juvenile, tarsus
Sex
  chromosome mosaics Q97.8

Sex — *continued*
  chromosome mosaics — *continued*
    lines with various numbers of X chromosomes Q97.2
  education Z70.8
  reassignment surgery status Z87.890
Sextuplet pregnancy — *see* Pregnancy, sextuplet
Sexual
  function, disorder of (psychogenic) F52.9
  immaturity (female) (male) E30.0
  impotence (psychogenic) organic origin NEC — *see* Dysfunction, sexual, male
  precocity (constitutional) (cryptogenic) (female) (idiopathic) (male) E30.1
Sexuality, pathologic — *see* Deviation, sexual
Sezary disease C84.1- ☑
Shadow, lung R91.8
Shaking palsy or paralysis — *see* Parkinsonism
Shallowness, acetabulum — *see* Derangement, joint, specified type NEC, hip
Shaver's disease J63.1
Sheath (tendon) — *see* condition
Sheathing, retinal vessels H35.01- ☑
Shedding
  nail L60.8
  premature, primary (deciduous) teeth K00.6
Sheehan's disease or syndrome E23.0
Shelf, rectal K62.89
Shell teeth K00.5
Shellshock (current) F43.0
  lasting state — *see* Disorder, post-traumatic stress
Shield kidney Q63.1
Shift
  auditory threshold (temporary) H93.24- ☑
  mediastinal R93.89
Shifting sleep-work schedule (affecting sleep) G47.26
Shiga (-Kruse) **dysentery** A03.0
Shiga's bacillus A03.0
Shigella (dysentery) — *see* Dysentery, bacillary
Shigellosis A03.9
  Group A A03.0
  Group B A03.1
  Group C A03.2
  Group D A03.3
Shin splints S86.89- ☑
Shingles — *see* Herpes, zoster
Shipyard disease or eye B30.0
Shirodkar suture, in pregnancy — *see* Pregnancy, complicated by, incompetent cervix
Shock R57.9
  with ectopic or molar pregnancy O08.3
  adrenal (cortical) (Addisonian) E27.2
  adverse food reaction (anaphylactic) — *see* Shock, anaphylactic, due to food
  allergic — *see* Shock, anaphylactic
  anaphylactic T78.2 ☑
    chemical — *see* Table of Drugs and Chemicals
    due to drug or medicinal substance
      correct substance properly administered T88.6 ☑
      overdose or wrong substance given or taken (by accident) — *see* Table of Drugs and Chemicals, by drug, poisoning
    due to food (nonpoisonous) T78.00 ☑
      additives T78.06 ☑
      dairy products T78.07 ☑
      eggs T78.08 ☑
      fish T78.03 ☑
        shellfish T78.02 ☑
      fruit T78.04 ☑
      milk T78.07 ☑
      nuts T78.05 ☑
        multiple types T78.05 ☑
        peanuts T78.01 ☑
      peanuts T78.01 ☑
      seeds T78.05 ☑
      specified type NEC T78.09 ☑
      vegetable T78.04 ☑
    following sting(s) — *see* Venom
    immunization T80.52 ☑
    serum T80.59 ☑
      blood and blood products T80.51 ☑
      immunization T80.52 ☑
      specified NEC T80.59 ☑
      vaccination T80.52 ☑
  anaphylactoid — *see* Shock, anaphylactic
  anesthetic
    correct substance properly administered T88.2 ☑

Shock — *continued*
  anesthetic — *continued*
    overdose or wrong substance given or taken — *see* Table of Drugs and Chemicals, by drug, poisoning
    specified anesthetic — *see* Table of Drugs and Chemicals, by drug, poisoning
  cardiogenic R57.0
  chemical substance — *see* Table of Drugs and Chemicals
  complicating ectopic or molar pregnancy O08.3
  culture — *see* Disorder, adjustment
  drug
    due to correct substance properly administered T88.6 ☑
    overdose or wrong substance given or taken (by accident) — *see* Table of Drugs and Chemicals, by drug, poisoning
  during or after labor and delivery O75.1
  electric T75.4 ☑
    (taser) T75.4 ☑
  endotoxic R65.21
    postprocedural (resulting from a procedure, not elsewhere classified) T81.12 ☑
  following
    ectopic or molar pregnancy O08.3
    injury (immediate) (delayed) T79.4 ☑
    labor and delivery O75.1
  food (anaphylactic) — *see* Shock, anaphylactic, due to food
  from electroshock gun (taser) T75.4 ☑
  gram-negative R65.21
    postprocedural (resulting from a procedure, not elsewhere classified) T81.12 ☑
  hematologic R57.8
  hemorrhagic R57.8
    surgery (intraoperative) (postoperative) T81.19 ☑
    trauma T79.4 ☑
  hypovolemic R57.1
    surgical T81.19 ☑
    traumatic T79.4 ☑
  insulin E15
    therapeutic misadventure — *see* subcategory T38.3 ☑
  kidney N17.0
    traumatic (following crushing) T79.5 ☑
  lightning T75.01 ☑
  liver K72.00
  lung J80
  obstetric O75.1
    with ectopic or molar pregnancy O08.3
    following ectopic or molar pregnancy O08.3
  pleural (surgical) T81.19 ☑
    due to trauma T79.4 ☑
  postprocedural (postoperative) T81.10 ☑
    with ectopic or molar pregnancy O08.3
    cardiogenic T81.11 ☑
    endotoxic T81.12 ☑
    following ectopic or molar pregnancy O08.3
    gram-negative T81.12 ☑
    hypovolemic T81.19 ☑
    septic T81.12 ☑
    specified type NEC T81.19 ☑
  psychic F43.0
  septic (due to severe sepsis) R65.21
  specified NEC R57.8
  surgical T81.10 ☑
  taser gun (taser) T75.4 ☑
  therapeutic misadventure NEC T81.10 ☑
  thyroxin
    overdose or wrong substance given or taken — *see* Table of Drugs and Chemicals, by drug, poisoning
  toxic, syndrome A48.3
  transfusion — *see* Complications, transfusion
  traumatic (immediate) (delayed) T79.4 ☑
Shoemaker's chest M95.4
Short, shortening, shortness
  arm (acquired) — *see also* Deformity, limb, unequal length
    congenital Q71.81- ☑
    forearm — *see* Deformity, limb, unequal length
  bowel syndrome K91.2
  breath R06.02
  cervical (complicating pregnancy) O26.87- ☑
    non-gravid uterus N88.3
  common bile duct, congenital Q44.5
  cord (umbilical), complicating delivery O69.3 ☑

Short, shortening, shortness — *continued*
  cystic duct, congenital Q44.5
  esophagus (congenital) Q39.8
  femur (acquired) — *see* Deformity, limb, unequal length, femur
    congenital — *see* Defect, reduction, lower limb, longitudinal, femur
  frenum, frenulum, linguae (congenital) Q38.1
  hip (acquired) — *see also* Deformity, limb, unequal length
    congenital Q65.89
  leg (acquired) — *see also* Deformity, limb, unequal length
    congenital Q72.81- ☑
    lower leg — *see also* Deformity, limb, unequal length
  limbed stature, with immunodeficiency D82.2
  lower limb (acquired) — *see also* Deformity, limb, unequal length
    congenital Q72.81- ☑
  organ or site, congenital NEC — *see* Distortion
  palate, congenital Q38.5
  radius (acquired) — *see also* Deformity, limb, unequal length
    congenital — *see* Defect, reduction, upper limb, longitudinal, radius
  rib syndrome Q77.2
  stature (child) (hereditary) (idiopathic) NEC R62.52
    constitutional E34.31
    due to
      endocrine disorder E34.30
        specified type NEC, due to endocrine dosorder E34.39
      genetic causes E34.329
        ACAN gene variant E34.328
        acid-labile subunit gene (IGFALS) defect E34.321
        aggrecan deficiency E34.328
        genetic syndrome with resistance to insulin-like growth factor-1 E34.322
        growth hormone gene 1 (GH1) defect with growth hormone neutralizing antibodies E34.321
        growth hormone insensitivity syndrome (GHIS) E34.321
        insulin-like growth factor 1 gene (IGF1) defect E34.321
        insulin-like growth factor-1 receptor (IGF-1R) defect E34.322
        insulin-like growth factor-1 (IGF-1) resistance E34.322
        NPR-2 gene variant E34.328
        post-insulin-like growth factor-1 receptor signaling defect E34.322
        primary insulin-like growth factor-1 (IGF-1) deficiency E34.321
        severe primary insulin-like growth factor-1 deficiency (SPIGFD) E34.321
        signal transducer and activator of transcription 5B gene (STAT5b) defect E34.321
        specified genetic cause NEC E34.328
      Laron-type E34.321
  tendon — *see also* Contraction, tendon
    with contracture of joint — *see* Contraction, joint
    Achilles (acquired) M67.0- ☑
      congenital Q66.89
    congenital Q79.8
  thigh (acquired) — *see also* Deformity, limb, unequal length, femur
    congenital — *see* Defect, reduction, lower limb, longitudinal, femur
  tibialis anterior (tendon) — *see* Contraction, tendon
  umbilical cord
    complicating delivery O69.3 ☑
  upper limb, congenital — *see* Defect, reduction, upper limb, specified type NEC
  urethra N36.8
  uvula, congenital Q38.5
  vagina (congenital) Q52.4
Shortsightedness — *see* Myopia
Shoshin (acute fulminating beriberi) E51.11
Shoulder — *see* condition
Shovel-shaped incisors K00.2
Shower, thromboembolic — *see* Embolism
Shunt
  arterial-venous (dialysis) Z99.2
  arteriovenous, pulmonary (acquired) I28.0
    congenital Q25.72
  cerebral ventricle (communicating) in situ Z98.2
  surgical, prosthetic, with complications — *see* Complications, cardiovascular, device or implant
Shutdown, renal N28.9

Shy-Drager syndrome G90.3
Sialadenitis, sialadenosis (any gland) (chronic) (periodic) (suppurative) — *see* Sialoadenitis
Sialectasia K11.8
Sialidosis E77.1
Sialitis, silitis (any gland) (chronic) (suppurative) — *see* Sialoadenitis
Sialoadenitis (any gland) (periodic) (suppurative) K11.20
  acute K11.21
    recurrent K11.22
  chronic K11.23
Sialoadenopathy K11.9
Sialoangitis — *see* Sialoadenitis
Sialodochitis (fibrinosa) — *see* Sialoadenitis
Sialodocholithiasis K11.5
Sialolithiasis K11.5
Sialometaplasia, necrotizing K11.8
Sialorrhea — *see also* Ptyalism
  periodic — *see* Sialoadenitis
Sialosis K11.7
Siamese twin Q89.4
Sibling rivalry Z62.891
Sicard's syndrome G52.7
Sicca syndrome — *see* Syndrome, Sjogren
Sick R69
  or handicapped person in family Z63.79
    needing care at home Z63.6
  sinus (syndrome) I49.5
Sick-euthyroid syndrome E07.81
Sickle-cell
  anemia — *see* Disease, sickle-cell
  beta plus — *see* Disease, sickle-cell, thalassemia, beta plus
  beta zero — *see* Disease, sickle-cell, thalassemia, beta zero
  trait D57.3
Sicklemia — *see also* Disease, sickle-cell
  trait D57.3
Sickness
  air (travel) T75.3 ☑
  airplane T75.3 ☑
  alpine T70.29 ☑
  altitude T70.20 ☑
  Andes T70.29 ☑
  aviator's T70.29 ☑
  balloon T70.29 ☑
  car T75.3 ☑
  compressed air T70.3 ☑
  decompression T70.3 ☑
  green D50.8
  milk — *see* Poisoning, food, noxious
  motion T75.3 ☑
  mountain T70.29 ☑
    acute D75.1
  protein — *see also* Reaction, serum T80.69 ☑
  radiation T66 ☑
  roundabout (motion) T75.3 ☑
  sea T75.3 ☑
  serum NEC — *see also* Reaction, serum T80.69 ☑
  sleeping (African) B56.9
    by Trypanosoma B56.9
      brucei
        gambiense B56.0
        rhodesiense B56.1
      East African B56.1
      Gambian B56.0
      Rhodesian B56.1
      West African B56.0
  swing (motion) T75.3 ☑
  train (railway) (travel) T75.3 ☑
  travel (any vehicle) T75.3 ☑
Sideropenia — *see* Anemia, iron deficiency
Siderosilicosis J62.8
Siderosis (lung) J63.4
  brain G93.89
  eye (globe) — *see* Disorder, globe, degenerative, siderosis
Siemens' syndrome (ectodermal dysplasia) Q82.8
Sighing R06.89
  psychogenic F45.8
Sigmoid — *see also* condition
  flexure — *see* condition
  kidney Q63.1
Sigmoiditis — *see also* Enteritis K52.9
  infectious A09
  noninfectious K52.9
Silfverskold's syndrome Q78.9
Silicosiderosis J62.8

☑ **Additional Character Required** — **Refer to the Tabular List for Character Selection**

Silicosis, silicotic (simple) (complicated) J62.8
  with tuberculosis J65
Silicotuberculosis J65
Silo-fillers' disease J68.8
  bronchitis J68.0
  pneumonitis J68.0
  pulmonary edema J68.1
Silver's syndrome Q87.19
Simian malaria B53.1
Simmonds' cachexia or disease E23.0
Simons' disease or syndrome (progressive lipodystrophy) E88.1
Simple, simplex — see condition
Simulation, conscious (of illness) Z76.5
Simultanagnosia (asimultagnosia) R48.3
Sin Nombre virus disease (Hantavirus) (cardio)-pulmonary syndrome) B33.4
Sinding-Larsen disease or osteochondrosis — see Osteochondrosis, juvenile, patella
Singapore hemorrhagic fever A91
Singer's node or nodule J38.2
Single
  atrium Q21.20
  coronary artery Q24.5
  umbilical artery Q27.0
  ventricle Q20.4
Singultus R06.6
  epidemicus B33.0
Sinus — see also Fistula
  abdominal K63.89
  arrest I45.5
  arrhythmia I49.8
  bradycardia R00.1
  branchial cleft (internal) (external) Q18.0
  coccygeal — see Sinus, pilonidal
  dental K04.6
  dermal (congenital) Q06.8
    with abscess Q06.8
    coccygeal, pilonidal — see Sinus, coccygeal
  infected, skin NEC L08.89
  marginal, ruptured or bleeding — see Hemorrhage, antepartum, specified cause NEC
  medial, face and neck Q18.8
  pause I45.5
  pericranii Q01.9
  pilonidal (infected) (rectum) L05.92
    with abscess L05.02
  preauricular Q18.1
  rectovaginal N82.3
  Rokitansky-Aschoff (gallbladder) K82.8
  sacrococcygeal (dermoid) (infected) — see Sinus, pilonidal
  tachycardia R00.0
    paroxysmal I47.19
  tarsi syndrome M25.57- ☑
  testis N50.89
  tract (postinfective) — see Fistula
  urachus Q64.4
Sinusitis (accessory) (chronic) (hyperplastic) (nasal) (nonpurulent) (purulent) J32.9
  acute J01.90
    ethmoidal J01.20
      recurrent J01.21
    frontal J01.10
      recurrent J01.11
    involving more than one sinus, other than pansinusitis J01.80
      recurrent J01.81
    maxillary J01.00
      recurrent J01.01
    pansinusitis J01.40
      recurrent J01.41
    recurrent J01.91
    specified NEC J01.80
      recurrent J01.81
    sphenoidal J01.30
      recurrent J01.31
  allergic — see Rhinitis, allergic
  due to high altitude T70.1 ☑
  ethmoidal J32.2
    acute J01.20
      recurrent J01.21
  frontal J32.1
    acute J01.10
      recurrent J01.11
  influenzal — see Influenza, with, respiratory manifestations NEC
  involving more than one sinus but not pansinusitis J32.8
    acute J01.80

Sinusitis — continued
  involving more than one sinus but not pansinusitis — continued
    acute — continued
      recurrent J01.81
    maxillary J32.0
      acute J01.00
        recurrent J01.01
    sphenoidal J32.3
      acute J01.30
        recurrent J01.31
    tuberculous, any sinus A15.8
Sinusitis-bronchiectasis-situs inversus (syndrome) (triad) Q89.3
Sipple's syndrome E31.22
Sirenomelia (syndrome) Q87.2
Siriasis T67.01 ☑
Sirkari's disease B55.0
Siti A65
Situation, psychiatric F99
Situational
  disturbance (transient) — see Disorder, adjustment
    acute F43.0
  maladjustment — see Disorder, adjustment
  reaction — see Disorder, adjustment
    acute F43.0
Situs inversus or transversus (abdominalis) (thoracis) Q89.3
Sixth disease B08.20
  due to human herpesvirus 6 B08.21
  due to human herpesvirus 7 B08.22
Sjogren-Larsson syndrome Q87.19
Sjogren's syndrome or disease — see Syndrome, Sjogren
Skeletal — see condition
Skene's gland — see condition
Skenitis — see Urethritis
Skerljevo A65
Skevas-Zerfus disease — see Toxicity, venom, marine animal, sea anemone
Skin — see also condition
  clammy R23.1
  donor — see Donor, skin
  dry L85.3
  hidebound M35.9
Slate-dressers' or slate-miners' lung J62.8
Sleep
  apnea — see Apnea, sleep
  deprivation Z72.820
  disorder or disturbance G47.9
    child F51.9
    nonorganic origin F51.9
    specified NEC G47.8
  disturbance G47.9
    nonorganic origin F51.9
  drunkenness F51.9
  rhythm inversion G47.2- ☑
  terrors F51.4
  walking F51.3
    hysterical F44.89
Sleep hygiene
  abuse Z72.821
  inadequate Z72.821
  poor Z72.821
Sleeping sickness — see Sickness, sleeping
Sleeplessness — see Insomnia
  menopausal N95.1
Sleep-wake schedule disorder G47.20
Slim disease (in HIV infection) B20
Slipped, slipping
  epiphysis (traumatic) — see also Osteochondropathy, specified type NEC
    capital femoral (traumatic) [SCFE]
      acute (on chronic) S79.01- ☑
      nontraumatic M93.00- ☑
    current traumatic — code as Fracture, by site
    upper femoral (nontraumatic) [SUFE] M93.00- ☑
      acute M93.01- ☑
        on chronic M93.03- ☑
      chronic M93.02- ☑
  intervertebral disc — see Displacement, intervertebral disc
  ligature, umbilical P51.8
  patella — see Disorder, patella, derangement NEC
  rib M89.8X8
  sacroiliac joint — see subcategory M53.2 ☑
  tendon — see Disorder, tendon
  ulnar nerve, nontraumatic — see Lesion, nerve, ulnar
  vertebra NEC — see Spondylolisthesis

Slocumb's syndrome E27.0
Sloughing (multiple) (phagedena) (skin) — see also Gangrene
  abscess — see Abscess
  appendix K38.8
  fascia — see Disorder, soft tissue, specified type NEC
  scrotum N50.89
  tendon — see Disorder, tendon
  transplanted organ — see Rejection, transplant
  ulcer — see Ulcer, skin
Slow
  feeding, newborn P92.2
  flow syndrome, coronary I20.89
  heart (beat) R00.1
Slowing, urinary stream R39.198
Sluder's neuralgia (syndrome) G44.89
Slurred, slurring speech R47.81
Small (ness)
  for gestational age — see Small for dates
  introitus, vagina N89.6
  kidney (unknown cause) N27.9
    bilateral N27.1
    unilateral N27.0
  ovary (congenital) Q50.39
  pelvis
    with disproportion (fetopelvic) O33.1
      causing obstructed labor O65.1
  uterus N85.8
  white kidney N03.9
Small-and-light-for-dates — see Small for dates
Small-for-dates (infant) P05.10
  with weight of
    499 grams or less P05.11
    500-749 grams P05.12
    750-999 grams P05.13
    1000-1249 grams P05.14
    1250-1499 grams P05.15
    1500-1749 grams P05.16
    1750-1999 grams P05.17
    2000-2499 grams P05.18
    2500 grams and over P05.19
  specified NEC P05.19
Smallpox B03
Smearing, fecal R15.1
SMEI (severe myoclonic epilepsy in infancy) G40.83- ☑
Smith-Lemli-Opitz syndrome E78.72
Smith's fracture S52.54- ☑
Smoker — see Dependence, drug, nicotine
Smoker's
  bronchitis J41.0
  cough J41.0
  palate K13.24
  throat J31.2
  tongue K13.24
Smoking
  passive Z77.22
Smothering spells R06.81
Snaggle teeth, tooth M26.39
Snapping
  finger — see Trigger finger
  hip — see Derangement, joint, specified type NEC, hip
    involving the iliotibial band M76.3- ☑
  knee — see Derangement, knee
    involving the iliotiblial band M76.3- ☑
Sneddon-Wilkinson disease or syndrome (sub-corneal pustular dermatosis) L13.1
Sneezing (intractable) R06.7
Sniffing
  cocaine
    abuse — see Abuse, drug, cocaine
    dependence — see Dependence, drug, cocaine
  gasoline
    abuse — see Abuse, drug, inhalant
    dependence — see Dependence, drug, inhalant
  glue (airplane)
    abuse — see Abuse, drug, inhalant
    drug dependence — see Dependence, drug, inhalant
Sniffles
  newborn P28.89
Snoring R06.83
Snow blindness — see Photokeratitis
Snuffles (non-syphilitic) R06.5
  newborn P28.89
  syphilitic (infant) A50.05 [J99]
Social
  exclusion Z60.4
    due to discrimination or persecution (perceived) Z60.5
  migrant Z59.00
    acculturation difficulty Z60.3

☑ **Additional Character Required — Refer to the Tabular List for Character Selection**

Social — continued
rejection Z60.4
due to discrimination or persecution Z60.5
role conflict NEC Z73.5
skills inadequacy NEC Z73.4
transplantation Z60.3
Sodoku A25.0
Soemmerring's ring — see Cataract, secondary
Soft — see also condition
nails L60.3
Softening
bone — see Osteomalacia
brain (necrotic) (progressive) G93.89
congenital Q04.8
embolic I63.4- ☑
hemorrhagic — see Hemorrhage, intracranial, intracerebral
occlusive I63.5- ☑
thrombotic I63.3- ☑
cartilage M94.2- ☑
patella M22.4- ☑
cerebellar — see Softening, brain
cerebral — see Softening, brain
cerebrospinal — see Softening, brain
myocardial, heart — see Degeneration, myocardial
spinal cord G95.89
stomach K31.89
Soldier's
heart F45.8
patches I31.0
Solitary
cyst, kidney N28.1
kidney, congenital Q60.0
Solvent abuse — see Abuse, drug, inhalant
dependence — see Dependence, drug, inhalant
Somatization reaction, somatic reaction — see Disorder, somatoform
Somnambulism F51.3
hysterical F44.89
Somnolence R40.0
nonorganic origin F51.11
Sonne dysentery A03.3
Soor B37.0
Sore
bed — see Ulcer, pressure, by site
chiclero B55.1
Delhi B55.1
desert — see Ulcer, skin
eye H57.1- ☑
Lahore B55.1
mouth K13.79
canker K12.0
muscle M79.10
Naga — see Ulcer, skin
of skin — see Ulcer, skin
oriental B55.1
pressure — see Ulcer, pressure, by site
skin L98.9
soft A57
throat (acute) — see also Pharyngitis
with influenza, flu, or grippe — see Influenza, with, respiratory manifestations NEC
chronic J31.2
coxsackie (virus) B08.5
diphtheritic A36.0
herpesviral B00.2
influenzal — see Influenza, with, respiratory manifestations NEC
septic J02.0
streptococcal (ulcerative) J02.0
viral NEC J02.8
coxsackie B08.5
tropical — see Ulcer, skin
veldt — see Ulcer, skin
Soto's syndrome (cerebral gigantism) Q87.3
South African cardiomyopathy syndrome I42.8
Southeast Asian hemorrhagic fever A91
Spacing
abnormal, tooth, teeth, fully erupted M26.30
excessive, tooth, fully erupted M26.32
Spade-like hand (congenital) Q68.1
Spading nail L60.8
congenital Q84.6
Spanish collar N47.1
Sparganosis B70.1
Spasm(s), spastic, spasticity — see also condition R25.2
accommodation — see Spasm, of accommodation
ampulla of Vater K83.4

Spasm(s), spastic, spasticity — continued
anus, ani (sphincter) (reflex) K59.4
psychogenic F45.8
artery I73.9
cerebral G45.9
Bell's G51.3- ☑
bladder (sphincter, external or internal) N32.89
psychogenic F45.8
bronchus, bronchiole J98.01
cardia K22.0
cardiac I20.1
carpopedal — see Tetany
cerebral (arteries) (vascular) G45.9
cervix, complicating delivery O62.4
ciliary body (of accommodation) — see Spasm, of accommodation
colon — see also Irritable, bowel K58.9
with diarrhea K58.0
psychogenic F45.8
common duct K83.8
compulsive — see Tic
conjugate H51.8
coronary (artery) I20.1
diaphragm (reflex) R06.6
epidemic B33.0
psychogenic F45.8
duodenum K59.89
epidemic diaphragmatic (transient) B33.0
esophagus (diffuse) K22.4
psychogenic F45.8
facial G51.3- ☑
fallopian tube N83.8
gastrointestinal (tract) K31.89
psychogenic F45.8
glottis J38.5
hysterical F44.4
psychogenic F45.8
conversion reaction F44.4
reflex through recurrent laryngeal nerve J38.5
habit — see Tic
heart I20.1
hemifacial (clonic) G51.3- ☑
hourglass — see Contraction, hourglass
hysterical F44.4
infantile — see Epilepsy, spasms
inferior oblique, eye H51.8
intestinal — see also Syndrome, irritable bowel K58.9
psychogenic F45.8
larynx, laryngeal J38.5
hysterical F44.4
psychogenic F45.8
conversion reaction F44.4
levator palpebrae superioris — see Disorder, eyelid function
muscle NEC M62.838
back M62.830
nerve, trigeminal G51.0
nervous F45.8
nodding F98.4
occupational F48.8
oculogyric H51.8
psychogenic F45.8
of accommodation H52.53- ☑
ophthalmic artery — see Occlusion, artery, retina
perineal, female N94.89
peroneo-extensor — see also Deformity, limb, flat foot
pharynx (reflex) J39.2
hysterical F45.8
psychogenic F45.8
psychogenic F45.8
pylorus NEC K31.3
adult hypertrophic K31.89
congenital or infantile Q40.0
psychogenic F45.8
rectum (sphincter) K59.4
psychogenic F45.8
retinal (artery) — see Occlusion, artery, retina
sigmoid — see also Syndrome, irritable bowel K58.9
psychogenic F45.8
sphincter of Oddi K83.4
stomach K31.89
neurotic F45.8
throat J39.2
hysterical F45.8
psychogenic F45.8
tic F95.9
chronic F95.1
transient of childhood F95.0
tongue K14.8

Spasm(s), spastic, spasticity — continued
torsion (progressive) G24.1
trigeminal nerve — see Neuralgia, trigeminal
ureter N13.5
urethra (sphincter) N35.919
uterus N85.8
complicating labor O62.4
vagina N94.2
psychogenic F52.5
vascular I73.9
vasomotor I73.9
vein NEC I87.8
viscera — see Pain, abdominal
Spasmodic — see condition
Spasmophilia — see Tetany
Spasmus nutans F98.4
Spastic, spasticity — see also Spasm
child (cerebral) (congenital) (paralysis) G80.1
Speaker's throat R49.8
Specific, specified — see condition
Speech
defect, disorder, disturbance, impediment — see Disorder, speech R47.9
psychogenic, in childhood and adolescence F98.8
slurring R47.81
specified NEC R47.89
Spells, transient oxygen desaturation of newborn — see also Apnea, newborn P28.40
during sleep — see also Apnea, newborn, sleep, primary P28.30
Spencer's disease A08.19
Spens' syndrome (syncope with heart block) I45.9
Sperm counts (fertility testing) Z31.41
postvasectomy Z30.8
reversal Z31.42
Spermatic cord — see condition
Spermatocele N43.40
congenital Q55.4
multiple N43.42
single N43.41
Spermatocystitis N49.0
Spermatocytoma C62.9- ☑
specified site — see Neoplasm, malignant, by site
Spermatorrhea N50.89
Sphacelus — see Gangrene
Sphenoidal — see condition
Sphenoiditis (chronic) — see Sinusitis, sphenoidal
Sphenopalatine ganglion neuralgia G90.09
Sphericity, increased, lens (congenital) Q12.4
Spherocytosis (congenital) (familial) (hereditary) D58.0
hemoglobin disease D58.0
sickle-cell (disease) D57.8- ☑
Spherophakia Q12.4
Sphincter — see condition
Sphincteritis, sphincter of Oddi — see Cholangitis
Sphingolipidosis E75.3
specified NEC E75.29
Sphingomyelinosis E75.3
Spicule tooth K00.2
Spider
bite — see Toxicity, venom, spider
nonvenomous — see Bite, by site, superficial, insect
fingers — see Syndrome, Marfan
nevus I78.1
toes — see Syndrome, Marfan
vascular I78.1
Spiegler-Fendt
benign lymphocytoma L98.8
sarcoid L08.89
Spielmeyer-Vogt disease E75.4
Spina bifida (aperta) Q05.9
with hydrocephalus NEC Q05.4
cervical Q05.5
with hydrocephalus Q05.0
dorsal Q05.6
with hydrocephalus Q05.1
lumbar Q05.7
with hydrocephalus Q05.2
lumbosacral Q05.7
with hydrocephalus Q05.2
occulta Q76.0
sacral Q05.8
with hydrocephalus Q05.3
thoracic Q05.6
with hydrocephalus Q05.1
thoracolumbar Q05.6
with hydrocephalus Q05.1
Spindle, Krukenberg's — see Pigmentation, cornea, posterior

☑ **Additional Character Required** — Refer to the Tabular List for Character Selection

Spine, spinal — *see* condition
Spiradenoma (eccrine) — *see* Neoplasm, skin, benign
Spirillosis A25.0
Spirillum
  minus A25.0
  obermeieri infection A68.0
Spirochetal — *see* condition
Spirochetosis A69.9
  arthritic, arthritica A69.9
  bronchopulmonary A69.8
  icterohemorrhagic A27.0
  lung A69.8
Spirometrosis B70.1
Spitting blood — *see* Hemoptysis
Splanchnoptosis K63.4
Spleen, splenic — *see* condition
Splenectasis — *see* Splenomegaly
Splenitis (interstitial) (malignant) (nonspecific) D73.89
  malarial — *see also* Malaria B54 *[D77]*
  tuberculous A18.85
Splenocele D73.89
Splenomegaly, splenomegalia (Bengal) (cryptogenic)
    (idiopathic) (tropical) R16.1
  with hepatomegaly R16.2
  cirrhotic D73.2
  congenital Q89.09
  congestive, chronic D73.2
  Egyptian B65.1
  Gaucher's E75.22
  malarial — *see also* Malaria B54 *[D77]*
  neutropenic D73.81
  Niemann-Pick — *see* Niemann-Pick disease or syndrome
  siderotic D73.2
  syphilitic A52.79
    congenital (early) A50.08 *[D77]*
Splenopathy D73.9
Splenoptosis D73.89
Splenosis D73.89
Splinter — *see* Foreign body, superficial, by site
Split, splitting
  foot Q72.7- ☑
  hand Q71.6 ☑
  heart sounds R01.2
  lip, congenital — *see* Cleft, lip
  nails L60.3
  urinary stream R39.13
Spondylarthrosis — *see* Spondylosis
Spondylitis (chronic) — *see also* Spondylopathy, inflammatory
  ankylopoietica — *see* Spondylitis, ankylosing
  ankylosing (chronic) M45.9
    with lung involvement M45.9 *[J99]*
    cervical region M45.2
    cervicothoracic region M45.3
    juvenile M08.1
    lumbar region M45.6
    lumbosacral region M45.7
    multiple sites M45.0
    occipito-atlanto-axial region M45.1
    sacrococcygeal region M45.8
    thoracic region M45.4
    thoracolumbar region M45.5
  atrophic (ligamentous) — *see* Spondylitis, ankylosing
  deformans (chronic) — *see* Spondylosis
  gonococcal A54.41
  gouty — *see also* Gout, by type, vertebrae M10.08
  in (due to)
    brucellosis A23.9 *[M49.80]*
      cervical region A23.9 *[M49.82]*
      cervicothoracic region A23.9 *[M49.83]*
      lumbar region A23.9 *[M49.86]*
      lumbosacral region A23.9 *[M49.87]*
      multiple sites A23.9 *[M49.89]*
      occipito-atlanto-axial region A23.9 *[M49.81]*
      sacrococcygeal region A23.9 *[M49.88]*
      thoracic region A23.9 *[M49.84]*
      thoracolumbar region A23.9 *[M49.85]*
    enterobacteria — *see also* subcategory M49.8 A04.9
    tuberculosis A18.01
  infectious NEC — *see* Spondylopathy, infective
  juvenile ankylosing (chronic) M08.1
  Kummell's — *see* Spondylopathy, traumatic
  Marie-Strumpell — *see* Spondylitis, ankylosing
  muscularis — *see* Spondylopathy, specified NEC
  psoriatic L40.53
  rheumatoid — *see* Spondylitis, ankylosing
  rhizomelica — *see* Spondylitis, ankylosing
  sacroiliac NEC M46.1
  senescent, senile — *see* Spondylosis

Spondylitis — *continued*
  traumatic (chronic) or post-traumatic — *see* Spondylopathy, traumatic
  tuberculous A18.01
  typhosa A01.05
Spondyloarthritis
  axial — *see also* Spondylitis, ankylosing
    non-radiographic M45.A0
      cervical M45.A2
      cervicothoracic M45.A3
      lumbar M45.A6
      lumbosacral M45.A7
      multiple sites M45.AB
      occipito-atlanto-axial region M45.A1
      sacral and sacrococcygeal M45.A8
      thoracic M45.A4
      thoracolumbar M45.A5
Spondylolisthesis (acquired) (degenerative) M43.10
  with disproportion (fetopelvic) O33.0
    causing obstructed labor O65.0
  cervical region M43.12
  cervicothoracic region M43.13
  congenital Q76.2
  lumbar region M43.16
  lumbosacral region M43.17
  multiple sites M43.19
  occipito-atlanto-axial region M43.11
  sacrococcygeal region M43.18
  thoracic region M43.14
  thoracolumbar region M43.15
  traumatic (old) M43.10
    acute
      fifth cervical (displaced) S12.430 ☑
        nondisplaced S12.431 ☑
        specified type NEC (displaced) S12.450 ☑
          nondisplaced S12.451 ☑
        type III S12.44 ☑
      fourth cervical (displaced) S12.330 ☑
        nondisplaced S12.331 ☑
        specified type NEC (displaced) S12.350 ☑
          nondisplaced S12.351 ☑
        type III S12.34 ☑
      second cervical (displaced) S12.130 ☑
        nondisplaced S12.131 ☑
        specified type NEC (displaced) S12.150 ☑
          nondisplaced S12.151 ☑
        type III S12.14 ☑
      seventh cervical (displaced) S12.630 ☑
        nondisplaced S12.631 ☑
        specified type NEC (displaced) S12.650 ☑
          nondisplaced S12.651 ☑
        type III S12.64 ☑
      sixth cervical (displaced) S12.530 ☑
        nondisplaced S12.531 ☑
        specified type NEC (displaced) S12.550 ☑
          nondisplaced S12.551 ☑
        type III S12.54 ☑
      third cervical (displaced) S12.230 ☑
        nondisplaced S12.231 ☑
        specified type NEC (displaced) S12.250 ☑
          nondisplaced S12.251 ☑
        type III S12.24 ☑
Spondylolysis (acquired) M43.00
  cervical region M43.02
  cervicothoracic region M43.03
  congenital Q76.2
  lumbar region M43.06
  lumbosacral region M43.07
    with disproportion (fetopelvic) O33.0
      causing obstructed labor O65.8
  multiple sites M43.09
  occipito-atlanto-axial region M43.01
  sacrococcygeal region M43.08
  thoracic region M43.04
  thoracolumbar region M43.05
Spondylopathy M48.9
  infective NEC M46.50
    cervical region M46.52
    cervicothoracic region M46.53
    lumbar region M46.56
    lumbosacral region M46.57
    multiple sites M46.59
    occipito-atlanto-axial region M46.51
    sacrococcygeal region M46.58
    thoracic region M46.54
    thoracolumbar region M46.55
  inflammatory M46.90

Spondylopathy — *continued*
  inflammatory — *continued*
    cervical region M46.92
    cervicothoracic region M46.93
    lumbar region M46.96
    lumbosacral region M46.97
    multiple sites M46.99
    occipito-atlanto-axial region M46.91
    sacrococcygeal region M46.98
    specified type NEC M46.80
      cervical region M46.82
      cervicothoracic region M46.83
      lumbar region M46.86
      lumbosacral region M46.87
      multiple sites M46.89
      occipito-atlanto-axial region M46.81
      sacrococcygeal region M46.88
      thoracic region M46.84
      thoracolumbar region M46.85
    thoracic region M46.94
    thoracolumbar region M46.95
  neuropathic, in
    syringomyelia and syringobulbia G95.0
    tabes dorsalis A52.11
  specified NEC — *see* subcategory M48.8 ☑
  traumatic M48.30
    cervical region M48.32
    cervicothoracic region M48.33
    lumbar region M48.36
    lumbosacral region M48.37
    occipito-atlanto-axial region M48.31
    sacrococcygeal region M48.38
    thoracic region M48.34
    thoracolumbar region M48.35
Spondylosis M47.9
  with
    disproportion (fetopelvic) O33.0
      causing obstructed labor O65.0
    myelopathy NEC M47.10
      cervical region M47.12
      cervicothoracic region M47.13
      lumbar region M47.16
      occipito-atlanto-axial region M47.11
      thoracic region M47.14
      thoracolumbar region M47.15
    radiculopathy M47.20
      cervical region M47.22
      cervicothoracic region M47.23
      lumbar region M47.26
      lumbosacral region M47.27
      occipito-atlanto-axial region M47.21
      sacrococcygeal region M47.28
      thoracic region M47.24
      thoracolumbar region M47.25
  specified NEC M47.899
    cervical region M47.892
    cervicothoracic region M47.893
    facet joint M47.819
    lumbar region M47.896
    lumbosacral region M47.897
    occipito-atlanto-axial region M47.891
    sacrococcygeal region M47.898
    thoracic region M47.894
    thoracolumbar region M47.895
  traumatic — *see* Spondylopathy, traumatic
  without myelopathy or radiculopathy M47.819
    cervical region M47.812
    cervicothoracic region M47.813
    lumbar region M47.816
    lumbosacral region M47.817
    occipito-atlanto-axial region M47.811
    sacrococcygeal region M47.818
    thoracic region M47.814
    thoracolumbar region M47.815
Sponge
  inadvertently left in operation wound — *see* Foreign body, accidentally left during a procedure
  kidney (medullary) Q61.5
Sponge-diver's disease — *see* Toxicity, venom, marine animal, sea anemone
Spongioblastoma (any type) — *see* Neoplasm, malignant, by site
  specified site — *see* Neoplasm, malignant, by site
  unspecified site C71.9
Spongioneuroblastoma — *see* Neoplasm, malignant, by site
Spontaneous — *see also* condition
  fracture (cause unknown) — *see* Fracture, pathological
Spoon nail L60.3

Spoon nail — continued
  congenital Q84.6
Sporadic — see condition
Sporothrix schenckii infection — see Sporotrichosis
Sporotrichosis B42.9
  arthritis B42.82
  disseminated B42.7
  generalized B42.7
  lymphocutaneous (fixed) (progressive) B42.1
  pulmonary B42.0
  specified NEC B42.89
Spots, spotting (in) (of)
  Bitot's — see also Pigmentation, conjunctiva
    in the young child E50.1
    vitamin A deficiency E50.1
  cafe, au lait L81.3
  Cayenne pepper I78.1
  cotton wool, retina — see Occlusion, artery, retina
  de Morgan's (senile angiomas) I78.1
  Fuchs' black (myopic) — see also Myopia, degenerative
    H44.2-
  intermenstrual (regular) N92.0
    irregular N92.1
  Koplik's B05.9
  liver L81.4
  pregnancy O26.85-
  purpuric R23.3
  ruby I78.1
Spotted fever — see Fever, spotted A77.9
Sprain (joint) (ligament)
  acromioclavicular joint or ligament S43.5-
  ankle S93.40-
    calcaneofibular ligament S93.41-
    deltoid ligament S93.42-
    internal collateral ligament — see Sprain, ankle,
      specified ligament NEC
    specified ligament NEC S93.49-
    talofibular ligament — see Sprain, ankle, specified
      ligament NEC
    tibiofibular ligament S93.43-
  anterior longitudinal, cervical S13.4
  atlas, atlanto-axial, atlanto-occipital S13.4
  breast bone — see Sprain, sternum
  calcaneofibular — see Sprain, ankle
  carpal — see Sprain, wrist
  carpometacarpal — see Sprain, hand, specified site NEC
  cartilage
    costal S23.41
    semilunar (knee) — see Sprain, knee, specified site
      NEC
      with current tear — see Tear, meniscus
    thyroid region S13.5
    xiphoid — see Sprain, sternum
  cervical, cervicodorsal, cervicothoracic S13.4
  chondrosternal S23.421
  coracoclavicular S43.8-
  coracohumeral S43.41-
  coronary, knee — see Sprain, knee, specified site NEC
  costal cartilage S23.41
  cricoarytenoid articulation or ligament S13.5
  cricothyroid articulation S13.5
  cruciate, knee — see Sprain, knee, cruciate
  deltoid, ankle — see Sprain, ankle
  dorsal (spine) S23.3
  elbow S53.40-
    radial collateral ligament S53.43-
    radiohumeral S53.41-
    rupture
      radial collateral ligament — see Rupture, traumatic, ligament, radial collateral
      ulnar collateral ligament — see Rupture, traumatic, ligament, ulnar collateral
    specified type NEC S53.49-
    ulnar collateral ligament S53.44-
    ulnohumeral S53.42-
  femur, head — see Sprain, hip
  fibular collateral, knee — see Sprain, knee, collateral
  fibulocalcaneal — see Sprain, ankle
  finger(s) S63.61-
    index S63.61-
    interphalangeal (joint) S63.63-
      index S63.63-
      little S63.63-
      middle S63.63-
      ring S63.63-
    little S63.61-
    metacarpophalangeal (joint) S63.65-

Sprain — continued
  finger(s) — continued
    middle S63.61-
    ring S63.61-
    specified site NEC S63.69-
      index S63.69-
      little S63.69-
      middle S63.69-
      ring S63.69-
  foot S93.60-
    specified ligament NEC S93.69-
    tarsal ligament S93.61-
    tarsometatarsal ligament S93.62-
    toe — see Sprain, toe
  hand S63.9-
    finger — see Sprain, finger
    specified site NEC — see subcategory S63.8
    thumb — see Sprain, thumb
  head S03.9
  hip S73.10-
    iliofemoral ligament S73.11-
    ischiocapsular (ligament) S73.12-
    specified NEC S73.19-
  iliofemoral — see Sprain, hip
  innominate
    acetabulum — see Sprain, hip
    sacral junction S33.6
  internal
    collateral, ankle — see Sprain, ankle
    semilunar cartilage — see Sprain, knee, specified site
      NEC
  interphalangeal
    finger — see Sprain, finger, interphalangeal (joint)
    toe — see Sprain, toe, interphalangeal joint
  ischiocapsular — see Sprain, hip
  ischiofemoral — see Sprain, hip
  jaw (articular disc) (cartilage) (meniscus) S03.4-
    old M26.69
  knee S83.9-
    collateral ligament S83.40-
      lateral (fibular) S83.42-
      medial (tibial) S83.41-
    cruciate ligament S83.50-
      anterior S83.51-
      posterior S83.52-
    lateral (fibular) collateral ligament S83.42-
    medial (tibial) collateral ligament S83.41-
    patellar ligament S76.11-
    specified site NEC S83.8X-
    superior tibiofibular joint (ligament) S83.6-
  lateral collateral, knee — see Sprain, knee, collateral
  lumbar (spine) S33.5
  lumbosacral S33.9
  mandible (articular disc) S03.4-
    old M26.69
  medial collateral, knee — see Sprain, knee, collateral
  meniscus
    jaw S03.4-
      old M26.69
    knee — see Sprain, knee, specified site NEC
      with current tear — see Tear, meniscus
        old — see Derangement, knee, meniscus, due
          to old tear
    mandible S03.4-
      old M26.69
  metacarpal (distal) (proximal) — see Sprain, hand, specified site NEC
  metacarpophalangeal — see Sprain, finger, metacarpophalangeal (joint)
  metatarsophalangeal — see Sprain, toe, metatarsophalangeal joint
  midcarpal — see Sprain, hand, specified site NEC
  midtarsal — see Sprain, foot, specified site NEC
  neck S13.9
    anterior longitudinal cervical ligament S13.4
    atlanto-axial joint S13.4
    atlanto-occipital joint S13.4
    cervical spine S13.4
    cricoarytenoid ligament S13.5
    cricothyroid ligament S13.5
    specified site NEC S13.8
    thyroid region (cartilage) S13.5
  nose S03.8
  orbicular, hip — see Sprain, hip
  patella — see Sprain, knee, specified site NEC
  patellar ligament S76.11-

Sprain — continued
  pelvis NEC S33.8
  phalanx
    finger — see Sprain, finger
    toe — see Sprain, toe
  pubofemoral — see Sprain, hip
  radiocarpal — see Sprain, wrist
  radiohumeral — see Sprain, elbow
  radius, collateral — see Rupture, traumatic, ligament, radial collateral
  rib (cage) S23.41
  rotator cuff (capsule) S43.42-
  sacroiliac (region)
    chronic or old — see subcategory M53.2
    joint S33.6
  scaphoid (hand) — see Sprain, hand, specified site NEC
  scapula (r) — see Sprain, shoulder girdle, specified site
    NEC
  semilunar cartilage (knee) — see Sprain, knee, specified
    site NEC
    with current tear — see Tear, meniscus
      old — see Derangement, knee, meniscus, due to
        old tear
  shoulder joint S43.40-
    acromioclavicular joint (ligament) — see Sprain,
      acromioclavicular joint
    blade — see Sprain, shoulder, girdle, specified site
      NEC
    coracoclavicular joint (ligament) — see Sprain, coracoclavicular joint
    coracohumeral ligament — see Sprain, coracohumeral
      joint
    girdle S43.9-
      specified site NEC S43.8-
    rotator cuff — see Sprain, rotator cuff
    specified site NEC S43.49-
    sternoclavicular joint (ligament) — see Sprain, sternoclavicular joint
  spine
    cervical S13.4
    lumbar S33.5
    thoracic S23.3
  sternoclavicular joint S43.6-
  sternum S23.429
    chondrosternal joint S23.421
    specified site NEC S23.428
    sternoclavicular (joint) (ligament) S43.6-
  symphysis
    jaw S03.4-
      old M26.69
    mandibular S03.4-
      old M26.69
  talofibular — see Sprain, ankle
  tarsal — see Sprain, foot, specified site NEC
  tarsometatarsal — see Sprain, foot, specified site NEC
  temporomandibular S03.4-
    old M26.69
  thorax S23.9
    ribs S23.41
    specified site NEC S23.8
    spine S23.3
    sternum — see Sprain, sternum
  thumb S63.60-
    interphalangeal (joint) S63.62-
    metacarpophalangeal (joint) S63.64-
    specified site NEC S63.68-
  thyroid cartilage or region S13.5
  tibia (proximal end) — see Sprain, knee, specified site
    NEC
  tibial collateral, knee — see Sprain, knee, collateral
  tibiofibular
    distal — see Sprain, ankle
    superior — see Sprain, knee, specified site NEC
  toe(s) S93.50-
    great S93.50-
    interphalangeal joint S93.51-
      great S93.51-
      lesser S93.51-
    lesser S93.50-
    metatarsophalangeal joint S93.52-
      great S93.52-
      lesser S93.52-
  ulna, collateral — see Rupture, traumatic, ligament, ulnar
    collateral
  ulnohumeral — see Sprain, elbow
  wrist S63.50-
    carpal S63.51-

Sprain — *continued*
  wrist — *continued*
    radiocarpal S63.52- ☑
    specified site NEC S63.59- ☑
    xiphoid cartilage — *see* Sprain, sternum
Sprengel's deformity (congenital) Q74.0
Sprue (tropical) K90.1
  celiac K90.0
  idiopathic K90.49
  meaning thrush B37.0
  nontropical K90.0
Spur, bone — *see also* Enthesopathy
  calcaneal M77.3- ☑
  iliac crest M76.2- ☑
  nose (septum) J34.89
Spurway's syndrome Q78.0
Sputum
  abnormal (amount) (color) (odor) (purulent) R09.3
  blood-stained R04.2
  excessive (cause unknown) R09.3
Squamous — *see also* condition
  epithelium in
    cervical canal (congenital) Q51.828
    uterine mucosa (congenital) Q51.818
Squashed nose M95.0
  congenital Q67.4
Squeeze, diver's T70.3 ☑
Squint — *see also* Strabismus
  accommodative — *see* Strabismus, convergent concomitant
SSADHD (succinic semialdehyde dehydrogenase deficiency) E72.81
St. Hubert's disease A82.9
Stab — *see also* Laceration
  internal organs — *see* Injury, by site
Stafne's cyst or cavity M27.0
Staggering gait R26.0
  hysterical F44.4
Staghorn calculus — *see* Calculus, kidney
Stahli's line (cornea) (pigment) — *see* Pigmentation, cornea, anterior
Stain, staining
  meconium (newborn) P96.83
  port wine Q82.5
  tooth, teeth (hard tissues) (extrinsic) K03.6
    due to
      accretions K03.6
      deposits (betel) (black) (green) (materia alba) (orange) (soft) (tobacco) K03.6
      metals (copper) (silver) K03.7
      nicotine K03.6
      pulpal bleeding K03.7
      tobacco K03.6
    intrinsic K00.8
Stammering — *see also* Disorder, fluency F80.81
Standstill
  auricular I45.5
  cardiac — *see* Arrest, cardiac
  sinoatrial I45.5
  ventricular — *see* Arrest, cardiac
Stannosis J63.5
Stanton's disease — *see* Melioidosis
Staphylitis (acute) (catarrhal) (chronic) (gangrenous) (membranous) (suppurative) (ulcerative) K12.2
Staphylococcal scalded skin syndrome L00
Staphylococcemia A41.2
Staphylococcus, staphylococcal — *see also* condition
  as cause of disease classified elsewhere B95.8
    aureus (methicillin susceptible) (MSSA) B95.61
      methicillin resistant (MRSA) B95.62
  specified NEC, as cause of disease classified elsewhere B95.7
Staphyloma (sclera)
  cornea H18.72- ☑
  equatorial H15.81- ☑
  localized (anterior) H15.82- ☑
  posticum H15.83- ☑
  ring H15.85- ☑
Stargardt's disease — *see* Dystrophy, retina
Starvation (inanition) (due to lack of food) T73.0 ☑
  edema — *see* Malnutrition, severe
Stasis
  bile (noncalculous) K83.1
  bronchus J98.09
    with infection — *see* Bronchitis
  cardiac — *see* Failure, heart, congestive
  cecum K59.89
  colon K59.89

Stasis — *continued*
  dermatitis I87.2
    with
      varicose ulcer — *see* Varix, leg, with ulcer, with inflammation
      varicose veins — *see* Varix, leg, with, inflammation
    due to postthrombotic syndrome — *see* Syndrome, postthrombotic
  duodenal K31.5
  eczema — *see* Varix, leg, with, inflammation
  edema — *see* Hypertension, venous (chronic), idiopathic
  foot T69.0- ☑
  ileocecal coil K59.89
  ileum K59.89
  intestinal K59.89
  jejunum K59.89
  kidney N19
  liver (cirrhotic) K76.1
  lymphatic I89.8
  pneumonia J18.2
  pulmonary — *see* Edema, lung
  rectal K59.89
  renal N19
    tubular N17.0
  ulcer — *see* Varix, leg, with, ulcer
    without varicose veins — *see also* Ulcer, by site I87.2
  urine — *see* Retention, urine
  venous I87.8
State (of)
  affective and paranoid, mixed, organic psychotic F06.8
  agitated R45.1
    acute reaction to stress F43.0
  anxiety (neurotic) F41.1
  apprehension F41.1
  burn-out Z73.0
  climacteric, female Z78.0
    symptomatic N95.1
  compulsive F42.8
    mixed with obsessional thoughts F42.2
  confusional (psychogenic) F44.89
    acute — *see also* Delirium
      with
        arteriosclerotic dementia — *see also* Dementia, vascular F01.50
          with behavioral disturbance — *see* Dementia, vascular
        senility or dementia F05
      alcoholic F10.231
    epileptic F05
    reactive (from emotional stress, psychological trauma) F44.89
    subacute — *see* Delirium
  convulsive — *see* Convulsions
  crisis F43.0
  depressive F32.A
    neurotic F34.1
  dissociative F44.9
  emotional shock (stress) R45.7
  hypercoagulation — *see* Hypercoagulable
  locked-in G83.5
  menopausal Z78.0
    symptomatic N95.1
  neurotic F48.9
    with depersonalization F48.1
  obsessional F42.8
  oneiroid (schizophrenia-like) F23
  organic
    hallucinatory (nonalcoholic) F06.0
    paranoid (-hallucinatory) F06.2
  panic F41.0
  paranoid F22
    climacteric F22
    involutional F22
    menopausal F22
    organic F06.2
    senile F03 ☑
    simple F22
  persistent vegetative R40.3
  phobic F40.9
  postleukotomy F07.0
  pregnant
    gestational carrier Z33.3
    incidental Z33.1
  psychogenic, twilight F44.89
  psychopathic (constitutional) F60.2
  psychotic, organic — *see also* Psychosis, organic
    mixed paranoid and affective F06.8
    senile or presenile F03 ☑
    transient NEC F06.8

State — *continued*
  psychotic, organic — *see also* Psychosis, organic — *continued*
    transient — *continued*
      with
        depression F06.31
        hallucinations F06.0
  residual schizophrenic F20.5
  restlessness R45.1
  stress (emotional) R45.7
  tension (mental) F48.9
    specified NEC F48.8
  transient organic psychotic NEC F06.8
    depressive type F06.31
    hallucinatory type F06.0
  twilight
    epileptic F05
    psychogenic F44.89
  vegetative, persistent R40.3
  vital exhaustion Z73.0
  withdrawal, — *see* Withdrawal, state
Status (post) — *see also* Presence (of)
  absence, epileptic — *see* Epilepsy, by type, with status epilepticus
  administration of tPA (rtPA) in a different facility within the last 24 hours prior to admission to current facility Z92.82
  adrenalectomy (unilateral) (bilateral) E89.6
  anastomosis Z98.0
  anginosus I20.9
  angioplasty (peripheral) Z98.62
    with implant Z95.820
    coronary artery Z98.61
      with implant Z95.5
  aortocoronary bypass Z95.1
  arthrodesis Z98.1
  artificial opening (of) Z93.9
    gastrointestinal tract Z93.4
    specified NEC Z93.8
    urinary tract Z93.6
    vagina Z93.8
  asthmaticus — *see* Asthma, by type, with status asthmaticus
  awaiting organ transplant Z76.82
  bariatric surgery Z98.84
  bed confinement Z74.01
  bleb, filtering (vitreous), after glaucoma surgery Z98.83
  breast implant Z98.82
    removal Z98.86
  cataract extraction Z98.4- ☑
  cholecystectomy Z90.49
  clitorectomy N90.811
    with excision of labia minora N90.812
  colectomy (complete) (partial) Z90.49
  colonization — *see* Carrier (suspected) of
  colostomy Z93.3
  combined receptor
    negative
      hormone receptor negative with human epidermal growth factor receptor 2 negative Z17.421
      hormone receptor negative with human epidermal growth factor receptor 2 positive Z17.420
    positive
      hormone receptor positive with human epidermal growth factor receptor 2 negative Z17.411
      hormone receptor positive with human epidermal growth factor receptor 2 positive Z17.410
  convulsivus idiopathicus — *see* Epilepsy, by type, with status epilepticus
  coronary artery angioplasty — *see* Status, angioplasty, coronary artery
  coronary artery bypass graft Z95.1
  cystectomy (urinary bladder) Z90.6
  cystostomy Z93.50
    appendico-vesicostomy Z93.52
    cutaneous Z93.51
    specified NEC Z93.59
  delinquent immunization Z28.39
    COVID-19 Z28.31- ☑
  dental Z98.818
    crown Z98.811
    fillings Z98.811
    restoration Z98.811
    sealant Z98.810
    specified NEC Z98.818
  deployment (current) (military) Z56.82
  dialysis (hemodialysis) (peritoneal) Z99.2
  do not resuscitate (DNR) Z66
  donor — *see* Donor

☑ **Additional Character Required** — **Refer to the Tabular List for Character Selection**

Index

Status — Stenosis, stenotic

Status — continued

embedded fragments — *see* Retained, foreign body fragments (type of)
embedded splinter — *see* Retained, foreign body fragments (type of)
enterostomy Z93.4
epileptic, epilepticus — *see also* Epilepsy, by type, with status epilepticus G40.901
estrogen receptor
    negative Z17.1
    positive Z17.0
female genital cutting — *see* Female genital mutilation status
female genital mutilation — *see* Female genital mutilation status
filtering (vitreous) bleb after glaucoma surgery Z98.83
gastrectomy (complete) (partial) Z90.3
gastric banding Z98.84
gastric bypass for obesity Z98.84
gastrostomy Z93.1
human epidermal growth factor 2 receptor
    negative Z17.32
    positive Z17.31
human immunodeficiency virus (HIV) infection, asymptomatic Z21
hysterectomy (complete) (total) Z90.710
    partial (with remaining cervical stump) Z90.711
ileostomy (ileal pouch) (Kock pouch) Z93.2
implant
    breast Z98.82
infibulation N90.813
intestinal bypass Z98.0
jejunostomy Z93.4
lapsed immunization schedule Z28.39
laryngectomy Z90.02
lymphaticus E32.8
malignancy
    castrate resistant prostate Z19.2
    hormone resistant Z19.2
    hormone sensitive Z19.1
marmoratus G80.3
mastectomy (unilateral) (bilateral) Z90.1- ☑
military deployment status (current) Z56.82
    in theater or in support of military war, peacekeeping and humanitarian operations Z56.82
nephrectomy (unilateral) (bilateral) Z90.5
nephrostomy Z93.6
obesity surgery Z98.84
oophorectomy
    bilateral Z90.722
    unilateral Z90.721
organ replacement
    by artificial or mechanical device or prosthesis of
        artery Z95.828
        bladder Z96.0
        blood vessel Z95.828
        breast Z97.8
        eye globe Z97.0
        heart Z95.812
            valve Z95.2
        intestine Z97.8
        joint Z96.60
            hip — *see* Presence, hip joint implant
            knee — *see* Presence, knee joint implant
            specified site NEC Z96.698
        kidney Z97.8
        larynx Z96.3
        lens Z96.1
        limbs — *see* Presence, artificial, limb
        liver Z97.8
        lung Z97.8
        pancreas Z97.8
    by organ transplant (heterologous) (homologous) — *see* Transplant
pacemaker
    brain Z96.89
    cardiac Z95.0
    specified NEC Z96.89
pancreatectomy Z90.410
    complete Z90.410
    partial Z90.411
    total Z90.410
physical restraint Z78.1
pneumonectomy (complete) (partial) Z90.2
pneumothorax, therapeutic Z98.3
postcommotio cerebri F07.81
postoperative (postprocedural) NEC Z98.890
    breast implant Z98.82
    dental Z98.818

Status — continued

postoperative — *continued*
    dental — *continued*
        crown Z98.811
        fillings Z98.811
        restoration Z98.811
        sealant Z98.810
        specified NEC Z98.818
    pneumothorax, therapeutic Z98.3
    uterine scar Z98.891
postpartum (routine follow-up) Z39.2
    care immediately after delivery Z39.0
postsurgical (postprocedural) NEC Z98.890
    pneumothorax, therapeutic Z98.3
pregnancy, incidental Z33.1
progesterone receptor
    negative Z17.22
    positive Z17.21
prosthesis coronary angioplasty Z95.5
pseudophakia Z96.1
renal dialysis (hemodialysis) (peritoneal) Z99.2
retained foreign body — *see* Retained, foreign body fragments (type of)
reversed jejunal transposition (for bypass) Z98.0
salpingo-oophorectomy
    bilateral Z90.722
    unilateral Z90.721
sex reassignment surgery status Z87.890
shunt
    arteriovenous (for dialysis) Z99.2
    cerebrospinal fluid Z98.2
    ventricular (communicating) (for drainage) Z98.2
splenectomy Z90.81
thymicolymphaticus E32.8
thymicus E32.8
thymolymphaticus E32.8
thyroidectomy (hypothyroidism) E89.0
tooth (teeth) extraction — *see also* Absence, teeth, acquired K08.409
tPA (rtPA) administration in a different facility within the last 24 hours prior to admission to current facility Z92.82
tracheostomy Z93.0
transplant — *see* Transplant
    organ removed Z98.85
tubal ligation Z98.51
underimmunization Z28.39
    COVID-19 Z28.31- ☑
        partially vaccinated (for) Z28.311
        unvaccinated (for) Z28.310
ureterostomy Z93.6
urethrostomy Z93.6
vagina, artificial Z93.8
vasectomy Z98.52
wheelchair confinement Z99.3

Stealing

child problem F91.8
    in company with others Z72.810
pathological (compulsive) F63.2
Steam burn — *see* Burn
Steatocystoma multiplex L72.2
Steatohepatitis (nonalcoholic) (NASH) K75.81
Steatoma L72.3
    eyelid (cystic) — *see* Dermatosis, eyelid
        infected — *see* Hordeolum
Steatorrhea (chronic) K90.9
    with lacteal obstruction K90.2
    idiopathic (adult) (infantile) K90.9
    pancreatic K90.3
    primary K90.0
    tropical K90.1
Steatosis E88.89
    heart — *see* Degeneration, myocardial
    kidney N28.89
    liver NEC K76.0
Steele-Richardson-Olszewski disease or syndrome G23.1
Steinbrocker's syndrome G90.89
Steinert's disease G71.11
Stein-Leventhal syndrome E28.2
Stein's syndrome E28.2
STEMI — *see also* Infarct, myocardium, ST elevation I21.3
Stenocardia I20.89
Stenocephaly Q75.8
Stenosis, stenotic (cicatricial) — *see also* Stricture
ampulla of Vater K83.1
anus, anal (canal) (sphincter) K62.4
    and rectum K62.4
    congenital Q42.3
        with fistula Q42.2

Stenosis, stenotic — continued

aorta (ascending) (supraventricular) (congenital) Q25.1
    arteriosclerotic I70.0
    calcified I70.0
    supravalvular Q25.3
aortic (valve) I35.0
    with insufficiency I35.2
    congenital Q23.0
    rheumatic I06.0
        with
            incompetency, insufficiency or regurgitation I06.2
                with mitral (valve) disease I08.0
                    with tricuspid (valve) disease I08.3
            mitral (valve) disease I08.0
                with tricuspid (valve) disease I08.3
            tricuspid (valve) disease I08.2
                with mitral (valve) disease I08.3
    specified cause NEC I35.0
    syphilitic A52.03
aqueduct of Sylvius (congenital) Q03.0
    with spina bifida — *see* Spina bifida, by site, with hydrocephalus
    acquired G91.1
artery NEC — *see also* Arteriosclerosis I77.1
    celiac (compression) I77.4
        arteriosclerotic I70.8
        atherosclerosis I70.8
    cerebral — *see* Occlusion, artery, cerebral
    extremities — *see* Arteriosclerosis, extremities
    precerebral — *see* Occlusion, artery, precerebral
    pulmonary (congenital) Q25.6
        acquired I28.8
    renal I70.1
    stent
        coronary T82.855 ☑
        peripheral T82.856 ☑
bile duct (common) (hepatic) K83.1
    congenital Q44.3
bladder-neck (acquired) N32.0
    congenital Q64.31
brain G93.89
bronchus J98.09
    congenital Q32.3
    syphilitic A52.72
cardia (stomach) K22.2
    congenital Q39.3
cardiovascular — *see* Disease, cardiovascular
caudal M48.08
cervix, cervical (canal) N88.2
    congenital Q51.828
    in pregnancy or childbirth — *see* Pregnancy, complicated by, abnormal cervix
colon — *see also* Obstruction, intestine
    congenital Q42.9
        specified NEC Q42.8
colostomy K94.03
common (bile) duct K83.1
    congenital Q44.3
coronary (artery) — *see* Disease, heart, ischemic, atherosclerotic
cystic duct — *see* Obstruction, gallbladder
due to presence of device, implant or graft — *see also* Complications, by site and type, specified NEC T85.858 ☑
    arterial graft NEC T82.858 ☑
    breast (implant) T85.858 ☑
    catheter T85.858 ☑
        dialysis (renal) T82.858 ☑
            intraperitoneal T85.858 ☑
        infusion NEC T82.858 ☑
            spinal (epidural) (subdural) T85.850 ☑
        urinary (indwelling) T83.85 ☑
    fixation, internal (orthopedic) NEC T84.85 ☑
    gastrointestinal (bile duct) (esophagus) T85.858 ☑
    genital NEC T83.85 ☑
    heart NEC T82.857 ☑
    joint prosthesis T84.85 ☑
    ocular (corneal graft) (orbital implant) NEC T85.858 ☑
    orthopedic NEC T84.85 ☑
    specified NEC T85.858 ☑
    urinary NEC T83.85 ☑
    vascular NEC T82.858 ☑
    ventricular intracranial shunt T85.850 ☑
duodenum K31.5
    congenital Q41.0
ejaculatory duct NEC N50.89

Stenosis, stenotic — *continued*
  ejaculatory duct — *continued*
    stent
      vascular
        end stent
          adjacent to stent — *see* Arteriosclerosis
          within the stent
            coronary T82.855 ☑
            peripheral T82.856 ☑
        in stent
          coronary vessel T82.855 ☑
          peripheral vessel T82.856 ☑
  endocervical os — *see* Stenosis, cervix
  enterostomy K94.13
  esophagus K22.2
    congenital Q39.3
    syphilitic A52.79
      congenital A50.59 *[K23]*
  eustachian tube — *see* Obstruction, eustachian tube
  external ear canal (acquired) H61.30- ☑
    congenital Q16.1
    due to
      inflammation H61.32- ☑
      trauma H61.31- ☑
    postprocedural H95.81- ☑
    specified cause NEC H61.39- ☑
  gallbladder — *see* Obstruction, gallbladder
  glottis J38.6
  heart valve — *see also* Endocarditis I38
    aortic — *see* Stenosis, aortic
    congenital Q24.8
    mitral — *see* Stenosis, mitral
    pulmonary — *see* Stenosis, pulmonary valve
    tricuspid — *see* Stenosis, tricuspid
  hepatic duct K83.1
  hymen N89.6
  hypertrophic subaortic (idiopathic) I42.1
  ileum — *see also* Obstruction, intestine, specified NEC K56.699
    congenital Q41.2
  infundibulum cardia Q24.3
  intervertebral foramina — *see also* Lesion, biomechanical, specified NEC
    connective tissue M99.79
      abdomen M99.79
      cervical region M99.71
      cervicothoracic M99.71
      head region M99.70
      lumbar region M99.73
      lumbosacral M99.73
      occipitocervical M99.70
      sacral region M99.74
      sacrococcygeal M99.74
      sacroiliac M99.74
      specified NEC M99.79
      thoracic region M99.72
      thoracolumbar M99.72
    disc M99.79
      abdomen M99.79
      cervical region M99.71
      cervicothoracic M99.71
      head region M99.70
      lower extremity M99.76
      lumbar region M99.73
      lumbosacral M99.73
      occipitocervical M99.70
      pelvic M99.75
      rib cage M99.78
      sacral region M99.74
      sacrococcygeal M99.74
      sacroiliac M99.74
      specified NEC M99.79
      thoracic region M99.72
      thoracolumbar M99.72
      upper extremity M99.77
    osseous M99.69
      abdomen M99.69
      cervical region M99.61
      cervicothoracic M99.61
      head region M99.60
      lower extremity M99.66
      lumbar region M99.63
      lumbosacral M99.63
      occipitocervical M99.60
      pelvic M99.65
      rib cage M99.68
      sacral region M99.64
      sacrococcygeal M99.64

Stenosis, stenotic — *continued*
  intervertebral foramina — *see also* Lesion, biomechanical, specified — *continued*
    osseous — *continued*
      sacroiliac M99.64
      specified NEC M99.69
      thoracic region M99.62
      thoracolumbar M99.62
      upper extremity M99.67
    subluxation — *see* Stenosis, intervertebral foramina, osseous
  intestine — *see also* Obstruction, intestine
    congenital (small) Q41.9
      large Q42.9
        specified NEC Q42.8
      specified NEC Q41.8
  jejunum — *see also* Obstruction, intestine, specified NEC K56.699
    congenital Q41.1
  lacrimal (passage)
    canaliculi H04.54- ☑
    congenital Q10.5
    duct H04.55- ☑
    punctum H04.56- ☑
    sac H04.57- ☑
  lacrimonasal duct — *see* Stenosis, lacrimal, duct
    congenital Q10.5
  larynx J38.6
    congenital NEC Q31.8
      subglottic Q31.1
    syphilitic A52.73
      congenital A50.59 *[J99]*
  mitral (chronic) (inactive) (valve) I05.0
    with
      aortic valve disease I08.0
      incompetency, insufficiency or regurgitation I05.2
    active or acute I01.1
      with rheumatic or Sydenham's chorea I02.0
    congenital Q23.2
    specified cause, except rheumatic I34.2
    syphilitic A52.03
  myocardium, myocardial — *see also* Degeneration, myocardial
    hypertrophic subaortic (idiopathic) I42.1
  nares (anterior) (posterior) J34.89
    congenital Q30.0
  nasal duct — *see also* Stenosis, lacrimal, duct
    congenital Q10.5
  nasolacrimal duct — *see also* Stenosis, lacrimal, duct
    congenital Q10.5
  neural canal — *see also* Lesion, biomechanical, specified NEC
    connective tissue M99.49
      abdomen M99.49
      cervical region M99.41
      cervicothoracic M99.41
      head region M99.40
      lower extremity M99.46
      lumbar region M99.43
      lumbosacral M99.43
      occipitocervical M99.40
      pelvic M99.45
      rib cage M99.48
      sacral region M99.44
      sacrococcygeal M99.44
      sacroiliac M99.44
      specified NEC M99.49
      thoracic region M99.42
      thoracolumbar M99.42
      upper extremity M99.47
    intervertebral disc M99.59
      abdomen M99.59
      cervical region M99.51
      cervicothoracic M99.51
      head region M99.50
      lower extremity M99.56
      lumbar region M99.53
      lumbosacral M99.53
      occipitocervical M99.50
      pelvic M99.55
      rib cage M99.58
      sacral region M99.54
      sacrococcygeal M99.54
      sacroiliac M99.54
      specified NEC M99.59
      thoracic region M99.52
      thoracolumbar M99.52
      upper extremity M99.57
    osseous M99.39

Stenosis, stenotic — *continued*
  neural canal — *see also* Lesion, biomechanical, specified — *continued*
    osseous — *continued*
      abdomen M99.39
      cervical region M99.31
      cervicothoracic M99.31
      head region M99.30
      lower extremity M99.36
      lumbar region M99.33
      lumbosacral M99.33
      occipitocervical M99.30
      pelvic M99.35
      rib cage M99.38
      sacral region M99.34
      sacrococcygeal M99.34
      sacroiliac M99.34
      specified NEC M99.39
      thoracic region M99.32
      thoracolumbar M99.32
      upper extremity M99.37
    subluxation M99.29
      cervical region M99.21
      cervicothoracic M99.21
      head region M99.20
      lower extremity M99.26
      lumbar region M99.23
      lumbosacral M99.23
      occipitocervical M99.20
      pelvic M99.25
      rib cage M99.28
      sacral region M99.24
      sacrococcygeal M99.24
      sacroiliac M99.24
      specified NEC M99.29
      thoracic region M99.22
      thoracolumbar M99.22
      upper extremity M99.27
  organ or site, congenital NEC — *see* Atresia, by site
  papilla of Vater K83.1
  pulmonary (artery) (congenital) Q25.6
    with ventricular septal defect, transposition of aorta, and hypertrophy of right ventricle Q21.3
    acquired I28.8
    in tetralogy of Fallot Q21.3
    infundibular Q24.3
    subvalvular Q24.3
    supravalvular Q25.6
    valve I37.0
      with insufficiency I37.2
      congenital Q22.1
      rheumatic I09.89
        with aortic, mitral or tricuspid (valve) disease I08.8
    vein, acquired I28.8
    vessel NEC I28.8
  pulmonic (congenital) Q22.1
    infundibular Q24.3
    subvalvular Q24.3
  pylorus (hypertrophic) (acquired) K31.1
    adult K31.1
    congenital Q40.0
    infantile Q40.0
  rectum (sphincter) — *see* Stricture, rectum
  renal artery I70.1
    congenital Q27.1
  salivary duct (any) K11.8
  sphincter of Oddi K83.1
  spinal M48.00
    cervical region M48.02
    cervicothoracic region M48.03
    lumbar region (NOS) (without neurogenic claudication) M48.061
      with neurogenic claudication M48.062
    lumbosacral region M48.07
    occipito-atlanto-axial region M48.01
    sacrococcygeal region M48.08
    thoracic region M48.04
    thoracolumbar region M48.05
  stomach, hourglass K31.2
  subaortic (congenital) Q24.4
    hypertrophic (idiopathic) I42.1
  subglottic J38.6
    congenital Q31.1
    postprocedural J95.5
  trachea J39.8
    congenital Q32.1
    syphilitic A52.73
    tuberculous NEC A15.5

Stenosis, stenotic — continued
tracheostomy J95.03
tricuspid (valve) I07.0
with
aortic (valve) disease I08.2
incompetency, insufficiency or regurgitation I07.2
with aortic (valve) disease I08.2
with mitral (valve) disease I08.3
mitral (valve) disease I08.1
with aortic (valve) disease I08.3
congenital Q22.4
nonrheumatic I36.0
with insufficiency I36.2
tubal N97.1
ureter — see Atresia, ureter
ureteropelvic junction, congenital Q62.11
ureterovesical orifice, congenital Q62.12
urethra (valve) see also Stricture, urethra
congenital Q64.32
urinary meatus, congenital Q64.33
vagina N89.5
congenital Q52.4
in pregnancy — see Pregnancy, complicated by, abnormal vagina
causing obstructed labor O65.5
valve (cardiac) (heart) — see also Endocarditis I38
congenital Q24.8
aortic Q23.0
mitral Q23.2
pulmonary Q22.1
tricuspid Q22.4
vena cava (inferior) (superior) I87.1
congenital Q26.0
vesicourethral orifice Q64.31
vulva N90.5
Stent jail T82.897 ☑
Stercolith (impaction) K56.41
appendix K38.1
Stercoraceous, stercoral ulcer K63.3
anus or rectum K62.6
Stereotypies NEC F98.4
Sterility — see Infertility
Sterilization — see Encounter (for), sterilization
Sternalgia — see Angina
Sternopagus Q89.4
Sternum bifidum Q76.7
Steroid
effects (adverse) (adrenocortical) (iatrogenic)
cushingoid E24.2
correct substance properly administered — see Table of Drugs and Chemicals, by drug, adverse effect
overdose or wrong substance given or taken — see Table of Drugs and Chemicals, by drug, poisoning
diabetes — see subcategory E09 ☑
correct substance properly administered — see Table of Drugs and Chemicals, by drug, adverse effect
overdose or wrong substance given or taken — see Table of Drugs and Chemicals, by drug, poisoning
fever R50.2
insufficiency E27.3
correct substance properly administered — see Table of Drugs and Chemicals, by drug, adverse effect
overdose or wrong substance given or taken — see Table of Drugs and Chemicals, by drug, poisoning
responder H40.04- ☑
Stevens-Johnson disease or syndrome L51.1
toxic epidermal necrolysis overlap L51.3
Stewart-Morel syndrome M85.2
Sticker's disease B08.3
Sticky eye — see Conjunctivitis, acute, mucopurulent
Stieda's disease — see Bursitis, tibial collateral
Stiff neck — see Torticollis
Stiff-man syndrome G25.82
Stiffness, joint NEC M25.60
ankle M25.67- ☑
ankylosis — see Ankylosis, joint
contracture — see Contraction, joint
elbow M25.62- ☑
foot M25.67- ☑
hand M25.64- ☑
hip M25.65- ☑
knee M25.66- ☑

Stiffness, joint — continued
shoulder M25.61- ☑
specified site NEC M25.69
wrist M25.63- ☑
Stigmata congenital syphilis A50.59
Stillbirth P95
Still-Felty syndrome — see Felty's syndrome
Still's disease or syndrome (juvenile) M08.20
adult-onset M06.1
ankle M08.27- ☑
elbow M08.22- ☑
foot joint M08.27- ☑
hand joint M08.24- ☑
hip M08.25- ☑
knee M08.26- ☑
multiple site M08.29
shoulder M08.21- ☑
specified site NEC M08.2A
vertebra M08.28
wrist M08.23- ☑
Stimulation, ovary E28.1
Sting (venomous) (with allergic or anaphylactic shock) — see Table of Drugs and Chemicals, by animal or substance, poisoning
Stippled epiphyses Q78.8
Stitch
abscess T81.41 ☑
burst (in operation wound) — see Disruption, wound, operation
Stokes' disease E05.00
with thyroid storm E05.01
Stokes-Adams disease or syndrome I45.9
Stokvis (-Talma) **disease** D74.8
Stoma malfunction
colostomy K94.03
enterostomy K94.13
gastrostomy K94.23
ileostomy K94.13
tracheostomy J95.03
Stomach — see condition
Stomatitis (denture) (ulcerative) K12.1
angular K13.0
due to dietary or vitamin deficiency E53.0
aphthous K12.0
bovine B08.61
candidal B37.0
catarrhal K12.1
diphtheritic A36.89
due to
dietary deficiency E53.0
thrush B37.0
vitamin deficiency
B group NEC E53.9
B2 (riboflavin) E53.0
epidemic B08.8
epizootic B08.8
follicular K12.1
gangrenous A69.0
Geotrichum B48.3
herpesviral, herpetic B00.2
herpetiformis K12.0
malignant K12.1
membranous acute K12.1
monilial B37.0
mycotic B37.0
necrotizing ulcerative A69.0
parasitic B37.0
septic K12.1
spirochetal A69.1
suppurative (acute) K12.2
ulceromembranous A69.1
vesicular K12.1
with exanthem (enteroviral) B08.4
virus disease A93.8
Vincent's A69.1
Stomatocytosis D58.8
Stomatomycosis B37.0
Stomatorrhagia K13.79
Stone(s) — see also Calculus
bladder (diverticulum) N21.0
cystine E72.09
heart syndrome I50.1
kidney N20.0
prostate N42.0
pulpal (dental) K04.2
renal N20.0
salivary gland or duct (any) K11.5
urethra (impacted) N21.1

Stone(s) — continued
urinary (duct) (impacted) (passage) N20.9
bladder (diverticulum) N21.0
lower tract N21.9
specified NEC N21.8
xanthine E79.82 [N22]
Stonecutter's lung J62.8
Stonemason's asthma, disease, lung or pneumoconiosis J62.8
Stoppage
heart — see Arrest, cardiac
urine — see Retention, urine
Storm, thyroid — see Thyrotoxicosis
Strabismus (congenital) (nonparalytic) H50.9
concomitant H50.40
convergent — see Strabismus, convergent concomitant
divergent — see Strabismus, divergent concomitant
convergent concomitant H50.00
accommodative component H50.43
alternating H50.05
with
A pattern H50.06
specified nonconcomitances NEC H50.08
V pattern H50.07
monocular H50.01- ☑
with
A pattern H50.02- ☑
specified nonconcomitances NEC H50.04- ☑
V pattern H50.03- ☑
intermittent H50.31- ☑
alternating H50.32
cyclotropia H50.41 ☑
divergent concomitant H50.10
alternating H50.15
with
A pattern H50.16
specified nonconcomitances NEC H50.18
V pattern H50.17
monocular H50.11- ☑
with
A pattern H50.12- ☑
specified nonconcomitances NEC H50.14- ☑
V pattern H50.13- ☑
intermittent H50.33 ☑
alternating H50.34
Duane's syndrome H50.81- ☑
due to adhesions, scars H50.69
heterophoria H50.50
alternating H50.55
cyclophoria H50.54
esophoria H50.51
exophoria H50.52
vertical H50.53
heterotropia H50.40
intermittent H50.30
hypertropia H50.2- ☑
hypotropia — see Hypertropia
latent H50.50
mechanical H50.60
Brown's sheath syndrome H50.61- ☑
specified type NEC H50.69
monofixation syndrome H50.42
paralytic H49.9
abducens nerve H49.2- ☑
fourth nerve H49.1- ☑
Kearns-Sayre syndrome H49.81- ☑
ophthalmoplegia (external)
progressive H49.4- ☑
with pigmentary retinopathy H49.81- ☑
total H49.3- ☑
sixth nerve H49.2- ☑
specified type NEC H49.88- ☑
third nerve H49.0- ☑
trochlear nerve H49.1- ☑
specified type NEC H50.89
vertical H50.2- ☑
Strain
back S39.012 ☑
cervical S16.1 ☑
eye NEC — see Disturbance, vision, subjective
heart — see Disease, heart
low back S39.012 ☑
mental NOS Z73.3
work-related Z56.6
muscle (tendon) — see Injury, muscle, by site, strain
neck S16.1 ☑

☑ **Additional Character Required — Refer to the Tabular List for Character Selection**

Strain — *continued*
  physical NOS Z73.3
    work-related Z56.6
  postural — *see also* Disorder, soft tissue, due to use
  psychological NEC Z73.3
  tendon — *see* Injury, muscle, by site, strain
Straining, on urination R39.16
Strand, vitreous — *see* Opacity, vitreous, membranes and
    strands
Strangulation, strangulated — *see also* Asphyxia, traumat-
    ic
  appendix K38.8
  bladder-neck N32.0
  bowel or colon K56.2
  food or foreign body — *see* Foreign body, by site
  hemorrhoids — *see* Hemorrhoids, with complication
  hernia — *see also* Hernia, by site, with obstruction
    with gangrene — *see* Hernia, by site, with gangrene
  intestine (large) (small) K56.2
    with hernia — *see also* Hernia, by site, with obstruc-
        tion
      with gangrene — *see* Hernia, by site, with gan-
          grene
  mesentery K56.2
  mucus — *see* Asphyxia, mucus
  omentum K56.2
  organ or site, congenital NEC — *see* Atresia, by site
  ovary — *see* Torsion, ovary
  penis N48.89
    foreign body T19.4 ☑
  rupture — *see* Hernia, by site, with obstruction
  stomach due to hernia — *see also* Hernia, by site, with
      obstruction
    with gangrene — *see* Hernia, by site, with gangrene
  vesicourethral orifice N32.0
Strangury R30.0
Straw itch B88.0
Strawberry
  gallbladder K82.4
  mark Q82.5
  tongue (red) (white) K14.3
Streak(s)
  macula, angioid H35.33
  ovarian Q50.32
Strephosymbolia F81.0
  secondary to organic lesion R48.8
Streptobacillary fever A25.1
Streptobacillosis A25.1
Streptobacillus moniliformis A25.1
Streptococcus, streptococcal — *see also* condition
  as cause of disease classified elsewhere B95.5
  group
    A, as cause of disease classified elsewhere B95.0
    B, as cause of disease classified elsewhere B95.1
    D, as cause of disease classified elsewhere B95.2
  pneumoniae, as cause of disease classified elsewhere
      B95.3
  specified NEC, as cause of disease classified elsewhere
      B95.4
Streptomycosis B47.1
Streptotrichosis A48.8
Stress F43.9
  family — *see* Disruption, family
  fetal P84
    complicating pregnancy O77.9
      due to drug administration O77.1
  mental NEC Z73.3
    work-related Z56.6
  physical NEC Z73.3
    work-related Z56.6
  polycythemia D75.1
  reaction — *see also* Reaction, stress F43.9
  work schedule Z56.3
Stretching, nerve — *see* Injury, nerve
Striae albicantes, atrophicae or distensae (cutis) L90.6
Stricture — *see also* Stenosis
  ampulla of Vater K83.1
  anus (sphincter) K62.4
    congenital Q42.3
      with fistula Q42.2
    infantile Q42.3
      with fistula Q42.2
  aorta (ascending) (congenital) Q25.1
    arteriosclerotic I70.0
    calcified I70.0
    supravalvular, congenital Q25.3
  aortic (valve) — *see* Stenosis, aortic
  aqueduct of Sylvius (congenital) Q03.0

Stricture — *continued*
  aqueduct of Sylvius — *continued*
    with spina bifida — *see* Spina bifida, by site, with hy-
        drocephalus
    acquired G91.1
  artery I77.1
    basilar — *see* Occlusion, artery, basilar
    carotid — *see* Occlusion, artery, carotid
    celiac (compression) I77.4
      arteriosclerotic I70.8
      atherosclerosis I70.8
    congenital (peripheral) Q27.8
      cerebral Q28.3
      coronary Q24.5
      digestive system Q27.8
      lower limb Q27.8
      retinal Q14.1
      specified site NEC Q27.8
      umbilical Q27.0
      upper limb Q27.8
    coronary — *see* Disease, heart, ischemic, atheroscle-
        rotic
      congenital Q24.5
    precerebral — *see* Occlusion, artery, precerebral
    pulmonary (congenital) Q25.6
      acquired I28.8
    renal I70.1
    vertebral — *see* Occlusion, artery, vertebral
  auditory canal (external) (congenital)
    acquired — *see* Stenosis, external ear canal
  bile duct (common) (hepatic) K83.1
    congenital Q44.3
    postoperative K91.89
  bladder N32.89
    neck N32.0
  bowel — *see* Obstruction, intestine
  brain G93.89
  bronchus J98.09
    congenital Q32.3
    syphilitic A52.72
  cardia (stomach) K22.2
    congenital Q39.3
  cardiac — *see also* Disease, heart
    orifice (stomach) K22.2
  cecum — *see* Obstruction, intestine
  cervix, cervical (canal) N88.2
    congenital Q51.828
    in pregnancy — *see* Pregnancy, complicated by, ab-
        normal cervix
      causing obstructed labor O65.5
  colon — *see also* Obstruction, intestine
    congenital Q42.9
      specified NEC Q42.8
  colostomy K94.03
  common (bile) duct K83.1
  coronary (artery) — *see* Disease, heart, ischemic,
      atherosclerotic
  cystic duct — *see* Obstruction, gallbladder
  digestive organs NEC, congenital Q45.8
  duodenum K31.5
    congenital Q41.0
  ear canal (external) (congenital) Q16.1
    acquired — *see* Stricture, auditory canal, acquired
  ejaculatory duct N50.89
  enterostomy K94.13
  esophagus K22.2
    congenital Q39.3
    syphilitic A52.79
      congenital A50.59 *[K23]*
  eustachian tube — *see also* Obstruction, eustachian tube
    congenital Q17.8
  fallopian tube N97.1
    gonococcal A54.24
    tuberculous A18.17
  gallbladder — *see* Obstruction, gallbladder
  glottis J38.6
  heart — *see also* Disease, heart
    valve — *see also* Endocarditis I38
      aortic Q23.0
      mitral Q23.2
      pulmonary Q22.1
      tricuspid Q22.4
  hepatic duct K83.1
  hourglass, of stomach K31.2
  hymen N89.6
  hypopharynx J39.2
  ileum — *see also* Obstruction, intestine, specified NEC
      K56.699
    congenital Q41.2

Stricture — *continued*
  intestine — *see also* Obstruction, intestine
    congenital (small) Q41.9
      large Q42.9
        specified NEC Q42.8
      specified NEC Q41.8
    ischemic K55.1
  jejunum — *see also* Obstruction, intestine, specified NEC
      K56.699
    congenital Q41.1
  lacrimal passages — *see also* Stenosis, lacrimal
    congenital Q10.5
  larynx J38.6
    congenital NEC Q31.8
      subglottic Q31.1
    syphilitic A52.73
      congenital A50.59 *[J99]*
  meatus
    ear (congenital) Q16.1
      acquired — *see* Stricture, auditory canal, acquired
    osseous (ear) (congenital) Q16.1
      acquired — *see* Stricture, auditory canal, acquired
    urinarius — *see also* Stricture, urethra
      congenital Q64.33
  mitral (valve) — *see* Stenosis, mitral
  myocardium, myocardial I51.5
    hypertrophic subaortic (idiopathic) I42.1
  nares (anterior) (posterior) J34.89
    congenital Q30.0
  nasal duct — *see also* Stenosis, lacrimal, duct
    congenital Q10.5
  nasolacrimal duct — *see also* Stenosis, lacrimal, duct
    congenital Q10.5
  nasopharynx J39.2
    syphilitic A52.73
  nose J34.89
    congenital Q30.0
  nostril (anterior) (posterior) J34.89
    congenital Q30.0
    syphilitic A52.73
      congenital A50.59 *[J99]*
  organ or site, congenital NEC — *see* Atresia, by site
  os uteri — *see* Stricture, cervix
  osseous meatus (ear) (congenital) Q16.1
    acquired — *see* Stricture, auditory canal, acquired
  oviduct — *see* Stricture, fallopian tube
  pelviureteric junction (congenital) Q62.11
    acquired, with hydronephrosis N13.0
  penis, by foreign body T19.4 ☑
  pharynx J39.2
  prostate N42.89
  pulmonary, pulmonic
    artery (congenital) Q25.6
      acquired I28.8
      noncongenital I28.8
    infundibulum (congenital) Q24.3
    valve I37.0
      congenital Q22.1
    vein, acquired I28.8
    vessel NEC I28.8
  punctum lacrimale — *see also* Stenosis, lacrimal, punc-
      tum
    congenital Q10.5
  pylorus (hypertrophic) K31.1
    adult K31.1
    congenital Q40.0
    infantile Q40.0
  rectosigmoid — *see also* Obstruction, intestine, specified
      NEC K56.699
  rectum (sphincter) K62.4
    congenital Q42.1
      with fistula Q42.0
    due to
      chlamydial lymphogranuloma A55
      irradiation K91.89
      lymphogranuloma venereum A55
    gonococcal A54.6
    inflammatory (chlamydial) A55
    syphilitic A52.74
    tuberculous A18.32
  renal artery I70.1
    congenital Q27.1
  salivary duct or gland (any) K11.8
  sigmoid (flexure) — *see* Obstruction, intestine
  spermatic cord N50.89
  stoma (following) (of)
    colostomy K94.03
    enterostomy K94.13
    gastrostomy K94.23

Stricture — *continued*
- stoma — *continued*
  - ileostomy K94.13
  - tracheostomy J95.03
- stomach K31.89
  - congenital Q40.2
  - hourglass K31.2
- subaortic Q24.4
  - hypertrophic (acquired) (idiopathic) I42.1
- subglottic J38.6
- syphilitic NEC A52.79
- trachea J39.8
  - congenital Q32.1
  - syphilitic A52.73
  - tuberculous NEC A15.5
- tracheostomy J95.03
- tricuspid (valve) — *see* Stenosis, tricuspid
- tunica vaginalis N50.89
- ureter (postoperative) N13.5
  - with
    - hydronephrosis N13.1
      - with infection N13.6
    - pyelonephritis (chronic) N11.1
  - congenital — *see* Atresia, ureter
  - tuberculous A18.11
- ureteropelvic junction (congenital) Q62.11
  - acquired, with hydronephrosis N13.0
- ureterovesical orifice N13.5
  - with infection N13.6
- urethra (organic) (spasmodic) — *see also* Stricture, urethra, male N35.919
  - associated with schistosomiasis B65.0 *[N37]*
  - congenital Q64.39
    - valvular (posterior) Q64.2
  - due to
    - infection — *see* Stricture, urethra, postinfective
    - trauma — *see* Stricture, urethra, post-traumatic
  - female N35.92
  - gonococcal, gonorrheal A54.01
  - infective NEC — *see* Stricture, urethra, postinfective
  - late effect (sequela) of injury — *see* Stricture, urethra, post-traumatic
  - male N35.919
    - anterior urethra N35.914
    - bulbous urethra N35.912
    - meatal N35.911
    - membranous urethra N35.913
    - overlapping sites N35.916
  - postcatheterization — *see* Stricture, urethra, postprocedural
  - postinfective NEC
    - female N35.12
    - male N35.119
      - anterior urethra N35.114
      - bulbous urethra N35.112
      - meatal N35.111
      - membranous urethra N35.113
      - overlapping sites N35.116
  - postobstetric N35.021
  - postoperative — *see* Stricture, urethra, postprocedural
  - postprocedural
    - female N99.12
    - male N99.114
      - anterior bulbous urethra N99.113
      - bulbous urethra N99.111
      - fossa navicularis N99.115
      - meatal N99.110
      - membranous urethra N99.112
      - overlapping sites N99.116
  - post-traumatic
    - female N35.028
      - due to childbirth N35.021
    - male N35.014
      - anterior urethra N35.013
      - bulbous urethra N35.011
      - meatal N35.010
      - membranous urethra N35.012
      - overlapping sites N35.016
  - sequela (late effect) of
    - childbirth N35.021
    - injury — *see* Stricture, urethra, post-traumatic
  - specified cause NEC
    - female N35.82
    - male N35.819
      - anterior urethra N35.814
      - bulbous urethra N35.812
      - meatal N35.811
      - membranous urethra N35.813
      - overlapping sites N35.816

Stricture — *continued*
- urethra — *see also* Stricture, urethra, male — *continued*
  - syphilitic A52.76
  - traumatic — *see* Stricture, urethra, post-traumatic
  - valvular (posterior), congenital Q64.2
- urinary meatus — *see* Stricture, urethra
- uterus, uterine (synechiae) N85.6
  - os (external) (internal) — *see* Stricture, cervix
- vagina (outlet) — *see* Stenosis, vagina
- valve (cardiac) (heart) — *see also* Endocarditis
  - congenital
    - aortic Q23.0
    - mitral Q23.2
    - pulmonary Q22.1
    - tricuspid Q22.4
- vas deferens N50.89
  - congenital Q55.4
- vein I87.1
- vena cava (inferior) (superior) NEC I87.1
  - congenital Q26.0
- vesicourethral orifice N32.0
  - congenital Q64.31
- vulva (acquired) N90.5

Stridor R06.1
- congenital (larynx) P28.89

Stridulous — *see* condition

Stroke (apoplectic) (brain) (ischemic) (paralytic) I63.9
- cerebral, perinatal P91.82- ☑
- cerebrovascular (ischemic) I63.9
  - chronic (old) (remote) (imaging) (without sequelae) Z86.73
    - with residual defects — *see* Sequelae, disease, cerebrovascular
  - embolic I63.- ☑
  - thrombolic I63.- ☑
- cryptogenic — *see also* infarction, cerebral I63.9
- epileptic — *see* Epilepsy
- heat T67.01 ☑
  - exertional T67.02 ☑
  - specified NEC T67.09 ☑
- in evolution I63.9
- intraoperative
  - during cardiac surgery I97.810
  - during other surgery I97.811
- ischemic, perinatal arterial P91.82- ☑
- lightning — *see* Lightning
- meaning
  - cerebral hemorrhage — *code to* Hemorrhage, intracranial
  - cerebral infarction — *code to* Infarction, cerebral
- neonatal P91.82- ☑
- postprocedural
  - following cardiac surgery I97.820
  - following other surgery I97.821
- sun T67.01 ☑
  - specified NEC T67.09 ☑
- unspecified (NOS) I63.9

Stromatosis, endometrial D39.0

Strongyloidiasis, strongyloidosis B78.9
- cutaneous B78.1
- disseminated B78.7
- intestinal B78.0

Strophulus pruriginosus L28.2

Struck by lightning — *see* Lightning

Struma — *see also* Goiter
- Hashimoto E06.3
- lymphomatosa E06.3
- nodosa (simplex) E04.9
  - endemic E01.2
    - multinodular E01.1
  - multinodular E04.2
    - iodine-deficiency related E01.1
  - toxic or with hyperthyroidism E05.20
    - with thyroid storm E05.21
    - multinodular E05.20
      - with thyroid storm E05.21
    - uninodular E05.10
      - with thyroid storm E05.11
  - toxicosa E05.20
    - with thyroid storm E05.21
    - multinodular E05.20
      - with thyroid storm E05.21
    - uninodular E05.10
      - with thyroid storm E05.11
  - uninodular E04.1
- ovarii D27.- ☑
- Riedel's E06.5

Strumipriva cachexia E03.4

Strumpell-Marie spine — *see* Spondylitis, ankylosing

Strumpell-Westphal pseudosclerosis E83.01

Stuart deficiency disease (factor X) D68.2

Stuart-Prower factor deficiency (factor X) D68.2

Student's elbow — *see* Bursitis, elbow, olecranon

Stump — *see* Amputation

Stunting, nutritional E45

Stupor (catatonic) R40.1
- depressive (single episode) F32.89
  - recurrent episode F33.8
- dissociative F44.2
- manic F30.2
- manic-depressive F31.89
- psychogenic (anergic) F44.2
- reaction to exceptional stress (transient) F43.0

Sturge (-Weber) (-Dimitri) (-Kalischer) **disease or syndrome** Q85.89

Stuttering F80.81
- adult onset F98.5
- childhood onset F80.81
- following cerebrovascular disease — *see* Disorder, fluency, following cerebrovascular disease
- in conditions classified elsewhere R47.82

Sty, stye (external) (internal) (meibomian) (zeisian) — *see* Hordeolum

Subacidity, gastric K31.89
- psychogenic F45.8

Subacute — *see* condition

Subarachnoid — *see* condition

Subcortical — *see* condition

Subcostal syndrome, nerve compression — *see* Mononeuropathy, upper limb, specified site NEC

Subcutaneous, subcuticular — *see* condition

Subdural — *see* condition

Subendocardium — *see* condition

Subependymoma
- specified site — *see* Neoplasm, uncertain behavior, by site
- unspecified site D43.2

Suberosis J67.3

Subglossitis — *see* Glossitis

Subhemophilia D66

Subinvolution
- breast (postlactational) (postpuerperal) N64.89
- puerperal O90.89
- uterus (chronic) (nonpuerperal) N85.3
  - puerperal O90.89

Sublingual — *see* condition

Sublinguitis — *see* Sialoadenitis

Subluxatable hip Q65.6

Subluxation — *see also* Dislocation
- acromioclavicular S43.11- ☑
- ankle S93.0- ☑
- atlantoaxial, recurrent M43.4
  - with myelopathy M43.3
- carpometacarpal (joint) NEC S63.05- ☑
  - thumb S63.04- ☑
- complex, vertebral — *see* Complex, subluxation
- congenital — *see also* Malposition, congenital
  - hip — *see* Dislocation, hip, congenital, partial
  - joint (excluding hip)
    - lower limb Q68.8
    - shoulder Q68.8
    - upper limb Q68.8
- elbow (traumatic) S53.10- ☑
  - anterior S53.11- ☑
  - lateral S53.14- ☑
  - medial S53.13- ☑
  - posterior S53.12- ☑
  - specified type NEC S53.19- ☑
- finger S63.20- ☑
  - index S63.20- ☑
  - interphalangeal S63.22- ☑
    - distal S63.24- ☑
      - index S63.24- ☑
      - little S63.24- ☑
      - middle S63.24- ☑
      - ring S63.24- ☑
    - index S63.22- ☑
    - little S63.22- ☑
    - middle S63.22- ☑
    - proximal S63.23- ☑
      - index S63.23- ☑
      - little S63.23- ☑
      - middle S63.23- ☑
      - ring S63.23- ☑

☑ **Additional Character Required** — Refer to the Tabular List for Character Selection

Subluxation — *continued*
- finger — *continued*
  - interphalangeal — *continued*
    - ring S63.22- ☑
  - little S63.20- ☑
  - metacarpophalangeal S63.21- ☑
    - index S63.21- ☑
    - little S63.21- ☑
    - middle S63.21- ☑
    - ring S63.21- ☑
  - middle S63.20- ☑
  - ring S63.20- ☑
- foot S93.30- ☑
  - specified site NEC S93.33- ☑
  - tarsal joint S93.31- ☑
  - tarsometatarsal joint S93.32- ☑
  - toe — *see* Subluxation, toe
- hip S73.00- ☑
  - anterior S73.03- ☑
    - obturator S73.02- ☑
  - central S73.04- ☑
  - posterior S73.01- ☑
- interphalangeal (joint)
  - finger S63.22- ☑
    - distal joint S63.24- ☑
      - index S63.24- ☑
      - little S63.24- ☑
      - middle S63.24- ☑
      - ring S63.24- ☑
    - index S63.22- ☑
    - little S63.22- ☑
    - middle S63.22- ☑
    - proximal joint S63.23- ☑
      - index S63.23- ☑
      - little S63.23- ☑
      - middle S63.23- ☑
      - ring S63.23- ☑
    - ring S63.22- ☑
  - thumb S63.12- ☑
  - toe S93.13- ☑
    - great S93.13- ☑
    - lesser S93.13- ☑
- joint prosthesis — *see* Complications, joint prosthesis, mechanical, displacement, by site
- knee S83.10- ☑
  - cap — *see* Subluxation, patella
  - patella — *see* Subluxation, patella
  - proximal tibia
    - anteriorly S83.11- ☑
    - laterally S83.14- ☑
    - medially S83.13- ☑
    - posteriorly S83.12- ☑
  - specified type NEC S83.19- ☑
- lens — *see* Dislocation, lens, partial
- ligament, traumatic — *see* Sprain, by site
- metacarpal (bone)
  - proximal end S63.06- ☑
- metacarpophalangeal (joint)
  - finger S63.21- ☑
    - index S63.21- ☑
    - little S63.21- ☑
    - middle S63.21- ☑
    - ring S63.21- ☑
  - thumb S63.11- ☑
- metatarsophalangeal joint S93.14- ☑
  - great toe S93.14- ☑
  - lesser toe S93.14- ☑
- midcarpal (joint) S63.03- ☑
- patella S83.00- ☑
  - lateral S83.01- ☑
  - recurrent (nontraumatic) — *see* Dislocation, patella, recurrent, incomplete
  - specified type NEC S83.09- ☑
- pathological — *see* Dislocation, pathological
- radial head S53.00- ☑
  - anterior S53.01- ☑
  - nursemaid's elbow S53.03- ☑
  - posterior S53.02- ☑
  - specified type NEC S53.09- ☑
- radiocarpal (joint) S63.02- ☑
- radioulnar (joint)
  - distal S63.01- ☑
  - proximal — *see* Subluxation, elbow
- shoulder
  - congenital Q68.8
  - girdle S43.30- ☑

Subluxation — *continued*
- shoulder — *continued*
  - girdle — *continued*
    - scapula S43.31- ☑
    - specified site NEC S43.39- ☑
  - traumatic S43.00- ☑
    - anterior S43.01- ☑
    - inferior S43.03- ☑
    - posterior S43.02- ☑
    - specified type NEC S43.08- ☑
- sternoclavicular (joint) S43.20- ☑
  - anterior S43.21- ☑
  - posterior S43.22- ☑
- symphysis (pubis) — *see also* Dislocation, symphysis pubis
- thumb S63.103 ☑
  - interphalangeal joint — *see* Subluxation, interphalangeal (joint), thumb
  - metacarpophalangeal joint — *see* Subluxation, metacarpophalangeal (joint), thumb
- toe(s) S93.10- ☑
  - great S93.10- ☑
    - interphalangeal joint S93.13- ☑
    - metatarsophalangeal joint S93.14- ☑
  - interphalangeal joint S93.13- ☑
  - lesser S93.10- ☑
    - interphalangeal joint S93.13- ☑
    - metatarsophalangeal joint S93.14- ☑
  - metatarsophalangeal joint S93.149 ☑
- ulna
  - distal end S63.07- ☑
  - proximal end — *see* Subluxation, elbow
- ulnohumeral joint — *see* Subluxation, elbow
- vertebral
  - recurrent NEC — *see* subcategory M43.5 ☑
  - traumatic
    - cervical S13.100 ☑
      - atlantoaxial joint S13.120 ☑
      - atlantooccipital joint S13.110 ☑
      - atloidooccipital joint S13.110 ☑
      - joint between
        - C0 and C1 S13.110 ☑
        - C1 and C2 S13.120 ☑
        - C2 and C3 S13.130 ☑
        - C3 and C4 S13.140 ☑
        - C4 and C5 S13.150 ☑
        - C5 and C6 S13.160 ☑
        - C6 and C7 S13.170 ☑
        - C7 and T1 S13.180 ☑
      - occipitoatloid joint S13.110 ☑
    - lumbar S33.100 ☑
      - joint between
        - L1 and L2 S33.110 ☑
        - L2 and L3 S33.120 ☑
        - L3 and L4 S33.130 ☑
        - L4 and L5 S33.140 ☑
    - thoracic S23.100 ☑
      - joint between
        - T1 and T2 S23.110 ☑
        - T2 and T3 S23.120 ☑
        - T3 and T4 S23.122 ☑
        - T4 and T5 S23.130 ☑
        - T5 and T6 S23.132 ☑
        - T6 and T7 S23.140 ☑
        - T7 and T8 S23.142 ☑
        - T8 and T9 S23.150 ☑
        - T9 and T10 S23.152 ☑
        - T10 and T11 S23.160 ☑
        - T11 and T12 S23.162 ☑
        - T12 and L1 S23.170 ☑
- wrist (carpal bone) S63.00- ☑
  - carpometacarpal joint — *see* Subluxation, carpometacarpal (joint)
  - distal radioulnar joint — *see* Subluxation, radioulnar (joint), distal
  - metacarpal bone, proximal — *see* Subluxation, metacarpal (bone), proximal end
  - midcarpal — *see* Subluxation, midcarpal (joint)
  - radiocarpal joint — *see* Subluxation, radiocarpal (joint)
  - recurrent — *see* Dislocation, recurrent, wrist
  - specified site NEC S63.09- ☑
  - ulna — *see* Subluxation, ulna, distal end

Submaxillary — *see* condition
Submersion (fatal) (nonfatal) T75.1 ☑
Submucous — *see* condition

Subnormal, subnormality
- accommodation (old age) H52.4
- mental — *see* Disability, intellectual
- temperature (accidental) T68 ☑

Subphrenic — *see* condition
Subscapular nerve — *see* condition
Subseptus uterus Q51.28
Subsiding appendicitis K36
Substance (other psychoactive) **-induced**
- anxiety disorder F19.980
- bipolar and related disorder F19.94
- delirium F19.921
- depressive disorder F19.94
- major neurocognitive disorder F19.97
- mild neurocognitive disorder F19.988
- obsessive-compulsive and related disorder F19.988
- psychotic disorder F19.959
- sexual dysfunction F19.981
- sleep disorder F19.982

Substernal thyroid E04.9
- congenital Q89.2

Substitution disorder F44.9
Subtentorial — *see* condition
Subthyroidism (acquired) — *see also* Hypothyroidism
- congenital E03.1

Succenturiate placenta O43.19- ☑
Sucking thumb, child (excessive) F98.8
Sudamen, sudamina L74.1
Sudanese kala-azar B55.0
Sudden
- hearing loss — *see* Deafness, sudden
- heart failure — *see* Failure, heart

Sudeck's atrophy, disease, or syndrome — *see* Algoneurodystrophy
Suffocation — *see* Asphyxia, traumatic
Sugar
- blood
  - high (transient) R73.9
  - low (transient) E16.2
- in urine R81

Suicide, suicidal (attempted) T14.91 ☑
- by poisoning — *see* Table of Drugs and Chemicals
- history of (personal) Z91.51
  - in family Z81.8
- ideation — *see* Ideation, suicidal
- risk
  - meaning personal history of attempted suicide Z91.51
  - meaning suicidal ideation — *see* Ideation, suicidal
- tendencies
  - meaning personal history of attempted suicide Z91.51
  - meaning suicidal ideation — *see* Ideation, suicidal
- trauma — *see* nature of injury by site

Suipestifer infection — *see* Infection, salmonella
Sulfhemoglobinemia, sulphemoglobinemia (acquired) (with methemoglobinemia) D74.8
Sumatran mite fever A75.3
Summer — *see* condition
Sunburn L55.9
- due to
  - tanning bed (acute) L56.8
    - chronic L57.8
  - ultraviolet radiation (acute) L56.8
    - chronic L57.8
- first degree L55.0
- second degree L55.1
- third degree L55.2

SUNCT (short lasting unilateral neuralgiform headache with conjunctival injection and tearing) G44.059
- intractable G44.051
- not intractable G44.059

Sundowning F05
Sunken acetabulum — *see* Derangement, joint, specified type NEC, hip
Sunstroke T67.01 ☑
- specified NEC T67.09 ☑

Superfecundation — *see* Pregnancy, multiple
Superfetation — *see* Pregnancy, multiple
Superinvolution (uterus) N85.8
Supernumerary (congenital)
- aortic cusps Q23.88
- auditory ossicles Q16.3
- bone Q79.8
- breast Q83.1
- carpal bones Q74.0
- cusps, heart valve NEC Q24.8
  - aortic Q23.88
  - mitral Q23.2
  - pulmonary Q22.3

☑ **Additional Character Required** — Refer to the Tabular List for Character Selection

Supernumerary — continued
  digit(s) Q69.9
  ear (lobule) Q17.0
  fallopian tube Q50.6
  finger Q69.0
  hymen Q52.4
  kidney Q63.0
  lacrimonasal duct Q10.6
  lobule (ear) Q17.0
  mitral cusps Q23.2
  muscle Q79.8
  nipple(s) Q83.3
  organ or site not listed — see Accessory
  ossicles, auditory Q16.3
  ovary Q50.31
  oviduct Q50.6
  pulmonary, pulmonic cusps Q22.3
  rib Q76.6
    cervical or first (syndrome) Q76.5
  roots (of teeth) K00.2
  spleen Q89.09
  tarsal bones Q74.2
  teeth K00.1
  testis Q55.29
  thumb Q69.1
  toe Q69.2
  uterus Q51.28
  vagina Q52.1 ☑
  vertebra Q76.49
Supervision (of)
  contraceptive — see Prescription, contraceptives
  dietary (for) Z71.3
    allergy (food) Z71.3
    colitis Z71.3
    diabetes mellitus Z71.3
    food allergy or intolerance Z71.3
    gastritis Z71.3
    hypercholesterolemia Z71.3
    hypoglycemia Z71.3
    intolerance (food) Z71.3
    obesity Z71.3
    specified NEC Z71.3
  healthy infant or child Z76.2
    foundling Z76.1
  high-risk pregnancy — see Pregnancy, supervision of, high-risk
  lactation Z39.1
  pregnancy — see Pregnancy, supervision of
Supplemental teeth K00.1
Suppression
  binocular vision H53.34
  lactation O92.5
  menstruation N94.89
  ovarian secretion E28.39
  renal N28.9
  urine, urinary secretion R34
Suppuration, suppurative — see also condition
  accessory sinus (chronic) — see Sinusitis
  adrenal gland
  antrum (chronic) — see Sinusitis, maxillary
  bladder — see Cystitis
  brain G06.0
    sequelae G09
  breast N61.1
    puerperal, postpartum or gestational — see Mastitis, obstetric, purulent
  dental periosteum M27.3
  ear (middle) — see also Otitis, media
    external NEC — see Otitis, externa, infective
    internal — see subcategory H83.0 ☑
  ethmoidal (chronic) (sinus) — see Sinusitis, ethmoidal
  fallopian tube — see Salpingo-oophoritis
  frontal (chronic) (sinus) — see Sinusitis, frontal
  gallbladder (acute) K81.0
  gum K05.20
    generalized — see Periodontitis, aggressive, generalized
    localized — see Periodontitis, aggressive, localized
  intracranial G06.0
  joint — see Arthritis, pyogenic or pyemic
  labyrinthine — see subcategory H83.0 ☑
  lung — see Abscess, lung
  mammary gland N61.1
    puerperal, postpartum O91.12
      associated with lactation O91.13
  maxilla, maxillary M27.2
    sinus (chronic) — see Sinusitis, maxillary
  muscle — see Myositis, infective
  nasal sinus (chronic) — see Sinusitis

Suppuration, suppurative — continued
  pancreas, acute — see also Pancreatitis, acute K85.80
  parotid gland — see Sialoadenitis
  pelvic, pelvic
    female — see Disease, pelvis, inflammatory
    male K65.0
  pericranial — see Osteomyelitis
  salivary duct or gland (any) — see Sialoadenitis
  sinus (accessory) (chronic) (nasal) — see Sinusitis
  sphenoidal sinus (chronic) — see Sinusitis, sphenoidal
  thymus (gland) E32.1
  thyroid (gland) E06.0
  tonsil — see Tonsillitis
  uterus — see Endometritis
Supraeruption of tooth (teeth) M26.34
Supraglottitis J04.30
  with obstruction J04.31
Suprarenal (gland) — see condition
Suprascapular nerve — see condition
Suprasellar — see condition
Surfer's knots or nodules S89.8- ☑
Surgical
  emphysema T81.82 ☑
  procedures, complication or misadventure — see Complications, surgical procedures
  shock T81.10 ☑
Surveillance (of) (for) — see also Observation
  alcohol abuse Z71.41
  contraceptive — see Prescription, contraceptives
  dietary Z71.3
  drug abuse Z71.51
  neoplasm — see Screening, neoplasm
Susceptibility to disease, genetic Z15.89
  malignant neoplasm Z15.09
    breast Z15.01
    endometrium Z15.04
    ovary Z15.02
    prostate Z15.03
    specified NEC Z15.09
  multiple endocrine neoplasia Z15.81
Suspected condition, ruled out — see also Observation, suspected
  amniotic cavity and membrane Z03.71
  cervical shortening Z03.75
  fetal anomaly Z03.73
  fetal growth Z03.74
  maternal and fetal conditions NEC Z03.79
  newborn — see also Observation, newborn, suspected condition ruled out Z05.9
  oligohydramnios Z03.71
  placental problem Z03.72
  polyhydramnios Z03.71
Suspended uterus
  in pregnancy or childbirth — see Pregnancy, complicated by, abnormal uterus
Sutton's nevus D22.9
Suture
  burst (in operation wound) T81.31 ☑
    external operation wound T81.31 ☑
    internal operation wound T81.329 ☑
  inadvertently left in operation wound — see Foreign body, accidentally left during a procedure
  removal Z48.02
Swab inadvertently left in operation wound — see Foreign body, accidentally left during a procedure
Swallowed, swallowing
  difficulty — see Dysphagia
  foreign body — see Foreign body, alimentary tract
Swan-neck deformity (finger) — see Deformity, finger, swan-neck
Swearing, compulsive F42.8
  in Gilles de la Tourette's syndrome F95.2
Sweat, sweats
  fetid L75.0
  night R61
Sweating, excessive R61
Sweeley-Klionsky disease E75.21
Sweet's disease or dermatosis L98.2
Swelling (of) R60.9
  abdomen, abdominal (not referable to any particular organ) — see Mass, abdominal
  ankle — see Effusion, joint, ankle
  arm M79.89
    forearm M79.89
  breast — see also Lump, breast N63.0
  Calabar B74.3
  cervical gland R59.0
  chest, localized R22.2

Swelling — continued
  ear H93.8- ☑
  extremity (lower) (upper) — see Disorder, soft tissue, specified type NEC
  finger M79.89
  foot M79.89
  glands R59.9
    generalized R59.1
    localized R59.0
  hand M79.89
  head (localized) R22.0
  inflammatory — see Inflammation
  intra-abdominal — see Mass, abdominal
  joint — see Effusion, joint
  leg M79.89
    lower M79.89
  limb — see Disorder, soft tissue, specified type NEC
  localized (skin) R22.9
    chest R22.2
    head R22.0
    limb
      lower — see Mass, localized, limb, lower
      upper — see Mass, localized, limb, upper
    neck R22.1
    trunk R22.2
  neck (localized) R22.1
  pelvic — see Mass, abdominal
  scrotum N50.89
  splenic — see Splenomegaly
  testis N50.89
  toe M79.89
  umbilical R19.09
  wandering, due to Gnathostoma (spinigerum) B83.1
  white — see Tuberculosis, arthritis
Swift (-Feer) disease
  overdose or wrong substance given or taken — see Table of Drugs and Chemicals, by drug, poisoning
Swimmer's
  cramp T75.1 ☑
  ear H60.33- ☑
  itch B65.3
Swimming in the head R42
Swollen — see Swelling
Swyer syndrome Q99.1
Sycosis L73.8
  barbae (not parasitic) L73.8
  contagiosa (mycotic) B35.0
  lupoides L73.8
  mycotic B35.0
  parasitic B35.0
  vulgaris L73.8
Sydenham's chorea — see Chorea, Sydenham's
Sylvatic yellow fever A95.0
Sylvest's disease B33.0
Symblepharon H11.23- ☑
  congenital Q10.3
Symond's syndrome G93.2
Sympathetic — see condition
Sympatheticotonia G90.89
Sympathicoblastoma
  specified site — see Neoplasm, malignant, by site
  unspecified site C74.90
Sympathogonioma — see Sympathicoblastoma
Symphalangy (fingers) (toes) Q70.9
Symptoms NEC R68.89
  breast NEC N64.59
  cold J00
  development NEC R63.8
  factitious, self-induced — see Disorder, factitious
  genital organs, female R10.2
  involving
    abdomen NEC R19.8
    appearance NEC R46.89
    awareness R41.9
      altered mental status R41.82
      amnesia — see Amnesia
      borderline intellectual functioning R41.83
      coma — see Coma
      disorientation R41.0
      neurologic neglect syndrome R41.4
      senile cognitive decline R41.81
      specified symptom NEC R41.89
    behavior NEC R46.89
    cardiovascular system NEC R09.89
    chest NEC R09.89
    circulatory system NEC R09.89
    cognitive functions R41.9
      altered mental status R41.82
      amnesia — see Amnesia

Symptoms — continued
  involving — continued
    cognitive functions — continued
      borderline intellectual functioning R41.83
      coma — see Coma
      disorientation R41.0
      neurologic neglect syndrome R41.4
      senile cognitive decline R41.81
      specified symptom NEC R41.89
    development NEC R62.50
    digestive system NEC R19.8
    emotional state NEC R45.89
      emotional lability R45.86
    food and fluid intake R63.8
    general perceptions and sensations R44.9
      specified NEC R44.8
    musculoskeletal system R29.91
      specified NEC R29.898
    nervous system R29.90
      specified NEC R29.818
    pelvis NEC R19.8
    respiratory system NEC R09.89
    skin and integument R23.9
    urinary system R39.9
  menopausal N95.1
  metabolism NEC R63.8
  neurotic F48.8
  of infancy R68.19
  pelvis NEC, female R10.2
  skin and integument NEC R23.9
  subcutaneous tissue NEC R23.9
  viral cold J00
Sympus Q74.2
Syncephalus Q89.4
Synchondrosis
  abnormal (congenital) Q78.8
  ischiopubic M91.0
Synchysis (scintillans) (senile) (vitreous body) H43.89
Syncope (near) (pre-) R55
  anginosa I20.89
  bradycardia R00.1
  cardiac R55
  carotid sinus G90.01
  due to spinal (lumbar) puncture G97.1
  heart R55
  heat T67.1 ☑
  laryngeal R05.4
  psychogenic F48.8
  tussive R05.8
  vasoconstriction R55
  vasodepressor R55
  vasomotor R55
  vasovagal R55
Syndactylism, syndactyly Q70.9
  complex (with synostosis)
    fingers Q70.0- ☑
    toes Q70.2- ☑
  simple (without synostosis)
    fingers Q70.1- ☑
    toes Q70.3- ☑
Syndrome — see also Disease
  22q13.3 deletion Q93.52
  48,XXXX Q97.1
  49,XXXXX Q97.1
  4H G11.5
  5q minus NOS D46.C (following D46.2)
  abdominal
    acute R10.0
    muscle deficiency Q79.4
  abnormal innervation H02.519
    left H02.516
      lower H02.515
      upper H02.514
    right H02.513
      lower H02.512
      upper H02.511
  abstinence, neonatal P96.1
  acid pulmonary aspiration, obstetric O74.0
  acquired immunodeficiency — see Human, immunode-
    ficiency virus (HIV) disease
  activated phosphoinositide 3-kinase delta syndrome
    [APDS] D81.82
  acute abdominal R10.0
  acute respiratory distress (adult) (child) J80
    idiopathic J84.114
  Adair-Dighton Q78.0
  Adams-Stokes (-Morgagni) I45.9
  adiposogenital E23.6

Syndrome — continued
  adrenal
    hemorrhage (meningococcal) A39.1
      meningococcic A39.1
  adrenocortical — see Cushing's, syndrome
  adrenogenital E25.9
    congenital, asscciated with enzyme deficiency E25.0
  afferent loop NEC K91.89
  Aicardi-Goutières E79.81
  Alagille (-Watson) Q44.71
  alcohol withdrawal (without convulsions) — see Depen-
    dence, alcohol, with, withdrawal
  Alder's D72.0
  Aldrich (-Wiskott) D82.0
  alien hand R41.4
  Alport Q87.81
  alveolar hypoventilation E66.2
  alveolocapillary block J84.10
  amnesic, amnestic (confabulatory) (due to) — see Disor-
    der, amnesic
  amyostatic (Wilson's disease) E83.01
  androgen insensitivity E34.50
    complete E34.51
    partial E34.52
  androgen resistance — see also Syndrome, androgen
    insensitivity E34.50
  Angelman Q93.51
  anginal — see Angina
  ankyloglossia superior Q38.1
  anterior
    chest wall R07.89
    cord G83.82
    spinal artery G95.19
      compression M47.019
        cervical region M47.012
        cervicothoracic region M47.013
        lumbar region M47.016
        occipito-atlanto-axial region M47.011
        thoracic region M47.014
        thoracolumbar region M47.015
    tibial M76.81- ☑
  antibody deficiency D80.9
    agammaglobulinemic D80.1
      hereditary D80.0
    congenital D80.9
    hypogammaglobulinemic D80.1
      hereditary D80.0
  anticardiolipin (-antibody) D68.61
  antidepressant discontinuation T43.205 ☑
  antiphospholipid (-antibody) D68.61
  aortic
    arch M31.4
    bifurcation I74.09
  aortomesenteric duodenum occlusion K31.5
  apical ballooning (transient left ventricular) I51.81
  arcuate ligament I77.4
  argentaffin, argintaffinoma E34.09
  Arnold-Chiari — see Arnold-Chiari disease
  Arrillaga-Ayerza I27.0
  arterial tortuosity Q87.82
  arteriovenous steal T82.898- ☑
  Asherman's N85.6
  aspiration, of newborn — see Aspiration, by substance,
    with pneumonia
    meconium P24.01
  ataxia-telangiectasia G11.3
  auriculotemporal G50.8
  autoerythrocyte sensitization (Gardner-Diamond) D69.2
  autoimmune lymphoproliferative [ALPS] D89.82
  autoimmune polyglandular E31.0
  autoinflammatory M04.9
    specified type NEC M04.8
  autosomal — see Abnormal, autosomes
  Avellis' G46.8
  Axenfeld-Rieger Q13.81
  Ayerza (-Arrillaga) I27.0
  Babinski-Nageotte G83.89
  Bakwin-Krida Q78.5
  Bardet-Biedl Q87.83
  bare lymphocyte D81.6
  Barre-Guillain G61.0
  Barre-Lieou M53.0
  Barrett's — see Barrett's, esophagus
  Barsony-Polgar K22.4
  Barsony-Teschendorf K22.4
  Barth E78.71
  Bartter's E26.81
  basal cell nevus Q87.89
  Basedow's E05.00

Syndrome — continued
  Basedow's — continued
    with thyroid storm E05.01
  basilar artery G45.0
  Batten-Steinert G71.11
  battered
    baby or child — see Maltreatment, child, physical
      abuse
    spouse — see Maltreatment, adult, physical abuse
  Beals Q87.40
  Beau's I51.5
  Beck's I65.8
  Benedikt's G46.3
  Bequez Cesar (-Steinbrinck-Chediak-Higashi) E70.330
  Bernhardt-Roth — see Meralgia paresthetica
  Bernheim's — see Failure, heart, right
  big spleen D73.1
  bilateral polycystic ovarian E28.2
  Bing-Horton's — see Horton's headache
  Birt-Hogg-Dube syndrome Q87.89
  Bjorck (-Thorsen) E34.09
  black
    lung J60
    widow spider bite — see Toxicity, venom, spider, black
      widow
  Blackfan-Diamond D61.01
  Blau M04.8
  blind loop K90.2
    congenital Q43.8
    postsurgical K91.2
  blue sclera Q78.0
  blue toe I75.02- ☑
  Boder-Sedgewick G11.3
  Boerhaave's K22.3
  Borjeson Forssman Lehmann Q89.8
  Bouillaud's I01.9
  Bourneville (-Pringle) Q85.1
  Bouveret (-Hoffman) I47.9
  brachial plexus G54.0
  bradycardia-tachycardia I49.5
  brain (nonpsychotic) F09
    with psychosis, psychotic reaction F09
    acute or subacute — see Delirium
    congenital — see Disability, intellectual
    organic F09
      post-traumatic (nonpsychotic) F07.81
        psychotic F09
    personality change F07.0
    postcontusional F07.81
    post-traumatic, nonpsychotic F07.81
    psycho-organic F09
    psychotic F06.8
  brain stem stroke G46.3
  Brandt's (acrodermatitis enteropathica) E83.2
  broad ligament laceration N83.8
  Brock's J98.11
  bronchiolitis obliterans — see also Bronchiolitis, obliter-
    ative J44.81
  bronze baby P83.88
  Brown-Sequard G83.81
  Brugada I49.8
  bubbly lung P27.0
  Buchem's M85.2
  Budd-Chiari I82.0
  bulbar (progressive) G12.22
  Burger-Grutz E78.3
  Burke's K86.89
  Burnett's (milk-alkali) E83.52
  burning feet E53.9
  Bywaters' T79.5 ☑
  Call-Fleming I67.841
  carbohydrate-deficient glycoprotein (CDGS) E77.8
  carcinogenic thrombophlebitis I82.1
  carcinoid E34.00
    heart E34.01
    specified NEC E34.09
  cardiac asthma I50.1
  cardiacos negros I27.0
  cardiofaciocutaneous Q87.89
  cardiopulmonary-obesity E66.2
  cardiorenal — see Hypertension, cardiorenal
  cardiorespiratory distress (idiopathic), newborn P22.0
  cardiovascular renal — see Hypertension, cardiorenal
  carotid
    artery (hemispheric) (internal) G45.1
    body G90.01
    sinus G90.01
  carpal tunnel G56.0- ☑
  Cassidy (-Scholte) E34.09

Index

Syndrome — Syndrome

Syndrome — *continued*
cat cry Q93.4
cat eye Q92.8
cauda equina G83.4
causalgia — *see* Causalgia
celiac K90.0
    artery compression I77.4
    axis I77.4
central pain G89.0
cerebellar
    hereditary G11.9
    stroke G46.4
cerebellomedullary malformation — *see* Spina bifida
cerebral
    artery
        anterior G46.1
        middle G46.0
        posterior G46.2
    gigantism E22.0
cervical (root) M53.1
    disc — *see* Disorder, disc, cervical, with neuritis
    fusion Q76.1
    posterior, sympathicus M53.0
    rib Q76.5
    sympathetic paralysis G90.2
cervicobrachial (diffuse) M53.1
cervicocranial M53.0
cervicodorsal outlet G54.2
cervicothoracic outlet — *see also* Syndrome, thoracic
        outlet G54.0
Cestan (-Raymond) I65.8
Charcot's (angina cruris) (intermittent claudication) I73.9
Charcot-Weiss-Baker G90.09
CHARGE Q89.8
Chediak-Higashi (-Steinbrinck) E70.330
chest wall R07.1
Chiari's (hepatic vein thrombosis) I82.0
Chilaiditi's Q43.3
child maltreatment — *see* Maltreatment, child
chondrocostal junction M94.0
chondroectodermal dysplasia Q77.6
chromosome 4 short arm deletion Q93.3
chromosome 5 short arm deletion Q93.4
chronic
    infantile neurological, cutaneous and articular (CINCA)
        M04.2
    pain G89.4
        personality F68.8
Churg-Strauss M30.1
Clarke-Hadfield K86.89
Clerambault's automatism G93.89
Clouston's (hidrotic ectodermal dysplasia) Q82.4
clumsiness, clumsy child F82
cluster headache G44.009
    intractable G44.001
    not intractable G44.009
Coffin-Lowry Q89.8
cold injury (newborn) P80.0
combined immunity deficiency D81.9
compartment (deep) (posterior) (traumatic) T79.A0 ☑
        (*following* T79.7)
    abdomen T79.A3 ☑ (*following* T79.7)
    lower extremity (hip, buttock, thigh, leg, foot, toes)
        T79.A2 ☑ (*following* T79.7)
    nontraumatic
        abdomen M79.A3 (*following* M79.7)
        lower extremity (hip, buttock, thigh, leg, foot, toes)
            M79.A2- ☑ (*following* M79.7)
        specified site NEC M79.A9 (*following* M79.7)
        upper extremity (shoulder, arm, forearm, wrist,
            hand, fingers) M79.A1- ☑ (*following* M79.7)
    postprocedural — *see* Syndrome, compartment,
        nontraumatic
    specified site NEC T79.A9 ☑ (*following* T79.7)
    upper extremity (shoulder, arm, forearm, wrist, hand,
        fingers) T79.A1 ☑ (*following* T79.7)
complex regional pain — *see* Syndrome, pain, complex
        regional
compression T79.5 ☑
    anterior spinal — *see* Syndrome, anterior, spinal
        artery, compression
    cauda equina G83.4
    celiac artery I77.4
    vertebral artery M47.029
        cervical region M47.022
        occipito-atlanto-axial region M47.021
concussion F07.81

Syndrome — *continued*
congenital
    affecting multiple systems NEC Q87.89
    central alveolar hypoventilation G47.35
    facial diplegia Q87.0
    muscular hypertrophy-cerebral Q87.89
    oculo-auriculovertebral Q87.89
    oculofacial diplegia (Moebius) Q87.0
    rubella (manifest) P35.0
congestion-fibrosis (pelvic), female N94.89
congestive dysmenorrhea N94.6
connective tissue M35.9
    overlap NEC M35.1
Conn's E26.01
conus medullaris G95.81
cord
    anterior G83.82
    posterior G83.83
coronary
    acute NEC I24.9
    insufficiency or intermediate I20.0
    slow flow I20.89
Costen's (complex) M26.69
costochondral junction M94.0
costoclavicular G54.0
costovertebral E22.0
Cowden
    PTEN related Q85.81
    specified NEC Q85.82
craniovertebral M53.0
Creutzfeldt-Jakob — *see* Creutzfeldt-Jakob disease or
        syndrome
crib death R99
cricopharyngeal — *see* Dysphagia
cri-du-chat Q93.4
croup J05.0
CRPS I — *see* Syndrome, pain, complex regional I
crush T79.5 ☑
cryopyrin-associated perodic M04.2
cryptophthalmos Q87.0
cubital tunnel — *see* Lesion, nerve, ulnar
Curschmann (-Batten) (-Steinert) G71.11
Cushing's E24.9
    alcohol-induced E24.4
    due to
        alcohol
        drugs E24.2
        ectopic ACTH E24.3
        overproduction of pituitary ACTH E24.0
    drug-induced E24.2
    overdose or wrong substance given or taken — *see*
        Table of Drugs and Chemicals, by drug, poison-
        ing
    pituitary-dependent E24.0
    specified type NEC E24.8
cystic duct stump K91.5
cytokine release D89.839
    grade 1 D89.831
    grade 2 D89.832
    grade 3 D89.833
    grade 4 D89.834
    grade 5 D89.835
Dana-Putnam D51.0
Danbolt (-Cross) (acrodermatitis enteropathica) E83.2
Dandy-Walker Q03.1
    with spina bifida Q07.01
Danlos' — *see also* Syndrome, Ehlers-Danlos Q79.60
De Quervain E34.51
de Toni-Fanconi (-Debre) E72.09
    with cystinosis E72.04
de Vivo syndrome E74.810
defibrination — *see also* Fibrinolysis
    with
        antepartum hemorrhage — *see* Hemorrhage, an-
            tepartum, with coagulation defect
        intrapartum hemorrhage — *see* Hemorrhage,
            complicating, delivery
    newborn P60
    postpartum O72.3
Degos' I77.89
Dejerine-Roussy G89.0
delayed sleep phase G47.21
demyelinating G37.9
dependence — *see* F10-F19 with fourth character .2
depersonalization (-derealization) F48.1
di George's D82.1
diabetes mellitus in newborn infant P70.2
diabetes mellitus-hypertension-nephrosis — *see* Dia-
        betes, nephrosis

Syndrome — *continued*
diabetes-nephrosis — *see* Diabetes, nephrosis
diabetic amyotrophy — *see* Diabetes, amyotrophy
dialysis associated steal T82.898- ☑
Diamond-Blackfan D61.01
Diamond-Gardener D69.2
DIC (diffuse or disseminated intravascular coagulopathy)
        D65
Dighton's Q78.0
disequilibrium E87.8
Dohle body-panmyelopathic D72.0
dorsolateral medullary G46.4
double athetosis G80.3
Down — *see also* Down syndrome Q90.9
Dravet (intractable) G40.834
    with status epilepticus G40.833
    without status epilepticus G40.834
Dresbach's (elliptocytosis) D58.1
DRESS (drug rash with eosinophilia and systemic symp-
        toms) D72.12
Dressler's (postmyocardial infarction) I24.1
    postcardiotomy I97.0
drug rash with eosinophilia and systemic symptoms
        (DRESS) D72.12
drug withdrawal, infant of dependent mother P96.1
dry eye H04.12- ☑
due to abnormality
    chromosomal Q99.9
        sex
            female phenotype Q97.9
            male phenotype Q98.9
        specified NEC Q99.8
dumping (postgastrectomy) K91.1
    nonsurgical K31.89
Dupre's (meningism) R29.1
dysmetabolic X E88.810
dyspraxia, developmental F82
Eagle-Barrett Q79.4
Eaton-Lambert — *see* Syndrome, Lambert-Eaton
Ebstein's Q22.5
ectopic ACTH E24.3
eczema-thrombocytopenia D82.0
Eddowes' Q78.0
effort (psychogenic) F45.8
Ehlers-Danlos Q79.60
    classical (cEDS) (classical EDS) Q79.61
    hypermobile (hEDS) (hypermobile EDS) Q79.62
    specified NEC Q79.69
    vascular (vascular EDS) (vEDS) Q79.63
Eisenmenger's I27.83
Ekman's Q78.0
electric feet E53.8
Ellis-van Creveld Q77.6
empty nest Z60.0
endocrine-hypertensive E27.0
entrapment — *see* Neuropathy, entrapment
eosinophilia-myalgia M35.89
epileptic — *see also* Epilepsy, by type
    absence G40.A09 (*following* G40.3)
        intractable G40.A19 (*following* G40.3)
            with status epilepticus G40.A11 (*following*
                G40.3)
            without status epilepticus G40.A19 (*following*
                G40.3)
        not intractable G40.A09 (*following* G40.3)
            with status epilepticus G40.A01 (*following*
                G40.3)
            without status epilepticus G40.A09 (*following*
                G40.3)
Erdheim-Chester (ECD) E88.89
Erdheim's E22.0
erythrocyte fragmentation D59.4
Evans D69.41
exhaustion F48.8
extrapyramidal G25.9
    specified NEC G25.89
eye retraction — *see* Strabismus
eyelid-malar-mandible Q87.0
Faber's D50.9
facet M47.89- ☑
facet joint — *see also* Spondylosis M47.819
facial pain, paroxysmal G50.0
Fallot's Q21.3
familial cold autoinflammatory M04.2
familial eczema-thrombocytopenia (Wiskott-Aldrich)
        D82.0
Fanconi (-de Toni) (-Debre) E72.09
    with cystinosis E72.04

☑ Additional Character Required — Refer to the Tabular List for Character Selection

Syndrome — continued

fatigue
  chronic G93.32
  postviral G93.31
  psychogenic F48.8
faulty bowel habit K59.39
Feil-Klippel (brevicollis) Q76.1
Felty's — see Felty's syndrome
fertile eunuch E23.0
fetal
  alcohol (dysmorphic) Q86.0
  hydantoin Q86.1
Fiedler's I40.1
first arch Q87.0
fish odor E72.89
Fisher's G61.0
Fitzhugh-Curtis
  due to
    Chlamydia trachomatis A74.81
    Neisseria gonorrhea (gonococcal peritonitis)
      A54.85
Fitz's — see also Pancreatitis, acute K85.80
Flajani (-Basedow) E05.00
  with thyroid storm E05.01
flatback — see Flatback syndrome
floppy
  baby P94.2
  iris (intraoeprative) (IFIS) H21.81
  mitral valve I34.1
flush E34.09
Foix-Alajouanine G95.19
Fong's Q87.2
food protein-induced enterocolitis (FPIES) K52.21
foramen magnum G93.5
Foster-Kennedy H47.14- ☑
Foville's (peduncular) G46.3
fragile X Q99.2
Franceschetti Q75.4
Frey's
  auriculotemporal G50.8
  hyperhidrosis L74.52
Friderichsen-Waterhouse A39.1
Froin's G95.89
frontal lobe F07.0
Fukuhara E88.49
functional
  bowel K59.9
  prepubertal castrate E29.1
Gaisbock's D75.1
ganglion (basal ganglia brain) G25.9
  geniculi G51.1
Gardner-Diamond D69.2
gastroesophageal
  junction K22.0
  laceration-hemorrhage K22.6
gastrojejunal loop obstruction K91.89
Gee-Herter-Heubner K90.0
Gelineau's G47.419
  with cataplexy G47.411
genito-anorectal A55
Gerstmann-Straussler-Scheinker (GSS) A81.82
Gianotti-Crosti L44.4
giant platelet (Bernard-Soulier) D69.1
Gilles de la Tourette's F95.2
Glass Q87.89
Gleich's D72.118
goiter-deafness E07.1
Goldberg Q89.8
Goldberg-Maxwell E34.51
Good's D83.8
Gopalan' (burning feet) E53.8
Gorlin's Q87.89
Gougerot-Blum L81.7
Gouley's I31.1
Gower's R55
gray or grey (newborn) P93.0
  platelet D69.1
Gubler-Millard G46.3
Guillain-Barre (-Strohl) G61.0
gustatory sweating G50.8
Hadfield-Clarke K86.89
hair tourniquet — see Constriction, external, by site
Hamman's J98.19
hand-foot L27.1
hand-shoulder G90.89
hantavirus (cardio)-pulmonary (HPS) (HCPS) B33.4
happy puppet Q93.51
Harada's H30.81- ☑
Hayem-Faber D50.9

Syndrome — continued

headache NEC G44.89
  complicated NEC G44.59
Heberden's I20.89
Hedinger's E34.01
Hegglin's D72.0
HELLP (hemolysis, elevated liver enzymes and low
    platelet count) O14.2- ☑
  complicating
    childbirth O14.24
    puerperium O14.25
hemolytic-uremic D59.30
  atypical D59.39
    genetic D59.32
    hereditary D59.32
    infection-associated D59.31
    secondary D59.39
    specified NEC D59.39
  due to genetic disorder D59.32
  familial D59.32
  hereditary D59.32
  infection-associated D59.31
  secondary D59.39
  Shiga toxin-producing E. coli [STEC] related D59.31
  specified NEC D59.39
  typical D59.31
hemophagocytic, infection-associated D76.2
Henoch-Schonlein D69.0
hepatic flexure K59.89
hepatopulmonary K76.81
hepatorenal K76.7
  following delivery O90.41
  postoperative or postprocedural K91.83
  postpartum, puerperal O90.41
hepatourologic K76.7
hereditary alpha tryptasemia D89.44
Herter (-Gee) (nontropical sprue) K90.0
Heubner-Herter K90.0
Heyd's K76.7
Hilger's G90.09
histamine-like (fish poisoning) — see Poisoning, fish
histiocytic D76.3
histiocytosis NEC D76.3
HIV infection, acute B20
Hoffmann-Werdnig G12.0
Hollander-Simons E88.1
Hoppe-Goldflam G70.00
  with exacerbation (acute) G70.01
  in crisis G70.01
Horner's G90.2
hungry bone E83.81
hunterian glossitis D51.0
Hunt's (herpetic geniculate ganglionitis) (neuralgia)
    B02.21
  dyssynergia cerebellaris myoclonica G11.19
Hutchinson's triad A50.53
hyperabduction G54.0
hyperammonemia-hyperornithinemia-homocitrullinemia
    E72.4
hypereosinophilic (HES) D72.119
  idiopathic (IHES) D72.110
  lymphocytic variant (LHES) D72.111
  myeloid D72.118
  specified NEC D72.118
hyperimmunoglobulin D M04.1
hyperimmunoglobulin E (IgE) D82.4
hyperkalemic E87.5
hyperkinetic — see Hyperkinesia
hypermobility M35.7
hypernatremia E87.0
hyperosmolarity — see also Diabetes, by type, with hy-
    perosmolarity E87.0
hyperperfusion G97.82
hypersplenic D73.1
hypertransfusion, newborn P61.1
hyperventilation F45.8
hyperviscosity (of serum)
  polycythemic D75.1
  sclerothymic D58.8
hypoglycemic (familial) (neonatal) E16.2
hypokalemic E87.6
hyponatremic E87.1
hypopituitarism E23.0
hypoplastic left-heart Q23.4
hypopotassemia E87.6
hyposmolality E87.1
hypotension, maternal O26.5- ☑
hypothenar hammer I73.89
hypoventilation, obesity (OHS) E66.2

Syndrome — continued

ICF (intravascular coagulation-fibrinolysis) D65
idiopathic
  cardiorespiratory distress, newborn P22.0
  nephrotic (infantile) N04.9
iliotibial band M76.3- ☑
immobility, immobilization (paraplegic) M62.3
immune effector cell-associated neurotoxicity (ICANS)
    G92.00
  grade
    1 G92.01
    2 G92.02
    3 G92.03
    4 G92.04
    5 G92.05
    unspecified G92.00
immune reconstitution D89.3
immune reconstitution inflammatory [IRIS] D89.3
immunity deficiency, combined D81.9
immunodeficiency
  acquired — see Human, immunodeficiency virus (HIV)
    disease
  combined D81.9
impending coronary I20.0
impingement, shoulder M75.4- ☑
inappropriate secretion of antidiuretic hormone E22.2
infant
  gestational diabetes P70.0
  of diabetic mother P70.1
infantilism (pituitary) E23.0
inferior vena cava I87.1
inspissated bile (newborn) P59.1
institutional (childhood) F94.2
insufficient sleep F51.12
insulin resistance
  type A E88.811
  type B E88.818
intermediate coronary (artery) I20.0
interspinous ligament — see Spondylopathy, specified
    NEC
intestinal
  carcinoid E34.09
  knot K56.2
intravascular coagulation-fibrinolysis (ICF) D65
iodine-deficiency, congenital E00.9
  type
    mixed E00.2
    myxedematous E00.1
    neurological E00.0
IRDS (idiopathic respiratory distress, newborn) P22.0
irritable
  bowel K58.9
    with
      constipation K58.1
      diarrhea K58.0
    mixed K58.2
    psychogenic F45.8
    specified NEC K58.8
  heart (psychogenic) F45.8
  weakness F48.8
ischemic
  bowel (transient) K55.9
    chronic K55.1
    due to mesenteric artery insufficiency K55.1
  steal T82.898 ☑
IVC (intravascular coagulopathy) D65
Ivemark's Q89.01
Jaccoud's — see Arthropathy, postrheumatic, chronic
Jackson's G83.89
Jakob-Creutzfeldt — see Creutzfeldt-Jakob disease or
    syndrome
jaw-winking Q07.8
Jervell-Lange-Nielsen I45.81
jet lag G47.25
Job's D71
Joseph-Diamond-Blackfan D61.01
jugular foramen G52.7
Kabuki Q89.8
Kanner's (autism) F84.0
Kartagener's Q89.3
Kelly's D50.1
Kimmelstiel-Wilson — see Diabetes, specified type, with
    Kimmelstiel-Wilson disease
Kleefstra Q87.86
Klein (e)-Levine G47.13
Klippel-Feil (brevicollis) Q76.1
Kohler-Pellegrini-Stieda — see Bursitis, tibial collateral
Konig's K59.89
Korsakoff (-Wernicke) (nonalcoholic) F04

Syndrome — *continued*
  Korsakoff — *continued*
    alcoholic F10.26
  Kostmann's D70.0
  Krabbe's congenital muscle hypoplasia Q79.8
  labyrinthine — *see* subcategory H83.2 ☑
  lacunar NEC G46.7
  Lambert-Eaton G70.80
    in
      neoplastic disease G73.1
      specified disease NEC G70.81
  Landau-Kleffner — *see* Epilepsy, specified NEC
  Larsen's Q74.8
  Lassueur Graham-Little Piccardi L66.19
  lateral
    cutaneous nerve of thigh G57.1- ☑
    medullary G46.4
  Launois' E22.0
  Laurence-Moon Q87.84
  lazy
    leukocyte D70.8
    posture M62.3
  Lemierre I80.8
  Lennox-Gastaut G40.812
    intractable G40.814
      with status epilepticus G40.813
      without status epilepticus G40.814
    not intractable G40.812
      with status epilepticus G40.811
      without status epilepticus G40.812
  lenticular, progressive E83.01
  Leopold-Levi's E05.90
  Lev's I44.2
  Lichtheim's D51.0
  Li-Fraumeni Z15.01
  Lightwood's N25.89
  Lignac (de Toni) (-Fanconi) (-Debre) E72.09
    with cystinosis E72.04
  Likoff's I20.89
  limbic epilepsy personality F07.0
  liver-kidney K76.7
  lobotomy F07.0
  Loffler's J82.89
  long arm 18 or 21 deletion Q93.89
  long QT I45.81
  Louis-Barre G11.3
  low
    atmospheric pressure T70.29 ☑
    back M54.50
    output (cardiac) I50.9
  lower radicular, newborn (birth injury) P14.8
  Luetscher's (dehydration) E86.0
  Lupus anticoagulant D68.62
  Lutembacher's Q21.19
  macrophage activation D76.1
    due to infection D76.2
  magnesium-deficiency R29.0
  Majeed M04.8
  Mal de Debarquement R42
  malabsorption K90.9
    postsurgical K91.2
  malformation, congenital, due to
    alcohol Q86.0
    exogenous cause NEC Q86.8
    hydantoin Q86.1
    warfarin Q86.2
  malignant
    carcinoid E34.00
    neuroleptic G21.0
  Mallory-Weiss K22.6
  mandibulofacial dysostosis Q75.4
  manic-depressive — *see* Disorder, bipolar
  maple-syrup-urine E71.0
  Marable's I77.4
  Marfan Q87.40
    with
      cardiovascular manifestations Q87.418
        aortic dilation Q87.410
      ocular manifestations Q87.42
      skeletal manifestations Q87.43
  Marie's (acromegaly) E22.0
  mast cell activation — *see* Activation, mast cell
  maternal hypotension — *see* Syndrome, hypotension, maternal
  May (-Hegglin) D72.0
  McArdle (-Schmidt) (-Pearson) E74.04
  McQuarrie's E16.2
  meconium plug (newborn) P76.0
  MED13L (mediator complex subunit 13L) Q87.85

Syndrome — *continued*
  median arcuate ligament I77.4
  mediator complex subunit 13L (MED13L) Q87.85
  Meekeren-Ehlers-Danlos Q79.6 ☑
  megavitamin-B6 E67.2
  Meige G24.4
  MELAS E88.41
  Mendelson's O74.0
  MERRF (myoclonic epilepsy associated with ragged-red fibers) E88.42
  mesenteric
    artery (superior) K55.1
    vascular insufficiency K55.1
  metabolic E88.810
  metastatic carcinoid E34.00
  micrognathia-glossoptosis Q87.0
  midbrain NEC G93.89
  middle lobe (lung) J98.19
  middle radicular G54.0
  migraine — *see also* Migraine G43.909
  Mikulicz' K11.8
  milk-alkali E83.52
  Millard-Gubler G46.3
  Miller-Dieker Q93.88
  Miller-Fisher G61.0
  Minkowski-Chauffard D58.0
  Mirizzi's K83.1
  MNGIE (Mitochondrial Neurogastrointestinal Encephalopathy) E88.49
  Mobius, ophthalmoplegic migraine — *see* Migraine, ophthalmoplegic
  monofixation H50.42
  Morel-Moore M85.2
  Morel-Morgagni M85.2
  Morgagni (-Morel) (-Stewart) M85.2
  Morgagni-Adams-Stokes I45.9
  Mounier-Kuhn Q32.4
    with bronchiectasis J47.9
      with
        exacerbation (acute) J47.1
        lower respiratory infection J47.0
    acquired J98.09
      with bronchiectasis J47.9
        with
          exacerbation (acute) J47.1
          lower respiratory infection J47.0
  Muckle-Wells M04.2
  mucocutaneous lymph node (acute febrile) (MCLS) M30.3
  multiple endocrine neoplasia (MEN) — *see* Neoplasia, endocrine, multiple (MEN)
  multiple operations — *see* Disorder, factitious
  multisystem inflammatory (in adults) (in children) M35.81
  myasthenic G70.9
    in
      diabetes mellitus — *see* Diabetes, amyotrophy
      endocrine disease NEC E34.9 *[G73.3]*
      neoplastic disease — *see also* Neoplasm D49.9 *[G73.3]*
      thyrotoxicosis (hyperthyroidism) E05.90 *[G73.3]*
        with thyroid storm E05.91 *[G73.3]*
  myelodysplastic D46.9
    with
      5q deletion D46.C (*following* D46.2)
      isolated del (5q) chromosomal abnormality D46.C (*following* D46.2)
      multilineage dysplasia D46.A (*following* D46.2)
        with ringed sideroblasts D46.B (*following* D46.2)
    lesions, low grade D46.20
    specified NEC D46.Z (*following* D46.4)
  myeloid hypereosinophilic D72.118
  myelopathic pain G89.0
  myeloproliferative (chronic) D47.1
  myofascial pain M79.18
  Naffziger's G54.0
  nail patella Q87.2
  NARP (Neuropathy, Ataxia and Retinitis pigmentosa) E88.49
  neonatal abstinence P96.1
  nephritic — *see also* Nephritis
    with edema — *see* Nephrosis
    acute N00.9
    chronic N03.9
    rapidly progressive N01.9
  nephrotic (congenital) — *see also* Nephrosis N04.9
    with
      C3
        glomerulonephritis N04.A
        glomerulopathy N04.A
          with dense deposit disease N04.6

Syndrome — *continued*
  nephrotic — *see also* Nephrosis — *continued*
    with — *continued*
      dense deposit disease N04.6
      diffuse
        crescentic glomerulonephritis N04.7
        endocapillary proliferative glomerulonephritis N04.4
        membranous glomerulonephritis N04.20
        mesangial proliferative glomerulonephritis N04.3
        mesangiocapillary glomerulonephritis N04.5
      focal and segmental glomerular lesions N04.1
      minor glomerular abnormality N04.0
      specified morphological changes NEC N04.8
    diabetic — *see* Diabetes, nephrosis
    specified type NEC with diffuse membranous glomerulonephritis N04.29
  neurologic neglect R41.4
  Nezelof's D81.4
  Nonne-Milroy-Meige Q82.0
  Nothnagel's vasomotor acroparesthesia I73.89
  obesity hypoventilation (OHS) E66.2
  obliterans
    bronchiolitis — *see also* Bronchiolitis, obliterative J44.81
  oculomotor H51.9
  Ogilvie K59.81
  Oliver-McFarlane Q87.89
  ophthalmoplegia-cerebellar ataxia — *see* Strabismus, paralytic, third nerve
  oral allergy T78.1 ☑
  oral-facial-digital Q87.0
  organic
    affective F06.30
    amnesic (not alcohol- or drug-induced) F04
    brain F09
    depressive F06.31
    hallucinosis F06.0
    personality F07.0
  Ormond's N13.5
  oro-facial-digital Q87.0
  os trigonum Q68.8
  Osler-Weber-Rendu I78.0
  osteoporosis-osteomalacia M83.8
  Osterreicher-Turner Q87.2
  otolith — *see* subcategory H81.8 ☑
  oto-palatal-digital Q87.0
  outlet (thoracic) — *see also* Syndrome, thoracic outlet G54.0
  ovary
    polycystic E28.2
    resistant E28.39
    sclerocystic E28.2
  Owren's D68.2
  Paget-Schroetter I82.890
  pain — *see also* Pain
    complex regional I G90.50
      lower limb G90.52- ☑
      specified site NEC G90.59
      upper limb G90.51- ☑
    complex regional II — *see* Causalgia
  painful
    bruising D69.2
    feet E53.8
    prostate N42.81
  paralysis agitans — *see* Parkinsonism
  paralytic G83.9
    specified NEC G83.89
  Parinaud's H51.0
  parkinsonian — *see* Parkinsonism
  Parkinson's — *see* Parkinsonism
  paroxysmal facial pain G50.0
  Parry's E05.00
    with thyroid storm E05.01
  Parsonage (-Aldren)-Turner G54.5
  patella clunk M25.86- ☑
  Paterson (-Brown) (-Kelly) D50.1
  pectoral girdle I77.89
  pectoralis minor I77.89
  pediatric autoimmune neuropsychiatric disorders associated with streptococcal infections (PANDAS) D89.89
  pediatric inflammatory multisystem M35.81
  Pelger-Huet D72.0
  pellagra-cerebellar ataxia-renal aminoaciduria E72.02
  pellagroid E52
  Pellegrini-Stieda — *see* Bursitis, tibial collateral

☑ **Additional Character Required** — **Refer to the Tabular List for Character Selection**

Syndrome — *continued*

pelvic congestion-fibrosis, female N94.89
penta X Q97.1
peptic ulcer — *see* Ulcer, peptic
perabduction I77.89
periodic fever M04.1
periodic fever, aphthous stomatitis, pharyngitis, and
    adenopathy [PFAPA] M04.8
periodic headache, in adults and children — *see*
    Headache, periodic syndromes in adults and chil-
    dren
periurethral fibrosis N13.5
Peutz-Jeghers Q85.89
phantom limb (without pain) G54.7
    with pain G54.6
pharyngeal pouch D82.1
Phelan-McDermid Q93.52
Pick's — *see* Disease, Pick's
Pickwickian E66.2
PIE (pulmonary infiltration with eosinophilia) — *see also*
    Eosinophilia, pulmonary J82.89
pigmentary pallidal degeneration (progressive) G23.0
pineal E34.8
pituitary E22.0
placental transfusion — *see* Pregnancy, complicated by,
    placental transfusion syndromes
plantar fascia M72.2
plateau iris (post-iridectomy) (postprocedural) H21.82
Plummer-Vinson D50.1
pluricarential of infancy E40
plurideficiency E40
pluriglandular (compensatory) E31.8
    autoimmune E31.0
pneumatic hammer T75.21 ☑
polyangiitis overlap M30.8
polycarential of infancy E40
polyglandular E31.8
    autoimmune E31.0
polysplenia Q89.09
pontine NEC G93.89
popliteal
    artery entrapment I77.89
    web Q87.89
post chemoembolization — *code to* associated conditions
post endometrial ablation N99.85
postbacterial fatigue G93.39
postcardiac injury
    postcardiotomy I97.0
    postmyocardial infarction I24.1
postcardiotomy I97.0
postcholecystectomy K91.5
postcommissurotomy I97.0
postconcussional F07.81
postcontusional F07.81
post-COVID (-19) U09.9
postencephalitic F07.89
posterior
    cervical sympathetic M53.0
    cord G83.83
    fossa compression G93.5
    reversible encephalopathy (PRES) I67.83
postgastrectomy (dumping) K91.1
postgastric surgery K91.1
postinfarction I24.1
postinfectious fatigue G93.39
postlaminectomy NEC M96.1
postleukotomy F07.0
postmastectomy lymphedema I97.2
postmyocardial infarction I24.1
postoperative NEC T81.9 ☑
    blind loop K90.2
postpartum panhypopituitary (Sheehan) E23.0
postpolio (myelitic) G14
postthrombotic I87.009
    with
        inflammation I87.02- ☑
            with ulcer I87.03- ☑
        specified complication NEC I87.09- ☑
        ulcer I87.01- ☑
            with inflammation I87.03- ☑
    asymptomatic I87.00- ☑
postural
    orthostatic tachycardia [POTS] G90.A
    tachycardia G90.A
postvagotomy K91.1
postvalvulotomy I97.0
postviral NEC G93.31
    fatigue G93.31

Syndrome — *continued*

Potain's K31.0
potassium intoxication E87.5
Prader-Willi Q87.11
Prader-Willi-like Q87.19
precerebral artery (multiple) (bilateral) G45.2
preinfarction I20.0
preleukemic D46.9
premature senility E34.8
premenstrual dysphoric F32.81
premenstrual tension N94.3
Prinzmetal-Massumi R07.1
prune belly Q79.4
pseudo-Turner's Q87.19
pseudocarpal tunnel (sublimis) — *see* Syndrome, carpal
    tunnel
pseudoparalytica G70.00
    with exacerbation (acute) G70.01
    in crisis G70.01
psycho-organic (nonpsychotic severity) F07.9
    acute or subacute F05
    depressive type F06.31
    hallucinatory type F06.0
    nonpsychotic severity F07.0
    specified NEC F07.89
PTEN (hamartoma) tumor Q85.81
pulmonary
    arteriosclerosis I27.0
    dysmaturity (Wilson-Mikity) P27.0
    hypoperfusion (idiopathic) P22.0
    renal (hemorrhagic) (Goodpasture's) M31.0
pure
    motor lacunar G46.5
    sensory lacunar G46.6
Putnam-Dana D51.0
pyogenic arthritis, pyoderma gangrenosum, and acne
    [PAPA] M04.8
pyramidopallidon gral G20.C
pyriformis — *see* Lesion, nerve, sciatic
QT interval prolongation I45.81
radicular NEC — *see* Radiculopathy
    upper limbs, newborn (birth injury) P14.3
rapid time-zone change G47.25
Rasmussen G04.81
Raymond (-Cestan) I65.8
Raynaud's I73.00
    with gangrene I73.01
RDS (respiratory distress syndrome, newborn) P22.0
reactive airways dysfunction J68.3
Refsum's G60.1
Reifenstein E34.52
renal glomerulohyalinosis-diabetic — *see* Diabetes,
    nephrosis
Rendu-Osler-Weber I78.0
residual ovary N99.83
resistant ovary E28.39
respiratory
    distress
        acute J80
            adult J80
            child J80
            idiopathic J84.114
        newborn (idiopathic) (type I) P22.0
            type II P22.1
restless legs G25.81
restrictive allograft J4A.0
retinoblastoma (familial) C69.2 ☑
retroperitoneal fibrosis K68.2
retroviral seroconversion (acute) Z21
Reye's G93.7
Richter — *see* Leukemia, chronic lymphocytic, B-cell type
Ridley's I50.1
right
    heart, hypoplastic Q22.6
    ventricular obstruction — *see* Failure, heart, right
Romano-Ward (prolonged QT interval) I45.81
rotator cuff, shoulder — *see also* Tear, rotator cuff
    M75.10- ☑
Rotes Querol — *see* Hyperostosis, ankylosing
Roth — *see* Meralgia paresthetica
rubella (congenital) P35.0
Ruvalcaba-Myhre-Smith E71.440
Rytand-Lipsitch I44.2
salt
    depletion E87.1
        due to heat NEC T67.8 ☑
            causing heat exhaustion or prostration T67.4 ☑
    low E87.1
salt-losing N28.89

Syndrome — *continued*

SATB2-associated Q87.89
Scaglietti-Dagnini E22.0
scalenus anticus (anterior) G54.0
scapulocostal — *see* Mononeuropathy, upper limb,
    specified site NEC
scapuloperoneal G71.09
schizophrenic, of childhood NEC F20.9
Schnitzler D47.2
Scholte's E34.09
Schroeder's E27.0
Schuller-Christian C96.5
Schwachman (-Diamond) D61.02
Schwartz (-Jampel) G71.13
Schwartz-Bartter E22.2
scimitar Q26.8
sclerocystic ovary E28.2
Seitelberger's G31.89
septicemic adrenal hemorrhage A39.1
seroconversion, retroviral (acute) Z21
serotonin G90.81
serous meningitis G93.2
severe acute respiratory (SARS) J12.81
    coronavirus 2 (*see also* COVID-19) U07.1
        pneumonia J12.82
shaken infant T74.4 ☑
shock (traumatic) T79.4 ☑
    kidney N17.0
        following crush injury T79.5 ☑
    toxic A48.3
shock-lung J80
Shone's — *code to* specific anomalies
short
    bowel K90.829
        with
            colon in continuity K90.821
            iliocolonic anastomosis K90.821
        without colon in continuity K90.822
    gut — *see* Syndrome, short, bowel
    rib Q77.2
shoulder-hand — *see* Algoneurodystrophy
Shwachman (-Diamond) D61.02
sicca — *see* Syndrome, Sjogren
sick
    cell E87.1
    sinus I49.5
sick-euthyroid E07.81
sideropenic D50.1
Siemens' ectodermal dysplasia Q82.4
Silfverskold's Q78.9
Simons' E88.1
sinus tarsi M25.57- ☑
sinusitis-bronchiectasis-situs inversus Q89.3
Sipple's E31.22
sirenomelia Q87.2
Sjogren M35.00
    with
        central nervous system involvement M35.07
        dental involvement M35.0C
        gastrointestinal involvement M35.08
        glomerular disease M35.0A
        inflammatory arthritis M35.05
        keratoconjunctivitis M35.01
        lung involvement M35.02
        myopathy M35.03
        peripheral nervous system involvement M35.06
        renal tubular acidosis M35.04
        specified organ involvement, NEC M35.09
        tubulo-interstitial nephropathy M35.04
        vasculitis M35.0B
Slocumb's E27.0
slow flow, coronary I20.89
Sluder's G44.89
Smith-Magenis Q93.88
Sneddon-Wilkinson L13.1
Snyder-Robinson Q87.89
Sotos' Q87.3
South African cardiomyopathy I42.8
spasmodic
    upward movement, eyes H51.8
    winking F95.8
Spen's I45.9
splenic
    agenesis Q89.01
    flexure K59.89
    neutropenia D73.81
Spurway's Q78.0
staphylococcal scalded skin L00

Syndrome — continued
  steal
    arteriovenous T82.898- ☑
    ischemic T82.898- ☑
    subclavian G45.8
  Stein-Leventhal E28.2
  Stein's E28.2
  Stevens-Johnson syndrome L51.1
    toxic epidermal necrolysis overlap L51.3
  Stewart-Morel M85.2
  Stickler Q89.8
  stiff baby Q89.8
  stiff man G25.82
  Still-Felty — see Felty's syndrome
  Stokes (-Adams) I45.9
  stone heart I50.1
  straight back, congenital Q76.49
  Sturge-Weber (-Dimitri) Q85.89
  subclavian steal G45.8
  subcoracoid-pectoralis minor G54.0
  subcostal nerve compression I77.89
  subphrenic interposition Q43.3
  superior
    cerebellar artery I63.89
    mesenteric artery K55.1
    semi-circular canal dehiscence H83.8X- ☑
    vena cava I87.1
  supine hypotensive (maternal) — see Syndrome, hypotension, maternal
  suprarenal cortical E27.0
  supraspinatus — see also Tear, rotator cuff M75.10- ☑
  Susac G93.49
  swallowed blood P78.2
  sweat retention L74.0
  Swyer Q99.1
  Symond's G93.2
  sympathetic
    cervical paralysis G90.2
    pelvic, female N94.89
  systemic inflammatory response (SIRS), of non-infectious origin (without organ dysfunction) R65.10
    with acute organ dysfunction R65.11
  tachycardia-bradycardia I49.5
  takotsubo I51.81
  TAR (thrombocytopenia with absent radius) Q87.2
  tarsal tunnel G57.5- ☑
  teething K00.7
  tegmental G93.89
  telangiectasic-pigmentation-cataract Q82.8
  temporal pyramidal apex — see Otitis, media, suppurative, acute
  temporomandibular joint-pain-dysfunction M26.62- ☑
  Terry's — see also Myopia, degenerative H44.2- ☑
  testicular feminization — see Syndrome, androgen insensitivity E34.51
  thalamic pain (hyperesthetic) G89.0
  thoracic outlet (compression) G54.0
    arterial I77.89
    neurogenic G54.0
    venous I87.1
  Thorson-Bjorck E34.09
  thrombocytopenia with absent radius (TAR) Q87.2
  thrombosis with thrombocytopenia D75.84
  thyroid-adrenocortical insufficiency E31.0
  tibial
    anterior M76.81- ☑
    posterior M76.82- ☑
  Tietze's M94.0
  time-zone (rapid) G47.25
  Toni-Fanconi E72.09
    with cystinosis E72.04
  Touraine's Q79.8
  tourniquet — see Constriction, external, by site
  toxic shock A48.3
  transient left ventricular apical ballooning I51.81
  traumatic vasospastic T75.22 ☑
  Treacher Collins Q75.4
  triple X, female Q97.0
  trisomy Q92.9
    13 Q91.7
      meiotic nondisjunction Q91.4
      mitotic nondisjunction Q91.5
      mosaicism Q91.5
      translocation Q91.6
    18 Q91.3
      meiotic nondisjunction Q91.0
      mitotic nondisjunction Q91.1
      mosaicism Q91.1

Syndrome — continued
  trisomy — continued
    18 — continued
      translocation Q91.2
    20 (q)(p) Q92.8
    21 Q90.9
      meiotic nondisjunction Q90.0
      mitotic nondisjunction Q90.1
      mosaicism Q90.1
      translocation Q90.2
    22 Q92.8
  tropical wet feet T69.0- ☑
  Trousseau's I82.1
  tumor lysis (following antineoplastic chemotherapy) (spontaneous) NEC E88.3
  tumor necrosis factor receptor associated periodic (TRAPS) M04.1
  Twiddler's (due to)
    automatic implantable defibrillator T82.198 ☑
    cardiac pacemaker T82.198 ☑
  Unverricht (-Lundborg) — see Epilepsy, generalized, idiopathic
  upward gaze H51.8
  uremia, chronic — see also Disease, kidney, chronic N18.9
  urethral N34.3
  urethro-oculo-articular — see Reiter's disease
  urohepatic K76.7
  vago-hypoglossal G52.7
  van Buchem's M85.2
  van der Hoeve's Q78.0
  vascular NEC in cerebrovascular disease G46.8
  vasoconstriction, reversible cerebrovascular I67.841
  vasomotor I73.9
  vasospastic (traumatic) T75.22 ☑
  vasovagal R55
  VATER Q87.2
  velo-cardio-facial Q93.81
  vena cava (inferior) (superior) (obstruction) I87.1
  vertebral
    artery G45.0
      compression — see Syndrome, anterior, spinal artery, compression
    steal G45.0
  vertebro-basilar artery G45.0
  vertebrogenic (pain) — see also Pain, vertebrogenic M54.89
  vertiginous — see Disorder, vestibular function
  Vinson-Plummer D50.1
  virus B34.9
  visceral larva migrans B83.0
  visual disorientation H53.8
  vitamin B6 deficiency E53.1
  vitreal corneal H59.01- ☑
  vitreous (touch) H59.01- ☑
  Vogt-Koyanagi H20.82- ☑
  Volkmann's T79.6 ☑
  von Hippel-Lindau Q85.83
  von Schroetter's I82.890
  von Willebrand (-Jurgen) — see Disease, von Willebrand
    acquired — see also Disease, von Willebrand D68.04
  Waldenstrom-Kjellberg D50.1
  Wallenberg's G46.3
  wasting (syndrome) due to underlying condition E88.A
  water retention E87.79
  Waterhouse (-Friderichsen) A39.1
  Weber-Gubler G46.3
  Weber-Leyden G46.3
  Weber's G46.3
  Wegener's M31.30
    with
      kidney involvement M31.31
      lung involvement M31.30
        with kidney involvement M31.31
  Weingarten's (tropical eosinophilia) J82.89
  Weiss-Baker G90.09
  Werdnig-Hoffman G12.0
  Wermer's E31.21
  Werner's E34.8
  Wernicke-Korsakoff (nonalcoholic) F04
    alcoholic F10.26
  Westphal-Strumpell E83.01
  West's — see Epilepsy, spasms
  wet
    feet (maceration) (tropical) T69.0- ☑
    lung, newborn P22.1
  whiplash S13.4 ☑
  whistling face Q87.0
  Wilkie's K55.1

Syndrome — continued
  Wilkinson-Sneddon L13.1
  Willebrand (-Jurgens) — see Disease, von Willebrand
  Williams Q93.82
  Wilson's (hepatolenticular degeneration) E83.01
  Wiskott-Aldrich D82.0
  withdrawal — see Withdrawal, state
    drug
      infant of dependent mother P96.1
      therapeutic use, newborn P96.2
  Woakes' (ethmoiditis) J33.1
  Wright's (hyperabduction) G54.0
  X I20.9
  XXXX Q97.1
  XXXXX Q97.1
  XXXXY Q98.1
  XXY Q98.0
  Yao M04.8
  yellow nail L60.5
  Zahorsky's B08.5
  Zellweger syndrome E71.510
  Zellweger-like syndrome E71.541
Synechia (anterior) (iris) (posterior) (pupil) — see also Adhesions, iris
  intra-uterine (traumatic) N85.6
Synesthesia R20.8
Syngamiasis, syngamosis B83.3
Synodontia K00.2
Synorchidism, synorchism Q55.1
Synostosis (congenital) Q78.8
  astragalo-scaphoid Q74.2
  radioulnar Q74.0
Synovial sarcoma — see Neoplasm, connective tissue, malignant
Synovioma (malignant) — see also Neoplasm, connective tissue, malignant
  benign — see Neoplasm, connective tissue, benign
Synoviosarcoma — see Neoplasm, connective tissue, malignant
Synovitis — see also Tenosynovitis M65.90
  ankle and foot M65.97- ☑
  arm, upper M65.92- ☑
  crepitant
    hand M70.0- ☑
    wrist M70.03- ☑
  forearm M65.93- ☑
  gonococcal A54.49
  gouty — see Gout
  hand M65.94- ☑
  in (due to)
    crystals M65.8- ☑
    gonorrhea A54.49
    syphilis (late) A52.78
    use, overuse, pressure — see Disorder, soft tissue, due to use
  infective NEC — see Tenosynovitis, infective NEC
  leg, lower M65.96- ☑
  multiple sites, unspecified type M65.99
  shoulder M65.91- ☑
  specified site, unspecified type M65.98
  specified NEC — see Tenosynovitis, specified type NEC
  syphilitic A52.78
    congenital (early) A50.02
  thigh M65.95- ☑
  toxic — see Synovitis, transient
  transient M67.3- ☑
    ankle M67.37- ☑
    elbow M67.32- ☑
    foot joint M67.37- ☑
    hand joint M67.34- ☑
    hip M67.35- ☑
    knee M67.36- ☑
    multiple site M67.39
    pelvic region M67.35- ☑
    shoulder M67.31- ☑
    specified joint NEC M67.38
    wrist M67.33- ☑
  traumatic, current — see Sprain
  tuberculous — see Tuberculosis, synovitis
  villonodular (pigmented) M12.2- ☑
    ankle M12.27- ☑
    elbow M12.22- ☑
    foot joint M12.27- ☑
    hand joint M12.24- ☑
    hip M12.25- ☑
    knee M12.26- ☑
    multiple site M12.29

☑ **Additional Character Required** — Refer to the Tabular List for Character Selection

Synovitis — *continued*
> villonodular — *continued*
>> pelvic region M12.25- ☑
>> shoulder M12.21- ☑
>> specified joint NEC M12.28
>> vertebrae M12.28
>> wrist M12.23- ☑

Syphilid A51.39
> congenital A50.06
> newborn A50.06
> tubercular (late) A52.79

Syphilis, syphilitic (acquired) A53.9
> abdomen (late) A52.79
> acoustic nerve A52.15
> adenopathy (secondary) A51.49
> adrenal (gland) (with cortical hypofunction) A52.79
> age under 2 years NOS — *see also* Syphilis, congenital, early
>> acquired A51.9
> alopecia (secondary) A51.32
> anemia (late) A52.79 [D63.8]
> aneurysm (aorta) (ruptured) A52.01
>> central nervous system A52.05
>> congenital A50.54 [I79.0]
> anus (late) A52.74
>> primary A51.1
>> secondary A51.39
> aorta (arch) (abdominal) (thoracic) A52.02
>> aneurysm A52.01
> aortic (insufficiency) (regurgitation) (stenosis) A52.03
>> aneurysm A52.01
> arachnoid (adhesive) (cerebral) (spinal) A52.13
> asymptomatic — *see* Syphilis, latent
> ataxia (locomotor) A52.11
> atrophoderma maculatum A51.39
> auricular fibrillation A52.06
> bladder (late) A52.76
> bone A52.77
>> secondary A51.46
> brain A52.17
> breast (late) A52.79
> bronchus (late) A52.72
> bubo (primary) A51.0
> bulbar palsy A52.19
> bursa (late) A52.78
> cardiac decompensation A52.06
> cardiovascular A52.00
> central nervous system (late) (recurrent) (relapse) (tertiary) A52.3
>> with
>>> ataxia A52.11
>>> general paralysis A52.17
>>>> juvenile A50.45
>>> paresis (general) A52.17
>>>> juvenile A50.45
>>> tabes (dorsalis) A52.11
>>>> juvenile A50.45
>>> taboparesis A52.17
>>>> juvenile A50.45
>> aneurysm A52.05
>> congenital A50.40
>> juvenile A50.40
>> remission in (sustained) A52.3
>> serology doubtful, negative, or positive A52.3
>> specified nature or site NEC A52.19
>> vascular A52.05
> cerebral A52.17
>> meningovascular A52.13
>> nerves (multiple palsies) A52.15
>> sclerosis A52.17
>> thrombosis A52.05
> cerebrospinal (tabetic type) A52.12
> cerebrovascular A52.05
> cervix (late) A52.76
> chancre (multiple) A51.0
>> extragenital A51.2
>> Rollet's A51.0
> Charcot's joint A52.16
> chorioretinitis A51.43
>> congenital A50.01
>> late A52.71
>> prenatal A50.01
> choroiditis — *see* Syphilitic chorioretinitis
> choroidoretinitis — *see* Syphilitic chorioretinitis
> ciliary body (secondary) A51.43
>> late A52.71
> colon (late) A52.74
> combined spinal sclerosis A52.11
> condyloma (latum) A51.31

Syphilis, syphilitic — *continued*
> congenital A50.9
>> with
>>> paresis (general) A50.45
>>> tabes (dorsalis) A50.45
>>> taboparesis A50.45
>> chorioretinitis, choroiditis A50.01 [H32]
>> early, or less than 2 years after birth NEC A50.2
>>> with manifestations — *see* Syphilis, congenital, early, symptomatic
>>> latent (without manifestations) A50.1
>>>> negative spinal fluid test A50.1
>>>> serology positive A50.1
>>> symptomatic A50.09
>>>> cutaneous A50.06
>>>> mucocutaneous A50.07
>>>> oculopathy A50.01
>>>> osteochondropathy A50.02
>>>> pharyngitis A50.03
>>>> pneumonia A50.04
>>>> rhinitis A50.05
>>>> visceral A50.08
>> interstitial keratitis A50.31
>> juvenile neurosyphilis A50.45
>> late, or 2 years or more after birth NEC A50.7
>>> chorioretinitis, choroiditis A50.32
>>> interstitial keratitis A50.31
>>> juvenile neurosyphilis A50.45
>>> latent (without manifestations) A50.6
>>>> negative spinal fluid test A50.6
>>>> serology positive A50.6
>>> symptomatic or with manifestations NEC A50.59
>>>> arthropathy A50.55
>>>> cardiovascular A50.54
>>>> Clutton's joints A50.51
>>>> Hutchinson's teeth A50.52
>>>> Hutchinson's triad A50.53
>>>> osteochondropathy A50.56
>>>> saddle nose A50.57
> conjugal A53.9
>> tabes A52.11
> conjunctiva (late) A52.71
> contact Z20.2
> cord bladder A52.19
> cornea, late A52.71
> coronary (artery) (sclerosis) A52.06
> coryza, congenital A50.05
> cranial nerve A52.15
>> multiple palsies A52.15
> cutaneous — *see* Syphilis, skin
> dacryocystitis (late) A52.71
> degeneration, spinal cord A52.12
> dementia paralytica A52.17
>> juvenilis A50.45
> destruction of bone A52.77
> dilatation, aorta A52.01
> due to blood transfusion A53.9
> dura mater A52.13
> ear A52.79
>> inner A52.79
>>> nerve (eighth) A52.15
>>> neurorecurrence A52.15
> early A51.9
>> cardiovascular A52.00
>> central nervous system A52.3
>> latent (without manifestations) (less than 2 years after infection) A51.5
>>> negative spinal fluid test A51.5
>>> serological relapse after treatment A51.5
>>> serology positive A51.5
>> relapse (treated, untreated) A51.9
>> skin A51.39
>> symptomatic A51.9
>>> extragenital chancre A51.2
>>> primary, except extragenital chancre A51.0
>>> secondary — *see also* Syphilis, secondary A51.39
>>>> relapse (treated, untreated) A51.49
>> ulcer A51.39
> eighth nerve (neuritis) A52.15
> endemic A65
> endocarditis A52.03
>> aortic A52.03
>> pulmonary A52.03
> epididymis (late) A52.76
> epiglottis (late) A52.73
> epiphysitis (congenital) (early) A50.02
> episcleritis (late) A52.71
> esophagus A52.79
> eustachian tube A52.73

Syphilis, syphilitic — *continued*
> exposure to Z20.2
> eye A52.71
> eyelid (late) (with gumma) A52.71
> fallopian tube (late) A52.76
> fracture A52.77
> gallbladder (late) A52.74
> gastric (polyposis) (late) A52.74
> general A53.9
>> paralysis A52.17
>>> juvenile A50.45
> genital (primary) A51.0
> glaucoma A52.71
> gumma NEC A52.79
>> cardiovascular system A52.00
>> central nervous system A52.3
>> congenital A50.59
> heart (block) (decompensation) (disease) (failure) A52.06 [I52]
>> valve NEC A52.03
> hemianesthesia A52.19
> hemianopsia A52.71
> hemiparesis A52.17
> hemiplegia A52.17
> hepatic artery A52.09
> hepatis A52.74
> hepatomegaly, congenital A50.08
> hereditaria tarda — *see* Syphilis, congenital, late
> hereditary — *see* Syphilis, congenital
> Hutchinson's teeth A50.52
> hyalitis A52.71
> inactive — *see* Syphilis, latent
> infantum — *see* Syphilis, congenital
> inherited — *see* Syphilis, congenital
> internal ear A52.79
> intestine (late) A52.74
> iris, iritis (secondary) A51.43
>> late A52.71
> joint (late) A52.77
> keratitis (congenital) (interstitial) (late) A50.31
> kidney (late) A52.75
> lacrimal passages (late) A52.71
> larynx (late) A52.73
> late A52.9
>> cardiovascular A52.00
>> central nervous system A52.3
>> kidney A52.75
>> latent or 2 years or more after infection (without manifestations) A52.8
>>> negative spinal fluid test A52.8
>>> serology positive A52.8
>> paresis A52.17
>> specified site NEC A52.79
>> symptomatic or with manifestations A52.79
>> tabes A52.11
> latent A53.0
>> with signs or symptoms — *code by* site and stage under Syphilis
>> central nervous system A52.2
>> date of infection unspecified A53.0
>> early, or less than 2 years after infection A51.5
>> follow-up of latent syphilis A53.0
>>> date of infection unspecified A53.0
>>> late, or 2 years or more after infection A52.8
>> late, or 2 years or more after infection A52.8
>> positive serology (only finding) A53.0
>>> date of infection unspecified A53.0
>>> early, or less than 2 years after infection A51.5
>>> late, or 2 years or more after infection A52.8
> lens (late) A52.71
> leukoderma A51.39
>> late A52.79
> lienitis A52.79
> lip A51.39
>> chancre (primary) A51.2
>> late A52.79
> Lissauer's paralysis A52.17
> liver A52.74
> locomotor ataxia A52.11
> lung A52.72
> lymph gland (early) (secondary) A51.49
>> late A52.79
> lymphadenitis (secondary) A51.49
> macular atrophy of skin A51.39
>> striated A52.79
> mediastinum (late) A52.73
> meninges (adhesive) (brain) (spinal cord) A52.13
> meningitis A52.13
>> acute (secondary) A51.41

☑ **Additional Character Required** — **Refer to the Tabular List for Character Selection**

meningitis — *continued*
congenital A50.41
meningoencephalitis A52.14
meningovascular A52.13
congenital A50.41
mesarteritis A52.09
brain A52.04
middle ear A52.77
mitral stenosis A52.03
monoplegia A52.17
mouth (secondary) A51.39
late A52.79
mucocutaneous (secondary) A51.39
late A52.79
mucous
membrane (secondary) A51.39
late A52.79
patches A51.39
congenital A50.07
mulberry molars A50.52
muscle A52.78
myocardium A52.06
nasal sinus (late) A52.73
neonatorum — *see* Syphilis, congenital
nephrotic syndrome (secondary) A51.44
nerve palsy (any cranial nerve) A52.15
multiple A52.15
nervous system, central A52.3
neuritis A52.15
acoustic A52.15
neurorecidive of retina A52.19
neuroretinitis A52.19
newborn — *see* Syphilis, congenital
nodular superficial (late) A52.79
nonvenereal A65
nose (late) A52.73
saddle back deformity A50.57
occlusive arterial disease A52.09
oculopathy A52.71
ophthalmic (late) A52.71
optic nerve (atrophy) (neuritis) (papilla) A52.15
orbit (late) A52.71
organic A53.9
osseous (late) A52.77
osteochondritis (congenital) (early) A50.02 *[M90.80]*
osteoporosis A52.77
ovary (late) A52.76
oviduct (late) A52.76
palate (late) A52.79
pancreas (late) A52.74
paralysis A52.17
general A52.17
juvenile A50.45
paresis (general) A52.17
juvenile A50.45
paresthesia A52.19
Parkinson's disease or syndrome A52.19
paroxysmal tachycardia A52.06
pemphigus (congenital) A50.06
penis (chancre) A51.0
late A52.76
pericardium A52.06
perichondritis, larynx (late) A52.73
periosteum (late) A52.77
congenital (early) A50.02 *[M90.80]*
early (secondary) A51.46
peripheral nerve A52.79
petrous bone (late) A52.77
pharynx (late) A52.73
secondary A51.39
pituitary (gland) A52.79
pleura (late) A52.73
pneumonia, white A50.04
pontine lesion A52.17
portal vein A52.09

primary A51.0
anal A51.1
and secondary — *see* Syphilis, secondary
central nervous system A52.3
extragenital chancre NEC A51.2
fingers A51.2
genital A51.0
lip A51.2
specified site NEC A51.2
tonsils A51.2
prostate (late) A52.76
ptosis (eyelid) A52.71
pulmonary (late) A52.72
artery A52.09
pyelonephritis (late) A52.75
recently acquired, symptomatic A51.9
rectum (late) A52.74
respiratory tract (late) A52.73
retina, late A52.71
retrobulbar neuritis A52.15
salpingitis A52.76
sclera (late) A52.71
sclerosis
cerebral A52.17
coronary A52.06
multiple A52.11
scotoma (central) A52.71
scrotum (late) A52.76
secondary (and primary) A51.49
adenopathy A51.49
anus A51.39
bone A51.46
chorioretinitis, choroiditis A51.43
hepatitis A51.45
liver A51.45
lymphadenitis A51.49
meningitis (acute) A51.41
mouth A51.39
mucous membranes A51.39
periosteum, periostitis A51.46
pharynx A51.39
relapse (treated, untreated) A51.49
skin A51.39
specified form NEC A51.49
tonsil A51.39
ulcer A51.39
viscera NEC A51.49
vulva A51.39
seminal vesicle (late) A52.76
seronegative with signs or symptoms — *code by* site and stage under Syphilis
seropositive
with signs or symptoms — *code by* site and stage under Syphilis
follow-up of latent syphilis — *see* Syphilis, latent
only finding — *see* Syphilis, latent
seventh nerve (paralysis) A52.15
sinus, sinusitis (late) A52.73
skeletal system A52.77
skin (with ulceration) (early) (secondary) A51.39
late or tertiary A52.79
small intestine A52.74
spastic spinal paralysis A52.17
spermatic cord (late) A52.76
spinal (cord) A52.12
spleen A52.79
splenomegaly A52.79
spondylitis A52.77
staphyloma A52.71
stigmata (congenital) A50.59
stomach A52.74
synovium A52.78
tabes dorsalis (late) A52.11
juvenile A50.45
tabetic type A52.11

tabetic type — *continued*
juvenile A50.45
taboparesis A52.17
juvenile A50.45
tachycardia A52.06
tendon (late) A52.78
tertiary A52.9
with symptoms NEC A52.79
cardiovascular A52.00
central nervous system A52.3
multiple NEC A52.79
specified site NEC A52.79
testis A52.76
thorax A52.73
throat A52.73
thymus (gland) (late) A52.79
thyroid (late) A52.79
tongue (late) A52.79
tonsil (lingual) (late) A52.73
primary A51.2
secondary A51.39
trachea (late) A52.73
tunica vaginalis (late) A52.76
ulcer (any site) (early) (secondary) A51.39
late A52.79
perforating A52.79
foot A52.11
urethra (late) A52.76
urogenital (late) A52.76
uterus (late) A52.76
uveal tract (secondary) A51.43
late A52.71
uveitis (secondary) A51.43
late A52.71
uvula (late) (perforated) A52.79
vagina A51.0
late A52.76
valvulitis NEC A52.03
vascular A52.00
brain (cerebral) A52.05
ventriculi A52.74
vesicae urinariae (late) A52.76
viscera (abdominal) (late) A52.74
secondary A51.49
vitreous (opacities) (late) A52.71
hemorrhage A52.71
vulva A51.0
late A52.76
secondary A51.39
Syphiloma A52.79
cardiovascular system A52.00
central nervous system A52.3
circulatory system A52.00
congenital A50.59
Syphilophobia F45.29
Syringadenoma — *see also* Neoplasm, skin, benign
papillary — *see* Neoplasm, skin, benign
Syringobulbia G95.0
Syringocystadenoma — *see* Neoplasm, skin, benign
papillary — *see* Neoplasm, skin, benign
Syringoma — *see also* Neoplasm, skin, benign
chondroid — *see* Neoplasm, skin, benign
Syringomyelia G95.0
Syringomyelitis — *see* Encephalitis
Syringomyelocele — *see* Spina bifida
Syringopontia G95.0
System, systemic — *see also* condition
disease, combined — *see* Degeneration, combined
inflammatory response syndrome (SIRS) of non-infectious origin (without organ dysfunction) R65.10
with acute organ dysfunction R65.11
lupus erythematosus M32.9
inhibitor present D68.62
Systemic exertion intolerance disease [SEID] G93.32

T

Tabacism, tabacosis, tabagism — see also Poisoning, tobacco
　　meaning dependence (without remission) F17.200
　　　with
　　　　disorder F17.299
　　　　　in remission F17.211
　　　　　specified disorder NEC F17.298
　　　　　withdrawal F17.203
Tabardillo A75.9
　　flea-borne A75.2
　　louse-borne A75.0
Tabes, tabetic A52.10
　　with
　　　central nervous system syphilis A52.10
　　　Charcot's joint A52.16
　　　cord bladder A52.19
　　　crisis, viscera (any) A52.19
　　　paralysis, general A52.17
　　　paresis (general) A52.17
　　　perforating ulcer (foot) A52.19
　　arthropathy (Charcot) A52.16
　　bladder A52.19
　　bone A52.11
　　cerebrospinal A52.12
　　congenital A50.45
　　conjugal A52.10
　　dorsalis A52.11
　　　juvenile A50.49
　　juvenile A50.49
　　latent A52.19
　　mesenterica A18.39
　　paralysis, insane, general A52.17
　　spasmodic A52.17
　　syphilis (cerebrospinal) A52.12
Taboparalysis A52.17
Taboparesis (remission) A52.17
　　juvenile A50.45
TAC (trigeminal autonomic cephalgia) **NEC** G44.099
　　intractable G44.091
　　not intractable G44.099
Tache noir S60.22- ☑
Tachyalimentation K91.2
Tachyarrhythmia, tachyrhythmia — see Tachycardia
Tachycardia R00.0
　　atrial (paroxysmal) I47.19
　　auricular I47.19
　　AV nodal re-entry (re-entrant) I47.19
　　junctional (paroxysmal) I47.19
　　newborn P29.11
　　nodal (paroxysmal) I47.19
　　non-paroxysmal AV nodal I45.89
　　paroxysmal (sustained) (nonsustained) I47.9
　　　with sinus bradycardia I49.5
　　　atrial (PAT) I47.19
　　　atrioventricular (AV) (re-entrant) I47.19
　　　　psychogenic F54
　　　junctional I47.19
　　　　ectopic I47.19
　　　nodal I47.19
　　　psychogenic (atrial) (supraventricular) (ventricular) F54
　　　supraventricular (sustained) I47.10
　　　　psychogenic F54
　　　ventricular I47.20
　　　　psychogenic F54
　　　　specified type NEC I47.29
　　psychogenic F45.8
　　sick sinus I49.5
　　sinoauricular NOS R00.0
　　　paroxysmal I47.19
　　sinus [sinusal] NOS R00.0
　　　inappropriate, so stated (IST) I47.11
　　　paroxysmal I47.19
　　supraventricular I47.10
　　ventricular (paroxysmal) (sustained) I47.20
　　　psychogenic F54
　　　specified NEC I47.29
Tachygastria K31.89
Tachypnea R06.82
　　hysterical F45.8
　　newborn (idiopathic) (transitory) P22.1
　　psychogenic F45.8
　　transitory, of newborn P22.1
TACO (transfusion associated circulatory overload) E87.71
TAD (transfusion-associated dyspnea) J95.87
Taenia (infection) (infestation) B68.9

Taenia — continued
　　diminuta B71.0
　　echinococcal infestation B67.90
　　mediocanellata B68.1
　　nana B71.0
　　saginata B68.1
　　solium (intestinal form) B68.0
　　　larval form — see Cysticercosis
Taeniasis (intestine) — see Taenia
Tag (hypertrophied skin) (infected) L91.8
　　adenoid J35.8
　　anus K64.4
　　hemorrhoidal K64.4
　　hymen N89.8
　　perineal N90.89
　　preauricular Q17.0
　　sentinel K64.4
　　skin L91.8
　　　accessory (congenital) Q82.8
　　　anus K64.4
　　　congenital Q82.8
　　　preauricular Q17.0
　　tonsil J35.8
　　urethra, urethral N36.8
　　vulva N90.89
Tahyna fever B33.8
Takahara's disease E80.3
Takayasu's disease or syndrome M31.4
Talaromycosis B48.4
Talcosis (pulmonary) J62.0
Talipes (congenital) Q66.89
　　acquired, planus — see Deformity, limb, flat foot
　　asymmetric Q66.89
　　calcaneovalgus Q66.4- ☑
　　calcaneovarus Q66.1- ☑
　　calcaneus Q66.89
　　cavus Q66.7- ☑
　　equinovalgus Q66.6
　　equinovarus Q66.0- ☑
　　equinus Q66.89
　　percavus Q66.7- ☑
　　planovalgus Q66.6
　　planus (acquired) (any degree) — see also Deformity, limb, flat foot
　　　congenital Q66.5- ☑
　　　due to rickets (sequelae) E64.3
　　valgus Q66.6
　　varus Q66.3- ☑
Tall stature, constitutional E34.4
Talma's disease M62.89
Talon noir S90.3- ☑
　　hand S60.22- ☑
　　heel S90.3- ☑
　　toe S90.1- ☑
Tamponade, heart I31.4
Tanapox (virus disease) B08.71
Tangier disease E78.6
Tantrum, child problem F91.8
Tapeworm (infection) (infestation) — see Infestation, tapeworm
Tapia's syndrome G52.7
TAR (thrombocytopenia with absent radius) **syndrome** Q87.2
Tarral-Besnier disease L44.0
Tarsal tunnel syndrome — see Syndrome, tarsal tunnel
Tarsalgia — see Pain, limb, lower
Tarsitis (eyelid) H01.3
　　syphilitic A52.71
　　tuberculous A18.4
Tartar (teeth) (dental calculus) K03.6
Tattoo (mark) L81.8
Tauri's disease E74.09
Taurodontism K00.2
Taussig-Bing syndrome Q20.1
Taybi's syndrome Q87.2
Tay-Sachs amaurotic familial idiocy or disease E75.02
TBI (traumatic brain injury) S06.9 ☑
Teacher's node or nodule J38.2
Tear, torn (traumatic) — see also Laceration
　　with abortion — see Abortion
　　annular fibrosis M51.35
　　anus, anal (sphincter) S31.831 ☑
　　　complicating delivery
　　　　with third degree perineal laceration — see also Delivery, complicated, by, laceration, perineum, third degree O70.20
　　　　　with mucosa O70.3
　　　　without third degree perineal laceration O70.4

Tear, torn — continued
　　anus, anal — continued
　　　nontraumatic (healed) (old) K62.81
　　articular cartilage, old — see Derangement, joint, articular cartilage, by site
　　bladder
　　　with ectopic or molar pregnancy O08.6
　　　following ectopic or molar pregnancy O08.6
　　　obstetrical O71.5
　　　traumatic — see Injury, bladder
　　bowel
　　　with ectopic or molar pregnancy O08.6
　　　following ectopic or molar pregnancy O08.6
　　　obstetrical trauma O71.5
　　broad ligament
　　　with ectopic or molar pregnancy O08.6
　　　following ectopic or molar pregnancy O08.6
　　　obstetrical trauma O71.6
　　bucket handle (knee) (meniscus) — see Tear, meniscus
　　capsule, joint — see Sprain
　　cartilage — see also Sprain
　　　articular, old — see Derangement, joint, articular cartilage, by site
　　cervix
　　　with ectopic or molar pregnancy O08.6
　　　following ectopic or molar pregnancy O08.6
　　　obstetrical trauma (current) O71.3
　　　old N88.1
　　　traumatic — see Injury, uterus
　　dural G97.41
　　　nontraumatic G96.11
　　internal organ — see Injury, by site
　　knee cartilage
　　　articular (current) S83.3- ☑
　　　old — see Derangement, knee, meniscus, due to old tear
　　ligament — see Sprain
　　meniscus (knee) (current injury) S83.209 ☑
　　　bucket-handle S83.20- ☑
　　　lateral
　　　　bucket-handle S83.25- ☑
　　　　complex S83.27- ☑
　　　　peripheral S83.26- ☑
　　　　specified type NEC S83.28- ☑
　　　medial
　　　　bucket-handle S83.21- ☑
　　　　complex S83.23- ☑
　　　　peripheral S83.22- ☑
　　　　specified type NEC S83.24- ☑
　　　old — see Derangement, knee, meniscus, due to old tear
　　　site other than knee — code as Sprain
　　　specified type NEC S83.20- ☑
　　muscle — see Strain
　　pelvic
　　　floor, complicating delivery O70.1
　　　organ NEC, obstetrical trauma O71.5
　　　　with ectopic or molar pregnancy O08.6
　　　　following ectopic or molar pregnancy O08.6
　　perineal, secondary O90.1
　　periurethral tissue, obstetrical trauma O71.82
　　　with ectopic or molar pregnancy O08.6
　　　following ectopic or molar pregnancy O08.6
　　rectovaginal septum — see Laceration, vagina
　　retina, retinal (without detachment) (horseshoe) — see also Break, retina, horseshoe
　　　with detachment — see Detachment, retina, with retinal, break
　　rotator cuff (nontraumatic) M75.10- ☑
　　　complete M75.12- ☑
　　　incomplete M75.11- ☑
　　　traumatic S46.01- ☑
　　　　capsule S43.42- ☑
　　semilunar cartilage, knee — see Tear, meniscus
　　supraspinatus (complete) (incomplete) (nontraumatic) — see also Tear, rotator cuff M75.10- ☑
　　tendon — see Strain
　　tentorial, at birth P10.4
　　umbilical cord
　　　complicating delivery O69.89 ☑
　　urethra
　　　with ectopic or molar pregnancy O08.6
　　　following ectopic or molar pregnancy O08.6
　　　obstetrical trauma O71.5
　　uterus — see Injury, uterus
　　vagina — see Laceration, vagina
　　vessel, from catheter — see Puncture, accidental complicating surgery

Tear, torn — *continued*
 vulva, complicating delivery O70.0
Tear-stone — *see* Dacryolith
Teeth — *see also* condition
 grinding
  psychogenic F45.8
  sleep related G47.63
Teething (syndrome) K00.7
Telangiectasia, telangiectasis (verrucous) I78.1
 ataxic (cerebellar) (Louis-Bar) G11.3
 familial I78.0
 hemorrhagic, hereditary (congenital) (senile) I78.0
 hereditary, hemorrhagic (congenital) (senile) I78.0
 juxtafoveal H35.07- ☑
 macular H35.07- ☑
 macularis eruptiva perstans D47.01
 parafoveal H35.07- ☑
 retinal (idiopathic) (juxtafoveal) (macular) (parafoveal) H35.07- ☑
 spider I78.1
Telephone scatologia F65.89
Telescoped bowel or intestine K56.1
 congenital Q43.8
Temperature
 body, high (of unknown origin) R50.9
 cold, trauma from T69.9 ☑
  newborn P80.0
  specified effect NEC T69.8 ☑
Temple — *see* condition
Temporal — *see* condition
Temporomandibular joint pain-dysfunction syndrome M26.62- ☑
Temporosphenoidal — *see* condition
Tendency
 bleeding — *see* Defect, coagulation
 suicide
  meaning personal history of attempted suicide Z91.51
  meaning suicidal ideation — *see* Ideation, suicidal
 to fall R29.6
Tenderness, abdominal R10.819
 epigastric R10.816
 generalized R10.817
 left lower quadrant R10.814
 left upper quadrant R10.812
 periumbilic R10.815
 rebound R10.829
  epigastric R10.826
  generalized R10.827
  left lower quadrant R10.824
  left upper quadrant R10.822
  periumbilic R10.825
  right lower quadrant R10.823
  right upper quadrant R10.821
 right lower quadrant R10.813
 right upper quadrant R10.811
Tendinitis, tendonitis — *see also* Enthesopathy
 Achilles M76.6- ☑
 adhesive — *see* Tenosynovitis, specified type NEC
  shoulder — *see* Capsulitis, adhesive
 bicipital M75.2- ☑
 calcific M65.2- ☑
  ankle M65.27- ☑
  foot M65.27- ☑
  forearm M65.23- ☑
  hand M65.24- ☑
  lower leg M65.26- ☑
  multiple sites M65.29
  pelvic region M65.25- ☑
  shoulder M75.3- ☑
  specified site NEC M65.28
  thigh M65.25- ☑
  upper arm M65.22- ☑
 due to use, overuse, pressure — *see also* Disorder, soft tissue, due to use
  specified NEC — *see* Disorder, soft tissue, due to use, specified NEC
 gluteal M76.0- ☑
 patellar M76.5- ☑
 peroneal M76.7- ☑
 psoas M76.1- ☑
 tibial (posterior) M76.82- ☑
  anterior M76.81- ☑
 trochanteric — *see* Bursitis, hip, trochanteric
Tendon — *see* condition
Tendosynovitis — *see* Tenosynovitis
Tenesmus (rectal) R19.8
 vesical R30.1
Tennis elbow — *see* Epicondylitis, lateral

Tenonitis — *see also* Tenosynovitis
 eye (capsule) H05.04- ☑
Tenontosynovitis — *see also* Tenosynovitis
Tenontothecitis — *see* Tenosynovitis
Tenophyte — *see* Disorder, synovium, specified type NEC
Tenosynovitis — *see also* Synovitis M65.90
 adhesive — *see* Tenosynovitis, specified type NEC
  shoulder — *see* Capsulitis, adhesive
 bicipital (calcifying) — *see* Tendinitis, bicipital
 gonococcal A54.49
 in (due to)
  crystals M65.8- ☑
  gonorrhea A54.49
  syphilis (late) A52.78
  use, overuse, pressure — *see also* Disorder, soft tissue, due to use
   specified NEC — *see* Disorder, soft tissue, due to use, specified NEC
 infective NEC M65.1- ☑
  ankle M65.17- ☑
  foot M65.17- ☑
  forearm M65.13- ☑
  hand M65.14- ☑
  lower leg M65.16- ☑
  multiple sites M65.19
  pelvic region M65.15- ☑
  shoulder region M65.11- ☑
  specified site NEC M65.18
  thigh M65.15- ☑
  upper arm M65.12- ☑
 radial styloid M65.4
 shoulder region M65.81- ☑
  adhesive — *see* Capsulitis, adhesive
 specified type NEC M65.88
  ankle M65.87- ☑
  foot M65.87- ☑
  forearm M65.83- ☑
  hand M65.84- ☑
  lower leg M65.86- ☑
  multiple sites M65.89
  pelvic region M65.85- ☑
  shoulder region M65.81- ☑
  specified site NEC M65.88
  thigh M65.85- ☑
  upper arm M65.82- ☑
 tuberculous — *see* Tuberculosis, tenosynovitis
Tenovaginitis — *see* Tenosynovitis
Tension
 arterial, high — *see also* Hypertension
  without diagnosis of hypertension R03.0
 headache G44.209
  intractable G44.201
  not intractable G44.209
 nervous R45.0
 pneumothorax J93.0
 premenstrual N94.3
 state (mental) F48.9
Tentorium — *see* condition
Teratencephalus Q89.8
Teratism Q89.7
Teratoblastoma (malignant) — *see* Neoplasm, malignant, by site
Teratocarcinoma — *see also* Neoplasm, malignant, by site
 liver C22.7
Teratoma (solid) — *see also* Neoplasm, uncertain behavior, by site
 with embryonal carcinoma, mixed — *see* Neoplasm, malignant, by site
 with malignant transformation — *see* Neoplasm, malignant, by site
 adult (cystic) — *see* Neoplasm, benign, by site
 benign — *see* Neoplasm, benign, by site
 combined with choriocarcinoma — *see* Neoplasm, malignant, by site
 cystic (adult) — *see* Neoplasm, benign, by site
 differentiated — *see* Neoplasm, benign, by site
 embryonal — *see also* Neoplasm, malignant, by site
  liver C22.7
 immature — *see* Neoplasm, malignant, by site
  liver C22.7
  adult, benign, cystic, differentiated type or mature D13.4
 malignant — *see also* Neoplasm, malignant, by site
  anaplastic — *see* Neoplasm, malignant, by site
  intermediate — *see* Neoplasm, malignant, by site
   specified site — *see* Neoplasm, malignant, by site
   unspecified site C62.90
  undifferentiated — *see* Neoplasm, malignant, by site

Teratoma — *continued*
 mature — *see* Neoplasm, uncertain behavior, by site
  malignant — *see* Neoplasm, by site, malignant, by site
 ovary D27.- ☑
  embryonal, immature or malignant C56- ☑
 solid — *see* Neoplasm, uncertain behavior, by site
 testis C62.9- ☑
  adult, benign, cystic, differentiated type or mature D29.2- ☑
  scrotal C62.1- ☑
  undescended C62.0- ☑
Termination
 anomalous — *see also* Malposition, congenital
  right pulmonary vein Q26.3
 pregnancy, elective Z33.2
Ternidens diminutus infestation B81.8
Ternidensiasis B81.8
Terror(s) night (child) F51.4
Terrorism, victim of Z65.4
Terry's syndrome — *see also* Myopia, degenerative H44.2- ☑
Tertiary — *see* condition
Test, tests, testing (for)
 adequacy (for dialysis)
  hemodialysis Z49.31
  peritoneal Z49.32
 blood pressure Z01.30
  abnormal reading — *see* Blood, pressure
 blood typing Z01.83
  Rh typing Z01.83
 blood-alcohol Z02.83
  positive — *see* Findings, abnormal, in blood
 blood-drug Z02.83
  positive — *see* Findings, abnormal, in blood
 cardiac pulse generator (battery) Z45.010
 fertility Z31.41
 genetic
  disease carrier status for procreative management
   female Z31.430
   male Z31.440
  male partner of patient with recurrent pregnancy loss Z31.441
  procreative management NEC
   female Z31.438
   male Z31.448
 hearing Z01.10
  with abnormal findings NEC Z01.118
  infant or child (over 28 days old) Z00.129
   with abnormal findings Z00.121
 HIV (human immunodeficiency virus)
  nonconclusive (in infants) R75
  positive Z21
  seropositive Z21
 immunity status Z01.84
 intelligence NEC Z01.89
 laboratory (as part of a general medical examination) Z00.00
  with abnormal finding Z00.01
  for medicolegal reason NEC Z04.89
 male partner of patient with recurrent pregnancy loss Z31.441
 Mantoux (for tuberculosis) Z11.1
  abnormal result R76.11
 pregnancy, positive first pregnancy — *see* Pregnancy, normal, first
 procreative Z31.49
  fertility Z31.41
 skin, diagnostic
  allergy Z01.82
   special screening examination — *see* Screening, by name of disease
  Mantoux Z11.1
  tuberculin Z11.1
 specified NEC Z01.89
 tuberculin Z11.1
  abnormal result R76.11
 vision Z01.00
  with abnormal findings Z01.01
  following failed vision screening Z01.020
   with abnormal findings Z01.021
  infant or child (over 28 days old) Z00.129
   with abnormal findings Z00.121
 Wassermann Z11.3
  positive — *see* Serology for syphilis, positive
Testicle, testicular, testis — *see also* condition
 feminization syndrome — *see also* Syndrome, androgen insensitivity E34.51

☑ **Additional Character Required** — **Refer to the Tabular List for Character Selection**

Testicle, testicular, testis — *continued*
  migrans Q55.29
Tetanus, tetanic (cephalic) (convulsions) A35
  with
    abortion A34
    ectopic or molar pregnancy O08.0
  following ectopic or molar pregnancy O08.0
  inoculation reaction (due to serum) — *see* Complications, vaccination
  neonatorum A33
  obstetrical A34
  puerperal, postpartum, childbirth A34
Tetany (due to) R29.0
  alkalosis E87.3
  associated with rickets E55.0
  convulsions R29.0
    hysterical F44.5
  functional (hysterical) F44.5
  hyperkinetic R29.0
    hysterical F44.5
  hyperpnea R06.4
    hysterical F44.5
    psychogenic F45.8
  hyperventilation — *see also* Hyperventilation R06.4
    hysterical F44.5
  neonatal (without calcium or magnesium deficiency) P71.3
  parathyroid (gland) E20.9
  parathyroprival E89.2
  post- (para)thyroidectomy E89.2
  postoperative E89.2
  pseudotetany R29.0
  psychogenic (conversion reaction) F44.5
Tetralogy of Fallot Q21.3
Tetraplegia (chronic) — *see also* Quadriplegia G82.50
Thailand hemorrhagic fever A91
Thalassanemia — *see* Thalassemia
Thalassemia (anemia) (disease) D56.9
  with other hemoglobinopathy D56.8
  alpha (major) (severe) (triple gene defect) D56.0
    minor D56.3
    silent carrier D56.3
    trait D56.3
  beta (severe) D56.1
    homozygous D56.1
    major D56.1
    minor D56.3
    trait D56.3
  delta-beta (homozygous) D56.2
    minor D56.3
    trait D56.3
  dominant D56.8
  hemoglobin
    C D56.8
    E-beta D56.5
  intermedia D56.1
  major D56.1
  minor D56.3
  mixed D56.8
  sickle-cell — *see* Disease, sickle-cell, thalassemia
  specified type NEC D56.8
  trait D56.3
  variants D56.8
Thanatophoric dwarfism or short stature Q77.1
Thaysen-Gee disease (nontropical sprue) K90.0
Thaysen's disease K90.0
Thecoma D27- ☑
  luteinized D27- ☑
  malignant C56- ☑
Thelarche, premature E30.8
Thelaziasis B83.8
Thelitis N61.0
  puerperal, postpartum or gestational — *see* Infection, nipple
Therapeutic — *see* condition
Therapy
  drug, long-term (current) (prophylactic)
    agents affecting estrogen receptors and estrogen levels NEC Z79.818
    anastrozole (Arimidex) Z79.811
    antibiotics Z79.2
      short-term use — *omit code*
    anticoagulants Z79.01
    anti-inflammatory Z79.1
    antiplatelet Z79.02
    antithrombotics Z79.02
    aromatase inhibitors Z79.811
    aspirin Z79.82
    birth control pill or patch Z79.3

Therapy — *continued*
  drug, long-term — *continued*
    bisphosphonates Z79.83
    contraceptive, oral Z79.3
    drug, specified NEC Z79.899
    estrogen receptor downregulators Z79.818
    Evista Z79.810
    exemestane (Aromasin) Z79.811
    Fareston Z79.810
    fulvestrant (Faslodex) Z79.818
    gonadotropin-releasing hormone (GnRH) agonist Z79.818
    goserelin acetate (Zoladex) Z79.818
    hormone replacement Z79.890
    insulin Z79.4
    letrozole (Femara) Z79.811
    leuprolide acetate (leuprorelin) (Lupron) Z79.818
    megestrol acetate (Megace) Z79.818
    methadone
      for pain management Z79.891
      maintenance therapy F11.20
    Nolvadex Z79.810
    opiate analgesic Z79.891
    oral antidiabetic Z79.84
    oral contraceptive Z79.3
    oral hypoglycemic Z79.84
    raloxifene (Evista) Z79.810
    selective estrogen receptor modulators (SERMs) Z79.810
    short term — *omit code*
    steroids
      inhaled Z79.51
      systemic Z79.52
    tamoxifen (Nolvadex) Z79.810
    toremifene (Fareston) Z79.810
Thermic — *see* condition
Thermography (abnormal) — *see also* Abnormal, diagnostic imaging R93.89
  breast R92.8
Thermoplegia T67.01 ☑
Thesaurismosis, glycogen — *see* Disease, glycogen storage
Thiamin deficiency E51.9
  specified NEC E51.8
Thiaminic deficiency with beriberi E51.11
Thibierge-Weissenbach syndrome — *see* Sclerosis, systemic
Thickening
  bone — *see* Hypertrophy, bone
  breast N64.59
  endometrium R93.89
  epidermal L85.9
    specified NEC L85.8
  hymen N89.6
  larynx J38.7
  nail L60.2
    congenital Q84.5
  periosteal — *see* Hypertrophy, bone
  pleura J92.9
    with asbestos J92.0
  skin R23.4
  subepiglottic J38.7
  tongue K14.8
  valve, heart — *see* Endocarditis
Thigh — *see* condition
Thinning vertebra — *see* Spondylopathy, specified NEC
Thirst, excessive R63.1
  due to deprivation of water T73.1 ☑
Thomsen disease G71.12
Thoracic — *see also* condition
  kidney Q63.2
  outlet syndrome — *see also* Syndrome, thoracic outlet G54.0
Thoracogastroschisis (congenital) Q79.8
Thoracopagus Q89.4
Thorax — *see* condition
Thorn's syndrome N28.89
Thorson-Bjorck syndrome E34.09
Threadworm (infection) (infestation) B80
Threatened
  abortion O20.0
    with subsequent abort on O03.9
  abuse (harm)
    adult — *see* Maltreatment, adult, threatened abuse
    child — *see* Maltreatment, child, threatened abuse
  job loss, anxiety concerning Z56.2
  labor (without delivery) O47.9
    at or after 37 completed weeks of gestation O47.1
    before 37 completed weeks of gestation O47.0- ☑
  loss of job, anxiety concerning Z56.2

Threatened — *continued*
  miscarriage O20.0
  unemployment, anxiety concerning Z56.2
Three-day fever A93.1
Threshers' lung J67.0
Thrix annulata (congenital) Q84.1
Throat — *see* condition
Thrombasthenia (Glanzmann) (hemorrhagic) (hereditary) D69.1
Thromboangiitis I73.1
  obliterans (general) I73.1
    cerebral I67.89
    vessels
      brain I67.89
      spinal cord I67.89
Thromboarteritis — *see* Arteritis
Thromboasthenia (Glanzmann) (hemorrhagic) (hereditary) D69.1
Thrombocytasthenia (Glanzmann) D69.1
Thrombocythemia (hemorrhagic) *see also* Thrombocytosis D75.839
  essential D47.3
  idiopathic D47.3
  primary D47.3
Thrombocytopathy (dystrophic) (granulopenic) D69.1
Thrombocytopenia, thrombocytopenic D69.6
  with absent radius (TAR) Q87.2
  congenital D69.42
  dilutional D69.59
  due to
    (massive) blood transfusion D69.59
    drugs D69.59
    extracorporeal circulation of blood D69.59
    platelet alloimmunization D69.59
  essential D69.3
  heparin induced (HIT) D75.829
    delayed-onset D75.828
    immune-mediated D75.822
    non-immune D75.821
    persisting D75.828
    syndrome
      autoimmune D75.828
      specified NEC D75.828
      spontaneous (without heparin exposure) D75.84
    type 1 D75.821
    type 2 D75.822
  heparin-associated D75.821
  hereditary D69.42
  idiopathic D69.3
  neonatal, transitory P61.0
    due to
      exchange transfusion P61.0
      idiopathic maternal thrombocytopenia P61.0
      isoimmunization P61.0
  primary NEC D69.49
    idiopathic D69.3
  puerperal, postpartum O72.3
  secondary D69.59
  transient neonatal P61.0
  vaccine-induced thrombotic D75.84
Thrombocytosis D75.839
  essential D47.3
  idiopathic D47.3
  primary D47.3
  reactive D75.838
  secondary D75.838
  specified NEC D75.838
Thromboembolism — *see* Embolism
Thrombopathy (Bernard-Soulier) D69.1
  constitutional — *see* Disease, von Willebrand
  Willebrand-Jurgens — *see* Disease, von Willebrand
Thrombopenia — *see* Thrombocytopenia
Thrombophilia D68.59
  primary NEC D68.59
  secondary NEC D68.69
  specified NEC D68.69
Thrombophlebitis I80.9
  antepartum O22.2- ☑
    deep O22.3- ☑
    superficial O22.2- ☑
  calf muscular vein (NOS) I80.25- ☑
  cavernous (venous) sinus G08
    complicating pregnancy O22.5- ☑
    nonpyogenic I67.6
  cerebral (sinus) (vein) G08
    nonpyogenic I67.6
    sequelae G09

Thrombophlebitis — *continued*
  due to implanted device — *see* Complications, by site and type, specified NEC
  during or resulting from a procedure NEC T81.72 ☑
  femoral vein (superficial) I80.1- ☑
  femoropopliteal vein I80.0- ☑
  gastrocnemial vein I80.25- ☑
  hepatic (vein) I80.8
  idiopathic, recurrent I82.1
  iliac vein (common) (external) (internal) I80.21- ☑
  iliofemoral I80.1- ☑
  intracranial venous sinus (any) G08
    nonpyogenic I67.6
    sequelae G09
  intraspinal venous sinuses and veins G08
    nonpyogenic G95.19
  lateral (venous) sinus G08
    nonpyogenic I67.6
  leg I80.3
    superficial I80.0- ☑
  longitudinal (venous) sinus G08
    nonpyogenic I67.6
  lower extremity I80.299
  migrans, migrating I82.1
  pelvic
    with ectopic or molar pregnancy O08.0
    following ectopic or molar pregnancy O08.0
    puerperal O87.1
  peroneal vein I80.24- ☑
  popliteal vein — *see* Phlebitis, leg, deep, popliteal
  portal (vein) K75.1
  postoperative T81.72 ☑
  pregnancy — *see* Thrombophlebitis, antepartum
  puerperal, postpartum, childbirth O87.0
    deep O87.1
    pelvic O87.1
    septic O86.81
    superficial O87.0
  saphenous (greater) (lesser) I80.0- ☑
  sinus (intracranial) G08
    nonpyogenic I67.6
  soleal vein I80.25- ☑
  specified site NEC I80.8
  tibial vein (anterior) (posterior) I80.23- ☑

Thrombosis, thrombotic (bland) (multiple) (progressive) (silent) (vessel) I82.90
  anal K64.5
  antepartum — *see* Thrombophlebitis, antepartum
  aorta, aortic I74.10
    abdominal I74.09
      saddle I74.01
    bifurcation I74.09
    saddle I74.01
    specified site NEC I74.19
    terminal I74.09
    thoracic I74.11
    valve — *see* Endocarditis, aortic
  apoplexy I63.3- ☑
  artery, arteries (postinfectional) I74.9
    auditory, internal — *see* Occlusion, artery, precerebral, specified NEC
    basilar — *see* Occlusion, artery, basilar
    carotid (common) (internal) — *see* Occlusion, artery, carotid
    cerebellar (anterior inferior) (posterior inferior) (superior) — *see* Occlusion, artery, cerebellar
    cerebral — *see* Occlusion, artery, cerebral
    choroidal (anterior) — *see* Occlusion, artery, precerebral, specified NEC
    communicating, posterior — *see* Occlusion, artery, precerebral, specified NEC
    coronary — *see also* Infarct, myocardium
      not resulting in infarction I24.0
    hepatic I74.8
    hypophyseal — *see* Occlusion, artery, precerebral, specified NEC
    iliac I74.5
    limb I74.4
      lower I74.3
      upper I74.2
    meningeal, anterior or posterior — *see* Occlusion, artery, cerebral, specified NEC
    mesenteric (with gangrene) — *see also* Infarct, intestine K55.069
    ophthalmic — *see* Occlusion, artery, retina
    pontine — *see* Occlusion, artery, precerebral, specified NEC
    precerebral — *see* Occlusion, artery, precerebral

Thrombosis, thrombotic — *continued*
  artery, arteries — *continued*
    pulmonary (iatrogenic) — *see* Embolism, pulmonary
    renal N28.0
    retinal — *see* Occlusion, artery, retina
    spinal, anterior or posterior G95.11
    traumatic NEC T14.8 ☑
    vertebral — *see* Occlusion, artery, vertebral
  atrium, auricular — *see also* Infarct, myocardium
    following acute myocardial infarction (current complication) I23.6
    not resulting in infarction I51.3
    old I51.3
  basilar (artery) — *see* Occlusion, artery, basilar
  brain (artery) (stem) — *see also* Occlusion, artery, cerebral
    due to syphilis A52.05
    puerperal O99.43
    sinus — *see* Thrombosis, intracranial, venous sinus
  capillary I78.8
  cardiac — *see also* Infarct, myocardium
    not resulting in infarction I51.3
    old I51.3
    valve — *see* Endocarditis
  carotid (artery) (common) (internal) — *see* Occlusion, artery, carotid
  cavernous (venous) sinus — *see* Thrombosis, intracranial, venous sinus
  cerebellar artery (anterior inferior) (posterior inferior) (superior) I66.3
  cerebral (artery) — *see* Occlusion, artery, cerebral
  cerebrovenous sinus — *see also* Thrombosis, intracranial, venous sinus
    puerperium O87.3
  chronic I82.91
  coronary (artery) (vein) — *see also* Infarct, myocardium
    not resulting in infarction I24.0
  corpus cavernosum N48.89
  cortical I66.9
  deep — *see* Embolism, vein, lower extremity
  due to device, implant or graft — *see also* Complications, by site and type, specified NEC T85.868 ☑
    arterial graft NEC T82.868 ☑
    breast (implant) T85.868 ☑
    catheter NEC T85.868 ☑
      dialysis (renal) T82.868 ☑
        intraperitoneal T85.868 ☑
      infusion NEC T82.868 ☑
        spinal (epidural) (subdural) T85.860 ☑
      urinary (indwelling) T83.86 ☑
    electronic (electrode) (pulse generator) (stimulator)
      bone T84.86 ☑
      cardiac T82.867 ☑
      nervous system (brain) (peripheral nerve) (spinal) T85.860 ☑
      urinary T83.86 ☑
    fixation, internal (orthopedic) NEC T84.86 ☑
    gastrointestinal (bile duct) (esophagus) T85.868 ☑
    genital NEC T83.86 ☑
    heart T82.867 ☑
    joint prosthesis T84.86 ☑
    ocular (corneal graft) (orbital implant) NEC T85.868 ☑
    orthopedic NEC T84.86 ☑
    specified NEC T85.868 ☑
    urinary NEC T83.86 ☑
    vascular NEC T82.868 ☑
    ventricular intracranial shunt T85.860 ☑
  during the puerperium — *see* Thrombosis, puerperal
  endocardial — *see also* Infarct, myocardium
    not resulting in infarction I51.3
  eye — *see* Occlusion, retina
  genital organ
    female NEC N94.89
      pregnancy — *see* Thrombophlebitis, antepartum
    male N50.1
  gestational — *see* Phlebopathy, gestational
  heart (chamber) — *see also* Infarct, myocardium
    not resulting in infarction I51.3
    old I51.3
  hepatic (vein) I82.0
    artery I74.8
  history (of) Z86.718
  intestine (with gangrene) — *see also* Infarct, intestine K55.069
  intracardiac NEC (apical) (atrial) (auricular) (ventricular) (old) I51.3
  intracranial (arterial) I66.9
    venous sinus (any) G08
      nonpyogenic I67.6

Thrombosis, thrombotic — *continued*
  intracranial — *continued*
    venous sinus — *continued*
      nonpyogenic origin I67.6
      puerperium O87.3
  intramural — *see also* Infarct, myocardium
    not resulting in infarction I51.3
    old I51.3
  intraspinal venous sinuses and veins G08
    nonpyogenic G95.19
  kidney (artery) N28.0
  lateral (venous) sinus — *see* Thrombosis, intracranial, venous sinus
  leg — *see* Thrombosis, vein, lower extremity
    arterial I74.3
  liver (venous) I82.0
    artery I74.8
    portal vein I81
  longitudinal (venous) sinus — *see* Thrombosis, intracranial, venous sinus
  lower limb — *see* Thrombosis, vein, lower extremity
  lung (iatrogenic) (postoperative) — *see* Embolism, pulmonary
  meninges (brain) (arterial) I66.8
  mesenteric (artery) (with gangrene) — *see also* Infarct, intestine K55.069
    vein (inferior) (superior) K55.0- ☑
  mitral I34.89
  mural — *see also* Infarct, myocardium
    due to syphilis A52.06
    not resulting in infarction I51.3
    old I51.3
  omentum (with gangrene) — *see also* Infarct, intestine K55.069
  ophthalmic — *see* Occlusion, retina
  pampiniform plexus (male) N50.1
  parietal — *see also* Infarct, myocardium
    not resulting in infarction I24.0
  penis, superficial vein N48.81
  perianal venous K64.5
  peripheral arteries I74.4
    upper I74.2
  personal history (of) Z86.718
  portal I81
    due to syphilis A52.09
  precerebral artery — *see* Occlusion, artery, precerebral
  puerperal, postpartum O87.0
    brain (artery) O99.43
      venous (sinus) O87.3
    cardiac O99.43
    cerebral (artery) O99.43
      venous (sinus) O87.3
    superficial O87.0
  pulmonary (artery) (iatrogenic) (postoperative) (vein) — *see* Embolism, pulmonary
  renal (artery) N28.0
    vein I82.3
  resulting from presence of device, implant or graft — *see* Complications, by site and type, specified NEC
  retina, retinal — *see* Occlusion, retina
  scrotum N50.1
  seminal vesicle N50.1
  sigmoid (venous) sinus — *see* Thrombosis, intracranial, venous sinus
  sinus, intracranial (any) — *see* Thrombosis, intracranial, venous sinus
  specified site NEC I82.890
    chronic I82.891
  spermatic cord N50.1
  spinal cord (arterial) G95.11
    due to syphilis A52.09
    pyogenic origin G06.1
  spleen, splenic D73.5
    artery I74.8
  testis N50.1
  traumatic NEC T14.8 ☑
  tricuspid I07.8
  tumor — *see* Neoplasm, unspecified behavior, by site
  tunica vaginalis N50.1
  umbilical cord (vessels), complicating delivery O69.5 ☑
  vas deferens N50.1
  vein (acute) I82.90
    antecubital I82.61- ☑
      chronic I82.71- ☑
    axillary I82.A1- ☑ (*following* I82.7)
      chronic I82.A2- ☑ (*following* I82.7)
    basilic I82.61- ☑
      chronic I82.71- ☑

☑ **Additional Character Required** — **Refer to the Tabular List for Character Selection**

Thrombosis, thrombotic — *continued*
  vein — *continued*
    brachial I82.62- ☑
      chronic I82.72- ☑
    brachiocephalic (innominate) I82.290
      chronic I82.291
    calf muscular I82.46- ☑
      chronic I82.56- ☑
    cephalic I82.61- ☑
      chronic I82.71- ☑
    cerebral, nonpyogenic I67.6
    chronic I82.91
    deep (DVT) I82.40- ☑
      calf I82.4Z- ☑
        chronic I82.5Z- ☑
      lower leg I82.4Z- ☑
        chronic I82.5Z- ☑
      thigh I82.4Y- ☑
        chronic I82.5Y- ☑
      upper leg I82.4Y- ☑
        chronic I82.5Y- ☑
    femoral I82.41- ☑
      chronic I82.51- ☑
    iliac (iliofemoral) I82.42- ☑
      chronic I82.52- ☑
    innominate I82.290
      chronic I82.291
    internal jugular I82.C1- ☑ (*following* I82.7)
      chronic I82.C2- ☑ (*following* I82.7)
    lower extremity
      deep I82.40- ☑
        chronic I82.50- ☑
        specified NEC I82.49- ☑
          chronic NEC I82.59- ☑
      distal
        deep I82.4Z- ☑
      proximal
        deep I82.4Y- ☑
          chronic I82.5Y- ☑
      superficial I82.81- ☑
    perianal K64.5
    peroneal I82.45- ☑
      chronic I82.55- ☑
    popliteal I82.43- ☑
      chronic I82.53- ☑
    radial I82.62- ☑
      chronic I82.72- ☑
    renal I82.3
    saphenous (greater) (lesser) I82.81- ☑
    specified NEC I82.890
      chronic NEC I82.891
    subclavian I82.B1- ☑ (*following* I82.7)
      chronic I82.B2- ☑ (*following* I82.7)
    thoracic NEC I82.290
      chronic I82.291
    tibial I82.44- ☑
      chronic I82.54- ☑
    ulnar I82.62- ☑
      chronic I82.72- ☑
    upper extremity I82.60- ☑
      chronic I82.70- ☑
      deep I82.62- ☑
        chronic I82.72- ☑
      superficial I82.61- ☑
        chronic I82.71- ☑
  vena cava
    inferior I82.220
      chronic I82.221
    superior I82.210
      chronic I82.211
  venous, perianal K64.5
  ventricle — *see also* Infarct, myocardium
    following acute myocardial infarction (current complication) I23.6
    not resulting in infarction I24.0
    old I51.3
Thrombus — *see* Thrombosis
Thrush — *see also* Candidiasis
  newborn P37.5
  oral B37.0
  vaginal (acute) B37.31
    chronic (recurrent) B37.32
Thumb — *see also* condition
  sucking (child problem) F98.8
Thymitis E32.8
Thymoma — *see also* Neoplasm, thymus, by type

Thymoma — *continued*
  malignant C37
  metaplastic C37
  microscopic D15.0
  sclerosing C37
  type A C37
  type AB C37
  type B1 C37
  type B2 C37
  type B3 C37
Thymus, thymic (gland) — *see* condition
Thyrocele — *see* Goiter
Thyroglossal — *see also* condition
  cyst Q89.2
  duct, persistent Q89.2
Thyroid (gland) (body) — *see also* condition
  hormone resistance E07.89
  lingual Q89.2
  nodule (cystic) (nontoxic) (single) E04.1
Thyroiditis E06.9
  acute (nonsuppurative) (pyogenic) (suppurative) E06.0
  autoimmune E06.3
  chronic (nonspecific) (sclerosing) E06.5
    with thyrotoxicosis, transient E06.2
    fibrous E06.5
    lymphadenoid E06.3
    lymphocytic E06.3
    lymphoid E06.3
  de Quervain's E06.1
  drug-induced E06.4
  fibrous (chronic) E06.5
  giant-cell (follicular) E06.1
  granulomatous (de Quervain) (subacute) E06.1
  Hashimoto's (struma lymphomatosa) E06.3
  iatrogenic E06.4
  ligneous E06.5
  lymphocytic (chronic) E06.3
  lymphoid E06.3
  lymphomatous E06.3
  nonsuppurative E06.1
  postpartum, puerperal O90.5
  pseudotuberculous E06.1
  pyogenic E06.0
  radiation E06.4
  Riedel's E06.5
  subacute (granulomatous) E06.1
  suppurative E06.0
  tuberculous A18.81
  viral E06.1
  woody E06.5
Thyrolingual duct, persistent Q89.2
Thyromegaly E01.0
Thyrotoxic
  crisis — *see* Thyrotoxicosis
  heart disease or failure — *see also* Thyrotoxicosis E05.90 [143]
    with thyroid storm E05.91 [143]
  storm — *see* Thyrotoxicosis
Thyrotoxicosis (recurrent) E05.90
  with
    goiter (diffuse) E05.00
      with thyroid storm E05.01
      adenomatous uninodular E05.10
        with thyroid storm E05.11
      multinodular E05.20
        with thyroid storm E05.21
      nodular E05.20
        with thyroid storm E05.21
      uninodular E05.10
        with thyroid storm E05.11
    infiltrative
      dermopathy E05.00
        with thyroid storm E05.01
      ophthalmopathy E05.00
        with thyroid storm E05.01
    single thyroid nodule E05.10
      with thyroid storm E05.11
    thyroid storm E05.91
  due to
    ectopic thyroid nodule or tissue E05.30
      with thyroid storm E05.31
    ingestion of (excessive) thyroid material E05.40
      with thyroid storm E05.41
    overproduction of thyroid-stimulating hormone E05.80
      with thyroid storm E05.81
    specified cause NEC E05.80
      with thyroid storm E05.81
  factitia E05.40

Thyrotoxicosis — *continued*
  factitia — *continued*
    with thyroid storm E05.41
  heart — *see also* Failure, heart, high-output E05.90 [143]
    with thyroid storm — *see also* Failure, heart, high-output E05.91 [143]
    failure — *see also* Failure, heart, high-output E05.90 [143]
  neonatal (transient) P72.1
  transient with chronic thyroiditis E06.2
Tibia vara M92.51- ☑
Tic (disorder) F95.9
  breathing F95.8
  child problem F95.9
  compulsive F95.1
  de la Tourette F95.2
  degenerative (generalized) (localized) G25.69
    facial G25.69
  disorder
    chronic
      motor F95.1
      vocal F95.1
    combined vocal and multiple motor F95.2
    transient F95.0
  douloureux G50.0
    atypical G50.1
    postherpetic, postzoster B02.22
  drug-induced G25.61
  eyelid F95.8
  habit F95.9
    chronic F95.1
    transient of childhood F95.0
  lid, transient of childhood F95.0
  motor-verbal F95.2
  occupational F48.8
  orbicularis F95.8
    transient of childhood F95.0
  organic origin G25.69
  postchoreic G25.69
  provisional F95.0
  psychogenic, compulsive F95.1
  salaam R25.8
  spasm (motor or vocal) F95.9
    chronic F95.1
    transient of childhood F95.0
  specified NEC F95.8
Tick-borne — *see* condition
Tietze's disease or syndrome M94.0
Tight, tightness
  anus K62.89
  chest R07.89
  fascia (lata) M62.89
  foreskin (congenital) N47.1
  hymen, hymenal ring N89.6
  introitus (acquired) (congenital) N89.6
  rectal sphincter K62.89
  tendon — *see* Short, tendon
  urethral sphincter N35.919
Tilting vertebra — *see* Dorsopathy, deforming, specified NEC
Timidity, child F93.8
Tinea (intersecta) (tarsi) B35.9
  amiantacea L44.8
  asbestina B35.0
  barbae B35.0
  beard B35.0
  black dot B35.0
  blanca B36.2
  capitis B35.0
  corporis B35.4
  cruris B35.6
  flava B36.0
  foot B35.3
  furfuracea B36.0
  imbricata (Tokelau) B35.5
  kerion B35.0
  manuum B35.2
  microsporic — *see* Dermatophytosis
  nigra B36.1
  nodosa — *see* Piedra
  pedis B35.3
  scalp B35.0
  specified NEC B35.8
  sycosis B35.0
  tonsurans B35.0
  trichophytic — *see* Dermatophytosis
  unguium B35.1
  versicolor B36.0
Tingling sensation (skin) R20.2

Tin-miner's lung J63.5
Tinnitus NOS H93.1- ☑
  audible H93.1- ☑
  aurium H93.1- ☑
  pulsatile H93.A- ☑
  subjective H93.1- ☑
Tipped tooth (teeth) M26.33
Tipping
  pelvis M95.5
    with disproportion (fetopelvic) O33.0
      causing obstructed labor O65.0
  tooth (teeth), fully erupted M26.33
Tiredness R53.83
Tissue — see condition
Tobacco (nicotine)
  abuse — see Tobacco, use
  dependence — see Dependence, drug, nicotine
  harmful use Z72.0
  heart — see Tobacco, toxic effect
  maternal use, affecting newborn P04.2
  toxic effect — see Table of Drugs and Chemicals, by
      substance, poisoning
    chewing tobacco — see Table of Drugs and Chemicals,
        by substance, poisoning
    cigarettes — see Table of Drugs and Chemicals, by
        substance, poisoning
  use Z72.0
    complicating
      childbirth O99.334
      pregnancy O99.33- ☑
      puerperium O99.335
    counseling and surveillance Z71.6
    history Z87.891
  withdrawal state — see also Dependence, drug, nicotine
      F17.203
Tocopherol deficiency E56.0
Todd's
  cirrhosis K74.3
  paralysis (postepileptic) (transitory) G83.84
Toe — see condition
Toilet, artificial opening — see Attention to, artificial,
    opening
Tokelau (ringworm) B35.5
Tollwut — see Rabies
Tommaselli's disease R31.9
  correct substance properly administered — see Table of
      Drugs and Chemicals, by drug, adverse effect
  overdose or wrong substance given or taken — see Table
      of Drugs and Chemicals, by drug, poisoning
Tongue — see also condition
  tie Q38.1
Tonic pupil — see Anomaly, pupil, function, tonic pupil
Toni-Fanconi syndrome (cystinosis) E72.09
  with cystinosis E72.04
Tonsil — see condition
Tonsillitis (acute) (catarrhal) (croupous) (follicular) (gan-
    grenous) (infective) (lacunar) (lingual) (malignant)
    (membranous) (parenchymatous) (phlegmonous)
    (pseudomembranous) (purulent) (septic) (subacute)
    (suppurative) (toxic) (ulcerative) (vesicular) (viral)
    J03.90
  chronic J35.01
    with adenoiditis J35.03
  diphtheritic A36.0
  hypertrophic J35.01
    with adenoiditis J35.03
  recurrent J03.91
  specified organism NEC J03.80
    recurrent J03.81
  staphylococcal J03.80
    recurrent J03.81
  streptococcal J03.00
    recurrent J03.01
  tuberculous A15.8
  Vincent's A69.1
Tooth, teeth — see condition
Toothache K08.89
Topagnosis R20.8
Tophi — see Gout, chronic
TORCH infection — see Infection, congenital
  without active infection P00.2
Torn — see Tear
Tornwaldt's cyst or disease J39.2
Torsades de pointes I47.21
Torsion
  accessory tube — see Torsion, fallopian tube
  adnexa (female) — see Torsion, fallopian tube
  aorta, acquired I77.1

Torsion — continued
  appendix epididymis N44.04
  appendix testis N44.03
  bile duct (common) (hepatic) K83.8
    congenital Q44.5
  bowel, colon or intestine K56.2
  cervix — see Malposition, uterus
  cystic duct K82.8
  dystonia — see Dystonia, torsion
  epididymis (appendix) N44.04
  fallopian tube N83.52- ☑
    with ovary N83.53
  gallbladder K82.8
    congenital Q44.1
  hydatid of Morgagni
    female N83.52- ☑
    male N44.03
  kidney (pedicle) (leading to infarction) N28.0
  Meckel's diverticulum (congenital) Q43.0
    malignant — see Table of Neoplasms, small intestine,
        malignant
  mesentery K56.2
  omentum K56.2
  organ or site, congenital NEC — see Anomaly, by site
  ovary (pedicle) N83.51- ☑
    with fallopian tube N83.53
    congenital Q50.2
  oviduct — see Torsion, fallopian tube
  penis (acquired) N48.82
    congenital Q55.63
  spasm — see Dystonia, torsion
  spermatic cord N44.02
    extravaginal N44.01
    intravaginal N44.02
  spleen D73.5
  testis, testicle N44.00
    appendix N44.03
  tibia — see Deformity, limb, specified type NEC, lower
      leg
  uterus — see Malposition, uterus
Torticollis (intermittent) (spastic) M43.6
  congenital (sternomastoid) Q68.0
  due to birth injury P15.8
  hysterical F44.4
  ocular R29.891
  psychogenic F45.8
    conversion reaction F44.4
  rheumatic M43.6
  rheumatoid M06.88
  spasmodic G24.3
  traumatic, current S13.4 ☑
Tortipelvis G24.1
Tortuous
  aortic arch Q25.46
  artery I77.1
  organ or site, congenital NEC — see Distortion
  retinal vessel, congenital Q14.1
  ureter N13.8
  urethra N36.8
  vein — see Varix
Torture, victim of Z65.4
Torula, torular (histolytica) (infection) — see Cryptococcosis
Torulosis — see Cryptococcosis
Torus (mandibularis) (palatinus) M27.0
  fracture — see Fracture, by site, torus
Touraine's syndrome Q79.8
Tourette's syndrome F95.2
Tourniquet syndrome — see Constriction, external, by site
Tower skull Q75.009
  with exophthalmos Q87.0
Toxemia R68.89
  bacterial — see Sepsis
  burn — see Burn
  eclamptic (with pre-existing hypertension) — see
      Eclampsia
  erysipelatous — see Erysipelas
  fatigue R68.89
  food — see Poisoning, food
  gastrointestinal K52.1
  intestinal K52.1
  kidney — see Uremia
  malarial — see Malaria
  myocardial — see Myocarditis, toxic
  of pregnancy — see Pre-eclampsia
  pre-eclamptic — see Pre-eclampsia
  small intestine K52.1
  staphylococcal, due to food A05.0
  stasis R68.89
  uremic — see Uremia

Toxemia — continued
  urinary — see Uremia
Toxemica cerebropathia psychica (nonalcoholic) F04
  alcoholic — see Alcohol, amnestic disorder
Toxic (poisoning) — see also condition T65.91 ☑
  effect — see Table of Drugs and Chemicals, by substance,
      poisoning
  shock syndrome A48.3
  thyroid (gland) — see Thyrotoxicosis
Toxicemia — see Toxemia
Toxicity — see Table of Drugs and Chemicals, by substance,
      poisoning
  fava bean D55.0
  food, noxious — see Poisoning, food
  from drug or nonmedicinal substance — see Table of
      Drugs and Chemicals, by drug
Toxicosis — see also Toxemia
  capillary, hemorrhagic D69.0
Toxinfection, gastrointestinal K52.1
Toxocariasis B83.0
Toxoplasma, toxoplasmosis (acquired) B58.9
  with
    hepatitis B58.1
    meningoencephalitis B58.2
    ocular involvement B58.00
    other organ involvement B58.89
    pneumonia, pneumonitis B58.3
  congenital (acute) (subacute) (chronic) P37.1
  maternal, manifest toxoplasmosis in infant (acute) (sub-
      acute) (chronic) P37.1
tPA (rtPA) **administration in a different facility within the
    last 24 hours prior to admission to current facility**
    Z92.82
Trabeculation, bladder N32.89
Trachea — see condition
Tracheitis (catarrhal) (infantile) (membranous) (plastic)
    (septal) (suppurative) (viral) J04.10
  with
    bronchitis (15 years of age and above) J40
      acute or subacute — see Bronchitis, acute
      chronic J42
      tuberculous NEC A15.5
      under 15 years of age J20.9
    laryngitis (acute) J04.2
      chronic J37.1
      tuberculous NEC A15.5
  acute J04.10
    with obstruction J04.11
  chronic J42
    with
      bronchitis (chronic) J42
      laryngitis (chronic) J37.1
  diphtheritic (membranous) A36.89
  due to external agent — see Inflammation, respiratory,
      upper, due to
  syphilitic A52.73
  tuberculous A15.5
Trachelitis (nonvenereal) — see Cervicitis
Tracheobronchial — see condition
Tracheobronchitis (15 years of age and above) — see also
    Bronchitis
  due to
    Bordetella bronchiseptica A37.80
      with pneumonia A37.81
    Francisella tularensis A21.8
Tracheobronchomegaly Q32.4
  with bronchiectasis J47.9
    with
      exacerbation (acute) J47.1
      lower respiratory infection J47.0
  acquired J98.09
    with bronchiectasis J47.9
      with
        exacerbation (acute) J47.1
        lower respiratory infection J47.0
Tracheobronchopneumonitis — see Pneumonia, broncho-
Tracheocele (external) (internal) J39.8
  congenital Q32.1
Tracheomalacia J39.8
  congenital Q32.0
Tracheopharyngitis (acute) J06.9
  chronic J42
  due to external agent — see Inflammation, respiratory,
      upper, due to
Tracheostenosis J39.8
Tracheostomy
  complication — see Complication, tracheostomy
  status Z93.0
    attention to Z43.0

Tracheostomy — *continued*
  status — *continued*
    malfunctioning J95.03
Trachoma, trachomatous A71.9
  active (stage) A71.1
  contraction of conjunctiva A71.1
  dubium A71.0
  healed or sequelae B94.0
  initial (stage) A71.0
  pannus A71.1
  Türck's J37.0
Traction, vitreomacular H43.82- ☑
Train sickness T75.3 ☑
Trait(s)
  Hb-S D57.3
  hemoglobin
    abnormal NEC D58.2
      with thalassemia D56.3
    C — *see* Disease, hemoglobin C
    S (Hb-S) D57.3
  Lepore D56.3
  personality, accentuated Z73.1
  sickle-cell D57.3
    with elliptocytosis or spherocytosis D57.3
  type A personality Z73.1
Tramp Z59.00
Trance R41.89
  hysterical F44.89
Transaminasemia R74.01
Transection
  abdomen (partial) S38.3 ☑
  aorta (incomplete) — *see also* Injury, aorta
    complete — *see* Injury, aorta, laceration, major
  carotid artery (incomplete) — *see also* Injury, blood vessel, carotid, laceration
    complete — *see* Injury, blood vessel, carotid, laceration, major
  celiac artery (incomplete) S35.211 ☑
    branch (incomplete) S35.291 ☑
      complete S35.292 ☑
    complete S35.212 ☑
  innominate
    artery (incomplete) — *see also* Injury, blood vessel, thoracic, innominate, artery, laceration
      complete — *see* Injury, blood vessel, thoracic, innominate, artery, laceration, major
    vein (incomplete) — *see also* Injury, blood vessel, thoracic, innominate, vein, laceration
      complete — *see* Injury, blood vessel, thoracic, innominate, vein, laceration, major
  jugular vein (external) (incomplete) — *see also* Injury, blood vessel, jugular vein, laceration
    complete — *see* Injury, blood vessel, jugular vein, laceration, major
    internal (incomplete) — *see also* Injury, blood vessel, jugular vein, internal, laceration
      complete — *see* Injury, blood vessel, jugular vein, internal, laceration, major
  mesenteric artery (incomplete) — *see also* Injury, mesenteric, artery, laceration
    complete — *see* Injury, mesenteric artery, laceration, major
  pulmonary vessel (incomplete) — *see also* Injury, blood vessel, thoracic, pulmonary, laceration
    complete — *see* Injury, blood vessel, thoracic, pulmonary, laceration, major
  subclavian — *see* Transection, innominate
  vena cava (incomplete) — *see also* Injury, vena cava
    complete — *see* Injury, vena cava, laceration, major
  vertebral artery (incomplete) — *see also* Injury, blood vessel, vertebral, laceration
    complete — *see* Injury, blood vessel, vertebral, laceration, major
Transfusion
  associated (red blood cell) hemochromatosis E83.111
  blood
    ABO incompatible — *see* Complication(s), transfusion, incompatibility reaction, ABO
    minor blood group (Duffy) (E) (K) (Kell) (Kidd) (Lewis) (M) (N) (P) (S) T80.89 ☑
    reaction or complication — *see* Complications, transfusion
  fetomaternal (mother) — *see* Pregnancy, complicated by, placenta, transfusion syndrome
  maternofetal (mother) — *see* Pregnancy, complicated by, placenta, transfusion syndrome
  placental (syndrome) (mother) — *see* Pregnancy, complicated by, placenta, transfusion syndrome

Transfusion — *continued*
  reaction (adverse) — *see* Complications, transfusion
  related acute lung injury (TRALI) J95.84
  twin-to-twin — *see* Pregnancy, complicated by, placenta, transfusion syndrome, fetus to fetus
Transgender F64.0
Transient (meaning homeless) — *see also* condition Z59.00
Translocation
  balanced autosomal Q95.9
    in normal individual Q95.0
  chromosomes NEC Q99.8
    balanced and insertion in normal individual Q95.0
  Down syndrome Q90.2
  trisomy
    13 Q91.6
    18 Q91.2
    21 Q90.2
Translucency, iris — *see* Degeneration, iris
Transmission of chemical substances through the placenta — *see* Absorption, chemical, through placenta
Transparency, lung, unilateral J43.0
Transplant (ed) (status) Z94.9
  awaiting organ Z76.82
  bone Z94.6
    marrow Z94.81
  candidate Z76.82
  complication — *see* Complication, transplant
  cornea Z94.7
  heart Z94.1
    and lung(s) Z94.3
    valve Z95.2
      prosthetic Z95.2
      specified NEC Z95.4
      xenogenic Z95.3
  intestine Z94.82
  kidney Z94.0
  liver Z94.4
  lung(s) Z94.2
    and heart Z94.3
  organ (failure) (infection) (rejection) Z94.9
    removal status Z98.85
  pancreas Z94.83
  skin Z94.5
  social Z60.3
  specified organ or tissue NEC Z94.89
  stem cells Z94.84
  tissue Z94.9
Transplants, ovarian, endometrial N80.10- ☑
Transposed — *see* Transposition
Transposition (congenital) — *see also* Malposition, congenital
  abdominal viscera Q89.3
  aorta (dextra) Q20.3
  appendix Q43.8
  colon Q43.8
  corrected Q20.5
  great vessels (complete) (partial) Q20.3
  heart Q24.0
    with complete transposition of viscera Q89.3
  intestine (large) (small) Q43.8
  reversed jejunal (for bypass) (status) Z98.0
  scrotum Q55.23
  stomach Q40.2
    with general transposition of viscera Q89.3
  tooth, teeth, fully erupted M26.30
  vessels, great (complete) (partial) Q20.3
  viscera (abdominal) (thoracic) Q89.3
Transsexualism F64.0
Transverse — *see also* condition
  arrest (deep), in labor O64.0 ☑
  lie (mother) O32.2 ☑
    causing obstructed labor O64.8 ☑
Transvestism, transvestitism (dual-role) F64.1
  fetishistic F65.1
Trapped placenta (with hemorrhage) O72.0
  without hemorrhage O73.0
TRAPS (tumor necrosis factor receptor associated periodic syndrome) M04.1
Trauma, traumatism — *see also* Injury
  acoustic — *see* subcategory H83.3 ☑
  birth — *see* Birth, injury
  complicating ectopic or molar pregnancy O08.6
  during delivery O71.9
  following ectopic or molar pregnancy O08.6
  non-accidental — *see* Abuse, physical
  obstetric O71.9
    specified NEC O71.89

Trauma, traumatism — *continued*
  occusal
    primary K08.81
    secondary K08.82
Traumatic — *see also* condition
  brain injury S06.9 ☑
Treacher Collins syndrome Q75.4
Treitz's hernia — *see* Hernia, abdomen, specified site NEC
Trematode infestation — *see* Infestation, fluke
Trematodiasis — *see* Infestation, fluke
Trembling paralysis — *see* Parkinsonism
Tremor(s) R25.1
  drug induced G25.1
  essential (benign) G25.0
  familial G25.0
  hereditary G25.0
  hysterical F44.4
  intention G25.2
  medication induced postural G25.1
  mercurial — *see* subcategory T56.1 ☑
  Parkinson's — *see* Parkinsonism
  psychogenic (conversion reaction) F44.4
  senilis R54
  specified type NEC G25.2
Trench
  fever A79.0
  foot — *see* Immersion, foot
  mouth A69.1
Treponema pallidum infection — *see* Syphilis
Treponematosis
  due to
    T. pallidum — *see* Syphilis
    T. pertenue — *see* Yaws
Triad
  Hutchinson's (congenital syphilis) A50.53
  Kartagener's Q89.3
  Saint's — *see* Hernia, diaphragm
Trichiasis (eyelid) H02.059
  with entropion — *see* Entropion
  left H02.056
    lower H02.055
    upper H02.054
  right H02.053
    lower H02.052
    upper H02.051
Trichinella spiralis (infection) (infestation) B75
Trichinellosis, trichiniasis, trichinelliasis, trichinosis B75
  with muscle disorder B75 *[M63.80]*
    ankle B75 *[M63.87-]* ☑
    foot B75 *[M63.87-]* ☑
    forearm B75 *[M63.83-]* ☑
    hand B75 *[M63.84-]* ☑
    lower leg B75 *[M63.86-]* ☑
    multiple sites B75 *[M63.89]*
    pelvic region B75 *[M63.85-]* ☑
    shoulder region B75 *[M63.81-]* ☑
    specified site NEC B75 *[M63.88]*
    thigh B75 *[M63.85-]* ☑
    upper arm B75 *[M63.82-]* ☑
Trichobezoar T18.9 ☑
  intestine T18.3 ☑
  stomach T18.2 ☑
Trichocephaliasis, trichocephalosis B79
Trichocephalus infestation B79
Trichoclasis L67.8
Trichoepithelioma — *see also* Neoplasm, skin, benign
  malignant — *see* Neoplasm, skin, malignant
Trichofolliculoma — *see* Neoplasm, skin, benign
Tricholemmoma — *see* Neoplasm, skin, benign
Trichomoniasis A59.9
  bladder A59.03
  cervix A59.09
  intestinal A07.8
  prostate A59.02
  seminal vesicles A59.09
  specified site NEC A59.8
  urethra A59.03
  urogenitalis A59.00
  vagina A59.01
  vulva A59.01
Trichomycosis
  axillaris A48.8
  nodosa, nodularis B36.8
Trichonodosis L67.8
Trichophytid, trichophyton infection — *see* Dermatophytosis
Trichophytobezoar T18.9 ☑
  intestine T18.3 ☑

Trichophytobezoar — *continued*
  stomach T18.2 ☑
Trichophytosis — *see* Dermatophytosis
Trichoptilosis L67.8
Trichorrhexis (nodosa) (invaginata) L67.0
Trichosis axillaris A48.8
Trichosporosis nodosa B36.2
Trichostasis spinulosa (congenital) Q84.1
Trichostrongyliasis, trichostrongylosis (small intestine) B81.2
Trichostrongylus infection B81.2
Trichotillomania F63.3
Trichromat, trichromatopsia, anomalous (congenital) H53.55
Trichuriasis B79
Trichuris trichiura (infection) (infestation) (any site) B79
Tricuspid (valve) — *see* condition
Trifid — *see also* Accessory
  kidney (pelvis) Q63.8
  tongue Q38.3
Trigeminal neuralgia — *see* Neuralgia, trigeminal
Trigeminy R00.8
Trigger finger (acquired) M65.30
  congenital Q74.0
  index finger M65.32- ☑
  little finger M65.35- ☑
  middle finger M65.33- ☑
  ring finger M65.34- ☑
  thumb M65.31- ☑
Trigonitis (bladder) (chronic) (pseudomembranous) N30.30
  with hematuria N30.31
Trigonocephaly Q75.03
Trilocular heart — *see* Cor triloculare
Trimethylaminuria E72.52
Tripartite placenta O43.19- ☑
Triphalangeal thumb Q74.0
Triple — *see also* Accessory
  kidneys Q63.0
  negative breast cancer (TNBC) Z17.421
  uteri Q51.818
  X, female Q97.0
Triple I O41.12- ☑
Triplegia G83.89
  congenital G80.8
Triplet (newborn) — *see also* Newborn, triplet
  complicating pregnancy — *see* Pregnancy, triplet
Triplication — *see* Accessory
Triploidy Q92.7
Trismus R25.2
  neonatorum A33
  newborn A33
Trisomy (syndrome) Q92.9
  13 (partial) Q91.7
    meiotic nondisjunction Q91.4
    mitotic nondisjunction Q91.5
    mosaicism Q91.5
    translocation Q91.6
  18 (partial) Q91.3
    meiotic nondisjunction Q91.0
    mitotic nondisjunction Q91.1
    mosaicism Q91.1
    translocation Q91.2
  20 Q92.8
  21 (partial) Q90.9
    meiotic nondisjunction Q90.0
    mitotic nondisjunction Q90.1
    mosaicism Q90.1
    translocation Q90.2
  22 Q92.8
  autosomes Q92.9
  chromosome specified NEC Q92.8
    partial Q92.2
      due to unbalanced translocation Q92.5
    specified NEC Q92.8
    whole (nonsex chromosome)
      meiotic nondisjunction Q92.0
      mitotic nondisjunction Q92.1
      mosaicism Q92.1
  due to
    dicentrics — *see* Extra, marker chromosomes
    extra rings — *see* Extra, marker chromosomes
    isochromosomes — *see* Extra, marker chromosomes
  specified NEC Q92.8
  whole chromosome Q92.9
    meiotic nondisjunction Q92.0
    mitotic nondisjunction Q92.1
    mosaicism Q92.1
    partial Q92.9

Trisomy — *continued*
  whole chromosome — *continued*
    specified NEC Q92.8
Tritanomaly, tritanopia H53.55
Trombiculosis, trombiculiasis, trombidiosis B88.0
Trophedema (congenital) (hereditary) Q82.0
Trophoblastic disease — *see also* Mole, hydatidiform O01.9
Tropholymphedema Q82.0
Trophoneurosis NEC G96.89
  disseminated M34.9
Tropical — *see* condition
Trouble — *see also* Disease
  heart — *see* Disease, heart
  kidney — *see* Disease, renal
  nervous R45.0
  sinus — *see* Sinusitis
Trousseau's syndrome (thrombophlebitis migrans) I82.1
Truancy, childhood
  from school Z72.810
Truncus
  arteriosus (persistent) Q20.0
  communis Q20.0
Trunk — *see* condition
Trypanosomiasis
  African B56.9
    by Trypanosoma brucei
      gambiense B56.0
      rhodesiense B56.1
  American — *see* Chagas' disease
  Brazilian — *see* Chagas' disease
  by Trypanosoma
    brucei gambiense B56.0
    brucei rhodesiense B56.1
    cruzi — *see* Chagas' disease
  gambiensis, Gambian B56.0
  rhodesiensis, Rhodesian B56.1
  South American — *see* Chagas' disease
  where
    African trypanosomiasis is prevalent B56.9
    Chagas' disease is prevalent B57.2
Tryptasemia, hereditary alpha D89.44
T-shaped incisors K00.2
Tsutsugamushi (disease) (fever) A75.3
Tube, tubal, tubular — *see* condition
Tubercle — *see also* Tuberculosis
  brain, solitary A17.81
  Darwin's Q17.8
  Ghon, primary infection A15.7
Tuberculid, tuberculide (indurating, subcutaneous) (lichenoid) (miliary) (papulonecrotic) (primary) (skin) A18.4
Tuberculoma — *see also* Tuberculosis
  brain A17.81
  meninges (cerebral) (spinal) A17.1
  spinal cord A17.81
Tuberculosis, tubercular, tuberculous (calcification) (calcified) (caseous) (chromogenic acid-fast bacilli) (degeneration) (fibrocaseous) (fistula) (interstitial) (isolated circumscribed lesions) (necrosis) (parenchymatous) (ulcerative) A15.9
  with pneumoconiosis (any condition in J60-J64) J65
  abdomen (lymph gland) A18.39
  abscess (respiratory) A15.9
    bone A18.03
      hip A18.02
      knee A18.02
      sacrum A18.01
      specified site NEC A18.03
      spinal A18.01
      vertebra A18.01
    brain A17.81
    breast A18.89
    Cowper's gland A18.15
    dura (mater) (cerebral) (spinal) A17.81
    epidural (cerebral) (spinal) A17.81
    female pelvis A18.17
    frontal sinus A15.8
    genital organs NEC A18.10
    genitourinary A18.10
    gland (lymphatic) — *see* Tuberculosis, lymph gland
    hip A18.02
    intestine A18.32
    ischiorectal A18.32
    joint NEC A18.02
      hip A18.02
      knee A18.02
      specified NEC A18.02
      vertebral A18.01
    kidney A18.11

Tuberculosis, tubercular, tuberculous — *continued*
  abscess — *continued*
    knee A18.02
    latent Z22.7
    lumbar (spine) A18.01
    lung — *see* Tuberculosis, pulmonary
    meninges (cerebral) (spinal) A17.0
    muscle A18.09
    perianal (fistula) A18.32
    perinephritic A18.11
    perirectal A18.32
    rectum A18.32
    retropharyngeal A15.8
    sacrum A18.01
    scrofulous A18.2
    scrotum A18.15
    skin (primary) A18.4
    spinal cord A17.81
    spine or vertebra (column) A18.01
    subdiaphragmatic A18.31
    testis A18.15
    urinary A18.13
    uterus A18.17
  accessory sinus — *see* Tuberculosis, sinus
  Addison's disease A18.7
  adenitis — *see* Tuberculosis, lymph gland
  adenoids A15.8
  adenopathy — *see* Tuberculosis, lymph gland
  adherent pericardium A18.84
  adnexa (uteri) A18.17
  adrenal (capsule) (gland) A18.7
  alimentary canal A18.32
  anemia A18.89
  ankle (joint) (bone) A18.02
  anus A18.32
  apex, apical — *see* Tuberculosis, pulmonary
  appendicitis, appendix A18.32
  arachnoid A17.0
  artery, arteritis A18.89
    cerebral A18.89
  arthritis (chronic) (synovial) A18.02
    spine or vertebra (column) A18.01
  articular — *see* Tuberculosis, joint
  ascites A18.31
  asthma — *see* Tuberculosis, pulmonary
  axilla, axillary (gland) A18.2
  bladder A18.12
  bone A18.03
    hip A18.02
    knee A18.02
    limb NEC A18.03
    sacrum A18.01
    spine or vertebral column A18.01
  bowel (miliary) A18.32
  brain A17.81
  breast A18.89
  broad ligament A18.17
  bronchi, bronchial, bronchus A15.5
    ectasia, ectasis (bronchiectasis) — *see* Tuberculosis, pulmonary
    fistula A15.5
      primary (progressive) A15.7
    gland or node A15.4
      primary (progressive) A15.7
    lymph gland or node A15.4
      primary (progressive) A15.7
  bronchiectasis — *see* Tuberculosis, pulmonary
  bronchitis A15.5
  bronchopleural A15.6
  bronchopneumonia, bronchopneumonic — *see* Tuberculosis, pulmonary
  bronchorrhagia A15.5
  bronchotracheal A15.5
  bronze disease A18.7
  buccal cavity A18.83
  bulbourethral gland A18.15
  bursa A18.09
  cachexia A15.9
  cardiomyopathy A18.84
  caries — *see* Tuberculosis, bone
  cartilage A18.02
    intervertebral A18.01
  catarrhal — *see* Tuberculosis, respiratory
  cecum A18.32
  cellulitis (primary) A18.4
  cerebellum A17.81
  cerebral, cerebrum A17.81
  cerebrospinal A17.81
    meninges A17.0

☑ **Additional Character Required** — **Refer to the Tabular List for Character Selection**

Tuberculosis, tubercular, tuberculous — *continued*

cervical (lymph gland or node) A18.2
cervicitis, cervix (uteri) A18.16
chest — *see* Tuberculosis, respiratory
chorioretinitis A18.53
choroid, choroiditis A18.53
ciliary body A18.54
colitis A18.32
collier's J65
colliquativa (primary) A18.4
colon A18.32
complex, primary A15.7
congenital P37.0
conjunctiva A18.59
connective tissue (systemic) A18.89
contact Z20.1
cornea (ulcer) A18.52
Cowper's gland A18.15
coxae A18.02
coxalgia A18.02
cul-de-sac of Douglas A18.17
curvature, spine A18.01
cutis (colliquativa) (primary) A18.4
cyst, ovary A18.18
cystitis A18.12
dactylitis A18.03
diarrhea A18.32
diffuse — *see* Tuberculosis, miliary
digestive tract A18.32
disseminated — *see* Tuberculosis, miliary
duodenum A18.32
dura (mater) (cerebral) (spinal) A17.0
    abscess (cerebral) (spinal) A17.81
dysentery A18.32
ear (inner) (middle) A18.6
    bone A18.03
    external (primary) A18.4
    skin (primary) A18.4
elbow A18.02
emphysema — *see* Tuberculosis, pulmonary
empyema A15.6
encephalitis A17.82
endarteritis A18.89
endocarditis A18.84
    aortic A18.84
    mitral A18.84
    pulmonary A18.84
    tricuspid A18.84
endocrine glands NEC A18.82
endometrium A18.17
enteric, enterica, enteritis A18.32
enterocolitis A18.32
epididymis, epididymitis A18.15
epidural abscess (cerebral) (spinal) A17.81
epiglottis A15.5
episcleritis A18.51
erythema (induratum) (nodosum) (primary) A18.4
esophagus A18.83
eustachian tube A18.6
exposure (to) Z20.1
exudative — *see* Tuberculosis, pulmonary
eye A18.50
eyelid (primary) (lupus) A18.4
fallopian tube (acute) (chronic) A18.17
fascia A18.09
fauces A15.8
female pelvic inflammatory disease A18.17
finger A18.03
first infection A15.7
gallbladder A18.83
ganglion A18.09
gastritis A18.83
gastrocolic fistula A18.32
gastroenteritis A18.32
gastrointestinal tract A18.32
general, generalized — *see* Tuberculosis, miliary
genital organs A18.10
genitourinary A18.10
genu A18.02
glandula suprarenalis A18.7
glandular, general A18.2
glottis A15.5
grinder's J65
gum A18.83
hand A18.03
heart A18.84
hematogenous — *see* Tuberculosis, miliary
hemoptysis — *see* Tuberculosis, pulmonary
hemorrhage NEC — *see* Tuberculosis, pulmonary

Tuberculosis, tubercular, tuberculous — *continued*

hemothorax A15.6
hepatitis A18.83
hilar lymph nodes A15.4
    primary (progressive) A15.7
hip (joint) (disease) (bone) A18.02
hydropneumothorax A15.6
hydrothorax A15.6
hypoadrenalism A18.7
hypopharynx A15.8
ileocecal (hyperplastic) A18.32
ileocolitis A18.32
ileum A18.32
iliac spine (superior) A18.03
immunological findings only A15.7
indurativa (primary) A18.4
infantile A15.7
infection A15.9
    without clinical manifestations A15.7
infraclavicular gland A18.2
inguinal gland A18.2
inguinalis A18.2
intestine (any part) A18.32
iridocyclitis A18.54
iris, iritis A18.54
ischiorectal A18.32
jaw A18.03
jejunum A18.32
joint A18.02
    vertebral A18.01
keratitis (interstitial) A18.52
keratoconjunctivitis A18.52
kidney A18.11
knee (joint) A18.02
kyphosis, kyphoscoliosis A18.01
laryngitis A15.5
larynx A15.5
latent Z22.7
leptomeninges, leptomeningitis (cerebral) (spinal) A17.0
lichenoides (primary) A18.4
linguae A18.83
lip A18.83
liver A18.83
lordosis A18.01
lung — *see* Tuberculosis, pulmonary
lupus vulgaris A18.4
lymph gland or node (peripheral) A18.2
    abdomen A18.39
    bronchial A15.4
        primary (progressive) A15.7
    cervical A18.2
    hilar A15.4
        primary (progressive) A15.7
    intrathoracic A15.4
        primary (progressive) A15.7
    mediastinal A15.4
        primary (progressive) A15.7
    mesenteric A18.39
    retroperitoneal A18.39
    tracheobronchial A15.4
        primary (progressive) A15.7
lymphadenitis — *see* Tuberculosis, lymph gland
lymphangitis — *see* Tuberculosis, lymph gland
lymphatic (gland) (vessel) — *see* Tuberculosis, lymph gland
mammary gland A18.89
marasmus A15.9
mastoiditis A18.03
mediastinal lymph gland or node A15.4
    primary (progressive) A15.7
mediastinitis A15.8
    primary (progressive) A15.7
mediastinum A15.8
    primary (progressive) A15.7
medulla A17.81
melanosis, Addisonian A18.7
meninges, meningitis (basilar) (cerebral) (cerebrospinal) (spinal) A17.0
meningoencephalitis A17.82
mesentery, mesenteric (gland or node) A18.39
miliary A19.9
    acute A19.2
        multiple sites A19.1
        single specified site A19.0
    chronic A19.8
    specified NEC A19.8
millstone makers' J65
miner's J65
molder's J65

Tuberculosis, tubercular, tuberculous — *continued*

mouth A18.83
multiple A19.9
    acute A19.1
    chronic A19.8
muscle A18.09
myelitis A17.82
myocardium, myocarditis A18.84
nasal (passage) (sinus) A15.8
nasopharynx A15.8
neck gland A18.2
nephritis A18.11
nerve (mononeuropathy) A17.83
nervous system A17.9
nose (septum) A15.8
ocular A18.50
omentum A18.31
oophoritis (acute) (chronic) A18.17
optic (nerve trunk) (papilla) A18.59
orbit A18.59
orchitis A18.15
organ, specified NEC A18.89
osseous — *see* Tuberculosis, bone
osteitis — *see* Tuberculosis, bone
osteomyelitis — *see* Tuberculosis, bone
otitis media A18.6
ovary, ovaritis (acute) (chronic) A18.17
oviduct (acute) (chronic) A18.17
pachymeningitis A17.0
palate (soft) A18.83
pancreas A18.83
papulonecrotic (a) (primary) A18.4
parathyroid glands A18.82
paronychia (primary) A18.4
parotid gland or region A18.83
pelvis (bony) A18.03
penis A18.15
peribronchitis A15.5
pericardium, pericarditis A18.84
perichondritis, larynx A15.5
periostitis — *see* Tuberculosis, bone
perirectal fistula A18.32
peritoneum NEC A18.31
peritonitis A18.31
pharynx, pharyngitis A15.8
phlyctenulosis (keratoconjunctivitis) A18.52
phthisis NEC — *see* Tuberculosis, pulmonary
pituitary gland A18.82
pleura, pleural, pleurisy, pleuritis (fibrinous) (obliterative) (purulent) (simple plastic) (with effusion) A15.6
    primary (progressive) A15.7
pneumonia, pneumonic — *see* Tuberculosis, pulmonary
pneumothorax (spontaneous) (tense valvular) — *see* Tuberculosis, pulmonary
polyneuropathy A17.89
polyserositis A19.9
    acute A19.1
    chronic A19.8
potter's J65
prepuce A18.15
primary (complex) A15.7
proctitis A18.32
prostate, prostatitis A18.14
pulmonalis — *see* Tuberculosis, pulmonary
pulmonary (cavitated) (fibrotic) (infiltrative) (nodular) A15.0
    childhood type or first infection A15.7
    primary (complex) A15.7
pyelitis A18.11
pyelonephritis A18.11
pyemia — *see* Tuberculosis, miliary
pyonephrosis A18.11
pyopneumothorax A15.6
pyothorax A15.6
rectum (fistula) (with abscess) A18.32
reinfection stage — *see* Tuberculosis, pulmonary
renal A18.11
renis A18.11
respiratory A15.9
    primary A15.7
    specified site NEC A15.8
retina, retinitis A18.53
retroperitoneal (lymph gland or node) A18.39
rheumatism NEC A18.09
rhinitis A15.8
sacroiliac (joint) A18.01
sacrum A18.01
salivary gland A18.83
salpingitis (acute) (chronic) A18.17

Tuberculosis, tubercular, tuberculous — *continued*
- sandblaster's J65
- sclera A18.51
- scoliosis A18.01
- scrofulous A18.2
- scrotum A18.15
- seminal tract or vesicle A18.15
- senile A15.9
- septic — *see* Tuberculosis, miliary
- shoulder (joint) A18.02
  - blade A18.03
- sigmoid A18.32
- sinus (any nasal) A15.8
  - bone A18.03
  - epididymis A18.15
- skeletal NEC A18.03
- skin (any site) (primary) A18.4
- small intestine A18.32
- soft palate A18.83
- spermatic cord A18.15
- spine, spinal (column) A18.01
  - cord A17.81
  - medulla A17.81
  - membrane A17.0
  - meninges A17.0
- spleen, splenitis A18.85
- spondylitis A18.01
- sternoclavicular joint A18.02
- stomach A18.83
- stonemason's J65
- subcutaneous tissue (cellular) (primary) A18.4
- subcutis (primary) A18.4
- subdeltoid bursa A18.83
- submaxillary (region) A18.83
- supraclavicular gland A18.2
- suprarenal (capsule) (gland) A18.7
- swelling, joint (*see also* category M01) — *see also* Tuberculosis, joint A18.02
- symphysis pubis A18.02
- synovitis A18.09
  - articular A18.02
  - spine or vertebra A18.01
- systemic — *see* Tuberculosis, miliary
- tarsitis A18.4
- tendon (sheath) — *see* Tuberculosis, tenosynovitis
- tenosynovitis A18.09
  - spine or vertebra A18.01
- testis A18.15
- throat A15.8
- thymus gland A18.82
- thyroid gland A18.81
- tongue A18.83
- tonsil, tonsillitis A15.8
- trachea, tracheal A15.5
  - lymph gland or node A15.4
    - primary (progressive) A15.7
- tracheobronchial A15.5
  - lymph gland or node A15.4
    - primary (progressive) A15.7
- tubal (acute) (chronic) A18.17
- tunica vaginalis A18.15
- ulcer (skin) (primary) A18.4
  - bowel or intestine A18.32
  - specified NEC — *see* Tuberculosis, by site
- unspecified site A15.9
- ureter A18.11
- urethra, urethral (gland) A18.13
- urinary organ or tract A18.13
- uterus A18.17
- uveal tract A18.54
- uvula A18.83
- vagina A18.18
- vas deferens A18.15
- verruca, verrucosa (cutis) (primary) A18.4
- vertebra (column) A18.01
- vesiculitis A18.15
- vulva A18.18
- wrist (joint) A18.02

Tuberculum
- Carabelli — *see* Excludes Note at K00.2
- occlusal — *see* Excludes Note at K00.2
- paramolare K00.2

Tuberosity, entire maxillary M26.07
Tuberous sclerosis (brain) Q85.1
Tubo-ovarian — *see* condition
Tuboplasty, after previous sterilization Z31.0
- aftercare Z31.42

Tubotympanitis, catarrhal (chronic) — *see* Otitis, media, nonsuppurative, chronic, serous

Tularemia A21.9
- with
  - conjunctivitis A21.1
  - pneumonia A21.2
- abdominal A21.3
- bronchopneumonic A21.2
- conjunctivitis A21.1
- cryptogenic A21.3
- enteric A21.3
- gastrointestinal A21.3
- generalized A21.7
- ingestion A21.3
- intestinal A21.3
- oculoglandular A21.1
- ophthalmic A21.1
- pneumonia (any), pneumonic A21.2
- pulmonary A21.2
- sepsis A21.7
- specified NEC A21.8
- typhoidal A21.7
- ulceroglandular A21.0
Tularensis conjunctivitis A21.1
Tumefaction — *see also* Swelling
- liver — *see* Hypertrophy, liver
Tumor — *see also* Neoplasm, unspecified behavior, by site
- acinar cell — *see* Neoplasm, uncertain behavior, by site
- acinic cell — *see* Neoplasm, uncertain behavior, by site
- adenocarcinoid — *see* Neoplasm, malignant, by site
- adenomatoid — *see also* Neoplasm, benign, by site
  - odontogenic — *see* Cyst, calcifying odontogenic
- adnexal (skin) — *see* Neoplasm, skin, benign, by site
- adrenal
  - cortical (benign) D35.0- ☑
    - malignant C74.0- ☑
  - rest — *see* Neoplasm, benign, by site
- alpha-cell
  - malignant
    - pancreas C25.4
    - specified site NEC — *see* Neoplasm, malignant, by site
    - unspecified site C25.4
  - pancreas D13.7
  - specified site NEC — *see* Neoplasm, benign, by site
  - unspecified site D13.7
- aneurysmal — *see* Aneurysm
- aortic body D44.7
  - malignant C75.5
- Askin's — *see* Neoplasm, connective tissue, malignant
- basal cell — *see also* Neoplasm, skin, uncertain behavior D48.5
- Bednar — *see* Neoplasm, skin, malignant
- benign (unclassified) — *see* Neoplasm, benign, by site
- beta-cell
  - malignant
    - pancreas C25.4
    - specified site NEC — *see* Neoplasm, malignant, by site
    - unspecified site C25.4
  - pancreas D13.7
  - specified site NEC — *see* Neoplasm, benign, by site
  - unspecified site D13.7
- Brenner D27.9
  - borderline malignancy D39.1- ☑
  - malignant C56- ☑
  - proliferating D39.1- ☑
- bronchial alveolar, intravascular D38.1
- Brooke's — *see* Neoplasm, skin, benign
- brown fat — *see* Lipoma
- Burkitt — *see* Lymphoma, Burkitt
- calcifying epithelial odontogenic — *see* Cyst, calcifying odontogenic
- carcinoid D3A.00 (*following* D36)
  - benign D3A.00 (*following* D36)
    - appendix D3A.020 (*following* D36)
    - ascending colon D3A.022 (*following* D36)
    - bronchus (lung) D3A.090 (*following* D36)
    - cecum D3A.021 (*following* D36)
    - colon D3A.029 (*following* D36)
    - descending colon D3A.024 (*following* D36)
    - duodenum D3A.010 (*following* D36)
    - foregut NOS D3A.094 (*following* D36)
    - hindgut NOS D3A.096 (*following* D36)
    - ileum D3A.012 (*following* D36)
    - jejunum D3A.011 (*following* D36)
    - kidney D3A.093 (*following* D36)
    - large intestine D3A.029 (*following* D36)
    - lung (bronchus) D3A.090 (*following* D36)
    - midgut NOS D3A.095 (*following* D36)

Tumor — *continued*
- carcinoid — *continued*
  - benign — *continued*
    - rectum D3A.026 (*following* D36)
    - sigmoid colon D3A.025 (*following* D36)
    - small intestine D3A.019 (*following* D36)
    - specified NEC D3A.098 (*following* D36)
    - stomach D3A.092 (*following* D36)
    - thymus D3A.091 (*following* D36)
    - transverse colon D3A.023 (*following* D36)
  - malignant C7A.00 (*following* C75)
    - appendix C7A.020 (*following* C75)
    - ascending colon C7A.022 (*following* C75)
    - bronchus (lung) C7A.090 (*following* C75)
    - cecum C7A.021 (*following* C75)
    - colon C7A.029 (*following* C75)
    - descending colon C7A.024 (*following* C75)
    - duodenum C7A.010 (*following* C75)
    - foregut NOS C7A.094 (*following* C75)
    - hindgut NOS C7A.096 (*following* C75)
    - ileum C7A.012 (*following* C75)
    - jejunum C7A.011 (*following* C75)
    - kidney C7A.093 (*following* C75)
    - large intestine C7A.029 (*following* C75)
    - lung (bronchus) C7A.090 (*following* C75)
    - midgut NOS C7A.095 (*following* C75)
    - rectum C7A.026 (*following* C75)
    - sigmoid colon C7A.025 (*following* C75)
    - small intestine C7A.019 (*following* C75)
    - specified NEC C7A.098 (*following* C75)
    - stomach C7A.092 (*following* C75)
    - thymus C7A.091 (*following* C75)
    - transverse colon C7A.023 (*following* C75)
  - mesentery metastasis C7B.04 (*following* C75)
  - secondary C7B.00 (*following* C75)
    - bone C7B.03 (*following* C75)
    - distant lymph nodes C7B.01 (*following* C75)
    - liver C7B.02 (*following* C75)
    - peritoneum C7B.04 (*following* C75)
    - specified NEC C7B.09 (*following* C75)
- carotid body D44.6
  - malignant C75.4
- cells — *see also* Neoplasm, unspecified behavior, by site
  - benign — *see* Neoplasm, benign, by site
  - malignant — *see* Neoplasm, malignant, by site
  - uncertain whether benign or malignant — *see* Neoplasm, uncertain behavior, by site
- cervix, in pregnancy or childbirth — *see* Pregnancy, complicated by, tumor, cervix
- chondromatous giant cell — *see* Neoplasm, bone, benign
- chromaffin — *see also* Neoplasm, benign, by site
  - malignant — *see* Neoplasm, malignant, by site
- Cock's peculiar L72.3
- Codman's — *see* Neoplasm, bone, benign
- dentigerous, mixed — *see* Cyst, calcifying odontogenic
- dermoid — *see* Neoplasm, benign, by site
  - with malignant transformation C56- ☑
- desmoid (extra-abdominal) — *see also* Neoplasm, connective tissue, uncertain behavior
  - abdominal — *see* Neoplasm, connective tissue, uncertain behavior
- embolus — *see* Neoplasm, secondary, by site
- embryonal (mixed) — *see also* Neoplasm, uncertain behavior, by site
  - liver C22.7
- endodermal sinus
  - specified site — *see* Neoplasm, malignant, by site
  - unspecified site
    - female C56.- ☑
    - male C62.90
- epithelial
  - benign — *see* Neoplasm, benign, by site
  - malignant — *see* Neoplasm, malignant, by site
- Ewing's — *see* Neoplasm, bone, malignant, by site
- fatty — *see* Lipoma
- fibroid — *see* Leiomyoma
- G cell
  - malignant
    - pancreas C25.4
    - specified site NEC — *see* Neoplasm, malignant, by site
    - unspecified site C25.4
  - specified site — *see* Neoplasm, uncertain behavior, by site
  - unspecified site D37.8
- germ cell — *see also* Neoplasm, malignant, by site
  - mixed — *see* Neoplasm, malignant, by site
- ghost cell, odontogenic — *see* Cyst, calcifying odontogenic

☑ **Additional Character Required — Refer to the Tabular List for Character Selection**

Index

Tumor — *continued*
  giant cell — *see also* Neoplasm, uncertain behavior, by site
    bone D48.0
      malignant — *see* Neoplasm, bone, malignant
    chondromatous — *see* Neoplasm, bone, benign
    malignant — *see* Neoplasm, malignant, by site
    soft parts — *see* Neoplasm, connective tissue, uncertain behavior
      malignant — *see* Neoplasm, connective tissue, malignant
  glomus D18.00
    intra-abdominal D18.03
    intracranial D18.02
    jugulare D44.7
      malignant C75.5
    skin D18.01
    specified site NEC D18.09
  gonadal stromal — *see* Neoplasm, uncertain behavior, by site
  granular cell — *see also* Neoplasm, connective tissue, benign
    malignant — *see* Neoplasm, connective tissue, malignant
  granulosa cell D39.1- ☑
    juvenile D39.1-
    malignant C56- ☑
  granulosa cell-theca cell D39.1- ☑
    malignant C56- ☑
  Grawitz's C64- ☑
  hemorrhoidal — *see* Hemorrhoids
  hilar cell D27- ☑
  hilus cell D27- ☑
  Hurthle cell (benign) D34
    malignant C73
  hydatid — *see* Echinococcus
  hypernephroid — *see also* Neoplasm, uncertain behavior, by site
  interstitial cell — *see also* Neoplasm, uncertain behavior, by site
    benign — *see* Neoplasm, benign, by site
    malignant — *see* Neoplasm, malignant, by site
  intravascular bronchial alveolar D38.1
  islet cell — *see* Neoplasm, benign, by site
    malignant — *see* Neoplasm, malignant, by site
      pancreas C25.4
      specified site NEC — *see* Neoplasm, malignant, by site
      unspecified site C25.4
    pancreas D13.7
    specified site NEC — *see* Neoplasm, benign, by site
    unspecified site D13.7
  juxtaglomerular D41.0- ☑
  Klatskin's C22.1
  Krukenberg's C79.6- ☑
  Leydig cell — *see* Neoplasm, uncertain behavior, by site
    benign — *see* Neoplasm, benign, by site
      specified site — *see* Neoplasm, benign, by site
      unspecified site
        female D27.9
        male D29.20
    malignant — *see* Neoplasm, malignant, by site
      specified site — *see* Neoplasm, malignant, by site
      unspecified site
        female C56.9
        male C62.90
    specified site — *see* Neoplasm, uncertain behavior, by site
    unspecified site
      female D39.10
      male D40.10
  lipid cell, ovary D27- ☑
  lipoid cell, ovary D27- ☑
  malignant — *see also* Neoplasm, malignant, by site C80.1
    fusiform cell (type) C80.1
    giant cell (type) C80.1
    localized, plasma cell — *see* Plasmacytoma, solitary
    mixed NEC C80.1
    small cell (type) C80.1
    spindle cell (type) C80.1
    unclassified C80.1
  mast cell D47.09
  melanotic, neuroectodermal — *see* Neoplasm, benign, by site
  Merkel cell — *see* Carcinoma, Merkel cell
  mesenchymal
    malignant — *see* Neoplasm, connective tissue, malignant

Tumor — *continued*
  mesenchymal — *continued*
    mixed — *see* Neoplasm, connective tissue, uncertain behavior
  mesodermal, mixed — *see also* Neoplasm, malignant, by site
    liver C22.4
  mesonephric — *see also* Neoplasm, uncertain behavior, by site
    malignant — *see* Neoplasm, malignant, by site
  metastatic
    from specified site — *see* Neoplasm, malignant, by site
    of specified site — *see* Neoplasm, malignant, by site
    to specified site — *see* Neoplasm, secondary, by site
  mixed NEC — *see also* Neoplasm, benign, by site
    malignant — *see* Neoplasm, malignant, by site
  mucinous of low malignant potential
    specified site — *see* Neoplasm, malignant, by site
    unspecified site C56.9
  mucocarcinoid
    specified site — *see* Neoplasm, malignant, by site
    unspecified site C18.1
  mucoepidermoid — *see* Neoplasm, uncertain behavior, by site
  Mullerian, mixed
    specified site — *see* Neoplasm, malignant, by site
    unspecified site C54.9
  myoepithelial — *see* Neoplasm, benign, by site
  neuroectodermal (peripheral) — *see* Neoplasm, malignant, by site
    primitive
      specified site — *see* Neoplasm, malignant, by site
      unspecified site C71.9
  neuroendocrine D3A.8 (*following* D36)
    malignant poorly differentiated C7A.1 (*following* C75)
    secondary NEC C7B.8 (*following* C75)
    specified NEC C7A.8 (*following* C75)
  neurogenic olfactory C30.0
  nonencapsulated sclerosing C73
  odontogenic (adenomatoid) (benign) (calcifying epithelial) (keratocystic) (squamous) — *see* Cyst, calcifying odontogenic
    malignant C41.1
      upper jaw (bone) C41.0
  ovarian stromal D39.1- ☑
  ovary, in pregnancy — *see* Pregnancy, complicated by
  pacinian — *see* Neoplasm, skin, benign
  Pancoast's — *see* Pancoast's syndrome
  papillary — *see also* Papilloma
    cystic D37.9
    mucinous of low malignant potential C56- ☑
      specified site — *see* Neoplasm, malignant, by site
      unspecified site C56.9
    serous of low malignant potential
      specified site — *see* Neoplasm, malignant, by site
      unspecified site C56.9
  pelvic, in pregnancy or childbirth — *see* Pregnancy, complicated by
  phantom F45.8
  phyllodes D48.6- ☑
    benign D24- ☑
    malignant — *see* Neoplasm, breast, malignant
  Pindborg — *see* Cyst, calcifying odontogenic
  placental site trophoblastic D39.2
  plasma cell (malignant) (localized) — *see* Plasmacytoma, solitary
  polyvesicular vitelline
    specified site — *see* Neoplasm, malignant, by site
    unspecified site
      female C56.9
      male C62.90
  Pott's puffy — *see* Osteomyelitis, specified NEC
  Rathke's pouch D44.3
  retinal anlage — *see* Neoplasm, benign, by site
  salivary gland or duct type, mixed — *see* Neoplasm, salivary gland or duct, benign
    malignant — *see* Neoplasm, salivary gland or duct, malignant
  Sampson's N80.10- ☑
  Schmincke's — *see* Neoplasm, nasopharynx, malignant
  sclerosing stromal D27- ☑
  sebaceous — *see* Cyst, sebaceous
  secondary — *see* Neoplasm, secondary, by site
    carcinoid C7B.00 (*following* C75)
      bone C7B.03 (*following* C75)
      distant lymph nodes C7B.01 (*following* C75)
      liver C7B.02 (*following* C75)

Tumor — *continued*
  secondary — *see* Neoplasm, secondary, by site — *continued*
    carcinoid — *continued*
      peritoneum C7B.04 (*following* C75)
      specified NEC C7B.09 (*following* C75)
    neuroendocrine NEC C7B.8 (*following* C75)
  serous of low malignant potential
    specified site — *see* Neoplasm, malignant, by site
    unspecified site C56.9
  Sertoli cell — *see* Neoplasm, benign, by site
    with lipid storage
      specified site — *see* Neoplasm, benign, by site
      unspecified site
        female D27.9
        male D29.20
    specified site — *see* Neoplasm, benign, by site
    unspecified site
      female D27.9
      male D29.20
  Sertoli-Leydig cell — *see* Neoplasm, benign, by site
    specified site — *see* Neoplasm, benign, by site
    unspecified site
      female D27.9
      male D29.20
  sex cord (-stromal) — *see* Neoplasm, uncertain behavior, by site
    with annular tubules D39.1- ☑
  skin appendage — *see* Neoplasm, skin, benign
  smooth muscle — *see* Neoplasm, connective tissue, uncertain behavior
  soft tissue
    benign — *see* Neoplasm, connective tissue, benign
    malignant — *see* Neoplasm, connective tissue, malignant
  sternomastoid (congenital) Q68.0
  stromal
    endometrial D39.0
    gastric D48.19
      benign D21.4
      malignant C49.A2
      uncertain behavior D48.19
    gastrointestinal C49.A- ☑
      benign D21.4
      esophagus C49.A1
      malignant C49.A0
        colon C49.A4
        duodenum C49.A3
        esophagus C49.A1
        ileum C49.A3
        jejunum C49.A3
        large intestine C49.A4
        Meckel diverticulum C49.A3
        omentum C49.A9
        peritoneum C49.A9
        rectum C49.A5
        small intestine C49.A3
        specified site NEC C49.A9
        stomach C49.A2
      rectum C49.A5
      small intestine C49.A3
      specified site NEC C49.A9
      stomach C49.A2
      uncertain behavior D48.19
    intestine
      benign D21.4
      malignant
        large C49.A4
        small C49.A3
      uncertain behavior D48.19
    ovarian D39.1- ☑
    stomach C49.A2
      benign D21.4
      malignant C49.A2
      uncertain behavior D48.19
  sweat gland — *see also* Neoplasm, skin, uncertain behavior
    benign — *see* Neoplasm, skin, benign
    malignant — *see* Neoplasm, skin, malignant
  syphilitic, brain A52.17
  testicular D40.10
  testicular stromal D40.1- ☑
  theca cell D27.- ☑
  theca cell-granulosa cell D39.1- ☑
  Triton, malignant — *see* Neoplasm, nerve, malignant
  trophoblastic, placental site D39.2
  turban D23.4

Tumor — Tumor

Tumor — *continued*
  uterus (body), in pregnancy or childbirth — *see* Pregnancy, complicated by, tumor, uterus
  vagina, in pregnancy or childbirth — *see* Pregnancy, complicated by
  varicose — *see* Varix
  von Recklinghausen's — *see* Neurofibromatosis
  vulva or perineum, in pregnancy or childbirth — *see* Pregnancy, complicated by
    causing obstructed labor O65.5
  Warthin's — *see* Neoplasm, salivary gland or duct, benign
  Wilms' C64- ☑
  yolk sac — *see* Neoplasm, malignant, by site
    specified site — *see* Neoplasm, malignant, by site
    unspecified site
      female C56.9
      male C62.90
Tumor lysis syndrome (following antineoplastic chemotherapy) (spontaneous) NEC E88.3
Tumorlet — *see* Neoplasm, uncertain behavior, by site
Tungiasis B88.1
Tunica vasculosa lentis Q12.2
Turban tumor D23.4
Türck's trachoma J37.0
Turner-Kieser syndrome Q87.2
Turner-like syndrome Q87.19
Turner's
  hypoplasia (tooth) K00.4
  syndrome Q96.9
    specified NEC Q96.8
  tooth K00.4
Turner-Ullrich syndrome Q96.9
Tussis convulsiva — *see* Whooping cough
Twiddler's syndrome (due to)
  automatic implantable defibrillator T82.198
  cardiac pacemaker T82.198 ☑
Twilight state
  epileptic F05
  psychogenic F44.89
Twin (newborn) — *see also* Newborn, twin
  conjoined Q89.4
  pregnancy — *see* Pregnancy, twin
Twinning, teeth K00.2
Twist, twisted
  bowel, colon or intestine K56.2
  hair (congenital) Q84.1
  mesentery K56.2
  omentum K56.2
  organ or site, congenital NEC — *see* Anomaly, by site
  ovarian pedicle — *see* Torsion, ovary
Twitching R25.3
Tylosis (acquired) L84
  buccalis K13.29
  linguae K13.29
  palmaris et plantaris (congenital) (inherited) Q82.8
    acquired L85.1
Tympanism R14.0
Tympanites (abdominal) (intestinal) R14.0
Tympanitis — *see* Myringitis
Tympanosclerosis H74.0 ☑
Tympanum — *see* condition
Tympany
  abdomen R14.0
  chest R09.89
Type A behavior pattern Z73.1
Typhlitis — *see* Cecitis
Typhoenteritis — *see* Typhoid
Typhoid (abortive) (ambulant) (any site) (clinical) (fever) (hemorrhagic) (infection) (intermittent) (malignant) (rheumatic) (Widal negative) A01.00
  with pneumonia A01.03
  abdominal A01.09
  arthritis A01.04
  carrier (suspected) of Z22.0
  cholecystitis (current) A01.09
  endocarditis A01.02
  heart involvement A01.02
  inoculation reaction — *see* Complications, vaccination
  meningitis A01.01
  mesenteric lymph nodes A01.09
  myocarditis A01.02
  osteomyelitis A01.05
  perichondritis, larynx A01.09
  pneumonia A01.03
  specified NEC A01.09
  spine A01.05
  ulcer (perforating) A01.09
Typhomalaria (fever) — *see* Malaria
Typhomania A01.00

Typhoperitonitis A01.09
Typhus (fever) A75.9
  abdominal, abdominalis — *see* Typhoid
  African tick A77.1
  amarillic A95.9
  brain A75.9 [G94]
  cerebral A75.9 [G94]
  classical A75.0
  due to Rickettsia
    prowazekii A75.0
      recrudescent A75.1
    tsutsugamushi A75.3
    typhi A75.2
  endemic (flea-borne) A75.2
  epidemic (louse-borne) A75.0
  exanthematicus SAI A75.0
    brillii SAI A75.1
    mexicanus SAI A75.2
    typhus murinus A75.2
  exanthematic NEC A75.0
  flea-borne A75.2
  India tick A77.1
  Kenya (tick) A77.1
  louse-borne A75.0
  Mexican A75.2
  mite-borne A75.3
  murine A75.2
  North Asian tick-borne A77.2
  Orientia Tsutsugamushi (scrub typhus) A75.3
  petechial A75.9
  Queensland tick A77.3
  rat A75.2
  recrudescent A75.1
  recurrens — *see* Fever, relapsing
  Sao Paulo A77.0
  scrub (China) (India) (Malaysia) (New Guinea) A75.3
  shop (of Malaysia) A75.2
  Siberian tick A77.2
  tick-borne A77.9
  tropical (mite-borne) A75.3
Tyrosinemia E70.21
  newborn, transitory P74.5
Tyrosinosis E70.21
Tyrosinuria E70.29

U

Uhl's anomaly or disease Q24.8
Ulcer, ulcerated, ulcerating, ulceration, ulcerative
  alveolar process M27.3
  amebic (intestine) A06.1
    skin A06.7
  anastomotic — *see* Ulcer, gastrojejunal
  anorectal K62.6
  antral — *see* Ulcer, stomach
  anus (sphincter) (solitary) K62.6
  aorta — *see* Aneurysm
  aphthous (oral) (recurrent) K12.0
    genital organ(s)
      female N76.6
      male N50.89
  artery I77.2
  atrophic — *see* Ulcer, skin
    decubitus — *see* Ulcer, pressure, by site
  back L98.429
    with
      bone involvement without evidence of necrosis L98.426
      bone necrosis L98.424
      exposed fat layer L98.422
      muscle involvement without evidence of necrosis L98.425
      muscle necrosis L98.423
      skin breakdown only L98.421
      specified severity NEC L98.428
  Barrett's (esophagus) K22.10
    with bleeding K22.11
  bile duct (common) (hepatic) K83.8
  bladder (solitary) (sphincter) NEC N32.89
    bilharzial B65.9 [N33]
    in schistosomiasis (bilharzial) B65.9 [N33]
    submucosal — *see* Cystitis, interstitial
    tuberculous A18.12
  bleeding K27.4
  bone — *see* Osteomyelitis, specified type NEC
  bowel — *see* Ulcer, intestine
  breast N61.1
  bronchus J98.09
  buccal (cavity) (traumatic) K12.1

Ulcer, ulcerated, ulcerating, ulceration, ulcerative — *continued*
  Buruli A31.1
  buttock L98.419
    with
      bone involvement without evidence of necrosis L98.416
      bone necrosis L98.414
      exposed fat layer L98.412
      muscle involvement without evidence of necrosis L98.415
      muscle necrosis L98.413
      skin breakdown only L98.411
      specified severity NEC L98.418
  cameron *see* Ulcer, stomach
  cancerous — *see* Neoplasm, malignant, by site
  cardia K22.10
    with bleeding K22.11
  cardioesophageal (peptic) K22.10
    with bleeding K22.11
  cecum — *see* Ulcer, intestine
  cervix (uteri) (decubitus) (trophic) N86
    with cervicitis N72
  chancroidal A57
  chiclero B55.1
  chronic (cause unknown) — *see* Ulcer, skin
  Cochin-China B55.1
  colon — *see* Ulcer, intestine
  conjunctiva H10.89
  cornea H16.00- ☑
    with hypopyon H16.03- ☑
    central H16.01- ☑
    dendritic (herpes simplex) B00.52
    marginal H16.04- ☑
    Mooren's H16.05- ☑
    mycotic H16.06- ☑
    perforated H16.07- ☑
    ring H16.02- ☑
    tuberculous (phlyctenular) A18.52
  corpus cavernosum (chronic) N48.5
  crural — *see* Ulcer, lower limb
  Curling's — *see* Ulcer, peptic, acute
  Cushing's — *see* Ulcer, peptic, acute
  cystic duct K82.8
  cystitis (interstitial) — *see* Cystitis, interstitial
  decubitus — *see* Ulcer, pressure, by site
  dendritic, cornea (herpes simplex) B00.52
  diabetes, diabetic — *see* Diabetes, ulcer
  Dieulafoy's K25.0
  due to
    infection NEC — *see* Ulcer, skin
    radiation NEC L59.8
    trophic disturbance (any region) — *see* Ulcer, skin
    X-ray L58.1
  duodenum, duodenal (eroded) (peptic) K26.9
    with
      hemorrhage K26.4
        and perforation K26.6
      perforation K26.5
    acute K26.3
      with
        hemorrhage K26.0
          and perforation K26.2
        perforation K26.1
    chronic (erosive) K26.7
      with
        hemorrhage K26.4
          and perforation K26.6
        perforation K26.5
  dysenteric A09
  elusive — *see* Cystitis, interstitial
  endocarditis (acute) (chronic) (subacute) I28.8
  epiglottis J38.7
  esophagus (peptic) K22.10
    with bleeding K22.11
    due to
      aspirin K22.10
        with bleeding K22.11
      gastrointestinal reflux disease (without bleeding) K21.00
        with bleeding K21.01
      ingestion of chemical or medicament K22.10
        with bleeding K22.11
    fungal K22.10
      with bleeding K22.11
    infective K22.10
      with bleeding K22.11
    varicose — *see* Varix, esophagus

Ulcer, ulcerated, ulcerating, ulceration, ulcerative — *continued*
  eyelid (region) H01.8
  fauces J39.2
  Fenwick (-Hunner) (solitary) — *see* Cystitis, interstitial
  fistulous — *see* Ulcer, skin
  foot (indolent) (trophic) — *see* Ulcer, lower limb
  frambesial, initial A66.0
  frenum (tongue) K14.0
  gallbladder or duct K82.8
  gangrenous — *see* Gangrene
  gastric — *see* Ulcer, stomach
  gastrocolic — *see* Ulcer, gastrojejunal
  gastroduodenal — *see* Ulcer, peptic
  gastroesophageal — *see* Ulcer, stomach
  gastrointestinal — *see* Ulcer, gastrojejunal
  gastrojejunal (peptic) K28.9
    with
      hemorrhage K28.4
        and perforation K28.6
      perforation K28.5
    acute K28.3
      with
        hemorrhage K28.0
          and perforation K28.2
        perforation K28.1
    chronic K28.7
      with
        hemorrhage K28.4
          and perforation K28.6
        perforation K28.5
  gastrojejunocolic — *see* Ulcer, gastrojejunal
  gingiva K06.8
  gingivitis K05.10
    nonplaque induced K05.11
    plaque induced K05.10
  glottis J38.7
  granuloma of pudenda A58
  gum K06.8
  gumma, due to yaws A66.4
  heel — *see* Ulcer, lower limb
  hemorrhoid — *see also* Hemorrhoids, by degree K64.8
  Hunner's — *see* Cystitis, interstitial
  hypopharynx J39.2
  hypopyon (chronic) (subacute) — *see* Ulcer, cornea, with hypopyon
  hypostaticum — *see* Ulcer, varicose
  ileum — *see* Ulcer, intestine
  intestine, intestinal K63.3
    with perforation K63.1
    amebic A06.1
    duodenal — *see* Ulcer, duodenum
    granulocytopenic (with hemorrhage) — *see* Neutropenia
    marginal — *see* Ulcer, gastrojejunal
    perforating K63.1
      newborn P78.0
    primary, small intestine K63.3
    rectum K62.6
    stercoraceous, stercoral K63.3
    tuberculous A18.32
    typhoid (fever) — *see* Typhoid
    varicose I86.8
  jejunum, jejunal — *see* Ulcer, gastrojejunal
  keratitis — *see* Ulcer, cornea
  knee — *see* Ulcer, lower limb
  labium (majus) (minus) N76.6
  laryngitis — *see* Laryngitis
  larynx (aphthous) (contact) J38.7
    diphtheritic A36.2
  leg — *see* Ulcer, lower limb
  lip K13.0
  Lipschütz's N76.6
  lower limb (atrophic) (chronic) (neurogenic) (perforating) (pyogenic) (trophic) (tropical) L97.909
    with
      bone involvement without evidence of necrosis L97.906
      bone necrosis L97.904
      exposed fat layer L97.902
      muscle involvement without evidence of necrosis L97.905
      muscle necrosis L97.903
      skin breakdown only L97.901
      specified severity NEC L97.908
    ankle L97.309
      with
        bone involvement without evidence of necrosis L97.306

Ulcer, ulcerated, ulcerating, ulceration, ulcerative — *continued*
  lower limb — *continued*
    ankle — *continued*
      with — *continued*
        bone necrosis L97.304
        exposed fat layer L97.302
        muscle involvement without evidence of necrosis L97.305
        muscle necrosis L97.303
        skin breakdown only L97.301
        specified severity NEC L97.308
      left L97.329
        with
          bone involvement without evidence of necrosis L97.326
          bone necrosis L97.324
          exposed fat layer L97.322
          muscle involvement without evidence of necrosis L97.325
          muscle necrosis L97.323
          skin breakdown only L97.321
          specified severity NEC L97.328
      right L97.319
        with
          bone involvement without evidence of necrosis L97.316
          bone necrosis L97.314
          exposed fat layer L97.312
          muscle involvement without evidence of necrosis L97.315
          muscle necrosis L97.313
          skin breakdown only L97.311
          specified severity NEC L97.318
    calf L97.209
      with
        bone involvement without evidence of necrosis L97.206
        bone necrosis L97.204
        exposed fat layer L97.202
        muscle involvement without evidence of necrosis L97.205
        muscle necrosis L97.203
        skin breakdown only L97.201
        specified severity NEC L97.208
      left L97.229
        with
          bone involvement without evidence of necrosis L97.226
          bone necrosis L97.224
          exposed fat layer L97.222
          muscle involvement without evidence of necrosis L97.225
          muscle necrosis L97.223
          skin breakdown only L97.221
          specified severity NEC L97.228
      right L97.219
        with
          bone involvement without evidence of necrosis L97.216
          bone necrosis L97.214
          exposed fat layer L97.212
          muscle involvement without evidence of necrosis L97.215
          muscle necrosis L97.213
          skin breakdown only L97.211
          specified severity NEC L97.218
    decubitus — *see* Ulcer, pressure, by site
    foot specified NEC L97.509
      with
        bone involvement without evidence of necrosis L97.506
        bone necrosis L97.504
        exposed fat layer L97.502
        muscle involvement without evidence of necrosis L97.505
        muscle necrosis L97.503
        skin breakdown only L97.501
        specified severity NEC L97.508
      left L97.529
        with
          bone involvement without evidence of necrosis L97.526
          bone necrosis L97.524
          exposed fat layer L97.522
          muscle involvement without evidence of necrosis L97.525
          muscle necrosis L97.523
          skin breakdown only L97.521

Ulcer, ulcerated, ulcerating, ulceration, ulcerative — *continued*
  lower limb — *continued*
    foot specified — *continued*
      left — *continued*
        with — *continued*
          specified severity NEC L97.528
      right L97.519
        with
          bone involvement without evidence of necrosis L97.516
          bone necrosis L97.514
          exposed fat layer L97.512
          muscle involvement without evidence of necrosis L97.515
          muscle necrosis L97.513
          skin breakdown only L97.511
          specified severity NEC L97.518
    heel L97.409
      with
        bone involvement without evidence of necrosis L97.406
        bone necrosis L97.404
        exposed fat layer L97.402
        muscle involvement without evidence of necrosis L97.405
        muscle necrosis L97.403
        skin breakdown only L97.401
        specified severity NEC L97.408
      left L97.429
        with
          bone involvement without evidence of necrosis L97.426
          bone necrosis L97.424
          exposed fat layer L97.422
          muscle involvement without evidence of necrosis L97.425
          muscle necrosis L97.423
          skin breakdown only L97.421
          specified severity NEC L97.428
      right L97.419
        with
          bone involvement without evidence of necrosis L97.416
          bone necrosis L97.414
          exposed fat layer L97.412
          muscle involvement without evidence of necrosis L97.415
          muscle necrosis L97.413
          skin breakdown only L97.411
          specified severity NEC L97.418
    left L97.929
      with
        bone involvement without evidence of necrosis L97.926
        bone necrosis L97.924
        exposed fat layer L97.922
        muscle involvement without evidence of necrosis L97.925
        muscle necrosis L97.923
        skin breakdown only L97.921
        specified severity NEC L97.928
    leprous A30.1
    lower leg NOS L97.909
      with
        bone involvement without evidence of necrosis L97.906
        bone necrosis L97.904
        exposed fat layer L97.902
        muscle involvement without evidence of necrosis L97.905
        muscle necrosis L97.903
        skin breakdown only L97.901
        specified severity NEC L97.908
      left L97.929
        with
          bone involvement without evidence of necrosis L97.926
          bone necrosis L97.924
          exposed fat layer L97.922
          muscle involvement without evidence of necrosis L97.925
          muscle necrosis L97.923
          skin breakdown only L97.921
          specified severity NEC L97.928
      right L97.919
        with
          bone involvement without evidence of necrosis L97.916

☑ **Additional Character Required — Refer to the Tabular List for Character Selection**

Ulcer, ulcerated, ulcerating, ulceration, ulcerative — *continued*
　lower limb — *continued*
　　lower leg — *continued*
　　　right — *continued*
　　　　with — *continued*
　　　　　bone necrosis L97.914
　　　　　exposed fat layer L97.912
　　　　　muscle involvement without evidence of necrosis L97.915
　　　　　muscle necrosis L97.913
　　　　　skin breakdown only L97.911
　　　　　specified severity NEC L97.918
　　　　specified site NEC L97.809
　　　　　with
　　　　　　bone involvement without evidence of necrosis L97.806
　　　　　　bone necrosis L97.804
　　　　　　exposed fat layer L97.802
　　　　　　muscle involvement without evidence of necrosis L97.805
　　　　　　muscle necrosis L97.803
　　　　　　skin breakdown only L97.801
　　　　　　specified severity NEC L97.808
　　　　　left L97.829
　　　　　　with
　　　　　　　bone involvement without evidence of necrosis L97.826
　　　　　　　bone necrosis L97.824
　　　　　　　exposed fat layer L97.822
　　　　　　　muscle involvement without evidence of necrosis L97.825
　　　　　　　muscle necrosis L97.823
　　　　　　　skin breakdown only L97.821
　　　　　　　specified severity NEC L97.828
　　　　　right L97.819
　　　　　　with
　　　　　　　bone involvement without evidence of necrosis L97.816
　　　　　　　bone necrosis L97.814
　　　　　　　exposed fat layer L97.812
　　　　　　　muscle involvement without evidence of necrosis L97.815
　　　　　　　muscle necrosis L97.813
　　　　　　　skin breakdown only L97.811
　　　　　　　specified severity NEC L97.818
　　　　midfoot L97.409
　　　　　with
　　　　　　bone involvement without evidence of necrosis L97.406
　　　　　　bone necrosis L97.404
　　　　　　exposed fat layer L97.402
　　　　　　muscle involvement without evidence of necrosis L97.405
　　　　　　muscle necrosis L97.403
　　　　　　skin breakdown only L97.401
　　　　　　specified severity NEC L97.408
　　　　　left L97.429
　　　　　　with
　　　　　　　bone involvement without evidence of necrosis L97.426
　　　　　　　bone necrosis L97.424
　　　　　　　exposed fat layer L97.422
　　　　　　　muscle involvement without evidence of necrosis L97.425
　　　　　　　muscle necrosis L97.423
　　　　　　　skin breakdown only L97.421
　　　　　　　specified severity NEC L97.428
　　　　　right L97.419
　　　　　　with
　　　　　　　bone involvement without evidence of necrosis L97.416
　　　　　　　bone necrosis L97.414
　　　　　　　exposed fat layer L97.412
　　　　　　　muscle involvement without evidence of necrosis L97.415
　　　　　　　muscle necrosis L97.413
　　　　　　　skin breakdown only L97.411
　　　　　　　specified severity NEC L97.418
　　　　right L97.919
　　　　　with
　　　　　　bone involvement without evidence of necrosis L97.916
　　　　　　bone necrosis L97.914
　　　　　　exposed fat layer L97.912
　　　　　　muscle involvement without evidence of necrosis L97.915
　　　　　　muscle necrosis L97.913
　　　　　　skin breakdown only L97.911

Ulcer, ulcerated, ulcerating, ulceration, ulcerative — *continued*
　lower limb — *continued*
　　right — *continued*
　　　with — *continued*
　　　　specified severity NEC L97.918
　　　syphilitic A52.19
　　　thigh L97.109
　　　　with
　　　　　bone involvement without evidence of necrosis L97.106
　　　　　bone necrosis L97.104
　　　　　exposed fat layer L97.102
　　　　　muscle involvement without evidence of necrosis L97.105
　　　　　muscle necrosis L97.103
　　　　　skin breakdown only L97.101
　　　　　specified severity NEC L97.108
　　　　left L97.129
　　　　　with
　　　　　　bone involvement without evidence of necrosis L97.126
　　　　　　bone necrosis L97.124
　　　　　　exposed fat layer L97.122
　　　　　　muscle involvement without evidence of necrosis L97.125
　　　　　　muscle necrosis L97.123
　　　　　　skin breakdown only L97.121
　　　　　　specified severity NEC L97.128
　　　　right L97.119
　　　　　with
　　　　　　bone involvement without evidence of necrosis L97.116
　　　　　　bone necrosis L97.114
　　　　　　exposed fat layer L97.112
　　　　　　muscle involvement without evidence of necrosis L97.115
　　　　　　muscle necrosis L97.113
　　　　　　skin breakdown only L97.111
　　　　　　specified severity NEC L97.118
　　　toe L97.509
　　　　with
　　　　　bone involvement without evidence of necrosis L97.506
　　　　　bone necrosis L97.504
　　　　　exposed fat layer L97.502
　　　　　muscle involvement without evidence of necrosis L97.505
　　　　　muscle necrosis L97.503
　　　　　skin breakdown only L97.501
　　　　　specified severity NEC L97.508
　　　　left L97.529
　　　　　with
　　　　　　bone involvement without evidence of necrosis L97.526
　　　　　　bone necrosis L97.524
　　　　　　exposed fat layer L97.522
　　　　　　muscle involvement without evidence of necrosis L97.525
　　　　　　muscle necrosis L97.523
　　　　　　skin breakdown only L97.521
　　　　　　specified severity NEC L97.528
　　　　right L97.519
　　　　　with
　　　　　　bone involvement without evidence of necrosis L97.516
　　　　　　bone necrosis L97.514
　　　　　　exposed fat layer L97.512
　　　　　　muscle involvement without evidence of necrosis L97.515
　　　　　　muscle necrosis L97.513
　　　　　　skin breakdown only L97.511
　　　　　　specified severity NEC L97.518
　　　varicose — *see* Varix, leg, with, ulcer
　luetic — *see* Ulcer, syphilitic
　lung J98.4
　　tuberculous — *see* Tuberculosis, pulmonary
　malignant — *see* Neoplasm, malignant, by site
　marginal NEC — *see* Ulcer, gastrojejunal
　meatus (urinarius) N34.2
　Meckel's diverticulum Q43.0
　　malignant — *see* Table of Neoplasms, small intestine, malignant
　Meleney's (chronic undermining) — *see* Ulcer, skin
　Mooren's (cornea) — *see* Ulcer, cornea, Mooren's
　mycobacterial (skin) A31.1
　nasopharynx J39.2
　neck, uterus N86
　neurogenic NEC — *see* Ulcer, skin

Ulcer, ulcerated, ulcerating, ulceration, ulcerative — *continued*
　nose, nasal (passage) (infective) (septum) J34.0
　　skin — *see* Ulcer, skin
　　spirochetal A69.8
　　varicose (bleeding) I86.8
　oral mucosa (traumatic) K12.1
　palate (soft) K12.1
　penis (chronic) N48.5
　peptic (site unspecified) K27.9
　　with
　　　hemorrhage K27.4
　　　　and perforation K27.6
　　　perforation K27.5
　　acute K27.3
　　　with
　　　　hemorrhage K27.0
　　　　　and perforation K27.2
　　　　perforation K27.1
　　chronic K27.7
　　　with
　　　　hemorrhage K27.4
　　　　　and perforation K27.6
　　　　perforation K27.5
　　esophagus K22.10
　　　with bleeding K22.11
　　newborn P78.82
　perforating K27.5
　　skin — *see* Ulcer, skin
　peritonsillar J35.8
　phagedenic (tropical) — *see* Ulcer, skin
　pharynx J39.2
　phlebitis — *see* Phlebitis
　plaster — *see* Ulcer, pressure, by site
　popliteal space — *see* Ulcer, lower limb
　postpyloric — *see* Ulcer, duodenum
　prepuce N47.7
　prepyloric — *see* Ulcer, stomach
　pressure (pressure area) L89.9- ☑
　　ankle L89.5- ☑
　　back L89.1- ☑
　　buttock L89.3- ☑
　　coccyx L89.15- ☑
　　contiguous site of back, buttock, hip L89.4- ☑
　　elbow L89.0- ☑
　　face L89.81- ☑
　　head L89.81- ☑
　　heel L89.6- ☑
　　hip L89.2- ☑
　　sacral region (tailbone) L89.15- ☑
　　specified site NEC L89.89- ☑
　　stage 1 (healing) (pre-ulcer skin changes limited to persistent focal edema)
　　　ankle L89.5- ☑
　　　back L89.1- ☑
　　　buttock L89.3- ☑
　　　coccyx L89.15- ☑
　　　contiguous site of back, buttock, hip L89.4- ☑
　　　elbow L89.0- ☑
　　　face L89.81- ☑
　　　head L89.81- ☑
　　　heel L89.6- ☑
　　　hip L89.2- ☑
　　　sacral region (tailbone) L89.15- ☑
　　　specified site NEC L89.89- ☑
　　stage 2 (healing) (abrasion, blister, partial thickness skin loss involving epidermis and/or dermis)
　　　ankle L89.5- ☑
　　　back L89.1- ☑
　　　buttock L89.3- ☑
　　　coccyx L89.15- ☑
　　　contiguous site of back, buttock, hip L89.4- ☑
　　　elbow L89.0- ☑
　　　face L89.81- ☑
　　　head L89.81- ☑
　　　heel L89.6- ☑
　　　hip L89.2- ☑
　　　sacral region (tailbone) L89.15- ☑
　　　specified site NEC L89.89- ☑
　　stage 3 (healing) (full thickness skin loss involving damage or necrosis of subcutaneous tissue)
　　　ankle L89.5- ☑
　　　back L89.1- ☑
　　　buttock L89.3- ☑
　　　coccyx L89.15- ☑
　　　contiguous site of back, buttock, hip L89.4- ☑
　　　elbow L89.0- ☑

Ulcer, ulcerated, ulcerating, ulceration, ulcerative — *continued*	**Ulcer, ulcerated, ulcerating, ulceration, ulcerative —** *continued*	**Ulcus** — *see also* Ulcer

Ulcer, ulcerated, ulcerating, ulceration, ulcerative — *continued*
  pressure — *continued*
    stage 3 — *continued*
      face L89.81- ☑
      head L89.81- ☑
      heel L89.6- ☑
      hip L89.2- ☑
      sacral region (tailbone) L89.15- ☑
      specified site NEC L89.89- ☑
    stage 4 (healing) (necrosis of soft tissues through to underlying muscle, tendon, or bone)
      ankle L89.5- ☑
      back L89.1- ☑
      buttock L89.3- ☑
      coccyx L89.15- ☑
      contiguous site of back, buttock, hip L89.4- ☑
      elbow L89.0- ☑
      face L89.81- ☑
      head L89.81- ☑
      heel L89.6- ☑
      hip L89.2- ☑
      sacral region (tailbone) L89.15- ☑
      specified site NEC L89.89- ☑
    unspecified stage
      ankle L89.5- ☑
      back L89.1- ☑
      buttock L89.3- ☑
      coccyx L89.15- ☑
      contiguous site of back, buttock, hip L89.4- ☑
      elbow L89.0- ☑
      face L89.81- ☑
      head L89.81- ☑
      heel L89.6- ☑
      hip L89.2- ☑
      sacral region (tailbone) L89.15- ☑
      specified site NEC L89.89- ☑
    unstageable
      ankle L89.5- ☑
      back L89.1- ☑
      buttock L89.3- ☑
      coccyx L89.15- ☑
      contiguous site of back, buttock, hip L89.4- ☑
      elbow L89.0- ☑
      face L89.81- ☑
      head L89.81- ☑
      heel L89.6- ☑
      hip L89.2- ☑
      sacral region (tailbone) L89.15- ☑
      specified site NEC L89.89- ☑
  primary of intestine K63.3
    with perforation K63.1
  prostate N41.9
  pyloric — *see* Ulcer, stomach
  rectosigmoid K63.3
    with perforation K63.1
  rectum (sphincter) (solitary) K62.6
    stercoraceous, stercoral K62.6
  retina — *see* Inflammation, chorioretinal
  rodent — *see also* Neoplasm, skin, malignant
  sclera — *see* Scleritis
  scrofulous (tuberculous) A18.2
  scrotum N50.89
    tuberculous A18.15
    varicose I86.1
  seminal vesicle N50.89
  sigmoid — *see* Ulcer, intestine
  skin (atrophic) (chronic) (neurogenic) (non-healing) (perforating) (pyogenic) (trophic) (tropical) L98.499
    with gangrene — *see* Gangrene
    amebic A06.7
    back — *see* Ulcer, back
    buttock — *see* Ulcer, buttock
    decubitus — *see* Ulcer, pressure
    lower limb — *see* Ulcer, lower limb
    mycobacterial A31.1
    specified site NEC L98.499
      with
        bone involvement without evidence of necrosis L98.496
        bone necrosis L98.494
        exposed fat layer L98.492
        muscle involvement without evidence of necrosis L98.495
        muscle necrosis L98.493
        skin breakdown only L98.491
        specified severity NEC L98.498

Ulcer, ulcerated, ulcerating, ulceration, ulcerative — *continued*
  skin — *continued*
    tuberculous (primary) A18.4
    varicose — *see* Ulcer, varicose
  sloughing — *see* Ulcer, skin
  solitary, anus or rectum (sphincter) K62.6
  sore throat J02.9
    streptococcal J02.0
  spermatic cord N50.89
  spine (tuberculous) A18.01
  stasis (venous) — *see* Varix, leg, with, ulcer
    without varicose veins — *see also* Ulcer, by site I87.2
  stercoraceous, stercoral K63.3
    with perforation K63.1
    anus or rectum K62.6
  stoma, stomal — *see* Ulcer, gastrojejunal
  stomach (eroded) (peptic) (round) K25.9
    with
      hemorrhage K25.4
        and perforation K25.6
      perforation K25.5
    acute K25.3
      with
        hemorrhage K25.0
          and perforation K25.2
        perforation K25.1
    chronic K25.7
      with
        hemorrhage K25.4
          and perforation K25.6
        perforation K25.5
  stomal — *see* Ulcer, gastrojejunal
  stomatitis K12.1
  stress — *see* Ulcer, peptic
  strumous (tuberculous) A18.2
  submucosal, bladder — *see* Cystitis, interstitial
  syphilitic (any site) (early) (secondary) A51.39
    late A52.79
    perforating A52.79
      foot A52.11
  testis N50.89
  thigh — *see* Ulcer, lower limb
  throat J39.2
    diphtheritic A36.0
  toe — *see* Ulcer, lower limb
  tongue (traumatic) K14.0
  tonsil J35.8
    diphtheritic A36.0
  trachea J39.8
  trophic — *see* Ulcer, skin
  tropical — *see* Ulcer, skin
  tuberculous — *see* Tuberculosis, ulcer
  tunica vaginalis N50.89
  turbinate J34.89
  typhoid (perforating) — *see* Typhoid
  unspecified site — *see* Ulcer, skin
  urethra (meatus) — *see* Urethritis
  uterus N85.8
    cervix N86
      with cervicitis N72
    neck N86
      with cervicitis N72
  vagina N76.5
    in Behcet's disease M35.2 [N77.0]
    pessary N89.8
  valve, heart I33.0
  varicose (lower limb, any part) — *see also* Varix, leg, with, ulcer
    broad ligament I86.2
    esophagus — *see* Varix, esophagus
    inflamed or infected — *see* Varix, leg, with ulcer, with inflammation
    nasal septum I86.8
    perineum I86.3
    scrotum I86.1
    specified site NEC I86.8
    sublingual I86.0
    vulva I86.3
  vas deferens N50.89
  vulva (acute) (infectional) N76.6
    in (due to)
      Behcet's disease M35.2 [N77.0]
      herpesviral (herpes simplex) infection A60.04
      tuberculosis A18.18
  vulvobuccal, recurring N76.6
  X-ray L58.1
  yaws A66.4
Ulcerosa scarlatina A38.8

Ulcus — *see also* Ulcer
  cutis tuberculosum A18.4
  duodeni — *see* Ulcer, duodenum
  durum (syphilitic) A51.0
    extragenital A51.2
  gastrojejunale — *see* Ulcer, gastrojejunal
  hypostaticum — *see* Ulcer, varicose
  molle (cutis) (skin) A57
  serpens corneae — *see* Ulcer, cornea, central
  ventriculi — *see* Ulcer, stomach
Ulegyria Q04.8
Ulerythema
  ophryogenes, congenital Q84.2
  sycosiforme L73.8
Ullrich (-Bonnevie) (-Turner) **syndrome** — *see also* Turner's syndrome Q87.19
Ullrich-Feichtiger syndrome Q87.0
Ulnar — *see* condition
Ulorrhagia, ulorrhea K06.8
Umbilicus, umbilical — *see* condition
Unable to
  make ends meet Z59.86
  obtain
    adequate
      childcare due to limited financial resources, specified NEC Z59.87
      clothing due to limited financial resources, specified NEC Z59.87
      utilities due to limited financial resources, specified NEC Z59.87
    basic
      needs due to limited financial resources, specified NEC Z59.87
      services in physical environment Z58.81
    internet service, due to unavailability in geographic area Z58.81
    telephone service, due to unavailability in geographic area Z58.81
    utilities, due to inadequate physical environment Z58.81
Unacceptable
  contours of tooth K08.54
  morphology of tooth K08.54
Unaffordable transportation Z59.82
Unavailability (of)
  bed at medical facility Z75.1
  health service-related agencies Z75.4
  medical facilities (at) Z75.3
    due to
      investigation by social service agency Z75.2
      lack of services at home Z75.0
      remoteness from facility Z75.3
      waiting list Z75.1
    home Z75.0
    outpatient clinic Z75.3
  schooling Z55.1
  social service agencies Z75.4
Uncinaria americana infestation B76.1
Uncinariasis B76.9
Uncongenial work Z56.5
Unconscious (ness) — *see* Coma
Under observation — *see* Observation
Underachievement in school Z55.3
Underdevelopment — *see also* Undeveloped
  nose Q30.1
  sexual E30.0
Underdosing — *see also* Table of Drugs and Chemicals, categories T36-T50, with final character 6 Z91.14 ☑
  intentional NEC Z91.128
    due to financial hardship of patient Z91.120
  unintentional NEC Z91.138
    due to patient's age related debility Z91.130
Underfeeding, newborn P92.3
Underfill, endodontic M27.53
Underimmunization status Z28.39
  COVID-19 Z28.31- ☑
    partially vaccinated (for) Z28.311
    unvaccinated (for) Z28.310
Undernourishment — *see* Malnutrition
Undernutrition — *see* Malnutrition
Underweight R63.6
  for gestational age — *see* Light for dates
Underwood's disease P83.0
Undescended — *see also* Malposition, congenital
  cecum Q43.3
  colon Q43.3
  testicle — *see* Cryptorchid
Undeveloped, undevelopment — *see also* Hypoplasia
  brain (congenital) Q02

Undeveloped, undevelopment — continued
  cerebral (congenital) Q02
  heart Q24.8
  lung Q33.6
  testis E29.1
  uterus E30.0
Undiagnosed (disease) R69
Undulant fever — see Brucellosis
Unemployment, anxiety concerning Z56.0
  threatened Z56.2
Unequal length (acquired) (limb) — see also Deformity, limb, unequal length
  leg — see also Deformity, limb, unequal length
    congenital Q72.9- ☑
Unextracted dental root K08.3
Unguis incarnatus L60.0
Unhappiness R45.2
Unicornate uterus Q51.4
  in pregnancy or childbirth O34.00
Unicuspid aortic valve (at birth) (congenital) Q23.81
Unilateral — see also condition
  development, breast N64.89
  organ or site, congenital NEC — see Agenesis, by site
Unilocular heart Q20.8
Unimmunized — see also Underimmunization status
  for COVID-19 Z28.310
Union, abnormal — see also Fusion
  larynx and trachea Q34.8
Universal mesentery Q43.3
Unreliable transportation Z59.82
Unrepairable overhanging of dental restorative materials K08.52
Unroofed coronary sinus Q21.13
Unsafe transportation Z59.82
Unsatisfactory
  restoration of tooth K08.50
    specified NEC K08.59
  sample of cytologic smear
    anus R85.615
    cervix R87.615
    vagina R87.625
  surroundings Z59.19
    work Z56.5
Unsoundness of mind — see Psychosis
Unstable
  back NEC — see Instability, joint, spine
  hip (congenital) Q65.6
    acquired — see Derangement, joint, specified type NEC, hip
  joint — see Instability, joint
    secondary to removal of joint prosthesis M96.89
  lie (mother) O32.0 ☑
  lumbosacral joint (congenital) — see subcategory M53.2
  sacroiliac — see subcategory M53.2 ☑
  spine NEC — see Instability, joint, spine
Unsteadiness on feet R26.81
Untruthfulness, child problem F91.8
Unvaccinated — see also Underimmunization status
  for COVID-19 Z28.310
Unverricht (-Lundborg) **disease or epilepsy** — see Epilepsy, generalized, idiopathic
Unwanted
  multiple moves in the last 12 months Z59.81- ☑
  pregnancy Z64.0
Upbringing, institutional Z62.22
  away from parents NEC Z62.29
  in care of non-parental family member Z62.21
  in foster care Z62.21
  in orphanage or group home Z62.22
  in welfare custody Z62.21
Upper respiratory — see condition
Upset
  gastric K30
  gastrointestinal K30
    psychogenic F45.8
  intestinal (large) (small) K59.9
    psychogenic F45.8
  menstruation N93.9
  mental F48.9
  stomach K30
    psychogenic F45.8
Urachus — see also condition
  patent or persistent Q64.4
Urbach-Oppenheim disease (necrobiosis lipoidica diabeticorum) — see E08-E13 with .620
Urbach's lipoid proteinosis E78.89
Urbach-Wiethe disease E78.89
Urban yellow fever A95.1

Urea
  blood, high — see Uremia
  cycle metabolism disorder — see Disorder, urea cycle metabolism
Uremia, uremic N19
  with
    ectopic or molar pregnancy O08.4
    polyneuropathy N18.9 [G63]
  chronic NOS — see also Disease, kidney, chronic N18.9
    due to hypertension — see Hypertensive, kidney
  complicating
    ectopic or molar pregnancy O08.4
  congenital P96.0
  extrarenal R39.2
  following ectopic or molar pregnancy O08.4
  newborn P96.0
  prerenal R39.2
Ureter, ureteral — see condition
Ureteralgia N23
Ureterectasis — see Hydroureter
Ureteritis N28.89
  cystica N28.86
  due to calculus N20.1
    with calculus, kidney N20.2
      with hydronephrosis N13.2
  gonococcal (acute) (chronic) A54.21
  nonspecific N28.89
Ureterocele N28.89
  congenital (orthotopic) Q62.31
  ectopic Q62.32
Ureterolith, ureterolithiasis — see Calculus, ureter
Ureterostomy
  attention to Z43.6
  status Z93.6
Urethra, urethral — see condition
Urethralgia R39.89
Urethritis (anterior) (posterior) N34.2
  calculous N21.1
  candidal B37.41
  chlamydial A56.01
  diplococcal (gonococcal) A54.01
    with abscess (accessory gland) (periurethral) A54.1
  gonococcal A54.01
    with abscess (accessory gland) (periurethral) A54.1
  nongonococcal N34.1
    Reiter's — see Reiter's disease
  nonspecific N34.1
  nonvenereal N34.1
  postmenopausal N34.2
  puerperal O86.22
  Reiter's — see Reiter's disease
  specified NEC N34.2
  trichomonal or due to Trichomonas (vaginalis) A59.03
Urethrocele N81.0
  with
    cystocele — see Cystocele
    prolapse of uterus — see Prolapse, uterus
Urethrolithiasis (with colic or infection) N21.1
Urethrorectal — see condition
Urethrorrhagia N36.8
Urethrorrhea R36.9
Urethrostomy
  attention to Z43.6
  status Z93.6
Urethrotrigonitis — see Trigonitis
Urethrovaginal — see condition
Urgency
  fecal R15.2
  hypertensive — see Hypertension
  urinary R39.15
Urhidrosis, uridrosis L74.8
Uric acid in blood (increased) E79.0
Uricacidemia (asymptomatic) E79.0
Uricemia (asymptomatic) E79.0
Uricosuria R82.998
Urinary — see condition
Urination
  frequent R35.0
  painful R30.9
Urine
  blood in — see Hematuria
  discharge, excessive R35.89
  enuresis, nonorganic origin F98.0
  extravasation R39.0
  frequency R35.0
  incontinence R32
    nonorganic origin F98.0
  intermittent stream R39.198
  pus in N39.0

Urine — continued
  retention or stasis R33.9
    organic R33.8
      drug-induced R33.0
    psychogenic F45.8
  secretion
    deficient R34
    excessive R35.89
    frequency R35.0
  stream
    intermittent R39.198
    slowing R39.198
    splitting R39.13
    weak R39.12
Urinemia — see Uremia
Urinoma, urethra N36.8
Uroarthritis, infectious (Reiter's) — see Reiter's disease
Urodialysis R34
Urolithiasis — see Calculus, urinary
Uronephrosis — see Hydronephrosis
Uropathy N39.9
  obstructive N13.9
    specified NEC N13.8
  reflux N13.9
    specified NEC N13.8
  vesicoureteral reflux-associated — see Reflux, vesicoureteral
Urosepsis — code to condition
Urticaria L50.9
  with angioneurotic edema T78.3 ☑
    hereditary D84.1
  allergic L50.0
  cholinergic L50.5
  chronic L50.8
  cold, familial L50.2
  contact L50.6
  dermatographic L50.3
  due to
    cold or heat L50.2
    drugs L50.0
    food L50.0
    inhalants L50.0
    plants L50.6
    serum — see also Reaction, serum T80.69 ☑
  factitial L50.3
  familial cold M04.2
  giant T78.3 ☑
    hereditary D84.1
  gigantea T78.3 ☑
  idiopathic L50.1
  larynx T78.3 ☑
    hereditary D84.1
  neonatorum P83.88
  nonallergic L50.1
  papulosa (Hebra) L28.2
  pigmentosa D47.01
    congenital Q82.2
    of neonatal onset Q82.2
    of newborn onset Q82.2
  recurrent periodic L50.8
  serum — see also Reaction, serum T80.69 ☑
  solar L56.3
  specified type NEC L50.8
  thermal (cold) (heat) L50.2
  vibratory L50.4
  xanthelasmoidea — see Urticaria pigmentosa
Use (of)
  alcohol — see also Alcohol, alcoholic, by disorder F10.90
    with
      anxiety disorder F10.980
      intoxication F10.929
      sleep disorder F10.982
      withdrawal F10.939
        with
          perceptual disturbance F10.932
        delirium F10.931
        uncomplicated F10.930
    harmful — see Abuse, alcohol
    in remission F10.91
  amphetamines — see Use, stimulant NEC
  caffeine — see Use, stimulant NEC
  cannabis F12.90
    with
      anxiety disorder F12.980
      intoxication F12.929
        with
          delirium F12.921
          perceptual disturbance F12.922

Use — *continued*
  cannabis — *continued*
    with — *continued*
      intoxication — *continued*
        uncomplicated F12.920
      other specified disorder F12.988
      psychosis F12.959
        delusions F12.950
        hallucinations F12.951
      unspecified disorder F12.99
      withdrawal F12.93
    in remission F12.91
  cocaine F14.90
    with
      anxiety disorder F14.980
      intoxication F14.929
        with
          delirium F14.921
          perceptual disturbance F14.922
        uncomplicated F14.920
      other specified disorder F14.988
      psychosis F14.959
        delusions F14.950
        hallucinations F14.951
      sexual dysfunction F14.981
      sleep disorder F14.982
      unspecified disorder F14.99
      withdrawal F14.93
    harmful — *see* Abuse, drug, cocaine
    in remission F14.91
  drug(s) NEC F19.90
    with sleep disorder F19.982
    harmful — *see* Abuse, drug, by type
  hallucinogen NEC F16.90
    with
      anxiety disorder F16.980
      intoxication F16.929
        with
          delirium F16.921
        uncomplicated F16.920
      mood disorder F16.94
      other specified disorder F16.988
      perception disorder (flashbacks) F16.983
      psychosis F16.959
        delusions F16.950
        hallucinations F16.951
      unspecified disorder F16.99
    harmful — *see* Abuse, drug, hallucinogen NEC
    in remission F16.91
  inhalants F18.90
    with
      anxiety disorder F18.980
      intoxication F18.929
        with delirium F18.921
        uncomplicated F18.920
      mood disorder F18.94
      other specified disorder F18.988
      persisting dementia F18.97
      psychosis F18.959
        delusions F18.950
        hallucinations F18.951
      unspecified disorder F18.99
    harmful — *see* Abuse, drug, inhalant
    in remission F18.91
  methadone — *see* Use, opioid
  nonprescribed drugs F19.90
    harmful — *see* Abuse, non-psychoactive substance
  opioid F11.90
    with
      disorder F11.99
        mood F11.94
        sleep F11.982
        specified type NEC F11.988
      intoxication F11.929
        with
          delirium F11.921
          perceptual disturbance F11.922
        uncomplicated F11.920
      opioid-associated amnestic syndrome F11.988
      withdrawal F11.93
    harmful — *see* Abuse, drug, opioid
    in remission F11.91
  patent medicines F19.90
    harmful — *see* Abuse, non-psychoactive substance
  psychoactive drug NEC F19.90
    with
      anxiety disorder F19.980
      intoxication F19.929

Use — *continued*
  psychoactive drug — *continued*
    with — *continued*
      intoxication — *continued*
        with
          delirium F19.921
          perceptual disturbance F19.922
        uncomplicated F19.920
      mood disorder F19.94
      other specified disorder F19.988
      persisting
        amnestic disorder F19.96
        dementia F19.97
      psychosis F19.959
        delusions F19.950
        hallucinations F19.951
      sexual dysfunction F19.981
      sleep disorder F19.982
      unspecified disorder F19.99
      withdrawal F19.939
        with
          delirium F19.931
          perceptual disturbance F19.932
        uncomplicated F19.930
    harmful — *see* Abuse, drug NEC, psychoactive NEC
    in remission F19.91
  sedative, hypnotic, or anxiolytic F13.90
    with
      anxiety disorder F13.980
      intoxication F13.929
        with
          delirium F13.921
        uncomplicated F13.920
      other specified disorder F13.988
      persisting
        amnestic disorder F13.96
        dementia F13.97
      psychosis F13.959
        delusions F13.950
        hallucinations F13.951
      sexual dysfunction F13.981
      sleep disorder F13.982
      unspecified disorder F13.99
    harmful — *see* Abuse, drug, sedative, hypnotic, or
      anxiolytic
    in remission F13.91
  stimulant NEC F15.90
    with
      anxiety disorder F15.980
      intoxication F15.929
        with
          delirium F15.921
          perceptual disturbance F15.922
        uncomplicated F15.920
      mood disorder F15.94
      other specified disorder F15.988
      psychosis F15.959
        delusions F15.950
        hallucinations F15.951
      sexual dysfunction F15.981
      sleep disorder F15.982
      unspecified disorder F15.99
      withdrawal F15.93
    harmful — *see* Abuse, drug, stimulant NEC
    in remission F15.91
  tobacco Z72.0
    with dependence — *see* Dependence, drug, nicotine
  volatile solvents — *see also* Use, inhalant F18.90
    harmful — *see* Abuse, drug, inhalant
Usher-Senear disease or syndrome L10.4
Uta B55.1
Uteromegaly N85.2
Uterovaginal — *see* condition
Uterovesical — *see* condition
Uveal — *see* condition
Uveitis (anterior) — *see also* Iridocyclitis
  acute — *see* Iridocyclitis, acute
  chronic — *see* Iridocyclitis, chronic
  due to toxoplasmosis (acquired) B58.09
    congenital P37.1
  granulomatous — *see* Iridocyclitis, chronic
  heterochromic — *see* Cyclitis, Fuchs' heterochromic
  lens-induced — *see* Iridocyclitis, lens-induced
  posterior — *see* Chorioretinitis
  sympathetic H44.13- ☑
  syphilitic (secondary) A51.43
    congenital (early) A50.01
    late A52.71
  tuberculous A18.54

Uveoencephalitis — *see* Inflammation, chorioretinal
Uveokeratitis — *see* Iridocyclitis
Uveoparotitis D86.89
Uvula — *see* condition
Uvulitis (acute) (catarrhal) (chronic) (membranous) (suppurative) (ulcerative) K12.2

V

Vaccination (prophylactic)
  complication or reaction — *see* Complications, vaccination
  delayed Z28.9
  encounter for Z23
  not done — *see* Immunization, not done
  partial — *see also* Underimmunization status
    for COVID-19 Z28.311
Vaccinia (generalized) (localized) T88.1 ☑
  congenital P35.8
  without vaccination B08.011
Vacuum, in sinus (accessory) (nasal) J34.89
Vagabond, vagabondage Z59.00
Vagabond's disease B85.1
Vagina, vaginal — *see* condition
Vaginalitis (tunica) (testis) N49.1
Vaginismus (reflex) N94.2
  functional F52.5
  nonorganic F52.5
  psychogenic F52.5
  secondary N94.2
Vaginitis (acute) (circumscribed) (diffuse) (emphysematous) (nonvenereal) (ulcerative) N76.0
  with ectopic or molar pregnancy O08.0
  amebic A06.82
  atrophic, postmenopausal N95.2
  bacterial N76.0
  blennorrhagic (gonococcal) A54.02
  candidal (acute) B37.31
    chronic (recurrent) B37.32
  chlamydial A56.02
  chronic N76.1
  due to Trichomonas (vaginalis) A59.01
  following ectopic or molar pregnancy O08.0
  gonococcal A54.02
    with abscess (accessory gland) (periurethral) A54.1
  granuloma A58
  in (due to)
    candidiasis (acute) B37.31
      chronic (recurrent) B37.32
    herpesviral (herpes simplex) infection A60.04
    pinworm infection B80 *[N77.1]*
  monilial (acute) B37.31
    chronic (recurrent) B37.32
  mycotic (candidal) (acute) B37.31
    chronic (recurrent) B37.32
  postmenopausal atrophic N95.2
  puerperal (postpartum) O86.13
  senile (atrophic) N95.2
  subacute or chronic N76.1
  syphilitic (early) A51.0
    late A52.76
  trichomonal A59.01
  tuberculous A18.18
Vaginosis — *see* Vaginitis
Vagotonia G52.2
Vagrancy Z59.00
VAIN — *see* Neoplasia, intraepithelial, vagina
Vallecula — *see* condition
Valley fever B38.0
Valsuani's disease O99.03
Valve, valvular (formation) — *see also* condition
  cerebral ventricle (communicating) in situ Z98.2
  cervix, internal os Q51.828
  congenital NEC — *see* Atresia, by site
  ureter (pelvic junction) (vesical orifice) Q62.39
  urethra (congenital) (posterior) Q64.2
Valvulitis (chronic) — *see* Endocarditis
Valvulopathy — *see* Endocarditis
Van Bogaert's leukoencephalopathy (sclerosing) (subacute) A81.1
Van Bogaert-Scherer-Epstein disease or syndrome E75.5
Van Buchem's syndrome M85.2
Van Creveld-von Gierke disease E74.01
Van der Hoeve (-de Kleyn) **syndrome** Q78.0
Van der Woude's syndrome Q38.0
Van Neck's disease or osteochondrosis M91.0
Vanishing lung J44.89
Vapor asphyxia or suffocation T59.9 ☑

Vapor asphyxia or suffocation — *continued*
  specified agent — *see* Table of Drugs and Chemicals
Variance, lethal ball, prosthetic heart valve T82.09 ☑
Variants, thalassemic D56.8
Variations in hair color L67.1
Varicella B01.9
  with
    complications NEC B01.89
    encephalitis B01.11
    encephalomyelitis B01.11
    meningitis B01.0
    myelitis B01.12
    pneumonia B01.2
  congenital P35.8
Varices — *see* Varix
Varicocele (scrotum) (thrombosed) I86.1
  ovary I86.2
  perineum I86.3
  spermatic cord (ulcerated) I86.1
Varicose
  aneurysm (ruptured) I77.0
  dermatitis — *see* Varix, leg, with, inflammation
  eczema — *see* Varix, leg, with, inflammation
  phlebitis — *see* Varix, with, inflammation
  tumor — *see* Varix
  ulcer (lower limb, any part) — *see also* Varix, leg, with, ulcer
    anus — *see also* Hemorrhoids K64.8
    esophagus — *see* Varix, esophagus
    inflamed or infected — *see* Varix, leg, with ulcer, with inflammation
    nasal septum I86.8
    perineum I86.3
    scrotum I86.1
    specified site NEC I86.8
  vein — *see* Varix
  vessel — *see* Varix, leg
Varicosis, varicosities, varicosity — *see* Varix
Variola (major) (minor) B03
Varioloid B03
Varix (lower limb) I83.90
  with
    bleeding I83.899
    edema I83.899
    inflammation I83.10
      with ulcer (venous) I83.209
    pain I83.819
    rupture I83.899
    specified complication NEC I83.899
    stasis dermatitis I83.10
      with ulcer (venous) I83.209
    swelling I83.899
    ulcer I83.009
      with inflammation I83.209
  aneurysmal I77.0
  asymptomatic I83.9- ☑
  bladder I86.2
  broad ligament I86.2
  complicating
    childbirth (lower extremity) O87.4
      anus or rectum O87.2
      genital (vagina, vulva or perineum) O87.8
    pregnancy (lower extremity) O22.0- ☑
      anus or rectum O22.4- ☑
      genital (vagina, vulva or perineum) O22.1- ☑
    puerperium (lower extremity) O87.4
      anus or rectum O87.2
      genital (vagina, vulva, perineum) O87.8
  congenital (any site) Q27.8
  esophagus (idiopathic) (primary) (ulcerated) I85.00
    bleeding I85.01
    congenital Q27.8
    in (due to)
      alcoholic liver disease I85.10
        bleeding I85.11
      cirrhosis of liver I85.10
        bleeding I85.11
      portal hypertension I85.10
        bleeding I85.11
      schistosomiasis I85.10
        bleeding I85.11
      toxic liver disease I85.10
        bleeding I85.11
    secondary I85.10
      bleeding I85.11
  gastric I86.4
  inflamed or infected I83.10
    ulcerated I83.209

Varix — *continued*
  labia (majora) I86.3
  leg (asymptomatic) I83.9- ☑
    with
      edema I83.899
      inflammation I83.10
        with ulcer — *see* Varix, leg, with, ulcer, with inflammation by site
      pain I83.819
      specified complication NEC I83.899
      swelling I83.899
      ulcer I83.0- ☑
        with inflammation I83.2- ☑
        ankle I83.003
          with inflammation I83.203
        calf I83.002
          with inflammation I83.202
        foot NEC I83.005
          with inflammation I83.205
        heel I83.004
          with inflammation I83.204
        lower leg NEC I83.008
          with inflammation I83.208
        midfoot I83.004
          with inflammation I83.204
        thigh I83.001
          with inflammation I83.201
    bilateral (asymptomatic) I83.93
      with
        edema I83.893
        pain I83.813
        specified complication NEC I83.893
        swelling I83.893
        ulcer I83.0- ☑
          with inflammation I83.209
    left (asymptomatic) I83.92
      with
        edema I83.892
        inflammation I83.12
          with ulcer — *see* Varix, leg, with, ulcer, with inflammation by site
        pain I83.812
        specified complication NEC I83.892
        swelling I83.892
        ulcer I83.029
          with inflammation I83.229
          ankle I83.023
            with inflammation I83.223
          calf I83.022
            with inflammation I83.222
          foot NEC I83.025
            with inflammation I83.225
          heel I83.024
            with inflammation I83.224
          lower leg NEC I83.028
            with inflammation I83.228
          midfoot I83.024
            with inflammation I83.224
          thigh I83.021
            with inflammation I83.221
    right (asymptomatic) I83.91
      with
        edema I83.891
        inflammation I83.11
          with ulcer — *see* Varix, leg, with, ulcer, with inflammation by site
        pain I83.811
        specified complication NEC I83.891
        swelling I83.891
        ulcer I83.019
          with inflammation I83.219
          ankle I83.013
            with inflammation I83.213
          calf I83.012
            with inflammation I83.212
          foot NEC I83.015
            with inflammation I83.215
          heel I83.014
            with inflammation I83.214
          lower leg NEC I83.018
            with inflammation I83.218
          midfoot I83.014
            with inflammation I83.214
          thigh I83.011
            with inflammation I83.211
  nasal septum I86.8
  orbit I86.8
    congenital Q27.8
  ovary I86.2

Varix — *continued*
  papillary I78.1
  pelvis I86.2
  perineum I86.3
  pharynx I86.8
  placenta O43.89- ☑
  renal papilla I86.8
  retina H35.09
  scrotum (ulcerated) I86.1
  sigmoid colon I86.8
  specified site NEC I86.8
  spinal (cord) (vessels) I86.8
  spleen, splenic (vein) (with phlebolith) I86.8
  stomach I86.4
  sublingual I86.0
  ulcerated I86.8
    inflamed or infected I83.209
  uterine ligament I86.2
  vagina I86.8
  vocal cord I86.8
  vulva I86.3
Vas deferens — *see* condition
Vas deferentitis N49.1
Vasa previa O69.4 ☑
  hemorrhage from, affecting newborn P50.0
Vascular — *see also* condition
  loop on optic papilla Q14.2
  spasm I73.9
  spider I78.1
Vascularization, cornea — *see* Neovascularization, cornea
Vasculitis I77.6
  allergic D69.0
  ANCA (antineutrophilic cytoplasmic antibody) associated I77.82
  ANCA (antineutrophilic cytoplasmic antibody) positive I77.82
  antineutrophilic cytoplasmic antibody [ANCA] I77.82
  cryoglobulinemic D89.1
  disseminated I77.6
  hypocomplementemic M31.8
  kidney I77.89
  leukocytoclastic M31.0
  livedoid L95.0
  nodular L95.8
  retina H35.06- ☑
  rheumatic — *see* Fever, rheumatic
  rheumatoid — *see* Rheumatoid, vasculitis
  skin (limited to) L95.9
    specified NEC L95.8
  systemic M31.8
Vasculopathy, necrotizing M31.9
  cardiac allograft T86.290
  specified NEC M31.8
Vasitis (nodosa) N49.1
  tuberculous A18.15
Vasodilation I73.9
Vasomotor — *see* condition
Vasoplasty, after previous sterilization Z31.0
  aftercare Z31.42
Vasospasm (vasoconstriction) — *see also* Angiospasm I73.9
  cerebral (cerebrovascular) (artery) I67.848
    reversible I67.841
  coronary I20.1
  nerve
    arm — *see* Mononeuropathy, upper limb
      brachial plexus G54.0
      cervical plexus G54.2
    leg — *see* Mononeuropathy, lower limb
  peripheral NOS I73.9
  retina (artery) — *see* Occlusion, artery, retina
Vasospastic — *see* condition
Vasovagal attack (paroxysmal) R55
  psychogenic F45.8
VATER syndrome Q87.2
Vater's ampulla — *see* condition
Vegetation, vegetative
  adenoid (nasal fossa) J35.8
  endocarditis (acute) (any valve) (subacute) I33.0
  heart (mycotic) (valve) I33.0
Veil
  Jackson's Q43.3
Vein, venous — *see* condition
Veldt sore — *see* Ulcer, skin
Velpeau's hernia — *see* Hernia, femoral
Venereal
  bubo A55
  disease A64
  granuloma inguinale A58
  lymphogranuloma (Durand-Nicolas-Favre) A55

Venofibrosis I87.8
Venom, venomous — *see* Table of Drugs and Chemicals, by animal or substance, poisoning
Venous — *see* condition
Ventilator lung, newborn P27.8
Ventral — *see* condition
Ventricle, ventricular — *see also* condition
    escape I49.3
    inversion Q20.5
Ventriculitis (cerebral) — *see also* Encephalitis G04.90
Ventriculostomy status Z98.2
Vernet's syndrome G52.7
Verneuil's disease (syphilitic bursitis) A52.78
Verruca (due to HPV) (filiformis) (simplex) (viral) (vulgaris) B07.9
    acuminata A63.0
    necrogenica (primary) (tuberculosa) A18.4
    plana B07.8
    plantaris B07.0
    seborrheica L82.1
        inflamed L82.0
    senile (seborrheic) L82.1
        inflamed L82.0
    tuberculosa (primary) A18.4
    venereal A63.0
Verrucosities — *see* Verruca
Verruga peruana, peruviana A44.1
Version
    cervix — *see* Malposition, uterus
    uterus (postinfectional) (postpartal, old) — *see* Malposition, uterus
Vertebra, vertebral — *see* condition
Vertical talus (congenital) Q66.80
    left foot Q66.82
    right foot Q66.81
Vertigo R42
    auditory — *see* Vertigo, aural
    aural H81.31- ☑
    benign paroxysmal (positional) H81.1- ☑
    central (origin) H81.4
    cerebral H81.4
    Dix and Hallpike (epidemic) — *see* Neuronitis, vestibular
    due to infrasound T75.23 ☑
    epidemic A88.1
        Dix and Hallpike — *see* Neuronitis, vestibular
        Pedersen's — *see* Neuronitis, vestibular
        vestibular neuronitis — *see* Neuronitis, vestibular
    hysterical F44.89
    infrasound T75.23 ☑
    labyrinthine — *see* subcategory H81.0 ☑
    laryngeal R05.4
    malignant positional H81.4
    Meniere's — *see* subcategory H81.0 ☑
    menopausal N95.1
    otogenic — *see* Vertigo, aural
    paroxysmal positional, benign — *see* Vertigo, benign paroxysmal
    Pedersen's (epidemic) — *see* Neuronitis, vestibular
    peripheral NEC H81.39- ☑
    positional
        benign paroxysmal — *see* Vertigo, benign paroxysmal
        malignant H81.4
Very-low-density-lipoprotein-type (VLDL) **hyperlipoproteinemia** E78.1
Vesania — *see* Psychosis
Vesical — *see* condition
Vesicle
    cutaneous R23.8
    seminal — *see* condition
    skin R23.8
Vesicocolic — *see* condition
Vesicoperineal — *see* condition
Vesicorectal — *see* condition
Vesicourethrorectal — *see* condition
Vesicovaginal — *see* condition
Vesicular — *see* condition
Vesiculitis (seminal) N49.0
    amebic A06.82
    gonorrheal (acute) (chronic) A54.23
    trichomonal A59.09
    tuberculous A18.15
Vestibulitis (ear) — *see also* subcategory H83.0 ☑
    nose (external) J34.89
    vulvar N94.810
Vestibulopathy , acute peripheral (recurrent) — *see* Neuronitis, vestibular
Vestige, vestigial — *see also* Persistence
    branchial Q18.0

Vestige, vestigial — *continued*
    structures in vitreous Q14.0
Vibration
    adverse effects T75.20 ☑
        pneumatic hammer syndrome T75.21 ☑
        specified effect NEC T75.29 ☑
        vasospastic syndrome T75.22 ☑
        vertigo from infrasound T75.23 ☑
    exposure (occupational) Z57.7
    vertigo T75.23 ☑
Vibriosis A28.9
Victim (of)
    crime Z65.4
    disaster Z65.5
    terrorism Z65.4
    torture Z65.4
    war Z65.5
Vidal's disease L28.0
Villaret's syndrome G52.7
Villous — *see* condition
VIN — *see* Neoplasia, intraepithelial, vulva
Vincent's infection (angina) (gingivitis) A69.1
    stomatitis NEC A69.1
Vinson-Plummer syndrome D50.1
Violence, physical R45.6
Viosterol deficiency — *see* Deficiency, calciferol
Vipoma — *see* Neoplasm, malignant, by site
Viremia B34.9
Virilism (adrenal) E25.9
    congenital E25.0
Virilization (female) (suprarenal) E25.9
    congenital E25.0
    isosexual E28.2
Virulent bubo A57
Virus, viral — *see also* condition
    as cause of disease classified elsewhere B97.89
        respiratory syncytial virus (RSV) — *see* Virus, respiratory syncytial (RSV)
    cytomegalovirus B25.9
    human immunodeficiency (HIV) — *see* Human, immunodeficiency virus (HIV) disease
    infection — *see* Infection, virus
    respiratory syncytial (RSV)
        as cause of disease classified elsewhere B97.4
        bronchiolitis J21.0
        bronchitis J20.5
        bronchopneumonia J12.1
        otitis media H65.- ☑ *[B97.4]*
        pneumonia J12.1
        upper respiratory infection J06.9 *[B97.4]*
    specified NEC B34.8
    swine influenza (viruses that normally cause infections in pigs) — *see also* Influenza, due to, identified novel influenza A virus J09.X2
    West Nile (fever) A92.30
        with
            complications NEC A92.39
            cranial nerve disorders A92.32
            encephalitis A92.31
            encephalomyelitis A92.31
            neurologic manifestation NEC A92.32
            optic neuritis A92.32
            polyradiculitis A92.32
Viscera, visceral — *see* condition
Visceroptosis K63.4
Visible peristalsis R19.2
Vision, visual
    binocular, suppression H53.34
    blurred, blurring H53.8
        hysterical F44.6
    defect, defective NEC H54.7
    disorientation (syndrome) H53.8
    disturbance H53.9
        hysterical F44.6
    double H53.2
    examination Z01.00
        with abnormal findings Z01.01
        following failed vision screening Z01.020
            with abnormal findings Z01.021
    field, limitation (defect) — *see* Defect, visual field
    hallucinations R44.1
    halos H53.19
    loss — *see* Loss, vision
        sudden — *see* Disturbance, vision, subjective, loss, sudden
    low (both eyes) — *see* Low, vision
    perception, simultaneous without fusion H53.33
Vitality, lack or want of R53.83

Vitality, lack or want of — *continued*
    newborn P96.89
Vitamin deficiency — *see* Deficiency, vitamin
Vitelline duct, persistent Q43.0
Vitiligo L80
    eyelid H02.739
        left H02.736
            lower H02.735
            upper H02.734
        right H02.733
            lower H02.732
            upper H02.731
    pinta A67.2
    vulva N90.89
Vitreal corneal syndrome H59.01- ☑
Vitreoretinopathy, proliferative — *see also* Retinopathy, proliferative
    with retinal detachment — *see* Detachment, retina, traction
Vitreous — *see also* condition
    touch syndrome — *see* Complication, postprocedural, following cataract surgery
Vocal cord — *see* condition
Vogt-Koyanagi syndrome H20.82- ☑
Vogt's disease or syndrome G80.3
Vogt-Spielmeyer amaurotic idiocy or disease E75.4
Voice
    change R49.9
        specified NEC R49.8
    loss — *see* Aphonia
Volhynian fever A79.0
Volkmann's ischemic contracture or paralysis (complicating trauma) T79.6 ☑
Volvulus (bowel) (colon) (intestine) K56.2
    with perforation K56.2
    congenital Q43.8
    duodenum K31.5
    fallopian tube — *see* Torsion, fallopian tube
    oviduct — *see* Torsion, fallopian tube
    stomach (due to absence of gastrocolic ligament) K31.89
Vomiting R11.10
    with nausea R11.2
    asphyxia — *see* Foreign body, by site, causing asphyxia, gastric contents
    bilious (cause unknown) R11.14
        following gastro-intestinal surgery K91.0
        in newborn P92.01
    blood — *see* Hematemesis
    causing asphyxia, choking, or suffocation — *see* Foreign body, by site
    cyclical, in migraine G43.A0 (*following* G43.7)
        with refractory migraine G43.A1 (*following* G43.7)
        intractable G43.A1 (*following* G43.7)
        not intractable G43.A0 (*following* G43.7)
        psychogenic F50.89
        without refractory migraine G43.A0 (*following* G43.7)
    cyclical syndrome NOS (unrelated to migraine) R11.15
    fecal matter R11.13
    following gastrointestinal surgery K91.0
        psychogenic F50.89
    functional K31.89
    hysterical F50.89
    nervous F50.89
    neurotic F50.89
    newborn NEC P92.09
        bilious P92.01
    periodic R11.10
        psychogenic F50.89
    persistent R11.15
    projectile R11.12
    psychogenic F50.89
    uremic — *see* Uremia
    without nausea R11.11
Vomito negro — *see* Fever, yellow
Von Bezold's abscess — *see* Mastoiditis, acute
Von Economo-Cruchet disease A85.8
Von Eulenburg's disease G71.19
Von Gierke's disease E74.01
Von Hippel (-Lindau) **disease or syndrome** Q85.83
Von Jaksch's anemia or disease D64.89
Von Recklinghausen
    disease (neurofibromatosis) Q85.01
        bones E21.0
Von Schroetter's syndrome I82.890
Von Willebrand (-Jurgens) (-Minot) **disease or syndrome** — *see* Disease, von Willebrand
Von Zumbusch's disease L40.1
Voyeurism F65.3
Vrolik's disease Q78.0

☑ **Additional Character Required** — Refer to the Tabular List for Character Selection

Vulva — see condition
Vulvismus N94.2
Vulvitis (acute) (allergic) (atrophic) (hypertrophic) (intertriginous) (senile) N76.2
  with ectopic or molar pregnancy O08.0
  adhesive, congenital Q52.79
  blennorrhagic (gonococcal) A54.02
  candidal (acute) B37.31
    chronic (recurrent) B37.32
  chlamydial A56.02
  due to Haemophilus ducreyi A57
  following ectopic or molar pregnancy O08.0
  gonococcal A54.02
    with abscess (accessory gland) (periurethral) A54.1
  herpesviral A60.04
  leukoplakic N90.4
  monilial (acute) B37.31
    chronic (recurrent) B37.32
  puerperal (postpartum) O86.19
  subacute or chronic N76.3
  syphilitic (early) A51.0
    late A52.76
  trichomonal A59.01
  tuberculous A18.18
Vulvodynia N94.819
  specified NEC N94.818
Vulvorectal — see condition
Vulvovaginitis (acute) — see Vaginitis

W

Waiting list, person on Z75.1
  for organ transplant Z76.82
  undergoing social agency investigation Z75.2
Waldenstrom
  hypergammaglobulinemia D89.0-
  syndrome or macroglobulinemia C88.0- ☑
Waldenstrom-Kjellberg syndrome D50.1
Walking
  difficulty R26.2
    psychogenic F44.4
  sleep F51.3
    hysterical F44.89
Wall, abdominal — see condition
Wallenberg's disease or syndrome G46.3
Wallgren's disease I87.8
Wandering
  gallbladder, congenital Q44.1
  in diseases classified elsewhere Z91.83
  kidney, congenital Q63.8
  organ or site, congenital NEC — see Malposition, congenital, by site
  pacemaker (heart) I49.8
  spleen D73.89
War neurosis F48.8
Wart (due to HPV) (filiform) (infectious) (viral) B07.9
  anogenital region (venereal) A63.0
  common B07.8
  external genital organs (venereal) A63.0
  flat B07.8
  Hassal-Henle's (of cornea) H18.49
  Peruvian A44.1
  plantar B07.0
  prosector (tuberculous) A18.4
  seborrheic L82.1
    inflamed L82.0
  senile (seborrheic) L82.1
    inflamed L82.0
  tuberculous A18.4
  venereal A63.0
Warthin's tumor — see Neoplasm, salivary gland or duct, benign
Wassilieff's disease A27.0
Wasting
  disease (syndrome) E88.A
    due to
      malnutrition E43
        with marasmus E41
      underlying condition E88.A
  extreme (due to malnutrition) E43
    with marasmus E41
  muscle NEC — see Atrophy, muscle
Water
  clefts (senile cataract) — see Cataract, senile, incipient
  deprivation of T73.1 ☑
  intoxication E87.79
  itch B76.9
  lack of T73.1 ☑

Water — continued
  lack of — continued
    safe drinking Z58.6
    loading E87.70
    on
      brain — see Hydrocephalus
      chest J94.8
    poisoning E87.79
Waterbrash R12
Waterhouse (-Friderichsen) **syndrome or disease** (meningococcal) A39.1
Water-losing nephritis N25.89
Watermelon stomach K31.819
  with hemorrhage K31.811
  without hemorrhage K31.819
Watsoniasis B66.8
Wax in ear — see Impaction, cerumen
Weak, weakening, weakness (generalized) R53.1
  arches (acquired) — see also Deformity, limb, flat foot
  bladder (sphincter) R32
  facial R29.810
    following
      cerebrovascular disease I69.992
        cerebral infarction I69.392
        intracerebral hemorrhage I69.192
        nontraumatic intracranial hemorrhage NEC I69.292
        specified disease NEC I69.892
        stroke I69.392
        subarachnoid hemorrhage I69.092
  foot (double) — see also Weak, arches
  heart, cardiac — see Failure, heart
  mind F70
  muscle M62.81
  myocardium — see Failure, heart
  newborn P96.89
  pelvic fundus N81.89
  pubocervical tissue N81.82
  rectovaginal tissue N81.83
  senile R54
  urinary stream R39.12
  valvular — see Endocarditis
Wear, worn (with normal or routine use)
  articular bearing surface of internal joint prosthesis — see Complications, joint prosthesis, mechanical, wear of articular bearing surfaces, by site
  device, implant or graft — see Complications, by site, mechanical complication
  tooth, teeth (approximal) (hard tissues) (interproximal) (occlusal) K03.0
Weather, weathered
  effects of
    cold T69.9 ☑
      specified effect NEC T69.8 ☑
    hot — see Heat
  skin L57.8
Weaver's syndrome Q87.3
Web, webbed (congenital)
  duodenal Q43.8
  esophagus Q39.4
  fingers Q70.1- ☑
  larynx (glottic) (subglottic) Q31.0
  neck (pterygium colli) Q18.3
  Paterson-Kelly D50.1
  popliteal syndrome Q87.89
  toes Q70.3- ☑
Weber-Christian disease M35.6
Weber-Cockayne syndrome (epidermolysis bullosa) Q81.8
Weber-Gubler syndrome G46.3
Weber-Leyden syndrome G46.3
Weber-Osler syndrome I78.0
Weber's paralysis or syndrome G46.3
Wedge-shaped or wedging vertebra — see Collapse, vertebra NEC
Wegener's granulomatosis or syndrome M31.30
  with
    kidney involvement M31.31
    lung involvement M31.30
      with kidney involvement M31.31
Wegner's disease A50.02
Weight
  1000-2499 grams at birth (low) — see Low, birthweight
  999 grams or less at birth (extremely low) — see Low, birthweight, extreme
  and length below 10th percentile for gestational age P05.1- ☑
  below but length above 10th percentile for gestational age P05.0- ☑

Weight — continued
  gain (abnormal) (excessive) R63.5
    in pregnancy — see Pregnancy, complicated by, excessive weight gain
    low — see Pregnancy, complicated by, insufficient, weight gain
  loss (abnormal) (cause unknown) R63.4
Weightlessness (effect of) T75.82 ☑
Weil (I)-**Marchesani syndrome** Q87.19
Weil's disease A27.0
Weingarten's syndrome J82.89
Weir Mitchell's disease I73.81
Weiss-Baker syndrome G90.09
Wells' disease L98.3
Wen — see Cyst, sebaceous
Wenckebach's block or phenomenon I44.1
Werdnig-Hoffmann syndrome (muscular atrophy) G12.0
Werlhof's disease D69.3
Wermer's disease or syndrome E31.21
Werner-His disease A79.0
Werner's disease or syndrome E34.8
Wernicke-Korsakoff's syndrome or psychosis (alcoholic) F10.96
  with dependence F10.26
  drug-induced
    due to drug abuse — see Abuse, drug, by type, with amnestic disorder
    due to drug dependence — see Dependence, drug, by type, with amnestic disorder
  nonalcoholic F04
Wernicke-Posadas disease B38.9
Wernicke's
  developmental aphasia F80.2
  disease or syndrome E51.2
  encephalopathy E51.2
  polioencephalitis, superior E51.2
West African fever B50.8
Westphal-Strumpell syndrome E83.01
West's syndrome — see Epilepsy, spasms
Wet
  feet, tropical (maceration) (syndrome) — see Immersion, foot
  lung (syndrome), newborn P22.1
Wharton's duct — see condition
Wheal — see Urticaria
Wheezing R06.2
Whiplash injury S13.4 ☑
Whipple's disease — see also subcategory M14.8- K90.81
Whipworm (disease) (infection) (infestation) B79
Whistling face Q87.0
White — see also condition
  kidney, small N03.9
  leg, puerperal, postpartum, childbirth O87.1
  mouth B37.0
  patches of mouth K13.29
  spot lesions, teeth
    chewing surface K02.51
    pit and fissure surface K02.51
    smooth surface K02.61
Whitehead L70.0
Whitlow — see also Cellulitis, digit
  with lymphangitis — see Lymphangitis, acute, digit
  herpesviral B00.89
Whitmore's disease or fever — see Melioidosis
Whooping cough A37.90
  with pneumonia A37.91
    due to Bordetella
      bronchiseptica A37.81
      parapertussis A37.11
      pertussis A37.01
    specified organism NEC A37.81
  due to
    Bordetella
      bronchiseptica A37.80
        with pneumonia A37.81
      parapertussis A37.10
        with pneumonia A37.11
      pertussis A37.00
        with pneumonia A37.01
    specified NEC A37.80
      with pneumonia A37.81
Wichman's asthma J38.5
Wide cranial sutures, newborn P96.3
Widening aorta — see Ectasia, aorta
  with aneurysm — see Aneurysm, aorta
Wilkie's disease or syndrome K55.1
Wilkinson-Sneddon disease or syndrome L13.1
Willebrand (-Jurgens) **thrombopathy** — see Disease, von Willebrand

☑ **Additional Character Required — Refer to the Tabular List for Character Selection**

Williams syndrome Q93.82
Willige-Hunt disease or syndrome G23.1
Wilms' tumor C64- ☑
Wilson-Mikity syndrome P27.0
Wilson's
    disease or syndrome E83.01
    hepatolenticular degeneration E83.01
    lichen ruber L43.9
Window — *see also* Imperfect, closure
    aorticopulmonary Q21.4
Winter — *see* condition
Wiskott-Aldrich syndrome D82.0
Withdrawal state — *see also* Dependence, drug by type, with withdrawal
    alcohol
        with perceptual disturbances F10.232
            due to alcohol abuse F10.132
            due to alcohol use F10.932
        abuse — *see* Abuse, alcohol, with, withdrawal
        dependence — *see* Dependence, alcohol, with, withdrawal
        use — *see* Use, alcohol, with, withdrawal
        without perceptual disturbances F10.239
            due to alcohol abuse F10.139
            due to alcohol use F10.939
    caffeine F15.93
    cannabis F12.23
    newborn
        correct therapeutic substance properly administered P96.2
        infant of dependent mother P96.1
    therapeutic substance, neonatal P96.2
Witts' anemia D50.8
Witzelsucht F07.0
Woakes' ethmoiditis or syndrome J33.1
Wolff-Hirschorn syndrome Q93.3
Wolff-Parkinson-White syndrome I45.6
Wolhynian fever A79.0
Wolman's disease E75.5
Wood lung or pneumonitis J67.8
Woolly, wooly hair (congenital) (nevus) Q84.1
Woolsorter's disease A22.1
Word
    blindness (congenital) (developmental) F81.0
    deafness (congenital) (developmental) H93.25
Worm(s) (infection) (infestation) — *see also* Infestation, helminth
    guinea B72
    in intestine NEC B82.0
Worm-eaten soles A66.3
Worn out — *see* Exhaustion
    cardiac
        defibrillator (with synchronous cardiac pacemaker) Z45.02
        pacemaker
            battery Z45.010
            lead Z45.018
    device, implant or graft — *see* Complications, by site, mechanical
Worried well Z71.1
Worries R45.82
Wound check Z48.0- ☑
    due to injury — *code to* Injury, by site, using appropriate seventh character for subsequent encounter
    postoperative — *see* Aftercare
Wound, open T14.8- ☑
    abdomen, abdominal
        wall S31.109 ☑
            with penetration into peritoneal cavity S31.609 ☑
            bite — *see* Bite, abdomen, wall
            epigastric region S31.102 ☑
                with penetration into peritoneal cavity S31.602 ☑
                bite — *see* Bite, abdomen, wall, epigastric region
                laceration — *see* Laceration, abdomen, wall, epigastric region
                puncture — *see* Puncture, abdomen, wall, epigastric region
            laceration — *see* Laceration, abdomen, wall
            left
                lower quadrant S31.104 ☑
                    with penetration into peritoneal cavity S31.604 ☑
                    bite — *see* Bite, abdomen, wall, left, lower quadrant
                    laceration — *see* Laceration, abdomen, wall, left, lower quadrant

Wound, open — *continued*
    abdomen, abdominal — *continued*
        wall — *continued*
            left — *continued*
                lower quadrant — *continued*
                    puncture — *see* Puncture, abdomen, wall, left, lower quadrant
                upper quadrant S31.101 ☑
                    with penetration into peritoneal cavity S31.601 ☑
                    bite — *see* Bite, abdomen, wall, left, upper quadrant
                    laceration — *see* Laceration, abdomen, wall, left, upper quadrant
                    puncture — *see* Puncture, abdomen, wall, left, upper quadrant
            periumbilic region S31.105 ☑
                with penetration into peritoneal cavity S31.605 ☑
                bite — *see* Bite, abdomen, wall, periumbilic region
                laceration — *see* Laceration, abdomen, wall, periumbilic region
                puncture — *see* Puncture, abdomen, wall, periumbilic region
            puncture — *see* Puncture, abdomen, wall
            right
                lower quadrant S31.103 ☑
                  with penetration into peritoneal cavity S31.603 ☑
                  bite — *see* Bite, abdomen, wall, right, lower quadrant
                  laceration — *see* Laceration, abdomen, wall, right, lower quadrant
                  puncture — *see* Puncture, abdomen, wall, right, lower quadrant
                upper quadrant S31.100 ☑
                  with penetration into peritoneal cavity S31.600 ☑
                  bite — *see* Bite, abdomen, wall, right, upper quadrant
                  laceration — *see* Laceration, abdomen, wall, right, upper quadrant
                  puncture — *see* Puncture, abdomen, wall, right, upper quadrant
    alveolar (process) — *see* Wound, open, oral cavity
    ankle S91.00- ☑
        bite — *see* Bite, ankle
        laceration — *see* Laceration, ankle
        puncture — *see* Puncture, ankle
    antecubital space — *see* Wound, open, elbow
    anterior chamber, eye — *see* Wound, open, ocular
    anus S31.839 ☑
        bite S31.835 ☑
        laceration — *see* Laceration, anus
        puncture — *see* Puncture, anus
    arm (upper) S41.10- ☑
        with amputation — *see* Amputation, traumatic, arm
        bite — *see* Bite, arm
        forearm — *see* Wound, open, forearm
        laceration — *see* Laceration, arm
        puncture — *see* Puncture, arm
    auditory canal (external) (meatus) — *see* Wound, open, ear
    auricle, ear — *see* Wound, open, ear
    axilla — *see* Wound, open, arm
    back — *see also* Wound, open, thorax, back
        lower S31.000 ☑
            with penetration into retroperitoneal space S31.001 ☑
            bite — *see* Bite, back, lower
            laceration — *see* Laceration, back, lower
            puncture — *see* Puncture, back, lower
    bite — *see* Bite
    blood vessel — *see* Injury, blood vessel
    breast S21.00- ☑
        with amputation — *see* Amputation, traumatic, breast
        bite — *see* Bite, breast
        laceration — *see* Laceration, breast
        puncture — *see* Puncture, breast
    buttock S31.809 ☑
        bite — *see* Bite, buttock
        laceration — *see* Laceration, buttock
        left S31.829 ☑
        puncture — *see* Puncture, buttock
        right S31.819 ☑
    calf — *see* Wound, open, leg
    canaliculus lacrimalis — *see* Wound, open, eyelid

Wound, open — *continued*
    canthus, eye — *see* Wound, open, eyelid
    cervical esophagus S11.20 ☑
        bite S11.25 ☑
        laceration — *see* Laceration, esophagus, traumatic, cervical
        puncture — *see* Puncture, cervical esophagus
    cheek (external) S01.40- ☑
        bite — *see* Bite, cheek
        internal — *see* Wound, open, oral cavity
        laceration — *see* Laceration, cheek
        puncture — *see* Puncture, cheek
    chest wall — *see* Wound, open, thorax
    chin — *see* Wound, open, head, specified site NEC
    choroid — *see* Wound, open, ocular
    ciliary body (eye) — *see* Wound, open, ocular
    clitoris S31.40 ☑
        with amputation — *see* Amputation, traumatic, clitoris
        bite S31.45 ☑
        laceration — *see* Laceration, vulva
        puncture — *see* Puncture, vulva
    conjunctiva — *see* Wound, open, ocular
    cornea — *see* Wound, open, ocular
    costal region — *see* Wound, open, thorax
    Descemet's membrane — *see* Wound, open, ocular
    digit(s)
        foot — *see* Wound, open, toe
        hand — *see* Wound, open, finger
    ear (canal) (external) S01.30- ☑
        with amputation — *see* Amputation, traumatic, ear
        bite — *see* Bite, ear
        drum S09.2- ☑
        laceration — *see* Laceration, ear
        puncture — *see* Puncture, ear
    elbow S51.00- ☑
        bite — *see* Bite, elbow
        laceration — *see* Laceration, elbow
        puncture — *see* Puncture, elbow
    epididymis — *see* Wound, open, testis
    epigastric region S31.102 ☑
        with penetration into peritoneal cavity S31.602 ☑
        bite — *see* Bite, abdomen, wall, epigastric region
        laceration — *see* Laceration, abdomen, wall, epigastric region
        puncture — *see* Puncture, abdomen, wall, epigastric region
    epiglottis — *see* Wound, open, neck, specified site NEC
    esophagus (thoracic) S27.819 ☑
        cervical — *see* Wound, open, cervical esophagus
        laceration S27.813 ☑
        specified type NEC S27.818 ☑
    eye — *see* Wound, open, ocular
    eyeball — *see* Wound, open, ocular
    eyebrow — *see* Wound, open, eyelid
    eyelid S01.10- ☑
        bite — *see* Bite, eyelid
        laceration — *see* Laceration, eyelid
        puncture — *see* Puncture, eyelid
    face NEC — *see* Wound, open, head, specified site NEC
    finger(s) S61.209 ☑
        with
            amputation — *see* Amputation, traumatic, finger
            damage to nail S61.309 ☑
        bite — *see* Bite, finger
        index S61.208 ☑
            with
                damage to nail S61.308 ☑
            left S61.201 ☑
                with
                    damage to nail S61.301 ☑
            right S61.200 ☑
                with
                    damage to nail S61.300 ☑
        laceration — *see* Laceration, finger
        little S61.208 ☑
            with
                damage to nail S61.308 ☑
            left S61.207 ☑
                with damage to nail S61.307 ☑
            right S61.206 ☑
                with damage to nail S61.306 ☑
        middle S61.208 ☑
            with
                damage to nail S61.308 ☑
            left S61.203 ☑
                with damage to nail S61.303 ☑
            right S61.202 ☑

Wound, open — *continued*
  finger(s) — *continued*
    middle — *continued*
      right — *continued*
        with damage to nail S61.302 ☑
      puncture — *see* Puncture, finger
    ring S61.208 ☑
      with
        damage to nail S61.308 ☑
      left S61.205 ☑
        with damage to nail S61.305 ☑
      right S61.204 ☑
        with damage to nail S61.304 ☑
  flank — *see* Wound, open, abdomen, wall
  foot (except toe(s) alone) S91.30- ☑
    with amputation — *see* Amputation, traumatic, foot
    bite — *see* Bite, foot
    laceration — *see* Laceration, foot
    puncture — *see* Puncture, foot
    toe — *see* Wound, open, toe
  forearm S51.80- ☑
    with
      amputation — *see* Amputation, traumatic, forearm
    bite — *see* Bite, forearm
    elbow only — *see* Wound, open, elbow
    laceration — *see* Laceration, forearm
    puncture — *see* Puncture, forearm
  forehead — *see* Wound, open, head, specified site NEC
  genital organs, external
    with amputation — *see* Amputation, traumatic, genital organs
    bite — *see* Bite, genital organ
    female S31.502 ☑
      vagina S31.40 ☑
      vulva S31.40 ☑
    laceration — *see* Laceration, genital organ
    male S31.501 ☑
      penis S31.20 ☑
      scrotum S31.30 ☑
      testes S31.30 ☑
    puncture — *see* Puncture, genital organ
  globe (eye) — *see* Wound, open, ocular
  groin — *see* Wound, open, abdomen, wall
  gum — *see* Wound, open, oral cavity
  hand S61.40- ☑
    with
      amputation — *see* Amputation, traumatic, hand
    bite — *see* Bite, hand
    finger(s) — *see* Wound, open, finger
    laceration — *see* Laceration, hand
    puncture — *see* Puncture, hand
    thumb — *see* Wound, open, thumb
  head S01.90 ☑
    bite — *see* Bite, head
    cheek — *see* Wound, open, cheek
    ear — *see* Wound, open, ear
    eyelid — *see* Wound, open, eyelid
    laceration — *see* Laceration, head
    lip — *see* Wound, open, lip
    nose S01.20 ☑
    oral cavity — *see* Wound, open, oral cavity
    puncture — *see* Puncture, head
    scalp — *see* Wound, open, scalp
    specified site NEC S01.80 ☑
    temporomandibular area — *see* Wound, open, cheek
  heel — *see* Wound, open, foot
  hip S71.00- ☑
    with amputation — *see* Amputation, traumatic, hip
    bite — *see* Bite, hip
    laceration — *see* Laceration, hip
    puncture — *see* Puncture, hip
  hymen S31.40 ☑
    bite — *see* Bite, vulva
    laceration — *see* Laceration, vagina
    puncture — *see* Puncture, vagina
  hypochondrium S31.109 ☑
    bite — *see* Bite, hypochondrium
    laceration — *see* Laceration, hypochondrium
    puncture — *see* Puncture, hypochondrium
  hypogastric region S31.109 ☑
    bite — *see* Bite, hypogastric region
    laceration — *see* Laceration, hypogastric region
    puncture — *see* Puncture, hypogastric region
  iliac (region) — *see* Wound, open, inguinal region
  inguinal region S31.109 ☑
    bite — *see* Bite, abdomen, wall, lower quadrant
    laceration — *see* Laceration, inguinal region
    puncture — *see* Puncture, inguinal region

Wound, open — *continued*
  instep — *see* Wound, open, foot
  interscapular region — *see* Wound, open, thorax, back
  intraocular — *see* Wound, open, ocular
  iris — *see* Wound, open, ocular
  jaw — *see* Wound, open, head, specified site NEC
  knee S81.00- ☑
    bite — *see* Bite, knee
    laceration — *see* Laceration, knee
    puncture — *see* Puncture, knee
  labium (majus) (minus) — *see* Wound, open, vulva
  laceration — *see* Laceration, by site
  lacrimal duct — *see* Wound, open, eyelid
  larynx S11.019 ☑
    bite — *see* Bite, larynx
    laceration — *see* Laceration, larynx
    puncture — *see* Puncture, larynx
  left
    lower quadrant S31.104 ☑
      with penetration into peritoneal cavity S31.604 ☑
      bite — *see* Bite, abdomen, wall, left, lower quadrant
      laceration — *see* Laceration, abdomen, wall, left, lower quadrant
      puncture — *see* Puncture, abdomen, wall, left, lower quadrant
    upper quadrant S31.101 ☑
      with penetration into peritoneal cavity S31.601 ☑
      bite — *see* Bite, abdomen, wall, left, upper quadrant
      laceration — *see* Laceration, abdomen, wall, left, upper quadrant
      puncture — *see* Puncture, abdomen, wall, left, upper quadrant
  leg (lower) S81.80- ☑
    with amputation — *see* Amputation, traumatic, leg
    ankle — *see* Wound, open, ankle
    bite — *see* Bite, leg
    foot — *see* Wound, open, foot
    knee — *see* Wound, open, knee
    laceration — *see* Laceration, leg
    puncture — *see* Puncture, leg
    toe — *see* Wound, open, toe
    upper — *see* Wound, open, thigh
  lip S01.501 ☑
    bite — *see* Bite, lip
    laceration — *see* Laceration, lip
    puncture — *see* Puncture, lip
  loin S31.109 ☑
    bite — *see* Bite, abdomen, wall
    laceration — *see* Laceration, loin
    puncture — *see* Puncture, loin
  lower back — *see* Wound, open, back, lower
  lumbar region — *see* Wound, open, back, lower
  malar region — *see* Wound, open, head, specified site NEC
  mammary — *see* Wound, open, breast
  mastoid region — *see* Wound, open, head, specified site NEC
  mouth — *see* Wound, open, oral cavity
  nail
    finger — *see* Wound, open, finger, with damage to nail
    toe — *see* Wound, open, toe, with damage to nail
  nape (neck) — *see* Wound, open, neck
  nasal (septum) (sinus) — *see* Wound, open, nose
  nasopharynx — *see* Wound, open, head, specified site NEC
  neck S11.90 ☑
    bite — *see* Bite, neck
    involving
      cervical esophagus S11.20 ☑
      larynx — *see* Wound, open, larynx
      pharynx S11.20 ☑
      thyroid S11.10 ☑
      trachea (cervical) S11.029 ☑
        bite — *see* Bite, trachea
        laceration S11.021 ☑
          with foreign body S11.022 ☑
        puncture S11.023 ☑
          with foreign body S11.024 ☑
    laceration — *see* Laceration, neck
    puncture — *see* Puncture, neck
    specified site NEC S11.80 ☑
      specified type NEC S11.89 ☑
  nose (septum) (sinus) S01.20 ☑
    with amputation — *see* Amputation, traumatic, nose
    bite — *see* Bite, nose

Wound, open — *continued*
  nose — *continued*
    laceration — *see* Laceration, nose
    puncture — *see* Puncture, nose
  ocular S05.90 ☑
    avulsion (traumatic enucleation) S05.7- ☑
    eyeball S05.6- ☑
      with foreign body S05.5- ☑
    eyelid — *see* Wound, open, eyelid
    laceration and rupture S05.3- ☑
      with prolapse or loss of intraocular tissue S05.2- ☑
    orbit (penetrating) (with or without foreign body) S05.4- ☑
    periocular area — *see* Wound, open, eyelid
    specified NEC S05.8X- ☑
  oral cavity S01.502 ☑
    bite S01.552 ☑
    laceration — *see* Laceration, oral cavity
    puncture — *see* Puncture, oral cavity
  orbit — *see* Wound, open, ocular, orbit
  palate — *see* Wound, open, oral cavity
  palm — *see* Wound, open, hand
  pelvis, pelvic — *see also* Wound, open, back, lower
    girdle — *see* Wound, open, hip
  penetrating — *see* Puncture, by site
  penis S31.20 ☑
    with amputation — *see* Amputation, traumatic, penis
    bite S31.25 ☑
    laceration — *see* Laceration, penis
    puncture — *see* Puncture, penis
  perineum
    bite — *see* Bite, perineum
    female S31.502 ☑
    laceration — *see* Laceration, perineum
    male S31.501 ☑
    puncture — *see* Puncture, perineum
  periocular area (with or without lacrimal passages) — *see* Wound, open, eyelid
  periumbilic region S31.105 ☑
    with penetration into peritoneal cavity S31.605 ☑
    bite — *see* Bite, abdomen, wall, periumbilic region
    laceration — *see* Laceration, abdomen, wall, periumbilic region
    puncture — *see* Puncture, abdomen, wall, periumbilic region
  phalanges
    finger — *see* Wound, open, finger
    toe — *see* Wound, open, toe
  pharynx S11.20 ☑
  pinna — *see* Wound, open, ear
  popliteal space — *see* Wound, open, knee
  prepuce — *see* Wound, open, penis
  pubic region — *see* Wound, open, back, lower
  pudendum — *see* Wound, open, genital organs, external
  puncture wound — *see* Puncture
  rectovaginal septum — *see* Wound, open, vagina
  right
    lower quadrant S31.103 ☑
      with penetration into peritoneal cavity S31.603 ☑
      bite — *see* Bite, abdomen, wall, right, lower quadrant
      laceration — *see* Laceration, abdomen, wall, right, lower quadrant
      puncture — *see* Puncture, abdomen, wall, right, lower quadrant
    upper quadrant S31.100 ☑
      with penetration into peritoneal cavity S31.600 ☑
      bite — *see* Bite, abdomen, wall, right, upper quadrant
      laceration — *see* Laceration, abdomen, wall, right, upper quadrant
      puncture — *see* Puncture, abdomen, wall, right, upper quadrant
  sacral region — *see* Wound, open, back, lower
  sacroiliac region — *see* Wound, open, back, lower
  salivary gland — *see* Wound, open, oral cavity
  scalp S01.00 ☑
    bite S01.05 ☑
    laceration — *see* Laceration, scalp
    puncture — *see* Puncture, scalp
  scalpel, newborn (birth injury) P15.8
  scapular region — *see* Wound, open, shoulder
  sclera — *see* Wound, open, ocular
  scrotum S31.30 ☑
    with amputation — *see* Amputation, traumatic, scrotum
    bite S31.35 ☑
    laceration — *see* Laceration, scrotum

☑ **Additional Character Required** — **Refer to the Tabular List for Character Selection**

Wound, open — *continued*
  scrotum — *continued*
    puncture — *see* Puncture, scrotum
  shin — *see* Wound, open, leg
  shoulder S41.00- ☑
    with amputation — *see* Amputation, traumatic, arm
    bite — *see* Bite, shoulder
    laceration — *see* Laceration, shoulder
    puncture — *see* Puncture, shoulder
  skin NOS T14.8 ☑
  spermatic cord — *see* Wound, open, testis
  sternal region — *see* Wound, open, thorax, front wall
  submaxillary region — *see* Wound, open, head, specified site NEC
  submental region — *see* Wound, open, head, specified site NEC
  subungual
    finger(s) — *see* Wound, open, finger
    toe(s) — *see* Wound, open, toe
  supraclavicular region — *see* Wound, open, neck, specified site NEC
  temple, temporal region — *see* Wound, open, head, specified site NEC
  temporomandibular area — *see* Wound, open, cheek
  testis S31.30 ☑
    with amputation — *see* Amputation, traumatic, testes
    bite S31.35 ☑
    laceration — *see* Laceration, testis
    puncture — *see* Puncture, testis
  thigh S71.10- ☑
    with amputation — *see* Amputation, traumatic, hip
    bite — *see* Bite, thigh
    laceration — *see* Laceration, thigh
    puncture — *see* Puncture, thigh
  thorax, thoracic (wall) S21.90 ☑
    back S21.20- ☑
      with penetration S21.40 ☑
    bite — *see* Bite, thorax
    breast — *see* Wound, open, breast
    front S21.10- ☑
      with penetration S21.30 ☑
    laceration — *see* Laceration, thorax
    puncture — *see* Puncture, thorax
  throat — *see* Wound, open, neck
  thumb S61.009 ☑
    with
      amputation — *see* Amputation, traumatic, thumb
      damage to nail S61.109 ☑
    bite — *see* Bite, thumb
    laceration — *see* Laceration, thumb
    left S61.002 ☑
      with
        damage to nail S61.102 ☑
    puncture — *see* Puncture, thumb
    right S61.001 ☑
      with
        damage to nail S61.101 ☑
  thyroid (gland) — *see* Wound, open, neck, thyroid
  toe(s) S91.109 ☑
    with
      amputation — *see* Amputation, traumatic, toe
      damage to nail S91.209 ☑
    bite — *see* Bite, toe
    great S91.103 ☑
      with
        damage to nail S91.203 ☑
      left S91.102 ☑
        with
          damage to nail S91.202 ☑
      right S91.101 ☑
        with
          damage to nail S91.201 ☑
    laceration — *see* Laceration, toe
    lesser S91.106 ☑
      with
        damage to nail S91.206 ☑
      left S91.105 ☑
        with
          damage to nail S91.205 ☑
      right S91.104 ☑
        with
          damage to nail S91.204 ☑
    puncture — *see* Puncture, toe
  tongue — *see* Wound, open, oral cavity
  trachea (cervical region) — *see* Wound, open, neck, trachea
  tunica vaginalis — *see* Wound, open, testis

Wound, open — *continued*
  tympanum, tympanic membrane S09.2- ☑
    laceration — *see* Laceration, ear, drum
    puncture — *see* Puncture, tympanum
  umbilical region — *see* Wound, open, abdomen, wall, periumbilic region
  uvula — *see* Wound, open, oral cavity
  vagina S31.40 ☑
    bite S31.45 ☑
    laceration — *see* Laceration, vagina
    puncture — *see* Puncture, vagina
  vitreous (humor) — *see* Wound, open, ocular
  vocal cord S11.039 ☑
    bite — *see* Bite, vocal cord
    laceration S11.031
      with foreign body S11.032 ☑
    puncture S11.033 ☑
      with foreign body S11.034 ☑
  vulva S31.40 ☑
    with amputation — *see* Amputation, traumatic, vulva
    bite S31.45 ☑
    laceration — *see* Laceration, vulva
    puncture — *see* Puncture, vulva
  wrist S61.50- ☑
    bite — *see* Bite, wrist
    laceration — *see* Laceration, wrist
    puncture — *see* Puncture, wrist
Wound, superficial — *see* Injury — *see also* specified injury type
Wright's syndrome G54.0
Wrist — *see* condition
Wrong drug (by accident) (given in error) — *see* Table of Drugs and Chemicals, by drug, poisoning
Wry neck — *see* Torticollis
Wuchereria (bancrofti) **infestation** B74.0
Wuchereriasis B74.0
Wuchernde Struma Langhans C73

X

Xanthelasma (eyelid) (palpebrarum) H02.60
  left H02.66
    lower H02.65
    upper H02.64
  right H02.63
    lower H02.62
    upper H02.61
Xanthelasmatosis (essential) E78.2
Xanthinuria, hereditary E79.82
Xanthoastrocytoma
  specified site — *see* Neoplasm, malignant, by site
  unspecified site C71.9
Xanthofibroma — *see* Neoplasm, connective tissue, benign
Xanthogranuloma D76.3
Xanthoma(s), xanthomatosis (primary) (familial) (hereditary) E75.5
  with
    hyperlipoproteinemia
      Type I E78.3
      Type III E78.2
      Type IV E78.1
      Type V E78.3
  bone (generalisata) C96.5
  cerebrotendinous E75.5
  cutaneotendinous E75.5
  disseminatum (skin) E78.2
  eruptive E78.2
  hypercholesterinemic E78.00
  hypercholesterolemic E78.00
  hyperlipidemic E78.5
  joint E75.5
  multiple (skin) E78.2
  tendon (sheath) E75.5
  tuberosum E78.2
  tuberous E78.2
  tubo-eruptive E78.2
  verrucous, oral mucosa K13.4
Xanthosis R23.8
Xenophobia F40.10
Xeroderma — *see also* Ichthyosis
  acquired L85.0
    eyelid H01.149
      left H01.146
        lower H01.145
        upper H01.144
      right H01.143
        lower H01.142
        upper H01.141

Xeroderma — *continued*
  pigmentosum Q82.1
  vitamin A deficiency E50.8
Xerophthalmia (vitamin A deficiency) E50.7
  unrelated to vitamin A deficiency — *see* Keratoconjunctivitis
Xerosis
  conjunctiva H11.14- ☑
    with Bitot's spots — *see also* Pigmentation, conjunctiva
      vitamin A deficiency E50.1
    vitamin A deficiency E50.0
  cornea H18.89- ☑
    with ulceration — *see* Ulcer, cornea
      vitamin A deficiency E50.3
    vitamin A deficiency E50.2
  cutis (dry skin) L85.3
  skin L85.3
Xerostomia K11.7
Xiphopagus Q89.4
XO syndrome Q96.9
X-ray (of)
  abnormal findings — *see* Abnormal, diagnostic imaging
  breast (mammogram) (routine) Z12.31
  chest
    routine (as part of a general medical examination) Z00.00
      with abnormal findings Z00.01
  routine (as part of a general medical examination) Z00.00
    with abnormal findings Z00.01
XXXXY syndrome Q98.1
XXY syndrome Q98.0

Y

Yaba pox (virus disease) B08.72
Yatapoxvirus B08.70
  specified NEC B08.79
Yawning R06.89
  psychogenic F45.8
Yaws A66.9
  bone lesions A66.6
  butter A66.1
  chancre A66.0
  cutaneous, less than five years after infection A66.2
  early (cutaneous) (macular) (maculopapular) (micropapular) (papular) A66.2
    frambeside A66.2
    skin lesions NEC A66.2
  eyelid A66.2
  ganglion A66.6
  gangosis, gangosa A66.5
  gumma, gummata A66.4
    bone A66.6
  gummatous
    frambeside A66.4
    osteitis A66.6
    periostitis A66.6
  hydrarthrosis — *see also* subcategory M14.8- A66.6
  hyperkeratosis (early) (late) A66.3
  initial lesions A66.0
  joint lesions — *see also* subcategory M14.8- A66.6
  juxta-articular nodules A66.7
  late nodular (ulcerated) A66.4
  latent (without clinical manifestations) (with positive serology) A66.8
  mother A66.0
  mucosal A66.7
  multiple papillomata A66.1
  nodular, late (ulcerated) A66.4
  osteitis A66.6
  papilloma, plantar or palmar A66.1
  periostitis (hypertrophic) A66.6
  specified NEC A66.7
  ulcers A66.4
  wet crab A66.1
Yeast infection — *see also* Candidiasis B37.9
Yellow
  atrophy (liver) — *see* Failure, hepatic
  fever — *see* Fever, yellow
  jack — *see* Fever, yellow
  jaundice — *see* Jaundice
  nail syndrome L60.5
Yersiniosis — *see also* Infection, Yersinia
  extraintestinal A28.2
  intestinal A04.6

Z

Zahorsky's syndrome (herpangina) B08.5
Zellweger's syndrome E71.510
Zenker's diverticulum (esophagus) K22.5

Ziehen-Oppenheim disease G24.1
Zieve's syndrome K70.0
Zika NOS A92.5
   congenital P35.4
Zinc
   deficiency, dietary E60
   metabolism disorder E83.2

Zollinger-Ellison syndrome E16.4
Zona — *see* Herpes, zoster
Zoophobia F40.218
Zoster (herpes) — *see* Herpes, zoster
Zygomycosis B46.9
   specified NEC B46.8
Zymotic — *see* condition

☑ **Additional Character Required — Refer to the Tabular List for Character Selection**

	Malignant Primary	Malignant Secondary	Ca in situ	Benign	Uncertain Behavior	Unspecified Behavior

Note: The list below gives the code number for neoplasms by anatomical site. For each site there are six possible code numbers according to whether the neoplasm in question is malignant, benign, in situ, of uncertain behavior, or of unspecified nature. The description of the neoplasm will often indicate which of the six columns is appropriate; e.g., malignant melanoma of skin, benign fibroadenoma of breast, carcinoma in situ of cervix uteri. Where such descriptors are not present, the remainder of the Index should be consulted where guidance is given to the appropriate column for each morphological (histological) variety listed; e.g., Mesonephroma – see Neoplasm, malignant; Embryoma — see also Neoplasm, uncertain behavior; Disease, Bowen's – see Neoplasm, skin, in situ. However, the guidance in the Index can be overridden if one of the descriptors mentioned above is present; e.g., malignant adenoma of colon is coded to C18.9 and not to D12.6 as the adjective "malignant" overrides the Index entry "Adenoma — see also Neoplasm, benign, by site." Codes listed with a dash -, following the code have a required additional character for laterality. The tabular list must be reviewed for the complete code.

	Malignant Primary	Malignant Secondary	Ca in situ	Benign	Uncertain Behavior	Unspecified Behavior
Neoplasm, neoplastic	C80.1	C79.9	D09.9	D36.9	D48.9	D49.9
abdomen,						
abdominal	C76.2	C79.8-☑	D09.8	D36.7	D48.7	D49.89
cavity	C76.2	C79.8-☑	D09.8	D36.7	D48.7	D49.89
organ	C76.2	C79.8-☑	D09.8	D36.7	D48.7	D49.89
viscera	C76.2	C79.8-☑	D09.8	D36.7	D48.7	D49.89
wall — see also						
Neoplasm, abdomen, wall, skin						
connective tissue	C44.509	C79.2	D04.5	D23.5	D48.5	D49.2
connective tissue	C49.4	C79.8-☑	—	D21.4	D48.1☑	D49.2
skin	C44.509	—	—	—	—	—
basal cell carcinoma	C44.519	—	—	—	—	—
specified type NEC	C44.599	—	—	—	—	—
squamous cell carcinoma	C44.529	—	—	—	—	—
abdominopelvic	C76.8	C79.8-☑	—	D36.7	D48.7	D49.89
accessory sinus — see Neoplasm, sinus						
acoustic nerve	C72.4-☑	C79.49	—	D33.3	D43.3	D49.7
adenoid (pharynx) (tissue)	C11.1	C79.89	D00.08	D10.6	D37.05	D49.0
adipose tissue — see also Neoplasm, connective tissue	C49.4	C79.89	—	D21.9	D48.1☑	D49.2
adnexa (uterine)	C57.4	C79.89	D07.39	D28.7	D39.8	D49.59
adrenal	C74.9-☑	C79.7-☑	D09.3	D35.0-☑	D44.1-☑	D49.7
capsule	C74.9-☑	C79.7-☑	D09.3	D35.0-☑	D44.1-☑	D49.7
cortex	C74.0-☑	C79.7-☑	D09.3	D35.0-☑	D44.1-☑	D49.7
gland	C74.9-☑	C79.7-☑	D09.3	D35.0-☑	D44.1-☑	D49.7
medulla	C74.1-☑	C79.7-☑	D09.3	D35.0-☑	D44.1-☑	D49.7
ala nasi (external) — see also Neoplasm, skin, nose	C44.301	C79.2	D04.39	D23.39	D48.5	D49.2
alimentary canal or tract NEC	C26.9	C78.80	D01.9	D13.99	D37.9	D49.0
alveolar	C03.9	C79.89	D00.03	D10.39	D37.09	D49.0
mucosa	C03.9	C79.89	D00.03	D10.39	D37.09	D49.0
lower	C03.1	C79.89	D00.03	D10.39	D37.09	D49.0
upper	C03.0	C79.89	D00.03	D10.39	D37.09	D49.0
ridge or process	C41.1	C79.51	—	D16.5	D48.0	D49.2
carcinoma	C03.9	C79.8-☑	—	—	—	—
lower	C03.1	C79.8-☑	—	—	—	—
upper	C03.0	C79.8-☑	—	—	—	—
lower	C41.1	C79.51	—	D16.5	D48.0	D49.2
mucosa	C03.9	C79.89	D00.03	D10.39	D37.09	D49.0
lower	C03.1	C79.89	D00.03	D10.39	D37.09	D49.0
upper	C03.0	C79.89	D00.03	D10.39	D37.09	D49.0
upper	C41.0	C79.51	—	D16.4	D48.0	D49.2
sulcus	C06.1	C79.89	D00.02	D10.39	D37.09	D49.0
alveolus	C03.9	C79.89	D00.03	D10.39	D37.09	D49.0
lower	C03.1	C79.89	D00.03	D10.39	D37.09	D49.0
upper	C03.0	C79.89	D00.03	D10.39	D37.09	D49.0
ampulla of Vater	C24.1	C78.89	D01.5	D13.5	D37.6	D49.0
ankle NEC	C76.5-☑	C79.89	D04.7-☑	D36.7	D48.7	D49.89
anorectum, anorectal (junction)	C21.8	C78.5	D01.3	D12.9	D37.8	D49.0
antecubital fossa or space	C76.4-☑	C79.89	D04.6-☑	D36.7	D48.7	D49.89

	Malignant Primary	Malignant Secondary	Ca in situ	Benign	Uncertain Behavior	Unspecified Behavior
Neoplasm, neoplastic						
— continued						
antrum (Highmore) (maxillary)	C31.0	C78.39	D02.3	D14.0	D38.5	D49.1
pyloric	C16.3	C78.89	D00.2	D13.1	D37.1	D49.0
tympanicum	C30.1	C78.39	D02.3	D14.0	D38.5	D49.1
anus, anal	C21.0	C78.5	D01.3	D12.9	D37.8	D49.0
canal	C21.1	C78.5	D01.3	D12.9	D37.8	D49.0
cloacogenic zone	C21.2	C78.5	D01.3	D12.9	D37.8	D49.0
margin — see also Neoplasm, anus, skin	C44.500	C79.2	D04.5	D23.5	D48.5	D49.2
overlapping lesion with rectosigmoid junction or rectum	C21.8	—	—	—	—	—
skin	C44.500	C79.2	D04.5	D23.5	D48.5	D49.2
basal cell carcinoma	C44.510	—	—	—	—	—
specified type NEC	C44.590	—	—	—	—	—
squamous cell carcinoma	C44.520	—	—	—	—	—
sphincter	C21.1	C78.5	D01.3	D12.9	D37.8	D49.0
aorta (thoracic)	C49.3	C79.89	—	D21.3	D48.1☑	D49.2
abdominal	C49.4	C79.89	—	D21.4	D48.1☑	D49.2
aortic body	C75.5	C79.89	—	D35.6	D44.7	D49.7
aponeurosis	C49.9	C79.89	—	D21.9	D48.1☑	D49.2
palmar	C49.1-☑	C79.89	—	D21.1-☑	D48.1☑	D49.2
plantar	C49.2-☑	C79.89	—	D21.2-☑	D48.1☑	D49.2
appendix	C18.1	C78.5	D01.0	D12.1	D37.3	D49.0
arachnoid	C70.9	C79.49	—	D32.9	D42.9	D49.7
cerebral	C70.0	C79.32	—	D32.0	D42.0	D49.7
spinal	C70.1	C79.49	—	D32.1	D42.1	D49.7
areola	C50.0-☑	C79.81	D05-☑	D24-☑	D48.6-☑	D49.3
arm NEC	C76.4-☑	C79.89	D04.6-☑	D36.7	D48.7	D49.89
artery — see Neoplasm, connective tissue						
aryepiglottic fold	C13.1	C79.89	D00.08	D10.7	D37.05	D49.0
hypopharyngeal aspect	C13.1	C79.89	D00.08	D10.7	D37.05	D49.0
laryngeal aspect	C32.1	C78.39	D02.0	D14.1	D38.0	D49.1
marginal zone	C13.1	C79.89	D00.08	D10.7	D37.05	D49.0
arytenoid (cartilage)	C32.3	C78.39	D02.0	D14.1	D38.0	D49.1
fold — see Neoplasm, aryepiglottic						
associated with transplanted organ	C80.2					
atlas	C41.2	C79.51	—	D16.6	D48.0	D49.2
atrium, cardiac	C38.0	C79.89	—	D15.1	D48.7	D49.89
auditory						
canal (external) (skin)	C44.20-☑	C79.2	D04.2-☑	D23.2-☑	D48.5	D49.2
internal	C30.1	C78.39	D02.3	D14.0	D38.5	D49.1
nerve	C72.4-☑	C79.49	—	D33.3	D43.3	D49.7
tube	C30.1	C78.39	D02.3	D14.0	D38.5	D49.1
opening	C11.2	C79.89	D00.08	D10.6	D37.05	D49.0
auricle, ear — see also Neoplasm, skin, ear	C44.20-☑	C79.2	D04.2-☑	D23.2-☑	D48.5	D49.2
auricular canal (external) — see also Neoplasm, skin, ear	C44.20-☑	C79.2	D04.2-☑	D23.2-☑	D48.5	D49.2
internal	C30.1	C78.39	D02.3	D14.0	D38.5	D49.2
autonomic nerve or nervous system NEC (see Neoplasm, nerve, peripheral)						
axilla, axillary	C76.1	C79.89	D09.8	D36.7	D48.7	D49.89
fold — see also Neoplasm, skin, trunk	C44.509	C79.2	D04.5	D23.5	D48.5	D49.2
back NEC	C76.8	C79.89	D04.5	D36.7	D48.7	D49.89
Bartholin's gland	C51.0	C79.82	D07.1	D28.0	D39.8	D49.59
basal ganglia	C71.0	C79.31	—	D33.0	D43.0	D49.6
basis pedunculi	C71.7	C79.31	—	D33.1	D43.1	D49.6
bile or biliary (tract)	C24.9	C78.89	D01.5	D13.5	D37.6	D49.0

Neoplasm, neoplastic — continued
bile or biliary — continued

	Malignant Primary	Malignant Secondary	Ca in situ	Benign	Uncertain Behavior	Unspecified Behavior
canaliculi (biliferi) (intrahepatic)	C22.1	C78.7	D01.5	D13.4	D37.6	D49.0
canals, interlobular	C22.1	C78.89	D01.5	D13.4	D37.6	D49.0
duct or passage (common) (cystic) (extrahepatic)	C24.0	C78.89	D01.5	D13.5	D37.6	D49.0
interlobular	C22.1	C78.89	D01.5	D13.4	D37.6	D49.0
intrahepatic	C22.1	C78.7	D01.5	D13.4	D37.6	D49.0
and extrahepatic	C24.8	C78.89	D01.5	D13.5	D37.6	D49.0
bladder (urinary)	C67.9	C79.11	D09.0	D30.3	D41.4	D49.4
dome	C67.1	C79.11	D09.0	D30.3	D41.4	D49.4
neck	C67.5	C79.11	D09.0	D30.3	D41.4	D49.4
orifice	C67.9	C79.11	D09.0	D30.3	D41.4	D49.4
ureteric	C67.6	C79.11	D09.0	D30.3	D41.4	D49.4
urethral	C67.5	C79.11	D09.0	D30.3	D41.4	D49.4
overlapping lesion	C67.8	—	—	—	—	—
sphincter	C67.8	C79.11	D09.0	D30.3	D41.4	D49.4
trigone	C67.0	C79.11	D09.0	D30.3	D41.4	D49.4
urachus	C67.7	C79.11	D09.0	D30.3	D41.4	D49.4
wall	C67.9	C79.11	D09.0	D30.3	D41.4	D49.4
anterior	C67.3	C79.11	D09.0	D30.3	D41.4	D49.4
lateral	C67.2	C79.11	D09.0	D30.3	D41.4	D49.4
posterior	C67.4	C79.11	D09.0	D30.3	D41.4	D49.4
blood vessel — see Neoplasm, connective tissue						
bone (periosteum)	C41.9	C79.51	—	D16.9-	D48.0	D49.2
acetabulum						
ankle	C40.3-☑	C79.51	—	D16.3-☑	—	—
arm NEC	C40.0-☑	C79.51	—	D16.0-☑	—	—
astragalus	C40.3-☑	C79.51	—	D16.3-☑	—	—
atlas	C41.2	C79.51	—	D16.6	D48.0	D49.2
axis	C41.2	C79.51	—	D16.6	D48.0	D49.2
back NEC	C41.2	C79.51	—	D16.6	D48.0	D49.2
calcaneus	C40.3-☑	C79.51	—	D16.3-☑	—	—
calvarium	C41.0	C79.51	—	D16.4	D48.0	D49.2
carpus (any)	C40.1-☑	C79.51	—	D16.1-☑	—	—
cartilage NEC	C41.9	C79.51	—	D16.9	D48.0	D49.2
clavicle	C41.3	C79.51	—	D16.7	D48.0	D49.2
clivus	C41.0	C79.51	—	D16.4	D48.0	D49.2
coccygeal vertebra	C41.4	C79.51	—	D16.8	D48.0	D49.2
coccyx	C41.4	C79.51	—	D16.8	D48.0	D49.2
costal cartilage	C41.3	C79.51	—	D16.7	D48.0	D49.2
costovertebral joint	C41.3	C79.51	—	D16.7	D48.0	D49.2
cranial	C41.0	C79.51	—	D16.4	D48.0	D49.2
cuboid	C40.3-☑	C79.51	—	D16.3-☑	—	—
cuneiform	C41.9	C79.51	—	D16.9	D48.0	D49.2
elbow	C40.0-☑	C79.51	—	D16.0-☑	—	—
ethmoid (labyrinth)	C41.0	C79.51	—	D16.4	D48.0	D49.2
face	C41.0	C79.51	—	D16.4	D48.0	D49.2
femur (any part)	C40.2-☑	C79.51	—	D16.2-☑	—	—
fibula (any part)	C40.2-☑	C79.51	—	D16.2-☑	—	—
finger (any)	C40.1-☑	C79.51	—	D16.1-☑	—	—
foot	C40.3-☑	C79.51	—	D16.3-☑	—	—
forearm	C40.0-☑	C79.51	—	D16.0-☑	—	—
frontal	C41.0	C79.51	—	D16.4	D48.0	D49.2
hand	C40.1-☑	C79.51	—	D16.1-☑	—	—
heel	C40.3-☑	C79.51	—	D16.3-☑	—	—
hip	C41.4	C79.51	—	D16.8	D48.0	D49.2
humerus (any part)	C40.0-☑	C79.51	—	D16.0-☑	—	—
hyoid	C41.0	C79.51	—	D16.4	D48.0	D49.2
ilium	C41.4	C79.51	—	D16.8	D48.0	D49.2
innominate	C41.4	C79.51	—	D16.8	D48.0	D49.2
intervertebral cartilage or disc	C41.2	C79.51	—	D16.6	D48.0	D49.2
ischium	C41.4	C79.51	—	D16.8	D48.0	D49.2
jaw (lower)	C41.1	C79.51	—	D16.5	D48.0	D49.2
knee	C40.2-☑	C79.51	—	D16.2-☑	—	—
leg NEC	C40.2-☑	C79.51	—	D16.2-☑	—	—
limb NEC	C40.9-☑	C79.51	—	D16.9	—	—

Neoplasm, neoplastic — continued
bone — continued
limb — continued

	Malignant Primary	Malignant Secondary	Ca in situ	Benign	Uncertain Behavior	Unspecified Behavior
lower (long bones)	C40.2-☑	C79.51	—	D16.2-☑	—	—
short bones	C40.3-☑	C79.51	—	D16.3-☑	—	—
upper (long bones)	C40.0-☑	C79.51	—	D16.0-☑	—	—
short bones	C40.1-☑	C79.51	—	D16.1-☑	—	—
malar	C41.0	C79.51	—	D16.4	D48.0	D49.2
mandible	C41.1	C79.51	—	D16.5	D48.0	D49.2
marrow NEC (any bone)	C96.9	C79.52	—	—	D47.9	D49.89
mastoid	C41.0	C79.51	—	D16.4	D48.0	D49.2
maxilla, maxillary (superior)	C41.0	C79.51	—	D16.4	D48.0	D49.2
inferior	C41.1	C79.51	—	D16.5	D48.0	D49.2
metacarpus (any)	C40.1-☑	C79.51	—	D16.1-☑	—	—
metatarsus (any)	C40.3-☑	C79.51	—	D16.3-☑	—	—
navicular						
ankle	C40.3-☑	C79.51	—	—	—	—
hand	C40.1-☑	C79.51	—	—	—	—
nose, nasal	C41.0	C79.51	—	D16.4	D48.0	D49.2
occipital	C41.0	C79.51	—	D16.4	D48.0	D49.2
orbit	C41.0	C79.51	—	D16.4	D48.0	D49.2
overlapping sites	C40.8-☑	—	—	—	—	—
parietal	C41.0	C79.51	—	D16.4	D48.0	D49.2
patella	C40.2-☑	C79.51	—	—	—	—
pelvic	C41.4	C79.51	—	D16.8	D48.0	D49.2
phalanges						
foot	C40.3-☑	C79.51	—	—	—	—
hand	C40.1-☑	C79.51	—	—	—	—
pubic	C41.4	C79.51	—	D16.8	D48.0	D49.2
radius (any part)	C40.0-☑	C79.51	—	D16.0-☑	—	—
rib	C41.3	C79.51	—	D16.7	D48.0	D49.2
sacral vertebra	C41.4	C79.51	—	D16.8	D48.0	D49.2
sacrum	C41.4	C79.51	—	D16.8	D48.0	D49.2
scaphoid						
of ankle	C40.3-☑	C79.51	—	—	—	—
of hand	C40.1-☑	C79.51	—	—	—	—
scapula (any part)	C40.0-☑	C79.51	—	D16.0-☑	—	—
sella turcica	C41.0	C79.51	—	D16.4	D48.0	D49.2
shoulder	C40.0-☑	C79.51	—	D16.0-☑	—	—
skull	C41.0	C79.51	—	D16.4	D48.0	D49.2
sphenoid	C41.0	C79.51	—	D16.4	D48.0	D49.2
spine, spinal (column)	C41.2	C79.51	—	D16.6	D48.0	D49.2
coccyx	C41.4	C79.51	—	D16.8	D48.0	D49.2
sacrum	C41.4	C79.51	—	D16.8	D48.0	D49.2
sternum	C41.3	C79.51	—	D16.7	D48.0	D49.2
tarsus (any)	C40.3-☑	C79.51	—	—	—	—
temporal	C41.0	C79.51	—	D16.4	D48.0	D49.2
thumb	C40.1-☑	C79.51	—	—	—	—
tibia (any part)	C40.2-☑	C79.51	—	—	—	—
toe (any)	C40.3-☑	C79.51	—	—	—	—
trapezium	C40.1-☑	C79.51	—	—	—	—
trapezoid	C40.1-☑	C79.51	—	—	—	—
turbinate	C41.0	C79.51	—	D16.4	D48.0	D49.2
ulna (any part)	C40.0-☑	C79.51	—	D16.0-☑	—	—
unciform	C40.1-☑	C79.51	—	—	—	—
vertebra (column)	C41.2	C79.51	—	D16.6	D48.0	D49.2
coccyx	C41.4	C79.51	—	D16.8	D48.0	D49.2
sacrum	C41.4	C79.51	—	D16.8	D48.0	D49.2
vomer	C41.0	C79.51	—	D16.4	D48.0	D49.2
wrist	C40.1-☑	C79.51	—	—	—	—
xiphoid process	C41.3	C79.51	—	D16.7	D48.0	D49.2
zygomatic	C41.0	C79.51	—	D16.4	D48.0	D49.2
book-leaf (mouth) — ventral surface of tongue and floor of mouth	C06.89	C79.89	D00.00	D10.39	D37.09	D49.0
bowel — see Neoplasm, intestine						
brachial plexus	C47.1-☑	C79.89	—	D36.12	D48.2	D49.2
brain NEC	C71.9	C79.31	—	D33.2	D43.2	D49.6

☑ **Additional Character Required — Refer to the Tabular List for Character Selection**

Neoplasm, neoplastic — continued

	Malignant Primary	Malignant Secondary	Ca in situ	Benign	Uncertain Behavior	Unspecified Behavior
brain — continued						
basal ganglia	C71.0	C79.31	—	D33.0	D43.0	D49.6
cerebellopontine angle	C71.6	C79.31	—	D33.1	D43.1	D49.6
cerebellum NOS	C71.6	C79.31	—	D33.1	D43.1	D49.6
cerebrum	C71.0	C79.31	—	D33.0	D43.0	D49.6
choroid plexus	C71.7	C79.31	—	D33.1	D43.1	D49.6
corpus callosum	C71.8	C79.31	—	D33.2	D43.2	D49.6
corpus striatum	C71.0	C79.31	—	D33.0	D43.0	D49.6
cortex (cerebral)	C71.0	C79.31	—	D33.0	D43.0	D49.6
frontal lobe	C71.1	C79.31	—	D33.0	D43.0	D49.6
globus pallidus	C71.0	C79.31	—	D33.0	D43.0	D49.6
hippocampus	C71.2	C79.31	—	D33.0	D43.0	D49.6
hypothalamus	C71.0	C79.31	—	D33.0	D43.0	D49.6
internal capsule	C71.0	C79.31	—	D33.0	D43.0	D49.6
medulla oblongata	C71.7	C79.31	—	D33.1	D43.1	D49.6
meninges	C70.0	C79.32	—	D32.0	D42.0	D49.7
midbrain	C71.7	C79.31	—	D33.1	D43.1	D49.6
occipital lobe	C71.4	C79.31	—	D33.0	D43.0	D49.6
overlapping lesion	C71.8	C79.31	—	—	—	—
parietal lobe	C71.3	C79.31	—	D33.0	D43.0	D49.6
peduncle	C71.7	C79.31	—	D33.1	D43.1	D49.6
pons	C71.7	C79.31	—	D33.1	D43.1	D49.6
stem	C71.7	C79.31	—	D33.1	D43.1	D49.6
tapetum	C71.8	C79.31	—	D33.2	D43.2	D49.6
temporal lobe	C71.2	C79.31	—	D33.0	D43.0	D49.6
thalamus	C71.0	C79.31	—	D33.0	D43.0	D49.6
uncus	C71.2	C79.31	—	D33.0	D43.0	D49.6
ventricle (floor)	C71.5	C79.31	—	D33.0	D43.0	D49.6
fourth	C71.7	C79.31	—	D33.1	D43.1	D49.6
branchial (cleft) (cyst) (vestiges)	C10.4	C79.89	D00.08	D10.5	D37.05	D49.0
breast (connective tissue) (glandular tissue) (soft parts)	C50.9-☑	C79.81	D05.-☑	D24.-☑	D48.6-☑	D49.3
areola	C50.0-☑	C79.81	D05.-☑	D24.-☑	D48.6-☑	D49.3
axillary tail	C50.6-☑	C79.81	D05.-☑	D24.-☑	D48.6-☑	D49.3
central portion	C50.1-☑	C79.81	D05.-☑	D24.-☑	D48.6-☑	D49.3
inner	C50.8-☑	C79.81	D05.-☑	D24.-☑	D48.6-☑	D49.3
lower	C50.8-☑	C79.81	D05.-☑	D24.-☑	D48.6-☑	D49.3
lower-inner quadrant	C50.3-☑	C79.81	D05.-☑	D24.-☑	D48.6-☑	D49.3
lower-outer quadrant	C50.5-☑	C79.81	D05.-☑	D24.-☑	D48.6-☑	D49.3
mastectomy site (skin) — see also Neoplasm, breast, skin	C44.501	C79.2	—	—	—	—
specified as breast tissue	C50.8-☑	C79.81	—	—	—	—
midline	C50.8-☑	C79.81	D05.-☑	D24.-☑	D48.6-☑	D49.3
nipple	C50.0-☑	C79.81	D05.-☑	D24.-☑	D48.6-☑	D49.3
outer	C50.8-☑	C79.81	D05.-☑	D24.-☑	D48.6-☑	D49.3
overlapping lesion	C50.8-☑	—	—	—	—	—
skin	C44.501	C79.2	D04.5	D23.5	D48.5	D49.2
basal cell carcinoma	C44.511	—	—	—	—	—
specified type NEC	C44.591	—	—	—	—	—
squamous cell carcinoma	C44.521	—	—	—	—	—
tail (axillary)	C50.6-☑	C79.81	D05.-☑	D24.-☑	D48.6-☑	D49.3
upper	C50.8-☑	C79.81	D05.-☑	D24.-☑	D48.6-☑	D49.3
upper-inner quadrant	C50.2-☑	C79.81	D05.-☑	D24.-☑	D48.6-☑	D49.3
upper-outer quadrant	C50.4-☑	C79.81	D05.-☑	D24.-☑	D48.6-☑	D49.3
broad ligament	C57.1-☑	C79.82	D07.39	D28.2	D39.8	D49.59
bronchiogenic, bronchogenic (lung)	C34.9-☑	C78.0-☑	D02.2-☑	D14.3-☑	D38.1	D49.1
bronchiole	C34.9-☑	C78.0-☑	D02.2-☑	D14.3-☑	D38.1	D49.1
bronchus	C34.9-☑	C78.0-☑	D02.2-☑	D14.3-☑	D38.1	D49.1
carina	C34.0-☑	C78.0-☑	D02.2-☑	D14.3-☑	D38.1	D49.1
lower lobe of lung	C34.3-☑	C78.0-☑	D02.2-☑	D14.3-☑	D38.1	D49.1

Neoplasm, neoplastic — continued

	Malignant Primary	Malignant Secondary	Ca in situ	Benign	Uncertain Behavior	Unspecified Behavior
bronchus — continued						
main	C34.0-☑	C78.0-☑	D02.2-☑	D14.3-☑	D38.1	D49.1
middle lobe of lung	C34.2	C78.0-☑	D02.21	D14.31	D38.1	D49.1
overlapping lesion	C34.8-☑	—	—	—	—	—
upper lobe of lung	C34.1-☑	C78.0-☑	D02.2-☑	D14.3-☑	D38.1	D49.1
brow	C44.309	C79.2	D04.39	D23.39	D48.5	D49.2
basal cell carcinoma	C44.319	—	—	—	—	—
specified type NEC	C44.399	—	—	—	—	—
squamous cell carcinoma	C44.329	—	—	—	—	—
buccal (cavity)	C06.9	C79.89	D00.00	D10.39	D37.09	D49.0
commissure	C06.0	C79.89	D00.02	D10.39	D37.09	D49.0
groove (lower) (upper)	C06.1	C79.89	D00.02	D10.39	D37.09	D49.0
mucosa	C06.0	C79.89	D00.02	D10.39	D37.09	D49.0
sulcus (lower) (upper)	C06.1	C79.89	D00.02	D10.39	D37.09	D49.0
bulbourethral gland	C68.0	C79.19	D09.19	D30.4	D41.3	D49.59
bursa — see Neoplasm, connective tissue						
buttock NEC	C76.3	C79.89	D04.5	D36.7	D48.7	D49.89
calf	C76.5-☑	C79.89	D04.7-☑	D36.7	D48.7	D49.89
calvarium	C41.0	C79.51	—	D16.4	D48.0	D49.2
calyx, renal	C65.-☑	C79.0-☑	D09.19	D30.1-☑	D41.1-☑	D49.51-☑
canal						
anal	C21.1	C78.5	D01.3	D12.9	D37.8	D49.0
auditory (external) — see also Neoplasm, skin, ear	C44.20-☑	C79.2	D04.2-☑	D23.2-☑	D48.5	D49.2
auricular (external) — see also Neoplasm, skin, ear	C44.20-☑	C79.2	D04.2-☑	D23.2-☑	D48.5	D49.2
canaliculi, biliary (biliferi) (intrahepatic)	C22.1	C78.7	D01.5	D13.4	D37.6	D49.0
canthus (eye) (inner) (outer)	C44.10-☑	C79.2	D04.1-☑	D23.1-☑	D48.5	D49.2
basal cell carcinoma	C44.11-☑	—	—	—	—	—
sebaceous cell	C44.13-☑	—	—	—	—	—
specified type NEC	C44.19-☑	—	—	—	—	—
squamous cell carcinoma	C44.12-☑	—	—	—	—	—
capillary — see Neoplasm, connective tissue						
caput coli	C18.0	C78.5	D01.0	D12.0	D37.4	D49.0
carcinoid — see Tumor, carcinoid						
cardia (gastric)	C16.0	C78.89	D00.2	D13.1	D37.1	D49.0
cardiac orifice (stomach)	C16.0	C78.89	D00.2	D13.1	D37.1	D49.0
cardio-esophageal junction	C16.0	C78.89	D00.2	D13.1	D37.1	D49.0
cardio-esophagus	C16.0	C78.89	D00.2	D13.1	D37.1	D49.0
carina (bronchus)	C34.0-☑	C78.0-☑	D02.2-☑	D14.3-☑	D38.1	D49.1
carotid (artery)	C49.0	C79.89	—	D21.0	D48.1☑	D49.2
body	C75.4	C79.89	—	D35.5	D44.6	D49.7
carpus (any bone)	C40.1-☑	C79.51	—	D16.1-☑	—	—
cartilage (articular) (joint) NEC — see also Neoplasm, bone	C41.9	C79.51	—	D16.9	D48.0	D49.2
arytenoid	C32.3	C78.39	D02.0	D14.1	D38.0	D49.1
auricular	C49.0	C79.89	—	D21.0	D48.1☑	D49.2
bronchi	C34.0-☑	C78.39	—	D14.3-☑	D38.1	D49.1
costal	C41.3	C79.51	—	D16.7	D48.0	D49.2
cricoid	C32.3	C78.39	D02.0	D14.1	D38.0	D49.1
cuneiform	C32.3	C78.39	D02.0	D14.1	D38.0	D49.1
ear (external)	C49.0	C79.89	—	D21.0	D48.1☑	D49.2
ensiform	C41.3	C79.51	—	D16.7	D48.0	D49.2
epiglottis	C32.1	C78.39	D02.0	D14.1	D38.0	D49.1

	Malignant Primary	Malignant Secondary	Ca in situ	Benign	Uncertain Behavior	Unspecified Behavior
Neoplasm, neoplastic						
— *continued*						
cartilage — *see also*						
Neoplasm, bone —						
continued						
epiglottis —						
continued						
anterior						
surface	C10.1	C79.89	D00.08	D10.5	D37.05	D49.0
eyelid	C49.0	C79.89	—	D21.0	D48.1☑	D49.2
intervertebral	C41.2	C79.51	—	D16.6	D48.0	D49.2
larynx, laryngeal	C32.3	C78.39	D02.0	D14.1	D38.0	D49.1
nose, nasal	C30.0	C78.39	D02.3	D14.0	D38.5	D49.1
pinna	C49.0	C79.89	—	D21.0	D48.1☑	D49.2
rib	C41.3	C79.51	—	D16.7	D48.0	D49.2
semilunar						
(knee)	C40.2-☑	C79.51	—	D16.2-☑	D48.0	D49.2
thyroid	C32.3	C78.39	D02.0	D14.1	D38.0	D49.1
trachea	C33	C78.39	D02.1	D14.2	D38.1	D49.1
cauda equina	C72.1	C79.49	—	D33.4	D43.4	D49.7
cavity						
buccal	C06.9	C79.89	D00.00	D10.30	D37.09	D49.0
nasal	C30.0	C78.39	D02.3	D14.0	D38.5	D49.1
oral	C06.9	C79.89	D00.00	D10.30	D37.09	D49.0
peritoneal	C48.2	C78.6	—	D20.1	D48.4	D49.0
tympanic	C30.1	C78.39	D02.3	D14.0	D38.5	D49.1
cecum	C18.0	C78.5	D01.0	D12.0	D37.4	D49.0
central nervous						
system	C72.9	C79.40	—	—	—	—
cerebellopontine						
(angle)	C71.6	C79.31	—	D33.1	D43.1	D49.6
cerebellum,						
cerebellar	C71.6	C79.31	—	D33.1	D43.1	D49.6
cerebrum, cerebra						
(cortex)						
(hemisphere)						
(white matter)	C71.0	C79.31	—	D33.0	D43.0	D49.6
meninges	C70.0	C79.32	—	D32.0	D42.0	D49.7
peduncle	C71.7	C79.31	—	D33.1	D43.1	D49.6
ventricle	C71.5	C79.31	—	D33.0	D43.0	D49.6
fourth	C71.7	C79.31	—	D33.1	D43.1	D49.6
cervical region	C76.0	C79.89	D09.8	D36.7	D48.7	D49.89
cervix (cervical) (uteri)						
(uterus)	C53.9	C79.82	D06.9	D26.0	D39.0	D49.59
canal	C53.0	C79.82	D06.0	D26.0	D39.0	D49.59
endocervix (canal)						
(gland)	C53.0	C79.82	D06.0	D26.0	D39.0	D49.59
exocervix	C53.1	C79.82	D06.1	D26.0	D39.0	D49.59
external os	C53.1	C79.82	D06.1	D26.0	D39.0	D49.59
internal os	C53.0	C79.82	D06.0	D26.0	D39.0	D49.59
nabothian gland	C53.0	C79.82	D06.0	D26.0	D39.0	D49.59
overlapping						
lesion	C53.8	—	—	—	—	—
squamocolumnar						
junction	C53.8	C79.82	D06.7	D26.0	D39.0	D49.59
stump	C53.8	C79.82	D06.7	D26.0	D39.0	D49.59
cheek	C76.0	C79.89	D09.8	D36.7	D48.7	D49.89
external	C44.309	C79.2	D04.39	D23.39	D48.5	D49.2
basal cell						
carcinoma	C44.319	—	—	—	—	—
specified type						
NEC	C44.399	—	—	—	—	—
squamous cell						
carcinoma	C44.329	—	—	—	—	—
inner aspect	C06.0	C79.89	D00.02	D10.39	D37.09	D49.0
internal	C06.0	C79.89	D00.02	D10.39	D37.09	D49.0
mucosa	C06.0	C79.89	D00.02	D10.39	D37.09	D49.0
chest (wall) NEC	C76.1	C79.89	D09.8	D36.7	D48.7	D49.89
chiasma opticum	C72.3-☑	C79.49	—	D33.3	D43.3	D49.7
chin	C44.309	C79.2	D04.39	D23.39	D48.5	D49.2
basal cell						
carcinoma	C44.319	—	—	—	—	—
specified type						
NEC	C44.399	—	—	—	—	—
squamous cell						
carcinoma	C44.329	—	—	—	—	—
choana	C11.3	C79.89	D00.08	D10.6	D37.05	D49.0
cholangiole	C22.1	C78.89	D01.5	D13.4	D37.6	D49.0
choledochal duct	C24.0	C78.89	D01.5	D13.5	D37.6	D49.0
choroid	C69.3-☑	C79.49	D09.2-☑	D31.3-☑	D48.7	D49.81
plexus	C71.5	C79.31	—	D33.0	D43.0	D49.6
ciliary body	C69.4-☑	C79.49	D09.2-☑	D31.4-☑	D48.7	D49.89
clavicle	C41.3	C79.51	—	D16.7	D48.0	D49.2

	Malignant Primary	Malignant Secondary	Ca in situ	Benign	Uncertain Behavior	Unspecified Behavior
Neoplasm, neoplastic						
— *continued*						
clitoris	C51.2	C79.82	D07.1	D28.0	D39.8	D49.59
clivus	C41.0	C79.51	—	D16.4	D48.0	D49.2
cloacogenic zone	C21.2	C78.5	D01.3	D12.9	D37.8	D49.0
coccygeal						
body or glomus	C49.5	C79.89	—	D21.5	D48.1☑	D49.2
vertebra	C41.4	C79.51	—	D16.8	D48.0	D49.2
coccyx	C41.4	C79.51	—	D16.8	D48.0	D49.2
colon — *see also*						
Neoplasm,						
intestine,						
large	C18.9	C78.5	—	—	—	—
with rectum	C19	C78.5	D01.1	D12.7	D37.5	D49.0
columnella — *see also*						
Neoplasm, skin,						
face	C44.390	C79.2	D04.39	D23.39	D48.5	D49.2
column, spinal — *see*						
Neoplasm, spine						
commissure						
labial, lip	C00.6	C79.89	D00.01	D10.39	D37.01	D49.0
laryngeal	C32.0	C78.39	D02.0	D14.1	D38.0	D49.1
common (bile)						
duct	C24.0	C78.89	D01.5	D13.5	D37.6	D49.0
concha — *see also*						
Neoplasm, skin,						
ear	C44.20-☑	C79.2	D04.2-☑	D23.2-☑	D48.5	D49.2
nose	C30.0	C78.39	D02.3	D14.0	D38.5	D49.1
conjunctiva	C69.0-☑	C79.49	D09.2-☑	D31.0-☑	D48.7	D49.89
connective tissue						
NEC	C49.9	C79.89	—	D21.9	D48.1☑	D49.2

> Note: For neoplasms of connective tissue (blood vessel, bursa, fascia, ligament, muscle, peripheral nerves, sympathetic and parasympathetic nerves and ganglia, synovia, tendon, etc.) or of morphological types that indicate connective tissue, code according to the list under "Neoplasm, connective tissue". For sites that do not appear in this list, code to neoplasm of that site; e.g., fibrosarcoma, pancreas (C25.9).

> Note: Morphological types that indicate connective tissue appear in their proper place in the alphabetic index with the instruction "see Neoplasm, connective tissue ...."

	Malignant Primary	Malignant Secondary	Ca in situ	Benign	Uncertain Behavior	Unspecified Behavior
abdomen	C49.4	C79.89	—	D21.4	D48.1☑	D49.2
abdominal wall	C49.4	C79.89	—	D21.4	D48.1☑	D49.2
ankle	C49.2-☑	C79.89	—	D21.2-☑	D48.1☑	D49.2
antecubital fossa or						
space	C49.1-☑	C79.89	—	D21.1-☑	D48.1☑	D49.2
arm	C49.1-☑	C79.89	—	D21.1-☑	D48.1☑	D49.2
auricle (ear)	C49.0	C79.89	—	D21.0	D48.1☑	D49.2
axilla	C49.3	C79.89	—	D21.3	D48.1☑	D49.2
back	C49.6	C79.89	—	D21.6	D48.1☑	D49.2
breast — *see*						
Neoplasm,						
breast						
buttock	C49.5	C79.89	—	D21.5	D48.1☑	D49.2
calf	C49.2-☑	C79.89	—	D21.2-☑	D48.1☑	D49.2
cervical region	C49.0	C79.89	—	D21.0	D48.1☑	D49.2
cheek	C49.0	C79.89	—	D21.0	D48.1☑	D49.2
chest (wall)	C49.3	C79.89	—	D21.3	D48.1☑	D49.2
chin	C49.0	C79.89	—	D21.0	D48.1☑	D49.2
diaphragm	C49.3	C79.89	—	D21.3	D48.1☑	D49.2
ear (external)	C49.0	C79.89	—	D21.0	D48.1☑	D49.2
elbow	C49.1-☑	C79.89	—	D21.1-☑	D48.1☑	D49.2
extrarectal	C49.5	C79.89	—	D21.5	D48.1☑	D49.2
extremity	C49.9	C79.89	—	D21.9	D48.1☑	D49.2
lower	C49.2-☑	C79.89	—	D21.2-☑	D48.1☑	D49.2
upper	C49.1-☑	C79.89	—	D21.1-☑	D48.1☑	D49.2
eyelid	C49.0	C79.89	—	D21.0	D48.1☑	D49.2
face	C49.0	C79.89	—	D21.0	D48.1☑	D49.2
finger	C49.1-☑	C79.89	—	D21.1-☑	D48.1☑	D49.2
flank	C49.6	C79.89	—	D21.6	D48.1☑	D49.2
foot	C49.2-☑	C79.89	—	D21.2-☑	D48.1☑	D49.2
forearm	C49.1-☑	C79.89	—	D21.1-☑	D48.1☑	D49.2
forehead	C49.0	C79.89	—	D21.0	D48.1☑	D49.2
gastric	C49.4	C79.89	—	D21.4	D48.1☑	D49.2
gastrointestinal	C49.4	C79.89	—	D21.4	D48.1☑	D49.2
gluteal region	C49.5	C79.89	—	D21.5	D48.1☑	D49.2
great vessels						
NEC	C49.3	C79.89	—	D21.3	D48.1☑	D49.2
groin	C49.5	C79.89	—	D21.5	D48.1☑	D49.2

☑ **Additional Character Required — Refer to the Tabular List for Character Selection**

Neoplasm, neoplastic — continued

connective tissue — continued	Malignant Primary	Malignant Secondary	Ca in situ	Benign	Uncertain Behavior	Unspecified Behavior
hand	C49.1-✓	C79.89	—	D21.1-✓	D48.1✓	D49.2
head	C49.0	C79.89	—	D21.0	D48.1✓	D49.2
heel	C49.2-✓	C79.89	—	D21.2-✓	D48.1✓	D49.2
hip	C49.2-✓	C79.89	—	D21.2-✓	D48.1✓	D49.2
hypochondrium	C49.4	C79.89	—	D21.4	D48.1✓	D49.2
iliopsoas muscle	C49.5	C79.89	—	D21.5	D48.1✓	D49.2
infraclavicular region	C49.3	C79.89	—	D21.3	D48.1✓	D49.2
inguinal (canal) (region)	C49.5	C79.89	—	D21.5	D48.1✓	D49.2
intestinal	C49.4	C79.89	—	D21.4	D48.1✓	D49.2
intrathoracic	C49.3	C79.89	—	D21.3	D48.1✓	D49.2
ischiorectal fossa	C49.5	C79.89	—	D21.5	D48.1✓	D49.2
jaw	C03.9	C79.89	D00.03	D10.39	D48.1✓	D49.0
knee	C49.2-✓	C79.89	—	D21.2-✓	D48.1✓	D49.2
leg	C49.2-✓	C79.89	—	D21.2-✓	D48.1✓	D49.2
limb NEC	C49.9	C79.89	—	D21.9	D48.1✓	D49.2
lower	C49.2-✓	C79.89	—	D21.2-✓	D48.1✓	D49.2
upper	C49.1-✓	C79.89	—	D21.1-✓	D48.1✓	D49.2
nates	C49.5	C79.89	—	D21.5	D48.1✓	D49.2
neck	C49.0	C79.89	—	D21.0	D48.1✓	D49.2
orbit	C69.6-✓	C79.49	D09.2-✓	D31.6-✓	D48.1✓	D49.89
overlapping lesion	C49.8	—	—	—	—	—
pararectal	C49.5	C79.89	—	D21.5	D48.1✓	D49.2
para-urethral	C49.5	C79.89	—	D21.5	D48.1✓	D49.2
paravaginal	C49.5	C79.89	—	D21.5	D48.1✓	D49.2
pelvis (floor)	C49.5	C79.89	—	D21.5	D48.1✓	D49.2
pelvo-abdominal	C49.8	C79.89	—	D21.6	D48.1✓	D49.2
perineum	C49.5	C79.89	—	D21.5	D48.1✓	D49.2
perirectal (tissue)	C49.5	C79.89	—	D21.5	D48.1✓	D49.2
periurethral (tissue)	C49.5	C79.89	—	D21.5	D48.1✓	D49.2
popliteal fossa or space	C49.2-✓	C79.89	—	D21.2-✓	D48.1✓	D49.2
presacral	C49.5	C79.89	—	D21.5	D48.1✓	D49.2
psoas muscle	C49.4	C79.89	—	D21.4	D48.1✓	D49.2
pterygoid fossa	C49.0	C79.89	—	D21.0	D48.1✓	D49.2
rectovaginal septum or wall	C49.5	C79.89	—	D21.5	D48.1✓	D49.2
rectovesical	C49.5	C79.89	—	D21.5	D48.1✓	D49.2
retroperitoneum	C48.0	C78.6	—	D20.0	D48.3	D49.0
sacrococcygeal region	C49.5	C79.89	—	D21.5	D48.1✓	D49.2
scalp	C49.0	C79.89	—	D21.0	D48.1✓	D49.2
scapular region	C49.3	C79.89	—	D21.3	D48.1✓	D49.2
shoulder	C49.1-✓	C79.89	—	D21.1-✓	D48.1✓	D49.2
skin (dermis) NEC — see also Neoplasm, skin, by site	C44.90	C79.2	D04.9	D23.9	D48.5	D49.2
stomach	C49.4	C79.89	—	D21.4	D48.1✓	D49.2
submental	C49.0	C79.89	—	D21.0	D48.1✓	D49.2
supraclavicular region	C49.0	C79.89	—	D21.0	D48.1✓	D49.2
temple	C49.0	C79.89	—	D21.0	D48.1✓	D49.2
temporal region	C49.0	C79.89	—	D21.0	D48.1✓	D49.2
thigh	C49.2-✓	C79.89	—	D21.2-✓	D48.1✓	D49.2
thoracic (duct) (wall)	C49.3	C79.89	—	D21.3	D48.1✓	D49.2
thorax	C49.3	C79.89	—	D21.3	D48.1✓	D49.2
thumb	C49.1-✓	C79.89	—	D21.1-✓	D48.1✓	D49.2
toe	C49.2-✓	C79.89	—	D21.2-✓	D48.1✓	D49.2
trunk	C49.6	C79.89	—	D21.6	D48.1✓	D49.2
umbilicus	C49.4	C79.89	—	D21.4	D48.1✓	D49.2
vesicorectal	C49.5	C79.89	—	D21.5	D48.1✓	D49.2
wrist	C49.1-✓	C79.89	—	D21.1-✓	D48.1✓	D49.2
conus medullaris	C72.0	C79.49	—	D33.4	D43.4	D49.7
cord (true) (vocal)	C32.0	C78.39	D02.0	D14.1	D38.0	D49.1
false	C32.1	C78.39	D02.0	D14.1	D38.0	D49.1
spermatic	C63.1-✓	C79.82	D07.69	D29.8	D40.8	D49.59
spinal (cervical) (lumbar) (thoracic)	C72.0	C79.49	—	D33.4	D43.4	D49.7

Neoplasm, neoplastic — continued

	Malignant Primary	Malignant Secondary	Ca in situ	Benign	Uncertain Behavior	Unspecified Behavior
cornea (limbus)	C69.1-✓	C79.49	D09.2-✓	D31.1-✓	D48.7	D49.89
corpus						
albicans	C56.-✓	C79.6-✓	D07.39	D27.-✓	D39.1-✓	D49.59
callosum, brain	C71.0	C79.31	—	D33.2	D43.2	D49.6
cavernosum	C60.2	C79.82	D07.4	D29.0	D40.8	D49.59
gastric	C16.2	C78.89	D00.2	D13.1	D37.1	D49.0
overlapping sites	C54.8	—	—	—	—	—
penis	C60.2	C79.82	D07.4	D29.0	D40.8	D49.59
striatum, cerebrum	C71.0	C79.31	—	D33.0	D43.0	D49.6
uteri	C54.9	C79.82	D07.0	D26.1	D39.0	D49.59
isthmus	C54.0	C79.82	D07.0	D26.1	D39.0	D49.59
cortex						
adrenal	C74.0-✓	C79.7-✓	D09.3	D35.0-✓	D44.1-✓	D49.7
cerebral	C71.0	C79.31	—	D33.0	D43.0	D49.6
costal cartilage	C41.3	C79.51	—	D16.7	D48.0	D49.2
costovertebral joint	C41.3	C79.51	—	D16.7	D48.0	D49.2
Cowper's gland	C68.0	C79.19	D09.19	D30.4	D41.3	D49.59
cranial (fossa, any)	C71.9	C79.31	—	D33.2	D43.2	D49.6
meninges	C70.0	C79.32	—	D32.0	D42.0	D49.7
nerve	C72.50	C79.49	—	D33.3	D43.3	D49.7
specified NEC	C72.59	C79.49	—	D33.3	D43.3	D49.7
craniobuccal pouch	C75.2	C79.89	D09.3	D35.2	D44.3	D49.7
craniopharyngeal (duct) (pouch)	C75.2	C79.89	D09.3	D35.3	D44.4	D49.7
cricoid	C13.0	C79.89	D00.08	D10.7	D37.05	D49.0
cartilage	C32.3	C78.39	D02.0	D14.1	D38.0	D49.1
cricopharynx	C13.0	C79.89	D00.08	D10.7	D37.05	D49.0
crypt of Morgagni	C21.8	C78.5	D01.3	D12.9	D37.8	D49.0
crystalline lens	C69.4-✓	C79.49	D09.2-✓	D31.4-✓	D48.7	D49.89
cul-de-sac (Douglas')	C48.1	C78.6	—	D20.1	D48.4	D49.0
cuneiform cartilage	C32.3	C78.39	D02.0	D14.1	D38.0	D49.1
cutaneous — see Neoplasm, skin						
cutis — see Neoplasm, skin						
cystic (bile) duct (common)	C24.0	C78.89	D01.5	D13.5	D37.6	D49.0
dermis — see Neoplasm, skin						
diaphragm	C49.3	C79.89	—	D21.3	D48.1✓	D49.2
digestive organs, system, tube, or tract NEC	C26.9	C78.89	D01.9	D13.99	D37.9	D49.0
disc, intervertebral	C41.2	C79.51	—	D16.6	D48.0	D49.2
disease, generalized	C80.0	—	—	—	—	—
disseminated	C80.0	—	—	—	—	—
Douglas' cul-de-sac or pouch	C48.1	C78.6	—	D20.1	D48.4	D49.0
duodenojejunal junction	C17.8	C78.4	D01.49	D13.39	D37.2	D49.0
duodenum	C17.0	C78.4	D01.49	D13.2	D37.2	D49.0
dura (cranial) (mater)	C70.9	C79.49	—	D32.9	D42.9	D49.7
cerebral	C70.0	C79.32	—	D32.0	D42.0	D49.7
spinal	C70.1	C79.49	—	D32.1	D42.1	D49.7
ear (external) — see also Neoplasm, skin, ear						
ear	C44.20-✓	C79.2	D04.2-✓	D23.2-✓	D48.5	D49.2
auricle or auris — see also Neoplasm, skin, ear	C44.20-✓	C79.2	D04.2-✓	D23.2-✓	D48.5	D49.2
canal, external — see also Neoplasm, skin, ear	C44.20-✓	C79.2	D04.2-✓	D23.2-✓	D48.5	D49.2
cartilage	C49.0	C79.89	—	D21.0	D48.1✓	D49.2
external meatus — see also Neoplasm, skin, ear	C44.20-✓	C79.2	D04.2-✓	D23.2-✓	D48.5	D49.2
inner	C30.1	C78.39	D02.3	D14.0	D38.5	D49.1
lobule — see also Neoplasm, skin, ear	C44.20-✓	C79.2	D04.2-✓	D23.2-✓	D48.5	D49.2

✓ **Additional Character Required — Refer to the Tabular List for Character Selection**

Neoplasm Table

Neoplasm, ear — Neoplasm, fourchette

	Malignant Primary	Malignant Secondary	Ca in situ	Benign	Uncertain Behavior	Unspecified Behavior
Neoplasm, neoplastic — *continued*						
ear — *see also* Neoplasm, skin, ear — *continued*						
middle	C30.1	C78.39	D02.3	D14.0	D38.5	D49.1
overlapping lesion with accessory sinuses	C31.8	—	—	—	—	—
skin	C44.20-✓	C79.2	D04.2-✓	D23.2-✓	D48.5	D49.2
basal cell carcinoma	C44.21-✓	—	—	—	—	—
specified type NEC	C44.29-✓	—	—	—	—	—
squamous cell carcinoma	C44.22-✓	—	—	—	—	—
earlobe	C44.20-✓	C79.2	D04.2-✓	D23.2-✓	D48.5	D49.2
basal cell carcinoma	C44.21-✓	—	—	—	—	—
specified type NEC	C44.29-✓	—	—	—	—	—
squamous cell carcinoma	C44.22-✓	—	—	—	—	—
ejaculatory duct	C63.7	C79.82	D07.69	D29.8	D40.8	D49.59
elbow NEC	C76.4-✓	C79.89	D04.6-✓	D36.7	D48.7	D49.89
endocardium	C38.0	C79.89	—	D15.1	D48.7	D49.89
endocervix (canal) (gland)	C53.0	C79.82	D06.0	D26.0	D39.0	D49.59
endocrine gland NEC	C75.9	C79.89	D09.3	D35.9	D44.9	D49.7
pluriglandular	C75.8	C79.89	D09.3	D35.7	D44.9	D49.7
endometrium (gland) (stroma)	C54.1	C79.82	D07.0	D26.1	D39.0	D49.59
ensiform cartilage	C41.3	C79.51	—	D16.7	D48.0	D49.2
enteric — *see* Neoplasm, intestine						
ependyma (brain)	C71.5	C79.31	—	D33.0	D43.0	D49.6
fourth ventricle	C71.7	C79.31	—	D33.1	D43.1	D49.6
epicardium	C38.0	C79.89	—	D15.1	D48.7	D49.89
epididymis	C63.0-✓	C79.82	D07.69	D29.3-✓	D40.8	D49.59
epidural	C72.9	C79.49	—	D33.9	D43.9	D49.7
epiglottis	C32.1	C78.39	D02.0	D14.1	D38.0	D49.1
anterior aspect or surface	C10.1	C79.89	D00.08	D10.5	D37.05	D49.0
cartilage	C32.3	C78.39	D02.0	D14.1	D38.0	D49.1
free border (margin)	C10.1	C79.89	D00.08	D10.5	D37.05	D49.0
junctional region	C10.8	C79.89	D00.08	D10.5	D37.05	D49.0
posterior (laryngeal) surface	C32.1	C78.39	D02.0	D14.1	D38.0	D49.1
suprahyoid portion	C32.1	C78.39	D02.0	D14.1	D38.0	D49.1
esophagogastric junction	C16.0	C78.89	D00.2	D13.1	D37.1	D49.0
esophagus	C15.9	C78.89	D00.1	D13.0	D37.8	D49.0
abdominal	C15.5	C78.89	D00.1	D13.0	D37.8	D49.0
cervical	C15.3	C78.89	D00.1	D13.0	D37.8	D49.0
distal (third)	C15.5	C78.89	D00.1	D13.0	D37.8	D49.0
lower (third)	C15.5	C78.89	D00.1	D13.0	D37.8	D49.0
middle (third)	C15.4	C78.89	D00.1	D13.0	D37.8	D49.0
overlapping lesion	C15.8	—	—	—	—	—
proximal (third)	C15.3	C78.89	D00.1	D13.0	D37.8	D49.0
thoracic	C15.4	C78.89	D00.1	D13.0	D37.8	D49.0
upper (third)	C15.3	C78.89	D00.1	D13.0	D37.8	D49.0
ethmoid (sinus)	C31.1	C78.39	D02.3	D14.0	D38.5	D49.1
bone or labyrinth	C41.0	C79.51	—	D16.4	D48.0	D49.2
eustachian tube	C30.1	C78.39	D02.3	D14.0	D38.5	D49.1
exocervix	C53.1	C79.82	D06.1	D26.0	D39.0	D49.59
external meatus (ear) — *see also* Neoplasm, skin, ear	C44.20-✓	C79.2	D04.2-✓	D23.2-✓	D48.5	D49.2
os, cervix uteri	C53.1	C79.82	D06.1	D26.0	D39.0	D49.59
extradural	C72.9	C79.49	—	D33.9	D43.9	D49.7
extrahepatic (bile) duct	C24.0	C78.89	D01.5	D13.5	D37.6	D49.0
overlapping lesion with gallbladder	C24.8	—	—	—	—	—
Neoplasm, neoplastic — *continued*						
extraocular muscle	C69.6-✓	C79.49	D09.2-✓	D31.6-✓	D48.7	D49.89
extrarectal	C76.3	C79.89	D09.8	D36.7	D48.7	D49.89
extremity	C76.8	C79.89	D04.8	D36.7	D48.7	D49.89
lower	C76.5-✓	C79.89	D04.7-✓	D36.7	D48.7	D49.89
upper	C76.4-✓	C79.89	D04.6-✓	D36.7	D48.7	D49.89
eyeball	C69.9-✓	C79.49	D09.2-✓	D31.9-✓	D48.7	D49.89
eyebrow	C44.309	C79.2	D04.39	D23.39	D48.5	D49.2
basal cell carcinoma	C44.319	—	—	—	—	—
specified type NEC	C44.399	—	—	—	—	—
squamous cell carcinoma	C44.329	—	—	—	—	—
eyelid (lower) (skin) (upper)	C44.10-✓	—	—	—	—	—
basal cell carcinoma	C44.11-✓	—	—	—	—	—
cartilage	C49.0	C79.89	—	D21.0	D48.1✓	D49.2
sebaceous cell	C44.13-✓	—	—	—	—	—
specified type NEC	C44.19-✓	—	—	—	—	—
squamous cell carcinoma	C44.12-✓	—	—	—	—	—
eye NEC	C69.9-✓	C79.49	D09.2-✓	D31.9-✓	D48.7	D49.89
overlapping sites	C69.8-✓	—	—	—	—	—
face NEC	C76.0	C79.89	D04.39	D36.7	D48.7	D49.89
fallopian tube (accessory)	C57.0-✓	C79.82	D07.39	D28.2	D39.8	D49.59
falx (cerebella) (cerebri)	C70.0	C79.32	—	D32.0	D42.0	D49.7
fascia — *see also* Neoplasm, connective tissue						
palmar	C49.1-✓	C79.89	—	D21.1-✓	D48.1✓	D49.2
plantar	C49.2-✓	C79.89	—	D21.2-✓	D48.1✓	D49.2
fatty tissue — *see* Neoplasm, connective tissue						
fauces, faucial NEC	C10.9	C79.89	D00.08	D10.5	D37.05	D49.0
pillars	C09.1	C79.89	D00.08	D10.5	D37.05	D49.0
tonsil	C09.9	C79.89	D00.08	D10.4	D37.05	D49.0
femur (any part)	C40.2-✓	—	—	D16.2-✓	—	—
fetal membrane	C58	C79.82	D07.0	D26.7	D39.2	D49.59
fibrous tissue — *see* Neoplasm, connective tissue						
fibula (any part)	C40.2-✓	C79.51	—	D16.2-✓	—	—
filum terminale	C72.0	C79.49	—	D33.4	D43.4	D49.7
finger NEC	C76.4-✓	C79.89	D04.6-✓	D36.7	D48.7	D49.89
flank NEC	C76.8	C79.89	D04.5	D36.7	D48.7	D49.89
follicle, nabothian	C53.0	C79.82	D06.0	D26.0	D39.0	D49.59
foot NEC	C76.5-✓	C79.89	D04.7-✓	D36.7	D48.7	D49.89
forearm NEC	C76.4-✓	C79.89	D04.6-✓	D36.7	D48.7	D49.89
forehead (skin)	C44.309	C79.2	D04.39	D23.39	D48.5	D49.2
basal cell carcinoma	C44.319	—	—	—	—	—
specified type NEC	C44.399	—	—	—	—	—
squamous cell carcinoma	C44.329	—	—	—	—	—
foreskin	C60.0	C79.82	D07.4	D29.0	D40.8	D49.59
fornix						
pharyngeal	C11.3	C79.89	D00.08	D10.6	D37.05	D49.0
vagina	C52	C79.82	D07.2	D28.1	D39.8	D49.59
fossa (of)						
anterior (cranial)	C71.9	C79.31	—	D33.2	D43.2	D49.6
cranial	C71.9	C79.31	—	D33.2	D43.2	D49.6
ischiorectal	C76.3	C79.89	D09.8	D36.7	D48.7	D49.89
middle (cranial)	C71.9	C79.31	—	D33.2	D43.2	D49.6
piriform	C12	C79.89	D00.08	D10.7	D37.05	D49.0
pituitary	C75.1	C79.89	D09.3	D35.2	D44.3	D49.7
posterior (cranial)	C71.9	C79.31	—	D33.2	D43.2	D49.6
pterygoid	C49.0	C79.89	—	D21.0	D48.1✓	D49.2
pyriform	C12	C79.89	D00.08	D10.7	D37.05	D49.0
Rosenmuller	C11.2	C79.89	D00.08	D10.6	D37.05	D49.0
tonsillar	C09.0	C79.89	D00.08	D10.5	D37.05	D49.0
fourchette	C51.9	C79.82	D07.1	D28.0	D39.8	D49.59

✓ Additional Character Required — Refer to the Tabular List for Character Selection

Neoplasm, neoplastic	Malignant Primary	Malignant Secondary	Ca in situ	Benign	Uncertain Behavior	Unspecified Behavior
— continued						
frenulum						
labii — see						
Neoplasm, lip, internal						
linguae	C02.2	C79.89	D00.07	D10.1	D37.02	D49.0
frontal						
bone	C41.0	C79.51	—	D16.4	D48.0	D49.2
lobe, brain	C71.1	C79.31	—	D33.0	D43.0	D49.6
pole	C71.1	C79.31	—	D33.0	D43.0	D49.6
sinus	C31.2	C78.39	D02.3	D14.0	D38.5	D49.1
fundus						
stomach	C16.1	C78.89	D00.2	D13.1	D37.1	D49.0
uterus	C54.3	C79.82	D07.0	D26.1	D39.0	D49.59
gallbladder	C23	C78.89	D01.5	D13.5	D37.6	D49.0
overlapping lesion with extrahepatic bile ducts	C24.8	—	—	—	—	—
gall duct (extrahepatic)	C24.0	C78.89	D01.5	D13.5	D37.6	D49.0
intrahepatic	C22.1	C78.7	D01.5	D13.4	D37.6	D49.0
ganglia — see also						
Neoplasm, nerve, peripheral	C47.9	C79.89	—	D36.10	D48.2	D49.2
basal	C71.0	C79.31	—	D33.0	D43.0	D49.6
cranial nerve	C72.50	C79.49	—	D33.3	D43.3	D49.7
Gartner's duct	C52	C79.82	D07.2	D28.1	D39.8	D49.59
gastric — see Neoplasm, stomach						
gastrocolic	C26.9	C78.89	D01.9	D13.99	D37.9	D49.0
gastroesophageal junction	C16.0	C78.89	D00.2	D13.1	D37.1	D49.0
gastrointestinal (tract) NEC	C26.9	C78.89	D01.9	D13.99	D37.9	D49.0
generalized	C80.0	—	—	—	—	—
genital organ or tract						
female NEC	C57.9	C79.82	D07.30	D28.9	D39.9	D49.59
overlapping lesion	C57.8	—	—	—	—	—
specified site NEC	C57.7	C79.82	D07.39	D28.7	D39.8	D49.59
male NEC	C63.9	C79.82	D07.60	D29.9	D40.9	D49.59
overlapping lesion	C63.8	—	—	—	—	—
specified site NEC	C63.7	C79.82	D07.69	D29.8	D40.8	D49.59
genitourinary tract						
female	C57.9	C79.82	D07.30	D28.9	D39.9	D49.59
male	C63.9	C79.82	D07.60	D29.9	D40.9	D49.59
gingiva (alveolar) (marginal)	C03.9	C79.89	D00.03	D10.39	D37.09	D49.0
lower	C03.1	C79.89	D00.03	D10.39	D37.09	D49.0
mandibular	C03.1	C79.89	D00.03	D10.39	D37.09	D49.0
maxillary	C03.0	C79.89	D00.03	D10.39	D37.09	D49.0
upper	C03.0	C79.89	D00.03	D10.39	D37.09	D49.0
gland, glandular (lymphatic) (system) — see also Neoplasm, lymph gland						
endocrine NEC	C75.9	C79.89	D09.3	D35.9	D44.9	D49.7
salivary — see Neoplasm, salivary gland						
glans penis	C60.1	C79.82	D07.4	D29.0	D40.8	D49.59
globus pallidus	C71.0	C79.31	—	D33.0	D43.0	D49.6
glomus						
coccygeal	C49.5	C79.89	—	D21.5	D48.1☑	D49.2
jugularis	C75.5	C79.89	—	D35.6	D44.7	D49.7
glosso-epiglottic fold(s)	C10.1	C79.89	D00.08	D10.5	D37.05	D49.0
glossopalatine fold	C09.1	C79.89	D00.08	D10.5	D37.05	D49.0
glossopharyngeal sulcus	C09.0	C79.89	D00.08	D10.5	D37.05	D49.0
glottis	C32.0	C78.39	D02.0	D14.1	D38.0	D49.1
gluteal region	C76.3	C79.89	D04.5	D36.7	D48.7	D49.89
great vessels NEC	C49.3	C79.89	—	D21.3	D48.1☑	D49.2
groin NEC	C76.3	C79.89	D04.5	D36.7	D48.7	D49.89
gum	C03.9	C79.89	D00.03	D10.39	D37.09	D49.0
lower	C03.1	C79.89	D00.03	D10.39	D37.09	D49.0
upper	C03.0	C79.89	D00.03	D10.39	D37.09	D49.0

Neoplasm, neoplastic	Malignant Primary	Malignant Secondary	Ca in situ	Benign	Uncertain Behavior	Unspecified Behavior
— continued						
hand NEC	C76.4-☑	C79.89	D04.6-☑	D36.7	D48.7	D49.89
head NEC	C76.0	C79.89	D04.4	D36.7	D48.7	D49.89
heart	C38.0	C79.89	—	D15.1	D48.7	D49.89
heel NEC	C76.5-☑	C79.89	D04.7-☑	D36.7	D48.7	D49.89
helix — see also Neoplasm, skin, ear	C44.20-☑	C79.2	D04.2-☑	D23.2-☑	D48.5	D49.2
hematopoietic, hemopoietic tissue NEC	C96.9	—	—	—	—	—
specified NEC	C96.Z	—	—	—	—	—
hemisphere, cerebral	C71.0	C79.31	—	D33.0	D43.0	D49.6
hemorrhoidal zone	C21.1	C78.5	D01.3	D12.9	D37.8	D49.0
hepatic — see also Index to disease, by histology	C22.9	C78.7	D01.5	D13.4	D37.6	D49.0
duct (bile)	C24.0	C78.89	D01.5	D13.5	D37.6	D49.0
flexure (colon)	C18.3	C78.5	D01.0	D12.3	D37.4	D49.0
primary	C22.8	C78.7	D01.5	D13.4	D37.6	D49.0
hepatobiliary	C24.9	C78.89	D01.5	D13.5	D37.6	D49.0
hepatoblastoma	C22.2	C78.7	D01.5	D13.4	D37.6	D49.0
hepatoma	C22.0	C78.7	D01.5	D13.4	D37.6	D49.0
hilus of lung	C34.0-☑	C78.0-☑	D02.2-☑	D14.3-☑	D38.1	D49.1
hippocampus, brain	C71.2	C79.31	—	D33.0	D43.0	D49.6
hip NEC	C76.5-☑	C79.89	D04.7-☑	D36.7	D48.7	D49.89
humerus (any part)	C40.0-☑	C79.51	—	D16.0-☑	—	—
hymen	C52	C79.82	D07.2	D28.1	D39.8	D49.59
hypopharynx, hypopharyngeal NEC	C13.9	C79.89	D00.08	D10.7	D37.05	D49.0
overlapping lesion	C13.8	—	—	—	—	—
postcricoid region	C13.0	C79.89	D00.08	D10.7	D37.05	D49.0
posterior wall	C13.2	C79.89	D00.08	D10.7	D37.05	D49.0
pyriform fossa (sinus)	C12	C79.89	D00.08	D10.7	D37.05	D49.0
hypophysis	C75.1	C79.89	D09.3	D35.2	D44.3	D49.7
hypothalamus	C71.0	C79.31	—	D33.0	D43.0	D49.6
ileocecum, ileocecal (coil) (junction) (valve)	C18.0	C78.5	D01.0	D12.0	D37.4	D49.0
ileum	C17.2	C78.4	D01.49	D13.39	D37.2	D49.0
ilium	C41.4	C79.51	—	D16.8	D48.0	D49.2
immunoproliferative NEC	C88.9☑	—	—	—	—	—
infraclavicular (region)	C76.1	C79.89	D04.5	D36.7	D48.7	D49.89
inguinal (region)	C76.3	C79.89	D04.5	D36.7	D48.7	D49.89
insula	C71.0	C79.31	—	D33.0	D43.0	D49.6
insular tissue (pancreas)	C25.4	C78.89	D01.7	D13.7	D37.8	D49.0
brain	C71.0	C79.31	—	D33.0	D43.0	D49.6
interarytenoid fold	C13.1	C78.39	D00.08	D10.7	D37.05	D49.0
hypopharyngeal aspect	C13.1	C79.89	D00.08	D10.7	D37.05	D49.0
laryngeal aspect	C32.1	C78.39	D02.0	D14.1	D38.0	D49.1
marginal zone	C13.1	C79.89	D00.08	D10.7	D37.05	D49.0
interdental papillae	C03.9	C79.89	D00.03	D10.39	D37.09	D49.0
lower	C03.1	C79.89	D00.03	D10.39	D37.09	D49.0
upper	C03.0	C79.89	D00.03	D10.39	D37.09	D49.0
internal						
capsule	C71.0	C79.31	—	D33.0	D43.0	D49.6
os (cervix)	C53.0	C79.82	D06.0	D26.0	D39.0	D49.59
intervertebral cartilage or disc	C41.2	C79.51	—	D16.6	D48.0	D49.2
intestine, intestinal	C26.0	C78.80	D01.40	D13.99	D37.8	D49.0
large	C18.9	C78.5	D01.0	D12.6	D37.4	D49.0
appendix	C18.1	C78.5	D01.0	D12.1	D37.3	D49.0
caput coli	C18.0	C78.5	D01.0	D12.0	D37.4	D49.0
cecum	C18.0	C78.5	D01.0	D12.0	D37.4	D49.0
colon	C18.9	C78.5	D01.0	D12.6	D37.4	D49.0
and rectum	C19	C78.5	D01.1	D12.7	D37.5	D49.0
ascending	C18.2	C78.5	D01.0	D12.2	D37.4	D49.0

☑ **Additional Character Required — Refer to the Tabular List for Character Selection**

	Malignant Primary	Malignant Secondary	Ca in situ	Benign	Uncertain Behavior	Unspecified Behavior
Neoplasm, neoplastic						
— *continued*						
intestine, intestinal —						
continued						
large — *continued*						
colon — *continued*						
caput	C18.0	C78.5	D01.0	D12.0	D37.4	D49.0
descending	C18.6	C78.5	D01.0	D12.4	D37.4	D49.0
distal	C18.6	C78.5	D01.0	D12.4	D37.4	D49.0
left	C18.6	C78.5	D01.0	D12.4	D37.4	D49.0
overlapping						
lesion	C18.8	—	—	—	—	—
pelvic	C18.7	C78.5	D01.0	D12.5	D37.4	D49.0
right	C18.2	C78.5	D01.0	D12.2	D37.4	D49.0
sigmoid						
(flexure)	C18.7	C78.5	D01.0	D12.5	D37.4	D49.0
transverse	C18.4	C78.5	D01.0	D12.3	D37.4	D49.0
hepatic						
flexure	C18.3	C78.5	D01.0	D12.3	D37.4	D49.0
ileocecum, ileocecal						
(coil)						
(valve)	C18.0	C78.5	D01.0	D12.0	D37.4	D49.0
overlapping						
lesion	C18.8	—	—	—	—	—
sigmoid flexure						
(lower)						
(upper)	C18.7	C78.5	D01.0	D12.5	D37.4	D49.0
splenic flexure	C18.5	C78.5	D01.0	D12.3	D37.4	D49.0
small	C17.9	C78.4	D01.40	D13.30	D37.2	D49.0
duodenum	C17.0	C78.4	D01.49	D13.2	D37.2	D49.0
ileum	C17.2	C78.4	D01.49	D13.39	D37.2	D49.0
jejunum	C17.1	C78.4	D01.49	D13.39	D37.2	D49.0
overlapping						
lesion	C17.8	—	—	—	—	—
tract NEC	C26.0	C78.89	D01.40	D13.99	D37.8	D49.0
intra-abdominal	C76.2	C79.89	D09.8	D36.7	D48.7	D49.89
intracranial NEC	C71.9	C79.31	—	D33.2	D43.2	D49.6
intrahepatic (bile)						
duct	C22.1	C78.7	D01.5	D13.4	D37.6	D49.0
intraocular	C69.9-☑	C79.49	D09.2-☑	D31.9-☑	D48.7	D49.89
intraorbital	C69.6-☑	C79.49	D09.2-☑	D31.6-☑	D48.7	D49.89
intrasellar	C75.1	C79.89	D09.3	D35.2	D44.3	D49.7
intrathoracic (cavity)						
(organs)	C76.1	C79.89	D09.8	D15.9	D48.7	D49.89
specified NEC	C76.1	C79.89	D09.8	D15.7	—	—
iris	C69.4-☑	C79.49	D09.2-☑	D31.4-☑	D48.7	D49.89
ischiorectal (fossa)	C76.3	C79.89	D09.8	D36.7	D48.7	D49.89
ischium	C41.4	C79.51	—	D16.8	D48.0	D49.2
island of Reil	C71.0	C79.31	—	D33.0	D43.0	D49.6
islands or islets of						
Langerhans	C25.4	C78.89	D01.7	D13.7	D37.8	D49.0
isthmus uteri	C54.0	C79.82	D07.0	D26.1	D39.0	D49.59
jaw	C76.0	C79.89	D09.8	D36.7	D48.7	D49.89
bone	C41.1	C79.51	—	D16.5	D48.0	D49.2
lower	C41.1	C79.51	—	D16.5	—	—
upper	C41.0	C79.51	—	D16.4	—	—
carcinoma (any type)						
(lower)						
(upper)	C76.0	C79.89	—	—	—	—
skin — *see also*						
Neoplasm, skin,						
face	C44.309	C79.2	D04.39	D23.39	D48.5	D49.2
soft tissues	C03.9	C79.89	D00.03	D10.39	D37.09	D49.0
lower	C03.1	C79.89	D00.03	D10.39	D37.09	D49.0
upper	C03.0	C79.89	D00.03	D10.39	D37.09	D49.0
jejunum	C17.1	C78.4	D01.49	D13.39	D37.2	D49.0
joint NEC — *see also*						
Neoplasm,						
bone	C41.9	C79.51	—	D16.9	D48.0	D49.2
acromioclavicular	C40.0-☑	C79.51	—	D16.0-☑	—	—
bursa or synovial						
membrane — *see*						
Neoplasm,						
connective						
tissue						
costovertebral	C41.3	C79.51	—	D16.7	D48.0	D49.2
sternocostal	C41.3	C79.51	—	D16.7	D48.0	D49.2
temporomandibular	C41.1	C79.51	—	D16.5	D48.0	D49.2
junction						
anorectal	C21.8	C78.5	D01.3	D12.9	D37.8	D49.0
cardioesophageal	C16.0	C78.89	D00.2	D13.1	D37.1	D49.0
esophagogastric	C16.0	C78.89	D00.2	D13.1	D37.1	D49.0
gastroesophageal	C16.0	C78.89	D00.2	D13.1	D37.1	D49.0

	Malignant Primary	Malignant Secondary	Ca in situ	Benign	Uncertain Behavior	Unspecified Behavior
Neoplasm, neoplastic						
— *continued*						
junction — *continued*						
hard and soft						
palate	C05.9	C79.89	D00.00	D10.39	D37.09	D49.0
ileocecal	C18.0	C78.5	D01.0	D12.0	D37.4	D49.0
pelvirectal	C19	C78.5	D01.1	D12.7	D37.5	D49.0
pelviureteric	C65.-☑	C79.0-☑	D09.19	D30.1-☑	D41.1-☑	D49.59
rectosigmoid	C19	C78.5	D01.1	D12.7	D37.5	D49.0
squamocolumnar, of						
cervix	C53.8	C79.82	D06.7	D26.0	D39.0	D49.59
Kaposi's sarcoma — *see*						
Kaposi's, sarcoma						
kidney						
(parenchymal)	C64.-☑	C79.0-☑	D09.19	D30.0-☑	D41.0-☑	D49.51-☑
calyx	C65.-☑	C79.0-☑	D09.19	D30.1-☑	D41.1-☑	D49.51-☑
hilus	C65.-☑	C79.0-☑	D09.19	D30.1-☑	D41.1-☑	D49.51-☑
pelvis	C65.-☑	C79.0-☑	D09.19	D30.1-☑	D41.1-☑	D49.51-☑
knee NEC	C76.5-☑	C79.89	D04.7-☑	D36.7	D48.7	D49.89
labia (skin)	C51.9	C79.82	D07.1	D28.0	D39.8	D49.59
majora	C51.0	C79.82	D07.1	D28.0	D39.8	D49.59
minora	C51.1	C79.82	D07.1	D28.0	D39.8	D49.59
labial — *see also*						
Neoplasm, lip	C00.9	C79.89	D00.01	D10.0	D37.01	D49.0
sulcus (lower)						
(upper)	C06.1	C79.89	D00.02	D10.39	D37.09	D49.0
labium (skin)	C51.9	C79.82	D07.1	D28.0	D39.8	D49.59
majus	C51.0	C79.82	D07.1	D28.0	D39.8	D49.59
minus	C51.1	C79.82	D07.1	D28.0	D39.8	D49.59
lacrimal						
canaliculi	C69.5-☑	C79.49	D09.2-☑	D31.5-☑	D48.7	D49.89
duct (nasal)	C69.5-☑	C79.49	D09.2-☑	D31.5-☑	D48.7	D49.89
gland	C69.5-☑	C79.49	D09.2-☑	D31.5-☑	D48.7	D49.89
punctum	C69.5-☑	C79.49	D09.2-☑	D31.5-☑	D48.7	D49.89
sac	C69.5-☑	C79.49	D09.2-☑	D31.5-☑	D48.7	D49.89
Langerhans, islands or						
islets	C25.4	C78.89	D01.7	D13.7	D37.8	D49.0
laryngopharynx	C13.9	C79.89	D00.08	D10.7	D37.05	D49.0
larynx, laryngeal						
NEC	C32.9	C78.39	D02.0	D14.1	D38.0	D49.1
aryepiglottic						
fold	C32.1	C78.39	D02.0	D14.1	D38.0	D49.1
cartilage (arytenoid)						
(cricoid)						
(cuneiform)						
(thyroid)	C32.3	C78.39	D02.0	D14.1	D38.0	D49.1
commissure (anterior)						
(posterior)	C32.0	C78.39	D02.0	D14.1	D38.0	D49.1
extrinsic NEC	C32.1	C78.39	D02.0	D14.1	D38.0	D49.1
meaning						
hypopharynx	C13.9	C79.89	D00.08	D10.7	D37.05	D49.0
interarytenoid						
fold	C32.1	C78.39	D02.0	D14.1	D38.0	D49.1
intrinsic	C32.0	C78.39	D02.0	D14.1	D38.0	D49.1
overlapping						
lesion	C32.8	—	—	—	—	—
ventricular band	C32.1	C78.39	D02.0	D14.1	D38.0	D49.1
leg NEC	C76.5-☑	C79.89	D04.7-☑	D36.7	D48.7	D49.89
lens, crystalline	C69.4-☑	C79.49	D09.2-☑	D31.4-☑	D48.7	D49.89
lid (lower) (upper)	C44.10-☑	C79.2	D04.1-☑	D23.1-☑	D48.5	D49.2
basal cell						
carcinoma	C44.11-☑					
sebaceous cell	C44.13-☑					
specified type						
NEC	C44.19-☑					
squamous cell						
carcinoma	C44.12-☑					
ligament — *see also*						
Neoplasm,						
connective tissue						
broad	C57.1-☑	C79.82	D07.39	D28.2	D39.8	D49.59
Mackenrodt's	C57.7	C79.82	D07.39	D28.7	D39.8	D49.59
non-uterine — *see*						
Neoplasm,						
connective						
tissue						
round	C57.2-☑	C79.82	—	D28.2	D39.8	D49.59
sacro-uterine	C57.3	C79.82	—	D28.2	D39.8	D49.59
uterine	C57.3	C79.82	—	D28.2	D39.8	D49.59
utero-ovarian	C57.7	C79.82	D07.39	D28.2	D39.8	D49.59
uterosacral	C57.3	C79.82	—	D28.2	D39.8	D49.59
limb	C76.8	C79.89	D04.8	D36.7	D48.7	D49.89

☑ **Additional Character Required — Refer to the Tabular List for Character Selection**

	Malignant Primary	Malignant Secondary	Ca in situ	Benign	Uncertain Behavior	Unspecified Behavior
Neoplasm, neoplastic						
— continued						
limb — continued						
lower	C76.5-☑	C79.89	D04.7-☑	D36.7	D48.7	D49.89
upper	C76.4-☑	C79.89	D04.6-☑	D36.7	D48.7	D49.89
limbus of cornea	C69.1-☑	C79.49	D09.2-☑	D31.1-☑	D48.7	D49.89
lingual NEC — see also Neoplasm, tongue	C02.9	C79.89	D00.07	D10.1	D37.02	D49.0
lingula, lung	C34.1-☑	C78.0-☑	D02.2-☑	D14.3-☑	D38.1	D49.1
lip	C00.9	C79.89	D00.01	D10.0	D37.01	D49.0
buccal aspect — see Neoplasm, lip, internal						
commissure	C00.6	C79.89	D00.01	D10.0	D37.01	D49.0
external	C00.2	C79.89	D00.01	D10.0	D37.01	D49.0
lower	C00.1	C79.89	D00.01	D10.0	D37.01	D49.0
upper	C00.0	C79.89	D00.01	D10.0	D37.01	D49.0
frenulum — see Neoplasm, lip, internal						
inner aspect — see Neoplasm, lip, internal						
internal	C00.5	C79.89	D00.01	D10.0	D37.01	D49.0
lower	C00.4	C79.89	D00.01	D10.0	D37.01	D49.0
upper	C00.3	C79.89	D00.01	D10.0	D37.01	D49.0
lipstick area	C00.2	C79.89	D00.01	D10.0	D37.01	D49.0
lower	C00.1	C79.89	D00.01	D10.0	D37.01	D49.0
upper	C00.0	C79.89	D00.01	D10.0	D37.01	D49.0
lower	C00.1	C79.89	D00.01	D10.0	D37.01	D49.0
internal	C00.4	C79.89	D00.01	D10.0	D37.01	D49.0
mucosa — see Neoplasm, lip, internal						
oral aspect — see Neoplasm, lip, internal						
overlapping lesion	C00.8	—	—	—	—	—
with oral cavity or pharynx	C14.8	—	—	—	—	—
skin (commissure) (lower) (upper)	C44.00	C79.2	D04.0	D23.0	D48.5	D49.2
basal cell carcinoma	C44.01	—	—	—	—	—
specified type NEC	C44.09					
squamous cell carcinoma	C44.02	—	—	—	—	—
upper	C00.0	C79.89	D00.01	D10.0	D37.01	D49.0
internal	C00.3	C79.89	D00.01	D10.0	D37.01	D49.0
vermilion border	C00.2	C79.89	D00.01	D10.0	D37.01	D49.0
lower	C00.1	C79.89	D00.01	D10.0	D37.01	D49.0
upper	C00.0	C79.89	D00.01	D10.0	D37.01	D49.0
lipomatous — see Lipoma, by site						
liver — see also Index to disease, by histology	C22.9	C78.7	D01.5	D13.4	D37.6	D49.0
primary	C22.8	C78.7	D01.5	D13.4	D37.6	D49.0
lumbosacral plexus	C47.5	C79.89	—	D36.16	D48.2	D49.2
lung	C34.9-☑	C78.0-☑	D02.2-☑	D14.3-☑	D38.1	D49.1
azygos lobe	C34.1-☑	C78.0-☑	D02.2-☑	D14.3-☑	D38.1	D49.1
carina	C34.0-☑	C78.0-☑	D02.2-☑	D14.3-☑	D38.1	D49.1
hilus	C34.0-☑	C78.0-☑	D02.2-☑	D14.3-☑	D38.1	D49.1
lingula	C34.1-☑	C78.0-☑	D02.2-☑	D14.3-☑	D38.1	D49.1
lobe NEC	C34.9-☑	C78.0-☑	D02.2-☑	D14.3-☑	D38.1	D49.1
lower lobe	C34.3-☑	C78.0-☑	D02.2-☑	D14.3-☑	D38.1	D49.1
main bronchus	C34.0-☑	C78.0-☑	D02.2-☑	D14.3-☑	D38.1	D49.1
mesothelioma — see Mesothelioma						
middle lobe	C34.2	C78.0-☑	D02.21	D14.31	D38.1	D49.1
overlapping lesion	C34.8-☑	—	—	—	—	—
upper lobe	C34.1-☑	C78.0-☑	D02.2-☑	D14.3-☑	D38.1	D49.1
lymph, lymphatic channel NEC	C49.9	C79.89	—	D21.9	D48.1☑	D49.2

	Malignant Primary	Malignant Secondary	Ca in situ	Benign	Uncertain Behavior	Unspecified Behavior
Neoplasm, neoplastic						
— continued						
lymph, lymphatic channel — continued						
gland (secondary)	—	C77.9	—	D36.0	D48.7	D49.89
abdominal	—	C77.2	—	D36.0	D48.7	D49.89
aortic	—	C77.2	—	D36.0	D48.7	D49.89
arm	—	C77.3	—	D36.0	D48.7	D49.89
auricular (anterior) (posterior)	—	C77.0	—	D36.0	D48.7	D49.89
axilla, axillary	—	C77.3	—	D36.0	D48.7	D49.89
brachial	—	C77.3	—	D36.0	D48.7	D49.89
bronchial	—	C77.1	—	D36.0	D48.7	D49.89
bronchopulmonary	—	C77.1	—	D36.0	D48.7	D49.89
celiac	—	C77.2	—	D36.0	D48.7	D49.89
cervical	—	C77.0	—	D36.0	D48.7	D49.89
cervicofacial	—	C77.0	—	D36.0	D48.7	D49.89
Cloquet	—	C77.4	—	D36.0	D48.7	D49.89
colic	—	C77.2	—	D36.0	D48.7	D49.89
common duct	—	C77.2	—	D36.0	D48.7	D49.89
cubital	—	C77.3	—	D36.0	D48.7	D49.89
diaphragmatic	—	C77.1	—	D36.0	D48.7	D49.89
epigastric, inferior	—	C77.1	—	D36.0	D48.7	D49.89
epitrochlear	—	C77.3	—	D36.0	D48.7	D49.89
esophageal	—	C77.1	—	D36.0	D48.7	D49.89
face	—	C77.0	—	D36.0	D48.7	D49.89
femoral	—	C77.4	—	D36.0	D48.7	D49.89
gastric	—	C77.2	—	D36.0	D48.7	D49.89
groin	—	C77.4	—	D36.0	D48.7	D49.89
head	—	C77.0	—	D36.0	D48.7	D49.89
hepatic	—	C77.2	—	D36.0	D48.7	D49.89
hilar (pulmonary)	—	C77.1	—	D36.0	D48.7	D49.89
splenic	—	C77.2	—	D36.0	D48.7	D49.89
hypogastric	—	C77.5	—	D36.0	D48.7	D49.89
ileocolic	—	C77.2	—	D36.0	D48.7	D49.89
iliac	—	C77.5	—	D36.0	D48.7	D49.89
infraclavicular	—	C77.3	—	D36.0	D48.7	D49.89
inguina, inguinal	—	C77.4	—	D36.0	D48.7	D49.89
innominate	—	C77.1	—	D36.0	D48.7	D49.89
intercostal	—	C77.1	—	D36.0	D48.7	D49.89
intestinal	—	C77.2	—	D36.0	D48.7	D49.89
intrabdominal	—	C77.2	—	D36.0	D48.7	D49.89
intrapelvic	—	C77.5	—	D36.0	D48.7	D49.89
intrathoracic	—	C77.1	—	D36.0	D48.7	D49.89
jugular	—	C77.0	—	D36.0	D48.7	D49.89
leg	—	C77.4	—	D36.0	D48.7	D49.89
limb						
lower	—	C77.4	—	D36.0	D48.7	D49.89
upper	—	C77.3	—	D36.0	D48.7	D49.89
lower limb	—	C77.4	—	D36.0	D48.7	D49.89
lumbar	—	C77.2	—	D36.0	D48.7	D49.89
mandibular	—	C77.0	—	D36.0	D48.7	D49.89
mediastinal	—	C77.1	—	D36.0	D48.7	D49.89
mesenteric (inferior) (superior)	—	C77.2	—	D36.0	D48.7	D49.89
midcolic	—	C77.2	—	D36.0	D48.7	D49.89
multiple sites in categories C77.0 - C77.5	—	C77.8	—	D36.0	D48.7	D49.89
neck	—	C77.0	—	D36.0	D48.7	D49.89
obturator	—	C77.5	—	D36.0	D48.7	D49.89
occipital	—	C77.0	—	D36.0	D48.7	D49.89
pancreatic	—	C77.2	—	D36.0	D48.7	D49.89
para-aortic	—	C77.2	—	D36.0	D48.7	D49.89
paracervical	—	C77.5	—	D36.0	D48.7	D49.89
parametrial	—	C77.5	—	D36.0	D48.7	D49.89
parasternal	—	C77.1	—	D36.0	D48.7	D49.89
parotid	—	C77.0	—	D36.0	D48.7	D49.89
pectoral	—	C77.3	—	D36.0	D48.7	D49.89
pelvic	—	C77.5	—	D36.0	D48.7	D49.89
peri-aortic	—	C77.2	—	D36.0	D48.7	D49.89
peripancreatic	—	C77.2	—	D36.0	D48.7	D49.89
popliteal	—	C77.4	—	D36.0	D48.7	D49.89
porta hepatis	—	C77.2	—	D36.0	D48.7	D49.89
portal	—	C77.2	—	D36.0	D48.7	D49.89
preauricular	—	C77.0	—	D36.0	D48.7	D49.89
prelaryngeal	—	C77.0	—	D36.0	D48.7	D49.89

☑ **Additional Character Required — Refer to the Tabular List for Character Selection**

	Malignant Primary	Malignant Secondary	Ca in situ	Benign	Uncertain Behavior	Unspecified Behavior
Neoplasm, neoplastic						
— *continued*						
lymph, lymphatic channel —						
continued						
gland — *continued*						
presymphysial	—	C77.5		D36.0	D48.7	D49.89
pretracheal	—	C77.0		D36.0	D48.7	D49.89
primary (any site) NEC	C96.9	—		—	—	—
pulmonary (hiler)	—	C77.1		D36.0	D48.7	D49.89
pyloric	—	C77.2		D36.0	D48.7	D49.89
retroperitoneal	—	C77.2		D36.0	D48.7	D49.89
retropharyngeal	—	C77.0		D36.0	D48.7	D49.89
Rosenmuller's	—	C77.4		D36.0	D48.7	D49.89
sacral	—	C77.5		D36.0	D48.7	D49.89
scalene	—	C77.0		D36.0	D48.7	D49.89
site NEC	—	C77.9		D36.0	D48.7	D49.89
splenic (hilar)	—	C77.2		D36.0	D48.7	D49.89
subclavicular	—	C77.3		D36.0	D48.7	D49.89
subinguinal	—	C77.4		D36.0	D48.7	D49.89
sublingual	—	C77.0		D36.0	D48.7	D49.89
submandibular	—	C77.0		D36.0	D48.7	D49.89
submaxillary	—	C77.0		D36.0	D48.7	D49.89
submental	—	C77.0		D36.0	D48.7	D49.89
subscapular	—	C77.3		D36.0	D48.7	D49.89
supraclavicular	—	C77.0		D36.0	D48.7	D49.89
thoracic	—	C77.1		D36.0	D48.7	D49.89
tibial	—	C77.4		D36.0	D48.7	D49.89
tracheal	—	C77.1		D36.0	D48.7	D49.89
tracheobronchial	—	C77.1		D36.0	D48.7	D49.89
upper limb	—	C77.3		D36.0	D48.7	D49.89
Virchow's	—	C77.0		D36.0	D48.7	D49.89
node — *see also* Neoplasm, lymph gland						
primary NEC	C96.9	—		—	—	—
vessel — *see also* Neoplasm, connective tissue	C49.9	C79.89	—	D21.9	D48.1 ☑	D49.2
Mackenrodt's ligament	C57.7	C79.82	D07.39	D28.7	D39.8	D49.59
malar	C41.0	C79.51		D16.4	D48.0	D49.2
region — *see* Neoplasm, cheek						
mammary gland — *see* Neoplasm, breast						
mandible	C41.1	C79.51	—	D16.5	D48.0	D49.2
alveolar						
mucosa (carcinoma)	C03.1	C79.89	D00.03	D10.39	D37.09	D49.0
ridge or process	C41.1	C79.51	—	D16.5	D48.0	D49.2
marrow (bone) NEC	C96.9	C79.52	—	—	D47.9	D49.89
mastectomy site (skin) — *see also* Neoplasm, breast, skin	C44.501	C79.2	—	—	—	—
specified as breast tissue	C50.8- ☑	C79.81	—	—	—	—
mastoid (air cells) (antrum) (cavity)	C30.1	C78.39	D02.3	D14.0	D38.5	D49.1
bone or process	C41.0	C79.51	—	D16.4	D48.0	D49.2
maxilla, maxillary (superior)	C41.0	C79.51	—	D16.4	D48.0	D49.2
alveolar						
mucosa	C03.0	C79.89	D00.03	D10.39	D37.09	D49.0
ridge or process (carcinoma)	C41.0	C79.51	—	D16.4	D48.0	D49.2
antrum	C31.0	C78.39	D02.3	D14.0	D38.5	D49.1
carcinoma	C03.0	C79.51	—	—	—	—
inferior — *see* Neoplasm, mandible						
sinus	C31.0	C78.39	D02.3	D14.0	D38.5	D49.1
meatus external (ear) — *see also* Neoplasm, skin, ear						
ear	C44.20- ☑	C79.2	D04.2- ☑	D23.2- ☑	D48.5	D49.2

	Malignant Primary	Malignant Secondary	Ca in situ	Benign	Uncertain Behavior	Unspecified Behavior
Neoplasm, neoplastic						
— *continued*						
Meckel diverticulum, malignant	C17.3	C78.4	D01.49	D13.39	D37.2	D49.0
mediastinum, mediastinal	C38.3	C78.1	—	D15.2	D38.3	D49.89
anterior	C38.1	C78.1	—	D15.2	D38.3	D49.89
posterior	C38.2	C78.1	—	D15.2	D38.3	D49.89
medulla						
adrenal	C74.1- ☑	C79.7- ☑	D09.3	D35.0- ☑	D44.1- ☑	D49.7
oblongata	C71.7	C79.31	—	D33.1	D43.1	D49.6
meibomian gland	C44.10- ☑	C79.2	D04.1- ☑	D23.1- ☑	D48.5	D49.2
basal cell carcinoma	C44.11- ☑			—	—	—
sebaceous cell	C44.13- ☑			—	—	—
specified type NEC	C44.19- ☑			—	—	—
squamous cell carcinoma	C44.12- ☑			—	—	—
melanoma — *see* Melanoma						
meninges	C70.9	C79.49	—	D32.9	D42.9	D49.7
brain	C70.0	C79.32	—	D32.0	D42.0	D49.7
cerebral	C70.0	C79.32	—	D32.0	D42.0	D49.7
crainial	C70.0	C79.32	—	D32.0	D42.0	D49.7
intracranial	C70.0	C79.32	—	D32.0	D42.0	D49.7
spinal (cord)	C70.1	C79.49	—	D32.1	D42.1	D49.7
meniscus, knee joint (lateral)						
(medial)	C40.2- ☑	C79.51	—	D16.2- ☑	D48.0	D49.2
Merkel cell — *see* Carcinoma, Merkel cell						
mesentery, mesenteric	C48.1	C78.6	—	D20.1	D48.4	D49.0
mesoappendix	C48.1	C78.6	—	D20.1	D48.4	D49.0
mesocolon	C48.1	C78.6	—	D20.1	D48.4	D49.0
mesopharynx — *see* Neoplasm, oropharynx						
mesosalpinx	C57.1- ☑	C79.82	D07.39	D28.2	D39.8	D49.59
mesothelial tissue — *see* Mesothelioma						
mesothelioma — *see* Mesothelioma						
mesovarium	C57.1- ☑	C79.82	D07.39	D28.2	D39.8	D49.59
metacarpus (any bone)	C40.1- ☑	C79.51	—	D16.1- ☑		
metastatic NEC — *see also* Neoplasm, by site, secondary	—	C79.9		—	—	—
metatarsus (any bone)	C40.3- ☑	C79.51	—	D16.3- ☑	—	—
midbrain	C71.7	C79.31	—	D33.1	D43.1	D49.6
milk duct — *see* Neoplasm, breast						
mons						
pubis	C51.9	C79.82	D07.1	D28.0	D39.8	D49.59
veneris	C51.9	C79.82	D07.1	D28.0	D39.8	D49.59
motor tract	C72.9	C79.49	—	D33.9	D43.9	D49.7
brain	C71.9	C79.31	—	D33.2	D43.2	D49.6
cauda equina	C72.1	C79.49	—	D33.4	D43.4	D49.7
spinal	C72.0	C79.49	—	D33.4	D43.4	D49.7
mouth	C06.9	C79.89	D00.00	D10.30	D37.09	D49.0
book-leaf	C06.89	C79.89	—	—	—	—
floor	C04.9	C79.89	D00.06	D10.2	D37.09	D49.0
anterior portion	C04.0	C79.89	D00.06	D10.2	D37.09	D49.0
lateral portion	C04.1	C79.89	D00.06	D10.2	D37.09	D49.0
overlapping lesion	C04.8					
overlapping NEC	C06.80	—		—	—	—
roof	C05.9	C79.89	D00.00	D10.39	D37.09	D49.0
specified part NEC	C06.89	C79.89	D00.00	D10.39	D37.09	D49.0
vestibule	C06.1	C79.89	D00.00	D10.39	D37.09	D49.0
mucosa						
alveolar (ridge or process)	C03.9	C79.89	D00.03	D10.39	D37.09	D49.0
lower	C03.1	C79.89	D00.03	D10.39	D37.09	D49.0
upper	C03.0	C79.89	D00.03	D10.39	D37.09	D49.0

☑ **Additional Character Required — Refer to the Tabular List for Character Selection**

Left column table

Neoplasm, neoplastic — continued	Malignant Primary	Malignant Secondary	Ca in situ	Benign	Uncertain Behavior	Unspecified Behavior
mucosa — continued						
buccal	C06.0	C79.89	D00.02	D10.39	D37.09	D49.0
cheek	C06.0	C79.89	D00.02	D10.39	D37.09	D49.0
lip — see Neoplasm, lip, internal						
nasal	C30.0	C78.39	D02.3	D14.0	D38.5	D49.1
oral	C06.0	C79.89	D00.02	D10.39	D37.09	D49.0
Mullerian duct						
female	C57.7	C79.82	D07.39	D28.7	D39.8	D49.59
male	C63.7	C79.82	D07.69	D29.8	D40.8	D49.59
muscle — see also Neoplasm, connective tissue						
extraocular	C69.6-☑	C79.49	D09.2-☑	D31.6-☑	D48.7	D49.89
myocardium	C38.0	C79.89		D15.1	D48.7	D49.89
myometrium	C54.2	C79.82	D07.0	D26.1	D39.0	D49.59
myopericardium	C38.0	C79.89	—	D15.1	D48.7	D49.89
nabothian gland (follicle)	C53.0	C79.82	D06.0	D26.0	D39.0	D49.59
nail — see also Neoplasm, skin, limb	C44.90	C79.2	D04.9	D23.9	D48.5	D49.2
finger — see also Neoplasm, skin, limb, upper	C44.60-☑	C79.2	D04.6-☑	D23.6-☑	D48.5	D49.2
toe — see also Neoplasm, skin, limb, lower	C44.70-☑	C79.2	D04.7-☑	D23.7-☑	D48.5	D49.2
nares, naris (anterior) (posterior)	C30.0	C78.39	D02.3	D14.0	D38.5	D49.1
nasal — see Neoplasm, nose						
nasolabial groove — see also Neoplasm, skin, face	C44.309	C79.2	D04.39	D23.39	D48.5	D49.2
nasolacrimal duct	C69.5-☑	C79.49	D09.2-☑	D31.5-☑	D48.7	D49.89
nasopharynx, nasopharyngeal	C11.9	C79.89	D00.08	D10.6	D37.05	D49.0
floor	C11.3	C79.89	D00.08	D10.6	D37.05	D49.0
overlapping lesion	C11.8	—	—	—	—	—
roof	C11.0	C79.89	D00.08	D10.6	D37.05	D49.0
wall	C11.9	C79.89	D00.08	D10.6	D37.05	D49.0
anterior	C11.3	C79.89	D00.08	D10.6	D37.05	D49.0
lateral	C11.2	C79.89	D00.08	D10.6	D37.05	D49.0
posterior	C11.1	C79.89	D00.08	D10.6	D37.05	D49.0
superior	C11.0	C79.89	D00.08	D10.6	D37.05	D49.0
nates — see also Neoplasm, skin, trunk	C44.509	C79.2	D04.5	D23.5	D48.5	D49.2
neck NEC	C76.0	C79.89	D09.8	D36.7	D48.7	D49.89
skin	C44.40	—	—	—	—	—
basal cell carcinoma	C44.41					
specified type NEC	C44.49	—	—	—	—	—
squamous cell carcinoma	C44.42	—	—	—	—	—
nerve (ganglion)	C47.9	C79.89	—	D36.10	D48.2	D49.2
abducens	C72.59	C79.49	—	D33.3	D43.3	D49.7
accessory (spinal)	C72.59	C79.49	—	D33.3	D43.3	D49.7
acoustic	C72.4-☑	C79.49	—	D33.3	D43.3	D49.7
auditory	C72.4-☑	C79.49	—	D33.3	D43.3	D49.7
autonomic NEC — see also Neoplasm, nerve, peripheral	C47.9	C79.89	—	D36.10	D48.2	D49.2
brachial	C47.1-☑	C79.89	—	D36.12	D48.2	D49.2
cranial	C72.50	C79.49	—	D33.3	D43.3	D49.7
specified NEC	C72.59	C79.49	—	D33.3	D43.3	D49.7
facial	C72.59	C79.49	—	D33.3	D43.3	D49.7
femoral	C47.2-☑	C79.89	—	D36.13	D48.2	D49.2
ganglion NEC — see also Neoplasm, nerve, peripheral	C47.9	C79.89	—	D36.10	D48.2	D49.2
glossopharyngeal	C72.59	C79.49	—	D33.3	D43.3	D49.7
hypoglossal	C72.59	C79.49	—	D33.3	D43.3	D49.7
intercostal	C47.3	C79.89	—	D36.14	D48.2	D49.2
lumbar	C47.6	C79.89	—	D36.17	D48.2	D49.2

Right column table

Neoplasm, neoplastic — continued	Malignant Primary	Malignant Secondary	Ca in situ	Benign	Uncertain Behavior	Unspecified Behavior
nerve — continued						
median	C47.1-☑	C79.89	—	D36.12	D48.2	D49.2
obturator	C47.2-☑	C79.89	—	D36.13	D48.2	D49.2
oculomotor	C72.59	C79.49	—	D33.3	D43.3	D49.7
olfactory	C47.2-☑	C79.49	—	D33.3	D43.3	D49.7
optic	C72.3-☑	C79.49	—	D33.3	D43.3	D49.7
parasympathetic NEC	C47.9	C79.89	—	D36.10	D48.2	D49.2
peripheral NEC	C47.9	C79.89	—	D36.10	D48.2	D49.2
abdomen	C47.4	C79.89	—	D36.15	D48.2	D49.2
abdominal wall	C47.4	C79.89	—	D36.15	D48.2	D49.2
ankle	C47.2-☑	C79.89	—	D36.13	D48.2	D49.2
antecubital fossa or space	C47.1-☑	C79.89	—	D36.12	D48.2	D49.2
arm	C47.1-☑	C79.89	—	D36.12	D48.2	D49.2
auricle (ear)	C47.0	C79.89	—	D36.11	D48.2	D49.2
axilla	C47.3	C79.89	—	D36.12	D48.2	D49.2
back	C47.6	C79.89	—	D36.17	D48.2	D49.2
buttock	C47.5	C79.89	—	D36.16	D48.2	D49.2
calf	C47.2-☑	C79.89	—	D36.13	D48.2	D49.2
cervical region	C47.0	C79.89	—	D36.11	D48.2	D49.2
cheek	C47.0	C79.89	—	D36.11	D48.2	D49.2
chest (wall)	C47.3	C79.89	—	D36.14	D48.2	D49.2
chin	C47.0	C79.89	—	D36.11	D48.2	D49.2
ear (external)	C47.0	C79.89	—	D36.11	D48.2	D49.2
elbow	C47.1-☑	C79.89	—	D36.12	D48.2	D49.2
extrarectal	C47.5	C79.89	—	D36.16	D48.2	D49.2
extremity	C47.9	C79.89	—	D36.10	D48.2	D49.2
lower	C47.2-☑	C79.89	—	D36.13	D48.2	D49.2
upper	C47.1-☑	C79.89	—	D36.12	D48.2	D49.2
eyelid	C47.0	C79.89	—	D36.11	D48.2	D49.2
face	C47.0	C79.89	—	D36.11	D48.2	D49.2
finger	C47.1-☑	C79.89	—	D36.12	D48.2	D49.2
flank	C47.6	C79.89	—	D36.17	D48.2	D49.2
foot	C47.2-☑	C79.89	—	D36.13	D48.2	D49.2
forearm	C47.1-☑	C79.89	—	D36.12	D48.2	D49.2
forehead	C47.0	C79.89	—	D36.11	D48.2	D49.2
gluteal region	C47.5	C79.89	—	D36.16	D48.2	D49.2
groin	C47.5	C79.89	—	D36.16	D48.2	D49.2
hand	C47.1-☑	C79.89	—	D36.12	D48.2	D49.2
head	C47.0	C79.89	—	D36.11	D48.2	D49.2
heel	C47.2-☑	C79.89	—	D36.13	D48.2	D49.2
hip	C47.2-☑	C79.89	—	D36.13	D48.2	D49.2
infraclavicular region	C47.3	C79.89	—	D36.14	D48.2	D49.2
inguinal (canal) (region)	C47.5	C79.89	—	D36.16	D48.2	D49.2
intrathoracic	C47.3	C79.89	—	D36.14	D48.2	D49.2
ischiorectal fossa	C47.5	C79.89	—	D36.16	D48.2	D49.2
knee	C47.2-☑	C79.89	—	D36.13	D48.2	D49.2
leg	C47.2-☑	C79.89	—	D36.13	D48.2	D49.2
limb NEC	C47.9	C79.89	—	D36.10	D48.2	D49.2
lower	C47.2-☑	C79.89	—	D36.13	D48.2	D49.2
upper	C47.1-☑	C79.89	—	D36.12	D48.2	D49.2
nates	C47.5	C79.89	—	D36.16	D48.2	D49.2
neck	C47.0	C79.89	—	D36.11	D48.2	D49.2
orbit	C69.6-☑	C79.49	—	D31.6-☑	D48.7	D49.2
pararectal	C47.5	C79.89	—	D36.16	D48.2	D49.2
paraurethral	C47.5	C79.89	—	D36.16	D48.2	D49.2
paravaginal	C47.5	C79.89	—	D36.16	D48.2	D49.2
pelvis (floor)	C47.5	C79.89	—	D36.16	D48.2	D49.2
pelvoabdominal	C47.8	C79.89	—	D36.17	D48.2	D49.2
perineum	C47.5	C79.89	—	D36.16	D48.2	D49.2
perirectal (tissue)	C47.5	C79.89	—	D36.16	D48.2	D49.2
periurethral (tissue)	C47.5	C79.89	—	D36.16	D48.2	D49.2
popliteal fossa or space	C47.2-☑	C79.89	—	D36.13	D48.2	D49.2
presacral	C47.5	C79.89	—	D36.16	D48.2	D49.2
pterygoid fossa	C47.0	C79.89	—	D36.11	D48.2	D49.2
rectovaginal septum or wall	C47.5	C79.89	—	D36.16	D48.2	D49.2
rectovesical	C47.5	C79.89	—	D36.16	D48.2	D49.2
sacrococcygeal region	C47.5	C79.89	—	D36.16	D48.2	D49.2

Neoplasm, neoplastic	Malignant Primary	Malignant Secondary	Ca in situ	Benign	Uncertain Behavior	Unspecified Behavior
— continued						
nerve — continued						
peripheral —						
continued						
scalp	C47.0	C79.89	—	D36.11	D48.2	D49.2
scapular						
region	C47.3	C79.89	—	D36.14	D48.2	D49.2
shoulder	C47.1-☑	C79.89	—	D36.12	D48.2	D49.2
submental	C47.0	C79.89	—	D36.11	D48.2	D49.2
supraclavicular						
region	C47.0	C79.89	—	D36.11	D48.2	D49.2
temple	C47.0	C79.89	—	D36.11	D48.2	D49.2
temporal						
region	C47.0	C79.89	—	D36.11	D48.2	D49.2
thigh	C47.2-☑	C79.89	—	D36.13	D48.2	D49.2
thoracic (duct)						
(wall)	C47.3	C79.89	—	D36.14	D48.2	D49.2
thorax	C47.3	C79.89	—	D36.14	D48.2	D49.2
thumb	C47.1-☑	C79.89	—	D36.12	D48.2	D49.2
toe	C47.2-☑	C79.89	—	D36.13	D48.2	D49.2
trunk	C47.6	C79.89	—	D36.17	D48.2	D49.2
umbilicus	C47.4	C79.89	—	D36.15	D48.2	D49.2
vesicorectal	C47.5	C79.89	—	D36.16	D48.2	D49.2
wrist	C47.1-☑	C79.89	—	D36.12	D48.2	D49.2
radial	C47.1-☑	C79.89	—	D36.12	D48.2	D49.2
sacral	C47.5	C79.89	—	D36.16	D48.2	D49.2
sciatic	C47.2-☑	C79.89	—	D36.13	D48.2	D49.2
spinal NEC	C47.9	C79.89	—	D36.10	D48.2	D49.2
accessory	C72.59	C79.49	—	D33.3	D43.3	D49.7
sympathetic NEC —						
see also						
Neoplasm, nerve,						
peripheral	C47.9	C79.89	—	D36.10	D48.2	D49.2
trigeminal	C72.59	C79.49	—	D33.3	D43.3	D49.7
trochlear	C72.59	C79.49	—	D33.3	D43.3	D49.7
ulnar	C47.1-☑	C79.89	—	D36.12	D48.2	D49.2
vagus	C72.59	C79.49	—	D33.3	D43.3	D49.7
nervous system						
(central)	C72.9	C79.40	—	D33.9	D43.9	D49.7
autonomic — see						
Neoplasm, nerve,						
peripheral						
parasympathetic —						
see Neoplasm,						
nerve, peripheral						
specified site						
NEC	—	C79.49	—	D33.7	D43.8	—
sympathetic — see						
Neoplasm, nerve,						
peripheral						
nevus — see Nevus						
nipple	C50.0-☑	C79.81	D05.-☑	D24.-☑	—	—
nose, nasal	C76.0	C79.89	D09.8	D36.7	D48.7	D49.89
ala (external) (nasi)						
— see also						
Neoplasm, nose,						
skin	C44.301	C79.2	D04.39	D23.39	D48.5	D49.2
bone	C41.0	C79.51	—	D16.4	D48.0	D49.2
cartilage	C30.0	C78.39	D02.3	D14.0	D38.5	D49.1
cavity	C30.0	C78.39	D02.3	D14.0	D38.5	D49.1
choana	C11.3	C79.89	D00.08	D10.6	D37.05	D49.0
external (skin) — see						
also Neoplasm,						
nose, skin	C44.301	C79.2	D04.39	D23.39	D48.5	D49.2
fossa	C30.0	C78.39	D02.3	D14.0	D38.5	D49.1
internal	C30.0	C78.39	D02.3	D14.0	D38.5	D49.1
mucosa	C30.0	C78.39	D02.3	D14.0	D38.5	D49.1
septum	C30.0	C78.39	D02.3	D14.0	D38.5	D49.1
posterior						
margin	C11.3	C79.89	D00.08	D10.6	D37.05	D49.0
sinus — see						
Neoplasm, sinus						
skin	C44.301	C79.2	D04.39	D23.39	D48.5	D49.2
basal cell						
carcinoma	C44.311	—	—	—	—	—
specified type						
NEC	C44.391	—	—	—	—	—
squamous cell						
carcinoma	C44.321	—	—	—	—	—
turbinate						
(mucosa)	C30.0	C78.39	D02.3	D14.0	D38.5	D49.1
bone	C41.0	C79.51	—	D16.4	D48.0	D49.2

Neoplasm, neoplastic	Malignant Primary	Malignant Secondary	Ca in situ	Benign	Uncertain Behavior	Unspecified Behavior
— continued						
nose, nasal —						
continued						
vestibule	C30.0	C78.39	D02.3	D14.0	D38.5	D49.1
nostril	C30.0	C78.39	D02.3	D14.0	D38.5	D49.1
nucleus pulposus	C41.2	C79.51	—	D16.6	D48.0	D49.2
occipital						
bone	C41.0	C79.51	—	D16.4	D48.0	D49.2
lobe or pole,						
brain	C71.4	C79.31	—	D33.0	D43.0	D49.6
odontogenic — see						
Neoplasm, jaw,						
bone						
olfactory nerve or						
bulb	C72.2-☑	C79.49	—	D33.3	D43.3	D49.7
olive (brain)	C71.7	C79.31	—	D33.1	D43.1	D49.6
omentum	C48.1	C78.6	—	D20.1	D48.4	D49.0
operculum (brain)	C71.0	C79.31	—	D33.0	D43.0	D49.6
optic nerve, chiasm, or						
tract	C72.3-☑	C79.49	—	D33.3	D43.3	D49.7
oral (cavity)	C06.9	C79.89	D00.00	D10.30	D37.09	D49.0
ill-defined	C14.8	C79.89	D00.00	D10.30	D37.09	D49.0
mucosa	C06.0	C79.89	D00.02	D10.39	D37.09	D49.0
orbit	C69.6-☑	C79.49	D09.2-☑	D31.6-☑	D48.7	D49.89
autonomic						
nerve	C69.6-☑	C79.49	—	D31.6-☑	D48.7	D49.2
bone	C41.0	C79.51	—	D16.4	D48.0	D49.2
eye	C69.6-☑	C79.49	D09.2-☑	D31.6-☑	D48.7	D49.89
peripheral						
nerves	C69.6-☑	C79.49	—	D31.6-☑	D48.7	D49.2
soft parts	C69.6-☑	C79.49	D09.2-☑	D31.6-☑	D48.7	D49.89
organ of						
Zuckerkandl	C75.5	C79.89	—	D35.6	D44.7	D49.7
oropharynx	C10.9	C79.89	D00.08	D10.5	D37.05	D49.0
branchial cleft						
(vestige)	C10.4	C79.89	D00.08	D10.5	D37.05	D49.0
junctional						
region	C10.8	C79.89	D00.08	D10.5	D37.05	D49.0
lateral wall	C10.2	C79.89	D00.08	D10.5	D37.05	D49.0
overlapping						
lesion	C10.8	—	—	—	—	—
pillars or fauces	C09.1	C79.89	D00.08	D10.5	D37.05	D49.0
posterior wall	C10.3	C79.89	D00.08	D10.5	D37.05	D49.0
vallecula	C10.0	C79.89	D00.08	D10.5	D37.05	D49.0
os						
external	C53.1	C79.82	D06.1	D26.0	D39.0	D49.59
internal	C53.0	C79.82	D06.0	D26.0	D39.0	D49.59
ovary	C56.-☑	C79.6-☑	D07.39	D27.-☑	D39.1-☑	D49.59
oviduct	C57.0-☑	C79.82	D07.39	D28.2	D39.8	D49.59
palate	C05.9	C79.89	D00.00	D10.39	D37.09	D49.0
hard	C05.0	C79.89	D00.05	D10.39	D37.09	D49.0
junction of hard and						
soft palate	C05.9	C79.89	D00.00	D10.39	D37.09	D49.0
overlapping						
lesions	C05.8	—	—	—	—	—
soft	C05.1	C79.89	D00.04	D10.39	D37.09	D49.0
nasopharyngeal						
surface	C11.3	C79.89	D00.08	D10.6	D37.05	D49.0
posterior						
surface	C11.3	C79.89	D00.08	D10.6	D37.05	D49.0
superior						
surface	C11.3	C79.89	D00.08	D10.6	D37.05	D49.0
palatoglossal arch	C09.1	C79.89	D00.00	D10.5	D37.09	D49.0
palatopharyngeal						
arch	C09.1	C79.89	D00.00	D10.5	D37.09	D49.0
pallium	C71.0	C79.31	—	D33.0	D43.0	D49.6
palpebra	C44.10-☑	C79.2	D04.1-☑	D23.1-☑	D48.5	D49.2
basal cell						
carcinoma	C44.11-☑	—	—	—	—	—
sebaceous cell	C44.13-☑	—	—	—	—	—
specified type						
NEC	C44.19-☑	—	—	—	—	—
squamous cell						
carcinoma	C44.12-☑	—	—	—	—	—
pancreas	C25.9	C78.89	D01.7	D13.6	D37.8	D49.0
body	C25.1	C78.89	D01.7	D13.6	D37.8	D49.0
duct (of Santorini) (of						
Wirsung)	C25.3	C78.89	D01.7	D13.6	D37.8	D49.0
ectopic tissue	C25.7	C78.89	—	D13.6	D37.8	D49.0
head	C25.0	C78.89	D01.7	D13.6	D37.8	D49.0
islet cells	C25.4	C78.89	D01.7	D13.7	D37.8	D49.0
neck	C25.7	C78.89	D01.7	D13.6	D37.8	D49.0

☑ **Additional Character Required** — Refer to the Tabular List for Character Selection

Neoplasm, neoplastic	Malignant Primary	Malignant Secondary	Ca in situ	Benign	Uncertain Behavior	Unspecified Behavior
— continued						
pancreas — continued						
overlapping lesion	C25.8	—	—	—	—	—
tail	C25.2	C78.89	D01.7	D13.6	D37.8	D49.0
para-aortic body	C75.5	C79.89	—	D35.6	D44.7	D49.7
paraganglion NEC	C75.5	C79.89	—	D35.6	D44.7	D49.7
parametrium	C57.3	C79.82	—	D28.2	D39.8	D49.59
paranephric	C48.0	C78.6	—	D20.0	D48.3	D49.0
pararectal	C76.3	C79.89	—	D36.7	D48.7	D49.89
parasagittal (region)	C76.0	C79.89	D09.8	D36.7	D48.7	D49.89
parasellar	C72.9	C79.49	—	D33.9	D43.8	D49.7
parathyroid (gland)	C75.0	C79.89	D09.3	D35.1	D44.2	D49.7
paraurethral	C76.3	C79.89	—	D36.7	D48.7	D49.89
gland	C68.1	C79.19	D09.19	D30.8	D41.8	D49.59
paravaginal	C76.3	C79.89	—	D36.7	D48.7	D49.89
parenchyma, kidney	C64.-☑	C79.0-☑	D09.19	D30.0-☑	D41.0-☑	D49.51-☑
parietal						
bone	C41.0	C79.51	—	D16.4	D48.0	D49.2
lobe, brain	C71.3	C79.31	—	D33.0	D43.0	D49.6
paroophoron	C57.1-☑	C79.82	D07.39	D28.2	D39.8	D49.59
parotid (duct) (gland)	C07	C79.89	D00.00	D11.0	D37.030	D49.0
parovarium	C57.1-☑	C79.82	D07.39	D28.2	D39.8	D49.59
patella	C40.20	C79.51	—	—	—	—
peduncle, cerebral	C71.7	C79.31	—	D33.1	D43.1	D49.6
pelvirectal junction	C19	C78.5	D01.1	D12.7	D37.5	D49.0
pelvis, pelvic	C76.3	C79.89	D09.8	D36.7	D48.7	D49.89
bone	C41.4	C79.51	—	D16.8	D48.0	D49.2
floor	C76.3	C79.89	D09.8	D36.7	D48.7	D49.89
renal	C65.-☑	C79.0-☑	D09.19	D30.1-☑	D41.1-☑	D49.51-☑
viscera	C76.3	C79.89	D09.8	D36.7	D48.7	D49.89
wall	C76.3	C79.89	D09.8	D36.7	D48.7	D49.89
pelvo-abdominal	C76.8	C79.89	D09.8	D36.7	D48.7	D49.89
penis	C60.9	C79.82	D07.4	D29.0	D40.8	D49.59
body	C60.2	C79.82	D07.4	D29.0	D40.8	D49.59
corpus (cavernosum)	C60.2	C79.82	D07.4	D29.0	D40.8	D49.59
glans	C60.1	C79.82	D07.4	D29.0	D40.8	D49.59
overlapping sites	C60.8	—	—	—	—	—
skin NEC	C60.9	C79.82	D07.4	D29.0	D40.8	D49.59
periadrenal (tissue)	C48.0	C78.6	—	D20.0	D48.3	D49.0
perianal (skin) — see also Neoplasm, anus, skin,	C44.500	C79.2	D04.5	D23.5	D48.5	D49.2
pericardium	C38.0	C79.89	—	D15.1	D48.7	D49.89
perinephric	C48.0	C78.6	—	D20.0	D48.3	D49.0
perineum	C76.3	C79.89	D09.8	D36.7	D48.7	D49.89
periodontal tissue NEC	C03.9	C79.89	D00.03	D10.39	D37.09	D49.0
periosteum — see Neoplasm, bone						
peripancreatic	C48.0	C78.6	—	D20.0	D48.3	D49.0
peripheral nerve NEC	C47.9	C79.89	—	D36.10	D48.2	D49.2
perirectal (tissue)	C76.3	C79.89	—	D36.7	D48.7	D49.89
perirenal (tissue)	C48.0	C78.6	—	D20.0	D48.3	D49.0
peritoneum, peritoneal (cavity)	C48.2	C78.6	—	D20.1	D48.4	D49.0
benign mesothelial tissue — see Mesothelioma, benign						
overlapping lesion	C48.8	—	—	—	—	—
with digestive organs	C26.9	—	—	—	—	—
parietal	C48.1	C78.6	—	D20.1	D48.4	D49.0
pelvic	C48.1	C78.6	—	D20.1	D48.4	D49.0
specified part NEC	C48.1	C78.6	—	D20.1	D48.4	D49.0
peritonsillar (tissue)	C76.0	C79.89	D09.8	D36.7	D48.7	D49.89
periurethral tissue	C76.3	C79.89	—	D36.7	D48.7	D49.89
phalanges						
foot	C40.3-☑	C79.51	—	D16.3-☑	—	—

Neoplasm, neoplastic	Malignant Primary	Malignant Secondary	Ca in situ	Benign	Uncertain Behavior	Unspecified Behavior
— continued						
phalanges — continued						
hand	C40.1-☑	C79.51	—	D16.1-☑	—	—
pharynx, pharyngeal	C14.0	C79.89	D00.08	D10.9	D37.05	D49.0
bursa	C11.1	C79.89	D00.08	D10.6	D37.05	D49.0
fornix	C11.3	C79.89	D00.08	D10.6	D37.05	D49.0
recess	C11.2	C79.89	D00.08	D10.6	D37.05	D49.0
region	C14.0	C79.89	D00.08	D10.9	D37.05	D49.0
tonsil	C11.1	C79.89	D00.08	D10.6	D37.05	D49.0
wall (lateral) (posterior)	C14.0	C79.89	D00.08	D10.9	D37.05	D49.0
pia mater	C70.9	C79.40	—	D32.9	D42.9	D49.7
cerebral	C70.0	C79.32	—	D32.0	D42.0	D49.7
cranial	C70.0	C79.32	—	D32.0	D42.0	D49.7
spinal	C70.1	C79.49	—	D32.1	D42.1	D49.7
pillars of fauces	C09.1	C79.89	D00.08	D10.5	D37.05	D49.0
pineal (body) (gland)	C75.3	C79.89	D09.3	D35.4	D44.5	D49.7
pinna (ear) NEC — see also Neoplasm, skin, ear	C44.20-☑	C79.2	D04.2-☑	D23.2-☑	D48.5	D49.2
piriform fossa or sinus	C12	C79.89	D00.08	D10.7	D37.05	D49.0
pituitary (body) (fossa) (gland) (lobe)	C75.1	C79.89	D09.3	D35.2	D44.3	D49.7
placenta	C58	C79.82	D07.0	D26.7	D39.2	D49.59
pleura, pleural (cavity)	C38.4	C78.2	—	D19.0	D38.2	D49.1
overlapping lesion with heart or mediastinum	C38.8	—	—	—	—	—
parietal	C38.4	C78.2	—	D19.0	D38.2	D49.1
visceral	C38.4	C78.2	—	D19.0	D38.2	D49.1
plexus						
brachial	C47.1-☑	C79.89	—	D36.12	D48.2	D49.2
cervical	C47.0	C79.89	—	D36.11	D48.2	D49.2
choroid	C71.5	C79.31	—	D33.0	D43.0	D49.6
lumbosacral	C47.5	C79.89	—	D36.16	D48.2	D49.2
sacral	C47.5	C79.89	—	D36.16	D48.2	D49.2
pluriendocrine	C75.8	C79.89	D09.3	D35.7	D44.9	D49.7
pole						
frontal	C71.1	C79.31	—	D33.0	D43.0	D49.6
occipital	C71.4	C79.31	—	D33.0	D43.0	D49.6
pons (varolii)	C71.7	C79.31	—	D33.1	D43.1	D49.6
popliteal fossa or space	C76.5-☑	C79.89	D04.7-☑	D36.7	D48.7	D49.89
postcricoid (region)	C13.0	C79.89	D00.08	D10.7	D37.05	D49.0
posterior fossa (cranial)	C71.9	C79.31	—	D33.2	D43.2	D49.6
postnasal space	C11.9	C79.89	D00.08	D10.6	D37.05	D49.0
prepuce	C60.9	C79.82	D07.4	D29.0	D40.8	D49.59
prepylorus	C16.4	C78.89	D00.2	D13.1	D37.1	D49.0
presacral (region)	C76.3	C79.89	—	D36.7	D48.7	D49.89
prostate (gland)	C61	C79.82	D07.5	D29.1	D40.0	D49.59
utricle	C68.0	C79.19	D09.19	D30.4	D41.3	D49.59
pterygoid fossa	C49.0	C79.89	—	D21.0	D48.1	D49.2
pubic bone	C41.4	C79.51	—	D16.8	D48.0	D49.2
pudenda, pudendum (femae)	C51.9	C79.82	D07.1	D28.0	D39.8	D49.59
pulmonary — see also Neoplasm, lung	C34.9-☑	C78.0-☑	D02.2-☑	D14.3-☑	D38.1	D49.1
putamen	C71.0	C79.31	—	D33.0	D43.0	D49.6
pyloric						
antrum	C16.3	C78.89	D00.2	D13.1	D37.1	D49.0
canal	C16.4	C78.89	D00.2	D13.1	D37.1	D49.0
pylorus	C16.4	C78.89	D00.2	D13.1	D37.1	D49.0
pyramid (brain)	C71.7	C79.31	—	D33.1	D43.1	D49.6
pyriform fossa or sinus	C12	C79.89	D00.08	D10.7	D37.05	D49.0
radius (any part)	C40.0-☑	C79.51	—	D16.0-☑	—	—
Rathke's pouch	C75.1	C79.89	D09.3	D35.2	D44.3	D49.7
rectosigmoid (junction)	C19	C78.5	D01.1	D12.7	D37.5	D49.0
overlapping lesion with anus or rectum	C21.8	—	—	—	—	—
rectouterine pouch	C48.1	C78.6	—	D20.1	D48.4	D49.0

Neoplasm Table

Neoplasm, rectovaginal septum or wall — Neoplasm, skin NOS

Neoplasm, neoplastic	Malignant Primary	Malignant Secondary	Ca in situ	Benign	Uncertain Behavior	Unspecified Behavior
— continued						
rectovaginal septum or wall	C76.3	C79.89	D09.8	D36.7	D48.7	D49.89
rectovesical septum	C76.3	C79.89	D09.8	D36.7	D48.7	D49.89
rectum (ampulla)	C20	C78.5	D01.2	D12.8	D37.5	D49.0
and colon	C19	C78.5	D01.1	D12.7	D37.5	D49.0
overlapping lesion with anus or rectosigmoid junction	C21.8	—	—	—	—	—
renal	C64.- ✓	C79.0- ✓	D09.19	D30.0- ✓	D41.0- ✓	D49.51- ✓
calyx	C65.- ✓	C79.0- ✓	D09.19	D30.1- ✓	D41.1- ✓	D49.51- ✓
hilus	C65.- ✓	C79.0- ✓	D09.19	D30.1- ✓	D41.1- ✓	D49.51- ✓
parenchyma	C64.- ✓	C79.0- ✓	D09.19	D30.0- ✓	D41.0- ✓	D49.51- ✓
pelvis	C65.- ✓	C79.0- ✓	D09.19	D30.1- ✓	D41.1- ✓	D49.51- ✓
respiratory organs or system NEC	C39.9	C78.30	D02.4	D14.4	D38.6	D49.1
tract NEC	C39.9	C78.30	D02.4	D14.4	D38.5	D49.1
upper	C39.0	C78.30	D02.4	D14.4	D38.5	D49.1
retina	C69.2- ✓	C79.49	D09.2- ✓	D31.2- ✓	D48.7	D49.81
retrobulbar	C69.6- ✓	C79.49	—	D31.6- ✓	D48.7	D49.89
retrocecal	C48.0	C78.6	—	D20.0	D48.3	D49.0
retromolar (area) (triangle) (trigone)	C06.2	C79.89	D00.00	D10.39	D37.09	D49.0
retro-orbital	C76.0	C79.89	D09.8	D36.7	D48.7	D49.89
retroperitoneal (space) (tissue)	C48.0	C78.6	—	D20.0	D48.3	D49.0
retroperitoneum	C48.0	C78.6	—	D20.0	D48.3	D49.0
retropharyngeal	C14.0	C79.89	D00.08	D10.9	D37.05	D49.0
retrovesical (septum)	C76.3	C79.89	D09.8	D36.7	D48.7	D49.89
rhinencephalon	C71.0	C79.31	—	D33.0	D43.0	D49.6
rib	C41.3	C79.51	—	D16.7	D48.0	D49.2
Rosenmuller's fossa	C11.2	C79.89	D00.08	D10.6	D37.05	D49.0
round ligament	C57.2- ✓	C79.82	—	D28.2	D39.8	D49.59
sacrococcyx, sacrococcygeal	C41.4	C79.51		D16.8	D48.0	D49.2
region	C76.3	C79.89	D09.8	D36.7	D48.7	D49.89
sacrouterine ligament	C57.3	C79.82		D28.2	D39.8	D49.59
sacrum, sacral (vertebra)	C41.4	C79.51		D16.8	D48.0	D49.2
salivary gland or duct (major)	C08.9	C79.89	D00.00	D11.9	D37.039	D49.0
minor NEC	C06.9	C79.89	D00.00	D10.39	D37.04	D49.0
overlapping lesion	C08.9	—	—	—	—	—
parotid	C07	C79.89	D00.00	D11.0	D37.030	D49.0
pluriglandular	C08.9	C79.89	D00.00	D11.9	D37.039	D49.0
sublingual	C08.1	C79.89	D00.00	D11.7	D37.031	D49.0
submandibular	C08.0	C79.89	D00.00	D11.7	D37.032	D49.0
submaxillary	C08.0	C79.89	D00.00	D11.7	D37.032	D49.0
salpinx (uterine)	C57.0- ✓	C79.82	D07.39	D28.2	D39.8	D49.59
Santorini's duct	C25.3	C78.89	D01.7	D13.6	D37.8	D49.0
scalp	C44.40	C79.2	D04.4	D23.4	D48.5	D49.2
basal cell carcinoma	C44.41	—	—	—	—	—
specified type NEC	C44.49	—	—	—	—	—
squamous cell carcinoma	C44.42	—	—	—	—	—
scapula (any part)	C40.0- ✓	C79.51	—	D16.0- ✓	—	—
scapular region	C76.1	C79.89	D09.8	D36.7	D48.7	D49.89
scar NEC — see also Neoplasm, skin, by site	C44.90	C79.2	D04.9	D23.9	D48.5	D49.2
sciatic nerve	C47.2- ✓	C79.89	—	D36.13	D48.2	D49.2
sclera	C69.4- ✓	C79.49	D09.2- ✓	D31.4- ✓	D48.7	D49.89
scrotum (skin)	C63.2	C79.82	D07.61	D29.4	D40.8	D49.59
sebaceous gland — see Neoplasm, skin						
sella turcica	C75.1	C79.89	D09.3	D35.2	D44.3	D49.7
bone	C41.0	C79.51		D16.4	D48.0	D49.2
semilunar cartilage (knee)	C40.2- ✓	C79.51	—	D16.2- ✓	D48.0	D49.2
seminal vesicle	C63.7	C79.82	D07.69	D29.8	D40.8	D49.59
septum nasal	C30.0	C78.39	D02.3	D14.0	D38.5	D49.1

Neoplasm, neoplastic	Malignant Primary	Malignant Secondary	Ca in situ	Benign	Uncertain Behavior	Unspecified Behavior
— continued						
septum — continued						
nasal — continued						
posterior margin	C11.3	C79.89	D00.08	D10.6	D37.05	D49.0
rectovaginal	C76.3	C79.89	D09.8	D36.7	D48.7	D49.89
rectovesical	C76.3	C79.89	D09.8	D36.7	D48.7	D49.89
urethrovaginal	C57.9	C79.82	D07.30	D28.9	D39.9	D49.59
vesicovaginal	C57.9	C79.82	D07.30	D28.9	D39.9	D49.59
shoulder NEC	C76.4- ✓	C79.89	D04.6- ✓	D36.7	D48.7	D49.89
sigmoid flexure (lower) (upper)	C18.7	C78.5	D01.0	D12.5	D37.4	D49.0
sinus (accessory)	C31.9	C78.39	D02.3	D14.0	D38.5	D49.1
bone (any)	C41.0	C79.51	—	D16.4	D48.0	D49.2
ethmoidal	C31.1	C78.39	D02.3	D14.0	D38.5	D49.1
frontal	C31.2	C78.39	D02.3	D14.0	D38.5	D49.1
maxillary	C31.0	C78.39	D02.3	D14.0	D38.5	D49.1
nasal, paranasal NEC	C31.9	C78.39	D02.3	D14.0	D38.5	D49.1
overlapping lesion	C31.8	—	—	—	—	—
pyriform	C12	C79.89	D00.08	D10.7	D37.05	D49.0
sphenoid	C31.3	C78.39	D02.3	D14.0	D38.5	D49.1
skeleton, skeletal NEC	C41.9	C79.51	—	D16.9	D48.0	D49.2
Skene's gland	C68.1	C79.19	D09.19	D30.8	D41.8	D49.59
skin NOS	C44.90	C79.2	D04.9	D23.9	D48.5	D49.2
abdominal wall	C44.509	C79.2	D04.5	D23.5	D48.5	D49.2
basal cell carcinoma	C44.519	—	—	—	—	—
specified type NEC	C44.599	—	—	—	—	—
squamous cell carcinoma	C44.529	—	—	—	—	—
ala nasi — see also Neoplasm, nose, skin	C44.301	C79.2	D04.39	D23.39	D48.5	D49.2
ankle — see also Neoplasm, skin, limb, lower	C44.70- ✓	C79.2	D04.7- ✓	D23.7- ✓	D48.5	D49.2
antecubital space — see also Neoplasm, skin, limb, upper	C44.60- ✓	C79.2	D04.6- ✓	D23.6- ✓	D48.5	D49.2
anus	C44.500	C79.2	D04.5	D23.5	D48.5	D49.2
basal cell carcinoma	C44.510	—	—	—	—	—
specified type NEC	C44.590	—	—	—	—	—
squamous cell carcinoma	C44.520	—	—	—	—	—
arm — see also Neoplasm, skin, limb, upper	C44.60- ✓	C79.2	D04.6- ✓	D23.6- ✓	D48.5	D49.2
auditory canal (external) — see also Neoplasm, skin, ear	C44.20- ✓	C79.2	D04.2- ✓	D23.2- ✓	D48.5	D49.2
auricle (ear) — see also Neoplasm, skin, ear	C44.20- ✓	C79.2	D04.2- ✓	D23.2- ✓	D48.5	D49.2
auricular canal (external) — see also Neoplasm, skin, ear	C44.20- ✓	C79.2	D04.2- ✓	D23.2- ✓	D48.5	D49.2
axilla, axillary fold — see also Neoplasm, skin, trunk	C44.509	C79.2	D04.5	D23.5	D48.5	D49.2
back — see also Neoplasm, skin, trunk	C44.509	C79.2	D04.5	D23.5	D48.5	D49.2
basal cell carcinoma	C44.91	—	—	—	—	—
breast	C44.501	C79.2	D04.5	D23.5	D48.5	D49.2
basal cell carcinoma	C44.511	—	—	—	—	—
specified type NEC	C44.591	—	—	—	—	—
squamous cell carcinoma	C44.521	—	—	—	—	—

☑ **Additional Character Required — Refer to the Tabular List for Character Selection**

Neoplasm, neoplastic	Malignant Primary	Malignant Secondary	Ca in situ	Benign	Uncertain Behavior	Unspecified Behavior
— continued						
skin — continued						
brow — see also Neoplasm, skin, face	C44.309	C79.2	D04.39	D23.39	D48.5	D49.2
buttock — see also Neoplasm, skin, trunk	C44.509	C79.2	D04.5	D23.5	D48.5	D49.2
calf — see also Neoplasm, skin, limb, lower	C44.70-☑	C79.2	D04.7-☑	D23.7-☑	D48.5	D49.2
canthus (eye) (inner) (outer)	C44.10-☑	C79.2	D04.1-☑	D23.1-☑	D48.5	D49.2
basal cell carcinoma	C44.11-☑	—	—	—	—	—
sebaceous cell	C44.13-☑	—	—	—	—	—
specified type NEC	C44.19-☑	—	—	—	—	—
squamous cell carcinoma	C44.12-☑	—	—	—	—	—
cervical region — see also Neoplasm, skin, neck	C44.40	C79.2	D04.4	D23.4	D48.5	D49.2
cheek (external) — see also Neoplasm, skin, face	C44.309	C79.2	D04.39	D23.39	D48.5	D49.2
chest (wall) — see also Neoplasm, skin, trunk	C44.509	C79.2	D04.5	D23.5	D48.5	D49.2
chin — see also Neoplasm, skin, face	C44.309	C79.2	D04.39	D23.39	D48.5	D49.2
clavicular area — see also Neoplasm, skin, trunk	C44.509	C79.2	D04.5	D23.5	D48.5	D49.2
clitoris	C51.2	C79.82	D07.1	D28.0	D39.8	D49.59
columnella — see also Neoplasm, skin, face	C44.309	C79.2	D04.39	D23.39	D48.5	D49.2
concha — see also Neoplasm, skin, ear	C44.20-☑	C79.2	D04.2-☑	D23.2-☑	D48.5	D49.2
ear (external)	C44.20-☑	C79.2	D04.2-☑	D23.2-☑	D48.5	D49.2
basal cell carcinoma	C44.21-☑	—	—	—	—	—
specified type NEC	C44.29-☑	—	—	—	—	—
squamous cell carcinoma	C44.22-☑	—	—	—	—	—
elbow — see also Neoplasm, skin, limb, upper	C44.60-☑	C79.2	D04.6-☑	D23.6-☑	D48.5	D49.2
eyebrow — see also Neoplasm, skin, face	C44.309	C79.2	D04.39	D23.39	D48.5	D49.2
eyelid	C44.10-☑	C79.2	D04.1-☑	D23.1-☑	D48.5	D49.2
basal cell carcinoma	C44.11-☑	—	—	—	—	—
sebaceous cell	C44.13-☑	—	—	—	—	—
specified type NEC	C44.19-☑	—	—	—	—	—
squamous cell carcinoma	C44.12-☑	—	—	—	—	—
face NOS	C44.300	C79.2	D04.30	D23.30	D48.5	D49.2
basal cell carcinoma	C44.310	—	—	—	—	—
specified type NEC	C44.390	—	—	—	—	—
squamous cell carcinoma	C44.320	—	—	—	—	—
female genital organs (external)	C51.9	C79.82	D07.1	D28.0	D39.8	D49.59
clitoris	C51.2	C79.82	D07.1	D28.0	D39.8	D49.59
labium NEC	C51.9	C79.82	D07.1	D28.0	D39.8	D49.59
majus	C51.0	C79.82	D07.1	D28.0	D39.8	D49.59
minus	C51.1	C79.82	D07.1	D28.0	D39.8	D49.59
pudendum	C51.9	C79.82	D07.1	D28.0	D39.8	D49.59
vulva	C51.9	C79.82	D07.1	D28.0	D39.8	D49.59
finger — see also Neoplasm, skin, limb, upper	C44.60-☑	C79.2	D04.6-☑	D23.6-☑	D48.5	D49.2

Neoplasm, neoplastic	Malignant Primary	Malignant Secondary	Ca in situ	Benign	Uncertain Behavior	Unspecified Behavior
— continued						
skin — continued						
flank — see also Neoplasm, skin, trunk	C44.509	C79.2	D04.5	D23.5	D48.5	D49.2
foot — see also Neoplasm, skin, limb, lower	C44.70-☑	C79.2	D04.7-☑	D23.7-☑	D48.5	D49.2
forearm — see also Neoplasm, skin, limb, upper	C44.60-☑	C79.2	D04.6-☑	D23.6-☑	D48.5	D49.2
forehead — see also Neoplasm, skin, face	C44.309	C79.2	D04.39	D23.39	D48.5	D49.2
glabella — see also Neoplasm, skin, face	C44.309	C79.2	D04.39	D23.39	D48.5	D49.2
gluteal region — see also Neoplasm, skin, trunk	C44.509	C79.2	D04.5	D23.5	D48.5	D49.2
groin — see also Neoplasm, skin, trunk	C44.509	C79.2	D04.5	D23.5	D48.5	D49.2
hand — see also Neoplasm, skin, limb, upper	C44.60-☑	C79.2	D04.6-☑	D23.6-☑	D48.5	D49.2
head NEC — see also Neoplasm, skin, scalp	C44.40	C79.2	D04.4	D23.4	D48.5	D49.2
heel — see also Neoplasm, skin, limb, lower	C44.70-☑	C79.2	D04.7-☑	D23.7-☑	D48.5	D49.2
helix — see also Neoplasm, skin, ear	C44.20-☑	C79.2	D04.2-☑	D23.2-☑	D48.5	D49.2
hip — see also Neoplasm, skin, limb, lower	C44.70-☑	C79.2	D04.7-☑	D23.7-☑	D48.5	D49.2
infraclavicular region — see also Neoplasm, skin, trunk	C44.509	C79.2	D04.5	D23.5	D48.5	D49.2
inguinal region — see also Neoplasm, skin, trunk	C44.509	C79.2	D04.5	D23.5	D48.5	D49.2
jaw — see also Neoplasm, skin, face	C44.309	C79.2	D04.39	D23.39	D48.5	D49.2
Kaposi's sarcoma — see Kaposi's, sarcoma, skin						
knee — see also Neoplasm, skin, limb, lower	C44.70-☑	C79.2	D04.7-☑	D23.7-☑	D48.5	D49.2
labia						
majora	C51.0	C79.82	D07.1	D28.0	D39.8	D49.59
minora	C51.1	C79.82	D07.1	D28.0	D39.8	D49.59
leg — see also Neoplasm, skin, limb, lower	C44.70-☑	C79.2	D04.7-☑	D23.7-☑	D48.5	D49.2
lid (lower) (upper)	C44.10-☑	C79.2	D04.1-☑	D23.1-☑	D48.5	D49.2
basal cell carcinoma	C44.11-☑	—	—	—	—	—
sebaceous cell	C44.13-☑	—	—	—	—	—
specified type NEC	C44.19-☑	—	—	—	—	—
squamous cell carcinoma	C44.12-☑	—	—	—	—	—
limb NEC	C44.90	C79.2	D04.9	D23.9	D48.5	D49.2
basal cell carcinoma	C44.91	—	—	—	—	—
lower	C44.70-☑	C79.2	D04.7-☑	D23.7-☑	D48.5	D49.2
basal cell carcinoma	C44.71-☑	—	—	—	—	—
specified type NEC	C44.79-☑	—	—	—	—	—
squamous cell carcinoma	C44.72-☑	—	—	—	—	—
upper	C44.60-☑	C79.2	D04.6-☑	D23.6-☑	D48.5	D49.2
basal cell carcinoma	C44.61-☑	—	—	—	—	—

Neoplasm Table

Neoplasm, skin NOS — Neoplasm, skin NOS

Neoplasm, neoplastic	Malignant Primary	Malignant Secondary	Ca in situ	Benign	Uncertain Behavior	Unspecified Behavior
— continued						
skin — continued						
limb — continued						
upper — continued						
specified type NEC	C44.69-✓	—	—	—	—	—
squamous cell carcinoma	C44.62-✓	—	—	—	—	—
lip (lower) (upper)	C44.00	C79.2	D04.0	D23.0	D48.5	D49.2
basal cell carcinoma	C44.01	—	—	—	—	—
specified type NEC	C44.09	—	—	—	—	—
squamous cell carcinoma	C44.02	—	—	—	—	—
male genital organs	C63.9	C79.82	D07.60	D29.9	D40.8	D49.59
penis	C60.9	C79.82	D07.4	D29.0	D40.8	D49.59
prepuce	C60.0	C79.82	D07.4	D29.0	D40.8	D49.59
scrotum	C63.2	C79.82	D07.61	D29.4	D40.8	D49.59
mastectomy site (skin) — see also Neoplasm, skin, breast	C44.501	C79.2	—	—	—	—
specified as breast tissue	C50.8-✓	C79.81	—	—	—	—
meatus, acoustic (external) — see also Neoplasm, skin, ear	C44.20-✓	C79.2	D04.2-✓	D23.2-✓	D48.5	D49.2
melanotic — see Melanoma						
Merkel cell — see Carcinoma, Merkel cell						
nates — see also Neoplasm, skin, trunk	C44.509	C79.2	D04.5	D23.5	D48.5	D49.2
neck	C44.40	C79.2	D04.4	D23.4	D48.5	D49.2
basal cell carcinoma	C44.41	—	—	—	—	—
specified type NEC	C44.49	—	—	—	—	—
squamous cell carcinoma	C44.42	—	—	—	—	—
nevus — see Nevus, skin						
nose (external) — see also Neoplasm, nose, skin	C44.301	C79.2	D04.39	D23.39	D48.5	D49.2
overlapping lesion	C44.80	—	—	—	—	—
basal cell carcinoma	C44.81	—	—	—	—	—
specified type NEC	C44.89	—	—	—	—	—
squamous cell carcinoma	C44.82	—	—	—	—	—
palm — see also Neoplasm, skin, limb, upper	C44.60-✓	C79.2	D04.6-✓	D23.6-✓	D48.5	D49.2
palpebra	C44.10-✓	C79.2	D04.1-✓	D23.1-✓	D48.5	D49.2
basal cell carcinoma	C44.11-✓	—	—	—	—	—
sebaceous cell	C44.13-✓	—	—	—	—	—
specified type NEC	C44.19-✓	—	—	—	—	—
squamous cell carcinoma	C44.12-✓	—	—	—	—	—
penis NEC	C60.9	C79.82	D07.4	D29.0	D40.8	D49.59
perianal — see also Neoplasm, skin, anus	C44.500	C79.2	D04.5	D23.5	D48.5	D49.2
perineum — see also Neoplasm, skin, anus	C44.500	C79.2	D04.5	D23.5	D48.5	D49.2
pinna — see also Neoplasm, skin, ear	C44.20-✓	C79.2	D04.2-✓	D23.2-✓	D48.5	D49.2
plantar — see also Neoplasm, skin, limb, lower	C44.70-✓	C79.2	D04.7-✓	D23.7-✓	D48.5	D49.2

Neoplasm, neoplastic	Malignant Primary	Malignant Secondary	Ca in situ	Benign	Uncertain Behavior	Unspecified Behavior
— continued						
skin — continued						
popliteal fossa or space — see also Neoplasm, skin, limb, lower	C44.70-✓	C79.2	D04.7-✓	D23.7-✓	D48.5	D49.2
prepuce	C60.0	C79.82	D07.4	D29.0	D40.8	D49.59
pubes — see also Neoplasm, skin, trunk	C44.509	C79.2	D04.5	D23.5	D48.5	D49.2
sacrococcygeal region — see also Neoplasm, skin, trunk	C44.509	C79.2	D04.5	D23.5	D48.5	D49.2
scalp	C44.40	C79.2	D04.4	D23.4	D48.5	D49.2
basal cell carcinoma	C44.41	—	—	—	—	—
specified type NEC	C44.49	—	—	—	—	—
squamous cell carcinoma	C44.42	—	—	—	—	—
scapular region — see also Neoplasm, skin, trunk	C44.509	C79.2	D04.5	D23.5	D48.5	D49.2
scrotum	C63.2	C79.82	D07.61	D29.4	D40.8	D49.59
shoulder — see also Neoplasm, skin, limb, upper	C44.60-✓	C79.2	D04.6-✓	D23.6-✓	D48.5	D49.2
sole (foot) — see also Neoplasm, skin, limb, lower	C44.70-✓	C79.2	D04.7-✓	D23.7-✓	D48.5	D49.2
specified sites NEC	C44.80	C79.2	D04.8	D23.9	D48.5	D49.2
basal cell carcinoma	C44.81	—	—	—	—	—
specified type NEC	C44.89	—	—	—	—	—
squamous cell carcinoma	C44.82	—	—	—	—	—
specified type NEC	C44.99	—	—	—	—	—
squamous cell carcinoma	C44.92	—	—	—	—	—
submammary fold — see also Neoplasm, skin, trunk	C44.509	C79.2	D04.5	D23.5	D48.5	D49.2
supraclavicular region — see also Neoplasm, skin, neck	C44.40	C79.2	D04.4	D23.4	D48.5	D49.2
temple — see also Neoplasm, skin, face	C44.309	C79.2	D04.39	D23.39	D48.5	D49.2
thigh — see also Neoplasm, skin, limb, lower	C44.70-✓	C79.2	D04.7-✓	D23.7-✓	D48.5	D49.2
thoracic wall — see also Neoplasm, skin, trunk	C44.509	C79.2	D04.5	D23.5	D48.5	D49.2
thumb — see also Neoplasm, skin, limb, upper	C44.60-✓	C79.2	D04.6-✓	D23.6-✓	D48.5	D49.2
toe — see also Neoplasm, skin, limb, lower	C44.70-✓	C79.2	D04.7-✓	D23.7-✓	D48.5	D49.2
tragus — see also Neoplasm, skin, ear	C44.20-✓	C79.2	D04.2-✓	D23.2-✓	D48.5	D49.2
trunk	C44.509	C79.2	D04.5	D23.5	D48.5	D49.2
basal cell carcinoma	C44.519	—	—	—	—	—
specified type NEC	C44.599	—	—	—	—	—
squamous cell carcinoma	C44.529	—	—	—	—	—
umbilicus — see also Neoplasm, skin, trunk	C44.509	C79.2	D04.5	D23.5	D48.5	D49.2
vulva	C51.9	C79.82	D07.1	D28.0	D39.8	D49.59
overlapping lesion	C51.8	—	—	—	—	—

✓ **Additional Character Required — Refer to the Tabular List for Character Selection**

Neoplasm, neoplastic	Malignant Primary	Malignant Secondary	Ca in situ	Benign	Uncertain Behavior	Unspecified Behavior
— continued						
skin — continued						
wrist — see also						
Neoplasm, skin,						
limb, upper	C44.60-☑	C79.2	D04.6-☑	D23.6-☑	D48.5	D49.2
skull	C41.0	C79.51	—	D16.4	D48.0	D49.2
soft parts or tissues —						
see Neoplasm,						
connective tissue						
specified site NEC	C76.8	C79.89	D09.8	D36.7	D48.7	D49.89
spermatic cord	C63.1-☑	C79.82	D07.69	D29.8	D40.8	D49.59
sphenoid	C31.3	C78.39	D02.3	D14.0	D38.5	D49.1
bone	C41.0	C79.51	—	D16.4	D48.0	D49.2
sinus	C31.3	C78.39	D02.3	D14.0	D38.5	D49.1
sphincter						
anal	C21.1	C78.5	D01.3	D12.9	D37.8	D49.0
of Oddi	C24.0	C78.89	D01.5	D13.5	D37.6	D49.0
spine, spinal						
(column)	C41.2	C79.51	—	D16.6	D48.0	D49.2
bulb	C71.7	C79.31	—	D33.1	D43.1	D49.6
coccyx	C41.4	C79.51	—	D16.8	D48.0	D49.2
cord (cervical)						
(lumbar) (sacral)						
(thoracic)	C72.0	C79.49	—	D33.4	D43.4	D49.7
dura mater	C70.1	C79.49	—	D32.1	D42.1	D49.7
lumbosacral	C41.2	C79.51	—	D16.6	D48.0	D49.2
marrow NEC	C96.9	C79.52	—	—	D47.9	D49.89
membrane	C70.1	C79.49	—	D32.1	D42.1	D49.7
meninges	C70.1	C79.49	—	D32.1	D42.1	D49.7
nerve (root)	C47.9	C79.89	—	D36.10	D48.2	D49.2
pia mater	C70.1	C79.49	—	D32.1	D42.1	D49.7
root	C47.9	C79.89	—	D36.10	D48.2	D49.2
sacrum	C41.4	C79.51	—	D16.8	D48.0	D49.2
spleen, splenic						
NEC	C26.1	C78.89	D01.7	D13.99	D37.8	D49.0
flexure (colon)	C18.5	C78.5	D01.0	D12.3	D37.4	D49.0
stem, brain	C71.7	C79.31	—	D33.1	D43.1	D49.6
Stensen's duct	C07	C79.89	D00.00	D11.0	D37.030	D49.0
sternum	C41.3	C79.51	—	D16.7	D48.0	D49.2
stomach	C16.9	C78.89	D00.2	D13.1	D37.1	D49.0
antrum (pyloric)	C16.3	C78.89	D00.2	D13.1	D37.1	D49.0
body	C16.2	C78.89	D00.2	D13.1	D37.1	D49.0
cardia	C16.0	C78.89	D00.2	D13.1	D37.1	D49.0
cardiac orifice	C16.0	C78.89	D00.2	D13.1	D37.1	D49.0
corpus	C16.2	C78.89	D00.2	D13.1	D37.1	D49.0
fundus	C16.1	C78.89	D00.2	D13.1	D37.1	D49.0
greater curvature						
NEC	C16.6	C78.89	D00.2	D13.1	D37.1	D49.0
lesser curvature						
NEC	C16.5	C78.89	D00.2	D13.1	D37.1	D49.0
overlapping						
lesion	C16.8	—	—	—	—	—
prepylorus	C16.4	C78.89	D00.2	D13.1	D37.1	D49.0
pylorus	C16.4	C78.89	D00.2	D13.1	D37.1	D49.0
wall NEC	C16.9	C78.89	D00.2	D13.1	D37.1	D49.0
anterior NEC	C16.8	C78.89	D00.2	D13.1	D37.1	D49.0
posterior NEC	C16.8	C78.89	D00.2	D13.1	D37.1	D49.0
stroma,						
endometrial	C54.1	C79.82	D07.0	D26.1	D39.0	D49.59
stump, cervical	C53.8	C79.82	D06.7	D26.0	D39.0	D49.59
subcutaneous (nodule)						
(tissue) NEC — see						
Neoplasm,						
connective tissue						
subdural	C70.9	C79.32	—	D32.9	D42.9	D49.7
subglottis,						
subglottic	C32.2	C78.39	D02.0	D14.1	D38.0	D49.1
sublingual	C04.9	C79.89	D00.06	D10.2	D37.09	D49.0
gland or duct	C08.1	C79.89	D00.00	D11.7	D37.031	D49.0
submandibular						
gland	C08.0	C79.89	D00.00	D11.7	D37.032	D49.0
submaxillary gland or						
duct	C08.0	C79.89	D00.00	D11.7	D37.032	D49.0
submental	C76.0	C79.89	D09.8	D36.7	D48.7	D49.89
subpleural	C34.9-☑	C78.0-☑	D02.2-☑	D14.3-☑	D38.1	D49.1
substernal	C38.1	C78.1	—	D15.2	D38.3	D49.89
sudoriferous,						
sudoriparous gland,						
site						
unspecified	C44.90	C79.2	D04.9	D23.9	D48.5	D49.2
specified site — see						
Neoplasm, skin						

Neoplasm, neoplastic	Malignant Primary	Malignant Secondary	Ca in situ	Benign	Uncertain Behavior	Unspecified Behavior
— continued						
supraclavicular						
region	C76.0	C79.89	D09.8	D36.7	D48.7	D49.89
supraglottis	C32.1	C78.39	D02.0	D14.1	D38.0	D49.1
suprarenal	C74.9-☑	C79.7-☑	D09.3	D35.0-☑	D44.1-☑	D49.7
capsule	C74.9-☑	C79.7-☑	D09.3	D35.0-☑	D44.1-☑	D49.7
cortex	C74.0-☑	C79.7-☑	D09.3	D35.0-☑	D44.1-☑	D49.7
gland	C74.9-☑	C79.7-☑	D09.3	D35.0-☑	D44.1-☑	D49.7
medulla	C74.1-☑	C79.7-☑	D09.3	D35.0-☑	D44.1-☑	D49.7
suprasellar						
(region)	C71.9	C79.31	—	D33.2	D43.2	D49.6
supratentorial (brain)						
NEC	C71.0	C79.31	—	D33.0	D43.0	D49.6
sweat gland (apocrine)						
(eccrine), site						
unspecified	C44.90	C79.2	D04.9	D23.9	D48.5	D49.2
specified site — see						
Neoplasm, skin						
sympathetic nerve or						
nervous system						
NEC	C47.9	C79.89	—	D36.10	D48.2	D49.2
symphysis pubis	C41.4	C79.51	—	D16.8	D48.0	D49.2
synovial membrane —						
see Neoplasm,						
connective tissue						
tapetum, brain	C71.8	C79.31	—	D33.2	D43.2	D49.6
tarsus (any bone)	C40.3-☑	C79.51	—	D16.3-☑	—	—
temple (skin) — see						
also Neoplasm, skin,						
face	C44.309	C79.2	D04.39	D23.39	D48.5	D49.2
temporal						
bone	C41.0	C79.51	—	D16.4	D48.0	D49.2
lobe or pole	C71.2	C79.31	—	D33.0	D43.0	D49.6
region	C76.0	C79.89	D09.8	D36.7	D48.7	D49.89
skin — see also						
Neoplasm, skin,						
face	C44.309	C79.2	D04.39	D23.39	D48.5	D49.2
tendon (sheath) — see						
Neoplasm,						
connective tissue						
tentorium						
(cerebelli)	C70.0	C79.32	—	D32.0	D42.0	D49.7
testis, testes	C62.9-☑	C79.82	D07.69	D29.2-☑	D40.1-☑	D49.59
descended	C62.1-☑	C79.82	D07.69	D29.2-☑	D40.1-☑	D49.59
ectopic	C62.0-☑	C79.82	D07.69	D29.2-☑	D40.1-☑	D49.59
retained	C62.0-☑	C79.82	D07.69	D29.2-☑	D40.1-☑	D49.59
scrotal	C62.1-☑	C79.82	D07.69	D29.2-☑	D40.1-☑	D49.59
undescended	C62.0-☑	C79.82	D07.69	D29.2-☑	D40.1-☑	D49.59
unspecified whether						
descended or						
undescended	C62.9-☑	C79.82	D07.69	D29.2-☑	D40.1-☑	D49.59
thalamus	C71.0	C79.31	—	D33.0	D43.0	D49.6
thigh NEC	C76.5-☑	C79.89	D04.7-☑	D36.7	D48.7	D49.89
thorax, thoracic (cavity)						
(organs NEC)	C76.1	C79.89	D09.8	D36.7	D48.7	D49.89
duct	C49.3	C79.89	—	D21.3	D48.1☑	D49.2
wall NEC	C76.1	C79.89	D09.8	D36.7	D48.7	D49.89
throat	C14.0	C79.89	D00.08	D10.9	D37.05	D49.0
thumb NEC	C76.4-☑	C79.89	D04.6-☑	D36.7	D48.7	D49.89
thymus (gland)	C37	C79.89	D09.3	D15.0	D38.4	D49.89
thyroglossal duct	C73	C79.89	D09.3	D34	D44.0	D49.7
thyroid (gland)	C73	C79.89	D09.3	D34	D44.0	D49.7
cartilage	C32.3	C78.39	D02.0	D14.1	D38.0	D49.1
tibia (any part)	C40.2-☑	C79.51	—	D16.2-☑	—	—
toe NEC	C76.5-☑	C79.89	D04.7-☑	D36.7	D48.7	D49.89
tongue	C02.9	C79.89	D00.07	D10.1	D37.02	D49.0
anterior (two-thirds)						
NEC	C02.3	C79.89	D00.07	D10.1	D37.02	D49.0
dorsal surface	C02.0	C79.89	D00.07	D10.1	D37.02	D49.0
ventral surface	C02.2	C79.89	D00.07	D10.1	D37.02	D49.0
base (dorsal						
surface)	C01	C79.89	D00.07	D10.1	D37.02	D49.0
border (lateral)	C02.1	C79.89	D00.07	D10.1	D37.02	D49.0
dorsal surface						
NEC	C02.0	C79.89	D00.07	D10.1	D37.02	D49.0
fixed part NEC	C01	C79.89	D00.07	D10.1	D37.02	D49.0
foreamen						
cecum	C02.0	C79.89	D00.07	D10.1	D37.02	D49.0
frenulum						
linguae	C02.2	C79.89	D00.07	D10.1	D37.02	D49.0
junctional zone	C02.8	C79.89	D00.07	D10.1	D37.02	D49.0

☑ Additional Character Required — Refer to the Tabular List for Character Selection

Neoplasm, neoplastic	Malignant Primary	Malignant Secondary	Ca in situ	Benign	Uncertain Behavior	Unspecified Behavior
— continued						
tongue — continued						
margin (lateral)	C02.1	C79.89	D00.07	D10.1	D37.02	D49.0
midline NEC	C02.0	C79.89	D00.07	D10.1	D37.02	D49.0
mobile part NEC	C02.3	C79.89	D00.07	D10.1	D37.02	D49.0
overlapping lesion	C02.8	—	—	—	—	—
posterior (third)	C01	C79.89	D00.07	D10.1	D37.02	D49.0
root	C01	C79.89	D00.07	D10.1	D37.02	D49.0
surface (dorsal)	C02.0	C79.89	D00.07	D10.1	D37.02	D49.0
base	C01	C79.89	D00.07	D10.1	D37.02	D49.0
ventral	C02.2	C79.89	D00.07	D10.1	D37.02	D49.0
tip	C02.1	C79.89	D00.07	D10.1	D37.02	D49.0
tonsil	C02.4	C79.89	D00.07	D10.1	D37.02	D49.0
tonsil	C09.9	C79.89	D00.08	D10.4	D37.05	D49.0
fauces, faucial	C09.9	C79.89	D00.08	D10.4	D37.05	D49.0
lingual	C02.4	C79.89	D00.07	D10.1	D37.02	D49.0
overlapping sites	C09.8	—	—	—	—	—
palatine	C09.9	C79.89	D00.08	D10.4	D37.05	D49.0
pharyngeal	C11.1	C79.89	D00.08	D10.6	D37.05	D49.0
pillar (anterior) (posterior)	C09.1	C79.89	D00.08	D10.5	D37.05	D49.0
tonsillar fossa	C09.0	C79.89	D00.08	D10.5	D37.05	D49.0
tooth socket NEC	C03.9	C79.89	D00.03	D10.39	D37.09	D49.0
trachea (cartilage) (mucosa)	C33	C78.39	D02.1	D14.2	D38.1	D49.1
overlapping lesion with bronchus or lung	C34.8-☑	—	—	—	—	—
tracheobronchial	C34.8-☑	C78.39	D02.1	D14.2	D38.1	D49.1
overlapping lesion with lung	C34.8-☑	—	—	—	—	—
tragus — see also Neoplasm, skin, ear	C44.20-☑	C79.2	D04.2-☑	D23.2-☑	D48.5	D49.2
trunk NEC	C76.8	C79.89	D04.5	D36.7	D48.7	D49.89
tubo-ovarian	C57.8	C79.82	D07.39	D28.7	D39.8	D49.59
tunica vaginalis	C63.7	C79.82	D07.69	D29.8	D40.8	D49.59
turbinate (bone)	C41.0	C79.51		D16.4	D48.0	D49.2
nasal	C30.0	C78.39	D02.3	D14.0	D38.5	D49.1
tympanic cavity	C30.1	C78.39	D02.3	D14.0	D38.5	D49.1
ulna (any part)	C40.0-☑	C79.51	—	D16.0-☑	—	—
umbilicus, umbilical — see also Neoplasm, skin, trunk	C44.509	C79.2	D04.5	D23.5	D48.5	D49.2
uncus, brain	C71.2	C79.31	—	D33.0	D43.0	D49.6
unknown site or unspecified	C80.1	C79.9	D09.9	D36.9	D48.9	D49.9
urachus	C67.7	C79.11	D09.0	D30.3	D41.4	D49.4
ureter-bladder (junction)	C67.6	C79.11	D09.0	D30.3	D41.4	D49.4
ureter, ureteral	C66.-☑	C79.19	D09.19	D30.2-☑	D41.2-☑	D49.59
orifice (bladder)	C67.6	C79.11	D09.0	D30.3	D41.4	D49.4
urethra, urethral (gland)	C68.0	C79.19	D09.19	D30.4	D41.3	D49.59
orifice, internal	C67.5	C79.11	D09.0	D30.3	D41.4	D49.4
urethrovaginal (septum)	C57.9	C79.82	D07.30	D28.9	D39.8	D49.59
urinary organ or system	C68.9	C79.10	D09.10	D30.9	D41.9	D49.59
bladder — see Neoplasm, bladder						
overlapping lesion	C68.8					
specified sites NEC	C68.8	C79.19	D09.19	D30.8	D41.8	D49.59
utero-ovarian	C57.8	C79.82	D07.39	D28.7	D39.8	D49.59
ligament	C57.1-☑	C79.82	D07.39	D28.2	D39.8	D49.59
uterosacral ligament	C57.3	C79.82	—	D28.2	D39.8	D49.59
uterus, uteri, uterine	C55	C79.82	D07.0	D26.9	D39.0	D49.59
adnexa NEC	C57.4	C79.82	D07.39	D28.7	D39.8	D49.59
body	C54.9	C79.82	D07.0	D26.1	D39.0	D49.59
cervix	C53.9	C79.82	D06.9	D26.0	D39.0	D49.59
cornu	C54.9	C79.82	D07.0	D26.1	D39.0	D49.59
corpus	C54.9	C79.82	D07.0	D26.1	D39.0	D49.59
endocervix (canal) (gland)	C53.0	C79.82	D06.0	D26.0	D39.0	D49.59
endometrium	C54.1	C79.82	D07.0	D26.1	D39.0	D49.59

Neoplasm, neoplastic	Malignant Primary	Malignant Secondary	Ca in situ	Benign	Uncertain Behavior	Unspecified Behavior
— continued						
uterus, uteri, uterine — continued						
exocervix	C53.1	C79.82	D06.1	D26.0	D39.0	D49.59
external os	C53.1	C79.82	D06.1	D26.0	D39.0	D49.59
fundus	C54.3	C79.82	D07.0	D26.1	D39.0	D49.59
internal os	C53.0	C79.82	D06.0	D26.0	D39.0	D49.59
isthmus	C54.0	C79.82	D07.0	D26.1	D39.0	D49.59
ligament	C57.3	C79.82	—	D28.2	D39.8	D49.59
broad	C57.1-☑	C79.82	D07.39	D28.2	D39.8	D49.59
round	C57.2-☑	C79.82	—	D28.2	D39.8	D49.59
lower segment	C54.0	C79.82	D07.0	D26.1	D39.0	D49.59
myometrium	C54.2	C79.82	D07.0	D26.1	D39.0	D49.59
overlapping sites	C54.8	—	—	—	—	—
squamocolumnar junction	C53.8	C79.82	D06.7	D26.0	D39.0	D49.59
tube	C57.0-☑	C79.82	D07.39	D28.2	D39.8	D49.59
utricle, prostatic	C68.0	C79.19	D09.19	D30.4	D41.3	D49.59
uveal tract	C69.4-☑	C79.49	D09.2-☑	D31.4-☑	D48.7	D49.89
uvula	C05.2	C79.89	D00.04	D10.39	D37.09	D49.0
vagina, vaginal (fornix) (vault) (wall)	C52	C79.82	D07.2	D28.1	D39.8	D49.59
vaginovesical	C57.9	C79.82	D07.30	D28.9	D39.9	D49.59
septum	C57.9	C79.82	D07.30	D28.9	D39.9	D49.59
vallecula (epigiottis)	C10.0	C79.89	D00.08	D10.5	D37.05	D49.0
vascular — see Neoplasm, connective tissue						
vas deferens	C63.1-☑	C79.82	D07.69	D29.8	D40.8	D49.59
Vater's ampulla	C24.1	C78.89	D01.5	D13.5	D37.6	D49.0
vein, venous — see Neoplasm, connective tissue						
vena cava (abdominal) (inferior)	C49.4	C79.89	—	D21.4	D48.1☑	D49.2
superior	C49.3	C79.89	—	D21.3	D48.1☑	D49.2
ventricle (cerebral) (floor) (lateral) (third)	C71.5	C79.31		D33.0	D43.0	D49.6
cardiac (left) (right)	C38.0	C79.89		D15.1	D48.7	D49.89
fourth	C71.7	C79.31		D33.1	D43.1	D49.6
ventricular band of larynx	C32.1	C78.39	D02.0	D14.1	D38.0	D49.1
ventriculus — see Neoplasm, stomach						
vermillion border — see Neoplasm, lip						
vermis, cerebellum	C71.6	C79.31	—	D33.1	D43.1	D49.6
vertebra (column)	C41.2	C79.51	—	D16.6	D48.0	D49.2
coccyx	C41.4	C79.51	—	D16.8	D48.0	D49.2
marrow NEC	C96.9	C79.52	—	—	D47.9	D49.89
sacrum	C41.4	C79.51	—	D16.8	D48.0	D49.2
vesical — see Neoplasm, bladder						
vesicle, seminal	C63.7	C79.82	D07.69	D29.8	D40.8	D49.59
vesicocervical tissue	C57.9	C79.82	D07.30	D28.9	D39.9	D49.59
vesicorectal	C76.3	C79.82	D09.8	D36.7	D48.7	D49.89
vesicovaginal	C57.9	C79.82	D07.30	D28.9	D39.9	D49.59
septum	C57.9	C79.82	D07.30	D28.9	D39.8	D49.59
vessel (blood) — see Neoplasm, connective tissue						
vestibular gland, greater	C51.0	C79.82	D07.1	D28.0	D39.8	D49.59
vestibule						
mouth	C06.1	C79.89	D00.00	D10.39	D37.09	D49.0
nose	C30.0	C78.39	D02.3	D14.0	D38.5	D49.1
Virchow's gland	C77.0	C77.0	—	D36.0	D48.7	D49.89
viscera NEC	C76.8	C79.89	D09.8	D36.7	D48.7	D49.89
vocal cords (true)	C32.0	C78.39	D02.0	D14.1	D38.0	D49.1
false	C32.1	C78.39	D02.0	D14.1	D38.0	D49.1
vomer	C41.0	C79.51	—	D16.4	D48.0	D49.2
vulva	C51.9	C79.82	D07.1	D28.0	D39.8	D49.59
vulvovaginal gland	C51.0	C79.82	D07.1	D28.0	D39.8	D49.59
Waldeyer's ring	C14.2	C79.89	D00.08	D10.9	D37.05	D49.0

☑ Additional Character Required — Refer to the Tabular List for Character Selection

Neoplasm, neoplastic	Malignant Primary	Malignant Secondary	Ca in situ	Benign	Uncertain Behavior	Unspecified Behavior
— *continued*						
Wharton's duct	C08.0	C79.89	D00.00	D11.7	D37.032	D49.0
white matter (central)						
(cerebral)	C71.0	C79.31	—	D33.0	D43.0	D49.6
windpipe	C33	C78.39	D02.1	D14.2	D38.1	D49.1
Wirsung's duct	C25.3	C78.89	D01.7	D13.6	D37.8	D49.0
wolffian (body) (duct)						
female	C57.7	C79.82	D07.39	D28.7	D39.8	D49.59
male	C63.7	C79.82	D07.69	D29.8	D40.8	D49.59
womb — *see*						
Neoplasm, uterus						
wrist NEC	C76.4-☑	C79.89	D04.6-☑	D36.7	D48.7	D49.89
xiphoid process	C41.3	C79.51	—	D16.7	D48.0	D49.2
Zuckerkandl						
organ	C75.5	C79.89	—	D35.6	D44.7	D49.7

Table of Drugs and Chemicals

14-hydroxydihydro-morphinone — Adrenochrome

Substance	Poisoning, Accidental (unintentional)	Poisoning, Intentional Self-harm	Poisoning, Assault	Poisoning, Undetermined	Adverse Effect	Under-dosing
14-hydroxydihydro-morphinone	T40.2X1	T40.2X2	T40.2X3	T40.2X4	T40.2X5	T40.2X6
1-Propanol	T51.3X1	T51.3X2	T51.3X3	T51.3X4	—	—
2,3,7,8-Tetrachlorodibenzo-p-dioxin	T53.7X1	T53.7X2	T53.7X3	T53.7X4	—	—
2,4,5-T (trichloro-phenoxyacetic acid)	T60.1X1	T60.1X2	T60.1X3	T60.1X4	—	—
2,4,5-Trichlorophen-oxyacetic acid	T60.3X1	T60.3X2	T60.3X3	T60.3X4	—	—
2,4-D (dichlorophen-oxyacetic acid)	T60.3X1	T60.3X2	T60.3X3	T60.3X4	—	—
2,4-Toluene diisocyanate	T65.0X1	T65.0X2	T65.0X3	T65.0X4	—	—
2-Deoxy-5-fluorouridine	T45.1X1	T45.1X2	T45.1X3	T45.1X4	T45.1X5	T45.1X6
2-Ethoxyethanol	T52.3X1	T52.3X2	T52.3X3	T52.3X4	—	—
2-Methoxyethanol	T52.3X1	T52.3X2	T52.3X3	T52.3X4	—	—
2-Propanol	T51.2X1	T51.2X2	T51.2X3	T51.2X4	—	—
3,4-methylenedioxymeth-amphetamine	T43.641	T43.642	T43.643	T43.644	—	—
4-Aminobutyric acid	T43.8X1	T43.8X2	T43.8X3	T43.8X4	T43.8X5	T43.8X6
4-Aminophenol derivatives	T39.1X1	T39.1X2	T39.1X3	T39.1X4	T39.1X5	T39.1X6
5-Deoxy-5-fluorouridine	T45.1X1	T45.1X2	T45.1X3	T45.1X4	T45.1X5	T45.1X6
5-Methoxypsoralen (5-MOP)	T50.991	T50.992	T50.993	T50.994	T50.995	T50.996
8-Aminoquinoline drugs	T37.2X1	T37.2X2	T37.2X3	T37.2X4	T37.2X5	T37.2X6
8-Methoxypsoralen (8-MOP)	T50.991	T50.992	T50.993	T50.994	T50.995	T50.996
9-hydroxyrisperidone*	T43.591	T43.592	T43.593	T43.594	T43.595	T43.596
ABOB	T37.5X1	T37.5X2	T37.5X3	T37.5X4	T37.5X5	T37.5X6
Abrine	T62.2X1	T62.2X2	T62.2X3	T62.2X4	—	—
Abrus (seed)	T62.2X1	T62.2X2	T62.2X3	T62.2X4	—	—
Absinthe	T51.0X1	T51.0X2	T51.0X3	T51.0X4	—	—
beverage	T51.0X1	T51.0X2	T51.0X3	T51.0X4	—	—
Acaricide	T60.8X1	T60.8X2	T60.8X3	T60.8X4	—	—
Acebutolol	T44.7X1	T44.7X2	T44.7X3	T44.7X4	T44.7X5	T44.7X6
Acecarbromal	T42.6X1	T42.6X2	T42.6X3	T42.6X4	T42.6X5	T42.6X6
Aceclidine	T44.1X1	T44.1X2	T44.1X3	T44.1X4	T44.1X5	T44.1X6
Acedapsone	T37.0X1	T37.0X2	T37.0X3	T37.0X4	T37.0X5	T37.0X6
Acefylline piperazine	T48.6X1	T48.6X2	T48.6X3	T48.6X4	T48.6X5	T48.6X6
Acemorphan	T40.2X1	T40.2X2	T40.2X3	T40.2X4	—	—
Acenocoumarin	T45.511	T45.512	T45.513	T45.514	T45.515	T45.516
Acenocoumarol	T45.511	T45.512	T45.513	T45.514	T45.515	T45.516
Aceon*	T46.4X1	T46.4X2	T46.4X3	T46.4X4	T46.4X5	T46.4X6
Acepifylline	T48.6X1	T48.6X2	T48.6X3	T48.6X4	T48.6X5	T48.6X6
Acepromazine	T43.3X1	T43.3X2	T43.3X3	T43.3X4	T43.3X5	T43.3X6
Acesulfamethoxypyridazine	T37.0X1	T37.0X2	T37.0X3	T37.0X4	T37.0X5	T37.0X6
Acetal	T52.8X1	T52.8X2	T52.8X3	T52.8X4	—	—
Acetaldehyde (vapor)	T52.8X1	T52.8X2	T52.8X3	T52.8X4	—	—
liquid	T65.891	T65.892	T65.893	T65.894	—	—
Acetaminophen	T39.1X1	T39.1X2	T39.1X3	T39.1X4	T39.1X5	T39.1X6
Acetaminosalol	T39.1X1	T39.1X2	T39.1X3	T39.1X4	T39.1X5	T39.1X6
Acetanilide	T39.1X1	T39.1X2	T39.1X3	T39.1X4	T39.1X5	T39.1X6
Acetarsol	T37.3X1	T37.3X2	T37.3X3	T37.3X4	T37.3X5	T37.3X6
Acetazolamide	T50.2X1	T50.2X2	T50.2X3	T50.2X4	T50.2X5	T50.2X6
Acetiamine	T45.2X1	T45.2X2	T45.2X3	T45.2X4	T45.2X5	T45.2X6
Acetic						
acid	T54.2X1	T54.2X2	T54.2X3	T54.2X4	—	—
with sodium acetate (ointment)	T49.3X1	T49.3X2	T49.3X3	T49.3X4	T49.3X5	T49.3X6
ester (solvent)(vapor)	T52.8X1	T52.8X2	T52.8X3	T52.8X4	—	—
irrigating solution	T50.3X1	T50.3X2	T50.3X3	T50.3X4	T50.3X5	T50.3X6
medicinal (lotion)	T49.2X1	T49.2X2	T49.2X3	T49.2X4	T49.2X5	T49.2X6
anhydride	T65.891	T65.892	T65.893	T65.894	—	—
ether (vapor)	T52.8X1	T52.8X2	T52.8X3	T52.8X4	—	—
Acetohexamide	T38.3X1	T38.3X2	T38.3X3	T38.3X4	T38.3X5	T38.3X6
Acetohydroxamic acid	T50.991	T50.992	T50.993	T50.994	T50.995	T50.996
Acetomenaphthone	T45.7X1	T45.7X2	T45.7X3	T45.7X4	T45.7X5	T45.7X6
Acetomorphine	T40.1X1	T40.1X2	T40.1X3	T40.1X4	—	—
Acetone (oils)	T52.4X1	T52.4X2	T52.4X3	T52.4X4	—	—
chlorinated	T52.4X1	T52.4X2	T52.4X3	T52.4X4	—	—
vapor	T52.4X1	T52.4X2	T52.4X3	T52.4X4	—	—
Acetonitrile	T52.8X1	T52.8X2	T52.8X3	T52.8X4	—	—
Acetophenazine	T43.3X1	T43.3X2	T43.3X3	T43.3X4	T43.3X5	T43.3X6
Acetophenetedin	T39.1X1	T39.1X2	T39.1X3	T39.1X4	T39.1X5	T39.1X6
Acetophenone	T52.4X1	T52.4X2	T52.4X3	T52.4X4	—	—
Acetorphine	T40.2X1	T40.2X2	T40.2X3	T40.2X4	—	—
Acetosulfone (sodium)	T37.1X1	T37.1X2	T37.1X3	T37.1X4	T37.1X5	T37.1X6
Acetrizoate (sodium)	T50.8X1	T50.8X2	T50.8X3	T50.8X4	T50.8X5	T50.8X6
Acetrizoic acid	T50.8X1	T50.8X2	T50.8X3	T50.8X4	T50.8X5	T50.8X6
Acetyl						
bromide	T53.6X1	T53.6X2	T53.6X3	T53.6X4	—	—
chloride	T53.6X1	T53.6X2	T53.6X3	T53.6X4	—	—
Acetylcarbromal	T42.6X1	T42.6X2	T42.6X3	T42.6X4	T42.6X5	T42.6X6
Acetylcholine						

Substance	Poisoning, Accidental (unintentional)	Poisoning, Intentional Self-harm	Poisoning, Assault	Poisoning, Undetermined	Adverse Effect	Under-dosing
Acetylcholine — continued						
chloride	T44.1X1	T44.1X2	T44.1X3	T44.1X4	T44.1X5	T44.1X6
derivative	T44.1X1	T44.1X2	T44.1X3	T44.1X4	T44.1X5	T44.1X6
Acetylcysteine	T48.4X1	T48.4X2	T48.4X3	T48.4X4	T48.4X5	T48.4X6
Acetyldigitoxin	T46.0X1	T46.0X2	T46.0X3	T46.0X4	T46.0X5	T46.0X6
Acetyldigoxin	T46.0X1	T46.0X2	T46.0X3	T46.0X4	T46.0X5	T46.0X6
Acetyldihydrocodeine	T40.2X1	T40.2X2	T40.2X3	T40.2X4	—	—
Acetyldihydrocodeinone	T40.2X1	T40.2X2	T40.2X3	T40.2X4	—	—
Acetylene (gas)	T59.891	T59.892	T59.893	T59.894	—	—
dichloride	T53.6X1	T53.6X2	T53.6X3	T53.6X4	—	—
incomplete combustion of	T58.11	T58.12	T58.13	T58.14	—	—
industrial	T59.891	T59.892	T59.893	T59.894	—	—
tetrachloride	T53.6X1	T53.6X2	T53.6X3	T53.6X4	—	—
vapor	T53.6X1	T53.6X2	T53.6X3	T53.6X4	—	—
Acetylpheneturide	T42.6X1	T42.6X2	T42.6X3	T42.6X4	T42.6X5	T42.6X6
Acetylphenylhydrazine	T39.8X1	T39.8X2	T39.8X3	T39.8X4	T39.8X5	T39.8X6
Acetylsalicylic acid (salts)	T39.011	T39.012	T39.013	T39.014	T39.015	T39.016
enteric coated	T39.011	T39.012	T39.013	T39.014	T39.015	T39.016
Acetylsulfamethoxypyridazine	T37.0X1	T37.0X2	T37.0X3	T37.0X4	T37.0X5	T37.0X6
Achromycin	T36.4X1	T36.4X2	T36.4X3	T36.4X4	T36.4X5	T36.4X6
ophthalmic preparation	T49.5X1	T49.5X2	T49.5X3	T49.5X4	T49.5X5	T49.5X6
topical NEC	T49.0X1	T49.0X2	T49.0X3	T49.0X4	T49.0X5	T49.0X6
Aciclovir	T37.5X1	T37.5X2	T37.5X3	T37.5X4	T37.5X5	T37.5X6
Acidifying agent NEC	T50.901	T50.902	T50.903	T50.904	T50.905	T50.906
Acid (corrosive) NEC	T54.2X1	T54.2X2	T54.2X3	T54.2X4	—	—
AcipHex*	T47.1X1	T47.1X2	T47.1X3	T47.1X4	T47.1X5	T47.1X6
Acipimox	T46.6X1	T46.6X2	T46.6X3	T46.6X4	T46.6X5	T46.6X6
Acitretin	T50.991	T50.992	T50.993	T50.994	T50.995	T50.996
Aclarubicin	T45.1X1	T45.1X2	T45.1X3	T45.1X4	T45.1X5	T45.1X6
Aclatonium napadisilate	T48.1X1	T48.1X2	T48.1X3	T48.1X4	T48.1X5	T48.1X6
Aconite (wild)	T46.991	T46.992	T46.993	T46.994	T46.995	T46.996
Aconitine	T46.991	T46.992	T46.993	T46.994	T46.995	T46.996
Aconitum ferox	T46.991	T46.992	T46.993	T46.994	T46.995	T46.996
Acridine	T65.6X1	T65.6X2	T65.6X3	T65.6X4	—	—
vapor	T59.891	T59.892	T59.893	T59.894	—	—
Acriflavine	T37.91	T37.92	T37.93	T37.94	T37.95	T37.96
Acriflavinium chloride	T49.0X1	T49.0X2	T49.0X3	T49.0X4	T49.0X5	T49.0X6
Acrinol	T49.0X1	T49.0X2	T49.0X3	T49.0X4	T49.0X5	T49.0X6
Acrisorcin	T49.0X1	T49.0X2	T49.0X3	T49.0X4	T49.0X5	T49.0X6
Acrivastine	T45.0X1	T45.0X2	T45.0X3	T45.0X4	T45.0X5	T45.0X6
Acrolein (gas)	T59.891	T59.892	T59.893	T59.894	—	—
liquid	T54.1X1	T54.1X2	T54.1X3	T54.1X4	—	—
Acrylamide	T65.891	T65.892	T65.893	T65.894	—	—
Acrylic resin	T49.3X1	T49.3X2	T49.3X3	T49.3X4	T49.3X5	T49.3X6
Acrylonitrile	T65.891	T65.892	T65.893	T65.894	—	—
Actaea spicata	T62.2X1	T62.2X2	T62.2X3	T62.2X4	—	—
berry	T62.1X1	T62.1X2	T62.1X3	T62.1X4	—	—
Acterol	T37.3X1	T37.3X2	T37.3X3	T37.3X4	T37.3X5	T37.3X6
ACTH	T38.811	T38.812	T38.813	T38.814	T38.815	T38.816
Acticlate*	T36.4X1	T36.4X2	T36.4X3	T36.4X4	T36.4X5	T36.4X6
Actinomycin C	T45.1X1	T45.1X2	T45.1X3	T45.1X4	T45.1X5	T45.1X6
Actinomycin D	T45.1X1	T45.1X2	T45.1X3	T45.1X4	T45.1X5	T45.1X6
Activated charcoal — see also Charcoal, medicinal	T47.6X1	T47.6X2	T47.6X3	T47.6X4	T47.6X5	T47.6X6
Activella*	T38.5X1	T38.5X2	T38.5X3	T38.5X4	T38.5X5	T38.5X6
Acyclovir	T37.5X1	T37.5X2	T37.5X3	T37.5X4	T37.5X5	T37.5X6
Adderall*	T43.621	T43.622	T43.623	T43.624	T43.625	T43.626
Adenine	T45.2X1	T45.2X2	T45.2X3	T45.2X4	T45.2X5	T45.2X6
arabinoside	T37.5X1	T37.5X2	T37.5X3	T37.5X4	T37.5X5	T37.5X6
Adenosine (phosphate)	T46.2X1	T46.2X2	T46.2X3	T46.2X4	T46.2X5	T46.2X6
ADH	T38.891	T38.892	T38.893	T38.894	T38.895	T38.896
Adhesive NEC	T65.891	T65.892	T65.893	T65.894	—	—
Adicillin	T36.0X1	T36.0X2	T36.0X3	T36.0X4	T36.0X5	T36.0X6
Adiphenine	T44.3X1	T44.3X2	T44.3X3	T44.3X4	T44.3X5	T44.3X6
Adipiodone	T50.8X1	T50.8X2	T50.8X3	T50.8X4	T50.8X5	T50.8X6
Adjunct, pharmaceutical	T50.901	T50.902	T50.903	T50.904	T50.905	T50.906
Adrenal (extract, cortex or medulla) (glucocorticoids) (hormones) (mineralocorticoids)	T38.0X1	T38.0X2	T38.0X3	T38.0X4	T38.0X5	T38.0X6
ENT agent	T49.6X1	T49.6X2	T49.6X3	T49.6X4	T49.6X5	T49.6X6
ophthalmic preparation	T49.5X1	T49.5X2	T49.5X3	T49.5X4	T49.5X5	T49.5X6
topical NEC	T49.0X1	T49.0X2	T49.0X3	T49.0X4	T49.0X5	T49.0X6
Adrenalin — see Adrenaline						
Adrenaline	T44.5X1	T44.5X2	T44.5X3	T44.5X4	T44.5X5	T44.5X6
Adrenergic NEC	T44.901	T44.902	T44.903	T44.904	T44.905	T44.906
blocking agent NEC	T44.8X1	T44.8X2	T44.8X3	T44.8X4	T44.8X5	T44.8X6
beta, heart	T44.7X1	T44.7X2	T44.7X3	T44.7X4	T44.7X5	T44.7X6
specified NEC	T44.991	T44.992	T44.993	T44.994	T44.995	T44.996
Adrenochrome						
derivative	T46.991	T46.992	T46.993	T46.994	T46.995	T46.996
(mono) semicarbazone	T46.991	T46.992	T46.993	T46.994	T46.995	T46.996

☑ Additional Character May Be Required — Refer to the Tabular List for Character Selection

*Optum Value-Add

Substance	Poisoning, Accidental (unintentional)	Poisoning, Intentional Self-harm	Poisoning, Assault	Poisoning, Undetermined	Adverse Effect	Underdosing
Adrenocorticotrophic hormone	T38.811	T38.812	T38.813	T38.814	T38.815	T38.816
Adrenocorticotrophin	T38.811	T38.812	T38.813	T38.814	T38.815	T38.816
Adriamycin	T45.1X1	T45.1X2	T45.1X3	T45.1X4	T45.1X5	T45.1X6
Adrucil*	T45.1X1	T45.1X2	T45.1X3	T45.1X4	T45.1X5	T45.1X6
Aerosol spray NEC	T65.91	T65.92	T65.93	T65.94	—	—
Aerosporin	T36.8X1	T36.8X2	T36.8X3	T36.8X4	T36.8X5	T36.8X6
ENT agent	T49.6X1	T49.6X2	T49.6X3	T49.6X4	T49.6X5	T49.6X6
ophthalmic preparation	T49.5X1	T49.5X2	T49.5X3	T49.5X4	T49.5X5	T49.5X6
topical NEC	T49.0X1	T49.0X2	T49.0X3	T49.0X4	T49.0X5	T49.0X6
Aethusa cynapium	T62.2X1	T62.2X2	T62.2X3	T62.2X4	—	—
Afghanistan black	T40.711	T40.712	T40.713	T40.714	T40.715	T40.716
Aflatoxin	T64.01	T64.02	T64.03	T64.04	—	—
Afloqualone	T42.8X1	T42.8X2	T42.8X3	T42.8X4	T42.8X5	T42.8X6
African boxwood	T62.2X1	T62.2X2	T62.2X3	T62.2X4	—	—
Agar	T47.4X1	T47.4X2	T47.4X3	T47.4X4	T47.4X5	T47.4X6
Agonist						
predominantly						
alpha-adrenoreceptor	T44.4X1	T44.4X2	T44.4X3	T44.4X4	T44.4X5	T44.4X6
beta-adrenoreceptor	T44.5X1	T44.5X2	T44.5X3	T44.5X4	T44.5X5	T44.5X6
Agricultural agent NEC	T65.91	T65.92	T65.93	T65.94	—	—
Agrypnal	T42.3X1	T42.3X2	T42.3X3	T42.3X4	T42.3X5	T42.3X6
AHLG	T50.Z11	T50.Z12	T50.Z13	T50.Z14	T50.Z15	T50.Z16
Air contaminant(s), source/type NOS	T65.91	T65.92	T65.93	T65.94	—	—
Ajmaline	T46.2X1	T46.2X2	T46.2X3	T46.2X4	T46.2X5	T46.2X6
Akee	T62.1X1	T62.1X2	T62.1X3	T62.1X4	—	—
Akne-Mycin*	T49.0X1	T49.0X2	T49.0X3	T49.0X4	T49.0X5	T49.0X6
Akrinol	T49.0X1	T49.0X2	T49.0X3	T49.0X4	T49.0X5	T49.0X6
Akritoin	T37.8X1	T37.8X2	T37.8X3	T37.8X4	T37.8X5	T37.8X6
Alacepril	T46.4X1	T46.4X2	T46.4X3	T46.4X4	T46.4X5	T46.4X6
Alantolactone	T37.4X1	T37.4X2	T37.4X3	T37.4X4	T37.4X5	T37.4X6
Albamycin	T36.8X1	T36.8X2	T36.8X3	T36.8X4	T36.8X5	T36.8X6
Albendazole	T37.4X1	T37.4X2	T37.4X3	T37.4X4	T37.4X5	T37.4X6
Albigutide*	T38.3X1	T38.3X2	T38.3X3	T38.3X4	T38.3X5	T38.3X6
Albumin						
bovine	T45.8X1	T45.8X2	T45.8X3	T45.8X4	T45.8X5	T45.8X6
human serum	T45.8X1	T45.8X2	T45.8X3	T45.8X4	T45.8X5	T45.8X6
salt-poor	T45.8X1	T45.8X2	T45.8X3	T45.8X4	T45.8X5	T45.8X6
normal human serum	T45.8X1	T45.8X2	T45.8X3	T45.8X4	T45.8X5	T45.8X6
Albuterol	T48.6X1	T48.6X2	T48.6X3	T48.6X4	T48.6X5	T48.6X6
Albutoin	T42.0X1	T42.0X2	T42.0X3	T42.0X4	T42.0X5	T42.0X6
Alclometasone	T49.0X1	T49.0X2	T49.0X3	T49.0X4	T49.0X5	T49.0X6
Alcohol	T51.91	T51.92	T51.93	T51.94	—	—
absolute	T51.0X1	T51.0X2	T51.0X3	T51.0X4	—	—
beverage	T51.0X1	T51.0X2	T51.0X3	T51.0X4	—	—
allyl	T51.8X1	T51.8X2	T51.8X3	T51.8X4	—	—
amyl	T51.3X1	T51.3X2	T51.3X3	T51.3X4	—	—
antifreeze	T51.1X1	T51.1X2	T51.1X3	T51.1X4	—	—
beverage	T51.0X1	T51.0X2	T51.0X3	T51.0X4	—	—
butyl	T51.3X1	T51.3X2	T51.3X3	T51.3X4	—	—
dehydrated	T51.0X1	T51.0X2	T51.0X3	T51.0X4	—	—
beverage	T51.0X1	T51.0X2	T51.0X3	T51.0X4	—	—
denatured	T51.0X1	T51.0X2	T51.0X3	T51.0X4	—	—
deterrent NEC	T50.6X1	T50.6X2	T50.6X3	T50.6X4	T50.6X5	T50.6X6
diagnostic (gastric function)	T50.8X1	T50.8X2	T50.8X3	T50.8X4	T50.8X5	T50.8X6
ethyl	T51.0X1	T51.0X2	T51.0X3	T51.0X4	—	—
beverage	T51.0X1	T51.0X2	T51.0X3	T51.0X4	—	—
grain	T51.0X1	T51.0X2	T51.0X3	T51.0X4	—	—
beverage	T51.0X1	T51.0X2	T51.0X3	T51.0X4	—	—
industrial	T51.0X1	T51.0X2	T51.0X3	T51.0X4	—	—
isopropyl	T51.2X1	T51.2X2	T51.2X3	T51.2X4	—	—
methyl	T51.1X1	T51.1X2	T51.1X3	T51.1X4	—	—
preparation for consumption	T51.0X1	T51.0X2	T51.0X3	T51.0X4	—	—
propyl	T51.3X1	T51.3X2	T51.3X3	T51.3X4	—	—
secondary	T51.2X1	T51.2X2	T51.2X3	T51.2X4	—	—
radiator	T51.1X1	T51.1X2	T51.1X3	T51.1X4	—	—
rubbing	T51.2X1	T51.2X2	T51.2X3	T51.2X4	—	—
specified type NEC	T51.8X1	T51.8X2	T51.8X3	T51.8X4	—	—
surgical	T51.0X1	T51.0X2	T51.0X3	T51.0X4	—	—
vapor (from any type of Alcohol)	T59.891	T59.892	T59.893	T59.894	—	—
wood	T51.1X1	T51.1X2	T51.1X3	T51.1X4	—	—
Alcuronium (chloride)	T48.1X1	T48.1X2	T48.1X3	T48.1X4	T48.1X5	T48.1X6
Aldactone	T50.0X1	T50.0X2	T50.0X3	T50.0X4	T50.0X5	T50.0X6
Aldesulfone sodium	T37.1X1	T37.1X2	T37.1X3	T37.1X4	T37.1X5	T37.1X6
Aldicarb	T60.0X1	T60.0X2	T60.0X3	T60.0X4	—	—
Aldomet	T46.5X1	T46.5X2	T46.5X3	T46.5X4	T46.5X5	T46.5X6
Aldosterone	T50.0X1	T50.0X2	T50.0X3	T50.0X4	T50.0X5	T50.0X6
Aldrin (dust)	T60.1X1	T60.1X2	T60.1X3	T60.1X4	—	—
Aleve — see Naproxen						

Substance	Poisoning, Accidental (unintentional)	Poisoning, Intentional Self-harm	Poisoning, Assault	Poisoning, Undetermined	Adverse Effect	Underdosing
Alexitol sodium	T47.1X1	T47.1X2	T47.1X3	T47.1X4	T47.1X5	T47.1X6
Alfacalcidol	T45.2X1	T45.2X2	T45.2X3	T45.2X4	T45.2X5	T45.2X6
Alfadolone	T41.1X1	T41.1X2	T41.1X3	T41.1X4	T41.1X5	T41.1X6
Alfaxalone	T41.1X1	T41.1X2	T41.1X3	T41.1X4	T41.1X5	T41.1X6
Alfentanil	T40.411	T40.412	T40.413	T40.414	T40.415	T40.416
Alfuzosin (hydrochloride)	T44.8X1	T44.8X2	T44.8X3	T44.8X4	T44.8X5	T44.8X6
Algae (harmful) (toxin)	T65.821	T65.822	T65.823	T65.824	—	—
Algeldrate	T47.1X1	T47.1X2	T47.1X3	T47.1X4	T47.1X5	T47.1X6
Algin	T47.8X1	T47.8X2	T47.8X3	T47.8X4	T47.8X5	T47.8X6
Alglucerase	T45.3X1	T45.3X2	T45.3X3	T45.3X4	T45.3X5	T45.3X6
Alidase	T45.3X1	T45.3X2	T45.3X3	T45.3X4	T45.3X5	T45.3X6
Alimemazine	T43.3X1	T43.3X2	T43.3X3	T43.3X4	T43.3X5	T43.3X6
Aliphatic thiocyanates	T65.0X1	T65.0X2	T65.0X3	T65.0X4	—	—
Alitretinoin*	T49.0X1	T49.0X2	T49.0X3	T49.0X4	T49.0X5	T49.0X6
Alizapride	T45.0X1	T45.0X2	T45.0X3	T45.0X4	T45.0X5	T45.0X6
Alkali (caustic)	T54.3X1	T54.3X2	T54.3X3	T54.3X4	—	—
Alkaline antiseptic solution (aromatic)	T49.6X1	T49.6X2	T49.6X3	T49.6X4	T49.6X5	T49.6X6
Alkalinizing agents (medicinal)	T50.901	T50.902	T50.903	T50.904	T50.905	T50.906
Alkalizing agent NEC	T50.901	T50.902	T50.903	T50.904	T50.905	T50.906
Alka-seltzer	T39.011	T39.012	T39.013	T39.014	T39.015	T39.016
Alkavervir	T46.5X1	T46.5X2	T46.5X3	T46.5X4	T46.5X5	T46.5X6
Alkeran*	T45.1X1	T45.1X2	T45.1X3	T45.1X4	T45.1X5	T45.1X6
Alkonium (bromide)	T49.0X1	T49.0X2	T49.0X3	T49.0X4	T49.0X5	T49.0X6
Alkylating drug NEC	T45.1X1	T45.1X2	T45.1X3	T45.1X4	T45.1X5	T45.1X6
antimyeloproliferative	T45.1X1	T45.1X2	T45.1X3	T45.1X4	T45.1X5	T45.1X6
lymphatic	T45.1X1	T45.1X2	T45.1X3	T45.1X4	T45.1X5	T45.1X6
Alkylisocyanate	T65.0X1	T65.0X2	T65.0X3	T65.0X4	—	—
Allantoin	T49.4X1	T49.4X2	T49.4X3	T49.4X4	T49.4X5	T49.4X6
Allegron	T43.011	T43.012	T43.013	T43.014	T43.015	T43.016
Allethrin	T49.0X1	T49.0X2	T49.0X3	T49.0X4	T49.0X5	T49.0X6
Allobarbital	T42.3X1	T42.3X2	T42.3X3	T42.3X4	T42.3X5	T42.3X6
Allopurinol	T50.4X1	T50.4X2	T50.4X3	T50.4X4	T50.4X5	T50.4X6
Allyl						
alcohol	T51.8X1	T51.8X2	T51.8X3	T51.8X4	—	—
disulfide	T46.6X1	T46.6X2	T46.6X3	T46.6X4	T46.6X5	T46.6X6
Allylestrenol	T38.5X1	T38.5X2	T38.5X3	T38.5X4	T38.5X5	T38.5X6
Allylisopropylacetylurea	T42.6X1	T42.6X2	T42.6X3	T42.6X4	T42.6X5	T42.6X6
Allylisopropylmalonylurea	T42.3X1	T42.3X2	T42.3X3	T42.3X4	T42.3X5	T42.3X6
Allylthiourea	T49.3X1	T49.3X2	T49.3X3	T49.3X4	T49.3X5	T49.3X6
Allyltribromide	T42.6X1	T42.6X2	T42.6X3	T42.6X4	T42.6X5	T42.6X6
Allypropymal	T42.3X1	T42.3X2	T42.3X3	T42.3X4	T42.3X5	T42.3X6
Almagate	T47.1X1	T47.1X2	T47.1X3	T47.1X4	T47.1X5	T47.1X6
Almasilate	T47.1X1	T47.1X2	T47.1X3	T47.1X4	T47.1X5	T47.1X6
Almitrine	T50.7X1	T50.7X2	T50.7X3	T50.7X4	T50.7X5	T50.7X6
Aloes	T47.2X1	T47.2X2	T47.2X3	T47.2X4	T47.2X5	T47.2X6
Aloglutamol	T47.1X1	T47.1X2	T47.1X3	T47.1X4	T47.1X5	T47.1X6
Aloin	T47.2X1	T47.2X2	T47.2X3	T47.2X4	T47.2X5	T47.2X6
Aloxidone	T42.2X1	T42.2X2	T42.2X3	T42.2X4	T42.2X5	T42.2X6
Alpha						
acetyldigoxin	T46.0X1	T46.0X2	T46.0X3	T46.0X4	T46.0X5	T46.0X6
adrenergic blocking drug	T44.6X1	T44.6X2	T44.6X3	T44.6X4	T44.6X5	T44.6X6
amylase	T45.3X1	T45.3X2	T45.3X3	T45.3X4	T45.3X5	T45.3X6
tocoferol (acetate)	T45.2X1	T45.2X2	T45.2X3	T45.2X4	T45.2X5	T45.2X6
tocopherol	T45.2X1	T45.2X2	T45.2X3	T45.2X4	T45.2X5	T45.2X6
Alphadolone	T41.1X1	T41.1X2	T41.1X3	T41.1X4	T41.1X5	T41.1X6
Alphaprodine	T40.491	T40.492	T40.493	T40.494	T40.495	T40.496
Alphaxalone	T41.1X1	T41.1X2	T41.1X3	T41.1X4	T41.1X5	T41.1X6
Alprazolam	T42.4X1	T42.4X2	T42.4X3	T42.4X4	T42.4X5	T42.4X6
Alprenolol	T44.7X1	T44.7X2	T44.7X3	T44.7X4	T44.7X5	T44.7X6
Alprostadil	T46.7X1	T46.7X2	T46.7X3	T46.7X4	T46.7X5	T46.7X6
Alsactide	T38.811	T38.812	T38.813	T38.814	T38.815	T38.816
Alseroxylon	T46.5X1	T46.5X2	T46.5X3	T46.5X4	T46.5X5	T46.5X6
Alteplase	T45.611	T45.612	T45.613	T45.614	T45.615	T45.616
Altizide	T50.2X1	T50.2X2	T50.2X3	T50.2X4	T50.2X5	T50.2X6
Altoprev*	T46.6X1	T46.6X2	T46.6X3	T46.6X4	T46.6X5	T46.6X6
Altretamine	T45.1X1	T45.1X2	T45.1X3	T45.1X4	T45.1X5	T45.1X6
Alum (medicinal)	T49.4X1	T49.4X2	T49.4X3	T49.4X4	T49.4X5	T49.4X6
nonmedicinal (ammonium) (potassium)	T56.891	T56.892	T56.893	T56.894	—	—
Aluminium, aluminum						
acetate	T49.2X1	T49.2X2	T49.2X3	T49.2X4	T49.2X5	T49.2X6
solution	T49.0X1	T49.0X2	T49.0X3	T49.0X4	T49.0X5	T49.0X6
aspirin	T39.011	T39.012	T39.013	T39.014	T39.015	T39.016
bis (acetylsalicylate)	T39.011	T39.012	T39.013	T39.014	T39.015	T39.016
carbonate (gel, basic)	T47.1X1	T47.1X2	T47.1X3	T47.1X4	T47.1X5	T47.1X6
chlorhydroxide-complex	T47.1X1	T47.1X2	T47.1X3	T47.1X4	T47.1X5	T47.1X6
chloride	T49.2X1	T49.2X2	T49.2X3	T49.2X4	T49.2X5	T49.2X6
clofibrate	T46.6X1	T46.6X2	T46.6X3	T46.6X4	T46.6X5	T46.6X6
diacetate	T49.2X1	T49.2X2	T49.2X3	T49.2X4	T49.2X5	T49.2X6
glycinate	T47.1X1	T47.1X2	T47.1X3	T47.1X4	T47.1X5	T47.1X6
hydroxide (gel)	T47.1X1	T47.1X2	T47.1X3	T47.1X4	T47.1X5	T47.1X6

Substance	Poisoning, Accidental (unintentional)	Poisoning, Intentional Self-harm	Poisoning, Assault	Poisoning, Undetermined	Adverse Effect	Under-dosing
Aluminium, aluminum — continued						
hydroxide-magnesium carb. gel	T47.1X1	T47.1X2	T47.1X3	T47.1X4	T47.1X5	T47.1X6
magnesium silicate	T47.1X1	T47.1X2	T47.1X3	T47.1X4	T47.1X5	T47.1X6
nicotinate	T46.7X1	T46.7X2	T46.7X3	T46.7X4	T46.7X5	T46.7X6
ointment (surgical) (topical)	T49.3X1	T49.3X2	T49.3X3	T49.3X4	T49.3X5	T49.3X6
phosphate	T47.1X1	T47.1X2	T47.1X3	T47.1X4	T47.1X5	T47.1X6
salicylate	T39.091	T39.092	T39.093	T39.094	T39.095	T39.096
silicate	T47.1X1	T47.1X2	T47.1X3	T47.1X4	T47.1X5	T47.1X6
sodium silicate	T47.1X1	T47.1X2	T47.1X3	T47.1X4	T47.1X5	T47.1X6
subacetate	T49.2X1	T49.2X2	T49.2X3	T49.2X4	T49.2X5	T49.2X6
sulfate	T49.0X1	T49.0X2	T49.0X3	T49.0X4	T49.0X5	T49.0X6
tannate	T47.6X1	T47.6X2	T47.6X3	T47.6X4	T47.6X5	T47.6X6
topical NEC	T49.3X1	T49.3X2	T49.3X3	T49.3X4	T49.3X5	T49.3X6
Alurate	T42.3X1	T42.3X2	T42.3X3	T42.3X4	T42.3X5	T42.3X6
Alverine	T44.3X1	T44.3X2	T44.3X3	T44.3X4	T44.3X5	T44.3X6
Alvodine	T40.2X1	T40.2X2	T40.2X3	T40.2X4	T40.2X5	T40.2X6
Amanita phalloides	T62.0X1	T62.0X2	T62.0X3	T62.0X4	—	—
Amanitine	T62.0X1	T62.0X2	T62.0X3	T62.0X4	—	—
Amantadine	T42.8X1	T42.8X2	T42.8X3	T42.8X4	T42.8X5	T42.8X6
Ambazone	T49.6X1	T49.6X2	T49.6X3	T49.6X4	T49.6X5	T49.6X6
Ambenonium (chloride)	T44.0X1	T44.0X2	T44.0X3	T44.0X4	T44.0X5	T44.0X6
Ambien*	T42.6X1	T42.6X2	T42.6X3	T42.6X4	T42.6X5	T42.6X6
Ambroxol	T48.4X1	T48.4X2	T48.4X3	T48.4X4	T48.4X5	T48.4X6
Ambuphylline	T48.6X1	T48.6X2	T48.6X3	T48.6X4	T48.6X5	T48.6X6
Ambutonium bromide	T44.3X1	T44.3X2	T44.3X3	T44.3X4	T44.3X5	T44.3X6
Amcinonide	T49.0X1	T49.0X2	T49.0X3	T49.0X4	T49.0X5	T49.0X6
Amdinocilline	T36.0X1	T36.0X2	T36.0X3	T36.0X4	T36.0X5	T36.0X6
Americaine*	T41.3X1	T41.3X2	T41.3X3	T41.3X4	T41.3X5	T41.3X6
Ametazole	T50.8X1	T50.8X2	T50.8X3	T50.8X4	T50.8X5	T50.8X6
Amethocaine	T41.3X1	T41.3X2	T41.3X3	T41.3X4	T41.3X5	T41.3X6
regional	T41.3X1	T41.3X2	T41.3X3	T41.3X4	T41.3X5	T41.3X6
spinal	T41.3X1	T41.3X2	T41.3X3	T41.3X4	T41.3X5	T41.3X6
Amethopterin	T45.1X1	T45.1X2	T45.1X3	T45.1X4	T45.1X5	T45.1X6
Amezinium metilsulfate	T44.991	T44.992	T44.993	T44.994	T44.995	T44.996
Amfebutamone	T43.291	T43.292	T43.293	T43.294	T43.295	T43.296
Amfepramone	T50.5X1	T50.5X2	T50.5X3	T50.5X4	T50.5X5	T50.5X6
Amfetamine	T43.621	T43.622	T43.623	T43.624	T43.625	T43.626
Amfetaminil	T43.621	T43.622	T43.623	T43.624	T43.625	T43.626
Amfomycin	T36.8X1	T36.8X2	T36.8X3	T36.8X4	T36.8X5	T36.8X6
Amidefrine mesilate	T48.5X1	T48.5X2	T48.5X3	T48.5X4	T48.5X5	T48.5X6
Amidone	T40.3X1	T40.3X2	T40.3X3	T40.3X4	T40.3X5	T40.3X6
Amidopyrine	T39.2X1	T39.2X2	T39.2X3	T39.2X4	T39.2X5	T39.2X6
Amidotrizoate	T50.8X1	T50.8X2	T50.8X3	T50.8X4	T50.8X5	T50.8X6
Amiflamine	T43.1X1	T43.1X2	T43.1X3	T43.1X4	T43.1X5	T43.1X6
Amikacin	T36.5X1	T36.5X2	T36.5X3	T36.5X4	T36.5X5	T36.5X6
Amikhelline	T46.3X1	T46.3X2	T46.3X3	T46.3X4	T46.3X5	T46.3X6
Amiloride	T50.2X1	T50.2X2	T50.2X3	T50.2X4	T50.2X5	T50.2X6
Aminacrine	T49.0X1	T49.0X2	T49.0X3	T49.0X4	T49.0X5	T49.0X6
Amineptine	T43.011	T43.012	T43.013	T43.014	T43.015	T43.016
Aminitrozole	T37.3X1	T37.3X2	T37.3X3	T37.3X4	T37.3X5	T37.3X6
Aminoacetic acid (derivatives)	T50.3X1	T50.3X2	T50.3X3	T50.3X4	T50.3X5	T50.3X6
Amino acids	T50.3X1	T50.3X2	T50.3X3	T50.3X4	T50.3X5	T50.3X6
Aminoacridine	T49.0X1	T49.0X2	T49.0X3	T49.0X4	T49.0X5	T49.0X6
Aminobenzoic acid (-p)	T49.3X1	T49.3X2	T49.3X3	T49.3X4	T49.3X5	T49.3X6
Aminocaproic acid	T45.621	T45.622	T45.623	T45.624	T45.625	T45.626
Aminoethylisothiourium	T45.8X1	T45.8X2	T45.8X3	T45.8X4	T45.8X5	T45.8X6
Aminofenazone	T39.2X1	T39.2X2	T39.2X3	T39.2X4	T39.2X5	T39.2X6
Aminoglutethimide	T45.1X1	T45.1X2	T45.1X3	T45.1X4	T45.1X5	T45.1X6
Aminoglycosides*	T36.5X1	T36.5X2	T36.5X3	T36.5X4	T36.5X5	T36.5X6
Aminohippuric acid	T50.8X1	T50.8X2	T50.8X3	T50.8X4	T50.8X5	T50.8X6
Aminometradine	T45.691	T45.692	T45.693	T45.694	T45.695	T45.696
Aminopentamide	T50.2X1	T50.2X2	T50.2X3	T50.2X4	T50.2X5	T50.2X6
Aminophenazone	T44.3X1	T44.3X2	T44.3X3	T44.3X4	T44.3X5	T44.3X6
Aminophenol	T39.2X1	T39.2X2	T39.2X3	T39.2X4	T39.2X5	T39.2X6
Aminophenylpyridone	T54.0X1	T54.0X2	T54.0X3	T54.0X4	—	—
Aminophylline	T43.591	T43.592	T43.593	T43.594	T43.595	T43.596
Aminopterin sodium	T48.6X1	T48.6X2	T48.6X3	T48.6X4	T48.6X5	T48.6X6
Aminopyrine	T45.1X1	T45.1X2	T45.1X3	T45.1X4	T45.1X5	T45.1X6
Aminorex	T39.2X1	T39.2X2	T39.2X3	T39.2X4	T39.2X5	T39.2X6
Aminosalicylic acid	T50.5X1	T50.5X2	T50.5X3	T50.5X4	T50.5X5	T50.5X6
Aminosalylum	T37.1X1	T37.1X2	T37.1X3	T37.1X4	T37.1X5	T37.1X6
Amiodarone	T37.1X1	T37.1X2	T37.1X3	T37.1X4	T37.1X5	T37.1X6
Amiphenazole	T46.2X1	T46.2X2	T46.2X3	T46.2X4	T46.2X5	T46.2X6
Amiquinsin	T50.7X1	T50.7X2	T50.7X3	T50.7X4	T50.7X5	T50.7X6
Amisometradine	T46.5X1	T46.5X2	T46.5X3	T46.5X4	T46.5X5	T46.5X6
Amisulpride	T50.2X1	T50.2X2	T50.2X3	T50.2X4	T50.2X5	T50.2X6
Amitriptyline	T43.591	T43.592	T43.593	T43.594	T43.595	T43.596
Amitriptylinoxide	T43.011	T43.012	T43.013	T43.014	T43.015	T43.016

Substance	Poisoning, Accidental (unintentional)	Poisoning, Intentional Self-harm	Poisoning, Assault	Poisoning, Undetermined	Adverse Effect	Under-dosing
Amlexanox	T48.6X1	T48.6X2	T48.6X3	T48.6X4	T48.6X5	T48.6X6
Amlodipine*	T46.1X1	T46.1X2	T46.1X3	T46.1X4	T46.1X5	T46.1X6
Ammonia (fumes) (gas) (vapor)	T59.891	T59.892	T59.893	T59.894	—	—
aromatic spirit	T48.991	T48.992	T48.993	T48.994	T48.995	T48.996
liquid (household)	T54.3X1	T54.3X2	T54.3X3	T54.3X4	—	—
Ammoniated mercury	T49.0X1	T49.0X2	T49.0X3	T49.0X4	T49.0X5	T49.0X6
Ammonium						
acid tartrate	T49.5X1	T49.5X2	T49.5X3	T49.5X4	T49.5X5	T49.5X6
bromide	T42.6X1	T42.6X2	T42.6X3	T42.6X4	T42.6X5	T42.6X6
carbonate	T54.3X1	T54.3X2	T54.3X3	T54.3X4	—	—
chloride	T50.991	T50.992	T50.993	T50.994	T50.995	T50.996
expectorant	T48.4X1	T48.4X2	T48.4X3	T48.4X4	T48.4X5	T48.4X6
compounds (household) NEC	T54.3X1	T54.3X2	T54.3X3	T54.3X4	—	—
fumes (any usage)	T59.891	T59.892	T59.893	T59.894	—	—
industrial	T54.3X1	T54.3X2	T54.3X3	T54.3X4	—	—
ichthyosulronate	T49.4X1	T49.4X2	T49.4X3	T49.4X4	T49.4X5	T49.4X6
mandelate	T37.91	T37.92	T37.93	T37.94	T37.95	T37.96
sulfamate	T60.3X1	T60.3X2	T60.3X3	T60.3X4	—	—
sulfonate resin	T47.8X1	T47.8X2	T47.8X3	T47.8X4	T47.8X5	T47.8X6
Amobarbital (sodium)	T42.3X1	T42.3X2	T42.3X3	T42.3X4	T42.3X5	T42.3X6
Amodiaquine	T37.2X1	T37.2X2	T37.2X3	T37.2X4	T37.2X5	T37.2X6
Amopyroquin (e)	T37.2X1	T37.2X2	T37.2X3	T37.2X4	T37.2X5	T37.2X6
Amoxapine	T43.011	T43.012	T43.013	T43.014	T43.015	T43.016
Amoxicillin	T36.0X1	T36.0X2	T36.0X3	T36.0X4	T36.0X5	T36.0X6
Amperozide	T43.591	T43.592	T43.593	T43.594	T43.595	T43.596
Amphenidone	T43.591	T43.592	T43.593	T43.594	T43.595	T43.596
Amphetamine NEC	T43.621	T43.622	T43.623	T43.624	T43.625	T43.626
Amphogel	T47.1X1	T47.1X2	T47.1X3	T47.1X4	T47.1X5	T47.1X6
Amphomycin	T36.8X1	T36.8X2	T36.8X3	T36.8X4	T36.8X5	T36.8X6
Amphotalide	T37.4X1	T37.4X2	T37.4X3	T37.4X4	T37.4X5	T37.4X6
Amphotericin B	T36.7X1	T36.7X2	T36.7X3	T36.7X4	T36.7X5	T36.7X6
topical	T49.0X1	T49.0X2	T49.0X3	T49.0X4	T49.0X5	T49.0X6
Ampicillin	T36.0X1	T36.0X2	T36.0X3	T36.0X4	T36.0X5	T36.0X6
Amprotropine	T44.3X1	T44.3X2	T44.3X3	T44.3X4	T44.3X5	T44.3X6
Amsacrine	T45.1X1	T45.1X2	T45.1X3	T45.1X4	T45.1X5	T45.1X6
Amygdaline	T62.2X1	T62.2X2	T62.2X3	T62.2X4	—	—
Amyl						
acetate	T52.8X1	T52.8X2	T52.8X3	T52.8X4	—	—
vapor	T59.891	T59.892	T59.893	T59.894	—	—
alcohol	T51.3X1	T51.3X2	T51.3X3	T51.3X4	—	—
chloride	T53.6X1	T53.6X2	T53.6X3	T53.6X4	—	—
formate	T52.8X1	T52.8X2	T52.8X3	T52.8X4	—	—
nitrite	T46.3X1	T46.3X2	T46.3X3	T46.3X4	T46.3X5	T46.3X6
propionate	T65.891	T65.892	T65.893	T65.894	—	—
Amylase	T47.5X1	T47.5X2	T47.5X3	T47.5X4	T47.5X5	T47.5X6
Amyleine, regional	T41.3X1	T41.3X2	T41.3X3	T41.3X4	T41.3X5	T41.3X6
Amylene						
dichloride	T53.6X1	T53.6X2	T53.6X3	T53.6X4	—	—
hydrate	T51.3X1	T51.3X2	T51.3X3	T51.3X4	—	—
Amylmetacresol	T49.6X1	T49.6X2	T49.6X3	T49.6X4	T49.6X5	T49.6X6
Amylobarbitone	T42.3X1	T42.3X2	T42.3X3	T42.3X4	T42.3X5	T42.3X6
Amylocaine, regional	T41.3X1	T41.3X2	T41.3X3	T41.3X4	T41.3X5	T41.3X6
infiltration (subcutaneous)	T41.3X1	T41.3X2	T41.3X3	T41.3X4	T41.3X5	T41.3X6
nerve block (peripheral) (plexus)	T41.3X1	T41.3X2	T41.3X3	T41.3X4	T41.3X5	T41.3X6
spinal	T41.3X1	T41.3X2	T41.3X3	T41.3X4	T41.3X5	T41.3X6
topical (surface)	T41.3X1	T41.3X2	T41.3X3	T41.3X4	T41.3X5	T41.3X6
Amylopectin	T47.6X1	T47.6X2	T47.6X3	T47.6X4	T47.6X5	T47.6X6
Amytal (sodium)	T42.3X1	T42.3X2	T42.3X3	T42.3X4	T42.3X5	T42.3X6
Anabolic steroid	T38.7X1	T38.7X2	T38.7X3	T38.7X4	T38.7X5	T38.7X6
Anacaine*	T41.3X1	T41.3X2	T41.3X3	T41.3X4	T41.3X5	T41.3X6
Analeptic NEC	T50.7X1	T50.7X2	T50.7X3	T50.7X4	T50.7X5	T50.7X6
Analgesic	T39.91	T39.92	T39.93	T39.94	T39.95	T39.96
anti-inflammatory NEC	T39.91	T39.92	T39.93	T39.94	T39.95	T39.96
propionic acid derivative	T39.311	T39.312	T39.313	T39.314	T39.315	T39.316
antirheumatic NEC	T39.4X1	T39.4X2	T39.4X3	T39.4X4	T39.4X5	T39.4X6
aromatic NEC	T39.1X1	T39.1X2	T39.1X3	T39.1X4	T39.1X5	T39.1X6
narcotic NEC	T40.601	T40.602	T40.603	T40.604	T40.605	T40.606
combination	T40.601	T40.602	T40.603	T40.604	T40.605	T40.606
obstetric	T40.601	T40.602	T40.603	T40.604	T40.605	T40.606
non-narcotic NEC	T39.91	T39.92	T39.93	T39.94	T39.95	T39.96
combination	T39.91	T39.92	T39.93	T39.94	T39.95	T39.96
pyrazole	T39.2X1	T39.2X2	T39.2X3	T39.2X4	T39.2X5	T39.2X6
specified NEC	T39.8X1	T39.8X2	T39.8X3	T39.8X4	T39.8X5	T39.8X6
Analgin	T39.2X1	T39.2X2	T39.2X3	T39.2X4	T39.2X5	T39.2X6
Anamirta cocculus	T62.1X1	T62.1X2	T62.1X3	T62.1X4	—	—
Ancillin	T36.0X1	T36.0X2	T36.0X3	T36.0X4	T36.0X5	T36.0X6
Ancrod	T45.691	T45.692	T45.693	T45.694	T45.695	T45.696
Androgen	T38.7X1	T38.7X2	T38.7X3	T38.7X4	T38.7X5	T38.7X6
Androgen-estrogen mixture	T38.7X1	T38.7X2	T38.7X3	T38.7X4	T38.7X5	T38.7X6

☑ Additional Character May Be Required — Refer to the Tabular List for Character Selection   *Optum Value-Add

Substance	Poisoning, Accidental (unintentional)	Poisoning, Intentional Self-harm	Poisoning, Assault	Poisoning, Undetermined	Adverse Effect	Under-dosing
Androstalone	T38.7X1	T38.7X2	T38.7X3	T38.7X4	T38.7X5	T38.7X6
Androstanolone	T38.7X1	T38.7X2	T38.7X3	T38.7X4	T38.7X5	T38.7X6
Androsterone	T38.7X1	T38.7X2	T38.7X3	T38.7X4	T38.7X5	T38.7X6
Anemone pulsatilla	T62.2X1	T62.2X2	T62.2X3	T62.2X4	—	—
Anesthesia						
caudal	T41.3X1	T41.3X2	T41.3X3	T41.3X4	T41.3X5	T41.3X6
endotracheal	T41.0X1	T41.0X2	T41.0X3	T41.0X4	T41.0X5	T41.0X6
epidural	T41.3X1	T41.3X2	T41.3X3	T41.3X4	T41.3X5	T41.3X6
inhalation	T41.0X1	T41.0X2	T41.0X3	T41.0X4	T41.0X5	T41.0X6
local	T41.3X1	T41.3X2	T41.3X3	T41.3X4	T41.3X5	T41.3X6
mucosal	T41.3X1	T41.3X2	T41.3X3	T41.3X4	T41.3X5	T41.3X6
muscle relaxation	T48.1X1	T48.1X2	T48.1X3	T48.1X4	T48.1X5	T48.1X6
nerve blocking	T41.3X1	T41.3X2	T41.3X3	T41.3X4	T41.3X5	T41.3X6
plexus blocking	T41.3X1	T41.3X2	T41.3X3	T41.3X4	T41.3X5	T41.3X6
potentiated	T41.201	T41.202	T41.203	T41.204	T41.205	T41.206
rectal	T41.201	T41.202	T41.203	T41.204	T41.205	T41.206
general	T41.201	T41.202	T41.203	T41.204	T41.205	T41.206
local	T41.3X1	T41.3X2	T41.3X3	T41.3X4	T41.3X5	T41.3X6
regional	T41.3X1	T41.3X2	T41.3X3	T41.3X4	T41.3X5	T41.3X6
surface	T41.3X1	T41.3X2	T41.3X3	T41.3X4	T41.3X5	T41.3X6
Anesthetic NEC — see also Anesthesia	T41.41	T41.42	T41.43	T41.44	T41.45	T41.46
with muscle relaxant	T41.201	T41.202	T41.203	T41.204	T41.205	T41.206
general	T41.201	T41.202	T41.203	T41.204	T41.205	T41.206
local	T41.3X1	T41.3X2	T41.3X3	T41.3X4	T41.3X5	T41.3X6
gaseous NEC	T41.0X1	T41.0X2	T41.0X3	T41.0X4	T41.0X5	T41.0X6
general NEC	T41.201	T41.202	T41.203	T41.204	T41.205	T41.206
halogenated hydrocarbon derivatives NEC	T41.0X1	T41.0X2	T41.0X3	T41.0X4	T41.0X5	T41.0X6
infiltration NEC	T41.3X1	T41.3X2	T41.3X3	T41.3X4	T41.3X5	T41.3X6
intravenous NEC	T41.1X1	T41.1X2	T41.1X3	T41.1X4	T41.1X5	T41.1X6
local NEC	T41.3X1	T41.3X2	T41.3X3	T41.3X4	T41.3X5	T41.3X6
rectal	T41.201	T41.202	T41.203	T41.204	T41.205	T41.206
general	T41.201	T41.202	T41.203	T41.204	T41.205	T41.206
local	T41.3X1	T41.3X2	T41.3X3	T41.3X4	T41.3X5	T41.3X6
regional NEC	T41.3X1	T41.3X2	T41.3X3	T41.3X4	T41.3X5	T41.3X6
spinal NEC	T41.3X1	T41.3X2	T41.3X3	T41.3X4	T41.3X5	T41.3X6
thiobarbiturate	T41.1X1	T41.1X2	T41.1X3	T41.1X4	T41.1X5	T41.1X6
topical	T41.3X1	T41.3X2	T41.3X3	T41.3X4	T41.3X5	T41.3X6
Aneurine	T45.2X1	T45.2X2	T45.2X3	T45.2X4	T45.2X5	T45.2X6
Angeliq*	T38.5X1	T38.5X2	T38.5X3	T38.5X4	T38.5X5	T38.5X6
Angio-Conray	T50.8X1	T50.8X2	T50.8X3	T50.8X4	T50.8X5	T50.8X6
Angiotensin	T44.5X1	T44.5X2	T44.5X3	T44.5X4	T44.5X5	T44.5X6
Angiotensinamide	T44.991	T44.992	T44.993	T44.994	T44.995	T44.996
Anhydrohydroxy-progesterone	T38.5X1	T38.5X2	T38.5X3	T38.5X4	T38.5X5	T38.5X6
Anhydron	T50.2X1	T50.2X2	T50.2X3	T50.2X4	T50.2X5	T50.2X6
Anileridine	T40.491	T40.492	T40.493	T40.494	T40.495	T40.496
Aniline (dye) (liquid)	T65.3X1	T65.3X2	T65.3X3	T65.3X4	—	—
analgesic	T39.1X1	T39.1X2	T39.1X3	T39.1X4	T39.1X5	T39.1X6
derivatives, therapeutic NEC	T39.1X1	T39.1X2	T39.1X3	T39.1X4	T39.1X5	T39.1X6
vapor	T65.3X1	T65.3X2	T65.3X3	T65.3X4	—	—
Aniscoropine	T44.3X1	T44.3X2	T44.3X3	T44.3X4	T44.3X5	T44.3X6
Anise oil	T47.5X1	T47.5X2	T47.5X3	T47.5X4	T47.5X5	T47.5X6
Anisidine	T65.3X1	T65.3X2	T65.3X3	T65.3X4	—	—
Anisindione	T45.511	T45.512	T45.513	T45.514	T45.515	T45.516
Anisotropine	T44.3X1	T44.3X2	T44.3X3	T44.3X4	T44.3X5	T44.3X6
methyl-bromide						
Anistreplase	T45.611	T45.612	T45.613	T45.614	T45.615	T45.616
Anorexiant (central)	T50.5X1	T50.5X2	T50.5X3	T50.5X4	T50.5X5	T50.5X6
Anorexic agents	T50.5X1	T50.5X2	T50.5X3	T50.5X4	T50.5X5	T50.5X6
Ansaid*	T39.311	T39.312	T39.313	T39.314	T39.315	T39.316
Ansamycin	T36.6X1	T36.6X2	T36.6X3	T36.6X4	T36.6X5	T36.6X6
Ant (bite) (sting)	T63.421	T63.422	T63.423	T63.424	—	—
Antabuse	T50.6X1	T50.6X2	T50.6X3	T50.6X4	T50.6X5	T50.6X6
Antacid NEC	T47.1X1	T47.1X2	T47.1X3	T47.1X4	T47.1X5	T47.1X6
Antagonist						
Aldosterone	T50.0X1	T50.0X2	T50.0X3	T50.0X4	T50.0X5	T50.0X6
alpha-adrenoreceptor	T44.6X1	T44.6X2	T44.6X3	T44.6X4	T44.6X5	T44.6X6
anticoagulant	T45.7X1	T45.7X2	T45.7X3	T45.7X4	T45.7X5	T45.7X6
beta-adrenoreceptor	T44.7X1	T44.7X2	T44.7X3	T44.7X4	T44.7X5	T44.7X6
extrapyramidal NEC	T44.3X1	T44.3X2	T44.3X3	T44.3X4	T44.3X5	T44.3X6
folic acid	T45.1X1	T45.1X2	T45.1X3	T45.1X4	T45.1X5	T45.1X6
H2 receptor	T47.0X1	T47.0X2	T47.0X3	T47.0X4	T47.0X5	T47.0X6
heavy metal	T45.8X1	T45.8X2	T45.8X3	T45.8X4	T45.8X5	T45.8X6
narcotic analgesic	T50.7X1	T50.7X2	T50.7X3	T50.7X4	T50.7X5	T50.7X6
opiate	T50.7X1	T50.7X2	T50.7X3	T50.7X4	T50.7X5	T50.7X6
pyrimidine	T45.1X1	T45.1X2	T45.1X3	T45.1X4	T45.1X5	T45.1X6
serotonin	T46.5X1	T46.5X2	T46.5X3	T46.5X4	T46.5X5	T46.5X6
Antazolin (e)	T45.0X1	T45.0X2	T45.0X3	T45.0X4	T45.0X5	T45.0X6
Anterior pituitary hormone NEC	T38.811	T38.812	T38.813	T38.814	T38.815	T38.816
Anthelmintic NEC	T37.4X1	T37.4X2	T37.4X3	T37.4X4	T37.4X5	T37.4X6

Substance	Poisoning, Accidental (unintentional)	Poisoning, Intentional Self-harm	Poisoning, Assault	Poisoning, Undetermined	Adverse Effect	Under-dosing
Anthiolimine	T37.4X1	T37.4X2	T37.4X3	T37.4X4	T37.4X5	T37.4X6
Anthralin	T49.4X1	T49.4X2	T49.4X3	T49.4X4	T49.4X5	T49.4X6
Anthramycin	T45.1X1	T45.1X2	T45.1X3	T45.1X4	T45.1X5	T45.1X6
Antiadrenergic NEC	T44.8X1	T44.8X2	T44.8X3	T44.8X4	T44.8X5	T44.8X6
Antiallergic NEC	T45.0X1	T45.0X2	T45.0X3	T45.0X4	T45.0X5	T45.0X6
Antiandrogen NEC	T38.6X1	T38.6X2	T38.6X3	T38.6X4	T38.6X5	T38.6X6
Anti-anemic (drug) (preparation)	T45.8X1	T45.8X2	T45.8X3	T45.8X4	T45.8X5	T45.8X6
Antianxiety drug NEC	T43.501	T43.502	T43.503	T43.504	T43.505	T43.506
Antiaris toxicaria	T65.891	T65.892	T65.893	T65.894	—	—
Antiarteriosclerotic drug	T46.6X1	T46.6X2	T46.6X3	T46.6X4	T46.6X5	T46.6X6
Antiasthmatic drug NEC	T48.6X1	T48.6X2	T48.6X3	T48.6X4	T48.6X5	T48.6X6
Antibiotic Otic Suspension (Solution)*	T49.6X1	T49.6X2	T49.6X3	T49.6X4	T49.6X5	T49.6X6
Antibiotic NEC	T36.91	T36.92	T36.93	T36.94	T36.95	T36.96
aminoglycoside	T36.5X1	T36.5X2	T36.5X3	T36.5X4	T36.5X5	T36.5X6
anticancer	T45.1X1	T45.1X2	T45.1X3	T45.1X4	T45.1X5	T45.1X6
antifungal	T36.7X1	T36.7X2	T36.7X3	T36.7X4	T36.7X5	T36.7X6
antimycobacterial	T36.5X1	T36.5X2	T36.5X3	T36.5X4	T36.5X5	T36.5X6
antineoplastic	T45.1X1	T45.1X2	T45.1X3	T45.1X4	T45.1X5	T45.1X6
b-lactam NEC	T36.1X1	T36.1X2	T36.1X3	T36.1X4	T36.1X5	T36.1X6
cephalosporin (group)	T36.1X1	T36.1X2	T36.1X3	T36.1X4	T36.1X5	T36.1X6
chloramphenicol (group)	T36.2X1	T36.2X2	T36.2X3	T36.2X4	T36.2X5	T36.2X6
ENT	T49.6X1	T49.6X2	T49.6X3	T49.6X4	T49.6X5	T49.6X6
eye	T49.5X1	T49.5X2	T49.5X3	T49.5X4	T49.5X5	T49.5X6
fungicidal (local)	T49.0X1	T49.0X2	T49.0X3	T49.0X4	T49.0X5	T49.0X6
intestinal	T36.8X1	T36.8X2	T36.8X3	T36.8X4	T36.8X5	T36.8X6
local	T49.0X1	T49.0X2	T49.0X3	T49.0X4	T49.0X5	T49.0X6
macrolides	T36.3X1	T36.3X2	T36.3X3	T36.3X4	T36.3X5	T36.3X6
polypeptide	T36.8X1	T36.8X2	T36.8X3	T36.8X4	T36.8X5	T36.8X6
specified NEC	T36.8X1	T36.8X2	T36.8X3	T36.8X4	T36.8X5	T36.8X6
tetracycline (group)	T36.4X1	T36.4X2	T36.4X3	T36.4X4	T36.4X5	T36.4X6
throat	T49.6X1	T49.6X2	T49.6X3	T49.6X4	T49.6X5	T49.6X6
Anticancer agents NEC	T45.1X1	T45.1X2	T45.1X3	T45.1X4	T45.1X5	T45.1X6
Anticholesterolemic drug NEC	T46.6X1	T46.6X2	T46.6X3	T46.6X4	T46.6X5	T46.6X6
Anticholinergic NEC	T44.3X1	T44.3X2	T44.3X3	T44.3X4	T44.3X5	T44.3X6
Anticholinesterase	T44.0X1	T44.0X2	T44.0X3	T44.0X4	T44.0X5	T44.0X6
organophosphorus	T44.0X1	T44.0X2	T44.0X3	T44.0X4	T44.0X5	T44.0X6
insecticide	T60.0X1	T60.0X2	T60.0X3	T60.0X4		
nerve gas	T59.891	T59.892	T59.893	T59.894	—	—
reversible	T44.0X1	T44.0X2	T44.0X3	T44.0X4	T44.0X5	T44.0X6
ophthalmological	T49.5X1	T49.5X2	T49.5X3	T49.5X4	T49.5X5	T49.5X6
Anticoagulant NEC	T45.511	T45.512	T45.513	T45.514	T45.515	T45.516
Antagonist	T45.7X1	T45.7X2	T45.7X3	T45.7X4	T45.7X5	T45.7X6
Anti-common-cold drug NEC	T48.5X1	T48.5X2	T48.5X3	T48.5X4	T48.5X5	T48.5X6
Anticonvulsant	T42.71	T42.72	T42.73	T42.74	T42.75	T42.76
barbiturate	T42.3X1	T42.3X2	T42.3X3	T42.3X4	T42.3X5	T42.3X6
combination (with barbiturate)	T42.3X1	T42.3X2	T42.3X3	T42.3X4	T42.3X5	T42.3X6
hydantoin	T42.0X1	T42.0X2	T42.0X3	T42.0X4	T42.0X5	T42.0X6
hypnotic NEC	T42.6X1	T42.6X2	T42.6X3	T42.6X4	T42.6X5	T42.6X6
oxazolidinedione	T42.2X1	T42.2X2	T42.2X3	T42.2X4	T42.2X5	T42.2X6
pyrimidinedione	T42.6X1	T42.6X2	T42.6X3	T42.6X4	T42.6X5	T42.6X6
specified NEC	T42.6X1	T42.6X2	T42.6X3	T42.6X4	T42.6X5	T42.6X6
succinimide	T42.2X1	T42.2X2	T42.2X3	T42.2X4	T42.2X5	T42.2X6
Antidepressant	T43.201	T43.202	T43.203	T43.204	T43.205	T43.206
monoamine oxidase inhibitor	T43.1X1	T43.1X2	T43.1X3	T43.1X4	T43.1X5	T43.1X6
selective serotonin norepinephrine reuptake inhibitor	T43.211	T43.212	T43.213	T43.214	T43.215	T43.216
selective serotonin reuptake inhibitor	T43.221	T43.222	T43.223	T43.224	T43.225	T43.226
specified NEC	T43.291	T43.292	T43.293	T43.294	T43.295	T43.296
tetracyclic	T43.021	T43.022	T43.023	T43.024	T43.025	T43.026
triazolopyridine	T43.211	T43.212	T43.213	T43.214	T43.215	T43.216
tricyclic	T43.011	T43.012	T43.013	T43.014	T43.015	T43.016
Antidiabetic NEC	T38.3X1	T38.3X2	T38.3X3	T38.3X4	T38.3X5	T38.3X6
biguanide	T38.3X1	T38.3X2	T38.3X3	T38.3X4	T38.3X5	T38.3X6
and sulfonyl combined	T38.3X1	T38.3X2	T38.3X3	T38.3X4	T38.3X5	T38.3X6
combined	T38.3X1	T38.3X2	T38.3X3	T38.3X4	T38.3X5	T38.3X6
sulfonylurea	T38.3X1	T38.3X2	T38.3X3	T38.3X4	T38.3X5	T38.3X6
Antidiarrheal drug NEC	T47.6X1	T47.6X2	T47.6X3	T47.6X4	T47.6X5	T47.6X6
absorbent	T47.6X1	T47.6X2	T47.6X3	T47.6X4	T47.6X5	T47.6X6
Anti-D immunoglobulin (human)	T50.Z11	T50.Z12	T50.Z13	T50.Z14	T50.Z15	T50.Z16
Antidiphtheria serum	T50.Z11	T50.Z12	T50.Z13	T50.Z14	T50.Z15	T50.Z16
Antidiuretic hormone	T38.891	T38.892	T38.893	T38.894	T38.895	T38.896
Antidote NEC	T50.6X1	T50.6X2	T50.6X3	T50.6X4	T50.6X5	T50.6X6
heavy metal	T45.8X1	T45.8X2	T45.8X3	T45.8X4	T45.8X5	T45.8X6
Antidysrhythmic NEC	T46.2X1	T46.2X2	T46.2X3	T46.2X4	T46.2X5	T46.2X6

Table of Drugs and Chemicals

Antiemetic drug — Apomorphine

Substance	Poisoning, Accidental (unintentional)	Poisoning, Intentional Self-harm	Poisoning, Assault	Poisoning, Undetermined	Adverse Effect	Underdosing
Antiemetic drug	T45.0X1	T45.0X2	T45.0X3	T45.0X4	T45.0X5	T45.0X6
Antiepilepsy agent	T42.71	T42.72	T42.73	T42.74	T42.75	T42.76
combination	T42.5X1	T42.5X2	T42.5X3	T42.5X4	T42.5X5	T42.5X6
mixed	T42.5X1	T42.5X2	T42.5X3	T42.5X4	T42.5X5	T42.5X6
specified, NEC	T42.6X1	T42.6X2	T42.6X3	T42.6X4	T42.6X5	T42.6X6
Antiestrogen NEC	T38.6X1	T38.6X2	T38.6X3	T38.6X4	T38.6X5	T38.6X6
Antifertility pill	T38.4X1	T38.4X2	T38.4X3	T38.4X4	T38.4X5	T38.4X6
Antifibrinolytic drug	T45.621	T45.622	T45.623	T45.624	T45.625	T45.626
Antifilarial drug	T37.4X1	T37.4X2	T37.4X3	T37.4X4	T37.4X5	T37.4X6
Antiflatulent	T47.5X1	T47.5X2	T47.5X3	T47.5X4	T47.5X5	T47.5X6
Antifreeze	T65.91	T65.92	T65.93	T65.94	—	—
alcohol	T51.1X1	T51.1X2	T51.1X3	T51.1X4	—	—
ethylene glycol	T51.8X1	T51.8X2	T51.8X3	T51.8X4	—	—
Antifungal						
antibiotic (systemic)	T36.7X1	T36.7X2	T36.7X3	T36.7X4	T36.7X5	T36.7X6
anti-infective NEC	T37.91	T37.92	T37.93	T37.94	T37.95	T37.96
disinfectant, local	T49.0X1	T49.0X2	T49.0X3	T49.0X4	T49.0X5	T49.0X6
nonmedicinal (spray)	T60.3X1	T60.3X2	T60.3X3	T60.3X4	—	—
topical	T49.0X1	T49.0X2	T49.0X3	T49.0X4	T49.0X5	T49.0X6
Anti-gastric-secretion drug NEC	T47.1X1	T47.1X2	T47.1X3	T47.1X4	T47.1X5	T47.1X6
Antigonadotrophin NEC	T38.6X1	T38.6X2	T38.6X3	T38.6X4	T38.6X5	T38.6X6
Antihallucinogen	T43.501	T43.502	T43.503	T43.504	T43.505	T43.506
Antihelmintics	T37.4X1	T37.4X2	T37.4X3	T37.4X4	T37.4X5	T37.4X6
Antihemophilic						
factor	T45.8X1	T45.8X2	T45.8X3	T45.8X4	T45.8X5	T45.8X6
fraction	T45.8X1	T45.8X2	T45.8X3	T45.8X4	T45.8X5	T45.8X6
globulin concentrate	T45.7X1	T45.7X2	T45.7X3	T45.7X4	T45.7X5	T45.7X6
human plasma	T45.8X1	T45.8X2	T45.8X3	T45.8X4	T45.8X5	T45.8X6
plasma, dried	T45.7X1	T45.7X2	T45.7X3	T45.7X4	T45.7X5	T45.7X6
Antihemorrhoidal preparation	T49.2X1	T49.2X2	T49.2X3	T49.2X4	T49.2X5	T49.2X6
Antiheparin drug	T45.7X1	T45.7X2	T45.7X3	T45.7X4	T45.7X5	T45.7X6
Antihistamine	T45.0X1	T45.0X2	T45.0X3	T45.0X4	T45.0X5	T45.0X6
Antihookworm drug	T37.4X1	T37.4X2	T37.4X3	T37.4X4	T37.4X5	T37.4X6
Anti-human lymphocytic globulin	T50.Z11	T50.Z12	T50.Z13	T50.Z14	T50.Z15	T50.Z16
Antihyperlipidemic drug	T46.6X1	T46.6X2	T46.6X3	T46.6X4	T46.6X5	T46.6X6
Antihypertensive drug NEC	T46.5X1	T46.5X2	T46.5X3	T46.5X4	T46.5X5	T46.5X6
Anti-infective NEC	T37.91	T37.92	T37.93	T37.94	T37.95	T37.96
anthelmintic	T37.4X1	T37.4X2	T37.4X3	T37.4X4	T37.4X5	T37.4X6
antibiotics	T36.91	T36.92	T36.93	T36.94	T36.95	T36.96
specified NEC	T36.8X1	T36.8X2	T36.8X3	T36.8X4	T36.8X5	T36.8X6
antimalarial	T37.2X1	T37.2X2	T37.2X3	T37.2X4	T37.2X5	T37.2X6
antimycobacterial NEC	T37.1X1	T37.1X2	T37.1X3	T37.1X4	T37.1X5	T37.1X6
antibiotics	T36.5X1	T36.5X2	T36.5X3	T36.5X4	T36.5X5	T36.5X6
antiprotozoal NEC	T37.3X1	T37.3X2	T37.3X3	T37.3X4	T37.3X5	T37.3X6
blood	T37.2X1	T37.2X2	T37.2X3	T37.2X4	T37.2X5	T37.2X6
antiviral	T37.5X1	T37.5X2	T37.5X3	T37.5X4	T37.5X5	T37.5X6
arsenical	T37.8X1	T37.8X2	T37.8X3	T37.8X4	T37.8X5	T37.8X6
bismuth, local	T49.0X1	T49.0X2	T49.0X3	T49.0X4	T49.0X5	T49.0X6
ENT	T49.6X1	T49.6X2	T49.6X3	T49.6X4	T49.6X5	T49.6X6
eye NEC	T49.5X1	T49.5X2	T49.5X3	T49.5X4	T49.5X5	T49.5X6
heavy metals NEC	T37.8X1	T37.8X2	T37.8X3	T37.8X4	T37.8X5	T37.8X6
local NEC	T49.0X1	T49.0X2	T49.0X3	T49.0X4	T49.0X5	T49.0X6
specified NEC	T49.0X1	T49.0X2	T49.0X3	T49.0X4	T49.0X5	T49.0X6
mixed	T37.91	T37.92	T37.93	T37.94	T37.95	T37.96
ophthalmic preparation	T49.5X1	T49.5X2	T49.5X3	T49.5X4	T49.5X5	T49.5X6
topical NEC	T49.0X1	T49.0X2	T49.0X3	T49.0X4	T49.0X5	T49.0X6
Anti-inflammatory drug NEC	T39.391	T39.392	T39.393	T39.394	T39.395	T39.396
local	T49.0X1	T49.0X2	T49.0X3	T49.0X4	T49.0X5	T49.0X6
nonsteroidal NEC	T39.391	T39.392	T39.393	T39.394	T39.395	T39.396
propionic acid derivative	T39.311	T39.312	T39.313	T39.314	T39.315	T39.316
specified NEC	T39.391	T39.392	T39.393	T39.394	T39.395	T39.396
Antikaluretic	T50.3X1	T50.3X2	T50.3X3	T50.3X4	T50.3X5	T50.3X6
Antiknock (tetraethyl lead)	T56.0X1	T56.0X2	T56.0X3	T56.0X4	—	—
Antilipemic drug NEC	T46.6X1	T46.6X2	T46.6X3	T46.6X4	T46.6X5	T46.6X6
Antilysin*	T45.621	T45.622	T45.623	T45.624	T45.625	T45.626
Antimalarial	T37.2X1	T37.2X2	T37.2X3	T37.2X4	T37.2X5	T37.2X6
prophylactic NEC	T37.2X1	T37.2X2	T37.2X3	T37.2X4	T37.2X5	T37.2X6
pyrimidine derivative	T37.2X1	T37.2X2	T37.2X3	T37.2X4	T37.2X5	T37.2X6
Antimetabolite	T45.1X1	T45.1X2	T45.1X3	T45.1X4	T45.1X5	T45.1X6
Antimitotic agent	T45.1X1	T45.1X2	T45.1X3	T45.1X4	T45.1X5	T45.1X6
Antimony (compounds) (vapor)	T56.891	T56.892	T56.893	T56.894	—	—
NEC						
anti-infectives	T37.8X1	T37.8X2	T37.8X3	T37.8X4	T37.8X5	T37.8X6
dimercaptosuccinate	T37.3X1	T37.3X2	T37.3X3	T37.3X4	T37.3X5	T37.3X6
hydride	T56.891	T56.892	T56.893	T56.894	—	—
pesticide (vapor)	T60.8X1	T60.8X2	T60.8X3	T60.8X4	—	—
potassium (sodium) tartrate	T37.8X1	T37.8X2	T37.8X3	T37.8X4	T37.8X5	T37.8X6

Substance	Poisoning, Accidental (unintentional)	Poisoning, Intentional Self-harm	Poisoning, Assault	Poisoning, Undetermined	Adverse Effect	Underdosing
Antimony (compounds) (vapor)						
NEC — continued						
sodium	T37.3X1	T37.3X2	T37.3X3	T37.3X4	T37.3X5	T37.3X6
dimercaptosuccinate						
tartrated	T37.8X1	T37.8X2	T37.8X3	T37.8X4	T37.8X5	T37.8X6
Antimuscarinic NEC	T44.3X1	T44.3X2	T44.3X3	T44.3X4	T44.3X5	T44.3X6
Antimycobacterial drug NEC	T37.1X1	T37.1X2	T37.1X3	T37.1X4	T37.1X5	T37.1X6
antibiotics	T36.5X1	T36.5X2	T36.5X3	T36.5X4	T36.5X5	T36.5X6
combination	T37.1X1	T37.1X2	T37.1X3	T37.1X4	T37.1X5	T37.1X6
Antinausea drug	T45.0X1	T45.0X2	T45.0X3	T45.0X4	T45.0X5	T45.0X6
Antinematode drug	T37.4X1	T37.4X2	T37.4X3	T37.4X4	T37.4X5	T37.4X6
Antineoplastic NEC	T45.1X1	T45.1X2	T45.1X3	T45.1X4	T45.1X5	T45.1X6
alkaloidal	T45.1X1	T45.1X2	T45.1X3	T45.1X4	T45.1X5	T45.1X6
antibiotics	T45.1X1	T45.1X2	T45.1X3	T45.1X4	T45.1X5	T45.1X6
combination	T45.1X1	T45.1X2	T45.1X3	T45.1X4	T45.1X5	T45.1X6
estrogen	T38.5X1	T38.5X2	T38.5X3	T38.5X4	T38.5X5	T38.5X6
steroid	T38.7X1	T38.7X2	T38.7X3	T38.7X4	T38.7X5	T38.7X6
Antiparasitic drug (systemic)	T37.91	T37.92	T37.93	T37.94	T37.95	T37.96
local	T49.0X1	T49.0X2	T49.0X3	T49.0X4	T49.0X5	T49.0X6
specified NEC	T37.8X1	T37.8X2	T37.8X3	T37.8X4	T37.8X5	T37.8X6
Antiparkinsonism drug NEC	T42.8X1	T42.8X2	T42.8X3	T42.8X4	T42.8X5	T42.8X6
Antiperspirant NEC	T49.2X1	T49.2X2	T49.2X3	T49.2X4	T49.2X5	T49.2X6
Antiphlogistic NEC	T39.4X1	T39.4X2	T39.4X3	T39.4X4	T39.4X5	T39.4X6
Antiplatyhelmintic drug	T37.4X1	T37.4X2	T37.4X3	T37.4X4	T37.4X5	T37.4X6
Antiprotozoal drug NEC	T37.3X1	T37.3X2	T37.3X3	T37.3X4	T37.3X5	T37.3X6
blood	T37.2X1	T37.2X2	T37.2X3	T37.2X4	T37.2X5	T37.2X6
local	T49.0X1	T49.0X2	T49.0X3	T49.0X4	T49.0X5	T49.0X6
Antipruritic drug NEC	T49.1X1	T49.1X2	T49.1X3	T49.1X4	T49.1X5	T49.1X6
Antipsychotic drug	T43.501	T43.502	T43.503	T43.504	T43.505	T43.506
specified NEC	T43.591	T43.592	T43.593	T43.594	T43.595	T43.596
Antipyretic	T39.91	T39.92	T39.93	T39.94	T39.95	T39.96
specified NEC	T39.8X1	T39.8X2	T39.8X3	T39.8X4	T39.8X5	T39.8X6
Antipyrine	T39.2X1	T39.2X2	T39.2X3	T39.2X4	T39.2X5	T39.2X6
Antirabies hyperimmune serum	T50.Z11	T50.Z12	T50.Z13	T50.Z14	T50.Z15	T50.Z16
Antirheumatic NEC	T39.4X1	T39.4X2	T39.4X3	T39.4X4	T39.4X5	T39.4X6
Antirigidity drug NEC	T42.8X1	T42.8X2	T42.8X3	T42.8X4	T42.8X5	T42.8X6
Antischistosomal drug	T37.4X1	T37.4X2	T37.4X3	T37.4X4	T37.4X5	T37.4X6
Antiscorpion sera	T50.Z11	T50.Z12	T50.Z13	T50.Z14	T50.Z15	T50.Z16
Antiseborrheics	T49.4X1	T49.4X2	T49.4X3	T49.4X4	T49.4X5	T49.4X6
Antiseptics (external) (medicinal)	T49.0X1	T49.0X2	T49.0X3	T49.0X4	T49.0X5	T49.0X6
Antistine	T45.0X1	T45.0X2	T45.0X3	T45.0X4	T45.0X5	T45.0X6
Antitapeworm drug	T37.4X1	T37.4X2	T37.4X3	T37.4X4	T37.4X5	T37.4X6
Antitetanus immunoglobulin	T50.Z11	T50.Z12	T50.Z13	T50.Z14	T50.Z15	T50.Z16
Antithrombin III*	T45.511	T45.512	T45.513	T45.514	T45.515	T45.516
Antithrombotic	T45.521	T45.522	T45.523	T45.524	T45.525	T45.526
Antithyroid drug NEC	T38.2X1	T38.2X2	T38.2X3	T38.2X4	T38.2X5	T38.2X6
Antitoxin	T50.Z11	T50.Z12	T50.Z13	T50.Z14	T50.Z15	T50.Z16
diphtheria	T50.Z11	T50.Z12	T50.Z13	T50.Z14	T50.Z15	T50.Z16
gas gangrene	T50.Z11	T50.Z12	T50.Z13	T50.Z14	T50.Z15	T50.Z16
tetanus	T50.Z11	T50.Z12	T50.Z13	T50.Z14	T50.Z15	T50.Z16
Antitrichomonal drug	T37.3X1	T37.3X2	T37.3X3	T37.3X4	T37.3X5	T37.3X6
Antituberculars	T37.1X1	T37.1X2	T37.1X3	T37.1X4	T37.1X5	T37.1X6
antibiotics	T36.5X1	T36.5X2	T36.5X3	T36.5X4	T36.5X5	T36.5X6
Antitussive NEC	T48.3X1	T48.3X2	T48.3X3	T48.3X4	T48.3X5	T48.3X6
codeine mixture	T40.2X1	T40.2X2	T40.2X3	T40.2X4	T40.2X5	T40.2X6
opiate	T40.2X1	T40.2X2	T40.2X3	T40.2X4	T40.2X5	T40.2X6
Antivaricose drug	T46.8X1	T46.8X2	T46.8X3	T46.8X4	T46.8X5	T46.8X6
Antivenin, antivenom (sera)	T50.Z11	T50.Z12	T50.Z13	T50.Z14	T50.Z15	T50.Z16
crotaline	T50.Z11	T50.Z12	T50.Z13	T50.Z14	T50.Z15	T50.Z16
spider bite	T50.Z11	T50.Z12	T50.Z13	T50.Z14	T50.Z15	T50.Z16
Antivert*	T45.0X1	T45.0X2	T45.0X3	T45.0X4	T45.0X5	T45.0X6
Antivertigo drug	T45.0X1	T45.0X2	T45.0X3	T45.0X4	T45.0X5	T45.0X6
Antiviral drug NEC	T37.5X1	T37.5X2	T37.5X3	T37.5X4	T37.5X5	T37.5X6
eye	T49.5X1	T49.5X2	T49.5X3	T49.5X4	T49.5X5	T49.5X6
Antiwhipworm drug	T37.4X1	T37.4X2	T37.4X3	T37.4X4	T37.4X5	T37.4X6
Ant poison — see also by Insecticide						
Antrol — see also by specific chemical substance	T60.91	T60.92	T60.93	T60.94	—	—
fungicide	T60.91	T60.92	T60.93	T60.94	—	—
ANTU (alpha naphthylthiourea)	T60.4X1	T60.4X2	T60.4X3	T60.4X4	—	—
Apalcillin	T36.0X1	T36.0X2	T36.0X3	T36.0X4	T36.0X5	T36.0X6
APC	T48.5X1	T48.5X2	T48.5X3	T48.5X4	T48.5X5	T48.5X6
Aplonidine	T44.4X1	T44.4X2	T44.4X3	T44.4X4	T44.4X5	T44.4X6
Apomorphine	T47.7X1	T47.7X2	T47.7X3	T47.7X4	T47.7X5	T47.7X6

Substance	Poisoning, Accidental (unintentional)	Poisoning, Intentional Self-harm	Poisoning, Assault	Poisoning, Undetermined	Adverse Effect	Under-dosing
Appetite depressants, central	T50.5X1	T50.5X2	T50.5X3	T50.5X4	T50.5X5	T50.5X6
Apraclonidine	T44.4X1	T44.4X2	T44.4X3	T44.4X4	T44.4X5	T44.4X6
(hydrochloride)						
Apresoline	T46.5X1	T46.5X2	T46.5X3	T46.5X4	T46.5X5	T46.5X6
Apri*	T38.4X1	T38.4X2	T38.4X3	T38.4X4	T38.4X5	T38.4X6
Aprindine	T46.2X1	T46.2X2	T46.2X3	T46.2X4	T46.2X5	T46.2X6
Aprobarbital	T42.3X1	T42.3X2	T42.3X3	T42.3X4	T42.3X5	T42.3X6
Apronalide	T42.6X1	T42.6X2	T42.6X3	T42.6X4	T42.6X5	T42.6X6
Aprotinin	T45.621	T45.622	T45.623	T45.624	T45.625	T45.626
Aptocaine	T41.3X1	T41.3X2	T41.3X3	T41.3X4	T41.3X5	T41.3X6
Aqua fortis	T54.2X1	T54.2X2	T54.2X3	T54.2X4	—	—
Ara-A	T37.5X1	T37.5X2	T37.5X3	T37.5X4	T37.5X5	T37.5X6
Ara-C	T45.1X1	T45.1X2	T45.1X3	T45.1X4	T45.1X5	T45.1X6
Arachis oil	T49.3X1	T49.3X2	T49.3X3	T49.3X4	T49.3X5	T49.3X6
cathartic	T47.4X1	T47.4X2	T47.4X3	T47.4X4	T47.4X5	T47.4X6
Aralen	T37.2X1	T37.2X2	T37.2X3	T37.2X4	T37.2X5	T37.2X6
Arecoline	T44.1X1	T44.1X2	T44.1X3	T44.1X4	T44.1X5	T44.1X6
Arginine	T50.991	T50.992	T50.993	T50.994	T50.995	T50.996
glutamate	T50.991	T50.992	T50.993	T50.994	T50.995	T50.996
Argyrol	T49.0X1	T49.0X2	T49.0X3	T49.0X4	T49.0X5	T49.0X6
ENT agent	T49.6X1	T49.6X2	T49.6X3	T49.6X4	T49.6X5	T49.6X6
ophthalmic preparation	T49.5X1	T49.5X2	T49.5X3	T49.5X4	T49.5X5	T49.5X6
Aristocort	T38.0X1	T38.0X2	T38.0X3	T38.0X4	T38.0X5	T38.0X6
ENT agent	T49.6X1	T49.6X2	T49.6X3	T49.6X4	T49.6X5	T49.6X6
ophthalmic preparation	T49.5X1	T49.5X2	T49.5X3	T49.5X4	T49.5X5	T49.5X6
topical NEC	T49.0X1	T49.0X2	T49.0X3	T49.0X4	T49.0X5	T49.0X6
Armour*	T38.1X1	T38.1X2	T38.1X3	T38.1X4	T38.1X5	T38.1X6
Aromatics, corrosive	T54.1X1	T54.1X2	T54.1X3	T54.1X4	—	—
disinfectants	T54.1X1	T54.1X2	T54.1X3	T54.1X4	—	—
Arsenate of lead	T57.0X1	T57.0X2	T57.0X3	T57.0X4	—	—
herbicide	T57.0X1	T57.0X2	T57.0X3	T57.0X4	—	—
Arsenic, arsenicals (compounds) (dust) (vapor) **NEC**	T57.0X1	T57.0X2	T57.0X3	T57.0X4	—	—
anti-infectives	T37.8X1	T37.8X2	T37.8X3	T37.8X4	T37.8X5	T37.8X6
pesticide (dust) (fumes)	T57.0X1	T57.0X2	T57.0X3	T57.0X4	—	—
Arsine (gas)	T57.0X1	T57.0X2	T57.0X3	T57.0X4	—	—
Arsobal*	T37.3X1	T37.3X2	T37.3X3	T37.3X4	T37.3X5	T37.3X6
Arsphenamine (silver)	T37.8X1	T37.8X2	T37.8X3	T37.8X4	T37.8X5	T37.8X6
Arsthinol	T37.3X1	T37.3X2	T37.3X3	T37.3X4	T37.3X5	T37.3X6
Artane	T44.3X1	T44.3X2	T44.3X3	T44.3X4	T44.3X5	T44.3X6
Arthropod (venomous) **NEC**	T63.481	T63.482	T63.483	T63.484	—	—
Articaine	T41.3X1	T41.3X2	T41.3X3	T41.3X4	T41.3X5	T41.3X6
Asbestos	T57.8X1	T57.8X2	T57.8X3	T57.8X4	—	—
Ascaridole	T37.4X1	T37.4X2	T37.4X3	T37.4X4	T37.4X5	T37.4X6
Ascorbic acid	T45.2X1	T45.2X2	T45.2X3	T45.2X4	T45.2X5	T45.2X6
Asiaticoside	T49.0X1	T49.0X2	T49.0X3	T49.0X4	T49.0X5	T49.0X6
Asparaginase	T45.1X1	T45.1X2	T45.1X3	T45.1X4	T45.1X5	T45.1X6
Aspidium (oleoresin)	T37.4X1	T37.4X2	T37.4X3	T37.4X4	T37.4X5	T37.4X6
Aspirin (aluminum) (soluble)	T39.011	T39.012	T39.013	T39.014	T39.015	T39.016
Aspoxicillin	T36.0X1	T36.0X2	T36.0X3	T36.0X4	T36.0X5	T36.0X6
Astemizole	T45.0X1	T45.0X2	T45.0X3	T45.0X4	T45.0X5	T45.0X6
Astringent (local)	T49.2X1	T49.2X2	T49.2X3	T49.2X4	T49.2X5	T49.2X6
specified NEC	T49.2X1	T49.2X2	T49.2X3	T49.2X4	T49.2X5	T49.2X6
Astromicin	T36.5X1	T36.5X2	T36.5X3	T36.5X4	T36.5X5	T36.5X6
Ataractic drug NEC	T43.501	T43.502	T43.503	T43.504	T43.505	T43.506
Atenolol	T44.7X1	T44.7X2	T44.7X3	T44.7X4	T44.7X5	T44.7X6
Atonia drug, intestinal	T47.4X1	T47.4X2	T47.4X3	T47.4X4	T47.4X5	T47.4X6
Atophan	T50.4X1	T50.4X2	T50.4X3	T50.4X4	T50.4X5	T50.4X6
Atorvastatin*	T46.6X1	T46.6X2	T46.6X3	T46.6X4	T46.6X5	T46.6X6
Atracurium besilate	T48.1X1	T48.1X2	T48.1X3	T48.1X4	T48.1X5	T48.1X6
Atropine	T44.3X1	T44.3X2	T44.3X3	T44.3X4	T44.3X5	T44.3X6
derivative	T44.3X1	T44.3X2	T44.3X3	T44.3X4	T44.3X5	T44.3X6
methonitrate	T44.3X1	T44.3X2	T44.3X3	T44.3X4	T44.3X5	T44.3X6
Atrovent*	T48.6X1	T48.6X2	T48.6X3	T48.6X4	T48.6X5	T48.6X6
Attapulgite	T47.6X1	T47.6X2	T47.6X3	T47.6X4	T47.6X5	T47.6X6
Augmentin (ES-600) (XR)*	T36.0X1	T36.0X2	T36.0X3	T36.0X4	T36.0X5	T36.0X6
Auramine	T65.891	T65.892	T65.893	T65.894	—	—
dye	T65.6X1	T65.6X2	T65.6X3	T65.6X4	—	—
fungicide	T60.3X1	T60.3X2	T60.3X3	T60.3X4	—	—
Auranofin	T39.4X1	T39.4X2	T39.4X3	T39.4X4	T39.4X5	T39.4X6
Aurantiin	T46.991	T46.992	T46.993	T46.994	T46.995	T46.996
Aureomycin	T36.4X1	T36.4X2	T36.4X3	T36.4X4	T36.4X5	T36.4X6
ophthalmic preparation	T49.5X1	T49.5X2	T49.5X3	T49.5X4	T49.5X5	T49.5X6
topical NEC	T49.0X1	T49.0X2	T49.0X3	T49.0X4	T49.0X5	T49.0X6
Aurothioglucose	T39.4X1	T39.4X2	T39.4X3	T39.4X4	T39.4X5	T39.4X6
Aurothioglycanide	T39.4X1	T39.4X2	T39.4X3	T39.4X4	T39.4X5	T39.4X6
Aurothiomalate sodium	T39.4X1	T39.4X2	T39.4X3	T39.4X4	T39.4X5	T39.4X6
Aurotioprol	T39.4X1	T39.4X2	T39.4X3	T39.4X4	T39.4X5	T39.4X6
Automobile fuel	T52.0X1	T52.0X2	T52.0X3	T52.0X4	—	—
Autonomic nervous system agent NEC	T44.901	T44.902	T44.903	T44.904	T44.905	T44.906
Avelox*	T36.8X1	T36.8X2	T36.8X3	T36.8X4	T36.8X5	T36.8X6
Avlosulfon	T37.1X1	T37.1X2	T37.1X3	T37.1X4	T37.1X5	T37.1X6
Avomine	T42.6X1	T42.6X2	T42.6X3	T42.6X4	T42.6X5	T42.6X6
Axerophthol	T45.2X1	T45.2X2	T45.2X3	T45.2X4	T45.2X5	T45.2X6
Azacitidine	T45.1X1	T45.1X2	T45.1X3	T45.1X4	T45.1X5	T45.1X6
Azacyclonol	T43.591	T43.592	T43.593	T43.594	T43.595	T43.596
Azadirachta	T60.2X1	T60.2X2	T60.2X3	T60.2X4	—	—
Azanidazole	T37.3X1	T37.3X2	T37.3X3	T37.3X4	T37.3X5	T37.3X6
Azapetine	T46.7X1	T46.7X2	T46.7X3	T46.7X4	T46.7X5	T46.7X6
Azapropazone	T39.2X1	T39.2X2	T39.2X3	T39.2X4	T39.2X5	T39.2X6
Azaribine	T45.1X1	T45.1X2	T45.1X3	T45.1X4	T45.1X5	T45.1X6
Azaserine	T45.1X1	T45.1X2	T45.1X3	T45.1X4	T45.1X5	T45.1X6
Azatadine	T45.0X1	T45.0X2	T45.0X3	T45.0X4	T45.0X5	T45.0X6
Azatepa	T45.1X1	T45.1X2	T45.1X3	T45.1X4	T45.1X5	T45.1X6
Azathioprine	T45.1X1	T45.1X2	T45.1X3	T45.1X4	T45.1X5	T45.1X6
Azelaic acid	T49.0X1	T49.0X2	T49.0X3	T49.0X4	T49.0X5	T49.0X6
Azelastine	T45.0X1	T45.0X2	T45.0X3	T45.0X4	T45.0X5	T45.0X6
Azidocillin	T36.0X1	T36.0X2	T36.0X3	T36.0X4	T36.0X5	T36.0X6
Azidothymidine	T37.5X1	T37.5X2	T37.5X3	T37.5X4	T37.5X5	T37.5X6
Azinphos (ethyl) (methyl)	T60.0X1	T60.0X2	T60.0X3	T60.0X4	—	—
Aziridine (chelating)	T54.1X1	T54.1X2	T54.1X3	T54.1X4	—	—
Azithromycin	T36.3X1	T36.3X2	T36.3X3	T36.3X4	T36.3X5	T36.3X6
Azlocillin	T36.0X1	T36.0X2	T36.0X3	T36.0X4	T36.0X5	T36.0X6
Azobenzene smoke	T65.3X1	T65.3X2	T65.3X3	T65.3X4	—	—
acaricide	T60.8X1	T60.8X2	T60.8X3	T60.8X4	—	—
Azo-Standard*	T49.0X1	T49.0X2	T49.0X3	T49.0X4	T49.0X5	T49.0X6
Azosulfamide	T37.0X1	T37.0X2	T37.0X3	T37.0X4	T37.0X5	T37.0X6
AZT	T37.5X1	T37.5X2	T37.5X3	T37.5X4	T37.5X5	T37.5X6
Aztreonam	T36.1X1	T36.1X2	T36.1X3	T36.1X4	T36.1X5	T36.1X6
Azulfidine	T37.0X1	T37.0X2	T37.0X3	T37.0X4	T37.0X5	T37.0X6
Azuresin	T50.8X1	T50.8X2	T50.8X3	T50.8X4	T50.8X5	T50.8X6
b-acetyldigoxin	T46.0X1	T46.0X2	T46.0X3	T46.0X4	T46.0X5	T46.0X6
P-Acetamidophenol	T39.1X1	T39.1X2	T39.1X3	T39.1X4	T39.1X5	T39.1X6
Bacampicillin	T36.0X1	T36.0X2	T36.0X3	T36.0X4	T36.0X5	T36.0X6
Bacillus						
lactobacillus	T47.8X1	T47.8X2	T47.8X3	T47.8X4	T47.8X5	T47.8X6
subtilis	T47.6X1	T47.6X2	T47.6X3	T47.6X4	T47.6X5	T47.6X6
Bacimycin	T49.0X1	T49.0X2	T49.0X3	T49.0X4	T49.0X5	T49.0X6
ophthalmic preparation	T49.5X1	T49.5X2	T49.5X3	T49.5X4	T49.5X5	T49.5X6
Bacitracin zinc	T49.0X1	T49.0X2	T49.0X3	T49.0X4	T49.0X5	T49.0X6
with neomycin	T49.0X1	T49.0X2	T49.0X3	T49.0X4	T49.0X5	T49.0X6
ENT agent	T49.6X1	T49.6X2	T49.6X3	T49.6X4	T49.6X5	T49.6X6
ophthalmic preparation	T49.5X1	T49.5X2	T49.5X3	T49.5X4	T49.5X5	T49.5X6
topical NEC	T49.0X1	T49.0X2	T49.0X3	T49.0X4	T49.0X5	T49.0X6
Baclofen	T42.8X1	T42.8X2	T42.8X3	T42.8X4	T42.8X5	T42.8X6
Bactrim*	T36.8X1	T36.8X2	T36.8X3	T36.8X4	T36.8X5	T36.8X6
Baking soda	T50.991	T50.992	T50.993	T50.994	T50.995	T50.996
BAL	T45.8X1	T45.8X2	T45.8X3	T45.8X4	T45.8X5	T45.8X6
Bambuterol	T48.6X1	T48.6X2	T48.6X3	T48.6X4	T48.6X5	T48.6X6
Bamethan (sulfate)	T46.7X1	T46.7X2	T46.7X3	T46.7X4	T46.7X5	T46.7X6
Bamifylline	T48.6X1	T48.6X2	T48.6X3	T48.6X4	T48.6X5	T48.6X6
Bamipine	T45.0X1	T45.0X2	T45.0X3	T45.0X4	T45.0X5	T45.0X6
Baneberry — *see* Actaea spicata						
Banewort — *see* Belladonna						
Barbenyl	T42.3X1	T42.3X2	T42.3X3	T42.3X4	T42.3X5	T42.3X6
Barbexaclone	T42.6X1	T42.6X2	T42.6X3	T42.6X4	T42.6X5	T42.6X6
Barbital	T42.3X1	T42.3X2	T42.3X3	T42.3X4	T42.3X5	T42.3X6
sodium	T42.3X1	T42.3X2	T42.3X3	T42.3X4	T42.3X5	T42.3X6
Barbitone	T42.3X1	T42.3X2	T42.3X3	T42.3X4	T42.3X5	T42.3X6
Barbiturate NEC	T42.3X1	T42.3X2	T42.3X3	T42.3X4	T42.3X5	T42.3X6
with tranquilizer	T42.3X1	T42.3X2	T42.3X3	T42.3X4	T42.3X5	T42.3X6
anesthetic (intravenous)	T41.1X1	T41.1X2	T41.1X3	T41.1X4	T41.1X5	T41.1X6
Barium (carbonate) (chloride) (sulfite)	T57.8X1	T57.8X2	T57.8X3	T57.8X4	—	—
diagnostic agent	T50.8X1	T50.8X2	T50.8X3	T50.8X4	T50.8X5	T50.8X6
pesticide	T60.4X1	T60.4X2	T60.4X3	T60.4X4	—	—
rodenticide	T60.4X1	T60.4X2	T60.4X3	T60.4X4	—	—
sulfate (medicinal)	T50.8X1	T50.8X2	T50.8X3	T50.8X4	T50.8X5	T50.8X6
Barrier cream	T49.3X1	T49.3X2	T49.3X3	T49.3X4	T49.3X5	T49.3X6
Basic fuchsin	T49.0X1	T49.0X2	T49.0X3	T49.0X4	T49.0X5	T49.0X6
Basiliximab*	T45.1X1	T45.1X2	T45.1X3	T45.1X4	T45.1X5	T45.1X6
Battery acid or fluid	T54.2X1	T54.2X2	T54.2X3	T54.2X4	—	—
Bay rum	T51.8X1	T51.8X2	T51.8X3	T51.8X4	—	—
b-benzalbutyramide	T46.6X1	T46.6X2	T46.6X3	T46.6X4	T46.6X5	T46.6X6
BCG (vaccine)	T50.A91	T50.A92	T50.A93	T50.A94	T50.A95	T50.A96
BCNU	T45.1X1	T45.1X2	T45.1X3	T45.1X4	T45.1X5	T45.1X6
Bearsfoot	T62.2X1	T62.2X2	T62.2X3	T62.2X4	—	—
Beclamide	T42.6X1	T42.6X2	T42.6X3	T42.6X4	T42.6X5	T42.6X6
Beclomethasone	T44.5X1	T44.5X2	T44.5X3	T44.5X4	T44.5X5	T44.5X6
Bee (sting) (venom)	T63.441	T63.442	T63.443	T63.444	—	—
Befunolol	T49.5X1	T49.5X2	T49.5X3	T49.5X4	T49.5X5	T49.5X6
Bekanamycin	T36.5X1	T36.5X2	T36.5X3	T36.5X4	T36.5X5	T36.5X6

Table of Drugs and Chemicals

Appetite depressants, central — Bekanamycin

Substance	Poisoning, Accidental (unintentional)	Poisoning, Intentional Self-harm	Poisoning, Assault	Poisoning, Undetermined	Adverse Effect	Under-dosing
Belladonna — see also						
Nightshade						
alkaloids	T44.3X1	T44.3X2	T44.3X3	T44.3X4	T44.3X5	T44.3X6
extract	T44.3X1	T44.3X2	T44.3X3	T44.3X4	T44.3X5	T44.3X6
herb	T44.3X1	T44.3X2	T44.3X3	T44.3X4	T44.3X5	T44.3X6
Belviq*	T50.5X1	T50.5X2	T50.5X3	T50.5X4	T50.5X5	T50.5X6
Bemegride	T50.7X1	T50.7X2	T50.7X3	T50.7X4	T50.7X5	T50.7X6
Benactyzine	T44.3X1	T44.3X2	T44.3X3	T44.3X4	T44.3X5	T44.3X6
Benadryl	T45.0X1	T45.0X2	T45.0X3	T45.0X4	T45.0X5	T45.0X6
Benaprizine	T44.3X1	T44.3X2	T44.3X3	T44.3X4	T44.3X5	T44.3X6
Benazepril	T46.4X1	T46.4X2	T46.4X3	T46.4X4	T46.4X5	T46.4X6
Bencyclane	T46.7X1	T46.7X2	T46.7X3	T46.7X4	T46.7X5	T46.7X6
Bendazol	T46.3X1	T46.3X2	T46.3X3	T46.3X4	T46.3X5	T46.3X6
Bendrofluazide	T50.2X1	T50.2X2	T50.2X3	T50.2X4	T50.2X5	T50.2X6
Bendroflumethiazide	T50.2X1	T50.2X2	T50.2X3	T50.2X4	T50.2X5	T50.2X6
Benemid	T50.4X1	T50.4X2	T50.4X3	T50.4X4	T50.4X5	T50.4X6
Benethamine penicillin	T36.0X1	T36.0X2	T36.0X3	T36.0X4	T36.0X5	T36.0X6
Benexate	T47.1X1	T47.1X2	T47.1X3	T47.1X4	T47.1X5	T47.1X6
Benfluorex	T46.6X1	T46.6X2	T46.6X3	T46.6X4	T46.6X5	T46.6X6
Benfotiamine	T45.2X1	T45.2X2	T45.2X3	T45.2X4	T45.2X5	T45.2X6
Benisone	T49.0X1	T49.0X2	T49.0X3	T49.0X4	T49.0X5	T49.0X6
Benomyl	T60.0X1	T60.0X2	T60.0X3	T60.0X4	—	—
Benoquin	T49.8X1	T49.8X2	T49.8X3	T49.8X4	T49.8X5	T49.8X6
Benoxinate	T41.3X1	T41.3X2	T41.3X3	T41.3X4	T41.3X5	T41.3X6
Benperidol	T43.4X1	T43.4X2	T43.4X3	T43.4X4	T43.4X5	T43.4X6
Benproperine	T48.3X1	T48.3X2	T48.3X3	T48.3X4	T48.3X5	T48.3X6
Benserazide	T42.8X1	T42.8X2	T42.8X3	T42.8X4	T42.8X5	T42.8X6
Bentazepam	T42.4X1	T42.4X2	T42.4X3	T42.4X4	T42.4X5	T42.4X6
Bentiromide	T50.8X1	T50.8X2	T50.8X3	T50.8X4	T50.8X5	T50.8X6
Bentonite	T49.3X1	T49.3X2	T49.3X3	T49.3X4	T49.3X5	T49.3X6
Benzalbutyramide	T46.6X1	T46.6X2	T46.6X3	T46.6X4	T46.6X5	T46.6X6
Benzalkonium (chloride)	T49.0X1	T49.0X2	T49.0X3	T49.0X4	T49.0X5	T49.0X6
ophthalmic preparation	T49.5X1	T49.5X2	T49.5X3	T49.5X4	T49.5X5	T49.5X6
Benzamidosalicylate (calcium)	T37.1X1	T37.1X2	T37.1X3	T37.1X4	T37.1X5	T37.1X6
Benzamine	T41.3X1	T41.3X2	T41.3X3	T41.3X4	T41.3X5	T41.3X6
lactate	T49.1X1	T49.1X2	T49.1X3	T49.1X4	T49.1X5	T49.1X6
Benzamphetamine	T50.5X1	T50.5X2	T50.5X3	T50.5X4	T50.5X5	T50.5X6
Benzapril hydrochloride	T46.5X1	T46.5X2	T46.5X3	T46.5X4	T46.5X5	T46.5X6
Benzathine benzylpenicillin	T36.0X1	T36.0X2	T36.0X3	T36.0X4	T36.0X5	T36.0X6
Benzathine penicillin	T36.0X1	T36.0X2	T36.0X3	T36.0X4	T36.0X5	T36.0X6
Benzatropine	T42.8X1	T42.8X2	T42.8X3	T42.8X4	T42.8X5	T42.8X6
Benzbromarone	T50.4X1	T50.4X2	T50.4X3	T50.4X4	T50.4X5	T50.4X6
Benzcarbimine	T45.1X1	T45.1X2	T45.1X3	T45.1X4	T45.1X5	T45.1X6
Benzedrex	T44.991	T44.992	T44.993	T44.994	T44.995	T44.996
Benzedrine (amphetamine)	T43.621	T43.622	T43.623	T43.624	T43.625	T43.626
Benzenamine	T65.3X1	T65.3X2	T65.3X3	T65.3X4	—	—
Benzene	T52.1X1	T52.1X2	T52.1X3	T52.1X4	—	—
homologues (acetyl) (dimethyl) (methyl) (solvent)	T52.2X1	T52.2X2	T52.2X3	T52.2X4	—	—
Benzethonium (chloride)	T49.0X1	T49.0X2	T49.0X3	T49.0X4	T49.0X5	T49.0X6
Benzfetamine	T50.5X1	T50.5X2	T50.5X3	T50.5X4	T50.5X5	T50.5X6
Benzhexol	T44.3X1	T44.3X2	T44.3X3	T44.3X4	T44.3X5	T44.3X6
Benzhydramine (chloride)	T45.0X1	T45.0X2	T45.0X3	T45.0X4	T45.0X5	T45.0X6
Benzidine	T65.891	T65.892	T65.893	T65.894	—	—
Benzilonium bromide	T44.3X1	T44.3X2	T44.3X3	T44.3X4	T44.3X5	T44.3X6
Benzimidazole	T60.3X1	T60.3X2	T60.3X3	T60.3X4	—	—
Benzin (e) — see Ligroin						
Benziodarone	T46.3X1	T46.3X2	T46.3X3	T46.3X4	T46.3X5	T46.3X6
Benznidazole	T37.3X1	T37.3X2	T37.3X3	T37.3X4	T37.3X5	T37.3X6
Benzocaine	T41.3X1	T41.3X2	T41.3X3	T41.3X4	T41.3X5	T41.3X6
Benzocol*	T41.3X1	T41.3X2	T41.3X3	T41.3X4	T41.3X5	T41.3X6
Benzodiapin	T42.4X1	T42.4X2	T42.4X3	T42.4X4	T42.4X5	T42.4X6
Benzodiazepine NEC	T42.4X1	T42.4X2	T42.4X3	T42.4X4	T42.4X5	T42.4X6
Benzoic acid	T49.0X1	T49.0X2	T49.0X3	T49.0X4	T49.0X5	T49.0X6
with salicylic acid	T49.0X1	T49.0X2	T49.0X3	T49.0X4	T49.0X5	T49.0X6
Benzoin (tincture)	T48.5X1	T48.5X2	T48.5X3	T48.5X4	T48.5X5	T48.5X6
Benzol (benzene)	T52.1X1	T52.1X2	T52.1X3	T52.1X4	—	—
vapor	T52.0X1	T52.0X2	T52.0X3	T52.0X4	—	—
Benzomorphan	T40.2X1	T40.2X2	T40.2X3	T40.2X4	T40.2X5	T40.2X6
Benzonatate	T48.3X1	T48.3X2	T48.3X3	T48.3X4	T48.3X5	T48.3X6
Benzophenones	T49.3X1	T49.3X2	T49.3X3	T49.3X4	T49.3X5	T49.3X6
Benzopyrone	T46.991	T46.992	T46.993	T46.994	T46.995	T46.996
Benzothiadiazides	T50.2X1	T50.2X2	T50.2X3	T50.2X4	T50.2X5	T50.2X6
Benzoxonium chloride	T49.0X1	T49.0X2	T49.0X3	T49.0X4	T49.0X5	T49.0X6
Benzoylpas calcium	T37.1X1	T37.1X2	T37.1X3	T37.1X4	T37.1X5	T37.1X6
Benzoyl peroxide	T49.0X1	T49.0X2	T49.0X3	T49.0X4	T49.0X5	T49.0X6
Benzperidin	T43.591	T43.592	T43.593	T43.594	T43.595	T43.596
Benzperidol	T43.591	T43.592	T43.593	T43.594	T43.595	T43.596
Benzphetamine	T50.5X1	T50.5X2	T50.5X3	T50.5X4	T50.5X5	T50.5X6
Benzpyrinium bromide	T44.1X1	T44.1X2	T44.1X3	T44.1X4	T44.1X5	T44.1X6
Benzquinamide	T45.0X1	T45.0X2	T45.0X3	T45.0X4	T45.0X5	T45.0X6

Substance	Poisoning, Accidental (unintentional)	Poisoning, Intentional Self-harm	Poisoning, Assault	Poisoning, Undetermined	Adverse Effect	Under-dosing
Benzthiazide	T50.2X1	T50.2X2	T50.2X3	T50.2X4	T50.2X5	T50.2X6
Benztropine						
anticholinergic	T44.3X1	T44.3X2	T44.3X3	T44.3X4	T44.3X5	T44.3X6
antiparkinson	T42.8X1	T42.8X2	T42.8X3	T42.8X4	T42.8X5	T42.8X6
Benzydamine	T49.0X1	T49.0X2	T49.0X3	T49.0X4	T49.0X5	T49.0X6
Benzyl						
acetate	T52.8X1	T52.8X2	T52.8X3	T52.8X4	—	—
alcohol	T49.0X1	T49.0X2	T49.0X3	T49.0X4	T49.0X5	T49.0X6
benzoate	T49.0X1	T49.0X2	T49.0X3	T49.0X4	T49.0X5	T49.0X6
Benzoic acid	T49.0X1	T49.0X2	T49.0X3	T49.0X4	T49.0X5	T49.0X6
hydroquinone*	T49.4X1	T49.4X2	T49.4X3	T49.4X4	T49.4X5	T49.4X6
morphine	T40.2X1	T40.2X2	T40.2X3	T40.2X4		
nicotinate	T46.6X1	T46.6X2	T46.6X3	T46.6X4	T46.6X5	T46.6X6
penicillin	T36.0X1	T36.0X2	T36.0X3	T36.0X4	T36.0X5	T36.0X6
Benzylhydrochlorthiazide	T50.2X1	T50.2X2	T50.2X3	T50.2X4	T50.2X5	T50.2X6
Benzylpenicillin	T36.0X1	T36.0X2	T36.0X3	T36.0X4	T36.0X5	T36.0X6
Benzylthiouracil	T38.2X1	T38.2X2	T38.2X3	T38.2X4	T38.2X5	T38.2X6
Bephenium hydroxynaphthoate	T37.4X1	T37.4X2	T37.4X3	T37.4X4	T37.4X5	T37.4X6
Bepridil	T46.1X1	T46.1X2	T46.1X3	T46.1X4	T46.1X5	T46.1X6
Bergamot oil	T65.891	T65.892	T65.893	T65.894	—	—
Bergapten	T50.991	T50.992	T50.993	T50.994	T50.995	T50.996
Berries, poisonous	T62.1X1	T62.1X2	T62.1X3	T62.1X4	—	—
Beryllium (compounds)	T56.7X1	T56.7X2	T56.7X3	T56.7X4	—	—
beta adrenergic blocking agent, heart	T44.7X1	T44.7X2	T44.7X3	T44.7X4	T44.7X5	T44.7X6
Betacarotene	T45.2X1	T45.2X2	T45.2X3	T45.2X4	T45.2X5	T45.2X6
Beta-Chlor	T42.6X1	T42.6X2	T42.6X3	T42.6X4	T42.6X5	T42.6X6
Betahistine	T46.7X1	T46.7X2	T46.7X3	T46.7X4	T46.7X5	T46.7X6
Betaine	T47.5X1	T47.5X2	T47.5X3	T47.5X4	T47.5X5	T47.5X6
Betamethasone	T49.0X1	T49.0X2	T49.0X3	T49.0X4	T49.0X5	T49.0X6
topical	T49.0X1	T49.0X2	T49.0X3	T49.0X4	T49.0X5	T49.0X6
Betamicin	T36.8X1	T36.8X2	T36.8X3	T36.8X4	T36.8X5	T36.8X6
Betanidine	T46.5X1	T46.5X2	T46.5X3	T46.5X4	T46.5X5	T46.5X6
Betaxolol	T44.7X1	T44.7X2	T44.7X3	T44.7X4	T44.7X5	T44.7X6
Betazole	T50.8X1	T50.8X2	T50.8X3	T50.8X4	T50.8X5	T50.8X6
Bethanechol	T44.1X1	T44.1X2	T44.1X3	T44.1X4	T44.1X5	T44.1X6
chloride	T44.1X1	T44.1X2	T44.1X3	T44.1X4	T44.1X5	T44.1X6
Bethanidine	T46.5X1	T46.5X2	T46.5X3	T46.5X4	T46.5X5	T46.5X6
Betoxycaine	T41.3X1	T41.3X2	T41.3X3	T41.3X4	T41.3X5	T41.3X6
Betula oil	T49.3X1	T49.3X2	T49.3X3	T49.3X4	T49.3X5	T49.3X6
Bevantolol	T44.7X1	T44.7X2	T44.7X3	T44.7X4	T44.7X5	T44.7X6
Bevonium metilsulfate	T44.3X1	T44.3X2	T44.3X3	T44.3X4	T44.3X5	T44.3X6
Bezafibrate	T46.6X1	T46.6X2	T46.6X3	T46.6X4	T46.6X5	T46.6X6
Bezitramide	T40.491	T40.492	T40.493	T40.494	T40.495	T40.496
BHA	T50.991	T50.992	T50.993	T50.994	T50.995	T50.996
Bhang	T40.711	T40.712	T40.713	T40.714	T40.715	T40.716
BHC (medicinal)	T49.0X1	T49.0X2	T49.0X3	T49.0X4	T49.0X5	T49.0X6
nonmedicinal (vapor)	T53.6X1	T53.6X2	T53.6X3	T53.6X4	—	—
Bialamicol	T37.3X1	T37.3X2	T37.3X3	T37.3X4	T37.3X5	T37.3X6
Bibenzonium bromide	T48.3X1	T48.3X2	T48.3X3	T48.3X4	T48.3X5	T48.3X6
Bibrocathol	T49.5X1	T49.5X2	T49.5X3	T49.5X4	T49.5X5	T49.5X6
Bichloride of mercury — see Mercury, chloride						
Bichromates (calcium) (potassium)(sodium) (crystals)	T57.8X1	T57.8X2	T57.8X3	T57.8X4		
fumes	T56.2X1	T56.2X2	T56.2X3	T56.2X4	—	—
Biclotymol	T49.6X1	T49.6X2	T49.6X3	T49.6X4	T49.6X5	T49.6X6
BiCNU*	T45.1X1	T45.1X2	T45.1X3	T45.1X4	T45.1X5	T45.1X6
Bicucculine	T50.7X1	T50.7X2	T50.7X3	T50.7X4	T50.7X5	T50.7X6
Bifemelane	T43.291	T43.292	T43.293	T43.294	T43.295	T43.296
Biguanide derivatives, oral	T38.3X1	T38.3X2	T38.3X3	T38.3X4	T38.3X5	T38.3X6
Bile salts	T47.5X1	T47.5X2	T47.5X3	T47.5X4	T47.5X5	T47.5X6
Biligrafin	T50.8X1	T50.8X2	T50.8X3	T50.8X4	T50.8X5	T50.8X6
Bilopaque	T50.8X1	T50.8X2	T50.8X3	T50.8X4	T50.8X5	T50.8X6
Binifibrate	T46.6X1	T46.6X2	T46.6X3	T46.6X4	T46.6X5	T46.6X6
Binitrobenzol	T65.3X1	T65.3X2	T65.3X3	T65.3X4	—	—
Bioflavonoid(s)	T46.991	T46.992	T46.993	T46.994	T46.995	T46.996
Biological substance NEC	T50.901	T50.902	T50.903	T50.904	T50.905	T50.906
Biotin	T45.2X1	T45.2X2	T45.2X3	T45.2X4	T45.2X5	T45.2X6
Biperiden	T44.3X1	T44.3X2	T44.3X3	T44.3X4	T44.3X5	T44.3X6
Bisacodyl	T47.2X1	T47.2X2	T47.2X3	T47.2X4	T47.2X5	T47.2X6
Bisbentiamine	T45.2X1	T45.2X2	T45.2X3	T45.2X4	T45.2X5	T45.2X6
Bisbutiamine	T45.2X1	T45.2X2	T45.2X3	T45.2X4	T45.2X5	T45.2X6
Bisdequalinium (salts) (diacetate)	T49.6X1	T49.6X2	T49.6X3	T49.6X4	T49.6X5	T49.6X6
Bishydroxycoumarin	T45.511	T45.512	T45.513	T45.514	T45.515	T45.516
Bismarsen	T37.8X1	T37.8X2	T37.8X3	T37.8X4	T37.8X5	T37.8X6
Bismuth salts	T47.6X1	T47.6X2	T47.6X3	T47.6X4	T47.6X5	T47.6X6
aluminate	T47.1X1	T47.1X2	T47.1X3	T47.1X4	T47.1X5	T47.1X6
anti-infectives	T37.8X1	T37.8X2	T37.8X3	T37.8X4	T37.8X5	T37.8X6

Substance	Poisoning, Accidental (unintentional)	Poisoning, Intentional Self-harm	Poisoning, Assault	Poisoning, Undetermined	Adverse Effect	Under-dosing
Bismuth salts — *continued*						
formic iodide	T49.0X1	T49.0X2	T49.0X3	T49.0X4	T49.0X5	T49.0X6
glycolylarsenate	T49.0X1	T49.0X2	T49.0X3	T49.0X4	T49.0X5	T49.0X6
nonmedicinal (compounds) NEC	T65.91	T65.92	T65.93	T65.94	—	—
subcarbonate	T47.6X1	T47.6X2	T47.6X3	T47.6X4	T47.6X5	T47.6X6
subsalicylate	T37.8X1	T37.8X2	T37.8X3	T37.8X4	T37.8X5	T37.8X6
sulfarsphenamine	T37.8X1	T37.8X2	T37.8X3	T37.8X4	T37.8X5	T37.8X6
Bisoprolol	T44.7X1	T44.7X2	T44.7X3	T44.7X4	T44.7X5	T44.7X6
Bisoxatin	T47.2X1	T47.2X2	T47.2X3	T47.2X4	T47.2X5	T47.2X6
Bisulepin (hydrochloride)	T45.0X1	T45.0X2	T45.0X3	T45.0X4	T45.0X5	T45.0X6
Bithionol	T37.8X1	T37.8X2	T37.8X3	T37.8X4	T37.8X5	T37.8X6
anthelminthic	T37.4X1	T37.4X2	T37.4X3	T37.4X4	T37.4X5	T37.4X6
Bitolterol	T48.6X1	T48.6X2	T48.6X3	T48.6X4	T48.6X5	T48.6X6
Bitoscanate	T37.4X1	T37.4X2	T37.4X3	T37.4X4	T37.4X5	T37.4X6
Bitter almond oil	T62.8X1	T62.8X2	T62.8X3	T62.8X4	—	—
Bittersweet	T62.2X1	T62.2X2	T62.2X3	T62.2X4	—	—
Bivalirudin*	T45.511	T45.512	T45.513	T45.514	T45.515	T45.516
Black						
flag	T60.91	T60.92	T60.93	T60.94	—	—
henbane	T62.2X1	T62.2X2	T62.2X3	T62.2X4	—	—
leaf (40)	T60.91	T60.92	T60.93	T60.94	—	—
widow spider (bite)	T63.311	T63.312	T63.313	T63.314	—	—
antivenin	T50.Z11	T50.Z12	T50.Z13	T50.Z14	T50.Z15	T50.Z16
Blast furnace gas (carbon monoxide from)	T58.8X1	T58.8X2	T58.8X3	T58.8X4	—	—
Bleach	T54.91	T54.92	T54.93	T54.94	—	—
Bleaching agent (medicinal)	T49.4X1	T49.4X2	T49.4X3	T49.4X4	T49.4X5	T49.4X6
Bleomycin	T45.1X1	T45.1X2	T45.1X3	T45.1X4	T45.1X5	T45.1X6
Blockain	T41.3X1	T41.3X2	T41.3X3	T41.3X4	T41.3X5	T41.3X6
infiltration (subcutaneous)	T41.3X1	T41.3X2	T41.3X3	T41.3X4	T41.3X5	T41.3X6
nerve block (peripheral) (plexus)	T41.3X1	T41.3X2	T41.3X3	T41.3X4	T41.3X5	T41.3X6
topical (surface)	T41.3X1	T41.3X2	T41.3X3	T41.3X4	T41.3X5	T41.3X6
Blockers, calcium channel	T46.1X1	T46.1X2	T46.1X3	T46.1X4	T46.1X5	T46.1X6
Blood (derivatives) (natural) (plasma) (whole)	T45.8X1	T45.8X2	T45.8X3	T45.8X4	T45.8X5	T45.8X6
dried	T45.8X1	T45.8X2	T45.8X3	T45.8X4	T45.8X5	T45.8X6
drug affecting NEC	T45.91	T45.92	T45.93	T45.94	T45.95	T45.96
expander NEC	T45.8X1	T45.8X2	T45.8X3	T45.8X4	T45.8X5	T45.8X6
fraction NEC	T45.8X1	T45.8X2	T45.8X3	T45.8X4	T45.8X5	T45.8X6
substitute (macromolecular)	T45.8X1	T45.8X2	T45.8X3	T45.8X4	T45.8X5	T45.8X6
Blue velvet	T40.2X1	T40.2X2	T40.2X3	T40.2X4	—	—
Bone meal	T62.8X1	T62.8X2	T62.8X3	T62.8X4	—	—
Bonine	T45.0X1	T45.0X2	T45.0X3	T45.0X4	T45.0X5	T45.0X6
Bontril*	T50.5X1	T50.5X2	T50.5X3	T50.5X4	T50.5X5	T50.5X6
Bopindolol	T44.7X1	T44.7X2	T44.7X3	T44.7X4	T44.7X5	T44.7X6
Boracic acid	T49.0X1	T49.0X2	T49.0X3	T49.0X4	T49.0X5	T49.0X6
ENT agent	T49.6X1	T49.6X2	T49.6X3	T49.6X4	T49.6X5	T49.6X6
ophthalmic preparation	T49.5X1	T49.5X2	T49.5X3	T49.5X4	T49.5X5	T49.5X6
Borane complex	T57.8X1	T57.8X2	T57.8X3	T57.8X4	—	—
Borate(s)	T57.8X1	T57.8X2	T57.8X3	T57.8X4	—	—
buffer	T50.991	T50.992	T50.993	T50.994	T50.995	T50.996
cleanser	T54.91	T54.92	T54.93	T54.94	—	—
sodium	T57.8X1	T57.8X2	T57.8X3	T57.8X4	—	—
Borax (cleanser)	T54.91	T54.92	T54.93	T54.94	—	—
Bordeaux mixture	T60.3X1	T60.3X2	T60.3X3	T60.3X4	—	—
Boric acid	T49.0X1	T49.0X2	T49.0X3	T49.0X4	T49.0X5	T49.0X6
ENT agent	T49.6X1	T49.6X2	T49.6X3	T49.6X4	T49.6X5	T49.6X6
ophthalmic preparation	T49.5X1	T49.5X2	T49.5X3	T49.5X4	T49.5X5	T49.5X6
Bornaprine	T44.3X1	T44.3X2	T44.3X3	T44.3X4	T44.3X5	T44.3X6
Boron	T57.8X1	T57.8X2	T57.8X3	T57.8X4	—	—
hydride NEC	T57.8X1	T57.8X2	T57.8X3	T57.8X4	—	—
fumes or gas	T57.8X1	T57.8X2	T57.8X3	T57.8X4	—	—
trifluoride	T59.891	T59.892	T59.893	T59.894	—	—
Botox	T48.291	T48.292	T48.293	T48.294	T48.295	T48.296
Botulinus anti-toxin (type A, B)	T50.Z11	T50.Z12	T50.Z13	T50.Z14	T50.Z15	T50.Z16
Brake fluid vapor	T59.891	T59.892	T59.893	T59.894	—	—
Brallobarbital	T42.3X1	T42.3X2	T42.3X3	T42.3X4	T42.3X5	T42.3X6
Bran (wheat)	T47.4X1	T47.4X2	T47.4X3	T47.4X4	T47.4X5	T47.4X6
Brass (fumes)	T56.891	T56.892	T56.893	T56.894	—	—
Brasso	T52.0X1	T52.0X2	T52.0X3	T52.0X4	—	—
Bretylium tosilate	T46.2X1	T46.2X2	T46.2X3	T46.2X4	T46.2X5	T46.2X6
Brevital (sodium)	T41.1X1	T41.1X2	T41.1X3	T41.1X4	T41.1X5	T41.1X6
Brinase	T45.3X1	T45.3X2	T45.3X3	T45.3X4	T45.3X5	T45.3X6
British antilewisite	T45.8X1	T45.8X2	T45.8X3	T45.8X4	T45.8X5	T45.8X6
Brodalumab*	T50.991	T50.992	T50.993	T50.994	T50.995	T50.996
Brodifacoum	T60.4X1	T60.4X2	T60.4X3	T60.4X4	—	—
Bromal (hydrate)	T42.6X1	T42.6X2	T42.6X3	T42.6X4	T42.6X5	T42.6X6
Bromazepam	T42.4X1	T42.4X2	T42.4X3	T42.4X4	T42.4X5	T42.4X6

Substance	Poisoning, Accidental (unintentional)	Poisoning, Intentional Self-harm	Poisoning, Assault	Poisoning, Undetermined	Adverse Effect	Under-dosing
Bromazine	T45.0X1	T45.0X2	T45.0X3	T45.0X4	T45.0X5	T45.0X6
Brombenzylcyanide	T59.3X1	T59.3X2	T59.3X3	T59.3X4	—	—
Bromelains	T45.3X1	T45.3X2	T45.3X3	T45.3X4	T45.3X5	T45.3X6
Bromethalin	T60.4X1	T60.4X2	T60.4X3	T60.4X4	—	—
Bromhexine	T48.4X1	T48.4X2	T48.4X3	T48.4X4	T48.4X5	T48.4X6
Bromide salts	T42.6X1	T42.6X2	T42.6X3	T42.6X4	T42.6X5	T42.6X6
Bromindione	T45.511	T45.512	T45.513	T45.514	T45.515	T45.516
Bromine						
compounds (medicinal)	T42.6X1	T42.6X2	T42.6X3	T42.6X4	T42.6X5	T42.6X6
sedative	T42.6X1	T42.6X2	T42.6X3	T42.6X4	T42.6X5	T42.6X6
vapor	T59.891	T59.892	T59.893	T59.894	—	—
Bromisoval	T42.6X1	T42.6X2	T42.6X3	T42.6X4	T42.6X5	T42.6X6
Bromisovalum	T42.6X1	T42.6X2	T42.6X3	T42.6X4	T42.6X5	T42.6X6
Bromobenzylcyanide	T59.3X1	T59.3X2	T59.3X3	T59.3X4	—	—
Bromochlorosalicylani-lide	T49.0X1	T49.0X2	T49.0X3	T49.0X4	T49.0X5	T49.0X6
Bromocriptine	T42.8X1	T42.8X2	T42.8X3	T42.8X4	T42.8X5	T42.8X6
Bromodiphenhydramine	T45.0X1	T45.0X2	T45.0X3	T45.0X4	T45.0X5	T45.0X6
Bromoform	T42.6X1	T42.6X2	T42.6X3	T42.6X4	T42.6X5	T42.6X6
Bromophenol blue reagent	T50.991	T50.992	T50.993	T50.994	T50.995	T50.996
Bromopride	T47.8X1	T47.8X2	T47.8X3	T47.8X4	T47.8X5	T47.8X6
Bromosalicylchloranitide	T49.0X1	T49.0X2	T49.0X3	T49.0X4	T49.0X5	T49.0X6
Bromosalicylhydroxamic acid	T37.1X1	T37.1X2	T37.1X3	T37.1X4	T37.1X5	T37.1X6
Bromo-seltzer	T39.1X1	T39.1X2	T39.1X3	T39.1X4	T39.1X5	T39.1X6
Bromoxynil	T60.3X1	T60.3X2	T60.3X3	T60.3X4	—	—
Bromperidol	T43.4X1	T43.4X2	T43.4X3	T43.4X4	—	T43.4X6
Brompheniramine	T45.0X1	T45.0X2	T45.0X3	T45.0X4	T45.0X5	T45.0X6
Bromsulfophthalein	T50.8X1	T50.8X2	T50.8X3	T50.8X4	T50.8X5	T50.8X6
Bromural	T42.6X1	T42.6X2	T42.6X3	T42.6X4	T42.6X5	T42.6X6
Bromvaletone	T42.6X1	T42.6X2	T42.6X3	T42.6X4	T42.6X5	T42.6X6
Bronchodilator NEC	T48.6X1	T48.6X2	T48.6X3	T48.6X4	T48.6X5	T48.6X6
Brotizolam	T42.4X1	T42.4X2	T42.4X3	T42.4X4	T42.4X5	T42.4X6
Brovincamine	T46.7X1	T46.7X2	T46.7X3	T46.7X4	T46.7X5	T46.7X6
Brown recluse spider (bite) (venom)	T63.331	T63.332	T63.333	T63.334	—	—
Brown spider (bite) (venom)	T63.391	T63.392	T63.393	T63.394	—	—
Broxaterol	T48.6X1	T48.6X2	T48.6X3	T48.6X4	T48.6X5	T48.6X6
Broxuridine	T45.1X1	T45.1X2	T45.1X3	T45.1X4	T45.1X5	T45.1X6
Broxyquinoline	T37.8X1	T37.8X2	T37.8X3	T37.8X4	T37.8X5	T37.8X6
Bruceine	T48.291	T48.292	T48.293	T48.294	T48.295	T48.296
Brucia	T62.2X1	T62.2X2	T62.2X3	T62.2X4	—	—
Brucine	T65.1X1	T65.1X2	T65.1X3	T65.1X4	—	—
Brunswick green — *see* Copper						
Bruten — *see* Ibuprofen						
Bryonia	T47.2X1	T47.2X2	T47.2X3	T47.2X4	T47.2X5	T47.2X6
Buclizine	T45.0X1	T45.0X2	T45.0X3	T45.0X4	T45.0X5	T45.0X6
Buclosamide	T49.0X1	T49.0X2	T49.0X3	T49.0X4	T49.0X5	T49.0X6
Budesonide	T44.5X1	T44.5X2	T44.5X3	T44.5X4	T44.5X5	T44.5X6
Budralazine	T46.5X1	T46.5X2	T46.5X3	T46.5X4	T46.5X5	T46.5X6
Bufferin	T39.011	T39.012	T39.013	T39.014	T39.015	T39.016
Buflomedil	T46.7X1	T46.7X2	T46.7X3	T46.7X4	T46.7X5	T46.7X6
Buformin	T38.3X1	T38.3X2	T38.3X3	T38.3X4	T38.3X5	T38.3X6
Bufotenine	T40.991	T40.992	T40.993	T40.994	—	—
Bufrolin	T48.6X1	T48.6X2	T48.6X3	T48.6X4	T48.6X5	T48.6X6
Bufylline	T48.6X1	T48.6X2	T48.6X3	T48.6X4	T48.6X5	T48.6X6
Bulgaricum IB*	T47.6X1	T47.6X2	T47.6X3	T47.6X4	T47.6X5	T47.6X6
Bulk filler	T50.5X1	T50.5X2	T50.5X3	T50.5X4	T50.5X5	T50.5X6
cathartic	T47.4X1	T47.4X2	T47.4X3	T47.4X4	T47.4X5	T47.4X6
Bumetanide	T50.1X1	T50.1X2	T50.1X3	T50.1X4	T50.1X5	T50.1X6
Bunaftine	T46.2X1	T46.2X2	T46.2X3	T46.2X4	T46.2X5	T46.2X6
Bunamiodyl	T50.8X1	T50.8X2	T50.8X3	T50.8X4	T50.8X5	T50.8X6
Bunazosin	T44.6X1	T44.6X2	T44.6X3	T44.6X4	T44.6X5	T44.6X6
Bunitrolol	T44.7X1	T44.7X2	T44.7X3	T44.7X4	T44.7X5	T44.7X6
Buphenine	T46.7X1	T46.7X2	T46.7X3	T46.7X4	T46.7X5	T46.7X6
Bupivacaine	T41.3X1	T41.3X2	T41.3X3	T41.3X4	T41.3X5	T41.3X6
infiltration (subcutaneous)	T41.3X1	T41.3X2	T41.3X3	T41.3X4	T41.3X5	T41.3X6
nerve block (peripheral) (plexus)	T41.3X1	T41.3X2	T41.3X3	T41.3X4	T41.3X5	T41.3X6
spinal	T41.3X1	T41.3X2	T41.3X3	T41.3X4	T41.3X5	T41.3X6
Bupranolol	T44.7X1	T44.7X2	T44.7X3	T44.7X4	T44.7X5	T44.7X6
Buprenorphine	T40.491	T40.492	T40.493	T40.494	T40.495	T40.496
Bupropion	T43.291	T43.292	T43.293	T43.294	T43.295	T43.296
Burimamide	T47.1X1	T47.1X2	T47.1X3	T47.1X4	T47.1X5	T47.1X6
Buserelin	T38.891	T38.892	T38.893	T38.894	T38.895	T38.896
Buspirone	T43.591	T43.592	T43.593	T43.594	T43.595	T43.596
Busulfan, busulphan	T45.1X1	T45.1X2	T45.1X3	T45.1X4	T45.1X5	T45.1X6
Busulfex*	T45.1X1	T45.1X2	T45.1X3	T45.1X4	T45.1X5	T45.1X6
Butabarbital (sodium)	T42.3X1	T42.3X2	T42.3X3	T42.3X4	T42.3X5	T42.3X6
Butabarbitone	T42.3X1	T42.3X2	T42.3X3	T42.3X4	T42.3X5	T42.3X6
Butabarpal	T42.3X1	T42.3X2	T42.3X3	T42.3X4	T42.3X5	T42.3X6
Butacaine	T41.3X1	T41.3X2	T41.3X3	T41.3X4	T41.3X5	T41.3X6

Substance	Poisoning, Accidental (unintentional)	Poisoning, Intentional Self-harm	Poisoning, Assault	Poisoning, Undetermined	Adverse Effect	Under-dosing
Butalamine	T46.7X1	T46.7X2	T46.7X3	T46.7X4	T46.7X5	T46.7X6
Butalbital	T42.3X1	T42.3X2	T42.3X3	T42.3X4	T42.3X5	T42.3X6
Butallylonal	T42.3X1	T42.3X2	T42.3X3	T42.3X4	T42.3X5	T42.3X6
Butamben	T41.3X1	T41.3X2	T41.3X3	T41.3X4	T41.3X5	T41.3X6
Butamirate	T48.3X1	T48.3X2	T48.3X3	T48.3X4	T48.3X5	T48.3X6
Butane (distributed in mobile container)	T59.891	T59.892	T59.893	T59.894	—	—
distributed through pipes	T59.891	T59.892	T59.893	T59.894	—	—
incomplete combustion	T58.11	T58.12	T58.13	T58.14	—	—
Butanilicaine	T41.3X1	T41.3X2	T41.3X3	T41.3X4	T41.3X5	T41.3X6
Butanol	T51.3X1	T51.3X2	T51.3X3	T51.3X4	—	—
Butanone, 2-butanone	T52.4X1	T52.4X2	T52.4X3	T52.4X4	—	—
Butantrone	T49.4X1	T49.4X2	T49.4X3	T49.4X4	T49.4X5	T49.4X6
Butaperazine	T43.3X1	T43.3X2	T43.3X3	T43.3X4	T43.3X5	T43.3X6
Butazolidin	T39.2X1	T39.2X2	T39.2X3	T39.2X4	T39.2X5	T39.2X6
Butetamate	T48.6X1	T48.6X2	T48.6X3	T48.6X4	T48.6X5	T48.6X6
Butethal	T42.3X1	T42.3X2	T42.3X3	T42.3X4	T42.3X5	T42.3X6
Butethamate	T44.3X1	T44.3X2	T44.3X3	T44.3X4	T44.3X5	T44.3X6
Buthalitone (sodium)	T41.1X1	T41.1X2	T41.1X3	T41.1X4	T41.1X5	T41.1X6
Butisol (sodium)	T42.3X1	T42.3X2	T42.3X3	T42.3X4	T42.3X5	T42.3X6
Butizide	T50.2X1	T50.2X2	T50.2X3	T50.2X4	T50.2X5	T50.2X6
Butobarbital	T42.3X1	T42.3X2	T42.3X3	T42.3X4	T42.3X5	T42.3X6
sodium	T42.3X1	T42.3X2	T42.3X3	T42.3X4	T42.3X5	T42.3X6
Butobarbitone	T42.3X1	T42.3X2	T42.3X3	T42.3X4	T42.3X5	T42.3X6
Butoconazole (nitrate)	T49.0X1	T49.0X2	T49.0X3	T49.0X4	T49.0X5	T49.0X6
Butorphanol	T40.491	T40.492	T40.493	T40.494	T40.495	T40.496
Butriptyline	T43.011	T43.012	T43.013	T43.014	T43.015	T43.016
Butropium bromide	T44.3X1	T44.3X2	T44.3X3	T44.3X4	T44.3X5	T44.3X6
Buttercups	T62.2X1	T62.2X2	T62.2X4	T62.2X4	—	—
Butter of antimony — see Antimony						
Butyl						
acetate (secondary)	T52.8X1	T52.8X2	T52.8X3	T52.8X4	—	—
alcohol	T51.3X1	T51.3X2	T51.3X3	T51.3X4	—	—
aminobenzoate	T41.3X1	T41.3X2	T41.3X3	T41.3X4	T41.3X5	T41.3X6
butyrate	T52.8X1	T52.8X2	T52.8X3	T52.8X4	—	—
carbinol	T51.3X1	T51.3X2	T51.3X3	T51.3X4	—	—
carbitol	T52.3X1	T52.3X2	T52.3X3	T52.3X4	—	—
cellosolve	T52.3X1	T52.3X2	T52.3X3	T52.3X4	—	—
chloral (hydrate)	T42.6X1	T42.6X2	T42.6X3	T42.6X4	T42.6X5	T42.6X6
formate	T52.8X1	T52.8X2	T52.8X3	T52.8X4	—	—
lactate	T52.8X1	T52.8X2	T52.8X3	T52.8X4	—	—
propionate	T52.8X1	T52.8X2	T52.8X3	T52.8X4	—	—
scopolamine bromide	T44.3X1	T44.3X2	T44.3X3	T44.3X4	T44.3X5	T44.3X6
thiobarbital sodium	T41.1X1	T41.1X2	T41.1X3	T41.1X4	T41.1X5	T41.1X6
Butylated hydroxyanisole	T50.991	T50.992	T50.993	T50.994	T50.995	T50.996
Butylchloral hydrate	T42.6X1	T42.6X2	T42.6X3	T42.6X4	T42.6X5	T42.6X6
Butyltoluene	T52.2X1	T52.2X2	T52.2X3	T52.2X4	—	—
Butyn	T41.3X1	T41.3X2	T41.3X3	T41.3X4	T41.3X5	T41.3X6
Butyrophenone (-based tranquilizers)	T43.4X1	T43.4X2	T43.4X3	T43.4X4	T43.4X5	T43.4X6
Cabazitaxel*	T45.1X1	T45.1X2	T45.1X3	T45.1X4	T45.1X5	T45.1X6
Cabergoline	T42.8X1	T42.8X2	T42.8X3	T42.8X4	T42.8X5	T42.8X6
Cacodyl, cacodylic acid	T57.0X1	T57.0X2	T57.0X3	T57.0X4	—	—
Cactinomycin	T45.1X1	T45.1X2	T45.1X3	T45.1X4	T45.1X5	T45.1X6
Cade oil	T49.4X1	T49.4X2	T49.4X3	T49.4X4	T49.4X5	T49.4X6
Cadexomer iodine	T49.0X1	T49.0X2	T49.0X3	T49.0X4	T49.0X5	T49.0X6
Cadmium (chloride) (fumes) (oxide)	T56.3X1	T56.3X2	T56.3X3	T56.3X4	—	—
sulfide (medicinal) NEC	T49.4X1	T49.4X2	T49.4X3	T49.4X4	T49.4X5	T49.4X6
Cadralazine	T46.5X1	T46.5X2	T46.5X3	T46.5X4	T46.5X5	T46.5X6
Caffeine	T43.611	T43.612	T43.613	T43.614	T43.615	T43.616
Calabar bean	T62.2X1	T62.2X2	T62.2X3	T62.2X4	—	—
Caladium seguinum	T62.2X1	T62.2X2	T62.2X3	T62.2X4	—	—
Calamine (lotion)	T49.3X1	T49.3X2	T49.3X3	T49.3X4	T49.3X5	T49.3X6
Calcifediol	T45.2X1	T45.2X2	T45.2X3	T45.2X4	T45.2X5	T45.2X6
Calciferol	T45.2X1	T45.2X2	T45.2X3	T45.2X4	T45.2X5	T45.2X6
Calcijex*	T45.2X1	T45.2X2	T45.2X3	T45.2X4	T45.2X5	T45.2X6
Calcitonin	T50.991	T50.992	T50.993	T50.994	T50.995	T50.996
Calcitriol	T45.2X1	T45.2X2	T45.2X3	T45.2X4	T45.2X5	T45.2X6
Calcium	T50.3X1	T50.3X2	T50.3X3	T50.3X4	T50.3X5	T50.3X6
actylsalicylate	T39.011	T39.012	T39.013	T39.014	T39.015	T39.016
benzamidosalicylate	T37.1X1	T37.1X2	T37.1X3	T37.1X4	T37.1X5	T37.1X6
bromide	T42.6X1	T42.6X2	T42.6X3	T42.6X4	T42.6X5	T42.6X6
bromolactobionate	T42.6X1	T42.6X2	T42.6X3	T42.6X4	T42.6X5	T42.6X6
carbaspirin	T39.011	T39.012	T39.013	T39.014	T39.015	T39.016
carbimide	T50.6X1	T50.6X2	T50.6X3	T50.6X4	T50.6X5	T50.6X6
carbonate	T47.1X1	T47.1X2	T47.1X3	T47.1X4	T47.1X5	T47.1X6
chloride	T50.991	T50.992	T50.993	T50.994	T50.995	T50.996
anhydrous	T50.991	T50.992	T50.993	T50.994	T50.995	T50.996
cyanide	T57.8X1	T57.8X2	T57.8X3	T57.8X4	—	—
dioctyl sulfosuccinate	T47.4X1	T47.4X2	T47.4X3	T47.4X4	T47.4X5	T47.4X6
disodium edathamil	T45.8X1	T45.8X2	T45.8X3	T45.8X4	T45.8X5	T45.8X6
Calcium — continued						
disodium edetate	T45.8X1	T45.8X2	T45.8X3	T45.8X4	T45.8X5	T45.8X6
dobesilate	T46.991	T46.992	T46.993	T46.994	T46.995	T46.996
EDTA	T45.8X1	T45.8X2	T45.8X3	T45.8X4	T45.8X5	T45.8X6
ferrous citrate	T45.4X1	T45.4X2	T45.4X3	T45.4X4	T45.4X5	T45.4X6
folinate	T45.8X1	T45.8X2	T45.8X3	T45.8X4	T45.8X5	T45.8X6
glubionate	T50.3X1	T50.3X2	T50.3X3	T50.3X4	T50.3X5	T50.3X6
gluconate	T50.3X1	T50.3X2	T50.3X3	T50.3X4	T50.3X5	T50.3X6
gluconogalactogluconate	T50.3X1	T50.3X2	T50.3X3	T50.3X4	T50.3X5	T50.3X6
hydrate, hydroxide	T54.3X1	T54.3X2	T54.3X3	T54.3X4	—	—
hypochlorite	T54.3X1	T54.3X2	T54.3X3	T54.3X4	—	—
iodide	T48.4X1	T48.4X2	T48.4X3	T48.4X4	T48.4X5	T48.4X6
ipodate	T50.8X1	T50.8X2	T50.8X3	T50.8X4	T50.8X5	T50.8X6
lactate	T50.3X1	T50.3X2	T50.3X3	T50.3X4	T50.3X5	T50.3X6
leucovorin	T45.8X1	T45.8X2	T45.8X3	T45.8X4	T45.8X5	T45.8X6
mandelate	T37.91	T37.92	T37.93	T37.94	T37.95	T37.96
oxide	T54.3X1	T54.3X2	T54.3X3	T54.3X4	—	—
pantothenate	T45.2X1	T45.2X2	T45.2X3	T45.2X4	T45.2X5	T45.2X6
phosphate	T50.3X1	T50.3X2	T50.3X3	T50.3X4	T50.3X5	T50.3X6
salicylate	T39.091	T39.092	T39.093	T39.094	T39.095	T39.096
salts	T50.3X1	T50.3X2	T50.3X3	T50.3X4	T50.3X5	T50.3X6
Calculus-dissolving drug	T50.991	T50.992	T50.993	T50.994	T50.995	T50.996
Calomel	T49.0X1	T49.0X2	T49.0X3	T49.0X4	T49.0X5	T49.0X6
Caloric agent	T50.3X1	T50.3X2	T50.3X3	T50.3X4	T50.3X5	T50.3X6
Calusterone	T38.7X1	T38.7X2	T38.7X3	T38.7X4	T38.7X5	T38.7X6
Camazepam	T42.4X1	T42.4X2	T42.4X3	T42.4X4	T42.4X5	T42.4X6
Camomile	T49.0X1	T49.0X2	T49.0X3	T49.0X4	T49.0X5	T49.0X6
Camoquin	T37.2X1	T37.2X2	T37.2X3	T37.2X4	T37.2X5	T37.2X6
Camphor						
insecticide	T60.2X1	T60.2X2	T60.2X3	T60.2X4	—	—
medicinal	T49.8X1	T49.8X2	T49.8X3	T49.8X4	T49.8X5	T49.8X6
Camylofin	T44.3X1	T44.3X2	T44.3X3	T44.3X4	T44.3X5	T44.3X6
Cancer chemotherapy drug regimen	T45.1X1	T45.1X2	T45.1X3	T45.1X4	T45.1X5	T45.1X6
Candeptin	T49.0X1	T49.0X2	T49.0X3	T49.0X4	T49.0X5	T49.0X6
Candicidin	T49.0X1	T49.0X2	T49.0X3	T49.0X4	T49.0X5	T49.0X6
Cankaid*	T49.6X1	T49.6X2	T49.6X3	T49.6X4	T49.6X5	T49.6X6
Cannabinoids, synthetic	T40.721	T40.722	T40.723	T40.724	T40.725	T40.726
Cannabinol	T40.711	T40.712	T40.713	T40.714	T40.715	T40.716
Cannabis (derivatives)	T40.711	T40.712	T40.713	T40.714	T40.715	T40.716
Canned heat	T51.1X1	T51.1X2	T51.1X3	T51.1X4	—	—
Canrenoic acid	T50.0X1	T50.0X2	T50.0X3	T50.0X4	T50.0X5	T50.0X6
Canrenone	T50.0X1	T50.0X2	T50.0X3	T50.0X4	T50.0X5	T50.0X6
Cantharides, cantharidin, cantharis	T49.8X1	T49.8X2	T49.8X3	T49.8X4	T49.8X5	T49.8X6
Canthaxanthin	T50.991	T50.992	T50.993	T50.994	T50.995	T50.996
Capillary-active drug NEC	T46.901	T46.902	T46.903	T46.904	T46.905	T46.906
Capreomycin	T36.8X1	T36.8X2	T36.8X3	T36.8X4	T36.8X5	T36.8X6
Capresla*	T45.1X1	T45.1X2	T45.1X3	T45.1X4	T45.1X5	T45.1X6
Capsicum	T49.4X1	T49.4X2	T49.4X3	T49.4X4	T49.4X5	T49.4X6
Captafol	T60.3X1	T60.3X2	T60.3X3	T60.3X4	—	—
Captan	T60.3X1	T60.3X2	T60.3X3	T60.3X4	—	—
Captodiame, captodiamine	T43.591	T43.592	T43.593	T43.594	T43.595	T43.596
Captopril	T46.4X1	T46.4X2	T46.4X3	T46.4X4	T46.4X5	T46.4X6
Caramiphen	T44.3X1	T44.3X2	T44.3X3	T44.3X4	T44.3X5	T44.3X6
Carazolol	T44.7X1	T44.7X2	T44.7X3	T44.7X4	T44.7X5	T44.7X6
Carbachol	T44.1X1	T44.1X2	T44.1X3	T44.1X4	T44.1X5	T44.1X6
Carbacrylamine (resin)	T50.3X1	T50.3X2	T50.3X3	T50.3X4	T50.3X5	T50.3X6
Carbamate (insecticide)	T60.0X1	T60.0X2	T60.0X3	T60.0X4	—	—
Carbamate (sedative)	T42.6X1	T42.6X2	T42.6X3	T42.6X4	T42.6X5	T42.6X6
herbicide	T60.0X1	T60.0X2	T60.0X3	T60.0X4	—	—
insecticide	T60.0X1	T60.0X2	T60.0X3	T60.0X4	—	—
Carbamazepine	T42.1X1	T42.1X2	T42.1X3	T42.1X4	T42.1X5	T42.1X6
Carbamide	T47.3X1	T47.3X2	T47.3X3	T47.3X4	T47.3X5	T47.3X6
peroxide	T49.0X1	T49.0X2	T49.0X3	T49.0X4	T49.0X5	T49.0X6
topical	T49.8X1	T49.8X2	T49.8X3	T49.8X4	T49.8X5	T49.8X6
Carbamylcholine chloride	T44.1X1	T44.1X2	T44.1X3	T44.1X4	T44.1X5	T44.1X6
Carbaril	T60.0X1	T60.0X2	T60.0X3	T60.0X4	—	—
Carbarsone	T37.3X1	T37.3X2	T37.3X3	T37.3X4	T37.3X5	T37.3X6
Carbaryl	T60.0X1	T60.0X2	T60.0X3	T60.0X4	—	—
Carbaspirin	T39.011	T39.012	T39.013	T39.014	T39.015	T39.016
Carbastat*	T49.5X1	T49.5X2	T49.5X3	T49.5X4	T49.5X5	T49.5X6
Carbazochrome (salicylate) (sodium sulfonate)	T49.4X1	T49.4X2	T49.4X3	T49.4X4	T49.4X5	T49.4X6
Carbenicillin	T36.0X1	T36.0X2	T36.0X3	T36.0X4	T36.0X5	T36.0X6
Carbenoxolone	T47.1X1	T47.1X2	T47.1X3	T47.1X4	T47.1X5	T47.1X6
Carbetapentane	T48.3X1	T48.3X2	T48.3X3	T48.3X4	T48.3X5	T48.3X6
Carbethyl salicylate	T39.091	T39.092	T39.093	T39.094	T39.095	T39.096
Carbidopa (with levodopa)	T42.8X1	T42.8X2	T42.8X3	T42.8X4	T42.8X5	T42.8X6
Carbimazole	T38.2X1	T38.2X2	T38.2X3	T38.2X4	T38.2X5	T38.2X6
Carbinol	T51.1X1	T51.1X2	T51.1X3	T51.1X4	—	—
Carbinoxamine	T45.0X1	T45.0X2	T45.0X3	T45.0X4	T45.0X5	T45.0X6

☑ **Additional Character May Be Required** — Refer to the Tabular List for Character Selection

*Optum Value-Add

Substance	Poisoning, Accidental (unintentional)	Poisoning, Intentional Self-harm	Poisoning, Assault	Poisoning, Undetermined	Adverse Effect	Under-dosing
Carbiphene	T39.8X1	T39.8X2	T39.8X3	T39.8X4	T39.8X5	T39.8X6
Carbitol	T52.3X1	T52.3X2	T52.3X3	T52.3X4	—	—
Carbocaine	T41.3X1	T41.3X2	T41.3X3	T41.3X4	T41.3X5	T41.3X6
infiltration (subcutaneous)	T41.3X1	T41.3X2	T41.3X3	T41.3X4	T41.3X5	T41.3X6
nerve block (peripheral) (plexus)	T41.3X1	T41.3X2	T41.3X3	T41.3X4	T41.3X5	T41.3X6
topical (surface)	T41.3X1	T41.3X2	T41.3X3	T41.3X4	T41.3X5	T41.3X6
Carbocisteine	T48.4X1	T48.4X2	T48.4X3	T48.4X4	T48.4X5	T48.4X6
Carbocromen	T46.3X1	T46.3X2	T46.3X3	T46.3X4	T46.3X5	T46.3X6
Carbol fuchsin	T49.0X1	T49.0X2	T49.0X3	T49.0X4	T49.0X5	T49.0X6
Carbolic acid — see also Phenol	T54.0X1	T54.0X2	T54.0X3	T54.0X4	—	—
Carbolonium (bromide)	T48.1X1	T48.1X2	T48.1X3	T48.1X4	T48.1X5	T48.1X6
Carbo medicinalis	T47.6X1	T47.6X2	T47.6X3	T47.6X4	T47.6X5	T47.6X6
Carbomycin	T36.8X1	T36.8X2	T36.8X3	T36.8X4	T36.8X5	T36.8X6
Carbon						
bisulfide (liquid)	T65.4X1	T65.4X2	T65.4X3	T65.4X4	—	—
vapor	T65.4X1	T65.4X2	T65.4X3	T65.4X4	—	—
dioxide (gas)	T59.7X1	T59.7X2	T59.7X3	T59.7X4	—	—
medicinal	T41.5X1	T41.5X2	T41.5X3	T41.5X4	T41.5X5	T41.5X6
nonmedicinal	T59.7X1	T59.7X2	T59.7X3	T59.7X4	—	—
snow	T49.4X1	T49.4X2	T49.4X3	T49.4X4	T49.4X5	T49.4X6
disulfide (liquid)	T65.4X1	T65.4X2	T65.4X3	T65.4X4	—	—
vapor	T65.4X1	T65.4X2	T65.4X3	T65.4X4	—	—
monoxide (from incomplete combustion)	T58.91	T58.92	T58.93	T58.94	—	—
blast furnace gas	T58.8X1	T58.8X2	T58.8X3	T58.8X4	—	—
butane (distributed in mobile container)	T58.11	T58.12	T58.13	T58.14	—	—
distributed through pipes	T58.11	T58.12	T58.13	T58.14	—	—
charcoal fumes	T58.2X1	T58.2X2	T58.2X3	T58.2X4	—	—
coal	T58.2X1	T58.2X2	T58.2X3	T58.2X4	—	—
coke (in domestic stoves, fireplaces)	T58.2X1	T58.2X2	T58.2X3	T58.2X4	—	—
exhaust gas (motor) not in transit	T58.01	T58.02	T58.03	T58.04	—	—
combustion engine, any not in watercraft	T58.01	T58.02	T58.03	T58.04	—	—
farm tractor, not in transit	T58.01	T58.02	T58.03	T58.04	—	—
gas engine	T58.01	T58.02	T58.03	T58.04	—	—
motor pump	T58.01	T58.02	T58.03	T58.04	—	—
motor vehicle, not in transit	T58.01	T58.02	T58.03	T58.04	—	—
fuel (in domestic use)	T58.2X1	T58.2X2	T58.2X3	T58.2X4	—	—
gas (piped)	T58.11	T58.12	T58.13	T58.14	—	—
in mobile container	T58.11	T58.12	T58.13	T58.14	—	—
piped (natural)	T58.11	T58.12	T58.13	T58.14	—	—
utility	T58.11	T58.12	T58.13	T58.14	—	—
in mobile container	T58.11	T58.12	T58.13	T58.14	—	—
gas (piped)	T58.11	T58.12	T58.13	T58.14	—	—
illuminating gas	T58.11	T58.12	T58.13	T58.14	—	—
industrial fuels or gases, any	T58.8X1	T58.8X2	T58.8X3	T58.8X4	—	—
kerosene (in domestic stoves, fireplaces)	T58.2X1	T58.2X2	T58.2X3	T58.2X4	—	—
kiln gas or vapor	T58.8X1	T58.8X2	T58.8X3	T58.8X4	—	—
motor exhaust gas, not in transit	T58.01	T58.02	T58.03	T58.04	—	—
piped gas (manufactured) (natural)	T58.11	T58.12	T58.13	T58.14	—	—
producer gas	T58.8X1	T58.8X2	T58.8X3	T58.8X4	—	—
propane (distributed in mobile container)	T58.11	T58.12	T58.13	T58.14	—	—
distributed through pipes	T58.11	T58.12	T58.13	T58.14	—	—
solid (in domestic stoves, fireplaces)	T58.2X1	T58.2X2	T58.2X3	T58.2X4	—	—
specified source NEC	T58.8X1	T58.8X2	T58.8X3	T58.8X4	—	—
stove gas	T58.11	T58.12	T58.13	T58.14	—	—
piped	T58.11	T58.12	T58.13	T58.14	—	—
utility gas	T58.11	T58.12	T58.13	T58.14	—	—
piped	T58.11	T58.12	T58.13	T58.14	—	—
water gas	T58.11	T58.12	T58.13	T58.14	—	—
wood (in domestic stoves, fireplaces)	T58.2X1	T58.2X2	T58.2X3	T58.2X4	—	—
tetrachloride (vapor) NEC	T53.0X1	T53.0X2	T53.0X3	T53.0X4	—	—
liquid (cleansing agent) NEC	T53.0X1	T53.0X2	T53.0X3	T53.0X4	—	—
solvent	T53.0X1	T53.0X2	T53.0X3	T53.0X4	—	—
Carbonic acid gas	T59.7X1	T59.7X2	T59.7X3	T59.7X4	—	—
anhydrase inhibitor NEC	T50.2X1	T50.2X2	T50.2X3	T50.2X4	T50.2X5	T50.2X6

Substance	Poisoning, Accidental (unintentional)	Poisoning, Intentional Self-harm	Poisoning, Assault	Poisoning, Undetermined	Adverse Effect	Under-dosing
Carbophenothion	T60.0X1	T60.0X2	T60.0X3	T60.0X4	—	—
Carboplatin	T45.1X1	T45.1X2	T45.1X3	T45.1X4	T45.1X5	T45.1X6
Carboprost	T48.0X1	T48.0X2	T48.0X3	T48.0X4	T48.0X5	T48.0X6
Carboquone	T45.1X1	T45.1X2	T45.1X3	T45.1X4	T45.1X5	T45.1X6
Carbowax	T49.3X1	T49.3X2	T49.3X3	T49.3X4	T49.3X5	T49.3X6
Carboxymethylcellulose	T47.4X1	T47.4X2	T47.4X3	T47.4X4	T47.4X5	T47.4X6
Carbrital	T42.3X1	T42.3X2	T42.3X3	T42.3X4	T42.3X5	T42.3X6
Carbromal	T42.6X1	T42.6X2	T42.6X3	T42.6X4	T42.6X5	T42.6X6
Carbutamide	T38.3X1	T38.3X2	T38.3X3	T38.3X4	T38.3X5	T38.3X6
Carbuterol	T48.6X1	T48.6X2	T48.6X3	T48.6X4	T48.6X5	T48.6X6
Cardiac						
depressants	T46.2X1	T46.2X2	T46.2X3	T46.2X4	T46.2X5	T46.2X6
rhythm regulator	T46.2X1	T46.2X2	T46.2X3	T46.2X4	T46.2X5	T46.2X6
specified NEC	T46.2X1	T46.2X2	T46.2X3	T46.2X4	T46.2X5	T46.2X6
Cardiografin	T50.8X1	T50.8X2	T50.8X3	T50.8X4	T50.8X5	T50.8X6
Cardiogreen	T50.8X1	T50.8X2	T50.8X3	T50.8X4	T50.8X5	T50.8X6
Cardiotonic (glycoside) NEC	T46.0X1	T46.0X2	T46.0X3	T46.0X4	T46.0X5	T46.0X6
Cardiovascular drug NEC	T46.901	T46.902	T46.903	T46.904	T46.905	T46.906
Cardizem*	T46.1X1	T46.1X2	T46.1X3	T46.1X4	T46.1X5	T46.1X6
Cardrase	T50.2X1	T50.2X2	T50.2X3	T50.2X4	T50.2X5	T50.2X6
Carfecillin	T36.0X1	T36.0X2	T36.0X3	T36.0X4	T36.0X5	T36.0X6
Carfenazine	T43.3X1	T43.3X2	T43.3X3	T43.3X4	T43.3X5	T43.3X6
Carfusin	T49.0X1	T49.0X2	T49.0X3	T49.0X4	T49.0X5	T49.0X6
Carindacillin	T36.0X1	T36.0X2	T36.0X3	T36.0X4	T36.0X5	T36.0X6
Carisoprodol	T42.8X1	T42.8X2	T42.8X3	T42.8X4	T42.8X5	T42.8X6
Carmellose	T47.4X1	T47.4X2	T47.4X3	T47.4X4	T47.4X5	T47.4X6
Carminative	T47.5X1	T47.5X2	T47.5X3	T47.5X4	T47.5X5	T47.5X6
Carmofur	T45.1X1	T45.1X2	T45.1X3	T45.1X4	T45.1X5	T45.1X6
Carmustine	T45.1X1	T45.1X2	T45.1X3	T45.1X4	T45.1X5	T45.1X6
Carotene	T45.2X1	T45.2X2	T45.2X3	T45.2X4	T45.2X5	T45.2X6
Carphenazine	T43.3X1	T43.3X2	T43.3X3	T43.3X4	T43.3X5	T43.3X6
Carpipramine	T42.4X1	T42.4X2	T42.4X3	T42.4X4	T42.4X5	T42.4X6
Carprofen	T39.311	T39.312	T39.313	T39.314	T39.315	T39.316
Carpronium chloride	T44.3X1	T44.3X2	T44.3X3	T44.3X4	T44.3X5	T44.3X6
Carrageenan	T47.8X1	T47.8X2	T47.8X3	T47.8X4	T47.8X5	T47.8X6
Carteolol	T44.7X1	T44.7X2	T44.7X3	T44.7X4	T44.7X5	T44.7X6
Carter's Little Pills	T47.2X1	T47.2X2	T47.2X3	T47.2X4	T47.2X5	T47.2X6
Cartia*	T46.1X1	T46.1X2	T46.1X3	T46.1X4	T46.1X5	T46.1X6
Cascara (sagrada)	T47.2X1	T47.2X2	T47.2X3	T47.2X4	T47.2X5	T47.2X6
Cassava	T62.2X1	T62.2X2	T62.2X3	T62.2X4	—	—
Castellani's paint	T49.0X1	T49.0X2	T49.0X3	T49.0X4	T49.0X5	T49.0X6
Castor						
bean	T62.2X1	T62.2X2	T62.2X3	T62.2X4	—	—
oil	T47.2X1	T47.2X2	T47.2X3	T47.2X4	T47.2X5	T47.2X6
Catalase	T45.3X1	T45.3X2	T45.3X3	T45.3X4	T45.3X5	T45.3X6
Caterpillar (sting)	T63.431	T63.432	T63.433	T63.434	—	—
Catha (edulis) (tea)	T43.691	T43.692	T43.693	T43.694	—	—
Cathartic NEC	T47.4X1	T47.4X2	T47.4X3	T47.4X4	T47.4X5	T47.4X6
anthacene derivative	T47.2X1	T47.2X2	T47.2X3	T47.2X4	T47.2X5	T47.2X6
bulk	T47.4X1	T47.4X2	T47.4X3	T47.4X4	T47.4X5	T47.4X6
contact	T47.2X1	T47.2X2	T47.2X3	T47.2X4	T47.2X5	T47.2X6
emollient NEC	T47.4X1	T47.4X2	T47.4X3	T47.4X4	T47.4X5	T47.4X6
irritant NEC	T47.2X1	T47.2X2	T47.2X3	T47.2X4	T47.2X5	T47.2X6
mucilage	T47.4X1	T47.4X2	T47.4X3	T47.4X4	T47.4X5	T47.4X6
saline	T47.3X1	T47.3X2	T47.3X3	T47.3X4	T47.3X5	T47.3X6
vegetable	T47.2X1	T47.2X2	T47.2X3	T47.2X4	T47.2X5	T47.2X6
Cathine	T50.5X1	T50.5X2	T50.5X3	T50.5X4	T50.5X5	T50.5X6
Cathomycin	T36.8X1	T36.8X2	T36.8X3	T36.8X4	T36.8X5	T36.8X6
Cation exchange resin	T50.3X1	T50.3X2	T50.3X3	T50.3X4	T50.3X5	T50.3X6
Caustic(s) NEC	T54.91	T54.92	T54.93	T54.94	—	—
alkali	T54.3X1	T54.3X2	T54.3X3	T54.3X4	—	—
hydroxide	T54.3X1	T54.3X2	T54.3X3	T54.3X4	—	—
potash	T54.3X1	T54.3X2	T54.3X3	T54.3X4	—	—
soda	T54.3X1	T54.3X2	T54.3X3	T54.3X4	—	—
specified NEC	T54.91	T54.92	T54.93	T54.94	—	—
Ceepryn	T49.0X1	T49.0X2	T49.0X3	T49.0X4	T49.0X5	T49.0X6
ENT agent	T49.6X1	T49.6X2	T49.6X3	T49.6X4	T49.6X5	T49.6X6
lozenges	T49.6X1	T49.6X2	T49.6X3	T49.6X4	T49.6X5	T49.6X6
Cefacetrile	T36.1X1	T36.1X2	T36.1X3	T36.1X4	T36.1X5	T36.1X6
Cefaclor	T36.1X1	T36.1X2	T36.1X3	T36.1X4	T36.1X5	T36.1X6
Cefadroxil	T36.1X1	T36.1X2	T36.1X3	T36.1X4	T36.1X5	T36.1X6
Cefalexin	T36.1X1	T36.1X2	T36.1X3	T36.1X4	T36.1X5	T36.1X6
Cefaloglycin	T36.1X1	T36.1X2	T36.1X3	T36.1X4	T36.1X5	T36.1X6
Cefaloridine	T36.1X1	T36.1X2	T36.1X3	T36.1X4	T36.1X5	T36.1X6
Cefalosporins	T36.1X1	T36.1X2	T36.1X3	T36.1X4	T36.1X5	T36.1X6
Cefalotin	T36.1X1	T36.1X2	T36.1X3	T36.1X4	T36.1X5	T36.1X6
Cefamandole	T36.1X1	T36.1X2	T36.1X3	T36.1X4	T36.1X5	T36.1X6
Cefamycin antibiotic	T36.1X1	T36.1X2	T36.1X3	T36.1X4	T36.1X5	T36.1X6
Cefapirin	T36.1X1	T36.1X2	T36.1X3	T36.1X4	T36.1X5	T36.1X6
Cefatrizine	T36.1X1	T36.1X2	T36.1X3	T36.1X4	T36.1X5	T36.1X6
Cefazedone	T36.1X1	T36.1X2	T36.1X3	T36.1X4	T36.1X5	T36.1X6
Cefazolin	T36.1X1	T36.1X2	T36.1X3	T36.1X4	T36.1X5	T36.1X6
Cefbuperazone	T36.1X1	T36.1X2	T36.1X3	T36.1X4	T36.1X5	T36.1X6

Table of Drugs and Chemicals

Cefetamet — Chlorimipramine

Substance	Poisoning, Accidental (unintentional)	Poisoning, Intentional Self-harm	Poisoning, Assault	Poisoning, Undetermined	Adverse Effect	Under-dosing
Cefetamet	T36.1X1	T36.1X2	T36.1X3	T36.1X4	T36.1X5	T36.1X6
Cefixime	T36.1X1	T36.1X2	T36.1X3	T36.1X4	T36.1X5	T36.1X6
Cefmenoxime	T36.1X1	T36.1X2	T36.1X3	T36.1X4	T36.1X5	T36.1X6
Cefmetazole	T36.1X1	T36.1X2	T36.1X3	T36.1X4	T36.1X5	T36.1X6
Cefminox	T36.1X1	T36.1X2	T36.1X3	T36.1X4	T36.1X5	T36.1X6
Cefonicid	T36.1X1	T36.1X2	T36.1X3	T36.1X4	T36.1X5	T36.1X6
Cefoperazone	T36.1X1	T36.1X2	T36.1X3	T36.1X4	T36.1X5	T36.1X6.
Ceforanide	T36.1X1	T36.1X2	T36.1X3	T36.1X4	T36.1X5	T36.1X6
Cefotaxime	T36.1X1	T36.1X2	T36.1X3	T36.1X4	T36.1X5	T36.1X6
Cefotetan	T36.1X1	T36.1X2	T36.1X3	T36.1X4	T36.1X5	T36.1X6
Cefotiam	T36.1X1	T36.1X2	T36.1X3	T36.1X4	T36.1X5	T36.1X6
Cefoxitin	T36.1X1	T36.1X2	T36.1X3	T36.1X4	T36.1X5	T36.1X6
Cefpimizole	T36.1X1	T36.1X2	T36.1X3	T36.1X4	T36.1X5	T36.1X6
Cefpiramide	T36.1X1	T36.1X2	T36.1X3	T36.1X4	T36.1X5	T36.1X6
Cefradine	T36.1X1	T36.1X2	T36.1X3	T36.1X4	T36.1X5	T36.1X6
Cefroxadine	T36.1X1	T36.1X2	T36.1X3	T36.1X4	T36.1X5	T36.1X6
Cefsulodin	T36.1X1	T36.1X2	T36.1X3	T36.1X4	T36.1X5	T36.1X6
Ceftazidime	T36.1X1	T36.1X2	T36.1X3	T36.1X4	T36.1X5	T36.1X6
Cefteram	T36.1X1	T36.1X2	T36.1X3	T36.1X4	T36.1X5	T36.1X6
Ceftezole	T36.1X1	T36.1X2	T36.1X3	T36.1X4	T36.1X5	T36.1X6
Ceftin*	T36.1X1	T36.1X2	T36.1X3	T36.1X4	T36.1X5	T36.1X6
Ceftizoxime	T36.1X1	T36.1X2	T36.1X3	T36.1X4	T36.1X5	T36.1X6
Ceftriaxone	T36.1X1	T36.1X2	T36.1X3	T36.1X4	T36.1X5	T36.1X6
Cefuroxime	T36.1X1	T36.1X2	T36.1X3	T36.1X4	T36.1X5	T36.1X6
Cefuzonam	T36.1X1	T36.1X2	T36.1X3	T36.1X4	T36.1X5	T36.1X6
Celestone	T38.0X1	T38.0X2	T38.0X3	T38.0X4	T38.0X5	T38.0X6
topical	T49.0X1	T49.0X2	T49.0X3	T49.0X4	T49.0X5	T49.0X6
Celexa*	T43.221	T43.222	T43.223	T43.224	T43.225	T43.226
Celiprolol	T44.7X1	T44.7X2	T44.7X3	T44.7X4	T44.7X5	T44.7X6
Cellosolve	T52.91	T52.92	T52.93	T52.94	—	—
Cell stimulants and proliferants	T49.8X1	T49.8X2	T49.8X3	T49.8X4	T49.8X5	T49.8X6
Cellulose						
cathartic	T47.4X1	T47.4X2	T47.4X3	T47.4X4	T47.4X5	T47.4X6
hydroxyethyl	T47.4X1	T47.4X2	T47.4X3	T47.4X4	T47.4X5	T47.4X6
nitrates (topical)	T49.3X1	T49.3X2	T49.3X3	T49.3X4	T49.3X5	T49.3X6
oxidized	T49.4X1	T49.4X2	T49.4X3	T49.4X4	T49.4X5	T49.4X6
Centipede (bite)	T63.411	T63.412	T63.413	T63.414	—	—
Central nervous system						
depressants	T42.71	T42.72	T42.73	T42.74	T42.75	T42.76
anesthetic (general) NEC	T41.201	T41.202	T41.203	T41.204	T41.205	T41.206
gases NEC	T41.0X1	T41.0X2	T41.0X3	T41.0X4	T41.0X5	T41.0X6
intravenous	T41.1X1	T41.1X2	T41.1X3	T41.1X4	T41.1X5	T41.1X6
barbiturates	T42.3X1	T42.3X2	T42.3X3	T42.3X4	T42.3X5	T42.3X6
benzodiazepines	T42.4X1	T42.4X2	T42.4X3	T42.4X4	T42.4X5	T42.4X6
bromides	T42.6X1	T42.6X2	T42.6X3	T42.6X4	T42.6X5	T42.6X6
cannabis sativa	T40.711	T40.712	T40.713	T40.714	T40.715	T40.716
chloral hydrate	T42.6X1	T42.6X2	T42.6X3	T42.6X4	T42.6X5	T42.6X6
ethanol	T51.0X1	T51.0X2	T51.0X3	T51.0X4	—	—
hallucinogenics	T40.901	T40.902	T40.903	T40.904	T40.905	T40.906
hypnotics	T42.71	T42.72	T42.73	T42.74	T42.75	T42.76
specified NEC	T42.6X1	T42.6X2	T42.6X3	T42.6X4	T42.6X5	T42.6X6
muscle relaxants	T42.8X1	T42.8X2	T42.8X3	T42.8X4	T42.8X5	T42.8X6
paraldehyde	T42.6X1	T42.6X2	T42.6X3	T42.6X4	T42.6X5	T42.6X6
sedatives; sedative-hypnotics mixed NEC	T42.71	T42.72	T42.73	T42.74	T42.75	T42.76
specified NEC	T42.6X1	T42.6X2	T42.6X3	T42.6X4	T42.6X5	T42.6X6
muscle-tone depressants	T42.8X1	T42.8X2	T42.8X3	T42.8X4	T42.8X5	T42.8X6
stimulants	T43.601	T43.602	T43.603	T43.604	T43.605	T43.606
amphetamines	T43.621	T43.622	T43.623	T43.624	T43.625	T43.626
analeptics	T50.7X1	T50.7X2	T50.7X3	T50.7X4	T50.7X5	T50.7X6
antidepressants	T43.201	T43.202	T43.203	T43.204	T43.205	T43.206
opiate antagonists	T50.7X1	T50.7X2	T50.7X3	T50.7X4	T50.7X5	T50.7X6
specified NEC	T43.691	T43.692	T43.693	T43.694	T43.695	T43.696
Cepacol*	T41.3X1	T41.3X2	T41.3X3	T41.3X4	T41.3X5	T41.3X6
Cephalexin	T36.1X1	T36.1X2	T36.1X3	T36.1X4	T36.1X5	T36.1X6
Cephaloglycin	T36.1X1	T36.1X2	T36.1X3	T36.1X4	T36.1X5	T36.1X6
Cephaloridine	T36.1X1	T36.1X2	T36.1X3	T36.1X4	T36.1X5	T36.1X6
Cephalosporins	T36.1X1	T36.1X2	T36.1X3	T36.1X4	T36.1X5	T36.1X6
N (adicillin)	T36.0X1	T36.0X2	T36.0X3	T36.0X4	T36.0X5	T36.0X6
Cephalothin	T36.1X1	T36.1X2	T36.1X3	T36.1X4	T36.1X5	T36.1X6
Cephalotin	T36.1X1	T36.1X2	T36.1X3	T36.1X4	T36.1X5	T36.1X6
Cephradine	T36.1X1	T36.1X2	T36.1X3	T36.1X4	T36.1X5	T36.1X6
Cerbera (odallam)	T62.2X1	T62.2X2	T62.2X3	T62.2X4	—	—
Cerberin	T46.0X1	T46.0X2	T46.0X3	T46.0X4	T46.0X5	T46.0X6
Cerebral stimulants	T43.601	T43.602	T43.603	T43.604	T43.605	T43.606
psychotherapeutic	T43.601	T43.602	T43.603	T43.604	T43.605	T43.606
specified NEC	T43.691	T43.692	T43.693	T43.694	T43.695	T43.696
Cerium oxalate	T45.0X1	T45.0X2	T45.0X3	T45.0X4	T45.0X5	T45.0X6
Cerous oxalate	T45.0X1	T45.0X2	T45.0X3	T45.0X4	T45.0X5	T45.0X6
Ceruletide	T50.8X1	T50.8X2	T50.8X3	T50.8X4	T50.8X5	T50.8X6
Cetacort*	T49.0X1	T49.0X2	T49.0X3	T49.0X4	T49.0X5	T49.0X6
Cetalkonium (chloride)	T49.0X1	T49.0X2	T49.0X3	T49.0X4	T49.0X5	T49.0X6
Cethexonium chloride	T49.0X1	T49.0X2	T49.0X3	T49.0X4	T49.0X5	T49.0X6
Cetiedil	T46.7X1	T46.7X2	T46.7X3	T46.7X4	T46.7X5	T46.7X6
Cetirizine	T45.0X1	T45.0X2	T45.0X3	T45.0X4	T45.0X5	T45.0X6
Cetomacrogol	T50.991	T50.992	T50.993	T50.994	T50.995	T50.996
Cetotiamine	T45.2X1	T45.2X2	T45.2X3	T45.2X4	T45.2X5	T45.2X6
Cetoxime	T45.0X1	T45.0X2	T45.0X3	T45.0X4	T45.0X5	T45.0X6
Cetraxate	T47.1X1	T47.1X2	T47.1X3	T47.1X4	T47.1X5	T47.1X6
Cetrimide	T49.0X1	T49.0X2	T49.0X3	T49.0X4	T49.0X5	T49.0X6
Cetrimonium (bromide)	T49.0X1	T49.0X2	T49.0X3	T49.0X4	T49.0X5	T49.0X6
Cetylpyridinium chloride	T49.0X1	T49.0X2	T49.0X3	T49.0X4	T49.0X5	T49.0X6
ENT agent	T49.6X1	T49.6X2	T49.6X3	T49.6X4	T49.6X5	T49.6X6
lozenges	T49.6X1	T49.6X2	T49.6X3	T49.6X4	T49.6X5	T49.6X6
Cevadilla — see Sabadilla						
Cevitamic acid	T45.2X1	T45.2X2	T45.2X3	T45.2X4	T45.2X5	T45.2X6
Chalk, precipitated	T47.1X1	T47.1X2	T47.1X3	T47.1X4	T47.1X5	T47.1X6
Chamomile	T49.0X1	T49.0X2	T49.0X3	T49.0X4	T49.0X5	T49.0X6
Ch'an su	T46.0X1	T46.0X2	T46.0X3	T46.0X4	T46.0X5	T46.0X6
Charcoal						
activated — see also Charcoal, medicinal						
fumes (Carbon monoxide)	T58.2X1	T58.2X2	T58.2X3	T58.2X4	—	—
industrial	T58.8X1	T58.8X2	T58.8X3	T58.8X4	—	—
medicinal (activated)	T47.6X1	T47.6X2	T47.6X3	T47.6X4	T47.6X5	T47.6X6
antidiarrheal	T47.6X1	T47.6X2	T47.6X3	T47.6X4	T47.6X5	T47.6X6
poison control	T47.8X1	T47.8X2	T47.8X3	T47.8X4	T47.8X5	T47.8X6
specified use other than for diarrhea	T47.8X1	T47.8X2	T47.8X3	T47.8X4	T47.8X5	T47.8X6
topical	T49.8X1	T49.8X2	T49.8X3	T49.8X4	T49.8X5	T49.8X6
Chaulmosulfone	T37.1X1	T37.1X2	T37.1X3	T37.1X4	T37.1X5	T37.1X6
Chelating agent NEC	T50.6X1	T50.6X2	T50.6X3	T50.6X4	T50.6X5	T50.6X6
Chelidonium majus	T62.2X1	T62.2X2	T62.2X3	T62.2X4	—	—
Chemical substance NEC	T65.91	T65.92	T65.93	T65.94	—	—
Chenodeoxycholic acid	T47.5X1	T47.5X2	T47.5X3	T47.5X4	T47.5X5	T47.5X6
Chenodiol	T47.5X1	T47.5X2	T47.5X3	T47.5X4	T47.5X5	T47.5X6
Chenopodium	T37.4X1	T37.4X2	T37.4X3	T37.4X4	T37.4X5	T37.4X6
Cherry laurel	T62.2X1	T62.2X2	T62.2X3	T62.2X4	—	—
Chiggertox*	T41.3X1	T41.3X2	T41.3X3	T41.3X4	T41.3X5	T41.3X6
Chinidin (e)	T46.2X1	T46.2X2	T46.2X3	T46.2X4	T46.2X5	T46.2X6
Chiniofon	T37.8X1	T37.8X2	T37.8X3	T37.8X4	T37.8X5	T37.8X6
Chlophedianol	T48.3X1	T48.3X2	T48.3X3	T48.3X4	T48.3X5	T48.3X6
Chloral	T42.6X1	T42.6X2	T42.6X3	T42.6X4	T42.6X5	T42.6X6
derivative	T42.6X1	T42.6X2	T42.6X3	T42.6X4	T42.6X5	T42.6X6
hydrate	T42.6X1	T42.6X2	T42.6X3	T42.6X4	T42.6X5	T42.6X6
Chloralamide	T42.6X1	T42.6X2	T42.6X3	T42.6X4	T42.6X5	T42.6X6
Chloralodol	T42.6X1	T42.6X2	T42.6X3	T42.6X4	T42.6X5	T42.6X6
Chloralose	T60.4X1	T60.4X2	T60.4X3	T60.4X4	—	—
Chlorambucil	T45.1X1	T45.1X2	T45.1X3	T45.1X4	T45.1X5	T45.1X6
Chloramine	T57.8X1	T57.8X2	T57.8X3	T57.8X4	—	—
T	T49.0X1	T49.0X2	T49.0X3	T49.0X4	T49.0X5	T49.0X6
topical	T49.0X1	T49.0X2	T49.0X3	T49.0X4	T49.0X5	T49.0X6
Chloramphenicol	T36.2X1	T36.2X2	T36.2X3	T36.2X4	T36.2X5	T36.2X6
ENT agent	T49.6X1	T49.6X2	T49.6X3	T49.6X4	T49.6X5	T49.6X6
ophthalmic preparation	T49.5X1	T49.5X2	T49.5X3	T49.5X4	T49.5X5	T49.5X6
topical NEC	T49.0X1	T49.0X2	T49.0X3	T49.0X4	T49.0X5	T49.0X6
Chlorate (potassium) (sodium) NEC	T60.3X1	T60.3X2	T60.3X3	T60.3X4	—	—
herbicide	T60.3X1	T60.3X2	T60.3X3	T60.3X4	—	—
Chlorazanil	T50.2X1	T50.2X2	T50.2X3	T50.2X4	T50.2X5	T50.2X6
Chlorbenzene, chlorbenzol	T53.7X1	T53.7X2	T53.7X3	T53.7X4	—	—
Chlorbenzoxamine	T44.3X1	T44.3X2	T44.3X3	T44.3X4	T44.3X5	T44.3X6
Chlorbutol	T42.6X1	T42.6X2	T42.6X3	T42.6X4	T42.6X5	T42.6X6
Chlorcyclizine	T45.0X1	T45.0X2	T45.0X3	T45.0X4	T45.0X5	T45.0X6
Chlordan (e) (dust)	T60.1X1	T60.1X2	T60.1X3	T60.1X4	—	—
Chlordantoin	T49.0X1	T49.0X2	T49.0X3	T49.0X4	T49.0X5	T49.0X6
Chlordiazepoxide	T42.4X1	T42.4X2	T42.4X3	T42.4X4	T42.4X5	T42.4X6
Chlordiethyl benzamide	T49.3X1	T49.3X2	T49.3X3	T49.3X4	T49.3X5	T49.3X6
Chloresium	T49.8X1	T49.8X2	T49.8X3	T49.8X4	T49.8X5	T49.8X6
Chlorethiazol	T42.6X1	T42.6X2	T42.6X3	T42.6X4	T42.6X5	T42.6X6
Chlorethyl — see Ethyl, chloride						
Chloretone	T42.6X1	T42.6X2	T42.6X3	T42.6X4	T42.6X5	T42.6X6
Chlorex	T53.6X1	T53.6X2	T53.6X3	T53.6X4	—	—
insecticide	T60.1X1	T60.1X2	T60.1X3	T60.1X4	—	—
Chlorfenvinphos	T60.0X1	T60.0X2	T60.0X3	T60.0X4	—	—
Chlorhexadol	T42.6X1	T42.6X2	T42.6X3	T42.6X4	T42.6X5	T42.6X6
Chlorhexamide	T45.1X1	T45.1X2	T45.1X3	T45.1X4	T45.1X5	T45.1X6
Chlorhexidine	T49.0X1	T49.0X2	T49.0X3	T49.0X4	T49.0X5	T49.0X6
Chlorhexidine Gluconate Oral Rinse*	T49.6X1	T49.6X2	T49.6X3	T49.6X4	T49.6X5	T49.6X6
Chlorhydroxyquinolin	T49.0X1	T49.0X2	T49.0X3	T49.0X4	T49.0X5	T49.0X6
Chloride of lime (bleach)	T54.3X1	T54.3X2	T54.3X3	T54.3X4	—	—
Chlorimipramine	T43.011	T43.012	T43.013	T43.014	T43.015	T43.016

☑ Additional Character May Be Required — Refer to the Tabular List for Character Selection

*Optum Value-Add

Table of Drugs and Chemicals

Chlorinated — Ciclonicate

Substance	Poisoning, Accidental (unintentional)	Poisoning, Intentional Self-harm	Poisoning, Assault	Poisoning, Undetermined	Adverse Effect	Under-dosing
Chlorinated						
camphene	T53.6X1	T53.6X2	T53.6X3	T53.6X4	—	—
diphenyl	T53.7X1	T53.7X2	T53.7X3	T53.7X4	—	—
hydrocarbons NEC	T53.91	T53.92	T53.93	T53.94	—	—
solvents	T53.91	T53.92	T53.93	T53.94	—	—
lime (bleach)	T54.3X1	T54.3X2	T54.3X3	T54.3X4	—	—
and boric acid solution	T49.0X1	T49.0X2	T49.0X3	T49.0X4	T49.0X5	T49.0X6
naphthalene (insecticide)	T60.1X1	T60.1X2	T60.1X3	T60.1X4	—	—
industrial (non-pesticide)	T53.7X1	T53.7X2	T53.7X3	T53.7X4	—	—
pesticide NEC	T60.8X1	T60.8X2	T60.8X3	T60.8X4	—	—
soda — see also sodium hypochlorite						
solution	T49.0X1	T49.0X2	T49.0X3	T49.0X4	T49.0X5	T49.0X6
Chlorine (fumes) (gas)	T59.4X1	T59.4X2	T59.4X3	T59.4X4	—	—
bleach	T54.3X1	T54.3X2	T54.3X3	T54.3X4	—	—
compound gas NEC	T59.4X1	T59.4X2	T59.4X3	T59.4X4	—	—
disinfectant	T59.4X1	T59.4X2	T59.4X3	T59.4X4	—	—
releasing agents NEC	T59.4X1	T59.4X2	T59.4X3	T59.4X4	—	—
Chlorisondamine chloride	T46.991	T46.992	T46.993	T46.994	T46.995	T46.996
Chlormadinone	T38.5X1	T38.5X2	T38.5X3	T38.5X4	T38.5X5	T38.5X6
Chlormephos	T60.0X1	T60.0X2	T60.0X3	T60.0X4	—	—
Chlormerodrin	T50.2X1	T50.2X2	T50.2X3	T50.2X4	T50.2X5	T50.2X6
Chlormethiazole	T42.6X1	T42.6X2	T42.6X3	T42.6X4	T42.6X5	T42.6X6
Chlormethine	T45.1X1	T45.1X2	T45.1X3	T45.1X4	T45.1X5	T45.1X6
Chlormethylenecycline	T36.4X1	T36.4X2	T36.4X3	T36.4X4	T36.4X5	T36.4X6
Chlormezanone	T42.6X1	T42.6X2	T42.6X3	T42.6X4	T42.6X5	T42.6X6
Chloroacetic acid	T60.3X1	T60.3X2	T60.3X3	T60.3X4	—	—
Chloroacetone	T59.3X1	T59.3X2	T59.3X3	T59.3X4	—	—
Chloroacetophenone	T59.3X1	T59.3X2	T59.3X3	T59.3X4	—	—
Chloroaniline	T53.7X1	T53.7X2	T53.7X3	T53.7X4	—	—
Chlorobenzene, chlorobenzol	T53.7X1	T53.7X2	T53.7X3	T53.7X4	—	—
Chlorobromomethane (fire extinguisher)	T53.6X1	T53.6X2	T53.6X3	T53.6X4	—	—
Chlorobutanol	T49.0X1	T49.0X2	T49.0X3	T49.0X4	T49.0X5	T49.0X6
Chlorocresol	T49.0X1	T49.0X2	T49.0X3	T49.0X4	T49.0X5	T49.0X6
Chlorodehydromethyltestosterone	T38.7X1	T38.7X2	T38.7X3	T38.7X4	T38.7X5	T38.7X6
Chlorodeoxyadenosine*	T45.1X1	T45.1X2	T45.1X3	T45.1X4	T45.1X5	T45.1X6
Chlorodinitrobenzene	T53.7X1	T53.7X2	T53.7X3	T53.7X4	—	—
dust or vapor	T53.7X1	T53.7X2	T53.7X3	T53.7X4	—	—
Chlorodiphenyl	T53.7X1	T53.7X2	T53.7X3	T53.7X4	—	—
Chloroethane — see Ethyl, chloride						
Chloroethylene	T53.6X1	T53.6X2	T53.6X3	T53.6X4	—	—
Chlorofluorocarbons	T53.5X1	T53.5X2	T53.5X3	T53.5X4	—	—
Chloroform (fumes) (vapor)	T53.1X1	T53.1X2	T53.1X3	T53.1X4	—	—
anesthetic	T41.0X1	T41.0X2	T41.0X3	T41.0X4	T41.0X5	T41.0X6
solvent	T53.1X1	T53.1X2	T53.1X3	T53.1X4	—	—
water, concentrated	T41.0X1	T41.0X2	T41.0X3	T41.0X4	T41.0X5	T41.0X6
Chloroguanide	T37.2X1	T37.2X2	T37.2X3	T37.2X4	T37.2X5	T37.2X6
Chloromycetin	T36.2X1	T36.2X2	T36.2X3	T36.2X4	T36.2X5	T36.2X6
ENT agent	T49.6X1	T49.6X2	T49.6X3	T49.6X4	T49.6X5	T49.6X6
ophthalmic preparation	T49.5X1	T49.5X2	T49.5X3	T49.5X4	T49.5X5	T49.5X6
otic solution	T49.6X1	T49.6X2	T49.6X3	T49.6X4	T49.6X5	T49.6X6
topical NEC	T49.0X1	T49.0X2	T49.0X3	T49.0X4	T49.0X5	T49.0X6
Chloronitrobenzene	T53.7X1	T53.7X2	T53.7X3	T53.7X4	—	—
dust or vapor	T53.7X1	T53.7X2	T53.7X3	T53.7X4	—	—
Chlorophacinone	T60.4X1	T60.4X2	T60.4X3	T60.4X4	—	—
Chlorophenol	T53.7X1	T53.7X2	T53.7X3	T53.7X4	—	—
Chlorophenothane	T60.1X1	T60.1X2	T60.1X3	T60.1X4	—	—
Chlorophyll	T50.991	T50.992	T50.993	T50.994	T50.995	T50.996
Chloropicrin (fumes)	T53.6X1	T53.6X2	T53.6X3	T53.6X4	—	—
fumigant	T60.8X1	T60.8X2	T60.8X3	T60.8X4	—	—
fungicide	T60.3X1	T60.3X2	T60.3X3	T60.3X4	—	—
pesticide	T60.8X1	T60.8X2	T60.8X3	T60.8X4	—	—
Chloroprocaine	T41.3X1	T41.3X2	T41.3X3	T41.3X4	T41.3X5	T41.3X6
infiltration (subcutaneous)	T41.3X1	T41.3X2	T41.3X3	T41.3X4	T41.3X5	T41.3X6
nerve block (peripheral) (plexus)	T41.3X1	T41.3X2	T41.3X3	T41.3X4	T41.3X5	T41.3X6
spinal	T41.3X1	T41.3X2	T41.3X3	T41.3X4	T41.3X5	T41.3X6
Chloroptic	T49.5X1	T49.5X2	T49.5X3	T49.5X4	T49.5X5	T49.5X6
Chloropurine	T45.1X1	T45.1X2	T45.1X3	T45.1X4	T45.1X5	T45.1X6
Chloropyramine	T45.0X1	T45.0X2	T45.0X3	T45.0X4	T45.0X5	T45.0X6
Chloropyrifos	T60.0X1	T60.0X2	T60.0X3	T60.0X4	—	—
Chloropyrilene	T45.0X1	T45.0X2	T45.0X3	T45.0X4	T45.0X5	T45.0X6
Chloroquine	T37.2X1	T37.2X2	T37.2X3	T37.2X4	T37.2X5	T37.2X6
Chlorostat*	T49.0X1	T49.0X2	T49.0X3	T49.0X4	T49.0X5	T49.0X6
Chlorothalonil	T60.3X1	T60.3X2	T60.3X3	T60.3X4	—	—
Chlorothen	T45.0X1	T45.0X2	T45.0X3	T45.0X4	T45.0X5	T45.0X6
Chlorothiazide	T50.2X1	T50.2X2	T50.2X3	T50.2X4	T50.2X5	T50.2X6
Chlorothymol	T49.4X1	T49.4X2	T49.4X3	T49.4X4	T49.4X5	T49.4X6
Chlorotrianisene	T38.5X1	T38.5X2	T38.5X3	T38.5X4	T38.5X5	T38.5X6
Chlorovinyldichloroarsine, not in war	T57.0X1	T57.0X2	T57.0X3	T57.0X4	—	—
Chloroxine	T49.4X1	T49.4X2	T49.4X3	T49.4X4	T49.4X5	T49.4X6
Chloroxylenol	T49.0X1	T49.0X2	T49.0X3	T49.0X4	T49.0X5	T49.0X6
Chlorphenamine	T45.0X1	T45.0X2	T45.0X3	T45.0X4	T45.0X5	T45.0X6
Chlorphenesin	T42.8X1	T42.8X2	T42.8X3	T42.8X4	T42.8X5	T42.8X6
topical (antifungal)	T49.0X1	T49.0X2	T49.0X3	T49.0X4	T49.0X5	T49.0X6
Chlorpheniramine	T45.0X1	T45.0X2	T45.0X3	T45.0X4	T45.0X5	T45.0X6
Chlorphenoxamine	T45.0X1	T45.0X2	T45.0X3	T45.0X4	T45.0X5	T45.0X6
Chlorphentermine	T50.5X1	T50.5X2	T50.5X3	T50.5X4	T50.5X5	T50.5X6
Chlorprocaine — see Chloroprocaine						
Chlorproguanil	T37.2X1	T37.2X2	T37.2X3	T37.2X4	T37.2X5	T37.2X6
Chlorpromazine	T43.3X1	T43.3X2	T43.3X3	T43.3X4	T43.3X5	T43.3X6
Chlorpropamide	T38.3X1	T38.3X2	T38.3X3	T38.3X4	T38.3X5	T38.3X6
Chlorprothixene	T43.4X1	T43.4X2	T43.4X3	T43.4X4	T43.4X5	T43.4X6
Chlorquinaldol	T49.0X1	T49.0X2	T49.0X3	T49.0X4	T49.0X5	T49.0X6
Chlorquinol	T49.0X1	T49.0X2	T49.0X3	T49.0X4	T49.0X5	T49.0X6
Chlortalidone	T50.2X1	T50.2X2	T50.2X3	T50.2X4	T50.2X5	T50.2X6
Chlortetracycline	T36.4X1	T36.4X2	T36.4X3	T36.4X4	T36.4X5	T36.4X6
Chlorthalidone	T50.2X1	T50.2X2	T50.2X3	T50.2X4	T50.2X5	T50.2X6
Chlorthion	T60.0X1	T60.0X2	T60.0X3	T60.0X4	—	—
Chlorthiophos	T60.0X1	T60.0X2	T60.0X3	T60.0X4	—	—
Chlortrianisene	T38.5X1	T38.5X2	T38.5X3	T38.5X4	T38.5X5	T38.5X6
Chlor-Trimeton	T45.0X1	T45.0X2	T45.0X3	T45.0X4	T45.0X5	T45.0X6
Chlorzoxazone	T42.8X1	T42.8X2	T42.8X3	T42.8X4	T42.8X5	T42.8X6
Choke damp	T59.7X1	T59.7X2	T59.7X3	T59.7X4	—	—
Cholagogues	T47.5X1	T47.5X2	T47.5X3	T47.5X4	T47.5X5	T47.5X6
Cholebrine	T50.8X1	T50.8X2	T50.8X3	T50.8X4	T50.8X5	T50.8X6
Cholecalciferol	T45.2X1	T45.2X2	T45.2X3	T45.2X4	T45.2X5	T45.2X6
Cholecystokinin	T50.8X1	T50.8X2	T50.8X3	T50.8X4	T50.8X5	T50.8X6
Cholera vaccine	T50.A91	T50.A92	T50.A93	T50.A94	T50.A95	T50.A96
Choleretic	T47.5X1	T47.5X2	T47.5X3	T47.5X4	T47.5X5	T47.5X6
Cholesterol-lowering agents	T46.6X1	T46.6X2	T46.6X3	T46.6X4	T46.6X5	T46.6X6
Cholestyramine (resin)	T46.6X1	T46.6X2	T46.6X3	T46.6X4	T46.6X5	T46.6X6
Cholic acid	T47.5X1	T47.5X2	T47.5X3	T47.5X4	T47.5X5	T47.5X6
Choline	T48.6X1	T48.6X2	T48.6X3	T48.6X4	T48.6X5	T48.6X6
chloride	T50.991	T50.992	T50.993	T50.994	T50.995	T50.996
dihydrogen citrate	T50.991	T50.992	T50.993	T50.994	T50.995	T50.996
salicylate	T39.091	T39.092	T39.093	T39.094	T39.095	T39.096
theophyllinate	T48.6X1	T48.6X2	T48.6X3	T48.6X4	T48.6X5	T48.6X6
Cholinergic (drug) **NEC**	T44.1X1	T44.1X2	T44.1X3	T44.1X4	T44.1X5	T44.1X6
muscle tone enhancer	T44.1X1	T44.1X2	T44.1X3	T44.1X4	T44.1X5	T44.1X6
organophosphorus	T44.0X1	T44.0X2	T44.0X3	T44.0X4	T44.0X5	T44.0X6
insecticide	T60.0X1	T60.0X2	T60.0X3	T60.0X4	—	—
nerve gas	T59.891	T59.892	T59.893	T59.894	—	—
trimethyl ammonium propanediol	T44.1X1	T44.1X2	T44.1X3	T44.1X4	T44.1X5	T44.1X6
Cholinesterase reactivator	T50.6X1	T50.6X2	T50.6X3	T50.6X4	T50.6X5	T50.6X6
Chologrfin	T50.8X1	T50.8X2	T50.8X3	T50.8X4	T50.8X5	T50.8X6
Chorionic gonadotropin	T38.891	T38.892	T38.893	T38.894	T38.895	T38.896
Chromate	T56.2X1	T56.2X2	T56.2X3	T56.2X4	—	—
dust or mist	T56.2X1	T56.2X2	T56.2X3	T56.2X4	—	—
lead — see also lead	T56.0X1	T56.0X2	T56.0X3	T56.0X4	—	—
paint	T56.0X1	T56.0X2	T56.0X3	T56.0X4	—	—
Chromelin*	T49.3X1	T49.3X2	T49.3X3	T49.3X4	T49.3X5	T49.3X6
Chromic						
acid	T56.2X1	T56.2X2	T56.2X3	T56.2X4	—	—
dust or mist	T56.2X1	T56.2X2	T56.2X3	T56.2X4	—	—
phosphate 32P	T45.1X1	T45.1X2	T45.1X3	T45.1X4	T45.1X5	T45.1X6
Chromium	T56.2X1	T56.2X2	T56.2X3	T56.2X4	—	—
compounds — see Chromate						
sesquioxide	T50.8X1	T50.8X2	T50.8X3	T50.8X4	T50.8X5	T50.8X6
Chromomycin A3	T45.1X1	T45.1X2	T45.1X3	T45.1X4	T45.1X5	T45.1X6
Chromonar	T46.3X1	T46.3X2	T46.3X3	T46.3X4	T46.3X5	T46.3X6
Chromyl chloride	T56.2X1	T56.2X2	T56.2X3	T56.2X4	—	—
Chrysarobin	T49.4X1	T49.4X2	T49.4X3	T49.4X4	T49.4X5	T49.4X6
Chrysazin	T47.2X1	T47.2X2	T47.2X3	T47.2X4	T47.2X5	T47.2X6
Chymar	T45.3X1	T45.3X2	T45.3X3	T45.3X4	T45.3X5	T45.3X6
ophthalmic preparation	T49.5X1	T49.5X2	T49.5X3	T49.5X4	T49.5X5	T49.5X6
Chymopapain	T45.3X1	T45.3X2	T45.3X3	T45.3X4	T45.3X5	T45.3X6
Chymotrypsin	T45.3X1	T45.3X2	T45.3X3	T45.3X4	T45.3X5	T45.3X6
ophthalmic preparation	T49.5X1	T49.5X2	T49.5X3	T49.5X4	T49.5X5	T49.5X6
Cialis*	T46.7X1	T46.7X2	T46.7X3	T46.7X4	T46.7X5	T46.7X6
Cianidanol	T50.991	T50.992	T50.993	T50.994	T50.995	T50.996
Cianopramine	T43.011	T43.012	T43.013	T43.014	T43.015	T43.016
Cibenzoline	T46.2X1	T46.2X2	T46.2X3	T46.2X4	T46.2X5	T46.2X6
Ciclacillin	T36.0X1	T36.0X2	T36.0X3	T36.0X4	T36.0X5	T36.0X6
Ciclobarbital — see Hexobarbital						
Ciclonicate	T46.7X1	T46.7X2	T46.7X3	T46.7X4	T46.7X5	T46.7X6

Substance	Poisoning, Accidental (unintentional)	Poisoning, Intentional Self-harm	Poisoning, Assault	Poisoning, Undetermined	Adverse Effect	Under-dosing
Ciclopirox (olamine)	T49.0X1	T49.0X2	T49.0X3	T49.0X4	T49.0X5	T49.0X6
Ciclosporin	T45.1X1	T45.1X2	T45.1X3	T45.1X4	T45.1X5	T45.1X6
Cicuta maculata or virosa	T62.2X1	T62.2X2	T62.2X3	T62.2X4	—	—
Cicutoxin	T62.2X1	T62.2X2	T62.2X3	T62.2X4	—	—
Cigarette lighter fluid	T52.0X1	T52.0X2	T52.0X3	T52.0X4	—	—
Cigarettes (tobacco)	T65.221	T65.222	T65.223	T65.224	—	—
Ciguatoxin	T61.01	T61.02	T61.03	T61.04	—	—
Cilazapril	T46.4X1	T46.4X2	T46.4X3	T46.4X4	T46.4X5	T46.4X6
Cimetidine	T47.0X1	T47.0X2	T47.0X3	T47.0X4	T47.0X5	T47.0X6
Cimetropium bromide	T44.3X1	T44.3X2	T44.3X3	T44.3X4	T44.3X5	T44.3X6
Cinchocaine	T41.3X1	T41.3X2	T41.3X3	T41.3X4	T41.3X5	T41.3X6
topical (surface)	T41.3X1	T41.3X2	T41.3X3	T41.3X4	T41.3X5	T41.3X6
Cinchona	T37.2X1	T37.2X2	T37.2X3	T37.2X4	T37.2X5	T37.2X6
Cinchonine alkaloids	T37.2X1	T37.2X2	T37.2X3	T37.2X4	T37.2X5	T37.2X6
Cinchophen	T50.4X1	T50.4X2	T50.4X3	T50.4X4	T50.4X5	T50.4X6
Cinepazide	T46.7X1	T46.7X2	T46.7X3	T46.7X4	T46.7X5	T46.7X6
Cinnamedrine	T48.5X1	T48.5X2	T48.5X3	T48.5X4	T48.5X5	T48.5X6
Cinnarizine	T45.0X1	T45.0X2	T45.0X3	T45.0X4	T45.0X5	T45.0X6
Cinoxacin	T37.8X1	T37.8X2	T37.8X3	T37.8X4	T37.8X5	T37.8X6
Ciprofibrate	T46.6X1	T46.6X2	T46.6X3	T46.6X4	T46.6X5	T46.6X6
Ciprofloxacin	T36.8X1	T36.8X2	T36.8X3	T36.8X4	T36.8X5	T36.8X6
Cisapride	T47.8X1	T47.8X2	T47.8X3	T47.8X4	T47.8X5	T47.8X6
Cisplatin	T45.1X1	T45.1X2	T45.1X3	T45.1X4	T45.1X5	T45.1X6
Citalopram	T43.221	T43.222	T43.223	T43.224	T43.225	T43.226
Citanest	T41.3X1	T41.3X2	T41.3X3	T41.3X4	T41.3X5	T41.3X6
infiltration (subcutaneous)	T41.3X1	T41.3X2	T41.3X3	T41.3X4	T41.3X5	T41.3X6
nerve block (peripheral) (plexus)	T41.3X1	T41.3X2	T41.3X3	T41.3X4	T41.3X5	T41.3X6
Citracel*	T50.3X1	T50.3X2	T50.3X3	T50.3X4	T50.3X5	T50.3X6
Citric acid	T47.5X1	T47.5X2	T47.5X3	T47.5X4	T47.5X5	T47.5X6
Citrovorum (factor)	T45.8X1	T45.8X2	T45.8X3	T45.8X4	T45.8X5	T45.8X6
Claviceps purpurea	T62.2X1	T62.2X2	T62.2X3	T62.2X4	—	—
Clavulanic acid	T36.1X1	T36.1X2	T36.1X3	T36.1X4	T36.1X5	T36.1X6
Cleaner, cleansing agent, type not specified	T65.891	T65.892	T65.893	T65.894	—	—
of paint or varnish	T52.91	T52.92	T52.93	T52.94	—	—
specified type NEC	T65.891	T65.892	T65.893	T65.894	—	—
Clebopride	T47.8X1	T47.8X2	T47.8X3	T47.8X4	T47.8X5	T47.8X6
Clefamide	T37.3X1	T37.3X2	T37.3X3	T37.3X4	T37.3X5	T37.3X6
Clemastine	T45.0X1	T45.0X2	T45.0X3	T45.0X4	T45.0X5	T45.0X6
Clematis vitalba	T62.2X1	T62.2X2	T62.2X3	T62.2X4	—	—
Clemizole	T45.0X1	T45.0X2	T45.0X3	T45.0X4	T45.0X5	T45.0X6
penicillin	T36.0X1	T36.0X2	T36.0X3	T36.0X4	T36.0X5	T36.0X6
Clenbuterol	T48.6X1	T48.6X2	T48.6X3	T48.6X4	T48.6X5	T48.6X6
Clidinium bromide	T44.3X1	T44.3X2	T44.3X3	T44.3X4	T44.3X5	T44.3X6
Climara*	T38.5X1	T38.5X2	T38.5X3	T38.5X4	T38.5X5	T38.5X6
Clinda-Derm*	T49.0X1	T49.0X2	T49.0X3	T49.0X4	T49.0X5	T49.0X6
Clindamycin	T36.8X1	T36.8X2	T36.8X3	T36.8X4	T36.8X5	T36.8X6
Clinofibrate	T46.6X1	T46.6X2	T46.6X3	T46.6X4	T46.6X5	T46.6X6
Clioquinol	T37.8X1	T37.8X2	T37.8X3	T37.8X4	T37.8X5	T37.8X6
Cliradon	T40.2X1	T40.2X2	T40.2X3	T40.2X4	—	—
Clobazam	T42.4X1	T42.4X2	T42.4X3	T42.4X4	T42.4X5	T42.4X6
Clobenzorex	T50.5X1	T50.5X2	T50.5X3	T50.5X4	T50.5X5	T50.5X6
Clobetasol	T49.0X1	T49.0X2	T49.0X3	T49.0X4	T49.0X5	T49.0X6
Clobetasone	T49.0X1	T49.0X2	T49.0X3	T49.0X4	T49.0X5	T49.0X6
Clobutinol	T48.3X1	T48.3X2	T48.3X3	T48.3X4	T48.3X5	T48.3X6
Clocortolone	T38.0X1	T38.0X2	T38.0X3	T38.0X4	T38.0X5	T38.0X6
Clodantoin	T49.0X1	T49.0X2	T49.0X3	T49.0X4	T49.0X5	T49.0X6
Clodronic acid	T50.991	T50.992	T50.993	T50.994	T50.995	T50.996
Clofazimine	T37.1X1	T37.1X2	T37.1X3	T37.1X4	T37.1X5	T37.1X6
Clofedanol	T48.3X1	T48.3X2	T48.3X3	T48.3X4	T48.3X5	T48.3X6
Clofenamide	T50.2X1	T50.2X2	T50.2X3	T50.2X4	T50.2X5	T50.2X6
Clofenotane	T49.0X1	T49.0X2	T49.0X3	T49.0X4	T49.0X5	T49.0X6
Clofezone	T39.2X1	T39.2X2	T39.2X3	T39.2X4	T39.2X5	T39.2X6
Clofibrate	T46.6X1	T46.6X2	T46.6X3	T46.6X4	T46.6X5	T46.6X6
Clofibride	T46.6X1	T46.6X2	T46.6X3	T46.6X4	T46.6X5	T46.6X6
Cloforex	T50.5X1	T50.5X2	T50.5X3	T50.5X4	T50.5X5	T50.5X6
Clomethiazole	T42.6X1	T42.6X2	T42.6X3	T42.6X4	T42.6X5	T42.6X6
Clometocillin	T36.0X1	T36.0X2	T36.0X3	T36.0X4	T36.0X5	T36.0X6
Clomifene	T38.5X1	T38.5X2	T38.5X3	T38.5X4	T38.5X5	T38.5X6
Clomiphene	T38.5X1	T38.5X2	T38.5X3	T38.5X4	T38.5X5	T38.5X6
Clomipramine	T43.011	T43.012	T43.013	T43.014	T43.015	T43.016
Clomocycline	T36.4X1	T36.4X2	T36.4X3	T36.4X4	T36.4X5	T36.4X6
Clonazepam	T42.4X1	T42.4X2	T42.4X3	T42.4X4	T42.4X5	T42.4X6
Clonidine	T46.5X1	T46.5X2	T46.5X3	T46.5X4	T46.5X5	T46.5X6
Clonixin	T39.8X1	T39.8X2	T39.8X3	T39.8X4	T39.8X5	T39.8X6
Clopamide	T50.2X1	T50.2X2	T50.2X3	T50.2X4	T50.2X5	T50.2X6
Clopenthixol	T43.4X1	T43.4X2	T43.4X3	T43.4X4	T43.4X5	T43.4X6
Cloperastine	T48.3X1	T48.3X2	T48.3X3	T48.3X4	T48.3X5	T48.3X6
Clophedianol	T48.3X1	T48.3X2	T48.3X3	T48.3X4	T48.3X5	T48.3X6
Cloponone	T36.2X1	T36.2X2	T36.2X3	T36.2X4	T36.2X5	T36.2X6
Cloprednol	T38.0X1	T38.0X2	T38.0X3	T38.0X4	T38.0X5	T38.0X6
Cloral betaine	T42.6X1	T42.6X2	T42.6X3	T42.6X4	T42.6X5	T42.6X6

Substance	Poisoning, Accidental (unintentional)	Poisoning, Intentional Self-harm	Poisoning, Assault	Poisoning, Undetermined	Adverse Effect	Under-dosing
Cloramfenicol	T36.2X1	T36.2X2	T36.2X3	T36.2X4	T36.2X5	T36.2X6
Clorazepate (dipotassium)	T42.4X1	T42.4X2	T42.4X3	T42.4X4	T42.4X5	T42.4X6
Clorexolone	T50.2X1	T50.2X2	T50.2X3	T50.2X4	T50.2X5	T50.2X6
Clorfenamine	T45.0X1	T45.0X2	T45.0X3	T45.0X4	T45.0X5	T45.0X6
Clorgiline	T43.1X1	T43.1X2	T43.1X3	T43.1X4	T43.1X5	T43.1X6
Clorotepine	T44.3X1	T44.3X2	T44.3X3	T44.3X4	T44.3X5	T44.3X6
Clorox (bleach)	T54.91	T54.92	T54.93	T54.94	—	—
Clorprenaline	T48.6X1	T48.6X2	T48.6X3	T48.6X4	T48.6X5	T48.6X6
Clortermine	T50.5X1	T50.5X2	T50.5X3	T50.5X4	T50.5X5	T50.5X6
Clotiapine	T43.591	T43.592	T43.593	T43.594	T43.595	T43.596
Clotiazepam	T42.4X1	T42.4X2	T42.4X3	T42.4X4	T42.4X5	T42.4X6
Clotibric acid	T46.6X1	T46.6X2	T46.6X3	T46.6X4	T46.6X5	T46.6X6
Clotrimazole	T49.0X1	T49.0X2	T49.0X3	T49.0X4	T49.0X5	T49.0X6
Cloxacillin	T36.0X1	T36.0X2	T36.0X3	T36.0X4	T36.0X5	T36.0X6
Cloxazolam	T42.4X1	T42.4X2	T42.4X3	T42.4X4	T42.4X5	T42.4X6
Cloxiquine	T49.0X1	T49.0X2	T49.0X3	T49.0X4	T49.0X5	T49.0X6
Clozapine	T42.4X1	T42.4X2	T42.4X3	T42.4X4	T42.4X5	T42.4X6
Coagulant NEC	T45.7X1	T45.7X2	T45.7X3	T45.7X4	T45.7X5	T45.7X6
Coal (carbon monoxide from) — see also Carbon, monoxide, coal	T58.2X1	T58.2X2	T58.2X3	T58.2X4		
oil — see Kerosene						
tar	T49.1X1	T49.1X2	T49.1X3	T49.1X4	T49.1X5	T49.1X6
fumes	T59.891	T59.892	T59.893	T59.894	—	—
medicinal (ointment)	T49.4X1	T49.4X2	T49.4X3	T49.4X4	T49.4X5	T49.4X6
analgesics NEC	T39.2X1	T39.2X2	T39.2X3	T39.2X4	T39.2X5	T39.2X6
naphtha (solvent)	T52.0X1	T52.0X2	T52.0X3	T52.0X4	—	—
Coartem*	T37.2X1	T37.2X2	T37.2X3	T37.2X4	T37.2X5	T37.2X6
Cobalamine	T45.2X1	T45.2X2	T45.2X3	T45.2X4	T45.2X5	T45.2X6
Cobalt (nonmedicinal) (fumes)	T56.891	T56.892	T56.893	T56.894	—	—
(industrial)						
medicinal (trace) (chloride)	T45.8X1	T45.8X2	T45.8X3	T45.8X4	T45.8X5	T45.8X6
Cobra (venom)	T63.041	T63.042	T63.043	T63.044	—	—
Coca (leaf)	T40.5X1	T40.5X2	T40.5X3	T40.5X4	T40.5X5	T40.5X6
Cocaine	T40.5X1	T40.5X2	T40.5X3	T40.5X4	T40.5X5	T40.5X6
topical anesthetic	T41.3X1	T41.3X2	T41.3X3	T41.3X4	T41.3X5	T41.3X6
Cocarboxylase	T45.3X1	T45.3X2	T45.3X3	T45.3X4	T45.3X5	T45.3X6
Coccidioidin	T50.8X1	T50.8X2	T50.8X3	T50.8X4	T50.8X5	T50.8X6
Cocculus indicus	T62.1X1	T62.1X2	T62.1X3	T62.1X4	—	—
Cochineal	T65.6X1	T65.6X2	T65.6X3	T65.6X4	—	—
medicinal products	T50.991	T50.992	T50.993	T50.994	T50.995	T50.996
Codeine	T40.2X1	T40.2X2	T40.2X3	T40.2X4	T40.2X5	T40.2X6
Cod-liver oil	T45.2X1	T45.2X2	T45.2X3	T45.2X4	T45.2X5	T45.2X6
Coenzyme A	T50.991	T50.992	T50.993	T50.994	T50.995	T50.996
Coffee	T62.8X1	T62.8X2	T62.8X3	T62.8X4	—	—
Cogalactoisomerase	T50.991	T50.992	T50.993	T50.994	T50.995	T50.996
Cogentin	T44.3X1	T44.3X2	T44.3X3	T44.3X4	T44.3X5	T44.3X6
Coke fumes or gas (carbon monoxide)	T58.2X1	T58.2X2	T58.2X3	T58.2X4		
industrial use	T58.8X1	T58.8X2	T58.8X3	T58.8X4		
Colace	T47.4X1	T47.4X2	T47.4X3	T47.4X4	T47.4X5	T47.4X6
Colaspase	T45.1X1	T45.1X2	T45.1X3	T45.1X4	T45.1X5	T45.1X6
Colazal*	T47.8X1	T47.8X2	T47.8X3	T47.8X4	T47.8X5	T47.8X6
Colchicine	T50.4X1	T50.4X2	T50.4X3	T50.4X4	T50.4X5	T50.4X6
Colchicum	T62.2X1	T62.2X2	T62.2X3	T62.2X4	—	—
Cold cream	T49.3X1	T49.3X2	T49.3X3	T49.3X4	T49.3X5	T49.3X6
Colecalciferol	T45.2X1	T45.2X2	T45.2X3	T45.2X4	T45.2X5	T45.2X6
Colestipol	T46.6X1	T46.6X2	T46.6X3	T46.6X4	T46.6X5	T46.6X6
Colestyramine	T46.6X1	T46.6X2	T46.6X3	T46.6X4	T46.6X5	T46.6X6
Colimycin	T36.8X1	T36.8X2	T36.8X3	T36.8X4	T36.8X5	T36.8X6
Colistimethate	T36.8X1	T36.8X2	T36.8X3	T36.8X4	T36.8X5	T36.8X6
Colistin	T36.8X1	T36.8X2	T36.8X3	T36.8X4	T36.8X5	T36.8X6
sulfate (eye preparation)	T49.5X1	T49.5X2	T49.5X3	T49.5X4	T49.5X5	T49.5X6
Collagen	T50.991	T50.992	T50.993	T50.994	T50.995	T50.996
Collagenase	T49.4X1	T49.4X2	T49.4X3	T49.4X4	T49.4X5	T49.4X6
Collodion	T49.3X1	T49.3X2	T49.3X3	T49.3X4	T49.3X5	T49.3X6
Colocynth	T47.2X1	T47.2X2	T47.2X3	T47.2X4	T47.2X5	T47.2X6
Colophony adhesive	T49.3X1	T49.3X2	T49.3X3	T49.3X4	T49.3X5	T49.3X6
Colorant — see also Dye	T50.991	T50.992	T50.993	T50.994	T50.995	T50.996
Coloring matter — see Dye(s)						
Combustion gas (after combustion) — see Carbon, monoxide						
prior to combustion	T59.891	T59.892	T59.893	T59.894	—	—
Cometriq*	T45.1X1	T45.1X2	T45.1X3	T45.1X4	T45.1X5	T45.1X6
Compazine	T43.3X1	T43.3X2	T43.3X3	T43.3X4	T43.3X5	T43.3X6
Compound						
1080 (sodium fluoroacetate)	T60.4X1	T60.4X2	T60.4X3	T60.4X4		
269 (endrin)	T60.1X1	T60.1X2	T60.1X3	T60.1X4		
3422 (parathion)	T60.0X1	T60.0X2	T60.0X3	T60.0X4		
3911 (phorate)	T60.0X1	T60.0X2	T60.0X3	T60.0X4		
3956 (toxaphene)	T60.1X1	T60.1X2	T60.1X3	T60.1X4		

☑ Additional Character May Be Required — Refer to the Tabular List for Character Selection

*Optum Value-Add

Substance	Poisoning, Accidental (unintentional)	Poisoning, Intentional Self-harm	Poisoning, Assault	Poisoning, Undetermined	Adverse Effect	Underdosing
Compound — *continued*						
4049 (malathion)	T60.0X1	T60.0X2	T60.0X3	T60.0X4	—	—
4069 (malathion)	T60.0X1	T60.0X2	T60.0X3	T60.0X4	—	—
4124 (dicapthon)	T60.0X1	T60.0X2	T60.0X3	T60.0X4	—	—
42 (warfarin)	T60.4X1	T60.4X2	T60.4X3	T60.4X4	—	—
497 (dieldrin)	T60.1X1	T60.1X2	T60.1X3	T60.1X4	—	—
E (cortisone)	T38.0X1	T38.0X2	T38.0X3	T38.0X4	T38.0X5	T38.0X6
F (hydrocortisone)	T38.0X1	T38.0X2	T38.0X3	T38.0X4	T38.0X5	T38.0X6
Comvax*	T50.A21	T50.A22	T50.A23	T50.A24	T50.A25	T50.A26
Congener, anabolic	T38.7X1	T38.7X2	T38.7X3	T38.7X4	T38.7X5	T38.7X6
Congo red	T50.8X1	T50.8X2	T50.8X3	T50.8X4	T50.8X5	T50.8X6
Coniine, conine	T62.2X1	T62.2X2	T62.2X3	T62.2X4	—	—
Conium (maculatum)	T62.2X1	T62.2X2	T62.2X3	T62.2X4	—	—
Conjugated estrogenic substances	T38.5X1	T38.5X2	T38.5X3	T38.5X4	T38.5X5	T38.5X6
Contac	T48.5X1	T48.5X2	T48.5X3	T48.5X4	T48.5X5	T48.5X6
Contact lens solution	T49.5X1	T49.5X2	T49.5X3	T49.5X4	T49.5X5	T49.5X6
Contraceptive (oral)	T38.4X1	T38.4X2	T38.4X3	T38.4X4	T38.4X5	T38.4X6
vaginal	T49.8X1	T49.8X2	T49.8X3	T49.8X4	T49.8X5	T49.8X6
Contrast medium, radiography	T50.8X1	T50.8X2	T50.8X3	T50.8X4	T50.8X5	T50.8X6
Convallaria glycosides	T46.0X1	T46.0X2	T46.0X3	T46.0X4	T46.0X5	T46.0X6
Convallaria majalis	T62.2X1	T62.2X2	T62.2X3	T62.2X4	—	—
berry	T62.1X1	T62.1X2	T62.1X3	T62.1X4	—	—
Copperhead snake (bite) (venom)	T63.061	T63.062	T63.063	T63.064	—	—
Copper (dust) (fumes) (nonmedicinal) **NEC**	T56.4X1	T56.4X2	T56.4X3	T56.4X4	—	—
arsenate, arsenite	T57.0X1	T57.0X2	T57.0X3	T57.0X4	—	—
insecticide	T60.2X1	T60.2X2	T60.2X3	T60.2X4	—	—
emetic	T47.7X1	T47.7X2	T47.7X3	T47.7X4	T47.7X5	T47.7X6
fungicide	T60.3X1	T60.3X2	T60.3X3	T60.3X4	—	—
gluconate	T49.0X1	T49.0X2	T49.0X3	T49.0X4	T49.0X5	T49.0X6
insecticide	T60.2X1	T60.2X2	T60.2X3	T60.2X4	—	—
medicinal (trace)	T45.8X1	T45.8X2	T45.8X3	T45.8X4	T45.8X5	T45.8X6
oleate	T49.0X1	T49.0X2	T49.0X3	T49.0X4	T49.0X5	T49.0X6
sulfate	T56.4X1	T56.4X2	T56.4X3	T56.4X4	—	—
cupric	T56.4X1	T56.4X2	T56.4X3	T56.4X4	—	—
fungicide	T60.3X1	T60.3X2	T60.3X3	T60.3X4	—	—
medicinal						
ear	T49.6X1	T49.6X2	T49.6X3	T49.6X4	T49.6X5	T49.6X6
emetic	T47.7X1	T47.7X2	T47.7X3	T47.7X4	T47.7X5	T47.7X6
eye	T49.5X1	T49.5X2	T49.5X3	T49.5X4	T49.5X5	T49.5X6
cuprous	T56.4X1	T56.4X2	T56.4X3	T56.4X4	—	—
fungicide	T60.3X1	T60.3X2	T60.3X3	T60.3X4	—	—
medicinal						
ear	T49.6X1	T49.6X2	T49.6X3	T49.6X4	T49.6X5	T49.6X6
emetic	T47.7X1	T47.7X2	T47.7X3	T47.7X4	T47.7X5	T47.7X6
eye	T49.5X1	T49.5X2	T49.5X3	T49.5X4	T49.5X5	T49.5X6
Coral (sting)	T63.691	T63.692	T63.693	T63.694	—	—
snake (bite) (venom)	T63.021	T63.022	T63.023	T63.024	—	—
Corbadrine	T49.6X1	T49.6X2	T49.6X3	T49.6X4	T49.6X5	T49.6X6
Cordite	T65.891	T65.892	T65.893	T65.894	—	—
vapor	T59.891	T59.892	T59.893	T59.894	—	—
Cordran	T49.0X1	T49.0X2	T49.0X3	T49.0X4	T49.0X5	T49.0X6
Coreg*	T44.7X1	T44.7X2	T44.7X3	T44.7X4	T44.7X5	T44.7X6
Cormax*	T49.0X1	T49.0X2	T49.0X3	T49.0X4	T49.0X5	T49.0X6
Corn cures	T49.4X1	T49.4X2	T49.4X3	T49.4X4	T49.4X5	T49.4X6
Cornhusker's lotion	T49.3X1	T49.3X2	T49.3X3	T49.3X4	T49.3X5	T49.3X6
Corn starch	T49.3X1	T49.3X2	T49.3X3	T49.3X4	T49.3X5	T49.3X6
Coronary vasodilator NEC	T46.3X1	T46.3X2	T46.3X3	T46.3X4	T46.3X5	T46.3X6
Corrosive NEC	T54.91	T54.92	T54.93	T54.94	—	—
acid NEC	T54.2X1	T54.2X2	T54.2X3	T54.2X4	—	—
aromatics	T54.1X1	T54.1X2	T54.1X3	T54.1X4	—	—
disinfectant	T54.1X1	T54.1X2	T54.1X3	T54.1X4	—	—
fumes NEC	T54.91	T54.92	T54.93	T54.94	—	—
specified NEC	T54.91	T54.92	T54.93	T54.94	—	—
sublimate	T56.1X1	T56.1X2	T56.1X3	T56.1X4	—	—
Cortate	T38.0X1	T38.0X2	T38.0X3	T38.0X4	T38.0X5	T38.0X6
Cort-Dome	T38.0X1	T38.0X2	T38.0X3	T38.0X4	T38.0X5	T38.0X6
ENT agent	T49.6X1	T49.6X2	T49.6X3	T49.6X4	T49.6X5	T49.6X6
ophthalmic preparation	T49.5X1	T49.5X2	T49.5X3	T49.5X4	T49.5X5	T49.5X6
topical NEC	T49.0X1	T49.0X2	T49.0X3	T49.0X4	T49.0X5	T49.0X6
Cortef	T38.0X1	T38.0X2	T38.0X3	T38.0X4	T38.0X5	T38.0X6
ENT agent	T49.6X1	T49.6X2	T49.6X3	T49.6X4	T49.6X5	T49.6X6
ophthalmic preparation	T49.5X1	T49.5X2	T49.5X3	T49.5X4	T49.5X5	T49.5X6
topical NEC	T49.0X1	T49.0X2	T49.0X3	T49.0X4	T49.0X5	T49.0X6
Corticosteroid	T38.0X1	T38.0X2	T38.0X3	T38.0X4	T38.0X5	T38.0X6
ENT agent	T49.6X1	T49.6X2	T49.6X3	T49.6X4	T49.6X5	T49.6X6
mineral	T50.0X1	T50.0X2	T50.0X3	T50.0X4	T50.0X5	T50.0X6
ophthalmic	T49.5X1	T49.5X2	T49.5X3	T49.5X4	T49.5X5	T49.5X6
topical NEC	T49.0X1	T49.0X2	T49.0X3	T49.0X4	T49.0X5	T49.0X6
Corticotropin	T38.811	T38.812	T38.813	T38.814	T38.815	T38.816
Cortisol	T49.0X1	T49.0X2	T49.0X3	T49.0X4	T49.0X5	T49.0X6
ENT agent	T49.6X1	T49.6X2	T49.6X3	T49.6X4	T49.6X5	T49.6X6
ophthalmic preparation	T49.5X1	T49.5X2	T49.5X3	T49.5X4	T49.5X5	T49.5X6
topical NEC	T49.0X1	T49.0X2	T49.0X3	T49.0X4	T49.0X5	T49.0X6
Cortisone (acetate)	T38.0X1	T38.0X2	T38.0X3	T38.0X4	T38.0X5	T38.0X6
ENT agent	T49.6X1	T49.6X2	T49.6X3	T49.6X4	T49.6X5	T49.6X6
ophthalmic preparation	T49.5X1	T49.5X2	T49.5X3	T49.5X4	T49.5X5	T49.5X6
topical NEC	T49.0X1	T49.0X2	T49.0X3	T49.0X4	T49.0X5	T49.0X6
Cortisporin*	T49.0X1	T49.0X2	T49.0X3	T49.0X4	T49.0X5	T49.0X6
Cortivazol	T38.0X1	T38.0X2	T38.0X3	T38.0X4	T38.0X5	T38.0X6
Cortogen	T38.0X1	T38.0X2	T38.0X3	T38.0X4	T38.0X5	T38.0X6
ENT agent	T49.6X1	T49.6X2	T49.6X3	T49.6X4	T49.6X5	T49.6X6
ophthalmic preparation	T49.5X1	T49.5X2	T49.5X3	T49.5X4	T49.5X5	T49.5X6
Cortone	T38.0X1	T38.0X2	T38.0X3	T38.0X4	T38.0X5	T38.0X6
ENT agent	T49.6X1	T49.6X2	T49.6X3	T49.6X4	T49.6X5	T49.6X6
ophthalmic preparation	T49.5X1	T49.5X2	T49.5X3	T49.5X4	T49.5X5	T49.5X6
Cortril	T38.0X1	T38.0X2	T38.0X3	T38.0X4	T38.0X5	T38.0X6
ENT agent	T49.6X1	T49.6X2	T49.6X3	T49.6X4	T49.6X5	T49.6X6
ophthalmic preparation	T49.5X1	T49.5X2	T49.5X3	T49.5X4	T49.5X5	T49.5X6
topical NEC	T49.0X1	T49.0X2	T49.0X3	T49.0X4	T49.0X5	T49.0X6
Corynebacterium parvum	T45.1X1	T45.1X2	T45.1X3	T45.1X4	T45.1X5	T45.1X6
Cosmetic preparation	T49.8X1	T49.8X2	T49.8X3	T49.8X4	T49.8X5	T49.8X6
Cosmetics	T49.8X1	T49.8X2	T49.8X3	T49.8X4	T49.8X5	T49.8X6
Cosyntropin	T38.811	T38.812	T38.813	T38.814	T38.815	T38.816
Cotarnine	T45.7X1	T45.7X2	T45.7X3	T45.7X4	T45.7X5	T45.7X6
Co-trimoxazole	T36.8X1	T36.8X2	T36.8X3	T36.8X4	T36.8X5	T36.8X6
Cottonseed oil	T49.3X1	T49.3X2	T49.3X3	T49.3X4	T49.3X5	T49.3X6
Cough mixture (syrup)	T48.4X1	T48.4X2	T48.4X3	T48.4X4	T48.4X5	T48.4X6
containing opiates	T40.2X1	T40.2X2	T40.2X3	T40.2X4	T40.2X5	T40.2X6
expectorants	T48.4X1	T48.4X2	T48.4X3	T48.4X4	T48.4X5	T48.4X6
Coumadin	T45.511	T45.512	T45.513	T45.514	T45.515	T45.516
rodenticide	T60.4X1	T60.4X2	T60.4X3	T60.4X4	—	—
Coumaphos	T60.0X1	T60.0X2	T60.0X3	T60.0X4	—	—
Coumarin	T45.511	T45.512	T45.513	T45.514	T45.515	T45.516
Coumetarol	T45.511	T45.512	T45.513	T45.514	T45.515	T45.516
Cowbane	T62.2X1	T62.2X2	T62.2X3	T62.2X4	—	—
Cozaar*	T46.5X1	T46.5X2	T46.5X3	T46.5X4	T46.5X5	T46.5X6
Cozyme	T45.2X1	T45.2X2	T45.2X3	T45.2X4	T45.2X5	T45.2X6
Crack	T40.5X1	T40.5X2	T40.5X3	T40.5X4	—	—
Crataegus extract	T46.0X1	T46.0X2	T46.0X3	T46.0X4	T46.0X5	T46.0X6
Creolin	T54.1X1	T54.1X2	T54.1X3	T54.1X4	—	—
disinfectant	T54.1X1	T54.1X2	T54.1X3	T54.1X4	—	—
Creosol (compound)	T49.0X1	T49.0X2	T49.0X3	T49.0X4	T49.0X5	T49.0X6
Creosote (coal tar) (beechwood)	T49.0X1	T49.0X2	T49.0X3	T49.0X4	T49.0X5	T49.0X6
medicinal (expectorant)	T48.4X1	T48.4X2	T48.4X3	T48.4X4	T48.4X5	T48.4X6
syrup	T48.4X1	T48.4X2	T48.4X3	T48.4X4	T48.4X5	T48.4X6
Cresol(s)	T49.0X1	T49.0X2	T49.0X3	T49.0X4	T49.0X5	T49.0X6
and soap solution	T49.0X1	T49.0X2	T49.0X3	T49.0X4	T49.0X5	T49.0X6
Crestor*	T46.6X1	T46.6X2	T46.6X3	T46.6X4	T46.6X5	T46.6X6
Cresyl acetate	T49.0X1	T49.0X2	T49.0X3	T49.0X4	T49.0X5	T49.0X6
Cresylic acid	T49.0X1	T49.0X2	T49.0X3	T49.0X4	T49.0X5	T49.0X6
Crimidine	T60.4X1	T60.4X2	T60.4X3	T60.4X4	—	—
Croconazole	T37.8X1	T37.8X2	T37.8X3	T37.8X4	T37.8X5	T37.8X6
Cromoglicic acid	T48.6X1	T48.6X2	T48.6X3	T48.6X4	T48.6X5	T48.6X6
Cromolyn	T48.6X1	T48.6X2	T48.6X3	T48.6X4	T48.6X5	T48.6X6
Cromonar	T46.3X1	T46.3X2	T46.3X3	T46.3X4	T46.3X5	T46.3X6
Cropropamide	T39.8X1	T39.8X2	T39.8X3	T39.8X4	T39.8X5	T39.8X6
with crotethamide	T50.7X1	T50.7X2	T50.7X3	T50.7X4	T50.7X5	T50.7X6
Crotamiton	T49.0X1	T49.0X2	T49.0X3	T49.0X4	T49.0X5	T49.0X6
Crotethamide	T39.8X1	T39.8X2	T39.8X3	T39.8X4	T39.8X5	T39.8X6
with cropropamide	T50.7X1	T50.7X2	T50.7X3	T50.7X4	T50.7X5	T50.7X6
Croton (oil)	T47.2X1	T47.2X2	T47.2X3	T47.2X4	T47.2X5	T47.2X6
chloral	T42.6X1	T42.6X2	T42.6X3	T42.6X4	T42.6X5	T42.6X6
Crude oil	T52.0X1	T52.0X2	T52.0X3	T52.0X4	—	—
Cryogenine	T39.8X1	T39.8X2	T39.8X3	T39.8X4	T39.8X5	T39.8X6
Cryolite (vapor)	T60.1X1	T60.1X2	T60.1X3	T60.1X4	—	—
insecticide	T60.1X1	T60.1X2	T60.1X3	T60.1X4	—	—
Cryptenamine (tannates)	T46.5X1	T46.5X2	T46.5X3	T46.5X4	T46.5X5	T46.5X6
Crystal violet	T49.0X1	T49.0X2	T49.0X3	T49.0X4	T49.0X5	T49.0X6
Cuckoopint	T62.2X1	T62.2X2	T62.2X3	T62.2X4	—	—
Cumetharol	T45.511	T45.512	T45.513	T45.514	T45.515	T45.516
Cupric						
acetate	T60.3X1	T60.3X2	T60.3X3	T60.3X4	—	—
acetoarsenite	T57.0X1	T57.0X2	T57.0X3	T57.0X4	—	—
arsenate	T57.0X1	T57.0X2	T57.0X3	T57.0X4	—	—
gluconate	T49.0X1	T49.0X2	T49.0X3	T49.0X4	T49.0X5	T49.0X6
oleate	T49.0X1	T49.0X2	T49.0X3	T49.0X4	T49.0X5	T49.0X6
sulfate	T56.4X1	T56.4X2	T56.4X3	T56.4X4	—	—
Cuprimine*	T50.6X1	T50.6X2	T50.6X3	T50.6X4	T50.6X5	T50.6X6
Cuprous sulfate — *see also* Copper, sulfate	T56.4X1	T56.4X2	T56.4X3	T56.4X4	—	—
Curare, curarine	T48.1X1	T48.1X2	T48.1X3	T48.1X4	T48.1X5	T48.1X6

Table of Drugs and Chemicals

Compound — Curare, curarine

Table of Drugs and Chemicals

Cyamemazine — Depressant

Substance	Poisoning, Accidental (unintentional)	Poisoning, Intentional Self-harm	Poisoning, Assault	Poisoning, Undetermined	Adverse Effect	Under-dosing
Cyamemazine	T43.3X1	T43.3X2	T43.3X3	T43.3X4	T43.3X5	T43.3X6
Cyamopsis tetragonoloba	T46.6X1	T46.6X2	T46.6X3	T46.6X4	T46.6X5	T46.6X6
Cyanacetic hydrazide	T37.1X1	T37.1X2	T37.1X3	T37.1X4	—	T37.1X6
Cyanic acid (gas)	T59.891	T59.892	T59.893	T59.894	—	—
Cyanide(s) (compounds) (potassium) (sodium)	T65.0X1	T65.0X2	T65.0X3	T65.0X4	—	—
NEC						
dust or gas (inhalation) NEC	T57.3X1	T57.3X2	T57.3X3	T57.3X4	—	—
fumigant	T65.0X1	T65.0X2	T65.0X3	T65.0X4	—	—
hydrogen	T57.3X1	T57.3X2	T57.3X3	T57.3X4	—	—
mercuric — see Mercury						
pesticide (dust) (fumes)	T65.0X1	T65.0X2	T65.0X3	T65.0X4	—	—
Cyanoacrylate adhesive	T49.3X1	T49.3X2	T49.3X3	T49.3X4	T49.3X5	T49.3X6
Cyanocobalamin	T45.8X1	T45.8X2	T45.8X3	T45.8X4	T45.8X5	T45.8X6
Cyanogen (chloride) (gas)	T59.891	T59.892	T59.893	T59.894	—	—
NEC						
Cyclacillin	T36.0X1	T36.0X2	T36.0X3	T36.0X4	T36.0X5	T36.0X6
Cyclaine	T41.3X1	T41.3X2	T41.3X3	T41.3X4	T41.3X5	T41.3X6
Cyclamate	T50.991	T50.992	T50.993	T50.994	T50.995	T50.996
Cyclamen europaeum	T62.2X1	T62.2X2	T62.2X3	T62.2X4	—	—
Cyclandelate	T46.7X1	T46.7X2	T46.7X3	T46.7X4	T46.7X5	T46.7X6
Cyclazocine	T50.7X1	T50.7X2	T50.7X3	T50.7X4	T50.7X5	T50.7X6
Cyclizine	T45.0X1	T45.0X2	T45.0X3	T45.0X4	T45.0X5	T45.0X6
Cyclobarbital	T42.3X1	T42.3X2	T42.3X3	T42.3X4	T42.3X5	T42.3X6
Cyclobarbitone	T42.3X1	T42.3X2	T42.3X3	T42.3X4	T42.3X5	T42.3X6
Cyclobenzaprine	T48.1X1	T48.1X2	T48.1X3	T48.1X4	T48.1X5	T48.1X6
Cyclodrine	T44.3X1	T44.3X2	T44.3X3	T44.3X4	T44.3X5	T44.3X6
Cycloguanil embonate	T37.2X1	T37.2X2	T37.2X3	T37.2X4	T37.2X5	T37.2X6
Cyclohexane	T52.8X1	T52.8X2	T52.8X3	T52.8X4	—	—
Cyclohexanol	T51.8X1	T51.8X2	T51.8X3	T51.8X4	—	—
Cyclohexanone	T52.4X1	T52.4X2	T52.4X3	T52.4X4	—	—
Cycloheximide	T60.3X1	T60.3X2	T60.3X3	T60.3X4	—	—
Cyclohexyl acetate	T52.8X1	T52.8X2	T52.8X3	T52.8X4	—	—
Cycloleucin	T45.1X1	T45.1X2	T45.1X3	T45.1X4	T45.1X5	T45.1X6
Cyclomethycaine	T41.3X1	T41.3X2	T41.3X3	T41.3X4	T41.3X5	T41.3X6
Cyclopentamine	T44.4X1	T44.4X2	T44.4X3	T44.4X4	T44.4X5	T44.4X6
Cyclopenthiazide	T50.2X1	T50.2X2	T50.2X3	T50.2X4	T50.2X5	T50.2X6
Cyclopentolate	T44.3X1	T44.3X2	T44.3X3	T44.3X4	T44.3X5	T44.3X6
Cyclophosphamide	T45.1X1	T45.1X2	T45.1X3	T45.1X4	T45.1X5	T45.1X6
Cycloplegic drug	T49.5X1	T49.5X2	T49.5X3	T49.5X4	T49.5X5	T49.5X6
Cyclopropane	T41.291	T41.292	T41.293	T41.294	T41.295	T41.296
Cyclopyrabital	T39.8X1	T39.8X2	T39.8X3	T39.8X4	T39.8X5	T39.8X6
Cycloserine	T37.1X1	T37.1X2	T37.1X3	T37.1X4	T37.1X5	T37.1X6
Cyclosporin	T45.1X1	T45.1X2	T45.1X3	T45.1X4	T45.1X5	T45.1X6
Cyclothiazide	T50.2X1	T50.2X2	T50.2X3	T50.2X4	T50.2X5	T50.2X6
Cycrimine	T44.3X1	T44.3X2	T44.3X3	T44.3X4	T44.3X5	T44.3X6
Cyhalothrin	T60.1X1	T60.1X2	T60.1X3	T60.1X4	—	—
Cymarin	T46.0X1	T46.0X2	T46.0X3	T46.0X4	T46.0X5	T46.0X6
Cymbalta*	T43.221	T43.222	T43.223	T43.224	T43.225	T43.226
Cypermethrin	T60.1X1	T60.1X2	T60.1X3	T60.1X4	—	—
Cyphenothrin	T60.2X1	T60.2X2	T60.2X3	T60.2X4	—	—
Cyproheptadine	T45.0X1	T45.0X2	T45.0X3	T45.0X4	T45.0X5	T45.0X6
Cyproterone	T38.6X1	T38.6X2	T38.6X3	T38.6X4	T38.6X5	T38.6X6
Cystaran*	T49.5X1	T49.5X2	T49.5X3	T49.5X4	T49.5X5	T49.5X6
Cysteamine	T50.6X1	T50.6X2	T50.6X3	T50.6X4	T50.6X5	T50.6X6
Cytarabine	T45.1X1	T45.1X2	T45.1X3	T45.1X4	T45.1X5	T45.1X6
Cytisus						
laburnum	T62.2X1	T62.2X2	T62.2X3	T62.2X4	—	—
scoparius	T62.2X1	T62.2X2	T62.2X3	T62.2X4	—	—
Cytochrome C	T47.5X1	T47.5X2	T47.5X3	T47.5X4	T47.5X5	T47.5X6
Cytomel	T38.1X1	T38.1X2	T38.1X3	T38.1X4	T38.1X5	T38.1X6
Cytosine arabinoside	T45.1X1	T45.1X2	T45.1X3	T45.1X4	T45.1X5	T45.1X6
Cytoxan	T45.1X1	T45.1X2	T45.1X3	T45.1X4	T45.1X5	T45.1X6
Cytozyme	T45.7X1	T45.7X2	T45.7X3	T45.7X4	T45.7X5	T45.7X6
S-Carboxymethylcysteine	T48.4X1	T48.4X2	T48.4X3	T48.4X4	T48.4X5	T48.4X6
Dabigatran*	T45.511	T45.512	T45.513	T45.514	T45.515	T45.516
Dacarbazine	T45.1X1	T45.1X2	T45.1X3	T45.1X4	T45.1X5	T45.1X6
Dactinomycin	T45.1X1	T45.1X2	T45.1X3	T45.1X4	T45.1X5	T45.1X6
DADPS	T37.1X1	T37.1X2	T37.1X3	T37.1X4	T37.1X5	T37.1X6
Dakin's solution	T49.0X1	T49.0X2	T49.0X3	T49.0X4	T49.0X5	T49.0X6
Dalapon (sodium)	T60.3X1	T60.3X2	T60.3X3	T60.3X4	—	—
Dalmane	T42.4X1	T42.4X2	T42.4X3	T42.4X4	T42.4X5	T42.4X6
Danazol	T38.6X1	T38.6X2	T38.6X3	T38.6X4	T38.6X5	T38.6X6
Danilone	T45.511	T45.512	T45.513	T45.514	T45.515	T45.516
Danthron	T47.2X1	T47.2X2	T47.2X3	T47.2X4	T47.2X5	T47.2X6
Dantrolene	T42.8X1	T42.8X2	T42.8X3	T42.8X4	T42.8X5	T42.8X6
Dantron	T47.2X1	T47.2X2	T47.2X3	T47.2X4	T47.2X5	T47.2X6
Daphne (gnidium) (mezereum)	T62.2X1	T62.2X2	T62.2X3	T62.2X4	—	—
berry	T62.1X1	T62.1X2	T62.1X3	T62.1X4	—	—
Dapsone	T37.1X1	T37.1X2	T37.1X3	T37.1X4	T37.1X5	T37.1X6
Daraprim	T37.2X1	T37.2X2	T37.2X3	T37.2X4	T37.2X5	T37.2X6

Substance	Poisoning, Accidental (unintentional)	Poisoning, Intentional Self-harm	Poisoning, Assault	Poisoning, Undetermined	Adverse Effect	Under-dosing
Darnel	T62.2X1	T62.2X2	T62.2X3	T62.2X4	—	—
Darvon	T39.8X1	T39.8X2	T39.8X3	T39.8X4	T39.8X5	T39.8X6
Daunomycin	T45.1X1	T45.1X2	T45.1X3	T45.1X4	T45.1X5	T45.1X6
Daunorubicin	T45.1X1	T45.1X2	T45.1X3	T45.1X4	T45.1X5	T45.1X6
DBI	T38.3X1	T38.3X2	T38.3X3	T38.3X4	T38.3X5	T38.3X6
D-Con	T60.91	T60.92	T60.93	T60.94	—	—
insecticide	T60.2X1	T60.2X2	T60.2X3	T60.2X4	—	—
rodenticide	T60.4X1	T60.4X2	T60.4X3	T60.4X4	—	—
DDAVP	T38.891	T38.892	T38.893	T38.894	T38.895	T38.896
DDE (bis(chlorophenyl)-dichloroethylene)	T60.2X1	T60.2X2	T60.2X3	T60.2X4	—	—
DDS	T37.1X1	T37.1X2	T37.1X3	T37.1X4	T37.1X5	T37.1X6
DDT (dust)	T60.1X1	T60.1X2	T60.1X3	T60.1X4	—	—
Deadly nightshade — see also Belladonna						
berry	T62.1X1	T62.1X2	T62.1X3	T62.1X4	—	—
Deamino-D-arginine vasopressin	T38.891	T38.892	T38.893	T38.894	T38.895	T38.896
Deanol (aceglumate)	T50.991	T50.992	T50.993	T50.994	T50.995	T50.996
Debrisoquine	T46.5X1	T46.5X2	T46.5X3	T46.5X4	T46.5X5	T46.5X6
Decaborane	T57.8X1	T57.8X2	T57.8X3	T57.8X4	—	—
fumes	T59.891	T59.892	T59.893	T59.894	—	—
Decadron	T38.0X1	T38.0X2	T38.0X3	T38.0X4	T38.0X5	T38.0X6
ENT agent	T49.6X1	T49.6X2	T49.6X3	T49.6X4	T49.6X5	T49.6X6
ophthalmic preparation	T49.5X1	T49.5X2	T49.5X3	T49.5X4	T49.5X5	T49.5X6
topical NEC	T49.0X1	T49.0X2	T49.0X3	T49.0X4	T49.0X5	T49.0X6
Decahydronaphthalene	T52.8X1	T52.8X2	T52.8X3	T52.8X4	—	—
Decalin	T52.8X1	T52.8X2	T52.8X3	T52.8X4	—	—
Decamethonium (bromide)	T48.1X1	T48.1X2	T48.1X3	T48.1X4	T48.1X5	T48.1X6
Decholin	T47.5X1	T47.5X2	T47.5X3	T47.5X4	T47.5X5	T47.5X6
Declomycin	T36.4X1	T36.4X2	T36.4X3	T36.4X4	T36.4X5	T36.4X6
Decongestant, nasal (mucosa)	T48.5X1	T48.5X2	T48.5X3	T48.5X4	T48.5X5	T48.5X6
combination	T48.5X1	T48.5X2	T48.5X3	T48.5X4	T48.5X5	T48.5X6
Deet	T60.8X1	T60.8X2	T60.8X3	T60.8X4	—	—
Deferoxamine	T45.8X1	T45.8X2	T45.8X3	T45.8X4	T45.8X5	T45.8X6
Deflazacort	T38.0X1	T38.0X2	T38.0X3	T38.0X4	T38.0X5	T38.0X6
Deglycyrrhizinized extract of licorice	T48.4X1	T48.4X2	T48.4X3	T48.4X4	T48.4X5	T48.4X6
Dehydrocholic acid	T47.5X1	T47.5X2	T47.5X3	T47.5X4	T47.5X5	T47.5X6
Dehydroemetine	T37.3X1	T37.3X2	T37.3X3	T37.3X4	T37.3X5	T37.3X6
Dekalin	T52.8X1	T52.8X2	T52.8X3	T52.8X4	—	—
Delafloxacin*	T36.8X1	T36.8X2	T36.8X3	T36.8X4	T36.8X5	T36.8X6
Delalutin	T38.5X1	T38.5X2	T38.5X3	T38.5X4	T38.5X5	T38.5X6
Delorazepam	T42.4X1	T42.4X2	T42.4X3	T42.4X4	T42.4X5	T42.4X6
Delphinium	T62.2X1	T62.2X2	T62.2X3	T62.2X4	—	—
Deltacortisone*	T38.0X1	T38.0X2	T38.0X3	T38.0X4	T38.0X5	T38.0X6
Deltamethrin	T60.1X1	T60.1X2	T60.1X3	T60.1X4	—	—
Deltasone	T38.0X1	T38.0X2	T38.0X3	T38.0X4	T38.0X5	T38.0X6
Deltra	T38.0X1	T38.0X2	T38.0X3	T38.0X4	T38.0X5	T38.0X6
Delvinal	T42.3X1	T42.3X2	T42.3X3	T42.3X4	T42.3X5	T42.3X6
Demecarium (bromide)	T49.5X1	T49.5X2	T49.5X3	T49.5X4	T49.5X5	T49.5X6
Demeclocycline	T36.4X1	T36.4X2	T36.4X3	T36.4X4	T36.4X5	T36.4X6
Demecolcine	T45.1X1	T45.1X2	T45.1X3	T45.1X4	T45.1X5	T45.1X6
Demegestone	T38.5X1	T38.5X2	T38.5X3	T38.5X4	T38.5X5	T38.5X6
Demelanizing agents	T49.8X1	T49.8X2	T49.8X3	T49.8X4	T49.8X5	T49.8X6
Demephion -O and -S	T60.0X1	T60.0X2	T60.0X3	T60.0X4	—	—
Demerol	T40.2X1	T40.2X2	T40.2X3	T40.2X4	T40.2X5	T40.2X6
Demethylchlortetracycline	T36.4X1	T36.4X2	T36.4X3	T36.4X4	T36.4X5	T36.4X6
Demethyltetracycline	T36.4X1	T36.4X2	T36.4X3	T36.4X4	T36.4X5	T36.4X6
Demeton -O and -S	T60.0X1	T60.0X2	T60.0X3	T60.0X4	—	—
Demulcent (external)	T49.3X1	T49.3X2	T49.3X3	T49.3X4	T49.3X5	T49.3X6
specified NEC	T49.3X1	T49.3X2	T49.3X3	T49.3X4	T49.3X5	T49.3X6
Demulen	T38.4X1	T38.4X2	T38.4X3	T38.4X4	T38.4X5	T38.4X6
Denatured alcohol	T51.0X1	T51.0X2	T51.0X3	T51.0X4	—	—
Dendrid	T49.5X1	T49.5X2	T49.5X3	T49.5X4	T49.5X5	T49.5X6
Dental drug, topical application NEC	T49.7X1	T49.7X2	T49.7X3	T49.7X4	T49.7X5	T49.7X6
Dentifrice	T49.7X1	T49.7X2	T49.7X3	T49.7X4	T49.7X5	T49.7X6
Deodorant spray (feminine hygiene)	T49.8X1	T49.8X2	T49.8X3	T49.8X4	T49.8X5	T49.8X6
Deoxycortone	T50.0X1	T50.0X2	T50.0X3	T50.0X4	T50.0X5	T50.0X6
Deoxyribonuclease (pancreatic)	T45.3X1	T45.3X2	T45.3X3	T45.3X4	T45.3X5	T45.3X6
Depilatory	T49.4X1	T49.4X2	T49.4X3	T49.4X4	T49.4X5	T49.4X6
Deprenalin	T42.8X1	T42.8X2	T42.8X3	T42.8X4	T42.8X5	T42.8X6
Deprenyl	T42.8X1	T42.8X2	T42.8X3	T42.8X4	T42.8X5	T42.8X6
Depressant						
appetite (central)	T50.5X1	T50.5X2	T50.5X3	T50.5X4	T50.5X5	T50.5X6
cardiac	T46.2X1	T46.2X2	T46.2X3	T46.2X4	T46.2X5	T46.2X6
central nervous system (anesthetic) — see also Central nervous system, depressants	T42.71	T42.72	T42.73	T42.74	T42.75	T42.76

Substance	Poisoning, Accidental (unintentional)	Poisoning, Intentional Self-harm	Poisoning, Assault	Poisoning, Undetermined	Adverse Effect	Under-dosing
Depressant — continued						
central nervous system — continued						
general anesthetic	T41.201	T41.202	T41.203	T41.204	T41.205	T41.206
muscle tone	T42.8X1	T42.8X2	T42.8X3	T42.8X4	T42.8X5	T42.8X6
muscle tone, central	T42.8X1	T42.8X2	T42.8X3	T42.8X4	T42.8X5	T42.8X6
psychotherapeutic	T43.501	T43.502	T43.503	T43.504	T43.505	T43.506
Depressant, appetite	T50.5X1	T50.5X2	T50.5X3	T50.5X4	T50.5X5	T50.5X6
Deptropine	T45.0X1	T45.0X2	T45.0X3	T45.0X4	T45.0X5	T45.0X6
Dequalinium (chloride)	T49.0X1	T49.0X2	T49.0X3	T49.0X4	T49.0X5	T49.0X6
Derris root	T60.2X1	T60.2X2	T60.2X3	T60.2X4	—	—
Deserpidine	T46.5X1	T46.5X2	T46.5X3	T46.5X4	T46.5X5	T46.5X6
Desferrioxamine	T45.8X1	T45.8X2	T45.8X3	T45.8X4	T45.8X5	T45.8X6
Desipramine	T43.011	T43.012	T43.013	T43.014	T43.015	T43.016
Deslanoside	T46.0X1	T46.0X2	T46.0X3	T46.0X4	T46.0X5	T46.0X6
Desloughing agent	T49.4X1	T49.4X2	T49.4X3	T49.4X4	T49.4X5	T49.4X6
Desmethylimipramine	T43.011	T43.012	T43.013	T43.014	T43.015	T43.016
Desmopressin	T38.891	T38.892	T38.893	T38.894	T38.895	T38.896
Desocodeine	T40.2X1	T40.2X2	T40.2X3	T40.2X4	T40.2X5	T40.2X6
Desogestrel	T38.5X1	T38.5X2	T38.5X3	T38.5X4	T38.5X5	T38.5X6
Desomorphine	T40.2X1	T40.2X2	T40.2X3	T40.2X4		
Desonide	T49.0X1	T49.0X2	T49.0X3	T49.0X4	T49.0X5	T49.0X6
Desoximetasone	T49.0X1	T49.0X2	T49.0X3	T49.0X4	T49.0X5	T49.0X6
Desoxycorticosteroid	T50.0X1	T50.0X2	T50.0X3	T50.0X4	T50.0X5	T50.0X6
Desoxycortone	T50.0X1	T50.0X2	T50.0X3	T50.0X4	T50.0X5	T50.0X6
Desoxyephedrine	T43.651	T43.652	T43.653	T43.654	T43.655	T43.656
Dessicated thyroid*	T38.1X1	T38.1X2	T38.1X3	T38.1X4	T38.1X5	T38.1X6
Detaxtran	T46.6X1	T46.6X2	T46.6X3	T46.6X4	T46.6X5	T46.6X6
Detergent	T49.2X1	T49.2X2	T49.2X3	T49.2X4	T49.2X5	T49.2X6
external medication	T49.2X1	T49.2X2	T49.2X3	T49.2X4	T49.2X5	T49.2X6
local	T49.2X1	T49.2X2	T49.2X3	T49.2X4	T49.2X5	T49.2X6
medicinal	T49.2X1	T49.2X2	T49.2X3	T49.2X4	T49.2X5	T49.2X6
nonmedicinal	T55.1X1	T55.1X2	T55.1X3	T55.1X4	—	—
specified NEC	T55.1X1	T55.1X2	T55.1X3	T55.1X4	—	—
Deterrent, alcohol	T50.6X1	T50.6X2	T50.6X3	T50.6X4	T50.6X5	T50.6X6
Detoxifying agent	T50.6X1	T50.6X2	T50.6X3	T50.6X4	T50.6X5	T50.6X6
Detrothyronine	T38.1X1	T38.1X2	T38.1X3	T38.1X4	T38.1X5	T38.1X6
Dettol (external medication)	T49.0X1	T49.0X2	T49.0X3	T49.0X4	T49.0X5	T49.0X6
Dexamethasone	T38.0X1	T38.0X2	T38.0X3	T38.0X4	T38.0X5	T38.0X6
ENT agent	T49.6X1	T49.6X2	T49.6X3	T49.6X4	T49.6X5	T49.6X6
ophthalmic preparation	T49.5X1	T49.5X2	T49.5X3	T49.5X4	T49.5X5	T49.5X6
topical NEC	T49.0X1	T49.0X2	T49.0X3	T49.0X4	T49.0X5	T49.0X6
Dexamfetamine	T43.621	T43.622	T43.623	T43.624	T43.625	T43.626
Dexamphetamine	T43.621	T43.622	T43.623	T43.624	T43.625	T43.626
Dexbrompheniramine	T45.0X1	T45.0X2	T45.0X3	T45.0X4	T45.0X5	T45.0X6
Dexchlorpheniramine	T45.0X1	T45.0X2	T45.0X3	T45.0X4	T45.0X5	T45.0X6
Dexedrine	T43.621	T43.622	T43.623	T43.624	T43.625	T43.626
Dexetimide	T44.3X1	T44.3X2	T44.3X3	T44.3X4	T44.3X5	T44.3X6
Dexfenfluramine	T50.5X1	T50.5X2	T50.5X3	T50.5X4	T50.5X5	T50.5X6
Dexpanthenol	T45.2X1	T45.2X2	T45.2X3	T45.2X4	T45.2X5	T45.2X6
Dextran (40) (70) (150)	T45.8X1	T45.8X2	T45.8X3	T45.8X4	T45.8X5	T45.8X6
Dextriferron	T45.4X1	T45.4X2	T45.4X3	T45.4X4	T45.4X5	T45.4X6
Dextroamphetamine	T43.621	T43.622	T43.623	T43.624	T43.625	T43.626
Dextro calcium pantothenate	T45.2X1	T45.2X2	T45.2X3	T45.2X4	T45.2X5	T45.2X6
Dextromethorphan	T48.3X1	T48.3X2	T48.3X3	T48.3X4	T48.3X5	T48.3X6
Dextromoramide	T40.491	T40.492	T40.493	T40.494	—	—
topical	T49.8X1	T49.8X2	T49.8X3	T49.8X4	T49.8X5	T49.8X6
Dextro pantothenyl alcohol	T45.2X1	T45.2X2	T45.2X3	T45.2X4	T45.2X5	T45.2X6
Dextropropoxyphene	T40.491	T40.492	T40.493	T40.494	T40.495	T40.496
Dextrorphan	T40.2X1	T40.2X2	T40.2X3	T40.2X4	T40.2X5	T40.2X6
Dextrose	T50.3X1	T50.3X2	T50.3X3	T50.3X4	T50.3X5	T50.3X6
concentrated solution, intravenous	T46.8X1	T46.8X2	T46.8X3	T46.8X4	T46.8X5	T46.8X6
Dextrothyroxin	T38.1X1	T38.1X2	T38.1X3	T38.1X4	T38.1X5	T38.1X6
Dextrothyroxine sodium	T38.1X1	T38.1X2	T38.1X3	T38.1X4	T38.1X5	T38.1X6
DFP	T44.0X1	T44.0X2	T44.0X3	T44.0X4	T44.0X5	T44.0X6
DHE	T37.3X1	T37.3X2	T37.3X3	T37.3X4	T37.3X5	T37.3X6
45	T46.5X1	T46.5X2	T46.5X3	T46.5X4	T46.5X5	T46.5X6
DiaBeta*	T38.3X1	T38.3X2	T38.3X3	T38.3X4	T38.3X5	T38.3X6
Diabinese	T38.3X1	T38.3X2	T38.3X3	T38.3X4	T38.3X5	T38.3X6
Diacetone alcohol	T52.4X1	T52.4X2	T52.4X3	T52.4X4	—	—
Diacetyl monoxime	T50.991	T50.992	T50.993	T50.994	—	—
Diacetylmorphine	T40.1X1	T40.1X2	T40.1X3	T40.1X4	—	—
Diachylon plaster	T49.4X1	T49.4X2	T49.4X3	T49.4X4	T49.4X5	T49.4X6
Diaethylstilboestrolum	T38.5X1	T38.5X2	T38.5X3	T38.5X4	T38.5X5	T38.5X6
Diagnostic agent NEC	T50.8X1	T50.8X2	T50.8X3	T50.8X4	T50.8X5	T50.8X6
Dial (soap)	T49.2X1	T49.2X2	T49.2X3	T49.2X4	T49.2X5	T49.2X6
sedative	T42.3X1	T42.3X2	T42.3X3	T42.3X4	T42.3X5	T42.3X6

Substance	Poisoning, Accidental (unintentional)	Poisoning, Intentional Self-harm	Poisoning, Assault	Poisoning, Undetermined	Adverse Effect	Under-dosing
Dialkyl carbonate	T52.91	T52.92	T52.93	T52.94	—	—
Diallylbarbituric acid	T42.3X1	T42.3X2	T42.3X3	T42.3X4	T42.3X5	T42.3X6
Diallymal	T42.3X1	T42.3X2	T42.3X3	T42.3X4	T42.3X5	T42.3X6
Dialysis solution (intraperitoneal)	T50.3X1	T50.3X2	T50.3X3	T50.3X4	T50.3X5	T50.3X6
Diaminodiphenylsulfone	T37.1X1	T37.1X2	T37.1X3	T37.1X4	T37.1X5	T37.1X6
Diamorphine	T40.1X1	T40.1X2	T40.1X3	T40.1X4	—	—
Diamox	T50.2X1	T50.2X2	T50.2X3	T50.2X4	T50.2X5	T50.2X6
Diamthazole	T49.0X1	T49.0X2	T49.0X3	T49.0X4	T49.0X5	T49.0X6
Dianthone	T47.2X1	T47.2X2	T47.2X3	T47.2X4	T47.2X5	T47.2X6
Diaphenylsulfone	T37.0X1	T37.0X2	T37.0X3	T37.0X4	T37.0X5	T37.0X6
Diasone (sodium)	T37.1X1	T37.1X2	T37.1X3	T37.1X4	T37.1X5	T37.1X6
Diastase	T47.5X1	T47.5X2	T47.5X3	T47.5X4	T47.5X5	T47.5X6
Diastat*	T42.4X1	T42.4X2	T42.4X3	T42.4X4	T42.4X5	T42.4X6
Diatrizoate	T50.8X1	T50.8X2	T50.8X3	T50.8X4	T50.8X5	T50.8X6
Diazepam	T42.4X1	T42.4X2	T42.4X3	T42.4X4	T42.4X5	T42.4X6
Diazinon	T60.0X1	T60.0X2	T60.0X3	T60.0X4	—	—
Diazomethane (gas)	T59.891	T59.892	T59.893	T59.894	—	—
Diazoxide	T46.5X1	T46.5X2	T46.5X3	T46.5X4	T46.5X5	T46.5X6
Dibekacin	T36.5X1	T36.5X2	T36.5X3	T36.5X4	T36.5X5	T36.5X6
Dibenamine	T44.6X1	T44.6X2	T44.6X3	T44.6X4	T44.6X5	T44.6X6
Dibenzepin	T43.011	T43.012	T43.013	T43.014	T43.015	T43.016
Dibenzheptropine	T45.0X1	T45.0X2	T45.0X3	T45.0X4	T45.0X5	T45.0X6
Dibenzyline	T44.6X1	T44.6X2	T44.6X3	T44.6X4	T44.6X5	T44.6X6
Diborane (gas)	T59.891	T59.892	T59.893	T59.894	—	—
Dibromochloropropane	T60.8X1	T60.8X2	T60.8X3	T60.8X4	—	—
Dibromodulcitol	T45.1X1	T45.1X2	T45.1X3	T45.1X4	T45.1X5	T45.1X6
Dibromoethane	T53.6X1	T53.6X2	T53.6X3	T53.6X4	—	—
Dibromomannitol	T45.1X1	T45.1X2	T45.1X3	T45.1X4	T45.1X5	T45.1X6
Dibromopropamidine isethionate	T49.0X1	T49.0X2	T49.0X3	T49.0X4	T49.0X5	T49.0X6
Dibrompropamidine	T49.0X1	T49.0X2	T49.0X3	T49.0X4	T49.0X5	T49.0X6
Dibucaine	T41.3X1	T41.3X2	T41.3X3	T41.3X4	T41.3X5	T41.3X6
topical (surface)	T41.3X1	T41.3X2	T41.3X3	T41.3X4	T41.3X5	T41.3X6
Dibunate sodium	T48.3X1	T48.3X2	T48.3X3	T48.3X4	T48.3X5	T48.3X6
Dibutoline sulfate	T44.3X1	T44.3X2	T44.3X3	T44.3X4	T44.3X5	T44.3X6
Dicamba	T60.3X1	T60.3X2	T60.3X3	T60.3X4	—	—
Dicapthon	T60.0X1	T60.0X2	T60.0X3	T60.0X4	—	—
Dichlobenil	T60.3X1	T60.3X2	T60.3X3	T60.3X4	—	—
Dichlone	T60.3X1	T60.3X2	T60.3X3	T60.3X4	—	—
Dichloralphenozone	T42.6X1	T42.6X2	T42.6X3	T42.6X4	T42.6X5	T42.6X6
Dichlorbenzidine	T65.3X1	T65.3X2	T65.3X3	T65.3X4	—	—
Dichlorhydrin	T52.8X1	T52.8X2	T52.8X3	T52.8X4	—	—
Dichlorhydroxyquinoline	T37.8X1	T37.8X2	T37.8X3	T37.8X4	T37.8X5	T37.8X6
Dichlorobenzene	T53.7X1	T53.7X2	T53.7X3	T53.7X4	—	—
Dichlorobenzyl alcohol	T49.6X1	T49.6X2	T49.6X3	T49.6X4	T49.6X5	T49.6X6
Dichlorodifluoromethane	T53.5X1	T53.5X2	T53.5X3	T53.5X4	—	—
Dichloroethane	T52.8X1	T52.8X2	T52.8X3	T52.8X4	—	—
Dichloroethylene	T53.6X1	T53.6X2	T53.6X3	T53.6X4	—	—
Dichloroethyl sulfide, not in war	T59.891	T59.892	T59.893	T59.894		
Dichloroformoxine, not in war	T59.891	T59.892	T59.893	T59.894		
Dichlorohydrin, alpha-dichlorohydrin	T52.8X1	T52.8X2	T52.8X3	T52.8X4		
Dichloromethane (solvent)	T53.4X1	T53.4X2	T53.4X3	T53.4X4	—	—
vapor	T53.4X1	T53.4X2	T53.4X3	T53.4X4	—	—
Dichloronaphthoquinone	T60.3X1	T60.3X2	T60.3X3	T60.3X4	—	—
Dichlorophen	T37.4X1	T37.4X2	T37.4X3	T37.4X4	T37.4X5	T37.4X6
Dichloropropene	T60.3X1	T60.3X2	T60.3X3	T60.3X4	—	—
Dichloropropionic acid	T60.3X1	T60.3X2	T60.3X3	T60.3X4	—	—
Dichlorphenamide	T50.2X1	T50.2X2	T50.2X3	T50.2X4	T50.2X5	T50.2X6
Dichlorvos	T60.0X1	T60.0X2	T60.0X3	T60.0X4	—	—
Dichysterol*	T45.2X1	T45.2X2	T45.2X3	T45.2X4	T45.2X5	T45.2X6
Diclofenac	T39.391	T39.392	T39.393	T39.394	T39.395	T39.396
Diclofenamide	T50.2X1	T50.2X2	T50.2X3	T50.2X4	T50.2X5	T50.2X6
Diclofensine	T43.291	T43.292	T43.293	T43.294	T43.295	T43.296
Diclonixine	T39.8X1	T39.8X2	T39.8X3	T39.8X4	T39.8X5	T39.8X6
Dicloxacillin	T36.0X1	T36.0X2	T36.0X3	T36.0X4	T36.0X5	T36.0X6
Dicophane	T49.0X1	T49.0X2	T49.0X3	T49.0X4	T49.0X5	T49.0X6
Dicoumarol, dicoumarin, dicumarol	T45.511	T45.512	T45.513	T45.514	T45.515	T45.516
Dicrotophos	T60.0X1	T60.0X2	T60.0X3	T60.0X4	—	—
Dicyanogen (gas)	T65.0X1	T65.0X2	T65.0X3	T65.0X4	—	—
Dicyclomine	T44.3X1	T44.3X2	T44.3X3	T44.3X4	T44.3X5	T44.3X6
Dicycloverine	T44.3X1	T44.3X2	T44.3X3	T44.3X4	T44.3X5	T44.3X6
Didanosine*	T37.5X1	T37.5X2	T37.5X3	T37.5X4	T37.5X5	T37.5X6
Dideoxycytidine	T37.5X1	T37.5X2	T37.5X3	T37.5X4	T37.5X5	T37.5X6
Dideoxyinosine	T37.5X1	T37.5X2	T37.5X3	T37.5X4	T37.5X5	T37.5X6
Dieldrin (vapor)	T60.1X1	T60.1X2	T60.1X3	T60.1X4	—	—
Diemal	T42.3X1	T42.3X2	T42.3X3	T42.3X4	T42.3X5	T42.3X6
Dienestrol	T38.5X1	T38.5X2	T38.5X3	T38.5X4	T38.5X5	T38.5X6
Dienoestrol	T38.5X1	T38.5X2	T38.5X3	T38.5X4	T38.5X5	T38.5X6

Table of Drugs and Chemicals

Dietetic drug NEC — Diphemanil

Substance	Poisoning, Accidental (unintentional)	Poisoning, Intentional Self-harm	Poisoning, Assault	Poisoning, Undetermined	Adverse Effect	Underdosing
Dietetic drug NEC	T50.901	T50.902	T50.903	T50.904	T50.905	T50.906
Diethazine	T42.8X1	T42.8X2	T42.8X3	T42.8X4	T42.8X5	T42.8X6
Diethyl						
barbituric acid	T42.3X1	T42.3X2	T42.3X3	T42.3X4	T42.3X5	T42.3X6
carbamazine	T37.4X1	T37.4X2	T37.4X3	T37.4X4	T37.4X5	T37.4X6
carbinol	T51.3X1	T51.3X2	T51.3X3	T51.3X4	—	—
carbonate	T52.8X1	T52.8X2	T52.8X3	T52.8X4	—	—
ether (vapor) — see also ether	T41.0X1	T41.0X2	T41.0X3	T41.0X4	T41.0X5	T41.0X6
oxide	T52.8X1	T52.8X2	T52.8X3	T52.8X4	—	—
propion	T50.5X1	T50.5X2	T50.5X3	T50.5X4	T50.5X5	T50.5X6
stilbestrol	T38.5X1	T38.5X2	T38.5X3	T38.5X4	T38.5X5	T38.5X6
toluamide (nonmedicinal)	T60.8X1	T60.8X2	T60.8X3	T60.8X4	—	—
medicinal	T49.3X1	T49.3X2	T49.3X3	T49.3X4	T49.3X5	T49.3X6
Diethylcarbamazine	T37.4X1	T37.4X2	T37.4X3	T37.4X4	T37.4X5	T37.4X6
Diethylene						
dioxide	T52.8X1	T52.8X2	T52.8X3	T52.8X4	—	—
glycol (monoacetate) (monobutyl ether) (monoethyl ether)	T52.3X1	T52.3X2	T52.3X3	T52.3X4	—	—
Diethylhexylphthalate	T65.891	T65.892	T65.893	T65.894	—	—
Diethylpropion	T50.5X1	T50.5X2	T50.5X3	T50.5X4	T50.5X5	T50.5X6
Diethylstilbestrol	T38.5X1	T38.5X2	T38.5X3	T38.5X4	T38.5X5	T38.5X6
Diethylstilboestrol	T38.5X1	T38.5X2	T38.5X3	T38.5X4	T38.5X5	T38.5X6
Diethylsulfone-diethyl-methane	T42.6X1	T42.6X2	T42.6X3	T42.6X4	T42.6X5	T42.6X6
Diethyltoluamide	T49.0X1	T49.0X2	T49.0X3	T49.0X4	T49.0X5	T49.0X6
Diethyltryptamine (DET)	T40.991	T40.992	T40.993	T40.994	—	—
Difebarbamate	T42.3X1	T42.3X2	T42.3X3	T42.3X4	T42.3X5	T42.3X6
Difencloxazine	T40.2X1	T40.2X2	T40.2X3	T40.2X4	T40.2X5	T40.2X6
Difenidol	T45.0X1	T45.0X2	T45.0X3	T45.0X4	T45.0X5	T45.0X6
Difenoxin	T47.6X1	T47.6X2	T47.6X3	T47.6X4	T47.6X5	T47.6X6
Difetarsone	T37.3X1	T37.3X2	T37.3X3	T37.3X4	T37.3X5	T37.3X6
Diffusin	T45.3X1	T45.3X2	T45.3X3	T45.3X4	T45.3X5	T45.3X6
Diflorasone	T49.0X1	T49.0X2	T49.0X3	T49.0X4	T49.0X5	T49.0X6
Diflos	T44.0X1	T44.0X2	T44.0X3	T44.0X4	T44.0X5	T44.0X6
Diflubenzuron	T60.1X1	T60.1X2	T60.1X3	T60.1X4	—	—
Diflucan*	T37.8X1	T37.8X2	T37.8X3	T37.8X4	T37.8X5	T37.8X6
Diflucortolone	T49.0X1	T49.0X2	T49.0X3	T49.0X4	T49.0X5	T49.0X6
Diflunisal	T39.091	T39.092	T39.093	T39.094	T39.095	T39.096
Difluoromethyldopa	T42.8X1	T42.8X2	T42.8X3	T42.8X4	T42.8X5	T42.8X6
Difluorophate	T44.0X1	T44.0X2	T44.0X3	T44.0X4	T44.0X5	T44.0X6
Digestant NEC	T47.5X1	T47.5X2	T47.5X3	T47.5X4	T47.5X5	T47.5X6
Digitalin (e)	T46.0X1	T46.0X2	T46.0X3	T46.0X4	T46.0X5	T46.0X6
Digitalis (leaf)(glycoside)	T46.0X1	T46.0X2	T46.0X3	T46.0X4	T46.0X5	T46.0X6
lanata	T46.0X1	T46.0X2	T46.0X3	T46.0X4	T46.0X5	T46.0X6
purpurea	T46.0X1	T46.0X2	T46.0X3	T46.0X4	T46.0X5	T46.0X6
Digitoxin	T46.0X1	T46.0X2	T46.0X3	T46.0X4	T46.0X5	T46.0X6
Digitoxose	T46.0X1	T46.0X2	T46.0X3	T46.0X4	T46.0X5	T46.0X6
Digoxin	T46.0X1	T46.0X2	T46.0X3	T46.0X4	T46.0X5	T46.0X6
Digoxine	T46.0X1	T46.0X2	T46.0X3	T46.0X4	T46.0X5	T46.0X6
Dihydralazine	T46.5X1	T46.5X2	T46.5X3	T46.5X4	T46.5X5	T46.5X6
Dihydrazine	T46.5X1	T46.5X2	T46.5X3	T46.5X4	T46.5X5	T46.5X6
Dihydrocodeine	T40.2X1	T40.2X2	T40.2X3	T40.2X4	T40.2X5	T40.2X6
Dihydrocodeinone	T40.2X1	T40.2X2	T40.2X3	T40.2X4	T40.2X5	T40.2X6
Dihydroergocornine	T46.7X1	T46.7X2	T46.7X3	T46.7X4	T46.7X5	T46.7X6
Dihydroergocristine (mesilate)	T46.7X1	T46.7X2	T46.7X3	T46.7X4	T46.7X5	T46.7X6
Dihydroergokryptine	T46.7X1	T46.7X2	T46.7X3	T46.7X4	T46.7X5	T46.7X6
Dihydroergotamine	T46.5X1	T46.5X2	T46.5X3	T46.5X4	T46.5X5	T46.5X6
Dihydroergotoxine	T46.7X1	T46.7X2	T46.7X3	T46.7X4	T46.7X5	T46.7X6
mesilate	T46.7X1	T46.7X2	T46.7X3	T46.7X4	T46.7X5	T46.7X6
Dihydrohydroxycodeinone	T40.2X1	T40.2X2	T40.2X3	T40.2X4	T40.2X5	T40.2X6
Dihydrohydroxymorphinone	T40.2X1	T40.2X2	T40.2X3	T40.2X4	T40.2X5	T40.2X6
Dihydroisocodeine	T40.2X1	T40.2X2	T40.2X3	T40.2X4	T40.2X5	T40.2X6
Dihydromorphine	T40.2X1	T40.2X2	T40.2X3	T40.2X4	—	—
Dihydromorphinone	T40.2X1	T40.2X2	T40.2X3	T40.2X4	T40.2X5	T40.2X6
Dihydrostreptomycin	T36.5X1	T36.5X2	T36.5X3	T36.5X4	T36.5X5	T36.5X6
Dihydrotachysterol	T45.2X1	T45.2X2	T45.2X3	T45.2X4	T45.2X5	T45.2X6
Dihydroxyacetone*	T49.3X1	T49.3X2	T49.3X3	T49.3X4	T49.3X5	T49.3X6
Dihydroxyaluminum aminoacetate	T47.1X1	T47.1X2	T47.1X3	T47.1X4	T47.1X5	T47.1X6
Dihydroxyaluminum sodium carbonate	T47.1X1	T47.1X2	T47.1X3	T47.1X4	T47.1X5	T47.1X6
Dihydroxyanthraquinone	T47.2X1	T47.2X2	T47.2X3	T47.2X4	T47.2X5	T47.2X6
Dihydroxycodeinone	T40.2X1	T40.2X2	T40.2X3	T40.2X4	T40.2X5	T40.2X6
Dihydroxypropyl theophylline	T50.2X1	T50.2X2	T50.2X3	T50.2X4	T50.2X5	T50.2X6
Diiodohydroxyquin	T37.8X1	T37.8X2	T37.8X3	T37.8X4	T37.8X5	T37.8X6
topical	T49.0X1	T49.0X2	T49.0X3	T49.0X4	T49.0X5	T49.0X6
Diiodohydroxyquinoline	T37.8X1	T37.8X2	T37.8X3	T37.8X4	T37.8X5	T37.8X6
Diiodotyrosine	T38.2X1	T38.2X2	T38.2X3	T38.2X4	T38.2X5	T38.2X6
Diisopromine	T44.3X1	T44.3X2	T44.3X3	T44.3X4	T44.3X5	T44.3X6

Substance	Poisoning, Accidental (unintentional)	Poisoning, Intentional Self-harm	Poisoning, Assault	Poisoning, Undetermined	Adverse Effect	Underdosing
Diisopropylamine	T46.3X1	T46.3X2	T46.3X3	T46.3X4	T46.3X5	T46.3X6
Diisopropylfluorophos-phonate	T44.0X1	T44.0X2	T44.0X3	T44.0X4	T44.0X5	T44.0X6
Dilantin	T42.0X1	T42.0X2	T42.0X3	T42.0X4	T42.0X5	T42.0X6
Dilatrate*	T46.3X1	T46.3X2	T46.3X3	T46.3X4	T46.3X5	T46.3X6
Dilaudid	T40.2X1	T40.2X2	T40.2X3	T40.2X4	T40.2X5	T40.2X6
Dilazep	T46.3X1	T46.3X2	T46.3X3	T46.3X4	T46.3X5	T46.3X6
Dill	T47.5X1	T47.5X2	T47.5X3	T47.5X4	T47.5X5	T47.5X6
Diloxanide	T37.3X1	T37.3X2	T37.3X3	T37.3X4	T37.3X5	T37.3X6
Diltiazem	T46.1X1	T46.1X2	T46.1X3	T46.1X4	T46.1X5	T46.1X6
Dimazole	T49.0X1	T49.0X2	T49.0X3	T49.0X4	T49.0X5	T49.0X6
Dimefline	T50.7X1	T50.7X2	T50.7X3	T50.7X4	T50.7X5	T50.7X6
Dimefox	T60.0X1	T60.0X2	T60.0X3	T60.0X4	—	—
Dimemorfan	T48.3X1	T48.3X2	T48.3X3	T48.3X4	T48.3X5	T48.3X6
Dimenhydrinate	T45.0X1	T45.0X2	T45.0X3	T45.0X4	T45.0X5	T45.0X6
Dimercaprol (British anti-lewisite)	T45.8X1	T45.8X2	T45.8X3	T45.8X4	T45.8X5	T45.8X6
Dimercaptopropanol	T45.8X1	T45.8X2	T45.8X3	T45.8X4	T45.8X5	T45.8X6
Dimestrol	T38.5X1	T38.5X2	T38.5X3	T38.5X4	T38.5X5	T38.5X6
Dimetane	T45.0X1	T45.0X2	T45.0X3	T45.0X4	T45.0X5	T45.0X6
Dimethicone	T47.1X1	T47.1X2	T47.1X3	T47.1X4	T47.1X5	T47.1X6
Dimethindene	T45.0X1	T45.0X2	T45.0X3	T45.0X4	T45.0X5	T45.0X6
Dimethisoquin	T49.1X1	T49.1X2	T49.1X3	T49.1X4	T49.1X5	T49.1X6
Dimethisterone	T38.5X1	T38.5X2	T38.5X3	T38.5X4	T38.5X5	T38.5X6
Dimethoate	T60.0X1	T60.0X2	T60.0X3	T60.0X4	—	—
Dimethocaine	T41.3X1	T41.3X2	T41.3X3	T41.3X4	T41.3X5	T41.3X6
Dimethoxanate	T48.3X1	T48.3X2	T48.3X3	T48.3X4	T48.3X5	T48.3X6
Dimethyl						
arsine, arsinic acid	T57.0X1	T57.0X2	T57.0X3	T57.0X4	—	—
carbinol	T51.2X1	T51.2X2	T51.2X3	T51.2X4	—	—
carbonate	T52.8X1	T52.8X2	T52.8X3	T52.8X4	—	—
diguanide	T38.3X1	T38.3X2	T38.3X3	T38.3X4	T38.3X5	T38.3X6
ketone	T52.4X1	T52.4X2	T52.4X3	T52.4X4	—	—
vapor	T52.4X1	T52.4X2	T52.4X3	T52.4X4	—	—
meperidine	T40.2X1	T40.2X2	T40.2X3	T40.2X4	T40.2X5	T40.2X6
parathion	T60.0X1	T60.0X2	T60.0X3	T60.0X4	—	—
phthlate	T49.3X1	T49.3X2	T49.3X3	T49.3X4	T49.3X5	T49.3X6
polysiloxane	T47.8X1	T47.8X2	T47.8X3	T47.8X4	T47.8X5	T47.8X6
sulfate (fumes)	T59.891	T59.892	T59.893	T59.894	—	—
liquid	T65.891	T65.892	T65.893	T65.894	—	—
sulfoxide (nonmedicinal)	T52.8X1	T52.8X2	T52.8X3	T52.8X4	—	—
medicinal	T49.4X1	T49.4X2	T49.4X3	T49.4X4	T49.4X5	T49.4X6
tryptamine	T40.991	T40.992	T40.993	T40.994	—	—
tubocurarine	T48.1X1	T48.1X2	T48.1X3	T48.1X4	T48.1X5	T48.1X6
Dimethylamine sulfate	T49.4X1	T49.4X2	T49.4X3	T49.4X4	T49.4X5	T49.4X6
Dimethylcysteine*	T50.6X1	T50.6X2	T50.6X3	T50.6X4	T50.6X5	T50.6X6
Dimethylformamide	T52.8X1	T52.8X2	T52.8X3	T52.8X4	—	—
Dimethyltubocurarinium chloride	T48.1X1	T48.1X2	T48.1X3	T48.1X4	T48.1X5	T48.1X6
Dimeticone	T47.1X1	T47.1X2	T47.1X3	T47.1X4	T47.1X5	T47.1X6
Dimetilan	T60.0X1	T60.0X2	T60.0X3	T60.0X4	—	—
Dimetindene	T45.0X1	T45.0X2	T45.0X3	T45.0X4	T45.0X5	T45.0X6
Dimetotiazine	T43.3X1	T43.3X2	T43.3X3	T43.3X4	T43.3X5	T43.3X6
Dimorpholamine	T50.7X1	T50.7X2	T50.7X3	T50.7X4	T50.7X5	T50.7X6
Dimoxyline	T46.3X1	T46.3X2	T46.3X3	T46.3X4	T46.3X5	T46.3X6
Dinitrobenzene	T65.3X1	T65.3X2	T65.3X3	T65.3X4	—	—
vapor	T59.891	T59.892	T59.893	T59.894	—	—
Dinitrobenzol	T65.3X1	T65.3X2	T65.3X3	T65.3X4	—	—
vapor	T59.891	T59.892	T59.893	T59.894	—	—
Dinitrobutylphenol	T65.3X1	T65.3X2	T65.3X3	T65.3X4	—	—
Dinitro (-ortho-)cresol (pesticide) (spray)	T65.3X1	T65.3X2	T65.3X3	T65.3X4	—	—
Dinitrocyclohexylphenol	T65.3X1	T65.3X2	T65.3X3	T65.3X4	—	—
Dinitrophenol	T65.3X1	T65.3X2	T65.3X3	T65.3X4	—	—
Dinoprost	T48.0X1	T48.0X2	T48.0X3	T48.0X4	T48.0X5	T48.0X6
Dinoprostone	T48.0X1	T48.0X2	T48.0X3	T48.0X4	T48.0X5	T48.0X6
Dinoseb	T60.3X1	T60.3X2	T60.3X3	T60.3X4	—	—
Dioctyl sulfosuccinate (calcium) (sodium)	T47.4X1	T47.4X2	T47.4X3	T47.4X4	T47.4X5	T47.4X6
Diodone	T50.8X1	T50.8X2	T50.8X3	T50.8X4	T50.8X5	T50.8X6
Diodoquin	T37.8X1	T37.8X2	T37.8X3	T37.8X4	T37.8X5	T37.8X6
Dionin	T40.2X1	T40.2X2	T40.2X3	T40.2X4	T40.2X5	T40.2X6
Diosmin	T46.991	T46.992	T46.993	T46.994	T46.995	T46.996
Diovan*	T46.5X1	T46.5X2	T46.5X3	T46.5X4	T46.5X5	T46.5X6
Dioxane	T52.8X1	T52.8X2	T52.8X3	T52.8X4	—	—
Dioxathion	T60.0X1	T60.0X2	T60.0X3	T60.0X4	—	—
Dioxin	T53.7X1	T53.7X2	T53.7X3	T53.7X4	—	—
Dioxopromethazine	T43.3X1	T43.3X2	T43.3X3	T43.3X4	T43.3X5	T43.3X6
Dioxyline	T46.3X1	T46.3X2	T46.3X3	T46.3X4	T46.3X5	T46.3X6
Dipentene	T52.8X1	T52.8X2	T52.8X3	T52.8X4	—	—
Diperodon	T41.3X1	T41.3X2	T41.3X3	T41.3X4	T41.3X5	T41.3X6
Diphacinone	T60.4X1	T60.4X2	T60.4X3	T60.4X4	—	—
Diphemanil	T44.3X1	T44.3X2	T44.3X3	T44.3X4	T44.3X5	T44.3X6

☑ Additional Character May Be Required — Refer to the Tabular List for Character Selection

*Optum Value-Add

Substance	Poisoning, Accidental (unintentional)	Poisoning, Intentional Self-harm	Poisoning, Assault	Poisoning, Undetermined	Adverse Effect	Under-dosing
Diphemanil — *continued*						
metilsulfate	T44.3X1	T44.3X2	T44.3X3	T44.3X4	T44.3X5	T44.3X6
Diphenadione	T45.511	T45.512	T45.513	T45.514	T45.515	T45.516
rodenticide	T60.4X1	T60.4X2	T60.4X3	T60.4X4	—	—
Diphenhydramine	T45.0X1	T45.0X2	T45.0X3	T45.0X4	T45.0X5	T45.0X6
Diphenidol	T45.0X1	T45.0X2	T45.0X3	T45.0X4	T45.0X5	T45.0X6
Diphenoxylate	T47.6X1	T47.6X2	T47.6X3	T47.6X4	T47.6X5	T47.6X6
Diphenylamine	T65.3X1	T65.3X2	T65.3X3	T65.3X4	—	—
Diphenylbutazone	T39.2X1	T39.2X2	T39.2X3	T39.2X4	T39.2X5	T39.2X6
Diphenylchloroarsine, not in war	T57.0X1	T57.0X2	T57.0X3	T57.0X4	—	—
Diphenylhydantoin	T42.0X1	T42.0X2	T42.0X3	T42.0X4	T42.0X5	T42.0X6
Diphenylmethane dye	T52.1X1	T52.1X2	T52.1X3	T52.1X4	—	—
Diphenylpyraline	T45.0X1	T45.0X2	T45.0X3	T45.0X4	T45.0X5	T45.0X6
Diphtheria						
antitoxin	T50.Z11	T50.Z12	T50.Z13	T50.Z14	T50.Z15	T50.Z16
toxoid	T50.A91	T50.A92	T50.A93	T50.A94	T50.A95	T50.A96
with tetanus toxoid	T50.A21	T50.A22	T50.A23	T50.A24	T50.A25	T50.A26
with pertussis component	T50.A11	T50.A12	T50.A13	T50.A14	T50.A15	T50.A16
vaccine	T50.A91	T50.A92	T50.A93	T50.A94	T50.A95	T50.A96
combination						
without pertussis	T50.A21	T50.A22	T50.A23	T50.A24	T50.A25	T50.A26
including pertussis	T50.A11	T50.A12	T50.A13	T50.A14	T50.A15	T50.A16
Diphylline	T50.2X1	T50.2X2	T50.2X3	T50.2X4	T50.2X5	T50.2X6
Dipipanone	T40.491	T40.492	T40.493	T40.494	—	—
Dipivefrine	T49.5X1	T49.5X2	T49.5X3	T49.5X4	T49.5X5	T49.5X6
Diplovax	T50.B91	T50.B92	T50.B93	T50.B94	T50.B95	T50.B96
Diprophylline	T50.2X1	T50.2X2	T50.2X3	T50.2X4	T50.2X5	T50.2X6
Dipropyline	T48.291	T48.292	T48.293	T48.294	T48.295	T48.296
Dipyridamole	T46.3X1	T46.3X2	T46.3X3	T46.3X4	T46.3X5	T46.3X6
Dipyrone	T39.2X1	T39.2X2	T39.2X3	T39.2X4	T39.2X5	T39.2X6
Diquat (dibromide)	T60.3X1	T60.3X2	T60.3X3	T60.3X4	—	—
Disinfectant	T65.891	T65.892	T65.893	T65.894	—	—
alkaline	T54.3X1	T54.3X2	T54.3X3	T54.3X4	—	—
aromatic	T54.1X1	T54.1X2	T54.1X3	T54.1X4	—	—
intestinal	T37.8X1	T37.8X2	T37.8X3	T37.8X4	T37.8X5	T37.8X6
Disipal	T42.8X1	T42.8X2	T42.8X3	T42.8X4	T42.8X5	T42.8X6
Disodium edetate	T50.6X1	T50.6X2	T50.6X3	T50.6X4	T50.6X5	T50.6X6
Disoprofol	T41.291	T41.292	T41.293	T41.294	T41.295	T41.296
Disopyramide*	T46.2X1	T46.2X2	T46.2X3	T46.2X4	T46.2X5	T46.2X6
Distigmine (bromide)	T44.0X1	T44.0X2	T44.0X3	T44.0X4	T44.0X5	T44.0X6
Disulfamide	T50.2X1	T50.2X2	T50.2X3	T50.2X4	T50.2X5	T50.2X6
Disulfanilamide	T37.0X1	T37.0X2	T37.0X3	T37.0X4	T37.0X5	T37.0X6
Disulfiram	T50.6X1	T50.6X2	T50.6X3	T50.6X4	T50.6X5	T50.6X6
Disulfoton	T60.0X1	T60.0X2	T60.0X3	T60.0X4	—	—
Dithiazanine iodide	T37.4X1	T37.4X2	T37.4X3	T37.4X4	T37.4X5	T37.4X6
Dithiocarbamate	T60.0X1	T60.0X2	T60.0X3	T60.0X4	—	—
Dithranol	T49.4X1	T49.4X2	T49.4X3	T49.4X4	T49.4X5	T49.4X6
Diucardin	T50.2X1	T50.2X2	T50.2X3	T50.2X4	T50.2X5	T50.2X6
Diupres	T50.2X1	T50.2X2	T50.2X3	T50.2X4	T50.2X5	T50.2X6
Diuretic NEC	T50.2X1	T50.2X2	T50.2X3	T50.2X4	T50.2X5	T50.2X6
benzothiadiazine	T50.2X1	T50.2X2	T50.2X3	T50.2X4	T50.2X5	T50.2X6
carbonic acid anhydrase inhibitors	T50.2X1	T50.2X2	T50.2X3	T50.2X4	T50.2X5	T50.2X6
furfuryl NEC	T50.2X1	T50.2X2	T50.2X3	T50.2X4	T50.2X5	T50.2X6
loop (high-ceiling)	T50.1X1	T50.1X2	T50.1X3	T50.1X4	T50.1X5	T50.1X6
mercurial NEC	T50.2X1	T50.2X2	T50.2X3	T50.2X4	T50.2X5	T50.2X6
osmotic	T50.2X1	T50.2X2	T50.2X3	T50.2X4	T50.2X5	T50.2X6
purine NEC	T50.2X1	T50.2X2	T50.2X3	T50.2X4	T50.2X5	T50.2X6
saluretic NEC	T50.2X1	T50.2X2	T50.2X3	T50.2X4	T50.2X5	T50.2X6
sulfonamide	T50.2X1	T50.2X2	T50.2X3	T50.2X4	T50.2X5	T50.2X6
thiazide NEC	T50.2X1	T50.2X2	T50.2X3	T50.2X4	T50.2X5	T50.2X6
xanthine	T50.2X1	T50.2X2	T50.2X3	T50.2X4	T50.2X5	T50.2X6
Diurgin	T50.2X1	T50.2X2	T50.2X3	T50.2X4	T50.2X5	T50.2X6
Diuril	T50.2X1	T50.2X2	T50.2X3	T50.2X4	T50.2X5	T50.2X6
Diuron	T60.3X1	T60.3X2	T60.3X3	T60.3X4	—	—
Divalproex	T42.6X1	T42.6X2	T42.6X3	T42.6X4	T42.6X5	T42.6X6
Divinyl ether	T41.0X1	T41.0X2	T41.0X3	T41.0X4	T41.0X5	T41.0X6
Dixanthogen	T49.0X1	T49.0X2	T49.0X3	T49.0X4	T49.0X5	T49.0X6
Dixyrazine	T43.3X1	T43.3X2	T43.3X3	T43.3X4	T43.3X5	T43.3X6
D-lysergic acid diethylamide	T40.8X1	T40.8X2	T40.8X3	T40.8X4	—	—
DMCT	T36.4X1	T36.4X2	T36.4X3	T36.4X4	T36.4X5	T36.4X6
DMSO — *see* Dimethyl, sulfoxide						
DNBP	T60.3X1	T60.3X2	T60.3X3	T60.3X4	—	—
DNOC	T65.3X1	T65.3X2	T65.3X3	T65.3X4	—	—
Dobutamine	T44.5X1	T44.5X2	T44.5X3	T44.5X4	T44.5X5	T44.5X6
DOCA	T38.0X1	T38.0X2	T38.0X3	T38.0X4	T38.0X5	T38.0X6
Docusate sodium	T47.4X1	T47.4X2	T47.4X3	T47.4X4	T47.4X5	T47.4X6
Dodicin	T49.0X1	T49.0X2	T49.0X3	T49.0X4	T49.0X5	T49.0X6
Dofamium chloride	T49.0X1	T49.0X2	T49.0X3	T49.0X4	T49.0X5	T49.0X6
Dolophine	T40.3X1	T40.3X2	T40.3X3	T40.3X4	T40.3X5	T40.3X6
Doloxene	T39.8X1	T39.8X2	T39.8X3	T39.8X4	T39.8X5	T39.8X6
Domestic gas (after combustion) — *see* Gas, utility						
prior to combustion	T59.891	T59.892	T59.893	T59.894	—	—
Domiodol	T48.4X1	T48.4X2	T48.4X3	T48.4X4	T48.4X5	T48.4X6
Domiphen (bromide)	T49.0X1	T49.0X2	T49.0X3	T49.0X4	T49.0X5	T49.0X6
Domperidone	T45.0X1	T45.0X2	T45.0X3	T45.0X4	T45.0X5	T45.0X6
Donepezil*	T44.0X1	T44.0X2	T44.0X3	T44.0X4	T44.0X5	T44.0X6
Dopa	T42.8X1	T42.8X2	T42.8X3	T42.8X4	T42.8X5	T42.8X6
Dopamine	T44.991	T44.992	T44.993	T44.994	T44.995	T44.996
Doriden	T42.6X1	T42.6X2	T42.6X3	T42.6X4	T42.6X5	T42.6X6
Dormiral	T42.3X1	T42.3X2	T42.3X3	T42.3X4	T42.3X5	T42.3X6
Dormison	T42.6X1	T42.6X2	T42.6X3	T42.6X4	T42.6X5	T42.6X6
Dornase	T48.4X1	T48.4X2	T48.4X3	T48.4X4	T48.4X5	T48.4X6
Dorsacaine	T41.3X1	T41.3X2	T41.3X3	T41.3X4	T41.3X5	T41.3X6
Dosulepin	T43.011	T43.012	T43.013	T43.014	T43.015	T43.016
Dothiepin	T43.011	T43.012	T43.013	T43.014	T43.015	T43.016
Doxantrazole	T48.6X1	T48.6X2	T48.6X3	T48.6X4	T48.6X5	T48.6X6
Doxapram	T50.7X1	T50.7X2	T50.7X3	T50.7X4	T50.7X5	T50.7X6
Doxazosin	T44.6X1	T44.6X2	T44.6X3	T44.6X4	T44.6X5	T44.6X6
Doxepin	T43.011	T43.012	T43.013	T43.014	T43.015	T43.016
Doxifluridine	T45.1X1	T45.1X2	T45.1X3	T45.1X4	T45.1X5	T45.1X6
Doxil*	T45.1X1	T45.1X2	T45.1X3	T45.1X4	T45.1X5	T45.1X6
Doxorubicin	T45.1X1	T45.1X2	T45.1X3	T45.1X4	T45.1X5	T45.1X6
Doxycycline	T36.4X1	T36.4X2	T36.4X3	T36.4X4	T36.4X5	T36.4X6
Doxylamine	T45.0X1	T45.0X2	T45.0X3	T45.0X4	T45.0X5	T45.0X6
Dramamine	T45.0X1	T45.0X2	T45.0X3	T45.0X4	T45.0X5	T45.0X6
Drano (drain cleaner)	T54.3X1	T54.3X2	T54.3X3	T54.3X4	—	—
Dressing, live pulp	T49.7X1	T49.7X2	T49.7X3	T49.7X4	T49.7X5	T49.7X6
Drocode	T40.2X1	T40.2X2	T40.2X3	T40.2X4	T40.2X5	T40.2X6
Dromoran	T40.2X1	T40.2X2	T40.2X3	T40.2X4	T40.2X5	T40.2X6
Dromostanolone	T38.7X1	T38.7X2	T38.7X3	T38.7X4	T38.7X5	T38.7X6
Dronabinol	T40.711	T40.712	T40.713	T40.714	T40.715	T40.716
Droperidol	T43.591	T43.592	T43.593	T43.594	T43.595	T43.596
Dropropizine	T48.3X1	T48.3X2	T48.3X3	T48.3X4	T48.3X5	T48.3X6
Drostanolone	T38.7X1	T38.7X2	T38.7X3	T38.7X4	T38.7X5	T38.7X6
Drotaverine	T44.3X1	T44.3X2	T44.3X3	T44.3X4	T44.3X5	T44.3X6
Drotrecogin alfa	T45.511	T45.512	T45.513	T45.514	T45.515	T45.516
Drug NEC	T50.901	T50.902	T50.903	T50.904	T50.905	T50.906
specified NEC	T50.991	T50.992	T50.993	T50.994	T50.995	T50.996
DTIC	T45.1X1	T45.1X2	T45.1X3	T45.1X4	T45.1X5	T45.1X6
Duboisine	T44.3X1	T44.3X2	T44.3X3	T44.3X4	T44.3X5	T44.3X6
Dulcolax	T47.2X1	T47.2X2	T47.2X3	T47.2X4	T47.2X5	T47.2X6
Duponol (C) (EP)	T49.2X1	T49.2X2	T49.2X3	T49.2X4	T49.2X5	T49.2X6
Durabolin	T38.7X1	T38.7X2	T38.7X3	T38.7X4	T38.7X5	T38.7X6
Durezol*	T49.5X1	T49.5X2	T49.5X3	T49.5X4	T49.5X5	T49.5X6
Dyclone	T41.3X1	T41.3X2	T41.3X3	T41.3X4	T41.3X5	T41.3X6
Dyclonine	T41.3X1	T41.3X2	T41.3X3	T41.3X4	T41.3X5	T41.3X6
Dydrogesterone	T38.5X1	T38.5X2	T38.5X3	T38.5X4	T38.5X5	T38.5X6
Dye NEC	T65.6X1	T65.6X2	T65.6X3	T65.6X4	—	—
antiseptic	T49.0X1	T49.0X2	T49.0X3	T49.0X4	T49.0X5	T49.0X6
diagnostic agents	T50.8X1	T50.8X2	T50.8X3	T50.8X4	T50.8X5	T50.8X6
pharmaceutical NEC	T50.901	T50.902	T50.903	T50.904	T50.905	T50.906
Dyflos	T44.0X1	T44.0X2	T44.0X3	T44.0X4	T44.0X5	T44.0X6
Dymelor	T38.3X1	T38.3X2	T38.3X3	T38.3X4	T38.3X5	T38.3X6
Dynamite	T65.3X1	T65.3X2	T65.3X3	T65.3X4	—	—
fumes	T59.891	T59.892	T59.893	T59.894	—	—
Dyphylline	T44.3X1	T44.3X2	T44.3X3	T44.3X4	T44.3X5	T44.3X6
b-eucaine	T49.1X1	T49.1X2	T49.1X3	T49.1X4	T49.1X5	T49.1X6
Ear drug NEC	T49.6X1	T49.6X2	T49.6X3	T49.6X4	T49.6X5	T49.6X6
Ear preparations	T49.6X1	T49.6X2	T49.6X3	T49.6X4	T49.6X5	T49.6X6
Echothiophate, echothiopate, ecothiopate	T49.5X1	T49.5X2	T49.5X3	T49.5X4	T49.5X5	T49.5X6
Econazole	T49.0X1	T49.0X2	T49.0X3	T49.0X4	T49.0X5	T49.0X6
Ecothiopate iodide	T49.5X1	T49.5X2	T49.5X3	T49.5X4	T49.5X5	T49.5X6
Ecstasy	T43.641	T43.642	T43.643	T43.644	—	—
Ectylurea	T42.6X1	T42.6X2	T42.6X3	T42.6X4	T42.6X5	T42.6X6
Edathamil disodium	T45.8X1	T45.8X2	T45.8X3	T45.8X4	T45.8X5	T45.8X6
Edecrin	T50.1X1	T50.1X2	T50.1X3	T50.1X4	T50.1X5	T50.1X6
Edetate, disodium (calcium)	T45.8X1	T45.8X2	T45.8X3	T45.8X4	T45.8X5	T45.8X6
Edoxudine	T49.5X1	T49.5X2	T49.5X3	T49.5X4	T49.5X5	T49.5X6
Edrophonium	T44.0X1	T44.0X2	T44.0X3	T44.0X4	T44.0X5	T44.0X6
chloride	T44.0X1	T44.0X2	T44.0X3	T44.0X4	T44.0X5	T44.0X6
EDTA	T50.6X1	T50.6X2	T50.6X3	T50.6X4	T50.6X5	T50.6X6
Effexor*	T43.221	T43.222	T43.223	T43.224	T43.225	T43.226
Eflornithine	T37.2X1	T37.2X2	T37.2X3	T37.2X4	T37.2X5	T37.2X6
Efloxate	T46.3X1	T46.3X2	T46.3X3	T46.3X4	T46.3X5	T46.3X6
Elase	T49.8X1	T49.8X2	T49.8X3	T49.8X4	T49.8X5	T49.8X6
Elastase	T47.5X1	T47.5X2	T47.5X3	T47.5X4	T47.5X5	T47.5X6
Elaterium	T47.2X1	T47.2X2	T47.2X3	T47.2X4	T47.2X5	T47.2X6
Elcatonin	T50.991	T50.992	T50.993	T50.994	T50.995	T50.996
Elder	T62.2X1	T62.2X2	T62.2X3	T62.2X4	—	—

Substance	Poisoning, Accidental (unintentional)	Poisoning, Intentional Self-harm	Poisoning, Assault	Poisoning, Undetermined	Adverse Effect	Under-dosing
Elder — *continued*						
berry, (unripe)	T62.1X1	T62.1X2	T62.1X3	T62.1X4	—	—
Electrolyte balance drug	T50.3X1	T50.3X2	T50.3X3	T50.3X4	T50.3X5	T50.3X6
Electrolytes NEC	T50.3X1	T50.3X2	T50.3X3	T50.3X4	T50.3X5	T50.3X6
Electrolytic agent NEC	T50.3X1	T50.3X2	T50.3X3	T50.3X4	T50.3X5	T50.3X6
Elemental diet	T50.901	T50.902	T50.903	T50.904	T50.905	T50.906
Elliptinium acetate	T45.1X1	T45.1X2	T45.1X3	T45.1X4	T45.1X5	T45.1X6
Elocon*	T49.0X1	T49.0X2	T49.0X3	T49.0X4	T49.0X5	T49.0X6
Embramine	T45.0X1	T45.0X2	T45.0X3	T45.0X4	T45.0X5	T45.0X6
Emepronium (salts)	T44.3X1	T44.3X2	T44.3X3	T44.3X4	T44.3X5	T44.3X6
bromide	T44.3X1	T44.3X2	T44.3X3	T44.3X4	T44.3X5	T44.3X6
Emetic NEC	T47.7X1	T47.7X2	T47.7X3	T47.7X4	T47.7X5	T47.7X6
Emetine	T37.3X1	T37.3X2	T37.3X3	T37.3X4	T37.3X5	T37.3X6
Emollient NEC	T49.3X1	T49.3X2	T49.3X3	T49.3X4	T49.3X5	T49.3X6
Emorfazone	T39.8X1	T39.8X2	T39.8X3	T39.8X4	T39.8X5	T39.8X6
Emylcamate	T43.591	T43.592	T43.593	T43.594	T43.595	T43.596
Enalapril	T46.4X1	T46.4X2	T46.4X3	T46.4X4	T46.4X5	T46.4X6
Enalaprilat	T46.4X1	T46.4X2	T46.4X3	T46.4X4	T46.4X5	T46.4X6
Enbrel*	T39.4X1	T39.4X2	T39.4X3	T39.4X4	T39.4X5	T39.4X6
Encainide	T46.2X1	T46.2X2	T46.2X3	T46.2X4	T46.2X5	T46.2X6
Endocaine	T41.3X1	T41.3X2	T41.3X3	T41.3X4	T41.3X5	T41.3X6
Endosulfan	T60.2X1	T60.2X2	T60.2X3	T60.2X4	—	—
Endothall	T60.3X1	T60.3X2	T60.3X3	T60.3X4	—	—
Endralazine	T46.5X1	T46.5X2	T46.5X3	T46.5X4	T46.5X5	T46.5X6
Endrin	T60.1X1	T60.1X2	T60.1X3	T60.1X4	—	—
Enflurane	T41.0X1	T41.0X2	T41.0X3	T41.0X4	T41.0X5	T41.0X6
Enfuvirtide*	T37.5X1	T37.5X2	T37.5X3	T37.5X4	T37.5X5	T37.5X6
Enhexymal	T42.3X1	T42.3X2	T42.3X3	T42.3X4	T42.3X5	T42.3X6
Enocitabine	T45.1X1	T45.1X2	T45.1X3	T45.1X4	T45.1X5	T45.1X6
Enovid	T38.4X1	T38.4X2	T38.4X3	T38.4X4	T38.4X5	T38.4X6
Enoxacin	T36.8X1	T36.8X2	T36.8X3	T36.8X4	T36.8X5	T36.8X6
Enoxaparin (sodium)	T45.511	T45.512	T45.513	T45.514	T45.515	T45.516
Enpiprazole	T43.591	T43.592	T43.593	T43.594	T43.595	T43.596
Enprofylline	T48.6X1	T48.6X2	T48.6X3	T48.6X4	T48.6X5	T48.6X6
Enprostil	T47.1X1	T47.1X2	T47.1X3	T47.1X4	T47.1X5	T47.1X6
Enterogastrone	T38.891	T38.892	T38.893	T38.894	T38.895	T38.896
ENT preparations (anti-infectives)	T49.6X1	T49.6X2	T49.6X3	T49.6X4	T49.6X5	T49.6X6
Enviomycin	T36.8X1	T36.8X2	T36.8X3	T36.8X4	T36.8X5	T36.8X6
Enzodase	T45.3X1	T45.3X2	T45.3X3	T45.3X4	T45.3X5	T45.3X6
Enzyme NEC	T45.3X1	T45.3X2	T45.3X3	T45.3X4	T45.3X5	T45.3X6
depolymerizing	T49.8X1	T49.8X2	T49.8X3	T49.8X4	T49.8X5	T49.8X6
fibrolytic	T45.3X1	T45.3X2	T45.3X3	T45.3X4	T45.3X5	T45.3X6
gastric	T47.5X1	T47.5X2	T47.5X3	T47.5X4	T47.5X5	T47.5X6
intestinal	T47.5X1	T47.5X2	T47.5X3	T47.5X4	T47.5X5	T47.5X6
local action	T49.4X1	T49.4X2	T49.4X3	T49.4X4	T49.4X5	T49.4X6
proteolytic	T49.4X1	T49.4X2	T49.4X3	T49.4X4	T49.4X5	T49.4X6
thrombolytic	T45.3X1	T45.3X2	T45.3X3	T45.3X4	T45.3X5	T45.3X6
EPAB	T41.3X1	T41.3X2	T41.3X3	T41.3X4	T41.3X5	T41.3X6
Epanutin	T42.0X1	T42.0X2	T42.0X3	T42.0X4	T42.0X5	T42.0X6
Ephedra	T44.991	T44.992	T44.993	T44.994	T44.995	T44.996
Ephedrine	T44.991	T44.992	T44.993	T44.994	T44.995	T44.996
Epichlorhydrin, epichlorohydrin	T52.8X1	T52.8X2	T52.8X3	T52.8X4	—	—
Epicillin	T36.0X1	T36.0X2	T36.0X3	T36.0X4	T36.0X5	T36.0X6
Epiestriol	T38.5X1	T38.5X2	T38.5X3	T38.5X4	T38.5X5	T38.5X6
Epilim — *see* Sodium, valproate						
Epimestrol	T38.5X1	T38.5X2	T38.5X3	T38.5X4	T38.5X5	T38.5X6
Epinephrine	T44.5X1	T44.5X2	T44.5X3	T44.5X4	T44.5X5	T44.5X6
EpiPen*	T44.5X1	T44.5X2	T44.5X3	T44.5X4	T44.5X5	T44.5X6
Epirubicin	T45.1X1	T45.1X2	T45.1X3	T45.1X4	T45.1X5	T45.1X6
Epitiostanol	T38.7X1	T38.7X2	T38.7X3	T38.7X4	T38.7X5	T38.7X6
Epitizide	T50.2X1	T50.2X2	T50.2X3	T50.2X4	T50.2X5	T50.2X6
EPN	T60.0X1	T60.0X2	T60.0X3	T60.0X4	—	—
EPO	T45.8X1	T45.8X2	T45.8X3	T45.8X4	T45.8X5	T45.8X6
Epoetin alpha	T45.8X1	T45.8X2	T45.8X3	T45.8X4	T45.8X5	T45.8X6
Epomediol	T50.991	T50.992	T50.993	T50.994	T50.995	T50.996
Epoprostenol	T45.521	T45.522	T45.523	T45.524	T45.525	T45.526
Epoxy resin	T65.891	T65.892	T65.893	T65.894	—	—
Eprazinone	T48.4X1	T48.4X2	T48.4X3	T48.4X4	T48.4X5	T48.4X6
Epsilon aminocaproic acid	T45.621	T45.622	T45.623	T45.624	T45.625	T45.626
Epsom salt	T47.3X1	T47.3X2	T47.3X3	T47.3X4	T47.3X5	T47.3X6
Eptazocine	T40.491	T40.492	T40.493	T40.494	T40.495	T40.496
Equanil	T43.591	T43.592	T43.593	T43.594	T43.595	T43.596
Equisetum	T62.2X1	T62.2X2	T62.2X3	T62.2X4	—	—
diuretic	T50.2X1	T50.2X2	T50.2X3	T50.2X4	T50.2X5	T50.2X6
Ergobasine	T48.0X1	T48.0X2	T48.0X3	T48.0X5	T48.0X6	
Ergocalciferol	T45.2X1	T45.2X2	T45.2X3	T45.2X4	T45.2X5	T45.2X6
Ergoloid mesylates	T46.7X1	T46.7X2	T46.7X3	T46.7X4	T46.7X5	T46.7X6
Ergometrine	T48.0X1	T48.0X2	T48.0X3	T48.0X4	T48.0X5	T48.0X6
Ergonovine	T48.0X1	T48.0X2	T48.0X3	T48.0X4	T48.0X5	T48.0X6
Ergotamine	T46.5X1	T46.5X2	T46.5X3	T46.5X4	T46.5X5	T46.5X6
Ergotocine	T48.0X1	T48.0X2	T48.0X3	T48.0X4	T48.0X5	T48.0X6

Substance	Poisoning, Accidental (unintentional)	Poisoning, Intentional Self-harm	Poisoning, Assault	Poisoning, Undetermined	Adverse Effect	Under-dosing
Ergotrate	T48.0X1	T48.0X2	T48.0X3	T48.0X4	T48.0X5	T48.0X6
Ergot NEC	T64.81	T64.82	T64.83	T64.84	—	—
derivative	T48.0X1	T48.0X2	T48.0X3	T48.0X4	T48.0X5	T48.0X6
medicinal (alkaloids)	T48.0X1	T48.0X2	T48.0X3	T48.0X4	T48.0X5	T48.0X6
prepared	T48.0X1	T48.0X2	T48.0X3	T48.0X4	T48.0X5	T48.0X6
Eritrityl tetranitrate	T46.3X1	T46.3X2	T46.3X3	T46.3X4	T46.3X5	T46.3X6
Erythrityl tetranitrate	T46.3X1	T46.3X2	T46.3X3	T46.3X4	T46.3X5	T46.3X6
Erythrol tetranitrate	T46.3X1	T46.3X2	T46.3X3	T46.3X4	T46.3X5	T46.3X6
Erythromycin (salts)	T36.3X1	T36.3X2	T36.3X3	T36.3X4	T36.3X5	T36.3X6
ophthalmic preparation	T49.5X1	T49.5X2	T49.5X3	T49.5X4	T49.5X5	T49.5X6
topical NEC	T49.0X1	T49.0X2	T49.0X3	T49.0X4	T49.0X5	T49.0X6
Erythropoietin	T45.8X1	T45.8X2	T45.8X3	T45.8X4	T45.8X5	T45.8X6
human	T45.8X1	T45.8X2	T45.8X3	T45.8X4	T45.8X5	T45.8X6
Esbriet*	T48.991	T48.992	T48.993	T48.994	T48.995	T48.996
Escin	T46.991	T46.992	T46.993	T46.994	T46.995	T46.996
Escitalopram*	T43.221	T43.222	T43.223	T43.224	T43.225	T43.226
Esculin	T45.2X1	T45.2X2	T45.2X3	T45.2X4	T45.2X5	T45.2X6
Esculoside	T45.2X1	T45.2X2	T45.2X3	T45.2X4	T45.2X5	T45.2X6
ESDT (ether-soluble tar distillate)	T49.1X1	T49.1X2	T49.1X3	T49.1X4	T49.1X5	T49.1X6
Eserine	T49.5X1	T49.5X2	T49.5X3	T49.5X4	T49.5X5	T49.5X6
Esflurbiprofen	T39.311	T39.312	T39.313	T39.314	T39.315	T39.316
Eskabarb	T42.3X1	T42.3X2	T42.3X3	T42.3X4	T42.3X5	T42.3X6
Eskalith	T43.8X1	T43.8X2	T43.8X3	T43.8X4	T43.8X5	T43.8X6
Esmolol	T44.7X1	T44.7X2	T44.7X3	T44.7X4	T44.7X5	T44.7X6
Estanozolol	T38.7X1	T38.7X2	T38.7X3	T38.7X4	T38.7X5	T38.7X6
Estazolam	T42.4X1	T42.4X2	T42.4X3	T42.4X4	T42.4X5	T42.4X6
Estradiol	T38.5X1	T38.5X2	T38.5X3	T38.5X4	T38.5X5	T38.5X6
with testosterone	T38.7X1	T38.7X2	T38.7X3	T38.7X4	T38.7X5	T38.7X6
benzoate	T38.5X1	T38.5X2	T38.5X3	T38.5X4	T38.5X5	T38.5X6
Estramustine	T45.1X1	T45.1X2	T45.1X3	T45.1X4	T45.1X5	T45.1X6
Estriol	T38.5X1	T38.5X2	T38.5X3	T38.5X4	T38.5X5	T38.5X6
Estrogen	T38.5X1	T38.5X2	T38.5X3	T38.5X4	T38.5X5	T38.5X6
with progesterone	T38.5X1	T38.5X2	T38.5X3	T38.5X4	T38.5X5	T38.5X6
conjugated	T38.5X1	T38.5X2	T38.5X3	T38.5X4	T38.5X5	T38.5X6
Estrone	T38.5X1	T38.5X2	T38.5X3	T38.5X4	T38.5X5	T38.5X6
Estropipate	T38.5X1	T38.5X2	T38.5X3	T38.5X4	T38.5X5	T38.5X6
Etacrynate sodium	T50.1X1	T50.1X2	T50.1X3	T50.1X4	T50.1X5	T50.1X6
Etacrynic acid	T50.1X1	T50.1X2	T50.1X3	T50.1X4	T50.1X5	T50.1X6
Etafedrine	T48.6X1	T48.6X2	T48.6X3	T48.6X4	T48.6X5	T48.6X6
Etafenone	T46.3X1	T46.3X2	T46.3X3	T46.3X4	T46.3X5	T46.3X6
Etambutol	T37.1X1	T37.1X2	T37.1X3	T37.1X4	T37.1X5	T37.1X6
Etamiphyllin	T48.6X1	T48.6X2	T48.6X3	T48.6X4	T48.6X5	T48.6X6
Etamivan	T50.7X1	T50.7X2	T50.7X3	T50.7X4	T50.7X5	T50.7X6
Etamsylate	T45.7X1	T45.7X2	T45.7X3	T45.7X4	T45.7X5	T45.7X6
Etebenecid	T50.4X1	T50.4X2	T50.4X3	T50.4X4	T50.4X5	T50.4X6
Ethacridine	T49.0X1	T49.0X2	T49.0X3	T49.0X4	T49.0X5	T49.0X6
Ethacrynate*	T50.1X1	T50.1X2	T50.1X3	T50.1X4	T50.1X5	T50.1X6
Ethacrynic acid	T50.1X1	T50.1X2	T50.1X3	T50.1X4	T50.1X5	T50.1X6
Ethadione	T42.2X1	T42.2X2	T42.2X3	T42.2X4	T42.2X5	T42.2X6
Ethambutol	T37.1X1	T37.1X2	T37.1X3	T37.1X4	T37.1X5	T37.1X6
Ethamide	T50.2X1	T50.2X2	T50.2X3	T50.2X4	T50.2X5	T50.2X6
Ethamivan	T50.7X1	T50.7X2	T50.7X3	T50.7X4	T50.7X5	T50.7X6
Ethamsylate	T45.7X1	T45.7X2	T45.7X3	T45.7X4	T45.7X5	T45.7X6
Ethanol	T51.0X1	T51.0X2	T51.0X3	T51.0X4	—	—
beverage	T51.0X1	T51.0X2	T51.0X3	T51.0X4	—	—
Ethanolamine oleate	T46.8X1	T46.8X2	T46.8X3	T46.8X4	T46.8X5	T46.8X6
Ethaverine	T44.3X1	T44.3X2	T44.3X3	T44.3X4	T44.3X5	T44.3X6
Ethchlorvynol	T42.6X1	T42.6X2	T42.6X3	T42.6X4	T42.6X5	T42.6X6
Ethebenecid	T50.4X1	T50.4X2	T50.4X3	T50.4X4	T50.4X5	T50.4X6
Ether (vapor)	T41.0X1	T41.0X2	T41.0X3	T41.0X4	T41.0X5	T41.0X6
anesthetic	T41.0X1	T41.0X2	T41.0X3	T41.0X4	T41.0X5	T41.0X6
divinyl	T41.0X1	T41.0X2	T41.0X3	T41.0X4	T41.0X5	T41.0X6
ethyl (medicinal)	T41.0X1	T41.0X2	T41.0X3	T41.0X4	T41.0X5	T41.0X6
nonmedicinal	T52.8X1	T52.8X2	T52.8X3	T52.8X4	—	—
petroleum — *see* Ligroin						
solvent	T52.8X1	T52.8X2	T52.8X3	T52.8X4	—	—
Ethiazide	T50.2X1	T50.2X2	T50.2X3	T50.2X4	T50.2X5	T50.2X6
Ethidium chloride (vapor)	T59.891	T59.892	T59.893	T59.894		
Ethinamate	T42.6X1	T42.6X2	T42.6X3	T42.6X4	T42.6X5	T42.6X6
Ethinylestradiol, ethinyloestradiol	T38.5X1	T38.5X2	T38.5X3	T38.5X4	T38.5X5	T38.5X6
with						
levonorgestrel	T38.4X1	T38.4X2	T38.4X3	T38.4X4	T38.4X5	T38.4X6
norethisterone	T38.4X1	T38.4X2	T38.4X3	T38.4X4	T38.4X5	T38.4X6
Ethiodized oil (131 I)	T50.8X1	T50.8X2	T50.8X3	T50.8X4	T50.8X5	T50.8X6
Ethiofos*	T50.991	T50.992	T50.993	T50.994	T50.995	T50.996
Ethion	T60.0X1	T60.0X2	T60.0X3	T60.0X4	—	—
Ethionamide	T37.1X1	T37.1X2	T37.1X3	T37.1X4	T37.1X5	T37.1X6
Ethioniamide	T37.1X1	T37.1X2	T37.1X3	T37.1X4	T37.1X5	T37.1X6
Ethisterone	T38.5X1	T38.5X2	T38.5X3	T38.5X4	T38.5X5	T38.5X6
Ethobral	T42.3X1	T42.3X2	T42.3X3	T42.3X4	T42.3X5	T42.3X6

☑ **Additional Character May Be Required** — Refer to the Tabular List for Character Selection

*Optum Value-Add

Substance	Poisoning, Accidental (unintentional)	Poisoning, Intentional Self-harm	Poisoning, Assault	Poisoning, Undetermined	Adverse Effect	Under-dosing
Ethocaine (infiltration) (topical)	T41.3X1	T41.3X2	T41.3X3	T41.3X4	T41.3X5	T41.3X6
nerve block (peripheral) (plexus)	T41.3X1	T41.3X2	T41.3X3	T41.3X4	T41.3X5	T41.3X6
spinal	T41.3X1	T41.3X2	T41.3X3	T41.3X4	T41.3X5	T41.3X6
Ethoheptazine	T40.491	T40.492	T40.493	T40.494	T40.495	T40.496
Ethopropazine	T44.3X1	T44.3X2	T44.3X3	T44.3X4	T44.3X5	T44.3X6
Ethosuximide	T42.2X1	T42.2X2	T42.2X3	T42.2X4	T42.2X5	T42.2X6
Ethotoin	T42.0X1	T42.0X2	T42.0X3	T42.0X4	T42.0X5	T42.0X6
Ethoxazene	T37.91	T37.92	T37.93	T37.94	T37.95	T37.96
Ethoxazorutoside	T46.991	T46.992	T46.993	T46.994	T46.995	T46.996
Ethoxzolamide	T50.2X1	T50.2X2	T50.2X3	T50.2X4	T50.2X5	T50.2X6
Ethyl						
acetate	T52.8X1	T52.8X2	T52.8X3	T52.8X4	—	—
alcohol	T51.0X1	T51.0X2	T51.0X3	T51.0X4	—	—
beverage	T51.0X1	T51.0X2	T51.0X3	T51.0X4	—	—
aldehyde (vapor)	T59.891	T59.892	T59.893	T59.894	—	—
liquid	T52.8X1	T52.8X2	T52.8X3	T52.8X4	—	—
aminobenzoate	T41.3X1	T41.3X2	T41.3X3	T41.3X4	T41.3X5	T41.3X6
aminophenothiazine	T43.3X1	T43.3X2	T43.3X3	T43.3X4	T43.3X5	T43.3X6
benzoate	T52.8X1	T52.8X2	T52.8X3	T52.8X4	—	—
biscoumacetate	T45.511	T45.512	T45.513	T45.514	T45.515	T45.516
bromide (anesthetic)	T41.0X1	T41.0X2	T41.0X3	T41.0X4	T41.0X5	T41.0X6
carbamate	T45.1X1	T45.1X2	T45.1X3	T45.1X4	T45.1X5	T45.1X6
carbinol	T51.3X1	T51.3X2	T51.3X3	T51.3X4	—	—
carbonate	T52.8X1	T52.8X2	T52.8X3	T52.8X4	—	—
chaulmoograte	T37.1X1	T37.1X2	T37.1X3	T37.1X4	T37.1X5	T37.1X6
chloride (anesthetic)	T41.0X1	T41.0X2	T41.0X3	T41.0X4	T41.0X5	T41.0X6
anesthetic (local)	T41.3X1	T41.3X2	T41.3X3	T41.3X4	T41.3X5	T41.3X6
inhaled	T41.0X1	T41.0X2	T41.0X3	T41.0X4	T41.0X5	T41.0X6
local	T49.4X1	T49.4X2	T49.4X3	T49.4X4	T49.4X5	T49.4X6
solvent	T53.6X1	T53.6X2	T53.6X3	T53.6X4	—	—
dibunate	T48.3X1	T48.3X2	T48.3X3	T48.3X4	T48.3X5	T48.3X6
dichloroarsine (vapor)	T57.0X1	T57.0X2	T57.0X3	T57.0X4	—	—
estranol	T38.7X1	T38.7X2	T38.7X3	T38.7X4	T38.7X5	T38.7X6
ether — *see also* ether						
formate NEC (solvent)	T52.0X1	T52.0X2	T52.0X3	T52.0X4	—	—
fumarate	T49.4X1	T49.4X2	T49.4X3	T49.4X4	T49.4X5	T49.4X6
hydroxyisobutyrate NEC (solvent)	T52.8X1	T52.8X2	T52.8X3	T52.8X4	—	—
iodoacetate	T59.3X1	T59.3X2	T59.3X3	T59.3X4	—	—
lactate NEC (solvent)	T52.8X1	T52.8X2	T52.8X3	T52.8X4	—	—
loflazepate	T42.4X1	T42.4X2	T42.4X3	T42.4X4	T42.4X5	T42.4X6
mercuric chloride	T56.1X1	T56.1X2	T56.1X3	T56.1X4	—	—
methylcarbinol	T51.8X1	T51.8X2	T51.8X3	T51.8X4	—	—
morphine	T40.2X1	T40.2X2	T40.2X3	T40.2X4	T40.2X5	T40.2X6
noradrenaline	T48.6X1	T48.6X2	T48.6X3	T48.6X4	T48.6X5	T48.6X6
oxybutyrate NEC (solvent)	T52.8X1	T52.8X2	T52.8X3	T52.8X4	—	—
Ethylene (gas)	T59.891	T59.892	T59.893	T59.894		
anesthetic (general)	T41.0X1	T41.0X2	T41.0X3	T41.0X4	T41.0X5	T41.0X6
chlorohydrin	T52.8X1	T52.8X2	T52.8X3	T52.8X4	—	—
vapor	T53.6X1	T53.6X2	T53.6X3	T53.6X4	—	—
dichloride	T52.8X1	T52.8X2	T52.8X3	T52.8X4	—	—
vapor	T53.6X1	T53.6X2	T53.6X3	T53.6X4	—	—
dinitrate	T52.3X1	T52.3X2	T52.3X3	T52.3X4	—	—
glycol(s)	T52.8X1	T52.8X2	T52.8X3	T52.8X4	—	—
dinitrate	T52.3X1	T52.3X2	T52.3X3	T52.3X4	—	—
monobutyl ether	T52.3X1	T52.3X2	T52.3X3	T52.3X4	—	—
imine	T54.1X1	T54.1X2	T54.1X3	T54.1X4	—	—
oxide (fumigant) (nonmedicinal)	T59.891	T59.892	T59.893	T59.894	—	—
medicinal	T49.0X1	T49.0X2	T49.0X3	T49.0X4	T49.0X5	T49.0X6
Ethylenediaminetetra-acetic acid	T50.6X1	T50.6X2	T50.6X3	T50.6X4	T50.6X5	T50.6X6
Ethylenediamine theophylline	T48.6X1	T48.6X2	T48.6X3	T48.6X4	T48.6X5	T48.6X6
Ethylenedinitrilotetra-acetate	T50.6X1	T50.6X2	T50.6X3	T50.6X4	T50.6X5	T50.6X6
Ethylestrenol	T38.7X1	T38.7X2	T38.7X3	T38.7X4	T38.7X5	T38.7X6
Ethylhydroxycellulose	T47.4X1	T47.4X2	T47.4X3	T47.4X4	T47.4X5	T47.4X6
Ethylidene						
chloride NEC	T53.6X1	T53.6X2	T53.6X3	T53.6X4	—	—
diacetate	T60.3X1	T60.3X2	T60.3X3	T60.3X4	—	—
dicoumarin	T45.511	T45.512	T45.513	T45.514	T45.515	T45.516
dicoumarol	T45.511	T45.512	T45.513	T45.514	T45.515	T45.516
diethyl ether	T52.0X1	T52.0X2	T52.0X3	T52.0X4	—	—
Ethylmorphine	T40.2X1	T40.2X2	T40.2X3	T40.2X4	T40.2X5	T40.2X6
Ethylnorepinephrine	T48.6X1	T48.6X2	T48.6X3	T48.6X4	T48.6X5	T48.6X6
Ethylparachlorophen-oxyisobutyrate	T46.6X1	T46.6X2	T46.6X3	T46.6X4	T46.6X5	T46.6X6
Ethynodiol	T38.4X1	T38.4X2	T38.4X3	T38.4X4	T38.4X5	T38.4X6
with mestranol diacetate	T38.4X1	T38.4X2	T38.4X3	T38.4X4	T38.4X5	T38.4X6
Ethyol*	T50.991	T50.992	T50.993	T50.994	T50.995	T50.995
Etidocaine	T41.3X1	T41.3X2	T41.3X3	T41.3X4	T41.3X5	T41.3X5

Substance	Poisoning, Accidental (unintentional)	Poisoning, Intentional Self-harm	Poisoning, Assault	Poisoning, Undetermined	Adverse Effect	Under-dosing
Etidocaine — *continued*						
infiltration (subcutaneous)	T41.3X1	T41.3X2	T41.3X3	T41.3X4	T41.3X5	T41.3X6
nerve (peripheral) (plexus)	T41.3X1	T41.3X2	T41.3X3	T41.3X4	T41.3X5	T41.3X6
Etidronate	T50.991	T50.992	T50.993	T50.994	T50.995	T50.996
Etidronic acid (disodium salt)	T50.991	T50.992	T50.993	T50.994	T50.995	T50.996
Etifoxine	T42.6X1	T42.6X2	T42.6X3	T42.6X4	T42.6X5	T42.6X6
Etilefrine	T44.4X1	T44.4X2	T44.4X3	T44.4X4	T44.4X5	T44.4X6
Etilfen	T42.3X1	T42.3X2	T42.3X3	T42.3X4	T42.3X5	T42.3X6
Etinodiol	T38.4X1	T38.4X2	T38.4X3	T38.4X4	T38.4X5	T38.4X6
Etiroxate	T46.6X1	T46.6X2	T46.6X3	T46.6X4	T46.6X5	T46.6X6
Etizolam	T42.4X1	T42.4X2	T42.4X3	T42.4X4	T42.4X5	T42.4X6
Etodolac	T39.391	T39.392	T39.393	T39.394	T39.395	T39.396
Etofamide	T37.3X1	T37.3X2	T37.3X3	T37.3X4	T37.3X5	T37.3X6
Etofibrate	T46.6X1	T46.6X2	T46.6X3	T46.6X4	T46.6X5	T46.6X6
Etofylline	T46.7X1	T46.7X2	T46.7X3	T46.7X4	T46.7X5	T46.7X6
clofibrate	T46.6X1	T46.6X2	T46.6X3	T46.6X4	T46.6X5	T46.6X6
Etoglucid	T45.1X1	T45.1X2	T45.1X3	T45.1X4	T45.1X5	T45.1X6
Etomidate	T41.1X1	T41.1X2	T41.1X3	T41.1X4	T41.1X5	T41.1X6
Etomide	T39.8X1	T39.8X2	T39.8X3	T39.8X4	T39.8X5	T39.8X6
Etomidoline	T44.3X1	T44.3X2	T44.3X3	T44.3X4	T44.3X5	T44.3X6
Etoposide	T45.1X1	T45.1X2	T45.1X3	T45.1X4	T45.1X5	T45.1X6
Etorphine	T40.2X1	T40.2X2	T40.2X3	T40.2X4	T40.2X5	T40.2X6
Etoval	T42.3X1	T42.3X2	T42.3X3	T42.3X4	T42.3X5	T42.3X6
Etozolin	T50.1X1	T50.1X2	T50.1X3	T50.1X4	T50.1X5	T50.1X6
Etravirine*	T37.5X1	T37.5X2	T37.5X3	T37.5X4	T37.5X5	T37.5X6
Etretinate	T50.991	T50.992	T50.993	T50.994	T50.995	T50.996
Etryptamine	T43.691	T43.692	T43.693	T43.694	T43.695	T43.696
Etybenzatropine	T44.3X1	T44.3X2	T44.3X3	T44.3X4	T44.3X5	T44.3X6
Etynodiol	T38.4X1	T38.4X2	T38.4X3	T38.4X4	T38.4X5	T38.4X6
Eucaine	T41.3X1	T41.3X2	T41.3X3	T41.3X4	T41.3X5	T41.3X6
Eucalyptus oil	T49.7X1	T49.7X2	T49.7X3	T49.7X4	T49.7X5	T49.7X6
Eucatropine	T49.5X1	T49.5X2	T49.5X3	T49.5X4	T49.5X5	T49.5X6
Eucodal	T40.2X1	T40.2X2	T40.2X3	T40.2X4	T40.2X5	T40.2X6
Euneryl	T42.3X1	T42.3X2	T42.3X3	T42.3X4	T42.3X5	T42.3X6
Euphthalmine	T44.3X1	T44.3X2	T44.3X3	T44.3X4	T44.3X5	T44.3X6
Eurax	T49.0X1	T49.0X2	T49.0X3	T49.0X4	T49.0X5	T49.0X6
Euresol	T49.4X1	T49.4X2	T49.4X3	T49.4X4	T49.4X5	T49.4X6
Euthroid	T38.1X1	T38.1X2	T38.1X3	T38.1X4	T38.1X5	T38.1X6
Evans blue	T50.8X1	T50.8X2	T50.8X3	T50.8X4	T50.8X5	T50.8X6
Evipal	T42.3X1	T42.3X2	T42.3X3	T42.3X4	T42.3X5	T42.3X6
sodium	T41.1X1	T41.1X2	T41.1X3	T41.1X4	T41.1X5	T41.1X6
Evipan	T42.3X1	T42.3X2	T42.3X3	T42.3X4	T42.3X5	T42.3X6
sodium	T41.1X1	T41.1X2	T41.1X3	T41.1X4	T41.1X5	T41.1X6
Exalamide	T49.0X1	T49.0X2	T49.0X3	T49.0X4	T49.0X5	T49.0X6
Exalgin	T39.1X1	T39.1X2	T39.1X3	T39.1X4	T39.1X5	T39.1X6
Excipients, pharmaceutical	T50.901	T50.902	T50.903	T50.904	T50.905	T50.906
Exhaust gas (engine) (motor vehicle)	T58.01	T58.02	T58.03	T58.04	—	—
Ex-Lax (phenolphthalein)	T47.2X1	T47.2X2	T47.2X3	T47.2X4	T47.2X5	T47.2X6
Expectorant NEC	T48.4X1	T48.4X2	T48.4X3	T48.4X4	T48.4X5	T48.4X6
Extended insulin zinc suspension	T38.3X1	T38.3X2	T38.3X3	T38.3X4	T38.3X5	T38.3X6
External medications (skin) (mucous membrane)	T49.91	T49.92	T49.93	T49.94	T49.95	T49.96
dental agent	T49.7X1	T49.7X2	T49.7X3	T49.7X4	T49.7X5	T49.7X6
ENT agent	T49.6X1	T49.6X2	T49.6X3	T49.6X4	T49.6X5	T49.6X6
ophthalmic preparation	T49.5X1	T49.5X2	T49.5X3	T49.5X4	T49.5X5	T49.5X6
specified NEC	T49.8X1	T49.8X2	T49.8X3	T49.8X4	T49.8X5	T49.8X6
Extina*	T49.0X1	T49.0X2	T49.0X3	T49.0X4	T49.0X5	T49.0X6
Extrapyramidal antagonist NEC	T44.3X1	T44.3X2	T44.3X3	T44.3X4	T44.3X5	T44.3X6
Eye agents (anti-infective)	T49.5X1	T49.5X2	T49.5X3	T49.5X4	T49.5X5	T49.5X6
Eye drug NEC	T49.5X1	T49.5X2	T49.5X3	T49.5X4	T49.5X5	T49.5X6
FAC (fluorouracil + doxorubicin + cyclophosphamide)	T45.1X1	T45.1X2	T45.1X3	T45.1X4	T45.1X5	T45.1X6
Factor						
I (fibrinogen)	T45.8X1	T45.8X2	T45.8X3	T45.8X4	T45.8X5	T45.8X6
III (thromboplastin)	T45.8X1	T45.8X2	T45.8X3	T45.8X4	T45.8X5	T45.8X6
IX complex	T45.7X1	T45.7X2	T45.7X3	T45.7X4	T45.7X5	T45.7X6
human	T45.8X1	T45.8X2	T45.8X3	T45.8X4	T45.8X5	T45.8X6
VIII (antihemophilic Factor) (concentrate)	T45.8X1	T45.8X2	T45.8X3	T45.8X4	T45.8X5	T45.8X6
Famotidine	T47.0X1	T47.0X2	T47.0X3	T47.0X4	T47.0X5	T47.0X6
Fat suspension, intravenous	T50.991	T50.992	T50.993	T50.994	T50.995	T50.996
Fazadinium bromide	T48.1X1	T48.1X2	T48.1X3	T48.1X4	T48.1X5	T48.1X6
Febarbamate	T42.3X1	T42.3X2	T42.3X3	T42.3X4	T42.3X5	T42.3X6
Fecal softener	T47.4X1	T47.4X2	T47.4X3	T47.4X4	T47.4X5	T47.4X6
Fedrilate	T48.3X1	T48.3X2	T48.3X3	T48.3X4	T48.3X5	T48.3X6
Felodipine	T46.1X1	T46.1X2	T46.1X3	T46.1X4	T46.1X5	T46.1X6
Felypressin	T38.891	T38.892	T38.893	T38.894	T38.895	T38.896

Table of Drugs and Chemicals

Substance	Poisoning, Accidental (unintentional)	Poisoning, Intentional Self-harm	Poisoning, Assault	Poisoning, Undetermined	Adverse Effect	Under-dosing
Femizol*	T49.0X1	T49.0X2	T49.0X3	T49.0X4	T49.0X5	T49.0X6
Femoxetine	T43.221	T43.222	T43.223	T43.224	T43.225	T43.226
Fenalcomine	T46.3X1	T46.3X2	T46.3X3	T46.3X4	T46.3X5	T46.3X6
Fenamisal	T37.1X1	T37.1X2	T37.1X3	T37.1X4	T37.1X5	T37.1X6
Fenazone	T39.2X1	T39.2X2	T39.2X3	T39.2X4	T39.2X5	T39.2X6
Fenbendazole	T37.4X1	T37.4X2	T37.4X3	T37.4X4	T37.4X5	T37.4X6
Fenbutrazate	T50.5X1	T50.5X2	T50.5X3	T50.5X4	T50.5X5	T50.5X6
Fencamfamine	T43.691	T43.692	T43.693	T43.694	T43.695	T43.696
Fendiline	T46.1X1	T46.1X2	T46.1X3	T46.1X4	T46.1X5	T46.1X6
Fenetylline	T43.691	T43.692	T43.693	T43.694	T43.695	T43.696
Fenflumizole	T39.391	T39.392	T39.393	T39.394	T39.395	T39.396
Fenfluramine	T50.5X1	T50.5X2	T50.5X3	T50.5X4	T50.5X5	T50.5X6
Fenobarbital	T42.3X1	T42.3X2	T42.3X3	T42.3X4	T42.3X5	T42.3X6
Fenofibrate	T46.6X1	T46.6X2	T46.6X3	T46.6X4	T46.6X5	T46.6X6
Fenoprofen	T39.311	T39.312	T39.313	T39.314	T39.315	T39.316
Fenoterol	T48.6X1	T48.6X2	T48.6X3	T48.6X4	T48.6X5	T48.6X6
Fenoverine	T44.3X1	T44.3X2	T44.3X3	T44.3X4	T44.3X5	T44.3X6
Fenoxazoline	T48.5X1	T48.5X2	T48.5X3	T48.5X4	T48.5X5	T48.5X6
Fenproporex	T50.5X1	T50.5X2	T50.5X3	T50.5X4	T50.5X5	T50.5X6
Fenquizone	T50.2X1	T50.2X2	T50.2X3	T50.2X4	T50.2X5	T50.2X6
Fentanyl (analogs)	T40.411	T40.412	T40.413	T40.414	T40.415	T40.416
Fentazin	T43.3X1	T43.3X2	T43.3X3	T43.3X4	T43.3X5	T43.3X6
Fenthion	T60.0X1	T60.0X2	T60.0X3	T60.0X4	—	—
Fenticlor	T49.0X1	T49.0X2	T49.0X3	T49.0X4	T49.0X5	T49.0X6
Fenylbutazone	T39.2X1	T39.2X2	T39.2X3	T39.2X4	T39.2X5	T39.2X6
Feprazone	T39.2X1	T39.2X2	T39.2X3	T39.2X4	T39.2X5	T39.2X6
Fer de lance (bite) (venom)	T63.061	T63.062	T63.063	T63.064	—	—
Ferrex*	T45.4X1	T45.4X2	T45.4X3	T45.4X4	T45.4X5	T45.4X6
Ferric — *see also* Iron						
chloride	T45.4X1	T45.4X2	T45.4X3	T45.4X4	T45.4X5	T45.4X6
citrate	T45.4X1	T45.4X2	T45.4X3	T45.4X4	T45.4X5	T45.4X6
hydroxide						
colloidal	T45.4X1	T45.4X2	T45.4X3	T45.4X4	T45.4X5	T45.4X6
polymaltose	T45.4X1	T45.4X2	T45.4X3	T45.4X4	T45.4X5	T45.4X6
pyrophosphate	T45.4X1	T45.4X2	T45.4X3	T45.4X4	T45.4X5	T45.4X6
Ferritin	T45.4X1	T45.4X2	T45.4X3	T45.4X4	T45.4X5	T45.4X6
Ferrocholinate	T45.4X1	T45.4X2	T45.4X3	T45.4X4	T45.4X5	T45.4X6
Ferrodextrane	T45.4X1	T45.4X2	T45.4X3	T45.4X4	T45.4X5	T45.4X6
Ferropolimaler	T45.4X1	T45.4X2	T45.4X3	T45.4X4	T45.4X5	T45.4X6
Ferrous — *see also* Iron						
phosphate	T45.4X1	T45.4X2	T45.4X3	T45.4X4	T45.4X5	T45.4X6
salt	T45.4X1	T45.4X2	T45.4X3	T45.4X4	T45.4X5	T45.4X6
with folic acid	T45.4X1	T45.4X2	T45.4X3	T45.4X4	T45.4X5	T45.4X6
Ferrous fumerate, gluconate, lactate, salt NEC, sulfate (medicinal)	T45.4X1	T45.4X2	T45.4X3	T45.4X4	T45.4X5	T45.4X6
Ferrovanadium (fumes)	T59.891	T59.892	T59.893	T59.894	—	—
Ferrum — *see* Iron						
Fertilizers NEC	T65.891	T65.892	T65.893	T65.894	—	—
with herbicide mixture	T60.3X1	T60.3X2	T60.3X3	T60.3X4	—	—
Fetoxilate	T47.6X1	T47.6X2	T47.6X3	T47.6X4	T47.6X5	T47.6X6
Fiber, dietary	T47.4X1	T47.4X2	T47.4X3	T47.4X4	T47.4X5	T47.4X6
Fiberglass	T65.831	T65.832	T65.833	T65.834	—	—
Fibrinogen (human)	T45.8X1	T45.8X2	T45.8X3	T45.8X4	T45.8X5	T45.8X6
Fibrinolysin (human)	T45.691	T45.692	T45.693	T45.694	T45.695	T45.696
Fibrinolysis						
affecting drug	T45.601	T45.602	T45.603	T45.604	T45.605	T45.606
inhibitor NEC	T45.621	T45.622	T45.623	T45.624	T45.625	T45.626
Fibrinolytic drug	T45.611	T45.612	T45.613	T45.614	T45.615	T45.616
Filix mas	T37.4X1	T37.4X2	T37.4X3	T37.4X4	T37.4X5	T37.4X6
Filtering cream	T49.3X1	T49.3X2	T49.3X3	T49.3X4	T49.3X5	T49.3X6
Finacea*	T49.0X1	T49.0X2	T49.0X3	T49.0X4	T49.0X5	T49.0X6
Fiorinal	T39.011	T39.012	T39.013	T39.014	T39.015	T39.016
Firedamp	T59.891	T59.892	T59.893	T59.894	—	—
Fish, noxious, nonbacterial	T61.91	T61.92	T61.93	T61.94	—	—
ciguatera	T61.01	T61.02	T61.03	T61.04	—	—
scombroid	T61.11	T61.12	T61.14	—	—	—
shell	T61.781	T61.782	T61.783	T61.784	—	—
specified NEC	T61.771	T61.772	T61.773	T61.774	—	—
Flagyl	T37.3X1	T37.3X2	T37.3X3	T37.3X4	T37.3X5	T37.3X6
Flavine adenine dinucleotide	T45.2X1	T45.2X2	T45.2X3	T45.2X4	T45.2X5	T45.2X6
Flavodic acid	T46.991	T46.992	T46.993	T46.994	T46.995	T46.996
Flavoxate	T44.3X1	T44.3X2	T44.3X4	T44.3X4	T44.3X5	T44.3X6
Flaxedil	T48.1X1	T48.1X2	T48.1X4	T48.1X4	T48.1X5	T48.1X6
Flaxseed (medicinal)	T49.3X1	T49.3X2	T49.3X3	T49.3X4	T49.3X5	T49.3X6
Flecainide	T46.2X1	T46.2X2	T46.2X3	T46.2X4	T46.2X5	T46.2X6
Fleroxacin	T36.8X1	T36.8X2	T36.8X3	T36.8X4	T36.8X5	T36.8X6
Floctafenine	T39.8X1	T39.8X2	T39.8X3	T39.8X4	T39.8X5	T39.8X6
Flomax	T44.6X1	T44.6X2	T44.6X3	T44.6X4	T44.6X5	T44.6X6
Flomoxef	T36.1X1	T36.1X2	T36.1X3	T36.1X4	T36.1X5	T36.1X6
Flonase*	T49.6X1	T49.6X2	T49.6X3	T49.6X4	T49.6X5	T49.6X6

Substance	Poisoning, Accidental (unintentional)	Poisoning, Intentional Self-harm	Poisoning, Assault	Poisoning, Undetermined	Adverse Effect	Under-dosing
Flopropione	T44.3X1	T44.3X2	T44.3X3	T44.3X4	T44.3X5	T44.3X6
FLORAjen*	T47.6X1	T47.6X2	T47.6X3	T47.6X4	T47.6X5	T47.6X6
Florantyrone	T47.5X1	T47.5X2	T47.5X3	T47.5X4	T47.5X5	T47.5X6
Floraquin	T37.8X1	T37.8X2	T37.8X3	T37.8X4	T37.8X5	T37.8X6
Florinef	T38.0X1	T38.0X2	T38.0X3	T38.0X4	T38.0X5	T38.0X6
ENT agent	T49.6X1	T49.6X2	T49.6X3	T49.6X4	T49.6X5	T49.6X6
ophthalmic preparation	T49.5X1	T49.5X2	T49.5X3	T49.5X4	T49.5X5	T49.5X6
topical NEC	T49.0X1	T49.0X2	T49.0X3	T49.0X4	T49.0X5	T49.0X6
Flovent*	T38.0X1	T38.0X2	T38.0X3	T38.0X4	T38.0X5	T38.0X6
Flowers of sulfur	T49.4X1	T49.4X2	T49.4X3	T49.4X4	T49.4X5	T49.4X6
Floxuridine	T45.1X1	T45.1X2	T45.1X3	T45.1X4	T45.1X5	T45.1X6
Fluanisone	T43.4X1	T43.4X2	T43.4X3	T43.4X4	T43.4X5	T43.4X6
Flubendazole	T37.4X1	T37.4X2	T37.4X3	T37.4X4	T37.4X5	T37.4X6
Fluclorolone acetonide	T49.0X1	T49.0X2	T49.0X3	T49.0X4	T49.0X5	T49.0X6
Flucloxacillin	T36.0X1	T36.0X2	T36.0X3	T36.0X4	T36.0X5	T36.0X6
Fluconazole	T37.8X1	T37.8X2	T37.8X3	T37.8X4	T37.8X5	T37.8X6
Flucytosine	T37.8X1	T37.8X2	T37.8X3	T37.8X4	T37.8X5	T37.8X6
Fludeoxyglucose (18F)	T50.8X1	T50.8X2	T50.8X3	T50.8X4	T50.8X5	T50.8X6
Fludiazepam	T42.4X1	T42.4X2	T42.4X3	T42.4X4	T42.4X5	T42.4X6
Fludrocortisone	T50.0X1	T50.0X2	T50.0X3	T50.0X4	T50.0X5	T50.0X6
ENT agent	T49.6X1	T49.6X2	T49.6X3	T49.6X4	T49.6X5	T49.6X6
ophthalmic preparation	T49.5X1	T49.5X2	T49.5X3	T49.5X4	T49.5X5	T49.5X6
topical NEC	T49.0X1	T49.0X2	T49.0X3	T49.0X4	T49.0X5	T49.0X6
Fludroxycortide	T49.0X1	T49.0X2	T49.0X3	T49.0X4	T49.0X5	T49.0X6
Flufenamic acid	T39.391	T39.392	T39.393	T39.394	T39.395	T39.396
Fluindione	T45.511	T45.512	T45.513	T45.514	T45.515	T45.516
Flumequine	T37.8X1	T37.8X2	T37.8X3	T37.8X4	T37.8X5	T37.8X6
Flumethasone	T49.0X1	T49.0X2	T49.0X3	T49.0X4	T49.0X5	T49.0X6
Flumethiazide	T50.2X1	T50.2X2	T50.2X3	T50.2X4	T50.2X5	T50.2X6
Flumidin	T37.5X1	T37.5X2	T37.5X3	T37.5X4	T37.5X5	T37.5X6
Flunarizine	T46.7X1	T46.7X2	T46.7X3	T46.7X4	T46.7X5	T46.7X6
Flunidazole	T37.8X1	T37.8X2	T37.8X3	T37.8X4	T37.8X5	T37.8X6
Flunisolide	T48.6X1	T48.6X2	T48.6X3	T48.6X4	T48.6X5	T48.6X6
Flunitrazepam	T42.4X1	T42.4X2	T42.4X3	T42.4X4	T42.4X5	T42.4X6
Fluocinolone (acetonide)	T49.0X1	T49.0X2	T49.0X3	T49.0X4	T49.0X5	T49.0X6
Fluocinonide	T49.0X1	T49.0X2	T49.0X3	T49.0X4	T49.0X5	T49.0X6
Fluocortin (butyl)	T49.0X1	T49.0X2	T49.0X3	T49.0X4	T49.0X5	T49.0X6
Fluocortolone	T49.0X1	T49.0X2	T49.0X3	T49.0X4	T49.0X5	T49.0X6
Fluohydrocortisone	T38.0X1	T38.0X2	T38.0X3	T38.0X4	T38.0X5	T38.0X6
ENT agent	T49.6X1	T49.6X2	T49.6X3	T49.6X4	T49.6X5	T49.6X6
ophthalmic preparation	T49.5X1	T49.5X2	T49.5X3	T49.5X4	T49.5X5	T49.5X6
topical NEC	T49.0X1	T49.0X2	T49.0X3	T49.0X4	T49.0X5	T49.0X6
Fluonid	T49.0X1	T49.0X2	T49.0X3	T49.0X4	T49.0X5	T49.0X6
Fluopromazine	T43.3X1	T43.3X2	T43.3X3	T43.3X4	T43.3X5	T43.3X6
Fluoracetate	T60.8X1	T60.8X2	T60.8X3	T60.8X4	—	—
Fluorescein	T50.8X1	T50.8X2	T50.8X3	T50.8X4	T50.8X5	T50.8X6
Fluorhydrocortisone	T50.0X1	T50.0X2	T50.0X3	T50.0X4	T50.0X5	T50.0X6
Fluoride (nonmedicinal) (pesticide) (sodium) **NEC**	T60.8X1	T60.8X2	T60.8X3	T60.8X4	—	—
hydrogen — *see* Hydrofluoric acid						
medicinal NEC	T50.991	T50.992	T50.993	T50.994	T50.995	T50.996
dental use	T49.7X1	T49.7X2	T49.7X3	T49.7X4	T49.7X5	T49.7X6
not pesticide NEC	T54.91	T54.92	T54.93	T54.94	—	—
stannous	T49.7X1	T49.7X2	T49.7X3	T49.7X4	T49.7X5	T49.7X6
Fluorigard*	T47.7X1	T47.7X2	T47.7X3	T47.7X4	T47.7X5	T47.7X6
Fluorinated corticosteroids	T38.0X1	T38.0X2	T38.0X3	T38.0X4	T38.0X5	T38.0X6
Fluorine (gas)	T59.5X1	T59.5X2	T59.5X3	T59.5X4	—	—
salt — *see* Fluoride(s)						
Fluoristan	T49.7X1	T49.7X2	T49.7X3	T49.7X4	T49.7X5	T49.7X6
Fluormetholone	T49.0X1	T49.0X2	T49.0X3	T49.0X4	T49.0X5	T49.0X6
Fluoroacetate	T60.8X1	T60.8X2	T60.8X3	T60.8X4	—	—
Fluorocarbon monomer	T53.6X1	T53.6X2	T53.6X3	T53.6X4	—	—
Fluorocytosine	T37.8X1	T37.8X2	T37.8X3	T37.8X4	T37.8X5	T37.8X6
Fluorodeoxyuridine	T45.1X1	T45.1X2	T45.1X3	T45.1X4	T45.1X5	T45.1X6
Fluorometholone	T49.0X1	T49.0X2	T49.0X3	T49.0X4	T49.0X5	T49.0X6
ophthalmic preparation	T49.5X1	T49.5X2	T49.5X3	T49.5X4	T49.5X5	T49.5X6
Fluorophosphate insecticide	T60.0X1	T60.0X2	T60.0X3	T60.0X4	—	—
Fluorosol	T46.3X1	T46.3X2	T46.3X3	T46.3X4	T46.3X5	T46.3X6
Fluorouracil	T45.1X1	T45.1X2	T45.1X3	T45.1X4	T45.1X5	T45.1X6
Fluorphenylalanine	T49.5X1	T49.5X2	T49.5X3	T49.5X4	T49.5X5	T49.5X6
Fluothane	T41.0X1	T41.0X2	T41.0X3	T41.0X4	T41.0X5	T41.0X6
Fluoxetine	T43.221	T43.222	T43.223	T43.224	T43.225	T43.226
Fluoxymesterone	T38.7X1	T38.7X2	T38.7X3	T38.7X4	T38.7X5	T38.7X6
Flupenthixol	T43.4X1	T43.4X2	T43.4X3	T43.4X4	T43.4X5	T43.4X6
Flupentixol	T43.4X1	T43.4X2	T43.4X3	T43.4X4	T43.4X5	T43.4X6
Fluphenazine	T43.3X1	T43.3X2	T43.3X3	T43.3X4	T43.3X5	T43.3X6
Fluprednidene	T49.0X1	T49.0X2	T49.0X3	T49.0X4	T49.0X5	T49.0X6
Fluprednisolone	T38.0X1	T38.0X2	T38.0X3	T38.0X4	T38.0X5	T38.0X6
Fluradoline	T39.8X1	T39.8X2	T39.8X3	T39.8X4	T39.8X5	T39.8X6
Flurandrenolide	T49.0X1	T49.0X2	T49.0X3	T49.0X4	T49.0X5	T49.0X6

☑ Additional Character May Be Required — Refer to the Tabular List for Character Selection

*Optum Value-Add

Femizol* — Flurandrenolide

Substance	Poisoning, Accidental (unintentional)	Poisoning, Intentional Self-harm	Poisoning, Assault	Poisoning, Undetermined	Adverse Effect	Under-dosing
Flurandrenolone	T49.0X1	T49.0X2	T49.0X3	T49.0X4	T49.0X5	T49.0X6
Flurazepam	T42.4X1	T42.4X2	T42.4X3	T42.4X4	T42.4X5	T42.4X6
Flurbiprofen	T39.311	T39.312	T39.313	T39.314	T39.315	T39.316
Flurobate	T49.0X1	T49.0X2	T49.0X3	T49.0X4	T49.0X5	T49.0X6
Fluroxene	T41.0X1	T41.0X2	T41.0X3	T41.0X4	T41.0X5	T41.0X6
Fluspirilene	T43.591	T43.592	T43.593	T43.594	T43.595	T43.596
Flutamide	T38.6X1	T38.6X2	T38.6X3	T38.6X4	T38.6X5	T38.6X6
Flutazolam	T38.0X1	T38.0X2	T38.0X3	T38.0X4	T38.0X5	T38.0X6
Fluticasone propionate	T38.0X1	T38.0X2	T38.0X3	T38.0X4	T38.0X5	T38.0X6
Flutoprazepam	T42.4X1	T42.4X2	T42.4X3	T42.4X4	T42.4X5	T42.4X6
Flutropium bromide	T48.6X1	T48.6X2	T48.6X3	T48.6X4	T48.6X5	T48.6X6
Fluvoxamine	T43.221	T43.222	T43.223	T43.224	T43.225	T43.226
Folacin	T45.8X1	T45.8X2	T45.8X3	T45.8X4	T45.8X5	T45.8X6
Folic acid	T45.8X1	T45.8X2	T45.8X3	T45.8X4	T45.8X5	T45.8X6
with ferrous salt	T45.2X1	T45.2X2	T45.2X3	T45.2X4	T45.2X5	T45.2X6
antagonist	T45.1X1	T45.1X2	T45.1X3	T45.1X4	T45.1X5	T45.1X6
Folinic acid	T45.8X1	T45.8X2	T45.8X3	T45.8X4	T45.8X5	T45.8X6
Folium stramoniae	T48.6X1	T48.6X2	T48.6X3	T48.6X4	T48.6X5	T48.6X6
Follicle-stimulating hormone, human	T38.811	T38.812	T38.813	T38.814	T38.815	T38.816
Folpet	T60.3X1	T60.3X2	T60.3X3	T60.3X4	—	—
Fomepizole*	T50.6X1	T50.6X2	T50.6X3	T50.6X4	T50.6X5	T50.6X6
Fominoben	T48.3X1	T48.3X2	T48.3X3	T48.3X4	T48.3X5	T48.3X6
Food, foodstuffs, noxious, nonbacterial, NEC	T62.91	T62.92	T62.93	T62.94	—	—
berries	T62.1X1	T62.1X2	T62.1X3	T62.1X4	—	—
fish — see also Fish	T61.91	T61.92	T61.93	T61.94	—	—
mushrooms	T62.0X1	T62.0X2	T62.0X3	T62.0X4	—	—
plants	T62.2X1	T62.2X2	T62.2X3	T62.2X4	—	—
seafood	T61.91	T61.92	T61.93	T61.94	—	—
specified NEC	T61.8X1	T61.8X2	T61.8X3	T61.8X4	—	—
seeds	T62.2X1	T62.2X2	T62.2X3	T62.2X4	—	—
shellfish	T61.781	T61.782	T61.783	T61.784	—	—
specified NEC	T62.8X1	T62.8X2	T62.8X3	T62.8X4	—	—
Fool's parsley	T62.2X1	T62.2X2	T62.2X3	T62.2X4	—	—
Formaldehyde (solution), gas or vapor	T59.2X1	T59.2X2	T59.2X3	T59.2X4	—	—
fungicide	T60.3X1	T60.3X2	T60.3X3	T60.3X4	—	—
Formalin	T59.2X1	T59.2X2	T59.2X3	T59.2X4	—	—
fungicide	T60.3X1	T60.3X2	T60.3X3	T60.3X4	—	—
vapor	T59.2X1	T59.2X2	T59.2X3	T59.2X4	—	—
Formic acid	T54.2X1	T54.2X2	T54.2X3	T54.2X4	—	—
vapor	T59.891	T59.892	T59.893	T59.894	—	—
Formoterol*	T48.6X1	T48.6X2	T48.6X3	T48.6X4	T48.6X5	T48.6X6
Fortaz*	T36.1X1	T36.1X2	T36.1X3	T36.1X4	T36.1X5	T36.1X6
Foscarnet sodium	T37.5X1	T37.5X2	T37.5X3	T37.5X4	T37.5X5	T37.5X6
Fosfestrol	T38.5X1	T38.5X2	T38.5X3	T38.5X4	T38.5X5	T38.5X6
Fosfomycin	T36.8X1	T36.8X2	T36.8X3	T36.8X4	T36.8X5	T36.8X6
Fosfonet sodium	T37.5X1	T37.5X2	T37.5X3	T37.5X4	T37.5X5	T37.5X6
Fosinopril	T46.4X1	T46.4X2	T46.4X3	T46.4X4	T46.4X5	T46.4X6
sodium	T46.4X1	T46.4X2	T46.4X3	T46.4X4	T46.4X5	T46.4X6
Fowler's solution	T57.0X1	T57.0X2	T57.0X3	T57.0X4	—	—
Foxglove	T62.2X1	T62.2X2	T62.2X3	T62.2X4	—	—
Framycetin	T36.5X1	T36.5X2	T36.5X3	T36.5X4	T36.5X5	T36.5X6
Frangula	T47.2X1	T47.2X2	T47.2X3	T47.2X4	T47.2X5	T47.2X6
extract	T47.2X1	T47.2X2	T47.2X3	T47.2X4	T47.2X5	T47.2X6
Frei antigen	T50.8X1	T50.8X2	T50.8X3	T50.8X4	T50.8X5	T50.8X6
Freon	T53.5X1	T53.5X2	T53.5X3	T53.5X4	—	—
Fructose	T50.3X1	T50.3X2	T50.3X3	T50.3X4	T50.3X5	T50.3X6
Frusemide	T50.1X1	T50.1X2	T50.1X3	T50.1X4	T50.1X5	T50.1X6
FSH	T38.811	T38.812	T38.813	T38.814	T38.815	T38.816
Ftorafur	T45.1X1	T45.1X2	T45.1X3	T45.1X4	T45.1X5	T45.1X6
Fuel						
automobile	T52.0X1	T52.0X2	T52.0X3	T52.0X4	—	—
exhaust gas, not in transit	T58.01	T58.02	T58.03	T58.04	—	—
vapor NEC	T52.0X1	T52.0X2	T52.0X3	T52.0X4	—	—
gas (domestic use) — see also Carbon, monoxide, fuel, utility	T59.891	T59.892	T59.893	T59.894	—	—
utility	T59.891	T59.892	T59.893	T59.894	—	—
incomplete combustion of — see Carbon, monoxide, fuel, utility						
in mobile container	T59.891	T59.892	T59.893	T59.894	—	—
piped (natural)	T59.891	T59.892	T59.893	T59.894	—	—
industrial, incomplete combustion	T58.8X1	T58.8X2	T58.8X3	T58.8X4	—	—
Fugillin	T36.8X1	T36.8X2	T36.8X3	T36.8X4	T36.8X5	T36.8X6
Fulminate of mercury	T56.1X1	T56.1X2	T56.1X3	T56.1X4	—	—
Fulvicin	T36.7X1	T36.7X2	T36.7X3	T36.7X4	T36.7X5	T36.7X6
Fumadil	T36.8X1	T36.8X2	T36.8X3	T36.8X4	T36.8X5	T36.8X6
Fumagillin	T36.8X1	T36.8X2	T36.8X3	T36.8X4	T36.8X5	T36.8X6

Substance	Poisoning, Accidental (unintentional)	Poisoning, Intentional Self-harm	Poisoning, Assault	Poisoning, Undetermined	Adverse Effect	Under-dosing
Fumaric acid	T49.4X1	T49.4X2	T49.4X3	T49.4X4	T49.4X5	T49.4X6
Fumes (from)	T59.91	T59.92	T59.93	T59.94	—	—
carbon monoxide — see Carbon, monoxide						
charcoal (domestic use) — see Charcoal, fumes						
chloroform — see Chloroform						
coke (in domestic stoves, fireplaces) — see Coke fumes						
corrosive NEC	T54.91	T54.92	T54.93	T54.94	—	—
ether — see ether						
freons	T53.5X1	T53.5X2	T53.5X3	T53.5X4	—	—
hydrocarbons	T59.891	T59.892	T59.893	T59.894	—	—
petroleum (liquefied)	T59.891	T59.892	T59.893	T59.894	—	—
distributed through pipes (pure or mixed with air)	T59.891	T59.892	T59.893	T59.894	—	—
lead — see lead						
metal — see Metals, or the specified metal						
nitrogen dioxide	T59.0X1	T59.0X2	T59.0X3	T59.0X4	—	—
pesticides — see Pesticide						
petroleum (liquefied)	T59.891	T59.892	T59.893	T59.894	—	—
distributed through pipes (pure or mixed with air)	T59.891	T59.892	T59.893	T59.894	—	—
polyester	T59.891	T59.892	T59.893	T59.894	—	—
specified source NEC — see also substance specified	T59.891	T59.892	T59.893	T59.894	—	—
sulfur dioxide	T59.1X1	T59.1X2	T59.1X3	T59.1X4	—	—
Fumigant NEC	T60.91	T60.92	T60.93	T60.94	—	—
Fungicide NEC (nonmedicinal)	T60.3X1	T60.3X2	T60.3X3	T60.3X4	—	—
Fungi, noxious, used as food	T62.0X1	T62.0X2	T62.0X3	T62.0X4	—	—
Fungizone	T36.7X1	T36.7X2	T36.7X3	T36.7X4	T36.7X5	T36.7X6
topical	T49.0X1	T49.0X2	T49.0X3	T49.0X4	T49.0X5	T49.0X6
Fungoid*	T49.0X1	T49.0X2	T49.0X3	T49.0X4	T49.0X5	T49.0X6
Furacin	T49.0X1	T49.0X2	T49.0X3	T49.0X4	T49.0X5	T49.0X6
Furadantin	T37.91	T37.92	T37.93	T37.94	T37.95	T37.96
Furazolidone	T37.8X1	T37.8X2	T37.8X3	T37.8X4	T37.8X5	T37.8X6
Furazolium chloride	T49.0X1	T49.0X2	T49.0X3	T49.0X4	T49.0X5	T49.0X6
Furfural	T52.8X1	T52.8X2	T52.8X3	T52.8X4	—	—
Furnace (coal burning) (domestic), gas from	T58.2X1	T58.2X2	T58.2X3	T58.2X4	—	—
industrial	T58.8X1	T58.8X2	T58.8X3	T58.8X4	—	—
Furniture polish	T65.891	T65.892	T65.893	T65.894	—	—
Furosemide	T50.1X1	T50.1X2	T50.1X3	T50.1X4	T50.1X5	T50.1X6
Furoxone	T37.91	T37.92	T37.93	T37.94	T37.95	T37.96
Fursultiamine	T45.2X1	T45.2X2	T45.2X3	T45.2X4	T45.2X5	T45.2X6
Fusafungine	T36.8X1	T36.8X2	T36.8X3	T36.8X4	T36.8X5	T36.8X6
Fusel oil (any) (amyl) (butyl) (propyl), vapor	T51.3X1	T51.3X2	T51.3X3	T51.3X4	—	—
Fusidate (ethanolamine) (sodium)	T36.8X1	T36.8X2	T36.8X3	T36.8X4	T36.8X5	T36.8X6
Fusidic acid	T36.8X1	T36.8X2	T36.8X3	T36.8X4	T36.8X5	T36.8X6
Fytic acid, nonasodium	T50.6X1	T50.6X2	T50.6X3	T50.6X4	T50.6X5	T50.6X6
b-Galactosidase	T47.5X1	T47.5X2	T47.5X3	T47.5X4	T47.5X5	T47.5X6
GABA	T43.8X1	T43.8X2	T43.8X3	T43.8X4	T43.8X5	T43.8X6
Gabapentin*	T42.6X1	T42.6X2	T42.6X3	T42.6X4	T42.6X5	T42.6X6
Gabitril*	T42.6X1	T42.6X2	T42.6X3	T42.6X4	T42.6X5	T42.6X6
Gadolinium	T56.821	T56.822	T56.823	T56.824	—	—
Gadopentetic acid	T50.8X1	T50.8X2	T50.8X3	T50.8X4	T50.8X5	T50.8X6
Galactose	T50.3X1	T50.3X2	T50.3X3	T50.3X4	T50.3X5	T50.3X6
Galantamine	T44.0X1	T44.0X2	T44.0X3	T44.0X4	T44.0X5	T44.0X6
Gallamine (triethiodide)	T48.1X1	T48.1X2	T48.1X3	T48.1X4	T48.1X5	T48.1X6
Gallium citrate	T50.991	T50.992	T50.993	T50.994	T50.995	T50.996
Gallopamil	T46.1X1	T46.1X2	T46.1X3	T46.1X4	T46.1X5	T46.1X6
Gamboge	T47.2X1	T47.2X2	T47.2X3	T47.2X4	T47.2X5	T47.2X6
Gamimune	T50.Z11	T50.Z12	T50.Z13	T50.Z14	T50.Z15	T50.Z16
Gamma-aminobutyric acid	T43.8X1	T43.8X2	T43.8X3	T43.8X4	T43.8X5	T43.8X6
Gamma-benzene hexachloride (medicinal)	T49.0X1	T49.0X2	T49.0X3	T49.0X4	T49.0X5	T49.0X6
nonmedicinal, vapor	T53.6X1	T53.6X2	T53.6X3	T53.6X4	—	—
Gamma-BHC (medicinal) — see also Gamma-benzene hexachloride	T49.0X1	T49.0X2	T49.0X3	T49.0X4	T49.0X5	T49.0X6
Gamma globulin	T50.Z11	T50.Z12	T50.Z13	T50.Z14	T50.Z15	T50.Z16
Gamulin	T50.Z11	T50.Z12	T50.Z13	T50.Z14	T50.Z15	T50.Z16
Ganciclovir (sodium)	T37.5X1	T37.5X2	T37.5X3	T37.5X4	T37.5X5	T37.5X6
Ganglionic blocking drug NEC	T44.2X1	T44.2X2	T44.2X3	T44.2X4	T44.2X5	T44.2X6

Table of Drugs and Chemicals

Ganglionic blocking drug NEC — Glutaral

Substance	Poisoning, Accidental (unintentional)	Poisoning, Intentional Self-harm	Poisoning, Assault	Poisoning, Undetermined	Adverse Effect	Under-dosing
Ganglionic blocking drug — *continued*						
specified NEC	T44.2X1	T44.2X2	T44.2X3	T44.2X4	T44.2X5	T44.2X6
Ganja	T40.711	T40.712	T40.713	T40.714	T40.715	T40.716
Garamycin	T36.5X1	T36.5X2	T36.5X3	T36.5X4	T36.5X5	T36.5X6
ophthalmic preparation	T49.5X1	T49.5X2	T49.5X3	T49.5X4	T49.5X5	T49.5X6
topical NEC	T49.0X1	T49.0X2	T49.0X3	T49.0X4	T49.0X5	T49.0X6
Gardenal	T42.3X1	T42.3X2	T42.3X3	T42.3X4	T42.3X5	T42.3X6
Gardepanyl	T42.3X1	T42.3X2	T42.3X3	T42.3X4	T42.3X5	T42.3X6
Gaseous substance — *see* Gas						
Gasoline	T52.0X1	T52.0X2	T52.0X3	T52.0X4	—	—
vapor	T52.0X1	T52.0X2	T52.0X3	T52.0X4	—	—
Gastric enzymes	T47.5X1	T47.5X2	T47.5X3	T47.5X4	T47.5X5	T47.5X6
Gastrografin	T50.8X1	T50.8X2	T50.8X3	T50.8X4	T50.8X5	T50.8X6
Gastrointestinal drug	T47.91	T47.92	T47.93	T47.94	T47.95	T47.96
biological	T47.8X1	T47.8X2	T47.8X3	T47.8X4	T47.8X5	T47.8X6
specified NEC	T47.8X1	T47.8X2	T47.8X3	T47.8X4	T47.8X5	T47.8X6
Gas NEC	T59.91	T59.92	T59.93	T59.94	—	—
acetylene	T59.891	T59.892	T59.893	T59.894	—	—
incomplete combustion of	T58.11	T58.12	T58.13	T58.14	—	—
air contaminants, source or type not specified	T59.91	T59.92	T59.93	T59.94	—	—
anesthetic	T41.0X1	T41.0X2	T41.0X3	T41.0X4	T41.0X5	T41.0X6
blast furnace	T58.8X1	T58.8X2	T58.8X3	T58.8X4	—	—
butane — *see* butane						
carbon monoxide — *see* Carbon, monoxide						
chlorine	T59.4X1	T59.4X2	T59.4X3	T59.4X4	—	—
coal	T58.2X1	T58.2X2	T58.2X3	T58.2X4	—	—
cyanide	T57.3X1	T57.3X2	T57.3X3	T57.3X4	—	—
dicyanogen	T65.0X1	T65.0X2	T65.0X3	T65.0X4	—	—
domestic — *see* Domestic gas						
exhaust	T58.01	T58.02	T58.03	T58.04	—	—
from utility (for cooking, heating, or lighting) (after combustion) — *see* Carbon, monoxide, fuel, utility						
prior to combustion	T59.891	T59.892	T59.893	T59.894	—	—
from wood- or coal-burning stove or fireplace	T58.2X1	T58.2X2	T58.2X3	T58.2X4	—	—
fuel (domestic use) (after combustion) — *see also* Carbon, monoxide, fuel						
industrial use	T58.8X1	T58.8X2	T58.8X3	T58.8X4	—	—
prior to combustion	T59.891	T59.892	T59.893	T59.894	—	—
utility	T59.891	T59.892	T59.893	T59.894	—	—
incomplete combustion of — *see* Carbon, monoxide, fuel, utility						
in mobile container	T59.891	T59.892	T59.893	T59.894	—	—
piped (natural)	T59.891	T59.892	T59.893	T59.894	—	—
garage	T58.01	T58.02	T58.03	T58.04	—	—
hydrocarbon NEC	T59.891	T59.892	T59.893	T59.894	—	—
incomplete combustion of — *see* Carbon, monoxide, fuel, utility						
liquefied — *see* butane						
piped	T59.891	T59.892	T59.893	T59.894	—	—
hydrocyanic acid	T65.0X1	T65.0X2	T65.0X3	T65.0X4	—	—
illuminating (after combustion)	T58.11	T58.12	T58.13	T58.14	—	—
prior to combustion	T59.891	T59.892	T59.893	T59.894	—	—
incomplete combustion, any — *see* Carbon, monoxide						
kiln	T58.8X1	T58.8X2	T58.8X3	T58.8X4	—	—
lacrimogenic	T59.3X1	T59.3X2	T59.3X3	T59.3X4	—	—
liquefied petroleum — *see* butane						
marsh	T59.891	T59.892	T59.893	T59.894	—	—
motor exhaust, not in transit	T58.01	T58.02	T58.03	T58.04	—	—
mustard, not in war	T59.891	T59.892	T59.893	T59.894	—	—
natural	T59.891	T59.892	T59.893	T59.894	—	—
nerve, not in war	T59.91	T59.92	T59.93	T59.94	—	—
oil	T52.0X1	T52.0X2	T52.0X3	T52.0X4	—	—
petroleum (liquefied) (distributed in mobile containers)	T59.891	T59.892	T59.893	T59.894	—	—
piped (pure or mixed with air)	T59.891	T59.892	T59.893	T59.894	—	—
piped (manufactured) (natural) NEC	T59.891	T59.892	T59.893	T59.894	—	—
Gas — *continued*						
producer	T58.8X1	T58.8X2	T58.8X3	T58.8X4	—	—
propane — *see* propane						
refrigerant (chlorofluoro-carbon)	T53.5X1	T53.5X2	T53.5X3	T53.5X4	—	—
not chlorofluoro-carbon	T59.891	T59.892	T59.893	T59.894	—	—
sewer	T59.91	T59.92	T59.93	T59.94	—	—
specified source NEC	T59.91	T59.92	T59.93	T59.94	—	—
stove (after combustion)	T58.11	T58.12	T58.13	T58.14	—	—
prior to combustion	T59.891	T59.892	T59.893	T59.894	—	—
tear	T59.3X1	T59.3X2	T59.3X3	T59.3X4	—	—
therapeutic	T41.5X1	T41.5X2	T41.5X3	T41.5X4	T41.5X5	T41.5X6
utility (for cooking, heating, or lighting) (piped) NEC	T59.891	T59.892	T59.893	T59.894	—	—
incomplete combustion of — *see* Carbon, monoxide, fuel, utility						
in mobile container	T59.891	T59.892	T59.893	T59.894	—	—
piped (natural)	T59.891	T59.892	T59.893	T59.894	—	—
water	T58.11	T58.12	T58.13	T58.14	—	—
incomplete combustion of — *see* Carbon, monoxide, fuel, utility						
Gaultheria procumbens	T62.2X1	T62.2X2	T62.2X3	T62.2X4	—	—
Gaviscon*	T47.1X1	T47.1X2	T47.1X3	T47.1X4	T47.1X5	T47.1X6
Gefarnate	T44.3X1	T44.3X2	T44.3X3	T44.3X4	T44.3X5	T44.3X6
Gelatin (intravenous)	T45.8X1	T45.8X2	T45.8X3	T45.8X4	T45.8X5	T45.8X6
absorbable (sponge)	T45.7X1	T45.7X2	T45.7X3	T45.7X4	T45.7X5	T45.7X6
Gelfilm	T49.8X1	T49.8X2	T49.8X3	T49.8X4	T49.8X5	T49.8X6
Gelfoam	T45.7X1	T45.7X2	T45.7X3	T45.7X4	T45.7X5	T45.7X6
Gelsemine	T50.991	T50.992	T50.993	T50.994	T50.995	T50.996
Gelsemium (sempervirens)	T62.2X1	T62.2X2	T62.2X3	T62.2X4	—	—
Gemeprost	T48.0X1	T48.0X2	T48.0X3	T48.0X4	T48.0X5	T48.0X6
Gemfibrozil	T46.6X1	T46.6X2	T46.6X3	T46.6X4	T46.6X5	T46.6X6
Gemonil	T42.3X1	T42.3X2	T42.3X3	T42.3X4	T42.3X5	T42.3X6
Gentamicin	T36.5X1	T36.5X2	T36.5X3	T36.5X4	T36.5X5	T36.5X6
ophthalmic preparation	T49.5X1	T49.5X2	T49.5X3	T49.5X4	T49.5X5	T49.5X6
topical NEC	T49.0X1	T49.0X2	T49.0X3	T49.0X4	T49.0X5	T49.0X6
Gentasol*	T49.5X1	T49.5X2	T49.5X3	T49.5X4	T49.5X5	T49.5X6
Gentian	T47.5X1	T47.5X2	T47.5X3	T47.5X4	T47.5X5	T47.5X6
violet	T49.0X1	T49.0X2	T49.0X3	T49.0X4	T49.0X5	T49.0X6
Gepefrine	T44.4X1	T44.4X2	T44.4X3	T44.4X4	T44.4X5	T44.4X6
Gestonorone caproate	T38.5X1	T38.5X2	T38.5X3	T38.5X4	T38.5X5	T38.5X6
Gexane	T49.0X1	T49.0X2	T49.0X3	T49.0X4	T49.0X5	T49.0X6
Gila monster (venom)	T63.111	T63.112	T63.113	T63.114	—	—
Ginger	T47.5X1	T47.5X2	T47.5X3	T47.5X4	—	T47.5X6
Jamaica — *see* Jamaica, ginger						
Gitalin	T46.0X1	T46.0X2	T46.0X3	T46.0X4	T46.0X5	T46.0X6
amorphous	T46.0X1	T46.0X2	T46.0X3	T46.0X4	T46.0X5	T46.0X6
Gitaloxin	T46.0X1	T46.0X2	T46.0X3	T46.0X4	T46.0X5	T46.0X6
Gitoxin	T46.0X1	T46.0X2	T46.0X3	T46.0X4	T46.0X5	T46.0X6
Glafenine	T39.8X1	T39.8X2	T39.8X3	T39.8X4	T39.8X5	T39.8X6
Glandular extract (medicinal) NEC	T50.Z91	T50.Z92	T50.Z93	T50.Z94	T50.Z95	T50.Z96
Glaucarubin	T37.3X1	T37.3X2	T37.3X3	T37.3X4	T37.3X5	T37.3X6
Glibenclamide	T38.3X1	T38.3X2	T38.3X3	T38.3X4	T38.3X5	T38.3X6
Glibornuride	T38.3X1	T38.3X2	T38.3X3	T38.3X4	T38.3X5	T38.3X6
Gliclazide	T38.3X1	T38.3X2	T38.3X3	T38.3X4	T38.3X5	T38.3X6
Glimidine	T38.3X1	T38.3X2	T38.3X3	T38.3X4	T38.3X5	T38.3X6
Glipizide	T38.3X1	T38.3X2	T38.3X3	T38.3X4	T38.3X5	T38.3X6
Gliquidone	T38.3X1	T38.3X2	T38.3X3	T38.3X4	T38.3X5	T38.3X6
Glisolamide	T38.3X1	T38.3X2	T38.3X3	T38.3X4	T38.3X5	T38.3X6
Glisoxepide	T38.3X1	T38.3X2	T38.3X3	T38.3X4	T38.3X5	T38.3X6
Globin zinc insulin	T38.3X1	T38.3X2	T38.3X3	T38.3X4	T38.3X5	T38.3X6
Globulin						
antilymphocytic	T50.Z11	T50.Z12	T50.Z13	T50.Z14	T50.Z15	T50.Z16
antirhesus	T50.Z11	T50.Z12	T50.Z13	T50.Z14	T50.Z15	T50.Z16
antivenin	T50.Z11	T50.Z12	T50.Z13	T50.Z14	T50.Z15	T50.Z16
antiviral	T50.Z11	T50.Z12	T50.Z13	T50.Z14	T50.Z15	T50.Z16
Glucagon	T38.3X1	T38.3X2	T38.3X3	T38.3X4	T38.3X5	T38.3X6
Glucocorticoids	T38.0X1	T38.0X2	T38.0X3	T38.0X4	T38.0X5	T38.0X6
Glucocorticosteroid	T38.0X1	T38.0X2	T38.0X3	T38.0X4	T38.0X5	T38.0X6
Gluconic acid	T50.991	T50.992	T50.993	T50.994	T50.995	T50.996
Glucosamine sulfate	T39.4X1	T39.4X2	T39.4X3	T39.4X4	T39.4X5	T39.4X6
Glucose	T50.3X1	T50.3X2	T50.3X3	T50.3X4	T50.3X5	T50.3X6
with sodium chloride	T50.3X1	T50.3X2	T50.3X3	T50.3X4	T50.3X5	T50.3X6
Glucosulfone sodium	T37.1X1	T37.1X2	T37.1X3	T37.1X4	T37.1X5	T37.1X6
Glucotrol*	T38.3X1	T38.3X2	T38.3X3	T38.3X4	T38.3X5	T38.3X6
Glucurolactone	T47.8X1	T47.8X2	T47.8X3	T47.8X4	T47.8X5	T47.8X6
Glue NEC	T52.8X1	T52.8X2	T52.8X3	T52.8X4	—	—
Glutamic acid	T47.5X1	T47.5X2	T47.5X3	T47.5X4	T47.5X5	T47.5X6
Glutaral (medicinal)	T49.0X1	T49.0X2	T49.0X3	T49.0X4	T49.0X5	T49.0X6
nonmedicinal	T65.891	T65.892	T65.893	T65.894	—	—

☑ Additional Character May Be Required — Refer to the Tabular List for Character Selection
*Optum Value-Add

Substance	Poisoning, Accidental (unintentional)	Poisoning, Intentional Self-harm	Poisoning, Assault	Poisoning, Undetermined	Adverse Effect	Under-dosing
Glutaraldehyde	T65.891	T65.892	T65.893	T65.894	—	—
(nonmedicinal)						
medicinal	T49.0X1	T49.0X2	T49.0X3	T49.0X4	T49.0X5	T49.0X6
Glutathione	T50.6X1	T50.6X2	T50.6X3	T50.6X4	T50.6X5	T50.6X6
Glutethimide	T42.6X1	T42.6X2	T42.6X3	T42.6X4	T42.6X5	T42.6X6
Glyburide	T38.3X1	T38.3X2	T38.3X3	T38.3X4	T38.3X5	T38.3X6
Glycerin	T47.4X1	T47.4X2	T47.4X3	T47.4X4	T47.4X5	T47.4X6
Glycerol	T47.4X1	T47.4X2	T47.4X3	T47.4X4	T47.4X5	T47.4X6
borax	T49.6X1	T49.6X2	T49.6X3	T49.6X4	T49.6X5	T49.6X6
intravenous	T50.3X1	T50.3X2	T50.3X3	T50.3X4	T50.3X5	T50.3X6
iodinated	T48.4X1	T48.4X2	T48.4X3	T48.4X4	T48.4X5	T48.4X6
Glycerophosphate	T50.991	T50.992	T50.993	T50.994	T50.995	T50.996
Glyceryl						
gualacolate	T48.4X1	T48.4X2	T48.4X3	T48.4X4	T48.4X5	T48.4X6
nitrate	T46.3X1	T46.3X2	T46.3X3	T46.3X4	T46.3X5	T46.3X6
triacetate (topical)	T49.0X1	T49.0X2	T49.0X3	T49.0X4	T49.0X5	T49.0X6
trinitrate	T46.3X1	T46.3X2	T46.3X3	T46.3X4	T46.3X5	T46.3X6
Glycine	T50.3X1	T50.3X2	T50.3X3	T50.3X4	T50.3X5	T50.3X6
Glyclopyramide	T38.3X1	T38.3X2	T38.3X3	T38.3X4	T38.3X5	T38.3X6
Glycobiarsol	T37.3X1	T37.3X2	T37.3X3	T37.3X4	T37.3X5	T37.3X6
Glycols (ether)	T52.3X1	T52.3X2	T52.3X3	T52.3X4	—	—
Glyconiazide	T37.1X1	T37.1X2	T37.1X3	T37.1X4	T37.1X5	T37.1X6
Glycopyrrolate	T44.3X1	T44.3X2	T44.3X3	T44.3X4	T44.3X5	T44.3X6
Glycopyrronium	T44.3X1	T44.3X2	T44.3X3	T44.3X4	T44.3X5	T44.3X6
bromide	T44.3X1	T44.3X2	T44.3X3	T44.3X4	T44.3X5	T44.3X6
Glycoside, cardiac	T46.0X1	T46.0X2	T46.0X3	T46.0X4	T46.0X5	T46.0X6
(stimulant)						
Glycyclamide	T38.3X1	T38.3X2	T38.3X3	T38.3X4	T38.3X5	T38.3X6
Glycyrrhiza extract	T48.4X1	T48.4X2	T48.4X3	T48.4X4	T48.4X5	T48.4X6
Glycyrrhizic acid	T48.4X1	T48.4X2	T48.4X3	T48.4X4	T48.4X5	T48.4X6
Glycyrrhizinate potassium	T48.4X1	T48.4X2	T48.4X3	T48.4X4	T48.4X5	T48.4X6
Glymidine sodium	T38.3X1	T38.3X2	T38.3X3	T38.3X4	T38.3X5	T38.3X6
Glyphosate	T60.3X1	T60.3X2	T60.3X3	T60.3X4	—	—
Glyphylline	T48.6X1	T48.6X2	T48.6X3	T48.6X4	T48.6X5	T48.6X6
Gold						
colloidal (I98Au)	T45.1X1	T45.1X2	T45.1X3	T45.1X4	T45.1X5	T45.1X6
salts	T39.4X1	T39.4X2	T39.4X3	T39.4X4	T39.4X5	T39.4X6
Golden sulfide of antimony	T56.891	T56.892	T56.893	T56.894	—	—
Goldylocks	T62.2X1	T62.2X2	T62.2X3	T62.2X4		
Gonadal tissue extract	T38.901	T38.902	T38.903	T38.904	T38.905	T38.906
female	T38.5X1	T38.5X2	T38.5X3	T38.5X4	T38.5X5	T38.5X6
male	T38.7X1	T38.7X2	T38.7X3	T38.7X4	T38.7X5	T38.7X6
Gonadorelin	T38.891	T38.892	T38.893	T38.894	T38.895	T38.896
Gonadotropin	T38.891	T38.892	T38.893	T38.894	T38.895	T38.896
chorionic	T38.891	T38.892	T38.893	T38.894	T38.895	T38.896
pituitary	T38.811	T38.812	T38.813	T38.814	T38.815	T38.816
Goserelin	T45.1X1	T45.1X2	T45.1X3	T45.1X4	T45.1X5	T45.1X6
Grain alcohol	T51.0X1	T51.0X2	T51.0X3	T51.0X4		
Gralise*	T42.6X1	T42.6X2	T42.6X3	T42.6X4	T42.6X5	T42.6X6
Gramicidin	T49.0X1	T49.0X2	T49.0X3	T49.0X4	T49.0X5	T49.0X6
Granisetron	T45.0X1	T45.0X2	T45.0X3	T45.0X4	T45.0X5	T45.0X6
Gratiola officinalis	T62.2X1	T62.2X2	T62.2X3	T62.2X4	—	—
Grease	T65.891	T65.892	T65.893	T65.894	—	—
Green hellebore	T62.2X1	T62.2X2	T62.2X3	T62.2X4	—	—
Green soap	T49.2X1	T49.2X2	T49.2X3	T49.2X4	T49.2X5	T49.2X6
Grifulvin	T36.7X1	T36.7X2	T36.7X3	T36.7X4	T36.7X5	T36.7X6
Griseofulvin	T36.7X1	T36.7X2	T36.7X3	T36.7X4	T36.7X5	T36.7X6
Growth hormone	T38.811	T38.812	T38.813	T38.814	T38.815	T38.816
Guaiacol derivatives	T48.4X1	T48.4X2	T48.4X3	T48.4X4	T48.4X5	T48.4X6
Guaiac reagent	T50.991	T50.992	T50.993	T50.994	T50.995	T50.996
Guaifenesin	T48.4X1	T48.4X2	T48.4X3	T48.4X4	T48.4X5	T48.4X6
Guaimesal	T48.4X1	T48.4X2	T48.4X3	T48.4X4	T48.4X5	T48.4X6
Guaiphenesin	T48.4X1	T48.4X2	T48.4X3	T48.4X4	T48.4X5	T48.4X6
Guaituss*	T48.4X1	T48.4X2	T48.4X3	T48.4X4	T48.4X5	T48.4X6
Guamecycline	T36.4X1	T36.4X2	T36.4X3	T36.4X4	T36.4X5	T36.4X6
Guanabenz	T46.5X1	T46.5X2	T46.5X3	T46.5X4	T46.5X5	T46.5X6
Guanacline	T46.5X1	T46.5X2	T46.5X3	T46.5X4	T46.5X5	T46.5X6
Guanadrel	T46.5X1	T46.5X2	T46.5X3	T46.5X4	T46.5X5	T46.5X6
Guanatol	T37.2X1	T37.2X2	T37.2X3	T37.2X4	T37.2X5	T37.2X6
Guanethidine	T46.5X1	T46.5X2	T46.5X3	T46.5X4	T46.5X5	T46.5X6
Guanfacine	T46.5X1	T46.5X2	T46.5X3	T46.5X4	T46.5X5	T46.5X6
Guano	T65.891	T65.892	T65.893	T65.894	—	—
Guanochlor	T46.5X1	T46.5X2	T46.5X3	T46.5X4	T46.5X5	T46.5X6
Guanoclor	T46.5X1	T46.5X2	T46.5X3	T46.5X4	T46.5X5	T46.5X6
Guanoctine	T46.5X1	T46.5X2	T46.5X3	T46.5X4	T46.5X5	T46.5X6
Guanoxabenz	T46.5X1	T46.5X2	T46.5X3	T46.5X4	T46.5X5	T46.5X6
Guanoxan	T46.5X1	T46.5X2	T46.5X3	T46.5X4	T46.5X5	T46.5X6
Guar gum (medicinal)	T46.6X1	T46.6X2	T46.6X3	T46.6X4	T46.6X5	T46.6X6
Hachimycin	T36.7X1	T36.7X2	T36.7X3	T36.7X4	T36.7X5	T36.7X6
Hair						
dye	T49.4X1	T49.4X2	T49.4X3	T49.4X4	T49.4X5	T49.4X6
preparation NEC	T49.4X1	T49.4X2	T49.4X3	T49.4X4	T49.4X5	T49.4X6
Halazepam	T42.4X1	T42.4X2	T42.4X3	T42.4X4	T42.4X5	T42.4X6
Halcinolone	T49.0X1	T49.0X2	T49.0X3	T49.0X4	T49.0X5	T49.0X6
Halcinonide	T49.0X1	T49.0X2	T49.0X3	T49.0X4	T49.0X5	T49.0X6
Halethazole	T49.0X1	T49.0X2	T49.0X3	T49.0X4	T49.0X5	T49.0X6
Hallucinogen NOS	T40.901	T40.902	T40.903	T40.904	T40.905	T40.906
specified NEC	T40.991	T40.992	T40.993	T40.994	T40.995	T40.996
Halofantrine	T37.2X1	T37.2X2	T37.2X3	T37.2X4	T37.2X5	T37.2X6
Halofenate	T46.6X1	T46.6X2	T46.6X3	T46.6X4	T46.6X5	T46.6X6
Halometasone	T49.0X1	T49.0X2	T49.0X3	T49.0X4	T49.0X5	T49.0X6
Haloperidol	T43.4X1	T43.4X2	T43.4X3	T43.4X4	T43.4X5	T43.4X6
Haloprogin	T49.0X1	T49.0X2	T49.0X3	T49.0X4	T49.0X5	T49.0X6
Halotex	T49.0X1	T49.0X2	T49.0X3	T49.0X4	T49.0X5	T49.0X6
Halothane	T41.0X1	T41.0X2	T41.0X3	T41.0X4	T41.0X5	T41.0X6
Haloxazolam	T42.4X1	T42.4X2	T42.4X3	T42.4X4	T42.4X5	T42.4X6
Halquinols	T49.0X1	T49.0X2	T49.0X3	T49.0X4	T49.0X5	T49.0X6
Hamamelis	T49.2X1	T49.2X2	T49.2X3	T49.2X4	T49.2X5	T49.2X6
Haptendextran	T45.8X1	T45.8X2	T45.8X3	T45.8X4	T45.8X5	T45.8X6
Harmonyl	T46.5X1	T46.5X2	T46.5X3	T46.5X4	T46.5X5	T46.5X6
Hartmann's solution	T50.3X1	T50.3X2	T50.3X3	T50.3X4	T50.3X5	T50.3X6
Hashish	T40.711	T40.712	T40.713	T40.714	T40.715	T40.716
Havrix*	T50.B91	T50.B92	T50.B93	T50.B94	T50.B95	T50.B96
Hawaiian Woodrose seeds	T40.991	T40.992	T40.993	T40.994	—	—
HCB	T60.3X1	T60.3X2	T60.3X3	T60.3X4	—	—
HCH	T53.6X1	T53.6X2	T53.6X3	T53.6X4	—	—
medicinal	T49.0X1	T49.0X2	T49.0X3	T49.0X4	T49.0X5	T49.0X6
HCN	T57.3X1	T57.3X2	T57.3X3	T57.3X4	—	—
Headache cures, drugs, powders NEC	T50.901	T50.902	T50.903	T50.904	T50.905	T50.906
Heavenly Blue (morning glory)	T40.991	T40.992	T40.993	T40.994		
Heavy metal antidote	T45.8X1	T45.8X2	T45.8X3	T45.8X4	T45.8X5	T45.8X6
Hedaquinium	T49.0X1	T49.0X2	T49.0X3	T49.0X4	T49.0X5	T49.0X6
Hedge hyssop	T62.2X1	T62.2X2	T62.2X3	T62.2X4	—	—
Heet	T49.8X1	T49.8X2	T49.8X3	T49.8X4	T49.8X5	T49.8X6
Helenin	T37.4X1	T37.4X2	T37.4X3	T37.4X4	T37.4X5	T37.4X6
Helium (nonmedicinal) **NEC**	T59.891	T59.892	T59.893	T59.894	—	—
medicinal	T48.991	T48.992	T48.993	T48.994	T48.995	T48.996
Hellebore (black) (green) (white)	T62.2X1	T62.2X2	T62.2X3	T62.2X4	—	—
Hematin	T45.8X1	T45.8X2	T45.8X3	T45.8X4	T45.8X5	T45.8X6
Hematinic preparation	T45.8X1	T45.8X2	T45.8X3	T45.8X4	T45.8X5	T45.8X6
Hematological agent	T45.91	T45.92	T45.93	T45.94	T45.95	T45.96
specified NEC	T45.8X1	T45.8X2	T45.8X3	T45.8X4	T45.8X5	T45.8X6
Hemlock	T62.2X1	T62.2X2	T62.2X3	T62.2X4	—	—
Hemostatic	T45.621	T45.622	T45.623	T45.624	T45.625	T45.626
drug, systemic	T45.621	T45.622	T45.623	T45.624	T45.625	T45.626
Hemostyptic	T49.4X1	T49.4X2	T49.4X3	T49.4X4	T49.4X5	T49.4X6
Henbane	T62.2X1	T62.2X2	T62.2X3	T62.2X4	—	—
Heparin (sodium)	T45.511	T45.512	T45.513	T45.514	T45.515	T45.516
action reverser	T45.7X1	T45.7X2	T45.7X3	T45.7X4	T45.7X5	T45.7X6
Heparin-fraction	T45.511	T45.512	T45.513	T45.514	T45.515	T45.516
Heparinoid (systemic)	T45.511	T45.512	T45.513	T45.514	T45.515	T45.516
Hepatic secretion stimulant	T47.8X1	T47.8X2	T47.8X3	T47.8X4	T47.8X5	T47.8X6
Hepatitis A vaccine*	T50.B91	T50.B92	T50.B93	T50.B94	T50.B95	T50.B96
Hepatitis B						
immune globulin	T50.Z11	T50.Z12	T50.Z13	T50.Z14	T50.Z15	T50.Z16
vaccine	T50.B91	T50.B92	T50.B93	T50.B94	T50.B95	T50.B96
Hepronicate	T46.7X1	T46.7X2	T46.7X3	T46.7X4	T46.7X5	T46.7X6
Heptabarb	T42.3X1	T42.3X2	T42.3X3	T42.3X4	T42.3X5	T42.3X6
Heptabarbital	T42.3X1	T42.3X2	T42.3X3	T42.3X4	T42.3X5	T42.3X6
Heptabarbitone	T42.3X1	T42.3X2	T42.3X3	T42.3X4	T42.3X5	T42.3X6
Heptachlor	T60.1X1	T60.1X2	T60.1X3	T60.1X4	—	—
Heptalgin	T40.2X1	T40.2X2	T40.2X3	T40.2X4	T40.2X5	T40.2X6
Heptaminol	T46.3X1	T46.3X2	T46.3X3	T46.3X4	T46.3X5	T46.3X6
Herbicide NEC	T60.3X1	T60.3X2	T60.3X3	T60.3X4	—	—
Heroin	T40.1X1	T40.1X2	T40.1X3	T40.1X4		
Herplex	T49.5X1	T49.5X2	T49.5X3	T49.5X4	T49.5X5	T49.5X6
HES	T45.8X1	T45.8X2	T45.8X3	T45.8X4	T45.8X5	T45.8X6
Hesperidin	T46.991	T46.992	T46.993	T46.994	T46.995	T46.996
Hetacillin	T36.0X1	T36.0X2	T36.0X3	T36.0X4	T36.0X5	T36.0X6
Hetastarch	T45.8X1	T45.8X2	T45.8X3	T45.8X4	T45.8X5	T45.8X6
HETP	T60.0X1	T60.0X2	T60.0X3	T60.0X4	—	—
Hexachlorobenzene	T60.3X1	T60.3X2	T60.3X3	T60.3X4	—	—
(vapor)						
Hexachlorocyclohexane	T53.6X1	T53.6X2	T53.6X3	T53.6X4	—	—
Hexachlorophene	T49.0X1	T49.0X2	T49.0X3	T49.0X4	T49.0X5	T49.0X6
Hexadiline	T46.3X1	T46.3X2	T46.3X3	T46.3X4	T46.3X5	T46.3X6
Hexadimethrine (bromide)	T45.7X1	T45.7X2	T45.7X3	T45.7X4	T45.7X5	T45.7X6
Hexadylamine	T46.3X1	T46.3X2	T46.3X3	T46.3X4	T46.3X5	T46.3X6
Hexaethyl tetraphosphate	T60.0X1	T60.0X2	T60.0X3	T60.0X4	—	—
Hexafluorenium bromide	T48.1X1	T48.1X2	T48.1X3	T48.1X4	T48.1X5	T48.1X6
Hexafluronium (bromide)	T48.1X1	T48.1X2	T48.1X3	T48.1X4	T48.1X5	T48.1X6

Table of Drugs and Chemicals

Hexa-germ — Hydroxyphenylbutazone

Substance	Poisoning, Accidental (unintentional)	Poisoning, Intentional Self-harm	Poisoning, Assault	Poisoning, Undetermined	Adverse Effect	Under-dosing
Hexa-germ	T49.2X1	T49.2X2	T49.2X3	T49.2X4	T49.2X5	T49.2X6
Hexahydrobenzol	T52.8X1	T52.8X2	T52.8X3	T52.8X4	—	—
Hexahydrocresol(s)	T51.8X1	T51.8X2	T51.8X3	T51.8X4	—	—
arsenide	T57.0X1	T57.0X2	T57.0X3	T57.0X4	—	—
arseniurated	T57.0X1	T57.0X2	T57.0X3	T57.0X4	—	—
cyanide	T57.3X1	T57.3X2	T57.3X3	T57.3X4	—	—
gas	T59.891	T59.892	T59.893	T59.894	—	—
Fluoride (liquid)	T57.8X1	T57.8X2	T57.8X3	T57.8X4	—	—
vapor	T59.891	T59.892	T59.893	T59.894	—	—
phophorated	T60.0X1	T60.0X2	T60.0X3	T60.0X4	—	—
sulfate	T57.8X1	T57.8X2	T57.8X3	T57.8X4	—	—
sulfide (gas)	T59.6X1	T59.6X2	T59.6X3	T59.6X4	—	—
arseniurated	T57.0X1	T57.0X2	T57.0X3	T57.0X4	—	—
sulfurated	T57.8X1	T57.8X2	T57.8X3	T57.8X4	—	—
Hexahydrophenol	T51.8X1	T51.8X2	T51.8X3	T51.8X4	—	—
Hexalen	T51.8X1	T51.8X2	T51.8X3	T51.8X4	—	—
Hexamethonium bromide	T44.2X1	T44.2X2	T44.2X3	T44.2X4	T44.2X5	T44.2X6
Hexamethylene	T52.8X1	T52.8X2	T52.8X3	T52.8X4	—	—
Hexamethylmelamine	T45.1X1	T45.1X2	T45.1X3	T45.1X4	T45.1X5	T45.1X6
Hexamidine	T49.0X1	T49.0X2	T49.0X3	T49.0X4	T49.0X5	T49.0X6
Hexamine (mandelate)	T37.8X1	T37.8X2	T37.8X3	T37.8X4	T37.8X5	T37.8X6
Hexanone, 2-hexanone	T52.4X1	T52.4X2	T52.4X3	T52.4X4	—	—
Hexanuorenium	T48.1X1	T48.1X2	T48.1X3	T48.1X4	T48.1X5	T48.1X6
Hexapropymate	T42.6X1	T42.6X2	T42.6X3	T42.6X4	T42.6X5	T42.6X6
Hexasonium iodide	T44.3X1	T44.3X2	T44.3X3	T44.3X4	T44.3X5	T44.3X6
Hexcarbacholine bromide	T48.1X1	T48.1X2	T48.1X3	T48.1X4	T48.1X5	T48.1X6
Hexemal	T42.3X1	T42.3X2	T42.3X3	T42.3X4	T42.3X5	T42.3X6
Hexestrol	T38.5X1	T38.5X2	T38.5X3	T38.5X4	T38.5X5	T38.5X6
Hexethal (sodium)	T42.3X1	T42.3X2	T42.3X3	T42.3X4	T42.3X5	T42.3X6
Hexetidine	T37.8X1	T37.8X2	T37.8X3	T37.8X4	T37.8X5	T37.8X6
Hexobarbital	T42.3X1	T42.3X2	T42.3X3	T42.3X4	T42.3X5	T42.3X6
rectal	T41.291	T41.292	T41.293	T41.294	T41.295	T41.296
sodium	T41.1X1	T41.1X2	T41.1X3	T41.1X4	T41.1X5	T41.1X6
Hexobendine	T46.3X1	T46.3X2	T46.3X3	T46.3X4	T46.3X5	T46.3X6
Hexocyclium	T44.3X1	T44.3X2	T44.3X3	T44.3X4	T44.3X5	T44.3X6
metilsulfate	T44.3X1	T44.3X2	T44.3X3	T44.3X4	T44.3X5	T44.3X6
Hexoestrol	T38.5X1	T38.5X2	T38.5X3	T38.5X4	T38.5X5	T38.5X6
Hexone	T52.4X1	T52.4X2	T52.4X3	T52.4X4	—	—
Hexoprenaline	T48.6X1	T48.6X2	T48.6X3	T48.6X4	T48.6X5	T48.6X6
Hexylcaine	T41.3X1	T41.3X2	T41.3X3	T41.3X4	T41.3X5	T41.3X6
Hexylresorcinol	T52.2X1	T52.2X2	T52.2X3	T52.2X4	—	—
HGH (human growth hormone)	T38.811	T38.812	T38.813	T38.814	T38.815	T38.816
Hibistat*	T49.0X1	T49.0X2	T49.0X3	T49.0X4	T49.0X5	T49.0X6
Hinkle's pills	T47.2X1	T47.2X2	T47.2X3	T47.2X4	T47.2X5	T47.2X6
Histalog	T50.8X1	T50.8X2	T50.8X3	T50.8X4	T50.8X5	T50.8X6
Histamine (phosphate)	T50.8X1	T50.8X2	T50.8X3	T50.8X4	T50.8X5	T50.8X6
Histolyn*	T50.8X1	T50.8X2	T50.8X3	T50.8X4	T50.8X5	T50.8X6
Histoplasmin	T50.8X1	T50.8X2	T50.8X3	T50.8X4	T50.8X5	T50.8X6
Holly berries	T62.2X1	T62.2X2	T62.2X3	T62.2X4	—	—
Homatropine	T44.3X1	T44.3X2	T44.3X3	T44.3X4	T44.3X5	T44.3X6
methylbromide	T44.3X1	T44.3X2	T44.3X3	T44.3X4	T44.3X5	T44.3X6
Homochlorcyclizine	T45.0X1	T45.0X2	T45.0X3	T45.0X4	T45.0X5	T45.0X6
Homosalate	T49.3X1	T49.3X2	T49.3X3	T49.3X4	T49.3X5	T49.3X6
Homo-tet	T50.Z11	T50.Z12	T50.Z13	T50.Z14	T50.Z15	T50.Z16
Hormone	T38.801	T38.802	T38.803	T38.804	T38.805	T38.806
adrenal cortical steroids	T38.0X1	T38.0X2	T38.0X3	T38.0X4	T38.0X5	T38.0X6
androgenic	T38.7X1	T38.7X2	T38.7X3	T38.7X4	T38.7X5	T38.7X6
anterior pituitary NEC	T38.811	T38.812	T38.813	T38.814	T38.815	T38.816
antidiabetic agents	T38.3X1	T38.3X2	T38.3X3	T38.3X4	T38.3X5	T38.3X6
antidiuretic	T38.891	T38.892	T38.893	T38.894	T38.895	T38.896
cancer therapy	T45.1X1	T45.1X2	T45.1X3	T45.1X4	T45.1X5	T45.1X6
follicle stimulating	T38.811	T38.812	T38.813	T38.814	T38.815	T38.816
gonadotropic	T38.891	T38.892	T38.893	T38.894	T38.895	T38.896
pituitary	T38.811	T38.812	T38.813	T38.814	T38.815	T38.816
growth	T38.811	T38.812	T38.813	T38.814	T38.815	T38.816
luteinizing	T38.811	T38.812	T38.813	T38.814	T38.815	T38.816
ovarian	T38.5X1	T38.5X2	T38.5X3	T38.5X4	T38.5X5	T38.5X6
oxytocic	T48.0X1	T48.0X2	T48.0X3	T48.0X4	T48.0X5	T48.0X6
parathyroid (derivatives)	T50.991	T50.992	T50.993	T50.994	T50.995	T50.996
pituitary (posterior) NEC	T38.891	T38.892	T38.893	T38.894	T38.895	T38.896
anterior	T38.811	T38.812	T38.813	T38.814	T38.815	T38.816
specified, NEC	T38.891	T38.892	T38.893	T38.894	T38.895	T38.896
thyroid	T38.1X1	T38.1X2	T38.1X3	T38.1X4	T38.1X5	T38.1X6
Hornet (sting)	T63.451	T63.452	T63.453	T63.454	—	—
Horse anti-human lymphocytic serum	T50.Z11	T50.Z12	T50.Z13	T50.Z14	T50.Z15	T50.Z16
Horticulture agent NEC	T65.91	T65.92	T65.93	T65.94	—	—
with pesticide	T60.91	T60.92	T60.93	T60.94	—	—
Human						
albumin	T45.8X1	T45.8X2	T45.8X3	T45.8X4	T45.8X5	T45.8X6
growth hormone (HGH)	T38.811	T38.812	T38.813	T38.814	T38.815	T38.816
immune serum	T50.Z11	T50.Z12	T50.Z13	T50.Z14	T50.Z15	T50.Z16

Substance	Poisoning, Accidental (unintentional)	Poisoning, Intentional Self-harm	Poisoning, Assault	Poisoning, Undetermined	Adverse Effect	Under-dosing
Hyaluronidase	T45.3X1	T45.3X2	T45.3X3	T45.3X4	T45.3X5	T45.3X6
Hyazyme	T45.3X1	T45.3X2	T45.3X3	T45.3X4	T45.3X5	T45.3X6
Hycodan	T40.2X1	T40.2X2	T40.2X3	T40.2X4	T40.2X5	T40.2X6
Hydantoin derivative NEC	T42.0X1	T42.0X2	T42.0X3	T42.0X4	T42.0X5	T42.0X6
Hydeltra	T38.0X1	T38.0X2	T38.0X3	T38.0X4	T38.0X5	T38.0X6
Hydergine	T44.6X1	T44.6X2	T44.6X3	T44.6X4	T44.6X5	T44.6X6
Hydrabamine penicillin	T36.0X1	T36.0X2	T36.0X3	T36.0X4	T36.0X5	T36.0X6
Hydralazine	T46.5X1	T46.5X2	T46.5X3	T46.5X4	T46.5X5	T46.5X6
Hydrargaphen	T49.0X1	T49.0X2	T49.0X3	T49.0X4	T49.0X5	T49.0X6
Hydrargyri aminochloridum	T49.0X1	T49.0X2	T49.0X3	T49.0X4	T49.0X5	T49.0X6
Hydrastine	T48.291	T48.292	T48.293	T48.294	T48.295	T48.296
Hydrazine	T54.1X1	T54.1X2	T54.1X3	T54.1X4	—	—
monoamine oxidase inhibitors	T43.1X1	T43.1X2	T43.1X3	T43.1X4	T43.1X5	T43.1X6
Hydrazoic acid, azides	T54.2X1	T54.2X2	T54.2X3	T54.2X4	—	—
Hydriodic acid	T48.4X1	T48.4X2	T48.4X3	T48.4X4	T48.4X5	T48.4X6
Hydrisalic*	T49.4X1	T49.4X2	T49.4X3	T49.4X4	T49.4X5	T49.4X6
Hydrocarbon gas	T59.891	T59.892	T59.893	T59.894	—	—
incomplete combustion of — see Carbon, monoxide, fuel, utility						
liquefied (mobile container)	T59.891	T59.892	T59.893	T59.894	—	—
piped (natural)	T59.891	T59.892	T59.893	T59.894	—	—
Hydrochloric acid (liquid)	T54.2X1	T54.2X2	T54.2X3	T54.2X4	—	—
medicinal (digestant)	T47.5X1	T47.5X2	T47.5X3	T47.5X4	T47.5X5	T47.5X6
vapor	T59.891	T59.892	T59.893	T59.894	—	—
Hydrochlorothiazide	T50.2X1	T50.2X2	T50.2X3	T50.2X4	T50.2X5	T50.2X6
Hydrocodone	T40.2X1	T40.2X2	T40.2X3	T40.2X4	T40.2X5	T40.2X6
Hydrocortisone	T38.0X1	T38.0X2	T38.0X3	T38.0X4	T38.0X5	T38.0X6
(derivatives)						
aceponate	T49.0X1	T49.0X2	T49.0X3	T49.0X4	T49.0X5	T49.0X6
ENT agent	T49.6X1	T49.6X2	T49.6X3	T49.6X4	T49.6X5	T49.6X6
ophthalmic preparation	T49.5X1	T49.5X2	T49.5X3	T49.5X4	T49.5X5	T49.5X6
topical NEC	T49.0X1	T49.0X2	T49.0X3	T49.0X4	T49.0X5	T49.0X6
Hydrocortone	T38.0X1	T38.0X2	T38.0X3	T38.0X4	T38.0X5	T38.0X6
ENT agent	T49.6X1	T49.6X2	T49.6X3	T49.6X4	T49.6X5	T49.6X6
ophthalmic preparation	T49.5X1	T49.5X2	T49.5X3	T49.5X4	T49.5X5	T49.5X6
topical NEC	T49.0X1	T49.0X2	T49.0X3	T49.0X4	T49.0X5	T49.0X6
Hydrocyanic acid (liquid)	T57.3X1	T57.3X2	T57.3X3	T57.3X4	—	—
gas	T65.0X1	T65.0X2	T65.0X3	T65.0X4	—	—
Hydroflumethiazide	T50.2X1	T50.2X2	T50.2X3	T50.2X4	T50.2X5	T50.2X6
Hydrofluoric acid (liquid)	T54.2X1	T54.2X2	T54.2X3	T54.2X4	—	—
vapor	T59.891	T59.892	T59.893	T59.894	—	—
Hydrogen	T59.891	T59.892	T59.893	T59.894	—	—
arsenide	T57.0X1	T57.0X2	T57.0X3	T57.0X4	—	—
arseniureted	T57.0X1	T57.0X2	T57.0X3	T57.0X4	—	—
chloride	T57.8X1	T57.8X2	T57.8X3	T57.8X4	—	—
cyanide (salts)	T57.3X1	T57.3X2	T57.3X3	T57.3X4	—	—
gas	T57.3X1	T57.3X2	T57.3X3	T57.3X4	—	—
Fluoride	T59.5X1	T59.5X2	T59.5X3	T59.5X4	—	—
vapor	T59.5X1	T59.5X2	T59.5X3	T59.5X4	—	—
peroxide	T49.0X1	T49.0X2	T49.0X3	T49.0X4	T49.0X5	T49.0X6
phosphureted	T57.1X1	T57.1X2	T57.1X3	T57.1X4	—	—
sulfide	T59.6X1	T59.6X2	T59.6X3	T59.6X4	—	—
arseniureted	T57.0X1	T57.0X2	T57.0X3	T57.0X4	—	—
sulfureted	T59.6X1	T59.6X2	T59.6X3	T59.6X4	—	—
Hydromethylpyridine	T46.7X1	T46.7X2	T46.7X3	T46.7X4	T46.7X5	T46.7X6
Hydromorphinol	T40.2X1	T40.2X2	T40.2X3	T40.2X4	—	—
Hydromorphinone	T40.2X1	T40.2X2	T40.2X3	T40.2X4	T40.2X5	T40.2X6
Hydromorphone	T40.2X1	T40.2X2	T40.2X3	T40.2X4	T40.2X5	T40.2X6
Hydromox	T50.2X1	T50.2X2	T50.2X3	T50.2X4	T50.2X5	T50.2X6
Hydrophilic lotion	T49.3X1	T49.3X2	T49.3X3	T49.3X4	T49.3X5	T49.3X6
Hydroquinidine	T46.2X1	T46.2X2	T46.2X3	T46.2X4	T46.2X5	T46.2X6
Hydroquinone	T52.2X1	T52.2X2	T52.2X3	T52.2X4	—	—
vapor	T59.891	T59.892	T59.893	T59.894	—	—
Hydro-ride*	T50.2X1	T50.2X2	T50.2X3	T50.2X4	T50.2X5	T50.2X6
Hydrosulfuric acid (gas)	T59.6X1	T59.6X2	T59.6X3	T59.6X4	—	—
Hydrotalcite	T47.1X1	T47.1X2	T47.1X3	T47.1X4	T47.1X5	T47.1X6
Hydrous wool fat	T49.3X1	T49.3X2	T49.3X3	T49.3X4	T49.3X5	T49.3X6
Hydroxide, caustic	T54.3X1	T54.3X2	T54.3X3	T54.3X4	—	—
Hydroxocobalamin	T45.8X1	T45.8X2	T45.8X3	T45.8X4	T45.8X5	T45.8X6
Hydroxyamphetamine	T49.5X1	T49.5X2	T49.5X3	T49.5X4	T49.5X5	T49.5X6
Hydroxycarbamide	T45.1X1	T45.1X2	T45.1X3	T45.1X4	T45.1X5	T45.1X6
Hydroxychloroquine	T37.8X1	T37.8X2	T37.8X3	T37.8X4	T37.8X5	T37.8X6
Hydroxydaunorubicin*	T45.1X1	T45.1X2	T45.1X3	T45.1X4	T45.1X5	T45.1X6
Hydroxydihydrocodeinone	T40.2X1	T40.2X2	T40.2X3	T40.2X4	T40.2X5	T40.2X6
Hydroxyestrone	T38.5X1	T38.5X2	T38.5X3	T38.5X4	T38.5X5	T38.5X6
Hydroxyethyl starch	T45.8X1	T45.8X2	T45.8X3	T45.8X4	T45.8X5	T45.8X6
Hydroxymethylpentanone	T52.4X1	T52.4X2	T52.4X3	T52.4X4	—	—
Hydroxyphenamate	T43.591	T43.592	T43.593	T43.594	T43.595	T43.596
Hydroxyphenylbutazone	T39.2X1	T39.2X2	T39.2X3	T39.2X4	T39.2X5	T39.2X6

☑ Additional Character May Be Required — Refer to the Tabular List for Character Selection

*Optum Value-Add

Substance	Poisoning, Accidental (unintentional)	Poisoning, Intentional Self-harm	Poisoning, Assault	Poisoning, Undetermined	Adverse Effect	Under-dosing
Hydroxyprogesterone	T38.5X1	T38.5X2	T38.5X3	T38.5X4	T38.5X5	T38.5X6
caproate	T38.5X1	T38.5X2	T38.5X3	T38.5X4	T38.5X5	T38.5X6
Hydroxyquinoline (derivatives) NEC	T37.8X1	T37.8X2	T37.8X3	T37.8X4	T37.8X5	T37.8X6
Hydroxystilbamidine	T37.3X1	T37.3X2	T37.3X3	T37.3X4	T37.3X5	T37.3X6
Hydroxytoluene (nonmedicinal)	T54.0X1	T54.0X2	T54.0X3	T54.0X4	—	—
medicinal	T49.0X1	T49.0X2	T49.0X3	T49.0X4	T49.0X5	T49.0X6
Hydroxyurea	T45.1X1	T45.1X2	T45.1X3	T45.1X4	T45.1X5	T45.1X6
Hydroxyzine	T43.591	T43.592	T43.593	T43.594	T43.595	T43.596
antiallergic	T45.0X1	T45.0X2	T45.0X3	T45.0X4	T45.0X5	T45.0X6
Hyoscine	T44.3X1	T44.3X2	T44.3X3	T44.3X4	T44.3X5	T44.3X6
Hyoscyamine	T44.3X1	T44.3X2	T44.3X3	T44.3X4	T44.3X5	T44.3X6
Hyoscyamus	T44.3X1	T44.3X2	T44.3X3	T44.3X4	T44.3X5	T44.3X6
dry extract	T44.3X1	T44.3X2	T44.3X3	T44.3X4	T44.3X5	T44.3X6
Hypaque	T50.8X1	T50.8X2	T50.8X3	T50.8X4	T50.8X5	T50.8X6
HyperRAB*	T50.Z11	T50.Z12	T50.Z13	T50.Z14	T50.Z15	T50.Z16
Hypertussis	T50.Z11	T50.Z12	T50.Z13	T50.Z14	T50.Z15	T50.Z16
Hypnotic	T42.71	T42.72	T42.73	T42.74	T42.75	T42.76
anticonvulsant	T42.71	T42.72	T42.73	T42.74	T42.75	T42.76
specified NEC	T42.6X1	T42.6X2	T42.6X3	T42.6X4	T42.6X5	T42.6X6
Hypochlorite	T49.0X1	T49.0X2	T49.0X3	T49.0X4	T49.0X5	T49.0X6
Hypophysis, posterior	T38.891	T38.892	T38.893	T38.894	T38.895	T38.896
Hypotensive NEC	T46.5X1	T46.5X2	T46.5X3	T46.5X4	T46.5X5	T46.5X6
Hypromellose	T49.5X1	T49.5X2	T49.5X3	T49.5X4	T49.5X5	T49.5X6
Ibacitabine	T37.5X1	T37.5X2	T37.5X3	T37.5X4	T37.5X5	T37.5X6
Ibopamine	T44.991	T44.992	T44.993	T44.994	T44.995	T44.996
Ibufenac	T39.311	T39.312	T39.313	T39.314	T39.315	T39.316
Ibuprofen	T39.311	T39.312	T39.313	T39.314	T39.315	T39.316
Ibuproxam	T39.311	T39.312	T39.313	T39.314	T39.315	T39.316
Ibuterol	T48.6X1	T48.6X2	T48.6X3	T48.6X4	T48.6X5	T48.6X6
Ichthammol	T49.0X1	T49.0X2	T49.0X3	T49.0X4	T49.0X5	T49.0X6
Ichthyol	T49.4X1	T49.4X2	T49.4X3	T49.4X4	T49.4X5	T49.4X6
Idarubicin	T45.1X1	T45.1X2	T45.1X3	T45.1X4	T45.1X5	T45.1X6
Idrocilamide	T42.8X1	T42.8X2	T42.8X3	T42.8X4	T42.8X5	T42.8X6
Ifenprodil	T46.7X1	T46.7X2	T46.7X3	T46.7X4	T46.7X5	T46.7X6
Ifosfamide	T45.1X1	T45.1X2	T45.1X3	T45.1X4	T45.1X5	T45.1X6
Iletin	T38.3X1	T38.3X2	T38.3X3	T38.3X4	T38.3X5	T38.3X6
Ilex	T62.2X1	T62.2X2	T62.2X3	T62.2X4	—	—
Illuminating gas (after combustion)	T58.11	T58.12	T58.13	T58.14	—	—
prior to combustion	T59.891	T59.892	T59.893	T59.894	—	—
Ilopan	T45.2X1	T45.2X2	T45.2X3	T45.2X4	T45.2X5	T45.2X6
Iloprost	T46.7X1	T46.7X2	T46.7X3	T46.7X4	T46.7X5	T46.7X6
Ilotycin	T36.3X1	T36.3X2	T36.3X3	T36.3X4	T36.3X5	T36.3X6
ophthalmic preparation	T49.5X1	T49.5X2	T49.5X3	T49.5X4	T49.5X5	T49.5X6
topical NEC	T49.0X1	T49.0X2	T49.0X3	T49.0X4	T49.0X5	T49.0X6
Imdur*	T46.3X1	T46.3X2	T46.3X3	T46.3X4	T46.3X5	T46.3X6
Imidazole-4-carboxamide	T45.1X1	T45.1X2	T45.1X3	T45.1X4	T45.1X5	T45.1X6
Iminostilbene	T42.1X1	T42.1X2	T42.1X3	T42.1X4	T42.1X5	T42.1X6
Imipenem	T36.0X1	T36.0X2	T36.0X3	T36.0X4	T36.0X5	T36.0X6
Imipramine	T43.011	T43.012	T43.013	T43.014	T43.015	T43.016
Immu-G	T50.Z11	T50.Z12	T50.Z13	T50.Z14	T50.Z15	T50.Z16
Immuglobin	T50.Z11	T50.Z12	T50.Z13	T50.Z14	T50.Z15	T50.Z16
Immune						
checkpoint inhibitors	T45.AX1	T45.AX2	T45.AX3	T45.AX4	T45.AX5	T45.AX6
globulin	T50.Z11	T50.Z12	T50.Z13	T50.Z14	T50.Z15	T50.Z16
serum globulin	T50.Z11	T50.Z12	T50.Z13	T50.Z14	T50.Z15	T50.Z16
Immunoglobin human (intravenous) (normal)	T50.Z11	T50.Z12	T50.Z13	T50.Z14	T50.Z15	T50.Z16
unmodified	T50.Z11	T50.Z12	T50.Z13	T50.Z14	T50.Z15	T50.Z16
Immunostimulant drug	T45.AX1	T45.AX2	T45.AX3	T45.AX4	T45.AX5	—
Immunosuppressive drug	T45.1X1	T45.1X2	T45.1X3	T45.1X4	T45.1X5	T45.1X6
Immu-tetanus	T50.Z11	T50.Z12	T50.Z13	T50.Z14	T50.Z15	T50.Z16
Indalpine	T43.221	T43.222	T43.223	T43.224	T43.225	T43.226
Indanazoline	T48.5X1	T48.5X2	T48.5X3	T48.5X4	T48.5X5	T48.5X6
Indandione (derivatives)	T45.511	T45.512	T45.513	T45.514	T45.515	T45.516
Indapamide	T46.5X1	T46.5X2	T46.5X3	T46.5X4	T46.5X5	T46.5X6
Indendione (derivatives)	T45.511	T45.512	T45.513	T45.514	T45.515	T45.516
Indenolol	T44.7X1	T44.7X2	T44.7X3	T44.7X4	T44.7X5	T44.7X6
Inderal	T44.7X1	T44.7X2	T44.7X3	T44.7X4	T44.7X5	T44.7X6
Indian						
hemp	T40.711	T40.712	T40.713	T40.714	T40.715	T40.716
tobacco	T62.2X1	T62.2X2	T62.2X3	T62.2X4	—	—
Indigo carmine	T50.8X1	T50.8X2	T50.8X3	T50.8X4	T50.8X5	T50.8X6
Indobufen	T45.521	T45.522	T45.523	T45.524	T45.525	T45.526
Indocin	T39.2X1	T39.2X2	T39.2X3	T39.2X4	T39.2X5	T39.2X6
Indocyanine green	T50.8X1	T50.8X2	T50.8X3	T50.8X4	T50.8X5	T50.8X6
Indometacin	T39.391	T39.392	T39.393	T39.394	T39.395	T39.396
Indomethacin	T39.391	T39.392	T39.393	T39.394	T39.395	T39.396
farnesil	T39.4X1	T39.4X2	T39.4X3	T39.4X4	T39.4X5	T39.4X6
Indoramin	T44.6X1	T44.6X2	T44.6X3	T44.6X4	T44.6X5	T44.6X6
Industrial						
alcohol	T51.0X1	T51.0X2	T51.0X3	T51.0X4	—	—
fumes	T59.891	T59.892	T59.893	T59.894	—	—
solvents (fumes) (vapors)	T52.91	T52.92	T52.93	T52.94	—	—
Inflectra*	T39.4X1	T39.4X2	T39.4X3	T39.4X4	T39.4X5	T39.4X6
Influenza vaccine	T50.B91	T50.B92	T50.B93	T50.B94	T50.B95	T50.B96
Ingested substance NEC	T65.91	T65.92	T65.93	T65.94	—	—
INH	T37.1X1	T37.1X2	T37.1X3	T37.1X4	T37.1X5	T37.1X6
Inhalation, gas (noxious) — see Gas						
Inhibitor						
angiotensin-converting enzyme	T46.4X1	T46.4X2	T46.4X3	T46.4X4	T46.4X5	T46.4X6
carbonic anhydrase	T50.2X1	T50.2X2	T50.2X3	T50.2X4	T50.2X5	T50.2X6
fibrinolysis	T45.621	T45.622	T45.623	T45.624	T45.625	T45.626
monoamine oxidase NEC	T43.1X1	T43.1X2	T43.1X3	T43.1X4	T43.1X5	T43.1X6
hydrazine	T43.1X1	T43.1X2	T43.1X3	T43.1X4	T43.1X5	T43.1X6
postsynaptic	T43.8X1	T43.8X2	T43.8X3	T43.8X4	T43.8X5	T43.8X6
prothrombin synthesis	T45.511	T45.512	T45.513	T45.514	T45.515	T45.516
Ink	T65.891	T65.892	T65.893	T65.894	—	—
Innopran*	T44.7X1	T44.7X2	T44.7X3	T44.7X4	T44.7X5	T44.7X6
Inorganic substance NEC	T57.91	T57.92	T57.93	T57.94	—	—
Inosine pranobex	T37.5X1	T37.5X2	T37.5X3	T37.5X4	T37.5X5	T37.5X6
Inositol	T50.991	T50.992	T50.993	T50.994	T50.995	T50.996
nicotinate	T46.7X1	T46.7X2	T46.7X3	T46.7X4	T46.7X5	T46.7X6
Inproquone	T45.1X1	T45.1X2	T45.1X3	T45.1X4	T45.1X5	T45.1X6
Insecticide NEC	T60.91	T60.92	T60.93	T60.94	—	—
carbamate	T60.0X1	T60.0X2	T60.0X3	T60.0X4	—	—
chlorinated	T60.1X1	T60.1X2	T60.1X3	T60.1X4	—	—
mixed	T60.91	T60.92	T60.93	T60.94	—	—
organochlorine	T60.1X1	T60.1X2	T60.1X3	T60.1X4	—	—
organophosphorus	T60.0X1	T60.0X2	T60.0X3	T60.0X4	—	—
Insect (sting), venomous	T63.481	T63.482	T63.483	T63.484	—	—
ant	T63.421	T63.422	T63.423	T63.424	—	—
bee	T63.441	T63.442	T63.443	T63.444	—	—
caterpillar	T63.431	T63.432	T63.433	T63.434	—	—
hornet	T63.451	T63.452	T63.453	T63.454	—	—
wasp	T63.461	T63.462	T63.463	T63.464	—	—
Insular tissue extract	T38.3X1	T38.3X2	T38.3X3	T38.3X4	T38.3X5	T38.3X6
Insulin (amorphous) (globin) (isophane) (Lente) (NPH) (Semilente) (Ultralente)	T38.3X1	T38.3X2	T38.3X3	T38.3X4	T38.3X5	T38.3X6
defalan	T38.3X1	T38.3X2	T38.3X3	T38.3X4	T38.3X5	T38.3X6
human	T38.3X1	T38.3X2	T38.3X3	T38.3X4	T38.3X5	T38.3X6
injection, soluble	T38.3X1	T38.3X2	T38.3X3	T38.3X4	T38.3X5	T38.3X6
biphasic	T38.3X1	T38.3X2	T38.3X3	T38.3X4	T38.3X5	T38.3X6
intermediate acting	T38.3X1	T38.3X2	T38.3X3	T38.3X4	T38.3X5	T38.3X6
protamine zinc	T38.3X1	T38.3X2	T38.3X3	T38.3X4	T38.3X5	T38.3X6
slow acting	T38.3X1	T38.3X2	T38.3X3	T38.3X4	T38.3X5	T38.3X6
zinc						
protamine injection	T38.3X1	T38.3X2	T38.3X3	T38.3X4	T38.3X5	T38.3X6
suspension (amorphous) (crystalline)	T38.3X1	T38.3X2	T38.3X3	T38.3X4	T38.3X5	T38.3X6
Interferon (alpha) (beta) (gamma)	T37.5X1	T37.5X2	T37.5X3	T37.5X4	T37.5X5	T37.5X6
Intestinal motility control drug	T47.6X1	T47.6X2	T47.6X3	T47.6X4	T47.6X5	T47.6X6
biological	T47.8X1	T47.8X2	T47.8X3	T47.8X4	T47.8X5	T47.8X6
Intranarcon	T41.1X1	T41.1X2	T41.1X3	T41.1X4	T41.1X5	T41.1X6
Intravenous						
amino acids	T50.991	T50.992	T50.993	T50.994	T50.995	T50.996
fat suspension	T50.991	T50.992	T50.993	T50.994	T50.995	T50.996
Inulin	T50.8X1	T50.8X2	T50.8X3	T50.8X4	T50.8X5	T50.8X6
Invanz*	T36.1X1	T36.1X2	T36.1X3	T36.1X4	T36.1X5	T36.1X6
Invert sugar	T50.3X1	T50.3X2	T50.3X3	T50.3X4	T50.3X5	T50.3X6
Inza — see Naproxen						
Iobenzamic acid	T50.8X1	T50.8X2	T50.8X3	T50.8X4	T50.8X5	T50.8X6
Iocarmic acid	T50.8X1	T50.8X2	T50.8X3	T50.8X4	T50.8X5	T50.8X6
Iocetamic acid	T50.8X1	T50.8X2	T50.8X3	T50.8X4	T50.8X5	T50.8X6
Iodamide	T50.8X1	T50.8X2	T50.8X3	T50.8X4	T50.8X5	T50.8X6
Iodide NEC — see also Iodine	T49.0X1	T49.0X2	T49.0X3	T49.0X4	T49.0X5	T49.0X6
mercury (ointment)	T49.0X1	T49.0X2	T49.0X3	T49.0X4	T49.0X5	T49.0X6
methylate	T49.0X1	T49.0X2	T49.0X3	T49.0X4	T49.0X5	T49.0X6
potassium (expectorant) NEC	T48.4X1	T48.4X2	T48.4X3	T48.4X4	T48.4X5	T48.4X6
Iodinated						
contrast medium	T50.8X1	T50.8X2	T50.8X3	T50.8X4	T50.8X5	T50.8X6
glycerol	T48.4X1	T48.4X2	T48.4X3	T48.4X4	T48.4X5	T48.4X6
human serum albumin (131I)	T50.8X1	T50.8X2	T50.8X3	T50.8X4	T50.8X5	T50.8X6
Iodine (antiseptic, external) (tincture) NEC	T49.0X1	T49.0X2	T49.0X3	T49.0X4	T49.0X5	T49.0X6

Table of Drugs and Chemicals

Hydroxyprogesterone — Iodine

Substance	Poisoning, Accidental (unintentional)	Poisoning, Intentional Self-harm	Poisoning, Assault	Poisoning, Undetermined	Adverse Effect	Underdosing
Iodine (antiseptic, external) (tincture) NEC — continued						
125 — see also Radiation sickness, and exposure to radioactive isotopes	T50.8X1	T50.8X2	T50.8X3	T50.8X4	T50.8X5	T50.8X6
therapeutic	T50.991	T50.992	T50.993	T50.994	T50.995	T50.996
131 — see also Radiation sickness, and exposure to radioactive isotopes	T50.8X1	T50.8X2	T50.8X3	T50.8X4	T50.8X5	T50.8X6
therapeutic	T38.2X1	T38.2X2	T38.2X3	T38.2X4	T38.2X5	T38.2X6
diagnostic	T50.8X1	T50.8X2	T50.8X3	T50.8X4	T50.8X5	T50.8X6
for thyroid conditions (antithyroid)	T38.2X1	T38.2X2	T38.2X3	T38.2X4	T38.2X5	T38.2X6
solution	T49.0X1	T49.0X2	T49.0X3	T49.0X4	T49.0X5	T49.0X6
vapor	T59.891	T59.892	T59.893	T59.894	—	—
Iodipamide	T50.8X1	T50.8X2	T50.8X3	T50.8X4	T50.8X5	T50.8X6
Iodized (poppy seed) oil	T50.8X1	T50.8X2	T50.8X3	T50.8X4	T50.8X5	T50.8X6
Iodobismitol	T37.8X1	T37.8X2	T37.8X3	T37.8X4	T37.8X5	T37.8X6
Iodochlorhydroxyquin	T37.8X1	T37.8X2	T37.8X3	T37.8X4	T37.8X5	T37.8X6
topical	T49.0X1	T49.0X2	T49.0X3	T49.0X4	T49.0X5	T49.0X6
Iodochlorhydroxyquinoline	T37.8X1	T37.8X2	T37.8X3	T37.8X4	T37.8X5	T37.8X6
Iodocholesterol (131I)	T50.8X1	T50.8X2	T50.8X3	T50.8X4	T50.8X5	T50.8X6
Iodoform	T49.0X1	T49.0X2	T49.0X3	T49.0X4	T49.0X5	T49.0X6
Iodohippuric acid	T50.8X1	T50.8X2	T50.8X3	T50.8X4	T50.8X5	T50.8X6
Iodopanoic acid	T50.8X1	T50.8X2	T50.8X3	T50.8X4	T50.8X5	T50.8X6
Iodophthalein (sodium)	T50.8X1	T50.8X2	T50.8X3	T50.8X4	T50.8X5	T50.8X6
Iodopyracet	T50.8X1	T50.8X2	T50.8X3	T50.8X4	T50.8X5	T50.8X6
Iodoquinol	T37.8X1	T37.8X2	T37.8X3	T37.8X4	T37.8X5	T37.8X6
Iodoxamic acid	T50.8X1	T50.8X2	T50.8X3	T50.8X4	T50.8X5	T50.8X6
Iofendylate	T50.8X1	T50.8X2	T50.8X3	T50.8X4	T50.8X5	T50.8X6
Ioglycamic acid	T50.8X1	T50.8X2	T50.8X3	T50.8X4	T50.8X5	T50.8X6
Iohexol	T50.8X1	T50.8X2	T50.8X3	T50.8X4	T50.8X5	T50.8X6
Ion exchange resin						
anion	T47.8X1	T47.8X2	T47.8X3	T47.8X4	T47.8X5	T47.8X6
cation	T50.3X1	T50.3X2	T50.3X3	T50.3X4	T50.3X5	T50.3X6
cholestyramine	T46.6X1	T46.6X2	T46.6X3	T46.6X4	T46.6X5	T46.6X6
intestinal	T47.8X1	T47.8X2	T47.8X3	T47.8X4	T47.8X5	T47.8X6
Iopamidol	T50.8X1	T50.8X2	T50.8X3	T50.8X4	T50.8X5	T50.8X6
Iopanoic acid	T50.8X1	T50.8X2	T50.8X3	T50.8X4	T50.8X5	T50.8X6
Iophenoic acid	T50.8X1	T50.8X2	T50.8X3	T50.8X4	T50.8X5	T50.8X6
Iopodate, sodium	T50.8X1	T50.8X2	T50.8X3	T50.8X4	T50.8X5	T50.8X6
Iopodic acid	T50.8X1	T50.8X2	T50.8X3	T50.8X4	T50.8X5	T50.8X6
Iopromide	T50.8X1	T50.8X2	T50.8X3	T50.8X4	T50.8X5	T50.8X6
Iopydol	T50.8X1	T50.8X2	T50.8X3	T50.8X4	T50.8X5	T50.8X6
Iotalamic acid	T50.8X1	T50.8X2	T50.8X3	T50.8X4	T50.8X5	T50.8X6
Iothalamate	T50.8X1	T50.8X2	T50.8X3	T50.8X4	T50.8X5	T50.8X6
Iothiouracil	T38.2X1	T38.2X2	T38.2X3	T38.2X4	T38.2X5	T38.2X6
Iotrol	T50.8X1	T50.8X2	T50.8X3	T50.8X4	T50.8X5	T50.8X6
Iotrolan	T50.8X1	T50.8X2	T50.8X3	T50.8X4	T50.8X5	T50.8X6
Iotroxate	T50.8X1	T50.8X2	T50.8X3	T50.8X4	T50.8X5	T50.8X6
Iotroxic acid	T50.8X1	T50.8X2	T50.8X3	T50.8X4	T50.8X5	T50.8X6
Ioversol	T50.8X1	T50.8X2	T50.8X3	T50.8X4	T50.8X5	T50.8X6
Ioxaglate	T50.8X1	T50.8X2	T50.8X3	T50.8X4	T50.8X5	T50.8X6
Ioxaglic acid	T50.8X1	T50.8X2	T50.8X3	T50.8X4	T50.8X5	T50.8X6
Ioxitalamic acid	T50.8X1	T50.8X2	T50.8X3	T50.8X4	T50.8X5	T50.8X6
Ipecac	T47.7X1	T47.7X2	T47.7X3	T47.7X4	T47.7X5	T47.7X6
Ipecacuanha	T48.4X1	T48.4X2	T48.4X3	T48.4X4	T48.4X5	T48.4X6
Ipodate, calcium	T50.8X1	T50.8X2	T50.8X3	T50.8X4	T50.8X5	T50.8X6
IPOL*	T50.B91	T50.B92	T50.B93	T50.B94	T50.B95	T50.B96
Ipral	T42.3X1	T42.3X2	T42.3X3	T42.3X4	T42.3X5	T42.3X6
Ipratropium (bromide)	T48.6X1	T48.6X2	T48.6X3	T48.6X4	T48.6X5	T48.6X6
Ipriflavone	T46.3X1	T46.3X2	T46.3X3	T46.3X4	T46.3X5	T46.3X6
Iprindole	T43.011	T43.012	T43.013	T43.014	T43.015	T43.016
Iproclozide	T43.1X1	T43.1X2	T43.1X3	T43.1X4	T43.1X5	T43.1X6
Iprofenin	T50.8X1	T50.8X2	T50.8X3	T50.8X4	T50.8X5	T50.8X6
Iproheptine	T49.2X1	T49.2X2	T49.2X3	T49.2X4	T49.2X5	T49.2X6
Iproniazid	T43.1X1	T43.1X2	T43.1X3	T43.1X4	T43.1X5	T43.1X6
Iproplatin	T45.1X1	T45.1X2	T45.1X3	T45.1X4	T45.1X5	T45.1X6
Iproveratril	T46.1X1	T46.1X2	T46.1X3	T46.1X4	T46.1X5	T46.1X6
Irinotecan*	T45.1X1	T45.1X2	T45.1X3	T45.1X4	T45.1X5	T45.1X6
Iron (compounds) (medicinal) NEC	T45.4X1	T45.4X2	T45.4X3	T45.4X4	T45.4X5	T45.4X6
ammonium	T45.4X1	T45.4X2	T45.4X3	T45.4X4	T45.4X5	T45.4X6
dextran injection	T45.4X1	T45.4X2	T45.4X3	T45.4X4	T45.4X5	T45.4X6
nonmedicinal	T56.891	T56.892	T56.893	T56.894	—	—
salts	T45.4X1	T45.4X2	T45.4X3	T45.4X4	T45.4X5	T45.4X6
sorbitex	T45.4X1	T45.4X2	T45.4X3	T45.4X4	T45.4X5	T45.4X6
sorbitol citric acid complex	T45.4X1	T45.4X2	T45.4X3	T45.4X4	T45.4X5	T45.4X6
Irrigating fluid (vaginal)	T49.8X1	T49.8X2	T49.8X3	T49.8X4	T49.8X5	T49.8X6
eye	T49.5X1	T49.5X2	T49.5X3	T49.5X4	T49.5X5	T49.5X6
Isepamicin	T36.5X1	T36.5X2	T36.5X3	T36.5X4	T36.5X5	T36.5X6
Isoaminile (citrate)	T48.3X1	T48.3X2	T48.3X3	T48.3X4	T48.3X5	T48.3X6
Isoamyl nitrite	T46.3X1	T46.3X2	T46.3X3	T46.3X4	T46.3X5	T46.3X6
Isobenzan	T60.1X1	T60.1X2	T60.1X3	T60.1X4		
Isobutyl acetate	T52.8X1	T52.8X2	T52.8X3	T52.8X4		
Isocarboxazid	T43.1X1	T43.1X2	T43.1X3	T43.1X4	T43.1X5	T43.1X6
Isoconazole	T49.0X1	T49.0X2	T49.0X3	T49.0X4	T49.0X5	T49.0X6
Isocyanate	T65.0X1	T65.0X2	T65.0X3	T65.0X4		
Isoephedrine	T44.991	T44.992	T44.993	T44.994	T44.995	T44.996
Isoetarine	T48.6X1	T48.6X2	T48.6X3	T48.6X4	T48.6X5	T48.6X6
Isoethadione	T42.2X1	T42.2X2	T42.2X3	T42.2X4	T42.2X5	T42.2X6
Isoetharine	T44.5X1	T44.5X2	T44.5X3	T44.5X4	T44.5X5	T44.5X6
Isoflurane	T41.0X1	T41.0X2	T41.0X3	T41.0X4	T41.0X5	T41.0X6
Isoflurophate	T44.0X1	T44.0X2	T44.0X3	T44.0X4	T44.0X5	T44.0X6
Isomaltose, ferric complex	T45.4X1	T45.4X2	T45.4X3	T45.4X4	T45.4X5	T45.4X6
Isometheptene	T44.3X1	T44.3X2	T44.3X3	T44.3X4	T44.3X5	T44.3X6
Isoniazid	T37.1X1	T37.1X2	T37.1X3	T37.1X4	T37.1X5	T37.1X6
with						
rifampicin	T36.6X1	T36.6X2	T36.6X3	T36.6X4	T36.6X5	T36.6X6
thioacetazone	T37.1X1	T37.1X2	T37.1X3	T37.1X4	T37.1X5	T37.1X6
Isonicotinic acid hydrazide	T37.1X1	T37.1X2	T37.1X3	T37.1X4	T37.1X5	T37.1X6
Isonipecaine	T40.491	T40.492	T40.493	T40.494	T40.495	T40.496
Isopentaquine	T37.2X1	T37.2X2	T37.2X3	T37.2X4	T37.2X5	T37.2X6
Isophane insulin	T38.3X1	T38.3X2	T38.3X3	T38.3X4	T38.3X5	T38.3X6
Isophorone	T65.891	T65.892	T65.893	T65.894		
Isophosphamide	T45.1X1	T45.1X2	T45.1X3	T45.1X4	T45.1X5	T45.1X6
Isopregnenone	T38.5X1	T38.5X2	T38.5X3	T38.5X4	T38.5X5	T38.5X6
Isoprenaline	T48.6X1	T48.6X2	T48.6X3	T48.6X4	T48.6X5	T48.6X6
Isopromethazine	T43.3X1	T43.3X2	T43.3X3	T43.3X4	T43.3X5	T43.3X6
Isopropamide	T44.3X1	T44.3X2	T44.3X3	T44.3X4	T44.3X5	T44.3X6
iodide	T44.3X1	T44.3X2	T44.3X3	T44.3X4	T44.3X5	T44.3X6
Isopropanol	T51.2X1	T51.2X2	T51.2X3	T51.2X4	—	—
Isopropyl						
acetate	T52.8X1	T52.8X2	T52.8X3	T52.8X4	—	—
alcohol	T51.2X1	T51.2X2	T51.2X3	T51.2X4	—	—
medicinal	T49.4X1	T49.4X2	T49.4X3	T49.4X4	T49.4X5	T49.4X6
ether	T52.8X1	T52.8X2	T52.8X3	T52.8X4	—	—
Isopropylaminophenazone	T39.2X1	T39.2X2	T39.2X3	T39.2X4	T39.2X5	T39.2X6
Isoproterenol	T48.6X1	T48.6X2	T48.6X3	T48.6X4	T48.6X5	T48.6X6
Isosorbide dinitrate	T46.3X1	T46.3X2	T46.3X3	T46.3X4	T46.3X5	T46.3X6
Isothipendyl	T45.0X1	T45.0X2	T45.0X3	T45.0X4	T45.0X5	T45.0X6
Isotretinoin	T50.991	T50.992	T50.993	T50.994	T50.995	T50.996
Isoxazolyl penicillin	T36.0X1	T36.0X2	T36.0X3	T36.0X4	T36.0X5	T36.0X6
Isoxicam	T39.391	T39.392	T39.393	T39.394	T39.395	T39.396
Isoxsuprine	T46.7X1	T46.7X2	T46.7X3	T46.7X4	T46.7X5	T46.7X6
Ispagula	T47.4X1	T47.4X2	T47.4X3	T47.4X4	T47.4X5	T47.4X6
husk	T47.4X1	T47.4X2	T47.4X3	T47.4X4	T47.4X5	T47.4X6
Isradipine	T46.1X1	T46.1X2	T46.1X3	T46.1X4	T46.1X5	T46.1X6
I-thyroxine sodium	T38.1X1	T38.1X2	T38.1X3	T38.1X4	T38.1X5	T38.1X6
Itraconazole	T37.8X1	T37.8X2	T37.8X3	T37.8X4	T37.8X5	T37.8X6
Itramin tosilate	T46.3X1	T46.3X2	T46.3X3	T46.3X4	T46.3X5	T46.3X6
Ivarest*	T41.3X1	T41.3X2	T41.3X3	T41.3X4	T41.3X5	T41.3X6
Ivermectin	T37.4X1	T37.4X2	T37.4X3	T37.4X4	T37.4X5	T37.4X6
Izoniazid	T37.1X1	T37.1X2	T37.1X3	T37.1X4	T37.1X5	T37.1X6
with thioacetazone	T37.1X1	T37.1X2	T37.1X3	T37.1X4	T37.1X5	T37.1X6
Jalap	T47.2X1	T47.2X2	T47.2X3	T47.2X4	T47.2X5	T47.2X6
Jamaica						
dogwood (bark)	T39.8X1	T39.8X2	T39.8X3	T39.8X4	T39.8X5	T39.8X6
ginger	T65.891	T65.892	T65.893	T65.894	—	—
root	T62.2X1	T62.2X2	T62.2X3	T62.2X4	—	—
Jantoven*	T45.511	T45.512	T45.513	T45.514	T45.515	T45.516
Jatropha	T62.2X1	T62.2X2	T62.2X3	T62.2X4	—	—
curcas	T62.2X1	T62.2X2	T62.2X3	T62.2X4	—	—
Jectofer	T45.4X1	T45.4X2	T45.4X3	T45.4X4	T45.4X5	T45.4X6
Jellyfish (sting)	T63.621	T63.622	T63.623	T63.624	—	—
Jequirity (bean)	T62.2X1	T62.2X2	T62.2X3	T62.2X4	—	—
Jimson weed (stramonium)	T62.2X1	T62.2X2	T62.2X3	T62.2X4	—	—
seeds	T62.2X1	T62.2X2	T62.2X3	T62.2X4	—	—
Josamycin	T36.3X1	T36.3X2	T36.3X3	T36.3X4	T36.3X5	T36.3X6
Juniper tar	T49.1X1	T49.1X2	T49.1X3	T49.1X4	T49.1X5	T49.1X6
Kaletra*	T37.5X1	T37.5X2	T37.5X3	T37.5X4	T37.5X5	T37.5X6
Kallidinogenase	T46.7X1	T46.7X2	T46.7X3	T46.7X4	T46.7X5	T46.7X6
Kallikrein	T46.7X1	T46.7X2	T46.7X3	T46.7X4	T46.7X5	T46.7X6
Kanamycin	T36.5X1	T36.5X2	T36.5X3	T36.5X4	T36.5X5	T36.5X6
Kantrex	T36.5X1	T36.5X2	T36.5X3	T36.5X4	T36.5X5	T36.5X6
Kaolin	T47.6X1	T47.6X2	T47.6X3	T47.6X4	T47.6X5	T47.6X6
light	T47.6X1	T47.6X2	T47.6X3	T47.6X4	T47.6X5	T47.6X6
Karaya (gum)	T47.4X1	T47.4X2	T47.4X3	T47.4X4	T47.4X5	T47.4X6
Kebuzone	T39.2X1	T39.2X2	T39.2X3	T39.2X4	T39.2X5	T39.2X6
Keflex*	T36.1X1	T36.1X2	T36.1X3	T36.1X4	T36.1X5	T36.1X6
Kelevan	T60.1X1	T60.1X2	T60.1X3	T60.1X4	—	—
Kemithal	T41.1X1	T41.1X2	T41.1X3	T41.1X4	T41.1X5	T41.1X6
Kenacort	T38.0X1	T38.0X2	T38.0X3	T38.0X4	T38.0X5	T38.0X6
Keratolytic drug NEC	T49.4X1	T49.4X2	T49.4X3	T49.4X4	T49.4X5	T49.4X6
anthracene	T49.4X1	T49.4X2	T49.4X3	T49.4X4	T49.4X5	T49.4X6
Keratoplastic NEC	T49.4X1	T49.4X2	T49.4X3	T49.4X4	T49.4X5	T49.4X6

☑ Additional Character May Be Required — Refer to the Tabular List for Character Selection

*Optum Value-Add

Substance	Poisoning, Accidental (unintentional)	Poisoning, Intentional Self-harm	Poisoning, Assault	Poisoning, Undetermined	Adverse Effect	Under-dosing
Kerosene, kerosine (fuel) (solvent) NEC	T52.0X1	T52.0X2	T52.0X3	T52.0X4	—	—
insecticide	T52.0X1	T52.0X2	T52.0X3	T52.0X4	—	—
vapor	T52.0X1	T52.0X2	T52.0X3	T52.0X4	—	—
Ketamine	T41.291	T41.292	T41.293	T41.294	T41.295	T41.296
Ketazolam	T42.4X1	T42.4X2	T42.4X3	T42.4X4	T42.4X5	T42.4X6
Ketazon	T39.2X1	T39.2X2	T39.2X3	T39.2X4	T39.2X5	T39.2X6
Ketobemidone	T40.491	T40.492	T40.493	T40.494		
Ketoconazole	T49.0X1	T49.0X2	T49.0X3	T49.0X4	T49.0X5	T49.0X6
Ketols	T52.4X1	T52.4X2	T52.4X3	T52.4X4	—	—
Ketone oils	T52.4X1	T52.4X2	T52.4X3	T52.4X4	—	—
Ketoprofen	T39.311	T39.312	T39.313	T39.314	T39.315	T39.316
Ketorolac	T39.8X1	T39.8X2	T39.8X3	T39.8X4	T39.8X5	T39.8X6
Ketotifen	T45.0X1	T45.0X2	T45.0X3	T45.0X4	T45.0X5	T45.0X6
Keytruda*	T45.1X1	T45.1X2	T45.1X3	T45.1X4	T45.1X5	T45.1X6
Khat	T43.691	T43.692	T43.693	T43.694		
Khellin	T46.3X1	T46.3X2	T46.3X3	T46.3X4	T46.3X5	T46.3X6
Khelloside	T46.3X1	T46.3X2	T46.3X3	T46.3X4	T46.3X5	T46.3X6
Kiln gas or vapor (carbon monoxide)	T58.8X1	T58.8X2	T58.8X3	T58.8X4	—	—
Kineret*	T39.4X1	T39.4X2	T39.4X3	T39.4X4	T39.4X5	T39.4X6
Kitasamycin	T36.3X1	T36.3X2	T36.3X3	T36.3X4	T36.3X5	T36.3X6
Klonopin*	T42.4X1	T42.4X2	T42.4X3	T42.4X4	T42.4X5	T42.4X6
Komgiblyze*	T38.3X1	T38.3X2	T38.3X3	T38.3X4	T38.3X5	T38.3X6
Konsyl	T47.4X1	T47.4X2	T47.4X3	T47.4X4	T47.4X5	T47.4X6
Kosam seed	T62.2X1	T62.2X2	T62.2X3	T62.2X4		
Krait (venom)	T63.091	T63.092	T63.093	T63.094		
Kwell (insecticide)	T60.1X1	T60.1X2	T60.1X3	T60.1X4	—	—
anti-infective (topical)	T49.0X1	T49.0X2	T49.0X3	T49.0X4	T49.0X5	T49.0X6
Labetalol	T44.8X1	T44.8X2	T44.8X3	T44.8X4	T44.8X5	T44.8X6
Laburnum (seeds)	T62.2X1	T62.2X2	T62.2X3	T62.2X4	—	—
leaves	T62.2X1	T62.2X2	T62.2X3	T62.2X4	—	—
Lachesine	T49.5X1	T49.5X2	T49.5X3	T49.5X4	T49.5X5	T49.5X6
Lacidipine	T46.5X1	T46.5X2	T46.5X3	T46.5X4	T46.5X5	T46.5X6
Lacquer	T65.6X1	T65.6X2	T65.6X3	T65.6X4	—	—
Lacrimogenic gas	T59.3X1	T59.3X2	T59.3X3	T59.3X4	—	—
Lactated potassic saline	T50.3X1	T50.3X2	T50.3X3	T50.3X4	T50.3X5	T50.3X6
Lactic acid	T49.8X1	T49.8X2	T49.8X3	T49.8X4	T49.8X5	T49.8X6
Lactobacillus						
acidophilus	T47.6X1	T47.6X2	T47.6X3	T47.6X4	T47.6X5	T47.6X6
compound	T47.6X1	T47.6X2	T47.6X3	T47.6X4	T47.6X5	T47.6X6
bifidus, lyophilized	T47.6X1	T47.6X2	T47.6X3	T47.6X4	T47.6X5	T47.6X6
bulgaricus	T47.6X1	T47.6X2	T47.6X3	T47.6X4	T47.6X5	T47.6X6
sporogenes	T47.6X1	T47.6X2	T47.6X3	T47.6X4	T47.6X5	T47.6X6
Lactoflavin	T45.2X1	T45.2X2	T45.2X3	T45.2X4	T45.2X5	T45.2X6
Lactose (as excipient)	T50.901	T50.902	T50.903	T50.904	T50.905	T50.906
Lactuca (virosa) (extract)	T42.6X1	T42.6X2	T42.6X3	T42.6X4	T42.6X5	T42.6X6
Lactucarium	T42.6X1	T42.6X2	T42.6X3	T42.6X4	T42.6X5	T42.6X6
Lactulose	T47.3X1	T47.3X2	T47.3X3	T47.3X4	T47.3X5	T47.3X6
Laevo — see Levo-						
Lanatosides	T46.0X1	T46.0X2	T46.0X3	T46.0X4	T46.0X5	T46.0X6
Lanolin	T49.3X1	T49.3X2	T49.3X3	T49.3X4	T49.3X5	T49.3X6
Lanoxin*	T46.0X1	T46.0X2	T46.0X3	T46.0X4	T46.0X5	T46.0X6
Largactil	T43.3X1	T43.3X2	T43.3X3	T43.3X4	T43.3X5	T43.3X6
Larkspur	T62.2X1	T62.2X2	T62.2X3	T62.2X4		
Laroxyl	T43.011	T43.012	T43.013	T43.014	T43.015	T43.016
Lasix	T50.1X1	T50.1X2	T50.1X3	T50.1X4	T50.1X5	T50.1X6
Lassar's paste	T49.4X1	T49.4X2	T49.4X3	T49.4X4	T49.4X5	T49.4X6
Latamoxef	T36.1X1	T36.1X2	T36.1X3	T36.1X4	T36.1X5	T36.1X6
Latex	T65.811	T65.812	T65.813	T65.814		
Lathyrus (seed)	T62.2X1	T62.2X2	T62.2X3	T62.2X4	—	—
Laudanum	T40.0X1	T40.0X2	T40.0X3	T40.0X4	T40.0X5	T40.0X6
Laudexium	T48.1X1	T48.1X2	T48.1X3	T48.1X4	T48.1X5	T48.1X6
Laughing gas	T41.0X1	T41.0X2	T41.0X3	T41.0X4	T41.0X5	T41.0X6
Laurel, black or cherry	T62.2X1	T62.2X2	T62.2X3	T62.2X4		
Laurolinium	T49.0X1	T49.0X2	T49.0X3	T49.0X4	T49.0X5	T49.0X6
Lauryl sulfoacetate	T49.2X1	T49.2X2	T49.2X3	T49.2X4	T49.2X5	T49.2X6
Laxative NEC	T47.4X1	T47.4X2	T47.4X3	T47.4X4	T47.4X5	T47.4X6
osmotic	T47.3X1	T47.3X2	T47.3X3	T47.3X4	T47.3X5	T47.3X6
saline	T47.3X1	T47.3X2	T47.3X3	T47.3X4	T47.3X5	T47.3X6
stimulant	T47.2X1	T47.2X2	T47.2X3	T47.2X4	T47.2X5	T47.2X6
L-dopa	T42.8X1	T42.8X2	T42.8X3	T42.8X4	T42.8X5	T42.8X6
Lead (dust) (fumes) (vapor) **NEC**	T56.0X1	T56.0X2	T56.0X3	T56.0X4	—	—
acetate	T49.2X1	T49.2X2	T49.2X3	T49.2X4	T49.2X5	T49.2X6
alkyl (fuel additive)	T56.0X1	T56.0X2	T56.0X3	T56.0X4	—	—
anti-infectives	T37.8X1	T37.8X2	T37.8X3	T37.8X4	T37.8X5	T37.8X6
antiknock compound (tetraethyl)	T56.0X1	T56.0X2	T56.0X3	T56.0X4	—	—
arsenate, arsenite (dust)(herbicide) (insecticide) (vapor)	T57.0X1	T57.0X2	T57.0X3	T57.0X4	—	—
carbonate	T56.0X1	T56.0X2	T56.0X3	T56.0X4	—	—

Substance	Poisoning, Accidental (unintentional)	Poisoning, Intentional Self-harm	Poisoning, Assault	Poisoning, Undetermined	Adverse Effect	Under-dosing
Lead (dust) (fumes) (vapor) **NEC** — continued						
carbonate — continued						
paint	T56.0X1	T56.0X2	T56.0X3	T56.0X4	—	—
chromate	T56.0X1	T56.0X2	T56.0X3	T56.0X4	—	—
paint	T56.0X1	T56.0X2	T56.0X3	T56.0X4	—	—
dioxide	T56.0X1	T56.0X2	T56.0X3	T56.0X4	—	—
inorganic	T56.0X1	T56.0X2	T56.0X3	T56.0X4	—	—
iodide	T56.0X1	T56.0X2	T56.0X3	T56.0X4	—	—
pigment (paint)	T56.0X1	T56.0X2	T56.0X3	T56.0X4	—	—
monoxide (dust)	T56.0X1	T56.0X2	T56.0X3	T56.0X4	—	—
paint	T56.0X1	T56.0X2	T56.0X3	T56.0X4	—	—
organic	T56.0X1	T56.0X2	T56.0X3	T56.0X4	—	—
oxide	T56.0X1	T56.0X2	T56.0X3	T56.0X4	—	—
paint	T56.0X1	T56.0X2	T56.0X3	T56.0X4	—	—
paint	T56.0X1	T56.0X2	T56.0X3	T56.0X4	—	—
salts	T56.0X1	T56.0X2	T56.0X3	T56.0X4	—	—
specified compound NEC	T56.0X1	T56.0X2	T56.0X3	T56.0X4	—	—
tetra-ethyl	T56.0X1	T56.0X2	T56.0X3	T56.0X4	—	—
Lebanese red	T40.711	T40.712	T40.713	T40.714	T40.715	T40.716
Lefetamine	T39.8X1	T39.8X2	T39.8X3	T39.8X4	T39.8X5	T39.8X6
Lenperone	T43.4X1	T43.4X2	T43.4X3	T43.4X4	T43.4X5	T43.4X6
Lente lietin (insulin)	T38.3X1	T38.3X2	T38.3X3	T38.3X4	T38.3X5	T38.3X6
Leptazol	T50.7X1	T50.7X2	T50.7X3	T50.7X4	T50.7X5	T50.7X6
Leptophos	T60.0X1	T60.0X2	T60.0X3	T60.0X4	—	—
Leritine	T40.2X1	T40.2X2	T40.2X3	T40.2X4	T40.2X5	T40.2X6
Lescol*	T46.6X1	T46.6X2	T46.6X3	T46.6X4	T46.6X5	T46.6X6
Letosteine	T48.4X1	T48.4X2	T48.4X3	T48.4X4	T48.4X5	T48.4X6
Letter	T38.1X1	T38.1X2	T38.1X3	T38.1X4	T38.1X5	T38.1X6
Lettuce opium	T42.6X1	T42.6X2	T42.6X3	T42.6X4	T42.6X5	T42.6X6
Leucinocaine	T41.3X1	T41.3X2	T41.3X3	T41.3X4	T41.3X5	T41.3X6
Leucocianidol	T46.991	T46.992	T46.993	T46.994	T46.995	T46.996
Leucovorin (factor)	T45.8X1	T45.8X2	T45.8X3	T45.8X4	T45.8X5	T45.8X6
Leukeran	T45.1X1	T45.1X2	T45.1X3	T45.1X4	T45.1X5	T45.1X6
Leuprolide	T38.891	T38.892	T38.893	T38.894	T38.895	T38.896
Levalbuterol	T48.6X1	T48.6X2	T48.6X3	T48.6X4	T48.6X5	T48.6X6
Levallorphan	T50.7X1	T50.7X2	T50.7X3	T50.7X4	T50.7X5	T50.7X6
Levamisole	T37.4X1	T37.4X2	T37.4X3	T37.4X4	T37.4X5	T37.4X6
Levanil	T42.6X1	T42.6X2	T42.6X3	T42.6X4	T42.6X5	T42.6X6
Levarterenol	T44.4X1	T44.4X2	T44.4X3	T44.4X4	T44.4X5	T44.4X6
Levdropropizine	T48.3X1	T48.3X2	T48.3X3	T48.3X4	T48.3X5	T48.3X6
Levobunolol	T49.5X1	T49.5X2	T49.5X3	T49.5X4	T49.5X5	T49.5X6
Levocabastine (hydrochloride)	T45.0X1	T45.0X2	T45.0X3	T45.0X4	T45.0X5	T45.0X6
Levocarnitine	T50.991	T50.992	T50.993	T50.994	T50.995	T50.996
Levodopa	T42.8X1	T42.8X2	T42.8X3	T42.8X4	T42.8X5	T42.8X6
with carbidopa	T42.8X1	T42.8X2	T42.8X3	T42.8X4	T42.8X5	T42.8X6
Levo-dromoran	T40.2X1	T40.2X2	T40.2X3	T40.2X4	T40.2X5	T40.2X6
Levoglutamide	T50.991	T50.992	T50.993	T50.994	T50.995	T50.996
Levoid	T38.1X1	T38.1X2	T38.1X3	T38.1X4	T38.1X5	T38.1X6
Levo-isomethadone	T40.3X1	T40.3X2	T40.3X3	T40.3X4	T40.3X5	T40.3X6
Levomepromazine	T43.3X1	T43.3X2	T43.3X3	T43.3X4	T43.3X5	T43.3X6
Levonordefrin	T49.6X1	T49.6X2	T49.6X3	T49.6X4	T49.6X5	T49.6X6
Levonorgestrel	T38.4X1	T38.4X2	T38.4X3	T38.4X4	T38.4X5	T38.4X6
with ethinylestradiol	T38.5X1	T38.5X2	T38.5X3	T38.5X4	T38.5X5	T38.5X6
Levopromazine	T43.3X1	T43.3X2	T43.3X3	T43.3X4	T43.3X5	T43.3X6
Levoprome	T42.6X1	T42.6X2	T42.6X3	T42.6X4	T42.6X5	T42.6X6
Levopropoxyphene	T40.491	T40.492	T40.493	T40.494	T40.495	T40.496
Levopropylhexedrine	T50.5X1	T50.5X2	T50.5X3	T50.5X4	T50.5X5	T50.5X6
Levoproxyphylline	T48.6X1	T48.6X2	T48.6X3	T48.6X4	T48.6X5	T48.6X6
Levorphanol	T40.491	T40.492	T40.493	T40.494	T40.495	T40.496
Levothroid*	T38.1X1	T38.1X2	T38.1X3	T38.1X4	T38.1X5	T38.1X6
Levothyroxine	T38.1X1	T38.1X2	T38.1X3	T38.1X4	T38.1X5	T38.1X6
sodium	T38.1X1	T38.1X2	T38.1X3	T38.1X4	T38.1X5	T38.1X6
Levoxyl*	T38.1X1	T38.1X2	T38.1X3	T38.1X4	T38.1X5	T38.1X6
Levsin	T44.3X1	T44.3X2	T44.3X3	T44.3X4	T44.3X5	T44.3X6
Levulose	T50.3X1	T50.3X2	T50.3X3	T50.3X4	T50.3X5	T50.3X6
Lewisite (gas), not in war	T57.0X1	T57.0X2	T57.0X3	T57.0X4	—	—
Lexapro*	T43.221	T43.222	T43.223	T43.224	T43.225	T43.226
Librium	T42.4X1	T42.4X2	T42.4X3	T42.4X4	T42.4X5	T42.4X6
Lidex	T49.0X1	T49.0X2	T49.0X3	T49.0X4	T49.0X5	T49.0X6
Lidocaine	T41.3X1	T41.3X2	T41.3X3	T41.3X4	T41.3X5	T41.3X6
regional	T41.3X1	T41.3X2	T41.3X3	T41.3X4	T41.3X5	T41.3X6
spinal	T41.3X1	T41.3X2	T41.3X3	T41.3X4	T41.3X5	T41.3X6
Lidofenin	T50.8X1	T50.8X2	T50.8X3	T50.8X4	T50.8X5	T50.8X6
Lidoflazine	T46.1X1	T46.1X2	T46.1X3	T46.1X4	T46.1X5	T46.1X6
Lighter fluid	T52.0X1	T52.0X2	T52.0X3	T52.0X4	—	—
Lignin hemicellulose	T47.6X1	T47.6X2	T47.6X3	T47.6X4	T47.6X5	T47.6X6
Lignocaine	T41.3X1	T41.3X2	T41.3X3	T41.3X4	T41.3X5	T41.3X6
regional	T41.3X1	T41.3X2	T41.3X3	T41.3X4	T41.3X5	T41.3X6
spinal	T41.3X1	T41.3X2	T41.3X3	T41.3X4	T41.3X5	T41.3X6
Ligroin (e) (solvent)	T52.0X1	T52.0X2	T52.0X3	T52.0X4	—	—
vapor	T59.891	T59.892	T59.893	T59.894	—	—

Substance	Poisoning, Accidental (unintentional)	Poisoning, Intentional Self-harm	Poisoning, Assault	Poisoning, Undetermined	Adverse Effect	Under-dosing
Ligustrum vulgare	T62.2X1	T62.2X2	T62.2X3	T62.2X4	—	—
Lily of the valley	T62.2X1	T62.2X2	T62.2X3	T62.2X4	—	—
Lime (chloride)	T54.3X1	T54.3X2	T54.3X3	T54.3X4	—	—
Limonene	T52.8X1	T52.8X2	T52.8X3	T52.8X4	—	—
Lincomycin	T36.8X1	T36.8X2	T36.8X3	T36.8X4	T36.8X5	T36.8X6
Lindane (insecticide) (nonmedicinal) (vapor)	T53.6X1	T53.6X2	T53.6X3	T53.6X4	—	—
medicinal	T49.0X1	T49.0X2	T49.0X3	T49.0X4	T49.0X5	T49.0X6
Liniments NEC	T49.91	T49.92	T49.93	T49.94	T49.95	T49.96
Linoleic acid	T46.6X1	T46.6X2	T46.6X3	T46.6X4	T46.6X5	T46.6X6
Linolenic acid	T46.6X1	T46.6X2	T46.6X3	T46.6X4	T46.6X5	T46.6X6
Linseed	T47.4X1	T47.4X2	T47.4X3	T47.4X4	T47.4X5	T47.4X6
Liothyronine	T38.1X1	T38.1X2	T38.1X3	T38.1X4	T38.1X5	T38.1X6
Liotrix	T38.1X1	T38.1X2	T38.1X3	T38.1X4	T38.1X5	T38.1X6
Lipancreatin	T47.5X1	T47.5X2	T47.5X3	T47.5X4	T47.5X5	T47.5X6
Lipitor*	T46.6X1	T46.6X2	T46.6X3	T46.6X4	T46.6X5	T46.6X6
Lipo-alprostadil	T46.7X1	T46.7X2	T46.7X3	T46.7X4	T46.7X5	T46.7X6
Lipo-Lutin	T38.5X1	T38.5X2	T38.5X3	T38.5X4	T38.5X5	T38.5X6
Lipotropic drug NEC	T50.901	T50.902	T50.903	T50.904	T50.905	T50.906
Liquefied petroleum gases	T59.891	T59.892	T59.893	T59.894	—	—
piped (pure or mixed with air)	T59.891	T59.892	T59.893	T59.894	—	—
Liquid						
paraffin	T47.4X1	T47.4X2	T47.4X3	T47.4X4	T47.4X5	T47.4X6
petrolatum	T47.4X1	T47.4X2	T47.4X3	T47.4X4	T47.4X5	T47.4X6
topical	T49.3X1	T49.3X2	T49.3X3	T49.3X4	T49.3X5	T49.3X6
specified NEC	T65.891	T65.892	T65.893	T65.894	—	—
substance	T65.91	T65.92	T65.93	T65.94	—	—
Liquor creosolis compositus	T65.891	T65.892	T65.893	T65.894	—	—
Liquorice	T48.4X1	T48.4X2	T48.4X3	T48.4X4	T48.4X5	T48.4X6
extract	T47.8X1	T47.8X2	T47.8X3	T47.8X4	T47.8X5	T47.8X6
Liraglutide*	T38.3X1	T38.3X2	T38.3X3	T38.3X4	T38.3X5	T38.3X6
Lisinopril	T46.4X1	T46.4X2	T46.4X3	T46.4X4	T46.4X5	T46.4X6
Lisuride	T42.8X1	T42.8X2	T42.8X3	T42.8X4	T42.8X5	T42.8X6
Lithane	T43.8X1	T43.8X2	T43.8X3	T43.8X4	T43.8X5	T43.8X6
Lithium	T56.891	T56.892	T56.893	T56.894	—	—
gluconate	T43.591	T43.592	T43.593	T43.594	T43.595	T43.596
salts (carbonate)	T43.591	T43.592	T43.593	T43.594	T43.595	T43.596
Lithonate	T43.8X1	T43.8X2	T43.8X3	T43.8X4	T43.8X5	T43.8X6
Liver						
extract	T45.8X1	T45.8X2	T45.8X3	T45.8X4	T45.8X5	T45.8X6
for parenteral use	T45.8X1	T45.8X2	T45.8X3	T45.8X4	T45.8X5	T45.8X6
fraction 1	T45.8X1	T45.8X2	T45.8X3	T45.8X4	T45.8X5	T45.8X6
hydrolysate	T45.8X1	T45.8X2	T45.8X3	T45.8X4	T45.8X5	T45.8X6
Lizard (bite) (venom)	T63.121	T63.122	T63.123	T63.124	—	—
LMD	T45.8X1	T45.8X2	T45.8X3	T45.8X4	T45.8X5	T45.8X6
Lobelia	T62.2X1	T62.2X2	T62.2X3	T62.2X4	—	—
Lobeline	T50.7X1	T50.7X2	T50.7X3	T50.7X4	T50.7X5	T50.7X6
Local action drug NEC	T49.8X1	T49.8X2	T49.8X3	T49.8X4	T49.8X5	T49.8X6
Locorten	T49.0X1	T49.0X2	T49.0X3	T49.0X4	T49.0X5	T49.0X6
Lofepramine	T43.011	T43.012	T43.013	T43.014	T43.015	T43.016
Lolium temulentum	T62.2X1	T62.2X2	T62.2X3	T62.2X4	—	—
Lomotil	T47.6X1	T47.6X2	T47.6X3	T47.6X4	T47.6X5	T47.6X6
Lomustine	T45.1X1	T45.1X2	T45.1X3	T45.1X4	T45.1X5	T45.1X6
Lonidamine	T45.1X1	T45.1X2	T45.1X3	T45.1X4	T45.1X5	T45.1X6
LoOvral*	T38.4X1	T38.4X2	T38.4X3	T38.4X4	T38.4X5	T38.4X6
Loperamide	T47.6X1	T47.6X2	T47.6X3	T47.6X4	T47.6X5	T47.6X6
Loprazolam	T42.4X1	T42.4X2	T42.4X3	T42.4X4	T42.4X5	T42.4X6
Lopressor*	T44.7X1	T44.7X2	T44.7X3	T44.7X4	T44.7X5	T44.7X6
Lorajmine	T46.2X1	T46.2X2	T46.2X3	T46.2X4	T46.2X5	T46.2X6
Loratidine	T45.0X1	T45.0X2	T45.0X3	T45.0X4	T45.0X5	T45.0X6
Lorazepam	T42.4X1	T42.4X2	T42.4X3	T42.4X4	T42.4X5	T42.4X6
Lorcainide	T46.2X1	T46.2X2	T46.2X3	T46.2X4	T46.2X5	T46.2X6
Lormetazepam	T42.4X1	T42.4X2	T42.4X3	T42.4X4	T42.4X5	T42.4X6
Losartan*	T46.5X1	T46.5X2	T46.5X3	T46.5X4	T46.5X5	T46.5X6
Lotions NEC	T49.91	T49.92	T49.93	T49.94	T49.95	T49.96
Lotrimin*	T49.0X1	T49.0X2	T49.0X3	T49.0X4	T49.0X5	T49.0X6
Lotusate	T42.3X1	T42.3X2	T42.3X3	T42.3X4	T42.3X5	T42.3X6
Lovastatin	T46.6X1	T46.6X2	T46.6X3	T46.6X4	T46.6X5	T46.6X6
Lowila	T49.2X1	T49.2X2	T49.2X3	T49.2X4	T49.2X5	T49.2X6
Loxapine	T43.591	T43.592	T43.593	T43.594	T43.595	T43.596
Lozenges (throat)	T49.6X1	T49.6X2	T49.6X3	T49.6X4	T49.6X5	T49.6X6
LSD	T40.8X1	T40.8X2	T40.8X3	T40.8X4	—	—
L-Tryptophan — see amino acid						
Lubricant, eye	T49.5X1	T49.5X2	T49.5X3	T49.5X4	T49.5X5	T49.5X6
Lubricating oil NEC	T52.0X1	T52.0X2	T52.0X3	T52.0X4	—	—
Lucanthone	T37.4X1	T37.4X2	T37.4X3	T37.4X4	T37.4X5	T37.4X6
Luminal	T42.3X1	T42.3X2	T42.3X3	T42.3X4	T42.3X5	T42.3X6
Lung irritant (gas) NEC	T59.91	T59.92	T59.93	T59.94	—	—
Luteinizing hormone	T38.811	T38.812	T38.813	T38.814	T38.815	T38.816
Lutocylol	T38.5X1	T38.5X2	T38.5X3	T38.5X4	T38.5X5	T38.5X6
Lutromone	T38.5X1	T38.5X2	T38.5X3	T38.5X4	T38.5X5	T38.5X6

Substance	Poisoning, Accidental (unintentional)	Poisoning, Intentional Self-harm	Poisoning, Assault	Poisoning, Undetermined	Adverse Effect	Under-dosing
Lututrin	T48.291	T48.292	T48.293	T48.294	T48.295	T48.296
Luveris*	T38.891	T38.892	T38.893	T38.894	T38.895	T38.896
Lye (concentrated)	T54.3X1	T54.3X2	T54.3X3	T54.3X4	—	—
Lygranum (skin test)	T50.8X1	T50.8X2	T50.8X3	T50.8X4	T50.8X5	T50.8X6
Lymecycline	T36.4X1	T36.4X2	T36.4X3	T36.4X4	T36.4X5	T36.4X6
Lymphogranuloma venereum antigen	T50.8X1	T50.8X2	T50.8X3	T50.8X4	T50.8X5	T50.8X6
Lynestrenol	T38.4X1	T38.4X2	T38.4X3	T38.4X4	T38.4X5	T38.4X6
Lyovac Sodium Edecrin	T50.1X1	T50.1X2	T50.1X3	T50.1X4	T50.1X5	T50.1X6
Lypressin	T38.891	T38.892	T38.893	T38.894	T38.895	T38.896
Lysergic acid diethylamide	T40.8X1	T40.8X2	T40.8X3	T40.8X4	—	—
Lysergide	T40.8X1	T40.8X2	T40.8X3	T40.8X4	—	—
Lysine vasopressin	T38.891	T38.892	T38.893	T38.894	T38.895	T38.896
Lysol	T54.1X1	T54.1X2	T54.1X3	T54.1X4	—	—
Lysozyme	T49.0X1	T49.0X2	T49.0X3	T49.0X4	T49.0X5	T49.0X6
Lytta (vitatta)	T49.8X1	T49.8X2	T49.8X3	T49.8X4	T49.8X5	T49.8X6
Mace	T59.3X1	T59.3X2	T59.3X3	T59.3X4	—	—
Macrogol	T50.991	T50.992	T50.993	T50.994	T50.995	T50.996
Macrolide						
anabolic drug	T38.7X1	T38.7X2	T38.7X3	T38.7X4	T38.7X5	T38.7X6
antibiotic	T36.3X1	T36.3X2	T36.3X3	T36.3X4	T36.3X5	T36.3X6
Mafenide	T49.0X1	T49.0X2	T49.0X3	T49.0X4	T49.0X5	T49.0X6
Magaldrate	T47.1X1	T47.1X2	T47.1X3	T47.1X4	T47.1X5	T47.1X6
Magic mushroom	T40.991	T40.992	T40.993	T40.994		
Magnamycin	T36.8X1	T36.8X2	T36.8X3	T36.8X4	T36.8X5	T36.8X6
Magnesia magma	T47.1X1	T47.1X2	T47.1X3	T47.1X4	T47.1X5	T47.1X6
Magnesium NEC	T56.891	T56.892	T56.893	T56.894		
carbonate	T47.1X1	T47.1X2	T47.1X3	T47.1X4	T47.1X5	T47.1X6
citrate	T47.4X1	T47.4X2	T47.4X3	T47.4X4	T47.4X5	T47.4X6
hydroxide	T47.1X1	T47.1X2	T47.1X3	T47.1X4	T47.1X5	T47.1X6
oxide	T47.1X1	T47.1X2	T47.1X3	T47.1X4	T47.1X5	T47.1X6
peroxide	T49.0X1	T49.0X2	T49.0X3	T49.0X4	T49.0X5	T49.0X6
salicylate	T39.091	T39.092	T39.093	T39.094	T39.095	T39.096
silicofluoride	T50.3X1	T50.3X2	T50.3X3	T50.3X4	T50.3X5	T50.3X6
sulfate	T47.4X1	T47.4X2	T47.4X3	T47.4X4	T47.4X5	T47.4X6
thiosulfate	T45.0X1	T45.0X2	T45.0X3	T45.0X4	T45.0X5	T45.0X6
trisilicate	T47.1X1	T47.1X2	T47.1X3	T47.1X4	T47.1X5	T47.1X6
Malathion (medicinal)	T49.0X1	T49.0X2	T49.0X3	T49.0X4	T49.0X5	T49.0X6
insecticide	T60.0X1	T60.0X2	T60.0X3	T60.0X4	—	—
Male fern extract	T37.4X1	T37.4X2	T37.4X3	T37.4X4	T37.4X5	T37.4X6
M-AMSA	T45.1X1	T45.1X2	T45.1X3	T45.1X4	T45.1X5	T45.1X6
Mandelic acid	T37.8X1	T37.8X2	T37.8X3	T37.8X4	T37.8X5	T37.8X6
Manganese (dioxide) (salts)	T57.2X1	T57.2X2	T57.2X3	T57.2X4	—	—
medicinal	T50.991	T50.992	T50.993	T50.994	T50.995	T50.996
Mannitol	T47.3X1	T47.3X2	T47.3X3	T47.3X4	T47.3X5	T47.3X6
hexanitrate	T46.3X1	T46.3X2	T46.3X3	T46.3X4	T46.3X5	T46.3X6
Mannomustine	T45.1X1	T45.1X2	T45.1X3	T45.1X4	T45.1X5	T45.1X6
MAO inhibitors	T43.1X1	T43.1X2	T43.1X3	T43.1X4	T43.1X5	T43.1X6
Mapharsen	T37.8X1	T37.8X2	T37.8X3	T37.8X4	T37.8X5	T37.8X6
Maphenide	T49.0X1	T49.0X2	T49.0X3	T49.0X4	T49.0X5	T49.0X6
Maprotiline	T43.021	T43.022	T43.023	T43.024	T43.025	T43.026
Marcaine	T41.3X1	T41.3X2	T41.3X3	T41.3X4	T41.3X5	T41.3X6
infiltration (subcutaneous)	T41.3X1	T41.3X2	T41.3X3	T41.3X4	T41.3X5	T41.3X6
nerve block (peripheral) (plexus)	T41.3X1	T41.3X2	T41.3X3	T41.3X4	T41.3X5	T41.3X6
Marezine	T45.0X1	T45.0X2	T45.0X3	T45.0X4	T45.0X5	T45.0X6
Marihuana	T40.711	T40.712	T40.713	T40.714	T40.715	T40.716
Marijuana	T40.711	T40.712	T40.713	T40.714	T40.715	T40.716
Marine (sting)	T63.691	T63.692	T63.693	T63.694	—	—
animals (sting)	T63.691	T63.692	T63.693	T63.694	—	—
plants (sting)	T63.711	T63.712	T63.713	T63.714	—	—
Marplan	T43.1X1	T43.1X2	T43.1X3	T43.1X4	T43.1X5	T43.1X6
Marsh gas	T59.891	T59.892	T59.893	T59.894	—	—
Marsilid	T43.1X1	T43.1X2	T43.1X3	T43.1X4	T43.1X5	T43.1X6
Massengill*	T49.0X1	T49.0X2	T49.0X3	T49.0X4	T49.0X5	T49.0X6
Matulane	T45.1X1	T45.1X2	T45.1X3	T45.1X4	T45.1X5	T45.1X6
Mazindol	T50.5X1	T50.5X2	T50.5X3	T50.5X4	T50.5X5	T50.5X6
MCPA	T60.3X1	T60.3X2	T60.3X3	T60.3X4	—	—
MDMA	T43.641	T43.642	T43.643	T43.644	—	—
Meadow saffron	T62.2X1	T62.2X2	T62.2X3	T62.2X4	—	—
Measles virus vaccine (attenuated)	T50.B91	T50.B92	T50.B93	T50.B94	T50.B95	T50.B96
Meat, noxious	T62.8X1	T62.8X2	T62.8X3	T62.8X4	—	—
Meballymal	T42.3X1	T42.3X2	T42.3X3	T42.3X4	T42.3X5	T42.3X6
Mebanazine	T43.1X1	T43.1X2	T43.1X3	T43.1X4	T43.1X5	T43.1X6
Mebaral	T42.3X1	T42.3X2	T42.3X3	T42.3X4	T42.3X5	T42.3X6
Mebendazole	T37.4X1	T37.4X2	T37.4X3	T37.4X4	T37.4X5	T37.4X6
Mebeverine	T44.3X1	T44.3X2	T44.3X3	T44.3X4	T44.3X5	T44.3X6
Mebhydrolin	T45.0X1	T45.0X2	T45.0X3	T45.0X4	T45.0X5	T45.0X6
Mebumal	T42.3X1	T42.3X2	T42.3X3	T42.3X4	T42.3X5	T42.3X6
Mebutamate	T43.591	T43.592	T43.593	T43.594	T43.595	T43.596
Mecamylamine	T44.2X1	T44.2X2	T44.2X3	T44.2X4	T44.2X5	T44.2X6
Mechlorethamine	T45.1X1	T45.1X2	T45.1X3	T45.1X4	T45.1X5	T45.1X6

☑ Additional Character May Be Required — Refer to the Tabular List for Character Selection

*Optum Value-Add

Substance	Poisoning, Accidental (unintentional)	Poisoning, Intentional Self-harm	Poisoning, Assault	Poisoning, Undetermined	Adverse Effect	Under-dosing
Mecillinam	T36.0X1	T36.0X2	T36.0X3	T36.0X4	T36.0X5	T36.0X6
Meclizine (hydrochloride)	T45.0X1	T45.0X2	T45.0X3	T45.0X4	T45.0X5	T45.0X6
Meclocycline	T36.4X1	T36.4X2	T36.4X3	T36.4X4	T36.4X5	T36.4X6
Meclofenamate	T39.391	T39.392	T39.393	T39.394	T39.395	T39.396
Meclofenamic acid	T39.391	T39.392	T39.393	T39.394	T39.395	T39.396
Meclofenoxate	T43.691	T43.692	T43.693	T43.694	T43.695	T43.696
Meclozine	T45.0X1	T45.0X2	T45.0X3	T45.0X4	T45.0X5	T45.0X6
Mecobalamin	T45.8X1	T45.8X2	T45.8X3	T45.8X4	T45.8X5	T45.8X6
Mecoprop	T60.3X1	T60.3X2	T60.3X3	T60.3X4	—	—
Mecrilate	T49.3X1	T49.3X2	T49.3X3	T49.3X4	T49.3X5	T49.3X6
Mecysteine	T48.4X1	T48.4X2	T48.4X3	T48.4X4	T48.4X5	T48.4X6
Medazepam	T42.4X1	T42.4X2	T42.4X3	T42.4X4	T42.4X5	T42.4X6
Medicament NEC	T50.901	T50.902	T50.903	T50.904	T50.905	T50.906
Medinal	T42.3X1	T42.3X2	T42.3X3	T42.3X4	T42.3X5	T42.3X6
Medomin	T42.3X1	T42.3X2	T42.3X3	T42.3X4	T42.3X5	T42.3X6
Medrogestone	T38.5X1	T38.5X2	T38.5X3	T38.5X4	T38.5X5	T38.5X6
Medrol*	T38.0X1	T38.0X2	T38.0X3	T38.0X4	T38.0X5	T38.0X6
Medroxalol	T44.8X1	T44.8X2	T44.8X3	T44.8X4	T44.8X5	T44.8X6
Medroxyprogesterone acetate (depot)	T38.5X1	T38.5X2	T38.5X3	T38.5X4	T38.5X5	T38.5X6
Medrysone	T49.0X1	T49.0X2	T49.0X3	T49.0X4	T49.0X5	T49.0X6
Mefenamic acid	T39.391	T39.392	T39.393	T39.394	T39.395	T39.396
Mefenorex	T50.5X1	T50.5X2	T50.5X3	T50.5X4	T50.5X5	T50.5X6
Mefloquine	T37.2X1	T37.2X2	T37.2X3	T37.2X4	T37.2X5	T37.2X6
Mefoxin*	T36.1X1	T36.1X2	T36.1X3	T36.1X4	T36.1X5	T36.1X6
Mefruside	T50.2X1	T50.2X2	T50.2X3	T50.2X4	T50.2X5	T50.2X6
Megahallucinogen	T40.901	T40.902	T40.903	T40.904	T40.905	T40.906
Megestrol	T38.5X1	T38.5X2	T38.5X3	T38.5X4	T38.5X5	T38.5X6
Meglumine						
antimoniate	T37.8X1	T37.8X2	T37.8X3	T37.8X4	T37.8X5	T37.8X6
diatrizoate	T50.8X1	T50.8X2	T50.8X3	T50.8X4	T50.8X5	T50.8X6
iodipamide	T50.8X1	T50.8X2	T50.8X3	T50.8X4	T50.8X5	T50.8X6
iotroxate	T50.8X1	T50.8X2	T50.8X3	T50.8X4	T50.8X5	T50.8X6
MEK (methyl ethyl ketone)	T52.4X1	T52.4X2	T52.4X3	T52.4X4	—	—
Meladinin	T49.3X1	T49.3X2	T49.3X3	T49.3X4	T49.3X5	T49.3X6
Meladrazine	T44.3X1	T44.3X2	T44.3X3	T44.3X4	T44.3X5	T44.3X6
Melaleuca alternifolia oil	T49.0X1	T49.0X2	T49.0X3	T49.0X4	T49.0X5	T49.0X6
Melanizing agents	T49.3X1	T49.3X2	T49.3X3	T49.3X4	T49.3X5	T49.3X6
Melanocyte-stimulating hormone	T38.891	T38.892	T38.893	T38.894	T38.895	T38.896
Melarsonyl potassium	T37.3X1	T37.3X2	T37.3X3	T37.3X4	T37.3X5	T37.3X6
Melarsoprol	T37.3X1	T37.3X2	T37.3X3	T37.3X4	T37.3X5	T37.3X6
Melia azedarach	T62.2X1	T62.2X2	T62.2X3	T62.2X4	—	—
Melitracen	T43.011	T43.012	T43.013	T43.014	T43.015	T43.016
Mellaril	T43.3X1	T43.3X2	T43.3X3	T43.3X4	T43.3X5	T43.3X6
Meloxicam*	T39.391	T39.392	T39.393	T39.394	T39.395	T39.396
Meloxine	T49.3X1	T49.3X2	T49.3X3	T49.3X4	T49.3X5	T49.3X6
Melperone	T43.4X1	T43.4X2	T43.4X3	T43.4X4	T43.4X5	T43.4X6
Melphalan	T45.1X1	T45.1X2	T45.1X3	T45.1X4	T45.1X5	T45.1X6
Memantine	T43.8X1	T43.8X2	T43.8X3	T43.8X4	T43.8X5	T43.8X6
Menadiol	T45.7X1	T45.7X2	T45.7X3	T45.7X4	T45.7X5	T45.7X6
sodium sulfate	T45.7X1	T45.7X2	T45.7X3	T45.7X4	T45.7X5	T45.7X6
Menadione	T45.7X1	T45.7X2	T45.7X3	T45.7X4	T45.7X5	T45.7X6
sodium bisulfite	T45.7X1	T45.7X2	T45.7X3	T45.7X4	T45.7X5	T45.7X6
Menaphthone	T45.7X1	T45.7X2	T45.7X3	T45.7X4	T45.7X5	T45.7X6
Menaquinone	T45.7X1	T45.7X2	T45.7X3	T45.7X4	T45.7X5	T45.7X6
Menatetrenone	T45.7X1	T45.7X2	T45.7X3	T45.7X4	T45.7X5	T45.7X6
Meningococcal vaccine	T50.A91	T50.A92	T50.A93	T50.A94	T50.A95	T50.A96
Menningovax (-AC) (-C)	T50.A91	T50.A92	T50.A93	T50.A94	T50.A95	T50.A96
Menotropins	T38.811	T38.812	T38.813	T38.814	T38.815	T38.816
Menthol	T48.5X1	T48.5X2	T48.5X3	T48.5X4	T48.5X5	T48.5X6
Mepacrine	T37.2X1	T37.2X2	T37.2X3	T37.2X4	T37.2X5	T37.2X6
Meparfynol	T42.6X1	T42.6X2	T42.6X3	T42.6X4	T42.6X5	T42.6X6
Mepartricin	T36.7X1	T36.7X2	T36.7X3	T36.7X4	T36.7X5	T36.7X6
Mepazine	T43.3X1	T43.3X2	T43.3X3	T43.3X4	T43.3X5	T43.3X6
Mepenzolate	T44.3X1	T44.3X2	T44.3X3	T44.3X4	T44.3X5	T44.3X6
bromide	T44.3X1	T44.3X2	T44.3X3	T44.3X4	T44.3X5	T44.3X6
Meperidine	T40.491	T40.492	T40.493	T40.494	T40.495	T40.496
Mephebarbital	T42.3X1	T42.3X2	T42.3X3	T42.3X4	T42.3X5	T42.3X6
Mephenamin (e)	T42.8X1	T42.8X2	T42.8X3	T42.8X4	T42.8X5	T42.8X6
Mephenesin	T42.8X1	T42.8X2	T42.8X3	T42.8X4	T42.8X5	T42.8X6
Mephenhydramine	T45.0X1	T45.0X2	T45.0X3	T45.0X4	T45.0X5	T45.0X6
Mephenoxalone	T42.8X1	T42.8X2	T42.8X3	T42.8X4	T42.8X5	T42.8X6
Mephentermine	T44.991	T44.992	T44.993	T44.994	T44.995	T44.996
Mephenytoin	T42.0X1	T42.0X2	T42.0X3	T42.0X4	T42.0X5	T42.0X6
with phenobarbital	T42.3X1	T42.3X2	T42.3X3	T42.3X4	T42.3X5	T42.3X6
Mephobarbital	T42.3X1	T42.3X2	T42.3X3	T42.3X4	T42.3X5	T42.3X6
Mephosfolan	T60.0X1	T60.0X2	T60.0X3	T60.0X4	—	—
Mepindolol	T44.7X1	T44.7X2	T44.7X3	T44.7X4	T44.7X5	T44.7X6
Mepiperphenidol	T44.3X1	T44.3X2	T44.3X3	T44.3X4	T44.3X5	T44.3X6
Mepitiostane	T38.7X1	T38.7X2	T38.7X3	T38.7X4	T38.7X5	T38.7X6
Mepivacaine	T41.3X1	T41.3X2	T41.3X3	T41.3X4	T41.3X5	T41.3X6
epidural	T41.3X1	T41.3X2	T41.3X3	T41.3X4	T41.3X5	T41.3X6

Substance	Poisoning, Accidental (unintentional)	Poisoning, Intentional Self-harm	Poisoning, Assault	Poisoning, Undetermined	Adverse Effect	Under-dosing
Meprednisone	T38.0X1	T38.0X2	T38.0X3	T38.0X4	T38.0X5	T38.0X6
Meprobam	T43.591	T43.592	T43.593	T43.594	T43.595	T43.596
Meprobamate	T43.591	T43.592	T43.593	T43.594	T43.595	T43.596
Meproscillarin	T46.0X1	T46.0X2	T46.0X3	T46.0X4	T46.0X5	T46.0X6
Meprylcaine	T41.3X1	T41.3X2	T41.3X3	T41.3X4	T41.3X5	T41.3X6
Meptazinol	T39.8X1	T39.8X2	T39.8X3	T39.8X4	T39.8X5	T39.8X6
Mepyramine	T45.0X1	T45.0X2	T45.0X3	T45.0X4	T45.0X5	T45.0X6
Mequinol*	T49.8X1	T49.8X2	T49.8X3	T49.8X4	T49.8X5	T49.8X6
Mequitazine	T43.3X1	T43.3X2	T43.3X3	T43.3X4	T43.3X5	T43.3X6
Meralluride	T50.2X1	T50.2X2	T50.2X3	T50.2X4	T50.2X5	T50.2X6
Merbaphen	T50.2X1	T50.2X2	T50.2X3	T50.2X4	T50.2X5	T50.2X6
Merbromin	T49.0X1	T49.0X2	T49.0X3	T49.0X4	T49.0X5	T49.0X6
Mercaptobenzothiazole salts	T49.0X1	T49.0X2	T49.0X3	T49.0X4	T49.0X5	T49.0X6
Mercaptomerin	T50.2X1	T50.2X2	T50.2X3	T50.2X4	T50.2X5	T50.2X6
Mercaptopurine	T45.1X1	T45.1X2	T45.1X3	T45.1X4	T45.1X5	T45.1X6
Mercumatilin	T50.2X1	T50.2X2	T50.2X3	T50.2X4	T50.2X5	T50.2X6
Mercuramide	T50.2X1	T50.2X2	T50.2X3	T50.2X4	T50.2X5	T50.2X6
Mercurochrome	T49.0X1	T49.0X2	T49.0X3	T49.0X4	T49.0X5	T49.0X6
Mercurophylline	T50.2X1	T50.2X2	T50.2X3	T50.2X4	T50.2X5	T50.2X6
Mercury, mercurial, mercuric, mercurous (compounds) (cyanide) (fumes) (nonmedicinal) (vapor)	T56.1X1	T56.1X2	T56.1X3	T56.1X4		
NEC						
ammoniated	T49.0X1	T49.0X2	T49.0X3	T49.0X4	T49.0X5	T49.0X6
anti-infective						
local	T49.0X1	T49.0X2	T49.0X3	T49.0X4	T49.0X5	T49.0X6
systemic	T37.8X1	T37.8X2	T37.8X3	T37.8X4	T37.8X5	T37.8X6
topical	T49.0X1	T49.0X2	T49.0X3	T49.0X4	T49.0X5	T49.0X6
chloride (ammoniated)	T49.0X1	T49.0X2	T49.0X3	T49.0X4	T49.0X5	T49.0X6
fungicide	T56.1X1	T56.1X2	T56.1X3	T56.1X4	—	—
diuretic NEC	T50.2X1	T50.2X2	T50.2X3	T50.2X4	T50.2X5	T50.2X6
fungicide	T56.1X1	T56.1X2	T56.1X3	T56.1X4	—	—
organic (fungicide)	T56.1X1	T56.1X2	T56.1X3	T56.1X4	—	—
oxide, yellow	T49.0X1	T49.0X2	T49.0X3	T49.0X4	T49.0X5	T49.0X6
Mersalyl	T50.2X1	T50.2X2	T50.2X3	T50.2X4	T50.2X5	T50.2X6
Merthiolate	T49.0X1	T49.0X2	T49.0X3	T49.0X4	T49.0X5	T49.0X6
ophthalmic preparation	T49.5X1	T49.5X2	T49.5X3	T49.5X4	T49.5X5	T49.5X6
Meruvax	T50.B91	T50.B92	T50.B93	T50.B94	T50.B95	T50.B96
Mesalazine	T47.8X1	T47.8X2	T47.8X3	T47.8X4	T47.8X5	T47.8X6
Mescal buttons	T40.991	T40.992	T40.993	T40.994	—	—
Mescaline	T40.991	T40.992	T40.993	T40.994	—	—
Mesna	T48.4X1	T48.4X2	T48.4X3	T48.4X4	T48.4X5	T48.4X6
Mesoglycan	T46.6X1	T46.6X2	T46.6X3	T46.6X4	T46.6X5	T46.6X6
Mesoridazine	T43.3X1	T43.3X2	T43.3X3	T43.3X4	T43.3X5	T43.3X6
Mestanolone	T38.7X1	T38.7X2	T38.7X3	T38.7X4	T38.7X5	T38.7X6
Mesterolone	T38.7X1	T38.7X2	T38.7X3	T38.7X4	T38.7X5	T38.7X6
Mestranol	T38.5X1	T38.5X2	T38.5X3	T38.5X4	T38.5X5	T38.5X6
Mesulergine	T42.8X1	T42.8X2	T42.8X3	T42.8X4	T42.8X5	T42.8X6
Mesulfen	T49.0X1	T49.0X2	T49.0X3	T49.0X4	T49.0X5	T49.0X6
Mesuximide	T42.2X1	T42.2X2	T42.2X3	T42.2X4	T42.2X5	T42.2X6
Metabutethamine	T41.3X1	T41.3X2	T41.3X3	T41.3X4	T41.3X5	T41.3X6
Metactesylacetate	T49.0X1	T49.0X2	T49.0X3	T49.0X4	T49.0X5	T49.0X6
Metacycline	T36.4X1	T36.4X2	T36.4X3	T36.4X4	T36.4X5	T36.4X6
Metaldehyde (snail killer) NEC	T60.8X1	T60.8X2	T60.8X3	T60.8X4	—	—
Metals (heavy) (nonmedicinal)	T56.91	T56.92	T56.93	T56.94	—	—
dust, fumes, or vapor NEC	T56.91	T56.92	T56.93	T56.94	—	—
gadolinium	T56.821	T56.822	T56.823	T56.824	—	—
light NEC	T56.91	T56.92	T56.93	T56.94	—	—
dust, fumes, or vapor NEC	T56.91	T56.92	T56.93	T56.94	—	—
specified NEC	T56.891	T56.892	T56.893	T56.894	—	—
thallium	T56.811	T56.812	T56.813	T56.814	—	—
Metamfetamine	T43.651	T43.652	T43.653	T43.654	T43.655	T43.656
Metamizole sodium	T39.2X1	T39.2X2	T39.2X3	T39.2X4	T39.2X5	T39.2X6
Metampicillin	T36.0X1	T36.0X2	T36.0X3	T36.0X4	T36.0X5	T36.0X6
Metamucil	T47.4X1	T47.4X2	T47.4X3	T47.4X4	T47.4X5	T47.4X6
Metandienone	T38.7X1	T38.7X2	T38.7X3	T38.7X4	T38.7X5	T38.7X6
Metandrostenolone	T38.7X1	T38.7X2	T38.7X3	T38.7X4	T38.7X5	T38.7X6
Metaphen	T49.0X1	T49.0X2	T49.0X3	T49.0X4	T49.0X5	T49.0X6
Metaphos	T60.0X1	T60.0X2	T60.0X3	T60.0X4	—	—
Metapramine	T43.011	T43.012	T43.013	T43.014	T43.015	T43.016
Metaproterenol	T48.291	T48.292	T48.293	T48.294	T48.295	T48.296
Metaraminol	T44.4X1	T44.4X2	T44.4X3	T44.4X4	T44.4X5	T44.4X6
Metaxalone	T42.8X1	T42.8X2	T42.8X3	T42.8X4	T42.8X5	T42.8X6
Meted*	T49.4X1	T49.4X2	T49.4X3	T49.4X4	T49.4X5	T49.4X6
Metenolone	T38.7X1	T38.7X2	T38.7X3	T38.7X4	T38.7X5	T38.7X6
Metergoline	T42.8X1	T42.8X2	T42.8X3	T42.8X4	T42.8X5	T42.8X6
Metescufylline	T46.991	T46.992	T46.993	T46.994	T46.995	T46.996
Metetoin	T42.0X1	T42.0X2	T42.0X3	T42.0X4	T42.0X5	T42.0X6

Substance	Poisoning, Accidental (unintentional)	Poisoning, Intentional Self-harm	Poisoning, Assault	Poisoning, Undetermined	Adverse Effect	Under-dosing
Metformin	T38.3X1	T38.3X2	T38.3X3	T38.3X4	T38.3X5	T38.3X6
Methacholine	T44.1X1	T44.1X2	T44.1X3	T44.1X4	T44.1X5	T44.1X6
Methacycline	T36.4X1	T36.4X2	T36.4X3	T36.4X4	T36.4X5	T36.4X6
Methadone*	T40.3X1	T40.3X2	T40.3X3	T40.3X4	T40.3X5	T40.3X6
Methadose*	T40.3X1	T40.3X2	T40.3X3	T40.3X4	T40.3X5	T40.3X6
Methallenestril	T38.5X1	T38.5X2	T38.5X3	T38.5X4	T38.5X5	T38.5X6
Methallenoestril	T38.5X1	T38.5X2	T38.5X3	T38.5X4	T38.5X5	T38.5X6
Methamphetamine	T43.651	T43.652	T43.653	T43.654	T43.655	T43.656
Methampyrone	T39.2X1	T39.2X2	T39.2X3	T39.2X4	T39.2X5	T39.2X6
Methandienone	T38.7X1	T38.7X2	T38.7X3	T38.7X4	T38.7X5	T38.7X6
Methandriol	T38.7X1	T38.7X2	T38.7X3	T38.7X4	T38.7X5	T38.7X6
Methandrostenolone	T38.7X1	T38.7X2	T38.7X3	T38.7X4	T38.7X5	T38.7X6
Methane	T59.891	T59.892	T59.893	T59.894	—	—
Methanethiol	T59.891	T59.892	T59.893	T59.894	—	—
Methaniazide	T37.1X1	T37.1X2	T37.1X3	T37.1X4	T37.1X5	T37.1X6
Methanol (vapor)	T51.1X1	T51.1X2	T51.1X3	T51.1X4	—	—
Methantheline	T44.3X1	T44.3X2	T44.3X3	T44.3X4	T44.3X5	T44.3X6
Methanthelinium bromide	T44.3X1	T44.3X2	T44.3X3	T44.3X4	T44.3X5	T44.3X6
Methaphenilene	T45.0X1	T45.0X2	T45.0X3	T45.0X4	T45.0X5	T45.0X6
Methapyrilene	T45.0X1	T45.0X2	T45.0X3	T45.0X4	T45.0X5	T45.0X6
Methaqualone (compound)	T42.6X1	T42.6X2	T42.6X3	T42.6X4	T42.6X5	T42.6X6
Metharbital	T42.3X1	T42.3X2	T42.3X3	T42.3X4	T42.3X5	T42.3X6
Methazolamide	T50.2X1	T50.2X2	T50.2X3	T50.2X4	T50.2X5	T50.2X6
Methdilazine	T43.3X1	T43.3X2	T43.3X3	T43.3X4	T43.3X5	T43.3X6
Methedrine	T43.651	T43.652	T43.653	T43.654	T43.655	T43.656
Methenamine (mandelate)	T37.8X1	T37.8X2	T37.8X3	T37.8X4	T37.8X5	T37.8X6
Methenolone	T38.7X1	T38.7X2	T38.7X3	T38.7X4	T38.7X5	T38.7X6
Methergine	T48.0X1	T48.0X2	T48.0X3	T48.0X4	T48.0X5	T48.0X6
Methetoin	T42.0X1	T42.0X2	T42.0X3	T42.0X4	T42.0X5	T42.0X6
Methiacil	T38.2X1	T38.2X2	T38.2X3	T38.2X4	T38.2X5	T38.2X6
Methicillin	T36.0X1	T36.0X2	T36.0X3	T36.0X4	T36.0X5	T36.0X6
Methimazole	T38.2X1	T38.2X2	T38.2X3	T38.2X4	T38.2X5	T38.2X6
Methiodal sodium	T50.8X1	T50.8X2	T50.8X3	T50.8X4	T50.8X5	T50.8X6
Methionine	T50.991	T50.992	T50.993	T50.994	T50.995	T50.996
Methisazone	T37.5X1	T37.5X2	T37.5X3	T37.5X4	T37.5X5	T37.5X6
Methisoprinol	T37.5X1	T37.5X2	T37.5X3	T37.5X4	T37.5X5	T37.5X6
Methitural	T42.3X1	T42.3X2	T42.3X3	T42.3X4	T42.3X5	T42.3X6
Methixene	T44.3X1	T44.3X2	T44.3X3	T44.3X4	T44.3X5	T44.3X6
Methobarbital, methobarbitone	T42.3X1	T42.3X2	T42.3X3	T42.3X4	T42.3X5	T42.3X6
Methocarbamol	T42.8X1	T42.8X2	T42.8X3	T42.8X4	T42.8X5	T42.8X6
skeletal muscle relaxant	T48.1X1	T48.1X2	T48.1X3	T48.1X4	T48.1X5	T48.1X6
Methohexital	T41.1X1	T41.1X2	T41.1X3	T41.1X4	T41.1X5	T41.1X6
Methohexitone	T41.1X1	T41.1X2	T41.1X3	T41.1X4	T41.1X5	T41.1X6
Methoin	T42.0X1	T42.0X2	T42.0X3	T42.0X4	T42.0X5	T42.0X6
Methopholine	T39.8X1	T39.8X2	T39.8X3	T39.8X4	T39.8X5	T39.8X6
Methopromazine	T43.3X1	T43.3X2	T43.3X3	T43.3X4	T43.3X5	T43.3X6
Methorate	T48.3X1	T48.3X2	T48.3X3	T48.3X4	T48.3X5	T48.3X6
Methoserpidine	T46.5X1	T46.5X2	T46.5X3	T46.5X4	T46.5X5	T46.5X6
Methotrexate	T45.1X1	T45.1X2	T45.1X3	T45.1X4	T45.1X5	T45.1X6
Methotrimeprazine	T43.3X1	T43.3X2	T43.3X3	T43.3X4	T43.3X5	T43.3X6
Methoxa-Dome	T49.3X1	T49.3X2	T49.3X3	T49.3X4	T49.3X5	T49.3X6
Methoxamine	T44.4X1	T44.4X2	T44.4X3	T44.4X4	T44.4X5	T44.4X6
Methoxsalen	T50.991	T50.992	T50.993	T50.994	T50.995	T50.996
Methoxyaniline	T65.3X1	T65.3X2	T65.3X3	T65.3X4	—	—
Methoxybenzyl penicillin	T36.0X1	T36.0X2	T36.0X3	T36.0X4	T36.0X5	T36.0X6
Methoxychlor	T53.7X1	T53.7X2	T53.7X3	T53.7X4	—	—
Methoxy-DDT	T53.7X1	T53.7X2	T53.7X3	T53.7X4	—	—
Methoxyflurane	T41.0X1	T41.0X2	T41.0X3	T41.0X4	T41.0X5	T41.0X6
Methoxyphenamine	T48.6X1	T48.6X2	T48.6X3	T48.6X4	T48.6X5	T48.6X6
Methoxypromazine	T43.3X1	T43.3X2	T43.3X3	T43.3X4	T43.3X5	T43.3X6
Methscopolamine bromide	T44.3X1	T44.3X2	T44.3X3	T44.3X4	T44.3X5	T44.3X6
Methsuximide	T42.2X1	T42.2X2	T42.2X3	T42.2X4	T42.2X5	T42.2X6
Methyclothiazide	T50.2X1	T50.2X2	T50.2X3	T50.2X4	T50.2X5	T50.2X6
Methyl						
acetate	T52.4X1	T52.4X2	T52.4X3	T52.4X4	—	—
acetone	T52.4X1	T52.4X2	T52.4X3	T52.4X4	—	—
acrylate	T65.891	T65.892	T65.893	T65.894	—	—
alcohol	T51.1X1	T51.1X2	T51.1X3	T51.1X4	—	—
aminophenol	T65.3X1	T65.3X2	T65.3X3	T65.3X4	—	—
amphetamine	T43.651	T43.652	T43.653	T43.654	T43.655	T43.656
androstanolone	T38.7X1	T38.7X2	T38.7X3	T38.7X4	T38.7X5	T38.7X6
atropine	T44.3X1	T44.3X2	T44.3X3	T44.3X4	T44.3X5	T44.3X6
benzene	T52.2X1	T52.2X2	T52.2X3	T52.2X4	—	—
benzoate	T52.8X1	T52.8X2	T52.8X3	T52.8X4	—	—
benzol	T52.2X1	T52.2X2	T52.2X3	T52.2X4	—	—
bromide (gas)	T59.891	T59.892	T59.893	T59.894	—	—
fumigant	T60.8X1	T60.8X2	T60.8X3	T60.8X4	—	—
butanol	T51.3X1	T51.3X2	T51.3X3	T51.3X4	—	—
carbinol	T51.1X1	T51.1X2	T51.1X3	T51.1X4	—	—
carbonate	T52.8X1	T52.8X2	T52.8X3	T52.8X4	—	—
CCNU	T45.1X1	T45.1X2	T45.1X3	T45.1X4	T45.1X5	T45.1X6
Methyl — *continued*						
cellosolve	T52.91	T52.92	T52.93	T52.94	—	—
cellulose	T47.4X1	T47.4X2	T47.4X3	T47.4X4	T47.4X5	T47.4X6
chloride (gas)	T59.891	T59.892	T59.893	T59.894	—	—
chloroformate	T59.3X1	T59.3X2	T59.3X3	T59.3X4	—	—
cyclohexane	T52.8X1	T52.8X2	T52.8X3	T52.8X4	—	—
cyclohexanol	T51.8X1	T51.8X2	T51.8X3	T51.8X4	—	—
cyclohexanone	T52.8X1	T52.8X2	T52.8X3	T52.8X4	—	—
cyclohexyl acetate	T52.8X1	T52.8X2	T52.8X3	T52.8X4	—	—
demeton	T60.0X1	T60.0X2	T60.0X3	T60.0X4	—	—
dihydromorphinone	T40.2X1	T40.2X2	T40.2X3	T40.2X4	T40.2X5	T40.2X6
ergometrine	T48.0X1	T48.0X2	T48.0X3	T48.0X4	T48.0X5	T48.0X6
ergonovine	T48.0X1	T48.0X2	T48.0X3	T48.0X4	T48.0X5	T48.0X6
ethyl ketone	T52.4X1	T52.4X2	T52.4X3	T52.4X4	—	—
glucamine antimonate	T37.8X1	T37.8X2	T37.8X3	T37.8X4	T37.8X5	T37.8X6
hydrazine	T65.891	T65.892	T65.893	T65.894	—	—
iodide	T65.891	T65.892	T65.893	T65.894	—	—
isobutyl ketone	T52.4X1	T52.4X2	T52.4X3	T52.4X4	—	—
isothiocyanate	T60.3X1	T60.3X2	T60.3X3	T60.3X4	—	—
mercaptan	T59.891	T59.892	T59.893	T59.894	—	—
morphine NEC	T40.2X1	T40.2X2	T40.2X3	T40.2X4	T40.2X5	T40.2X6
nicotinate	T49.4X1	T49.4X2	T49.4X3	T49.4X4	T49.4X5	T49.4X6
paraben	T49.0X1	T49.0X2	T49.0X3	T49.0X4	T49.0X5	T49.0X6
parafynol	T42.6X1	T42.6X2	T42.6X3	T42.6X4	T42.6X5	T42.6X6
parathion	T60.0X1	T60.0X2	T60.0X3	T60.0X4	—	—
peridol	T43.4X1	T43.4X2	T43.4X3	T43.4X4	T43.4X5	T43.4X6
phenidate	T43.631	T43.632	T43.633	T43.634	T43.635	T43.636
prednisolone	T38.0X1	T38.0X2	T38.0X3	T38.0X4	T38.0X5	T38.0X6
ENT agent	T49.6X1	T49.6X2	T49.6X3	T49.6X4	T49.6X5	T49.6X6
ophthalmic preparation	T49.5X1	T49.5X2	T49.5X3	T49.5X4	T49.5X5	T49.5X6
topical NEC	T49.0X1	T49.0X2	T49.0X3	T49.0X4	T49.0X5	T49.0X6
propylcarbinol	T51.3X1	T51.3X2	T51.3X3	T51.3X4	—	—
rosaniline NEC	T49.0X1	T49.0X2	T49.0X3	T49.0X4	T49.0X5	T49.0X6
salicylate	T49.2X1	T49.2X2	T49.2X3	T49.2X4	T49.2X5	T49.2X6
sulfate (fumes)	T59.891	T59.892	T59.893	T59.894	—	—
liquid	T52.8X1	T52.8X2	T52.8X3	T52.8X4	—	—
sulfonal	T42.6X1	T42.6X2	T42.6X3	T42.6X4	T42.6X5	T42.6X6
testosterone	T38.7X1	T38.7X2	T38.7X3	T38.7X4	T38.7X5	T38.7X6
thiouracil	T38.2X1	T38.2X2	T38.2X3	T38.2X4	T38.2X5	T38.2X6
Methylacetoxyprogesterone*	T38.5X1	T38.5X2	T38.5X3	T38.5X4	T38.5X5	T38.5X6
Methylamphetamine	T43.651	T43.652	T43.653	T43.654	T43.655	T43.656
Methylated spirit	T51.1X1	T51.1X2	T51.1X3	T51.1X4	—	—
Methylatropine nitrate	T44.3X1	T44.3X2	T44.3X3	T44.3X4	T44.3X5	T44.3X6
Methylbenactyzium bromide	T44.3X1	T44.3X2	T44.3X3	T44.3X4	T44.3X5	T44.3X6
Methylbenzethonium chloride	T49.0X1	T49.0X2	T49.0X3	T49.0X4	T49.0X5	T49.0X6
Methylcellulose	T47.4X1	T47.4X2	T47.4X3	T47.4X4	T47.4X5	T47.4X6
laxative	T47.4X1	T47.4X2	T47.4X3	T47.4X4	T47.4X5	T47.4X6
Methylchlorophenoxyacetic acid	T60.3X1	T60.3X2	T60.3X3	T60.3X4	—	—
Methyldopa	T46.5X1	T46.5X2	T46.5X3	T46.5X4	T46.5X5	T46.5X6
Methyldopate	T46.5X1	T46.5X2	T46.5X3	T46.5X4	T46.5X5	T46.5X6
Methylene						
blue	T50.6X1	T50.6X2	T50.6X3	T50.6X4	T50.6X5	T50.6X6
chloride or dichloride (solvent) NEC	T53.4X1	T53.4X2	T53.4X3	T53.4X4	—	—
Methylenedioxyamphetamine	T43.621	T43.622	T43.623	T43.624	T43.625	T43.626
Methylenedioxymeth-amphetamine	T43.641	T43.642	T43.643	T43.644	—	—
Methylergometrine	T48.0X1	T48.0X2	T48.0X3	T48.0X4	T48.0X5	T48.0X6
Methylergonovine	T48.0X1	T48.0X2	T48.0X3	T48.0X4	T48.0X5	T48.0X6
Methylestrenolone	T38.5X1	T38.5X2	T38.5X3	T38.5X4	T38.5X5	T38.5X6
Methylethyl cellulose	T50.991	T50.992	T50.993	T50.994	T50.995	T50.996
Methylhexabital	T42.3X1	T42.3X2	T42.3X3	T42.3X4	T42.3X5	T42.3X6
Methylmorphine	T40.2X1	T40.2X2	T40.2X3	T40.2X4	T40.2X5	T40.2X6
Methylparaben (ophthalmic)	T49.5X1	T49.5X2	T49.5X3	T49.5X4	T49.5X5	T49.5X6
Methylparafynol	T42.6X1	T42.6X2	T42.6X3	T42.6X4	T42.6X5	T42.6X6
Methylpentynol, methylpenthynol	T42.6X1	T42.6X2	T42.6X3	T42.6X4	T42.6X5	T42.6X6
Methylphenidate	T43.631	T43.632	T43.633	T43.634	T43.635	T43.636
Methylphenobarbital	T42.3X1	T42.3X2	T42.3X3	T42.3X4	T42.3X5	T42.3X6
Methylpolysiloxane	T47.1X1	T47.1X2	T47.1X3	T47.1X4	T47.1X5	T47.1X6
Methylprednisolone — *see* Methyl, prednisolone						
Methylrosaniline	T49.0X1	T49.0X2	T49.0X3	T49.0X4	T49.0X5	T49.0X6
Methylrosanilinium chloride	T49.0X1	T49.0X2	T49.0X3	T49.0X4	T49.0X5	T49.0X6
Methyltestosterone	T38.7X1	T38.7X2	T38.7X3	T38.7X4	T38.7X5	T38.7X6
Methylthionine chloride	T50.6X1	T50.6X2	T50.6X3	T50.6X4	T50.6X5	T50.6X6
Methylthioninium chloride	T50.6X1	T50.6X2	T50.6X3	T50.6X4	T50.6X5	T50.6X6

Substance	Poisoning, Accidental (unintentional)	Poisoning, Intentional Self-harm	Poisoning, Assault	Poisoning, Undetermined	Adverse Effect	Under-dosing
Methylthiouracil	T38.2X1	T38.2X2	T38.2X3	T38.2X4	T38.2X5	T38.2X6
Methyprylon	T42.6X1	T42.6X2	T42.6X3	T42.6X4	T42.6X5	T42.6X6
Methysergide	T46.5X1	T46.5X2	T46.5X3	T46.5X4	T46.5X5	T46.5X6
Metiamide	T47.1X1	T47.1X2	T47.1X3	T47.1X4	T47.1X5	T47.1X6
Meticillin	T36.0X1	T36.0X2	T36.0X3	T36.0X4	T36.0X5	T36.0X6
Meticrane	T50.2X1	T50.2X2	T50.2X3	T50.2X4	T50.2X5	T50.2X6
Metildigoxin	T46.0X1	T46.0X2	T46.0X3	T46.0X4	T46.0X5	T46.0X6
Metipranolol	T49.5X1	T49.5X2	T49.5X3	T49.5X4	T49.5X5	T49.5X6
Metirosine	T46.5X1	T46.5X2	T46.5X3	T46.5X4	T46.5X5	T46.5X6
Metisazone	T37.5X1	T37.5X2	T37.5X3	T37.5X4	T37.5X5	T37.5X6
Metixene	T44.3X1	T44.3X2	T44.3X3	T44.3X4	T44.3X5	T44.3X6
Metizoline	T48.5X1	T48.5X2	T48.5X3	T48.5X4	T48.5X5	T48.5X6
Metoclopramide	T45.0X1	T45.0X2	T45.0X3	T45.0X4	T45.0X5	T45.0X6
Metofenazate	T43.3X1	T43.3X2	T43.3X3	T43.3X4	T43.3X5	T43.3X6
Metofoline	T39.8X1	T39.8X2	T39.8X3	T39.8X4	T39.8X5	T39.8X6
Metolazone	T50.2X1	T50.2X2	T50.2X3	T50.2X4	T50.2X5	T50.2X6
Metopon	T40.2X1	T40.2X2	T40.2X3	T40.2X4	T40.2X5	T40.2X6
Metoprine	T45.1X1	T45.1X2	T45.1X3	T45.1X4	T45.1X5	T45.1X6
Metoprolol	T44.7X1	T44.7X2	T44.7X3	T44.7X4	T44.7X5	T44.7X6
Metrifonate	T60.0X1	T60.0X2	T60.0X3	T60.0X4	—	—
Metrizamide	T50.8X1	T50.8X2	T50.8X3	T50.8X4	T50.8X5	T50.8X6
Metrizoic acid	T50.8X1	T50.8X2	T50.8X3	T50.8X4	T50.8X5	T50.8X6
MetroGel*	T49.0X1	T49.0X2	T49.0X3	T49.0X4	T49.0X5	T49.0X6
Metronidazole	T37.8X1	T37.8X2	T37.8X3	T37.8X4	T37.8X5	T37.8X6
Metycaine	T41.3X1	T41.3X2	T41.3X3	T41.3X4	T41.3X5	T41.3X6
infiltration (subcutaneous)	T41.3X1	T41.3X2	T41.3X3	T41.3X4	T41.3X5	T41.3X6
nerve block (peripheral) (plexus)	T41.3X1	T41.3X2	T41.3X3	T41.3X4	T41.3X5	T41.3X6
topical (surface)	T41.3X1	T41.3X2	T41.3X3	T41.3X4	T41.3X5	T41.3X6
Metyrapone	T50.8X1	T50.8X2	T50.8X3	T50.8X4	T50.8X5	T50.8X6
Mevacor*	T46.6X1	T46.6X2	T46.6X3	T46.6X4	T46.6X5	T46.6X6
Mevinphos	T60.0X1	T60.0X2	T60.0X3	T60.0X4	—	—
Mexazolam	T42.4X1	T42.4X2	T42.4X3	T42.4X4	T42.4X5	T42.4X6
Mexenone	T49.3X1	T49.3X2	T49.3X3	T49.3X4	T49.3X5	T49.3X6
Mexiletine	T46.2X1	T46.2X2	T46.2X3	T46.2X4	T46.2X5	T46.2X6
Mezereon	T62.2X1	T62.2X2	T62.2X3	T62.2X4	—	—
berries	T62.1X1	T62.1X2	T62.1X3	T62.1X4	—	—
Mezlocillin	T36.0X1	T36.0X2	T36.0X3	T36.0X4	T36.0X5	T36.0X6
Mianserin	T43.021	T43.022	T43.023	T43.024	T43.025	T43.026
Micatin	T49.0X1	T49.0X2	T49.0X3	T49.0X4	T49.0X5	T49.0X6
Miconazole	T49.0X1	T49.0X2	T49.0X3	T49.0X4	T49.0X5	T49.0X6
Micronomicin	T36.5X1	T36.5X2	T36.5X3	T36.5X4	T36.5X5	T36.5X6
Microzide*	T50.2X1	T50.2X2	T50.2X3	T50.2X4	T50.2X5	T50.2X6
Midazolam	T42.4X1	T42.4X2	T42.4X3	T42.4X4	T42.4X5	T42.4X6
Midecamycin	T36.3X1	T36.3X2	T36.3X3	T36.3X4	T36.3X5	T36.3X6
Mifepristone	T38.6X1	T38.6X2	T38.6X3	T38.6X4	T38.6X5	T38.6X6
Milk of magnesia	T47.1X1	T47.1X2	T47.1X3	T47.1X4	T47.1X5	T47.1X6
Millipede (tropical) (venomous)	T63.411	T63.412	T63.413	T63.414	—	—
Miltown	T43.591	T43.592	T43.593	T43.594	T43.595	T43.596
Milverine	T44.3X1	T44.3X2	T44.3X3	T44.3X4	T44.3X5	T44.3X6
Minaprine	T43.291	T43.292	T43.293	T43.294	T43.295	T43.296
Minaxolone	T41.291	T41.292	T41.293	T41.294	T41.295	T41.296
Mineral						
acids	T54.2X1	T54.2X2	T54.2X3	T54.2X4	—	—
oil (laxative)(medicinal)	T47.4X1	T47.4X2	T47.4X3	T47.4X4	T47.4X5	T47.4X6
emulsion	T47.2X1	T47.2X2	T47.2X3	T47.2X4	T47.2X5	T47.2X6
nonmedicinal	T52.0X1	T52.0X2	T52.0X3	T52.0X4	—	—
topical	T49.3X1	T49.3X2	T49.3X3	T49.3X4	T49.3X5	T49.3X6
salt NEC	T50.3X1	T50.3X2	T50.3X3	T50.3X4	T50.3X5	T50.3X6
spirits	T52.0X1	T52.0X2	T52.0X3	T52.0X4	—	—
Mineralocorticosteroid	T50.0X1	T50.0X2	T50.0X3	T50.0X4	T50.0X5	T50.0X6
Minocycline	T36.4X1	T36.4X2	T36.4X3	T36.4X4	T36.4X5	T36.4X6
Minoxidil	T46.7X1	T46.7X2	T46.7X3	T46.7X4	T46.7X5	T46.7X6
Miokamycin	T36.3X1	T36.3X2	T36.3X3	T36.3X4	T36.3X5	T36.3X6
Miotic drug	T49.5X1	T49.5X2	T49.5X3	T49.5X4	T49.5X5	T49.5X6
Mipafox	T60.0X1	T60.0X2	T60.0X3	T60.0X4	—	—
Mipomerson*	T46.6X1	T46.6X2	T46.6X3	T46.6X4	T46.6X5	T46.6X6
Mirex	T60.1X1	T60.1X2	T60.1X3	T60.1X4	—	—
Mirtazapine	T43.021	T43.022	T43.023	T43.024	T43.025	T43.026
Misonidazole	T37.3X1	T37.3X2	T37.3X3	T37.3X4	T37.3X5	T37.3X6
Misoprostol	T47.1X1	T47.1X2	T47.1X3	T47.1X4	T47.1X5	T47.1X6
Mithramycin	T45.1X1	T45.1X2	T45.1X3	T45.1X4	T45.1X5	T45.1X6
Mitobronitol	T45.1X1	T45.1X2	T45.1X3	T45.1X4	T45.1X5	T45.1X6
Mitoguazone	T45.1X1	T45.1X2	T45.1X3	T45.1X4	T45.1X5	T45.1X6
Mitolactol	T45.1X1	T45.1X2	T45.1X3	T45.1X4	T45.1X5	T45.1X6
Mitomycin	T45.1X1	T45.1X2	T45.1X3	T45.1X4	T45.1X5	T45.1X6
Mitopodozide	T45.1X1	T45.1X2	T45.1X3	T45.1X4	T45.1X5	T45.1X6
Mitotane	T45.1X1	T45.1X2	T45.1X3	T45.1X4	T45.1X5	T45.1X6
Mitoxantrone	T45.1X1	T45.1X2	T45.1X3	T45.1X4	T45.1X5	T45.1X6
Mivacurium chloride	T48.1X1	T48.1X2	T48.1X3	T48.1X4	T48.1X5	T48.1X6
Miyari bacteria	T47.6X1	T47.6X2	T47.6X3	T47.6X4	T47.6X5	T47.6X6
Mobic*	T39.391	T39.392	T39.393	T39.394	T39.395	T39.396

Substance	Poisoning, Accidental (unintentional)	Poisoning, Intentional Self-harm	Poisoning, Assault	Poisoning, Undetermined	Adverse Effect	Under-dosing
Moclobemide	T43.1X1	T43.1X2	T43.1X3	T43.1X4	T43.1X5	T43.1X6
Moderil	T46.5X1	T46.5X2	T46.5X3	T46.5X4	T46.5X5	T46.5X6
Mofebutazone	T39.2X1	T39.2X2	T39.2X3	T39.2X4	T39.2X5	T39.2X6
Mogadon — see Nitrazepam						
Molindone	T43.591	T43.592	T43.593	T43.594	T43.595	T43.596
Molsidomine	T46.3X1	T46.3X2	T46.3X3	T46.3X4	T46.3X5	T46.3X6
Mometasone	T49.0X1	T49.0X2	T49.0X3	T49.0X4	T49.0X5	T49.0X6
Monistat	T49.0X1	T49.0X2	T49.0X3	T49.0X4	T49.0X5	T49.0X6
Monkshood	T62.2X1	T62.2X2	T62.2X3	T62.2X4	—	—
Monoamine oxidase inhibitor NEC	T43.1X1	T43.1X2	T43.1X3	T43.1X4	T43.1X5	T43.1X6
hydrazine	T43.1X1	T43.1X2	T43.1X3	T43.1X4	T43.1X5	T43.1X6
Monobenzone	T49.4X1	T49.4X2	T49.4X3	T49.4X4	T49.4X5	T49.4X6
Monochloroacetic acid	T60.3X1	T60.3X2	T60.3X3	T60.3X4	—	—
Monochlorobenzene	T53.7X1	T53.7X2	T53.7X3	T53.7X4	—	—
Monoethanolamine	T46.8X1	T46.8X2	T46.8X3	T46.8X4	T46.8X5	T46.8X6
oleate	T46.8X1	T46.8X2	T46.8X3	T46.8X4	T46.8X5	T46.8X6
Monooctanoin	T50.991	T50.992	T50.993	T50.994	T50.995	T50.996
Monophenylbutazone	T39.2X1	T39.2X2	T39.2X3	T39.2X4	T39.2X5	T39.2X6
Monopril*	T46.4X1	T46.4X2	T46.4X3	T46.4X4	T46.4X5	T46.4X6
Monosodium glutamate	T65.891	T65.892	T65.893	T65.894	—	—
Monosulfiram	T49.0X1	T49.0X2	T49.0X3	T49.0X4	T49.0X5	T49.0X6
Monoxide, carbon — see Carbon, monoxide						
Monoxidine hydrochloride	T46.1X1	T46.1X2	T46.1X3	T46.1X4	T46.1X5	T46.1X6
Montelukast*	T48.6X1	T48.6X2	T48.6X3	T48.6X4	T48.6X5	T48.6X6
Monuron	T60.3X1	T60.3X2	T60.3X3	T60.3X4	—	—
Moperone	T43.4X1	T43.4X2	T43.4X3	T43.4X4	T43.4X5	T43.4X6
Mopidamol	T45.1X1	T45.1X2	T45.1X3	T45.1X4	T45.1X5	T45.1X6
MOPP (mechloreth-amine + vincristine + prednisone + procarba-zine)	T45.1X1	T45.1X2	T45.1X3	T45.1X4	T45.1X5	T45.1X6
Morfin	T40.2X1	T40.2X2	T40.2X3	T40.2X4	T40.2X5	T40.2X6
Morinamide	T37.1X1	T37.1X2	T37.1X3	T37.1X4	T37.1X5	T37.1X6
Morning glory seeds	T40.991	T40.992	T40.993	T40.994		
Moroxydine	T37.5X1	T37.5X2	T37.5X3	T37.5X4	T37.5X5	T37.5X6
Morphazinamide	T37.1X1	T37.1X2	T37.1X3	T37.1X4	T37.1X5	T37.1X6
Morphine	T40.2X1	T40.2X2	T40.2X3	T40.2X4	T40.2X5	T40.2X6
antagonist	T50.7X1	T50.7X2	T50.7X3	T50.7X4	T50.7X5	T50.7X6
Morpholinylethylmorphine	T40.2X1	T40.2X2	T40.2X3	T40.2X4	T40.2X5	T40.2X6
Morsuximide	T42.2X1	T42.2X2	T42.2X3	T42.2X4	T42.2X5	T42.2X6
Mosapramine	T43.591	T43.592	T43.593	T43.594	T43.595	T43.596
Moth balls — see also Pesticide	T60.2X1	T60.2X2	T60.2X3	T60.2X4	—	—
naphthalene	T60.2X1	T60.2X2	T60.2X3	T60.2X4	—	—
paradichlorobenzene	T60.1X1	T60.1X2	T60.1X3	T60.1X4	—	—
Motor exhaust gas	T58.01	T58.02	T58.03	T58.04	—	—
Motrin*	T39.311	T39.312	T39.313	T39.314	T39.315	T39.316
Mouthwash (antiseptic) (zinc chloride)	T49.6X1	T49.6X2	T49.6X3	T49.6X4	T49.6X5	T49.6X6
Moxastine	T45.0X1	T45.0X2	T45.0X3	T45.0X4	T45.0X5	T45.0X6
Moxaverine	T44.3X1	T44.3X2	T44.3X3	T44.3X4	T44.3X5	T44.3X6
Moxisylyte	T46.7X1	T46.7X2	T46.7X3	T46.7X4	T46.7X5	T46.7X6
Mucilage, plant	T47.4X1	T47.4X2	T47.4X3	T47.4X4	T47.4X5	T47.4X6
Mucolytic drug	T48.4X1	T48.4X2	T48.4X3	T48.4X4	T48.4X5	T48.4X6
Mucomyst	T48.4X1	T48.4X2	T48.4X3	T48.4X4	T48.4X5	T48.4X6
Mucous membrane agents (external)	T49.91	T49.92	T49.93	T49.94	T49.95	T49.96
specified NEC	T49.8X1	T49.8X2	T49.8X3	T49.8X4	T49.8X5	T49.8X6
Multaq*	T46.2X1	T46.2X2	T46.2X3	T46.2X4	T46.2X5	T46.2X6
Multiple unspecified drugs, medicaments and biological substances	T50.911	T50.912	T50.913	T50.914	T50.915	T50.916
Mumps						
immune globulin (human)	T50.Z11	T50.Z12	T50.Z13	T50.Z14	T50.Z15	T50.Z16
skin test antigen	T50.8X1	T50.8X2	T50.8X3	T50.8X4	T50.8X5	T50.8X6
vaccine	T50.B91	T50.B92	T50.B93	T50.B94	T50.B95	T50.B96
Mumpsvax	T50.B91	T50.B92	T50.B93	T50.B94	T50.B95	T50.B96
Mupirocin	T49.0X1	T49.0X2	T49.0X3	T49.0X4	T49.0X5	T49.0X6
Muriatic acid — see Hydrochloric acid						
Muromonab-CD3	T45.1X1	T45.1X2	T45.1X3	T45.1X4	T45.1X5	T45.1X6
Muscle-action drug NEC	T48.201	T48.202	T48.203	T48.204	T48.205	T48.206
Muscle affecting agents NEC	T48.201	T48.202	T48.203	T48.204	T48.205	T48.206
oxytocic	T48.0X1	T48.0X2	T48.0X3	T48.0X4	T48.0X5	T48.0X6
relaxants	T48.201	T48.202	T48.203	T48.204	T48.205	T48.206
central nervous system	T42.8X1	T42.8X2	T42.8X3	T42.8X4	T42.8X5	T42.8X6
skeletal	T48.1X1	T48.1X2	T48.1X3	T48.1X4	T48.1X5	T48.1X6
smooth	T44.3X1	T44.3X2	T44.3X3	T44.3X4	T44.3X5	T44.3X6
Muscle relaxant — see Relaxant, muscle						

Table of Drugs and Chemicals

Muscle-tone depressant, central NEC — Nilstat

Substance	Poisoning, Accidental (unintentional)	Poisoning, Intentional Self-harm	Poisoning, Assault	Poisoning, Undetermined	Adverse Effect	Under-dosing
Muscle-tone depressant, central NEC	T42.8X1	T42.8X2	T42.8X3	T42.8X4	T42.8X5	T42.8X6
specified NEC	T42.8X1	T42.8X2	T42.8X3	T42.8X4	T42.8X5	T42.8X6
Mushroom, noxious	T62.0X1	T62.0X2	T62.0X3	T62.0X4	—	—
Mussel, noxious	T61.781	T61.782	T61.783	T61.784	—	—
Mustard (emetic)	T47.7X1	T47.7X2	T47.7X3	T47.7X4	T47.7X5	T47.7X6
black	T47.7X1	T47.7X2	T47.7X3	T47.7X4	T47.7X5	T47.7X6
gas, not in war	T59.91	T59.92	T59.93	T59.94		
nitrogen	T45.1X1	T45.1X2	T45.1X3	T45.1X4	T45.1X5	T45.1X6
Mustine	T45.1X1	T45.1X2	T45.1X3	T45.1X4	T45.1X5	T45.1X6
M-vac	T45.1X1	T45.1X2	T45.1X3	T45.1X4	T45.1X5	T45.1X6
Mycifradin	T36.5X1	T36.5X2	T36.5X3	T36.5X4	T36.5X5	T36.5X6
topical	T49.0X1	T49.0X2	T49.0X3	T49.0X4	T49.0X5	T49.0X6
Mycitracin	T36.8X1	T36.8X2	T36.8X3	T36.8X4	T36.8X5	T36.8X6
ophthalmic preparation	T49.5X1	T49.5X2	T49.5X3	T49.5X4	T49.5X5	T49.5X6
Mycostatin	T36.7X1	T36.7X2	T36.7X3	T36.7X4	T36.7X5	T36.7X6
topical	T49.0X1	T49.0X2	T49.0X3	T49.0X4	T49.0X5	T49.0X6
Mycotoxins	T64.81	T64.82	T64.83	T64.84	—	—
aflatoxin	T64.01	T64.02	T64.03	T64.04	—	—
specified NEC	T64.81	T64.82	T64.83	T64.84	—	—
Mydriacyl	T44.3X1	T44.3X2	T44.3X3	T44.3X4	T44.3X5	T44.3X6
Mydriatic drug	T49.5X1	T49.5X2	T49.5X3	T49.5X4	T49.5X5	T49.5X6
Myelobromal	T45.1X1	T45.1X2	T45.1X3	T45.1X4	T45.1X5	T45.1X6
Myleran	T45.1X1	T45.1X2	T45.1X3	T45.1X4	T45.1X5	T45.1X6
Myochrysin (e)	T39.2X1	T39.2X2	T39.2X3	T39.2X4	T39.2X5	T39.2X6
Myoneural blocking agents	T48.1X1	T48.1X2	T48.1X3	T48.1X4	T48.1X5	T48.1X6
Myrac*	T36.4X1	T36.4X2	T36.4X3	T36.4X4	T36.4X5	T36.4X6
Myralact	T49.0X1	T49.0X2	T49.0X3	T49.0X4	T49.0X5	T49.0X6
Myristica fragrans	T62.2X1	T62.2X2	T62.2X3	T62.2X4	—	—
Myristicin	T65.891	T65.892	T65.893	T65.894	—	—
Mysoline	T42.3X1	T42.3X2	T42.3X3	T42.3X4	T42.3X5	T42.3X6
Nabilone	T40.711	T40.712	T40.713	T40.714	T40.715	T40.716
Nabumetone	T39.391	T39.392	T39.393	T39.394	T39.395	T39.396
Nadolol	T44.7X1	T44.7X2	T44.7X3	T44.7X4	T44.7X5	T44.7X6
Nafcillin	T36.0X1	T36.0X2	T36.0X3	T36.0X4	T36.0X5	T36.0X6
Nafoxidine	T38.6X1	T38.6X2	T38.6X3	T38.6X4	T38.6X5	T38.6X6
Naftazone	T46.991	T46.992	T46.993	T46.994	T46.995	T46.996
Naftidrofuryl (oxalate)	T46.7X1	T46.7X2	T46.7X3	T46.7X4	T46.7X5	T46.7X6
Naftifine	T49.0X1	T49.0X2	T49.0X3	T49.0X4	T49.0X5	T49.0X6
Nail polish remover	T52.91	T52.92	T52.93	T52.94	—	—
Nalbuphine	T40.491	T40.492	T40.493	T40.494	T40.495	T40.496
Naled	T60.0X1	T60.0X2	T60.0X3	T60.0X4	—	—
Nalidixic acid	T37.8X1	T37.8X2	T37.8X3	T37.8X4	T37.8X5	T37.8X6
Nalorphine	T50.7X1	T50.7X2	T50.7X3	T50.7X4	T50.7X5	T50.7X6
Naloxone	T50.7X1	T50.7X2	T50.7X3	T50.7X4	T50.7X5	T50.7X6
Naltrexone	T50.7X1	T50.7X2	T50.7X3	T50.7X4	T50.7X5	T50.7X6
Namenda	T43.8X1	T43.8X2	T43.8X3	T43.8X4	T43.8X5	T43.8X6
Nandrolone	T38.7X1	T38.7X2	T38.7X3	T38.7X4	T38.7X5	T38.7X6
Naphazoline	T48.5X1	T48.5X2	T48.5X3	T48.5X4	T48.5X5	T48.5X6
Naphtha (painters') (petroleum)	T52.0X1	T52.0X2	T52.0X3	T52.0X4		
solvent	T52.0X1	T52.0X2	T52.0X3	T52.0X4		
vapor	T52.0X1	T52.0X2	T52.0X3	T52.0X4		
Naphthalene (non-chlorinated)	T60.2X1	T60.2X2	T60.2X3	T60.2X4	—	—
chlorinated	T60.1X1	T60.1X2	T60.1X3	T60.1X4	—	—
vapor	T60.1X1	T60.1X2	T60.1X3	T60.1X4	—	—
insecticide or moth repellent	T60.2X1	T60.2X2	T60.2X3	T60.2X4	—	—
chlorinated	T60.1X1	T60.1X2	T60.1X3	T60.1X4	—	—
vapor	T60.2X1	T60.2X2	T60.2X3	T60.2X4	—	—
chlorinated	T60.1X1	T60.1X2	T60.1X3	T60.1X4	—	—
Naphthol	T65.891	T65.892	T65.893	T65.894	—	—
Naphthylamine	T65.891	T65.892	T65.893	T65.894	—	—
Naphthylthiourea (ANTU)	T60.4X1	T60.4X2	T60.4X3	T60.4X4	—	—
Naprosyn — see Naproxen						
Naproxen	T39.311	T39.312	T39.313	T39.314	T39.315	T39.316
Narcotic (drug)	T40.601	T40.602	T40.603	T40.604	T40.605	T40.606
analgesic NEC	T40.601	T40.602	T40.603	T40.604	T40.605	T40.606
antagonist	T50.7X1	T50.7X2	T50.7X3	T50.7X4	T50.7X5	T50.7X6
specified NEC	T40.691	T40.692	T40.693	T40.694	T40.695	T40.696
synthetic	T40.491	T40.492	T40.493	T40.494	T40.495	T40.496
Narcotine	T48.3X1	T48.3X2	T48.3X3	T48.3X4	T48.3X5	T48.3X6
Nardil	T43.1X1	T43.1X2	T43.1X3	T43.1X4	T43.1X5	T43.1X6
Nasacort*	T49.5X1	T49.5X2	T49.5X3	T49.5X4	T49.5X5	T49.5X6
Nasal drug NEC	T49.6X1	T49.6X2	T49.6X3	T49.6X4	T49.6X5	T49.6X6
Natamycin	T49.0X1	T49.0X2	T49.0X3	T49.0X4	T49.0X5	T49.0X6
Natrium cyanide — see Cyanide(s)						
Natural						
blood (product)	T45.8X1	T45.8X2	T45.8X3	T45.8X4	T45.8X5	T45.8X6
gas (piped)	T59.891	T59.892	T59.893	T59.894	—	—

Substance	Poisoning, Accidental (unintentional)	Poisoning, Intentional Self-harm	Poisoning, Assault	Poisoning, Undetermined	Adverse Effect	Under-dosing
Natural — continued						
gas — continued						
incomplete combustion	T58.11	T58.12	T58.13	T58.14	—	—
Nealbarbital	T42.3X1	T42.3X2	T42.3X3	T42.3X4	T42.3X5	T42.3X6
Nectadon	T48.3X1	T48.3X2	T48.3X3	T48.3X4	T48.3X5	T48.3X6
Nedocromil	T48.6X1	T48.6X2	T48.6X3	T48.6X4	T48.6X5	T48.6X6
Nefopam	T39.8X1	T39.8X2	T39.8X3	T39.8X4	T39.8X5	T39.8X6
Nematocyst (sting)	T63.691	T63.692	T63.693	T63.694	—	—
Nembutal	T42.3X1	T42.3X2	T42.3X3	T42.3X4	T42.3X5	T42.3X6
Nemonapride	T43.591	T43.592	T43.593	T43.594	T43.595	T43.596
Neoarsphenamine	T37.8X1	T37.8X2	T37.8X3	T37.8X4	T37.8X5	T37.8X6
Neocinchophen	T50.4X1	T50.4X2	T50.4X3	T50.4X4	T50.4X5	T50.4X6
Neomycin (derivatives)	T36.5X1	T36.5X2	T36.5X3	T36.5X4	T36.5X5	T36.5X6
with						
bacitracin	T49.0X1	T49.0X2	T49.0X3	T49.0X4	T49.0X5	T49.0X6
neostigmine	T44.0X1	T44.0X2	T44.0X3	T44.0X4	T44.0X5	T44.0X6
ENT agent	T49.6X1	T49.6X2	T49.6X3	T49.6X4	T49.6X5	T49.6X6
ophthalmic preparation	T49.5X1	T49.5X2	T49.5X3	T49.5X4	T49.5X5	T49.5X6
topical NEC	T49.0X1	T49.0X2	T49.0X3	T49.0X4	T49.0X5	T49.0X6
Neonal	T42.3X1	T42.3X2	T42.3X3	T42.3X4	T42.3X5	T42.3X6
Neopham*	T50.3X1	T50.3X2	T50.3X3	T50.3X4	T50.3X5	T50.3X6
Neoprontosil	T37.0X1	T37.0X2	T37.0X3	T37.0X4	T37.0X5	T37.0X6
Neosalvarsan	T37.8X1	T37.8X2	T37.8X3	T37.8X4	T37.8X5	T37.8X6
Neosilversalvarsan	T37.8X1	T37.8X2	T37.8X3	T37.8X4	T37.8X5	T37.8X6
Neosporin	T36.8X1	T36.8X2	T36.8X3	T36.8X4	T36.8X5	T36.8X6
ENT agent	T49.6X1	T49.6X2	T49.6X3	T49.6X4	T49.6X5	T49.6X6
ophthalmic preparation	T49.5X1	T49.5X2	T49.5X3	T49.5X4	T49.5X5	T49.5X6
topical NEC	T49.0X1	T49.0X2	T49.0X3	T49.0X4	T49.0X5	T49.0X6
Neostigmine bromide	T44.0X1	T44.0X2	T44.0X3	T44.0X4	T44.0X5	T44.0X6
Neraval	T42.3X1	T42.3X2	T42.3X3	T42.3X4	T42.3X5	T42.3X6
Neravan	T42.3X1	T42.3X2	T42.3X3	T42.3X4	T42.3X5	T42.3X6
Nerium oleander	T62.2X1	T62.2X2	T62.2X3	T62.2X4	—	—
Nerlynx*	T45.1X1	T45.1X2	T45.1X3	T45.1X4	T45.1X5	T45.1X6
Nerve gas, not in war	T59.91	T59.92	T59.93	T59.94	—	—
Nesacaine	T41.3X1	T41.3X2	T41.3X3	T41.3X4	T41.3X5	T41.3X6
infiltration (subcutaneous)	T41.3X1	T41.3X2	T41.3X3	T41.3X4	T41.3X5	T41.3X6
nerve block (peripheral) (plexus)	T41.3X1	T41.3X2	T41.3X3	T41.3X4	T41.3X5	T41.3X6
Netilmicin	T36.5X1	T36.5X2	T36.5X3	T36.5X4	T36.5X5	T36.5X6
Neurobarb	T42.3X1	T42.3X2	T42.3X3	T42.3X4	T42.3X5	T42.3X6
Neuroleptic drug NEC	T43.501	T43.502	T43.503	T43.504	T43.505	T43.506
Neuromuscular blocking drug	T48.1X1	T48.1X2	T48.1X3	T48.1X4	T48.1X5	T48.1X6
Neurontin*	T42.6X1	T42.6X2	T42.6X3	T42.6X4	T42.6X5	T42.6X6
Neutral insulin injection	T38.3X1	T38.3X2	T38.3X3	T38.3X4	T38.3X5	T38.3X6
Neutral spirits	T51.0X1	T51.0X2	T51.0X3	T51.0X4		
beverage	T51.0X1	T51.0X2	T51.0X3	T51.0X4	—	—
Niacin	T46.7X1	T46.7X2	T46.7X3	T46.7X4	T46.7X5	T46.7X6
Niacinamide	T45.2X1	T45.2X2	T45.2X3	T45.2X4	T45.2X5	T45.2X6
Nialamide	T43.1X1	T43.1X2	T43.1X3	T43.1X4	T43.1X5	T43.1X6
Niaprazine	T42.6X1	T42.6X2	T42.6X3	T42.6X4	T42.6X5	T42.6X6
Nicamete	T46.7X1	T46.7X2	T46.7X3	T46.7X4	T46.7X5	T46.7X6
Nicardipine	T46.1X1	T46.1X2	T46.1X3	T46.1X4	T46.1X5	T46.1X6
Nicergoline	T46.7X1	T46.7X2	T46.7X3	T46.7X4	T46.7X5	T46.7X6
Nickel (carbonyl) (tetra-carbonyl) (fumes) (vapor)	T56.891	T56.892	T56.893	T56.894		
Nickelocene	T56.891	T56.892	T56.893	T56.894		
Niclosamide	T37.4X1	T37.4X2	T37.4X3	T37.4X4	T37.4X5	T37.4X6
Nicofuranose	T46.7X1	T46.7X2	T46.7X3	T46.7X4	T46.7X5	T46.7X6
Nicomorphine	T40.2X1	T40.2X2	T40.2X3	T40.2X4		
Nicorandil	T46.3X1	T46.3X2	T46.3X3	T46.3X4	T46.3X5	T46.3X6
Nicotiana (plant)	T62.2X1	T62.2X2	T62.2X3	T62.2X4	—	—
Nicotinamide	T45.2X1	T45.2X2	T45.2X3	T45.2X4	T45.2X5	T45.2X6
Nicotine (insecticide) (spray) (sulfate) NEC	T60.2X1	T60.2X2	T60.2X3	T60.2X4	—	—
from tobacco	T65.291	T65.292	T65.293	T65.294	—	—
cigarettes	T65.221	T65.222	T65.223	T65.224	—	—
not insecticide	T65.291	T65.292	T65.293	T65.294	—	—
Nicotinic acid	T46.7X1	T46.7X2	T46.7X3	T46.7X4	T46.7X5	T46.7X6
Nicotinyl alcohol	T46.7X1	T46.7X2	T46.7X3	T46.7X4	T46.7X5	T46.7X6
Nicoumalone	T45.511	T45.512	T45.513	T45.514	T45.515	T45.516
Nifedipine	T46.1X1	T46.1X2	T46.1X3	T46.1X4	T46.1X5	T46.1X6
Nifenazone	T39.2X1	T39.2X2	T39.2X3	T39.2X4	T39.2X5	T39.2X6
Nifuraldezone	T37.91	T37.92	T37.93	T37.94	T37.95	T37.96
Nifuratel	T37.8X1	T37.8X2	T37.8X3	T37.8X4	T37.8X5	T37.8X6
Nifurtimox	T37.3X1	T37.3X2	T37.3X3	T37.3X4	T37.3X5	T37.3X6
Nifurtoinol	T37.8X1	T37.8X2	T37.8X3	T37.8X4	T37.8X5	T37.8X6
Nightshade, deadly (solanum) — see also Belladonna	T62.2X1	T62.2X2	T62.2X3	T62.2X4		
berry	T62.1X1	T62.1X2	T62.1X3	T62.1X4		
Nikethamide	T50.7X1	T50.7X2	T50.7X3	T50.7X4	T50.7X5	T50.7X6
Nilstat	T36.7X1	T36.7X2	T36.7X3	T36.7X4	T36.7X5	T36.7X6
topical	T49.0X1	T49.0X2	T49.0X3	T49.0X4	T49.0X5	T49.0X6

☑ Additional Character May Be Required — Refer to the Tabular List for Character Selection

*Optum Value-Add

Substance	Poisoning, Accidental (unintentional)	Poisoning, Intentional Self-harm	Poisoning, Assault	Poisoning, Undetermined	Adverse Effect	Underdosing
Nilutamide	T38.6X1	T38.6X2	T38.6X3	T38.6X4	T38.6X5	T38.6X6
Nimesulide	T39.391	T39.392	T39.393	T39.394	T39.395	T39.396
Nimetazepam	T42.4X1	T42.4X2	T42.4X3	T42.4X4	T42.4X5	T42.4X6
Nimodipine	T46.1X1	T46.1X2	T46.1X3	T46.1X4	T46.1X5	T46.1X6
Nimorazole	T37.3X1	T37.3X2	T37.3X3	T37.3X4	T37.3X5	T37.3X6
Nimustine	T45.1X1	T45.1X2	T45.1X3	T45.1X4	T45.1X5	T45.1X6
Nipent*	T45.1X1	T45.1X2	T45.1X3	T45.1X4	T45.1X5	T45.1X6
Niridazole	T37.4X1	T37.4X2	T37.4X3	T37.4X4	T37.4X5	T37.4X6
Nisentil	T40.2X1	T40.2X2	T40.2X3	T40.2X4	T40.2X5	T40.2X6
Nisoldipine	T46.1X1	T46.1X2	T46.1X3	T46.1X4	T46.1X5	T46.1X6
Nitramine	T65.3X1	T65.3X2	T65.3X3	T65.3X4	—	—
Nitrate, organic	T46.3X1	T46.3X2	T46.3X3	T46.3X4	T46.3X5	T46.3X6
Nitrazepam	T42.4X1	T42.4X2	T42.4X3	T42.4X4	T42.4X5	T42.4X6
Nitrefazole	T50.6X1	T50.6X2	T50.6X3	T50.6X4	T50.6X5	T50.6X6
Nitrendipine	T46.1X1	T46.1X2	T46.1X3	T46.1X4	T46.1X5	T46.1X6
Nitric						
acid (liquid)	T54.2X1	T54.2X2	T54.2X3	T54.2X4	—	—
vapor	T59.891	T59.892	T59.893	T59.894	—	—
oxide (gas)	T59.0X1	T59.0X2	T59.0X3	T59.0X4	—	—
Nitrimidazine	T37.3X1	T37.3X2	T37.3X3	T37.3X4	T37.3X5	T37.3X6
Nitrite, amyl (medicinal)	T46.3X1	T46.3X2	T46.3X3	T46.3X4	T46.3X5	T46.3X6
(vapor)						
Nitroaniline	T65.3X1	T65.3X2	T65.3X3	T65.3X4	—	—
vapor	T59.891	T59.892	T59.893	T59.894	—	—
Nitrobenzene, nitrobenzol	T65.3X1	T65.3X2	T65.3X3	T65.3X4	—	—
vapor	T65.3X1	T65.3X2	T65.3X3	T65.3X4	—	—
Nitrocellulose	T65.891	T65.892	T65.893	T65.894	—	—
lacquer	T65.891	T65.892	T65.893	T65.894	—	—
Nitrodiphenyl	T65.3X1	T65.3X2	T65.3X3	T65.3X4	—	—
Nitrofural	T49.0X1	T49.0X2	T49.0X3	T49.0X4	T49.0X5	T49.0X6
Nitrofurantoin	T37.8X1	T37.8X2	T37.8X3	T37.8X4	T37.8X5	T37.8X6
Nitrofurazone	T49.0X1	T49.0X2	T49.0X3	T49.0X4	T49.0X5	T49.0X6
Nitrogen	T59.0X1	T59.0X2	T59.0X3	T59.0X4	—	—
mustard	T45.1X1	T45.1X2	T45.1X3	T45.1X4	T45.1X5	T45.1X6
Nitroglycerin, nitroglycerol	T46.3X1	T46.3X2	T46.3X3	T46.3X4	T46.3X5	T46.3X6
(medicinal)						
nonmedicinal	T65.5X1	T65.5X2	T65.5X3	T65.5X4	—	—
fumes	T65.5X1	T65.5X2	T65.5X3	T65.5X4	—	—
Nitroglycol	T52.3X1	T52.3X2	T52.3X3	T52.3X4	—	—
Nitrohydrochloric acid	T54.2X1	T54.2X2	T54.2X3	T54.2X4	—	—
Nitromersol	T49.0X1	T49.0X2	T49.0X3	T49.0X4	T49.0X5	T49.0X6
Nitronaphthalene	T65.891	T65.892	T65.893	T65.894	—	—
Nitrophenol	T54.0X1	T54.0X2	T54.0X3	T54.0X4	—	—
Nitropropane	T52.8X1	T52.8X2	T52.8X3	T52.8X4	—	—
Nitroprusside	T46.5X1	T46.5X2	T46.5X3	T46.5X4	T46.5X5	T46.5X6
Nitrosodimethylamine	T65.3X1	T65.3X2	T65.3X3	T65.3X4	—	—
Nitrothiazol	T37.4X1	T37.4X2	T37.4X3	T37.4X4	T37.4X5	T37.4X6
Nitrotoluene, nitrotoluol	T65.3X1	T65.3X2	T65.3X3	T65.3X4	—	—
vapor	T65.3X1	T65.3X2	T65.3X3	T65.3X4	—	—
Nitrous						
acid (liquid)	T54.2X1	T54.2X2	T54.2X3	T54.2X4	—	—
fumes	T59.891	T59.892	T59.893	T59.894	—	—
ether spirit	T46.3X1	T46.3X2	T46.3X3	T46.3X4	T46.3X5	T46.3X6
oxide	T41.0X1	T41.0X2	T41.0X3	T41.0X4	T41.0X5	T41.0X6
Nitroxoline	T37.8X1	T37.8X2	T37.8X3	T37.8X4	T37.8X5	T37.8X6
Nitrozone	T49.0X1	T49.0X2	T49.0X3	T49.0X4	T49.0X5	T49.0X6
Nizatidine	T47.0X1	T47.0X2	T47.0X3	T47.0X4	T47.0X5	T47.0X6
Nizofenone	T43.8X1	T43.8X2	T43.8X3	T43.8X4	T43.8X5	T43.8X6
Noctec	T42.6X1	T42.6X2	T42.6X3	T42.6X4	T42.6X5	T42.6X6
No Doz*	T43.611	T43.612	T43.613	T43.614	T43.615	T43.616
Noludar	T42.6X1	T42.6X2	T42.6X3	T42.6X4	T42.6X5	T42.6X6
Nomegestrol	T38.5X1	T38.5X2	T38.5X3	T38.5X4	T38.5X5	T38.5X6
Nomifensine	T43.291	T43.292	T43.293	T43.294	T43.295	T43.296
Nonoxinol	T49.8X1	T49.8X2	T49.8X3	T49.8X4	T49.8X5	T49.8X6
Nonylphenoxy	T49.8X1	T49.8X2	T49.8X3	T49.8X4	T49.8X5	T49.8X6
(polyethoxyethanol)						
Noptil	T42.3X1	T42.3X2	T42.3X3	T42.3X4	T42.3X5	T42.3X6
Noradrenaline	T44.4X1	T44.4X2	T44.4X3	T44.4X4	T44.4X5	T44.4X6
Noramidopyrine	T39.2X1	T39.2X2	T39.2X3	T39.2X4	T39.2X5	T39.2X6
methanesulfonate sodium	T39.2X1	T39.2X2	T39.2X3	T39.2X4	T39.2X5	T39.2X6
Norbormide	T60.4X1	T60.4X2	T60.4X3	T60.4X4	—	—
Nordazepam	T42.4X1	T42.4X2	T42.4X3	T42.4X4	T42.4X5	T42.4X6
Norepinephrine	T44.4X1	T44.4X2	T44.4X3	T44.4X4	T44.4X5	T44.4X6
Norethandrolone	T38.7X1	T38.7X2	T38.7X3	T38.7X4	T38.7X5	T38.7X6
Norethindrone	T38.4X1	T38.4X2	T38.4X3	T38.4X4	T38.4X5	T38.4X6
Norethisterone (acetate)	T38.4X1	T38.4X2	T38.4X3	T38.4X4	T38.4X5	T38.4X6
(enantate)						
with ethinylestradiol	T38.5X1	T38.5X2	T38.5X3	T38.5X4	T38.5X5	T38.5X6
Noretynodrel	T38.5X1	T38.5X2	T38.5X3	T38.5X4	T38.5X5	T38.5X6
Norfenefrine	T44.4X1	T44.4X2	T44.4X3	T44.4X4	T44.4X5	T44.4X6
Norfloxacin	T36.8X1	T36.8X2	T36.8X3	T36.8X4	T36.8X5	T36.8X6
Norgestrel	T38.4X1	T38.4X2	T38.4X3	T38.4X4	T38.4X5	T38.4X6
Norgestrienone	T38.4X1	T38.4X2	T38.4X3	T38.4X4	T38.4X5	T38.4X6

Substance	Poisoning, Accidental (unintentional)	Poisoning, Intentional Self-harm	Poisoning, Assault	Poisoning, Undetermined	Adverse Effect	Underdosing
Norlestrin	T38.4X1	T38.4X2	T38.4X3	T38.4X4	T38.4X5	T38.4X6
Norlutin	T38.4X1	T38.4X2	T38.4X3	T38.4X4	T38.4X5	T38.4X6
Normal serum albumin	T45.8X1	T45.8X2	T45.8X3	T45.8X4	T45.8X5	T45.8X6
(human), salt-poor						
Normethandrone	T38.5X1	T38.5X2	T38.5X3	T38.5X4	T38.5X5	T38.5X6
Normison — see Benzodiazepines						
Normorphine	T40.2X1	T40.2X2	T40.2X3	T40.2X4	—	—
Norpseudoephedrine	T50.5X1	T50.5X2	T50.5X3	T50.5X4	T50.5X5	T50.5X6
Nortestosterone	T38.7X1	T38.7X2	T38.7X3	T38.7X4	T38.7X5	T38.7X6
(furanpropionate)						
Nortriptyline	T43.011	T43.012	T43.013	T43.014	T43.015	T43.016
Norvasc*	T46.1X1	T46.1X2	T46.1X3	T46.1X4	T46.1X5	T46.1X6
Noscapine	T48.3X1	T48.3X2	T48.3X3	T48.3X4	T48.3X5	T48.3X6
Nose preparations	T49.6X1	T49.6X2	T49.6X3	T49.6X4	T49.6X5	T49.6X6
Novobiocin	T36.5X1	T36.5X2	T36.5X3	T36.5X4	T36.5X5	T36.5X6
Novocain (infiltration)	T41.3X1	T41.3X2	T41.3X3	T41.3X4	T41.3X5	T41.3X6
(topical)						
nerve block (peripheral)	T41.3X1	T41.3X2	T41.3X3	T41.3X4	T41.3X5	T41.3X6
(plexus)						
spinal	T41.3X1	T41.3X2	T41.3X3	T41.3X4	T41.3X5	T41.3X6
Noxious foodstuff	T62.91	T62.92	T62.93	T62.94	—	—
specified NEC	T62.8X1	T62.8X2	T62.8X3	T62.8X4	—	—
Noxiptiline	T43.011	T43.012	T43.013	T43.014	T43.015	T43.016
Noxytiolin	T49.0X1	T49.0X2	T49.0X3	T49.0X4	T49.0X5	T49.0X6
NPH Iletin (insulin)	T38.3X1	T38.3X2	T38.3X3	T38.3X4	T38.3X5	T38.3X6
Numorphan	T40.2X1	T40.2X2	T40.2X3	T40.2X4	T40.2X5	T40.2X6
Nunol	T42.3X1	T42.3X2	T42.3X3	T42.3X4	T42.3X5	T42.3X6
Nupercaine (spinal anesthetic)	T41.3X1	T41.3X2	T41.3X3	T41.3X4	T41.3X5	T41.3X6
topical (surface)	T41.3X1	T41.3X2	T41.3X3	T41.3X4	T41.3X5	T41.3X6
Nutmeg oil (liniment)	T49.3X1	T49.3X2	T49.3X3	T49.3X4	T49.3X5	T49.3X6
Nutrilipid*	T50.991	T50.992	T50.993	T50.994	T50.995	T50.996
Nutritional supplement	T50.901	T50.902	T50.903	T50.904	T50.905	T50.906
Nux vomica	T65.1X1	T65.1X2	T65.1X3	T65.1X4	—	—
Nydrazid	T37.1X1	T37.1X2	T37.1X3	T37.1X4	T37.1X5	T37.1X6
Nylidrin	T46.7X1	T46.7X2	T46.7X3	T46.7X4	T46.7X5	T46.7X6
Nystatin	T36.7X1	T36.7X2	T36.7X3	T36.7X4	T36.7X5	T36.7X6
topical	T49.0X1	T49.0X2	T49.0X3	T49.0X4	T49.0X5	T49.0X6
Nytol	T45.0X1	T45.0X2	T45.0X3	T45.0X4	T45.0X5	T45.0X6
Obidoxime chloride	T50.6X1	T50.6X2	T50.6X3	T50.6X4	T50.6X5	T50.6X6
Octafonium (chloride)	T49.3X1	T49.3X2	T49.3X3	T49.3X4	T49.3X5	T49.3X6
Octamethyl pyrophosphoramide	T60.0X1	T60.0X2	T60.0X3	T60.0X4	—	—
Octanoin	T50.991	T50.992	T50.993	T50.994	T50.995	T50.996
Octatropine methylbromide	T44.3X1	T44.3X2	T44.3X3	T44.3X4	T44.3X5	T44.3X6
Octotiamine	T45.2X1	T45.2X2	T45.2X3	T45.2X4	T45.2X5	T45.2X6
Octoxinol (9)	T49.8X1	T49.8X2	T49.8X3	T49.8X4	T49.8X5	T49.8X6
Octreotide	T38.991	T38.992	T38.993	T38.994	T38.995	T38.996
Octyl nitrite	T46.3X1	T46.3X2	T46.3X3	T46.3X4	T46.3X5	T46.3X6
Oestradiol	T38.5X1	T38.5X2	T38.5X3	T38.5X4	T38.5X5	T38.5X6
Oestriol	T38.5X1	T38.5X2	T38.5X3	T38.5X4	T38.5X5	T38.5X6
Oestrogen	T38.5X1	T38.5X2	T38.5X3	T38.5X4	T38.5X5	T38.5X6
Oestrone	T38.5X1	T38.5X2	T38.5X3	T38.5X4	T38.5X5	T38.5X6
Ofloxacin	T36.8X1	T36.8X2	T36.8X3	T36.8X4	T36.8X5	T36.8X6
Oil (of)	T65.891	T65.892	T65.893	T65.894	—	—
bitter almond	T62.8X1	T62.8X2	T62.8X3	T62.8X4	—	—
cloves	T49.7X1	T49.7X2	T49.7X3	T49.7X4	T49.7X5	T49.7X6
colors	T65.6X1	T65.6X2	T65.6X3	T65.6X4	—	—
fumes	T59.891	T59.892	T59.893	T59.894	—	—
lubricating	T52.0X1	T52.0X2	T52.0X3	T52.0X4	—	—
Niobe	T52.8X1	T52.8X2	T52.8X3	T52.8X4	—	—
vitriol (liquid)	T54.2X1	T54.2X2	T54.2X3	T54.2X4	—	—
fumes	T54.2X1	T54.2X2	T54.2X3	T54.2X4	—	—
wintergreen (bitter) NEC	T49.3X1	T49.3X2	T49.3X3	T49.3X4	T49.3X5	T49.3X6
Oily preparation (for skin)	T49.3X1	T49.3X2	T49.3X3	T49.3X4	T49.3X5	T49.3X6
Ointment NEC	T49.3X1	T49.3X2	T49.3X3	T49.3X4	T49.3X5	T49.3X6
Olanzapine	T43.591	T43.592	T43.593	T43.594	T43.595	T43.596
Oleander	T62.2X1	T62.2X2	T62.2X3	T62.2X4	—	—
Oleandomycin	T36.3X1	T36.3X2	T36.3X3	T36.3X4	T36.3X5	T36.3X6
Oleandrin	T46.0X1	T46.0X2	T46.0X3	T46.0X4	T46.0X5	T46.0X6
Oleic acid	T46.6X1	T46.6X2	T46.6X3	T46.6X4	T46.6X5	T46.6X6
Oleovitamin A	T45.2X1	T45.2X2	T45.2X3	T45.2X4	T45.2X5	T45.2X6
Oleum ricini	T47.2X1	T47.2X2	T47.2X3	T47.2X4	T47.2X5	T47.2X6
Olive oil (medicinal) NEC	T47.4X1	T47.4X2	T47.4X3	T47.4X4	T47.4X5	T47.4X6
Olivomycin	T45.1X1	T45.1X2	T45.1X3	T45.1X4	T45.1X5	T45.1X6
Olodaterol*	T48.6X1	T48.6X2	T48.6X3	T48.6X4	T48.6X5	T48.6X6
Olsalazine	T47.8X1	T47.8X2	T47.8X3	T47.8X4	T47.8X5	T47.8X6
Omeprazole	T47.1X1	T47.1X2	T47.1X3	T47.1X4	T47.1X5	T47.1X6
OMPA	T60.0X1	T60.0X2	T60.0X3	T60.0X4	—	—
Oncovin	T45.1X1	T45.1X2	T45.1X3	T45.1X4	T45.1X5	T45.1X6
Ondansetron	T45.0X1	T45.0X2	T45.0X3	T45.0X4	T45.0X5	T45.0X6

Substance	Poisoning, Accidental (unintentional)	Poisoning, Intentional Self-harm	Poisoning, Assault	Poisoning, Undetermined	Adverse Effect	Under-dosing
Ophthaine	T41.3X1	T41.3X2	T41.3X3	T41.3X4	T41.3X5	T41.3X6
Ophthetic	T41.3X1	T41.3X2	T41.3X3	T41.3X4	T41.3X5	T41.3X6
Opiate NEC	T40.601	T40.602	T40.603	T40.604	T40.605	T40.606
antagonists	T50.7X1	T50.7X2	T50.7X3	T50.7X4	T50.7X5	T50.7X6
Opioid NEC	T40.2X1	T40.2X2	T40.2X3	T40.2X4	T40.2X5	T40.2X6
Opipramol	T43.011	T43.012	T43.013	T43.014	T43.015	T43.016
Opium alkaloids (total)	T40.0X1	T40.0X2	T40.0X3	T40.0X4	T40.0X5	T40.0X6
standardized powdered	T40.0X1	T40.0X2	T40.0X3	T40.0X4	T40.0X5	T40.0X6
tincture (camphorated)	T40.0X1	T40.0X2	T40.0X3	T40.0X4	T40.0X5	T40.0X6
Optivar*	T49.5X1	T49.5X2	T49.5X3	T49.5X4	T49.5X5	T49.5X6
Oracon	T38.4X1	T38.4X2	T38.4X3	T38.4X4	T38.4X5	T38.4X6
Oragrafin	T50.8X1	T50.8X2	T50.8X3	T50.8X4	T50.8X5	T50.8X6
Oral contraceptives	T38.4X1	T38.4X2	T38.4X3	T38.4X4	T38.4X5	T38.4X6
Oral rehydration salts	T50.3X1	T50.3X2	T50.3X3	T50.3X4	T50.3X5	T50.3X6
Orazamide	T50.991	T50.992	T50.993	T50.994	T50.995	T50.996
Orciprenaline	T48.291	T48.292	T48.293	T48.294	T48.295	T48.296
Organidin	T48.4X1	T48.4X2	T48.4X3	T48.4X4	T48.4X5	T48.4X6
Organonitrate NEC	T46.3X1	T46.3X2	T46.3X3	T46.3X4	T46.3X5	T46.3X6
Organophosphates	T60.0X1	T60.0X2	T60.0X3	T60.0X4	—	—
Orimune	T50.B91	T50.B92	T50.B93	T50.B94	T50.B95	T50.B96
Orinase	T38.3X1	T38.3X2	T38.3X3	T38.3X4	T38.3X5	T38.3X6
Ormeloxifene	T38.6X1	T38.6X2	T38.6X3	T38.6X4	T38.6X5	T38.6X6
Ornidazole	T37.3X1	T37.3X2	T37.3X3	T37.3X4	T37.3X5	T37.3X6
Ornithine aspartate	T50.991	T50.992	T50.993	T50.994	T50.995	T50.996
Ornoprostil	T47.1X1	T47.1X2	T47.1X3	T47.1X4	T47.1X5	T47.1X6
Orphenadrine	T42.8X1	T42.8X2	T42.8X3	T42.8X4	T42.8X5	T42.8X6
(hydrochloride)						
Ortal (sodium)	T42.3X1	T42.3X2	T42.3X3	T42.3X4	T42.3X5	T42.3X6
Orthoboric acid	T49.0X1	T49.0X2	T49.0X3	T49.0X4	T49.0X5	T49.0X6
ENT agent	T49.6X1	T49.6X2	T49.6X3	T49.6X4	T49.6X5	T49.6X6
ophthalmic preparation	T49.5X1	T49.5X2	T49.5X3	T49.5X4	T49.5X5	T49.5X6
Orthocaine	T41.3X1	T41.3X2	T41.3X3	T41.3X4	T41.3X5	T41.3X6
Orthodichlorobenzene	T53.7X1	T53.7X2	T53.7X3	T53.7X4	—	—
Ortho-Novum	T38.4X1	T38.4X2	T38.4X3	T38.4X4	T38.4X5	T38.4X6
Orthotolidine (reagent)	T54.2X1	T54.2X2	T54.2X3	T54.2X4	—	—
Osmic acid (liquid)	T54.2X1	T54.2X2	T54.2X3	T54.2X4	—	—
fumes	T54.2X1	T54.2X2	T54.2X3	T54.2X4	—	—
Osmotic diuretics	T50.2X1	T50.2X2	T50.2X3	T50.2X4	T50.2X5	T50.2X6
Otilonium bromide	T44.3X1	T44.3X2	T44.3X3	T44.3X4	T44.3X5	T44.3X6
Otorhinolaryngological drug NEC	T49.6X1	T49.6X2	T49.6X3	T49.6X4	T49.6X5	T49.6X6
Ouabain (e)	T46.0X1	T46.0X2	T46.0X3	T46.0X4	T46.0X5	T46.0X6
Ovarian						
hormone	T38.5X1	T38.5X2	T38.5X3	T38.5X4	T38.5X5	T38.5X6
stimulant	T38.5X1	T38.5X2	T38.5X3	T38.5X4	T38.5X5	T38.5X6
Ovide*	T49.0X1	T49.0X2	T49.0X3	T49.0X4	T49.0X5	T49.0X6
Ovral	T38.4X1	T38.4X2	T38.4X3	T38.4X4	T38.4X5	T38.4X6
Ovulen	T38.4X1	T38.4X2	T38.4X3	T38.4X4	T38.4X5	T38.4X6
Oxacillin	T36.0X1	T36.0X2	T36.0X3	T36.0X4	T36.0X5	T36.0X6
Oxalic acid	T54.2X1	T54.2X2	T54.2X3	T54.2X4	—	—
ammonium salt	T50.991	T50.992	T50.993	T50.994	T50.995	T50.996
Oxamniquine	T37.4X1	T37.4X2	T37.4X3	T37.4X4	T37.4X5	T37.4X6
Oxanamide	T43.591	T43.592	T43.593	T43.594	T43.595	T43.596
Oxandrolone	T38.7X1	T38.7X2	T38.7X3	T38.7X4	T38.7X5	T38.7X6
Oxantel	T37.4X1	T37.4X2	T37.4X3	T37.4X4	T37.4X5	T37.4X6
Oxapium iodide	T44.3X1	T44.3X2	T44.3X3	T44.3X4	T44.3X5	T44.3X6
Oxaprotiline	T43.021	T43.022	T43.023	T43.024	T43.025	T43.026
Oxaprozin	T39.311	T39.312	T39.313	T39.314	T39.315	T39.316
Oxatomide	T45.0X1	T45.0X2	T45.0X3	T45.0X4	T45.0X5	T45.0X6
Oxazepam	T42.4X1	T42.4X2	T42.4X3	T42.4X4	T42.4X5	T42.4X6
Oxazimedrine	T50.5X1	T50.5X2	T50.5X3	T50.5X4	T50.5X5	T50.5X6
Oxazolam	T42.4X1	T42.4X2	T42.4X3	T42.4X4	T42.4X5	T42.4X6
Oxazolidine derivatives	T42.2X1	T42.2X2	T42.2X3	T42.2X4	T42.2X5	T42.2X6
Oxazolidinedione (derivative)	T42.2X1	T42.2X2	T42.2X3	T42.2X4	T42.2X5	T42.2X6
Ox bile extract	T47.5X1	T47.5X2	T47.5X3	T47.5X4	T47.5X5	T47.5X6
Oxcarbazepine	T42.1X1	T42.1X2	T42.1X3	T42.1X4	T42.1X5	T42.1X6
Oxedrine	T44.4X1	T44.4X2	T44.4X3	T44.4X4	T44.4X5	T44.4X6
Oxeladin (citrate)	T48.3X1	T48.3X2	T48.3X3	T48.3X4	T48.3X5	T48.3X6
Oxendolone	T38.5X1	T38.5X2	T38.5X3	T38.5X4	T38.5X5	T38.5X6
Oxetacaine	T41.3X1	T41.3X2	T41.3X3	T41.3X4	T41.3X5	T41.3X6
Oxethazine	T41.3X1	T41.3X2	T41.3X3	T41.3X4	T41.3X5	T41.3X6
Oxetorone	T39.8X1	T39.8X2	T39.8X3	T39.8X4	T39.8X5	T39.8X6
Oxiconazole	T49.0X1	T49.0X2	T49.0X3	T49.0X4	T49.0X5	T49.0X6
Oxidizing agent NEC	T54.91	T54.92	T54.93	T54.94	—	—
Oxipurinol	T50.4X1	T50.4X2	T50.4X3	T50.4X4	T50.4X5	T50.4X6
Oxitriptan	T43.291	T43.292	T43.293	T43.294	T43.295	T43.296
Oxitropium bromide	T48.6X1	T48.6X2	T48.6X3	T48.6X4	T48.6X5	T48.6X6
Oxodipine	T46.1X1	T46.1X2	T46.1X3	T46.1X4	T46.1X5	T46.1X6
Oxolamine	T48.3X1	T48.3X2	T48.3X3	T48.3X4	T48.3X5	T48.3X6
Oxolinic acid	T37.8X1	T37.8X2	T37.8X3	T37.8X4	T37.8X5	T37.8X6
Oxomemazine	T43.3X1	T43.3X2	T43.3X3	T43.3X4	T43.3X5	T43.3X6
Oxophenarsine	T37.3X1	T37.3X2	T37.3X3	T37.3X4	T37.3X5	T37.3X6

Substance	Poisoning, Accidental (unintentional)	Poisoning, Intentional Self-harm	Poisoning, Assault	Poisoning, Undetermined	Adverse Effect	Under-dosing
Oxprenolol	T44.7X1	T44.7X2	T44.7X3	T44.7X4	T44.7X5	T44.7X6
Oxsoralen	T49.3X1	T49.3X2	T49.3X3	T49.3X4	T49.3X5	T49.3X6
Oxtriphylline	T48.6X1	T48.6X2	T48.6X3	T48.6X4	T48.6X5	T48.6X6
Oxybate sodium	T41.291	T41.292	T41.293	T41.294	T41.295	T41.296
Oxybuprocaine	T41.3X1	T41.3X2	T41.3X3	T41.3X4	T41.3X5	T41.3X6
Oxybutynin	T44.3X1	T44.3X2	T44.3X3	T44.3X4	T44.3X5	T44.3X6
Oxychlorosene	T49.0X1	T49.0X2	T49.0X3	T49.0X4	T49.0X5	T49.0X6
Oxycodone	T40.2X1	T40.2X2	T40.2X3	T40.2X4	T40.2X5	T40.2X6
OxyContin*	T40.2X1	T40.2X2	T40.2X3	T40.2X4	T40.2X5	T40.2X6
Oxyfedrine	T46.3X1	T46.3X2	T46.3X3	T46.3X4	T46.3X5	T46.3X6
Oxygen	T41.5X1	T41.5X2	T41.5X3	T41.5X4	T41.5X5	T41.5X6
Oxylone	T49.0X1	T49.0X2	T49.0X3	T49.0X4	T49.0X5	T49.0X6
ophthalmic preparation	T49.5X1	T49.5X2	T49.5X3	T49.5X4	T49.5X5	T49.5X6
Oxymesterone	T38.7X1	T38.7X2	T38.7X3	T38.7X4	T38.7X5	T38.7X6
Oxymetazoline	T48.5X1	T48.5X2	T48.5X3	T48.5X4	T48.5X5	T48.5X6
Oxymetholone	T38.7X1	T38.7X2	T38.7X3	T38.7X4	T38.7X5	T38.7X6
Oxymorphone	T40.2X1	T40.2X2	T40.2X3	T40.2X4	T40.2X5	T40.2X6
Oxypertine	T43.591	T43.592	T43.593	T43.594	T43.595	T43.596
Oxyphenbutazone	T39.2X1	T39.2X2	T39.2X3	T39.2X4	T39.2X5	T39.2X6
Oxyphencyclimine	T44.3X1	T44.3X2	T44.3X3	T44.3X4	T44.3X5	T44.3X6
Oxyphenisatine	T47.2X1	T47.2X2	T47.2X3	T47.2X4	T47.2X5	T47.2X6
Oxyphenonium bromide	T44.3X1	T44.3X2	T44.3X3	T44.3X4	T44.3X5	T44.3X6
Oxypolygelatin	T45.8X1	T45.8X2	T45.8X3	T45.8X4	T45.8X5	T45.8X6
Oxyquinoline (derivatives)	T37.8X1	T37.8X2	T37.8X3	T37.8X4	T37.8X5	T37.8X6
Oxytetracycline	T36.4X1	T36.4X2	T36.4X3	T36.4X4	T36.4X5	T36.4X6
Oxytocic drug NEC	T48.0X1	T48.0X2	T48.0X3	T48.0X4	T48.0X5	T48.0X6
Oxytocin (synthetic)	T48.0X1	T48.0X2	T48.0X3	T48.0X4	T48.0X5	T48.0X6
Oxytrol*	T44.3X1	T44.3X2	T44.3X3	T44.3X4	T44.3X5	T44.3X6
Ozone	T59.891	T59.892	T59.893	T59.894	—	—
PABA	T49.3X1	T49.3X2	T49.3X3	T49.3X4	T49.3X5	T49.3X6
Packed red cells	T45.8X1	T45.8X2	T45.8X3	T45.8X4	T45.8X5	T45.8X6
Padimate	T49.3X1	T49.3X2	T49.3X3	T49.3X4	T49.3X5	T49.3X6
Paint NEC	T65.6X1	T65.6X2	T65.6X3	T65.6X4	—	—
cleaner	T52.91	T52.92	T52.93	T52.94	—	—
fumes NEC	T59.891	T59.892	T59.893	T59.894	—	—
lead (fumes)	T56.0X1	T56.0X2	T56.0X3	T56.0X4	—	—
solvent NEC	T52.8X1	T52.8X2	T52.8X3	T52.8X4	—	—
stripper	T52.8X1	T52.8X2	T52.8X3	T52.8X4	—	—
Palfium	T40.2X1	T40.2X2	T40.2X3	T40.2X4	—	—
Palm kernel oil	T50.991	T50.992	T50.993	T50.994	T50.995	T50.996
Paludrine	T37.2X1	T37.2X2	T37.2X3	T37.2X4	T37.2X5	T37.2X6
PAM (pralidoxime)	T50.6X1	T50.6X2	T50.6X3	T50.6X4	T50.6X5	T50.6X6
Pamaquine (naphthoute)	T37.2X1	T37.2X2	T37.2X3	T37.2X4	T37.2X5	T37.2X6
Panadol	T39.1X1	T39.1X2	T39.1X3	T39.1X4	T39.1X5	T39.1X6
Pancreatic						
digestive secretion stimulant	T47.8X1	T47.8X2	T47.8X3	T47.8X4	T47.8X5	T47.8X6
dornase	T45.3X1	T45.3X2	T45.3X3	T45.3X4	T45.3X5	T45.3X6
Pancreatin	T47.5X1	T47.5X2	T47.5X3	T47.5X4	T47.5X5	T47.5X6
Pancrelipase	T47.5X1	T47.5X2	T47.5X3	T47.5X4	T47.5X5	T47.5X6
Pancuronium (bromide)	T48.1X1	T48.1X2	T48.1X3	T48.1X4	T48.1X5	T48.1X6
Pangamic acid	T45.2X1	T45.2X2	T45.2X3	T45.2X4	T45.2X5	T45.2X6
Panthenol	T45.2X1	T45.2X2	T45.2X3	T45.2X4	T45.2X5	T45.2X6
topical	T49.8X1	T49.8X2	T49.8X3	T49.8X4	T49.8X5	T49.8X6
Pantopon	T40.0X1	T40.0X2	T40.0X3	T40.0X4	T40.0X5	T40.0X6
Pantoprazole*	T47.1X1	T47.1X2	T47.1X3	T47.1X4	T47.1X5	T47.1X6
Pantothenic acid	T45.2X1	T45.2X2	T45.2X3	T45.2X4	T45.2X5	T45.2X6
Panwarfin	T45.511	T45.512	T45.513	T45.514	T45.515	T45.516
Papain	T47.5X1	T47.5X2	T47.5X3	T47.5X4	T47.5X5	T47.5X6
digestant	T47.5X1	T47.5X2	T47.5X3	T47.5X4	T47.5X5	T47.5X6
Papaveretum	T40.0X1	T40.0X2	T40.0X3	T40.0X4	T40.0X5	T40.0X6
Papaverine	T44.3X1	T44.3X2	T44.3X3	T44.3X4	T44.3X5	T44.3X6
Para-acetamidophenol	T39.1X1	T39.1X2	T39.1X3	T39.1X4	T39.1X5	T39.1X6
Para-aminobenzoic acid	T49.3X1	T49.3X2	T49.3X3	T49.3X4	T49.3X5	T49.3X6
Para-aminophenol derivatives	T39.1X1	T39.1X2	T39.1X3	T39.1X4	T39.1X5	T39.1X6
Para-aminosalicylic acid	T37.1X1	T37.1X2	T37.1X3	T37.1X4	T37.1X5	T37.1X6
Paracetaldehyde	T42.6X1	T42.6X2	T42.6X3	T42.6X4	T42.6X5	T42.6X6
Paracetamol	T39.1X1	T39.1X2	T39.1X3	T39.1X4	T39.1X5	T39.1X6
Parachlorophenol (camphorated)	T49.0X1	T49.0X2	T49.0X3	T49.0X4	T49.0X5	T49.0X6
Paracodin	T40.2X1	T40.2X2	T40.2X3	T40.2X4	T40.2X5	T40.2X6
Paradione	T42.2X1	T42.2X2	T42.2X3	T42.2X4	T42.2X5	T42.2X6
Paraffin(s) (wax)	T52.0X1	T52.0X2	T52.0X3	T52.0X4	—	—
liquid (medicinal)	T47.4X1	T47.4X2	T47.4X3	T47.4X4	T47.4X5	T47.4X6
nonmedicinal	T52.0X1	T52.0X2	T52.0X3	T52.0X4	—	—
Paraformaldehyde	T60.3X1	T60.3X2	T60.3X3	T60.3X4	—	—
Paraldehyde	T42.6X1	T42.6X2	T42.6X3	T42.6X4	T42.6X5	T42.6X6
Paramethadione	T42.2X1	T42.2X2	T42.2X3	T42.2X4	T42.2X5	T42.2X6
Paramethasone	T38.0X1	T38.0X2	T38.0X3	T38.0X4	T38.0X5	T38.0X6
acetate	T49.0X1	T49.0X2	T49.0X3	T49.0X4	T49.0X5	T49.0X6
Paraoxon	T60.0X1	T60.0X2	T60.0X3	T60.0X4	—	—
Paraquat	T60.3X1	T60.3X2	T60.3X3	T60.3X4	—	—

☑ Additional Character May Be Required — Refer to the Tabular List for Character Selection *Optum Value-Add

Substance	Poisoning, Accidental (unintentional)	Poisoning, Intentional Self-harm	Poisoning, Assault	Poisoning, Undetermined	Adverse Effect	Under-dosing
Parasympatholytic NEC	T44.3X1	T44.3X2	T44.3X3	T44.3X4	T44.3X5	T44.3X6
Parasympathomimetic drug NEC	T44.1X1	T44.1X2	T44.1X3	T44.1X4	T44.1X5	T44.1X6
Parathion	T60.0X1	T60.0X2	T60.0X3	T60.0X4	—	—
Parathormone	T50.991	T50.992	T50.993	T50.994	T50.995	T50.996
Parathyroid extract	T50.991	T50.992	T50.993	T50.994	T50.995	T50.996
Paratyphoid vaccine	T50.A91	T50.A92	T50.A93	T50.A94	T50.A95	T50.A96
Paredrine	T44.4X1	T44.4X2	T44.4X3	T44.4X4	T44.4X5	T44.4X6
Paregoric	T40.0X1	T40.0X2	T40.0X3	T40.0X4	T40.0X5	T40.0X6
Pargyline	T46.5X1	T46.5X2	T46.5X3	T46.5X4	T46.5X5	T46.5X6
Paris green	T57.0X1	T57.0X2	T57.0X3	T57.0X4	—	—
insecticide	T57.0X1	T57.0X2	T57.0X3	T57.0X4	—	—
Parnate	T43.1X1	T43.1X2	T43.1X3	T43.1X4	T43.1X5	T43.1X6
Paromomycin	T36.5X1	T36.5X2	T36.5X3	T36.5X4	T36.5X5	T36.5X6
Paroxypropione	T45.1X1	T45.1X2	T45.1X3	T45.1X4	T45.1X5	T45.1X6
Parsabiv*	T50.991	T50.992	T50.993	T50.994	T50.995	T50.996
Parzone	T40.2X1	T40.2X2	T40.2X3	T40.2X4	T40.2X5	T40.2X6
PAS	T37.1X1	T37.1X2	T37.1X3	T37.1X4	T37.1X5	T37.1X6
Pasiniazid	T37.1X1	T37.1X2	T37.1X3	T37.1X4	T37.1X5	T37.1X6
PBB (polybrominated biphenyls)	T65.891	T65.892	T65.893	T65.894	—	—
PCB	T65.891	T65.892	T65.893	T65.894	—	—
PCP						
meaning pentachlorophenol	T60.1X1	T60.1X2	T60.1X3	T60.1X4	—	—
fungicide	T60.3X1	T60.3X2	T60.3X3	T60.3X4	—	—
herbicide	T60.3X1	T60.3X2	T60.3X3	T60.3X4	—	—
insecticide	T60.1X1	T60.1X2	T60.1X3	T60.1X4	—	—
meaning phencyclidine	T40.991	T40.992	T40.993	T40.994	—	—
Peach kernel oil (emulsion)	T47.4X1	T47.4X2	T47.4X3	T47.4X4	T47.4X5	T47.4X6
Peanut oil (emulsion) NEC	T47.4X1	T47.4X2	T47.4X3	T47.4X4	T47.4X5	T47.4X6
topical	T49.3X1	T49.3X2	T49.3X3	T49.3X4	T49.3X5	T49.3X6
Pearly Gates (morning glory seeds)	T40.991	T40.992	T40.993	T40.994	—	—
Pecazine	T43.3X1	T43.3X2	T43.3X3	T43.3X4	T43.3X5	T43.3X6
Pectin	T47.6X1	T47.6X2	T47.6X3	T47.6X4	T47.6X5	T47.6X6
Pediaflor*	T49.7X1	T49.7X2	T49.7X3	T49.7X4	T49.7X5	T49.7X6
Pefloxacin	T37.8X1	T37.8X2	T37.8X3	T37.8X4	T37.8X5	T37.8X6
Pegademase, bovine	T50.Z91	T50.Z92	T50.Z93	T50.Z94	T50.Z95	T50.Z96
Pelletierine tannate	T37.4X1	T37.4X2	T37.4X3	T37.4X4	T37.4X5	T37.4X6
Pemirolast (potassium)	T48.6X1	T48.6X2	T48.6X3	T48.6X4	T48.6X5	T48.6X6
Pemoline	T50.7X1	T50.7X2	T50.7X3	T50.7X4	T50.7X5	T50.7X6
Pempidine	T44.2X1	T44.2X2	T44.2X3	T44.2X4	T44.2X5	T44.2X6
Penamecillin	T36.0X1	T36.0X2	T36.0X3	T36.0X4	T36.0X5	T36.0X6
Penbutolol	T44.7X1	T44.7X2	T44.7X3	T44.7X4	T44.7X5	T44.7X6
Penethamate	T36.0X1	T36.0X2	T36.0X3	T36.0X4	T36.0X5	T36.0X6
Penfluridol	T43.591	T43.592	T43.593	T43.594	T43.595	T43.596
Penflutizide	T50.2X1	T50.2X2	T50.2X3	T50.2X4	T50.2X5	T50.2X6
Pengitoxin	T46.0X1	T46.0X2	T46.0X3	T46.0X4	T46.0X5	T46.0X6
Penicillamine	T50.6X1	T50.6X2	T50.6X3	T50.6X4	T50.6X5	T50.6X6
Penicillin (any)	T36.0X1	T36.0X2	T36.0X3	T36.0X4	T36.0X5	T36.0X6
Penicillinase	T45.3X1	T45.3X2	T45.3X3	T45.3X4	T45.3X5	T45.3X6
Penicilloyl polylysine	T50.8X1	T50.8X2	T50.8X3	T50.8X4	T50.8X5	T50.8X6
Penimepicycline	T36.4X1	T36.4X2	T36.4X3	T36.4X4	T36.4X5	T36.4X6
Pentacel*	T50.A11	T50.A12	T50.A13	T50.A14	T50.A15	T50.A16
Pentachloroethane	T53.6X1	T53.6X2	T53.6X3	T53.6X4	—	—
Pentachloronaphthalene	T53.7X1	T53.7X2	T53.7X3	T53.7X4	—	—
Pentachlorophenol (pesticide)	T60.1X1	T60.1X2	T60.1X3	T60.1X4	—	—
fungicide	T60.3X1	T60.3X2	T60.3X3	T60.3X4	—	—
herbicide	T60.3X1	T60.3X2	T60.3X3	T60.3X4	—	—
insecticide	T60.1X1	T60.1X2	T60.1X3	T60.1X4	—	—
Pentaerythritol	T46.3X1	T46.3X2	T46.3X3	T46.3X4	T46.3X5	T46.3X6
chloral	T42.6X1	T42.6X2	T42.6X3	T42.6X4	T42.6X5	T42.6X6
tetranitrate NEC	T46.3X1	T46.3X2	T46.3X3	T46.3X4	T46.3X5	T46.3X6
Pentaerythrityl tetranitrate	T46.3X1	T46.3X2	T46.3X3	T46.3X4	T46.3X5	T46.3X6
Pentagastrin	T50.8X1	T50.8X2	T50.8X3	T50.8X4	T50.8X5	T50.8X6
Pentalin	T53.6X1	T53.6X2	T53.6X3	T53.6X4	—	—
Pentamethonium bromide	T44.2X1	T44.2X2	T44.2X3	T44.2X4	T44.2X5	T44.2X6
Pentamidine	T37.3X1	T37.3X2	T37.3X3	T37.3X4	T37.3X5	T37.3X6
Pentanol	T51.3X1	T51.3X2	T51.3X3	T51.3X4	—	—
Pentapyrrolinium (bitartrate)	T44.2X1	T44.2X2	T44.2X3	T44.2X4	T44.2X5	T44.2X6
Pentaquine	T37.2X1	T37.2X2	T37.2X3	T37.2X4	T37.2X5	T37.2X6
Pentazocine	T40.491	T40.492	T40.493	T40.494	T40.495	T40.496
Pentetrazole	T50.7X1	T50.7X2	T50.7X3	T50.7X4	T50.7X5	T50.7X6
Penthienate bromide	T44.3X1	T44.3X2	T44.3X3	T44.3X4	T44.3X5	T44.3X6
Pentifylline	T46.7X1	T46.7X2	T46.7X3	T46.7X4	T46.7X5	T46.7X6
Pentobarbital	T42.3X1	T42.3X2	T42.3X3	T42.3X4	T42.3X5	T42.3X6
sodium	T42.3X1	T42.3X2	T42.3X3	T42.3X4	T42.3X5	T42.3X6
Pentobarbitone	T42.3X1	T42.3X2	T42.3X3	T42.3X4	T42.3X5	T42.3X6
Pentolonium tartrate	T44.2X1	T44.2X2	T44.2X3	T44.2X4	T44.2X5	T44.2X6

Substance	Poisoning, Accidental (unintentional)	Poisoning, Intentional Self-harm	Poisoning, Assault	Poisoning, Undetermined	Adverse Effect	Under-dosing
Pentosan polysulfate (sodium)	T39.8X1	T39.8X2	T39.8X3	T39.8X4	T39.8X5	T39.8X6
Pentostatin	T45.1X1	T45.1X2	T45.1X3	T45.1X4	T45.1X5	T45.1X6
Pentothal	T41.1X1	T41.1X2	T41.1X3	T41.1X4	T41.1X5	T41.1X6
Pentoxifylline	T46.7X1	T46.7X2	T46.7X3	T46.7X4	T46.7X5	T46.7X6
Pentoxyverine	T48.3X1	T48.3X2	T48.3X3	T48.3X4	T48.3X5	T48.3X6
Pentrinat	T46.3X1	T46.3X2	T46.3X3	T46.3X4	T46.3X5	T46.3X6
Pentylenetetrazole	T50.7X1	T50.7X2	T50.7X3	T50.7X4	T50.7X5	T50.7X6
Pentylsalicylamide	T37.1X1	T37.1X2	T37.1X3	T37.1X4	T37.1X5	T37.1X6
Pentymal	T42.3X1	T42.3X2	T42.3X3	T42.3X4	T42.3X5	T42.3X6
Pepcid*	T47.0X1	T47.0X2	T47.0X3	T47.0X4	T47.0X5	T47.0X6
Peplomycin	T45.1X1	T45.1X2	T45.1X3	T45.1X4	T45.1X5	T45.1X6
Peppermint (oil)	T47.5X1	T47.5X2	T47.5X3	T47.5X4	T47.5X5	T47.5X6
Pepsin	T47.5X1	T47.5X2	T47.5X3	T47.5X4	T47.5X5	T47.5X6
digestant	T47.5X1	T47.5X2	T47.5X3	T47.5X4	T47.5X5	T47.5X6
Pepstatin	T47.1X1	T47.1X2	T47.1X3	T47.1X4	T47.1X5	T47.1X6
Peptavlon	T50.8X1	T50.8X2	T50.8X3	T50.8X4	T50.8X5	T50.8X6
Perazine	T43.3X1	T43.3X2	T43.3X3	T43.3X4	T43.3X5	T43.3X6
Percaine (spinal)	T41.3X1	T41.3X2	T41.3X3	T41.3X4	T41.3X5	T41.3X6
topical (surface)	T41.3X1	T41.3X2	T41.3X3	T41.3X4	T41.3X5	T41.3X6
Perchloroethylene	T53.3X1	T53.3X2	T53.3X3	T53.3X4	—	—
medicinal	T37.4X1	T37.4X2	T37.4X3	T37.4X4	T37.4X5	T37.4X6
vapor	T53.3X1	T53.3X2	T53.3X3	T53.3X4	—	—
Percodan	T40.2X1	T40.2X2	T40.2X3	T40.2X4	T40.2X5	T40.2X6
Percogesic — see also acetaminophen	T45.0X1	T45.0X2	T45.0X3	T45.0X4	T45.0X5	T45.0X6
Percorten	T38.0X1	T38.0X2	T38.0X3	T38.0X4	T38.0X5	T38.0X6
Pergolide	T42.8X1	T42.8X2	T42.8X3	T42.8X4	T42.8X5	T42.8X6
Pergonal	T38.811	T38.812	T38.813	T38.814	T38.815	T38.816
Perhexilene	T46.3X1	T46.3X2	T46.3X3	T46.3X4	T46.3X5	T46.3X6
Perhexiline (maleate)	T46.3X1	T46.3X2	T46.3X3	T46.3X4	T46.3X5	T46.3X6
Periactin	T45.0X1	T45.0X2	T45.0X3	T45.0X4	T45.0X5	T45.0X6
Periciazine	T43.3X1	T43.3X2	T43.3X3	T43.3X4	T43.3X5	T43.3X6
Periclor	T42.6X1	T42.6X2	T42.6X3	T42.6X4	T42.6X5	T42.6X6
Perindopril	T46.4X1	T46.4X2	T46.4X3	T46.4X4	T46.4X5	T46.4X6
Perisoxal	T39.8X1	T39.8X2	T39.8X3	T39.8X4	T39.8X5	T39.8X6
Peritoneal dialysis solution	T50.3X1	T50.3X2	T50.3X3	T50.3X4	T50.3X5	T50.3X6
Peritrate	T46.3X1	T46.3X2	T46.3X3	T46.3X4	T46.3X5	T46.3X6
Perlapine	T42.4X1	T42.4X2	T42.4X3	T42.4X4	T42.4X5	T42.4X6
Permanganate	T65.891	T65.892	T65.893	T65.894	—	—
Permapen*	T36.0X1	T36.0X2	T36.0X3	T36.0X4	T36.0X5	T36.0X6
Permethrin	T60.1X1	T60.1X2	T60.1X3	T60.1X4	—	—
Pernocton	T42.3X1	T42.3X2	T42.3X3	T42.3X4	T42.3X5	T42.3X6
Pernoston	T42.3X1	T42.3X2	T42.3X3	T42.3X4	T42.3X5	T42.3X6
Peronine	T40.2X1	T40.2X2	T40.2X3	T40.2X4	—	—
Perphenazine	T43.3X1	T43.3X2	T43.3X3	T43.3X4	T43.3X5	T43.3X6
Pertofrane	T43.011	T43.012	T43.013	T43.014	T43.015	T43.016
Pertussis						
immune serum (human)	T50.Z11	T50.Z12	T50.Z13	T50.Z14	T50.Z15	T50.Z16
vaccine (with diphtheria toxoid) (with tetanus toxoid)	T50.A11	T50.A12	T50.A13	T50.A14	T50.A15	T50.A16
Peruvian balsam	T49.0X1	T49.0X2	T49.0X3	T49.0X4	T49.0X5	T49.0X6
Peruvoside	T46.0X1	T46.0X2	T46.0X3	T46.0X4	T46.0X5	T46.0X6
Pesticide (dust) (fumes) (vapor) NEC	T60.91	T60.92	T60.93	T60.94	—	—
arsenic	T57.0X1	T57.0X2	T57.0X3	T57.0X4	—	—
chlorinated	T60.1X1	T60.1X2	T60.1X3	T60.1X4	—	—
cyanide	T65.0X1	T65.0X2	T65.0X3	T65.0X4	—	—
kerosene	T52.0X1	T52.0X2	T52.0X3	T52.0X4	—	—
mixture (of compounds)	T60.91	T60.92	T60.93	T60.94	—	—
naphthalene	T60.2X1	T60.2X2	T60.2X3	T60.2X4	—	—
organochlorine (compounds)	T60.1X1	T60.1X2	T60.1X3	T60.1X4	—	—
petroleum (distillate) (products) NEC	T60.8X1	T60.8X2	T60.8X3	T60.8X4	—	—
specified ingredient NEC	T60.8X1	T60.8X2	T60.8X3	T60.8X4	—	—
strychnine	T65.1X1	T65.1X2	T65.1X3	T65.1X4	—	—
thallium	T60.4X1	T60.4X2	T60.4X3	T60.4X4	—	—
Pethidine	T40.491	T40.492	T40.493	T40.494	T40.495	T40.496
Petrichloral	T42.6X1	T42.6X2	T42.6X3	T42.6X4	T42.6X5	T42.6X6
Petrol	T52.0X1	T52.0X2	T52.0X3	T52.0X4	—	—
vapor	T52.0X1	T52.0X2	T52.0X3	T52.0X4	—	—
Petrolatum	T49.3X1	T49.3X2	T49.3X3	T49.3X4	T49.3X5	T49.3X6
hydrophilic	T49.3X1	T49.3X2	T49.3X3	T49.3X4	T49.3X5	T49.3X6
liquid	T47.4X1	T47.4X2	T47.4X3	T47.4X4	T47.4X5	T47.4X6
topical	T49.3X1	T49.3X2	T49.3X3	T49.3X4	T49.3X5	T49.3X6
nonmedicinal	T52.0X1	T52.0X2	T52.0X3	T52.0X4	—	—
red veterinary	T49.3X1	T49.3X2	T49.3X3	T49.3X4	T49.3X5	T49.3X6
white	T49.3X1	T49.3X2	T49.3X3	T49.3X4	T49.3X5	T49.3X6
Petroleum (products) NEC	T52.0X1	T52.0X2	T52.0X3	T52.0X4	—	—
benzine(s) — see Ligroin						
ether — see Ligroin						

*Optum Value-Add   ☑ Additional Character May Be Required — Refer to the Tabular List for Character Selection

Substance	Poisoning, Accidental (unintentional)	Poisoning, Intentional Self-harm	Poisoning, Assault	Poisoning, Undetermined	Adverse Effect	Under-dosing
Petroleum (products) NEC — *continued*						
jelly — *see* Petrolatum						
naphtha — *see* Ligroin						
pesticide	T60.8X1	T60.8X2	T60.8X3	T60.8X4	—	—
solids	T52.0X1	T52.0X2	T52.0X3	T52.0X4	—	—
solvents	T52.0X1	T52.0X2	T52.0X3	T52.0X4	—	—
vapor	T52.0X1	T52.0X2	T52.0X3	T52.0X4	—	—
Peyote	T40.991	T40.992	T40.993	T40.994	—	—
Phanodorm, phanodorn	T42.3X1	T42.3X2	T42.3X3	T42.3X4	T42.3X5	T42.3X6
Phanquinone	T37.3X1	T37.3X2	T37.3X3	T37.3X4	T37.3X5	T37.3X6
Phanquone	T37.3X1	T37.3X2	T37.3X3	T37.3X4	T37.3X5	T37.3X6
Pharmaceutical						
adjunct NEC	T50.901	T50.902	T50.903	T50.904	T50.905	T50.906
excipient NEC	T50.901	T50.902	T50.903	T50.904	T50.905	T50.906
sweetener	T50.901	T50.902	T50.903	T50.904	T50.905	T50.906
viscous agent	T50.901	T50.902	T50.903	T50.904	T50.905	T50.906
Phazyme*	T47.1X1	T47.1X2	T47.1X3	T47.1X4	T47.1X5	T47.1X6
Phemitone	T42.3X1	T42.3X2	T42.3X3	T42.3X4	T42.3X5	T42.3X6
Phenacaine	T41.3X1	T41.3X2	T41.3X3	T41.3X4	T41.3X5	T41.3X6
Phenacemide	T42.6X1	T42.6X2	T42.6X3	T42.6X4	T42.6X5	T42.6X6
Phenacetin	T39.1X1	T39.1X2	T39.1X3	T39.1X4	T39.1X5	T39.1X6
Phenadoxone	T40.2X1	T40.2X2	T40.2X3	T40.2X4	—	—
Phenaglycodol	T43.591	T43.592	T43.593	T43.594	T43.595	T43.596
Phenantoin	T42.0X1	T42.0X2	T42.0X3	T42.0X4	T42.0X5	T42.0X6
Phenaphthazine reagent	T50.991	T50.992	T50.993	T50.994	T50.995	T50.996
Phenazocine	T40.491	T40.492	T40.493	T40.494	T40.495	T40.496
Phenazone	T39.2X1	T39.2X2	T39.2X3	T39.2X4	T39.2X5	T39.2X6
Phenazopyridine	T39.8X1	T39.8X2	T39.8X3	T39.8X4	T39.8X5	T39.8X6
Phenbenicillin	T36.0X1	T36.0X2	T36.0X3	T36.0X4	T36.0X5	T36.0X6
Phenbutrazate	T50.5X1	T50.5X2	T50.5X3	T50.5X4	T50.5X5	T50.5X6
Phencyclidine	T40.991	T40.992	T40.993	T40.994	T40.995	T40.996
Phendimetrazine	T50.5X1	T50.5X2	T50.5X3	T50.5X4	T50.5X5	T50.5X6
Phenelzine	T43.1X1	T43.1X2	T43.1X3	T43.1X4	T43.1X5	T43.1X6
Phenemal	T42.3X1	T42.3X2	T42.3X3	T42.3X4	T42.3X5	T42.3X6
Phenergan	T42.6X1	T42.6X2	T42.6X3	T42.6X4	T42.6X5	T42.6X6
Pheneticillin	T36.0X1	T36.0X2	T36.0X3	T36.0X4	T36.0X5	T36.0X6
Pheneturide	T42.6X1	T42.6X2	T42.6X3	T42.6X4	T42.6X5	T42.6X6
Phenformin	T38.3X1	T38.3X2	T38.3X3	T38.3X4	T38.3X5	T38.3X6
Phenglutarimide	T44.3X1	T44.3X2	T44.3X3	T44.3X4	T44.3X5	T44.3X6
Phenicarbazide	T39.8X1	T39.8X2	T39.8X3	T39.8X4	T39.8X5	T39.8X6
Phenindamine	T45.0X1	T45.0X2	T45.0X3	T45.0X4	T45.0X5	T45.0X6
Phenindione	T45.511	T45.512	T45.513	T45.514	T45.515	T45.516
Pheniprazine	T43.1X1	T43.1X2	T43.1X3	T43.1X4	T43.1X5	T43.1X6
Pheniramine	T45.0X1	T45.0X2	T45.0X3	T45.0X4	T45.0X5	T45.0X6
Phenisatin	T47.2X1	T47.2X2	T47.2X3	T47.2X4	T47.2X5	T47.2X6
Phenmetrazine	T50.5X1	T50.5X2	T50.5X3	T50.5X4	T50.5X5	T50.5X6
Phenobal	T42.3X1	T42.3X2	T42.3X3	T42.3X4	T42.3X5	T42.3X6
Phenobarbital	T42.3X1	T42.3X2	T42.3X3	T42.3X4	T42.3X5	T42.3X6
with						
mephenytoin	T42.3X1	T42.3X2	T42.3X3	T42.3X4	T42.3X5	T42.3X6
phenytoin	T42.3X1	T42.3X2	T42.3X3	T42.3X4	T42.3X5	T42.3X6
sodium	T42.3X1	T42.3X2	T42.3X3	T42.3X4	T42.3X5	T42.3X6
Phenobarbitone	T50.8X1	T50.8X2	T50.8X3	T50.8X4	T50.8X5	T50.8X6
Phenobutiodil	T50.8X1	T50.8X2	T50.8X3	T50.8X4	T50.8X5	T50.8X6
Phenoctide	T49.0X1	T49.0X2	T49.0X3	T49.0X4	T49.0X5	T49.0X6
Phenol	T49.0X1	T49.0X2	T49.0X3	T49.0X4	T49.0X5	T49.0X6
disinfectant	T54.0X1	T54.0X2	T54.0X3	T54.0X4	—	—
in oil injection	T46.8X1	T46.8X2	T46.8X3	T46.8X4	T46.8X5	T46.8X6
medicinal	T49.1X1	T49.1X2	T49.1X3	T49.1X4	T49.1X5	T49.1X6
nonmedicinal NEC	T54.0X1	T54.0X2	T54.0X3	T54.0X4	—	—
pesticide	T60.8X1	T60.8X2	T60.8X3	T60.8X4	—	—
red	T50.8X1	T50.8X2	T50.8X3	T50.8X4	T50.8X5	T50.8X6
Phenolic preparation	T49.1X1	T49.1X2	T49.1X3	T49.1X4	T49.1X5	T49.1X6
Phenolphthalein	T47.2X1	T47.2X2	T47.2X3	T47.2X4	T47.2X5	T47.2X6
Phenolsulfonphthalein	T50.8X1	T50.8X2	T50.8X3	T50.8X4	T50.8X5	T50.8X6
Phenomorphan	T40.2X1	T40.2X2	T40.2X3	T40.2X4	—	—
Phenonyl	T42.3X1	T42.3X2	T42.3X3	T42.3X4	T42.3X5	T42.3X6
Phenoperidine	T40.491	T40.492	T40.493	T40.494	—	—
Phenopyrazone	T46.991	T46.992	T46.993	T46.994	T46.995	T46.996
Phenoquin	T50.4X1	T50.4X2	T50.4X3	T50.4X4	T50.4X5	T50.4X6
Phenothiazine (psychotropic)	T43.3X1	T43.3X2	T43.3X3	T43.3X4	T43.3X5	T43.3X6
NEC						
insecticide	T60.2X1	T60.2X2	T60.2X3	T60.2X4	—	—
Phenothrin	T49.0X1	T49.0X2	T49.0X3	T49.0X4	T49.0X5	T49.0X6
Phenoxybenzamine	T46.7X1	T46.7X2	T46.7X3	T46.7X4	T46.7X5	T46.7X6
Phenoxyethanol	T49.0X1	T49.0X2	T49.0X3	T49.0X4	T49.0X5	T49.0X6
Phenoxymethyl penicillin	T36.0X1	T36.0X2	T36.0X3	T36.0X4	T36.0X5	T36.0X6
Phenprobamate	T42.8X1	T42.8X2	T42.8X3	T42.8X4	T42.8X5	T42.8X6
Phenprocoumon	T45.511	T45.512	T45.513	T45.514	T45.515	T45.516
Phensuximide	T42.2X1	T42.2X2	T42.2X3	T42.2X4	T42.2X5	T42.2X6
Phentermine	T50.5X1	T50.5X2	T50.5X3	T50.5X4	T50.5X5	T50.5X6
Phenthicillin	T36.0X1	T36.0X2	T36.0X3	T36.0X4	T36.0X5	T36.0X6
Phentolamine	T46.7X1	T46.7X2	T46.7X3	T46.7X4	T46.7X5	T46.7X6
Phenyl						
butazone	T39.2X1	T39.2X2	T39.2X3	T39.2X4	T39.2X5	T39.2X6
enediamine	T65.3X1	T65.3X2	T65.3X3	T65.3X4	—	—
hydrazine	T65.3X1	T65.3X2	T65.3X3	T65.3X4	—	—
antineoplastic	T45.1X1	T45.1X2	T45.1X3	T45.1X4	T45.1X5	T45.1X6
mercuric compounds — *see* Mercury						
salicylate	T49.3X1	T49.3X2	T49.3X3	T49.3X4	T49.3X5	T49.3X6
Phenylalanine mustard	T45.1X1	T45.1X2	T45.1X3	T45.1X4	T45.1X5	T45.1X6
Phenylbutazone	T39.2X1	T39.2X2	T39.2X3	T39.2X4	T39.2X5	T39.2X6
Phenylenediamine	T65.3X1	T65.3X2	T65.3X3	T65.3X4	—	—
Phenylephrine	T44.4X1	T44.4X2	T44.4X3	T44.4X4	T44.4X5	T44.4X6
Phenylethylbiguanide	T38.3X1	T38.3X2	T38.3X3	T38.3X4	T38.3X5	T38.3X6
Phenylmercuric						
acetate	T49.0X1	T49.0X2	T49.0X3	T49.0X4	T49.0X5	T49.0X6
borate	T49.0X1	T49.0X2	T49.0X3	T49.0X4	T49.0X5	T49.0X6
nitrate	T49.0X1	T49.0X2	T49.0X3	T49.0X4	T49.0X5	T49.0X6
Phenylmethylbarbitone	T42.3X1	T42.3X2	T42.3X3	T42.3X4	T42.3X5	T42.3X6
Phenylpropanol	T47.5X1	T47.5X2	T47.5X3	T47.5X4	T47.5X5	T47.5X6
Phenylpropanolamine	T44.991	T44.992	T44.993	T44.994	T44.995	T44.996
Phenylsulfthion	T60.0X1	T60.0X2	T60.0X3	T60.0X4	—	—
Phenyltoloxamine	T45.0X1	T45.0X2	T45.0X3	T45.0X4	T45.0X5	T45.0X6
Phenyramidol, phenyramidon	T39.8X1	T39.8X2	T39.8X3	T39.8X4	T39.8X5	T39.8X6
Phenytek*	T42.0X1	T42.0X2	T42.0X3	T42.0X4	T42.0X5	T42.0X6
Phenytoin	T42.0X1	T42.0X2	T42.0X3	T42.0X4	T42.0X5	T42.0X6
with Phenobarbital	T42.3X1	T42.3X2	T42.3X3	T42.3X4	T42.3X5	T42.3X6
pHisoHex	T49.2X1	T49.2X2	T49.2X3	T49.2X4	T49.2X5	T49.2X6
Pholcodine	T48.3X1	T48.3X2	T48.3X3	T48.3X4	T48.3X5	T48.3X6
Pholedrine	T46.991	T46.992	T46.993	T46.994	T46.995	T46.996
Phorate	T60.0X1	T60.0X2	T60.0X3	T60.0X4	—	—
Phosdrin	T60.0X1	T60.0X2	T60.0X3	T60.0X4	—	—
Phosfolan	T60.0X1	T60.0X2	T60.0X3	T60.0X4	—	—
Phosgene (gas)	T59.891	T59.892	T59.893	T59.894	—	—
Phosphamidon	T60.0X1	T60.0X2	T60.0X3	T60.0X4	—	—
Phosphate	T65.891	T65.892	T65.893	T65.894	—	—
laxative	T47.4X1	T47.4X2	T47.4X3	T47.4X4	T47.4X5	T47.4X6
organic	T60.0X1	T60.0X2	T60.0X3	T60.0X4	—	—
solvent	T52.91	T52.92	T52.93	T52.94	—	—
tricresyl	T65.891	T65.892	T65.893	T65.894	—	—
Phosphine	T57.1X1	T57.1X2	T57.1X3	T57.1X4	—	—
fumigant	T57.1X1	T57.1X2	T57.1X3	T57.1X4	—	—
Phospholine	T49.5X1	T49.5X2	T49.5X3	T49.5X4	T49.5X5	T49.5X6
Phosphoric acid	T54.2X1	T54.2X2	T54.2X3	T54.2X4	—	—
Phosphorus (compound) NEC	T57.1X1	T57.1X2	T57.1X3	T57.1X4	—	—
pesticide	T60.0X1	T60.0X2	T60.0X3	T60.0X4	—	—
Photrexa*	T49.5X1	T49.5X2	T49.5X3	T49.5X4	T49.5X5	T49.5X6
Phthalates	T65.891	T65.892	T65.893	T65.894	—	—
Phthalic anhydride	T65.891	T65.892	T65.893	T65.894	—	—
Phthalimidoglutarimide	T42.6X1	T42.6X2	T42.6X3	T42.6X4	T42.6X5	T42.6X6
Phthalylsulfathiazole	T37.0X1	T37.0X2	T37.0X3	T37.0X4	T37.0X5	T37.0X6
Phylloquinone	T45.7X1	T45.7X2	T45.7X3	T45.7X4	T45.7X5	T45.7X6
Physeptone	T40.3X1	T40.3X2	T40.3X3	T40.3X4	T40.3X5	T40.3X6
Physostigma venenosum	T62.2X1	T62.2X2	T62.2X3	T62.2X4	—	—
Physostigmine	T49.5X1	T49.5X2	T49.5X3	T49.5X4	T49.5X5	T49.5X6
Phytolacca decandra	T62.2X1	T62.2X2	T62.2X3	T62.2X4	—	—
berries	T62.1X1	T62.1X2	T62.1X3	T62.1X4	—	—
Phytomenadione	T45.7X1	T45.7X2	T45.7X3	T45.7X4	T45.7X5	T45.7X6
Phytonadione	T45.7X1	T45.7X2	T45.7X3	T45.7X4	T45.7X5	T45.7X6
Picoperine	T48.3X1	T48.3X2	T48.3X3	T48.3X4	T48.3X5	T48.3X6
Picosulfate (sodium)	T47.2X1	T47.2X2	T47.2X3	T47.2X4	T47.2X5	T47.2X6
Picric (acid)	T54.2X1	T54.2X2	T54.2X3	T54.2X4	—	—
Picrotoxin	T50.7X1	T50.7X2	T50.7X3	T50.7X4	T50.7X5	T50.7X6
Piketoprofen	T49.0X1	T49.0X2	T49.0X3	T49.0X4	T49.0X5	T49.0X6
Pilocarpine	T44.1X1	T44.1X2	T44.1X3	T44.1X4	T44.1X5	T44.1X6
Pilocarpus (jaborandi)	T44.1X1	T44.1X2	T44.1X3	T44.1X4	T44.1X5	T44.1X6
extract						
Pilsicainide (hydrochloride)	T46.2X1	T46.2X2	T46.2X3	T46.2X4	T46.2X5	T46.2X6
Pimaricin	T36.7X1	T36.7X2	T36.7X3	T36.7X4	T36.7X5	T36.7X6
Pimeclone	T50.7X1	T50.7X2	T50.7X3	T50.7X4	T50.7X5	T50.7X6
Pimelic ketone	T52.8X1	T52.8X2	T52.8X3	T52.8X4	—	—
Pimethixene	T45.0X1	T45.0X2	T45.0X3	T45.0X4	T45.0X5	T45.0X6
Piminodine	T40.2X1	T40.2X2	T40.2X3	T40.2X4	T40.2X5	T40.2X6
Pimozide	T43.591	T43.592	T43.593	T43.594	T43.595	T43.596
Pinacidil	T46.5X1	T46.5X2	T46.5X3	T46.5X4	T46.5X5	T46.5X6
Pinaverium bromide	T44.3X1	T44.3X2	T44.3X3	T44.3X4	T44.3X5	T44.3X6
Pinazepam	T42.4X1	T42.4X2	T42.4X3	T42.4X4	T42.4X5	T42.4X6
Pindolol	T44.7X1	T44.7X2	T44.7X3	T44.7X4	T44.7X5	T44.7X6
Pindone	T60.4X1	T60.4X2	T60.4X3	T60.4X4	—	—
Pine oil (disinfectant)	T65.891	T65.892	T65.893	T65.894	—	—
Pinkroot	T37.4X1	T37.4X2	T37.4X3	T37.4X4	T37.4X5	T37.4X6

Substance	Poisoning, Accidental (unintentional)	Poisoning, Intentional Self-harm	Poisoning, Assault	Poisoning, Undetermined	Adverse Effect	Underdosing
Pipadone	T40.2X1	T40.2X2	T40.2X3	T40.2X4	—	—
Pipamazine	T45.0X1	T45.0X2	T45.0X3	T45.0X4	T45.0X5	T45.0X6
Pipamperone	T43.4X1	T43.4X2	T43.4X3	T43.4X4	T43.4X5	T43.4X6
Pipazetate	T48.3X1	T48.3X2	T48.3X3	T48.3X4	T48.3X5	T48.3X6
Pipemidic acid	T37.8X1	T37.8X2	T37.8X3	T37.8X4	T37.8X5	T37.8X6
Pipenzolate bromide	T44.3X1	T44.3X2	T44.3X3	T44.3X4	T44.3X5	T44.3X6
Piperacetazine	T43.3X1	T43.3X2	T43.3X3	T43.3X4	T43.3X5	T43.3X6
Piperacillin	T36.0X1	T36.0X2	T36.0X3	T36.0X4	T36.0X5	T36.0X6
Piperazine	T37.4X1	T37.4X2	T37.4X3	T37.4X4	T37.4X5	T37.4X6
estrone sulfate	T38.5X1	T38.5X2	T38.5X3	T38.5X4	T38.5X5	T38.5X6
Piper cubeba	T62.2X1	T62.2X2	T62.2X3	T62.2X4	—	—
Piperidione	T48.3X1	T48.3X2	T48.3X3	T48.3X4	T48.3X5	T48.3X6
Piperidolate	T44.3X1	T44.3X2	T44.3X3	T44.3X4	T44.3X5	T44.3X6
Piperocaine	T41.3X1	T41.3X2	T41.3X3	T41.3X4	T41.3X5	T41.3X6
infiltration (subcutaneous)	T41.3X1	T41.3X2	T41.3X3	T41.3X4	T41.3X5	T41.3X6
nerve block (peripheral) (plexus)	T41.3X1	T41.3X2	T41.3X3	T41.3X4	T41.3X5	T41.3X6
topical (surface)	T41.3X1	T41.3X2	T41.3X3	T41.3X4	T41.3X5	T41.3X6
Piperonyl butoxide	T60.8X1	T60.8X2	T60.8X3	T60.8X4	—	—
Pipethanate	T44.3X1	T44.3X2	T44.3X3	T44.3X4	T44.3X5	T44.3X6
Pipobroman	T45.1X1	T45.1X2	T45.1X3	T45.1X4	T45.1X5	T45.1X6
Pipotiazine	T43.3X1	T43.3X2	T43.3X3	T43.3X4	T43.3X5	T43.3X6
Pipoxizine	T45.0X1	T45.0X2	T45.0X3	T45.0X4	T45.0X5	T45.0X6
Pipradrol	T43.691	T43.692	T43.693	T43.694	T43.695	T43.696
Piprinhydrinate	T45.0X1	T45.0X2	T45.0X3	T45.0X4	T45.0X5	T45.0X6
Pirarubicin	T45.1X1	T45.1X2	T45.1X3	T45.1X4	T45.1X5	T45.1X6
Pirazinamide	T37.1X1	T37.1X2	T37.1X3	T37.1X4	T37.1X5	T37.1X6
Pirbuterol	T48.6X1	T48.6X2	T48.6X3	T48.6X4	T48.6X5	T48.6X6
Pirenzepine	T47.1X1	T47.1X2	T47.1X3	T47.1X4	T47.1X5	T47.1X6
Piretanide	T50.1X1	T50.1X2	T50.1X3	T50.1X4	T50.1X5	T50.1X6
Pirfenidone*	T48.991	T48.992	T48.993	T48.994	T48.995	T48.996
Piribedil	T42.8X1	T42.8X2	T42.8X3	T42.8X4	T42.8X5	T42.8X6
Piridoxilate	T46.3X1	T46.3X2	T46.3X3	T46.3X4	T46.3X5	T46.3X6
Piritramide	T40.491	T40.492	T40.493	T40.494	—	—
Piromidic acid	T37.8X1	T37.8X2	T37.8X3	T37.8X4	T37.8X5	T37.8X6
Piroxicam	T39.391	T39.392	T39.393	T39.394	T39.395	T39.396
beta-cyclodextrin complex	T39.8X1	T39.8X2	T39.8X3	T39.8X4	T39.8X5	T39.8X6
Pirozadil	T46.6X1	T46.6X2	T46.6X3	T46.6X4	T46.6X5	T46.6X6
Piscidia (bark) (erythrina)	T39.8X1	T39.8X2	T39.8X3	T39.8X4	T39.8X5	T39.8X6
Pitch	T65.891	T65.892	T65.893	T65.894	—	—
Pitkin's solution	T41.3X1	T41.3X2	T41.3X3	T41.3X4	T41.3X5	T41.3X6
Pitocin	T48.0X1	T48.0X2	T48.0X3	T48.0X4	T48.0X5	T48.0X6
Pitressin (tannate)	T38.891	T38.892	T38.893	T38.894	T38.895	T38.896
Pituitary extracts (posterior)	T38.891	T38.892	T38.893	T38.894	T38.895	T38.896
anterior	T38.811	T38.812	T38.813	T38.814	T38.815	T38.816
Pituitrin	T38.891	T38.892	T38.893	T38.894	T38.895	T38.896
Pivampicillin	T36.0X1	T36.0X2	T36.0X3	T36.0X4	T36.0X5	T36.0X6
Pivmecillinam	T36.0X1	T36.0X2	T36.0X3	T36.0X4	T36.0X5	T36.0X6
Placental hormone	T38.891	T38.892	T38.893	T38.894	T38.895	T38.896
Placidyl	T42.6X1	T42.6X2	T42.6X3	T42.6X4	T42.6X5	T42.6X6
Plague vaccine	T50.A91	T50.A92	T50.A93	T50.A94	T50.A95	T50.A96
Plant						
food or fertilizer NEC	T65.891	T65.892	T65.893	T65.894	—	—
containing herbicide	T60.3X1	T60.3X2	T60.3X3	T60.3X4	—	—
noxious, used as food	T62.2X1	T62.2X2	T62.2X3	T62.2X4	—	—
berries	T62.1X1	T62.1X2	T62.1X3	T62.1X4	—	—
seeds	T62.2X1	T62.2X2	T62.2X3	T62.2X4	—	—
specified type NEC	T62.2X1	T62.2X2	T62.2X3	T62.2X4	—	—
Plasma	T45.8X1	T45.8X2	T45.8X3	T45.8X4	T45.8X5	T45.8X6
expander NEC	T45.8X1	T45.8X2	T45.8X3	T45.8X4	T45.8X5	T45.8X6
protein fraction (human)	T45.8X1	T45.8X2	T45.8X3	T45.8X4	T45.8X5	T45.8X6
Plasmanate	T45.8X1	T45.8X2	T45.8X3	T45.8X4	T45.8X5	T45.8X6
Plasminogen (tissue) activator	T45.611	T45.612	T45.613	T45.614	T45.615	T45.616
Plaster dressing	T49.3X1	T49.3X2	T49.3X3	T49.3X4	T49.3X5	T49.3X6
Plastic dressing	T49.3X1	T49.3X2	T49.3X3	T49.3X4	T49.3X5	T49.3X6
Plavix*	T45.521	T45.522	T45.523	T45.524	T45.525	T45.526
Plegicil	T43.3X1	T43.3X2	T43.3X3	T43.3X4	T43.3X5	T43.3X6
Plicamycin	T45.1X1	T45.1X2	T45.1X3	T45.1X4	T45.1X5	T45.1X6
Podophyllotoxin	T49.8X1	T49.8X2	T49.8X3	T49.8X4	T49.8X5	T49.8X6
Podophyllum (resin)	T49.4X1	T49.4X2	T49.4X3	T49.4X4	T49.4X5	T49.4X6
Poisonous berries	T62.1X1	T62.1X2	T62.1X3	T62.1X4	—	—
Poison NEC	T65.91	T65.92	T65.93	T65.94	—	—
Pokeweed (any part)	T62.2X1	T62.2X2	T62.2X3	T62.2X4	—	—
Poldine metilsulfate	T44.3X1	T44.3X2	T44.3X3	T44.3X4	T44.3X5	T44.3X6
Polidexide (sulfate)	T46.6X1	T46.6X2	T46.6X3	T46.6X4	T46.6X5	T46.6X6
Polidocanol	T46.8X1	T46.8X2	T46.8X3	T46.8X4	T46.8X5	T46.8X6
Poliomyelitis vaccine	T50.B91	T50.B92	T50.B93	T50.B94	T50.B95	T50.B96
Polish (car) (floor) (furniture) (metal) (porcelain) (silver)	T65.891	T65.892	T65.893	T65.894	—	—
abrasive	T65.891	T65.892	T65.893	T65.894	—	—

Substance	Poisoning, Accidental (unintentional)	Poisoning, Intentional Self-harm	Poisoning, Assault	Poisoning, Undetermined	Adverse Effect	Underdosing
Polish — continued						
porcelain	T65.891	T65.892	T65.893	T65.894	—	—
Poloxalkol	T47.4X1	T47.4X2	T47.4X3	T47.4X4	T47.4X5	T47.4X6
Poloxamer	T47.4X1	T47.4X2	T47.4X3	T47.4X4	T47.4X5	T47.4X6
Polyaminostyrene resins	T50.3X1	T50.3X2	T50.3X3	T50.3X4	T50.3X5	T50.3X6
Polycarbophil	T47.4X1	T47.4X2	T47.4X3	T47.4X4	T47.4X5	T47.4X6
Polychlorinated biphenyl	T65.891	T65.892	T65.893	T65.894	—	—
Polycycline	T36.4X1	T36.4X2	T36.4X3	T36.4X4	T36.4X5	T36.4X6
Polyester fumes	T59.891	T59.892	T59.893	T59.894	—	—
Polyester resin hardener	T52.91	T52.92	T52.93	T52.94	—	—
fumes	T59.891	T59.892	T59.893	T59.894	—	—
Polyestradiol phosphate	T38.5X1	T38.5X2	T38.5X3	T38.5X4	T38.5X5	T38.5X6
Polyethanolamine alkyl sulfate	T49.2X1	T49.2X2	T49.2X3	T49.2X4	T49.2X5	T49.2X6
Polyethylene adhesive	T49.3X1	T49.3X2	T49.3X3	T49.3X4	T49.3X5	T49.3X6
Polyferose	T45.4X1	T45.4X2	T45.4X3	T45.4X4	T45.4X5	T45.4X6
Polygeline	T45.8X1	T45.8X2	T45.8X3	T45.8X4	T45.8X5	T45.8X6
Polymyxin	T36.8X1	T36.8X2	T36.8X3	T36.8X4	T36.8X5	T36.8X6
B	T36.8X1	T36.8X2	T36.8X3	T36.8X4	T36.8X5	T36.8X6
ENT agent	T49.6X1	T49.6X2	T49.6X3	T49.6X4	T49.6X5	T49.6X6
ophthalmic preparation	T49.5X1	T49.5X2	T49.5X3	T49.5X4	T49.5X5	T49.5X6
topical NEC	T49.0X1	T49.0X2	T49.0X3	T49.0X4	T49.0X5	T49.0X6
E sulfate (eye preparation)	T49.5X1	T49.5X2	T49.5X3	T49.5X4	T49.5X5	T49.5X6
Polynoxylin	T49.0X1	T49.0X2	T49.0X3	T49.0X4	T49.0X5	T49.0X6
Polyoestradiol phosphate	T38.5X1	T38.5X2	T38.5X3	T38.5X4	T38.5X5	T38.5X6
Polyoxymethyleneurea	T49.0X1	T49.0X2	T49.0X3	T49.0X4	T49.0X5	T49.0X6
Poly-Pred*	T49.5X1	T49.5X2	T49.5X3	T49.5X4	T49.5X5	T49.5X6
Polysilane	T47.8X1	T47.8X2	T47.8X3	T47.8X4	T47.8X5	T47.8X6
Polytetrafluoroethylene (inhaled)	T59.891	T59.892	T59.893	T59.894	—	—
Polythiazide	T50.2X1	T50.2X2	T50.2X3	T50.2X4	T50.2X5	T50.2X6
Polyvidone	T45.8X1	T45.8X2	T45.8X3	T45.8X4	T45.8X5	T45.8X6
Polyvinylpyrrolidone	T45.8X1	T45.8X2	T45.8X3	T45.8X4	T45.8X5	T45.8X6
Pontocaine (hydrochloride) (infiltration) (topical)	T41.3X1	T41.3X2	T41.3X3	T41.3X4	T41.3X5	T41.3X6
nerve block (peripheral) (plexus)	T41.3X1	T41.3X2	T41.3X3	T41.3X4	T41.3X5	T41.3X6
spinal	T41.3X1	T41.3X2	T41.3X3	T41.3X4	T41.3X5	T41.3X6
Porfiromycin	T45.1X1	T45.1X2	T45.1X3	T45.1X4	T45.1X5	T45.1X6
Portactant alfa*	T48.991	T48.992	T48.993	T48.994	T48.995	T48.996
Posterior pituitary hormone NEC	T38.891	T38.892	T38.893	T38.894	T38.895	T38.896
Pot	T40.711	T40.712	T40.713	T40.714	T40.715	T40.716
Potash (caustic)	T54.3X1	T54.3X2	T54.3X3	T54.3X4	—	—
Potassic saline injection (lactated)	T50.3X1	T50.3X2	T50.3X3	T50.3X4	T50.3X5	T50.3X6
Potassium (salts) NEC	T50.3X1	T50.3X2	T50.3X3	T50.3X4	T50.3X5	T50.3X6
aminobenzoate	T45.8X1	T45.8X2	T45.8X3	T45.8X4	T45.8X5	T45.8X6
aminosalicylate	T37.1X1	T37.1X2	T37.1X3	T37.1X4	T37.1X5	T37.1X6
antimony ' tartrate'	T37.8X1	T37.8X2	T37.8X3	T37.8X4	T37.8X5	T37.8X6
arsenite (solution)	T57.0X1	T57.0X2	T57.0X3	T57.0X4	—	—
bichromate	T56.2X1	T56.2X2	T56.2X3	T56.2X4	—	—
bisulfate	T47.3X1	T47.3X2	T47.3X3	T47.3X4	T47.3X5	T47.3X6
bromide	T42.6X1	T42.6X2	T42.6X3	T42.6X4	T42.6X5	T42.6X6
canrenoate	T50.0X1	T50.0X2	T50.0X3	T50.0X4	T50.0X5	T50.0X6
carbonate	T54.3X1	T54.3X2	T54.3X3	T54.3X4	—	—
chlorate NEC	T65.891	T65.892	T65.893	T65.894	—	—
chloride	T50.3X1	T50.3X2	T50.3X3	T50.3X4	T50.3X5	T50.3X6
citrate	T50.991	T50.992	T50.993	T50.994	T50.995	T50.996
cyanide	T65.0X1	T65.0X2	T65.0X3	T65.0X4	—	—
ferric hexacyanoferrate (medicinal)	T50.6X1	T50.6X2	T50.6X3	T50.6X4	T50.6X5	T50.6X6
nonmedicinal	T65.891	T65.892	T65.893	T65.894	—	—
Fluoride	T57.8X1	T57.8X2	T57.8X3	T57.8X4	—	—
glucaldrate	T47.1X1	T47.1X2	T47.1X3	T47.1X4	T47.1X5	T47.1X6
hydroxide	T54.3X1	T54.3X2	T54.3X3	T54.3X4	—	—
iodate	T49.0X1	T49.0X2	T49.0X3	T49.0X4	T49.0X5	T49.0X6
iodide	T48.4X1	T48.4X2	T48.4X3	T48.4X4	T48.4X5	T48.4X6
nitrate	T57.8X1	T57.8X2	T57.8X3	T57.8X4	—	—
oxalate	T65.891	T65.892	T65.893	T65.894	—	—
perchlorate (nonmedicinal) NEC	T65.891	T65.892	T65.893	T65.894	—	—
antithyroid	T38.2X1	T38.2X2	T38.2X3	T38.2X4	T38.2X5	T38.2X6
medicinal	T38.2X1	T38.2X2	T38.2X3	T38.2X4	T38.2X5	T38.2X6
Permanganate (nonmedicinal)	T65.891	T65.892	T65.893	T65.894	—	—
medicinal	T49.0X1	T49.0X2	T49.0X3	T49.0X4	T49.0X5	T49.0X6
sulfate	T47.2X1	T47.2X2	T47.2X3	T47.2X4	T47.2X5	T47.2X6
Potassium-removing resin	T50.3X1	T50.3X2	T50.3X3	T50.3X4	T50.3X5	T50.3X6
Potassium-retaining drug	T50.3X1	T50.3X2	T50.3X3	T50.3X4	T50.3X5	T50.3X6
Povidone	T45.8X1	T45.8X2	T45.8X3	T45.8X4	T45.8X5	T45.8X6
iodine	T49.0X1	T49.0X2	T49.0X3	T49.0X4	T49.0X5	T49.0X6
Practolol	T44.7X1	T44.7X2	T44.7X3	T44.7X4	T44.7X5	T44.7X6

Substance	Poisoning, Accidental (unintentional)	Poisoning, Intentional Self-harm	Poisoning, Assault	Poisoning, Undetermined	Adverse Effect	Under-dosing
Prajmalium bitartrate	T46.2X1	T46.2X2	T46.2X3	T46.2X4	T46.2X5	T46.2X6
Pralidoxime (iodide)	T50.6X1	T50.6X2	T50.6X3	T50.6X4	T50.6X5	T50.6X6
chloride	T50.6X1	T50.6X2	T50.6X3	T50.6X4	T50.6X5	T50.6X6
Pramiverine	T44.3X1	T44.3X2	T44.3X3	T44.3X4	T44.3X5	T44.3X6
Pramlintide*	T38.3X1	T38.3X2	T38.3X3	T38.3X4	T38.3X5	T38.3X6
Pramocaine	T49.1X1	T49.1X2	T49.1X3	T49.1X4	T49.1X5	T49.1X6
Pramoxine	T49.1X1	T49.1X2	T49.1X3	T49.1X4	T49.1X5	T49.1X6
Prasterone	T38.7X1	T38.7X2	T38.7X3	T38.7X4	T38.7X5	T38.7X6
Pravachol*	T46.6X1	T46.6X2	T46.6X3	T46.6X4	T46.6X5	T46.6X6
Pravastatin	T46.6X1	T46.6X2	T46.6X3	T46.6X4	T46.6X5	T46.6X6
Prazepam	T42.4X1	T42.4X2	T42.4X3	T42.4X4	T42.4X5	T42.4X6
Praziquantel	T37.4X1	T37.4X2	T37.4X3	T37.4X4	T37.4X5	T37.4X6
Prazitone	T43.291	T43.292	T43.293	T43.294	T43.295	T43.296
Prazosin	T44.6X1	T44.6X2	T44.6X3	T44.6X4	T44.6X5	T44.6X6
Prednicarbate	T49.0X1	T49.0X2	T49.0X3	T49.0X4	T49.0X5	T49.0X6
Prednimustine	T45.1X1	T45.1X2	T45.1X3	T45.1X4	T45.1X5	T45.1X6
Prednisolone	T38.0X1	T38.0X2	T38.0X3	T38.0X4	T38.0X5	T38.0X6
ENT agent	T49.6X1	T49.6X2	T49.6X3	T49.6X4	T49.6X5	T49.6X6
ophthalmic preparation	T49.5X1	T49.5X2	T49.5X3	T49.5X4	T49.5X5	T49.5X6
steaglate	T49.0X1	T49.0X2	T49.0X3	T49.0X4	T49.0X5	T49.0X6
topical NEC	T49.0X1	T49.0X2	T49.0X3	T49.0X4	T49.0X5	T49.0X6
Prednisone	T38.0X1	T38.0X2	T38.0X3	T38.0X4	T38.0X5	T38.0X6
Prednylidene	T38.0X1	T38.0X2	T38.0X3	T38.0X4	T38.0X5	T38.0X6
Pregnandiol	T38.5X1	T38.5X2	T38.5X3	T38.5X4	T38.5X5	T38.5X6
Pregneninolone	T38.5X1	T38.5X2	T38.5X3	T38.5X4	T38.5X5	T38.5X6
Preludin	T43.691	T43.692	T43.693	T43.694	T43.695	T43.696
Premarin	T38.5X1	T38.5X2	T38.5X3	T38.5X4	T38.5X5	T38.5X6
Premedication anesthetic	T41.201	T41.202	T41.203	T41.204	T41.205	T41.206
Prenalterol	T44.5X1	T44.5X2	T44.5X3	T44.5X4	T44.5X5	T44.5X6
Prenoxdiazine	T48.3X1	T48.3X2	T48.3X3	T48.3X4	T48.3X5	T48.3X6
Prenylamine	T46.3X1	T46.3X2	T46.3X3	T46.3X4	T46.3X5	T46.3X6
Preparation H	T49.8X1	T49.8X2	T49.8X3	T49.8X4	T49.8X5	T49.8X6
Preparation, local	T49.4X1	T49.4X2	T49.4X3	T49.4X4	T49.4X5	T49.4X6
Preservative	T65.891	T65.892	T65.893	T65.894	—	—
(nonmedicinal)						
medicinal	T50.901	T50.902	T50.903	T50.904	T50.905	T50.906
wood	T60.91	T60.92	T60.93	T60.94	—	—
Prethcamide	T50.7X1	T50.7X2	T50.7X3	T50.7X4	T50.7X5	T50.7X6
Prevacid*	T47.1X1	T47.1X2	T47.1X3	T47.1X4	T47.1X5	T47.1X6
Pride of China	T62.2X1	T62.2X2	T62.2X3	T62.2X4	—	—
Pridinol	T44.3X1	T44.3X2	T44.3X3	T44.3X4	T44.3X5	T44.3X6
Prifinium bromide	T44.3X1	T44.3X2	T44.3X3	T44.3X4	T44.3X5	T44.3X6
Prilocaine	T41.3X1	T41.3X2	T41.3X3	T41.3X4	T41.3X5	T41.3X6
infiltration (subcutaneous)	T41.3X1	T41.3X2	T41.3X3	T41.3X4	T41.3X5	T41.3X6
nerve block (peripheral)	T41.3X1	T41.3X2	T41.3X3	T41.3X4	T41.3X5	T41.3X6
(plexus)						
regional	T41.3X1	T41.3X2	T41.3X3	T41.3X4	T41.3X5	T41.3X6
Prilosec*	T47.1X1	T47.1X2	T47.1X3	T47.1X4	T47.1X5	T47.1X6
Primaquine	T37.2X1	T37.2X2	T37.2X3	T37.2X4	T37.2X5	T37.2X6
Primidone	T42.6X1	T42.6X2	T42.6X3	T42.6X4	T42.6X5	T42.6X6
Primula (veris)	T62.2X1	T62.2X2	T62.2X3	T62.2X4	—	—
Prinadol	T40.2X1	T40.2X2	T40.2X3	T40.2X4	T40.2X5	T40.2X6
Prinivil*	T46.4X1	T46.4X2	T46.4X3	T46.4X4	T46.4X5	T46.4X6
Priscol, Priscoline	T44.6X1	T44.6X2	T44.6X3	T44.6X4	T44.6X5	T44.6X6
Pristinamycin	T36.3X1	T36.3X2	T36.3X3	T36.3X4	T36.3X5	T36.3X6
Pristiq*	T43.211	T43.212	T43.213	T43.214	T43.215	T43.216
Privet	T62.2X1	T62.2X2	T62.2X3	T62.2X4	—	—
berries	T62.1X1	T62.1X2	T62.1X3	T62.1X4	—	—
Privine	T44.4X1	T44.4X2	T44.4X3	T44.4X4	T44.4X5	T44.4X6
Pro-Banthine	T44.3X1	T44.3X2	T44.3X3	T44.3X4	T44.3X5	T44.3X6
Probarbital	T42.3X1	T42.3X2	T42.3X3	T42.3X4	T42.3X5	T42.3X6
Probenecid	T50.4X1	T50.4X2	T50.4X3	T50.4X4	T50.4X5	T50.4X6
Probucol	T46.6X1	T46.6X2	T46.6X3	T46.6X4	T46.6X5	T46.6X6
Procainamide	T46.2X1	T46.2X2	T46.2X3	T46.2X4	T46.2X5	T46.2X6
Procaine	T41.3X1	T41.3X2	T41.3X3	T41.3X4	T41.3X5	T41.3X6
benzylpenicillin	T36.0X1	T36.0X2	T36.0X3	T36.0X4	T36.0X5	T36.0X6
nerve block (periphreal)	T41.3X1	T41.3X2	T41.3X3	T41.3X4	T41.3X5	T41.3X6
(plexus)						
penicillin G	T36.0X1	T36.0X2	T36.0X3	T36.0X4	T36.0X5	T36.0X6
regional	T41.3X1	T41.3X2	T41.3X3	T41.3X4	T41.3X5	T41.3X6
spinal	T41.3X1	T41.3X2	T41.3X3	T41.3X4	T41.3X5	T41.3X6
Procalmidol	T43.591	T43.592	T43.593	T43.594	T43.595	T43.596
Procarbazine	T45.1X1	T45.1X2	T45.1X3	T45.1X4	T45.1X5	T45.1X6
Procaterol	T44.5X1	T44.5X2	T44.5X3	T44.5X4	T44.5X5	T44.5X6
Prochlorperazine	T43.3X1	T43.3X2	T43.3X3	T43.3X4	T43.3X5	T43.3X6
Procyclidine	T44.3X1	T44.3X2	T44.3X3	T44.3X4	T44.3X5	T44.3X6
Producer gas	T58.8X1	T58.8X2	T58.8X3	T58.8X4	—	—
Profadol	T40.491	T40.492	T40.493	T40.494	T40.495	T40.496
Profenamine	T44.3X1	T44.3X2	T44.3X3	T44.3X4	T44.3X5	T44.3X6
Profenil	T44.3X1	T44.3X2	T44.3X3	T44.3X4	T44.3X5	T44.3X6
Proflavine	T49.0X1	T49.0X2	T49.0X3	T49.0X4	T49.0X5	T49.0X6
Progabide	T42.6X1	T42.6X2	T42.6X3	T42.6X4	T42.6X5	T42.6X6
Progesterone	T38.5X1	T38.5X2	T38.5X3	T38.5X4	T38.5X5	T38.5X6
Progestin	T38.5X1	T38.5X2	T38.5X3	T38.5X4	T38.5X5	T38.5X6
oral contraceptive	T38.4X1	T38.4X2	T38.4X3	T38.4X4	T38.4X5	T38.4X6
Progestogen NEC	T38.5X1	T38.5X2	T38.5X3	T38.5X4	T38.5X5	T38.5X6
Progestone	T38.5X1	T38.5X2	T38.5X3	T38.5X4	T38.5X5	T38.5X6
Proglumide	T47.1X1	T47.1X2	T47.1X3	T47.1X4	T47.1X5	T47.1X6
Prograf*	T45.1X1	T45.1X2	T45.1X3	T45.1X4	T45.1X5	T45.1X6
Proguanil	T37.2X1	T37.2X2	T37.2X3	T37.2X4	T37.2X5	T37.2X6
Prolactin	T38.811	T38.812	T38.813	T38.814	T38.815	T38.816
Prolintane	T43.691	T43.692	T43.693	T43.694	T43.695	T43.696
Proloid	T38.1X1	T38.1X2	T38.1X3	T38.1X4	T38.1X5	T38.1X6
Proluton	T38.5X1	T38.5X2	T38.5X3	T38.5X4	T38.5X5	T38.5X6
Promacetin	T37.1X1	T37.1X2	T37.1X3	T37.1X4	T37.1X5	T37.1X6
Promazine	T43.3X1	T43.3X2	T43.3X3	T43.3X4	T43.3X5	T43.3X6
Promedol	T40.2X1	T40.2X2	T40.2X3	T40.2X4	—	T38.5X6
Promegestone	T38.5X1	T38.5X2	T38.5X3	T38.5X4	T38.5X5	T38.5X6
Promethazine (teoclate)	T43.3X1	T43.3X2	T43.3X3	T43.3X4	T43.3X5	T43.3X6
Promin	T37.1X1	T37.1X2	T37.1X3	T37.1X4	T37.1X5	T37.1X6
Pronase	T45.3X1	T45.3X2	T45.3X3	T45.3X4	T45.3X5	T45.3X6
Pronestyl (hydrochloride)	T46.2X1	T46.2X2	T46.2X3	T46.2X4	T46.2X5	T46.2X6
Pronetalol	T44.7X1	T44.7X2	T44.7X3	T44.7X4	T44.7X5	T44.7X6
Prontosil	T37.0X1	T37.0X2	T37.0X3	T37.0X4	T37.0X5	T37.0X6
Propachlor	T60.3X1	T60.3X2	T60.3X3	T60.3X4	—	—
Propafenone	T46.2X1	T46.2X2	T46.2X3	T46.2X4	T46.2X5	T46.2X6
Propallylonal	T42.3X1	T42.3X2	T42.3X3	T42.3X4	T42.3X5	T42.3X6
Propamidine	T49.0X1	T49.0X2	T49.0X3	T49.0X4	T49.0X5	T49.0X6
Propane (distributed in mobile	T59.891	T59.892	T59.893	T59.894	—	—
container)						
distributed through pipes	T59.891	T59.892	T59.893	T59.894	—	—
incomplete combustion	T58.11	T58.12	T58.13	T58.14	—	—
Propanidid	T41.291	T41.292	T41.293	T41.294	T41.295	T41.296
Propanil	T60.3X1	T60.3X2	T60.3X3	T60.3X4	—	—
Propantheline	T44.3X1	T44.3X2	T44.3X3	T44.3X4	T44.3X5	T44.3X6
bromide	T44.3X1	T44.3X2	T44.3X3	T44.3X4	T44.3X5	T44.3X6
Proparacaine	T41.3X1	T41.3X2	T41.3X3	T41.3X4	T41.3X5	T41.3X6
Propatylnitrate	T46.3X1	T46.3X2	T46.3X3	T46.3X4	T46.3X5	T46.3X6
Propicillin	T36.0X1	T36.0X2	T36.0X3	T36.0X4	T36.0X5	T36.0X6
Propine*	T49.5X1	T49.5X2	T49.5X3	T49.5X4	T49.5X5	T49.5X6
Propiolactone	T49.0X1	T49.0X2	T49.0X3	T49.0X4	T49.0X5	T49.0X6
Propiomazine	T45.0X1	T45.0X2	T45.0X3	T45.0X4	T45.0X5	T45.0X6
Propionaldehyde	T42.6X1	T42.6X2	T42.6X3	T42.6X4	T42.6X5	T42.6X6
(medicinal)						
Propionate (calcium)	T49.0X1	T49.0X2	T49.0X3	T49.0X4	T49.0X5	T49.0X6
(sodium)						
Propion gel	T49.0X1	T49.0X2	T49.0X3	T49.0X4	T49.0X5	T49.0X6
Propitocaine	T41.3X1	T41.3X2	T41.3X3	T41.3X4	T41.3X5	T41.3X6
infiltration (subcutaneous)	T41.3X1	T41.3X2	T41.3X3	T41.3X4	T41.3X5	T41.3X6
nerve block (peripheral)	T41.3X1	T41.3X2	T41.3X3	T41.3X4	T41.3X5	T41.3X6
(plexus)						
Propofol	T41.291	T41.292	T41.293	T41.294	T41.295	T41.296
Propoxur	T60.0X1	T60.0X2	T60.0X3	T60.0X4	—	—
Propoxycaine	T41.3X1	T41.3X2	T41.3X3	T41.3X4	T41.3X5	T41.3X6
infiltration (subcutaneous)	T41.3X1	T41.3X2	T41.3X3	T41.3X4	T41.3X5	T41.3X6
nerve block (peripheral)	T41.3X1	T41.3X2	T41.3X3	T41.3X4	T41.3X5	T41.3X6
(plexus)						
topical (surface)	T41.3X1	T41.3X2	T41.3X3	T41.3X4	T41.3X5	T41.3X6
Propoxyphene	T40.491	T40.492	T40.493	T40.494	T40.495	T40.496
Propranolol	T44.7X1	T44.7X2	T44.7X3	T44.7X4	T44.7X5	T44.7X6
Propyl						
alcohol	T51.3X1	T51.3X2	T51.3X3	T51.3X4	—	—
carbinol	T51.3X1	T51.3X2	T51.3X3	T51.3X4	—	—
hexadrine	T44.4X1	T44.4X2	T44.4X3	T44.4X4	T44.4X5	T44.4X6
iodone	T50.8X1	T50.8X2	T50.8X3	T50.8X4	T50.8X5	T50.8X6
thiouracil	T38.2X1	T38.2X2	T38.2X3	T38.2X4	T38.2X5	T38.2X6
Propylaminophenothiazine	T43.3X1	T43.3X2	T43.3X3	T43.3X4	T43.3X5	T43.3X6
Propylene	T59.891	T59.892	T59.893	T59.894	—	—
Propylhexedrine	T48.5X1	T48.5X2	T48.5X3	T48.5X4	T48.5X5	T48.5X6
Propyliodone	T50.8X1	T50.8X2	T50.8X3	T50.8X4	T50.8X5	T50.8X6
Propylparaben	T49.5X1	T49.5X2	T49.5X3	T49.5X4	T49.5X5	T49.5X6
(ophthalmic)						
Propylthiouracil	T38.2X1	T38.2X2	T38.2X3	T38.2X4	T38.2X5	T38.2X6
Propyphenazone	T39.2X1	T39.2X2	T39.2X3	T39.2X4	T39.2X5	T39.2X6
Proquazone	T39.391	T39.392	T39.393	T39.394	T39.395	T39.396
Proscar*	T38.6X1	T38.6X2	T38.6X3	T38.6X4	T38.6X5	T38.6X6
Proscillaridin	T46.0X1	T46.0X2	T46.0X3	T46.0X4	T46.0X5	T46.0X6
Prostacyclin	T45.521	T45.522	T45.523	T45.524	T45.525	T45.526
Prostaglandin (I2)	T45.521	T45.522	T45.523	T45.524	T45.525	T45.526
E1	T46.7X1	T46.7X2	T46.7X3	T46.7X4	T46.7X5	T46.7X6
E2	T48.0X1	T48.0X2	T48.0X3	T48.0X4	T48.0X5	T48.0X6
F2 alpha	T48.0X1	T48.0X2	T48.0X3	T48.0X4	T48.0X5	T48.0X6
Prostigmin	T44.0X1	T44.0X2	T44.0X3	T44.0X4	T44.0X5	T44.0X6
Prosultiamine	T45.2X1	T45.2X2	T45.2X3	T45.2X4	T45.2X5	T45.2X6
Protamine sulfate	T45.7X1	T45.7X2	T45.7X3	T45.7X4	T45.7X5	T45.7X6
zinc insulin	T38.3X1	T38.3X2	T38.3X3	T38.3X4	T38.3X5	T38.3X6

☑ **Additional Character May Be Required — Refer to the Tabular List for Character Selection**

*Optum Value-Add

Substance	Poisoning, Accidental (unintentional)	Poisoning, Intentional Self-harm	Poisoning, Assault	Poisoning, Undetermined	Adverse Effect	Underdosing
Protease	T47.5X1	T47.5X2	T47.5X3	T47.5X4	T47.5X5	T47.5X6
Protectant, skin NEC	T49.3X1	T49.3X2	T49.3X3	T49.3X4	T49.3X5	T49.3X6
Protein hydrolysate	T50.991	T50.992	T50.993	T50.994	T50.995	T50.996
Prothiaden — see Dothiepin hydrochloride						
Prothionamide	T37.1X1	T37.1X2	T37.1X3	T37.1X4	T37.1X5	T37.1X6
Prothipendyl	T43.591	T43.592	T43.593	T43.594	T43.595	T43.596
Prothoate	T60.0X1	T60.0X2	T60.0X3	T60.0X4	—	—
Prothrombin						
activator	T45.7X1	T45.7X2	T45.7X3	T45.7X4	T45.7X5	T45.7X6
synthesis inhibitor	T45.511	T45.512	T45.513	T45.514	T45.515	T45.516
Protionamide	T37.1X1	T37.1X2	T37.1X3	T37.1X4	T37.1X5	T37.1X6
Protirelin	T38.891	T38.892	T38.893	T38.894	T38.895	T38.896
Protokylol	T48.6X1	T48.6X2	T48.6X3	T48.6X4	T48.6X5	T48.6X6
Protonix*	T47.1X1	T47.1X2	T47.1X3	T47.1X4	T47.1X5	T47.1X6
Protopam	T50.6X1	T50.6X2	T50.6X3	T50.6X4	T50.6X5	T50.6X6
Protoveratrine(s) (A) (B)	T46.5X1	T46.5X2	T46.5X3	T46.5X4	T46.5X5	T46.5X6
Protriptyline	T43.011	T43.012	T43.013	T43.014	T43.015	T43.016
Proventil*	T48.6X1	T48.6X2	T48.6X3	T48.6X4	T48.6X5	T48.6X6
Provera	T38.5X1	T38.5X2	T38.5X3	T38.5X4	T38.5X5	T38.5X6
Provitamin A	T45.2X1	T45.2X2	T45.2X3	T45.2X4	T45.2X5	T45.2X6
Proxibarbal	T42.3X1	T42.3X2	T42.3X3	T42.3X4	T42.3X5	T42.3X6
Proxymetacaine	T41.3X1	T41.3X2	T41.3X3	T41.3X4	T41.3X5	T41.3X6
Proxyphylline	T48.6X1	T48.6X2	T48.6X3	T48.6X4	T48.6X5	T48.6X6
Prozac — see Fluoxetine hydrochloride						
Prunus						
laurocerasus	T62.2X1	T62.2X2	T62.2X3	T62.2X4	—	—
virginiana	T62.2X1	T62.2X2	T62.2X3	T62.2X4	—	—
Prussian blue						
commercial	T65.891	T65.892	T65.893	T65.894	—	—
therapeutic	T50.6X1	T50.6X2	T50.6X3	T50.6X4	T50.6X5	T50.6X6
Prussic acid	T65.0X1	T65.0X2	T65.0X3	T65.0X4	—	—
vapor	T57.3X1	T57.3X2	T57.3X3	T57.3X4	—	—
Pseudoephedrine	T44.991	T44.992	T44.993	T44.994	T44.995	T44.996
Psilocin	T40.991	T40.992	T40.993	T40.994	—	—
Psilocybin	T40.991	T40.992	T40.993	T40.994	—	—
Psilocybine	T40.991	T40.992	T40.993	T40.994	—	—
Psoralene (nonmedicinal)	T65.891	T65.892	T65.893	T65.894	—	—
Psoralens (medicinal)	T50.991	T50.992	T50.993	T50.994	T50.995	T50.996
PSP (phenolsulfonphthalein)	T50.8X1	T50.8X2	T50.8X3	T50.8X4	T50.8X5	T50.8X6
Psychodysleptic drug NOS	T40.901	T40.902	T40.903	T40.904	T40.905	T40.906
specified NEC	T40.991	T40.992	T40.993	T40.994	T40.995	T40.996
Psychostimulant	T43.601	T43.602	T43.603	T43.604	T43.605	T43.606
amphetamine	T43.621	T43.622	T43.623	T43.624	T43.625	T43.626
caffeine	T43.611	T43.612	T43.613	T43.614	T43.615	T43.616
methylphenidate	T43.631	T43.632	T43.633	T43.634	T43.635	T43.636
specified NEC	T43.691	T43.692	T43.693	T43.694	T43.695	T43.696
Psychotherapeutic drug NEC	T43.91	T43.92	T43.93	T43.94	T43.95	T43.96
antidepressants — see also Antidepressant	T43.201	T43.202	T43.203	T43.204	T43.205	T43.206
specified NEC	T43.8X1	T43.8X2	T43.8X3	T43.8X4	T43.8X5	T43.8X6
tranquilizers NEC	T43.501	T43.502	T43.503	T43.504	T43.505	T43.506
Psychotomimetic agents	T40.901	T40.902	T40.903	T40.904	T40.905	T40.906
Psychotropic drug NEC	T43.91	T43.92	T43.93	T43.94	T43.95	T43.96
specified NEC	T43.8X1	T43.8X2	T43.8X3	T43.8X4	T43.8X5	T43.8X6
Psyllium hydrophilic mucilloid	T47.4X1	T47.4X2	T47.4X3	T47.4X4	T47.4X5	T47.4X6
Pteroylglutamic acid	T45.8X1	T45.8X2	T45.8X3	T45.8X4	T45.8X5	T45.8X6
Pteroyltriglutamate	T45.1X1	T45.1X2	T45.1X3	T45.1X4	T45.1X5	T45.1X6
PTFE — see Polytetrafluoroethylene						
Pulmicort*	T44.5X1	T44.5X2	T44.5X3	T44.5X4	T44.5X5	T44.5X6
Pulp						
devitalizing paste	T49.7X1	T49.7X2	T49.7X3	T49.7X4	T49.7X5	T49.7X6
dressing	T49.7X1	T49.7X2	T49.7X3	T49.7X4	T49.7X5	T49.7X6
Pulsatilla	T62.2X1	T62.2X2	T62.2X3	T62.2X4	—	—
Pumpkin seed extract	T37.4X1	T37.4X2	T37.4X3	T37.4X4	T37.4X5	T37.4X6
Purex (bleach)	T54.91	T54.92	T54.93	T54.94	—	—
Purgative NEC — see also Cathartic	T47.4X1	T47.4X2	T47.4X3	T47.4X4	T47.4X5	T47.4X6
Purine analogue (antineoplastic)	T45.1X1	T45.1X2	T45.1X3	T45.1X4	T45.1X5	T45.1X6
Purine diuretics	T50.2X1	T50.2X2	T50.2X3	T50.2X4	T50.2X5	T50.2X6
Purinethol	T45.1X1	T45.1X2	T45.1X3	T45.1X4	T45.1X5	T45.1X6
PVP	T45.8X1	T45.8X2	T45.8X3	T45.8X4	T45.8X5	T45.8X6
Pyrabital	T39.8X1	T39.8X2	T39.8X3	T39.8X4	T39.8X5	T39.8X6
Pyramidon	T39.2X1	T39.2X2	T39.2X3	T39.2X4	T39.2X5	T39.2X6
Pyrantel	T37.4X1	T37.4X2	T37.4X3	T37.4X4	T37.4X5	T37.4X6
Pyrathiazine	T45.0X1	T45.0X2	T45.0X3	T45.0X4	T45.0X5	T45.0X6
Pyrazinamide	T37.1X1	T37.1X2	T37.1X3	T37.1X4	T37.1X5	T37.1X6
Pyrazinoic acid (amide)	T37.1X1	T37.1X2	T37.1X3	T37.1X4	T37.1X5	T37.1X6
Pyrazole (derivatives)	T39.2X1	T39.2X2	T39.2X3	T39.2X4	T39.2X5	T39.2X6
Pyrazolone analgesic NEC	T39.2X1	T39.2X2	T39.2X3	T39.2X4	T39.2X5	T39.2X6
Pyrethrin, pyrethrum (nonmedicinal)	T60.2X1	T60.2X2	T60.2X3	T60.2X4	—	—
Pyrethrum extract	T49.0X1	T49.0X2	T49.0X3	T49.0X4	T49.0X5	T49.0X6
Pyribenzamine	T45.0X1	T45.0X2	T45.0X3	T45.0X4	T45.0X5	T45.0X6
Pyridine	T52.8X1	T52.8X2	T52.8X3	T52.8X4	—	—
aldoxime methiodide	T50.6X1	T50.6X2	T50.6X3	T50.6X4	T50.6X5	T50.6X6
aldoxime methyl chloride	T50.6X1	T50.6X2	T50.6X3	T50.6X4	T50.6X5	T50.6X6
vapor	T59.891	T59.892	T59.893	T59.894	—	—
Pyridium	T39.8X1	T39.8X2	T39.8X3	T39.8X4	T39.8X5	T39.8X6
Pyridostigmine bromide	T44.0X1	T44.0X2	T44.0X3	T44.0X4	T44.0X5	T44.0X6
Pyridoxal phosphate	T45.2X1	T45.2X2	T45.2X3	T45.2X4	T45.2X5	T45.2X6
Pyridoxine	T45.2X1	T45.2X2	T45.2X3	T45.2X4	T45.2X5	T45.2X6
Pyrilamine	T45.0X1	T45.0X2	T45.0X3	T45.0X4	T45.0X5	T45.0X6
Pyrimethamine	T37.2X1	T37.2X2	T37.2X3	T37.2X4	T37.2X5	T37.2X6
with sulfadoxine	T37.2X1	T37.2X2	T37.2X3	T37.2X4	T37.2X5	T37.2X6
Pyrimidine antagonist	T45.1X1	T45.1X2	T45.1X3	T45.1X4	T45.1X5	T45.1X6
Pyriminil	T60.4X1	T60.4X2	T60.4X3	T60.4X4	—	—
Pyrithione zinc	T49.4X1	T49.4X2	T49.4X3	T49.4X4	T49.4X5	T49.4X6
Pyrithyldione	T42.6X1	T42.6X2	T42.6X3	T42.6X4	T42.6X5	T42.6X6
Pyrogallic acid	T49.0X1	T49.0X2	T49.0X3	T49.0X4	T49.0X5	T49.0X6
Pyrogallol	T49.0X1	T49.0X2	T49.0X3	T49.0X4	T49.0X5	T49.0X6
Pyroxylin	T49.3X1	T49.3X2	T49.3X3	T49.3X4	T49.3X5	T49.3X6
Pyrrobutamine	T45.0X1	T45.0X2	T45.0X3	T45.0X4	T45.0X5	T45.0X6
Pyrrolizidine alkaloids	T62.8X1	T62.8X2	T62.8X3	T62.8X4	—	—
Pyrvinium chloride	T37.4X1	T37.4X2	T37.4X3	T37.4X4	T37.4X5	T37.4X6
PZI	T38.3X1	T38.3X2	T38.3X3	T38.3X4	T38.3X5	T38.3X6
Qbrelis*	T46.4X1	T46.4X2	T46.4X3	T46.4X4	T46.4X5	T46.4X6
Quaalude	T42.6X1	T42.6X2	T42.6X3	T42.6X4	T42.6X5	T42.6X6
Quarternary ammonium						
anti-infective	T49.0X1	T49.0X2	T49.0X3	T49.0X4	T49.0X5	T49.0X6
ganglion blocking	T44.2X1	T44.2X2	T44.2X3	T44.2X4	T44.2X5	T44.2X6
parasympatholytic	T44.3X1	T44.3X2	T44.3X3	T44.3X4	T44.3X5	T44.3X6
Quazepam	T42.4X1	T42.4X2	T42.4X3	T42.4X4	T42.4X5	T42.4X6
Quicklime	T54.3X1	T54.3X2	T54.3X3	T54.3X4	—	—
Quilbron-T*	T48.6X1	T48.6X2	T48.6X3	T48.6X4	T48.6X5	T48.6X6
Quillaja extract	T48.4X1	T48.4X2	T48.4X3	T48.4X4	T48.4X5	T48.4X6
Quinacrine	T37.2X1	T37.2X2	T37.2X3	T37.2X4	T37.2X5	T37.2X6
Quinaglute	T46.2X1	T46.2X2	T46.2X3	T46.2X4	T46.2X5	T46.2X6
Quinalbarbital	T42.3X1	T42.3X2	T42.3X3	T42.3X4	T42.3X5	T42.3X6
Quinalbarbitone sodium	T42.3X1	T42.3X2	T42.3X3	T42.3X4	T42.3X5	T42.3X6
Quinalphos	T60.0X1	T60.0X2	T60.0X3	T60.0X4	—	—
Quinapril	T46.4X1	T46.4X2	T46.4X3	T46.4X4	T46.4X5	T46.4X6
Quinestradiol	T38.5X1	T38.5X2	T38.5X3	T38.5X4	T38.5X5	T38.5X6
Quinestradol	T38.5X1	T38.5X2	T38.5X3	T38.5X4	T38.5X5	T38.5X6
Quinestrol	T38.5X1	T38.5X2	T38.5X3	T38.5X4	T38.5X5	T38.5X6
Quinethazone	T50.2X1	T50.2X2	T50.2X3	T50.2X4	T50.2X5	T50.2X6
Quingestanol	T38.4X1	T38.4X2	T38.4X3	T38.4X4	T38.4X5	T38.4X6
Quinidine	T46.2X1	T46.2X2	T46.2X3	T46.2X4	T46.2X5	T46.2X6
Quinine	T37.2X1	T37.2X2	T37.2X3	T37.2X4	T37.2X5	T37.2X6
Quiniobine	T37.8X1	T37.8X2	T37.8X3	T37.8X4	T37.8X5	T37.8X6
Quinisocaine	T49.1X1	T49.1X2	T49.1X3	T49.1X4	T49.1X5	T49.1X6
Quinocide	T37.2X1	T37.2X2	T37.2X3	T37.2X4	T37.2X5	T37.2X6
Quinoline (derivatives) NEC	T37.8X1	T37.8X2	T37.8X3	T37.8X4	T37.8X5	T37.8X6
Quinupramine	T43.011	T43.012	T43.013	T43.014	T43.015	T43.016
Quixin*	T49.5X1	T49.5X2	T49.5X3	T49.5X4	T49.5X5	T49.5X6
Quotane	T41.3X1	T41.3X2	T41.3X3	T41.3X4	T41.3X5	T41.3X6
Rabies						
immune globulin (human)	T50.Z11	T50.Z12	T50.Z13	T50.Z14	T50.Z15	T50.Z16
vaccine	T50.B91	T50.B92	T50.B93	T50.B94	T50.B95	T50.B96
Racemoramide	T40.2X1	T40.2X2	T40.2X3	T40.2X4	—	—
Racemorphan	T40.2X1	T40.2X2	T40.2X3	T40.2X4	T40.2X5	T40.2X6
Racepinefrin	T44.5X1	T44.5X2	T44.5X3	T44.5X4	T44.5X5	T44.5X6
Raclopride	T43.591	T43.592	T43.593	T43.594	T43.595	T43.596
Radiator alcohol	T51.1X1	T51.1X2	T51.1X3	T51.1X4	—	—
Radioactive drug NEC	T50.8X1	T50.8X2	T50.8X3	T50.8X4	T50.8X5	T50.8X6
Radio-opaque (drugs) (materials)	T50.8X1	T50.8X2	T50.8X3	T50.8X4	T50.8X5	T50.8X6
Ramifenazone	T39.2X1	T39.2X2	T39.2X3	T39.2X4	T39.2X5	T39.2X6
Ramipril	T46.4X1	T46.4X2	T46.4X3	T46.4X4	T46.4X5	T46.4X6
Ranitidine	T47.0X1	T47.0X2	T47.0X3	T47.0X4	T47.0X5	T47.0X6
Ranunculus	T62.2X1	T62.2X2	T62.2X3	T62.2X4	—	—
Rat poison NEC	T60.4X1	T60.4X2	T60.4X3	T60.4X4	—	—
Rattlesnake (venom)	T63.011	T63.012	T63.013	T63.014	—	—
Raubasine	T46.7X1	T46.7X2	T46.7X3	T46.7X4	T46.7X5	T46.7X6
Raudixin	T46.5X1	T46.5X2	T46.5X3	T46.5X4	T46.5X5	T46.5X6
Rautensin	T46.5X1	T46.5X2	T46.5X3	T46.5X4	T46.5X5	T46.5X6
Rautina	T46.5X1	T46.5X2	T46.5X3	T46.5X4	T46.5X5	T46.5X6
Rautotal	T46.5X1	T46.5X2	T46.5X3	T46.5X4	T46.5X5	T46.5X6
Rauwiloid	T46.5X1	T46.5X2	T46.5X3	T46.5X4	T46.5X5	T46.5X6
Rauwoldin	T46.5X1	T46.5X2	T46.5X3	T46.5X4	T46.5X5	T46.5X6

Protease — Rauwoldin

Substance	Poisoning, Accidental (unintentional)	Poisoning, Intentional Self-harm	Poisoning, Assault	Poisoning, Undetermined	Adverse Effect	Under-dosing
Rauwolfia (alkaloids)	T46.5X1	T46.5X2	T46.5X3	T46.5X4	T46.5X5	T46.5X6
Razadyne*	T44.0X1	T44.0X2	T44.0X3	T44.0X4	T44.0X5	T44.0X6
Razoxane	T45.1X1	T45.1X2	T45.1X3	T45.1X4	T45.1X5	T45.1X6
Realgar	T57.0X1	T57.0X2	T57.0X3	T57.0X4	—	—
Recombinant (R) — see specific protein						
Red blood cells, packed	T45.8X1	T45.8X2	T45.8X3	T45.8X4	T45.8X5	T45.8X6
Red squill (scilliroside)	T60.4X1	T60.4X2	T60.4X3	T60.4X4	—	—
Reducing agent, industrial NEC	T65.891	T65.892	T65.893	T65.894	—	—
Refrigerant gas (chlorofluorocarbon)	T53.5X1	T53.5X2	T53.5X3	T53.5X4	—	—
not chlorofluorocarbon	T59.891	T59.892	T59.893	T59.894	—	—
Regroton	T50.2X1	T50.2X2	T50.2X3	T50.2X4	T50.2X5	T50.2X6
Rehydration salts (oral)	T50.3X1	T50.3X2	T50.3X3	T50.3X4	T50.3X5	T50.3X6
Rela	T42.8X1	T42.8X2	T42.8X3	T42.8X4	T42.8X5	T42.8X6
Relaxant, muscle						
anesthetic	T48.1X1	T48.1X2	T48.1X3	T48.1X4	T48.1X5	T48.1X6
central nervous system	T42.8X1	T42.8X2	T42.8X3	T42.8X4	T42.8X5	T42.8X6
skeletal NEC	T48.1X1	T48.1X2	T48.1X3	T48.1X4	T48.1X5	T48.1X6
smooth NEC	T44.3X1	T44.3X2	T44.3X3	T44.3X4	T44.3X5	T44.3X6
Remoxipride	T43.591	T43.592	T43.593	T43.594	T43.595	T43.596
Renese	T50.2X1	T50.2X2	T50.2X3	T50.2X4	T50.2X5	T50.2X6
Renografin	T50.8X1	T50.8X2	T50.8X3	T50.8X4	T50.8X5	T50.8X6
Replacement solution	T50.3X1	T50.3X2	T50.3X3	T50.3X4	T50.3X5	T50.3X6
Reproterol	T48.6X1	T48.6X2	T48.6X3	T48.6X4	T48.6X5	T48.6X6
Rescinnamine	T46.5X1	T46.5X2	T46.5X3	T46.5X4	T46.5X5	T46.5X6
Reserpin (e)	T46.5X1	T46.5X2	T46.5X3	T46.5X4	T46.5X5	T46.5X6
Resorcin, resorcinol (nonmedicinal)	T65.891	T65.892	T65.893	T65.894	—	—
medicinal	T49.4X1	T49.4X2	T49.4X3	T49.4X4	T49.4X5	T49.4X6
Respaire	T48.4X1	T48.4X2	T48.4X3	T48.4X4	T48.4X5	T48.4X6
Respiratory drug NEC	T48.901	T48.902	T48.903	T48.904	T48.905	T48.906
antiasthmatic NEC	T48.6X1	T48.6X2	T48.6X3	T48.6X4	T48.6X5	T48.6X6
anti-common-cold NEC	T48.5X1	T48.5X2	T48.5X3	T48.5X4	T48.5X5	T48.5X6
expectorant NEC	T48.4X1	T48.4X2	T48.4X3	T48.4X4	T48.4X5	T48.4X6
stimulant	T48.901	T48.902	T48.903	T48.904	T48.905	T48.906
Restoril*	T42.4X1	T42.4X2	T42.4X3	T42.4X4	T42.4X5	T42.4X6
Retinoic acid	T49.0X1	T49.0X2	T49.0X3	T49.0X4	T49.0X5	T49.0X6
Retinol	T45.2X1	T45.2X2	T45.2X3	T45.2X4	T45.2X5	T45.2X6
Revatio*	T46.7X1	T46.7X2	T46.7X3	T46.7X4	T46.7X5	T46.7X6
Rh (D) **immune globulin** (human)	T50.Z11	T50.Z12	T50.Z13	T50.Z14	T50.Z15	T50.Z16
Rhodine	T39.011	T39.012	T39.013	T39.014	T39.015	T39.016
RhoGAM	T50.Z11	T50.Z12	T50.Z13	T50.Z14	T50.Z15	T50.Z16
Rhubarb						
dry extract	T47.2X1	T47.2X2	T47.2X3	T47.2X4	T47.2X5	T47.2X6
tincture, compound	T47.2X1	T47.2X2	T47.2X3	T47.2X4	T47.2X5	T47.2X6
Ribavirin	T37.5X1	T37.5X2	T37.5X3	T37.5X4	T37.5X5	T37.5X6
Riboflavin	T45.2X1	T45.2X2	T45.2X3	T45.2X4	T45.2X5	T45.2X6
Ribostamycin	T36.5X1	T36.5X2	T36.5X3	T36.5X4	T36.5X5	T36.5X6
Ricin	T62.2X1	T62.2X2	T62.2X3	T62.2X4	—	—
Ricinus communis	T62.2X1	T62.2X2	T62.2X3	T62.2X4	—	—
Rickettsial vaccine NEC	T50.A91	T50.A92	T50.A93	T50.A94	T50.A95	T50.A96
Rifabutin	T36.6X1	T36.6X2	T36.6X3	T36.6X4	T36.6X5	T36.6X6
Rifamide	T36.6X1	T36.6X2	T36.6X3	T36.6X4	T36.6X5	T36.6X6
Rifampicin	T36.6X1	T36.6X2	T36.6X3	T36.6X4	T36.6X5	T36.6X6
with isoniazid	T37.1X1	T37.1X2	T37.1X3	T37.1X4	T37.1X5	T37.1X6
Rifampin	T36.6X1	T36.6X2	T36.6X3	T36.6X4	T36.6X5	T36.6X6
Rifamycin	T36.6X1	T36.6X2	T36.6X3	T36.6X4	T36.6X5	T36.6X6
Rifaximin	T36.6X1	T36.6X2	T36.6X3	T36.6X4	T36.6X5	T36.6X6
Rimantadine	T37.5X1	T37.5X2	T37.5X3	T37.5X4	T37.5X5	T37.5X6
Rimazolium metilsulfate	T39.8X1	T39.8X2	T39.8X3	T39.8X4	T39.8X5	T39.8X6
Rimifon	T37.1X1	T37.1X2	T37.1X3	T37.1X4	T37.1X5	T37.1X6
Rimiterol	T48.6X1	T48.6X2	T48.6X3	T48.6X4	T48.6X5	T48.6X6
Ringer (lactate) **solution**	T50.3X1	T50.3X2	T50.3X3	T50.3X4	T50.3X5	T50.3X6
Riomet*	T38.3X1	T38.3X2	T38.3X3	T38.3X4	T38.3X5	T38.3X6
Risperdal*	T43.591	T43.592	T43.593	T43.594	T43.595	T43.596
Ristocetin	T36.8X1	T36.8X2	T36.8X3	T36.8X4	T36.8X5	T36.8X6
Ritalin	T43.631	T43.632	T43.633	T43.634	T43.635	T43.636
Ritodrine	T44.5X1	T44.5X2	T44.5X3	T44.5X4	T44.5X5	T44.5X6
Roach killer — see Insecticide						
Robaxin*	T48.1X1	T48.1X2	T48.1X3	T48.1X4	T48.1X5	T48.1X6
Robitussin*	T48.3X1	T48.3X2	T48.3X3	T48.3X4	T48.3X5	T48.3X6
Rociverine	T44.3X1	T44.3X2	T44.3X3	T44.3X4	T44.3X5	T44.3X6
Rocky Mountain spotted fever vaccine	T50.A91	T50.A92	T50.A93	T50.A94	T50.A95	T50.A96
Rodenticide NEC	T60.4X1	T60.4X2	T60.4X3	T60.4X4	—	—
Rohypnol	T42.4X1	T42.4X2	T42.4X3	T42.4X4	T42.4X5	T42.4X6
Rokitamycin	T36.3X1	T36.3X2	T36.3X3	T36.3X4	T36.3X5	T36.3X6
Rolaids	T47.1X1	T47.1X2	T47.1X3	T47.1X4	T47.1X5	T47.1X6
Rolitetracycline	T36.4X1	T36.4X2	T36.4X3	T36.4X4	T36.4X5	T36.4X6
Romilar	T48.3X1	T48.3X2	T48.3X3	T48.3X4	T48.3X5	T48.3X6
Ronifibrate	T46.6X1	T46.6X2	T46.6X3	T46.6X4	T46.6X5	T46.6X6
Rosaprostol	T47.1X1	T47.1X2	T47.1X3	T47.1X4	T47.1X5	T47.1X6
Rose bengal sodium (131I)	T50.8X1	T50.8X2	T50.8X3	T50.8X4	T50.8X5	T50.8X6
Rose water ointment	T49.3X1	T49.3X2	T49.3X3	T49.3X4	T49.3X5	T49.3X6
Rosoxacin	T37.8X1	T37.8X2	T37.8X3	T37.8X4	T37.8X5	T37.8X6
Rotenone	T60.2X1	T60.2X2	T60.2X3	T60.2X4	—	—
Rotoxamine	T45.0X1	T45.0X2	T45.0X3	T45.0X4	T45.0X5	T45.0X6
Rough-on-rats	T60.4X1	T60.4X2	T60.4X3	T60.4X4	—	—
Roxatidine	T47.0X1	T47.0X2	T47.0X3	T47.0X4	T47.0X5	T47.0X6
Roxithromycin	T36.3X1	T36.3X2	T36.3X3	T36.3X4	T36.3X5	T36.3X6
Rt-PA	T45.611	T45.612	T45.613	T45.614	T45.615	T45.616
Rubbing alcohol	T51.2X1	T51.2X2	T51.2X3	T51.2X4	—	—
Rubefacient	T49.4X1	T49.4X2	T49.4X3	T49.4X4	T49.4X5	T49.4X6
Rubella vaccine	T50.B91	T50.B92	T50.B93	T50.B94	T50.B95	T50.B96
Rubeola vaccine	T50.B91	T50.B92	T50.B93	T50.B94	T50.B95	T50.B96
Rubidium chloride Rb82	T50.8X1	T50.8X2	T50.8X3	T50.8X4	T50.8X5	T50.8X6
Rubidomycin	T45.1X1	T45.1X2	T45.1X3	T45.1X4	T45.1X5	T45.1X6
Rue	T62.2X1	T62.2X2	T62.2X3	T62.2X4	—	—
Rufocromomycin	T45.1X1	T45.1X2	T45.1X3	T45.1X4	T45.1X5	T45.1X6
Russel's viper venin	T45.7X1	T45.7X2	T45.7X3	T45.7X4	T45.7X5	T45.7X6
Ruta (graveolens)	T62.2X1	T62.2X2	T62.2X3	T62.2X4	—	—
Rutinum	T46.991	T46.992	T46.993	T46.994	T46.995	T46.996
Rutoside	T46.991	T46.992	T46.993	T46.994	T46.995	T46.996
b-sitosterol(s)	T46.6X1	T46.6X2	T46.6X3	T46.6X4	T46.6X5	T46.6X6
Sabadilla (plant)	T62.2X1	T62.2X2	T62.2X3	T62.2X4	—	—
pesticide	T60.2X1	T60.2X2	T60.2X3	T60.2X4	—	—
Sabril*	T42.6X1	T42.6X2	T42.6X3	T42.6X4	T42.6X5	T42.6X6
Saccharated iron oxide	T45.8X1	T45.8X2	T45.8X3	T45.8X4	T45.8X5	T45.8X6
Saccharin	T50.901	T50.902	T50.903	T50.904	T50.905	T50.906
Saccharomyces boulardii	T47.6X1	T47.6X2	T47.6X3	T47.6X4	T47.6X5	T47.6X6
Safflower oil	T46.6X1	T46.6X2	T46.6X3	T46.6X4	T46.6X5	T46.6X6
Safrazine	T43.1X1	T43.1X2	T43.1X3	T43.1X4	T43.1X5	T43.1X6
Salazosulfapyridine	T37.0X1	T37.0X2	T37.0X3	T37.0X4	T37.0X5	T37.0X6
Salbutamol	T48.6X1	T48.6X2	T48.6X3	T48.6X4	T48.6X5	T48.6X6
Salicylamide	T39.091	T39.092	T39.093	T39.094	T39.095	T39.096
Salicylate NEC	T39.091	T39.092	T39.093	T39.094	T39.095	T39.096
methyl	T49.3X1	T49.3X2	T49.3X3	T49.3X4	T49.3X5	T49.3X6
theobromine calcium	T50.2X1	T50.2X2	T50.2X3	T50.2X4	T50.2X5	T50.2X6
Salicylazosulfapyridine	T37.0X1	T37.0X2	T37.0X3	T37.0X4	T37.0X5	T37.0X6
Salicylhydroxamic acid	T49.0X1	T49.0X2	T49.0X3	T49.0X4	T49.0X5	T49.0X6
Salicylic acid	T49.4X1	T49.4X2	T49.4X3	T49.4X4	T49.4X5	T49.4X6
with benzoic acid	T49.4X1	T49.4X2	T49.4X3	T49.4X4	T49.4X5	T49.4X6
congeners	T39.091	T39.092	T39.093	T39.094	T39.095	T39.096
derivative	T39.091	T39.092	T39.093	T39.094	T39.095	T39.096
salts	T39.091	T39.092	T39.093	T39.094	T39.095	T39.096
Salinazid	T37.1X1	T37.1X2	T37.1X3	T37.1X4	T37.1X5	T37.1X6
Salmeterol	T48.6X1	T48.6X2	T48.6X3	T48.6X4	T48.6X5	T48.6X6
Salol	T49.3X1	T49.3X2	T49.3X3	T49.3X4	T49.3X5	T49.3X6
Salsalate	T39.091	T39.092	T39.093	T39.094	T39.095	T39.096
Salt-replacing drug	T50.901	T50.902	T50.903	T50.904	T50.905	T50.906
Salt-retaining mineralocorticoid	T50.0X1	T50.0X2	T50.0X3	T50.0X4	T50.0X5	T50.0X6
Salt substitute	T50.901	T50.902	T50.903	T50.904	T50.905	T50.906
Saluretic NEC	T50.2X1	T50.2X2	T50.2X3	T50.2X4	T50.2X5	T50.2X6
Saluron	T50.2X1	T50.2X2	T50.2X3	T50.2X4	T50.2X5	T50.2X6
Salvarsan 606 (neosilver) (silver)	T37.8X1	T37.8X2	T37.8X3	T37.8X4	T37.8X5	T37.8X6
Sambucus canadensis	T62.2X1	T62.2X2	T62.2X3	T62.2X4	—	—
berry	T62.1X1	T62.1X2	T62.1X3	T62.1X4	—	—
Sandril	T46.5X1	T46.5X2	T46.5X3	T46.5X4	T46.5X5	T46.5X6
Sanguinaria canadensis	T62.2X1	T62.2X2	T62.2X3	T62.2X4	—	—
Saniflush (cleaner)	T54.2X1	T54.2X2	T54.2X3	T54.2X4	—	—
Santonin	T37.4X1	T37.4X2	T37.4X3	T37.4X4	T37.4X5	T37.4X6
Santyl	T49.8X1	T49.8X2	T49.8X3	T49.8X4	T49.8X5	T49.8X6
Saralasin	T46.5X1	T46.5X2	T46.5X3	T46.5X4	T46.5X5	T46.5X6
Sarcolysin	T45.1X1	T45.1X2	T45.1X3	T45.1X4	T45.1X5	T45.1X6
Sarilumab*	T39.4X1	T39.4X2	T39.4X3	T39.4X4	T39.4X5	T39.4X6
Sarkomycin	T45.1X1	T45.1X2	T45.1X3	T45.1X4	T45.1X5	T45.1X6
Saroten	T43.011	T43.012	T43.013	T43.014	T43.015	T43.016
Saturnine — see Lead						
Savin (oil)	T49.4X1	T49.4X2	T49.4X3	T49.4X4	T49.4X5	T49.4X6
Scammony	T47.2X1	T47.2X2	T47.2X3	T47.2X4	T47.2X5	T47.2X6
Scarlet red	T49.8X1	T49.8X2	T49.8X3	T49.8X4	T49.8X5	T49.8X6
Scheele's green	T57.0X1	T57.0X2	T57.0X3	T57.0X4	—	—
insecticide	T57.0X1	T57.0X2	T57.0X3	T57.0X4	—	—
Schizontozide (blood) (tissue)	T37.2X1	T37.2X2	T37.2X3	T37.2X4	T37.2X5	T37.2X6
Schradan	T60.0X1	T60.0X2	T60.0X3	T60.0X4	—	—
Schweinfurth green	T57.0X1	T57.0X2	T57.0X3	T57.0X4	—	—
insecticide	T57.0X1	T57.0X2	T57.0X3	T57.0X4	—	—
Scilla, rat poison	T60.4X1	T60.4X2	T60.4X3	T60.4X4	—	—
Scillaren	T60.4X1	T60.4X2	T60.4X3	T60.4X4	—	—
Sclerosing agent	T46.8X1	T46.8X2	T46.8X3	T46.8X4	T46.8X5	T46.8X6

Substance	Poisoning, Accidental (unintentional)	Poisoning, Intentional Self-harm	Poisoning, Assault	Poisoning, Undetermined	Adverse Effect	Under-dosing
Scombrotoxin	T61.11	T61.12	T61.13	T61.14	—	—
Scopolamine	T44.3X1	T44.3X2	T44.3X3	T44.3X4	T44.3X5	T44.3X6
Scopolia extract	T44.3X1	T44.3X2	T44.3X3	T44.3X4	T44.3X5	T44.3X6
Scouring powder	T65.891	T65.892	T65.893	T65.894	—	—
Sea						
anemone (sting)	T63.631	T63.632	T63.633	T63.634	—	—
cucumber (sting)	T63.691	T63.692	T63.693	T63.694	—	—
snake (bite) (venom)	T63.091	T63.092	T63.093	T63.094	—	—
urchin spine (puncture)	T63.691	T63.692	T63.693	T63.694	—	—
Seafood	T61.91	T61.92	T61.93	T61.94	—	—
specified NEC	T61.8X1	T61.8X2	T61.8X3	T61.8X4	—	—
Secbutabarbital	T42.3X1	T42.3X2	T42.3X3	T42.3X4	T42.3X5	T42.3X6
Secbutabarbitone	T42.3X1	T42.3X2	T42.3X3	T42.3X4	T42.3X5	T42.3X6
Secnidazole	T37.3X1	T37.3X2	T37.3X3	T37.3X4	T37.3X5	T37.3X6
Secobarbital	T42.3X1	T42.3X2	T42.3X3	T42.3X4	T42.3X5	T42.3X6
Seconal	T42.3X1	T42.3X2	T42.3X3	T42.3X4	T42.3X5	T42.3X6
Secretin	T50.8X1	T50.8X2	T50.8X3	T50.8X4	T50.8X5	T50.8X6
Sectral*	T44.7X1	T44.7X2	T44.7X3	T44.7X4	T44.7X5	T44.7X6
Sedative NEC	T42.71	T42.72	T42.73	T42.74	T42.75	T42.76
mixed NEC	T42.6X1	T42.6X2	T42.6X3	T42.6X4	T42.6X5	T42.6X6
Sedormid	T42.6X1	T42.6X2	T42.6X3	T42.6X4	T42.6X5	T42.6X6
Seed disinfectant or dressing	T60.8X1	T60.8X2	T60.8X3	T60.8X4	—	—
Seeds (poisonous)	T62.2X1	T62.2X2	T62.2X3	T62.2X4	—	—
Selegiline	T42.8X1	T42.8X2	T42.8X3	T42.8X4	T42.8X5	T42.8X6
Selenium NEC	T56.891	T56.892	T56.893	T56.894	—	—
disulfide or sulfide	T49.4X1	T49.4X2	T49.4X3	T49.4X4	T49.4X5	T49.4X6
fumes	T59.891	T59.892	T59.893	T59.894	—	—
sulfide	T49.4X1	T49.4X2	T49.4X3	T49.4X4	T49.4X5	T49.4X6
Selenomethionine (75Se)	T50.8X1	T50.8X2	T50.8X3	T50.8X4	T50.8X5	T50.8X6
Selsun	T49.4X1	T49.4X2	T49.4X3	T49.4X4	T49.4X5	T49.4X6
Semustine	T45.1X1	T45.1X2	T45.1X3	T45.1X4	T45.1X5	T45.1X6
Senega syrup	T48.4X1	T48.4X2	T48.4X3	T48.4X4	T48.4X5	T48.4X6
Senna	T47.2X1	T47.2X2	T47.2X3	T47.2X4	T47.2X5	T47.2X6
Sennoside A+B	T47.2X1	T47.2X2	T47.2X3	T47.2X4	T47.2X5	T47.2X6
Septisol	T49.2X1	T49.2X2	T49.2X3	T49.2X4	T49.2X5	T49.2X6
Seractide	T38.811	T38.812	T38.813	T38.814	T38.815	T38.816
Serax	T42.4X1	T42.4X2	T42.4X3	T42.4X4	T42.4X5	T42.4X6
Serenesil	T42.6X1	T42.6X2	T42.6X3	T42.6X4	T42.6X5	T42.6X6
Serenium (hydrochloride)	T37.91	T37.92	T37.93	T37.94	T37.95	T37.96
Serepax — see Oxazepam						
Serevent*	T48.6X1	T48.6X2	T48.6X3	T48.6X4	T48.6X5	T48.6X6
Sermorelin	T38.891	T38.892	T38.893	T38.894	T38.895	T38.896
Sernyl	T41.1X1	T41.1X2	T41.1X3	T41.1X4	T41.1X5	T41.1X6
Serotonin	T50.991	T50.992	T50.993	T50.994	T50.995	T50.996
Serpasil	T46.5X1	T46.5X2	T46.5X3	T46.5X4	T46.5X5	T46.5X6
Serrapeptase	T45.3X1	T45.3X2	T45.3X3	T45.3X4	T45.3X5	T45.3X6
Sertraline*	T43.221	T43.222	T43.223	T43.224	T43.225	T43.226
Serum						
antibotulinus	T50.Z11	T50.Z12	T50.Z13	T50.Z14	T50.Z15	T50.Z16
anticytotoxic	T50.Z11	T50.Z12	T50.Z13	T50.Z14	T50.Z15	T50.Z16
antidiphtheria	T50.Z11	T50.Z12	T50.Z13	T50.Z14	T50.Z15	T50.Z16
antimeningococcus	T50.Z11	T50.Z12	T50.Z13	T50.Z14	T50.Z15	T50.Z16
anti-Rh	T50.Z11	T50.Z12	T50.Z13	T50.Z14	T50.Z15	T50.Z16
anti-snake-bite	T50.Z11	T50.Z12	T50.Z13	T50.Z14	T50.Z15	T50.Z16
antitetanic	T50.Z11	T50.Z12	T50.Z13	T50.Z14	T50.Z15	T50.Z16
antitoxic	T50.Z11	T50.Z12	T50.Z13	T50.Z14	T50.Z15	T50.Z16
complement (inhibitor)	T45.8X1	T45.8X2	T45.8X3	T45.8X4	T45.8X5	T45.8X6
convalescent	T50.Z11	T50.Z12	T50.Z13	T50.Z14	T50.Z15	T50.Z16
hemolytic complement	T45.8X1	T45.8X2	T45.8X3	T45.8X4	T45.8X5	T45.8X6
immune (human)	T50.Z11	T50.Z12	T50.Z13	T50.Z14	T50.Z15	T50.Z16
protective NEC	T50.Z11	T50.Z12	T50.Z13	T50.Z14	T50.Z15	T50.Z16
Setastine	T45.0X1	T45.0X2	T45.0X3	T45.0X4	T45.0X5	T45.0X6
Setoperone	T43.591	T43.592	T43.593	T43.594	T43.595	T43.596
Sewer gas	T59.91	T59.92	T59.93	T59.94	—	—
Shampoo	T55.0X1	T55.0X2	T55.0X3	T55.0X4	—	—
Shellfish, noxious, nonbacterial	T61.781	T61.782	T61.783	T61.784	—	—
Sildenafil	T46.7X1	T46.7X2	T46.7X3	T46.7X4	T46.7X5	T46.7X6
Silibinin	T50.991	T50.992	T50.993	T50.994	T50.995	T50.996
Silicone NEC	T65.891	T65.892	T65.893	T65.894	—	—
medicinal	T49.3X1	T49.3X2	T49.3X3	T49.3X4	T49.3X5	T49.3X6
Silvadene	T49.0X1	T49.0X2	T49.0X3	T49.0X4	T49.0X5	T49.0X6
Silver	T49.0X1	T49.0X2	T49.0X3	T49.0X4	T49.0X5	T49.0X6
anti-infectives	T49.0X1	T49.0X2	T49.0X3	T49.0X4	T49.0X5	T49.0X6
arsphenamine	T37.8X1	T37.8X2	T37.8X3	T37.8X4	T37.8X5	T37.8X6
colloidal	T49.0X1	T49.0X2	T49.0X3	T49.0X4	T49.0X5	T49.0X6
nitrate	T49.0X1	T49.0X2	T49.0X3	T49.0X4	T49.0X5	T49.0X6
ophthalmic preparation	T49.5X1	T49.5X2	T49.5X3	T49.5X4	T49.5X5	T49.5X6
toughened (keratolytic)	T49.4X1	T49.4X2	T49.4X3	T49.4X4	T49.4X5	T49.4X6
nonmedicinal (dust)	T56.891	T56.892	T56.893	T56.894	—	—
protein	T49.5X1	T49.5X2	T49.5X3	T49.5X4	T49.5X5	T49.5X6
salvarsan	T37.8X1	T37.8X2	T37.8X3	T37.8X4	T37.8X5	T37.8X6

Substance	Poisoning, Accidental (unintentional)	Poisoning, Intentional Self-harm	Poisoning, Assault	Poisoning, Undetermined	Adverse Effect	Under-dosing
Silver — continued						
sulfadiazine	T49.4X1	T49.4X2	T49.4X3	T49.4X4	T49.4X5	T49.4X6
Silymarin	T50.991	T50.992	T50.993	T50.994	T50.995	T50.996
Simaldrate	T47.1X1	T47.1X2	T47.1X3	T47.1X4	T47.1X5	T47.1X6
Simazine	T60.3X1	T60.3X2	T60.3X3	T60.3X4	—	—
Simethicone	T47.1X1	T47.1X2	T47.1X3	T47.1X4	T47.1X5	T47.1X6
Simfibrate	T46.6X1	T46.6X2	T46.6X3	T46.6X4	T46.6X5	T46.6X6
Simvastatin	T46.6X1	T46.6X2	T46.6X3	T46.6X4	T46.6X5	T46.6X6
Sincalide	T50.8X1	T50.8X2	T50.8X3	T50.8X4	T50.8X5	T50.8X6
Sinequan	T43.011	T43.012	T43.013	T43.014	T43.015	T43.016
Singoserp	T46.5X1	T46.5X2	T46.5X3	T46.5X4	T46.5X5	T46.5X6
Singulair*	T48.6X1	T48.6X2	T48.6X3	T48.6X4	T48.6X5	T48.6X6
Sintrom	T45.511	T45.512	T45.513	T45.514	T45.515	T45.516
Sisomicin	T36.5X1	T36.5X2	T36.5X3	T36.5X4	T36.5X5	T36.5X6
Sitosterols	T46.6X1	T46.6X2	T46.6X3	T46.6X4	T46.6X5	T46.6X6
Skeletal muscle relaxants	T48.1X1	T48.1X2	T48.1X3	T48.1X4	T48.1X5	T48.1X6
Skin						
agents (external)	T49.91	T49.92	T49.93	T49.94	T49.95	T49.96
specified NEC	T49.8X1	T49.8X2	T49.8X3	T49.8X4	T49.8X5	T49.8X6
test antigen	T50.8X1	T50.8X2	T50.8X3	T50.8X4	T50.8X5	T50.8X6
Sleep-eze	T45.0X1	T45.0X2	T45.0X3	T45.0X4	T45.0X5	T45.0X6
Sleeping draught, pill	T42.71	T42.72	T42.73	T42.74	T42.75	T42.76
Smallpox vaccine	T50.B11	T50.B12	T50.B13	T50.B14	T50.B15	T50.B16
Smelter fumes NEC	T56.91	T56.92	T56.93	T56.94	—	—
Smog	T59.1X1	T59.1X2	T59.1X3	T59.1X4	—	—
Smoke NEC	T59.811	T59.812	T59.813	T59.814	—	—
Smooth muscle relaxant	T44.3X1	T44.3X2	T44.3X3	T44.3X4	T44.3X5	T44.3X6
Snail killer NEC	T60.8X1	T60.8X2	T60.8X3	T60.8X4	—	—
Snake venom or bite	T63.001	T63.002	T63.003	T63.004	—	—
hemocoagulase	T45.7X1	T45.7X2	T45.7X3	T45.7X4	T45.7X5	T45.7X6
Snuff	T65.211	T65.212	T65.213	T65.214	—	—
Soap (powder) (product)	T55.0X1	T55.0X2	T55.0X3	T55.0X4	—	—
enema	T47.4X1	T47.4X2	T47.4X3	T47.4X4	T47.4X5	T47.4X6
medicinal, soft	T49.2X1	T49.2X2	T49.2X3	T49.2X4	T49.2X5	T49.2X6
superfatted	T49.2X1	T49.2X2	T49.2X3	T49.2X4	T49.2X5	T49.2X6
Sobrerol	T48.4X1	T48.4X2	T48.4X3	T48.4X4	T48.4X5	T48.4X6
Soda (caustic)	T54.3X1	T54.3X2	T54.3X3	T54.3X4	—	—
bicarb	T47.1X1	T47.1X2	T47.1X3	T47.1X4	T47.1X5	T47.1X6
chlorinated — see Sodium, hypochlorite						
Sodium						
acetosulfone	T37.1X1	T37.1X2	T37.1X3	T37.1X4	T37.1X5	T37.1X6
acetrizoate	T50.8X1	T50.8X2	T50.8X3	T50.8X4	T50.8X5	T50.8X6
acid phosphate	T50.3X1	T50.3X2	T50.3X3	T50.3X4	T50.3X5	T50.3X6
alginate	T47.8X1	T47.8X2	T47.8X3	T47.8X4	T47.8X5	T47.8X6
amidotrizoate	T50.8X1	T50.8X2	T50.8X3	T50.8X4	T50.8X5	T50.8X6
aminohippurate*	T50.8X1	T50.8X2	T50.8X3	T50.8X4	T50.8X5	T50.8X6
aminopterin	T45.1X1	T45.1X2	T45.1X3	T45.1X4	T45.1X5	T45.1X6
amylosulfate	T47.8X1	T47.8X2	T47.8X3	T47.8X4	T47.8X5	T47.8X6
amytal	T42.3X1	T42.3X2	T42.3X3	T42.3X4	T42.3X5	T42.3X6
antimony gluconate	T37.3X1	T37.3X2	T37.3X3	T37.3X4	T37.3X5	T37.3X6
arsenate	T57.0X1	T57.0X2	T57.0X3	T57.0X4	—	—
aurothiomalate	T39.4X1	T39.4X2	T39.4X3	T39.4X4	T39.4X5	T39.4X6
aurothiosulfate	T39.4X1	T39.4X2	T39.4X3	T39.4X4	T39.4X5	T39.4X6
barbiturate	T42.3X1	T42.3X2	T42.3X3	T42.3X4	T42.3X5	T42.3X6
basic phosphate	T47.4X1	T47.4X2	T47.4X3	T47.4X4	T47.4X5	T47.4X6
bicarbonate	T47.1X1	T47.1X2	T47.1X3	T47.1X4	T47.1X5	T47.1X6
bichromate	T57.8X1	T57.8X2	T57.8X3	T57.8X4	—	—
biphosphate	T50.3X1	T50.3X2	T50.3X3	T50.3X4	T50.3X5	T50.3X6
bisulfate	T65.891	T65.892	T65.893	T65.894	—	—
borate						
cleanser	T57.8X1	T57.8X2	T57.8X3	T57.8X4	—	—
eye	T49.5X1	T49.5X2	T49.5X3	T49.5X4	T49.5X5	T49.5X6
therapeutic	T49.8X1	T49.8X2	T49.8X3	T49.8X4	T49.8X5	T49.8X6
bromide	T42.6X1	T42.6X2	T42.6X3	T42.6X4	T42.6X5	T42.6X6
cacodylate (nonmedicinal) NEC	T50.8X1	T50.8X2	T50.8X3	T50.8X4	T50.8X5	T50.8X6
anti-infective	T37.8X1	T37.8X2	T37.8X3	T37.8X4	T37.8X5	T37.8X6
herbicide	T60.3X1	T60.3X2	T60.3X3	T60.3X4	—	—
calcium edetate	T45.8X1	T45.8X2	T45.8X3	T45.8X4	T45.8X5	T45.8X6
carbonate NEC	T54.3X1	T54.3X2	T54.3X3	T54.3X4	—	—
chlorate NEC	T65.891	T65.892	T65.893	T65.894	—	—
herbicide	T54.91	T54.92	T54.93	T54.94	—	—
chloride	T50.3X1	T50.3X2	T50.3X3	T50.3X4	T50.3X5	T50.3X6
with glucose	T50.3X1	T50.3X2	T50.3X3	T50.3X4	T50.3X5	T50.3X6
chromate	T65.891	T65.892	T65.893	T65.894	—	—
citrate	T50.991	T50.992	T50.993	T50.994	T50.995	T50.996
cromoglicate	T48.6X1	T48.6X2	T48.6X3	T48.6X4	T48.6X5	T48.6X6
cyanide	T65.0X1	T65.0X2	T65.0X3	T65.0X4	—	—
cyclamate	T50.3X1	T50.3X2	T50.3X3	T50.3X4	T50.3X5	T50.3X6
dehydrocholate	T45.8X1	T45.8X2	T45.8X3	T45.8X4	T45.8X5	T45.8X6
diatrizoate	T50.8X1	T50.8X2	T50.8X3	T50.8X4	T50.8X5	T50.8X6
dibunate	T48.4X1	T48.4X2	T48.4X3	T48.4X4	T48.4X5	T48.4X6

Table of Drugs and Chemicals

Sodium — Spurge flax

Substance	Poisoning, Accidental (unintentional)	Poisoning, Intentional Self-harm	Poisoning, Assault	Poisoning, Undetermined	Adverse Effect	Under-dosing
Sodium — *continued*						
dioctyl sulfosuccinate	T47.4X1	T47.4X2	T47.4X3	T47.4X4	T47.4X5	T47.4X6
dipantoyl ferrate	T45.8X1	T45.8X2	T45.8X3	T45.8X4	T45.8X5	T45.8X6
edetate	T45.8X1	T45.8X2	T45.8X3	T45.8X4	T45.8X5	T45.8X6
ethacrynate	T50.1X1	T50.1X2	T50.1X3	T50.1X4	T50.1X5	T50.1X6
etidronate*	T50.991	T50.992	T50.993	T50.994	T50.995	T50.996
feredetate	T45.8X1	T45.8X2	T45.8X3	T45.8X4	T45.8X5	T45.8X6
Fluoride — *see* Fluoride						
fluoroacetate (dust) (pesticide)	T60.4X1	T60.4X2	T60.4X3	T60.4X4	—	—
free salt	T50.3X1	T50.3X2	T50.3X3	T50.3X4	T50.3X5	T50.3X6
fusidate	T36.8X1	T36.8X2	T36.8X3	T36.8X4	T36.8X5	T36.8X6
glucaldrate	T47.1X1	T47.1X2	T47.1X3	T47.1X4	T47.1X5	T47.1X6
glucosulfone	T37.1X1	T37.1X2	T37.1X3	T37.1X4	T37.1X5	T37.1X6
glutamate	T45.8X1	T45.8X2	T45.8X3	T45.8X4	T45.8X5	T45.8X6
hydrogen carbonate	T50.3X1	T50.3X2	T50.3X3	T50.3X4	T50.3X5	T50.3X6
hydroxide	T54.3X1	T54.3X2	T54.3X3	T54.3X4	—	—
hypochlorite (bleach) NEC	T54.3X1	T54.3X2	T54.3X3	T54.3X4	—	—
disinfectant	T54.3X1	T54.3X2	T54.3X3	T54.3X4	—	—
medicinal (anti-infective) (external)	T49.0X1	T49.0X2	T49.0X3	T49.0X4	T49.0X5	T49.0X6
vapor	T54.3X1	T54.3X2	T54.3X3	T54.3X4	—	—
hyposulfite	T49.0X1	T49.0X2	T49.0X3	T49.0X4	T49.0X5	T49.0X6
indigotin disulfonate	T50.8X1	T50.8X2	T50.8X3	T50.8X4	T50.8X5	T50.8X6
iodide	T50.991	T50.992	T50.993	T50.994	T50.995	T50.996
I-131	T50.8X1	T50.8X2	T50.8X3	T50.8X4	T50.8X5	T50.8X6
therapeutic	T38.2X1	T38.2X2	T38.2X3	T38.2X4	T38.2X5	T38.2X6
iodohippurate (131I)	T50.8X1	T50.8X2	T50.8X3	T50.8X4	T50.8X5	T50.8X6
iopodate	T50.8X1	T50.8X2	T50.8X3	T50.8X4	T50.8X5	T50.8X6
iothalamate	T50.8X1	T50.8X2	T50.8X3	T50.8X4	T50.8X5	T50.8X6
iron edetate	T45.4X1	T45.4X2	T45.4X3	T45.4X4	T45.4X5	T45.4X6
lactate (compound solution)	T45.8X1	T45.8X2	T45.8X3	T45.8X4	T45.8X5	T45.8X6
lauryl (sulfate)	T49.2X1	T49.2X2	T49.2X3	T49.2X4	T49.2X5	T49.2X6
L-triiodothyronine	T38.1X1	T38.1X2	T38.1X3	T38.1X4	T38.1X5	T38.1X6
magnesium citrate	T50.991	T50.992	T50.993	T50.994	T50.995	T50.996
mersalate	T50.2X1	T50.2X2	T50.2X3	T50.2X4	T50.2X5	T50.2X6
metasilicate	T65.891	T65.892	T65.893	T65.894	—	—
metrizoate	T50.8X1	T50.8X2	T50.8X3	T50.8X4	T50.8X5	T50.8X6
monofluoroacetate (pesticide)	T60.1X1	T60.1X2	T60.1X3	T60.1X4		
morrhuate	T46.8X1	T46.8X2	T46.8X3	T46.8X4	T46.8X5	T46.8X6
nafcillin	T36.0X1	T36.0X2	T36.0X3	T36.0X4	T36.0X5	T36.0X6
nitrate (oxidizing agent)	T65.891	T65.892	T65.893	T65.894	—	—
nitrite	T50.6X1	T50.6X2	T50.6X3	T50.6X4	T50.6X5	T50.6X6
nitroferricyanide	T46.5X1	T46.5X2	T46.5X3	T46.5X4	T46.5X5	T46.5X6
nitroprusside	T46.5X1	T46.5X2	T46.5X3	T46.5X4	T46.5X5	T46.5X6
oxalate	T65.891	T65.892	T65.893	T65.894	—	—
oxide/peroxide	T65.891	T65.892	T65.893	T65.894	—	—
oxybate	T41.291	T41.292	T41.293	T41.294	T41.295	T41.296
para-aminohippurate	T50.8X1	T50.8X2	T50.8X3	T50.8X4	T50.8X5	T50.8X6
perborate (nonmedicinal) NEC	T65.891	T65.892	T65.893	T65.894	—	—
medicinal	T49.0X1	T49.0X2	T49.0X3	T49.0X4	T49.0X5	T49.0X6
soap	T55.0X1	T55.0X2	T55.0X3	T55.0X4	—	—
percarbonate — *see* Sodium, perborate						
pertechnetate Tc99m	T50.8X1	T50.8X2	T50.8X3	T50.8X4	T50.8X5	T50.8X6
phosphate						
cellulose	T45.8X1	T45.8X2	T45.8X3	T45.8X4	T45.8X5	T45.8X6
dibasic	T47.2X1	T47.2X2	T47.2X3	T47.2X4	T47.2X5	T47.2X6
monobasic	T47.2X1	T47.2X2	T47.2X3	T47.2X4	T47.2X5	T47.2X6
phytate	T50.6X1	T50.6X2	T50.6X3	T50.6X4	T50.6X5	T50.6X6
picosulfate	T47.2X1	T47.2X2	T47.2X3	T47.2X4	T47.2X5	T47.2X6
polyhydroxyaluminium monocarbonate	T47.1X1	T47.1X2	T47.1X3	T47.1X4	T47.1X5	T47.1X6
polystyrene sulfonate	T50.3X1	T50.3X2	T50.3X3	T50.3X4	T50.3X5	T50.3X6
propionate	T49.0X1	T49.0X2	T49.0X3	T49.0X4	T49.0X5	T49.0X6
propyl hydroxybenzoate	T50.991	T50.992	T50.993	T50.994	T50.995	T50.996
psylliate	T46.8X1	T46.8X2	T46.8X3	T46.8X4	T46.8X5	T46.8X6
removing resins	T50.3X1	T50.3X2	T50.3X3	T50.3X4	T50.3X5	T50.3X6
salicylate	T39.091	T39.092	T39.093	T39.094	T39.095	T39.096
salt NEC	T50.3X1	T50.3X2	T50.3X3	T50.3X4	T50.3X5	T50.3X6
selenate	T60.2X1	T60.2X2	T60.2X3	T60.2X4	—	—
stibogluconate	T37.3X1	T37.3X2	T37.3X3	T37.3X4	T37.3X5	T37.3X6
sulfate	T47.4X1	T47.4X2	T47.4X3	T47.4X4	T47.4X5	T47.4X6
sulfoxone	T37.1X1	T37.1X2	T37.1X3	T37.1X4	T37.1X5	T37.1X6
tetradecyl sulfate	T46.8X1	T46.8X2	T46.8X3	T46.8X4	T46.8X5	T46.8X6
thiopental	T41.1X1	T41.1X2	T41.1X3	T41.1X4	T41.1X5	T41.1X6
thiosalicylate	T39.091	T39.092	T39.093	T39.094	T39.095	T39.096
thiosulfate	T50.6X1	T50.6X2	T50.6X3	T50.6X4	T50.6X5	T50.6X6
tolbutamide	T38.3X1	T38.3X2	T38.3X3	T38.3X4	T38.3X5	T38.3X6
(L)-triiodothyronine	T38.1X1	T38.1X2	T38.1X3	T38.1X4	T38.1X5	T38.1X6

Substance	Poisoning, Accidental (unintentional)	Poisoning, Intentional Self-harm	Poisoning, Assault	Poisoning, Undetermined	Adverse Effect	Under-dosing
Sodium — *continued*						
tyropanoate	T50.8X1	T50.8X2	T50.8X3	T50.8X4	T50.8X5	T50.8X6
valproate	T42.6X1	T42.6X2	T42.6X3	T42.6X4	T42.6X5	T42.6X6
versenate	T50.6X1	T50.6X2	T50.6X3	T50.6X4	T50.6X5	T50.6X6
Sodium-free salt	T50.901	T50.902	T50.903	T50.904	T50.905	T50.906
Sodium-removing resin	T50.3X1	T50.3X2	T50.3X3	T50.3X4	T50.3X5	T50.3X6
Soft soap	T55.0X1	T55.0X2	T55.0X3	T55.0X4	—	—
Solanine	T62.2X1	T62.2X2	T62.2X3	T62.2X4	—	—
berries	T62.1X1	T62.1X2	T62.1X3	T62.1X4	—	—
Solanum dulcamara	T62.2X1	T62.2X2	T62.2X3	T62.2X4	—	—
berries	T62.1X1	T62.1X2	T62.1X3	T62.1X4	—	—
Solapsone	T37.1X1	T37.1X2	T37.1X3	T37.1X4	T37.1X5	T37.1X6
Solaquin*	T49.8X1	T49.8X2	T49.8X3	T49.8X4	T49.8X5	T49.8X6
Solar lotion	T49.3X1	T49.3X2	T49.3X3	T49.3X4	T49.3X5	T49.3X6
Solasulfone	T37.1X1	T37.1X2	T37.1X3	T37.1X4	T37.1X5	T37.1X6
Soldering fluid	T65.891	T65.892	T65.893	T65.894	—	—
Solid substance	T65.91	T65.92	T65.93	T65.94	—	—
specified NEC	T65.891	T65.892	T65.893	T65.894	—	—
Solvent, industrial NEC	T52.91	T52.92	T52.93	T52.94	—	—
naphtha	T52.0X1	T52.0X2	T52.0X3	T52.0X4	—	—
petroleum	T52.0X1	T52.0X2	T52.0X3	T52.0X4	—	—
specified NEC	T52.8X1	T52.8X2	T52.8X3	T52.8X4	—	—
Soma	T42.8X1	T42.8X2	T42.8X3	T42.8X4	T42.8X5	T42.8X6
Somatorelin	T38.891	T38.892	T38.893	T38.894	T38.895	T38.896
Somatostatin	T38.991	T38.992	T38.993	T38.994	T38.995	T38.996
Somatotropin	T38.811	T38.812	T38.813	T38.814	T38.815	T38.816
Somatrem	T38.811	T38.812	T38.813	T38.814	T38.815	T38.816
Somatropin	T38.811	T38.812	T38.813	T38.814	T38.815	T38.816
Sominex	T45.0X1	T45.0X2	T45.0X3	T45.0X4	T45.0X5	T45.0X6
Somnos	T42.6X1	T42.6X2	T42.6X3	T42.6X4	T42.6X5	T42.6X6
Somonal	T42.3X1	T42.3X2	T42.3X3	T42.3X4	T42.3X5	T42.3X6
Soneryl	T42.3X1	T42.3X2	T42.3X3	T42.3X4	T42.3X5	T42.3X6
Soothing syrup	T50.901	T50.902	T50.903	T50.904	T50.905	T50.906
Sopor	T42.6X1	T42.6X2	T42.6X3	T42.6X4	T42.6X5	T42.6X6
Soporific	T42.71	T42.72	T42.73	T42.74	T42.75	T42.76
Soporific drug	T42.71	T42.72	T42.73	T42.74	T42.75	T42.76
specified type NEC	T42.6X1	T42.6X2	T42.6X3	T42.6X4	T42.6X5	T42.6X6
Sorbide nitrate	T46.3X1	T46.3X2	T46.3X3	T46.3X4	T46.3X5	T46.3X6
Sorbitol	T47.4X1	T47.4X2	T47.4X3	T47.4X4	T47.4X5	T47.4X6
Sotalol	T44.7X1	T44.7X2	T44.7X3	T44.7X4	T44.7X5	T44.7X6
Sotradecol	T46.8X1	T46.8X2	T46.8X3	T46.8X4	T46.8X5	T46.8X6
Soysterol	T46.6X1	T46.6X2	T46.6X3	T46.6X4	T46.6X5	T46.6X6
Spacoline	T44.3X1	T44.3X2	T44.3X3	T44.3X4	T44.3X5	T44.3X6
Spanish fly	T49.8X1	T49.8X2	T49.8X3	T49.8X4	T49.8X5	T49.8X6
Sparine	T43.3X1	T43.3X2	T43.3X3	T43.3X4	T43.3X5	T43.3X6
Sparteine	T48.0X1	T48.0X2	T48.0X3	T48.0X4	T48.0X5	T48.0X6
Spasmolytic						
anticholinergics	T44.3X1	T44.3X2	T44.3X3	T44.3X4	T44.3X5	T44.3X6
autonomic	T44.3X1	T44.3X2	T44.3X3	T44.3X4	T44.3X5	T44.3X6
bronchial NEC	T48.6X1	T48.6X2	T48.6X3	T48.6X4	T48.6X5	T48.6X6
quaternary ammonium	T44.3X1	T44.3X2	T44.3X3	T44.3X4	T44.3X5	T44.3X6
skeletal muscle NEC	T48.1X1	T48.1X2	T48.1X3	T48.1X4	T48.1X5	T48.1X6
Spectinomycin	T36.5X1	T36.5X2	T36.5X3	T36.5X4	T36.5X5	T36.5X6
Spectracef*	T36.1X1	T36.1X2	T36.1X3	T36.1X4	T36.1X5	T36.1X6
Speed	T43.651	T43.652	T43.653	T43.654	T43.655	T43.656
Spermicide	T49.8X1	T49.8X2	T49.8X3	T49.8X4	T49.8X5	T49.8X6
Spider (bite) (venom)	T63.391	T63.392	T63.393	T63.394	—	—
antivenin	T50.Z11	T50.Z12	T50.Z13	T50.Z14	T50.Z15	T50.Z16
Spigelia (root)	T37.4X1	T37.4X2	T37.4X3	T37.4X4	T37.4X5	T37.4X6
Spindle inactivator	T50.4X1	T50.4X2	T50.4X3	T50.4X4	T50.4X5	T50.4X6
Spiperone	T43.4X1	T43.4X2	T43.4X3	T43.4X4	T43.4X5	T43.4X6
Spiramycin	T36.3X1	T36.3X2	T36.3X3	T36.3X4	T36.3X5	T36.3X6
Spirapril	T46.4X1	T46.4X2	T46.4X3	T46.4X4	T46.4X5	T46.4X6
Spirilene	T43.591	T43.592	T43.593	T43.594	T43.595	T43.596
Spirit(s) (neutral) **NEC**	T51.0X1	T51.0X2	T51.0X3	T51.0X4	—	—
beverage	T51.0X1	T51.0X2	T51.0X3	T51.0X4	—	—
industrial	T51.0X1	T51.0X2	T51.0X3	T51.0X4	—	—
mineral	T52.0X1	T52.0X2	T52.0X3	T52.0X4	—	—
of salt — *see* Hydrochloric acid						
surgical	T51.0X1	T51.0X2	T51.0X3	T51.0X4	—	—
Spiriva*	T44.3X1	T44.3X2	T44.3X3	T44.3X4	T44.3X5	T44.3X6
Spironolactone	T50.0X1	T50.0X2	T50.0X3	T50.0X4	T50.0X5	T50.0X6
Spiroperidol	T43.4X1	T43.4X2	T43.4X3	T43.4X4	T43.4X5	T43.4X6
Sponge, absorbable (gelatin)	T45.7X1	T45.7X2	T45.7X3	T45.7X4	T45.7X5	T45.7X6
Sporostacin	T49.0X1	T49.0X2	T49.0X3	T49.0X4	T49.0X5	T49.0X6
Spray (aerosol)	T65.91	T65.92	T65.93	T65.94	—	—
cosmetic	T65.891	T65.892	T65.893	T65.894	—	—
medicinal NEC	T50.901	T50.902	T50.903	T50.904	T50.905	T50.906
pesticides — *see* Pesticide						
specified content — *see* specific substance						
Spurge flax	T62.2X1	T62.2X2	T62.2X3	T62.2X4	—	—

Substance	Poisoning, Accidental (unintentional)	Poisoning, Intentional Self-harm	Poisoning, Assault	Poisoning, Undetermined	Adverse Effect	Under-dosing
Spurges	T62.2X1	T62.2X2	T62.2X3	T62.2X4	—	—
Sputum viscosity-lowering drug	T48.4X1	T48.4X2	T48.4X3	T48.4X4	T48.4X5	T48.4X6
Squill	T46.0X1	T46.0X2	T46.0X3	T46.0X4	T46.0X5	T46.0X6
rat poison	T60.4X1	T60.4X2	T60.4X3	T60.4X4	—	—
Squirting cucumber (cathartic)	T47.2X1	T47.2X2	T47.2X3	T47.2X4	T47.2X5	T47.2X6
Stains	T65.6X1	T65.6X2	T65.6X3	T65.6X4	—	—
Stannous fluoride	T49.7X1	T49.7X2	T49.7X3	T49.7X4	T49.7X5	T49.7X6
Stanolone	T38.7X1	T38.7X2	T38.7X3	T38.7X4	T38.7X5	T38.7X6
Stanozolol	T38.7X1	T38.7X2	T38.7X3	T38.7X4	T38.7X5	T38.7X6
Staphisagria or stavesacre (pediculicide)	T49.0X1	T49.0X2	T49.0X3	T49.0X4	T49.0X5	T49.0X6
Starch	T50.901	T50.902	T50.903	T50.904	T50.905	T50.906
Stavzor*	T42.6X1	T42.6X2	T42.6X3	T42.6X4	T42.6X5	T42.6X6
Stelazine	T43.3X1	T43.3X2	T43.3X3	T43.3X4	T43.3X5	T43.3X6
Stemetil	T43.3X1	T43.3X2	T43.3X3	T43.3X4	T43.3X5	T43.3X6
Stepronin	T48.4X1	T48.4X2	T48.4X3	T48.4X4	T48.4X5	T48.4X6
Sterculia	T47.4X1	T47.4X2	T47.4X3	T47.4X4	T47.4X5	T47.4X6
Sternutator gas	T59.891	T59.892	T59.893	T59.894	—	—
Steroid	T38.0X1	T38.0X2	T38.0X3	T38.0X4	T38.0X5	T38.0X6
anabolic	T38.7X1	T38.7X2	T38.7X3	T38.7X4	T38.7X5	T38.7X6
androgenic	T38.7X1	T38.7X2	T38.7X3	T38.7X4	T38.7X5	T38.7X6
antineoplastic, hormone	T38.7X1	T38.7X2	T38.7X3	T38.7X4	T38.7X5	T38.7X6
estrogen	T38.5X1	T38.5X2	T38.5X3	T38.5X4	T38.5X5	T38.5X6
ENT agent	T49.6X1	T49.6X2	T49.6X3	T49.6X4	T49.6X5	T49.6X6
ophthalmic preparation	T49.5X1	T49.5X2	T49.5X3	T49.5X4	T49.5X5	T49.5X6
topical NEC	T49.0X1	T49.0X2	T49.0X3	T49.0X4	T49.0X5	T49.0X6
Stibine	T56.891	T56.892	T56.893	T56.894	—	—
Stibogluconate	T37.3X1	T37.3X2	T37.3X3	T37.3X4	T37.3X5	T37.3X6
Stibophen	T37.4X1	T37.4X2	T37.4X3	T37.4X4	T37.4X5	T37.4X6
Stilbamidine (isetionate)	T37.3X1	T37.3X2	T37.3X3	T37.3X4	T37.3X5	T37.3X6
Stilbestrol	T38.5X1	T38.5X2	T38.5X3	T38.5X4	T38.5X5	T38.5X6
Stilboestrol	T38.5X1	T38.5X2	T38.5X3	T38.5X4	T38.5X5	T38.5X6
Stimulant						
central nervous system — see also Psychostimulant	T43.601	T43.602	T43.603	T43.604	T43.605	T43.606
analeptics	T50.7X1	T50.7X2	T50.7X3	T50.7X4	T50.7X5	T50.7X6
opiate antagonist	T50.7X1	T50.7X2	T50.7X3	T50.7X4	T50.7X5	T50.7X6
psychotherapeutic NEC — see also Psychotherapeutic drug	T43.601	T43.602	T43.603	T43.604	T43.605	T43.606
specified NEC	T43.691	T43.692	T43.693	T43.694	T43.695	T43.696
respiratory	T48.901	T48.902	T48.903	T48.904	T48.905	T48.906
Stone-dissolving drug	T50.901	T50.902	T50.903	T50.904	T50.905	T50.906
Storage battery (cells) (acid)	T54.2X1	T54.2X2	T54.2X3	T54.2X4	—	—
Stovaine	T41.3X1	T41.3X2	T41.3X3	T41.3X4	T41.3X5	T41.3X6
infiltration (subcutaneous)	T41.3X1	T41.3X2	T41.3X3	T41.3X4	T41.3X5	T41.3X6
nerve block (peripheral) (plexus)	T41.3X1	T41.3X2	T41.3X3	T41.3X4	T41.3X5	T41.3X6
spinal	T41.3X1	T41.3X2	T41.3X3	T41.3X4	T41.3X5	T41.3X6
topical (surface)	T41.3X1	T41.3X2	T41.3X3	T41.3X4	T41.3X5	T41.3X6
Stovarsol	T37.8X1	T37.8X2	T37.8X3	T37.8X4	T37.8X5	T37.8X6
Stove gas — see Gas, stove						
Stoxil	T49.5X1	T49.5X2	T49.5X3	T49.5X4	T49.5X5	T49.5X6
Stramonium	T48.6X1	T48.6X2	T48.6X3	T48.6X4	T48.6X5	T48.6X6
natural state	T62.2X1	T62.2X2	T62.2X3	T62.2X4	—	—
Streptodornase	T45.3X1	T45.3X2	T45.3X3	T45.3X4	T45.3X5	T45.3X6
Streptoduocin	T36.5X1	T36.5X2	T36.5X3	T36.5X4	T36.5X5	T36.5X6
Streptokinase	T45.611	T45.612	T45.613	T45.614	T45.615	T45.616
Streptomycin (derivative)	T36.5X1	T36.5X2	T36.5X3	T36.5X4	T36.5X5	T36.5X6
Streptonivicin	T36.5X1	T36.5X2	T36.5X3	T36.5X4	T36.5X5	T36.5X6
Streptovarycin	T36.5X1	T36.5X2	T36.5X3	T36.5X4	T36.5X5	T36.5X6
Streptozocin	T45.1X1	T45.1X2	T45.1X3	T45.1X4	T45.1X5	T45.1X6
Streptozotocin	T45.1X1	T45.1X2	T45.1X3	T45.1X4	T45.1X5	T45.1X6
Stripper (paint) (solvent)	T52.8X1	T52.8X2	T52.8X3	T52.8X4	—	—
Strobane	T60.1X1	T60.1X2	T60.1X3	T60.1X4	—	—
Strofantina	T46.0X1	T46.0X2	T46.0X3	T46.0X4	T46.0X5	T46.0X6
Stromectol*	T37.4X1	T37.4X2	T37.4X3	T37.4X4	T37.4X5	T37.4X6
Strophanthin (g) (k)	T46.0X1	T46.0X2	T46.0X3	T46.0X4	T46.0X5	T46.0X6
Strophanthus	T46.0X1	T46.0X2	T46.0X3	T46.0X4	T46.0X5	T46.0X6
Strophantin	T46.0X1	T46.0X2	T46.0X3	T46.0X4	T46.0X5	T46.0X6
Strophantin-g	T46.0X1	T46.0X2	T46.0X3	T46.0X4	T46.0X5	T46.0X6
Strychnine (nonmedicinal) (pesticide) (salts)	T65.1X1	T65.1X2	T65.1X3	T65.1X4	—	—
medicinal	T48.291	T48.292	T48.293	T48.294	T48.295	T48.296
Strychnos (ignatii) — see Strychnine						
Styramate	T42.8X1	T42.8X2	T42.8X3	T42.8X4	T42.8X5	T42.8X6
Styrene	T65.891	T65.892	T65.893	T65.894	—	—
Succinimide, antiepileptic or anticonvulsant	T42.2X1	T42.2X2	T42.2X3	T42.2X4	T42.2X5	T42.2X6

Substance	Poisoning, Accidental (unintentional)	Poisoning, Intentional Self-harm	Poisoning, Assault	Poisoning, Undetermined	Adverse Effect	Under-dosing
Succinimide, antiepileptic or anticonvulsant — continued mercuric — see Mercury						
Succinylcholine	T48.1X1	T48.1X2	T48.1X3	T48.1X4	T48.1X5	T48.1X6
Succinylsulfathiazole	T37.0X1	T37.0X2	T37.0X3	T37.0X4	T37.0X5	T37.0X6
Sucralfate	T47.1X1	T47.1X2	T47.1X3	T47.1X4	T47.1X5	T47.1X6
Sucrose	T50.3X1	T50.3X2	T50.3X3	T50.3X4	T50.3X5	T50.3X6
Sufentanil	T40.411	T40.412	T40.413	T40.414	T40.415	T40.416
Sulbactam	T36.0X1	T36.0X2	T36.0X3	T36.0X4	T36.0X5	T36.0X6
Sulbenicillin	T36.0X1	T36.0X2	T36.0X3	T36.0X4	T36.0X5	T36.0X6
Sulbentine	T49.0X1	T49.0X2	T49.0X3	T49.0X4	T49.0X5	T49.0X6
Sulconazole*	T49.0X1	T49.0X2	T49.0X3	T49.0X4	T49.0X5	T49.0X6
Sulfacetamide	T49.0X1	T49.0X2	T49.0X3	T49.0X4	T49.0X5	T49.0X6
ophthalmic preparation	T49.5X1	T49.5X2	T49.5X3	T49.5X4	T49.5X5	T49.5X6
Sulfachlorpyridazine	T37.0X1	T37.0X2	T37.0X3	T37.0X4	T37.0X5	T37.0X6
Sulfacitine	T37.0X1	T37.0X2	T37.0X3	T37.0X4	T37.0X5	T37.0X6
Sulfadiasulfone sodium	T37.0X1	T37.0X2	T37.0X3	T37.0X4	T37.0X5	T37.0X6
Sulfadiazine	T37.0X1	T37.0X2	T37.0X3	T37.0X4	T37.0X5	T37.0X6
silver (topical)	T49.0X1	T49.0X2	T49.0X3	T49.0X4	T49.0X5	T49.0X6
Sulfadimethoxine	T37.0X1	T37.0X2	T37.0X3	T37.0X4	T37.0X5	T37.0X6
Sulfadimidine	T37.0X1	T37.0X2	T37.0X3	T37.0X4	T37.0X5	T37.0X6
Sulfadoxine	T37.0X1	T37.0X2	T37.0X3	T37.0X4	T37.0X5	T37.0X6
with pyrimethamine	T37.2X1	T37.2X2	T37.2X3	T37.2X4	T37.2X5	T37.2X6
Sulfaethidole	T37.0X1	T37.0X2	T37.0X3	T37.0X4	T37.0X5	T37.0X6
Sulfafurazole	T37.0X1	T37.0X2	T37.0X3	T37.0X4	T37.0X5	T37.0X6
Sulfaguanidine	T37.0X1	T37.0X2	T37.0X3	T37.0X4	T37.0X5	T37.0X6
Sulfalene	T37.0X1	T37.0X2	T37.0X3	T37.0X4	T37.0X5	T37.0X6
Sulfaloxate	T37.0X1	T37.0X2	T37.0X3	T37.0X4	T37.0X5	T37.0X6
Sulfaloxic acid	T37.0X1	T37.0X2	T37.0X3	T37.0X4	T37.0X5	T37.0X6
Sulfamazone	T39.2X1	T39.2X2	T39.2X3	T39.2X4	T39.2X5	T39.2X6
Sulfamerazine	T37.0X1	T37.0X2	T37.0X3	T37.0X4	T37.0X5	T37.0X6
Sulfameter	T37.0X1	T37.0X2	T37.0X3	T37.0X4	T37.0X5	T37.0X6
Sulfamethazine	T37.0X1	T37.0X2	T37.0X3	T37.0X4	T37.0X5	T37.0X6
Sulfamethizole	T37.0X1	T37.0X2	T37.0X3	T37.0X4	T37.0X5	T37.0X6
Sulfamethoxazole	T37.0X1	T37.0X2	T37.0X3	T37.0X4	T37.0X5	T37.0X6
with trimethoprim	T36.8X1	T36.8X2	T36.8X3	T36.8X4	T36.8X5	T36.8X6
Sulfamethoxydiazine	T37.0X1	T37.0X2	T37.0X3	T37.0X4	T37.0X5	T37.0X6
Sulfamethoxypyridazine	T37.0X1	T37.0X2	T37.0X3	T37.0X4	T37.0X5	T37.0X6
Sulfamethylthiazole	T37.0X1	T37.0X2	T37.0X3	T37.0X4	T37.0X5	T37.0X6
Sulfametoxydiazine	T37.0X1	T37.0X2	T37.0X3	T37.0X4	T37.0X5	T37.0X6
Sulfamidopyrine	T39.2X1	T39.2X2	T39.2X3	T39.2X4	T39.2X5	T39.2X6
Sulfamonomethoxine	T37.0X1	T37.0X2	T37.0X3	T37.0X4	T37.0X5	T37.0X6
Sulfamoxole	T37.0X1	T37.0X2	T37.0X3	T37.0X4	T37.0X5	T37.0X6
Sulfamylon	T49.0X1	T49.0X2	T49.0X3	T49.0X4	T49.0X5	T49.0X6
Sulfan blue (diagnostic dye)	T50.8X1	T50.8X2	T50.8X3	T50.8X4	T50.8X5	T50.8X6
Sulfanilamide	T37.0X1	T37.0X2	T37.0X3	T37.0X4	T37.0X5	T37.0X6
Sulfanilylguanidine	T37.0X1	T37.0X2	T37.0X3	T37.0X4	T37.0X5	T37.0X6
Sulfaperin	T37.0X1	T37.0X2	T37.0X3	T37.0X4	T37.0X5	T37.0X6
Sulfaphenazole	T37.0X1	T37.0X2	T37.0X3	T37.0X4	T37.0X5	T37.0X6
Sulfaphenylthiazole	T37.0X1	T37.0X2	T37.0X3	T37.0X4	T37.0X5	T37.0X6
Sulfaproxyline	T37.0X1	T37.0X2	T37.0X3	T37.0X4	T37.0X5	T37.0X6
Sulfapyridine	T37.0X1	T37.0X2	T37.0X3	T37.0X4	T37.0X5	T37.0X6
Sulfapyrimidine	T37.0X1	T37.0X2	T37.0X3	T37.0X4	T37.0X5	T37.0X6
Sulfarsphenamine	T37.8X1	T37.8X2	T37.8X3	T37.8X4	T37.8X5	T37.8X6
Sulfasalazine	T37.0X1	T37.0X2	T37.0X3	T37.0X4	T37.0X5	T37.0X6
Sulfasuxidine	T37.0X1	T37.0X2	T37.0X3	T37.0X4	T37.0X5	T37.0X6
Sulfasymazine	T37.0X1	T37.0X2	T37.0X3	T37.0X4	T37.0X5	T37.0X6
Sulfated amylopectin	T47.8X1	T47.8X2	T47.8X3	T47.8X4	T47.8X5	T47.8X6
Sulfathiazole	T37.0X1	T37.0X2	T37.0X3	T37.0X4	T37.0X5	T37.0X6
Sulfatostearate	T49.2X1	T49.2X2	T49.2X3	T49.2X4	T49.2X5	T49.2X6
Sulfatrim*	T36.8X1	T36.8X2	T36.8X3	T36.8X4	T36.8X5	T36.8X6
Sulfinpyrazone	T50.4X1	T50.4X2	T50.4X3	T50.4X4	T50.4X5	T50.4X6
Sulfiram	T49.0X1	T49.0X2	T49.0X3	T49.0X4	T49.0X5	T49.0X6
Sulfisomidine	T37.0X1	T37.0X2	T37.0X3	T37.0X4	T37.0X5	T37.0X6
Sulfisoxazole	T37.0X1	T37.0X2	T37.0X3	T37.0X4	T37.0X5	T37.0X6
ophthalmic preparation	T49.5X1	T49.5X2	T49.5X3	T49.5X4	T49.5X5	T49.5X6
Sulfobromophthalein (sodium)	T50.8X1	T50.8X2	T50.8X3	T50.8X4	T50.8X5	T50.8X6
Sulfobromphthalein	T50.8X1	T50.8X2	T50.8X3	T50.8X4	T50.8X5	T50.8X6
Sulfogaiacol	T48.4X1	T48.4X2	T48.4X3	T48.4X4	T48.4X5	T48.4X6
Sulfomyxin	T36.8X1	T36.8X2	T36.8X3	T36.8X4	T36.8X5	T36.8X6
Sulfonal	T42.6X1	T42.6X2	T42.6X3	T42.6X4	T42.6X5	T42.6X6
Sulfonamide NEC	T37.0X1	T37.0X2	T37.0X3	T37.0X4	T37.0X5	T37.0X6
eye	T49.5X1	T49.5X2	T49.5X3	T49.5X4	T49.5X5	T49.5X6
Sulfonazide	T37.1X1	T37.1X2	T37.1X3	T37.1X4	T37.1X5	T37.1X6
Sulfones	T37.1X1	T37.1X2	T37.1X3	T37.1X4	T37.1X5	T37.1X6
Sulfonethylmethane	T42.6X1	T42.6X2	T42.6X3	T42.6X4	T42.6X5	T42.6X6
Sulfonmethane	T42.6X1	T42.6X2	T42.6X3	T42.6X4	T42.6X5	T42.6X6
Sulfonphthal, sulfonphthol	T50.8X1	T50.8X2	T50.8X3	T50.8X4	T50.8X5	T50.8X6
Sulfonylurea derivatives, oral	T38.3X1	T38.3X2	T38.3X3	T38.3X4	T38.3X5	T38.3X6
Sulforidazine	T43.3X1	T43.3X2	T43.3X3	T43.3X4	T43.3X5	T43.3X6

Table of Drugs and Chemicals

Spurges — Sulforidazine

Substance	Poisoning, Accidental (unintentional)	Poisoning, Intentional Self-harm	Poisoning, Assault	Poisoning, Undetermined	Adverse Effect	Under-dosing
Sulfoxone	T37.1X1	T37.1X2	T37.1X3	T37.1X4	T37.1X5	T37.1X6
Sulfuric acid	T54.2X1	T54.2X2	T54.2X3	T54.2X4	—	—
Sulfur, sulfurated, sulfuric, sulfurous, sulfuryl	T49.4X1	T49.4X2	T49.4X3	T49.4X4	T49.4X5	T49.4X6
(compounds NEC) (medicinal)						
acid	T54.2X1	T54.2X2	T54.2X3	T54.2X4	—	—
dioxide (gas)	T59.1X1	T59.1X2	T59.1X3	T59.1X4	—	—
ether — see Ether(s)						
hydrogen	T59.6X1	T59.6X2	T59.6X3	T59.6X4	—	—
medicinal (keratolytic) (ointment) NEC	T49.4X1	T49.4X2	T49.4X3	T49.4X4	T49.4X5	T49.4X6
ointment	T49.0X1	T49.0X2	T49.0X3	T49.0X4	T49.0X5	T49.0X6
pesticide (vapor)	T60.91	T60.92	T60.93	T60.94	—	—
vapor NEC	T59.891	T59.892	T59.893	T59.894	—	—
Sulglicotide	T47.1X1	T47.1X2	T47.1X3	T47.1X4	T47.1X5	T47.1X6
Sulindac	T39.391	T39.392	T39.393	T39.394	T39.395	T39.396
Sulisatin	T47.2X1	T47.2X2	T47.2X3	T47.2X4	T47.2X5	T47.2X6
Sulisobenzone	T49.3X1	T49.3X2	T49.3X3	T49.3X4	T49.3X5	T49.3X6
Sulkowitch's reagent	T50.8X1	T50.8X2	T50.8X3	T50.8X4	T50.8X5	T50.8X6
Sulmetozine	T44.3X1	T44.3X2	T44.3X3	T44.3X4	T44.3X5	T44.3X6
Suloctidil	T46.7X1	T46.7X2	T46.7X3	T46.7X4	T46.7X5	T46.7X6
Sulph- — see also Sulf-						
Sulphadiazine	T37.0X1	T37.0X2	T37.0X3	T37.0X4	T37.0X5	T37.0X6
Sulphadimethoxine	T37.0X1	T37.0X2	T37.0X3	T37.0X4	T37.0X5	T37.0X6
Sulphadimidine	T37.0X1	T37.0X2	T37.0X3	T37.0X4	T37.0X5	T37.0X6
Sulphadione	T37.1X1	T37.1X2	T37.1X3	T37.1X4	T37.1X5	T37.1X6
Sulphafurazole	T37.0X1	T37.0X2	T37.0X3	T37.0X4	T37.0X5	T37.0X6
Sulphamethizole	T37.0X1	T37.0X2	T37.0X3	T37.0X4	T37.0X5	T37.0X6
Sulphamethoxazole	T37.0X1	T37.0X2	T37.0X3	T37.0X4	T37.0X5	T37.0X6
Sulphan blue	T50.8X1	T50.8X2	T50.8X3	T50.8X4	T50.8X5	T50.8X6
Sulphaphenazole	T37.0X1	T37.0X2	T37.0X3	T37.0X4	T37.0X5	T37.0X6
Sulphapyridine	T37.0X1	T37.0X2	T37.0X3	T37.0X4	T37.0X5	T37.0X6
Sulphasalazine	T37.0X1	T37.0X2	T37.0X3	T37.0X4	T37.0X5	T37.0X6
Sulphinpyrazone	T50.4X1	T50.4X2	T50.4X3	T50.4X4	T50.4X5	T50.4X6
Sulpiride	T43.591	T43.592	T43.593	T43.594	T43.595	T43.596
Sulprostone	T48.0X1	T48.0X2	T48.0X3	T48.0X4	T48.0X5	T48.0X6
Sulpyrine	T39.2X1	T39.2X2	T39.2X3	T39.2X4	T39.2X5	T39.2X6
Sultamicillin	T36.0X1	T36.0X2	T36.0X3	T36.0X4	T36.0X5	T36.0X6
Sulthiame	T42.6X1	T42.6X2	T42.6X3	T42.6X4	T42.6X5	T42.6X6
Sultiame	T42.6X1	T42.6X2	T42.6X3	T42.6X4	T42.6X5	T42.6X6
Sultopride	T43.591	T43.592	T43.593	T43.594	T43.595	T43.596
Sumatriptan	T39.8X1	T39.8X2	T39.8X3	T39.8X4	T39.8X5	T39.8X6
Sumavel*	T39.8X1	T39.8X2	T39.8X3	T39.8X4	T39.8X5	T39.8X6
Sunflower seed oil	T46.6X1	T46.6X2	T46.6X3	T46.6X4	T46.6X5	T46.6X6
Superinone	T48.4X1	T48.4X2	T48.4X3	T48.4X4	T48.4X5	T48.4X6
Suprofen	T39.311	T39.312	T39.313	T39.314	T39.315	T39.316
Suramin (sodium)	T37.4X1	T37.4X2	T37.4X3	T37.4X4	T37.4X5	T37.4X6
Surfacaine	T41.3X1	T41.3X2	T41.3X3	T41.3X4	T41.3X5	T41.3X6
Surital	T41.1X1	T41.1X2	T41.1X3	T41.1X4	T41.1X5	T41.1X6
Sutilains	T45.3X1	T45.3X2	T45.3X3	T45.3X4	T45.3X5	T45.3X6
Suxamethonium (chloride)	T48.1X1	T48.1X2	T48.1X3	T48.1X4	T48.1X5	T48.1X6
Suxethonium (chloride)	T48.1X1	T48.1X2	T48.1X3	T48.1X4	T48.1X5	T48.1X6
Suxibuzone	T39.2X1	T39.2X2	T39.2X3	T39.2X4	T39.2X5	T39.2X6
Sweetener	T50.901	T50.902	T50.903	T50.904	T50.905	T50.906
Sweet niter spirit	T46.3X1	T46.3X2	T46.3X3	T46.3X4	T46.3X5	T46.3X6
Sweet oil (birch)	T49.3X1	T49.3X2	T49.3X3	T49.3X4	T49.3X5	T49.3X6
Sylvant*	T45.1X1	T45.1X2	T45.1X3	T45.1X4	T45.1X5	T45.1X6
Sym-dichloroethyl ether	T53.6X1	T53.6X2	T53.6X3	T53.6X4	—	—
Sympatholytic NEC	T44.8X1	T44.8X2	T44.8X3	T44.8X4	T44.8X5	T44.8X6
haloalkylamine	T44.8X1	T44.8X2	T44.8X3	T44.8X4	T44.8X5	T44.8X6
Sympathomimetic NEC	T44.901	T44.902	T44.903	T44.904	T44.905	T44.906
anti-common-cold	T48.5X1	T48.5X2	T48.5X3	T48.5X4	T48.5X5	T48.5X6
bronchodilator	T48.6X1	T48.6X2	T48.6X3	T48.6X4	T48.6X5	T48.6X6
specified NEC	T44.991	T44.992	T44.993	T44.994	T44.995	T44.996
Synagis	T50.B91	T50.B92	T50.B93	T50.B94	T50.B95	T50.B96
Synalar	T49.0X1	T49.0X2	T49.0X3	T49.0X4	T49.0X5	T49.0X6
Synthetic cannabinoids	T40.721	T40.722	T40.723	T40.724	T40.725	T40.726
Synthroid	T38.1X1	T38.1X2	T38.1X3	T38.1X4	T38.1X5	T38.1X6
Syntocinon	T48.0X1	T48.0X2	T48.0X3	T48.0X4	T48.0X5	T48.0X6
Syrosingopine	T46.5X1	T46.5X2	T46.5X3	T46.5X4	T46.5X5	T46.5X6
Systemic drug	T45.91	T45.92	T45.93	T45.94	T45.95	T45.96
specified NEC	T45.8X1	T45.8X2	T45.8X3	T45.8X4	T45.8X5	T45.8X6
Tablets — see also specified substance	T50.901	T50.902	T50.903	T50.904	T50.905	T50.906
Tace	T38.5X1	T38.5X2	T38.5X3	T38.5X4	T38.5X5	T38.5X6
Tacrine	T44.0X1	T44.0X2	T44.0X3	T44.0X4	T44.0X5	T44.0X6
Tadalafil	T46.7X1	T46.7X2	T46.7X3	T46.7X4	T46.7X5	T46.7X6
Talampicillin	T36.0X1	T36.0X2	T36.0X3	T36.0X4	T36.0X5	T36.0X6
Talbutal	T42.3X1	T42.3X2	T42.3X3	T42.3X4	T42.3X5	T42.3X6
Talc powder	T49.3X1	T49.3X2	T49.3X3	T49.3X4	T49.3X5	T49.3X6
Talcum	T49.3X1	T49.3X2	T49.3X3	T49.3X4	T49.3X5	T49.3X6
Taleranol	T38.6X1	T38.6X2	T38.6X3	T38.6X4	T38.6X5	T38.6X6

Substance	Poisoning, Accidental (unintentional)	Poisoning, Intentional Self-harm	Poisoning, Assault	Poisoning, Undetermined	Adverse Effect	Under-dosing
Taltz*	T39.391	T39.392	T39.393	T39.394	T39.395	T39.396
Tamoxifen	T38.6X1	T38.6X2	T38.6X3	T38.6X4	T38.6X5	T38.6X6
Tamsulosin	T44.6X1	T44.6X2	T44.6X3	T44.6X4	T44.6X5	T44.6X6
Tandearil, tanderil	T39.2X1	T39.2X2	T39.2X3	T39.2X4	T39.2X5	T39.2X6
Tannic acid	T49.2X1	T49.2X2	T49.2X3	T49.2X4	T49.2X5	T49.2X6
medicinal (astringent)	T49.2X1	T49.2X2	T49.2X3	T49.2X4	T49.2X5	T49.2X6
Tannin — see Tannic acid						
Tansy	T62.2X1	T62.2X2	T62.2X3	T62.2X4	—	—
TAO	T36.3X1	T36.3X2	T36.3X3	T36.3X4	T36.3X5	T36.3X6
Tapazole	T38.2X1	T38.2X2	T38.2X3	T38.2X4	T38.2X5	T38.2X6
Taractan	T43.591	T43.592	T43.593	T43.594	T43.595	T43.596
Tarantula (venomous)	T63.321	T63.322	T63.323	T63.324	—	—
Tartar emetic	T37.8X1	T37.8X2	T37.8X3	T37.8X4	T37.8X5	—
Tartaric acid	T65.891	T65.892	T65.893	T65.894	—	—
Tartrated antimony (anti-infective)	T37.8X1	T37.8X2	T37.8X3	T37.8X4	T37.8X5	—
Tartrate, laxative	T47.4X1	T47.4X2	T47.4X3	T47.4X4	T47.4X5	T47.4X6
Tar NEC	T52.0X1	T52.0X2	T52.0X3	T52.0X4	—	—
camphor	T60.1X1	T60.1X2	T60.1X3	T60.1X4	—	—
distillate	T49.1X1	T49.1X2	T49.1X3	T49.1X4	T49.1X5	T49.1X6
fumes	T59.891	T59.892	T59.893	T59.894	—	—
medicinal	T49.1X1	T49.1X2	T49.1X3	T49.1X4	T49.1X5	T49.1X6
ointment	T49.1X1	T49.1X2	T49.1X3	T49.1X4	T49.1X5	T49.1X6
Tauromustine	T45.1X1	T45.1X2	T45.1X3	T45.1X4	T45.1X5	T45.1X6
TCA — see Trichloroacetic acid						
TCDD	T53.7X1	T53.7X2	T53.7X3	T53.7X4	—	—
TDI (vapor)	T65.0X1	T65.0X2	T65.0X3	T65.0X4	—	—
Tear						
gas	T59.3X1	T59.3X2	T59.3X3	T59.3X4	—	—
solution	T49.5X1	T49.5X2	T49.5X3	T49.5X4	T49.5X5	T49.5X6
Tecentriq*	T45.1X1	T45.1X2	T45.1X3	T45.1X4	T45.1X5	T45.1X6
Teclothiazide	T50.2X1	T50.2X2	T50.2X3	T50.2X4	T50.2X5	T50.2X6
Teclozan	T37.3X1	T37.3X2	T37.3X3	T37.3X4	T37.3X5	T37.3X6
Tegafur	T45.1X1	T45.1X2	T45.1X3	T45.1X4	T45.1X5	T45.1X6
Tegretol	T42.1X1	T42.1X2	T42.1X3	T42.1X4	T42.1X5	T42.1X6
Teicoplanin	T36.8X1	T36.8X2	T36.8X3	T36.8X4	T36.8X5	T36.8X6
Telepaque	T50.8X1	T50.8X2	T50.8X3	T50.8X4	T50.8X5	T50.8X6
Tellurium	T56.891	T56.892	T56.893	T56.894	—	—
fumes	T56.891	T56.892	T56.893	T56.894	—	—
TEM	T45.1X1	T45.1X2	T45.1X3	T45.1X4	T45.1X5	T45.1X6
Temazepam	T42.4X1	T42.4X2	T42.4X3	T42.4X4	T42.4X5	T42.4X6
Temocillin	T36.0X1	T36.0X2	T36.0X3	T36.0X4	T36.0X5	T36.0X6
Tenamfetamine	T43.621	T43.622	T43.623	T43.624	T43.625	T43.626
Tenecteplase*	T45.611	T45.612	T45.613	T45.614	T45.615	T45.616
Teniposide	T45.1X1	T45.1X2	T45.1X3	T45.1X4	T45.1X5	T45.1X6
Tenitramine	T46.3X1	T46.3X2	T46.3X3	T46.3X4	T46.3X5	T46.3X6
Tenoglicin	T48.4X1	T48.4X2	T48.4X3	T48.4X4	T48.4X5	T48.4X6
Tenonitrozole	T37.3X1	T37.3X2	T37.3X3	T37.3X4	T37.3X5	T37.3X6
Tenormin*	T44.7X1	T44.7X2	T44.7X3	T44.7X4	T44.7X5	T44.7X6
Tenoxicam	T39.391	T39.392	T39.393	T39.394	T39.395	T39.396
TEPA	T45.1X1	T45.1X2	T45.1X3	T45.1X4	T45.1X5	T45.1X6
TEPP	T60.0X1	T60.0X2	T60.0X3	T60.0X4	—	—
Teprotide	T46.5X1	T46.5X2	T46.5X3	T46.5X4	T46.5X5	T46.5X6
Terazosin	T44.6X1	T44.6X2	T44.6X3	T44.6X4	T44.6X5	T44.6X6
Terbufos	T60.0X1	T60.0X2	T60.0X3	T60.0X4	—	—
Terbutaline	T48.6X1	T48.6X2	T48.6X3	T48.6X4	T48.6X5	T48.6X6
Terconazole	T49.0X1	T49.0X2	T49.0X3	T49.0X4	T49.0X5	T49.0X6
Terfenadine	T45.0X1	T45.0X2	T45.0X3	T45.0X4	T45.0X5	T45.0X6
Teriparatide (acetate)	T50.991	T50.992	T50.993	T50.994	T50.995	T50.996
Terizidone	T37.1X1	T37.1X2	T37.1X3	T37.1X4	T37.1X5	T37.1X6
Terlipressin	T38.891	T38.892	T38.893	T38.894	T38.895	T38.896
Terodiline	T46.3X1	T46.3X2	T46.3X3	T46.3X4	T46.3X5	T46.3X6
Teroxalene	T37.4X1	T37.4X2	T37.4X3	T37.4X4	T37.4X5	T37.4X6
Terpin (cis) hydrate	T48.4X1	T48.4X2	T48.4X3	T48.4X4	T48.4X5	T48.4X6
Terramycin	T36.4X1	T36.4X2	T36.4X3	T36.4X4	T36.4X5	T36.4X6
Tertatolol	T44.7X1	T44.7X2	T44.7X3	T44.7X4	T44.7X5	T44.7X6
Tessalon	T48.3X1	T48.3X2	T48.3X3	T48.3X4	T48.3X5	T48.3X6
Testolactone	T38.7X1	T38.7X2	T38.7X3	T38.7X4	T38.7X5	T38.7X6
Testosterone	T38.7X1	T38.7X2	T38.7X3	T38.7X4	T38.7X5	T38.7X6
Tetanus toxoid or vaccine	T50.A91	T50.A92	T50.A93	T50.A94	T50.A95	T50.A96
antitoxin	T50.Z11	T50.Z12	T50.Z13	T50.Z14	T50.Z15	T50.Z16
immune globulin (human)	T50.Z11	T50.Z12	T50.Z13	T50.Z14	T50.Z15	T50.Z16
toxoid	T50.A91	T50.A92	T50.A93	T50.A94	T50.A95	T50.A96
with diphtheria toxoid	T50.A21	T50.A22	T50.A23	T50.A24	T50.A25	T50.A26
with pertussis	T50.A11	T50.A12	T50.A13	T50.A14	T50.A15	T50.A16
Tetrabenazine	T43.591	T43.592	T43.593	T43.594	T43.595	T43.596
Tetracaine	T41.3X1	T41.3X2	T41.3X3	T41.3X4	T41.3X5	T41.3X6
nerve block (peripheral) (plexus)	T41.3X1	T41.3X2	T41.3X3	T41.3X4	T41.3X5	T41.3X6
regional	T41.3X1	T41.3X2	T41.3X3	T41.3X4	T41.3X5	T41.3X6
spinal	T41.3X1	T41.3X2	T41.3X3	T41.3X4	T41.3X5	T41.3X6
Tetrachlorethylene — see Tetrachloroethylene						

☑ Additional Character May Be Required — Refer to the Tabular List for Character Selection   *Optum Value-Add

Substance	Poisoning, Accidental (unintentional)	Poisoning, Intentional Self-harm	Poisoning, Assault	Poisoning, Undetermined	Adverse Effect	Under-dosing
Tetrachlormethiazide	T50.2X1	T50.2X2	T50.2X3	T50.2X4	T50.2X5	T50.2X6
Tetrachloroethane	T53.6X1	T53.6X2	T53.6X3	T53.6X4	—	—
vapor	T53.6X1	T53.6X2	T53.6X3	T53.6X4	—	—
paint or varnish	T53.6X1	T53.6X2	T53.6X3	T53.6X4	—	—
Tetrachloroethylene (liquid)	T53.3X1	T53.3X2	T53.3X3	T53.3X4	—	—
medicinal	T37.4X1	T37.4X2	T37.4X3	T37.4X4	T37.4X5	T37.4X6
vapor	T53.3X1	T53.3X2	T53.3X3	T53.3X4	—	—
Tetrachloromethane — see Carbon tetrachloride						
Tetracosactide	T38.811	T38.812	T38.813	T38.814	T38.815	T38.816
Tetracosactrin	T38.811	T38.812	T38.813	T38.814	T38.815	T38.816
Tetracycline	T36.4X1	T36.4X2	T36.4X3	T36.4X4	T36.4X5	T36.4X6
ophthalmic preparation	T49.5X1	T49.5X2	T49.5X3	T49.5X4	T49.5X5	T49.5X6
topical NEC	T49.0X1	T49.0X2	T49.0X3	T49.0X4	T49.0X5	T49.0X6
Tetradifon	T60.8X1	T60.8X2	T60.8X3	T60.8X4	—	—
Tetradotoxin	T61.771	T61.772	T61.773	T61.774	—	—
Tetraethyl						
lead	T56.0X1	T56.0X2	T56.0X3	T56.0X4	—	—
pyrophosphate	T60.0X1	T60.0X2	T60.0X3	T60.0X4	—	—
Tetraethylammonium chloride	T44.2X1	T44.2X2	T44.2X3	T44.2X4	T44.2X5	T44.2X6
Tetraethylthiuram disulfide	T50.6X1	T50.6X2	T50.6X3	T50.6X4	T50.6X5	T50.6X6
Tetrahydroaminoacridine	T44.0X1	T44.0X2	T44.0X3	T44.0X4	T44.0X5	T44.0X6
Tetrahydrocannabinol	T40.711	T40.712	T40.713	T40.714	T40.715	T40.716
Tetrahydrofuran	T52.8X1	T52.8X2	T52.8X3	T52.8X4	—	—
Tetrahydrolipstatin*	T47.8X1	T47.8X2	T47.8X3	T47.8X4	T47.8X5	T47.8X6
Tetrahydronaphthalene	T52.8X1	T52.8X2	T52.8X3	T52.8X4	—	—
Tetrahydrozoline	T49.5X1	T49.5X2	T49.5X3	T49.5X4	T49.5X5	T49.5X6
Tetralin	T52.8X1	T52.8X2	T52.8X3	T52.8X4	—	—
Tetramethrin	T60.2X1	T60.2X2	T60.2X3	T60.2X4	—	—
Tetramethylthiuram (disulfide) NEC	T60.3X1	T60.3X2	T60.3X3	T60.3X4	—	—
medicinal	T49.0X1	T49.0X2	T49.0X3	T49.0X4	T49.0X5	T49.0X6
Tetramisole	T37.4X1	T37.4X2	T37.4X3	T37.4X4	T37.4X5	T37.4X6
Tetranicotinoyl fructose	T46.7X1	T46.7X2	T46.7X3	T46.7X4	T46.7X5	T46.7X6
Tetrazepam	T42.4X1	T42.4X2	T42.4X3	T42.4X4	T42.4X5	T42.4X6
Tetronal	T42.6X1	T42.6X2	T42.6X3	T42.6X4	T42.6X5	T42.6X6
Tetryl	T65.3X1	T65.3X2	T65.3X3	T65.3X4	—	—
Tetrylammonium chloride	T44.2X1	T44.2X2	T44.2X3	T44.2X4	T44.2X5	T44.2X6
Tetryzoline	T49.5X1	T49.5X2	T49.5X3	T49.5X4	T49.5X5	T49.5X6
Thalidomide	T45.1X1	T45.1X2	T45.1X3	T45.1X4	T45.1X5	T45.1X6
Thallium (compounds) (dust) NEC	T56.811	T56.812	T56.813	T56.814	—	—
pesticide	T60.4X1	T60.4X2	T60.4X3	T60.4X4	—	—
THC	T40.711	T40.712	T40.713	T40.714	T40.715	T40.716
Thebacon	T48.3X1	T48.3X2	T48.3X3	T48.3X4	T48.3X5	T48.3X6
Thebaine	T40.2X1	T40.2X2	T40.2X3	T40.2X4	T40.2X5	T40.2X6
Thenoic acid	T49.6X1	T49.6X2	T49.6X3	T49.6X4	T49.6X5	T49.6X6
Thenyldiamine	T45.0X1	T45.0X2	T45.0X3	T45.0X4	T45.0X5	T45.0X6
Theobromine (calcium salicylate)	T48.6X1	T48.6X2	T48.6X3	T48.6X4	T48.6X5	T48.6X6
sodium salicylate	T48.6X1	T48.6X2	T48.6X3	T48.6X4	T48.6X5	T48.6X6
Theolair*	T48.6X1	T48.6X2	T48.6X3	T48.6X4	T48.6X5	T48.6X6
Theophyllamine	T48.6X1	T48.6X2	T48.6X3	T48.6X4	T48.6X5	T48.6X6
Theophylline	T48.6X1	T48.6X2	T48.6X3	T48.6X4	T48.6X5	T48.6X6
aminobenzoic acid	T48.6X1	T48.6X2	T48.6X3	T48.6X4	T48.6X5	T48.6X6
ethylenediamine	T48.6X1	T48.6X2	T48.6X3	T48.6X4	T48.6X5	T48.6X6
piperazine	T48.6X1	T48.6X2	T48.6X3	T48.6X4	T48.6X5	T48.6X6
p-amino-benzoate	T47.4X1	T47.4X2	T47.4X3	T47.4X4	T47.4X5	T47.4X6
Therevac*	T47.4X1	T47.4X2	T47.4X3	T47.4X4	T47.4X5	T47.4X6
Thiabendazole	T37.4X1	T37.4X2	T37.4X3	T37.4X4	T37.4X5	T37.4X6
Thialbarbital	T41.1X1	T41.1X2	T41.1X3	T41.1X4	T41.1X5	T41.1X6
Thiamazole	T38.2X1	T38.2X2	T38.2X3	T38.2X4	T38.2X5	T38.2X6
Thiambutosine	T37.1X1	T37.1X2	T37.1X3	T37.1X4	T37.1X5	T37.1X6
Thiamine	T45.2X1	T45.2X2	T45.2X3	T45.2X4	T45.2X5	T45.2X6
Thiamphenicol	T36.2X1	T36.2X2	T36.2X3	T36.2X4	T36.2X5	T36.2X6
Thiamylal	T41.1X1	T41.1X2	T41.1X3	T41.1X4	T41.1X5	T41.1X6
sodium	T41.1X1	T41.1X2	T41.1X3	T41.1X4	T41.1X5	T41.1X6
Thiazesim	T43.291	T43.292	T43.293	T43.294	T43.295	T43.296
Thiazides (diuretics)	T50.2X1	T50.2X2	T50.2X3	T50.2X4	T50.2X5	T50.2X6
Thiazinamium metilsulfate	T43.3X1	T43.3X2	T43.3X3	T43.3X4	T43.3X5	T43.3X6
Thiethylperazine	T43.3X1	T43.3X2	T43.3X3	T43.3X4	T43.3X5	T43.3X6
Thimerosal	T49.0X1	T49.0X2	T49.0X3	T49.0X4	T49.0X5	T49.0X6
ophthalmic preparation	T49.5X1	T49.5X2	T49.5X3	T49.5X4	T49.5X5	T49.5X6
Thioacetazone	T37.1X1	T37.1X2	T37.1X3	T37.1X4	T37.1X5	T37.1X6
with isoniazid	T37.1X1	T37.1X2	T37.1X3	T37.1X4	T37.1X5	T37.1X6
Thiobarbital sodium	T41.1X1	T41.1X2	T41.1X3	T41.1X4	T41.1X5	T41.1X6
Thiobarbiturate anesthetic	T41.1X1	T41.1X2	T41.1X3	T41.1X4	T41.1X5	T41.1X6
Thiobismol	T37.8X1	T37.8X2	T37.8X3	T37.8X4	T37.8X5	T37.8X6

Substance	Poisoning, Accidental (unintentional)	Poisoning, Intentional Self-harm	Poisoning, Assault	Poisoning, Undetermined	Adverse Effect	Under-dosing
Thiobutabarbital sodium	T41.1X1	T41.1X2	T41.1X3	T41.1X4	T41.1X5	T41.1X6
Thiocarbamate (insecticide)	T60.0X1	T60.0X2	T60.0X3	T60.0X4	—	—
Thiocarbamide	T38.2X1	T38.2X2	T38.2X3	T38.2X4	T38.2X5	T38.2X6
Thiocarbarsone	T37.8X1	T37.8X2	T37.8X3	T37.8X4	T37.8X5	T37.8X6
Thiocarlide	T37.1X1	T37.1X2	T37.1X3	T37.1X4	T37.1X5	T37.1X6
Thioctamide	T50.991	T50.992	T50.993	T50.994	T50.995	T50.996
Thioctic acid	T50.991	T50.992	T50.993	T50.994	T50.995	T50.996
Thiofos	T60.0X1	T60.0X2	T60.0X3	T60.0X4	—	—
Thioglycolate	T49.4X1	T49.4X2	T49.4X3	T49.4X4	T49.4X5	T49.4X6
Thioglycolic acid	T65.891	T65.892	T65.893	T65.894	—	—
Thioguanine	T45.1X1	T45.1X2	T45.1X3	T45.1X4	T45.1X5	T45.1X6
Thiomercaptomerin	T50.2X1	T50.2X2	T50.2X3	T50.2X4	T50.2X5	T50.2X6
Thiomerin	T50.2X1	T50.2X2	T50.2X3	T50.2X4	T50.2X5	T50.2X6
Thiomersal	T49.0X1	T49.0X2	T49.0X3	T49.0X4	T49.0X5	T49.0X6
Thionazin	T60.0X1	T60.0X2	T60.0X3	T60.0X4	—	—
Thiopental (sodium)	T41.1X1	T41.1X2	T41.1X3	T41.1X4	T41.1X5	T41.1X6
Thiopentone (sodium)	T41.1X1	T41.1X2	T41.1X3	T41.1X4	T41.1X5	T41.1X6
Thiopropazate	T43.3X1	T43.3X2	T43.3X3	T43.3X4	T43.3X5	T43.3X6
Thioproperazine	T43.3X1	T43.3X2	T43.3X3	T43.3X4	T43.3X5	T43.3X6
Thioridazine	T43.3X1	T43.3X2	T43.3X3	T43.3X4	T43.3X5	T43.3X6
Thiosinamine	T49.3X1	T49.3X2	T49.3X3	T49.3X4	T49.3X5	T49.3X6
Thiotepa	T45.1X1	T45.1X2	T45.1X3	T45.1X4	T45.1X5	T45.1X6
Thiothixene	T43.4X1	T43.4X2	T43.4X3	T43.4X4	T43.4X5	T43.4X6
Thiouracil (benzyl) (methyl) (propyl)	T38.2X1	T38.2X2	T38.2X3	T38.2X4	T38.2X5	T38.2X6
Thiourea	T38.2X1	T38.2X2	T38.2X3	T38.2X4	T38.2X5	T38.2X6
Thiphenamil	T44.3X1	T44.3X2	T44.3X3	T44.3X4	T44.3X5	T44.3X6
Thiram	T60.3X1	T60.3X2	T60.3X3	T60.3X4	—	—
medicinal	T49.2X1	T49.2X2	T49.2X3	T49.2X4	T49.2X5	T49.2X6
Thonzylamine (systemic)	T45.0X1	T45.0X2	T45.0X3	T45.0X4	T45.0X5	T45.0X6
mucosal decongestant	T48.5X1	T48.5X2	T48.5X3	T48.5X4	T48.5X5	T48.5X6
Thorazine	T43.3X1	T43.3X2	T43.3X3	T43.3X4	T43.3X5	T43.3X6
Thorium dioxide suspension	T50.8X1	T50.8X2	T50.8X3	T50.8X4	T50.8X5	T50.8X6
Thornapple	T62.2X1	T62.2X2	T62.2X3	T62.2X4	—	—
Throat drug NEC	T49.6X1	T49.6X2	T49.6X3	T49.6X4	T49.6X5	T49.6X6
Thrombate 111*	T45.511	T45.512	T45.513	T45.514	T45.515	T45.516
Thrombin	T45.7X1	T45.7X2	T45.7X3	T45.7X4	T45.7X5	T45.7X6
Thrombolysin	T45.611	T45.612	T45.613	T45.614	T45.615	T45.616
Thromboplastin	T45.7X1	T45.7X2	T45.7X3	T45.7X4	T45.7X5	T45.7X6
Thurfyl nicotinate	T46.7X1	T46.7X2	T46.7X3	T46.7X4	T46.7X5	T46.7X6
Thymol	T49.0X1	T49.0X2	T49.0X3	T49.0X4	T49.0X5	T49.0X6
Thymopentin	T37.5X1	T37.5X2	T37.5X3	T37.5X4	T37.5X5	T37.5X6
Thymoxamine	T46.7X1	T46.7X2	T46.7X3	T46.7X4	T46.7X5	T46.7X6
Thymus extract	T38.891	T38.892	T38.893	T38.894	T38.895	T38.896
Thyreotrophic hormone	T38.811	T38.812	T38.813	T38.814	T38.815	T38.816
Thyroglobulin	T38.1X1	T38.1X2	T38.1X3	T38.1X4	T38.1X5	T38.1X6
Thyroid (hormone)	T38.1X1	T38.1X2	T38.1X3	T38.1X4	T38.1X5	T38.1X6
Thyrolar	T38.1X1	T38.1X2	T38.1X3	T38.1X4	T38.1X5	T38.1X6
Thyrotrophin	T38.811	T38.812	T38.813	T38.814	T38.815	T38.816
Thyrotropic hormone	T38.811	T38.812	T38.813	T38.814	T38.815	T38.816
Thyroxine	T38.1X1	T38.1X2	T38.1X3	T38.1X4	T38.1X5	T38.1X6
Tiabendazole	T37.4X1	T37.4X2	T37.4X3	T37.4X4	T37.4X5	T37.4X6
Tiamizide	T50.2X1	T50.2X2	T50.2X3	T50.2X4	T50.2X5	T50.2X6
Tianeptine	T43.291	T43.292	T43.293	T43.294	T43.295	T43.296
Tiapamil	T46.1X1	T46.1X2	T46.1X3	T46.1X4	T46.1X5	T46.1X6
Tiapride	T43.591	T43.592	T43.593	T43.594	T43.595	T43.596
Tiaprofenic acid	T39.311	T39.312	T39.313	T39.314	T39.315	T39.316
Tiaramide	T39.8X1	T39.8X2	T39.8X3	T39.8X4	T39.8X5	T39.8X6
Ticagrelor*	T45.521	T45.522	T45.523	T45.524	T45.525	T45.526
Ticarcillin	T36.0X1	T36.0X2	T36.0X3	T36.0X4	T36.0X5	T36.0X6
Ticlatone	T49.0X1	T49.0X2	T49.0X3	T49.0X4	T49.0X5	T49.0X6
Ticlopidine	T45.521	T45.522	T45.523	T45.524	T45.525	T45.526
Ticrynafen	T50.1X1	T50.1X2	T50.1X3	T50.1X4	T50.1X5	T50.1X6
Tidiacic	T50.991	T50.992	T50.993	T50.994	T50.995	T50.996
Tiemonium	T44.3X1	T44.3X2	T44.3X3	T44.3X4	T44.3X5	T44.3X6
iodide	T44.3X1	T44.3X2	T44.3X3	T44.3X4	T44.3X5	T44.3X6
Tienilic acid	T50.1X1	T50.1X2	T50.1X3	T50.1X4	T50.1X5	T50.1X6
Tifenamil	T44.3X1	T44.3X2	T44.3X3	T44.3X4	T44.3X5	T44.3X6
Tigan	T45.0X1	T45.0X2	T45.0X3	T45.0X4	T45.0X5	T45.0X6
Tigloidine	T44.3X1	T44.3X2	T44.3X3	T44.3X4	T44.3X5	T44.3X6
Tilactase	T47.5X1	T47.5X2	T47.5X3	T47.5X4	T47.5X5	T47.5X6
Tiletamine	T41.291	T41.292	T41.293	T41.294	T41.295	T41.296
Tilidine	T40.491	T40.492	T40.493	T40.494	—	—
Timepidium bromide	T44.3X1	T44.3X2	T44.3X3	T44.3X4	T44.3X5	T44.3X6
Timiperone	T43.4X1	T43.4X2	T43.4X3	T43.4X4	T43.4X5	T43.4X6
Timolol	T44.7X1	T44.7X2	T44.7X3	T44.7X4	T44.7X5	T44.7X6
Tincture, iodine — see Iodine						
Tindal	T43.3X1	T43.3X2	T43.3X3	T43.3X4	T43.3X5	T43.3X6
Tinidazole	T37.3X1	T37.3X2	T37.3X3	T37.3X4	T37.3X5	T37.3X6
Tin (chloride) (dust) (oxide) NEC	T56.6X1	T56.6X2	T56.6X3	T56.6X4	—	—

Table of Drugs and Chemicals

Tetrachlormethiazide — Tin

Substance	Poisoning, Accidental (unintentional)	Poisoning, Intentional Self-harm	Poisoning, Assault	Poisoning, Undetermined	Adverse Effect	Under-dosing
Tin (chloride) (dust) (oxide) **NEC**						
— continued						
anti-infectives	T37.8X1	T37.8X2	T37.8X3	T37.8X4	T37.8X5	T37.8X6
Tinoridine	T39.8X1	T39.8X2	T39.8X3	T39.8X4	T39.8X5	T39.8X6
Tiocarlide	T37.1X1	T37.1X2	T37.1X3	T37.1X4	T37.1X5	T37.1X6
Tioclomarol	T45.511	T45.512	T45.513	T45.514	T45.515	T45.516
Tioconazole	T49.0X1	T49.0X2	T49.0X3	T49.0X4	T49.0X5	T49.0X6
Tioguanine	T45.1X1	T45.1X2	T45.1X3	T45.1X4	T45.1X5	T45.1X6
Tiopronin	T50.991	T50.992	T50.993	T50.994	T50.995	T50.996
Tiotixene	T43.4X1	T43.4X2	T43.4X3	T43.4X4	T43.4X5	T43.4X6
Tioxolone	T49.4X1	T49.4X2	T49.4X3	T49.4X4	T49.4X5	T49.4X6
Tipepidine	T48.3X1	T48.3X2	T48.3X3	T48.3X4	T48.3X5	T48.3X6
Tiquizium bromide	T44.3X1	T44.3X2	T44.3X3	T44.3X4	T44.3X5	T44.3X6
Tiratricol	T38.1X1	T38.1X2	T38.1X3	T38.1X4	T38.1X5	T38.1X6
Tisopurine	T50.4X1	T50.4X2	T50.4X3	T50.4X4	T50.4X5	T50.4X6
Titanium (compounds)	T56.891	T56.892	T56.893	T56.894	—	—
(vapor)						
dioxide	T49.3X1	T49.3X2	T49.3X3	T49.3X4	T49.3X5	T49.3X6
ointment	T49.3X1	T49.3X2	T49.3X3	T49.3X4	T49.3X5	T49.3X6
oxide	T49.3X1	T49.3X2	T49.3X3	T49.3X4	T49.3X5	T49.3X6
tetrachloride	T56.891	T56.892	T56.893	T56.894	—	—
Titanocene	T56.891	T56.892	T56.893	T56.894	—	—
Titroid	T38.1X1	T38.1X2	T38.1X3	T38.1X4	T38.1X5	T38.1X6
Tizanidine	T42.8X1	T42.8X2	T42.8X3	T42.8X4	T42.8X5	T42.8X6
TMTD	T60.3X1	T60.3X2	T60.3X3	T60.3X4	—	—
TNT (fumes)	T65.3X1	T65.3X2	T65.3X3	T65.3X4	—	—
Toadstool	T62.0X1	T62.0X2	T62.0X3	T62.0X4	—	—
Tobacco NEC	T65.291	T65.292	T65.293	T65.294	—	—
cigarettes	T65.221	T65.222	T65.223	T65.224	—	—
Indian	T62.2X1	T62.2X2	T62.2X3	T62.2X4	—	—
smoke, second-hand	T65.221	T65.222	T65.223	T65.224	—	—
Tobraflex*	T49.5X1	T49.5X2	T49.5X3	T49.5X4	T49.5X5	T49.5X6
Tobramycin	T36.5X1	T36.5X2	T36.5X3	T36.5X4	T36.5X5	T36.5X6
Tocainide	T46.2X1	T46.2X2	T46.2X3	T46.2X4	T46.2X5	T46.2X6
Tocoferol	T45.2X1	T45.2X2	T45.2X3	T45.2X4	T45.2X5	T45.2X6
Tocopherol	T45.2X1	T45.2X2	T45.2X3	T45.2X4	T45.2X5	T45.2X6
acetate	T45.2X1	T45.2X2	T45.2X3	T45.2X4	T45.2X5	T45.2X6
Tocosamine	T48.0X1	T48.0X2	T48.0X3	T48.0X4	T48.0X5	T48.0X6
Todralazine	T46.5X1	T46.5X2	T46.5X3	T46.5X4	T46.5X5	T46.5X6
Tofisopam	T42.4X1	T42.4X2	T42.4X3	T42.4X4	T42.4X5	T42.4X6
Tofranil	T43.011	T43.012	T43.013	T43.014	T43.015	T43.016
Toilet deodorizer	T65.891	T65.892	T65.893	T65.894	—	—
Tolamolol	T44.7X1	T44.7X2	T44.7X3	T44.7X4	T44.7X5	T44.7X6
Tolazamide	T38.3X1	T38.3X2	T38.3X3	T38.3X4	T38.3X5	T38.3X6
Tolazoline	T46.7X1	T46.7X2	T46.7X3	T46.7X4	T46.7X5	T46.7X6
Tolbutamide (sodium)	T38.3X1	T38.3X2	T38.3X3	T38.3X4	T38.3X5	T38.3X6
Tolciclate	T49.0X1	T49.0X2	T49.0X3	T49.0X4	T49.0X5	T49.0X6
Tolmetin	T39.391	T39.392	T39.393	T39.394	T39.395	T39.396
Tolnaftate	T49.0X1	T49.0X2	T49.0X3	T49.0X4	T49.0X5	T49.0X6
Tolonidine	T46.5X1	T46.5X2	T46.5X3	T46.5X4	T46.5X5	T46.5X6
Toloxatone	T42.6X1	T42.6X2	T42.6X3	T42.6X4	T42.6X5	T42.6X6
Tolperisone	T44.3X1	T44.3X2	T44.3X3	T44.3X4	T44.3X5	T44.3X6
Tolserol	T42.8X1	T42.8X2	T42.8X3	T42.8X4	T42.8X5	T42.8X6
Toluene (liquid)	T52.2X1	T52.2X2	T52.2X3	T52.2X4	—	—
diisocyanate	T65.0X1	T65.0X2	T65.0X3	T65.0X4	—	—
Toluidine	T65.891	T65.892	T65.893	T65.894	—	—
vapor	T59.891	T59.892	T59.893	T59.894	—	—
Toluol (liquid)	T52.2X1	T52.2X2	T52.2X3	T52.2X4	—	—
vapor	T52.2X1	T52.2X2	T52.2X3	T52.2X4	—	—
Toluylenediamine	T65.3X1	T65.3X2	T65.3X3	T65.3X4	—	—
Tolylene-2,4-diisocyanate	T65.0X1	T65.0X2	T65.0X3	T65.0X4	—	—
Tonic NEC	T50.901	T50.902	T50.903	T50.904	T50.905	T50.906
Topical action drug NEC	T49.91	T49.92	T49.93	T49.94	T49.95	T49.96
ear, nose or throat	T49.6X1	T49.6X2	T49.6X3	T49.6X4	T49.6X5	T49.6X6
eye	T49.5X1	T49.5X2	T49.5X3	T49.5X4	T49.5X5	T49.5X6
skin	T49.91	T49.92	T49.93	T49.94	T49.95	T49.96
specified NEC	T49.8X1	T49.8X2	T49.8X3	T49.8X4	T49.8X5	T49.8X6
Toprol*	T44.7X1	T44.7X2	T44.7X3	T44.7X4	T44.7X5	T44.7X6
Toquizine	T44.3X1	T44.3X2	T44.3X3	T44.3X4	T44.3X5	T44.3X6
Toremifene	T38.6X1	T38.6X2	T38.6X3	T38.6X4	T38.6X5	T38.6X6
Tosylchloramide sodium	T49.8X1	T49.8X2	T49.8X3	T49.8X4	T49.8X5	T49.8X6
Toxaphene (dust) (spray)	T60.1X1	T60.1X2	T60.1X3	T60.1X4	—	—
Toxin, diphtheria (Schick Test)	T50.8X1	T50.8X2	T50.8X3	T50.8X4	T50.8X5	T50.8X6
Toxoid						
combined	T50.A21	T50.A22	T50.A23	T50.A24	T50.A25	T50.A26
diphtheria	T50.A91	T50.A92	T50.A93	T50.A94	T50.A95	T50.A96
tetanus	T50.A91	T50.A92	T50.A93	T50.A94	T50.A95	T50.A96
Trace element NEC	T45.8X1	T45.8X2	T45.8X3	T45.8X4	T45.8X5	T45.8X6
Tractor fuel NEC	T52.0X1	T52.0X2	T52.0X3	T52.0X4	—	—
Tragacanth	T50.991	T50.992	T50.993	T50.994	T50.995	T50.996
Tramadol	T40.421	T40.422	T40.423	T40.424	T40.425	T40.426
Tramazoline	T48.5X1	T48.5X2	T48.5X3	T48.5X4	T48.5X5	T48.5X6

Substance	Poisoning, Accidental (unintentional)	Poisoning, Intentional Self-harm	Poisoning, Assault	Poisoning, Undetermined	Adverse Effect	Under-dosing
Tranexamic acid	T45.621	T45.622	T45.623	T45.624	T45.625	T45.626
Tranilast	T45.0X1	T45.0X2	T45.0X3	T45.0X4	T45.0X5	T45.0X6
Tranquilizer NEC	T43.501	T43.502	T43.503	T43.504	T43.505	T43.506
with hypnotic or sedative	T42.6X1	T42.6X2	T42.6X3	T42.6X4	T42.6X5	T42.6X6
benzodiazepine NEC	T42.4X1	T42.4X2	T42.4X3	T42.4X4	T42.4X5	T42.4X6
butyrophenone NEC	T43.4X1	T43.4X2	T43.4X3	T43.4X4	T43.4X5	T43.4X6
carbamate	T43.591	T43.592	T43.593	T43.594	T43.595	T43.596
dimethylamine	T43.3X1	T43.3X2	T43.3X3	T43.3X4	T43.3X5	T43.3X6
ethylamine	T43.3X1	T43.3X2	T43.3X3	T43.3X4	T43.3X5	T43.3X6
hydroxyzine	T43.591	T43.592	T43.593	T43.594	T43.595	T43.596
major NEC	T43.501	T43.502	T43.503	T43.504	T43.505	T43.506
penothiazine NEC	T43.3X1	T43.3X2	T43.3X3	T43.3X4	T43.3X5	T43.3X6
phenothiazine-based	T43.3X1	T43.3X2	T43.3X3	T43.3X4	T43.3X5	T43.3X6
piperazine NEC	T43.3X1	T43.3X2	T43.3X3	T43.3X4	T43.3X5	T43.3X6
piperidine	T43.3X1	T43.3X2	T43.3X3	T43.3X4	T43.3X5	T43.3X6
propylamine	T43.3X1	T43.3X2	T43.3X3	T43.3X4	T43.3X5	T43.3X6
specified NEC	T43.591	T43.592	T43.593	T43.594	T43.595	T43.596
thioxanthene NEC	T43.591	T43.592	T43.593	T43.594	T43.595	T43.596
Tranxene	T42.4X1	T42.4X2	T42.4X3	T42.4X4	T42.4X5	T42.4X6
Tranylcypromine	T43.1X1	T43.1X2	T43.1X3	T43.1X4	T43.1X5	T43.1X6
Trapidil	T46.3X1	T46.3X2	T46.3X3	T46.3X4	T46.3X5	T46.3X6
Trasentine	T44.3X1	T44.3X2	T44.3X3	T44.3X4	T44.3X5	T44.3X6
Travert	T50.3X1	T50.3X2	T50.3X3	T50.3X4	T50.3X5	T50.3X6
Trazodone	T43.211	T43.212	T43.213	T43.214	T43.215	T43.216
Treanda*	T45.1X1	T45.1X2	T45.1X3	T45.1X4	T45.1X5	T45.1X6
Trecator	T37.1X1	T37.1X2	T37.1X3	T37.1X4	T37.1X5	T37.1X6
Treosulfan	T45.1X1	T45.1X2	T45.1X3	T45.1X4	T45.1X5	T45.1X6
Tretamine	T45.1X1	T45.1X2	T45.1X3	T45.1X4	T45.1X5	T45.1X6
Tretinoin	T49.0X1	T49.0X2	T49.0X3	T49.0X4	T49.0X5	T49.0X6
Tretoquinol	T48.6X1	T48.6X2	T48.6X3	T48.6X4	T48.6X5	T48.6X6
Triacetin	T49.0X1	T49.0X2	T49.0X3	T49.0X4	T49.0X5	T49.0X6
Triacetoxyanthracene	T49.4X1	T49.4X2	T49.4X3	T49.4X4	T49.4X5	T49.4X6
Triacetyloleandomycin	T36.3X1	T36.3X2	T36.3X3	T36.3X4	T36.3X5	T36.3X6
Triamcinolone	T38.0X1	T38.0X2	T38.0X3	T38.0X4	T38.0X5	T38.0X6
ENT agent	T49.6X1	T49.6X2	T49.6X3	T49.6X4	T49.6X5	T49.6X6
hexacetonide	T49.0X1	T49.0X2	T49.0X3	T49.0X4	T49.0X5	T49.0X6
ophthalmic preparation	T49.5X1	T49.5X2	T49.5X3	T49.5X4	T49.5X5	T49.5X6
topical NEC	T49.0X1	T49.0X2	T49.0X3	T49.0X4	T49.0X5	T49.0X6
Triampyzine	T44.3X1	T44.3X2	T44.3X3	T44.3X4	T44.3X5	T44.3X6
Triamterene	T50.2X1	T50.2X2	T50.2X3	T50.2X4	T50.2X5	T50.2X6
Triazine (herbicide)	T60.3X1	T60.3X2	T60.3X3	T60.3X4	—	—
Triaziquone	T45.1X1	T45.1X2	T45.1X3	T45.1X4	T45.1X5	T45.1X6
Triazolam	T42.4X1	T42.4X2	T42.4X3	T42.4X4	T42.4X5	T42.4X6
Triazole (herbicide)	T60.3X1	T60.3X2	T60.3X3	T60.3X4	—	—
Tribavirin*	T37.5X1	T37.5X2	T37.5X3	T37.5X4	T37.5X5	T37.5X6
Tribenoside	T46.991	T46.992	T46.993	T46.994	T46.995	T46.996
Tribromacetaldehyde	T42.6X1	T42.6X2	T42.6X3	T42.6X4	T42.6X5	T42.6X6
Tribromoethanol, rectal	T41.291	T41.292	T41.293	T41.294	T41.295	T41.296
Tribromomethane	T42.6X1	T42.6X2	T42.6X3	T42.6X4	T42.6X5	T42.6X6
Trichlorethane	T53.2X1	T53.2X2	T53.2X3	T53.2X4	—	—
Trichlorethylene	T53.2X1	T53.2X2	T53.2X3	T53.2X4	—	—
Trichlorfon	T60.0X1	T60.0X2	T60.0X3	T60.0X4	—	—
Trichlormethiazide	T50.2X1	T50.2X2	T50.2X3	T50.2X4	T50.2X5	T50.2X6
Trichlormethine	T45.1X1	T45.1X2	T45.1X3	T45.1X4	T45.1X5	T45.1X6
Trichloroacetic acid, Trichloracetic acid	T54.2X1	T54.2X2	T54.2X3	T54.2X4	—	—
medicinal	T49.4X1	T49.4X2	T49.4X3	T49.4X4	T49.4X5	T49.4X6
Trichloroethane	T53.2X1	T53.2X2	T53.2X3	T53.2X4	—	—
Trichloroethanol	T42.6X1	T42.6X2	T42.6X3	T42.6X4	T42.6X5	T42.6X6
Trichloroethylene (liquid)	T53.2X1	T53.2X2	T53.2X3	T53.2X4	—	—
(vapor)						
anesthetic (gas)	T41.0X1	T41.0X2	T41.0X3	T41.0X4	T41.0X5	T41.0X6
vapor NEC	T53.2X1	T53.2X2	T53.2X3	T53.2X4	—	—
Trichloroethyl phosphate	T42.6X1	T42.6X2	T42.6X3	T42.6X4	T42.6X5	T42.6X6
Trichlorofluoromethane NEC	T53.5X1	T53.5X2	T53.5X3	T53.5X4	—	—
Trichloronate	T60.0X1	T60.0X2	T60.0X3	T60.0X4	—	—
Trichloropropane	T53.6X1	T53.6X2	T53.6X3	T53.6X4	—	—
Trichlorotriethylamine	T45.1X1	T45.1X2	T45.1X3	T45.1X4	T45.1X5	T45.1X6
Trichomonacides NEC	T37.3X1	T37.3X2	T37.3X3	T37.3X4	T37.3X5	T37.3X6
Trichomycin	T36.7X1	T36.7X2	T36.7X3	T36.7X4	T36.7X5	T36.7X6
Triclobisonium chloride	T49.0X1	T49.0X2	T49.0X3	T49.0X4	T49.0X5	T49.0X6
Triclocarban	T49.0X1	T49.0X2	T49.0X3	T49.0X4	T49.0X5	T49.0X6
Triclofos	T42.6X1	T42.6X2	T42.6X3	T42.6X4	T42.6X5	T42.6X6
Triclosan	T49.0X1	T49.0X2	T49.0X3	T49.0X4	T49.0X5	T49.0X6
Tricosal*	T39.091	T39.092	T39.093	T39.094	T39.095	T39.096
Tricresyl phosphate	T65.891	T65.892	T65.893	T65.894	—	—
solvent	T52.91	T52.92	T52.93	T52.94	—	—
Tricyclamol chloride	T44.3X1	T44.3X2	T44.3X3	T44.3X4	T44.3X5	T44.3X6
Tridesilon	T49.0X1	T49.0X2	T49.0X3	T49.0X4	T49.0X5	T49.0X6
Tridihexethyl iodide	T44.3X1	T44.3X2	T44.3X3	T44.3X4	T44.3X5	T44.3X6
Tridione	T42.2X1	T42.2X2	T42.2X3	T42.2X4	T42.2X5	T42.2X6
Trientine	T45.8X1	T45.8X2	T45.8X3	T45.8X4	T45.8X5	T45.8X6

☑ Additional Character May Be Required — Refer to the Tabular List for Character Selection

*Optum Value-Add

Substance	Poisoning, Accidental (unintentional)	Poisoning, Intentional Self-harm	Poisoning, Assault	Poisoning, Undetermined	Adverse Effect	Under-dosing
Triethanolamine NEC	T54.3X1	T54.3X2	T54.3X3	T54.3X4	—	—
detergent	T54.3X1	T54.3X2	T54.3X3	T54.3X4	—	—
trinitrate (biphosphate)	T46.3X1	T46.3X2	T46.3X3	T46.3X4	T46.3X5	T46.3X6
Triethanomelamine	T45.1X1	T45.1X2	T45.1X3	T45.1X4	T45.1X5	T45.1X6
Triethylenemelamine	T45.1X1	T45.1X2	T45.1X3	T45.1X4	T45.1X5	T45.1X6
Triethylenephosphoramide	T45.1X1	T45.1X2	T45.1X3	T45.1X4	T45.1X5	T45.1X6
Triethylenethiophosphora-mide	T45.1X1	T45.1X2	T45.1X3	T45.1X4	T45.1X5	T45.1X6
Trifluoperazine	T43.3X1	T43.3X2	T43.3X3	T43.3X4	T43.3X5	T43.3X6
Trifluoroethyl vinyl ether	T41.0X1	T41.0X2	T41.0X3	T41.0X4	T41.0X5	T41.0X6
Trifluperidol	T43.4X1	T43.4X2	T43.4X3	T43.4X4	T43.4X5	T43.4X6
Triflupromazine	T43.3X1	T43.3X2	T43.3X3	T43.3X4	T43.3X5	T43.3X6
Trifluridine	T37.5X1	T37.5X2	T37.5X3	T37.5X4	T37.5X5	T37.5X6
Triflusal	T45.521	T45.522	T45.523	T45.524	T45.525	T45.526
Trihexyphenidyl	T44.3X1	T44.3X2	T44.3X3	T44.3X4	T44.3X5	T44.3X6
Triiodothyronine	T38.1X1	T38.1X2	T38.1X3	T38.1X4	T38.1X5	T38.1X6
Trilene	T41.0X1	T41.0X2	T41.0X3	T41.0X4	T41.0X5	T41.0X6
Trilostane	T38.991	T38.992	T38.993	T38.994	T38.995	T38.996
Trimebutine	T44.3X1	T44.3X2	T44.3X3	T44.3X4	T44.3X5	T44.3X6
Trimecaine	T41.3X1	T41.3X2	T41.3X3	T41.3X4	T41.3X5	T41.3X6
Trimeprazine (tartrate)	T44.3X1	T44.3X2	T44.3X3	T44.3X4	T44.3X5	T44.3X6
Trimetaphan camsilate	T44.2X1	T44.2X2	T44.2X3	T44.2X4	T44.2X5	T44.2X6
Trimetazidine	T46.7X1	T46.7X2	T46.7X3	T46.7X4	T46.7X5	T46.7X6
Trimethadione	T42.2X1	T42.2X2	T42.2X3	T42.2X4	T42.2X5	T42.2X6
Trimethaphan	T44.2X1	T44.2X2	T44.2X3	T44.2X4	T44.2X5	T44.2X6
Trimethidinium	T44.2X1	T44.2X2	T44.2X3	T44.2X4	T44.2X5	T44.2X6
Trimethobenzamide	T45.0X1	T45.0X2	T45.0X3	T45.0X4	T45.0X5	T45.0X6
Trimethoprim	T37.8X1	T37.8X2	T37.8X3	T37.8X4	T37.8X5	T37.8X6
with sulfamethoxazole	T36.8X1	T36.8X2	T36.8X3	T36.8X4	T36.8X5	T36.8X6
Trimethylcarbinol	T51.3X1	T51.3X2	T51.3X3	T51.3X4	—	—
Trimethylpsoralen	T49.3X1	T49.3X2	T49.3X3	T49.3X4	T49.3X5	T49.3X6
Trimeton	T45.0X1	T45.0X2	T45.0X3	T45.0X4	T45.0X5	T45.0X6
Trimetrexate	T45.1X1	T45.1X2	T45.1X3	T45.1X4	T45.1X5	T45.1X6
Trimipramine	T43.011	T43.012	T43.013	T43.014	T43.015	T43.016
Trimox*	T36.0X1	T36.0X2	T36.0X3	T36.0X4	T36.0X5	T36.0X6
Trimustine	T45.1X1	T45.1X2	T45.1X3	T45.1X4	T45.1X5	T45.1X6
Trinitrine	T46.3X1	T46.3X2	T46.3X3	T46.3X4	T46.3X5	T46.3X6
Trinitrobenzol	T65.3X1	T65.3X2	T65.3X3	T65.3X4	—	—
Trinitrophenol	T65.3X1	T65.3X2	T65.3X3	T65.3X4	—	—
Trinitrotoluene (fumes)	T65.3X1	T65.3X2	T65.3X3	T65.3X4	—	—
Trional	T42.6X1	T42.6X2	T42.6X3	T42.6X4	T42.6X5	T42.6X6
Triorthocresyl phosphate	T65.891	T65.892	T65.893	T65.894	—	—
Trioxide of arsenic	T57.0X1	T57.0X2	T57.0X3	T57.0X4	—	—
Trioxysalen	T49.4X1	T49.4X2	T49.4X3	T49.4X4	T49.4X5	T49.4X6
Tripamide	T50.2X1	T50.2X2	T50.2X3	T50.2X4	T50.2X5	T50.2X6
Triparanol	T46.6X1	T46.6X2	T46.6X3	T46.6X4	T46.6X5	T46.6X6
Tripelennamine	T45.0X1	T45.0X2	T45.0X3	T45.0X4	T45.0X5	T45.0X6
Triperiden	T44.3X1	T44.3X2	T44.3X3	T44.3X4	T44.3X5	T44.3X6
Triperidol	T43.4X1	T43.4X2	T43.4X3	T43.4X4	T43.4X5	T43.4X6
Triphenylphosphate	T65.891	T65.892	T65.893	T65.894	—	—
Triple						
bromides	T42.6X1	T42.6X2	T42.6X3	T42.6X4	T42.6X5	T42.6X6
carbonate	T47.1X1	T47.1X2	T47.1X3	T47.1X4	T47.1X5	T47.1X6
vaccine						
DPT	T50.A11	T50.A12	T50.A13	T50.A14	T50.A15	T50.A16
including pertussis	T50.A11	T50.A12	T50.A13	T50.A14	T50.A15	T50.A16
MMR	T50.B91	T50.B92	T50.B93	T50.B94	T50.B95	T50.B96
Triprolidine	T45.0X1	T45.0X2	T45.0X3	T45.0X4	T45.0X5	T45.0X6
Trisodium hydrogen edetate	T50.6X1	T50.6X2	T50.6X3	T50.6X4	T50.6X5	T50.6X6
Trisoralen	T49.3X1	T49.3X2	T49.3X3	T49.3X4	T49.3X5	T49.3X6
Trisulfapyrimidines	T37.0X1	T37.0X2	T37.0X3	T37.0X4	T37.0X5	T37.0X6
Trithiozine	T44.3X1	T44.3X2	T44.3X3	T44.3X4	T44.3X5	T44.3X6
Tritiozine	T44.3X1	T44.3X2	T44.3X3	T44.3X4	T44.3X5	T44.3X6
Tritoqualine	T45.0X1	T45.0X2	T45.0X3	T45.0X4	T45.0X5	T45.0X6
Trizivir*	T37.5X1	T37.5X2	T37.5X3	T37.5X4	T37.5X5	T37.5X6
Trofosfamide	T45.1X1	T45.1X2	T45.1X3	T45.1X4	T45.1X5	T45.1X6
Troleandomycin	T36.3X1	T36.3X2	T36.3X3	T36.3X4	T36.3X5	T36.3X6
Trolnitrate (phosphate)	T46.3X1	T46.3X2	T46.3X3	T46.3X4	T46.3X5	T46.3X6
Tromantadine	T37.5X1	T37.5X2	T37.5X3	T37.5X4	T37.5X5	T37.5X6
Trometamol	T50.2X1	T50.2X2	T50.2X3	T50.2X4	T50.2X5	T50.2X6
Tromethamine	T50.2X1	T50.2X2	T50.2X3	T50.2X4	T50.2X5	T50.2X6
Tronothane	T41.3X1	T41.3X2	T41.3X3	T41.3X4	T41.3X5	T41.3X6
Tropacine	T44.3X1	T44.3X2	T44.3X3	T44.3X4	T44.3X5	T44.3X6
Tropatepine	T44.3X1	T44.3X2	T44.3X3	T44.3X4	T44.3X5	T44.3X6
Tropicamide	T44.3X1	T44.3X2	T44.3X3	T44.3X4	T44.3X5	T44.3X6
Trospium chloride	T44.3X1	T44.3X2	T44.3X3	T44.3X4	T44.3X5	T44.3X6
Troxerutin	T46.991	T46.992	T46.993	T46.994	T46.995	T46.996
Troxidone	T42.2X1	T42.2X2	T42.2X3	T42.2X4	T42.2X5	T42.2X6
Tryparsamide	T37.3X1	T37.3X2	T37.3X3	T37.3X4	T37.3X5	T37.3X6
Trypsin	T45.3X1	T45.3X2	T45.3X3	T45.3X4	T45.3X5	T45.3X6
Tryptizol	T43.011	T43.012	T43.013	T43.014	T43.015	T43.016
TSH	T38.811	T38.812	T38.813	T38.814	T38.815	T38.816

Substance	Poisoning, Accidental (unintentional)	Poisoning, Intentional Self-harm	Poisoning, Assault	Poisoning, Undetermined	Adverse Effect	Under-dosing
Tuaminoheptane	T48.5X1	T48.5X2	T48.5X3	T48.5X4	T48.5X5	T48.5X6
Tuberculin, purified protein derivative (PPD)	T50.8X1	T50.8X2	T50.8X3	T50.8X4	T50.8X5	T50.8X6
Tubocurare	T48.1X1	T48.1X2	T48.1X3	T48.1X4	T48.1X5	T48.1X6
Tubocurarine (chloride)	T48.1X1	T48.1X2	T48.1X3	T48.1X4	T48.1X5	T48.1X6
Tulobuterol	T48.6X1	T48.6X2	T48.6X3	T48.6X4	T48.6X5	T48.6X6
Turpentine (spirits of)	T52.8X1	T52.8X2	T52.8X3	T52.8X4	—	—
vapor	T52.8X1	T52.8X2	T52.8X3	T52.8X4	—	—
Twinrix*	T50.B91	T50.B92	T50.B93	T50.B94	T50.B95	T50.B96
Tybamate	T43.591	T43.592	T43.593	T43.594	T43.595	T43.596
Tygacil*	T36.4X1	T36.4X2	T36.4X3	T36.4X4	T36.4X5	T36.4X6
Tyloxapol	T48.4X1	T48.4X2	T48.4X3	T48.4X4	T48.4X5	T48.4X6
Tymazoline	T48.5X1	T48.5X2	T48.5X3	T48.5X4	T48.5X5	T48.5X6
Tymlos*	T50.991	T50.992	T50.993	T50.994	T50.995	T50.996
Typhoid-paratyphoid vaccine	T50.A91	T50.A92	T50.A93	T50.A94	T50.A95	T50.A96
Typhus vaccine	T50.A91	T50.A92	T50.A93	T50.A94	T50.A95	T50.A96
Tyropanoate	T50.8X1	T50.8X2	T50.8X3	T50.8X4	T50.8X5	T50.8X6
Tyrothricin	T49.6X1	T49.6X2	T49.6X3	T49.6X4	T49.6X5	T49.6X6
ENT agent	T49.6X1	T49.6X2	T49.6X3	T49.6X4	T49.6X5	T49.6X6
ophthalmic preparation	T49.5X1	T49.5X2	T49.5X3	T49.5X4	T49.5X5	T49.5X6
Ufenamate	T39.391	T39.392	T39.393	T39.394	T39.395	T39.396
Ultraviolet light protectant	T49.3X1	T49.3X2	T49.3X3	T49.3X4	T49.3X5	T49.3X6
Unasyn*	T36.0X1	T36.0X2	T36.0X3	T36.0X4	T36.0X5	T36.0X6
Undecenoic acid	T49.0X1	T49.0X2	T49.0X3	T49.0X4	T49.0X5	T49.0X6
Undecoylium	T49.0X1	T49.0X2	T49.0X3	T49.0X4	T49.0X5	T49.0X6
Undecylenic acid (derivatives)	T49.0X1	T49.0X2	T49.0X3	T49.0X4	T49.0X5	T49.0X6
Unithroid*	T38.1X1	T38.1X2	T38.1X3	T38.1X4	T38.1X5	T38.1X6
Unna's boot	T49.3X1	T49.3X2	T49.3X3	T49.3X4	T49.3X5	T49.3X6
Unsaturated fatty acid	T46.6X1	T46.6X2	T46.6X3	T46.6X4	T46.6X5	T46.6X6
Uracil mustard	T45.1X1	T45.1X2	T45.1X3	T45.1X4	T45.1X5	T45.1X6
Uramustine	T45.1X1	T45.1X2	T45.1X3	T45.1X4	T45.1X5	T45.1X6
Urapidil	T46.5X1	T46.5X2	T46.5X3	T46.5X4	T46.5X5	T46.5X6
Urari	T48.1X1	T48.1X2	T48.1X3	T48.1X4	T48.1X5	T48.1X6
Urate oxidase	T50.4X1	T50.4X2	T50.4X3	T50.4X4	T50.4X5	T50.4X6
Urea	T47.3X1	T47.3X2	T47.3X3	T47.3X4	T47.3X5	T47.3X6
peroxide	T49.0X1	T49.0X2	T49.0X3	T49.0X4	T49.0X5	T49.0X6
stibamine	T37.4X1	T37.4X2	T37.4X3	T37.4X4	T37.4X5	T37.4X6
topical	T49.8X1	T49.8X2	T49.8X3	T49.8X4	T49.8X5	T49.8X6
Ureaphil*	T48.0X1	T48.0X2	T48.0X3	T48.0X4	T48.0X5	T48.0X6
Urethane	T45.1X1	T45.1X2	T45.1X3	T45.1X4	T45.1X5	T45.1X6
Urginea (maritima) (scilla) — see Squill						
Uric acid metabolism drug NEC	T50.4X1	T50.4X2	T50.4X3	T50.4X4	T50.4X5	T50.4X6
Uricosuric agent	T50.4X1	T50.4X2	T50.4X3	T50.4X4	T50.4X5	T50.4X6
Urinary anti-infective	T37.8X1	T37.8X2	T37.8X3	T37.8X4	T37.8X5	T37.8X6
Urofollitropin	T38.811	T38.812	T38.813	T38.814	T38.815	T38.816
Urokinase	T45.611	T45.612	T45.613	T45.614	T45.615	T45.616
Urokon	T50.8X1	T50.8X2	T50.8X3	T50.8X4	T50.8X5	T50.8X6
Ursodeoxycholic acid	T50.991	T50.992	T50.993	T50.994	T50.995	T50.996
Ursodiol	T50.991	T50.992	T50.993	T50.994	T50.995	T50.996
Urtica	T62.2X1	T62.2X2	T62.2X3	T62.2X4	—	—
Utility gas — see Gas, utility						
Vaccine NEC	T50.Z91	T50.Z92	T50.Z93	T50.Z94	T50.Z95	T50.Z96
antineoplastic	T50.Z91	T50.Z92	T50.Z93	T50.Z94	T50.Z95	T50.Z96
bacterial NEC	T50.A91	T50.A92	T50.A93	T50.A94	T50.A95	T50.A96
with						
other bacterial component	T50.A21	T50.A22	T50.A23	T50.A24	T50.A25	T50.A26
pertussis component	T50.A11	T50.A12	T50.A13	T50.A14	T50.A15	T50.A16
viral-rickettsial component	T50.A21	T50.A22	T50.A23	T50.A24	T50.A25	T50.A26
mixed NEC	T50.A21	T50.A22	T50.A23	T50.A24	T50.A25	T50.A26
BCG	T50.A91	T50.A92	T50.A93	T50.A94	T50.A95	T50.A96
cholera	T50.A91	T50.A92	T50.A93	T50.A94	T50.A95	T50.A96
diphtheria	T50.A91	T50.A92	T50.A93	T50.A94	T50.A95	T50.A96
with tetanus	T50.A21	T50.A22	T50.A23	T50.A24	T50.A25	T50.A26
and pertussis	T50.A11	T50.A12	T50.A13	T50.A14	T50.A15	T50.A16
influenza	T50.B91	T50.B92	T50.B93	T50.B94	T50.B95	T50.B96
measles	T50.B91	T50.B92	T50.B93	T50.B94	T50.B95	T50.B96
with mumps and rubella	T50.B91	T50.B92	T50.B93	T50.B94	T50.B95	T50.B96
meningococcal	T50.A91	T50.A92	T50.A93	T50.A94	T50.A95	T50.A96
mumps	T50.B91	T50.B92	T50.B93	T50.B94	T50.B95	T50.B96
paratyphoid	T50.A91	T50.A92	T50.A93	T50.A94	T50.A95	T50.A96
pertussis	T50.A11	T50.A12	T50.A13	T50.A14	T50.A15	T50.A16
with diphtheria	T50.A11	T50.A12	T50.A13	T50.A14	T50.A15	T50.A16
and tetanus	T50.A11	T50.A12	T50.A13	T50.A14	T50.A15	T50.A16
with other component	T50.A11	T50.A12	T50.A13	T50.A14	T50.A15	T50.A16
plague	T50.A91	T50.A92	T50.A93	T50.A94	T50.A95	T50.A96
poliomyelitis	T50.B91	T50.B92	T50.B93	T50.B94	T50.B95	T50.B96

Substance	Poisoning, Accidental (unintentional)	Poisoning, Intentional Self-harm	Poisoning, Assault	Poisoning, Undetermined	Adverse Effect	Under-dosing
Vaccine — continued						
poliovirus	T50.B91	T50.B92	T50.B93	T50.B94	T50.B95	T50.B96
rabies	T50.B91	T50.B92	T50.B93	T50.B94	T50.B95	T50.B96
respiratory syncytial virus	T50.B91	T50.B92	T50.B93	T50.B94	T50.B95	T50.B96
rickettsial NEC	T50.A91	T50.A92	T50.A93	T50.A94	T50.A95	T50.A96
with						
bacterial component	T50.A21	T50.A22	T50.A23	T50.A24	T50.A25	T50.A26
Rocky Mountain spotted	T50.A91	T50.A92	T50.A93	T50.A94	T50.A95	T50.A96
fever						
rubella	T50.B91	T50.B92	T50.B93	T50.B94	T50.B95	T50.B96
sabin oral	T50.B91	T50.B92	T50.B93	T50.B94	T50.B95	T50.B96
smallpox	T50.B11	T50.B12	T50.B13	T50.B14	T50.B15	T50.B16
TAB	T50.A91	T50.A92	T50.A93	T50.A94	T50.A95	T50.A96
tetanus	T50.A91	T50.A92	T50.A93	T50.A94	T50.A95	T50.A96
typhoid	T50.A91	T50.A92	T50.A93	T50.A94	T50.A95	T50.A96
typhus	T50.A91	T50.A92	T50.A93	T50.A94	T50.A95	T50.A96
viral NEC	T50.B91	T50.B92	T50.B93	T50.B94	T50.B95	T50.B96
yellow fever	T50.B91	T50.B92	T50.B93	T50.B94	T50.B95	T50.B96
Vaccinia immune globulin	T50.Z11	T50.Z12	T50.Z13	T50.Z14	T50.Z15	T50.Z16
Vaginal contraceptives	T49.8X1	T49.8X2	T49.8X3	T49.8X4	T49.8X5	T49.8X6
Valacyclovir*	T37.5X1	T37.5X2	T37.5X3	T37.5X4	T37.5X5	T37.5X6
Valerian						
root	T42.6X1	T42.6X2	T42.6X3	T42.6X4	T42.6X5	T42.6X6
tincture	T42.6X1	T42.6X2	T42.6X3	T42.6X4	T42.6X5	T42.6X6
Valethamate bromide	T44.3X1	T44.3X2	T44.3X3	T44.3X4	T44.3X5	T44.3X6
Valisone	T49.0X1	T49.0X2	T49.0X3	T49.0X4	T49.0X5	T49.0X6
Valium	T42.4X1	T42.4X2	T42.4X3	T42.4X4	T42.4X5	T42.4X6
Valmid	T42.6X1	T42.6X2	T42.6X3	T42.6X4	T42.6X5	T42.6X6
Valnoctamide	T42.6X1	T42.6X2	T42.6X3	T42.6X4	T42.6X5	T42.6X6
Valproate (sodium)	T42.6X1	T42.6X2	T42.6X3	T42.6X4	T42.6X5	T42.6X6
Valproic acid	T42.6X1	T42.6X2	T42.6X3	T42.6X4	T42.6X5	T42.6X6
Valpromide	T42.6X1	T42.6X2	T42.6X3	T42.6X4	T42.6X5	T42.6X6
Vanadium	T56.891	T56.892	T56.893	T56.894	—	—
Vancomycin	T36.8X1	T36.8X2	T36.8X3	T36.8X4	T36.8X5	T36.8X6
Vandazole*	T49.0X1	T49.0X2	T49.0X3	T49.0X4	T49.0X5	T49.0X6
Vapor — see also Gas	T59.91	T59.92	T59.93	T59.94	—	—
kiln (carbon monoxide)	T58.8X1	T58.8X2	T58.8X3	T58.8X4	—	—
lead — see lead						
specified source NEC	T59.891	T59.892	T59.893	T59.894	—	—
Vardenafil	T46.7X1	T46.7X2	T46.7X3	T46.7X4	T46.7X5	T46.7X6
Varicose reduction drug	T46.8X1	T46.8X2	T46.8X3	T46.8X4	T46.8X5	T46.8X6
Varnish	T65.4X1	T65.4X2	T65.4X3	T65.4X4	—	—
cleaner	T52.91	T52.92	T52.93	T52.94	—	—
Vaseline	T49.3X1	T49.3X2	T49.3X3	T49.3X4	T49.3X5	T49.3X6
Vasodilan	T46.7X1	T46.7X2	T46.7X3	T46.7X4	T46.7X5	T46.7X6
Vasodilator						
coronary NEC	T46.3X1	T46.3X2	T46.3X3	T46.3X4	T46.3X5	T46.3X6
peripheral NEC	T46.7X1	T46.7X2	T46.7X3	T46.7X4	T46.7X5	T46.7X6
Vasopressin	T38.892	T38.892	T38.893	T38.894	T38.895	T38.896
Vasopressor drugs	T38.891	T38.892	T38.893	T38.894	T38.895	T38.896
Vecuronium bromide	T48.1X1	T48.1X2	T48.1X3	T48.1X4	T48.1X5	T48.1X6
Vegetable extract, astringent	T49.2X1	T49.2X2	T49.2X3	T49.2X4	T49.2X5	T49.2X6
Venlafaxine	T43.211	T43.212	T43.213	T43.214	T43.215	T43.216
Venom, venomous (bite) (sting)	T63.91	T63.92	T63.93	T63.94	—	—
amphibian NEC	T63.831	T63.832	T63.833	T63.834	—	—
animal NEC	T63.891	T63.892	T63.893	T63.894	—	—
ant	T63.421	T63.422	T63.423	T63.424	—	—
arthropod NEC	T63.481	T63.482	T63.483	T63.484	—	—
bee	T63.441	T63.442	T63.443	T63.444	—	—
centipede	T63.411	T63.412	T63.413	T63.414	—	—
fish	T63.591	T63.592	T63.593	T63.594	—	—
frog	T63.811	T63.812	T63.813	T63.814	—	—
hornet	T63.451	T63.452	T63.453	T63.454	—	—
insect NEC	T63.481	T63.482	T63.483	T63.484	—	—
lizard	T63.121	T63.122	T63.123	T63.124	—	—
marine						
animals	T63.691	T63.692	T63.693	T63.694	—	—
bluebottle	T63.611	T63.612	T63.613	T63.614	—	—
jellyfish NEC	T63.621	T63.622	T63.623	T63.624	—	—
Portuguese Man-o-war	T63.611	T63.612	T63.613	T63.614	—	—
sea anemone	T63.631	T63.632	T63.633	T63.634	—	—
specified NEC	T63.691	T63.692	T63.693	T63.694	—	—
fish	T63.591	T63.592	T63.593	T63.594	—	—
plants	T63.711	T63.712	T63.713	T63.714	—	—
sting ray	T63.511	T63.512	T63.513	T63.514	—	—
millipede (tropical)	T63.411	T63.412	T63.413	T63.414	—	—
plant NEC	T63.791	T63.792	T63.793	T63.794	—	—
marine	T63.711	T63.712	T63.713	T63.714	—	—
reptile	T63.191	T63.192	T63.193	T63.194	—	—
gila monster	T63.111	T63.112	T63.113	T63.114	—	—
lizard NEC	T63.121	T63.122	T63.123	T63.124	—	—

Substance	Poisoning, Accidental (unintentional)	Poisoning, Intentional Self-harm	Poisoning, Assault	Poisoning, Undetermined	Adverse Effect	Under-dosing
Venom, venomous — continued						
scorpion	T63.2X1	T63.2X2	T63.2X3	T63.2X4	—	—
snake	T63.001	T63.002	T63.003	T63.004	—	—
African NEC	T63.081	T63.082	T63.083	T63.084	—	—
American (North) (South) NEC	T63.061	T63.062	T63.063	T63.064	—	—
Asian	T63.081	T63.082	T63.083	T63.084	—	—
Australian	T63.071	T63.072	T63.073	T63.074	—	—
cobra	T63.041	T63.042	T63.043	T63.044	—	—
coral snake	T63.021	T63.022	T63.023	T63.024	—	—
rattlesnake	T63.011	T63.012	T63.013	T63.014	—	—
specified NEC	T63.091	T63.092	T63.093	T63.094	—	—
taipan	T63.031	T63.032	T63.033	T63.034	—	—
specified NEC	T63.891	T63.892	T63.893	T63.894	—	—
spider	T63.301	T63.302	T63.303	T63.304	—	—
black widow	T63.311	T63.312	T63.313	T63.314	—	—
brown recluse	T63.331	T63.332	T63.333	T63.334	—	—
specified NEC	T63.391	T63.392	T63.393	T63.394	—	—
tarantula	T63.321	T63.322	T63.323	T63.324	—	—
sting ray	T63.511	T63.512	T63.513	T63.514	—	—
toad	T63.821	T63.822	T63.823	T63.824	—	—
wasp	T63.461	T63.462	T63.463	T63.464	—	—
Venous sclerosing drug NEC	T46.8X1	T46.8X2	T46.8X3	T46.8X4	T46.8X5	T46.8X6
Ventavis*	T46.7X1	T46.7X2	T46.7X3	T46.7X4	T46.7X5	T46.7X6
Ventolin — see Albuterol						
Veramon	T42.3X1	T42.3X2	T42.3X3	T42.3X4	T42.3X5	T42.3X6
Verapamil	T46.1X1	T46.1X2	T46.1X3	T46.1X4	T46.1X5	T46.1X6
Veratrine	T46.5X1	T46.5X2	T46.5X3	T46.5X4	T46.5X5	T46.5X6
Veratrum						
album	T62.2X1	T62.2X2	T62.2X3	T62.2X4	—	—
alkaloids	T46.5X1	T46.5X2	T46.5X3	T46.5X4	T46.5X5	T46.5X6
viride	T62.2X1	T62.2X2	T62.2X3	T62.2X4	—	—
Verdigris	T60.3X1	T60.3X2	T60.3X3	T60.3X4	—	—
Veronal	T42.3X1	T42.3X2	T42.3X3	T42.3X4	T42.3X5	T42.3X6
Veroxil	T37.4X1	T37.4X2	T37.4X3	T37.4X4	T37.4X5	T37.4X6
Versenate	T50.6X1	T50.6X2	T50.6X3	T50.6X4	T50.6X5	T50.6X6
Versidyne	T39.8X1	T39.8X2	T39.8X3	T39.8X4	T39.8X5	T39.8X6
Vetrabutine	T48.0X1	T48.0X2	T48.0X3	T48.0X4	T48.0X5	T48.0X6
Vexol*	T49.5X1	T49.5X2	T49.5X3	T49.5X4	T49.5X5	T49.5X6
Viagra*	T46.7X1	T46.7X2	T46.7X3	T46.7X4	T46.7X5	T46.7X6
Vibramycin*	T36.4X1	T36.4X2	T36.4X3	T36.4X4	T36.4X5	T36.4X6
Victrelis*	T37.5X1	T37.5X2	T37.5X3	T37.5X4	T37.5X5	T37.5X6
Vidarabine	T37.5X1	T37.5X2	T37.5X3	T37.5X4	T37.5X5	T37.5X6
Vienna						
green	T57.0X1	T57.0X2	T57.0X3	T57.0X4	—	—
insecticide	T60.2X1	T60.2X2	T60.2X3	T60.2X4	—	—
red	T57.0X1	T57.0X2	T57.0X3	T57.0X4	—	—
pharmaceutical dye	T50.991	T50.992	T50.993	T50.994	T50.995	T50.996
Vigabatrin	T42.6X1	T42.6X2	T42.6X3	T42.6X4	T42.6X5	T42.6X6
Viloxazine	T43.291	T43.292	T43.293	T43.294	T43.295	T43.296
Viminol	T39.8X1	T39.8X2	T39.8X3	T39.8X4	T39.8X5	T39.8X6
Vinbarbital, vinbarbitone	T42.3X1	T42.3X2	T42.3X3	T42.3X4	T42.3X5	T42.3X6
Vinblastine	T45.1X1	T45.1X2	T45.1X3	T45.1X4	T45.1X5	T45.1X6
Vinburnine	T46.7X1	T46.7X2	T46.7X3	T46.7X4	T46.7X5	T46.7X6
Vincamine	T45.1X1	T45.1X2	T45.1X3	T45.1X4	T45.1X5	T45.1X6
Vincristine	T45.1X1	T45.1X2	T45.1X3	T45.1X4	T45.1X5	T45.1X6
Vindesine	T45.1X1	T45.1X2	T45.1X3	T45.1X4	T45.1X5	T45.1X6
Vinesthene, vinethene	T41.0X1	T41.0X2	T41.0X3	T41.0X4	T41.0X5	T41.0X6
Vinorelbine tartrate	T45.1X1	T45.1X2	T45.1X3	T45.1X4	T45.1X5	T45.1X6
Vinpocetine	T46.7X1	T46.7X2	T46.7X3	T46.7X4	T46.7X5	T46.7X6
Vinyl						
acetate	T65.891	T65.892	T65.893	T65.894	—	—
bital	T42.3X1	T42.3X2	T42.3X3	T42.3X4	T42.3X5	T42.3X6
bromide	T65.891	T65.892	T65.893		—	—
chloride	T59.891	T59.892	T59.893	T59.894	—	—
ether	T41.0X1	T41.0X2	T41.0X3	T41.0X4	T41.0X5	T41.0X6
Vinylbital	T42.3X1	T42.3X2	T42.3X3	T42.3X4	T42.3X5	T42.3X6
Vinylidene chloride	T65.891	T65.892	T65.893		—	—
Vioform	T37.8X1	T37.8X2	T37.8X3	T37.8X4	T37.8X5	T37.8X6
topical	T49.0X1	T49.0X2	T49.0X3	T49.0X4	T49.0X5	T49.0X6
Viokase*	T47.5X1	T47.5X2	T47.5X3	T47.5X4	T47.5X5	T47.5X6
Viomycin	T36.8X1	T36.8X2	T36.8X3	T36.8X4	T36.8X5	T36.8X6
Viosterol	T45.2X1	T45.2X2	T45.2X3	T45.2X4	T45.2X5	T45.2X6
Viper (venom)	T63.091	T63.092	T63.093	T63.094	—	—
Viprynium	T37.4X1	T37.4X2	T37.4X3	T37.4X4	T37.4X5	T37.4X6
Viquidil	T46.7X1	T46.7X2	T46.7X3	T46.7X4	T46.7X5	T46.7X6
Viral vaccine NEC	T50.B91	T50.B92	T50.B93	T50.B94	T50.B95	T50.B96
Virginiamycin	T36.8X1	T36.8X2	T36.8X3	T36.8X4	T36.8X5	T36.8X6
Virugon	T37.5X1	T37.5X2	T37.5X3	T37.5X4	T37.5X5	T37.5X6
Viscous agent	T50.901	T50.902	T50.903	T50.904	T50.905	T50.906
Visine	T49.5X1	T49.5X2	T49.5X3	T49.5X4	T49.5X5	T49.5X6
Visnadine	T46.3X1	T46.3X2	T46.3X3	T46.3X4	T46.3X5	T46.3X6

☑ Additional Character May Be Required — Refer to the Tabular List for Character Selection

*Optum Value-Add

Substance	Poisoning, Accidental (unintentional)	Poisoning, Intentional Self-harm	Poisoning, Assault	Poisoning, Undetermined	Adverse Effect	Under-dosing
Vitamin NEC	T45.2X1	T45.2X2	T45.2X3	T45.2X4	T45.2X5	T45.2X6
A	T45.2X1	T45.2X2	T45.2X3	T45.2X4	T45.2X5	T45.2X6
B1	T45.2X1	T45.2X2	T45.2X3	T45.2X4	T45.2X5	T45.2X6
B2	T45.2X1	T45.2X2	T45.2X3	T45.2X4	T45.2X5	T45.2X6
B6	T45.2X1	T45.2X2	T45.2X3	T45.2X4	T45.2X5	T45.2X6
B12	T45.2X1	T45.2X2	T45.2X3	T45.2X4	T45.2X5	T45.2X6
B15	T45.2X1	T45.2X2	T45.2X3	T45.2X4	T45.2X5	T45.2X6
B NEC	T45.2X1	T45.2X2	T45.2X3	T45.2X4	T45.2X5	T45.2X6
nicotinic acid	T46.7X1	T46.7X2	T46.7X3	T46.7X4	T46.7X5	T46.7X6
C	T45.2X1	T45.2X2	T45.2X3	T45.2X4	T45.2X5	T45.2X6
D	T45.2X1	T45.2X2	T45.2X3	T45.2X4	T45.2X5	T45.2X6
D2	T45.2X1	T45.2X2	T45.2X3	T45.2X4	T45.2X5	T45.2X6
D3	T45.2X1	T45.2X2	T45.2X3	T45.2X4	T45.2X5	T45.2X6
E	T45.2X1	T45.2X2	T45.2X3	T45.2X4	T45.2X5	T45.2X6
E acetate	T45.2X1	T45.2X2	T45.2X3	T45.2X4	T45.2X5	T45.2X6
hematopoietic	T45.8X1	T45.8X2	T45.8X3	T45.8X4	T45.8X5	T45.8X6
K1	T45.7X1	T45.7X2	T45.7X3	T45.7X4	T45.7X5	T45.7X6
K2	T45.7X1	T45.7X2	T45.7X3	T45.7X4	T45.7X5	T45.7X6
K NEC	T45.7X1	T45.7X2	T45.7X3	T45.7X4	T45.7X5	T45.7X6
PP	T45.2X1	T45.2X2	T45.2X3	T45.2X4	T45.2X5	T45.2X6
ulceroprotectant	T47.1X1	T47.1X2	T47.1X3	T47.1X4	T47.1X5	T47.1X6
Vleminckx's solution	T49.4X1	T49.4X2	T49.4X3	T49.4X4	T49.4X5	T49.4X6
Voltaren — see Diclofenac sodium						
Voraxaze*	T50.6X1	T50.6X2	T50.6X3	T50.6X4	T50.6X5	T50.6X6
Warfarin	T45.511	T45.512	T45.513	T45.514	T45.515	T45.516
rodenticide	T60.4X1	T60.4X2	T60.4X3	T60.4X4	—	—
sodium	T45.511	T45.512	T45.513	T45.514	T45.515	T45.516
Wasp (sting)	T63.461	T63.462	T63.463	T63.464	—	—
Water						
balance drug	T50.3X1	T50.3X2	T50.3X3	T50.3X4	T50.3X5	T50.3X6
distilled	T50.3X1	T50.3X2	T50.3X3	T50.3X4	T50.3X5	T50.3X6
gas — see Gas, water						
incomplete combustion of — see Carbon, monoxide, fuel, utility						
hemlock	T62.2X1	T62.2X2	T62.2X3	T62.2X4	—	—
moccasin (venom)	T63.061	T63.062	T63.063	T63.064	—	—
purified	T50.3X1	T50.3X2	T50.3X3	T50.3X4	T50.3X5	T50.3X6
Wax (paraffin) (petroleum)	T52.0X1	T52.0X2	T52.0X3	T52.0X4	—	—
automobile	T65.891	T65.892	T65.893	T65.894	—	—
floor	T52.0X1	T52.0X2	T52.0X3	T52.0X4	—	—
Weed killers NEC	T60.3X1	T60.3X2	T60.3X3	T60.3X4	—	—
Wellbutrin*	T43.291	T43.292	T43.293	T43.294	T43.295	T43.296
Welldorm	T42.6X1	T42.6X2	T42.6X3	T42.6X4	T42.6X5	T42.6X6
Westcort*	T49.0X1	T49.0X2	T49.0X3	T49.0X4	T49.0X5	T49.0X6
White						
arsenic	T57.0X1	T57.0X2	T57.0X3	T57.0X4	—	—
hellebore	T62.2X1	T62.2X2	T62.2X3	T62.2X4	—	—
lotion (keratolytic)	T49.4X1	T49.4X2	T49.4X3	T49.4X4	T49.4X5	T49.4X6
spirit	T52.0X1	T52.0X2	T52.0X3	T52.0X4	—	—
Whitewash	T65.891	T65.892	T65.893	T65.894	—	—
Whole blood (human)	T45.8X1	T45.8X2	T45.8X3	T45.8X4	T45.8X5	T45.8X6
Wild						
black cherry	T62.2X1	T62.2X2	T62.2X3	T62.2X4	—	—
poisonous plants NEC	T62.2X1	T62.2X2	T62.2X3	T62.2X4	—	—
Window cleaning fluid	T65.891	T65.892	T65.893	T65.894	—	—
Wintergreen (oil)	T49.3X1	T49.3X2	T49.3X3	T49.3X4	T49.3X5	T49.3X6
Wisterine	T62.2X1	T62.2X2	T62.2X3	T62.2X4	—	—
Witch hazel	T49.2X1	T49.2X2	T49.2X3	T49.2X4	T49.2X5	T49.2X6
Wood alcohol or spirit	T51.1X1	T51.1X2	T51.1X3	T51.1X4	—	—
Wool fat (hydrous)	T49.3X1	T49.3X2	T49.3X3	T49.3X4	T49.3X5	T49.3X6
Woorali	T48.1X1	T48.1X2	T48.1X3	T48.1X4	T48.1X5	T48.1X6
Wormseed, American	T37.4X1	T37.4X2	T37.4X3	T37.4X4	T37.4X5	T37.4X6
Xamoterol	T44.5X1	T44.5X2	T44.5X3	T44.5X4	T44.5X5	T44.5X6
Xanax*	T42.4X1	T42.4X2	T42.4X3	T42.4X4	T42.4X5	T42.4X6
Xanthine diuretics	T50.2X1	T50.2X2	T50.2X3	T50.2X4	T50.2X5	T50.2X6
Xanthinol nicotinate	T46.7X1	T46.7X2	T46.7X3	T46.7X4	T46.7X5	T46.7X6
Xanthotoxin	T49.3X1	T49.3X2	T49.3X3	T49.3X4	T49.3X5	T49.3X6
Xantinol nicotinate	T46.7X1	T46.7X2	T46.7X3	T46.7X4	T46.7X5	T46.7X6
Xantocillin	T36.0X1	T36.0X2	T36.0X3	T36.0X4	T36.0X5	T36.0X6
Xenon (127Xe) (133Xe)	T50.8X1	T50.8X2	T50.8X3	T50.8X4	T50.8X5	T50.8X6
Xenysalate	T49.4X1	T49.4X2	T49.4X3	T49.4X4	T49.4X5	T49.4X6
Xibornol	T37.8X1	T37.8X2	T37.8X3	T37.8X4	T37.8X5	T37.8X6
Xigris	T45.511	T45.512	T45.513	T45.514	T45.515	T45.516
Xipamide	T50.2X1	T50.2X2	T50.2X3	T50.2X4	T50.2X5	T50.2X6
Xylene (vapor)	T52.2X1	T52.2X2	T52.2X3	T52.2X4	—	—
Xylocaine (infiltration) (topical)	T41.3X1	T41.3X2	T41.3X3	T41.3X4	T41.3X5	T41.3X6
nerve block (peripheral) (plexus)	T41.3X1	T41.3X2	T41.3X3	T41.3X4	T41.3X5	T41.3X6
spinal	T41.3X1	T41.3X2	T41.3X3	T41.3X4	T41.3X5	T41.3X6
Xylol (vapor)	T52.2X1	T52.2X2	T52.2X3	T52.2X4	—	—

Substance	Poisoning, Accidental (unintentional)	Poisoning, Intentional Self-harm	Poisoning, Assault	Poisoning, Undetermined	Adverse Effect	Under-dosing
Xylometazoline	T48.5X1	T48.5X2	T48.5X3	T48.5X4	T48.5X5	T48.5X6
Xylose*	T50.8X1	T50.8X2	T50.8X3	T50.8X4	T50.8X5	T50.8X6
Yaz*	T38.4X1	T38.4X2	T38.4X3	T38.4X4	T38.4X5	T38.4X6
Yeast	T45.2X1	T45.2X2	T45.2X3	T45.2X4	T45.2X5	T45.2X6
dried	T45.2X1	T45.2X2	T45.2X3	T45.2X4	T45.2X5	T45.2X6
Yellow						
fever vaccine	T50.B91	T50.B92	T50.B93	T50.B94	T50.B95	T50.B96
jasmine	T62.2X1	T62.2X2	T62.2X3	T62.2X4	—	—
phenolphthalein	T47.2X1	T47.2X2	T47.2X3	T47.2X4	T47.2X5	T47.2X6
Yervoy*	T45.1X1	T45.1X2	T45.1X3	T45.1X4	T45.1X5	T45.1X6
Yew	T62.2X1	T62.2X2	T62.2X3	T62.2X4	—	—
Yohimbic acid	T40.991	T40.992	T40.993	T40.994	T40.995	T40.996
Zactane	T39.8X1	T39.8X2	T39.8X3	T39.8X4	T39.8X5	T39.8X6
Zalcitabine	T37.5X1	T37.5X2	T37.5X3	T37.5X4	T37.5X5	T37.5X6
Zanaflex*	T48.1X1	T48.1X2	T48.1X3	T48.1X4	T48.1X5	T48.1X6
Zaroxolyn	T50.2X1	T50.2X2	T50.2X3	T50.2X4	T50.2X5	T50.2X6
Zephiran (topical)	T49.0X1	T49.0X2	T49.0X3	T49.0X4	T49.0X5	T49.0X6
ophthalmic preparation	T49.5X1	T49.5X2	T49.5X3	T49.5X4	T49.5X5	T49.5X6
Zeranol	T38.7X1	T38.7X2	T38.7X3	T38.7X4	T38.7X5	T38.7X6
Zerone	T51.1X1	T51.1X2	T51.1X3	T51.1X4	—	—
Zestril*	T46.4X1	T46.4X2	T46.4X3	T46.4X4	T46.4X5	T46.4X6
Zidovudine	T37.5X1	T37.5X2	T37.5X3	T37.5X4	T37.5X5	T37.5X6
Zilactin*	T41.3X1	T41.3X2	T41.3X3	T41.3X4	T41.3X5	T41.3X6
Zimeldine	T43.221	T43.222	T43.223	T43.224	T43.225	T43.226
Zinc (compounds) (fumes) (vapor)	T56.5X1	T56.5X2	T56.5X3	T56.5X4	—	—
NEC	T49.0X1	T49.0X2	T49.0X3	T49.0X4	T49.0X5	T49.0X6
anti-infectives	T49.0X1	T49.0X2	T49.0X3	T49.0X4	T49.0X5	T49.0X6
antivaricose	T46.8X1	T46.8X2	T46.8X3	T46.8X4	T46.8X5	T46.8X6
bacitracin	T49.0X1	T49.0X2	T49.0X3	T49.0X4	T49.0X5	T49.0X6
chloride (mouthwash)	T49.6X1	T49.6X2	T49.6X3	T49.6X4	T49.6X5	T49.6X6
chromate	T56.5X1	T56.5X2	T56.5X3	T56.5X4	—	—
gelatin	T49.3X1	T49.3X2	T49.3X3	T49.3X4	T49.3X5	T49.3X6
oxide	T49.3X1	T49.3X2	T49.3X3	T49.3X4	T49.3X5	T49.3X6
plaster	T49.3X1	T49.3X2	T49.3X3	T49.3X4	T49.3X5	T49.3X6
peroxide	T49.0X1	T49.0X2	T49.0X3	T49.0X4	T49.0X5	T49.0X6
pesticides	T56.5X1	T56.5X2	T56.5X3	T56.5X4	—	—
phosphide	T60.4X1	T60.4X2	T60.4X3	T60.4X4	—	—
pyrithionate	T49.4X1	T49.4X2	T49.4X3	T49.4X4	T49.4X5	T49.4X6
stearate	T49.3X1	T49.3X2	T49.3X3	T49.3X4	T49.3X5	T49.3X6
sulfate	T49.5X1	T49.5X2	T49.5X3	T49.5X4	T49.5X5	T49.5X6
ENT agent	T49.6X1	T49.6X2	T49.6X3	T49.6X4	T49.6X5	T49.6X6
ophthalmic solution	T49.5X1	T49.5X2	T49.5X3	T49.5X4	T49.5X5	T49.5X6
topical NEC	T49.0X1	T49.0X2	T49.0X3	T49.0X4	T49.0X5	T49.0X6
undecylenate	T49.0X1	T49.0X2	T49.0X3	T49.0X4	T49.0X5	T49.0X6
Zineb	T60.0X1	T60.0X2	T60.0X3	T60.0X4	—	—
Zinostatin	T45.1X1	T45.1X2	T45.1X3	T45.1X4	T45.1X5	T45.1X6
Zipeprol	T48.3X1	T48.3X2	T48.3X3	T48.3X4	T48.3X5	T48.3X6
Zithromax*	T36.3X1	T36.3X2	T36.3X3	T36.3X4	T36.3X5	T36.3X6
Zocor*	T46.6X1	T46.6X2	T46.6X3	T46.6X4	T46.6X5	T46.6X6
Zofenopril	T46.4X1	T46.4X2	T46.4X3	T46.4X4	T46.4X5	T46.4X6
Zoloft*	T43.221	T43.222	T43.223	T43.224	T43.225	T43.226
Zolpidem	T42.6X1	T42.6X2	T42.6X3	T42.6X4	T42.6X5	T42.6X6
Zolpimist*	T42.6X1	T42.6X2	T42.6X3	T42.6X4	T42.6X5	T42.6X6
Zomepirac	T39.391	T39.392	T39.393	T39.394	T39.395	T39.396
Zopiclone	T42.6X1	T42.6X2	T42.6X3	T42.6X4	T42.6X5	T42.6X6
Zorubicin	T45.1X1	T45.1X2	T45.1X3	T45.1X4	T45.1X5	T45.1X6
Zotepine	T43.591	T43.592	T43.593	T43.594	T43.595	T43.596
Zovant	T45.511	T45.512	T45.513	T45.514	T45.515	T45.516
Zoxazolamine	T42.8X1	T42.8X2	T42.8X3	T42.8X4	T42.8X5	T42.8X6
Zuclopenthixol	T43.4X1	T43.4X2	T43.4X3	T43.4X4	T43.4X5	T43.4X6
Zyban*	T43.291	T43.292	T43.293	T43.294	T43.295	T43.296
Zyflo*	T48.6X1	T48.6X2	T48.6X3	T48.6X4	T48.6X5	T48.6X6
Zygadenus (venenosus)	T62.2X1	T62.2X2	T62.2X3	T62.2X4	—	—
Zyprexa	T43.591	T43.592	T43.593	T43.594	T43.595	T43.596
Zyzal*	T45.0X1	T45.0X2	T45.0X3	T45.0X4	T45.0X5	T45.0X6

A

Abandonment (causing exposure to weather conditions) (with intent to injure or kill) NEC X58 ☑
Abuse (adult) (child) (mental) (physical) (sexual) X58 ☑
Accident (to) X58 ☑
  aircraft (in transit) (powered) — *see also* Accident, transport, aircraft
    due to, caused by cataclysm — *see* Forces of nature, by type
  animal-drawn vehicle — *see* Accident, transport, animal-drawn vehicle occupant
  animal-rider — *see* Accident, transport, animal-rider
  automobile — *see* Accident, transport, car occupant
  bare foot water skier V94.4 ☑
  boat, boating — *see also* Accident, watercraft
    striking swimmer
      powered V94.11 ☑
      unpowered V94.12 ☑
  bus — *see* Accident, transport, bus occupant
  cable car, not on rails V98.0 ☑
    on rails — *see* Accident, transport, streetcar occupant
  car — *see* Accident, transport, car occupant
  caused by, due to
    animal NEC W64 ☑
    chain hoist W24.0 ☑
    cold (excessive) — *see* Exposure, cold
    corrosive liquid, substance — *see* Table of Drugs and Chemicals
    cutting or piercing instrument — *see* Contact, with, by type of instrument
    drive belt W24.0 ☑
    electric
      current — *see* Exposure, electric current
      motor — *see also* Contact, with, by type of machine W31.3 ☑
      current (of) W86.8 ☑
    environmental factor NEC X58 ☑
    explosive material — *see* Explosion
    fire, flames — *see* Exposure, fire
    firearm missile — *see* Discharge, firearm by type
    heat (excessive) — *see* Heat
    hot — *see* Contact, with, hot
    ignition — *see* Ignition
    lifting device W24.0 ☑
    lightning — *see* subcategory T75.0 ☑
      causing fire — *see* Exposure, fire
    machine, machinery — *see* Contact, with, by type of machine
    natural factor NEC X58 ☑
    pulley (block) W24.0 ☑
    radiation — *see* Radiation
    steam X13.1 ☑
      inhalation X13.0 ☑
      pipe X16 ☑
    thunderbolt — *see* subcategory T75.0 ☑
      causing fire — *see* Exposure, fire
    transmission device W24.1 ☑
  coach — *see* Accident, transport, bus occupant
  coal car — *see* Accident, transport, industrial vehicle occupant
  diving — *see also* Fall, into, water
    with
      drowning or submersion — *see* Drowning
  forklift — *see* Accident, transport, industrial vehicle occupant
  heavy transport vehicle NOS — *see* Accident, transport, truck occupant
  ice yacht V98.2 ☑
  in
    medical, surgical procedure
      as, or due to misadventure — *see* Misadventure
      causing an abnormal reaction or later complication without mention of misadventure — *see also* Complication of or following, by type of procedure Y84.9
  land yacht V98.1 ☑
  late effect of — *see* W00-X58 with 7th character S
  logging car — *see* Accident, transport, industrial vehicle occupant
  machine, machinery — *see also* Contact, with, by type of machine
    on board watercraft V93.69 ☑
      explosion — *see* Explosion, in, watercraft
      fire — *see* Burn, on board watercraft
      powered craft V93.63 ☑

Accident — *continued*
  machine, machinery — *see also* Contact, with, by type of machine — *continued*
    on board watercraft — *continued*
      powered craft — *continued*
        ferry boat V93.61 ☑
        fishing boat V93.62 ☑
        jetskis V93.63 ☑
        liner V93.61 ☑
        merchant ship V93.60 ☑
        passenger ship V93.61 ☑
        sailboat V93.64 ☑
  mine tram — *see* Accident, transport, industrial vehicle occupant
  mobility scooter (motorized) — *see* Accident, transport, pedestrian, conveyance, specified type NEC
  motor scooter — *see* Accident, transport, motorcycle
  motor vehicle NOS (traffic) — *see also* Accident, transport V89.2 ☑
    nontraffic V89.0 ☑
    three-wheeled NOS — *see* Accident, transport, three-wheeled motor vehicle occupant
  motorcycle NOS — *see* Accident, transport, motorcycle
  nonmotor vehicle NOS (nontraffic) — *see also* Accident, transport V89.1 ☑
    traffic NOS V89.3 ☑
  nontraffic (victim's mode of transport NOS) V88.9 ☑
    collision (between) V88.7 ☑
      bus and truck V88.5 ☑
      car and:
        bus V88.3 ☑
        pickup V88.2 ☑
        three-wheeled motor vehicle V88.0 ☑
        train V88.6 ☑
        truck V88.4 ☑
        two-wheeled motor vehicle V88.0 ☑
        van V88.2 ☑
      specified vehicle NEC and:
        three-wheeled motor vehicle V88.1 ☑
        two-wheeled motor vehicle V88.1 ☑
    known mode of transport — *see* Accident, transport, by type of vehicle
    noncollision V88.8 ☑
  on board watercraft V93.89 ☑
    powered craft V93.83 ☑
      ferry boat V93.81 ☑
      fishing boat V93.82 ☑
      jetskis V93.83 ☑
      liner V93.81 ☑
      merchant ship V93.80 ☑
      passenger ship V93.81 ☑
    unpowered craft V93.88 ☑
      canoe V93.85 ☑
      inflatable V93.86 ☑
        in tow
          recreational V94.31 ☑
          specified NEC V94.32 ☑
      kayak V93.85 ☑
      sailboat V93.84 ☑
      surf-board V93.88 ☑
      water skis V93.87 ☑
      windsurfer V93.88 ☑
  parachutist V97.29 ☑
    entangled in object V97.21 ☑
    injured on landing V97.22 ☑
  pedal cycle — *see* Accident, transport, pedal cyclist
  pedestrian (on foot)
    with
      another pedestrian W51 ☑
        on pedestrian conveyance NEC V00.09 ☑
        with fall W03 ☑
          due to ice or snow W00.0 ☑
      rider of
        hoverboard V00.038 ☑
        Segway V00.038 ☑
        standing
          electric scooter V00.031 ☑
          micro-mobility pedestrian conveyance NEC V00.038 ☑
      roller skater (in-line) V00.01 ☑
      skate boarder V00.02 ☑
      transport vehicle — *see* Accident, transport
    on pedestrian conveyance — *see* Accident, transport, pedestrian, conveyance
  pick-up truck or van — *see* Accident, transport, pickup truck occupant

Accident — *continued*
  quarry truck — *see* Accident, transport, industrial vehicle occupant
  railway vehicle (any) (in motion) — *see* Accident, transport, railway vehicle occupant
    due to cataclysm — *see* Forces of nature, by type
  scooter (non-motorized) — *see* Accident, transport, pedestrian, conveyance, scooter
  sequelae of — *see* categories W00-X58 with 7th character S
  skateboard — *see* Accident, transport, pedestrian, conveyance, skateboard
  ski(ing) — *see* Accident, transport, pedestrian, conveyance
    lift V98.3 ☑
  specified cause NEC X58 ☑
  streetcar — *see* Accident, transport, streetcar occupant
  traffic (victim's mode of transport NOS) V87.9 ☑
    collision (between) V87.7 ☑
      bus and truck V87.5 ☑
      car and:
        bus V87.3 ☑
        pickup V87.2 ☑
        three-wheeled motor vehicle V87.0 ☑
        train V87.6 ☑
        truck V87.4 ☑
        two-wheeled motor vehicle V87.0 ☑
        van V87.2 ☑
      specified vehicle NEC V86.39 ☑
        and
          three-wheeled motor vehicle V87.1 ☑
          two-wheeled motor vehicle V87.1 ☑
        driver V86.09 ☑
        passenger V86.19 ☑
        person on outside V86.29 ☑
        while boarding or alighting V86.49 ☑
    known mode of transport — *see* Accident, transport, by type of vehicle
    noncollision V87.8 ☑
  transport (involving injury to) V99 ☑
    18 wheeler — *see* Accident, transport, truck occupant
    agricultural vehicle occupant (nontraffic) V84.9 ☑
      driver V84.5 ☑
      hanger-on V84.7 ☑
      passenger V84.6 ☑
      traffic V84.3 ☑
        driver V84.0 ☑
        hanger-on V84.2 ☑
        passenger V84.1 ☑
      while boarding or alighting V84.4 ☑
    aircraft NEC V97.89 ☑
      military NEC V97.818 ☑
        civilian injured by V97.811 ☑
        with civilian aircraft V97.810 ☑
      occupant injured (in)
        nonpowered craft accident V96.9 ☑
          balloon V96.00 ☑
            collision V96.03 ☑
            crash V96.01 ☑
            explosion V96.05 ☑
            fire V96.04 ☑
            forced landing V96.02 ☑
            specified type NEC V96.09 ☑
          glider V96.20 ☑
            collision V96.23 ☑
            crash V96.21 ☑
            explosion V96.25 ☑
            fire V96.24 ☑
            forced landing V96.22 ☑
            specified type NEC V96.29 ☑
          hang glider V96.10 ☑
            collision V96.13 ☑
            crash V96.11 ☑
            explosion V96.15 ☑
            fire V96.14 ☑
            forced landing V96.12 ☑
            specified type NEC V96.19 ☑
          specified craft NEC V96.8 ☑
        powered craft accident V95.9 ☑
          fixed wing NEC
            commercial V95.30 ☑
              collision V95.33 ☑
              crash V95.31 ☑
              explosion V95.35 ☑
              fire V95.34 ☑
              forced landing V95.32 ☑

☑ **Additional Character Required — Refer to the Tabular List for Character Selection**

Accident — *continued*
  transport — *continued*
    aircraft — *continued*
      occupant injured — *continued*
        powered craft accident — *continued*
          fixed wing — *continued*
            commercial — *continued*
              specified type NEC V95.39 ☑
            private V95.20 ☑
              collision V95.23 ☑
              crash V95.21 ☑
              explosion V95.25 ☑
              fire V95.24 ☑
              forced landing V95.22 ☑
              specified type NEC V95.29 ☑
          glider V95.10 ☑
            collision V95.13 ☑
            crash V95.11 ☑
            explosion V95.15 ☑
            fire V95.14 ☑
            forced landing V95.12 ☑
            specified type NEC V95.19 ☑
          helicopter V95.00 ☑
            collision V95.03 ☑
            crash V95.01 ☑
            explosion V95.05 ☑
            fire V95.04 ☑
            forced landing V95.02 ☑
            specified type NEC V95.09 ☑
          spacecraft V95.40 ☑
            collision V95.43 ☑
            crash V95.41 ☑
            explosion V95.45 ☑
            fire V95.44 ☑
            forced landing V95.42 ☑
            specified type NEC V95.49 ☑
          specified craft NEC V95.8 ☑
          ultralight V95.10 ☑
            collision V95.13 ☑
            crash V95.11 ☑
            explosion V95.15 ☑
            fire V95.14 ☑
            forced landing V95.12 ☑
            specified type NEC V95.19 ☑
        specified accident NEC V97.0 ☑
        while boarding or alighting V97.1 ☑
      person (injured by)
        falling from, in or on aircraft V97.0 ☑
        machinery on aircraft V97.89 ☑
        on ground with aircraft involvement V97.39 ☑
        rotating propeller V97.32 ☑
        struck by object falling from aircraft V97.31 ☑
        sucked into aircraft jet V97.33 ☑
        while boarding or alighting aircraft V97.1 ☑
    airport (battery-powered) passenger vehicle — *see* Accident, transport, industrial vehicle occupant
    all-terrain vehicle occupant (nontraffic) V86.95 ☑
      driver V86.55 ☑
      dune buggy — *see* Accident, transport, dune buggy occupant
      hanger-on V86.75 ☑
      passenger V86.65 ☑
      snowmobile — *see* Accident, transport, snowmobile occupant
      specified type NEC V86.99 ☑
        driver V86.59 ☑
        passenger V86.69 ☑
        person on outside V86.79 ☑
      traffic V86.35 ☑
        driver V86.05 ☑
        hanger-on V86.25 ☑
        passenger V86.15 ☑
      while boarding or alighting V86.45 ☑
    ambulance occupant (traffic) V86.31 ☑
      driver V86.01 ☑
      hanger-on V86.21 ☑
      nontraffic V86.91 ☑
        driver V86.51 ☑
        hanger-on V86.71 ☑
        passenger V86.61 ☑
      passenger V86.11 ☑
      while boarding or alighting V86.41 ☑
    animal-drawn vehicle occupant (in) V80.929 ☑
      collision (with)
        animal V80.12 ☑

Accident — *continued*
  transport — *continued*
    animal-drawn vehicle occupant — *continued*
      collision — *continued*
        animal — *continued*
          being ridden V80.711 ☑
        animal-drawn vehicle V80.721 ☑
        bus V80.42 ☑
        car V80.42 ☑
        fixed or stationary object V80.82 ☑
        military vehicle V80.920 ☑
        nonmotor vehicle V80.791 ☑
        pedal cycle V80.22 ☑
        pedestrian V80.12 ☑
        pickup V80.42 ☑
        railway train or vehicle V80.62 ☑
        specified motor vehicle NEC V80.52 ☑
        streetcar V80.73 ☑
        truck V80.42 ☑
        two- or three-wheeled motor vehicle V80.32 ☑
        van V80.42 ☑
      noncollision V80.02 ☑
      specified circumstance NEC V80.928 ☑
    animal-rider V80.919 ☑
      collision (with)
        animal V80.11 ☑
          being ridden V80.710 ☑
        animal-drawn vehicle V80.720 ☑
        bus V80.41 ☑
        car V80.41 ☑
        fixed or stationary object V80.81 ☑
        military vehicle V80.910 ☑
        nonmotor vehicle V80.790 ☑
        pedal cycle V80.21 ☑
        pedestrian V80.11 ☑
        pickup V80.41 ☑
        railway train or vehicle V80.61 ☑
        specified motor vehicle NEC V80.51 ☑
        streetcar V80.730 ☑
        truck V80.41 ☑
        two- or three-wheeled motor vehicle V80.31 ☑
        van V80.41 ☑
      noncollision V80.013 ☑
        specified as horse rider V80.010 ☑
      specified circumstance NEC V80.918 ☑
    armored car — *see* Accident, transport, truck occupant
    battery-powered truck (baggage) (mail) — *see* Accident, transport, industrial vehicle occupant
    bus occupant V79.9 ☑
      collision (with)
        animal (traffic) V70.9 ☑
          being ridden (traffic) V76.9 ☑
            nontraffic V76.3 ☑
              while boarding or alighting V76.4 ☑
          nontraffic V70.3 ☑
            while boarding or alighting V70.4 ☑
        animal-drawn vehicle (traffic) V76.9 ☑
          nontraffic V76.3 ☑
            while boarding or alighting V76.4 ☑
        bus (traffic) V74.9 ☑
          nontraffic V74.3 ☑
            while boarding or alighting V74.4 ☑
        car (traffic) V73.9 ☑
          nontraffic V73.3 ☑
            while boarding or alighting V73.4 ☑
        motor vehicle NOS (traffic) V79.60 ☑
          nontraffic V79.20 ☑
          specified type NEC (traffic) V79.69 ☑
            nontraffic V79.29 ☑
        pedal cycle (traffic) V71.9 ☑
          nontraffic V71.3 ☑
            while boarding or alighting V71.4 ☑
        pickup truck (traffic) V73.9 ☑
          nontraffic V73.3 ☑
            while boarding or alighting V73.4 ☑
        railway vehicle (traffic) V75.9 ☑
          nontraffic V75.3 ☑
            while boarding or alighting V75.4 ☑
        specified vehicle NEC (traffic) V76.9 ☑
          nontraffic V75.3 ☑
            while boarding or alighting V76.4 ☑
        stationary object (traffic) V77.9 ☑
          nontraffic V77.3 ☑
            while boarding or alighting V77.4 ☑
        streetcar (traffic) V76.9 ☑

Accident — *continued*
  transport — *continued*
    bus occupant — *continued*
      collision — *continued*
        streetcar — *continued*
          nontraffic V76.3 ☑
            while boarding or alighting V76.4 ☑
        three wheeled motor vehicle (traffic) V72.9 ☑
          nontraffic V72.3 ☑
            while boarding or alighting V72.4 ☑
        truck (traffic) V74.9 ☑
          nontraffic V74.3 ☑
            while boarding or alighting V74.4 ☑
        two wheeled motor vehicle (traffic) V72.9 ☑
          nontraffic V72.3 ☑
            while boarding or alighting V72.4 ☑
        van (traffic) V73.9 ☑
          nontraffic V73.3 ☑
            while boarding or alighting V73.4 ☑
      driver
        collision (with)
          animal (traffic) V70.5 ☑
            being ridden (traffic) V76.5 ☑
              nontraffic V76.0 ☑
            nontraffic V70.0 ☑
          animal-drawn vehicle (traffic) V76.5 ☑
            nontraffic V76.0 ☑
          bus (traffic) V74.5 ☑
            nontraffic V74.0 ☑
          car (traffic) V73.5 ☑
            nontraffic V73.0 ☑
          motor vehicle NOS (traffic) V79.40 ☑
            nontraffic V79.00 ☑
            specified type NEC (traffic) V79.49 ☑
              nontraffic V79.09 ☑
          pedal cycle (traffic) V71.5 ☑
            nontraffic V71.0 ☑
          pickup truck (traffic) V73.5 ☑
            nontraffic V73.0 ☑
          railway vehicle (traffic) V75.5 ☑
            nontraffic V75.0 ☑
          specified vehicle NEC (traffic) V76.5 ☑
            nontraffic V76.0 ☑
          stationary object (traffic) V77.5 ☑
            nontraffic V77.0 ☑
          streetcar (traffic) V76.5 ☑
            nontraffic V76.0 ☑
          three wheeled motor vehicle (traffic) V72.5 ☑
            nontraffic V72.0 ☑
          truck (traffic) V74.5 ☑
            nontraffic V74.0 ☑
          two wheeled motor vehicle (traffic) V72.5 ☑
            nontraffic V72.0 ☑
          van (traffic) V73.5 ☑
            nontraffic V73.0 ☑
        noncollision accident (traffic) V78.5 ☑
          nontraffic V78.0 ☑
      hanger-on
        collision (with)
          animal (traffic) V70.7 ☑
            being ridden (traffic) V76.7 ☑
              nontraffic V76.2 ☑
            nontraffic V70.2 ☑
          animal-drawn vehicle (traffic) V76.7 ☑
            nontraffic V76.2 ☑
          bus (traffic) V74.7 ☑
            nontraffic V74.2 ☑
          car (traffic) V73.7 ☑
            nontraffic V73.2 ☑
          pedal cycle (traffic) V71.7 ☑
            nontraffic V71.2 ☑
          pickup truck (traffic) V73.7 ☑
            nontraffic V73.2 ☑
          railway vehicle (traffic) V75.7 ☑
            nontraffic V75.2 ☑
          specified vehicle NEC (traffic) V76.7 ☑
            nontraffic V76.2 ☑
          stationary object (traffic) V77.7 ☑
            nontraffic V77.2 ☑
          streetcar (traffic) V76.7 ☑
            nontraffic V76.2 ☑
          three wheeled motor vehicle (traffic) V72.7 ☑

External Causes Index

Accident — *continued*
  transport — *continued*
    bus occupant — *continued*
      hanger-on — *continued*
        collision — *continued*
          three wheeled motor vehicle — *continued*
            nontraffic V72.2 ☑
            truck (traffic) V74.7 ☑
              nontraffic V74.2 ☑
          two wheeled motor vehicle (traffic) V72.7 ☑
            nontraffic V72.2 ☑
          van (traffic) V73.7 ☑
            nontraffic V73.2 ☑
        noncollision accident (traffic) V78.7 ☑
          nontraffic V78.2 ☑
      noncollision accident (traffic) V78.9 ☑
        nontraffic V78.3 ☑
        while boarding or alighting V78.4 ☑
      nontraffic V79.3 ☑
      passenger
        collision (with)
          animal (traffic) V70.6 ☑
            being ridden (traffic) V76.6 ☑
              nontraffic V76.1 ☑
            nontraffic V70.1 ☑
          animal-drawn vehicle (traffic) V76.6 ☑
            nontraffic V76.1 ☑
          bus (traffic) V74.6 ☑
            nontraffic V74.1 ☑
          car (traffic) V73.6 ☑
            nontraffic V73.1 ☑
          motor vehicle NOS (traffic) V79.50 ☑
            nontraffic V79.10 ☑
            specified type NEC (traffic) V79.59 ☑
              nontraffic V79.19 ☑
          pedal cycle (traffic) V71.6 ☑
            nontraffic V71.1 ☑
          pickup truck (traffic) V73.6 ☑
            nontraffic V73.1 ☑
          railway vehicle (traffic) V75.6 ☑
            nontraffic V75.1 ☑
          specified vehicle NEC (traffic) V76.6 ☑
            nontraffic V76.1 ☑
          stationary object (traffic) V77.6 ☑
            nontraffic V77.1 ☑
          streetcar (traffic) V76.6 ☑
            nontraffic V76.1 ☑
          three wheeled motor vehicle (traffic) V72.6 ☑
            nontraffic V72.1 ☑
          truck (traffic) V74.6 ☑
            nontraffic V74.1 ☑
          two wheeled motor vehicle (traffic) V72.6 ☑
            nontraffic V72.1 ☑
          van (traffic) V73.6 ☑
            nontraffic V73.1 ☑
        noncollision accident (traffic) V78.6 ☑
          nontraffic V78.1 ☑
      specified type NEC V79.88 ☑
      military vehicle V79.81 ☑
    cable car, not on rails V98.0 ☑
      on rails — *see* Accident, transport, streetcar occupant
    car occupant V49.9 ☑
      ambulance occupant — *see* Accident, transport, ambulance occupant
      collision (with)
        animal (traffic) V40.9 ☑
          being ridden (traffic) V46.9 ☑
            nontraffic V46.3 ☑
              while boarding or alighting V46.4 ☑
          nontraffic V40.3 ☑
          while boarding or alighting V40.4 ☑
        animal-drawn vehicle (traffic) V46.9 ☑
          nontraffic V46.3 ☑
          while boarding or alighting V46.4 ☑
        bus (traffic) V44.9 ☑
          nontraffic V44.3 ☑
          while boarding or alighting V44.4 ☑
        car (traffic) V43.92 ☑
          nontraffic V43.32 ☑
          while boarding or alighting V43.42 ☑

Accident — *continued*
  transport — *continued*
    car occupant — *continued*
      collision — *continued*
        motor vehicle NOS (traffic) V49.60 ☑
          nontraffic V49.20 ☑
          specified type NEC (traffic) V49.69 ☑
            nontraffic V49.29 ☑
        pedal cycle (traffic) V41.9 ☑
          nontraffic V41.3 ☑
          while boarding or alighting V41.4 ☑
        pickup truck (traffic) V43.93 ☑
          nontraffic V43.33 ☑
          while boarding or alighting V43.43 ☑
        railway vehicle (traffic) V45.9 ☑
          nontraffic V45.3 ☑
          while boarding or alighting V45.4 ☑
        specified vehicle NEC (traffic) V46.9 ☑
          nontraffic V46.3 ☑
          while boarding or alighting V46.4 ☑
        sport utility vehicle (traffic) V43.91 ☑
          nontraffic V43.31 ☑
          while boarding or alighting V43.41 ☑
        stationary object (traffic) V47.9 ☑
          nontraffic V47.3 ☑
          while boarding or alighting V47.4 ☑
        streetcar (traffic) V46.9 ☑
          nontraffic V46.3 ☑
          while boarding or alighting V46.4 ☑
        three wheeled motor vehicle (traffic) V42.9 ☑
          nontraffic V42.3 ☑
          while boarding or alighting V42.4 ☑
        truck (traffic) V44.9 ☑
          nontraffic V44.3 ☑
          while boarding or alighting V44.4 ☑
        two wheeled motor vehicle (traffic) V42.9 ☑
          nontraffic V42.3 ☑
          while boarding or alighting V42.4 ☑
        van (traffic) V43.94 ☑
          nontraffic V43.34 ☑
          while boarding or alighting V43.44 ☑
      driver
        collision (with)
          animal (traffic) V40.5 ☑
            being ridden (traffic) V46.5 ☑
              nontraffic V46.0 ☑
            nontraffic V40.0 ☑
          animal-drawn vehicle (traffic) V46.5 ☑
            nontraffic V46.0 ☑
          bus (traffic) V44.5 ☑
            nontraffic V44.0 ☑
          car (traffic) V43.52 ☑
            nontraffic V43.02 ☑
          motor vehicle NOS (traffic) V49.40 ☑
            nontraffic V49.00 ☑
            specified type NEC (traffic) V49.49 ☑
              nontraffic V49.09 ☑
          pedal cycle (traffic) V41.5 ☑
            nontraffic V41.0 ☑
          pickup truck (traffic) V43.53 ☑
            nontraffic V43.03 ☑
          railway vehicle (traffic) V45.5 ☑
            nontraffic V45.0 ☑
          specified vehicle NEC (traffic) V46.5 ☑
            nontraffic V46.0 ☑
          sport utility vehicle (traffic) V43.51 ☑
            nontraffic V43.01 ☑
          stationary object (traffic) V47.5 ☑
            nontraffic V47.0 ☑
          streetcar (traffic) V46.5 ☑
            nontraffic V46.0 ☑
          three wheeled motor vehicle (traffic) V42.5 ☑
            nontraffic V42.0 ☑
          truck (traffic) V44.5 ☑
            nontraffic V44.0 ☑
          two wheeled motor vehicle (traffic) V42.5 ☑
            nontraffic V42.0 ☑
          van (traffic) V43.54 ☑
            nontraffic V43.04 ☑
        noncollision accident (traffic) V48.5 ☑
          nontraffic V48.0 ☑

Accident — *continued*
  transport — *continued*
    car occupant — *continued*
      hanger-on
        collision (with)
          animal (traffic) V40.7 ☑
            being ridden (traffic) V46.7 ☑
              nontraffic V46.2 ☑
            nontraffic V40.2 ☑
          animal-drawn vehicle (traffic) V46.7 ☑
            nontraffic V46.2 ☑
          bus (traffic) V44.7 ☑
            nontraffic V44.2 ☑
          car (traffic) V43.72 ☑
            nontraffic V43.22 ☑
          pedal cycle (traffic) V41.7 ☑
            nontraffic V41.2 ☑
          pickup truck (traffic) V43.73 ☑
            nontraffic V43.23 ☑
          railway vehicle (traffic) V45.7 ☑
            nontraffic V45.2 ☑
          specified vehicle NEC (traffic) V46.7 ☑
            nontraffic V46.2 ☑
          sport utility vehicle (traffic) V43.71 ☑
            nontraffic V43.21 ☑
          stationary object (traffic) V47.7 ☑
            nontraffic V47.2 ☑
          streetcar (traffic) V46.7 ☑
            nontraffic V46.2 ☑
          three wheeled motor vehicle (traffic) V42.7 ☑
            nontraffic V42.2 ☑
          truck (traffic) V44.7 ☑
            nontraffic V44.2 ☑
          two wheeled motor vehicle (traffic) V42.7 ☑
            nontraffic V42.2 ☑
          van (traffic) V43.74 ☑
            nontraffic V43.24 ☑
        noncollision accident (traffic) V48.7 ☑
          nontraffic V48.2 ☑
      noncollision accident (traffic) V48.9 ☑
        nontraffic V48.3 ☑
        while boarding or alighting V48.4 ☑
      nontraffic V49.3 ☑
      passenger
        collision (with)
          animal (traffic) V40.6 ☑
            being ridden (traffic) V46.6 ☑
              nontraffic V46.1 ☑
            nontraffic V40.1 ☑
          animal-drawn vehicle (traffic) V46.6 ☑
            nontraffic V46.1 ☑
          bus (traffic) V44.6 ☑
            nontraffic V44.1 ☑
          car (traffic) V43.62 ☑
            nontraffic V43.12 ☑
          motor vehicle NOS (traffic) V49.50 ☑
            nontraffic V49.10 ☑
            specified type NEC (traffic) V49.59 ☑
              nontraffic V49.19 ☑
          pedal cycle (traffic) V41.6 ☑
            nontraffic V41.1 ☑
          pickup truck (traffic) V43.63 ☑
            nontraffic V43.13 ☑
          railway vehicle (traffic) V45.6 ☑
            nontraffic V45.1 ☑
          specified vehicle NEC (traffic) V46.6 ☑
            nontraffic V46.1 ☑
          sport utility vehicle (traffic) V43.61 ☑
            nontraffic V43.11 ☑
          stationary object (traffic) V47.6 ☑
            nontraffic V47.1 ☑
          streetcar (traffic) V46.6 ☑
            nontraffic V46.1 ☑
          three wheeled motor vehicle (traffic) V42.6 ☑
            nontraffic V42.1 ☑
          truck (traffic) V44.6 ☑
            nontraffic V44.1 ☑
          two wheeled motor vehicle (traffic) V42.6 ☑
            nontraffic V42.1 ☑
          van (traffic) V43.64 ☑
            nontraffic V43.14 ☑

Accident — Accident

Accident — *continued*
 transport — *continued*
  car occupant — *continued*
   passenger — *continued*
    noncollision accident (traffic) V48.6 ☑
     nontraffic V48.1 ☑
    specified type NEC V49.88 ☑
    military vehicle V49.81 ☑
  coal car — *see* Accident, transport, industrial vehicle occupant
  construction vehicle occupant (nontraffic) V85.9 ☑
   driver V85.5 ☑
   hanger-on V85.7 ☑
   passenger V85.6 ☑
   traffic V85.3 ☑
    driver V85.0 ☑
    hanger-on V85.2 ☑
    passenger V85.1 ☑
   while boarding or alighting V85.4 ☑
  dirt bike rider (nontraffic) V86.96 ☑
   driver V86.56 ☑
   hanger-on V86.76 ☑
   passenger V86.66 ☑
   traffic V86.36 ☑
    driver V86.06 ☑
    hanger-on V86.26 ☑
    passenger V86.16 ☑
   while boarding or alighting V86.46 ☑
  due to cataclysm — *see* Forces of nature, by type
  dune buggy occupant (nontraffic) V86.93 ☑
   driver V86.53 ☑
   hanger-on V86.73 ☑
   passenger V86.63 ☑
   traffic V86.33 ☑
    driver V86.03 ☑
    hanger-on V86.23 ☑
    passenger V86.13 ☑
   while boarding or alighting V86.43 ☑
  e-bicycle — *see* Accident, transport, electric (assisted) bicyclist
  e-bike — *see* Accident, transport, electric (assisted) bicyclist
  electric (assisted) bicyclist V29.91 ☑
   collision (with)
    animal (traffic) V20.91 ☑
     being ridden (traffic) V26.91 ☑
      nontraffic V26.21 ☑
       while boarding or alighting V26.31 ☑
     nontraffic V20.21 ☑
      while boarding or alighting V20.31 ☑
    animal-drawn vehicle (traffic) V26.91 ☑
     nontraffic V26.21 ☑
      while boarding or alighting V26.31 ☑
    bus (traffic) V24.91 ☑
     nontraffic V24.21 ☑
      while boarding or alighting V24.31 ☑
    car (traffic) V23.91 ☑
     nontraffic V23.21 ☑
      while boarding or alighting V23.31 ☑
    motor vehicle NOS (traffic) V29.601 ☑
     nontraffic V29.201 ☑
      specified type NEC (traffic) V29.691 ☑
       nontraffic V29.291 ☑
    pedal cycle (traffic) V21.91 ☑
     nontraffic V21.21 ☑
      while boarding or alighting V21.31 ☑
    pedestrian V20.91 ☑
     nontraffic V20.01 ☑
      while boarding or alighting V20.31 ☑
    pickup truck (traffic) V23.91 ☑
     nontraffic V23.21 ☑
      while boarding or alighting V23.31 ☑
    railway vehicle (traffic) V25.91 ☑
     nontraffic V25.21 ☑
      while boarding or alighting V25.31 ☑
    specified vehicle NEC (traffic) V26.91 ☑
     nontraffic V26.21 ☑
      while boarding or alighting V26.31 ☑
    stationary object (traffic) V27.91 ☑
     nontraffic V27.21 ☑
      while boarding or alighting V27.31 ☑
    streetcar (traffic) V26.91 ☑
     nontraffic V26.21 ☑
      while boarding or alighting V26.31 ☑
    three wheeled motor vehicle (traffic) V22.91 ☑

Accident — *continued*
 transport — *continued*
  electric bicyclist — *continued*
   collision — *continued*
    three wheeled motor vehicle — *continued*
     nontraffic V22.21 ☑
      while boarding or alighting V22.31 ☑
    truck (traffic) V24.91 ☑
     nontraffic V24.21 ☑
      while boarding or alighting V24.31 ☑
    two wheeled motor vehicle (traffic) V22.91 ☑
     nontraffic V22.21 ☑
      while boarding or alighting V22.31 ☑
    van (traffic) V23.91 ☑
     nontraffic V23.21 ☑
      while boarding or alighting V23.31 ☑
   driver
    collision (with)
     animal (traffic) V20.41 ☑
      being ridden (traffic) V26.41 ☑
       nontraffic V26.01 ☑
      nontraffic V20.01 ☑
     animal-drawn vehicle (traffic) V26.41 ☑
      nontraffic V26.01 ☑
     bus (traffic) V24.41 ☑
      nontraffic V24.01 ☑
     car (traffic) V23.41 ☑
      nontraffic V23.01 ☑
     motor vehicle NOS (traffic) V29.401 ☑
      nontraffic V29.001 ☑
      specified type NEC (traffic) V29.491 ☑
       nontraffic V29.091 ☑
     pedal cycle (traffic) V21.41 ☑
      nontraffic V21.01 ☑
     pedestrian
      nontraffic V20.01 ☑
      traffic V20.41 ☑
     pickup truck (traffic) V23.41 ☑
      nontraffic V23.01 ☑
     railway vehicle (traffic) V25.41 ☑
      nontraffic V25.01 ☑
     specified vehicle NEC (traffic) V26.41 ☑
      nontraffic V26.01 ☑
     stationary object (traffic) V27.41 ☑
      nontraffic V27.01 ☑
     streetcar (traffic) V26.41 ☑
      nontraffic V26.01 ☑
     three wheeled motor vehicle (traffic) V22.41 ☑
      nontraffic V22.01 ☑
     truck (traffic) V24.41 ☑
      nontraffic V24.01 ☑
     two wheeled motor vehicle (traffic) V22.41 ☑
      nontraffic V22.01 ☑
     van (traffic) V23.41 ☑
      nontraffic V23.01 ☑
    noncollision accident (traffic) V28.41 ☑
     nontraffic V28.01 ☑
   noncollision accident (traffic) V28.91 ☑
    nontraffic V28.21 ☑
     while boarding or alighting V28.31 ☑
   nontraffic V29.31 ☑
   passenger
    collision (with)
     animal (traffic) V20.51 ☑
      being ridden (traffic) V26.51 ☑
       nontraffic V26.11 ☑
      nontraffic V20.11 ☑
     animal-drawn vehicle (traffic) V26.51 ☑
      nontraffic V26.11 ☑
     bus (traffic) V24.51 ☑
      nontraffic V24.11 ☑
     car (traffic) V23.51 ☑
      nontraffic V23.11 ☑
     motor vehicle NOS (traffic) V29.501 ☑
      nontraffic V29.101 ☑
      specified type NEC (traffic) V29.591 ☑
       nontraffic V29.191 ☑
     pedal cycle (traffic) V21.51 ☑
      nontraffic V21.11 ☑
     pedestrian
      nontraffic V20.11 ☑
      traffic V20.51 ☑
     pickup truck (traffic) V23.51 ☑

Accident — *continued*
 transport — *continued*
  electric bicyclist — *continued*
   passenger — *continued*
    collision — *continued*
     pickup truck — *continued*
      nontraffic V23.11 ☑
     railway vehicle (traffic) V25.51 ☑
      nontraffic V25.11 ☑
     specified vehicle NEC (traffic) V26.51 ☑
      nontraffic V26.11 ☑
     stationary object (traffic) V27.51 ☑
      nontraffic V27.11 ☑
     streetcar (traffic) V26.51 ☑
      nontraffic V26.11 ☑
     three wheeled motor vehicle (traffic) V22.51 ☑
      nontraffic V22.11 ☑
     truck (traffic) V24.51 ☑
      nontraffic V24.11 ☑
     two wheeled motor vehicle (traffic) V22.51 ☑
      nontraffic V22.11 ☑
     van (traffic) V23.51 ☑
      nontraffic V23.11 ☑
    noncollision accident (traffic) V28.51 ☑
     nontraffic V28.11 ☑
   specified type NEC V29.881 ☑
   military vehicle V29.811 ☑
  forklift — *see* Accident, transport, industrial vehicle occupant
  go cart — *see* Accident, transport, all-terrain vehicle occupant
  golf cart — *see* Accident, transport, all-terrain vehicle occupant
  heavy transport vehicle occupant — *see* Accident, transport, truck occupant
  hoverboard V00.848 ☑
  ice yacht V98.2 ☑
  industrial vehicle occupant (nontraffic) V83.9 ☑
   driver V83.5 ☑
   hanger-on V83.7 ☑
   passenger V83.6 ☑
   traffic V83.3 ☑
    driver V83.0 ☑
    hanger-on V83.2 ☑
    passenger V83.1 ☑
   while boarding or alighting V83.4 ☑
  interurban electric car — *see* Accident, transport, streetcar
  land yacht V98.1 ☑
  logging car — *see* Accident, transport, industrial vehicle occupant
  military vehicle occupant (traffic) V86.34 ☑
   driver V86.04 ☑
   hanger-on V86.24 ☑
   nontraffic V86.94 ☑
    driver V86.54 ☑
    hanger-on V86.74 ☑
    passenger V86.64 ☑
   passenger V86.14 ☑
   while boarding or alighting V86.44 ☑
  mine tram — *see* Accident, transport, industrial vehicle occupant
  motor vehicle NEC occupant (traffic) V89.2 ☑
  motorcoach — *see* Accident, transport, bus occupant
  motor/cross bike rider — *see also* Accident, transport, dirt bike rider V86.96 ☑
  motorcycle V29.99 ☑
   collision (with)
    animal (traffic) V20.99 ☑
     being ridden (traffic) V26.99 ☑
      nontraffic V26.29 ☑
       while boarding or alighting V26.39 ☑
     nontraffic V20.29 ☑
      while boarding or alighting V20.39 ☑
    animal-drawn vehicle (traffic) V26.99 ☑
     nontraffic V26.29 ☑
      while boarding or alighting V26.39 ☑
    bus (traffic) V24.99 ☑
     nontraffic V24.29 ☑
      while boarding or alighting V24.39 ☑
    car (traffic) V23.99 ☑
     nontraffic V23.29 ☑
      while boarding or alighting V23.39 ☑
    motor vehicle NOS (traffic) V29.608 ☑

External Causes Index

Accident — Accident

Accident — *continued*
  transport — *continued*
    motorcycle — *continued*
      collision — *continued*
        motor vehicle — *continued*
          nontraffic V29.208 ☑
          specified type NEC (traffic) V29.698 ☑
            nontraffic V29.298 ☑
        pedal cycle (traffic) V21.99 ☑
          nontraffic V21.29 ☑
          while boarding or alighting V21.39 ☑
        pickup truck (traffic) V23.99 ☑
          nontraffic V23.29 ☑
          while boarding or alighting V23.39 ☑
        railway vehicle (traffic) V25.99 ☑
          nontraffic V25.29 ☑
          while boarding or alighting V25.39 ☑
        specified vehicle NEC (traffic) V26.99 ☑
          nontraffic V26.29 ☑
          while boarding or alighting V26.39 ☑
        stationary object (traffic) V27.99 ☑
          nontraffic V27.29 ☑
          while boarding or alighting V27.39 ☑
        streetcar (traffic) V26.99 ☑
          nontraffic V26.29 ☑
          while boarding or alighting V26.39 ☑
        three wheeled motor vehicle (traffic) V22.99 ☑
          nontraffic V22.29 ☑
          while boarding or alighting V22.39 ☑
        truck (traffic) V24.99 ☑
          nontraffic V24.29 ☑
          while boarding or alighting V24.39 ☑
        two wheeled motor vehicle (traffic) V22.99 ☑
          nontraffic V22.29 ☑
          while boarding or alighting V22.39 ☑
        van (traffic) V23.99 ☑
          nontraffic V23.29 ☑
          while boarding or alighting V23.39 ☑
      driver
        collision (with)
          animal (traffic) V20.49 ☑
            being ridden (traffic) V26.49 ☑
              nontraffic V26.09 ☑
            nontraffic V20.09 ☑
          animal-drawn vehicle (traffic) V26.49 ☑
            nontraffic V26.09 ☑
          bus (traffic) V24.49 ☑
            nontraffic V24.09 ☑
          car (traffic) V23.49 ☑
            nontraffic V23.09 ☑
          motor vehicle NOS (traffic) V29.408 ☑
            nontraffic V29.008 ☑
            specified type NEC (traffic) V29.498 ☑
              nontraffic V29.098 ☑
          pedal cycle (traffic) V21.49 ☑
            nontraffic V21.09 ☑
          pedestrian
            nontraffic V20.09 ☑
            traffic V20.49 ☑
          pickup truck (traffic) V23.49 ☑
            nontraffic V23.09 ☑
          railway vehicle (traffic) V25.49 ☑
            nontraffic V25.09 ☑
          specified vehicle NEC (traffic) V26.49 ☑
            nontraffic V26.09 ☑
          stationary object (traffic) V27.49 ☑
            nontraffic V27.09 ☑
          streetcar (traffic) V26.49 ☑
            nontraffic V26.09 ☑
          three wheeled motor vehicle (traffic) V22.49 ☑
            nontraffic V22.09 ☑
          truck (traffic) V24.49 ☑
            nontraffic V24.09 ☑
          two wheeled motor vehicle (traffic) V22.49 ☑
            nontraffic V22.09 ☑
          van (traffic) V23.49 ☑
            nontraffic V23.09 ☑
        noncollision accident (traffic) V28.49 ☑
          nontraffic V28.09 ☑
      noncollision accident (traffic) V28.99 ☑
        nontraffic V28.29 ☑
        while boarding or alighting V28.39 ☑
      nontraffic V29.39 ☑

Accident — *continued*
  transport — *continued*
    motorcycle — *continued*
      passenger
        collision (with)
          animal (traffic) V20.59 ☑
            being ridden (traffic) V26.59 ☑
              nontraffic V26.19 ☑
            nontraffic V20.19 ☑
          animal-drawn vehicle (traffic) V26.59 ☑
            nontraffic V26.19 ☑
          bus (traffic) V24.59 ☑
            nontraffic V24.19 ☑
          car (traffic) V23.59 ☑
            nontraffic V23.19 ☑
          motor vehicle NOS (traffic) V29.508 ☑
            nontraffic V29.108 ☑
            specified type NEC (traffic) V29.598 ☑
              nontraffic V29.198 ☑
          pedal cycle (traffic) V21.59 ☑
            nontraffic V21.19 ☑
          pedestrian
            nontraffic V20.19 ☑
            traffic V20.59 ☑
          pickup truck (traffic) V23.59 ☑
            nontraffic V23.19 ☑
          railway vehicle (traffic) V25.59 ☑
            nontraffic V25.19 ☑
          specified vehicle NEC (traffic) V26.59 ☑
            nontraffic V26.19 ☑
          stationary object (traffic) V27.59 ☑
            nontraffic V27.19 ☑
          streetcar (traffic) V26.59 ☑
            nontraffic V26.19 ☑
          three wheeled motor vehicle (traffic) V22.59 ☑
            nontraffic V22.19 ☑
          truck (traffic) V24.59 ☑
            nontraffic V24.19 ☑
          two wheeled motor vehicle (traffic) V22.59 ☑
            nontraffic V22.19 ☑
          van (traffic) V23.59 ☑
            nontraffic V23.19 ☑
        noncollision accident (traffic) V28.59 ☑
          nontraffic V28.19 ☑
      specified type NEC V29.888 ☑
      military vehicle V29.818 ☑
    occupant (of)
      aircraft (powered) V95.9 ☑
        fixed wing
          commercial — *see* Accident, transport, aircraft, occupant, powered, fixed wing, commercial
          private — *see* Accident, transport, aircraft, occupant, powered, fixed wing, private
        nonpowered V96.9 ☑
        specified NEC V95.8 ☑
      airport battery-powered vehicle — *see* Accident, transport, industrial vehicle occupant
      all-terrain vehicle (ATV) — *see* Accident, transport, all-terrain vehicle occupant
      animal-drawn vehicle — *see* Accident, transport, animal-drawn vehicle occupant
      automobile — *see* Accident, transport, car occupant
      balloon V96.00 ☑
      battery-powered vehicle — *see* Accident, transport, industrial vehicle occupant
      bicycle — *see* Accident, transport, pedal cyclist
        motorized — *see* Accident, transport, motorcycle rider
      boat NEC — *see* Accident, watercraft
      bulldozer — *see* Accident, transport, construction vehicle occupant
      bus — *see* Accident, transport, bus occupant
      cable car (on rails) — *see also* Accident, transport, streetcar occupant
        not on rails V98.0 ☑
      car — *see also* Accident, transport, car occupant
        cable (on rails) — *see also* Accident, transport, streetcar occupant
        not on rails V98.0 ☑
      coach — *see* Accident, transport, bus occupant
      coal-car — *see* Accident, transport, industrial vehicle occupant

Accident — *continued*
  transport — *continued*
    occupant — *continued*
      digger — *see* Accident, transport, construction vehicle occupant
      dump truck — *see* Accident, transport, construction vehicle occupant
      earth-leveler — *see* Accident, transport, construction vehicle occupant
      farm machinery (self-propelled) — *see* Accident, transport, agricultural vehicle occupant
      forklift — *see* Accident, transport, industrial vehicle occupant
      glider (unpowered) V96.20 ☑
        hang V96.10 ☑
        powered (microlight) (ultralight) — *see* Accident, transport, aircraft, occupant, powered, glider
      glider (unpowered) NEC V96.20 ☑
      hang-glider V96.10 ☑
      harvester — *see* Accident, transport, agricultural vehicle occupant
      heavy (transport) vehicle — *see* Accident, transport, truck occupant
      helicopter — *see* Accident, transport, aircraft, occupant, helicopter
      ice-yacht V98.2 ☑
      kite (carrying person) V96.8 ☑
      land-yacht V98.1 ☑
      logging car — *see* Accident, transport, industrial vehicle occupant
      mechanical shovel — *see* Accident, transport, construction vehicle occupant
      microlight — *see* Accident, transport, aircraft, occupant, powered, glider
      minibus — *see* Accident, transport, pickup truck occupant
      minivan — *see* Accident, transport, pickup truck occupant
      moped — *see* Accident, transport, motorcycle
      motor scooter — *see* Accident, transport, motorcycle
      motorcycle (with sidecar) — *see* Accident, transport, motorcycle
      off-road motor-vehicle — *see also* Accident, transport, all-terrain vehicle occupant V86.99 ☑
      pedal cycle — *see also* Accident, transport, pedal cyclist
      pick-up (truck) — *see* Accident, transport, pickup truck occupant
      railway (train) (vehicle) (subterranean) (elevated) — *see* Accident, transport, railway vehicle occupant
      rickshaw — *see* Accident, transport, pedal cycle
        motorized — *see* Accident, transport, three-wheeled motor vehicle
        pedal driven — *see* Accident, transport, pedal cyclist
      road-roller — *see* Accident, transport, construction vehicle occupant
      ship NOS V94.9 ☑
      ski-lift (chair) (gondola) V98.3 ☑
      snowmobile — *see* Accident, transport, snowmobile occupant
      spacecraft, spaceship — *see* Accident, transport, aircraft, occupant, spacecraft
      sport utility vehicle — *see* Accident, transport, pickup truck occupant
      streetcar (interurban) (operating on public street or highway) — *see* Accident, transport, streetcar occupant
      SUV — *see* Accident, transport, pickup truck occupant
      téléférique V98.0 ☑
      three-wheeled vehicle (motorized) — *see also* Accident, transport, three-wheeled motor vehicle occupant
        nonmotorized — *see* Accident, transport, pedal cycle
      tractor (farm) (and trailer) — *see* Accident, transport, agricultural vehicle occupant
      train — *see* Accident, transport, railway vehicle occupant
      tram — *see* Accident, transport, streetcar occupant
        in mine or quarry — *see* Accident, transport, industrial vehicle occupant
      tricycle — *see* Accident, transport, pedal cycle

☑ **Additional Character Required — Refer to the Tabular List for Character Selection**

Accident — *continued*
  transport — *continued*
    occupant — *continued*
      tricycle — *see* Accident, transport, pedal cycle — *continued*
        motorized — *see* Accident, transport, three-wheeled motor vehicle
      trolley — *see* Accident, transport, streetcar occupant
      in mine or quarry — *see* Accident, transport, industrial vehicle occupant
      tub, in mine or quarry — *see* Accident, transport, industrial vehicle occupant
      ultralight — *see* Accident, transport, aircraft, occupant, powered, glider
      van — *see* Accident, transport, van occupant
      vehicle NEC V89.9 ☑
        heavy transport — *see* Accident, transport, truck occupant
        motor (traffic) NEC V89.2 ☑
        nontraffic NEC V89.0 ☑
      watercraft NOS V94.9 ☑
        causing drowning — *see* Drowning, resulting from accident to boat
      off-road motor-vehicle — *see also* Accident, transport, all-terrain vehicle occupant V86.99 ☑
    parachutist V97.29 ☑
      after accident to aircraft — *see* Accident, transport, aircraft
      entangled in object V97.21 ☑
      injured on landing V97.22 ☑
    pedal cyclist V19.9 ☑
      collision (with)
        animal (traffic) V10.9 ☑
          being ridden (traffic) V16.9 ☑
            nontraffic V16.2 ☑
              while boarding or alighting V16.3 ☑
          nontraffic V10.2 ☑
            while boarding or alighting V10.3 ☑
        animal-drawn vehicle (traffic) V16.9 ☑
          nontraffic V16.2 ☑
            while boarding or alighting V16.3 ☑
        bus (traffic) V14.9 ☑
          nontraffic V14.2 ☑
            while boarding or alighting V14.3 ☑
        car (traffic) V13.9 ☑
          nontraffic V13.2 ☑
            while boarding or alighting V13.3 ☑
        motor vehicle NOS (traffic) V19.60 ☑
          nontraffic V19.20 ☑
          specified type NEC (traffic) V19.69 ☑
            nontraffic V19.29 ☑
        pedal cycle (traffic) V11.9 ☑
          nontraffic V11.2 ☑
            while boarding or alighting V11.3 ☑
        pickup truck (traffic) V13.9 ☑
          nontraffic V13.2 ☑
            while boarding or alighting V13.3 ☑
        railway vehicle (traffic) V15.9 ☑
          nontraffic V15.2 ☑
            while boarding or alighting V15.3 ☑
        specified vehicle NEC (traffic) V16.9 ☑
          nontraffic V16.2 ☑
            while boarding or alighting V16.3 ☑
        stationary object (traffic) V17.9 ☑
          nontraffic V17.2 ☑
            while boarding or alighting V17.3 ☑
        streetcar (traffic) V16.9 ☑
          nontraffic V16.2 ☑
            while boarding or alighting V16.3 ☑
        three wheeled motor vehicle (traffic) V12.9 ☑
          nontraffic V12.2 ☑
            while boarding or alighting V12.3 ☑
        truck (traffic) V14.9 ☑
          nontraffic V14.2 ☑
            while boarding or alighting V14.3 ☑
        two wheeled motor vehicle (traffic) V12.9 ☑
          nontraffic V12.2 ☑
            while boarding or alighting V12.3 ☑
        van (traffic) V13.9 ☑
          nontraffic V13.2 ☑
            while boarding or alighting V13.3 ☑
      driver
        collision (with)
          animal (traffic) V10.4 ☑
            being ridden (traffic) V16.4 ☑

Accident — *continued*
  transport — *continued*
    pedal cyclist — *continued*
      driver — *continued*
        collision — *continued*
          animal — *continued*
            being ridden — *continued*
              nontraffic V16.0 ☑
              nontraffic V10.0 ☑
          animal-drawn vehicle (traffic) V16.4 ☑
            nontraffic V16.0 ☑
          bus (traffic) V14.4 ☑
            nontraffic V14.0 ☑
          car (traffic) V13.4 ☑
            nontraffic V13.0 ☑
          motor vehicle NOS (traffic) V19.40 ☑
            nontraffic V19.00 ☑
            specified type NEC (traffic) V19.49 ☑
              nontraffic V19.09 ☑
          pedal cycle (traffic) V11.4 ☑
            nontraffic V11.0 ☑
          pickup truck (traffic) V13.4 ☑
            nontraffic V13.0 ☑
          railway vehicle (traffic) V15.4 ☑
            nontraffic V15.0 ☑
          specified vehicle NEC (traffic) V16.4 ☑
            nontraffic V16.0 ☑
          stationary object (traffic) V17.4 ☑
            nontraffic V17.0 ☑
          streetcar (traffic) V16.4 ☑
            nontraffic V16.0 ☑
          three wheeled motor vehicle (traffic) V12.4 ☑
            nontraffic V12.0 ☑
          truck (traffic) V14.4 ☑
            nontraffic V14.0 ☑
          two wheeled motor vehicle (traffic) V12.4 ☑
            nontraffic V12.0 ☑
          van (traffic) V13.4 ☑
            nontraffic V13.0 ☑
        noncollision accident (traffic) V18.4 ☑
          nontraffic V18.0 ☑
      noncollision accident (traffic) V18.9 ☑
        nontraffic V18.2 ☑
          while boarding or alighting V18.3 ☑
      nontraffic V19.3 ☑
      passenger
        collision (with)
          animal (traffic) V10.5 ☑
            being ridden (traffic) V16.5 ☑
              nontraffic V16.1 ☑
              nontraffic V10.1 ☑
          animal-drawn vehicle (traffic) V16.5 ☑
            nontraffic V16.1 ☑
          bus (traffic) V14.5 ☑
            nontraffic V14.1 ☑
          car (traffic) V13.5 ☑
            nontraffic V13.1 ☑
          motor vehicle NOS (traffic) V19.50 ☑
            nontraffic V19.10 ☑
            specified type NEC (traffic) V19.59 ☑
              nontraffic V19.19 ☑
          pedal cycle (traffic) V11.5 ☑
            nontraffic V11.1 ☑
          pickup truck (traffic) V13.5 ☑
            nontraffic V13.1 ☑
          railway vehicle (traffic) V15.5 ☑
            nontraffic V15.1 ☑
          specified vehicle NEC (traffic) V16.5 ☑
            nontraffic V16.1 ☑
          stationary object (traffic) V17.5 ☑
            nontraffic V17.1 ☑
          streetcar (traffic) V16.5 ☑
            nontraffic V16.1 ☑
          three wheeled motor vehicle (traffic) V12.5 ☑
            nontraffic V12.1 ☑
          truck (traffic) V14.5 ☑
            nontraffic V14.1 ☑
          two wheeled motor vehicle (traffic) V12.5 ☑
            nontraffic V12.1 ☑
          van (traffic) V13.5 ☑
            nontraffic V13.1 ☑

Accident — *continued*
  transport — *continued*
    pedal cyclist — *continued*
      passenger — *continued*
        noncollision accident (traffic) V18.5 ☑
          nontraffic V18.1 ☑
      specified type NEC V19.88 ☑
        military vehicle V19.81 ☑
    pedestrian
      conveyance (occupant) V09.9 ☑
        baby stroller V00.828 ☑
        collision (with) V09.9 ☑
          animal being ridden or animal drawn vehicle V06.99 ☑
            nontraffic V06.09 ☑
            traffic V06.19 ☑
          bus or heavy transport V04.99 ☑
            nontraffic V04.09 ☑
            traffic V04.19 ☑
          car V03.99 ☑
            nontraffic V03.09 ☑
            traffic V03.19 ☑
          pedal cycle V01.99 ☑
            nontraffic V01.09 ☑
            traffic V01.19 ☑
          pick-up truck or van V03.99 ☑
            nontraffic V03.09 ☑
            traffic V03.19 ☑
          railway (train) (vehicle) V05.99 ☑
            nontraffic V05.09 ☑
            traffic V05.19 ☑
          stationary object V00.822 ☑
          streetcar V06.99 ☑
            nontraffic V06.09 ☑
            traffic V06.19 ☑
          two- or three-wheeled motor vehicle V02.99 ☑
            nontraffic V02.09 ☑
            traffic V02.19 ☑
          vehicle V09.9 ☑
            animal-drawn V06.99 ☑
              nontraffic V06.09 ☑
              traffic V06.19 ☑
            motor
              nontraffic V09.00 ☑
              traffic V09.20 ☑
        fall V00.821 ☑
        nontraffic V09.1 ☑
          involving motor vehicle NEC V09.00 ☑
        traffic V09.3 ☑
          involving motor vehicle NEC V09.20 ☑
      flat-bottomed NEC V00.388 ☑
        collision (with) V09.9 ☑
          animal being ridden or animal drawn vehicle V06.99 ☑
            nontraffic V06.09 ☑
            traffic V06.19 ☑
          bus or heavy transport V04.99 ☑
            nontraffic V04.09 ☑
            traffic V04.19 ☑
          car V03.99 ☑
            nontraffic V03.09 ☑
            traffic V03.19 ☑
          pedal cycle V01.99 ☑
            nontraffic V01.09 ☑
            traffic V01.19 ☑
          pick-up truck or van V03.99 ☑
            nontraffic V03.09 ☑
            traffic V03.19 ☑
          railway (train) (vehicle) V05.99 ☑
            nontraffic V05.09 ☑
            traffic V05.19 ☑
          stationary object V00.382 ☑
          streetcar V06.99 ☑
            nontraffic V06.09 ☑
            traffic V06.19 ☑
          two- or three-wheeled motor vehicle V02.99 ☑
            nontraffic V02.09 ☑
            traffic V02.19 ☑
          vehicle V09.9 ☑
            animal-drawn V06.99 ☑
              nontraffic V06.09 ☑
              traffic V06.19 ☑

Accident — *continued*
  transport — *continued*
    pedestrian — *continued*
      conveyance — *continued*
        flat-bottomed — *continued*
          collision — *continued*
            vehicle — *continued*
              motor
                nontraffic V09.00 ☑
                traffic V09.20 ☑
          fall V00.381 ☑
          nontraffic V09.1 ☑
            involving motor vehicle NEC V09.00 ☑
          snow
            board — *see* Accident, transport, pedestrian, conveyance, snow board
            ski — *see* Accident, transport, pedestrian, conveyance, skis (snow)
          traffic V09.3 ☑
            involving motor vehicle NEC V09.20 ☑
        gliding type NEC V00.288 ☑
          collision (with) V09.9 ☑
            animal being ridden or animal drawn vehicle V06.99 ☑
              nontraffic V06.09 ☑
              traffic V06.19 ☑
            bus or heavy transport V04.99 ☑
              nontraffic V04.09 ☑
              traffic V04.19 ☑
            car V03.99 ☑
              nontraffic V03.09 ☑
              traffic V03.19 ☑
            pedal cycle V01.99 ☑
              nontraffic V01.09 ☑
              traffic V01.19 ☑
            pick-up truck or van V03.99 ☑
              nontraffic V03.09 ☑
              traffic V03.19 ☑
            railway (train) (vehicle) V05.99 ☑
              nontraffic V05.09 ☑
              traffic V05.19 ☑
            stationary object V00.282 ☑
            streetcar V06.99 ☑
              nontraffic V06.09 ☑
              traffic V02.19 ☑
            two- or three-wheeled motor vehicle V02.99 ☑
              nontraffic V02.09 ☑
              traffic V02.19 ☑
            vehicle V09.9 ☑
              animal-drawn V06.99 ☑
                nontraffic V06.09 ☑
                traffic V06.19 ☑
              motor
                nontraffic V09.00 ☑
                traffic V09.20 ☑
          fall V00.281 ☑
          heelies — *see* Accident, transport, pedestrian, conveyance, heelies
          ice skate — *see* Accident, transport, pedestrian, conveyance, ice skate
          nontraffic V09.1 ☑
            involving motor vehicle NEC V09.00 ☑
          sled — *see* Accident, transport, pedestrian, conveyance, sled
          traffic V09.3 ☑
            involving motor vehicle NEC V09.20 ☑
          wheelies — *see* Accident, transport, pedestrian, conveyance, heelies
        heelies V00.158 ☑
          colliding with stationary object V00.152 ☑
          fall V00.151 ☑
        hoverboard
          collision with
            animal being ridden or animal drawn vehicle V06.938 ☑
              nontraffic V06.038 ☑
              traffic V06.138 ☑
            bus or heavy transport V04.938 ☑
              nontraffic V04.038 ☑
              traffic V04.138 ☑
            car V03.938 ☑
              nontraffic V03.038 ☑
              traffic V03.138 ☑
            pedal cycle V01.938 ☑

Accident — *continued*
  transport — *continued*
    pedestrian — *continued*
      conveyance — *continued*
        hoverboard — *continued*
          collision with — *continued*
            pedal cycle — *continued*
              nontraffic V01.038 ☑
              traffic V01.138 ☑
            pick-up or van V03.938 ☑
              nontraffic V03.038 ☑
              traffic V03.138 ☑
            railway (train) (vehicle) V05.938 ☑
              nontraffic V05.038 ☑
              traffic V05.138 ☑
            streetcar V06.938 ☑
              nontraffic V06.038 ☑
              traffic V06.138 ☑
            three-wheeled motor vehicle V02.938 ☑
              nontraffic V02.038 ☑
              traffic V02.138 ☑
            two-wheeled motor vehicle V02.938 ☑
              nontraffic V02.038 ☑
              traffic V02.138 ☑
            vehicle, nonmotor, specified NEC V06.938 ☑
              nontraffic V06.038 ☑
              traffic V06.138 ☑
          fall V00.848 ☑
        ice skates V00.218 ☑
          collision (with) V09.9 ☑
            animal being ridden or animal drawn vehicle V06.99 ☑
              nontraffic V06.09 ☑
              traffic V06.19 ☑
            bus or heavy transport V04.99 ☑
              nontraffic V04.09 ☑
              traffic V04.19 ☑
            car V03.99 ☑
              nontraffic V03.09 ☑
              traffic V03.19 ☑
            pedal cycle V01.99 ☑
              nontraffic V01.09 ☑
              traffic V01.19 ☑
            pick-up truck or van V03.99 ☑
              nontraffic V03.09 ☑
              traffic V03.19 ☑
            railway (train) (vehicle) V05.99 ☑
              nontraffic V05.09 ☑
              traffic V05.19 ☑
            stationary object V00.212 ☑
            streetcar V06.99 ☑
              nontraffic V06.09 ☑
              traffic V06.19 ☑
            two- or three-wheeled motor vehicle V02.99 ☑
              nontraffic V02.09 ☑
              traffic V02.19 ☑
            vehicle V09.9 ☑
              animal-drawn V06.99 ☑
                nontraffic V06.09 ☑
                traffic V06.19 ☑
              motor
                nontraffic V09.00 ☑
                traffic V09.20 ☑
          fall V00.211 ☑
          nontraffic V09.1 ☑
            involving motor vehicle NEC V09.00 ☑
          traffic V09.3 ☑
            involving motor vehicle NEC V09.20 ☑
        motorized mobility scooter V00.838 ☑
          collision with stationary object V00.832 ☑
          fall from V00.831 ☑
        nontraffic V09.1 ☑
          involving motor vehicle V09.00 ☑
            military V09.01 ☑
            specified type NEC V09.09 ☑
        roller skates (non in-line) V00.128 ☑
          collision (with) V09.9 ☑
            animal being ridden or animal drawn vehicle V06.91 ☑
              nontraffic V06.01 ☑
              traffic V06.11 ☑
            bus or heavy transport V04.91 ☑

Accident — *continued*
  transport — *continued*
    pedestrian — *continued*
      conveyance — *continued*
        roller skates — *continued*
          collision — *continued*
            bus or heavy transport — *continued*
              nontraffic V04.01 ☑
              traffic V04.11 ☑
            car V03.91 ☑
              nontraffic V03.01 ☑
              traffic V03.11 ☑
            pedal cycle V01.91 ☑
              nontraffic V01.01 ☑
              traffic V01.11 ☑
            pick-up truck or van V03.91 ☑
              nontraffic V03.01 ☑
              traffic V03.11 ☑
            railway (train) (vehicle) V05.91 ☑
              nontraffic V05.01 ☑
              traffic V05.11 ☑
            stationary object V00.122 ☑
            streetcar V06.91 ☑
              nontraffic V06.01 ☑
              traffic V06.11 ☑
            two- or three-wheeled motor vehicle V02.91 ☑
              nontraffic V02.01 ☑
              traffic V02.11 ☑
            vehicle V09.9 ☑
              animal-drawn V06.91 ☑
                nontraffic V06.01 ☑
                traffic V06.11 ☑
              motor
                nontraffic V09.00 ☑
                traffic V09.20 ☑
          fall V00.121 ☑
          in-line V00.118 ☑
            collision — *see also* Accident, transport, pedestrian, conveyance occupant, roller skates, collision with stationary object V00.112 ☑
            fall V00.111 ☑
          nontraffic V09.1 ☑
            involving motor vehicle NEC V09.00 ☑
          traffic V09.3 ☑
            involving motor vehicle NEC V09.20 ☑
        rolling shoes V00.158 ☑
          colliding with stationary object V00.152 ☑
          fall V00.151 ☑
        rolling type NEC V00.188 ☑
          collision (with) V09.9 ☑
            animal being ridden or animal drawn vehicle V06.99 ☑
              nontraffic V06.09 ☑
              traffic V06.19 ☑
            bus or heavy transport V04.99 ☑
              nontraffic V04.09 ☑
              traffic V04.19 ☑
            car V03.99 ☑
              nontraffic V03.09 ☑
              traffic V03.19 ☑
            pedal cycle V01.99 ☑
              nontraffic V01.09 ☑
              traffic V01.19 ☑
            pick-up truck or van V03.99 ☑
              nontraffic V03.09 ☑
              traffic V03.19 ☑
            railway (train) (vehicle) V05.99 ☑
              nontraffic V05.09 ☑
              traffic V05.19 ☑
            stationary object V00.182 ☑
            streetcar V06.99 ☑
              nontraffic V06.09 ☑
              traffic V06.19 ☑
            two- or three-wheeled motor vehicle V02.99 ☑
              nontraffic V02.09 ☑
              traffic V02.19 ☑
            vehicle V09.9 ☑
              animal-drawn V06.99 ☑
                nontraffic V06.09 ☑
                traffic V06.19 ☑
              motor
                nontraffic V09.00 ☑

Accident — *continued*
  transport — *continued*
    pedestrian — *continued*
      conveyance — *continued*
        rolling type — *continued*
          collision — *continued*
            vehicle — *continued*
              motor — *continued*
                traffic V09.20 ☑
          fall V00.181
          in-line roller skate — *see* Accident, transport, pedestrian, conveyance, roller skate, in-line
          nontraffic V09.1 ☑
            involving motor vehicle NEC V09.00 ☑
          roller skate — *see* Accident, transport, pedestrian, conveyance, roller skate
          scooter (non-motorized) — *see* Accident, transport, pedestrian, conveyance, scooter
          skateboard — *see* Accident, transport, pedestrian, conveyance, skateboard
          traffic V09.3 ☑
            involving motor vehicle NEC V09.20 ☑
        scooter (non-motorized) V00.148 ☑
          collision (with) V09.9 ☑
            animal being ridden or animal drawn vehicle V06.99 ☑
              nontraffic V06.09 ☑
              traffic V06.19 ☑
            bus or heavy transport V04.99 ☑
              nontraffic V04.09 ☑
              traffic V04.19 ☑
            car V03.99 ☑
              nontraffic V03.09 ☑
              traffic V03.19 ☑
            pedal cycle V01.99 ☑
              nontraffic V01.09 ☑
              traffic V01.19 ☑
            pick-up truck or van V03.99 ☑
              nontraffic V03.09 ☑
              traffic V03.19 ☑
            railway (train) (vehicle) V05.99 ☑
              nontraffic V05.09 ☑
              traffic V05.19 ☑
            stationary object V00.142 ☑
            streetcar V06.99 ☑
              nontraffic V06.09 ☑
              traffic V06.19 ☑
            two- or three-wheeled motor vehicle V02.99 ☑
              nontraffic V02.09 ☑
              traffic V02.19 ☑
            vehicle V09.9 ☑
              animal-drawn V06.99 ☑
                nontraffic V06.09 ☑
                traffic V06.19 ☑
              motor
                nontraffic V09.00 ☑
                traffic V09.20 ☑
           fall V00.141 ☑
          nontraffic V09.1 ☑
            involving motor vehicle NEC V09.00 ☑
          traffic V09.3 ☑
            involving motor vehicle NEC V09.20 ☑
        Segway
          collision with
            animal being ridden or animal drawn vehicle V06.938 ☑
              nontraffic V06.038 ☑
              traffic V06.138 ☑
            bus or heavy transport V04.938 ☑
              nontraffic V04.038 ☑
              traffic V04.138 ☑
            car V03.938 ☑
              nontraffic V03.038 ☑
              traffic V03.138 ☑
            pedal cycle V01.938 ☑
              nontraffic V01.038 ☑
              traffic V01.138 ☑
            pick-up or van V03.938 ☑
              nontraffic V03.038 ☑
              traffic V03.138 ☑
            railway (train) (vehicle) V05.938 ☑
              nontraffic V05.038 ☑
              traffic V05.138 ☑

Accident — *continued*
  transport — *continued*
    pedestrian — *continued*
      conveyance — *continued*
        Segway — *continued*
          collision with — *continued*
            streetcar V06.938 ☑
              nontraffic V06.038 ☑
              traffic V06.138 ☑
            three-wheeled vehicle V02.938 ☑
              nontraffic V02.038 ☑
              traffic V02.138 ☑
            two-wheeled vehicle V02.938 ☑
              nontraffic V02.038 ☑
              traffic V02.138 ☑
            vehicle, nonmotor, specified NEC V06.938 ☑
              nontraffic V06.038 ☑
              traffic V06.138 ☑
          fall V00.848 ☑
        skateboard V00.138 ☑
          collision (with) V09.9 ☑
            animal being ridden or animal drawn vehicle V06.92 ☑
              nontraffic V06.02 ☑
              traffic V06.12 ☑
            bus or heavy transport V04.92 ☑
              nontraffic V04.02 ☑
              traffic V04.12 ☑
            car V03.92 ☑
              nontraffic V03.02 ☑
              traffic V03.12 ☑
            pedal cycle V01.92 ☑
              nontraffic V01.02 ☑
              traffic V01.12 ☑
            pick-up truck or van V03.92 ☑
              nontraffic V03.02 ☑
              traffic V03.12 ☑
            railway (train) (vehicle) V05.92 ☑
              nontraffic V05.02 ☑
              traffic V05.12 ☑
            stationary object V00.132 ☑
            streetcar V06.92 ☑
              nontraffic V06.02 ☑
              traffic V06.12 ☑
            two- or three-wheeled motor vehicle V02.92 ☑
              nontraffic V02.02 ☑
              traffic V02.12 ☑
            vehicle V09.9 ☑
              animal-drawn V06.92 ☑
                nontraffic V06.02 ☑
                traffic V06.12 ☑
              motor
                nontraffic V09.00 ☑
                traffic V09.20 ☑
         fall V00.131 ☑
        nontraffic V09.1 ☑
          involving motor vehicle NEC V09.00 ☑
        traffic V09.3 ☑
          involving motor vehicle NEC V09.20 ☑
        skis (snow) V00.328 ☑
          collision (with) V09.9 ☑
            animal being ridden or animal drawn vehicle V06.99 ☑
              nontraffic V06.09 ☑
              traffic V06.19 ☑
            bus or heavy transport V04.99 ☑
              nontraffic V04.09 ☑
              traffic V04.19 ☑
            car V03.99 ☑
              nontraffic V03.09 ☑
              traffic V03.19 ☑
            pedal cycle V01.99 ☑
              nontraffic V01.09 ☑
              traffic V01.19 ☑
            pick-up truck or van V03.99 ☑
              nontraffic V03.09 ☑
              traffic V03.19 ☑
            railway (train) (vehicle) V05.99 ☑
              nontraffic V05.09 ☑
              traffic V05.19 ☑
            stationary object V00.322 ☑
            streetcar V06.99 ☑
              nontraffic V06.09 ☑

Accident — *continued*
  transport — *continued*
    pedestrian — *continued*
      conveyance — *continued*
        skis — *continued*
          collision — *continued*
            streetcar — *continued*
              traffic V06.19 ☑
            two- or three-wheeled motor vehicle V02.99 ☑
              nontraffic V02.09 ☑
              traffic V02.19 ☑
            vehicle V09.9 ☑
              animal-drawn V06.99 ☑
                nontraffic V06.09 ☑
                traffic V06.19 ☑
              motor
                nontraffic V09.00 ☑
                traffic V09.20 ☑
         fall V00.321 ☑
        nontraffic V09.1 ☑
          involving motor vehicle NEC V09.00 ☑
        traffic V09.3 ☑
          involving motor vehicle NEC V09.20 ☑
        sled V00.228 ☑
          collision (with) V09.9 ☑
            animal being ridden or animal drawn vehicle V06.99 ☑
              nontraffic V06.09 ☑
              traffic V06.19 ☑
            bus or heavy transport V04.99 ☑
              nontraffic V04.09 ☑
              traffic V04.19 ☑
            car V03.99 ☑
              nontraffic V03.09 ☑
              traffic V03.19 ☑
            pedal cycle V01.99 ☑
              nontraffic V01.09 ☑
              traffic V01.19 ☑
            pick-up truck or van V03.99 ☑
              nontraffic V03.09 ☑
              traffic V03.19 ☑
            railway (train) (vehicle) V05.99 ☑
              nontraffic V05.09 ☑
              traffic V05.19 ☑
            stationary object V00.222 ☑
            streetcar V06.99 ☑
              nontraffic V06.09 ☑
              traffic V06.19 ☑
            two- or three-wheeled motor vehicle V02.99 ☑
              nontraffic V02.09 ☑
              traffic V02.19 ☑
            vehicle V09.9 ☑
              animal-drawn V06.99 ☑
                nontraffic V06.09 ☑
                traffic V06.19 ☑
              motor
                nontraffic V09.00 ☑
                traffic V09.20 ☑
        fall V00.221 ☑
        nontraffic V09.1 ☑
          involving motor vehicle NEC V09.00 ☑
        traffic V09.3 ☑
          involving motor vehicle NEC V09.20 ☑
        snow board V00.318 ☑
          collision (with) V09.9 ☑
            animal being ridden or animal drawn vehicle V06.99 ☑
              nontraffic V06.09 ☑
              traffic V06.19 ☑
            bus or heavy transport V04.99 ☑
              nontraffic V04.09 ☑
              traffic V04.19 ☑
            car V03.99 ☑
              nontraffic V03.09 ☑
              traffic V03.19 ☑
            pedal cycle V01.99 ☑
              nontraffic V01.09 ☑
              traffic V01.19 ☑
            pick-up truck or van V03.99 ☑
              nontraffic V03.09 ☑
              traffic V03.19 ☑
            railway (train) (vehicle) V05.99 ☑
              nontraffic V05.09 ☑

Accident — *continued*
  transport — *continued*
    pedestrian — *continued*
      conveyance — *continued*
        snow board — *continued*
          collision — *continued*
            railway — *continued*
              traffic V05.19 ☑
            stationary object V00.312 ☑
            streetcar V06.99 ☑
              nontraffic V06.09 ☑
              traffic V06.19 ☑
            two- or three-wheeled motor vehicle V02.99 ☑
              nontraffic V02.09 ☑
              traffic V02.19 ☑
            vehicle V09.9 ☑
              animal-drawn V06.99 ☑
                nontraffic V06.09 ☑
                traffic V06.19 ☑
              motor
                nontraffic V09.00 ☑
                traffic V09.20 ☑
           fall V00.311 ☑
          nontraffic V09.1 ☑
            involving motor vehicle NEC V09.00 ☑
          traffic V09.3 ☑
            involving motor vehicle NEC V09.20 ☑
         specified type NEC V00.898 ☑
          collision (with) V09.9 ☑
            animal being ridden or animal drawn vehicle V06.99 ☑
              nontraffic V06.09 ☑
              traffic V06.19 ☑
            bus or heavy transport V04.99 ☑
              nontraffic V04.09 ☑
              traffic V04.19 ☑
            car V03.99 ☑
              nontraffic V03.09 ☑
              traffic V03.19 ☑
            pedal cycle V01.99 ☑
              nontraffic V01.09 ☑
              traffic V01.19 ☑
            pick-up truck or van V03.99 ☑
              nontraffic V03.09 ☑
              traffic V03.19 ☑
            railway (train) (vehicle) V05.99 ☑
              nontraffic V05.09 ☑
              traffic V05.19 ☑
            stationary object V00.892 ☑
            streetcar V06.99 ☑
              nontraffic V06.09 ☑
              traffic V06.19 ☑
            two- or three-wheeled motor vehicle V02.99 ☑
              nontraffic V02.09 ☑
              traffic V02.19 ☑
            vehicle V09.9 ☑
              animal-drawn V06.99 ☑
                nontraffic V06.09 ☑
                traffic V06.19 ☑
              motor
                nontraffic V09.00 ☑
                traffic V09.20 ☑
           fall V00.891 ☑
          nontraffic V09.1 ☑
            involving motor vehicle NEC V09.00 ☑
          traffic V09.3 ☑
            involving motor vehicle NEC V09.20 ☑
        standing
          electric scooter
            collision with
              animal being ridden or animal drawn vehicle V06.931 ☑
                nontraffic V06.031 ☑
                traffic V06.131 ☑
              bus or heavy transport V04.931 ☑
                nontraffic V04.031 ☑
                traffic V04.131 ☑
              car V03.931 ☑
                nontraffic V04.031 ☑
                traffic V04.131 ☑
              pedal cycle V01.931 ☑
                nontraffic V01.031 ☑
                traffic V01.131 ☑

Accident — *continued*
  transport — *continued*
    pedestrian — *continued*
      conveyance — *continued*
        standing — *continued*
          electric scooter — *continued*
            collision with — *continued*
              pick-up or van V03.931 ☑
                nontraffic V03.031 ☑
                traffic V03.131 ☑
              railway (train) (vehicle) V05.931 ☑
                nontraffic V05.031 ☑
                traffic V05.131 ☑
              streetcar V06.931 ☑
                nontraffic V06.031 ☑
                traffic V06.131 ☑
              three-wheeled motor vehicle V02.931 ☑
                nontraffic V02.031 ☑
                traffic V02.131 ☑
              two-wheeled motor vehicle V02.931 ☑
                nontraffic V02.031 ☑
                traffic V02.131 ☑
              vehicle, nonmotor, specified NEC V06.931 ☑
                nontraffic V06.031 ☑
                traffic V06.131 ☑
             fall V00.841 ☑
          micro-mobility pedestrian conveyance
            collision with
              animal being ridden or animal drawn vehicle V06.938 ☑
                nontraffic V06.038 ☑
                traffic V06.138 ☑
              bus or heavy transport V04.938 ☑
                nontraffic V04.038 ☑
                traffic V04.138 ☑
              car V03.938 ☑
                nontraffic V03.038 ☑
                traffic V03.138 ☑
              pedal cycle V01.938 ☑
                nontraffic V01.038 ☑
                traffic V01.138 ☑
              pick-up or van V03.938 ☑
                nontraffic V03.038 ☑
                traffic V03.138 ☑
              railway (train) (vehicle) V05.938 ☑
                nontraffic V05.038 ☑
                traffic V05.138 ☑
              stationary object V00.842 ☑
              streetcar V06.938 ☑
                nontraffic V06.038 ☑
                traffic V06.138 ☑
              three-wheeled motor vehicle V02.938 ☑
                nontraffic V02.038 ☑
                traffic V02.138 ☑
              two-wheeled motor vehicle V02.938 ☑
                nontraffic V02.038 ☑
                traffic V02.138 ☑
              vehicle, nonmotor, specified NEC V06.938 ☑
                nontraffic V06.038 ☑
                traffic V06.138 ☑
             fall V00.848 ☑
          traffic V09.3 ☑
            involving motor vehicle V09.20 ☑
              military V09.21 ☑
              specified type NEC V09.29 ☑
         wheelchair (powered) V00.818 ☑
          collision (with) V09.9 ☑
            animal being ridden or animal drawn vehicle V06.99 ☑
              nontraffic V06.09 ☑
              traffic V06.19 ☑
            bus or heavy transport V04.99 ☑
              nontraffic V04.09 ☑
              traffic V04.19 ☑
            car V03.99 ☑
              nontraffic V03.09 ☑
              traffic V03.19 ☑
            pedal cycle V01.99 ☑
              nontraffic V01.09 ☑

Accident — *continued*
  transport — *continued*
    pedestrian — *continued*
      conveyance — *continued*
        wheelchair — *continued*
          collision — *continued*
            pedal cycle — *continued*
              traffic V01.19 ☑
            pick-up truck or van V03.99 ☑
              nontraffic V03.09 ☑
              traffic V03.19 ☑
            railway (train) (vehicle) V05.99 ☑
              nontraffic V05.09 ☑
              traffic V05.19 ☑
            stationary object V00.812 ☑
            streetcar V06.99 ☑
              nontraffic V06.09 ☑
              traffic V06.19 ☑
            two- or three-wheeled motor vehicle V02.99 ☑
              nontraffic V02.09 ☑
              traffic V02.19 ☑
            vehicle V09.9 ☑
              animal-drawn V06.99 ☑
                nontraffic V06.09 ☑
                traffic V06.19 ☑
              motor
                nontraffic V09.00 ☑
                traffic V09.20 ☑
           fall V00.811 ☑
          nontraffic V09.1 ☑
            involving motor vehicle NEC V09.00 ☑
          traffic V09.3 ☑
            involving motor vehicle NEC V09.20 ☑
         wheeled shoe V00.158 ☑
          colliding with stationary object V00.152 ☑
          fall V00.151 ☑
      on foot — *see also* Accident, pedestrian
        collision (with)
          animal being ridden or animal drawn vehicle V06.90 ☑
            nontraffic V06.00 ☑
            traffic V06.10 ☑
          bus or heavy transport V04.90 ☑
            nontraffic V04.00 ☑
            traffic V04.10 ☑
          car V03.90 ☑
            nontraffic V03.00 ☑
            traffic V03.10 ☑
          pedal cycle V01.90 ☑
            nontraffic V01.00 ☑
            traffic V01.10 ☑
          pick-up truck or van V03.90 ☑
            nontraffic V03.00 ☑
            traffic V03.10 ☑
          railway (train) (vehicle) V05.90 ☑
            nontraffic V05.00 ☑
            traffic V05.10 ☑
          streetcar V06.90 ☑
            nontraffic V06.00 ☑
            traffic V06.10 ☑
          two- or three-wheeled motor vehicle V02.90 ☑
            nontraffic V02.00 ☑
            traffic V02.10 ☑
          vehicle V09.9 ☑
            animal-drawn V06.90 ☑
              nontraffic V06.00 ☑
              traffic V06.10 ☑
            motor
        nontraffic V09.1 ☑
          involving motor vehicle V09.00 ☑
            military V09.01 ☑
            specified type NEC V09.09 ☑
         traffic V09.3 ☑
          involving motor vehicle V09.20 ☑
            military V09.21 ☑
            specified type NEC V09.29 ☑
    person NEC (unknown way or transportation) V99 ☑
      collision (between)
        bus (with)
          heavy transport vehicle (traffic) V87.5 ☑
            nontraffic V88.5 ☑
        car (with)
          bus (traffic) V87.3 ☑

☑ **Additional Character Required** — **Refer to the Tabular List for Character Selection**

Accident — *continued*
transport — *continued*
person — *continued*
collision — *continued*
car — *continued*
bus — *continued*
nontraffic V88.3 ☑
heavy transport vehicle (traffic) V87.4 ☑
nontraffic V88.4 ☑
nontraffic V88.5 ☑
pick-up truck or van (traffic) V87.2 ☑
nontraffic V88.2 ☑
train or railway vehicle (traffic) V87.6 ☑
nontraffic V88.6 ☑
two-or three-wheeled motor vehicle (traffic) V87.0 ☑
nontraffic V88.0 ☑
motor vehicle (traffic) NEC V87.7 ☑
nontraffic V88.7 ☑
two-or three-wheeled vehicle (with) (traffic)
motor vehicle NEC V87.1 ☑
nontraffic V88.1 ☑
nonmotor vehicle (collision) (noncollision) (traffic) V87.9 ☑
nontraffic V88.9 ☑
pickup truck occupant V59.9 ☑
collision (with)
animal (traffic) V50.9 ☑
being ridden (traffic) V56.9 ☑
nontraffic V56.3 ☑
while boarding or alighting V56.4 ☑
nontraffic V50.3 ☑
while boarding or alighting V50.4 ☑
animal-drawn vehicle (traffic) V56.9 ☑
nontraffic V56.3 ☑
while boarding or alighting V56.4 ☑
bus (traffic) V54.9 ☑
nontraffic V54.3 ☑
while boarding or alighting V54.4 ☑
car (traffic) V53.9 ☑
nontraffic V53.3 ☑
while boarding or alighting V53.4 ☑
motor vehicle NOS (traffic) V59.60 ☑
nontraffic V59.20 ☑
specified type NEC (traffic) V59.69 ☑
nontraffic V59.29 ☑
pedal cycle (traffic) V51.9 ☑
nontraffic V51.3 ☑
while boarding or alighting V51.4 ☑
pickup truck (traffic) V53.9 ☑
nontraffic V53.3 ☑
while boarding or alighting V53.4 ☑
railway vehicle (traffic) V55.9 ☑
nontraffic V55.3 ☑
while boarding or alighting V55.4 ☑
specified vehicle NEC (traffic) V56.9 ☑
nontraffic V56.3 ☑
while boarding or alighting V56.4 ☑
stationary object (traffic) V57.9 ☑
nontraffic V57.3 ☑
while boarding or alighting V57.4 ☑
streetcar (traffic) V56.9 ☑
nontraffic V56.3 ☑
while boarding or alighting V56.4 ☑
three wheeled motor vehicle (traffic) V52.9 ☑
nontraffic V52.3 ☑
while boarding or alighting V52.4 ☑
truck (traffic) V54.9 ☑
nontraffic V54.3 ☑
while boarding or alighting V54.4 ☑
two wheeled motor vehicle (traffic) V52.9 ☑
nontraffic V52.3 ☑
while boarding or alighting V52.4 ☑
van (traffic) V53.9 ☑
nontraffic V53.3 ☑
while boarding or alighting V53.4 ☑
driver
collision (with)
animal (traffic) V50.5 ☑
being ridden (traffic) V56.5 ☑
nontraffic V56.0 ☑
nontraffic V50.0 ☑
animal-drawn vehicle (traffic) V56.5 ☑
nontraffic V56.0 ☑
bus (traffic) V54.5 ☑

Accident — *continued*
transport — *continued*
pickup truck occupant — *continued*
driver — *continued*
collision — *continued*
bus — *continued*
nontraffic V54.0 ☑
car (traffic) V53.5 ☑
nontraffic V53.0 ☑
motor vehicle NOS (traffic) V59.40 ☑
nontraffic V59.00 ☑
specified type NEC (traffic) V59.49 ☑
nontraffic V59.09 ☑
pedal cycle (traffic) V51.5 ☑
nontraffic V51.0 ☑
pickup truck (traffic) V53.5 ☑
nontraffic V53.0 ☑
railway vehicle (traffic) V55.5 ☑
nontraffic V55.0 ☑
specified vehicle NEC (traffic) V56.5 ☑
nontraffic V56.0 ☑
stationary object (traffic) V57.5 ☑
nontraffic V57.0 ☑
streetcar (traffic) V56.5 ☑
nontraffic V56.0 ☑
three wheeled motor vehicle (traffic) V52.5 ☑
nontraffic V52.0 ☑
truck (traffic) V54.5 ☑
nontraffic V54.0 ☑
two wheeled motor vehicle (traffic) V52.5 ☑
nontraffic V52.0 ☑
van (traffic) V53.5 ☑
nontraffic V53.0 ☑
noncollision accident (traffic) V58.5 ☑
nontraffic V58.0 ☑
hanger-on
collision (with)
animal (traffic) V50.7 ☑
being ridden (traffic) V56.7 ☑
nontraffic V56.2 ☑
nontraffic V50.2 ☑
animal-drawn vehicle (traffic) V56.7 ☑
nontraffic V56.2 ☑
bus (traffic) V54.7 ☑
nontraffic V54.2 ☑
car (traffic) V53.7 ☑
nontraffic V53.2 ☑
pedal cycle (traffic) V51.7 ☑
nontraffic V51.2 ☑
pickup truck (traffic) V53.7 ☑
nontraffic V53.2 ☑
railway vehicle (traffic) V55.7 ☑
nontraffic V55.2 ☑
specified vehicle NEC (traffic) V56.7 ☑
nontraffic V56.2 ☑
stationary object (traffic) V57.7 ☑
nontraffic V57.2 ☑
streetcar (traffic) V56.7 ☑
nontraffic V56.2 ☑
three wheeled motor vehicle (traffic) V52.7 ☑
nontraffic V52.2 ☑
truck (traffic) V54.7 ☑
nontraffic V54.2 ☑
two wheeled motor vehicle (traffic) V52.7 ☑
nontraffic V52.2 ☑
van (traffic) V53.7 ☑
nontraffic V53.2 ☑
noncollision accident (traffic) V58.7 ☑
nontraffic V58.2 ☑
noncollision accident (traffic) V58.9 ☑
nontraffic V58.3 ☑
while boarding or alighting V58.4 ☑
nontraffic V59.3 ☑
passenger
collision (with)
animal (traffic) V50.6 ☑
being ridden (traffic) V56.6 ☑
nontraffic V56.1 ☑
nontraffic V50.1 ☑
animal-drawn vehicle (traffic) V56.6 ☑
nontraffic V56.1 ☑

Accident — *continued*
transport — *continued*
pickup truck occupant — *continued*
passenger — *continued*
collision — *continued*
bus (traffic) V54.6 ☑
nontraffic V54.1 ☑
car (traffic) V53.6 ☑
nontraffic V53.1 ☑
motor vehicle NOS (traffic) V59.50 ☑
nontraffic V59.10 ☑
specified type NEC (traffic) V59.59 ☑
nontraffic V59.19 ☑
pedal cycle (traffic) V51.6 ☑
nontraffic V51.1 ☑
pickup truck (traffic) V53.6 ☑
nontraffic V53.1 ☑
railway vehicle (traffic) V55.6 ☑
nontraffic V55.1 ☑
specified vehicle NEC (traffic) V56.6 ☑
nontraffic V56.1 ☑
stationary object (traffic) V57.6 ☑
nontraffic V57.1 ☑
streetcar (traffic) V56.6 ☑
nontraffic V56.1 ☑
three wheeled motor vehicle (traffic) V52.6 ☑
nontraffic V52.1 ☑
truck (traffic) V54.6 ☑
nontraffic V54.1 ☑
two wheeled motor vehicle (traffic) V52.6 ☑
nontraffic V52.1 ☑
van (traffic) V53.6 ☑
nontraffic V53.1 ☑
noncollision accident (traffic) V58.6 ☑
nontraffic V58.1 ☑
specified type NEC V59.88 ☑
military vehicle V59.81 ☑
quarry truck — *see* Accident, transport, industrial vehicle occupant
race car — *see* Accident, transport, motor vehicle NEC occupant
railway vehicle occupant V81.9 ☑
collision (with) V81.3 ☑
motor vehicle (non-military) (traffic) V81.1 ☑
military V81.83 ☑
nontraffic V81.0 ☑
rolling stock V81.2 ☑
specified object NEC V81.3 ☑
during derailment V81.7 ☑
with antecedent collision — *see* Accident, transport, railway vehicle occupant, collision
explosion V81.81 ☑
fall (in railway vehicle) V81.5 ☑
during derailment V81.7 ☑
with antecedent collision — *see* Accident, transport, railway vehicle occupant, collision
from railway vehicle V81.6 ☑
during derailment V81.7 ☑
with antecedent collision — *see* Accident, transport, railway vehicle occupant, collision
while boarding or alighting V81.4 ☑
fire V81.81 ☑
object falling onto train V81.82 ☑
specified type NEC V81.89 ☑
while boarding or alighting V81.4 ☑
Segway V00.848 ☑
ski lift V98.3 ☑
snowmobile occupant (nontraffic) V86.92 ☑
driver V86.52 ☑
hanger-on V86.72 ☑
passenger V86.62 ☑
traffic V86.32 ☑
driver V86.02 ☑
hanger-on V86.22 ☑
passenger V86.12 ☑
while boarding or alighting V86.42 ☑
specified NEC V98.8 ☑
sport utility vehicle occupant — *see also* Accident, transport, pickup truck occupant
streetcar occupant V82.9 ☑
collision (with) V82.3 ☑

Accident — *continued*
  transport — *continued*
    streetcar occupant — *continued*
      collision — *continued*
        motor vehicle (traffic) V82.1 ☑
          nontraffic V82.0 ☑
        rolling stock V82.2 ☑
        during derailment V82.7 ☑
          with antecedent collision — *see* Accident, transport, streetcar occupant, collision
      fall (in streetcar) V82.5 ☑
        during derailment V82.7 ☑
          with antecedent collision — *see* Accident, transport, streetcar occupant, collision
        from streetcar V82.6 ☑
          during derailment V82.7 ☑
            with antecedent collision — *see* Accident, transport, streetcar occupant, collision
        while boarding or alighting V82.4 ☑
      while boarding or alighting V82.4 ☑
      specified type NEC V82.8 ☑
      while boarding or alighting V82.4 ☑
    three-wheeled motor vehicle occupant V39.9 ☑
      collision (with)
        animal (traffic) V30.9 ☑
          being ridden (traffic) V36.9 ☑
            nontraffic V36.3 ☑
              while boarding or alighting V36.4 ☑
          nontraffic V30.3 ☑
          while boarding or alighting V30.4 ☑
        animal-drawn vehicle (traffic) V36.9 ☑
          nontraffic V36.3 ☑
          while boarding or alighting V36.4 ☑
        bus (traffic) V34.9 ☑
          nontraffic V34.3 ☑
          while boarding or alighting V34.4 ☑
        car (traffic) V33.9 ☑
          nontraffic V33.3 ☑
          while boarding or alighting V33.4 ☑
        motor vehicle NOS (traffic) V39.60 ☑
          nontraffic V39.20 ☑
          specified type NEC (traffic) V39.69 ☑
            nontraffic V39.29 ☑
        pedal cycle (traffic) V31.9 ☑
          nontraffic V31.3 ☑
          while boarding or alighting V31.4 ☑
        pickup truck (traffic) V33.9 ☑
          nontraffic V33.3 ☑
          while boarding or alighting V33.4 ☑
        railway vehicle (traffic) V35.9 ☑
          nontraffic V35.3 ☑
          while boarding or alighting V35.4 ☑
        specified vehicle NEC (traffic) V36.9 ☑
          nontraffic V36.3 ☑
          while boarding or alighting V36.4 ☑
        stationary object (traffic) V37.9 ☑
          nontraffic V37.3 ☑
          while boarding or alighting V37.4 ☑
        streetcar (traffic) V36.9 ☑
          nontraffic V36.3 ☑
          while boarding or alighting V36.4 ☑
        three wheeled motor vehicle (traffic) V32.9 ☑
          nontraffic V32.3 ☑
          while boarding or alighting V32.4 ☑
        truck (traffic) V34.9 ☑
          nontraffic V34.3 ☑
          while boarding or alighting V34.4 ☑
        two wheeled motor vehicle (traffic) V32.9 ☑
          nontraffic V32.3 ☑
          while boarding or alighting V32.4 ☑
        van (traffic) V33.9 ☑
          nontraffic V33.3 ☑
          while boarding or alighting V33.4 ☑
      driver
        collision (with)
          animal (traffic) V30.5 ☑
            being ridden (traffic) V36.5 ☑
              nontraffic V36.0 ☑
            nontraffic V30.0 ☑
          animal-drawn vehicle (traffic) V36.5 ☑
            nontraffic V36.0 ☑
          bus (traffic) V34.5 ☑
            nontraffic V34.0 ☑

Accident — *continued*
  transport — *continued*
    three-wheeled motor vehicle occupant — *continued*
      driver — *continued*
        collision — *continued*
          car (traffic) V33.5 ☑
            nontraffic V33.0 ☑
          motor vehicle NOS (traffic) V39.40 ☑
            nontraffic V39.00 ☑
            specified type NEC (traffic) V39.49 ☑
              nontraffic V39.09 ☑
          pedal cycle (traffic) V31.5 ☑
            nontraffic V31.0 ☑
          pickup truck (traffic) V33.5 ☑
            nontraffic V33.0 ☑
          railway vehicle (traffic) V35.5 ☑
            nontraffic V35.0 ☑
          specified vehicle NEC (traffic) V36.5 ☑
            nontraffic V36.0 ☑
          stationary object (traffic) V37.5 ☑
            nontraffic V37.0 ☑
          streetcar (traffic) V36.5 ☑
            nontraffic V36.0 ☑
          three wheeled motor vehicle (traffic) V32.5 ☑
            nontraffic V32.0 ☑
          truck (traffic) V34.5 ☑
            nontraffic V34.0 ☑
          two wheeled motor vehicle (traffic) V32.5 ☑
            nontraffic V32.0 ☑
          van (traffic) V33.5 ☑
            nontraffic V33.0 ☑
        noncollision accident (traffic) V38.5 ☑
          nontraffic V38.0 ☑
      hanger-on
        collision (with)
          animal (traffic) V30.7 ☑
            being ridden (traffic) V36.7 ☑
              nontraffic V36.2 ☑
            nontraffic V30.2 ☑
          animal-drawn vehicle (traffic) V36.7 ☑
            nontraffic V36.2 ☑
          bus (traffic) V34.7 ☑
            nontraffic V34.2 ☑
          car (traffic) V33.7 ☑
            nontraffic V33.2 ☑
          pedal cycle (traffic) V31.7 ☑
            nontraffic V31.2 ☑
          pickup truck (traffic) V33.7 ☑
            nontraffic V33.2 ☑
          railway vehicle (traffic) V35.7 ☑
            nontraffic V35.2 ☑
          specified vehicle NEC (traffic) V36.7 ☑
            nontraffic V36.2 ☑
          stationary object (traffic) V37.7 ☑
            nontraffic V37.2 ☑
          streetcar (traffic) V36.7 ☑
            nontraffic V36.2 ☑
          three wheeled motor vehicle (traffic) V32.7 ☑
            nontraffic V32.2 ☑
          truck (traffic) V34.7 ☑
            nontraffic V34.2 ☑
          two wheeled motor vehicle (traffic) V32.7 ☑
            nontraffic V32.2 ☑
          van (traffic) V33.7 ☑
            nontraffic V33.2 ☑
        noncollision accident (traffic) V38.7 ☑
          nontraffic V38.2 ☑
      noncollision accident (traffic) V38.9 ☑
        nontraffic V38.3 ☑
        while boarding or alighting V38.4 ☑
      nontraffic V39.3 ☑
      passenger
        collision (with)
          animal (traffic) V30.6 ☑
            being ridden (traffic) V36.6 ☑
              nontraffic V36.1 ☑
            nontraffic V30.1 ☑
          animal-drawn vehicle (traffic) V36.6 ☑
            nontraffic V36.1 ☑
          bus (traffic) V34.6 ☑

Accident — *continued*
  transport — *continued*
    three-wheeled motor vehicle occupant — *continued*
      passenger — *continued*
        collision — *continued*
          bus — *continued*
            nontraffic V34.1 ☑
          car (traffic) V33.6 ☑
            nontraffic V33.1 ☑
          motor vehicle NOS (traffic) V39.50 ☑
            nontraffic V39.10 ☑
            specified type NEC (traffic) V39.59 ☑
              nontraffic V39.19 ☑
          pedal cycle (traffic) V31.6 ☑
            nontraffic V31.1 ☑
          pickup truck (traffic) V33.6 ☑
            nontraffic V33.1 ☑
          railway vehicle (traffic) V35.6 ☑
            nontraffic V35.1 ☑
          specified vehicle NEC (traffic) V36.6 ☑
            nontraffic V36.1 ☑
          stationary object (traffic) V37.6 ☑
            nontraffic V37.1 ☑
          streetcar (traffic) V36.6 ☑
            nontraffic V36.1 ☑
          three wheeled motor vehicle (traffic) V32.6 ☑
            nontraffic V32.1 ☑
          truck (traffic) V34.6 ☑
            nontraffic V34.1 ☑
          two wheeled motor vehicle (traffic) V32.6 ☑
            nontraffic V32.1 ☑
          van (traffic) V33.6 ☑
            nontraffic V33.1 ☑
        noncollision accident (traffic) V38.6 ☑
          nontraffic V38.1 ☑
      specified type NEC V39.89 ☑
      military vehicle V39.81 ☑
    tractor (farm) (and trailer) — *see* Accident, transport, agricultural vehicle occupant
    tram — *see* Accident, transport, streetcar
      in mine or quarry — *see* Accident, transport, industrial vehicle occupant
    trolley — *see* Accident, transport, streetcar
      in mine or quarry — *see* Accident, transport, industrial vehicle occupant
    truck (heavy) occupant V69.9 ☑
      collision (with)
        animal (traffic) V60.9 ☑
          being ridden (traffic) V66.9 ☑
            nontraffic V66.3 ☑
              while boarding or alighting V66.4 ☑
          nontraffic V60.3 ☑
          while boarding or alighting V60.4 ☑
        animal-drawn vehicle (traffic) V66.9 ☑
          nontraffic V66.3 ☑
          while boarding or alighting V66.4 ☑
        bus (traffic) V64.9 ☑
          nontraffic V64.3 ☑
          while boarding or alighting V64.4 ☑
        car (traffic) V63.9 ☑
          nontraffic V63.3 ☑
          while boarding or alighting V63.4 ☑
        motor vehicle NOS (traffic) V69.60 ☑
          nontraffic V69.20 ☑
          specified type NEC (traffic) V69.69 ☑
            nontraffic V69.29 ☑
        pedal cycle (traffic) V61.9 ☑
          nontraffic V61.3 ☑
          while boarding or alighting V61.4 ☑
        pickup truck (traffic) V63.9 ☑
          nontraffic V63.3 ☑
          while boarding or alighting V63.4 ☑
        railway vehicle (traffic) V65.9 ☑
          nontraffic V65.3 ☑
          while boarding or alighting V65.4 ☑
        specified vehicle NEC (traffic) V66.9 ☑
          nontraffic V66.3 ☑
          while boarding or alighting V66.4 ☑
        stationary object (traffic) V67.9 ☑
          nontraffic V67.3 ☑
          while boarding or alighting V67.4 ☑
        streetcar (traffic) V66.9 ☑
          nontraffic V66.3 ☑

Accident — *continued*
  transport — *continued*
    truck occupant — *continued*
      collision — *continued*
        streetcar — *continued*
          while boarding or alighting V66.4 ☑
        three wheeled motor vehicle (traffic) V62.9 ☑
          nontraffic V62.3 ☑
          while boarding or alighting V62.4 ☑
        truck (traffic) V64.9 ☑
          nontraffic V64.3 ☑
          while boarding or alighting V64.4 ☑
        two wheeled motor vehicle (traffic) V62.9 ☑
          nontraffic V62.3 ☑
          while boarding or alighting V62.4 ☑
        van (traffic) V63.9 ☑
          nontraffic V63.3 ☑
          while boarding or alighting V63.4 ☑
      driver
        collision (with)
          animal (traffic) V60.5 ☑
            being ridden (traffic) V66.5 ☑
              nontraffic V66.0 ☑
            nontraffic V60.0 ☑
          animal-drawn vehicle (traffic) V66.5 ☑
            nontraffic V66.0 ☑
          bus (traffic) V64.5 ☑
            nontraffic V64.0 ☑
          car (traffic) V63.5 ☑
            nontraffic V63.0 ☑
          motor vehicle NOS (traffic) V69.40 ☑
            nontraffic V69.00 ☑
            specified type NEC (traffic) V69.49 ☑
              nontraffic V69.09 ☑
          pedal cycle (traffic) V61.5 ☑
            nontraffic V61.0 ☑
          pickup truck (traffic) V63.5 ☑
            nontraffic V63.0 ☑
          railway vehicle (traffic) V65.5 ☑
            nontraffic V65.0 ☑
          specified vehicle NEC (traffic) V66.5 ☑
            nontraffic V66.0 ☑
          stationary object (traffic) V67.5 ☑
            nontraffic V67.0 ☑
          streetcar (traffic) V66.5 ☑
            nontraffic V66.0 ☑
          three wheeled motor vehicle (traffic)
            V62.5 ☑
            nontraffic V62.0 ☑
          truck (traffic) V64.5 ☑
            nontraffic V64.0 ☑
          two wheeled motor vehicle (traffic)
            V62.5 ☑
            nontraffic V62.0 ☑
          van (traffic) V63.5 ☑
            nontraffic V63.0 ☑
        noncollision accident (traffic) V68.5 ☑
          nontraffic V68.0 ☑
      dump — *see* Accident, transport, construction
        vehicle occupant
      hanger-on
        collision (with)
          animal (traffic) V60.7 ☑
            being ridden (traffic) V66.7 ☑
              nontraffic V66.2 ☑
            nontraffic V60.2 ☑
          animal-drawn vehicle (traffic) V66.7 ☑
            nontraffic V66.2 ☑
          bus (traffic) V64.7 ☑
            nontraffic V64.2 ☑
          car (traffic) V63.7 ☑
            nontraffic V63.2 ☑
          pedal cycle (traffic) V61.7 ☑
            nontraffic V61.2 ☑
          pickup truck (traffic) V63.7 ☑
            nontraffic V63.2 ☑
          railway vehicle (traffic) V65.7 ☑
            nontraffic V65.2 ☑
          specified vehicle NEC (traffic) V66.7 ☑
            nontraffic V66.2 ☑
          stationary object (traffic) V67.7 ☑
            nontraffic V67.2 ☑
          streetcar (traffic) V66.7 ☑
            nontraffic V66.2 ☑

Accident — *continued*
  transport — *continued*
    truck occupant — *continued*
      hanger-on — *continued*
        collision — *continued*
          three wheeled motor vehicle (traffic)
            V62.7 ☑
            nontraffic V62.2 ☑
          truck (traffic) V64.7 ☑
            nontraffic V64.2 ☑
          two wheeled motor vehicle (traffic)
            V62.7 ☑
            nontraffic V62.2 ☑
          van (traffic) V63.7 ☑
            nontraffic V63.2 ☑
        noncollision accident (traffic) V68.7 ☑
          nontraffic V68.2 ☑
      noncollision accident (traffic) V68.9 ☑
        nontraffic V68.3 ☑
        while boarding or alighting V68.4 ☑
      nontraffic V59.3 ☑
      passenger
        collision (with)
          animal (traffic) V60.6 ☑
            being ridden (traffic) V66.6 ☑
              nontraffic V66.1- ☑
            nontraffic V60.1 ☑
          animal-drawn vehicle (traffic) V66.6 ☑
            nontraffic V66.1 ☑
          bus (traffic) V64.6 ☑
            nontraffic V64.1 ☑
          car (traffic) V63.6 ☑
            nontraffic V63.1 ☑
          motor vehicle NOS (traffic) V69.50 ☑
            nontraffic V69.10 ☑
            specified type NEC (traffic) V69.59 ☑
              nontraffic V69.19 ☑
          pedal cycle (traffic) V61.6 ☑
            nontraffic V61.1 ☑
          pickup truck (traffic) V63.6 ☑
            nontraffic V63.1 ☑
          railway vehicle (traffic) V65.6 ☑
            nontraffic V65.1 ☑
          specified vehicle NEC (traffic) V66.6 ☑
            nontraffic V66.1 ☑
          stationary object (traffic) V67.6 ☑
            nontraffic V67.1 ☑
          streetcar (traffic) V66.6 ☑
            nontraffic V66.1 ☑
          three wheeled motor vehicle (traffic)
            V62.6 ☑
            nontraffic V62.1 ☑
          truck (traffic) V64.6 ☑
            nontraffic V64.1 ☑
          two wheeled motor vehicle (traffic)
            V62.6 ☑
            nontraffic V62.1 ☑
          van (traffic) V63.6 ☑
            nontraffic V63.1 ☑
        noncollision accident (traffic) V68.6 ☑
          nontraffic V68.1 ☑
      pickup — *see* Accident, transport, pickup truck
        occupant
      specified type NEC V59.88 ☑
      military vehicle V69.81 ☑
    van occupant V59.9 ☑
      collision (with)
        animal (traffic) V50.9 ☑
          being ridden (traffic) V56.9 ☑
            nontraffic V56.3 ☑
            while boarding or alighting V56.4 ☑
          nontraffic V50.3 ☑
          while boarding or alighting V50.4 ☑
          animal-drawn vehicle (traffic) V56.9 ☑
            nontraffic V56.3 ☑
            while boarding or alighting V56.4 ☑
          bus (traffic) V54.9 ☑
            nontraffic V54.3 ☑
            while boarding or alighting V54.4 ☑
          car (traffic) V53.9 ☑
            nontraffic V53.3 ☑
            while boarding or alighting V53.4 ☑
          motor vehicle NOS (traffic) V59.60 ☑
            nontraffic V59.20 ☑
            specified type NEC (traffic) V59.69 ☑

Accident — *continued*
  transport — *continued*
    van occupant — *continued*
      collision — *continued*
        motor vehicle — *continued*
          specified type — *continued*
            nontraffic V59.29 ☑
        pedal cycle (traffic) V51.9 ☑
          nontraffic V51.3 ☑
          while boarding or alighting V51.4 ☑
        pickup truck (traffic) V53.9 ☑
          nontraffic V53.3 ☑
          while boarding or alighting V53.4 ☑
        railway vehicle (traffic) V55.9 ☑
          nontraffic V55.3 ☑
          while boarding or alighting V55.4 ☑
        specified vehicle NEC (traffic) V56.9 ☑
          nontraffic V56.3 ☑
          while boarding or alighting V56.4 ☑
        stationary object (traffic) V57.9 ☑
          nontraffic V57.3 ☑
          while boarding or alighting V57.4 ☑
        streetcar (traffic) V56.9 ☑
          nontraffic V56.3 ☑
          while boarding or alighting V56.4 ☑
        three wheeled motor vehicle (traffic) V52.9 ☑
          nontraffic V52.3 ☑
          while boarding or alighting V52.4 ☑
        truck (traffic) V54.9 ☑
          nontraffic V54.3 ☑
          while boarding or alighting V54.4 ☑
        two wheeled motor vehicle (traffic) V52.9 ☑
          nontraffic V52.3 ☑
          while boarding or alighting V52.4 ☑
        van (traffic) V53.9 ☑
          nontraffic V53.3 ☑
          while boarding or alighting V53.4 ☑
      driver
        collision (with)
          animal (traffic) V50.5 ☑
            being ridden (traffic) V56.5 ☑
              nontraffic V56.0 ☑
            nontraffic V50.0 ☑
          animal-drawn vehicle (traffic) V56.5 ☑
            nontraffic V56.0 ☑
          bus (traffic) V54.5 ☑
            nontraffic V54.0 ☑
          car (traffic) V53.5 ☑
            nontraffic V53.0 ☑
          motor vehicle NOS (traffic) V59.40 ☑
            nontraffic V59.00 ☑
            specified type NEC (traffic) V59.49 ☑
              nontraffic V59.09 ☑
          pedal cycle (traffic) V51.5 ☑
            nontraffic V51.0 ☑
          pickup truck (traffic) V53.5 ☑
            nontraffic V53.0 ☑
          railway vehicle (traffic) V55.5 ☑
            nontraffic V55.0 ☑
          specified vehicle NEC (traffic) V56.5 ☑
            nontraffic V56.0 ☑
          stationary object (traffic) V57.5 ☑
            nontraffic V57.0 ☑
          streetcar (traffic) V56.5 ☑
            nontraffic V56.0 ☑
          three wheeled motor vehicle (traffic)
            V52.5 ☑
            nontraffic V52.0 ☑
          truck (traffic) V54.5 ☑
            nontraffic V54.0 ☑
          two wheeled motor vehicle (traffic)
            V52.5 ☑
            nontraffic V52.0 ☑
          van (traffic) V53.5 ☑
            nontraffic V53.0 ☑
        noncollision accident (traffic) V58.5 ☑
          nontraffic V58.0 ☑
      hanger-on
        collision (with)
          animal (traffic) V50.7 ☑
            being ridden (traffic) V56.7 ☑
              nontraffic V56.2 ☑
            nontraffic V50.2 ☑
          animal-drawn vehicle (traffic) V56.7 ☑
            nontraffic V56.2 ☑

Accident — *continued*
transport — *continued*
van occupant — *continued*
hanger-on — *continued*
collision — *continued*
bus (traffic) V54.7 ☑
nontraffic V54.2 ☑
car (traffic) V53.7 ☑
nontraffic V53.2 ☑
pedal cycle (traffic) V51.7 ☑
nontraffic V51.2 ☑
pickup truck (traffic) V53.7 ☑
nontraffic V53.2 ☑
railway vehicle (traffic) V55.7 ☑
nontraffic V55.2 ☑
specified vehicle NEC (traffic) V56.7 ☑
nontraffic V56.2 ☑
stationary object (traffic) V57.7 ☑
nontraffic V57.2 ☑
streetcar (traffic) V56.7 ☑
nontraffic V56.2 ☑
three wheeled motor vehicle (traffic) V52.7 ☑
nontraffic V52.2 ☑
truck (traffic) V54.7 ☑
nontraffic V54.2 ☑
two wheeled motor vehicle (traffic) V52.7 ☑
nontraffic V52.2 ☑
van (traffic) V53.7 ☑
nontraffic V53.2 ☑
noncollision accident (traffic) V58.7 ☑
nontraffic V58.2 ☑
noncollision accident (traffic) V58.9 ☑
nontraffic V58.3 ☑
while boarding or alighting V58.4 ☑
nontraffic V59.3 ☑
passenger
collision (with)
animal (traffic) V50.6 ☑
being ridden (traffic) V56.6 ☑
nontraffic V56.1 ☑
nontraffic V50.1 ☑
animal-drawn vehicle (traffic) V56.6 ☑
nontraffic V56.1 ☑
bus (traffic) V54.6 ☑
nontraffic V54.1 ☑
car (traffic) V53.6 ☑
nontraffic V53.1 ☑
motor vehicle NOS (traffic) V59.50 ☑
nontraffic V59.10 ☑
specified type NEC (traffic) V59.59 ☑
nontraffic V59.19 ☑
pedal cycle (traffic) V51.6 ☑
nontraffic V51.1 ☑
pickup truck (traffic) V53.6 ☑
nontraffic V53.1 ☑
railway vehicle (traffic) V55.6 ☑
nontraffic V55.1 ☑
specified vehicle NEC (traffic) V56.6 ☑
nontraffic V56.1 ☑
stationary object (traffic) V57.6 ☑
nontraffic V57.1 ☑
streetcar (traffic) V56.6 ☑
nontraffic V56.1 ☑
three wheeled motor vehicle (traffic) V52.6 ☑
nontraffic V52.1 ☑
truck (traffic) V54.6 ☑
nontraffic V54.1 ☑
two wheeled motor vehicle (traffic) V52.6 ☑
nontraffic V52.1 ☑
van (traffic) V53.6 ☑
nontraffic V53.1 ☑
noncollision accident (traffic) V58.6 ☑
nontraffic V58.1 ☑
specified type NEC V59.88 ☑
military vehicle V59.81 ☑
watercraft occupant — *see* Accident, watercraft
vehicle NEC V89.9 ☑
animal-drawn NEC — *see* Accident, transport, animal-drawn vehicle occupant

Accident — *continued*
vehicle — *continued*
special
agricultural — *see* Accident, transport, agricultural vehicle occupant
construction — *see* Accident, transport, construction vehicle occupant
industrial — *see* Accident, transport, industrial vehicle occupant
three-wheeled NEC (motorized) — *see* Accident, transport, three-wheeled motor vehicle occupant
watercraft V94.9 ☑
causing
drowning — *see* Drowning, due to, accident to, watercraft
injury NEC V91.89 ☑
crushed between craft and object V91.19 ☑
powered craft V91.13 ☑
ferry boat V91.11 ☑
fishing boat V91.12 ☑
jetskis V91.13 ☑
liner V91.11 ☑
merchant ship V91.10 ☑
passenger ship V91.11 ☑
unpowered craft V91.18 ☑
canoe V91.15 ☑
inflatable V91.16 ☑
kayak V91.15 ☑
sailboat V91.14 ☑
surf-board V91.18 ☑
windsurfer V91.18 ☑
fall on board V91.29 ☑
powered craft V91.23 ☑
ferry boat V91.21 ☑
fishing boat V91.22 ☑
jetskis V91.23 ☑
liner V91.21 ☑
merchant ship V91.20 ☑
passenger ship V91.21 ☑
unpowered craft
canoe V91.25 ☑
inflatable V91.26 ☑
kayak V91.25 ☑
sailboat V91.24 ☑
fire on board causing burn V91.09 ☑
powered craft V91.03 ☑
ferry boat V91.01 ☑
fishing boat V91.02 ☑
jetskis V91.03 ☑
liner V91.01 ☑
merchant ship V91.00 ☑
passenger ship V91.01 ☑
unpowered craft V91.08 ☑
canoe V91.05 ☑
inflatable V91.06 ☑
kayak V91.05 ☑
sailboat V91.04 ☑
surf-board V91.08 ☑
water skis V91.07 ☑
windsurfer V91.08 ☑
hit by falling object V91.39 ☑
powered craft V91.33 ☑
ferry boat V91.31 ☑
fishing boat V91.32 ☑
jetskis V91.33 ☑
liner V91.31 ☑
merchant ship V91.30 ☑
passenger ship V91.31 ☑
unpowered craft V91.38 ☑
canoe V91.35 ☑
inflatable V91.36 ☑
kayak V91.35 ☑
sailboat V91.34 ☑
surf-board V91.38 ☑
water skis V91.37 ☑
windsurfer V91.38 ☑
specified type NEC V91.89 ☑
powered craft V91.83 ☑
ferry boat V91.81 ☑
fishing boat V91.82 ☑
jetskis V91.83 ☑
liner V91.81 ☑
merchant ship V91.80 ☑
passenger ship V91.81 ☑

Accident — *continued*
watercraft — *continued*
causing — *continued*
injury — *continued*
specified type — *continued*
unpowered craft V91.88 ☑
canoe V91.85 ☑
inflatable V91.86 ☑
kayak V91.85 ☑
sailboat V91.84 ☑
surf-board V91.88 ☑
water skis V91.87 ☑
windsurfer V91.88 ☑
due to, caused by cataclysm — *see* Forces of nature, by type
military NEC V94.818 ☑
civilian in water injured by V94.811 ☑
with civilian watercraft V94.810 ☑
nonpowered, struck by
nonpowered vessel V94.22 ☑
powered vessel V94.21 ☑
specified type NEC V94.89 ☑
striking swimmer
powered V94.11 ☑
unpowered V94.12 ☑
Acid throwing (assault) Y08.89 ☑
Activity (involving) (of victim at time of event) Y93.9
aerobic and step exercise (class) Y93.A3 (*following* Y93.7)
alpine skiing Y93.23
animal care NEC Y93.K9 (*following* Y93.7)
arts and handcrafts NEC Y93.D9 (*following* Y93.7)
athletics played as a team or group NEC Y93.69
athletics played individually NEC Y93.59
athletics NEC Y93.79
baking Y93.G3 (*following* Y93.7)
ballet Y93.41
barbells Y93.B3 (*following* Y93.7)
BASE (Building, Antenna, Span, Earth) jumping Y93.33
baseball Y93.64
basketball Y93.67
bathing (personal) Y93.E1 (*following* Y93.7)
beach volleyball Y93.68
bike riding Y93.55
blackout game Y93.85
boogie boarding Y93.18
bowling Y93.54
boxing Y93.71
brass instrument playing Y93.J4 (*following* Y93.7)
building construction Y93.H3 (*following* Y93.7)
bungee jumping Y93.34
calisthenics Y93.A2 (*following* Y93.7)
canoeing (in calm and turbulent water) Y93.16
capture the flag Y93.6A
cardiorespiratory exercise NEC Y93.A9 (*following* Y93.7)
caregiving (providing) NEC Y93.F9 (*following* Y93.7)
bathing Y93.F1 (*following* Y93.7)
lifting Y93.F2 (*following* Y93.7)
cellular
communication device Y93.C2 (*following* Y93.7)
telephone Y93.C2 (*following* Y93.7)
challenge course Y93.A5 (*following* Y93.7)
cheerleading Y93.45
choking game Y93.85
circuit training Y93.A4 (*following* Y93.7)
cleaning
floor Y93.E5 (*following* Y93.7)
climbing NEC Y93.39
mountain Y93.31
rock Y93.31
wall Y93.31
clothing care and maintenance NEC Y93.E9 (*following* Y93.7)
combatives Y93.75
computer
keyboarding Y93.C1 (*following* Y93.7)
technology NEC Y93.C9 (*following* Y93.7)
confidence course Y93.A5 (*following* Y93.7)
construction (building) Y93.H3 (*following* Y93.7)
cooking and baking Y93.G3 (*following* Y93.7)
cool down exercises Y93.A2 (*following* Y93.7)
cricket Y93.69
crocheting Y93.D1 (*following* Y93.7)
cross country skiing Y93.24
dancing (all types) Y93.41
digging
dirt Y93.H1 (*following* Y93.7)
dirt digging Y93.H1 (*following* Y93.7)
dishwashing Y93.G1 (*following* Y93.7)

☑ Additional Character Required — Refer to the Tabular List for Character Selection

Activity — *continued*

diving (platform) (springboard) Y93.12
  underwater Y93.15
dodge ball Y93.6A
downhill skiing Y93.23
drum playing Y93.J2 (*following* Y93.7)
dumbbells Y93.B3 (*following* Y93.7)
electronic
  devices NEC Y93.C9 (*following* Y93.7)
    hand held interactive Y93.C2 (*following* Y93.7)
  game playing (using) (with)
    interactive device Y93.C2 (*following* Y93.7)
    keyboard or other stationary device Y93.C1 (*following* Y93.7)
elliptical machine Y93.A1 (*following* Y93.7)
exercise(s)
  machines ((primarily) for)
    cardiorespiratory conditioning Y93.A1 (*following* Y93.7)
    muscle strengthening Y93.B1 (*following* Y93.7)
  muscle strengthening (non-machine) NEC Y93.B9 (*following* Y93.7)
  external motion NEC Y93.I9 (*following* Y93.7)
  rollercoaster Y93.I1 (*following* Y93.7)
fainting game Y93.85
field hockey Y93.65
figure skating (pairs) (singles) Y93.21
flag football Y93.62
floor mopping and cleaning Y93.E5 (*following* Y93.7)
food preparation and clean up Y93.G1 (*following* Y93.7)
football (American) NOS Y93.61
  flag Y93.62
  tackle Y93.61
  touch Y93.62
four square Y93.6A
free weights Y93.B3 (*following* Y93.7)
frisbee (ultimate) Y93.74
furniture
  building Y93.D3 (*following* Y93.7)
  finishing Y93.D3 (*following* Y93.7)
  repair Y93.D3 (*following* Y93.7)
game playing (electronic)
  using interactive device Y93.C2 (*following* Y93.7)
  using keyboard or other stationary device Y93.C1 (*following* Y93.7)
gardening Y93.H2 (*following* Y93.7)
golf Y93.53
grass drills Y93.A6 (*following* Y93.7)
grilling and smoking food Y93.G2 (*following* Y93.7)
grooming and shearing an animal Y93.K3 (*following* Y93.7)
guerilla drills Y93.A6 (*following* Y93.7)
gymnastics (rhythmic) Y93.43
hand held interactive electronic device Y93.C2 (*following* Y93.7)
handball Y93.73
handcrafts NEC Y93.D9 (*following* Y93.7)
hang gliding Y93.35
hiking (on level or elevated terrain) Y93.01
hockey (ice) Y93.22
  field Y93.65
horseback riding Y93.52
household (interior) maintenance NEC Y93.E9 (*following* Y93.7)
ice NEC Y93.29
  dancing Y93.21
  hockey Y93.22
  skating Y93.21
inline roller skating Y93.51
ironing Y93.E4 (*following* Y93.7)
judo Y93.75
jumping jacks Y93.A2 (*following* Y93.7)
jumping rope Y93.56
jumping (off) NEC Y93.39
  BASE (Building, Antenna, Span, Earth) Y93.33
  bungee Y93.34
  jacks Y93.A2 (*following* Y93.7)
  rope Y93.56
karate Y93.75
kayaking (in calm and turbulent water) Y93.16
keyboarding (computer) Y93.C1 (*following* Y93.7)
kickball Y93.6A
knitting Y93.D1 (*following* Y93.7)
lacrosse Y93.65
land maintenance NEC Y93.H9 (*following* Y93.7)
landscaping Y93.H2 (*following* Y93.7)
laundry Y93.E2 (*following* Y93.7)

Activity — *continued*

machines (exercise)
  primarily for cardiorespiratory conditioning Y93.A1 (*following* Y93.7)
  primarily for muscle strengthening Y93.B1 (*following* Y93.7)
maintenance
  exterior building NEC Y93.H9 (*following* Y93.7)
  household (interior) NEC Y93.E9 (*following* Y93.7)
  land Y93.H9 (*following* Y93.7)
  property Y93.H9 (*following* Y93.7)
marching (on level or elevated terrain) Y93.01
martial arts Y93.75
microwave oven Y93.G3 (*following* Y93.7)
milking an animal Y93.K2 (*following* Y93.7)
mopping (floor) Y93.E5 (*following* Y93.7)
mountain climbing Y93.31
muscle strengthening
  exercises (non-machine) NEC Y93.B9 (*following* Y93.7)
  machines Y93.B1 (*following* Y93.7)
musical keyboard (electronic) playing Y93.J1 (*following* Y93.7)
nordic skiing Y93.24
obstacle course Y93.A5 (*following* Y93.7)
oven (microwave) Y93.G3 (*following* Y93.7)
packing up and unpacking in moving to a new residence Y93.E6 (*following* Y93.7)
parasailing Y93.19
pass out game Y93.85
percussion instrument playing NEC Y93.J2 (*following* Y93.7)
personal
  bathing and showering Y93.E1 (*following* Y93.7)
  hygiene NEC Y93.E8 (*following* Y93.7)
  showering Y93.E1 (*following* Y93.7)
physical games generally associated with school recess, summer camp and children Y93.6A
physical training NEC Y93.A9 (*following* Y93.7)
piano playing Y93.J1 (*following* Y93.7)
pilates Y93.B4 (*following* Y93.7)
platform diving Y93.12
playing musical instrument
  brass instrument Y93.J4 (*following* Y93.7)
  drum Y93.J2 (*following* Y93.7)
  musical keyboard (electronic) Y93.J1 (*following* Y93.7)
  percussion instrument NEC Y93.J2 (*following* Y93.7)
  piano Y93.J1 (*following* Y93.7)
  string instrument Y93.J3 (*following* Y93.7)
  winds instrument Y93.J4 (*following* Y93.7)
property maintenance
  exterior NEC Y93.H9 (*following* Y93.7)
  interior NEC Y93.E9 (*following* Y93.7)
pruning (garden and lawn) Y93.H2 (*following* Y93.7)
pull-ups Y93.B2 (*following* Y93.7)
push-ups Y93.B2 (*following* Y93.7)
racquetball Y93.73
rafting (in calm and turbulent water) Y93.16
raking (leaves) Y93.H1 (*following* Y93.7)
rappelling Y93.32
refereeing a sports activity Y93.81
residential relocation Y93.E6 (*following* Y93.7)
rhythmic gymnastics Y93.43
rhythmic movement NEC Y93.49
riding
  horseback Y93.52
  rollercoaster Y93.I1 (*following* Y93.7)
rock climbing Y93.31
roller skating (inline) Y93.51
rollercoaster riding Y93.I1 (*following* Y93.7)
rough housing and horseplay Y93.83
rowing (in calm and turbulent water) Y93.16
rugby Y93.63
running Y93.02
SCUBA diving Y93.15
sewing Y93.D2 (*following* Y93.7)
shoveling Y93.H1 (*following* Y93.7)
  dirt Y93.H1 (*following* Y93.7)
  snow Y93.H1 (*following* Y93.7)
showering (personal) Y93.E1 (*following* Y93.7)
sit-ups Y93.B2 (*following* Y93.7)
skateboarding Y93.51
skating (ice) Y93.21
  roller Y93.51
skiing (alpine) (downhill) Y93.23
  cross country Y93.24
  nordic Y93.24
  water Y93.17
sledding (snow) Y93.23
sleeping (sleep) Y93.84

Activity — *continued*

smoking and grilling food Y93.G2 (*following* Y93.7)
snorkeling Y93.15
snow NEC Y93.29
  boarding Y93.23
  shoveling Y93.H1 (*following* Y93.7)
  sledding Y93.23
  tubing Y93.23
soccer Y93.66
softball Y93.64
specified NEC Y93.89
spectator at an event Y93.82
sports NEC Y93.79
  sports played as a team or group NEC Y93.69
  sports played individually NEC Y93.59
springboard diving Y93.12
squash Y93.73
stationary bike Y93.A1 (*following* Y93.7)
step (stepping) exercise (class) Y93.A3 (*following* Y93.7)
stepper machine Y93.A1 (*following* Y93.7)
stove Y93.G3 (*following* Y93.7)
string instrument playing Y93.J3 (*following* Y93.7)
surfing Y93.18
  wind Y93.18
swimming Y93.11
tackle football Y93.61
tap dancing Y93.41
tennis Y93.73
tobogganing Y93.23
touch football Y93.62
track and field events (non-running) Y93.57
  running Y93.02
trampoline Y93.44
treadmill Y93.A1 (*following* Y93.7)
trimming shrubs Y93.H2 (*following* Y93.7)
tubing (in calm and turbulent water) Y93.16
  snow Y93.23
ultimate frisbee Y93.74
underwater diving Y93.15
unpacking in moving to a new residence Y93.E6 (*following* Y93.7)
use of stove, oven and microwave oven Y93.G3 (*following* Y93.7)
vacuuming Y93.E3 (*following* Y93.7)
volleyball (beach) (court) Y93.68
wake boarding Y93.17
walking (on level or elevated terrain) Y93.01
  an animal Y93.K1 (*following* Y93.7)
walking an animal Y93.K1 (*following* Y93.7)
wall climbing Y93.31
warm up and cool down exercises Y93.A2 (*following* Y93.7)
water NEC Y93.19
  aerobics Y93.14
  craft NEC Y93.19
  exercise Y93.14
  polo Y93.13
  skiing Y93.17
  sliding Y93.18
  survival training and testing Y93.19
weeding (garden and lawn) Y93.H2 (*following* Y93.7)
wind instrument playing Y93.J4 (*following* Y93.7)
windsurfing Y93.18
wrestling Y93.72
yoga Y93.42
Adverse effect of drugs — *see* Table of Drugs and Chemicals
Aerosinusitis — *see* Air, pressure
After-effect, late — *see* Sequelae
Air
  blast in war operations — *see* War operations, air blast
  pressure
    change, rapid
      during
        ascent W94.29 ☑
          while (in) (surfacing from)
            aircraft W94.23 ☑
            deep water diving W94.21 ☑
            underground W94.22 ☑
        descent W94.39 ☑
          in
            aircraft W94.31 ☑
            water W94.32 ☑
      high, prolonged W94.0 ☑
      low, prolonged W94.12 ☑
        due to residence or long visit at high altitude W94.11 ☑
Alpine sickness W94.11 ☑

Altitude sickness W94.11 ☑
Anaphylactic shock, anaphylaxis — *see* Table of Drugs and Chemicals
Andes disease W94.11 ☑
Arachnidism, arachnoidism X58 ☑
Arson (with intent to injure or kill) X97 ☑
Asphyxia, asphyxiation
  by
    food (bone) (seed) — *see* categories T17 and T18 ☑
    gas — *see also* Table of Drugs and Chemicals
      legal
        execution — *see* Legal, intervention, gas
        intervention — *see* Legal, intervention, gas
  from
    fire — *see also* Exposure, fire
      in war operations — *see* War operations, fire
    ignition — *see* Ignition
    vomitus T17.81 ☑
  in war operations — *see* War operations, restriction of airway
Aspiration
  food (any type) (into respiratory tract) (with asphyxia, obstruction respiratory tract, suffocation) — *see* categories T17 and T18 ☑
  foreign body — *see* Foreign body, aspiration
  vomitus (with asphyxia, obstruction respiratory tract, suffocation) T17.81 ☑
Assassination (attempt) — *see* Assault
Assault (homicidal) (by) (in) Y09
  arson X97 ☑
  bite (of human being) Y04.1 ☑
  bodily force Y04.8 ☑
    bite Y04.1 ☑
    bumping into Y04.2 ☑
    sexual (confirmed) T74.2- ☑
      suspected T76.2- ☑
    unarmed fight Y04.0 ☑
  bomb X96.9 ☑
    antipersonnel X96.0 ☑
    fertilizer X96.3 ☑
    gasoline X96.1 ☑
    letter X96.2 ☑
    petrol X96.1 ☑
    pipe X96.3 ☑
    specified NEC X96.8 ☑
  brawl (hand) (fists) (foot) (unarmed) Y04.0 ☑
  burning, burns (by fire) NEC X97 ☑
    acid Y08.89 ☑
    caustic, corrosive substance Y08.89 ☑
    chemical from swallowing caustic, corrosive substance — *see* Table of Drugs and Chemicals
    cigarette(s) X97 ☑
    hot object X98.9 ☑
      fluid NEC X98.2 ☑
      household appliance X98.3 ☑
      specified NEC X98.8 ☑
      steam X98.0 ☑
      tap water X98.1 ☑
      vapors X98.0 ☑
    scalding — *see* Assault, burning
    steam X98.0 ☑
    vitriol Y08.89 ☑
  caustic, corrosive substance (gas) Y08.89 ☑
  crashing of
    aircraft Y08.81 ☑
    motor vehicle Y03.8 ☑
      pushed in front of Y02.0 ☑
      run over Y03.0 ☑
      specified NEC Y03.8 ☑
  cutting or piercing instrument X99.9 ☑
    dagger X99.2 ☑
    glass X99.0 ☑
    knife X99.1 ☑
    specified NEC X99.8 ☑
    sword X99.2 ☑
  dagger X99.2 ☑
  drowning (in) X92.9 ☑
    bathtub X92.0 ☑
    natural water X92.3 ☑
    specified NEC X92.8 ☑
    swimming pool X92.1 ☑
      following fall X92.2 ☑
  dynamite X96.8 ☑
  explosive(s) (material) X96.9 ☑
  fight (hand) (fists) (foot) (unarmed) Y04.0 ☑
    with weapon — *see* Assault, by type of weapon

Assault — *continued*
  fire X97 ☑
  firearm X95.9 ☑
    airgun X95.01 ☑
    handgun X93 ☑
    hunting rifle X94.1 ☑
    larger X94.9 ☑
      specified NEC X94.8 ☑
    machine gun X94.2 ☑
    shotgun X94.0 ☑
    specified NEC X95.8 ☑
  from high place Y01 ☑
  gunshot (wound) NEC — *see* Assault, firearm, by type
  incendiary device X97 ☑
  injury Y09
    to child due to criminal abortion attempt NEC Y08.89 ☑
  knife X99.1 ☑
  late effect of — *see* categories X92-Y08 with 7th character S
  placing before moving object NEC Y02.8 ☑
    motor vehicle Y02.0 ☑
  poisoning — *see* categories T36-T65 with 7th character S
  puncture, any part of body — *see* Assault, cutting or piercing instrument
  pushing
    before moving object NEC Y02.8 ☑
      motor vehicle Y02.0 ☑
      subway train Y02.1 ☑
      train Y02.1 ☑
    from high place Y01 ☑
  rape (confirmed) T74.2- ☑
    suspected T76.2- ☑
  scalding — *see* Assault, burning
  sequelae of — *see* categories X92-Y08 with 7th character S
  sexual (by bodily force) T74.2- ☑
    suspected T76.2- ☑
  shooting — *see* Assault, firearm
  specified means NEC Y08.89 ☑
  stab, any part of body — *see* Assault, cutting or piercing instrument
  steam X98.0 ☑
  striking against
    other person Y04.2 ☑
    sports equipment Y08.09 ☑
      baseball bat Y08.02 ☑
      hockey stick Y08.01 ☑
  struck by
    sports equipment Y08.09 ☑
      baseball bat Y08.02 ☑
      hockey stick Y08.01 ☑
  submersion — *see* Assault, drowning
  violence Y09
  weapon Y09
    blunt Y00 ☑
    cutting or piercing — *see* Assault, cutting or piercing instrument
    firearm — *see* Assault, firearm
  wound Y09
    cutting — *see* Assault, cutting or piercing instrument
    gunshot — *see* Assault, firearm
    knife X99.1 ☑
    piercing — *see* Assault, cutting or piercing instrument
    puncture — *see* Assault, cutting or piercing instrument
    stab — *see* Assault, cutting or piercing instrument
Attack by mammals NEC W55.89 ☑
Avalanche — *see* Landslide
Aviator's disease — *see* Air, pressure

B

Barotitis, barodontalgia, barosinusitis, barotrauma (otitic) (sinus) — *see* Air, pressure
Battered (baby) (child) (person) (syndrome) X58 ☑
Bayonet wound W26.1 ☑
  in
    legal intervention — *see* Legal, intervention, sharp object, bayonet
    war operations — *see* War operations, combat
  stated as undetermined whether accidental or intentional Y28.8 ☑
  suicide (attempt) X78.2 ☑
Bean in nose — *see* categories T17 and T18 ☑

Bed set on fire NEC — *see* Exposure, fire, uncontrolled, building, bed
Beheading (by guillotine)
  homicide X99.9 ☑
  legal execution — *see* Legal, intervention
Bending, injury in (prolonged) (static) X50.1 ☑
Bends — *see* Air, pressure, change
Bite, bitten by
  alligator W58.01 ☑
  arthropod (nonvenomous) NEC W57 ☑
  bull W55.21 ☑
  cat W55.01 ☑
  cow W55.21 ☑
  crocodile W58.11 ☑
  dog W54.0 ☑
  goat W55.31 ☑
  hoof stock NEC W55.31 ☑
  horse W55.11 ☑
  human being (accidentally) W50.3 ☑
    with intent to injure or kill Y04.1 ☑
    as, or caused by, a crowd or human stampede (with fall) W52 ☑
    assault Y04.1 ☑
    homicide (attempt) Y04.1 ☑
    in
      fight Y04.1 ☑
  insect (nonvenomous) W57 ☑
  lizard (nonvenomous) W59.01 ☑
  mammal NEC W55.81 ☑
    marine W56.31 ☑
  marine animal (nonvenomous) W56.81 ☑
  millipede W57 ☑
  moray eel W56.51 ☑
  mouse W53.01 ☑
  person(s) (accidentally) W50.3 ☑
    with intent to injure or kill Y04.1 ☑
    as, or caused by, a crowd or human stampede (with fall) W52 ☑
    assault Y04.1 ☑
    homicide (attempt) Y04.1 ☑
    in
      fight Y04.1 ☑
  pig W55.41 ☑
  raccoon W55.51 ☑
  rat W53.11 ☑
  reptile W59.81 ☑
    lizard W59.01 ☑
    snake W59.11 ☑
    turtle W59.21 ☑
      terrestrial W59.81 ☑
  rodent W53.81 ☑
    mouse W53.01 ☑
    rat W53.11 ☑
    specified NEC W53.81 ☑
    squirrel W53.21 ☑
  shark W56.41 ☑
  sheep W55.31 ☑
  snake (nonvenomous) W59.11 ☑
  spider (nonvenomous) W57 ☑
  squirrel W53.21 ☑
Blast (air) in war operations — *see* War operations, blast
Blizzard X37.2 ☑
Blood alcohol level Y90.9
  less than 20mg/100ml Y90.0
  presence in blood, level not specified Y90.9
  20-39mg/100ml Y90.1
  40-59mg/100ml Y90.2
  60-79mg/100ml Y90.3
  80-99mg/100ml Y90.4
  100-119mg/100ml Y90.5
  120-199mg/100ml Y90.6
  200-239mg/100ml Y90.7
Blow X58 ☑
  by law-enforcing agent, police (on duty) — *see* Legal, intervention, manhandling
  blunt object — *see* Legal, intervention, blunt object
Blowing up — *see* Explosion
Brawl (hand) (fists) (foot) Y04.0 ☑
Breakage (accidental) (part of)
  ladder (causing fall) W11 ☑
  scaffolding (causing fall) W12 ☑
Broken
  glass, contact with — *see* Contact, with, glass
  power line (causing electric shock) W85 ☑
Bumping against, into (accidentally)
  object NEC W22.8 ☑

Bumping against, into — *continued*
- object — *continued*
  - caused by crowd or human stampede (with fall) W52 ☑
  - sports equipment W21.9 ☑
    - with fall — *see* Fall, due to, bumping against, object
- person(s) W51 ☑
  - with fall W03 ☑
    - due to ice or snow W00.0 ☑
  - assault Y04.2 ☑
  - caused by, a crowd or human stampede (with fall) W52 ☑
  - homicide (attempt) Y04.2 ☑
- sports equipment W21.9 ☑

Burn, burned, burning (accidental) (by) (from) (on)
- acid NEC — *see* Table of Drugs and Chemicals
- bed linen — *see* Exposure, fire, uncontrolled, in building, bed
- blowtorch X08.8 ☑
  - with ignition of clothing NEC X06.2 ☑
    - nightwear X05 ☑
- bonfire, campfire (controlled) — *see also* Exposure, fire, controlled, not in building)
  - uncontrolled — *see* Exposure, fire, uncontrolled, not in building
- candle X08.8 ☑
  - with ignition of clothing NEC X06.2 ☑
    - nightwear X05 ☑
- caustic liquid, substance (external) (internal) NEC — *see* Table of Drugs and Chemicals
- chemical (external) (internal) — *see also* Table of Drugs and Chemicals
  - in war operations — *see* War operations. fire
- cigar(s) or cigarette(s) X08.8 ☑
  - with ignition of clothing NEC X06.2 ☑
    - nightwear X05 ☑
- clothes, clothing NEC (from controlled fire) X06.2 ☑
  - with conflagration — *see* Exposure, fire, uncontrolled, building
    - not in building or structure — *see* Exposure, fire, uncontrolled, not in building
- cooker (hot) X15.8 ☑
  - stated as undetermined whether accidental or intentional Y27.3 ☑
  - suicide (attempt) X77.3 ☑
- electric blanket X16 ☑
- engine (hot) X17 ☑
- fire, flames — *see* Exposure, fire
- flare, Very pistol — *see* Discharge, firearm NEC
- heat
  - from appliance (electrical) (household) X15.8 ☑
    - cooker X15.8 ☑
    - hotplate X15.2 ☑
    - kettle X15.8 ☑
    - light bulb X15.8 ☑
    - saucepan X15.3 ☑
    - skillet X15.3 ☑
    - stated as undetermined whether accidental or intentional Y27.3 ☑
    - stove X15.0 ☑
    - suicide (attempt) X77.3 ☑
    - toaster X15.1 ☑
  - in local application or packing during medical or surgical procedure Y63.5
- heating
  - appliance, radiator or pipe X16 ☑
- homicide (attempt) — *see* Assault, burning
- hot
  - air X14.1 ☑
  - cooker X15.8 ☑
  - drink X10.0 ☑
  - engine X17 ☑
  - fat X10.2 ☑
  - fluid NEC X12 ☑
  - food X10.1 ☑
  - gases X14.1 ☑
  - heating appliance X16 ☑
  - household appliance NEC X15.8 ☑
  - kettle X15.8 ☑
  - liquid NEC X12 ☑
  - machinery X17 ☑
  - metal (molten) (liquid) NEC X18 ☑
  - object (not producing fire or flames) NEC X19 ☑
  - oil (cooking) X10.2 ☑
  - pipe(s) X16 ☑
  - radiator X16 ☑

Burn, burned, burning — *continued*
- hot — *continued*
  - saucepan (glass) (metal) X15.3 ☑
  - stove (kitchen) X15.0 ☑
  - substance NEC X19 ☑
    - caustic or corrosive NEC — *see* Table of Drugs and Chemicals
  - toaster X15.1 ☑
  - tool X17 ☑
  - vapor X13.1 ☑
  - water (tap) — *see* Contact, with, hot, tap water
- hotplate X15.2 ☑
  - suicide (attempt) X77.3 ☑
- ignition — *see* Ignition
- in war operations — *see* War operations, fire
- inflicted by other person X97 ☑
  - by hot objects, hot vapor, and steam — *see* Assault, burning, hot object
- internal, from swallowed caustic, corrosive liquid, substance — *see* Table of Drugs and Chemicals
- iron (hot) X15.8 ☑
  - stated as undetermined whether accidental or intentional Y27.3 ☑
  - suicide (attempt) X77.3 ☑
- kettle (hot) X15.8 ☑
  - stated as undetermined whether accidental or intentional Y27.3 ☑
  - suicide (attempt) X77.3 ☑
- lamp (flame) X08.8 ☑
  - with ignition of clothing NEC X06.2 ☑
    - nightwear X05 ☑
- lighter (cigar) (cigarette) X08.8 ☑
  - with ignition of clothing NEC X06.2 ☑
    - nightwear X05 ☑
- lightning — *see* subcategory T75.0 ☑
  - causing fire — *see* Exposure, fire
- liquid (boiling) (hot) NEC X12 ☑
  - stated as undetermined whether accidental or intentional Y27.2 ☑
  - suicide (attempt) X77.2 ☑
- local application of externally applied substance in medical or surgical care Y63.5
- machinery (hot) X17 ☑
- matches X08.8 ☑
  - with ignition of clothing NEC X06.2 ☑
    - nightwear X05 ☑
- mattress — *see* Exposure, fire, uncontrolled, building, bed
- medicament, externally applied Y63.5
- metal (hot) (liquid) (molten) NEC X18 ☑
- nightwear (nightclothes, nightdress, gown, pajamas, robe) X05 ☑
- object (hot) NEC X19 ☑
- on board watercraft
  - due to
    - accident to watercraft V91.09 ☑
      - powered craft V91.03 ☑
        - ferry boat V91.01 ☑
        - fishing boat V91.02 ☑
        - jetskis V91.03 ☑
        - liner V91.01 ☑
        - merchant ship V91.00 ☑
        - passenger ship V91.01 ☑
      - unpowered craft V91.08 ☑
        - canoe V91.05 ☑
        - inflatable V91.06 ☑
        - kayak V91.05 ☑
        - sailboat V91.04 ☑
        - surf-board V91.08 ☑
        - water skis V91.07 ☑
        - windsurfer V91.08 ☑
    - fire on board V93.09 ☑
      - ferry boat V93.01 ☑
      - fishing boat V93.02 ☑
      - jetskis V93.03 ☑
      - liner V93.01 ☑
      - merchant ship V93.00 ☑
      - passenger ship V93.01 ☑
      - powered craft NEC V93.03 ☑
      - sailboat V93.04 ☑
    - specified heat source NEC on board V93.19 ☑
      - ferry boat V93.11 ☑
      - fishing boat V93.12 ☑
      - jetskis V93.13 ☑
      - liner V93.11 ☑
      - merchant ship V93.10 ☑

Burn, burned, burning — *continued*
- on board watercraft — *continued*
  - due to — *continued*
    - specified heat source on board — *continued*
      - passenger ship V93.11 ☑
      - powered craft NEC V93.13 ☑
      - sailboat V93.14 ☑
- pipe (hot) X16 ☑
  - smoking X08.8 ☑
    - with ignition of clothing NEC X06.2 ☑
      - nightwear X05 ☑
- powder — *see* Powder burn
- radiator (hot) X16 ☑
- saucepan (hot) (glass) (metal) X15.3 ☑
  - stated as undetermined whether accidental or intentional Y27.3 ☑
  - suicide (attempt) X77.3 ☑
- self-inflicted X76 ☑
  - stated as undetermined whether accidental or intentional Y26 ☑
- stated as undetermined whether accidental or intentional Y27.0 ☑
- steam X13.1 ☑
  - pipe X16 ☑
    - stated as undetermined whether accidental or intentional Y27.8 ☑
  - stated as undetermined whether accidental or intentional Y27.0 ☑
  - suicide (attempt) X77.0 ☑
- stove (hot) (kitchen) X15.0 ☑
  - stated as undetermined whether accidental or intentional Y27.3 ☑
  - suicide (attempt) X77.3 ☑
- substance (hot) NEC X19 ☑
  - boiling X12 ☑
    - stated as undetermined whether accidental or intentional Y27.2 ☑
    - suicide (attempt) X77.2 ☑
  - molten (metal) X18 ☑
- suicide (attempt) NEC X76 ☑
  - hot
    - household appliance X77.3 ☑
    - object X77.9 ☑
- therapeutic misadventure
  - heat in local application or packing during medical or surgical procedure Y63.5
  - overdose of radiation Y63.2
- toaster (hot) X15.1 ☑
  - stated as undetermined whether accidental or intentional Y27.3 ☑
  - suicide (attempt) X77.3 ☑
- tool (hot) X17 ☑
- torch, welding X08.8 ☑
  - with ignition of clothing NEC X06.2 ☑
    - nightwear X05 ☑
- trash fire (controlled) — *see* Exposure, fire, controlled, not in building
  - uncontrolled — *see* Exposure, fire, uncontrolled, not in building
- vapor (hot) X13.1 ☑
  - stated as undetermined whether accidental or intentional Y27.0 ☑
  - suicide (attempt) X77.0 ☑
- Very pistol — *see* Discharge, firearm NEC

Butted by animal W55.82 ☑
- bull W55.22 ☑
- cow W55.22 ☑
- goat W55.32 ☑
- horse W55.12 ☑
- pig W55.42 ☑
- sheep W55.32 ☑

C

Caisson disease — *see* Air, pressure, change
Campfire (exposure to) (controlled) — *see also* Exposure, fire, controlled, not in building
- uncontrolled — *see* Exposure, fire, uncontrolled, not in building
Capital punishment (any means) — *see* Legal, intervention
Car sickness T75.3 ☑
Casualty (not due to war) NEC X58 ☑
- war — *see* War operations
Cat
- bite W55.01 ☑
- scratch W55.03 ☑

☑ **Additional Character Required** — Refer to the Tabular List for Character Selection

Cataclysm, cataclysmic (any injury) NEC — *see* Forces of nature
Catching fire — *see* Exposure, fire
Caught
  between
    folding object W23.Ø ☑
    objects (moving) W23.Ø ☑
      and
        machinery — *see* Contact, with, by type of machine
        stationary W23.2 ☑
      stationary W23.1 ☑
        and moving W23.2 ☑
    sliding door and door frame W23.Ø ☑
  by, in
    machinery (moving parts of) — *see* Contact, with, by type of machine
    washing-machine wringer W23.Ø ☑
  under packing crate (due to losing grip) W23.1 ☑
Cave-in caused by cataclysmic earth surface movement or eruption — *see* Landslide
Change(s) in air pressure — *see* Air, pressure, change
Choked, choking (on) (any object except food or vomitus)
  food (bone) (seed) — *see* categories T17 and T18 ☑
  vomitus T17.81- ☑
Civil insurrection — *see* War operations
Cloudburst (any injury) X37.8 ☑
Cold, exposure to (accidental) (excessive) (extreme) (natural) (place) NEC — *see* Exposure, cold
Collapse
  building W2Ø.1 ☑
    burning (uncontrolled fire) XØØ.2 ☑
  dam or man-made structure (causing earth movement) X36.Ø ☑
  machinery — *see* Contact, with, by type of machine
  structure W2Ø.1 ☑
    burning (uncontrolled fire) XØØ.2 ☑
Collision (accidental) NEC — *see also* Accident, transport V89.9 ☑
  pedestrian W51 ☑
    with fall WØ3 ☑
      due to ice or snow WØØ.Ø ☑
      involving pedestrian conveyance — *see* Accident, transport, pedestrian, conveyance
    and
      crowd or human stampede (with fall) W52 ☑
      object W22.8 ☑
        with fall — *see* Fall, due to, bumping against, object
  person(s) — *see* Collision, pedestrian
  transport vehicle NEC V89.9 ☑
    and
      avalanche, fallen or not moving — *see* Accident, transport
        falling or moving — *see* Landslide
      landslide, fallen or not moving — *see* Accident, transport
        falling or moving — *see* Landslide
      due to cataclysm — *see* Forces of nature, by type
      intentional, purposeful suicide (attempt) — *see* Suicide, collision
Combustion, spontaneous — *see* Ignition
Complication (delayed) **of or following** (medical or surgical procedure) Y84.9
  with misadventure — *see* Misadventure
  amputation of limb(s) Y83.5
  anastomosis (arteriovenous) (blood vessel) (gastrojejunal) (tendon) (natural or artificial material) Y83.2
  aspiration (of fluid) Y84.4
    tissue Y84.8
  biopsy Y84.8
  blood
    sampling Y84.7
    transfusion
      procedure Y84.8
  bypass Y83.2
  catheterization (urinary) Y84.6
    cardiac Y84.Ø
  colostomy Y83.3
  cystostomy Y83.3
  dialysis (kidney) Y84.1
  drug — *see* Table of Drugs and Chemicals
    due to misadventure — *see* Misadventure
  duodenostomy Y83.3
  electroshock therapy Y84.3
  external stoma, creation of Y83.3
  formation of external stoma Y83.3
  gastrostomy Y83.3

Complication (delayed) **of or following** — *continued*
  graft Y83.2
  hypothermia (medically-induced) Y84.8
  implant, implantation (of)
    artificial
      internal device (cardiac pacemaker) (electrodes in brain) (heart valve prosthesis) (orthopedic) Y83.1
      material or tissue (for anastomosis or bypass) Y83.2
        with creation of external stoma Y83.3
      natural tissues (for anastomosis or bypass) Y83.2
        with creation of external stoma Y83.3
  infusion
    procedure Y84.8
  injection — *see* Table of Drugs and Chemicals
    procedure Y84.8
  insertion of gastric or duodenal sound Y84.5
  insulin-shock therapy Y84.3
  paracentesis (abdominal) (thoracic) (aspirative) Y84.4
  procedures other than surgical operation — *see* Complication of or following, by type of procedure
  radiological procedure or therapy Y84.2
  removal of organ (partial) (total) NEC Y83.6
  sampling
    blood Y84.7
    fluid NEC Y84.4
    tissue Y84.8
  shock therapy Y84.3
  surgical operation NEC — *see also* Complication of or following, by type of operation Y83.9
    reconstructive NEC Y83.4
      with
        anastomosis, bypass or graft Y83.2
        formation of external stoma Y83.3
    specified NEC Y83.8
  transfusion — *see also* Table of Drugs and Chemicals
    procedure Y84.8
  transplant, transplantation (heart) (kidney) (liver) (whole organ, any) Y83.Ø
    partial organ Y83.4
  ureterostomy Y83.3
  vaccination — *see also* Table of Drugs and Chemicals
    procedure Y84.8
Compression
  divers' squeeze — *see* Air, pressure, change
  trachea by
    food (lodged in esophagus) — *see* categories T17 and T18 ☑
    vomitus (lodged in esophagus) T17.81- ☑
Conflagration — *see* Exposure, fire, uncontrolled
Constriction (external)
  hair W49.Ø1 ☑
  jewelry W49.Ø4 ☑
  ring W49.Ø4 ☑
  rubber band W49.Ø3 ☑
  specified item NEC W49.Ø9 ☑
  string W49.Ø2 ☑
  thread W49.Ø2 ☑
Contact (accidental)
  with
    abrasive wheel (metalworking) W31.1 ☑
    alligator W58.Ø9 ☑
      bite W58.Ø1 ☑
      crushing W58.Ø3 ☑
      strike W58.Ø2 ☑
    amphibian W62.9 ☑
      frog W62.Ø ☑
      toad W62.1 ☑
    animal (nonvenomous) NEC W64 ☑
      marine W56.89 ☑
        bite W56.81 ☑
        dolphin — *see* Contact, with, dolphin
        fish NEC — *see* Contact, with, fish
        mammal — *see* Contact, with, mammal, marine
        orca — *see* Contact, with, orca
        sea lion — *see* Contact, with, sea lion
        shark — *see* Contact, with, shark
        strike W56.82 ☑
    animate mechanical force NEC W64 ☑
    arrow W21.89 ☑
      not thrown, projected or falling W45.8 ☑
    arthropods (nonvenomous) W57 ☑
    axe W27.Ø ☑
    band-saw (industrial) W31.2 ☑
    bayonet — *see* Bayonet wound
    bee(s) X58 ☑
    bench-saw (industrial) W31.2 ☑

Contact — *continued*
  with — *continued*
    bird W61.99 ☑
      bite W61.91 ☑
      chicken — *see* Contact, with, chicken
      duck — *see* Contact, with, duck
      goose — *see* Contact, with, goose
      macaw — *see* Contact, with, macaw
      parrot — *see* Contact, with, parrot
      psittacine — *see* Contact, with, psittacine
      strike W61.92 ☑
      turkey — *see* Contact, with, turkey
    blender W29.Ø ☑
    boiling water X12 ☑
      stated as undetermined whether accidental or intentional Y27.2 ☑
      suicide (attempt) X77.2 ☑
    bore, earth-drilling or mining (land) (seabed) W31.Ø ☑
    buffalo — *see* Contact, with, hoof stock NEC
    bull W55.29 ☑
      bite W55.21 ☑
      gored W55.22 ☑
      strike W55.22 ☑
    bumper cars W31.81 ☑
    camel — *see* Contact, with, hoof stock NEC
    can
      lid W26.8 ☑
      opener W27.4 ☑
        powered W29.Ø ☑
    cat W55.Ø9 ☑
      bite W55.Ø1 ☑
      scratch W55.Ø3 ☑
    caterpillar (venomous) X58 ☑
    centipede (venomous) X58 ☑
    chain
      hoist W24.Ø ☑
        agricultural operations W3Ø.89 ☑
      saw W29.3 ☑
    chicken W61.39 ☑
      peck W61.33 ☑
      strike W61.32 ☑
    chisel W27.Ø ☑
    circular saw W31.2 ☑
    cobra X58 ☑
    combine (harvester) W3Ø.Ø ☑
    conveyer belt W24.1 ☑
    cooker (hot) X15.8 ☑
      stated as undetermined whether accidental or intentional Y27.3 ☑
      suicide (attempt) X77.3 ☑
    coral X58 ☑
    cotton gin W31.82 ☑
    cow W55.29 ☑
      bite W55.21 ☑
      strike W55.22 ☑
    crane W24.Ø ☑
      agricultural operations W3Ø.89 ☑
    crocodile W58.19 ☑
      bite W58.11 ☑
      crushing W58.13 ☑
      strike W58.12 ☑
    dagger W26.1 ☑
      stated as undetermined whether accidental or intentional Y28.2 ☑
      suicide (attempt) X78.2 ☑
    dairy equipment W31.82 ☑
    dart W21.89 ☑
      not thrown, projected or falling W45.8 ☑
    deer — *see* Contact, with, hoof stock NEC
    derrick W24.Ø ☑
      agricultural operations W3Ø.89 ☑
        hay W3Ø.2 ☑
    dog W54.8 ☑
      bite W54.Ø ☑
      strike W54.1 ☑
    dolphin W56.Ø9 ☑
      bite W56.Ø1 ☑
      strike W56.Ø2 ☑
    donkey — *see* Contact, with, hoof stock NEC
    drill (powered) W29.8 ☑
      earth (land) (seabed) W31.Ø ☑
      nonpowered W27.8 ☑
    drive belt W24.Ø ☑
      agricultural operations W3Ø.89 ☑
    dry ice — *see* Exposure, cold, man-made

☑ **Additional Character Required** — Refer to the Tabular List for Character Selection

Contact — *continued*
  with — *continued*
    dryer (clothes) (powered) (spin) W29.2 ☑
    duck W61.69 ☑
      bite W61.61 ☑
      strike W61.62 ☑
    earth (-)
      drilling machine (industrial) W31.0 ☑
      scraping machine in stationary use W31.83 ☑
    edge of stiff paper W26.2 ☑
    electric
      beater W29.0 ☑
      blanket X16 ☑
      fan W29.2 ☑
        commercial W31.82 ☑
      knife W29.1 ☑
      mixer W29.0 ☑
    elevator (building) W24.0 ☑
      agricultural operations W30.89 ☑
        grain W30.3 ☑
    engine(s), hot NEC X17 ☑
    excavating machine W31.0 ☑
    farm machine W30.9 ☑
    feces — *see* Contact, with, by type of animal
    fer de lance X58 ☑
    fish W56.59 ☑
      bite W56.51 ☑
      shark — *see* Contact, with, shark
      strike W56.52 ☑
    flying horses W31.81 ☑
    forging (metalworking) machine W31.1 ☑
    fork W27.4 ☑
    forklift (truck) W24.0 ☑
      agricultural operations W30.89 ☑
    frog W62.0 ☑
    garden
      cultivator (powered) W29.3 ☑
        riding W30.89 ☑
      fork W27.1 ☑
    gas turbine W31.3 ☑
    Gila monster X58 ☑
    giraffe — *see* Contact, with, hoof stock NEC
    glass (sharp) (broken) W25 ☑
      assault X99.0 ☑
      due to fall — *see* Fall, by type
      stated as undetermined whether accidental or intentional Y28.0 ☑
      suicide (attempt) X78.0 ☑
      with subsequent fall W18.02 ☑
    goat W55.39 ☑
      bite W55.31 ☑
      strike W55.32 ☑
    goose W61.59 ☑
      bite W61.51 ☑
      strike W61.52 ☑
    hand
      saw W27.0 ☑
      tool (not powered) NEC W27.8 ☑
        powered W29.8 ☑
    harvester W30.0 ☑
    hay-derrick W30.2 ☑
    heating
      appliance (hot) X16 ☑
      pad (electric) X16 ☑
    heat NEC X19 ☑
      from appliance (electrical) (household) — *see* Contact, with, hot, household appliance heating appliance X16 ☑
    hedge-trimmer (powered) W29.3 ☑
    hoe W27.1 ☑
    hoist (chain) (shaft) NEC W24.0 ☑
      agricultural W30.89 ☑
    hoof stock NEC W55.39 ☑
      bite W55.31 ☑
      strike W55.32 ☑
    hornet(s) X58 ☑
    horse W55.19 ☑
      bite W55.11 ☑
      strike W55.12 ☑
    hot
      air X14.1 ☑
        inhalation X14.0 ☑
      cooker X15.8 ☑
      cooking
        pan X15.3 ☑

Contact — *continued*
  with — *continued*
    hot — *continued*
      cooking — *continued*
        pot X15.3 ☑
      drinks X10.0 ☑
      engine X17 ☑
      fats X10.2 ☑
      fluids NEC X12 ☑
        assault X98.2 ☑
        suicide (attempt) X77.2 ☑
        undetermined whether accidental or intentional Y27.2 ☑
      food X10.1 ☑
      gases X14.1 ☑
        inhalation X14.0 ☑
      heating appliance X16 ☑
      household appliance X15.8 ☑
        assault X98.3 ☑
        cooker X15.8 ☑
        hotplate X15.2 ☑
        kettle X15.8 ☑
        light bulb X15.8 ☑
        object NEC X19 ☑
          assault X98.8 ☑
          stated as undetermined whether accidental or intentional Y27.9 ☑
          suicide (attempt) X77.8 ☑
        saucepan X15.3 ☑
        skillet X15.3 ☑
        stated as undetermined whether accidental or intentional Y27.3 ☑
        stove X15.0 ☑
        suicide (attempt) X77.3 ☑
        toaster X15.1 ☑
      kettle X15.8 ☑
      light bulb X15.8 ☑
      liquid NEC — *see also* Burn X12 ☑
        drinks X10.0 ☑
        stated as undetermined whether accidental or intentional Y27.2 ☑
        suicide (attempt) X77.2 ☑
        tap water X11.8 ☑
          stated as undetermined whether accidental or intentional Y27.1 ☑
          suicide (attempt) X77.1 ☑
      machinery X17 ☑
      metal (molten) (liquid) NEC X18 ☑
      object (not producing fire or flames) NEC X19 ☑
      oil (cooking) X10.2 ☑
      pipe X16 ☑
      plate X15.2 ☑
      radiator X16 ☑
      saucepan (glass) (metal) X15.3 ☑
      skillet X15.3 ☑
      stove (kitchen) X15.0 ☑
      substance NEC X19 ☑
      tap-water X11.8 ☑
        assault X98.1 ☑
        heated on stove X12 ☑
          stated as undetermined whether accidental or intentional Y27.2 ☑
          suicide (attempt) X77.2 ☑
        in bathtub X11.0 ☑
        running X11.1 ☑
        stated as undetermined whether accidental or intentional Y27.1 ☑
        suicide (attempt) X77.1 ☑
      toaster X15.1 ☑
      tool X17 ☑
      vapors X13.1 ☑
        inhalation X13.0 ☑
      water (tap) X11.8 ☑
        boiling X12 ☑
          stated as undetermined whether accidental or intentional Y27.2 ☑
          suicide (attempt) X77.2 ☑
        heated on stove X12 ☑
          stated as undetermined whether accidental or intentional Y27.2 ☑
          suicide (attempt) X77.2 ☑
        in bathtub X11.0 ☑
        running X11.1 ☑
        stated as undetermined whether accidental or intentional Y27.1 ☑

Contact — *continued*
  with — *continued*
    hot — *continued*
      water — *continued*
        suicide (attempt) X77.1 ☑
      hotplate X15.2 ☑
      ice-pick W27.4 ☑
      insect (nonvenomous) NEC W57 ☑
      kettle (hot) X15.8 ☑
      knife W26.0 ☑
        assault X99.1 ☑
        electric W29.1 ☑
        stated as undetermined whether accidental or intentional Y28.1 ☑
        suicide (attempt) X78.1 ☑
      lathe (metalworking) W31.1 ☑
        turnings W45.8 ☑
        woodworking W31.2 ☑
      lawnmower (powered) (ridden) W28 ☑
        causing electrocution W86.8 ☑
          suicide (attempt) X83.1 ☑
        unpowered W27.1 ☑
      lift, lifting (devices) W24.0 ☑
        agricultural operations W30.89 ☑
        shaft W24.0 ☑
      liquefied gas — *see* Exposure, cold, man-made
      liquid air, hydrogen, nitrogen — *see* Exposure, cold, man-made
      lizard (nonvenomous) W59.09 ☑
        bite W59.01 ☑
        strike W59.02 ☑
      llama — *see* Contact, with, hoof stock NEC
      macaw W61.19 ☑
        bite W61.11 ☑
        strike W61.12 ☑
      machine, machinery W31.9 ☑
        abrasive wheel W31.1 ☑
        agricultural including animal-powered W30.9 ☑
          combine harvester W30.0 ☑
          grain storage elevator W30.3 ☑
          hay derrick W30.2 ☑
          power take-off device W30.1 ☑
          reaper W30.0 ☑
          specified NEC W30.89 ☑
          thresher W30.0 ☑
          transport vehicle, stationary W30.81 ☑
        band saw W31.2 ☑
        bench saw W31.2 ☑
        circular saw W31.2 ☑
        commercial NEC W31.82 ☑
        drilling, metal (industrial) W31.1 ☑
        earth-drilling W31.0 ☑
        earthmoving or scraping W31.89 ☑
        excavating W31.89 ☑
        forging machine W31.1 ☑
        gas turbine W31.3 ☑
        hot X17 ☑
        internal combustion engine W31.3 ☑
        land drill W31.0 ☑
        lathe W31.1 ☑
        lifting (devices) W24.0 ☑
        metal drill W31.1 ☑
        metalworking (industrial) W31.1 ☑
        milling, metal W31.1 ☑
        mining W31.0 ☑
        molding W31.2 ☑
        overhead plane W31.2 ☑
        power press, metal W31.1 ☑
        prime mover W31.3 ☑
        printing W31.89 ☑
        radial saw W31.2 ☑
        recreational W31.81 ☑
        roller-coaster W31.81 ☑
        rolling mill, metal W31.1 ☑
        sander W31.2 ☑
        seabed drill W31.0 ☑
        shaft
          hoist W31.0 ☑
          lift W31.0 ☑
        specified NEC W31.89 ☑
        spinning W31.89 ☑
        steam engine W31.3 ☑
        transmission W24.1 ☑
        undercutter W31.0 ☑
        water driven turbine W31.3 ☑

☑ **Additional Character Required — Refer to the Tabular List for Character Selection**

Contact — *continued*
  with — *continued*
    machine, machinery — *continued*
      weaving W31.89 ☑
      woodworking or forming (industrial) W31.2 ☑
    mammal (feces) (urine) W55.89 ☑
      bull — *see* Contact, with, bull
      cat — *see* Contact, with, cat
      cow — *see* Contact, with, cow
      goat — *see* Contact, with, goat
      hoof stock — *see* Contact, with, hoof stock
      horse — *see* Contact, with, horse
      marine W56.39 ☑
        dolphin — *see* Contact, with, dolphin
        orca — *see* Contact, with, orca
        sea lion — *see* Contact, with, sea lion
        specified NEC W56.39 ☑
          bite W56.31 ☑
          strike W56.32 ☑
      pig — *see* Contact, with, pig
      raccoon — *see* Contact, with, raccoon
      rodent — *see* Contact, with, rodent
      sheep — *see* Contact, with, sheep
      specified NEC W55.89 ☑
        bite W55.81 ☑
        strike W55.82 ☑
    marine
      animal W56.89 ☑
        bite W56.81 ☑
        dolphin — *see* Contact, with, dolphin
        fish NEC — *see* Contact, with, fish
        mammal — *see* Contact, with, mammal, marine
        orca — *see* Contact, with, orca
        sea lion — *see* Contact, with, sea lion
        shark — *see* Contact, with, shark
        strike W56.82 ☑
    meat
      grinder (domestic) W29.0 ☑
        industrial W31.82 ☑
        nonpowered W27.4 ☑
      slicer (domestic) W29.0 ☑
        industrial W31.82 ☑
    merry go round W31.81 ☑
    metal, hot (liquid) (molten) NEC X18 ☑
    millipede W57 ☑
    nail W45.0 ☑
      gun W29.4 ☑
    needle (sewing) W27.3 ☑
      hypodermic W46.0 ☑
        contaminated W46.1 ☑
    object (blunt) NEC
      hot NEC X19 ☑
      legal intervention — *see* Legal, intervention, blunt object
      sharp NEC W45.8 ☑
        inflicted by other person NEC W45.8 ☑
          stated as
            intentional homicide (attempt) — *see* Assault, cutting or piercing instrument
        legal intervention — *see* Legal, intervention, sharp object
        self-inflicted X78.9 ☑
    orca W56.29 ☑
      bite W56.21 ☑
      strike W56.22 ☑
    overhead plane W31.2 ☑
    paper (as sharp object) W26.2 ☑
    paper-cutter W27.5 ☑
    parrot W61.09 ☑
      bite W61.01 ☑
      strike W61.02 ☑
    pig W55.49 ☑
      bite W55.41 ☑
      strike W55.42 ☑
    pipe, hot X16 ☑
    pitchfork W27.1 ☑
    plane (metal) (wood) W27.0 ☑
      overhead W31.2 ☑
    plant thorns, spines, sharp leaves or other mechanisms W60 ☑
    powered
      garden cultivator W29.3 ☑
      household appliance, implement, or machine W29.8 ☑
      saw (industrial) W31.2 ☑

Contact — *continued*
  with — *continued*
    powered — *continued*
      saw — *continued*
        hand W29.8 ☑
    printing machine W31.89 ☑
    psittacine bird W61.29 ☑
      bite W61.21 ☑
      macaw — *see* Contact, with, macaw
      parrot — *see* Contact, with, parrot
      strike W61.22 ☑
    pulley (block) (transmission) W24.0 ☑
      agricultural operations W30.89 ☑
    raccoon W55.59 ☑
      bite W55.51 ☑
      strike W55.52 ☑
    radial-saw (industrial) W31.2 ☑
    radiator (hot) X16 ☑
    rake W27.1 ☑
    rattlesnake X58 ☑
    reaper W30.0 ☑
    reptile W59.89 ☑
      lizard — *see* Contact, with, lizard
      snake — *see* Contact, with, snake
      specified NEC W59.89 ☑
        bite W59.81 ☑
        crushing W59.83 ☑
        strike W59.82 ☑
      turtle — *see* Contact, with, turtle
    rivet gun (powered) W29.4 ☑
    road scraper — *see* Accident, transport, construction vehicle
    rodent (feces) (urine) W53.89 ☑
      bite W53.81 ☑
      mouse W53.09 ☑
        bite W53.01 ☑
      rat W53.19 ☑
        bite W53.11 ☑
      specified NEC W53.89 ☑
        bite W53.81 ☑
      squirrel W53.29 ☑
        bite W53.21 ☑
    roller coaster W31.81 ☑
    rope NEC W24.0 ☑
      agricultural operations W30.89 ☑
    saliva — *see* Contact, with, by type of animal
    sander W29.8 ☑
      industrial W31.2 ☑
    saucepan (hot) (glass) (metal) X15.3 ☑
    saw W27.0 ☑
      band (industrial) W31.2 ☑
      bench (industrial) W31.2 ☑
      chain W29.3 ☑
      hand W27.0 ☑
    sawing machine, metal W31.1 ☑
    scissors W27.2 ☑
    scorpion X58 ☑
    screwdriver W27.0 ☑
      powered W29.8 ☑
    sea
      anemone, cucumber or urchin (spine) X58 ☑
      lion W56.19 ☑
        bite W56.11 ☑
        strike W56.12 ☑
    serpent — *see* Contact, with, snake, by type
    sewing-machine (electric) (powered) W29.2 ☑
      not powered W27.8 ☑
    shaft (hoist) (lift) (transmission) NEC W24.0 ☑
      agricultural W30.89 ☑
    shark W56.49 ☑
      bite W56.41 ☑
      strike W56.42 ☑
    sharp object(s) W26.9 ☑
      specified NEC W26.8 ☑
    shears (hand) W27.2 ☑
      powered (industrial) W31.1 ☑
        domestic W29.2 ☑
    sheep W55.39 ☑
      bite W55.31 ☑
      strike W55.32 ☑
    shovel W27.8 ☑
      steam — *see* Accident, transport, construction vehicle
    snake (nonvenomous) W59.19 ☑
      bite W59.11 ☑

Contact — *continued*
  with — *continued*
    snake — *continued*
      crushing W59.13 ☑
      strike W59.12 ☑
    spade W27.1 ☑
    spider (venomous) X58 ☑
    spin-drier W29.2 ☑
    spinning machine W31.89 ☑
    splinter W45.8 ☑
    sports equipment W21.9 ☑
    staple gun (powered) W29.8 ☑
    steam X13.1 ☑
      engine W31.3 ☑
      inhalation X13.0 ☑
      pipe X16 ☑
      shovel W31.89 ☑
    stove (hot) (kitchen) X15.0 ☑
    substance, hot NEC X19 ☑
      molten (metal) X18 ☑
    sword W26.1 ☑
      assault X99.2 ☑
      stated as undetermined whether accidental or intentional Y28.2 ☑
      suicide (attempt) X78.2 ☑
    tarantula X58 ☑
    thresher W30.0 ☑
    tin can lid W26.8 ☑
    toad W62.1 ☑
    toaster (hot) X15.1 ☑
    tool W27.8 ☑
      hand (not powered) W27.8 ☑
        auger W27.0 ☑
        axe W27.0 ☑
        can opener W27.4 ☑
        chisel W27.0 ☑
        fork W27.4 ☑
        garden W27.1 ☑
        handsaw W27.0 ☑
        hoe W27.1 ☑
        ice-pick W27.4 ☑
        kitchen utensil W27.4 ☑
        manual
          lawn mower W27.1 ☑
          sewing machine W27.8 ☑
        meat grinder W27.4 ☑
        needle (sewing) W27.3 ☑
          hypodermic W46.0 ☑
            contaminated W46.1 ☑
        paper cutter W27.5 ☑
        pitchfork W27.1 ☑
        rake W27.1 ☑
        scissors W27.2 ☑
        screwdriver W27.0 ☑
        specified NEC W27.8 ☑
        workbench W27.0 ☑
      hot X17 ☑
      powered W29.8 ☑
        blender W29.0 ☑
          commercial W31.82 ☑
        can opener W29.0 ☑
          commercial W31.82 ☑
        chainsaw W29.3 ☑
        clothes dryer W29.2 ☑
          commercial W31.82 ☑
        dishwasher W29.2 ☑
          commercial W31.82 ☑
        edger W29.3 ☑
        electric fan W29.2 ☑
          commercial W31.82 ☑
        electric knife W29.1 ☑
        food processor W29.0 ☑
          commercial W31.82 ☑
        garbage disposal W29.0 ☑
          commercial W31.82 ☑
        garden tool W29.3 ☑
        hedge trimmer W29.3 ☑
        ice maker W29.0 ☑
          commercial W31.82 ☑
        kitchen appliance W29.0 ☑
          commercial W31.82 ☑
        lawn mower W28 ☑
        meat grinder W29.0 ☑
          commercial W31.82 ☑
        mixer W29.0 ☑

☑ **Additional Character Required** — **Refer to the Tabular List for Character Selection**

Contact — *continued*	**Crash** — *continued*	**Discharge** — *continued*
with — *continued*	transport vehicle — *see also* Accident, transport — *continued*	firearm — *continued*
tool — *continued*	homicide (attempt) Y03.8 ☑	assault X95.9 ☑
powered — *continued*	motor NEC (traffic) V89.2 ☑	handgun (pistol) (revolver) W32.0 ☑
mixer — *continued*	homicide (attempt) Y03.8 ☑	assault X93 ☑
commercial W31.82 ☑	suicide (attempt) — *see* Suicide, collision	homicide (attempt) X93 ☑
rototiller W29.3 ☑	**Cruelty** (mental) (physical) (sexual) X58 ☑	legal intervention — *see* Legal, intervention, firearm, handgun
sewing machine W29.2 ☑	**Crushed** (accidentally) X58 ☑	stated as undetermined whether accidental or intentional Y22 ☑
commercial W31.82 ☑	between objects (moving) (stationary and moving) W23.0 ☑	suicide (attempt) X72 ☑
washing machine W29.2 ☑	stationary W23.1 ☑	homicide (attempt) X95.9 ☑
commercial W31.82 ☑	by	hunting rifle W33.02 ☑
transmission device (belt, cable, chain, gear, pinion, shaft) W24.1 ☑	alligator W58.03 ☑	assault X94.1 ☑
agricultural operations W30.89 ☑	avalanche NEC — *see* Landslide	homicide (attempt) X94.1 ☑
turbine (gas) (water-driven) W31.3 ☑	cave-in W20.0 ☑	legal intervention
turkey W61.49 ☑	caused by cataclysmic earth surface movement — *see* Landslide	injuring
peck W61.43 ☑	crocodile W58.13 ☑	bystander Y35.032 ☑
strike W61.42 ☑	crowd or human stampede W52 ☑	law enforcement personnel Y35.031 ☑
turtle (nonvenomous) W59.29 ☑	falling	suspect Y35.033 ☑
bite W59.21 ☑	aircraft W97.39 ☑	unspecified person Y35.039 ☑
strike W59.22 ☑	in war operations — *see* War operations, destruction of aircraft	stated as undetermined whether accidental or intentional Y23.1 ☑
terrestrial W59.89 ☑	earth, material W20.0 ☑	suicide (attempt) X73.1 ☑
bite W59.81 ☑	caused by cataclysmic earth surface movement — *see* Landslide	larger W33.00 ☑
crushing W59.83 ☑	object NEC W20.8 ☑	assault X94.9 ☑
strike W59.82 ☑	landslide NEC — *see* Landslide	homicide (attempt) X94.9 ☑
under-cutter W31.0 ☑	lizard (nonvenomous) W59.09 ☑	hunting rifle — *see* Discharge, firearm, hunting rifle
urine — *see* Contact, with, by type of animal	machinery — *see* Contact, with, by type of machine	legal intervention — *see* Legal, intervention, firearm by type of firearm
vehicle	reptile NEC W59.89 ☑	machine gun — *see* Discharge, firearm, machine gun
agricultural use (transport) — *see* Accident, transport, agricultural vehicle	snake (nonvenomous) W59.13 ☑	shotgun — *see* Discharge, firearm, shotgun
not on public highway W30.81 ☑	in	specified NEC W33.09 ☑
industrial use (transport) — *see* Accident, transport, industrial vehicle	machinery — *see* Contact, with, by type of machine	assault X94.8 ☑
not on public highway W31.83 ☑	**Cut, cutting** (any part of body) (accidental) — *see also* Contact, with, by object or machine	homicide (attempt) X94.8 ☑
off-road use (transport) — *see* Accident, transport, all-terrain or off-road vehicle	during medical or surgical treatment as misadventure — *see* Index to Diseases and Injuries, Complications	legal intervention
not on public highway W31.83 ☑	homicide (attempt) — *see* Assault, cutting or piercing instrument	injuring
special construction use (transport) — *see* Accident, transport, construction vehicle	inflicted by other person — *see* Assault, cutting or piercing instrument	bystander Y35.092 ☑
not on public highway W31.83 ☑	legal	law enforcement personnel Y35.091 ☑
venomous	execution — *see* Legal, intervention	suspect Y35.093 ☑
animal X58 ☑	intervention — *see* Legal, intervention, sharp object	unspecified person Y35.099 ☑
arthropods X58 ☑	machine NEC — *see also* Contact, with, by type of machine W31.9 ☑	stated as undetermined whether accidental or intentional Y23.8 ☑
lizard X58 ☑	self-inflicted — *see* Suicide, cutting or piercing instrument	suicide (attempt) X73.8 ☑
marine animal NEC X58 ☑	suicide (attempt) — *see* Suicide, cutting or piercing instrument	stated as undetermined whether accidental or intentional Y23.9 ☑
marine plant NEC X58 ☑	**Cyclone** (any injury) X37.1 ☑	suicide (attempt) X73.9 ☑
millipedes (tropical) X58 ☑		legal intervention
plant(s) X58 ☑		injuring
snake X58 ☑	**D**	bystander Y35.002 ☑
spider X58 ☑		law enforcement personnel Y35.001 ☑
viper X58 ☑	**Decapitation** (accidental circumstances) NEC X58 ☑	suspect Y35.03 ☑
washing-machine (powered) W29.2 ☑	homicide X99.9 ☑	unspecified person Y35.009 ☑
wasp X58 ☑	legal execution — *see* Legal, intervention	using rubber bullet
weaving-machine W31.89 ☑	**Dehydration from lack of water** X58 ☑	injuring
winch W24.0 ☑	**Deprivation** X58 ☑	bystander Y35.042 ☑
agricultural operations W30.89 ☑	**Derailment** (accidental)	law enforcement personnel Y35.041 ☑
wire NEC W24.0 ☑	railway (rolling stock) (train) (vehicle) (without antecedent collision) V81.7 ☑	suspect Y35.043 ☑
agricultural operations W30.89 ☑	with antecedent collision — *see* Accident, transport, railway vehicle occupant	unspecified person Y35.049 ☑
wood slivers W45.8 ☑	streetcar (without antecedent collision) V82.7 ☑	machine gun W33.03 ☑
yellow jacket X58 ☑	with antecedent collision — *see* Accident, transport, streetcar occupant	assault X94.2 ☑
zebra — *see* Contact, with, hoof stock NEC	**Descent**	homicide (attempt) X94.2 ☑
pressure X50.9 ☑	parachute (voluntary) (without accident to aircraft) V97.29 ☑	legal intervention — *see* Legal, intervention, firearm, machine gun
stress X50.9 ☑	due to accident to aircraft — *see* Accident, transport, aircraft	stated as undetermined whether accidental or intentional Y23.3 ☑
Coup de soleil X32 ☑	**Desertion** X58 ☑	suicide (attempt) X73.2 ☑
Crash	**Destitution** X58 ☑	pellet gun — *see* Discharge, airgun
aircraft (in transit) (powered) V95.9 ☑	**Disability, late effect or sequela of injury** — *see* Sequelae	shotgun W33.01 ☑
balloon V96.01 ☑	**Discharge** (accidental)	assault X94.0 ☑
fixed wing NEC (private) V95.21 ☑	airgun W34.010 ☑	homicide (attempt) X94.0 ☑
commercial V95.31 ☑	assault X95.01 ☑	legal intervention — *see* Legal, intervention, firearm, specified NEC
glider V96.21 ☑	homicide (attempt) X95.01 ☑	stated as undetermined whether accidental or intentional Y23.0 ☑
hang V96.11 ☑	stated as undetermined whether accidental or intentional Y24.0 ☑	suicide (attempt) X73.0 ☑
powered V95.11 ☑	suicide (attempt) X74.01 ☑	specified NEC W34.09 ☑
helicopter V95.01 ☑	BB gun — *see* Discharge, airgun	assault X95.8 ☑
in war operations — *see* War operations, destruction of aircraft	firearm (accidental) W34.00 ☑	homicide (attempt) X95.8 ☑
microlight V95.11 ☑		legal intervention — *see* Legal, intervention, firearm, specified NEC
nonpowered V96.9 ☑		stated as undetermined whether accidental or intentional Y24.8 ☑
specified NEC V96.8 ☑		suicide (attempt) X74.8 ☑
powered NEC V95.8 ☑		
stated as		
homicide (attempt) Y08.81 ☑		
suicide (attempt) X83.0 ☑		
ultralight V95.11 ☑		
spacecraft V95.41 ☑		
transport vehicle NEC — *see also* Accident, transport V89.9 ☑		

Discharge — *continued*
- firearm — *continued*
  - stated as undetermined whether accidental or intentional Y24.9 ☑
  - suicide (attempt) X74.9 ☑
  - Very pistol W34.09 ☑
    - assault X95.8 ☑
    - homicide (attempt) X95.8 ☑
    - stated as undetermined whether accidental or intentional Y24.8 ☑
    - suicide (attempt) X74.8 ☑
- firework(s) W39 ☑
  - stated as undetermined whether accidental or intentional Y25 ☑
- gas-operated gun NEC W34.018 ☑
  - airgun — *see* Discharge, airgun
  - assault X95.09 ☑
  - homicide (attempt) X95.09 ☑
  - paintball gun — *see* Discharge, paintball gun
  - stated as undetermined whether accidental or intentional Y24.8 ☑
  - suicide (attempt) X74.09 ☑
- gun NEC — *see also* Discharge, firearm NEC
  - air — *see* Discharge, airgun
  - BB — *see* Discharge, airgun
  - for single hand use — *see* Discharge, firearm, handgun
  - hand — *see* Discharge, firearm, handgun
  - machine — *see* Discharge, firearm, machine gun
  - other specified — *see* Discharge, firearm NEC
  - paintball — *see* Discharge, paintball gun
  - pellet — *see* Discharge, airgun
- handgun — *see* Discharge, firearm, handgun
- machine gun — *see* Discharge, firearm, machine gun
- paintball gun W34.011 ☑
  - assault X95.02 ☑
  - homicide (attempt) X95.02 ☑
  - stated as undetermined whether accidental or intentional Y24.8 ☑
  - suicide (attempt) X74.02 ☑
- pistol — *see* Discharge, firearm, handgun
  - flare — *see* Discharge, firearm, Very pistol
  - pellet — *see* Discharge, airgun
  - Very — *see* Discharge, firearm, Very pistol
- revolver — *see* Discharge, firearm, handgun
- rifle (hunting) — *see* Discharge, firearm, hunting rifle
- shotgun — *see* Discharge, firearm, shotgun
- spring-operated gun NEC W34.018 ☑
  - assault X95.09 ☑
  - homicide (attempt) X95.09 ☑
  - stated as undetermined whether accidental or intentional Y24.8 ☑
  - suicide (attempt) X74.09 ☑

Disease
- Andes W94.11 ☑
- aviator's — *see* Air, pressure
- range W94.11 ☑

Diver's disease, palsy, paralysis, squeeze — *see* Air, pressure

Diving (into water) — *see* Accident, diving

Dog bite W54.0 ☑

Dragged by transport vehicle NEC — *see also* Accident, transport V09.9 ☑

Drinking poison (accidental) — *see* Table of Drugs and Chemicals

Dropped (accidentally) **while being carried or supported by other person** W04 ☑

Drowning (accidental) W74 ☑
- assault X92.9 ☑
- due to
  - accident (to)
    - machinery — *see* Contact, with, by type of machine
    - watercraft V90.89 ☑
      - burning V90.29 ☑
        - powered V90.23 ☑
          - fishing boat V90.22 ☑
          - jetskis V90.23 ☑
          - merchant ship V90.20 ☑
          - passenger ship V90.21 ☑
        - unpowered V90.28 ☑
          - canoe V90.25 ☑
          - inflatable V90.26 ☑
          - kayak V90.25 ☑
          - sailboat V90.24 ☑
          - water skis V90.27 ☑
        - crushed V90.39 ☑

Drowning — *continued*
- due to — *continued*
  - accident — *continued*
    - watercraft — *continued*
      - crushed — *continued*
        - powered V90.33 ☑
          - fishing boat V90.32 ☑
          - jetskis V90.33 ☑
          - merchant ship V90.30 ☑
          - passenger ship V90.31 ☑
        - unpowered V90.38 ☑
          - canoe V90.35 ☑
          - inflatable V90.36 ☑
          - kayak V90.35 ☑
          - sailboat V90.34 ☑
          - water skis V90.37 ☑
      - overturning V90.09 ☑
        - powered V90.03 ☑
          - fishing boat V90.02 ☑
          - jetskis V90.03 ☑
          - merchant ship V90.00 ☑
          - passenger ship V90.01 ☑
        - unpowered V90.08 ☑
          - canoe V90.05 ☑
          - inflatable V90.06 ☑
          - kayak V90.05 ☑
          - sailboat V90.04 ☑
      - sinking V90.19 ☑
        - powered V90.13 ☑
          - fishing boat V90.12 ☑
          - jetskis V90.13 ☑
          - merchant ship V90.10 ☑
          - passenger ship V90.11 ☑
        - unpowered V90.18 ☑
          - canoe V90.15 ☑
          - inflatable V90.16 ☑
          - kayak V90.15 ☑
          - sailboat V90.14 ☑
      - specified type NEC V90.89 ☑
        - powered V90.83 ☑
          - fishing boat V90.82 ☑
          - jetskis V90.83 ☑
          - merchant ship V90.80 ☑
          - passenger ship V90.81 ☑
        - unpowered V90.88 ☑
          - canoe V90.85 ☑
          - inflatable V90.86 ☑
          - kayak V90.85 ☑
          - sailboat V90.84 ☑
          - water skis V90.87 ☑
  - avalanche — *see* Landslide
  - cataclysmic
    - earth surface movement NEC — *see* Forces of nature, earth movement
    - storm — *see* Forces of nature, cataclysmic storm
  - cloudburst X37.8 ☑
  - cyclone X37.1 ☑
  - fall overboard (from) V92.09 ☑
    - powered craft V92.03 ☑
      - ferry boat V92.01 ☑
      - fishing boat V92.02 ☑
      - jetskis V92.03 ☑
      - liner V92.01 ☑
      - merchant ship V92.00 ☑
      - passenger ship V92.01 ☑
    - resulting from
      - accident to watercraft — *see* Drowning, due to, accident to, watercraft
      - being washed overboard (from) V92.29 ☑
        - powered craft V92.23 ☑
          - ferry boat V92.21 ☑
          - fishing boat V92.22 ☑
          - jetskis V92.23 ☑
          - liner V92.21 ☑
          - merchant ship V92.20 ☑
          - passenger ship V92.21 ☑
        - unpowered craft V92.28 ☑
          - canoe V92.25 ☑
          - inflatable V92.26 ☑
          - kayak V92.25 ☑
          - sailboat V92.24 ☑
          - surf-board V92.28 ☑
          - water skis V92.27 ☑
          - windsurfer V92.28 ☑
      - motion of watercraft V92.19 ☑

Drowning — *continued*
- due to — *continued*
  - fall overboard — *continued*
    - resulting from — *continued*
      - motion of watercraft — *continued*
        - powered craft V92.13 ☑
          - ferry boat V92.11 ☑
          - fishing boat V92.12 ☑
          - jetskis V92.13 ☑
          - liner V92.11 ☑
          - merchant ship V92.10 ☑
          - passenger ship V92.11 ☑
        - unpowered craft
          - canoe V92.15 ☑
          - inflatable V92.16 ☑
          - kayak V92.15 ☑
          - sailboat V92.14 ☑
    - unpowered craft V92.08 ☑
      - canoe V92.05 ☑
      - inflatable V92.06 ☑
      - kayak V92.05 ☑
      - sailboat V92.04 ☑
      - surf-board V92.08 ☑
      - water skis V92.07 ☑
      - windsurfer V92.08 ☑
  - hurricane X37.0 ☑
  - jumping into water from watercraft (involved in accident) — *see also* Drowning, due to, accident to, watercraft
    - without accident to or on watercraft W16.711 ☑
  - tidal wave NEC — *see* Forces of nature, tidal wave
  - torrential rain X37.8 ☑
- following
  - fall
    - into
      - bathtub W16.211 ☑
      - bucket W16.221 ☑
      - fountain — *see* Drowning, following, fall, into, water, specified NEC
      - quarry — *see* Drowning, following, fall, into, water, specified NEC
      - reservoir — *see* Drowning, following, fall, into, water, specified NEC
      - swimming-pool W16.011 ☑
        - stated as undetermined whether accidental or intentional Y21.3 ☑
        - striking
          - bottom W16.021 ☑
          - wall W16.031 ☑
        - suicide (attempt) X71.2 ☑
      - water NOS W16.41 ☑
        - natural (lake) (open sea) (river) (stream) (pond) W16.111 ☑
          - striking
            - bottom W16.121 ☑
            - side W16.131 ☑
        - specified NEC W16.311 ☑
          - striking
            - bottom W16.321 ☑
            - wall W16.331 ☑
    - overboard NEC — *see* Drowning, due to, fall overboard
  - jump or dive
    - from boat W16.711 ☑
      - striking bottom W16.721 ☑
    - into
      - fountain — *see* Drowning, following, jump or dive, into, water, specified NEC
      - quarry — *see* Drowning, following, jump or dive, into, water, specified NEC
      - reservoir — *see* Drowning, following, jump or dive, into, water, specified NEC
      - swimming-pool W16.511 ☑
        - striking
          - bottom W16.521 ☑
          - wall W16.531 ☑
        - suicide (attempt) X71.2 ☑
      - water NOS W16.91 ☑
        - natural (lake) (open sea) (river) (stream) (pond) W16.611 ☑
        - specified NEC W16.811 ☑
          - bottom W16.821 ☑
          - striking
            - bottom W16.821 ☑
            - wall W16.831 ☑

☑ **Additional Character Required** — **Refer to the Tabular List for Character Selection**

Drowning — *continued*
 following — *continued*
  jump or dive — *continued*
   into — *continued*
    water — *continued*
     striking
      bottom W16.821 ☑
       wall W16.831 ☑
      striking bottom W16.621 ☑
 homicide (attempt) X92.9 ☑
 in
  bathtub (accidental) W65 ☑
   assault X92.0 ☑
   following fall W16.211 ☑
    stated as undetermined whether accidental or
     intentional Y21.1 ☑
   stated as undetermined whether accidental or in-
    tentional Y21.0 ☑
   suicide (attempt) X71.0 ☑
  lake — *see* Drowning, in, natural water
  natural water (lake) (open sea) (river) (stream) (pond)
    W69 ☑
   assault X92.3 ☑
   following
    dive or jump W16.611 ☑
     striking bottom W16.621 ☑
    fall W16.111 ☑
     striking
      bottom W16.121 ☑
       side W16.131 ☑
   stated as undetermined whether accidental or in-
    tentional Y21.4 ☑
   suicide (attempt) X71.3 ☑
  quarry — *see* Drowning, in, specified place NEC
  quenching tank — *see* Drowning, in, specified place
    NEC
  reservoir — *see* Drowning, in, specified place NEC
  river — *see* Drowning, in, natural water
  sea — *see* Drowning, in, natural water
  specified place NEC W73 ☑
   assault X92.8 ☑
   following
    dive or jump W16.811 ☑
     striking
      bottom W16.821 ☑
       wall W16.831 ☑
    fall W16.311 ☑
     striking
      bottom W16.321 ☑
       wall W16.331 ☑
   stated as undetermined whether accidental or in-
    tentional Y21.8 ☑
   suicide (attempt) X71.8 ☑
  stream — *see* Drowning, in, natural water
  swimming-pool W67 ☑
   assault X92.1 ☑
    following fall X92.2 ☑
   following
    dive or jump W16.511 ☑
     striking
      bottom W16.521 ☑
       wall W16.531 ☑
    fall W16.011 ☑
     striking
      bottom W16.021 ☑
       wall W16.031 ☑
   stated as undetermined whether accidental or in-
    tentional Y21.2 ☑
    following fall Y21.3 ☑
   suicide (attempt) X71.1 ☑
    following fall X71.2 ☑
 war operations — *see* War operations, restriction of
   airway
 resulting from accident to watercraft — *see* Drowning,
   due to, accident, watercraft
 self-inflicted X71.9 ☑
 stated as undetermined whether accidental or intentional
   Y21.9 ☑
 suicide (attempt) X71.9 ☑

E

Earth falling (on) W20.0 ☑
 caused by cataclysmic earth surface movement or eruption — *see* Landslide

Earth (surface) **movement NEC** — *see* Forces of nature,
   earth movement
Earthquake (any injury) X34 ☑
Effect(s) (adverse) **of**
 air pressure (any) — *see* Air, pressure
 cold, excessive (exposure to) — *see* Exposure, cold
 heat (excessive) — *see* Heat
 hot place (weather) — *see* Heat
 insolation X30 ☑
 late — *see* Sequelae
 motion — *see* Motion
 nuclear explosion or weapon in war operations — *see*
   War operations, nuclear weapon
 radiation — *see* Radiation
 travel — *see* Travel
Electric shock (accidental) (by) (in) — *see* Exposure, electric
   current
Electrocution (accidental) — *see* Exposure, electric current
**Endotracheal tube wrongly placed during anesthetic
   procedure**
Entanglement
 in
  bed linen, causing suffocation T71 ☑
  wheel of pedal cycle V19.88 ☑
Entry of foreign body or material — *see* Foreign body
Environmental pollution related condition — *see* category Z57 ☑
Execution, legal (any method) — *see* Legal, intervention
Exhaustion
 cold — *see* Exposure, cold
 due to excessive exertion — *see also* Overexertion
   X50.9 ☑
 heat — *see* Heat
Explosion (accidental) (of) (with secondary fire) W40.9 ☑
 acetylene W40.1 ☑
 aerosol can W36.1 ☑
 air tank (compressed) (in machinery) W36.2 ☑
 aircraft (in transit) (powered) NEC V95.9 ☑
  balloon V96.05 ☑
  fixed wing NEC (private) V95.25 ☑
   commercial V95.35 ☑
  glider V96.25 ☑
   hang V96.15 ☑
   powered V95.15 ☑
  helicopter V95.05 ☑
  in war operations — *see* War operations, destruction
   of aircraft
  microlight V95.15 ☑
  nonpowered V96.9 ☑
   specified NEC V96.8 ☑
  powered NEC V95.8 ☑
  stated as
   homicide (attempt) Y08.81 ☑
   suicide (attempt) X83.0 ☑
  ultralight V95.15 ☑
 anesthetic gas in operating room W40.1 ☑
 antipersonnel bomb W40.8 ☑
  assault X96.0 ☑
  homicide (attempt) X96.0 ☑
  suicide (attempt) X75 ☑
 assault X96.9 ☑
 bicycle tire W37.0 ☑
 blasting (cap) (materials) W40.0 ☑
 boiler (machinery), not on transport vehicle W35 ☑
  on watercraft — *see* Explosion, in, watercraft
 butane W40.1 ☑
 caused by other person X96.9 ☑
 coal gas W40.1 ☑
 detonator W40.0 ☑
 dump (munitions) W40.8 ☑
 dynamite W40.0 ☑
  in
   assault X96.8 ☑
   homicide (attempt) X96.8 ☑
   legal intervention
    injuring
     bystander Y35.112 ☑
     law enforcement personnel Y35.111 ☑
     suspect Y35.113 ☑
     unspecified person Y35.119 ☑
    suicide (attempt) X75 ☑
 explosive (material) W40.9 ☑
  gas W40.1 ☑
  in blasting operation W40.0 ☑
  specified NEC W40.8 ☑

Explosion — *continued*
 explosive — *continued*
  specified — *continued*
   in
    assault X96.8 ☑
    homicide (attempt) X96.8 ☑
    legal intervention
     injuring
      bystander Y35.192 ☑
      law enforcement personnel Y35.191 ☑
      suspect Y35.193 ☑
      unspecified person Y35.199 ☑
    suicide (attempt) X75 ☑
 factory (munitions) W40.8 ☑
 fertilizer bomb W40.8 ☑
  assault X96.3 ☑
  homicide (attempt) X96.3 ☑
  suicide (attempt) X75 ☑
 firearm (parts) NEC W34.19 ☑
  airgun W34.110 ☑
  BB gun W34.110 ☑
  gas, air or spring-operated gun NEC W34.118 ☑
  handgun W32.1 ☑
  hunting rifle W33.12 ☑
  larger firearm W33.10 ☑
   specified NEC W33.19 ☑
  machine gun W33.13 ☑
  paintball gun W34.111 ☑
  pellet gun W34.110 ☑
  shotgun W33.11 ☑
  Very pistol [flare] W34.19 ☑
 fire-damp W40.1 ☑
 fireworks W39 ☑
 gas (coal) (explosive) W40.1 ☑
  cylinder W36.9 ☑
   aerosol can W36.1 ☑
   air tank W36.2 ☑
   pressurized W36.3 ☑
   specified NEC W36.8 ☑
 gasoline (fumes) (tank) not in moving motor vehicle
   W40.1 ☑
  bomb W40.8 ☑
   assault X96.1 ☑
   homicide (attempt) X96.1 ☑
   suicide (attempt) X75 ☑
  in motor vehicle — *see* Accident, transport, by type
   of vehicle
 grain store W40.8 ☑
 grenade W40.8 ☑
  in
   assault X96.8 ☑
   homicide (attempt) X96.8 ☑
   legal intervention
    injuring
     bystander Y35.192 ☑
     law enforcement personnel Y35.191 ☑
     suspect Y35.193 ☑
     unspecified person Y35.199 ☑
    suicide (attempt) X75 ☑
 handgun (parts) — *see* Explosion, firearm, handgun
   (parts)
 homicide (attempt) X96.9 ☑
  antipersonnel bomb — *see* Explosion, antipersonnel
   bomb
  fertilizer bomb — *see* Explosion, fertilizer bomb
  gasoline bomb — *see* Explosion, gasoline bomb
  letter bomb — *see* Explosion, letter bomb
  pipe bomb — *see* Explosion, pipe bomb
  specified NEC X96.8 ☑
 hose, pressurized W37.8 ☑
 hot water heater, tank (in machinery) W35 ☑
  on watercraft — *see* Explosion, in, watercraft
 in, on
  dump W40.8 ☑
  factory W40.8 ☑
  mine (of explosive gases) NEC W40.1 ☑
  watercraft V93.59 ☑
   powered craft V93.53 ☑
    ferry boat V93.51 ☑
    fishing boat V93.52 ☑
    jetskis V93.53 ☑
    liner V93.51 ☑
    merchant ship V93.50 ☑
    passenger ship V93.51 ☑
    sailboat V93.54 ☑
 letter bomb W40.8 ☑

☑ **Additional Character Required — Refer to the Tabular List for Character Selection**

Explosion — *continued*
- letter bomb — *continued*
  - assault X96.2 ☑
  - homicide (attempt) X96.2 ☑
  - suicide (attempt) X75 ☑
- machinery — *see also* Contact, with, by type of machine
  - on board watercraft — *see* Explosion, in, watercraft
  - pressure vessel — *see* Explosion, by type of vessel
- methane W40.1 ☑
- mine W40.1 ☑
- missile NEC W40.8 ☑
- mortar bomb W40.8 ☑
  - in
    - assault X96.8 ☑
    - homicide (attempt) X96.8 ☑
    - legal intervention
      - injuring
        - bystander Y35.192 ☑
        - law enforcement personnel Y35.191 ☑
        - suspect Y35.193 ☑
        - unspecified person Y35.199 ☑
  - suicide (attempt) X75 ☑
- munitions (dump) (factory) W40.8 ☑
- pipe, pressurized W37.8 ☑
  - bomb W40.8 ☑
    - assault X96.4 ☑
    - homicide (attempt) X96.4 ☑
    - suicide (attempt) X75 ☑
- pressure, pressurized
  - cooker W38 ☑
  - gas tank (in machinery) W36.3 ☑
  - hose W37.8 ☑
  - pipe W37.8 ☑
  - specified device NEC W38 ☑
  - tire W37.8 ☑
    - bicycle W37.0 ☑
  - vessel (in machinery) W38 ☑
- propane W40.1 ☑
- self-inflicted X75 ☑
- shell (artillery) NEC W40.8 ☑
  - during war operations — *see* War operations, explosion
  - in
    - legal intervention
      - injuring
        - bystander Y35.122 ☑
        - law enforcement personnel Y35.121 ☑
        - suspect Y35.123 ☑
        - unspecified person Y35.129 ☑
    - war — *see* War operations, explosion
- spacecraft V95.45 ☑
- stated as undetermined whether accidental or intentional Y25 ☑
- steam or water lines (in machinery) W37.8 ☑
- stove W40.9 ☑
- suicide (attempt) X75 ☑
- tire, pressurized W37.8 ☑
  - bicycle W37.0 ☑
- undetermined whether accidental or intentional Y25 ☑
- vehicle tire NEC W37.8 ☑
  - bicycle W37.0 ☑
- war operations — *see* War operations, explosion

Exposure (to) X58 ☑
- air pressure change — *see* Air, pressure
- cold (accidental) (excessive) (extreme) (natural) (place) X31 ☑
  - assault Y08.89 ☑
  - due to
    - man-made conditions W93.8 ☑
      - dry ice (contact) W93.01 ☑
        - inhalation W93.02 ☑
      - liquid air (contact) (hydrogen) (nitrogen) W93.11 ☑
        - inhalation W93.12 ☑
      - refrigeration unit (deep freeze) W93.2 ☑
    - suicide (attempt) X83.2 ☑
    - weather (conditions) X31 ☑
  - homicide (attempt) Y08.89 ☑
  - self-inflicted X83.2 ☑
- due to abandonment or neglect X58 ☑
- electric current W86.8 ☑
  - appliance (faulty) W86.8 ☑
    - domestic W86.0 ☑
  - caused by other person Y08.89 ☑
  - conductor (faulty) W86.1 ☑
  - control apparatus (faulty) W86.1 ☑

Exposure — *continued*
- electric current — *continued*
  - electric power generating plant, distribution station W86.1 ☑
  - electroshock gun — *see* Exposure, electric current, taser
  - high-voltage cable W85 ☑
  - homicide (attempt) Y08.89 ☑
  - legal execution — *see* Legal, intervention, specified means NEC
  - lightning — *see* subcategory T75.0 ☑
  - live rail W86.8 ☑
  - misadventure in medical or surgical procedure in electroshock therapy Y63.4
  - motor (electric) (faulty) W86.8 ☑
    - domestic W86.0 ☑
  - self-inflicted X83.1 ☑
  - specified NEC W86.8 ☑
    - domestic W86.0 ☑
  - stun gun — *see* Exposure, electric current, taser
  - suicide (attempt) X83.1 ☑
  - taser W86.8 ☑
    - assault Y08.89 ☑
    - legal intervention — *see* category Y35 ☑
    - self-harm (intentional) X83.8 ☑
    - undetermined intent Y33 ☑
  - third rail W86.8 ☑
  - transformer (faulty) W86.1 ☑
  - transmission lines W85 ☑
- environmental tobacco smoke X58 ☑
- excessive
  - cold — *see* Exposure, cold
  - heat (natural) NEC X30 ☑
    - man-made W92 ☑
- factor(s) NOS X58 ☑
  - environmental NEC X58 ☑
    - man-made NEC W99 ☑
    - natural NEC — *see* Forces of nature
  - specified NEC X58 ☑
- fire, flames (accidental) X08.8 ☑
  - assault X97 ☑
  - campfire — *see* Exposure, fire, controlled, not in building
  - controlled (in)
    - with ignition (of) clothing — *see also* Ignition, clothes X06.2 ☑
      - nightwear X05 ☑
    - bonfire — *see* Exposure, fire, controlled, not in building
    - brazier (in building or structure) — *see also* Exposure, fire, controlled, building
      - not in building or structure — *see* Exposure, fire, controlled, not in building
    - building or structure X02.0 ☑
      - with
        - fall from building X02.3 ☑
        - from building X02.5 ☑
        - injury due to building collapse X02.2 ☑
        - smoke inhalation X02.1 ☑
        - hit by object from building X02.4 ☑
        - specified mode of injury NEC X02.8 ☑
    - fireplace, furnace or stove — *see* Exposure, fire, controlled, building
    - not in building or structure X03.0 ☑
      - with
        - fall X03.3 ☑
        - smoke inhalation X03.1 ☑
        - hit by object X03.4 ☑
        - specified mode of injury NEC X03.8 ☑
    - trash — *see* Exposure, fire, controlled, not in building
  - fireplace — *see* Exposure, fire, controlled, building
  - fittings or furniture (in building or structure) (uncontrolled) — *see* Exposure, fire, uncontrolled, building
  - forest (uncontrolled) — *see* Exposure, fire, uncontrolled, not in building
  - grass (uncontrolled) — *see* Exposure, fire, uncontrolled, not in building
  - hay (uncontrolled) — *see* Exposure, fire, uncontrolled, not in building
  - homicide (attempt) X97 ☑
  - ignition of highly flammable material X04 ☑
  - in, of, on, starting in
    - machinery — *see* Contact, with, by type of machine

Exposure — *continued*
- fire, flames — *continued*
  - in, of, on, starting in — *continued*
    - motor vehicle (in motion) — *see also* Accident, transport, occupant by type of vehicle V87.8 ☑
      - with collision — *see* Collision
    - railway rolling stock, train, vehicle V81.81 ☑
      - with collision — *see* Accident, transport, railway vehicle occupant
    - streetcar (in motion) V82.8 ☑
      - with collision — *see* Accident, transport, streetcar occupant
    - transport vehicle NEC — *see also* Accident, transport
      - with collision — *see* Collision
    - war operations — *see also* War operations, fire
      - from nuclear explosion — *see* War operations, nuclear weapons
    - watercraft (in transit) (not in transit) V91.09 ☑
      - localized — *see* Burn, on board watercraft, due to, fire on board
      - powered craft V91.03 ☑
        - ferry boat V91.01 ☑
        - fishing boat V91.02 ☑
        - jet skis V91.03 ☑
        - liner V91.01 ☑
        - merchant ship V91.00 ☑
        - passenger ship V91.01 ☑
      - unpowered craft V91.08 ☑
        - canoe V91.05 ☑
        - inflatable V91.06 ☑
        - kayak V91.05 ☑
        - sailboat V91.04 ☑
        - surf-board V91.08 ☑
        - waterskis V91.07 ☑
        - windsurfer V91.08 ☑
  - lumber (uncontrolled) — *see* Exposure, fire, uncontrolled, not in building
  - mine (uncontrolled) — *see* Exposure, fire, uncontrolled, not in building
  - prairie (uncontrolled) — *see* Exposure, fire, uncontrolled, not in building
  - resulting from
    - explosion — *see* Explosion
    - lightning X08.8 ☑
  - self-inflicted X76 ☑
  - specified NEC X08.8 ☑
  - started by other person X97 ☑
  - stated as undetermined whether accidental or intentional Y26 ☑
  - stove — *see* Exposure, fire, controlled, building
  - suicide (attempt) X76 ☑
  - tunnel (uncontrolled) — *see* Exposure, fire, uncontrolled, not in building
  - uncontrolled
    - in building or structure X00.0 ☑
      - with
        - fall from building X00.3 ☑
        - injury due to building collapse X00.2 ☑
        - jump from building X00.5 ☑
        - smoke inhalation X00.1 ☑
      - bed X08.00 ☑
        - due to
          - cigarette X08.01 ☑
          - specified material NEC X08.09 ☑
      - furniture NEC X08.20 ☑
        - due to
          - cigarette X08.21 ☑
          - specified material NEC X08.29 ☑
      - hit by object from building X00.4 ☑
      - sofa X08.10 ☑
        - due to
          - cigarette X08.11 ☑
          - specified material NEC X08.19 ☑
      - specified mode of injury NEC X00.8 ☑
    - not in building or structure (any) X01.0 ☑
      - with
        - fall X01.3 ☑
        - smoke inhalation X01.1 ☑
        - hit by object X01.4 ☑
        - specified mode of injury NEC X01.8 ☑
    - undetermined whether accidental or intentional Y26 ☑
- forces of nature NEC — *see* Forces of nature
- G-forces (abnormal) W49.9 ☑

Exposure — *continued*
gravitational forces (abnormal) W49.9 ☑
heat (natural) NEC — *see* Heat
high-pressure jet (hydraulic) (pneumatic) W49.9 ☑
hydraulic jet W49.9 ☑
inanimate mechanical force W49.9 ☑
jet, high-pressure (hydraulic) (pneumatic) W49.9 ☑
lightning — *see* subcategory T75.0 ☑
   causing fire — *see* Exposure, fire
mechanical forces NEC W49.9 ☑
   animate NEC W64 ☑
   inanimate NEC W49.9 ☑
noise W42.9 ☑
   supersonic W42.0 ☑
noxious substance — *see* Table of Drugs and Chemicals
pneumatic jet W49.9 ☑
prolonged in deep-freeze unit or refrigerator W93.2 ☑
radiation — *see* Radiation
smoke — *see also* Exposure, fire
   tobacco, second hand Z77.22
specified factors NEC X58 ☑
sunlight X32 ☑
   man-made (sun lamp) W89.8 ☑
      tanning bed W89.1 ☑
supersonic waves W42.0 ☑
transmission line(s), electric W85 ☑
vibration W49.9 ☑
waves
   infrasound W49.9 ☑
   sound W42.9 ☑
   supersonic — *see* Forces of nature
weather NEC — *see* Forces of nature

External cause status Y99.9
child assisting in compensated work for family Y99.8
civilian activity done for financial or other compensation Y99.0
civilian activity done for income or pay Y99.0
family member assisting in compensated work for other family member Y99.8
hobby not done for income Y99.8
leisure activity Y99.8
military activity Y99.1
off-duty activity of military personnel Y99.8
recreation or sport not for income or while a student Y99.8
specified NEC Y99.8
student activity Y99.8
volunteer activity Y99.2

F

Factors, supplemental
alcohol
   blood level
      less than 20mg/100ml Y90.0
      presence in blood, level not specified Y90.9
      20-39mg/100ml Y90.1
      40-59mg/100ml Y90.2
      60-79mg/100ml Y90.3
      80-99mg/100ml Y90.4
      100-119mg/100ml Y90.5
      120-199mg/100ml Y90.6
      200-239mg/100ml Y90.7
      240mg/100ml or more Y90.8
   presence in blood, but level not specified Y90.9
environmental-pollution-related condition- see Z57 ☑
nosocomial condition Y95
work-related condition Y99.0

Failure
in suture or ligature during surgical procedure Y65.2
mechanical, of instrument or apparatus (any) (during any medical or surgical procedure) Y65.8
sterile precautions (during medical and surgical care) — *see* Misadventure, failure, sterile precautions, by type of procedure
to
   introduce tube or instrument Y65.4
      endotracheal tube during anesthesia Y65.3
   make curve (transport vehicle) NEC — *see* Accident, transport
   remove tube or instrument Y65.4

Fall, falling (accidental) W19 ☑
building W20.1 ☑
   burning (uncontrolled fire) X00.3 ☑
down
   embankment W17.81 ☑
   escalator W10.0 ☑

Fall, falling — *continued*
down — *continued*
   hill W17.81 ☑
   ladder W11 ☑
   ramp W10.2 ☑
   stairs, steps W10.9 ☑
due to
   bumping against
      object W18.00 ☑
         sharp glass W18.02 ☑
         specified NEC W18.09 ☑
         sports equipment W18.01 ☑
      person W03 ☑
         due to ice or snow W00.0 ☑
         on pedestrian conveyance — *see* Accident, transport, pedestrian, conveyance
   collision with another person W03 ☑
      due to ice or snow W00.0 ☑
      involving pedestrian conveyance — *see* Accident, transport, pedestrian, conveyance
   grocery cart tipping over W17.82 ☑
   ice or snow W00.9 ☑
      from one level to another W00.2 ☑
      on stairs or steps W00.1 ☑
      involving pedestrian conveyance — *see* Accident, transport, pedestrian, conveyance
      on same level W00.0 ☑
   slipping (on moving sidewalk) W01.0 ☑
      with subsequent striking against object W01.10 ☑
         furniture W01.190 ☑
         sharp object W01.119 ☑
            glass W01.110 ☑
            power tool or machine W01.111 ☑
            specified NEC W01.118 ☑
         specified NEC W01.198 ☑
   striking against
      object W18.00 ☑
         sharp glass W18.02 ☑
         specified NEC W18.09 ☑
         sports equipment W18.01 ☑
      person W03 ☑
         due to ice or snow W00.0 ☑
         on pedestrian conveyance — *see* Accident, transport, pedestrian, conveyance
earth (with asphyxia or suffocation (by pressure)) — *see* Earth, falling
from, off, out of
   aircraft NEC (with accident to aircraft NEC) V97.0 ☑
      while boarding or alighting V97.1 ☑
   balcony W13.0 ☑
   bed W06 ☑
   boat, ship, watercraft NEC (with drowning or submersion) — *see* Drowning, due to, fall overboard
      with hitting bottom or object V94.0 ☑
   bridge W13.1 ☑
   building W13.9 ☑
      burning (uncontrolled fire) X00.3 ☑
   cavity W17.2 ☑
   chair W07 ☑
   cherry picker W17.89 ☑
   cliff W15 ☑
   dock W17.4 ☑
   embankment W17.81 ☑
   escalator W10.0 ☑
   flagpole W13.8 ☑
   furniture NEC W08 ☑
   grocery cart W17.82 ☑
   haystack W17.89 ☑
   high place NEC W17.89 ☑
      stated as undetermined whether accidental or intentional Y30 ☑
   hole W17.2 ☑
   incline W10.2 ☑
   ladder W11 ☑
   lifting device W17.89 ☑
   machine, machinery — *see also* Contact, with, by type of machine
      not in operation W17.89 ☑
   manhole W17.1 ☑
   mobile elevated work platform [MEWP] W17.89 ☑
   motorized mobility scooter W05.2 ☑
   one level to another NEC W17.89 ☑
      intentional, purposeful, suicide (attempt) X80 ☑
      stated as undetermined whether accidental or intentional Y30 ☑
   pit W17.2 ☑

Fall, falling — *continued*
from, off, out of — *continued*
   playground equipment W09.8 ☑
      jungle gym W09.2 ☑
      slide W09.0 ☑
      swing W09.1 ☑
   quarry W17.89 ☑
   railing W13.9 ☑
   ramp W10.2 ☑
   roof W13.2 ☑
   scaffolding W12 ☑
   scooter (nonmotorized) W05.1 ☑
      motorized mobility W05.2 ☑
   sky lift W17.89 ☑
   stairs, steps W10.9 ☑
      curb W10.1 ☑
      due to ice or snow W00.1 ☑
      escalator W10.0 ☑
      incline W10.2 ☑
      ramp W10.2 ☑
      sidewalk curb W10.1 ☑
      specified NEC W10.8 ☑
      standing
         electric scooter V00.841 ☑
         micro-mobility pedestrian conveyance V00.848 ☑
   stepladder W11 ☑
   stool W08 ☑
   storm drain W17.1 ☑
   streetcar NEC V82.6 ☑
      while boarding or alighting V82.4 ☑
      with antecedent collision — *see* Accident, transport, streetcar occupant
   structure NEC W13.8 ☑
      burning (uncontrolled fire) X00.3 ☑
   table W08 ☑
   toilet W18.11 ☑
      with subsequent striking against object W18.12 ☑
   train NEC V81.6 ☑
      during derailment (without antecedent collision) V81.7 ☑
      with antecedent collision — *see* Accident, transport, railway vehicle occupant
      while boarding or alighting V81.4 ☑
   transport vehicle after collision — *see* Accident, transport, by type of vehicle, collision
   tree W14 ☑
   vehicle (in motion) NEC — *see also* Accident, transport V89.9 ☑
      motor NEC — *see also* Accident, transport, occupant, by type of vehicle V87.8 ☑
      stationary W17.89 ☑
         while boarding or alighting — *see* Accident, transport, by type of vehicle, while boarding or alighting
   viaduct W13.8 ☑
   wall W13.8 ☑
   watercraft — *see also* Drowning, due to, fall overboard
      with hitting bottom or object V94.0 ☑
   well W17.0 ☑
   wheelchair, non-moving W05.0 ☑
      powered — *see* Accident, transport, pedestrian, conveyance occupant, specified type NEC
   window W13.4 ☑
in, on
   aircraft NEC V97.0 ☑
      while boarding or alighting V97.1 ☑
      with accident to aircraft V97.0 ☑
   bathtub (empty) W18.2 ☑
      filled W16.212 ☑
         causing drowning W16.211 ☑
   escalator W10.0 ☑
   incline W10.2 ☑
   ladder W11 ☑
   machine, machinery — *see* Contact, with, by type of machine
   object, edged, pointed or sharp (with cut) — *see* Fall, by type
   playground equipment W09.8 ☑
      jungle gym W09.2 ☑
      slide W09.0 ☑
      swing W09.1 ☑
   ramp W10.2 ☑
   scaffolding W12 ☑
   shower W18.2 ☑
      causing drowning W16.211 ☑

Fall, falling — *continued*
  in, on — *continued*
    staircase, stairs, steps W10.9 ☑
      curb W10.1 ☑
      due to ice or snow W00.1 ☑
      escalator W10.0 ☑
      incline W10.2 ☑
      specified NEC W10.8 ☑
    streetcar (without antecedent collision) V82.5 ☑
      with antecedent collision — *see* Accident, transport, streetcar occupant
      while boarding or alighting V82.4 ☑
    train (without antecedent collision) V81.5 ☑
      with antecedent collision — *see* Accident, transport, railway vehicle occupant
      during derailment (without antecedent collision) V81.7 ☑
        with antecedent collision — *see* Accident, transport, railway vehicle occupant
      while boarding or alighting V81.4 ☑
    transport vehicle after collision — *see* Accident, transport, by type of vehicle, collision
    watercraft V93.39 ☑
      due to
        accident to craft V91.29 ☑
          powered craft V91.23 ☑
            ferry boat V91.21 ☑
            fishing boat V91.22 ☑
            jetskis V91.23 ☑
            liner V91.21 ☑
            merchant ship V91.20 ☑
            passenger ship V91.21 ☑
          unpowered craft
            canoe V91.25 ☑
            inflatable V91.26 ☑
            kayak V91.25 ☑
            sailboat V91.24 ☑
      powered craft V93.33 ☑
        ferry boat V93.31 ☑
        fishing boat V93.32 ☑
        jetskis V93.33 ☑
        liner V93.31 ☑
        merchant ship V93.30 ☑
        passenger ship V93.31 ☑
      unpowered craft V93.38 ☑
        canoe V93.35 ☑
        inflatable V93.36 ☑
        kayak V93.35 ☑
        sailboat V93.34 ☑
        surf-board V93.38 ☑
        windsurfer V93.38 ☑
  into
    cavity W17.2 ☑
    dock W17.4 ☑
    fire — *see* Exposure, fire, by type
    haystack W17.89 ☑
    hole W17.2 ☑
    lake — *see* Fall, into, water
    manhole W17.1 ☑
    moving part of machinery — *see* Contact, with, by type of machine
    ocean — *see* Fall, into, water
    opening in surface NEC W17.89 ☑
    pit W17.2 ☑
    pond — *see* Fall, into, water
    quarry W17.89 ☑
    river — *see* Fall, into, water
    shaft W17.89 ☑
    storm drain W17.1 ☑
    stream — *see* Fall, into, water
    swimming pool — *see also* Fall, into, water, in, swimming pool
      empty W17.3 ☑
    tank W17.89 ☑
    water W16.42 ☑
      causing drowning W16.41 ☑
      from watercraft — *see* Drowning, due to, fall overboard
      hitting diving board W21.4 ☑
      in
        bathtub W16.212 ☑
          causing drowning W16.211 ☑
        bucket W16.222 ☑
          causing drowning W16.221 ☑
        natural body of water W16.112 ☑
          causing drowning W16.111 ☑

Fall, falling — *continued*
  into — *continued*
    water — *continued*
      in — *continued*
        natural body of water — *continued*
          striking
            bottom W16.122 ☑
              causing drowning W16.121 ☑
            side W16.132 ☑
              causing drowning W16.131 ☑
        specified water NEC W16.312 ☑
          causing drowning W16.311 ☑
          striking
            bottom W16.322 ☑
              causing drowning W16.321 ☑
            wall W16.332 ☑
              causing drowning W16.331 ☑
        swimming pool W16.012 ☑
          causing drowning W16.011 ☑
          striking
            bottom W16.022 ☑
              causing drowning W16.031 ☑
            wall W16.032 ☑
              causing drowning W16.021 ☑
        utility bucket W16.222 ☑
          causing drowning W16.221 ☑
    well W17.0 ☑
  involving
    bed W06 ☑
    chair W07 ☑
    furniture NEC W08 ☑
    glass — *see* Fall, by type
    playground equipment W09.8 ☑
      jungle gym W09.2 ☑
      slide W09.0 ☑
      swing W09.1 ☑
    roller blades — *see* Accident, transport, pedestrian, conveyance
    skateboard(s) — *see* Accident, transport, pedestrian, conveyance
    skates (ice) (in line) (roller) — *see* Accident, transport, pedestrian, conveyance
    skis — *see* Accident, transport, pedestrian, conveyance
    table W08 ☑
    wheelchair, non-moving W05.0 ☑
      powered — *see* Accident, transport, pedestrian, conveyance, specified type NEC
  object — *see* Struck by, object, falling
  off
    toilet W18.11 ☑
      with subsequent striking against object W18.12 ☑
  on same level W18.30 ☑
    due to
      specified NEC W18.39 ☑
      stepping on an object W18.31 ☑
  out of
    bed W06 ☑
    building NEC W13.8 ☑
    chair W07 ☑
    furniture NEC W08 ☑
    wheelchair, non-moving W05.0 ☑
      powered — *see* Accident, transport, pedestrian, conveyance, specified type NEC
    window W13.4 ☑
  over
    animal W01.0 ☑
    cliff W15 ☑
    embankment W17.81 ☑
    small object W01.0 ☑
  rock W20.8 ☑
  same level W18.30 ☑
    from
      being crushed, pushed, or stepped on by a crowd or human stampede W52 ☑
      collision, pushing, shoving, by or with other person W03 ☑
      slipping, stumbling, tripping W01.0 ☑
    involving ice or snow W00.0 ☑
      involving skates (ice) (roller), skateboard, skis — *see* Accident, transport, pedestrian, conveyance
  snowslide (avalanche) — *see* Landslide
  stone W20.8 ☑
  structure W20.1 ☑
    burning (uncontrolled fire) X00.3 ☑

Fall, falling — *continued*
  through
    bridge W13.1 ☑
    floor W13.3 ☑
    roof W13.2 ☑
    wall W13.8 ☑
    window W13.4 ☑
  timber W20.8 ☑
  tree (caused by lightning) W20.8 ☑
  while being carried or supported by other person(s) W04 ☑
Fallen on by
  animal (not being ridden) NEC W55.89 ☑
Felo-de-se — *see* Suicide
Fight (hand) (fists) (foot) — *see* Assault, fight
Fire (accidental) — *see* Exposure, fire
Firearm discharge — *see* Discharge, firearm
Fireball effects from nuclear explosion in war operations
      — *see* War operations, nuclear weapons
Fireworks (explosion) W39 ☑
Flash burns from explosion — *see* Explosion
Flood (any injury) (caused by) X38 ☑
  collapse of man-made structure causing earth movement X36.0 ☑
  tidal wave — *see* Forces of nature, tidal wave
Food (any type) **in**
  air passages (with asphyxia, obstruction, or suffocation) — *see* categories T17 and T18 ☑
  alimentary tract causing asphyxia (due to compression of trachea) — *see* categories T17 and T18 ☑
Forces of nature X39.8 ☑
  avalanche X36.1 ☑
    causing transport accident — *see* Accident, transport, by type of vehicle
  blizzard X37.2 ☑
  cataclysmic storm X37.9 ☑
    with flood X38 ☑
    blizzard X37.2 ☑
    cloudburst X37.8 ☑
    cyclone X37.1 ☑
    dust storm X37.3 ☑
    hurricane X37.0 ☑
    specified storm NEC X37.8 ☑
    storm surge X37.0 ☑
    tornado X37.1 ☑
    twister X37.1 ☑
    typhoon X37.0 ☑
  cloudburst X37.8 ☑
  cold (natural) X31 ☑
  cyclone X37.1 ☑
  dam collapse causing earth movement X36.0 ☑
  dust storm X37.3 ☑
  earth movement X36.1 ☑
    caused by dam or structure collapse X36.0 ☑
    earthquake X34 ☑
  earthquake X34 ☑
  flood (caused by) X38 ☑
    dam collapse X36.0 ☑
    tidal wave — *see* Forces of nature, tidal wave
  heat (natural) X30 ☑
  hurricane X37.0 ☑
  landslide X36.1 ☑
    causing transport accident — *see* Accident, transport, by type of vehicle
  lightning — *see* subcategory T75.0 ☑
    causing fire — *see* Exposure, fire
  mudslide X36.1 ☑
    causing transport accident — *see* Accident, transport, by type of vehicle
  radiation (natural) X39.08 ☑
    radon X39.01 ☑
  radon X39.01 ☑
  specified force NEC X39.8 ☑
  storm surge X37.0 ☑
  structure collapse causing earth movement X36.0 ☑
  sunlight X32 ☑
  tidal wave X37.41 ☑
    due to
      earthquake X37.41 ☑
      landslide X37.43 ☑
      storm X37.42 ☑
      volcanic eruption X37.41 ☑
  tornado X37.1 ☑
  tsunami X37.41 ☑
  twister X37.1 ☑
  typhoon X37.0 ☑

Forces of nature — *continued*
  volcanic eruption X35 ☑
Foreign body
  aspiration — *see* Index to Diseases and Injuries, Foreign body, respiratory tract
  embedded in skin W45 ☑
  entering through
    natural orifice W44.9 ☑
      audio device W44.G1 ☑
      battery W44.A0 ☑
        button W44.A1 ☑
        cylindrical W44.A9 ☑
        other specified NEC W44.A9 ☑
      bezoar W44.F1 ☑
      bottle cap W44.E9 ☑
      can lid W44.E9 ☑
      combination metal and plastic
        jewelry W44.G3 ☑
        toy and toy part W44.G2 ☑
      dagger W44.H2 ☑
      dart W44.H1 ☑
      ear buds W44.G1 ☑
      food W44.F3 ☑
      glass W44.C0 ☑
        intact W44.C2 ☑
          bottle W44.C2 ☑
        shard W44.C1 ☑
        sharp W44.C1 ☑
      hearing aids W44.G1 ☑
      insect W44.F4 ☑
      knife W44.H2 ☑
      magnetic metal W44.D0 ☑
        bead W44.D1 ☑
        coin W44.D2 ☑
        jewelry W44.D4 ☑
        object specified NEC W44.D9 ☑
        toy W44.D3 ☑
      needle (hypodermic) (sewing) W44.H1 ☑
      non-magnetic metal W44.E0 ☑
        bead W44.E1 ☑
        coin W44.E2 ☑
        jewelry W44.E4 ☑
        object specified NEC W44.E9 ☑
        toy W44.E3 ☑
      objects of natural or organic material W44.F0 ☑
        specified NEC W44.F9 ☑
      other
        non-organic objects W44.G0 ☑
          specified NEC W44.G9 ☑
        sharp object unspecified W44.H0 ☑
      plastic
        bead W44.B1 ☑
        bottle W44.B5 ☑
        coin W44.B2 ☑
        jewelry W44.B4 ☑
        object W44.B0 ☑
          specified NEC W44.B9 ☑
        toy and toy part W44.B3 ☑
      pull tab W44.E9 ☑
      rubber band W44.F2 ☑
      safety pin W44.H1 ☑
      specified NEC W44.8 ☑
      sword W44.H2 ☑
    skin W45.8 ☑
      can lid W26.8 ☑
      nail W45.0 ☑
      paper W26.2 ☑
      specified NEC W45.8 ☑
      splinter W45.8 ☑
Forest fire (exposure to) — *see* Exposure, fire, uncontrolled, not in building
Found injured X58 ☑
  from exposure (to) — *see* Exposure
  on
    highway, road(way), street V89.9 ☑
    railway right of way V81.9 ☑
Fracture (circumstances unknown or unspecified) X58 ☑
  due to specified cause NEC X58 ☑
Freezing — *see* Exposure, cold
Frostbite X31 ☑
  due to man-made conditions — *see* Exposure, cold, man-made
Frozen — *see* Exposure, cold

G

Gored by bull W55.22 ☑
Gunshot wound W34.00 ☑

H

Hailstones, injured by X39.8 ☑
Hanged herself or himself — *see* Hanging, self-inflicted
Hanging (accidental) — *see also* category T71 ☑
  legal execution — *see* Legal, intervention, specified means NEC
Heat (effects of) (excessive) X30 ☑
  due to
    man-made conditions W92 ☑
      on board watercraft V93.29 ☑
        fishing boat V93.22 ☑
        merchant ship V93.20 ☑
        passenger ship V93.21 ☑
        sailboat V93.24 ☑
        specified powered craft NEC V93.23 ☑
    weather (conditions) X30 ☑
  from
    electric heating apparatus causing burning X16 ☑
    nuclear explosion in war operations — *see* War operations, nuclear weapons
  inappropriate in local application or packing in medical or surgical procedure Y63.5
Hemorrhage
  delayed following medical or surgical treatment without mention of misadventure — *see* Index to Diseases and Injuries, Complication(s)
  during medical or surgical treatment as misadventure — *see* Index to Diseases and Injuries, Complication(s)
High
  altitude (effects) — *see* Air, pressure, low
  level of radioactivity, effects — *see* Radiation
  pressure (effects) — *see* Air, pressure, high
  temperature, effects — *see* Heat
Hit, hitting (accidental) by — *see* Struck by
Hitting against — *see* Striking against
Homicide (attempt) (justifiable) — *see* Assault
Hot
  place, effects — *see also* Heat
  weather, effects X30 ☑
House fire (uncontrolled) — *see* Exposure, fire, uncontrolled, building
Humidity, causing problem X39.8 ☑
Hunger X58 ☑
Hurricane (any injury) X37.0 ☑
Hypobarism, hypobaropathy — *see* Air, pressure, low

I

Ictus
  caloris — *see also* Heat
  solaris X30 ☑
Ignition (accidental) — *see also* Exposure, fire X08.8 ☑
  anesthetic gas in operating room W40.1 ☑
  apparel X06.2 ☑
    from highly flammable material X04 ☑
    nightwear X05 ☑
  bed linen (sheets) (spreads) (pillows) (mattress) — *see* Exposure, fire, uncontrolled, building, bed
  benzine X04 ☑
  clothes, clothing NEC (from controlled fire) X06.2 ☑
    from
      highly flammable material X04 ☑
  ether X04 ☑
    in operating room W40.1 ☑
  explosive material — *see* Explosion
  gasoline X04 ☑
  jewelry (plastic) (any) X06.0 ☑
  kerosene X04 ☑
  material
    explosive — *see* Explosion
    highly flammable with secondary explosion X04 ☑
  nightwear X05 ☑
  paraffin X04 ☑
  petrol X04 ☑
Immersion (accidental) — *see also* Drowning
  hand or foot due to cold (excessive) X31 ☑
Implantation of quills of porcupine W55.89 ☑
Inanition (from) (hunger) X58 ☑

Inanition — *continued*
  thirst X58 ☑
Inappropriate operation performed
  correct operation on wrong side or body part (wrong side) (wrong site) Y65.53
  operation intended for another patient done on wrong patient Y65.52
  wrong operation performed on correct patient Y65.51
Inattention after, at birth (homicidal intent) (infanticidal intent) X58 ☑
Incident, adverse
  device
    anesthesiology Y70.8
      accessory Y70.2
      diagnostic Y70.0
      miscellaneous Y70.8
      monitoring Y70.0
      prosthetic Y70.2
      rehabilitative Y70.1
      surgical Y70.3
      therapeutic Y70.1
    cardiovascular Y71.8
      accessory Y71.2
      diagnostic Y71.0
      miscellaneous Y71.8
      monitoring Y71.0
      prosthetic Y71.2
      rehabilitative Y71.1
      surgical Y71.3
      therapeutic Y71.1
    gastroenterology Y73.8
      accessory Y73.2
      diagnostic Y73.0
      miscellaneous Y73.8
      monitoring Y73.0
      prosthetic Y73.2
      rehabilitative Y73.1
      surgical Y73.3
      therapeutic Y73.1
    general
      hospital Y74.8
        accessory Y74.2
        diagnostic Y74.0
        miscellaneous Y74.8
        monitoring Y74.0
        prosthetic Y74.2
        rehabilitative Y74.1
        surgical Y74.3
        therapeutic Y74.1
      surgical Y81.8
        accessory Y81.2
        diagnostic Y81.0
        miscellaneous Y81.8
        monitoring Y81.0
        prosthetic Y81.2
        rehabilitative Y81.1
        surgical Y81.3
        therapeutic Y81.1
    gynecological Y76.8
      accessory Y76.2
      diagnostic Y76.0
      miscellaneous Y76.8
      monitoring Y76.0
      prosthetic Y76.2
      rehabilitative Y76.1
      surgical Y76.3
      therapeutic Y76.1
    medical Y82.9
      specified type NEC Y82.8
    neurological Y75.8
      accessory Y75.2
      diagnostic Y75.0
      miscellaneous Y75.8
      monitoring Y75.0
      prosthetic Y75.2
      rehabilitative Y75.1
      surgical Y75.3
      therapeutic Y75.1
    obstetrical Y76.8
      accessory Y76.2
      diagnostic Y76.0
      miscellaneous Y76.8
      monitoring Y76.0
      prosthetic Y76.2
      rehabilitative Y76.1
      surgical Y76.3
      therapeutic Y76.1
    ophthalmic Y77.8
      accessory Y77.2

Incident, adverse — *continued*
 device — *continued*
  ophthalmic — *continued*
   contact lens (rigid gas permeable) (soft (hy-
    drophilic)) Y77.11
   diagnostic Y77.0
   miscellaneous Y77.8
   monitoring Y77.0
   prosthetic Y77.2
   rehabilitative Y77.19
   surgical Y77.3
   therapeutic Y77.19
  orthopedic Y79.8
   accessory Y79.2
   diagnostic Y79.0
   miscellaneous Y79.8
   monitoring Y79.0
   prosthetic Y79.2
   rehabilitative Y79.1
   surgical Y79.3
   therapeutic Y79.1
  otorhinolaryngological Y72.8
   accessory Y72.2
   diagnostic Y72.0
   miscellaneous Y72.8
   monitoring Y72.0
   prosthetic Y72.2
   rehabilitative Y72.1
   surgical Y72.3
   therapeutic Y72.1
  personal use Y74.8
   accessory Y74.2
   diagnostic Y74.0
   miscellaneous Y74.8
   monitoring Y74.0
   prosthetic Y74.2
   rehabilitative Y74.1
   surgical Y74.3
   therapeutic Y74.1
  physical medicine Y80.8
   accessory Y80.2
   diagnostic Y80.0
   miscellaneous Y80.8
   monitoring Y80.0
   prosthetic Y80.2
   rehabilitative Y80.1
   surgical Y80.3
   therapeutic Y80.1
  plastic surgical Y81.8
   accessory Y81.2
   diagnostic Y81.0
   miscellaneous Y81.8
   monitoring Y81.0
   prosthetic Y81.2
   rehabilitative Y81.1
   surgical Y81.3
   therapeutic Y81.1
  radiological Y78.8
   accessory Y78.2
   diagnostic Y78.0
   miscellaneous Y78.8
   monitoring Y78.0
   prosthetic Y78.2
   rehabilitative Y78.1
   surgical Y78.3
   therapeutic Y78.1
  urology Y73.8
   accessory Y73.2
   diagnostic Y73.0
   miscellaneous Y73.8
   monitoring Y73.0
   prosthetic Y73.2
   rehabilitative Y73.1
   surgical Y73.3
   therapeutic Y73.1
Incineration (accidental) — *see* Exposure, fire
Infanticide — *see* Assault
Infrasound waves (causing injury) W49.9 ✓
Ingestion
 foreign body (causing injury) (with obstruction) — *see*
  Foreign body, alimentary canal
 poisonous
  plant(s) X58 ✓
  substance NEC — *see* Table of Drugs and Chemicals
Inhalation
 excessively cold substance, man-made — *see* Exposure,
  cold, man-made

Inhalation — *continued*
 food (any type) (into respiratory tract) (with asphyxia,
  obstruction respiratory tract, suffocation) — *see*
  categories T17 and T18 ✓
 foreign body — *see* Foreign body, aspiration
 gastric contents (with asphyxia, obstruction respiratory
  passage, suffocation) T17.81- ✓
 hot air or gases X14.0 ✓
 liquid air, hydrogen, nitrogen W93.12 ✓
  suicide (attempt) X83.2 ✓
 steam X13.0 ✓
  assault X98.0 ✓
  stated as undetermined whether accidental or intentional Y27.0 ✓
  suicide (attempt) X77.0 ✓
 toxic gas — *see* Table of Drugs and Chemicals
 vomitus (with asphyxia, obstruction respiratory passage,
  suffocation) T17.81- ✓
Injury, injured (accidental(ly)) NOS X58 ✓
 by, caused by, from
  assault — *see* Assault
  law-enforcing agent, police, in course of legal intervention — *see* Legal intervention
  suicide (attempt) X83.8 ✓
 due to, in
  civil insurrection — *see* War operations
  fight — *see also* Assault, fight Y04.0 ✓
  war operations — *see* War operations
 homicide — *see also* Assault Y09
 inflicted (by)
  in course of arrest (attempted), suppression of disturbance, maintenance of order, by law-enforcing
   agents — *see* Legal intervention
  other person
   stated as
    accidental X58 ✓
    intentional, homicide (attempt) — *see* Assault
    undetermined whether accidental or intention-
     al Y33 ✓
  purposely (inflicted) by other person(s) — *see* Assault
  self-inflicted X83.8 ✓
   stated as accidental X58 ✓
  specified cause NEC X58 ✓
  undetermined whether accidental or intentional Y33 ✓
Insolation, effects X30 ✓
Insufficient nourishment X58 ✓
Interruption of respiration (by)
 food (lodged in esophagus) — *see* categories T17 and
  T18 ✓
 vomitus (lodged in esophagus) T17.81- ✓
Intervention, legal — *see* Legal intervention
Intoxication
 drug — *see* Table of Drugs and Chemicals
 poison — *see* Table of Drugs and Chemicals

J

Jammed (accidentally)
 between objects (moving) (stationary and moving)
  W23.0 ✓
  stationary W23.1 ✓
Jumped, jumping
 before moving object NEC X81.8 ✓
  motor vehicle X81.0 ✓
  subway train X81.1 ✓
  train X81.1 ✓
  undetermined whether accidental or intentional
   Y31 ✓
 from
  boat (into water) voluntarily, without accident (to or
   on boat) W16.712 ✓
   striking bottom W16.722 ✓
    causing drowning W16.721 ✓
   with
    accident to or on boat — *see* Accident, water-
     craft
    drowning or submersion W16.711 ✓
     suicide (attempt) X71.3 ✓
  building — *see also* Jumped, from, high place
   W13.9 ✓
   burning (uncontrolled fire) X00.5 ✓
  high place NEC W17.89 ✓
   suicide (attempt) X80 ✓
   undetermined whether accidental or intentional
    Y30 ✓
  structure — *see also* Jumped, from, high place
   W13.9 ✓

Jumped, jumping — *continued*
 from — *continued*
  structure — *see also* Jumped, from, high place —
   continued
   burning (uncontrolled fire) X00.5 ✓
 into water W16.92 ✓
  causing drowning W16.91 ✓
  from, off watercraft — *see* Jumped, from, boat
  in
   natural body W16.612 ✓
    causing drowning W16.611 ✓
    striking bottom W16.622 ✓
     causing drowning W16.621 ✓
   specified place NEC W16.812 ✓
    causing drowning W16.811 ✓
    striking
     bottom W16.822 ✓
      causing drowning W16.821 ✓
     wall W16.832 ✓
      causing drowning W16.831 ✓
   swimming pool W16.512 ✓
    causing drowning W16.511 ✓
    striking
     bottom W16.522 ✓
      causing drowning W16.521 ✓
     wall W16.532 ✓
      causing drowning W16.531 ✓
  suicide (attempt) X71.3 ✓

K

Kicked by
 animal NEC W55.82 ✓
 person(s) (accidentally) W50.1 ✓
  with intent to injure or kill Y04.0 ✓
  as, or caused by, a crowd or human stampede (with
   fall) W52 ✓
  assault Y04.0 ✓
  homicide (attempt) Y04.0 ✓
  in
   fight Y04.0 ✓
   legal intervention
    injuring
     bystander Y35.812 ✓
     law enforcement personnel Y35.811 ✓
     suspect Y35.813 ✓
     unspecified person Y35.819 ✓
Kicking
 against
  object W22.8 ✓
   sports equipment W21.9 ✓
   stationary W22.09 ✓
    sports equipment W21.89 ✓
  person — *see* Striking against, person
  sports equipment W21.9 ✓
 carpet stretcher with knee X50.3 ✓
Killed, killing (accidentally) NOS — *see also* Injury X58 ✓
 in
  action — *see* War operations
  brawl, fight (hand) (fists) (foot) Y04.0 ✓
   by weapon — *see also* Assault
    cutting, piercing — *see* Assault, cutting or
     piercing instrument
    firearm — *see* Discharge, firearm, by type,
     homicide
 self
  stated as
   accident NOS X58 ✓
   suicide — *see* Suicide
   undetermined whether accidental or intentional
    Y33 ✓
Kneeling (prolonged (static)) X50.1 ✓
Knocked down (accidentally) (by) NOS X58 ✓
 animal (not being ridden) NEC — *see also* Struck by, by
  type of animal
 crowd or human stampede W52 ✓
 person W51 ✓
  in brawl, fight Y04.0 ✓
 transport vehicle NEC — *see also* Accident, transport
  V09.9 ✓

L

Laceration NEC — *see* Injury
Lack of
 care (helpless person) (infant) (newborn) X58 ✓

✓ **Additional Character Required — Refer to the Tabular List for Character Selection**

Lack of — *continued*
  food except as result of abandonment or neglect X58 ☑
    due to abandonment or neglect X58 ☑
  water except as result of transport accident X58 ☑
    due to transport accident — *see* Accident, transport, by type
  helpless person, infant, newborn X58 ☑
Landslide (falling on transport vehicle) X36.1 ☑
  caused by collapse of man-made structure X36.0 ☑
Late effect — *see* Sequelae
Legal
  execution (any method) — *see* Legal, intervention
  intervention (by)
    baton — *see* Legal, intervention, blunt object, baton
    bayonet — *see* Legal, intervention, sharp object, bayonet
    blow — *see* Legal, intervention, manhandling
    blunt object
      baton
        injuring
          bystander Y35.312 ☑
          law enforcement personnel Y35.311 ☑
          suspect Y35.313 ☑
          unspecified person Y35.319 ☑
      injuring
        bystander Y35.302 ☑
        law enforcement personnel Y35.301 ☑
        suspect Y35.303 ☑
        unspecified person Y35.309 ☑
      specified NEC
        injuring
          bystander Y35.392 ☑
          law enforcement personnel Y35.391 ☑
          suspect Y35.393 ☑
          unspecified person Y35.399 ☑
      stave
        injuring
          bystander Y35.392 ☑
          law enforcement personnel Y35.391 ☑
          suspect Y35.393 ☑
          unspecified person Y35.399 ☑
    bomb — *see* Legal, intervention, explosive
    conducted energy device
      injuring
        bystander Y35.832 ☑
        law enforcement personnel Y35.831 ☑
        suspect Y35.833 ☑
        unspecified person Y35.839 ☑
    cutting or piercing instrument — *see* Legal, intervention, sharp object
    dynamite — *see* Legal, intervention, explosive, dynamite
    electroshock device (taser)
      injuring
        bystander Y35.832 ☑
        law enforcement personnel Y35.831 ☑
        suspect Y35.833 ☑
        unspecified person Y35.839 ☑
    explosive(s)
      dynamite
        injuring
          bystander Y35.112 ☑
          law enforcement personnel Y35.111 ☑
          suspect Y35.113 ☑
          unspecified person Y35.119 ☑
      grenade
        injuring
          bystander Y35.192 ☑
          law enforcement personnel Y35.191 ☑
          suspect Y35.193 ☑
          unspecified person Y35.199 ☑
      injuring
        bystander Y35.102 ☑
        law enforcement personnel Y35.101 ☑
        suspect Y35.103 ☑
        unspecified person Y35.109 ☑
      mortar bomb
        injuring
          bystander Y35.192 ☑
          law enforcement personnel Y35.191 ☑
          suspect Y35.193 ☑
          unspecified person Y35.199 ☑
      shell
        injuring
          bystander Y35.122 ☑
          law enforcement personnel Y35.121 ☑

Legal — *continued*
  intervention — *continued*
    explosive(s) — *continued*
      shell — *continued*
        injuring — *continued*
          suspect Y35.123 ☑
          unspecified person Y35.129 ☑
      specified NEC
        injuring
          bystander Y35.192 ☑
          law enforcement personnel Y35.191 ☑
          suspect Y35.193 ☑
          unspecified person Y35.199 ☑
    firearm(s) (discharge)
      handgun
        injuring
          bystander Y35.022 ☑
          law enforcement personnel Y35.021 ☑
          suspect Y35.023 ☑
          unspecified person Y35.029 ☑
      injuring
        bystander Y35.002 ☑
        law enforcement personnel Y35.001 ☑
        suspect Y35.003 ☑
        unspecified person Y35.009 ☑
      machine gun
        injuring
          bystander Y35.012 ☑
          law enforcement personnel Y35.011 ☑
          suspect Y35.013 ☑
          unspecified person Y35.019 ☑
      rifle pellet
        injuring
          bystander Y35.032 ☑
          law enforcement personnel Y35.031 ☑
          suspect Y35.033 ☑
          unspecified person Y35.039 ☑
      rubber bullet
        injuring
          bystander Y35.042 ☑
          law enforcement personnel Y35.041 ☑
          suspect Y35.043 ☑
          unspecified person Y35.049 ☑
      shotgun — *see* Legal, intervention, firearm, specified NEC
      specified NEC
        injuring
          bystander Y35.092 ☑
          law enforcement personnel Y35.091 ☑
          suspect Y35.093 ☑
          unspecified person Y35.099 ☑
    gas (asphyxiation) (poisoning)
      injuring
        bystander Y35.202 ☑
        law enforcement personnel Y35.201 ☑
        suspect Y35.203 ☑
        unspecified person Y35.209 ☑
      specified NEC
        injuring
          bystander Y35.292 ☑
          law enforcement personnel Y35.291 ☑
          suspect Y35.293 ☑
          unspecified person Y35.299 ☑
      tear gas
        injuring
          bystander Y35.212 ☑
          law enforcement personnel Y35.211 ☑
          suspect Y35.213 ☑
          unspecified person Y35.219 ☑
    grenade — *see* Legal, intervention, explosive, grenade
    injuring
      bystander Y35.92 ☑
      law enforcement personnel Y35.91 ☑
      suspect Y35.93 ☑
      unspecified person Y35.99 ☑
    late effect (of) — *see* with 7th character S Y35 ☑
    manhandling
      injuring
        bystander Y35.812 ☑
        law enforcement personnel Y35.811 ☑
        suspect Y35.813 ☑
        unspecified person Y35.819 ☑
    sequelae (of) — *see* with 7th character S Y35 ☑

Legal — *continued*
  intervention — *continued*
    sharp objects
      bayonet
        injuring
          bystander Y35.412 ☑
          law enforcement personnel Y35.411 ☑
          suspect Y35.413 ☑
          unspecified person Y35.419 ☑
      injuring
        bystander Y35.402 ☑
        law enforcement personnel Y35.401 ☑
        suspect Y35.403 ☑
        unspecified person Y35.409 ☑
      specified NEC
        injuring
          bystander Y35.492 ☑
          law enforcement personnel Y35.491 ☑
          suspect Y35.493 ☑
          unspecified person Y35.499 ☑
    specified means NEC
      injuring
        bystander Y35.892 ☑
        law enforcement personnel Y35.891 ☑
        suspect Y35.893 ☑
        unspecified person Y35.899 ☑
    stabbing — *see* Legal, intervention, sharp object
    stave — *see* Legal, intervention, blunt object, stave
    stun gun
      injuring
        bystander Y35.832 ☑
        law enforcement personnel Y35.831 ☑
        suspect Y35.833 ☑
        unspecified person Y35.839 ☑
    taser
      injuring
        bystander Y35.832 ☑
        law enforcement personnel Y35.831 ☑
        suspect Y35.833 ☑
        unspecified person Y35.839 ☑
    tear gas — *see* Legal, intervention, gas, tear gas
    truncheon — *see* Legal, intervention, blunt object, stave
Lifting — *see also* Overexertion
  heavy objects X50.0 ☑
  weights X50.0 ☑
Lightning (shock) (stroke) (struck by) — *see* subcategory T75.0 ☑
  causing fire — *see* Exposure, fire
Loss of control (transport vehicle) NEC — *see* Accident, transport
Lost at sea NOS — *see* Drowning, due to, fall overboard
Low
  pressure (effects) — *see* Air, pressure, low
  temperature (effects) — *see* Exposure, cold
Lying before train, vehicle or other moving object X81.8 ☑
  subway train X81.1 ☑
  train X81.1 ☑
  undetermined whether accidental or intentional Y31 ☑
Lynching — *see* Assault

M

Malfunction (mechanism or component) (of)
  firearm W34.10 ☑
    airgun W34.110 ☑
    BB gun W34.110 ☑
    gas, air or spring-operated gun NEC W34.118 ☑
    handgun W32.1 ☑
    hunting rifle W33.12 ☑
    larger firearm W33.10 ☑
      specified NEC W33.19 ☑
    machine gun W33.13 ☑
    paintball gun W34.111 ☑
    pellet gun W34.110 ☑
    shotgun W33.11 ☑
    specified NEC W34.19 ☑
    Very pistol [flare] W34.19 ☑
  handgun — *see* Malfunction, firearm, handgun
Maltreatment — *see* Perpetrator
Mangled (accidentally) NOS X58 ☑
Manhandling (in brawl, fight) Y04.0 ☑
  legal intervention — *see* Legal, intervention, manhandling
Manslaughter (nonaccidental) — *see* Assault

Mauled by animal NEC W55.89 ☑
Medical procedure, complication of (delayed or as an
    abnormal reaction without mention of misadventure)
    — *see* Complication of or following, by specified type
    of procedure
  due to or as a result of misadventure — *see* Misadventure
Melting (due to fire) — *see also* Exposure, fire
  apparel NEC X06.3 ☑
  clothes, clothing NEC X06.3 ☑
    nightwear X05 ☑
  fittings or furniture (burning building) (uncontrolled fire)
    X00.8 ☑
  nightwear X05 ☑
  plastic jewelry X06.1 ☑
Mental cruelty X58 ☑
Military operations (injuries to military and civilians occur-
    ing during peacetime on military property and during
    routine military exercises and operations) (by) (from)
    (involving) Y37.90- ☑
  air blast Y37.20- ☑
  aircraft
    destruction — *see* Military operations, destruction of
      aircraft
    airway restriction — *see* Military operations, restriction
      of airways
    asphyxiation — *see* Military operations, restriction of
      airways
  biological weapons Y37.6X- ☑
  blast Y37.20- ☑
  blast fragments Y37.20- ☑
  blast wave Y37.20- ☑
  blast wind Y37.20- ☑
  bomb Y37.20- ☑
    dirty Y37.50- ☑
    gasoline Y37.31- ☑
    incendiary Y37.31- ☑
    petrol Y37.31- ☑
  bullet Y37.43- ☑
    incendiary Y37.32- ☑
    rubber Y37.41- ☑
  chemical weapons Y37.7X- ☑
  combat
    hand to hand (unarmed) combat Y37.44- ☑
    using blunt or piercing object Y37.45- ☑
  conflagration — *see* Military operations, fire
  conventional warfare NEC Y37.49- ☑
  depth-charge Y37.01- ☑
  destruction of aircraft Y37.10- ☑
    due to
      air to air missile Y37.11- ☑
      collision with other aircraft Y37.12- ☑
      detonation (accidental) of onboard munitions and
        explosives Y37.14- ☑
      enemy fire or explosives Y37.11- ☑
      explosive placed on aircraft Y37.11- ☑
      onboard fire Y37.13- ☑
      rocket propelled grenade [RPG] Y37.11- ☑
      small arms fire Y37.11- ☑
      surface to air missile Y37.11- ☑
    specified NEC Y37.19- ☑
  detonation (accidental) of
    onboard marine weapons Y37.05- ☑
    own munitions or munitions launch device Y37.24- ☑
  dirty bomb Y37.50- ☑
  explosion (of) Y37.20- ☑
    aerial bomb Y37.21- ☑
    bomb NOS — *see also* Military operations, bomb(s)
      Y37.20- ☑
    fragments Y37.20- ☑
    grenade Y37.29- ☑
    guided missile Y37.22- ☑
    improvised explosive device [IED] (person-borne)
      (roadside) (vehicle-borne) Y37.23- ☑
    land mine Y37.29- ☑
    marine mine (at sea) (in harbor) Y37.02- ☑
    marine weapon Y37.00- ☑
      specified NEC Y37.09- ☑
    own munitions or munitions launch device (acciden-
      tal) Y37.24- ☑
    sea-based artillery shell Y37.03- ☑
    specified NEC Y37.29- ☑
    torpedo Y37.04- ☑
  fire Y37.30- ☑
    specified NEC Y37.39- ☑
  firearms
    discharge Y37.43- ☑

Military operations — *continued*
  firearms — *continued*
    pellets Y37.42- ☑
  flamethrower Y37.33- ☑
  fragments (from) (of)
    improvised explosive device [IED] (person-borne)
      (roadside) (vehicle-borne) Y37.26- ☑
    munitions Y37.25- ☑
    specified NEC Y37.29- ☑
    weapons Y37.27- ☑
  friendly fire Y37.92- ☑
  hand to hand (unarmed) combat Y37.44- ☑
  hot substances — *see* Military operations, fire
  incendiary bullet Y37.32- ☑
  nuclear weapon (effects of) Y37.50- ☑
    acute radiation exposure Y37.54- ☑
    blast pressure Y37.51- ☑
    direct blast Y37.51- ☑
    direct heat Y37.53- ☑
    fallout exposure Y37.54- ☑
    fireball Y37.53- ☑
    indirect blast (struck or crushed by blast debris) (being
      thrown by blast) Y37.52- ☑
    ionizing radiation (immediate exposure) Y37.54- ☑
    nuclear radiation Y37.54- ☑
    radiation
      ionizing (immediate exposure) Y37.54- ☑
      nuclear Y37.54- ☑
      thermal Y37.53- ☑
    secondary effects Y37.54- ☑
    specified NEC Y37.59- ☑
    thermal radiation Y37.53- ☑
  restriction of air (airway)
    intentional Y37.46- ☑
    unintentional Y37.47- ☑
  rubber bullets Y37.41- ☑
  shrapnel NOS Y37.29- ☑
  suffocation — *see* Military operations, restriction of air-
    ways
  unconventional warfare NEC Y37.7X- ☑
  underwater blast NOS Y37.00- ☑
  warfare
    conventional NEC Y37.49- ☑
    unconventional NEC Y37.7X- ☑
  weapon of mass destruction [WMD] Y37.91- ☑
  weapons
    biological weapons Y37.6X- ☑
    chemical Y37.7X- ☑
    nuclear (effects of) Y37.50- ☑
      acute radiation exposure Y37.54- ☑
      blast pressure Y37.51- ☑
      direct blast Y37.51- ☑
      direct heat Y37.53- ☑
      fallout exposure Y37.54- ☑
      fireball Y37.53- ☑
      radiation
        ionizing (immediate exposure) Y37.54- ☑
        nuclear Y37.54- ☑
        thermal Y37.53- ☑
      secondary effects Y37.54- ☑
      specified NEC Y37.59- ☑
    of mass destruction [WMD] Y37.91- ☑
Misadventure(s) **to patient**(s) **during surgical or medical
  care** Y69
  contaminated medical or biological substance (blood,
    drug, fluid) Y64.9
    administered (by) NEC Y64.9
      immunization Y64.1
      infusion Y64.0
      injection Y64.1
      specified means NEC Y64.8
      transfusion Y64.0
      vaccination Y64.1
  excessive amount of blood or other fluid during transfu-
    sion or infusion Y63.0
  failure
    in dosage Y63.9
      electroshock therapy Y63.4
      inappropriate temperature (too hot or too cold)
        in local application and packing Y63.5
      infusion
        excessive amount of fluid Y63.0
        incorrect dilution of fluid Y63.1
      insulin-shock therapy Y63.4
      nonadministration of necessary drug or biological
        substance Y63.6

Misadventure(s) **to patient**(s) **during surgical or medical
  care** — *continued*
  failure — *continued*
    in dosage — *continued*
      overdose — *see* Table of Drugs and Chemicals
        radiation, in therapy Y63.2
      radiation
        overdose Y63.2
      specified procedure NEC Y63.8
      transfusion
        excessive amount of blood Y63.0
    mechanical, of instrument or apparatus (any) (during
      any procedure) Y65.8
    sterile precautions (during procedure) Y62.9
      aspiration of fluid or tissue (by puncture or
        catheterization, except heart) Y62.6
      biopsy (except needle aspiration) Y62.8
        needle (aspirating) Y62.6
      blood sampling Y62.6
      catheterization Y62.6
        heart Y62.5
      dialysis (kidney) Y62.2
      endoscopic examination Y62.4
      enema Y62.8
      immunization Y62.3
      infusion Y62.1
      injection Y62.3
      needle biopsy Y62.6
      paracentesis (abdominal) (thoracic) Y62.6
      perfusion Y62.2
      puncture (lumbar) Y62.6
      removal of catheter or packing Y62.8
      specified procedure NEC Y62.8
      surgical operation Y62.0
      transfusion Y62.1
      vaccination Y62.3
    suture or ligature during surgical procedure Y65.2
    to introduce or to remove tube or instrument — *see*
      Failure, to
  hemorrhage — *see* Index to Diseases and Injuries, Com-
    plication(s)
  inadvertent exposure of patient to radiation Y63.3
  inappropriate
    operation performed — *see* Inappropriate operation
      performed
    temperature (too hot or too cold) in local application
      or packing Y63.5
  infusion — *see also* Misadventure, by type, infusion Y69
    excessive amount of fluid Y63.0
    incorrect dilution of fluid Y63.1
    wrong fluid Y65.1
  mismatched blood in transfusion Y65.0
  nonadministration of necessary drug or biological sub-
    stance Y63.6
  overdose — *see* Table of Drugs and Chemicals
    radiation (in therapy) Y63.2
  perforation — *see* Index to Diseases and Injuries, Compli-
    cation(s)
  performance of inappropriate operation — *see* Inappro-
    priate operation performed
  puncture — *see* Index to Diseases and Injuries, Compli-
    cation(s)
  specified type NEC Y65.8
    failure
      suture or ligature during surgical operation Y65.2
      to introduce or to remove tube or instrument —
        see Failure, to
    infusion of wrong fluid Y65.1
    performance of inappropriate operation — *see* Inap-
      propriate operation performed
    transfusion of mismatched blood Y65.0
    wrong
      fluid in infusion Y65.1
      placement of endotracheal tube during anesthetic
        procedure Y65.3
  transfusion — *see* Misadventure, by type, transfusion
    excessive amount of blood Y63.0
    mismatched blood Y65.0
  wrong
    drug given in error — *see* Table of Drugs and Chemi-
      cals
    fluid in infusion Y65.1
    placement of endotracheal tube during anesthetic
      procedure Y65.3
Mismatched blood in transfusion Y65.0
Motion sickness T75.3 ☑
Mountain sickness W94.11 ☑
Mudslide (of cataclysmic nature) — *see* Landslide
Murder (attempt) — *see* Assault

☑ **Additional Character Required — Refer to the Tabular List for Character Selection**

N

Nail
  contact with W45.0 ☑
    gun W29.4 ☑
  embedded in skin W45.0 ☑
Neglect (criminal) (homicidal intent) X58 ☑
Noise (causing injury) (pollution) W42.9 ☑
  supersonic W42.0 ☑
Nonadministration (of)
  drug or biological substance (necessary) Y63.6
  surgical and medical care Y66
Nosocomial condition Y95

O

Object
  falling
    from, in, on, hitting
      machinery — see Contact, with, by type of machine
  set in motion by
    accidental explosion or rupture of pressure vessel W38 ☑
    firearm — see Discharge, firearm, by type
    machine(ry) — see Contact, with, by type of machine
Overdose (drug) — see Table of Drugs and Chemicals
  radiation Y63.2
Overexertion X50.9 ☑
  from
    prolonged static or awkward postures X50.1 ☑
    repetitive movements X50.3 ☑
    specified strenuous movements or postures NEC X50.9 ☑
    strenuous movement or load X50.0 ☑
Overexposure (accidental) (to)
  cold — see also Exposure, cold X31 ☑
    due to man-made conditions — see Exposure, cold, man-made
  heat — see also Heat X30 ☑
  radiation — see Radiation
  radioactivity W88.0 ☑
  sun (sunburn) X32 ☑
  weather NEC — see Forces of nature
  wind NEC — see Forces of nature
Overheated — see Heat
Overturning (accidental)
  machinery — see Contact, with, by type of machine
  transport vehicle NEC — see also Accident, transport V89.9 ☑
  watercraft (causing drowning, submersion) — see also Drowning, due to, accident to, watercraft, overturning
    causing injury except drowning or submersion — see Accident, watercraft, causing, injury NEC

P

Parachute descent (voluntary) (without accident to aircraft) V97.29 ☑
  due to accident to aircraft — see Accident, transport, aircraft
Pecked by bird W61.99 ☑
Perforation during medical or surgical treatment as misadventure — see Index to Diseases and Injuries, Complication(s)
Perpetrator, perpetration, of assault, maltreatment and neglect (by) Y07.9
  acquaintance Y07.54
  aunt Y07.47
  boyfriend
    current Y07.030
    former Y07.031
  brother Y07.410
    stepbrother Y07.435
  child (adopted) (biological) (foster) (in-law) (step) Y07.44
  coach Y07.53
  cousin
    female Y07.491
    male Y07.490
  daughter (adopted) (biological) (foster) (in-law) (step) Y07.44
  daycare provider Y07.519
    at-home
      adult care Y07.512
      childcare Y07.510

Perpetrator, perpetration, of assault, maltreatment and neglect — continued
  daycare provider — continued
    care center
      adult care Y07.513
      childcare Y07.511
  family member NEC Y07.499
  father Y07.11
    adoptive Y07.13
    foster Y07.420
    stepfather Y07.430
  foster father Y07.420
  foster mother Y07.421
  friend Y07.54
  girl friend
    current Y07.040
    former Y07.041
  grandchild (adopted) (biological) (foster) (in-law) (step) Y07.45
  granddaughter (adopted) (biological) (foster) (in-law) (step) Y07.45
  grandfather Y07.46
  grandmother Y07.46
  grandparent Y07.45
  grandson (adopted) (biological) (foster) (in-law) (step) Y07.45
  healthcare provider Y07.529
    mental health Y07.521
    specified NEC Y07.528
  husband
    current Y07.010
    former Y07.011
  instructor Y07.53
  mother Y07.12
    adoptive Y07.14
    foster Y07.421
    stepmother Y07.433
  multiple perpetrators Y07.6
  non-binary
    child (adopted) (biological) (foster) (in-law) (step) Y07.44
    grandchild (adopted) (biological) (foster) (in-law) (step) Y07.45
    grandparent Y07.46
    parental sibling Y07.47
  nonfamily member Y07.50
    specified NEC Y07.59
  nurse Y07.528
  occupational therapist Y07.528
  parental sibling Y07.47
  partner
    female (dating) (intimate)
      current Y07.040
      former Y07.041
    gender non-conforming
      current Y07.050
      former Y07.051
    male (dating) (intimate)
      current Y07.030
      former Y07.031
    non-binary
      current Y07.050
      former Y07.051
    of parent
      female Y07.434
      male Y07.432
  physical therapist Y07.528
  sister Y07.411
  son (adopted) (biological) (foster) (in-law) (step) Y07.44
  speech therapist Y07.528
  stepbrother Y07.435
  stepfather Y07.430
  stepmother Y07.433
  stepsister Y07.436
  teacher Y07.53
  uncle Y07.47
  wife
    current Y07.020
    former Y07.021
Piercing — see Contact, with, by type of object or machine
Pinched
  between objects (moving) (stationary and moving) W23.0 ☑
    stationary W23.1 ☑
Pinned under machine(ry) — see Contact, with, by type of machine
Place of occurrence Y92.9
  abandoned house Y92.89
  airplane Y92.813

Place of occurrence — continued
  airport Y92.520
  ambulatory health services establishment NEC Y92.538
  ambulatory surgery center Y92.530
  amusement park Y92.831
  apartment (co-op) — see Place of occurrence, residence, apartment
  assembly hall Y92.29
  bank Y92.510
  bar Y92.59
  barn Y92.71
  baseball field Y92.320
  basketball court Y92.310
  beach Y92.832
  boarding house — see Place of occurrence, residence, boarding house
  boat Y92.814
  bowling alley Y92.39
  bridge Y92.89
  building under construction Y92.61
  bus Y92.811
    station Y92.521
  cafe Y92.511
  campsite Y92.833
  campus — see Place of occurrence, school
  canal Y92.89
  car Y92.810
  casino Y92.59
  children's home — see Place of occurrence, residence, institutional, orphanage
  church Y92.22
  cinema Y92.26
  clubhouse Y92.29
  coal pit Y92.64
  college (community) Y92.214
  condominium — see Place of occurrence, residence, apartment
  construction area — see Place of occurrence, industrial and construction area
  convalescent home — see Place of occurrence, residence, institutional, nursing home
  court-house Y92.240
  cricket ground Y92.328
  cultural building Y92.258
    art gallery Y92.250
    museum Y92.251
    music hall Y92.252
    opera house Y92.253
    specified NEC Y92.258
    theater Y92.254
  dancehall Y92.252
  day nursery Y92.210
  dentist office Y92.531
  derelict house Y92.89
  desert Y92.820
  dockyard Y92.62
  dock NOS Y92.89
  doctor's office Y92.531
  dormitory — see Place of occurrence, residence, institutional, school dormitory
  dry dock Y92.62
  factory (building) (premises) Y92.63
  farm (land under cultivation) (outbuildings) Y92.79
    barn Y92.71
    chicken coop Y92.72
    field Y92.73
    hen house Y92.72
    house — see Place of occurrence, residence, house
    orchard Y92.74
    specified NEC Y92.79
  football field Y92.321
  forest Y92.821
  freeway Y92.411
  gallery Y92.250
  garage (commercial) Y92.59
    boarding house Y92.044
    military base Y92.135
    mobile home Y92.025
    nursing home Y92.124
    orphanage Y92.114
    private house Y92.015
    reform school Y92.155
  gas station Y92.524
  gasworks Y92.69
  golf course Y92.39
  gravel pit Y92.64
  grocery Y92.512
  gymnasium Y92.39
  handball court Y92.318

☑ Additional Character Required — Refer to the Tabular List for Character Selection

Place of occurrence — Place of occurrence

External Causes Index

Place of occurrence — *continued*
- shipyard Y92.62
- shop (commercial) Y92.513
- sidewalk Y92.480
- silo Y92.79
- skating rink (roller) Y92.331
  - ice Y92.330
- slaughter house Y92.86
- soccer field Y92.322
- specified place NEC Y92.89
- sports area Y92.39
  - athletic
    - court Y92.318
      - basketball Y92.310
      - specified NEC Y92.318
      - squash Y92.311
      - tennis Y92.312
    - field Y92.328
      - baseball Y92.320
      - cricket ground Y92.328
      - football Y92.321
      - hockey Y92.328
      - soccer Y92.322
      - specified NEC Y92.328
  - golf course Y92.39
  - gymnasium Y92.39
  - riding school Y92.39
  - skating rink (roller) Y92.331
    - ice Y92.330
  - stadium Y92.39
  - swimming pool Y92.34
- squash court Y92.311
- stadium Y92.39
- steeplechasing course Y92.39
- store Y92.512
- stream Y92.828
- street and highway Y92.410
  - bike path Y92.482
  - freeway Y92.411
  - highway ramp Y92.415
  - interstate highway Y92.411
  - local residential or business street Y92.414
  - motorway Y92.411
  - parking lot Y92.481
  - parkway Y92.412
  - sidewalk Y92.480
  - specified NEC Y92.488
  - state road Y92.413
- subway car Y92.816
- supermarket Y92.512
- swamp Y92.828
- swimming pool (public) Y92.34
  - private (at) Y92.095
    - boarding house Y92.045
    - military base Y92.136
    - mobile home Y92.026
    - nursing home Y92.125
    - orphanage Y92.115
    - prison Y92.146
    - reform school Y92.156
    - single family residence Y92.016
- synagogue Y92.22
- tavern Y92.59
- television station Y92.59
- tennis court Y92.312
- theater Y92.254
- trade area Y92.59
  - bank Y92.510
  - cafe Y92.511
  - casino Y92.59
  - garage Y92.59
  - hotel Y92.59
  - market Y92.512
  - office building Y92.59
  - radio station Y92.59
  - restaurant Y92.511
  - shop Y92.513
  - shopping mall Y92.59
  - store Y92.512
  - supermarket Y92.512
  - television station Y92.59
  - warehouse Y92.59
- trailer park, residential — *see* Place of occurrence, residence, mobile home
- trailer site NOS Y92.89
- train Y92.815
  - station Y92.522
- truck Y92.812
- tunnel under construction Y92.69

Place of occurrence — *continued*
- university Y92.214
- urgent (health) care center Y92.532
- vehicle (transport) Y92.818
  - airplane Y92.813
  - boat Y92.814
  - bus Y92.811
  - car Y92.810
  - specified NEC Y92.818
  - subway car Y92.816
  - train Y92.815
  - truck Y92.812
- warehouse Y92.59
- water reservoir Y92.89
- wilderness area Y92.828
  - desert Y92.820
  - forest Y92.821
  - marsh Y92.828
  - mountain Y92.828
  - prairie Y92.828
  - specified NEC Y92.828
  - swamp Y92.828
- workshop Y92.69
- yard, private Y92.096
  - boarding house Y92.046
  - mobile home Y92.027
  - single family house Y92.017
- youth center Y92.29
- zoo (zoological garden) Y92.834

Plumbism — *see* Table of Drugs and Chemicals, lead

Poisoning (accidental) (by) — *see also* Table of Drugs and Chemicals
- by plant, thorns, spines, sharp leaves or other mechanisms NEC X58 ☑
- carbon monoxide
  - generated by
    - motor vehicle — *see* Accident, transport
    - watercraft (in transit) (not in transit) V93.89 ☑
      - ferry boat V93.81 ☑
      - fishing boat V93.82 ☑
      - jet skis V93.83 ☑
      - liner V93.81 ☑
      - merchant ship V93.80 ☑
      - passenger ship V93.81 ☑
      - powered craft NEC V93.83 ☑
- caused by injection of poisons into skin by plant thorns, spines, sharp leaves X58 ☑
- marine or sea plants (venomous) X58 ☑
- execution — *see* Legal, intervention, gas
- intervention
  - by gas — *see* Legal, intervention, gas
  - other specified means — *see* Legal, intervention, specified means NEC
- exhaust gas
  - generated by
    - motor vehicle — *see* Accident, transport
    - watercraft (in transit) (not in transit) V93.89 ☑
      - ferry boat V93.81 ☑
      - fishing boat V93.82 ☑
      - jet skis V93.83 ☑
      - liner V93.81 ☑
      - merchant ship V93.80 ☑
      - passenger ship V93.81 ☑
      - powered craft NEC V93.83 ☑
- fumes or smoke due to
  - explosion — *see also* Explosion W40.9 ☑
  - fire — *see* Exposure, fire
  - ignition — *see* Ignition
- gas
  - in legal intervention — *see* Legal, intervention, gas
  - legal execution — *see* Legal, intervention, gas
- in war operations — *see* War operations
- legal

Powder burn (by) (from)
- airgun W34.110 ☑
- BB gun W34.110 ☑
- firearm NEC W34.19 ☑
- gas, air or spring-operated gun NEC W34.118 ☑
- handgun W32.1 ☑
- hunting rifle W33.12 ☑
- larger firearm W33.10 ☑
  - specified NEC W33.19 ☑
- machine gun W33.13 ☑
- paintball gun W34.111 ☑
- pellet gun W34.110 ☑
- shotgun W33.11 ☑
- Very pistol [flare] W34.19 ☑

Premature cessation (of) **surgical and medical care** Y66
Privation (food) (water) X58 ☑
Procedure (operation)
- correct, on wrong side or body part (wrong side) (wrong site) Y65.53
- intended for another patient done on wrong patient Y65.52
- performed on patient not scheduled for surgery Y65.52
- performed on wrong patient Y65.52
- wrong, performed on correct patient Y65.51

Prolonged
- sitting in transport vehicle — *see* Sitting
- stay in
  - high altitude as cause of anoxia, barodontalgia, barotitis or hypoxia W94.11 ☑
  - weightless environment X52 ☑

Pulling, excessive — *see also* Overexertion X50.9- ☑
Puncture, puncturing — *see also* Contact, with, by type of object or machine
- by
  - plant thorns, spines, sharp leaves or other mechanisms NEC W60 ☑
- during medical or surgical treatment as misadventure — *see* Index to Diseases and Injuries, Complication(s)

Pushed, pushing (accidental) (injury in)
- by other person(s) (accidental) W51 ☑
- as, or caused by, a crowd or human stampede (with fall) W52 ☑
  - before moving object NEC Y02.8 ☑
    - motor vehicle Y02.0 ☑
    - subway train Y02.1 ☑
    - train Y02.1 ☑
  - from
    - high place NEC
      - in accidental circumstances W17.89 ☑
      - stated as
        - intentional, homicide (attempt) Y01 ☑
        - undetermined whether accidental or intentional Y30 ☑
    - transport vehicle NEC — *see also* Accident, transport V89.9 ☑
      - stated as
        - intentional, homicide (attempt) Y08.89 ☑
  - with fall W03 ☑
    - due to ice or snow W00.0 ☑
- overexertion X50.9 ☑

R

Radiation (exposure to)
- arc lamps W89.0 ☑
- atomic power plant (malfunction) NEC W88.1 ☑
- complication of or abnormal reaction to medical radiotherapy Y84.2
- electromagnetic, ionizing W88.0 ☑
- gamma rays W88.1 ☑
- in
  - war operations (from or following nuclear explosion) — *see* War operations
- inadvertent exposure of patient (receiving test or therapy) Y63.3
- infrared (heaters and lamps) W90.1 ☑
  - excessive heat from W92 ☑
- ionized, ionizing (particles, artificially accelerated)
  - radioisotopes W88.1 ☑
  - specified NEC W88.8 ☑
  - x-rays W88.0 ☑
- isotopes, radioactive — *see* Radiation, radioactive isotopes
- laser(s) W90.2 ☑
  - in war operations — *see* War operations
  - misadventure in medical care Y63.2
- light sources (man-made visible and ultraviolet) W89.9 ☑
  - natural X32 ☑
  - specified NEC W89.8 ☑
  - tanning bed W89.1 ☑
  - welding light W89.0 ☑
- man-made visible light W89.9 ☑
  - specified NEC W89.8 ☑
  - tanning bed W89.1 ☑
  - welding light W89.0 ☑
- microwave W90.8 ☑
- misadventure in medical or surgical procedure Y63.2
- natural NEC X39.08 ☑
  - radon X39.01 ☑
- overdose (in medical or surgical procedure) Y63.2

Radiation — *continued*
  radar W90.0 ☑
  radioactive isotopes (any) W88.1 ☑
    atomic power plant malfunction W88.1 ☑
    misadventure in medical or surgical treatment Y63.2
  radiofrequency W90.0 ☑
  radium NEC W88.1 ☑
  sun X32 ☑
  ultraviolet (light) (man-made) W89.9 ☑
    natural X32 ☑
    specified NEC W89.8 ☑
    tanning bed W89.1 ☑
    welding light W89.0 ☑
  welding arc, torch, or light W89.0 ☑
    excessive heat from W92 ☑
  x-rays (hard) (soft) W88.0 ☑
Range disease W94.11 ☑
Rape (attempted) (confirmed) T74.2- ☑
  suspected T76.2- ☑
Rat bite W53.11 ☑
Reaching (prolonged) (static) X50.1 ☑
Reaction, abnormal to medical procedure — *see also*
    Complication of or following, by type of procedure
    Y84.9
  biologicals — *see* Table of Drugs and Chemicals
  drugs — *see* Table of Drugs and Chemicals
  vaccine — *see* Table of Drugs and Chemicals
  with misadventure — *see* Misadventure
Recoil
  airgun W34.110 ☑
  BB gun W34.110 ☑
  firearm NEC W34.19 ☑
  gas, air or spring-operated gun NEC W34.118 ☑
  handgun W32.1 ☑
  hunting rifle W33.12 ☑
  larger firearm W33.10 ☑
    specified NEC W33.19 ☑
  machine gun W33.13 ☑
  paintball gun W34.111 ☑
  pellet W34.110 ☑
  shotgun W33.11 ☑
  Very pistol [flare] W34.19 ☑
Reduction in
  atmospheric pressure — *see* Air, pressure, change
Rock falling on or hitting (accidentally) (person) W20.8 ☑
  in cave-in W20.0 ☑
Run over (accidentally) (by)
  animal (not being ridden) NEC W55.89 ☑
  machinery — *see* Contact, with, by specified type of
    machine
  transport vehicle NEC — *see also* Accident, transport
    V09.9 ☑
    intentional homicide (attempt) Y03.0 ☑
    motor NEC V09.20 ☑
      intentional homicide (attempt) Y03.0 ☑
Running
  before moving object X81.8 ☑
    motor vehicle X81.0 ☑
Running off, away
  animal (being ridden) — *see also* Accident, transport
    V80.918 ☑
    not being ridden W55.89 ☑
  animal-drawn vehicle NEC — *see also* Accident, transport
    V80.928 ☑
  highway, road(way), street
    transport vehicle NEC — *see also* Accident, transport
    V89.9 ☑
Rupture pressurized devices — *see* Explosion, by type of
    device

S

Saturnism — *see* Table of Drugs and Chemicals, lead
Scald, scalding (accidental) (by) (from) (in) X19 ☑
  air (hot) X14.1 ☑
  gases (hot) X14.1 ☑
  homicide (attempt) — *see* Assault, burning, hot object
  inflicted by other person
    stated as intentional, homicide (attempt) — *see* As-
      sault, burning, hot object
  liquid (boiling) (hot) NEC X12 ☑
    stated as undetermined whether accidental or inten-
      tional Y27.2 ☑
    suicide (attempt) X77.2 ☑
  local application of externally applied substance in
    medical or surgical care Y63.5

Scald, scalding — *continued*
  metal (molten) (liquid) (hot) NEC X18 ☑
  self-inflicted X77.9 ☑
  stated as undetermined whether accidental or intentional
    Y27.8 ☑
  steam X13.1 ☑
    assault X98.0 ☑
    stated as undetermined whether accidental or inten-
      tional Y27.0 ☑
    suicide (attempt) X77.0 ☑
  suicide (attempt) X77.9 ☑
  vapor (hot) X13.1 ☑
    assault X98.0 ☑
    stated as undetermined whether accidental or inten-
      tional Y27.0 ☑
    suicide (attempt) X77.0 ☑
Scratched by
  cat W55.03 ☑
  person(s) (accidentally) W50.4 ☑
    with intent to injure or kill Y04.0 ☑
    as, or caused by, a crowd or human stampede (with
      fall) W52 ☑
    assault Y04.0 ☑
    homicide (attempt) Y04.0 ☑
    in
      fight Y04.0 ☑
      legal intervention
        injuring
          bystander Y35.892 ☑
          law enforcement personnel Y35.891 ☑
          suspect Y35.893 ☑
          unspecified person Y35.899 ☑
Seasickness T75.3 ☑
Self-harm NEC — *see also* External cause by type, undeter-
    mined whether accidental or intentional
  intentional — *see* Suicide
  poisoning NEC — *see* Table of Drugs and Chemicals,
    poisoning, accidental
Self-inflicted (injury) **NEC** — *see also* External cause by
    type, undetermined whether accidental or intentional
  intentional — *see* Suicide
  poisoning NEC — *see* Table of Drugs and Chemicals,
    poisoning, accidental
Sequelae (of)
  accident NEC — *see* W00-X58 with 7th character S
  assault (homicidal) (any means) — *see* X92-Y08 with 7th
    character S
  homicide, attempt (any means) — *see* X92-Y08 with 7th
    character S
  injury undetermined whether accidentally or purposely
    inflicted — *see* Y21-Y33 with 7th character S
  intentional self-harm (classifiable to X71-X83) — *see* X71-
    X83 with 7th character S
  legal intervention — *see* with 7th character S Y35 ☑
  motor vehicle accident — *see* V00-V99 with 7th character
    S
  suicide, attempt (any means) — *see* X71-X83 with 7th
    character S
  transport accident — *see* V00-V99 with 7th character S
  war operations — *see* War operations
Shock
  electric — *see* Exposure, electric current
  from electric appliance (any) (faulty) W86.8 ☑
    domestic W86.0 ☑
    suicide (attempt) X83.1 ☑
Shooting, shot (accidental(ly)) — *see also* Discharge,
    firearm, by type
  herself or himself — *see* Discharge, firearm by type, self-
    inflicted
  homicide (attempt) — *see* Discharge, firearm by type,
    homicide
  in war operations — *see* War operations
  inflicted by other person — *see* Discharge, firearm by
    type, homicide
    accidental — *see* Discharge, firearm, by type of firearm
  legal
    execution — *see* Legal, intervention, firearm
    intervention — *see* Legal, intervention, firearm
  self-inflicted — *see* Discharge, firearm by type, suicide
    accidental — *see* Discharge, firearm, by type of firearm
  suicide (attempt) — *see* Discharge, firearm by type, sui-
    cide
Shoving (accidentally) **by other person** — *see* Pushed, by
    other person
Sickness
  alpine W94.11 ☑
  motion — *see* Motion

Sickness — *continued*
  mountain W94.11 ☑
Sinking (accidental)
  watercraft (causing drowning, submersion) — *see also*
    Drowning, due to, accident to, watercraft, sinking
  causing injury except drowning or submersion — *see*
    Accident, watercraft, causing, injury NEC
Siriasis X32 ☑
Sitting (prolonged) (static) X50.1 ☑
Slashed wrists — *see* Cut, self-inflicted
Slipping (accidental) (on same level) (with fall) W01.0 ☑
  on
    ice W00.0 ☑
      with skates — *see* Accident, transport, pedestrian,
        conveyance
    mud W01.0 ☑
    oil W01.0 ☑
    snow W00.0 ☑
      with skis — *see* Accident, transport, pedestrian,
        conveyance
    surface (slippery) (wet) NEC W01.0 ☑
  without fall W18.40 ☑
    due to
      specified NEC W18.49 ☑
      stepping from one level to another W18.43 ☑
      stepping into hole or opening W18.42 ☑
      stepping on object W18.41 ☑
Sliver, wood, contact with W45.8 ☑
Smoldering (due to fire) — *see* Exposure, fire
Sodomy (attempted) **by force** T74.2 ☑
Sound waves (causing injury) W42.9 ☑
  supersonic W42.0 ☑
Splinter, contact with W45.8 ☑
Stab, stabbing — *see* Cut
Standing (prolonged) (static) X50.1 ☑
Starvation X58 ☑
Status of external cause Y99.9
  child assisting in compensated work for family Y99.8
  civilian activity done for financial or other compensation
    Y99.0
  civilian activity done for income or pay Y99.0
  family member assisting in compensated work for other
    family member Y99.8
  hobby not done for income Y99.8
  leisure activity Y99.8
  military activity Y99.1
  off-duty activity of military personnel Y99.8
  recreation or sport not for income or while a student
    Y99.8
  specified NEC Y99.8
  student activity Y99.8
  volunteer activity Y99.2
Stepped on
  by
    animal (not being ridden) NEC W55.89 ☑
    crowd or human stampede W52 ☑
    person W50.0 ☑
Stepping on
  object W22.8 ☑
    sports equipment W21.9 ☑
    stationary W22.09 ☑
      sports equipment W21.89 ☑
    with fall W18.31 ☑
  person W51 ☑
    by crowd or human stampede W52 ☑
  sports equipment W21.9 ☑
Sting
  arthropod, nonvenomous W57 ☑
  insect, nonvenomous W57 ☑
Storm (cataclysmic) — *see* Forces of nature, cataclysmic
    storm
Straining, excessive — *see also* Overexertion X50.9 ☑
Strangling — *see* Strangulation
Strangulation (accidental) T71 ☑
Strenuous movements — *see also* Overexertion X50.9 ☑
Striking against
  airbag (automobile) W22.10 ☑
    driver side W22.11 ☑
    front passenger side W22.12 ☑
    specified NEC W22.19 ☑
  bottom when
    diving or jumping into water (in) W16.822 ☑
      causing drowning W16.821 ☑
      from boat W16.722 ☑
        causing drowning W16.721 ☑
      natural body W16.622 ☑
        causing drowning W16.821 ☑

☑ **Additional Character Required — Refer to the Tabular List for Character Selection**

Striking against — *continued*
  bottom when — *continued*
    diving or jumping into water — *continued*
      swimming pool W16.522 ☑
        causing drowning W16.521 ☑
      falling into water (in) W16.322 ☑
        causing drowning W16.321 ☑
        fountain — *see* Striking against, bottom when, falling into water, specified NEC
      natural body W16.122 ☑
        causing drowning W16.121 ☑
      reservoir — *see* Striking against, bottom when, falling into water, specified NEC
    specified NEC W16.322 ☑
      causing drowning W16.321 ☑
    swimming pool W16.022 ☑
      causing drowning W16.021 ☑
  diving board (swimming-pool) W21.4 ☑
  object W22.8 ☑
    caused by crowd or human stampede (with fall) W52 ☑
    furniture W22.03 ☑
    lamppost W22.02 ☑
    sports equipment W21.9 ☑
    stationary W22.09 ☑
      sports equipment W21.89 ☑
    wall W22.01 ☑
    with
      drowning or submersion — *see* Drowning
      fall — *see* Fall, due to, bumping against, object
  person(s) W51 ☑
    as, or caused by, a crowd or human stampede (with fall) W52 ☑
    assault Y04.2 ☑
    homicide (attempt) Y04.2 ☑
    with fall W03 ☑
      due to ice or snow W00.0 ☑
  sports equipment W21.9 ☑
  wall (when) W22.01 ☑
    diving or jumping into water (in) W16.832 ☑
      causing drowning W16.831 ☑
      swimming pool W16.532 ☑
        causing drowning W16.531 ☑
    falling into water (in) W16.332 ☑
      causing drowning W16.331 ☑
      fountain — *see* Striking against, wall when, falling into water, specified NEC
    natural body W16.132 ☑
      causing drowning W16.131 ☑
      reservoir — *see* Striking against, wall when, falling into water, specified NEC
    specified NEC W16.332 ☑
      causing drowning W16.331 ☑
    swimming pool W16.032 ☑
      causing drowning W16.031 ☑
    swimming pool (when) W22.042 ☑
      causing drowning W22.041 ☑
      diving or jumping into water W16.532 ☑
        causing drowning W16.531 ☑
      falling into water W16.032 ☑
        causing drowning W16.031 ☑

Struck (accidentally) **by**
  airbag (automobile) W22.10 ☑
    driver side W22.11 ☑
    front passenger side W22.12 ☑
    specified NEC W22.19 ☑
  alligator W58.02 ☑
  animal (not being ridden) NEC W55.89 ☑
  avalanche — *see* Landslide
  ball (hit) (thrown) W21.00 ☑
    assault Y08.09 ☑
    baseball W21.03 ☑
    basketball W21.05 ☑
    football W21.01 ☑
    golf ball W21.04 ☑
    soccer W21.02 ☑
    softball W21.07 ☑
    specified NEC W21.09 ☑
    volleyball W21.06 ☑
  bat or racquet
    baseball bat W21.11 ☑
      assault Y08.02 ☑
    golf club W21.13 ☑
      assault Y08.09 ☑
    specified NEC W21.19 ☑
      assault Y08.09 ☑

Struck (accidentally) **by** — *continued*
  bat or racquet — *continued*
    tennis racquet W21.12 ☑
      assault Y08.09 ☑
  bullet — *see also* Discharge, firearm by type
    in war operations — *see* War operations
  crocodile W58.12 ☑
  dog W54.1 ☑
  flare, Very pistol — *see* Discharge, firearm NEC
  hailstones X39.8 ☑
  hockey (ice)
    field
      puck W21.221 ☑
      stick W21.211 ☑
    puck W21.220 ☑
    stick W21.210 ☑
      assault Y08.01 ☑
  landslide — *see* Landslide
  law-enforcement agent (on duty) — *see* Legal, intervention, manhandling
    with blunt object — *see* Legal, intervention, blunt object
  lightning T75.0 ☑
    causing fire — *see* Exposure, fire
  machine — *see* Contact, with, by type of machine
  mammal NEC W55.89 ☑
    marine W56.32 ☑
  marine animal W56.82 ☑
  missile
    firearm — *see* Discharge, firearm by type
    in war operations — *see* War operations, missile
  object W22.8 ☑
    blunt W22.8 ☑
      assault Y00 ☑
      suicide (attempt) X79 ☑
      undetermined whether accidental or intentional Y29 ☑
    falling W20.8 ☑
      from, in, on
        building W20.1 ☑
          burning (uncontrolled fire) X00.4 ☑
        cataclysmic
          earth surface movement NEC — *see* Landslide
          storm — *see* Forces of nature, cataclysmic storm
        cave-in W20.0 ☑
        earthquake X34 ☑
        machine (in operation) — *see* Contact, with, by type of machine
        structure W20.1 ☑
          burning X00.4 ☑
        transport vehicle (in motion) — *see* Accident, transport, by type of vehicle
        watercraft V93.49 ☑
          due to
            accident to craft V91.39 ☑
              powered craft V91.33 ☑
                ferry boat V91.31 ☑
                fishing boat V91.32 ☑
                jetskis V91.33 ☑
                liner V91.31 ☑
                merchant ship V91.30 ☑
                passenger ship V91.31 ☑
              unpowered craft V91.38 ☑
                canoe V91.35 ☑
                inflatable V91.36 ☑
                kayak V91.35 ☑
                sailboat V91.34 ☑
                surf-board V91.38 ☑
                windsurfer V91.38 ☑
            powered craft V93.43 ☑
              ferry boat V93.41 ☑
              fishing boat V93.42 ☑
              jetskis V93.43 ☑
              liner V93.41 ☑
              merchant ship V93.40 ☑
              passenger ship V93.41 ☑
            unpowered craft V93.48 ☑
              sailboat V93.44 ☑
              surf-board V93.48 ☑
              windsurfer V93.48 ☑
      moving NEC W20.8 ☑
      projected W20.8 ☑
        assault Y00 ☑
        in sports W21.9 ☑

Struck (accidentally) **by** — *continued*
  object — *continued*
    projected — *continued*
      in sports — *continued*
        assault Y08.09 ☑
        ball W21.00 ☑
          baseball W21.03 ☑
          basketball W21.05 ☑
          football W21.01 ☑
          golf ball W21.04 ☑
          soccer W21.02 ☑
          softball W21.07 ☑
          specified NEC W21.09 ☑
          volleyball W21.06 ☑
        bat or racquet
          baseball bat W21.11 ☑
            assault Y08.02 ☑
          golf club W21.13 ☑
            assault Y08.09 ☑
          specified NEC W21.19 ☑
            assault Y08.09 ☑
          tennis racquet W21.12 ☑
            assault Y08.09 ☑
        hockey (ice)
          field
            puck W21.221 ☑
            stick W21.211 ☑
          puck W21.220 ☑
          stick W21.210 ☑
            assault Y08.01 ☑
          specified NEC W21.89 ☑
      set in motion by explosion — *see* Explosion
    thrown W20.8 ☑
      assault Y00 ☑
      in sports W21.9 ☑
        assault Y08.09 ☑
        ball W21.00 ☑
          baseball W21.03 ☑
          basketball W21.05 ☑
          football W21.01 ☑
          golf ball W21.04 ☑
          soccer W21.02 ☑
          soft ball W21.07 ☑
          specified NEC W21.09 ☑
          volleyball W21.06 ☑
        bat or racquet
          baseball bat W21.11 ☑
            assault Y08.02 ☑
          golf club W21.13 ☑
            assault Y08.09 ☑
          specified NEC W21.19 ☑
            assault Y08.09 ☑
          tennis racquet W21.12 ☑
            assault Y08.09 ☑
        hockey (ice)
          field
            puck W21.221 ☑
            stick W21.211 ☑
          puck W21.220 ☑
          stick W21.210 ☑
            assault Y08.01 ☑
          specified NEC W21.89 ☑
  other person(s) W50.0 ☑
    with
      blunt object W22.8 ☑
        intentional, homicide (attempt) Y00 ☑
        sports equipment W21.9 ☑
        undetermined whether accidental or intentional Y29 ☑
      fall W03 ☑
        due to ice or snow W00.0 ☑
    as, or caused by, a crowd or human stampede (with fall) W52 ☑
    assault Y04.2 ☑
    homicide (attempt) Y04.2 ☑
    in legal intervention
      injuring
        bystander Y35.812 ☑
        law enforcement personnel Y35.811 ☑
        suspect Y35.813 ☑
        unspecified person Y35.819 ☑
    sports equipment W21.9 ☑
  police (on duty) — *see* Legal, intervention, manhandling
    with blunt object — *see* Legal, intervention, blunt object
  sports equipment W21.9 ☑

Struck (accidentally) **by** — *continued*
  sports equipment — *continued*
    assault Y08.09 ☑
    ball W21.00 ☑
      baseball W21.03 ☑
      basketball W21.05 ☑
      football W21.01 ☑
      golf ball W21.04 ☑
      soccer W21.02 ☑
      soft ball W21.07 ☑
      specified NEC W21.09 ☑
      volleyball W21.06 ☑
    bat or racquet
      baseball bat W21.11 ☑
        assault Y08.02 ☑
      golf club W21.13 ☑
        assault Y08.09 ☑
      specified NEC W21.19 ☑
      tennis racquet W21.12 ☑
        assault Y08.09 ☑
    cleats (shoe) W21.31 ☑
    foot wear NEC W21.39 ☑
    football helmet W21.81 ☑
    hockey (ice)
      field
        puck W21.221 ☑
        stick W21.211 ☑
      puck W21.220 ☑
      stick W21.210 ☑
        assault Y08.01 ☑
    skate blades W21.32 ☑
    specified NEC W21.89 ☑
      assault Y08.09 ☑
  thunderbolt — *see* subcategory T75.0 ☑
    causing fire — *see* Exposure, fire
  transport vehicle NEC — *see also* Accident, transport
      V09.9 ☑
    intentional, homicide (attempt) Y03.0 ☑
    motor NEC — *see also* Accident, transport V09.20 ☑
      homicide Y03.0 ☑
  vehicle (transport) NEC — *see* Accident, transport, by
      type of vehicle
  stationary (falling from jack, hydraulic lift, ramp)
      W20.8 ☑
Stumbling
  over
    animal NEC W01.0 ☑
      with fall W18.09 ☑
    carpet, rug or (small) object W22.8 ☑
      with fall W18.09 ☑
    person W51 ☑
      with fall W03 ☑
        due to ice or snow W00.0 ☑
  without fall W18.40 ☑
    due to
      specified NEC W18.49 ☑
      stepping from one level to another W18.43 ☑
      stepping into hole or opening W18.42 ☑
      stepping on object W18.41 ☑
Submersion (accidental) — *see* Drowning
Suffocation (accidental) (by external means) (by pressure)
    (mechanical) — *see also* category T71 ☑
  due to, by
    avalanche — *see* Landslide
    explosion — *see* Explosion
    fire — *see* Exposure, fire
    food, any type (aspiration) (ingestion) (inhalation) —
        see categories T17 and T18 ☑
    ignition — *see* Ignition
    landslide — *see* Landslide
    machine(ry) — *see* Contact, with, by type of machine
    vomitus (aspiration) (inhalation) T17.81- ☑
  in
    burning building X00.8 ☑
Suicide, suicidal (attempted) (by) X83.8 ☑
  blunt object X79 ☑
  burning, burns X76 ☑
    hot object X77.9 ☑
      fluid NEC X77.2 ☑
      household appliance X77.3 ☑
      specified NEC X77.8 ☑
      steam X77.0 ☑
      tap water X77.1 ☑
      vapors X77.0 ☑
  caustic substance — *see* Table of Drugs and Chemicals
  cold, extreme X83.2 ☑

Suicide, suicidal — *continued*
  collision of motor vehicle with
    motor vehicle X82.0 ☑
    specified NEC X82.8 ☑
    train X82.1 ☑
    tree X82.2 ☑
  crashing of aircraft X83.0 ☑
  cut (any part of body) X78.9 ☑
  cutting or piercing instrument X78.9 ☑
    dagger X78.2 ☑
    glass X78.0 ☑
    knife X78.1 ☑
    specified NEC X78.8 ☑
    sword X78.2 ☑
  drowning (in) X71.9 ☑
    bathtub X71.0 ☑
    natural water X71.3 ☑
    specified NEC X71.8 ☑
    swimming pool X71.1 ☑
      following fall X71.2 ☑
  electrocution X83.1 ☑
  explosive(s) (material) X75 ☑
  fire, flames X76 ☑
  firearm X74.9 ☑
    airgun X74.01 ☑
    handgun X72 ☑
    hunting rifle X73.1 ☑
    larger X73.9 ☑
      specified NEC X73.8 ☑
    machine gun X73.2 ☑
    shotgun X73.0 ☑
    specified NEC X74.8 ☑
  hanging X83.8 ☑
  hot object — *see* Suicide, burning, hot object
  jumping
    before moving object X81.8 ☑
      motor vehicle X81.0 ☑
      subway train X81.1 ☑
      train X81.1 ☑
    from high place X80 ☑
  late effect of attempt — *see* X71-X83 with 7th character
      S
  lying before moving object, train, vehicle X81.8 ☑
  poisoning — *see* Table of Drugs and Chemicals
  puncture (any part of body) — *see* Suicide, cutting or
      piercing instrument
  scald — *see* Suicide, burning, hot object
  sequelae of attempt — *see* X71-X83 with 7th character
      S
  sharp object (any) — *see* Suicide, cutting or piercing in-
      strument
  shooting — *see* Suicide, firearm
  specified means NEC X83.8 ☑
  stab (any part of body) — *see* Suicide, cutting or piercing
      instrument
  steam, hot vapors X77.0 ☑
  strangulation X83.8 ☑
  submersion — *see* Suicide, drowning
  suffocation X83.8 ☑
  wound NEC X83.8 ☑
Sunstroke X32 ☑
Supersonic waves (causing injury) W42.0 ☑
Surgical procedure, complication of (delayed or as an
      abnormal reaction without mention of misadventure)
      — *see also* Complication of or following, by type of
      procedure
    due to or as a result of misadventure — *see* Misadventure
Swallowed, swallowing
  foreign body — *see* Foreign body, alimentary canal
  poison — *see* Table of Drugs and Chemicals
  substance
    caustic or corrosive — *see* Table of Drugs and Chemi-
        cals
    poisonous — *see* Table of Drugs and Chemicals

T

Tackle in sport W03 ☑
Terrorism (involving) Y38.80 ☑
  biological weapons Y38.6X- ☑
  chemical weapons Y38.7X- ☑
  conflagration Y38.3X- ☑
  drowning and submersion Y38.89- ☑
  explosion Y38.2X- ☑
    destruction of aircraft Y38.1X- ☑
    marine weapons Y38.0X- ☑

Terrorism — *continued*
  fire Y38.3X- ☑
  firearms Y38.4X- ☑
  hot substances Y38.3X- ☑
  lasers Y38.89- ☑
  nuclear weapons Y38.5X- ☑
  piercing or stabbing instruments Y38.89- ☑
  secondary effects Y38.9X- ☑
  specified method NEC Y38.89- ☑
  suicide bomber Y38.81- ☑
Thirst X58 ☑
Threat to breathing
  aspiration — *see* Aspiration
  due to cave-in, falling earth or substance NEC T71 ☑
Thrown (accidentally)
  against part (any) of or object in transport vehicle (in
      motion) NEC — *see also* Accident, transport
  from
    high place, homicide (attempt) Y01 ☑
    machinery — *see* Contact, with, by type of machine
    transport vehicle NEC — *see also* Accident, transport
        V89.9 ☑
  off — *see* Thrown, from
Thunderbolt — *see* subcategory T75.0 ☑
  causing fire — *see* Exposure, fire
Tidal wave (any injury) **NEC** — *see* Forces of nature, tidal
      wave
Took
  overdose (drug) — *see* Table of Drugs and Chemicals
  poison — *see* Table of Drugs and Chemicals
Tornado (any injury) X37.1 ☑
Torrential rain (any injury) X37.8 ☑
Torture X58 ☑
Trampled by animal NEC W55.89 ☑
Trapped (accidentally)
  between objects (moving) (stationary and moving) —
      see Caught
  by part (any) of
    electric (assisted) bicycle V29.881 ☑
    motorcycle V29.888 ☑
    pedal cycle V19.88 ☑
    transport vehicle NEC — *see also* Accident, transport
        V89.9 ☑
Travel (effects) (sickness) T75.3 ☑
Tree falling on or hitting (accidentally) (person) W20.8 ☑
Tripping
  over
    animal W01.0 ☑
      with fall W01.0 ☑
    carpet, rug or (small) object W22.8 ☑
      with fall W18.09 ☑
    person W51 ☑
      with fall W03 ☑
        due to ice or snow W00.0 ☑
  without fall W18.40 ☑
    due to
      specified NEC W18.49 ☑
      stepping from one level to another W18.43 ☑
      stepping into hole or opening W18.42 ☑
      stepping on object W18.41 ☑
Twisted by person(s) (accidentally) W50.2 ☑
  with intent to injure or kill Y04.0 ☑
  as, or caused by, a crowd or human stampede (with fall)
      W52 ☑
  assault Y04.0 ☑
  homicide (attempt) Y04.0 ☑
  in
    fight Y04.0 ☑
    legal intervention — *see* Legal, intervention, manhan-
        dling
Twisting (prolonged) (static) X50.1- ☑

U

**Underdosing of necessary drugs, medicaments or bio-
      logical substances** Y63.6 ☑
Undetermined intent (contact) (exposure)
  automobile collision Y32 ☑
  blunt object Y29 ☑
  drowning (submersion) (in) Y21.9 ☑
    bathtub Y21.0 ☑
      after fall Y21.1 ☑
    natural water (lake) (ocean) (pond) (river) (stream)
        Y21.4 ☑
    specified place NEC Y21.8 ☑
    swimming pool Y21.2 ☑

Undetermined intent — *continued*
  drowning — *continued*
    swimming pool — *continued*
      after fall Y21.3 ☑
  explosive material Y25 ☑
  fall, jump or push from high place Y30 ☑
  falling, lying or running before moving object Y31 ☑
  fire Y26 ☑
  firearm discharge Y24.9 ☑
    airgun (BB) (pellet) Y24.0 ☑
    handgun (pistol) (revolver) Y22 ☑
    hunting rifle Y23.1 ☑
    larger Y23.9 ☑
      hunting rifle Y23.1 ☑
      machine gun Y23.3 ☑
      military Y23.2 ☑
      shotgun Y23.0 ☑
      specified type NEC Y23.8 ☑
    machine gun Y23.3 ☑
    military Y23.2 ☑
    shotgun Y23.0 ☑
    specified type NEC Y24.8 ☑
    Very pistol Y24.8 ☑
  hot object Y27.9 ☑
    fluid NEC Y27.2 ☑
    household appliance Y27.3 ☑
    specified object NEC Y27.8 ☑
    steam Y27.0 ☑
    tap water Y27.1 ☑
    vapor Y27.0 ☑
  jump, fall or push from high place Y30 ☑
  lying, falling or running before moving object Y31 ☑
  motor vehicle crash Y32 ☑
  push, fall or jump from high place Y30 ☑
  running, falling or lying before moving object Y31 ☑
  sharp object Y28.9 ☑
    dagger Y28.2 ☑
    glass Y28.0 ☑
    knife Y28.1 ☑
    specified object NEC Y28.8 ☑
    sword Y28.2 ☑
  smoke Y26 ☑
  specified event NEC Y33 ☑
Use of hand as hammer X50.3 ☑

V

Vibration (causing injury) W49.9 ☑
Victim (of)
  avalanche — *see* Landslide
  earth movements NEC — *see* Forces of nature, earth movement
  earthquake X34 ☑
  flood — *see* Flood
  landslide — *see* Landslide
  lightning — *see* subcategory T75.0 ☑
    causing fire — *see* Exposure, fire
  storm (cataclysmic) NEC — *see* Forces of nature, cataclysmic storm
  volcanic eruption X35 ☑
Volcanic eruption (any injury) X35 ☑
Vomitus, gastric contents in air passages (with asphyxia, obstruction or suffocation) T17.81- ☑

W

Walked into stationary object (any) W22.09 ☑
  furniture W22.03 ☑
  lamppost W22.02 ☑
  wall W22.01 ☑
War operations (injuries to military personnel and civilians during war, civil insurrection and peacekeeping missions) (by) (from) (involving) Y36.90 ☑
  after cessation of hostilities Y36.89- ☑
    explosion (of)
      bomb placed during war operations Y36.82- ☑

War operations — *continued*
  after cessation of hostilities — *continued*
    explosion — *continued*
      mine placed during war operations Y36.81- ☑
      specified NEC Y36.88- ☑
  air blast Y36.20- ☑
  aircraft
    destruction — *see* War operations, destruction of aircraft
  airway restriction — *see* War operations, restriction of airways
  asphyxiation — *see* War operations, restriction of airways
  biological weapons Y36.6X- ☑
  blast Y36.20- ☑
  blast fragments Y36.20- ☑
  blast wave Y36.20- ☑
  blast wind Y36.20- ☑
  bomb Y36.20- ☑
    dirty Y36.50- ☑
    gasoline Y36.31- ☑
    incendiary Y36.31- ☑
    petrol Y36.31- ☑
  bullet Y36.43- ☑
    incendiary Y36.32- ☑
    rubber Y36.41- ☑
  chemical weapons Y36.7X- ☑
  combat
    hand to hand (unarmed) combat Y36.44- ☑
    using blunt or piercing object Y36.45- ☑
  conflagration — *see* War operations, fire
  conventional warfare NEC Y36.49- ☑
  depth-charge Y36.01- ☑
  destruction of aircraft Y36.10- ☑
    due to
      air to air missile Y36.11- ☑
      collision with other aircraft Y36.12- ☑
      detonation (accidental) of onboard munitions and explosives Y36.14- ☑
      enemy fire or explosives Y36.11- ☑
      explosive placed on aircraft Y36.11- ☑
      onboard fire Y36.13- ☑
      rocket propelled grenade [RPG] Y36.11- ☑
      small arms fire Y36.11- ☑
      surface to air missile Y36.11- ☑
    specified NEC Y36.19- ☑
  detonation (accidental) of
    onboard marine weapons Y36.05- ☑
    own munitions or munitions launch device Y36.24- ☑
  dirty bomb Y36.50- ☑
  explosion (of) Y36.20- ☑
    aerial bomb Y36.21- ☑
    after cessation of hostilities
      bomb placed during war operations Y36.82- ☑
      mine placed during war operations Y36.81- ☑
    bomb NOS — *see also* War operations, bomb(s) Y36.20- ☑
    fragments Y36.20- ☑
    grenade Y36.29- ☑
    guided missile Y36.22- ☑
    improvised explosive device [IED] (person-borne) (roadside) (vehicle-borne) Y36.23- ☑
    land mine Y36.29- ☑
    marine mine (at sea) (in harbor) Y36.02- ☑
    marine weapon Y36.00- ☑
      specified NEC Y36.09- ☑
    own munitions or munitions launch device (accidental) Y36.24- ☑
    sea-based artillery shell Y36.03- ☑
    specified NEC Y36.29- ☑
    torpedo Y36.04- ☑
  fire Y36.30- ☑
    specified NEC Y36.39- ☑
  firearms
    discharge Y36.43- ☑
    pellets Y36.42- ☑
  flamethrower Y36.33- ☑

War operations — *continued*
  fragments (from) (of)
    improvised explosive device [IED] (person-borne) (roadside) (vehicle-borne) Y36.26- ☑
    munitions Y36.25- ☑
    specified NEC Y36.29- ☑
    weapons Y36.27- ☑
  friendly fire Y36.92 ☑
  hand to hand (unarmed) combat Y36.44- ☑
  hot substances — *see* War operations, fire
  incendiary bullet Y36.32- ☑
  nuclear weapon (effects of) Y36.50- ☑
    acute radiation exposure Y36.54- ☑
    blast pressure Y36.51- ☑
    direct blast Y36.51- ☑
    direct heat Y36.53- ☑
    fallout exposure Y36.54- ☑
    fireball Y36.53- ☑
    indirect blast (struck or crushed by blast debris) (being thrown by blast) Y36.52- ☑
    ionizing radiation (immediate exposure) Y36.54- ☑
    nuclear radiation Y36.54- ☑
    radiation
      ionizing (immediate exposure) Y36.54- ☑
      nuclear Y36.54- ☑
      thermal Y36.53- ☑
    secondary effects Y36.54- ☑
    specified NEC Y36.59- ☑
    thermal radiation Y36.53- ☑
  restriction of air (airway)
    intentional Y36.46- ☑
    unintentional Y36.47- ☑
  rubber bullets Y36.41- ☑
  shrapnel NOS Y36.29- ☑
  suffocation — *see* War operations, restriction of airways
  unconventional warfare NEC Y36.7X- ☑
  underwater blast NOS Y36.00- ☑
  warfare
    conventional NEC Y36.49- ☑
    unconventional NEC Y36.7X- ☑
  weapon of mass destruction [WMD] Y36.91 ☑
  weapons
    biological weapons Y36.6X- ☑
    chemical Y36.7X- ☑
    nuclear (effects of) Y36.50- ☑
      acute radiation exposure Y36.54- ☑
      blast pressure Y36.51- ☑
      direct blast Y36.51- ☑
      direct heat Y36.53- ☑
      fallout exposure Y36.54- ☑
      fireball Y36.53- ☑
      radiation
        ionizing (immediate exposure) Y36.54- ☑
        nuclear Y36.54- ☑
        thermal Y36.53- ☑
      secondary effects Y36.54- ☑
      specified NEC Y36.59- ☑
  of mass destruction [WMD] Y36.91 ☑
Washed
  away by flood — *see* Flood
  off road by storm (transport vehicle) — *see* Forces of nature, cataclysmic storm
Weather exposure NEC — *see* Forces of nature
Weightlessness (causing injury) (effects of) (in spacecraft, real or simulated) X52 ☑
Work related condition Y99.0
Wound (accidental) NEC — *see also* Injury X58 ☑
  battle — *see also* War operations Y36.90 ☑
  gunshot — *see* Discharge, firearm by type
Wreck transport vehicle NEC — *see also* Accident, transport V89.9 ☑
Wrong
  device implanted into correct surgical site Y65.51
  fluid in infusion Y65.1
  patient, procedure performed on Y65.52
  procedure (operation) on correct patient Y65.51

ICD-10-CM Tabular List of Diseases and Injuries

Chapter 1. Certain Infectious and Parasitic Diseases (A00–B99), U07.1, U09.9

Chapter-specific Guidelines with Coding Examples

The chapter-specific guidelines from the ICD-10-CM Official Guidelines for Coding and Reporting have been provided below. Along with these guidelines are coding examples, contained in the shaded boxes, that have been developed to help illustrate the coding and/or sequencing guidance found in these guidelines.

a. Human immunodeficiency virus (HIV) infections

1) Code only confirmed cases

Code only confirmed cases of HIV infection/illness. This is an exception to the hospital inpatient guideline Section II, H.

In this context, "confirmation" does not require documentation of positive serology or culture for HIV; the provider's diagnostic statement that the patient is HIV positive or has an HIV-related illness is sufficient.

Patient admitted with anemia with possible HIV infection

D64.9   Anemia, unspecified

Explanation: Only the anemia is coded in this scenario because it has not been confirmed that an HIV infection is present. This is an exception to the guideline Section II, H for hospital inpatient coding.

---

2) Selection and sequencing of HIV codes

(a) Patient admitted for HIV-related condition

If a patient is admitted for an HIV-related condition, the principal diagnosis should be B20, Human immunodeficiency virus [HIV] disease followed by additional diagnosis codes for all reported HIV-related conditions.

An exception to this guideline is if the reason for admission is hemolytic-uremic syndrome associated with HIV disease. Assign code D59.31, Infection-associated hemolytic-uremic syndrome, followed by code B20, Human immunodeficiency virus [HIV] disease.

(b) Patient with HIV disease admitted for unrelated condition

If a patient with HIV disease is admitted for an unrelated condition (such as a traumatic injury), the code for the unrelated condition (e.g., the nature of injury code) should be the principal diagnosis. Other diagnoses would be B20 followed by additional diagnosis codes for all reported HIV-related conditions.

Unstable angina, native coronary artery atherosclerosis, HIV

I25.110   Atherosclerotic heart disease of native coronary artery with unstable angina pectoris

B20   Human immunodeficiency virus [HIV] disease

Explanation: The arteriosclerotic coronary artery disease and the unstable angina are not related to HIV, so those conditions are reported first using a combination code, and HIV is reported secondarily.

(c) Whether the patient is newly diagnosed

Whether the patient is newly diagnosed or has had previous admissions/encounters for HIV conditions is irrelevant to the sequencing decision.

(d) Asymptomatic human immunodeficiency virus

Z21, Asymptomatic human immunodeficiency virus [HIV] infection status, is to be applied when the patient without any documentation of symptoms is listed as being "HIV positive," "known HIV," "HIV test positive," or similar terminology. Do not use this code if the term "AIDS" or "HIV disease" is used or if the patient is treated for any HIV-related illness or is described as having any condition(s) resulting from his/her HIV positive status; use B20 in these cases.

(e) Patients with inconclusive HIV serology

Patients with inconclusive HIV serology, but no definitive diagnosis or manifestations of the illness, may be assigned code R75, Inconclusive laboratory evidence of human immunodeficiency virus [HIV].

(f) Previously diagnosed HIV-related illness

Patients with any known prior diagnosis of an HIV-related illness should be coded to B20. Once a patient has developed an HIV-related illness, the patient should always be assigned code B20 on every subsequent admission/encounter. Patients previously diagnosed with any HIV illness (B20) should never be assigned to R75 or Z21, Asymptomatic human immunodeficiency virus [HIV] infection status.

(g) HIV infection in pregnancy, childbirth and the puerperium

During pregnancy, childbirth or the puerperium, a patient admitted (or presenting for a health care encounter) because of an HIV-related illness should receive a principal diagnosis code of O98.7-, Human

immunodeficiency [HIV] disease complicating pregnancy, childbirth and the puerperium, followed by B20 and the code(s) for the HIV-related illness(es). Codes from Chapter 15 always take sequencing priority.

Patients with asymptomatic HIV infection status admitted (or presenting for a health care encounter) during pregnancy, childbirth, or the puerperium should receive codes of O98.7- and Z21.

(h) Encounters for testing for HIV

If a patient is being seen to determine his/her HIV status, use code Z11.4, Encounter for screening for human immunodeficiency virus [HIV]. Use additional codes for any associated high-risk behavior, if applicable.

If a patient with signs or symptoms is being seen for HIV testing, code the signs and symptoms. An additional counseling code Z71.7, Human immunodeficiency virus [HIV] counseling, may be used if counseling is provided during the encounter for the test.

When a patient returns to be informed of his/her HIV test results and the test result is negative, use code Z71.7, Human immunodeficiency virus [HIV] counseling.

If the results are positive, see previous guidelines and assign codes as appropriate.

(i) HIV managed by antiretroviral medication

If a patient with documented HIV disease, HIV-related illness or AIDS is currently managed on antiretroviral medications, assign code B20, Human immunodeficiency virus [HIV] disease. Code Z79.899, Other long term (current) drug therapy, may be assigned as an additional code to identify the long-term (current) use of antiretroviral medications.

(j) Encounter for HIV Prophylaxis Measure

When a patient is seen for administration of pre-exposure prophylaxis medication for HIV, assign code Z29.81, Encounter for HIV pre-exposure prophylaxis. Pre-exposure prophylaxis (PrEP) is intended to prevent infection in people who are at risk for getting HIV through sex or injection drug use. Any risk factors for HIV should also be coded.

b. Infectious agents as the cause of diseases classified to other chapters

Certain infections are classified in chapters other than Chapter 1 and no organism is identified as part of the infection code. In these instances, it is necessary to use an additional code from Chapter 1 to identify the organism. A code from category B95, Streptococcus, Staphylococcus, and Enterococcus as the cause of diseases classified to other chapters, B96, Other bacterial agents as the cause of diseases classified to other chapters, or B97, Viral agents as the cause of diseases classified to other chapters, is to be used as an additional code to identify the organism. An instructional note will be found at the infection code advising that an additional organism code is required.

c. Infections resistant to antibiotics

Many bacterial infections are resistant to current antibiotics. It is necessary to identify all infections documented as antibiotic resistant. Assign a code from category Z16, Resistance to antimicrobial drugs, following the infection code only if the infection code does not identify drug resistance.

d. Sepsis, severe sepsis, and septic shock infections resistant to antibiotics

1) Coding of sepsis and severe sepsis

(a) Sepsis

For a diagnosis of sepsis, assign the appropriate code for the underlying systemic infection. If the type of infection or causal organism is not further specified, assign code A41.9, Sepsis, unspecified organism.

A code from subcategory R65.2, Severe sepsis, should not be assigned unless severe sepsis or an associated acute organ dysfunction is documented.

(i) Negative or inconclusive blood cultures and sepsis

Negative or inconclusive blood cultures do not preclude a diagnosis of sepsis in patients with clinical evidence of the condition; however, the provider should be queried.

(ii) Urosepsis

The term urosepsis is a nonspecific term. It is not to be considered synonymous with sepsis. It has no default code in the Alphabetic Index. Should a provider use this term, he/she must be queried for clarification.

(iii) Sepsis with organ dysfunction

If a patient has sepsis and associated acute organ dysfunction or multiple organ dysfunction (MOD), follow the instructions for coding severe sepsis.

(iv) Acute organ dysfunction that is not clearly associated with the sepsis

If a patient has sepsis and an acute organ dysfunction, but the medical record documentation indicates that the acute organ dysfunction is related to a medical condition other than the sepsis, do not assign a code from subcategory R65.2, Severe sepsis. An acute organ dysfunction must be associated with the sepsis in order to assign the severe sepsis code. If the documentation is not clear as to whether an acute organ dysfunction is related to the sepsis or another medical condition, query the provider.

Sepsis and acute respiratory failure due to COPD exacerbation	
A41.9	Sepsis, unspecified organism
J44.1	Chronic obstructive pulmonary disease with (acute) exacerbation
J96.00	Acute respiratory failure, unspecified whether with hypoxia or hypercapnia

Explanation: Although acute organ dysfunction is present in the form of acute respiratory failure, severe sepsis (R65.2) is not coded in this example, as the acute respiratory failure is attributed to the COPD exacerbation rather than the sepsis. Sequencing of these codes would be determined by the circumstances of the admission.

(b) Severe sepsis

The coding of severe sepsis requires a minimum of 2 codes: first a code for the underlying systemic infection, followed by a code from subcategory R65.2, Severe sepsis. If the causal organism is not documented, assign code A41.9, Sepsis, unspecified organism, for the infection. Additional code(s) for the associated acute organ dysfunction are also required.

Due to the complex nature of severe sepsis, some cases may require querying the provider prior to assignment of the codes.

2) Septic shock

Septic shock generally refers to circulatory failure associated with severe sepsis, and therefore, it represents a type of acute organ dysfunction.

For cases of septic shock, the code for the systemic infection should be sequenced first, followed by code R65.21, Severe sepsis with septic shock or code T81.12, Postprocedural septic shock. Any additional codes for the other acute organ dysfunctions should also be assigned. As noted in the sequencing instructions in the Tabular List, the code for septic shock cannot be assigned as a principal diagnosis.

Sepsis with septic shock	
A41.9	Sepsis, unspecified organism
R65.21	Severe sepsis with septic shock

Explanation: Documentation of septic shock automatically implies severe sepsis as it is a form of acute organ dysfunction. Septic shock is not coded as the principal diagnosis; it is always preceded by the code for the systemic infection.

3) Sequencing of severe sepsis

If severe sepsis is present on admission, and meets the definition of principal diagnosis, the underlying systemic infection should be assigned as principal diagnosis followed by the appropriate code from subcategory R65.2 as required by the sequencing rules in the Tabular List. A code from subcategory R65.2 can never be assigned as a principal diagnosis.

When severe sepsis develops during an encounter (it was not present on admission), the underlying systemic infection and the appropriate code from subcategory R65.2 should be assigned as secondary diagnoses.

Severe sepsis may be present on admission, but the diagnosis may not be confirmed until sometime after admission. If the documentation is not clear whether severe sepsis was present on admission, the provider should be queried.

For infection-associated hemolytic-uremic syndrome with severe sepsis, see guideline I.C.1.d.9.

4) Sepsis or severe sepsis with a localized infection

If the reason for admission is sepsis or severe sepsis and a localized infection, such as pneumonia or cellulitis, a code(s) for the underlying systemic infection should be assigned first and the code for the localized infection should be assigned as a secondary diagnosis. If the patient has severe sepsis, a code from subcategory R65.2 should also be assigned as a secondary diagnosis. If the patient is admitted with a localized infection, such as pneumonia, and sepsis/severe sepsis doesn't develop until after admission, the localized infection should be assigned first, followed by the appropriate sepsis/severe sepsis codes.

For hemolytic-uremic syndrome associated with sepsis, see guideline I.C.1.d.9.

Patient presents with acute renal failure due to severe sepsis from *Pseudomonas* pneumonia	
A41.52	Sepsis due to Pseudomonas
J15.1	Pneumonia due to Pseudomonas
R65.20	Severe sepsis without septic shock
N17.9	Acute kidney failure, unspecified

Explanation: If all conditions are present on admission, the systemic infection (sepsis) is sequenced first followed by the codes for the localized infection (pneumonia), severe sepsis and any organ dysfunction. If only the pneumonia was present on admission with the sepsis and resulting renal failure developing later in the admission, then the pneumonia would be sequenced first.

5) Sepsis due to a postprocedural infection

(a) Documentation of causal relationship

As with all postprocedural complications, code assignment is based on the provider's documentation of the relationship between the infection and the procedure.

(b) Sepsis due to a postprocedural infection

For sepsis following a postprocedural wound (surgical site) infection, a code from T81.41 to T81.43, Infection following a procedure, T81.49, Infection following a procedure, other surgical site, or a code from O86.00 to O86.03, Infection of obstetric surgical wound, or code O86.09, Infection of obstetric surgical wound, other surgical site, that identifies the site of the infection should be sequenced first, if known. Assign an additional code for sepsis following a procedure (T81.44) or sepsis following an obstetrical procedure (O86.04). Use an additional code to identify the infectious agent. If the patient has severe sepsis, the appropriate code from subcategory R65.2 should also be assigned with the additional code(s) for any acute organ dysfunction.

For infections following infusion, transfusion, therapeutic injection, or immunization, a code from subcategory T80.2, Infections following infusion, transfusion, and therapeutic injection, or code T88.0-, Infection following immunization, should be coded first, followed by the code for the specific infection. If the patient has severe sepsis, the appropriate code from subcategory R65.2 should also be assigned, with the additional codes(s) for any acute organ dysfunction.

(c) Postprocedural infection and postprocedural septic shock

If a postprocedural infection has resulted in postprocedural septic shock, assign the codes indicated above for sepsis due to a postprocedural infection, followed by code T81.12-, Postprocedural septic shock. Do not assign code R65.21, Severe sepsis with septic shock. Additional code(s) should be assigned for any acute organ dysfunction.

Septic shock following abdominal procedure with intramuscular abscess	
T81.42XA	Infection following a procedure, deep incisional surgical site, initial encounter
T81.44XA	Sepsis following a procedure, initial encounter
A41.9	Sepsis, unspecified organism
T81.12XA	Postprocedural septic shock, initial encounter

Explanation: The first code reported identifies the site of the postprocedural infection with intramuscular abscess coded to "deep incisional surgical site." If sepsis occurred as a result of the postprocedural infection, code T81.44- should be coded as a secondary diagnosis, followed by a code for the specific type of sepsis. Postprocedural septic shock is captured by code T81.12- and not with code R65.21. If any other acute organ dysfunction was documented as associated with the postprocedural sepsis, additional codes could be assigned to represent those conditions.

6) Sepsis and severe sepsis associated with a noninfectious process (condition)

In some cases, a noninfectious process (condition) such as trauma, may lead to an infection which can result in sepsis or severe sepsis. If sepsis or severe sepsis is documented as associated with a noninfectious condition, such as a burn or serious injury, and this condition meets the definition for principal diagnosis, the code for the noninfectious condition should be sequenced first, followed by the code for the resulting infection. If severe sepsis is present, a code from subcategory R65.2 should also be assigned with any associated organ dysfunction(s) codes. It is not necessary to assign a code from subcategory R65.1, Systemic inflammatory response syndrome (SIRS) of non-infectious origin, for these cases.

If the infection meets the definition of principal diagnosis, it should be sequenced before the non-infectious condition. When both the associated non-infectious condition and the infection meet the definition of principal diagnosis, either may be assigned as principal diagnosis.

Only one code from category R65, Symptoms and signs specifically associated with systemic inflammation and infection, should be assigned. Therefore, when a non-infectious condition leads to an infection resulting in severe sepsis, assign the appropriate code from subcategory R65.2, Severe sepsis. Do not additionally assign a code from subcategory R65.1, Systemic inflammatory response syndrome (SIRS) of non-infectious origin.

See Section I.C.18. SIRS due to non-infectious process.

> Patient admitted with multiple third-degree burns of right upper arm develops severe MSSA sepsis with septic shock, three days into admission
>
> | T22.391A | Burn of third degree of multiple sites of right shoulder and upper arm limb, except wrist and hand, initial encounter |
> |---|---|
> | A41.01 | Sepsis due to Methicillin susceptible Staphylococcus aureus |
> | R65.21 | Severe sepsis with septic shock |
>
> *Explanation:* Severe sepsis is coded rather than SIRS from R65 because it is documented as a severe systemic infectious response with septic shock to a noninfectious condition. The code for the systemic infection is not used as the principal diagnosis because it was not present on admission. The patient was admitted for the burn injury.

7) Sepsis and septic shock complicating abortion, pregnancy, childbirth, and the puerperium

See Section I.C.15. Sepsis and septic shock complicating abortion, pregnancy, childbirth and the puerperium

8) Newborn sepsis

See Section I.C.16. f. Bacterial sepsis of Newborn

9) Hemolytic-uremic syndrome associated with sepsis

If the reason for admission is hemolytic-uremic syndrome that is associated with sepsis, assign code D59.31, Infection-associated hemolytic-uremic syndrome, as the principal diagnosis. Codes for the underlying systemic infection and any other conditions (such as severe sepsis) should be assigned as secondary diagnoses.

e. Methicillin resistant Staphylococcus aureus (MRSA) conditions

1) Selection and sequencing of MRSA codes

(a) Combination codes for MRSA infection

When a patient is diagnosed with an infection that is due to methicillin resistant *Staphylococcus aureus* (MRSA), and that infection has a combination code that includes the causal organism (e.g., sepsis, pneumonia) assign the appropriate combination code for the condition (e.g., code A41.02, Sepsis due to Methicillin resistant Staphylococcus aureus or code J15.212, Pneumonia due to Methicillin resistant Staphylococcus aureus). Do not assign code B95.62, Methicillin resistant Staphylococcus aureus infection as the cause of diseases classified elsewhere, as an additional code, because the combination code includes the type of infection and the MRSA organism. Do not assign a code from subcategory Z16.11, Resistance to penicillins, as an additional diagnosis.

See Section C.1. for instructions on coding and sequencing of sepsis and severe sepsis.

(b) Other codes for MRSA infection

When there is documentation of a current infection (e.g., wound infection, stitch abscess, urinary tract infection) due to MRSA, and that infection does not have a combination code that includes the causal organism, assign the appropriate code to identify the condition along with code B95.62, Methicillin resistant Staphylococcus aureus infection as the cause of diseases classified elsewhere for the MRSA infection. Do not assign a code from subcategory Z16.11, Resistance to penicillins.

(c) Methicillin susceptible Staphylococcus aureus (MSSA) and MRSA colonization

The condition or state of being colonized or carrying MSSA or MRSA is called colonization or carriage, while an individual person is described as being colonized or being a carrier.

Colonization means that MSSA or MSRA is present on or in the body without necessarily causing illness. A positive MRSA colonization test might be documented by the provider as "MRSA screen positive" or "MRSA nasal swab positive".

Assign code Z22.322, Carrier or suspected carrier of Methicillin resistant Staphylococcus aureus, for patients documented as having MRSA colonization. Assign code Z22.321, Carrier or suspected carrier

of Methicillin susceptible Staphylococcus aureus, for patients documented as having MSSA colonization. Colonization is not necessarily indicative of a disease process or as the cause of a specific condition the patient may have unless documented as such by the provider.

(d) MRSA colonization and infection

If a patient is documented as having both MRSA colonization and infection during a hospital admission, code Z22.322, Carrier or suspected carrier of Methicillin resistant Staphylococcus aureus, and a code for the MRSA infection may both be assigned.

f. Zika virus infections

1) Code only confirmed cases

Code only a confirmed diagnosis of Zika virus (A92.5, Zika virus disease) as documented by the provider. This is an exception to the hospital inpatient guideline Section II, H. In this context, "confirmation" does not require documentation of the type of test performed; the provider's diagnostic statement that the condition is confirmed is sufficient. This code should be assigned regardless of the stated mode of transmission.

If the provider documents "suspected", "possible" or "probable" Zika, do not assign code A92.5. Assign a code(s) explaining the reason for encounter (such as fever, rash, or joint pain) or Z20.821, Contact with and (suspected) exposure to Zika virus.

g. Coronavirus infections

1) COVID-19 infection (infection due to SARS-CoV-2)

(a) Code only confirmed cases

Code only a confirmed diagnosis of the 2019 novel coronavirus disease (COVID-19) as documented by the provider, or documentation of a positive COVID-19 test result. For a confirmed diagnosis, assign code U07.1, COVID-19. This is an exception to the hospital inpatient guideline Section II, H. In this context, "confirmation" does not require documentation of a positive test result for COVID-19; the provider's documentation that the individual has COVID-19 is sufficient.

If the provider documents "suspected," "possible," "probable," or "inconclusive" COVID-19, do not assign code U07.1. Instead, code the signs and symptoms reported. See guideline I.C.1.g.1.g.

> An elderly patient who is a former smoker is admitted with a productive cough, fatigue, and chest discomfort. CXR and PFTs indicate acute bronchitis. Treatment includes cough suppressants and anti-inflammatory medication, along with isolation precautions. The provider documents acute bronchitis likely due to COVID-19. Laboratory tests were inconclusive.
>
> | J20.9 | Acute bronchitis, unspecified |
> |---|---|
> | Z87.891 | History of tobacco dependence |
>
> *Explanation:* Because the COVID-19 diagnosis was documented as likely by the provider, code U07.1 cannot be assigned. Instead a code explaining the reason for the encounter is used, in this case the acute bronchitis. Code J20.9 Acute bronchitis, unspecified, is used because the causative organism, specifically that which causes COVID-19, is not confirmed. Without further documentation of COVID-19 or another causative organism being present, code J20.8 Acute bronchitis due to other specified organisms, does not apply.

(b) Sequencing of codes

When COVID-19 meets the definition of principal diagnosis, code U07.1, COVID-19, should be sequenced first, followed by the appropriate codes for associated manifestations, except when another guideline requires that certain codes be sequenced first, such as obstetrics, sepsis, or transplant complications.

> The patient presents with acute hypoxic respiratory failure due to sepsis from COVID-19 related pneumonia.
>
> | A41.89 | Other specified sepsis |
> |---|---|
> | U07.1 | COVID-19 |
> | J12.82 | Pneumonia due to coronavirus disease 2019 |
> | J96.01 | Acute respiratory failure with hypoxia |
> | R65.20 | Severe sepsis without septic shock |
>
> *Explanation:* If all conditions are present on admission, the systemic infection (sepsis) is sequenced first, followed by the code(s) for the localized infection (COVID-19 and pneumonia). The acute respiratory failure (acute organ dysfunction) is clearly documented as being associated with the sepsis, and therefore a severe sepsis code from subcategory R65.2- can also be assigned. If the sepsis had developed later in the admission, with or without any associated respiratory failure, the COVID-19 code would be sequenced first.

For a COVID-19 infection that progresses to sepsis, see Section I.C.1.d. Sepsis, Severe Sepsis, and Septic Shock

See Section I.C.15.s. for COVID-19 infection in pregnancy, childbirth, and the puerperium

See Section I.C.16.h. for COVID-19 infection in newborn

For a COVID-19 infection in a lung transplant patient, see Section I.C.19.g.3.a. Transplant complications other than kidney.

(c) Acute respiratory manifestations of COVID-19

When the reason for the encounter/admission is a respiratory manifestation of COVID-19, assign code U07.1, COVID-19, as the principal/first-listed diagnosis and assign code(s) for the respiratory manifestation(s) as additional diagnoses.

The following conditions are examples of common respiratory manifestations of COVID-19.

(i) Pneumonia

For a patient with pneumonia confirmed as due to COVID-19, assign codes U07.1, COVID-19, and J12.82, Pneumonia due to coronavirus disease 2019.

(ii) Acute bronchitis

For a patient with acute bronchitis confirmed as due to COVID-19, assign codes U07.1, and J20.8, Acute bronchitis due to other specified organisms.

Bronchitis not otherwise specified (NOS) due to COVID-19 should be coded using code U07.1 and J40, Bronchitis, not specified as acute or chronic.

(iii) Lower respiratory infection

If the COVID-19 is documented as being associated with a lower respiratory infection, not otherwise specified (NOS), or an acute respiratory infection, NOS, codes U07.1 and J22, Unspecified acute lower respiratory infection, should be assigned.

If the COVID-19 is documented as being associated with a respiratory infection, NOS, codes U07.1 and J98.8, Other specified respiratory disorders, should be assigned.

(iv) Acute respiratory distress syndrome

For acute respiratory distress syndrome (ARDS) due to COVID-19, assign codes U07.1, and J80, Acute respiratory distress syndrome.

(v) Acute respiratory failure

For acute respiratory failure due to COVID-19, assign code U07.1, and J96.0-, Acute respiratory failure.

(d) Non-respiratory manifestations of COVID-19

When the reason for the encounter/admission is a non-respiratory manifestation (e.g., viral enteritis) of COVID-19, assign code U07.1, COVID-19, as the principal/first-listed diagnosis and assign code(s) for the manifestation(s) as additional diagnoses.

(e) Exposure to COVID-19

For asymptomatic individuals with actual or suspected exposure to COVID-19, assign code Z20.822, Contact with and (suspected) exposure to COVID-19.

For symptomatic individuals with actual or suspected exposure to COVID-19 and the infection has been ruled out, or test results are inconclusive or unknown, assign code Z20.822, Contact with and (suspected) exposure to COVID-19. See guideline I.C.21.c.1, Contact/Exposure, for additional guidance regarding the use of category Z20 codes.

If COVID-19 is confirmed, see guideline I.C.1.g.1.a.

(f) Screening for COVID-19

For screening for COVID-19, including preoperative testing, assign code Z11.52, Encounter for screening for COVID-19.

(g) Signs and symptoms without definitive diagnosis of COVID-19

For patients presenting with any signs/symptoms associated with COVID-19 (such as fever, etc.) but a definitive diagnosis has not been established, assign the appropriate code(s) for each of the presenting signs and symptoms such as:

- R05.1, Acute cough, or R05.9, Cough, unspecified
- R06.02 Shortness of breath
- R50.9 Fever, unspecified

If a patient with signs/symptoms associated with COVID-19 also has an actual or suspected contact with or exposure to COVID-19, assign Z20.822, Contact with and (suspected) exposure to COVID19, as an additional code.

(h) Asymptomatic individuals who test positive for COVID-19

For asymptomatic individuals who test positive for COVID-19, see guideline I.C.1.g.1.a. Although the individual is asymptomatic, the individual has tested positive and is considered to have the COVID-19 infection.

(i) Personal history of COVID-19

For patients with a history of COVID-19, assign code Z86.16, Personal history of COVID-19.

(j) Follow-up visits after COVID-19 infection has resolved

For individuals who previously had COVID-19, without residual symptom(s) or condition(s), and are being seen for follow-up evaluation, and COVID-19 test results are negative, assign codes Z09, Encounter for follow-up examination after completed treatment for conditions other than malignant neoplasm, and Z86.16, Personal history of COVID-19.

For follow-up visits for individuals with symptom(s) or condition(s) related to a previous COVID-19 infection, see guideline I.C.1.g.1.m.

See Section I.C.21.c.8, Factors influencing health states and contact with health services, Follow-up

(k) Encounter for antibody testing

For an encounter for antibody testing that is not being performed to confirm a current COVID-19 infection, nor is a follow-up test after resolution of COVID-19, assign Z01.84, Encounter for antibody response examination.

Follow the applicable guidelines above if the individual is being tested to confirm a current COVID-19 infection.

For follow-up testing after a COVID-19 infection, see guideline I.C.1.g.1.j.

(l) Multisystem inflammatory syndrome

For individuals with multisystem inflammatory syndrome (MIS) and COVID-19, assign code U07.1, COVID-19, as the principal/first-listed diagnosis and assign code M35.81, Multisystem inflammatory syndrome, as an additional diagnosis.

If an individual with a history of COVID-19 develops MIS, assign codes M35.81, Multisystem inflammatory syndrome, and U09.9, Post COVID-19 condition, unspecified.

If an individual with a known or suspected exposure to COVID-19, and no current COVID-19 infection or history of COVID-19, develops MIS, assign codes M35.81, Multisystem inflammatory syndrome, and Z20.822, Contact with and (suspected) exposure to COVID-19.

Additional codes should be assigned for any associated complications of MIS.

(m) Post COVID-19 condition

For sequela of COVID-19, or associated symptoms or conditions that develop following a previous COVID-19 infection, assign a code(s) for the specific symptom(s) or condition(s) related to the previous COVID-19 infection, if known, and code U09.9, Post COVID-19 condition, unspecified.

Code U09.9 should not be assigned for manifestations of an active (current) COVID-19 infection.

If a patient has a condition(s) associated with a previous COVID-19 infection and develops a new active (current) COVID-19 infection, code U09.9 may be assigned in conjunction with code U07.1, COVID-19, to identify that the patient also has a condition(s) associated with a previous COVID-19 infection. Code(s) for the specific condition(s) associated with the previous COVID-19 infection and code(s) for manifestation(s) of the new active (current) COVID-19 infection should also be assigned.

(n) Underimmunization for COVID-19 Status

Code Z28.310, Unvaccinated for COVID-19, may be assigned when the patient has not received a COVID-19 vaccine of any type. Code Z28.311, Partially vaccinated for COVID-19, may be assigned when the patient has been partially vaccinated for COVID-19 as per the recommendations of the Centers for Disease Control and Prevention (CDC) in place at the time of the encounter. For information, visit the CDC's website https://www.cdc.gov/coronavirus/2019-ncov/vaccines/.

See Section I.B.14. for underimmunization documentation by clinicians other than patient's provider.

Chapter 1. Certain Infectious and Parasitic Diseases (A00-B99)

INCLUDES diseases generally recognized as communicable or transmissible
Use additional code to identify resistance to antimicrobial drugs (Z16.-)
EXCLUDES 1 certain localized infections - see body system-related chapters
EXCLUDES 2 carrier or suspected carrier of infectious disease (Z22.-)
infectious and parasitic diseases complicating pregnancy, childbirth and the puerperium (O98.-)
infectious and parasitic diseases specific to the perinatal period (P35-P39)
influenza and other acute respiratory infections (J00-J22)

This chapter contains the following blocks:

A00-A09 Intestinal infectious diseases
A15-A19 Tuberculosis
A20-A28 Certain zoonotic bacterial diseases
A30-A49 Other bacterial diseases
A50-A64 Infections with a predominantly sexual mode of transmission
A65-A69 Other spirochetal diseases
A70-A74 Other diseases caused by chlamydiae
A75-A79 Rickettsioses
A80-A89 Viral and prion infections of the central nervous system
A90-A99 Arthropod-borne viral fevers and viral hemorrhagic fevers
B00-B09 Viral infections characterized by skin and mucous membrane lesions
B10 Other human herpesviruses
B15-B19 Viral hepatitis
B20 Human immunodeficiency virus [HIV] disease
B25-B34 Other viral diseases
B35-B49 Mycoses
B50-B64 Protozoal diseases
B65-B83 Helminthiases
B85-B89 Pediculosis, acariasis and other infestations
B90-B94 Sequelae of infectious and parasitic diseases
B95-B97 Bacterial and viral infectious agents
B99 Other infectious diseases

Intestinal infectious diseases (A00-A09)

✓4ᵗʰ A00 Cholera

DEF: Acute infection of the bowel due to *Vibrio cholerae* that presents with profuse diarrhea, cramps, and vomiting, resulting in severe dehydration, electrolyte imbalance, and death. It is spread through ingestion of food or water contaminated with feces of infected persons.

A00.0 **Cholera due to Vibrio cholerae 01, biovar cholerae** `CC`
Classical cholera

A00.1 **Cholera due to Vibrio cholerae 01, biovar eltor** `CC`
Cholera eltor

A00.9 **Cholera, unspecified** `CC`

✓4ᵗʰ A01 Typhoid and paratyphoid fevers

DEF: Typhoid fever: Acute generalized illness caused by *Salmonella typhi*. Clinical features include fever, headache, abdominal pain, cough, toxemia, leukopenia, abnormal pulse, rose spots on the skin, bacteremia, hyperplasia of intestinal lymph nodes, mesenteric lymphadenopathy, and Peyer's patches in the intestines.
DEF: Paratyphoid fever: Prolonged febrile illness, caused by *Salmonella* serotypes other than *S. typhi*, especially *S. enterica* serotypes paratyphi A, B, and C.

✓5ᵗʰ A01.0 Typhoid fever
Infection due to Salmonella typhi

A01.00 **Typhoid fever, unspecified** `CC`

A01.01 **Typhoid meningitis** `CC`

A01.02 **Typhoid fever with heart involvement** `CC`
Typhoid endocarditis
Typhoid myocarditis

A01.03 **Typhoid pneumonia** `CC`

A01.04 **Typhoid arthritis** `CC` `HCC`

A01.05 **Typhoid osteomyelitis** `CC` `HCC`

A01.09 **Typhoid fever with other complications** `CC`

A01.1 **Paratyphoid fever A** `CC`

A01.2 **Paratyphoid fever B** `CC`

A01.3 **Paratyphoid fever C** `CC`

A01.4 **Paratyphoid fever, unspecified** `CC`
Infection due to Salmonella paratyphi NOS

✓4ᵗʰ A02 Other salmonella infections

INCLUDES infection or foodborne intoxication due to any Salmonella species other than S. typhi and S. paratyphi

A02.0 **Salmonella enteritis**
Salmonellosis
TIP: Dehydration (E86.0) is a complication of salmonella enteritis and may be reported separately.

A02.1 **Salmonella sepsis** `HIV` `MCC` `HCC`

✓5ᵗʰ A02.2 Localized salmonella infections

A02.20 **Localized salmonella infection, unspecified** `HIV`

A02.21 **Salmonella meningitis** `HIV` `MCC`

A02.22 **Salmonella pneumonia** `HIV` `MCC`

A02.23 **Salmonella arthritis** `HIV` `CC` `HCC`

A02.24 **Salmonella osteomyelitis** `HIV` `CC` `HCC`

A02.25 **Salmonella pyelonephritis** `HIV` `CC`
Salmonella tubulo-interstitial nephropathy

A02.29 **Salmonella with other localized infection** `HIV` `CC`

A02.8 **Other specified salmonella infections** `HIV` `CC`

A02.9 **Salmonella infection, unspecified** `HIV` `CC`

✓4ᵗʰ A03 Shigellosis

DEF: Infection caused by the genus *Shigella*, of the family *Enterobacteriaceae* that is known to cause an acute dysenteric infection of the bowel with fever, drowsiness, anorexia, nausea, vomiting, bloody diarrhea, abdominal cramps, and distention.

A03.0 **Shigellosis due to Shigella dysenteriae** `CC`
Group A shigellosis [Shiga-Kruse dysentery]

A03.1 **Shigellosis due to Shigella flexneri**
Group B shigellosis

A03.2 **Shigellosis due to Shigella boydii**
Group C shigellosis

A03.3 **Shigellosis due to Shigella sonnei**
Group D shigellosis

A03.8 **Other shigellosis**

A03.9 **Shigellosis, unspecified**
Bacillary dysentery NOS

✓4ᵗʰ A04 Other bacterial intestinal infections

EXCLUDES 1 bacterial foodborne intoxications, NEC (A05.-)
tuberculous enteritis (A18.32)

DEF: *Escherichia coli*: Gram-negative, anaerobic bacteria of the family *Enterobacteriaceae* found in the large intestine of warm-blooded animals, generally as a nonpathologic entity aiding in digestion. They become pathogenic when an opportunity to grow somewhere outside this relationship presents itself, such as ingestion of fecal-contaminated food or water.

A04.0 **Enteropathogenic Escherichia coli infection** `CC`

A04.1 **Enterotoxigenic Escherichia coli infection** `CC`

A04.2 **Enteroinvasive Escherichia coli infection** `CC`

A04.3 **Enterohemorrhagic Escherichia coli infection** `CC`
DEF: *E. coli* infection penetrating the intestinal mucosa, producing microscopic ulceration and bleeding.

A04.4 **Other intestinal Escherichia coli infections** `CC`
Escherichia coli enteritis NOS

A04.5 **Campylobacter enteritis** `CC`
TIP: For Guillain-Barre syndrome occurring as a sequela of *Campylobacter enteritis*, assign code G61.0 as the first-listed diagnosis followed by B94.8 for the sequelae.

A04.6 **Enteritis due to Yersinia enterocolitica** `CC`
EXCLUDES 1 extraintestinal yersiniosis (A28.2)

✓5ᵗʰ A04.7 Enterocolitis due to Clostridium difficile
▶Clostridioides difficile colitis◀
Foodborne intoxication by Clostridium difficile
Pseudomembranous colitis
AHA: 2017,4Q,4

A04.71 **Enterocolitis due to Clostridium difficile, recurrent**
AHA: 2020,1Q,18

A04.72 **Enterocolitis due to Clostridium difficile, not specified as recurrent** `CC`

A04.8 **Other specified bacterial intestinal infections** `CC`

A04.9 **Bacterial intestinal infection, unspecified** `CC`
Bacterial enteritis NOS

✓4ᵗʰ A05 Other bacterial foodborne intoxications, not elsewhere classified

EXCLUDES 1 Clostridium difficile foodborne intoxication and infection (A04.7-)
Escherichia coli infection (A04.0-A04.4)
listeriosis (A32.-)
salmonella foodborne intoxication and infection (A02.-)
toxic effect of noxious foodstuffs (T61-T62)

A05.0 **Foodborne staphylococcal intoxication** `CC`
TIP: Assign code A04.8 to report a staphylococcal infection when it is caused by the ingestion of contaminated food but not caused by *S. aureus* toxins.

✅ Additional Character Required ✓ₓ7ᵗʰ Placeholder Questionable PDx Manifestation Unspecified `UPD` Unacceptable PDx `H1`-`H14` HAC `HCC` CMS-HCC Dx `HIV` HIV Dx

A05.1 Botulism food poisoning `CC`
Botulism NOS
Classical foodborne intoxication due to Clostridium botulinum
EXCLUDES 1   *infant botulism (A48.51)*
wound botulism (A48.52)
DEF: Muscle-paralyzing neurotoxic disease caused by ingesting pre-formed toxin from the bacterium *Clostridium botulinum*. It causes vomiting and diarrhea, vision problems, slurred speech, difficulty swallowing, paralysis, and death.

A05.2 Foodborne Clostridium perfringens [Clostridium welchii] intoxication `CC`
Enteritis necroticans
Pig-bel

A05.3 Foodborne Vibrio parahaemolyticus intoxication `CC`

A05.4 Foodborne Bacillus cereus intoxication `CC`

A05.5 Foodborne Vibrio vulnificus intoxication `CC`

A05.8 Other specified bacterial foodborne intoxications `CC`

A05.9 Bacterial foodborne intoxication, unspecified

√4th A06 Amebiasis
INCLUDES   infection due to Entamoeba histolytica
EXCLUDES 1   *other protozoal intestinal diseases (A07.-)*
EXCLUDES 2   *acanthamebiasis (B60.1-)*
Naegleriasis (B60.2)
DEF: Infection with a single cell protozoan known as the amoeba. Transmission occurs through ingestion of feces, contaminated food or water, use of human feces as fertilizer, or person-to-person contact.

A06.0 Acute amebic dysentery `CC`
Acute amebiasis
Intestinal amebiasis NOS

A06.1 Chronic intestinal amebiasis `CC`

A06.2 Amebic nondysenteric colitis `CC`

A06.3 Ameboma of intestine `CC`
Ameboma NOS

A06.4 Amebic liver abscess `MCC`
Hepatic amebiasis

A06.5 Amebic lung abscess `MCC` `HCC`
Amebic abscess of lung (and liver)

A06.6 Amebic brain abscess `MCC`
Amebic abscess of brain (and liver) (and lung)

A06.7 Cutaneous amebiasis

√5th A06.8 Amebic infection of other sites
A06.81 Amebic cystitis `CC`
A06.82 Other amebic genitourinary infections `CC`
Amebic balanitis
Amebic vesiculitis
Amebic vulvovaginitis
A06.89 Other amebic infections `CC`
Amebic appendicitis
Amebic splenic abscess

A06.9 Amebiasis, unspecified

√4th A07 Other protozoal intestinal diseases
DEF: Protozoa: Group comprised of the simplest, single celled organisms, ranging in size from micro to macroscopic. They can live alone or in colonies, and do not show any differentiation in tissues. Most are motile and can live free in nature, but some are parasitic, causing disease in the variety of hosts they inhabit.

A07.0 Balantidiasis
Balantidial dysentery

A07.1 Giardiasis [lambliasis] `CC`
DEF: Infection caused by the flagellate protozoan *Giardia lamblia* causing gastrointestinal problems such as vomiting, chronic diarrhea, and weight loss. The most common parasite in the U.S., this is usually transmitted by ingesting contaminated water while in the cyst state, after which it latches onto the wall of the small intestine.

A07.2 Cryptosporidiosis `CC` `HCC`
DEF: Microscopic parasite found in water and one of the most common causes of waterborne gastrointestinal infectious disease in the United States. It is usually transmitted by ingesting contaminated drinking water or recreational water and causes profuse watery diarrhea, flatulence, abdominal pain, and cramping.

A07.3 Isosporiasis `HIV` `CC`
Infection due to Isospora belli and Isospora hominis
Intestinal coccidiosis
Isosporosis

A07.4 Cyclosporiasis `CC`

A07.8 Other specified protozoal intestinal diseases `CC`
Intestinal microsporidiosis
Intestinal trichomoniasis
Sarcocystosis
Sarcosporidiosis

A07.9 Protozoal intestinal disease, unspecified `CC`
Flagellate diarrhea
Protozoal colitis
Protozoal diarrhea
Protozoal dysentery

√4th A08 Viral and other specified intestinal infections
EXCLUDES 1   *influenza with involvement of gastrointestinal tract (J09.X3, J10.2, J11.2)*

A08.0 Rotaviral enteritis `CC`

√5th A08.1 Acute gastroenteropathy due to Norwalk agent and other small round viruses
A08.11 Acute gastroenteropathy due to Norwalk agent `CC`
Acute gastroenteropathy due to Norovirus
Acute gastroenteropathy due to Norwalk-like agent
A08.19 Acute gastroenteropathy due to other small round viruses `CC`
Acute gastroenteropathy due to small round virus [SRV] NOS

A08.2 Adenoviral enteritis `CC`

√5th A08.3 Other viral enteritis
A08.31 Calicivirus enteritis `CC`
A08.32 Astrovirus enteritis `CC`
A08.39 Other viral enteritis `CC`
Coxsackie virus enteritis
Echovirus enteritis
Enterovirus enteritis NEC
Torovirus enteritis

A08.4 Viral intestinal infection, unspecified
Viral enteritis NOS
Viral gastroenteritis NOS
Viral gastroenteropathy NOS
AHA: 2016,3Q,12

A08.8 Other specified intestinal infections

A09 Infectious gastroenteritis and colitis, unspecified `CC`
Infectious colitis NOS
Infectious enteritis NOS
Infectious gastroenteritis NOS
EXCLUDES 1   *colitis NOS (K52.9)*
diarrhea NOS (R19.7)
enteritis NOS (K52.9)
gastroenteritis NOS (K52.9)
noninfective gastroenteritis and colitis, unspecified (K52.9)
DEF: Colitis: Inflammation of mucous membranes of the colon.
DEF: Enteritis: Inflammation of mucous membranes of the small intestine.
DEF: Gastroenteritis: Inflammation of mucous membranes of the stomach and intestines.

Tuberculosis (A15-A19)

INCLUDES   infections due to Mycobacterium tuberculosis and Mycobacterium bovis

EXCLUDES 1   *congenital tuberculosis (P37.0)*
nonspecific reaction to test for tuberculosis without active tuberculosis (R76.1-)
pneumoconiosis associated with tuberculosis, any type in A15 (J65)
positive PPD (R76.11)
positive tuberculin skin test without active tuberculosis (R76.11)
sequelae of tuberculosis (B90.-)
silicotuberculosis (J65)

DEF: Bacterial infection that typically spreads by inhalation of an airborne agent that usually attacks the lungs, but may also affect other organs.

✓4ᵗʰ A15   Respiratory tuberculosis

A15.0   Tuberculosis of lung   `HIV` `CC`
    Tuberculous bronchiectasis
    Tuberculous fibrosis of lung
    Tuberculous pneumonia
    Tuberculous pneumothorax

Tuberculosis of Lung

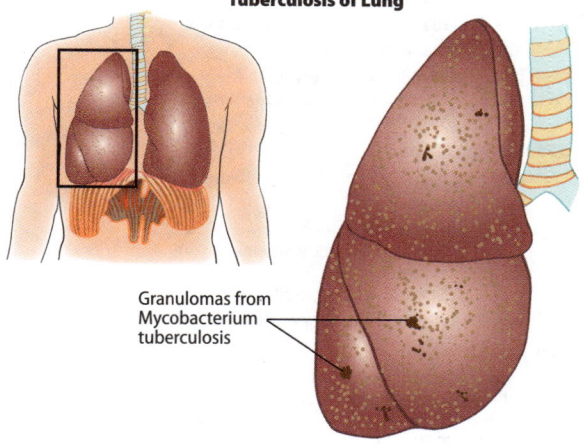

Granulomas from Mycobacterium tuberculosis

A15.4   Tuberculosis of intrathoracic lymph nodes   `HIV` `CC`
    Tuberculosis of hilar lymph nodes
    Tuberculosis of mediastinal lymph nodes
    Tuberculosis of tracheobronchial lymph nodes
    EXCLUDES 1   *tuberculosis specified as primary (A15.7)*

A15.5   Tuberculosis of larynx, trachea and bronchus   `HIV` `CC`
    Tuberculosis of bronchus
    Tuberculosis of glottis
    Tuberculosis of larynx
    Tuberculosis of trachea

A15.6   Tuberculous pleurisy   `HIV` `CC`
    Tuberculosis of pleura Tuberculous empyema
    EXCLUDES 1   *primary respiratory tuberculosis (A15.7)*

A15.7   Primary respiratory tuberculosis   `HIV` `CC`

A15.8   Other respiratory tuberculosis   `HIV` `CC`
    Mediastinal tuberculosis
    Nasopharyngeal tuberculosis
    Tuberculosis of nose
    Tuberculosis of sinus [any nasal]

A15.9   Respiratory tuberculosis unspecified   `HIV` `CC`

✓4ᵗʰ A17   Tuberculosis of nervous system

A17.0   Tuberculous meningitis   `HIV` `MCC`
    Tuberculosis of meninges (cerebral)(spinal)
    Tuberculous leptomeningitis
    EXCLUDES 1   *tuberculous meningoencephalitis (A17.82)*

A17.1   Meningeal tuberculoma   `HIV` `MCC`
    Tuberculoma of meninges (cerebral) (spinal)
    EXCLUDES 2   *tuberculoma of brain and spinal cord (A17.81)*

✓5ᵗʰ A17.8   Other tuberculosis of nervous system

A17.81   Tuberculoma of brain and spinal cord   `HIV` `MCC`
    Tuberculous abscess of brain and spinal cord

A17.82   Tuberculous meningoencephalitis   `HIV` `MCC`
    Tuberculous myelitis

A17.83   Tuberculous neuritis   `HIV` `MCC`
    Tuberculous mononeuropathy

A17.89   Other tuberculosis of nervous system   `HIV` `MCC`
    Tuberculous polyneuropathy

A17.9   Tuberculosis of nervous system, unspecified   `HIV` `CC`

✓4ᵗʰ A18   Tuberculosis of other organs

✓5ᵗʰ A18.0   Tuberculosis of bones and joints

A18.01   Tuberculosis of spine   `HIV` `CC`
    Pott's disease or curvature of spine
    Tuberculous arthritis
    Tuberculous osteomyelitis of spine
    Tuberculous spondylitis

A18.02   Tuberculous arthritis of other joints   `HIV` `CC`
    Tuberculosis of hip (joint)
    Tuberculosis of knee (joint)

A18.03   Tuberculosis of other bones   `HIV` `CC`
    Tuberculous mastoiditis
    Tuberculous osteomyelitis

A18.09   Other musculoskeletal tuberculosis   `HIV` `CC`
    Tuberculous myositis
    Tuberculous synovitis
    Tuberculous tenosynovitis

✓5ᵗʰ A18.1   Tuberculosis of genitourinary system

A18.10   Tuberculosis of genitourinary system, unspecified   `HIV` `CC`

A18.11   Tuberculosis of kidney and ureter   `HIV` `CC`

A18.12   Tuberculosis of bladder   `HIV` `CC`

A18.13   Tuberculosis of other urinary organs   `HIV` `CC`
    Tuberculous urethritis

A18.14   Tuberculosis of prostate   `HIV` `CC` `A`

A18.15   Tuberculosis of other male genital organs   `HIV` `CC`

A18.16   Tuberculosis of cervix   `HIV` `CC`

A18.17   Tuberculous female pelvic inflammatory disease   `HIV` `CC`
    Tuberculous endometritis
    Tuberculous oophoritis and salpingitis

A18.18   Tuberculosis of other female genital organs   `HIV` `CC`
    Tuberculous ulceration of vulva

A18.2   Tuberculous peripheral lymphadenopathy   `HIV` `CC`
    Tuberculous adenitis
    EXCLUDES 2   *tuberculosis of bronchial and mediastinal lymph nodes (A15.4)*
    tuberculosis of mesenteric and retroperitoneal lymph nodes (A18.39)
    tuberculous tracheobronchial adenopathy (A15.4)

✓5ᵗʰ A18.3   Tuberculosis of intestines, peritoneum and mesenteric glands

A18.31   Tuberculous peritonitis   `HIV` `MCC`
    Tuberculous ascites
    DEF: Tuberculous inflammation of the membrane lining the abdomen.

A18.32   Tuberculous enteritis   `HIV` `CC`
    Tuberculosis of anus and rectum
    Tuberculosis of intestine (large) (small)

A18.39   Retroperitoneal tuberculosis   `HIV` `CC`
    Tuberculosis of mesenteric glands
    Tuberculosis of retroperitoneal (lymph glands)

A18.4   Tuberculosis of skin and subcutaneous tissue   `HIV` `CC`
    Erythema induratum, tuberculous
    ▶Lupus exedens◀
    Lupus vulgaris NOS
    Lupus vulgaris of eyelid
    Scrofuloderma
    Tuberculosis of external ear
    EXCLUDES 2   *lupus erythematosus (L93.-)*
    systemic lupus erythematosus (M32.-)

✓5ᵗʰ A18.5   Tuberculosis of eye
    EXCLUDES 2   *lupus vulgaris of eyelid (A18.4)*

A18.50   Tuberculosis of eye, unspecified   `HIV` `CC`

A18.51   Tuberculous episcleritis   `HIV` `CC`

A18.52   Tuberculous keratitis   `HIV` `CC`
    Tuberculous interstitial keratitis
    Tuberculous keratoconjunctivitis (interstitial) (phlyctenular)

A18.53   Tuberculous chorioretinitis   `HIV` `CC`

A18.54   Tuberculous iridocyclitis   `HIV` `CC`

A18.59   Other tuberculosis of eye   `HIV` `CC`
    Tuberculous conjunctivitis

✔ Additional Character Required   `✗7ᵗʰ` Placeholder   `Questionable PDx`   `Manifestation`   `Unspecified`   `UPD` Unacceptable PDx   `H1`-`H14` HAC   `HCC` CMS-HCC Dx   `HIV` HIV Dx

ICD-10-CM 2025   **451**

A18.6   **Tuberculosis of (inner) (middle) ear**   `HIV` `CC`
Tuberculous otitis media
EXCLUDES 2   *tuberculosis of external ear (A18.4)*
tuberculous mastoiditis (A18.03)

A18.7   **Tuberculosis of adrenal glands**   `HIV` `CC`
Tuberculous Addison's disease

✓5th **A18.8**   **Tuberculosis of other specified organs**

A18.81   **Tuberculosis of thyroid gland**   `HIV` `CC`

A18.82   **Tuberculosis of other endocrine glands**   `HIV` `CC`
Tuberculosis of pituitary gland
Tuberculosis of thymus gland

A18.83   **Tuberculosis of digestive tract organs, not elsewhere classified**   `HIV` `CC`
EXCLUDES 1   *tuberculosis of intestine (A18.32)*

A18.84   **Tuberculosis of heart**   `HIV` `CC`
Tuberculous cardiomyopathy
Tuberculous endocarditis
Tuberculous myocarditis
Tuberculous pericarditis

A18.85   **Tuberculosis of spleen**   `HIV` `CC`

A18.89   **Tuberculosis of other sites**   `HIV` `CC`
Tuberculosis of muscle
Tuberculous cerebral arteritis

✓4th **A19**   **Miliary tuberculosis**
INCLUDES   disseminated tuberculosis
generalized tuberculosis
tuberculous polyserositis

A19.0   **Acute miliary tuberculosis of a single specified site**   `HIV` `MCC`

A19.1   **Acute miliary tuberculosis of multiple sites**   `HIV` `MCC`

A19.2   **Acute miliary tuberculosis, unspecified**   `HIV` `MCC`

A19.8   **Other miliary tuberculosis**   `HIV` `MCC`

A19.9   **Miliary tuberculosis, unspecified**   `HIV` `MCC`

Certain zoonotic bacterial diseases (A20-A28)

✓4th **A20**   **Plague**
INCLUDES   infection due to Yersinia pestis

A20.0   **Bubonic plague**   `MCC`

A20.1   **Cellulocutaneous plague**   `MCC`

A20.2   **Pneumonic plague**   `MCC`

A20.3   **Plague meningitis**   `MCC`

A20.7   **Septicemic plague**   `MCC` `HCC`

A20.8   **Other forms of plague**   `MCC`
Abortive plague
Asymptomatic plague
Pestis minor

A20.9   **Plague, unspecified**   `MCC`

✓4th **A21**   **Tularemia**
INCLUDES   deer-fly fever
infection due to Francisella tularensis
rabbit fever
DEF: Febrile disease transmitted to humans by the bites of deer flies, fleas, and ticks, by inhaling aerosolized *F. tularensis*, or by ingesting contaminated food or water. Patients quickly develop fever, chills, weakness, headache, backache, and malaise.

A21.0   **Ulceroglandular tularemia**   `CC`

A21.1   **Oculoglandular tularemia**   `CC`
Ophthalmic tularemia

A21.2   **Pulmonary tularemia**   `CC`

A21.3   **Gastrointestinal tularemia**   `CC`
Abdominal tularemia

A21.7   **Generalized tularemia**   `CC`

A21.8   **Other forms of tularemia**   `CC`

A21.9   **Tularemia, unspecified**   `CC`

✓4th **A22**   **Anthrax**
INCLUDES   infection due to Bacillus anthracis

A22.0   **Cutaneous anthrax**   `CC`
Malignant carbuncle
Malignant pustule

A22.1   **Pulmonary anthrax**   `MCC`
Inhalation anthrax
Ragpicker's disease
Woolsorter's disease

A22.2   **Gastrointestinal anthrax**   `CC`

A22.7   **Anthrax sepsis**   `MCC` `HCC`

A22.8   **Other forms of anthrax**   `CC`
Anthrax meningitis

A22.9   **Anthrax, unspecified**   `CC`

✓4th **A23**   **Brucellosis**
INCLUDES   Malta fever
Mediterranean fever
undulant fever

A23.0   **Brucellosis due to Brucella melitensis**

A23.1   **Brucellosis due to Brucella abortus**

A23.2   **Brucellosis due to Brucella suis**

A23.3   **Brucellosis due to Brucella canis**

A23.8   **Other brucellosis**   `CC`

A23.9   **Brucellosis, unspecified**   `CC`

✓4th **A24**   **Glanders and melioidosis**

A24.0   **Glanders**   `CC`
Infection due to Pseudomonas mallei
Malleus

A24.1   **Acute and fulminating melioidosis**   `CC`
Melioidosis pneumonia
Melioidosis sepsis

A24.2   **Subacute and chronic melioidosis**   `CC`

A24.3   **Other melioidosis**   `CC`

A24.9   **Melioidosis, unspecified**   `CC`
Infection due to Pseudomonas pseudomallei NOS
Whitmore's disease

✓4th **A25**   **Rat-bite fevers**

A25.0   **Spirillosis**   `CC`
Sodoku

A25.1   **Streptobacillosis**   `CC`
Epidemic arthritic erythema
Haverhill fever
Streptobacillary rat-bite fever

A25.9   **Rat-bite fever, unspecified**   `CC`

✓4th **A26**   **Erysipeloid**
DEF: Acute cutaneous infection typically caused by trauma to the skin. Presenting as cellulitis, it may become systemic, affecting other organs. It is a gram-positive bacillus and mainly acquired by those who routinely handle meat.

A26.0   **Cutaneous erysipeloid**
Erythema migrans

A26.7   **Erysipelothrix sepsis**   `MCC` `HCC`

A26.8   **Other forms of erysipeloid**

A26.9   **Erysipeloid, unspecified**

✓4th **A27**   **Leptospirosis**

A27.0   **Leptospirosis icterohemorrhagica**   `CC`
Leptospiral or spirochetal jaundice (hemorrhagic)
Weil's disease

✓5th **A27.8**   **Other forms of leptospirosis**

A27.81   **Aseptic meningitis in leptospirosis**   `MCC`

A27.89   **Other forms of leptospirosis**   `CC`

A27.9   **Leptospirosis, unspecified**   `CC`

✓4th **A28**   **Other zoonotic bacterial diseases, not elsewhere classified**

A28.0   **Pasteurellosis**   `CC`

A28.1   **Cat-scratch disease**   `CC`
Cat-scratch fever

A28.2   **Extraintestinal yersiniosis**   `CC`
EXCLUDES 1   *enteritis due to Yersinia enterocolitica (A04.6)*
plague (A20.-)

A28.8   **Other specified zoonotic bacterial diseases, not elsewhere classified**   `CC`

A28.9   **Zoonotic bacterial disease, unspecified**   `CC`

Other bacterial diseases (A30-A49)

AHA: 2016,3Q,8-14

✓4th **A30**   **Leprosy [Hansen's disease]**
INCLUDES   infection due to Mycobacterium leprae
EXCLUDES 1   *sequelae of leprosy (B92)*

A30.0   **Indeterminate leprosy**   `CC`
I leprosy

A30.1   **Tuberculoid leprosy**   `CC`
TT leprosy

`N` Newborn: 0   `P` Pediatric: 0-17   `M` Maternity: 9-64   `A` Adult: 15-124   `UNS` Unspecified Site   `MCC` Major Complication/Comorbidity   `CC` Complication/Comorbidity   `PE` POA Exempt

452   ICD-10-CM 2025

A30.2 **Borderline tuberculoid** leprosy `CC`
BT leprosy

A30.3 **Borderline** leprosy `CC`
BB leprosy

A30.4 **Borderline lepromatous** leprosy `CC`
BL leprosy

A30.5 **Lepromatous** leprosy `CC`
LL leprosy

A30.8 Other forms of leprosy `CC`

A30.9 Leprosy, unspecified `CC`

✓4th **A31** **Infection due to other mycobacteria**
EXCLUDES 2   leprosy (A30.-)
tuberculosis (A15-A19)

A31.0 **Pulmonary** mycobacterial infection `CC` `HCC`
Infection due to Mycobacterium avium
Infection due to Mycobacterium intracellulare [Battey bacillus]
Infection due to Mycobacterium kansasii

A31.1 **Cutaneous** mycobacterial infection `CC`
Buruli ulcer
Infection due to Mycobacterium marinum
Infection due to Mycobacterium ulcerans

A31.2 **Disseminated mycobacterium avium-intracellulare complex (DMAC)** `HIV` `CC` `HCC`
MAC sepsis

A31.8 **Other mycobacterial infections** `HIV` `CC`

A31.9 Mycobacterial infection, unspecified `HIV` `CC`
Atypical mycobacterial infection NOS
Mycobacteriosis NOS

✓4th **A32** **Listeriosis**
INCLUDES   listerial foodborne infection
EXCLUDES 1   neonatal (disseminated) listeriosis (P37.2)

A32.0 **Cutaneous** listeriosis `CC`

✓5th **A32.1** **Listerial meningitis and meningoencephalitis**
A32.11 **Listerial meningitis** `CC`
A32.12 **Listerial meningoencephalitis** `CC`

A32.7 **Listerial sepsis** `MCC` `HCC`

✓5th **A32.8** **Other forms of listeriosis**
A32.81 **Oculoglandular** listeriosis `CC`
A32.82 **Listerial endocarditis** `CC`
A32.89 **Other forms of listeriosis** `CC`
Listerial cerebral arteritis

A32.9 **Listeriosis, unspecified** `CC`

A33 **Tetanus neonatorum** `MCC` `N`

A34 **Obstetrical tetanus** `CC` `M`

A35 **Other tetanus** `MCC`
Tetanus NOS
EXCLUDES 1   obstetrical tetanus (A34)
tetanus neonatorum (A33)
DEF: Tetanus: Acute, often fatal, infectious disease caused by the anaerobic, spore-forming bacillus *Clostridium tetani*. The bacillus enters the body through a contaminated wound, burns, surgical wounds, or cutaneous ulcers. Symptoms include lockjaw, spasms, seizures, and paralysis.

✓4th **A36** **Diphtheria**

A36.0 **Pharyngeal** diphtheria `CC`
Diphtheritic membranous angina
Tonsillar diphtheria

A36.1 **Nasopharyngeal** diphtheria `CC`

A36.2 **Laryngeal** diphtheria `CC`
Diphtheritic laryngotracheitis

A36.3 **Cutaneous** diphtheria `CC`
EXCLUDES 2   erythrasma (L08.1)

✓5th **A36.8** **Other diphtheria**
A36.81 **Diphtheritic cardiomyopathy** `CC` `HCC`
Diphtheritic myocarditis
A36.82 **Diphtheritic radiculomyelitis** `CC`
A36.83 **Diphtheritic polyneuritis** `CC`
A36.84 **Diphtheritic tubulo-interstitial nephropathy** `CC`
A36.85 **Diphtheritic cystitis** `CC`
A36.86 **Diphtheritic conjunctivitis** `CC`
A36.89 **Other diphtheritic complications** `CC`
Diphtheritic peritonitis

A36.9 Diphtheria, unspecified `CC`

✓4th **A37** **Whooping cough**
DEF: Acute, highly contagious respiratory tract infection caused by *Bordetella pertussis* and *B. bronchiseptica*. Whooping cough is known by its characteristic paroxysmal cough.

✓5th **A37.0** **Whooping cough due to Bordetella pertussis**
A37.00 **Whooping cough due to Bordetella pertussis without pneumonia** `CC`
Paroxysmal cough due to Bordetella pertussis without pneumonia
A37.01 **Whooping cough due to Bordetella pertussis with pneumonia** `MCC`
Paroxysmal cough due to Bordetella pertussis with pneumonia

✓5th **A37.1** **Whooping cough due to Bordetella parapertussis**
A37.10 **Whooping cough due to Bordetella parapertussis without pneumonia** `CC`
A37.11 **Whooping cough due to Bordetella parapertussis with pneumonia** `MCC`

✓5th **A37.8** **Whooping cough due to other Bordetella species**
A37.80 **Whooping cough due to other Bordetella species without pneumonia** `CC`
A37.81 **Whooping cough due to other Bordetella species with pneumonia** `MCC`

✓5th **A37.9** **Whooping cough, unspecified species**
A37.90 **Whooping cough, unspecified species without pneumonia** `CC`
A37.91 **Whooping cough, unspecified species with pneumonia** `MCC`

✓4th **A38** **Scarlet fever**
INCLUDES   scarlatina
EXCLUDES 2   streptococcal sore throat (J02.0)
DEF: Acute contagious disease caused by Group A bacteria, the same bacterium that causes strep throat. Individuals with strep throat can develop scarlet fever particularly if the infection is not treated with antibiotics. It is characterized by a red blush to the skin of the chest and abdomen and swelling of the nose, throat, and mouth.

A38.0 **Scarlet fever with otitis media** `CC`
A38.1 **Scarlet fever with myocarditis** `CC`
A38.8 **Scarlet fever with other complications** `CC`
A38.9 **Scarlet fever, uncomplicated** `CC`
Scarlet fever, NOS

✓4th **A39** **Meningococcal infection**
DEF: Condition caused by *Neisseria meningitidis*, a bacteria that may invade the spinal cord, brain, heart, joints, optic nerve, or bloodstream.

A39.0 **Meningococcal meningitis** `MCC`
A39.1 **Waterhouse-Friderichsen** syndrome `MCC`
Meningococcal hemorrhagic adrenalitis
Meningococcic adrenal syndrome
A39.2 **Acute meningococcemia** `MCC` `HCC`
A39.3 **Chronic meningococcemia** `MCC` `HCC`
A39.4 **Meningococcemia, unspecified** `MCC` `HCC`

✓5th **A39.5** **Meningococcal heart disease**
A39.50 **Meningococcal carditis, unspecified** `MCC`
A39.51 **Meningococcal endocarditis** `MCC`
A39.52 **Meningococcal myocarditis** `MCC`
A39.53 **Meningococcal pericarditis** `MCC`

✓5th **A39.8** **Other meningococcal infections**
A39.81 **Meningococcal encephalitis** `MCC`
A39.82 **Meningococcal retrobulbar neuritis** `CC`
A39.83 **Meningococcal arthritis** `CC` `HCC`
A39.84 **Postmeningococcal arthritis** `CC` `HCC`
A39.89 **Other meningococcal infections** `CC`
Meningococcal conjunctivitis

A39.9 **Meningococcal infection, unspecified** `CC`
Meningococcal disease NOS

✔ Additional Character Required   ✓x7th Placeholder   Questionable PDx   Manifestation   Unspecified   UPD Unacceptable PDx   H1 - H14 HAC   HCC CMS-HCC Dx   HIV HIV Dx

ICD-10-CM 2025   453   A30.2-A39.9

✓4th **A40 Streptococcal sepsis**

Code first, if applicable, postprocedural sepsis (T81.44-)
sepsis due to central venous catheter (T80.211-)
streptococcal sepsis during labor (O75.3)
streptococcal sepsis following abortion or ectopic or molar pregnancy
(O03.37, O03.87, O04.87, O07.37, O08.82)
streptococcal sepsis following immunization (T88.0-)
streptococcal sepsis following infusion, transfusion or therapeutic
injection (T80.22-, T80.29-)

EXCLUDES 1   neonatal (P36.0-P36.1)
puerperal sepsis (O85)
sepsis due to Streptococcus, group D (A41.81)

AHA: 2020,2Q,8,28; 2019,4Q,65; 2018,4Q,89; 2018,1Q,16; 2016,1Q,32

A40.0 Sepsis due to streptococcus, group A   `MCC` `HCC`

A40.1 Sepsis due to streptococcus, group B   `MCC` `HCC`
AHA: 2019,1Q,14

A40.3 Sepsis due to Streptococcus pneumoniae   `MCC` `HCC`
Pneumococcal sepsis

A40.8 Other streptococcal sepsis   `MCC` `HCC`

A40.9 Streptococcal sepsis, unspecified   `HIV` `MCC` `HCC`

✓4th **A41 Other sepsis**

Code first, if applicable, postprocedural sepsis (T81.44-)
sepsis due to central venous catheter (T80.211-)
sepsis during labor (O75.3)
sepsis following abortion, ectopic or molar pregnancy (O03.37, O03.87,
O04.87, O07.37, O08.82)
sepsis following immunization (T88.0-)
sepsis following infusion, transfusion or therapeutic injection (T80.22-,
T80.29-)

EXCLUDES 1   bacteremia NOS (R78.81)
neonatal (P36.-)
puerperal sepsis (O85)
streptococcal sepsis (A40.-)

EXCLUDES 2   sepsis (due to) (in) actinomycotic (A42.7)
sepsis (due to) (in) anthrax (A22.7)
sepsis (due to) (in) candidal (B37.7)
sepsis (due to) (in) Erysipelothrix (A26.7)
sepsis (due to) (in) extraintestinal yersiniosis (A28.2)
sepsis (due to) (in) gonococcal (A54.86)
sepsis (due to) (in) herpesviral (B00.7)
sepsis (due to) (in) listerial (A32.7)
sepsis (due to) (in) melioidosis (A24.1)
sepsis (due to) (in) meningococcal (A39.2-A39.4)
sepsis (due to) (in) plague (A20.7)
sepsis (due to) (in) tularemia (A21.7)
toxic shock syndrome (A48.3)

AHA: 2020,2Q,8,28; 2019,4Q,65; 2019,3Q,17; 2018,4Q,18; 2018,1Q,16;
2016,1Q,32; 2014,2Q,13

✓5th **A41.0 Sepsis due to Staphylococcus aureus**

**A41.01 Sepsis due to Methicillin susceptible Staphylococcus
aureus**   `HIV` `MCC` `HCC`
MSSA sepsis
Staphylococcus aureus sepsis NOS
AHA: 2020,2Q,17

**A41.02 Sepsis due to Methicillin resistant Staphylococcus
aureus**   `HIV` `MCC` `HCC`

A41.1 Sepsis due to other specified staphylococcus   `HIV` `MCC` `HCC`
Coagulase negative staphylococcus sepsis
AHA: 2024,1Q,19

A41.2 Sepsis due to unspecified staphylococcus   `HIV` `MCC` `HCC`

A41.3 Sepsis due to Hemophilus influenzae   `HIV` `MCC` `HCC`

A41.4 Sepsis due to anaerobes   `HIV` `MCC` `HCC`
EXCLUDES 1   gas gangrene (A48.0)

✓5th **A41.5 Sepsis due to other Gram-negative organisms**

A41.50 Gram-negative sepsis, unspecified   `HIV` `MCC` `HCC`
Gram-negative sepsis NOS
AHA: 2020,2Q,28

A41.51 Sepsis due to Escherichia coli [E. coli]   `HIV` `MCC` `HCC`
AHA: 2020,2Q,17

A41.52 Sepsis due to Pseudomonas   `HIV` `MCC` `HCC`
Pseudomonas aeruginosa

A41.53 Sepsis due to Serratia   `HIV` `MCC` `HCC`

A41.54 Sepsis due to Acinetobacter baumannii   `MCC` `HCC`
AHA: 2023,4Q,4

A41.59 Other Gram-negative sepsis   `HIV` `MCC` `HCC`

✓5th **A41.8 Other specified sepsis**

A41.81 Sepsis due to Enterococcus   `HIV` `MCC` `HCC`
TIP: E. faecium, is a species of Enterococcus that is
highly resistant to multiple antibiotics. Assign a code
from category Z16 when resistance to antimicrobial
drugs is documented.

A41.89 Other specified sepsis   `HIV` `MCC` `HCC`
AHA: 2020,2Q,8; 2017,1Q,51; 2016,3Q,8-14
TIP: Viral sepsis is coded here; assign an additional code
to identify the specific viral agent or illness.

A41.9 Sepsis, unspecified organism   `HIV` `MCC` `HCC`
Septicemia NOS
AHA: 2022,2Q,5; 2022,1Q,35; 2020,2Q,28

✓4th **A42 Actinomycosis**

EXCLUDES 1   actinomycetoma (B47.1)

A42.0 Pulmonary actinomycosis   `HIV` `CC`

A42.1 Abdominal actinomycosis   `HIV` `CC`

A42.2 Cervicofacial actinomycosis   `HIV` `CC`

A42.7 Actinomycotic sepsis   `HIV` `MCC` `HCC`

✓5th **A42.8 Other forms of actinomycosis**

A42.81 Actinomycotic meningitis   `HIV` `CC`

A42.82 Actinomycotic encephalitis   `HIV` `CC`

A42.89 Other forms of actinomycosis   `HIV` `CC`

A42.9 Actinomycosis, unspecified   `HIV` `CC`

✓4th **A43 Nocardiosis**

DEF: Rare bacterial infection occurring most often in those with weakened
immune systems. Can be acquired in soil, decaying plants, or standing
water. It typically begins in the lungs and has a tendency to spread to
other body systems.

A43.0 Pulmonary nocardiosis   `HIV` `CC`

A43.1 Cutaneous nocardiosis   `HIV` `CC`

A43.8 Other forms of nocardiosis   `HIV` `CC`

A43.9 Nocardiosis, unspecified   `HIV` `CC`

✓4th **A44 Bartonellosis**

A44.0 Systemic bartonellosis   `CC`
Oroya fever

A44.1 Cutaneous and mucocutaneous bartonellosis   `CC`
Verruga peruana

A44.8 Other forms of bartonellosis   `CC`

A44.9 Bartonellosis, unspecified   `CC`

A46 Erysipelas

EXCLUDES 1   postpartum or puerperal erysipelas (O86.89)

DEF: Skin infection affecting the upper dermis and superficial dermal
lymphatics. Lesion edges are well-demarcated with distinct raised borders.
It is often caused by group A Streptococci.

✓4th **A48 Other bacterial diseases, not elsewhere classified**

EXCLUDES 1   actinomycetoma (B47.1)

A48.0 Gas gangrene   `MCC` `HCC`
Clostridial cellulitis
Clostridial myonecrosis
AHA: 2017,4Q,102

A48.1 Legionnaires' disease   `HIV` `MCC` `HCC`
DEF: Severe and often fatal infection by Legionella pneumophila.
Symptoms include high fever, gastrointestinal pain, headache,
myalgia, dry cough, and pneumonia and it is usually transmitted
through airborne water droplets via air conditioning systems or
hot tubs.

A48.2 Nonpneumonic Legionnaires' disease [Pontiac fever]

A48.3 Toxic shock syndrome   `MCC` `HCC`
Use additional code to identify the organism (B95, B96)
EXCLUDES 1   endotoxic shock NOS (R57.8)
sepsis NOS (A41.9)
AHA: 2022,1Q,35
DEF: Bacteria producing an endotoxin, such as Staphylococci,
flood the body with the toxins producing a high fever, vomiting
and diarrhea, decreasing blood pressure, a skin rash, and shock.
Synonym(s): TSS.

A48.4 Brazilian purpuric fever
Systemic Hemophilus aegyptius infection

✓5th **A48.5**   **Other specified botulism**
Non-foodborne intoxication due to toxins of Clostridium
botulinum [C. botulinum]

> *EXCLUDES 1*   *food poisoning due to toxins of Clostridium botulinum (A05.1)*

    A48.51   **Infant** botulism   `CC` `P`
    A48.52   **Wound** botulism   `CC`
      Non-foodborne botulism NOS
      Use additional code for associated wound

A48.8   **Other specified bacterial diseases**

✓4th **A49**   **Bacterial infection of unspecified site**

> *EXCLUDES 1*   *bacterial agents as the cause of diseases classified elsewhere (B95-B96)*
> *chlamydial infection NOS (A74.9)*
> *meningococcal infection NOS (A39.9)*
> *rickettsial infection NOS (A79.9)*
> *spirochetal infection NOS (A69.9)*

✓5th **A49.0**   **Staphylococcal** infection, unspecified site

    A49.01   **Methicillin susceptible** Staphylococcus aureus
      infection, unspecified site
      Methicillin susceptible Staphylococcus aureus (MSSA)
      infection
      Staphylococcus aureus infection NOS

    A49.02   **Methicillin resistant** Staphylococcus aureus infection,
      unspecified site
      Methicillin resistant Staphylococcus aureus (MRSA)
      infection

    A49.1   **Streptococcal** infection, unspecified site
    A49.2   **Hemophilus influenzae** infection, unspecified site
    A49.3   **Mycoplasma** infection, unspecified site
    A49.8   **Other bacterial infections of unspecified site**
    A49.9   **Bacterial infection, unspecified**

> *EXCLUDES 1*   *bacteremia NOS (R78.81)*

Infections with a predominantly sexual mode of transmission (A50-A64)

> *EXCLUDES 1*   *nonspecific and nongonococcal urethritis (N34.1)*
> *Reiter's disease (M02.3-)*
> *EXCLUDES 2*   *human immunodeficiency virus [HIV] disease (B20)*
> **AHA:** 2021,2Q,6

✓4th **A50**   **Congenital syphilis**

✓5th **A50.0**   **Early congenital syphilis, symptomatic**
Any congenital syphilitic condition specified as early or manifest
less than two years after birth.

    A50.01   **Early congenital syphilitic oculopathy**   `CC`
    A50.02   **Early congenital syphilitic osteochondropathy**   `CC`
    A50.03   **Early congenital syphilitic pharyngitis**   `CC`
      Early congenital syphilitic laryngitis
    A50.04   **Early congenital syphilitic pneumonia**   `CC`
    A50.05   **Early congenital syphilitic rhinitis**   `CC`
    A50.06   **Early cutaneous congenital syphilis**   `CC`
    A50.07   **Early mucocutaneous congenital syphilis**   `CC`
    A50.08   **Early visceral congenital syphilis**   `CC`
    A50.09   **Other early congenital syphilis, symptomatic**   `CC`

    A50.1   **Early congenital syphilis, latent**
Congenital syphilis without clinical manifestations, with positive
serological reaction and negative spinal fluid test, less than
two years after birth.

    A50.2   **Early congenital syphilis, unspecified**   `CC`
Congenital syphilis NOS less than two years after birth.

✓5th **A50.3**   **Late congenital syphilitic oculopathy**

> *EXCLUDES 1*   *Hutchinson's triad (A50.53)*

    A50.30   **Late congenital syphilitic oculopathy,**
      unspecified   `CC`
    A50.31   **Late congenital syphilitic interstitial keratitis**   `CC`
    A50.32   **Late congenital syphilitic chorioretinitis**   `CC`
    A50.39   **Other late congenital syphilitic oculopathy**   `CC`

✓5th **A50.4**   **Late congenital neurosyphilis [juvenile neurosyphilis]**
Use additional code to identify any associated mental disorder

> *EXCLUDES 1*   *Hutchinson's triad (A50.53)*

    A50.40   **Late congenital neurosyphilis, unspecified**   `CC`
      Juvenile neurosyphilis NOS
    A50.41   **Late congenital syphilitic meningitis**   `MCC`
    A50.42   **Late congenital syphilitic encephalitis**   `MCC`
    A50.43   **Late congenital syphilitic polyneuropathy**   `CC`

    A50.44   **Late congenital syphilitic optic nerve atrophy**   `CC`
    A50.45   **Juvenile general paresis**   `CC`
      Dementia paralytica juvenilis
      ▶Juvenile taboparetic neurosyphilis◀
    A50.49   **Other late congenital neurosyphilis**   `CC`
      Juvenile tabes dorsalis

✓5th **A50.5**   **Other late congenital syphilis, symptomatic**
Any congenital syphilitic condition specified as late or manifest
two years or more after birth.

    A50.51   **Clutton's joints**   `CC`
    A50.52   **Hutchinson's teeth**   `CC`
    A50.53   **Hutchinson's triad**   `CC`
    A50.54   **Late congenital cardiovascular syphilis**   `CC`
    A50.55   **Late congenital syphilitic arthropathy**   `CC` `HCC`
    A50.56   **Late congenital syphilitic osteochondropathy**   `CC`
    A50.57   **Syphilitic saddle nose**   `CC`
    A50.59   **Other late congenital syphilis, symptomatic**   `CC`

    A50.6   **Late congenital syphilis, latent**
Congenital syphilis without clinical manifestations, with positive
serological reaction and negative spinal fluid test, two years
or more after birth.

    A50.7   **Late congenital syphilis, unspecified**
Congenital syphilis NOS two years or more after birth.

    A50.9   **Congenital syphilis, unspecified**

✓4th **A51**   **Early syphilis**

> **DEF:** Syphilis: Sexually transmitted disease caused by the *Treponema
> pallidum* spirochete. Syphilis usually exhibits cutaneous manifestations
> and may exist for years without symptoms.

    A51.0   **Primary genital syphilis**
      Syphilitic chancre NOS
    A51.1   **Primary anal syphilis**
    A51.2   **Primary syphilis of other sites**

✓5th **A51.3**   **Secondary syphilis of skin and mucous membranes**

> **DEF:** Transitory or chronic cutaneous eruptions that present within
> two to 10 weeks following an initial syphilis infection that may
> include nontender lymphadenopathy along with alopecia and
> condylomata lata.

    A51.31   **Condyloma latum**   `CC`
    A51.32   **Syphilitic alopecia**   `CC`
    A51.39   **Other secondary syphilis of skin**   `CC`
      Syphilitic leukoderma
      Syphilitic mucous patch
>   *EXCLUDES 1*   *late syphilitic leukoderma (A52.79)*

✓5th **A51.4**   **Other secondary syphilis**

    A51.41   **Secondary syphilitic meningitis**   `MCC`
    A51.42   **Secondary syphilitic female pelvic disease**
    A51.43   **Secondary syphilitic oculopathy**   `CC`
      Secondary syphilitic chorioretinitis
      Secondary syphilitic iridocyclitis, iritis
      Secondary syphilitic uveitis
    A51.44   **Secondary syphilitic nephritis**   `CC`
    A51.45   **Secondary syphilitic hepatitis**   `CC`
    A51.46   **Secondary syphilitic osteopathy**   `CC`
    A51.49   **Other secondary syphilitic conditions**   `CC`
      Secondary syphilitic lymphadenopathy
      Secondary syphilitic myositis

    A51.5   **Early syphilis, latent**
Syphilis (acquired) without clinical manifestations, with positive
serological reaction and negative spinal fluid test, less than
two years after infection.

    A51.9   **Early syphilis, unspecified**

✓4th **A52**   **Late syphilis**

✓5th **A52.0**   **Cardiovascular and cerebrovascular syphilis**

    A52.00   **Cardiovascular syphilis, unspecified**   `CC`
    A52.01   **Syphilitic aneurysm of aorta**   `CC`
    A52.02   **Syphilitic aortitis**   `CC`
    A52.03   **Syphilitic endocarditis**   `CC`
      Syphilitic aortic valve incompetence or stenosis
      Syphilitic mitral valve stenosis
      Syphilitic pulmonary valve regurgitation
    A52.04   **Syphilitic cerebral arteritis**   `CC`
    A52.05   **Other cerebrovascular syphilis**   `CC`
      Syphilitic cerebral aneurysm (ruptured) (non-ruptured)
      Syphilitic cerebral thrombosis

✔ Additional Character Required   ✓x7th Placeholder   Questionable PDx   Manifestation   Unspecified   UPD Unacceptable PDx   H1 - H14 HAC   HCC CMS-HCC Dx   HIV HIV Dx

ICD-10-CM 2025   455

Chapter 1. Certain Infectious and Parasitic Diseases

A52.06 Other syphilitic heart involvement `CC`
Syphilitic coronary artery disease
Syphilitic myocarditis
Syphilitic pericarditis

A52.09 Other cardiovascular syphilis `CC`

✓5th **A52.1 Symptomatic neurosyphilis**

A52.10 Symptomatic neurosyphilis, unspecified `CC`

A52.11 Tabes dorsalis `CC`
Locomotor ataxia (progressive)
Tabetic neurosyphilis

A52.12 Other cerebrospinal syphilis `CC`

A52.13 Late syphilitic meningitis `MCC`

A52.14 Late syphilitic encephalitis `MCC`

A52.15 Late syphilitic neuropathy `CC`
Late syphilitic acoustic neuritis
Late syphilitic optic (nerve) atrophy
Late syphilitic polyneuropathy
Late syphilitic retrobulbar neuritis

A52.16 Charcôt's arthropathy (tabetic) `CC`
DEF: Progressive neurologic arthropathy in which chronic degeneration of joints in the weight-bearing areas with peripheral hypertrophy occurs as a complication of a neuropathy disorder. Supporting structures relax from a loss of sensation resulting in chronic joint instability.

A52.17 General paresis `CC`
Dementia paralytica

A52.19 Other symptomatic neurosyphilis `CC`
Syphilitic parkinsonism

A52.2 Asymptomatic neurosyphilis `CC`

A52.3 Neurosyphilis, unspecified `CC`
Gumma (syphilitic)
Syphilis (late)
Syphiloma
AHA: 2021,2Q,6

✓5th **A52.7 Other symptomatic late syphilis**

A52.71 Late syphilitic oculopathy `CC`
Late syphilitic chorioretinitis
Late syphilitic episcleritis

A52.72 Syphilis of lung and bronchus `CC`

A52.73 Symptomatic late syphilis of other respiratory organs `CC`

A52.74 Syphilis of liver and other viscera `CC`
Late syphilitic peritonitis

A52.75 Syphilis of kidney and ureter `CC`
Syphilitic glomerular disease

A52.76 Other genitourinary symptomatic late syphilis `CC`
Late syphilitic female pelvic inflammatory disease

A52.77 Syphilis of bone and joint `CC`

A52.78 Syphilis of other musculoskeletal tissue `CC`
Late syphilitic bursitis
Syphilis [stage unspecified] of bursa
Syphilis [stage unspecified] of muscle
Syphilis [stage unspecified] of synovium
Syphilis [stage unspecified] of tendon

A52.79 Other symptomatic late syphilis `CC`
Late syphilitic leukoderma
Syphilis of adrenal gland
Syphilis of pituitary gland
Syphilis of thyroid gland
Syphilitic splenomegaly
EXCLUDES 1 syphilitic leukoderma (secondary) (A51.39)

A52.8 Late syphilis, latent
Syphilis (acquired) without clinical manifestations, with positive serological reaction and negative spinal fluid test, two years or more after infection

A52.9 Late syphilis, unspecified

✓4th **A53 Other and unspecified syphilis**

A53.0 Latent syphilis, unspecified as early or late
Latent syphilis NOS
Positive serological reaction for syphilis

A53.9 Syphilis, unspecified
Infection due to Treponema pallidum NOS
Syphilis (acquired) NOS
EXCLUDES 1 syphilis NOS under two years of age (A50.2)

✓4th **A54 Gonococcal infection**
DEF: Sexually transmitted bacterial infection caused by *Neisseria gonorrhoeae*. Women are often asymptomatic, while men tend to develop urinary symptoms quickly.

✓5th **A54.0 Gonococcal infection of lower genitourinary tract without periurethral or accessory gland abscess**
EXCLUDES 1 gonococcal infection with genitourinary gland abscess (A54.1)
gonococcal infection with periurethral abscess (A54.1)

A54.00 Gonococcal infection of lower genitourinary tract, unspecified

A54.01 Gonococcal cystitis and urethritis, unspecified `CC`

A54.02 Gonococcal vulvovaginitis, unspecified `CC`

A54.03 Gonococcal cervicitis, unspecified `CC`

A54.09 Other gonococcal infection of lower genitourinary tract `CC`

A54.1 Gonococcal infection of lower genitourinary tract with periurethral and accessory gland abscess
Gonococcal Bartholin's gland abscess

✓5th **A54.2 Gonococcal pelviperitonitis and other gonococcal genitourinary infection**

A54.21 Gonococcal infection of kidney and ureter `CC`

A54.22 Gonococcal prostatitis `CC`

A54.23 Gonococcal infection of other male genital organs `CC`
Gonococcal epididymitis
Gonococcal orchitis

A54.24 Gonococcal female pelvic inflammatory disease `CC`
Gonococcal pelviperitonitis
EXCLUDES 1 gonococcal peritonitis (A54.85)

A54.29 Other gonococcal genitourinary infections `CC`

✓5th **A54.3 Gonococcal infection of eye**

A54.30 Gonococcal infection of eye, unspecified `CC`

A54.31 Gonococcal conjunctivitis `CC`
Ophthalmia neonatorum due to gonococcus

A54.32 Gonococcal iridocyclitis `CC`

A54.33 Gonococcal keratitis `CC`

A54.39 Other gonococcal eye infection `CC`
Gonococcal endophthalmia

✓5th **A54.4 Gonococcal infection of musculoskeletal system**

A54.40 Gonococcal infection of musculoskeletal system, unspecified `CC` `HCC`

A54.41 Gonococcal spondylopathy `CC` `HCC`

A54.42 Gonococcal arthritis `CC` `HCC`
EXCLUDES 2 gonococcal infection of spine (A54.41)

A54.43 Gonococcal osteomyelitis `CC` `HCC`
EXCLUDES 2 gonococcal infection of spine (A54.41)

A54.49 Gonococcal infection of other musculoskeletal tissue `CC` `HCC`
Gonococcal bursitis
Gonococcal myositis
Gonococcal synovitis
Gonococcal tenosynovitis

A54.5 Gonococcal pharyngitis

A54.6 Gonococcal infection of anus and rectum

✓5th **A54.8 Other gonococcal infections**

A54.81 Gonococcal meningitis `MCC`

A54.82 Gonococcal brain abscess `CC`

A54.83 Gonococcal heart infection `CC`
Gonococcal endocarditis
Gonococcal myocarditis
Gonococcal pericarditis

A54.84 Gonococcal pneumonia `CC`

A54.85 Gonococcal peritonitis `CC` `HCC`
EXCLUDES 1 gonococcal pelviperitonitis (A54.24)

A54.86 Gonococcal sepsis `MCC` `HCC`

A54.89 Other gonococcal infections `CC`
Gonococcal keratoderma
Gonococcal lymphadenitis

A54.9 Gonococcal infection, unspecified `CC`

A55 Chlamydial lymphogranuloma (venereum)
Climatic or tropical bubo
Durand-Nicolas-Favre disease
Esthiomene
Lymphogranuloma inguinale

✓4th A56 Other sexually transmitted chlamydial diseases
INCLUDES   sexually transmitted diseases due to Chlamydia trachomatis
EXCLUDES 1   neonatal chlamydial conjunctivitis (P39.1)
neonatal chlamydial pneumonia (P23.1)
EXCLUDES 2   chlamydial lymphogranuloma (A55)
conditions classified to A74.-
DEF: *Chlamydia trachomatis*: Bacterium that causes a common venereal disease. Symptoms of chlamydia are usually mild or absent, however, serious complications may cause irreversible damage, including cystitis, pelvic inflammatory disease, and infertility in women and discharge from the penis, prostatitis, and infertility in men. Genital chlamydial infection can cause arthritis, skin lesions, and inflammation of the eye and urethra.
Synonym(s): *Reiter's syndrome.*

✓5th **A56.0 Chlamydial infection of lower genitourinary tract**
   A56.00 Chlamydial infection of lower genitourinary tract, unspecified
   A56.01 Chlamydial cystitis and urethritis
   A56.02 Chlamydial vulvovaginitis
   A56.09 Other chlamydial infection of lower genitourinary tract
     Chlamydial cervicitis

✓5th **A56.1 Chlamydial infection of pelviperitoneum and other genitourinary organs**
   A56.11 Chlamydial female pelvic inflammatory disease
   A56.19 Other chlamydial genitourinary infection
     Chlamydial epididymitis
     Chlamydial orchitis

A56.2 Chlamydial infection of genitourinary tract, unspecified
A56.3 Chlamydial infection of anus and rectum
A56.4 Chlamydial infection of pharynx
A56.8 Sexually transmitted chlamydial infection of other sites

A57 Chancroid
Ulcus molle
DEF: Localized infection by *Haemophilus ducreyi,* causing genital ulcers and infecting the inguinal lymph nodes.

A58 Granuloma inguinale
Donovanosis

✓4th A59 Trichomoniasis
EXCLUDES 2   intestinal trichomoniasis (A07.8)
DEF: Infection with the parasitic, flagellated protozoa of the genus *Trichomonas.* This protozoon is found in the intestinal and genitourinary tracts of humans and in the mouth around tartar, cavities, and areas of periodontal disease.

✓5th **A59.0 Urogenital trichomoniasis**
   A59.00 Urogenital trichomoniasis, unspecified
     Fluor (vaginalis) due to Trichomonas
     Leukorrhea (vaginalis) due to Trichomonas
   A59.01 Trichomonal vulvovaginitis
   A59.02 Trichomonal prostatitis
   A59.03 Trichomonal cystitis and urethritis
   A59.09 Other urogenital trichomoniasis
     Trichomonas cervicitis

A59.8 Trichomoniasis of other sites
A59.9 Trichomoniasis, unspecified

✓4th A60 Anogenital herpesviral [herpes simplex] infections

✓5th **A60.0 Herpesviral infection of genitalia and urogenital tract**
   A60.00 Herpesviral infection of urogenital system, unspecified HIV
   A60.01 Herpesviral infection of penis HIV
   A60.02 Herpesviral infection of other male genital organs
   A60.03 Herpesviral cervicitis
   A60.04 Herpesviral vulvovaginitis HIV
     Herpesviral [herpes simplex] ulceration
     Herpesviral [herpes simplex] vaginitis
     Herpesviral [herpes simplex] vulvitis
   A60.09 Herpesviral infection of other urogenital tract HIV
     AHA: 2020,1Q,20

A60.1 Herpesviral infection of perianal skin and rectum HIV
A60.9 Anogenital herpesviral infection, unspecified HIV

✓4th A63 Other predominantly sexually transmitted diseases, not elsewhere classified
EXCLUDES 2   molluscum contagiosum (B08.1)
papilloma of cervix (D26.0)

A63.0 Anogenital (venereal) warts
Anogenital warts due to (human) papillomavirus [HPV]
Condyloma acuminatum

A63.8 Other specified predominantly sexually transmitted diseases

A64 Unspecified sexually transmitted disease

Other spirochetal diseases (A65-A69)

EXCLUDES 2   leptospirosis (A27.-)
syphilis (A50-A53)

A65 Nonvenereal syphilis
Bejel
Endemic syphilis
Njovera

✓4th A66 Yaws
INCLUDES   bouba
frambesia (tropica)
pian

A66.0 Initial lesions of yaws
Chancre of yaws
Frambesia, initial or primary
Initial frambesial ulcer
Mother yaw

A66.1 Multiple papillomata and wet crab yaws
Frambesioma
Pianoma
Plantar or palmar papilloma of yaws

A66.2 Other early skin lesions of yaws
Cutaneous yaws, less than five years after infection
Early yaws (cutaneous) (macular) (maculopapular) (micropapular) (papular)
Frambeside of early yaws

A66.3 Hyperkeratosis of yaws
Ghoul hand
Hyperkeratosis, palmar or plantar (early) (late) due to yaws
Worm-eaten soles

A66.4 Gummata and ulcers of yaws
Gummatous frambeside
Nodular late yaws (ulcerated)

A66.5 Gangosa
Rhinopharyngitis mutilans

A66.6 Bone and joint lesions of yaws HCC
Yaws ganglion
Yaws goundou
Yaws gumma, bone
Yaws gummatous osteitis or periostitis
Yaws hydrarthrosis
Yaws osteitis
Yaws periostitis (hypertrophic)

A66.7 Other manifestations of yaws
Juxta-articular nodules of yaws
Mucosal yaws

A66.8 Latent yaws
Yaws without clinical manifestations, with positive serology

A66.9 Yaws, unspecified

✓4th A67 Pinta [carate]

A67.0 Primary lesions of pinta
Chancre (primary) of pinta
Papule (primary) of pinta

A67.1 Intermediate lesions of pinta
Erythematous plaques of pinta
Hyperchromic lesions of pinta
Hyperkeratosis of pinta
Pintids

A67.2 Late lesions of pinta
Achromic skin lesions of pinta
Cicatricial skin lesions of pinta
Dyschromic skin lesions of pinta

A67.3 Mixed lesions of pinta
Achromic with hyperchromic skin lesions of pinta [carate]

A67.9 Pinta, unspecified

✔ Additional Character Required   ✓x7th Placeholder   Questionable PDx   Manifestation   Unspecified   UPD Unacceptable PDx   H1 - H14 HAC   HCC CMS-HCC Dx   HIV HIV Dx

Chapter 1. Certain Infectious and Parasitic Diseases

√4th **A68 Relapsing fevers**

    INCLUDES recurrent fever

    EXCLUDES 2 *Lyme disease (A69.2-)*

    A68.0 Louse-borne relapsing fever   CC

         Relapsing fever due to Borrelia recurrentis

    A68.1 Tick-borne relapsing fever   CC

         Relapsing fever due to any Borrelia species other than Borrelia recurrentis

    A68.9 Relapsing fever, unspecified   CC

√4th **A69 Other spirochetal infections**

    A69.0 Necrotizing ulcerative stomatitis

         Cancrum oris

         Fusospirochetal gangrene

         Noma

         Stomatitis gangrenosa

    A69.1 Other Vincent's infections   CC

         Fusospirochetal pharyngitis

         Necrotizing ulcerative (acute) gingivitis

         Necrotizing ulcerative (acute) gingivostomatitis

         Spirochetal stomatitis

         Trench mouth

         Vincent's angina

         Vincent's gingivitis

   √5th **A69.2 Lyme disease**

         Erythema chronicum migrans due to Borrelia burgdorferi

         DEF: Recurrent multisystem disorder through tick bites that begins with lesions of erythema chronicum migrans and is followed by arthritis of the large joints, myalgia, malaise, and neurological and cardiac manifestations.

        A69.20 Lyme disease, unspecified   CC

             AHA: 2021,4Q,5

        A69.21 Meningitis due to Lyme disease   CC

        A69.22 Other neurologic disorders in Lyme disease   CC

             Cranial neuritis

             Meningoencephalitis

             Polyneuropathy

        A69.23 Arthritis due to Lyme disease   CC HCC

        A69.29 Other conditions associated with Lyme disease   CC

             Myopericarditis due to Lyme disease

             AHA: 2016,3Q,12

    A69.8 Other specified spirochetal infections

    A69.9 Spirochetal infection, unspecified

Other diseases caused by chlamydiae (A70-A74)

    EXCLUDES 1 *sexually transmitted chlamydial diseases (A55-A56)*

A70 Chlamydia psittaci infections   CC

     Ornithosis

     Parrot fever

     Psittacosis

√4th **A71 Trachoma**

    EXCLUDES 1 *sequelae of trachoma (B94.0)*

    A71.0 Initial stage of trachoma

         Trachoma dubium

    A71.1 Active stage of trachoma

         Granular conjunctivitis (trachomatous)

         Trachomatous follicular conjunctivitis

         Trachomatous pannus

    A71.9 Trachoma, unspecified

√4th **A74 Other diseases caused by chlamydiae**

    EXCLUDES 1 *neonatal chlamydial conjunctivitis (P39.1)*

                   neonatal chlamydial pneumonia (P23.1)

                   Reiter's disease (M02.3-)

                   sexually transmitted chlamydial diseases (A55-A56)

    EXCLUDES 2 *chlamydial pneumonia (J16.0)*

    A74.0 Chlamydial conjunctivitis

         Paratrachoma

   √5th **A74.8 Other chlamydial diseases**

        A74.81 Chlamydial peritonitis

        A74.89 Other chlamydial diseases

    A74.9 Chlamydial infection, unspecified

         Chlamydiosis NOS

Rickettsioses (A75-A79)

DEF: Rickettsia: Condition caused by bacteria that live in lice/ticks transmitted to humans through bites.

√4th **A75 Typhus fever**

    EXCLUDES 1 *rickettsiosis due to Ehrlichia sennetsu (A79.81)*

    A75.0 Epidemic louse-borne typhus fever due to Rickettsia prowazekii   CC

         Classical typhus (fever)

         Epidemic (louse-borne) typhus

    A75.1 Recrudescent typhus [Brill's disease]   CC

         Brill-Zinsser disease

    A75.2 Typhus fever due to Rickettsia typhi   CC

         Murine (flea-borne) typhus

    A75.3 Typhus fever due to Rickettsia tsutsugamushi   CC

         Scrub (mite-borne) typhus

         Tsutsugamushi fever

         Typhus fever due to Orientia Tsutsugamushi (scrub typhus)

    A75.9 Typhus fever, unspecified   CC

         Typhus (fever) NOS

√4th **A77 Spotted fever [tick-borne rickettsioses]**

    A77.0 Spotted fever due to Rickettsia rickettsii   CC

         Rocky Mountain spotted fever

         Sao Paulo fever

    A77.1 Spotted fever due to Rickettsia conorii   CC

         African tick typhus

         Boutonneuse fever

         India tick typhus

         Kenya tick typhus

         Marseilles fever

         Mediterranean tick fever

    A77.2 Spotted fever due to Rickettsia siberica   CC

         North Asian tick fever

         Siberian tick typhus

    A77.3 Spotted fever due to Rickettsia australis   CC

         Queensland tick typhus

   √5th **A77.4 Ehrlichiosis**

        EXCLUDES 1 *anaplasmosis [A. phagocytophilum] (A79.82)*

                   rickettsiosis due to Ehrlichia sennetsu (A79.81)

         AHA: 2021,4Q,5

        A77.40 Ehrlichiosis, unspecified   CC

        A77.41 Ehrlichiosis chaffeensis [E. chaffeensis]   CC

        A77.49 Other ehrlichiosis   CC

             Ehrlichiosis due to E. ewingii

             Ehrlichiosis due to E. muris euclairensis

    A77.8 Other spotted fevers   CC

         Rickettsia 364D/R. philipii (Pacific Coast tick fever)

         Spotted fever due to Rickettsia africae (African tick bite fever)

         Spotted fever due to Rickettsia parkeri

    A77.9 Spotted fever, unspecified   CC

         Tick-borne typhus NOS

A78 Q fever   CC

     Infection due to Coxiella burnetii

     Nine Mile fever

     Quadrilateral fever

√4th **A79 Other rickettsioses**

    A79.0 Trench fever   CC

         Quintan fever

         Wolhynian fever

    A79.1 Rickettsialpox due to Rickettsia akari   CC

         Kew Garden fever

         Vesicular rickettsiosis

   √5th **A79.8 Other specified rickettsioses**

        A79.81 Rickettsiosis due to Ehrlichia sennetsu   CC

             Rickettsiosis due to Neorickettsia sennetsu

        A79.82 Anaplasmosis [A. phagocytophilum]   CC

             Transfusion transmitted A. phagocytophilum

             AHA: 2021,4Q,4-5

        A79.89 Other specified rickettsioses   CC

    A79.9 Rickettsiosis, unspecified   CC

         Rickettsial infection NOS

N Newborn: 0   P Pediatric: 0-17   M Maternity: 9-64   A Adult: 15-124   UNS Unspecified Site   MCC Major Complication/Comorbidity   CC Complication/Comorbidity   PE POA Exempt

458   ICD-10-CM 2025

Viral and prion infections of the central nervous system (A80-A89)

EXCLUDES 1   postpolio syndrome (G14)
sequelae of poliomyelitis (B91)
sequelae of viral encephalitis (B94.1)

✓4ᵗʰ **A80** **Acute poliomyelitis**

EXCLUDES 1   acute flaccid myelitis (G04.82)

A80.0 **Acute paralytic poliomyelitis, vaccine-associated** `MCC`

A80.1 **Acute paralytic poliomyelitis, wild virus, imported** `MCC`

A80.2 **Acute paralytic poliomyelitis, wild virus, indigenous** `MCC`

✓5ᵗʰ **A80.3** **Acute paralytic poliomyelitis, other and unspecified**

A80.30 **Acute paralytic poliomyelitis, unspecified** `MCC`

A80.39 **Other acute paralytic poliomyelitis** `MCC`

A80.4 **Acute nonparalytic poliomyelitis**

A80.9 **Acute poliomyelitis, unspecified**

✓4ᵗʰ **A81** **Atypical virus infections of central nervous system**

INCLUDES   diseases of the central nervous system caused by prions
Use additional code, if applicable, to identify:
dementia with anxiety (F02.84, F02.A4, F02.B4, F02.C4)
dementia with behavioral disturbance (F02.81-, F02.A1-, F02.B1-, F02.C1-)
dementia with mood disturbance (F02.83, F02.A3, F02.B3, F02.C3)
dementia with psychotic disturbance (F02.82, F02.A2, F02.B2, F02.C2)
dementia without behavioral disturbance (F02.80, F02.A0, F02.B0, F02.C0)
mild neurocognitive disorder due to known physiological condition (F06.7-)

✓5ᵗʰ **A81.0** **Creutzfeldt-Jakob disease**

DEF: Communicable, rare spongiform encephalopathy occurring later in life with progressive destruction of the pyramidal and extrapyramidal systems eventually leading to death. Progressive dementia, wasting of muscles, tremor, and other symptoms are present.

A81.00 **Creutzfeldt-Jakob disease, unspecified** `CC` `HCC`
Jakob-Creutzfeldt disease, unspecified

A81.01 **Variant Creutzfeldt-Jakob disease** `CC` `HCC`
vCJD

A81.09 **Other Creutzfeldt-Jakob disease** `CC` `HCC`
CJD
Familial Creutzfeldt-Jakob disease
Iatrogenic Creutzfeldt-Jakob disease
Sporadic Creutzfeldt-Jakob disease
Subacute spongiform encephalopathy (with dementia)

A81.1 **Subacute sclerosing panencephalitis** `CC` `HCC`
Dawson's inclusion body encephalitis
Van Bogaert's sclerosing leukoencephalopathy

A81.2 **Progressive multifocal leukoencephalopathy** `HIV` `CC` `HCC`
Multifocal leukoencephalopathy NOS

✓5ᵗʰ **A81.8** **Other atypical virus infections of central nervous system**

A81.81 **Kuru** `CC` `HCC`

A81.82 **Gerstmann-Straussler-Scheinker syndrome** `HIV` `CC` `HCC`
GSS syndrome

A81.83 **Fatal familial insomnia** `HIV` `CC` `HCC`
FFI

A81.89 **Other atypical virus infections of central nervous system** `HIV` `CC` `HCC`

A81.9 **Atypical virus infection of central nervous system, unspecified** `HIV` `CC` `HCC`
Prion diseases of the central nervous system NOS

✓4ᵗʰ **A82** **Rabies**

A82.0 **Sylvatic rabies** `CC`

A82.1 **Urban rabies** `CC`

A82.9 **Rabies, unspecified** `CC`

✓4ᵗʰ **A83** **Mosquito-borne viral encephalitis**

INCLUDES   mosquito-borne viral meningoencephalitis
EXCLUDES 2   Venezuelan equine encephalitis (A92.2)
West Nile fever (A92.3-)
West Nile virus (A92.3-)

A83.0 **Japanese encephalitis** `MCC`

A83.1 **Western equine encephalitis** `MCC`

A83.2 **Eastern equine encephalitis** `MCC`

A83.3 **St Louis encephalitis** `MCC`

A83.4 **Australian encephalitis** `MCC`
Kunjin virus disease

A83.5 **California encephalitis** `MCC`
California meningoencephalitis
La Crosse encephalitis

A83.6 **Rocio virus disease** `MCC`

A83.8 **Other mosquito-borne viral encephalitis** `MCC`

A83.9 **Mosquito-borne viral encephalitis, unspecified** `MCC`

✓4ᵗʰ **A84** **Tick-borne viral encephalitis**

INCLUDES   tick-borne viral meningoencephalitis

A84.0 **Far Eastern tick-borne encephalitis [Russian spring-summer encephalitis]** `MCC`

A84.1 **Central European tick-borne encephalitis** `MCC`

✓5ᵗʰ **A84.8** **Other tick-borne viral encephalitis**
AHA: 2020,4Q,4-5

A84.81 **Powassan virus disease** `MCC`

A84.89 **Other tick-borne viral encephalitis** `MCC`
Louping ill
Code first, if applicable, transfusion related infection (T80.22-)

A84.9 **Tick-borne viral encephalitis, unspecified** `MCC`

✓4ᵗʰ **A85** **Other viral encephalitis, not elsewhere classified**

INCLUDES   specified viral encephalomyelitis NEC
specified viral meningoencephalitis NEC
EXCLUDES 1   encephalitis due to cytomegalovirus (B25.8)
encephalitis due to herpesvirus NEC (B10.0-)
encephalitis due to herpesvirus [herpes simplex] (B00.4)
encephalitis due to measles virus (B05.0)
encephalitis due to mumps virus (B26.2)
encephalitis due to poliomyelitis virus (A80.-)
encephalitis due to zoster (B02.0)
lymphocytic choriomeningitis (A87.2)
myalgic encephalomyelitis (G93.32)

A85.0 **Enteroviral encephalitis** `HIV` `CC`
Enteroviral encephalomyelitis

A85.1 **Adenoviral encephalitis** `HIV` `CC`
Adenoviral meningoencephalitis

A85.2 **Arthropod-borne viral encephalitis, unspecified** `MCC`
EXCLUDES 1   West nile virus with encephalitis (A92.31)

A85.8 **Other specified viral encephalitis** `HIV` `CC`
Encephalitis lethargica
Von Economo-Cruchet disease

A86 **Unspecified viral encephalitis** `HIV` `CC`
Viral encephalomyelitis NOS
Viral meningoencephalitis NOS

✓4ᵗʰ **A87** **Viral meningitis**

EXCLUDES 1   meningitis due to herpesvirus [herpes simplex] (B00.3)
meningitis due to measles virus (B05.1)
meningitis due to mumps virus (B26.1)
meningitis due to poliomyelitis virus (A80.-)
meningitis due to zoster (B02.1)

DEF: Meningitis: Inflammation of the meningeal layers of the brain and spine.

A87.0 **Enteroviral meningitis** `CC`
Coxsackievirus meningitis
Echovirus meningitis

A87.1 **Adenoviral meningitis** `CC`

A87.2 **Lymphocytic choriomeningitis** `CC`
Lymphocytic meningoencephalitis

A87.8 **Other viral meningitis** `CC`

A87.9 **Viral meningitis, unspecified** `CC`

✓4ᵗʰ **A88** **Other viral infections of central nervous system, not elsewhere classified**

EXCLUDES 1   viral encephalitis NOS (A86)
viral meningitis NOS (A87.9)

A88.0 **Enteroviral exanthematous fever [Boston exanthem]** `CC`

A88.1 **Epidemic vertigo**

A88.8 **Other specified viral infections of central nervous system** `HIV` `CC`

A89 **Unspecified viral infection of central nervous system** `HIV` `CC`

☑ Additional Character Required   ✓x7ᵗʰ Placeholder   Questionable PDx   Manifestation   Unspecified   UPD Unacceptable PDx   H1-H14 HAC   HCC CMS-HCC Dx   HIV HIV Dx

ICD-10-CM 2025   459

Arthropod-borne viral fevers and viral hemorrhagic fevers (A90-A99)

A90 **Dengue fever [classical dengue]** `CC`
> EXCLUDES 1   *dengue hemorrhagic fever (A91)*
> **AHA:** 2016,3Q,13

A91 **Dengue hemorrhagic fever** `CC`

✓4ᵗʰ **A92** **Other mosquito-borne viral fevers**
> EXCLUDES 1   *Ross River disease (B33.1)*

  A92.0 **Chikungunya virus disease** `CC`
    Chikungunya (hemorrhagic) fever

  A92.1 **O'nyong-nyong fever** `CC`

  A92.2 **Venezuelan equine fever** `CC`
    Venezuelan equine encephalitis
    Venezuelan equine encephalomyelitis virus disease

✓5ᵗʰ **A92.3** **West Nile virus infection**
    West Nile fever
    AHA: 2016,3Q,12

    A92.30 **West Nile virus infection, unspecified** `MCC`
      West Nile fever NOS
      West Nile fever without complications
      West Nile virus NOS

    A92.31 **West Nile virus infection with encephalitis** `MCC`
      West Nile encephalitis
      West Nile encephalomyelitis

    A92.32 **West Nile virus infection with other neurologic manifestation** `MCC`
      Use additional code to specify the neurologic manifestation

    A92.39 **West Nile virus infection with other complications** `MCC`
      Use additional code to specify the other conditions

  A92.4 **Rift Valley fever** `CC`

  A92.5 **Zika virus disease** `CC`
    Zika virus fever
    Zika virus infection
    Zika NOS
    EXCLUDES 1   *congenital Zika virus disease (P35.4)*
    AHA: 2016,4Q,4-7
    DEF: Virus transmitted via a bite from an infected Aedes species mosquito. Common symptoms of the virus include fever, rash, joint pain, and conjunctivitis; they are usually mild in nature and may last from several days to a week. Most people who have the Zika virus do not require medical attention; however, in pregnant women, the Zika virus can cause a serious birth defect called microcephaly, as well as other severe fetal brain defects.
    TIP: Code only confirmed diagnoses of Zika virus; documentation by the physician that the disease is confirmed is sufficient.

  A92.8 **Other specified mosquito-borne viral fevers** `CC`

  A92.9 **Mosquito-borne viral fever, unspecified** `CC`

✓4ᵗʰ **A93** **Other arthropod-borne viral fevers, not elsewhere classified**

  A93.0 **Oropouche virus disease** `CC`
    Oropouche fever

  A93.1 **Sandfly fever** `CC`
    Pappataci fever
    Phlebotomus fever

  A93.2 **Colorado tick fever** `CC`

  A93.8 **Other specified arthropod-borne viral fevers** `CC`
    Piry virus disease
    Vesicular stomatitis virus disease [Indiana fever]

A94 **Unspecified arthropod-borne viral fever**
  Arboviral fever NOS
  Arbovirus infection NOS

✓4ᵗʰ **A95** **Yellow fever**

  A95.0 **Sylvatic yellow fever** `CC`
    Jungle yellow fever

  A95.1 **Urban yellow fever** `CC`

  A95.9 **Yellow fever, unspecified** `CC`

✓4ᵗʰ **A96** **Arenaviral hemorrhagic fever**

  A96.0 **Junin hemorrhagic fever** `CC`
    Argentinian hemorrhagic fever

  A96.1 **Machupo hemorrhagic fever** `CC`
    Bolivian hemorrhagic fever

  A96.2 **Lassa fever** `CC`

  A96.8 **Other arenaviral hemorrhagic fevers** `CC`

  A96.9 **Arenaviral hemorrhagic fever, unspecified** `CC`

✓4ᵗʰ **A98** **Other viral hemorrhagic fevers, not elsewhere classified**
> EXCLUDES 1   *chikungunya hemorrhagic fever (A92.0)*
> *dengue hemorrhagic fever (A91)*

  A98.0 **Crimean-Congo hemorrhagic fever** `CC`
    Central Asian hemorrhagic fever

  A98.1 **Omsk hemorrhagic fever** `CC`

  A98.2 **Kyasanur Forest disease** `CC`

  A98.3 **Marburg virus disease**

  A98.4 **Ebola virus disease**

  A98.5 **Hemorrhagic fever with renal syndrome** `CC`
    Epidemic hemorrhagic fever
    Korean hemorrhagic fever
    Russian hemorrhagic fever
    Hantaan virus disease
    Hantavirus disease with renal manifestations
    Nephropathia epidemica
    Songo fever
    EXCLUDES 1   *hantavirus (cardio)-pulmonary syndrome (B33.4)*

  A98.8 **Other specified viral hemorrhagic fevers** `CC`

A99 **Unspecified viral hemorrhagic fever** `CC`

Viral infections characterized by skin and mucous membrane lesions (B00-B09)

✓4ᵗʰ **B00** **Herpesviral [herpes simplex] infections**
> EXCLUDES 1   *congenital herpesviral infections (P35.2)*
> EXCLUDES 2   *anogenital herpesviral infection (A60.-)*
> *gammaherpesviral mononucleosis (B27.0-)*
> *herpangina (B08.5)*

  B00.0 **Eczema herpeticum** `HIV`
    Kaposi's varicelliform eruption

  B00.1 **Herpesviral vesicular dermatitis** `HIV`
    Herpes simplex facialis
    Herpes simplex labialis
    Herpes simplex otitis externa
    Vesicular dermatitis of ear
    Vesicular dermatitis of lip

  B00.2 **Herpesviral gingivostomatitis and pharyngotonsillitis** `HIV` `CC`
    Herpesviral pharyngitis

  B00.3 **Herpesviral meningitis** `HIV` `MCC`

  B00.4 **Herpesviral encephalitis** `HIV` `MCC`
    Herpesviral meningoencephalitis
    Simian B disease
    EXCLUDES 1   *herpesviral encephalitis due to herpesvirus 6 and 7 (B10.01, B10.09)*
    non-simplex herpesviral encephalitis (B10.0-)

✓5ᵗʰ **B00.5** **Herpesviral ocular disease**

    B00.50 **Herpesviral ocular disease, unspecified** `HIV` `CC`

    B00.51 **Herpesviral iridocyclitis** `HIV` `CC`
      Herpesviral iritis
      Herpesviral uveitis, anterior

    B00.52 **Herpesviral keratitis** `HIV` `CC`
      Herpesviral keratoconjunctivitis

    B00.53 **Herpesviral conjunctivitis** `HIV` `CC`

    B00.59 **Other herpesviral disease of eye** `HIV` `CC`
      Herpesviral dermatitis of eyelid

  B00.7 **Disseminated herpesviral disease** `HIV` `MCC` `HCC`
    Herpesviral sepsis

✓5ᵗʰ **B00.8** **Other forms of herpesviral infections**

    B00.81 **Herpesviral hepatitis** `HIV` `CC`

    B00.82 **Herpes simplex myelitis** `MCC` `HCC`

    B00.89 **Other herpesviral infection** `HIV` `CC`
      Herpesviral whitlow

  B00.9 **Herpesviral infection, unspecified** `HIV`
    Herpes simplex infection NOS

✓4ᵗʰ **B01** **Varicella [chickenpox]**

  B01.0 **Varicella meningitis** `CC`

✓5ᵗʰ **B01.1** **Varicella encephalitis, myelitis and encephalomyelitis**
    Postchickenpox encephalitis, myelitis and encephalomyelitis

    B01.11 **Varicella encephalitis and encephalomyelitis** `MCC`
      Postchickenpox encephalitis and encephalomyelitis

B01.12   **Varicella myelitis**   `MCC` `HCC`
     Postchickenpox myelitis

B01.2   **Varicella pneumonia**   `MCC`

√5ᵗʰ **B01.8**   **Varicella with other complications**

     B01.81   **Varicella keratitis**   `CC`

     B01.89   **Other varicella complications**   `CC`

B01.9   **Varicella without complication**   `CC`
     Varicella NOS

√4ᵗʰ **B02**   **Zoster [herpes zoster]**

     `INCLUDES`   shingles
                 zona

B02.0   **Zoster encephalitis**   `HIV` `CC`
     Zoster meningoencephalitis

B02.1   **Zoster meningitis**   `HIV` `MCC`
     AHA: 2019,1Q,18

√5ᵗʰ **B02.2**   **Zoster with other nervous system involvement**

     B02.21   **Postherpetic geniculate ganglionitis**   `HIV` `CC`

     B02.22   **Postherpetic trigeminal neuralgia**   `HIV` `CC`

     B02.23   **Postherpetic polyneuropathy**   `HIV` `CC`

     B02.24   **Postherpetic myelitis**   `MCC` `HCC`
          Herpes zoster myelitis

     B02.29   **Other postherpetic nervous system involvement**   `HIV` `CC`
          Postherpetic radiculopathy

√5ᵗʰ **B02.3**   **Zoster ocular disease**

     B02.30   **Zoster ocular disease, unspecified**   `HIV` `CC`

     B02.31   **Zoster conjunctivitis**   `HIV` `CC`

     B02.32   **Zoster iridocyclitis**   `HIV` `CC`

     B02.33   **Zoster keratitis**   `HIV` `CC`
          Herpes zoster keratoconjunctivitis

     B02.34   **Zoster scleritis**   `HIV` `CC`

     B02.39   **Other herpes zoster eye disease**   `HIV` `CC`
          Zoster blepharitis

B02.7   **Disseminated zoster**   `HIV` `CC`

B02.8   **Zoster with other complications**   `HIV` `CC`
     Herpes zoster otitis externa

B02.9   **Zoster without complications**   `HIV`
     Zoster NOS

B03   **Smallpox**   `CC`

     `NOTE`   In 1980 the 33rd World Health Assembly declared that smallpox had been eradicated.

          The classification is maintained for surveillance purposes.

B04   **Monkeypox**   `CC`
     ▶Mpox◀
     AHA: 2022,3Q,3-4

√4ᵗʰ **B05**   **Measles**

     `INCLUDES`   morbilli
     `EXCLUDES 1`   subacute sclerosing panencephalitis (A81.1)

B05.0   **Measles complicated by encephalitis**   `MCC`
     Postmeasles encephalitis

B05.1   **Measles complicated by meningitis**   `CC`
     Postmeasles meningitis

B05.2   **Measles complicated by pneumonia**   `MCC`
     Postmeasles pneumonia

B05.3   **Measles complicated by otitis media**
     Postmeasles otitis media

B05.4   **Measles with intestinal complications**   `CC`

√5ᵗʰ **B05.8**   **Measles with other complications**

     B05.81   **Measles keratitis and keratoconjunctivitis**   `CC`

     B05.89   **Other measles complications**   `CC`

B05.9   **Measles without complication**
     Measles NOS

√4ᵗʰ **B06**   **Rubella [German measles]**

     `EXCLUDES 1`   congenital rubella (P35.0)
     DEF: Highly contagious virus in which the symptoms are mild and short-lived in most people. Rubella during pregnancy, however, can result in abortion, stillbirth, or congenital defects.

√5ᵗʰ **B06.0**   **Rubella with neurological complications**

     B06.00   **Rubella with neurological complication, unspecified**   `CC`

B06.01   **Rubella encephalitis**   `MCC`
     Rubella meningoencephalitis

B06.02   **Rubella meningitis**   `CC`

B06.09   **Other neurological complications of rubella**   `CC`

√5ᵗʰ **B06.8**   **Rubella with other complications**

     B06.81   **Rubella pneumonia**   `CC`

     B06.82   **Rubella arthritis**   `CC` `HCC`

     B06.89   **Other rubella complications**   `CC`

B06.9   **Rubella without complication**
     Rubella NOS

√4ᵗʰ **B07**   **Viral warts**

     `INCLUDES`   verruca simplex
                  verruca vulgaris
                  viral warts due to human papillomavirus
     `EXCLUDES 2`   anogenital (venereal) warts (A63.0)
                  papilloma of bladder (D41.4)
                  papilloma of cervix (D26.0)
                  papilloma larynx (D14.1)

B07.0   **Plantar wart**
     Verruca plantaris

B07.8   **Other viral warts**
     Common wart
     Flat wart
     Verruca plana

B07.9   **Viral wart, unspecified**

√4ᵗʰ **B08**   **Other viral infections characterized by skin and mucous membrane lesions, not elsewhere classified**

     `EXCLUDES 1`   vesicular stomatitis virus disease (A93.8)

√5ᵗʰ **B08.0**   **Other orthopoxvirus infections**

     `EXCLUDES 2`   monkeypox (B04)

√6ᵗʰ   **B08.01**   **Cowpox and vaccinia not from vaccine**

         B08.010   **Cowpox**
              DEF: Disease contracted by milking infected cows. The vesicles usually appear on the fingers, hands, and adjacent areas and usually disappear without scarring. Other symptoms include local edema, lymphangitis, and regional lymphadenitis with or without fever.

         B08.011   **Vaccinia not from vaccine**
              `EXCLUDES 1`   vaccinia (from vaccination) (generalized) (T88.1)

     B08.02   **Orf virus disease**
          Contagious pustular dermatitis
          Ecthyma contagiosum

     B08.03   **Pseudocowpox [milker's node]**

     B08.04   **Paravaccinia, unspecified**

     B08.09   **Other orthopoxvirus infections**
          Orthopoxvirus infection NOS

B08.1   **Molluscum contagiosum**
     DEF: Benign poxvirus infection causing small bumps on the skin or conjunctiva, transmitted by close contact.

√5ᵗʰ **B08.2**   **Exanthema subitum [sixth disease]**
     Roseola infantum

     B08.20   **Exanthema subitum [sixth disease], unspecified**   `P`
          Roseola infantum, unspecified

     B08.21   **Exanthema subitum [sixth disease] due to human herpesvirus 6**   `P`
          Roseola infantum due to human herpesvirus 6

     B08.22   **Exanthema subitum [sixth disease] due to human herpesvirus 7**   `P`
          Roseola infantum due to human herpesvirus 7

B08.3   **Erythema infectiosum [fifth disease]**   `CC`
     DEF: Infection with human parvovirus B19, mainly occurring in children. Symptoms include a low-grade fever, malaise, or a "cold" a few days before the appearance of a mild rash illness that presents as a "slapped-cheek" rash on the face and a lacy red rash on the trunk and limbs.

B08.4   **Enteroviral vesicular stomatitis with exanthem**
     Hand, foot and mouth disease

B08.5   **Enteroviral vesicular pharyngitis**
     Herpangina
     DEF: Acute infectious Coxsackie virus infection causing throat lesions, fever, and vomiting that generally affects children in the summer.

√5ᵗʰ **B08.6**   **Parapoxvirus infections**

     B08.60   **Parapoxvirus infection, unspecified**

| ✔ Additional Character Required | √x7ᵗʰ Placeholder | Questionable PDx | Manifestation | Unspecified | `UPD` Unacceptable PDx | `H1`-`H14` HAC | `HCC` CMS-HCC Dx | `HIV` HIV Dx |

ICD-10-CM 2025   461

Chapter 1. Certain Infectious and Parasitic Diseases

             B08.61   **Bovine stomatitis**

             B08.62   **Sealpox**

             B08.69   **Other parapoxvirus infections**

   ✓5th   **B08.7**   **Yatapoxvirus infections**

             B08.70   **Yatapoxvirus infection, unspecified**

             B08.71   **Tanapox virus disease**   `CC`

             B08.72   **Yaba pox virus disease**
                    Yaba monkey tumor disease

             B08.79   **Other yatapoxvirus infections**

      B08.8   **Other specified viral infections characterized by skin and mucous membrane lesions**
             Enteroviral lymphonodular pharyngitis
             Foot-and-mouth disease
             Poxvirus NEC

   B09   **Unspecified viral infection characterized by skin and mucous membrane lesions**
          Viral enanthema NOS
          Viral exanthema NOS

Other human herpesviruses (B10)

  ✓4th   **B10**   **Other human herpesviruses**

       EXCLUDES 2   *cytomegalovirus (B25.9)*
              Epstein-Barr virus (B27.0-)
              herpes NOS (B00.9)
              herpes simplex (B00.-)
              herpes zoster (B02.-)
              human herpesvirus NOS (B00.-)
              human herpesvirus 1 and 2 (B00.-)
              human herpesvirus 3 (B01.-, B02.-)
              human herpesvirus 4 (B27.0-)
              human herpesvirus 5 (B25.-)
              varicella (B01.-)
              zoster (B02.-)

   ✓5th   **B10.0**   **Other human herpesvirus encephalitis**

       EXCLUDES 2   *herpes encephalitis NOS (B00.4)*
              herpes simplex encephalitis (B00.4)
              human herpesvirus encephalitis (B00.4)
              simian B herpes virus encephalitis (B00.4)

          B10.01   **Human herpesvirus 6 encephalitis**   `HIV` `MCC`

          B10.09   **Other human herpesvirus encephalitis**   `HIV` `MCC`
                Human herpesvirus 7 encephalitis
                AHA: AHA:2024,2Q,21

   ✓5th   **B10.8**   **Other human herpesvirus infection**

          B10.81   **Human herpesvirus 6 infection**

          B10.82   **Human herpesvirus 7 infection**

          B10.89   **Other human herpesvirus infection**
                Human herpesvirus 8 infection
                Kaposi's sarcoma-associated herpesvirus infection

Viral hepatitis (B15-B19)

  EXCLUDES 1   *sequelae of viral hepatitis (B94.2)*
  EXCLUDES 2   *cytomegaloviral hepatitis (B25.1)*
             herpesviral [herpes simplex] hepatitis (B00.81)

DEF: Hepatitis A: HAV infection that is self-limiting with flulike symptoms. Transmission is fecal-oral.

DEF: Hepatitis B: HBV infection that can be chronic and systemic. Transmission is bodily fluids.

DEF: Hepatitis C: HCV infection that can be chronic and systemic. Transmission is blood transfusion and unidentified agents.

DEF: Hepatitis D (delta): HDV that occurs only in the presence of hepatitis B virus. Transmission is contaminated blood in contact with mucous membranes.

DEF: Hepatitis E: HEV is an epidemic form. Transmission is fecal-oral, most often from contaminated water.

  ✓4th   **B15**   **Acute hepatitis A**

          B15.0   **Hepatitis A with hepatic coma**   `MCC`

          B15.9   **Hepatitis A without hepatic coma**   `CC`
                Hepatitis A (acute)(viral) NOS

  ✓4th   **B16**   **Acute hepatitis B**

       AHA: 2016,3Q,13

          B16.0   **Acute hepatitis B with delta-agent with hepatic coma**   `MCC`

          B16.1   **Acute hepatitis B with delta-agent without hepatic coma**   `CC`

          B16.2   **Acute hepatitis B without delta-agent with hepatic coma**   `MCC`

          B16.9   **Acute hepatitis B without delta-agent and without hepatic coma**   `CC`
                Hepatitis B (acute) (viral) NOS

  ✓4th   **B17**   **Other acute viral hepatitis**

          B17.0   **Acute delta-(super) infection of hepatitis B carrier**   `CC`

   ✓5th   **B17.1**   **Acute hepatitis C**

          B17.10   **Acute hepatitis C without hepatic coma**   `CC`
                Acute hepatitis C NOS

          B17.11   **Acute hepatitis C with hepatic coma**   `MCC`

          B17.2   **Acute hepatitis E**   `CC`

          B17.8   **Other specified acute viral hepatitis**   `CC`
                Hepatitis non-A non-B (acute) (viral) NEC

          B17.9   **Acute viral hepatitis, unspecified**   `CC`
                Acute hepatitis NOS
                Acute infectious hepatitis NOS

  ✓4th   **B18**   **Chronic viral hepatitis**

       INCLUDES   carrier of viral hepatitis

       AHA: 2017,1Q,41

          B18.0   **Chronic viral hepatitis B with delta-agent**   `CC` `HCC`

          B18.1   **Chronic viral hepatitis B without delta-agent**   `CC` `HCC`
                Carrier of viral hepatitis B
                Chronic (viral) hepatitis B

          B18.2   **Chronic viral hepatitis C**   `HCC`
                Carrier of viral hepatitis C
                AHA: 2018,1Q,4

          B18.8   **Other chronic viral hepatitis**   `CC` `HCC`
                Carrier of other viral hepatitis

          B18.9   **Chronic viral hepatitis, unspecified**   `CC` `HCC`
                Carrier of unspecified viral hepatitis

  ✓4th   **B19**   **Unspecified viral hepatitis**

          B19.0   **Unspecified viral hepatitis with hepatic coma**   `MCC`

   ✓5th   **B19.1**   **Unspecified viral hepatitis B**

          B19.10   **Unspecified viral hepatitis B without hepatic coma**   `CC`
                Unspecified viral hepatitis B NOS

          B19.11   **Unspecified viral hepatitis B with hepatic coma**   `MCC`

   ✓5th   **B19.2**   **Unspecified viral hepatitis C**

          B19.20   **Unspecified viral hepatitis C without hepatic coma**
                Viral hepatitis C NOS

          B19.21   **Unspecified viral hepatitis C with hepatic coma**   `MCC`

          B19.9   **Unspecified viral hepatitis without hepatic coma**   `CC`
                Viral hepatitis NOS

Human immunodeficiency virus [HIV] disease (B20)

   B20   **Human immunodeficiency virus [HIV] disease**   `CC` `HCC`

       INCLUDES   acquired immune deficiency syndrome [AIDS]
              AIDS-related complex [ARC]
              HIV infection, symptomatic

      Code first human immunodeficiency virus [HIV] disease complicating pregnancy, childbirth and the puerperium, if applicable (O98.7-)
      Use additional code(s) to identify all manifestations of HIV infection

       EXCLUDES 1   *asymptomatic human immunodeficiency virus [HIV] infection status (Z21)*
              exposure to HIV virus (Z20.6)
              inconclusive serologic evidence of HIV (R75)

       AHA: 2022,1Q,36; 2021,2Q,6; 2021,1Q,52; 2020,4Q,97; 2020,2Q,12; 2019,1Q,8-11

Other viral diseases (B25-B34)

  ✓4th   **B25**   **Cytomegaloviral disease**

       EXCLUDES 1   *congenital cytomegalovirus infection (P35.1)*
              cytomegaloviral mononucleosis (B27.1-)

          B25.0   **Cytomegaloviral pneumonitis**   `MCC` `HCC`

          B25.1   **Cytomegaloviral hepatitis**   `CC` `HCC`

          B25.2   **Cytomegaloviral pancreatitis**   `MCC` `HCC`

          B25.8   **Other cytomegaloviral diseases**   `HIV` `CC` `HCC`
                Cytomegaloviral encephalitis

          B25.9   **Cytomegaloviral disease, unspecified**   `HIV` `CC` `HCC`

N Newborn: 0   P Pediatric: 0-17   M Maternity: 9-64   A Adult: 15-124   UNS Unspecified Site   MCC Major Complication/Comorbidity   CC Complication/Comorbidity   PE POA Exempt

462

ICD-10-CM 2025

☑4ᵗʰ B26 Mumps

INCLUDES   epidemic parotitis
     infectious parotitis

B26.0 Mumps orchitis   CC
B26.1 Mumps meningitis   MCC
B26.2 Mumps encephalitis   MCC
B26.3 Mumps pancreatitis   CC
☑5ᵗʰ B26.8 Mumps with other complications

     B26.81 Mumps hepatitis   CC
     B26.82 Mumps myocarditis   CC
     B26.83 Mumps nephritis   CC
     B26.84 Mumps polyneuropathy   CC
     B26.85 Mumps arthritis   CC HCC
     B26.89 Other mumps complications   CC

B26.9 Mumps without complication
     Mumps NOS
     Mumps parotitis NOS

☑4ᵗʰ B27 Infectious mononucleosis

INCLUDES   glandular fever
     monocytic angina
     Pfeiffer's disease

☑5ᵗʰ B27.0 Gammaherpesviral mononucleosis

     Mononucleosis due to Epstein-Barr virus

     B27.00 Gammaherpesviral mononucleosis without complication
     B27.01 Gammaherpesviral mononucleosis with polyneuropathy
     B27.02 Gammaherpesviral mononucleosis with meningitis
     B27.09 Gammaherpesviral mononucleosis with other complications
       Hepatomegaly in gammaherpesviral mononucleosis
       AHA: AHA:2024,2Q,21

☑5ᵗʰ B27.1 Cytomegaloviral mononucleosis

     B27.10 Cytomegaloviral mononucleosis without complications
     B27.11 Cytomegaloviral mononucleosis with polyneuropathy
     B27.12 Cytomegaloviral mononucleosis with meningitis
     B27.19 Cytomegaloviral mononucleosis with other complication
       Hepatomegaly in cytomegaloviral mononucleosis

☑5ᵗʰ B27.8 Other infectious mononucleosis

     B27.80 Other infectious mononucleosis without complication
     B27.81 Other infectious mononucleosis with polyneuropathy
     B27.82 Other infectious mononucleosis with meningitis
     B27.89 Other infectious mononucleosis with other complication
       Hepatomegaly in other infectious mononucleosis

☑5ᵗʰ B27.9 Infectious mononucleosis, unspecified

     B27.90 Infectious mononucleosis, unspecified without complication
     B27.91 Infectious mononucleosis, unspecified with polyneuropathy
     B27.92 Infectious mononucleosis, unspecified with meningitis
     B27.99 Infectious mononucleosis, unspecified with other complication
       Hepatomegaly in unspecified infectious mononucleosis

☑4ᵗʰ B30 Viral conjunctivitis

EXCLUDES 1   *herpesviral [herpes simplex] ocular disease (B00.5)*
     ocular zoster (B02.3)

Viral Conjunctivitis

Inflamed conjunctiva

Normal conjunctiva

B30.0 Keratoconjunctivitis due to adenovirus
     Epidemic keratoconjunctivitis
     Shipyard eye

B30.1 Conjunctivitis due to adenovirus
     Acute adenoviral follicular conjunctivitis
     Swimming-pool conjunctivitis

B30.2 Viral pharyngoconjunctivitis

B30.3 Acute epidemic hemorrhagic conjunctivitis (enteroviral)
     Conjunctivitis due to coxsackievirus 24
     Conjunctivitis due to enterovirus 70
     Hemorrhagic conjunctivitis (acute)(epidemic)

B30.8 Other viral conjunctivitis
     Newcastle conjunctivitis

B30.9 Viral conjunctivitis, unspecified

☑4ᵗʰ B33 Other viral diseases, not elsewhere classified

B33.0 Epidemic myalgia
     Bornholm disease

B33.1 Ross River disease   CC
     Epidemic polyarthritis and exanthema
     Ross River fever

☑5ᵗʰ B33.2 Viral carditis

     Coxsackie (virus) carditis

     B33.20 Viral carditis, unspecified   CC
     B33.21 Viral endocarditis   CC
     B33.22 Viral myocarditis   CC
     B33.23 Viral pericarditis   CC
     B33.24 Viral cardiomyopathy   HCC

B33.3 Retrovirus infections, not elsewhere classified
     Retrovirus infection NOS

B33.4 Hantavirus (cardio)-pulmonary syndrome [HPS] [HCPS]   CC
     Hantavirus disease with pulmonary manifestations
     Sin nombre virus disease
     Use additional code to identify any associated acute kidney failure (N17.9)
     EXCLUDES 1   *hantavirus disease with renal manifestations (A98.5)*
         hemorrhagic fever with renal manifestations (A98.5)

B33.8 Other specified viral diseases
     EXCLUDES 1   *anogenital human papillomavirus infection (A63.0)*
         viral warts due to human papillomavirus infection (B07)

☑4ᵗʰ B34 Viral infection of unspecified site

EXCLUDES 1   *anogenital human papillomavirus infection (A63.0)*
     cytomegaloviral disease NOS (B25.9)
     herpesvirus [herpes simplex] infection NOS (B00.9)
     retrovirus infection NOS (B33.3)
     viral agents as the cause of diseases classified elsewhere (B97.-)
     viral warts due to human papillomavirus infection (B07)

B34.0 Adenovirus infection, unspecified

B34.1 Enterovirus infection, unspecified
     Coxsackievirus infection NOS
     Echovirus infection NOS

B34.2 Coronavirus infection, unspecified
     EXCLUDES 1   *COVID-19 (U07.1)*
         pneumonia due to SARS-associated coronavirus (J12.81)
     AHA: 2020,1Q,34-36

B34.3 Parvovirus infection, unspecified   CC
B34.4 Papovavirus infection, unspecified
B34.8 Other viral infections of unspecified site
B34.9 Viral infection, unspecified
     Viremia NOS
     AHA: 2016,3Q,10

Mycoses (B35-B49)

EXCLUDES 2   *hypersensitivity pneumonitis due to organic dust (J67.-)*
     mycosis fungoides (C84.0-)

☑4ᵗʰ B35 Dermatophytosis

INCLUDES   favus
     infections due to species of Epidermophyton, Micro-sporum and Trichophyton
     tinea, any type except those in B36.-

DEF: Contagious superficial fungal infection of the skin that invades and grows in dead keratin.

B35.0 Tinea barbae and tinea capitis
     Beard ringworm
     Kerion
     Scalp ringworm
     Sycosis, mycotic

☑ Additional Character Required   ☑x7ᵗʰ Placeholder   Questionable PDx   Manifestation   Unspecified   UPD Unacceptable PDx   H1-H14 HAC   HCC CMS-HCC Dx   HIV HIV Dx

ICD-10-CM 2025   463

B35.1 Tinea unguium
Dermatophytic onychia
Dermatophytosis of nail
Onychomycosis
Ringworm of nails

B35.2 Tinea manuum
Dermatophytosis of hand
Hand ringworm

B35.3 Tinea pedis
Athlete's foot
Dermatophytosis of foot
Foot ringworm

B35.4 Tinea corporis
Ringworm of the body

B35.5 Tinea imbricata
Tokelau

B35.6 Tinea cruris
Dhobi itch
Groin ringworm
Jock itch

B35.8 Other dermatophytoses
Disseminated dermatophytosis
Granulomatous dermatophytosis

B35.9 Dermatophytosis, unspecified
Ringworm NOS

✓4ᵗʰ B36 Other superficial mycoses

B36.0 Pityriasis versicolor
Tinea flava
Tinea versicolor

B36.1 Tinea nigra
Keratomycosis nigricans palmaris
Microsporosis nigra
Pityriasis nigra

B36.2 White piedra
Tinea blanca

B36.3 Black piedra

B36.8 Other specified superficial mycoses

B36.9 Superficial mycosis, unspecified

✓4ᵗʰ B37 Candidiasis

INCLUDES　candidosis
moniliasis

EXCLUDES 1　neonatal candidiasis (P37.5)

DEF: *Candida:* Genus of yeast-like fungi that are commonly found in the mouth, skin, intestinal tract, and vagina. It may cause a white, cheesy discharge.

B37.0 Candidal stomatitis `HIV` `CC`
Oral thrush

B37.1 Pulmonary candidiasis `HIV` `MCC` `HCC`
Candidal bronchitis
Candidal pneumonia

B37.2 Candidiasis of skin and nail `HIV`
Candidal onychia
Candidal paronychia
EXCLUDES 2　diaper dermatitis (L22)

✓5ᵗʰ B37.3 Candidiasis of vulva and vagina
Candidal vulvovaginitis
Monilial vulvovaginitis
Vaginal thrush
AHA: 2022,4Q,4-5

B37.31 Acute candidiasis of vulva and vagina
Candidiasis of vulva and vagina NOS

B37.32 Chronic candidiasis of vulva and vagina
Recurrent candidiasis of vulva and vagina

✓5ᵗʰ B37.4 Candidiasis of other urogenital sites

B37.41 Candidal cystitis and urethritis `CC` `H6`
B37.42 Candidal balanitis
B37.49 Other urogenital candidiasis `CC` `H6`
Candidal pyelonephritis

B37.5 Candidal meningitis `HIV` `MCC`
B37.6 Candidal endocarditis `HIV` `MCC`
B37.7 Candidal sepsis `MCC` `HCC`
Disseminated candidiasis
Systemic candidiasis
AHA: 2014,4Q,46

✓5ᵗʰ B37.8 Candidiasis of other sites

B37.81 Candidal esophagitis `HIV` `CC` `HCC`

B37.82 Candidal enteritis `HIV` `CC`
Candidal proctitis

B37.83 Candidal cheilitis `HIV` `CC`
B37.84 Candidal otitis externa `HIV` `CC`
B37.89 Other sites of candidiasis `HIV` `CC`
Candidal osteomyelitis

B37.9 Candidiasis, unspecified `HIV`
Thrush NOS

✓4ᵗʰ B38 Coccidioidomycosis

B38.0 Acute pulmonary coccidioidomycosis `HIV` `CC`
B38.1 Chronic pulmonary coccidioidomycosis `HIV` `CC`
B38.2 Pulmonary coccidioidomycosis, unspecified `HIV` `CC`
B38.3 Cutaneous coccidioidomycosis `HIV` `CC`
B38.4 Coccidioidomycosis meningitis `HIV` `MCC`
DEF: *Coccidioides immitis* infection of the lining of the brain and/or spinal cord.

B38.7 Disseminated coccidioidomycosis `HIV` `CC`
Generalized coccidioidomycosis

✓5ᵗʰ B38.8 Other forms of coccidioidomycosis

B38.81 Prostatic coccidioidomycosis `HIV` `CC`
B38.89 Other forms of coccidioidomycosis `HIV` `CC`

B38.9 Coccidioidomycosis, unspecified `HIV` `CC`

✓4ᵗʰ B39 Histoplasmosis

Code first associated AIDS (B20)
Use additional code for any associated manifestations, such as:
endocarditis (I39)
meningitis (G02)
pericarditis (I32)
retinitis (H32)
DEF: Type of lung infection caused by breathing in fungal spores often found in the droppings of bats and birds or soil contaminated by their droppings.

Histoplasmosis

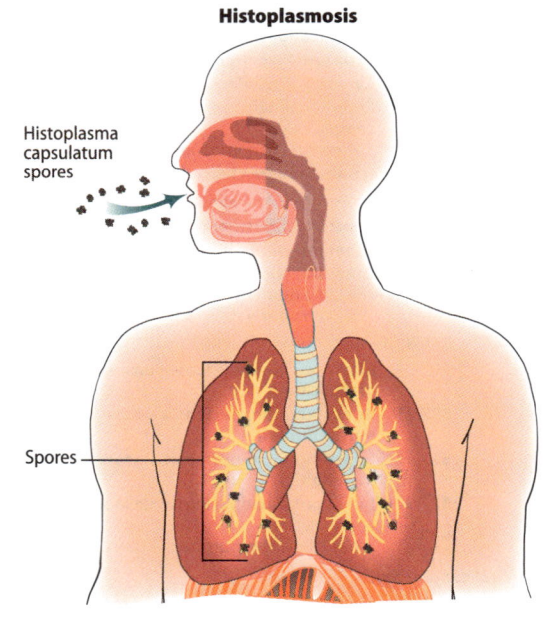

Histoplasma capsulatum spores

Spores

B39.0 Acute pulmonary histoplasmosis capsulati `HIV` `MCC`
B39.1 Chronic pulmonary histoplasmosis capsulati `HIV` `MCC`
B39.2 Pulmonary histoplasmosis capsulati, unspecified `HIV` `MCC`
B39.3 Disseminated histoplasmosis capsulati `HIV` `CC`
Generalized histoplasmosis capsulati

B39.4 Histoplasmosis capsulati, unspecified `HIV`
American histoplasmosis

B39.5 Histoplasmosis duboisii `HIV`
African histoplasmosis

B39.9 Histoplasmosis, unspecified `HIV`

✓4ᵗʰ B40 Blastomycosis

EXCLUDES 1　Brazilian blastomycosis (B41.-)
keloidal blastomycosis (B48.0)

B40.0 Acute pulmonary blastomycosis `CC`
B40.1 Chronic pulmonary blastomycosis `CC`

N Newborn: 0　P Pediatric: 0-17　M Maternity: 9-64　A Adult: 15-124　UNS Unspecified Site　MCC Major Complication/Comorbidity　CC Complication/Comorbidity　PE POA Exempt

464

ICD-10-CM 2025

B40.2   **Pulmonary** blastomycosis, unspecified   `CC`

B40.3   **Cutaneous** blastomycosis   `CC`

B40.7   **Disseminated** blastomycosis   `CC`
    Generalized blastomycosis

✓5ᵗʰ **B40.8**   **Other forms** of blastomycosis

     B40.81   **Blastomycotic meningoencephalitis**   `CC`
        Meningomyelitis due to blastomycosis

     B40.89   **Other forms** of blastomycosis   `CC`

B40.9   **Blastomycosis, unspecified**   `CC`

✓4ᵗʰ **B41**   **Paracoccidioidomycosis**

    INCLUDES   Brazilian blastomycosis
           Lutz' disease

B41.0   **Pulmonary** paracoccidioidomycosis   `CC`

B41.7   **Disseminated** paracoccidioidomycosis   `CC`
    Generalized paracoccidioidomycosis

B41.8   **Other forms** of paracoccidioidomycosis   `CC`

B41.9   **Paracoccidioidomycosis, unspecified**   `CC`

✓4ᵗʰ **B42**   **Sporotrichosis**

B42.0   **Pulmonary** sporotrichosis

B42.1   **Lymphocutaneous** sporotrichosis

B42.7   **Disseminated** sporotrichosis
    Generalized sporotrichosis

✓5ᵗʰ **B42.8**   **Other forms** of sporotrichosis

     B42.81   **Cerebral** sporotrichosis
        Meningitis due to sporotrichosis

     B42.82   **Sporotrichosis arthritis**   `HCC`

     B42.89   **Other forms** of sporotrichosis

B42.9   **Sporotrichosis, unspecified**

✓4ᵗʰ **B43**   **Chromomycosis and pheomycotic abscess**

B43.0   **Cutaneous** chromomycosis
    Dermatitis verrucosa

B43.1   **Pheomycotic brain abscess**
    Cerebral chromomycosis

B43.2   **Subcutaneous** pheomycotic **abscess and cyst**

B43.8   **Other forms** of chromomycosis

B43.9   **Chromomycosis, unspecified**

✓4ᵗʰ **B44**   **Aspergillosis**

    INCLUDES   aspergilloma

B44.0   **Invasive pulmonary** aspergillosis   `MCC` `HCC`

B44.1   **Other pulmonary** aspergillosis   `CC` `HCC`

B44.2   **Tonsillar** aspergillosis   `CC` `HCC`

B44.7   **Disseminated** aspergillosis   `CC` `HCC`
    Generalized aspergillosis

✓5ᵗʰ **B44.8**   **Other forms** of aspergillosis

     B44.81   **Allergic bronchopulmonary** aspergillosis   `CC` `HCC`

     B44.89   **Other forms** of aspergillosis   `CC` `HCC`

B44.9   **Aspergillosis, unspecified**   `CC` `HCC`

✓4ᵗʰ **B45**   **Cryptococcosis**

B45.0   **Pulmonary** cryptococcosis   `HIV` `CC` `HCC`

B45.1   **Cerebral** cryptococcosis   `MCC` `HCC`
    Cryptococcal meningitis
    Cryptococcosis meningocerebralis

B45.2   **Cutaneous** cryptococcosis   `HIV` `CC` `HCC`

B45.3   **Osseous** cryptococcosis   `HIV` `CC` `HCC`

B45.7   **Disseminated** cryptococcosis   `HIV` `CC` `HCC`
    Generalized cryptococcosis

B45.8   **Other forms** of cryptococcosis   `HIV` `CC` `HCC`

B45.9   **Cryptococcosis, unspecified**   `HIV` `CC` `HCC`

✓4ᵗʰ **B46**   **Zygomycosis**

B46.0   **Pulmonary** mucormycosis   `MCC` `HCC`

B46.1   **Rhinocerebral** mucormycosis   `MCC` `HCC`

B46.2   **Gastrointestinal** mucormycosis   `MCC` `HCC`

B46.3   **Cutaneous** mucormycosis   `MCC` `HCC`
    Subcutaneous mucormycosis

B46.4   **Disseminated** mucormycosis   `MCC` `HCC`
    Generalized mucormycosis

B46.5   **Mucormycosis, unspecified**   `MCC` `HCC`

B46.8   **Other zygomycoses**   `MCC` `HCC`
    Entomophthoromycosis

B46.9   **Zygomycosis, unspecified**   `MCC` `HCC`
    Phycomycosis NOS

✓4ᵗʰ **B47**   **Mycetoma**

B47.0   **Eumycetoma**   `CC`
    Madura foot, mycotic
    Maduromycosis

B47.1   **Actinomycetoma**   `HIV` `CC`

B47.9   **Mycetoma, unspecified**   `HIV` `CC`
    Madura foot NOS

✓4ᵗʰ **B48**   **Other mycoses, not elsewhere classified**

B48.0   **Lobomycosis**
    Keloidal blastomycosis
    Lobo's disease

B48.1   **Rhinosporidiosis**

B48.2   **Allescheriasis**   `CC`
    Infection due to Pseudallescheria boydii
    EXCLUDES 1   eumycetoma (B47.0)

B48.3   **Geotrichosis**   `CC`
    Geotrichum stomatitis

B48.4   **Penicillosis**   `CC` `HCC`
    Talaromycosis

B48.8   **Other specified mycoses**   `HIV` `CC` `HCC`
    Adiaspiromycosis
    Infection of tissue and organs by Alternaria
    Infection of tissue and organs by Drechslera
    Infection of tissue and organs by Fusarium
    Infection of tissue and organs by saprophytic fungi NEC
    AHA: 2014,4Q,46; 2014,2Q,13

B49   **Unspecified mycosis**   `CC`
    Fungemia NOS

Protozoal diseases (B50-B64)

EXCLUDES 1   amebiasis (A06.-)
          other protozoal intestinal diseases (A07.-)

✓4ᵗʰ **B50**   **Plasmodium falciparum malaria**

    INCLUDES   mixed infections of Plasmodium falciparum with any other
           Plasmodium species

B50.0   **Plasmodium falciparum malaria with cerebral complications**   `CC`
    Cerebral malaria NOS

B50.8   **Other severe and complicated Plasmodium falciparum malaria**   `CC`
    Severe or complicated Plasmodium falciparum malaria NOS

B50.9   **Plasmodium falciparum malaria, unspecified**   `MCC`

✓4ᵗʰ **B51**   **Plasmodium vivax malaria**

    INCLUDES   mixed infections of Plasmodium vivax with other Plasmodium
           species, except Plasmodium falciparum
    EXCLUDES 1   Plasmodium vivax with Plasmodium falciparum (B50.-)

B51.0   **Plasmodium vivax malaria with rupture of spleen**   `CC`

B51.8   **Plasmodium vivax malaria with other complications**   `CC`

B51.9   **Plasmodium vivax malaria without complication**   `CC`
    Plasmodium vivax malaria NOS

✓4ᵗʰ **B52**   **Plasmodium malariae malaria**

    INCLUDES   mixed infections of Plasmodium malariae with other
           Plasmodium species, except Plasmodium falciparum
           and Plasmodium vivax
    EXCLUDES 1   Plasmodium falciparum (B50.-)
               Plasmodium vivax (B51.-)

B52.0   **Plasmodium malariae malaria with nephropathy**   `CC`

B52.8   **Plasmodium malariae malaria with other complications**   `CC`

B52.9   **Plasmodium malariae malaria without complication**   `CC`
    Plasmodium malariae malaria NOS

✓4ᵗʰ **B53**   **Other specified malaria**

B53.0   **Plasmodium ovale malaria**   `CC`
    EXCLUDES 1   Plasmodium ovale with Plasmodium falciparum (B50.-)
               Plasmodium ovale with Plasmodium malariae (B52.-)
               Plasmodium ovale with Plasmodium vivax (B51.-)

Chapter 1. Certain Infectious and Parasitic Diseases

B40.2–B53.0

✔ Additional Character Required   ✓7ᵗʰ Placeholder   Questionable PDx   Manifestation   Unspecified   `UPD` Unacceptable PDx   `H1`-`H14` HAC   `HCC` CMS-HCC Dx   `HIV` HIV Dx

ICD-10-CM 2025   **465**

Chapter 1. Certain Infectious and Parasitic Diseases

B53.1 Malaria due to simian plasmodia `CC`
> **EXCLUDES 1**   *malaria due to simian plasmodia with Plasmodium falciparum (B50.-)*
> *malaria due to simian plasmodia with Plasmodium malariae (B52.-)*
> *malaria due to simian plasmodia with Plasmodium ovale (B53.0)*
> *malaria due to simian plasmodia with Plasmodium vivax (B51.-)*

B53.8 Other malaria, not elsewhere classified `CC`

B54 Unspecified malaria `CC`

✓4ᵗʰ **B55 Leishmaniasis**
> **B55.0 Visceral leishmaniasis** `CC`
> Kala-azar
> Post-kala-azar dermal leishmaniasis
>
> **B55.1 Cutaneous leishmaniasis** `CC`
> **B55.2 Mucocutaneous leishmaniasis** `CC`
> **B55.9 Leishmaniasis, unspecified** `CC`

✓4ᵗʰ **B56 African trypanosomiasis**
> **B56.0 Gambiense trypanosomiasis** `CC`
> Infection due to Trypanosoma brucei gambiense
> West African sleeping sickness
>
> **B56.1 Rhodesiense trypanosomiasis** `CC`
> East African sleeping sickness
> Infection due to Trypanosoma brucei rhodesiense
>
> **B56.9 African trypanosomiasis, unspecified** `CC`
> Sleeping sickness NOS

✓4ᵗʰ **B57 Chagas' disease**
> **INCLUDES**   American trypanosomiasis
> infection due to Trypanosoma cruzi
>
> **B57.0 Acute Chagas' disease with heart involvement** `CC`
> Acute Chagas' disease with myocarditis
>
> **B57.1 Acute Chagas' disease without heart involvement** `CC`
> Acute Chagas' disease NOS
>
> **B57.2 Chagas' disease (chronic) with heart involvement** `CC`
> American trypanosomiasis NOS
> Chagas' disease (chronic) NOS
> Chagas' disease (chronic) with myocarditis
> Trypanosomiasis NOS
>
> ✓5ᵗʰ **B57.3 Chagas' disease (chronic) with digestive system involvement**
>> **B57.30 Chagas' disease with digestive system involvement, unspecified** `CC`
>> **B57.31 Megaesophagus in Chagas' disease** `CC`
>> **B57.32 Megacolon in Chagas' disease** `CC`
>> **B57.39 Other digestive system involvement in Chagas' disease** `CC`
>
> ✓5ᵗʰ **B57.4 Chagas' disease (chronic) with nervous system involvement**
>> **B57.40 Chagas' disease with nervous system involvement, unspecified** `CC`
>> **B57.41 Meningitis in Chagas' disease** `CC`
>> **B57.42 Meningoencephalitis in Chagas' disease** `CC`
>> **B57.49 Other nervous system involvement in Chagas' disease** `CC`
>
> **B57.5 Chagas' disease (chronic) with other organ involvement** `CC`

✓4ᵗʰ **B58 Toxoplasmosis**
> **INCLUDES**   infection due to Toxoplasma gondii
> **EXCLUDES 1**   *congenital toxoplasmosis (P37.1)*
>
> ✓5ᵗʰ **B58.0 Toxoplasma oculopathy**
>> **B58.00 Toxoplasma oculopathy, unspecified** `HIV` `CC`
>> **B58.01 Toxoplasma chorioretinitis** `HIV` `CC`
>> **B58.09 Other toxoplasma oculopathy** `HIV` `CC`
>> Toxoplasma uveitis
>
> **B58.1 Toxoplasma hepatitis** `HIV` `CC`
> **B58.2 Toxoplasma meningoencephalitis** `HIV` `MCC` `HCC`
> **B58.3 Pulmonary toxoplasmosis** `HIV` `MCC` `HCC`
>
> ✓5ᵗʰ **B58.8 Toxoplasmosis with other organ involvement**
>> **B58.81 Toxoplasma myocarditis** `HIV` `MCC`
>> **B58.82 Toxoplasma myositis** `HIV` `CC`
>> **B58.83 Toxoplasma tubulo-interstitial nephropathy** `HIV` `CC`
>> Toxoplasma pyelonephritis
>> **B58.89 Toxoplasmosis with other organ involvement** `HIV` `CC`

B58.9 Toxoplasmosis, unspecified `HIV` `CC`

B59 Pneumocystosis `HIV` `MCC` `HCC`
Pneumonia due to Pneumocystis carinii
Pneumonia due to Pneumocystis jiroveci

✓4ᵗʰ **B60 Other protozoal diseases, not elsewhere classified**
> **EXCLUDES 1**   *cryptosporidiosis (A07.2)*
> *intestinal microsporidiosis (A07.8)*
> *isosporiasis (A07.3)*
>
> ✓5ᵗʰ **B60.0 Babesiosis**
> **AHA:** 2020,4Q,5-6
>> **B60.00 Babesiosis, unspecified** `CC`
>> Babesiosis due to unspecified Babesia species
>> Piroplasmosis, unspecified
>>
>> **B60.01 Babesiosis due to Babesia microti** `CC`
>> Infection due to B. microti
>>
>> **B60.02 Babesiosis due to Babesia duncani** `CC`
>> Infection due to B. duncani and B. duncani-type species
>>
>> **B60.03 Babesiosis due to Babesia divergens** `CC`
>> Babesiosis due to Babesia MO-1
>> Infection due to B. divergens and B. divergens-like strains
>>
>> **B60.09 Other babesiosis** `CC`
>> Babesiosis due to Babesia KO-1
>> Babesiosis due to Babesia venatorum
>> Infection due to other Babesia species
>> Infection due to other protozoa of the order Piroplasmida
>> Other piroplasmosis
>
> ✓5ᵗʰ **B60.1 Acanthamebiasis**
>> **B60.10 Acanthamebiasis, unspecified** `CC`
>> **B60.11 Meningoencephalitis due to Acanthamoeba (culbertsoni)**
>> **B60.12 Conjunctivitis due to Acanthamoeba**
>> **B60.13 Keratoconjunctivitis due to Acanthamoeba**
>> **B60.19 Other acanthamebic disease** `CC`
>
> **B60.2 Naegleriasis** `CC`
> Primary amebic meningoencephalitis
>
> **B60.8 Other specified protozoal diseases** `HIV`
> Microsporidiosis

B64 Unspecified protozoal disease `CC`

Helminthiases (B65-B83)

✓4ᵗʰ **B65 Schistosomiasis [bilharziasis]**
> **INCLUDES**   snail fever
>
> **B65.0 Schistosomiasis due to Schistosoma haematobium [urinary schistosomiasis]** `CC`
> **B65.1 Schistosomiasis due to Schistosoma mansoni [intestinal schistosomiasis]** `CC`
> **B65.2 Schistosomiasis due to Schistosoma japonicum** `CC`
> Asiatic schistosomiasis
>
> **B65.3 Cercarial dermatitis** `CC`
> Swimmer's itch
>
> **B65.8 Other schistosomiasis** `CC`
> Infection due to Schistosoma intercalatum
> Infection due to Schistosoma mattheei
> Infection due to Schistosoma mekongi
>
> **B65.9 Schistosomiasis, unspecified** `CC`

✓4ᵗʰ **B66 Other fluke infections**
> **B66.0 Opisthorchiasis** `CC`
> Infection due to cat liver fluke
> Infection due to Opisthorchis (felineus)(viverrini)
>
> **B66.1 Clonorchiasis**
> Chinese liver fluke disease
> Infection due to Clonorchis sinensis
> Oriental liver fluke disease
>
> **B66.2 Dicroceliasis** `CC`
> Infection due to Dicrocoelium dendriticum
> Lancet fluke infection
>
> **B66.3 Fascioliasis** `CC`
> Infection due to Fasciola gigantica
> Infection due to Fasciola hepatica
> Infection due to Fasciola indica
> Sheep liver fluke disease

N Newborn: 0   **P** Pediatric: 0-17   **M** Maternity: 9-64   **A** Adult: 15-124   **UNS** Unspecified Site   **MCC** Major Complication/Comorbidity   **CC** Complication/Comorbidity   **PE** POA Exempt

466   ICD-10-CM 2025

B66.4 Paragonimiasis `CC`
Infection due to Paragonimus species
Lung fluke disease
Pulmonary distomiasis

B66.5 Fasciolopsiasis `CC`
Infection due to Fasciolopsis buski
Intestinal distomiasis

B66.8 Other specified fluke infections `CC`
Echinostomiasis
Heterophyiasis
Metagonimiasis
Nanophyetiasis
Watsoniasis

B66.9 Fluke infection, unspecified

√4th **B67 Echinococcosis**
INCLUDES   hydatidosis

B67.0 Echinococcus granulosus infection of liver `CC`

B67.1 Echinococcus granulosus infection of lung `CC`

B67.2 Echinococcus granulosus infection of bone `CC`

√5th **B67.3 Echinococcus granulosus infection, other and multiple sites**

   B67.31 Echinococcus granulosus infection, thyroid gland `CC`

   B67.32 Echinococcus granulosus infection, multiple sites `CC`

   B67.39 Echinococcus granulosus infection, other sites `CC`

B67.4 Echinococcus granulosus infection, unspecified `CC`
Dog tapeworm (infection)

B67.5 Echinococcus multilocularis infection of liver `CC`

√5th **B67.6 Echinococcus multilocularis infection, other and multiple sites**

   B67.61 Echinococcus multilocularis infection, multiple sites `CC`

   B67.69 Echinococcus multilocularis infection, other sites

B67.7 Echinococcus multilocularis infection, unspecified `CC`

B67.8 Echinococcosis, unspecified, of liver `CC`

√5th **B67.9 Echinococcosis, other and unspecified**

   B67.90 Echinococcosis, unspecified `CC`
Echinococcosis NOS

   B67.99 Other echinococcosis `CC`

√4th **B68 Taeniasis**
EXCLUDES 1   cysticercosis (B69.-)

B68.0 Taenia solium taeniasis `CC`
Pork tapeworm (infection)

B68.1 Taenia saginata taeniasis `CC`
Beef tapeworm (infection)
Infection due to adult tapeworm Taenia saginata

B68.9 Taeniasis, unspecified `CC`

√4th **B69 Cysticercosis**
INCLUDES   cysticerciasis infection due to larval form of Taenia solium
DEF: Condition that is developed when larvae or eggs of the tapeworm *Taenia solium* are ingested, most commonly in fecally contaminated water or undercooked pork.

B69.0 Cysticercosis of central nervous system `CC`

B69.1 Cysticercosis of eye `CC`

√5th **B69.8 Cysticercosis of other sites**

   B69.81 Myositis in cysticercosis `CC`

   B69.89 Cysticercosis of other sites `CC`

B69.9 Cysticercosis, unspecified `CC`

√4th **B70 Diphyllobothriasis and sparganosis**

B70.0 Diphyllobothriasis `CC`
Diphyllobothrium (adult) (latum) (pacificum) infection
Fish tapeworm (infection)
EXCLUDES 2   larval diphyllobothriasis (B70.1)

B70.1 Sparganosis `CC`
Infection due to Sparganum (mansoni) (proliferum)
Infection due to Spirometra larva
Larval diphyllobothriasis
Spirometrosis

√4th **B71 Other cestode infections**

B71.0 Hymenolepiasis `CC`
Dwarf tapeworm infection
Rat tapeworm (infection)

B71.1 Dipylidiasis `CC`

B71.8 Other specified cestode infections `CC`
Coenurosis

B71.9 Cestode infection, unspecified `CC`
Tapeworm (infection) NOS

B72 Dracunculiasis `CC`
INCLUDES   guinea worm infection
         infection due to Dracunculus medinensis

√4th **B73 Onchocerciasis**
INCLUDES   onchocerca volvulus infection
         onchocercosis
         river blindness

√5th **B73.0 Onchocerciasis with eye disease**

   B73.00 Onchocerciasis with eye involvement, unspecified `CC`

   B73.01 Onchocerciasis with endophthalmitis `CC`

   B73.02 Onchocerciasis with glaucoma `CC`

   B73.09 Onchocerciasis with other eye involvement `CC`
Infestation of eyelid due to onchocerciasis

B73.1 Onchocerciasis without eye disease `CC`

√4th **B74 Filariasis**
EXCLUDES 2   *onchocerciasis (B73)*
         tropical (pulmonary) eosinophilia NOS (J82.89)

B74.0 Filariasis due to Wuchereria bancrofti `CC`
Bancroftian elephantiasis
Bancroftian filariasis

B74.1 Filariasis due to Brugia malayi `CC`

B74.2 Filariasis due to Brugia timori `CC`

B74.3 Loiasis
Calabar swelling
Eyeworm disease of Africa
Loa loa infection

B74.4 Mansonelliasis `CC`
Infection due to Mansonella ozzardi
Infection due to Mansonella perstans
Infection due to Mansonella streptocerca

B74.8 Other filariases `CC`
Dirofilariasis

B74.9 Filariasis, unspecified `CC`

B75 Trichinellosis `CC`
INCLUDES   infection due to Trichinella species
         trichiniasis
DEF: Infection by *Trichinella spiralis,* the smallest of the parasitic nematodes, that is transmitted by eating undercooked pork or bear meat. **Synonym(s):** Trichinosis.

√4th **B76 Hookworm diseases**
INCLUDES   uncinariasis

B76.0 Ancylostomiasis `CC`
Infection due to Ancylostoma species

B76.1 Necatoriasis
Infection due to Necator americanus

B76.8 Other hookworm diseases `CC`

B76.9 Hookworm disease, unspecified `CC`
Cutaneous larva migrans NOS

√4th **B77 Ascariasis**
INCLUDES   ascaridiasis
         roundworm infection

B77.0 Ascariasis with intestinal complications `CC`

√5th **B77.8 Ascariasis with other complications**

   B77.81 Ascariasis pneumonia `MCC`

   B77.89 Ascariasis with other complications `CC`

B77.9 Ascariasis, unspecified `CC`

√4th **B78 Strongyloidiasis**
EXCLUDES 1   *trichostrongyliasis (B81.2)*

B78.0 Intestinal strongyloidiasis `HIV` `CC`

B78.1 Cutaneous strongyloidiasis

B78.7 Disseminated strongyloidiasis `HIV` `CC`

B78.9 Strongyloidiasis, unspecified `HIV` `CC`

B79 Trichuriasis `CC`
INCLUDES   trichocephaliasis
         whipworm (disease)(infection)

☑ Additional Character Required   √x7th Placeholder   Questionable PDx   Manifestation   Unspecified   UPD Unacceptable PDx   H1-H14 HAC   HCC CMS-HCC Dx   HIV HIV Dx

B80 Enterobiasis `CC`
> INCLUDES   oxyuriasis
> pinworm infection
> threadworm infection

✓4ᵗʰ B81 Other intestinal helminthiases, not elsewhere classified
> EXCLUDES 1   angiostrongyliasis due to:
>   angiostrongylus cantonensis (B83.2)
>   parastrongylus cantonensis (B83.2)

B81.0 Anisakiasis `CC`
> Infection due to Anisakis larva

B81.1 Intestinal capillariasis `CC`
> Capillariasis NOS
> Infection due to Capillaria philippinensis
> EXCLUDES 2   hepatic capillariasis (B83.8)

B81.2 Trichostrongyliasis `CC`

B81.3 Intestinal angiostrongyliasis `CC`
> Angiostrongyliasis due to:
> Angiostrongylus costaricensis
> Parastrongylus costaricensis

B81.4 Mixed intestinal helminthiases `CC`
> Infection due to intestinal helminths classified to more than one
>   of the categories B65.0-B81.3 and B81.8
> Mixed helminthiasis NOS

B81.8 Other specified intestinal helminthiases `CC`
> Infection due to Oesophagostomum species [esophagostomiasis]
> Infection due to Ternidens diminutus [ternidensiasis]

✓4ᵗʰ B82 Unspecified intestinal parasitism
> **B82.0 Intestinal helminthiasis, unspecified** `CC`
> **B82.9 Intestinal parasitism, unspecified**

✓4ᵗʰ B83 Other helminthiases
> EXCLUDES 1   capillariasis NOS (B81.1)
> EXCLUDES 2   intestinal capillariasis (B81.1)

B83.0 Visceral larva migrans
> Toxocariasis

B83.1 Gnathostomiasis
> Wandering swelling

B83.2 Angiostrongyliasis due to Parastrongylus cantonensis
> Eosinophilic meningoencephalitis due to Parastrongylus
>   cantonensis
> EXCLUDES 2   intestinal angiostrongyliasis (B81.3)

B83.3 Syngamiasis
> Syngamosis

B83.4 Internal hirudiniasis
> EXCLUDES 2   external hirudiniasis (B88.3)

B83.8 Other specified helminthiases
> Acanthocephaliasis
> Gongylonemiasis
> Hepatic capillariasis
> Metastrongyliasis
> Thelaziasis

B83.9 Helminthiasis, unspecified
> Worms NOS
> EXCLUDES 1   intestinal helminthiasis NOS (B82.0)

Pediculosis, acariasis and other infestations (B85-B89)

✓4ᵗʰ B85 Pediculosis and phthiriasis
> **B85.0 Pediculosis due to Pediculus humanus capitis**
> Head-louse infestation

B85.1 Pediculosis due to Pediculus humanus corporis
> Body-louse infestation

B85.2 Pediculosis, unspecified

B85.3 Phthiriasis
> Infestation by crab-louse
> Infestation by Phthirus pubis

B85.4 Mixed pediculosis and phthiriasis
> Infestation classifiable to more than one of the categories
>   B85.0-B85.3

B86 Scabies
> Sarcoptic itch
> DEF: Mite infestation that is caused by Sarcoptes scabiei. Scabies causes
> intense itching and sometimes secondary infection.

✓4ᵗʰ B87 Myiasis
> INCLUDES   infestation by larva of flies
> **B87.0 Cutaneous myiasis**
> Creeping myiasis

B87.1 Wound myiasis
> Traumatic myiasis

B87.2 Ocular myiasis

B87.3 Nasopharyngeal myiasis
> Laryngeal myiasis

B87.4 Aural myiasis

✓5ᵗʰ B87.8 Myiasis of other sites
> **B87.81 Genitourinary myiasis**
> **B87.82 Intestinal myiasis**
> **B87.89 Myiasis of other sites**

B87.9 Myiasis, unspecified

✓4ᵗʰ B88 Other infestations
> **B88.0 Other acariasis**
> Acarine dermatitis
> Dermatitis due to Demodex species
> Dermatitis due to Dermanyssus gallinae
> Dermatitis due to Liponyssoides sanguineus
> Trombiculosis
> EXCLUDES 2   scabies (B86)

B88.1 Tungiasis [sandflea infestation]

B88.2 Other arthropod infestations
> Scarabiasis

B88.3 External hirudiniasis
> Leech infestation NOS
> EXCLUDES 2   internal hirudiniasis (B83.4)

B88.8 Other specified infestations
> Ichthyoparasitism due to Vandellia cirrhosa
> Linguatulosis
> Porocephaliasis

B88.9 Infestation, unspecified
> Infestation (skin) NOS
> Infestation by mites NOS
> Skin parasites NOS

B89 Unspecified parasitic disease

Sequelae of infectious and parasitic diseases (B90-B94)

> NOTE   Categories B90-B94 are to be used to indicate conditions in categories
> A00-B89 as the cause of sequelae, which are themselves classified
> elsewhere. The "sequelae" include conditions specified as such; they
> also include residuals of diseases classifiable to the above categories
> if there is evidence that the disease itself is no longer present. Codes
> from these categories are not to be used for chronic infections. Code
> chronic current infections to active infectious disease as appropriate.

Code first condition resulting from (sequela) the infectious or parasitic disease

✓4ᵗʰ B90 Sequelae of tuberculosis
> **B90.0 Sequelae of central nervous system tuberculosis** `PE`
> **B90.1 Sequelae of genitourinary tuberculosis** `PE`
> **B90.2 Sequelae of tuberculosis of bones and joints** `PE`
> **B90.8 Sequelae of tuberculosis of other organs** `PE`
> EXCLUDES 2   sequelae of respiratory tuberculosis (B90.9)
> **B90.9 Sequelae of respiratory and unspecified tuberculosis** `PE`
> Sequelae of tuberculosis NOS

B91 Sequelae of poliomyelitis `PE`
> EXCLUDES 1   postpolio syndrome (G14)

B92 Sequelae of leprosy `PE`

✓4ᵗʰ B94 Sequelae of other and unspecified infectious and parasitic diseases
> **B94.0 Sequelae of trachoma** `PE`
> **B94.1 Sequelae of viral encephalitis** `PE`
> **B94.2 Sequelae of viral hepatitis** `PE`
> **B94.8 Sequelae of other specified infectious and parasitic diseases** `PE`
> AHA: 2021,1Q,25-30,31-49; 2020,3Q,10-14; 2017,4Q,109
> **B94.9 Sequelae of unspecified infectious and parasitic disease** `PE`
> EXCLUDES 1   post COVID-19 condition (U09.9)

Bacterial and viral infectious agents (B95-B97)

> NOTE   These categories are provided for use as supplementary or additional
> codes to identify the infectious agent(s) in diseases classified
> elsewhere.

AHA: 2020,2Q,18; 2018,4Q,34; 2018,1Q,16

✓4ᵗʰ B95 Streptococcus, Staphylococcus, and Enterococcus as the cause of diseases classified elsewhere
> **B95.0 Streptococcus, group A, as the cause of diseases classified elsewhere** `UPD`

N Newborn: 0   P Pediatric: 0-17   M Maternity: 9-64   A Adult: 15-124   UNS Unspecified Site   MCC Major Complication/Comorbidity   CC Complication/Comorbidity   PE POA Exempt

468   ICD-10-CM 2025

B95.1 **Streptococcus, group B,** as the cause of diseases classified elsewhere `UPD`
    AHA: 2020,1Q,10; 2019,2Q,8-10

B95.2 **Enterococcus** as the cause of diseases classified elsewhere `UPD`

B95.3 **Streptococcus pneumoniae** as the cause of diseases classified elsewhere `UPD`

B95.4 **Other streptococcus** as the cause of diseases classified elsewhere

B95.5 Unspecified streptococcus as the cause of diseases classified elsewhere `UPD`

✓5th **B95.6** **Staphylococcus aureus** as the cause of diseases classified elsewhere

    B95.61 **Methicillin susceptible** Staphylococcus aureus infection as the cause of diseases classified elsewhere `UPD`
        Methicillin susceptible Staphylococcus aureus (MSSA) infection as the cause of diseases classified elsewhere
        Staphylococcus aureus infection NOS as the cause of diseases classified elsewhere

    B95.62 **Methicillin resistant** Staphylococcus aureus infection as the cause of diseases classified elsewhere `UPD`
        Methicillin resistant staphylococcus aureus (MRSA) infection as the cause of diseases classified elsewhere
        AHA: 2016,1Q,12

B95.7 **Other staphylococcus** as the cause of diseases classified elsewhere `UPD`

B95.8 Unspecified staphylococcus as the cause of diseases classified elsewhere `UPD`

✓4th **B96** **Other bacterial agents as the cause of diseases classified elsewhere**

B96.0 **Mycoplasma pneumoniae [M. pneumoniae]** as the cause of diseases classified elsewhere `UPD`
    Pleuro-pneumonia-like-organism [PPLO]

B96.1 **Klebsiella pneumoniae [K. pneumoniae]** as the cause of diseases classified elsewhere `UPD`

✓5th **B96.2** **Escherichia coli [E. coli]** as the cause of diseases classified elsewhere
    AHA: 2022,1Q,31

    B96.20 Unspecified Escherichia coli [E. coli] as the cause of diseases classified elsewhere `UPD`
        Escherichia coli [E. coli] NOS

    B96.21 **Shiga toxin-producing** Escherichia coli [E. coli] [STEC] O157 as the cause of diseases classified elsewhere `UPD`
        E. coli O157:H- (nonmotile) with confirmation of Shiga toxin
        E. coli O157 with confirmation of Shiga toxin when H antigen is unknown, or is not H7
        O157:H7 Escherichia coli [E.coli] with or without confirmation of Shiga toxin-production
        Shiga toxin-producing Escherichia coli [E.coli] O157:H7 with or without confirmation of Shiga toxin-production
        STEC O157:H7 with or without confirmation of Shiga toxin-production

    B96.22 Other specified **Shiga toxin-producing** Escherichia coli [E. coli] [STEC] as the cause of diseases classified elsewhere `UPD`
        Non-O157 Shiga toxin-producing Escherichia coli [E.coli]
        Non-O157 Shiga toxin-producing Escherichia coli [E.coli] with known O group

    B96.23 Unspecified **Shiga toxin-producing** Escherichia coli [E. coli] [STEC] as the cause of diseases classified elsewhere `UPD`
        Shiga toxin-producing Escherichia coli [E. coli] with unspecified O group
        STEC NOS

    B96.29 Other Escherichia coli [E. coli] as the cause of diseases classified elsewhere `UPD`
        Non-Shiga toxin-producing E. coli

B96.3 **Hemophilus influenzae [H. influenzae]** as the cause of diseases classified elsewhere `UPD`

B96.4 **Proteus** (mirabilis) (morganii) as the cause of diseases classified elsewhere `UPD`

B96.5 **Pseudomonas** (aeruginosa) (mallei) (pseudomallei) as the cause of diseases classified elsewhere `UPD`
    AHA: 2015,1Q,18

B96.6 **Bacteroides fragilis [B. fragilis]** as the cause of diseases classified elsewhere `UPD`

B96.7 **Clostridium perfringens [C. perfringens]** as the cause of diseases classified elsewhere `UPD`

✓5th **B96.8** Other specified bacterial agents as the cause of diseases classified elsewhere

    B96.81 **Helicobacter pylori [H. pylori]** as the cause of diseases classified elsewhere `UPD`

    B96.82 **Vibrio vulnificus** as the cause of diseases classified elsewhere `UPD`

    B96.83 **Acinetobacter baumannii** as the cause of diseases classified elsewhere `UPD`
        AHA: 2023,4Q,4

    B96.89 **Other specified** bacterial agents as the cause of diseases classified elsewhere `UPD`

✓4th **B97** **Viral agents as the cause of diseases classified elsewhere**
    AHA: 2016,3Q,8-10,14

B97.0 **Adenovirus** as the cause of diseases classified elsewhere `UPD`

✓5th **B97.1** **Enterovirus** as the cause of diseases classified elsewhere

    B97.10 Unspecified enterovirus as the cause of diseases classified elsewhere `UPD`

    B97.11 **Coxsackievirus** as the cause of diseases classified elsewhere `UPD`

    B97.12 **Echovirus** as the cause of diseases classified elsewhere `UPD`

    B97.19 **Other enterovirus** as the cause of diseases classified elsewhere `UPD`

✓5th **B97.2** **Coronavirus as the cause of diseases classified elsewhere**

    B97.21 **SARS-associated** coronavirus as the cause of diseases classified elsewhere `CC` `UPD`
        EXCLUDES 1   *pneumonia due to SARS-associated coronavirus (J12.81)*

    B97.29 **Other coronavirus** as the cause of diseases classified elsewhere `UPD`
        AHA: 2020,2Q,5; 2020,1Q,34-36

✓5th **B97.3** **Retrovirus as the cause of diseases classified elsewhere**
    EXCLUDES 1   *human immunodeficiency virus [HIV] disease (B20)*

    B97.30 Unspecified retrovirus as the cause of diseases classified elsewhere `UPD`

    B97.31 **Lentivirus** as the cause of diseases classified elsewhere `UPD`

    B97.32 **Oncovirus** as the cause of diseases classified elsewhere `UPD`

    B97.33 **Human T-cell lymphotrophic virus, type I [HTLV-I]** as the cause of diseases classified elsewhere `CC` `UPD`

    B97.34 **Human T-cell lymphotrophic virus, type II [HTLV-II]** as the cause of diseases classified elsewhere `CC` `UPD`

    B97.35 **Human immunodeficiency virus, type 2 [HIV 2]** as the cause of diseases classified elsewhere `CC` `UPD` `HCC`

    B97.39 **Other retrovirus** as the cause of diseases classified elsewhere `UPD`

B97.4 **Respiratory syncytial** virus as the cause of diseases classified elsewhere `UPD`
    RSV as the cause of diseases classified elsewhere
    Code first related disorders, such as:
      otitis media (H65.-)
      upper respiratory infection (J06.9)
    EXCLUDES 1   *acute bronchiolitis due to respiratory syncytial virus (RSV) (J21.0)*
        acute bronchitis due to respiratory syncytial virus (RSV) (J20.5)
        respiratory syncytial virus (RSV) pneumonia (J12.1)

B97.5 **Reovirus** as the cause of diseases classified elsewhere `UPD`

B97.6 **Parvovirus** as the cause of diseases classified elsewhere `UPD`

B97.7 **Papillomavirus** as the cause of diseases classified elsewhere `UPD`

✓5th **B97.8** **Other viral agents as the cause of diseases classified elsewhere**

    B97.81 **Human metapneumovirus** as the cause of diseases classified elsewhere `UPD`

    B97.89 **Other viral agents** as the cause of diseases classified elsewhere `UPD`

Other infectious diseases (B99)

✓4th **B99** **Other and unspecified infectious diseases**

B99.8 Other infectious disease `HIV`

B99.9 Unspecified infectious disease

✔ Additional Character Required   ✓x 7th Placeholder   Questionable PDx   Manifestation   Unspecified   `UPD` Unacceptable PDx   `H1`-`H14` HAC   `HCC` CMS-HCC Dx   `HIV` HIV Dx

Chapter 2. Neoplasms (C00–D49)

Chapter-specific Guidelines with Coding Examples

The chapter-specific guidelines from the ICD-10-CM Official Guidelines for Coding and Reporting have been provided below. Along with these guidelines are coding examples, contained in the shaded boxes, that have been developed to help illustrate the coding and/or sequencing guidance found in these guidelines.

General guidelines

Chapter 2 of the ICD-10-CM contains the codes for most benign and all malignant neoplasms. Certain benign neoplasms, such as prostatic adenomas, may be found in the specific body system chapters. To properly code a neoplasm, it is necessary to determine from the record if the neoplasm is benign, in-situ, malignant, or of uncertain histologic behavior. If malignant, any secondary (metastatic) sites should also be determined.

Primary malignant neoplasms overlapping site boundaries

A primary malignant neoplasm that overlaps two or more contiguous (next to each other) sites should be classified to the subcategory/code .8 ('overlapping lesion'), unless the combination is specifically indexed elsewhere. For multiple neoplasms of the same site that are not contiguous such as tumors in different quadrants of the same breast, codes for each site should be assigned.

> A 73-year-old white female with a large rapidly growing malignant tumor in the left breast extending from the upper outer quadrant into the axillary tail
>
> **C50.812**   **Malignant neoplasm of overlapping sites of left female breast**
>
> *Explanation*: Because this is a single large tumor that overlaps two contiguous sites, a single code for overlapping sites is assigned.

> A 52-year old white female with two distinct lesions of the right breast, one (0.5 cm) in the upper outer quadrant and a second (1.5 cm) in the lower outer quadrant; path report indicates both lesions are malignant
>
> **C50.411**   **Malignant neoplasm of upper-outer quadrant of right female breast**
>
> **C50.511**   **Malignant neoplasm of lower-outer quadrant of right female breast**
>
> *Explanation*: This patient has two distinct malignant lesions of right breast in adjacent quadrants. Because the lesions are not contiguous, two codes are reported.

Malignant neoplasm of ectopic tissue

Malignant neoplasms of ectopic tissue are to be coded to the site of origin mentioned, e.g., ectopic pancreatic malignant neoplasms involving the stomach are coded to malignant neoplasm of pancreas, unspecified (C25.9).

The neoplasm table in the Alphabetic Index should be referenced first. However, if the histological term is documented, that term should be referenced first, rather than going immediately to the Neoplasm Table, in order to determine which column in the Neoplasm Table is appropriate. For example, if the documentation indicates "adenoma," refer to the term in the Alphabetic Index to review the entries under this term and the instructional note to "see also neoplasm, by site, benign." The table provides the proper code based on the type of neoplasm and the site. It is important to select the proper column in the table that corresponds to the type of neoplasm. The Tabular List should then be referenced to verify that the correct code has been selected from the table and that a more specific site code does not exist.

See Section I.C.21. Factors influencing health status and contact with health services, Status, for information regarding Z15.0, codes for genetic susceptibility to cancer.

a. Admission/Encounter for treatment of primary site

If the malignancy is chiefly responsible for occasioning the patient admission/encounter and treatment is directed at the primary site, designate the primary malignancy as the principal/first-listed diagnosis.

The only exception to this guideline is if the administration of chemotherapy, immunotherapy or external beam radiation therapy is chiefly responsible for occasioning the admission/encounter. In that case, assign the appropriate Z51.-- code as the first-listed or principal diagnosis, and the underlying diagnosis or problem for which the service is being performed as a secondary diagnosis.

b. Admission/Encounter for treatment of secondary site

When a patient is admitted because of a primary neoplasm with metastasis and treatment is directed toward the secondary site only, the secondary neoplasm is designated as the principal diagnosis even though the primary malignancy is still present.

> Patient with primary prostate cancer with metastasis to lungs admitted for wedge resection of mass in right lung
>
> **C78.01**   **Secondary malignant neoplasm of right lung**
>
> **C61**   **Malignant neoplasm of prostate**
>
> *Explanation*: Since the admission is for treatment of the lung metastasis, the secondary lung metastasis is sequenced before the primary prostate cancer.

c. Coding and sequencing of complications

Coding and sequencing of complications associated with the malignancies or with the therapy thereof are subject to the following guidelines:

1) Anemia associated with malignancy

When admission/encounter is for management of an anemia associated with the malignancy, and the treatment is only for anemia, the appropriate code for the malignancy is sequenced as the principal or first-listed diagnosis followed by the appropriate code for the anemia (such as code D63.0, Anemia in neoplastic disease).

> Patient is admitted for treatment of anemia in advanced colon cancer
>
> **C18.9**   **Malignant neoplasm of colon, unspecified**
>
> **D63.0**   **Anemia in neoplastic disease**
>
> *Explanation*: Even though the admission was solely to treat the anemia, this guideline indicates that the code for the malignancy is sequenced first.

2) Anemia associated with chemotherapy, immunotherapy and radiation therapy

When the admission/encounter is for management of an anemia associated with an adverse effect of the administration of chemotherapy or immunotherapy and the only treatment is for the anemia, the anemia code is sequenced first followed by the appropriate codes for the neoplasm and the adverse effect (T45.1X5, Adverse effect of antineoplastic and immunosuppressive drugs).

> A 56-year-old Hispanic male with grade II follicular lymphoma involving multiple lymph node sites referred for blood transfusion to treat anemia due to chemotherapy
>
> **D64.81**   **Anemia due to antineoplastic chemotherapy**
>
> **C82.18**   **Follicular lymphoma grade II, lymph nodes of multiple sites**
>
> **T45.1X5A**   **Adverse effect of antineoplastic and immunosuppressive drugs, initial encounter**
>
> *Explanation*: The code for the anemia is sequenced first followed by the code for the malignant neoplasm and lastly the code for the adverse effect.

When the admission/encounter is for management of an anemia associated with an adverse effect of radiotherapy, the anemia code should be sequenced first, followed by the appropriate neoplasm code and code Y84.2, Radiological procedure and radiotherapy as the cause of abnormal reaction of the patient, or of later complication, without mention of misadventure at the time of the procedure.

> A 55-year-old male with a large malignant rectal tumor has been receiving external radiation therapy to shrink the tumor prior to planned surgery. He is admitted today for a blood transfusion to treat anemia related to radiation therapy.
>
> **D64.89**   **Other specified anemias**
>
> **C20**   **Malignant neoplasm of rectum**
>
> **Y84.2**   **Radiological procedure and radiotherapy as the cause of abnormal reaction of the patient, or of later complication, without mention of misadventure at the time of the procedure**
>
> *Explanation*: The code for the anemia is sequenced first, followed by the code for the malignancy, and lastly the code for the abnormal reaction due to radiotherapy.

3) Management of dehydration due to the malignancy

When the admission/encounter is for management of dehydration due to the malignancy and only the dehydration is being treated (intravenous rehydration), the dehydration is sequenced first, followed by the code(s) for the malignancy.

4) Treatment of a complication resulting from a surgical procedure

When the admission/encounter is for treatment of a complication resulting from a surgical procedure, designate the complication as the principal or first-listed diagnosis if treatment is directed at resolving the complication.

d. Primary malignancy previously excised

When a primary malignancy has been previously excised or eradicated from its site and there is no further treatment directed to that site and there is no evidence of any existing primary malignancy at that site, a code from category Z85, Personal history of malignant neoplasm, should be used to indicate the former site of the malignancy. Any mention of extension, invasion, or metastasis to another site is coded as a secondary malignant neoplasm to that site. The secondary site may be the principal or first-listed diagnosis with the Z85 code used as a secondary code.

See section I.C.2.t. Secondary malignant neoplasm of lymphoid tissue.

> History of breast cancer, left radical mastectomy 18 months ago with no current treatment; bronchoscopy with lung biopsy shows metastatic disease in the right lung
>
> **C78.Ø1**   **Secondary malignant neoplasm of right lung**
>
> **Z85.3**   **Personal history of malignant neoplasm of breast**
>
> *Explanation*: The patient has undergone a diagnostic procedure that revealed metastatic breast cancer in the right lung. The code for the secondary (metastatic) site is sequenced first followed by a personal history code to identify the former site of the primary malignancy.

e. Admissions/encounters involving chemotherapy, immunotherapy and radiation therapy

1) Episode of care involves surgical removal of neoplasm

When an episode of care involves the surgical removal of a neoplasm, primary or secondary site, followed by adjunct chemotherapy or radiation treatment during the same episode of care, the code for the neoplasm should be assigned as principal or first-listed diagnosis.

2) Patient admission/encounter chiefly for administration of chemotherapy, immunotherapy and radiation therapy

If a patient admission/encounter is chiefly for the administration of chemotherapy, immunotherapy or external beam radiation therapy assign code Z51.Ø, Encounter for antineoplastic radiation therapy, or Z51.11, Encounter for antineoplastic chemotherapy, or Z51.12, Encounter for antineoplastic immunotherapy as the first-listed or principal diagnosis. If a patient receives more than one of these therapies during the same admission, more than one of these codes may be assigned, in any sequence.

The malignancy for which the therapy is being administered should be assigned as a secondary diagnosis.

If a patient admission/encounter is for the insertion or implantation of radioactive elements (e.g., brachytherapy) the appropriate code for the malignancy is sequenced as the principal or first-listed diagnosis. Code Z51.Ø should not be assigned.

3) Patient admitted for radiation therapy, chemotherapy or immunotherapy and develops complications

When a patient is admitted for the purpose of external beam radiotherapy, immunotherapy or chemotherapy and develops complications such as uncontrolled nausea and vomiting or dehydration, the principal or first-listed diagnosis is Z51.Ø, Encounter for antineoplastic radiation therapy, or Z51.11, Encounter for antineoplastic chemotherapy, or Z51.12, Encounter for antineoplastic immunotherapy followed by any codes for the complications.

When a patient is admitted for the purpose of insertion or implantation of radioactive elements (e.g., brachytherapy) and develops complications such as uncontrolled nausea and vomiting or dehydration, the principal or first-listed diagnosis is the appropriate code for the malignancy followed by any codes for the complications.

> A patient with prostate cancer was admitted for brachytherapy seed implantation and consequently developed urinary retention.
>
> **C61**   **Malignant neoplasm of prostate**
>
> **R33.9**   **Retention of urine, unspecified**
>
> *Explanation*: A code for the malignancy should be listed as the principal diagnosis when insertion of a radioactive element is the reason for admission, even when a complication related to that radioactive element occurs. Codes describing the complications should be listed as secondary codes.

f. Admission/encounter to determine extent of malignancy

When the reason for admission/encounter is to determine the extent of the malignancy, or for a procedure such as paracentesis or thoracentesis, the primary malignancy or appropriate metastatic site is designated as the principal or first-listed diagnosis, even though chemotherapy or radiotherapy is administered.

> Patient with left lung cancer with malignant pleural effusion admitted for paracentesis and initiation/administration of chemotherapy
>
> **C34.92**   **Malignant neoplasm of unspecified part of left bronchus or lung**
>
> **J91.Ø**   **Malignant pleural effusion**
>
> **Z51.11**   **Encounter for antineoplastic chemotherapy**
>
> *Explanation*: The lung cancer is sequenced before the chemotherapy in this instance because the paracentesis for the malignant effusion is also being performed. An instructional note under the malignant effusion instructs that the lung cancer be sequenced first.

g. Symptoms, signs, and abnormal findings listed in Chapter 18 associated with neoplasms

Symptoms, signs, and ill-defined conditions listed in Chapter 18 characteristic of, or associated with, an existing primary or secondary site malignancy cannot be used to replace the malignancy as principal or first-listed diagnosis, regardless of the number of admissions or encounters for treatment and care of the neoplasm.

See Section I.C.21. Factors influencing health status and contact with health services, Encounter for prophylactic organ removal.

h. Admission/encounter for pain control/management

See Section I.C.6. for information on coding admission/encounter for pain control/management.

i. Malignancy in two or more noncontiguous sites

A patient may have more than one malignant tumor in the same organ. These tumors may represent different primaries or metastatic disease, depending on the site. Should the documentation be unclear, the provider should be queried as to the status of each tumor so that the correct codes can be assigned.

j. Disseminated malignant neoplasm, unspecified

Code C80.Ø, Disseminated malignant neoplasm, unspecified, is for use only in those cases where the patient has advanced metastatic disease and no known primary or secondary sites are specified. It should not be used in place of assigning codes for the primary site and all known secondary sites.

> Patient who has had no medical care for many years is seen today and diagnosed with carcinomatosis
>
> **C80.Ø**   **Disseminated malignant neoplasm, unspecified**
>
> *Explanation*: Carcinomatosis NOS is an "includes" note under this code. Should seldom be used but is available for use in cases such as this.

k. Malignant neoplasm without specification of site

Code C80.1, Malignant (primary) neoplasm, unspecified, equates to Cancer, unspecified. This code should only be used when no determination can be made as to the primary site of a malignancy. This code should rarely be used in the inpatient setting.

l. Sequencing of neoplasm codes

1) Encounter for treatment of primary malignancy

If the reason for the encounter is for treatment of a primary malignancy, assign the malignancy as the principal/first-listed diagnosis. The primary site is to be sequenced first, followed by any metastatic sites.

2) Encounter for treatment of secondary malignancy

When an encounter is for a primary malignancy with metastasis and treatment is directed toward the metastatic (secondary) site(s) only, the metastatic site(s) is designated as the principal/first-listed diagnosis. The primary malignancy is coded as an additional code.

> Patient has primary colon cancer with metastasis to rib and is evaluated for possible excision of portion of rib bone
>
> **C79.51**   **Secondary malignant neoplasm of bone**
>
> **C18.9**   **Malignant neoplasm of colon, unspecified**
>
> *Explanation*: The treatment for this encounter is focused on the metastasis to the rib bone rather than the primary colon cancer, thus indicating that the bone metastasis is sequenced as the first-listed code.

3) Malignant neoplasm in a pregnant patient

When a pregnant patient has a malignant neoplasm, a code from subcategory O9A.1-, Malignant neoplasm complicating pregnancy, childbirth, and the puerperium, should be sequenced first, followed by the appropriate code from Chapter 2 to indicate the type of neoplasm.

> A 30-year-old pregnant female in second trimester evaluated for thyroid malignancy
>
> **O9A.112**   **Malignant neoplasm complicating pregnancy, second trimester**
>
> **C73**   **Malignant neoplasm of thyroid gland**
>
> *Explanation*: Codes from chapter 15 describing complications of pregnancy are sequenced as first-listed codes, further specified by codes from other chapters such as neoplastic, unless the pregnancy is documented as incidental to the condition. See also guideline 1.C.15.a.1.

4) Encounter for complication associated with a neoplasm

When an encounter is for management of a complication associated with a neoplasm, such as dehydration, and the treatment is only for the complication, the complication is coded first, followed by the appropriate code(s) for the neoplasm.

The exception to this guideline is anemia. When the admission/encounter is for management of an anemia associated with the malignancy, and the treatment is only for anemia, the appropriate code for the malignancy is sequenced as the principal or first-listed diagnosis followed by code D63.0, Anemia in neoplastic disease.

> Patient with pancreatic cancer is seen for initiation of TPN for cancer-related moderate protein-calorie malnutrition
>
> **E44.0**   **Moderate protein-calorie malnutrition**
>
> **C25.9**   **Malignant neoplasm of pancreas, unspecified**
>
> *Explanation*: The encounter is to initiate treatment for malnutrition, a common complication of many types of neoplasms, and is sequenced first.

5) Complication from surgical procedure for treatment of a neoplasm

When an encounter is for treatment of a complication resulting from a surgical procedure performed for the treatment of the neoplasm, designate the complication as the principal/first-listed diagnosis. See the guideline regarding the coding of a current malignancy versus personal history to determine if the code for the neoplasm should also be assigned

6) Pathologic fracture due to a neoplasm

When an encounter is for a pathological fracture due to a neoplasm, and the focus of treatment is the fracture, a code from subcategory M84.5, Pathological fracture in neoplastic disease, should be sequenced first, followed by the code for the neoplasm.

If the focus of treatment is the neoplasm with an associated pathological fracture, the neoplasm code should be sequenced first, followed by a code from M84.5 for the pathological fracture.

m. Current malignancy versus personal history of malignancy

When a primary malignancy has been excised but further treatment, such as an additional surgery for the malignancy, radiation therapy or chemotherapy is directed to that site, the primary malignancy code should be used until treatment is completed.

> Female patient with ongoing chemotherapy after right mastectomy for breast cancer
>
> **C50.911**   **Malignant neoplasm of unspecified site of right female breast**
>
> **Z90.11**   **Acquired absence of right breast and nipple**
>
> *Explanation*: Even though the breast has been removed, the breast cancer is still being treated with chemotherapy and therefore is still coded as a current condition rather than personal history.

When a primary malignancy has been previously excised or eradicated from its site, there is no further treatment (of the malignancy) directed to that site, and there is no evidence of any existing primary malignancy at that site, a code from category Z85, Personal history of malignant neoplasm, should be used to indicate the former site of the malignancy.

Codes from subcategories Z85.0 – Z85.85 should only be assigned for the former site of a primary malignancy, not the site of a secondary malignancy. Code Z85.89 may be assigned for the former site(s) of either a primary or secondary malignancy.

See Section I.C.21. Factors influencing health status and contact with health services, History (of)

n. Leukemia, multiple myeloma, and malignant plasma cell neoplasms in remission versus personal history

The categories for leukemia, and category C90, Multiple myeloma and malignant plasma cell neoplasms, have codes indicating whether or not the leukemia has achieved remission. There are also codes Z85.6, Personal history of leukemia, and Z85.79, Personal history of other malignant neoplasms of lymphoid, hematopoietic and related tissues. If the documentation is unclear as to whether the leukemia has achieved remission, the provider should be queried.

See Section I.C.21. Factors influencing health status and contact with health services, History (of)

o. Aftercare following surgery for neoplasm

See Section I.C.21. Factors influencing health status and contact with health services, Aftercare

p. Follow-up care for completed treatment of a malignancy

See Section I.C.21. Factors influencing health status and contact with health services, Follow-up

q. Prophylactic organ removal for prevention of malignancy

See Section I.C. 21, Factors influencing health status and contact with health services, Prophylactic organ removal

r. Malignant neoplasm associated with transplanted organ

A malignant neoplasm of a transplanted organ should be coded as a transplant complication. Assign first the appropriate code from category T86.-, Complications of transplanted organs and tissue, followed by code C80.2, Malignant neoplasm associated with transplanted organ. Use an additional code for the specific malignancy.

s. Breast Implant Associated Anaplastic Large Cell Lymphoma

Breast implant associated anaplastic large cell lymphoma (BIA-ALCL) is a type of lymphoma that can develop around breast implants. Assign code C84.7A, Anaplastic large cell lymphoma, ALK-negative, breast, for BIA-ALCL **or C84.7B, Anaplastic large cell lymphoma, ALK-negative, in remission, for BIA-ALCL in remission**. Do not assign a complication code from chapter 19.

t. Secondary malignant neoplasm of lymphoid tissue

When a malignant neoplasm of lymphoid tissue metastasizes beyond the lymph nodes, a code from categories C81-C85 with a final character identifying "extranodal and solid organ sites" **should be assigned** rather than a code for the secondary neoplasm of the affected solid organ. For example, for metastasis of diffuse large B-cell lymphoma to the lung, brain and left adrenal gland, assign code C83.39**8**, Diffuse large B-cell lymphoma **of other** extranodal and solid organ sites.

Chapter 2. Neoplasms (C00-D49)

NOTE

Functional activity

All neoplasms are classified in this chapter, whether they are functionally active or not. An additional code from Chapter 4 may be used, to identify functional activity associated with any neoplasm.

Morphology [Histology]

Chapter 2 classifies neoplasms primarily by site (topography), with broad groupings for behavior, malignant, in situ, benign, etc. The Table of Neoplasms should be used to identify the correct topography code. In a few cases, such as for malignant melanoma and certain neuroendocrine tumors, the morphology (histologic type) is included in the category and codes.

Primary malignant neoplasms overlapping site boundaries

A primary malignant neoplasm that overlaps two or more contiguous (next to each other) sites should be classified to the subcategory/code .8 ("overlapping lesion"), unless the combination is specifically indexed elsewhere. For multiple neoplasms of the same site that are not contiguous, such as tumors in different quadrants of the same breast, codes for each site should be assigned.

Malignant neoplasm of ectopic tissue

Malignant neoplasms of ectopic tissue are to be coded to the site mentioned, e.g., ectopic pancreatic malignant neoplasms are coded to pancreas, unspecified (C25.9).

AHA: 2024,1Q,24; 2023,2Q,6; 2017,4Q,103; 2017,1Q,4,5-6,8

This chapter contains the following blocks:

C00-C14	Malignant neoplasms of lip, oral cavity and pharynx
C15-C26	Malignant neoplasms of digestive organs
C30-C39	Malignant neoplasms of respiratory and intrathoracic organs
C40-C41	Malignant neoplasms of bone and articular cartilage
C43-C44	Melanoma and other malignant neoplasms of skin
C45-C49	Malignant neoplasms of mesothelial and soft tissue
C50	Malignant neoplasms of breast
C51-C58	Malignant neoplasms of female genital organs
C60-C63	Malignant neoplasms of male genital organs
C64-C68	Malignant neoplasms of urinary tract
C69-C72	Malignant neoplasms of eye, brain and other parts of central nervous system
C73-C75	Malignant neoplasms of thyroid and other endocrine glands
C7A	Malignant neuroendocrine tumors
C7B	Secondary neuroendocrine tumors
C76-C80	Malignant neoplasms of ill-defined, other secondary and unspecified sites
C81-C96	Malignant neoplasms of lymphoid, hematopoietic and related tissue
D00-D09	In situ neoplasms
D10-D36	Benign neoplasms, except benign neuroendocrine tumors
D3A	Benign neuroendocrine tumors
D37-D48	Neoplasms of uncertain behavior, polycythemia vera and myelodysplastic syndromes
D49	Neoplasms of unspecified behavior

MALIGNANT NEOPLASMS (C00-C96)

Malignant neoplasms, stated or presumed to be primary (of specified sites), and certain specified histologies, except neuroendocrine, and of lymphoid, hematopoietic and related tissue (C00-C75)

AHA: 2022,1Q,16

Malignant neoplasms of lip, oral cavity and pharynx (C00-C14)

√4th C00 Malignant neoplasm of lip

Use additional code to identify:
alcohol abuse and dependence (F10.-)
history of tobacco dependence (Z87.891)
tobacco dependence (F17.-)
tobacco use (Z72.0)

EXCLUDES 1   malignant melanoma of lip (C43.0)

Merkel cell carcinoma of lip (C4A.0)

other and unspecified malignant neoplasm of skin of lip (C44.0-)

C00.0 Malignant neoplasm of external upper lip
Malignant neoplasm of lipstick area of upper lip
Malignant neoplasm of upper lip NOS
Malignant neoplasm of vermilion border of upper lip

C00.1 Malignant neoplasm of external lower lip
Malignant neoplasm of lower lip NOS
Malignant neoplasm of lipstick area of lower lip
Malignant neoplasm of vermilion border of lower lip

C00.2 Malignant neoplasm of external lip, unspecified
Malignant neoplasm of vermilion border of lip NOS

C00.3 Malignant neoplasm of upper lip, inner aspect
Malignant neoplasm of buccal aspect of upper lip
Malignant neoplasm of frenulum of upper lip
Malignant neoplasm of mucosa of upper lip
Malignant neoplasm of oral aspect of upper lip

C00.4 Malignant neoplasm of lower lip, inner aspect
Malignant neoplasm of buccal aspect of lower lip
Malignant neoplasm of frenulum of lower lip
Malignant neoplasm of mucosa of lower lip
Malignant neoplasm of oral aspect of lower lip

C00.5 Malignant neoplasm of lip, unspecified, inner aspect
Malignant neoplasm of buccal aspect of lip, unspecified
Malignant neoplasm of frenulum of lip, unspecified
Malignant neoplasm of mucosa of lip, unspecified
Malignant neoplasm of oral aspect of lip, unspecified

C00.6 Malignant neoplasm of commissure of lip, unspecified

C00.8 Malignant neoplasm of overlapping sites of lip

C00.9 Malignant neoplasm of lip, unspecified

C01 Malignant neoplasm of base of tongue   HCC
Malignant neoplasm of dorsal surface of base of tongue
Malignant neoplasm of fixed part of tongue NOS
Malignant neoplasm of posterior third of tongue

Use additional code to identify:
alcohol abuse and dependence (F10.-)
history of tobacco dependence (Z87.891)
tobacco dependence (F17.-)
tobacco use (Z72.0)

Malignant Neoplasm of Tongue

Circumvallate papillae — Dorsal surface — Tip of tongue — Base of the tongue — Ventral (underside) surface

√4th C02 Malignant neoplasm of other and unspecified parts of tongue

Use additional code to identify:
alcohol abuse and dependence (F10.-)
history of tobacco dependence (Z87.891)
tobacco dependence (F17.-)
tobacco use (Z72.0)

C02.0 Malignant neoplasm of dorsal surface of tongue   HCC
Malignant neoplasm of anterior two-thirds of tongue, dorsal surface
EXCLUDES 2   malignant neoplasm of dorsal surface of base of tongue (C01)

C02.1 Malignant neoplasm of border of tongue   HCC
Malignant neoplasm of tip of tongue

C02.2 Malignant neoplasm of ventral surface of tongue   HCC
Malignant neoplasm of anterior two-thirds of tongue, ventral surface
Malignant neoplasm of frenulum linguae

C02.3 Malignant neoplasm of anterior two-thirds of tongue, part unspecified   HCC
Malignant neoplasm of middle third of tongue NOS
Malignant neoplasm of mobile part of tongue NOS

C02.4 Malignant neoplasm of lingual tonsil   HCC
EXCLUDES 2   malignant neoplasm of tonsil NOS (C09.9)

C02.8 Malignant neoplasm of overlapping sites of tongue   HCC
Malignant neoplasm of two or more contiguous sites of tongue

C02.9 Malignant neoplasm of tongue, unspecified   HCC

N Newborn: 0   P Pediatric: 0-17   M Maternity: 9-64   A Adult: 15-124   UNS Unspecified Site   MCC Major Complication/Comorbidity   CC Complication/Comorbidity   PE POA Exempt

474   ICD-10-CM 2025

Chapter 2. Neoplasms

✓4ᵗʰ C03 Malignant neoplasm of gum

> **INCLUDES**   malignant neoplasm of alveolar (ridge) mucosa
> malignant neoplasm of gingiva

Use additional code to identify:
alcohol abuse and dependence (F10.-)
history of tobacco dependence (Z87.891)
tobacco dependence (F17.-)
tobacco use (Z72.0)

> **EXCLUDES 2**   *malignant odontogenic neoplasms (C41.0-C41.1)*

C03.0   Malignant neoplasm of upper gum   `HCC`
C03.1   Malignant neoplasm of lower gum   `HCC`
C03.9   Malignant neoplasm of gum, unspecified   `HCC`

✓4ᵗʰ C04 Malignant neoplasm of floor of mouth

Use additional code to identify:
alcohol abuse and dependence (F10.-)
history of tobacco dependence (Z87.891)
tobacco dependence (F17.-)
tobacco use (Z72.0)

C04.0   Malignant neoplasm of anterior floor of mouth   `HCC`
     Malignant neoplasm of anterior to the premolar-canine junction
C04.1   Malignant neoplasm of lateral floor of mouth   `HCC`
C04.8   Malignant neoplasm of overlapping sites of floor of mouth   `HCC`
C04.9   Malignant neoplasm of floor of mouth, unspecified   `HCC`

✓4ᵗʰ C05 Malignant neoplasm of palate

Use additional code to identify:
alcohol abuse and dependence (F10.-)
history of tobacco dependence (Z87.891)
tobacco dependence (F17.-)
tobacco use (Z72.0)

> **EXCLUDES 1**   *Kaposi's sarcoma of palate (C46.2)*

C05.0   Malignant neoplasm of hard palate   `HCC`
C05.1   Malignant neoplasm of soft palate   `HCC`
> **EXCLUDES 2**   *malignant neoplasm of nasopharyngeal surface of soft palate (C11.3)*

C05.2   Malignant neoplasm of uvula   `HCC`
C05.8   Malignant neoplasm of overlapping sites of palate   `HCC`
C05.9   Malignant neoplasm of palate, unspecified   `HCC`
     Malignant neoplasm of roof of mouth

✓4ᵗʰ C06 Malignant neoplasm of other and unspecified parts of mouth

Use additional code to identify:
alcohol abuse and dependence (F10.-)
history of tobacco dependence (Z87.891)
tobacco dependence (F17.-)
tobacco use (Z72.0)

C06.0   Malignant neoplasm of cheek mucosa   `HCC`
     Malignant neoplasm of buccal mucosa NOS
     Malignant neoplasm of internal cheek
C06.1   Malignant neoplasm of vestibule of mouth   `HCC`
     Malignant neoplasm of buccal sulcus (upper) (lower)
     Malignant neoplasm of labial sulcus (upper) (lower)
C06.2   Malignant neoplasm of retromolar area   `HCC`
✓5ᵗʰ C06.8   Malignant neoplasm of overlapping sites of other and unspecified parts of mouth
     C06.80   Malignant neoplasm of overlapping sites of unspecified parts of mouth   `HCC`
     C06.89   Malignant neoplasm of overlapping sites of other parts of mouth   `HCC`
         "book leaf" neoplasm [ventral surface of tongue and floor of mouth]
C06.9   Malignant neoplasm of mouth, unspecified   `HCC`
     Malignant neoplasm of minor salivary gland, unspecified site
     Malignant neoplasm of oral cavity NOS

C07 Malignant neoplasm of parotid gland   `HCC`

Use additional code to identify:
alcohol abuse and dependence (F10.-)
exposure to environmental tobacco smoke (Z77.22)
exposure to tobacco smoke in the perinatal period (P96.81)
history of tobacco dependence (Z87.891)
occupational exposure to environmental tobacco smoke (Z57.31)
tobacco dependence (F17.-)
tobacco use (Z72.0)

✓4ᵗʰ C08 Malignant neoplasm of other and unspecified major salivary glands

> **INCLUDES**   malignant neoplasm of salivary ducts

Use additional code to identify:
alcohol abuse and dependence (F10.-)
exposure to environmental tobacco smoke (Z77.22)
exposure to tobacco smoke in the perinatal period (P96.81)
history of tobacco dependence (Z87.891)
occupational exposure to environmental tobacco smoke (Z57.31)
tobacco dependence (F17.-)
tobacco use (Z72.0)

> **EXCLUDES 1**   *malignant neoplasms of specified minor salivary glands which are classified according to their anatomical location*
> **EXCLUDES 2**   *malignant neoplasms of minor salivary glands NOS (C06.9)*
> *malignant neoplasm of parotid gland (C07)*

C08.0   Malignant neoplasm of submandibular gland   `HCC`
     Malignant neoplasm of submaxillary gland
C08.1   Malignant neoplasm of sublingual gland   `HCC`
C08.9   Malignant neoplasm of major salivary gland, unspecified   `HCC`
     Malignant neoplasm of salivary gland (major) NOS

✓4ᵗʰ C09 Malignant neoplasm of tonsil

Use additional code to identify:
alcohol abuse and dependence (F10.-)
exposure to environmental tobacco smoke (Z77.22)
exposure to tobacco smoke in the perinatal period (P96.81)
history of tobacco dependence (Z87.891)
occupational exposure to environmental tobacco smoke (Z57.31)
tobacco dependence (F17.-)
tobacco use (Z72.0)

> **EXCLUDES 2**   *malignant neoplasm of lingual tonsil (C02.4)*
> *malignant neoplasm of pharyngeal tonsil (C11.1)*

C09.0   Malignant neoplasm of tonsillar fossa   `HCC`
C09.1   Malignant neoplasm of tonsillar pillar (anterior) (posterior)   `HCC`
C09.8   Malignant neoplasm of overlapping sites of tonsil   `HCC`
C09.9   Malignant neoplasm of tonsil, unspecified   `HCC`
     Malignant neoplasm of faucial tonsils
     Malignant neoplasm of palatine tonsils
     Malignant neoplasm of tonsil NOS

✓4ᵗʰ C10 Malignant neoplasm of oropharynx

Use additional code to identify:
alcohol abuse and dependence (F10.-)
exposure to environmental tobacco smoke (Z77.22)
exposure to tobacco smoke in the perinatal period (P96.81)
history of tobacco dependence (Z87.891)
occupational exposure to environmental tobacco smoke (Z57.31)
tobacco dependence (F17.-)
tobacco use (Z72.0)

> **EXCLUDES 2**   *malignant neoplasm of tonsil (C09.-)*

DEF: Oropharynx: Middle portion of pharynx (throat); communicates with the oral cavity, nasopharynx and laryngopharynx.

C10.0   Malignant neoplasm of vallecula   `HCC`
C10.1   Malignant neoplasm of anterior surface of epiglottis   `HCC`
     Malignant neoplasm of epiglottis, free border [margin]
     Malignant neoplasm of glossoepiglottic fold(s)
> **EXCLUDES 2**   *malignant neoplasm of epiglottis (suprahyoid portion) NOS (C32.1)*

C10.2   Malignant neoplasm of lateral wall of oropharynx   `HCC`
C10.3   Malignant neoplasm of posterior wall of oropharynx   `HCC`
C10.4   Malignant neoplasm of branchial cleft   `HCC`
     Malignant neoplasm of branchial cyst [site of neoplasm]
C10.8   Malignant neoplasm of overlapping sites of oropharynx   `HCC`
     Malignant neoplasm of junctional region of oropharynx
C10.9   Malignant neoplasm of oropharynx, unspecified   `HCC`

✅ Additional Character Required   ✓x7ᵗʰ Placeholder   Questionable PDx   Manifestation   Unspecified   UPD Unacceptable PDx   H1-H14 HAC   HCC CMS-HCC Dx   HIV HIV Dx

ICD-10-CM 2025   475

C11 **Malignant neoplasm of nasopharynx**

Use additional code to identify:

exposure to environmental tobacco smoke (Z77.22)

exposure to tobacco smoke in the perinatal period (P96.81)

history of tobacco dependence (Z87.891)

occupational exposure to environmental tobacco smoke (Z57.31)

tobacco dependence (F17.-)

tobacco use (Z72.0)

DEF: Nasopharynx: Upper portion of pharynx (throat); communicates with the nasal cavities, oropharynx and tympanic cavities.

C11.0 **Malignant neoplasm of superior wall of nasopharynx** HCC

Malignant neoplasm of roof of nasopharynx

C11.1 **Malignant neoplasm of posterior wall of nasopharynx** HCC

Malignant neoplasm of adenoid

Malignant neoplasm of pharyngeal tonsil

C11.2 **Malignant neoplasm of lateral wall of nasopharynx** HCC

Malignant neoplasm of fossa of Rosenmuller

Malignant neoplasm of opening of auditory tube

Malignant neoplasm of pharyngeal recess

C11.3 **Malignant neoplasm of anterior wall of nasopharynx** HCC

Malignant neoplasm of floor of nasopharynx

Malignant neoplasm of nasopharyngeal (anterior) (posterior) surface of soft palate

Malignant neoplasm of posterior margin of nasal choana

Malignant neoplasm of posterior margin of nasal septum

C11.8 **Malignant neoplasm of overlapping sites of nasopharynx** HCC

C11.9 **Malignant neoplasm of nasopharynx, unspecified** HCC

Malignant neoplasm of nasopharyngeal wall NOS

C12 **Malignant neoplasm of pyriform sinus** HCC

Malignant neoplasm of pyriform fossa

Use additional code to identify:

exposure to environmental tobacco smoke (Z77.22)

exposure to tobacco smoke in the perinatal period (P96.81)

history of tobacco dependence (Z87.891)

occupational exposure to environmental tobacco smoke (Z57.31)

tobacco dependence (F17.-)

tobacco use (Z72.0)

C13 **Malignant neoplasm of hypopharynx**

Use additional code to identify:

exposure to environmental tobacco smoke (Z77.22)

exposure to tobacco smoke in the perinatal period (P96.81)

history of tobacco dependence (Z87.891)

occupational exposure to environmental tobacco smoke (Z57.31)

tobacco dependence (F17.-)

tobacco use (Z72.0)

EXCLUDES 2 *malignant neoplasm of pyriform sinus (C12)*

DEF: Hypopharynx: Lower portion of pharynx (throat); communicates with the oropharynx and the esophagus. *Synonym(s): laryngopharynx.*

C13.0 **Malignant neoplasm of postcricoid region** HCC

C13.1 **Malignant neoplasm of aryepiglottic fold, hypopharyngeal aspect** HCC

Malignant neoplasm of aryepiglottic fold, marginal zone

Malignant neoplasm of aryepiglottic fold NOS

Malignant neoplasm of interarytenoid fold, marginal zone

Malignant neoplasm of interarytenoid fold NOS

EXCLUDES 2 *malignant neoplasm of aryepiglottic fold or interarytenoid fold, laryngeal aspect (C32.1)*

C13.2 **Malignant neoplasm of posterior wall of hypopharynx** HCC

C13.8 **Malignant neoplasm of overlapping sites of hypopharynx** HCC

C13.9 **Malignant neoplasm of hypopharynx, unspecified** HCC

Malignant neoplasm of hypopharyngeal wall NOS

C14 **Malignant neoplasm of other and ill-defined sites in the lip, oral cavity and pharynx**

Use additional code to identify:

alcohol abuse and dependence (F10.-)

exposure to environmental tobacco smoke (Z77.22)

exposure to tobacco smoke in the perinatal period (P96.81)

history of tobacco dependence (Z87.891)

occupational exposure to environmental tobacco smoke (Z57.31)

tobacco dependence (F17.-)

tobacco use (Z72.0)

EXCLUDES 1 *malignant neoplasm of oral cavity NOS (C06.9)*

C14.0 **Malignant neoplasm of pharynx, unspecified** HCC

C14.2 **Malignant neoplasm of Waldeyer's ring** HCC

DEF: Waldeyer's ring: Ring of lymphoid tissue that is made up of the two palatine tonsils, the pharyngeal tonsil (adenoid), and the lingual tonsil. It functions as the defense against infection and assists with the development of the immune system.

C14.8 **Malignant neoplasm of overlapping sites of lip, oral cavity and pharynx** HCC

Primary malignant neoplasm of two or more contiguous sites of lip, oral cavity and pharynx

EXCLUDES 1 *"book leaf" neoplasm [ventral surface of tongue and floor of mouth] (C06.89)*

Malignant neoplasms of digestive organs (C15-C26)

EXCLUDES 1 *Kaposi's sarcoma of gastrointestinal sites (C46.4)*

EXCLUDES 2 *gastrointestinal stromal tumors (C49.A-)*

C15 **Malignant neoplasm of esophagus**

Use additional code to identify:

alcohol abuse and dependence (F10.-)

AHA: 2022,3Q,10

C15.3 **Malignant neoplasm of upper third of esophagus** CC HCC

C15.4 **Malignant neoplasm of middle third of esophagus** CC HCC

C15.5 **Malignant neoplasm of lower third of esophagus** CC HCC

EXCLUDES 1 *malignant neoplasm of cardio-esophageal junction (C16.0)*

C15.8 **Malignant neoplasm of overlapping sites of esophagus** CC HCC

C15.9 **Malignant neoplasm of esophagus, unspecified** CC HCC

C16 **Malignant neoplasm of stomach**

Use additional code to identify:

alcohol abuse and dependence (F10.-)

EXCLUDES 2 *malignant carcinoid tumor of the stomach (C7A.092)*

C16.0 **Malignant neoplasm of cardia** CC HCC

Malignant neoplasm of cardiac orifice

Malignant neoplasm of cardio-esophageal junction

Malignant neoplasm of esophagus and stomach

Malignant neoplasm of gastro-esophageal junction

C16.1 **Malignant neoplasm of fundus of stomach** CC HCC

C16.2 **Malignant neoplasm of body of stomach** CC HCC

C16.3 **Malignant neoplasm of pyloric antrum** CC HCC

Malignant neoplasm of gastric antrum

C16.4 **Malignant neoplasm of pylorus** CC HCC

Malignant neoplasm of prepylorus

Malignant neoplasm of pyloric canal

C16.5 **Malignant neoplasm of lesser curvature of stomach, unspecified** CC HCC

Malignant neoplasm of lesser curvature of stomach, not classifiable to C16.1-C16.4

C16.6 **Malignant neoplasm of greater curvature of stomach, unspecified** CC HCC

Malignant neoplasm of greater curvature of stomach, not classifiable to C16.0-C16.4

C16.8 **Malignant neoplasm of overlapping sites of stomach** CC HCC

C16.9 **Malignant neoplasm of stomach, unspecified** CC HCC

Gastric cancer NOS

C17 **Malignant neoplasm of small intestine**

EXCLUDES 1 *malignant carcinoid tumors of the small intestine (C7A.01)*

AHA: 2016,1Q,19

C17.0 **Malignant neoplasm of duodenum** CC HCC

C17.1 **Malignant neoplasm of jejunum** CC HCC

C17.2 **Malignant neoplasm of ileum** CC HCC

EXCLUDES 1 *malignant neoplasm of ileocecal valve (C18.0)*

C17.3 **Meckel's diverticulum, malignant** CC HCC

EXCLUDES 1 *Meckel's diverticulum, congenital (Q43.0)*

DEF: Congenital, abnormal remnant of embryonic digestive system development that leaves a sacculation or outpouching from the wall of the small intestine near the terminal part of the ileum made of acid-secreting tissue as in the stomach.

C17.8 **Malignant neoplasm of overlapping sites of small intestine** CC HCC

C17.9 **Malignant neoplasm of small intestine, unspecified** CC HCC

N Newborn: 0   P Pediatric: 0-17   M Maternity: 9-64   A Adult: 15-124   UNS Unspecified Site   MCC Major Complication/Comorbidity   CC Complication/Comorbidity   PE POA Exempt

476   ICD-10-CM 2025

✓4th C18 Malignant neoplasm of colon

> EXCLUDES 1   *malignant carcinoid tumors of the colon (C7A.Ø2-)*

Colon

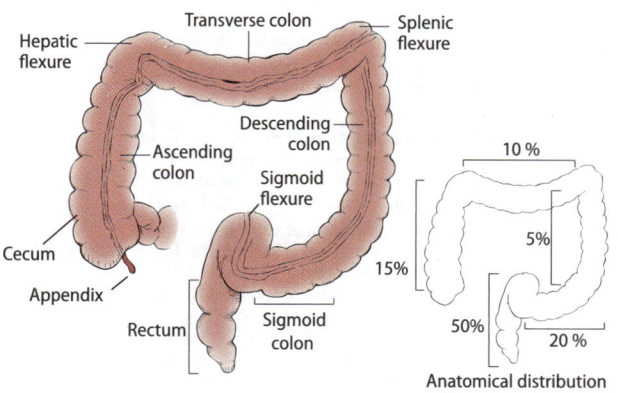

Anatomical distribution of large bowel cancers

C18.Ø Malignant neoplasm of cecum   CC HCC
Malignant neoplasm of ileocecal valve

C18.1 Malignant neoplasm of appendix   CC HCC

C18.2 Malignant neoplasm of ascending colon   CC HCC

C18.3 Malignant neoplasm of hepatic flexure   CC HCC

C18.4 Malignant neoplasm of transverse colon   CC HCC

C18.5 Malignant neoplasm of splenic flexure   CC HCC

C18.6 Malignant neoplasm of descending colon   CC HCC

C18.7 Malignant neoplasm of sigmoid colon   CC HCC
Malignant neoplasm of sigmoid (flexure)
> EXCLUDES 1   *malignant neoplasm of rectosigmoid junction (C19)*

C18.8 Malignant neoplasm of overlapping sites of colon   CC HCC

C18.9 Malignant neoplasm of colon, unspecified   CC HCC
Malignant neoplasm of large intestine NOS

C19 Malignant neoplasm of rectosigmoid junction   CC HCC
Malignant neoplasm of colon with rectum
Malignant neoplasm of rectosigmoid (colon)
> EXCLUDES 1   *malignant carcinoid tumors of the colon (C7A.Ø2-)*

C2Ø Malignant neoplasm of rectum   CC HCC
Malignant neoplasm of rectal ampulla
> EXCLUDES 1   *malignant carcinoid tumor of the rectum (C7A.Ø26)*

✓4th C21 Malignant neoplasm of anus and anal canal
> EXCLUDES 2   *malignant carcinoid tumors of the colon (C7A.Ø2-)*
> *malignant melanoma of anal margin (C43.51)*
> *malignant melanoma of anal skin (C43.51)*
> *malignant melanoma of perianal skin (C43.51)*
> *other and unspecified malignant neoplasm of anal margin (C44.5ØØ, C44.51Ø, C44.52Ø, C44.59Ø)*
> *other and unspecified malignant neoplasm of anal skin (C44.5ØØ, C44.51Ø, C44.52Ø, C44.59Ø)*
> *other and unspecified malignant neoplasm of perianal skin (C44.5ØØ, C44.51Ø, C44.52Ø, C44.59Ø)*

C21.Ø Malignant neoplasm of anus, unspecified   CC HCC

C21.1 Malignant neoplasm of anal canal   CC HCC
Malignant neoplasm of anal sphincter

C21.2 Malignant neoplasm of cloacogenic zone   CC HCC

C21.8 Malignant neoplasm of overlapping sites of rectum, anus and anal canal   CC HCC
Malignant neoplasm of anorectal junction
Malignant neoplasm of anorectum
Primary malignant neoplasm of two or more contiguous sites of rectum, anus and anal canal

✓4th C22 Malignant neoplasm of liver and intrahepatic bile ducts
> EXCLUDES 1   *malignant neoplasm of biliary tract NOS (C24.9)*
> *secondary malignant neoplasm of liver and intrahepatic bile duct (C78.7)*

Use additional code to identify:
   alcohol abuse and dependence (F1Ø.-)
   hepatitis B (B16.-, B18.Ø-B18.1)
   hepatitis C (B17.1-, B18.2)

C22.Ø Liver cell carcinoma   CC HCC
Hepatocellular carcinoma
Hepatoma
AHA: 2016,1Q,18

C22.1 Intrahepatic bile duct carcinoma   CC HCC
Cholangiocarcinoma
> EXCLUDES 1   *malignant neoplasm of hepatic duct (C24.Ø)*
AHA: 2023,1Q,24

C22.2 Hepatoblastoma   CC HCC

C22.3 Angiosarcoma of liver   CC HCC
Kupffer cell sarcoma

C22.4 Other sarcomas of liver   CC HCC

C22.7 Other specified carcinomas of liver   CC HCC

C22.8 Malignant neoplasm of liver, primary, unspecified as to type   CC HCC

C22.9 Malignant neoplasm of liver, not specified as primary or secondary   CC HCC

C23 Malignant neoplasm of gallbladder   CC HCC

✓4th C24 Malignant neoplasm of other and unspecified parts of biliary tract
> EXCLUDES 1   *malignant neoplasm of intrahepatic bile duct (C22.1)*

C24.Ø Malignant neoplasm of extrahepatic bile duct   CC HCC
Malignant neoplasm of biliary duct or passage NOS
Malignant neoplasm of common bile duct
Malignant neoplasm of cystic duct
Malignant neoplasm of hepatic duct

C24.1 Malignant neoplasm of ampulla of Vater   CC HCC
DEF: Malignant neoplasm in the area of dilation at the juncture of the common bile and pancreatic ducts near the opening into the lumen of the duodenum.

C24.8 Malignant neoplasm of overlapping sites of biliary tract   CC HCC
Malignant neoplasm involving both intrahepatic and extrahepatic bile ducts
Primary malignant neoplasm of two or more contiguous sites of biliary tract

C24.9 Malignant neoplasm of biliary tract, unspecified   CC HCC

✓4th C25 Malignant neoplasm of pancreas

Code also if applicable exocrine pancreatic insufficiency (K86.81)
Use additional code to identify:
   alcohol abuse and dependence (F1Ø.-)

Pancreas

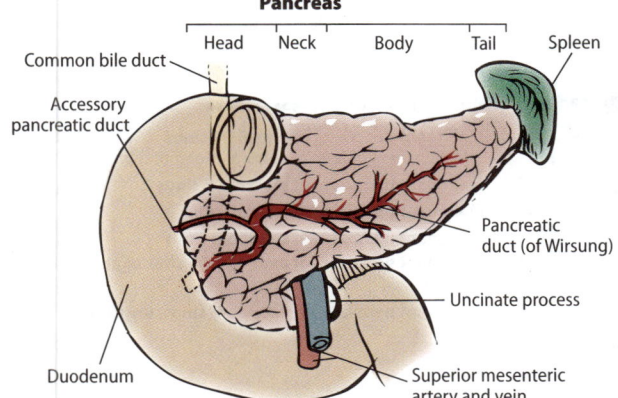

C25.Ø Malignant neoplasm of head of pancreas   CC HCC

C25.1 Malignant neoplasm of body of pancreas   CC HCC

C25.2 Malignant neoplasm of tail of pancreas   CC HCC

C25.3 Malignant neoplasm of pancreatic duct   CC HCC

C25.4 Malignant neoplasm of endocrine pancreas   CC HCC
Malignant neoplasm of islets of Langerhans
Use additional code to identify any functional activity

✓ Additional Character Required   ✓x7th Placeholder   Questionable PDx   Manifestation   Unspecified   UPD Unacceptable PDx   H1-H14 HAC   HCC CMS-HCC Dx   HIV HIV Dx

ICD-10-CM 2025   477

C25.7 **Malignant neoplasm of other parts of pancreas** `CC` `HCC`
Malignant neoplasm of neck of pancreas

C25.8 **Malignant neoplasm of overlapping sites of pancreas** `CC` `HCC`

C25.9 **Malignant neoplasm of pancreas, unspecified** `CC` `HCC`

✓4ᵗʰ **C26** **Malignant neoplasm of other and ill-defined digestive organs**
EXCLUDES 1   *malignant neoplasm of peritoneum and retroperitoneum (C48.-)*

C26.0 **Malignant neoplasm of intestinal tract, part unspecified** `HCC`
Malignant neoplasm of intestine NOS

C26.1 **Malignant neoplasm of spleen** `HCC`
EXCLUDES 1   *Hodgkin lymphoma (C81.-)*
non-Hodgkin lymphoma (C82-C85)

C26.9 **Malignant neoplasm of ill-defined sites within the digestive system** `HCC`
Malignant neoplasm of alimentary canal or tract NOS
Malignant neoplasm of gastrointestinal tract NOS
EXCLUDES 1   *malignant neoplasm of abdominal NOS (C76.2)*
malignant neoplasm of intra-abdominal NOS (C76.2)

Malignant neoplasms of respiratory and intrathoracic organs (C30-C39)

INCLUDES   malignant neoplasm of middle ear
EXCLUDES 1   mesothelioma (C45.-)

✓4ᵗʰ **C30** **Malignant neoplasm of nasal cavity and middle ear**

C30.0 **Malignant neoplasm of nasal cavity** `HCC`
Malignant neoplasm of cartilage of nose
Malignant neoplasm of nasal concha
Malignant neoplasm of internal nose
Malignant neoplasm of septum of nose
Malignant neoplasm of vestibule of nose
EXCLUDES 1   *malignant neoplasm of nasal bone (C41.0)*
malignant neoplasm of nose NOS (C76.0)
malignant neoplasm of olfactory bulb (C72.2)
malignant neoplasm of posterior margin of nasal septum and choana (C11.3)
malignant melanoma of skin of nose (C43.31)
malignant neoplasm of turbinates (C41.0)
other and unspecified malignant neoplasm of skin of nose (C44.301, C44.311, C44.321, C44.391)

C30.1 **Malignant neoplasm of middle ear** `HCC`
Malignant neoplasm of antrum tympanicum
Malignant neoplasm of auditory tube
Malignant neoplasm of eustachian tube
Malignant neoplasm of inner ear
Malignant neoplasm of mastoid air cells
Malignant neoplasm of tympanic cavity
EXCLUDES 1   *malignant neoplasm of auricular canal (external) (C43.2-,C44.2-)*
malignant neoplasm of bone of ear (meatus) (C41.0)
malignant neoplasm of cartilage of ear (C49.0)
malignant melanoma of skin of (external) ear (C43.2-)
other and unspecified malignant neoplasm of skin of (external) ear (C44.2-)

✓4ᵗʰ **C31** **Malignant neoplasm of accessory sinuses**

C31.0 **Malignant neoplasm of maxillary sinus** `HCC`
Malignant neoplasm of antrum (Highmore) (maxillary)

C31.1 **Malignant neoplasm of ethmoidal sinus** `HCC`

C31.2 **Malignant neoplasm of frontal sinus** `HCC`

C31.3 **Malignant neoplasm of sphenoid sinus** `HCC`

C31.8 **Malignant neoplasm of overlapping sites of accessory sinuses** `HCC`

C31.9 **Malignant neoplasm of accessory sinus, unspecified** `HCC`

✓4ᵗʰ **C32** **Malignant neoplasm of larynx**
Use additional code to identify:
   alcohol abuse and dependence (F10.-)
   exposure to environmental tobacco smoke (Z77.22)
   exposure to tobacco smoke in the perinatal period (P96.81)
   history of tobacco dependence (Z87.891)
   occupational exposure to environmental tobacco smoke (Z57.31)
   tobacco dependence (F17.-)
   tobacco use (Z72.0)

C32.0 **Malignant neoplasm of glottis** `HCC`
Malignant neoplasm of intrinsic larynx
Malignant neoplasm of laryngeal commissure (anterior)(posterior)
Malignant neoplasm of vocal cord (true) NOS

C32.1 **Malignant neoplasm of supraglottis** `HCC`
Malignant neoplasm of aryepiglottic fold or interarytenoid fold, laryngeal aspect
Malignant neoplasm of epiglottis (suprahyoid portion) NOS
Malignant neoplasm of extrinsic larynx
Malignant neoplasm of false vocal cord
Malignant neoplasm of posterior (laryngeal) surface of epiglottis
Malignant neoplasm of ventricular bands
EXCLUDES 2   *malignant neoplasm of anterior surface of epiglottis (C10.1)*
malignant neoplasm of aryepiglottic fold or interarytenoid fold, hypopharyngeal aspect (C13.1)
malignant neoplasm of aryepiglottic fold or interarytenoid fold, marginal zone (C13.1)
malignant neoplasm of aryepiglottic fold or interarytenoid fold NOS (C13.1)

C32.2 **Malignant neoplasm of subglottis** `HCC`

C32.3 **Malignant neoplasm of laryngeal cartilage** `HCC`

C32.8 **Malignant neoplasm of overlapping sites of larynx** `HCC`

C32.9 **Malignant neoplasm of larynx, unspecified** `HCC`

C33 **Malignant neoplasm of trachea** `CC` `HCC`
Use additional code to identify:
   exposure to environmental tobacco smoke (Z77.22)
   exposure to tobacco smoke in the perinatal period (P96.81)
   history of tobacco dependence (Z87.891)
   occupational exposure to environmental tobacco smoke (Z57.31)
   tobacco dependence (F17.-)
   tobacco use (Z72.0)

✓4ᵗʰ **C34** **Malignant neoplasm of bronchus and lung**
Use additional code to identify:
   exposure to environmental tobacco smoke (Z77.22)
   exposure to tobacco smoke in the perinatal period (P96.81)
   history of tobacco dependence (Z87.891)
   occupational exposure to environmental tobacco smoke (Z57.31)
   tobacco dependence (F17.-)
   tobacco use (Z72.0)
EXCLUDES 1   *Kaposi's sarcoma of lung (C46.5-)*
malignant carcinoid tumor of the bronchus and lung (C7A.090)
AHA: 2023,1Q,20-21; 2022,4Q,22; 2019,1Q,16
TIP: When documented, assign code I31.31 for associated malignant pericardial effusion. The neoplasm code should be sequenced first.

✓5ᵗʰ **C34.0** **Malignant neoplasm of main bronchus**
Malignant neoplasm of carina
Malignant neoplasm of hilus (of lung)

C34.00 **Malignant neoplasm of unspecified main bronchus** `CC` `HCC`

C34.01 **Malignant neoplasm of right main bronchus** `CC` `HCC`

C34.02 **Malignant neoplasm of left main bronchus** `CC` `HCC`

✓5ᵗʰ **C34.1** **Malignant neoplasm of upper lobe, bronchus or lung**

C34.10 **Malignant neoplasm of upper lobe, unspecified bronchus or lung** `CC` `HCC`

C34.11 **Malignant neoplasm of upper lobe, right bronchus or lung** `CC` `HCC`

C34.12 **Malignant neoplasm of upper lobe, left bronchus or lung** `CC` `HCC`

C34.2 **Malignant neoplasm of middle lobe, bronchus or lung** `CC` `HCC`

✓5ᵗʰ **C34.3** **Malignant neoplasm of lower lobe, bronchus or lung**

C34.30 **Malignant neoplasm of lower lobe, unspecified bronchus or lung** `CC` `HCC`

C34.31 Malignant neoplasm of lower lobe, right bronchus or lung `CC` `HCC`

C34.32 Malignant neoplasm of lower lobe, left bronchus or lung `CC` `HCC`

✓5th **C34.8** Malignant neoplasm of overlapping sites of bronchus and lung

   C34.80 Malignant neoplasm of overlapping sites of unspecified bronchus and lung `CC` `HCC`

   C34.81 Malignant neoplasm of overlapping sites of right bronchus and lung `CC` `HCC`

   C34.82 Malignant neoplasm of overlapping sites of left bronchus and lung `CC` `HCC`

✓5th **C34.9** Malignant neoplasm of unspecified part of bronchus or lung

   C34.90 Malignant neoplasm of unspecified part of unspecified bronchus or lung `CC` `HCC`
      Lung cancer NOS

   C34.91 Malignant neoplasm of unspecified part of right bronchus or lung `CC` `HCC`

   C34.92 Malignant neoplasm of unspecified part of left bronchus or lung `CC` `HCC`

C37 Malignant neoplasm of thymus `CC` `HCC`
   EXCLUDES 1 malignant carcinoid tumor of the thymus (C7A.091)

✓4th **C38** Malignant neoplasm of heart, mediastinum and pleura
   EXCLUDES 1 mesothelioma (C45.-)

   C38.0 Malignant neoplasm of heart `CC` `HCC`
      Malignant neoplasm of pericardium
      EXCLUDES 1 malignant neoplasm of great vessels (C49.3)

   C38.1 Malignant neoplasm of anterior mediastinum `CC` `HCC`

   C38.2 Malignant neoplasm of posterior mediastinum `CC` `HCC`

   C38.3 Malignant neoplasm of mediastinum, part unspecified `CC` `HCC`

   C38.4 Malignant neoplasm of pleura `CC` `HCC`

   C38.8 Malignant neoplasm of overlapping sites of heart, mediastinum and pleura `CC` `HCC`

✓4th **C39** Malignant neoplasm of other and ill-defined sites in the respiratory system and intrathoracic organs
   Use additional code to identify:
     exposure to environmental tobacco smoke (Z77.22)
     exposure to tobacco smoke in the perinatal period (P96.81)
     history of tobacco dependence (Z87.891)
     occupational exposure to environmental tobacco smoke (Z57.31)
     tobacco dependence (F17.-)
     tobacco use (Z72.0)
   EXCLUDES 1 intrathoracic malignant neoplasm NOS (C76.1)
            thoracic malignant neoplasm NOS (C76.1)

   C39.0 Malignant neoplasm of upper respiratory tract, part unspecified `HCC`

   C39.9 Malignant neoplasm of lower respiratory tract, part unspecified `HCC`
      Malignant neoplasm of respiratory tract NOS

Malignant neoplasms of bone and articular cartilage (C40-C41)

`INCLUDES` malignant neoplasm of cartilage (articular) (joint)
         malignant neoplasm of periosteum
`EXCLUDES 1` malignant neoplasm of bone marrow NOS (C96.9)
         malignant neoplasm of synovia (C49.-)

✓4th **C40** Malignant neoplasm of bone and articular cartilage of limbs
   Use additional code to identify major osseous defect, if applicable (M89.7-)

✓5th **C40.0** Malignant neoplasm of scapula and long bones of upper limb

   C40.00 Malignant neoplasm of scapula and long bones of unspecified upper limb `CC` `HCC`

   C40.01 Malignant neoplasm of scapula and long bones of right upper limb `CC` `HCC`

   C40.02 Malignant neoplasm of scapula and long bones of left upper limb `CC` `HCC`

✓5th **C40.1** Malignant neoplasm of short bones of upper limb

   C40.10 Malignant neoplasm of short bones of unspecified upper limb `CC` `HCC`

   C40.11 Malignant neoplasm of short bones of right upper limb `CC` `HCC`

   C40.12 Malignant neoplasm of short bones of left upper limb `CC` `HCC`

✓5th **C40.2** Malignant neoplasm of long bones of lower limb

   C40.20 Malignant neoplasm of long bones of unspecified lower limb `CC` `HCC`

C40.21 Malignant neoplasm of long bones of right lower limb `CC` `HCC`

C40.22 Malignant neoplasm of long bones of left lower limb `CC` `HCC`

✓5th **C40.3** Malignant neoplasm of short bones of lower limb

   C40.30 Malignant neoplasm of short bones of unspecified lower limb `CC` `HCC`

   C40.31 Malignant neoplasm of short bones of right lower limb `CC` `HCC`

   C40.32 Malignant neoplasm of short bones of left lower limb `CC` `HCC`

✓5th **C40.8** Malignant neoplasm of overlapping sites of bone and articular cartilage of limb

   C40.80 Malignant neoplasm of overlapping sites of bone and articular cartilage of unspecified limb `CC` `HCC`

   C40.81 Malignant neoplasm of overlapping sites of bone and articular cartilage of right limb `CC` `HCC`

   C40.82 Malignant neoplasm of overlapping sites of bone and articular cartilage of left limb `CC` `HCC`

✓5th **C40.9** Malignant neoplasm of unspecified bones and articular cartilage of limb

   C40.90 Malignant neoplasm of unspecified bones and articular cartilage of unspecified limb `CC` `HCC`

   C40.91 Malignant neoplasm of unspecified bones and articular cartilage of right limb `CC` `HCC`

   C40.92 Malignant neoplasm of unspecified bones and articular cartilage of left limb `CC` `HCC`

✓4th **C41** Malignant neoplasm of bone and articular cartilage of other and unspecified sites
   EXCLUDES 1 malignant neoplasm of bones of limbs (C40.-)
         malignant neoplasm of cartilage of ear (C49.0)
         malignant neoplasm of cartilage of eyelid (C49.0)
         malignant neoplasm of cartilage of larynx (C32.3)
         malignant neoplasm of cartilage of limbs (C40.-)
         malignant neoplasm of cartilage of nose (C30.0)

   C41.0 Malignant neoplasm of bones of skull and face `CC` `HCC`
      Malignant neoplasm of maxilla (superior)
      Malignant neoplasm of orbital bone
      EXCLUDES 2 carcinoma, any type except intraosseous or odontogenic of:
           maxillary sinus (C31.0)
           upper jaw (C03.0)
           malignant neoplasm of jaw bone (lower) (C41.1)

   C41.1 Malignant neoplasm of mandible `CC` `HCC`
      Malignant neoplasm of inferior maxilla
      Malignant neoplasm of lower jaw bone
      EXCLUDES 2 carcinoma, any type except intraosseous or odontogenic of:
           jaw NOS (C03.9)
           lower (C03.1)
           malignant neoplasm of upper jaw bone (C41.0)

   C41.2 Malignant neoplasm of vertebral column `CC` `HCC`
      EXCLUDES 1 malignant neoplasm of sacrum and coccyx (C41.4)

   C41.3 Malignant neoplasm of ribs, sternum and clavicle `CC` `HCC`

   C41.4 Malignant neoplasm of pelvic bones, sacrum and coccyx `CC` `HCC`

   C41.9 Malignant neoplasm of bone and articular cartilage, unspecified `CC` `HCC`

Melanoma and other malignant neoplasms of skin (C43-C44)

✓4th **C43** Malignant melanoma of skin
   EXCLUDES 1 melanoma in situ (D03.-)
   EXCLUDES 2 malignant melanoma of skin of genital organs (C51-C52, C60.-, C63.-)
         Merkel cell carcinoma (C4A.-)
         sites other than skin - code to malignant neoplasm of the site

   C43.0 Malignant melanoma of lip `HCC`
      EXCLUDES 1 malignant neoplasm of vermilion border of lip (C00.0-C00.2)

✓5th **C43.1** Malignant melanoma of eyelid, including canthus
      AHA: 2018,4Q,4

   C43.10 Malignant melanoma of unspecified eyelid, including canthus `HCC`

✅ Additional Character Required   ✓x7th Placeholder   Questionable PDx   Manifestation   Unspecified   `UPD` Unacceptable PDx   `H1`-`H14` HAC   `HCC` CMS-HCC Dx   `HIV` HIV Dx

ICD-10-CM 2025   479

Chapter 2. Neoplasms

C34.31–C43.10

☑6ᵗʰ **C43.11** **Malignant melanoma** of **right** eyelid, including canthus

    C43.111 Malignant melanoma of right **upper** eyelid, including canthus `HCC`

    C43.112 Malignant melanoma of right **lower** eyelid, including canthus `HCC`

☑6ᵗʰ **C43.12** Malignant melanoma of **left** eyelid, including canthus

    C43.121 Malignant melanoma of left **upper** eyelid, including canthus `HCC`

    C43.122 Malignant melanoma of left **lower** eyelid, including canthus `HCC`

☑5ᵗʰ **C43.2** Malignant melanoma of **ear and external auricular canal**

    C43.20 Malignant melanoma of unspecified ear and external auricular canal `HCC`

    C43.21 Malignant melanoma of **right** ear and external auricular canal

    C43.22 Malignant melanoma of **left** ear and external auricular canal `HCC`

☑5ᵗʰ **C43.3** Malignant melanoma of other and unspecified **parts of face**

    C43.30 Malignant melanoma of unspecified part of face `HCC`

    C43.31 Malignant melanoma of **nose** `HCC`

    C43.39 Malignant melanoma of other parts of face `HCC`

C43.4 Malignant melanoma of **scalp and neck** `HCC`

☑5ᵗʰ **C43.5** Malignant melanoma of **trunk**

    EXCLUDES 2 *malignant neoplasm of anus NOS (C21.0)*
                malignant neoplasm of scrotum (C63.2)

    C43.51 Malignant melanoma of **anal skin** `HCC`
        Malignant melanoma of anal margin
        Malignant melanoma of perianal skin

    C43.52 Malignant melanoma of **skin of breast** `HCC`

    C43.59 Malignant melanoma of other part of trunk `HCC`

☑5ᵗʰ **C43.6** Malignant melanoma of **upper limb, including shoulder**

    C43.60 Malignant melanoma of unspecified upper limb, including shoulder `HCC`

    C43.61 Malignant melanoma of **right** upper limb, including shoulder `HCC`

    C43.62 Malignant melanoma of **left** upper limb, including shoulder `HCC`

☑5ᵗʰ **C43.7** Malignant melanoma of **lower limb, including hip**

    C43.70 Malignant melanoma of unspecified lower limb, including hip `HCC`

    C43.71 Malignant melanoma of **right** lower limb, including hip `HCC`

    C43.72 Malignant melanoma of **left** lower limb, including hip `HCC`

C43.8 Malignant melanoma of **overlapping sites** of skin `HCC`

C43.9 Malignant melanoma of skin, unspecified `HCC`
    Malignant melanoma of unspecified site of skin
    Melanoma (malignant) NOS

☑4ᵗʰ **C4A** **Merkel cell carcinoma**

    DEF: Malignant cutaneous cancer predominantly found in elderly patients with sun exposure that usually presents as a flesh-colored or bluish-red lump typically seen on the neck, head, and face.

C4A.0 Merkel cell carcinoma of **lip** `HCC`

    EXCLUDES 1 *malignant neoplasm of vermilion border of lip (C00.0-C00.2)*

☑5ᵗʰ **C4A.1** Merkel cell carcinoma of **eyelid, including canthus**

    AHA: 2018,4Q,4

    C4A.10 Merkel cell carcinoma of unspecified eyelid, including canthus `HCC`

☑6ᵗʰ **C4A.11** Merkel cell carcinoma of **right** eyelid, including canthus

    C4A.111 Merkel cell carcinoma of right **upper** eyelid, including canthus `HCC`

    C4A.112 Merkel cell carcinoma of right **lower** eyelid, including canthus `HCC`

☑6ᵗʰ **C4A.12** Merkel cell carcinoma of **left** eyelid, including canthus

    C4A.121 Merkel cell carcinoma of left **upper** eyelid, including canthus `HCC`

    C4A.122 Merkel cell carcinoma of left **lower** eyelid, including canthus `HCC`

☑5ᵗʰ **C4A.2** Merkel cell carcinoma of **ear and external auricular canal**

    C4A.20 Merkel cell carcinoma of unspecified ear and external auricular canal `HCC`

    C4A.21 Merkel cell carcinoma of **right** ear and external auricular canal `HCC`

    C4A.22 Merkel cell carcinoma of **left** ear and external auricular canal `HCC`

☑5ᵗʰ **C4A.3** Merkel cell carcinoma of other and unspecified **parts of face**

    C4A.30 Merkel cell carcinoma of unspecified part of face `HCC`

    C4A.31 Merkel cell carcinoma of **nose** `HCC`

    C4A.39 Merkel cell carcinoma of other parts of face `HCC`

C4A.4 Merkel cell carcinoma of **scalp and neck** `HCC`

☑5ᵗʰ **C4A.5** Merkel cell carcinoma of **trunk**

    EXCLUDES 2 *malignant neoplasm of anus NOS (C21.0)*
                malignant neoplasm of scrotum (C63.2)

    C4A.51 Merkel cell carcinoma of **anal skin**
        Merkel cell carcinoma of anal margin
        Merkel cell carcinoma of perianal skin

    C4A.52 Merkel cell carcinoma of **skin of breast** `HCC`

    C4A.59 Merkel cell carcinoma of other part of trunk `HCC`

☑5ᵗʰ **C4A.6** Merkel cell carcinoma of **upper limb, including shoulder**

    C4A.60 Merkel cell carcinoma of unspecified upper limb, including shoulder `HCC`

    C4A.61 Merkel cell carcinoma of **right** upper limb, including shoulder `HCC`

    C4A.62 Merkel cell carcinoma of **left** upper limb, including shoulder `HCC`

☑5ᵗʰ **C4A.7** Merkel cell carcinoma of **lower limb, including hip**

    C4A.70 Merkel cell carcinoma of unspecified lower limb, including hip `HCC`

    C4A.71 Merkel cell carcinoma of **right** lower limb, including hip `HCC`

    C4A.72 Merkel cell carcinoma of **left** lower limb, including hip `HCC`

C4A.8 Merkel cell carcinoma of **overlapping sites** `HCC`

C4A.9 Merkel cell carcinoma, unspecified `HCC`
    Merkel cell carcinoma of unspecified site
    Merkel cell carcinoma NOS

☑4ᵗʰ **C44** **Other and unspecified malignant neoplasm of skin**

    INCLUDES malignant neoplasm of sebaceous glands
              malignant neoplasm of sweat glands

    EXCLUDES 1 *Kaposi's sarcoma of skin (C46.0)*
                malignant melanoma of skin (C43.-)
                malignant neoplasm of skin of genital organs (C51-C52, C60.-, C63.2)
                Merkel cell carcinoma (C4A.-)

    DEF: Basal cell carcinoma: Abnormal growth of skin cells that arises from the deepest layer of the epidermis and may present as an open sore, red patches, pink growth, or scar. Typically caused by sun exposure, it is one of the most common forms of skin cancer.

    DEF: Squamous cell carcinoma: Uncontrolled growth of abnormal skin cells that arises from the outer layers of the skin (epidermis) and may present as an open sore. It is characterized by a firm, red nodule, elevated growth with a central depression, or a flat sore with a scaly crust.

☑5ᵗʰ **C44.0** **Other and unspecified malignant neoplasm of skin of lip**

    EXCLUDES 1 *malignant neoplasm of lip (C00.-)*

    C44.00 Unspecified malignant neoplasm of skin of lip

    C44.01 **Basal cell carcinoma** of skin of lip

    C44.02 **Squamous cell carcinoma** of skin of lip

    C44.09 Other specified malignant neoplasm of skin of lip

☑5ᵗʰ **C44.1** **Other and unspecified malignant neoplasm of skin of eyelid, including canthus**

    EXCLUDES 1 *connective tissue of eyelid (C49.0)*

    AHA: 2018,4Q,4

☑6ᵗʰ **C44.10** Unspecified malignant neoplasm of skin of eyelid, including canthus

    C44.101 Unspecified malignant neoplasm of skin of unspecified eyelid, including canthus

    ☑7ᵗʰ **C44.102** Unspecified malignant neoplasm of skin of **right** eyelid, including canthus

        C44.1021 Unspecified malignant neoplasm of skin of right **upper** eyelid, including canthus

        C44.1022 Unspecified malignant neoplasm of skin of right **lower** eyelid, including canthus

    ☑7ᵗʰ **C44.109** Unspecified malignant neoplasm of skin of **left** eyelid, including canthus

N Newborn: 0   P Pediatric: 0-17   M Maternity: 9-64   A Adult: 15-124   UNS Unspecified Site   MCC Major Complication/Comorbidity   CC Complication/Comorbidity   PE POA Exempt

480   ICD-10-CM 2025

C44.1091 Unspecified malignant neoplasm of skin of left upper eyelid, including canthus

C44.1092 Unspecified malignant neoplasm of skin of left lower eyelid, including canthus

✓6ᵗʰ **C44.11** Basal cell carcinoma of skin of eyelid, including canthus

    C44.111 Basal cell carcinoma of skin of unspecified eyelid, including canthus

    ✓7ᵗʰ **C44.112** Basal cell carcinoma of skin of right eyelid, including canthus

        C44.1121 Basal cell carcinoma of skin of right upper eyelid, including canthus

        C44.1122 Basal cell carcinoma of skin of right lower eyelid, including canthus

    ✓7ᵗʰ **C44.119** Basal cell carcinoma of skin of left eyelid, including canthus

        C44.1191 Basal cell carcinoma of skin of left upper eyelid, including canthus

        C44.1192 Basal cell carcinoma of skin of left lower eyelid, including canthus

✓6ᵗʰ **C44.12** Squamous cell carcinoma of skin of eyelid, including canthus

    C44.121 Squamous cell carcinoma of skin of unspecified eyelid, including canthus

    ✓7ᵗʰ **C44.122** Squamous cell carcinoma of skin of right eyelid, including canthus

        C44.1221 Squamous cell carcinoma of skin of right upper eyelid, including canthus

        C44.1222 Squamous cell carcinoma of skin of right lower eyelid, including canthus

    ✓7ᵗʰ **C44.129** Squamous cell carcinoma of skin of left eyelid, including canthus

        C44.1291 Squamous cell carcinoma of skin of left upper eyelid, including canthus

        C44.1292 Squamous cell carcinoma of skin of left lower eyelid, including canthus

✓6ᵗʰ **C44.13** Sebaceous cell carcinoma of skin of eyelid, including canthus

    C44.131 Sebaceous cell carcinoma of skin of unspecified eyelid, including canthus

    ✓7ᵗʰ **C44.132** Sebaceous cell carcinoma of skin of right eyelid, including canthus

        C44.1321 Sebaceous cell carcinoma of skin of right upper eyelid, including canthus

        C44.1322 Sebaceous cell carcinoma of skin of right lower eyelid, including canthus

    ✓7ᵗʰ **C44.139** Sebaceous cell carcinoma of skin of left eyelid, including canthus

        C44.1391 Sebaceous cell carcinoma of skin of left upper eyelid, including canthus

        C44.1392 Sebaceous cell carcinoma of skin of left lower eyelid, including canthus

✓6ᵗʰ **C44.19** Other specified malignant neoplasm of skin of eyelid, including canthus

    C44.191 Other specified malignant neoplasm of skin of unspecified eyelid, including canthus

    ✓7ᵗʰ **C44.192** Other specified malignant neoplasm of skin of right eyelid, including canthus

        C44.1921 Other specified malignant neoplasm of skin of right upper eyelid, including canthus

        C44.1922 Other specified malignant neoplasm of skin of right lower eyelid, including canthus

    ✓7ᵗʰ **C44.199** Other specified malignant neoplasm of skin of left eyelid, including canthus

        C44.1991 Other specified malignant neoplasm of skin of left upper eyelid, including canthus

C44.1992 Other specified malignant neoplasm of skin of left lower eyelid, including canthus

✓5ᵗʰ **C44.2** Other and unspecified malignant neoplasm of skin of ear and external auricular canal

    EXCLUDES 1   connective tissue of ear (C49.0)

  ✓6ᵗʰ **C44.20** Unspecified malignant neoplasm of skin of ear and external auricular canal

    C44.201 Unspecified malignant neoplasm of skin of unspecified ear and external auricular canal

    C44.202 Unspecified malignant neoplasm of skin of right ear and external auricular canal

    C44.209 Unspecified malignant neoplasm of skin of left ear and external auricular canal

  ✓6ᵗʰ **C44.21** Basal cell carcinoma of skin of ear and external auricular canal

    C44.211 Basal cell carcinoma of skin of unspecified ear and external auricular canal

    C44.212 Basal cell carcinoma of skin of right ear and external auricular canal

    C44.219 Basal cell carcinoma of skin of left ear and external auricular canal

  ✓6ᵗʰ **C44.22** Squamous cell carcinoma of skin of ear and external auricular canal

    C44.221 Squamous cell carcinoma of skin of unspecified ear and external auricular canal

    C44.222 Squamous cell carcinoma of skin of right ear and external auricular canal

    C44.229 Squamous cell carcinoma of skin of left ear and external auricular canal

  ✓6ᵗʰ **C44.29** Other specified malignant neoplasm of skin of ear and external auricular canal

    C44.291 Other specified malignant neoplasm of skin of unspecified ear and external auricular canal

    C44.292 Other specified malignant neoplasm of skin of right ear and external auricular canal

    C44.299 Other specified malignant neoplasm of skin of left ear and external auricular canal

✓5ᵗʰ **C44.3** Other and unspecified malignant neoplasm of skin of other and unspecified parts of face

  ✓6ᵗʰ **C44.30** Unspecified malignant neoplasm of skin of other and unspecified parts of face

    C44.300 Unspecified malignant neoplasm of skin of unspecified part of face

    C44.301 Unspecified malignant neoplasm of skin of nose

    C44.309 Unspecified malignant neoplasm of skin of other parts of face

  ✓6ᵗʰ **C44.31** Basal cell carcinoma of skin of other and unspecified parts of face

    C44.310 Basal cell carcinoma of skin of unspecified parts of face

    C44.311 Basal cell carcinoma of skin of nose

    C44.319 Basal cell carcinoma of skin of other parts of face

  ✓6ᵗʰ **C44.32** Squamous cell carcinoma of skin of other and unspecified parts of face

    C44.320 Squamous cell carcinoma of skin of unspecified parts of face

    C44.321 Squamous cell carcinoma of skin of nose

    C44.329 Squamous cell carcinoma of skin of other parts of face

  ✓6ᵗʰ **C44.39** Other specified malignant neoplasm of skin of other and unspecified parts of face

    C44.390 Other specified malignant neoplasm of skin of unspecified parts of face

    C44.391 Other specified malignant neoplasm of skin of nose

    C44.399 Other specified malignant neoplasm of skin of other parts of face

✓5ᵗʰ **C44.4** Other and unspecified malignant neoplasm of skin of scalp and neck

    C44.40 Unspecified malignant neoplasm of skin of scalp and neck

    C44.41 Basal cell carcinoma of skin of scalp and neck

    C44.42 Squamous cell carcinoma of skin of scalp and neck

    C44.49 Other specified malignant neoplasm of skin of scalp and neck

✓ Additional Character Required   ✓x7ᵗʰ Placeholder   Questionable PDx   Manifestation   Unspecified   UPD Unacceptable PDx   H1 - H14 HAC   HCC CMS-HCC Dx   HIV HIV Dx

ICD-10-CM 2025   481

✓5th **C44.5** **Other and unspecified malignant neoplasm of skin of trunk**

    EXCLUDES 1   *anus NOS (C21.0)*
                scrotum (C63.2)

    ✓6th **C44.50** **Unspecified malignant neoplasm of skin of trunk**

       C44.500 **Unspecified malignant neoplasm of anal skin**
            Unspecified malignant neoplasm of anal margin
            Unspecified malignant neoplasm of perianal skin

       C44.501 **Unspecified malignant neoplasm of skin of breast**

       C44.509 **Unspecified malignant neoplasm of skin of other part of trunk**

    ✓6th **C44.51** **Basal cell carcinoma of skin of trunk**

       C44.510 **Basal cell carcinoma of anal skin**
            Basal cell carcinoma of anal margin
            Basal cell carcinoma of perianal skin

       C44.511 **Basal cell carcinoma of skin of breast**

       C44.519 **Basal cell carcinoma of skin of other part of trunk**

    ✓6th **C44.52** **Squamous cell carcinoma of skin of trunk**

       C44.520 **Squamous cell carcinoma of anal skin**
            Squamous cell carcinoma of anal margin
            Squamous cell carcinoma of perianal skin

       C44.521 **Squamous cell carcinoma of skin of breast**

       C44.529 **Squamous cell carcinoma of skin of other part of trunk**

    ✓6th **C44.59** **Other specified malignant neoplasm of skin of trunk**

       C44.590 **Other specified malignant neoplasm of anal skin**
            Other specified malignant neoplasm of anal margin
            Other specified malignant neoplasm of perianal skin

       C44.591 **Other specified malignant neoplasm of skin of breast**

       C44.599 **Other specified malignant neoplasm of skin of other part of trunk**

✓5th **C44.6** **Other and unspecified malignant neoplasm of skin of upper limb, including shoulder**

    ✓6th **C44.60** **Unspecified malignant neoplasm of skin of upper limb, including shoulder**

       C44.601 **Unspecified malignant neoplasm of skin of unspecified upper limb, including shoulder**

       C44.602 **Unspecified malignant neoplasm of skin of right upper limb, including shoulder**

       C44.609 **Unspecified malignant neoplasm of skin of left upper limb, including shoulder**

    ✓6th **C44.61** **Basal cell carcinoma of skin of upper limb, including shoulder**

       C44.611 **Basal cell carcinoma of skin of unspecified upper limb, including shoulder**

       C44.612 **Basal cell carcinoma of skin of right upper limb, including shoulder**

       C44.619 **Basal cell carcinoma of skin of left upper limb, including shoulder**

    ✓6th **C44.62** **Squamous cell carcinoma of skin of upper limb, including shoulder**

       C44.621 **Squamous cell carcinoma of skin of unspecified upper limb, including shoulder**

       C44.622 **Squamous cell carcinoma of skin of right upper limb, including shoulder**

       C44.629 **Squamous cell carcinoma of skin of left upper limb, including shoulder**

    ✓6th **C44.69** **Other specified malignant neoplasm of skin of upper limb, including shoulder**

       C44.691 **Other specified malignant neoplasm of skin of unspecified upper limb, including shoulder**

       C44.692 **Other specified malignant neoplasm of skin of right upper limb, including shoulder**

       C44.699 **Other specified malignant neoplasm of skin of left upper limb, including shoulder**

✓5th **C44.7** **Other and unspecified malignant neoplasm of skin of lower limb, including hip**

    ✓6th **C44.70** **Unspecified malignant neoplasm of skin of lower limb, including hip**

       C44.701 **Unspecified malignant neoplasm of skin of unspecified lower limb, including hip**

       C44.702 **Unspecified malignant neoplasm of skin of right lower limb, including hip**

       C44.709 **Unspecified malignant neoplasm of skin of left lower limb, including hip**

    ✓6th **C44.71** **Basal cell carcinoma of skin of lower limb, including hip**

       C44.711 **Basal cell carcinoma of skin of unspecified lower limb, including hip**

       C44.712 **Basal cell carcinoma of skin of right lower limb, including hip**

       C44.719 **Basal cell carcinoma of skin of left lower limb, including hip**

    ✓6th **C44.72** **Squamous cell carcinoma of skin of lower limb, including hip**

       C44.721 **Squamous cell carcinoma of skin of unspecified lower limb, including hip**

       C44.722 **Squamous cell carcinoma of skin of right lower limb, including hip**

       C44.729 **Squamous cell carcinoma of skin of left lower limb, including hip**

    ✓6th **C44.79** **Other specified malignant neoplasm of skin of lower limb, including hip**

       C44.791 **Other specified malignant neoplasm of skin of unspecified lower limb, including hip**

       C44.792 **Other specified malignant neoplasm of skin of right lower limb, including hip**

       C44.799 **Other specified malignant neoplasm of skin of left lower limb, including hip**

✓5th **C44.8** **Other and unspecified malignant neoplasm of overlapping sites of skin**

       C44.80 **Unspecified malignant neoplasm of overlapping sites of skin**

       C44.81 **Basal cell carcinoma of overlapping sites of skin**

       C44.82 **Squamous cell carcinoma of overlapping sites of skin**

       C44.89 **Other specified malignant neoplasm of overlapping sites of skin**

✓5th **C44.9** **Other and unspecified malignant neoplasm of skin, unspecified**

       C44.90 **Unspecified malignant neoplasm of skin, unspecified**
            Malignant neoplasm of unspecified site of skin

       C44.91 **Basal cell carcinoma of skin, unspecified**

       C44.92 **Squamous cell carcinoma of skin, unspecified**

       C44.99 **Other specified malignant neoplasm of skin, unspecified**

Malignant neoplasms of mesothelial and soft tissue (C45-C49)

✓4th **C45** **Mesothelioma**

    DEF: Rare type of cancer that forms in the thin layer of protective tissue that covers the majority of internal organs (mesothelium).

    C45.0 **Mesothelioma of pleura**   CC   HCC
       EXCLUDES 1   *other malignant neoplasm of pleura (C38.4)*
       AHA: 2017,2Q,11
       TIP: For pleural mesothelioma that has metastasized to the chest wall, assign this code for the primary site along with C79.89 for metastatic cancer in the chest wall.

    C45.1 **Mesothelioma of peritoneum**   CC   HCC
       Mesothelioma of cul-de-sac
       Mesothelioma of mesentery
       Mesothelioma of mesocolon
       Mesothelioma of omentum
       Mesothelioma of peritoneum (parietal) (pelvic)
       EXCLUDES 1   *other malignant neoplasm of soft tissue of peritoneum (C48.-)*

    C45.2 **Mesothelioma of pericardium**   CC   HCC
       EXCLUDES 1   *other malignant neoplasm of pericardium (C38.0)*

    C45.7 **Mesothelioma of other sites**   HCC

    C45.9 **Mesothelioma, unspecified**   HCC

✓4th **C46** **Kaposi's sarcoma**

    Code first any human immunodeficiency virus [HIV] disease (B20)
    DEF: Malignant neoplasm that causes patches of abnormal tissue to grow under the skin, in the lining of the mouth, nose, and throat, in lymph nodes, or in other visceral organs. Kaposi's sarcoma is caused by human herpesvirus8 (HHV8).

    C46.0 **Kaposi's sarcoma of skin**   HIV   CC   HCC

N Newborn: 0   P Pediatric: 0-17   M Maternity: 9-64   A Adult: 15-124   UNS Unspecified Site   MCC Major Complication/Comorbidity   CC Complication/Comorbidity   PE POA Exempt

482   ICD-10-CM 2025

C46.1   **Kaposi's sarcoma of soft tissue**   `HIV` `CC` `HCC`
Kaposi's sarcoma of blood vessel
Kaposi's sarcoma of connective tissue
Kaposi's sarcoma of fascia
Kaposi's sarcoma of ligament
Kaposi's sarcoma of lymphatic(s) NEC
Kaposi's sarcoma of muscle
> *EXCLUDES 2*   *Kaposi's sarcoma of lymph glands and nodes (C46.3)*

C46.2   **Kaposi's sarcoma of palate**   `HIV` `CC` `HCC`

C46.3   **Kaposi's sarcoma of lymph nodes**   `HIV` `CC` `HCC`

C46.4   **Kaposi's sarcoma of gastrointestinal sites**   `HIV` `CC` `HCC`

✓5th **C46.5**   **Kaposi's sarcoma of lung**
AHA: 2019,1Q,16
TIP: When documented, assign code I31.31 for associated malignant pericardial effusion. The neoplasm code should be sequenced first.

     C46.50   **Kaposi's sarcoma of unspecified lung**   `HIV` `CC` `HCC`

     C46.51   **Kaposi's sarcoma of right lung**   `HIV` `CC` `HCC`

     C46.52   **Kaposi's sarcoma of left lung**   `HIV` `CC` `HCC`

C46.7   **Kaposi's sarcoma of other sites**   `HIV` `CC` `HCC`

C46.9   **Kaposi's sarcoma, unspecified**   `HIV` `CC` `HCC`
Kaposi's sarcoma of unspecified site

✓4th **C47**   **Malignant neoplasm of peripheral nerves and autonomic nervous system**
> *INCLUDES*   malignant neoplasm of sympathetic and parasympathetic nerves and ganglia
> *EXCLUDES 1*   *Kaposi's sarcoma of soft tissue (C46.1)*

C47.0   **Malignant neoplasm of peripheral nerves of head, face and neck**   `CC` `HCC`
> *EXCLUDES 1*   *malignant neoplasm of peripheral nerves of orbit (C69.6-)*

✓5th **C47.1**   **Malignant neoplasm of peripheral nerves of upper limb, including shoulder**

     C47.10   **Malignant neoplasm of peripheral nerves of unspecified upper limb, including shoulder**   `CC` `HCC`

     C47.11   **Malignant neoplasm of peripheral nerves of right upper limb, including shoulder**   `CC` `HCC`

     C47.12   **Malignant neoplasm of peripheral nerves of left upper limb, including shoulder**   `CC` `HCC`

✓5th **C47.2**   **Malignant neoplasm of peripheral nerves of lower limb, including hip**

     C47.20   **Malignant neoplasm of peripheral nerves of unspecified lower limb, including hip**   `CC` `HCC`

     C47.21   **Malignant neoplasm of peripheral nerves of right lower limb, including hip**   `CC` `HCC`

     C47.22   **Malignant neoplasm of peripheral nerves of left lower limb, including hip**   `CC` `HCC`

C47.3   **Malignant neoplasm of peripheral nerves of thorax**   `CC` `HCC`

C47.4   **Malignant neoplasm of peripheral nerves of abdomen**   `CC` `HCC`

C47.5   **Malignant neoplasm of peripheral nerves of pelvis**   `CC` `HCC`

C47.6   **Malignant neoplasm of peripheral nerves of trunk, unspecified**   `CC` `HCC`
Malignant neoplasm of peripheral nerves of unspecified part of trunk

C47.8   **Malignant neoplasm of overlapping sites of peripheral nerves and autonomic nervous system**   `CC` `HCC`

C47.9   **Malignant neoplasm of peripheral nerves and autonomic nervous system, unspecified**   `CC` `HCC`
Malignant neoplasm of unspecified site of peripheral nerves and autonomic nervous system

✓4th **C48**   **Malignant neoplasm of retroperitoneum and peritoneum**
> *EXCLUDES 1*   *Kaposi's sarcoma of connective tissue (C46.1)*
>   *mesothelioma (C45.-)*

C48.0   **Malignant neoplasm of retroperitoneum**   `CC` `HCC`

C48.1   **Malignant neoplasm of specified parts of peritoneum**   `CC` `HCC`
Malignant neoplasm of cul-de-sac
Malignant neoplasm of mesentery
Malignant neoplasm of mesocolon
Malignant neoplasm of omentum
Malignant neoplasm of parietal peritoneum
Malignant neoplasm of pelvic peritoneum

C48.2   **Malignant neoplasm of peritoneum, unspecified**   `CC` `HCC`

C48.8   **Malignant neoplasm of overlapping sites of retroperitoneum and peritoneum**   `CC` `HCC`

✓4th **C49**   **Malignant neoplasm of other connective and soft tissue**
> *INCLUDES*   malignant neoplasm of blood vessel
>   malignant neoplasm of bursa
>   malignant neoplasm of cartilage
>   malignant neoplasm of fascia
>   malignant neoplasm of fat
>   malignant neoplasm of ligament, except uterine
>   malignant neoplasm of lymphatic vessel
>   malignant neoplasm of muscle
>   malignant neoplasm of synovia
>   malignant neoplasm of tendon (sheath)
> *EXCLUDES 1*   *malignant neoplasm of cartilage (of):*
>   *articular (C40-C41)*
>   *larynx (C32.3)*
>   *nose (C30.0)*
>   *malignant neoplasm of connective tissue of breast (C50.-)*
> *EXCLUDES 2*   *Kaposi's sarcoma of soft tissue (C46.1)*
>   *malignant neoplasm of heart (C38.0)*
>   *malignant neoplasm of peripheral nerves and autonomic nervous system (C47.-)*
>   *malignant neoplasm of peritoneum (C48.2)*
>   *malignant neoplasm of retroperitoneum (C48.0)*
>   *malignant neoplasm of uterine ligament (C57.3)*
>   *mesothelioma (C45.-)*

C49.0   **Malignant neoplasm of connective and soft tissue of head, face and neck**   `CC` `HCC`
Malignant neoplasm of connective tissue of ear
Malignant neoplasm of connective tissue of eyelid
> *EXCLUDES 1*   *connective tissue of orbit (C69.6-)*

✓5th **C49.1**   **Malignant neoplasm of connective and soft tissue of upper limb, including shoulder**

     C49.10   **Malignant neoplasm of connective and soft tissue of unspecified upper limb, including shoulder**   `CC` `HCC`

     C49.11   **Malignant neoplasm of connective and soft tissue of right upper limb, including shoulder**   `CC` `HCC`

     C49.12   **Malignant neoplasm of connective and soft tissue of left upper limb, including shoulder**   `CC` `HCC`

✓5th **C49.2**   **Malignant neoplasm of connective and soft tissue of lower limb, including hip**

     C49.20   **Malignant neoplasm of connective and soft tissue of unspecified lower limb, including hip**   `CC` `HCC`

     C49.21   **Malignant neoplasm of connective and soft tissue of right lower limb, including hip**   `CC` `HCC`

     C49.22   **Malignant neoplasm of connective and soft tissue of left lower limb, including hip**   `CC` `HCC`

C49.3   **Malignant neoplasm of connective and soft tissue of thorax**   `CC` `HCC`
Malignant neoplasm of axilla
Malignant neoplasm of diaphragm
Malignant neoplasm of great vessels
> *EXCLUDES 1*   *malignant neoplasm of breast (C50.-)*
>   *malignant neoplasm of heart (C38.0)*
>   *malignant neoplasm of mediastinum (C38.1-C38.3)*
>   *malignant neoplasm of thymus (C37)*

     AHA: 2015,3Q,19

C49.4   **Malignant neoplasm of connective and soft tissue of abdomen**   `CC` `HCC`
Malignant neoplasm of abdominal wall
Malignant neoplasm of hypochondrium

C49.5   **Malignant neoplasm of connective and soft tissue of pelvis**   `CC` `HCC`
Malignant neoplasm of buttock
Malignant neoplasm of groin
Malignant neoplasm of perineum

C49.6   **Malignant neoplasm of connective and soft tissue of trunk, unspecified**   `CC` `HCC`
Malignant neoplasm of back NOS

C49.8   **Malignant neoplasm of overlapping sites of connective and soft tissue**   `CC` `HCC`
Primary malignant neoplasm of two or more contiguous sites of connective and soft tissue

C49.9   **Malignant neoplasm of connective and soft tissue, unspecified**   `CC` `HCC`

✔ Additional Character Required   ✓x7th Placeholder   Questionable PDx   Manifestation   Unspecified   `UPD` Unacceptable PDx   `H1`-`H14` HAC   `HCC` CMS-HCC Dx   `HIV` HIV Dx

ICD-10-CM 2025   483

Chapter 2. Neoplasms

C46.1–C49.9

✓5th **C49.A**   **Gastrointestinal stromal tumor**

AHA: 2016,4Q,8

DEF: Uncommon malignant tumor found in the GI tract that originates from interstitial cells of the autonomic nervous system. Most occur in the stomach or small intestine but can originate anywhere in the GI tract.

  C49.A0   Gastrointestinal stromal tumor, unspecified site   `CC` `HCC`

  C49.A1   Gastrointestinal stromal tumor of esophagus   `CC` `HCC`

  C49.A2   Gastrointestinal stromal tumor of stomach   `CC` `HCC`

  C49.A3   Gastrointestinal stromal tumor of small intestine   `CC` `HCC`

  C49.A4   Gastrointestinal stromal tumor of large intestine   `CC` `HCC`

  C49.A5   Gastrointestinal stromal tumor of rectum   `CC` `HCC`

  C49.A9   Gastrointestinal stromal tumor of other sites   `CC` `HCC`

Malignant neoplasms of breast (C50)

✓4th **C50**   **Malignant neoplasm of breast**

  `INCLUDES`   connective tissue of breast
            Paget's disease of breast
            Paget's disease of nipple

▶Use additional code to identify estrogen, and other hormones and factors receptor status (Z17.-)◀

  `EXCLUDES 1`   *skin of breast (C44.501, C44.511, C44.521, C44.591)*

AHA: 2017,4Q,19

Female Breast

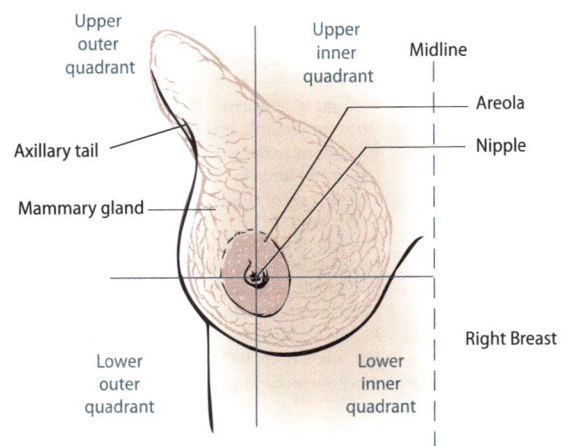

Upper outer quadrant

Upper inner quadrant

Midline

Areola

Nipple

Axillary tail

Mammary gland

Right Breast

Lower outer quadrant

Lower inner quadrant

✓5th **C50.0**   **Malignant neoplasm of nipple and areola**

  ✓6th **C50.01**   Malignant neoplasm of nipple and areola, female

    C50.011   Malignant neoplasm of nipple and areola, right female breast   `HCC`

    C50.012   Malignant neoplasm of nipple and areola, left female breast   `HCC`

    C50.019   Malignant neoplasm of nipple and areola, unspecified female breast   `HCC`

  ✓6th **C50.02**   Malignant neoplasm of nipple and areola, male

    C50.021   Malignant neoplasm of nipple and areola, right male breast   `HCC`

    C50.022   Malignant neoplasm of nipple and areola, left male breast   `HCC`

    C50.029   Malignant neoplasm of nipple and areola, unspecified male breast   `HCC`

✓5th **C50.1**   **Malignant neoplasm of central portion of breast**

  ✓6th **C50.11**   Malignant neoplasm of central portion of breast, female

    C50.111   Malignant neoplasm of central portion of right female breast   `HCC`

    C50.112   Malignant neoplasm of central portion of left female breast   `HCC`

    C50.119   Malignant neoplasm of central portion of unspecified female breast   `HCC`

  ✓6th **C50.12**   Malignant neoplasm of central portion of breast, male

    C50.121   Malignant neoplasm of central portion of right male breast   `HCC`

    C50.122   Malignant neoplasm of central portion of left male breast   `HCC`

    C50.129   Malignant neoplasm of central portion of unspecified male breast   `HCC`

✓5th **C50.2**   **Malignant neoplasm of upper-inner quadrant of breast**

  ✓6th **C50.21**   Malignant neoplasm of upper-inner quadrant of breast, female

    C50.211   Malignant neoplasm of upper-inner quadrant of right female breast   `HCC`

    C50.212   Malignant neoplasm of upper-inner quadrant of left female breast   `HCC`

    C50.219   Malignant neoplasm of upper-inner quadrant of unspecified female breast   `HCC`

  ✓6th **C50.22**   Malignant neoplasm of upper-inner quadrant of breast, male

    C50.221   Malignant neoplasm of upper-inner quadrant of right male breast   `HCC`

    C50.222   Malignant neoplasm of upper-inner quadrant of left male breast   `HCC`

    C50.229   Malignant neoplasm of upper-inner quadrant of unspecified male breast   `HCC`

✓5th **C50.3**   **Malignant neoplasm of lower-inner quadrant of breast**

  ✓6th **C50.31**   Malignant neoplasm of lower-inner quadrant of breast, female

    C50.311   Malignant neoplasm of lower-inner quadrant of right female breast   `HCC`

    C50.312   Malignant neoplasm of lower-inner quadrant of left female breast   `HCC`

    C50.319   Malignant neoplasm of lower-inner quadrant of unspecified female breast   `HCC`

  ✓6th **C50.32**   Malignant neoplasm of lower-inner quadrant of breast, male

    C50.321   Malignant neoplasm of lower-inner quadrant of right male breast   `HCC`

    C50.322   Malignant neoplasm of lower-inner quadrant of left male breast   `HCC`

    C50.329   Malignant neoplasm of lower-inner quadrant of unspecified male breast   `HCC`

✓5th **C50.4**   **Malignant neoplasm of upper-outer quadrant of breast**

  ✓6th **C50.41**   Malignant neoplasm of upper-outer quadrant of breast, female

    C50.411   Malignant neoplasm of upper-outer quadrant of right female breast   `HCC`

    C50.412   Malignant neoplasm of upper-outer quadrant of left female breast   `HCC`

    C50.419   Malignant neoplasm of upper-outer quadrant of unspecified female breast   `HCC`

  ✓6th **C50.42**   Malignant neoplasm of upper-outer quadrant of breast, male

    C50.421   Malignant neoplasm of upper-outer quadrant of right male breast   `HCC`

    C50.422   Malignant neoplasm of upper-outer quadrant of left male breast   `HCC`

    C50.429   Malignant neoplasm of upper-outer quadrant of unspecified male breast   `HCC`

✓5th **C50.5**   **Malignant neoplasm of lower-outer quadrant of breast**

  ✓6th **C50.51**   Malignant neoplasm of lower-outer quadrant of breast, female

    C50.511   Malignant neoplasm of lower-outer quadrant of right female breast   `HCC`

    C50.512   Malignant neoplasm of lower-outer quadrant of left female breast   `HCC`

    C50.519   Malignant neoplasm of lower-outer quadrant of unspecified female breast   `HCC`

  ✓6th **C50.52**   Malignant neoplasm of lower-outer quadrant of breast, male

    C50.521   Malignant neoplasm of lower-outer quadrant of right male breast   `HCC`

`N` Newborn: 0   `P` Pediatric: 0-17   `M` Maternity: 9-64   `A` Adult: 15-124   `UNS` Unspecified Site   `MCC` Major Complication/Comorbidity   `CC` Complication/Comorbidity   `PE` POA Exempt

484   ICD-10-CM 2025

C50.522 Malignant neoplasm of lower-outer quadrant of **left** male breast `HCC`

C50.529 Malignant neoplasm of lower-outer quadrant of unspecified male breast `HCC`

✓5th **C50.6** Malignant neoplasm of **axillary tail** of breast

   ✓6th **C50.61** Malignant neoplasm of axillary tail of breast, **female**

     C50.611 Malignant neoplasm of axillary tail of **right** female breast `HCC`

     C50.612 Malignant neoplasm of axillary tail of **left** female breast `HCC`

     C50.619 Malignant neoplasm of axillary tail of unspecified female breast `HCC`

   ✓6th **C50.62** Malignant neoplasm of axillary tail of breast, **male**

     C50.621 Malignant neoplasm of axillary tail of **right** male breast `HCC`

     C50.622 Malignant neoplasm of axillary tail of **left** male breast `HCC`

     C50.629 Malignant neoplasm of axillary tail of unspecified male breast `HCC`

✓5th **C50.8** Malignant neoplasm of **overlapping sites** of breast

   ✓6th **C50.81** Malignant neoplasm of overlapping sites of breast, **female**

     C50.811 Malignant neoplasm of overlapping sites of **right** female breast `HCC`

     C50.812 Malignant neoplasm of overlapping sites of **left** female breast `HCC`

     C50.819 Malignant neoplasm of overlapping sites of unspecified female breast `HCC`

   ✓6th **C50.82** Malignant neoplasm of overlapping sites of breast, **male**

     C50.821 Malignant neoplasm of overlapping sites of **right** male breast `HCC`

     C50.822 Malignant neoplasm of overlapping sites of **left** male breast `HCC`

     C50.829 Malignant neoplasm of overlapping sites of unspecified male breast `HCC`

✓5th **C50.9** Malignant neoplasm of breast of unspecified site

   ✓6th **C50.91** Malignant neoplasm of breast of unspecified site, **female**

     AHA: 2022,3Q,10,14

     C50.911 Malignant neoplasm of unspecified site of **right** female breast `HCC`

     C50.912 Malignant neoplasm of unspecified site of **left** female breast `HCC`

     C50.919 Malignant neoplasm of unspecified site of unspecified female breast `HCC`

   ✓6th **C50.92** Malignant neoplasm of breast of unspecified site, **male**

     C50.921 Malignant neoplasm of unspecified site of **right** male breast `HCC`

     C50.922 Malignant neoplasm of unspecified site of **left** male breast `HCC`

     C50.929 Malignant neoplasm of unspecified site of unspecified male breast `HCC`

Malignant neoplasms of female genital organs (C51-C58)

`INCLUDES` malignant neoplasm of skin of female genital organs

✓4th **C51** Malignant neoplasm of **vulva**

   `EXCLUDES 1` carcinoma in situ of vulva (D07.1)

   C51.0 Malignant neoplasm of **labium majus** `HCC`
     Malignant neoplasm of Bartholin's [greater vestibular] gland

   C51.1 Malignant neoplasm of **labium minus** `HCC`

   C51.2 Malignant neoplasm of **clitoris** `HCC`

   C51.8 Malignant neoplasm of **overlapping sites** of vulva `HCC`

   C51.9 Malignant neoplasm of vulva, unspecified `HCC`
     Malignant neoplasm of external female genitalia NOS
     Malignant neoplasm of pudendum

C52 Malignant neoplasm of **vagina** `HCC`
   `EXCLUDES 1` carcinoma in situ of vagina (D07.2)

✓4th **C53** Malignant neoplasm of **cervix uteri**

   `EXCLUDES 1` carcinoma in situ of cervix uteri (D06.-)

   AHA: 2017,4Q,103

   C53.0 Malignant neoplasm of **endocervix** `HCC`

   C53.1 Malignant neoplasm of **exocervix** `HCC`

   C53.8 Malignant neoplasm of **overlapping sites** of cervix uteri `HCC`

C53.9 Malignant neoplasm of cervix uteri, unspecified `HCC`

✓4th **C54** Malignant neoplasm of **corpus uteri**

   C54.0 Malignant neoplasm of **isthmus uteri** `HCC`
     Malignant neoplasm of lower uterine segment

   C54.1 Malignant neoplasm of **endometrium** `HCC`

   C54.2 Malignant neoplasm of **myometrium** `HCC`

   C54.3 Malignant neoplasm of **fundus uteri** `HCC`

   C54.8 Malignant neoplasm of **overlapping sites** of corpus uteri `HCC`
     AHA: 2023,3Q,14

   C54.9 Malignant neoplasm of corpus uteri, unspecified `HCC`

C55 Malignant neoplasm of uterus, part unspecified `HCC`

✓4th **C56** Malignant neoplasm of **ovary**

   Use additional code to identify any functional activity

   C56.1 Malignant neoplasm of **right** ovary `CC` `HCC`

   C56.2 Malignant neoplasm of **left** ovary `CC` `HCC`

   C56.3 Malignant neoplasm of **bilateral** ovaries `CC` `HCC`

   C56.9 Malignant neoplasm of unspecified ovary `CC` `HCC`

✓4th **C57** Malignant neoplasm of **other and unspecified female genital organs**

   ✓5th **C57.0** Malignant neoplasm of **fallopian tube**
     Malignant neoplasm of oviduct
     Malignant neoplasm of uterine tube

     C57.00 Malignant neoplasm of unspecified fallopian tube `HCC`

     C57.01 Malignant neoplasm of **right** fallopian tube `HCC`

     C57.02 Malignant neoplasm of **left** fallopian tube `HCC`

   ✓5th **C57.1** Malignant neoplasm of **broad ligament**

     C57.10 Malignant neoplasm of unspecified broad ligament `HCC`

     C57.11 Malignant neoplasm of **right** broad ligament `HCC`

     C57.12 Malignant neoplasm of **left** broad ligament `HCC`

   ✓5th **C57.2** Malignant neoplasm of **round ligament**

     C57.20 Malignant neoplasm of unspecified round ligament `HCC`

     C57.21 Malignant neoplasm of **right** round ligament `HCC`

     C57.22 Malignant neoplasm of **left** round ligament `HCC`

   C57.3 Malignant neoplasm of **parametrium** `HCC`
     Malignant neoplasm of uterine ligament NOS

   C57.4 Malignant neoplasm of **uterine adnexa**, unspecified `HCC`

   C57.7 Malignant neoplasm of other specified female genital organs `HCC`
     Malignant neoplasm of wolffian body or duct

   C57.8 Malignant neoplasm of **overlapping sites** of female genital organs `HCC`
     Primary malignant neoplasm of two or more contiguous sites of the female genital organs whose point of origin cannot be determined
     Primary tubo-ovarian malignant neoplasm whose point of origin cannot be determined
     Primary utero-ovarian malignant neoplasm whose point of origin cannot be determined

   C57.9 Malignant neoplasm of female genital organ, unspecified `HCC`
     Malignant neoplasm of female genitourinary tract NOS

C58 Malignant neoplasm of **placenta** `HCC` `M`
   `INCLUDES` choriocarcinoma NOS
     chorionepithelioma NOS
   `EXCLUDES 1` chorioadenoma (destruens) (D39.2)
     hydatidiform mole NOS (O01.9)
     invasive hydatidiform mole (D39.2)
     male choriocarcinoma NOS (C62.9-)
     malignant hydatidiform mole (D39.2)

Malignant neoplasms of male genital organs (C60-C63)

`INCLUDES` malignant neoplasm of skin of male genital organs

✓4th **C60** Malignant neoplasm of **penis**

   C60.0 Malignant neoplasm of **prepuce** `HCC`
     Malignant neoplasm of foreskin

   C60.1 Malignant neoplasm of **glans** penis `HCC`

   C60.2 Malignant neoplasm of **body** of penis `HCC`
     Malignant neoplasm of corpus cavernosum

   C60.8 Malignant neoplasm of **overlapping sites** of penis `HCC`

✔ Additional Character Required   ✓x7th Placeholder   Questionable PDx   Manifestation   Unspecified   `UPD` Unacceptable PDx   `H1`-`H14` HAC   `HCC` CMS-HCC Dx   `HIV` HIV Dx

ICD-10-CM 2025   485

Chapter 2. Neoplasms

C60.9   **Malignant neoplasm of penis, unspecified**   HCC
    Malignant neoplasm of skin of penis NOS

C61   **Malignant neoplasm of prostate**   HCC
   Use additional code, if applicable, to identify:
     hormone sensitivity status (Z19.1-Z19.2)
     rising PSA following treatment for malignant neoplasm of prostate (R97.21)
   EXCLUDES 1   *malignant neoplasm of seminal vesicle (C63.7)*
   AHA: 2017,1Q,17

✓4th **C62**   **Malignant neoplasm of testis**
   Use additional code to identify any functional activity

✓5th   **C62.0**   **Malignant neoplasm of undescended testis**
     Malignant neoplasm of ectopic testis
     Malignant neoplasm of retained testis

     C62.00   **Malignant neoplasm of unspecified undescended testis**   HCC

     C62.01   **Malignant neoplasm of undescended right testis**   HCC

     C62.02   **Malignant neoplasm of undescended left testis**   HCC

✓5th   **C62.1**   **Malignant neoplasm of descended testis**
     Malignant neoplasm of scrotal testis

     C62.10   **Malignant neoplasm of unspecified descended testis**   HCC

     C62.11   **Malignant neoplasm of descended right testis**   HCC

     C62.12   **Malignant neoplasm of descended left testis**   HCC

✓5th   **C62.9**   **Malignant neoplasm of testis, unspecified whether descended or undescended**

     C62.90   **Malignant neoplasm of unspecified testis, unspecified whether descended or undescended**   HCC
       Malignant neoplasm of testis NOS

     C62.91   **Malignant neoplasm of right testis, unspecified whether descended or undescended**   HCC

     C62.92   **Malignant neoplasm of left testis, unspecified whether descended or undescended**   HCC

✓4th **C63**   **Malignant neoplasm of other and unspecified male genital organs**

✓5th   **C63.0**   **Malignant neoplasm of epididymis**

     C63.00   **Malignant neoplasm of unspecified epididymis**   HCC

     C63.01   **Malignant neoplasm of right epididymis**   HCC

     C63.02   **Malignant neoplasm of left epididymis**   HCC

✓5th   **C63.1**   **Malignant neoplasm of spermatic cord**

     C63.10   **Malignant neoplasm of unspecified spermatic cord**   HCC

     C63.11   **Malignant neoplasm of right spermatic cord**   HCC

     C63.12   **Malignant neoplasm of left spermatic cord**   HCC

   C63.2   **Malignant neoplasm of scrotum**   HCC
     Malignant neoplasm of skin of scrotum

   C63.7   **Malignant neoplasm of other specified male genital organs**   HCC
     Malignant neoplasm of seminal vesicle
     Malignant neoplasm of tunica vaginalis

   C63.8   **Malignant neoplasm of overlapping sites of male genital organs**   HCC
     Primary malignant neoplasm of two or more contiguous sites of male genital organs whose point of origin cannot be determined

   C63.9   **Malignant neoplasm of male genital organ, unspecified**   HCC
     Malignant neoplasm of male genitourinary tract NOS

Malignant neoplasms of urinary tract (C64-C68)

✓4th **C64**   **Malignant neoplasm of kidney, except renal pelvis**
   EXCLUDES 1   *malignant carcinoid tumor of the kidney (C7A.093)*
     malignant neoplasm of renal calyces (C65.-)
     malignant neoplasm of renal pelvis (C65.-)

   C64.1   **Malignant neoplasm of right kidney, except renal pelvis**   CC HCC

   C64.2   **Malignant neoplasm of left kidney, except renal pelvis**   CC HCC

   C64.9   **Malignant neoplasm of unspecified kidney, except renal pelvis**   CC HCC

✓4th **C65**   **Malignant neoplasm of renal pelvis**
   INCLUDES   malignant neoplasm of pelviureteric junction
     malignant neoplasm of renal calyces

   C65.1   **Malignant neoplasm of right renal pelvis**   CC HCC

   C65.2   **Malignant neoplasm of left renal pelvis**   CC HCC

   C65.9   **Malignant neoplasm of unspecified renal pelvis**   CC HCC

✓4th **C66**   **Malignant neoplasm of ureter**
   EXCLUDES 1   *malignant neoplasm of ureteric orifice of bladder (C67.6)*

   C66.1   **Malignant neoplasm of right ureter**   CC HCC

   C66.2   **Malignant neoplasm of left ureter**   CC HCC

   C66.9   **Malignant neoplasm of unspecified ureter**   CC HCC

✓4th **C67**   **Malignant neoplasm of bladder**
   AHA: 2023,3Q,15

   C67.0   **Malignant neoplasm of trigone of bladder**   HCC

   C67.1   **Malignant neoplasm of dome of bladder**   HCC

   C67.2   **Malignant neoplasm of lateral wall of bladder**   HCC

   C67.3   **Malignant neoplasm of anterior wall of bladder**   HCC

   C67.4   **Malignant neoplasm of posterior wall of bladder**   HCC

   C67.5   **Malignant neoplasm of bladder neck**   HCC
     Malignant neoplasm of internal urethral orifice

   C67.6   **Malignant neoplasm of ureteric orifice**   HCC

   C67.7   **Malignant neoplasm of urachus**   HCC

   C67.8   **Malignant neoplasm of overlapping sites of bladder**   HCC

   C67.9   **Malignant neoplasm of bladder, unspecified**   HCC
     AHA: 2016,1Q,19

✓4th **C68**   **Malignant neoplasm of other and unspecified urinary organs**
   EXCLUDES 1   *malignant neoplasm of female genitourinary tract NOS (C57.9)*
     malignant neoplasm of male genitourinary tract NOS (C63.9)

   C68.0   **Malignant neoplasm of urethra**   CC HCC
     EXCLUDES 1   *malignant neoplasm of urethral orifice of bladder (C67.5)*

   C68.1   **Malignant neoplasm of paraurethral glands**   CC HCC

   C68.8   **Malignant neoplasm of overlapping sites of urinary organs**   CC HCC
     Primary malignant neoplasm of two or more contiguous sites of urinary organs whose point of origin cannot be determined

   C68.9   **Malignant neoplasm of urinary organ, unspecified**   CC HCC
     Malignant neoplasm of urinary system NOS

Malignant neoplasms of eye, brain and other parts of central nervous system (C69-C72)

✓4th **C69**   **Malignant neoplasm of eye and adnexa**
   EXCLUDES 1   *malignant neoplasm of connective tissue of eyelid (C49.0)*
     malignant neoplasm of eyelid (skin) (C43.1-, C44.1-)
     malignant neoplasm of optic nerve (C72.3-)

✓5th   **C69.0**   **Malignant neoplasm of conjunctiva**

     C69.00   **Malignant neoplasm of unspecified conjunctiva**   HCC

     C69.01   **Malignant neoplasm of right conjunctiva**   HCC

     C69.02   **Malignant neoplasm of left conjunctiva**   HCC

✓5th   **C69.1**   **Malignant neoplasm of cornea**

     C69.10   **Malignant neoplasm of unspecified cornea**   HCC

     C69.11   **Malignant neoplasm of right cornea**   HCC

     C69.12   **Malignant neoplasm of left cornea**   HCC

✓5th   **C69.2**   **Malignant neoplasm of retina**
     EXCLUDES 1   *dark area on retina (D49.81)*
       neoplasm of unspecified behavior of retina and choroid (D49.81)
       retinal freckle (D49.81)

     C69.20   **Malignant neoplasm of unspecified retina**   HCC

     C69.21   **Malignant neoplasm of right retina**   HCC

     C69.22   **Malignant neoplasm of left retina**   HCC

✓5th   **C69.3**   **Malignant neoplasm of choroid**

     C69.30   **Malignant neoplasm of unspecified choroid**   HCC

     C69.31   **Malignant neoplasm of right choroid**   HCC

     C69.32   **Malignant neoplasm of left choroid**   HCC

✓5th   **C69.4**   **Malignant neoplasm of ciliary body**

     C69.40   **Malignant neoplasm of unspecified ciliary body**   HCC

     C69.41   **Malignant neoplasm of right ciliary body**   HCC

N Newborn: 0   **P** Pediatric: 0-17   **M** Maternity: 9-64   **A** Adult: 15-124   **UNS** Unspecified Site   **MCC** Major Complication/Comorbidity   **CC** Complication/Comorbidity   **PE** POA Exempt

486   ICD-10-CM 2025

C69.42 Malignant neoplasm of left ciliary body `HCC`

✓5ᵗʰ **C69.5** Malignant neoplasm of lacrimal gland and duct

Malignant neoplasm of lacrimal sac
Malignant neoplasm of nasolacrimal duct

C69.50 Malignant neoplasm of unspecified lacrimal gland and duct `HCC`

C69.51 Malignant neoplasm of right lacrimal gland and duct `HCC`

C69.52 Malignant neoplasm of left lacrimal gland and duct `HCC`

✓5ᵗʰ **C69.6** Malignant neoplasm of orbit

Malignant neoplasm of connective tissue of orbit
Malignant neoplasm of extraocular muscle
Malignant neoplasm of peripheral nerves of orbit
Malignant neoplasm of retrobulbar tissue
Malignant neoplasm of retro-ocular tissue

> *EXCLUDES 1*   *malignant neoplasm of orbital bone (C41.0)*

C69.60 Malignant neoplasm of unspecified orbit `HCC`

C69.61 Malignant neoplasm of right orbit `HCC`

C69.62 Malignant neoplasm of left orbit `HCC`

✓5ᵗʰ **C69.8** Malignant neoplasm of overlapping sites of eye and adnexa

C69.80 Malignant neoplasm of overlapping sites of unspecified eye and adnexa `HCC`

C69.81 Malignant neoplasm of overlapping sites of right eye and adnexa `HCC`

C69.82 Malignant neoplasm of overlapping sites of left eye and adnexa `HCC`

✓5ᵗʰ **C69.9** Malignant neoplasm of unspecified site of eye

Malignant neoplasm of eyeball

C69.90 Malignant neoplasm of unspecified site of unspecified eye `HCC`

C69.91 Malignant neoplasm of unspecified site of right eye `HCC`

C69.92 Malignant neoplasm of unspecified site of left eye `HCC`

✓4ᵗʰ **C70** Malignant neoplasm of meninges

C70.0 Malignant neoplasm of cerebral meninges `CC` `HCC`

C70.1 Malignant neoplasm of spinal meninges `CC` `HCC`

C70.9 Malignant neoplasm of meninges, unspecified `CC` `HCC`

✓4ᵗʰ **C71** Malignant neoplasm of brain

> *EXCLUDES 1*   *malignant neoplasm of cranial nerves (C72.2-C72.5)*
> *retrobulbar malignant neoplasm (C69.6-)*

Lobes of the Brain

Frontal lobe
Parietal lobe
Occipital lobe
Temporal lobe
Brain stem
Cerebellum

C71.0 Malignant neoplasm of cerebrum, except lobes and ventricles `CC` `HCC`

Malignant neoplasm of supratentorial NOS

C71.1 Malignant neoplasm of frontal lobe `CC` `HCC`

C71.2 Malignant neoplasm of temporal lobe `CC` `HCC`

C71.3 Malignant neoplasm of parietal lobe `CC` `HCC`

C71.4 Malignant neoplasm of occipital lobe `CC` `HCC`

C71.5 Malignant neoplasm of cerebral ventricle `CC` `HCC`

> *EXCLUDES 1*   *malignant neoplasm of fourth cerebral ventricle (C71.7)*

C71.6 Malignant neoplasm of cerebellum `CC` `HCC`

C71.7 Malignant neoplasm of brain stem `CC` `HCC`

Malignant neoplasm of fourth cerebral ventricle
Infratentorial malignant neoplasm NOS

C71.8 Malignant neoplasm of overlapping sites of brain `CC` `HCC`

C71.9 Malignant neoplasm of brain, unspecified `CC` `HCC`

> **AHA:** 2014,3Q,3

✓4ᵗʰ **C72** Malignant neoplasm of spinal cord, cranial nerves and other parts of central nervous system

> *EXCLUDES 1*   *malignant neoplasm of meninges (C70.-)*
> *malignant neoplasm of peripheral nerves and autonomic nervous system (C47.-)*

C72.0 Malignant neoplasm of spinal cord `CC` `HCC`

C72.1 Malignant neoplasm of cauda equina `CC` `HCC`

✓5ᵗʰ **C72.2** Malignant neoplasm of olfactory nerve

Malignant neoplasm of olfactory bulb

C72.20 Malignant neoplasm of unspecified olfactory nerve `CC` `HCC`

C72.21 Malignant neoplasm of right olfactory nerve `CC` `HCC`

C72.22 Malignant neoplasm of left olfactory nerve `CC` `HCC`

✓5ᵗʰ **C72.3** Malignant neoplasm of optic nerve

C72.30 Malignant neoplasm of unspecified optic nerve `CC` `HCC`

C72.31 Malignant neoplasm of right optic nerve `CC` `HCC`

C72.32 Malignant neoplasm of left optic nerve `CC` `HCC`

✓5ᵗʰ **C72.4** Malignant neoplasm of acoustic nerve

C72.40 Malignant neoplasm of unspecified acoustic nerve `CC` `HCC`

C72.41 Malignant neoplasm of right acoustic nerve `CC` `HCC`

C72.42 Malignant neoplasm of left acoustic nerve `CC` `HCC`

✓5ᵗʰ **C72.5** Malignant neoplasm of other and unspecified cranial nerves

C72.50 Malignant neoplasm of unspecified cranial nerve `CC` `HCC`

Malignant neoplasm of cranial nerve NOS

C72.59 Malignant neoplasm of other cranial nerves `CC` `HCC`

C72.9 Malignant neoplasm of central nervous system, unspecified `CC` `HCC`

Malignant neoplasm of unspecified site of central nervous system
Malignant neoplasm of nervous system NOS

Malignant neoplasms of thyroid and other endocrine glands (C73-C75)

C73 Malignant neoplasm of thyroid gland `HCC`

> Use additional code to identify any functional activity

✓4ᵗʰ **C74** Malignant neoplasm of adrenal gland

> **TIP:** If an adrenal gland tumor is described as functioning (producing too much of a hormone), additional codes should be assigned to report the functional activity.

✓5ᵗʰ **C74.0** Malignant neoplasm of cortex of adrenal gland

C74.00 Malignant neoplasm of cortex of unspecified adrenal gland `CC` `HCC`

C74.01 Malignant neoplasm of cortex of right adrenal gland `CC` `HCC`

C74.02 Malignant neoplasm of cortex of left adrenal gland `CC` `HCC`

✓5ᵗʰ **C74.1** Malignant neoplasm of medulla of adrenal gland

C74.10 Malignant neoplasm of medulla of unspecified adrenal gland `CC` `HCC`

C74.11 Malignant neoplasm of medulla of right adrenal gland `CC` `HCC`

C74.12 Malignant neoplasm of medulla of left adrenal gland `CC` `HCC`

✓5ᵗʰ **C74.9** Malignant neoplasm of unspecified part of adrenal gland

C74.90 Malignant neoplasm of unspecified part of unspecified adrenal gland `CC` `HCC`

C74.91 Malignant neoplasm of unspecified part of right adrenal gland `CC` `HCC`

C74.92 Malignant neoplasm of unspecified part of left adrenal gland `CC` `HCC`

✔ Additional Character Required   ✓7ᵗʰ Placeholder   Questionable PDx   Manifestation   Unspecified   **UPD** Unacceptable PDx   **H1**-**H14** HAC   **HCC** CMS-HCC Dx   **HIV** HIV Dx

ICD-10-CM 2025   487

C69.42–C74.92

✓4th **C75 Malignant neoplasm of other endocrine glands and related structures**

> EXCLUDES 1   *malignant carcinoid tumors (C7A.Ø-)*
> *malignant neoplasm of adrenal gland (C74.-)*
> *malignant neoplasm of endocrine pancreas (C25.4)*
> *malignant neoplasm of islets of Langerhans (C25.4)*
> *malignant neoplasm of ovary (C56.-)*
> *malignant neoplasm of testis (C62.-)*
> *malignant neoplasm of thymus (C37)*
> *malignant neoplasm of thyroid gland (C73)*
> *malignant neuroendocrine tumors (C7A.-)*

C75.Ø Malignant neoplasm of parathyroid gland `CC` `HCC`

C75.1 Malignant neoplasm of pituitary gland `CC` `HCC`

C75.2 Malignant neoplasm of craniopharyngeal duct `CC` `HCC`

C75.3 Malignant neoplasm of pineal gland `CC` `HCC`

C75.4 Malignant neoplasm of carotid body `CC` `HCC`

C75.5 Malignant neoplasm of aortic body and other paraganglia `CC` `HCC`

C75.8 Malignant neoplasm with pluriglandular involvement, unspecified `CC` `HCC`

C75.9 Malignant neoplasm of endocrine gland, unspecified `CC` `HCC`

Malignant neuroendocrine tumors (C7A)

✓4th **C7A Malignant neuroendocrine tumors**

> Code also any associated multiple endocrine neoplasia [MEN] syndromes (E31.2-)
> Use additional code to identify any associated endocrine syndrome, such as:
> carcinoid syndrome ▶(E34.ØØ)◄
>
> EXCLUDES 2   *malignant pancreatic islet cell tumors (C25.4)*
> *Merkel cell carcinoma (C4A.-)*

AHA: 2019,3Q,7
DEF: Tumors comprised of cells that are capable of producing hormonal syndromes in which the normal hormonal balance required to support body system function is adversely affected.

✓5th **C7A.Ø Malignant carcinoid tumors**

> **AHA:** 2019,3Q,7
> **DEF:** Specific type of slow-growing neuroendocrine tumors. Carcinoid tumors occur most commonly in the hormone producing cells of the gastrointestinal tracts and can also occur in the pancreas, testes, ovaries, or lungs.

C7A.ØØ Malignant carcinoid tumor of unspecified site `CC` `HCC`

✓6th **C7A.Ø1 Malignant carcinoid tumors of the small intestine**

     C7A.Ø1Ø Malignant carcinoid tumor of the duodenum `CC` `HCC`

     C7A.Ø11 Malignant carcinoid tumor of the jejunum `CC` `HCC`

     C7A.Ø12 Malignant carcinoid tumor of the ileum `CC` `HCC`

     C7A.Ø19 Malignant carcinoid tumor of the small intestine, unspecified portion `CC` `HCC`

✓6th **C7A.Ø2 Malignant carcinoid tumors of the appendix, large intestine, and rectum**

     C7A.Ø2Ø Malignant carcinoid tumor of the appendix `CC` `HCC`

     C7A.Ø21 Malignant carcinoid tumor of the cecum `CC` `HCC`

     C7A.Ø22 Malignant carcinoid tumor of the ascending colon `CC` `HCC`

     C7A.Ø23 Malignant carcinoid tumor of the transverse colon `CC` `HCC`

     C7A.Ø24 Malignant carcinoid tumor of the descending colon `CC` `HCC`

     C7A.Ø25 Malignant carcinoid tumor of the sigmoid colon `CC` `HCC`

     C7A.Ø26 Malignant carcinoid tumor of the rectum `CC` `HCC`

     C7A.Ø29 Malignant carcinoid tumor of the large intestine, unspecified portion `CC` `HCC`
         Malignant carcinoid tumor of the colon NOS

✓6th **C7A.Ø9 Malignant carcinoid tumors of other sites**

     C7A.Ø9Ø Malignant carcinoid tumor of the bronchus and lung `CC` `HCC`
         AHA: 2019,1Q,16
         TIP: When documented, assign code I31.31 for associated malignant pericardial effusion. The neoplasm code should be sequenced first.

     C7A.Ø91 Malignant carcinoid tumor of the thymus `CC` `HCC`

     C7A.Ø92 Malignant carcinoid tumor of the stomach `CC` `HCC`

     C7A.Ø93 Malignant carcinoid tumor of the kidney `CC` `HCC`

     C7A.Ø94 Malignant carcinoid tumor of the foregut, unspecified `CC` `HCC`

     C7A.Ø95 Malignant carcinoid tumor of the midgut, unspecified `CC` `HCC`

     C7A.Ø96 Malignant carcinoid tumor of the hindgut, unspecified `CC` `HCC`

     C7A.Ø98 Malignant carcinoid tumors of other sites `CC` `HCC`

C7A.1 Malignant poorly differentiated neuroendocrine tumors `CC` `HCC`
     Malignant poorly differentiated neuroendocrine tumor NOS
     Malignant poorly differentiated neuroendocrine carcinoma, any site
     High grade neuroendocrine carcinoma, any site
     AHA: 2023,1Q,20-21

C7A.8 Other malignant neuroendocrine tumors `CC` `HCC`
     AHA: 2019,3Q,7

Secondary neuroendocrine tumors (C7B)

✓4th **C7B Secondary neuroendocrine tumors**

> Use additional code to identify any functional activity

✓5th **C7B.Ø Secondary carcinoid tumors**

> **AHA:** 2019,3Q,7
> **DEF:** Specific type of slow-growing neuroendocrine tumors. Carcinoid tumors occur most commonly in the hormone producing cells of the gastrointestinal tracts and can also occur in the pancreas, testes, ovaries, or lungs.

C7B.ØØ Secondary carcinoid tumors, unspecified site `HCC`

C7B.Ø1 Secondary carcinoid tumors of distant lymph nodes `CC` `HCC`

C7B.Ø2 Secondary carcinoid tumors of liver `CC` `HCC`

C7B.Ø3 Secondary carcinoid tumors of bone `CC` `HCC`

C7B.Ø4 Secondary carcinoid tumors of peritoneum `CC` `HCC`
     Mesentary metastasis of carcinoid tumor

C7B.Ø9 Secondary carcinoid tumors of other sites `CC` `HCC`

C7B.1 Secondary Merkel cell carcinoma `HCC`
     Merkel cell carcinoma nodal presentation
     Merkel cell carcinoma visceral metastatic presentation

C7B.8 Other secondary neuroendocrine tumors `CC` `HCC`
     AHA: 2024,2Q,10; 2023,1Q,20; 2019,3Q,7

Malignant neoplasms of ill-defined, other secondary and unspecified sites (C76-C8Ø)

✓4th **C76 Malignant neoplasm of other and ill-defined sites**

> EXCLUDES 1   *malignant neoplasm of female genitourinary tract NOS (C57.9)*
> *malignant neoplasm of lymphoid, hematopoietic and related tissue (C81-C96)*
> *malignant neoplasm of male genitourinary tract NOS (C63.9)*
> *malignant neoplasm of skin (C44.-)*
> *malignant neoplasm of unspecified site NOS (C8Ø.1)*

C76.Ø Malignant neoplasm of head, face and neck `HCC`
     Malignant neoplasm of cheek NOS
     Malignant neoplasm of nose NOS

C76.1 Malignant neoplasm of thorax `HCC`
     Intrathoracic malignant neoplasm NOS
     Malignant neoplasm of axilla NOS
     Thoracic malignant neoplasm NOS

C76.2 Malignant neoplasm of abdomen `HCC`

C76.3 **Malignant neoplasm of pelvis** `HCC`
Malignant neoplasm of groin NOS
Malignant neoplasm of sites overlapping systems within the pelvis
Rectovaginal (septum) malignant neoplasm
Rectovesical (septum) malignant neoplasm

√5th **C76.4** **Malignant neoplasm of upper limb**

C76.40 **Malignant neoplasm of unspecified upper limb** `HCC`

C76.41 **Malignant neoplasm of right upper limb** `HCC`

C76.42 **Malignant neoplasm of left upper limb** `HCC`

√5th **C76.5** **Malignant neoplasm of lower limb**

C76.50 **Malignant neoplasm of unspecified lower limb** `HCC`

C76.51 **Malignant neoplasm of right lower limb** `HCC`

C76.52 **Malignant neoplasm of left lower limb** `HCC`

C76.8 **Malignant neoplasm of other specified ill-defined sites** `HCC`
Malignant neoplasm of overlapping ill-defined sites

√4th **C77** **Secondary and unspecified malignant neoplasm of lymph nodes**

> EXCLUDES 1   *malignant neoplasm of lymph nodes, specified as primary (C81-C86, C88, C96.-)*
> *mesentary metastasis of carcinoid tumor (C7B.04)*
> *secondary carcinoid tumors of distant lymph nodes (C7B.01)*

C77.0 **Secondary and unspecified malignant neoplasm of lymph nodes of head, face and neck** `CC` `HCC`
Secondary and unspecified malignant neoplasm of supraclavicular lymph nodes
AHA: 2022,3Q,14

C77.1 **Secondary and unspecified malignant neoplasm of intrathoracic lymph nodes** `CC` `HCC`

C77.2 **Secondary and unspecified malignant neoplasm of intra-abdominal lymph nodes** `CC` `HCC`

C77.3 **Secondary and unspecified malignant neoplasm of axilla and upper limb lymph nodes** `CC` `HCC`
Secondary and unspecified malignant neoplasm of pectoral lymph nodes

C77.4 **Secondary and unspecified malignant neoplasm of inguinal and lower limb lymph nodes** `CC` `HCC`

C77.5 **Secondary and unspecified malignant neoplasm of intrapelvic lymph nodes** `CC` `HCC`

C77.8 **Secondary and unspecified malignant neoplasm of lymph nodes of multiple regions** `CC` `HCC`

C77.9 **Secondary and unspecified malignant neoplasm of lymph node, unspecified** `CC` `HCC`

√4th **C78** **Secondary malignant neoplasm of respiratory and digestive organs**

> EXCLUDES 1   *secondary carcinoid tumors of liver (C7B.02)*
> *secondary carcinoid tumors of peritoneum (C7B.04)*
> EXCLUDES 2   *lymph node metastases (C77.0)*
> **AHA:** 2023,1Q,22

√5th **C78.0** **Secondary malignant neoplasm of lung**
AHA: 2024,2Q,11; 2022,3Q,9; 2019,1Q,16

C78.00 **Secondary malignant neoplasm of unspecified lung** `CC` `HCC`

C78.01 **Secondary malignant neoplasm of right lung** `CC` `HCC`

C78.02 **Secondary malignant neoplasm of left lung** `CC` `HCC`

C78.1 **Secondary malignant neoplasm of mediastinum** `CC` `HCC`

C78.2 **Secondary malignant neoplasm of pleura** `CC` `HCC`

√5th **C78.3** **Secondary malignant neoplasm of other and unspecified respiratory organs**

C78.30 **Secondary malignant neoplasm of unspecified respiratory organ** `CC` `HCC`

C78.39 **Secondary malignant neoplasm of other respiratory organs** `CC` `HCC`

C78.4 **Secondary malignant neoplasm of small intestine** `CC` `HCC`

C78.5 **Secondary malignant neoplasm of large intestine and rectum** `CC` `HCC`

C78.6 **Secondary malignant neoplasm of retroperitoneum and peritoneum** `CC` `HCC`
AHA: 2017,2Q,12

C78.7 **Secondary malignant neoplasm of liver and intrahepatic bile duct** `CC` `HCC`
AHA: 2024,1Q,25; 2022,3Q,14

√5th **C78.8** **Secondary malignant neoplasm of other and unspecified digestive organs**

C78.80 **Secondary malignant neoplasm of unspecified digestive organ** `CC` `HCC`

C78.89 **Secondary malignant neoplasm of other digestive organs** `CC` `HCC`
Code also exocrine pancreatic insufficiency (K86.81)

√4th **C79** **Secondary malignant neoplasm of other and unspecified sites**

> EXCLUDES 1   *secondary carcinoid tumors (C7B.-)*
> *secondary neuroendocrine tumors (C7B.-)*
> **AHA:** 2023,1Q,22

√5th **C79.0** **Secondary malignant neoplasm of kidney and renal pelvis**

C79.00 **Secondary malignant neoplasm of unspecified kidney and renal pelvis** `CC` `HCC`

C79.01 **Secondary malignant neoplasm of right kidney and renal pelvis** `CC` `HCC`

C79.02 **Secondary malignant neoplasm of left kidney and renal pelvis** `CC` `HCC`

√5th **C79.1** **Secondary malignant neoplasm of bladder and other and unspecified urinary organs**

C79.10 **Secondary malignant neoplasm of unspecified urinary organs** `CC` `HCC`

C79.11 **Secondary malignant neoplasm of bladder** `CC` `HCC`
> EXCLUDES 2   *lymph node metastases (C77.0)*

C79.19 **Secondary malignant neoplasm of other urinary organs** `CC` `HCC`

C79.2 **Secondary malignant neoplasm of skin** `CC` `HCC`
> EXCLUDES 1   *secondary Merkel cell carcinoma (C7B.1)*

√5th **C79.3** **Secondary malignant neoplasm of brain and cerebral meninges**

C79.31 **Secondary malignant neoplasm of brain** `CC` `HCC`
AHA: 2022,3Q,9-10

C79.32 **Secondary malignant neoplasm of cerebral meninges** `CC` `HCC`
AHA: 2020,1Q,13

√5th **C79.4** **Secondary malignant neoplasm of other and unspecified parts of nervous system**

C79.40 **Secondary malignant neoplasm of unspecified part of nervous system** `CC` `HCC`

C79.49 **Secondary malignant neoplasm of other parts of nervous system** `CC` `HCC`

√5th **C79.5** **Secondary malignant neoplasm of bone and bone marrow**

> EXCLUDES 1   *secondary carcinoid tumors of bone (C7B.03)*

C79.51 **Secondary malignant neoplasm of bone** `CC` `HCC`
AHA: 2022,3Q,14
TIP: Do not assign in addition to a code from subcategory C90.0 when multiple myeloma is described as metastatic to the bone; bone involvement is integral to multiple myeloma.

C79.52 **Secondary malignant neoplasm of bone marrow** `CC` `HCC`

√5th **C79.6** **Secondary malignant neoplasm of ovary**

C79.60 **Secondary malignant neoplasm of unspecified ovary** `CC` `HCC`

C79.61 **Secondary malignant neoplasm of right ovary** `CC` `HCC`

C79.62 **Secondary malignant neoplasm of left ovary** `CC` `HCC`

C79.63 **Secondary malignant neoplasm of bilateral ovaries** `CC` `HCC`

√5th **C79.7** **Secondary malignant neoplasm of adrenal gland**

C79.70 **Secondary malignant neoplasm of unspecified adrenal gland** `CC` `HCC`

C79.71 **Secondary malignant neoplasm of right adrenal gland** `CC` `HCC`

C79.72 **Secondary malignant neoplasm of left adrenal gland** `CC` `HCC`

√5th **C79.8** **Secondary malignant neoplasm of other specified sites**

C79.81 **Secondary malignant neoplasm of breast** `CC` `HCC`

C79.82 **Secondary malignant neoplasm of genital organs** `CC` `HCC`

C79.89 **Secondary malignant neoplasm of other specified sites** `CC` `HCC`
AHA: 2017,2Q,11

| ✔ Additional Character Required | √x 7th Placeholder | Questionable PDx | Manifestation | Unspecified | UPD Unacceptable PDx | H1 - H14 HAC | HCC CMS-HCC Dx | HIV HIV Dx |

ICD-10-CM 2025   489

Chapter 2. Neoplasms

C76.3–C79.89

C79.9 **Secondary malignant neoplasm of unspecified site** `CC` `HCC`
Metastatic cancer NOS
Metastatic disease NOS
EXCLUDES 1   *carcinomatosis NOS (C80.0)*
generalized cancer NOS (C80.0)
malignant (primary) neoplasm of unspecified site (C80.1)
AHA: 2023,2Q,5

✓4ᵗʰ **C80** **Malignant neoplasm without specification of site**
EXCLUDES 1   *malignant carcinoid tumor of unspecified site (C7A.00)*
malignant neoplasm of specified multiple sites - code to each site

C80.0 **Disseminated malignant neoplasm, unspecified** `CC` `HCC`
Carcinomatosis NOS
Generalized cancer, unspecified site (primary) (secondary)
Generalized malignancy, unspecified site (primary) (secondary)

C80.1 **Malignant (primary) neoplasm, unspecified** `HCC`
Cancer NOS
Cancer unspecified site (primary)
Carcinoma unspecified site (primary)
Malignancy unspecified site (primary)
EXCLUDES 1   *secondary malignant neoplasm of unspecified site (C79.9)*

C80.2 **Malignant neoplasm associated with transplanted organ** `CC` `UPD` `HCC`
Code first complication of transplanted organ (T86.-)
Use additional code to identify the specific malignancy

Malignant neoplasms of lymphoid, hematopoietic and related tissue (C81-C96)

EXCLUDES 2   *Kaposi's sarcoma of lymph nodes (C46.3)*
secondary and unspecified neoplasm of lymph nodes (C77.-)
secondary neoplasm of bone marrow (C79.52)
secondary neoplasm of spleen (C78.89)

✓4ᵗʰ **C81** **Hodgkin lymphoma**
EXCLUDES 1   *personal history of Hodgkin lymphoma (Z85.71)*
AHA: 2023,1Q,22
DEF: Malignant disorder of lymphoid cells characterized by the presence of progressively swollen lymph nodes and spleen that may also involve the liver. A diagnosis of Hodgkin's lymphoma can be confirmed by the presence of Reed-Sternberg cells. *Synonym(s): Hodgkin disease.*

✓5ᵗʰ **C81.0** **Nodular lymphocyte predominant Hodgkin lymphoma**

C81.00 Nodular lymphocyte predominant Hodgkin lymphoma, unspecified site `CC` `HCC`

C81.01 Nodular lymphocyte predominant Hodgkin lymphoma, lymph nodes of head, face, and neck `CC` `HCC`

C81.02 Nodular lymphocyte predominant Hodgkin lymphoma, intrathoracic lymph nodes `CC` `HCC`

C81.03 Nodular lymphocyte predominant Hodgkin lymphoma, intra-abdominal lymph nodes `CC` `HCC`

C81.04 Nodular lymphocyte predominant Hodgkin lymphoma, lymph nodes of axilla and upper limb `CC` `HCC`

C81.05 Nodular lymphocyte predominant Hodgkin lymphoma, lymph nodes of inguinal region and lower limb `CC` `HCC`

C81.06 Nodular lymphocyte predominant Hodgkin lymphoma, intrapelvic lymph nodes `CC` `HCC`

C81.07 Nodular lymphocyte predominant Hodgkin lymphoma, spleen `CC` `HCC`

C81.08 Nodular lymphocyte predominant Hodgkin lymphoma, lymph nodes of multiple sites `CC` `HCC`

C81.09 Nodular lymphocyte predominant Hodgkin lymphoma, extranodal and solid organ sites `CC` `HCC`

C81.0A Nodular lymphocyte predominant Hodgkin lymphoma, in remission `CC`

✓5ᵗʰ **C81.1** **Nodular sclerosis Hodgkin lymphoma**
Nodular sclerosis classical Hodgkin lymphoma

C81.10 Nodular sclerosis Hodgkin lymphoma, unspecified site `CC` `HCC`

C81.11 Nodular sclerosis Hodgkin lymphoma, lymph nodes of head, face, and neck `CC` `HCC`

C81.12 Nodular sclerosis Hodgkin lymphoma, intrathoracic lymph nodes `CC` `HCC`

C81.13 Nodular sclerosis Hodgkin lymphoma, intra-abdominal lymph nodes `CC` `HCC`

C81.14 Nodular sclerosis Hodgkin lymphoma, lymph nodes of axilla and upper limb `CC` `HCC`

C81.15 Nodular sclerosis Hodgkin lymphoma, lymph nodes of inguinal region and lower limb `CC` `HCC`

C81.16 Nodular sclerosis Hodgkin lymphoma, intrapelvic lymph nodes `CC` `HCC`

C81.17 Nodular sclerosis Hodgkin lymphoma, spleen `CC` `HCC`

C81.18 Nodular sclerosis Hodgkin lymphoma, lymph nodes of multiple sites `CC` `HCC`

C81.19 Nodular sclerosis Hodgkin lymphoma, extranodal and solid organ sites `CC` `HCC`

C81.1A Nodular sclerosis Hodgkin lymphoma, in remission `CC`

✓5ᵗʰ **C81.2** **Mixed cellularity Hodgkin lymphoma**
Mixed cellularity classical Hodgkin lymphoma

C81.20 Mixed cellularity Hodgkin lymphoma, unspecified site `CC` `HCC`

C81.21 Mixed cellularity Hodgkin lymphoma, lymph nodes of head, face, and neck `CC` `HCC`

C81.22 Mixed cellularity Hodgkin lymphoma, intrathoracic lymph nodes `CC` `HCC`

C81.23 Mixed cellularity Hodgkin lymphoma, intra-abdominal lymph nodes `CC` `HCC`

C81.24 Mixed cellularity Hodgkin lymphoma, lymph nodes of axilla and upper limb `CC` `HCC`

C81.25 Mixed cellularity Hodgkin lymphoma, lymph nodes of inguinal region and lower limb `CC` `HCC`

C81.26 Mixed cellularity Hodgkin lymphoma, intrapelvic lymph nodes `CC` `HCC`

C81.27 Mixed cellularity Hodgkin lymphoma, spleen `CC` `HCC`

C81.28 Mixed cellularity Hodgkin lymphoma, lymph nodes of multiple sites `CC` `HCC`

C81.29 Mixed cellularity Hodgkin lymphoma, extranodal and solid organ sites `CC` `HCC`

C81.2A Mixed cellularity Hodgkin lymphoma, in remission `CC`

✓5ᵗʰ **C81.3** **Lymphocyte depleted Hodgkin lymphoma**
Lymphocyte depleted classical Hodgkin lymphoma

C81.30 Lymphocyte depleted Hodgkin lymphoma, unspecified site `CC` `HCC`

C81.31 Lymphocyte depleted Hodgkin lymphoma, lymph nodes of head, face, and neck `CC` `HCC`

C81.32 Lymphocyte depleted Hodgkin lymphoma, intrathoracic lymph nodes `CC` `HCC`

C81.33 Lymphocyte depleted Hodgkin lymphoma, intra-abdominal lymph nodes `CC` `HCC`

C81.34 Lymphocyte depleted Hodgkin lymphoma, lymph nodes of axilla and upper limb `CC` `HCC`

C81.35 Lymphocyte depleted Hodgkin lymphoma, lymph nodes of inguinal region and lower limb `CC` `HCC`

C81.36 Lymphocyte depleted Hodgkin lymphoma, intrapelvic lymph nodes `CC` `HCC`

C81.37 Lymphocyte depleted Hodgkin lymphoma, spleen `CC` `HCC`

C81.38 Lymphocyte depleted Hodgkin lymphoma, lymph nodes of multiple sites `CC` `HCC`

C81.39 Lymphocyte depleted Hodgkin lymphoma, extranodal and solid organ sites `CC` `HCC`

C81.3A Lymphocyte depleted Hodgkin lymphoma, in remission `CC`

✓5ᵗʰ **C81.4** **Lymphocyte-rich Hodgkin lymphoma**
Lymphocyte-rich classical Hodgkin lymphoma
EXCLUDES 1   *nodular lymphocyte predominant Hodgkin lymphoma (C81.0-)*

C81.40 Lymphocyte-rich Hodgkin lymphoma, unspecified site `CC` `HCC`

C81.41 Lymphocyte-rich Hodgkin lymphoma, lymph nodes of head, face, and neck `CC` `HCC`

C81.42 Lymphocyte-rich Hodgkin lymphoma, intrathoracic lymph nodes `CC` `HCC`

C81.43 Lymphocyte-rich Hodgkin lymphoma, intra-abdominal lymph nodes `CC` `HCC`

C81.44 Lymphocyte-rich Hodgkin lymphoma, lymph nodes of axilla and upper limb `CC` `HCC`

C81.45 Lymphocyte-rich Hodgkin lymphoma, lymph nodes of inguinal region and lower limb `CC` `HCC`

C81.46 Lymphocyte-rich Hodgkin lymphoma, intrapelvic lymph nodes `CC` `HCC`

C81.47 Lymphocyte-rich Hodgkin lymphoma, spleen `CC` `HCC`

C81.48 Lymphocyte-rich Hodgkin lymphoma, lymph nodes of multiple sites `CC` `HCC`

C81.49 Lymphocyte-rich Hodgkin lymphoma, extranodal and solid organ sites `CC` `HCC`

C81.4A Lymphocyte-rich Hodgkin lymphoma, in remission `CC`

√5th **C81.7** Other Hodgkin lymphoma

Classical Hodgkin lymphoma NOS
Other classical Hodgkin lymphoma

C81.70 Other Hodgkin lymphoma, unspecified site `CC` `HCC`

C81.71 Other Hodgkin lymphoma, lymph nodes of head, face, and neck `CC` `HCC`

C81.72 Other Hodgkin lymphoma, intrathoracic lymph nodes `CC` `HCC`

C81.73 Other Hodgkin lymphoma, intra-abdominal lymph nodes `CC` `HCC`

C81.74 Other Hodgkin lymphoma, lymph nodes of axilla and upper limb `CC` `HCC`

C81.75 Other Hodgkin lymphoma, lymph nodes of inguinal region and lower limb `CC` `HCC`

C81.76 Other Hodgkin lymphoma, intrapelvic lymph nodes `CC` `HCC`

C81.77 Other Hodgkin lymphoma, spleen `CC` `HCC`

C81.78 Other Hodgkin lymphoma, lymph nodes of multiple sites `CC` `HCC`

C81.79 Other Hodgkin lymphoma, extranodal and solid organ sites `CC` `HCC`

C81.7A Other Hodgkin lymphoma, in remission `CC`

√5th **C81.9** Hodgkin lymphoma, unspecified

C81.90 Hodgkin lymphoma, unspecified, unspecified site `CC` `HCC`

C81.91 Hodgkin lymphoma, unspecified, lymph nodes of head, face, and neck `CC` `HCC`

C81.92 Hodgkin lymphoma, unspecified, intrathoracic lymph nodes `CC` `HCC`

C81.93 Hodgkin lymphoma, unspecified, intra-abdominal lymph nodes `CC` `HCC`

C81.94 Hodgkin lymphoma, unspecified, lymph nodes of axilla and upper limb `CC` `HCC`

C81.95 Hodgkin lymphoma, unspecified, lymph nodes of inguinal region and lower limb `CC` `HCC`

C81.96 Hodgkin lymphoma, unspecified, intrapelvic lymph nodes `CC` `HCC`

C81.97 Hodgkin lymphoma, unspecified, spleen `CC` `HCC`

C81.98 Hodgkin lymphoma, unspecified, lymph nodes of multiple sites `CC` `HCC`

C81.99 Hodgkin lymphoma, unspecified, extranodal and solid organ sites `CC` `HCC`

C81.9A Hodgkin lymphoma, unspecified, in remission `CC`

√4th **C82** Follicular lymphoma

INCLUDES   follicular lymphoma with or without diffuse areas
EXCLUDES 1   *mature T/NK-cell lymphomas (C84.-)*
    personal history of non-Hodgkin lymphoma (Z85.72)

AHA: 2023,1Q,22
DEF: Most common subgroup of non-Hodgkin lymphomas (NHL), accounting for 20 to 30 percent of all NHLs. NHL is a B-cell lymphoma that is slow growing and characterized by the circular pattern of malignant cell growth with the cells clustered into identifiable nodules or follicles.

√5th **C82.0** Follicular lymphoma grade I

C82.00 Follicular lymphoma grade I, unspecified site `CC` `HCC`

C82.01 Follicular lymphoma grade I, lymph nodes of head, face, and neck `CC` `HCC`

C82.02 Follicular lymphoma grade I, intrathoracic lymph nodes `CC` `HCC`

C82.03 Follicular lymphoma grade I, intra-abdominal lymph nodes `CC` `HCC`

C82.04 Follicular lymphoma grade I, lymph nodes of axilla and upper limb `CC` `HCC`

C82.05 Follicular lymphoma grade I, lymph nodes of inguinal region and lower limb `CC` `HCC`

C82.06 Follicular lymphoma grade I, intrapelvic lymph nodes `CC` `HCC`

C82.07 Follicular lymphoma grade I, spleen `CC` `HCC`

C82.08 Follicular lymphoma grade I, lymph nodes of multiple sites `CC` `HCC`

C82.09 Follicular lymphoma grade I, extranodal and solid organ sites `CC` `HCC`

C82.0A Follicular lymphoma grade I, in remission `CC`

√5th **C82.1** Follicular lymphoma grade II

C82.10 Follicular lymphoma grade II, unspecified site `CC` `HCC`

C82.11 Follicular lymphoma grade II, lymph nodes of head, face, and neck `CC` `HCC`

C82.12 Follicular lymphoma grade II, intrathoracic lymph nodes `CC` `HCC`

C82.13 Follicular lymphoma grade II, intra-abdominal lymph nodes `CC` `HCC`

C82.14 Follicular lymphoma grade II, lymph nodes of axilla and upper limb `CC` `HCC`

C82.15 Follicular lymphoma grade II, lymph nodes of inguinal region and lower limb `CC` `HCC`

C82.16 Follicular lymphoma grade II, intrapelvic lymph nodes `CC` `HCC`

C82.17 Follicular lymphoma grade II, spleen `CC` `HCC`

C82.18 Follicular lymphoma grade II, lymph nodes of multiple sites `CC` `HCC`

C82.19 Follicular lymphoma grade II, extranodal and solid organ sites `CC` `HCC`

C82.1A Follicular lymphoma grade II, in remission `CC`

√5th **C82.2** Follicular lymphoma grade III, unspecified

C82.20 Follicular lymphoma grade III, unspecified, unspecified site `CC` `HCC`

C82.21 Follicular lymphoma grade III, unspecified, lymph nodes of head, face, and neck `CC` `HCC`

C82.22 Follicular lymphoma grade III, unspecified, intrathoracic lymph nodes `CC` `HCC`

C82.23 Follicular lymphoma grade III, unspecified, intra-abdominal lymph nodes `CC` `HCC`

C82.24 Follicular lymphoma grade III, unspecified, lymph nodes of axilla and upper limb `CC` `HCC`

C82.25 Follicular lymphoma grade III, unspecified, lymph nodes of inguinal region and lower limb `CC` `HCC`

C82.26 Follicular lymphoma grade III, unspecified, intrapelvic lymph nodes `CC` `HCC`

C82.27 Follicular lymphoma grade III, unspecified, spleen `CC` `HCC`

C82.28 Follicular lymphoma grade III, unspecified, lymph nodes of multiple sites `CC` `HCC`

C82.29 Follicular lymphoma grade III, unspecified, extranodal and solid organ sites `CC` `HCC`

C82.2A Follicular lymphoma grade III, unspecified, in remission `CC`

√5th **C82.3** Follicular lymphoma grade IIIa

C82.30 Follicular lymphoma grade IIIa, unspecified site `CC` `HCC`

C82.31 Follicular lymphoma grade IIIa, lymph nodes of head, face, and neck `CC` `HCC`

C82.32 Follicular lymphoma grade IIIa, intrathoracic lymph nodes `CC` `HCC`

C82.33 Follicular lymphoma grade IIIa, intra-abdominal lymph nodes `CC` `HCC`

C82.34 Follicular lymphoma grade IIIa, lymph nodes of axilla and upper limb `CC` `HCC`

C82.35 Follicular lymphoma grade IIIa, lymph nodes of inguinal region and lower limb `CC` `HCC`

C82.36 Follicular lymphoma grade IIIa, intrapelvic lymph nodes `CC` `HCC`

C82.37 Follicular lymphoma grade IIIa, spleen `CC` `HCC`

C82.38 Follicular lymphoma grade IIIa, lymph nodes of multiple sites `CC` `HCC`

C82.39 Follicular lymphoma grade IIIa, extranodal and solid organ sites `CC` `HCC`

C82.3A Follicular lymphoma grade IIIa, in remission `CC`

√5th **C82.4** Follicular lymphoma grade IIIb

C82.40 Follicular lymphoma grade IIIb, unspecified site `CC` `HCC`

✓ Additional Character Required   √x7th Placeholder   **Questionable PDx**   Manifestation   Unspecified   `UPD` Unacceptable PDx   `H1`-`H14` HAC   `HCC` CMS-HCC Dx   `HIV` HIV Dx

Chapter 2. Neoplasms

C82.41–C83.14

C82.41 Follicular lymphoma grade IIIb, lymph nodes of head, face, and neck `CC` `HCC`

C82.42 Follicular lymphoma grade IIIb, intrathoracic lymph nodes

C82.43 Follicular lymphoma grade IIIb, intra-abdominal lymph nodes `CC` `HCC`

C82.44 Follicular lymphoma grade IIIb, lymph nodes of axilla and upper limb `CC` `HCC`

C82.45 Follicular lymphoma grade IIIb, lymph nodes of inguinal region and lower limb

C82.46 Follicular lymphoma grade IIIb, intrapelvic lymph nodes

C82.47 Follicular lymphoma grade IIIb, spleen `CC` `HCC`

C82.48 Follicular lymphoma grade IIIb, lymph nodes of multiple sites `CC` `HCC`

C82.49 Follicular lymphoma grade IIIb, extranodal and solid organ sites `CC` `HCC`

C82.4A Follicular lymphoma grade IIIb, in remission `CC`

√5th **C82.5 Diffuse follicle center lymphoma**

C82.50 Diffuse follicle center lymphoma, unspecified site `HIV` `CC` `HCC`

C82.51 Diffuse follicle center lymphoma, lymph nodes of head, face, and neck `HIV` `CC` `HCC`

C82.52 Diffuse follicle center lymphoma, intrathoracic lymph nodes `HIV` `CC`

C82.53 Diffuse follicle center lymphoma, intra-abdominal lymph nodes

C82.54 Diffuse follicle center lymphoma, lymph nodes of axilla and upper limb `HIV` `CC` `HCC`

C82.55 Diffuse follicle center lymphoma, lymph nodes of inguinal region and lower limb `HIV` `CC` `HCC`

C82.56 Diffuse follicle center lymphoma, intrapelvic lymph nodes `HIV` `CC` `HCC`

C82.57 Diffuse follicle center lymphoma, spleen `HIV` `CC` `HCC`

C82.58 Diffuse follicle center lymphoma, lymph nodes of multiple sites `HIV` `CC` `HCC`

C82.59 Diffuse follicle center lymphoma, extranodal and solid organ sites `HIV` `CC` `HCC`

C82.5A Diffuse follicle center lymphoma, in remission `CC`

√5th **C82.6 Cutaneous follicle center lymphoma**

C82.60 Cutaneous follicle center lymphoma, unspecified site `CC` `HCC`

C82.61 Cutaneous follicle center lymphoma, lymph nodes of head, face, and neck

C82.62 Cutaneous follicle center lymphoma, intrathoracic lymph nodes

C82.63 Cutaneous follicle center lymphoma, intra-abdominal lymph nodes

C82.64 Cutaneous follicle center lymphoma, lymph nodes of axilla and upper limb

C82.65 Cutaneous follicle center lymphoma, lymph nodes of inguinal region and lower limb

C82.66 Cutaneous follicle center lymphoma, intrapelvic lymph nodes `CC` `HCC`

C82.67 Cutaneous follicle center lymphoma, spleen `CC` `HCC`

C82.68 Cutaneous follicle center lymphoma, lymph nodes of multiple sites `CC` `HCC`

C82.69 Cutaneous follicle center lymphoma, extranodal and solid organ sites `CC` `HCC`

C82.6A Cutaneous follicle center lymphoma, in remission `CC`

√5th **C82.8 Other types of follicular lymphoma**

C82.80 Other types of follicular lymphoma, unspecified site `CC` `HCC`

C82.81 Other types of follicular lymphoma, lymph nodes of head, face, and neck `CC` `HCC`

C82.82 Other types of follicular lymphoma, intrathoracic lymph nodes `CC` `HCC`

C82.83 Other types of follicular lymphoma, intra-abdominal lymph nodes `CC` `HCC`

C82.84 Other types of follicular lymphoma, lymph nodes of axilla and upper limb `CC` `HCC`

C82.85 Other types of follicular lymphoma, lymph nodes of inguinal region and lower limb `CC` `HCC`

C82.86 Other types of follicular lymphoma, intrapelvic lymph nodes `CC` `HCC`

C82.87 Other types of follicular lymphoma, spleen `CC` `HCC`

C82.88 Other types of follicular lymphoma, lymph nodes of multiple sites `CC` `HCC`

C82.89 Other types of follicular lymphoma, extranodal and solid organ sites `CC` `HCC`

C82.8A Other types of follicular lymphoma, in remission `CC`

√5th **C82.9 Follicular lymphoma, unspecified**

C82.90 Follicular lymphoma, unspecified, unspecified site `CC` `HCC`

C82.91 Follicular lymphoma, unspecified, lymph nodes of head, face, and neck `CC` `HCC`

C82.92 Follicular lymphoma, unspecified, intrathoracic lymph nodes `CC` `HCC`

C82.93 Follicular lymphoma, unspecified, intra-abdominal lymph nodes `CC` `HCC`

C82.94 Follicular lymphoma, unspecified, lymph nodes of axilla and upper limb `CC` `HCC`

C82.95 Follicular lymphoma, unspecified, lymph nodes of inguinal region and lower limb `CC` `HCC`

C82.96 Follicular lymphoma, unspecified, intrapelvic lymph nodes `CC` `HCC`

C82.97 Follicular lymphoma, unspecified, spleen `CC` `HCC`

C82.98 Follicular lymphoma, unspecified, lymph nodes of multiple sites `CC` `HCC`

C82.99 Follicular lymphoma, unspecified, extranodal and solid organ sites `CC` `HCC`

C82.9A Follicular lymphoma, unspecified, in remission `CC`

√4th **C83 Non-follicular lymphoma**

     EXCLUDES 1   personal history of non-Hodgkin lymphoma (Z85.72)

     AHA: 2023,1Q,22

√5th **C83.0 Small cell B-cell lymphoma**

     Lymphoplasmacytic lymphoma
     Nodal marginal zone lymphoma
     Non-leukemic variant of B-CLL
     Splenic marginal zone lymphoma

     EXCLUDES 1   chronic lymphocytic leukemia (C91.1)
                 mature T/NK-cell lymphomas (C84.-)
                 Waldenstrom macroglobulinemia ►(C88.00)◄

     AHA: 2023,1Q,18
     DEF: Nonfollicular lymphoma that is rare, slow growing, and usually found in the older population.

C83.00 Small cell B-cell lymphoma, unspecified site `HIV` `CC` `HCC`

C83.01 Small cell B-cell lymphoma, lymph nodes of head, face, and neck `HIV` `CC` `HCC`

C83.02 Small cell B-cell lymphoma, intrathoracic lymph nodes `HIV` `CC` `HCC`

C83.03 Small cell B-cell lymphoma, intra-abdominal lymph nodes `HIV` `CC` `HCC`

C83.04 Small cell B-cell lymphoma, lymph nodes of axilla and upper limb `HIV` `CC` `HCC`

C83.05 Small cell B-cell lymphoma, lymph nodes of inguinal region and lower limb `HIV` `CC` `HCC`

C83.06 Small cell B-cell lymphoma, intrapelvic lymph nodes `HIV` `CC` `HCC`

C83.07 Small cell B-cell lymphoma, spleen `HIV` `CC` `HCC`

C83.08 Small cell B-cell lymphoma, lymph nodes of multiple sites `HIV` `CC` `HCC`

C83.09 Small cell B-cell lymphoma, extranodal and solid organ sites `HIV` `CC` `HCC`

C83.0A Small cell B-cell lymphoma, in remission `CC`

√5th **C83.1 Mantle cell lymphoma**

     Centrocytic lymphoma
     Malignant lymphomatous polyposis
     DEF: Rare form of B-cell non-Hodgkin lymphoma named for the location of the tumor cell production, the mantle zone of the lymph nodes.

C83.10 Mantle cell lymphoma, unspecified site `HIV` `CC` `HCC`

C83.11 Mantle cell lymphoma, lymph nodes of head, face, and neck `HIV` `CC` `HCC`

C83.12 Mantle cell lymphoma, intrathoracic lymph nodes `HIV` `CC` `HCC`

C83.13 Mantle cell lymphoma, intra-abdominal lymph nodes `HIV` `CC` `HCC`

C83.14 Mantle cell lymphoma, lymph nodes of axilla and upper limb `HIV` `CC` `HCC`

N Newborn: 0   P Pediatric: 0-17   M Maternity: 9-64   A Adult: 15-124   UNS Unspecified Site   MCC Major Complication/Comorbidity   CC Complication/Comorbidity   PE POA Exempt

492   ICD-10-CM 2025

C83.15   **Mantle cell lymphoma, lymph nodes of inguinal region and lower limb** `HIV` `CC` `HCC`

C83.16   **Mantle cell lymphoma, intrapelvic lymph nodes** `HIV` `CC` `HCC`

C83.17   **Mantle cell lymphoma, spleen** `HIV` `CC` `HCC`

C83.18   **Mantle cell lymphoma, lymph nodes of multiple sites** `HIV` `CC` `HCC`

C83.19   **Mantle cell lymphoma, extranodal and solid organ sites** `HIV` `CC` `HCC`

● **C83.1A**   **Mantle cell lymphoma, in remission** `CC`
Centrocytic lymphoma, in remission

√5th **C83.3**   **Diffuse large B-cell lymphoma**

Anaplastic diffuse large B-cell lymphoma
CD30-positive diffuse large B-cell lymphoma
Centroblastic diffuse large B-cell lymphoma
Diffuse large B-cell lymphoma, subtype not specified
Immunoblastic diffuse large B-cell lymphoma
Plasmablastic diffuse large B-cell lymphoma
T-cell rich diffuse large B-cell lymphoma

> **EXCLUDES 1**   *mediastinal (thymic) large B-cell lymphoma (C85.2-)*
> *mature T/NK-cell lymphomas (C84.-)*

DEF: Nonfollicular lymphoma that is one of the more common types of lymphoma. This cancer is fast growing and affects any age but is found mostly in the older population.

C83.30   **Diffuse large B-cell lymphoma, unspecified site** `HIV` `CC` `HCC`

C83.31   **Diffuse large B-cell lymphoma, lymph nodes of head, face, and neck** `HIV` `CC` `HCC`

C83.32   **Diffuse large B-cell lymphoma, intrathoracic lymph nodes** `HIV` `CC` `HCC`

C83.33   **Diffuse large B-cell lymphoma, intra-abdominal lymph nodes** `HIV` `CC` `HCC`

C83.34   **Diffuse large B-cell lymphoma, lymph nodes of axilla and upper limb** `HIV` `CC` `HCC`

C83.35   **Diffuse large B-cell lymphoma, lymph nodes of inguinal region and lower limb** `HIV` `CC` `HCC`

C83.36   **Diffuse large B-cell lymphoma, intrapelvic lymph nodes** `HIV` `CC` `HCC`

C83.37   **Diffuse large B-cell lymphoma, spleen** `HIV` `CC` `HCC`

C83.38   **Diffuse large B-cell lymphoma, lymph nodes of multiple sites** `HIV` `CC` `HCC`
AHA: 2023,1Q,22

▲   √6th **C83.39**   **Diffuse large B-cell lymphoma, extranodal and solid organ sites**
AHA: 2023,1Q,22

● **C83.390**   **Primary central nervous system lymphoma** `CC`
PCNSL of brain
PCNSL of meninges
PCNSL of spinal cord
PCNSL NOS

> **EXCLUDES 1**   *primary central nervous system lymphoma, Burkitt (C83.79)*
> *primary central nervous system lymphoma, lymphoblastic (C83.59)*
> *primary central nervous system lymphoma, other (C83.89)*
> *primary central nervous system lymphoma, peripheral T-cell (C84.49)*

● **C83.398**   **Diffuse large B-cell lymphoma of other extranodal and solid organ sites** `CC`

● **C83.3A**   **Diffuse large B-cell lymphoma, in remission** `CC`

√5th **C83.5**   **Lymphoblastic (diffuse) lymphoma**

B-precursor lymphoma
Lymphoblastic B-cell lymphoma
Lymphoblastic lymphoma NOS
Lymphoblastic T-cell lymphoma
T-precursor lymphoma

DEF: Type of non-Hodgkin lymphoma considered lymphoma or leukemia—the determination is made based on the amount of bone marrow involvement. The cells are small to medium immature T-cells that often originate in the thymus where many of the T-cells are made.

C83.50   **Lymphoblastic (diffuse) lymphoma, unspecified site** `CC` `HCC`

C83.51   **Lymphoblastic (diffuse) lymphoma, lymph nodes of head, face, and neck** `CC` `HCC`

C83.52   **Lymphoblastic (diffuse) lymphoma, intrathoracic lymph nodes** `CC` `HCC`

C83.53   **Lymphoblastic (diffuse) lymphoma, intra-abdominal lymph nodes** `CC` `HCC`

C83.54   **Lymphoblastic (diffuse) lymphoma, lymph nodes of axilla and upper limb** `CC` `HCC`

C83.55   **Lymphoblastic (diffuse) lymphoma, lymph nodes of inguinal region and lower limb** `CC` `HCC`

C83.56   **Lymphoblastic (diffuse) lymphoma, intrapelvic lymph nodes** `CC` `HCC`

C83.57   **Lymphoblastic (diffuse) lymphoma, spleen** `CC` `HCC`

C83.58   **Lymphoblastic (diffuse) lymphoma, lymph nodes of multiple sites** `CC` `HCC`

C83.59   **Lymphoblastic (diffuse) lymphoma, extranodal and solid organ sites** `CC` `HCC`

● **C83.5A**   **Lymphoblastic (diffuse) lymphoma, in remission** `CC`

√5th **C83.7**   **Burkitt lymphoma**

Atypical Burkitt lymphoma
Burkitt-like lymphoma

> **EXCLUDES 1**   *mature B-cell leukemia Burkitt type (C91.A-)*

DEF: Malignancy of the lymphatic system, most often seen as a large bone-deteriorating lesion within the jaw or as an abdominal mass. It is a form of non-Hodgkin's lymphoma and is recognized as the fastest growing human tumor.

C83.70   **Burkitt lymphoma, unspecified site** `HIV` `CC` `HCC`

C83.71   **Burkitt lymphoma, lymph nodes of head, face, and neck** `HIV` `CC` `HCC`

C83.72   **Burkitt lymphoma, intrathoracic lymph nodes** `HIV` `CC` `HCC`

C83.73   **Burkitt lymphoma, intra-abdominal lymph nodes** `HIV` `CC` `HCC`

C83.74   **Burkitt lymphoma, lymph nodes of axilla and upper limb** `HIV` `CC` `HCC`

C83.75   **Burkitt lymphoma, lymph nodes of inguinal region and lower limb** `HIV` `CC` `HCC`

C83.76   **Burkitt lymphoma, intrapelvic lymph nodes** `HIV` `CC` `HCC`

C83.77   **Burkitt lymphoma, spleen** `HIV` `CC` `HCC`

C83.78   **Burkitt lymphoma, lymph nodes of multiple sites** `HIV` `CC` `HCC`

C83.79   **Burkitt lymphoma, extranodal and solid organ sites** `HIV` `CC` `HCC`

● **C83.7A**   **Burkitt lymphoma, in remission** `CC`

√5th **C83.8**   **Other non-follicular lymphoma**

Intravascular large B-cell lymphoma
Lymphoid granulomatosis
Primary effusion B-cell lymphoma

> **EXCLUDES 1**   *mediastinal (thymic) large B-cell lymphoma (C85.2-)*
> *T-cell rich B-cell lymphoma (C83.3-)*

C83.80   **Other non-follicular lymphoma, unspecified site** `HIV` `CC` `HCC`

C83.81   **Other non-follicular lymphoma, lymph nodes of head, face, and neck** `HIV` `CC` `HCC`

C83.82   **Other non-follicular lymphoma, intrathoracic lymph nodes** `HIV` `CC` `HCC`

C83.83   **Other non-follicular lymphoma, intra-abdominal lymph nodes** `HIV` `CC` `HCC`

C83.84   **Other non-follicular lymphoma, lymph nodes of axilla and upper limb** `HIV` `CC` `HCC`

C83.85   **Other non-follicular lymphoma, lymph nodes of inguinal region and lower limb** `HIV` `CC` `HCC`

C83.86   **Other non-follicular lymphoma, intrapelvic lymph nodes** `HIV` `CC` `HCC`

C83.87   **Other non-follicular lymphoma, spleen** `HIV` `CC` `HCC`

C83.88   **Other non-follicular lymphoma, lymph nodes of multiple sites** `HIV` `CC` `HCC`

C83.89   **Other non-follicular lymphoma, extranodal and solid organ sites** `HIV` `CC` `HCC`

● **C83.8A**   **Other non-follicular lymphoma, in remission** `CC`

√5th **C83.9**   **Non-follicular (diffuse) lymphoma, unspecified**

C83.90   **Non-follicular (diffuse) lymphoma, unspecified, unspecified site** `HIV` `CC` `HCC`

C83.91   **Non-follicular (diffuse) lymphoma, unspecified, lymph nodes of head, face, and neck** `HIV` `CC` `HCC`

C83.92 Non-follicular (diffuse) lymphoma, unspecified, intrathoracic lymph nodes `HIV` `CC` `HCC`

C83.93 Non-follicular (diffuse) lymphoma, unspecified, intra-abdominal lymph nodes `HIV` `CC` `HCC`

C83.94 Non-follicular (diffuse) lymphoma, unspecified, lymph nodes of axilla and upper limb `HIV` `CC` `HCC`

C83.95 Non-follicular (diffuse) lymphoma, unspecified, lymph nodes of inguinal region and lower limb `HIV` `CC` `HCC`

C83.96 Non-follicular (diffuse) lymphoma, unspecified, intrapelvic lymph nodes `HIV` `CC` `HCC`

C83.97 Non-follicular (diffuse) lymphoma, unspecified, spleen `HIV` `CC` `HCC`

C83.98 Non-follicular (diffuse) lymphoma, unspecified, lymph nodes of multiple sites `HIV` `CC` `HCC`

C83.99 Non-follicular (diffuse) lymphoma, unspecified, extranodal and solid organ sites `HIV` `CC` `HCC`

● **C83.9A** Non-follicular (diffuse) lymphoma, unspecified, in remission `CC`

√4th **C84** **Mature T/NK-cell lymphomas**

     EXCLUDES 1   *personal history of non-Hodgkin lymphoma (Z85.72)*

     AHA: 2023,1Q,22

√5th **C84.0** **Mycosis fungoides**

     EXCLUDES 1   *peripheral T-cell lymphoma, not elsewhere classified (C84.4-)*

     DEF: Most common form of cutaneous T-cell lymphoma. A type of non-Hodgkin lymphoma in which white blood cells become cancerous and affect the skin and sometimes internal organs. *Synonym(s): Alibert-Bazin syndrome.*

C84.00 Mycosis fungoides, unspecified site `CC` `HCC`

C84.01 Mycosis fungoides, lymph nodes of head, face, and neck `CC` `HCC`

C84.02 Mycosis fungoides, intrathoracic lymph nodes `CC` `HCC`

C84.03 Mycosis fungoides, intra-abdominal lymph nodes `CC` `HCC`

C84.04 Mycosis fungoides, lymph nodes of axilla and upper limb `CC` `HCC`

C84.05 Mycosis fungoides, lymph nodes of inguinal region and lower limb `CC` `HCC`

C84.06 Mycosis fungoides, intrapelvic lymph nodes `CC` `HCC`

C84.07 Mycosis fungoides, spleen `CC` `HCC`

C84.08 Mycosis fungoides, lymph nodes of multiple sites `CC` `HCC`

C84.09 Mycosis fungoides, extranodal and solid organ sites `CC` `HCC`

● **C84.0A** Mycosis fungoides, in remission `CC`

√5th **C84.1** **Sezary disease**

     DEF: Extension of mycosis fungoides that affects the blood and all of the skin, appearing as sunburn, rather than patches. It spreads to the lymph nodes and is often linked to a weakened immune system.

C84.10 Sezary disease, unspecified site `CC` `HCC`

C84.11 Sezary disease, lymph nodes of head, face, and neck `CC` `HCC`

C84.12 Sezary disease, intrathoracic lymph nodes `CC` `HCC`

C84.13 Sezary disease, intra-abdominal lymph nodes `CC` `HCC`

C84.14 Sezary disease, lymph nodes of axilla and upper limb `CC` `HCC`

C84.15 Sezary disease, lymph nodes of inguinal region and lower limb `CC` `HCC`

C84.16 Sezary disease, intrapelvic lymph nodes `CC` `HCC`

C84.17 Sezary disease, spleen `CC` `HCC`

C84.18 Sezary disease, lymph nodes of multiple sites `CC` `HCC`

C84.19 Sezary disease, extranodal and solid organ sites `CC` `HCC`

C84.1A Sezary disease, in remission `CC`

√5th **C84.4** **Peripheral T-cell lymphoma, not elsewhere classified**

     Lennert's lymphoma
     Lymphoepithelioid lymphoma
     Mature T-cell lymphoma, not elsewhere classified

C84.40 Peripheral T-cell lymphoma, not elsewhere classified, unspecified site `HIV` `CC` `HCC`

C84.41 Peripheral T-cell lymphoma, not elsewhere classified, lymph nodes of head, face, and neck `HIV` `CC` `HCC`

C84.42 Peripheral T-cell lymphoma, not elsewhere classified, intrathoracic lymph nodes `HIV` `CC` `HCC`

C84.43 Peripheral T-cell lymphoma, not elsewhere classified, intra-abdominal lymph nodes `HIV` `CC` `HCC`

C84.44 Peripheral T-cell lymphoma, not elsewhere classified, lymph nodes of axilla and upper limb `HIV` `CC` `HCC`

C84.45 Peripheral T-cell lymphoma, not elsewhere classified, lymph nodes of inguinal region and lower limb `HIV` `CC` `HCC`

C84.46 Peripheral T-cell lymphoma, not elsewhere classified, intrapelvic lymph nodes `HIV` `CC` `HCC`

C84.47 Peripheral T-cell lymphoma, not elsewhere classified, spleen `HIV` `CC` `HCC`

C84.48 Peripheral T-cell lymphoma, not elsewhere classified, lymph nodes of multiple sites `HIV` `CC` `HCC`

C84.49 Peripheral T-cell lymphoma, not elsewhere classified, extranodal and solid organ sites `HIV` `CC` `HCC`

● **C84.4A** Peripheral T-cell lymphoma, not elsewhere classified, in remission `CC`

√5th **C84.6** **Anaplastic large cell lymphoma, ALK-positive**

     Anaplastic large cell lymphoma, CD30-positive

C84.60 Anaplastic large cell lymphoma, ALK-positive, unspecified site `HIV` `CC` `HCC`

C84.61 Anaplastic large cell lymphoma, ALK-positive, lymph nodes of head, face, and neck `HIV` `CC` `HCC`

C84.62 Anaplastic large cell lymphoma, ALK-positive, intrathoracic lymph nodes `HIV` `CC` `HCC`

C84.63 Anaplastic large cell lymphoma, ALK-positive, intra-abdominal lymph nodes `HIV` `CC` `HCC`

C84.64 Anaplastic large cell lymphoma, ALK-positive, lymph nodes of axilla and upper limb `HIV` `CC` `HCC`

C84.65 Anaplastic large cell lymphoma, ALK-positive, lymph nodes of inguinal region and lower limb `HIV` `CC` `HCC`

C84.66 Anaplastic large cell lymphoma, ALK-positive, intrapelvic lymph nodes `HIV` `CC` `HCC`

C84.67 Anaplastic large cell lymphoma, ALK-positive, spleen `HIV` `CC` `HCC`

C84.68 Anaplastic large cell lymphoma, ALK-positive, lymph nodes of multiple sites `HIV` `CC` `HCC`

C84.69 Anaplastic large cell lymphoma, ALK-positive, extranodal and solid organ sites `HIV` `CC` `HCC`

● **C84.6A** Anaplastic large cell lymphoma, ALK-positive, in remission `CC`

√5th **C84.7** **Anaplastic large cell lymphoma, ALK-negative**

     EXCLUDES 1   *primary cutaneous CD30-positive T-cell proliferations (C86.6-)*

C84.70 Anaplastic large cell lymphoma, ALK-negative, unspecified site `HIV` `CC` `HCC`

C84.71 Anaplastic large cell lymphoma, ALK-negative, lymph nodes of head, face, and neck `HIV` `CC` `HCC`

C84.72 Anaplastic large cell lymphoma, ALK-negative, intrathoracic lymph nodes `HIV` `CC` `HCC`

C84.73 Anaplastic large cell lymphoma, ALK-negative, intra-abdominal lymph nodes `HIV` `CC` `HCC`

C84.74 Anaplastic large cell lymphoma, ALK-negative, lymph nodes of axilla and upper limb `HIV` `CC` `HCC`

C84.75 Anaplastic large cell lymphoma, ALK-negative, lymph nodes of inguinal region and lower limb `HIV` `CC` `HCC`

C84.76 Anaplastic large cell lymphoma, ALK-negative, intrapelvic lymph nodes `HIV` `CC` `HCC`

C84.77 Anaplastic large cell lymphoma, ALK-negative, spleen `HIV` `CC` `HCC`

C84.78 Anaplastic large cell lymphoma, ALK-negative, lymph nodes of multiple sites `HIV` `CC` `HCC`

C84.79 Anaplastic large cell lymphoma, ALK-negative, extranodal and solid organ sites `HIV` `CC` `HCC`

C84.7A Anaplastic large cell lymphoma, ALK-negative, breast `HIV` `CC` `HCC`

     Breast implant associated anaplastic large cell lymphoma (BIA-ALCL)

     Use additional code to identify:
       breast implant status (Z98.82)
       personal history of breast implant removal (Z98.86)

     AHA: 2021,4Q,6

C84.7B   Anaplastic large cell lymphoma, ALK-negative, in remission   `CC`

✓5ᵗʰ C84.A   Cutaneous T-cell lymphoma, unspecified
    AHA: 2021,2Q,6

C84.A0   Cutaneous T-cell lymphoma, unspecified, unspecified site   `HIV` `CC` `HCC`

C84.A1   Cutaneous T-cell lymphoma, unspecified lymph nodes of head, face, and neck   `HIV` `CC` `HCC`

C84.A2   Cutaneous T-cell lymphoma, unspecified, intrathoracic lymph nodes   `HIV` `CC` `HCC`

C84.A3   Cutaneous T-cell lymphoma, unspecified, intra-abdominal lymph nodes   `HIV` `CC` `HCC`

C84.A4   Cutaneous T-cell lymphoma, unspecified, lymph nodes of axilla and upper limb   `HIV` `CC` `HCC`

C84.A5   Cutaneous T-cell lymphoma, unspecified, lymph nodes of inguinal region and lower limb   `HIV` `CC` `HCC`

C84.A6   Cutaneous T-cell lymphoma, unspecified, intrapelvic lymph nodes   `HIV` `CC` `HCC`

C84.A7   Cutaneous T-cell lymphoma, unspecified, spleen   `HIV` `CC` `HCC`

C84.A8   Cutaneous T-cell lymphoma, unspecified, lymph nodes of multiple sites   `HIV` `CC` `HCC`

C84.A9   Cutaneous T-cell lymphoma, unspecified, extranodal and solid organ sites   `HIV` `CC` `HCC`

C84.AA   Cutaneous T-cell lymphoma, unspecified, in remission   `CC`

✓5ᵗʰ C84.Z   Other mature T/NK-cell lymphomas

> **NOTE**   If T-cell lineage or involvement is mentioned in conjunction with a specific lymphoma, code to the more specific description.
>
> *EXCLUDES 1*   angioimmunoblastic T-cell lymphoma ▶(C86.50)◀
> blastic NK-cell lymphoma ▶(C86.40)◀
> enteropathy-type T-cell lymphoma ▶(C86.20)◀
> extranodal NK-cell lymphoma, nasal type ▶(C86.00)◀
> hepatosplenic T-cell lymphoma ▶(C86.10)◀
> primary cutaneous CD30-positive T-cell proliferations ▶(C86.60)◀
> subcutaneous panniculitis-like T-cell lymphoma ▶(C86.30)◀
> T-cell leukemia (C91.1-)

C84.Z0   Other mature T/NK-cell lymphomas, unspecified site   `HIV` `CC` `HCC`

C84.Z1   Other mature T/NK-cell lymphomas, lymph nodes of head, face, and neck   `HIV` `CC` `HCC`

C84.Z2   Other mature T/NK-cell lymphomas, intrathoracic lymph nodes   `HIV` `CC` `HCC`

C84.Z3   Other mature T/NK-cell lymphomas, intra-abdominal lymph nodes   `HIV` `CC` `HCC`

C84.Z4   Other mature T/NK-cell lymphomas, lymph nodes of axilla and upper limb   `HIV` `CC` `HCC`

C84.Z5   Other mature T/NK-cell lymphomas, lymph nodes of inguinal region and lower limb   `HIV` `CC` `HCC`

C84.Z6   Other mature T/NK-cell lymphomas, intrapelvic lymph nodes   `HIV` `CC` `HCC`

C84.Z7   Other mature T/NK-cell lymphomas, spleen   `HIV` `CC` `HCC`

C84.Z8   Other mature T/NK-cell lymphomas, lymph nodes of multiple sites   `HIV` `CC` `HCC`

C84.Z9   Other mature T/NK-cell lymphomas, extranodal and solid organ sites   `HIV` `CC` `HCC`

C84.ZA   Other mature T/NK-cell lymphomas, in remission   `CC`

✓5ᵗʰ C84.9   Mature T/NK-cell lymphomas, unspecified
    NK/T cell lymphoma NOS

> *EXCLUDES 1*   mature T-cell lymphoma, not elsewhere classified (C84.4-)

C84.90   Mature T/NK-cell lymphomas, unspecified, unspecified site   `HIV` `CC` `HCC`

C84.91   Mature T/NK-cell lymphomas, unspecified, lymph nodes of head, face, and neck   `HIV` `CC` `HCC`

C84.92   Mature T/NK-cell lymphomas, unspecified, intrathoracic lymph nodes   `HIV` `CC` `HCC`

C84.93   Mature T/NK-cell lymphomas, unspecified, intra-abdominal lymph nodes   `HIV` `CC` `HCC`

C84.94   Mature T/NK-cell lymphomas, unspecified, lymph nodes of axilla and upper limb   `HIV` `CC` `HCC`

C84.95   Mature T/NK-cell lymphomas, unspecified, lymph nodes of inguinal region and lower limb   `HIV` `CC` `HCC`

C84.96   Mature T/NK-cell lymphomas, unspecified, intrapelvic lymph nodes   `HIV` `CC` `HCC`

C84.97   Mature T/NK-cell lymphomas, unspecified, spleen   `HIV` `CC` `HCC`

C84.98   Mature T/NK-cell lymphomas, unspecified, lymph nodes of multiple sites   `HIV` `CC` `HCC`

C84.99   Mature T/NK-cell lymphomas, unspecified, extranodal and solid organ sites   `HIV` `CC` `HCC`

C84.9A   Mature T/NK-cell lymphomas, unspecified, in remission   `CC`

✓4ᵗʰ C85   Other specified and unspecified types of non-Hodgkin lymphoma

> *EXCLUDES 1*   other specified types of T/NK-cell lymphoma (C86.-)
> personal history of non-Hodgkin lymphoma (Z85.72)

    AHA: 2023,1Q,22

✓5ᵗʰ C85.1   Unspecified B-cell lymphoma

> **NOTE**   If B-cell lineage or involvement is mentioned in conjunction with a specific lymphoma, code to the more specific description.

C85.10   Unspecified B-cell lymphoma, unspecified site   `HIV` `CC` `HCC`

C85.11   Unspecified B-cell lymphoma, lymph nodes of head, face, and neck   `HIV` `CC` `HCC`

C85.12   Unspecified B-cell lymphoma, intrathoracic lymph nodes   `HIV` `CC` `HCC`

C85.13   Unspecified B-cell lymphoma, intra-abdominal lymph nodes   `HIV` `CC` `HCC`

C85.14   Unspecified B-cell lymphoma, lymph nodes of axilla and upper limb   `HIV` `CC` `HCC`

C85.15   Unspecified B-cell lymphoma, lymph nodes of inguinal region and lower limb   `HIV` `CC` `HCC`

C85.16   Unspecified B-cell lymphoma, intrapelvic lymph nodes   `HIV` `CC` `HCC`

C85.17   Unspecified B-cell lymphoma, spleen   `HIV` `CC` `HCC`

C85.18   Unspecified B-cell lymphoma, lymph nodes of multiple sites   `HIV` `CC` `HCC`

C85.19   Unspecified B-cell lymphoma, extranodal and solid organ sites   `HIV` `CC` `HCC`

C85.1A   Unspecified B-cell lymphoma, in remission   `CC`

✓5ᵗʰ C85.2   Mediastinal (thymic) large B-cell lymphoma

C85.20   Mediastinal (thymic) large B-cell lymphoma, unspecified site   `HIV` `CC` `HCC`

C85.21   Mediastinal (thymic) large B-cell lymphoma, lymph nodes of head, face, and neck   `HIV` `CC` `HCC`

C85.22   Mediastinal (thymic) large B-cell lymphoma, intrathoracic lymph nodes   `HIV` `CC` `HCC`

C85.23   Mediastinal (thymic) large B-cell lymphoma, intra-abdominal lymph nodes   `HIV` `CC` `HCC`

C85.24   Mediastinal (thymic) large B-cell lymphoma, lymph nodes of axilla and upper limb   `HIV` `CC` `HCC`

C85.25   Mediastinal (thymic) large B-cell lymphoma, lymph nodes of inguinal region and lower limb   `HIV` `CC` `HCC`

C85.26   Mediastinal (thymic) large B-cell lymphoma, intrapelvic lymph nodes   `HIV` `CC` `HCC`

C85.27   Mediastinal (thymic) large B-cell lymphoma, spleen   `HIV` `CC` `HCC`

C85.28   Mediastinal (thymic) large B-cell lymphoma, lymph nodes of multiple sites   `HIV` `CC` `HCC`

C85.29   Mediastinal (thymic) large B-cell lymphoma, extranodal and solid organ sites   `HIV` `CC` `HCC`

C85.2A   Mediastinal (thymic) large B-cell lymphoma, in remission   `CC`

✓5ᵗʰ C85.8   Other specified types of non-Hodgkin lymphoma

C85.80   Other specified types of non-Hodgkin lymphoma, unspecified site   `HIV` `CC` `HCC`

C85.81   Other specified types of non-Hodgkin lymphoma, lymph nodes of head, face, and neck   `HIV` `CC` `HCC`

C85.82   Other specified types of non-Hodgkin lymphoma, intrathoracic lymph nodes   `HIV` `CC` `HCC`

C85.83   Other specified types of non-Hodgkin lymphoma, intra-abdominal lymph nodes   `HIV` `CC` `HCC`

C85.84   Other specified types of non-Hodgkin lymphoma, lymph nodes of axilla and upper limb   `HIV` `CC` `HCC`

✔ Additional Character Required   ✓x7ᵗʰ Placeholder   Questionable PDx   Manifestation   Unspecified   `UPD` Unacceptable PDx   `H1`-`H14` HAC   `HCC` CMS-HCC Dx   `HIV` HIV Dx

Chapter 2. Neoplasms

C85.85 Other specified types of non-Hodgkin lymphoma, lymph nodes of inguinal region and lower limb `HIV` `CC` `HCC`

C85.86 Other specified types of non-Hodgkin lymphoma, intrapelvic lymph nodes `HIV` `CC` `HCC`

C85.87 Other specified types of non-Hodgkin lymphoma, spleen `HIV` `CC` `HCC`

C85.88 Other specified types of non-Hodgkin lymphoma, lymph nodes of multiple sites `HIV` `CC` `HCC`

C85.89 Other specified types of non-Hodgkin lymphoma, extranodal and solid organ sites `HIV` `CC` `HCC`

C85.8A Other specified types of non-Hodgkin lymphoma, in remission `CC`

✓5ᵗʰ **C85.9** Non-Hodgkin lymphoma, unspecified
    Lymphoma NOS
    Malignant lymphoma NOS
    Non-Hodgkin lymphoma NOS

C85.90 Non-Hodgkin lymphoma, unspecified, unspecified site `HIV` `CC` `HCC`

C85.91 Non-Hodgkin lymphoma, unspecified, lymph nodes of head, face, and neck `HIV` `CC` `HCC`

C85.92 Non-Hodgkin lymphoma, unspecified, intrathoracic lymph nodes `HIV` `CC` `HCC`

C85.93 Non-Hodgkin lymphoma, unspecified, intra-abdominal lymph nodes `HIV` `CC` `HCC`

C85.94 Non-Hodgkin lymphoma, unspecified, lymph nodes of axilla and upper limb `HIV` `CC` `HCC`

C85.95 Non-Hodgkin lymphoma, unspecified, lymph nodes of inguinal region and lower limb `HIV` `CC` `HCC`

C85.96 Non-Hodgkin lymphoma, unspecified, intrapelvic lymph nodes `HIV` `CC` `HCC`

C85.97 Non-Hodgkin lymphoma, unspecified, spleen `HIV` `CC` `HCC`

C85.98 Non-Hodgkin lymphoma, unspecified, lymph nodes of multiple sites `HIV` `CC` `HCC`

C85.99 Non-Hodgkin lymphoma, unspecified, extranodal and solid organ sites `HIV` `CC` `HCC`

C85.9A Non-Hodgkin lymphoma, unspecified, in remission `CC`

✓4ᵗʰ **C86** Other specified types of T/NK-cell lymphoma

    EXCLUDES 1   anaplastic large cell lymphoma, ALK negative (C84.7-)
                    anaplastic large cell lymphoma, ALK positive (C84.6-)
                    mature T/NK-cell lymphomas (C84.-)
                    other specified types of non-Hodgkin lymphoma (C85.8-)

▲ ✓5ᵗʰ **C86.0** Extranodal NK/T-cell lymphoma, nasal type

C86.00 Extranodal NK/T-cell lymphoma, nasal type not having achieved remission `CC`
    Extranodal NK/T-cell lymphoma, nasal type NOS
    Extranodal NK/T-cell lymphoma, nasal type with failed remission

C86.01 Extranodal NK/T-cell lymphoma, nasal type, in remission `CC`

▲ ✓5ᵗʰ **C86.1** Hepatosplenic T-cell lymphoma
    Alpha-beta and gamma delta types

C86.10 Hepatosplenic T-cell lymphoma not having achieved remission `CC`
    Hepatosplenic T-cell lymphoma NOS
    Hepatosplenic T-cell lymphoma with failed remission

C86.11 Hepatosplenic T-cell lymphoma, in remission `CC`

▲ ✓5ᵗʰ **C86.2** Enteropathy-type (intestinal) T-cell lymphoma
    Enteropathy associated T-cell lymphoma

C86.20 Enteropathy-type (intestinal) T-cell lymphoma not having achieved remission `CC`
    Enteropathy associated T-cell lymphoma NOS
    Enteropathy associated T-cell lymphoma not having achieved remission
    Enteropathy associated T-cell lymphoma with failed remission
    Enteropathy-type (intestinal) T-cell lymphoma NOS
    Enteropathy-type (intestinal) T-cell lymphoma with failed remission

C86.21 Enteropathy-type (intestinal) T-cell lymphoma, in remission `CC`
    Enteropathy associated T-cell lymphoma, in remission

▲ ✓5ᵗʰ **C86.3** Subcutaneous panniculitis-like T-cell lymphoma

C86.30 Subcutaneous panniculitis-like T-cell lymphoma not having achieved remission `CC`
    Subcutaneous panniculitis-like T-cell lymphoma NOS
    Subcutaneous panniculitis-like T-cell lymphoma with failed remission

C86.31 Subcutaneous panniculitis-like T-cell lymphoma, in remission `CC`

▲ ✓5ᵗʰ **C86.4** Blastic NK-cell lymphoma
    Blastic plasmacytoid dendritic cell neoplasm (BPDCN)

C86.40 Blastic NK-cell lymphoma not having achieved remission `CC`
    Blastic NK-cell lymphoma NOS
    Blastic NK-cell lymphoma with failed remission
    Blastic plasmacytoid dendritic cell neoplasm (BPDCN) NOS
    Blastic plasmacytoid dendritic cell neoplasm (BPDCN) not having achieved remission
    Blastic plasmacytoid dendritic cell neoplasm (BPDCN) with failed remission

C86.41 Blastic NK-cell lymphoma, in remission `CC`
    Blastic plasmacytoid dendritic cell neoplasm (BPDCN), in remission

▲ ✓5ᵗʰ **C86.5** Angioimmunoblastic T-cell lymphoma
    Angioimmunoblastic lymphadenopathy with dysproteinemia (AILD)

C86.50 Angioimmunoblastic T-cell lymphoma not having achieved remission `CC`
    Angioimmunoblastic lymphadenopathy with dysproteinemia (AILD) NOS
    Angioimmunoblastic lymphadenopathy with dysproteinemia (AILD) not having achieved remission
    Angioimmunoblastic lymphadenopathy with dysproteinemia (AILD) with failed remission
    Angioimmunoblastic T-cell lymphoma NOS
    Angioimmunoblastic T-cell lymphoma with failed remission

C86.51 Angioimmunoblastic T-cell lymphoma, in remission `CC`
    Angioimmunoblastic lymphadenopathy with dysproteinemia (AILD), in remission

▲ ✓5ᵗʰ **C86.6** Primary cutaneous CD30-positive T-cell proliferations
    Lymphomatoid papulosis
    Primary cutaneous anaplastic large cell lymphoma
    Primary cutaneous CD30-positive large T-cell lymphoma

C86.60 Primary cutaneous CD30-positive T-cell proliferations not having achieved remission `CC`
    Lymphomatoid papulosis NOS
    Lymphomatoid papulosis not having achieved remission
    Lymphomatoid papulosis with failed remission
    Primary cutaneous anaplastic large cell lymphoma NOS
    Primary cutaneous anaplastic large cell lymphoma not having achieved remission
    Primary cutaneous anaplastic large cell lymphoma with failed remission
    Primary cutaneous CD30-positive large T-cell lymphoma NOS
    Primary cutaneous CD30-positive large T-cell lymphoma not having achieved remission
    Primary cutaneous CD30-positive large T-cell lymphoma with failed remission
    Primary cutaneous CD30-positive T-cell proliferations NOS
    Primary cutaneous CD30-positive T-cell proliferations with failed remission

C86.61 Primary cutaneous CD30-positive T-cell proliferations, in remission `CC`

N Newborn: 0   P Pediatric: 0-17   M Maternity: 9-64   A Adult: 15-124   UNS Unspecified Site   MCC Major Complication/Comorbidity   CC Complication/Comorbidity   PE POA Exempt

496   ICD-10-CM 2025

✓4ᵗʰ C88 Malignant immunoproliferative diseases and certain other B-cell lymphomas

> EXCLUDES 1   B-cell lymphoma, unspecified (C85.1-)
>
> personal history of other malignant neoplasms of lymphoid, hematopoietic and related tissues (Z85.79)

▲   ✓5ᵗʰ **C88.0 Waldenstrom macroglobulinemia**

Lymphoplasmacytic lymphoma with IgM-production
Macroglobulinemia (idiopathic) (primary)

> EXCLUDES 1   small cell B-cell lymphoma (C83.0)

●   **C88.00 Waldenstrom macroglobulinemia not having achieved remission**

Lymphoplasmacytic lymphoma with IgM-production, NOS
Lymphoplasmacytic lymphoma with IgM-production not having achieved remission
Lymphoplasmacytic lymphoma with IgM-production with failed remission
Macroglobulinemia (idiopathic) (primary) NOS
Macroglobulinemia (idiopathic) (primary) not having achieved remission
Macroglobulinemia (idiopathic) (primary) with failed remission
Waldenstrom macroglobulinemia NOS
Waldenstrom macroglobulinemia with failed remission

●   **C88.01 Waldenstrom macroglobulinemia, in remission**

▲   ✓5ᵗʰ **C88.2 Heavy chain disease**

Franklin disease
Gamma heavy chain disease
Mu heavy chain disease

●   **C88.20 Heavy chain disease not having achieved remission** `CC`

Franklin disease NOS
Franklin disease not having achieved remission
Franklin disease with failed remission
Gamma heavy chain disease NOS
Gamma heavy chain disease not having achieved remission
Gamma heavy chain disease with failed remission
Heavy chain disease NOS
Heavy chain disease with failed remission
Mu heavy chain disease NOS
Mu heavy chain disease not having achieved remission
Mu heavy chain disease with failed remission

●   **C88.21 Heavy chain disease, in remission** `CC`

▲   ✓5ᵗʰ **C88.3 Immunoproliferative small intestinal disease**

Alpha heavy chain disease
Mediterranean lymphoma

●   **C88.30 Immunoproliferative small intestinal disease not having achieved remission** `CC`

Alpha heavy chain disease NOS
Alpha heavy chain disease not having achieved remission
Alpha heavy chain disease with failed remission
Immunoproliferative small intestinal disease NOS
Immunoproliferative small intestinal disease with failed remission
Mediterranean lymphoma NOS
Mediterranean lymphoma not having achieved remission
Mediterranean lymphoma with failed remission

●   **C88.31 Immunoproliferative small intestinal disease, in remission** `CC`

▲   ✓5ᵗʰ **C88.4 Extranodal marginal zone B-cell lymphoma of mucosa-associated lymphoid tissue [MALT-lymphoma]**

Lymphoma of skin-associated lymphoid tissue [SALT-lymphoma]
Lymphoma of bronchial-associated lymphoid tissue [BALT-lymphoma]

> EXCLUDES 1   high malignant (diffuse large B-cell) lymphoma (C83.3-)

●   **C88.40 Extranodal marginal zone B-cell lymphoma of mucosa-associated lymphoid tissue [MALT-lymphoma] not having achieved remission** `CC`

Extranodal marginal zone B-cell lymphoma of mucosa-associated lymphoid tissue [MALT-lymphoma] NOS
Extranodal marginal zone B-cell lymphoma of mucosa-associated lymphoid tissue [MALT-lymphoma] with failed remission
Lymphoma of bronchial-associated lymphoid tissue [BALT-lymphoma] NOS
Lymphoma of bronchial-associated lymphoid tissue [BALT-lymphoma] not having achieved remission
Lymphoma of bronchial-associated lymphoid tissue [BALT-lymphoma] with failed remission
Lymphoma of skin-associated lymphoid tissue [SALT-lymphoma] NOS
Lymphoma of skin-associated lymphoid tissue [SALT-lymphoma] not having achieved remission
Lymphoma of skin-associated lymphoid tissue [SALT-lymphoma] with failed remission

●   **C88.41 Extranodal marginal zone B-cell lymphoma of mucosa-associated lymphoid tissue [MALT-lymphoma], in remission** `CC`

▲   ✓5ᵗʰ **C88.8 Other malignant immunoproliferative diseases**

●   **C88.80 Other malignant immunoproliferative diseases not having achieved remission** `CC`

Other malignant immunoproliferative diseases NOS
Other malignant immunoproliferative diseases with failed remission

●   **C88.81 Other malignant immunoproliferative diseases, in remission** `CC`

▲   ✓5ᵗʰ **C88.9 Malignant immunoproliferative disease, unspecified**

Immunoproliferative disease NOS

●   **C88.90 Malignant immunoproliferative disease, unspecified not having achieved remission** `CC`

Immunoproliferative disease NOS
Immunoproliferative disease NOS not having achieved remission
Immunoproliferative disease NOS with failed remission
Malignant immunoproliferative disease, unspecified NOS
Malignant immunoproliferative disease, unspecified with failed remission

●   **C88.91 Malignant immunoproliferative disease, unspecified, in remission** `CC`

✓4ᵗʰ C90 Multiple myeloma and malignant plasma cell neoplasms

> EXCLUDES 1   personal history of other malignant neoplasms of lymphoid, hematopoietic and related tissues (Z85.79)

AHA: 2019,2Q,30

✓5ᵗʰ C90.0 Multiple myeloma

Kahler's disease
Medullary plasmacytoma
Myelomatosis
Plasma cell myeloma

> EXCLUDES 1   solitary myeloma (C90.3-)
>
> solitary plasmactyoma (C90.3-)

AHA: 2021,3Q,5

TIP: Smoldering multiple myeloma (SMM) is a plasma cell disorder that has not yet progressed to active multiple myeloma. Code D47.2 should be used when only SMM is documented.

TIP: Do not assign an additional code for bone metastasis (C79.51) when multiple myeloma is described as metastatic to the bone; bone involvement is integral to this disease process.

   C90.00 Multiple myeloma not having achieved remission `CC` `HCC`

Multiple myeloma with failed remission
Multiple myeloma NOS

   C90.01 Multiple myeloma in remission `CC` `HCC`

   C90.02 Multiple myeloma in relapse `CC` `HCC`

Chapter 2. Neoplasms

C90.1–C91.92

√5th **C90.1 Plasma cell leukemia**

Plasmacytic leukemia

AHA: 2019,2Q,30

C90.10 Plasma cell leukemia not having achieved remission CC HCC

Plasma cell leukemia with failed remission

Plasma cell leukemia NOS

C90.11 Plasma cell leukemia in remission CC HCC

C90.12 Plasma cell leukemia in relapse CC HCC

√5th **C90.2 Extramedullary plasmacytoma**

C90.20 Extramedullary plasmacytoma not having achieved remission CC HCC

Extramedullary plasmacytoma with failed remission

Extramedullary plasmacytoma NOS

C90.21 Extramedullary plasmacytoma in remission CC HCC

C90.22 Extramedullary plasmacytoma in relapse CC HCC

√5th **C90.3 Solitary plasmacytoma**

Localized malignant plasma cell tumor NOS

Plasmacytoma NOS

Solitary myeloma

C90.30 Solitary plasmacytoma not having achieved remission CC HCC

Solitary plasmacytoma with failed remission

Solitary plasmacytoma NOS

C90.31 Solitary plasmacytoma in remission CC HCC

C90.32 Solitary plasmacytoma in relapse CC HCC

√4th **C91 Lymphoid leukemia**

EXCLUDES 1   *personal history of leukemia (Z85.6)*

AHA: 2020,1Q,13

DEF: Malignant proliferation of immature lymphocytes (white blood cells that make up lymphoid tissue), called lymphoblasts, that originate in the bone marrow. Can be acute (ALL) or chronic (CLL).

√5th **C91.0 Acute lymphoblastic leukemia [ALL]**

NOTE   Codes in subcategory C91.0- should only be used for T-cell and B-cell precursor leukemia

C91.00 Acute lymphoblastic leukemia not having achieved remission CC HCC

Acute lymphoblastic leukemia with failed remission

Acute lymphoblastic leukemia NOS

C91.01 Acute lymphoblastic leukemia, in remission CC HCC

C91.02 Acute lymphoblastic leukemia, in relapse CC HCC

√5th **C91.1 Chronic lymphocytic leukemia of B-cell type**

Lymphoplasmacytic leukemia

Richter syndrome

EXCLUDES 1   *lymphoplasmacytic lymphoma (C83.0-)*

AHA: 2023,1Q,18

C91.10 Chronic lymphocytic leukemia of B-cell type not having achieved remission CC HCC

Chronic lymphocytic leukemia of B-cell type with failed remission

Chronic lymphocytic leukemia of B-cell type NOS

C91.11 Chronic lymphocytic leukemia of B-cell type in remission CC HCC

C91.12 Chronic lymphocytic leukemia of B-cell type in relapse CC HCC

√5th **C91.3 Prolymphocytic leukemia of B-cell type**

C91.30 Prolymphocytic leukemia of B-cell type not having achieved remission CC HCC

Prolymphocytic leukemia of B-cell type with failed remission

Prolymphocytic leukemia of B-cell type NOS

C91.31 Prolymphocytic leukemia of B-cell type, in remission CC HCC

C91.32 Prolymphocytic leukemia of B-cell type, in relapse CC HCC

√5th **C91.4 Hairy cell leukemia**

Leukemic reticuloendotheliosis

DEF: Rare type of leukemia that is slow growing and often also considered a type of lymphoma. The small B-cell lymphocytes appear with "hairy" projections under a microscope and are found mostly in the bone marrow, spleen, and blood.

C91.40 Hairy cell leukemia not having achieved remission CC HCC

Hairy cell leukemia with failed remission

Hairy cell leukemia NOS

C91.41 Hairy cell leukemia, in remission CC HCC

C91.42 Hairy cell leukemia, in relapse CC HCC

√5th **C91.5 Adult T-cell lymphoma/leukemia (HTLV-1-associated)**

Acute variant of adult T-cell lymphoma/leukemia (HTLV-1-associated)

Chronic variant of adult T-cell lymphoma/leukemia (HTLV-1-associated)

Lymphomatoid variant of adult T-cell lymphoma/leukemia (HTLV-1-associated)

Smouldering variant of adult T-cell lymphoma/leukemia (HTLV-1-associated)

C91.50 Adult T-cell lymphoma/leukemia (HTLV-1-associated) not having achieved remission CC HCC A

Adult T-cell lymphoma/leukemia (HTLV-1-associated) with failed remission

Adult T-cell lymphoma/leukemia (HTLV-1-associated) NOS

C91.51 Adult T-cell lymphoma/leukemia (HTLV-1-associated), in remission CC HCC A

C91.52 Adult T-cell lymphoma/leukemia (HTLV-1-associated), in relapse CC HCC A

√5th **C91.6 Prolymphocytic leukemia of T-cell type**

C91.60 Prolymphocytic leukemia of T-cell type not having achieved remission CC HCC

Prolymphocytic leukemia of T-cell type with failed remission

Prolymphocytic leukemia of T-cell type NOS

C91.61 Prolymphocytic leukemia of T-cell type, in remission CC HCC

C91.62 Prolymphocytic leukemia of T-cell type, in relapse CC HCC

√5th **C91.A Mature B-cell leukemia Burkitt-type**

EXCLUDES 1   *Burkitt lymphoma (C83.7-)*

C91.A0 Mature B-cell leukemia Burkitt-type not having achieved remission CC HCC

Mature B-cell leukemia Burkitt-type with failed remission

Mature B-cell leukemia Burkitt-type NOS

C91.A1 Mature B-cell leukemia Burkitt-type, in remission CC HCC

C91.A2 Mature B-cell leukemia Burkitt-type, in relapse CC HCC

√5th **C91.Z Other lymphoid leukemia**

T-cell large granular lymphocytic leukemia (associated with rheumatoid arthritis)

C91.Z0 Other lymphoid leukemia not having achieved remission CC HCC

Other lymphoid leukemia with failed remission

Other lymphoid leukemia NOS

C91.Z1 Other lymphoid leukemia, in remission CC HCC

C91.Z2 Other lymphoid leukemia, in relapse CC HCC

√5th **C91.9 Lymphoid leukemia, unspecified**

C91.90 Lymphoid leukemia, unspecified not having achieved remission CC HCC

Lymphoid leukemia with failed remission

Lymphoid leukemia NOS

C91.91 Lymphoid leukemia, unspecified, in remission CC HCC

C91.92 Lymphoid leukemia, unspecified, in relapse CC HCC

N Newborn: 0   P Pediatric: 0-17   M Maternity: 9-64   A Adult: 15-124   UNS Unspecified Site   MCC Major Complication/Comorbidity   CC Complication/Comorbidity   PE POA Exempt

498   ICD-10-CM 2025

Chapter 2. Neoplasms

✓4ᵗʰ **C92 Myeloid leukemia**

INCLUDES   granulocytic leukemia
         myelogenous leukemia

Code also, if applicable, pancytopenia (acquired) (D61.818)

EXCLUDES 1   personal history of leukemia (Z85.6)

AHA: 2020,1Q,13; 2019,1Q,16

DEF: Cancer that develops in immature myelocytes called myeloblasts. These are the cells that become white blood cells (except lymphocytes), red blood cells, or platelet-making cells. Can be acute (AML) or chronic (CML).

TIP: Pancytopenia, although common in some types of myeloid leukemias, is not always inherent. When it is documented, code D61.818 can be assigned in addition to a code from this category.

✓5ᵗʰ **C92.0 Acute myeloblastic leukemia**

Acute myeloblastic leukemia, minimal differentiation
Acute myeloblastic leukemia (with maturation)
Acute myeloblastic leukemia 1/ETO
Acute myeloblastic leukemia M0
Acute myeloblastic leukemia M1
Acute myeloblastic leukemia M2
Acute myeloblastic leukemia with t(8;21)
Acute myeloblastic leukemia (without a FAB classification) NOS
Refractory anemia with excess blasts in transformation [RAEBT]

EXCLUDES 1   acute exacerbation of chronic myeloid leukemia (C92.10)
           refractory anemia with excess of blasts not in transformation (D46.2-)

AHA: 2018,4Q,87

C92.00 Acute myeloblastic leukemia, not having achieved remission CC HCC
     Acute myeloblastic leukemia with failed remission
     Acute myeloblastic leukemia NOS

C92.01 Acute myeloblastic leukemia, in remission CC HCC
     AHA: 2021,3Q,4

C92.02 Acute myeloblastic leukemia, in relapse CC HCC
     AHA: 2023,1Q,23

✓5ᵗʰ **C92.1 Chronic myeloid leukemia, BCR/ABL-positive**

Chronic myelogenous leukemia, Philadelphia chromosome (Ph1) positive
Chronic myelogenous leukemia, t(9;22) (q34;q11)
Chronic myelogenous leukemia with crisis of blast cells

EXCLUDES 1   atypical chronic myeloid leukemia BCR/ABL-negative (C92.2-)
           chronic myelomonocytic leukemia (C93.1-)
           chronic myeloproliferative disease (D47.1)

C92.10 Chronic myeloid leukemia, BCR/ABL-positive, not having achieved remission CC HCC
     Chronic myeloid leukemia, BCR/ABL-positive with failed remission
     Chronic myeloid leukemia, BCR/ABL-positive NOS

C92.11 Chronic myeloid leukemia, BCR/ABL-positive, in remission CC HCC

C92.12 Chronic myeloid leukemia, BCR/ABL-positive, in relapse CC HCC

✓5ᵗʰ **C92.2 Atypical chronic myeloid leukemia, BCR/ABL-negative**

C92.20 Atypical chronic myeloid leukemia, BCR/ABL-negative, not having achieved remission CC HCC
     Atypical chronic myeloid leukemia, BCR/ABL-negative with failed remission
     Atypical chronic myeloid leukemia, BCR/ABL-negative NOS

C92.21 Atypical chronic myeloid leukemia, BCR/ABL-negative, in remission CC HCC

C92.22 Atypical chronic myeloid leukemia, BCR/ABL-negative, in relapse CC HCC

✓5ᵗʰ **C92.3 Myeloid sarcoma**

A malignant tumor of immature myeloid cells
Chloroma
Granulocytic sarcoma

C92.30 Myeloid sarcoma, not having achieved remission CC HCC
     Myeloid sarcoma with failed remission
     Myeloid sarcoma NOS

C92.31 Myeloid sarcoma, in remission CC HCC

C92.32 Myeloid sarcoma, in relapse CC HCC

✓5ᵗʰ **C92.4 Acute promyelocytic leukemia**

AML M3
AML Me with t(15;17) and variants

C92.40 Acute promyelocytic leukemia, not having achieved remission CC HCC
     Acute promyelocytic leukemia with failed remission
     Acute promyelocytic leukemia NOS

C92.41 Acute promyelocytic leukemia, in remission CC HCC

C92.42 Acute promyelocytic leukemia, in relapse CC HCC

✓5ᵗʰ **C92.5 Acute myelomonocytic leukemia**

AML M4
AML M4 Eo with inv(16) or t(16;16)

C92.50 Acute myelomonocytic leukemia, not having achieved remission CC HCC
     Acute myelomonocytic leukemia with failed remission
     Acute myelomonocytic leukemia NOS

C92.51 Acute myelomonocytic leukemia, in remission CC HCC

C92.52 Acute myelomonocytic leukemia, in relapse CC HCC

✓5ᵗʰ **C92.6 Acute myeloid leukemia with 11q23-abnormality**

Acute myeloid leukemia with variation of MLL-gene

C92.60 Acute myeloid leukemia with 11q23-abnormality not having achieved remission CC HCC
     Acute myeloid leukemia with 11q23-abnormality with failed remission
     Acute myeloid leukemia with 11q23-abnormality NOS

C92.61 Acute myeloid leukemia with 11q23-abnormality in remission CC HCC

C92.62 Acute myeloid leukemia with 11q23-abnormality in relapse CC HCC

✓5ᵗʰ **C92.A Acute myeloid leukemia with multilineage dysplasia**

Acute myeloid leukemia with dysplasia of remaining haematopoesis and/or myelodysplastic disease in its history

C92.A0 Acute myeloid leukemia with multilineage dysplasia, not having achieved remission CC HCC
     Acute myeloid leukemia with multilineage dysplasia with failed remission
     Acute myeloid leukemia with multilineage dysplasia NOS

C92.A1 Acute myeloid leukemia with multilineage dysplasia, in remission CC HCC

C92.A2 Acute myeloid leukemia with multilineage dysplasia, in relapse CC HCC

✓5ᵗʰ **C92.Z Other myeloid leukemia**

C92.Z0 Other myeloid leukemia not having achieved remission CC HCC
     Myeloid leukemia NEC with failed remission
     Myeloid leukemia NEC

C92.Z1 Other myeloid leukemia, in remission CC HCC

C92.Z2 Other myeloid leukemia, in relapse CC HCC

✓5ᵗʰ **C92.9 Myeloid leukemia, unspecified**

C92.90 Myeloid leukemia, unspecified, not having achieved remission CC HCC
     Myeloid leukemia, unspecified with failed remission
     Myeloid leukemia, unspecified NOS

C92.91 Myeloid leukemia, unspecified in remission CC HCC

C92.92 Myeloid leukemia, unspecified in relapse CC HCC

✓4ᵗʰ **C93 Monocytic leukemia**

INCLUDES   monocytoid leukemia

EXCLUDES 1   personal history of leukemia (Z85.6)

AHA: 2020,1Q,13

✓5ᵗʰ **C93.0 Acute monoblastic/monocytic leukemia**

AML M5
AML M5a
AML M5b

C93.00 Acute monoblastic/monocytic leukemia, not having achieved remission CC HCC
     Acute monoblastic/monocytic leukemia with failed remission
     Acute monoblastic/monocytic leukemia NOS

C93.01 Acute monoblastic/monocytic leukemia, in remission CC HCC

C93.02 Acute monoblastic/monocytic leukemia, in relapse CC HCC

✓ Additional Character Required   ✓x7ᵗʰ Placeholder   Questionable PDx   Manifestation   Unspecified   UPD Unacceptable PDx   H1 - H14 HAC   HCC CMS-HCC Dx   HIV HIV Dx

ICD-10-CM 2025   499

√5ᵗʰ C93.1 Chronic myelomonocytic leukemia
Chronic monocytic leukemia
CMML-1
CMML-2
CMML with eosinophilia
Code also, if applicable, eosinophilia (D72.18)

    C93.1Ø Chronic myelomonocytic leukemia not having achieved remission `CC` `HCC`
Chronic myelomonocytic leukemia with failed remission
Chronic myelomonocytic leukemia NOS

    C93.11 Chronic myelomonocytic leukemia, in remission `CC` `HCC`

    C93.12 Chronic myelomonocytic leukemia, in relapse `CC` `HCC`

√5ᵗʰ C93.3 Juvenile myelomonocytic leukemia

    C93.3Ø Juvenile myelomonocytic leukemia, not having achieved remission `CC` `HCC` `P`
Juvenile myelomonocytic leukemia with failed remission
Juvenile myelomonocytic leukemia NOS

    C93.31 Juvenile myelomonocytic leukemia, in remission `CC` `HCC` `P`

    C93.32 Juvenile myelomonocytic leukemia, in relapse `CC` `HCC` `P`

√5ᵗʰ C93.Z Other monocytic leukemia

    C93.ZØ Other monocytic leukemia, not having achieved remission `CC` `HCC`
Other monocytic leukemia NOS

    C93.Z1 Other monocytic leukemia, in remission `CC` `HCC`

    C93.Z2 Other monocytic leukemia, in relapse `CC` `HCC`

√5ᵗʰ C93.9 Monocytic leukemia, unspecified

    C93.9Ø Monocytic leukemia, unspecified, not having achieved remission `CC` `HCC`
Monocytic leukemia, unspecified with failed remission
Monocytic leukemia, unspecified NOS

    C93.91 Monocytic leukemia, unspecified in remission `CC` `HCC`

    C93.92 Monocytic leukemia, unspecified in relapse `CC` `HCC`

√4ᵗʰ C94 Other leukemias of specified cell type
EXCLUDES 1 *leukemic reticuloendotheliosis (C91.4-)*
myelodysplastic syndromes (D46.-)
personal history of leukemia (Z85.6)
plasma cell leukemia (C9Ø.1-)
AHA: 2020,1Q,13

√5ᵗʰ C94.Ø Acute erythroid leukemia
Acute myeloid leukemia M6(a)(b)
Erythroleukemia
DEF: Erythroleukemia: Malignant blood dyscrasia (a myeloproliferative disorder).

    C94.ØØ Acute erythroid leukemia, not having achieved remission `CC` `HCC`
Acute erythroid leukemia with failed remission
Acute erythroid leukemia NOS

    C94.Ø1 Acute erythroid leukemia, in remission `CC` `HCC`

    C94.Ø2 Acute erythroid leukemia, in relapse `CC` `HCC`

√5ᵗʰ C94.2 Acute megakaryoblastic leukemia
Acute megakaryocytic leukemia
Acute myeloid leukemia M7

    C94.2Ø Acute megakaryoblastic leukemia not having achieved remission `CC` `HCC`
Acute megakaryoblastic leukemia with failed remission
Acute megakaryoblastic leukemia NOS

    C94.21 Acute megakaryoblastic leukemia, in remission `CC` `HCC`

    C94.22 Acute megakaryoblastic leukemia, in relapse `CC` `HCC`

√5ᵗʰ C94.3 Mast cell leukemia
AHA: 2017,4Q,5

    C94.3Ø Mast cell leukemia not having achieved remission `CC` `HCC`
Mast cell leukemia with failed remission
Mast cell leukemia NOS

    C94.31 Mast cell leukemia, in remission `CC` `HCC`

    C94.32 Mast cell leukemia, in relapse `CC` `HCC`

√5ᵗʰ C94.4 Acute panmyelosis with myelofibrosis
Acute myelofibrosis
EXCLUDES 1 *myelofibrosis NOS (D75.81)*
secondary myelofibrosis NOS (D75.81)

    C94.4Ø Acute panmyelosis with myelofibrosis not having achieved remission `CC` `HCC`
Acute myelofibrosis NOS
Acute panmyelosis with myelofibrosis with failed remission
Acute panmyelosis NOS

    C94.41 Acute panmyelosis with myelofibrosis, in remission `CC` `HCC`

    C94.42 Acute panmyelosis with myelofibrosis, in relapse `CC` `HCC`

    C94.6 Myelodysplastic disease, not elsewhere classified `CC` `HCC`
Myelodysplastic/myeloproliferative neoplasm, unclassifiable
Myeloproliferative disease, not elsewhere classified

√5ᵗʰ C94.8 Other specified leukemias
Aggressive NK-cell leukemia
Acute basophilic leukemia
Code also, if applicable, eosinophilia (D72.18)

    C94.8Ø Other specified leukemias not having achieved remission `CC` `HCC`
Other specified leukemia with failed remission
Other specified leukemias NOS

    C94.81 Other specified leukemias, in remission `CC` `HCC`

    C94.82 Other specified leukemias, in relapse `CC` `HCC`

√4ᵗʰ C95 Leukemia of unspecified cell type
EXCLUDES 1 *personal history of leukemia (Z85.6)*
AHA: 2020,1Q,13

√5ᵗʰ C95.Ø Acute leukemia of unspecified cell type
Acute bilineal leukemia
Acute mixed lineage leukemia
Biphenotypic acute leukemia
Stem cell leukemia of unclear lineage
EXCLUDES 1 *acute exacerbation of unspecified chronic leukemia (C95.1Ø)*

    C95.ØØ Acute leukemia of unspecified cell type not having achieved remission `CC` `HCC`
Acute leukemia of unspecified cell type with failed remission
Acute leukemia NOS

    C95.Ø1 Acute leukemia of unspecified cell type, in remission `CC` `HCC`

    C95.Ø2 Acute leukemia of unspecified cell type, in relapse `CC` `HCC`

√5ᵗʰ C95.1 Chronic leukemia of unspecified cell type

    C95.1Ø Chronic leukemia of unspecified cell type not having achieved remission `CC` `HCC`
Chronic leukemia of unspecified cell type with failed remission
Chronic leukemia NOS

    C95.11 Chronic leukemia of unspecified cell type, in remission `CC` `HCC`

    C95.12 Chronic leukemia of unspecified cell type, in relapse `CC` `HCC`

√5ᵗʰ C95.9 Leukemia, unspecified

    C95.9Ø Leukemia, unspecified not having achieved remission `CC` `HCC`
Leukemia, unspecified with failed remission
Leukemia NOS

    C95.91 Leukemia, unspecified, in remission `CC` `HCC`

    C95.92 Leukemia, unspecified, in relapse `CC` `HCC`

√4ᵗʰ C96 Other and unspecified malignant neoplasms of lymphoid, hematopoietic and related tissue
EXCLUDES 1 *personal history of other malignant neoplasms of lymphoid, hematopoietic and related tissues (Z85.79)*

    C96.Ø Multifocal and multisystemic (disseminated) Langerhans-cell histiocytosis `CC` `HCC`
Histiocytosis X, multisystemic
Letterer-Siwe disease
EXCLUDES 1 *adult pulmonary Langerhans cell histiocytosis (J84.82)*
multifocal and unisystemic Langerhans-cell histiocytosis (C96.5)
unifocal Langerhans-cell histiocytosis (C96.6)

`N` Newborn: 0   `P` Pediatric: 0-17   `M` Maternity: 9-64   `A` Adult: 15-124   `UNS` Unspecified Site   `MCC` Major Complication/Comorbidity   `CC` Complication/Comorbidity   `PE` POA Exempt

500   ICD-10-CM 2025

✓5ᵗʰ **C96.2 Malignant mast cell neoplasm**

> EXCLUDES 1   *indolent mastocytosis (D47.02)*
> *mast cell leukemia (C94.30)*
> *mastocytosis (congenital) (cutaneous) (Q82.2)*

AHA: 2017,4Q,5
DEF: Mast cell: Type of white blood cell found in the loose connective tissue of blood vessels and bronchioles responsible for acute hypersensitivity reactions, including anaphylactic shock. The IgE receptors on these cells bind with allergens causing cell degranulation and diffuse, widespread histamine release that results in airway constriction and vasodilation with decreased systemic blood pressure.

   C96.20 Malignant mast cell neoplasm, unspecified CC HCC
   C96.21 Aggressive systemic mastocytosis CC HCC
   C96.22 Mast cell sarcoma CC HCC
   C96.29 Other malignant mast cell neoplasm CC HCC

C96.4 Sarcoma of dendritic cells (accessory cells) CC HCC
   Follicular dendritic cell sarcoma
   Interdigitating dendritic cell sarcoma
   Langerhans cell sarcoma

C96.5 Multifocal and unisystemic Langerhans-cell histiocytosis CC HCC
   Hand-Schuller-Christian disease
   Histiocytosis X, multifocal

> EXCLUDES 1   *multifocal and multisystemic (disseminated) Langerhans-cell histiocytosis (C96.0)*
> *unifocal Langerhans-cell histiocytosis (C96.6)*

C96.6 Unifocal Langerhans-cell histiocytosis CC HCC
   Eosinophilic granuloma
   Histiocytosis X, unifocal
   Histiocytosis X NOS
   Langerhans-cell histiocytosis NOS

> EXCLUDES 1   *multifocal and multisysemic (disseminated) Langerhans-cell histiocytosis (C96.0)*
> *multifocal and unisysemic Langerhans-cell histiocytosis (C96.5)*

C96.A Histiocytic sarcoma CC HCC
   Malignant histiocytosis

C96.Z Other specified malignant neoplasms of lymphoid, hematopoietic and related tissue CC HCC

C96.9 Malignant neoplasm of lymphoid, hematopoietic and related tissue, unspecified CC HCC

In situ neoplasms (D00-D09)

INCLUDES   Bowen's disease
     erythroplasia
     grade III intraepithelial neoplasia
     Queyrat's erythroplasia

AHA: 2023,3Q,15
TIP: When carcinoma in situ and malignant carcinoma are present at the same site, only the malignant carcinoma code should be assigned.

✓4ᵗʰ **D00 Carcinoma in situ of oral cavity, esophagus and stomach**

> EXCLUDES 1   *melanoma in situ (D03.-)*

✓5ᵗʰ **D00.0 Carcinoma in situ of lip, oral cavity and pharynx**

Use additional code to identify:
exposure to environmental tobacco smoke (Z77.22)
exposure to tobacco smoke in the perinatal period (F96.81)
history of tobacco dependence (Z87.891)
occupational exposure to environmental tobacco smoke (Z57.31)
tobacco dependence (F17.-)
tobacco use (Z72.0)

> EXCLUDES 1   *carcinoma in situ of aryepiglottic fold or interarytenoid fold, laryngeal aspect (D02.0)*
> *carcinoma in situ of epiglottis NOS (D02.0)*
> *carcinoma in situ of epiglottis suprahyoid portion (D02.0)*
> *carcinoma in situ of skin of lip (D03.0, D04.0)*

   D00.00 Carcinoma in situ of oral cavity, unspecified site
   D00.01 Carcinoma in situ of labial mucosa and vermilion border
   D00.02 Carcinoma in situ of buccal mucosa
   D00.03 Carcinoma in situ of gingiva and edentulous alveolar ridge
   D00.04 Carcinoma in situ of soft palate
   D00.05 Carcinoma in situ of hard palate
   D00.06 Carcinoma in situ of floor of mouth
   D00.07 Carcinoma in situ of tongue

   D00.08 Carcinoma in situ of pharynx
     Carcinoma in situ of aryepiglottic fold NOS
     Carcinoma in situ of hypopharyngeal aspect of aryepiglottic fold
     Carcinoma in situ of marginal zone of aryepiglottic fold

D00.1 Carcinoma in situ of esophagus
D00.2 Carcinoma in situ of stomach

✓4ᵗʰ **D01 Carcinoma in situ of other and unspecified digestive organs**

> EXCLUDES 1   *melanoma in situ (D03.-)*

D01.0 Carcinoma in situ of colon

> EXCLUDES 1   *carcinoma in situ of rectosigmoid junction (D01.1)*

D01.1 Carcinoma in situ of rectosigmoid junction
D01.2 Carcinoma in situ of rectum
D01.3 Carcinoma in situ of anus and anal canal
   Anal intraepithelial neoplasia III [AIN III]
   Severe dysplasia of anus

> EXCLUDES 1   *anal intraepithelial neoplasia I and II [AIN I and AIN II] (K62.82)*
> *carcinoma in situ of anal margin (D04.5)*
> *carcinoma in situ of anal skin (D04.5)*
> *carcinoma in situ of perianal skin (D04.5)*

✓5ᵗʰ **D01.4 Carcinoma in situ of other and unspecified parts of intestine**

> EXCLUDES 1   *carcinoma in situ of ampulla of Vater (D01.5)*

   D01.40 Carcinoma in situ of unspecified part of intestine
   D01.49 Carcinoma in situ of other parts of intestine

D01.5 Carcinoma in situ of liver, gallbladder and bile ducts
   Carcinoma in situ of ampulla of Vater

D01.7 Carcinoma in situ of other specified digestive organs
   Carcinoma in situ of pancreas

   D01.9 Carcinoma in situ of digestive organ, unspecified

✓4ᵗʰ **D02 Carcinoma in situ of middle ear and respiratory system**

Use additional code to identify:
exposure to environmental tobacco smoke (Z77.22)
exposure to tobacco smoke in the perinatal period (P96.81)
history of tobacco dependence (Z87.891)
occupational exposure to environmental tobacco smoke (Z57.31)
tobacco dependence (F17.-)
tobacco use (Z72.0)

> EXCLUDES 1   *melanoma in situ (D03.-)*

D02.0 Carcinoma in situ of larynx
   Carcinoma in situ of aryepiglottic fold or interarytenoid fold, laryngeal aspect
   Carcinoma in situ of epiglottis (suprahyoid portion)

> EXCLUDES 1   *carcinoma in situ of aryepiglottic fold or interarytenoid fold NOS (D00.08)*
> *carcinoma in situ of hypopharyngeal aspect (D00.08)*
> *carcinoma in situ of marginal zone (D00.08)*

D02.1 Carcinoma in situ of trachea

✓5ᵗʰ **D02.2 Carcinoma in situ of bronchus and lung**

   D02.20 Carcinoma in situ of unspecified bronchus and lung
   D02.21 Carcinoma in situ of right bronchus and lung
   D02.22 Carcinoma in situ of left bronchus and lung

D02.3 Carcinoma in situ of other parts of respiratory system
   Carcinoma in situ of accessory sinuses
   Carcinoma in situ of middle ear
   Carcinoma in situ of nasal cavities

> EXCLUDES 1   *carcinoma in situ of ear (external) (skin) (D04.2-)*
> *carcinoma in situ of nose NOS (D09.8)*
> *carcinoma in situ of skin of nose (D04.3)*

   D02.4 Carcinoma in situ of respiratory system, unspecified

✓4ᵗʰ **D03 Melanoma in situ**

D03.0 Melanoma in situ of lip HCC
✓5ᵗʰ **D03.1 Melanoma in situ of eyelid, including canthus**

   AHA: 2018,4Q,4

   D03.10 Melanoma in situ of unspecified eyelid, including canthus HCC
✓6ᵗʰ   **D03.11 Melanoma in situ of right eyelid, including canthus**
     D03.111 Melanoma in situ of right upper eyelid, including canthus HCC
     D03.112 Melanoma in situ of right lower eyelid, including canthus HCC
✓6ᵗʰ   **D03.12 Melanoma in situ of left eyelid, including canthus**
     D03.121 Melanoma in situ of left upper eyelid, including canthus HCC

D03.122 Melanoma in situ of left **lower** eyelid, including canthus `HCC`

√5th **D03.2** Melanoma in situ of **ear and external auricular canal**

D03.20 Melanoma in situ of unspecified ear and external auricular canal `HCC`

D03.21 Melanoma in situ of **right** ear and external auricular canal `HCC`

D03.22 Melanoma in situ of **left** ear and external auricular canal `HCC`

√5th **D03.3** Melanoma in situ of other and unspecified parts of **face**

D03.30 Melanoma in situ of unspecified part of face `HCC`

D03.39 Melanoma in situ of other parts of face `HCC`

D03.4 Melanoma in situ of **scalp and neck** `HCC`

√5th **D03.5** Melanoma in situ of **trunk**

D03.51 Melanoma in situ of **anal skin** `HCC`
Melanoma in situ of anal margin
Melanoma in situ of perianal skin

D03.52 Melanoma in situ of **breast (skin) (soft tissue)** `HCC`

D03.59 Melanoma in situ of other part of trunk `HCC`

√5th **D03.6** Melanoma in situ of **upper limb, including shoulder**

D03.60 Melanoma in situ of unspecified upper limb, including shoulder `HCC`

D03.61 Melanoma in situ of **right** upper limb, including shoulder `HCC`

D03.62 Melanoma in situ of **left** upper limb, including shoulder `HCC`

√5th **D03.7** Melanoma in situ of **lower limb, including hip**

D03.70 Melanoma in situ of unspecified lower limb, including hip `HCC`

D03.71 Melanoma in situ of **right** lower limb, including hip `HCC`

D03.72 Melanoma in situ of **left** lower limb, including hip `HCC`

D03.8 Melanoma in situ of other sites `HCC`
Melanoma in situ of scrotum
> EXCLUDES 1   carcinoma in situ of scrotum (D07.61)

D03.9 Melanoma in situ, unspecified `HCC`

√4th **D04** Carcinoma in situ of **skin**
> EXCLUDES 1   erythroplasia of Queyrat (penis) NOS (D07.4)
> melanoma in situ (D03.-)

D04.0 Carcinoma in situ of skin of **lip**
> EXCLUDES 2   carcinoma in situ of vermilion border of lip (D00.01)

√5th **D04.1** Carcinoma in situ of skin of **eyelid, including canthus**
AHA: 2018,4Q,4

D04.10 Carcinoma in situ of skin of unspecified eyelid, including canthus

√6th **D04.11** Carcinoma in situ of skin of **right** eyelid, including canthus

D04.111 Carcinoma in situ of skin of right **upper** eyelid, including canthus

D04.112 Carcinoma in situ of skin of right **lower** eyelid, including canthus

√6th **D04.12** Carcinoma in situ of skin of **left** eyelid, including canthus

D04.121 Carcinoma in situ of skin of left **upper** eyelid, including canthus

D04.122 Carcinoma in situ of skin of left **lower** eyelid, including canthus

√5th **D04.2** Carcinoma in situ of skin of **ear and external auricular canal**

D04.20 Carcinoma in situ of skin of unspecified ear and external auricular canal

D04.21 Carcinoma in situ of skin of **right** ear and external auricular canal

D04.22 Carcinoma in situ of skin of **left** ear and external auricular canal

√5th **D04.3** Carcinoma in situ of skin of other and unspecified **parts of face**

D04.30 Carcinoma in situ of skin of unspecified part of face

D04.39 Carcinoma in situ of skin of other parts of face

D04.4 Carcinoma in situ of skin of **scalp and neck**

D04.5 Carcinoma in situ of skin of **trunk**
Carcinoma in situ of anal margin
Carcinoma in situ of anal skin
Carcinoma in situ of perianal skin
Carcinoma in situ of skin of breast
> EXCLUDES 1   carcinoma in situ of anus NOS (D01.3)
> carcinoma in situ of scrotum (D07.61)
> carcinoma in situ of skin of genital organs (D07.-)

√5th **D04.6** Carcinoma in situ of skin of **upper limb, including shoulder**

D04.60 Carcinoma in situ of skin of unspecified upper limb, including shoulder

D04.61 Carcinoma in situ of skin of **right** upper limb, including shoulder

D04.62 Carcinoma in situ of skin of **left** upper limb, including shoulder

√5th **D04.7** Carcinoma in situ of skin of **lower limb, including hip**

D04.70 Carcinoma in situ of skin of unspecified lower limb, including hip

D04.71 Carcinoma in situ of skin of **right** lower limb, including hip

D04.72 Carcinoma in situ of skin of **left** lower limb, including hip

D04.8 Carcinoma in situ of skin of other sites

D04.9 Carcinoma in situ of skin, unspecified

√4th **D05** Carcinoma in situ of **breast**
> EXCLUDES 1   carcinoma in situ of skin of breast (D04.5)
> melanoma in situ of breast (skin) (D03.5)
> Paget's disease of breast or nipple (C50.-)
> EXCLUDES 2   ▶malignant neoplasm of breast (C50.-)◀

√5th **D05.0** **Lobular** carcinoma in situ of breast

D05.00 Lobular carcinoma in situ of unspecified breast

D05.01 Lobular carcinoma in situ of **right** breast

D05.02 Lobular carcinoma in situ of **left** breast

√5th **D05.1** **Intraductal** carcinoma in situ of breast

D05.10 Intraductal carcinoma in situ of unspecified breast

D05.11 Intraductal carcinoma in situ of **right** breast

D05.12 Intraductal carcinoma in situ of **left** breast

√5th **D05.8** Other specified type of carcinoma in situ of breast

D05.80 Other specified type of carcinoma in situ of unspecified breast

D05.81 Other specified type of carcinoma in situ of **right** breast

D05.82 Other specified type of carcinoma in situ of **left** breast

√5th **D05.9** Unspecified type of carcinoma in situ of breast

D05.90 Unspecified type of carcinoma in situ of unspecified breast

D05.91 Unspecified type of carcinoma in situ of **right** breast

D05.92 Unspecified type of carcinoma in situ of **left** breast

√4th **D06** Carcinoma in situ of **cervix uteri**
> INCLUDES   cervical adenocarcinoma in situ
> cervical intraepithelial glandular neoplasia
> cervical intraepithelial neoplasia III [CIN III]
> severe dysplasia of cervix uteri
> EXCLUDES 1   cervical intraepithelial neoplasia II [CIN II] (N87.1)
> cytologic evidence of malignancy of cervix without histologic confirmation (R87.614)
> high grade squamous intraepithelial lesion (HGSIL) of cervix (R87.613)
> melanoma in situ of cervix (D03.5)
> moderate cervical dysplasia (N87.1)

D06.0 Carcinoma in situ of **endocervix**

D06.1 Carcinoma in situ of **exocervix**

D06.7 Carcinoma in situ of other **parts of cervix**

D06.9 Carcinoma in situ of cervix, unspecified

√4th **D07** Carcinoma in situ of other and unspecified **genital organs**
> EXCLUDES 1   melanoma in situ of trunk (D03.5)

D07.0 Carcinoma in situ of **endometrium**

D07.1 Carcinoma in situ of **vulva**
Severe dysplasia of vulva
Vulvar intraepithelial neoplasia III [VIN III]
> EXCLUDES 1   moderate dysplasia of vulva (N90.1)
> vulvar intraepithelial neoplasia II [VIN II] (N90.1)

D07.2 **Carcinoma in situ of vagina**
Severe dysplasia of vagina
Vaginal intraepithelial neoplasia III [VAIN III]
> **EXCLUDES 1**   moderate dysplasia of vagina (N89.1)
>   vaginal intraepithelial neoplasia II [VIN II] (N89.1)

✓5th **D07.3** **Carcinoma in situ of other and unspecified female genital organs**
> **D07.30** **Carcinoma in situ of unspecified female genital organs**
> **D07.39** **Carcinoma in situ of other female genital organs**

D07.4 **Carcinoma in situ of penis**
Erythroplasia of Queyrat NOS

D07.5 **Carcinoma in situ of prostate**
Prostatic intraepithelial neoplasia III (PIN III)
Severe dysplasia of prostate
> **EXCLUDES 1**   dysplasia (mild) (moderate) of prostate (N42.3-)
>   prostatic intraepithelial neoplasia II [PIN II] (N42.3-)

✓5th **D07.6** **Carcinoma in situ of other and unspecified male genital organs**
> **D07.60** **Carcinoma in situ of unspecified male genital organs**
> **D07.61** **Carcinoma in situ of scrotum**
> **D07.69** **Carcinoma in situ of other male genital organs**

✓4th **D09** **Carcinoma in situ of other and unspecified sites**
> **EXCLUDES 1**   melanoma in situ (D03.-)

D09.0 **Carcinoma in situ of bladder**

✓5th **D09.1** **Carcinoma in situ of other and unspecified urinary organs**
> **D09.10** **Carcinoma in situ of unspecified urinary organ**
> **D09.19** **Carcinoma in situ of other urinary organs**

✓5th **D09.2** **Carcinoma in situ of eye**
> **EXCLUDES 1**   carcinoma in situ of skin of eyelid (D04.1-)
> **D09.20** **Carcinoma in situ of unspecified eye**
> **D09.21** **Carcinoma in situ of right eye**
> **D09.22** **Carcinoma in situ of left eye**

D09.3 **Carcinoma in situ of thyroid and other endocrine glands**
> **EXCLUDES 1**   carcinoma in situ of endocrine pancreas (D01.7)
>   carcinoma in situ of ovary (D07.39)
>   carcinoma in situ of testis (D07.69)

D09.8 **Carcinoma in situ of other specified sites**
D09.9 **Carcinoma in situ, unspecified**

Benign neoplasms, except benign neuroendocrine tumors (D10-D36)

✓4th **D10** **Benign neoplasm of mouth and pharynx**

D10.0 **Benign neoplasm of lip**
Benign neoplasm of lip (frenulum) (inner aspect) (mucosa) (vermilion border)
> **EXCLUDES 1**   benign neoplasm of skin of lip (D22.0, D23.0)

D10.1 **Benign neoplasm of tongue**
Benign neoplasm of lingual tonsil

D10.2 **Benign neoplasm of floor of mouth**

✓5th **D10.3** **Benign neoplasm of other and unspecified parts of mouth**
> **D10.30** **Benign neoplasm of unspecified part of mouth**
> **D10.39** **Benign neoplasm of other parts of mouth**
> Benign neoplasm of minor salivary gland NOS
> > **EXCLUDES 1**   benign odontogenic neoplasms (D16.4-D16.5)
> >   benign neoplasm of mucosa of lip (D10.0)
> >   benign neoplasm of nasopharyngeal surface of soft palate (D10.6)

D10.4 **Benign neoplasm of tonsil**
Benign neoplasm of tonsil (faucial) (palatine)
> **EXCLUDES 1**   benign neoplasm of lingual tonsil (D10.1)
>   benign neoplasm of pharyngeal tonsil (D10.6)
>   benign neoplasm of tonsillar fossa (D10.5)
>   benign neoplasm of tonsillar pillars (D10.5)

D10.5 **Benign neoplasm of other parts of oropharynx**
Benign neoplasm of epiglottis, anterior aspect
Benign neoplasm of tonsillar fossa
Benign neoplasm of tonsillar pillars
Benign neoplasm of vallecula
> **EXCLUDES 1**   benign neoplasm of epiglottis NOS (D14.1)
>   benign neoplasm of epiglottis, suprahyoid portion (D14.1)

DEF: Oropharynx: Middle portion of pharynx (throat); communicates with the oral cavity, nasopharynx and laryngopharynx.

D10.6 **Benign neoplasm of nasopharynx**
Benign neoplasm of pharyngeal tonsil
Benign neoplasm of posterior margin of septum and choanae
DEF: Nasopharynx: Upper portion of pharynx (throat); communicates with the nasal cavities, oropharynx and tympanic cavities.

D10.7 **Benign neoplasm of hypopharynx**
DEF: Hypopharynx: Lower portion of pharynx (throat); communicates with the oropharynx and the esophagus.
***Synonym(s):** laryngopharynx.*

D10.9 **Benign neoplasm of pharynx, unspecified**

✓4th **D11** **Benign neoplasm of major salivary glands**
> **EXCLUDES 1**   benign neoplasms of specified minor salivary glands which are classified according to their anatomical location
>   benign neoplasms of minor salivary glands NOS (D10.39)

D11.0 **Benign neoplasm of parotid gland**

D11.7 **Benign neoplasm of other major salivary glands**
Benign neoplasm of sublingual salivary gland
Benign neoplasm of submandibular salivary gland

D11.9 **Benign neoplasm of major salivary gland, unspecified**

✓4th **D12** **Benign neoplasm of colon, rectum, anus and anal canal**
> **EXCLUDES 2**   benign carcinoid tumors of the large intestine, and rectum (D3A.02-)
>   polyp of colon NOS (K63.5)

AHA: 2018,2Q,14; 2017,1Q,15; 2015,2Q,14
TIP: Code K63.5 Polyp of colon, is assigned when documentation states hyperplastic colon polyps, regardless of the site in the colon. Slow-growing, hyperplastic polyps are not precancerous and are classified differently from benign or adenomatous polyps.

D12.0 **Benign neoplasm of cecum**
Benign neoplasm of ileocecal valve

D12.1 **Benign neoplasm of appendix**
> **EXCLUDES 1**   benign carcinoid tumor of the appendix (D3A.020)

D12.2 **Benign neoplasm of ascending colon**

D12.3 **Benign neoplasm of transverse colon**
Benign neoplasm of hepatic flexure
Benign neoplasm of splenic flexure
AHA: 2017,1Q,16

D12.4 **Benign neoplasm of descending colon**

D12.5 **Benign neoplasm of sigmoid colon**

D12.6 **Benign neoplasm of colon, unspecified**
Adenomatosis of colon
Benign neoplasm of large intestine NOS
Polyposis (hereditary) of colon
> **EXCLUDES 1**   inflammatory polyp of colon (K51.4-)

D12.7 **Benign neoplasm of rectosigmoid junction**

D12.8 **Benign neoplasm of rectum**
> **EXCLUDES 1**   benign carcinoid tumor of the rectum (D3A.026)

AHA: 2018,1Q,6

D12.9 **Benign neoplasm of anus and anal canal**
Benign neoplasm of anus NOS
> **EXCLUDES 1**   benign neoplasm of anal margin (D22.5, D23.5)
>   benign neoplasm of anal skin (D22.5, D23.5)
>   benign neoplasm of perianal skin (D22.5, D23.5)

✓4th **D13** **Benign neoplasm of other and ill-defined parts of digestive system**
> **EXCLUDES 1**   benign stromal tumors of digestive system (D21.4)

D13.0 **Benign neoplasm of esophagus**

D13.1 **Benign neoplasm of stomach**
> **EXCLUDES 1**   benign carcinoid tumor of the stomach (D3A.092)

D13.2 **Benign neoplasm of duodenum**
> **EXCLUDES 1**   benign carcinoid tumor of the duodenum (D3A.010)

☑5ᵗʰ D13.3 Benign neoplasm of other and unspecified parts of small intestine

> **EXCLUDES 1**   *benign carcinoid tumors of the small intestine (D3A.01-)*
>
> *benign neoplasm of ileocecal valve (D12.0)*

    D13.30 Benign neoplasm of unspecified part of small intestine

    D13.39 Benign neoplasm of other parts of small intestine

D13.4 Benign neoplasm of liver
Benign neoplasm of intrahepatic bile ducts

D13.5 Benign neoplasm of extrahepatic bile ducts

D13.6 Benign neoplasm of pancreas

> **EXCLUDES 1**   *benign neoplasm of endocrine pancreas (D13.7)*

D13.7 Benign neoplasm of endocrine pancreas
Benign neoplasm of islets of Langerhans
Islet cell tumor
Use additional code to identify any functional activity

☑5ᵗʰ D13.9 Benign neoplasm of ill-defined sites within the digestive system
    AHA: 2023,4Q,4-5

    D13.91 Familial adenomatous polyposis
    Code also associated conditions, such as:
      benign neoplasm of colon (D12.6)
      malignant neoplasm of colon (C18.-)

    D13.99 Benign neoplasm of ill-defined sites within the digestive system
    Benign neoplasm of digestive system NOS
    Benign neoplasm of intestine NOS
    Benign neoplasm of spleen

☑4ᵗʰ D14 Benign neoplasm of middle ear and respiratory system

D14.0 Benign neoplasm of middle ear, nasal cavity and accessory sinuses
Benign neoplasm of cartilage of nose

> **EXCLUDES 1**   *benign neoplasm of auricular canal (external) (D22.2-, D23.2-)*
>
> *benign neoplasm of bone of ear (D16.4)*
>
> *benign neoplasm of bone of nose (D16.4)*
>
> *benign neoplasm of cartilage of ear (D21.0)*
>
> *benign neoplasm of ear (external)(skin) (D22.2-, D23.2-)*
>
> *benign neoplasm of nose NOS (D36.7)*
>
> *benign neoplasm of skin of nose (D22.39, D23.39)*
>
> *benign neoplasm of olfactory bulb (D33.3)*
>
> *benign neoplasm of posterior margin of septum and choanae (D10.6)*
>
> *polyp of accessory sinus (J33.8)*
>
> *polyp of ear (middle) (H74.4)*
>
> *polyp of nasal (cavity) (J33.-)*

D14.1 Benign neoplasm of larynx
Adenomatous polyp of larynx
Benign neoplasm of epiglottis (suprahyoid portion)

> **EXCLUDES 1**   *benign neoplasm of epiglottis, anterior aspect (D10.5)*
>
> *polyp (nonadenomatous) of vocal cord or larynx (J38.1)*

D14.2 Benign neoplasm of trachea

☑5ᵗʰ D14.3 Benign neoplasm of bronchus and lung

> **EXCLUDES 1**   *benign carcinoid tumor of the bronchus and lung (D3A.090)*

    D14.30 Benign neoplasm of unspecified bronchus and lung
    D14.31 Benign neoplasm of right bronchus and lung
    D14.32 Benign neoplasm of left bronchus and lung
    D14.4 Benign neoplasm of respiratory system, unspecified

☑4ᵗʰ D15 Benign neoplasm of other and unspecified intrathoracic organs

> **EXCLUDES 1**   *benign neoplasm of mesothelial tissue (D19.-)*

D15.0 Benign neoplasm of thymus

> **EXCLUDES 1**   *benign carcinoid tumor of the thymus (D3A.091)*

D15.1 Benign neoplasm of heart

> **EXCLUDES 1**   *benign neoplasm of great vessels (D21.3)*

D15.2 Benign neoplasm of mediastinum

D15.7 Benign neoplasm of other specified intrathoracic organs

D15.9 Benign neoplasm of intrathoracic organ, unspecified

☑4ᵗʰ D16 Benign neoplasm of bone and articular cartilage

> **EXCLUDES 1**   *benign neoplasm of connective tissue of ear (D21.0)*
>
> *benign neoplasm of connective tissue of eyelid (D21.0)*
>
> *benign neoplasm of connective tissue of larynx (D14.1)*
>
> *benign neoplasm of connective tissue of nose (D14.0)*
>
> *benign neoplasm of synovia (D21.-)*

☑5ᵗʰ D16.0 Benign neoplasm of scapula and long bones of upper limb

    D16.00 Benign neoplasm of scapula and long bones of unspecified upper limb
    D16.01 Benign neoplasm of scapula and long bones of right upper limb
    D16.02 Benign neoplasm of scapula and long bones of left upper limb

☑5ᵗʰ D16.1 Benign neoplasm of short bones of upper limb

    D16.10 Benign neoplasm of short bones of unspecified upper limb
    D16.11 Benign neoplasm of short bones of right upper limb
    D16.12 Benign neoplasm of short bones of left upper limb

☑5ᵗʰ D16.2 Benign neoplasm of long bones of lower limb

    D16.20 Benign neoplasm of long bones of unspecified lower limb
    D16.21 Benign neoplasm of long bones of right lower limb
    D16.22 Benign neoplasm of long bones of left lower limb

☑5ᵗʰ D16.3 Benign neoplasm of short bones of lower limb

    D16.30 Benign neoplasm of short bones of unspecified lower limb
    D16.31 Benign neoplasm of short bones of right lower limb
    D16.32 Benign neoplasm of short bones of left lower limb

D16.4 Benign neoplasm of bones of skull and face
Benign neoplasm of maxilla (superior)
Benign neoplasm of orbital bone
Keratocyst of maxilla
Keratocystic odontogenic tumor of maxilla

> **EXCLUDES 2**   *benign neoplasm of lower jaw bone (D16.5)*

D16.5 Benign neoplasm of lower jaw bone
Keratocyst of mandible
Keratocystic odontogenic tumor of mandible

D16.6 Benign neoplasm of vertebral column

> **EXCLUDES 1**   *benign neoplasm of sacrum and coccyx (D16.8)*

D16.7 Benign neoplasm of ribs, sternum and clavicle

D16.8 Benign neoplasm of pelvic bones, sacrum and coccyx

D16.9 Benign neoplasm of bone and articular cartilage, unspecified

☑4ᵗʰ D17 Benign lipomatous neoplasm

D17.0 Benign lipomatous neoplasm of skin and subcutaneous tissue of head, face and neck

D17.1 Benign lipomatous neoplasm of skin and subcutaneous tissue of trunk

☑5ᵗʰ D17.2 Benign lipomatous neoplasm of skin and subcutaneous tissue of limb

    D17.20 Benign lipomatous neoplasm of skin and subcutaneous tissue of unspecified limb
    D17.21 Benign lipomatous neoplasm of skin and subcutaneous tissue of right arm
    D17.22 Benign lipomatous neoplasm of skin and subcutaneous tissue of left arm
    D17.23 Benign lipomatous neoplasm of skin and subcutaneous tissue of right leg
    D17.24 Benign lipomatous neoplasm of skin and subcutaneous tissue of left leg

☑5ᵗʰ D17.3 Benign lipomatous neoplasm of skin and subcutaneous tissue of other and unspecified sites

    D17.30 Benign lipomatous neoplasm of skin and subcutaneous tissue of unspecified sites
    D17.39 Benign lipomatous neoplasm of skin and subcutaneous tissue of other sites

D17.4 Benign lipomatous neoplasm of intrathoracic organs

D17.5 Benign lipomatous neoplasm of intra-abdominal organs

> **EXCLUDES 1**   *benign lipomatous neoplasm of peritoneum and retroperitoneum (D17.79)*

D17.6 Benign lipomatous neoplasm of spermatic cord

☑5ᵗʰ D17.7 Benign lipomatous neoplasm of other sites

    D17.71 Benign lipomatous neoplasm of kidney
    D17.72 Benign lipomatous neoplasm of other genitourinary organ
    D17.79 Benign lipomatous neoplasm of other sites
    Benign lipomatous neoplasm of peritoneum
    Benign lipomatous neoplasm of retroperitoneum

Chapter 2. Neoplasms   **D13.3–D17.79**

N Newborn: 0   **P** Pediatric: 0-17   **M** Maternity: 9-64   **A** Adult: 15-124   **UNS** Unspecified Site   **MCC** Major Complication/Comorbidity   **CC** Complication/Comorbidity   **PE** POA Exempt

504   ICD-10-CM 2025

Chapter 2. Neoplasms

D17.9   **Benign lipomatous neoplasm, unspecified**
Lipoma NOS

✓4th **D18**   **Hemangioma and lymphangioma, any site**
> EXCLUDES 1   *benign neoplasm of glomus jugulare (D35.6)*
> *blue or pigmented nevus (D22.-)*
> *nevus NOS (D22.-)*
> *vascular nevus (Q82.5)*

✓5th **D18.0**   **Hemangioma**
Angioma NOS
Cavernous nevus
DEF: Common benign tumor usually occurring in infancy that is composed of newly formed blood vessels due to malformation of the angioblastic tissue.

D18.00   **Hemangioma unspecified site**
D18.01   **Hemangioma of skin and subcutaneous tissue**
D18.02   **Hemangioma of intracranial structures**   HCC
D18.03   **Hemangioma of intra-abdominal structures**
D18.09   **Hemangioma of other sites**

D18.1   **Lymphangioma, any site**
AHA: 2018,3Q,31; 2018,2Q,13

✓4th **D19**   **Benign neoplasm of mesothelial tissue**

D19.0   **Benign neoplasm of mesothelial tissue of pleura**
D19.1   **Benign neoplasm of mesothelial tissue of peritoneum**
D19.7   **Benign neoplasm of mesothelial tissue of other sites**
D19.9   **Benign neoplasm of mesothelial tissue, unspecified**
Benign mesothelioma NOS

✓4th **D20**   **Benign neoplasm of soft tissue of retroperitoneum and peritoneum**
> EXCLUDES 1   *benign lipomatous neoplasm of peritoneum and retroperitoneum (D17.79)*
> *benign neoplasm of mesothelial tissue (D19.-)*

D20.0   **Benign neoplasm of soft tissue of retroperitoneum**
D20.1   **Benign neoplasm of soft tissue of peritoneum**

✓4th **D21**   **Other benign neoplasms of connective and other soft tissue**
> INCLUDES   benign neoplasm of blood vessel
> benign neoplasm of bursa
> benign neoplasm of cartilage
> benign neoplasm of fascia
> benign neoplasm of fat
> benign neoplasm of ligament, except uterine
> benign neoplasm of lymphatic channel
> benign neoplasm of muscle
> benign neoplasm of synovia
> benign neoplasm of tendon (sheath)
> benign stromal tumors

> EXCLUDES 1   *benign neoplasm of articular cartilage (D16.-)*
> *benign neoplasm of cartilage of larynx (D14.1)*
> *benign neoplasm of cartilage of nose (D14.0)*
> *benign neoplasm of connective tissue of breast (D24.-)*
> *benign neoplasm of peripheral nerves and autonomic nervous system (D36.1-)*
> *benign neoplasm of peritoneum (D20.1)*
> *benign neoplasm of retroperitoneum (D20.0)*
> *benign neoplasm of uterine ligament, any (D28.2)*
> *benign neoplasm of vascular tissue (D18.-)*
> *hemangioma (D18.0-)*
> *lipomatous neoplasm (D17.-)*
> *lymphangioma (D18.1)*
> *uterine leiomyoma (D25.-)*

D21.0   **Benign neoplasm of connective and other soft tissue of head, face and neck**
Benign neoplasm of connective tissue of ear
Benign neoplasm of connective tissue of eyelid
> EXCLUDES 1   *benign neoplasm of connective tissue of orbit (D31.5-)*

✓5th **D21.1**   **Benign neoplasm of connective and other soft tissue of upper limb, including shoulder**
D21.10   **Benign neoplasm of connective and other soft tissue of unspecified upper limb, including shoulder**
D21.11   **Benign neoplasm of connective and other soft tissue of right upper limb, including shoulder**
D21.12   **Benign neoplasm of connective and other soft tissue of left upper limb, including shoulder**

✓5th **D21.2**   **Benign neoplasm of connective and other soft tissue of lower limb, including hip**
D21.20   **Benign neoplasm of connective and other soft tissue of unspecified lower limb, including hip**

D21.21   **Benign neoplasm of connective and other soft tissue of right lower limb, including hip**
D21.22   **Benign neoplasm of connective and other soft tissue of left lower limb, including hip**

D21.3   **Benign neoplasm of connective and other soft tissue of thorax**
Benign neoplasm of axilla
Benign neoplasm of diaphragm
Benign neoplasm of great vessels
> EXCLUDES 1   *benign neoplasm of heart (D15.1)*
> *benign neoplasm of mediastinum (D15.2)*
> *benign neoplasm of thymus (D15.0)*

D21.4   **Benign neoplasm of connective and other soft tissue of abdomen**
Benign stromal tumors of abdomen

D21.5   **Benign neoplasm of connective and other soft tissue of pelvis**
> EXCLUDES 1   *benign neoplasm of any uterine ligament (D28.2)*
> *uterine leiomyoma (D25.-)*

D21.6   **Benign neoplasm of connective and other soft tissue of trunk, unspecified**
Benign neoplasm of connective and other soft tissue of back NOS

D21.9   **Benign neoplasm of connective and other soft tissue, unspecified**

✓4th **D22**   **Melanocytic nevi**
> INCLUDES   atypical nevus
> blue hairy pigmented nevus
> nevus NOS

D22.0   **Melanocytic nevi of lip**

✓5th **D22.1**   **Melanocytic nevi of eyelid, including canthus**
AHA: 2018,4Q,4

D22.10   **Melanocytic nevi of unspecified eyelid, including canthus**
✓6th **D22.11**   **Melanocytic nevi of right eyelid, including canthus**
D22.111   **Melanocytic nevi of right upper eyelid, including canthus**
D22.112   **Melanocytic nevi of right lower eyelid, including canthus**
✓6th **D22.12**   **Melanocytic nevi of left eyelid, including canthus**
D22.121   **Melanocytic nevi of left upper eyelid, including canthus**
D22.122   **Melanocytic nevi of left lower eyelid, including canthus**

✓5th **D22.2**   **Melanocytic nevi of ear and external auricular canal**
D22.20   **Melanocytic nevi of unspecified ear and external auricular canal**
D22.21   **Melanocytic nevi of right ear and external auricular canal**
D22.22   **Melanocytic nevi of left ear and external auricular canal**

✓5th **D22.3**   **Melanocytic nevi of other and unspecified parts of face**
D22.30   **Melanocytic nevi of unspecified part of face**
D22.39   **Melanocytic nevi of other parts of face**

D22.4   **Melanocytic nevi of scalp and neck**

D22.5   **Melanocytic nevi of trunk**
Melanocytic nevi of anal margin
Melanocytic nevi of anal skin
Melanocytic nevi of perianal skin
Melanocytic nevi of skin of breast

✓5th **D22.6**   **Melanocytic nevi of upper limb, including shoulder**
D22.60   **Melanocytic nevi of unspecified upper limb, including shoulder**
D22.61   **Melanocytic nevi of right upper limb, including shoulder**
D22.62   **Melanocytic nevi of left upper limb, including shoulder**

✓5th **D22.7**   **Melanocytic nevi of lower limb, including hip**
D22.70   **Melanocytic nevi of unspecified lower limb, including hip**
D22.71   **Melanocytic nevi of right lower limb, including hip**
D22.72   **Melanocytic nevi of left lower limb, including hip**
D22.9   **Melanocytic nevi, unspecified**

✓ Additional Character Required   ✓x7th Placeholder   Questionable PDx   Manifestation   Unspecified   UPD Unacceptable PDx   H1 - H14 HAC   HCC CMS-HCC Dx   HIV HIV Dx

Chapter 2. Neoplasms

D23–D29.3Ø

✓4th **D23 Other benign neoplasms of skin**

INCLUDES   benign neoplasm of hair follicles
       benign neoplasm of sebaceous glands
       benign neoplasm of sweat glands

EXCLUDES 1   *benign lipomatous neoplasms of skin (D17.Ø-D17.3)*

EXCLUDES 2   *melanocytic nevi (D22.-)*

D23.Ø Other benign neoplasm of skin of lip

    EXCLUDES 1   *benign neoplasm of vermilion border of lip (D1Ø.Ø)*

✓5th **D23.1 Other benign neoplasm of skin of eyelid, including canthus**

    AHA: 2018,4Q,4

    D23.1Ø Other benign neoplasm of skin of unspecified eyelid, including canthus

    ✓6th **D23.11 Other benign neoplasm of skin of right eyelid, including canthus**

        D23.111 Other benign neoplasm of skin of right upper eyelid, including canthus

        D23.112 Other benign neoplasm of skin of right lower eyelid, including canthus

    ✓6th **D23.12 Other benign neoplasm of skin of left eyelid, including canthus**

        D23.121 Other benign neoplasm of skin of left upper eyelid, including canthus

        D23.122 Other benign neoplasm of skin of left lower eyelid, including canthus

✓5th **D23.2 Other benign neoplasm of skin of ear and external auricular canal**

    D23.2Ø Other benign neoplasm of skin of unspecified ear and external auricular canal

    D23.21 Other benign neoplasm of skin of right ear and external auricular canal

    D23.22 Other benign neoplasm of skin of left ear and external auricular canal

✓5th **D23.3 Other benign neoplasm of skin of other and unspecified parts of face**

    D23.3Ø Other benign neoplasm of skin of unspecified part of face

    D23.39 Other benign neoplasm of skin of other parts of face

D23.4 Other benign neoplasm of skin of scalp and neck

D23.5 Other benign neoplasm of skin of trunk

    Other benign neoplasm of anal margin
    Other benign neoplasm of anal skin
    Other benign neoplasm of perianal skin
    Other benign neoplasm of skin of breast

    EXCLUDES 1   *benign neoplasm of anus NOS (D12.9)*

✓5th **D23.6 Other benign neoplasm of skin of upper limb, including shoulder**

    D23.6Ø Other benign neoplasm of skin of unspecified upper limb, including shoulder

    D23.61 Other benign neoplasm of skin of right upper limb, including shoulder

    D23.62 Other benign neoplasm of skin of left upper limb, including shoulder

✓5th **D23.7 Other benign neoplasm of skin of lower limb, including hip**

    D23.7Ø Other benign neoplasm of skin of unspecified lower limb, including hip

    D23.71 Other benign neoplasm of skin of right lower limb, including hip

    D23.72 Other benign neoplasm of skin of left lower limb, including hip

D23.9 Other benign neoplasm of skin, unspecified

✓4th **D24 Benign neoplasm of breast**

INCLUDES   benign neoplasm of connective tissue of breast
       benign neoplasm of soft parts of breast
       fibroadenoma of breast

EXCLUDES 2   *adenofibrosis of breast (N6Ø.2)*
       benign cyst of breast (N6Ø.-)
       benign mammary dysplasia (N6Ø.-)
       benign neoplasm of skin of breast (D22.5, D23.5)
       fibrocystic disease of breast (N6Ø.-)

D24.1 Benign neoplasm of right breast

D24.2 Benign neoplasm of left breast

D24.9 Benign neoplasm of unspecified breast

✓4th **D25 Leiomyoma of uterus**

INCLUDES   uterine fibroid
       uterine fibromyoma
       uterine myoma

Uterine Leiomyomas (Fibroids)

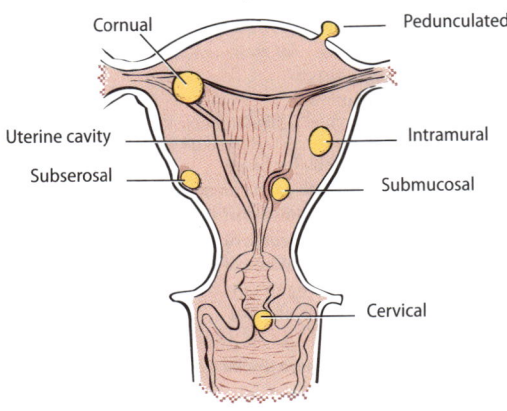

D25.Ø Submucous leiomyoma of uterus

D25.1 Intramural leiomyoma of uterus

    Interstitial leiomyoma of uterus

D25.2 Subserosal leiomyoma of uterus

    Subperitoneal leiomyoma of uterus

D25.9 Leiomyoma of uterus, unspecified

✓4th **D26 Other benign neoplasms of uterus**

D26.Ø Other benign neoplasm of cervix uteri

D26.1 Other benign neoplasm of corpus uteri

D26.7 Other benign neoplasm of other parts of uterus

D26.9 Other benign neoplasm of uterus, unspecified

✓4th **D27 Benign neoplasm of ovary**

Use additional code to identify any functional activity

EXCLUDES 2   *corpus albicans cyst (N83.2-)*
       corpus luteum cyst (N83.1-)
       endometrial cyst (N8Ø.1-)
       follicular (atretic) cyst (N83.Ø-)
       graafian follicle cyst (N83.Ø-)
       ovarian cyst NEC (N83.2-)
       ovarian retention cyst (N83.2-)

D27.Ø Benign neoplasm of right ovary

D27.1 Benign neoplasm of left ovary

D27.9 Benign neoplasm of unspecified ovary

✓4th **D28 Benign neoplasm of other and unspecified female genital organs**

INCLUDES   adenomatous polyp
       benign neoplasm of skin of female genital organs
       benign teratoma

EXCLUDES 1   *epoophoron cyst (Q5Ø.5)*
       fimbrial cyst (Q5Ø.4)
       Gartner's duct cyst (Q52.4)
       parovarian cyst (Q5Ø.5)

D28.Ø Benign neoplasm of vulva

D28.1 Benign neoplasm of vagina

D28.2 Benign neoplasm of uterine tubes and ligaments

    Benign neoplasm of fallopian tube
    Benign neoplasm of uterine ligament (broad) (round)

D28.7 Benign neoplasm of other specified female genital organs

D28.9 Benign neoplasm of female genital organ, unspecified

✓4th **D29 Benign neoplasm of male genital organs**

INCLUDES   benign neoplasm of skin of male genital organs

D29.Ø Benign neoplasm of penis

D29.1 Benign neoplasm of prostate

    EXCLUDES 1   *enlarged prostate (N4Ø.-)*

✓5th **D29.2 Benign neoplasm of testis**

Use additional code to identify any functional activity

    D29.2Ø Benign neoplasm of unspecified testis

    D29.21 Benign neoplasm of right testis

    D29.22 Benign neoplasm of left testis

✓5th **D29.3 Benign neoplasm of epididymis**

    D29.3Ø Benign neoplasm of unspecified epididymis

N Newborn: 0   P Pediatric: 0-17   M Maternity: 9-64   A Adult: 15-124   UNS Unspecified Site   MCC Major Complication/Comorbidity   CC Complication/Comorbidity   PE POA Exempt

506   ICD-10-CM 2025

D29.31   Benign neoplasm of right epididymis

D29.32   Benign neoplasm of left epididymis

D29.4   **Benign neoplasm of scrotum**
Benign neoplasm of skin of scrotum

D29.8   **Benign neoplasm of other specified male genital organs**
Benign neoplasm of seminal vesicle
Benign neoplasm of spermatic cord
Benign neoplasm of tunica vaginalis

D29.9   **Benign neoplasm of male genital organ, unspecified**

✓4th **D30**   **Benign neoplasm of urinary organs**

   ✓5th **D30.0**   **Benign neoplasm of kidney**
     EXCLUDES 1   benign carcinoid tumor of the kidney (D3A.093)
           benign neoplasm of renal calyces (D30.1-)
           benign neoplasm of renal pelvis (D30.1-)

     D30.00   **Benign neoplasm of unspecified kidney**

     D30.01   Benign neoplasm of right kidney

     D30.02   Benign neoplasm of left kidney

   ✓5th **D30.1**   **Benign neoplasm of renal pelvis**

     D30.10   **Benign neoplasm of unspecified renal pelvis**

     D30.11   Benign neoplasm of right renal pelvis

     D30.12   Benign neoplasm of left renal pelvis

   ✓5th **D30.2**   **Benign neoplasm of ureter**
     EXCLUDES 1   benign neoplasm of ureteric orifice of bladder (D30.3)

     D30.20   **Benign neoplasm of unspecified ureter**

     D30.21   Benign neoplasm of right ureter

     D30.22   Benign neoplasm of left ureter

   D30.3   **Benign neoplasm of bladder**
Benign neoplasm of ureteric orifice of bladder
Benign neoplasm of urethral orifice of bladder

   D30.4   **Benign neoplasm of urethra**
     EXCLUDES 1   benign neoplasm of urethral orifice of bladder (D30.3)

   D30.8   **Benign neoplasm of other specified urinary organs**
Benign neoplasm of paraurethral glands

   D30.9   **Benign neoplasm of urinary organ, unspecified**
Benign neoplasm of urinary system NOS

✓4th **D31**   **Benign neoplasm of eye and adnexa**
     EXCLUDES 1   benign neoplasm of connective tissue of eyelid (D21.0)
           benign neoplasm of optic nerve (D33.3)
           benign neoplasm of skin of eyelid (D22.1-, D23.1-)

   ✓5th **D31.0**   **Benign neoplasm of conjunctiva**

     D31.00   **Benign neoplasm of unspecified conjunctiva**

     D31.01   Benign neoplasm of right conjunctiva

     D31.02   Benign neoplasm of left conjunctiva

   ✓5th **D31.1**   **Benign neoplasm of cornea**

     D31.10   **Benign neoplasm of unspecified cornea**

     D31.11   Benign neoplasm of right cornea

     D31.12   Benign neoplasm of left cornea

   ✓5th **D31.2**   **Benign neoplasm of retina**
     EXCLUDES 1   dark area on retina (D49.81)
           hemangioma of retina (D49.81)
           neoplasm of unspecified behavior of retina and choroid (D49.81)
           retinal freckle (D49.81)

     D31.20   **Benign neoplasm of unspecified retina**

     D31.21   Benign neoplasm of right retina

     D31.22   Benign neoplasm of left retina

   ✓5th **D31.3**   **Benign neoplasm of choroid**

     D31.30   **Benign neoplasm of unspecified choroid**

     D31.31   Benign neoplasm of right choroid

     D31.32   Benign neoplasm of left choroid

   ✓5th **D31.4**   **Benign neoplasm of ciliary body**

     D31.40   **Benign neoplasm of unspecified ciliary body**

     D31.41   Benign neoplasm of right ciliary body

     D31.42   Benign neoplasm of left ciliary body

   ✓5th **D31.5**   **Benign neoplasm of lacrimal gland and duct**
Benign neoplasm of lacrimal sac
Benign neoplasm of nasolacrimal duct

     D31.50   **Benign neoplasm of unspecified lacrimal gland and duct**

     D31.51   Benign neoplasm of right lacrimal gland and duct

     D31.52   Benign neoplasm of left lacrimal gland and duct

   ✓5th **D31.6**   **Benign neoplasm of unspecified site of orbit**
Benign neoplasm of connective tissue of orbit
Benign neoplasm of extraocular muscle
Benign neoplasm of peripheral nerves of orbit
Benign neoplasm of retrobulbar tissue
Benign neoplasm of retro-ocular tissue
     EXCLUDES 1   benign neoplasm of orbital bone (D16.4)

     D31.60   **Benign neoplasm of unspecified site of unspecified orbit**

     D31.61   **Benign neoplasm of unspecified site of right orbit**

     D31.62   **Benign neoplasm of unspecified site of left orbit**

   ✓5th **D31.9**   **Benign neoplasm of unspecified part of eye**
Benign neoplasm of eyeball

     D31.90   **Benign neoplasm of unspecified part of unspecified eye**

     D31.91   Benign neoplasm of unspecified part of right eye

     D31.92   Benign neoplasm of unspecified part of left eye

✓4th **D32**   **Benign neoplasm of meninges**

   D32.0   **Benign neoplasm of cerebral meninges**   `HCC`

   D32.1   **Benign neoplasm of spinal meninges**   `HCC`

   D32.9   **Benign neoplasm of meninges, unspecified**   `HCC`
Meningioma NOS

✓4th **D33**   **Benign neoplasm of brain and other parts of central nervous system**
     EXCLUDES 1   angioma (D18.0-)
           benign neoplasm of meninges (D32.-)
           benign neoplasm of peripheral nerves and autonomic nervous system (D36.1-)
           hemangioma (D18.0-)
           neurofibromatosis (Q85.0-)
           retro-ocular benign neoplasm (D31.6-)

   D33.0   **Benign neoplasm of brain, supratentorial**   `HCC`
Benign neoplasm of cerebral ventricle
Benign neoplasm of cerebrum
Benign neoplasm of frontal lobe
Benign neoplasm of occipital lobe
Benign neoplasm of parietal lobe
Benign neoplasm of temporal lobe
     EXCLUDES 1   benign neoplasm of fourth ventricle (D33.1)

   D33.1   **Benign neoplasm of brain, infratentorial**   `HCC`
Benign neoplasm of brain stem
Benign neoplasm of cerebellum
Benign neoplasm of fourth ventricle

   D33.2   **Benign neoplasm of brain, unspecified**   `HCC`

   D33.3   **Benign neoplasm of cranial nerves**   `HCC`
Benign neoplasm of olfactory bulb

   D33.4   **Benign neoplasm of spinal cord**   `HCC`

   D33.7   **Benign neoplasm of other specified parts of central nervous system**   `HCC`

   D33.9   **Benign neoplasm of central nervous system, unspecified**   `HCC`
Benign neoplasm of nervous system (central) NOS

D34   **Benign neoplasm of thyroid gland**
Use additional code to identify any functional activity

✓4th **D35**   **Benign neoplasm of other and unspecified endocrine glands**
Use additional code to identify any functional activity
     EXCLUDES 1   benign neoplasm of endocrine pancreas (D13.7)
           benign neoplasm of ovary (D27.-)
           benign neoplasm of testis (D29.2.-)
           benign neoplasm of thymus (D15.0)

   ✓5th **D35.0**   **Benign neoplasm of adrenal gland**

     D35.00   **Benign neoplasm of unspecified adrenal gland**

     D35.01   Benign neoplasm of right adrenal gland

     D35.02   Benign neoplasm of left adrenal gland

   D35.1   **Benign neoplasm of parathyroid gland**

   D35.2   **Benign neoplasm of pituitary gland**   `HCC`
AHA: 2014,3Q,22

   D35.3   **Benign neoplasm of craniopharyngeal duct**   `HCC`

   D35.4   **Benign neoplasm of pineal gland**   `HCC`

   D35.5   **Benign neoplasm of carotid body**

   D35.6   **Benign neoplasm of aortic body and other paraganglia**
Benign tumor of glomus jugulare

   D35.7   **Benign neoplasm of other specified endocrine glands**

   D35.9   **Benign neoplasm of endocrine gland, unspecified**
Benign neoplasm of unspecified endocrine gland

☑ Additional Character Required   ✓x7th Placeholder   Questionable PDx   Manifestation   Unspecified   `UPD` Unacceptable PDx   `H1`-`H14` HAC   `HCC` CMS-HCC Dx   `HIV` HIV Dx

ICD-10-CM 2025   **507**

Chapter 2. Neoplasms

D36–D37.6

√4th **D36 Benign neoplasm of other and unspecified sites**

D36.0 Benign neoplasm of lymph nodes
> EXCLUDES 1   *lymphangioma (D18.1)*

√5th **D36.1 Benign neoplasm of peripheral nerves and autonomic nervous system**
> EXCLUDES 1   *benign neoplasm of peripheral nerves of orbit (D31.6-)*
> *neurofibromatosis (Q85.0-)*

D36.10 Benign neoplasm of peripheral nerves and autonomic nervous system, unspecified

D36.11 Benign neoplasm of peripheral nerves and autonomic nervous system of face, head, and neck

D36.12 Benign neoplasm of peripheral nerves and autonomic nervous system, upper limb, including shoulder

D36.13 Benign neoplasm of peripheral nerves and autonomic nervous system of lower limb, including hip

D36.14 Benign neoplasm of peripheral nerves and autonomic nervous system of thorax

D36.15 Benign neoplasm of peripheral nerves and autonomic nervous system of abdomen

D36.16 Benign neoplasm of peripheral nerves and autonomic nervous system of pelvis

D36.17 Benign neoplasm of peripheral nerves and autonomic nervous system of trunk, unspecified

D36.7 Benign neoplasm of other specified sites
Benign neoplasm of back NOS
Benign neoplasm of nose NOS

D36.9 Benign neoplasm, unspecified site

Benign neuroendocrine tumors (D3A)

√4th **D3A Benign neuroendocrine tumors**
Code also any associated multiple endocrine neoplasia [MEN] syndromes (E31.2-)
Use additional code to identify any associated endocrine syndrome, such as:
carcinoid syndrome ▶(E34.00)◀
> EXCLUDES 2   *benign pancreatic islet cell tumors (D13.7)*

√5th **D3A.0 Benign carcinoid tumors**
DEF: Specific type of slow-growing neuroendocrine tumors. Carcinoid tumors occur most commonly in the hormone producing cells of the gastrointestinal tracts and can also occur in the pancreas, testes, ovaries, or lungs.

D3A.00 Benign carcinoid tumor of unspecified site HCC
Carcinoid tumor NOS

√6th **D3A.01 Benign carcinoid tumors of the small intestine**

D3A.010 Benign carcinoid tumor of the duodenum HCC

D3A.011 Benign carcinoid tumor of the jejunum HCC

D3A.012 Benign carcinoid tumor of the ileum HCC

D3A.019 Benign carcinoid tumor of the small intestine, unspecified portion HCC

√6th **D3A.02 Benign carcinoid tumors of the appendix, large intestine, and rectum**

D3A.020 Benign carcinoid tumor of the appendix HCC

D3A.021 Benign carcinoid tumor of the cecum HCC

D3A.022 Benign carcinoid tumor of the ascending colon HCC

D3A.023 Benign carcinoid tumor of the transverse colon HCC

D3A.024 Benign carcinoid tumor of the descending colon HCC

D3A.025 Benign carcinoid tumor of the sigmoid colon HCC

D3A.026 Benign carcinoid tumor of the rectum HCC

D3A.029 Benign carcinoid tumor of the large intestine, unspecified portion HCC
Benign carcinoid tumor of the colon NOS

√6th **D3A.09 Benign carcinoid tumors of other sites**

D3A.090 Benign carcinoid tumor of the bronchus and lung HCC

D3A.091 Benign carcinoid tumor of the thymus HCC

D3A.092 Benign carcinoid tumor of the stomach HCC

D3A.093 Benign carcinoid tumor of the kidney HCC

D3A.094 Benign carcinoid tumor of the foregut, unspecified HCC

D3A.095 Benign carcinoid tumor of the midgut, unspecified HCC

D3A.096 Benign carcinoid tumor of the hindgut, unspecified HCC

D3A.098 Benign carcinoid tumors of other sites HCC

D3A.8 Other benign neuroendocrine tumors HCC
Neuroendocrine tumor NOS

Neoplasms of uncertain behavior, polycythemia vera and myelodysplastic syndromes (D37-D48)

> NOTE   Categories D37-D44, and D48 classify by site neoplasms of uncertain behavior, i.e., histologic confirmation whether the neoplasm is malignant or benign cannot be made.

> EXCLUDES 1   *neoplasms of unspecified behavior (D49.-)*

√4th **D37 Neoplasm of uncertain behavior of oral cavity and digestive organs**
> EXCLUDES 1   *stromal tumors of uncertain behavior of digestive system (D48.1-)*

√5th **D37.0 Neoplasm of uncertain behavior of lip, oral cavity and pharynx**
> EXCLUDES 1   *neoplasm of uncertain behavior of aryepiglottic fold or interarytenoid fold, laryngeal aspect (D38.0)*
> *neoplasm of uncertain behavior of epiglottis NOS (D38.0)*
> *neoplasm of uncertain behavior of skin of lip (D48.5)*
> *neoplasm of uncertain behavior of suprahyoid portion of epiglottis (D38.0)*

D37.01 Neoplasm of uncertain behavior of lip
Neoplasm of uncertain behavior of vermilion border of lip

D37.02 Neoplasm of uncertain behavior of tongue

√6th **D37.03 Neoplasm of uncertain behavior of the major salivary glands**

D37.030 Neoplasm of uncertain behavior of the parotid salivary glands

D37.031 Neoplasm of uncertain behavior of the sublingual salivary glands

D37.032 Neoplasm of uncertain behavior of the submandibular salivary glands

D37.039 Neoplasm of uncertain behavior of the major salivary glands, unspecified

D37.04 Neoplasm of uncertain behavior of the minor salivary glands
Neoplasm of uncertain behavior of submucosal salivary glands of cheek
Neoplasm of uncertain behavior of submucosal salivary glands of hard palate
Neoplasm of uncertain behavior of submucosal salivary glands of lip
Neoplasm of uncertain behavior of submucosal salivary glands of soft palate

D37.05 Neoplasm of uncertain behavior of pharynx
Neoplasm of uncertain behavior of aryepiglottic fold of pharynx NOS
Neoplasm of uncertain behavior of hypopharyngeal aspect of aryepiglottic fold of pharynx
Neoplasm of uncertain behavior of marginal zone of aryepiglottic fold of pharynx

D37.09 Neoplasm of uncertain behavior of other specified sites of the oral cavity

D37.1 Neoplasm of uncertain behavior of stomach

D37.2 Neoplasm of uncertain behavior of small intestine

D37.3 Neoplasm of uncertain behavior of appendix

D37.4 Neoplasm of uncertain behavior of colon

D37.5 Neoplasm of uncertain behavior of rectum
Neoplasm of uncertain behavior of rectosigmoid junction

D37.6 Neoplasm of uncertain behavior of liver, gallbladder and bile ducts
Neoplasm of uncertain behavior of ampulla of Vater

D37.8 **Neoplasm of uncertain behavior of other specified digestive organs**
Neoplasm of uncertain behavior of anal canal
Neoplasm of uncertain behavior of anal sphincter
Neoplasm of uncertain behavior of anus NOS
Neoplasm of uncertain behavior of esophagus
Neoplasm of uncertain behavior of intestine NOS
Neoplasm of uncertain behavior of pancreas
EXCLUDES 1   *neoplasm of uncertain behavior of anal margin (D48.5)*
neoplasm of uncertain behavior of anal skin (D48.5)
neoplasm of uncertain behavior of perianal skin (D48.5)

D37.9 **Neoplasm of uncertain behavior of digestive organ, unspecified**

✓4ᵗʰ D38 **Neoplasm of uncertain behavior of middle ear and respiratory and intrathoracic organs**
EXCLUDES 1   *neoplasm of uncertain behavior of heart (D48.7)*

D38.0 **Neoplasm of uncertain behavior of larynx**
Neoplasm of uncertain behavior of aryepiglottic fold or interarytenoid fold, laryngeal aspect
Neoplasm of uncertain behavior of epiglottis (suprahyoid portion)
EXCLUDES 1   *neoplasm of uncertain behavior of aryepiglottic fold or interarytenoid fold NOS (D37.05)*
neoplasm of uncertain behavior of hypopharyngeal aspect of aryepiglottic fold (D37.05)
neoplasm of uncertain behavior of marginal zone of aryepiglottic fold (D37.05)

D38.1 **Neoplasm of uncertain behavior of trachea, bronchus and lung**

D38.2 **Neoplasm of uncertain behavior of pleura**

D38.3 **Neoplasm of uncertain behavior of mediastinum**

D38.4 **Neoplasm of uncertain behavior of thymus**

D38.5 **Neoplasm of uncertain behavior of other respiratory organs**
Neoplasm of uncertain behavior of accessory sinuses
Neoplasm of uncertain behavior of cartilage of nose
Neoplasm of uncertain behavior of middle ear
Neoplasm of uncertain behavior of nasal cavities
EXCLUDES 1   *neoplasm of uncertain behavior of ear (external) (skin) (D48.5)*
neoplasm of uncertain behavior of nose NOS (D48.7)
neoplasm of uncertain behavior of skin of nose (D48.5)

D38.6 **Neoplasm of uncertain behavior of respiratory organ, unspecified**

✓4ᵗʰ D39 **Neoplasm of uncertain behavior of female genital organs**

D39.0 **Neoplasm of uncertain behavior of uterus**

✓5ᵗʰ D39.1 **Neoplasm of uncertain behavior of ovary**
Use additional code to identify any functional activity

D39.10 **Neoplasm of uncertain behavior of unspecified ovary**

D39.11 **Neoplasm of uncertain behavior of right ovary**

D39.12 **Neoplasm of uncertain behavior of left ovary**

D39.2 **Neoplasm of uncertain behavior of placenta** Ⓜ
Chorioadenoma destruens
Invasive hydatidiform mole
Malignant hydatidiform mole
EXCLUDES 1   *hydatidiform mole NOS (O01.9)*
AHA: 2023,3Q,14

D39.8 **Neoplasm of uncertain behavior of other specified female genital organs**
Neoplasm of uncertain behavior of skin of female genital organs

D39.9 **Neoplasm of uncertain behavior of female genital organ, unspecified**

✓4ᵗʰ D40 **Neoplasm of uncertain behavior of male genital organs**

D40.0 **Neoplasm of uncertain behavior of prostate**

✓5ᵗʰ D40.1 **Neoplasm of uncertain behavior of testis**

D40.10 **Neoplasm of uncertain behavior of unspecified testis**

D40.11 **Neoplasm of uncertain behavior of right testis**

D40.12 **Neoplasm of uncertain behavior of left testis**

D40.8 **Neoplasm of uncertain behavior of other specified male genital organs**
Neoplasm of uncertain behavior of skin of male genital organs

D40.9 **Neoplasm of uncertain behavior of male genital organ, unspecified**

✓4ᵗʰ D41 **Neoplasm of uncertain behavior of urinary organs**

✓5ᵗʰ D41.0 **Neoplasm of uncertain behavior of kidney**
EXCLUDES 1   *neoplasm of uncertain behavior of renal pelvis (D41.1-)*

D41.00 **Neoplasm of uncertain behavior of unspecified kidney**

D41.01 **Neoplasm of uncertain behavior of right kidney**

D41.02 **Neoplasm of uncertain behavior of left kidney**

✓5ᵗʰ D41.1 **Neoplasm of uncertain behavior of renal pelvis**

D41.10 **Neoplasm of uncertain behavior of unspecified renal pelvis**

D41.11 **Neoplasm of uncertain behavior of right renal pelvis**

D41.12 **Neoplasm of uncertain behavior of left renal pelvis**

✓5ᵗʰ D41.2 **Neoplasm of uncertain behavior of ureter**

D41.20 **Neoplasm of uncertain behavior of unspecified ureter**

D41.21 **Neoplasm of uncertain behavior of right ureter**

D41.22 **Neoplasm of uncertain behavior of left ureter**

D41.3 **Neoplasm of uncertain behavior of urethra**

D41.4 **Neoplasm of uncertain behavior of bladder**

D41.8 **Neoplasm of uncertain behavior of other specified urinary organs**

D41.9 **Neoplasm of uncertain behavior of unspecified urinary organ**

✓4ᵗʰ D42 **Neoplasm of uncertain behavior of meninges**

D42.0 **Neoplasm of uncertain behavior of cerebral meninges** HCC

D42.1 **Neoplasm of uncertain behavior of spinal meninges** HCC

D42.9 **Neoplasm of uncertain behavior of meninges, unspecified** HCC

✓4ᵗʰ D43 **Neoplasm of uncertain behavior of brain and central nervous system**
EXCLUDES 1   *neoplasm of uncertain behavior of peripheral nerves and autonomic nervous system (D48.2)*

D43.0 **Neoplasm of uncertain behavior of brain, supratentorial** HCC
Neoplasm of uncertain behavior of cerebral ventricle
Neoplasm of uncertain behavior of cerebrum
Neoplasm of uncertain behavior of frontal lobe
Neoplasm of uncertain behavior of occipital lobe
Neoplasm of uncertain behavior of parietal lobe
Neoplasm of uncertain behavior of temporal lobe
EXCLUDES 1   *neoplasm of uncertain behavior of fourth ventricle (D43.1)*

D43.1 **Neoplasm of uncertain behavior of brain, infratentorial** HCC
Neoplasm of uncertain behavior of brain stem
Neoplasm of uncertain behavior of cerebellum
Neoplasm of uncertain behavior of fourth ventricle
AHA: 2023,2Q,16

D43.2 **Neoplasm of uncertain behavior of brain, unspecified** HCC

D43.3 **Neoplasm of uncertain behavior of cranial nerves** HCC

D43.4 **Neoplasm of uncertain behavior of spinal cord** HCC

D43.8 **Neoplasm of uncertain behavior of other specified parts of central nervous system** HCC

D43.9 **Neoplasm of uncertain behavior of central nervous system, unspecified** HCC
Neoplasm of uncertain behavior of nervous system (central) NOS

✓4ᵗʰ D44 **Neoplasm of uncertain behavior of endocrine glands**
EXCLUDES 1   *multiple endocrine adenomatosis (E31.2-)*
multiple endocrine neoplasia (E31.2-)
neoplasm of uncertain behavior of endocrine pancreas (D37.8)
neoplasm of uncertain behavior of ovary (D39.1-)
neoplasm of uncertain behavior of testis (D40.1-)
neoplasm of uncertain behavior of thymus (D38.4)

D44.0 **Neoplasm of uncertain behavior of thyroid gland**

✓5ᵗʰ D44.1 **Neoplasm of uncertain behavior of adrenal gland**
Use additional code to identify any functional activity

D44.10 **Neoplasm of uncertain behavior of unspecified adrenal gland**

D44.11 **Neoplasm of uncertain behavior of right adrenal gland**

D44.12 **Neoplasm of uncertain behavior of left adrenal gland**

D44.2 **Neoplasm of uncertain behavior of parathyroid gland**

D44.3 **Neoplasm of uncertain behavior of pituitary gland** HCC
Use additional code to identify any functional activity

D44.4 **Neoplasm of uncertain behavior of craniopharyngeal duct** HCC

D44.5 **Neoplasm of uncertain behavior of pineal gland** HCC

D44.6 **Neoplasm of uncertain behavior of carotid body** HCC

D44.7 **Neoplasm of uncertain behavior of aortic body and other paraganglia** HCC
AHA: 2021,2Q,7; 2016,4Q,26

D44.9 **Neoplasm of uncertain behavior of unspecified endocrine gland**

D45 Polycythemia vera `HCC`

> **EXCLUDES 1**   familial polycythemia (D75.0)
>
>   secondary polycythemia (D75.1)
>
> **DEF:** Abnormal proliferation of all bone marrow elements, increased red cell mass, and total blood volume. The etiology is unknown, but it is frequently associated with splenomegaly, leukocytosis, and thrombocythemia.

✓4th D46 Myelodysplastic syndromes

> Use additional code for adverse effect, if applicable, to identify drug (T36-T50 with fifth or sixth character 5)
>
> **EXCLUDES 2**   drug-induced aplastic anemia (D61.1)

D46.0 Refractory anemia without ring sideroblasts, so stated `HCC`
> Refractory anemia without sideroblasts, without excess of blasts

D46.1 Refractory anemia with ring sideroblasts `HCC`
> RARS

✓5th D46.2 Refractory anemia with excess of blasts [RAEB]

> **D46.20 Refractory anemia with excess of blasts, unspecified** `HCC`
> > RAEB NOS
>
> **D46.21 Refractory anemia with excess of blasts 1** `HCC`
> > RAEB 1
>
> **D46.22 Refractory anemia with excess of blasts 2** `CC` `HCC`
> > RAEB 2

D46.A Refractory cytopenia with multilineage dysplasia `HCC`

D46.B Refractory cytopenia with multilineage dysplasia and ring sideroblasts `HCC`
> RCMD RS

D46.C Myelodysplastic syndrome with isolated del(5q) chromosomal abnormality `CC` `HCC`
> Myelodysplastic syndrome with 5q deletion
> 5q minus syndrome NOS

D46.4 Refractory anemia, unspecified `HCC`

D46.Z Other myelodysplastic syndromes `HCC`
> **EXCLUDES 1**   chronic myelomonocytic leukemia (C93.1-)

D46.9 Myelodysplastic syndrome, unspecified `HCC`
> Myelodysplasia NOS

✓4th D47 Other neoplasms of uncertain behavior of lymphoid, hematopoietic and related tissue

✓5th D47.0 Mast cell neoplasms of uncertain behavior

> **EXCLUDES 1**   congenital cutaneous mastocytosis (Q82.2)
>
>   histiocytic neoplasms of uncertain behavior (D47.Z9)
>
>   malignant mast cell neoplasm (C96.2-)
>
> **AHA:** 2017,4Q,5

> **D47.01 Cutaneous mastocytosis** `CC`
> > Diffuse cutaneous mastocytosis
> > Maculopapular cutaneous mastocytosis
> > Solitary mastocytoma
> > Telangiectasia macularis eruptiva perstans
> > Urticaria pigmentosa
> >
> > **EXCLUDES 1**   congenital (diffuse) (maculopapular) cutaneous mastocytosis (Q82.2)
> >   congenital urticaria pigmentosa (Q82.2)
> >   extracutaneous mastocytoma (D47.09)

> **D47.02 Systemic mastocytosis** `CC`
> > Indolent systemic mastocytosis
> > Isolated bone marrow mastocytosis
> > Smoldering systemic mastocytosis
> > Systemic mastocytosis, with an associated hematological non-mast cell lineage disease (SM-AHNMD)
> >
> > Code also, if applicable, any associated hematological non-mast cell lineage disease, such as:
> > > acute myeloid leukemia (C92.6-, C92.A-)
> > > chronic myelomonocytic leukemia (C93.1-)
> > > essential thrombocytosis (D47.3)
> > > hypereosinophilic syndrome (D72.1)
> > > myelodysplastic syndrome (D46.9)
> > > myeloproliferative syndrome (D47.1)
> > > non-Hodgkin lymphoma (C82-C85)
> > > plasma cell myeloma (C90.0-)
> > > polycythemia vera (D45)
> >
> > **EXCLUDES 1**   aggressive systemic mastocytosis (C96.21)
> >   mast cell leukemia (C94.3-)

D47.09 Other mast cell neoplasms of uncertain behavior `CC`
> Extracutaneous mastocytoma
> Mast cell tumor NOS
> Mastocytoma NOS
> Mastocytosis NOS

D47.1 Chronic myeloproliferative disease `CC` `HCC`
> Chronic neutrophilic leukemia
> Myeloproliferative disease, unspecified
>
> **EXCLUDES 1**   atypical chronic myeloid leukemia BCR/ABL-negative (C92.2-)
>   chronic myeloid leukemia BCR/ABL-positive (C92.1-)
>   myelofibrosis NOS (D75.81)
>   myelophthisic anemia (D61.82)
>   myelophthisis (D61.82)
>   secondary myelofibrosis NOS (D75.81)

D47.2 Monoclonal gammopathy
> Monoclonal gammopathy of undetermined significance [MGUS]
>
> **AHA:** 2021,3Q,5
>
> **TIP:** Smoldering multiple myeloma (SMM) is coded here.

D47.3 Essential (hemorrhagic) thrombocythemia `HCC`
> Essential thrombocytosis
> Idiopathic hemorrhagic thrombocythemia
> Primary thrombocytosis
>
> **EXCLUDES 2**   reactive thrombocytosis (D75.838)
>   secondary thrombocytosis (D75.838)
>   thrombocythemia NOS (D75.839)
>   thrombocytosis NOS (D75.839)
>
> **DEF:** Chronic myeloproliferative neoplasm involving production of excess blood platelets that may result in abnormal clotting or hemorrhaging.

D47.4 Osteomyelofibrosis `HCC`
> Chronic idiopathic myelofibrosis
> Myelofibrosis (idiopathic) (with myeloid metaplasia)
> Myelosclerosis (megakaryocytic) with myeloid metaplasia
> Secondary myelofibrosis in myeloproliferative disease
>
> **EXCLUDES 1**   acute myelofibrosis (C94.4-)

✓5th D47.Z Other specified neoplasms of uncertain behavior of lymphoid, hematopoietic and related tissue
> **AHA:** 2016,4Q,8

> **D47.Z1 Post-transplant lymphoproliferative disorder (PTLD)** `CC` `UPD` `HCC`
> > Code first complications of transplanted organs and tissue (T86.-)
> >
> > **DEF:** Excessive proliferation of B-cell lymphocytes following Epstein-Barr virus infection in organ transplant patients. It may progress to non-Hodgkin lymphoma.

> **D47.Z2 Castleman disease** `CC` `HCC`
> > Code also, if applicable, human herpesvirus 8 infection (B10.89)
> >
> > **EXCLUDES 2**   Kaposi's sarcoma (C46.-)
> >
> > **DEF:** Rare disease of the lymph nodes and lymphoid tissues that closely mimics lymphoma.

> **D47.Z9 Other specified neoplasms of uncertain behavior of lymphoid, hematopoietic and related tissue** `CC` `HCC`
> > Histiocytic tumors of uncertain behavior

D47.9 Neoplasm of uncertain behavior of lymphoid, hematopoietic and related tissue, unspecified `CC` `HCC`
> Lymphoproliferative disease NOS

✓4th D48 Neoplasm of uncertain behavior of other and unspecified sites
> **EXCLUDES 1**   neurofibromatosis (nonmalignant) (Q85.0-)

D48.0 Neoplasm of uncertain behavior of bone and articular cartilage
> **EXCLUDES 1**   neoplasm of uncertain behavior of cartilage of ear (D48.1-)
>   neoplasm of uncertain behavior of cartilage of larynx (D38.0)
>   neoplasm of uncertain behavior of cartilage of nose (D38.5)
>   neoplasm of uncertain behavior of connective tissue of eyelid (D48.1-)
>   neoplasm of uncertain behavior of synovia (D48.1-)

N Newborn: 0   **P** Pediatric: 0-17   **M** Maternity: 9-64   **A** Adult: 15-124   **UNS** Unspecified Site   **MCC** Major Complication/Comorbidity   **CC** Complication/Comorbidity   **PE** POA Exempt

510   ICD-10-CM 2025

☑5th **D48.1** **Neoplasm of uncertain behavior of connective and other soft tissue**
Neoplasm of uncertain behavior of connective tissue of ear
Neoplasm of uncertain behavior of connective tissue of eyelid
Stromal tumors of uncertain behavior of digestive system
> EXCLUDES 1   *neoplasm of uncertain behavior of articular cartilage (D48.0)*
> *neoplasm of uncertain behavior of cartilage of larynx (D38.0)*
> *neoplasm of uncertain behavior of cartilage of nose (D38.5)*
> *neoplasm of uncertain behavior of connective tissue of breast (D48.6-)*

    AHA: 2023,4Q,5-6

☑6th **D48.11** **Desmoid tumor**
    D48.110 **Desmoid tumor of head and neck**
    D48.111 **Desmoid tumor of chest wall**
    D48.112 **Desmoid tumor, intrathoracic**
    D48.113 **Desmoid tumor of abdominal wall**
    D48.114 **Desmoid tumor, intraabdominal**
        Desmoid tumor of pelvic cavity
        Desmoid tumor, peritoneal, retroperitoneal
    D48.115 **Desmoid tumor of upper extremity and shoulder girdle**
    D48.116 **Desmoid tumor of lower extremity and pelvic girdle**
        Desmoid tumor of buttock
    D48.117 **Desmoid tumor of back**
    D48.118 **Desmoid tumor of other site**
    D48.119 **Desmoid tumor of unspecified site**
D48.19 **Other specified neoplasm of uncertain behavior of connective and other soft tissue**

D48.2 **Neoplasm of uncertain behavior of peripheral nerves and autonomic nervous system**
> EXCLUDES 1   *neoplasm of uncertain behavior of peripheral nerves of orbit (D48.7)*

D48.3 **Neoplasm of uncertain behavior of retroperitoneum**

D48.4 **Neoplasm of uncertain behavior of peritoneum**

D48.5 **Neoplasm of uncertain behavior of skin**
Neoplasm of uncertain behavior of anal margin
Neoplasm of uncertain behavior of anal skin
Neoplasm of uncertain behavior of perianal skin
Neoplasm of uncertain behavior of skin of breast
> EXCLUDES 1   *neoplasm of uncertain behavior of anus NOS (D37.8)*
> *neoplasm of uncertain behavior of skin of genital organs (D39.8, D40.8)*
> *neoplasm of uncertain behavior of vermilion border of lip (D37.0)*

☑5th **D48.6** **Neoplasm of uncertain behavior of breast**
Cystosarcoma phyllodes
Neoplasm of uncertain behavior of connective tissue of breast
> EXCLUDES 1   *neoplasm of uncertain behavior of skin of breast (D48.5)*

    D48.60 **Neoplasm of uncertain behavior of unspecified breast**
    D48.61 **Neoplasm of uncertain behavior of right breast**
    D48.62 **Neoplasm of uncertain behavior of left breast**

D48.7 **Neoplasm of uncertain behavior of other specified sites**
Neoplasm of uncertain behavior of eye
Neoplasm of uncertain behavior of heart
Neoplasm of uncertain behavior of peripheral nerves of orbit
> EXCLUDES 1   *neoplasm of uncertain behavior of connective tissue (D48.1-)*
> *neoplasm of uncertain behavior of skin of eyelid (D48.5)*

D48.9 **Neoplasm of uncertain behavior, unspecified**

Neoplasms of unspecified behavior (D49)

☑4th **D49** **Neoplasms of unspecified behavior**

> NOTE   Category D49 classifies by site neoplasms of unspecified morphology and behavior. The term "mass", unless otherwise stated, is not to be regarded as a neoplastic growth.

> INCLUDES   "growth" NOS
> neoplasm NOS
> new growth NOS
> tumor NOS

> EXCLUDES 1   *neoplasms of uncertain behavior (D37-D44, D48)*

D49.0 **Neoplasm of unspecified behavior of digestive system**
> EXCLUDES 1   *neoplasm of unspecified behavior of margin of anus (D49.2)*
> *neoplasm of unspecified behavior of perianal skin (D49.2)*
> *neoplasm of unspecified behavior of skin of anus (D49.2)*

D49.1 **Neoplasm of unspecified behavior of respiratory system**

D49.2 **Neoplasm of unspecified behavior of bone, soft tissue, and skin**
> EXCLUDES 1   *neoplasm of unspecified behavior of anal canal (D49.0)*
> *neoplasm of unspecified behavior of anus NOS (D49.0)*
> *neoplasm of unspecified behavior of bone marrow (D49.89)*
> *neoplasm of unspecified behavior of cartilage of larynx (D49.1)*
> *neoplasm of unspecified behavior of cartilage of nose (D49.1)*
> *neoplasm of unspecified behavior of connective tissue of breast (D49.3)*
> *neoplasm of unspecified behavior of skin of genital organs (D49.59)*
> *neoplasm of unspecified behavior of vermilion border of lip (D49.0)*

D49.3 **Neoplasm of unspecified behavior of breast**
> EXCLUDES 1   *neoplasm of unspecified behavior of skin of breast (D49.2)*

D49.4 **Neoplasm of unspecified behavior of bladder**

☑5th **D49.5** **Neoplasm of unspecified behavior of other genitourinary organs**
    AHA: 2016,4Q,9

☑6th **D49.51** **Neoplasm of unspecified behavior of kidney**
    D49.511 **Neoplasm of unspecified behavior of right kidney**
    D49.512 **Neoplasm of unspecified behavior of left kidney**
    D49.519 **Neoplasm of unspecified behavior of unspecified kidney**
D49.59 **Neoplasm of unspecified behavior of other genitourinary organ**

D49.6 **Neoplasm of unspecified behavior of brain**   HCC
> EXCLUDES 1   *neoplasm of unspecified behavior of cerebral meninges (D49.7)*
> *neoplasm of unspecified behavior of cranial nerves (D49.7)*

D49.7 **Neoplasm of unspecified behavior of endocrine glands and other parts of nervous system**
> EXCLUDES 1   *neoplasm of unspecified behavior of peripheral, sympathetic, and parasympathetic nerves and ganglia (D49.2)*

☑5th **D49.8** **Neoplasm of unspecified behavior of other specified sites**
> EXCLUDES 1   *neoplasm of unspecified behavior of eyelid (skin) (D49.2)*
> *neoplasm of unspecified behavior of eyelid cartilage (D49.2)*
> *neoplasm of unspecified behavior of great vessels (D49.2)*
> *neoplasm of unspecified behavior of optic nerve (D49.7)*

    D49.81 **Neoplasm of unspecified behavior of retina and choroid**
        Dark area on retina
        Retinal freckle

☑ Additional Character Required   ☑x7th Placeholder   Questionable PDx   Manifestation   Unspecified   UPD Unacceptable PDx   H1-H4 HAC   HCC CMS-HCC Dx   HIV HIV Dx

ICD-10-CM 2025   **511**

       D49.89   **Neoplasm of unspecified behavior of other specified sites**

D49.9   **Neoplasm of unspecified behavior of unspecified site**

🅝 Newborn: 0   🅟 Pediatric: 0-17   🅜 Maternity: 9-64   🅐 Adult: 15-124   UNS Unspecified Site   MCC Major Complication/Comorbidity   CC Complication/Comorbidity   PE POA Exempt

512   ICD-10-CM 2025

Chapter 3. Diseases of the Blood and Blood-forming Organs and Certain Disorders Involving the Immune Mechanism (D5Ø–D89)

Chapter-specific Guidelines with Coding Examples
Reserved for future guideline expansion

Chapter 3. Diseases of the Blood and Blood-forming Organs and Certain Disorders Involving the Immune Mechanism (D50-D89)

EXCLUDES 2   autoimmune disease (systemic) NOS (M35.9)
certain conditions originating in the perinatal period (P00-P96)
complications of pregnancy, childbirth and the puerperium (O00-O9A)
congenital malformations, deformations and chromosomal abnormalities (Q00-Q99)
endocrine, nutritional and metabolic diseases (E00-E88)
human immunodeficiency virus [HIV] disease (B20)
injury, poisoning and certain other consequences of external causes (S00-T88)
neoplasms (C00-D49)
symptoms, signs and abnormal clinical and laboratory findings, not elsewhere classified (R00-R94)

This chapter contains the following blocks:

D50-D53   Nutritional anemias
D55-D59   Hemolytic anemias
D60-D64   Aplastic and other anemias and other bone marrow failure syndromes
D65-D69   Coagulation defects, purpura and other hemorrhagic conditions
D70-D77   Other disorders of blood and blood-forming organs
D78   Intraoperative and postprocedural complications of the spleen
D80-D89   Certain disorders involving the immune mechanism

Nutritional anemias (D50-D53)

DEF: Nutritional anemia: The result of inadequate intake or absorption of a vitamin or mineral that impacts the production of red blood cells or causes them to develop abnormally affecting the size and shape.
TIP: Documentation must identify a link between anemia and the nutritional deficiency; low levels of a particular nutrient may occur concurrently with anemia but not cause the anemia.

√4th **D50**   **Iron deficiency anemia**

   INCLUDES   asiderotic anemia
hypochromic anemia

   D50.0   **Iron deficiency anemia secondary to blood loss (chronic)**
Posthemorrhagic anemia (chronic)
EXCLUDES 1   acute posthemorrhagic anemia (D62)
congenital anemia from fetal blood loss (P61.3)
AHA: 2019,3Q,17

   D50.1   **Sideropenic dysphagia**
Kelly-Paterson syndrome
Plummer-Vinson syndrome

   D50.8   **Other iron deficiency anemias**
Iron deficiency anemia due to inadequate dietary iron intake

   D50.9   **Iron deficiency anemia, unspecified**

√4th **D51**   **Vitamin B12 deficiency anemia**

   EXCLUDES 1   vitamin B12 deficiency (E53.8)

   D51.0   **Vitamin B12 deficiency anemia due to intrinsic factor deficiency**
Addison anemia
Biermer anemia
Congenital intrinsic factor deficiency
Pernicious (congenital) anemia
DEF: Chronic progressive anemia due to vitamin B12 malabsorption, caused by lack of secretion of intrinsic factor, which is produced by the gastric mucosa of the stomach.

   D51.1   **Vitamin B12 deficiency anemia due to selective vitamin B12 malabsorption with proteinuria**
Imerslund (Gräsbeck) syndrome
Megaloblastic hereditary anemia

   D51.2   **Transcobalamin II deficiency**

   D51.3   **Other dietary vitamin B12 deficiency anemia**
Vegan anemia

   D51.8   **Other vitamin B12 deficiency anemias**

   D51.9   **Vitamin B12 deficiency anemia, unspecified**

√4th **D52**   **Folate deficiency anemia**

   EXCLUDES 1   folate deficiency without anemia (E53.8)

   DEF: Deficiency in a B complex vitamin needed for the production of healthy red blood cells. Lack of folate, or folic acid, and other absorption conditions can cause anemia resulting in large, misshapen red blood cells called megaloblasts.

   D52.0   **Dietary folate deficiency anemia**
Nutritional megaloblastic anemia
DEF: Result of a poor diet with inadequate intake of folate, which is needed to produce healthy red blood cells.

   D52.1   **Drug-induced folate deficiency anemia**
Use additional code for adverse effect, if applicable, to identify drug (T36-T50 with fifth or sixth character 5)

   D52.8   **Other folate deficiency anemias**

   D52.9   **Folate deficiency anemia, unspecified**
Folic acid deficiency anemia NOS

√4th **D53**   **Other nutritional anemias**

   INCLUDES   megaloblastic anemia unresponsive to vitamin B12 or folate therapy

   D53.0   **Protein deficiency anemia**
Amino-acid deficiency anemia
Orotaciduric anemia
EXCLUDES 1   Lesch-Nyhan syndrome (E79.1)

   D53.1   **Other megaloblastic anemias, not elsewhere classified**
Megaloblastic anemia NOS
EXCLUDES 1   Di Guglielmo's disease (C94.0)

   D53.2   **Scorbutic anemia**
EXCLUDES 1   scurvy (E54)

   D53.8   **Other specified nutritional anemias**
Anemia associated with deficiency of copper
Anemia associated with deficiency of molybdenum
Anemia associated with deficiency of zinc
EXCLUDES 1   nutritional deficiencies without anemia, such as:
copper deficiency NOS (E61.0)
molybdenum deficiency NOS (E61.5)
zinc deficiency NOS (E60)

   D53.9   **Nutritional anemia, unspecified**
Simple chronic anemia
EXCLUDES 1   anemia NOS (D64.9)
AHA: 2018,4Q,88

Hemolytic anemias (D55-D59)

√4th **D55**   **Anemia due to enzyme disorders**

   EXCLUDES 1   drug-induced enzyme deficiency anemia (D59.2)

   D55.0   **Anemia due to glucose-6-phosphate dehydrogenase [G6PD] deficiency**
Favism
G6PD deficiency anemia
EXCLUDES 1   glucose-6-phosphate dehydrogenase (G6PD) deficiency without anemia (D75.A)

   D55.1   **Anemia due to other disorders of glutathione metabolism**
Anemia (due to) enzyme deficiencies, except G6PD, related to the hexose monophosphate [HMP] shunt pathway
Anemia (due to) hemolytic nonspherocytic (hereditary), type I

√5th **D55.2**   **Anemia due to disorders of glycolytic enzymes**
EXCLUDES 1   disorders of glycolysis not associated with anemia (E74.81-)
AHA: 2021,4Q,6-7

     D55.21   **Anemia due to pyruvate kinase deficiency**
PK deficiency anemia
Pyruvate kinase deficiency anemia

     D55.29   **Anemia due to other disorders of glycolytic enzymes**
Hexokinase deficiency anemia
Triose-phosphate isomerase deficiency anemia

   D55.3   **Anemia due to disorders of nucleotide metabolism**

   D55.8   **Other anemias due to enzyme disorders**

   D55.9   **Anemia due to enzyme disorder, unspecified**

N Newborn: 0   **P** Pediatric: 0-17   **M** Maternity: 9-64   **A** Adult: 15-124   **UNS** Unspecified Site   **MCC** Major Complication/Comorbidity   **CC** Complication/Comorbidity   **PE** POA Exempt

514   ICD-10-CM 2025

✓4ᵗʰ D56 Thalassemia

> **EXCLUDES 1**   *sickle-cell thalassemia (D57.4-)*
>
> **DEF:** Group of inherited disorders of hemoglobin metabolism causing mild to severe anemia. It is usually found in people of Mediterranean, African, Chinese, or Asian descent.

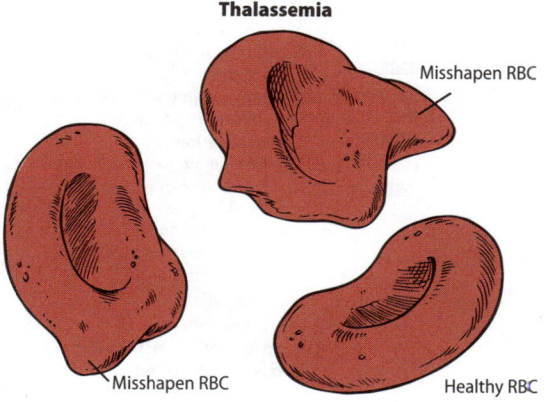

Thalassemia

Misshapen RBC

Misshapen RBC

Healthy RBC

D56.0 Alpha thalassemia

Alpha thalassemia major
Hemoglobin H Constant Spring
Hemoglobin H disease
Hydrops fetalis due to alpha thalassemia
Severe alpha thalassemia
Triple gene defect alpha thalassemia

Use additional code, if applicable, for hydrops fetalis due to alpha thalassemia (P56.99)

> **EXCLUDES 1**   *alpha thalassemia trait or minor (D56.3)*
> *asymptomatic alpha thalassemia (D56.3)*
> *hydrops fetalis due to isoimmunization (P56.0)*
> *hydrops fetalis not due to immune hemolysis (P83.2)*

DEF: HBA1 and HBA2 genetic variant of chromosome 16 prevalent among those of African and Southeast Asian descent. Alpha thalassemia is associated with a wide spectrum of anemic presentation and includes hemoglobin H disease subtypes.

D56.1 Beta thalassemia   `HCC`

Beta thalassemia major
Cooley's anemia
Homozygous beta thalassemia
Severe beta thalassemia
Thalassemia intermedia
Thalassemia major

> **EXCLUDES 1**   *beta thalassemia minor (D56.3)*
> *beta thalassemia trait (D56.3)*
> *delta-beta thalassemia (D56.2)*
> *hemoglobin E-beta thalassemia (D56.5)*
> *sickle-cell beta thalassemia (D57.4-)*

D56.2 Delta-beta thalassemia   `HCC`

Homozygous delta-beta thalassemia

> **EXCLUDES 1**   *delta-beta thalassemia minor (D56.3)*
> *delta-beta thalassemia trait (D56.3)*

D56.3 Thalassemia minor

Alpha thalassemia minor
Alpha thalassemia silent carrier
Alpha thalassemia trait
Beta thalassemia minor
Beta thalassemia trait
Delta-beta thalassemia minor
Delta-beta thalassemia trait
Thalassemia trait NOS

> **EXCLUDES 1**   *alpha thalassemia (D56.0)*
> *beta thalassemia (D56.1)*
> *delta-beta thalassemia (D56.2)*
> *hemoglobin E-beta thalassemia (D56.5)*
> *sickle-cell trait (D57.3)*

DEF: Solitary abnormal gene that identifies a carrier of the disease, yet with an absence of symptoms or a clinically mild anemic presentation.

D56.4 Hereditary persistence of fetal hemoglobin [HPFH]

D56.5 Hemoglobin E-beta thalassemia   `HCC`

> **EXCLUDES 1**   *beta thalassemia (D56.1)*
> *beta thalassemia minor (D56.3)*
> *beta thalassemia trait (D56.3)*
> *delta-beta thalassemia (D56.2)*
> *delta-beta thalassemia trait (D56.3)*
> *hemoglobin E disease (D58.2)*
> *other hemoglobinopathies (D58.2)*
> *sickle-cell beta thalassemia (D57.4-)*

D56.8 Other thalassemias

Dominant thalassemia
Hemoglobin C thalassemia
Mixed thalassemia
Thalassemia with other hemoglobinopathy

> **EXCLUDES 1**   *hemoglobin C disease (D58.2)*
> *hemoglobin E disease (D58.2)*
> *other hemoglobinopathies (D58.2)*
> *sickle-cell anemia (D57.-)*
> *sickle-cell thalassemia (D57.4-)*

D56.9 Thalassemia, unspecified

Mediterranean anemia (with other hemoglobinopathy)

✓4ᵗʰ D57 Sickle-cell disorders

Use additional code for any associated fever (R50.81)

> **EXCLUDES 1**   *other hemoglobinopathies (D58.-)*

AHA: 2023,4Q,6-7; 2022,2Q,28

DEF: Severe, chronic inherited diseases caused by a genetic variation in hemoglobin protein of the red blood cell. The gene mutation causes the red blood cell to become hard, sticky, and crescent or sickle shaped, making it harder for red blood cells to travel through the bloodstream, disrupting blood flow and decreasing oxygen transport to tissues.

Sickle cell

Sickle cells

Normal RBCs

✓5ᵗʰ D57.0 Hb-SS disease with crisis

Sickle-cell disease with crisis
Hb-SS disease with (vaso-occlusive) pain

AHA: 2020,4Q,6-7

> **D57.00 Hb-SS disease with crisis, unspecified**   `MCC` `HCC`
> Hb-SS disease with (painful) crisis NOS
> Hb-SS disease with (vaso-occlusive) pain NOS

> **D57.01 Hb-SS disease with acute chest syndrome**   `MCC` `HCC`

> **D57.02 Hb-SS disease with splenic sequestration**   `MCC` `HCC`

> **D57.03 Hb-SS disease with cerebral vascular involvement**   `MCC` `HCC`
> Code also, if applicable, cerebral infarction (I63.-)

> **D57.04 Hb-SS disease with dactylitis**   `MCC` `HCC`

> **D57.09 Hb-SS disease with crisis with other specified complication**   `MCC` `HCC`
> Use additional code to identify complications, such as:
> cholelithiasis (K80.-)
> priapism (N48.32)

D57.1 Sickle-cell disease without crisis   `HCC`

Hb-SS disease without crisis
Sickle-cell anemia NOS
Sickle-cell disease NOS
Sickle-cell disorder NOS

✓5ᵗʰ D57.2 Sickle-cell/Hb-C disease

Hb-SC disease
Hb-S/Hb-C disease

AHA: 2020,4Q,6-7

> **D57.20 Sickle-cell/Hb-C disease without crisis**   `HCC`

> **✓6ᵗʰ D57.21 Sickle-cell/Hb-C disease with crisis**

> > **D57.211 Sickle-cell/Hb-C disease with acute chest syndrome**   `MCC` `HCC`

> > **D57.212 Sickle-cell/Hb-C disease with splenic sequestration**   `MCC` `HCC`

✓ Additional Character Required   ✓x7ᵗʰ Placeholder   Questionable PDx   Manifestation   Unspecified   UPD Unacceptable PDx   H1-H14 HAC   HCC CMS-HCC Dx   HIV HIV Dx

ICD-10-CM 2025   515

D57.213 Sickle-cell/Hb-C disease **with cerebral vascular involvement** `MCC` `HCC`
Code also, if applicable, cerebral infarction (I63.-)

D57.214 Sickle-cell/Hb-C disease **with dactylitis** `MCC` `HCC`

D57.218 Sickle-cell/Hb-C disease with crisis with other specified complication `MCC` `HCC`
Use additional code to identify complications, such as:
cholelithiasis (K80.-)
priapism (N48.32)

D57.219 Sickle-cell/Hb-C disease with crisis, unspecified `MCC` `HCC`
Sickle-cell/Hb-C disease with crisis NOS
Sickle-cell/Hb-C disease with (vaso-occlusive) pain NOS

D57.3 **Sickle-cell trait**
Hb-S trait
Heterozygous hemoglobin S
DEF: Heterozygous genetic makeup characterized by one gene for normal hemoglobin and one for sickle-cell hemoglobin. The clinical disease is rarely present.

✓5th **D57.4** **Sickle-cell thalassemia**
Sickle-cell beta thalassemia
Thalassemia Hb-S disease
AHA: 2020,4Q,6-7

D57.40 **Sickle-cell thalassemia without crisis** `HCC`
Microdrepanocytosis
Sickle-cell thalassemia NOS

✓6th **D57.41** **Sickle-cell thalassemia, unspecified, with crisis**
Sickle-cell thalassemia with (painful) crisis NOS
Sickle-cell thalassemia with (vaso-occlusive) pain NOS

D57.411 Sickle-cell thalassemia, unspecified, **with acute chest syndrome** `MCC` `HCC`

D57.412 Sickle-cell thalassemia, unspecified, **with splenic sequestration** `MCC` `HCC`

D57.413 Sickle-cell thalassemia, unspecified, **with cerebral vascular involvement** `MCC` `HCC`
Code also, if applicable cerebral infarction (I63.-)

D57.414 Sickle-cell thalassemia, unspecified, **with dactylitis** `MCC` `HCC`

D57.418 Sickle-cell thalassemia, unspecified, **with crisis with other specified complication** `MCC` `HCC`
Use additional code to identify complications, such as:
cholelithiasis (K80.-)
priapism (N48.32)

D57.419 Sickle-cell thalassemia, unspecified, with crisis `MCC` `HCC`
Sickle-cell thalassemia with (painful) crisis NOS
Sickle-cell thalassemia with (vaso-occlusive) pain NOS

D57.42 **Sickle-cell thalassemia beta zero without crisis** `HCC`
HbS-beta zero without crisis
Sickle-cell beta zero without crisis

✓6th **D57.43** **Sickle-cell thalassemia beta zero with crisis**
HbS-beta zero with crisis
Sickle-cell beta zero with crisis

D57.431 Sickle-cell thalassemia beta zero **with acute chest syndrome** `MCC` `HCC`
HbS-beta zero with acute chest syndrome
Sickle-cell beta zero with acute chest syndrome

D57.432 Sickle-cell thalassemia beta zero **with splenic sequestration** `MCC` `HCC`
HbS-beta zero with splenic sequestration
Sickle-cell beta zero with splenic sequestration

D57.433 Sickle-cell thalassemia beta zero **with cerebral vascular involvement** `MCC` `HCC`
HbS-beta zero with cerebral vascular involvement
Sickle-cell beta zero with cerebral vascular involvement
Code also, if applicable cerebral infarction (I63.-)

D57.434 Sickle-cell thalassemia beta zero **with dactylitis** `MCC` `HCC`

D57.438 Sickle-cell thalassemia beta zero with crisis with other specified complication `MCC` `HCC`
HbS-beta zero with other specified complication
Sickle-cell beta zero with other specified complication
Use additional code to identify complications, such as:
cholelithiasis (K80.-)
priapism (N48.32)

D57.439 Sickle-cell thalassemia beta zero with crisis, unspecified `MCC` `HCC`
HbS-beta zero with other specified complication
Sickle-cell beta zero with crisis unspecified
Sickle-cell thalassemia beta zero with (painful) crisis NOS
Sickle-cell thalassemia beta zero with (vaso-occlusive) pain NOS

D57.44 **Sickle-cell thalassemia beta plus without crisis** `HCC`
HbS-beta plus without crisis
Sickle-cell beta plus without crisis

✓6th **D57.45** **Sickle-cell thalassemia beta plus with crisis**
HbS-beta plus with crisis
Sickle-cell beta plus with crisis

D57.451 Sickle-cell thalassemia beta plus **with acute chest syndrome** `MCC` `HCC`
HbS-beta plus with acute chest syndrome
Sickle-cell beta plus with acute chest syndrome

D57.452 Sickle-cell thalassemia beta plus **with splenic sequestration** `MCC` `HCC`
HbS-beta plus with splenic sequestration
Sickle-cell beta plus with splenic sequestration

D57.453 Sickle-cell thalassemia beta plus **with cerebral vascular involvement** `MCC` `HCC`
HbS-beta plus with cerebral vascular involvement
Sickle-cell beta plus with cerebral vascular involvement
Code also, if applicable cerebral infarction (I63.-)

D57.454 Sickle-cell thalassemia beta plus **with dactylitis** `MCC` `HCC`

D57.458 Sickle-cell thalassemia beta plus with crisis with other specified complication `MCC` `HCC`
HbS-beta plus with crisis with other specified complication
Sickle-cell beta plus with crisis with other specified complication
Use additional code to identify complications, such as:
cholelithiasis (K80.-)
priapism (N48.32)

D57.459 Sickle-cell thalassemia beta plus with crisis, unspecified `MCC` `HCC`
HbS-beta plus with crisis with unspecified complication
Sickle-cell beta plus with crisis with unspecified complication
Sickle-cell thalassemia beta plus with (painful) crisis NOS
Sickle-cell thalassemia beta plus with (vaso-occlusive) pain NOS

✓5ᵗʰ **D57.8** **Other sickle-cell disorders**
Hb-SD disease
Hb-SE disease
AHA: 2020,4Q,6-7

    D57.80   **Other sickle-cell disorders without crisis**   HCC

✓6ᵗʰ   **D57.81**   **Other sickle-cell disorders with crisis**

       D57.811   **Other sickle-cell disorders with acute chest syndrome**   MCC HCC

       D57.812   **Other sickle-cell disorders with splenic sequestration**   MCC HCC

       D57.813   **Other sickle-cell disorders with cerebral vascular involvement**   MCC HCC
         Code also, if applicable: cerebral infarction (I63.-)

       D57.814   **Other sickle-cell disorders with dactylitis**   MCC HCC

       D57.818   **Other sickle-cell disorders with crisis with other specified complication**   MCC HCC
         Use additional code to identify complications, such as:
         cholelithiasis (K80.-)
         priapism (N48.32)

       D57.819   **Other sickle-cell disorders with crisis, unspecified**   MCC HCC
         Other sickle-cell disorders with crisis NOS
         Other sickle-cell disorders with (vaso-occlusive) pain NOS

✓4ᵗʰ **D58** **Other hereditary hemolytic anemias**
    EXCLUDES 1   hemolytic anemia of the newborn (P55.-)

    D58.0   **Hereditary spherocytosis**
      Acholuric (familial) jaundice
      Congenital (spherocytic) hemolytic icterus
      Minkowski-Chauffard syndrome
      DEF: Inherited condition caused by mutations to genes responsible for the production of proteins that form the membranes of red blood cells. The shape and flexibility of the red blood cell membrane is altered, diminishing the cell's ability to traverse the spleen, therefore becoming trapped and destroyed before the red blood cell has reached maturity.

    D58.1   **Hereditary elliptocytosis**
      Elliptocytosis (congenital)
      Ovalocytosis (congenital) (hereditary)

    D58.2   **Other hemoglobinopathies**
      Abnormal hemoglobin NOS
      Congenital Heinz body anemia
      Hb-C disease
      Hb-D disease
      Hb-E disease
      Hemoglobinopathy NOS
      Unstable hemoglobin hemolytic disease
      EXCLUDES 1   familial polycythemia (D75.0)
         Hb-M disease (D74.0)
         hemoglobin E-beta thalassemia (D56.5)
         hereditary persistence of fetal hemoglobin [HPFH] (D56.4)
         high-altitude polycythemia (D75.1)
         methemoglobinemia (D74.-)
         other hemoglobinopathies with thalassemia (D56.8)

    D58.8   **Other specified hereditary hemolytic anemias**   CC
      Stomatocytosis

    D58.9   **Hereditary hemolytic anemia, unspecified**   CC

✓4ᵗʰ **D59** **Acquired hemolytic anemia**
    DEF: Non-hereditary anemia characterized by premature destruction of red blood cells caused by infectious organisms, poisons, and physical agents.

    D59.0   **Drug-induced autoimmune hemolytic anemia**   CC
      Use additional code for adverse effect, if applicable, to identify drug (T36-T50 with fifth or sixth character 5)

✓5ᵗʰ   **D59.1**   **Other autoimmune hemolytic anemias**
      EXCLUDES 2   Evans syndrome (D69.41)
         hemolytic disease of newborn (P55.-)
         paroxysmal cold hemoglobinuria (D59.6)
      AHA: 2020,4Q,7-8

       D59.10   **Autoimmune hemolytic anemia, unspecified**   CC HCC

       D59.11   **Warm autoimmune hemolytic anemia**   CC HCC
         Warm type (primary) (secondary) (symptomatic) autoimmune hemolytic anemia
         Warm type autoimmune hemolytic disease

       D59.12   **Cold autoimmune hemolytic anemia**   CC HCC
         Chronic cold hemagglutinin disease
         Cold agglutinin disease
         Cold agglutinin hemoglobinuria
         Cold type (primary) (secondary) (symptomatic) autoimmune hemolytic anemia
         Cold type autoimmune hemolytic disease

       D59.13   **Mixed type autoimmune hemolytic anemia**   CC HCC
         Mixed type autoimmune hemolytic disease
         Mixed type, cold and warm, (primary) (secondary) (symptomatic) autoimmune hemolytic anemia

       D59.19   **Other autoimmune hemolytic anemia**   CC HCC

    D59.2   **Drug-induced nonautoimmune hemolytic anemia**   CC
      Drug-induced enzyme deficiency anemia
      Use additional code for adverse effect, if applicable, to identify drug (T36-T50 with fifth or sixth character 5)

✓5ᵗʰ   **D59.3**   **Hemolytic-uremic syndrome**
      Code also, if applicable, any associated:
        acute kidney failure (N17.-)
        chronic kidney disease (N18.-)
      AHA: 2022,4Q,5-6
      DEF: Condition typically precipitated by infection causing low platelets and destruction of red blood cells resulting in hemolytic anemia. This cell damage and blockage of renal capillaries lead to kidney failure. Mainly affects children.

       D59.30   **Hemolytic-uremic syndrome, unspecified**   MCC HCC
         Hemolytic-uremic syndrome NOS

       D59.31   **Infection-associated hemolytic-uremic syndrome**   MCC HCC
         Shiga toxin-producing E. coli [STEC] related hemolytic uremic syndrome
         Typical hemolytic uremic syndrome
         Use additional code to identify associated infection, such as:
           E. coli infection (B96.2-)
           human immunodeficiency virus [HIV] disease (B20)
           pneumococcal meningitis (G00.1)
           pneumococcal pneumonia (J13)
           sepsis due to Streptococcus pneumoniae (A40.3)
           Shigella dysenteriae (A03.9)
           streptococcus pneumoniae as the cause of diseases classified elsewhere (B95.3)

       D59.32   **Hereditary hemolytic-uremic syndrome**   MCC HCC
         Atypical hemolytic uremic syndrome with an identified genetic cause
         Code also, if applicable:
           defects in the complement system (D84.1)
           methylmalonic acidemia (E71.120)

       D59.39   **Other hemolytic-uremic syndrome**   MCC HCC
         Atypical (nongenetic) hemolytic uremic syndrome
         Secondary hemolytic-uremic syndrome
         Code first, if applicable, any associated:
           COVID-19 (U07.1)
           complications of heart transplant (T86.2-)
           complications of kidney transplant (T86.1-)
           complications of liver transplant (T86.4-)
         Code also, if applicable, any associated condition, such as:
           hypertensive emergency (I16.1)
           malignant neoplasm (C00-C96)
           systemic lupus erythematosus (M32.-)
         Use additional code, if applicable, for adverse effect to identify drug (T36-T50 with fifth or sixth character 5)
         AHA: 2022,4Q,6

    D59.4   **Other nonautoimmune hemolytic anemias**   CC HCC
      Mechanical hemolytic anemia
      Microangiopathic hemolytic anemia
      Toxic hemolytic anemia

    D59.5   **Paroxysmal nocturnal hemoglobinuria [Marchiafava-Micheli]**   HCC
      EXCLUDES 1   hemoglobinuria NOS (R82.3)

✔ Additional Character Required   ✓x7ᵗʰ Placeholder   Questionable PDx   Manifestation   Unspecified   UPD Unacceptable PDx   H1-H14 HAC   HCC CMS-HCC Dx   HIV HIV Dx

ICD-10-CM 2025   517

D59.6 Hemoglobinuria due to hemolysis from other external causes   HCC
  Hemoglobinuria from exertion
  March hemoglobinuria
  Paroxysmal cold hemoglobinuria
  Use additional code (Chapter 20) to identify external cause
  EXCLUDES 1   hemoglobinuria NOS (R82.3)

D59.8 Other acquired hemolytic anemias   HCC

D59.9 Acquired hemolytic anemia, unspecified   CC HCC
  Idiopathic hemolytic anemia, chronic

Aplastic and other anemias and other bone marrow failure syndromes (D60-D64)

✓4th D60 Acquired pure red cell aplasia [erythroblastopenia]
  INCLUDES   red cell aplasia (acquired) (adult) (with thymoma)
  EXCLUDES 1   congenital red cell aplasia (D61.01)
  DEF: Bone marrow failure characterized by underproduction of red blood cells while white blood cell and platelet production remains normal.

D60.0 Chronic acquired pure red cell aplasia   MCC HCC
D60.1 Transient acquired pure red cell aplasia   MCC
D60.8 Other acquired pure red cell aplasias   MCC HCC
D60.9 Acquired pure red cell aplasia, unspecified   MCC HCC

✓4th D61 Other aplastic anemias and other bone marrow failure syndromes
  EXCLUDES 2   neutropenia (D70.-)
  AHA: 2020,3Q,22; 2014,4Q,22
  DEF: Aplastic anemia: Bone marrow failure characterized by underproduction of red bloods cells, white blood cells and platelets.

✓5th D61.0 Constitutional aplastic anemia
  D61.01 Constitutional (pure) red blood cell aplasia   CC HCC
    Blackfan-Diamond syndrome
    Congenital (pure) red cell aplasia
    Familial hypoplastic anemia
    Primary (pure) red cell aplasia
    Red cell (pure) aplasia of infants
    EXCLUDES 1   acquired red cell aplasia (D60.9)

  D61.02 Shwachman-Diamond syndrome   CC HCC
    Code also, if applicable, associated conditions such as:
      acute myeloblastic leukemia (C92.0-)
      exocrine pancreatic insufficiency (K86.81)
      myelodysplastic syndrome (D46.-)
    Use additional code, if applicable, for genetic susceptibility to other malignant neoplasm (Z15.09)
    AHA: 2023,4Q,8

  D61.03 Fanconi anemia   CC
    Fanconi pancytopenia
    Fanconi's anemia
    EXCLUDES 1   Fanconi syndrome (E72.0-)

  D61.09 Other constitutional aplastic anemia   CC HCC
    ~~Fanconi's anemia~~
    Pancytopenia with malformations

D61.1 Drug-induced aplastic anemia   MCC
  Use additional code for adverse effect, if applicable, to identify drug (T36-T50 with fifth or sixth character 5)

D61.2 Aplastic anemia due to other external agents   MCC HCC
  Code first, if applicable, toxic effects of substances chiefly nonmedicinal as to source (T51-T65)

D61.3 Idiopathic aplastic anemia   MCC HCC

✓5th D61.8 Other specified aplastic anemias and other bone marrow failure syndromes
  ✓6th D61.81 Pancytopenia
    EXCLUDES 1   pancytopenia (due to) (with) aplastic anemia (D61.9)
      pancytopenia (due to) (with) bone marrow infiltration (D61.82)
      pancytopenia (due to) (with) congenital (pure) red cell aplasia (D61.01)
      pancytopenia (due to) (with) hairy cell leukemia (C91.4-)
      pancytopenia (due to) (with) human immunodeficiency virus disease (B20)
      pancytopenia (due to) (with) leukoerythroblastic anemia (D61.82)
      pancytopenia (due to) (with) myeloproliferative disease (D47.1)
    EXCLUDES 2   pancytopenia (due to) (with) myelodysplastic syndromes (D46.-)
    DEF: Shortage of all three blood cells: white, red, and platelets.

    D61.810 Antineoplastic chemotherapy induced pancytopenia   MCC
      EXCLUDES 2   aplastic anemia due to antineoplastic chemotherapy (D61.1)
      AHA: 2020,3Q,22

    D61.811 Other drug-induced pancytopenia   MCC
      EXCLUDES 2   aplastic anemia due to drugs (D61.1)
      AHA: 2023,3Q,4

    D61.818 Other pancytopenia   CC HCC
      AHA: 2023,1Q,23; 2020,3Q,24; 2019,1Q,16
      TIP: Assign this code in addition to myeloid leukemia codes (C92.-) when pancytopenia is documented. Although common in some types of myeloid leukemia, pancytopenia is not always inherent.

  D61.82 Myelophthisis   CC HCC
    Leukoerythroblastic anemia
    Myelophthisic anemia
    Panmyelophthisis
    Code also the underlying disorder, such as:
      malignant neoplasm of breast (C50.-)
      tuberculosis (A15.-)
    EXCLUDES 1   idiopathic myelofibrosis (D47.1)
      myelofibrosis NOS (D75.81)
      myelofibrosis with myeloid metaplasia (D47.4)
      primary myelofibrosis (D47.1)
      secondary myelofibrosis (D75.81)
    DEF: Condition that occurs when normal hematopoietic tissue in the bone marrow is replaced with abnormal tissue, such as fibrous tissue or tumors. Most commonly seen during the advanced stages of cancer.

  D61.89 Other specified aplastic anemias and other bone marrow failure syndromes   MCC HCC

D61.9 Aplastic anemia, unspecified   CC
  Hypoplastic anemia NOS
  Medullary hypoplasia

D62 Acute posthemorrhagic anemia   CC
  EXCLUDES 1   anemia due to chronic blood loss (D50.0)
    blood loss anemia NOS (D50.0)
    congenital anemia from fetal blood loss (P61.3)
  AHA: 2023,1Q,15,16; 2019,3Q,11,17

✓4th D63 Anemia in chronic diseases classified elsewhere
  D63.0 Anemia in neoplastic disease
    Code first neoplasm (C00-D49)
    EXCLUDES 1   aplastic anemia due to antineoplastic chemotherapy (D61.1)
    EXCLUDES 2   anemia due to antineoplastic chemotherapy (D64.81)

  D63.1 Anemia in chronic kidney disease
    Erythropoietin resistant anemia (EPO resistant anemia)
    Code first underlying chronic kidney disease (CKD) (N18.-)

N Newborn: 0   P Pediatric: 0-17   M Maternity: 9-64   A Adult: 15-124   UNS Unspecified Site   MCC Major Complication/Comorbidity   CC Complication/Comorbidity   PE POA Exempt

518   **ICD-10-CM 2025**

D63.8   **Anemia in other chronic diseases classified elsewhere**
    Code first underlying disease, such as:
      diphyllobothriasis (B70.0)
      hookworm disease (B76.0-B76.9)
      hypothyroidism (E00.0-E03.9)
      malaria (B50.0-B54)
      symptomatic late syphilis (A52.79)
      tuberculosis (A18.89)

✓4ᵗʰ **D64**   **Other anemias**

   EXCLUDES 1   *refractory anemia (D46.-)*
          refractory anemia with excess blasts in transformation [RAEB T] (C92.0-)

   DEF: Sideroblastic anemia: Hereditary or secondary disorder in which the red blood cells cannot effectively use iron, a nutrient needed to make hemoglobin. Although the iron can enter the red blood cell it is not assimilated into the hemoglobin molecule and builds up ringed sideroblasts around the cell nucleus.

   D64.0   **Hereditary sideroblastic anemia**   HCC
      Sex-linked hypochromic sideroblastic anemia

   D64.1   *Secondary sideroblastic anemia due to disease*   HCC
      Code first underlying disease

   D64.2   **Secondary sideroblastic anemia due to drugs and toxins**
      Code first poisoning due to drug or toxin, if applicable (T36-T65 with fifth or sixth character 1-4)
      Use additional code for adverse effect, if applicable, to identify drug (T36-T50 with fifth or sixth character 5)

   D64.3   **Other sideroblastic anemias**   HCC
      Sideroblastic anemia NOS
      Pyridoxine-responsive sideroblastic anemia NEC

   D64.4   **Congenital dyserythropoietic anemia**   HCC
      Dyshematopoietic anemia (congenital)
     EXCLUDES 1   *Blackfan-Diamond syndrome (D61.01)*
          Di Guglielmo's disease (C94.0)

✓5ᵗʰ **D64.8**   **Other specified anemias**

     D64.81   **Anemia due to antineoplastic chemotherapy**
        Antineoplastic chemotherapy induced anemia
       EXCLUDES 2   *anemia in neoplastic disease (D63.0)*
            aplastic anemia due to antineoplastic chemotherapy (D61.1)
        AHA: 2023,2Q,17; 2021,3Q,4; 2014,4Q,22

     D64.89   **Other specified anemias**
        Infantile pseudoleukemia

   D64.9   **Anemia, unspecified**
      AHA: 2020,3Q,24; 2018,4Q,88; 2017,1Q,7

Coagulation defects, purpura and other hemorrhagic conditions (D65-D69)

D65   **Disseminated intravascular coagulation [defibrination syndrome]**   MCC
     Afibrinogenemia, acquired
     Consumption coagulopathy
     COVID-19 associated diffuse or disseminated intravascular coagulopathy
     Diffuse or disseminated intravascular coagulation [DIC]
     Fibrinolytic hemorrhage, acquired
     Fibrinolytic purpura
     Purpura fulminans
     Code also, if applicable, associated condition
    EXCLUDES 1   *disseminated intravascular coagulation (complicating):*
         abortion or ectopic or molar pregnancy (O00-O07, O08.1)
         in newborn (P60)
         pregnancy, childbirth and the puerperium (O45.0, O46.0, O67.0, O72.3)
    AHA: 2021,1Q,39

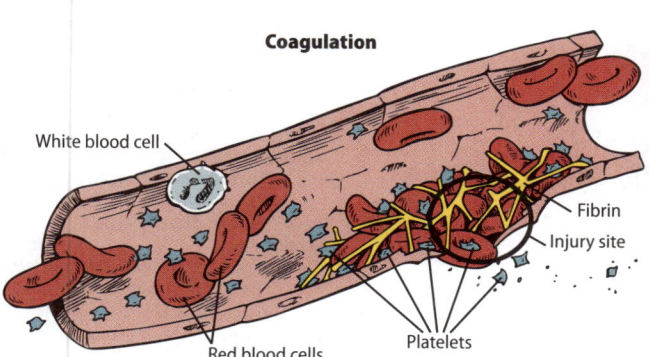

Coagulation

White blood cell — Fibrin — Injury site — Platelets — Red blood cells

D66   **Hereditary factor VIII deficiency**   MCC HCC
     Classical hemophilia
     Deficiency factor VIII (with functional defect)
     Hemophilia A
     Hemophilia NOS
    EXCLUDES 1   *factor VIII deficiency with vascular defect (D68.0-)*
    AHA: 2022,4Q,9
    DEF: Hereditary, sex-linked lack of antihemophilic globulin (AHG) (factor VIII) that causes abnormal coagulation characterized by increased bleeding; large bruises of skin; bleeding in the mouth, nose, and gastrointestinal tract; and hemorrhages into joints, resulting in swelling and impaired function.
    TIP: Factor VIII deficiency may also be documented in patients with VWD. Only a code for the VWD should be reported; do not report code D66.

D67   **Hereditary factor IX deficiency**   MCC HCC
     Christmas disease
     Factor IX deficiency (with functional defect)
     Hemophilia B
     Plasma thromboplastin component [PTC] deficiency

✓4ᵗʰ **D68**   **Other coagulation defects**

    EXCLUDES 1   *abnormal coagulation profile NOS (R79.1)*
    EXCLUDES 2   *coagulation defects complicating abortion or ectopic or molar pregnancy (O00-O07, O08.1)*
         coagulation defects complicating pregnancy, childbirth and the puerperium (O45.0, O46.0, O67.0, O72.3)
    AHA: 2016,1Q,14

✓5ᵗʰ **D68.0**   **Von Willebrand disease**

     EXCLUDES 1   *capillary fragility (hereditary) (D69.8)*
         factor VIII deficiency NOS (D66)
         factor VIII deficiency with functional defect (D66)

     AHA: 2022,4Q,7-9
     DEF: Congenital, abnormal blood coagulation caused by deficient blood factor VII. Symptoms include excess or prolonged bleeding.
     TIP: Factor VIII deficiency may also be documented in patients with VWD. Only a code for the VWD should be reported; do not report code D66.

     D68.00   **Von Willebrand disease, unspecified**   CC HCC

     D68.01   **Von Willebrand disease, type 1**   CC HCC
        Partial quantitative deficiency of von Willebrand factor
        Type 1C von Willebrand disease
        AHA: 2022,4Q,9

Chapter 3. Diseases of the Blood and Blood-forming Organs

✓6th **D68.02   Von Willebrand disease, type 2**
Qualitative defects of von Willebrand factor

     D68.020   Von Willebrand disease, type 2A CC HCC
Qualitative defects of von Willebrand factor with decreased platelet adhesion and selective deficiency of high-molecular-weight multimers

     D68.021   Von Willebrand disease, type 2B CC HCC
Qualitative defects of von Willebrand factor with high-molecular-weight von Willebrand factor loss
Qualitative defects of von Willebrand factor with hyper-adhesive forms
Qualitative defects of von Willebrand factor with increased affinity for platelet glycoprotein Ib

     D68.022   Von Willebrand disease, type 2M CC HCC
Qualitative defects of von Willebrand factor with defective platelet adhesion with a normal size distribution of von Willebrand factor multimers

     D68.023   Von Willebrand disease, type 2N CC HCC
Qualitative defects of von Willebrand factor with defective von Willebrand factor to factor VIII binding
Qualitative defects of von Willebrand factor with markedly decreased affinity for factor VIII

     D68.029   Von Willebrand disease, type 2, unspecified CC HCC
Qualitative defect in von Willebrand factor function, with no further subtyping

D68.03   Von Willebrand disease, type 3 CC HCC
(Near) complete absence of von Willebrand factor
Total quantitative deficiency of von Willebrand factor

D68.04   Acquired von Willebrand disease CC HCC
Acquired von Willebrand syndrome

D68.09   Other von Willebrand disease CC HCC
Platelet-type von Willebrand disease
Pseudo-von Willebrand disease
Code also, if applicable, qualitative platelet defects (D69.1)

D68.1   Hereditary factor XI deficiency CC HCC
Hemophilia C
Plasma thromboplastin antecedent [PTA] deficiency
Rosenthal's disease

D68.2   Hereditary deficiency of other clotting factors CC HCC
AC globulin deficiency
Congenital afibrinogenemia
Deficiency of factor I [fibrinogen]
Deficiency of factor II [prothrombin]
Deficiency of factor V [labile]
Deficiency of factor VII [stable]
Deficiency of factor X [Stuart-Prower]
Deficiency of factor XII [Hageman]
Deficiency of factor XIII [fibrin stabilizing]
Dysfibrinogenemia (congenital)
Hypoproconvertinemia
Owren's disease
Proaccelerin deficiency

✓5th **D68.3   Hemorrhagic disorder due to circulating anticoagulants**

✓6th   **D68.31   Hemorrhagic disorder due to intrinsic circulating anticoagulants, antibodies, or inhibitors**

     D68.311   Acquired hemophilia CC HCC
Autoimmune hemophilia
Autoimmune inhibitors to clotting factors
Secondary hemophilia

     D68.312   Antiphospholipid antibody with hemorrhagic disorder CC
Lupus anticoagulant (LAC) with hemorrhagic disorder
Systemic lupus erythematosus [SLE] inhibitor with hemorrhagic disorder
EXCLUDES 1   *antiphospholipid antibody, finding without diagnosis (R76.0)*
antiphospholipid antibody syndrome (D68.61)
antiphospholipid antibody with hypercoagulable state (D68.61)
lupus anticoagulant (LAC) finding without diagnosis (R76.0)
lupus anticoagulant (LAC) with hypercoagulable state (D68.62)
systemic lupus erythematosus [SLE] inhibitor finding without diagnosis (R76.0)
systemic lupus erythematosus [SLE] inhibitor with hypercoagulable state (D68.62)

     D68.318   Other hemorrhagic disorder due to intrinsic circulating anticoagulants, antibodies, or inhibitors CC
Antithromboplastinemia
Antithromboplastinogenemia
Hemorrhagic disorder due to intrinsic increase in antithrombin
Hemorrhagic disorder due to intrinsic increase in anti-VIIIa
Hemorrhagic disorder due to intrinsic increase in anti-IXa
Hemorrhagic disorder due to intrinsic increase in anti-XIa

   D68.32   Hemorrhagic disorder due to extrinsic circulating anticoagulants CC
Drug-induced hemorrhagic disorder
Hemorrhagic disorder due to increase in anti-IIa
Hemorrhagic disorder due to increase in anti-Xa
Hyperheparinemia
Use additional code for adverse effect, if applicable, to identify drug (T45.515, T45.525)
AHA: 2021,1Q,4; 2016,1Q,14-15
TIP: Do not assign to identify routine therapeutic anticoagulation effects; assign only for documented adverse effects.

D68.4   Acquired coagulation factor deficiency CC
Deficiency of coagulation factor due to liver disease
Deficiency of coagulation factor due to vitamin K deficiency
EXCLUDES 1   *vitamin K deficiency of newborn (P53)*

✓5th **D68.5   Primary thrombophilia**
Primary hypercoagulable states
EXCLUDES 1   *antiphospholipid syndrome (D68.61)*
lupus anticoagulant (D68.62)
secondary activated protein C resistance (D68.69)
secondary antiphospholipid antibody syndrome (D68.69)
secondary lupus anticoagulant with hypercoagulable state (D68.69)
secondary systemic lupus erythematosus [SLE] inhibitor with hypercoagulable state (D68.69)
systemic lupus erythematosus [SLE] inhibitor finding without diagnosis (R76.0)
systemic lupus erythematosus [SLE] inhibitor with hemorrhagic disorder (D68.312)
thrombotic thrombocytopenic purpura (M31.19)
DEF: Thrombophilia: Increased tendency of the blood to clot, which can lead to thrombus or embolus formation.

D68.51   Activated protein C resistance CC
Factor V Leiden mutation

D68.52   Prothrombin gene mutation CC

N Newborn: 0   P Pediatric: 0-17   M Maternity: 9-64   A Adult: 15-124   UNS Unspecified Site   MCC Major Complication/Comorbidity   CC Complication/Comorbidity   PE POA Exempt

520   ICD-10-CM 2025

D68.59   **Other primary thrombophilia**   `CC`
Antithrombin III deficiency
Hypercoagulable state NOS
Primary hypercoagulable state NEC
Primary thrombophilia NEC
Protein C deficiency
Protein S deficiency
Thrombophilia NOS
AHA: 2021,2Q,8

`√5th` **D68.6**   **Other thrombophilia**
Other hypercoagulable states
EXCLUDES 1   *diffuse or disseminated intravascular coagulation [DIC] (D65)*
    heparin induced thrombocytopenia (HIT) (D75.82-)
    hyperhomocysteinemia (E72.11)

D68.61   **Antiphospholipid syndrome**   `CC`
Anticardiolipin syndrome
Antiphospholipid antibody syndrome
EXCLUDES 1   *anti-phospholipid antibody, finding without diagnosis (R76.0)*
    anti-phospholipid antibody with hemorrhagic disorder (D68.312)
    lupus anticoagulant syndrome (D68.62)

D68.62   **Lupus anticoagulant syndrome**   `CC`
Lupus anticoagulant
Presence of systemic lupus erythematosus [SLE] inhibitor
EXCLUDES 1   *anticardiolipin syndrome (D68.61)*
    antiphospholipid syndrome (D68.61)
    lupus anticoagulant (LAC) finding without diagnosis (R76.0)
    lupus anticoagulant (LAC) with hemorrhagic disorder (D68.312)

D68.69   **Other thrombophilia**   `CC`
COVID-19 associated hypercoagulability
Hypercoagulable states NEC
Secondary hypercoagulable state NOS
Code also, if applicable, associated condition
AHA: 2021,2Q,8

D68.8   **Other specified coagulation defects**   `CC`
COVID-19 associated coagulopathy
Code also, if applicable, associated condition
EXCLUDES 1   *hemorrhagic disease of newborn (P53)*
AHA: 2021,1Q,39

D68.9   **Coagulation defect, unspecified**   `CC`

`√4th` **D69**   **Purpura and other hemorrhagic conditions**
EXCLUDES 1   *benign hypergammaglobulinemic purpura (D89.0)*
    cryoglobulinemic purpura (D89.1)
    essential (hemorrhagic) thrombocythemia (D47.3)
    hemorrhagic thrombocythemia (D47.3)
    purpura fulminans (D65)
    thrombotic thrombocytopenic purpura (M31.19)
    Waldenstrom hypergammaglobulinemic purpura (D89.0)

D69.0   **Allergic purpura**   `CC`
Allergic vasculitis
Nonthrombocytopenic hemorrhagic purpura
Nonthrombocytopenic idiopathic purpura
Purpura anaphylactoid
Purpura Henoch(-Schonlein)
Purpura rheumatica
Vascular purpura
EXCLUDES 1   *thrombocytopenic hemorrhagic purpura (D69.3)*
AHA: 2020,3Q,26
DEF: Any hemorrhagic condition, thrombocytic or nonthrombocytopenic in origin, caused by a presumed allergic reaction.

D69.1   **Qualitative platelet defects**   `HCC`
Bernard-Soulier [giant platelet] syndrome
Glanzmann's disease
Grey platelet syndrome
Thromboasthenia (hemorrhagic) (hereditary)
Thrombocytopathy
EXCLUDES 1   *hemolytic-uremic syndrome (D59.3-)*
EXCLUDES 2   *von Willebrand disease (D68.0-)*

D69.2   **Other nonthrombocytopenic purpura**
Purpura NOS
Purpura simplex
Senile purpura

D69.3   **Immune thrombocytopenic purpura**   `CC` `HCC`
Hemorrhagic (thrombocytopenic) purpura
Idiopathic thrombocytopenic purpura
Tidal platelet dysgenesis
DEF: Tidal platelet dysgenesis: Fluctuation of platelet counts from normal to very low within periods of 20 to 40 days and may involve autoimmune platelet destruction.

`√5th` **D69.4**   **Other primary thrombocytopenia**
EXCLUDES 1   *transient neonatal thrombocytopenia (P61.0)*
    Wiskott-Aldrich syndrome (D82.0)

D69.41   **Evans syndrome**   `CC` `HCC`

D69.42   **Congenital and hereditary thrombocytopenia purpura**   `CC` `HCC`
Congenital thrombocytopenia
Hereditary thrombocytopenia
Code first congenital or hereditary disorder, such as: thrombocytopenia with absent radius (TAR syndrome) (Q87.2)

D69.49   **Other primary thrombocytopenia**   `HCC`
Megakaryocytic hypoplasia
Primary thrombocytopenia NOS

`√5th` **D69.5**   **Secondary thrombocytopenia**
EXCLUDES 1   *heparin induced thrombocytopenia (HIT) (D75.82-)*
    transient thrombocytopenia of newborn (P61.0)

D69.51   **Posttransfusion purpura**
Posttransfusion purpura from whole blood (fresh) or blood products
PTP

D69.59   **Other secondary thrombocytopenia**
AHA: 2014,4Q,22

D69.6   **Thrombocytopenia, unspecified**
AHA: 2020,3Q,24

D69.8   **Other specified hemorrhagic conditions**
Capillary fragility (hereditary)
Vascular pseudohemophilia

D69.9   **Hemorrhagic condition, unspecified**

Other disorders of blood and blood-forming organs (D70-D77)

`√4th` **D70**   **Neutropenia**
INCLUDES   agranulocytosis
    decreased absolute neurophile count (ANC)
Use additional code for any associated:
    fever (R50.81)
Code also, if applicable, mucositis (J34.81, K12.3-, K92.81, N76.81)
EXCLUDES 1   *neutropenic splenomegaly (D73.81)*
    transient neonatal neutropenia (P61.5)
DEF: Abnormally low number of neutrophils. Neutrophils are phagocytic, meaning they surround and consume harmful pathogens, primarily bacteria. When neutrophil counts decrease the risk of infection increases.

D70.0   **Congenital agranulocytosis**   `HCC`
Congenital neutropenia
Infantile genetic agranulocytosis
Kostmann's disease

D70.1   **Agranulocytosis secondary to cancer chemotherapy**
Code also underlying neoplasm
Use additional code for adverse effect, if applicable, to identify drug (T45.1X5)
AHA: 2020,3Q,22; 2014,4Q,22

D70.2   **Other drug-induced agranulocytosis**
Use additional code for adverse effect, if applicable, to identify drug (T36-T50 with fifth or sixth character 5)

D70.3   **Neutropenia due to infection**

D70.4   **Cyclic neutropenia**   `HCC`
Cyclic hematopoiesis
Periodic neutropenia

D70.8   **Other neutropenia**

D70.9   **Neutropenia, unspecified**
AHA: 2020,3Q,24

Chapter 3. Diseases of the Blood and Blood-forming Organs

D71 **Functional disorders of polymorphonuclear neutrophils** `HCC`
Cell membrane receptor complex [CR3] defect
Chronic (childhood) granulomatous disease
Congenital dysphagocytosis
Progressive septic granulomatosis

✓4th **D72** **Other disorders of white blood cells**
     EXCLUDES 1   *basophilia (D72.824)*
         immunity disorders (D80-D89)
         neutropenia (D70)
         preleukemia (syndrome) (D46.9)

D72.0 **Genetic anomalies of leukocytes** `HCC`
Alder (granulation) (granulocyte) anomaly
Alder syndrome
Hereditary leukocytic hypersegmentation
Hereditary leukocytic hyposegmentation
Hereditary leukomelanopathy
May-Hegglin (granulation) (granulocyte) anomaly
May-Hegglin syndrome
Pelger-Huet (granulation) (granulocyte) anomaly
Pelger-Huet syndrome
     EXCLUDES 1   *Chediak (-Steinbrinck)-Higashi syndrome (E70.330)*

✓5th **D72.1** **Eosinophilia**
     EXCLUDES 2   *Loffler's syndrome (J82.89)*
         pulmonary eosinophilia (J82.-)
     AHA: 2020,4Q,8-10
     DEF: Abnormally large accumulation or formation of eosinophils (nucleated, granular leukocytes) in the blood, characteristic of allergic states and infection.

     D72.10 **Eosinophilia, unspecified**

     ✓6th **D72.11** **Hypereosinophilic syndrome [HES]**
         D72.110 **Idiopathic hypereosinophilic syndrome [IHES]**
         D72.111 **Lymphocytic Variant Hypereosinophilic Syndrome [LHES]**
             Lymphocyte variant hypereosinophilia
             Code also, if applicable, any associated lymphocytic neoplastic disorder
         D72.118 **Other hypereosinophilic syndrome**
             Episodic angioedema with eosinophilia
             Gleich's syndrome
         D72.119 **Hypereosinophilic syndrome [HES], unspecified**

     D72.12 **Drug rash with eosinophilia and systemic symptoms syndrome**
         DRESS syndrome
         Use additional code for adverse effect, if applicable, to identify drug (T36-T50 with fifth or sixth character 5)

     D72.18 *Eosinophilia in diseases classified elsewhere*
         Code first underlying disease, such as:
         chronic myelomonocytic leukemia (C93.1-)

     D72.19 **Other eosinophilia**
         Familial eosinophilia
         Hereditary eosinophilia

✓5th **D72.8** **Other specified disorders of white blood cells**
     EXCLUDES 1   *leukemia (C91-C95)*

     ✓6th **D72.81** **Decreased white blood cell count**
         EXCLUDES 1   *neutropenia (D70.-)*
         D72.810 **Lymphocytopenia**
             Decreased lymphocytes
         D72.818 **Other decreased white blood cell count**
             Basophilic leukopenia
             Eosinophilic leukopenia
             Monocytopenia
             Other decreased leukocytes
             Plasmacytopenia
         D72.819 **Decreased white blood cell count, unspecified**
             Decreased leukocytes, unspecified
             Leukocytopenia, unspecified
             Leukopenia
             EXCLUDES 1   *malignant leukopenia (D70.9)*

     ✓6th **D72.82** **Elevated white blood cell count**
         EXCLUDES 1   *eosinophilia (D72.1)*
         D72.820 **Lymphocytosis (symptomatic)**
             Elevated lymphocytes
         D72.821 **Monocytosis (symptomatic)**
             EXCLUDES 1   *infectious mononucleosis (B27.-)*
         D72.822 **Plasmacytosis**

         D72.823 **Leukemoid reaction**
             Basophilic leukemoid reaction
             Leukemoid reaction NOS
             Lymphocytic leukemoid reaction
             Monocytic leukemoid reaction
             Myelocytic leukemoid reaction
             Neutrophilic leukemoid reaction

         D72.824 **Basophilia**
             DEF: Increase in the basophils of the blood, a type of white blood cell, often seen in conjunction with neoplastic disorders.

         D72.825 **Bandemia**
             Bandemia without diagnosis of specific infection
             EXCLUDES 1   *confirmed infection - code to infection*
                 leukemia (C91.-, C92.-, C93.-, C94.-, C95.-)
             DEF: Increase in early neutrophil cells, called band cells, that may indicate infection.

         D72.828 **Other elevated white blood cell count**
         D72.829 **Elevated white blood cell count, unspecified**
             Elevated leukocytes, unspecified
             Leukocytosis, unspecified

     D72.89 **Other specified disorders of white blood cells**
         Abnormality of white blood cells NEC

D72.9 **Disorder of white blood cells, unspecified**
     Abnormal leukocyte differential NOS

✓4th **D73** **Diseases of spleen**

     D73.0 **Hyposplenism**
         Atrophy of spleen
         EXCLUDES 1   *asplenia (congenital) (Q89.01)*
             postsurgical absence of spleen (Z90.81)

     D73.1 **Hypersplenism**
         EXCLUDES 1   *neutropenic splenomegaly (D73.81)*
             primary splenic neutropenia (D73.81)
             splenitis, splenomegaly in late syphilis (A52.79)
             splenitis, splenomegaly in tuberculosis (A18.85)
             splenomegaly NOS (R16.1)
             splenomegaly congenital (Q89.0)

     D73.2 **Chronic congestive splenomegaly**
     D73.3 **Abscess of spleen**
     D73.4 **Cyst of spleen**
     D73.5 **Infarction of spleen**
         Splenic rupture, nontraumatic
         Torsion of spleen
         EXCLUDES 1   *rupture of spleen due to Plasmodium vivax malaria (B51.0)*
             traumatic rupture of spleen (S36.03-)

     ✓5th **D73.8** **Other diseases of spleen**
         D73.81 **Neutropenic splenomegaly**
             Werner-Schultz disease
         D73.89 **Other diseases of spleen**
             Fibrosis of spleen NOS
             Perisplenitis
             Splenitis NOS

     D73.9 **Disease of spleen, unspecified**

✓4th **D74** **Methemoglobinemia**

     D74.0 **Congenital methemoglobinemia** `CC`
         Congenital NADH-methemoglobin reductase deficiency
         Hemoglobin-M [Hb-M] disease
         Methemoglobinemia, hereditary

     D74.8 **Other methemoglobinemias** `CC`
         Acquired methemoglobinemia (with sulfhemoglobinemia)
         Toxic methemoglobinemia

     D74.9 **Methemoglobinemia, unspecified** `CC`

N Newborn: 0   P Pediatric: 0-17   M Maternity: 9-64   A Adult: 15-124   UNS Unspecified Site   MCC Major Complication/Comorbidity   CC Complication/Comorbidity   PE POA Exempt

522   ICD-10-CM 2025

✓4ᵗʰ D75 Other and unspecified diseases of blood and blood-forming organs

EXCLUDES 2   *acute lymphadenitis (LØ4.-)*
chronic lymphadenitis (I88.1)
enlarged lymph nodes (R59.-)
hypergammaglobulinemia NOS (D89.2)
lymphadenitis NOS (I88.9)
mesenteric lymphadenitis (acute) (chronic) (I88.Ø)

D75.Ø Familial erythrocytosis
Benign polycythemia
Familial polycythemia
EXCLUDES 1   *hereditary ovalocytosis (D58.1)*

D75.1 Secondary polycythemia
Acquired polycythemia
Emotional polycythemia
Erythrocytosis NOS
Hypoxemic polycythemia
Nephrogenous polycythemia
Polycythemia due to erythropoietin
Polycythemia due to fall in plasma volume
Polycythemia due to high altitude
Polycythemia due to stress
Polycythemia NOS
Relative polycythemia
EXCLUDES 1   *polycythemia neonatorum (P61.1)*
polycythemia vera (D45)
DEF: Elevated number of red blood cells in circulating blood as a result of reduced oxygen supply to the tissues.

✓5ᵗʰ D75.8 Other specified diseases of blood and blood-forming organs

D75.81 *Myelofibrosis*   `CC` `HCC`
Myelofibrosis NOS
Secondary myelofibrosis NOS
Code first the underlying disorder, such as:
    malignant neoplasm of breast (C5Ø.-)
Use additional code, if applicable, for associated therapy-related myelodysplastic syndrome (D46.-)
Use additional code for adverse effect, if applicable, to identify drug (T45.1X5)
EXCLUDES 1   *acute myelofibrosis (C94.4-)*
idiopathic myelofibrosis (D47.1)
leukoerythroblastic anemia (D61.82)
myelofibrosis with myeloid metaplasia (D47.4)
myelophthisic anemia (D61.82)
myelophthisis (D61.82)
primary myelofibrosis (D47.1)

✓6ᵗʰ D75.82 Heparin induced thrombocytopenia (HIT)
Use additional code, if applicable, for adverse effect of heparin (T45.515-)
AHA: 2022,4Q,9-10
DEF: Immune-mediated reaction to heparin therapy causing an abrupt fall in platelet count and serious complications such as pulmonary embolism, stroke, AMI, or DVT.

D75.821 Non-immune heparin-induced thrombocytopenia
Non-immune HIT
Type 1 heparin-induced thrombocytopenia

D75.822 Immune-mediated heparin-induced thrombocytopenia
Immune-mediated HIT
Type 2 heparin-induced thrombocytopenia

D75.828 Other heparin-induced thrombocytopenia syndrome
Autoimmune heparin-induced thrombocytopenia syndrome
Delayed-onset heparin-induced thrombocytopenia
Persisting heparin-induced thrombocytopenia

D75.829 Heparin-induced thrombocytopenia, unspecified

✓6ᵗʰ D75.83 Thrombocytosis
EXCLUDES 2   *essential thrombocythemia (D47.3)*
AHA: 2021,4Q,7-8

D75.838 Other thrombocytosis
Reactive thrombocytosis
Secondary thrombocytosis
Code also underlying condition, if known and applicable

D75.839 Thrombocytosis, unspecified
Thrombocythemia NOS
Thrombocytosis NOS

D75.84 Other platelet-activating anti-PF4 disorders   `HCC`
Spontaneous heparin-induced thrombocytopenia syndrome (without heparin exposure)
Thrombosis with thrombocytopenia syndrome
Vaccine-induced thrombotic thrombocytopenia
Use additional code, if applicable, for adverse effect of other viral vaccine (T5Ø.B95-)
AHA: 2022,4Q,9-10

D75.89 Other specified diseases of blood and blood-forming organs

D75.9 Disease of blood and blood-forming organs, unspecified

D75.A Glucose-6-phosphate dehydrogenase (G6PD) deficiency without anemia
EXCLUDES 1   *glucose-6-phosphate dehydrogenase (G6PD) deficiency with anemia (D55.Ø)*
AHA: 2019,4Q,4-5

✓4ᵗʰ D76 Other specified diseases with participation of lymphoreticular and reticulohistiocytic tissue
EXCLUDES 1   *(Abt-) Letterer-Siwe disease (C96.Ø)*
eosinophilic granuloma (C96.6)
Hand-Schuller-Christian disease (C96.5)
histiocytic medullary reticulosis (C96.9)
histiocytic sarcoma (C96.A)
histiocytosis X, multifocal (C96.5)
histiocytosis X, unifocal (C96.6)
Langerhans-cell histiocytosis, multifocal (C96.5)
Langerhans-cell histiocytosis NOS (C96.6)
Langerhans-cell histiocytosis, unifocal (C96.6)
leukemic reticuloendotheliosis (C91.4-)
lipomelanotic reticulosis (I89.8)
malignant histiocytosis (C96.A)
malignant reticulosis (C86.Ø)
nonlipid reticuloendotheliosis (C96.Ø)

D76.1 Hemophagocytic lymphohistiocytosis   `CC` `HCC`
Familial hemophagocytic reticulosis
Histiocytoses of mononuclear phagocytes

D76.2 Hemophagocytic syndrome, infection-associated   `CC`
Use additional code to identify infectious agent or disease

D76.3 Other histiocytosis syndromes   `CC` `HCC`
Reticulohistiocytoma (giant-cell)
Sinus histiocytosis with massive lymphadenopathy
Xanthogranuloma

D77 *Other disorders of blood and blood-forming organs in diseases classified elsewhere*
Code first underlying disease, such as:
    amyloidosis (E85.-)
    congenital early syphilis (A5Ø.Ø-)
    echinococcosis (B67.Ø-B67.9)
    malaria (B5Ø.Ø-B54)
    schistosomiasis [bilharziasis] (B65.Ø-B65.9)
    vitamin C deficiency (E54)
EXCLUDES 1   *rupture of spleen due to Plasmodium vivax malaria (B51.Ø)*
splenitis, splenomegaly in late syphilis (A52.79)
splenitis, splenomegaly in tuberculosis (A18.85)

✔ Additional Character Required   ✓x7ᵗʰ Placeholder   Questionable PDx   Manifestation   Unspecified   UPD Unacceptable PDx   H1 - H14 HAC   HCC CMS-HCC Dx   HIV HIV Dx

ICD-10-CM 2025   **523**

Chapter 3. Diseases of the Blood and Blood-forming Organs

D78–D82.Ø

Intraoperative and postprocedural complications of the spleen (D78)

✓4th D78 Intraoperative and postprocedural complications of the spleen
AHA: 2016,4Q,9-10

  ✓5th **D78.Ø Intraoperative hemorrhage and hematoma** of the spleen complicating a procedure
      EXCLUDES 1   *intraoperative hemorrhage and hematoma of the spleen due to accidental puncture or laceration during a procedure (D78.1-)*

     D78.Ø1   Intraoperative hemorrhage and hematoma of the spleen complicating a **procedure on the spleen**   CC
     D78.Ø2   Intraoperative hemorrhage and hematoma of the spleen complicating other procedure   CC

  ✓5th **D78.1 Accidental puncture and laceration** of the spleen during a procedure
     D78.11   Accidental puncture and laceration of the spleen during a **procedure on the spleen**   CC
     D78.12   Accidental puncture and laceration of the spleen during other procedure   CC
       AHA: 2022,1Q,22

  ✓5th **D78.2 Postprocedural hemorrhage** of the spleen following a procedure
     D78.21   Postprocedural hemorrhage of the spleen following a **procedure on the spleen**   CC
     D78.22   Postprocedural hemorrhage of the spleen following other procedure   CC

  ✓5th **D78.3 Postprocedural hematoma and seroma** of the spleen following a procedure
     D78.31   Postprocedural **hematoma** of the spleen following a **procedure on the spleen**   CC
     D78.32   Postprocedural **hematoma** of the spleen following other procedure   CC
     D78.33   Postprocedural **seroma** of the spleen following a **procedure on the spleen**   CC
     D78.34   Postprocedural **seroma** of the spleen following other procedure   CC

  ✓5th **D78.8 Other intraoperative and postprocedural complications of the spleen**
       Use additional code, if applicable, to further specify disorder
     D78.81   Other **intraoperative** complications of the spleen   CC
     D78.89   Other **postprocedural** complications of the spleen   CC

Certain disorders involving the immune mechanism (D8Ø-D89)

INCLUDES   defects in the complement system
      immunodeficiency disorders, except human immunodeficiency virus [HIV] disease
      sarcoidosis
EXCLUDES 1   *autoimmune disease (systemic) NOS (M35.9)*
      functional disorders of polymorphonuclear neutrophils (D71)
      human immunodeficiency virus [HIV] disease (B2Ø)

✓4th D8Ø Immunodeficiency with predominantly antibody defects

   D8Ø.Ø Hereditary hypogammaglobulinemia   CC HCC
      Autosomal recessive agammaglobulinemia (Swiss type)
      X-linked agammaglobulinemia [Bruton] (with growth hormone deficiency)

   D8Ø.1 Nonfamilial hypogammaglobulinemia   CC
      Agammaglobulinemia with immunoglobulin-bearing B-lymphocytes
      Common variable agammaglobulinemia [CVAgamma]
      Hypogammaglobulinemia NOS

   D8Ø.2 Selective deficiency of immunoglobulin A [IgA]   CC HCC
   D8Ø.3 Selective deficiency of immunoglobulin G [IgG] subclasses   CC HCC
   D8Ø.4 Selective deficiency of immunoglobulin M [IgM]   CC HCC
   D8Ø.5 Immunodeficiency with increased immunoglobulin M [IgM]   CC HCC
   D8Ø.6 Antibody deficiency with near-normal immunoglobulins or with hyperimmunoglobulinemia   CC
   D8Ø.7 Transient hypogammaglobulinemia of infancy   CC
   D8Ø.8 Other immunodeficiencies with predominantly antibody defects   CC
      Kappa light chain deficiency
   D8Ø.9 Immunodeficiency with predominantly antibody defects, unspecified   CC

✓4th D81 Combined immunodeficiencies
     EXCLUDES 1   *autosomal recessive agammaglobulinemia (Swiss type) (D8Ø.Ø)*

   D81.Ø Severe combined immunodeficiency [SCID] with reticular dysgenesis   CC HCC
   D81.1 Severe combined immunodeficiency [SCID] with low T- and B-cell numbers
   D81.2 Severe combined immunodeficiency [SCID] with low or normal B-cell numbers   CC HCC

  ✓5th **D81.3 Adenosine deaminase [ADA] deficiency**
      AHA: 2019,4Q,5-6
     D81.3Ø   Adenosine deaminase deficiency, unspecified   CC HCC
       ADA deficiency NOS
     D81.31   Severe combined immunodeficiency due to adenosine deaminase deficiency   CC HCC
       ADA deficiency with SCID
       Adenosine deaminase [ADA] deficiency with severe combined immunodeficiency
     D81.32   Adenosine deaminase 2 deficiency   CC HCC
       ADA2 deficiency
       Adenosine deaminase deficiency type 2
       Code also, if applicable, any associated manifestations, such as:
         polyarteritis nodosa (M3Ø.Ø)
         stroke (I63.-)
     D81.39   Other adenosine deaminase deficiency   CC HCC
       Adenosine deaminase [ADA] deficiency type 1, NOS
       Adenosine deaminase [ADA] deficiency type 1, without SCID
       Adenosine deaminase [ADA] deficiency type 1, without severe combined immunodeficiency
       Partial ADA deficiency (type 1)
       Partial adenosine deaminase deficiency (type 1)

   D81.4 Nezelof's syndrome   CC HCC
   D81.5 Purine nucleoside phosphorylase [PNP] deficiency   CC HCC
   D81.6 Major histocompatibility complex class I deficiency   CC HCC
      Bare lymphocyte syndrome
   D81.7 Major histocompatibility complex class II deficiency   CC HCC

  ✓5th **D81.8 Other combined immunodeficiencies**
    ✓6th **D81.81 Biotin-dependent carboxylase deficiency**
       Multiple carboxylase deficiency
       EXCLUDES 1   *biotin-dependent carboxylase deficiency due to dietary deficiency of biotin (E53.8)*
       D81.81Ø   Biotinidase deficiency
       D81.818   Other biotin-dependent carboxylase deficiency
         Holocarboxylase synthetase deficiency
         Other multiple carboxylase deficiency
       D81.819   Biotin-dependent carboxylase deficiency, unspecified
         Multiple carboxylase deficiency, unspecified
     D81.82   Activated Phosphoinositide 3-kinase Delta Syndrome [APDS]
       p11Ød-activating mutation causing senescent T cells, lymphadenopathy, and immunodeficiency [PASLI] disease
       Code also, if applicable, any associated manifestations, such as:
         bronchiectasis (J47.-)
         herpes virus infections (BØØ.-)
         other acute respiratory tract infections (JØØ-JØ6; J2Ø-J22)
         other infections (AØØ-B99)
         pneumonia (J12-J18)
       AHA: 2022,4Q,11
     D81.89   Other combined immunodeficiencies   CC HCC
   D81.9 Combined immunodeficiency, unspecified   CC HCC
      Severe combined immunodeficiency disorder [SCID] NOS

✓4th D82 Immunodeficiency associated with other major defects
     EXCLUDES 1   *ataxia telangiectasia [Louis-Bar] (G11.3)*

   D82.Ø Wiskott-Aldrich syndrome   CC HCC
      Immunodeficiency with thrombocytopenia and eczema

N Newborn: 0   P Pediatric: 0-17   M Maternity: 9-64   A Adult: 15-124   UNS Unspecified Site   MCC Major Complication/Comorbidity   CC Complication/Comorbidity   PE POA Exempt

524   ICD-10-CM 2025

D82.1 **Di George's syndrome**   `CC` `HCC`
Pharyngeal pouch syndrome
Thymic alymphoplasia
Thymic aplasia or hypoplasia with immunodeficiency
AHA: 2019,3Q,14

D82.2 **Immunodeficiency with short-limbed stature**

D82.3 **Immunodeficiency following hereditary defective response to Epstein-Barr virus**
X-linked lymphoproliferative disease

D82.4 **Hyperimmunoglobulin E [IgE] syndrome**

D82.8 **Immunodeficiency associated with other specified major defects**

D82.9 **Immunodeficiency associated with major defect, unspecified**

✓4ᵗʰ **D83** **Common variable immunodeficiency**

D83.0 **Common variable immunodeficiency with predominant abnormalities of B-cell numbers and function**   `CC` `HCC`

D83.1 **Common variable immunodeficiency with predominant immunoregulatory T-cell disorders**   `CC` `HCC`

D83.2 **Common variable immunodeficiency with autoantibodies to B- or T-cells**   `CC` `HCC`

D83.8 **Other common variable immunodeficiencies**   `CC` `HCC`

D83.9 **Common variable immunodeficiency, unspecified**   `CC` `HCC`

✓4ᵗʰ **D84** **Other immunodeficiencies**

D84.0 **Lymphocyte function antigen-1 [LFA-1] defect**

D84.1 **Defects in the complement system**   `HCC`
C1 esterase inhibitor [C1-INH] deficiency

✓5ᵗʰ **D84.8** **Other specified immunodeficiencies**
AHA: 2020,4Q,10-12

D84.81 *Immunodeficiency due to conditions classified elsewhere*   `CC`
Code first underlying condition, such as:
chromosomal abnormalities (Q90-Q99)
diabetes mellitus (E08-E13)
malignant neoplasms (C00-C96)
EXCLUDES 1 *certain disorders involving the immune mechanism (D80-D83, D84.0, D84.1, D84.9)*
human immunodeficiency virus [HIV] disease (B20)
AHA: 2021,1Q,52

✓6ᵗʰ **D84.82** **Immunodeficiency due to drugs and external causes**

D84.821 **Immunodeficiency due to drugs**   `CC`
Immunodeficiency due to (current or past) medication
Use additional code for adverse effect if applicable, to identify adverse effect of drug (T36-T50 with fifth or six character 5)
Use additional code, if applicable, for associated long term (current) drug therapy drug or medication such as:
long term (current) drug therapy systemic steroids (Z79.52)
other long term (current) drug therapy (Z79.899)

D84.822 **Immunodeficiency due to external causes**   `CC`
Code also, if applicable, radiological procedure and radiotherapy (Y84.2)
Use additional code for external cause such as:
exposure to ionizing radiation (W88)

D84.89 **Other immunodeficiencies**   `CC`

D84.9 **Immunodeficiency, unspecified**   `CC`
Immunocompromised NOS
Immunodeficient NOS
Immunosuppressed NOS
AHA: 2020,4Q,10

✓4ᵗʰ **D86** **Sarcoidosis**
DEF: Clustering of immune cells resulting in granuloma formation. Often affects the lungs and lymphatic system but can occur in other body sites.

D86.0 **Sarcoidosis of lung**

D86.1 **Sarcoidosis of lymph nodes**

D86.2 **Sarcoidosis of lung with sarcoidosis of lymph nodes**

D86.3 **Sarcoidosis of skin**   `HCC`

✓5ᵗʰ **D86.8** **Sarcoidosis of other sites**

D86.81 **Sarcoid meningitis**

D86.82 **Multiple cranial nerve palsies in sarcoidosis**

D86.83 **Sarcoid iridocyclitis**

D86.84 **Sarcoid pyelonephritis**
Tubulo-interstitial nephropathy in sarcoidosis

D86.85 **Sarcoid myocarditis**

D86.86 **Sarcoid arthropathy**   `HCC`
Polyarthritis in sarcoidosis

D86.87 **Sarcoid myositis**   `HCC`

D86.89 **Sarcoidosis of other sites**
Hepatic granuloma
Uveoparotid fever [Heerfordt]

D86.9 **Sarcoidosis, unspecified**

✓4ᵗʰ **D89** **Other disorders involving the immune mechanism, not elsewhere classified**
EXCLUDES 1 *hyperglobulinemia NOS (R77.1)*
monoclonal gammopathy (of undetermined significance) (D47.2)
EXCLUDES 2 *transplant failure and rejection (T86.-)*

D89.0 **Polyclonal hypergammaglobulinemia**
Benign hypergammaglobulinemic purpura
Polyclonal gammopathy NOS

D89.1 **Cryoglobulinemia**
Cryoglobulinemic purpura
Cryoglobulinemic vasculitis
Essential cryoglobulinemia
Idiopathic cryoglobulinemia
Mixed cryoglobulinemia
Primary cryoglobulinemia
Secondary cryoglobulinemia

D89.2 **Hypergammaglobulinemia, unspecified**

D89.3 **Immune reconstitution syndrome**
Immune reconstitution inflammatory syndrome [IRIS]
Use additional code for adverse effect, if applicable, to identify drug (T36-T50 with fifth or sixth character 5)

✓5ᵗʰ **D89.4** **Mast cell activation syndrome and related disorders**
EXCLUDES 1 *aggressive systemic mastocytosis (C96.21)*
congenital cutaneous mastocytosis (Q82.2)
(non-congenital) cutaneous mastocytosis (D47.01)
(indolent) systemic mastocytosis (D47.02)
malignant mast cell neoplasm (C96.2-)
malignant mastocytoma (C96.29)
mast cell leukemia (C94.3-)
mast cell sarcoma (C96.22)
mastocytoma NOS (D47.09)
other mast cell neoplasms of uncertain behavior (D47.09)
systemic mastocytosis associated with a clonal hematologic non-mast cell lineage disease (SM-AHNMD) (D47.02)
AHA: 2016,4Q,11

D89.40 **Mast cell activation, unspecified**
Mast cell activation disorder, unspecified
Mast cell activation syndrome, NOS

D89.41 **Monoclonal mast cell activation syndrome**

D89.42 **Idiopathic mast cell activation syndrome**

D89.43 **Secondary mast cell activation**
Secondary mast cell activation syndrome
Code also underlying etiology, if known

D89.44 **Hereditary alpha tryptasemia**
Use additional code, if applicable, for:
allergy status, other than to drugs and biological substances (Z91.0-)
personal history of anaphylaxis (Z87.892)
AHA: 2021,4Q,8

D89.49 **Other mast cell activation disorder**
Other mast cell activation syndrome

☑ Additional Character Required	✓x7ᵗʰ Placeholder	Questionable PDx	Manifestation	Unspecified	UPD Unacceptable PDx	H1 - H14 HAC	HCC CMS-HCC Dx	HIV HIV Dx

ICD-10-CM 2025   525

✓5ᵗʰ **D89.8**   **Other specified disorders involving the immune mechanism, not elsewhere classified**

     ✓6ᵗʰ **D89.81**   **Graft-versus-host disease**

         Code first underlying cause, such as:
            complications of blood transfusion (T80.89)
            complications of transplanted organs and tissue (T86.-)
         Use additional code to identify associated manifestations, such as:
            desquamative dermatitis (L30.8)
            diarrhea (R19.7)
            elevated bilirubin (R17)
            hair loss (L65.9)
         AHA: 2023,3Q,19

         D89.810   **Acute** graft-versus-host disease   `CC` `UPD` `HCC`

         D89.811   **Chronic** graft-versus-host disease   `CC` `UPD` `HCC`

         D89.812   **Acute on chronic** graft-versus-host disease   `CC` `UPD` `HCC`

         D89.813   **Graft-versus-host disease, unspecified**   `CC` `UPD` `HCC`

     D89.82   **Autoimmune lymphoproliferative syndrome [ALPS]**

         DEF: Rare genetic alteration of the Fas protein that impairs normal cellular apoptosis (normal cell death), causing abnormal accumulation of lymphocytes in the lymph glands, liver, and spleen. Symptoms include neutropenia, anemia, and thrombocytopenia.

     ✓6ᵗʰ **D89.83**   **Cytokine release syndrome**

         Code first underlying cause, such as:
            complications following infusion, transfusion and therapeutic injection (T80.89-)
            complications of transplanted organs and tissue (T86.-)
         ▶Use additional code for adverse effect, if applicable, to identify immune checkpoint inhibitors and immunostimulant drugs (T45.AX5)◀
         Use additional code to identify associated manifestations
         AHA: 2020,4Q,12-15
         DEF: Form of systemic inflammatory response syndrome (SIRS) in which immune substances (cytokines) are released rapidly and in large amounts from the affected immune cells into the blood. The severity of associated symptoms or manifestations varies based on the underlying cause. This syndrome occurs as a complication of a disease, infection, or drug (often an adverse effect of immunotherapy in the form of treatment receiving monoclonal antibodies or Chimeric Antigen Receptor T [CAR-T] cells).

         D89.831   **Cytokine release syndrome, grade 1**   `UPD`

         D89.832   **Cytokine release syndrome, grade 2**   `UPD`

         D89.833   **Cytokine release syndrome, grade 3**   `CC` `UPD`

         D89.834   **Cytokine release syndrome, grade 4**   `CC` `UPD`

         D89.835   **Cytokine release syndrome, grade 5**   `CC` `UPD`

         D89.839   **Cytokine release syndrome, grade unspecified**   `UPD`

     D89.84   **IgG4-related disease**   `HCC`
         Immunoglobulin G4-related disease
         AHA: 2023,4Q,9

     D89.89   **Other specified disorders involving the immune mechanism, not elsewhere classified**
         `EXCLUDES 1`   *human immunodeficiency virus disease (B20)*
         AHA: 2017,4Q,109

D89.9   **Disorder involving the immune mechanism, unspecified**
     Immune disease NOS
     AHA: 2015,3Q,22

`N` Newborn: 0   `P` Pediatric: 0-17   `M` Maternity: 9-64   `A` Adult: 15-124   `UNS` Unspecified Site   `MCC` Major Complication/Comorbidity   `CC` Complication/Comorbidity   `PE` POA Exempt

526   ICD-10-CM 2025

Chapter 4. Endocrine, Nutritional, and Metabolic Diseases (E00–E89)

Chapter-specific Guidelines with Coding Examples

The chapter-specific guidelines from the ICD-10-CM Official Guidelines for Coding and Reporting have been provided below. Along with these guidelines are coding examples, contained in the shaded boxes, that have been developed to help illustrate the coding and/or sequencing guidance found in these guidelines.

a. Diabetes mellitus

The diabetes mellitus codes are combination codes that include the type of diabetes mellitus, the body system affected, and the complications affecting that body system. As many codes within a particular category as are necessary to describe all of the complications of the disease may be used. They should be sequenced based on the reason for a particular encounter. Assign as many codes from categories E08–E13 as needed to identify all of the associated conditions that the patient has.

> Patient is seen for poorly controlled diabetes, type 2, with diabetic polyneuropathy and diabetic retinopathy with macular edema
>
> **E11.65**   **Type 2 diabetes mellitus with hyperglycemia**
>
> **E11.311**   **Type 2 diabetes mellitus with unspecified diabetic retinopathy with macular edema**
>
> **E11.42**   **Type 2 diabetes mellitus with diabetic polyneuropathy**
>
> *Explanation*: Use as many codes to describe the diabetic complications as needed. Many are combination codes that describe more than one condition. Code first the reason for the encounter. "Poorly controlled" is described as "with hyperglycemia." Diabetes documented as "uncontrolled" is not assumed to be hyperglycemic but can be classified to either hyperglycemia or hypoglycemia. If documentation is not clear, the provider must be queried so that the appropriate code can be reported.

1) Type of diabetes

The age of a patient is not the sole determining factor, though most type 1 diabetics develop the condition before reaching puberty. For this reason, type 1 diabetes mellitus is also referred to as juvenile diabetes.

(a) Presymptomatic Type 1 Diabetes Mellitus

Codes E10.A-, Type 1 diabetes mellitus, presymptomatic, are assigned for early-stage type 1 diabetes that predates the onset of symptoms.

2) Type of diabetes mellitus not documented

If the type of diabetes mellitus is not documented in the medical record the default is E11.-, Type 2 diabetes mellitus.

> H & P lists diabetes and hypertension on patient problem list
>
> **E11.9**   **Type 2 diabetes mellitus without complications**
>
> **I10**   **Essential (primary) hypertension**
>
> *Explanation*: Since the type of diabetes was not documented and no complications were noted, the default code is E11.9.

3) Diabetes mellitus and the use of insulin, oral hypoglycemics, and injectable non-insulin drugs

If the documentation in a medical record does not indicate the type of diabetes but does indicate that the patient uses insulin, code E11-, Type 2 diabetes mellitus, should be assigned. Additional code(s) should be assigned from category Z79 to identify the long-term (current) use of insulin, oral hypoglycemic drugs, or injectable non-insulin antidiabetic, as follows:

If the patient is treated with both oral hypoglycemic drugs and insulin, both code Z79.4, Long term (current) use of insulin, and code Z79.84, Long term (current) use of oral hypoglycemic drugs, should be assigned.

If the patient is treated with both insulin and an injectable non-insulin antidiabetic drug, assign codes Z79.4, Long term (current) use of insulin, and Z79.85, Long-term (current) use of injectable non-insulin antidiabetic drugs.

If the patient is treated with both oral hypoglycemic drugs and an injectable non-insulin antidiabetic drug, assign codes Z79.84, Long term (current) use of oral hypoglycemic drugs, and Z79.85, Long-term (current) use of injectable non-insulin antidiabetic drugs.

Code Z79.4 should not be assigned if insulin is given temporarily to bring a type 2 patient's blood sugar under control during an encounter.

> Type 2 diabetic patient on daily metformin and Victoza is admitted in ketoacidosis, insulin given to stabilize blood sugars and discontinued at discharge
>
> **E11.10**   **Type 2 diabetes mellitus with ketoacidosis without coma**
>
> **Z79.84**   **Long term (current) use of oral hypoglycemic drugs**
>
> **Z79.85**   **Long term (current) use of injectable non-insulin anti-diabetic drugs**
>
> *Explanation*: Documentation indicates the patient is on an oral antidiabetic medication (metformin) and an injectable noninsulin antidiabetic medication (Victoza). Although insulin was given to the patient during the encounter, it was discontinued at discharge, indicating that the patient does not regularly use insulin. A Z code representing long-term use of the oral drug and long-term use of the injectable medication can be applied. Applying code Z79.4 to represent long-term use of insulin would be inappropriate.

4) Diabetes mellitus in pregnancy and gestational diabetes

See Section I.C.15. Diabetes mellitus in pregnancy.

See Section I.C.15. Gestational (pregnancy induced) diabetes

5) Complications due to insulin pump malfunction

(a) Underdose of insulin due to insulin pump failure

An underdose of insulin due to an insulin pump failure should be assigned to a code from subcategory T85.6, Mechanical complication of other specified internal and external prosthetic devices, implants and grafts, that specifies the type of pump malfunction, as the principal or first-listed code, followed by code T38.3X6-, Underdosing of insulin and oral hypoglycemic [antidiabetic] drugs. Additional codes for the type of diabetes mellitus and any associated complications due to the underdosing should also be assigned.

> A 24-year-old type 1 diabetic male treated in ED for hyperglycemia; insulin pump found to be malfunctioning and underdosing
>
> **T85.614A**   **Breakdown (mechanical) of insulin pump, initial encounter**
>
> **T38.3X6A**   **Underdosing of insulin and oral hypoglycemic [antidiabetic] drugs, initial encounter**
>
> **E10.65**   **Type 1 diabetes mellitus with hyperglycemia**
>
> *Explanation*: The complication code for the mechanical breakdown of the pump is sequenced first, followed by the underdosing code and type of diabetes with complication. Code all other diabetic complication codes necessary to describe the patient's condition.

(b) Overdose of insulin due to insulin pump failure

The principal or first-listed code for an encounter due to an insulin pump malfunction resulting in an overdose of insulin, should also be T85.6-, Mechanical complication of other specified internal and external prosthetic devices, implants and grafts, followed by code T38.3X1-, Poisoning by insulin and oral hypoglycemic [antidiabetic] drugs, accidental (unintentional).

> A 24-year-old type 1 diabetic male found down with diabetic coma, brought into ED and treated for hypoglycemia; insulin pump found to be malfunctioning and overdosing
>
> **T85.614A**   **Breakdown (mechanical) of insulin pump, initial encounter**
>
> **T38.3X1A**   **Poisoning by insulin and oral hypoglycemic [antidiabetic] drugs, accidental (unintentional), initial encounter**
>
> **E10.641**   **Type 1 diabetes mellitus with hypoglycemia with coma**
>
> *Explanation*: The complication code for the mechanical breakdown of the pump is sequenced first, followed by the poisoning code and type of diabetes with complication. All the characters in the combination code must be used to form a valid code and to fully describe the type of diabetes, the hypoglycemia, and the coma.

Chapter 4. Endocrine, Nutritional, and Metabolic Diseases

6) Secondary diabetes mellitus

Codes under categories E08, Diabetes mellitus due to underlying condition, E09, Drug or chemical induced diabetes mellitus, and E13, Other specified diabetes mellitus, identify complications/manifestations associated with secondary diabetes mellitus. Secondary diabetes is always caused by another condition or event (e.g., cystic fibrosis, malignant neoplasm of pancreas, pancreatectomy, adverse effect of drug, or poisoning).

(a) Secondary diabetes mellitus and the use of insulin or oral hypoglycemic drugs

For patients with secondary diabetes mellitus who routinely use insulin, oral hypoglycemic drugs, or injectable non-insulin drugs, additional code(s) from category Z79 should be assigned to identify the long-term (current) use of insulin, oral hypoglycemic drugs, or non-injectable non-insulin drugs as follows:

If the patient is treated with both oral hypoglycemic drugs and insulin, both code Z79.4, Long term (current) use of insulin, and code Z79.84, Long term (current) use of oral hypoglycemic drugs, should be assigned.

If the patient is treated with both insulin and an injectable non-insulin antidiabetic drug, assign codes Z79.4, Long-term (current) use of insulin, and Z79.85, Long-term (current) use of injectable non-insulin antidiabetic drugs.

If the patient is treated with both oral hypoglycemic drugs and an injectable non-insulin antidiabetic drug, assign codes Z79.84, Long-term (current) use of oral hypoglycemic drugs, and Z79.85, Long-term (current) use of injectable non-insulin antidiabetic drugs.

Code Z79.4 should not be assigned if insulin is given temporarily to bring a secondary diabetic patient's blood sugar under control during an encounter

---

The patient, maintained on metformin and insulin, was admitted for treatment of diabetic gangrene. The patient developed diabetes secondary to Nelson's syndrome.

E24.1   **Nelson's syndrome**

E08.52   **Diabetes mellitus due to underlying condition with diabetic peripheral angiopathy with gangrene**

Z79.4   **Long term (current) use of insulin**

Z79.84   **Long term (current) use of oral hypoglycemic drugs**

Explanation: When diabetes is caused by an underlying condition, the underlying condition should always be sequenced before any codes representing the diabetes. Patients with secondary diabetes may be maintained on both insulin and an oral hypoglycemic. When maintained on both, report a code for the long term use of insulin and a code for the long term use of oral hypoglycemic.

(b) Assigning and sequencing secondary diabetes codes and its causes

The sequencing of the secondary diabetes codes in relationship to codes for the cause of the diabetes is based on the Tabular List instructions for categories E08, E09 and E13.

(i) Secondary diabetes mellitus due to pancreatectomy

For postpancreatectomy diabetes mellitus (lack of insulin due to the surgical removal of all or part of the pancreas), assign code E89.1, Postprocedural hypoinsulinemia. Assign a code from category E13 as the principal or first-listed diagnosis and a code from subcategory Z90.41, Acquired absence of pancreas, as an additional code.

(ii) Secondary diabetes due to drugs

Secondary diabetes may be caused by an adverse effect of correctly administered medications, poisoning or sequela of poisoning.

See section I.C.19.e. for coding of adverse effects and poisoning, and section I.C.20 for external cause code reporting.

Initial encounter for corticosteroid-induced diabetes mellitus

E09.9   **Drug or chemical induced diabetes mellitus without complications**

T38.0X5A   **Adverse effect of glucocorticoids and synthetic analogues, initial encounter**

Explanation: If the diabetes is caused by an adverse effect of a drug, the diabetic condition is coded first. If it occurs from a poisoning or overdose, the poisoning code causing the diabetes is sequenced first.

Chapter 4. Endocrine, Nutritional and Metabolic Diseases (E00-E89)

NOTE   All neoplasms, whether functionally active or not, are classified in Chapter 2. Appropriate codes in this chapter (i.e. E05.8, E07.0, E16-E31, E34.-) may be used as additional codes to indicate either functional activity by neoplasms and ectopic endocrine tissue or hyperfunction and hypofunction of endocrine glands associated with neoplasms and other conditions classified elsewhere.

EXCLUDES 1   *transitory endocrine and metabolic disorders specific to newborn (P70-P74)*

AHA: 2018,2Q,6

This chapter contains the following blocks:

E00-E07	Disorders of thyroid gland
E08-E13	Diabetes mellitus
E15-E16	Other disorders of glucose regulation and pancreatic internal secretion
E20-E35	Disorders of other endocrine glands
E36	Intraoperative complications of endocrine system
E40-E46	Malnutrition
E50-E64	Other nutritional deficiencies
E65-E68	Overweight, obesity and other hyperalimentation
E70-E88	Metabolic disorders
E89	Postprocedural endocrine and metabolic complications and disorders, not elsewhere classified

Disorders of thyroid gland (E00-E07)

✓4ᵗʰ E00 Congenital iodine-deficiency syndrome
Use additional code (F70-F79) to identify associated intellectual disabilities
EXCLUDES 1   *subclinical iodine-deficiency hypothyroidism (E02)*

E00.0 Congenital iodine-deficiency syndrome, neurological type
Endemic cretinism, neurological type

E00.1 Congenital iodine-deficiency syndrome, myxedematous type
Endemic hypothyroid cretinism
Endemic cretinism, myxedematous type

E00.2 Congenital iodine-deficiency syndrome, mixed type
Endemic cretinism, mixed type

E00.9 Congenital iodine-deficiency syndrome, unspecified
Congenital iodine-deficiency hypothyroidism NOS
Endemic cretinism NOS

✓4ᵗʰ E01 Iodine-deficiency related thyroid disorders and allied conditions
EXCLUDES 1   *congenital iodine-deficiency syndrome (E00.-)*
subclinical iodine-deficiency hypothyroidism (E02)

E01.0 Iodine-deficiency related diffuse (endemic) goiter

E01.1 Iodine-deficiency related multinodular (endemic) goiter
Iodine-deficiency related nodular goiter

E01.2 Iodine-deficiency related (endemic) goiter, unspecified
Endemic goiter NOS

E01.8 Other iodine-deficiency related thyroid disorders and allied conditions
Acquired iodine-deficiency hypothyroidism NOS

E02 Subclinical iodine-deficiency hypothyroidism
AHA: 2021,1Q,8

✓4ᵗʰ E03 Other hypothyroidism
EXCLUDES 1   *iodine-deficiency related hypothyroidism (E00-E02)*
postprocedural hypothyroidism (E89.0)
DEF: Hypothyroidism: Underproduction of thyroid hormone.

E03.0 Congenital hypothyroidism with diffuse goiter
Congenital parenchymatous goiter (nontoxic)
Congenital goiter (nontoxic) NOS
EXCLUDES 1   *transitory congenital goiter with normal function (P72.0)*

E03.1 Congenital hypothyroidism without goiter
Aplasia of thyroid (with myxedema)
Congenital atrophy of thyroid
Congenital hypothyroidism NOS

E03.2 Hypothyroidism due to medicaments and other exogenous substances
Code first poisoning due to drug or toxin, if applicable (T36-T65 with fifth or sixth character 1-4)
Use additional code for adverse effect, if applicable, to identify drug (T36-T50 with fifth or sixth character 5)

E03.3 Postinfectious hypothyroidism

E03.4 Atrophy of thyroid (acquired)
EXCLUDES 1   *congenital atrophy of thyroid (E03.1)*

E03.5 Myxedema coma   **MCC** **HCC**

E03.8 Other specified hypothyroidism
AHA: 2021,1Q,8

E03.9 Hypothyroidism, unspecified
Myxedema NOS
AHA: 2024,1Q,14

✓4ᵗʰ E04 Other nontoxic goiter
EXCLUDES 1   *congenital goiter (NOS) (diffuse) (parenchymatous) (E03.0)*
iodine-deficiency related goiter (E00-E02)

E04.0 Nontoxic diffuse goiter
Diffuse (colloid) nontoxic goiter
Simple nontoxic goiter

E04.1 Nontoxic single thyroid nodule
Colloid nodule (cystic) (thyroid)
Nontoxic uninodular goiter
Thyroid (cystic) nodule NOS
DEF: Enlarged thyroid, commonly due to decreased thyroid production, with a single nodule. No clinical hypothyroidism.

E04.2 Nontoxic multinodular goiter
Cystic goiter NOS
Multinodular (cystic) goiter NOS
DEF: Enlarged thyroid, commonly due to decreased thyroid production with multiple nodules. No clinical hypothyroidism.

E04.8 Other specified nontoxic goiter

E04.9 Nontoxic goiter, unspecified
Goiter NOS
Nodular goiter (nontoxic) NOS

✓4ᵗʰ E05 Thyrotoxicosis [hyperthyroidism]
EXCLUDES 1   *chronic thyroiditis with transient thyrotoxicosis (E06.2)*
neonatal thyrotoxicosis (P72.1)
DEF: Excessive quantities of hormones from the thyroid gland caused by overproduction or loss of storage ability.

✓5ᵗʰ E05.0 Thyrotoxicosis with diffuse goiter
Exophthalmic or toxic goiter NOS
Graves' disease
Toxic diffuse goiter
DEF: Diffuse thyroid enlargement accompanied by hyperthyroidism, bulging eyes, and dermopathy.

E05.00 Thyrotoxicosis with diffuse goiter without thyrotoxic crisis or storm

E05.01 Thyrotoxicosis with diffuse goiter with thyrotoxic crisis or storm   **MCC**

Goiter

Pyramidal lobe
Thyroid cartilage
Healthy thyroid
Goiter (hyperfunctioning thyroid)

✓5ᵗʰ E05.1 Thyrotoxicosis with toxic single thyroid nodule
Thyrotoxicosis with toxic uninodular goiter
DEF: Symptomatic hyperthyroidism with a single nodule on the enlarged thyroid gland. Onset of symptoms can be abrupt and include extreme nervousness, insomnia, weight loss, tremors, and psychosis or coma.

E05.10 Thyrotoxicosis with toxic single thyroid nodule without thyrotoxic crisis or storm

E05.11 Thyrotoxicosis with toxic single thyroid nodule with thyrotoxic crisis or storm   **MCC**

✓5ᵗʰ E05.2 Thyrotoxicosis with toxic multinodular goiter
Toxic nodular goiter NOS

E05.20 Thyrotoxicosis with toxic multinodular goiter without thyrotoxic crisis or storm

E05.21 Thyrotoxicosis with toxic multinodular goiter with thyrotoxic crisis or storm   **MCC**

✓5ᵗʰ E05.3 Thyrotoxicosis from ectopic thyroid tissue

E05.30 Thyrotoxicosis from ectopic thyroid tissue without thyrotoxic crisis or storm

E05.31 Thyrotoxicosis from ectopic thyroid tissue with thyrotoxic crisis or storm   **MCC**

✔ Additional Character Required   ✓x7ᵗʰ Placeholder   Questionable PDx   Manifestation   Unspecified   UPD Unacceptable PDx   H1-H14 HAC   HCC CMS-HCC Dx   HIV HIV Dx

ICD-10-CM 2025   529

✓5ᵗʰ E05.4 Thyrotoxicosis factitia

E05.40   **Thyrotoxicosis factitia** without thyrotoxic crisis or storm

E05.41   **Thyrotoxicosis factitia** with thyrotoxic crisis or storm   `MCC`

✓5ᵗʰ E05.8 Other thyrotoxicosis

Overproduction of thyroid-stimulating hormone

E05.80   **Other thyrotoxicosis** without thyrotoxic crisis or storm

E05.81   **Other thyrotoxicosis** with thyrotoxic crisis or storm   `MCC`

✓5ᵗʰ E05.9 Thyrotoxicosis, unspecified

Hyperthyroidism NOS

E05.90   **Thyrotoxicosis, unspecified** without thyrotoxic crisis or storm

E05.91   **Thyrotoxicosis, unspecified** with thyrotoxic crisis or storm   `MCC`

✓4ᵗʰ E06 Thyroiditis

EXCLUDES 1   postpartum thyroiditis (O90.5)

DEF: Inflammation of the thyroid gland.

E06.0   **Acute thyroiditis**   `CC`

Abscess of thyroid
Pyogenic thyroiditis
Suppurative thyroiditis
Use additional code (B95-B97) to identify infectious agent

E06.1   **Subacute thyroiditis**

de Quervain thyroiditis
Giant-cell thyroiditis
Granulomatous thyroiditis
Nonsuppurative thyroiditis
Viral thyroiditis
EXCLUDES 1   autoimmune thyroiditis (E06.3)

E06.2   **Chronic thyroiditis with transient thyrotoxicosis**

EXCLUDES 1   autoimmune thyroiditis (E06.3)

E06.3   **Autoimmune thyroiditis**

Hashimoto's thyroiditis
Hashitoxicosis (transient)
Lymphadenoid goiter
Lymphocytic thyroiditis
Struma lymphomatosa
AHA: 2024,1Q,14

E06.4   **Drug-induced thyroiditis**

Use additional code for adverse effect, if applicable, to identify drug (T36-T50 with fifth or sixth character 5)

E06.5   **Other chronic thyroiditis**

Chronic fibrous thyroiditis
Chronic thyroiditis NOS
Ligneous thyroiditis
Riedel thyroiditis

E06.9   **Thyroiditis, unspecified**

✓4ᵗʰ E07 Other disorders of thyroid

E07.0   **Hypersecretion of calcitonin**

C-cell hyperplasia of thyroid
Hypersecretion of thyrocalcitonin

E07.1   **Dyshormogenetic goiter**

▶Dyshormonogenetic goiter◀
Familial dyshormogenetic goiter
▶Familial dyshormonogenetic goiter◀
Pendred's syndrome
EXCLUDES 1   transitory congenital goiter with normal function (P72.0)

✓5ᵗʰ E07.8 Other specified disorders of thyroid

E07.81   **Sick-euthyroid syndrome**

Euthyroid sick-syndrome
DEF: Thyroid dysfunction caused by abnormal levels of thyroid hormones T3 and/or T4. This syndrome is often associated with starvation or critical illness.

E07.89   **Other specified disorders of thyroid**

Abnormality of thyroid-binding globulin
Hemorrhage of thyroid
Infarction of thyroid

E07.9   **Disorder of thyroid, unspecified**

Diabetes mellitus (E08-E13)

AHA: 2020,1Q,12; 2018,2Q,6; 2017,4Q,100-101; 2016,2Q,36; 2016,1Q,11-13; 2013,4Q,114; 2013,3Q,20

✓4ᵗʰ E08 Diabetes mellitus due to underlying condition

Code first the underlying condition, such as:
   congenital rubella (P35.0)
   Cushing's syndrome (E24.-)
   cystic fibrosis (E84.-)
   malignant neoplasm (C00-C96)
   malnutrition (E40-E46)
   pancreatitis and other diseases of the pancreas (K85-K86.-)
Use additional code to identify control using:
   ▶injectable non-insulin antidiabetic drugs (Z79.85)◀
   insulin (Z79.4)
   oral antidiabetic drugs (Z79.84)
   oral hypoglycemic drugs (Z79.84)

EXCLUDES 1   drug or chemical induced diabetes mellitus (E09.-)
   gestational diabetes (O24.4-)
   neonatal diabetes mellitus (P70.2)
   postpancreatectomy diabetes mellitus (E13.-)
   postprocedural diabetes mellitus (E13.-)
   secondary diabetes mellitus NEC (E13.-)
   type 1 diabetes mellitus (E10.-)
   type 2 diabetes mellitus (E11.-)

✓5ᵗʰ E08.0 Diabetes mellitus due to underlying condition with hyperosmolarity

DEF: Diabetic hyperosmolarity: Extremely high levels of glucose in the blood without ketones.

E08.00   *Diabetes mellitus due to underlying condition with hyperosmolarity without nonketotic hyperglycemic-hyperosmolar coma (NKHHC)*   `MCC` `H9` `HCC`

E08.01   *Diabetes mellitus due to underlying condition with hyperosmolarity with coma*   `MCC` `H9` `HCC`

✓5ᵗʰ E08.1 Diabetes mellitus due to underlying condition with ketoacidosis

DEF: Diabetic ketoacidosis: Potentially life-threatening complication due to a shortage of insulin in which the body switches to burning fatty acids and producing acidic ketone bodies.

E08.10   *Diabetes mellitus due to underlying condition with ketoacidosis without coma*   `MCC` `H9` `HCC`

E08.11   *Diabetes mellitus due to underlying condition with ketoacidosis with coma*   `MCC` `H9` `HCC`

✓5ᵗʰ E08.2 Diabetes mellitus due to underlying condition with kidney complications

AHA: 2019,3Q,3; 2018,4Q,88

E08.21   *Diabetes mellitus due to underlying condition with diabetic nephropathy*   `HCC`

Diabetes mellitus due to underlying condition with intercapillary glomerulosclerosis
Diabetes mellitus due to underlying condition with intracapillary glomerulonephrosis
Diabetes mellitus due to underlying condition with Kimmelstiel-Wilson disease

E08.22   *Diabetes mellitus due to underlying condition with diabetic chronic kidney disease*   `HCC`

Use additional code to identify stage of chronic kidney disease (N18.1-N18.6)

E08.29   *Diabetes mellitus due to underlying condition with other diabetic kidney complication*   `HCC`

Renal tubular degeneration in diabetes mellitus due to underlying condition

---

`N` Newborn: 0   `P` Pediatric: 0-17   `M` Maternity: 9-64   `A` Adult: 15-124   `UNS` Unspecified Site   `MCC` Major Complication/Comorbidity   `CC` Complication/Comorbidity   `PE` POA Exempt

530

ICD-10-CM 2025

√5ᵗʰ **E08.3** **Diabetes mellitus due to underlying condition with ophthalmic complications**

AHA: 2016,4Q,11-13

One of the following 7th characters is to be assigned to codes in subcategories E08.32, E08.33, E08.34, E08.35, and E08.37 to designate laterality of the disease:

1   right eye
2   left eye
3   bilateral
9   unspecified eye

√6ᵗʰ **E08.31** **Diabetes mellitus due to underlying condition with unspecified diabetic retinopathy**

DEF: Diabetic retinopathy: Diabetic complication from damage to the retinal vessels resulting in vision problems that can progress to blindness.

E08.311 *Diabetes mellitus due to underlying condition with unspecified diabetic retinopathy with macular edema* `HCC`

E08.319 *Diabetes mellitus due to underlying condition with unspecified diabetic retinopathy without macular edema* `HCC`

√6ᵗʰ **E08.32** **Diabetes mellitus due to underlying condition with mild nonproliferative diabetic retinopathy**

Diabetes mellitus due to underlying condition with nonproliferative diabetic retinopathy NOS

√7ᵗʰ *E08.321* *Diabetes mellitus due to underlying condition with mild nonproliferative diabetic retinopathy with macular edema* `HCC`

√7ᵗʰ *E08.329* *Diabetes mellitus due to underlying condition with mild nonproliferative diabetic retinopathy without macular edema* `HCC`

√6ᵗʰ **E08.33** **Diabetes mellitus due to underlying condition with moderate nonproliferative diabetic retinopathy**

√7ᵗʰ *E08.331* *Diabetes mellitus due to underlying condition with moderate nonproliferative diabetic retinopathy with macular edema* `HCC`

√7ᵗʰ *E08.339* *Diabetes mellitus due to underlying condition with moderate nonproliferative diabetic retinopathy without macular edema* `HCC`

√6ᵗʰ **E08.34** **Diabetes mellitus due to underlying condition with severe nonproliferative diabetic retinopathy**

√7ᵗʰ *E08.341* *Diabetes mellitus due to underlying condition with severe nonproliferative diabetic retinopathy with macular edema* `HCC`

√7ᵗʰ *E08.349* *Diabetes mellitus due to underlying condition with severe nonproliferative diabetic retinopathy without macular edema* `HCC`

√6ᵗʰ **E08.35** **Diabetes mellitus due to underlying condition with proliferative diabetic retinopathy**

√7ᵗʰ *E08.351* *Diabetes mellitus due to underlying condition with proliferative diabetic retinopathy with macular edema* `HCC`

√7ᵗʰ *E08.352* *Diabetes mellitus due to underlying condition with proliferative diabetic retinopathy with traction retinal detachment involving the macula* `HCC`

√7ᵗʰ *E08.353* *Diabetes mellitus due to underlying condition with proliferative diabetic retinopathy with traction retinal detachment not involving the macula* `HCC`

√7ᵗʰ *E08.354* *Diabetes mellitus due to underlying condition with proliferative diabetic retinopathy with combined traction retinal detachment and rhegmatogenous retinal detachment* `HCC`

√7ᵗʰ *E08.355* *Diabetes mellitus due to underlying condition with stable proliferative diabetic retinopathy* `HCC`

√7ᵗʰ *E08.359* *Diabetes mellitus due to underlying condition with proliferative diabetic retinopathy without macular edema* `HCC`

E08.36 *Diabetes mellitus due to underlying condition with diabetic cataract* `HCC`

AHA: 2019,2Q,30-31; 2016,4Q,142

√x7ᵗʰ *E08.37* *Diabetes mellitus due to underlying condition with diabetic macular edema, resolved following treatment* `HCC`

E08.39 *Diabetes mellitus due to underlying condition with other diabetic ophthalmic complication* `HCC`

Use additional code to identify manifestation, such as: diabetic glaucoma (H40-H42)

AHA: 2023,3Q,19

√5ᵗʰ **E08.4** **Diabetes mellitus due to underlying condition with neurological complications**

E08.40 *Diabetes mellitus due to underlying condition with diabetic neuropathy, unspecified* `HCC`

E08.41 *Diabetes mellitus due to underlying condition with diabetic mononeuropathy* `HCC`

E08.42 *Diabetes mellitus due to underlying condition with diabetic polyneuropathy* `HCC`

Diabetes mellitus due to underlying condition with diabetic neuralgia

E08.43 *Diabetes mellitus due to underlying condition with diabetic autonomic (poly)neuropathy* `HCC`

Diabetes mellitus due to underlying condition with diabetic gastroparesis

AHA: 2013,4Q,114

E08.44 *Diabetes mellitus due to underlying condition with diabetic amyotrophy* `HCC`

E08.49 *Diabetes mellitus due to underlying condition with other diabetic neurological complication* `HCC`

√5ᵗʰ **E08.5** **Diabetes mellitus due to underlying condition with circulatory complications**

E08.51 *Diabetes mellitus due to underlying condition with diabetic peripheral angiopathy without gangrene* `HCC`

AHA: 2018,3Q,3-4; 2018,2Q,7

E08.52 *Diabetes mellitus due to underlying condition with diabetic peripheral angiopathy with gangrene* `CC` `HCC`

Diabetes mellitus due to underlying condition with diabetic gangrene

AHA: 2020,2Q,18; 2018,3Q,3; 2018,2Q,7; 2017,4Q,102

E08.59 *Diabetes mellitus due to underlying condition with other circulatory complications* `HCC`

√5ᵗʰ **E08.6** **Diabetes mellitus due to underlying condition with other specified complications**

√6ᵗʰ **E08.61** **Diabetes mellitus due to underlying condition with diabetic arthropathy**

E08.610 *Diabetes mellitus due to underlying condition with diabetic neuropathic arthropathy* `HCC`

Diabetes mellitus due to underlying condition with Charcôt's joints

DEF: Charcot's joint: Progressive neurologic arthropathy in which chronic degeneration of joints in the weight-bearing areas with peripheral hypertrophy occurs as a complication of a neuropathy disorder. Supporting structures relax from a loss of sensation resulting in chronic joint instability.

E08.618 *Diabetes mellitus due to underlying condition with other diabetic arthropathy* `HCC`

AHA: 2018,2Q,6

√6ᵗʰ **E08.62** **Diabetes mellitus due to underlying condition with skin complications**

E08.620 *Diabetes mellitus due to underlying condition with diabetic dermatitis* `HCC`

Diabetes mellitus due to underlying condition with diabetic necrobiosis lipoidica

E08.621 *Diabetes mellitus due to underlying condition with foot ulcer* `HCC`

Use additional code to identify site of ulcer (L97.4-, L97.5-)

AHA: 2020,2Q,19

E08.622 *Diabetes mellitus due to underlying condition with other skin ulcer* `HCC`

Use additional code to identify site of ulcer (L97.1-L97.9, L98.41-L98.49)

AHA: 2021,1Q,7; 2017,4Q,17

E08.628 *Diabetes mellitus due to underlying condition with other skin complications* `HCC`

| ✔ Additional Character Required | √x7ᵗʰ Placeholder | Questionable PDx | Manifestation | Unspecified | `UPD` Unacceptable PDx | `H1`-`H14` HAC | `HCC` CMS-HCC Dx | `HIV` HIV Dx |

ICD-10-CM 2025   531

✓6ᵗʰ E08.63 Diabetes mellitus due to underlying condition with oral complications

    E08.630 Diabetes mellitus due to underlying condition with periodontal disease   **HCC**

    E08.638 Diabetes mellitus due to underlying condition with other oral complications   **HCC**

✓6ᵗʰ E08.64 Diabetes mellitus due to underlying condition with hypoglycemia

▶ Use additional code for hypoglycemia level, if applicable (E16.A-) ◀

AHA: 2017,1Q,42

    E08.641 Diabetes mellitus due to underlying condition with hypoglycemia with coma   **MCC HCC**

    E08.649 Diabetes mellitus due to underlying condition with hypoglycemia without coma   **HCC**

       AHA: 2016,3Q,42; 2015,3Q,21

    E08.65 *Diabetes mellitus due to underlying condition with hyperglycemia*   **HCC**

       AHA: 2017,1Q,42; 2013,3Q,20

    E08.69 *Diabetes mellitus due to underlying condition with other specified complication*   **HCC**

       Use additional code to identify complication

       AHA: 2016,4Q,141; 2016,1Q,13

E08.8 *Diabetes mellitus due to underlying condition with unspecified complications*   **HCC**

E08.9 *Diabetes mellitus due to underlying condition without complications*   **HCC**

     AHA: 2023,3Q,19; 2020,2Q,18

✓4ᵗʰ E09 Drug or chemical induced diabetes mellitus

Code first poisoning due to drug or toxin, if applicable (T36-T65 with fifth or sixth character 1-4)

Use additional code for adverse effect, if applicable, to identify drug (T36-T50 with fifth or sixth character 5)

Use additional code to identify control using:
▶ injectable non-insulin antidiabetic drugs (Z79.85) ◀
   insulin (Z79.4)
   oral antidiabetic drugs (Z79.84)
   oral hypoglycemic drugs (Z79.84)

EXCLUDES 1   diabetes mellitus due to underlying condition (E08.-)
       gestational diabetes (O24.4-)
       neonatal diabetes mellitus (P70.2)
       postpancreatectomy diabetes mellitus (E13.-)
       postprocedural diabetes mellitus (E13.-)
       secondary diabetes mellitus NEC (E13.-)
       type 1 diabetes mellitus (E10.-)
       type 2 diabetes mellitus (E11.-)

✓5ᵗʰ E09.0 Drug or chemical induced diabetes mellitus with hyperosmolarity

   DEF: Diabetic hyperosmolarity: Extremely high levels of glucose in the blood without ketones.

    E09.00 Drug or chemical induced diabetes mellitus with hyperosmolarity without nonketotic hyperglycemic-hyperosmolar coma (NKHHC)   **MCC H9**

    E09.01 Drug or chemical induced diabetes mellitus with hyperosmolarity with coma   **MCC H9**

✓5ᵗʰ E09.1 Drug or chemical induced diabetes mellitus with ketoacidosis

   DEF: Diabetic ketoacidosis: Potentially life-threatening complication due to a shortage of insulin in which the body switches to burning fatty acids and producing acidic ketone bodies.

    E09.10 Drug or chemical induced diabetes mellitus with ketoacidosis without coma   **MCC H9**

    E09.11 Drug or chemical induced diabetes mellitus with ketoacidosis with coma   **MCC H9**

✓5ᵗʰ E09.2 Drug or chemical induced diabetes mellitus with kidney complications

   AHA: 2019,3Q,3; 2018,4Q,88

    E09.21 Drug or chemical induced diabetes mellitus with diabetic nephropathy

       Drug or chemical induced diabetes mellitus with intercapillary glomerulosclerosis

       Drug or chemical induced diabetes mellitus with intracapillary glomerulonephrosis

       Drug or chemical induced diabetes mellitus with Kimmelstiel-Wilson disease

    E09.22 Drug or chemical induced diabetes mellitus with diabetic chronic kidney disease

       Use additional code to identify stage of chronic kidney disease (N18.1-N18.6)

    E09.29 Drug or chemical induced diabetes mellitus with other diabetic kidney complication

       Drug or chemical induced diabetes mellitus with renal tubular degeneration

✓5ᵗʰ E09.3 Drug or chemical induced diabetes mellitus with ophthalmic complications

   AHA: 2016,4Q,11-13

   One of the following 7th characters is to be assigned to codes in subcategories E09.32, E09.33, E09.34, E09.35, and E09.37 to designate laterality of the disease:
     1   right eye
     2   left eye
     3   bilateral
     9   unspecified eye

✓6ᵗʰ E09.31 Drug or chemical induced diabetes mellitus with unspecified diabetic retinopathy

     DEF: Diabetic retinopathy: Diabetic complication from damage to the retinal vessels resulting in vision problems that can progress to blindness.

    E09.311 Drug or chemical induced diabetes mellitus with unspecified diabetic retinopathy with macular edema

    E09.319 Drug or chemical induced diabetes mellitus with unspecified diabetic retinopathy without macular edema

✓6ᵗʰ E09.32 Drug or chemical induced diabetes mellitus with mild nonproliferative diabetic retinopathy

     Drug or chemical induced diabetes mellitus with nonproliferative diabetic retinopathy NOS

    ✓7ᵗʰ E09.321 Drug or chemical induced diabetes mellitus with mild nonproliferative diabetic retinopathy with macular edema

    ✓7ᵗʰ E09.329 Drug or chemical induced diabetes mellitus with mild nonproliferative diabetic retinopathy without macular edema

✓6ᵗʰ E09.33 Drug or chemical induced diabetes mellitus with moderate nonproliferative diabetic retinopathy

    ✓7ᵗʰ E09.331 Drug or chemical induced diabetes mellitus with moderate nonproliferative diabetic retinopathy with macular edema

    ✓7ᵗʰ E09.339 Drug or chemical induced diabetes mellitus with moderate nonproliferative diabetic retinopathy without macular edema

✓6ᵗʰ E09.34 Drug or chemical induced diabetes mellitus with severe nonproliferative diabetic retinopathy

    ✓7ᵗʰ E09.341 Drug or chemical induced diabetes mellitus with severe nonproliferative diabetic retinopathy with macular edema

    ✓7ᵗʰ E09.349 Drug or chemical induced diabetes mellitus with severe nonproliferative diabetic retinopathy without macular edema

✓6ᵗʰ E09.35 Drug or chemical induced diabetes mellitus with proliferative diabetic retinopathy

    ✓7ᵗʰ E09.351 Drug or chemical induced diabetes mellitus with proliferative diabetic retinopathy with macular edema

    ✓7ᵗʰ E09.352 Drug or chemical induced diabetes mellitus with proliferative diabetic retinopathy with traction retinal detachment involving the macula

    ✓7ᵗʰ E09.353 Drug or chemical induced diabetes mellitus with proliferative diabetic retinopathy with traction retinal detachment not involving the macula

    ✓7ᵗʰ E09.354 Drug or chemical induced diabetes mellitus with proliferative diabetic retinopathy with combined traction retinal detachment and rhegmatogenous retinal detachment

N Newborn: 0   **P** Pediatric: 0-17   **M** Maternity: 9-64   **A** Adult: 15-124   **UNS** Unspecified Site   **MCC** Major Complication/Comorbidity   **CC** Complication/Comorbidity   **PE** POA Exempt

532   ICD-10-CM 2025

✓7ᵗʰ **E09.355** **Drug or chemical induced diabetes mellitus with stable proliferative diabetic retinopathy**

✓7ᵗʰ **E09.359** **Drug or chemical induced diabetes mellitus with proliferative diabetic retinopathy without macular edema**

E09.36 **Drug or chemical induced diabetes mellitus with diabetic cataract**
    AHA: 2019,2Q,30-31; 2016,4Q,142

✓x7ᵗʰ **E09.37** **Drug or chemical induced diabetes mellitus with diabetic macular edema, resolved following treatment**

E09.39 **Drug or chemical induced diabetes mellitus with other diabetic ophthalmic complication**
    Use additional code to identify manifestation, such as: diabetic glaucoma (H40-H42)
    AHA: 2023,3Q,19

✓5ᵗʰ **E09.4** **Drug or chemical induced diabetes mellitus with neurological complications**

E09.40 **Drug or chemical induced diabetes mellitus with neurological complications with diabetic neuropathy, unspecified**

E09.41 **Drug or chemical induced diabetes mellitus with neurological complications with diabetic mononeuropathy**

E09.42 **Drug or chemical induced diabetes mellitus with neurological complications with diabetic polyneuropathy**
    Drug or chemical induced diabetes mellitus with diabetic neuralgia

E09.43 **Drug or chemical induced diabetes mellitus with neurological complications with diabetic autonomic (poly)neuropathy**
    Drug or chemical induced diabetes mellitus with diabetic gastroparesis
    AHA: 2013,4Q,114

E09.44 **Drug or chemical induced diabetes mellitus with neurological complications with diabetic amyotrophy**

E09.49 **Drug or chemical induced diabetes mellitus with neurological complications with other diabetic neurological complication**

✓5ᵗʰ **E09.5** **Drug or chemical induced diabetes mellitus with circulatory complications**

E09.51 **Drug or chemical induced diabetes mellitus with diabetic peripheral angiopathy without gangrene**
    AHA: 2018,3Q,3-4; 2018,2Q,7

E09.52 **Drug or chemical induced diabetes mellitus with diabetic peripheral angiopathy with gangrene** CC
    Drug or chemical induced diabetes mellitus with diabetic gangrene
    AHA: 2020,2Q,18; 2018,3Q,3; 2018,2Q,7; 2017,4Q,102

E09.59 **Drug or chemical induced diabetes mellitus with other circulatory complications**

✓5ᵗʰ **E09.6** **Drug or chemical induced diabetes mellitus with other specified complications**

✓6ᵗʰ **E09.61** **Drug or chemical induced diabetes mellitus with diabetic arthropathy**

E09.610 **Drug or chemical induced diabetes mellitus with diabetic neuropathic arthropathy**
    Drug or chemical induced diabetes mellitus with Charcôt's joints
    DEF: Charcot's joint: Progressive neurologic arthropathy in which chronic degeneration of joints in the weight-bearing areas with peripheral hypertrophy occurs as a complication of a neuropathy disorder. Supporting structures relax from a loss of sensation resulting in chronic joint instability.

E09.618 **Drug or chemical induced diabetes mellitus with other diabetic arthropathy**
    AHA: 2018,2Q,6

✓6ᵗʰ **E09.62** **Drug or chemical induced diabetes mellitus with skin complications**

E09.620 **Drug or chemical induced diabetes mellitus with diabetic dermatitis**
    Drug or chemical induced diabetes mellitus with diabetic necrobiosis lipoidica

E09.621 **Drug or chemical induced diabetes mellitus with foot ulcer**
    Use additional code to identify site of ulcer (L97.4-, L97.5-)
    AHA: 2020,2Q,19

E09.622 **Drug or chemical induced diabetes mellitus with other skin ulcer**
    Use additional code to identify site of ulcer (L97.1-L97.9, L98.41-L98.49)
    AHA: 2021,1Q,7; 2017,4Q,17

E09.628 **Drug or chemical induced diabetes mellitus with other skin complications**

✓6ᵗʰ **E09.63** **Drug or chemical induced diabetes mellitus with oral complications**

E09.630 **Drug or chemical induced diabetes mellitus with periodontal disease**

E09.638 **Drug or chemical induced diabetes mellitus with other oral complications**

✓6ᵗʰ **E09.64** **Drug or chemical induced diabetes mellitus with hypoglycemia**
    ▶Use additional code for hypoglycemia level, if applicable (E16.A-)◀
    AHA: 2017,1Q,42

E09.641 **Drug or chemical induced diabetes mellitus with hypoglycemia with coma** MCC

E09.649 **Drug or chemical induced diabetes mellitus with hypoglycemia without coma**
    AHA: 2016,3Q,42; 2015,3Q,21

E09.65 **Drug or chemical induced diabetes mellitus with hyperglycemia**
    AHA: 2017,1Q,42; 2013,3Q,20

E09.69 **Drug or chemical induced diabetes mellitus with other specified complication**
    Use additional code to identify complication
    AHA: 2016,4Q,141; 2016,1Q,13

E09.8 **Drug or chemical induced diabetes mellitus with unspecified complications**

E09.9 **Drug or chemical induced diabetes mellitus without complications**
    AHA: 2023,3Q,19; 2020,2Q,18

✓4ᵗʰ **E10** **Type 1 diabetes mellitus**

    INCLUDES   brittle diabetes (mellitus)
      diabetes (mellitus) due to autoimmune process
      diabetes (mellitus) due to immune mediated pancreatic islet beta-cell destruction
      idiopathic diabetes (mellitus)
      juvenile onset diabetes (mellitus)
      ketosis-prone diabetes (mellitus)

    EXCLUDES 1   *diabetes mellitus due to underlying condition (E08.-)*
      drug or chemical induced diabetes mellitus (E09.-)
      gestational diabetes (O24.4-)
      hyperglycemia NOS (R73.9)
      neonatal diabetes mellitus (P70.2)
      postpancreatectomy diabetes mellitus (E13.-)
      postprocedural diabetes mellitus (E13.-)
      secondary diabetes mellitus NEC (E13.-)
      type 2 diabetes mellitus (E11.-)

    AHA: 2023,2Q,10; 2020,3Q,30

✓5ᵗʰ **E10.1** **Type 1 diabetes mellitus with ketoacidosis**
    AHA: 2013,3Q,20
    DEF: Diabetic ketoacidosis: Potentially life-threatening complication due to a shortage of insulin in which the body switches to burning fatty acids and producing acidic ketone bodies.

E10.10 **Type 1 diabetes mellitus with ketoacidosis without coma** MCC H9 HCC

E10.11 **Type 1 diabetes mellitus with ketoacidosis with coma** MCC H9 HCC

✔ Additional Character Required   ✓x7ᵗʰ Placeholder   Questionable PDx   Manifestation   Unspecified   UPD Unacceptable PDx   H1-H14 HAC   HCC CMS-HCC Dx   HIV HIV Dx

ICD-10-CM 2025   533

√5th **E10.2** **Type 1 diabetes mellitus with kidney complications**
     AHA: 2019,3Q,3; 2018,4Q,88

E10.21 **Type 1 diabetes mellitus with diabetic nephropathy** HCC
     Type 1 diabetes mellitus with intercapillary glomerulosclerosis
     Type 1 diabetes mellitus with intracapillary glomerulonephrosis
     Type 1 diabetes mellitus with Kimmelstiel-Wilson disease

E10.22 **Type 1 diabetes mellitus with diabetic chronic kidney disease** HCC
     Use additional code to identify stage of chronic kidney disease (N18.1-N18.6)

E10.29 **Type 1 diabetes mellitus with other diabetic kidney complication** HCC
     Type 1 diabetes mellitus with renal tubular degeneration
     AHA: 2016,1Q,13

√5th **E10.3** **Type 1 diabetes mellitus with ophthalmic complications**
     AHA: 2016,4Q,11-13

> One of the following 7th characters is to be assigned to codes in subcategories E10.32, E10.33, E10.34, E10.35, and E10.37 to designate laterality of the disease:
> 1   right eye
> 2   left eye
> 3   bilateral
> 9   unspecified eye

√6th **E10.31** **Type 1 diabetes mellitus with unspecified diabetic retinopathy**
     DEF: Diabetic retinopathy: Diabetic complication from damage to the retinal vessels resulting in vision problems that can progress to blindness.

     E10.311 **Type 1 diabetes mellitus with unspecified diabetic retinopathy with macular edema** HCC

     E10.319 **Type 1 diabetes mellitus with unspecified diabetic retinopathy without macular edema** HCC

√6th **E10.32** **Type 1 diabetes mellitus with mild nonproliferative diabetic retinopathy**
     Type 1 diabetes mellitus with nonproliferative diabetic retinopathy NOS

     √7th **E10.321** **Type 1 diabetes mellitus with mild nonproliferative diabetic retinopathy with macular edema** HCC

     √7th **E10.329** **Type 1 diabetes mellitus with mild nonproliferative diabetic retinopathy without macular edema** HCC

√6th **E10.33** **Type 1 diabetes mellitus with moderate nonproliferative diabetic retinopathy**

     √7th **E10.331** **Type 1 diabetes mellitus with moderate nonproliferative diabetic retinopathy with macular edema**

     √7th **E10.339** **Type 1 diabetes mellitus with moderate nonproliferative diabetic retinopathy without macular edema** HCC

√6th **E10.34** **Type 1 diabetes mellitus with severe nonproliferative diabetic retinopathy**

     √7th **E10.341** **Type 1 diabetes mellitus with severe nonproliferative diabetic retinopathy with macular edema** HCC

     √7th **E10.349** **Type 1 diabetes mellitus with severe nonproliferative diabetic retinopathy without macular edema** HCC

√6th **E10.35** **Type 1 diabetes mellitus with proliferative diabetic retinopathy**

     √7th **E10.351** **Type 1 diabetes mellitus with proliferative diabetic retinopathy with macular edema** HCC

     √7th **E10.352** **Type 1 diabetes mellitus with proliferative diabetic retinopathy with traction retinal detachment involving the macula** HCC

     √7th **E10.353** **Type 1 diabetes mellitus with proliferative diabetic retinopathy with traction retinal detachment not involving the macula** HCC

     √7th **E10.354** **Type 1 diabetes mellitus with proliferative diabetic retinopathy with combined traction retinal detachment and rhegmatogenous retinal detachment** HCC

     √7th **E10.355** **Type 1 diabetes mellitus with stable proliferative diabetic retinopathy** HCC

     √7th **E10.359** **Type 1 diabetes mellitus with proliferative diabetic retinopathy without macular edema** HCC

E10.36 **Type 1 diabetes mellitus with diabetic cataract** HCC
     AHA: 2019,2Q,30-31; 2016,4Q,142

√x 7th **E10.37** **Type 1 diabetes mellitus with diabetic macular edema, resolved following treatment** HCC

E10.39 **Type 1 diabetes mellitus with other diabetic ophthalmic complication** HCC
     Use additional code to identify manifestation, such as: diabetic glaucoma (H40-H42)
     AHA: 2023,3Q,19

√5th **E10.4** **Type 1 diabetes mellitus with neurological complications**

E10.40 **Type 1 diabetes mellitus with diabetic neuropathy, unspecified** HCC

E10.41 **Type 1 diabetes mellitus with diabetic mononeuropathy** HCC

E10.42 **Type 1 diabetes mellitus with diabetic polyneuropathy** HCC
     Type 1 diabetes mellitus with diabetic neuralgia

E10.43 **Type 1 diabetes mellitus with diabetic autonomic (poly)neuropathy** HCC
     Type 1 diabetes mellitus with diabetic gastroparesis
     AHA: 2013,4Q,114

E10.44 **Type 1 diabetes mellitus with diabetic amyotrophy** HCC

E10.49 **Type 1 diabetes mellitus with other diabetic neurological complication** HCC

√5th **E10.5** **Type 1 diabetes mellitus with circulatory complications**

E10.51 **Type 1 diabetes mellitus with diabetic peripheral angiopathy without gangrene** HCC
     AHA: 2018,3Q,3-4; 2018,2Q,7

E10.52 **Type 1 diabetes mellitus with diabetic peripheral angiopathy with gangrene** CC HCC
     Type 1 diabetes mellitus with diabetic gangrene
     AHA: 2020,2Q,18; 2018,3Q,3; 2018,2Q,7; 2017,4Q,102

E10.59 **Type 1 diabetes mellitus with other circulatory complications** HCC

√5th **E10.6** **Type 1 diabetes mellitus with other specified complications**

√6th **E10.61** **Type 1 diabetes mellitus with diabetic arthropathy**

     E10.610 **Type 1 diabetes mellitus with diabetic neuropathic arthropathy** HCC
     Type 1 diabetes mellitus with Charcôt's joints
     DEF: Charcot's joint: Progressive neurologic arthropathy in which chronic degeneration of joints in the weight-bearing areas with peripheral hypertrophy occurs as a complication of a neuropathy disorder. Supporting structures relax from a loss of sensation resulting in chronic joint instability.

     E10.618 **Type 1 diabetes mellitus with other diabetic arthropathy**
     AHA: 2018,2Q,6

√6th **E10.62** **Type 1 diabetes mellitus with skin complications**

     E10.620 **Type 1 diabetes mellitus with diabetic dermatitis** HCC
     Type 1 diabetes mellitus with diabetic necrobiosis lipoidica

     E10.621 **Type 1 diabetes mellitus with foot ulcer** HCC
     Use additional code to identify site of ulcer (L97.4-, L97.5-)
     AHA: 2020,2Q,19

     E10.622 **Type 1 diabetes mellitus with other skin ulcer**
     Use additional code to identify site of ulcer (L97.1-L97.9, L98.41-L98.49)
     AHA: 2021,1Q,7; 2017,4Q,17

N Newborn: 0   P Pediatric: 0-17   M Maternity: 9-64   A Adult: 15-124   UNS Unspecified Site   MCC Major Complication/Comorbidity   CC Complication/Comorbidity   PE POA Exempt

534   ICD-10-CM 2025

E10.628   Type 1 diabetes mellitus with other skin complications   `HCC`

✓6ᵗʰ **E10.63**   Type 1 diabetes mellitus with **oral complications**

E10.630   Type 1 diabetes mellitus with **periodontal disease**   `HCC`

E10.638   Type 1 diabetes mellitus with other oral complications   `HCC`

✓6ᵗʰ **E10.64**   Type 1 diabetes mellitus with **hypoglycemia**

▶Use additional code for hypoglycemia level, if applicable (E16.A-)◀

AHA: 2017,1Q,42

E10.641   Type 1 diabetes mellitus with hypoglycemia **with coma**   `MCC` `HCC`

E10.649   Type 1 diabetes mellitus with hypoglycemia **without coma**   `HCC`

AHA: 2016,3Q,42; 2016,1Q,13; 2015,3Q,21

E10.65   Type 1 diabetes mellitus with **hyperglycemia**   `HCC`

AHA: 2022,1Q,28; 2017,1Q,42; 2013,3Q,20

E10.69   Type 1 diabetes mellitus with other specified complication   `HCC`

Use additional code to identify complication

AHA: 2022,1Q,28; 2016,4Q,141; 2016,1Q,13

E10.8   Type 1 diabetes mellitus with unspecified complications   `HCC`

E10.9   Type 1 diabetes mellitus **without complications**   `HCC`

AHA: 2023,3Q,19; 2020,2Q,18

● ✓5ᵗʰ **E10.A**   Type 1 diabetes mellitus, **presymptomatic**

Early-stage type 1 diabetes mellitus

● **E10.A0**   Type 1 diabetes mellitus, presymptomatic, unspecified

● **E10.A1**   Type 1 diabetes mellitus, presymptomatic, **Stage 1**

Multiple confirmed islet autoantibodies with normoglycemia

● **E10.A2**   Type 1 diabetes mellitus, presymptomatic, **Stage 2**

Confirmed islet autoimmunity with dysglycemia

✓4ᵗʰ **E11**   **Type 2 diabetes mellitus**

INCLUDES   diabetes (mellitus) due to insulin secretory defect
diabetes NOS
insulin resistant diabetes (mellitus)

Use additional code to identify control using:
▶injectable non-insulin antidiabetic drugs (Z79.85)◀
insulin (Z79.4)
oral antidiabetic drugs (Z79.84)
oral hypoglycemic drugs (Z79.84)

EXCLUDES 1   diabetes mellitus due to underlying condition (E08.-)
drug or chemical induced diabetes mellitus (E09.-)
gestational diabetes (O24.4-)
neonatal diabetes mellitus (P70.2)
postpancreatectomy diabetes mellitus (E13.-)
postprocedural diabetes mellitus (E13.-)
secondary diabetes mellitus NEC (E13.-)
type 1 diabetes mellitus (E10.-)

AHA: 2020,3Q,30; 2020,1Q,12; 2016,2Q,10; 2013,1Q,26

✓5ᵗʰ **E11.0**   Type 2 diabetes mellitus with **hyperosmolarity**

DEF: Diabetic hyperosmolarity: Extremely high levels of glucose in the blood without ketones.

E11.00   Type 2 diabetes mellitus with hyperosmolarity without nonketotic hyperglycemic-hyperosmolar coma (NKHHC)   `MCC` `H9` `HCC`

AHA: 2022,1Q,28

E11.01   Type 2 diabetes mellitus with hyperosmolarity **with coma**   `MCC` `H9` `HCC`

✓5ᵗʰ **E11.1**   Type 2 diabetes mellitus with **ketoacidosis**

AHA: 2017,4Q,6

DEF: Diabetic ketoacidosis: Potentially life-threatening complication due to a shortage of insulin in which the body switches to burning fatty acids and producing acidic ketone bodies.

E11.10   Type 2 diabetes mellitus with ketoacidosis **without coma**   `MCC` `H9` `HCC`

E11.11   Type 2 diabetes mellitus with ketoacidosis **with coma**   `MCC` `H9` `HCC`

✓5ᵗʰ **E11.2**   Type 2 diabetes mellitus with **kidney complications**

AHA: 2019,3Q,3; 2018,4Q,88

E11.21   Type 2 diabetes mellitus with diabetic **nephropathy**   `HCC`

Type 2 diabetes mellitus with intercapillary glomerulosclerosis
Type 2 diabetes mellitus with intracapillary glomerulonephrosis
Type 2 diabetes mellitus with Kimmelstiel-Wilson disease

E11.22   Type 2 diabetes mellitus with diabetic **chronic kidney disease**   `HCC`

Use additional code to identify stage of chronic kidney disease (N18.1-N18.6)

AHA: 2022,3Q,15

E11.29   Type 2 diabetes mellitus with other diabetic kidney complication   `HCC`

Type 2 diabetes mellitus with renal tubular degeneration

✓5ᵗʰ **E11.3**   Type 2 diabetes mellitus with **ophthalmic complications**

AHA: 2016,4Q,11-13

One of the following 7th characters is to be assigned to codes in subcategories E11.32, E11.33, E11.34, E11.35, and E11.37 to designate laterality of the disease:
1   right eye
2   left eye
3   bilateral
9   unspecified eye

✓6ᵗʰ **E11.31**   Type 2 diabetes mellitus with unspecified diabetic **retinopathy**

DEF: Diabetic retinopathy: Diabetic complication from damage to the retinal vessels resulting in vision problems that can progress to blindness.

E11.311   Type 2 diabetes mellitus with unspecified diabetic retinopathy **with macular edema**   `HCC`

E11.319   Type 2 diabetes mellitus with unspecified diabetic retinopathy **without macular edema**   `HCC`

✓6ᵗʰ **E11.32**   Type 2 diabetes mellitus with **mild nonproliferative** diabetic **retinopathy**

Type 2 diabetes mellitus with nonproliferative diabetic retinopathy NOS

✓7ᵗʰ **E11.321**   Type 2 diabetes mellitus with mild nonproliferative diabetic retinopathy **with macular edema**   `HCC`

✓7ᵗʰ **E11.329**   Type 2 diabetes mellitus with mild nonproliferative diabetic retinopathy **without macular edema**   `HCC`

✓6ᵗʰ **E11.33**   Type 2 diabetes mellitus with **moderate nonproliferative** diabetic **retinopathy**

✓7ᵗʰ **E11.331**   Type 2 diabetes mellitus with moderate nonproliferative diabetic retinopathy **with macular edema**   `HCC`

✓7ᵗʰ **E11.339**   Type 2 diabetes mellitus with moderate nonproliferative diabetic retinopathy **without macular edema**   `HCC`

✓6ᵗʰ **E11.34**   Type 2 diabetes mellitus with **severe nonproliferative** diabetic **retinopathy**

✓7ᵗʰ **E11.341**   Type 2 diabetes mellitus with severe nonproliferative diabetic retinopathy **with macular edema**   `HCC`

✓7ᵗʰ **E11.349**   Type 2 diabetes mellitus with severe nonproliferative diabetic retinopathy **without macular edema**   `HCC`

✓6ᵗʰ **E11.35**   Type 2 diabetes mellitus with **proliferative** diabetic **retinopathy**

✓7ᵗʰ **E11.351**   Type 2 diabetes mellitus with proliferative diabetic retinopathy **with macular edema**   `HCC`

✓7ᵗʰ **E11.352**   Type 2 diabetes mellitus with proliferative diabetic retinopathy **with traction retinal detachment involving the macula**   `HCC`

✓7ᵗʰ **E11.353**   Type 2 diabetes mellitus with proliferative diabetic retinopathy **with traction retinal detachment not involving the macula**   `HCC`

✔ Additional Character Required   ✓x7ᵗʰ Placeholder   Questionable PDx   Manifestation   Unspecified   UPD Unacceptable PDx   H1-H14 HAC   HCC CMS-HCC Dx   HIV HIV Dx

ICD-10-CM 2025   535

√7th **E11.354** **Type 2 diabetes mellitus with proliferative diabetic retinopathy with combined traction retinal detachment and rhegmatogenous retinal detachment** HCC

√7th **E11.355** **Type 2 diabetes mellitus with stable proliferative diabetic retinopathy** HCC

√7th **E11.359** **Type 2 diabetes mellitus with proliferative diabetic retinopathy without macular edema** HCC

E11.36 **Type 2 diabetes mellitus with diabetic cataract** HCC
AHA: 2019,2Q,30-31; 2016,4Q,142

√x7th **E11.37** **Type 2 diabetes mellitus with diabetic macular edema, resolved following treatment** HCC

E11.39 **Type 2 diabetes mellitus with other diabetic ophthalmic complication** HCC
Use additional code to identify manifestation, such as: diabetic glaucoma (H40-H42)
AHA: 2023,3Q,19

√5th **E11.4** **Type 2 diabetes mellitus with neurological complications**
AHA: 2022,3Q,15

E11.40 **Type 2 diabetes mellitus with diabetic neuropathy, unspecified** HCC
AHA: 2013,4Q,129

E11.41 **Type 2 diabetes mellitus with diabetic mononeuropathy** HCC

E11.42 **Type 2 diabetes mellitus with diabetic polyneuropathy** HCC
Type 2 diabetes mellitus with diabetic neuralgia
AHA: 2020,1Q,12

E11.43 **Type 2 diabetes mellitus with diabetic autonomic (poly)neuropathy** HCC
Type 2 diabetes mellitus with diabetic gastroparesis
AHA: 2023,2Q,8; 2013,4Q,114

E11.44 **Type 2 diabetes mellitus with diabetic amyotrophy** HCC

E11.49 **Type 2 diabetes mellitus with other diabetic neurological complication** HCC

√5th **E11.5** **Type 2 diabetes mellitus with circulatory complications**

E11.51 **Type 2 diabetes mellitus with diabetic peripheral angiopathy without gangrene** HCC
AHA: 2018,3Q,3-4; 2018,2Q,7

E11.52 **Type 2 diabetes mellitus with diabetic peripheral angiopathy with gangrene** CC HCC
Type 2 diabetes mellitus with diabetic gangrene
AHA: 2020,2Q,18; 2018,3Q,3; 2018,2Q,7; 2017,4Q,102

E11.59 **Type 2 diabetes mellitus with other circulatory complications** HCC

√5th **E11.6** **Type 2 diabetes mellitus with other specified complications**

√6th **E11.61** **Type 2 diabetes mellitus with diabetic arthropathy**

E11.610 **Type 2 diabetes mellitus with diabetic neuropathic arthropathy** HCC
Type 2 diabetes mellitus with Charcôt's joints
DEF: Charcot's joint: Progressive neurologic arthropathy in which chronic degeneration of joints in the weight-bearing areas with peripheral hypertrophy occurs as a complication of a neuropathy disorder. Supporting structures relax from a loss of sensation resulting in chronic joint instability.

E11.618 **Type 2 diabetes mellitus with other diabetic arthropathy** HCC
AHA: 2018,2Q,6

√6th **E11.62** **Type 2 diabetes mellitus with skin complications**

E11.620 **Type 2 diabetes mellitus with diabetic dermatitis** HCC
Type 2 diabetes mellitus with diabetic necrobiosis lipoidica

E11.621 **Type 2 diabetes mellitus with foot ulcer** HCC
Use additional code to identify site of ulcer (L97.4-, L97.5-)
AHA: 2020,2Q,19; 2020,1Q,12

E11.622 **Type 2 diabetes mellitus with other skin ulcer** HCC
Use additional code to identify site of ulcer (L97.1-L97.9, L98.41-L98.49)
AHA: 2021,1Q,7; 2017,4Q,17

E11.628 **Type 2 diabetes mellitus with other skin complications** HCC

√6th **E11.63** **Type 2 diabetes mellitus with oral complications**

E11.630 **Type 2 diabetes mellitus with periodontal disease** HCC

E11.638 **Type 2 diabetes mellitus with other oral complications** HCC

√6th **E11.64** **Type 2 diabetes mellitus with hypoglycemia**
▶Use additional code for hypoglycemia level, if applicable (E16.A-)◀
AHA: 2017,1Q,42

E11.641 **Type 2 diabetes mellitus with hypoglycemia with coma** MCC HCC

E11.649 **Type 2 diabetes mellitus with hypoglycemia without coma** HCC
AHA: 2016,3Q,42; 2015,3Q,21

E11.65 **Type 2 diabetes mellitus with hyperglycemia** HCC
AHA: 2023,2Q,10; 2022,1Q,28; 2017,1Q,42; 2013,3Q,20

E11.69 **Type 2 diabetes mellitus with other specified complication** HCC
Use additional code to identify complication
AHA: 2020,1Q,12; 2016,4Q,141; 2016,1Q,13

E11.8 **Type 2 diabetes mellitus with unspecified complications** HCC

E11.9 **Type 2 diabetes mellitus without complications** HCC
AHA: 2023,3Q,19; 2020,2Q,18

√4th **E13** **Other specified diabetes mellitus**
INCLUDES diabetes mellitus due to genetic defects of beta-cell function
diabetes mellitus due to genetic defects in insulin action
postpancreatectomy diabetes mellitus
postprocedural diabetes mellitus
secondary diabetes mellitus NEC
Use additional code to identify control using:
▶injectable non-insulin antidiabetic drugs (Z79.85)◀
insulin (Z79.4)
oral antidiabetic drugs (Z79.84)
oral hypoglycemic drugs (Z79.84)
EXCLUDES 1 diabetes (mellitus) due to autoimmune process (E10.-)
diabetes (mellitus) due to immune mediated pancreatic islet beta-cell destruction (E10.-)
diabetes mellitus due to underlying condition (E08.-)
drug or chemical induced diabetes mellitus (E09.-)
gestational diabetes (O24.4-)
neonatal diabetes mellitus (P70.2)
type 1 diabetes mellitus (E10.-)
AHA: 2018,3Q,4; 2016,1Q,11-13
TIP: Use this category when the diabetes is documented as diabetes type 1.5. Synonymous terms used in the documentation may also include combined diabetes type 1 and type 2, latent autoimmune diabetes of adults (LADA), slow-progressing type 1 diabetes, or double diabetes.
TIP: When postprocedural or postpancreatectomy hypoinsulinemia (E89.1) is documented with postprocedural or postpancreatectomy diabetes mellitus (E13.-), code E89.1 should be sequenced first.

√5th **E13.0** **Other specified diabetes mellitus with hyperosmolarity**
DEF: Diabetic hyperosmolarity: Extremely high levels of glucose in the blood without ketones.

E13.00 **Other specified diabetes mellitus with hyperosmolarity without nonketotic hyperglycemic-hyperosmolar coma (NKHHC)** MCC H9 HCC

E13.01 **Other specified diabetes mellitus with hyperosmolarity with coma** MCC H9 HCC

√5th **E13.1** **Other specified diabetes mellitus with ketoacidosis**
AHA: 2016,2Q,10; 2013,1Q,26
DEF: Diabetic ketoacidosis: Potentially life-threatening complication due to a shortage of insulin in which the body switches to burning fatty acids and producing acidic ketone bodies.

E13.10 **Other specified diabetes mellitus with ketoacidosis without coma** MCC H9 HCC

E13.11 **Other specified diabetes mellitus with ketoacidosis with coma** MCC H9 HCC

√5ᵗʰ **E13.2** **Other specified diabetes mellitus with kidney complications**
    AHA: 2019,3Q,3; 2018,4Q,88

    E13.21 **Other specified diabetes mellitus with diabetic nephropathy** `HCC`
        Other specified diabetes mellitus with intercapillary glomerulosclerosis
        Other specified diabetes mellitus with intracapillary glomerulonephrosis
        Other specified diabetes mellitus with Kimmelstiel-Wilson disease

    E13.22 **Other specified diabetes mellitus with diabetic chronic kidney disease** `HCC`
        Use additional code to identify stage of chronic kidney disease (N18.1-N18.6)

    E13.29 **Other specified diabetes mellitus with other diabetic kidney complication** `HCC`
        Other specified diabetes mellitus with renal tubular degeneration

√5ᵗʰ **E13.3** **Other specified diabetes mellitus with ophthalmic complications**
    AHA: 2016,4Q,11-13

> One of the following 7th characters is to be assigned to codes in subcategories E13.32, E13.33, E13.34, E13.35, and E13.37 to designate laterality of the disease:
> 1   right eye
> 2   left eye
> 3   bilateral
> 9   unspecified eye

    √6ᵗʰ **E13.31** **Other specified diabetes mellitus with unspecified diabetic retinopathy**
        DEF: Diabetic retinopathy: Diabetic complication from damage to the retinal vessels resulting in vision problems that can progress to blindness.
        E13.311 **Other specified diabetes mellitus with unspecified diabetic retinopathy with macular edema** `HCC`
        E13.319 **Other specified diabetes mellitus with unspecified diabetic retinopathy without macular edema** `HCC`

    √6ᵗʰ **E13.32** **Other specified diabetes mellitus with mild nonproliferative diabetic retinopathy**
        Other specified diabetes mellitus with nonproliferative diabetic retinopathy NOS
        √7ᵗʰ **E13.321** **Other specified diabetes mellitus with mild nonproliferative diabetic retinopathy with macular edema** `HCC`
        √7ᵗʰ **E13.329** **Other specified diabetes mellitus with mild nonproliferative diabetic retinopathy without macular edema** `HCC`

    √6ᵗʰ **E13.33** **Other specified diabetes mellitus with moderate nonproliferative diabetic retinopathy**
        √7ᵗʰ **E13.331** **Other specified diabetes mellitus with moderate nonproliferative diabetic retinopathy with macular edema** `HCC`
        √7ᵗʰ **E13.339** **Other specified diabetes mellitus with moderate nonproliferative diabetic retinopathy without macular edema** `HCC`

    √6ᵗʰ **E13.34** **Other specified diabetes mellitus with severe nonproliferative diabetic retinopathy**
        √7ᵗʰ **E13.341** **Other specified diabetes mellitus with severe nonproliferative diabetic retinopathy with macular edema** `HCC`
        √7ᵗʰ **E13.349** **Other specified diabetes mellitus with severe nonproliferative diabetic retinopathy without macular edema** `HCC`

    √6ᵗʰ **E13.35** **Other specified diabetes mellitus with proliferative diabetic retinopathy**
        √7ᵗʰ **E13.351** **Other specified diabetes mellitus with proliferative diabetic retinopathy with macular edema** `HCC`
        √7ᵗʰ **E13.352** **Other specified diabetes mellitus with proliferative diabetic retinopathy with traction retinal detachment involving the macula** `HCC`
        √7ᵗʰ **E13.353** **Other specified diabetes mellitus with proliferative diabetic retinopathy with traction retinal detachment not involving the macula** `HCC`
        √7ᵗʰ **E13.354** **Other specified diabetes mellitus with proliferative diabetic retinopathy with combined traction retinal detachment and rhegmatogenous retinal detachment** `HCC`
        √7ᵗʰ **E13.355** **Other specified diabetes mellitus with stable proliferative diabetic retinopathy** `HCC`
        √7ᵗʰ **E13.359** **Other specified diabetes mellitus with proliferative diabetic retinopathy without macular edema** `HCC`

    E13.36 **Other specified diabetes mellitus with diabetic cataract** `HCC`
        AHA: 2019,2Q,30-31; 2016,4Q,142

√x 7ᵗʰ **E13.37** **Other specified diabetes mellitus with diabetic macular edema, resolved following treatment** `HCC`

    E13.39 **Other specified diabetes mellitus with other diabetic ophthalmic complication** `HCC`
        Use additional code to identify manifestation, such as: diabetic glaucoma (H40-H42)
        AHA: 2023,3Q,19

√5ᵗʰ **E13.4** **Other specified diabetes mellitus with neurological complications**

    E13.40 **Other specified diabetes mellitus with diabetic neuropathy, unspecified** `HCC`

    E13.41 **Other specified diabetes mellitus with diabetic mononeuropathy** `HCC`

    E13.42 **Other specified diabetes mellitus with diabetic polyneuropathy** `HCC`
        Other specified diabetes mellitus with diabetic neuralgia

    E13.43 **Other specified diabetes mellitus with diabetic autonomic (poly)neuropathy** `HCC`
        Other specified diabetes mellitus with diabetic gastroparesis
        AHA: 2013,4Q,114

    E13.44 **Other specified diabetes mellitus with diabetic amyotrophy** `HCC`

    E13.49 **Other specified diabetes mellitus with other diabetic neurological complication** `HCC`

√5ᵗʰ **E13.5** **Other specified diabetes mellitus with circulatory complications**

    E13.51 **Other specified diabetes mellitus with diabetic peripheral angiopathy without gangrene** `HCC`
        AHA: 2018,3Q,3-4; 2018,2Q,7

    E13.52 **Other specified diabetes mellitus with diabetic peripheral angiopathy with gangrene** `CC` `HCC`
        Other specified diabetes mellitus with diabetic gangrene
        AHA: 2020,2Q,18; 2018,3Q,3; 2018,2Q,7; 2017,4Q,102

    E13.59 **Other specified diabetes mellitus with other circulatory complications** `HCC`

√5ᵗʰ **E13.6** **Other specified diabetes mellitus with other specified complications**

    √6ᵗʰ **E13.61** **Other specified diabetes mellitus with diabetic arthropathy**
        E13.610 **Other specified diabetes mellitus with diabetic neuropathic arthropathy** `HCC`
        Other specified diabetes mellitus with Charcôt's joints
        DEF: Charcot's joint: Progressive neurologic arthropathy in which chronic degeneration of joints in the weight-bearing areas with peripheral hypertrophy occurs as a complication of a neuropathy disorder. Supporting structures relax from a loss of sensation resulting in chronic joint instability.
        E13.618 **Other specified diabetes mellitus with other diabetic arthropathy** `HCC`
        AHA: 2018,2Q,6

    √6ᵗʰ **E13.62** **Other specified diabetes mellitus with skin complications**
        E13.620 **Other specified diabetes mellitus with diabetic dermatitis** `HCC`
        Other specified diabetes mellitus with diabetic necrobiosis lipoidica

E13.621 Other specified diabetes mellitus with foot ulcer HCC
Use additional code to identify site of ulcer (L97.4-, L97.5-)
AHA: 2020,2Q,19

E13.622 Other specified diabetes mellitus with other skin ulcer HCC
Use additional code to identify site of ulcer (L97.1-L97.9, L98.41-L98.49)
AHA: 2021,1Q,7; 2017,4Q,17

E13.628 Other specified diabetes mellitus with other skin complications HCC

✓6th **E13.63 Other specified diabetes mellitus with oral complications**

E13.630 Other specified diabetes mellitus with periodontal disease HCC

E13.638 Other specified diabetes mellitus with other oral complications HCC

✓6th **E13.64 Other specified diabetes mellitus with hypoglycemia**
▶Use additional code for hypoglycemia level, if applicable (E16.A-)◀
AHA: 2017,1Q,42

E13.641 Other specified diabetes mellitus with hypoglycemia with coma MCC HCC

E13.649 Other specified diabetes mellitus with hypoglycemia without coma HCC
AHA: 2016,3Q,42; 2015,3Q,21

E13.65 Other specified diabetes mellitus with hyperglycemia HCC
AHA: 2017,1Q,42; 2013,3Q,20

E13.69 Other specified diabetes mellitus with other specified complication HCC
Use additional code to identify complication
AHA: 2016,4Q,141; 2016,1Q,13

E13.8 Other specified diabetes mellitus with unspecified complications HCC

E13.9 Other specified diabetes mellitus without complications HCC
AHA: 2023,3Q,19; 2020,2Q,18

Other disorders of glucose regulation and pancreatic internal secretion (E15-E16)

E15 Nondiabetic hypoglycemic coma CC H9
INCLUDES drug-induced insulin coma in nondiabetic
hyperinsulinism with hypoglycemic coma
hypoglycemic coma NOS

✓4th **E16 Other disorders of pancreatic internal secretion**

E16.0 Drug-induced hypoglycemia without coma
EXCLUDES 1 diabetes with hypoglycemia without coma (E09.649)
Use additional code for adverse effect, if applicable, to identify drug (T36-T50 with fifth or sixth character 5)
▶Use additional code for hypoglycemia level, if applicable (E16.A-)◀

E16.1 Other hypoglycemia
Functional hyperinsulinism
Functional nonhyperinsulinemic hypoglycemia
Hyperinsulinism NOS
Hyperplasia of pancreatic islet beta cells NOS
▶Use additional code for hypoglycemia level, if applicable (E16.A-)◀
EXCLUDES 1 diabetes with hypoglycemia (E08.649, E10.649, E11.649, E13.649)
hypoglycemia in infant of diabetic mother (P70.1)
neonatal hypoglycemia (P70.4)
AHA: AHA:2024,2Q,10

E16.2 Hypoglycemia, unspecified
▶Use additional code for hypoglycemia level, if applicable (E16.A-)◀
EXCLUDES 1 diabetes with hypoglycemia (E08.649, E10.649, E11.649, E13.649)
AHA: 2016,3Q,42
TIP: Assign for nondiabetic hypoglycemic encephalopathy not further clarified in the documentation.

E16.3 Increased secretion of glucagon
Hyperplasia of pancreatic endocrine cells with glucagon excess

E16.4 Increased secretion of gastrin
Hypergastrinemia
Hyperplasia of pancreatic endocrine cells with gastrin excess
Zollinger-Ellison syndrome

E16.8 Other specified disorders of pancreatic internal secretion
Increased secretion from endocrine pancreas of growth hormone-releasing hormone
Increased secretion from endocrine pancreas of pancreatic polypeptide
Increased secretion from endocrine pancreas of somatostatin
Increased secretion from endocrine pancreas of vasoactive-intestinal polypeptide

E16.9 Disorder of pancreatic internal secretion, unspecified
Islet-cell hyperplasia NOS
Pancreatic endocrine cell hyperplasia NOS

● ✓5th **E16.A Hypoglycemia level**

● **E16.A1 Hypoglycemia level 1**
Decreased blood glucose level 1

E16.A2 Hypoglycemia level 2
Decreased blood glucose level 2

● **E16.A3 Hypoglycemia level 3**
Decreased blood glucose level 3

Disorders of other endocrine glands (E20-E35)

EXCLUDES 1 galactorrhea (N64.3)
gynecomastia (N62)

✓4th **E20 Hypoparathyroidism**
EXCLUDES 1 Di George's syndrome (D82.1)
postprocedural hypoparathyroidism (E89.2)
tetany NOS (R29.0)
transitory neonatal hypoparathyroidism (P71.4)

E20.0 Idiopathic hypoparathyroidism
DEF: Abnormally low secretion of parathyroid hormones, with unknown cause, which triggers decreased calcium and increased phosphorus in the blood that can result in cataracts, muscle cramps, tetany, tingling, or burning in the lips, fingers, and toes.

E20.1 Pseudohypoparathyroidism

✓5th **E20.8 Other hypoparathyroidism**

✓6th **E20.81 Hypoparathyroidism due to impaired parathyroid hormone secretion**
AHA: 2023,4Q,9-11

E20.810 Autosomal dominant hypocalcemia
Autosomal dominant hypocalcemia type 1 (ADH1)
Autosomal dominant hypocalcemia type 2 (ADH2)
Code also, if applicable, any associated conditions, such as:
calculus of kidney (N20.0)
chronic kidney disease (N18.-)
respiratory distress (J80, R06.-)
seizure disorder (G40.-, R56.9)

E20.811 Secondary hypoparathyroidism in diseases classified elsewhere
Code first underlying condition, if known

E20.812 Autoimmune hypoparathyroidism
Code first, if applicable, underlying condition such as:
autoimmune polyglandular failure (E31.0)
Schmidt's syndrome (E31.0)

E20.818 Other specified hypoparathyroidism due to impaired parathyroid hormone secretion
Familial isolated hypoparathyroidism

E20.819 Hypoparathyroidism due to impaired parathyroid hormone secretion, unspecified

E20.89 Other specified hypoparathyroidism
Familial hypoparathyroidism

E20.9 Hypoparathyroidism, unspecified
Parathyroid tetany

N Newborn: 0   P Pediatric: 0-17   M Maternity: 9-64   A Adult: 15-124   UNS Unspecified Site   MCC Major Complication/Comorbidity   CC Complication/Comorbidity   PE POA Exempt

538

ICD-10-CM 2025

✓4th **E21 Hyperparathyroidism and other disorders of parathyroid gland**

> EXCLUDES 1   *adult osteomalacia (M83.-)*
> *ectopic hyperparathyroidism (E34.2)*
> *hungry bone syndrome (E83.81)*
> *infantile and juvenile osteomalacia (E55.0)*
> EXCLUDES 2   *familial hypocalciuric hypercalcemia (E83.52)*

E21.0 Primary hyperparathyroidism
Hyperplasia of parathyroid
Osteitis fibrosa cystica generalisata [von Recklinghauser's disease of bone]
> **DEF:** Parathyroid dysfunction commonly caused by hyperplasia of two or more glands. Symptoms include hypercalcemia and increased parathyroid hormone levels.

E21.1 Secondary hyperparathyroidism, not elsewhere classified
> EXCLUDES 1   *secondary hyperparathyroidism of renal origin (N25.81)*

E21.2 Other hyperparathyroidism
Tertiary hyperparathyroidism
> EXCLUDES 1   *familial hypocalciuric hypercalcemia (E83.52)*

E21.3 Hyperparathyroidism, unspecified

E21.4 Other specified disorders of parathyroid gland

E21.5 Disorder of parathyroid gland, unspecified

✓4th **E22 Hyperfunction of pituitary gland**

> EXCLUDES 1   *Cushing's syndrome (E24.-)*
> *Nelson's syndrome (E24.1)*
> *overproduction of ACTH not associated with Cushing's disease (E27.0)*
> *overproduction of pituitary ACTH (E24.0)*
> *overproduction of thyroid-stimulating hormone (E05.8-)*

E22.0 Acromegaly and pituitary gigantism   HCC
Overproduction of growth hormone
> EXCLUDES 1   *constitutional gigantism (E34.4)*
> *constitutional tall stature (E34.4)*
> *increased secretion from endocrine pancreas of growth hormone-releasing hormone (E16.8)*

> **DEF:** Acromegaly: Chronic condition caused by overproduction of the pituitary growth hormone resulting in enlarged skeletal parts and facial features.

E22.1 Hyperprolactinemia   CC
Use additional code for adverse effect, if applicable, to identify drug (T36-T50 with fifth or sixth character 5)

E22.2 Syndrome of inappropriate secretion of antidiuretic hormone   CC

E22.8 Other hyperfunction of pituitary gland   CC
Central precocious puberty

E22.9 Hyperfunction of pituitary gland, unspecified   CC

✓4th **E23 Hypofunction and other disorders of the pituitary gland**

> INCLUDES   the listed conditions whether the disorder is in the pituitary or the hypothalamus
> EXCLUDES 1   *postprocedural hypopituitarism (E89.3)*
> *short stature due to endocrine disorder (E34.3-)*

E23.0 Hypopituitarism   CC
Fertile eunuch syndrome
Hypogonadotropic hypogonadism
Idiopathic growth hormone deficiency
Isolated deficiency of gonadotropin
Isolated deficiency of growth hormone
Isolated deficiency of pituitary hormone
Kallmann's syndrome
Lorain-Levi short stature
Necrosis of pituitary gland (postpartum)
Panhypopituitarism
Pituitary cachexia
Pituitary insufficiency NOS
Pituitary short stature
Sheehan's syndrome
Simmonds' disease
AHA: 2024,1Q,15

E23.1 Drug-induced hypopituitarism
Use additional code for adverse effect, if applicable, to identify drug (T36-T50 with fifth or sixth character 5)

E23.2 Diabetes insipidus   CC
> EXCLUDES 1   *nephrogenic diabetes insipidus (N25.1)*

E23.3 Hypothalamic dysfunction, not elsewhere classified
> EXCLUDES 1   *Prader-Willi syndrome (Q87.11)*
> *Russell-Silver syndrome (Q87.19)*
> **AHA:** 2024,1Q,15

E23.6 Other disorders of pituitary gland
Abscess of pituitary
Adiposogenital dystrophy

E23.7 Disorder of pituitary gland, unspecified

✓4th **E24 Cushing's syndrome**

> EXCLUDES 1   *congenital adrenal hyperplasia (E25.0)*
> **DEF:** Abdominal striae, acne, hypertension, decreased carbohydrate tolerance, moon face, obesity, protein catabolism, and psychiatric disturbances resulting from increased adrenocortical secretion of cortisol caused by ACTH-dependent adrenocortical hyperplasia or tumor, or by steroid effects.

E24.0 Pituitary-dependent Cushing's disease   CC HCC
Overproduction of pituitary ACTH
Pituitary-dependent hypercorticalism

E24.1 Nelson's syndrome

E24.2 Drug-induced Cushing's syndrome   CC
Use additional code for adverse effect, if applicable, to identify drug (T36-T50 with fifth or sixth character 5)

E24.3 Ectopic ACTH syndrome   CC

E24.4 Alcohol-induced pseudo-Cushing's syndrome   CC

E24.8 Other Cushing's syndrome   CC

E24.9 Cushing's syndrome, unspecified   CC

✓4th **E25 Adrenogenital disorders**

> INCLUDES   adrenogenital syndromes, virilizing or feminizing, whether acquired or due to adrenal hyperplasia consequent on inborn enzyme defects in hormone synthesis
> female adrenal pseudohermaphroditism
> female heterosexual precocious pseudopuberty
> male isosexual precocious pseudopuberty
> male macrogenitosomia praecox
> male sexual precocity with adrenal hyperplasia
> male virilization (female)
> EXCLUDES 1   *chromosomal abnormalities (Q90-Q99)*
> *indeterminate sex and pseudohermaphroditism (Q56)*

E25.0 Congenital adrenogenital disorders associated with enzyme deficiency
Congenital adrenal hyperplasia
21-Hydroxylase deficiency
Salt-losing congenital adrenal hyperplasia

E25.8 Other adrenogenital disorders
Idiopathic adrenogenital disorder
Use additional code for adverse effect, if applicable, to identify drug (T36-T50 with fifth or sixth character 5)

E25.9 Adrenogenital disorder, unspecified
Adrenogenital syndrome NOS

✓4th **E26 Hyperaldosteronism**

✓5th **E26.0 Primary hyperaldosteronism**

> **E26.01 Conn's syndrome**
> Code also adrenal adenoma (D35.0-)

> **E26.02 Glucocorticoid-remediable aldosteronism**
> Familial aldosteronism type I
> **DEF:** Rare autosomal dominant familial form of primary aldosteronism in which the secretion of aldosterone is under the influence of adrenocorticotrophic hormone (ACTH) rather than the renin-angiotensin mechanism. Moderate hypersecretion of aldosterone and suppressed plasma renin activity that are rapidly reversed by administration of glucosteroids. Symptoms include hypertension and mild hypokalemia.

> **E26.09 Other primary hyperaldosteronism**
> Primary aldosteronism due to adrenal hyperplasia (bilateral)

E26.1 Secondary hyperaldosteronism

✓5th **E26.8 Other hyperaldosteronism**

> **E26.81 Bartter's syndrome**
> **E26.89 Other hyperaldosteronism**

E26.9 Hyperaldosteronism, unspecified
Aldosteronism NOS
Hyperaldosteronism NOS

✔ Additional Character Required   ✓x7th Placeholder   Questionable PDx   Manifestation   Unspecified   UPD Unacceptable PDx   H1-H14 HAC   HCC CMS-HCC Dx   HIV HIV Dx

ICD-10-CM 2025   539

Chapter 4. Endocrine, Nutritional and Metabolic Diseases

E27–E32.9

✓4th **E27 Other disorders of adrenal gland**

E27.0 Other adrenocortical overactivity   CC
     Overproduction of ACTH, not associated with Cushing's disease
     Premature adrenarche
     EXCLUDES 1   *Cushing's syndrome (E24.-)*

E27.1 Primary adrenocortical insufficiency   CC HCC
     Addison's disease
     Autoimmune adrenalitis
     EXCLUDES 1   *Addison only phenotype adrenoleukodystrophy*
             (E71.528)
             amyloidosis (E85.-)
             tuberculous Addison's disease (A18.7)
             Waterhouse-Friderichsen syndrome (A39.1)

E27.2 Addisonian crisis   CC
     Adrenal crisis
     Adrenocortical crisis
     DEF: Life-threatening condition that occurs when there is not enough cortisol excreted from the adrenal glands. This condition may be due to injury to the adrenal glands or to the pituitary gland, which controls adrenal hormone secretion, or when a patient stops hydrocortisone treatment too quickly or too early.

E27.3 Drug-induced adrenocortical insufficiency   CC
     Use additional code for adverse effect, if applicable, to identify drug (T36-T50 with fifth or sixth character 5)

✓5th **E27.4 Other and unspecified adrenocortical insufficiency**
     EXCLUDES 1   *adrenoleukodystrophy [Addison-Schilder] (E71.528)*
             Waterhouse-Friderichsen syndrome (A39.1)

     E27.40 Unspecified adrenocortical insufficiency   CC
         Adrenocortical insufficiency NOS
         Hypoaldosteronism

     E27.49 Other adrenocortical insufficiency   CC
         Adrenal hemorrhage
         Adrenal infarction
         AHA: 2024,1Q,15

E27.5 Adrenomedullary hyperfunction   CC
     Adrenomedullary hyperplasia
     Catecholamine hypersecretion

E27.8 Other specified disorders of adrenal gland
     Abnormality of cortisol-binding globulin

E27.9 Disorder of adrenal gland, unspecified

✓4th **E28 Ovarian dysfunction**
     EXCLUDES 1   *isolated gonadotropin deficiency (E23.0)*
             postprocedural ovarian failure (E89.4-)

E28.0 Estrogen excess
     Use additional code for adverse effect, if applicable, to identify drug (T36-T50 with fifth or sixth character 5)

E28.1 Androgen excess
     Hypersecretion of ovarian androgens
     Use additional code for adverse effect, if applicable, to identify drug (T36-T50 with fifth or sixth character 5)

E28.2 Polycystic ovarian syndrome
     Sclerocystic ovary syndrome
     Stein-Leventhal syndrome
     AHA: 2022,2Q,16
     DEF: Common hormonal disorder among women of reproductive age that involves enlarged ovaries with numerous small cysts located along the outer ovarian edge.

✓5th **E28.3 Primary ovarian failure**
     EXCLUDES 1   *pure gonadal dysgenesis (Q99.1)*
             Turner's syndrome (Q96.-)

     ✓6th **E28.31 Premature menopause**

         E28.310 Symptomatic premature menopause   A
             Symptoms such as flushing, sleeplessness, headache, lack of concentration, associated with premature menopause

         E28.319 Asymptomatic premature menopause   A
             Premature menopause NOS

     E28.39 Other primary ovarian failure
         Decreased estrogen
         Resistant ovary syndrome

E28.8 Other ovarian dysfunction
     Ovarian hyperfunction NOS
     EXCLUDES 1   *postprocedural ovarian failure (E89.4-)*

E28.9 Ovarian dysfunction, unspecified

✓4th **E29 Testicular dysfunction**
     EXCLUDES 1   *androgen insensitivity syndrome (E34.5-)*
             azoospermia or oligospermia NOS (N46.0-N46.1)
             isolated gonadotropin deficiency (E23.0)
             Klinefelter's syndrome (Q98.0-Q98.1, Q98.4)

E29.0 Testicular hyperfunction
     Hypersecretion of testicular hormones

E29.1 Testicular hypofunction
     Defective biosynthesis of testicular androgen NOS
     5-delta-Reductase deficiency (with male pseudohermaphroditism)
     Testicular hypogonadism NOS
     Use additional code for adverse effect, if applicable, to identify drug (T36-T50 with fifth or sixth character 5)
     EXCLUDES 1   *postprocedural testicular hypofunction (E89.5)*

E29.8 Other testicular dysfunction

E29.9 Testicular dysfunction, unspecified

✓4th **E30 Disorders of puberty, not elsewhere classified**

E30.0 Delayed puberty
     Constitutional delay of puberty
     Delayed sexual development

E30.1 Precocious puberty   P
     Precocious menstruation
     EXCLUDES 1   *Albright (-McCune) (-Sternberg) syndrome (Q78.1)*
             central precocious puberty (E22.8)
             congenital adrenal hyperplasia (E25.0)
             female heterosexual precocious pseudopuberty (E25.-)
             male isosexual precocious pseudopuberty (E25.-)

E30.8 Other disorders of puberty   P
     Premature thelarche

E30.9 Disorder of puberty, unspecified

✓4th **E31 Polyglandular dysfunction**
     EXCLUDES 1   *ataxia telangiectasia [Louis-Bar] (G11.3)*
             dystrophia myotonica [Steinert] (G71.11)
             pseudohypoparathyroidism (E20.1)

E31.0 Autoimmune polyglandular failure   HCC
     Schmidt's syndrome

E31.1 Polyglandular hyperfunction   HCC
     EXCLUDES 1   *multiple endocrine adenomatosis (E31.2-)*
             multiple endocrine neoplasia (E31.2-)

✓5th **E31.2 Multiple endocrine neoplasia [MEN] syndromes**
     Multiple endocrine adenomatosis
     Code also any associated malignancies and other conditions associated with the syndromes
     DEF: Group of conditions in which several endocrine glands grow excessively (such as in adenomatous hyperplasia) and/or develop benign or malignant tumors. Tumors and hyperplasia associated with MEN often produce excess hormones, which impede normal physiology. There is no comprehensive cure known for MEN syndrome. Treatment is directed at the hyperplasia or tumors in each individual gland. Tumors are usually surgically removed and oral medications or hormonal injections are used to correct hormone imbalances.

     E31.20 Multiple endocrine neoplasia [MEN] syndrome, unspecified   HCC
         Multiple endocrine adenomatosis NOS
         Multiple endocrine neoplasia [MEN] syndrome NOS

     E31.21 Multiple endocrine neoplasia [MEN] type I   HCC
         Wermer's syndrome

     E31.22 Multiple endocrine neoplasia [MEN] type IIA   HCC
         Sipple's syndrome

     E31.23 Multiple endocrine neoplasia [MEN] type IIB   HCC

E31.8 Other polyglandular dysfunction   HCC

E31.9 Polyglandular dysfunction, unspecified   HCC

✓4th **E32 Diseases of thymus**
     EXCLUDES 1   *aplasia or hypoplasia of thymus with immunodeficiency (D82.1)*
             myasthenia gravis (G70.0)

E32.0 Persistent hyperplasia of thymus
     Hypertrophy of thymus

E32.1 Abscess of thymus   CC

E32.8 Other diseases of thymus
     EXCLUDES 1   *aplasia or hypoplasia with immunodeficiency (D82.1)*
             thymoma (D15.0)

E32.9 Disease of thymus, unspecified

N Newborn: 0   P Pediatric: 0-17   M Maternity: 9-64   A Adult: 15-124   UNS Unspecified Site   MCC Major Complication/Comorbidity   CC Complication/Comorbidity   PE POA Exempt

540   ICD-10-CM 2025

✓4th **E34 Other endocrine disorders**

     EXCLUDES 1   *pseudohypoparathyroidism (E20.1)*

▲   ✓5th **E34.0 Carcinoid syndrome**

     NOTE   May be used as an additional code to identify functional activity associated with a carcinoid tumor.

     ▶Code also the underlying disorder, such as:◀
       ▶primary neuroendocrine tumors (C7A.-)◀
       ▶secondary neuroendocrine tumors (C7B.-)◀

●   **E34.00 Carcinoid syndrome, unspecified**   CC
       Carcinoid disease, unspecified

●   **E34.01 Carcinoid heart syndrome**   CC
       Carcinoid heart disease
       Hedinger syndrome

●   **E34.09 Other carcinoid syndrome**   CC
       Carcinoid disease NEC
       Carcinoid syndrome NEC
       Other carcinoid disease

   E34.1 Other hypersecretion of intestinal hormones

   E34.2 Ectopic hormone secretion, not elsewhere classified
     EXCLUDES 1   *ectopic ACTH syndrome (E24.3)*

✓5th **E34.3 Short stature due to endocrine disorder**
     EXCLUDES 1   *achondroplastic short stature (Q77.4)*
       hypochondroplastic short stature (Q77.4)
       nutritional short stature (E45)
       pituitary short stature (E23.0)
       progeria (E34.8)
       renal short stature (N25.0)
       Russell-Silver syndrome (Q87.19)
       short-limbed stature with immunodeficiency (D82.2)
       short stature (child) (R62.52)
       short stature in specific dysmorphic syndromes - code to syndrome - see Alphabetical Index
       short stature NOS (R62.52)

     AHA: 2022,4Q,11-13

     E34.30 Short stature due to endocrine disorder, unspecified

     E34.31 Constitutional short stature
       Constitutional delay of growth, puberty, or maturation

✓6th   **E34.32 Genetic causes of short stature**

       E34.321 Primary insulin-like growth factor-1 (IGF-1) deficiency
         Acid-labile subunit gene (IGFALS) defect
         Growth hormone gene 1 (GH1) defect with growth hormone neutralizing antibodies
         Growth hormone insensitivity syndrome (GHIS)
         Insulin-like growth factor 1 gene (IGF1) defect
         Laron type short stature
         Severe primary insulin-like growth factor-1 deficiency (SPIGFD)
         Signal transducer and activator of transcription 5B gene (STAT5b) defect

       E34.322 Insulin-like growth factor-1 (IGF-1) resistance
         Genetic syndrome with resistance to insulin-like growth factor-1
         Insulin-like growth factor-1 receptor (IGF-1R) defect
         Post-insulin-like growth factor-1 receptor signaling defect

       E34.328 Other genetic causes of short stature
         Short stature due to ACAN gene variant
         Short stature due to aggrecan deficiency
         Short stature due to NPR-2 gene variant

       E34.329 Unspecified genetic causes of short stature

     E34.39 Other short stature due to endocrine disorder

   E34.4 Constitutional tall stature
       Constitutional gigantism

✓5th **E34.5 Androgen insensitivity syndrome**
     DEF: X-linked recessive condition in which individuals that are chromosomally male fail to develop normal male external genitalia due to an abnormality on the X chromosome that prohibits the body, completely or in part, from recognizing the androgens produced. ***Synonym(s):*** AIS

     E34.50 Androgen insensitivity syndrome, unspecified
       Androgen insensitivity NOS

     E34.51 Complete androgen insensitivity syndrome
       Complete androgen insensitivity
       de Quervain syndrome
       Goldberg-Maxwell syndrome

     E34.52 Partial androgen insensitivity syndrome
       Partial androgen insensitivity
       Reifenstein syndrome

   E34.8 Other specified endocrine disorders
       Pineal gland dysfunction
       Progeria
     EXCLUDES 2   *pseudohypoparathyroidism (E20.1)*

   E34.9 Endocrine disorder, unspecified
       Endocrine disturbance NOS
       Hormone disturbance NOS

E35 Disorders of endocrine glands in diseases classified elsewhere

   Code first underlying disease, such as:
     late congenital syphilis of thymus gland [Dubois disease] (A50.59)
   Use additional code, if applicable, to identify:
     sequelae of tuberculosis of other organs (B90.8)
     EXCLUDES 1   *Echinococcus granulosus infection of thyroid gland (B67.3)*
       meningococcal hemorrhagic adrenalitis (A39.1)
       syphilis of endocrine gland (A52.79)
       tuberculosis of adrenal gland, except calcification (A18.7)
       tuberculosis of endocrine gland NEC (A18.82)
       tuberculosis of thyroid gland (A18.81)
       Waterhouse-Friderichsen syndrome (A39.1)

Intraoperative complications of endocrine system (E36)

✓4th **E36 Intraoperative complications of endocrine system**

     EXCLUDES 2   *postprocedural endocrine and metabolic complications and disorders, not elsewhere classified (E89.-)*

✓5th **E36.0 Intraoperative hemorrhage and hematoma of an endocrine system organ or structure complicating a procedure**
     EXCLUDES 1   *intraoperative hemorrhage and hematoma of an endocrine system organ or structure due to accidental puncture or laceration during a procedure (E36.1-)*

     E36.01 Intraoperative hemorrhage and hematoma of an endocrine system organ or structure complicating an endocrine system procedure   CC
       AHA: 2020,1Q,19

     E36.02 Intraoperative hemorrhage and hematoma of an endocrine system organ or structure complicating other procedure   CC

✓5th **E36.1 Accidental puncture and laceration of an endocrine system organ or structure during a procedure**

     E36.11 Accidental puncture and laceration of an endocrine system organ or structure during an endocrine system procedure   CC

     E36.12 Accidental puncture and laceration of an endocrine system organ or structure during other procedure   CC

   E36.8 Other intraoperative complications of endocrine system
     Use additional code, if applicable, to further specify disorder

Malnutrition (E40-E46)

     EXCLUDES 1   *intestinal malabsorption (K90.-)*
       sequelae of protein-calorie malnutrition (E64.0)
     EXCLUDES 2   *nutritional anemias (D50-D53)*
       starvation (T73.0)

AHA: 2020,1Q,4-7; 2017,4Q,108; 2017,3Q,25

TIP: Assign additional code for BMI from category Z68, when documented. BMI can be based on documentation from clinicians who are not the patient's provider.

TIP: Malnutrition is not considered integral to cancer; assign the appropriate code in addition to the code for the specific type of cancer.

E40 Kwashiorkor   MCC
     Severe malnutrition with nutritional edema with dyspigmentation of skin and hair
     EXCLUDES 1   *marasmic kwashiorkor (E42)*

E41 Nutritional marasmus   MCC
     Severe malnutrition with marasmus
     EXCLUDES 1   *marasmic kwashiorkor (E42)*
     AHA: 2017,3Q,24
     DEF: Protein-calorie malabsorption or malnutrition in children characterized by tissue wasting, dehydration, and subcutaneous fat depletion. It may occur with infectious disease.

✓ Additional Character Required   ✓x7th Placeholder   Questionable PDx   Manifestation   Unspecified   UPD Unacceptable PDx   H1 - H14 HAC   HCC CMS-HCC Dx   HIV HIV Dx

ICD-10-CM 2025   541

E34–E41

E42 Marasmic kwashiorkor `MCC`
Intermediate form severe protein-calorie malnutrition
Severe protein-calorie malnutrition with signs of both kwashiorkor and marasmus

E43 Unspecified severe protein-calorie malnutrition `MCC`
Starvation edema
AHA: 2022,1Q,13; 2020,1Q,5,6; 2017,4Q,108

✓4ᵗʰ **E44 Protein-calorie malnutrition of moderate and mild degree**
AHA: 2020,1Q,5

     E44.0 Moderate protein-calorie malnutrition `CC`
     E44.1 Mild protein-calorie malnutrition `CC`

E45 Retarded development following protein-calorie malnutrition `CC`
Nutritional short stature
Nutritional stunting
Physical retardation due to malnutrition

E46 Unspecified protein-calorie malnutrition `CC`
Malnutrition NOS
Protein-calorie imbalance NOS
EXCLUDES 1   nutritional deficiency NOS (E63.9)
AHA: 2018,4Q,82

Other nutritional deficiencies (E50-E64)

EXCLUDES 2   nutritional anemias (D50–D53)

✓4ᵗʰ **E50 Vitamin A deficiency**
     EXCLUDES 1   sequelae of vitamin A deficiency (E64.1)

     E50.0 Vitamin A deficiency with conjunctival xerosis
     E50.1 Vitamin A deficiency with Bitot's spot and conjunctival xerosis
       Bitot's spot in the young child
       DEF: Vitamin A deficiency with conjunctival dryness and superficial spots of keratinized epithelium.
     E50.2 Vitamin A deficiency with corneal xerosis
     E50.3 Vitamin A deficiency with corneal ulceration and xerosis
     E50.4 Vitamin A deficiency with keratomalacia
       DEF: Vitamin A deficiency creating corneal dryness that progresses to corneal insensitivity, softness, and necrosis. It is usually bilateral.
     E50.5 Vitamin A deficiency with night blindness
     E50.6 Vitamin A deficiency with xerophthalmic scars of cornea
     E50.7 Other ocular manifestations of vitamin A deficiency
       Xerophthalmia NOS
     E50.8 Other manifestations of vitamin A deficiency
       Follicular keratosis
       Xeroderma
     E50.9 Vitamin A deficiency, unspecified
       Hypovitaminosis A NOS

✓4ᵗʰ **E51 Thiamine deficiency**
     EXCLUDES 1   sequelae of thiamine deficiency (E64.8)

     ✓5ᵗʰ **E51.1 Beriberi**
       E51.11 Dry beriberi `CC`
         Beriberi NOS
         Beriberi with polyneuropathy
       E51.12 Wet beriberi `CC`
         Beriberi with cardiovascular manifestations
         Cardiovascular beriberi
         Shoshin disease
     E51.2 Wernicke's encephalopathy `CC`
       DEF: Deficiency of vitamin B1 resulting in a triad of acute mental confusion, ataxia, and ophthalmoplegia. The vast majority of affected patients are alcoholics.
     E51.8 Other manifestations of thiamine deficiency `CC`
     E51.9 Thiamine deficiency, unspecified `CC`

E52 Niacin deficiency [pellagra]
Niacin (-tryptophan) deficiency
Nicotinamide deficiency
Pellagra (alcoholic)
EXCLUDES 1   sequelae of niacin deficiency (E64.8)

✓4ᵗʰ **E53 Deficiency of other B group vitamins**
     EXCLUDES 1   sequelae of vitamin B deficiency (E64.8)

     E53.0 Riboflavin deficiency `CC`
       Ariboflavinosis
       Vitamin B2 deficiency
     E53.1 Pyridoxine deficiency
       Vitamin B6 deficiency
       EXCLUDES 1   pyridoxine-responsive sideroblastic anemia (D64.3)

     E53.8 Deficiency of other specified B group vitamins
       Biotin deficiency
       Cyanocobalamin deficiency
       Folate deficiency
       Folic acid deficiency
       Pantothenic acid deficiency
       Vitamin B12 deficiency
       EXCLUDES 1   folate deficiency anemia (D52.-)
                 vitamin B12 deficiency anemia (D51.-)
     E53.9 Vitamin B deficiency, unspecified

E54 Ascorbic acid deficiency
Deficiency of vitamin C
Scurvy
EXCLUDES 1   scorbutic anemia (D53.2)
             sequelae of vitamin C deficiency (E64.2)
DEF: Vitamin C deficiency causing swollen gums, myalgia, weight loss, and weakness.

✓4ᵗʰ **E55 Vitamin D deficiency**
     EXCLUDES 1   adult osteomalacia (M83.-)
             osteoporosis (M80.-)
             sequelae of rickets (E64.3)

     E55.0 Rickets, active `CC`
       Infantile osteomalacia
       Juvenile osteomalacia
       EXCLUDES 1   celiac rickets (K90.0)
                 Crohn's rickets (K50.-)
                 hereditary vitamin D-dependent rickets (E83.32)
                 inactive rickets (E64.3)
                 renal rickets (N25.0)
                 sequelae of rickets (E64.3)
                 vitamin D-resistant rickets (E83.31)
       DEF: Rickets: Softening or weakening of the bones due to a lack of vitamin D, calcium, and phosphate.
     E55.9 Vitamin D deficiency, unspecified
       Avitaminosis D

✓4ᵗʰ **E56 Other vitamin deficiencies**
     EXCLUDES 1   sequelae of other vitamin deficiencies (E64.8)

     E56.0 Deficiency of vitamin E
     E56.1 Deficiency of vitamin K
       EXCLUDES 1   deficiency of coagulation factor due to vitamin K deficiency (D68.4)
                 vitamin K deficiency of newborn (P53)
     E56.8 Deficiency of other vitamins
     E56.9 Vitamin deficiency, unspecified

E58 Dietary calcium deficiency
EXCLUDES 1   disorders of calcium metabolism (E83.5-)
             sequelae of calcium deficiency (E64.8)

E59 Dietary selenium deficiency
Keshan disease
EXCLUDES 1   sequelae of selenium deficiency (E64.8)

E60 Dietary zinc deficiency

✓4ᵗʰ **E61 Deficiency of other nutrient elements**
Use additional code for adverse effect, if applicable, to identify drug (T36-T50 with fifth or sixth character 5)
EXCLUDES 1   disorders of mineral metabolism (E83.-)
             iodine deficiency related thyroid disorders (E00-E02)
             sequelae of malnutrition and other nutritional deficiencies (E64.-)

     E61.0 Copper deficiency
     E61.1 Iron deficiency
       EXCLUDES 1   iron deficiency anemia (D50.-)
     E61.2 Magnesium deficiency
     E61.3 Manganese deficiency
     E61.4 Chromium deficiency
     E61.5 Molybdenum deficiency
     E61.6 Vanadium deficiency
     E61.7 Deficiency of multiple nutrient elements
     E61.8 Deficiency of other specified nutrient elements
     E61.9 Deficiency of nutrient element, unspecified

`N` Newborn: 0   `P` Pediatric: 0-17   `M` Maternity: 9-64   `A` Adult: 15-124   `UNS` Unspecified Site   `MCC` Major Complication/Comorbidity   `CC` Complication/Comorbidity   `PE` POA Exempt

542   ICD-10-CM 2025

✓4ᵗʰ **E63 Other nutritional deficiencies**

     EXCLUDES 2   dehydration (E86.0)
                failure to thrive, adult (R62.7)
                failure to thrive, child (R62.51)
                feeding problems in newborn (P92.-)
                sequelae of malnutrition and other nutritional deficiencies
                (E64.-)

   E63.0 **Essential fatty acid [EFA] deficiency**
   E63.1 **Imbalance of constituents of food intake**
   E63.8 **Other specified nutritional deficiencies**
   E63.9 **Nutritional deficiency, unspecified**

✓4ᵗʰ **E64 Sequelae of malnutrition and other nutritional deficiencies**

     NOTE   This category is to be used to indicate conditions in categories E43, E44, E46, E50-E63 as the cause of sequelae, which are themselves classified elsewhere. The 'sequelae' include conditions specified as such; they also include the late effects of diseases classifiable to the above categories if the disease itself is no longer present

     Code first condition resulting from (sequela) of malnutrition and other nutritional deficiencies

   E64.0 **Sequelae of protein-calorie malnutrition**   CC PE
       EXCLUDES 2   retarded development following protein-calorie malnutrition (E45)
   E64.1 **Sequelae of vitamin A deficiency**   PE
   E64.2 **Sequelae of vitamin C deficiency**   PE
   E64.3 **Sequelae of rickets**   PE
   E64.8 **Sequelae of other nutritional deficiencies**   PE
   E64.9 **Sequelae of unspecified nutritional deficiency**   PE

Overweight, obesity and other hyperalimentation (E65-E68)

   E65 Localized adiposity
         Fat pad

✓4ᵗʰ **E66 Overweight and obesity**

     Code first obesity complicating pregnancy, childbirth and the puerperium, if applicable (O99.21-)
     ▶Use additional code to identify body mass index (BMI), if known, for adults (Z68.1-Z68.45) or pediatrics (Z68.5-)◀
     EXCLUDES 1   adiposogenital dystrophy (E23.6)
               lipomatosis NOS (E88.2)
               lipomatosis dolorosa [Dercum] (E88.2)
               Prader-Willi syndrome (Q87.11)
     EXCLUDES 2   ▶adiposogenital dystrophy (E23.6)◀
               ▶lipomatosis dolorosa [Dercum] (E88.2)◀
               ▶lipomatosis NOS (E88.2)◀
               ▶Prader-Willi syndrome (Q87.11)◀
     AHA: 2022,3Q,6; 2018,4Q,77,79-80
     TIP: Do not assign a BMI code (Z68.-) when a pregnant patient is documented as being overweight or obese. Only a code from subcategory O99.21- and a code from this category should be assigned.

✓5ᵗʰ   E66.0 **Obesity due to excess calories**
       E66.01 **Morbid (severe) obesity due to excess calories**   H11 HCC
          EXCLUDES 1   morbid (severe) obesity with alveolar hypoventilation (E66.2)
          AHA: 2022,3Q,6; 2022,2Q,9
          TIP: Assign this code when Class 3 obesity is documented. Class 3 obesity is synonymous with morbid obesity.
       E66.09 **Other obesity due to excess calories**
   E66.1 **Drug-induced obesity**
       Use additional code for adverse effect, if applicable, to identify drug (T36-T50 with fifth or sixth character 5)
   E66.2 **Morbid (severe) obesity with alveolar hypoventilation**   CC HCC
       Obesity hypoventilation syndrome (OHS)
       Pickwickian syndrome
   E66.3 **Overweight**
       AHA: 2018,4Q,78
▲ ✓5ᵗʰ   E66.8 **Other obesity**
● ✓6ᵗʰ   E66.81 **Obesity class**
●   E66.811 **Obesity, class 1**
●   E66.812 **Obesity, class 2**
●   E66.813 **Obesity, class 3**

●   E66.89 **Other obesity not elsewhere classified**
   E66.9 **Obesity, unspecified**
       Obesity NOS
       AHA: 2021,2Q,10

✓4ᵗʰ **E67 Other hyperalimentation**

     EXCLUDES 1   hyperalimentation NOS (R63.2)
               sequelae of hyperalimentation (E68)

   E67.0 **Hypervitaminosis A**
   E67.1 **Hypercarotenemia**
       DEF: Elevated blood carotene level as a result of excessive carotenoid ingestion or an inability to convert carotenoids to vitamin A. Characteristics often include yellow discoloration of the skin, which may follow overeating of carotenoid-rich foods such as carrots, sweet potatoes, or squash.
   E67.2 **Megavitamin-B6 syndrome**
   E67.3 **Hypervitaminosis D**
   E67.8 **Other specified hyperalimentation**

   E68 Sequelae of hyperalimentation
     Code first condition resulting from (sequela) of hyperalimentation

Metabolic disorders (E70-E88)

   EXCLUDES 1   androgen insensitivity syndrome (E34.5-)
               congenital adrenal hyperplasia (E25.0)
               hemolytic anemias attributable to enzyme disorders (D55.-)
               Marfan syndrome (Q87.4-)
               5-alpha-reductase deficiency (E29.1)
   EXCLUDES 2   Ehlers-Danlos syndromes (Q79.6-)
   AHA: 2018,2Q,6

✓4ᵗʰ **E70 Disorders of aromatic amino-acid metabolism**

   E70.0 **Classical phenylketonuria**   CC
   E70.1 **Other hyperphenylalaninemias**   CC
✓5ᵗʰ   E70.2 **Disorders of tyrosine metabolism**
       EXCLUDES 1   transitory tyrosinemia of newborn (P74.5)
       E70.20 **Disorder of tyrosine metabolism, unspecified**   CC
       E70.21 **Tyrosinemia**   CC
          Hypertyrosinemia
       E70.29 **Other disorders of tyrosine metabolism**
          Alkaptonuria
          Ochronosis
✓5ᵗʰ   E70.3 **Albinism**
       DEF: Absence of pigment in skin, hair, and eyes. This genetic condition is often accompanied by astigmatism, photophobia, and nystagmus.
       E70.30 **Albinism, unspecified**   CC
✓6ᵗʰ   E70.31 **Ocular albinism**
         E70.310 **X-linked ocular albinism**   CC
         E70.311 **Autosomal recessive ocular albinism**   CC
         E70.318 **Other ocular albinism**   CC
         E70.319 **Ocular albinism, unspecified**   CC
✓6ᵗʰ   E70.32 **Oculocutaneous albinism**
          EXCLUDES 1   Chediak-Higashi syndrome (E70.330)
                 Hermansky-Pudlak syndrome (E70.331)
         E70.320 **Tyrosinase negative oculocutaneous albinism**   CC
            Albinism I
            Oculocutaneous albinism ty-neg
         E70.321 **Tyrosinase positive oculocutaneous albinism**   CC
            Albinism II
            Oculocutaneous albinism ty-pos
         E70.328 **Other oculocutaneous albinism**   CC
            Cross syndrome
         E70.329 **Oculocutaneous albinism, unspecified**   CC
✓6ᵗʰ   E70.33 **Albinism with hematologic abnormality**
         E70.330 **Chediak-Higashi syndrome**   CC
         E70.331 **Hermansky-Pudlak syndrome**   CC
         E70.338 **Other albinism with hematologic abnormality**   CC
         E70.339 **Albinism with hematologic abnormality, unspecified**   CC
       E70.39 **Other specified albinism**   CC
          Piebaldism

✔ Additional Character Required   ✓x7ᵗʰ Placeholder   Questionable PDx   Manifestation   Unspecified   UPD Unacceptable PDx   H1 - H14 HAC   HCC CMS-HCC Dx   HIV HIV Dx

ICD-10-CM 2025   543

√5th **E70.4** Disorders of **histidine** metabolism

     E70.40 Disorders of histidine metabolism, unspecified `CC`

     E70.41 Histidinemia `CC`

     E70.49 Other disorders of histidine metabolism `CC`

E70.5 Disorders of **tryptophan** metabolism `CC`

√5th **E70.8** Other disorders of aromatic amino-acid metabolism

     AHA: 2020,4Q,15-16

     E70.81 Aromatic L-amino acid decarboxylase deficiency `CC`
       AADC deficiency

     E70.89 Other disorders of aromatic amino-acid metabolism `CC`

E70.9 Disorder of aromatic amino-acid metabolism, unspecified `CC`

√4th **E71** Disorders of branched-chain amino-acid metabolism and fatty-acid metabolism

E71.0 Maple-syrup-urine disease `CC`

√5th **E71.1** Other disorders of **branched-chain amino-acid** metabolism

     √6th **E71.11** Branched-chain **organic acidurias**

       E71.110 Isovaleric acidemia `CC`

       E71.111 3-methylglutaconic aciduria `CC`

       E71.118 Other branched-chain organic acidurias `CC`

     √6th **E71.12** Disorders of **propionate** metabolism

       E71.120 Methylmalonic acidemia `CC`

       E71.121 Propionic acidemia `CC`

       E71.128 Other disorders of propionate metabolism `CC`

     E71.19 Other disorders of branched-chain amino-acid metabolism `CC`
       Hyperleucine-isoleucinemia
       Hypervalinemia

E71.2 Disorder of branched-chain amino-acid metabolism, unspecified `CC`

√5th **E71.3** Disorders of fatty-acid metabolism

     EXCLUDES 1   peroxisomal disorders (E71.5)
         Refsum's disease (G60.1)
         Schilder's disease (G37.0)

     EXCLUDES 2   carnitine deficiency due to inborn error of metabolism (E71.42)

     E71.30 Disorder of fatty-acid metabolism, unspecified

     √6th **E71.31** Disorders of fatty-acid **oxidation**

       E71.310 Long chain/very long chain acyl CoA dehydrogenase deficiency `CC`
         LCAD deficiency
         VLCAD deficiency

       E71.311 Medium chain acyl CoA dehydrogenase deficiency `CC`
         MCAD deficiency

       E71.312 Short chain acyl CoA dehydrogenase deficiency `CC`
         SCAD deficiency

       E71.313 Glutaric aciduria type II `CC`
         Glutaric aciduria type II A
         Glutaric aciduria type II B
         Glutaric aciduria type II C

         EXCLUDES 1   glutaric aciduria (type 1) NOS (E72.3)

       E71.314 Muscle carnitine palmitoyltransferase deficiency `CC`

       E71.318 Other disorders of fatty-acid oxidation `CC`

     E71.32 Disorders of **ketone metabolism** `CC`

     E71.39 Other disorders of fatty-acid metabolism `CC`

√5th **E71.4** Disorders of **carnitine metabolism**

     EXCLUDES 1   muscle carnitine palmitoyltransferase deficiency (E71.314)

     E71.40 Disorder of carnitine metabolism, unspecified

     E71.41 Primary carnitine deficiency

     E71.42 Carnitine deficiency due to **inborn errors of metabolism**
       Code also associated inborn error or metabolism

     E71.43 Iatrogenic carnitine deficiency
       Carnitine deficiency due to hemodialysis
       Carnitine deficiency due to Valproic acid therapy

√6th **E71.44** Other **secondary** carnitine deficiency

     E71.440 Ruvalcaba-Myhre-Smith syndrome

     E71.448 Other secondary carnitine deficiency

√5th **E71.5** Peroxisomal disorders

     EXCLUDES 1   Schilder's disease (G37.0)

     E71.50 Peroxisomal disorder, unspecified `CC`

     √6th **E71.51** Disorders of peroxisome **biogenesis**
       Group 1 peroxisomal disorders

       EXCLUDES 1   Refsum's disease (G60.1)

       E71.510 Zellweger syndrome `CC`

       E71.511 Neonatal adrenoleukodystrophy `CC`

         EXCLUDES 1   X-linked adrenoleukodystrophy (E71.42-)

       E71.518 Other disorders of peroxisome biogenesis `CC`

     √6th **E71.52** X-linked adrenoleukodystrophy

       E71.520 Childhood cerebral X-linked adrenoleukodystrophy `CC`

       E71.521 Adolescent X-linked adrenoleukodystrophy `CC`

       E71.522 Adrenomyeloneuropathy `CC`

       E71.528 Other X-linked adrenoleukodystrophy `CC`
         Addison only phenotype adrenoleukodystrophy
         Addison-Schilder adrenoleukodystrophy

       E71.529 X-linked adrenoleukodystrophy, unspecified type `CC`

     E71.53 Other **group 2** peroxisomal disorders `CC`

     √6th **E71.54** Other peroxisomal disorders

       E71.540 Rhizomelic chondrodysplasia punctata `CC`

       EXCLUDES 1   chondrodysplasia punctata NOS (Q77.3)

       E71.541 Zellweger-like syndrome `CC`

       E71.542 Other group 3 peroxisomal disorders `CC`

       E71.548 Other peroxisomal disorders `CC`

√4th **E72** Other disorders of amino-acid metabolism

     EXCLUDES 1   disorders of:
       aromatic amino-acid metabolism (E70.-)
       branched-chain amino-acid metabolism (E71.0-E71.2)
       fatty-acid metabolism (E71.3)
       purine and pyrimidine metabolism (E79.-)
       gout (M1A.-, M10.-)

√5th **E72.0** Disorders of amino-acid **transport**

     EXCLUDES 1   disorders of tryptophan metabolism (E70.5)

     E72.00 Disorders of amino-acid transport, unspecified `CC`

     E72.01 Cystinuria `CC`

     E72.02 Hartnup's disease `CC`

     E72.03 Lowe's syndrome `CC`
       Use additional code for associated glaucoma (H42)

     E72.04 Cystinosis `CC`
       Fanconi (-de Toni) (-Debre) syndrome with cystinosis

       EXCLUDES 1   Fanconi (-de Toni) (-Debre) syndrome without cystinosis (E72.09)

     E72.09 Other disorders of amino-acid transport `CC`
       Fanconi (-de Toni) (-Debre) syndrome, unspecified

√5th **E72.1** Disorders of **sulfur-bearing** amino-acid metabolism

     EXCLUDES 1   cystinosis (E72.04)
       cystinuria (E72.01)
       transcobalamin II deficiency (D51.2)

     E72.10 Disorders of sulfur-bearing amino-acid metabolism, unspecified `CC`

     E72.11 Homocystinuria `CC`
       Cystathionine synthase deficiency
       AHA: 2021,4Q,28

     E72.12 Methylenetetrahydrofolate reductase deficiency `CC`

     E72.19 Other disorders of sulfur-bearing amino-acid metabolism `CC`
       Cystathioninuria
       Methioninemia
       Sulfite oxidase deficiency

N Newborn: 0   **P** Pediatric: 0-17   **M** Maternity: 9-64   **A** Adult: 15-124   **UNS** Unspecified Site   **MCC** Major Complication/Comorbidity   **CC** Complication/Comorbidity   **PE** POA Exempt

544
ICD-10-CM 2025

√5ᵗʰ E72.2 **Disorders of urea cycle metabolism**

> **EXCLUDES 1**   *disorders of ornithine metabolism (E72.4)*

    E72.20 **Disorder of urea cycle metabolism, unspecified** `CC`
        Hyperammonemia

> **EXCLUDES 1**   *hyperammonemia- hyperornithinemia-*
> *homocitrullinemia syndrome E72.4*
> *transient hyperammonemia of newborn*
> *(P74.6)*

    E72.21 **Argininemia** `CC`
    E72.22 **Arginosuccinic aciduria** `CC`
    E72.23 **Citrullinemia** `CC`
    E72.29 **Other disorders of urea cycle metabolism** `CC`

E72.3 **Disorders of lysine and hydroxylysine metabolism** `CC`
        Glutaric aciduria NOS
        Glutaric aciduria (type I)
        Hydroxylysinemia
        Hyperlysinemia

> **EXCLUDES 1**   *glutaric aciduria type II (E71.313)*
> *Refsum's disease (G60.1)*
> *Zellweger syndrome (E71.510)*

E72.4 **Disorders of ornithine metabolism** `CC`
        Hyperammonemia-Hyperornithinemia-Homocitrullinemia
        syndrome
        Ornithinemia (types I, II)
        Ornithine transcarbamylase deficiency

> **EXCLUDES 1**   *hereditary choroidal dystrophy (H31.2-)*

√5ᵗʰ E72.5 **Disorders of glycine metabolism**

    E72.50 **Disorder of glycine metabolism, unspecified** `CC`
    E72.51 **Non-ketotic hyperglycinemia** `CC`
    E72.52 **Trimethylaminuria** `CC`
    E72.53 **Primary hyperoxaluria** `CC` `HCC`
        Oxalosis
        Oxaluria
        AHA: 2018,4Q,29
    E72.59 **Other disorders of glycine metabolism** `CC`
        D-glycericacidemia
        Hyperhydroxyprolinemia
        Hyperprolinemia (types I, II)
        Sarcosinemia

√5ᵗʰ E72.8 **Other specified disorders of amino-acid metabolism**
        AHA: 2018,4Q,5

    E72.81 **Disorders of gamma aminobutyric acid metabolism** `CC`
        4-hydroxybutyric aciduria
        Disorders of GABA metabolism
        GABA metabolic defect
        GABA transaminase deficiency
        GABA-T deficiency
        Gamma-hydroxybutyric aciduria
        SSADHD
        Succinic semialdehyde dehydrogenase deficiency
    E72.89 **Other specified disorders of amino-acid metabolism** `CC`
        Disorders of beta-amino-acid metabolism
        Disorders of gamma-glutamyl cycle

E72.9 **Disorder of amino-acid metabolism, unspecified** `CC`

√4ᵗʰ E73 **Lactose intolerance**
        DEF: Inability to break down sugar in dairy products due to a deficiency in the enzyme lactase.

    E73.0 **Congenital lactase deficiency**
    E73.1 **Secondary lactase deficiency**
    E73.8 **Other lactose intolerance**
    E73.9 **Lactose intolerance, unspecified**

√4ᵗʰ E74 **Other disorders of carbohydrate metabolism**

> **EXCLUDES 1**   *diabetes mellitus (E08-E13)*
> *hypoglycemia NOS (E16.2)*
> *increased secretion of glucagon (E16.3)*
> *mucopolysaccharidosis (E76.0-E76.3)*

√5ᵗʰ E74.0 **Glycogen storage disease**

    E74.00 **Glycogen storage disease, unspecified** `CC` `HCC`
    E74.01 **von Gierke disease** `CC` `HCC`
        Type I glycogen storage disease
    E74.02 **Pompe disease** `CC` `HCC`
        Cardiac glycogenosis
        Type II glycogen storage disease

    E74.03 **Cori disease** `CC` `HCC`
        Forbes disease
        Type III glycogen storage disease
    E74.04 **McArdle disease** `CC` `HCC`
        Type V glycogen storage disease
    E74.05 **Lysosome-associated membrane protein 2 [LAMP2] deficiency** `CC` `HCC`
        Danon disease
        Code also, if applicable, associated manifestations such as:
          dilated cardiomyopathy (I42.0)
          obstructive hypertrophic cardiomyopathy (I42.1)
        AHA: 2023,4Q,11
    E74.09 **Other glycogen storage disease** `CC` `HCC`
        Andersen disease
        Glycogen storage disease, types 0, IV, VI-XI
        Hers disease
        Liver phosphorylase deficiency
        Muscle phosphofructokinase deficiency
        Tauri disease

√5ᵗʰ E74.1 **Disorders of fructose metabolism**

> **EXCLUDES 1**   *muscle phosphofructokinase deficiency (E74.09)*

    E74.10 **Disorder of fructose metabolism, unspecified**
    E74.11 **Essential fructosuria**
        Fructokinase deficiency
    E74.12 **Hereditary fructose intolerance**
        Fructosemia
    E74.19 **Other disorders of fructose metabolism**
        Fructose-1, 6-diphosphatase deficiency

√5ᵗʰ E74.2 **Disorders of galactose metabolism**

    E74.20 **Disorders of galactose metabolism, unspecified** `CC`
    E74.21 **Galactosemia** `CC`
        DEF: Any of three genetic disorders caused by a defective galactose metabolism. Symptoms include failure to thrive in infancy, jaundice, liver and spleen damage, cataracts, and mental retardation.
    E74.29 **Other disorders of galactose metabolism** `CC`
        Galactokinase deficiency

√5ᵗʰ E74.3 **Other disorders of intestinal carbohydrate absorption**

> **EXCLUDES 2**   *lactose intolerance (E73.-)*

    E74.31 **Sucrase-isomaltase deficiency**
    E74.39 **Other disorders of intestinal carbohydrate absorption**
        Disorder of intestinal carbohydrate absorption NOS
        Glucose-galactose malabsorption
        Sucrase deficiency

E74.4 **Disorders of pyruvate metabolism and gluconeogenesis** `CC`
        Deficiency of phosphoenolpyruvate carboxykinase
        Deficiency of pyruvate carboxylase
        Deficiency of pyruvate dehydrogenase

> **EXCLUDES 1**   *disorders of pyruvate metabolism and gluconeogenesis*
> *with anemia (D55.-)*
> *Leigh's syndrome (G31.82)*

√5ᵗʰ E74.8 **Other specified disorders of carbohydrate metabolism**
        AHA: 2020,4Q,16

    √6ᵗʰ E74.81 **Disorders of glucose transport, not elsewhere classified**
        E74.810 **Glucose transporter protein type 1 deficiency** `CC`
           De Vivo syndrome
           Glucose transport defect, blood-brain barrier
           Glut1 deficiency
           GLUT1 deficiency syndrome 1, infantile onset
           GLUT1 deficiency syndrome 2, childhood onset
        E74.818 **Other disorders of glucose transport** `CC`
           (Familial) renal glycosuria
        E74.819 **Disorders of glucose transport, unspecified** `CC`
    √6ᵗʰ E74.82 **Disorders of citrate metabolism**
        E74.820 **SLC13A5 Citrate Transporter Disorder** `CC`
        E74.829 **Other disorders of citrate metabolism** `CC`

☑ Additional Character Required   √7ᵗʰ Placeholder   Questionable PDx   Manifestation   Unspecified   **UPD** Unacceptable PDx   **H1 - H14** HAC   **HCC** CMS-HCC Dx   **HIV** HIV Dx

ICD-10-CM 2025   545

Chapter 4. Endocrine, Nutritional and Metabolic Diseases

E74.89   **Other specified disorders of carbohydrate metabolism**   CC
Essential pentosuria
AHA: 2023,3Q,3

E74.9   **Disorder of carbohydrate metabolism, unspecified**

√4th **E75** **Disorders of sphingolipid metabolism and other lipid storage disorders**
> EXCLUDES 1   mucolipidosis, types I-III (E77.0-E77.1)
> Refsum's disease (G60.1)

√5th **E75.0** **GM2 gangliosidosis**

E75.00   **GM2 gangliosidosis, unspecified**   CC

E75.01   **Sandhoff disease**   CC

E75.02   **Tay-Sachs disease**   CC
DEF: Genetic mutation of the HEXA gene that inhibits the breakdown of a toxic substance called ganglioside. The accumulation of ganglioside results in destruction of the neurons in the brain and spinal cord.

Tay-Sachs Disease

E75.09   **Other GM2 gangliosidosis**   CC
Adult GM2 gangliosidosis
Juvenile GM2 gangliosidosis

√5th **E75.1** **Other and unspecified gangliosidosis**

E75.10   **Unspecified gangliosidosis**   CC
Gangliosidosis NOS

E75.11   **Mucolipidosis IV**   CC

E75.19   **Other gangliosidosis**   CC
GM1 gangliosidosis
GM3 gangliosidosis

√5th **E75.2** **Other sphingolipidosis**
> EXCLUDES 1   adrenoleukodystrophy [Addison-Schilder] (E71.528)

E75.21   **Fabry (-Anderson) disease**   HCC

E75.22   **Gaucher disease**   HCC

E75.23   **Krabbe disease**   CC

√6th **E75.24** **Niemann-Pick disease**
Acid sphingomyelinase deficiency (ASMD)

E75.240   **Niemann-Pick disease type A**
Acid sphingomyelinase deficiency type A (ASMD type A)
Infantile neurovisceral acid sphingomyelinase deficiency

E75.241   **Niemann-Pick disease type B**
Acid sphingomyelinase deficiency type B (ASMD type B)
Chronic visceral acid sphingomyelinase deficiency

E75.242   **Niemann-Pick disease type C**

E75.243   **Niemann-Pick disease type D**

E75.244   **Niemann-Pick disease type A/B**
Acid sphingomyelinase deficiency type A/B (ASMD type A/B)
Chronic neurovisceral acid sphingomyelinase deficiency
AHA: 2021,4Q,8-9

E75.248   **Other Niemann-Pick disease**

E75.249   **Niemann-Pick disease, unspecified**
Acid sphingomyelinase deficiency (ASMD) NOS

E75.25   **Metachromatic leukodystrophy**   CC

E75.26   **Sulfatase deficiency**   CC
Multiple sulfatase deficiency (MSD)
AHA: 2018,4Q,5-6

E75.27   **Pelizaeus-Merzbacher disease**   CC
AHA: 2023,4Q,12-13

E75.28   **Canavan disease**   CC
AHA: 2023,4Q,12-13

E75.29   **Other sphingolipidosis**   CC
Farber's syndrome
Sulfatide lipidosis

E75.3   **Sphingolipidosis, unspecified**

E75.4   **Neuronal ceroid lipofuscinosis**   CC
Batten disease
Bielschowsky-Jansky disease
Kufs disease
Spielmeyer-Vogt disease

E75.5   **Other lipid storage disorders**
Cerebrotendinous cholesterosis [van Bogaert-Scherer-Epstein]
Wolman's disease

E75.6   **Lipid storage disorder, unspecified**

√4th **E76** **Disorders of glycosaminoglycan metabolism**

√5th **E76.0** **Mucopolysaccharidosis, type I**

E76.01   **Hurler's syndrome**   CC HCC

E76.02   **Hurler-Scheie syndrome**   CC HCC

E76.03   **Scheie's syndrome**   CC HCC

E76.1   **Mucopolysaccharidosis, type II**   CC HCC
Hunter's syndrome

√5th **E76.2** **Other mucopolysaccharidoses**

√6th **E76.21** **Morquio mucopolysaccharidoses**

E76.210   **Morquio A mucopolysaccharidoses**   CC HCC
Classic Morquio syndrome
Morquio syndrome A
Mucopolysaccharidosis, type IVA

E76.211   **Morquio B mucopolysaccharidoses**   CC HCC
Morquio-like mucopolysaccharidoses
Morquio-like syndrome
Morquio syndrome B
Mucopolysaccharidosis, type IVB

E76.219   **Morquio mucopolysaccharidoses, unspecified**   CC HCC
Morquio syndrome
Mucopolysaccharidosis, type IV

E76.22   **Sanfilippo mucopolysaccharidoses**   CC HCC
Mucopolysaccharidosis, type III (A) (B) (C) (D)
Sanfilippo A syndrome
Sanfilippo B syndrome
Sanfilippo C syndrome
Sanfilippo D syndrome

E76.29   **Other mucopolysaccharidoses**   CC HCC
beta-Glucuronidase deficiency
Maroteaux-Lamy (mild) (severe) syndrome
Mucopolysaccharidosis, types VI, VII

E76.3   **Mucopolysaccharidosis, unspecified**   CC HCC

E76.8   **Other disorders of glycosaminoglycan metabolism**   CC

E76.9   **Glucosaminoglycan metabolism disorder, unspecified**   CC

√4th **E77** **Disorders of glycoprotein metabolism**

E77.0   **Defects in post-translational modification of lysosomal enzymes**
Mucolipidosis II [I-cell disease]
Mucolipidosis III [pseudo-Hurler polydystrophy]

E77.1   **Defects in glycoprotein degradation**
Aspartylglucosaminuria
Fucosidosis
Mannosidosis
Sialidosis [mucolipidosis I]

E77.8   **Other disorders of glycoprotein metabolism**

E77.9   **Disorder of glycoprotein metabolism, unspecified**

N Newborn: 0   P Pediatric: 0-17   M Maternity: 9-64   A Adult: 15-124   UNS Unspecified Site   MCC Major Complication/Comorbidity   CC Complication/Comorbidity   PE POA Exempt

546   ICD-10-CM 2025

✓4ᵗʰ **E78 Disorders of lipoprotein metabolism and other lipidemias**

   EXCLUDES 1   *sphingolipidosis (E75.0-E75.3)*

✓5ᵗʰ **E78.0 Pure hypercholesterolemia**
   AHA: 2016,4Q,13-14

   E78.00 Pure hypercholesterolemia, unspecified
   Fredrickson's hyperlipoproteinemia, type IIa
   Hyperbetalipoproteinemia
   Low-density-lipoprotein-type [LDL]
      hyperlipoproteinemia
   (Pure) hypercholesterolemia NOS
   AHA: 2023,2Q,9; 2022,2Q,5-6

   E78.01 Familial hypercholesterolemia

E78.1 Pure hyperglyceridemia
   Elevated fasting triglycerides
   Endogenous hyperglyceridemia
   Fredrickson's hyperlipoproteinemia, type IV
   Hyperlipidemia, group B
   Hyperprebetalipoproteinemia
   Very-low-density-lipoprotein-type [VLDL] hyperlipoprcteinemia

E78.2 Mixed hyperlipidemia
   Broad- or floating-betalipoproteinemia
   Combined hyperlipidemia NOS
   Elevated cholesterol with elevated triglycerides NEC
   Fredrickson's hyperlipoproteinemia, type IIb or III
   Hyperbetalipoproteinemia with prebetalipoproteinemia
   Hypercholesteremia with endogenous hyperglyceridemia
   Hyperlipidemia, group C
   Tubo-eruptive xanthoma
   Xanthoma tuberosum
      EXCLUDES 1   *cerebrotendinous cholesterosis [van Bogaert-Scherer-Epstein] (E75.5)*
      familial combined hyperlipidemia (E78.49)
   AHA: 2023,2Q,9; 2022,2Q,6

E78.3 Hyperchylomicronemia
   Chylomicron retention disease
   Fredrickson's hyperlipoproteinemia, type I or V
   Hyperlipidemia, group D
   Mixed hyperglyceridemia

✓5ᵗʰ **E78.4 Other hyperlipidemia**
   AHA: 2018,4Q,6

   E78.41 Elevated Lipoprotein(a)
   Elevated Lp(a)

   E78.49 Other hyperlipidemia
   Familial combined hyperlipidemia

E78.5 Hyperlipidemia, unspecified
   AHA: 2022,2Q,5

E78.6 Lipoprotein deficiency
   Abetalipoproteinemia
   Depressed HDL cholesterol
   High-density lipoprotein deficiency
   Hypoalphalipoproteinemia
   Hypobetalipoproteinemia (familial)
   Lecithin cholesterol acyltransferase deficiency
   Tangier disease

✓5ᵗʰ **E78.7 Disorders of bile acid and cholesterol metabolism**
      EXCLUDES 1   *Niemann-Pick disease type C (E75.242)*

   E78.70 Disorder of bile acid and cholesterol metabolism, unspecified

   E78.71 Barth syndrome   CC

   E78.72 Smith-Lemli-Opitz syndrome   CC

   E78.79 Other disorders of bile acid and cholesterol metabolism
   AHA: 2023,1Q,26

✓5ᵗʰ **E78.8 Other disorders of lipoprotein metabolism**

   E78.81 Lipoid dermatoarthritis

   E78.89 Other lipoprotein metabolism disorders

E78.9 Disorder of lipoprotein metabolism, unspecified

✓4ᵗʰ **E79 Disorders of purine and pyrimidine metabolism**

   EXCLUDES 1   *Ataxia-telangiectasia (Q87.19)*
   Bloom's syndrome (Q82.8)
   Cockayne's syndrome (Q87.19)
   calculus of kidney (N20.0)
   combined immunodeficiency disorders (D81.-)
   Fanconi's anemia (D61.09)
   gout (M1A.-, M10.-)
   orotaciduric anemia (D53.0)
   progeria (E34.8)
   Werner's syndrome (E34.8)
   xeroderma pigmentosum (Q82.1)

E79.0 Hyperuricemia without signs of inflammatory arthritis and tophaceous disease
   Asymptomatic hyperuricemia

E79.1 Lesch-Nyhan syndrome   CC HCC
   HGPRT deficiency

E79.2 Myoadenylate deaminase deficiency   CC

✓5ᵗʰ **E79.8 Other disorders of purine and pyrimidine metabolism**
   AHA: 2023,4Q,12-13

   E79.81 Aicardi-Goutieres syndrome   CC

   E79.82 Hereditary xanthinuria   CC

   E79.89 Other specified disorders of purine and pyrimidine metabolism   CC

E79.9 Disorder of purine and pyrimidine metabolism, unspecified   CC

✓4ᵗʰ **E80 Disorders of porphyrin and bilirubin metabolism**

   INCLUDES   defects of catalase and peroxidase

E80.0 Hereditary erythropoietic porphyria   CC HCC
   Congenital erythropoietic porphyria
   Erythropoietic protoporphyria

E80.1 Porphyria cutanea tarda   CC HCC

✓5ᵗʰ **E80.2 Other and unspecified porphyria**

   E80.20 Unspecified porphyria   CC HCC
   Porphyria NOS

   E80.21 Acute intermittent (hepatic) porphyria   CC HCC

   E80.29 Other porphyria   CC HCC
   Hereditary coproporphyria

E80.3 Defects of catalase and peroxidase   CC HCC
   Acatalasia [Takahara]

E80.4 Gilbert syndrome

E80.5 Crigler-Najjar syndrome

E80.6 Other disorders of bilirubin metabolism
   Dubin-Johnson syndrome
   Rotor's syndrome
   AHA: 2022,3Q,7
   TIP: Assign codes E80.6 and K76.89 to report benign recurrent intrahepatic cholestasis (BRIC) or progressive familial intrahepatic cholestasis (PFIC).

E80.7 Disorder of bilirubin metabolism, unspecified

✓4ᵗʰ **E83 Disorders of mineral metabolism**

   EXCLUDES 1   *dietary mineral deficiency (E58-E61)*
   parathyroid disorders (E20-E21)
   vitamin D deficiency (E55.-)

✓5ᵗʰ **E83.0 Disorders of copper metabolism**

   E83.00 Disorder of copper metabolism, unspecified   HCC

   E83.01 Wilson's disease   HCC
   Code also associated Kayser Fleischer ring (H18.04-)

   E83.09 Other disorders of copper metabolism   HCC
   Menkes' (kinky hair) (steely hair) disease

✓5ᵗʰ **E83.1 Disorders of iron metabolism**

      EXCLUDES 1   *iron deficiency anemia (D50.-)*
      sideroblastic anemia (D64.0-D64.3)

   E83.10 Disorder of iron metabolism, unspecified

✓6ᵗʰ **E83.11 Hemochromatosis**

      EXCLUDES 1   *GALD (P78.84)*
      gestational alloimmune liver disease (P78.84)
      neonatal hemochromatosis (P78.84)

   E83.110 Hereditary hemochromatosis
   Bronzed diabetes
   Pigmentary cirrhosis (of liver)
   Primary (hereditary) hemochromatosis

☑ Additional Character Required   ✓x7ᵗʰ Placeholder   **Questionable PDx**   Manifestation   Unspecified   UPD Unacceptable PDx   H1 - H14 HAC   HCC CMS-HCC Dx   HIV HIV Dx

ICD-10-CM 2025   **547**

E83.111   **Hemochromatosis due to repeated red blood cell transfusions**
Iron overload due to repeated red blood cell transfusions
Transfusion (red blood cell) associated hemochromatosis

    E83.118   **Other hemochromatosis**

    E83.119   **Hemochromatosis, unspecified**

E83.19   **Other disorders of iron metabolism**
Use additional code, if applicable, for idiopathic pulmonary hemosiderosis (J84.03)

E83.2   Disorders of zinc metabolism
Acrodermatitis enteropathica

✓5th **E83.3   Disorders of phosphorus metabolism and phosphatases**
    EXCLUDES 1   *adult osteomalacia (M83.-)*
              osteoporosis (M80.-)

    E83.30   **Disorder of phosphorus metabolism, unspecified**

    E83.31   **Familial hypophosphatemia**   HCC
Vitamin D-resistant osteomalacia
Vitamin D-resistant rickets
    EXCLUDES 1   *vitamin D-deficiency rickets (E55.0)*

    E83.32   **Hereditary vitamin D-dependent rickets (type 1) (type 2)**
25-hydroxyvitamin D 1-alpha-hydroxylase deficiency
Pseudovitamin D deficiency
Vitamin D receptor defect

    E83.39   **Other disorders of phosphorus metabolism**
Acid phosphatase deficiency
Hypophosphatasia

✓5th **E83.4   Disorders of magnesium metabolism**

    E83.40   **Disorders of magnesium metabolism, unspecified**

    E83.41   **Hypermagnesemia**
AHA: 2016,4Q,54

    E83.42   **Hypomagnesemia**

    E83.49   **Other disorders of magnesium metabolism**

✓5th **E83.5   Disorders of calcium metabolism**
    EXCLUDES 1   *autoimmune hypoparathyroidism (E20.812)*
              autosomal dominant hypocalcemia (E20.810)
              chondrocalcinosis (M11.1-M11.2)
              hungry bone syndrome (E83.81)
              hyperparathyroidism (E21.0-E21.3)
              secondary hypoparathyroidism in diseases classified elsewhere (E20.811)

    E83.50   **Unspecified disorder of calcium metabolism**

    E83.51   **Hypocalcemia**

    E83.52   **Hypercalcemia**
Familial hypocalciuric hypercalcemia

    E83.59   **Other disorders of calcium metabolism**

✓5th **E83.8   Other disorders of mineral metabolism**

    E83.81   **Hungry bone syndrome**

    E83.89   **Other disorders of mineral metabolism**

E83.9   Disorder of mineral metabolism, unspecified

✓4th **E84   Cystic fibrosis**
    INCLUDES   mucoviscidosis
Code also exocrine pancreatic insufficiency (K86.81)
DEF: Genetic disorder affecting the respiratory, digestive, and reproductive systems in infants to young adults by disturbing exocrine gland function and causing chronic pulmonary disease with excess mucus production and pancreatic deficiency.

    E84.0   Cystic fibrosis with pulmonary manifestations   MCC HCC
Use additional code to identify any infectious organism present, such as:
Pseudomonas (B96.5)
AHA: 2021,1Q,23

✓5th   **E84.1   Cystic fibrosis with intestinal manifestations**

       E84.11   **Meconium ileus in cystic fibrosis**   MCC HCC N
       EXCLUDES 1   *meconium ileus not due to cystic fibrosis (P76.0)*

       E84.19   **Cystic fibrosis with other intestinal manifestations**   CC HCC
Distal intestinal obstruction syndrome

    E84.8   Cystic fibrosis with other manifestations   CC HCC

    E84.9   Cystic fibrosis, unspecified   CC HCC

✓4th **E85   Amyloidosis**
    EXCLUDES 2   *Alzheimer's disease (G30.0-)*
DEF: Conditions of diverse etiologies characterized by the accumulation of insoluble fibrillar proteins (amyloid) in various organs and tissues of the body, compromising vital functions.

    E85.0   Non-neuropathic heredofamilial amyloidosis   CC HCC
Hereditary amyloid nephropathy
Code also associated disorders, such as:
autoinflammatory syndromes (M04.-)
    EXCLUDES 2   *transthyretin-related (ATTR) familial amyloid cardiomyopathy (E85.4)*

    E85.1   Neuropathic heredofamilial amyloidosis   CC HCC
Amyloid polyneuropathy (Portuguese)
Transthyretin-related (ATTR) familial amyloid polyneuropathy
AHA: 2012,4Q,99

    E85.2   Heredofamilial amyloidosis, unspecified   CC HCC

    E85.3   Secondary systemic amyloidosis   CC HCC
Hemodialysis-associated amyloidosis

    E85.4   Organ-limited amyloidosis   CC HCC
Localized amyloidosis
Transthyretin-related (ATTR) familial amyloid cardiomyopathy

✓5th   **E85.8   Other amyloidosis**
AHA: 2017,4Q,7

       E85.81   **Light chain (AL) amyloidosis**   CC HCC
AHA: AHA:2024,2Q,9

       E85.82   **Wild-type transthyretin-related (ATTR) amyloidosis**   CC HCC
Senile systemic amyloidosis (SSA)

       E85.89   **Other amyloidosis**   CC HCC

    E85.9   Amyloidosis, unspecified   CC HCC

✓4th **E86   Volume depletion**
Use additional code(s) for any associated disorders of electrolyte and acid-base balance (E87.-)
    EXCLUDES 1   *dehydration of newborn (P74.1)*
              postprocedural hypovolemic shock (T81.19)
              traumatic hypovolemic shock (T79.4)
    EXCLUDES 2   *hypovolemic shock NOS (R57.1)*
AHA: 2019,2Q,7; 2018,2Q,6

    E86.0   Dehydration
AHA: 2019,2Q,7; 2019,1Q,12; 2014,1Q,7
TIP: Can be assigned in addition to hypernatremia (E87.0) or hyponatremia (E87.1), when documented.

    E86.1   Hypovolemia
Depletion of volume of plasma

    E86.9   Volume depletion, unspecified
DEF: Depletion of total body water (dehydration) and/or contraction of total intravascular plasma (hypovolemia).

✓4th **E87   Other disorders of fluid, electrolyte and acid-base balance**
    EXCLUDES 1   *diabetes insipidus (E23.2)*
              electrolyte imbalance associated with hyperemesis gravidarum (O21.1)
              electrolyte imbalance following ectopic or molar pregnancy (O08.5)
              familial periodic paralysis (G72.3)
              metabolic acidemia in newborn, unspecified (P19.9)
AHA: 2018,2Q,6

    E87.0   Hyperosmolality and hypernatremia   CC
Sodium [Na] excess
Sodium [Na] overload
    EXCLUDES 1   ~~*diabetes with hyperosmolarity (E08, E09, E11, E13 with final characters .00 or .01)*~~
    EXCLUDES 2   ▶*diabetes with hyperosmolarity (E08, E09, E11, E13 with final characters .00 or .01)*◀
AHA: 2022,1Q,28; 2014,1Q,7
TIP: Assign an additional code for dehydration (E86.0), when documented.

    E87.1   Hypo-osmolality and hyponatremia   CC
Sodium [Na] deficiency
    EXCLUDES 1   *syndrome of inappropriate secretion of antidiuretic hormone (E22.2)*
AHA: 2014,1Q,7
TIP: Assign an additional code for dehydration (E86.0), when documented.

☑5ᵗʰ **E87.2** Acidosis

    EXCLUDES 1   *diabetic acidosis - see categories E08-E10, E11, E13 with ketoacidosis*

    AHA: 2022,4Q,13-14; 2020,3Q,30

    DEF: Reduction of alkaline in the blood and tissues caused by an increase in acid and decrease in bicarbonate.

    E87.20   **Acidosis, unspecified**   CC

        Lactic acidosis NOS

        Metabolic acidosis NOS

        Code also, if applicable, respiratory failure with hypercapnia (J96. with 5th character 2)

    E87.21   **Acute** metabolic acidosis   CC

        Acute lactic acidosis

    E87.22   **Chronic** metabolic acidosis   CC

        Chronic lactic acidosis

        Code first underlying etiology, if applicable

        AHA: 2022,4Q,14

    E87.29   **Other acidosis**   CC

        Respiratory acidosis NOS

        EXCLUDES 2   *acute respiratory acidosis (J96.02)*

                  chronic respiratory acidosis (J96.12)

E87.3 Alkalosis   CC

     Alkalosis NOS

     Metabolic alkalosis

     Respiratory alkalosis

E87.4 Mixed disorder of acid-base balance   CC

E87.5 Hyperkalemia

     Potassium [K] excess

     Potassium [K] overload

E87.6 Hypokalemia

     Potassium [K] deficiency

☑5ᵗʰ **E87.7** Fluid overload

    EXCLUDES 1   *edema NOS (R60.9)*

               fluid retention (R60.9)

    E87.70   **Fluid overload, unspecified**

        AHA: 2023,1Q,19

    E87.71   **Transfusion associated** circulatory overload

        Fluid overload due to transfusion (blood) (blood components)

        TACO

    E87.79   **Other fluid overload**

E87.8 Other disorders of electrolyte and fluid balance, not elsewhere classified

     Electrolyte imbalance NOS

     Hyperchloremia

     Hypochloremia

☑4ᵗʰ **E88** **Other and unspecified metabolic disorders**

     Use additional codes for associated conditions

    EXCLUDES 1   *histiocytosis X (chronic) (C96.6)*

☑5ᵗʰ **E88.0** Disorders of plasma-protein metabolism, not elsewhere classified

    EXCLUDES 1   *monoclonal gammopathy (of undetermined significance) (D47.2)*

               polyclonal hypergammaglobulinemia (D89.0)

               Waldenstrom macroglobulinemia ▶(C88.00)◀

    EXCLUDES 2   *disorder of lipoprotein metabolism (E78.-)*

    E88.01   **Alpha-1-antitrypsin deficiency**   HCC

        AAT deficiency

    E88.02   **Plasminogen deficiency**   CC

        Dysplasminogenemia

        Hypoplasminogenemia

        Type 1 plasminogen deficiency

        Type 2 plasminogen deficiency

        Code also, if applicable, ligneous conjunctivitis (H10.51)

        Use additional code for associated findings, such as:

          hydrocephalus (G91.4)

          otitis media (H67.-)

          respiratory disorder related to plasminogen deficiency (J99)

        AHA: 2018,4Q,6-7

    E88.09   **Other disorders of plasma-protein metabolism, not elsewhere classified**

        Bisalbuminemia

E88.1 Lipodystrophy, not elsewhere classified

     Lipodystrophy NOS

    EXCLUDES 1   *Whipple's disease (K90.81)*

E88.2 Lipomatosis, not elsewhere classified

     Lipomatosis NOS

     Lipomatosis (Check) dolorosa [Dercum]

E88.3 Tumor lysis syndrome   MCC

     Tumor lysis syndrome (spontaneous)

     Tumor lysis syndrome following antineoplastic drug chemotherapy

     Use additional code for adverse effect, if applicable, to identify drug (T45.1X5)

     AHA: 2020,1Q,37; 2019,2Q,24

     DEF: Potentially fatal metabolic complication of tumor necrosis caused by spontaneous or treatment-related accumulation of byproducts from dying cancer cells. Symptoms include hyperkalemia, hyperphosphatemia, hypocalcemia, hyperuricemia, and hyperuricosuria.

☑5ᵗʰ **E88.4** Mitochondrial metabolism disorders

    EXCLUDES 1   *disorders of pyruvate metabolism (E74.4)*

               Kearns-Sayre syndrome (H49.81)

               Leber's disease (H47.22)

               Leigh's encephalopathy (G31.82)

               mitochondrial myopathy, NEC (G71.3)

               Reye's syndrome (G93.7)

    E88.40   **Mitochondrial metabolism disorder, unspecified**   CC

    E88.41   **MELAS syndrome**   CC

        Mitochondrial myopathy, encephalopathy, lactic acidosis and stroke-like episodes

    E88.42   **MERRF syndrome**   CC

        Myoclonic epilepsy associated with ragged-red fibers

        Code also progressive myoclonic epilepsy (G40.3-)

    E88.43   **Disorders of mitochondrial tRNA synthetases**   CC

        AHA: 2023,4Q,12-13

    E88.49   **Other mitochondrial metabolism disorders**   CC

☑5ᵗʰ **E88.8** Other specified metabolic disorders

    ☑6ᵗʰ **E88.81**   **Metabolic syndrome and other insulin resistance**

        Use additional codes for associated manifestations, such as:

          obesity (E66.-)

        AHA: 2023,4Q,13-14; 2022,3Q,6

        DEF: Group of health risks that increase the likelihood of developing heart disease, stroke, and diabetes. These risks include certain parameters for blood pressure, cholesterol, and glucose levels.

       E88.810   **Metabolic syndrome**

           Dysmetabolic syndrome

       E88.811   **Insulin resistance syndrome, Type A**

       E88.818   **Other insulin resistance**

           Insulin resistance syndrome, Type B

       E88.819   **Insulin resistance, unspecified**

    E88.82   **Obesity due to disruption of MC4R pathway**

        Use additional code, if applicable, to identify associated manifestations, such as polyphagia (R63.2)

        Use additional code to identify body mass index (BMI), if known (Z68.-)

    E88.89   **Other specified metabolic disorders**   HCC

        Launois-Bensaude adenolipomatosis

        EXCLUDES 1   *adult pulmonary Langerhans cell histiocytosis (J84.82)*

E88.9 Metabolic disorder, unspecified

E88.A Wasting disease (syndrome) due to underlying condition   UPD

     Cachexia due to underlying condition

     Code first underlying condition

    EXCLUDES 1   *cachexia NOS (R64)*

               nutritional marasmus (E41)

    EXCLUDES 2   *failure to thrive (R62.51, R62.7)*

     AHA: 2023,4Q,14-15

☑ Additional Character Required   ☑x7ᵗʰ Placeholder   Questionable PDx   Manifestation   Unspecified   UPD Unacceptable PDx   H1-H14 HAC   HCC CMS-HCC Dx   HIV HIV Dx

ICD-10-CM 2025   549

Postprocedural endocrine and metabolic complications and disorders, not elsewhere classified (E89)

√4ᵗʰ E89 Postprocedural endocrine and metabolic complications and disorders, not elsewhere classified
> **EXCLUDES 2**   *intraoperative complications of endocrine system organ or structure (E36.0-, E36.1-, E36.8)*

E89.0 Postprocedural hypothyroidism
Postirradiation hypothyroidism
Postsurgical hypothyroidism

E89.1 Postprocedural hypoinsulinemia   `CC`
Postpancreatectomy hyperglycemia
Postsurgical hypoinsulinemia
▶Code first, if applicable, diabetes mellitus (postpancreatectomy) (postprocedural) (E13.-)◀
Use additional code, if applicable, to identify:
   acquired absence of pancreas (Z90.41-)
   ~~diabetes mellitus (postpancreatectomy) (postprocedural) (E13.-)~~
   insulin use (Z79.4)
> **EXCLUDES 1**   *transient postprocedural hyperglycemia (R73.9)*
> *transient postprocedural hypoglycemia (E16.2)*

E89.2 Postprocedural hypoparathyroidism
Parathyroprival tetany
AHA: 2023,3Q,13

E89.3 Postprocedural hypopituitarism
Postirradiation hypopituitarism

√5ᵗʰ E89.4 Postprocedural ovarian failure

    E89.40 Asymptomatic postprocedural ovarian failure
      Postprocedural ovarian failure NOS

    E89.41 Symptomatic postprocedural ovarian failure
      Symptoms such as flushing, sleeplessness, headache, lack of concentration, associated with postprocedural menopause

E89.5 Postprocedural testicular hypofunction

E89.6 Postprocedural adrenocortical (-medullary) hypofunction   `CC`

√5ᵗʰ E89.8 Other postprocedural endocrine and metabolic complications and disorders
   AHA: 2016,4Q,9-10

   √6ᵗʰ E89.81 Postprocedural hemorrhage of an endocrine system organ or structure following a procedure

     E89.810 Postprocedural hemorrhage of an endocrine system organ or structure following an endocrine system procedure   `CC`

     E89.811 Postprocedural hemorrhage of an endocrine system organ or structure following other procedure   `CC`

   √6ᵗʰ E89.82 Postprocedural hematoma and seroma of an endocrine system organ or structure

     E89.820 Postprocedural hematoma of an endocrine system organ or structure following an endocrine system procedure   `CC`

     E89.821 Postprocedural hematoma of an endocrine system organ or structure following other procedure   `CC`

     E89.822 Postprocedural seroma of an endocrine system organ or structure following an endocrine system procedure   `CC`

     E89.823 Postprocedural seroma of an endocrine system organ or structure following other procedure   `CC`

   E89.89 Other postprocedural endocrine and metabolic complications and disorders   `CC`
     Use additional code, if applicable, to further specify disorder

Chapter 5. Mental, Behavioral and Neurodevelopmental Disorders (FØ1–F99)

Chapter-specific Guidelines with Coding Examples

The chapter-specific guidelines from the ICD-10-CM Official Guidelines for Coding and Reporting have been provided below. Along with these guidelines are coding examples, contained in the shaded boxes, that have been developed to help illustrate the coding and/or sequencing guidance found in these guidelines.

a. Pain disorders related to psychological factors

Assign code F45.41, for pain that is exclusively related to psychological disorders. As indicated by the Excludes 1 note under category G89, a code from category G89 should not be assigned with code F45.41.

> Perceived abdominal pain determined to be persistent somatoform pain disorder
>
> **F45.41   Pain disorder exclusively related to psychological factors**
>
> *Explanation*: This pain was diagnosed as being exclusively psychological; therefore, no code from category G89 is added.

Code F45.42, Pain disorders with related psychological factors, should be used with a code from category G89, Pain, not elsewhere classified, if there is documentation of a psychological component for a patient with acute or chronic pain.

See Section I.C.6. Pain

b. Mental and behavioral disorders due to psychoactive substance use

1) In remission

Selection of codes describing "in remission" for categories F10–F19, Mental and behavioral disorders due to psychoactive substance use (categories F10–F19 with -.11, -.21, -.91) requires the provider's clinical judgment and are assigned only on the basis of provider documentation (as defined in the Official Guidelines for Coding and Reporting), unless otherwise instructed by the classification.

Mild substance use disorders in early or sustained remission are classified to the appropriate codes for substance abuse in remission, and moderate or severe substance use disorders in early or sustained remission are classified to the appropriate codes for substance dependence in remission.

> Insomnia in patient with history of methamphetamine abuse; lab results indicate no current drug use
>
> **G47.00   Insomnia, unspecified**
>
> **F15.10   Other stimulant abuse, uncomplicated**
>
> *Explanation*: Insomnia is a common side-effect of stimulant use, such as methamphetamines. Although lab tests do not indicate that the patient is currently using methamphetamines, there is no specific documentation stating that the stimulant abuse is in remission. "History of" abuse does not equate to "in remission" in this instance.

2) Psychoactive substance use, abuse and dependence

When the provider documentation refers to use, abuse and dependence of the same substance (e.g. alcohol, opioid, cannabis, etc.), only one code should be assigned to identify the pattern of use based on the following hierarchy:

- If both use and abuse are documented, assign only the code for abuse
- If both abuse and dependence are documented, assign only the code for dependence
- If use, abuse and dependence are all documented, assign only the code for dependence
- If both use and dependence are documented, assign only the code for dependence.

> History and physical notes cannabis dependence; progress note says cannabis abuse
>
> **F12.20   Cannabis dependence, uncomplicated**
>
> *Explanation*: In the hierarchy, the dependence code is used if both abuse and dependence are documented.

> Discharge summary says cocaine abuse; progress notes list cocaine use
>
> **F14.10   Cocaine abuse, uncomplicated**
>
> *Explanation*: In the hierarchy, the abuse code is used if both abuse and use are documented.

3) Psychoactive substance use, unspecified

As with all other unspecified diagnoses, the codes for unspecified psychoactive substance use (F10.9-, F11.9-, F12.9-, F13.9-, F14.9-, F15.9-, F16.9-, F18.9-, F19.9-) should only be assigned based on provider documentation and when they meet the definition of a reportable diagnosis (see Section III, Reporting Additional Diagnoses). These codes are to be used only when the psychoactive substance use is associated with a substance related disorder (chapter 5 disorders such as sexual dysfunction, sleep disorder, or a mental or behavioral disorder) or medical condition, and such a relationship is documented by the provider.

4) Medical conditions due to psychoactive substance use, abuse and dependence

Medical conditions due to substance use, abuse, and dependence are not classified as substance-induced disorders. Assign the diagnosis code for the medical condition as directed by the Alphabetical Index along with the appropriate psychoactive substance use, abuse or dependence code. For example, for alcoholic pancreatitis due to alcohol dependence, assign the appropriate code from subcategory K85.2, Alcohol induced acute pancreatitis, and the appropriate code from subcategory F10.2, such as code F10.20, Alcohol dependence, uncomplicated. It would not be appropriate to assign code F10.288, Alcohol dependence with other alcohol-induced disorder.

5) Blood alcohol level

A code from category Y90, Evidence of alcohol involvement determined by blood alcohol level, may be assigned when this information is documented and the patient's provider has documented a condition classifiable to category F10, Alcohol related disorders. The blood alcohol level does not need to be documented by the patient's provider in order for it to be coded.

See Section I.B.14. for blood alcohol level documentation by clinicians other than patient's provider.

c. Factitious disorder

Factitious disorder imposed on self or Munchausen's syndrome is a disorder in which a person falsely reports or causes his or her own physical or psychological signs or symptoms. For patients with documented factitious disorder on self or Munchausen's syndrome, assign the appropriate code from subcategory F68.1-, Factitious disorder imposed on self.

Munchausen's syndrome by proxy (MSBP) is a disorder in which a caregiver (perpetrator) falsely reports or causes an illness or injury in another person (victim) under his or her care, such as a child, an elderly adult, or a person who has a disability. The condition is also referred to as "factitious disorder imposed on another" or "factitious disorder by proxy." The perpetrator, not the victim, receives this diagnosis. Assign code F68.A, Factitious disorder imposed on another, to the perpetrator's record. For the victim of a patient suffering from MSBP, assign the appropriate code from categories T74, Adult and child abuse, neglect and other maltreatment, confirmed, or T76, Adult and child abuse, neglect and other maltreatment, suspected.

See Section I.C.19.f. Adult and child abuse, neglect and other maltreatment

d. Dementia

The ICD-10-CM classifies dementia (categories F01, F02, and F03) on the basis of the etiology and severity (unspecified, mild, moderate or severe). Selection of the appropriate severity level requires the provider's clinical judgment and codes should be assigned only on the basis of provider documentation (as defined in the *Official Guidelines for Coding and Reporting*), unless otherwise instructed by the classification. If the documentation does not provide information about the severity of the dementia, assign the appropriate code for unspecified severity.

If a patient is admitted to an inpatient acute care hospital or other inpatient facility setting with dementia at one severity level and it progresses to a higher severity level, assign one code for the highest severity level reported during the stay.

Chapter 5. Mental, Behavioral and Neurodevelopmental Disorders (F01-F99)

> **INCLUDES**   disorders of psychological development
>
> **EXCLUDES 2**   symptoms, signs and abnormal clinical laboratory findings, not elsewhere classified (R00-R99)

This chapter contains the following blocks:

F01-F09	Mental disorders due to known physiological conditions
F10-F19	Mental and behavioral disorders due to psychoactive substance use
F20-F29	Schizophrenia, schizotypal, delusional, and other non-mood psychotic disorders
F30-F39	Mood [affective] disorders
F40-F48	Anxiety, dissociative, stress-related, somatoform and other nonpsychotic mental disorders
F50-F59	Behavioral syndromes associated with physiological disturbances and physical factors
F60-F69	Disorders of adult personality and behavior
F70-F79	Intellectual disabilities
F80-F89	Pervasive and specific developmental disorders
F90-F98	Behavioral and emotional disorders with onset usually occurring in childhood and adolescence
F99	Unspecified mental disorder

Mental disorders due to known physiological conditions (F01-F09)

> **NOTE**   This block comprises a range of mental disorders grouped together on the basis of their having in common a demonstrable etiology in cerebral disease, brain injury, or other insult leading to cerebral dysfunction. The dysfunction may be primary, as in diseases, injuries, and insults that affect the brain directly and selectively; or secondary, as in systemic diseases and disorders that attack the brain only as one of the multiple organs or systems of the body that are involved.

☑4ᵗʰ **F01**   **Vascular dementia**

Vascular dementia as a result of infarction of the brain due to vascular disease, including hypertensive cerebrovascular disease.

> **INCLUDES**   arteriosclerotic dementia
> major neurocognitive disorder due to vascular disease
> multi-infarct dementia

▶Code first, if applicable, any causal condition◀

AHA: 2022,4Q,14-15

   ☑5ᵗʰ **F01.5**   **Vascular dementia, unspecified severity**

     F01.50   **Vascular dementia, unspecified severity, without behavioral disturbance, psychotic disturbance, mood disturbance, and anxiety**   HCC A

       Major neurocognitive disorder due to vascular disease NOS

       Vascular dementia NOS

       AHA: 2021,2Q,4

     ☑6ᵗʰ **F01.51**   **Vascular dementia, unspecified severity, with behavioral disturbance**

       F01.511   **Vascular dementia, unspecified severity, with agitation**   CC HCC A

         Major neurocognitive disorder due to vascular disease, unspecified severity, with aberrant motor behavior such as restlessness, rocking, pacing, or exit-seeking

         Major neurocognitive disorder due to vascular disease, unspecified severity, with verbal or physical behaviors such as profanity, shouting, threatening, anger, aggression, combativeness, or violence

         Vascular dementia, unspecified severity, with aberrant motor behavior such as restlessness, rocking, pacing, or exit-seeking

         Vascular dementia, unspecified severity, with verbal or physical behaviors such as profanity, shouting, threatening, anger, aggression, combativeness, or violence

     F01.518   **Vascular dementia, unspecified severity, with other behavioral disturbance**   CC HCC A

       Major neurocognitive disorder due to vascular disease, unspecified severity, with behavioral disturbances such as sleep disturbance, social disinhibition, or sexual disinhibition

       Vascular dementia, unspecified severity, with behavioral disturbances such as sleep disturbance, social disinhibition, or sexual disinhibition

       Use additional code, if applicable, to identify wandering in vascular dementia (Z91.83)

     F01.52   **Vascular dementia, unspecified severity, with psychotic disturbance**   CC HCC A

       Major neurocognitive disorder due to vascular disease, unspecified severity, with psychotic disturbance such as hallucinations, paranoia, suspiciousness, or delusional state

       Vascular dementia, unspecified severity, with psychotic disturbance such as hallucinations, paranoia, suspiciousness, or delusional state

     F01.53   **Vascular dementia, unspecified severity, with mood disturbance**   CC HCC A

       Major neurocognitive disorder due to vascular disease, unspecified severity, with mood disturbance such as depression, apathy, or anhedonia

       Vascular dementia, unspecified severity, with mood disturbance such as depression, apathy, or anhedonia

     F01.54   **Vascular dementia, unspecified severity, with anxiety**   CC HCC A

       Major neurocognitive disorder due to vascular disease, unspecified severity, with anxiety

   ☑5ᵗʰ **F01.A**   **Vascular dementia, mild**

> **EXCLUDES 1**   mild neurocognitive disorder due to known physiological condition with or without behavioral disturbance (F06.7-)

     F01.A0   **Vascular dementia, mild, without behavioral disturbance, psychotic disturbance, mood disturbance, and anxiety**   HCC A

       Major neurocognitive disorder due to vascular disease, mild, NOS

       Vascular dementia, mild, NOS

     ☑6ᵗʰ **F01.A1**   **Vascular dementia, mild, with behavioral disturbance**

       F01.A11   **Vascular dementia, mild, with agitation**   CC HCC A

         Major neurocognitive disorder due to vascular disease, mild, with aberrant motor behavior such as restlessness, rocking, pacing, or exit-seeking

         Major neurocognitive disorder due to vascular disease, mild, with verbal or physical behaviors such as profanity, shouting, threatening, anger, aggression, combativeness, or violence

         Vascular dementia, mild, with aberrant motor behavior such as restlessness, rocking, pacing, or exit-seeking

         Vascular dementia, mild, with verbal or physical behaviors such as profanity, shouting, threatening, anger, aggression, combativeness, or violence

       F01.A18   **Vascular dementia, mild, with other behavioral disturbance**   CC HCC A

         Major neurocognitive disorder due to vascular disease, mild, with behavioral disturbances such as sleep disturbance, social disinhibition, or sexual disinhibition

         Vascular dementia, mild, with behavioral disturbances such as sleep disturbance, social disinhibition, or sexual disinhibition

         Use additional code, if applicable, to identify wandering in vascular dementia (Z91.83)

N Newborn: 0   **P** Pediatric: 0-17   **M** Maternity: 9-64   **A** Adult: 15-124   **UNS** Unspecified Site   **MCC** Major Complication/Comorbidity   **CC** Complication/Comorbidity   **PE** POA Exempt

552

ICD-10-CM 2025

F01.A2   **Vascular dementia, mild, with psychotic disturbance**   CC HCC A
> Major neurocognitive disorder due to vascular disease, mild, with psychotic disturbance such as hallucinations, paranoia, suspiciousness, or delusional state
> Vascular dementia, mild, with psychotic disturbance such as hallucinations, paranoia, suspiciousness, or delusional state

F01.A3   **Vascular dementia, mild, with mood disturbance**   CC HCC A
> Major neurocognitive disorder due to vascular disease, mild, with mood disturbance such as depression, apathy, or anhedonia
> Vascular dementia, mild, with mood disturbance such as depression, apathy, or anhedonia

F01.A4   **Vascular dementia, mild, with anxiety**   CC HCC A
> Major neurocognitive disorder due to vascular disease, mild, with anxiety

✓5th **F01.B**   **Vascular dementia, moderate**

F01.B0   **Vascular dementia, moderate, without behavioral disturbance, psychotic disturbance, mood disturbance, and anxiety**   HCC A
> Major neurocognitive disorder due to vascular disease, moderate, NOS
> Vascular dementia, moderate, NOS

✓6th **F01.B1**   **Vascular dementia, moderate, with behavioral disturbance**

     F01.B11   **Vascular dementia, moderate, with agitation**   CC HCC A
> Major neurocognitive disorder due to vascular disease, moderate, with aberrant motor behavior such as restlessness, rocking, pacing, or exit-seeking
> Major neurocognitive disorder due to vascular disease, moderate, with verbal or physical behaviors such as profanity, shouting, threatening, anger, aggression, combativeness, or violence
> Vascular dementia, moderate, with aberrant motor behavior such as restlessness, rocking, pacing, or exit-seeking
> Vascular dementia, moderate, with verbal or physical behaviors such as profanity, shouting, threatening, anger, aggression, combativeness, or violence

     F01.B18   **Vascular dementia, moderate, with other behavioral disturbance**   CC HCC A
> Major neurocognitive disorder due to vascular disease, moderate, with behavioral disturbances such as sleep disturbance, social disinhibition, or sexual disinhibition
> Vascular dementia, moderate, with behavioral disturbances such as sleep disturbance, social disinhibition, or sexual disinhibition
> Use additional code, if applicable, to identify wandering in vascular dementia (Z91.83)

F01.B2   **Vascular dementia, moderate, with psychotic disturbance**   CC HCC A
> Major neurocognitive disorder due to vascular disease, moderate, with psychotic disturbance such as hallucinations, paranoia, suspiciousness, or delusional state
> Vascular dementia, moderate, with psychotic disturbance such as hallucinations, paranoia, suspiciousness, or delusional state

F01.B3   **Vascular dementia, moderate, with mood disturbance**   CC HCC A
> Major neurocognitive disorder due to vascular disease, moderate, with mood disturbance such as depression, apathy, or anhedonia
> Vascular dementia, moderate, with mood disturbance such as depression, apathy, or anhedonia

F01.B4   **Vascular dementia, moderate, with anxiety**   CC HCC A
> Major neurocognitive disorder due to vascular disease, moderate, with anxiety

✓5th **F01.C**   **Vascular dementia, severe**

F01.C0   **Vascular dementia, severe, without behavioral disturbance, psychotic disturbance, mood disturbance, and anxiety**   HCC A
> Major neurocognitive disorder due to vascular disease, severe, NOS
> Vascular dementia, severe, NOS

✓6th **F01.C1**   **Vascular dementia, severe, with behavioral disturbance**

     F01.C11   **Vascular dementia, severe, with agitation**   CC HCC A
> Major neurocognitive disorder due to vascular disease, severe, with aberrant motor behavior such as restlessness, rocking, pacing, or exit-seeking
> Major neurocognitive disorder due to vascular disease, severe, with verbal or physical behaviors such as profanity, shouting, threatening, anger, aggression, combativeness, or violence
> Vascular dementia, severe, with aberrant motor behavior such as restlessness, rocking, pacing, or exit-seeking
> Vascular dementia, severe, with verbal or physical behaviors such as profanity, shouting, threatening, anger, aggression, combativeness, or violence

     F01.C18   **Vascular dementia, severe, with other behavioral disturbance**   CC HCC A
> Major neurocognitive disorder due to vascular disease, severe, with behavioral disturbances such as sleep disturbance, social disinhibition, or sexual disinhibition
> Vascular dementia, severe, with behavioral disturbances such as sleep disturbance, social disinhibition, or sexual disinhibition
> Use additional code, if applicable, to identify wandering in vascular dementia (Z91.83)

F01.C2   **Vascular dementia, severe, with psychotic disturbance**   CC HCC A
> Major neurocognitive disorder due to vascular disease, severe, with psychotic disturbance such as hallucinations, paranoia, suspiciousness, or delusional state
> Vascular dementia, severe, with psychotic disturbance such as hallucinations, paranoia, suspiciousness, or delusional state

F01.C3   **Vascular dementia, severe, with mood disturbance**   CC HCC A
> Major neurocognitive disorder due to vascular disease, severe, with mood disturbance such as depression, apathy, or anhedonia
> Vascular dementia, severe, with mood disturbance such as depression, apathy, or anhedonia

F01.C4   **Vascular dementia, severe, with anxiety**   CC HCC A
> Major neurocognitive disorder due to vascular disease, severe, with anxiety

Chapter 5. Mental, Behavioral and Neurodevelopmental Disorders

F02–F02.A11

✓4ᵗʰ **F02 Dementia in other diseases classified elsewhere**

INCLUDES   major neurocognitive disorder in other diseases classified elsewhere

Code first the underlying physiological condition, such as:
- Alzheimer's (G30.-)
- cerebral lipidosis (E75.4)
- Creutzfeldt-Jakob disease (A81.0-)
- ~~dementia with Lewy bodies (G31.83)~~
- ~~dementia with Parkinsonism (G31.83)~~
- epilepsy and recurrent seizures (G40.-)
- frontotemporal dementia (G31.09)
- hepatolenticular degeneration (E83.01)
- human immunodeficiency virus [HIV] disease (B20)
- Huntington's disease (G10)
- hypercalcemia (E83.52)
- hypothyroidism, acquired (E00-E03.-)
- intoxications (T36-T65)
- Jakob-Creutzfeldt disease (A81.0-)
- multiple sclerosis (G35)
- ▶neurocognitive disorder with Lewy bodies (G31.83)◀
- neurosyphilis (A52.17)
- niacin deficiency [pellagra] (E52)
- ▶other frontotemporal neurocognitive disorder (G31.90)◀
- Parkinson's disease (G20.-)
- Pick's disease (G31.01)
- polyarteritis nodosa (M30.0)
- prion disease (A81.9)
- systemic lupus erythematosus (M32.-)
- traumatic brain injury (S06.-)
- trypanosomiasis (B56.-, B57.-)
- vitamin B deficiency (E53.8)

EXCLUDES 1   mild neurocognitive disorder due to known physiological condition with or without behavioral disturbance (F06.7-)

EXCLUDES 2   dementia in alcohol and psychoactive substance disorders (F10-F19, with .17, .27, .97)
vascular dementia (F01.5-, F01.A-, F01.B-, F01.C-)

AHA: 2022,4Q,14-15

✓5ᵗʰ **F02.8 Dementia in other diseases classified elsewhere, unspecified severity**

AHA: 2024,2Q,8; 2022,4Q,15; 2022,1Q,25; 2017,2Q,7; 2016,4Q,141; 2016,2Q,6

    F02.80 Dementia in other diseases classified elsewhere, unspecified severity, without behavioral disturbance, psychotic disturbance, mood disturbance, and anxiety HCC

Dementia in other diseases classified elsewhere NOS
Major neurocognitive disorder in other diseases classified elsewhere NOS

✓6ᵗʰ   **F02.81 Dementia in other diseases classified elsewhere, unspecified severity, with behavioral disturbance**

    F02.811 Dementia in other diseases classified elsewhere, unspecified severity, with agitation CC HCC

Dementia in other diseases classified elsewhere, unspecified severity, with aberrant motor behavior such as restlessness, rocking, pacing, or exit-seeking

Dementia in other diseases classified elsewhere, unspecified severity, with verbal or physical behaviors such as profanity, shouting, threatening, anger, aggression, combativeness, or violence

Major neurocognitive disorder in other diseases classified elsewhere, unspecified severity, with aberrant motor behavior such as restlessness, rocking, pacing, or exit-seeking

Major neurocognitive disorder in other diseases classified elsewhere, unspecified severity, with verbal or physical behaviors such as profanity, shouting, threatening, anger, aggression, combativeness, or violence

    F02.818 Dementia in other diseases classified elsewhere, unspecified severity, with other behavioral disturbance CC HCC

Dementia in other diseases classified elsewhere with sleep disturbance, social disinhibition, or sexual disinhibition

Major neurocognitive disorder in other diseases classified elsewhere with sleep disturbance, social disinhibition, or sexual disinhibition

Use additional code, if applicable, to identify wandering in dementia in conditions classified elsewhere (Z91.83)

    F02.82 Dementia in other diseases classified elsewhere, unspecified severity, with psychotic disturbance CC HCC

Dementia in other diseases classified elsewhere, unspecified severity, with psychotic disturbance such as hallucinations, paranoia, suspiciousness, or delusional state

Major neurocognitive disorder in other diseases classified elsewhere, unspecified, with psychotic disturbance such as hallucinations, paranoia, suspiciousness, or delusional state

    F02.83 Dementia in other diseases classified elsewhere, unspecified severity, with mood disturbance CC HCC

Dementia in other diseases classified elsewhere, unspecified severity, with mood disturbance such as depression, apathy, or anhedonia

Major neurocognitive disorder in other diseases classified elsewhere unspecified severity, with mood disturbance such as with depression, apathy, or anhedonia

    F02.84 Dementia in other diseases classified elsewhere, unspecified severity, with anxiety CC HCC

Major neurocognitive disorder in other diseases classified elsewhere unspecified severity, with anxiety

✓5ᵗʰ **F02.A Dementia in other diseases classified elsewhere, mild**

EXCLUDES 1   mild neurocognitive disorder due to known physiological condition with or without behavioral disturbance (F06.7-)

    F02.A0 Dementia in other diseases classified elsewhere, mild, without behavioral disturbance, psychotic disturbance, mood disturbance, and anxiety HCC

Dementia in other diseases classified elsewhere, mild, NOS

Major neurocognitive disorder in other diseases classified elsewhere, mild, NOS

✓6ᵗʰ   **F02.A1 Dementia in other diseases classified elsewhere, mild, with behavioral disturbance**

    F02.A11 Dementia in other diseases classified elsewhere, mild, with agitation CC HCC

Dementia in other diseases classified elsewhere, mild, with aberrant motor behavior such as restlessness, rocking, pacing, or exit-seeking

Dementia in other diseases classified elsewhere, mild, with verbal or physical behaviors such as profanity, shouting, threatening, anger, aggression, combativeness, or violence

Major neurocognitive disorder in other diseases classified elsewhere, mild, with aberrant motor behavior such as restlessness, rocking, pacing, or exit-seeking

Major neurocognitive disorder in other diseases classified elsewhere, mild, with verbal or physical behaviors such as profanity, shouting, threatening, anger, aggression, combativeness, or violence

N Newborn: 0   P Pediatric: 0-17   M Maternity: 9-64   A Adult: 15-124   UNS Unspecified Site   MCC Major Complication/Comorbidity   CC Complication/Comorbidity   PE POA Exempt

554

ICD-10-CM 2025

F02.A18   ***Dementia in other diseases classified elsewhere, mild, with other behavioral disturbance*** `CC` `HCC`

Dementia in other diseases classified elsewhere, mild, with behavioral disturbances such as sleep disturbance, social disinhibition, or sexual disinhibition

Major neurocognitive disorder in other diseases classified elsewhere, mild, with behavioral disturbances such as sleep disturbance, social disinhibition, or sexual disinhibition

Use additional code, if applicable, to identify wandering in dementia in conditions classified elsewhere (Z91.83)

F02.A2   ***Dementia in other diseases classified elsewhere, mild, with psychotic disturbance*** `CC` `HCC`

Dementia in other diseases classified elsewhere, mild, with psychotic disturbance such as hallucinations, paranoia, suspiciousness, or delusional state

Major neurocognitive disorder in other diseases classified elsewhere, mild, with psychotic disturbance such as hallucinations, paranoia, suspiciousness, or delusional state

F02.A3   ***Dementia in other diseases classified elsewhere, mild, with mood disturbance*** `CC` `HCC`

Dementia in other diseases classified elsewhere, mild, with mood disturbance such as depression, apathy, or anhedonia

Major neurocognitive disorder in other diseases classified elsewhere, mild, with mood disturbance such as depression, apathy, or anhedonia

F02.A4   ***Dementia in other diseases classified elsewhere, mild, with anxiety*** `CC` `HCC`

Major neurocognitive disorder in other diseases classified elsewhere, mild, with anxiety

√5th   **F02.B**   **Dementia in other diseases classified elsewhere, moderate**

F02.B0   ***Dementia in other diseases classified elsewhere, moderate, without behavioral disturbance, psychotic disturbance, mood disturbance, and anxiety*** `HCC`

Dementia in other diseases classified elsewhere, moderate, NOS

Major neurocognitive disorder in other diseases classified elsewhere, moderate, NOS

√6th   **F02.B1**   **Dementia in other diseases classified elsewhere, moderate, with behavioral disturbance**

F02.B11   ***Dementia in other diseases classified elsewhere, moderate, with agitation*** `CC` `HCC`

Dementia in other diseases classified elsewhere, moderate, with aberrant motor behavior such as restlessness, rocking, pacing, or exit-seeking

Dementia in other diseases classified elsewhere, moderate, with verbal or physical behaviors such as profanity, shouting, threatening, anger, aggression, combativeness, or violence

Major neurocognitive disorder in other diseases classified elsewhere, moderate, with aberrant motor behavior such as restlessness, rocking, pacing, or exit-seeking

Major neurocognitive disorder in other diseases classified elsewhere, moderate, with verbal or physical behaviors such as profanity, shouting, threatening, anger, aggression, combativeness, or violence

F02.B18   ***Dementia in other diseases classified elsewhere, moderate, with other behavioral disturbance*** `CC` `HCC`

Dementia in other diseases classified elsewhere, moderate, with behavioral disturbances such as sleep disturbance, social disinhibition, or sexual disinhibition

Major neurocognitive disorder in other diseases classified elsewhere, moderate, with behavioral disturbance such as sleep disturbance, social disinhibition, or sexual disinhibition

Use additional code, if applicable, to identify wandering in dementia in conditions classified elsewhere (Z91.83)

F02.B2   ***Dementia in other diseases classified elsewhere, moderate, with psychotic disturbance*** `CC` `HCC`

Dementia in other diseases classified elsewhere, moderate, with psychotic disturbance such as hallucinations, paranoia, suspiciousness, or delusional state

Major neurocognitive disorder in other diseases classified elsewhere, moderate, with psychotic disturbance such as hallucinations, paranoia, suspiciousness, or delusional state

F02.B3   ***Dementia in other diseases classified elsewhere, moderate, with mood disturbance*** `CC` `HCC`

Dementia in other diseases classified elsewhere, moderate, with mood disturbance such as depression, apathy, or anhedonia

Major neurocognitive disorder in other diseases classified elsewhere, moderate, with mood disturbance such as depression, apathy, or anhedonia

F02.B4   ***Dementia in other diseases classified elsewhere, moderate, with anxiety*** `CC` `HCC`

Major neurocognitive disorder in other diseases classified elsewhere, moderate, with anxiety

√5th   **F02.C**   **Dementia in other diseases classified elsewhere, severe**

F02.C0   ***Dementia in other diseases classified elsewhere, severe, without behavioral disturbance, psychotic disturbance, mood disturbance, and anxiety*** `HCC`

Dementia in other diseases classified elsewhere, severe, NOS

Major neurocognitive disorder in other diseases classified elsewhere, severe, NOS

√6th   **F02.C1**   **Dementia in other diseases classified elsewhere, severe, with behavioral disturbance**

F02.C11   ***Dementia in other diseases classified elsewhere, severe, with agitation*** `CC` `HCC`

Dementia in other diseases classified elsewhere, severe, with aberrant motor behavior such as restlessness, rocking, pacing, or exit-seeking

Dementia in other diseases classified elsewhere, severe, with verbal or physical behaviors such as profanity, shouting, threatening, anger, aggression, combativeness, or violence

Major neurocognitive disorder in other diseases classified elsewhere, severe, with aberrant motor behavior such as restlessness, rocking, pacing, or exit-seeking

Major neurocognitive disorder in other diseases classified elsewhere, severe, with verbal or physical behaviors such as profanity, shouting, threatening, anger, aggression, combativeness, or violence

☑ Additional Character Required   √x7th Placeholder   Questionable PDx   Manifestation   Unspecified   UPD Unacceptable PDx   H1-H14 HAC   HCC CMS-HCC Dx   HIV HIV Dx

ICD-10-CM 2025   555

Chapter 5. Mental, Behavioral and Neurodevelopmental Disorders

F02.C18   *Dementia in other diseases classified elsewhere, severe, with other behavioral disturbance*   **CC** **HCC**

Dementia in other diseases classified elsewhere, severe, with behavioral disturbances such as sleep disturbance, social disinhibition, or sexual disinhibition

Major neurocognitive disorder in other diseases classified elsewhere, severe, with behavioral disturbances such as sleep disturbance, social disinhibition, or sexual disinhibition

Use additional code, if applicable, to identify wandering in dementia in conditions classified elsewhere (Z91.83)

F02.C2   *Dementia in other diseases classified elsewhere, severe, with psychotic disturbance*   **CC** **HCC**

Dementia in other diseases classified elsewhere, severe, with psychotic disturbance such as hallucinations, paranoia, suspiciousness, or delusional state

Major neurocognitive disorder in other diseases classified elsewhere, severe, with psychotic disturbance such as hallucinations, paranoia, suspiciousness, or delusional state

F02.C3   *Dementia in other diseases classified elsewhere, severe, with mood disturbance*   **CC** **HCC**

Dementia in other diseases classified elsewhere, severe, with mood disturbance such as depression, apathy, or anhedonia

Major neurocognitive disorder in other diseases classified elsewhere, severe, with mood disturbance such as depression, apathy, or anhedonia

F02.C4   *Dementia in other diseases classified elsewhere, severe, with anxiety*   **CC** **HCC**

Major neurocognitive disorder in other diseases classified elsewhere, severe, with anxiety

✓4th **F03**   **Unspecified dementia**

Major neurocognitive disorder NOS
Presenile dementia NOS
Presenile psychosis NOS
Primary degenerative dementia NOS
Senile dementia NOS
Senile dementia depressed or paranoid type
Senile psychosis NOS

EXCLUDES 1   *senility NOS (R41.81)*

EXCLUDES 2   ▶*dementia with delirium or acute confusional state (F05)*◀
     mild memory disturbance due to known physiological condition (F06.8)

AHA: 2022,4Q,14-15

✓5th **F03.9**   **Unspecified dementia, unspecified severity**

F03.90   Unspecified dementia, unspecified severity, without behavioral disturbance, psychotic disturbance, mood disturbance, and anxiety   **HIV** **HCC** **A**

Dementia NOS

AHA: 2024,2Q,8; 2021,2Q,4; 2012,4Q,92

✓6th **F03.91**   Unspecified dementia, unspecified severity, with behavioral disturbance

F03.911   Unspecified dementia, unspecified severity, with agitation   **CC** **HCC** **A**

Unspecified dementia, unspecified severity, with aberrant motor behavior such as restlessness, rocking, pacing, or exit-seeking

Unspecified dementia, unspecified severity, with verbal or physical behaviors such as profanity, shouting, threatening, anger, aggression, combativeness, or violence

F03.918   Unspecified dementia, unspecified severity, with other behavioral disturbance   **CC** **HCC** **A**

Unspecified dementia, unspecified severity, with behavioral disturbances such as sleep disturbance, social disinhibition, or sexual disinhibition

Use additional code, if applicable, to identify wandering in unspecified dementia (Z91.83)

F03.92   Unspecified dementia, unspecified severity, with psychotic disturbance   **CC** **HCC** **A**

Unspecified dementia, unspecified severity, with psychotic disturbance such as hallucinations, paranoia, suspiciousness, or delusional state

F03.93   Unspecified dementia, unspecified severity, with mood disturbance   **CC** **HCC** **A**

Unspecified dementia, unspecified severity, with mood disturbance such as depression, apathy, or anhedonia

F03.94   Unspecified dementia, unspecified severity, with anxiety   **CC** **HCC** **A**

✓5th **F03.A**   **Unspecified dementia, mild**

EXCLUDES 1   *mild neurocognitive disorder due to known physiological condition with or without behavioral disturbance (F06.7-)*

F03.A0   Unspecified dementia, mild, without behavioral disturbance, psychotic disturbance, mood disturbance, and anxiety   **HCC** **A**

Dementia, mild, NOS

✓6th **F03.A1**   Unspecified dementia, mild, with behavioral disturbance

F03.A11   Unspecified dementia, mild, with agitation   **CC** **HCC** **A**

Unspecified dementia, mild, with aberrant motor behavior such as restlessness, rocking, pacing, or exit-seeking

Unspecified dementia, mild, with verbal or physical behaviors such as profanity, shouting, threatening, anger, aggression, combativeness, or violence

F03.A18   Unspecified dementia, mild, with other behavioral disturbance   **CC** **HCC** **A**

Unspecified dementia, mild, with behavioral disturbances such as sleep disturbance, social disinhibition, or sexual disinhibition

Use additional code, if applicable, to identify wandering in unspecified dementia (Z91.83)

F03.A2   Unspecified dementia, mild, with psychotic disturbance   **CC** **HCC** **A**

Unspecified dementia, mild, with psychotic disturbance such as hallucinations, paranoia, suspiciousness, or delusional state

F03.A3   Unspecified dementia, mild, with mood disturbance   **CC** **HCC** **A**

Unspecified dementia, mild, with mood disturbance such as depression, apathy, or anhedonia

F03.A4   Unspecified dementia, mild, with anxiety   **CC** **HCC** **A**

✓5th **F03.B**   **Unspecified dementia, moderate**

F03.B0   Unspecified dementia, moderate, without behavioral disturbance, psychotic disturbance, mood disturbance, and anxiety   **HCC** **A**

Dementia, moderate, NOS

✓6th **F03.B1**   Unspecified dementia, moderate, with behavioral disturbance

F03.B11   Unspecified dementia, moderate, with agitation   **CC** **HCC** **A**

Unspecified dementia, moderate, with aberrant motor behavior such as restlessness, rocking, pacing, or exit-seeking

Unspecified dementia, moderate, with verbal or physical behaviors such as profanity, shouting, threatening, anger, aggression, combativeness, or violence

F03.B18   Unspecified dementia, moderate, with other behavioral disturbance   **CC** **HCC** **A**

Unspecified dementia, moderate, with behavioral disturbances such as sleep disturbance, social disinhibition, or sexual disinhibition

Use additional code, if applicable, to identify wandering in unspecified dementia (Z91.83)

F03.B2   **Unspecified dementia, moderate, with psychotic disturbance**   `CC` `HCC` `A`
Unspecified dementia, moderate, with psychotic disturbance such as hallucinations, paranoia, suspiciousness, or delusional state

F03.B3   **Unspecified dementia, moderate, with mood disturbance**   `CC` `HCC` `A`
Unspecified dementia, moderate, with mood disturbance such as depression, apathy, or anhedonia

F03.B4   **Unspecified dementia, moderate, with anxiety**   `CC` `HCC` `A`

✓5th   **F03.C**   **Unspecified dementia, severe**

F03.C0   **Unspecified dementia, severe, without behavioral disturbance, psychotic disturbance, mood disturbance, and anxiety**   `HCC` `A`
Dementia, severe, NOS

✓6th   **F03.C1**   **Unspecified dementia, severe, with behavioral disturbance**

F03.C11   **Unspecified dementia, severe, with agitation**   `CC` `HCC` `A`
Unspecified dementia, severe, with aberrant motor behavior such as restlessness, rocking, pacing, or exit-seeking
Unspecified dementia, severe, with verbal or physical behaviors such as profanity, shouting, threatening, anger, aggression, combativeness, or violence

F03.C18   **Unspecified dementia, severe, with other behavioral disturbance**   `CC` `HCC` `A`
Unspecified dementia, severe, with behavioral disturbances such as sleep disturbance, social disinhibition, or sexual disinhibition

Use additional code, if applicable, to identify wandering in unspecified dementia (Z91.83)

F03.C2   **Unspecified dementia, severe, with psychotic disturbance**   `CC` `HCC` `A`
Unspecified dementia, severe, with psychotic disturbance such as hallucinations, paranoia, suspiciousness, or delusional state

F03.C3   **Unspecified dementia, severe, with mood disturbance**   `CC` `HCC` `A`
Unspecified dementia, severe, with mood disturbance such as depression, apathy, or anhedonia
AHA: 2023,4Q,14

F03.C4   **Unspecified dementia, severe, with anxiety**   `CC` `HCC` `A`

F04   **Amnestic disorder due to known physiological condition**
Korsakov's psychosis or syndrome, nonalcoholic
Code first the underlying physiological condition
EXCLUDES 1   amnesia NOS (R41.3)
anterograde amnesia (R41.1)
dissociative amnesia (F44.0)
retrograde amnesia (R41.2)
EXCLUDES 2   alcohol-induced or unspecified Korsakov's syndrome (F10.26, F10.96)
Korsakov's syndrome induced by other psychoactive substances (F13.26, F13.96, F19.16, F19.26, F19.96)

F05   **Delirium due to known physiological condition**   `CC` `UPD`
Acute or subacute brain syndrome
Acute or subacute confusional state (nonalcoholic)
Acute or subacute infective psychosis
Acute or subacute organic reaction
Acute or subacute psycho-organic syndrome
Delirium of mixed etiology
Delirium superimposed on dementia
Sundowning
Code first the underlying physiological condition, such as:
dementia (F03.9-)
EXCLUDES 1   delirium NOS (R41.0)
EXCLUDES 2   delirium tremens alcohol-induced or unspecified (F10.231, F10.921)

AHA: 2019,2Q,34

✓4th   **F06**   **Other mental disorders due to known physiological condition**
INCLUDES   mental disorders due to endocrine disorder
mental disorders due to exogenous hormone
mental disorders due to exogenous toxic substance
mental disorders due to primary cerebral disease
mental disorders due to somatic illness
mental disorders due to systemic disease affecting the brain
Code first the underlying physiological condition
EXCLUDES 1   unspecified dementia ▶(F03.-)◀
EXCLUDES 2   delirium due to known physiological condition (F05)
dementia as classified in F01-F02
other mental disorders associated with alcohol and other psychoactive substances (F10-F19)

F06.0   **Psychotic disorder with hallucinations due to known physiological condition**   `CC`
Organic hallucinatory state (nonalcoholic)
EXCLUDES 2   hallucinations and perceptual disturbance induced by alcohol and other psychoactive substances (F10-F19 with .151, .251, .951)
schizophrenia (F20.-)

F06.1   **Catatonic disorder due to known physiological condition**
Catatonia associated with another mental disorder
Catatonia NOS
EXCLUDES 1   catatonic stupor (R40.1)
stupor NOS (R40.1)
EXCLUDES 2   catatonic schizophrenia (F20.2)
dissociative stupor (F44.2)

DEF: Catatonic: Abnormal neuropsychiatric state characterized by stupor, immobility or purposeless movements, or unresponsiveness in a person who otherwise appears awake.

F06.2   **Psychotic disorder with delusions due to known physiological condition**   `CC`
Paranoid and paranoid-hallucinatory organic states
Schizophrenia-like psychosis in epilepsy
EXCLUDES 2   alcohol and drug-induced psychotic disorder (F10-F19 with .150, .250, .950)
brief psychotic disorder (F23)
delusional disorder (F22)
schizophrenia (F20.-)

✓5th   **F06.3**   **Mood disorder due to known physiological condition**
EXCLUDES 2   mood disorders due to alcohol and other psychoactive substances (F10-F19 with .14, .24, .94)
mood disorders, not due to known physiological condition or unspecified (F30-F39)

F06.30   **Mood disorder due to known physiological condition, unspecified**

F06.31   **Mood disorder due to known physiological condition with depressive features**
Depressive disorder due to known physiological condition, with depressive features

F06.32   **Mood disorder due to known physiological condition with major depressive-like episode**
Depressive disorder due to known physiological condition, with major depressive-like episode

F06.33   **Mood disorder due to known physiological condition with manic features**
Bipolar and related disorder due to a known physiological condition, with manic features
Bipolar and related disorder due to known physiological condition, with manic- or hypomanic-like episodes

F06.34   **Mood disorder due to known physiological condition with mixed features**
Bipolar and related disorder due to known physiological condition, with mixed features
Depressive disorder due to known physiological condition, with mixed features

F06.4   **Anxiety disorder due to known physiological condition**
EXCLUDES 2   anxiety disorders due to alcohol and other psychoactive substances (F10-F19 with .180, .280, .980)
anxiety disorders, not due to known physiological condition or unspecified (F40.-, F41.-)

✓ Additional Character Required   ✓x7th Placeholder   Questionable PDx   Manifestation   Unspecified   `UPD` Unacceptable PDx   `H1`-`H14` HAC   `HCC` CMS-HCC Dx   `HIV` HIV Dx

✓5ᵗʰ **F06.7 Mild neurocognitive disorder due to known physiological condition**

Mild neurocognitive impairment due to a known physiological condition

Code first the underlying physiological condition, such as:
Alzheimer's disease (G30.-)
human immunodeficiency virus [HIV] disease (B20)
Huntington's disease (G10)
neurocognitive disorder with Lewy bodies (G31.83)
▶other frontotemporal neurocognitive disorder (G31.09)◀
Parkinson's disease (G20.-)
systemic lupus erythematosus (M32.-)
traumatic brain injury (S06.-)
vitamin B deficiency (E53.-)

EXCLUDES 1   *age related cognitive decline (R41.81)*
altered mental status (R41.82)
cerebral degeneration (G31.9)
change in mental status (R41.82)
cognitive deficits following (sequelae of) cerebral hemorrhage or infarction (I69.01-I69.11-, I69.21-I69.31-, I69.81- I69.91-)
dementia ▶(F01.-, F02.-, F03.-)◀
mild cognitive impairment due to unknown or unspecified etiology (G31.84)
neurologic neglect syndrome (R41.4)
personality change, nonpsychotic (F68.8)

AHA: 2022,4Q,16

F06.70 Mild neurocognitive disorder due to known physiological condition without behavioral disturbance HIV UPD

Mild neurocognitive disorder due to known physiological condition, NOS

F06.71 Mild neurocognitive disorder due to known physiological condition with behavioral disturbance HIV CC UPD

F06.8 Other specified mental disorders due to known physiological condition HIV

Epileptic psychosis NOS
Obsessive-compulsive and related disorder due to a known physiological condition
Organic dissociative disorder
Organic emotionally labile [asthenic] disorder

✓4ᵗʰ **F07 Personality and behavioral disorders due to known physiological condition**

Code first the underlying physiological condition

F07.0 Personality change due to known physiological condition

Frontal lobe syndrome
Limbic epilepsy personality syndrome
Lobotomy syndrome
Organic personality disorder
Organic pseudopsychopathic personality
Organic pseudoretarded personality
Postleucotomy syndrome

EXCLUDES 1   *mild cognitive impairment (G31.84)*
postconcussional syndrome (F07.81)
postencephalitic syndrome (F07.89)
signs and symptoms involving emotional state (R45.-)

EXCLUDES 2   *specific personality disorder (F60.-)*

✓5ᵗʰ **F07.8 Other personality and behavioral disorders due to known physiological condition**

F07.81 Postconcussional syndrome

Postcontusional syndrome (encephalopathy)
Post-traumatic brain syndrome, nonpsychotic
Use additional code to identify associated post-traumatic headache, if applicable (G44.3-)

EXCLUDES 1   *current concussion (brain) (S06.0-)*
postencephalitic syndrome (F07.89)

DEF: Concussion symptoms that persist for weeks or months after a head injury. These symptoms may include headache, giddiness, fatigue, insomnia, mood fluctuation, and a subjective feeling of impaired intellectual function with extreme reaction to normal stressors.

F07.89 Other personality and behavioral disorders due to known physiological condition UPD

Postencephalitic syndrome
Right hemispheric organic affective disorder

F07.9 Unspecified personality and behavioral disorder due to known physiological condition HIV

Organic psychosyndrome

F09 Unspecified mental disorder due to known physiological condition HIV

Mental disorder NOS due to known physiological condition
Organic brain syndrome NOS
Organic mental disorder NOS
Organic psychosis NOS
Symptomatic psychosis NOS

Code first the underlying physiological condition

EXCLUDES 1   *mild neurocognitive disorder due to known physiological condition (F06.7-)*
psychosis NOS (F29)

Mental and behavioral disorders due to psychoactive substance use (F10-F19)

AHA: 2022,4Q,16-17; 2022,1Q,34; 2020,1Q,9; 2018,4Q,69-70; 2017,4Q,8; 2017,2Q,27
TIP: Psychoactive substance withdrawal can occur in individuals who do not have a diagnosis of dependence but who use the substance regularly (i.e., use or abuse) and then reduce or cease the use.

✓4ᵗʰ **F10 Alcohol related disorders**

Use additional code for blood alcohol level, if applicable (Y90.-)
AHA: 2019,3Q,8

✓5ᵗʰ **F10.1 Alcohol abuse**

EXCLUDES 1   *alcohol dependence (F10.2-)*
alcohol use, unspecified (F10.9-)

AHA: 2018,1Q,16; 2015,2Q,15

F10.10 Alcohol abuse, uncomplicated

Alcohol use disorder, mild

F10.11 Alcohol abuse, in remission

Alcohol use disorder, mild, in early remission
Alcohol use disorder, mild, in sustained remission

AHA: 2022,1Q,25

✓6ᵗʰ **F10.12 Alcohol abuse with intoxication**

F10.120 Alcohol abuse with intoxication, uncomplicated

F10.121 Alcohol abuse with intoxication delirium CC

F10.129 Alcohol abuse with intoxication, unspecified

✓6ᵗʰ **F10.13 Alcohol abuse, with withdrawal**

AHA: 2020,4Q,16-17

F10.130 Alcohol abuse with withdrawal, uncomplicated CC HCC

F10.131 Alcohol abuse with withdrawal delirium CC HCC

F10.132 Alcohol abuse with withdrawal with perceptual disturbance CC HCC

F10.139 Alcohol abuse with withdrawal, unspecified CC HCC

F10.14 Alcohol abuse with alcohol-induced mood disorder CC HCC

Alcohol use disorder, mild, with alcohol-induced bipolar or related disorder
Alcohol use disorder, mild, with alcohol-induced depressive disorder

✓6ᵗʰ **F10.15 Alcohol abuse with alcohol-induced psychotic disorder**

F10.150 Alcohol abuse with alcohol-induced psychotic disorder with delusions HCC

F10.151 Alcohol abuse with alcohol-induced psychotic disorder with hallucinations CC HCC

DEF: Psychosis lasting less than six months with slight or no clouding of consciousness in which auditory hallucinations predominate.

F10.159 Alcohol abuse with alcohol-induced psychotic disorder, unspecified CC HCC

✓6ᵗʰ **F10.18 Alcohol abuse with other alcohol-induced disorders**

AHA: 2022,1Q,33

F10.180 Alcohol abuse with alcohol-induced anxiety disorder CC HCC

AHA: 2022,1Q,25,33

F10.181 Alcohol abuse with alcohol-induced sexual dysfunction CC HCC

F10.182 Alcohol abuse with alcohol-induced sleep disorder HCC

N Newborn: 0   P Pediatric: 0-17   M Maternity: 9-64   A Adult: 15-124   UNS Unspecified Site   MCC Major Complication/Comorbidity   CC Complication/Comorbidity   PE POA Exempt

Chapter 5. Mental, Behavioral and Neurodevelopmental Disorders

F10.188–F10.97

      F10.188   **Alcohol abuse with other alcohol-induced disorder** `CC` `HCC`
         AHA: 2022,1Q,25

   F10.19   **Alcohol abuse with unspecified alcohol-induced disorder** `CC`

`✓5ᵗʰ` **F10.2**   **Alcohol dependence**

     `EXCLUDES 1`   *alcohol abuse (F10.1-)*
                alcohol use, unspecified (F10.9-)
     `EXCLUDES 2`   *toxic effect of alcohol (T51.0-)*

   F10.20   **Alcohol dependence, uncomplicated** `HCC`
        Alcohol use disorder, moderate
        Alcohol use disorder, severe
        AHA: 2020,1Q,9

   F10.21   **Alcohol dependence, in remission** `HCC`
        Alcohol use disorder, moderate, in early remission
        Alcohol use disorder, moderate, in sustained remission
        Alcohol use disorder, severe, in early remission
        Alcohol use disorder, severe, in sustained remission

`✓6ᵗʰ` **F10.22**   **Alcohol dependence with intoxication**
        Acute drunkenness (in alcoholism)
      `EXCLUDES 2`   *alcohol dependence with withdrawal (F10.23-)*

    F10.220   **Alcohol dependence with intoxication, uncomplicated** `HCC`

    F10.221   **Alcohol dependence with intoxication delirium** `CC` `HCC`

    F10.229   **Alcohol dependence with intoxication, unspecified** `HCC`

`✓6ᵗʰ` **F10.23**   **Alcohol dependence with withdrawal**
      `EXCLUDES 2`   *alcohol dependence with intoxication (F10.22-)*
        AHA: 2018,1Q,16; 2015,2Q,15

    F10.230   **Alcohol dependence with withdrawal, uncomplicated** `CC` `HCC`

    F10.231   **Alcohol dependence with withdrawal delirium** `CC` `HCC`

    F10.232   **Alcohol dependence with withdrawal with perceptual disturbance** `CC` `HCC`

    F10.239   **Alcohol dependence with withdrawal, unspecified** `CC` `HCC`

   F10.24   **Alcohol dependence with alcohol-induced mood disorder** `CC` `HCC`
        Alcohol use disorder, moderate, with alcohol-induced bipolar or related disorder
        Alcohol use disorder, moderate, with alcohol-induced depressive disorder
        Alcohol use disorder, severe, with alcohol-induced bipolar or related disorder
        Alcohol use disorder, severe, with alcohol-induced depressive disorder

`✓6ᵗʰ` **F10.25**   **Alcohol dependence with alcohol-induced psychotic disorder**

    F10.250   **Alcohol dependence with alcohol-induced psychotic disorder with delusions** `HCC`

    F10.251   **Alcohol dependence with alcohol-induced psychotic disorder with hallucinations** `CC` `HCC`

    F10.259   **Alcohol dependence with alcohol-induced psychotic disorder, unspecified** `CC` `HCC`

   F10.26   **Alcohol dependence with alcohol-induced persisting amnestic disorder** `HCC`
        Alcohol use disorder, moderate, with alcohol-induced major neurocognitive disorder, amnestic-confabulatory type
        Alcohol use disorder, severe, with alcohol-induced major neurocognitive disorder, amnestic-confabulatory type
        DEF: Prominent and lasting reduced memory span and disordered time appreciation and confabulation that occurs in alcoholics as sequel to acute alcoholic psychosis.

   F10.27   **Alcohol dependence with alcohol-induced persisting dementia** `CC` `HCC`
        Alcohol use disorder, moderate, with alcohol-induced major neurocognitive disorder, nonamnestic-confabulatory type
        Alcohol use disorder, severe, with alcohol-induced major neurocognitive disorder, nonamnestic-confabulatory type

`✓6ᵗʰ` **F10.28**   **Alcohol dependence with other alcohol-induced disorders**

    F10.280   **Alcohol dependence with alcohol-induced anxiety disorder** `CC` `HCC`

    F10.281   **Alcohol dependence with alcohol-induced sexual dysfunction** `CC` `HCC`

    F10.282   **Alcohol dependence with alcohol-induced sleep disorder** `HCC`

    F10.288   **Alcohol dependence with other alcohol-induced disorder** `CC` `HCC`
          Alcohol use disorder, moderate, with alcohol-induced mild neurocognitive disorder
          Alcohol use disorder, severe, with alcohol-induced mild neurocognitive disorder
          AHA: 2020,1Q,9

   F10.29   **Alcohol dependence with unspecified alcohol-induced disorder** `CC` `HCC`

`✓5ᵗʰ` **F10.9**   **Alcohol use, unspecified**
     `EXCLUDES 1`   *alcohol abuse (F10.1-)*
                alcohol dependence (F10.2-)
     AHA: 2018,2Q,10-11
     TIP: Assign a substance use code only when the provider documents a relationship between the use and an associated physical, mental, or behavioral disorder. As with all diagnoses, substance use codes must meet the definition of a reportable diagnosis.

   F10.90   **Alcohol use, unspecified, uncomplicated**

   F10.91   **Alcohol use, unspecified, in remission**

`✓6ᵗʰ` **F10.92**   **Alcohol use, unspecified with intoxication**

    F10.920   **Alcohol use, unspecified with intoxication, uncomplicated**
         AHA: 2018,2Q,10-11

    F10.921   **Alcohol use, unspecified with intoxication delirium** `CC`

    F10.929   **Alcohol use, unspecified with intoxication, unspecified**

`✓6ᵗʰ` **F10.93**   **Alcohol use, unspecified with withdrawal**
        AHA: 2020,4Q,16-17

    F10.930   **Alcohol use, unspecified with withdrawal, uncomplicated** `CC` `HCC`

    F10.931   **Alcohol use, unspecified with withdrawal delirium** `CC` `HCC`

    F10.932   **Alcohol use, unspecified with withdrawal with perceptual disturbance** `CC` `HCC`

    F10.939   **Alcohol use, unspecified with withdrawal, unspecified** `CC` `HCC`

   F10.94   **Alcohol use, unspecified with alcohol-induced mood disorder** `CC` `HCC`
        Alcohol induced bipolar or related disorder, without use disorder
        Alcohol induced depressive disorder, without use disorder

`✓6ᵗʰ` **F10.95**   **Alcohol use, unspecified with alcohol-induced psychotic disorder**

    F10.950   **Alcohol use, unspecified with alcohol-induced psychotic disorder with delusions** `HCC`

    F10.951   **Alcohol use, unspecified with alcohol-induced psychotic disorder with hallucinations** `CC` `HCC`

    F10.959   **Alcohol use, unspecified with alcohol-induced psychotic disorder, unspecified** `CC` `HCC`
         Alcohol-induced psychotic disorder without use disorder

   F10.96   **Alcohol use, unspecified with alcohol-induced persisting amnestic disorder** `HCC`
        Alcohol-induced major neurocognitive disorder, amnestic-confabulatory type, without use disorder

   F10.97   **Alcohol use, unspecified with alcohol-induced persisting dementia** `HCC`
        Alcohol-induced major neurocognitive disorder, nonamnestic-confabulatory type, without use disorder

---

`✓` Additional Character Required   `✓x7ᵗʰ` Placeholder   Questionable PDx   Manifestation   Unspecified   `UPD` Unacceptable PDx   `H1`-`H14` HAC   `HCC` CMS-HCC Dx   `HIV` HIV Dx

✓6th **F10.98 Alcohol use, unspecified with other alcohol-induced disorders**

F10.980 Alcohol use, unspecified with alcohol-induced anxiety disorder CC HCC
Alcohol induced anxiety disorder, without use disorder

F10.981 Alcohol use, unspecified with alcohol-induced sexual dysfunction CC HCC
Alcohol induced sexual dysfunction, without use disorder

F10.982 Alcohol use, unspecified with alcohol-induced sleep disorder HCC
Alcohol induced sleep disorder, without use disorder

F10.988 Alcohol use, unspecified with other alcohol-induced disorder CC HCC
Alcohol induced mild neurocognitive disorder, without use disorder

F10.99 Alcohol use, unspecified with unspecified alcohol-induced disorder CC

✓4th **F11 Opioid related disorders**

✓5th **F11.1 Opioid abuse**
EXCLUDES 1   *opioid dependence (F11.2-)*
           opioid use, unspecified (F11.9-)

F11.10 Opioid abuse, uncomplicated HCC
Opioid use disorder, mild

F11.11 Opioid abuse, in remission HCC
Opioid use disorder, mild, in early remission
Opioid use disorder, mild, in sustained remission

✓6th **F11.12 Opioid abuse with intoxication**

F11.120 Opioid abuse with intoxication, uncomplicated

F11.121 Opioid abuse with intoxication delirium

F11.122 Opioid abuse with intoxication with perceptual disturbance HCC

F11.129 Opioid abuse with intoxication, unspecified HCC

F11.13 Opioid abuse with withdrawal CC HCC
AHA: 2020,4Q,16-17

F11.14 Opioid abuse with opioid-induced mood disorder HCC
Opioid use disorder, mild, with opioid-induced depressive disorder

✓6th **F11.15 Opioid abuse with opioid-induced psychotic disorder**

F11.150 Opioid abuse with opioid-induced psychotic disorder with delusions CC HCC

F11.151 Opioid abuse with opioid-induced psychotic disorder with hallucinations CC HCC

F11.159 Opioid abuse with opioid-induced psychotic disorder, unspecified HCC

✓6th **F11.18 Opioid abuse with other opioid-induced disorder**

F11.181 Opioid abuse with opioid-induced sexual dysfunction HCC

F11.182 Opioid abuse with opioid-induced sleep disorder HCC

F11.188 Opioid abuse with other opioid-induced disorder HCC
Opioid-associated amnestic syndrome with opioid abuse

F11.19 Opioid abuse with unspecified opioid-induced disorder HCC

✓5th **F11.2 Opioid dependence**
EXCLUDES 1   *opioid abuse (F11.1-)*
           opioid use, unspecified (F11.9-)
EXCLUDES 2   *opioid poisoning (T40.0-T40.2-)*

F11.20 Opioid dependence, uncomplicated CC HCC
Opioid use disorder, moderate
Opioid use disorder, severe

F11.21 Opioid dependence, in remission HCC
Opioid use disorder, moderate, in early remission
Opioid use disorder, moderate, in sustained remission
Opioid use disorder, severe, in early remission
Opioid use disorder, severe, in sustained remission

✓6th **F11.22 Opioid dependence with intoxication**
EXCLUDES 1   *opioid dependence with withdrawal (F11.23)*

F11.220 Opioid dependence with intoxication, uncomplicated HCC

F11.221 Opioid dependence with intoxication delirium CC HCC

F11.222 Opioid dependence with intoxication with perceptual disturbance CC HCC

F11.229 Opioid dependence with intoxication, unspecified

F11.23 Opioid dependence with withdrawal CC HCC
EXCLUDES 1   *opioid dependence with intoxication (F11.22-)*

F11.24 Opioid dependence with opioid-induced mood disorder HCC
Opioid use disorder, moderate, with opioid induced depressive disorder

✓6th **F11.25 Opioid dependence with opioid-induced psychotic disorder**

F11.250 Opioid dependence with opioid-induced psychotic disorder with delusions CC HCC

F11.251 Opioid dependence with opioid-induced psychotic disorder with hallucinations CC HCC

F11.259 Opioid dependence with opioid-induced psychotic disorder, unspecified CC HCC

✓6th **F11.28 Opioid dependence with other opioid-induced disorder**

F11.281 Opioid dependence with opioid-induced sexual dysfunction CC HCC

F11.282 Opioid dependence with opioid-induced sleep disorder CC HCC

F11.288 Opioid dependence with other opioid-induced disorder CC HCC
Opioid-associated amnestic syndrome with opioid dependence

F11.29 Opioid dependence with unspecified opioid-induced disorder HCC

✓5th **F11.9 Opioid use, unspecified**
EXCLUDES 1   *opioid abuse (F11.1-)*
           opioid dependence (F11.2-)

TIP: Assign a substance use code only when the provider documents a relationship between the use and an associated physical, mental, or behavioral disorder. As with all diagnoses, substance use codes must meet the definition of a reportable diagnosis.

F11.90 Opioid use, unspecified, uncomplicated
AHA: 2018,2Q,10-11

F11.91 Opioid use, unspecified, in remission

✓6th **F11.92 Opioid use, unspecified with intoxication**
EXCLUDES 1   *opioid use, unspecified with withdrawal (F11.93)*

F11.920 Opioid use, unspecified with intoxication, uncomplicated HCC

F11.921 Opioid use, unspecified with intoxication delirium CC HCC
Opioid-induced delirium

F11.922 Opioid use, unspecified with intoxication with perceptual disturbance HCC

F11.929 Opioid use, unspecified with intoxication, unspecified HCC

F11.93 Opioid use, unspecified with withdrawal CC HCC
EXCLUDES 1   *opioid use, unspecified with intoxication (F11.92-)*

F11.94 Opioid use, unspecified with opioid-induced mood disorder HCC
Opioid induced depressive disorder, without use disorder

✓6th **F11.95 Opioid use, unspecified with opioid-induced psychotic disorder**

F11.950 Opioid use, unspecified with opioid-induced psychotic disorder with delusions CC HCC

F11.951 Opioid use, unspecified with opioid-induced psychotic disorder with hallucinations CC HCC

N Newborn: 0   P Pediatric: 0-17   M Maternity: 9-64   A Adult: 15-124   UNS Unspecified Site   MCC Major Complication/Comorbidity   CC Complication/Comorbidity   PE POA Exempt

560   ICD-10-CM 2025

F11.959 Opioid use, unspecified with opioid-induced psychotic disorder, unspecified `HCC`

✓6ᵗʰ **F11.98** Opioid use, unspecified with other specified opioid-induced disorder

    F11.981 Opioid use, unspecified with opioid-induced **sexual dysfunction** `HCC`
        Opioid induced sexual dysfunction, without use disorder

    F11.982 Opioid use, unspecified with opioid-induced **sleep disorder** `HCC`
        Opioid induced sleep disorder, without use disorder

    F11.988 Opioid use, unspecified with other opioid-induced disorder `HCC`
        Opioid-associated amnestic syndrome without use disorder
        Opioid induced anxiety disorder, without use disorder

F11.99 Opioid use, unspecified with unspecified opioid-induced disorder `HCC`

✓4ᵗʰ **F12** **Cannabis** related disorders
    `INCLUDES` marijuana
    AHA: 2020,1Q,8

✓5ᵗʰ **F12.1** Cannabis **abuse**
    `EXCLUDES 1` *cannabis dependence (F12.2-)*
        cannabis use, unspecified (F12.9-)

    F12.10 Cannabis abuse, **uncomplicated**
        Cannabis use disorder, mild

    F12.11 Cannabis abuse, **in remission**
        Cannabis use disorder, mild, in early remission
        Cannabis use disorder, mild, in sustained remission

✓6ᵗʰ **F12.12** Cannabis abuse with **intoxication**
    F12.120 Cannabis abuse with intoxication, **uncomplicated**
    F12.121 Cannabis abuse with intoxication **delirium** `CC`
    F12.122 Cannabis abuse with intoxication with **perceptual disturbance**
    F12.129 Cannabis abuse with intoxication, unspecified

    F12.13 Cannabis abuse with **withdrawal** `HCC`
        AHA: 2020,4Q,16-17

✓6ᵗʰ **F12.15** Cannabis abuse with **psychotic disorder**
    F12.150 Cannabis abuse with psychotic disorder with **delusions** `CC` `HCC`
    F12.151 Cannabis abuse with psychotic disorder with **hallucinations** `CC` `HCC`
    F12.159 Cannabis abuse with psychotic disorder, unspecified `HCC`

✓6ᵗʰ **F12.18** Cannabis abuse with other cannabis-induced disorder
    F12.180 Cannabis abuse with cannabis-induced **anxiety disorder** `HCC`
    F12.188 Cannabis abuse with other cannabis-induced disorder `HCC`
        Cannabis use disorder, mild, with cannabis-induced sleep disorder

    F12.19 Cannabis abuse with unspecified cannabis-induced disorder

✓5ᵗʰ **F12.2** Cannabis **dependence**
    `EXCLUDES 1` *cannabis abuse (F12.1-)*
        cannabis use, unspecified (F12.9-)
    `EXCLUDES 2` *cannabis poisoning (T40.7-)*

    F12.20 Cannabis dependence, **uncomplicated** `HCC`
        Cannabis use disorder, moderate
        Cannabis use disorder, severe

    F12.21 Cannabis dependence, **in remission** `HCC`
        Cannabis use disorder, moderate, in early remission
        Cannabis use disorder, moderate, in sustained remission
        Cannabis use disorder, severe, in early remission
        Cannabis use disorder, severe, in sustained remission

✓6ᵗʰ **F12.22** Cannabis dependence with **intoxication**
    F12.220 Cannabis dependence with intoxication, **uncomplicated** `HCC`
    F12.221 Cannabis dependence with intoxication **delirium** `CC` `HCC`
    F12.222 Cannabis dependence with intoxication with **perceptual disturbance** `HCC`

F12.229 Cannabis dependence with intoxication, unspecified `HCC`

F12.23 Cannabis dependence with **withdrawal** `HCC`
    AHA: 2018,4Q,7

✓6ᵗʰ **F12.25** Cannabis dependence with **psychotic disorder**
    F12.250 Cannabis dependence with psychotic disorder with **delusions** `CC` `HCC`
    F12.251 Cannabis dependence with psychotic disorder with **hallucinations** `CC` `HCC`
    F12.259 Cannabis dependence with psychotic disorder, unspecified `HCC`

✓6ᵗʰ **F12.28** Cannabis dependence with other cannabis-induced disorder
    F12.280 Cannabis dependence with cannabis-induced **anxiety disorder** `HCC`
    F12.288 Cannabis dependence with other cannabis-induced disorder `HCC`
        Cannabis use disorder, moderate, with cannabis-induced sleep disorder
        Cannabis use disorder, severe, with cannabis-induced sleep disorder

F12.29 Cannabis dependence with unspecified cannabis-induced disorder `HCC`

✓5ᵗʰ **F12.9** Cannabis use, unspecified
    `EXCLUDES 1` *cannabis abuse (F12.1-)*
        cannabis dependence (F12.2-)
    TIP: Assign a substance use code only when the provider documents a relationship between the use and an associated physical, mental, or behavioral disorder. As with all diagnoses, substance use codes must meet the definition of a reportable diagnosis.

    F12.90 Cannabis use, unspecified, **uncomplicated**
        AHA: 2023,3Q,18; 2018,2Q,10-11

    F12.91 Cannabis use, unspecified, **in remission**

✓6ᵗʰ **F12.92** Cannabis use, unspecified with **intoxication**
    F12.920 Cannabis use, unspecified with intoxication, **uncomplicated**
    F12.921 Cannabis use, unspecified with intoxication **delirium** `CC`
    F12.922 Cannabis use, unspecified with intoxication with **perceptual disturbance**
    F12.929 Cannabis use, unspecified with intoxication, unspecified

    F12.93 Cannabis use, unspecified with **withdrawal** `HCC`
        AHA: 2018,4Q,7

✓6ᵗʰ **F12.95** Cannabis use, unspecified with **psychotic disorder**
    F12.950 Cannabis use, unspecified with psychotic disorder with **delusions** `CC` `HCC`
    F12.951 Cannabis use, unspecified with psychotic disorder with **hallucinations** `CC` `HCC`
    F12.959 Cannabis use, unspecified with psychotic disorder, unspecified `HCC`
        Cannabis induced psychotic disorder, without use disorder

✓6ᵗʰ **F12.98** Cannabis use, unspecified with other cannabis-induced disorder
    F12.980 Cannabis use, unspecified with **anxiety disorder** `HCC`
        Cannabis induced anxiety disorder, without use disorder
    F12.988 Cannabis use, unspecified with other cannabis-induced disorder `HCC`
        Cannabis induced sleep disorder, without use disorder

F12.99 Cannabis use, unspecified with unspecified cannabis-induced disorder

✓4ᵗʰ **F13** **Sedative, hypnotic, or anxiolytic** related disorders

✓5ᵗʰ **F13.1** Sedative, hypnotic or anxiolytic-related **abuse**
    `EXCLUDES 1` *sedative, hypnotic or anxiolytic-related dependence (F13.2-)*
        sedative, hypnotic, or anxiolytic use, unspecified (F13.9-)

    F13.10 Sedative, hypnotic or anxiolytic abuse, **uncomplicated** `HCC`
        Sedative, hypnotic, or anxiolytic use disorder, mild

☑ Additional Character Required   ✓x7ᵗʰ Placeholder   `Questionable PDx`   Manifestation   Unspecified   `UPD` Unacceptable PDx   `H1`-`H14` HAC   `HCC` CMS-HCC Dx   `HIV` HIV Dx

F13.11 Sedative, hypnotic or anxiolytic abuse, in remission **HCC**
    Sedative, hypnotic or anxiolytic use disorder, mild, in early remission
    Sedative, hypnotic or anxiolytic use disorder, mild, in sustained remission

✓6th **F13.12** Sedative, hypnotic or anxiolytic abuse with intoxication
    F13.120 Sedative, hypnotic or anxiolytic abuse with intoxication, uncomplicated **HCC**
    F13.121 Sedative, hypnotic or anxiolytic abuse with intoxication delirium **CC** **HCC**
    F13.129 Sedative, hypnotic or anxiolytic abuse with intoxication, unspecified **HCC**

✓6th **F13.13** Sedative, hypnotic or anxiolytic abuse with withdrawal
    AHA: 2020,4Q,16-17
    F13.130 Sedative, hypnotic or anxiolytic abuse with withdrawal, uncomplicated **CC** **HCC**
    F13.131 Sedative, hypnotic or anxiolytic abuse with withdrawal delirium **CC** **HCC**
    F13.132 Sedative, hypnotic or anxiolytic abuse with withdrawal with perceptual disturbance **CC** **HCC**
    F13.139 Sedative, hypnotic or anxiolytic abuse with withdrawal, unspecified **CC** **HCC**

F13.14 Sedative, hypnotic or anxiolytic abuse with sedative, hypnotic or anxiolytic-induced mood disorder **HCC**
    Sedative, hypnotic, or anxiolytic use disorder, mild, with sedative, hypnotic, or anxiolytic-induced bipolar or related disorder
    Sedative, hypnotic, or anxiolytic use disorder, mild, with sedative, hypnotic, or anxiolytic-induced depressive disorder

✓6th **F13.15** Sedative, hypnotic or anxiolytic abuse with sedative, hypnotic or anxiolytic-induced psychotic disorder
    F13.150 Sedative, hypnotic or anxiolytic abuse with sedative, hypnotic or anxiolytic-induced psychotic disorder with delusions **CC** **HCC**
    F13.151 Sedative, hypnotic or anxiolytic abuse with sedative, hypnotic or anxiolytic-induced psychotic disorder with hallucinations **CC** **HCC**
    F13.159 Sedative, hypnotic or anxiolytic abuse with sedative, hypnotic or anxiolytic-induced psychotic disorder, unspecified **HCC**

✓6th **F13.18** Sedative, hypnotic or anxiolytic abuse with other sedative, hypnotic or anxiolytic-induced disorders
    F13.180 Sedative, hypnotic or anxiolytic abuse with sedative, hypnotic or anxiolytic-induced anxiety disorder **HCC**
    F13.181 Sedative, hypnotic or anxiolytic abuse with sedative, hypnotic or anxiolytic-induced sexual dysfunction **HCC**
    F13.182 Sedative, hypnotic or anxiolytic abuse with sedative, hypnotic or anxiolytic-induced sleep disorder **HCC**
    F13.188 Sedative, hypnotic or anxiolytic abuse with other sedative, hypnotic or anxiolytic-induced disorder **HCC**

F13.19 Sedative, hypnotic or anxiolytic abuse with unspecified sedative, hypnotic or anxiolytic-induced disorder **HCC**

✓5th **F13.2** Sedative, hypnotic or anxiolytic-related dependence
    EXCLUDES 1 sedative, hypnotic or anxiolytic-related abuse (F13.1-)
       sedative, hypnotic, or anxiolytic use, unspecified (F13.9-)
    EXCLUDES 2 sedative, hypnotic, or anxiolytic poisoning (T42.-)

    F13.20 Sedative, hypnotic or anxiolytic dependence, uncomplicated **CC** **HCC**
    F13.21 Sedative, hypnotic or anxiolytic dependence, in remission **HCC**
       Sedative, hypnotic or anxiolytic use disorder, moderate, in early remission
       Sedative, hypnotic or anxiolytic use disorder, moderate, in sustained remission
       Sedative, hypnotic or anxiolytic use disorder, severe, in early remission
       Sedative, hypnotic or anxiolytic use disorder, severe, in sustained remission

✓6th **F13.22** Sedative, hypnotic or anxiolytic dependence with intoxication
    EXCLUDES 1 sedative, hypnotic or anxiolytic dependence with withdrawal (F13.23-)
    F13.220 Sedative, hypnotic or anxiolytic dependence with intoxication, uncomplicated **HCC**
    F13.221 Sedative, hypnotic or anxiolytic dependence with intoxication delirium **CC** **HCC**
    F13.229 Sedative, hypnotic or anxiolytic dependence with intoxication, unspecified **HCC**

✓6th **F13.23** Sedative, hypnotic or anxiolytic dependence with withdrawal
    Sedative, hypnotic, or anxiolytic use disorder, moderate
    Sedative, hypnotic, or anxiolytic use disorder, severe
    EXCLUDES 1 sedative, hypnotic or anxiolytic dependence with intoxication (F13.22-)
    F13.230 Sedative, hypnotic or anxiolytic dependence with withdrawal, uncomplicated **CC** **HCC**
    F13.231 Sedative, hypnotic or anxiolytic dependence with withdrawal delirium **CC** **HCC**
    F13.232 Sedative, hypnotic or anxiolytic dependence with withdrawal with perceptual disturbance **CC** **HCC**
       Sedative, hypnotic, or anxiolytic withdrawal with perceptual disturbances
    F13.239 Sedative, hypnotic or anxiolytic dependence with withdrawal, unspecified **CC** **HCC**
       Sedative, hypnotic, or anxiolytic withdrawal without perceptual disturbances

F13.24 Sedative, hypnotic or anxiolytic dependence with sedative, hypnotic or anxiolytic-induced mood disorder **HCC**
    Sedative, hypnotic, or anxiolytic use disorder, moderate, with sedative, hypnotic, or anxiolytic-induced bipolar or related disorder
    Sedative, hypnotic, or anxiolytic use disorder, moderate, with sedative, hypnotic, or anxiolytic-induced depressive disorder
    Sedative, hypnotic, or anxiolytic use disorder, severe, with sedative, hypnotic, or anxiolytic-induced bipolar or related disorder
    Sedative, hypnotic, or anxiolytic use disorder, severe, with sedative, hypnotic, or anxiolytic-induced depressive disorder

✓6th **F13.25** Sedative, hypnotic or anxiolytic dependence with sedative, hypnotic or anxiolytic-induced psychotic disorder
    F13.250 Sedative, hypnotic or anxiolytic dependence with sedative, hypnotic or anxiolytic-induced psychotic disorder with delusions **CC** **HCC**
    F13.251 Sedative, hypnotic or anxiolytic dependence with sedative, hypnotic or anxiolytic-induced psychotic disorder with hallucinations **CC** **HCC**
    F13.259 Sedative, hypnotic or anxiolytic dependence with sedative, hypnotic or anxiolytic-induced psychotic disorder, unspecified **CC** **HCC**

F13.26 Sedative, hypnotic or anxiolytic dependence with sedative, hypnotic or anxiolytic-induced persisting amnestic disorder **CC** **HCC**

F13.27 Sedative, hypnotic or anxiolytic dependence with sedative, hypnotic or anxiolytic-induced persisting dementia **CC** **HCC**
    Sedative, hypnotic, or anxiolytic use disorder, moderate, with sedative, hypnotic, or anxiolytic induced major neurocognitive disorder
    Sedative, hypnotic, or anxiolytic use disorder, severe, with sedative, hypnotic, or anxiolytic-induced major neurocognitive disorder

✓6th **F13.28** Sedative, hypnotic or anxiolytic dependence with other sedative, hypnotic or anxiolytic-induced disorders
    F13.280 Sedative, hypnotic or anxiolytic dependence with sedative, hypnotic or anxiolytic-induced anxiety disorder **CC** **HCC**

F13.281 Sedative, hypnotic or anxiolytic dependence with sedative, hypnotic or anxiolytic-induced **sexual dysfunction** `CC` `HCC`

F13.282 Sedative, hypnotic or anxiolytic dependence with sedative, hypnotic or anxiolytic-induced **sleep disorder** `CC` `HCC`

F13.288 Sedative, hypnotic or anxiolytic dependence with other sedative, hypnotic or anxiolytic-induced disorder `CC` `HCC`
> Sedative, hypnotic, or anxiolytic use disorder, moderate, with sedative, hypnotic, or anxiolytic-induced mild neurocognitive disorder
> Sedative, hypnotic, or anxiolytic use disorder, severe, with sedative, hypnotic, or anxiolytic-induced mild neurocognitive disorder

F13.29 Sedative, hypnotic or anxiolytic dependence with unspecified sedative, hypnotic or anxiolytic-induced disorder `HCC`

✓5th **F13.9** Sedative, hypnotic or anxiolytic-related use, unspecified
> `EXCLUDES 1`   *sedative, hypnotic or anxiolytic-related abuse (F13.1-)*
> *sedative, hypnotic or anxiolytic-related dependence (F13.2-)*

> **TIP:** Assign a substance use code only when the provider documents a relationship between the use and an associated physical, mental, or behavioral disorder. As with all diagnoses, substance use codes must meet the definition of a reportable diagnosis.

F13.90 Sedative, hypnotic, or anxiolytic use, unspecified, **uncomplicated**
> **AHA:** 2018,2Q,10-11

F13.91 Sedative, hypnotic or anxiolytic use, unspecified, **in remission**

✓6th **F13.92** Sedative, hypnotic or anxiolytic use, unspecified with **intoxication**
> `EXCLUDES 1`   *sedative, hypnotic or anxiolytic use, unspecified with withdrawal (F13.93-)*

F13.920 Sedative, hypnotic or anxiolytic use, unspecified with intoxication, **uncomplicated** `HCC`

F13.921 Sedative, hypnotic or anxiolytic use, unspecified with intoxication **delirium** `CC` `HCC`
> Sedative, hypnotic, or anxiolytic-induced delirium

F13.929 Sedative, hypnotic or anxiolytic use, unspecified with intoxication, **unspecified** `HCC`

✓6th **F13.93** Sedative, hypnotic or anxiolytic use, unspecified with **withdrawal**
> `EXCLUDES 1`   *sedative, hypnotic or anxiolytic use, unspecified with intoxication (F13.92-)*

F13.930 Sedative, hypnotic or anxiolytic use, unspecified with withdrawal, **uncomplicated** `CC` `HCC`

F13.931 Sedative, hypnotic or anxiolytic use, unspecified with withdrawal **delirium** `CC` `HCC`

F13.932 Sedative, hypnotic or anxiolytic use, unspecified with withdrawal with **perceptual disturbances** `CC` `HCC`

F13.939 Sedative, hypnotic or anxiolytic use, unspecified with withdrawal, **unspecified** `CC` `HCC`

F13.94 Sedative, hypnotic or anxiolytic use, unspecified with sedative, hypnotic or anxiolytic-induced **mood disorder** `HCC`
> Sedative, hypnotic, or anxiolytic-induced bipolar or related disorder, without use disorder
> Sedative, hypnotic, or anxiolytic-induced depressive disorder, without use disorder

✓6th **F13.95** Sedative, hypnotic or anxiolytic use, unspecified with sedative, hypnotic or anxiolytic-induced **psychotic disorder**

F13.950 Sedative, hypnotic or anxiolytic use, unspecified with sedative, hypnotic or anxiolytic-induced psychotic disorder with **delusions** `CC` `HCC`

F13.951 Sedative, hypnotic or anxiolytic use, unspecified with sedative, hypnotic or anxiolytic-induced psychotic disorder with **hallucinations** `CC` `HCC`

F13.959 Sedative, hypnotic or anxiolytic use, unspecified with sedative, hypnotic or anxiolytic-induced psychotic disorder, **unspecified** `HCC`
> Sedative, hypnotic, or anxiolytic-induced psychotic disorder, without use disorder

F13.96 Sedative, hypnotic or anxiolytic use, unspecified with sedative, hypnotic or anxiolytic-induced **persisting amnestic disorder** `HCC`

F13.97 Sedative, hypnotic or anxiolytic use, unspecified with sedative, hypnotic or anxiolytic-induced **persisting dementia** `CC` `HCC`
> Sedative, hypnotic, or anxiolytic-induced major neurocognitive disorder, without use disorder

✓6th **F13.98** Sedative, hypnotic or anxiolytic use, unspecified with other sedative, hypnotic or anxiolytic-induced disorders

F13.980 Sedative, hypnotic or anxiolytic use, unspecified with sedative, hypnotic or anxiolytic-induced **anxiety disorder** `HCC`
> Sedative, hypnotic, or anxiolytic-induced anxiety disorder, without use disorder

F13.981 Sedative, hypnotic or anxiolytic use, unspecified with sedative, hypnotic or anxiolytic-induced **sexual dysfunction** `HCC`
> Sedative, hypnotic, or anxiolytic-induced sexual dysfunction disorder, without use disorder

F13.982 Sedative, hypnotic or anxiolytic use, unspecified with sedative, hypnotic or anxiolytic-induced **sleep disorder** `HCC`
> Sedative, hypnotic, or anxiolytic-induced sleep disorder, without use disorder

F13.988 Sedative, hypnotic or anxiolytic use, unspecified with other sedative, hypnotic or anxiolytic-induced disorder `HCC`
> Sedative, hypnotic, or anxiolytic-induced mild neurocognitive disorder

F13.99 Sedative, hypnotic or anxiolytic use, unspecified with unspecified sedative, hypnotic or anxiolytic-induced disorder `HCC`

✓4th **F14** **Cocaine** related disorders
> `EXCLUDES 2`   *other stimulant-related disorders (F15.-)*

✓5th **F14.1** Cocaine **abuse**
> `EXCLUDES 1`   *cocaine dependence (F14.2-)*
> *cocaine use, unspecified (F14.9-)*

F14.10 Cocaine abuse, **uncomplicated** `HCC`
> Cocaine use disorder, mild

F14.11 Cocaine abuse, **in remission** `HCC`
> Cocaine use disorder, mild, in early remission
> Cocaine use disorder, mild, in sustained remission

✓6th **F14.12** Cocaine abuse with **intoxication**

F14.120 Cocaine abuse with intoxication, **uncomplicated** `HCC`

F14.121 Cocaine abuse with intoxication with **delirium** `CC` `HCC`

F14.122 Cocaine abuse with intoxication with **perceptual disturbance** `HCC`

F14.129 Cocaine abuse with intoxication, **unspecified** `HCC`

F14.13 Cocaine abuse, unspecified with **withdrawal** `CC` `HCC`
> **AHA:** 2020,4Q,16-17

F14.14 Cocaine abuse with cocaine-induced **mood disorder** `HCC`
> Cocaine use disorder, mild, with cocaine-induced bipolar or related disorder
> Cocaine use disorder, mild, with cocaine-induced depressive disorder

✓6th **F14.15** Cocaine abuse with cocaine-induced **psychotic disorder**

F14.150 Cocaine abuse with cocaine-induced psychotic disorder with **delusions** `CC` `HCC`

☑ Additional Character Required   ✓x7th Placeholder   Questionable PDx   Manifestation   Unspecified   `UPD` Unacceptable PDx   `H1`-`H14` HAC   `HCC` CMS-HCC Dx   `HIV` HIV Dx

Chapter 5. Mental, Behavioral and Neurodevelopmental Disorders

F14.151–F14.99

F14.151   Cocaine abuse with cocaine-induced psychotic disorder with hallucinations   `CC` `HCC`

F14.159   Cocaine abuse with cocaine-induced psychotic disorder, unspecified   `HCC`

✓6th   **F14.18**   Cocaine abuse with other cocaine-induced disorder

F14.180   Cocaine abuse with cocaine-induced anxiety disorder   `HCC`

F14.181   Cocaine abuse with cocaine-induced sexual dysfunction   `HCC`

F14.182   Cocaine abuse with cocaine-induced sleep disorder   `HCC`

F14.188   Cocaine abuse with other cocaine-induced disorder   `HCC`
Cocaine use disorder, mild, with cocaine-induced obsessive compulsive or related disorder

F14.19   Cocaine abuse with unspecified cocaine-induced disorder   `HCC`

✓5th   **F14.2**   Cocaine **dependence**

    `EXCLUDES 1`   *cocaine abuse (F14.1-)*
            cocaine use, unspecified (F14.9-)
    `EXCLUDES 2`   *cocaine poisoning (T40.5-)*

F14.20   **Cocaine dependence, uncomplicated**   `CC` `HCC`
Cocaine use disorder, moderate
Cocaine use disorder, severe

F14.21   **Cocaine dependence, in remission**   `HCC`
Cocaine use disorder, moderate, in early remission
Cocaine use disorder, moderate, in sustained remission
Cocaine use disorder, severe, in early remission
Cocaine use disorder, severe, in sustained remission

✓6th   **F14.22**   **Cocaine dependence with intoxication**

    `EXCLUDES 1`   *cocaine dependence with withdrawal (F14.23)*

F14.220   Cocaine dependence with intoxication, uncomplicated   `HCC`

F14.221   Cocaine dependence with intoxication delirium   `CC` `HCC`

F14.222   Cocaine dependence with intoxication with perceptual disturbance   `CC` `HCC`

F14.229   Cocaine dependence with intoxication, unspecified   `CC` `HCC`

F14.23   **Cocaine dependence with withdrawal**   `CC` `HCC`

    `EXCLUDES 1`   *cocaine dependence with intoxication (F14.22-)*

F14.24   Cocaine dependence with cocaine-induced mood disorder   `HCC`
Cocaine use disorder, moderate, with cocaine-induced bipolar or related disorder
Cocaine use disorder, moderate, with cocaine-induced depressive disorder
Cocaine use disorder, severe, with cocaine-induced bipolar or related disorder
Cocaine use disorder, severe, with cocaine-induced depressive disorder

✓6th   **F14.25**   Cocaine dependence with cocaine-induced psychotic disorder

F14.250   Cocaine dependence with cocaine-induced psychotic disorder with delusions   `CC` `HCC`

F14.251   Cocaine dependence with cocaine-induced psychotic disorder with hallucinations   `CC` `HCC`

F14.259   Cocaine dependence with cocaine-induced psychotic disorder, unspecified   `CC` `HCC`

✓6th   **F14.28**   Cocaine dependence with other cocaine-induced disorder

F14.280   Cocaine dependence with cocaine-induced anxiety disorder   `CC` `HCC`

F14.281   Cocaine dependence with cocaine-induced sexual dysfunction   `CC` `HCC`

F14.282   Cocaine dependence with cocaine-induced sleep disorder   `CC` `HCC`

F14.288   Cocaine dependence with other cocaine-induced disorder   `CC` `HCC`
Cocaine use disorder, moderate, with cocaine-induced obsessive compulsive or related disorder
Cocaine use disorder, severe, with cocaine-induced obsessive compulsive or related disorder

F14.29   Cocaine dependence with unspecified cocaine-induced disorder   `HCC`

✓5th   **F14.9**   Cocaine use, unspecified

    `EXCLUDES 1`   *cocaine abuse (F14.1-)*
            cocaine dependence (F14.2-)

TIP: Assign a substance use code only when the provider documents a relationship between the use and an associated physical, mental, or behavioral disorder. As with all diagnoses, substance use codes must meet the definition of a reportable diagnosis.

F14.90   **Cocaine use, unspecified, uncomplicated**
    AHA: 2018,2Q,10-11

F14.91   **Cocaine use, unspecified, in remission**

✓6th   **F14.92**   **Cocaine use, unspecified with intoxication**

F14.920   Cocaine use, unspecified with intoxication, uncomplicated   `HCC`

F14.921   Cocaine use, unspecified with intoxication delirium   `CC` `HCC`

F14.922   Cocaine use, unspecified with intoxication with perceptual disturbance   `HCC`

F14.929   Cocaine use, unspecified with intoxication, unspecified   `HCC`

F14.93   **Cocaine use, unspecified with withdrawal**   `CC` `HCC`
    AHA: 2020,4Q,16-17

F14.94   Cocaine use, unspecified with cocaine-induced mood disorder   `HCC`
Cocaine induced bipolar or related disorder, without use disorder
Cocaine induced depressive disorder, without use disorder

✓6th   **F14.95**   Cocaine use, unspecified with cocaine-induced psychotic disorder

F14.950   Cocaine use, unspecified with cocaine-induced psychotic disorder with delusions   `CC` `HCC`

F14.951   Cocaine use, unspecified with cocaine-induced psychotic disorder with hallucinations   `CC` `HCC`

F14.959   Cocaine use, unspecified with cocaine-induced psychotic disorder, unspecified   `HCC`
Cocaine induced psychotic disorder, without use disorder

✓6th   **F14.98**   Cocaine use, unspecified with other specified cocaine-induced disorder

F14.980   Cocaine use, unspecified with cocaine-induced anxiety disorder   `HCC`
Cocaine induced anxiety disorder, without use disorder

F14.981   Cocaine use, unspecified with cocaine-induced sexual dysfunction   `HCC`
Cocaine induced sexual dysfunction, without use disorder

F14.982   Cocaine use, unspecified with cocaine-induced sleep disorder   `HCC`
Cocaine induced sleep disorder, without use disorder

F14.988   Cocaine use, unspecified with other cocaine-induced disorder   `HCC`
Cocaine induced obsessive compulsive or related disorder

F14.99   Cocaine use, unspecified with unspecified cocaine-induced disorder   `HCC`

✓4th F15 Other stimulant related disorders

    INCLUDES   amphetamine-related disorders
            caffeine
    EXCLUDES 2   cocaine-related disorders (F14.-)

✓5th F15.1 Other stimulant abuse

    EXCLUDES 1   other stimulant dependence (F15.2-)
               other stimulant use, unspecified (F15.9-)

  F15.10 Other stimulant abuse, uncomplicated `HCC`
    Amphetamine type substance use disorder, mild
    Other or unspecified stimulant use disorder, mild

  F15.11 Other stimulant abuse, in remission `HCC`
    Amphetamine type substance use disorder, mild, in early remission
    Amphetamine type substance use disorder, mild, in sustained remission
    Other or unspecified stimulant use disorder, mild, in early remission
    Other or unspecified stimulant use disorder, mild, in sustained remission
    AHA: 2021,3Q,8

  ✓6th F15.12 Other stimulant abuse with intoxication

    F15.120 Other stimulant abuse with intoxication, uncomplicated `HCC`
    F15.121 Other stimulant abuse with intoxication delirium `CC` `HCC`
    F15.122 Other stimulant abuse with intoxication with perceptual disturbance `HCC`
      Amphetamine or other stimulant use disorder, mild, with amphetamine or other stimulant intoxication, with perceptual disturbances
    F15.129 Other stimulant abuse with intoxication, unspecified `HCC`
      Amphetamine or other stimulant use disorder, mild, with amphetamine or other stimulant intoxication, without perceptual disturbances

  F15.13 Other stimulant abuse with withdrawal `CC` `HCC`
    AHA: 2020,4Q,16-17

  F15.14 Other stimulant abuse with stimulant-induced mood disorder `HCC`
    Amphetamine or other stimulant use disorder, mild, with amphetamine or other stimulant induced bipolar or related disorder
    Amphetamine or other stimulant use disorder, mild, with amphetamine or other stimulant induced depressive disorder

  ✓6th F15.15 Other stimulant abuse with stimulant-induced psychotic disorder

    F15.150 Other stimulant abuse with stimulant-induced psychotic disorder with delusions `CC` `HCC`
    F15.151 Other stimulant abuse with stimulant-induced psychotic disorder with hallucinations `CC` `HCC`
    F15.159 Other stimulant abuse with stimulant-induced psychotic disorder, unspecified `HCC`

  ✓6th F15.18 Other stimulant abuse with other stimulant-induced disorder

    F15.180 Other stimulant abuse with stimulant-induced anxiety disorder `HCC`
    F15.181 Other stimulant abuse with stimulant-induced sexual dysfunction `HCC`
    F15.182 Other stimulant abuse with stimulant-induced sleep disorder `HCC`
    F15.188 Other stimulant abuse with other stimulant-induced disorder `HCC`
      Amphetamine or other stimulant use disorder, mild, with amphetamine or other stimulant induced obsessive-compulsive or related disorder

    F15.19 Other stimulant abuse with unspecified stimulant-induced disorder `HCC`

✓5th F15.2 Other stimulant dependence

    EXCLUDES 1   other stimulant abuse (F15.1-)
               other stimulant use, unspecified (F15.9-)

  F15.20 Other stimulant dependence, uncomplicated `CC` `HCC`
    Amphetamine type substance use disorder, moderate
    Amphetamine type substance use disorder, severe
    Other or unspecified stimulant use disorder, moderate
    Other or unspecified stimulant use disorder, severe

  F15.21 Other stimulant dependence, in remission `HCC`
    Amphetamine type substance use disorder, moderate, in early remission
    Amphetamine type substance use disorder, moderate, in sustained remission
    Amphetamine type substance use disorder, severe, in early remission
    Amphetamine type substance use disorder, severe, in sustained remission
    Other or unspecified stimulant use disorder, moderate, in early remission
    Other or unspecified stimulant use disorder, moderate, in sustained remission
    Other or unspecified stimulant use disorder, severe, in early remission
    Other or unspecified stimulant use disorder, severe, in sustained remission

  ✓6th F15.22 Other stimulant dependence with intoxication

    EXCLUDES 1   other stimulant dependence with withdrawal (F15.23)

    F15.220 Other stimulant dependence with intoxication, uncomplicated `HCC`
    F15.221 Other stimulant dependence with intoxication delirium `CC` `HCC`
    F15.222 Other stimulant dependence with intoxication with perceptual disturbance `CC` `HCC`
      Amphetamine or other stimulant use disorder, moderate, with amphetamine or other stimulant intoxication, with perceptual disturbances
      Amphetamine or other stimulant use disorder, severe, with amphetamine or other stimulant intoxication, with perceptual disturbances
    F15.229 Other stimulant dependence with intoxication, unspecified `HCC`
      Amphetamine or other stimulant use disorder, moderate, with amphetamine or other stimulant intoxication, without perceptual disturbances
      Amphetamine or other stimulant use disorder, severe, with amphetamine or other stimulant intoxication, without perceptual disturbances

  F15.23 Other stimulant dependence with withdrawal `CC` `HCC`
    Amphetamine or other stimulant withdrawal
    EXCLUDES 1   other stimulant dependence with intoxication (F15.22-)

  F15.24 Other stimulant dependence with stimulant-induced mood disorder `HCC`
    Amphetamine or other stimulant use disorder, moderate, with amphetamine or other stimulant-induced bipolar or related disorder
    Amphetamine or other stimulant use disorder, moderate, with amphetamine or other stimulant induced depressive disorder
    Amphetamine or other stimulant use disorder, severe, with amphetamine or other stimulant-induced bipolar or related disorder
    Amphetamine or other stimulant use disorder, severe, with amphetamine or other stimulant-induced depressive disorder

  ✓6th F15.25 Other stimulant dependence with stimulant-induced psychotic disorder

    F15.250 Other stimulant dependence with stimulant-induced psychotic disorder with delusions `CC` `HCC`
    F15.251 Other stimulant dependence with stimulant-induced psychotic disorder with hallucinations `CC` `HCC`

✓ Additional Character Required   ✓x7th Placeholder   Questionable PDx   Manifestation   Unspecified   UPD Unacceptable PDx   H1-H14 HAC   HCC CMS-HCC Dx   HIV HIV Dx

ICD-10-CM 2025   565

Chapter 5. Mental, Behavioral and Neurodevelopmental Disorders

F15–F15.251

Chapter 5. Mental, Behavioral and Neurodevelopmental Disorders

F15.259 Other stimulant dependence with stimulant-induced psychotic disorder, unspecified `CC` `HCC`

√6ᵗʰ **F15.28 Other stimulant dependence with other stimulant-induced disorder**

     F15.280 Other stimulant dependence with stimulant-induced anxiety disorder `CC` `HCC`

     F15.281 Other stimulant dependence with stimulant-induced sexual dysfunction `CC` `HCC`

     F15.282 Other stimulant dependence with stimulant-induced sleep disorder `CC` `HCC`

     F15.288 Other stimulant dependence with other stimulant-induced disorder `CC` `HCC`
         Amphetamine or other stimulant use disorder, moderate, with amphetamine orother stimulant induced obsessive compulsive or related disorder
         Amphetamine or other stimulant use disorder, severe, with amphetamine or otherstimulant induced obsessive compulsive or related disorder

     F15.29 Other stimulant dependence with unspecified stimulant-induced disorder `HCC`

√5ᵗʰ **F15.9 Other stimulant use, unspecified**

     `EXCLUDES 1`   *other stimulant abuse (F15.1-)*
                 other stimulant dependence (F15.2-)

     TIP: Assign a substance use code only when the provider documents a relationship between the use and an associated physical, mental, or behavioral disorder. As with all diagnoses, substance use codes must meet the definition of a reportable diagnosis.

     F15.90 Other stimulant use, unspecified, uncomplicated
         AHA: 2018,2Q,10-11

     F15.91 Other stimulant use, unspecified, in remission

√6ᵗʰ **F15.92 Other stimulant use, unspecified with intoxication**

     `EXCLUDES 1`   *other stimulant use, unspecified with withdrawal (F15.93)*

     F15.920 Other stimulant use, unspecified with intoxication, uncomplicated `HCC`

     F15.921 Other stimulant use, unspecified with intoxication delirium `CC` `HCC`
         Amphetamine or other stimulant-induced delirium

     F15.922 Other stimulant use, unspecified with intoxication with perceptual disturbance `HCC`

     F15.929 Other stimulant use, unspecified with intoxication, unspecified `HCC`
         Caffeine intoxication

     F15.93 Other stimulant use, unspecified with withdrawal `CC` `HCC`
         Caffeine withdrawal
         `EXCLUDES 1`   *other stimulant use, unspecified with intoxication (F15.92-)*

     F15.94 Other stimulant use, unspecified with stimulant-induced mood disorder `HCC`
         Amphetamine or other stimulant-induced bipolar or related disorder, without use disorder
         Amphetamine or other stimulant-induced depressive disorder, without use disorder

√6ᵗʰ **F15.95 Other stimulant use, unspecified with stimulant-induced psychotic disorder**

     F15.950 Other stimulant use, unspecified with stimulant-induced psychotic disorder with delusions `CC` `HCC`

     F15.951 Other stimulant use, unspecified with stimulant-induced psychotic disorder with hallucinations `CC` `HCC`

     F15.959 Other stimulant use, unspecified with stimulant-induced psychotic disorder, unspecified `HCC`
         Amphetamine or other stimulant-induced psychotic disorder, without use disorder

√6ᵗʰ **F15.98 Other stimulant use, unspecified with other stimulant-induced disorder**

     F15.980 Other stimulant use, unspecified with stimulant-induced anxiety disorder `HCC`
         Amphetamine or other stimulant-induced anxiety disorder, without use disorder
         Caffeine induced anxiety disorder, without use disorder

     F15.981 Other stimulant use, unspecified with stimulant-induced sexual dysfunction `HCC`
         Amphetamine or other stimulant-induced sexual dysfunction, without use disorder

     F15.982 Other stimulant use, unspecified with stimulant-induced sleep disorder `HCC`
         Amphetamine or other stimulant-induced sleep disorder, without use disorder
         Caffeine induced sleep disorder, without use disorder

     F15.988 Other stimulant use, unspecified with other stimulant-induced disorder `HCC`
         Amphetamine or other stimulant-induced obsessive compulsive or related disorder, without use disorder

     F15.99 Other stimulant use, unspecified with unspecified stimulant-induced disorder `HCC`

√4ᵗʰ **F16 Hallucinogen related disorders**

     `INCLUDES`   ecstasy
               PCP
               phencyclidine
     AHA: 2018,4Q,31

√5ᵗʰ **F16.1 Hallucinogen abuse**

     `EXCLUDES 1`   *hallucinogen dependence (F16.2-)*
                 hallucinogen use, unspecified (F16.9-)

     F16.10 Hallucinogen abuse, uncomplicated `HCC`
         Other hallucinogen use disorder, mild
         Phencyclidine use disorder, mild

     F16.11 Hallucinogen abuse, in remission `HCC`
         Other hallucinogen use disorder, mild, in early remission
         Other hallucinogen use disorder, mild, in sustained remission
         Phencyclidine use disorder, mild, in early remission
         Phencyclidine use disorder, mild, in sustained remission

√6ᵗʰ **F16.12 Hallucinogen abuse with intoxication**

     F16.120 Hallucinogen abuse with intoxication, uncomplicated `HCC`

     F16.121 Hallucinogen abuse with intoxication with delirium `CC` `HCC`

     F16.122 Hallucinogen abuse with intoxication with perceptual disturbance `HCC`

     F16.129 Hallucinogen abuse with intoxication, unspecified `HCC`

     F16.14 Hallucinogen abuse with hallucinogen-induced mood disorder `HCC`
         Other hallucinogen use disorder, mild, with other hallucinogen induced bipolar or related disorder
         Other hallucinogen use disorder, mild, with other hallucinogen induced depressive disorder
         Phencyclidine use disorder, mild, with phencyclidine induced bipolar or related disorder
         Phencyclidine use disorder, mild, with phencyclidine induced depressive disorder

√6ᵗʰ **F16.15 Hallucinogen abuse with hallucinogen-induced psychotic disorder**

     F16.150 Hallucinogen abuse with hallucinogen-induced psychotic disorder with delusions `CC` `HCC`

     F16.151 Hallucinogen abuse with hallucinogen-induced psychotic disorder with hallucinations `CC` `HCC`

     F16.159 Hallucinogen abuse with hallucinogen-induced psychotic disorder, unspecified `HCC`

√6ᵗʰ **F16.18 Hallucinogen abuse with other hallucinogen-induced disorder**

     F16.180 Hallucinogen abuse with hallucinogen-induced anxiety disorder `HCC`

N Newborn: 0   P Pediatric: 0-17   M Maternity: 9-64   A Adult: 15-124   UNS Unspecified Site   MCC Major Complication/Comorbidity   CC Complication/Comorbidity   PE POA Exempt

566   ICD-10-CM 2025

F16.183   **Hallucinogen abuse with hallucinogen persisting perception disorder (flashbacks)**   `HCC`

F16.188   **Hallucinogen abuse with other hallucinogen-induced disorder**   `HCC`

F16.19   **Hallucinogen abuse with unspecified hallucinogen-induced disorder**   `HCC`

✓5th F16.2   **Hallucinogen dependence**

    EXCLUDES 1   *hallucinogen abuse (F16.1-)*

                    hallucinogen use, unspecified (F16.9-)

F16.20   **Hallucinogen dependence, uncomplicated**   `CC` `HCC`
Other hallucinogen use disorder, moderate
Other hallucinogen use disorder, severe
Phencyclidine use disorder, moderate
Phencyclidine use disorder, severe

F16.21   **Hallucinogen dependence, in remission**   `HCC`
Other hallucinogen use disorder, moderate, in early remission
Other hallucinogen use disorder, moderate, in sustained remission
Other hallucinogen use disorder, severe, in early remission
Other hallucinogen use disorder, severe, in sustained remission
Phencyclidine use disorder, moderate, in early remission
Phencyclidine use disorder, moderate, in sustained remission
Phencyclidine use disorder, severe, in early remission
Phencyclidine use disorder, severe, in sustained remission

✓6th F16.22   **Hallucinogen dependence with intoxication**

F16.220   **Hallucinogen dependence with intoxication, uncomplicated**   `HCC`

F16.221   **Hallucinogen dependence with intoxication with delirium**   `CC` `HCC`

F16.229   **Hallucinogen dependence with intoxication, unspecified**   `HCC`

F16.24   **Hallucinogen dependence with hallucinogen-induced mood disorder**   `HCC`
Other hallucinogen use disorder, moderate, with other hallucinogen induced bipolar or related disorder
Other hallucinogen use disorder, moderate, with other hallucinogen induced depressive disorder
Other hallucinogen use disorder, severe, with other hallucinogen-induced bipolar or related disorder
Other hallucinogen use disorder, severe, with other hallucinogen-induced depressive disorder
Phencyclidine use disorder, moderate, with phencyclidine induced bipolar or related disorder
Phencyclidine use disorder, moderate, with phencyclidine induced depressive disorder
Phencyclidine use disorder, severe, with phencyclidine induced bipolar or related disorder
Phencyclidine use disorder, severe, with phencyclidine-induced depressive disorder

✓6th F16.25   **Hallucinogen dependence with hallucinogen-induced psychotic disorder**

F16.250   **Hallucinogen dependence with hallucinogen-induced psychotic disorder with delusions**   `CC` `HCC`

F16.251   **Hallucinogen dependence with hallucinogen-induced psychotic disorder with hallucinations**   `CC` `HCC`

F16.259   **Hallucinogen dependence with hallucinogen-induced psychotic disorder, unspecified**   `CC` `HCC`

✓6th F16.28   **Hallucinogen dependence with other hallucinogen-induced disorder**

F16.280   **Hallucinogen dependence with hallucinogen-induced anxiety disorder**   `CC` `HCC`

F16.283   **Hallucinogen dependence with hallucinogen persisting perception disorder (flashbacks)**   `CC` `HCC`

F16.288   **Hallucinogen dependence with other hallucinogen-induced disorder**   `CC` `HCC`

F16.29   **Hallucinogen dependence with unspecified hallucinogen-induced disorder**   `HCC`

✓5th F16.9   **Hallucinogen use, unspecified**

    EXCLUDES 1   *hallucinogen abuse (F16.1-)*

                    hallucinogen dependence (F16.2-)

TIP: Assign a substance use code only when the provider documents a relationship between the use and an associated physical, mental, or behavioral disorder. As with all diagnoses, substance use codes must meet the definition of a reportable diagnosis.

F16.90   **Hallucinogen use, unspecified, uncomplicated**
      AHA: 2018,2Q,10-11

F16.91   **Hallucinogen use, unspecified, in remission**

✓6th F16.92   **Hallucinogen use, unspecified with intoxication**

F16.920   **Hallucinogen use, unspecified with intoxication, uncomplicated**   `HCC`

F16.921   **Hallucinogen use, unspecified with intoxication with delirium**   `CC` `HCC`
Other hallucinogen intoxication delirium

F16.929   **Hallucinogen use, unspecified with intoxication, unspecified**   `HCC`

F16.94   **Hallucinogen use, unspecified with hallucinogen-induced mood disorder**   `HCC`
Other hallucinogen induced bipolar or related disorder, without use disorder
Other hallucinogen induced depressive disorder, without use disorder
Phencyclidine induced bipolar or related disorder, without use disorder
Phencyclidine induced depressive disorder, without use disorder

✓6th F16.95   **Hallucinogen use, unspecified with hallucinogen-induced psychotic disorder**

F16.950   **Hallucinogen use, unspecified with hallucinogen-induced psychotic disorder with delusions**   `CC` `HCC`

F16.951   **Hallucinogen use, unspecified with hallucinogen-induced psychotic disorder with hallucinations**   `CC` `HCC`

F16.959   **Hallucinogen use, unspecified with hallucinogen-induced psychotic disorder, unspecified**   `HCC`
Other hallucinogen induced psychotic disorder, without use disorder
Phencyclidine induced psychotic disorder, without use disorder

✓6th F16.98   **Hallucinogen use, unspecified with other specified hallucinogen-induced disorder**

F16.980   **Hallucinogen use, unspecified with hallucinogen-induced anxiety disorder**   `HCC`
Other hallucinogen-induced anxiety disorder, without use disorder
Phencyclidine induced anxiety disorder, without use disorder

F16.983   **Hallucinogen use, unspecified with hallucinogen persisting perception disorder (flashbacks)**   `HCC`

F16.988   **Hallucinogen use, unspecified with other hallucinogen-induced disorder**   `HCC`

F16.99   **Hallucinogen use, unspecified with unspecified hallucinogen-induced disorder**   `HCC`

✓4th **F17   Nicotine dependence**

    EXCLUDES 1   *history of tobacco dependence (Z87.891)*

                    tobacco use NOS (Z72.0)

    EXCLUDES 2   *tobacco use (smoking) during pregnancy, childbirth and the puerperium (O99.33-)*

                    toxic effect of nicotine (T65.2-)

    AHA: 2013,4Q,108-109

✓5th **F17.2   Nicotine dependence**

✓6th F17.20   **Nicotine dependence, unspecified**

F17.200   **Nicotine dependence, unspecified, uncomplicated**   `UPD`
Tobacco use disorder, mild
Tobacco use disorder, moderate
Tobacco use disorder, severe
     AHA: 2016,1Q,36
     TIP: Assign when provider documentation indicates "smoker" without further specification.

| ✔ Additional Character Required | ✔x7th Placeholder | Questionable PDx | Manifestation | Unspecified | UPD Unacceptable PDx | H1-H14 HAC | HCC CMS-HCC Dx | HIV HIV Dx |

ICD-10-CM 2025   **567**

F17.201 Nicotine dependence, unspecified, in remission **UPD**
   Tobacco use disorder, mild, in early remission
   Tobacco use disorder, mild, in sustained remission
   Tobacco use disorder, moderate, in early remission
   Tobacco use disorder, moderate, in sustained remission
   Tobacco use disorder, severe, in early remission
   Tobacco use disorder, severe, in sustained remission

F17.203 Nicotine dependence unspecified, with withdrawal **CC**
   Tobacco withdrawal

F17.208 Nicotine dependence, unspecified, with other nicotine-induced disorders

F17.209 Nicotine dependence, unspecified, with unspecified nicotine-induced disorders

√6th **F17.21** Nicotine dependence, cigarettes

F17.210 Nicotine dependence, cigarettes, uncomplicated **UPD**
   AHA: 2017,2Q,28-29

F17.211 Nicotine dependence, cigarettes, in remission **UPD**
   Tobacco use disorder, cigarettes, mild, in early remission
   Tobacco use disorder, cigarettes, mild, in sustained remission
   Tobacco use disorder, cigarettes, moderate, in early remission
   Tobacco use disorder, cigarettes, moderate, in sustained remission
   Tobacco use disorder, cigarettes, severe, in early remission
   Tobacco use disorder, cigarettes, severe, in sustained remission

F17.213 Nicotine dependence, cigarettes, with withdrawal **CC**

F17.218 Nicotine dependence, cigarettes, with other nicotine-induced disorders

F17.219 Nicotine dependence, cigarettes, with unspecified nicotine-induced disorders

√6th **F17.22** Nicotine dependence, chewing tobacco

F17.220 Nicotine dependence, chewing tobacco, uncomplicated **UPD**

F17.221 Nicotine dependence, chewing tobacco, in remission **UPD**
   Tobacco use disorder, chewing tobacco, mild, in early remission
   Tobacco use disorder, chewing tobacco, mild, in sustained remission
   Tobacco use disorder, chewing tobacco, moderate, in early remission
   Tobacco use disorder, chewing tobacco, moderate, in sustained remission
   Tobacco use disorder, chewing tobacco, severe, in early remission
   Tobacco use disorder, chewing tobacco, severe, in sustained remission

F17.223 Nicotine dependence, chewing tobacco, with withdrawal **CC**

F17.228 Nicotine dependence, chewing tobacco, with other nicotine-induced disorders

F17.229 Nicotine dependence, chewing tobacco, with unspecified nicotine-induced disorders

√6th **F17.29** Nicotine dependence, other tobacco product

F17.290 Nicotine dependence, other tobacco product, uncomplicated **UPD**
   AHA: 2017,2Q,28-29

F17.291 Nicotine dependence, other tobacco product, in remission **UPD**
   Tobacco use disorder, other tobacco product, mild, in early remission
   Tobacco use disorder, other tobacco product, mild, in sustained remission
   Tobacco use disorder, other tobacco product, moderate, in early remission
   Tobacco use disorder, other tobacco product, moderate, in sustained remission
   Tobacco use disorder, other tobacco product, severe, in early remission
   Tobacco use disorder, other tobacco product, severe, in sustained remission

F17.293 Nicotine dependence, other tobacco product, with withdrawal **CC**

F17.298 Nicotine dependence, other tobacco product, with other nicotine-induced disorders

F17.299 Nicotine dependence, other tobacco product, with unspecified nicotine-induced disorders

√4th **F18** Inhalant related disorders
   INCLUDES volatile solvents

√5th **F18.1** Inhalant abuse
   EXCLUDES 1 inhalant dependence (F18.2-)
         inhalant use, unspecified (F18.9-)

F18.10 Inhalant abuse, uncomplicated **HCC**
   Inhalant use disorder, mild

F18.11 Inhalant abuse, in remission **HCC**
   Inhalant use disorder, mild, in early remission
   Inhalant use disorder, mild, in sustained remission

√6th **F18.12** Inhalant abuse with intoxication

F18.120 Inhalant abuse with intoxication, uncomplicated **HCC**

F18.121 Inhalant abuse with intoxication delirium **CC** **HCC**

F18.129 Inhalant abuse with intoxication, unspecified **HCC**

F18.14 Inhalant abuse with inhalant-induced mood disorder **HCC**
   Inhalant use disorder, mild, with inhalant induced depressive disorder

√6th **F18.15** Inhalant abuse with inhalant-induced psychotic disorder

F18.150 Inhalant abuse with inhalant-induced psychotic disorder with delusions **CC** **HCC**

F18.151 Inhalant abuse with inhalant-induced psychotic disorder with hallucinations **CC** **HCC**

F18.159 Inhalant abuse with inhalant-induced psychotic disorder, unspecified **HCC**

F18.17 Inhalant abuse with inhalant-induced dementia **CC** **HCC**
   Inhalant use disorder, mild, with inhalant induced major neurocognitive disorder

√6th **F18.18** Inhalant abuse with other inhalant-induced disorders

F18.180 Inhalant abuse with inhalant-induced anxiety disorder **HCC**

F18.188 Inhalant abuse with other inhalant-induced disorder **HCC**
   Inhalant use disorder, mild, with inhalant induced mild neurocognitive disorder

F18.19 Inhalant abuse with unspecified inhalant-induced disorder **HCC**

√5th **F18.2** Inhalant dependence
   EXCLUDES 1 inhalant abuse (F18.1-)
         inhalant use, unspecified (F18.9-)

F18.20 Inhalant dependence, uncomplicated **CC** **HCC**
   Inhalant use disorder, moderate
   Inhalant use disorder, severe

F18.21 Inhalant dependence, in remission **HCC**
   Inhalant use disorder, moderate, in early remission
   Inhalant use disorder, moderate, in sustained remission
   Inhalant use disorder, severe, in early remission
   Inhalant use disorder, severe, in sustained remission

N Newborn: 0   **P** Pediatric: 0-17   **M** Maternity: 9-64   **A** Adult: 15-124   **UNS** Unspecified Site   **MCC** Major Complication/Comorbidity   **CC** Complication/Comorbidity   **PE** POA Exempt

568

ICD-10-CM 2025

✓6ᵗʰ **F18.22 Inhalant dependence with intoxication**

    F18.22Ø Inhalant dependence with intoxication, uncomplicated `HCC`

    F18.221 Inhalant dependence with intoxication delirium `CC` `HCC`

    F18.229 Inhalant dependence with intoxication, unspecified `HCC`

F18.24 Inhalant dependence with inhalant-induced mood disorder `HCC`
    Inhalant use disorder, moderate, with inhalant induced depressive disorder
    Inhalant use disorder, severe, with inhalant induced depressive disorder

✓6ᵗʰ **F18.25 Inhalant dependence with inhalant-induced psychotic disorder**

    F18.25Ø Inhalant dependence with inhalant-induced psychotic disorder with delusions `CC` `HCC`

    F18.251 Inhalant dependence with inhalant-induced psychotic disorder with hallucinations `CC` `HCC`

    F18.259 Inhalant dependence with inhalant-induced psychotic disorder, unspecified `CC` `HCC`

F18.27 Inhalant dependence with inhalant-induced dementia `CC` `HCC`
    Inhalant use disorder, moderate, with inhalant induced major neurocognitive disorder
    Inhalant use disorder, severe, with inhalant induced major neurocognitive disorder

✓6ᵗʰ **F18.28 Inhalant dependence with other inhalant-induced disorders**

    F18.28Ø Inhalant dependence with inhalant-induced anxiety disorder `CC` `HCC`

    F18.288 Inhalant dependence with other inhalant-induced disorder `CC` `HCC`
        Inhalant use disorder, moderate, with inhalant-induced mild neurocognitive disorder
        Inhalant use disorder, severe, with inhalant-induced mild neurocognitive disorder

F18.29 Inhalant dependence with unspecified inhalant-induced disorder `HCC`

✓5ᵗʰ **F18.9 Inhalant use, unspecified**

    EXCLUDES 1   *inhalant abuse (F18.1-)*
             inhalant dependence (F18.2-)

    TIP: Assign a substance use code only when the provider documents a relationship between the use and an associated physical, mental, or behavioral disorder. As with all diagnoses, substance use codes must meet the definition of a reportable diagnosis.

    F18.9Ø Inhalant use, unspecified, uncomplicated
        AHA: 2018,2Q,10-11

    F18.91 Inhalant use, unspecified, in remission

✓6ᵗʰ   **F18.92 Inhalant use, unspecified with intoxication**

        F18.92Ø Inhalant use, unspecified with intoxication, uncomplicated `HCC`

        F18.921 Inhalant use, unspecified with intoxication with delirium `CC` `HCC`

        F18.929 Inhalant use, unspecified with intoxication, unspecified `HCC`

    F18.94 Inhalant use, unspecified with inhalant-induced mood disorder `HCC`
        Inhalant induced depressive disorder

✓6ᵗʰ   **F18.95 Inhalant use, unspecified with inhalant-induced psychotic disorder**

        F18.95Ø Inhalant use, unspecified with inhalant-induced psychotic disorder with delusions `CC` `HCC`

        F18.951 Inhalant use, unspecified with inhalant-induced psychotic disorder with hallucinations `CC` `HCC`

        F18.959 Inhalant use, unspecified with inhalant-induced psychotic disorder, unspecified `HCC`

    F18.97 Inhalant use, unspecified with inhalant-induced persisting dementia `CC` `HCC`
        Inhalant-induced major neurocognitive disorder

✓6ᵗʰ **F18.98 Inhalant use, unspecified with other inhalant-induced disorders**

    F18.98Ø Inhalant use, unspecified with inhalant-induced anxiety disorder `HCC`

    F18.988 Inhalant use, unspecified with other inhalant-induced disorder `HCC`
        Inhalant-induced mild neurocognitive disorder

    F18.99 Inhalant use, unspecified with unspecified inhalant-induced disorder `HCC`

✓4ᵗʰ **F19 Other psychoactive substance related disorders**

    INCLUDES   polysubstance drug use (indiscriminate drug use)

✓5ᵗʰ **F19.1 Other psychoactive substance abuse**

    EXCLUDES 1   *other psychoactive substance dependence (F19.2-)*
             other psychoactive substance use, unspecified (F19.9-)

    F19.1Ø Other psychoactive substance abuse, uncomplicated `HCC`
        Other (or unknown) substance use disorder, mild

    F19.11 Other psychoactive substance abuse, in remission `HCC`
        Other (or unknown) substance use disorder, mild, in early remission
        Other (or unknown) substance use disorder, mild, in sustained remission

✓6ᵗʰ   **F19.12 Other psychoactive substance abuse with intoxication**

        F19.12Ø Other psychoactive substance abuse with intoxication, uncomplicated `HCC`

        F19.121 Other psychoactive substance abuse with intoxication delirium `CC` `HCC`

        F19.122 Other psychoactive substance abuse with intoxication with perceptual disturbances `HCC`

        F19.129 Other psychoactive substance abuse with intoxication, unspecified `HCC`

✓6ᵗʰ   **F19.13 Other psychoactive substance abuse with withdrawal**
        AHA: 2020,4Q,16-17

        F19.13Ø Other psychoactive substance abuse with withdrawal, uncomplicated `CC` `HCC`

        F19.131 Other psychoactive substance abuse with withdrawal delirium `CC` `HCC`

        F19.132 Other psychoactive substance abuse with withdrawal with perceptual disturbance `CC` `HCC`

        F19.139 Other psychoactive substance abuse with withdrawal, unspecified `CC` `HCC`
        AHA: 2023,3Q,16

    F19.14 Other psychoactive substance abuse with psychoactive substance-induced mood disorder `HCC`
        Other (or unknown) substance use disorder, mild, with other (or unknown) substance-induced bipolar or related disorder
        Other (or unknown) substance use disorder, mild, with other (or unknown) substance-induced depressive disorder

✓6ᵗʰ   **F19.15 Other psychoactive substance abuse with psychoactive substance-induced psychotic disorder**

        F19.15Ø Other psychoactive substance abuse with psychoactive substance-induced psychotic disorder with delusions `CC` `HCC`

        F19.151 Other psychoactive substance abuse with psychoactive substance-induced psychotic disorder with hallucinations `CC` `HCC`

        F19.159 Other psychoactive substance abuse with psychoactive substance-induced psychotic disorder, unspecified `HCC`

    F19.16 Other psychoactive substance abuse with psychoactive substance-induced persisting amnestic disorder `HCC`

    F19.17 Other psychoactive substance abuse with psychoactive substance-induced persisting dementia `CC` `HCC`
        Other (or unknown) substance use disorder, mild, with other (or unknown) substance-induced major neurocognitive disorder

✓6ᵗʰ   **F19.18 Other psychoactive substance abuse with other psychoactive substance-induced disorders**

        F19.18Ø Other psychoactive substance abuse with psychoactive substance-induced anxiety disorder `HCC`

☑ Additional Character Required   ✓x7ᵗʰ Placeholder   Questionable PDx   Manifestation   Unspecified   `UPD` Unacceptable PDx   `H1`-`H14` HAC   `HCC` CMS-HCC Dx   `HIV` HIV Dx

F19.181 **Other psychoactive substance abuse with psychoactive substance-induced sexual dysfunction** `HCC`

F19.182 **Other psychoactive substance abuse with psychoactive substance-induced sleep disorder** `HCC`

F19.188 **Other psychoactive substance abuse with other psychoactive substance-induced disorder** `HCC`

Other (or unknown) substance use disorder, mild, with other (or unknown) substance induced mild neurocognitive disorder

Other (or unknown) substance use disorder, mild, with other (or unknown) substance induced obsessive-compulsive or related disorder

F19.19 **Other psychoactive substance abuse with unspecified psychoactive substance-induced disorder** `HCC`

✓5ᵗʰ **F19.2** **Other psychoactive substance dependence**

EXCLUDES 1   *other psychoactive substance abuse (F19.1-)*
other psychoactive substance use, unspecified (F19.9-)

F19.20 **Other psychoactive substance dependence, uncomplicated** `CC` `HCC`

Other (or unknown) substance use disorder, moderate
Other (or unknown) substance use disorder, severe

F19.21 **Other psychoactive substance dependence, in remission** `HCC`

Other (or unknown) substance use disorder, moderate, in early remission
Other (or unknown) substance use disorder, moderate, in sustained remission
Other (or unknown) substance use disorder, severe, in early remission
Other (or unknown) substance use disorder, severe, in sustained remission

✓6ᵗʰ **F19.22** **Other psychoactive substance dependence with intoxication**

EXCLUDES 1   *other psychoactive substance dependence with withdrawal (F19.23-)*

F19.220 **Other psychoactive substance dependence with intoxication, uncomplicated** `HCC`

F19.221 **Other psychoactive substance dependence with intoxication delirium** `CC` `HCC`

F19.222 **Other psychoactive substance dependence with intoxication with perceptual disturbance** `CC` `HCC`

F19.229 **Other psychoactive substance dependence with intoxication, unspecified** `HCC`

✓6ᵗʰ **F19.23** **Other psychoactive substance dependence with withdrawal**

EXCLUDES 1   *other psychoactive substance dependence with intoxication (F19.22-)*

F19.230 **Other psychoactive substance dependence with withdrawal, uncomplicated** `CC` `HCC`

F19.231 **Other psychoactive substance dependence with withdrawal delirium** `CC` `HCC`

F19.232 **Other psychoactive substance dependence with withdrawal with perceptual disturbance** `CC` `HCC`

F19.239 **Other psychoactive substance dependence with withdrawal, unspecified** `CC` `HCC`

F19.24 **Other psychoactive substance dependence with psychoactive substance-induced mood disorder** `HCC`

Other (or unknown) substance use disorder, moderate, with other (or unknown) substance induced bipolar or related disorder
Other (or unknown) substance use disorder, moderate, with other (or unknown) substance induced depressive disorder
Other (or unknown) substance use disorder, severe, with other (or unknown) substance induced bipolar or related disorder
Other (or unknown) substance use disorder, severe, with other (or unknown) substance induced depressive disorder

✓6ᵗʰ **F19.25** **Other psychoactive substance dependence with psychoactive substance-induced psychotic disorder**

F19.250 **Other psychoactive substance dependence with psychoactive substance-induced psychotic disorder with delusions** `CC` `HCC`

F19.251 **Other psychoactive substance dependence with psychoactive substance-induced psychotic disorder with hallucinations** `CC` `HCC`

F19.259 **Other psychoactive substance dependence with psychoactive substance-induced psychotic disorder, unspecified** `CC` `HCC`

F19.26 **Other psychoactive substance dependence with psychoactive substance-induced persisting amnestic disorder** `CC` `HCC`

F19.27 **Other psychoactive substance dependence with psychoactive substance-induced persisting dementia** `CC` `HCC`

Other (or unknown) substance use disorder, moderate, with other (or unknown) substance induced major neurocognitive disorder
Other (or unknown) substance use disorder, severe, with other (or unknown) substance induced major neurocognitive disorder

✓6ᵗʰ **F19.28** **Other psychoactive substance dependence with other psychoactive substance-induced disorders**

F19.280 **Other psychoactive substance dependence with psychoactive substance-induced anxiety disorder** `CC` `HCC`

F19.281 **Other psychoactive substance dependence with psychoactive substance-induced sexual dysfunction** `CC` `HCC`

F19.282 **Other psychoactive substance dependence with psychoactive substance-induced sleep disorder** `CC` `HCC`

F19.288 **Other psychoactive substance dependence with other psychoactive substance-induced disorder** `CC` `HCC`

Other (or unknown) substance use disorder, moderate, with other (or unknown) substance induced mild neurocognitive disorder
Other (or unknown) substance use disorder, severe, with other (or unknown) substance induced mild neurocognitive disorder
Other (or unknown) substance use disorder, moderate, with other (or unknown) substance induced obsessive compulsive or related disorder
Other (or unknown) substance use disorder, severe, with other (or unknown) substance induced obsessive-compulsive or related disorder

F19.29 **Other psychoactive substance dependence with unspecified psychoactive substance-induced disorder** `HCC`

✓5ᵗʰ **F19.9** **Other psychoactive substance use, unspecified**

EXCLUDES 1   *other psychoactive substance abuse (F19.1-)*
other psychoactive substance dependence (F19.2-)

TIP: Assign a substance use code only when the provider documents a relationship between the use and an associated physical, mental, or behavioral disorder. As with all diagnoses, substance use codes must meet the definition of a reportable diagnosis.

F19.90 **Other psychoactive substance use, unspecified, uncomplicated**

AHA: 2018,2Q,10-11

F19.91 **Other psychoactive substance use, unspecified, in remission**

✓6ᵗʰ **F19.92** **Other psychoactive substance use, unspecified with intoxication**

EXCLUDES 1   *other psychoactive substance use, unspecified with withdrawal (F19.93)*

F19.920 **Other psychoactive substance use, unspecified with intoxication, uncomplicated** `HCC`

`N` Newborn: 0   `P` Pediatric: 0-17   `M` Maternity: 9-64   `A` Adult: 15-124   `UNS` Unspecified Site   `MCC` Major Complication/Comorbidity   `CC` Complication/Comorbidity   `PE` POA Exempt

570

ICD-10-CM 2025

F19.921 Other psychoactive substance use, unspecified with intoxication with **delirium** `CC` `HCC`
　Other (or unknown) substance-induced delirium

F19.922 Other psychoactive substance use, unspecified with intoxication with **perceptual disturbance** `HCC`

F19.929 Other psychoactive substance use, unspecified with intoxication, unspecified `HCC`

✓6ᵗʰ **F19.93** Other psychoactive substance use, unspecified with **withdrawal**
　　EXCLUDES 1　*other psychoactive substance use, unspecified with intoxication (F19.92-)*

F19.930 Other psychoactive substance use, unspecified with withdrawal, **uncomplicated** `CC` `HCC`

F19.931 Other psychoactive substance use, unspecified with withdrawal **delirium** `CC` `HCC`

F19.932 Other psychoactive substance use, unspecified with withdrawal with **perceptual disturbance** `CC` `HCC`

F19.939 Other psychoactive substance use, unspecified with withdrawal, unspecified `CC` `HCC`

F19.94 Other psychoactive substance use, unspecified with psychoactive substance-induced **mood disorder** `HCC`
　Other (or unknown) substance-induced bipolar or related disorder, without use disorder
　Other (or unknown) substance-induced depressive disorder, without use disorder

✓6ᵗʰ **F19.95** Other psychoactive substance use, unspecified with psychoactive substance-induced **psychotic disorder**

F19.950 Other psychoactive substance use, unspecified with psychoactive substance-induced psychotic disorder with **delusions** `CC` `HCC`

F19.951 Other psychoactive substance use, unspecified with psychoactive substance-induced psychotic disorder with **hallucinations** `CC` `HCC`

F19.959 Other psychoactive substance use, unspecified with psychoactive substance-induced psychotic disorder, **unspecified** `HCC`
　Other or unknown substance-induced psychotic disorder, without use disorder

F19.96 Other psychoactive substance use, unspecified with psychoactive substance-induced **persisting amnestic disorder** `HCC`

F19.97 Other psychoactive substance use, unspecified with psychoactive substance-induced **persisting dementia** `CC` `HCC`
　Other (or unknown) substance-induced major neurocognitive disorder, without use disorder

✓6ᵗʰ **F19.98** Other psychoactive substance use, unspecified with other psychoactive substance-induced disorders

F19.980 Other psychoactive substance use, unspecified with psychoactive substance-induced **anxiety disorder** `HCC`
　Other (or unknown) substance-induced anxiety disorder, without use disorder

F19.981 Other psychoactive substance use, unspecified with psychoactive substance-induced **sexual dysfunction** `HCC`
　Other (or unknown) substance-induced sexual dysfunction, without use disorder

F19.982 Other psychoactive substance use, unspecified with psychoactive substance-induced **sleep disorder** `HCC`
　Other (or unknown) substance-induced sleep disorder, without use disorder

F19.988 Other psychoactive substance use, unspecified with other psychoactive substance-induced disorder `HCC`
　Other (or unknown) substance-induced mild neurocognitive disorder, without use disorder
　Other (or unknown) substance-induced obsessive-compulsive or related disorder, without use disorder

F19.99 Other psychoactive substance use, unspecified with unspecified psychoactive substance-induced disorder `HCC`

Schizophrenia, schizotypal, delusional, and other non-mood psychotic disorders (F20-F29)

✓4ᵗʰ **F20　Schizophrenia**
　▶Use additional code, if applicable, to identify:◀
　▶other specified cognitive deficit (R41.84-)◀
　　EXCLUDES 1　*brief psychotic disorder (F23)*
　　　　cyclic schizophrenia (F25.0)
　　　　mood [affective] disorders with psychotic symptoms (F30.2, F31.2, F31.5, F31.64, F32.3, F33.3)
　　　　schizoaffective disorder (F25.-)
　　　　schizophrenic reaction NOS (F23)
　　EXCLUDES 2　*schizophrenic reaction in:*
　　　　alcoholism (F10.15-, F10.25-, F10.95-)
　　　　brain disease (F06.2)
　　　　epilepsy (F06.2)
　　　　psychoactive drug use (F11-F19 with .15, .25, .95)
　　　　schizotypal disorder (F21)
　DEF: Group of disorders with disturbances in thought (delusions, hallucinations), mood (blunted, flattened, inappropriate affect), and sense of self. Schizophrenia also includes bizarre, purposeless behavior, repetitious activity, or inactivity.

F20.0　Paranoid schizophrenia `CC` `HCC`
　Paraphrenic schizophrenia
　　EXCLUDES 1　*involutional paranoid state (F22)*
　　　　paranoia (F22)
　DEF: Preoccupied with delusional suspicions and auditory hallucinations related to a single theme. This type of schizophrenia is usually hostile, grandiose, threatening, persecutory, and occasionally hypochondriacal.

F20.1　Disorganized schizophrenia `CC` `HCC`
　Hebephrenic schizophrenia
　Hebephrenia

F20.2　Catatonic schizophrenia `CC` `HCC`
　Schizophrenic catalepsy
　Schizophrenic catatonia
　Schizophrenic flexibilitas cerea
　　EXCLUDES 1　*catatonic stupor (R40.1)*
　DEF: Extreme changes in motor activity. One extreme is a decreased response or reaction to the environment and the other is spontaneous activity.

F20.3　Undifferentiated schizophrenia `HCC`
　Atypical schizophrenia
　　EXCLUDES 1　*acute schizophrenia-like psychotic disorder (F23)*
　　EXCLUDES 2　*post-schizophrenic depression (F32.89)*

F20.5　Residual schizophrenia `CC` `HCC`
　Restzustand (schizophrenic)
　Schizophrenic residual state

✓5ᵗʰ **F20.8　Other schizophrenia**

F20.81　Schizophreniform disorder `CC` `HCC`
　Schizophreniform psychosis NOS

F20.89　Other schizophrenia `CC` `HCC`
　Cenesthopathic schizophrenia
　Simple schizophrenia

F20.9　Schizophrenia, unspecified `HCC`
　AHA: 2019,2Q,32

☑ Additional Character Required　✓x7ᵗʰ Placeholder　`Questionable PDx`　Manifestation　Unspecified　`UPD` Unacceptable PDx　`H1`-`H14` HAC　`HCC` CMS-HCC Dx　`HIV` HIV Dx

ICD-10-CM 2025　　　　571

F21　Schizotypal disorder　　HCC
Borderline schizophrenia
Latent schizophrenia
Latent schizophrenic reaction
Prepsychotic schizophrenia
Prodromal schizophrenia
Pseudoneurotic schizophrenia
Pseudopsychopathic schizophrenia
Schizotypal personality disorder
> EXCLUDES 2　Asperger's syndrome (F84.5)
> schizoid personality disorder (F60.1)

DEF: Disorder characterized by various oddities of thinking, perception, communication, and behavior that may be manifested as magical thinking, ideas of reference, paranoid ideation, recurrent illusions and derealization (depersonalization), or social isolation.

F22　Delusional disorders　　HCC
Delusional dysmorphophobia
Involutional paranoid state
Paranoia
Paranoia querulans
Paranoid psychosis
Paranoid state
Paraphrenia (late)
Sensitiver Beziehungswahn
> EXCLUDES 1　mood [affective] disorders with psychotic symptoms (F30.2, F31.2, F31.5, F31.64, F32.3, F33.3)
> paranoid schizophrenia (F20.0)
> EXCLUDES 2　paranoid personality disorder (F60.0)
> paranoid psychosis, psychogenic (F23)
> paranoid reaction (F23)

F23　Brief psychotic disorder　　CC HCC
Paranoid reaction
Psychogenic paranoid psychosis
> EXCLUDES 2　mood [affective] disorders with psychotic symptoms (F30.2, F31.2, F31.5, F31.64, F32.3, F33.3)

AHA: 2019,2Q,32

F24　Shared psychotic disorder　　HCC
Folie a deux
Induced paranoid disorder
Induced psychotic disorder

F25　Schizoaffective disorders
> EXCLUDES 1　mood [affective] disorders with psychotic symptoms (F30.2, F31.2, F31.5, F31.64, F32.3, F33.3)
> schizophrenia (F20.-)

F25.0　Schizoaffective disorder, bipolar type　　HCC
Cyclic schizophrenia
Schizoaffective disorder, manic type
Schizoaffective disorder, mixed type
Schizoaffective psychosis, bipolar type

F25.1　Schizoaffective disorder, depressive type　　HCC
Schizoaffective psychosis, depressive type

F25.8　Other schizoaffective disorders　　HCC

F25.9　Schizoaffective disorder, unspecified　　HCC
Schizoaffective psychosis NOS

F28　Other psychotic disorder not due to a substance or known physiological condition　　HIV HCC
Chronic hallucinatory psychosis
Other specified schizophrenia spectrum and other psychotic disorder

F29　Unspecified psychosis not due to a substance or known physiological condition　　HIV HCC
Psychosis NOS
Unspecified schizophrenia spectrum and other psychotic disorder
> EXCLUDES 1　mental disorder NOS (F99)
> unspecified mental disorder due to known physiological condition (F09)

Mood [affective] disorders (F30-F39)

F30　Manic episode
> INCLUDES　bipolar disorder, single manic episode
> mixed affective episode
> EXCLUDES 1　bipolar disorder (F31.-)
> major depressive disorder, recurrent (F33.-)
> major depressive disorder, single episode (F32.-)

DEF: Mania: Characterized by abnormal states of elation or excitement out of keeping with the individual's circumstances and varying from enhanced liveliness (hypomania) to violent, almost uncontrollable, excitement. Aggression and anger, flight of ideas, distractibility, impaired judgment, and grandiose ideas are common.

F30.1　Manic episode without psychotic symptoms
F30.10　Manic episode without psychotic symptoms, unspecified　　CC HCC
F30.11　Manic episode without psychotic symptoms, mild　　CC HCC
F30.12　Manic episode without psychotic symptoms, moderate　　CC HCC
F30.13　Manic episode, severe, without psychotic symptoms　　CC HCC

F30.2　Manic episode, severe with psychotic symptoms　　CC HCC
Manic stupor
Mania with mood-congruent psychotic symptoms
Mania with mood-incongruent psychotic symptoms

F30.3　Manic episode in partial remission　　HCC

F30.4　Manic episode in full remission

F30.8　Other manic episodes　　HCC
Hypomania

F30.9　Manic episode, unspecified　　CC HCC
Mania NOS

F31　Bipolar disorder
> INCLUDES　bipolar I disorder
> bipolar type I disorder
> manic-depressive illness
> manic-depressive psychosis
> manic-depressive reaction
> seasonal bipolar disorder
> EXCLUDES 1　bipolar disorder, single manic episode (F30.-)
> major depressive disorder, recurrent (F33.-)
> major depressive disorder, single episode (F32.-)
> EXCLUDES 2　cyclothymia (F34.0)

AHA: 2020,1Q,23

F31.0　Bipolar disorder, current episode hypomanic　　CC HCC

F31.1　Bipolar disorder, current episode manic without psychotic features
F31.10　Bipolar disorder, current episode manic without psychotic features, unspecified　　CC HCC
F31.11　Bipolar disorder, current episode manic without psychotic features, mild　　CC HCC
F31.12　Bipolar disorder, current episode manic without psychotic features, moderate　　CC HCC
F31.13　Bipolar disorder, current episode manic without psychotic features, severe　　CC HCC

F31.2　Bipolar disorder, current episode manic severe with psychotic features　　CC HCC
Bipolar disorder, current episode manic with mood-congruent psychotic symptoms
Bipolar disorder, current episode manic with mood-incongruent psychotic symptoms
Bipolar I disorder, current or most recent episode manic with psychotic features

F31.3　Bipolar disorder, current episode depressed, mild or moderate severity
F31.30　Bipolar disorder, current episode depressed, mild or moderate severity, unspecified　　CC HCC
F31.31　Bipolar disorder, current episode depressed, mild　　CC HCC
F31.32　Bipolar disorder, current episode depressed, moderate　　CC HCC

F31.4　Bipolar disorder, current episode depressed, severe, without psychotic features　　CC HCC

F31.5   **Bipolar disorder, current episode depressed, severe, with psychotic features**   `CC` `HCC`
> Bipolar disorder, current episode depressed with mood-congruent psychotic symptoms
> Bipolar disorder, current episode depressed with mood-incongruent psychotic symptoms
> Bipolar I disorder, current or most recent episode depressed, with psychotic features

√5th **F31.6**   **Bipolar disorder, current episode mixed**

     F31.60   **Bipolar disorder, current episode mixed, unspecified**   `CC` `HCC`

     F31.61   **Bipolar disorder, current episode mixed, mild**   `CC` `HCC`

     F31.62   **Bipolar disorder, current episode mixed, moderate**   `CC` `HCC`

     F31.63   **Bipolar disorder, current episode mixed, severe, without psychotic features**   `CC` `HCC`

     F31.64   **Bipolar disorder, current episode mixed, severe, with psychotic features**   `CC` `HCC`
> Bipolar disorder, current episode mixed with mood-congruent psychotic symptoms
> Bipolar disorder, current episode mixed with mood-incongruent psychotic symptoms

√5th **F31.7**   **Bipolar disorder, currently in remission**

     F31.70   **Bipolar disorder, currently in remission, most recent episode unspecified**

     F31.71   **Bipolar disorder, in partial remission, most recent episode hypomanic**   `HCC`

     F31.72   **Bipolar disorder, in full remission, most recent episode hypomanic**

     F31.73   **Bipolar disorder, in partial remission, most recent episode manic**   `HCC`

     F31.74   **Bipolar disorder, in full remission, most recent episode manic**

     F31.75   **Bipolar disorder, in partial remission, most recent episode depressed**   `HCC`

     F31.76   **Bipolar disorder, in full remission, most recent episode depressed**

     F31.77   **Bipolar disorder, in partial remission, most recent episode mixed**   `HCC`

     F31.78   **Bipolar disorder, in full remission, most recent episode mixed**

√5th **F31.8**   **Other bipolar disorders**

     F31.81   **Bipolar II disorder**   `CC` `HCC`
> Bipolar disorder, type 2

     F31.89   **Other bipolar disorder**   `CC` `HCC`
> Recurrent manic episodes NOS

F31.9   **Bipolar disorder, unspecified**   `HCC`
> Manic depression
> **AHA:** 2020,1Q,23

√4th **F32**   **Depressive episode**

> `INCLUDES`   single episode of agitated depression
> single episode of depressive reaction
> single episode of major depression
> single episode of psychogenic depression
> single episode of reactive depression
> single episode of vital depression

> `EXCLUDES 1`   bipolar disorder (F31.-)
> manic episode (F30.-)
> recurrent depressive disorder (F33.-)

> `EXCLUDES 2`   adjustment disorder (F43.2)

> **AHA:** 2020,1Q,23
> **DEF:** Mood disorder that produces depression that may exhibit as sadness, low self-esteem, or guilt feelings. Other manifestations may be withdrawal from friends and family and interrupted sleep.

F32.0   **Major depressive disorder, single episode, mild**   `CC`

F32.1   **Major depressive disorder, single episode, moderate**   `CC` `HCC`

F32.2   **Major depressive disorder, single episode, severe without psychotic features**   `CC` `HCC`

F32.3   **Major depressive disorder, single episode, severe with psychotic features**   `CC` `HCC`
> Single episode of major depression with mood-congruent psychotic symptoms
> Single episode of major depression with mood-incongruent psychotic symptoms
> Single episode of major depression with psychotic symptoms
> Single episode of psychogenic depressive psychosis
> Single episode of psychotic depression
> Single episode of reactive depressive psychosis

F32.4   **Major depressive disorder, single episode, in partial remission**

F32.5   **Major depressive disorder, single episode, in full remission**

√5th **F32.8**   **Other depressive episodes**
> **AHA:** 2016,4Q,14

     F32.81   **Premenstrual dysphoric disorder**
> `EXCLUDES 1`   premenstrual tension syndrome (N94.3)
> **DEF:** Severe manifestation of premenstrual syndrome (PMS) that can be disabling and destructive to day-to-day activities. It can exacerbate pre-existing emotional disorders, like depression and anxiety, and cause feelings of loss of control, fatigue, and irritability.

     F32.89   **Other specified depressive episodes**
> Atypical depression
> Post-schizophrenic depression
> Single episode of 'masked' depression NOS

F32.9   **Major depressive disorder, single episode, unspecified**
> Major depression NOS
> **AHA:** 2021,4Q,10; 2021,1Q,10; 2013,4Q,107

F32.A   **Depression, unspecified**
> Depression NOS
> Depressive disorder NOS
> **AHA:** 2021,4Q,9-10

√4th **F33**   **Major depressive disorder, recurrent**

> `INCLUDES`   recurrent episodes of depressive reaction
> recurrent episodes of endogenous depression
> recurrent episodes of major depression
> recurrent episodes of psychogenic depression
> recurrent episodes of reactive depression
> recurrent episodes of seasonal affective disorder
> recurrent episodes of seasonal depressive disorder
> recurrent episodes of vital depression

> `EXCLUDES 1`   bipolar disorder (F31.-)
> manic episode (F30.-)

> **AHA:** 2020,1Q,23
> **DEF:** Mood disorder that produces depression that may exhibit as sadness, low self-esteem, or guilt feelings. Other manifestations may be withdrawal from friends and family and interrupted sleep.

F33.0   **Major depressive disorder, recurrent, mild**   `CC`

F33.1   **Major depressive disorder, recurrent, moderate**   `CC` `HCC`

F33.2   **Major depressive disorder, recurrent, severe without psychotic features**   `CC` `HCC`

F33.3   **Major depressive disorder, recurrent, severe with psychotic symptoms**   `CC` `HCC`
> Endogenous depression with psychotic symptoms
> Major depressive disorder, recurrent, with psychotic features
> Recurrent severe episodes of major depression with mood-congruent psychotic symptoms
> Recurrent severe episodes of major depression with mood-incongruent psychotic symptoms
> Recurrent severe episodes of major depression with psychotic symptoms
> Recurrent severe episodes of psychogenic depressive psychosis
> Recurrent severe episodes of psychotic depression
> Recurrent severe episodes of reactive depressive psychosis

√5th **F33.4**   **Major depressive disorder, recurrent, in remission**

     F33.40   **Major depressive disorder, recurrent, in remission, unspecified**   `CC`

     F33.41   **Major depressive disorder, recurrent, in partial remission**

     F33.42   **Major depressive disorder, recurrent, in full remission**

F33.8   **Other recurrent depressive disorders**   `CC`
> Recurrent brief depressive episodes

F33.9   **Major depressive disorder, recurrent, unspecified**   `CC`
> Monopolar depression NOS

✔ Additional Character Required   ✔x7th Placeholder   `Questionable PDx`   Manifestation   Unspecified   `UPD` Unacceptable PDx   `H1`-`H14` HAC   `HCC` CMS-HCC Dx   `HIV` HIV Dx

ICD-10-CM 2025   573

✓4th F34 Persistent mood [affective] disorders

F34.0 Cyclothymic disorder
Affective personality disorder
Cycloid personality
Cyclothymia
Cyclothymic personality
DEF: Mood disorder characterized by fast and repeated alterations between hypomanic and depressed moods.

F34.1 Dysthymic disorder
Depressive neurosis
Depressive personality disorder
Dysthymia
Neurotic depression
Persistent anxiety depression
Persistent depressive disorder
EXCLUDES 2 anxiety depression (mild or not persistent) (F41.8)
DEF: Depression without psychosis. It is a less severe but persistent depression and is considered a mild to moderate chronic form of depression.

✓5th F34.8 Other persistent mood [affective] disorders
AHA: 2016,4Q,14

F34.81 Disruptive mood dysregulation disorder CC
F34.89 Other specified persistent mood disorders CC
F34.9 Persistent mood [affective] disorder, unspecified CC

F39 Unspecified mood [affective] disorder
Affective psychosis NOS

Anxiety, dissociative, stress-related, somatoform and other nonpsychotic mental disorders (F40-F48)

✓4th F40 Phobic anxiety disorders
DEF: Phobia: Broad-range anxiety with abnormally intense dread of certain objects or specific situations that would not normally have that effect.

✓5th F40.0 Agoraphobia
DEF: Profound anxiety or fear of leaving familiar settings like home, or being in unfamiliar locations or with strangers or crowds. Agoraphobia may or may not be preceded by recurrent panic attacks.

F40.00 Agoraphobia, unspecified
F40.01 Agoraphobia with panic disorder
Panic disorder with agoraphobia
EXCLUDES 1 panic disorder without agoraphobia (F41.0)
F40.02 Agoraphobia without panic disorder

✓5th F40.1 Social phobias
Anthropophobia
Social anxiety disorder
Social anxiety disorder of childhood
Social neurosis
F40.10 Social phobia, unspecified
F40.11 Social phobia, generalized

✓5th F40.2 Specific (isolated) phobias
EXCLUDES 2 dysmorphophobia (nondelusional) (F45.22)
nosophobia (F45.22)

✓6th F40.21 Animal type phobia
F40.210 Arachnophobia
Fear of spiders
F40.218 Other animal type phobia

✓6th F40.22 Natural environment type phobia
F40.220 Fear of thunderstorms
F40.228 Other natural environment type phobia

✓6th F40.23 Blood, injection, injury type phobia
F40.230 Fear of blood
F40.231 Fear of injections and transfusions
F40.232 Fear of other medical care
F40.233 Fear of injury

✓6th F40.24 Situational type phobia
F40.240 Claustrophobia
F40.241 Acrophobia
F40.242 Fear of bridges
F40.243 Fear of flying
F40.248 Other situational type phobia

✓6th F40.29 Other specified phobia
F40.290 Androphobia
Fear of men
F40.291 Gynephobia
Fear of women
F40.298 Other specified phobia

F40.8 Other phobic anxiety disorders
Phobic anxiety disorder of childhood
F40.9 Phobic anxiety disorder, unspecified
Phobia NOS
Phobic state NOS

✓4th F41 Other anxiety disorders
EXCLUDES 2 anxiety in:
acute stress reaction (F43.0)
neurasthenia (F48.8)
psychophysiologic disorders (F45.-)
transient adjustment reaction (F43.2)
separation anxiety (F93.0)

F41.0 Panic disorder [episodic paroxysmal anxiety]
Panic attack
Panic state
EXCLUDES 1 panic disorder with agoraphobia (F40.01)
DEF: Neurotic disorder characterized by recurrent panic or anxiety, apprehension, fear, or terror. Symptoms include shortness of breath, palpitations, dizziness, and shakiness; fear of dying may persist.

F41.1 Generalized anxiety disorder
Anxiety neurosis
Anxiety reaction
Anxiety state
Overanxious disorder
EXCLUDES 2 neurasthenia (F48.8)

F41.3 Other mixed anxiety disorders
F41.8 Other specified anxiety disorders
Anxiety depression (mild or not persistent)
Anxiety hysteria
Mixed anxiety and depressive disorder
AHA: 2021,1Q,10

F41.9 Anxiety disorder, unspecified
Anxiety NOS
AHA: 2021,1Q,10

✓4th F42 Obsessive-compulsive disorder
EXCLUDES 2 obsessive-compulsive personality (disorder) (F60.5)
obsessive-compulsive symptoms occurring in depression (F32-F33)
obsessive-compulsive symptoms occurring in schizophrenia (F20.-)
AHA: 2016,4Q,14-15

F42.2 Mixed obsessional thoughts and acts
F42.3 Hoarding disorder
F42.4 Excoriation (skin-picking) disorder
EXCLUDES 1 factitial dermatitis (L98.1)
other specified behavioral and emotional disorders with onset usually occurring in early childhood and adolescence (F98.8)

F42.8 Other obsessive-compulsive disorder
Anancastic neurosis
Obsessive-compulsive neurosis

F42.9 Obsessive-compulsive disorder, unspecified

✓4th F43 Reaction to severe stress, and adjustment disorders
F43.0 Acute stress reaction
Acute crisis reaction
Acute reaction to stress
Combat and operational stress reaction
Combat fatigue
Crisis state
Psychic shock

✓5th F43.1 Post-traumatic stress disorder (PTSD)
Traumatic neurosis
DEF: Preoccupation with traumatic events beyond normal experience (i.e., rape, personal assault, etc.) that may also include recurring flashbacks of the trauma. Symptoms include difficulty remembering, sleeping, or concentrating, and guilt feelings for surviving.
F43.10 Post-traumatic stress disorder, unspecified
F43.11 Post-traumatic stress disorder, acute
F43.12 Post-traumatic stress disorder, chronic

✓5th F43.2 Adjustment disorders
Culture shock
Grief reaction
Hospitalism in children
EXCLUDES 2 separation anxiety disorder of childhood (F93.0)
F43.20 Adjustment disorder, unspecified

F43.21	**Adjustment disorder with depressed mood**	

        AHA: 2014,1Q,25

F43.22   **Adjustment disorder with anxiety**

F43.23   **Adjustment disorder with mixed anxiety and depressed mood**

F43.24   **Adjustment disorder with disturbance of conduct**

F43.25   **Adjustment disorder with mixed disturbance of emotions and conduct**

F43.29   **Adjustment disorder with other symptoms**

✓5th **F43.8**   **Other reactions to severe stress**

      Other specified trauma and stressor-related disorder

      AHA: 2022,4Q,17

    F43.81   **Prolonged grief disorder**

        Complicated grief

        Complicated grief disorder

        Persistent complex bereavement disorder

    F43.89   **Other reactions to severe stress**

F43.9   **Reaction to severe stress, unspecified**

      Trauma and stressor-related disorder, NOS

      Unspecified trauma and stressor-related disorder

✓4th **F44**   **Dissociative and conversion disorders**

    INCLUDES   conversion hysteria

             conversion reaction

             hysteria

             hysterical psychosis

    EXCLUDES 2   *malingering [conscious simulation] (Z76.5)*

    F44.0   **Dissociative amnesia**   HCC

        EXCLUDES 1   *amnesia NOS (R41.3)*

               anterograde amnesia (R41.1)

               dissociative amnesia with dissociative fugue (F44.1)

               retrograde amnesia (R41.2)

        EXCLUDES 2   *alcohol-or other psychoactive substance-induced amnestic disorder (F10, F13, F19 with .26, .96)*

               amnestic disorder due to known physiological condition (F04)

               postictal amnesia in epilepsy (G40.-)

    F44.1   **Dissociative fugue**   HCC

        Dissociative amnesia with dissociative fugue

        EXCLUDES 2   *postictal fugue in epilepsy (G40.-)*

        DEF: Dissociative hysteria identified by memory loss and flight from familiar surroundings to a completely separate environment. Episodes may last hours or days. Conscious activity is not associated with perception of surroundings and there is no later memory of the episode.

    F44.2   **Dissociative stupor**

        EXCLUDES 1   *catatonic stupor (R40.1)*

                stupor NOS (R40.1)

        EXCLUDES 2   *catatonic disorder due to known physiological condition (F06.1)*

                depressive stupor (F32, F33)

                manic stupor (F30, F31)

    F44.4   **Conversion disorder with motor symptom or deficit**

        Conversion disorder with abnormal movement

        Conversion disorder with speech symptoms

        Conversion disorder with swallowing symptoms

        Conversion disorder with weakness/paralysis

        Dissociative motor disorders

        Psychogenic aphonia

        Psychogenic dysphonia

    F44.5   **Conversion disorder with seizures or convulsions**

        Conversion disorder with attacks or seizures

        Dissociative convulsions

        AHA: 2021,1Q,3; 2019,1Q,19

    F44.6   **Conversion disorder with sensory symptom or deficit**

        Conversion disorder with anesthesia or sensory loss

        Conversion disorder with special sensory symptoms

        Dissociative anesthesia and sensory loss

        Psychogenic deafness

    F44.7   **Conversion disorder with mixed symptom presentation**

✓5th **F44.8**   **Other dissociative and conversion disorders**

    F44.81   **Dissociative identity disorder**   HCC

        Multiple personality disorder

    F44.89   **Other dissociative and conversion disorders**

        Ganser's syndrome

        Psychogenic confusion

        Psychogenic twilight state

        Trance and possession disorders

    F44.9   **Dissociative and conversion disorder, unspecified**

        Dissociative disorder NOS

✓4th **F45**   **Somatoform disorders**

    EXCLUDES 2   *dissociative and conversion disorders (F44.-)*

               factitious disorders (F68.1-, F68.A)

               hair-plucking (F63.3)

               lalling (F80.0)

               lisping (F80.0)

               malingering [conscious simulation] (Z76.5)

               nail-biting (F98.8)

               psychological or behavioral factors associated with disorders or diseases classified elsewhere (F54)

               sexual dysfunction, not due to a substance or known physiological condition (F52.-)

               thumb-sucking (F98.8)

               tic disorders (in childhood and adolescence) (F95.-)

               Tourette's syndrome (F95.2)

               trichotillomania (F63.3)

    DEF: Types of disorders causing inconsistent physical symptoms that cannot be explained.

    F45.0   **Somatization disorder**

        Briquet's disorder

        Multiple psychosomatic disorder

    F45.1   **Undifferentiated somatoform disorder**

        Somatic symptom disorder

        Undifferentiated psychosomatic disorder

✓5th **F45.2**   **Hypochondriacal disorders**

        EXCLUDES 2   *delusional dysmorphophobia (F22)*

                fixed delusions about bodily functions or shape (F22)

    F45.20   **Hypochondriacal disorder, unspecified**

    F45.21   **Hypochondriasis**

        Hypochondriacal neurosis

        Illness anxiety disorder

    F45.22   **Body dysmorphic disorder**

        ▶Bigorexia◀

        Dysmorphophobia (nondelusional)

        ▶Muscle dysmorphia◀

        Nosophobia

    F45.29   **Other hypochondriacal disorders**

✓5th **F45.4**   **Pain disorders related to psychological factors**

        EXCLUDES 1   *pain NOS (R52)*

    F45.41   **Pain disorder exclusively related to psychological factors**

        Somatoform pain disorder (persistent)

    F45.42   **Pain disorder with related psychological factors**

        Code also associated acute or chronic pain (G89.-)

    F45.8   **Other somatoform disorders**

        Psychogenic dysmenorrhea

        Psychogenic dysphagia, including 'globus hystericus'

        Psychogenic pruritus

        Psychogenic torticollis

        Somatoform autonomic dysfunction

        Teeth grinding

        EXCLUDES 1   *sleep related teeth grinding (G47.63)*

    F45.9   **Somatoform disorder, unspecified**

        Psychosomatic disorder NOS

✓4th **F48**   **Other nonpsychotic mental disorders**

    F48.1   **Depersonalization-derealization syndrome**   HCC

    F48.2   **Pseudobulbar affect**

        Involuntary emotional expression disorder

        Code first underlying cause, if known, such as:

           amyotrophic lateral sclerosis (G12.21)

           multiple sclerosis (G35)

           sequelae of cerebrovascular disease (I69.-)

           sequelae of traumatic intracranial injury (S06.-)

    F48.8   **Other specified nonpsychotic mental disorders**

        Dhat syndrome

        Neurasthenia

        Occupational neurosis, including writer's cramp

        Psychasthenia

        Psychasthenic neurosis

        Psychogenic syncope

    F48.9   **Nonpsychotic mental disorder, unspecified**

        Neurosis NOS

✔ Additional Character Required   ✓x7th Placeholder   Questionable PDx   Manifestation   Unspecified   UPD Unacceptable PDx   H1 - H14 HAC   HCC CMS-HCC Dx   HIV HIV Dx

ICD-10-CM 2025   575

Chapter 5. Mental, Behavioral and Neurodevelopmental Disorders

F5Ø–F5Ø.9

Behavioral syndromes associated with physiological disturbances and physical factors (F5Ø-F59)

✓4th F5Ø Eating disorders

EXCLUDES 1   anorexia NOS (R63.Ø)
       feeding problems of newborn (P92.-)
       polyphagia (R63.2)

EXCLUDES 2   feeding difficulties (R63.3-)
       feeding disorder in infancy or childhood (F98.2-)

AHA: 2022,1Q,13; 2018,4Q,82

TIP: Assign additional code for BMI from category Z68, when documented. BMI can be based on documentation from clinicians who are not the patient's provider.

✓5th F5Ø.Ø Anorexia nervosa

EXCLUDES 1   loss of appetite (R63.Ø)
       psychogenic loss of appetite (F5Ø.89)

DEF: Psychological eating disorder characterized by an intense fear of gaining weight and an unrealistic perception of body image that perpetuates the feeling of being fat or having too much fat. Avoidance of food and restrictive or unhealthy eating are common.

F5Ø.ØØ Anorexia nervosa, unspecified   CC HCC

✓6th F5Ø.Ø1 Anorexia nervosa, restricting type

   F5Ø.Ø1Ø Anorexia nervosa, restricting type, mild   CC
     Anorexia nervosa, restricting type, with a body mass index greater than or equal to 17 kg/m2

   F5Ø.Ø11 Anorexia nervosa, restricting type, moderate   CC
     Anorexia nervosa, restricting type, with a body mass index of 16.Ø-16.99 kg/m2

   F5Ø.Ø12 Anorexia nervosa, restricting type, severe   CC
     Anorexia nervosa, restricting type, with a body mass index of 15.Ø-15.99 kg/m2

   F5Ø.Ø13 Anorexia nervosa, restricting type, extreme   CC
     Anorexia nervosa, restricting type, with a body mass index of less than 15.Ø kg/m2

   F5Ø.Ø14 Anorexia nervosa, restricting type, in remission   CC
     Anorexia nervosa, restricting type, in full remission
     Anorexia nervosa, restricting type, in partial remission

   F5Ø.Ø19 Anorexia nervosa, restricting type, unspecified   CC

✓6th F5Ø.Ø2 Anorexia nervosa, binge eating/purging type

EXCLUDES 1   bulimia nervosa ▶(F5Ø.2-)◄

   F5Ø.Ø2Ø Anorexia nervosa, binge eating/purging type, mild   CC
     Anorexia nervosa, binge eating/purging type, with a body mass index greater than or equal to 17 kg/m2

   F5Ø.Ø21 Anorexia nervosa, binge eating/purging type, moderate   CC
     Anorexia nervosa, binge eating/purging type, with a body mass index of 16.Ø-16.99 kg/m2

   F5Ø.Ø22 Anorexia nervosa, binge eating/purging type, severe   CC
     Anorexia nervosa, binge eating/purging type, with a body mass index of 15.Ø-15.99 kg/m2

   F5Ø.Ø23 Anorexia nervosa, binge eating/purging type, extreme   CC
     Anorexia nervosa, binge eating/purging type, with a body mass index of less than 15.Ø kg/m2

   F5Ø.Ø24 Anorexia nervosa, binge eating/purging type, in remission   CC
     Anorexia nervosa, binge eating/purging type, in full remission
     Anorexia nervosa, binge eating/purging type, in partial remission

   F5Ø.Ø29 Anorexia nervosa, binge eating/purging type, unspecified   CC

✓5th F5Ø.2 Bulimia nervosa

Bulimia NOS
Hyperorexia nervosa

EXCLUDES 1   anorexia nervosa, binge eating/purging type ▶(F5Ø.Ø2-)◄

DEF: Episodic pattern of overeating (binge eating) followed by purging or extreme exercise accompanied by an awareness of the abnormal eating pattern with a fear of not being able to stop eating.

F5Ø.2Ø Bulimia nervosa, unspecified   CC

F5Ø.21 Bulimia nervosa, mild   CC
   Bulimia nervosa with 1-3 episodes of inappropriate compensatory behavior per week

F5Ø.22 Bulimia nervosa, moderate   CC
   Bulimia nervosa with 4-7 episodes of inappropriate compensatory behavior per week

F5Ø.23 Bulimia nervosa, severe   CC
   Bulimia nervosa with 8-13 episodes of inappropriate compensatory behavior per week

F5Ø.24 Bulimia nervosa, extreme   CC
   Bulimia nervosa with 14 or more episodes of inappropriate compensatory behavior per week

F5Ø.25 Bulimia nervosa, in remission   CC
   Bulimia nervosa, in full remission
   Bulimia nervosa, in partial remission

✓5th F5Ø.8 Other eating disorders

EXCLUDES 2   pica of infancy and childhood (F98.3)

AHA: 2017,4Q,9; 2016,4Q,15-16

✓6th F5Ø.81 Binge eating disorder

   F5Ø.81Ø Binge eating disorder, mild
     Binge eating disorder with 1-3 binge eating episodes per week

   F5Ø.811 Binge eating disorder, moderate
     Binge eating disorder with 4-7 binge eating episodes per week

   F5Ø.812 Binge eating disorder, severe
     Binge eating disorder with 8-13 binge eating episodes per week

   F5Ø.813 Binge eating disorder, extreme
     Binge eating disorder with 14 or more eating episodes per week

   F5Ø.814 Binge eating disorder, in remission
     Binge eating disorder, in full remission
     Binge eating disorder, in partial remission

   F5Ø.819 Binge eating disorder, unspecified

F5Ø.82 Avoidant/restrictive food intake disorder
   ▶Avoidant/restrictive food intake disorder, in remission◄

F5Ø.83 Pica in adults   A
   Pica in adults, in remission

EXCLUDES 1   pica in infancy and childhood (F98.3)

F5Ø.84 Rumination disorder in adults   A
   Rumination disorder in adults, in remission

EXCLUDES 1   rumination disorder in infancy and childhood (F98.21)

F5Ø.89 Other specified eating disorder
   ~~Pica in adults~~
   Psychogenic loss of appetite

F5Ø.9 Eating disorder, unspecified
   Atypical anorexia nervosa
   Atypical bulimia nervosa
   Feeding or eating disorder, unspecified
   Other specified feeding disorder

N Newborn: 0   P Pediatric: 0-17   M Maternity: 9-64   A Adult: 15-124   UNS Unspecified Site   MCC Major Complication/Comorbidity   CC Complication/Comorbidity   PE POA Exempt

576   ICD-10-CM 2025

✓4th F51　Sleep disorders not due to a substance or known physiological condition
　　EXCLUDES 2　*organic sleep disorders (G47.-)*

✓5th F51.0　Insomnia not due to a substance or known physiological condition
　　　EXCLUDES 2　*alcohol related insomnia (F10.182, F10.282, F10.982)*
　　　　　drug-related insomnia (F11.182, F11.282, F11.982, F13.182, F13.282, F13.982, F14.182, F14.282, F14.982, F15.182, F15.282, F15.982, F19.182, F19.282, F19.982)
　　　　　insomnia NOS (G47.0-)
　　　　　insomnia due to known physiological condition (G47.0-)
　　　　　organic insomnia (G47.0-)
　　　　　sleep deprivation (Z72.820)

F51.01　Primary insomnia
　　Idiopathic insomnia
F51.02　Adjustment insomnia
F51.03　Paradoxical insomnia
F51.04　Psychophysiologic insomnia
F51.05　Insomnia due to other mental disorder
　　Code also associated mental disorder
F51.09　Other insomnia not due to a substance or known physiological condition

✓5th F51.1　Hypersomnia not due to a substance or known physiological condition
　　　EXCLUDES 2　*alcohol related hypersomnia (F10.182, F10.282, F10.982)*
　　　　　drug-related hypersomnia (F11.182, F11.282, F11.982, F13.182, F13.282, F13.982, F14.182, F14.282, F14.982, F15.182, F15.282, F15.982, F19.182, F19.282, F19.982)
　　　　　hypersomnia NOS (G47.10)
　　　　　hypersomnia due to known physiological condition (G47.10)
　　　　　idiopathic hypersomnia (G47.11, G47.12)
　　　　　narcolepsy (G47.4-)

F51.11　Primary hypersomnia
F51.12　Insufficient sleep syndrome
　　　EXCLUDES 1　*sleep deprivation (Z72.820)*
F51.13　Hypersomnia due to other mental disorder
　　Code also associated mental disorder
F51.19　Other hypersomnia not due to a substance or known physiological condition

F51.3　Sleepwalking [somnambulism]
　　Non-rapid eye movement sleep arousal disorders, sleepwalking type
F51.4　Sleep terrors [night terrors]
　　Non-rapid eye movement sleep arousal disorders, sleep terror type
F51.5　Nightmare disorder
　　Dream anxiety disorder
F51.8　Other sleep disorders not due to a substance or known physiological condition
F51.9　Sleep disorder not due to a substance or known physiological condition, unspecified
　　Emotional sleep disorder NOS

✓4th F52　Sexual dysfunction not due to a substance or known physiological condition
　　EXCLUDES 2　*Dhat syndrome (F48.8)*

F52.0　Hypoactive sexual desire disorder
　　Lack or loss of sexual desire
　　Male hypoactive sexual desire disorder
　　Sexual anhedonia
　　　EXCLUDES 1　*decreased libido (R68.82)*
F52.1　Sexual aversion disorder
　　Sexual aversion and lack of sexual enjoyment
✓5th F52.2　Sexual arousal disorders
　　Failure of genital response
F52.21　Male erectile disorder
　　Erectile disorder
　　Psychogenic impotence
　　　EXCLUDES 1　*impotence of organic origin (N52.-)*
　　　　　impotence NOS (N52.-)
F52.22　Female sexual arousal disorder
　　Female sexual interest/arousal disorder

✓5th F52.3　Orgasmic disorder
　　Inhibited orgasm
　　Psychogenic anorgasmia
F52.31　Female orgasmic disorder
F52.32　Male orgasmic disorder
　　Delayed ejaculation
F52.4　Premature ejaculation
F52.5　Vaginismus not due to a substance or known physiological condition
　　Psychogenic vaginismus
　　　EXCLUDES 2　*vaginismus (due to a known physiological condition) (N94.2)*
　　DEF: Psychogenic response resulting in painful contractions of the vaginal canal muscles. This condition can be severe enough to prevent sexual intercourse.
F52.6　Dyspareunia not due to a substance or known physiological condition
　　Genito-pelvic pain penetration disorder
　　Psychogenic dyspareunia
　　　EXCLUDES 2　*dyspareunia (due to a known physiological condition) (N94.1-)*
F52.8　Other sexual dysfunction not due to a substance or known physiological condition
　　Excessive sexual drive
　　Nymphomania
　　Satyriasis
F52.9　Unspecified sexual dysfunction not due to a substance or known physiological condition　UPD
　　Sexual dysfunction NOS

✓4th F53　Mental and behavioral disorders associated with the puerperium, not elsewhere classified
　　EXCLUDES 1　*mood disorders with psychotic features (F30.2, F31.2, F31.5, F31.64, F32.3, F33.3)*
　　　　　postpartum dysphoria (O90.6)
　　　　　psychosis in schizophrenia, schizotypal, delusional, and other psychotic disorders (F20-F29)
　　AHA: 2018,4Q,8

F53.0　Postpartum depression　M
　　Postnatal depression, NOS
　　Postpartum depression, NOS
F53.1　Puerperal psychosis　HCC　M
　　Postpartum psychosis
　　Puerperal psychosis, NOS

F54　*Psychological and behavioral factors associated with disorders or diseases classified elsewhere*
　　Psychological factors affecting physical conditions
　　Code first the associated physical disorder, such as:
　　　asthma (J45.-)
　　　dermatitis (L23-L25)
　　　gastric ulcer (K25.-)
　　　mucous colitis (K58.-)
　　　ulcerative colitis (K51.-)
　　　urticaria (L50.-)
　　　EXCLUDES 2　*tension-type headache (G44.2)*

✓4th F55　Abuse of non-psychoactive substances
　　EXCLUDES 2　*abuse of psychoactive substances (F10-F19)*

F55.0　Abuse of antacids
F55.1　Abuse of herbal or folk remedies
　　AHA: 2023,3Q,16
F55.2　Abuse of laxatives
F55.3　Abuse of steroids or hormones
F55.4　Abuse of vitamins
F55.8　Abuse of other non-psychoactive substances

F59　Unspecified behavioral syndromes associated with physiological disturbances and physical factors
　　Psychogenic physiological dysfunction NOS

Chapter 5. Mental, Behavioral and Neurodevelopmental Disorders

Disorders of adult personality and behavior (F60-F69)

✓4ᵗʰ F60 Specific personality disorders

  F60.0 Paranoid personality disorder   HCC
    Expansive paranoid personality (disorder)
    Fanatic personality (disorder)
    Paranoid personality (disorder)
    Querulant personality (disorder)
    Sensitive paranoid personality (disorder)
    EXCLUDES 2   *paranoia (F22)*
        paranoia querulans (F22)
        paranoid psychosis (F22)
        paranoid schizophrenia (F20.0)
        paranoid state (F22)

  F60.1 Schizoid personality disorder   HCC
    EXCLUDES 2   *Asperger's syndrome (F84.5)*
        delusional disorder (F22)
        schizoid disorder of childhood (F84.5)
        schizophrenia (F20.-)
        schizotypal disorder (F21)

  F60.2 Antisocial personality disorder   HCC
    Amoral personality (disorder)
    Asocial personality (disorder)
    Dissocial personality disorder
    Psychopathic personality (disorder)
    Sociopathic personality (disorder)
    EXCLUDES 1   *conduct disorders (F91.-)*
    EXCLUDES 2   *borderline personality disorder (F60.3)*

  F60.3 Borderline personality disorder   HCC
    Aggressive personality (disorder)
    Emotionally unstable personality disorder
    Explosive personality (disorder)
    EXCLUDES 2   *antisocial personality disorder (F60.2)*

  F60.4 Histrionic personality disorder   HCC
    Hysterical personality (disorder)
    Psychoinfantile personality (disorder)

  F60.5 Obsessive-compulsive personality disorder   HCC
    Anankastic personality (disorder)
    Compulsive personality (disorder)
    Obsessional personality (disorder)
    EXCLUDES 2   *obsessive-compulsive disorder (F42.-)*

  F60.6 Avoidant personality disorder   HCC
    Anxious personality disorder

  F60.7 Dependent personality disorder   HCC
    Asthenic personality (disorder)
    Inadequate personality (disorder)
    Passive personality (disorder)
    DEF: Lack of self-confidence, fear of abandonment, and an obsessive need to be taken care of.

  ✓5ᵗʰ F60.8 Other specific personality disorders

    F60.81 Narcissistic personality disorder   HCC
    F60.89 Other specific personality disorders   HCC
      Eccentric personality disorder
      "Haltlose" type personality disorder
      Immature personality disorder
      Passive-aggressive personality disorder
      Psychoneurotic personality disorder
      Self-defeating personality disorder

  F60.9 Personality disorder, unspecified   HCC
    Character disorder NOS
    Character neurosis NOS
    Pathological personality NOS

✓4ᵗʰ F63 Impulse disorders

  EXCLUDES 2   *habitual excessive use of alcohol or psychoactive substances (F10-F19)*
        impulse disorders involving sexual behavior (F65.-)

  F63.0 Pathological gambling
    Compulsive gambling
    Gambling disorder
    EXCLUDES 1   *gambling and betting NOS (Z72.6)*
    EXCLUDES 2   *excessive gambling by manic patients (F30, F31)*
        gambling in antisocial personality disorder (F60.2)

  F63.1 Pyromania
    Pathological fire-setting
    EXCLUDES 2   *fire-setting (by) (in):*
        adult with antisocial personality disorder (F60.2)
        alcohol or psychoactive substance intoxication (F10-F19)
        conduct disorders (F91.-)
        mental disorders due to known physiological condition (F01-F09)
        schizophrenia (F20.-)

  F63.2 Kleptomania
    Pathological stealing
    EXCLUDES 1   *shoplifting as the reason for observation for suspected mental disorder (Z03.8)*
    EXCLUDES 2   *depressive disorder with stealing (F31-F33)*
        stealing due to underlying mental condition - code to mental condition
        stealing in mental disorders due to known physiological condition (F01-F09)

  F63.3 Trichotillomania
    Hair plucking
    EXCLUDES 2   *other stereotyped movement disorder (F98.4)*

  ✓5ᵗʰ F63.8 Other impulse disorders

    F63.81 Intermittent explosive disorder
    F63.89 Other impulse disorders

  F63.9 Impulse disorder, unspecified
    Impulse control disorder NOS

✓4ᵗʰ F64 Gender identity disorders
  AHA: 2016,4Q,16

  F64.0 Transsexualism
    Gender dysphoria in adolescents and adults
    Gender identity disorder in adolescence and adulthood
    Gender incongruence in adolescents and adults
    Transgender
    EXCLUDES 1   *gender identity disorder of childhood (F64.2)*

  F64.1 Dual role transvestism
    Use additional code to identify sex reassignment status (Z87.890)
    EXCLUDES 1   *gender identity disorder in childhood (F64.2)*
    EXCLUDES 2   *fetishistic transvestism (F65.1)*

  F64.2 Gender identity disorder of childhood   P
    Gender dysphoria in children
    Gender incongruence of childhood
    EXCLUDES 1   *gender identity disorder in adolescence and adulthood (F64.0)*
    EXCLUDES 2   *sexual maturation disorder (F66)*

  F64.8 Other gender identity disorders
    Other specified gender dysphoria

  F64.9 Gender identity disorder, unspecified
    Gender dysphoria, unspecified
    Gender incongruence, unspecified
    Gender-role disorder NOS

✓4ᵗʰ F65 Paraphilias

  F65.0 Fetishism
    Fetishistic disorder

  F65.1 Transvestic fetishism
    Fetishistic transvestism
    Transvestic disorder

  F65.2 Exhibitionism
    Exhibitionistic disorder

  F65.3 Voyeurism
    Voyeuristic disorder

  F65.4 Pedophilia
    Pedophilic disorder

  ✓5ᵗʰ F65.5 Sadomasochism

    F65.50 Sadomasochism, unspecified
    F65.51 Sexual masochism
      Sexual masochism disorder
    F65.52 Sexual sadism
      Sexual sadism disorder

  ✓5ᵗʰ F65.8 Other paraphilias

    F65.81 Frotteurism
      Frotteuristic disorder
    F65.89 Other paraphilias
      Necrophilia
      Other specified paraphilic disorder

F65.9   **Paraphilia, unspecified**
Paraphilic disorder, unspecified
Sexual deviation NOS

F66   **Other sexual disorders**
Sexual maturation disorder
Sexual relationship disorder

✓4ᵗʰ **F68**   **Other disorders of adult personality and behavior**
AHA: 2018,4Q,9,65

   ✓5ᵗʰ **F68.1**   **Factitious disorder imposed on self**
Compensation neurosis
Elaboration of physical symptoms for psychological reasons
Hospital hopper syndrome
Münchausen's syndrome
Peregrinating patient
     EXCLUDES 2   *factitial dermatitis (L98.1)*
             person feigning illness (with obvious motivation) (Z76.5)

      F68.10   **Factitious disorder imposed on self, unspecified**   CC

      F68.11   **Factitious disorder imposed on self, with predominantly psychological signs and symptoms**

      F68.12   **Factitious disorder imposed on self, with predominantly physical signs and symptoms**   CC

      F68.13   **Factitious disorder imposed on self, with combined psychological and physical signs and symptoms**

    F68.A   **Factitious disorder imposed on another**   CC
Factitious disorder by proxy
Münchausen's by proxy

    F68.8   **Other specified disorders of adult personality and behavior**

F69   **Unspecified disorder of adult personality and behavior**   A

Intellectual disabilities (F70-F79)

Code first any associated physical or developmental disorders
EXCLUDES 1   *borderline intellectual functioning, IQ above 70 to 84 (R41.83)*

F70   **Mild intellectual disabilities**
IQ level 50-55 to approximately 70
Mild mental subnormality

F71   **Moderate intellectual disabilities**
IQ level 35-40 to 50-55
Moderate mental subnormality

F72   **Severe intellectual disabilities**   CC
IQ 20-25 to 35-40
Severe mental subnormality

F73   **Profound intellectual disabilities**   CC
IQ level below 20-25
Profound mental subnormality

✓4ᵗʰ **F78**   **Other intellectual disabilities**

   ✓5ᵗʰ **F78.A**   **Other genetic related intellectual disabilities**
AHA: 2021,4Q,10-11

      F78.A1   **SYNGAP1-related intellectual disability**
Code also, if applicable, any associated:
autism spectrum disorder (F84.0)
autistic disorder (F84.0)
encephalopathy (G93.4-)
epilepsy and recurrent seizures (G40.-)
other pervasive developmental disorders (F84.8)
pervasive developmental disorder, NOS (F84.9)

      F78.A9   **Other genetic related intellectual disability**
Code also, if applicable, any associated disorders

F79   **Unspecified intellectual disabilities**
Mental deficiency NOS
Mental subnormality NOS

Pervasive and specific developmental disorders (F80-F89)

✓4ᵗʰ **F80**   **Specific developmental disorders of speech and language**

    F80.0   **Phonological disorder**
Dyslalia
Functional speech articulation disorder
Lalling
Lisping
Phonological developmental disorder
Speech articulation developmental disorder
Speech-sound disorder
     EXCLUDES 1   *speech articulation impairment due to aphasia NOS (R47.01)*
             speech articulation impairment due to apraxia (R48.2)
     EXCLUDES 2   *speech articulation impairment due to hearing loss (F80.4)*
             speech articulation impairment due to intellectual disabilities (F70-F79)
             speech articulation impairment with expressive language developmental disorder (F80.1)
             speech articulation impairment with mixed receptive expressive language developmental disorder (F80.2)

    F80.1   **Expressive language disorder**
Developmental dysphasia or aphasia, expressive type
     EXCLUDES 1   *mixed receptive-expressive language disorder (F80.2)*
             dysphasia and aphasia NOS (R47.-)
     EXCLUDES 2   *acquired aphasia with epilepsy [Landau-Kleffner] (G40.80-)*
             intellectual disabilities (F70-F79)
             pervasive developmental disorders (F84.-)
             selective mutism (F94.0)

    F80.2   **Mixed receptive-expressive language disorder**
Developmental dysphasia or aphasia, receptive type
Developmental Wernicke's aphasia
     EXCLUDES 1   *central auditory processing disorder (H93.25)*
             dysphasia or aphasia NOS (R47.-)
             expressive language disorder (F80.1)
             expressive type dysphasia or aphasia (F80.1)
             word deafness (H93.25)
     EXCLUDES 2   *acquired aphasia with epilepsy [Landau-Kleffner] (G40.80-)*
             intellectual disabilities (F70-F79)
             pervasive developmental disorders (F84.-)
             selective mutism (F94.0)

    F80.4   **Speech and language development delay due to hearing loss**
Code also type of hearing loss (H90.-, H91.-)

   ✓5ᵗʰ **F80.8**   **Other developmental disorders of speech and language**
AHA: 2017,1Q,27

      F80.81   **Childhood onset fluency disorder**
Cluttering NOS
Stuttering NOS
       EXCLUDES 1   *adult onset fluency disorder (F98.5)*
               fluency disorder in conditions classified elsewhere (R47.82)
               fluency disorder (stuttering) following cerebrovascular disease (I69. with final characters -23)

      F80.82   **Social pragmatic communication disorder**
       EXCLUDES 1   *Asperger's syndrome (F84.5)*
               autistic disorder (F84.0)
       AHA: 2016,4Q,16

      F80.89   **Other developmental disorders of speech and language**

    F80.9   **Developmental disorder of speech and language, unspecified**
Communication disorder NOS
Language disorder NOS

Chapter 5. Mental, Behavioral and Neurodevelopmental Disorders

F81–F93.9

✓4ᵗʰ **F81 Specific developmental disorders of scholastic skills**

F81.0 Specific reading disorder
"Backward reading"
Developmental dyslexia
Specific learning disorder, with impairment in reading
Specific reading retardation
> **EXCLUDES 1**   *alexia NOS (R48.0)*
>   *dyslexia NOS (R48.0)*
> **DEF:** Serious impairment of reading skills unexplained in relation to general intelligence and teaching processes.

F81.2 Mathematics disorder
Developmental acalculia
Developmental arithmetical disorder
Developmental Gerstmann's syndrome
Specific learning disorder, with impairment in mathematics
> **EXCLUDES 1**   *acalculia NOS (R48.8)*
> **EXCLUDES 2**   *arithmetical difficulties associated with a reading disorder (F81.0)*
>   *arithmetical difficulties associated with a spelling disorder (F81.81)*
>   *arithmetical difficulties due to inadequate teaching (Z55.8)*

✓5ᵗʰ **F81.8 Other developmental disorders of scholastic skills**

F81.81 Disorder of written expression
Specific learning disorder, with impairment in written expression
Specific spelling disorder

F81.89 Other developmental disorders of scholastic skills

F81.9 Developmental disorder of scholastic skills, unspecified   UPD
Knowledge acquisition disability NOS
Learning disability NOS
Learning disorder NOS

F82 Specific developmental disorder of motor function
Clumsy child syndrome
Developmental coordination disorder
Developmental dyspraxia
> **EXCLUDES 1**   *abnormalities of gait and mobility (R26.-)*
>   *lack of coordination (R27.-)*
> **EXCLUDES 2**   *lack of coordination secondary to intellectual disabilities (F70-F79)*

✓4ᵗʰ **F84 Pervasive developmental disorders**
Code also any associated medical condition and intellectual disabilities

F84.0 Autistic disorder   CC
Autism spectrum disorder
Infantile autism
Infantile psychosis
Kanner's syndrome
> **EXCLUDES 1**   *Asperger's syndrome (F84.5)*
> **AHA:** 2017,1Q,27

F84.2 Rett's syndrome   CC
> **EXCLUDES 1**   *Asperger's syndrome (F84.5)*
>   *autistic disorder (F84.0)*
>   *other childhood disintegrative disorder (F84.3)*

F84.3 Other childhood disintegrative disorder   CC P
Dementia infantilis
Disintegrative psychosis
Heller's syndrome
Symbiotic psychosis
Use additional code to identify any associated neurological condition
> **EXCLUDES 1**   *Asperger's syndrome (F84.5)*
>   *autistic disorder (F84.0)*
>   *Rett's syndrome (F84.2)*

F84.5 Asperger's syndrome   CC
Asperger's disorder
Autistic psychopathy
Schizoid disorder of childhood
> **DEF:** High-functioning form of autism. Children with this syndrome usually develop speech on schedule, are generally very intelligent, and communicate well, but have considerable social shortcomings. *Synonym(s): AS.*

F84.8 Other pervasive developmental disorders   CC
Overactive disorder associated with intellectual disabilities and stereotyped movements

F84.9 Pervasive developmental disorder, unspecified   CC
Atypical autism

F88 Other disorders of psychological development
Developmental agnosia
Global developmental delay
Other specified neurodevelopmental disorder

F89 Unspecified disorder of psychological development
Developmental disorder NOS
Neurodevelopmental disorder NOS

Behavioral and emotional disorders with onset usually occurring in childhood and adolescence (F90-F98)

> **NOTE**   Codes within categories F90-F98 may be used regardless of the age of a patient. These disorders generally have onset within the childhood or adolescent years, but may continue throughout life or not be diagnosed until adulthood

✓4ᵗʰ **F90 Attention-deficit hyperactivity disorders**
> **INCLUDES**   attention deficit disorder with hyperactivity
>   attention deficit syndrome with hyperactivity
> **EXCLUDES 2**   *anxiety disorders (F40.-, F41.-)*
>   *mood [affective] disorders (F30-F39)*
>   *pervasive developmental disorders (F84.-)*
>   *schizophrenia (F20.-)*

F90.0 Attention-deficit hyperactivity disorder, predominantly inattentive type
Attention-deficit/hyperactivity disorder, predominantly inattentive presentation

F90.1 Attention-deficit hyperactivity disorder, predominantly hyperactive type
Attention-deficit/hyperactivity disorder, predominantly hyperactive impulsive presentation

F90.2 Attention-deficit hyperactivity disorder, combined type
Attention-deficit/hyperactivity disorder, combined presentation

F90.8 Attention-deficit hyperactivity disorder, other type

F90.9 Attention-deficit hyperactivity disorder, unspecified type
Attention-deficit hyperactivity disorder of childhood or adolescence NOS
Attention-deficit hyperactivity disorder NOS

✓4ᵗʰ **F91 Conduct disorders**
> **EXCLUDES 1**   *antisocial behavior (Z72.81-)*
>   *antisocial personality disorder (F60.2)*
> **EXCLUDES 2**   *conduct problems associated with attention-deficit hyperactivity disorder (F90.-)*
>   *mood [affective] disorders (F30-F39)*
>   *pervasive developmental disorders (F84.-)*
>   *schizophrenia (F20.-)*

F91.0 Conduct disorder confined to family context

F91.1 Conduct disorder, childhood-onset type
Unsocialized conduct disorder
Conduct disorder, solitary aggressive type
Unsocialized aggressive disorder

F91.2 Conduct disorder, adolescent-onset type
Socialized conduct disorder
Conduct disorder, group type

F91.3 Oppositional defiant disorder

F91.8 Other conduct disorders
Other specified conduct disorder
Other specified disruptive disorder

F91.9 Conduct disorder, unspecified
Behavioral disorder NOS
Conduct disorder NOS
Disruptive behavior disorder NOS
Disruptive disorder NOS

✓4ᵗʰ **F93 Emotional disorders with onset specific to childhood**

F93.0 Separation anxiety disorder of childhood
> **EXCLUDES 2**   *mood [affective] disorders (F30-F39)*
>   *nonpsychotic mental disorders (F40-F48)*
>   *phobic anxiety disorder of childhood (F40.8)*
>   *social phobia (F40.1)*

F93.8 Other childhood emotional disorders
Identity disorder
> **EXCLUDES 2**   *gender identity disorder of childhood (F64.2)*

F93.9 Childhood emotional disorder, unspecified

✓4th **F94 Disorders of social functioning with onset specific to childhood and adolescence**

    F94.0 Selective mutism
        Elective mutism
        EXCLUDES 2   *pervasive developmental disorders (F84.-)*
                     schizophrenia (F20.-)
                     specific developmental disorders of speech and language (F80.-)
                     transient mutism as part of separation anxiety in young children (F93.0)

    F94.1 Reactive attachment disorder of childhood
        Use additional code to identify any associated failure to thrive or growth retardation
        EXCLUDES 1   *disinhibited attachment disorder of childhood (F94.2)*
                     normal variation in pattern of selective attachment
        EXCLUDES 2   *Asperger's syndrome (F84.5)*
                     maltreatment syndromes (T74.-)
                     sexual or physical abuse in childhood, resulting in psychosocial problems (Z62.81-)

    F94.2 Disinhibited attachment disorder of childhood
        Affectionless psychopathy
        Institutional syndrome
        EXCLUDES 1   *reactive attachment disorder of childhood (F94.1)*
        EXCLUDES 2   *Asperger's syndrome (F84.5)*
                     attention-deficit hyperactivity disorders (F90.-)
                     hospitalism in children (F43.2-)

    F94.8 Other childhood disorders of social functioning
    F94.9 Childhood disorder of social functioning, unspecified

✓4th **F95 Tic disorder**

    F95.0 Transient tic disorder
        Provisional tic disorder

    F95.1 Chronic motor or vocal tic disorder

    F95.2 Tourette's disorder
        Combined vocal and multiple motor tic disorder [de la Tourette]
        Tourette's syndrome

    F95.8 Other tic disorders
    F95.9 Tic disorder, unspecified
        Tic NOS

✓4th **F98 Other behavioral and emotional disorders with onset usually occurring in childhood and adolescence**
        EXCLUDES 2   *breath-holding spells (R06.89)*
                     gender identity disorder of childhood (F64.2)
                     Kleine-Levin syndrome (G47.13)
                     obsessive-compulsive disorder (F42.-)
                     sleep disorders not due to a substance or known physiological condition (F51.-)

    F98.0 Enuresis not due to a substance or known physiological condition
        Enuresis (primary) (secondary) of nonorganic origin
        Functional enuresis
        Psychogenic enuresis
        Urinary incontinence of nonorganic origin
        EXCLUDES 1   *enuresis NOS (R32)*

    F98.1 Encopresis not due to a substance or known physiological condition
        Functional encopresis
        Incontinence of feces of nonorganic origin
        Psychogenic encopresis
        Use additional code to identify the cause of any coexisting constipation
        EXCLUDES 1   *encopresis NOS (R15.-)*

✓5th **F98.2 Other feeding disorders of infancy and childhood**
        EXCLUDES 2   *anorexia nervosa and other eating disorders (F50.-)*
                     feeding difficulties (R63.3-)
                     feeding problems of newborn (P92.-)
                     pica of infancy or childhood (F98.3)

▲   **F98.21 Rumination disorder of infancy and childhood**
            ►Rumination disorder in infancy or childhood, in remission◄
            EXCLUDES 1 ►*rumination disorder in adults (F50.84)*◄
        F98.29 Other feeding disorders of infancy and early childhood

    F98.3 Pica of infancy and childhood
        ►Pica in infancy or childhood, in remission◄
        EXCLUDES 1 ►*pica in adults (F50.83)*◄

    F98.4 Stereotyped movement disorders
        Stereotype/habit disorder
        EXCLUDES 1   *abnormal involuntary movements (R25.-)*
        EXCLUDES 2   *compulsions in obsessive-compulsive disorder (F42.-)*
                     hair plucking (F63.3)
                     movement disorders of organic origin (G20-G25)
                     nail-biting (F98.8)
                     nose-picking (F98.8)
                     stereotypies that are part of a broader psychiatric condition (F01-F95)
                     thumb-sucking (F98.8)
                     tic disorders (F95.-)
                     trichotillomania (F63.3)

    F98.5 Adult onset fluency disorder
        EXCLUDES 1   *childhood onset fluency disorder (F80.81)*
                     dysphasia (R47.02)
                     fluency disorder in conditions classified elsewhere (R47.82)
                     fluency disorder (stuttering) following cerebrovascular disease (I69. with final characters -23)
                     tic disorders (F95.-)

    F98.8 Other specified behavioral and emotional disorders with onset usually occurring in childhood and adolescence
        Excessive masturbation
        Nail-biting
        Nose-picking
        Thumb-sucking

    F98.9 Unspecified behavioral and emotional disorders with onset usually occurring in childhood and adolescence

Unspecified mental disorder (F99)

F99 Mental disorder, not otherwise specified
    Mental illness NOS
    EXCLUDES 1   *unspecified mental disorder due to known physiological condition (F09)*

Chapter 6. Diseases of the Nervous System (G00–G99)

Chapter-specific Guidelines with Coding Examples

The chapter-specific guidelines from the ICD-10-CM Official Guidelines for Coding and Reporting have been provided below. Along with these guidelines are coding examples, contained in the shaded boxes, that have been developed to help illustrate the coding and/or sequencing guidance found in these guidelines.

a. Dominant/nondominant side

Codes from category G81, Hemiplegia and hemiparesis, and subcategories G83.1, Monoplegia of lower limb, G83.2, Monoplegia of upper limb, and G83.3, Monoplegia, unspecified, identify whether the dominant or nondominant side is affected. Should the affected side be documented, but not specified as dominant or nondominant, and the classification system does not indicate a default, code selection is as follows:

- For ambidextrous patients, the default should be dominant.
- If the left side is affected, the default is non-dominant.
- If the right side is affected, the default is dominant.

> Hemiplegia affecting left side of ambidextrous patient
>
> **G81.92**   **Hemiplegia, unspecified affecting left dominant side**
>
> *Explanation*: Documentation states that the left side is affected and dominant is used for ambidextrous persons.

> Right spastic hemiplegia, unknown whether patient is right- or left-handed
>
> **G81.11**   **Spastic hemiplegia affecting right dominant side**
>
> *Explanation*: Since it is unknown whether the patient is right- or left-handed, if the right side is affected, the default is dominant.

b. Pain—category G89

1) General coding information

Codes in category G89, Pain, not elsewhere classified, may be used in conjunction with codes from other categories and chapters to provide more detail about acute or chronic pain and neoplasm-related pain, unless otherwise indicated below.

If the pain is not specified as acute or chronic, post-thoracotomy, postprocedural, or neoplasm-related, do not assign codes from category G89.

A code from category G89 should not be assigned if the underlying (definitive) diagnosis is known, unless the reason for the encounter is pain control/ management and not management of the underlying condition.

When an admission or encounter is for a procedure aimed at treating the underlying condition (e.g., spinal fusion, kyphoplasty), a code for the underlying condition (e.g., vertebral fracture, spinal stenosis) should be assigned as the principal diagnosis. No code from category G89 should be assigned.

> Elderly patient with back pain is admitted for kyphoplasty for age-related osteopathic compression fracture at vertebra T3
>
> **M80.08XA**   **Age-related osteoporosis with current pathological fracture, vertebra(e), initial encounter for fracture**
>
> *Explanation*: No code is assigned for the pain as it is inherent in the underlying condition being treated.

(a) Category G89 codes as principal or first-listed diagnosis

Category G89 codes are acceptable as principal diagnosis or the first-listed code:

- When pain control or pain management is the reason for the admission/encounter (e.g., a patient with displaced intervertebral disc, nerve impingement and severe back pain presents for injection of steroid into the spinal canal). The underlying cause of the pain should be reported as an additional diagnosis, if known.

- When a patient is admitted for the insertion of a neurostimulator for pain control, assign the appropriate pain code as the principal or first-listed diagnosis. When an admission or encounter is for a procedure aimed at treating the underlying condition and a neurostimulator is inserted for pain control during the same admission/encounter, a code for the underlying condition should be assigned as the principal diagnosis and the appropriate pain code should be assigned as a secondary diagnosis.

> Patient with chronic pain from lumbar spondylosis with radiculopathy not relieved by surgery is admitted for insertion of neurostimulator.
>
> **G89.29**   **Other chronic pain**
>
> **M47.26**   **Other spondylosis with radiculopathy, lumbar region**
>
> *Explanation*: Since the patient is admitted specifically for a neurostimulator implantation for pain management and not to treat the underlying spondylosis, the chronic pain code is sequenced first, followed by the underlying condition. Neither code M54.16 nor M54.5 is necessary because M47.26 describes the radiculopathy and the site.

(b) Use of category G89 codes in conjunction with site specific pain codes

(i) Assigning category G89 and site-specific pain codes

Codes from category G89 may be used in conjunction with codes that identify the site of pain (including codes from chapter 18) if the category G89 code provides additional information. For example, if the code describes the site of the pain, but does not fully describe whether the pain is acute or chronic, then both codes should be assigned.

> During hospital stay, patient is seen by orthopaedics to evaluate chronic left shoulder pain.
>
> **M25.512**   **Pain in left shoulder**
>
> **G89.29**   **Other chronic pain**
>
> *Explanation*: No underlying condition has been determined yet so the pain would be the reason for the visit. The M25 pain code in this instance does not fully describe the condition as it does not represent that the pain is chronic. The G89 chronic pain code is assigned to provide specificity.

(ii) Sequencing of category G89 codes with site-specific pain codes

The sequencing of category G89 codes with site-specific pain codes (including chapter 18 codes), is dependent on the circumstances of the encounter/admission as follows:

- If the encounter is for pain control or pain management, assign the code from category G89 followed by the code identifying the specific site of pain (e.g., encounter for pain management for acute neck pain from trauma is assigned code G89.11, Acute pain due to trauma, followed by code M54.2, Cervicalgia, to identify the site of pain).

> Management of acute, traumatic right knee pain
>
> **G89.11**   **Acute pain due to trauma**
>
> **M25.561**   **Pain in right knee**
>
> *Explanation*: The reason for the encounter is to manage or control the pain, not to treat or evaluate an underlying condition. The G89 pain code is assigned as the principal diagnosis but in this instance does not fully describe the condition as it does not include the site and laterality. The M25 pain code is added to provide this information.

- If the encounter is for any other reason except pain control or pain management, and a related definitive diagnosis has not been established (confirmed) by the provider, assign the code for the specific site of pain first, followed by the appropriate code from category G89.

> Tests are performed to investigate the source of the patient's chronic epigastric abdominal pain
>
> **R10.13**   **Epigastric pain**
>
> **G89.29**   **Other chronic pain**
>
> *Explanation*: In this instance the patient's epigastric pain is not being treated; rather the source of the pain is being investigated. A code from chapter 18 for epigastric pain is sequenced before the additional specificity of the G89 code for the chronic pain.

2) Pain due to devices, implants and grafts
See Section I.C.19. Pain due to medical devices

3) Postoperative pain
The provider's documentation should be used to guide the coding of postoperative pain, as well as *Section III. Reporting Additional Diagnoses* and *Section IV. Diagnostic Coding and Reporting in the Outpatient Setting*.

The default for post-thoracotomy and other postoperative pain not specified as acute or chronic is the code for the acute form.

Routine or expected postoperative pain immediately after surgery should not be coded.

> Pain pump dose is increased for the patient's unexpected, extreme pain post-thoracotomy
>
> **G89.12**   **Acute post-thoracotomy pain**
>
> *Explanation*: When acute or chronic is not documented, default to acute. The use of "unexpected, extreme" and the increase of medication dosage indicate that the pain was more than routine or expected.

(a) Postoperative pain not associated with specific postoperative complication

Postoperative pain not associated with a specific postoperative complication is assigned to the appropriate postoperative pain code in category G89.

(b) Postoperative pain associated with specific postoperative complication

Postoperative pain associated with a specific postoperative complication (such as painful wire sutures) is assigned to the appropriate code(s) found in Chapter 19, Injury, poisoning, and certain other consequences of external causes. If appropriate, use additional code(s) from category G89 to identify acute or chronic pain (G89.18 or G89.28).

4) Chronic pain
Chronic pain is classified to subcategory G89.2. There is no time frame defining when pain becomes chronic pain. The provider's documentation should be used to guide use of these codes.

5) Neoplasm related pain
Code G89.3 is assigned to pain documented as being related, associated or due to cancer, primary or secondary malignancy, or tumor. This code is assigned regardless of whether the pain is acute or chronic.

This code may be assigned as the principal or first-listed code when the stated reason for the admission/encounter is documented as pain control/pain management. The underlying neoplasm should be reported as an additional diagnosis.

> Pain medication adjustment for chronic pain from bone metastasis
>
> **G89.3**   **Neoplasm related pain (acute)(chronic)**
>
> **C79.51**   **Secondary malignant neoplasm of bone**
>
> *Explanation*: Since the encounter was for pain medication management, the pain, rather than the neoplasm, was the reason for the encounter and is sequenced first. This "neoplasm-related pain" code includes both acute and chronic pain.

When the reason for the admission/encounter is management of the neoplasm and the pain associated with the neoplasm is also documented, code G89.3 may be assigned as an additional diagnosis. It is not necessary to assign an additional code for the site of the pain.

See Section I.C.2. for instructions on the sequencing of neoplasms for all other stated reasons for the admission/encounter (except for pain control/pain management).

> Patient with lung cancer presents with acute hip pain and is evaluated and found to have iliac bone metastasis
>
> **C79.51**   **Secondary malignant neoplasm of bone**
>
> **C34.90**   **Malignant neoplasm of unspecified part of unspecified bronchus or lung**
>
> **G89.3**   **Neoplasm related pain (acute)(chronic)**
>
> *Explanation*: The reason for the encounter was the evaluation and diagnosis of the bone metastasis, whose code would be assigned as first-listed, followed by codes for the primary neoplasm and the pain due to the iliac bone metastasis.

6) Chronic pain syndrome
Central pain syndrome (G89.0) and chronic pain syndrome (G89.4) are different than the term "chronic pain," and therefore codes should only be used when the provider has specifically documented this condition.

See Section I.C.5. Pain disorders related to psychological factors

Chapter 6. Diseases of the Nervous System (G00-G99)

EXCLUDES 2   *certain conditions originating in the perinatal period (P04-P96)*
certain infectious and parasitic diseases (A00-B99)
complications of pregnancy, childbirth and the puerperium (O00-O9A)
congenital malformations, deformations, and chromosomal abnormalities (Q00-Q99)
endocrine, nutritional and metabolic diseases (E00-E88)
injury, poisoning and certain other consequences of external causes (S00-T88)
neoplasms (C00-D49)
symptoms, signs and abnormal clinical and laboratory findings, not elsewhere classified (R00-R94)

This chapter contains the following blocks:

G00-G09   Inflammatory diseases of the central nervous system
G10-G14   Systemic atrophies primarily affecting the central nervous system
G20-G26   Extrapyramidal and movement disorders
G30-G32   Other degenerative diseases of the nervous system
G35-G37   Demyelinating diseases of the central nervous system
G40-G47   Episodic and paroxysmal disorders
G50-G59   Nerve, nerve root and plexus disorders
G60-G65   Polyneuropathies and other disorders of the peripheral nervous system
G70-G73   Diseases of myoneural junction and muscle
G80-G83   Cerebral palsy and other paralytic syndromes
G89-G99   Other disorders of the nervous system

Inflammatory diseases of the central nervous system (G00-G09)

✓4ᵗʰ G00   **Bacterial** meningitis, not elsewhere classified

INCLUDES   bacterial arachnoiditis
bacterial leptomeningitis
bacterial meningitis
bacterial pachymeningitis

EXCLUDES 1   *bacterial meningoencephalitis (G04.2)*
bacterial meningomyelitis (G04.2)

DEF: Inflammation of meningeal layers of the brain and spinal cord due to a bacterial infection.

G00.0   **Hemophilus** meningitis   MCC
Meningitis due to Hemophilus influenzae

G00.1   **Pneumococcal** meningitis   MCC
Meningitis due to Streptococcal pneumoniae

G00.2   **Streptococcal** meningitis   MCC
Use additional code to further identify organism (B95.0-B95.5)

G00.3   **Staphylococcal** meningitis   MCC
Use additional code to further identify organism (B95.61-B95.8)

G00.8   **Other bacterial** meningitis   MCC
Meningitis due to Escherichia coli
Meningitis due to Friedlander's bacillus
Meningitis due to Klebsiella
Use additional code to further identify organism (B96.-)

G00.9   **Bacterial meningitis, unspecified**   MCC
Meningitis due to gram-negative bacteria, unspecified
Purulent meningitis NOS
Pyogenic meningitis NOS
Suppurative meningitis NOS

G01   *Meningitis in bacterial diseases classified elsewhere*   MCC

Code first underlying disease

EXCLUDES 1   *meningitis (in):*
gonococcal (A54.81)
leptospirosis (A27.81)
listeriosis (A32.11)
Lyme disease (A69.21)
meningococcal (A39.0)
neurosyphilis (A52.13)
tuberculosis (A17.0)
meningoencephalitis and meningomyelitis in bacterial diseases classified elsewhere (G05)

G02   *Meningitis in other infectious and parasitic diseases classified elsewhere*   MCC

Code first underlying disease, such as:
African trypanosomiasis (B56.-)
poliovirus infection (A80.-)

EXCLUDES 1   *candidal meningitis (B37.5)*
coccidioidomycosis meningitis (B38.4)
cryptococcal meningitis (B45.1)
herpesviral [herpes simplex] meningitis (B00.3)
infectious mononucleosis complicated by meningitis (B27.- with fifth character 2)
measles complicated by meningitis (B05.1)
meningoencephalitis and meningomyelitis in other infectious and parasitic diseases classified elsewhere (G05)
mumps meningitis (B26.1)
rubella meningitis (B06.02)
varicella [chickenpox] meningitis (B01.0)
zoster meningitis (B02.1)

✓4ᵗʰ G03   **Meningitis due to other and unspecified causes**

INCLUDES   arachnoiditis NOS
leptomeningitis NOS
meningitis NOS
pachymeningitis NOS

EXCLUDES 1   *meningoencephalitis (G04.-)*
meningomyelitis (G04.-)

G03.0   **Nonpyogenic** meningitis   MCC
Aseptic meningitis
Nonbacterial meningitis
DEF: Type of meningitis where no bacterial, viral, or other infectious source exists that explains the meningitis symptomology.

G03.1   **Chronic** meningitis   CC

G03.2   **Benign recurrent** meningitis **[Mollaret]**   CC
DEF: Aseptic or noninfectious inflammation of the meninges with the presence of Mollaret cells in the spinal fluid. The patient experiences recurrent bouts of inflammation, lasting anywhere from two to five days.

G03.8   **Meningitis due to other specified causes**   MCC

G03.9   **Meningitis, unspecified**   MCC
Arachnoiditis (spinal) NOS

✓4ᵗʰ G04   **Encephalitis, myelitis and encephalomyelitis**

INCLUDES   acute ascending myelitis
meningoencephalitis
meningomyelitis

EXCLUDES 1   *encephalopathy NOS (G93.40)*

EXCLUDES 2   *acute transverse myelitis (G37.3)*
alcoholic encephalopathy (G31.2)
multiple sclerosis (G35)
myalgic encephalomyelitis (G93.32)
subacute necrotizing myelitis (G37.4)
toxic encephalitis (G92.8)
toxic encephalopathy (G92.8)

DEF: Encephalitis: Inflammation of the brain, often caused by viral or bacterial infection.
DEF: Encephalomyelitis: Inflammatory disease, often viral in nature, that affects the brain and spinal cord.
DEF: Myelitis: Inflammation of the spinal cord.

✓5ᵗʰ **G04.0**   **Acute disseminated encephalitis and encephalomyelitis (ADEM)**

EXCLUDES 1   *acute necrotizing hemorrhagic encephalopathy (G04.3-)*
other noninfectious acute disseminated encephalomyelitis (noninfectious ADEM) (G04.81)

G04.00   **Acute disseminated encephalitis and encephalomyelitis, unspecified**   MCC

G04.01   **Postinfectious** acute disseminated encephalitis and encephalomyelitis (postinfectious ADEM)   MCC
EXCLUDES 1   *post chickenpox encephalitis (B01.1)*
post measles encephalitis (B05.0)
post measles myelitis (B05.1)

G04.02   **Postimmunization** acute disseminated encephalitis, myelitis and encephalomyelitis   MCC
Encephalitis, post immunization
Encephalomyelitis, post immunization
Use additional code to identify the vaccine (T50.A-, T50.B-, T50.Z-)

G04.1   **Tropical spastic paraplegia**   CC   HCC

✓ Additional Character Required   ✓x7ᵗʰ Placeholder   Questionable PDx   Manifestation   Unspecified   UPD Unacceptable PDx   H1-H14 HAC   HCC CMS-HCC Dx   HIV HIV Dx

ICD-10-CM 2025   585

Chapter 6. Diseases of the Nervous System

G04.2   **Bacterial meningoencephalitis and meningomyelitis, not elsewhere classified** `MCC`

✓5ᵗʰ G04.3   **Acute necrotizing hemorrhagic encephalopathy**

> **EXCLUDES 1**   acute disseminated encephalitis and encephalomyelitis (G04.0-)

    G04.30   **Acute necrotizing hemorrhagic encephalopathy, unspecified** `MCC`

    G04.31   **Postinfectious acute necrotizing hemorrhagic encephalopathy** `MCC`

    G04.32   **Postimmunization acute necrotizing hemorrhagic encephalopathy** `MCC`

> Use additional code to identify the vaccine (T50.A-, T50.B-, T50.Z-)

    G04.39   **Other acute necrotizing hemorrhagic encephalopathy** `MCC`

> Code also underlying etiology, if applicable

✓5ᵗʰ G04.8   **Other encephalitis, myelitis and encephalomyelitis**

> Code also any associated seizure (G40.-, R56.9)

    G04.81   **Other encephalitis and encephalomyelitis** `HIV` `MCC`
> Noninfectious acute disseminated encephalomyelitis (noninfectious ADEM)

    G04.82   **Acute flaccid myelitis** `MCC` `HCC`
> **EXCLUDES 1**   transverse myelitis (G37.3)
> **AHA:** 2021,4Q,11

    G04.89   **Other myelitis** `HIV` `MCC` `HCC`
> **AHA:** 2020,1Q,14

✓5ᵗʰ G04.9   **Encephalitis, myelitis and encephalomyelitis, unspecified**

    G04.90   **Encephalitis and encephalomyelitis, unspecified** `HIV` `MCC`
> Ventriculitis (cerebral) NOS

    G04.91   **Myelitis, unspecified** `HIV` `MCC` `HCC`

✓4ᵗʰ G05   **Encephalitis, myelitis and encephalomyelitis in diseases classified elsewhere**

> Code first underlying disease, such as:
> congenital toxoplasmosis encephalitis, myelitis and encephalomyelitis (P37.1)
> cytomegaloviral encephalitis, myelitis and encephalomyelitis (B25.8)
> encephalitis, myelitis and encephalomyelitis (in) systemic lupus erythematosus (M32.19)
> eosinophilic meningoencephalitis (B83.2)
> human immunodeficiency virus [HIV] disease (B20)
> poliovirus (A80.-)
> suppurative otitis media (H66.01-H66.4)
> systemic lupus erythematosus (M32.19)
> trichinellosis (B75)

> **EXCLUDES 1**   adenoviral encephalitis, myelitis and encephalomyelitis (A85.1)
> encephalitis, myelitis and encephalomyelitis (in) measles (B05.0)
> enteroviral encephalitis, myelitis and encephalomyelitis (A85.0)
> herpesviral [herpes simplex] encephalitis, myelitis and encephalomyelitis (B00.4)
> listerial encephalitis, myelitis and encephalomyelitis (A32.12)
> meningococcal encephalitis, myelitis and encephalomyelitis (A39.81)
> mumps encephalitis, myelitis and encephalomyelitis (B26.2)
> postchickenpox encephalitis, myelitis and encephalomyelitis (B01.1-)
> rubella encephalitis, myelitis and encephalomyelitis (B06.01)
> toxoplasmosis encephalitis, myelitis and encephalomyelitis (B58.2)
> zoster encephalitis, myelitis and encephalomyelitis (B02.0)

    G05.3   *Encephalitis and encephalomyelitis in diseases classified elsewhere* `MCC`
> Meningoencephalitis in diseases classified elsewhere
> Code first underlying disease

    G05.4   *Myelitis in diseases classified elsewhere* `MCC` `HCC`
> Meningomyelitis in diseases classified elsewhere

✓4ᵗʰ G06   **Intracranial and intraspinal abscess and granuloma**

> Use additional code (B95-B97) to identify infectious agent
> **DEF:** Abscess: Circumscribed collection of pus resulting from bacteria, frequently associated with swelling and other signs of inflammation.
> **DEF:** Granuloma: Abnormal, dense collections of cells forming a mass or nodule of chronically inflamed tissue with granulations that is usually associated with an infective process.

    G06.0   **Intracranial abscess and granuloma** `MCC`
> Brain [any part] abscess (embolic)
> Cerebellar abscess (embolic)
> Cerebral abscess (embolic)
> Intracranial epidural abscess or granuloma
> Intracranial extradural abscess or granuloma
> Intracranial subdural abscess or granuloma
> Otogenic abscess (embolic)
> **EXCLUDES 1**   tuberculous intracranial abscess and granuloma (A17.81)

    G06.1   **Intraspinal abscess and granuloma** `MCC`
> Abscess (embolic) of spinal cord [any part]
> Intraspinal epidural abscess or granuloma
> Intraspinal extradural abscess or granuloma
> Intraspinal subdural abscess or granuloma
> **EXCLUDES 1**   tuberculous intraspinal abscess and granuloma (A17.81)

    G06.2   **Extradural and subdural abscess, unspecified** `MCC`

G07   *Intracranial and intraspinal abscess and granuloma in diseases classified elsewhere* `MCC`

> Code first underlying disease, such as:
> schistosomiasis granuloma of brain (B65.-)

> **EXCLUDES 1**   abscess of brain:
> amebic (A06.6)
> chromomycotic (B43.1)
> gonococcal (A54.82)
> tuberculous (A17.81)
> tuberculoma of meninges (A17.1)

G08   **Intracranial and intraspinal phlebitis and thrombophlebitis** `MCC`

> Septic embolism of intracranial or intraspinal venous sinuses and veins
> Septic endophlebitis of intracranial or intraspinal venous sinuses and veins
> Septic phlebitis of intracranial or intraspinal venous sinuses and veins
> Septic thrombophlebitis of intracranial or intraspinal venous sinuses and veins
> Septic thrombosis of intracranial or intraspinal venous sinuses and veins

> **EXCLUDES 1**   intracranial phlebitis and thrombophlebitis complicating:
> abortion, ectopic or molar pregnancy (O00-O07, O08.7)
> pregnancy, childbirth and the puerperium (O22.5, O87.3)
> nonpyogenic intracranial phlebitis and thrombophlebitis (I67.6)

> **EXCLUDES 2**   intracranial phlebitis and thrombophlebitis complicating nonpyogenic intraspinal phlebitis and thrombophlebitis (G95.1)

> **DEF:** Inflammation and formation of a blood clot in a vein within the brain or spine, or their linings.

G09   **Sequelae of inflammatory diseases of central nervous system**

> **NOTE**   Category G09 is to be used to indicate conditions whose primary classification is to G00-G08 as the cause of sequelae, themselves classifiable elsewhere. The "sequelae" include conditions specified as residuals.

> Code first condition resulting from (sequela) of inflammatory diseases of central nervous system

N Newborn: 0   **P** Pediatric: 0-17   **M** Maternity: 9-64   **A** Adult: 15-124   **UNS** Unspecified Site   **MCC** Major Complication/Comorbidity   **CC** Complication/Comorbidity   **PE** POA Exempt

586   ICD-10-CM 2025

Systemic atrophies primarily affecting the central nervous system (G10-G14)

G10   **Huntington's disease** `CC` `HCC`
Huntington's chorea
Huntington's dementia
Use additional code, if applicable, to identify:
  dementia with anxiety (F02.84, F02.A4, F02.B4, F02.C4)
  dementia with behavioral disturbance (F02.81-, F02.A1-, F02.B1-, F02.C1-)
  dementia with mood disturbance (F02.83, F02.A3, F02.B3, F02.C3)
  dementia with psychotic disturbance (F02.82, F02.A2, F02.B2, F02.C2)
  dementia without behavioral disturbance (F02.80, F02.A0, F02.B0, F02.C0)
  mild neurocognitive disorder due to known physiological condition (F06.7-)
DEF: Genetic disease caused by degeneration of nerve cells in the brain, characterized by chronic progressive mental deterioration. Dementia and death occur within 15 to 20 years of onset.

✓4ᵗʰ **G11**   **Hereditary ataxia**
    EXCLUDES 2   *cerebral palsy (G80.-)*
              hereditary and idiopathic neuropathy (G60.-)
              metabolic disorders (E70-E88)
DEF: Ataxia: Defect in muscular control or coordination due to a central nervous system disorder, particularly when voluntary muscular movements are attempted.

G11.0   **Congenital nonprogressive ataxia** `CC` `HCC`

✓5ᵗʰ **G11.1**   **Early-onset cerebellar ataxia**
    AHA: 2020,4Q,17-18

    G11.10   **Early-onset cerebellar ataxia, unspecified** `CC` `HCC`

    G11.11   **Friedreich ataxia** `CC` `HCC`
       Autosomal recessive Friedreich ataxia
       Friedreich ataxia with retained reflexes

    G11.19   **Other early-onset cerebellar ataxia** `CC` `HCC`
       Early-onset cerebellar ataxia with essential tremor
       Early-onset cerebellar ataxia with myoclonus [Hunt's ataxia]
       Early-onset cerebellar ataxia with retained tendon reflexes
       X-linked recessive spinocerebellar ataxia

G11.2   **Late-onset cerebellar ataxia** `CC` `HCC` `A`

G11.3   **Cerebellar ataxia with defective DNA repair** `CC` `HCC`
    Ataxia telangiectasia [Louis-Bar]
    EXCLUDES 2   *Cockayne's syndrome (Q87.19)*
              other disorders of purine and pyrimidine metabolism (E79.-)
              xeroderma pigmentosum (Q82.1)

G11.4   **Hereditary spastic paraplegia** `CC` `HCC`

G11.5   **Hypomyelination - hypogonadotropic hypogonadism - hypodontia** `CC` `HCC`
    4H syndrome
    Pol III-related leukodystrophy
    AHA: 2023,4Q,12-13

G11.6   **Leukodystrophy with vanishing white matter disease** `CC` `HCC`
    AHA: 2023,4Q,12-13

G11.8   **Other hereditary ataxias** `CC` `HCC`

G11.9   **Hereditary ataxia, unspecified** `CC` `HCC`
    Hereditary cerebellar ataxia NOS
    Hereditary cerebellar degeneration
    Hereditary cerebellar disease
    Hereditary cerebellar syndrome

✓4ᵗʰ **G12**   **Spinal muscular atrophy and related syndromes**

G12.0   **Infantile spinal muscular atrophy, type I [Werdnig-Hoffman]** `CC` `HCC`

G12.1   **Other inherited spinal muscular atrophy** `CC` `HCC`
    Adult form spinal muscular atrophy
    Childhood form, type II spinal muscular atrophy
    Distal spinal muscular atrophy
    Juvenile form, type III spinal muscular atrophy [Kugelberg-Welander]
    Progressive bulbar palsy of childhood [Fazio-Londe]
    Scapuloperoneal form spinal muscular atrophy

✓5ᵗʰ **G12.2**   **Motor neuron disease**
    AHA: 2017,4Q,9-10

    G12.20   **Motor neuron disease, unspecified** `CC` `HCC`

G12.21   **Amyotrophic lateral sclerosis** `CC` `HCC` `A`
G12.22   **Progressive bulbar palsy** `CC` `HCC`
G12.23   **Primary lateral sclerosis** `CC` `HCC`
G12.24   **Familial motor neuron disease** `CC` `HCC`
G12.25   **Progressive spinal muscle atrophy** `CC` `HCC`
G12.29   **Other motor neuron disease** `CC` `HCC`

G12.8   **Other spinal muscular atrophies and related syndromes** `CC` `HCC`

G12.9   **Spinal muscular atrophy, unspecified** `CC` `HCC`

✓4ᵗʰ **G13**   **Systemic atrophies primarily affecting central nervous system in diseases classified elsewhere**

G13.0   *Paraneoplastic neuromyopathy and neuropathy*
    Carcinomatous neuromyopathy
    Sensorial paraneoplastic neuropathy [Denny Brown]
    Code first underlying neoplasm (C00-D49)

G13.1   *Other systemic atrophy primarily affecting central nervous system in neoplastic disease*
    Paraneoplastic limbic encephalopathy
    Code first underlying neoplasm (C00-D49)

G13.2   *Systemic atrophy primarily affecting the central nervous system in myxedema*
    Code first underlying disease, such as:
       hypothyroidism (E03.-)
       myxedematous congenital iodine deficiency (E00.1)

G13.8   *Systemic atrophy primarily affecting central nervous system in other diseases classified elsewhere*
    Code first underlying disease

G14   **Postpolio syndrome** `HCC`
    INCLUDES   postpolio myelitic syndrome
    EXCLUDES 1   *sequelae of poliomyelitis (B91)*

Extrapyramidal and movement disorders (G20-G26)

✓4ᵗʰ **G20**   **Parkinson's disease**
Hemiparkinsonism
Idiopathic Parkinsonism or Parkinson's disease
Paralysis agitans
Primary Parkinsonism or Parkinson's disease
Use additional code, if applicable, to identify:
  dementia with anxiety (F02.84, F02.A4, F02.B4, F02.C4)
  dementia with behavioral disturbance (F02.81-, F02.A1-, F02.B1-, F02.C1-)
  dementia with mood disturbance (F02.83, F02.A3, F02.B3, F02.C3)
  dementia with psychotic disturbance (F02.82, F02.A2, F02.B2, F02.C2)
  dementia without behavioral disturbance (F02.80, F02.A0, F02.B0, F02.C0)
  mild neurocognitive disorder due to known physiological condition (F06.7-)
AHA: 2023,4Q,15-17; 2017,2Q,7; 2016,2Q,6
TIP: Repeated falls (R29.6) are not integral to Parkinson's disease and can be separately coded.

✓5ᵗʰ **G20.A**   **Parkinson's disease without dyskinesia**

    G20.A1   **Parkinson's disease without dyskinesia, without mention of fluctuations** `HCC`
       Parkinson's disease NOS
       Parkinson's disease without dyskinesia, without mention of OFF episodes

    G20.A2   **Parkinson's disease without dyskinesia, with fluctuations** `HCC`
       Parkinson's disease without dyskinesia, with OFF episodes

✓5ᵗʰ **G20.B**   **Parkinson's disease with dyskinesia**
    EXCLUDES 1   *drug induced dystonia (G24.0-)*

    G20.B1   **Parkinson's disease with dyskinesia, without mention of fluctuations** `HCC`
       Parkinson's disease with dyskinesia, without mention of OFF episodes

    G20.B2   **Parkinson's disease with dyskinesia, with fluctuations** `HCC`
       Parkinson's disease with dyskinesia, with OFF episodes

    G20.C   **Parkinsonism, unspecified** `HCC`
       Parkinsonism, NOS
    EXCLUDES 1   *Parkinson's disease NOS (G20.A1)*
              Parkinson's disease with dyskinesia (G20.B-)
              Parkinson's disease without dyskinesia (G20.A-)
              secondary parkinsonism ▶(G21.-)◀

☑ Additional Character Required   ✓x7ᵗʰ Placeholder   Questionable PDx   Manifestation   Unspecified   UPD Unacceptable PDx   H1-H14 HAC   HCC CMS-HCC Dx   HIV HIV Dx

ICD-10-CM 2025   587

Chapter 6. Diseases of the Nervous System

G10–G20.C

Chapter 6. Diseases of the Nervous System

G21 Secondary parkinsonism ✓4th

EXCLUDES 1   *dementia with Parkinsonism (G31.83)*
       Huntington's disease (G10)
       ▶*neurocognitive disorder with Lewy bodies (G31.83)*◀
       Shy-Drager syndrome (G90.3)
       syphilitic Parkinsonism (A52.19)

G21.0 Malignant neuroleptic syndrome   MCC
   Use additional code for adverse effect, if applicable, to identify drug (T43.3X5, T43.4X5, T43.5Ø5, T43.595)
     EXCLUDES 1   *neuroleptic induced parkinsonism (G21.11)*

G21.1 Other drug-induced secondary parkinsonism ✓5th

   G21.11 Neuroleptic induced parkinsonism   CC
     Use additional code for adverse effect, if applicable, to identify drug (T43.3X5, T43.4X5, T43.5Ø5, T43.595)
      EXCLUDES 1   *malignant neuroleptic syndrome (G21.0)*

   G21.19 Other drug induced secondary parkinsonism   CC
     Other medication-induced parkinsonism
     Use additional code for adverse effect, if applicable, to identify drug (T36-T5Ø with fifth or sixth character 5)

G21.2 Secondary parkinsonism due to other external agents   CC
   Code first (T51-T65) to identify external agent

G21.3 Postencephalitic parkinsonism   CC HCC

G21.4 Vascular parkinsonism   HCC

G21.8 Other secondary parkinsonism   CC HCC

G21.9 Secondary parkinsonism, unspecified   CC HCC

G23 Other degenerative diseases of basal ganglia ✓4th

   EXCLUDES 2   *multi-system degeneration of the autonomic nervous system (G90.3)*

G23.0 Hallervorden-Spatz disease   CC HCC
   Pigmentary pallidal degeneration

G23.1 Progressive supranuclear ophthalmoplegia [Steele-Richardson-Olszewski]   CC HCC
   Progressive supranuclear palsy

G23.2 Striatonigral degeneration   CC HCC

G23.3 Hypomyelination with atrophy of the basal ganglia and cerebellum   CC HCC
   H-ABC
   AHA: 2023,4Q,12-13

G23.8 Other specified degenerative diseases of basal ganglia   CC HCC
   Calcification of basal ganglia

G23.9 Degenerative disease of basal ganglia, unspecified   CC HCC

G24 Dystonia ✓4th

   INCLUDES   dyskinesia
   EXCLUDES 2   *athetoid cerebral palsy (G80.3)*
   DEF: Disorder of abnormal muscle tone, excessive or inadequate. Involuntary movements and prolonged muscle contractions result in tremors, abnormalities in posture, and twisting body motions that affect an isolated area or the whole body.

G24.0 Drug induced dystonia ✓5th
   Use additional code for adverse effect, if applicable, to identify drug (T36-T5Ø with fifth or sixth character 5)

   G24.01 Drug induced subacute dyskinesia
     Drug induced blepharospasm
     Drug induced orofacial dyskinesia
     Neuroleptic induced tardive dyskinesia
     Tardive dyskinesia

   G24.02 Drug induced acute dystonia   CC
     Acute dystonic reaction to drugs
     Neuroleptic induced acute dystonia

   G24.09 Other drug induced dystonia   CC

G24.1 Genetic torsion dystonia
   Dystonia deformans progressiva
   Dystonia musculorum deformans
   Familial torsion dystonia
   Idiopathic familial dystonia
   Idiopathic (torsion) dystonia NOS
   (Schwalbe-) Ziehen-Oppenheim disease

G24.2 Idiopathic nonfamilial dystonia   CC

G24.3 Spasmodic torticollis
   EXCLUDES 1   *congenital torticollis (Q68.0)*
       hysterical torticollis (F44.4)
       ocular torticollis (R29.891)
       psychogenic torticollis (F45.8)
       torticollis NOS (M43.6)
       traumatic recurrent torticollis (S13.4)
   DEF: Twisted, unnatural position of the neck due to contracted cervical muscles that pull the head to one side or cause involuntary shaking of the head.

G24.4 Idiopathic orofacial dystonia
   Orofacial dyskinesia
   EXCLUDES 1   *drug induced orofacial dyskinesia (G24.01)*

G24.5 Blepharospasm
   EXCLUDES 1   *drug induced blepharospasm (G24.01)*
   DEF: Involuntary contraction of the orbicularis oculi muscle, resulting in the eyelids being completely closed.

G24.8 Other dystonia   CC
   Acquired torsion dystonia NOS

G24.9 Dystonia, unspecified
   Dyskinesia NOS

G25 Other extrapyramidal and movement disorders ✓4th

   EXCLUDES 2   *sleep related movement disorders (G47.6-)*

G25.0 Essential tremor
   Familial tremor
   EXCLUDES 1   *tremor NOS (R25.1)*

G25.1 Drug-induced tremor
   Use additional code for adverse effect, if applicable, to identify drug (T36-T5Ø with fifth or sixth character 5)

G25.2 Other specified forms of tremor
   Intention tremor

G25.3 Myoclonus
   Drug-induced myoclonus
   Palatal myoclonus
   Use additional code for adverse effect, if applicable, to identify drug (T36-T5Ø with fifth or sixth character 5)
   EXCLUDES 1   *facial myokymia (G51.4)*
       myoclonic epilepsy (G40.-)
   DEF: Spasmodic, brief, involuntary muscle contractions that can be due to an undetermined etiology, drug-induced, or caused by a disease process.

G25.4 Drug-induced chorea
   Use additional code for adverse effect, if applicable, to identify drug (T36-T5Ø with fifth or sixth character 5)

G25.5 Other chorea
   Chorea NOS
   EXCLUDES 1   *chorea NOS with heart involvement (I02.0)*
       Huntington's chorea (G10)
       rheumatic chorea (I02.-)
       Sydenham's chorea (I02.-)

G25.6 Drug induced tics and other tics of organic origin ✓5th

   G25.61 Drug induced tics
     Use additional code for adverse effect, if applicable, to identify drug (T36-T5Ø with fifth or sixth character 5)

   G25.69 Other tics of organic origin
     EXCLUDES 1   *habit spasm (F95.9)*
       tic NOS (F95.9)
       Tourette's syndrome (F95.2)

G25.7 Other and unspecified drug induced movement disorders ✓5th
   Use additional code for adverse effect, if applicable, to identify drug (T36-T5Ø with fifth or sixth character 5)

   G25.70 Drug induced movement disorder, unspecified

   G25.71 Drug induced akathisia
     Drug induced acathisia
     Neuroleptic induced acute akathisia
     Tardive akathisia

   G25.79 Other drug induced movement disorders

G25.8 Other specified extrapyramidal and movement disorders ✓5th

   G25.81 Restless legs syndrome
     DEF: Neurological disorder of unknown etiology creating an irresistible urge to move the legs, which may temporarily relieve the symptoms. This syndrome is accompanied by motor restlessness and sensations of pain, burning, prickling, or tingling.

   G25.82 Stiff-man syndrome   CC

   G25.83 Benign shuddering attacks

N Newborn: 0   P Pediatric: 0-17   M Maternity: 9-64   A Adult: 15-124   UNS Unspecified Site   MCC Major Complication/Comorbidity   CC Complication/Comorbidity   PE POA Exempt

588   ICD-10-CM 2025

G25.89 **Other specified extrapyramidal and movement disorders**

G25.9 **Extrapyramidal and movement disorder, unspecified** CC

G26 *Extrapyramidal and movement disorders in diseases classified elsewhere*
  Code first underlying disease

Other degenerative diseases of the nervous system (G30-G32)

✓4th G30 **Alzheimer's disease**

INCLUDES Alzheimer's dementia senile and presenile forms
Use additional code, if applicable, to identify:
  delirium, if applicable (F05)
  dementia with anxiety (F02.84, F02.A4, F02.B4, F02.C4)
  dementia with behavioral disturbance (F02.81-, F02.A1-, F02.B1-, F02.C1-)
  dementia with mood disturbance (F02.83, F02.A3, F02.B3, F02.C3)
  dementia with psychotic disturbance (F02.82, F02.A2, F02.B2, F02.C2)
  dementia without behavioral disturbance (F02.80, F02.A0, F02.B0, F02.C0)
  mild neurocognitive disorder due to known physiological condition (F06.7-)

EXCLUDES 1 *senile degeneration of brain NEC (G31.1)*
senile dementia NOS ▶(F03.-)◀
senility NOS (R41.81)

AHA: 2022,4Q,15; 2017,1Q,43
TIP: A code from category F02 should always be assigned with a code from this category, even in the absence of documented dementia.
TIP: Functional quadriplegia (R53.2) is not integral to Alzheimer's disease and can be coded in addition to codes from category G30.

G30.0 **Alzheimer's disease with early onset** HCC
G30.1 **Alzheimer's disease with late onset** HCC A
G30.8 **Other Alzheimer's disease** HCC
G30.9 **Alzheimer's disease, unspecified** HCC
  AHA: 2016,2Q,6; 2012,4Q,95

✓4th G31 **Other degenerative diseases of nervous system, not elsewhere classified**

Use additional code, if applicable, for codes G31.0-G31.83, G31.85-G31.9, to identify:
  dementia with anxiety (F02.84, F02.A4, F02.B4, F02.C4)
  dementia with behavioral disturbance (F02.81-, F02.A1-, F02.B1-, F02.C1-)
  dementia with mood disturbance (F02.83, F02.A3, F02.B3, F02.C3)
  dementia with psychotic disturbance (F02.82, F02.A2, F02.B2, F02.C2)
  dementia without behavioral disturbance (F02.80, F02.A0, F02.B0, F02.C0)
  mild neurocognitive disorder due to known physiological condition (F06.7-)

EXCLUDES 2 *Reye's syndrome (G93.7)*

✓5th G31.0 **Frontotemporal dementia**

G31.01 **Pick's disease** HCC
  Primary progressive aphasia
  Progressive isolated aphasia
  DEF: Progressive frontotemporal dementia with asymmetrical atrophy of the frontal and temporal regions of the cerebral cortex and abnormal rounded brain cells called Pick cells with the presence of abnormal staining of protein (called tau). Symptoms include prominent apathy, behavioral changes such as disinhibition and restlessness, echolalia, impairment of language, memory, and intellect, increased carelessness, poor personal hygiene, and decreased attention span.

G31.09 **Other frontotemporal neurocognitive disorder** HCC
  Frontal dementia
  Use additional code, if applicable, to identify mild neurocognitive disorders due to known physiological condition (F06.7-)

G31.1 **Senile degeneration of brain, not elsewhere classified**
  EXCLUDES 1 *Alzheimer's disease (G30.-)*
  senility NOS (R41.81)

G31.2 **Degeneration of nervous system due to alcohol**
  Alcoholic cerebellar ataxia
  Alcoholic cerebellar degeneration
  Alcoholic cerebral degeneration
  Alcoholic encephalopathy
  Dysfunction of the autonomic nervous system due to alcohol
  Code also associated alcoholism (F10.-)

✓5th G31.8 **Other specified degenerative diseases of nervous system**

G31.80 **Leukodystrophy, unspecified** HCC
  AHA: 2023,4Q,12-13

G31.81 **Alpers disease** CC HCC
  Grey-matter degeneration

G31.82 **Leigh's disease** CC HCC
  Subacute necrotizing encephalopathy

G31.83 **Neurocognitive disorder with Lewy bodies** HCC
  Lewy body dementia
  Lewy body disease
  Use additional code, if applicable, to identify mild neurocognitive disorders due to known physiological condition (F06.7-)
  AHA: 2017,2Q,7; 2016,4Q,141
  DEF: Cerebral dementia with neurophysiologic changes, increased hippocampal volume, hypoperfusion in the occipital lobes, beta amyloid deposits with neurofibrillary tangles, and atrophy of the cortex and brainstem. Hallmark neuropsychological characteristics include fluctuating cognition with pronounced variation in attention and alertness, recurrent hallucinations, and Parkinsonism.

G31.84 **Mild cognitive impairment of uncertain or unknown etiology**
  Mild cognitive disorder NOS
  Mild neurocognitive disorder of uncertain or unknown etiology
  Use additional code to identify presence of:
    alcohol abuse and dependence (F10.-)
    exposure to environmental tobacco smoke (Z77.22)
    history of tobacco dependence (Z87.891)
    hypertension (I10-I1A)
    occupational exposure to environmental tobacco smoke (Z57.31)
    tobacco dependence (F17.-)
    tobacco use (Z72.0)
  EXCLUDES 1 *age related cognitive decline (R41.81)*
    altered mental status (R41.82)
    cerebral degeneration (G31.9)
    cerebrovascular diseases (I60-I69)
    change in mental status (R41.82)
    cognitive deficits following (sequelae of) cerebral hemorrhage or infarction (I69.01-, I69.11-, I69.21-, I69.31-, I69.81-, I69.91-)
    cognitive impairment due to intracranial or head injury (S06.-)
    dementia ▶(F01.-, F02.-, F03.-)◀
    mild neurocognitive disorder due to a known physiological condition (F06.7-)
    neurologic neglect syndrome (R41.4)
    personality change, nonpsychotic (F68.8)
  AHA: 2021,3Q,3

G31.85 **Corticobasal degeneration**

G31.86 **Alexander disease** HCC
  AHA: 2023,4Q,12-13

G31.89 **Other specified degenerative diseases of nervous system**

G31.9 **Degenerative disease of nervous system, unspecified**
  AHA: 2021,3Q,3

✓ Additional Character Required   ✓x7th Placeholder   Questionable PDx   Manifestation   Unspecified   UPD Unacceptable PDx   H1 - H14 HAC   HCC CMS-HCC Dx   HIV HIV Dx

✓4ᵗʰ **G32 Other degenerative disorders of nervous system in diseases classified elsewhere**

    G32.0 Subacute combined degeneration of spinal cord in diseases classified elsewhere `CC` `HCC`
        Dana-Putnam syndrome
        Sclerosis of spinal cord (combined) (dorsolateral) (posterolateral)
        Code first underlying disease, such as:
          other dietary vitamin B12 deficiency anemia (D51.3)
          vitamin B12 deficiency anemia due to intrinsic factor deficiency (D51.0)
          vitamin B12 deficiency anemia, unspecified (D51.8)
          vitamin B12 deficiency (E53.8)
        EXCLUDES 1   *syphilitic combined degeneration of spinal cord (A52.11)*

   ✓5ᵗʰ **G32.8 Other specified degenerative disorders of nervous system in diseases classified elsewhere**
        Code first underlying disease, such as:
          amyloidosis cerebral degeneration (E85.-)
          cerebral degeneration (due to) hypothyroidism (E00.0-E03.9)
          cerebral degeneration (due to) neoplasm (C00-D49)
          cerebral degeneration (due to) vitamin B deficiency, except thiamine (E52-E53.-)
        EXCLUDES 1   *superior hemorrhagic polioencephalitis [Wernicke's encephalopathy] (E51.2)*

      G32.81 Cerebellar ataxia in diseases classified elsewhere `CC` `HCC`
        Code first underlying disease, such as:
          celiac disease (with gluten ataxia) (K90.0)
          cerebellar ataxia (in) neoplastic disease (paraneoplastic cerebellar degeneration) (C00-D49)
          non-celiac gluten ataxia (M35.9)
         EXCLUDES 1   *systemic atrophy primarily affecting the central nervous system in alcoholic cerebellar ataxia (G31.2)*
             systemic atrophy primarily affecting the central nervous system in myxedema (G13.2)

      G32.89 Other specified degenerative disorders of nervous system in diseases classified elsewhere
        Degenerative encephalopathy in diseases classified elsewhere

Demyelinating diseases of the central nervous system (G35-G37)

G35 Multiple sclerosis `HCC`
    Disseminated multiple sclerosis
    Generalized multiple sclerosis
    Multiple sclerosis NOS
    Multiple sclerosis of brain stem
    Multiple sclerosis of cord
    AHA: 2021,1Q,7

✓4ᵗʰ **G36 Other acute disseminated demyelination**
    EXCLUDES 1   *postinfectious encephalitis and encephalomyelitis NOS (G04.01)*
    DEF: Demyelination: Abnormal loss of myelin, the protective white matter that insulates nerve endings and facilitates neuroreception and neurotransmission. When this substance is damaged, the nerve is short-circuited, resulting in impaired or loss of function.

   G36.0 Neuromyelitis optica [Devic] `CC` `HCC`
        Demyelination in optic neuritis
        EXCLUDES 1   *optic neuritis NOS (H46)*

   G36.1 Acute and subacute hemorrhagic leukoencephalitis [Hurst] `CC` `HCC`

   G36.8 Other specified acute disseminated demyelination `CC` `HCC`

   G36.9 Acute disseminated demyelination, unspecified `HIV` `CC` `HCC`

✓4ᵗʰ **G37 Other demyelinating diseases of central nervous system**

   G37.0 Diffuse sclerosis of central nervous system `CC` `HCC`
        Periaxial encephalitis
        Schilder's disease
        EXCLUDES 1   *X linked adrenoleukodystrophy (E71.52-)*

   G37.1 Central demyelination of corpus callosum `CC` `HCC`

   G37.2 Central pontine myelinolysis `CC` `HCC`
        AHA: 2022,2Q,10

   G37.3 Acute transverse myelitis in demyelinating disease of central nervous system `CC` `HCC`
        Acute transverse myelitis NOS
        Acute transverse myelopathy
        EXCLUDES 1   *acute flaccid myelitis (G04.82)*
             multiple sclerosis (G35)
             neuromyelitis optica [Devic] (G36.0)

   G37.4 Subacute necrotizing myelitis of central nervous system `HIV` `MCC` `HCC`

   G37.5 Concentric sclerosis [Balo] of central nervous system `CC` `HCC`

   ✓5ᵗʰ **G37.8 Other specified demyelinating diseases of central nervous system**
        AHA: 2023,4Q,18
      G37.81 Myelin oligodendrocyte glycoprotein antibody disease `CC` `HCC`
        MOG antibody disease
        Code also associated manifestations, if known, such as:
          noninfectious acute disseminated encephalomyelitis (G04.81)
          neuromyelitis optica (G36.0)
      G37.89 Other specified demyelinating diseases of central nervous system `CC` `HCC`

   G37.9 Demyelinating disease of central nervous system, unspecified `HIV` `CC` `HCC`

Episodic and paroxysmal disorders (G40-G47)

✓4ᵗʰ **G40 Epilepsy and recurrent seizures**
    NOTE   The following terms are to be considered equivalent to intractable: pharmacoresistant (pharmacologically resistant), treatment resistant, refractory (medically) and poorly controlled
    EXCLUDES 1   *conversion disorder with seizures (F44.5)*
             convulsions NOS (R56.9)
             post traumatic seizures (R56.1)
             seizure (convulsive) NOS (R56.9)
             seizure of newborn (P90)
    EXCLUDES 2   *hippocampal sclerosis (G93.81)*
             mesial temporal sclerosis (G93.81)
             temporal sclerosis (G93.81)
             Todd's paralysis (G83.84)

   ✓5ᵗʰ **G40.0 Localization-related (focal) (partial) idiopathic epilepsy and epileptic syndromes with seizures of localized onset**
        Benign childhood epilepsy with centrotemporal EEG spikes
        Childhood epilepsy with occipital EEG paroxysms
        EXCLUDES 1   *adult onset localization-related epilepsy (G40.1-, G40.2-)*

    ✓6ᵗʰ **G40.00 Localization-related (focal) (partial) idiopathic epilepsy and epileptic syndromes with seizures of localized onset, not intractable**
        Localization-related (focal) (partial) idiopathic epilepsy and epileptic syndromes with seizures of localized onset without intractability
      G40.001 Localization-related (focal) (partial) idiopathic epilepsy and epileptic syndromes with seizures of localized onset, not intractable, with status epilepticus `CC` `HCC`
      G40.009 Localization-related (focal) (partial) idiopathic epilepsy and epileptic syndromes with seizures of localized onset, not intractable, without status epilepticus `CC` `HCC`
        Localization-related (focal) (partial) idiopathic epilepsy and epileptic syndromes with seizures of localized onset NOS

    ✓6ᵗʰ **G40.01 Localization-related (focal) (partial) idiopathic epilepsy and epileptic syndromes with seizures of localized onset, intractable**
      G40.011 Localization-related (focal) (partial) idiopathic epilepsy and epileptic syndromes with seizures of localized onset, intractable, with status epilepticus `CC` `HCC`
      G40.019 Localization-related (focal) (partial) idiopathic epilepsy and epileptic syndromes with seizures of localized onset, intractable, without status epilepticus `CC` `HCC`

✓5th **G40.1** **Localization-related (focal) (partial) symptomatic epilepsy and epileptic syndromes with simple partial seizures**
> Attacks without alteration of consciousness
> Epilepsia partialis continua [Kozhevnikof]
> Simple partial seizures developing into secondarily generalized seizures
>
> **AHA:** 2023,3Q,4

     ✓6th **G40.10** **Localization-related (focal) (partial) symptomatic epilepsy and epileptic syndromes with simple partial seizures, not intractable**
> Localization-related (focal) (partial) symptomatic epilepsy and epileptic syndromes with simple partial seizures without intractability

         G40.101 **Localization-related (focal) (partial) symptomatic epilepsy and epileptic syndromes with simple partial seizures, not intractable, with status epilepticus** `CC` `HCC`

         G40.109 **Localization-related (focal) (partial) symptomatic epilepsy and epileptic syndromes with simple partial seizures, not intractable, without status epilepticus** `CC` `HCC`
> Localization-related (focal) (partial) symptomatic epilepsy and epileptic syndromes with simple partial seizures NOS

     ✓6th **G40.11** **Localization-related (focal) (partial) symptomatic epilepsy and epileptic syndromes with simple partial seizures, intractable**

         G40.111 **Localization-related (focal) (partial) symptomatic epilepsy and epileptic syndromes with simple partial seizures, intractable, with status epilepticus** `CC` `HCC`

         G40.119 **Localization-related (focal) (partial) symptomatic epilepsy and epileptic syndromes with simple partial seizures, intractable, without status epilepticus** `CC` `HCC`

✓5th **G40.2** **Localization-related (focal) (partial) symptomatic epilepsy and epileptic syndromes with complex partial seizures**
> Attacks with alteration of consciousness, often with automatisms
> Complex partial seizures developing into secondarily generalized seizures

     ✓6th **G40.20** **Localization-related (focal) (partial) symptomatic epilepsy and epileptic syndromes with complex partial seizures, not intractable**
> Localization-related (focal) (partial) symptomatic epilepsy and epileptic syndromes with complex partial seizures without intractability

         G40.201 **Localization-related (focal) (partial) symptomatic epilepsy and epileptic syndromes with complex partial seizures, not intractable, with status epilepticus** `CC` `HCC`

         G40.209 **Localization-related (focal) (partial) symptomatic epilepsy and epileptic syndromes with complex partial seizures, not intractable, without status epilepticus** `CC` `HCC`
> Localization-related (focal) (partial) symptomatic epilepsy and epileptic syndromes with complex partial seizures NOS

     ✓6th **G40.21** **Localization-related (focal) (partial) symptomatic epilepsy and epileptic syndromes with complex partial seizures, intractable**

         G40.211 **Localization-related (focal) (partial) symptomatic epilepsy and epileptic syndromes with complex partial seizures, intractable, with status epilepticus** `CC` `HCC`

         G40.219 **Localization-related (focal) (partial) symptomatic epilepsy and epileptic syndromes with complex partial seizures, intractable, without status epilepticus** `CC` `HCC`

✓5th **G40.3** **Generalized idiopathic epilepsy and epileptic syndromes**
> Code also MERRF syndrome, if applicable (E88.42)

     ✓6th **G40.30** **Generalized idiopathic epilepsy and epileptic syndromes, not intractable**
> Generalized idiopathic epilepsy and epileptic syndromes without intractability

         G40.301 **Generalized idiopathic epilepsy and epileptic syndromes, not intractable, with status epilepticus** `MCC` `HCC`

         G40.309 **Generalized idiopathic epilepsy and epileptic syndromes, not intractable, without status epilepticus** `HCC`
> Generalized idiopathic epilepsy and epileptic syndromes NOS

     ✓6th **G40.31** **Generalized idiopathic epilepsy and epileptic syndromes, intractable**

         G40.311 **Generalized idiopathic epilepsy and epileptic syndromes, intractable, with status epilepticus** `MCC` `HCC`

         G40.319 **Generalized idiopathic epilepsy and epileptic syndromes, intractable, without status epilepticus** `MCC` `HCC`

✓5th **G40.A** **Absence epileptic syndrome**
> Childhood absence epilepsy [pyknolepsy]
> Juvenile absence epilepsy
> Absence epileptic syndrome, NOS

     ✓6th **G40.A0** **Absence epileptic syndrome, not intractable**

         G40.A01 **Absence epileptic syndrome, not intractable, with status epilepticus** `HCC`

         G40.A09 **Absence epileptic syndrome, not intractable, without status epilepticus** `HCC`

     ✓6th **G40.A1** **Absence epileptic syndrome, intractable**

         G40.A11 **Absence epileptic syndrome, intractable, with status epilepticus** `CC` `HCC`

         G40.A19 **Absence epileptic syndrome, intractable, without status epilepticus** `CC` `HCC`

✓5th **G40.B** **Juvenile myoclonic epilepsy [impulsive petit mal]**

     ✓6th **G40.B0** **Juvenile myoclonic epilepsy, not intractable**

         G40.B01 **Juvenile myoclonic epilepsy, not intractable, with status epilepticus** `CC` `HCC`

         G40.B09 **Juvenile myoclonic epilepsy, not intractable, without status epilepticus** `CC` `HCC`

     ✓6th **G40.B1** **Juvenile myoclonic epilepsy, intractable**

         G40.B11 **Juvenile myoclonic epilepsy, intractable, with status epilepticus** `CC` `HCC`

         G40.B19 **Juvenile myoclonic epilepsy, intractable, without status epilepticus** `CC` `HCC`

✓5th **G40.C** **Lafora progressive myoclonus epilepsy**
> Lafora body disease
> Code also, if applicable, associated conditions such as dementia (F02.8-)
>
> **AHA:** 2023,4Q,18-19

     ✓6th **G40.C0** **Lafora progressive myoclonus epilepsy, not intractable**

         G40.C01 **Lafora progressive myoclonus epilepsy, not intractable, with status epilepticus** `CC` `HCC`

         G40.C09 **Lafora progressive myoclonus epilepsy, not intractable, without status epilepticus** `CC` `HCC`
> Lafora progressive myoclonus epilepsy NOS

     ✓6th **G40.C1** **Lafora progressive myoclonus epilepsy, intractable**

         G40.C11 **Lafora progressive myoclonus epilepsy, intractable, with status epilepticus** `CC` `HCC`

         G40.C19 **Lafora progressive myoclonus epilepsy, intractable, without status epilepticus** `CC` `HCC`

Chapter 6. Diseases of the Nervous System

G40.1–G40.C19

✅ Additional Character Required   ✓x7th Placeholder   `Questionable PDx`   `Manifestation`   `Unspecified`   `UPD` Unacceptable PDx   `H1`-`H4` HAC   `HCC` CMS-HCC Dx   `HIV` HIV Dx

ICD-10-CM 2025   **591**

Chapter 6. Diseases of the Nervous System

✓5ᵗʰ **G40.4** **Other generalized epilepsy and epileptic syndromes**

Epilepsy with grand mal seizures on awakening
Epilepsy with myoclonic absences
Epilepsy with myoclonic-astatic seizures
Grand mal seizure NOS
Nonspecific atonic epileptic seizures
Nonspecific clonic epileptic seizures
Nonspecific myoclonic epileptic seizures
Nonspecific tonic epileptic seizures
Nonspecific tonic-clonic epileptic seizures
Symptomatic early myoclonic encephalopathy

  ✓6ᵗʰ **G40.40** **Other generalized epilepsy and epileptic syndromes, not intractable**

Other generalized epilepsy and epileptic syndromes without intractability
Other generalized epilepsy and epileptic syndromes NOS

    G40.401 **Other generalized epilepsy and epileptic syndromes, not intractable, with status epilepticus** HCC

    G40.409 **Other generalized epilepsy and epileptic syndromes, not intractable, without status epilepticus** HCC

  ✓6ᵗʰ **G40.41** **Other generalized epilepsy and epileptic syndromes, intractable**

    G40.411 **Other generalized epilepsy and epileptic syndromes, intractable, with status epilepticus** CC HCC

    G40.419 **Other generalized epilepsy and epileptic syndromes, intractable, without status epilepticus** CC HCC

  G40.42 **Cyclin-Dependent Kinase-Like 5 Deficiency Disorder** HCC
CDKL5
Use additional code, if known, to identify associated manifestations, such as:
  cortical blindness (H47.61-)
  global development delay (F88)
AHA: 2020,4Q,18-19

✓5ᵗʰ **G40.5** **Epileptic seizures related to external causes**

Epileptic seizures related to alcohol
Epileptic seizures related to drugs
Epileptic seizures related to hormonal changes
Epileptic seizures related to sleep deprivation
Epileptic seizures related to stress
Code also, if applicable, associated epilepsy and recurrent seizures (G40.-)
Use additional code for adverse effect, if applicable, to identify drug (T36-T50 with fifth or sixth character 5)

  ✓6ᵗʰ **G40.50** **Epileptic seizures related to external causes, not intractable**

    G40.501 **Epileptic seizures related to external causes, not intractable, with status epilepticus** CC HCC

    G40.509 **Epileptic seizures related to external causes, not intractable, without status epilepticus** CC HCC
Epileptic seizures related to external causes, NOS

✓5ᵗʰ **G40.8** **Other epilepsy and recurrent seizures**

Epilepsies and epileptic syndromes undetermined as to whether they are focal or generalized
Landau-Kleffner syndrome

  ✓6ᵗʰ **G40.80** **Other epilepsy**

    G40.801 **Other epilepsy, not intractable, with status epilepticus** CC HCC
Other epilepsy without intractability with status epilepticus

    G40.802 **Other epilepsy, not intractable, without status epilepticus** CC HCC
Other epilepsy NOS
Other epilepsy without intractability without status epilepticus

    G40.803 **Other epilepsy, intractable, with status epilepticus** CC HCC

    G40.804 **Other epilepsy, intractable, without status epilepticus** CC HCC

✓6ᵗʰ **G40.81** **Lennox-Gastaut syndrome**

DEF: Severe form of epilepsy with usual onset in early childhood. Seizures are frequent and difficult to treat, causing falls and intellectual impairment.

  G40.811 **Lennox-Gastaut syndrome, not intractable, with status epilepticus** CC HCC

  G40.812 **Lennox-Gastaut syndrome, not intractable, without status epilepticus** CC HCC

  G40.813 **Lennox-Gastaut syndrome, intractable, with status epilepticus** CC HCC

  G40.814 **Lennox-Gastaut syndrome, intractable, without status epilepticus** CC HCC

✓6ᵗʰ **G40.82** **Epileptic spasms**

Infantile spasms
Salaam attacks
West's syndrome

  G40.821 **Epileptic spasms, not intractable, with status epilepticus** CC HCC

  G40.822 **Epileptic spasms, not intractable, without status epilepticus** CC HCC

  G40.823 **Epileptic spasms, intractable, with status epilepticus** CC HCC

  G40.824 **Epileptic spasms, intractable, without status epilepticus** CC HCC

✓6ᵗʰ **G40.83** **Dravet syndrome**

Polymorphic epilepsy in infancy (PMEI)
Severe myoclonic epilepsy in infancy (SMEI)
AHA: 2020,4Q,19

  G40.833 **Dravet syndrome, intractable, with status epilepticus** CC HCC

  G40.834 **Dravet syndrome, intractable, without status epilepticus** CC HCC
Dravet syndrome NOS

● ✓6ᵗʰ **G40.84** **KCNQ2-related epilepsy**

●   **G40.841** **KCNQ2-related epilepsy, not intractable, with status epilepticus** CC

●   **G40.842** **KCNQ2-related epilepsy, not intractable, without status epilepticus** CC
KCNQ2-related epilepsy NOS

●   **G40.843** **KCNQ2-related epilepsy, intractable, with status epilepticus** CC

●   **G40.844** **KCNQ2-related epilepsy, intractable, without status epilepticus** CC

G40.89 **Other seizures** CC HCC
EXCLUDES 1   post traumatic seizures (R56.1)
       recurrent seizures NOS (G40.909)
       seizure NOS (R56.9)

✓5ᵗʰ **G40.9** **Epilepsy, unspecified**
AHA: 2019,1Q,19

  ✓6ᵗʰ **G40.90** **Epilepsy, unspecified, not intractable**
Epilepsy, unspecified, without intractability

    G40.901 **Epilepsy, unspecified, not intractable, with status epilepticus** HCC

    G40.909 **Epilepsy, unspecified, not intractable, without status epilepticus** HCC
Epilepsy NOS
Epileptic convulsions NOS
Epileptic fits NOS
Epileptic seizures NOS
Recurrent seizures NOS
Seizure disorder NOS
AHA: 2024,2Q,8; 2021,2Q,3; 2021,1Q,3

  ✓6ᵗʰ **G40.91** **Epilepsy, unspecified, intractable**
Intractable seizure disorder NOS

    G40.911 **Epilepsy, unspecified, intractable, with status epilepticus** CC HCC

    G40.919 **Epilepsy, unspecified, intractable, without status epilepticus** CC HCC

N Newborn: 0   **P** Pediatric: 0-17   **M** Maternity: 9-64   **A** Adult: 15-124   **UNS** Unspecified Site   **MCC** Major Complication/Comorbidity   **CC** Complication/Comorbidity   **PE** POA Exempt

592
ICD-10-CM 2025

✓4th **G43 Migraine**

NOTE The following terms are to be considered equivalent to intractable: pharmacoresistant (pharmacologically resistant), treatment resistant, refractory (medically) and poorly controlled

Use additional code for adverse effect, if applicable, to identify drug (T36-T50 with fifth or sixth character 5)

EXCLUDES 1   headache NOS (R51.9)

          lower half migraine (G44.00)

EXCLUDES 2   headache syndromes (G44.-)

DEF: Headaches that occur periodically on one or both sides of the head that may be associated with nausea and vomiting, sensitivity to light and sound, dizziness, distorted vision, and cognitive disturbances.

✓5th **G43.Ø Migraine without aura**

Common migraine

EXCLUDES 1   chronic migraine without aura (G43.7-)

✓6th **G43.ØØ Migraine without aura, not intractable**

Migraine without aura without mention of refractory migraine

     G43.ØØ1 Migraine without aura, not intractable, with status migrainosus

     G43.ØØ9 Migraine without aura, not intractable, without status migrainosus

          Migraine without aura NOS

✓6th **G43.Ø1 Migraine without aura, intractable**

Migraine without aura with refractory migraine

     G43.Ø11 Migraine without aura, intractable, with status migrainosus

     G43.Ø19 Migraine without aura, intractable, without status migrainosus

✓5th **G43.1 Migraine with aura**

Basilar migraine

Classical migraine

Migraine equivalents

Migraine preceded or accompanied by transient focal neurological phenomena

Migraine triggered seizures

Migraine with acute-onset aura

Migraine with aura without headache (migraine equivalents)

Migraine with prolonged aura

Migraine with typical aura

Retinal migraine

Code also any associated seizure (G40.-, R56.9)

EXCLUDES 1   chronic migraine with aura (G43.E-)

          persistent migraine aura (G43.5-, G43.6-)

✓6th **G43.1Ø Migraine with aura, not intractable**

Migraine with aura without mention of refractory migraine

     G43.1Ø1 Migraine with aura, not intractable, with status migrainosus

     G43.1Ø9 Migraine with aura, not intractable, without status migrainosus

          Migraine with aura NOS

✓6th **G43.11 Migraine with aura, intractable**

Migraine with aura with refractory migraine

     G43.111 Migraine with aura, intractable, with status migrainosus

     G43.119 Migraine with aura, intractable, without status migrainosus

✓5th **G43.4 Hemiplegic migraine**

Familial migraine

Sporadic migraine

✓6th **G43.4Ø Hemiplegic migraine, not intractable**

Hemiplegic migraine without refractory migraine

     G43.4Ø1 Hemiplegic migraine, not intractable, with status migrainosus

     G43.4Ø9 Hemiplegic migraine, not intractable, without status migrainosus

          Hemiplegic migraine NOS

✓6th **G43.41 Hemiplegic migraine, intractable**

Hemiplegic migraine with refractory migraine

     G43.411 Hemiplegic migraine, intractable, with status migrainosus

     G43.419 Hemiplegic migraine, intractable, without status migrainosus

✓5th **G43.5 Persistent migraine aura without cerebral infarction**

✓6th **G43.5Ø Persistent migraine aura without cerebral infarction, not intractable**

Persistent migraine aura without cerebral infarction, without refractory migraine

     G43.5Ø1 Persistent migraine aura without cerebral infarction, not intractable, with status migrainosus

     G43.5Ø9 Persistent migraine aura without cerebral infarction, not intractable, without status migrainosus

          Persistent migraine aura NOS

✓6th **G43.51 Persistent migraine aura without cerebral infarction, intractable**

Persistent migraine aura without cerebral infarction, with refractory migraine

     G43.511 Persistent migraine aura without cerebral infarction, intractable, with status migrainosus

     G43.519 Persistent migraine aura without cerebral infarction, intractable, without status migrainosus

✓5th **G43.6 Persistent migraine aura with cerebral infarction**

Code also the type of cerebral infarction (I63.-)

✓6th **G43.6Ø Persistent migraine aura with cerebral infarction, not intractable**

Persistent migraine aura with cerebral infarction, without refractory migraine

     G43.6Ø1 Persistent migraine aura with cerebral infarction, not intractable, with status migrainosus   CC

     G43.6Ø9 Persistent migraine aura with cerebral infarction, not intractable, without status migrainosus   CC

✓6th **G43.61 Persistent migraine aura with cerebral infarction, intractable**

Persistent migraine aura with cerebral infarction, with refractory migraine

     G43.611 Persistent migraine aura with cerebral infarction, intractable, with status migrainosus   CC

     G43.619 Persistent migraine aura with cerebral infarction, intractable, without status migrainosus   CC

✓5th **G43.7 Chronic migraine without aura**

Transformed migraine

EXCLUDES 1   migraine without aura (G43.Ø-)

✓6th **G43.7Ø Chronic migraine without aura, not intractable**

Chronic migraine without aura, without refractory migraine

     G43.7Ø1 Chronic migraine without aura, not intractable, with status migrainosus

     G43.7Ø9 Chronic migraine without aura, not intractable, without status migrainosus

          Chronic migraine without aura NOS

✓6th **G43.71 Chronic migraine without aura, intractable**

Chronic migraine without aura, with refractory migraine

     G43.711 Chronic migraine without aura, intractable, with status migrainosus

     G43.719 Chronic migraine without aura, intractable, without status migrainosus

✓5th **G43.A Cyclical vomiting**

EXCLUDES 1   cyclical vomiting syndrome unrelated to migraine (R11.15)

AHA: 2019,4Q,15

     G43.AØ Cyclical vomiting, in migraine, not intractable

          Cyclical vomiting, without refractory migraine

     G43.A1 Cyclical vomiting, in migraine, intractable

          Cyclical vomiting, with refractory migraine

✓5th **G43.B Ophthalmoplegic migraine**

     G43.BØ Ophthalmoplegic migraine, not intractable

          Ophthalmoplegic migraine, without refractory migraine

     G43.B1 Ophthalmoplegic migraine, intractable

          Ophthalmoplegic migraine, with refractory migraine

✓5th **G43.C Periodic headache syndromes in child or adult**

     G43.CØ Periodic headache syndromes in child or adult, not intractable

          Periodic headache syndromes in child or adult, without refractory migraine

✓ Additional Character Required   ✓7th Placeholder   Questionable PDx   Manifestation   Unspecified   UPD Unacceptable PDx   H1-H14 HAC   HCC CMS-HCC Dx   HIV HIV Dx

ICD-10-CM 2025   593

Chapter 6. Diseases of the Nervous System

G43.C1   **Periodic headache syndromes in child or adult, intractable**
Periodic headache syndromes in child or adult, with refractory migraine

✓5th **G43.D**   **Abdominal migraine**

     G43.D0   **Abdominal migraine, not intractable**
     Abdominal migraine, without refractory migraine

     G43.D1   **Abdominal migraine, intractable**
     Abdominal migraine, with refractory migraine

✓5th **G43.8**   **Other migraine**

   ✓6th **G43.80**   **Other migraine, not intractable**
     Other migraine, without refractory migraine

     G43.801   **Other migraine, not intractable, with status migrainosus**

     G43.809   **Other migraine, not intractable, without status migrainosus**

   ✓6th **G43.81**   **Other migraine, intractable**
     Other migraine, with refractory migraine

     G43.811   **Other migraine, intractable, with status migrainosus**

     G43.819   **Other migraine, intractable, without status migrainosus**

   ✓6th **G43.82**   **Menstrual migraine, not intractable**
     Menstrual headache, not intractable
     Menstrual migraine, without refractory migraine
     Menstrually related migraine, not intractable
     Pre-menstrual headache, not intractable
     Pre-menstrual migraine, not intractable
     Pure menstrual migraine, not intractable
     Code also associated premenstrual tension syndrome (N94.3)

     G43.821   **Menstrual migraine, not intractable, with status migrainosus**

     G43.829   **Menstrual migraine, not intractable, without status migrainosus**
     Menstrual migraine NOS

   ✓6th **G43.83**   **Menstrual migraine, intractable**
     Menstrual headache, intractable
     Menstrual migraine, with refractory migraine
     Menstrually related migraine, intractable
     Pre-menstrual headache, intractable
     Pre-menstrual migraine, intractable
     Pure menstrual migraine, intractable
     Code also associated premenstrual tension syndrome (N94.3)

     G43.831   **Menstrual migraine, intractable, with status migrainosus**

     G43.839   **Menstrual migraine, intractable, without status migrainosus**

✓5th **G43.9**   **Migraine, unspecified**

   ✓6th **G43.90**   **Migraine, unspecified, not intractable**
     Migraine, unspecified, without refractory migraine

     G43.901   **Migraine, unspecified, not intractable, with status migrainosus**
     Status migrainosus NOS

     G43.909   **Migraine, unspecified, not intractable, without status migrainosus**
     Migraine NOS

   ✓6th **G43.91**   **Migraine, unspecified, intractable**
     Migraine, unspecified, with refractory migraine

     G43.911   **Migraine, unspecified, intractable, with status migrainosus**

     G43.919   **Migraine, unspecified, intractable, without status migrainosus**

✓5th **G43.E**   **Chronic migraine with aura**
     EXCLUDES 1   *migraine with aura (G43.1-)*
     AHA: 2023,4Q,19-20

   ✓6th **G43.E0**   **Chronic migraine with aura, not intractable**
     Chronic migraine with aura, without refractory migraine

     G43.E01   **Chronic migraine with aura, not intractable, with status migrainosus**

     G43.E09   **Chronic migraine with aura, not intractable, without status migrainosus**
     Chronic migraine with aura NOS

   ✓6th **G43.E1**   **Chronic migraine with aura, intractable**
     Chronic migraine with aura, with refractory migraine

     G43.E11   **Chronic migraine with aura, intractable, with status migrainosus**

     G43.E19   **Chronic migraine with aura, intractable, without status migrainosus**

✓4th **G44**   **Other headache syndromes**
     EXCLUDES 1   *headache NOS (R51.9)*
     EXCLUDES 2   *atypical facial pain (G50.1)*
     headache due to lumbar puncture (G97.1)
     migraines (G43.-)
     trigeminal neuralgia (G50.0)

✓5th **G44.0**   **Cluster headaches and other trigeminal autonomic cephalgias (TAC)**
     DEF: Cluster headache: Characteristic grouping or clustering of headaches that can last for a number of weeks or months and then completely disappear for months or years. They are typically not associated with gastrointestinal upset or light sensitivity as experienced in migraines.

   ✓6th **G44.00**   **Cluster headache syndrome, unspecified**
     Ciliary neuralgia
     Cluster headache NOS
     Histamine cephalgia
     Lower half migraine
     Migrainous neuralgia

     G44.001   **Cluster headache syndrome, unspecified, intractable**

     G44.009   **Cluster headache syndrome, unspecified, not intractable**
     Cluster headache syndrome NOS

   ✓6th **G44.01**   **Episodic cluster headache**

     G44.011   **Episodic cluster headache, intractable**

     G44.019   **Episodic cluster headache, not intractable**
     Episodic cluster headache NOS

   ✓6th **G44.02**   **Chronic cluster headache**

     G44.021   **Chronic cluster headache, intractable**

     G44.029   **Chronic cluster headache, not intractable**
     Chronic cluster headache NOS

   ✓6th **G44.03**   **Episodic paroxysmal hemicrania**
     Paroxysmal hemicrania NOS

     G44.031   **Episodic paroxysmal hemicrania, intractable**

     G44.039   **Episodic paroxysmal hemicrania, not intractable**
     Episodic paroxysmal hemicrania NOS

   ✓6th **G44.04**   **Chronic paroxysmal hemicrania**

     G44.041   **Chronic paroxysmal hemicrania, intractable**

     G44.049   **Chronic paroxysmal hemicrania, not intractable**
     Chronic paroxysmal hemicrania NOS

   ✓6th **G44.05**   **Short lasting unilateral neuralgiform headache with conjunctival injection and tearing (SUNCT)**

     G44.051   **Short lasting unilateral neuralgiform headache with conjunctival injection and tearing (SUNCT), intractable**

     G44.059   **Short lasting unilateral neuralgiform headache with conjunctival injection and tearing (SUNCT), not intractable**
     Short lasting unilateral neuralgiform headache with conjunctival injection and tearing (SUNCT) NOS

   ✓6th **G44.09**   **Other trigeminal autonomic cephalgias (TAC)**

     G44.091   **Other trigeminal autonomic cephalgias (TAC), intractable**

     G44.099   **Other trigeminal autonomic cephalgias (TAC), not intractable**

G44.1   **Vascular headache, not elsewhere classified**
     EXCLUDES 2   *cluster headache (G44.0)*
     complicated headache syndromes (G44.5-)
     drug-induced headache (G44.4-)
     migraine (G43.-)
     other specified headache syndromes (G44.8-)
     post-traumatic headache (G44.3-)
     tension-type headache (G44.2-)

✓5th **G44.2**   **Tension-type headache**

   ✓6th **G44.20**   **Tension-type headache, unspecified**

     G44.201   **Tension-type headache, unspecified, intractable**

     G44.209   **Tension-type headache, unspecified, not intractable**
     Tension headache NOS

   ✓6th **G44.21**   **Episodic tension-type headache**

     G44.211   **Episodic tension-type headache, intractable**

N Newborn: 0   P Pediatric: 0-17   M Maternity: 9-64   A Adult: 15-124   UNS Unspecified Site   MCC Major Complication/Comorbidity   CC Complication/Comorbidity   PE POA Exempt

594

ICD-10-CM 2025

        G44.219   Episodic tension-type headache, not intractable
            Episodic tension-type headache NOS

✓6ᵗʰ **G44.22   Chronic tension-type headache**
        G44.221   Chronic tension-type headache, intractable
        G44.229   Chronic tension-type headache, not intractable
            Chronic tension-type headache NOS

✓5ᵗʰ **G44.3   Post-traumatic headache**
     ✓6ᵗʰ **G44.30   Post-traumatic headache, unspecified**
        G44.301   Post-traumatic headache, unspecified, intractable
        G44.309   Post-traumatic headache, unspecified, not intractable
            Post-traumatic headache NOS

     ✓6ᵗʰ **G44.31   Acute post-traumatic headache**
        G44.311   Acute post-traumatic headache, intractable
        G44.319   Acute post-traumatic headache, not intractable
            Acute post-traumatic headache NOS

     ✓6ᵗʰ **G44.32   Chronic post-traumatic headache**
        G44.321   Chronic post-traumatic headache, intractable
        G44.329   Chronic post-traumatic headache, not intractable
            Chronic post-traumatic headache NOS

✓5ᵗʰ **G44.4   Drug-induced headache, not elsewhere classified**
     Medication overuse headache
     Use additional code for adverse effect, if applicable, to identify drug (T36-T50 with fifth or sixth character 5)
    G44.40   Drug-induced headache, not elsewhere classified, not intractable
    G44.41   Drug-induced headache, not elsewhere classified, intractable

✓5ᵗʰ **G44.5   Complicated headache syndromes**
    G44.51   Hemicrania continua
        DEF: Persistent primary headache of unknown causation occurring on one side of the face and head. May last for more than three months, with daily and continuous pain of moderate intensity with severe exacerbations.
    G44.52   New daily persistent headache (NDPH)
    G44.53   Primary thunderclap headache
    G44.59   Other complicated headache syndrome

✓5ᵗʰ **G44.8   Other specified headache syndromes**
     EXCLUDES 2   headache with orthostatic or positional component, not elsewhere classifed (R51.0)
    G44.81   Hypnic headache
    G44.82   Headache associated with sexual activity
         Orgasmic headache
         Preorgasmic headache
    G44.83   Primary cough headache
    G44.84   Primary exertional headache
    G44.85   Primary stabbing headache
    G44.86   Cervicogenic headache
         Code also associated cervical spinal condition, if known
         AHA: 2021,4Q,11-12
    G44.89   Other headache syndrome

✓4ᵗʰ **G45   Transient cerebral ischemic attacks and related syndromes**
     EXCLUDES 1   neonatal cerebral ischemia (P91.0)
              transient retinal artery occlusion (H34.0-)
     AHA: 2023,1Q,37; 2018,2Q,9
     DEF: Transient cerebral ischemic attack: Intermittent or brief cerebral dysfunction from lack of oxygenation with no persistent neurological deficits associated with occlusive vascular disease. TIA may denote an impending cerebrovascular accident.
    G45.0   Vertebro-basilar artery syndrome   cc
    G45.1   Carotid artery syndrome (hemispheric)   cc
    G45.2   Multiple and bilateral precerebral artery syndromes   cc
    G45.3   Amaurosis fugax   cc
    G45.4   Transient global amnesia
         EXCLUDES 1   amnesia NOS (R41.3)
    G45.8   Other transient cerebral ischemic attacks and related syndromes   cc

G45.9   Transient cerebral ischemic attack, unspecified   cc
     Spasm of cerebral artery
     TIA
     Transient cerebral ischemia NOS

✓4ᵗʰ **G46   Vascular syndromes of brain in cerebrovascular diseases**
     Code first underlying cerebrovascular disease (I60-I69)
    G46.0   Middle cerebral artery syndrome   cc
    G46.1   Anterior cerebral artery syndrome   cc
    G46.2   Posterior cerebral artery syndrome   cc
    G46.3   Brain stem stroke syndrome
         Benedikt syndrome
         Claude syndrome
         Foville syndrome
         Millard-Gubler syndrome
         Wallenberg syndrome
         Weber syndrome
    G46.4   Cerebellar stroke syndrome
    G46.5   Pure motor lacunar syndrome
    G46.6   Pure sensory lacunar syndrome
    G46.7   Other lacunar syndromes
    G46.8   Other vascular syndromes of brain in cerebrovascular diseases

✓4ᵗʰ **G47   Sleep disorders**
     EXCLUDES 2   nightmares (F51.5)
              nonorganic sleep disorders (F51.-)
              sleep terrors (F51.4)
              sleepwalking (F51.3)

✓5ᵗʰ **G47.0   Insomnia**
     EXCLUDES 2   alcohol related insomnia (F10.182, F10.282, F10.982)
              drug-related insomnia (F11.182, F11.282, F11.982, F13.182, F13.282, F13.982, F14.182, F14.282, F14.982, F15.182, F15.282, F15.982, F19.182, F19.282, F19.982)
              idiopathic insomnia (F51.01)
              insomnia due to a mental disorder (F51.05)
              insomnia not due to a substance or known physiological condition (F51.0-)
              nonorganic insomnia (F51.0-)
              primary insomnia (F51.01)
              sleep apnea (G47.3-)
    G47.00   Insomnia, unspecified
         Insomnia NOS
    G47.01   Insomnia due to medical condition
         Code also associated medical condition
    G47.09   Other insomnia

✓5ᵗʰ **G47.1   Hypersomnia**
     EXCLUDES 2   alcohol-related hypersomnia (F10.182, F10.282, F10.982)
              drug-related hypersomnia (F11.182, F11.282, F11.982, F13.182, F13.282, F13.982, F14.182, F14.282, F14.982, F15.182, F15.282, F15.982, F19.182, F19.282, F19.982)
              hypersomnia due to a mental disorder (F51.13)
              hypersomnia not due to a substance or known physiological condition (F51.1-)
              primary hypersomnia (F51.11)
              sleep apnea (G47.3-)
    G47.10   Hypersomnia, unspecified
         Hypersomnia NOS
    G47.11   Idiopathic hypersomnia with long sleep time
         Idiopathic hypersomnia NOS
    G47.12   Idiopathic hypersomnia without long sleep time
    G47.13   Recurrent hypersomnia
         Kleine-Levin syndrome
         Menstrual related hypersomnia
    G47.14   Hypersomnia due to medical condition
         Code also associated medical condition
    G47.19   Other hypersomnia

✔ Additional Character Required   ✔x7ᵗʰ Placeholder   Questionable PDx   Manifestation   Unspecified   UPD Unacceptable PDx   H1 -H14 HAC   HCC CMS-HCC Dx   HIV HIV Dx

ICD-10-CM 2025   595

Chapter 6. Diseases of the Nervous System

☑5ᵗʰ **G47.2 Circadian rhythm sleep disorders**
Disorders of the sleep wake schedule
Inversion of nyctohemeral rhythm
Inversion of sleep rhythm
DEF: Circadian rhythm: Daily cycle (24-hour period) of physical, mental, and behavioral changes. It is largely influenced by environmental cues, such as changes in light or temperature.
Synonym(s): sleep/wake cycle.

G47.20 Circadian rhythm sleep disorder, unspecified type
Sleep wake schedule disorder NOS

G47.21 Circadian rhythm sleep disorder, delayed sleep phase type
Delayed sleep phase syndrome

G47.22 Circadian rhythm sleep disorder, advanced sleep phase type

G47.23 Circadian rhythm sleep disorder, irregular sleep wake type
Irregular sleep-wake pattern

G47.24 Circadian rhythm sleep disorder, free running type
Circadian rhythm sleep disorder, non-24-hour sleep-wake type

G47.25 Circadian rhythm sleep disorder, jet lag type

G47.26 Circadian rhythm sleep disorder, shift work type

G47.27 Circadian rhythm sleep disorder in conditions classified elsewhere
Code first underlying condition

G47.29 Other circadian rhythm sleep disorder

☑5ᵗʰ **G47.3 Sleep apnea**
Code also any associated underlying condition
EXCLUDES 1 apnea NOS (R06.81)
Cheyne-Stokes breathing (R06.3)
pickwickian syndrome (E66.2)
sleep apnea of newborn (P28.3-)

G47.30 Sleep apnea, unspecified
Sleep apnea NOS

G47.31 Primary central sleep apnea
Idiopathic central sleep apnea

G47.32 High altitude periodic breathing

G47.33 Obstructive sleep apnea (adult) (pediatric)
Obstructive sleep apnea hypopnea
EXCLUDES 1 obstructive sleep apnea of newborn (P28.3-)

G47.34 Idiopathic sleep related nonobstructive alveolar hypoventilation
Sleep related hypoxia

G47.35 Congenital central alveolar hypoventilation syndrome

G47.36 Sleep related hypoventilation in conditions classified elsewhere
Sleep related hypoxemia in conditions classified elsewhere
Code first underlying condition

G47.37 Central sleep apnea in conditions classified elsewhere
Code first underlying condition

G47.39 Other sleep apnea

☑5ᵗʰ **G47.4 Narcolepsy and cataplexy**

☑6ᵗʰ **G47.41 Narcolepsy**

G47.411 Narcolepsy with cataplexy

G47.419 Narcolepsy without cataplexy
Narcolepsy NOS

☑6ᵗʰ **G47.42 Narcolepsy in conditions classified elsewhere**
Code first underlying condition

G47.421 Narcolepsy in conditions classified elsewhere with cataplexy

G47.429 Narcolepsy in conditions classified elsewhere without cataplexy

☑5ᵗʰ **G47.5 Parasomnia**
EXCLUDES 1 alcohol induced parasomnia (F10.182, F10.282, F10.982)
drug induced parasomnia (F11.182, F11.282, F11.982, F13.182, F13.282, F13.982, F14.182, F14.282, F14.982, F15.182, F15.282, F15.982, F19.182, F19.282, F19.982)
parasomnia not due to a substance or known physiological condition (F51.8)

G47.50 Parasomnia, unspecified
Parasomnia NOS

G47.51 Confusional arousals

G47.52 REM sleep behavior disorder

G47.53 Recurrent isolated sleep paralysis

G47.54 Parasomnia in conditions classified elsewhere
Code first underlying condition

G47.59 Other parasomnia

☑5ᵗʰ **G47.6 Sleep related movement disorders**
EXCLUDES 2 restless legs syndrome (G25.81)

G47.61 Periodic limb movement disorder

G47.62 Sleep related leg cramps

G47.63 Sleep related bruxism
EXCLUDES 1 psychogenic bruxism (F45.8)

G47.69 Other sleep related movement disorders

G47.8 Other sleep disorders
Other specified sleep-wake disorder

G47.9 Sleep disorder, unspecified
Sleep disorder NOS
Unspecified sleep-wake disorder

Nerve, nerve root and plexus disorders (G50-G59)

EXCLUDES 1 current traumatic nerve, nerve root and plexus disorders - see Injury, nerve by body region
neuralgia NOS (M79.2)
neuritis NOS (M79.2)
peripheral neuritis in pregnancy (O26.82-)
radiculitis NOS (M54.1-)

☑4ᵗʰ **G50 Disorders of trigeminal nerve**
INCLUDES disorders of 5th cranial nerve

G50.0 Trigeminal neuralgia
Syndrome of paroxysmal facial pain
Tic douloureux

G50.1 Atypical facial pain

G50.8 Other disorders of trigeminal nerve

G50.9 Disorder of trigeminal nerve, unspecified

☑4ᵗʰ **G51 Facial nerve disorders**
INCLUDES disorders of 7th cranial nerve

G51.0 Bell's palsy
Facial palsy

G51.1 Geniculate ganglionitis
EXCLUDES 1 postherpetic geniculate ganglionitis (B02.21)

G51.2 Melkersson's syndrome
Melkersson-Rosenthal syndrome

☑5ᵗʰ **G51.3 Clonic hemifacial spasm**
AHA: 2018,4Q,10

G51.31 Clonic hemifacial spasm, right

G51.32 Clonic hemifacial spasm, left

G51.33 Clonic hemifacial spasm, bilateral

G51.39 Clonic hemifacial spasm, unspecified

G51.4 Facial myokymia

G51.8 Other disorders of facial nerve

G51.9 Disorder of facial nerve, unspecified

☑4ᵗʰ **G52 Disorders of other cranial nerves**
EXCLUDES 2 disorders of acoustic [8th] nerve (H93.3)
disorders of optic [2nd] nerve (H46, H47.0)
paralytic strabismus due to nerve palsy (H49.0-H49.2)

G52.0 Disorders of olfactory nerve
Disorders of 1st cranial nerve

G52.1 Disorders of glossopharyngeal nerve
Disorder of 9th cranial nerve
Glossopharyngeal neuralgia

G52.2 Disorders of vagus nerve
Disorders of pneumogastric [10th] nerve

G52.3 Disorders of hypoglossal nerve
Disorders of 12th cranial nerve

G52.7 Disorders of multiple cranial nerves
Polyneuritis cranialis

G52.8 Disorders of other specified cranial nerves

G52.9 Cranial nerve disorder, unspecified

G53 Cranial nerve disorders in diseases classified elsewhere
Code first underlying disease, such as:
neoplasm (C00-D49)
EXCLUDES 1 multiple cranial nerve palsy in sarcoidosis (D86.82)
multiple cranial nerve palsy in syphilis (A52.15)
postherpetic geniculate ganglionitis (B02.21)
postherpetic trigeminal neuralgia (B02.22)

✅**4th** **G54** **Nerve root and plexus disorders**

> EXCLUDES 1   *current traumatic nerve root and plexus disorders - see nerve injury by body region*
> *intervertebral disc disorders (M50-M51)*
> *neuralgia or neuritis NOS (M79.2)*
> *neuritis or radiculitis brachial NOS (M54.13)*
> *neuritis or radiculitis lumbar NOS (M54.16)*
> *neuritis or radiculitis lumbosacral NOS (M54.17)*
> *neuritis or radiculitis thoracic NOS (M54.14)*
> *radiculitis NOS (M54.10)*
> *radiculopathy NOS (M54.10)*
> *spondylosis (M47.-)*

G54.0 **Brachial plexus disorders**
Thoracic outlet syndrome
AHA: 2023,2Q,8
DEF: Acquired disorder affecting the spinal nerves that send signals to the shoulder, arm, and hand, causing corresponding motor and sensory dysfunction. This disorder is characterized by regional paresthesia, pain, muscle weakness, and in severe cases paralysis.

G54.1 **Lumbosacral plexus disorders**

G54.2 **Cervical root disorders, not elsewhere classified**

G54.3 **Thoracic root disorders, not elsewhere classified**

G54.4 **Lumbosacral root disorders, not elsewhere classified**

G54.5 **Neuralgic amyotrophy**
Parsonage-Aldren-Turner syndrome
Shoulder-girdle neuritis
> EXCLUDES 1   *neuralgic amyotrophy in diabetes mellitus (E08-E13 with .44)*

G54.6 **Phantom limb syndrome with pain**   HCC

G54.7 **Phantom limb syndrome without pain**   HCC
Phantom limb syndrome NOS

G54.8 **Other nerve root and plexus disorders**

G54.9 **Nerve root and plexus disorder, unspecified**

G55 *Nerve root and plexus compressions in diseases classified elsewhere*
Code first underlying disease, such as:
neoplasm (C00-D49)
> EXCLUDES 1   *nerve root compression (due to) (in) ankylosing spondylitis (M45.-)*
> *nerve root compression (due to) (in) dorsopathies (M53.-, M54.-)*
> *nerve root compression (due to) (in) intervertebral disc disorders (M50.1-, M51.1-)*
> *nerve root compression (due to) (in) spondylopathies (M46.-M48.-)*
> *nerve root compression (due to) (in) spondylosis (M47.0-, M47.2-)*

✅**4th** **G56** **Mononeuropathies of upper limb**
> EXCLUDES 1   *current traumatic nerve disorder - see nerve injury by body region*

AHA: 2016,4Q,17-18

✅**5th** **G56.0** **Carpal tunnel syndrome**
DEF: Swelling and inflammation in the tendons or bursa surrounding the median nerve caused by repetitive activity. The resulting compression on the nerve causes pain, numbness, and tingling especially to the palm, index, middle finger, and thumb.

  G56.00 **Carpal tunnel syndrome, unspecified upper limb**
  G56.01 **Carpal tunnel syndrome, right upper limb**
  G56.02 **Carpal tunnel syndrome, left upper limb**
  G56.03 **Carpal tunnel syndrome, bilateral upper limbs**

✅**5th** **G56.1** **Other lesions of median nerve**
  G56.10 **Other lesions of median nerve, unspecified upper limb**
  G56.11 **Other lesions of median nerve, right upper limb**
  G56.12 **Other lesions of median nerve, left upper limb**
  G56.13 **Other lesions of median nerve, bilateral upper limbs**

✅**5th** **G56.2** **Lesion of ulnar nerve**
Tardy ulnar nerve palsy
  G56.20 **Lesion of ulnar nerve, unspecified upper limb**
  G56.21 **Lesion of ulnar nerve, right upper limb**
  G56.22 **Lesion of ulnar nerve, left upper limb**
  G56.23 **Lesion of ulnar nerve, bilateral upper limbs**

✅**5th** **G56.3** **Lesion of radial nerve**
  G56.30 **Lesion of radial nerve, unspecified upper limb**
  G56.31 **Lesion of radial nerve, right upper limb**
  G56.32 **Lesion of radial nerve, left upper limb**

  G56.33 **Lesion of radial nerve, bilateral upper limbs**

✅**5th** **G56.4** **Causalgia of upper limb**
Complex regional pain syndrome II of upper limb
> EXCLUDES 1   *complex regional pain syndrome I of lower limb (G90.52-)*
> *complex regional pain syndrome I of upper limb (G90.51-)*
> *complex regional pain syndrome II of lower limb (G57.7-)*
> *reflex sympathetic dystrophy of lower limb (G90.52-)*
> *reflex sympathetic dystrophy of upper limb (G90.51-)*

  G56.40 **Causalgia of unspecified upper limb**
  G56.41 **Causalgia of right upper limb**
  G56.42 **Causalgia of left upper limb**
  G56.43 **Causalgia of bilateral upper limbs**

✅**5th** **G56.8** **Other specified mononeuropathies of upper limb**
Interdigital neuroma of upper limb
  G56.80 **Other specified mononeuropathies of unspecified upper limb**
  G56.81 **Other specified mononeuropathies of right upper limb**
  G56.82 **Other specified mononeuropathies of left upper limb**
  G56.83 **Other specified mononeuropathies of bilateral upper limbs**

✅**5th** **G56.9** **Unspecified mononeuropathy of upper limb**
  G56.90 **Unspecified mononeuropathy of unspecified upper limb**
  G56.91 **Unspecified mononeuropathy of right upper limb**
  G56.92 **Unspecified mononeuropathy of left upper limb**
  G56.93 **Unspecified mononeuropathy of bilateral upper limbs**

✅**4th** **G57** **Mononeuropathies of lower limb**
> EXCLUDES 1   *current traumatic nerve disorder - see nerve injury by body region*

AHA: 2016,4Q,17-18

✅**5th** **G57.0** **Lesion of sciatic nerve**
> EXCLUDES 1   *sciatica NOS (M54.3-)*
> EXCLUDES 2   *sciatica attributed to intervertebral disc disorder (M51.1.-)*

  G57.00 **Lesion of sciatic nerve, unspecified lower limb**
  G57.01 **Lesion of sciatic nerve, right lower limb**
  G57.02 **Lesion of sciatic nerve, left lower limb**
  G57.03 **Lesion of sciatic nerve, bilateral lower limbs**

✅**5th** **G57.1** **Meralgia paresthetica**
Lateral cutaneous nerve of thigh syndrome
  G57.10 **Meralgia paresthetica, unspecified lower limb**
  G57.11 **Meralgia paresthetica, right lower limb**
  G57.12 **Meralgia paresthetica, left lower limb**
  G57.13 **Meralgia paresthetica, bilateral lower limbs**

✅**5th** **G57.2** **Lesion of femoral nerve**
  G57.20 **Lesion of femoral nerve, unspecified lower limb**
  G57.21 **Lesion of femoral nerve, right lower limb**
  G57.22 **Lesion of femoral nerve, left lower limb**
  G57.23 **Lesion of femoral nerve, bilateral lower limbs**

✅**5th** **G57.3** **Lesion of lateral popliteal nerve**
Peroneal nerve palsy
AHA: 2020,3Q,12
  G57.30 **Lesion of lateral popliteal nerve, unspecified lower limb**
  G57.31 **Lesion of lateral popliteal nerve, right lower limb**
  G57.32 **Lesion of lateral popliteal nerve, left lower limb**
  G57.33 **Lesion of lateral popliteal nerve, bilateral lower limbs**

✅**5th** **G57.4** **Lesion of medial popliteal nerve**
  G57.40 **Lesion of medial popliteal nerve, unspecified lower limb**
  G57.41 **Lesion of medial popliteal nerve, right lower limb**
  G57.42 **Lesion of medial popliteal nerve, left lower limb**
  G57.43 **Lesion of medial popliteal nerve, bilateral lower limbs**

✅**5th** **G57.5** **Tarsal tunnel syndrome**
  G57.50 **Tarsal tunnel syndrome, unspecified lower limb**
  G57.51 **Tarsal tunnel syndrome, right lower limb**
  G57.52 **Tarsal tunnel syndrome, left lower limb**
  G57.53 **Tarsal tunnel syndrome, bilateral lower limbs**

✅**5th** **G57.6** **Lesion of plantar nerve**
Morton's metatarsalgia
  G57.60 **Lesion of plantar nerve, unspecified lower limb**

✅ Additional Character Required   ✓x7th Placeholder   Questionable PDx   Manifestation   Unspecified   UPD Unacceptable PDx   H1-H4 HAC   HCC CMS-HCC Dx   HIV HIV Dx

ICD-10-CM 2025   597

Chapter 6. Diseases of the Nervous System

G57.61   Lesion of plantar nerve, **right** lower limb
G57.62   Lesion of plantar nerve, **left** lower limb
G57.63   Lesion of plantar nerve, **bilateral** lower limbs

√5ᵗʰ   **G57.7**   **Causalgia of lower limb**

Complex regional pain syndrome II of lower limb

EXCLUDES 1   *complex regional pain syndrome I of lower limb (G90.52-)*
complex regional pain syndrome I of upper limb (G90.51-)
complex regional pain syndrome II of upper limb (G56.4-)
reflex sympathetic dystrophy of lower limb (G90.52-)
reflex sympathetic dystrophy of upper limb (G90.51-)

G57.70   Causalgia of unspecified lower limb
G57.71   Causalgia of **right** lower limb
G57.72   Causalgia of **left** lower limb
G57.73   Causalgia of **bilateral** lower limbs

√5ᵗʰ   **G57.8**   **Other specified mononeuropathies of lower limb**

Interdigital neuroma of lower limb

G57.80   Other specified mononeuropathies of unspecified lower limb
G57.81   Other specified mononeuropathies of **right** lower limb
G57.82   Other specified mononeuropathies of **left** lower limb
G57.83   Other specified mononeuropathies of **bilateral** lower limbs

√5ᵗʰ   **G57.9**   **Unspecified mononeuropathy of lower limb**

G57.90   Unspecified mononeuropathy of unspecified lower limb
G57.91   Unspecified mononeuropathy of **right** lower limb
G57.92   Unspecified mononeuropathy of **left** lower limb
G57.93   Unspecified mononeuropathy of **bilateral** lower limbs

√4ᵗʰ   **G58**   **Other mononeuropathies**

G58.0   **Intercostal neuropathy**
G58.7   **Mononeuritis multiplex**
G58.8   Other specified mononeuropathies
G58.9   Mononeuropathy, unspecified

G59   *Mononeuropathy in diseases classified elsewhere*

Code first underlying disease

EXCLUDES 1   *diabetic mononeuropathy (E08-E13 with .41)*
syphilitic nerve paralysis (A52.19)
syphilitic neuritis (A52.15)
tuberculous mononeuropathy (A17.83)

Polyneuropathies and other disorders of the peripheral nervous system (G60-G65)

EXCLUDES 1   *neuralgia NOS (M79.2)*
neuritis NOS (M79.2)
peripheral neuritis in pregnancy (O26.82-)
radiculitis NOS (M54.10)

√4ᵗʰ   **G60**   **Hereditary and idiopathic neuropathy**

G60.0   **Hereditary motor and sensory neuropathy**

Charcôt-Marie-Tooth disease
Dejerine-Sottas disease
Hereditary motor and sensory neuropathy, types I-IV
Hypertrophic neuropathy of infancy
Peroneal muscular atrophy (axonal type) (hypertrophic type)
Roussy-Levy syndrome

G60.1   **Refsum's disease**   CC

Infantile Refsum disease

DEF: Genetic disorder of the lipid metabolism characterized by retinitis pigmentosa, degenerative nerve disease, ataxia, and dry, rough, scaly skin.

G60.2   **Neuropathy in association with hereditary ataxia**
G60.3   **Idiopathic progressive neuropathy**
G60.8   **Other hereditary and idiopathic neuropathies**

Dominantly inherited sensory neuropathy
Morvan's disease
Nelaton's syndrome
Recessively inherited sensory neuropathy

G60.9   **Hereditary and idiopathic neuropathy, unspecified**

√4ᵗʰ   **G61**   **Inflammatory polyneuropathy**

G61.0   **Guillain-Barre syndrome**   CC

Acute (post-)infective polyneuritis
Miller Fisher syndrome

AHA: 2020,3Q,12; 2014,2Q,4

DEF: Autoimmune disorder due to an immune response to foreign antigens with paraplegia of limbs, flaccid paralysis, ophthalmoplegia, ataxia, and areflexia. In most cases, this disorder is triggered by a mild viral infection, surgery, or following an immunization.

TIP: Guillain-Barre syndrome can occur as a sequela of *Campylobacter* enteritis. Assign code B94.8 for the sequelae as an additional diagnosis.

G61.1   **Serum neuropathy**

Use additional code for adverse effect, if applicable, to identify serum (T50.-)

√5ᵗʰ   **G61.8**   **Other inflammatory polyneuropathies**

G61.81   **Chronic inflammatory demyelinating polyneuritis**   CC HCC
G61.82   **Multifocal motor neuropathy**   HCC

MMN

AHA: 2016,4Q,18

G61.89   Other inflammatory polyneuropathies

G61.9   Inflammatory polyneuropathy, unspecified

√4ᵗʰ   **G62**   **Other and unspecified polyneuropathies**

G62.0   **Drug-induced polyneuropathy**

Use additional code for adverse effect, if applicable, to identify drug (T36-T50 with fifth or sixth character 5)

G62.1   **Alcoholic polyneuropathy**

AHA: 2019,3Q,8

G62.2   **Polyneuropathy due to other toxic agents**

Code first (T51-T65) to identify toxic agent

√5ᵗʰ   **G62.8**   **Other specified polyneuropathies**

G62.81   **Critical illness polyneuropathy**   CC

Acute motor neuropathy

G62.82   **Radiation-induced polyneuropathy**

Use additional external cause code (W88-W90, X39.0-) to identify cause

G62.89   Other specified polyneuropathies

AHA: 2016,2Q,11

G62.9   **Polyneuropathy, unspecified**

Neuropathy NOS

G63   *Polyneuropathy in diseases classified elsewhere*

Code first underlying disease, such as:
amyloidosis (E85.-)
endocrine disease, except diabetes (E00-E07, E15-E16, E20-E34)
metabolic diseases (E70-E88)
neoplasm (C00-D49)
nutritional deficiency (E40-E64)

EXCLUDES 1   *polyneuropathy (in):*
diabetes mellitus (E08-E13 with .42)
diphtheria (A36.83)
infectious mononucleosis complicated by polyneuropathy (B27.0-B27.9 with fifth character 1)
Lyme disease (A69.22)
mumps (B26.84)
postherpetic (B02.23)
rheumatoid arthritis (M05.5-)
scleroderma (M34.83)
systemic lupus erythematosus (M32.19)

AHA: 2023,3Q,19; 2021,1Q,7; 2012,4Q,99

G64   **Other disorders of peripheral nervous system**

Disorder of peripheral nervous system NOS

√4ᵗʰ   **G65**   **Sequelae of inflammatory and toxic polyneuropathies**

Code first condition resulting from (sequela) of inflammatory and toxic polyneuropathies

G65.0   Sequelae of **Guillain-Barre syndrome**
G65.1   Sequelae of other **inflammatory** polyneuropathy
G65.2   Sequelae of **toxic** polyneuropathy

Ⓝ Newborn: 0   Ⓟ Pediatric: 0-17   Ⓜ Maternity: 9-64   Ⓐ Adult: 15-124   UNS Unspecified Site   MCC Major Complication/Comorbidity   CC Complication/Comorbidity   PE POA Exempt

598

ICD-10-CM 2025

Diseases of myoneural junction and muscle (G70-G73)

✓4ᵗʰ G70 Myasthenia gravis and other myoneural disorders

> **EXCLUDES 1**   botulism (A05.1, A48.51-A48.52)
>
>   transient neonatal myasthenia gravis (P94.0)

✓5ᵗʰ G70.0 Myasthenia gravis

> **AHA:** 2022,3Q,15
>
> **DEF:** Autoimmune neuromuscular disorder caused by antibodies to the acetylcholine receptors at the neuromuscular junction, interfering with proper binding of the neurotransmitter from the neuron to the target muscle, causing muscle weakness, fatigue, and exhaustion, without pain or atrophy.

     G70.00 Myasthenia gravis without (acute) exacerbation   `HCC`

         Myasthenia gravis NOS

     G70.01 Myasthenia gravis with (acute) exacerbation   `MCC` `HCC`

         Myasthenia gravis in crisis

G70.1 Toxic myoneural disorders   `HCC`

> Code first (T51-T65) to identify toxic agent

G70.2 Congenital and developmental myasthenia   `HCC`

✓5ᵗʰ G70.8 Other specified myoneural disorders

     G70.80 Lambert-Eaton syndrome, unspecified   `CC` `HCC`

         Lambert-Eaton syndrome NOS

     G70.81 *Lambert-Eaton syndrome in disease classified elsewhere*   `CC` `HCC`

         Code first underlying disease

>   **EXCLUDES 1**   Lambert-Eaton syndrome in neoplastic disease (G73.1)

     G70.89 Other specified myoneural disorders   `HCC`

G70.9 Myoneural disorder, unspecified   `HCC`

✓4ᵗʰ G71 Primary disorders of muscles

> **EXCLUDES 2**   arthrogryposis multiplex congenita (Q74.3)
>
>   metabolic disorders (E70-E88)
>
>   myositis (M60.-)

✓5ᵗʰ G71.0 Muscular dystrophy

> **AHA:** 2022,4Q,17-18; 2018,4Q,11-12

     G71.00 Muscular dystrophy, unspecified   `HCC`

     G71.01 Duchenne or Becker muscular dystrophy   `HCC`

         Autosomal recessive, childhood type, muscular dystrophy resembling Duchenne or Becker muscular dystrophy

         Benign [Becker] muscular dystrophy

         Severe [Duchenne] muscular dystrophy

     G71.02 Facioscapulohumeral muscular dystrophy   `HCC`

         Scapulohumeral muscular dystrophy

     ✓6ᵗʰ G71.03 Limb girdle muscular dystrophies

         G71.031 Autosomal dominant limb girdle muscular dystrophy   `HCC`

             LGMD D4 calpain-3-related

             LGMD D5 collagen 6-related

             Limb girdle muscular dystrophy type 1

         G71.032 Autosomal recessive limb girdle muscular dystrophy due to calpain-3 dysfunction   `HCC`

             Limb girdle muscular dystrophy type 2A

             LGMD R1 calpain-3-related

             Primary calpainopathy

         G71.033 Limb girdle muscular dystrophy due to dysferlin dysfunction   `HCC`

             Dysferlinopathy

             LGMD R2 dysferlin-related

             Limb girdle muscular dystrophy type 2B

             Miyoshi Myopathy type 1

         ✓7ᵗʰ G71.034 Limb girdle muscular dystrophy due to sarcoglycan dysfunction

             G71.0340 Limb girdle muscular dystrophy due to sarcoglycan dysfunction, unspecified   `HCC`

                Sarcoglycanopathy, NOS

             G71.0341 Limb girdle muscular dystrophy due to alpha sarcoglycan dysfunction   `HCC`

                Alpha sarcoglycanopathy

                Limb-girdle muscular dystrophy due to alpha-sarcoglycan deficiency

                Limb girdle muscular dystrophy type 2D

             G71.0342 Limb girdle muscular dystrophy due to beta sarcoglycan dysfunction   `HCC`

                Beta sarcoglycanopathy

                Limb girdle muscular dystrophy due to beta-sarcoglycan deficiency

                Limb girdle muscular dystrophy type 2E

             G71.0349 Limb girdle muscular dystrophy due to other sarcoglycan dysfunction   `HCC`

                Delta sarcoglycanopathy

                Delta-sarcoglycan-related LGMD R6

                Gamma sarcoglycanopathy

                Gamma-sarcoglycan-related LGMD R5

                Limb girdle muscular dystrophy type 2C

                Limb girdle muscular dystrophy type 2F

         G71.035 Limb girdle muscular dystrophy due to anoctamin-5 dysfunction   `HCC`

             Anoctamin-5-related LGMD R12

             Anoctaminopathy

             Autosomal recessive limb girdle muscular dystrophy type 2L

             Miyoshi myopathy type 3

         G71.038 Other limb girdle muscular dystrophy   `HCC`

             LGMD R9 FKRP-related

             LGMD R22 collagen 6-related

             Limb girdle muscular dystrophy due to fukutin related protein dysfunction

             Limb girdle muscular dystrophy type 2I

             Other autosomal recessive limb girdle muscular dystrophy

         G71.039 Limb girdle muscular dystrophy, unspecified   `HCC`

     G71.09 Other specified muscular dystrophies   `HCC`

         Benign scapuloperoneal muscular dystrophy with early contractures [Emery-Dreifuss]

         Congenital muscular dystrophy NOS

         Congenital muscular dystrophy with specific morphological abnormalities of the muscle fiber

         Distal muscular dystrophy

         Ocular muscular dystrophy

         Oculopharyngeal muscular dystrophy

         Scapuloperoneal muscular dystrophy

✓5ᵗʰ G71.1 Myotonic disorders

     G71.11 Myotonic muscular dystrophy   `HCC`

         Dystrophia myotonica [Steinert]

         Myotonia atrophica

         Myotonic dystrophy

         Proximal myotonic myopathy (PROMM)

         Steinert disease

     G71.12 Myotonia congenita

         Acetazolamide responsive myotonia congenita

         Dominant myotonia congenita [Thomsen disease]

         Myotonia levior

         Recessive myotonia congenita [Becker disease]

     G71.13 Myotonic chondrodystrophy

         Chondrodystrophic myotonia

         Congenital myotonic chondrodystrophy

         Schwartz-Jampel disease

     G71.14 Drug induced myotonia

> Use additional code for adverse effect, if applicable, to identify drug (T36-T50 with fifth or sixth character 5)

☑ Additional Character Required   ✓x7ᵗʰ Placeholder   Questionable PDx   Manifestation   Unspecified   `UPD` Unacceptable PDx   `H1`-`H14` HAC   `HCC` CMS-HCC Dx   `HIV` HIV Dx

ICD-10-CM 2025   599

G71.19 Other specified myotonic disorders
Myotonia fluctuans
Myotonia permanens
Neuromyotonia [Isaacs]
Paramyotonia congenita (of von Eulenburg)
Pseudomyotonia
Symptomatic myotonia

✓5th **G71.2 Congenital myopathies**
> EXCLUDES 2 arthrogryposis multiplex congenita (Q74.3)
> **AHA:** 2020,4Q,19-21

G71.20 **Congenital myopathy, unspecified** CC HCC
G71.21 **Nemaline myopathy** CC HCC
✓6th G71.22 **Centronuclear myopathy**

G71.220 **X-linked myotubular myopathy** CC HCC
Myotubular (centronuclear) myopathy
G71.228 **Other centronuclear myopathy** CC HCC
Autosomal centronuclear myopathy
Autosomal dominant centronuclear myopathy
Autosomal recessive centronuclear myopathy
Centronuclear myopathy, NOS

G71.29 **Other congenital myopathy** CC HCC
Central core disease
Minicore disease
Multicore disease
Multiminicore disease

G71.3 Mitochondrial myopathy, not elsewhere classified
> EXCLUDES 1 Kearns-Sayre syndrome (H49.81)
> Leber's disease (H47.21)
> Leigh's encephalopathy (G31.82)
> mitochondrial metabolism disorders (E88.4.-)
> Reye's syndrome (G93.7)

G71.8 Other primary disorders of muscles
G71.9 **Primary disorder of muscle, unspecified**
Hereditary myopathy NOS

✓4th **G72 Other and unspecified myopathies**
> EXCLUDES 1 arthrogryposis multiplex congenita (Q74.3)
> dermatopolymyositis (M33.-)
> ischemic infarction of muscle (M62.2-)
> myositis (M60.-)
> polymyositis (M33.2.-)

G72.0 **Drug-induced myopathy** CC
> Use additional code for adverse effect, if applicable, to identify drug (T36-T50 with fifth or sixth character 5)
G72.1 **Alcoholic myopathy** CC
> Use additional code to identify alcoholism (F10.-)
G72.2 **Myopathy due to other toxic agents** CC
> Code first (T51-T65) to identify toxic agent
G72.3 **Periodic paralysis**
Familial periodic paralysis
Hyperkalemic periodic paralysis (familial)
Hypokalemic periodic paralysis (familial)
Myotonic periodic paralysis (familial)
Normokalemic paralysis (familial)
Potassium sensitive periodic paralysis
> EXCLUDES 1 paramyotonia (of von Eulenburg) (G71.19)

✓5th G72.4 **Inflammatory and immune myopathies, not elsewhere classified**
G72.41 **Inclusion body myositis [IBM]** HCC
G72.49 **Other inflammatory and immune myopathies, not elsewhere classified**
Inflammatory myopathy NOS

✓5th G72.8 **Other specified myopathies**
G72.81 **Critical illness myopathy** CC
Acute necrotizing myopathy
Acute quadriplegic myopathy
Intensive care (ICU) myopathy
Myopathy of critical illness
> **AHA:** 2020,3Q,12
G72.89 **Other specified myopathies**
G72.9 **Myopathy, unspecified**

✓4th **G73 Disorders of myoneural junction and muscle in diseases classified elsewhere**
G73.1 *Lambert-Eaton syndrome in neoplastic disease* CC UPD HCC
> Code first underlying neoplasm (C00-D49)
> EXCLUDES 1 Lambert-Eaton syndrome not associated with neoplasm (G70.80-G70.81)

G73.3 *Myasthenic syndromes in other diseases classified elsewhere* CC HCC
> Code first underlying disease, such as:
> neoplasm (C00-D49)
> thyrotoxicosis (E05.-)

G73.7 *Myopathy in diseases classified elsewhere*
> Code first underlying disease, such as:
> glycogen storage disease (E74.0-)
> hyperparathyroidism (E21.0, E21.3)
> hypoparathyroidism (E20.-)
> lipid storage disorders (E75.-)
> EXCLUDES 1 myopathy in:
> rheumatoid arthritis (M05.32)
> sarcoidosis (D86.87)
> scleroderma (M34.82)
> Sjogren syndrome (M35.03)
> systemic lupus erythematosus (M32.19)

Cerebral palsy and other paralytic syndromes (G80-G83)

✓4th **G80 Cerebral palsy**
> EXCLUDES 1 hereditary spastic paraplegia (G11.4)

G80.0 **Spastic quadriplegic cerebral palsy** MCC HCC
Congenital spastic paralysis (cerebral)
G80.1 **Spastic diplegic cerebral palsy** CC HCC
Spastic cerebral palsy NOS
G80.2 **Spastic hemiplegic cerebral palsy** CC HCC
G80.3 **Athetoid cerebral palsy** CC HCC
Double athetosis (syndrome)
Dyskinetic cerebral palsy
Dystonic cerebral palsy
Vogt disease
G80.4 **Ataxic cerebral palsy** HCC
G80.8 **Other cerebral palsy** HCC
Mixed cerebral palsy syndromes
G80.9 **Cerebral palsy, unspecified** HCC
Cerebral palsy NOS

✓4th **G81 Hemiplegia and hemiparesis**
> **NOTE** This category is to be used only when hemiplegia (complete)(incomplete) is reported without further specification, or is stated to be old or longstanding but of unspecified cause. The category is also for use in multiple coding to identify these types of hemiplegia resulting from any cause.
> EXCLUDES 1 congenital cerebral palsy (G80.-)
> hemiplegia and hemiparesis due to sequela of cerebrovascular disease (I69.05-, I69.15-, I69.25-, I69.35-, I69.85-, I69.95-)
> **AHA:** 2015,1Q,25
> **TIP:** If the documentation specifies the affected side but not whether it is the dominant or nondominant side, the default is as follows: for ambidextrous patients, the default is dominant; when the left side is affected, the default is nondominant; and when the right side is affected, the default is dominant.

✓5th G81.0 **Flaccid hemiplegia**
G81.00 **Flaccid hemiplegia affecting unspecified side** CC UNS HCC
G81.01 **Flaccid hemiplegia affecting right dominant side** CC HCC
G81.02 **Flaccid hemiplegia affecting left dominant side** CC HCC
G81.03 **Flaccid hemiplegia affecting right nondominant side** CC HCC
G81.04 **Flaccid hemiplegia affecting left nondominant side** CC HCC

✓5th G81.1 **Spastic hemiplegia**
G81.10 **Spastic hemiplegia affecting unspecified side** CC UNS HCC
G81.11 **Spastic hemiplegia affecting right dominant side** CC HCC

G81.12 Spastic hemiplegia affecting **left dominant** `CC` `HCC`

G81.13 Spastic hemiplegia affecting **right nondominant** side `CC` `HCC`

G81.14 Spastic hemiplegia affecting **left nondominant** side `CC` `HCC`

√5th **G81.9** **Hemiplegia**, unspecified

    AHA: 2014,1Q,23

G81.90 Hemiplegia, unspecified affecting unspecified side `CC` `UNS` `HCC`

G81.91 Hemiplegia, unspecified affecting **right dominant** side `CC` `HCC`

G81.92 Hemiplegia, unspecified affecting **left dominant** side `CC` `HCC`

G81.93 Hemiplegia, unspecified affecting **right nondominant** side `CC` `HCC`

G81.94 Hemiplegia, unspecified affecting **left nondominant** side `CC` `HCC`

√4th **G82** **Paraplegia (paraparesis) and quadriplegia (quadriparesis)**

    `NOTE` This category is to be used only when the listed conditions are reported without further specification, or are stated to be old or longstanding but of unspecified cause. The category is also for use in multiple coding to identify these conditions resulting from any cause

    `EXCLUDES 1` *congenital cerebral palsy (G80.-)*
                 functional quadriplegia (R53.2)
                 hysterical paralysis (F44.4)

√5th **G82.2** **Paraplegia**

    Paralysis of both lower limbs NOS
    Paraparesis (lower) NOS
    Paraplegia (lower) NOS
    AHA: 2017,3Q,3

G82.20 **Paraplegia, unspecified** `CC` `HCC`

G82.21 **Paraplegia, complete** `CC` `HCC`

G82.22 **Paraplegia, incomplete** `CC` `HCC`

√5th **G82.5** **Quadriplegia**

    AHA: AHA:2024,2Q,23

G82.50 **Quadriplegia, unspecified** `MCC` `HCC`

G82.51 **Quadriplegia, C1-C4 complete** `MCC` `HCC`

G82.52 **Quadriplegia, C1-C4 incomplete** `MCC` `HCC`

G82.53 **Quadriplegia, C5-C7 complete** `MCC` `HCC`

G82.54 **Quadriplegia, C5-C7 incomplete** `MCC` `HCC`

√4th **G83** **Other paralytic syndromes**

    `NOTE` This category is to be used only when the listed conditions are reported without further specification, or are stated to be old or longstanding but of unspecified cause. The category is also for use in multiple coding to identify these conditions resulting from any cause.

    `INCLUDES` paralysis (complete) (incomplete), except as in G80-G82

G83.0 **Diplegia of upper limbs** `CC` `HCC`

    Diplegia (upper)
    Paralysis of both upper limbs

√5th **G83.1** **Monoplegia of lower limb**

    Paralysis of lower limb

    `EXCLUDES 1` *monoplegia of lower limbs due to sequela of cerebrovascular disease (I69.04-, I69.14-, I69.24-, I69.34-, I69.84-, I69.94-)*

    TIP: If the documentation specifies the affected side but not whether it is the dominant or nondominant side, the default is as follows: for ambidextrous patients, the default is dominant; when the left side is affected, the default is nondominant; and when the right side is affected, the default is dominant.

G83.10 Monoplegia of lower limb affecting **unspecified** side `HCC`

G83.11 Monoplegia of lower limb affecting **right dominant** side `HCC`

G83.12 Monoplegia of lower limb affecting **left dominant** side `HCC`

G83.13 Monoplegia of lower limb affecting **right nondominant** side `HCC`

G83.14 Monoplegia of lower limb affecting **left nondominant** side `HCC`

√5th **G83.2** **Monoplegia of upper limb**

    Paralysis of upper limb

    `EXCLUDES 1` *monoplegia of upper limbs due to sequela of cerebrovascular disease (I69.03-, I69.13-, I69.23-, I69.33-, I69.83-, I69.93-)*

    TIP: If the documentation specifies the affected side but not whether it is the dominant or nondominant side, the default is as follows: for ambidextrous patients, the default is dominant; when the left side is affected, the default is nondominant; and when the right side is affected, the default is dominant.

G83.20 Monoplegia of upper limb affecting **unspecified** side `HCC`

G83.21 Monoplegia of upper limb affecting **right dominant** side `HCC`

G83.22 Monoplegia of upper limb affecting **left dominant** side `HCC`

G83.23 Monoplegia of upper limb affecting **right nondominant** side `HCC`

G83.24 Monoplegia of upper limb affecting **left nondominant** side `HCC`

√5th **G83.3** **Monoplegia, unspecified**

    TIP: If the documentation specifies the affected side but not whether it is the dominant or nondominant side, the default is as follows: for ambidextrous patients, the default is dominant; when the left side is affected, the default is nondominant; and when the right side is affected, the default is dominant.

G83.30 Monoplegia, unspecified affecting **unspecified** side `HCC`

G83.31 Monoplegia, unspecified affecting **right dominant** side `HCC`

G83.32 Monoplegia, unspecified affecting **left dominant** side `HCC`

G83.33 Monoplegia, unspecified affecting **right nondominant** side `HCC`

G83.34 Monoplegia, unspecified affecting **left nondominant** side `HCC`

G83.4 **Cauda equina syndrome** `CC` `HCC`

    Neurogenic bladder due to cauda equina syndrome

    `EXCLUDES 1` *cord bladder NOS (G95.89)*
                 neurogenic bladder NOS (N31.9)

    AHA: 2024,1Q,17; 2020,3Q,24

    DEF: Compression of the spinal nerve roots presenting with pain and tingling radiating down the buttocks, back of the thigh and calf, and into the foot in a sciatic manner with aching in the bladder, perineum, and sacrum. Loss of bowel and bladder control may also occur.

G83.5 **Locked-in state** `MCC` `HCC`

    AHA: 2022,2Q,10

√5th **G83.8** **Other specified paralytic syndromes**

    `EXCLUDES 1` *paralytic syndromes due to current spinal cord injury - code to spinal cord injury (S14, S24, S34)*

G83.81 **Brown-Sequard syndrome** `HCC`

G83.82 **Anterior cord syndrome** `HCC`

G83.83 **Posterior cord syndrome** `HCC`

G83.84 **Todd's paralysis (postepileptic)** `HCC`

G83.89 **Other specified paralytic syndromes** `HCC`

G83.9 **Paralytic syndrome, unspecified** `HCC`

✔ Additional Character Required   √x7th Placeholder   Questionable PDx   Manifestation   Unspecified   `UPD` Unacceptable PDx   `H1`-`H14` HAC   `HCC` CMS-HCC Dx   `HIV` HIV Dx

ICD-10-CM 2025   601

Chapter 6. Diseases of the Nervous System

Other disorders of the nervous system (G89-G99)

✓4th G89   Pain, not elsewhere classified

Code also related psychological factors associated with pain (F45.42)

EXCLUDES 1   generalized pain NOS (R52)

pain disorders exclusively related to psychological factors (F45.41)

pain NOS (R52)

EXCLUDES 2   atypical face pain (G50.1)

headache syndromes (G44.-)

localized pain, unspecified type - code to pain by site, such as:

     abdomen pain (R10.-)

     back pain (M54.9)

     breast pain (N64.4)

     chest pain (R07.1-R07.9)

     ear pain (H92.0-)

     eye pain (H57.1)

     headache (R51.9)

     joint pain (M25.5-)

     limb pain (M79.6-)

     lumbar region pain (M54.5-)

     painful urination (R30.9)

     pelvic and perineal pain (R10.2)

     renal colic (N23)

     shoulder pain (M25.51-)

     spine pain (M54.-)

     throat pain (R07.0)

     tongue pain (K14.6)

     tooth pain (K08.8)

migraines (G43.-)

myalgia (M79.1-)

pain from prosthetic devices, implants, and grafts (T82.84, T83.84, T84.84, T85.84-)

phantom limb syndrome with pain (G54.6)

vulvar vestibulitis (N94.810)

vulvodynia (N94.81-)

G89.0   Central pain syndrome

Dejerine-Roussy syndrome

Myelopathic pain syndrome

Thalamic pain syndrome (hyperesthetic)

✓5th G89.1   Acute pain, not elsewhere classified

G89.11   Acute pain due to trauma

G89.12   Acute post-thoracotomy pain

Post-thoracotomy pain NOS

G89.18   Other acute postprocedural pain

Postoperative pain NOS

Postprocedural pain NOS

✓5th G89.2   Chronic pain, not elsewhere classified

EXCLUDES 1   causalgia, lower limb (G57.7-)

causalgia, upper limb (G56.4-)

central pain syndrome (G89.0)

chronic pain syndrome (G89.4)

complex regional pain syndrome II, lower limb (G57.7-)

complex regional pain syndrome II, upper limb (G56.4-)

neoplasm related chronic pain (G89.3)

reflex sympathetic dystrophy (G90.5-)

G89.21   Chronic pain due to trauma

G89.22   Chronic post-thoracotomy pain

G89.28   Other chronic postprocedural pain

Other chronic postoperative pain

G89.29   Other chronic pain

AHA: 2023,3Q,17

G89.3   Neoplasm related pain (acute) (chronic)

Cancer associated pain

Pain due to malignancy (primary) (secondary)

Tumor associated pain

G89.4   Chronic pain syndrome

Chronic pain associated with significant psychosocial dysfunction

✓4th G90   Disorders of autonomic nervous system

EXCLUDES 1   dysfunction of the autonomic nervous system due to alcohol (G31.2)

✓5th G90.0   Idiopathic peripheral autonomic neuropathy

G90.01   Carotid sinus syncope

Carotid sinus syndrome

DEF: Vagal activation caused by pressure on the carotid sinus baroreceptors. Sympathetic nerve impulses may cause sinus arrest or AV block.

G90.09   Other idiopathic peripheral autonomic neuropathy

Idiopathic peripheral autonomic neuropathy NOS

G90.1   Familial dysautonomia [Riley-Day]   HCC

G90.2   Horner's syndrome

Bernard(-Horner) syndrome

Cervical sympathetic dystrophy or paralysis

G90.3   Multi-system degeneration of the autonomic nervous system   CC HCC

Neurogenic orthostatic hypotension [Shy-Drager]

EXCLUDES 1   orthostatic hypotension NOS (I95.1)

G90.4   Autonomic dysreflexia

Use additional code to identify the cause, such as:

fecal impaction (K56.41)

pressure ulcer (pressure area) (L89.-)

urinary tract infection (N39.0)

✓5th G90.5   Complex regional pain syndrome I (CRPS I)

Reflex sympathetic dystrophy

EXCLUDES 1   causalgia of lower limb (G57.7-)

causalgia of upper limb (G56.4-)

complex regional pain syndrome II of lower limb (G57.7-)

complex regional pain syndrome II of upper limb (G56.4-)

G90.50   Complex regional pain syndrome I, unspecified   CC UNS

✓6th G90.51   Complex regional pain syndrome I of upper limb

G90.511   Complex regional pain syndrome I of right upper limb   CC

G90.512   Complex regional pain syndrome I of left upper limb   CC

G90.513   Complex regional pain syndrome I of upper limb, bilateral   CC

G90.519   Complex regional pain syndrome I of unspecified upper limb   CC UNS

✓6th G90.52   Complex regional pain syndrome I of lower limb

G90.521   Complex regional pain syndrome I of right lower limb   CC

G90.522   Complex regional pain syndrome I of left lower limb   CC

G90.523   Complex regional pain syndrome I of lower limb, bilateral   CC

G90.529   Complex regional pain syndrome I of unspecified lower limb   CC UNS

G90.59   Complex regional pain syndrome I of other specified site   CC

N Newborn: 0   P Pediatric: 0-17   M Maternity: 9-64   A Adult: 15-124   UNS Unspecified Site   MCC Major Complication/Comorbidity   CC Complication/Comorbidity   PE POA Exempt

602

ICD-10-CM 2025

▲ ✓5th **G90.8** **Other disorders of autonomic nervous system**

    AHA: 2023,2Q,8

●   **G90.81**   **Serotonin syndrome**

         Serotonin toxicity

         Code first poisoning due to drug or toxin, such as:

             linezolid (T36.8X- with sixth character 1-4)

             monoamine oxidase inhibitors (T43.1X with sixth character 1-4)

             selective serotonin and norepinephrine reuptake inhibitors [SSNRI] (T43.21 with sixth character 1-4)

             selective serotonin reuptake inhibitors [SSRI] (T43.22 with sixth character 1-4)

         Use additional code for adverse effect, if applicable, to identify drug, such as:

             linezolid (T36.8X5)

             monoamine oxidase inhibitors (T43.1X5)

             selective serotonin and norepinephrine reuptake inhibitors [SSNRI] (T43.215)

             selective serotonin reuptake inhibitors [SSRI] (T43.225)

         Use additional code, if applicable, to identify:

             disseminated intravascular coagulation (D65)

             hypertensive crisis (I16.-)

             metabolic acidosis (E87.2-)

             shock, not elsewhere classified (R57.-)

             toxic encephalopathy (G92.-)

             ventricular tachycardia (I47.2-)

●   **G90.89**   **Other disorders of autonomic nervous system**

G90.9 **Disorder of the autonomic nervous system, unspecified**

G90.A **Postural orthostatic tachycardia syndrome** [POTS]

     Chronic orthostatic intolerance

     Postural tachycardia syndrome

    AHA: 2022,4Q,19-20

G90.B **LMNB1-related autosomal dominant leukodystrophy** `HCC`

    AHA: 2023,4Q,12-13

✓4th **G91** **Hydrocephalus**

     `INCLUDES`   acquired hydrocephalus

     `EXCLUDES 1`   *Arnold-Chiari syndrome with hydrocephalus (Q07.-)*

                 congenital hydrocephalus (Q03.-)

                 spina bifida with hydrocephalus (Q05.-)

    DEF: Abnormal buildup of cerebrospinal fluid in the brain causing dilation of the ventricles.

Hydrocephalus (Acquired)

Normal ventricles   Hydrocephalic ventricles

G91.0 **Communicating hydrocephalus** `CC` `HCC`

     Secondary normal pressure hydrocephalus

G91.1 **Obstructive hydrocephalus** `CC` `HCC`

    DEF: Obstruction of the cerebrospinal fluid passage from the brain into the spinal canal characterized by headaches, drowsiness, poor coordination, urinary incontinence, nausea, vomiting, and papilledema.

G91.2 **(Idiopathic) normal pressure hydrocephalus** `CC` `HCC`

     Normal pressure hydrocephalus NOS

G91.3 **Post-traumatic hydrocephalus, unspecified** `CC` `HCC`

G91.4   *Hydrocephalus in diseases classified elsewhere* `HCC`

     Code first underlying condition, such as:

         congenital syphilis (A50.4-)

         neoplasm (C00-D49)

         plasminogen deficiency (E88.02)

     `EXCLUDES 1`   *hydrocephalus due to congenital toxoplasmosis (P37.1)*

    AHA: 2014,3Q,3

G91.8 **Other hydrocephalus** `CC` `HCC`

G91.9 **Hydrocephalus, unspecified** `CC` `HCC`

✓4th **G92** **Toxic encephalopathy**

    AHA: 2022,1Q,52; 2021,4Q,12-14; 2021,1Q,13; 2017,1Q,39-40

    DEF: Brain tissue degeneration due to a toxic substance.

✓5th **G92.0** **Immune effector cell-associated neurotoxicity syndrome**

     Code first underlying cause such as:

         complications of immune effector cellular therapy (T80.82)

     Code also, if applicable, associated signs and symptoms, such as:

         cerebral edema (G93.6)

         unspecified convulsions (R56.9)

     G92.00   **Immune effector cell-associated neurotoxicity syndrome, grade unspecified** `UPD`

         ICANS, grade unspecified

     G92.01   **Immune effector cell-associated neurotoxicity syndrome, grade 1** `UPD`

         ICANS, grade 1

     G92.02   **Immune effector cell-associated neurotoxicity syndrome, grade 2** `UPD`

         ICANS, grade 2

     G92.03   **Immune effector cell-associated neurotoxicity syndrome, grade 3** `CC` `UPD`

         ICANS, grade 3

     G92.04   **Immune effector cell-associated neurotoxicity syndrome, grade 4** `CC` `UPD`

         ICANS, grade 4

     G92.05   **Immune effector cell-associated neurotoxicity syndrome, grade 5** `CC` `UPD`

         ICANS, grade 5

G92.8 **Other toxic encephalopathy** `MCC`

     Toxic encephalitis

     Toxic metabolic encephalopathy

     Code first poisoning due to drug or toxin, if applicable, (T36-T65 with fifth or sixth character 1-4)

     Use additional code for adverse effect, if applicable, to identify drug (T36-T50 with fifth or sixth character 5)

    AHA: 2024,2Q,14; 2022,1Q,52

G92.9 **Unspecified toxic encephalopathy** `MCC`

     Code first poisoning due to drug or toxin, if applicable, (T36-T65 with fifth or sixth character 1-4)

     Use additional code for adverse effect, if applicable, to identify drug (T36-T50 with fifth or sixth character 5)

✓4th **G93** **Other disorders of brain**

G93.0 **Cerebral cysts**

     Arachnoid cyst

     Porencephalic cyst, acquired

     `EXCLUDES 1`   *acquired periventricular cysts of newborn (P91.1)*

                 congenital cerebral cysts (Q04.6)

G93.1 **Anoxic brain damage, not elsewhere classified** `CC` `HCC`

     `EXCLUDES 1`   *cerebral anoxia due to anesthesia during labor and delivery (O74.3)*

                 cerebral anoxia due to anesthesia during the puerperium (O89.2)

                 neonatal anoxia (P84)

    DEF: Brain injury not resulting from birth trauma that is due to lack of oxygen. Brain cells, when deprived of oxygen, begin to expire after four minutes.

G93.2 **Benign intracranial hypertension**

     Pseudotumor

     `EXCLUDES 1`   *hypertensive encephalopathy (I67.4)*

                 obstructive hydrocephalus (G91.1)

✓5th **G93.3** **Postviral and related fatigue syndromes**

     Use additional code, if applicable, for post COVID-19 condition, unspecified (U09.9)

     `EXCLUDES 1`   *chronic fatigue NOS (R53.82)*

                 neurasthenia (F48.8)

    AHA: 2022,4Q,20

     G93.31   **Postviral fatigue syndrome**

✓ Additional Character Required   ✓x7th Placeholder   `Questionable PDx`   `Manifestation`   `Unspecified`   `UPD` Unacceptable PDx   `H1`-`H14` HAC   `HCC` CMS-HCC Dx   `HIV` HIV Dx

ICD-10-CM 2025   **603**

G93.32 Myalgic encephalomyelitis/chronic fatigue syndrome
Chronic fatigue syndrome
ME/CFS
Myalgic encephalomyelitis

G93.39 Other post infection and related fatigue syndromes

√5th **G93.4 Other and unspecified encephalopathy**

EXCLUDES 2   *alcoholic encephalopathy (G31.2)*
encephalopathy in diseases classified elsewhere (G94)
hypertensive encephalopathy (I67.4)
toxic (metabolic) encephalopathy (G92.8)

G93.40 Encephalopathy, unspecified HIV CC
AHA: 2017,2Q,8

G93.41 Metabolic encephalopathy HIV MCC
Septic encephalopathy
AHA: 2024,2Q,14; 2017,2Q,8; 2016,3Q,42; 2015,3Q,21
TIP: Assign separately when documented with diabetic hypoglycemia (E08.649, E09.649, E10.649, E11.649, E13.649).

▲ **G93.42 Megalencephalic leukoencephalopathy with subcortical cysts** CC HCC
AHA: 2023,4Q,12-13

G93.43 Leukoencephalopathy with calcifications and cysts CC HCC
AHA: 2023,4Q,12-13

G93.44 Adult-onset leukodystrophy with axonal spheroids CC HCC A
Adult-onset leukoencephalopathy with axonal spheroids and pigmented glia
AHA: 2023,4Q,12-13

● **G93.45 Developmental and epileptic encephalopathy** CC
Early infantile epileptic encephalopathy
Code also, if applicable, associated disorders such as:
developmental disorders of scholastic skills (F81.-)
developmental disorder of speech and language (F80.-)
epilepsy, by specific type (G40.-)
intellectual disabilities (F70-F79)
other neurodevelopmental disorder (F88)
pervasive developmental disorders (F84.-)

G93.49 Other encephalopathy HIV CC
Encephalopathy NEC
AHA: 2021,2Q,3; 2018,4Q,16; 2018,2Q,22,24; 2017,2Q,9

G93.5 Compression of brain MCC HCC
Arnold-Chiari type 1 compression of brain
Compression of brain (stem)
Herniation of brain (stem)
EXCLUDES 1   *traumatic compression of brain (S06.A-)*
AHA: 2020,2Q,31

G93.6 Cerebral edema MCC HCC
EXCLUDES 1   *cerebral edema due to birth injury (P11.0)*
traumatic cerebral edema (S06.1-)
AHA: 2022,3Q,9-10

G93.7 Reye's syndrome MCC HCC P
Code first poisoning due to salicylates, if applicable (T39.0-, with sixth character 1-4)
Use additional code for adverse effect due to salicylates, if applicable (T39.0-, with sixth character 5)
DEF: Rare childhood illness often developed after a viral upper respiratory infection. Symptoms include vomiting, elevated serum transaminase, brain swelling, disturbances of consciousness, seizures, and changes in liver and other viscera; it can be fatal.

√5th **G93.8 Other specified disorders of brain**

G93.81 Temporal sclerosis
Hippocampal sclerosis
Mesial temporal sclerosis

G93.82 Brain death MCC

G93.89 Other specified disorders of brain
Postradiation encephalopathy
AHA: 2024,2Q,15; 2020,2Q,24; 2019,3Q,8

G93.9 Disorder of brain, unspecified HIV

G94 Other disorders of brain in diseases classified elsewhere
Code first underlying disease
EXCLUDES 1   *encephalopathy in congenital syphilis (A50.49)*
encephalopathy in influenza (J09.X9, J10.81, J11.81)
encephalopathy in syphilis (A52.19)
hydrocephalus in diseases classified elsewhere (G91.4)
AHA: 2018,2Q,22; 2017,2Q,8-9

√4th **G95 Other and unspecified diseases of spinal cord**
EXCLUDES 2   *myelitis (G04.-)*

G95.0 Syringomyelia and syringobulbia CC HCC

√5th **G95.1 Vascular myelopathies**
EXCLUDES 2   *intraspinal phlebitis and thrombophlebitis, except non-pyogenic (G08)*

G95.11 Acute infarction of spinal cord (embolic) (nonembolic) MCC HCC
Anoxia of spinal cord
Arterial thrombosis of spinal cord

G95.19 Other vascular myelopathies MCC HCC
Edema of spinal cord
Hematomyelia
Nonpyogenic intraspinal phlebitis and thrombophlebitis
Subacute necrotic myelopathy
AHA: 2023,3Q,21

√5th **G95.2 Other and unspecified cord compression**

G95.20 Unspecified cord compression HIV CC HCC
G95.29 Other cord compression HIV CC HCC

√5th **G95.8 Other specified diseases of spinal cord**
EXCLUDES 1   *neurogenic bladder NOS (N31.9)*
neurogenic bladder due to cauda equina syndrome (G83.4)
neuromuscular dysfunction of bladder without spinal cord lesion (N31.-)

G95.81 Conus medullaris syndrome CC HCC
G95.89 Other specified diseases of spinal cord CC HCC
Cord bladder NOS
Drug-induced myelopathy
Radiation-induced myelopathy
EXCLUDES 1   *myelopathy NOS (G95.9)*

G95.9 Disease of spinal cord, unspecified HIV CC HCC
Myelopathy NOS

√4th **G96 Other disorders of central nervous system**

√5th **G96.0 Cerebrospinal fluid leak**
Code also if applicable:
intracranial hypotension (G96.81-)
EXCLUDES 1   *cerebrospinal fluid leak from spinal puncture (G97.0)*
AHA: 2020,4Q,21-22; 2018,2Q,13

G96.00 Cerebrospinal fluid leak, unspecified CC
Code also if applicable:
head injury (S00-S09)

G96.01 Cranial cerebrospinal fluid leak, spontaneous CC
Otorrhea due to spontaneous cerebrospinal fluid CSF leak
Rhinorrhea due to spontaneous cerebrospinal fluid CSF leak
Spontaneous cerebrospinal fluid leak from skull base

G96.02 Spinal cerebrospinal fluid leak, spontaneous CC
Spontaneous cerebrospinal fluid leak from spine

G96.08 Other cranial cerebrospinal fluid leak CC
Postoperative cranial cerebrospinal fluid leak
Traumatic cranial cerebrospinal fluid leak
Code also if applicable:
head injury (S00 - S09)

G96.09 Other spinal cerebrospinal fluid leak CC
Other spinal CSF leak
Postoperative spinal cerebrospinal fluid leak
Traumatic spinal cerebrospinal fluid leak
Code also if applicable:
head injury (S00 - S09)
AHA: 2022,3Q,24

√5ᵗʰ **G96.1**   **Disorders of meninges, not elsewhere classified**

     G96.11   **Dural tear**   `CC`

         Code also intracranial hypotension, if applicable (G96.81-)

         EXCLUDES 1   accidental puncture or laceration of dura during a procedure (G97.41)

         AHA: 2014,4Q,24

     G96.12   **Meningeal adhesions (cerebral) (spinal)**

√6ᵗʰ   **G96.19**   **Other disorders of meninges, not elsewhere classified**

         AHA: 2020,4Q,22

         G96.191   **Perineural cyst**

              Cervical nerve root cyst

              Lumbar nerve root cyst

              Sacral nerve root cyst

              Tarlov cyst

              Thoracic nerve root cyst

         G96.198   **Other disorders of meninges, not elsewhere classified**

√5ᵗʰ   **G96.8**   **Other specified disorders of central nervous system**

         AHA: 2020,4Q,21,23-24

     √6ᵗʰ   **G96.81**   **Intracranial hypotension**

         Code also any associated diagnoses, such as:

            brachial amyotrophy (G54.5)

            cerebrospinal fluid leak from spine (G96.02)

            cranial nerve disorders in diseases classified elsewhere (G53)

            nerve root and compressions in diseases classified elsewhere (G55)

            nonpyogenic thrombosis of intracranial venous system (I67.6)

            nontraumatic intracerebral hemorrhage (I61.-)

            nontraumatic subdural hemorrhage (I62.0-)

            other and unspecified cord compression (G95.2-)

            other secondary parkinsonism (G21.8)

            reversible cerebrovascular vasoconstriction syndrome (I67.841)

            spinal cord herniation (G95.89)

            stroke (I63.-)

            syringomyelia (G95.0)

         DEF: Central nervous system disorder resulting from a loss of cerebrospinal fluid (CSF) volume. More often associated with CSF leak at the level of the spine rather than the skull base, causes can be spontaneous, iatrogenic or traumatic spinal dura defects or holes, or overdrainage of CSF shunt devices. The most common symptom is headache.

         G96.810   **Intracranial hypotension, unspecified**

         G96.811   **Intracranial hypotension, spontaneous**

         G96.819   **Other intracranial hypotension**

     G96.89   **Other specified disorders of central nervous system**

G96.9   **Disorder of central nervous system, unspecified**   `HIV`

√4ᵗʰ   **G97**   **Intraoperative and postprocedural complications and disorders of nervous system, not elsewhere classified**

     EXCLUDES 2   intraoperative and postprocedural cerebrovascular infarction (I97.81-, I97.82-)

     AHA: 2016,4Q,9-10

     G97.0   **Cerebrospinal fluid leak from spinal puncture**   `CC`

         Code also any associated diagnoses or complications, such as: intracranial hypotension following a procedure (G97.83-G97.84)

Spinal Puncture

- Spinal cord
- Epidural space
- Subarachnoid space
- Vertebra
- Spinal needle

Lumbar area

     G97.1   **Other reaction to spinal and lumbar puncture**

         Headache due to lumbar puncture

         Other reaction to spinal dural puncture

         Code also, if applicable, any associated headache with orthostatic component (R51.0)

     G97.2   **Intracranial hypotension following ventricular shunting**   `CC`

         Code also any associated diagnoses or complications

√5ᵗʰ   **G97.3**   **Intraoperative hemorrhage and hematoma of a nervous system organ or structure complicating a procedure**

         EXCLUDES 1   intraoperative hemorrhage and hematoma of a nervous system organ or structure due to accidental puncture and laceration during a procedure (G97.4-)

     G97.31   **Intraoperative hemorrhage and hematoma of a nervous system organ or structure complicating a nervous system procedure**   `CC`

     G97.32   **Intraoperative hemorrhage and hematoma of a nervous system organ or structure complicating other procedure**

√5ᵗʰ   **G97.4**   **Accidental puncture and laceration of a nervous system organ or structure during a procedure**

     G97.41   **Accidental puncture or laceration of dura during a procedure**   `CC`

         Incidental (inadvertent) durotomy

         Code also any associated diagnoses or complications

         AHA: 2024,1Q,20-21; 2014,4Q,24

         TIP: Dural tears are always clinically significant and should be coded when documented by the provider.

     G97.48   **Accidental puncture and laceration of other nervous system organ or structure during a nervous system procedure**   `CC`

     G97.49   **Accidental puncture and laceration of other nervous system organ or structure during other procedure**   `CC`

√5ᵗʰ   **G97.5**   **Postprocedural hemorrhage of a nervous system organ or structure following a procedure**

     G97.51   **Postprocedural hemorrhage of a nervous system organ or structure following a nervous system procedure**   `CC`

     G97.52   **Postprocedural hemorrhage of a nervous system organ or structure following other procedure**   `CC`

√5ᵗʰ   **G97.6**   **Postprocedural hematoma and seroma of a nervous system organ or structure following a procedure**

     G97.61   **Postprocedural hematoma of a nervous system organ or structure following a nervous system procedure**   `CC`

         AHA: 2020,3Q,24

     G97.62   **Postprocedural hematoma of a nervous system organ or structure following other procedure**   `CC`

☑ Additional Character Required   √x7ᵗʰ Placeholder   Questionable PDx   Manifestation   Unspecified   UPD Unacceptable PDx   H1-H14 HAC   HCC CMS-HCC Dx   HIV HIV Dx

ICD-10-CM 2025   **605**

Chapter 6. Diseases of the Nervous System

    G97.63   Postprocedural seroma of a nervous system organ or structure following a nervous system procedure   `CC`

    G97.64   Postprocedural seroma of a nervous system organ or structure following other procedure   `CC`

✓5ᵗʰ **G97.8**   **Other intraoperative and postprocedural complications and disorders of nervous system**
     Use additional code to further specify disorder
     AHA: 2020,4Q,23

    G97.81   Other intraoperative complications of nervous system   `CC`

    G97.82   Other postprocedural complications and disorders of nervous system   `CC`
         AHA: 2022,1Q,34

    G97.83   Intracranial hypotension following lumbar cerebrospinal fluid shunting   `CC`
         Code also any associated diagnoses or complications

    G97.84   Intracranial hypotension following other procedure   `CC`
         Code also, if applicable:
             accidental puncture or laceration of dura during a procedure (G97.41)
             cerebrospinal fluid leak from spinal puncture (G97.0)

✓4ᵗʰ **G98**   **Other disorders of nervous system not elsewhere classified**
     [INCLUDES]   nervous system disorder NOS

    G98.0   **Neurogenic arthritis, not elsewhere classified**
         Nonsyphilitic neurogenic arthropathy NEC
         Nonsyphilitic neurogenic spondylopathy NEC
         [EXCLUDES 1]   spondylopathy (in):
                syringomyelia and syringobulbia (G95.0)
                tabes dorsalis (A52.11)

    G98.8   **Other disorders of nervous system**   `HIV`
         Nervous system disorder NOS

✓4ᵗʰ **G99**   **Other disorders of nervous system in diseases classified elsewhere**

    G99.0   *Autonomic neuropathy in diseases classified elsewhere*   `CC`
         Code first underlying disease, such as:
             amyloidosis (E85.-)
             gout (M1A.-, M10.-)
             hyperthyroidism (E05.-)
         [EXCLUDES 1]   diabetic autonomic neuropathy (E08-E13 with .43)

    G99.2   *Myelopathy in diseases classified elsewhere*   `CC` `HCC`
         Code first underlying disease, such as:
             neoplasm (C00-D49)
         [EXCLUDES 1]   myelopathy in:
                intervertebral disease (M50.0-, M51.0-)
                spondylosis (M47.0-, M47.1-)
         AHA: 2018,3Q,18-19
         TIP: Use this code in addition to a spondylolisthesis code (M43.1-) or a spinal stenosis code (M48.0-) when either of these disorders is documented as the cause of the myelopathy.

    G99.8   *Other specified disorders of nervous system in diseases classified elsewhere*
         Code first underlying disorder, such as:
             amyloidosis (E85.-)
             avitaminosis (E56.-)
         [EXCLUDES 1]   nervous system involvement in:
                cysticercosis (B69.0)
                rubella (B06.0-)
                syphilis (A52.1-)

N Newborn: 0   P Pediatric: 0-17   M Maternity: 9-64   A Adult: 15-124   UNS Unspecified Site   MCC Major Complication/Comorbidity   CC Complication/Comorbidity   PE POA Exempt

606   ICD-10-CM 2025

Chapter 7. Diseases of the Eye and Adnexa (H00–H59)

Chapter-specific Guidelines with Coding Examples

The chapter-specific guidelines from the ICD-10-CM Official Guidelines for Coding and Reporting have been provided below. Along with these guidelines are coding examples, contained in the shaded boxes, that have been developed to help illustrate the coding and/or sequencing guidance found in these guidelines.

a. Glaucoma

1) Assigning glaucoma codes

Assign as many codes from category H40, Glaucoma, as needed to identify the type of glaucoma, the affected eye, and the glaucoma stage.

2) Bilateral glaucoma with same type and stage

When a patient has bilateral glaucoma and both eyes are documented as being the same type and stage, and there is a code for bilateral glaucoma, report only the code for the type of glaucoma, bilateral, with the seventh character for the stage.

> Bilateral severe stage pigmentary glaucoma
>
> **H40.1333   Pigmentary glaucoma, bilateral, severe stage**
>
> *Explanation*: In this scenario, the patient has the same type and stage of glaucoma in both eyes. As this type of glaucoma has a code for bilateral, assign only the code for the bilateral glaucoma with the seventh character for the stage.

When a patient has bilateral glaucoma and both eyes are documented as being the same type and stage, and the classification does not provide a code for bilateral glaucoma (i.e. subcategories H40.10 and H40.20) report only one code for the type of glaucoma with the appropriate seventh character for the stage.

> Bilateral open-angle glaucoma; not specified as to type and stage indeterminate in both eyes
>
> **H40.10X4   Unspecified open-angle glaucoma, indeterminate stage**
>
> *Explanation*: In this scenario, the patient has glaucoma of the same type and stage of both eyes, but there is no code specifically for bilateral glaucoma. Only one code is assigned with the appropriate seventh character for the stage.

3) Bilateral glaucoma stage with different types or stages

When a patient has bilateral glaucoma and each eye is documented as having a different type or stage, and the classification distinguishes laterality, assign the appropriate code for each eye rather than the code for bilateral glaucoma.

When a patient has bilateral glaucoma and each eye is documented as having a different type, and the classification does not distinguish laterality (i.e. subcategories H40.10 and H40.20), assign one code for each type of glaucoma with the appropriate seventh character for the stage.

> Documentation relates mild, unspecified primary angle-closure glaucoma of the left eye with mild unspecified open-angle glaucoma of the right eye
>
> **H40.20X1   Unspecified primary angle-closure glaucoma, mild stage**
>
> **H40.10X1   Unspecified open-angle glaucoma, mild stage**
>
> *Explanation*: In this scenario the patient has a different type of glaucoma in each eye and the classification does not distinguish laterality. A code for each type of glaucoma is assigned, each with the appropriate seventh character for the stage.

When a patient has bilateral glaucoma and each eye is documented as having the same type, but different stage, and the classification does not distinguish laterality (i.e. subcategories H40.10 and H40.20), assign a code for the type of glaucoma for each eye with the seventh character for the specific glaucoma stage documented for each eye.

> Bilateral open-angle glaucoma, not specified as to type; the right eye is documented to be in mild stage and the left eye as being in moderate stage
>
> **H40.10X1   Unspecified open-angle glaucoma, mild stage**
>
> **H40.10X2   Unspecified open-angle glaucoma, moderate stage**
>
> *Explanation*: In this scenario the patient has the same type of glaucoma in each eye but each eye is at a different stage, and the classification does not distinguish laterality at this subcategory level. Two codes are assigned; both codes represent the same type of glaucoma but each has a different seventh character identifying the appropriate stage for each eye.

4) Patient admitted with glaucoma and stage evolves during the admission

If a patient is admitted with glaucoma and the stage progresses during the admission, assign the code for highest stage documented.

> Patient admitted with mild low-tension glaucoma of the right eye, which progresses to moderate stage during the patient's stay
>
> **H40.1212   Low-tension glaucoma, right eye, moderate stage**
>
> *Explanation*: When the glaucoma stage progresses during an admission, assign only the code for the highest stage documented.

5) Indeterminate stage glaucoma

Assignment of the seventh character "4" for "indeterminate stage" should be based on the clinical documentation. The seventh character "4" is used for glaucomas whose stage cannot be clinically determined. This seventh character should not be confused with the seventh character "0", unspecified, which should be assigned when there is no documentation regarding the stage of the glaucoma.

b. Blindness

If "blindness" or "low vision" of both eyes is documented but the visual impairment category is not documented, assign code H54.3, Unqualified visual loss, both eyes. If "blindness" or "low vision" in one eye is documented but the visual impairment category is not documented, assign a code from H54.6-, Unqualified visual loss, one eye. If "blindness" or "visual loss" is documented without any information about whether one or both eyes are affected, assign code H54.7, Unspecified visual loss.

> Blindness in 89-year-old male
>
> **H54.7   Unspecified visual loss**
>
> *Explanation*: Blindness is stated, but there is no mention of whether one or both eyes are affected or the severity of this visual impairment.

Chapter 7. Diseases of the Eye and Adnexa

Chapter 7. Diseases of the Eye and Adnexa (H00–H59)

NOTE   Use an external cause code following the code for the eye condition, if applicable, to identify the cause of the eye condition

EXCLUDES 2   certain conditions originating in the perinatal period (P04-P96)
certain infectious and parasitic diseases (A00-B99)
complications of pregnancy, childbirth and the puerperium (O00-O9A)
congenital malformations, deformations, and chromosomal abnormalities (Q00-Q99)
diabetes mellitus related eye conditions (E09.3-, E10.3-, E11.3-, E13.3-)
endocrine, nutritional and metabolic diseases (E00-E88)
injury (trauma) of eye and orbit (S05.-)
injury, poisoning and certain other consequences of external causes (S00-T88)
neoplasms (C00-D49)
symptoms, signs and abnormal clinical and laboratory findings, not elsewhere classified (R00-R94)
syphilis related eye disorders (A50.01, A50.3-, A51.43, A52.71)

This chapter contains the following blocks:
H00-H05   Disorders of eyelid, lacrimal system and orbit
H10-H11   Disorders of conjunctiva
H15-H22   Disorders of sclera, cornea, iris and ciliary body
H25-H28   Disorders of lens
H30-H36   Disorders of choroid and retina
H40-H42   Glaucoma
H43-H44   Disorders of vitreous body and globe
H46-H47   Disorders of optic nerve and visual pathways
H49-H52   Disorders of ocular muscles, binocular movement, accommodation and refraction
H53-H54   Visual disturbances and blindness
H55-H57   Other disorders of eye and adnexa
H59   Intraoperative and postprocedural complications and disorders of eye and adnexa, not elsewhere classified

Disorders of eyelid, lacrimal system and orbit (H00–H05)

EXCLUDES 2   open wound of eyelid (S01.1-)
superficial injury of eyelid (S00.1-, S00.2-)

✓4ᵗʰ H00 Hordeolum and chalazion

  ✓5ᵗʰ H00.0 Hordeolum (externum) (internum) of eyelid

    DEF: Acute localized infection of the gland of Zeis (external hordeolum) or Molt or of the meibomian glands (internal hordeolum) of the orbit.

    ✓6ᵗʰ H00.01 Hordeolum externum

      Hordeolum NOS
      Stye
      H00.011 Hordeolum externum right upper eyelid
      H00.012 Hordeolum externum right lower eyelid
      H00.013 Hordeolum externum right eye, unspecified eyelid
      H00.014 Hordeolum externum left upper eyelid
      H00.015 Hordeolum externum left lower eyelid
      H00.016 Hordeolum externum left eye, unspecified eyelid
      H00.019 Hordeolum externum unspecified eye, unspecified eyelid

    ✓6ᵗʰ H00.02 Hordeolum internum

      Infection of meibomian gland
      H00.021 Hordeolum internum right upper eyelid
      H00.022 Hordeolum internum right lower eyelid
      H00.023 Hordeolum internum right eye, unspecified eyelid
      H00.024 Hordeolum internum left upper eyelid
      H00.025 Hordeolum internum left lower eyelid
      H00.026 Hordeolum internum left eye, unspecified eyelid
      H00.029 Hordeolum internum unspecified eye, unspecified eyelid

    ✓6ᵗʰ H00.03 Abscess of eyelid

      Furuncle of eyelid
      H00.031 Abscess of right upper eyelid
      H00.032 Abscess of right lower eyelid
      H00.033 Abscess of eyelid right eye, unspecified eyelid
      H00.034 Abscess of left upper eyelid
      H00.035 Abscess of left lower eyelid
      H00.036 Abscess of eyelid left eye, unspecified eyelid
      H00.039 Abscess of eyelid unspecified eye, unspecified eyelid

✓5ᵗʰ H00.1 Chalazion

  Meibomian (gland) cyst
  EXCLUDES 2   infected meibomian gland (H00.02-)
  DEF: Noninfectious, obstructive mass in the oil gland of the eyelid that results in a small chronic lump or inflammation.
  H00.11 Chalazion right upper eyelid
  H00.12 Chalazion right lower eyelid
  H00.13 Chalazion right eye, unspecified eyelid
  H00.14 Chalazion left upper eyelid
  H00.15 Chalazion left lower eyelid
  H00.16 Chalazion left eye, unspecified eyelid
  H00.19 Chalazion unspecified eye, unspecified eyelid

✓4ᵗʰ H01 Other inflammation of eyelid

  ✓5ᵗʰ H01.0 Blepharitis

    EXCLUDES 1   blepharoconjunctivitis (H10.5-)

    ✓6ᵗʰ H01.00 Unspecified blepharitis

      AHA: 2018,4Q,13
      H01.001 Unspecified blepharitis right upper eyelid
      H01.002 Unspecified blepharitis right lower eyelid
      H01.003 Unspecified blepharitis right eye, unspecified eyelid
      H01.004 Unspecified blepharitis left upper eyelid
      H01.005 Unspecified blepharitis left lower eyelid
      H01.006 Unspecified blepharitis left eye, unspecified eyelid
      H01.009 Unspecified blepharitis unspecified eye, unspecified eyelid
      H01.00A Unspecified blepharitis right eye, upper and lower eyelids
      H01.00B Unspecified blepharitis left eye, upper and lower eyelids

    ✓6ᵗʰ H01.01 Ulcerative blepharitis

      AHA: 2018,4Q,13
      H01.011 Ulcerative blepharitis right upper eyelid
      H01.012 Ulcerative blepharitis right lower eyelid
      H01.013 Ulcerative blepharitis right eye, unspecified eyelid
      H01.014 Ulcerative blepharitis left upper eyelid
      H01.015 Ulcerative blepharitis left lower eyelid
      H01.016 Ulcerative blepharitis left eye, unspecified eyelid
      H01.019 Ulcerative blepharitis unspecified eye, unspecified eyelid
      H01.01A Ulcerative blepharitis right eye, upper and lower eyelids
      H01.01B Ulcerative blepharitis left eye, upper and lower eyelids

    ✓6ᵗʰ H01.02 Squamous blepharitis

      AHA: 2018,4Q,13
      H01.021 Squamous blepharitis right upper eyelid
      H01.022 Squamous blepharitis right lower eyelid
      H01.023 Squamous blepharitis right eye, unspecified eyelid
      H01.024 Squamous blepharitis left upper eyelid
      H01.025 Squamous blepharitis left lower eyelid
      H01.026 Squamous blepharitis left eye, unspecified eyelid
      H01.029 Squamous blepharitis unspecified eye, unspecified eyelid
      H01.02A Squamous blepharitis right eye, upper and lower eyelids
      H01.02B Squamous blepharitis left eye, upper and lower eyelids

  ✓5ᵗʰ H01.1 Noninfectious dermatoses of eyelid

    ✓6ᵗʰ H01.11 Allergic dermatitis of eyelid

      Contact dermatitis of eyelid
      H01.111 Allergic dermatitis of right upper eyelid
      H01.112 Allergic dermatitis of right lower eyelid
      H01.113 Allergic dermatitis of right eye, unspecified eyelid
      H01.114 Allergic dermatitis of left upper eyelid
      H01.115 Allergic dermatitis of left lower eyelid
      H01.116 Allergic dermatitis of left eye, unspecified eyelid
      H01.119 Allergic dermatitis of unspecified eye, unspecified eyelid

    ✓6ᵗʰ H01.12 Discoid lupus erythematosus of eyelid

      H01.121 Discoid lupus erythematosus of right upper eyelid

H01.122   Discoid lupus erythematosus of **right lower** eyelid

H01.123   Discoid lupus erythematosus of **right eye,** unspecified eyelid

H01.124   Discoid lupus erythematosus of **left upper** eyelid

H01.125   Discoid lupus erythematosus of **left lower** eyelid

H01.126   Discoid lupus erythematosus of **left eye,** unspecified eyelid

H01.129   Discoid lupus erythematosus of unspecified eye, unspecified eyelid

√6th   **H01.13**   **Eczematous dermatitis of eyelid**

H01.131   Eczematous dermatitis of **right upper** eyelid

H01.132   Eczematous dermatitis of **right lower** eyelid

H01.133   Eczematous dermatitis of **right eye,** unspecified eyelid

H01.134   Eczematous dermatitis of **left upper** eyelid

H01.135   Eczematous dermatitis of **left lower** eyelid

H01.136   Eczematous dermatitis of **left eye,** unspecified eyelid

H01.139   Eczematous dermatitis of unspecified eye, unspecified eyelid

√6th   **H01.14**   **Xeroderma of eyelid**

H01.141   Xeroderma of **right upper** eyelid

H01.142   Xeroderma of **right lower** eyelid

H01.143   Xeroderma of **right eye,** unspecified eyelid

H01.144   Xeroderma of **left upper** eyelid

H01.145   Xeroderma of **left lower** eyelid

H01.146   Xeroderma of **left eye,** unspecified eyelid

H01.149   Xeroderma of unspecified eye, unspecified eyelid

H01.8   **Other specified inflammations of eyelid**

H01.9   **Unspecified inflammation of eyelid**
Inflammation of eyelid NOS

√4th   **H02**   **Other disorders of eyelid**

     EXCLUDES 1   congenital malformations of eyelid (Q10.0-Q10.3)

Entropion and Ectropion

Normal eyelid   Entropion   Ectropion

√5th   **H02.0**   **Entropion and trichiasis of eyelid**

     DEF: Entropion: Inversion of the eyelid, turning the edge in toward the eyeball and causing irritation from contact of the lashes with the surface of the eye.
     DEF: Trichiasis: Condition wherein the eyelid is in a normal position but lashes are ingrown or misdirected in their growth so that they irritate the tissues of the eye.

√6th   **H02.00**   **Unspecified entropion of eyelid**

H02.001   Unspecified entropion of **right upper** eyelid

H02.002   Unspecified entropion of **right lower** eyelid

H02.003   Unspecified entropion of **right eye,** unspecified eyelid

H02.004   Unspecified entropion of **left upper** eyelid

H02.005   Unspecified entropion of **left lower** eyelid

H02.006   Unspecified entropion of **left eye,** unspecified eyelid

H02.009   Unspecified entropion of unspecified eye, unspecified eyelid

√6th   **H02.01**   **Cicatricial entropion of eyelid**

H02.011   Cicatricial entropion of **right upper** eyelid

H02.012   Cicatricial entropion of **right lower** eyelid

H02.013   Cicatricial entropion of **right eye,** unspecified eyelid

H02.014   Cicatricial entropion of **left upper** eyelid

H02.015   Cicatricial entropion of **left lower** eyelid

H02.016   Cicatricial entropion of **left eye,** unspecified eyelid

H02.019   Cicatricial entropion of unspecified eye, unspecified eyelid

√6th   **H02.02**   **Mechanical entropion of eyelid**

H02.021   Mechanical entropion of **right upper** eyelid

H02.022   Mechanical entropion of **right lower** eyelid

H02.023   Mechanical entropion of **right eye,** unspecified eyelid

H02.024   Mechanical entropion of **left upper** eyelid

H02.025   Mechanical entropion of **left lower** eyelid

H02.026   Mechanical entropion of **left eye,** unspecified eyelid

H02.029   Mechanical entropion of unspecified eye, unspecified eyelid

√6th   **H02.03**   **Senile entropion of eyelid**

H02.031   Senile entropion of **right upper** eyelid   Ⓐ

H02.032   Senile entropion of **right lower** eyelid   Ⓐ

H02.033   Senile entropion of **right eye,** unspecified eyelid   Ⓐ

H02.034   Senile entropion of **left upper** eyelid   Ⓐ

H02.035   Senile entropion of **left lower** eyelid   Ⓐ

H02.036   Senile entropion of **left eye,** unspecified eyelid   Ⓐ

H02.039   Senile entropion of unspecified eye, unspecified eyelid   Ⓐ

√6th   **H02.04**   **Spastic entropion of eyelid**

H02.041   Spastic entropion of **right upper** eyelid

H02.042   Spastic entropion of **right lower** eyelid

H02.043   Spastic entropion of **right eye,** unspecified eyelid

H02.044   Spastic entropion of **left upper** eyelid

H02.045   Spastic entropion of **left lower** eyelid

H02.046   Spastic entropion of **left eye,** unspecified eyelid

H02.049   Spastic entropion of unspecified eye, unspecified eyelid

√6th   **H02.05**   **Trichiasis without entropion**

H02.051   Trichiasis without entropion **right upper** eyelid

H02.052   Trichiasis without entropion **right lower** eyelid

H02.053   Trichiasis without entropion **right eye,** unspecified eyelid

H02.054   Trichiasis without entropion **left upper** eyelid

H02.055   Trichiasis without entropion **left lower** eyelid

H02.056   Trichiasis without entropion **left eye,** unspecified eyelid

H02.059   Trichiasis without entropion unspecified eye, unspecified eyelid

√5th   **H02.1**   **Ectropion of eyelid**

     DEF: Drooping of the lower eyelid away from the eye or outward turning or eversion of the edge of the eyelid, exposing the palpebral conjunctiva and causing irritation.

√6th   **H02.10**   **Unspecified ectropion of eyelid**

H02.101   Unspecified ectropion of **right upper** eyelid

H02.102   Unspecified ectropion of **right lower** eyelid

H02.103   Unspecified ectropion of **right eye,** unspecified eyelid

H02.104   Unspecified ectropion of **left upper** eyelid

H02.105   Unspecified ectropion of **left lower** eyelid

H02.106   Unspecified ectropion of **left eye,** unspecified eyelid

H02.109   Unspecified ectropion of unspecified eye, unspecified eyelid

√6th   **H02.11**   **Cicatricial ectropion of eyelid**

H02.111   Cicatricial ectropion of **right upper** eyelid

H02.112   Cicatricial ectropion of **right lower** eyelid

H02.113   Cicatricial ectropion of **right eye,** unspecified eyelid

H02.114   Cicatricial ectropion of **left upper** eyelid

H02.115   Cicatricial ectropion of **left lower** eyelid

H02.116   Cicatricial ectropion of **left eye,** unspecified eyelid

H02.119   Cicatricial ectropion of unspecified eye, unspecified eyelid

Chapter 7. Diseases of the Eye and Adnexa

H02.12–H02.432

✓6ᵗʰ **H02.12 Mechanical** ectropion of eyelid

H02.121 Mechanical ectropion of **right upper** eyelid

H02.122 Mechanical ectropion of **right lower** eyelid

H02.123 Mechanical ectropion of **right eye,** unspecified eyelid

H02.124 Mechanical ectropion of **left upper** eyelid

H02.125 Mechanical ectropion of **left lower** eyelid

H02.126 Mechanical ectropion of **left eye,** unspecified eyelid

H02.129 Mechanical ectropion of unspecified eye, unspecified eyelid

✓6ᵗʰ **H02.13 Senile** ectropion of eyelid

H02.131 Senile ectropion of **right upper** eyelid 🅐

H02.132 Senile ectropion of **right lower** eyelid 🅐

H02.133 Senile ectropion of **right eye,** unspecified eyelid 🅐

H02.134 Senile ectropion of **left upper** eyelid 🅐

H02.135 Senile ectropion of **left lower** eyelid 🅐

H02.136 Senile ectropion of **left eye,** unspecified eyelid 🅐

H02.139 Senile ectropion of unspecified eye, unspecified eyelid 🅐

✓6ᵗʰ **H02.14 Spastic** ectropion of eyelid

H02.141 Spastic ectropion of **right upper** eyelid

H02.142 Spastic ectropion of **right lower** eyelid

H02.143 Spastic ectropion of **right eye,** unspecified eyelid

H02.144 Spastic ectropion of **left upper** eyelid

H02.145 Spastic ectropion of **left lower** eyelid

H02.146 Spastic ectropion of **left eye,** unspecified eyelid

H02.149 Spastic ectropion of unspecified eye, unspecified eyelid

✓6ᵗʰ **H02.15 Paralytic** ectropion of eyelid

AHA: 2018,4Q,13

H02.151 Paralytic ectropion of **right upper** eyelid

H02.152 Paralytic ectropion of **right lower** eyelid

H02.153 Paralytic ectropion of **right eye,** unspecified eyelid

H02.154 Paralytic ectropion of **left upper** eyelid

H02.155 Paralytic ectropion of **left lower** eyelid

H02.156 Paralytic ectropion of **left eye,** unspecified eyelid

H02.159 Paralytic ectropion of unspecified eye, unspecified eyelid

✓5ᵗʰ **H02.2 Lagophthalmos**

AHA: 2018,4Q,14

DEF: Condition of the eye that prevents it from closing completely.

✓6ᵗʰ **H02.20 Unspecified lagophthalmos**

H02.201 Unspecified lagophthalmos **right upper** eyelid

H02.202 Unspecified lagophthalmos **right lower** eyelid

H02.203 Unspecified lagophthalmos **right eye,** unspecified eyelid

H02.204 Unspecified lagophthalmos **left upper** eyelid

H02.205 Unspecified lagophthalmos **left lower** eyelid

H02.206 Unspecified lagophthalmos **left eye,** unspecified eyelid

H02.209 Unspecified lagophthalmos unspecified eye, unspecified eyelid

H02.20A Unspecified lagophthalmos **right eye, upper and lower** eyelids

H02.20B Unspecified lagophthalmos **left eye, upper and lower** eyelids

H02.20C Unspecified lagophthalmos, **bilateral, upper and lower** eyelids

✓6ᵗʰ **H02.21 Cicatricial** lagophthalmos

H02.211 Cicatricial lagophthalmos **right upper** eyelid

H02.212 Cicatricial lagophthalmos **right lower** eyelid

H02.213 Cicatricial lagophthalmos **right eye,** unspecified eyelid

H02.214 Cicatricial lagophthalmos **left upper** eyelid

H02.215 Cicatricial lagophthalmos **left lower** eyelid

H02.216 Cicatricial lagophthalmos **left eye,** unspecified eyelid

H02.219 Cicatricial lagophthalmos unspecified eye, unspecified eyelid

H02.21A Cicatricial lagophthalmos **right eye, upper and lower** eyelids

H02.21B Cicatricial lagophthalmos **left eye, upper and lower** eyelids

H02.21C Cicatricial lagophthalmos, **bilateral, upper and lower** eyelids

✓6ᵗʰ **H02.22 Mechanical** lagophthalmos

H02.221 Mechanical lagophthalmos **right upper** eyelid

H02.222 Mechanical lagophthalmos **right lower** eyelid

H02.223 Mechanical lagophthalmos **right eye,** unspecified eyelid

H02.224 Mechanical lagophthalmos **left upper** eyelid

H02.225 Mechanical lagophthalmos **left lower** eyelid

H02.226 Mechanical lagophthalmos **left eye,** unspecified eyelid

H02.229 Mechanical lagophthalmos unspecified eye, unspecified eyelid

H02.22A Mechanical lagophthalmos **right eye, upper and lower** eyelids

H02.22B Mechanical lagophthalmos **left eye, upper and lower** eyelids

H02.22C Mechanical lagophthalmos, **bilateral, upper and lower** eyelids

✓6ᵗʰ **H02.23 Paralytic** lagophthalmos

H02.231 Paralytic lagophthalmos **right upper** eyelid

H02.232 Paralytic lagophthalmos **right lower** eyelid

H02.233 Paralytic lagophthalmos **right eye,** unspecified eyelid

H02.234 Paralytic lagophthalmos **left upper** eyelid

H02.235 Paralytic lagophthalmos **left lower** eyelid

H02.236 Paralytic lagophthalmos **left eye,** unspecified eyelid

H02.239 Paralytic lagophthalmos unspecified eye, unspecified eyelid

H02.23A Paralytic lagophthalmos **right eye, upper and lower** eyelids

H02.23B Paralytic lagophthalmos **left eye, upper and lower** eyelids

H02.23C Paralytic lagophthalmos, **bilateral, upper and lower** eyelids

✓5ᵗʰ **H02.3 Blepharochalasis**

Pseudoptosis

DEF: Loss of elasticity and relaxation of skin of the eyelid, thickened or indurated skin on the eyelid associated with recurrent episodes of edema, and intracellular atrophy.

H02.30 Blepharochalasis unspecified eye, unspecified eyelid

H02.31 Blepharochalasis **right upper** eyelid

H02.32 Blepharochalasis **right lower** eyelid

H02.33 Blepharochalasis **right eye,** unspecified eyelid

H02.34 Blepharochalasis **left upper** eyelid

H02.35 Blepharochalasis **left lower** eyelid

H02.36 Blepharochalasis **left eye,** unspecified eyelid

✓5ᵗʰ **H02.4 Ptosis of eyelid**

✓6ᵗʰ **H02.40 Unspecified ptosis of eyelid**

H02.401 Unspecified ptosis of **right** eyelid

H02.402 Unspecified ptosis of **left** eyelid

H02.403 Unspecified ptosis of **bilateral** eyelids

H02.409 Unspecified ptosis of unspecified eyelid

✓6ᵗʰ **H02.41 Mechanical** ptosis of eyelid

H02.411 Mechanical ptosis of **right** eyelid

H02.412 Mechanical ptosis of **left** eyelid

H02.413 Mechanical ptosis of **bilateral** eyelids

H02.419 Mechanical ptosis of unspecified eyelid

✓6ᵗʰ **H02.42 Myogenic** ptosis of eyelid

H02.421 Myogenic ptosis of **right** eyelid

H02.422 Myogenic ptosis of **left** eyelid

H02.423 Myogenic ptosis of **bilateral** eyelids

H02.429 Myogenic ptosis of unspecified eyelid

✓6ᵗʰ **H02.43 Paralytic** ptosis of eyelid

Neurogenic ptosis of eyelid

H02.431 Paralytic ptosis of **right** eyelid

H02.432 Paralytic ptosis of **left** eyelid

H02.433   **Paralytic ptosis of bilateral eyelids**

H02.439   **Paralytic ptosis unspecified eyelid**

✓5th   **H02.5**   **Other disorders affecting eyelid function**

EXCLUDES 2   *blepharospasm (G24.5)*

organic tic (G25.69)

psychogenic tic (F95.-)

✓6th   **H02.51**   **Abnormal innervation syndrome**

H02.511   **Abnormal innervation syndrome right upper eyelid**

H02.512   **Abnormal innervation syndrome right lower eyelid**

H02.513   **Abnormal innervation syndrome right eye, unspecified eyelid**

H02.514   **Abnormal innervation syndrome left upper eyelid**

H02.515   **Abnormal innervation syndrome left lower eyelid**

H02.516   **Abnormal innervation syndrome left eye, unspecified eyelid**

H02.519   **Abnormal innervation syndrome unspecified eye, unspecified eyelid**

✓6th   **H02.52**   **Blepharophimosis**

Ankyloblepharon

H02.521   **Blepharophimosis right upper eyelid**

H02.522   **Blepharophimosis right lower eyelid**

H02.523   **Blepharophimosis right eye, unspecified eyelid**

H02.524   **Blepharophimosis left upper eyelid**

H02.525   **Blepharophimosis left lower eyelid**

H02.526   **Blepharophimosis left eye, unspecified eyelid**

H02.529   **Blepharophimosis unspecified eye, unspecified lid**

✓6th   **H02.53**   **Eyelid retraction**

Eyelid lag

H02.531   **Eyelid retraction right upper eyelid**

H02.532   **Eyelid retraction right lower eyelid**

H02.533   **Eyelid retraction right eye, unspecified eyelid**

H02.534   **Eyelid retraction left upper eyelid**

H02.535   **Eyelid retraction left lower eyelid**

H02.536   **Eyelid retraction left eye, unspecified eyelid**

H02.539   **Eyelid retraction unspecified eye, unspecified lid**

H02.59   **Other disorders affecting eyelid function**

Deficient blink reflex

Sensory disorders

✓5th   **H02.6**   **Xanthelasma of eyelid**

DEF: Condition in which there are small yellow tumors that occur on the eyelid, usually appearing near the nose.

H02.60   **Xanthelasma of unspecified eye, unspecified eyelid**

H02.61   **Xanthelasma of right upper eyelid**

H02.62   **Xanthelasma of right lower eyelid**

H02.63   **Xanthelasma of right eye, unspecified eyelid**

H02.64   **Xanthelasma of left upper eyelid**

H02.65   **Xanthelasma of left lower eyelid**

H02.66   **Xanthelasma of left eye, unspecified eyelid**

✓5th   **H02.7**   **Other and unspecified degenerative disorders of eyelid and periocular area**

H02.70   **Unspecified degenerative disorders of eyelid and periocular area**

✓6th   **H02.71**   **Chloasma of eyelid and periocular area**

Dyspigmentation of eyelid

Hyperpigmentation of eyelid

H02.711   **Chloasma of right upper eyelid and periocular area**

H02.712   **Chloasma of right lower eyelid and periocular area**

H02.713   **Chloasma of right eye, unspecified eyelid and periocular area**

H02.714   **Chloasma of left upper eyelid and periocular area**

H02.715   **Chloasma of left lower eyelid and periocular area**

H02.716   **Chloasma of left eye, unspecified eyelid and periocular area**

H02.719   **Chloasma of unspecified eye, unspecified eyelid and periocular area**

✓6th   **H02.72**   **Madarosis of eyelid and periocular area**

Hypotrichosis of eyelid

H02.721   **Madarosis of right upper eyelid and periocular area**

H02.722   **Madarosis of right lower eyelid and periocular area**

H02.723   **Madarosis of right eye, unspecified eyelid and periocular area**

H02.724   **Madarosis of left upper eyelid and periocular area**

H02.725   **Madarosis of left lower eyelid and periocular area**

H02.726   **Madarosis of left eye, unspecified eyelid and periocular area**

H02.729   **Madarosis of unspecified eye, unspecified eyelid and periocular area**

✓6th   **H02.73**   **Vitiligo of eyelid and periocular area**

Hypopigmentation of eyelid

H02.731   **Vitiligo of right upper eyelid and periocular area**

H02.732   **Vitiligo of right lower eyelid and periocular area**

H02.733   **Vitiligo of right eye, unspecified eyelid and periocular area**

H02.734   **Vitiligo of left upper eyelid and periocular area**

H02.735   **Vitiligo of left lower eyelid and periocular area**

H02.736   **Vitiligo of left eye, unspecified eyelid and periocular area**

H02.739   **Vitiligo of unspecified eye, unspecified eyelid and periocular area**

H02.79   **Other degenerative disorders of eyelid and periocular area**

✓5th   **H02.8**   **Other specified disorders of eyelid**

✓6th   **H02.81**   **Retained foreign body in eyelid**

Use additional code to identify the type of retained foreign body (Z18.-)

EXCLUDES 1   *laceration of eyelid with foreign body (S01.12-)*

retained intraocular foreign body (H44.6-, H44.7-)

superficial foreign body of eyelid and periocular area (S00.25-)

H02.811   **Retained foreign body in right upper eyelid**

H02.812   **Retained foreign body in right lower eyelid**

H02.813   **Retained foreign body in right eye, unspecified eyelid**

H02.814   **Retained foreign body in left upper eyelid**

H02.815   **Retained foreign body in left lower eyelid**

H02.816   **Retained foreign body in left eye, unspecified eyelid**

H02.819   **Retained foreign body in unspecified eye, unspecified eyelid**

✓6th   **H02.82**   **Cysts of eyelid**

Sebaceous cyst of eyelid

H02.821   **Cysts of right upper eyelid**

H02.822   **Cysts of right lower eyelid**

H02.823   **Cysts of right eye, unspecified eyelid**

H02.824   **Cysts of left upper eyelid**

H02.825   **Cysts of left lower eyelid**

H02.826   **Cysts of left eye, unspecified eyelid**

H02.829   **Cysts of unspecified eye, unspecified eyelid**

✓6th   **H02.83**   **Dermatochalasis of eyelid**

DEF: Acquired form of connective tissue disorder associated with decreased elastic tissue and abnormal elastin formation, resulting in loss of elasticity of the skin of the eyelid. It is generally associated with aging.

H02.831   **Dermatochalasis of right upper eyelid**

H02.832   **Dermatochalasis of right lower eyelid**

H02.833   **Dermatochalasis of right eye, unspecified eyelid**

H02.834   **Dermatochalasis of left upper eyelid**

H02.835   **Dermatochalasis of left lower eyelid**

H02.836   **Dermatochalasis of left eye, unspecified eyelid**

H02.839   **Dermatochalasis of unspecified eye, unspecified eyelid**

✔ Additional Character Required   ✓x7th Placeholder   Questionable PDx   Manifestation   Unspecified   UPD Unacceptable PDx   H1-H14 HAC   HCC CMS-HCC Dx   HIV HIV Dx

ICD-10-CM 2025   611

Chapter 7. Diseases of the Eye and Adnexa

H02.84–H04.203

√6th **H02.84** **Edema** of eyelid
　　　Hyperemia of eyelid
　　H02.841 Edema of **right upper** eyelid
　　H02.842 Edema of **right lower** eyelid
　　H02.843 Edema of **right eye,** unspecified eyelid
　　H02.844 Edema of **left upper** eyelid
　　H02.845 Edema of **left lower** eyelid
　　H02.846 Edema of **left eye,** unspecified eyelid
　　H02.849 Edema of unspecified eye, unspecified eyelid

√6th **H02.85** **Elephantiasis** of eyelid
　　H02.851 Elephantiasis of **right upper** eyelid
　　H02.852 Elephantiasis of **right lower** eyelid
　　H02.853 Elephantiasis of **right eye,** unspecified eyelid
　　H02.854 Elephantiasis of **left upper** eyelid
　　H02.855 Elephantiasis of **left lower** eyelid
　　H02.856 Elephantiasis of **left eye,** unspecified eyelid
　　H02.859 Elephantiasis of unspecified eye, unspecified eyelid

√6th **H02.86** **Hypertrichosis** of eyelid
　　H02.861 Hypertrichosis of **right upper** eyelid
　　H02.862 Hypertrichosis of **right lower** eyelid
　　H02.863 Hypertrichosis of **right eye,** unspecified eyelid
　　H02.864 Hypertrichosis of **left upper** eyelid
　　H02.865 Hypertrichosis of **left lower** eyelid
　　H02.866 Hypertrichosis of **left eye,** unspecified eyelid
　　H02.869 Hypertrichosis of unspecified eye, unspecified eyelid

√6th **H02.87** **Vascular anomalies** of eyelid
　　H02.871 Vascular anomalies of **right upper** eyelid
　　H02.872 Vascular anomalies of **right lower** eyelid
　　H02.873 Vascular anomalies of **right eye,** unspecified eyelid
　　H02.874 Vascular anomalies of **left upper** eyelid
　　H02.875 Vascular anomalies of **left lower** eyelid
　　H02.876 Vascular anomalies of **left eye,** unspecified eyelid
　　H02.879 Vascular anomalies of unspecified eye, unspecified eyelid

√6th **H02.88** **Meibomian gland dysfunction** of eyelid
　　AHA: 2018,4Q,14-15
　　H02.881 Meibomian gland dysfunction **right upper** eyelid
　　H02.882 Meibomian gland dysfunction **right lower** eyelid
　　H02.883 Meibomian gland dysfunction of **right eye,** unspecified eyelid
　　H02.884 Meibomian gland dysfunction **left upper** eyelid
　　H02.885 Meibomian gland dysfunction **left lower** eyelid
　　H02.886 Meibomian gland dysfunction of **left eye,** unspecified eyelid
　　H02.889 Meibomian gland dysfunction of unspecified eye, unspecified eyelid
　　H02.88A Meibomian gland dysfunction **right eye, upper and lower** eyelids
　　H02.88B Meibomian gland dysfunction **left eye, upper and lower** eyelids
　　H02.89 **Other specified disorders** of eyelid
　　　Hemorrhage of eyelid

H02.9 **Unspecified disorder of eyelid**
　　Disorder of eyelid NOS

√4th **H04** **Disorders of lacrimal system**
　　EXCLUDES 1 congenital malformations of lacrimal system (Q10.4-Q10.6)

√5th **H04.0** **Dacryoadenitis**
　　DEF: Inflammation of the lacrimal gland.

√6th **H04.00** **Unspecified dacryoadenitis**
　　H04.001 Unspecified dacryoadenitis, **right** lacrimal gland
　　H04.002 Unspecified dacryoadenitis, **left** lacrimal gland
　　H04.003 Unspecified dacryoadenitis, **bilateral** lacrimal glands
　　H04.009 Unspecified dacryoadenitis, unspecified lacrimal gland

√6th **H04.01** **Acute** dacryoadenitis
　　H04.011 Acute dacryoadenitis, **right** lacrimal gland
　　H04.012 Acute dacryoadenitis, **left** lacrimal gland
　　H04.013 Acute dacryoadenitis, **bilateral** lacrimal glands
　　H04.019 Acute dacryoadenitis, unspecified lacrimal gland

√6th **H04.02** **Chronic** dacryoadenitis
　　H04.021 Chronic dacryoadenitis, **right** lacrimal
　　H04.022 Chronic dacryoadenitis, **left** lacrimal gland
　　H04.023 Chronic dacryoadenitis, **bilateral** lacrimal gland
　　H04.029 Chronic dacryoadenitis, unspecified lacrimal gland

√6th **H04.03** **Chronic enlargement** of lacrimal gland
　　H04.031 Chronic enlargement of **right** lacrimal gland
　　H04.032 Chronic enlargement of **left** lacrimal gland
　　H04.033 Chronic enlargement of **bilateral** lacrimal glands
　　H04.039 Chronic enlargement of unspecified lacrimal gland

√5th **H04.1** **Other disorders of lacrimal gland**

√6th **H04.11** **Dacryops**
　　H04.111 Dacryops of **right** lacrimal gland
　　H04.112 Dacryops of **left** lacrimal gland
　　H04.113 Dacryops of **bilateral** lacrimal glands
　　H04.119 Dacryops of unspecified lacrimal gland

√6th **H04.12** **Dry eye syndrome**
　　　Tear film insufficiency, NOS
　　H04.121 Dry eye syndrome of **right** lacrimal gland
　　H04.122 Dry eye syndrome of **left** lacrimal gland
　　H04.123 Dry eye syndrome of **bilateral** lacrimal glands
　　H04.129 Dry eye syndrome of unspecified lacrimal gland

√6th **H04.13** **Lacrimal cyst**
　　　Lacrimal cystic degeneration
　　H04.131 Lacrimal cyst, **right** lacrimal gland
　　H04.132 Lacrimal cyst, **left** lacrimal gland
　　H04.133 Lacrimal cyst, **bilateral** lacrimal glands
　　H04.139 Lacrimal cyst, unspecified lacrimal gland

√6th **H04.14** **Primary** lacrimal gland atrophy
　　H04.141 Primary lacrimal gland atrophy, **right** lacrimal gland
　　H04.142 Primary lacrimal gland atrophy, **left** lacrimal gland
　　H04.143 Primary lacrimal gland atrophy, **bilateral** lacrimal glands
　　H04.149 Primary lacrimal gland atrophy, unspecified lacrimal gland

√6th **H04.15** **Secondary** lacrimal gland atrophy
　　H04.151 Secondary lacrimal gland atrophy, **right** lacrimal gland
　　H04.152 Secondary lacrimal gland atrophy, **left** lacrimal gland
　　H04.153 Secondary lacrimal gland atrophy, **bilateral** lacrimal glands
　　H04.159 Secondary lacrimal gland atrophy, unspecified lacrimal gland

√6th **H04.16** **Lacrimal gland dislocation**
　　H04.161 Lacrimal gland dislocation, **right** lacrimal gland
　　H04.162 Lacrimal gland dislocation, **left** lacrimal gland
　　H04.163 Lacrimal gland dislocation, **bilateral** lacrimal glands
　　H04.169 Lacrimal gland dislocation, unspecified lacrimal gland

　　H04.19 **Other specified disorders** of lacrimal gland

√5th **H04.2** **Epiphora**
　　DEF: Excessive tearing or overflow of tears down the cheeks often due to a stricture in the lacrimal passages but can be caused by other conditions.

√6th **H04.20** **Unspecified epiphora**
　　H04.201 Unspecified epiphora, **right** side
　　H04.202 Unspecified epiphora, **left** side
　　H04.203 Unspecified epiphora, **bilateral**

N Newborn: 0   **P** Pediatric: 0-17   **M** Maternity: 9-64   **A** Adult: 15-124   **UNS** Unspecified Site   **MCC** Major Complication/Comorbidity   **CC** Complication/Comorbidity   **PE** POA Exempt

612

ICD-10-CM 2025

H04.209   Unspecified epiphora, unspecified side

✓6ᵗʰ   **H04.21**   Epiphora **due to excess lacrimation**

    H04.211   Epiphora due to excess lacrimation, **right** lacrimal gland

    H04.212   Epiphora due to excess lacrimation, **left** lacrimal gland

    H04.213   Epiphora due to excess lacrimation, **bilateral** lacrimal glands

    H04.219   Epiphora due to excess lacrimation, unspecified lacrimal gland

✓6ᵗʰ   **H04.22**   Epiphora **due to insufficient drainage**

    H04.221   Epiphora due to insufficient drainage, **right** side

    H04.222   Epiphora due to insufficient drainage, **left** side

    H04.223   Epiphora due to insufficient drainage, **bilateral**

    H04.229   Epiphora due to insufficient drainage, unspecified side

✓5ᵗʰ   **H04.3**   **Acute and unspecified inflammation of lacrimal passages**

    EXCLUDES 1   *neonatal dacryocystitis (P39.1)*

   ✓6ᵗʰ   **H04.30**   **Unspecified dacryocystitis**

      H04.301   Unspecified dacryocystitis of **right** lacrimal passage

      H04.302   Unspecified dacryocystitis of **left** lacrimal passage

      H04.303   Unspecified dacryocystitis of **bilateral** lacrimal passages

      H04.309   Unspecified dacryocystitis of unspecified lacrimal passage

   ✓6ᵗʰ   **H04.31**   **Phlegmonous** dacryocystitis

      H04.311   Phlegmonous dacryocystitis of **right** lacrimal passage

      H04.312   Phlegmonous dacryocystitis of **left** lacrimal passage

      H04.313   Phlegmonous dacryocystitis of **bilateral** lacrimal passages

      H04.319   Phlegmonous dacryocystitis of unspecified lacrimal passage

   ✓6ᵗʰ   **H04.32**   **Acute** dacryocystitis

      Acute dacryopericystitis

      H04.321   Acute dacryocystitis of **right** lacrimal passage

      H04.322   Acute dacryocystitis of **left** lacrimal passage

      H04.323   Acute dacryocystitis of **bilateral** lacrimal passages

      H04.329   Acute dacryocystitis of unspecified lacrimal passage

   ✓6ᵗʰ   **H04.33**   **Acute** lacrimal **canaliculitis**

      H04.331   Acute lacrimal canaliculitis of **right** lacrimal passage

      H04.332   Acute lacrimal canaliculitis of **left** lacrimal passage

      H04.333   Acute lacrimal canaliculitis of **bilateral** lacrimal passages

      H04.339   Acute lacrimal canaliculitis of unspecified lacrimal passage

✓5ᵗʰ   **H04.4**   **Chronic inflammation of lacrimal passages**

   ✓6ᵗʰ   **H04.41**   **Chronic dacryocystitis**

      H04.411   Chronic dacryocystitis of **right** lacrimal passage

      H04.412   Chronic dacryocystitis of **left** lacrimal passage

      H04.413   Chronic dacryocystitis of **bilateral** lacrimal passages

      H04.419   Chronic dacryocystitis of unspecified lacrimal passage

   ✓6ᵗʰ   **H04.42**   **Chronic** lacrimal **canaliculitis**

      H04.421   Chronic lacrimal canaliculitis of **right** lacrimal passage

      H04.422   Chronic lacrimal canaliculitis of **left** lacrimal passage

      H04.423   Chronic lacrimal canaliculitis of **bilateral** lacrimal passages

      H04.429   Chronic lacrimal canaliculitis of unspecified lacrimal passage

   ✓6ᵗʰ   **H04.43**   **Chronic** lacrimal **mucocele**

      H04.431   Chronic lacrimal mucocele of **right** lacrimal passage

H04.432   Chronic lacrimal mucocele of **left** lacrimal passage

H04.433   Chronic lacrimal mucocele of **bilateral** lacrimal passages

H04.439   Chronic lacrimal mucocele of unspecified lacrimal passage

✓5ᵗʰ   **H04.5**   **Stenosis and insufficiency of lacrimal passages**

   ✓6ᵗʰ   **H04.51**   **Dacryolith**

      H04.511   Dacryolith of **right** lacrimal passage

      H04.512   Dacryolith of **left** lacrimal passage

      H04.513   Dacryolith of **bilateral** lacrimal passages

      H04.519   Dacryolith of unspecified lacrimal passage

   ✓6ᵗʰ   **H04.52**   **Eversion** of lacrimal **punctum**

      H04.521   Eversion of **right** lacrimal punctum

      H04.522   Eversion of **left** lacrimal punctum

      H04.523   Eversion of **bilateral** lacrimal punctum

      H04.529   Eversion of unspecified lacrimal punctum

   ✓6ᵗʰ   **H04.53**   **Neonatal obstruction** of nasolacrimal duct

      EXCLUDES 1   *congenital stenosis and stricture of lacrimal duct (Q10.5)*

      H04.531   Neonatal obstruction of **right** nasolacrimal duct   N

      H04.532   Neonatal obstruction of **left** nasolacrimal duct   N

      H04.533   Neonatal obstruction of **bilateral** nasolacrimal duct   N

      H04.539   Neonatal obstruction of unspecified nasolacrimal duct   N

   ✓6ᵗʰ   **H04.54**   **Stenosis of lacrimal canaliculi**

      H04.541   Stenosis of **right** lacrimal canaliculi

      H04.542   Stenosis of **left** lacrimal canaliculi

      H04.543   Stenosis of **bilateral** lacrimal canaliculi

      H04.549   Stenosis of unspecified lacrimal canaliculi

   ✓6ᵗʰ   **H04.55**   **Acquired stenosis of nasolacrimal duct**

      H04.551   Acquired stenosis of **right** nasolacrimal duct

      H04.552   Acquired stenosis of **left** nasolacrimal duct

      H04.553   Acquired stenosis of **bilateral** nasolacrimal duct

      H04.559   Acquired stenosis of unspecified nasolacrimal duct

   ✓6ᵗʰ   **H04.56**   **Stenosis of lacrimal punctum**

      H04.561   Stenosis of **right** lacrimal punctum

      H04.562   Stenosis of **left** lacrimal punctum

      H04.563   Stenosis of **bilateral** lacrimal punctum

      H04.569   Stenosis of unspecified lacrimal punctum

   ✓6ᵗʰ   **H04.57**   **Stenosis of lacrimal sac**

      H04.571   Stenosis of **right** lacrimal sac

      H04.572   Stenosis of **left** lacrimal sac

      H04.573   Stenosis of **bilateral** lacrimal sac

      H04.579   Stenosis of unspecified lacrimal sac

✓5ᵗʰ   **H04.6**   **Other changes of lacrimal passages**

   ✓6ᵗʰ   **H04.61**   **Lacrimal fistula**

      H04.611   Lacrimal fistula **right** lacrimal passage

      H04.612   Lacrimal fistula **left** lacrimal passage

      H04.613   Lacrimal fistula **bilateral** lacrimal passages

      H04.619   Lacrimal fistula unspecified lacrimal passage

      H04.69   Other changes of lacrimal passages

✓5ᵗʰ   **H04.8**   **Other disorders of lacrimal system**

   ✓6ᵗʰ   **H04.81**   **Granuloma of lacrimal passages**

      H04.811   Granuloma of **right** lacrimal passage

      H04.812   Granuloma of **left** lacrimal passage

      H04.813   Granuloma of **bilateral** lacrimal passages

      H04.819   Granuloma of unspecified lacrimal passage

      H04.89   Other disorders of lacrimal system

   H04.9   Disorder of lacrimal system, unspecified

✓4ᵗʰ   **H05**   **Disorders of orbit**

      EXCLUDES 1   *congenital malformation of orbit (Q10.7)*

   ✓5ᵗʰ   **H05.0**   **Acute inflammation** of orbit

      H05.00   Unspecified acute inflammation of orbit

    ✓6ᵗʰ   **H05.01**   **Cellulitis** of orbit

       Abscess of orbit

       H05.011   Cellulitis of **right** orbit   CC

       H05.012   Cellulitis of **left** orbit   CC

       H05.013   Cellulitis of **bilateral** orbits   CC

✔ Additional Character Required   ✓x7ᵗʰ Placeholder   Questionable PDx   Manifestation   Unspecified   UPD Unacceptable PDx   H1-H14 HAC   HCC CMS-HCC Dx   HIV HIV Dx

ICD-10-CM 2025   613

H05.019   **Cellulitis** of unspecified orbit   `CC` `UNS`

√6ᵗʰ   H05.02   **Osteomyelitis** of orbit

    H05.021   Osteomyelitis of **right** orbit   `CC`
    H05.022   Osteomyelitis of **left** orbit   `CC`
    H05.023   Osteomyelitis of **bilateral** orbits   `CC`
    H05.029   Osteomyelitis of unspecified orbit   `CC` `UNS`

√6ᵗʰ   H05.03   **Periostitis** of orbit

    H05.031   Periostitis of **right** orbit   `CC`
    H05.032   Periostitis of **left** orbit   `CC`
    H05.033   Periostitis of **bilateral** orbits   `CC`
    H05.039   Periostitis of unspecified orbit   `CC` `UNS`

√6ᵗʰ   H05.04   **Tenonitis** of orbit

    H05.041   Tenonitis of **right** orbit
    H05.042   Tenonitis of **left** orbit
    H05.043   Tenonitis of **bilateral** orbits
    H05.049   Tenonitis of unspecified orbit

√5ᵗʰ   H05.1   **Chronic inflammatory** disorders of orbit

    H05.10   Unspecified chronic inflammatory disorders of orbit

√6ᵗʰ   H05.11   **Granuloma** of orbit
      Pseudotumor (inflammatory) of orbit
    H05.111   Granuloma of **right** orbit
    H05.112   Granuloma of **left** orbit
    H05.113   Granuloma of **bilateral** orbits
    H05.119   Granuloma of unspecified orbit

√6ᵗʰ   H05.12   Orbital **myositis**
    H05.121   Orbital myositis, **right** orbit
    H05.122   Orbital myositis, **left** orbit
    H05.123   Orbital myositis, **bilateral**
    H05.129   Orbital myositis, unspecified orbit

√5ᵗʰ   H05.2   **Exophthalmic conditions**

    H05.20   Unspecified exophthalmos

√6ᵗʰ   H05.21   Displacement (lateral) of globe
    H05.211   Displacement (lateral) of globe, **right** eye
    H05.212   Displacement (lateral) of globe, **left** eye
    H05.213   Displacement (lateral) of globe, **bilateral**
    H05.219   Displacement (lateral) of globe, unspecified eye

√6ᵗʰ   H05.22   **Edema** of orbit
      Orbital congestion
    H05.221   Edema of **right** orbit
    H05.222   Edema of **left** orbit
    H05.223   Edema of **bilateral** orbit
    H05.229   Edema of unspecified orbit

√6ᵗʰ   H05.23   **Hemorrhage** of orbit
    H05.231   Hemorrhage of **right** orbit
    H05.232   Hemorrhage of **left** orbit
    H05.233   Hemorrhage of **bilateral** orbit
    H05.239   Hemorrhage of unspecified orbit

√6ᵗʰ   H05.24   **Constant** exophthalmos
    H05.241   Constant exophthalmos, **right** eye
    H05.242   Constant exophthalmos, **left** eye
    H05.243   Constant exophthalmos, **bilateral**
    H05.249   Constant exophthalmos, unspecified eye

√6ᵗʰ   H05.25   **Intermittent** exophthalmos
    H05.251   Intermittent exophthalmos, **right** eye
    H05.252   Intermittent exophthalmos, **left** eye
    H05.253   Intermittent exophthalmos, **bilateral**
    H05.259   Intermittent exophthalmos, unspecified eye

√6ᵗʰ   H05.26   **Pulsating** exophthalmos
    H05.261   Pulsating exophthalmos, **right** eye
    H05.262   Pulsating exophthalmos, **left** eye
    H05.263   Pulsating exophthalmos, **bilateral**
    H05.269   Pulsating exophthalmos, unspecified eye

√5ᵗʰ   H05.3   **Deformity of orbit**

    `EXCLUDES 1`   *congenital deformity of orbit (Q10.7)*
            hypertelorism (Q75.2)

    H05.30   Unspecified deformity of orbit

√6ᵗʰ   H05.31   **Atrophy** of orbit
    H05.311   Atrophy of **right** orbit
    H05.312   Atrophy of **left** orbit
    H05.313   Atrophy of **bilateral** orbit
    H05.319   Atrophy of unspecified orbit

√6ᵗʰ   H05.32   **Deformity of orbit** due to bone disease
      Code also associated bone disease
    H05.321   Deformity of **right** orbit due to bone disease
    H05.322   Deformity of **left** orbit due to bone disease
    H05.323   Deformity of **bilateral** orbits due to bone disease
    H05.329   Deformity of unspecified orbit due to bone disease

√6ᵗʰ   H05.33   **Deformity of orbit** due to trauma or surgery
    H05.331   Deformity of **right** orbit due to trauma or surgery
    H05.332   Deformity of **left** orbit due to trauma or surgery
    H05.333   Deformity of **bilateral** orbits due to trauma or surgery
    H05.339   Deformity of unspecified orbit due to trauma or surgery

√6ᵗʰ   H05.34   **Enlargement** of orbit
    H05.341   Enlargement of **right** orbit
    H05.342   Enlargement of **left** orbit
    H05.343   Enlargement of **bilateral** orbits
    H05.349   Enlargement of unspecified orbit

√6ᵗʰ   H05.35   **Exostosis** of orbit
    H05.351   Exostosis of **right** orbit
    H05.352   Exostosis of **left** orbit
    H05.353   Exostosis of **bilateral** orbits
    H05.359   Exostosis of unspecified orbit

√5ᵗʰ   H05.4   **Enophthalmos**

√6ᵗʰ   H05.40   Unspecified enophthalmos
    H05.401   Unspecified enophthalmos, **right** eye
    H05.402   Unspecified enophthalmos, **left** eye
    H05.403   Unspecified enophthalmos, **bilateral**
    H05.409   Unspecified enophthalmos, unspecified eye

√6ᵗʰ   H05.41   **Enophthalmos** due to atrophy of orbital tissue
    H05.411   Enophthalmos due to atrophy of orbital tissue, **right** eye
    H05.412   Enophthalmos due to atrophy of orbital tissue, **left** eye
    H05.413   Enophthalmos due to atrophy of orbital tissue, **bilateral**
    H05.419   Enophthalmos due to atrophy of orbital tissue, unspecified eye

√6ᵗʰ   H05.42   **Enophthalmos** due to trauma or surgery
    H05.421   Enophthalmos due to trauma or surgery, **right** eye
    H05.422   Enophthalmos due to trauma or surgery, **left** eye
    H05.423   Enophthalmos due to trauma or surgery, **bilateral**
    H05.429   Enophthalmos due to trauma or surgery, unspecified eye

√5ᵗʰ   H05.5   **Retained (old) foreign body following penetrating wound of orbit**
      Retrobulbar foreign body
      Use additional code to identify the type of retained foreign body (Z18.-)
    `EXCLUDES 1`   *current penetrating wound of orbit (S05.4-)*
    `EXCLUDES 2`   *retained foreign body of eyelid (H02.81-)*
            retained intraocular foreign body (H44.6-, H44.7-)

    H05.50   Retained (old) foreign body following penetrating wound of unspecified orbit
    H05.51   Retained (old) foreign body following penetrating wound of **right** orbit
    H05.52   Retained (old) foreign body following penetrating wound of **left** orbit
    H05.53   Retained (old) foreign body following penetrating wound of **bilateral** orbits

√5ᵗʰ   H05.8   **Other disorders of orbit**

√6ᵗʰ   H05.81   Cyst of orbit
      Encephalocele of orbit
    H05.811   Cyst of **right** orbit
    H05.812   Cyst of **left** orbit
    H05.813   Cyst of **bilateral** orbits
    H05.819   Cyst of unspecified orbit

√6ᵗʰ   H05.82   Myopathy of extraocular muscles
    H05.821   Myopathy of extraocular muscles, **right** orbit

`N` Newborn: 0   `P` Pediatric: 0-17   `M` Maternity: 9-64   `A` Adult: 15-124   `UNS` Unspecified Site   `MCC` Major Complication/Comorbidity   `CC` Complication/Comorbidity   `PE` POA Exempt

614

ICD-10-CM 2025

        H05.822   Myopathy of extraocular muscles, **left** orbit

        H05.823   Myopathy of extraocular muscles, **bilateral**

        H05.829   Myopathy of extraocular muscles, unspecified orbit

    H05.89   Other disorders of orbit

    H05.9   Unspecified disorder of orbit

Disorders of conjunctiva (H10–H11)

√4ᵗʰ **H10**   **Conjunctivitis**

    EXCLUDES 1   *keratoconjunctivitis (H16.2-)*

    √5ᵗʰ   **H10.0**   **Mucopurulent** conjunctivitis

       √6ᵗʰ   **H10.01**   Acute follicular conjunctivitis

         H10.011   Acute follicular conjunctivitis, **right** eye

         H10.012   Acute follicular conjunctivitis, **left** eye

         H10.013   Acute follicular conjunctivitis, **bilateral**

         H10.019   Acute follicular conjunctivitis, unspecified eye

       √6ᵗʰ   **H10.02**   Other mucopurulent conjunctivitis

         H10.021   Other mucopurulent conjunctivitis, **right** eye

         H10.022   Other mucopurulent conjunctivitis, **left** eye

         H10.023   Other mucopurulent conjunctivitis, **bilateral**

         H10.029   Other mucopurulent conjunctivitis, unspecified eye

    √5ᵗʰ   **H10.1**   **Acute atopic** conjunctivitis

       Acute papillary conjunctivitis

       H10.10   Acute atopic conjunctivitis, unspecified eye

       H10.11   Acute atopic conjunctivitis, **right** eye

       H10.12   Acute atopic conjunctivitis, **left** eye

       H10.13   Acute atopic conjunctivitis, **bilateral**

    √5ᵗʰ   **H10.2**   Other **acute** conjunctivitis

       √6ᵗʰ   **H10.21**   Acute **toxic** conjunctivitis

        Acute chemical conjunctivitis

        Code first (T51-T65) to identify chemical and intent

        EXCLUDES 1   *burn and corrosion of eye and adnexa (T26.-)*

         H10.211   Acute toxic conjunctivitis, **right** eye

         H10.212   Acute toxic conjunctivitis, **left** eye

         H10.213   Acute toxic conjunctivitis, **bilateral**

         H10.219   Acute toxic conjunctivitis, unspecified eye

       √6ᵗʰ   **H10.22**   **Pseudomembranous** conjunctivitis

         H10.221   Pseudomembranous conjunctivitis, **right** eye

         H10.222   Pseudomembranous conjunctivitis, **left** eye

         H10.223   Pseudomembranous conjunctivitis, **bilateral**

         H10.229   Pseudomembranous conjunctivitis, unspecified eye

       √6ᵗʰ   **H10.23**   **Serous** conjunctivitis, except viral

        EXCLUDES 1   *viral conjunctivitis (B30.-)*

         H10.231   Serous conjunctivitis, except viral, **right** eye

         H10.232   Serous conjunctivitis, except viral, **left** eye

         H10.233   Serous conjunctivitis, except viral, **bilateral**

         H10.239   Serous conjunctivitis, except viral, unspecified eye

    √5ᵗʰ   **H10.3**   Unspecified **acute** conjunctivitis

       EXCLUDES 1   *ophthalmia neonatorum NOS (P39.1)*

       H10.30   Unspecified acute conjunctivitis, unspecified eye

       H10.31   Unspecified acute conjunctivitis, **right** eye

       H10.32   Unspecified acute conjunctivitis, **left** eye

       H10.33   Unspecified acute conjunctivitis, **bilateral**

    √5ᵗʰ   **H10.4**   **Chronic** conjunctivitis

       √6ᵗʰ   **H10.40**   Unspecified chronic conjunctivitis

         H10.401   Unspecified chronic conjunctivitis, **right** eye

         H10.402   Unspecified chronic conjunctivitis, **left** eye

         H10.403   Unspecified chronic conjunctivitis, **bilateral**

         H10.409   Unspecified chronic conjunctivitis, unspecified eye

       √6ᵗʰ   **H10.41**   Chronic **giant papillary** conjunctivitis

         H10.411   Chronic giant papillary conjunctivitis, **right** eye

         H10.412   Chronic giant papillary conjunctivitis, **left** eye

         H10.413   Chronic giant papillary conjunctivitis, **bilateral**

         H10.419   Chronic giant papillary conjunctivitis, unspecified eye

       √6ᵗʰ   **H10.42**   **Simple** chronic conjunctivitis

         H10.421   Simple chronic conjunctivitis, **right** eye

         H10.422   Simple chronic conjunctivitis, **left** eye

         H10.423   Simple chronic conjunctivitis, **bilateral**

         H10.429   Simple chronic conjunctivitis, unspecified eye

       √6ᵗʰ   **H10.43**   Chronic **follicular** conjunctivitis

         H10.431   Chronic follicular conjunctivitis, **right** eye

         H10.432   Chronic follicular conjunctivitis, **left** eye

         H10.433   Chronic follicular conjunctivitis, **bilateral**

         H10.439   Chronic follicular conjunctivitis, unspecified eye

       H10.44   **Vernal** conjunctivitis

        EXCLUDES 1   *vernal keratoconjunctivitis with limbar and corneal involvement (H16.26-)*

       H10.45   Other chronic **allergic** conjunctivitis

    √5ᵗʰ   **H10.5**   **Blepharoconjunctivitis**

       √6ᵗʰ   **H10.50**   Unspecified blepharoconjunctivitis

         H10.501   Unspecified blepharoconjunctivitis, **right** eye

         H10.502   Unspecified blepharoconjunctivitis, **left** eye

         H10.503   Unspecified blepharoconjunctivitis, **bilateral**

         H10.509   Unspecified blepharoconjunctivitis, unspecified eye

       √6ᵗʰ   **H10.51**   **Ligneous** conjunctivitis

        Code also underlying condition if known, such as: plasminogen deficiency (E88.02)

         H10.511   Ligneous conjunctivitis, **right** eye

         H10.512   Ligneous conjunctivitis, **left** eye

         H10.513   Ligneous conjunctivitis, **bilateral**

         H10.519   Ligneous conjunctivitis, unspecified eye

       √6ᵗʰ   **H10.52**   **Angular** blepharoconjunctivitis

         H10.521   Angular blepharoconjunctivitis, **right** eye

         H10.522   Angular blepharoconjunctivitis, **left** eye

         H10.523   Angular blepharoconjunctivitis, **bilateral**

         H10.529   Angular blepharoconjunctivitis, unspecified eye

       √6ᵗʰ   **H10.53**   **Contact** blepharoconjunctivitis

         H10.531   Contact blepharoconjunctivitis, **right** eye

         H10.532   Contact blepharoconjunctivitis, **left** eye

         H10.533   Contact blepharoconjunctivitis, **bilateral**

         H10.539   Contact blepharoconjunctivitis, unspecified eye

    √5ᵗʰ   **H10.8**   Other conjunctivitis

       √6ᵗʰ   **H10.81**   **Pingueculitis**

        EXCLUDES 1   *pinguecula (H11.15-)*

         H10.811   Pingueculitis, **right** eye

         H10.812   Pingueculitis, **left** eye

         H10.813   Pingueculitis, **bilateral**

         H10.819   Pingueculitis, unspecified eye

       √6ᵗʰ   **H10.82**   **Rosacea** conjunctivitis

        Code first underlying rosacea dermatitis (L71.-)

        AHA: 2018,4Q,15

         H10.821   Rosacea conjunctivitis, **right** eye

         H10.822   Rosacea conjunctivitis, **left** eye

         H10.823   Rosacea conjunctivitis, **bilateral**

         H10.829   Rosacea conjunctivitis, unspecified eye

       H10.89   Other conjunctivitis

    H10.9   **Unspecified conjunctivitis**

✔ Additional Character Required   √x7ᵗʰ Placeholder   Questionable PDx   Manifestation   Unspecified   UPD Unacceptable PDx   H1 - H14 HAC   HCC CMS-HCC Dx   HIV HIV Dx

✓4ᵗʰ **H11 Other disorders of conjunctiva**

    EXCLUDES 1   keratoconjunctivitis (H16.2-)

✓5ᵗʰ **H11.0 Pterygium of eye**

    EXCLUDES 1   pseudopterygium (H11.81-)

    DEF: Benign, wedge-shaped, conjunctival thickening that advances from the inner corner of the eye toward the cornea.

Pterygium

Pterygium

✓6ᵗʰ **H11.00 Unspecified pterygium of eye**

    H11.001 Unspecified pterygium of **right** eye
    H11.002 Unspecified pterygium of **left** eye
    H11.003 Unspecified pterygium of eye, **bilateral**
    H11.009 Unspecified pterygium of unspecified eye

✓6ᵗʰ **H11.01 Amyloid pterygium**

    H11.011 Amyloid pterygium of **right** eye
    H11.012 Amyloid pterygium of **left** eye
    H11.013 Amyloid pterygium of eye, **bilateral**
    H11.019 Amyloid pterygium of unspecified eye

✓6ᵗʰ **H11.02 Central pterygium of eye**

    H11.021 Central pterygium of **right** eye
    H11.022 Central pterygium of **left** eye
    H11.023 Central pterygium of eye, **bilateral**
    H11.029 Central pterygium of unspecified eye

✓6ᵗʰ **H11.03 Double pterygium of eye**

    H11.031 Double pterygium of **right** eye
    H11.032 Double pterygium of **left** eye
    H11.033 Double pterygium of eye, **bilateral**
    H11.039 Double pterygium of unspecified eye

✓6ᵗʰ **H11.04 Peripheral pterygium of eye, stationary**

    H11.041 Peripheral pterygium, stationary, **right** eye
    H11.042 Peripheral pterygium, stationary, **left** eye
    H11.043 Peripheral pterygium, stationary, **bilateral**
    H11.049 Peripheral pterygium, stationary, unspecified eye

✓6ᵗʰ **H11.05 Peripheral pterygium of eye, progressive**

    H11.051 Peripheral pterygium, progressive, **right** eye
    H11.052 Peripheral pterygium, progressive, **left** eye
    H11.053 Peripheral pterygium, progressive, **bilateral**
    H11.059 Peripheral pterygium, progressive, unspecified eye

✓6ᵗʰ **H11.06 Recurrent pterygium of eye**

    H11.061 Recurrent pterygium of **right** eye
    H11.062 Recurrent pterygium of **left** eye
    H11.063 Recurrent pterygium of eye, **bilateral**
    H11.069 Recurrent pterygium of unspecified eye

✓5ᵗʰ **H11.1 Conjunctival degenerations and deposits**

    EXCLUDES 2   pseudopterygium (H11.81)

    H11.10 Unspecified conjunctival degenerations

✓6ᵗʰ **H11.11 Conjunctival deposits**

    H11.111 Conjunctival deposits, **right** eye
    H11.112 Conjunctival deposits, **left** eye
    H11.113 Conjunctival deposits, **bilateral**
    H11.119 Conjunctival deposits, unspecified eye

✓6ᵗʰ **H11.12 Conjunctival concretions**

    H11.121 Conjunctival concretions, **right** eye
    H11.122 Conjunctival concretions, **left** eye
    H11.123 Conjunctival concretions, **bilateral**
    H11.129 Conjunctival concretions, unspecified eye

✓6ᵗʰ **H11.13 Conjunctival pigmentations**

    Conjunctival argyrosis [argyria]

    H11.131 Conjunctival pigmentations, **right** eye
    H11.132 Conjunctival pigmentations, **left** eye

    H11.133 Conjunctival pigmentations, **bilateral**
    H11.139 Conjunctival pigmentations, unspecified eye

✓6ᵗʰ **H11.14 Conjunctival xerosis, unspecified**

    EXCLUDES 1   xerosis of conjunctiva due to vitamin A deficiency (E50.0, E50.1)

    DEF: Abnormal dryness of the conjunctiva due to lack of sufficient tears or conjunctival secretions.

    H11.141 Conjunctival xerosis, unspecified, **right** eye
    H11.142 Conjunctival xerosis, unspecified, **left** eye
    H11.143 Conjunctival xerosis, unspecified, **bilateral**
    H11.149 Conjunctival xerosis, unspecified, unspecified eye

✓6ᵗʰ **H11.15 Pinguecula**

    EXCLUDES 1   pingueculitis (H10.81-)

    DEF: Proliferation on the conjunctiva near the sclerocorneal junction, usually of the side of the nose and usually in older patients.

Pinguecula

Pinguecula

    H11.151 Pinguecula, **right** eye
    H11.152 Pinguecula, **left** eye
    H11.153 Pinguecula, **bilateral**
    H11.159 Pinguecula, unspecified eye

✓5ᵗʰ **H11.2 Conjunctival scars**

✓6ᵗʰ **H11.21 Conjunctival adhesions and strands (localized)**

    H11.211 Conjunctival adhesions and strands (localized), **right** eye
    H11.212 Conjunctival adhesions and strands (localized), **left** eye
    H11.213 Conjunctival adhesions and strands (localized), **bilateral**
    H11.219 Conjunctival adhesions and strands (localized), unspecified eye

✓6ᵗʰ **H11.22 Conjunctival granuloma**

    H11.221 Conjunctival granuloma, **right** eye
    H11.222 Conjunctival granuloma, **left** eye
    H11.223 Conjunctival granuloma, **bilateral**
    H11.229 Conjunctival granuloma, unspecified

✓6ᵗʰ **H11.23 Symblepharon**

    H11.231 Symblepharon, **right** eye
    H11.232 Symblepharon, **left** eye
    H11.233 Symblepharon, **bilateral**
    H11.239 Symblepharon, unspecified eye

✓6ᵗʰ **H11.24 Scarring of conjunctiva**

    H11.241 Scarring of conjunctiva, **right** eye
    H11.242 Scarring of conjunctiva, **left** eye
    H11.243 Scarring of conjunctiva, **bilateral**
    H11.249 Scarring of conjunctiva, unspecified eye

✓5ᵗʰ **H11.3 Conjunctival hemorrhage**

    Subconjunctival hemorrhage

    H11.30 Conjunctival hemorrhage, unspecified eye
    H11.31 Conjunctival hemorrhage, **right** eye
    H11.32 Conjunctival hemorrhage, **left** eye
    H11.33 Conjunctival hemorrhage, **bilateral**

✓5ᵗʰ **H11.4 Other conjunctival vascular disorders and cysts**

✓6ᵗʰ **H11.41 Vascular abnormalities of conjunctiva**

    Conjunctival aneurysm

    H11.411 Vascular abnormalities of conjunctiva, **right** eye
    H11.412 Vascular abnormalities of conjunctiva, **left** eye
    H11.413 Vascular abnormalities of conjunctiva, **bilateral**
    H11.419 Vascular abnormalities of conjunctiva, unspecified eye

N Newborn: 0   **P** Pediatric: 0-17   **M** Maternity: 9-64   **A** Adult: 15-124   **UNS** Unspecified Site   **MCC** Major Complication/Comorbidity   **CC** Complication/Comorbidity   **PE** POA Exempt

616   ICD-10-CM 2025

√6ᵗʰ **H11.42** **Conjunctival** edema

    H11.421 **Conjunctival edema, right** eye
    H11.422 **Conjunctival edema, left** eye
    H11.423 **Conjunctival edema, bilateral**
    H11.429 **Conjunctival edema, unspecified eye**

√6ᵗʰ **H11.43** **Conjunctival** hyperemia

    H11.431 **Conjunctival hyperemia, right** eye
    H11.432 **Conjunctival hyperemia, left** eye
    H11.433 **Conjunctival hyperemia, bilateral**
    H11.439 **Conjunctival hyperemia, unspecified eye**

√6ᵗʰ **H11.44** **Conjunctival** cysts

    H11.441 **Conjunctival cysts, right** eye
    H11.442 **Conjunctival cysts, left** eye
    H11.443 **Conjunctival cysts, bilateral**
    H11.449 **Conjunctival cysts, unspecified eye**

√5ᵗʰ **H11.8** **Other specified disorders of conjunctiva**

√6ᵗʰ **H11.81** **Pseudopterygium of conjunctiva**

    H11.811 **Pseudopterygium of conjunctiva, right** eye
    H11.812 **Pseudopterygium of conjunctiva, left** eye
    H11.813 **Pseudopterygium of conjunctiva, bilateral**
    H11.819 **Pseudopterygium of conjunctiva, unspecified eye**

√6ᵗʰ **H11.82** **Conjunctivochalasis**

    H11.821 **Conjunctivochalasis, right** eye
    H11.822 **Conjunctivochalasis, left** eye
    H11.823 **Conjunctivochalasis, bilateral**
    H11.829 **Conjunctivochalasis, unspecified eye**

  H11.89 **Other specified disorders of conjunctiva**

H11.9 **Unspecified disorder of conjunctiva**

Disorders of sclera, cornea, iris and ciliary body (H15-H22)

√4ᵗʰ **H15** **Disorders of sclera**

√5ᵗʰ **H15.0** **Scleritis**

√6ᵗʰ **H15.00** **Unspecified scleritis**

    H15.001 **Unspecified scleritis, right** eye
    H15.002 **Unspecified scleritis, left** eye
    H15.003 **Unspecified scleritis, bilateral**
    H15.009 **Unspecified scleritis, unspecified eye**

√6ᵗʰ **H15.01** **Anterior** scleritis

    H15.011 **Anterior scleritis, right** eye
    H15.012 **Anterior scleritis, left** eye
    H15.013 **Anterior scleritis, bilateral**
    H15.019 **Anterior scleritis, unspecified eye**

√6ᵗʰ **H15.02** **Brawny** scleritis

    H15.021 **Brawny scleritis, right** eye
    H15.022 **Brawny scleritis, left** eye
    H15.023 **Brawny scleritis, bilateral**
    H15.029 **Brawny scleritis, unspecified eye**

√6ᵗʰ **H15.03** **Posterior** scleritis

   Sclerotenonitis
    H15.031 **Posterior scleritis, right** eye
    H15.032 **Posterior scleritis, left** eye
    H15.033 **Posterior scleritis, bilateral**
    H15.039 **Posterior scleritis, unspecified eye**

√6ᵗʰ **H15.04** **Scleritis with** corneal involvement

    H15.041 **Scleritis with corneal involvement, right** eye
    H15.042 **Scleritis with corneal involvement, left** eye
    H15.043 **Scleritis with corneal involvement, bilateral**
    H15.049 **Scleritis with corneal involvement, unspecified eye**

√6ᵗʰ **H15.05** **Scleromalacia perforans**

    H15.051 **Scleromalacia perforans, right** eye
    H15.052 **Scleromalacia perforans, left** eye
    H15.053 **Scleromalacia perforans, bilateral**
    H15.059 **Scleromalacia perforans, unspecified eye**

√6ᵗʰ **H15.09** **Other scleritis**

   Scleral abscess
    H15.091 **Other scleritis, right** eye
    H15.092 **Other scleritis, left** eye
    H15.093 **Other scleritis, bilateral**
    H15.099 **Other scleritis, unspecified eye**

√5ᵗʰ **H15.1** **Episcleritis**

√6ᵗʰ **H15.10** **Unspecified episcleritis**

    H15.101 **Unspecified episcleritis, right** eye
    H15.102 **Unspecified episcleritis, left** eye
    H15.103 **Unspecified episcleritis, bilateral**
    H15.109 **Unspecified episcleritis, unspecified eye**

√6ᵗʰ **H15.11** **Episcleritis** periodica fugax

    H15.111 **Episcleritis periodica fugax, right** eye
    H15.112 **Episcleritis periodica fugax, left** eye
    H15.113 **Episcleritis periodica fugax, bilateral**
    H15.119 **Episcleritis periodica fugax, unspecified eye**

√6ᵗʰ **H15.12** **Nodular** episcleritis

    H15.121 **Nodular episcleritis, right** eye
    H15.122 **Nodular episcleritis, left** eye
    H15.123 **Nodular episcleritis, bilateral**
    H15.129 **Nodular episcleritis, unspecified eye**

√5ᵗʰ **H15.8** **Other disorders of sclera**

    EXCLUDES 2   blue sclera (Q13.5)
              degenerative myopia (H44.2-)

√6ᵗʰ **H15.81** **Equatorial** staphyloma

    H15.811 **Equatorial staphyloma, right** eye
    H15.812 **Equatorial staphyloma, left** eye
    H15.813 **Equatorial staphyloma, bilateral**
    H15.819 **Equatorial staphyloma, unspecified eye**

√6ᵗʰ **H15.82** **Localized anterior** staphyloma

    H15.821 **Localized anterior staphyloma, right** eye
    H15.822 **Localized anterior staphyloma, left** eye
    H15.823 **Localized anterior staphyloma, bilateral**
    H15.829 **Localized anterior staphyloma, unspecified eye**

√6ᵗʰ **H15.83** **Staphyloma posticum**

    H15.831 **Staphyloma posticum, right** eye
    H15.832 **Staphyloma posticum, left** eye
    H15.833 **Staphyloma posticum, bilateral**
    H15.839 **Staphyloma posticum, unspecified eye**

√6ᵗʰ **H15.84** **Scleral** ectasia

    H15.841 **Scleral ectasia, right** eye
    H15.842 **Scleral ectasia, left** eye
    H15.843 **Scleral ectasia, bilateral**
    H15.849 **Scleral ectasia, unspecified eye**

√6ᵗʰ **H15.85** **Ring** staphyloma

    H15.851 **Ring staphyloma, right** eye
    H15.852 **Ring staphyloma, left** eye
    H15.853 **Ring staphyloma, bilateral**
    H15.859 **Ring staphyloma, unspecified eye**

  H15.89 **Other disorders of sclera**

H15.9 **Unspecified disorder of sclera**

√4ᵗʰ **H16** **Keratitis**

  DEF: Condition in which the cornea becomes inflamed and irritated.

√5ᵗʰ **H16.0** **Corneal ulcer**

√6ᵗʰ **H16.00** **Unspecified corneal ulcer**

    H16.001 **Unspecified corneal ulcer, right** eye
    H16.002 **Unspecified corneal ulcer, left** eye
    H16.003 **Unspecified corneal ulcer, bilateral**
    H16.009 **Unspecified corneal ulcer, unspecified eye**

√6ᵗʰ **H16.01** **Central** corneal ulcer

    H16.011 **Central corneal ulcer, right** eye
    H16.012 **Central corneal ulcer, left** eye
    H16.013 **Central corneal ulcer, bilateral**
    H16.019 **Central corneal ulcer, unspecified eye**

√6ᵗʰ **H16.02** **Ring** corneal ulcer

    H16.021 **Ring corneal ulcer, right** eye
    H16.022 **Ring corneal ulcer, left** eye
    H16.023 **Ring corneal ulcer, bilateral**
    H16.029 **Ring corneal ulcer, unspecified eye**

√6ᵗʰ **H16.03** **Corneal ulcer with** hypopyon

    H16.031 **Corneal ulcer with hypopyon, right** eye
    H16.032 **Corneal ulcer with hypopyon, left** eye
    H16.033 **Corneal ulcer with hypopyon, bilateral**
    H16.039 **Corneal ulcer with hypopyon, unspecified eye**

√6ᵗʰ **H16.04** **Marginal** corneal ulcer

    H16.041 **Marginal corneal ulcer, right** eye
    H16.042 **Marginal corneal ulcer, left** eye

✔ Additional Character Required   ✓x7ᵗʰ Placeholder   Questionable PDx   Manifestation   Unspecified   UPD Unacceptable PDx   H1-H14 HAC   HCC CMS-HCC Dx   HIV HIV Dx

ICD-10-CM 2025   617

H16.043　Marginal corneal ulcer, **bilateral**
H16.049　Marginal corneal ulcer, unspecified eye

✓6th　H16.05　**Mooren's** corneal ulcer
H16.051　Mooren's corneal ulcer, **right** eye
H16.052　Mooren's corneal ulcer, **left** eye
H16.053　Mooren's corneal ulcer, **bilateral**
H16.059　Mooren's corneal ulcer, unspecified eye

✓6th　H16.06　**Mycotic** corneal ulcer
H16.061　Mycotic corneal ulcer, **right** eye
H16.062　Mycotic corneal ulcer, **left** eye
H16.063　Mycotic corneal ulcer, **bilateral**
H16.069　Mycotic corneal ulcer, unspecified eye

✓6th　H16.07　**Perforated** corneal ulcer
H16.071　Perforated corneal ulcer, **right** eye
H16.072　Perforated corneal ulcer, **left** eye
H16.073　Perforated corneal ulcer, **bilateral**
H16.079　Perforated corneal ulcer, unspecified eye

✓5th　H16.1　**Other and unspecified superficial keratitis without conjunctivitis**
✓6th　H16.10　Unspecified **superficial** keratitis
H16.101　Unspecified superficial keratitis, **right** eye
H16.102　Unspecified superficial keratitis, **left** eye
H16.103　Unspecified superficial keratitis, **bilateral**
H16.109　Unspecified superficial keratitis, unspecified eye

✓6th　H16.11　**Macular** keratitis
Areolar keratitis
Nummular keratitis
Stellate keratitis
Striate keratitis
H16.111　Macular keratitis, **right** eye
H16.112　Macular keratitis, **left** eye
H16.113　Macular keratitis, **bilateral**
H16.119　Macular keratitis, unspecified eye

✓6th　H16.12　**Filamentary** keratitis
H16.121　Filamentary keratitis, **right** eye
H16.122　Filamentary keratitis, **left** eye
H16.123　Filamentary keratitis, **bilateral**
H16.129　Filamentary keratitis, unspecified eye

✓6th　H16.13　**Photokeratitis**
Snow blindness
Welders keratitis
H16.131　Photokeratitis, **right** eye
H16.132　Photokeratitis, **left** eye
H16.133　Photokeratitis, **bilateral**
H16.139　Photokeratitis, unspecified eye

✓6th　H16.14　**Punctate** keratitis
H16.141　Punctate keratitis, **right** eye
H16.142　Punctate keratitis, **left** eye
H16.143　Punctate keratitis, **bilateral**
H16.149　Punctate keratitis, unspecified eye

✓5th　H16.2　**Keratoconjunctivitis**
✓6th　H16.20　Unspecified keratoconjunctivitis
Superficial keratitis with conjunctivitis NOS
H16.201　Unspecified keratoconjunctivitis, **right** eye
H16.202　Unspecified keratoconjunctivitis, **left** eye
H16.203　Unspecified keratoconjunctivitis, **bilateral**
H16.209　Unspecified keratoconjunctivitis, unspecified eye

✓6th　H16.21　**Exposure** keratoconjunctivitis
H16.211　Exposure keratoconjunctivitis, **right** eye
H16.212　Exposure keratoconjunctivitis, **left** eye
H16.213　Exposure keratoconjunctivitis, **bilateral**
H16.219　Exposure keratoconjunctivitis, unspecified eye

✓6th　H16.22　**Keratoconjunctivitis sicca, not specified as Sjögren's**
EXCLUDES 1　Sjögren's syndrome (M35.01)
H16.221　Keratoconjunctivitis sicca, not specified as Sjögren's, **right** eye
H16.222　Keratoconjunctivitis sicca, not specified as Sjögren's, **left** eye
H16.223　Keratoconjunctivitis sicca, not specified as Sjögren's, **bilateral**
H16.229　Keratoconjunctivitis sicca, not specified as Sjögren's, unspecified eye

✓6th　H16.23　**Neurotrophic** keratoconjunctivitis
H16.231　Neurotrophic keratoconjunctivitis, **right** eye
H16.232　Neurotrophic keratoconjunctivitis, **left** eye
H16.233　Neurotrophic keratoconjunctivitis, **bilateral**
H16.239　Neurotrophic keratoconjunctivitis, unspecified eye

✓6th　H16.24　**Ophthalmia nodosa**
H16.241　Ophthalmia nodosa, **right** eye
H16.242　Ophthalmia nodosa, **left** eye
H16.243　Ophthalmia nodosa, **bilateral**
H16.249　Ophthalmia nodosa, unspecified eye

✓6th　H16.25　**Phlyctenular** keratoconjunctivitis
H16.251　Phlyctenular keratoconjunctivitis, **right** eye
H16.252　Phlyctenular keratoconjunctivitis, **left** eye
H16.253　Phlyctenular keratoconjunctivitis, **bilateral**
H16.259　Phlyctenular keratoconjunctivitis, unspecified eye

✓6th　H16.26　**Vernal** keratoconjunctivitis, with **limbar and corneal** involvement
EXCLUDES 1　vernal conjunctivitis without limbar and corneal involvement (H10.44)
H16.261　Vernal keratoconjunctivitis, with limbar and corneal involvement, **right** eye
H16.262　Vernal keratoconjunctivitis, with limbar and corneal involvement, **left** eye
H16.263　Vernal keratoconjunctivitis, with limbar and corneal involvement, **bilateral**
H16.269　Vernal keratoconjunctivitis, with limbar and corneal involvement, unspecified eye

✓6th　H16.29　Other keratoconjunctivitis
H16.291　Other keratoconjunctivitis, **right** eye
H16.292　Other keratoconjunctivitis, **left** eye
H16.293　Other keratoconjunctivitis, **bilateral**
H16.299　Other keratoconjunctivitis, unspecified eye

✓5th　H16.3　**Interstitial and deep keratitis**
✓6th　H16.30　Unspecified interstitial keratitis
H16.301　Unspecified interstitial keratitis, **right** eye
H16.302　Unspecified interstitial keratitis, **left** eye
H16.303　Unspecified interstitial keratitis, **bilateral**
H16.309　Unspecified interstitial keratitis, unspecified eye

✓6th　H16.31　**Corneal** abscess
H16.311　Corneal abscess, **right** eye
H16.312　Corneal abscess, **left** eye
H16.313　Corneal abscess, **bilateral**
H16.319　Corneal abscess, unspecified eye

✓6th　H16.32　**Diffuse** interstitial keratitis
Cogan's syndrome
H16.321　Diffuse interstitial keratitis, **right** eye
H16.322　Diffuse interstitial keratitis, **left** eye
H16.323　Diffuse interstitial keratitis, **bilateral**
H16.329　Diffuse interstitial keratitis, unspecified eye

✓6th　H16.33　**Sclerosing** keratitis
H16.331　Sclerosing keratitis, **right** eye
H16.332　Sclerosing keratitis, **left** eye
H16.333　Sclerosing keratitis, **bilateral**
H16.339　Sclerosing keratitis, unspecified eye

✓6th　H16.39　Other interstitial and deep keratitis
H16.391　Other interstitial and deep keratitis, **right** eye
H16.392　Other interstitial and deep keratitis, **left** eye
H16.393　Other interstitial and deep keratitis, **bilateral**
H16.399　Other interstitial and deep keratitis, unspecified eye

✓5th　H16.4　**Corneal neovascularization**
✓6th　H16.40　Unspecified corneal neovascularization
H16.401　Unspecified corneal neovascularization, **right** eye
H16.402　Unspecified corneal neovascularization, **left** eye

H16.403   Unspecified corneal neovascularization, bilateral

H16.409   Unspecified corneal neovascularization, unspecified eye

√6th H16.41   **Ghost vessels** (corneal)

    H16.411   Ghost vessels (corneal), right eye

    H16.412   Ghost vessels (corneal), left eye

    H16.413   Ghost vessels (corneal), bilateral

    H16.419   Ghost vessels (corneal), unspecified eye

√6th H16.42   **Pannus** (corneal)

    H16.421   Pannus (corneal), right eye

    H16.422   Pannus (corneal), left eye

    H16.423   Pannus (corneal), bilateral

    H16.429   Pannus (corneal), unspecified eye

√6th H16.43   **Localized vascularization** of cornea

    H16.431   Localized vascularization of cornea, right eye

    H16.432   Localized vascularization of cornea, left eye

    H16.433   Localized vascularization of cornea, bilateral

    H16.439   Localized vascularization of cornea, unspecified eye

√6th H16.44   **Deep vascularization** of cornea

    H16.441   Deep vascularization of cornea, right eye

    H16.442   Deep vascularization of cornea, left eye

    H16.443   Deep vascularization of cornea, bilateral

    H16.449   Deep vascularization of cornea, unspecified eye

H16.8   Other keratitis   **UPD**

H16.9   Unspecified keratitis

√4th **H17**   **Corneal scars and opacities**

  √5th H17.0   **Adherent leukoma**

     H17.00   Adherent leukoma, unspecified eye

     H17.01   Adherent leukoma, right eye

     H17.02   Adherent leukoma, left eye

     H17.03   Adherent leukoma, bilateral

  √5th H17.1   **Central corneal opacity**

     H17.10   Central corneal opacity, unspecified eye

     H17.11   Central corneal opacity, right eye

     H17.12   Central corneal opacity, left eye

     H17.13   Central corneal opacity, bilateral

  √5th H17.8   **Other corneal scars and opacities**

   √6th H17.81   **Minor** opacity of cornea

      Corneal nebula

      H17.811   Minor opacity of cornea, right eye

      H17.812   Minor opacity of cornea, left eye

      H17.813   Minor opacity of cornea, bilateral

      H17.819   Minor opacity of cornea, unspecified eye

   √6th H17.82   **Peripheral** opacity of cornea

      H17.821   Peripheral opacity of cornea, right eye

      H17.822   Peripheral opacity of cornea, left eye

      H17.823   Peripheral opacity of cornea, bilateral

      H17.829   Peripheral opacity of cornea, unspecified eye

     H17.89   Other corneal scars and opacities

    H17.9   Unspecified corneal scar and opacity

√4th **H18**   **Other disorders of cornea**

  √5th H18.0   **Corneal pigmentations and deposits**

   √6th H18.00   **Unspecified corneal deposit**

      H18.001   Unspecified corneal deposit, right eye

      H18.002   Unspecified corneal deposit, left eye

      H18.003   Unspecified corneal deposit, bilateral

      H18.009   Unspecified corneal deposit, unspecified eye

   √6th H18.01   **Anterior** corneal pigmentations

      Staehli's line

      H18.011   Anterior corneal pigmentations, right eye

      H18.012   Anterior corneal pigmentations, left eye

      H18.013   Anterior corneal pigmentations, bilateral

      H18.019   Anterior corneal pigmentations, unspecified eye

   √6th H18.02   **Argentous** corneal deposits

      H18.021   Argentous corneal deposits, right eye

      H18.022   Argentous corneal deposits, left eye

      H18.023   Argentous corneal deposits, bilateral

      H18.029   Argentous corneal deposits, unspecified eye

  √6th H18.03   **Corneal deposits in metabolic disorders**

     Code also associated metabolic disorder

     H18.031   Corneal deposits in metabolic disorders, right eye

     H18.032   Corneal deposits in metabolic disorders, left eye

     H18.033   Corneal deposits in metabolic disorders, bilateral

     H18.039   Corneal deposits in metabolic disorders, unspecified eye

  √6th H18.04   **Kayser-Fleischer ring**

     Code also associated Wilson's disease (E83.01)

     H18.041   Kayser-Fleischer ring, right eye

     H18.042   Kayser-Fleischer ring, left eye

     H18.043   Kayser-Fleischer ring, bilateral

     H18.049   Kayser-Fleischer ring, unspecified eye

  √6th H18.05   **Posterior** corneal pigmentations

     Krukenberg's spindle

     H18.051   Posterior corneal pigmentations, right eye

     H18.052   Posterior corneal pigmentations, left eye

     H18.053   Posterior corneal pigmentations, bilateral

     H18.059   Posterior corneal pigmentations, unspecified eye

  √6th H18.06   **Stromal** corneal pigmentations

     Hematocornea

     H18.061   Stromal corneal pigmentations, right eye

     H18.062   Stromal corneal pigmentations, left eye

     H18.063   Stromal corneal pigmentations, bilateral

     H18.069   Stromal corneal pigmentations, unspecified eye

  √5th H18.1   **Bullous keratopathy**

     DEF: Corneal swelling due to a damaged corneal endothelium. Bullous keratopathy is characterized by recurring, rupturing epithelial blisters causing glaucoma, iridocyclitis, and Fuchs' dystrophy.

     H18.10   Bullous keratopathy, unspecified eye

     H18.11   Bullous keratopathy, right eye

     H18.12   Bullous keratopathy, left eye

     H18.13   Bullous keratopathy, bilateral

  √5th H18.2   **Other and unspecified corneal edema**

     H18.20   Unspecified corneal edema

   √6th H18.21   **Corneal edema secondary to contact lens**

      EXCLUDES 2   other corneal disorders due to contact lens (H18.82-)

      H18.211   Corneal edema secondary to contact lens, right eye

      H18.212   Corneal edema secondary to contact lens, left eye

      H18.213   Corneal edema secondary to contact lens, bilateral

      H18.219   Corneal edema secondary to contact lens, unspecified eye

   √6th H18.22   **Idiopathic** corneal edema

      H18.221   Idiopathic corneal edema, right eye

      H18.222   Idiopathic corneal edema, left eye

      H18.223   Idiopathic corneal edema, bilateral

      H18.229   Idiopathic corneal edema, unspecified eye

   √6th H18.23   **Secondary** corneal edema

      H18.231   Secondary corneal edema, right eye

      H18.232   Secondary corneal edema, left eye

      H18.233   Secondary corneal edema, bilateral

      H18.239   Secondary corneal edema, unspecified eye

  √5th H18.3   **Changes of corneal membranes**

     H18.30   Unspecified corneal membrane change

   √6th H18.31   **Folds and rupture in Bowman's membrane**

      H18.311   Folds and rupture in Bowman's membrane, right eye

      H18.312   Folds and rupture in Bowman's membrane, left eye

      H18.313   Folds and rupture in Bowman's membrane, bilateral

      H18.319   Folds and rupture in Bowman's membrane, unspecified eye

   √6th H18.32   **Folds in Descemet's membrane**

      H18.321   Folds in Descemet's membrane, right eye

      H18.322   Folds in Descemet's membrane, left eye

✔ Additional Character Required   √x7th Placeholder   Questionable PDx   Manifestation   Unspecified   **UPD** Unacceptable PDx   **H1-H14** HAC   **HCC** CMS-HCC Dx   **HIV** HIV Dx

Chapter 7. Diseases of the Eye and Adnexa

H18.323–H18.821

H18.323   **Folds in Descemet's membrane, bilateral**
H18.329   **Folds in Descemet's membrane, unspecified eye**

✓6th   H18.33   **Rupture in Descemet's membrane**

H18.331   **Rupture in Descemet's membrane, right eye**
H18.332   **Rupture in Descemet's membrane, left eye**
H18.333   **Rupture in Descemet's membrane, bilateral**
H18.339   **Rupture in Descemet's membrane, unspecified eye**

✓5th   H18.4   **Corneal degeneration**

> EXCLUDES 1   Mooren's ulcer (H16.0-)
> recurrent erosion of cornea (H18.83-)

H18.40   **Unspecified corneal degeneration**

✓6th   H18.41   **Arcus senilis**

Senile corneal changes

H18.411   **Arcus senilis, right eye**
H18.412   **Arcus senilis, left eye**
H18.413   **Arcus senilis, bilateral**
H18.419   **Arcus senilis, unspecified eye**

✓6th   H18.42   **Band keratopathy**

H18.421   **Band keratopathy, right eye**
H18.422   **Band keratopathy, left eye**
H18.423   **Band keratopathy, bilateral**
H18.429   **Band keratopathy, unspecified eye**

H18.43   **Other calcerous corneal degeneration**

✓6th   H18.44   **Keratomalacia**

> EXCLUDES 1   keratomalacia due to vitamin A deficiency (E50.4)

H18.441   **Keratomalacia, right eye**
H18.442   **Keratomalacia, left eye**
H18.443   **Keratomalacia, bilateral**
H18.449   **Keratomalacia, unspecified eye**

✓6th   H18.45   **Nodular corneal degeneration**

H18.451   **Nodular corneal degeneration, right eye**
H18.452   **Nodular corneal degeneration, left eye**
H18.453   **Nodular corneal degeneration, bilateral**
H18.459   **Nodular corneal degeneration, unspecified eye**

✓6th   H18.46   **Peripheral corneal degeneration**

H18.461   **Peripheral corneal degeneration, right eye**
H18.462   **Peripheral corneal degeneration, left eye**
H18.463   **Peripheral corneal degeneration, bilateral**
H18.469   **Peripheral corneal degeneration, unspecified eye**

H18.49   **Other corneal degeneration**

✓5th   H18.5   **Hereditary corneal dystrophies**

AHA: 2020,4Q,24

✓6th   H18.50   **Unspecified hereditary corneal dystrophies**

H18.501   **Unspecified hereditary corneal dystrophies, right eye**
H18.502   **Unspecified hereditary corneal dystrophies, left eye**
H18.503   **Unspecified hereditary corneal dystrophies, bilateral**
H18.509   **Unspecified hereditary corneal dystrophies, unspecified eye**

✓6th   H18.51   **Endothelial corneal dystrophy**

Fuchs' dystrophy

H18.511   **Endothelial corneal dystrophy, right eye**
H18.512   **Endothelial corneal dystrophy, left eye**
H18.513   **Endothelial corneal dystrophy, bilateral**
H18.519   **Endothelial corneal dystrophy, unspecified eye**

✓6th   H18.52   **Epithelial (juvenile) corneal dystrophy**

H18.521   **Epithelial (juvenile) corneal dystrophy, right eye**
H18.522   **Epithelial (juvenile) corneal dystrophy, left eye**
H18.523   **Epithelial (juvenile) corneal dystrophy, bilateral**
H18.529   **Epithelial (juvenile) corneal dystrophy, unspecified eye**

✓6th   H18.53   **Granular corneal dystrophy**

H18.531   **Granular corneal dystrophy, right eye**
H18.532   **Granular corneal dystrophy, left eye**
H18.533   **Granular corneal dystrophy, bilateral**

H18.539   **Granular corneal dystrophy, unspecified eye**

✓6th   H18.54   **Lattice corneal dystrophy**

H18.541   **Lattice corneal dystrophy, right eye**
H18.542   **Lattice corneal dystrophy, left eye**
H18.543   **Lattice corneal dystrophy, bilateral**
H18.549   **Lattice corneal dystrophy, unspecified eye**

✓6th   H18.55   **Macular corneal dystrophy**

H18.551   **Macular corneal dystrophy, right eye**
H18.552   **Macular corneal dystrophy, left eye**
H18.553   **Macular corneal dystrophy, bilateral**
H18.559   **Macular corneal dystrophy, unspecified eye**

✓6th   H18.59   **Other hereditary corneal dystrophies**

H18.591   **Other hereditary corneal dystrophies, right eye**
H18.592   **Other hereditary corneal dystrophies, left eye**
H18.593   **Other hereditary corneal dystrophies, bilateral**
H18.599   **Other hereditary corneal dystrophies, unspecified eye**

✓5th   H18.6   **Keratoconus**

✓6th   H18.60   **Keratoconus, unspecified**

H18.601   **Keratoconus, unspecified, right eye**
H18.602   **Keratoconus, unspecified, left eye**
H18.603   **Keratoconus, unspecified, bilateral**
H18.609   **Keratoconus, unspecified, unspecified eye**

✓6th   H18.61   **Keratoconus, stable**

H18.611   **Keratoconus, stable, right eye**
H18.612   **Keratoconus, stable, left eye**
H18.613   **Keratoconus, stable, bilateral**
H18.619   **Keratoconus, stable, unspecified eye**

✓6th   H18.62   **Keratoconus, unstable**

Acute hydrops

H18.621   **Keratoconus, unstable, right eye**
H18.622   **Keratoconus, unstable, left eye**
H18.623   **Keratoconus, unstable, bilateral**
H18.629   **Keratoconus, unstable, unspecified eye**

✓5th   H18.7   **Other and unspecified corneal deformities**

> EXCLUDES 1   congenital malformations of cornea (Q13.3-Q13.4)

H18.70   **Unspecified corneal deformity**

✓6th   H18.71   **Corneal ectasia**

H18.711   **Corneal ectasia, right eye**
H18.712   **Corneal ectasia, left eye**
H18.713   **Corneal ectasia, bilateral**
H18.719   **Corneal ectasia, unspecified eye**

✓6th   H18.72   **Corneal staphyloma**

H18.721   **Corneal staphyloma, right eye**
H18.722   **Corneal staphyloma, left eye**
H18.723   **Corneal staphyloma, bilateral**
H18.729   **Corneal staphyloma, unspecified eye**

✓6th   H18.73   **Descemetocele**

H18.731   **Descemetocele, right eye**
H18.732   **Descemetocele, left eye**
H18.733   **Descemetocele, bilateral**
H18.739   **Descemetocele, unspecified eye**

✓6th   H18.79   **Other corneal deformities**

H18.791   **Other corneal deformities, right eye**
H18.792   **Other corneal deformities, left eye**
H18.793   **Other corneal deformities, bilateral**
H18.799   **Other corneal deformities, unspecified eye**

✓5th   H18.8   **Other specified disorders of cornea**

✓6th   H18.81   **Anesthesia and hypoesthesia of cornea**

H18.811   **Anesthesia and hypoesthesia of cornea, right eye**
H18.812   **Anesthesia and hypoesthesia of cornea, left eye**
H18.813   **Anesthesia and hypoesthesia of cornea, bilateral**
H18.819   **Anesthesia and hypoesthesia of cornea, unspecified eye**

✓6th   H18.82   **Corneal disorder due to contact lens**

> EXCLUDES 2   corneal edema due to contact lens (H18.21-)

H18.821   **Corneal disorder due to contact lens, right eye**

N Newborn: 0   P Pediatric: 0-17   M Maternity: 9-64   A Adult: 15-124   UNS Unspecified Site   MCC Major Complication/Comorbidity   CC Complication/Comorbidity   PE POA Exempt

620   ICD-10-CM 2025

H18.822 **Corneal disorder due to contact lens, left eye**

H18.823 **Corneal disorder due to contact lens, bilateral**

H18.829 **Corneal disorder due to contact lens, unspecified eye**

✓6th H18.83 **Recurrent erosion of cornea**

H18.831 **Recurrent erosion of cornea, right eye**

H18.832 **Recurrent erosion of cornea, left eye**

H18.833 **Recurrent erosion of cornea, bilateral**

H18.839 **Recurrent erosion of cornea, unspecified eye**

✓6th H18.89 **Other specified disorders of cornea**

H18.891 **Other specified disorders of cornea, right eye**

H18.892 **Other specified disorders of cornea, left eye**

H18.893 **Other specified disorders of cornea, bilateral**

H18.899 **Other specified disorders of cornea, unspecified eye**

H18.9 **Unspecified disorder of cornea**

✓4th H20 **Iridocyclitis**

✓5th H20.0 **Acute and subacute iridocyclitis**

Acute anterior uveitis
Acute cyclitis
Acute iritis
Subacute anterior uveitis
Subacute cyclitis
Subacute iritis

EXCLUDES 1   *iridocyclitis, iritis, uveitis (due to) (in) diabetes mellitus (E08-E13 with .39)*

iridocyclitis, iritis, uveitis (due to) (in) diphtheria (A36.89)

iridocyclitis, iritis, uveitis (due to) (in) gonococcal (A54.32)

iridocyclitis, iritis, uveitis (due to) (in) herpes (simplex) (B00.51)

iridocyclitis, iritis, uveitis (due to) (in) herpes zoster (B02.32)

iridocyclitis, iritis, uveitis (due to) (in) late congenital syphilis (A50.39)

iridocyclitis, iritis, uveitis (due to) (in) late syphilis (A52.71)

iridocyclitis, iritis, uveitis (due to) (in) sarcoidosis (D86.83)

iridocyclitis, iritis, uveitis (due to) (in) syphilis (A51.43)

iridocyclitis, iritis, uveitis (due to) (in) toxoplasmosis (B58.09)

iridocyclitis, iritis, uveitis (due to) (in) tuberculosis (A18.54)

H20.00 **Unspecified acute and subacute iridocyclitis** CC

✓6th H20.01 **Primary iridocyclitis**

H20.011 **Primary iridocyclitis, right eye** CC

H20.012 **Primary iridocyclitis, left eye** CC

H20.013 **Primary iridocyclitis, bilateral** CC

H20.019 **Primary iridocyclitis, unspecified eye** CC UPD

✓6th H20.02 **Recurrent acute iridocyclitis**

H20.021 **Recurrent acute iridocyclitis, right eye** CC

H20.022 **Recurrent acute iridocyclitis, left eye** CC

H20.023 **Recurrent acute iridocyclitis, bilateral** CC

H20.029 **Recurrent acute iridocyclitis, unspecified eye** CC UPD

✓6th H20.03 **Secondary infectious iridocyclitis**

H20.031 **Secondary infectious iridocyclitis, right eye**

H20.032 **Secondary infectious iridocyclitis, left eye**

H20.033 **Secondary infectious iridocyclitis, bilateral**

H20.039 **Secondary infectious iridocyclitis, unspecified eye** CC UPD

✓6th H20.04 **Secondary noninfectious iridocyclitis**

H20.041 **Secondary noninfectious iridocyclitis, right eye**

H20.042 **Secondary noninfectious iridocyclitis, left eye**

H20.043 **Secondary noninfectious iridocyclitis, bilateral**

H20.049 **Secondary noninfectious iridocyclitis, unspecified eye**

✓6th H20.05 **Hypopyon**

H20.051 **Hypopyon, right eye**

H20.052 **Hypopyon, left eye**

H20.053 **Hypopyon, bilateral**

H20.059 **Hypopyon, unspecified eye**

✓5th H20.1 **Chronic iridocyclitis**

Use additional code for any associated cataract (H26.21-)

EXCLUDES 2   *posterior cyclitis (H30.2-)*

H20.10 **Chronic iridocyclitis, unspecified eye**

H20.11 **Chronic iridocyclitis, right eye**

H20.12 **Chronic iridocyclitis, left eye**

H20.13 **Chronic iridocyclitis, bilateral**

✓5th H20.2 **Lens-induced iridocyclitis**

H20.20 **Lens-induced iridocyclitis, unspecified eye**

H20.21 **Lens-induced iridocyclitis, right eye**

H20.22 **Lens-induced iridocyclitis, left eye**

H20.23 **Lens-induced iridocyclitis, bilateral**

✓5th H20.8 **Other iridocyclitis**

EXCLUDES 2   *glaucomatocyclitis crises (H40.4-)*
posterior cyclitis (H30.2-)
sympathetic uveitis (H44.13-)

✓6th H20.81 **Fuchs' heterochromic cyclitis**

H20.811 **Fuchs' heterochromic cyclitis, right eye**

H20.812 **Fuchs' heterochromic cyclitis, left eye**

H20.813 **Fuchs' heterochromic cyclitis, bilateral**

H20.819 **Fuchs' heterochromic cyclitis, unspecified eye**

✓6th H20.82 **Vogt-Koyanagi syndrome**

H20.821 **Vogt-Koyanagi syndrome, right eye**

H20.822 **Vogt-Koyanagi syndrome, left eye**

H20.823 **Vogt-Koyanagi syndrome, bilateral**

H20.829 **Vogt-Koyanagi syndrome, unspecified eye**

H20.9 **Unspecified iridocyclitis** CC

Uveitis NOS

✓4th H21 **Other disorders of iris and ciliary body**

EXCLUDES 2   *sympathetic uveitis (H44.1-)*

✓5th H21.0 **Hyphema**

EXCLUDES 1   *traumatic hyphema (S05.1-)*

Hyphema

- Iris
- Cornea
- Hyphema

H21.00 **Hyphema, unspecified eye**

H21.01 **Hyphema, right eye**

H21.02 **Hyphema, left eye**

H21.03 **Hyphema, bilateral**

✓5th H21.1 **Other vascular disorders of iris and ciliary body**

Neovascularization of iris or ciliary body
Rubeosis iridis
Rubeosis of iris

✓6th H21.1X **Other vascular disorders of iris and ciliary body**

H21.1X1 **Other vascular disorders of iris and ciliary body, right eye**

H21.1X2 **Other vascular disorders of iris and ciliary body, left eye**

✓ Additional Character Required   **✓x7th Placeholder**   **Questionable PDx**   **Manifestation**   **Unspecified**   **UPD Unacceptable PDx**   **H1-H4 HAC**   **HCC CMS-HCC Dx**   **HIV HIV Dx**

H21.1X3   **Other vascular disorders of iris and ciliary body, bilateral**

H21.1X9   **Other vascular disorders of iris and ciliary body, unspecified eye**

✓5ᵗʰ **H21.2**   **Degeneration of iris and ciliary body**

    ✓6ᵗʰ **H21.21**   **Degeneration of chamber angle**

        H21.211   **Degeneration of chamber angle, right eye**

        H21.212   **Degeneration of chamber angle, left eye**

        H21.213   **Degeneration of chamber angle, bilateral**

        H21.219   **Degeneration of chamber angle, unspecified eye**

    ✓6ᵗʰ **H21.22**   **Degeneration of ciliary body**

        H21.221   **Degeneration of ciliary body, right eye**

        H21.222   **Degeneration of ciliary body, left eye**

        H21.223   **Degeneration of ciliary body, bilateral**

        H21.229   **Degeneration of ciliary body, unspecified eye**

    ✓6ᵗʰ **H21.23**   **Degeneration of iris (pigmentary)**

        Translucency of iris

        H21.231   **Degeneration of iris (pigmentary), right eye**

        H21.232   **Degeneration of iris (pigmentary), left eye**

        H21.233   **Degeneration of iris (pigmentary), bilateral**

        H21.239   **Degeneration of iris (pigmentary), unspecified eye**

    ✓6ᵗʰ **H21.24**   **Degeneration of pupillary margin**

        H21.241   **Degeneration of pupillary margin, right eye**

        H21.242   **Degeneration of pupillary margin, left eye**

        H21.243   **Degeneration of pupillary margin, bilateral**

        H21.249   **Degeneration of pupillary margin, unspecified eye**

    ✓6ᵗʰ **H21.25**   **Iridoschisis**

        H21.251   **Iridoschisis, right eye**

        H21.252   **Iridoschisis, left eye**

        H21.253   **Iridoschisis, bilateral**

        H21.259   **Iridoschisis, unspecified eye**

    ✓6ᵗʰ **H21.26**   **Iris atrophy (essential) (progressive)**

        H21.261   **Iris atrophy (essential) (progressive), right eye**

        H21.262   **Iris atrophy (essential) (progressive), left eye**

        H21.263   **Iris atrophy (essential) (progressive), bilateral**

        H21.269   **Iris atrophy (essential) (progressive), unspecified eye**

    ✓6ᵗʰ **H21.27**   **Miotic pupillary cyst**

        H21.271   **Miotic pupillary cyst, right eye**

        H21.272   **Miotic pupillary cyst, left eye**

        H21.273   **Miotic pupillary cyst, bilateral**

        H21.279   **Miotic pupillary cyst, unspecified eye**

    H21.29   **Other iris atrophy**

✓5ᵗʰ **H21.3**   **Cyst of iris, ciliary body and anterior chamber**

    EXCLUDES 2   miotic pupillary cyst (H21.27-)

    ✓6ᵗʰ **H21.30**   **Idiopathic cysts of iris, ciliary body or anterior chamber**

        Cyst of iris, ciliary body or anterior chamber NOS

        H21.301   **Idiopathic cysts of iris, ciliary body or anterior chamber, right eye**

        H21.302   **Idiopathic cysts of iris, ciliary body or anterior chamber, left eye**

        H21.303   **Idiopathic cysts of iris, ciliary body or anterior chamber, bilateral**

        H21.309   **Idiopathic cysts of iris, ciliary body or anterior chamber, unspecified eye**

    ✓6ᵗʰ **H21.31**   **Exudative cysts of iris or anterior chamber**

        H21.311   **Exudative cysts of iris or anterior chamber, right eye**

        H21.312   **Exudative cysts of iris or anterior chamber, left eye**

        H21.313   **Exudative cysts of iris or anterior chamber, bilateral**

        H21.319   **Exudative cysts of iris or anterior chamber, unspecified eye**

    ✓6ᵗʰ **H21.32**   **Implantation cysts of iris, ciliary body or anterior chamber**

        H21.321   **Implantation cysts of iris, ciliary body or anterior chamber, right eye**

        H21.322   **Implantation cysts of iris, ciliary body or anterior chamber, left eye**

        H21.323   **Implantation cysts of iris, ciliary body or anterior chamber, bilateral**

        H21.329   **Implantation cysts of iris, ciliary body or anterior chamber, unspecified eye**

    ✓6ᵗʰ **H21.33**   **Parasitic cyst of iris, ciliary body or anterior chamber**

        H21.331   **Parasitic cyst of iris, ciliary body or anterior chamber, right eye**   CC

        H21.332   **Parasitic cyst of iris, ciliary body or anterior chamber, left eye**   CC

        H21.333   **Parasitic cyst of iris, ciliary body or anterior chamber, bilateral**   CC

        H21.339   **Parasitic cyst of iris, ciliary body or anterior chamber, unspecified eye**   CC UNS

    ✓6ᵗʰ **H21.34**   **Primary cyst of pars plana**

        H21.341   **Primary cyst of pars plana, right eye**

        H21.342   **Primary cyst of pars plana, left eye**

        H21.343   **Primary cyst of pars plana, bilateral**

        H21.349   **Primary cyst of pars plana, unspecified eye**

    ✓6ᵗʰ **H21.35**   **Exudative cyst of pars plana**

        DEF: Protein, fatty-filled bullous elevation of the nonpigmented outermost ciliary epithelium of pars plana, due to fluid leak from blood vessels.

        H21.351   **Exudative cyst of pars plana, right eye**

        H21.352   **Exudative cyst of pars plana, left eye**

        H21.353   **Exudative cyst of pars plana, bilateral**

        H21.359   **Exudative cyst of pars plana, unspecified eye**

✓5ᵗʰ **H21.4**   **Pupillary membranes**

    Iris bombé

    Pupillary occlusion

    Pupillary seclusion

    EXCLUDES 1   congenital pupillary membranes (Q13.8)

    H21.40   **Pupillary membranes, unspecified eye**

    H21.41   **Pupillary membranes, right eye**

    H21.42   **Pupillary membranes, left eye**

    H21.43   **Pupillary membranes, bilateral**

✓5ᵗʰ **H21.5**   **Other and unspecified adhesions and disruptions of iris and ciliary body**

    EXCLUDES 1   corectopia (Q13.2)

    ✓6ᵗʰ **H21.50**   **Unspecified adhesions of iris**

        Synechia (iris) NOS

        H21.501   **Unspecified adhesions of iris, right eye**

        H21.502   **Unspecified adhesions of iris, left eye**

        H21.503   **Unspecified adhesions of iris, bilateral**

        H21.509   **Unspecified adhesions of iris and ciliary body, unspecified eye**

    ✓6ᵗʰ **H21.51**   **Anterior synechiae (iris)**

        H21.511   **Anterior synechiae (iris), right eye**

        H21.512   **Anterior synechiae (iris), left eye**

        H21.513   **Anterior synechiae (iris), bilateral**

        H21.519   **Anterior synechiae (iris), unspecified eye**

    ✓6ᵗʰ **H21.52**   **Goniosynechiae**

        H21.521   **Goniosynechiae, right eye**

        H21.522   **Goniosynechiae, left eye**

        H21.523   **Goniosynechiae, bilateral**

        H21.529   **Goniosynechiae, unspecified eye**

    ✓6ᵗʰ **H21.53**   **Iridodialysis**

        H21.531   **Iridodialysis, right eye**

        H21.532   **Iridodialysis, left eye**

        H21.533   **Iridodialysis, bilateral**

        H21.539   **Iridodialysis, unspecified eye**

    ✓6ᵗʰ **H21.54**   **Posterior synechiae (iris)**

        H21.541   **Posterior synechiae (iris), right eye**

        H21.542   **Posterior synechiae (iris), left eye**

        H21.543   **Posterior synechiae (iris), bilateral**

        H21.549   **Posterior synechiae (iris), unspecified eye**

    ✓6ᵗʰ **H21.55**   **Recession of chamber angle**

        H21.551   **Recession of chamber angle, right eye**

        H21.552   **Recession of chamber angle, left eye**

        H21.553   **Recession of chamber angle, bilateral**

        H21.559   **Recession of chamber angle, unspecified eye**

N Newborn: 0   P Pediatric: 0-17   M Maternity: 9-64   A Adult: 15-124   UNS Unspecified Site   MCC Major Complication/Comorbidity   CC Complication/Comorbidity   PE POA Exempt

622

ICD-10-CM 2025

☑6th H21.56 Pupillary abnormalities
Deformed pupil
Ectopic pupil
Rupture of sphincter, pupil
EXCLUDES 1   congenital deformity of pupil (Q13.2-)

    H21.561 Pupillary abnormality, right eye
    H21.562 Pupillary abnormality, left eye
    H21.563 Pupillary abnormality, bilateral
    H21.569 Pupillary abnormality, unspecified eye

☑5th H21.8 Other specified disorders of iris and ciliary body

    H21.81 Floppy iris syndrome
    Intraoperative floppy iris syndrome (IFIS)
    Use additional code for adverse effect, if applicable, to identify drug (T36-T50 with fifth or sixth character 5)

    H21.82 Plateau iris syndrome (post-iridectomy) (postprocedural)

    H21.89 Other specified disorders of iris and ciliary body

H21.9 Unspecified disorder of iris and ciliary body

H22 Disorders of iris and ciliary body in diseases classified elsewhere
Code first underlying disease, such as:
    gout (M1A.-, M10.-)
    leprosy (A30.-)
    parasitic disease (B89)

Disorders of lens (H25-H28)

☑4th H25 Age-related cataract
Senile cataract
EXCLUDES 2   capsular glaucoma with pseudoexfoliation of lens (H40.1-)

Cataracts

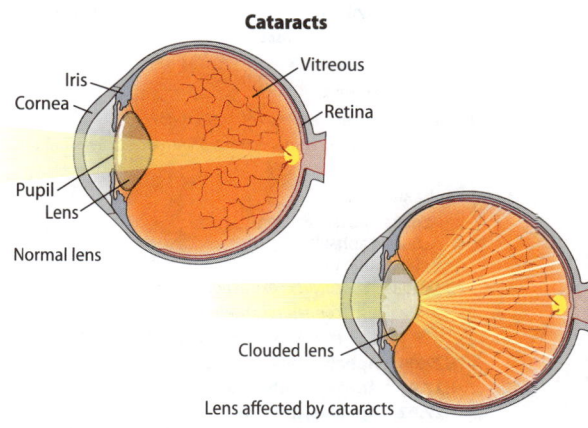

Lens affected by cataracts

☑5th H25.0 Age-related incipient cataract

    ☑6th H25.01 Cortical age-related cataract
        H25.011 Cortical age-related cataract, right eye A
        H25.012 Cortical age-related cataract, left eye A
        H25.013 Cortical age-related cataract, bilateral A
        H25.019 Cortical age-related cataract, unspecified eye A

    ☑6th H25.03 Anterior subcapsular polar age-related cataract
        H25.031 Anterior subcapsular polar age-related cataract, right eye A
        H25.032 Anterior subcapsular polar age-related cataract, left eye A
        H25.033 Anterior subcapsular polar age-related cataract, bilateral A
        H25.039 Anterior subcapsular polar age-related cataract, unspecified eye A

    ☑6th H25.04 Posterior subcapsular polar age-related cataract
        H25.041 Posterior subcapsular polar age-related cataract, right eye A
        H25.042 Posterior subcapsular polar age-related cataract, left eye A
        H25.043 Posterior subcapsular polar age-related cataract, bilateral A
        H25.049 Posterior subcapsular polar age-related cataract, unspecified eye A

☑6th H25.09 Other age-related incipient cataract
Coronary age-related cataract
Punctate age-related cataract
Water clefts
    H25.091 Other age-related incipient cataract, right eye A
    H25.092 Other age-related incipient cataract, left eye A
    H25.093 Other age-related incipient cataract, bilateral A
    H25.099 Other age-related incipient cataract, unspecified eye A

☑5th H25.1 Age-related nuclear cataract
Cataracta brunescens
Nuclear sclerosis cataract
AHA: 2019,2Q,31; 2016,1Q,32
    H25.10 Age-related nuclear cataract, unspecified eye A
    H25.11 Age-related nuclear cataract, right eye A
    H25.12 Age-related nuclear cataract, left eye A
    H25.13 Age-related nuclear cataract, bilateral A

☑5th H25.2 Age-related cataract, morgagnian type
Age-related hypermature cataract
    H25.20 Age-related cataract, morgagnian type, unspecified eye A
    H25.21 Age-related cataract, morgagnian type, right eye A
    H25.22 Age-related cataract, morgagnian type, left eye A
    H25.23 Age-related cataract, morgagnian type, bilateral A

☑5th H25.8 Other age-related cataract

    ☑6th H25.81 Combined forms of age-related cataract
    AHA: 2019,2Q,30
        H25.811 Combined forms of age-related cataract, right eye A
        H25.812 Combined forms of age-related cataract, left eye A
        H25.813 Combined forms of age-related cataract, bilateral A
        H25.819 Combined forms of age-related cataract, unspecified eye A

    H25.89 Other age-related cataract A

H25.9 Unspecified age-related cataract A

☑4th H26 Other cataract
EXCLUDES 1   congenital cataract (Q12.0)

☑5th H26.0 Infantile and juvenile cataract

    ☑6th H26.00 Unspecified infantile and juvenile cataract
        H26.001 Unspecified infantile and juvenile cataract, right eye P
        H26.002 Unspecified infantile and juvenile cataract, left eye P
        H26.003 Unspecified infantile and juvenile cataract, bilateral P
        H26.009 Unspecified infantile and juvenile cataract, unspecified eye P

    ☑6th H26.01 Infantile and juvenile cortical, lamellar, or zonular cataract
        H26.011 Infantile and juvenile cortical, lamellar, or zonular cataract, right eye P
        H26.012 Infantile and juvenile cortical, lamellar, or zonular cataract, left eye P
        H26.013 Infantile and juvenile cortical, lamellar, or zonular cataract, bilateral P
        H26.019 Infantile and juvenile cortical, lamellar, or zonular cataract, unspecified eye P

    ☑6th H26.03 Infantile and juvenile nuclear cataract
        H26.031 Infantile and juvenile nuclear cataract, right eye P
        H26.032 Infantile and juvenile nuclear cataract, left eye P
        H26.033 Infantile and juvenile nuclear cataract, bilateral P
        H26.039 Infantile and juvenile nuclear cataract, unspecified eye P

    ☑6th H26.04 Anterior subcapsular polar infantile and juvenile cataract
        H26.041 Anterior subcapsular polar infantile and juvenile cataract, right eye P

☑ Additional Character Required   ☑x7th Placeholder   Questionable PDx   Manifestation   Unspecified   UPD Unacceptable PDx   H1 - H4 HAC   HCC CMS-HCC Dx   HIV HIV Dx

ICD-10-CM 2025   623

Chapter 7. Diseases of the Eye and Adnexa

H21.56-H26.041

H26.042   Anterior subcapsular polar infantile and juvenile cataract, **left** eye   **P**

H26.043   Anterior subcapsular polar infantile and juvenile cataract, **bilateral**   **P**

H26.049   Anterior subcapsular polar infantile and juvenile cataract, unspecified eye   **P**

√6ᵗʰ   H26.05   **Posterior subcapsular polar** infantile and juvenile cataract

H26.051   Posterior subcapsular polar infantile and juvenile cataract, **right** eye   **P**

H26.052   Posterior subcapsular polar infantile and juvenile cataract, **left** eye   **P**

H26.053   Posterior subcapsular polar infantile and juvenile cataract, **bilateral**   **P**

H26.059   Posterior subcapsular polar infantile and juvenile cataract, unspecified eye   **P**

√6ᵗʰ   H26.06   **Combined forms** of infantile and juvenile cataract

H26.061   Combined forms of infantile and juvenile cataract, **right** eye   **P**

H26.062   Combined forms of infantile and juvenile cataract, **left** eye   **P**

H26.063   Combined forms of infantile and juvenile cataract, **bilateral**   **P**

H26.069   Combined forms of infantile and juvenile cataract, unspecified eye   **P**

H26.09   Other infantile and juvenile cataract   **P**

√5ᵗʰ   H26.1   **Traumatic** cataract

Use additional code (Chapter 20) to identify external cause

√6ᵗʰ   H26.10   Unspecified traumatic cataract

H26.101   Unspecified traumatic cataract, **right** eye

H26.102   Unspecified traumatic cataract, **left** eye

H26.103   Unspecified traumatic cataract, **bilateral**

H26.109   Unspecified traumatic cataract, unspecified eye

√6ᵗʰ   H26.11   **Localized** traumatic opacities

H26.111   Localized traumatic opacities, **right** eye

H26.112   Localized traumatic opacities, **left** eye

H26.113   Localized traumatic opacities, **bilateral**

H26.119   Localized traumatic opacities, unspecified eye

√6ᵗʰ   H26.12   **Partially resolved** traumatic cataract

H26.121   Partially resolved traumatic cataract, **right** eye

H26.122   Partially resolved traumatic cataract, **left** eye

H26.123   Partially resolved traumatic cataract, **bilateral**

H26.129   Partially resolved traumatic cataract, unspecified eye

√6ᵗʰ   H26.13   **Total** traumatic cataract

H26.131   Total traumatic cataract, **right** eye

H26.132   Total traumatic cataract, **left** eye

H26.133   Total traumatic cataract, **bilateral**

H26.139   Total traumatic cataract, unspecified eye

√5ᵗʰ   H26.2   **Complicated** cataract

H26.20   Unspecified complicated cataract

Cataracta complicata NOS

√6ᵗʰ   H26.21   Cataract **with neovascularization**

Code also, if applicable, associated condition, such as: chronic iridocyclitis (H20.1-)

H26.211   Cataract with neovascularization, **right** eye

H26.212   Cataract with neovascularization, **left** eye

H26.213   Cataract with neovascularization, **bilateral**

H26.219   Cataract with neovascularization, unspecified eye

√6ᵗʰ   H26.22   Cataract **secondary to ocular disorders** (degenerative) (inflammatory)

Code also associated ocular disorder

H26.221   Cataract secondary to ocular disorders (degenerative) (inflammatory), **right** eye

H26.222   Cataract secondary to ocular disorders (degenerative) (inflammatory), **left** eye

H26.223   Cataract secondary to ocular disorders (degenerative) (inflammatory), **bilateral**

H26.229   Cataract secondary to ocular disorders (degenerative) (inflammatory), unspecified eye

√6ᵗʰ   H26.23   **Glaucomatous flecks** (subcapsular)

Code first underlying glaucoma (H40-H42)

H26.231   Glaucomatous flecks (subcapsular), **right** eye

H26.232   Glaucomatous flecks (subcapsular), **left** eye

H26.233   Glaucomatous flecks (subcapsular), **bilateral**

H26.239   Glaucomatous flecks (subcapsular), unspecified eye

√5ᵗʰ   H26.3   **Drug-induced** cataract

Toxic cataract

Use additional code for adverse effect, if applicable, to identify drug (T36-T50 with fifth or sixth character 5)

H26.30   Drug-induced cataract, unspecified eye

H26.31   Drug-induced cataract, **right** eye

H26.32   Drug-induced cataract, **left** eye

H26.33   Drug-induced cataract, **bilateral**

√5ᵗʰ   H26.4   **Secondary** cataract

H26.40   Unspecified secondary cataract

√6ᵗʰ   H26.41   **Soemmering's ring**

H26.411   Soemmering's ring, **right** eye

H26.412   Soemmering's ring, **left** eye

H26.413   Soemmering's ring, **bilateral**

H26.419   Soemmering's ring, unspecified eye

√6ᵗʰ   H26.49   **Other secondary cataract**

AHA: 2018,2Q,14

H26.491   Other secondary cataract, **right** eye

H26.492   Other secondary cataract, **left** eye

H26.493   Other secondary cataract, **bilateral**

H26.499   Other secondary cataract, unspecified eye

H26.8   Other specified cataract

H26.9   Unspecified cataract

√4ᵗʰ   **H27**   **Other disorders of lens**

EXCLUDES 1   *congenital lens malformations (Q12.-)*

mechanical complications of intraocular lens implant (T85.2)

pseudophakia (Z96.1)

√5ᵗʰ   H27.0   **Aphakia**

Acquired absence of lens

Acquired aphakia

Aphakia due to trauma

EXCLUDES 1   *cataract extraction status (Z98.4-)*

congenital absence of lens (Q12.3)

congenital aphakia (Q12.3)

H27.00   Aphakia, unspecified eye

H27.01   Aphakia, **right** eye

H27.02   Aphakia, **left** eye

H27.03   Aphakia, **bilateral**

√5ᵗʰ   H27.1   **Dislocation of lens**

H27.10   Unspecified dislocation of lens

√6ᵗʰ   H27.11   Subluxation of lens

H27.111   Subluxation of lens, **right** eye

H27.112   Subluxation of lens, **left** eye

H27.113   Subluxation of lens, **bilateral**

H27.119   Subluxation of lens, unspecified eye

√6ᵗʰ   H27.12   Anterior dislocation of lens

H27.121   Anterior dislocation of lens, **right** eye

H27.122   Anterior dislocation of lens, **left** eye

H27.123   Anterior dislocation of lens, **bilateral**

H27.129   Anterior dislocation of lens, unspecified eye

√6ᵗʰ   H27.13   Posterior dislocation of lens

H27.131   Posterior dislocation of lens, **right** eye

H27.132   Posterior dislocation of lens, **left** eye

H27.133   Posterior dislocation of lens, **bilateral**

H27.139   Posterior dislocation of lens, unspecified eye

H27.8   Other specified disorders of lens

H27.9   Unspecified disorder of lens

N Newborn: 0   **P** Pediatric: 0-17   **M** Maternity: 9-64   **A** Adult: 15-124   **UNS** Unspecified Site   **MCC** Major Complication/Comorbidity   **CC** Complication/Comorbidity   **PE** POA Exempt

624

ICD-10-CM 2025

H28   *Cataract in diseases classified elsewhere*

Code first underlying disease, such as:
hypoparathyroidism (E20.-)
myotonia (G71.1-)
myxedema (E03.-)
protein-calorie malnutrition (E40-E46)

EXCLUDES 1   cataract in diabetes mellitus (E08.36, E09.36, E10.36, E11.36, E13.36)

Disorders of choroid and retina (H30-H36)

✓4th **H30**   **Chorioretinal inflammation**

   ✓5th **H30.0**   **Focal chorioretinal inflammation**

Focal chorioretinitis
Focal choroiditis
Focal retinitis
Focal retinochoroiditis

    ✓6th **H30.00**   **Unspecified focal chorioretinal inflammation**

Focal chorioretinitis NOS
Focal choroiditis NOS
Focal retinitis NOS
Focal retinochoroiditis NOS

     H30.001   Unspecified focal chorioretinal inflammation, **right** eye
     H30.002   Unspecified focal chorioretinal inflammation, **left** eye
     H30.003   Unspecified focal chorioretinal inflammation, **bilateral**
     H30.009   Unspecified focal chorioretinal inflammation, unspecified eye

    ✓6th **H30.01**   **Focal chorioretinal inflammation, juxtapapillary**

     H30.011   Focal chorioretinal inflammation, juxtapapillary, **right** eye
     H30.012   Focal chorioretinal inflammation, juxtapapillary, **left** eye
     H30.013   Focal chorioretinal inflammation, juxtapapillary, **bilateral**
     H30.019   Focal chorioretinal inflammation, juxtapapillary, unspecified eye

    ✓6th **H30.02**   **Focal chorioretinal inflammation of posterior pole**

     H30.021   Focal chorioretinal inflammation of posterior pole, **right** eye
     H30.022   Focal chorioretinal inflammation of posterior pole, **left** eye
     H30.023   Focal chorioretinal inflammation of posterior pole, **bilateral**
     H30.029   Focal chorioretinal inflammation of posterior pole, unspecified eye

    ✓6th **H30.03**   **Focal chorioretinal inflammation, peripheral**

     H30.031   Focal chorioretinal inflammation, peripheral, **right** eye
     H30.032   Focal chorioretinal inflammation, peripheral, **left** eye
     H30.033   Focal chorioretinal inflammation, peripheral, **bilateral**
     H30.039   Focal chorioretinal inflammation, peripheral, unspecified eye

    ✓6th **H30.04**   **Focal chorioretinal inflammation, macular or paramacular**

     H30.041   Focal chorioretinal inflammation, macular or paramacular, **right** eye
     H30.042   Focal chorioretinal inflammation, macular or paramacular, **left** eye
     H30.043   Focal chorioretinal inflammation, macular or paramacular, **bilateral**
     H30.049   Focal chorioretinal inflammation, macular or paramacular, unspecified eye

   ✓5th **H30.1**   **Disseminated chorioretinal inflammation**

Disseminated chorioretinitis
Disseminated choroiditis
Disseminated retinitis
Disseminated retinochoroiditis

EXCLUDES 2   exudative retinopathy (H35.02-)

    ✓6th **H30.10**   **Unspecified disseminated chorioretinal inflammation**

Disseminated chorioretinitis NOS
Disseminated choroiditis NOS
Disseminated retinitis NOS
Disseminated retinochoroiditis NOS

     H30.101   Unspecified disseminated chorioretinal inflammation, **right** eye   CC

     H30.102   Unspecified disseminated chorioretinal inflammation, **left** eye   CC
     H30.103   Unspecified disseminated chorioretinal inflammation, **bilateral**   CC
     H30.109   Unspecified disseminated chorioretinal inflammation, unspecified eye   CC UNS

    ✓6th **H30.11**   **Disseminated chorioretinal inflammation of posterior pole**

     H30.111   Disseminated chorioretinal inflammation of posterior pole, **right** eye   CC
     H30.112   Disseminated chorioretinal inflammation of posterior pole, **left** eye   CC
     H30.113   Disseminated chorioretinal inflammation of posterior pole, **bilateral**   CC
     H30.119   Disseminated chorioretinal inflammation of posterior pole, unspecified eye   CC UNS

    ✓6th **H30.12**   **Disseminated chorioretinal inflammation, peripheral**

     H30.121   Disseminated chorioretinal inflammation, peripheral **right** eye   CC
     H30.122   Disseminated chorioretinal inflammation, peripheral, **left** eye   CC
     H30.123   Disseminated chorioretinal inflammation, peripheral, **bilateral**   CC
     H30.129   Disseminated chorioretinal inflammation, peripheral, unspecified eye   CC UNS

    ✓6th **H30.13**   **Disseminated chorioretinal inflammation, generalized**

     H30.131   Disseminated chorioretinal inflammation, generalized, **right** eye   CC
     H30.132   Disseminated chorioretinal inflammation, generalized, **left** eye   CC
     H30.133   Disseminated chorioretinal inflammation, generalized, **bilateral**   CC
     H30.139   Disseminated chorioretinal inflammation, generalized, unspecified eye   CC UNS

    ✓6th **H30.14**   **Acute posterior multifocal placoid pigment epitheliopathy**

     H30.141   Acute posterior multifocal placoid pigment epitheliopathy, **right** eye   CC
     H30.142   Acute posterior multifocal placoid pigment epitheliopathy, **left** eye   CC
     H30.143   Acute posterior multifocal placoid pigment epitheliopathy, **bilateral**   CC
     H30.149   Acute posterior multifocal placoid pigment epitheliopathy, unspecified eye   CC UNS

   ✓5th **H30.2**   **Posterior cyclitis**

Pars planitis

    H30.20   Posterior cyclitis, unspecified eye
    H30.21   Posterior cyclitis, **right** eye
    H30.22   Posterior cyclitis, **left** eye
    H30.23   Posterior cyclitis, **bilateral**

   ✓5th **H30.8**   **Other chorioretinal inflammations**

    ✓6th **H30.81**   **Harada's disease**

     H30.811   Harada's disease, **right** eye
     H30.812   Harada's disease, **left** eye
     H30.813   Harada's disease, **bilateral**
     H30.819   Harada's disease, unspecified eye

    ✓6th **H30.89**   **Other chorioretinal inflammations**

     H30.891   Other chorioretinal inflammations, **right** eye   CC
     H30.892   Other chorioretinal inflammations, **left** eye   CC
     H30.893   Other chorioretinal inflammations, **bilateral**   CC
     H30.899   Other chorioretinal inflammations, unspecified eye   CC UNS

   ✓5th **H30.9**   **Unspecified chorioretinal inflammation**

Chorioretinitis NOS
Choroiditis NOS
Neuroretinitis NOS
Retinitis NOS
Retinochoroiditis NOS

    H30.90   Unspecified chorioretinal inflammation, unspecified eye   CC UNS
    H30.91   Unspecified chorioretinal inflammation, **right** eye   CC
    H30.92   Unspecified chorioretinal inflammation, **left** eye   CC

✔ Additional Character Required   ✓x7th Placeholder   Questionable PDx   Manifestation   Unspecified   UPD Unacceptable PDx   H1-H14 HAC   HCC CMS-HCC Dx   HIV HIV Dx

ICD-10-CM 2025   625

H30.93 Unspecified chorioretinal inflammation, **bilateral**   CC

✓4ᵗʰ **H31 Other disorders of choroid**

  ✓5ᵗʰ **H31.0 Chorioretinal scars**

      EXCLUDES 2   *postsurgical chorioretinal scars (H59.81-)*

    ✓6ᵗʰ **H31.00 Unspecified chorioretinal scars**

      H31.001 Unspecified chorioretinal scars, **right** eye

      H31.002 Unspecified chorioretinal scars, **left** eye

      H31.003 Unspecified chorioretinal scars, **bilateral**

      H31.009 Unspecified chorioretinal scars, unspecified eye

    ✓6ᵗʰ **H31.01 Macula scars of posterior pole (postinflammatory) (post-traumatic)**

      EXCLUDES 1   *postprocedural chorioretinal scar (H59.81-)*

      H31.011 Macula scars of posterior pole (postinflammatory) (post-traumatic), **right** eye

      H31.012 Macula scars of posterior pole (postinflammatory) (post-traumatic), **left** eye

      H31.013 Macula scars of posterior pole (postinflammatory) (post-traumatic), **bilateral**

      H31.019 Macula scars of posterior pole (postinflammatory) (post-traumatic), unspecified eye

    ✓6ᵗʰ **H31.02 Solar retinopathy**

      H31.021 Solar retinopathy, **right** eye

      H31.022 Solar retinopathy, **left** eye

      H31.023 Solar retinopathy, **bilateral**

      H31.029 Solar retinopathy, unspecified eye

    ✓6ᵗʰ **H31.09 Other chorioretinal scars**

      H31.091 Other chorioretinal scars, **right** eye

      H31.092 Other chorioretinal scars, **left** eye

      H31.093 Other chorioretinal scars, **bilateral**

      H31.099 Other chorioretinal scars, unspecified eye

  ✓5ᵗʰ **H31.1 Choroidal degeneration**

      EXCLUDES 2   *angioid streaks of macula (H35.33)*

    ✓6ᵗʰ **H31.10 Unspecified choroidal degeneration**

      Choroidal sclerosis NOS

      H31.101 Choroidal degeneration, unspecified, **right** eye

      H31.102 Choroidal degeneration, unspecified, **left** eye

      H31.103 Choroidal degeneration, unspecified, **bilateral**

      H31.109 Choroidal degeneration, unspecified, unspecified eye

    ✓6ᵗʰ **H31.11 Age-related choroidal atrophy**

      H31.111 Age-related choroidal atrophy, **right** eye   A

      H31.112 Age-related choroidal atrophy, **left** eye   A

      H31.113 Age-related choroidal atrophy, **bilateral**   A

      H31.119 Age-related choroidal atrophy, unspecified eye   A

    ✓6ᵗʰ **H31.12 Diffuse secondary atrophy of choroid**

      H31.121 Diffuse secondary atrophy of choroid, **right** eye

      H31.122 Diffuse secondary atrophy of choroid, **left** eye

      H31.123 Diffuse secondary atrophy of choroid, **bilateral**

      H31.129 Diffuse secondary atrophy of choroid, unspecified eye

  ✓5ᵗʰ **H31.2 Hereditary choroidal dystrophy**

      EXCLUDES 2   *hyperornithinemia (E72.4)*

               ornithinemia (E72.4)

    H31.20 Hereditary choroidal dystrophy, unspecified

    H31.21 Choroideremia

    H31.22 Choroidal dystrophy (central areolar) (generalized) (peripapillary)

    H31.23 Gyrate atrophy, choroid

    H31.29 Other hereditary choroidal dystrophy

  ✓5ᵗʰ **H31.3 Choroidal hemorrhage and rupture**

    ✓6ᵗʰ **H31.30 Unspecified choroidal hemorrhage**

      H31.301 Unspecified choroidal hemorrhage, **right** eye

      H31.302 Unspecified choroidal hemorrhage, **left** eye

      H31.303 Unspecified choroidal hemorrhage, **bilateral**

      H31.309 Unspecified choroidal hemorrhage, unspecified eye

    ✓6ᵗʰ **H31.31 Expulsive choroidal hemorrhage**

      H31.311 Expulsive choroidal hemorrhage, **right** eye

      H31.312 Expulsive choroidal hemorrhage, **left** eye

      H31.313 Expulsive choroidal hemorrhage, **bilateral**

      H31.319 Expulsive choroidal hemorrhage, unspecified eye

    ✓6ᵗʰ **H31.32 Choroidal rupture**

      H31.321 Choroidal rupture, **right** eye   CC

      H31.322 Choroidal rupture, **left** eye   CC

      H31.323 Choroidal rupture, **bilateral**   CC

      H31.329 Choroidal rupture, unspecified eye   CC UNS

  ✓5ᵗʰ **H31.4 Choroidal detachment**

    ✓6ᵗʰ **H31.40 Unspecified choroidal detachment**

      H31.401 Unspecified choroidal detachment, **right** eye   CC

      H31.402 Unspecified choroidal detachment, **left** eye   CC

      H31.403 Unspecified choroidal detachment, **bilateral**   CC

      H31.409 Unspecified choroidal detachment, unspecified eye   CC UNS

    ✓6ᵗʰ **H31.41 Hemorrhagic choroidal detachment**

      H31.411 Hemorrhagic choroidal detachment, **right** eye   CC

      H31.412 Hemorrhagic choroidal detachment, **left** eye   CC

      H31.413 Hemorrhagic choroidal detachment, **bilateral**   CC

      H31.419 Hemorrhagic choroidal detachment, unspecified eye   CC UNS

    ✓6ᵗʰ **H31.42 Serous choroidal detachment**

      H31.421 Serous choroidal detachment, **right** eye   CC

      H31.422 Serous choroidal detachment, **left** eye   CC

      H31.423 Serous choroidal detachment, **bilateral**   CC

      H31.429 Serous choroidal detachment, unspecified eye   CC UNS

  H31.8 Other specified disorders of choroid

  H31.9 Unspecified disorder of choroid

H32 ***Chorioretinal disorders in diseases classified elsewhere***

Code first underlying disease, such as:
  congenital toxoplasmosis (P37.1)
  histoplasmosis (B39.-)
  leprosy (A30.-)

    EXCLUDES 1   *chorioretinitis (in):*
               toxoplasmosis (acquired) (B58.01)
               tuberculosis (A18.53)

N Newborn: 0   **P** Pediatric: 0-17   **M** Maternity: 9-64   **A** Adult: 15-124   **UNS** Unspecified Site   **MCC** Major Complication/Comorbidity   **CC** Complication/Comorbidity   **PE** POA Exempt

626   ICD-10-CM 2025

✓4ᵗʰ H33   Retinal detachments and breaks

> EXCLUDES 1   *detachment of retinal pigment epithelium (H35.72-, H35.73-)*

Retinal Detachment

Labeled: Vitreous, Choroid, Area of detachment, Retina, Sclera, Cornea, Lens, Iris

✓5ᵗʰ H33.0   Retinal detachment with retinal break

Rhegmatogenous retinal detachment

> EXCLUDES 1   *serous retinal detachment (without retinal break) (H33.2-)*

✓6ᵗʰ H33.00   Unspecified retinal detachment with retinal break

- H33.001   Unspecified retinal detachment with retinal break, **right** eye
- H33.002   Unspecified retinal detachment with retinal break, **left** eye
- H33.003   Unspecified retinal detachment with retinal break, **bilateral**
- H33.009   Unspecified retinal detachment with retinal break, unspecified eye

✓6ᵗʰ H33.01   Retinal detachment with single break

- H33.011   Retinal detachment with single break, **right** eye
- H33.012   Retinal detachment with single break, **left** eye
- H33.013   Retinal detachment with single break, **bilateral**
- H33.019   Retinal detachment with single break, unspecified eye

✓6ᵗʰ H33.02   Retinal detachment with multiple breaks

- H33.021   Retinal detachment with multiple breaks, **right** eye
- H33.022   Retinal detachment with multiple breaks, **left** eye
- H33.023   Retinal detachment with multiple breaks, **bilateral**
- H33.029   Retinal detachment with multiple breaks, unspecified eye

✓6ᵗʰ H33.03   Retinal detachment with giant retinal tear

- H33.031   Retinal detachment with giant retinal tear, **right** eye
- H33.032   Retinal detachment with giant retinal tear, **left** eye
- H33.033   Retinal detachment with giant retinal tear, **bilateral**
- H33.039   Retinal detachment with giant retinal tear, unspecified eye

✓6ᵗʰ H33.04   Retinal detachment with retinal dialysis

- H33.041   Retinal detachment with retinal dialysis, **right** eye
- H33.042   Retinal detachment with retinal dialysis, **left** eye
- H33.043   Retinal detachment with retinal dialysis, **bilateral**
- H33.049   Retinal detachment with retinal dialysis, unspecified eye

✓6ᵗʰ H33.05   Total retinal detachment

- H33.051   Total retinal detachment, **right** eye
- H33.052   Total retinal detachment, **left** eye
- H33.053   Total retinal detachment, **bilateral**
- H33.059   Total retinal detachment, unspecified eye

✓5ᵗʰ H33.1   Retinoschisis and retinal cysts

> EXCLUDES 1   *congenital retinoschisis (Q14.1)*
> *microcystoid degeneration of retina (H35.42-)*

✓6ᵗʰ H33.10   Unspecified retinoschisis

- H33.101   Unspecified retinoschisis, **right** eye
- H33.102   Unspecified retinoschisis, **left** eye
- H33.103   Unspecified retinoschisis, **bilateral**
- H33.109   Unspecified retinoschisis, unspecified eye

✓6ᵗʰ H33.11   Cyst of ora serrata

- H33.111   Cyst of ora serrata, **right** eye
- H33.112   Cyst of ora serrata, **left** eye
- H33.113   Cyst of ora serrata, **bilateral**
- H33.119   Cyst of ora serrata, unspecified eye

✓6ᵗʰ H33.12   Parasitic cyst of retina

- H33.121   Parasitic cyst of retina, **right** eye   CC
- H33.122   Parasitic cyst of retina, **left** eye   CC
- H33.123   Parasitic cyst of retina, **bilateral**   CC
- H33.129   Parasitic cyst of retina, unspecified eye   CC UNS

✓6ᵗʰ H33.19   Other retinoschisis and retinal cysts

Pseudocyst of retina

- H33.191   Other retinoschisis and retinal cysts, **right** eye
- H33.192   Other retinoschisis and retinal cysts, **left** eye
- H33.193   Other retinoschisis and retinal cysts, **bilateral**
- H33.199   Other retinoschisis and retinal cysts, unspecified eye

✓5ᵗʰ H33.2   Serous retinal detachment

Retinal detachment NOS
Retinal detachment without retinal break

> EXCLUDES 1   *central serous chorioretinopathy (H35.71-)*

- H33.20   Serous retinal detachment, unspecified eye   CC UNS
- H33.21   Serous retinal detachment, **right** eye   CC
- H33.22   Serous retinal detachment, **left** eye   CC
- H33.23   Serous retinal detachment, **bilateral**   CC

✓5ᵗʰ H33.3   Retinal breaks without detachment

> EXCLUDES 1   *chorioretinal scars after surgery for detachment (H59.81-)*
> *peripheral retinal degeneration without break (H35.4-)*

✓6ᵗʰ H33.30   Unspecified retinal break

- H33.301   Unspecified retinal break, **right** eye
- H33.302   Unspecified retinal break, **left** eye
- H33.303   Unspecified retinal break, **bilateral**
- H33.309   Unspecified retinal break, unspecified eye

✓6ᵗʰ H33.31   Horseshoe tear of retina without detachment

Operculum of retina without detachment

- H33.311   Horseshoe tear of retina without detachment, **right** eye
- H33.312   Horseshoe tear of retina without detachment, **left** eye
- H33.313   Horseshoe tear of retina without detachment, **bilateral**
- H33.319   Horseshoe tear of retina without detachment, unspecified eye

✓6ᵗʰ H33.32   Round hole of retina without detachment

- H33.321   Round hole, **right** eye
- H33.322   Round hole, **left** eye
- H33.323   Round hole, **bilateral**
- H33.329   Round hole, unspecified eye

✓6ᵗʰ H33.33   Multiple defects of retina without detachment

- H33.331   Multiple defects of retina without detachment, **right** eye
- H33.332   Multiple defects of retina without detachment, **left** eye
- H33.333   Multiple defects of retina without detachment, **bilateral**
- H33.339   Multiple defects of retina without detachment, unspecified eye

✓5ᵗʰ H33.4   Traction detachment of retina

Proliferative vitreo-retinopathy with retinal detachment

- H33.40   Traction detachment of retina, unspecified eye   CC UNS
- H33.41   Traction detachment of retina, **right** eye   CC
- H33.42   Traction detachment of retina, **left** eye   CC
- H33.43   Traction detachment of retina, **bilateral**   CC

H33.8   Other retinal detachments   CC

☑ Additional Character Required   ✓x7ᵗʰ Placeholder   Questionable PDx   Manifestation   Unspecified   UPD Unacceptable PDx   H1-H14 HAC   HCC CMS-HCC Dx   HIV HIV Dx

ICD-10-CM 2025   627

✓4ᵗʰ H34 Retinal vascular occlusions

> **EXCLUDES 1**   *amaurosis fugax (G45.3)*

✓5ᵗʰ H34.0 Transient retinal artery occlusion

     H34.00 Transient retinal artery occlusion, unspecified eye CC UNS

     H34.01 Transient retinal artery occlusion, **right** eye CC

     H34.02 Transient retinal artery occlusion, **left** eye CC

     H34.03 Transient retinal artery occlusion, **bilateral** CC

✓5ᵗʰ H34.1 Central retinal artery occlusion

     H34.10 Central retinal artery occlusion, unspecified eye CC UNS

     H34.11 Central retinal artery occlusion, **right** eye CC

     H34.12 Central retinal artery occlusion, **left** eye CC

     H34.13 Central retinal artery occlusion, **bilateral** CC

✓5ᵗʰ H34.2 Other retinal artery occlusions

     ✓6ᵗʰ H34.21 Partial retinal artery occlusion

         Hollenhorst's plaque
         Retinal microembolism

         H34.211 Partial retinal artery occlusion, **right** eye CC

         H34.212 Partial retinal artery occlusion, **left** eye CC

         H34.213 Partial retinal artery occlusion, **bilateral** CC

         H34.219 Partial retinal artery occlusion, unspecified eye CC UNS

     ✓6ᵗʰ H34.23 Retinal artery branch occlusion

         H34.231 Retinal artery branch occlusion, **right** eye CC

         H34.232 Retinal artery branch occlusion, **left** eye CC

         H34.233 Retinal artery branch occlusion, **bilateral** CC

         H34.239 Retinal artery branch occlusion, unspecified eye CC UNS

✓5ᵗʰ H34.8 Other retinal vascular occlusions

     AHA: 2016,4Q,19

     ✓6ᵗʰ H34.81 Central retinal vein occlusion

> One of the following 7th characters is to be assigned to codes in subcategory H34.81 to designate the severity of the occlusion:
> 0   with macular edema
> 1   with retinal neovascularization
> 2   stable
>   old central retinal vein occlusion

         ✓7ᵗʰ H34.811 Central retinal vein occlusion, right eye CC HCC

         ✓7ᵗʰ H34.812 Central retinal vein occlusion, left eye CC HCC

         ✓7ᵗʰ H34.813 Central retinal vein occlusion, bilateral CC HCC

         ✓7ᵗʰ H34.819 Central retinal vein occlusion, unspecified eye CC UNS HCC

     ✓6ᵗʰ H34.82 Venous engorgement

         Incipient retinal vein occlusion
         Partial retinal vein occlusion

         H34.821 Venous engorgement, **right** eye

         H34.822 Venous engorgement, **left** eye

         H34.823 Venous engorgement, **bilateral**

         H34.829 Venous engorgement, unspecified eye

     ✓6ᵗʰ H34.83 Tributary (branch) retinal vein occlusion

> One of the following 7th characters is to be assigned to codes in subcategory H34.83 to designate the severity of the occlusion:
> 0   with macular edema
> 1   with retinal neovascularization
> 2   stable
>   old tributary (branch) retinal vein occlusion

         ✓7ᵗʰ H34.831 Tributary (branch) retinal vein occlusion, right eye HCC

         ✓7ᵗʰ H34.832 Tributary (branch) retinal vein occlusion, left eye HCC

         ✓7ᵗʰ H34.833 Tributary (branch) retinal vein occlusion, bilateral HCC

         ✓7ᵗʰ H34.839 Tributary (branch) retinal vein occlusion, unspecified eye HCC

H34.9 Unspecified retinal vascular occlusion CC

✓4ᵗʰ H35 Other retinal disorders

> **EXCLUDES 2**   *diabetic retinal disorders (E08.311-E08.359, E09.311-E09.359, E10.311-E10.359, E11.311-E11.359, E13.311-E13.359)*

✓5ᵗʰ H35.0 Background retinopathy and retinal vascular changes

     Code also any associated hypertension (I10)

     H35.00 Unspecified background retinopathy

     ✓6ᵗʰ H35.01 Changes in retinal vascular appearance

         Retinal vascular sheathing

         H35.011 Changes in retinal vascular appearance, **right** eye

         H35.012 Changes in retinal vascular appearance, **left** eye

         H35.013 Changes in retinal vascular appearance, **bilateral**

         H35.019 Changes in retinal vascular appearance, unspecified eye

     ✓6ᵗʰ H35.02 Exudative retinopathy

         Coats retinopathy

         H35.021 Exudative retinopathy, **right** eye

         H35.022 Exudative retinopathy, **left** eye

         H35.023 Exudative retinopathy, **bilateral**

         H35.029 Exudative retinopathy, unspecified eye

     ✓6ᵗʰ H35.03 Hypertensive retinopathy

         H35.031 Hypertensive retinopathy, **right** eye

         H35.032 Hypertensive retinopathy, **left** eye

         H35.033 Hypertensive retinopathy, **bilateral**

         H35.039 Hypertensive retinopathy, unspecified eye

     ✓6ᵗʰ H35.04 Retinal micro-aneurysms, unspecified

         H35.041 Retinal micro-aneurysms, unspecified, right eye

         H35.042 Retinal micro-aneurysms, unspecified, left eye

         H35.043 Retinal micro-aneurysms, unspecified, bilateral

         H35.049 Retinal micro-aneurysms, unspecified, unspecified eye

     ✓6ᵗʰ H35.05 Retinal neovascularization, unspecified

         H35.051 Retinal neovascularization, unspecified, right eye

         H35.052 Retinal neovascularization, unspecified, left eye

         H35.053 Retinal neovascularization, unspecified, bilateral

         H35.059 Retinal neovascularization, unspecified, unspecified eye

     ✓6ᵗʰ H35.06 Retinal vasculitis

         Eales disease
         Retinal perivasculitis
         DEF: Sight-threatening intraocular inflammation of the retinal blood vessels that causes minimal, partial, or even complete blindness.

         H35.061 Retinal vasculitis, **right** eye

         H35.062 Retinal vasculitis, **left** eye

         H35.063 Retinal vasculitis, **bilateral**

         H35.069 Retinal vasculitis, unspecified eye

     ✓6ᵗʰ H35.07 Retinal telangiectasis

         H35.071 Retinal telangiectasis, **right** eye

         H35.072 Retinal telangiectasis, **left** eye

         H35.073 Retinal telangiectasis, **bilateral**

         H35.079 Retinal telangiectasis, unspecified eye

     H35.09 Other intraretinal microvascular abnormalities

         Retinal varices

✓5ᵗʰ H35.1 Retinopathy of prematurity

     ✓6ᵗʰ H35.10 Retinopathy of prematurity, unspecified

         Retinopathy of prematurity NOS

         H35.101 Retinopathy of prematurity, unspecified, right eye

         H35.102 Retinopathy of prematurity, unspecified, left eye

         H35.103 Retinopathy of prematurity, unspecified, bilateral

         H35.109 Retinopathy of prematurity, unspecified, unspecified eye

---

N Newborn: 0   P Pediatric: 0-17   M Maternity: 9-64   A Adult: 15-124   UNS Unspecified Site   MCC Major Complication/Comorbidity   CC Complication/Comorbidity   PE POA Exempt

628   ICD-10-CM 2025

✓6th **H35.11** **Retinopathy of prematurity, stage 0**

     H35.111   **Retinopathy of prematurity, stage 0, right eye**

     H35.112   **Retinopathy of prematurity, stage 0, left eye**

     H35.113   **Retinopathy of prematurity, stage 0, bilateral**

     H35.119   **Retinopathy of prematurity, stage 0, unspecified eye**

✓6th **H35.12** **Retinopathy of prematurity, stage 1**

     H35.121   **Retinopathy of prematurity, stage 1, right eye**

     H35.122   **Retinopathy of prematurity, stage 1, left eye**

     H35.123   **Retinopathy of prematurity, stage 1, bilateral**

     H35.129   **Retinopathy of prematurity, stage 1, unspecified eye**

✓6th **H35.13** **Retinopathy of prematurity, stage 2**

     H35.131   **Retinopathy of prematurity, stage 2, right eye**

     H35.132   **Retinopathy of prematurity, stage 2, left eye**

     H35.133   **Retinopathy of prematurity, stage 2, bilateral**

     H35.139   **Retinopathy of prematurity, stage 2, unspecified eye**

✓6th **H35.14** **Retinopathy of prematurity, stage 3**

     H35.141   **Retinopathy of prematurity, stage 3, right eye**

     H35.142   **Retinopathy of prematurity, stage 3, left eye**

     H35.143   **Retinopathy of prematurity, stage 3, bilateral**

     H35.149   **Retinopathy of prematurity, stage 3, unspecified eye**

✓6th **H35.15** **Retinopathy of prematurity, stage 4**

     H35.151   **Retinopathy of prematurity, stage 4, right eye**

     H35.152   **Retinopathy of prematurity, stage 4, left eye**

     H35.153   **Retinopathy of prematurity, stage 4, bilateral**

     H35.159   **Retinopathy of prematurity, stage 4, unspecified eye**

✓6th **H35.16** **Retinopathy of prematurity, stage 5**

     H35.161   **Retinopathy of prematurity, stage 5, right eye**

     H35.162   **Retinopathy of prematurity, stage 5, left eye**

     H35.163   **Retinopathy of prematurity, stage 5, bilateral**

     H35.169   **Retinopathy of prematurity, stage 5, unspecified eye**

✓6th **H35.17** **Retrolental fibroplasia**

     H35.171   **Retrolental fibroplasia, right eye**

     H35.172   **Retrolental fibroplasia, left eye**

     H35.173   **Retrolental fibroplasia, bilateral**

     H35.179   **Retrolental fibroplasia, unspecified eye**

✓5th **H35.2** **Other non-diabetic proliferative retinopathy**

     Proliferative vitreo-retinopathy

     Thalassemia proliferative retinopathy

     EXCLUDES 1   proliferative vitreo-retinopathy with retinal detachment (H33.4-)

     EXCLUDES 2   proliferative sickle-cell retinopathy (H36.82-)

     H35.20   **Other non-diabetic proliferative retinopathy, unspecified eye**

     H35.21   **Other non-diabetic proliferative retinopathy, right eye**

     H35.22   **Other non-diabetic proliferative retinopathy, left eye**

     H35.23   **Other non-diabetic proliferative retinopathy, bilateral**

✓5th **H35.3** **Degeneration of macula and posterior pole**

     H35.30   **Unspecified macular degeneration**   A

         Age-related macular degeneration

✓6th **H35.31** **Nonexudative age-related macular degeneration**

     Atrophic age-related macular degeneration

     Dry age-related macular degeneration

     AHA: 2016,4Q,20-21

> One of the following 7th characters is to be assigned to each code in subcategory H35.31 to designate the stage of the disease:
> 0   stage unspecified
> 1   early dry stage
> 2   intermediate dry stage
> 3   advanced atrophic without subfoveal involvement
>   advanced dry stage
> 4   advanced atrophic with subfoveal involvement

   ✓7th **H35.311** **Nonexudative age-related macular degeneration, right eye**   A

   ✓7th **H35.312** **Nonexudative age-related macular degeneration, left eye**   A

   ✓7th **H35.313** **Nonexudative age-related macular degeneration, bilateral**   A

   ✓7th **H35.319** **Nonexudative age-related macular degeneration, unspecified eye**   A

✓6th **H35.32** **Exudative age-related macular degeneration**

     Wet age-related macular degeneration

     AHA: 2016,4Q,20-21

> One of the following 7th characters is to be assigned to each code in subcategory H35.32 to designate the stage of the disease:
> 0   stage unspecified
> 1   with active choroidal neovascularization
> 2   with inactive choroidal neovascularization
>   with involuted or regressed neovascularization
> 3   with inactive scar

   ✓7th **H35.321** **Exudative age-related macular degeneration, right eye**   HCC A

   ✓7th **H35.322** **Exudative age-related macular degeneration, left eye**   HCC A

   ✓7th **H35.323** **Exudative age-related macular degeneration, bilateral**   HCC A

   ✓7th **H35.329** **Exudative age-related macular degeneration, unspecified eye**   HCC A

H35.33 **Angioid streaks of macula**

     DEF: Degeneration of the choroid, characterized by broad, irregular, dark brown streaks radiating from the optic disc; occurs with pseudoxanthoma elasticum or Paget's disease.

✓6th **H35.34** **Macular cyst, hole, or pseudohole**

     H35.341   **Macular cyst, hole, or pseudohole, right eye**

     H35.342   **Macular cyst, hole, or pseudohole, left eye**

     H35.343   **Macular cyst, hole, or pseudohole, bilateral**

     H35.349   **Macular cyst, hole, or pseudohole, unspecified eye**

✓6th **H35.35** **Cystoid macular degeneration**

     EXCLUDES 1   cystoid macular edema following cataract surgery (H59.03-)

     H35.351   **Cystoid macular degeneration, right eye**

     H35.352   **Cystoid macular degeneration, left eye**

     H35.353   **Cystoid macular degeneration, bilateral**

     H35.359   **Cystoid macular degeneration, unspecified eye**

✓6th **H35.36** **Drusen (degenerative) of macula**

     AHA: 2017,1Q,51; 2016,4Q,21

     H35.361   **Drusen (degenerative) of macula, right eye**

     H35.362   **Drusen (degenerative) of macula, left eye**

     H35.363   **Drusen (degenerative) of macula, bilateral**

     H35.369   **Drusen (degenerative) of macula, unspecified eye**

✓6th **H35.37** **Puckering of macula**

     H35.371   **Puckering of macula, right eye**

     H35.372   **Puckering of macula, left eye**

     H35.373   **Puckering of macula, bilateral**

     H35.379   **Puckering of macula, unspecified eye**

✓ Additional Character Required   ✓x7th Placeholder   Questionable PDx   Manifestation   Unspecified   UPD Unacceptable PDx   H1-H14 HAC   HCC CMS-HCC Dx   HIV HIV Dx

√6th H35.38　Toxic maculopathy

Code first poisoning due to drug or toxin, if applicable (T36-T65 with fifth or sixth character 1-4)

Use additional code for adverse effect, if applicable, to identify drug (T36-T50 with fifth or sixth character 5)

H35.381　Toxic maculopathy, **right** eye
H35.382　Toxic maculopathy, **left** eye
H35.383　Toxic maculopathy, **bilateral**
H35.389　Toxic maculopathy, unspecified eye

√5th H35.4　Peripheral retinal degeneration

EXCLUDES 1　*hereditary retinal degeneration (dystrophy) (H35.5-)*
peripheral retinal degeneration with retinal break (H33.3-)

H35.40　Unspecified peripheral retinal degeneration

√6th H35.41　Lattice degeneration of retina

Palisade degeneration of retina
DEF: Degeneration of the retina, often bilateral, that is usually benign. It is characterized by lines intersecting at irregular intervals in the peripheral retina. Retinal thinning and retinal holes may occur.

H35.411　Lattice degeneration of retina, **right** eye
H35.412　Lattice degeneration of retina, **left** eye
H35.413　Lattice degeneration of retina, **bilateral**
H35.419　Lattice degeneration of retina, unspecified eye

√6th H35.42　Microcystoid degeneration of retina

H35.421　Microcystoid degeneration of retina, **right** eye
H35.422　Microcystoid degeneration of retina, **left** eye
H35.423　Microcystoid degeneration of retina, **bilateral**
H35.429　Microcystoid degeneration of retina, unspecified eye

√6th H35.43　Paving stone degeneration of retina

H35.431　Paving stone degeneration of retina, **right** eye
H35.432　Paving stone degeneration of retina, **left** eye
H35.433　Paving stone degeneration of retina, **bilateral**
H35.439　Paving stone degeneration of retina, unspecified eye

√6th H35.44　Age-related reticular degeneration of retina

H35.441　Age-related reticular degeneration of retina, **right** eye　A
H35.442　Age-related reticular degeneration of retina, **left** eye　A
H35.443　Age-related reticular degeneration of retina, **bilateral**　A
H35.449　Age-related reticular degeneration of retina, unspecified eye　A

√6th H35.45　Secondary pigmentary degeneration

H35.451　Secondary pigmentary degeneration, **right** eye
H35.452　Secondary pigmentary degeneration, **left** eye
H35.453　Secondary pigmentary degeneration, **bilateral**
H35.459　Secondary pigmentary degeneration, unspecified eye

√6th H35.46　Secondary vitreoretinal degeneration

H35.461　Secondary vitreoretinal degeneration, **right** eye
H35.462　Secondary vitreoretinal degeneration, **left** eye
H35.463　Secondary vitreoretinal degeneration, **bilateral**
H35.469　Secondary vitreoretinal degeneration, unspecified eye

√5th H35.5　Hereditary retinal dystrophy

EXCLUDES 1　*dystrophies primarily involving Bruch's membrane (H31.1-)*

H35.50　Unspecified hereditary retinal dystrophy
H35.51　**Vitreoretinal** dystrophy

H35.52　Pigmentary retinal dystrophy

Albipunctate retinal dystrophy
Retinitis pigmentosa
Tapetoretinal dystrophy

H35.53　Other dystrophies primarily involving the sensory retina

Stargardt's disease

H35.54　Dystrophies primarily involving the retinal pigment epithelium

Vitelliform retinal dystrophy

√5th H35.6　Retinal hemorrhage

H35.60　Retinal hemorrhage, unspecified eye
H35.61　Retinal hemorrhage, **right** eye
H35.62　Retinal hemorrhage, **left** eye
H35.63　Retinal hemorrhage, **bilateral**

√5th H35.7　Separation of retinal layers

EXCLUDES 1　*retinal detachment (serous) (H33.2-)*
rhegmatogenous retinal detachment (H33.0-)

H35.70　Unspecified separation of retinal layers　CC

√6th H35.71　Central serous chorioretinopathy

H35.711　Central serous chorioretinopathy, **right** eye
H35.712　Central serous chorioretinopathy, **left** eye
H35.713　Central serous chorioretinopathy, **bilateral**
H35.719　Central serous chorioretinopathy, unspecified eye

√6th H35.72　Serous detachment of retinal pigment epithelium

H35.721　Serous detachment of retinal pigment epithelium, **right** eye　CC
H35.722　Serous detachment of retinal pigment epithelium, **left** eye　CC
H35.723　Serous detachment of retinal pigment epithelium, **bilateral**　CC
H35.729　Serous detachment of retinal pigment epithelium, unspecified eye　CC UNS

√6th H35.73　Hemorrhagic detachment of retinal pigment epithelium

H35.731　Hemorrhagic detachment of retinal pigment epithelium, **right** eye　CC
H35.732　Hemorrhagic detachment of retinal pigment epithelium, **left** eye　CC
H35.733　Hemorrhagic detachment of retinal pigment epithelium, **bilateral**　CC
H35.739　Hemorrhagic detachment of retinal pigment epithelium, unspecified eye　CC UNS

√5th H35.8　Other specified retinal disorders

EXCLUDES 2　*retinal hemorrhage (H35.6-)*

H35.81　Retinal edema
Retinal cotton wool spots
H35.82　Retinal ischemia　CC
H35.89　Other specified retinal disorders

H35.9　Unspecified retinal disorder

√4th H36　Retinal disorders in diseases classified elsewhere

Code first underlying disease, such as:
lipid storage disorders (E75.-)
sickle-cell disorders (D57.-)

EXCLUDES 1　*arteriosclerotic retinopathy (H35.0-)*
diabetic retinopathy (E08.3-, E09.3-, E10.3-, E11.3-, E13.3-)

AHA: 2023,4Q,20-21

√5th H36.8　Other retinal disorders in diseases classified elsewhere

√6th H36.81　Nonproliferative sickle-cell retinopathy

H36.811　Nonproliferative sickle-cell retinopathy, **right** eye　UPD HCC
H36.812　Nonproliferative sickle-cell retinopathy, **left** eye　UPD HCC
H36.813　Nonproliferative sickle-cell retinopathy, **bilateral**　UPD HCC
H36.819　Nonproliferative sickle-cell retinopathy, unspecified eye　UPD HCC

√6th H36.82　Proliferative sickle-cell retinopathy

H36.821　Proliferative sickle-cell retinopathy, **right** eye　UPD HCC
H36.822　Proliferative sickle-cell retinopathy, **left** eye　UPD HCC
H36.823　Proliferative sickle-cell retinopathy, **bilateral**　UPD HCC

N Newborn: 0　P Pediatric: 0-17　M Maternity: 9-64　A Adult: 15-124　UNS Unspecified Site　MCC Major Complication/Comorbidity　CC Complication/Comorbidity　PE POA Exempt

630　　　ICD-10-CM 2025

    H36.829   Proliferative sickle-cell retinopathy, unspecified eye   `UPD` `HCC`

H36.89   *Other retinal disorders in diseases classified elsewhere*
     Retinal dystrophy in lipid storage disorders

Glaucoma (H40-H42)

✓4th H40 Glaucoma

> **EXCLUDES 1**   absolute glaucoma (H44.51-)
> congenital glaucoma (Q15.0)
> traumatic glaucoma due to birth injury (P15.3)

Open Angle/Angle Closure Glaucoma

Open angle   Closed angle
Fluid flow
Lens   Lens
Iris
Cornea   Fluid flow
Drainage canal

✓5th H40.0 Glaucoma suspect

  ✓6th H40.00 Preglaucoma, unspecified
     H40.001 Preglaucoma, unspecified, **right** eye
     H40.002 Preglaucoma, unspecified, **left** eye
     H40.003 Preglaucoma, unspecified, **bilateral**
     H40.009 Preglaucoma, unspecified, unspecified eye

  ✓6th H40.01 Open angle with borderline findings, low risk
     Open angle, low risk
     H40.011 Open angle with borderline findings, low risk, **right** eye
     H40.012 Open angle with borderline findings, low risk, **left** eye
     H40.013 Open angle with borderline findings, low risk, **bilateral**
     H40.019 Open angle with borderline findings, low risk, unspecified eye

  ✓6th H40.02 Open angle with borderline findings, high risk
     Open angle, high risk
     H40.021 Open angle with borderline findings, high risk, **right** eye
     H40.022 Open angle with borderline findings, high risk, **left** eye
     H40.023 Open angle with borderline findings, high risk, **bilateral**
     H40.029 Open angle with borderline findings, high risk, unspecified eye

  ✓6th H40.03 Anatomical narrow angle
     Primary angle closure suspect
     H40.031 Anatomical narrow angle, **right** eye
     H40.032 Anatomical narrow angle, **left** eye
     H40.033 Anatomical narrow angle, **bilateral**
     H40.039 Anatomical narrow angle, unspecified eye

  ✓6th H40.04 Steroid responder
     H40.041 Steroid responder, **right** eye
     H40.042 Steroid responder, **left** eye
     H40.043 Steroid responder, **bilateral**
     H40.049 Steroid responder, unspecified eye

  ✓6th H40.05 Ocular hypertension
     H40.051 Ocular hypertension, **right** eye
     H40.052 Ocular hypertension, **left** eye
     H40.053 Ocular hypertension, **bilateral**
     H40.059 Ocular hypertension, unspecified eye

  ✓6th H40.06 Primary angle closure without glaucoma damage
     H40.061 Primary angle closure without glaucoma damage, **right** eye
     H40.062 Primary angle closure without glaucoma damage, **left** eye
     H40.063 Primary angle closure without glaucoma damage, **bilateral**
     H40.069 Primary angle closure without glaucoma damage, unspecified eye

✓5th H40.1 Open-angle glaucoma

> One of the following 7th characters is to be assigned to each code in subcategories H40.10, H40.11, H40.12, H40.13, and H40.14 to designate the stage of glaucoma.
> 0   stage unspecified
> 1   mild stage
> 2   moderate stage
> 3   severe stage
> 4   indeterminate stage

  ✓x7th H40.10 Unspecified open-angle glaucoma
     TIP: Only one code from this subcategory should be assigned when both left and right eyes are the same stage.

  ✓6th H40.11 Primary open-angle glaucoma
     Chronic simple glaucoma
     AHA: 2016,4Q,22
     ✓7th H40.111 Primary open-angle glaucoma, **right** eye
     ✓7th H40.112 Primary open-angle glaucoma, **left** eye
     ✓7th H40.113 Primary open-angle glaucoma, **bilateral**
     ✓7th H40.119 Primary open-angle glaucoma, unspecified eye

  ✓6th H40.12 Low-tension glaucoma
     ✓7th H40.121 Low-tension glaucoma, **right** eye   `UPD`
     ✓7th H40.122 Low-tension glaucoma, **left** eye   `UPD`
     ✓7th H40.123 Low-tension glaucoma, **bilateral**   `UPD`
     ✓7th H40.129 Low-tension glaucoma, unspecified eye   `UPD`

  ✓6th H40.13 Pigmentary glaucoma
     ✓7th H40.131 Pigmentary glaucoma, **right** eye   `UPD`
     ✓7th H40.132 Pigmentary glaucoma, **left** eye   `UPD`
     ✓7th H40.133 Pigmentary glaucoma, **bilateral**   `UPD`
     ✓7th H40.139 Pigmentary glaucoma, unspecified eye   `UPD`

  ✓6th H40.14 Capsular glaucoma with pseudoexfoliation of lens
     ✓7th H40.141 Capsular glaucoma with pseudoexfoliation of lens, **right** eye
     ✓7th H40.142 Capsular glaucoma with pseudoexfoliation of lens, **left** eye
     ✓7th H40.143 Capsular glaucoma with pseudoexfoliation of lens, **bilateral**
     ✓7th H40.149 Capsular glaucoma with pseudoexfoliation of lens, unspecified eye

  ✓6th H40.15 Residual stage of open-angle glaucoma
     H40.151 Residual stage of open-angle glaucoma, **right** eye   `UPD`
     H40.152 Residual stage of open-angle glaucoma, **left** eye   `UPD`
     H40.153 Residual stage of open-angle glaucoma, **bilateral**   `UPD`
     H40.159 Residual stage of open-angle glaucoma, unspecified eye   `UPD`

✓5th H40.2 Primary angle-closure glaucoma

> **EXCLUDES 1**   aqueous misdirection (H40.83-)
> malignant glaucoma (H40.83-)

> One of the following 7th characters is to be assigned to code H40.20 and H40.22 to designate the stage of glaucoma.
> 0   stage unspecified
> 1   mild stage
> 2   moderate stage
> 3   severe stage
> 4   indeterminate stage

  ✓x7th H40.20 Unspecified primary angle-closure glaucoma
     TIP: Only one code from this subcategory should be assigned when both left and right eyes are the same stage.

  ✓6th H40.21 Acute angle-closure glaucoma
     Acute angle-closure glaucoma attack
     Acute angle-closure glaucoma crisis
     H40.211 Acute angle-closure glaucoma, **right** eye   `CC`
     H40.212 Acute angle-closure glaucoma, **left** eye   `CC`
     H40.213 Acute angle-closure glaucoma, **bilateral**   `CC`

✔ Additional Character Required   ✓x7th Placeholder   Questionable PDx   Manifestation   Unspecified   `UPD` Unacceptable PDx   `H1`-`H14` HAC   `HCC` CMS-HCC Dx   `HIV` HIV Dx

ICD-10-CM 2025   631

Chapter 7. Diseases of the Eye and Adnexa

H40.219–H43.312

H40.219 **Acute** angle-closure glaucoma, unspecified eye `CC` `UNS`

✓6ᵗʰ H40.22 **Chronic** angle-closure glaucoma

Chronic primary angle closure glaucoma

✓7ᵗʰ H40.221 **Chronic** angle-closure glaucoma, **right** eye

✓7ᵗʰ H40.222 **Chronic** angle-closure glaucoma, **left** eye

✓7ᵗʰ H40.223 **Chronic** angle-closure glaucoma, **bilateral**

✓7ᵗʰ H40.229 **Chronic** angle-closure glaucoma, unspecified eye

✓6ᵗʰ H40.23 **Intermittent** angle-closure glaucoma

H40.231 Intermittent angle-closure glaucoma, **right** eye

H40.232 Intermittent angle-closure glaucoma, **left** eye

H40.233 Intermittent angle-closure glaucoma, **bilateral**

H40.239 Intermittent angle-closure glaucoma, unspecified eye

✓6ᵗʰ H40.24 **Residual stage** of angle-closure glaucoma

H40.241 Residual stage of angle-closure glaucoma, **right** eye

H40.242 Residual stage of angle-closure glaucoma, **left** eye

H40.243 Residual stage of angle-closure glaucoma, **bilateral**

H40.249 Residual stage of angle-closure glaucoma, unspecified eye

✓5ᵗʰ H40.3 Glaucoma **secondary** to eye **trauma**

Code also underlying condition

One of the following 7th characters is to be assigned to each code in subcategory H40.3 to designate the stage of glaucoma.
0 stage unspecified
1 mild stage
2 moderate stage
3 severe stage
4 indeterminate stage

✓x7ᵗʰ H40.30 Glaucoma secondary to eye trauma, unspecified eye

✓x7ᵗʰ H40.31 Glaucoma secondary to eye trauma, **right** eye

✓x7ᵗʰ H40.32 Glaucoma secondary to eye trauma, **left** eye

✓x7ᵗʰ H40.33 Glaucoma secondary to eye trauma, **bilateral**

✓5ᵗʰ H40.4 Glaucoma **secondary** to eye **inflammation**

Code also underlying condition

One of the following 7th characters is to be assigned to each code in subcategory H40.4 to designate the stage of glaucoma.
0 stage unspecified
1 mild stage
2 moderate stage
3 severe stage
4 indeterminate stage

✓x7ᵗʰ H40.40 Glaucoma secondary to eye inflammation, unspecified eye

✓x7ᵗʰ H40.41 Glaucoma secondary to eye inflammation, **right** eye

✓x7ᵗʰ H40.42 Glaucoma secondary to eye inflammation, **left** eye

✓x7ᵗʰ H40.43 Glaucoma secondary to eye inflammation, **bilateral**

✓5ᵗʰ H40.5 Glaucoma **secondary** to other **eye disorders**

Code also underlying eye disorder

One of the following 7th characters is to be assigned to each code in subcategory H40.5 to designate the stage of glaucoma.
0 stage unspecified
1 mild stage
2 moderate stage
3 severe stage
4 indeterminate stage

✓x7ᵗʰ H40.50 Glaucoma secondary to other eye disorders, unspecified eye

✓x7ᵗʰ H40.51 Glaucoma secondary to other eye disorders, **right** eye

✓x7ᵗʰ H40.52 Glaucoma secondary to other eye disorders, **left** eye

✓x7ᵗʰ H40.53 Glaucoma secondary to other eye disorders, **bilateral**

✓5ᵗʰ H40.6 Glaucoma **secondary** to **drugs**

Use additional code for adverse effect, if applicable, to identify drug (T36-T50 with fifth or sixth character 5)

One of the following 7th characters is to be assigned to each code in subcategory H40.6 to designate the stage of glaucoma
0 stage unspecified
1 mild stage
2 moderate stage
3 severe stage
4 indeterminate stage

✓x7ᵗʰ H40.60 Glaucoma secondary to drugs, unspecified eye

✓x7ᵗʰ H40.61 Glaucoma secondary to drugs, **right** eye

✓x7ᵗʰ H40.62 Glaucoma secondary to drugs, **left** eye

✓x7ᵗʰ H40.63 Glaucoma secondary to drugs, **bilateral**

✓5ᵗʰ H40.8 Other glaucoma

✓6ᵗʰ H40.81 Glaucoma with **increased episcleral venous pressure**

H40.811 Glaucoma with increased episcleral venous pressure, **right** eye

H40.812 Glaucoma with increased episcleral venous pressure, **left** eye

H40.813 Glaucoma with increased episcleral venous pressure, **bilateral**

H40.819 Glaucoma with increased episcleral venous pressure, unspecified eye

✓6ᵗʰ H40.82 **Hypersecretion** glaucoma

H40.821 Hypersecretion glaucoma, **right** eye

H40.822 Hypersecretion glaucoma, **left** eye

H40.823 Hypersecretion glaucoma, **bilateral**

H40.829 Hypersecretion glaucoma, unspecified eye

✓6ᵗʰ H40.83 **Aqueous misdirection**

Malignant glaucoma

H40.831 Aqueous misdirection, **right** eye

H40.832 Aqueous misdirection, **left** eye

H40.833 Aqueous misdirection, **bilateral**

H40.839 Aqueous misdirection, unspecified eye

H40.89 Other specified glaucoma

H40.9 Unspecified glaucoma

H42 *Glaucoma in diseases classified elsewhere*

Code first underlying condition, such as:
amyloidosis (E85.-)
aniridia (Q13.1)
glaucoma (in) diabetes mellitus (E08.39, E09.39, E10.39, E11.39, E13.39)
Lowe's syndrome (E72.03)
▶Rieger anomaly◄ (Q13.81)
specified metabolic disorder (E70-E88)

EXCLUDES 1 *glaucoma (in) onchocerciasis (B73.02)*
glaucoma (in) syphilis (A52.71)
glaucoma (in) tuberculous (A18.59)

Disorders of vitreous body and globe (H43-H44)

✓4ᵗʰ H43 **Disorders of vitreous body**

✓5ᵗʰ H43.0 Vitreous **prolapse**

EXCLUDES 1 *traumatic vitreous prolapse (S05.2-)*
vitreous syndrome following cataract surgery (H59.0-)

H43.00 Vitreous prolapse, unspecified eye

H43.01 Vitreous prolapse, **right** eye

H43.02 Vitreous prolapse, **left** eye

H43.03 Vitreous prolapse, **bilateral**

✓5ᵗʰ H43.1 Vitreous **hemorrhage**

H43.10 Vitreous hemorrhage, unspecified eye `HCC`

H43.11 Vitreous hemorrhage, **right** eye `HCC`

H43.12 Vitreous hemorrhage, **left** eye `HCC`

H43.13 Vitreous hemorrhage, **bilateral** `HCC`

✓5ᵗʰ H43.2 **Crystalline deposits** in vitreous body

H43.20 Crystalline deposits in vitreous body, unspecified eye

H43.21 Crystalline deposits in vitreous body, **right** eye

H43.22 Crystalline deposits in vitreous body, **left** eye

H43.23 Crystalline deposits in vitreous body, **bilateral**

✓5ᵗʰ H43.3 Other vitreous opacities

✓6ᵗʰ H43.31 Vitreous **membranes and strands**

H43.311 Vitreous membranes and strands, **right** eye

H43.312 Vitreous membranes and strands, **left** eye

| H43.313 | Vitreous membranes and strands, **bilateral** |
| H43.319 | Vitreous membranes and strands, unspecified eye |

✓6ᵗʰ H43.39 Other vitreous opacities

Vitreous floaters

H43.391	Other vitreous opacities, **right** eye
H43.392	Other vitreous opacities, **left** eye
H43.393	Other vitreous opacities, **bilateral**
H43.399	Other vitreous opacities, unspecified eye

✓5ᵗʰ H43.8 Other disorders of vitreous body

EXCLUDES 1   *proliferative vitreo-retinopathy with retinal detachment (H33.4-)*

EXCLUDES 2   *vitreous abscess (H44.02-)*

✓6ᵗʰ H43.81 Vitreous degeneration

Vitreous detachment

H43.811	Vitreous degeneration, **right** eye
H43.812	Vitreous degeneration, **left** eye
H43.813	Vitreous degeneration, **bilateral**
H43.819	Vitreous degeneration, unspecified eye

✓6ᵗʰ H43.82 Vitreomacular adhesion

Vitreomacular traction

H43.821	Vitreomacular adhesion, **right** eye	A
H43.822	Vitreomacular adhesion, **left** eye	A
H43.823	Vitreomacular adhesion, **bilateral**	A
H43.829	Vitreomacular adhesion, unspecified eye	A

| H43.89 | Other disorders of vitreous body |
| H43.9 | Unspecified disorder of vitreous body |

✓4ᵗʰ H44 Disorders of globe

INCLUDES   disorders affecting multiple structures of eye

✓5ᵗʰ H44.0 Purulent endophthalmitis ▲

Use additional code to identify organism

EXCLUDES 1   *bleb associated endophthalmitis (H59.4-)*

✓6ᵗʰ H44.00 Unspecified purulent endophthalmitis

H44.001	Unspecified purulent endophthalmitis, **right** eye	CC
H44.002	Unspecified purulent endophthalmitis, **left** eye	CC
H44.003	Unspecified purulent endophthalmitis, **bilateral**	CC
H44.009	Unspecified purulent endophthalmitis, unspecified eye ▲	CC UNS

✓6ᵗʰ H44.01 Panophthalmitis (acute)

H44.011	Panophthalmitis (acute), **right** eye	CC
H44.012	Panophthalmitis (acute), **left** eye	CC
H44.013	Panophthalmitis (acute), **bilateral**	CC
H44.019	Panophthalmitis (acute), unspecified eye	CC UNS

✓6ᵗʰ H44.02 Vitreous abscess (chronic) ▲

H44.021	Vitreous abscess (chronic), **right** eye	CC
H44.022	Vitreous abscess (chronic), **left** eye	CC
H44.023	Vitreous abscess (chronic), **bilateral**	CC
H44.029	Vitreous abscess (chronic), unspecified eye	CC UNS

✓5ᵗʰ H44.1 Other endophthalmitis

EXCLUDES 1   *bleb associated endophthalmitis (H59.4-)*

EXCLUDES 2   *ophthalmia nodosa (H16.2-)*

✓6ᵗʰ H44.11 Panuveitis ▲

DEF: Inflammation of all layers of the uvea of the eye, including the choroid, iris, and ciliary body. It also typically involves the lens, retina, optic nerve, and vitreous and causes reduced vision or blindness.

H44.111	Panuveitis, **right** eye	CC
H44.112	Panuveitis, **left** eye	CC
H44.113	Panuveitis, **bilateral**	CC
H44.119	Panuveitis, unspecified eye	CC UNS

✓6ᵗʰ H44.12 Parasitic endophthalmitis, unspecified

H44.121	Parasitic endophthalmitis, unspecified, **right** eye	CC
H44.122	Parasitic endophthalmitis, unspecified, **left** eye	CC
H44.123	Parasitic endophthalmitis, unspecified, **bilateral**	CC
H44.129	Parasitic endophthalmitis, unspecified, unspecified eye	CC UNS

✓6ᵗʰ H44.13 Sympathetic uveitis

H44.131	Sympathetic uveitis, **right** eye	CC
H44.132	Sympathetic uveitis, **left** eye	CC
H44.133	Sympathetic uveitis, **bilateral**	CC
H44.139	Sympathetic uveitis, unspecified eye	CC UNS

| H44.19 | Other endophthalmitis | CC |

✓5ᵗʰ H44.2 Degenerative myopia

Malignant myopia

AHA: 2017,4Q,10-11

H44.20	Degenerative myopia, unspecified eye
H44.21	Degenerative myopia, **right** eye
H44.22	Degenerative myopia, **left** eye
H44.23	Degenerative myopia, **bilateral**

✓6ᵗʰ H44.2A Degenerative myopia with choroidal neovascularization

Use additional code for any associated choroid disorders (H31.-)

H44.2A1	Degenerative myopia with choroidal neovascularization, **right** eye
H44.2A2	Degenerative myopia with choroidal neovascularization, **left** eye
H44.2A3	Degenerative myopia with choroidal neovascularization, **bilateral**
H44.2A9	Degenerative myopia with choroidal neovascularization, unspecified eye

✓6ᵗʰ H44.2B Degenerative myopia with macular hole

H44.2B1	Degenerative myopia with macular hole, **right** eye
H44.2B2	Degenerative myopia with macular hole, **left** eye
H44.2B3	Degenerative myopia with macular hole, **bilateral**
H44.2B9	Degenerative myopia with macular hole, unspecified eye

✓6ᵗʰ H44.2C Degenerative myopia with retinal detachment

Use additional code to identify the retinal detachment (H33.-)

H44.2C1	Degenerative myopia with retinal detachment, **right** eye
H44.2C2	Degenerative myopia with retinal detachment, **left** eye
H44.2C3	Degenerative myopia with retinal detachment, **bilateral**
H44.2C9	Degenerative myopia with retinal detachment, unspecified eye

✓6ᵗʰ H44.2D Degenerative myopia with foveoschisis

H44.2D1	Degenerative myopia with foveoschisis, **right** eye
H44.2D2	Degenerative myopia with foveoschisis, **left** eye
H44.2D3	Degenerative myopia with foveoschisis, **bilateral**
H44.2D9	Degenerative myopia with foveoschisis, unspecified eye

✓6ᵗʰ H44.2E Degenerative myopia with other maculopathy

H44.2E1	Degenerative myopia with other maculopathy, **right** eye
H44.2E2	Degenerative myopia with other maculopathy, **left** eye
H44.2E3	Degenerative myopia with other maculopathy, **bilateral**
H44.2E9	Degenerative myopia with other maculopathy, unspecified eye

✓5ᵗʰ H44.3 Other and unspecified degenerative disorders of globe

| H44.30 | Unspecified degenerative disorder of globe |

✓6ᵗʰ H44.31 Chalcosis

H44.311	Chalcosis, **right** eye
H44.312	Chalcosis, **left** eye
H44.313	Chalcosis, **bilateral**
H44.319	Chalcosis, unspecified eye

✓6ᵗʰ H44.32 Siderosis of eye

DEF: Iron pigment deposits within tissue of the eyeball caused by high iron content of the blood. Symptoms include cataracts, rust-colored anterior subcapsular deposits, iris heterochromia, pupillary mydriasis, and depressed electroretinogram amplitudes.

| H44.321 | Siderosis of eye, **right** eye |
| H44.322 | Siderosis of eye, **left** eye |

H44.323 **Siderosis of eye, bilateral**

H44.329 Siderosis of eye, unspecified eye

✓6ᵗʰ H44.39 **Other degenerative disorders of globe**

H44.391 **Other degenerative disorders of globe, right eye**

H44.392 **Other degenerative disorders of globe, left eye**

H44.393 **Other degenerative disorders of globe, bilateral**

H44.399 Other degenerative disorders of globe, unspecified eye

✓5ᵗʰ H44.4 **Hypotony of eye**

H44.40 Unspecified hypotony of eye

✓6ᵗʰ H44.41 **Flat anterior chamber hypotony of eye**

H44.411 **Flat anterior chamber hypotony of right eye**

H44.412 **Flat anterior chamber hypotony of left eye**

H44.413 **Flat anterior chamber hypotony of eye, bilateral**

H44.419 Flat anterior chamber hypotony of unspecified eye

✓6ᵗʰ H44.42 **Hypotony of eye due to ocular fistula**

H44.421 **Hypotony of right eye due to ocular fistula**

H44.422 **Hypotony of left eye due to ocular fistula**

H44.423 **Hypotony of eye due to ocular fistula, bilateral**

H44.429 Hypotony of unspecified eye due to ocular fistula

✓6ᵗʰ H44.43 **Hypotony of eye due to other ocular disorders**

H44.431 **Hypotony of eye due to other ocular disorders, right eye**

H44.432 **Hypotony of eye due to other ocular disorders, left eye**

H44.433 **Hypotony of eye due to other ocular disorders, bilateral**

H44.439 Hypotony of eye due to other ocular disorders, unspecified eye

✓6ᵗʰ H44.44 **Primary hypotony of eye**

H44.441 **Primary hypotony of right eye**

H44.442 **Primary hypotony of left eye**

H44.443 **Primary hypotony of eye, bilateral**

H44.449 Primary hypotony of unspecified eye

✓5ᵗʰ H44.5 **Degenerated conditions of globe**

H44.50 Unspecified degenerated conditions of globe

✓6ᵗʰ H44.51 **Absolute glaucoma**

H44.511 **Absolute glaucoma, right eye**

H44.512 **Absolute glaucoma, left eye**

H44.513 **Absolute glaucoma, bilateral**

H44.519 Absolute glaucoma, unspecified eye

✓6ᵗʰ H44.52 **Atrophy of globe**

Phthisis bulbi

H44.521 **Atrophy of globe, right eye**

H44.522 **Atrophy of globe, left eye**

H44.523 **Atrophy of globe, bilateral**

H44.529 Atrophy of globe, unspecified eye

✓6ᵗʰ H44.53 **Leucocoria**

H44.531 **Leucocoria, right eye**

H44.532 **Leucocoria, left eye**

H44.533 **Leucocoria, bilateral**

H44.539 Leucocoria, unspecified eye

✓5ᵗʰ H44.6 **Retained (old) intraocular foreign body, magnetic**

Use additional code to identify magnetic foreign body (Z18.11)

EXCLUDES 1 *current intraocular foreign body (S05.-)*

EXCLUDES 2 *retained foreign body in eyelid (H02.81-)*

retained (old) foreign body following penetrating wound of orbit (H05.5-)

retained (old) intraocular foreign body, nonmagnetic (H44.7-)

✓6ᵗʰ H44.60 **Unspecified retained (old) intraocular foreign body, magnetic**

H44.601 **Unspecified retained (old) intraocular foreign body, magnetic, right eye**

H44.602 **Unspecified retained (old) intraocular foreign body, magnetic, left eye**

H44.603 **Unspecified retained (old) intraocular foreign body, magnetic, bilateral**

H44.609 Unspecified retained (old) intraocular foreign body, magnetic, unspecified eye

✓6ᵗʰ H44.61 **Retained (old) magnetic foreign body in anterior chamber**

H44.611 **Retained (old) magnetic foreign body in anterior chamber, right eye**

H44.612 **Retained (old) magnetic foreign body in anterior chamber, left eye**

H44.613 **Retained (old) magnetic foreign body in anterior chamber, bilateral**

H44.619 Retained (old) magnetic foreign body in anterior chamber, unspecified eye

✓6ᵗʰ H44.62 **Retained (old) magnetic foreign body in iris or ciliary body**

H44.621 **Retained (old) magnetic foreign body in iris or ciliary body, right eye**

H44.622 **Retained (old) magnetic foreign body in iris or ciliary body, left eye**

H44.623 **Retained (old) magnetic foreign body in iris or ciliary body, bilateral**

H44.629 Retained (old) magnetic foreign body in iris or ciliary body, unspecified eye

✓6ᵗʰ H44.63 **Retained (old) magnetic foreign body in lens**

H44.631 **Retained (old) magnetic foreign body in lens, right eye**

H44.632 **Retained (old) magnetic foreign body in lens, left eye**

H44.633 **Retained (old) magnetic foreign body in lens, bilateral**

H44.639 Retained (old) magnetic foreign body in lens, unspecified eye

✓6ᵗʰ H44.64 **Retained (old) magnetic foreign body in posterior wall of globe**

H44.641 **Retained (old) magnetic foreign body in posterior wall of globe, right eye**

H44.642 **Retained (old) magnetic foreign body in posterior wall of globe, left eye**

H44.643 **Retained (old) magnetic foreign body in posterior wall of globe, bilateral**

H44.649 Retained (old) magnetic foreign body in posterior wall of globe, unspecified eye

✓6ᵗʰ H44.65 **Retained (old) magnetic foreign body in vitreous body**

H44.651 **Retained (old) magnetic foreign body in vitreous body, right eye**

H44.652 **Retained (old) magnetic foreign body in vitreous body, left eye**

H44.653 **Retained (old) magnetic foreign body in vitreous body, bilateral**

H44.659 Retained (old) magnetic foreign body in vitreous body, unspecified eye

✓6ᵗʰ H44.69 **Retained (old) intraocular foreign body, magnetic, in other or multiple sites**

H44.691 **Retained (old) intraocular foreign body, magnetic, in other or multiple sites, right eye**

H44.692 **Retained (old) intraocular foreign body, magnetic, in other or multiple sites, left eye**

H44.693 **Retained (old) intraocular foreign body, magnetic, in other or multiple sites, bilateral**

H44.699 Retained (old) intraocular foreign body, magnetic, in other or multiple sites, unspecified eye

✓5ᵗʰ H44.7 **Retained (old) intraocular foreign body, nonmagnetic**

Use additional code to identify nonmagnetic foreign body (Z18.01-Z18.10, Z18.12, Z18.2-Z18.9)

EXCLUDES 1 *current intraocular foreign body (S05.-)*

EXCLUDES 2 *retained foreign body in eyelid (H02.81-)*

retained (old) foreign body following penetrating wound of orbit (H05.5-)

retained (old) intraocular foreign body, magnetic (H44.6-)

✓6ᵗʰ H44.70 **Unspecified retained (old) intraocular foreign body, nonmagnetic**

H44.701 **Unspecified retained (old) intraocular foreign body, nonmagnetic, right eye**

H44.702 **Unspecified retained (old) intraocular foreign body, nonmagnetic, left eye**

H44.703 **Unspecified retained (old) intraocular foreign body, nonmagnetic, bilateral**

N Newborn: 0 P Pediatric: 0-17 M Maternity: 9-64 A Adult: 15-124 UNS Unspecified Site MCC Major Complication/Comorbidity CC Complication/Comorbidity PE POA Exempt

634

ICD-10-CM 2025

H44.709 Unspecified retained (old) intraocular foreign body, nonmagnetic, unspecified eye

Retained (old) intraocular foreign body NOS

√6th **H44.71** Retained (nonmagnetic) (old) foreign body in anterior chamber

H44.711 Retained (nonmagnetic) (old) foreign body in anterior chamber, right eye

H44.712 Retained (nonmagnetic) (old) foreign body in anterior chamber, left eye

H44.713 Retained (nonmagnetic) (old) foreign body in anterior chamber, bilateral

H44.719 Retained (nonmagnetic) (old) foreign body in anterior chamber, unspecified eye

√6th **H44.72** Retained (nonmagnetic) (old) foreign body in iris or ciliary body

H44.721 Retained (nonmagnetic) (old) foreign body in iris or ciliary body, right eye

H44.722 Retained (nonmagnetic) (old) foreign body in iris or ciliary body, left eye

H44.723 Retained (nonmagnetic) (old) foreign body in iris or ciliary body, bilateral

H44.729 Retained (nonmagnetic) (old) foreign body in iris or ciliary body, unspecified eye

√6th **H44.73** Retained (nonmagnetic) (old) foreign body in lens

H44.731 Retained (nonmagnetic) (old) foreign body in lens, right eye

H44.732 Retained (nonmagnetic) (old) foreign body in lens, left eye

H44.733 Retained (nonmagnetic) (old) foreign body in lens, bilateral

H44.739 Retained (nonmagnetic) (old) foreign body in lens, unspecified eye

√6th **H44.74** Retained (nonmagnetic) (old) foreign body in posterior wall of globe

H44.741 Retained (nonmagnetic) (old) foreign body in posterior wall of globe, right eye

H44.742 Retained (nonmagnetic) (old) foreign body in posterior wall of globe, left eye

H44.743 Retained (nonmagnetic) (old) foreign body in posterior wall of globe, bilateral

H44.749 Retained (nonmagnetic) (old) foreign body in posterior wall of globe, unspecified eye

√6th **H44.75** Retained (nonmagnetic) (old) foreign body in vitreous body

H44.751 Retained (nonmagnetic) (old) foreign body in vitreous body, right eye

H44.752 Retained (nonmagnetic) (old) foreign body in vitreous body, left eye

H44.753 Retained (nonmagnetic) (old) foreign body in vitreous body, bilateral

H44.759 Retained (nonmagnetic) (old) foreign body in vitreous body, unspecified eye

√6th **H44.79** Retained (old) intraocular foreign body, nonmagnetic, in other or multiple sites

H44.791 Retained (old) intraocular foreign body, nonmagnetic, in other or multiple sites, right eye

H44.792 Retained (old) intraocular foreign body, nonmagnetic, in other or multiple sites, left eye

H44.793 Retained (old) intraocular foreign body, nonmagnetic, in other or multiple sites, bilateral

H44.799 Retained (old) intraocular foreign body, nonmagnetic, in other or multiple sites, unspecified eye

√5th **H44.8** Other disorders of globe

√6th **H44.81** Hemophthalmos

DEF: Pool of blood within the eyeball, not from a current injury.

H44.811 Hemophthalmos, right eye

H44.812 Hemophthalmos, left eye

H44.813 Hemophthalmos, bilateral

H44.819 Hemophthalmos, unspecified eye

√6th **H44.82** Luxation of globe

H44.821 Luxation of globe, right eye

H44.822 Luxation of globe, left eye

H44.823 Luxation of globe, bilateral

H44.829 Luxation of globe, unspecified eye

H44.89 Other disorders of globe

AHA: 2022,1Q,33

H44.9 Unspecified disorder of globe

Disorders of optic nerve and visual pathways (H46-H47)

√4th **H46** Optic neuritis

EXCLUDES 2   ischemic optic neuropathy (H47.01-)

neuromyelitis optica [Devic] (G36.0)

√5th **H46.0** Optic papillitis

H46.00 Optic papillitis, unspecified eye   CC UNS

H46.01 Optic papillitis, right eye   CC

H46.02 Optic papillitis, left eye   CC

H46.03 Optic papillitis, bilateral   CC

√5th **H46.1** Retrobulbar neuritis

Retrobulbar neuritis NOS

EXCLUDES 1   syphilitic retrobulbar neuritis (A52.15)

H46.10 Retrobulbar neuritis, unspecified eye   CC UNS

H46.11 Retrobulbar neuritis, right eye   CC

H46.12 Retrobulbar neuritis, left eye   CC

H46.13 Retrobulbar neuritis, bilateral   CC

H46.2 Nutritional optic neuropathy

H46.3 Toxic optic neuropathy

Code first (T51-T65) to identify cause

H46.8 Other optic neuritis   CC

H46.9 Unspecified optic neuritis   CC

AHA: 2023,3Q,19

√4th **H47** Other disorders of optic [2nd] nerve and visual pathways

√5th **H47.0** Disorders of optic nerve, not elsewhere classified

√6th **H47.01** Ischemic optic neuropathy

H47.011 Ischemic optic neuropathy, right eye

H47.012 Ischemic optic neuropathy, left eye

H47.013 Ischemic optic neuropathy, bilateral

H47.019 Ischemic optic neuropathy, unspecified eye

√6th **H47.02** Hemorrhage in optic nerve sheath

H47.021 Hemorrhage in optic nerve sheath, right eye

H47.022 Hemorrhage in optic nerve sheath, left eye

H47.023 Hemorrhage in optic nerve sheath, bilateral

H47.029 Hemorrhage in optic nerve sheath, unspecified eye

√6th **H47.03** Optic nerve hypoplasia

H47.031 Optic nerve hypoplasia, right eye

H47.032 Optic nerve hypoplasia, left eye

H47.033 Optic nerve hypoplasia, bilateral

H47.039 Optic nerve hypoplasia, unspecified eye

√6th **H47.09** Other disorders of optic nerve, not elsewhere classified

Compression of optic nerve

H47.091 Other disorders of optic nerve, not elsewhere classified, right eye

H47.092 Other disorders of optic nerve, not elsewhere classified, left eye

H47.093 Other disorders of optic nerve, not elsewhere classified, bilateral

H47.099 Other disorders of optic nerve, not elsewhere classified, unspecified eye

√5th **H47.1** Papilledema

DEF: Swelling of the optic papilla, the raised area connected to the optic disk made up of nerves that enter the eyeball. It may be caused by increased intracranial pressure, decreased ocular pressure, or a retinal disorder.

H47.10 Unspecified papilledema   CC

H47.11 Papilledema associated with increased intracranial pressure   CC

H47.12 Papilledema associated with decreased ocular pressure

H47.13 Papilledema associated with retinal disorder

√6th **H47.14** Foster-Kennedy syndrome

H47.141 Foster-Kennedy syndrome, right eye

H47.142 Foster-Kennedy syndrome, left eye

H47.143 Foster-Kennedy syndrome, bilateral

H47.149 Foster-Kennedy syndrome, unspecified eye

☑ Additional Character Required   √x7th Placeholder   Questionable PDx   Manifestation   Unspecified   UPD Unacceptable PDx   H1-H14 HAC   HCC CMS-HCC Dx   HIV HIV Dx

ICD-10-CM 2025   635

✓5th **H47.2 Optic atrophy**

   H47.20 Unspecified optic atrophy

  ✓6th **H47.21 Primary optic atrophy**

     H47.211 **Primary optic atrophy, right eye**

     H47.212 **Primary optic atrophy, left eye**

     H47.213 **Primary optic atrophy, bilateral**

     H47.219 **Primary optic atrophy, unspecified eye**

   H47.22 Hereditary optic atrophy

     Leber's optic atrophy

  ✓6th **H47.23 Glaucomatous optic atrophy**

     H47.231 **Glaucomatous optic atrophy, right eye**

     H47.232 **Glaucomatous optic atrophy, left eye**

     H47.233 **Glaucomatous optic atrophy, bilateral**

     H47.239 **Glaucomatous optic atrophy, unspecified eye**

  ✓6th **H47.29 Other optic atrophy**

     Temporal pallor of optic disc

     H47.291 **Other optic atrophy, right eye**

     H47.292 **Other optic atrophy, left eye**

     H47.293 **Other optic atrophy, bilateral**

     H47.299 **Other optic atrophy, unspecified eye**

✓5th **H47.3 Other disorders of optic disc**

  ✓6th **H47.31 Coloboma of optic disc**

     H47.311 **Coloboma of optic disc, right eye**

     H47.312 **Coloboma of optic disc, left eye**

     H47.313 **Coloboma of optic disc, bilateral**

     H47.319 **Coloboma of optic disc, unspecified eye**

  ✓6th **H47.32 Drusen of optic disc**

     H47.321 **Drusen of optic disc, right eye**

     H47.322 **Drusen of optic disc, left eye**

     H47.323 **Drusen of optic disc, bilateral**

     H47.329 **Drusen of optic disc, unspecified eye**

  ✓6th **H47.33 Pseudopapilledema of optic disc**

     H47.331 **Pseudopapilledema of optic disc, right eye**

     H47.332 **Pseudopapilledema of optic disc, left eye**

     H47.333 **Pseudopapilledema of optic disc, bilateral**

     H47.339 **Pseudopapilledema of optic disc, unspecified eye**

  ✓6th **H47.39 Other disorders of optic disc**

     H47.391 **Other disorders of optic disc, right eye**

     H47.392 **Other disorders of optic disc, left eye**

     H47.393 **Other disorders of optic disc, bilateral**

     H47.399 **Other disorders of optic disc, unspecified eye**

✓5th **H47.4 Disorders of optic chiasm**

   Code also underlying condition

   H47.41 Disorders of optic chiasm in (due to) inflammatory disorders CC

   H47.42 Disorders of optic chiasm in (due to) neoplasm CC

   H47.43 Disorders of optic chiasm in (due to) vascular disorders CC

   H47.49 Disorders of optic chiasm in (due to) other disorders CC

✓5th **H47.5 Disorders of other visual pathways**

   Disorders of optic tracts, geniculate nuclei and optic radiations

   Code also underlying condition

  ✓6th **H47.51 Disorders of visual pathways in (due to) inflammatory disorders**

     H47.511 **Disorders of visual pathways in (due to) inflammatory disorders, right side** CC

     H47.512 **Disorders of visual pathways in (due to) inflammatory disorders, left side** CC

     H47.519 **Disorders of visual pathways in (due to) inflammatory disorders, unspecified side** CC UNS

  ✓6th **H47.52 Disorders of visual pathways in (due to) neoplasm**

     H47.521 **Disorders of visual pathways in (due to) neoplasm, right side** CC

     H47.522 **Disorders of visual pathways in (due to) neoplasm, left side** CC

     H47.529 **Disorders of visual pathways in (due to) neoplasm, unspecified side** CC UNS

  ✓6th **H47.53 Disorders of visual pathways in (due to) vascular disorders**

     H47.531 **Disorders of visual pathways in (due to) vascular disorders, right side** CC

     H47.532 **Disorders of visual pathways in (due to) vascular disorders, left side** CC

     H47.539 **Disorders of visual pathways in (due to) vascular disorders, unspecified side** CC UNS

✓5th **H47.6 Disorders of visual cortex**

   Code also underlying condition

   EXCLUDES 1 *injury to visual cortex S04.04-*

  ✓6th **H47.61 Cortical blindness**

     H47.611 **Cortical blindness, right side of brain**

     H47.612 **Cortical blindness, left side of brain**

     H47.619 **Cortical blindness, unspecified side of brain**

  ✓6th **H47.62 Disorders of visual cortex in (due to) inflammatory disorders**

     H47.621 **Disorders of visual cortex in (due to) inflammatory disorders, right side of brain** CC

     H47.622 **Disorders of visual cortex in (due to) inflammatory disorders, left side of brain** CC

     H47.629 **Disorders of visual cortex in (due to) inflammatory disorders, unspecified side of brain** CC UNS

  ✓6th **H47.63 Disorders of visual cortex in (due to) neoplasm**

     H47.631 **Disorders of visual cortex in (due to) neoplasm, right side of brain** CC

     H47.632 **Disorders of visual cortex in (due to) neoplasm, left side of brain** CC

     H47.639 **Disorders of visual cortex in (due to) neoplasm, unspecified side of brain** CC UNS

  ✓6th **H47.64 Disorders of visual cortex in (due to) vascular disorders**

     H47.641 **Disorders of visual cortex in (due to) vascular disorders, right side of brain** CC

     H47.642 **Disorders of visual cortex in (due to) vascular disorders, left side of brain** CC

     H47.649 **Disorders of visual cortex in (due to) vascular disorders, unspecified side of brain** CC UNS

   H47.9 Unspecified disorder of visual pathways

Disorders of ocular muscles, binocular movement, accommodation and refraction (H49-H52)

EXCLUDES 2 *nystagmus and other irregular eye movements (H55)*

✓4th **H49 Paralytic strabismus**

   EXCLUDES 2 *internal ophthalmoplegia (H52.51-)*

          internuclear ophthalmoplegia (H51.2-)

          progressive supranuclear ophthalmoplegia (G23.1)

   DEF: Strabismus: Misalignment of the eyes with the inability to move and focus in the same direction due to conditions affecting the muscles controlling them.

  ✓5th **H49.0 Third [oculomotor] nerve palsy**

     H49.00 **Third [oculomotor] nerve palsy, unspecified eye**

     H49.01 **Third [oculomotor] nerve palsy, right eye**

     H49.02 **Third [oculomotor] nerve palsy, left eye**

     H49.03 **Third [oculomotor] nerve palsy, bilateral**

  ✓5th **H49.1 Fourth [trochlear] nerve palsy**

     H49.10 **Fourth [trochlear] nerve palsy, unspecified eye**

     H49.11 **Fourth [trochlear] nerve palsy, right eye**

     H49.12 **Fourth [trochlear] nerve palsy, left eye**

     H49.13 **Fourth [trochlear] nerve palsy, bilateral**

  ✓5th **H49.2 Sixth [abducent] nerve palsy**

     H49.20 **Sixth [abducent] nerve palsy, unspecified eye**

     H49.21 **Sixth [abducent] nerve palsy, right eye**

     H49.22 **Sixth [abducent] nerve palsy, left eye**

     H49.23 **Sixth [abducent] nerve palsy, bilateral**

  ✓5th **H49.3 Total (external) ophthalmoplegia**

     H49.30 **Total (external) ophthalmoplegia, unspecified eye**

     H49.31 **Total (external) ophthalmoplegia, right eye**

     H49.32 **Total (external) ophthalmoplegia, left eye**

     H49.33 **Total (external) ophthalmoplegia, bilateral**

N Newborn: 0   P Pediatric: 0-17   M Maternity: 9-64   A Adult: 15-124   UNS Unspecified Site   MCC Major Complication/Comorbidity   CC Complication/Comorbidity   PE POA Exempt

636   ICD-10-CM 2025

√5ᵗʰ **H49.4** **Progressive** external ophthalmoplegia

    EXCLUDES 1   *Kearns-Sayre syndrome (H49.81-)*

    H49.40   Progressive external ophthalmoplegia, unspecified eye

    H49.41   Progressive external ophthalmoplegia, **right** eye

    H49.42   Progressive external ophthalmoplegia, **left** eye

    H49.43   Progressive external ophthalmoplegia, **bilateral**

√5ᵗʰ **H49.8** **Other paralytic strabismus**

    √6ᵗʰ **H49.81**   **Kearns-Sayre syndrome**

        Progressive external ophthalmoplegia with pigmentary retinopathy

        Code also, if applicable, other manifestations, such as: heart block (I45.9)

        H49.811   Kearns-Sayre syndrome, **right** eye   **CC**

        H49.812   Kearns-Sayre syndrome, **left** eye   **CC**

        H49.813   Kearns-Sayre syndrome, **bilateral**   **CC**

        H49.819   Kearns-Sayre syndrome, unspecified eye   **CC** **UNS**

    √6ᵗʰ **H49.88**   **Other paralytic strabismus**

        External ophthalmoplegia NOS

        H49.881   Other paralytic strabismus, **right** eye

        H49.882   Other paralytic strabismus, **left** eye

        H49.883   Other paralytic strabismus, **bilateral**

        H49.889   Other paralytic strabismus, unspecified eye

    H49.9   **Unspecified paralytic strabismus**

√4ᵗʰ **H50** **Other strabismus**

    DEF: Strabismus: Misalignment of the eyes with the inability to move and focus in the same direction due to conditions affecting the muscles controlling them.

    √5ᵗʰ **H50.0**   **Esotropia**

        Convergent concomitant strabismus

        EXCLUDES 1   *intermittent esotropia (H50.31-, H50.32)*

        H50.00   Unspecified esotropia

        √6ᵗʰ **H50.01**   **Monocular** esotropia

           H50.011   Monocular esotropia, **right** eye

           H50.012   Monocular esotropia, **left** eye

        √6ᵗʰ **H50.02**   Monocular esotropia with **A pattern**

           H50.021   Monocular esotropia with A pattern, **right** eye

           H50.022   Monocular esotropia with A pattern, **left** eye

        √6ᵗʰ **H50.03**   Monocular esotropia with **V pattern**

           H50.031   Monocular esotropia with V pattern, **right** eye

           H50.032   Monocular esotropia with V pattern, **left** eye

        √6ᵗʰ **H50.04**   Monocular esotropia with **other noncomitancies**

           H50.041   Monocular esotropia with other noncomitancies, **right** eye

           H50.042   Monocular esotropia with other noncomitancies, **left** eye

        H50.05   **Alternating** esotropia

        H50.06   Alternating esotropia with **A pattern**

        H50.07   Alternating esotropia with **V pattern**

        H50.08   Alternating esotropia with other noncomitancies

Eye Muscle Diseases

R.   L.
Monocular (one eye only) esotropia (inward)

Monocular exotropia (outward)

Monocular hypertropia (upward)

√5ᵗʰ **H50.1** **Exotropia**

    Divergent concomitant strabismus

    EXCLUDES 1   *intermittent exotropia (H50.33-, H50.34)*

    H50.10   Unspecified exotropia

    √6ᵗʰ **H50.11**   **Monocular** exotropia

        H50.111   Monocular exotropia, **right** eye

        H50.112   Monocular exotropia, **left** eye

    √6ᵗʰ **H50.12**   Monocular exotropia with **A pattern**

        H50.121   Monocular exotropia with A pattern, **right** eye

        H50.122   Monocular exotropia with A pattern, **left** eye

    √6ᵗʰ **H50.13**   Monocular exotropia with **V pattern**

        H50.131   Monocular exotropia with V pattern, **right** eye

        H50.132   Monocular exotropia with V pattern, **left** eye

    √6ᵗʰ **H50.14**   Monocular exotropia with other noncomitancies

        H50.141   Monocular exotropia with other noncomitancies, **right** eye

        H50.142   Monocular exotropia with other noncomitancies, **left** eye

    H50.15   **Alternating** exotropia

    H50.16   Alternating exotropia with **A pattern**

    H50.17   Alternating exotropia with **V pattern**

    H50.18   Alternating exotropia with other noncomitancies

√5ᵗʰ **H50.2** **Vertical strabismus**

    Hypertropia

    H50.21   Vertical strabismus, **right** eye

    H50.22   Vertical strabismus, **left** eye

√5ᵗʰ **H50.3** **Intermittent heterotropia**

    H50.30   Unspecified intermittent heterotropia

    √6ᵗʰ **H50.31**   Intermittent **monocular esotropia**

        H50.311   Intermittent monocular esotropia, **right** eye

        H50.312   Intermittent monocular esotropia, **left** eye

    H50.32   Intermittent **alternating** esotropia

    √6ᵗʰ **H50.33**   Intermittent **monocular exotropia**

        H50.331   Intermittent monocular exotropia, **right** eye

        H50.332   Intermittent monocular exotropia, **left** eye

    H50.34   Intermittent **alternating** exotropia

√5ᵗʰ **H50.4** **Other and unspecified heterotropia**

    H50.40   Unspecified heterotropia

    √6ᵗʰ **H50.41**   **Cyclotropia**

        H50.411   Cyclotropia, **right** eye

        H50.412   Cyclotropia, **left** eye

    H50.42   **Monofixation** syndrome

    H50.43   Accommodative component in esotropia

√5ᵗʰ **H50.5** **Heterophoria**

    H50.50   Unspecified heterophoria

    H50.51   **Esophoria**

    H50.52   **Exophoria**

✔ Additional Character Required   √x7ᵗʰ Placeholder   Questionable PDx   Manifestation   Unspecified   **UPD** Unacceptable PDx   **H1**-**H14** HAC   **HCC** CMS-HCC Dx   **HIV** HIV Dx

ICD-10-CM 2025   637

H50.53 **Vertical** heterophoria
H50.54 **Cyclophoria**
H50.55 **Alternating** heterophoria
✓5th H50.6 Mechanical strabismus
AHA: 2023,4Q,21-23
H50.60 Mechanical strabismus, unspecified
✓6th H50.61 **Brown's sheath** syndrome
H50.611 Brown's sheath syndrome, **right** eye
H50.612 Brown's sheath syndrome, **left** eye
✓6th H50.62 **Inferior oblique** muscle entrapment
H50.621 Inferior oblique muscle entrapment, **right** eye
H50.622 Inferior oblique muscle entrapment, **left** eye
H50.629 Inferior oblique muscle entrapment, unspecified eye
✓6th H50.63 **Inferior rectus** muscle entrapment
H50.631 Inferior rectus muscle entrapment, **right** eye
H50.632 Inferior rectus muscle entrapment, **left** eye
H50.639 Inferior rectus muscle entrapment, unspecified eye
✓6th H50.64 **Lateral rectus** muscle entrapment
H50.641 Lateral rectus muscle entrapment, **right** eye
H50.642 Lateral rectus muscle entrapment, **left** eye
H50.649 Lateral rectus muscle entrapment, unspecified eye
✓6th H50.65 **Medial rectus** muscle entrapment
H50.651 Medial rectus muscle entrapment, **right** eye
H50.652 Medial rectus muscle entrapment, **left** eye
H50.659 Medial rectus muscle entrapment, unspecified eye
✓6th H50.66 **Superior oblique** muscle entrapment
H50.661 Superior oblique muscle entrapment, **right** eye
H50.662 Superior oblique muscle entrapment, **left** eye
H50.669 Superior oblique muscle entrapment, unspecified eye
✓6th H50.67 **Superior rectus** muscle entrapment
H50.671 Superior rectus muscle entrapment, **right** eye
H50.672 Superior rectus muscle entrapment, **left** eye
H50.679 Superior rectus muscle entrapment, unspecified eye
✓6th H50.68 Extraocular muscle entrapment, unspecified
H50.681 Extraocular muscle entrapment, unspecified, **right** eye
H50.682 Extraocular muscle entrapment, unspecified, **left** eye
H50.689 Extraocular muscle entrapment, unspecified, unspecified eye
H50.69 **Other mechanical strabismus**
Strabismus due to adhesions
Traumatic limitation of duction of eye muscle
✓5th H50.8 Other specified strabismus
✓6th H50.81 **Duane's syndrome**
H50.811 Duane's syndrome, **right** eye
H50.812 Duane's syndrome, **left** eye
H50.89 Other specified strabismus
H50.9 Unspecified strabismus
✓4th H51 **Other disorders of binocular movement**
H51.0 **Palsy (spasm) of conjugate gaze**
✓5th H51.1 Convergence insufficiency and excess
H51.11 Convergence **insufficiency**
H51.12 Convergence **excess**
✓5th H51.2 Internuclear ophthalmoplegia
H51.20 Internuclear ophthalmoplegia, unspecified eye
H51.21 Internuclear ophthalmoplegia, **right** eye
H51.22 Internuclear ophthalmoplegia, **left** eye
H51.23 Internuclear ophthalmoplegia, **bilateral**
H51.8 **Other specified disorders of binocular movement**
H51.9 Unspecified disorder of binocular movement

✓4th H52 **Disorders of refraction and accommodation**
✓5th H52.0 Hypermetropia
H52.00 Hypermetropia, unspecified eye
H52.01 Hypermetropia, **right** eye
H52.02 Hypermetropia, **left** eye
H52.03 Hypermetropia, **bilateral**
✓5th H52.1 Myopia
EXCLUDES 1   degenerative myopia (H44.2-)
H52.10 Myopia, unspecified eye
H52.11 Myopia, **right** eye
H52.12 Myopia, **left** eye
H52.13 Myopia, **bilateral**
✓5th H52.2 Astigmatism
✓6th H52.20 Unspecified astigmatism
H52.201 Unspecified astigmatism, **right** eye
H52.202 Unspecified astigmatism, **left** eye
H52.203 Unspecified astigmatism, **bilateral**
H52.209 Unspecified astigmatism, unspecified eye
✓6th H52.21 **Irregular** astigmatism
H52.211 Irregular astigmatism, **right** eye
H52.212 Irregular astigmatism, **left** eye
H52.213 Irregular astigmatism, **bilateral**
H52.219 Irregular astigmatism, unspecified eye
✓6th H52.22 **Regular** astigmatism
H52.221 Regular astigmatism, **right** eye
H52.222 Regular astigmatism, **left** eye
H52.223 Regular astigmatism, **bilateral**
H52.229 Regular astigmatism, unspecified eye
✓5th H52.3 **Anisometropia and aniseikonia**
H52.31 **Anisometropia**
H52.32 **Aniseikonia**
H52.4 **Presbyopia**
✓5th H52.5 Disorders of accommodation
✓6th H52.51 **Internal ophthalmoplegia** (complete) (total)
H52.511 Internal ophthalmoplegia (complete) (total), **right** eye
H52.512 Internal ophthalmoplegia (complete) (total), **left** eye
H52.513 Internal ophthalmoplegia (complete) (total), **bilateral**
H52.519 Internal ophthalmoplegia (complete) (total), unspecified eye
✓6th H52.52 **Paresis** of accommodation
H52.521 Paresis of accommodation, **right** eye
H52.522 Paresis of accommodation, **left** eye
H52.523 Paresis of accommodation, **bilateral**
H52.529 Paresis of accommodation, unspecified eye
✓6th H52.53 **Spasm** of accommodation
H52.531 Spasm of accommodation, **right** eye
H52.532 Spasm of accommodation, **left** eye
H52.533 Spasm of accommodation, **bilateral**
H52.539 Spasm of accommodation, unspecified eye
H52.6 **Other disorders of refraction**
H52.7 Unspecified disorder of refraction

Visual disturbances and blindness (H53-H54)

✓4th H53 **Visual disturbances**
✓5th H53.0 Amblyopia ex anopsia
EXCLUDES 1   amblyopia due to vitamin A deficiency (E50.5)
✓6th H53.00 **Unspecified amblyopia**
H53.001 Unspecified amblyopia, **right** eye
H53.002 Unspecified amblyopia, **left** eye
H53.003 Unspecified amblyopia, **bilateral**
H53.009 Unspecified amblyopia, unspecified eye
✓6th H53.01 **Deprivation** amblyopia
H53.011 Deprivation amblyopia, **right** eye
H53.012 Deprivation amblyopia, **left** eye
H53.013 Deprivation amblyopia, **bilateral**
H53.019 Deprivation amblyopia, unspecified eye
✓6th H53.02 **Refractive** amblyopia
H53.021 Refractive amblyopia, **right** eye
H53.022 Refractive amblyopia, **left** eye
H53.023 Refractive amblyopia, **bilateral**
H53.029 Refractive amblyopia, unspecified eye

N Newborn: 0   P Pediatric: 0-17   M Maternity: 9-64   A Adult: 15-124   UNS Unspecified Site   MCC Major Complication/Comorbidity   CC Complication/Comorbidity   PE POA Exempt

638   ICD-10-CM 2025

√6ᵗʰ H53.03 Strabismic amblyopia

> **EXCLUDES 1**   *strabismus (H50.-)*

     H53.031   Strabismic amblyopia, **right** eye
     H53.032   Strabismic amblyopia, **left** eye
     H53.033   Strabismic amblyopia, **bilateral**
     H53.039   Strabismic amblyopia, unspecified eye

√6ᵗʰ H53.04 Amblyopia suspect

> **AHA:** 2016,4Q,22-23

     H53.041   Amblyopia suspect, **right** eye
     H53.042   Amblyopia suspect, **left** eye
     H53.043   Amblyopia suspect, **bilateral**
     H53.049   Amblyopia suspect, unspecified eye

√5ᵗʰ H53.1 Subjective visual disturbances

> **EXCLUDES 1**   *subjective visual disturbances due to vitamin A deficiency (E50.5)*
> *visual hallucinations (R44.1)*

     H53.10   Unspecified subjective visual disturbances
     H53.11   **Day blindness**
         Hemeralopia

√6ᵗʰ H53.12 Transient visual loss

     Scintillating scotoma

> **EXCLUDES 1**   *amaurosis fugax (G45.3-)*
> *transient retinal artery occlusion (H34.0-)*
> **AHA:** 2022,1Q,30

     H53.121   Transient visual loss, **right** eye   `CC`
     H53.122   Transient visual loss, **left** eye   `CC`
     H53.123   Transient visual loss, **bilateral**   `CC`
     H53.129   Transient visual loss, unspecified eye   `CC` `UNS`

√6ᵗʰ H53.13 Sudden visual loss

     H53.131   Sudden visual loss, **right** eye   `CC`
     H53.132   Sudden visual loss, **left** eye   `CC`
     H53.133   Sudden visual loss, **bilateral**   `CC`
     H53.139   Sudden visual loss, unspecified eye   `CC` `UNS`

√6ᵗʰ H53.14 Visual discomfort

     Asthenopia
     Photophobia

     H53.141   Visual discomfort, **right** eye
     H53.142   Visual discomfort, **left** eye
     H53.143   Visual discomfort, **bilateral**
     H53.149   Visual discomfort, unspecified

     H53.15   Visual **distortions** of shape and size
         Metamorphopsia
     H53.16   **Psychophysical** visual disturbances
     H53.19   Other subjective visual disturbances
         Visual halos
> **AHA:** 2022,1Q,30

H53.2 Diplopia

     Double vision

√5ᵗʰ H53.3 Other and unspecified disorders of binocular vision

     H53.30   Unspecified disorder of binocular vision
     H53.31   Abnormal retinal correspondence
     H53.32   Fusion with defective stereopsis
     H53.33   Simultaneous visual perception without fusion
     H53.34   Suppression of binocular vision

√5ᵗʰ H53.4 Visual field defects

     H53.40   Unspecified visual field defects

√6ᵗʰ H53.41 Scotoma involving central area

     Central scotoma
> **AHA:** 2022,1Q,30

     H53.411   Scotoma involving central area, **right** eye
     H53.412   Scotoma involving central area, **left** eye
     H53.413   Scotoma involving central area, **bilateral**
     H53.419   Scotoma involving central area, unspecified eye

√6ᵗʰ H53.42 Scotoma of blind spot area

     Enlarged blind spot

     H53.421   Scotoma of blind spot area, **right** eye
     H53.422   Scotoma of blind spot area, **left** eye
     H53.423   Scotoma of blind spot area, **bilateral**
     H53.429   Scotoma of blind spot area, unspecified eye

√6ᵗʰ H53.43 Sector or arcuate defects

     Arcuate scotoma
     Bjerrum scotoma

     H53.431   Sector or arcuate defects, **right** eye
     H53.432   Sector or arcuate defects, **left** eye
     H53.433   Sector or arcuate defects, **bilateral**
     H53.439   Sector or arcuate defects, unspecified eye

√6ᵗʰ H53.45 Other localized visual field defect

     Peripheral visual field defect
     Ring scotoma NOS
     Scotoma NOS

     H53.451   Other localized visual field defect, **right** eye
     H53.452   Other localized visual field defect, **left** eye
     H53.453   Other localized visual field defect, **bilateral**
     H53.459   Other localized visual field defect, unspecified eye

√6ᵗʰ H53.46 Homonymous bilateral field defects

     Homonymous hemianopia
     Homonymous hemianopsia
     Quadrant anopia
     Quadrant anopsia

     H53.461   Homonymous bilateral field defects, **right** side
     H53.462   Homonymous bilateral field defects, **left** side
     H53.469   Homonymous bilateral field defects, unspecified side
         Homonymous bilateral field defects NOS

     H53.47   **Heteronymous** bilateral field defects
         Heteronymous hemianop(s)ia

√6ᵗʰ H53.48 Generalized contraction of visual field

     H53.481   Generalized contraction of visual field, **right** eye
     H53.482   Generalized contraction of visual field, **left** eye
     H53.483   Generalized contraction of visual field, **bilateral**
     H53.489   Generalized contraction of visual field, unspecified eye

√5ᵗʰ H53.5 Color vision deficiencies

     Color blindness

> **EXCLUDES 2**   *day blindness (H53.11)*

     H53.50   Unspecified color vision deficiencies
         Color blindness NOS
     H53.51   Achromatopsia
>   **DEF:** Nonprogressive genetic visual disorder characterized by complete color blindness, decreased vision, and light sensitivity.
     H53.52   Acquired color vision deficiency
     H53.53   Deuteranomaly
         Deuteranopia
>   **DEF:** Male-only genetic disorder causing difficulty in distinguishing green and red; no shortened spectrum.
     H53.54   Protanomaly
         Protanopia
     H53.55   Tritanomaly
         Tritanopia
     H53.59   Other color vision deficiencies

√5ᵗʰ H53.6 Night blindness

> **EXCLUDES 1**   *night blindness due to vitamin A deficiency (E50.5)*

     H53.60   Unspecified night blindness
     H53.61   **Abnormal dark adaptation curve**
     H53.62   **Acquired** night blindness
     H53.63   **Congenital** night blindness
     H53.69   Other night blindness

√5ᵗʰ H53.7 Vision sensitivity deficiencies

     H53.71   **Glare** sensitivity
     H53.72   **Impaired contrast** sensitivity

H53.8 Other visual disturbances

H53.9 Unspecified visual disturbance

✅ Additional Character Required   √x7ᵗʰ Placeholder   Questionable PDx   Manifestation   Unspecified   `UPD` Unacceptable PDx   `H1`-`H14` HAC   `HCC` CMS-HCC Dx   `HIV` HIV Dx

Chapter 7. Diseases of the Eye and Adnexa (side tab)

H54–H54.7 (side tab)

√4th **H54 Blindness and low vision**

> **NOTE** For definition of visual impairment categories see table below
>
> Code first any associated underlying cause of the blindness
>
> **EXCLUDES 1** *amaurosis fugax (G45.3)*
>
> **AHA:** 2017,4Q,11-12

√5th **H54.0 Blindness, both eyes**

Visual impairment categories 3, 4, 5 in both eyes.

√6th **H54.0X Blindness, both eyes, different category levels**

√7th **H54.0X3 Blindness right eye, category 3**

H54.0X33 Blindness right eye category 3, blindness left eye category 3

H54.0X34 Blindness right eye category 3, blindness left eye category 4

H54.0X35 Blindness right eye category 3, blindness left eye category 5

√7th **H54.0X4 Blindness right eye, category 4**

H54.0X43 Blindness right eye category 4, blindness left eye category 3

H54.0X44 Blindness right eye category 4, blindness left eye category 4

H54.0X45 Blindness right eye category 4, blindness left eye category 5

√7th **H54.0X5 Blindness right eye, category 5**

H54.0X53 Blindness right eye category 5, blindness left eye category 3

H54.0X54 Blindness right eye category 5, blindness left eye category 4

H54.0X55 Blindness right eye category 5, blindness left eye category 5

√5th **H54.1 Blindness, one eye, low vision other eye**

Visual impairment categories 3, 4, 5 in one eye, with categories 1 or 2 in the other eye.

H54.10 Blindness, one eye, low vision other eye, unspecified eyes

√6th **H54.11 Blindness, right eye, low vision left eye**

√7th **H54.113 Blindness right eye category 3, low vision left eye**

H54.1131 Blindness right eye category 3, low vision left eye category 1

H54.1132 Blindness right eye category 3, low vision left eye category 2

√7th **H54.114 Blindness right eye category 4, low vision left eye**

H54.1141 Blindness right eye category 4, low vision left eye category 1

H54.1142 Blindness right eye category 4, low vision left eye category 2

√7th **H54.115 Blindness right eye category 5, low vision left eye**

H54.1151 Blindness right eye category 5, low vision left eye category 1

H54.1152 Blindness right eye category 5, low vision left eye category 2

√6th **H54.12 Blindness, left eye, low vision right eye**

√7th **H54.121 Low vision right eye category 1, blindness left eye**

H54.1213 Low vision right eye category 1, blindness left eye category 3

H54.1214 Low vision right eye category 1, blindness left eye category 4

H54.1215 Low vision right eye category 1, blindness left eye category 5

√7th **H54.122 Low vision right eye category 2, blindness left eye**

H54.1223 Low vision right eye category 2, blindness left eye category 3

H54.1224 Low vision right eye category 2, blindness left eye category 4

H54.1225 Low vision right eye category 2, blindness left eye category 5

√5th **H54.2 Low vision, both eyes**

Visual impairment categories 1 or 2 in both eyes.

√6th **H54.2X Low vision, both eyes, different category levels**

√7th **H54.2X1 Low vision, right eye, category 1**

H54.2X11 Low vision right eye category 1, low vision left eye category 1

H54.2X12 Low vision right eye category 1, low vision left eye category 2

√7th **H54.2X2 Low vision, right eye, category 2**

H54.2X21 Low vision right eye category 2, low vision left eye category 1

H54.2X22 Low vision right eye category 2, low vision left eye category 2

H54.3 Unqualified visual loss, both eyes

Visual impairment category 9 in both eyes.

TIP: Assign only when both eyes are documented as affected by blindness or low vision but the visual impairment category is not documented.

√5th **H54.4 Blindness, one eye**

Visual impairment categories 3, 4, 5 in one eye [normal vision in other eye]

H54.40 Blindness, one eye, unspecified eye

√6th **H54.41 Blindness, right eye, normal vision left eye**

√7th **H54.413 Blindness, right eye, category 3**

H54.413A Blindness right eye category 3, normal vision left eye

√7th **H54.414 Blindness, right eye, category 4**

H54.414A Blindness right eye category 4, normal vision left eye

√7th **H54.415 Blindness, right eye, category 5**

H54.415A Blindness right eye category 5, normal vision left eye

√6th **H54.42 Blindness, left eye, normal vision right eye**

√7th **H54.42A Blindness, left eye, category 3-5**

H54.42A3 Blindness left eye category 3, normal vision right eye

H54.42A4 Blindness left eye category 4, normal vision right eye

H54.42A5 Blindness left eye category 5, normal vision right eye

√5th **H54.5 Low vision, one eye**

Visual impairment categories 1 or 2 in one eye [normal vision in other eye].

H54.50 Low vision, one eye, unspecified eye

√6th **H54.51 Low vision, right eye, normal vision left eye**

√7th **H54.511 Low vision, right eye, category 1**

H54.511A Low vision right eye category 1, normal vision left eye

√7th **H54.512 Low vision, right eye, category 2**

H54.512A Low vision right eye category 2, normal vision left eye

√7th **H54.52 Low vision, left eye, normal vision right eye**

√7th **H54.52A Low vision, left eye, category 1-2**

H54.52A1 Low vision left eye category 1, normal vision right eye

H54.52A2 Low vision left eye category 2, normal vision right eye

√5th **H54.6 Unqualified visual loss, one eye**

Visual impairment category 9 in one eye [normal vision in other eye].

TIP: Assign a code from this category only when one eye is documented as affected by blindness or low vision but the visual impairment category is not documented.

H54.60 Unqualified visual loss, one eye, unspecified

H54.61 Unqualified visual loss, right eye, normal vision left eye

H54.62 Unqualified visual loss, left eye, normal vision right eye

H54.7 Unspecified visual loss UPD

Visual impairment category 9 NOS

TIP: Assign only when documentation specifies blindness, visual loss, or low vision but not whether one or both eyes are affected or the visual impairment category.

N Newborn: 0   P Pediatric: 0-17   M Maternity: 9-64   A Adult: 15-124   UNS Unspecified Site   MCC Major Complication/Comorbidity   CC Complication/Comorbidity   PE POA Exempt

640   ICD-10-CM 2025

H54.8 Legal blindness, as defined in USA
Blindness NOS according to USA definition

EXCLUDES 1   *legal blindness with specification of impairment level (H54.0-H54.7)*

NOTE   The table below gives a classification of severity of visual impairment recommended by a WHO Study Group on the Prevention of Blindness, Geneva, 6-10 November 1972.

The term "low vision" in category H54 comprises categories 1 and 2 of the table, the term "blindness" categories 3, 4 and 5, and the term "unqualified visual loss" category 9.

If the extent of the visual field is taken into account, patients with a field no greater than 10 but greater than 5 around central fixation should be placed in category 3 and patients with a field no greater than 5 around central fixation should be placed in category 4, even if the central acuity is not impaired.

Category of visual impairment	Visual acuity with best possible correction	
	Maximum less than:	**Minimum equal to or better than:**
1	6/18 3/10 (0.3) 20/70	6/60 1/10 (0.1) 20/200
2	6/60 1/10 (0.1) 20/200	3/60 1/20 (0.05) 20/400
3	3/60 1/200 (0.05) 20/400	1/60 (finger counting at one meter) 1/50 (0.02) 5/300 (20/1200)
4	1/60 (finger counting at one meter) 1/50 (0.02) 5/300	Light perception
5	No light perception	
9	Undetermined or unspecified	

Other disorders of eye and adnexa (H55-H57)

√4th H55 Nystagmus and other irregular eye movements

   √5th H55.0 Nystagmus

     DEF: Rapid, rhythmic, involuntary movements of the eyeball in vertical, horizontal, rotational, or mixed directions.

     H55.00   Unspecified nystagmus
     H55.01   Congenital nystagmus
     H55.02   Latent nystagmus
     H55.03   Visual deprivation nystagmus
     H55.04   Dissociated nystagmus
     H55.09   Other forms of nystagmus

   √5th H55.8 Other irregular eye movements

     AHA: 2020,4Q,25

     H55.81   Deficient saccadic eye movements
     H55.82   Deficient smooth pursuit eye movements
     H55.89   Other irregular eye movements

√4th H57 Other disorders of eye and adnexa

   √5th H57.0 Anomalies of pupillary function

     H57.00   Unspecified anomaly of pupillary function
     H57.01   Argyll Robertson pupil, atypical
       EXCLUDES 1   *syphilitic Argyll Robertson pupil (A52.19)*
     H57.02   Anisocoria
     H57.03   Miosis
     H57.04   Mydriasis
     √6th H57.05 Tonic pupil

       H57.051   Tonic pupil, right eye
       H57.052   Tonic pupil, left eye
       H57.053   Tonic pupil, bilateral
       H57.059   Tonic pupil, unspecified eye
     H57.09   Other anomalies of pupillary function

   √5th H57.1 Ocular pain

     H57.10   Ocular pain, unspecified eye

H57.11   Ocular pain, right eye
H57.12   Ocular pain, left eye
H57.13   Ocular pain, bilateral

√5th H57.8 Other specified disorders of eye and adnexa

   AHA: 2018,4Q,15-16

   √6th H57.81 Brow ptosis

     H57.811   Brow ptosis, right
     H57.812   Brow ptosis, left
     H57.813   Brow ptosis, bilateral
     H57.819   Brow ptosis, unspecified
   H57.89   Other specified disorders of eye and adnexa

   √6th H57.8A Foreign body sensation eye (ocular)

     AHA: 2023,4Q,23

     H57.8A1   Foreign body sensation, right eye
     H57.8A2   Foreign body sensation, left eye
     H57.8A3   Foreign body sensation, bilateral eyes
     H57.8A9   Foreign body sensation, unspecified eye

   H57.9   Unspecified disorder of eye and adnexa   UPD

Intraoperative and postprocedural complications and disorders of eye and adnexa, not elsewhere classified (H59)

√4th H59 Intraoperative and postprocedural complications and disorders of eye and adnexa, not elsewhere classified

   EXCLUDES 1   *mechanical complication of intraocular lens (T85.2)*
       mechanical complication of other ocular prosthetic devices, implants and grafts (T85.3)
       pseudophakia (Z96.1)
       secondary cataracts (H26.4-)

   √5th H59.0 Disorders of the eye following cataract surgery

     √6th H59.01 Keratopathy (bullous aphakic) following cataract surgery
       Vitreal corneal syndrome
       Vitreous (touch) syndrome

       H59.011   Keratopathy (bullous aphakic) following cataract surgery, right eye   CC
       H59.012   Keratopathy (bullous aphakic) following cataract surgery, left eye   CC
       H59.013   Keratopathy (bullous aphakic) following cataract surgery, bilateral   CC
       H59.019   Keratopathy (bullous aphakic) following cataract surgery, unspecified eye   CC UNS

     √6th H59.02 Cataract (lens) fragments in eye following cataract surgery
       H59.021   Cataract (lens) fragments in eye following cataract surgery, right eye
       H59.022   Cataract (lens) fragments in eye following cataract surgery, left eye
       H59.023   Cataract (lens) fragments in eye following cataract surgery, bilateral
       H59.029   Cataract (lens) fragments in eye following cataract surgery, unspecified eye

     √6th H59.03 Cystoid macular edema following cataract surgery
       H59.031   Cystoid macular edema following cataract surgery, right eye   CC
       H59.032   Cystoid macular edema following cataract surgery, left eye   CC
       H59.033   Cystoid macular edema following cataract surgery, bilateral   CC
       H59.039   Cystoid macular edema following cataract surgery, unspecified eye   CC UNS

     √6th H59.09 Other disorders of the eye following cataract surgery
       H59.091   Other disorders of the right eye following cataract surgery   CC
       H59.092   Other disorders of the left eye following cataract surgery   CC
       H59.093   Other disorders of the eye following cataract surgery, bilateral   CC
       H59.099   Other disorders of unspecified eye following cataract surgery   CC UNS

✔ Additional Character Required   √x7th Placeholder   Questionable PDx   Manifestation   Unspecified   UPD Unacceptable PDx   H1-H14 HAC   HCC CMS-HCC Dx   HIV HIV Dx

ICD-10-CM 2025   641

✓5ᵗʰ **H59.1** **Intraoperative hemorrhage and hematoma** of eye and adnexa complicating a procedure

     EXCLUDES 1   *intraoperative hemorrhage and hematoma of eye and adnexa due to accidental puncture or laceration during a procedure (H59.2-)*

   ✓6ᵗʰ **H59.11** Intraoperative hemorrhage and hematoma of eye and adnexa complicating an **ophthalmic procedure**

     H59.111 Intraoperative hemorrhage and hematoma of **right** eye and adnexa complicating an ophthalmic procedure   CC

     H59.112 Intraoperative hemorrhage and hematoma of **left** eye and adnexa complicating an ophthalmic procedure   CC

     H59.113 Intraoperative hemorrhage and hematoma of eye and adnexa complicating an ophthalmic procedure, **bilateral**   CC

     H59.119 Intraoperative hemorrhage and hematoma of unspecified eye and adnexa complicating an ophthalmic procedure   CC UNS

   ✓6ᵗʰ **H59.12** Intraoperative hemorrhage and hematoma of eye and adnexa complicating **other procedure**

     H59.121 Intraoperative hemorrhage and hematoma of **right** eye and adnexa complicating other procedure   CC

     H59.122 Intraoperative hemorrhage and hematoma of **left** eye and adnexa complicating other procedure   CC

     H59.123 Intraoperative hemorrhage and hematoma of eye and adnexa complicating other procedure, **bilateral**   CC

     H59.129 Intraoperative hemorrhage and hematoma of unspecified eye and adnexa complicating other procedure   CC UNS

✓5ᵗʰ **H59.2** **Accidental puncture and laceration** of eye and adnexa during a procedure

   ✓6ᵗʰ **H59.21** Accidental puncture and laceration of eye and adnexa during an **ophthalmic procedure**

     H59.211 Accidental puncture and laceration of **right** eye and adnexa during an ophthalmic procedure   CC

     H59.212 Accidental puncture and laceration of **left** eye and adnexa during an ophthalmic procedure   CC

     H59.213 Accidental puncture and laceration of eye and adnexa during an ophthalmic procedure, **bilateral**   CC

     H59.219 Accidental puncture and laceration of unspecified eye and adnexa during an ophthalmic procedure   CC UNS

   ✓6ᵗʰ **H59.22** Accidental puncture and laceration of eye and adnexa during **other procedure**

     H59.221 Accidental puncture and laceration of **right** eye and adnexa during other procedure   CC

     H59.222 Accidental puncture and laceration of **left** eye and adnexa during other procedure   CC

     H59.223 Accidental puncture and laceration of eye and adnexa during other procedure, **bilateral**   CC

     H59.229 Accidental puncture and laceration of unspecified eye and adnexa during other procedure   CC UNS

✓5ᵗʰ **H59.3** **Postprocedural hemorrhage, hematoma, and seroma** of eye and adnexa following a procedure

     AHA: 2016,4Q,9-10

   ✓6ᵗʰ **H59.31** Postprocedural **hemorrhage** of eye and adnexa following an **ophthalmic procedure**

     H59.311 Postprocedural hemorrhage of **right** eye and adnexa following an ophthalmic procedure   CC

     H59.312 Postprocedural hemorrhage of **left** eye and adnexa following an ophthalmic procedure   CC

     H59.313 Postprocedural hemorrhage of eye and adnexa following an ophthalmic procedure, **bilateral**   CC

     H59.319 Postprocedural hemorrhage of unspecified eye and adnexa following an ophthalmic procedure   CC UNS

   ✓6ᵗʰ **H59.32** Postprocedural **hemorrhage** of eye and adnexa following **other procedure**

     H59.321 Postprocedural hemorrhage of **right** eye and adnexa following other procedure   CC

     H59.322 Postprocedural hemorrhage of **left** eye and adnexa following other procedure   CC

     H59.323 Postprocedural hemorrhage of eye and adnexa following other procedure, **bilateral**   CC

     H59.329 Postprocedural hemorrhage of unspecified eye and adnexa following other procedure   CC UNS

   ✓6ᵗʰ **H59.33** Postprocedural **hematoma** of eye and adnexa following an **ophthalmic procedure**

     H59.331 Postprocedural hematoma of **right** eye and adnexa following an ophthalmic procedure   CC

     H59.332 Postprocedural hematoma of **left** eye and adnexa following an ophthalmic procedure   CC

     H59.333 Postprocedural hematoma of eye and adnexa following an ophthalmic procedure, **bilateral**   CC

     H59.339 Postprocedural hematoma of unspecified eye and adnexa following an ophthalmic procedure   CC UNS

   ✓6ᵗʰ **H59.34** Postprocedural **hematoma** of eye and adnexa following **other procedure**

     H59.341 Postprocedural hematoma of **right** eye and adnexa following other procedure   CC

     H59.342 Postprocedural hematoma of **left** eye and adnexa following other procedure   CC

     H59.343 Postprocedural hematoma of eye and adnexa following other procedure, **bilateral**   CC

     H59.349 Postprocedural hematoma of unspecified eye and adnexa following other procedure   CC UNS

   ✓6ᵗʰ **H59.35** Postprocedural **seroma** of eye and adnexa following an **ophthalmic procedure**

     H59.351 Postprocedural seroma of **right** eye and adnexa following an ophthalmic procedure   CC

     H59.352 Postprocedural seroma of **left** eye and adnexa following an ophthalmic procedure   CC

     H59.353 Postprocedural seroma of eye and adnexa following an ophthalmic procedure, **bilateral**   CC

     H59.359 Postprocedural seroma of unspecified eye and adnexa following an ophthalmic procedure   CC UNS

   ✓6ᵗʰ **H59.36** Postprocedural **seroma** of eye and adnexa following **other procedure**

     H59.361 Postprocedural seroma of **right** eye and adnexa following other procedure   CC

     H59.362 Postprocedural seroma of **left** eye and adnexa following other procedure   CC

     H59.363 Postprocedural seroma of eye and adnexa following other procedure, **bilateral**   CC

     H59.369 Postprocedural seroma of unspecified eye and adnexa following other procedure   CC UNS

✓5ᵗʰ **H59.4** **Inflammation (infection)** of **postprocedural bleb**

     Postprocedural blebitis

     EXCLUDES 1   *filtering (vitreous) bleb after glaucoma surgery status (Z98.83)*

     H59.40 Inflammation (infection) of postprocedural bleb, unspecified

     H59.41 Inflammation (infection) of postprocedural bleb, **stage 1**

     H59.42 Inflammation (infection) of postprocedural bleb, **stage 2**

     H59.43 Inflammation (infection) of postprocedural bleb, **stage 3**

       Bleb endophthalmitis

N Newborn: 0   **P** Pediatric: 0-17   **M** Maternity: 9-64   **A** Adult: 15-124   **UNS** Unspecified Site   **MCC** Major Complication/Comorbidity   **CC** Complication/Comorbidity   **PE** POA Exempt

642   ICD-10-CM 2025

☑5ᵗʰ **H59.8 Other intraoperative and postprocedural complications and disorders of eye and adnexa, not elsewhere classified**

☑6ᵗʰ **H59.81 Chorioretinal scars after surgery for detachment**

H59.811 Chorioretinal scars after surgery for detachment, right eye `CC`

H59.812 Chorioretinal scars after surgery for detachment, left eye `CC`

H59.813 Chorioretinal scars after surgery for detachment, bilateral `CC`

H59.819 Chorioretinal scars after surgery for detachment, unspecified eye `CC` `UNS`

H59.88 Other intraoperative complications of eye and adnexa, not elsewhere classified `CC`

H59.89 Other postprocedural complications and disorders of eye and adnexa, not elsewhere classified `CC`

AHA: 2020,3Q,29

☑ Additional Character Required   ☑x7ᵗʰ Placeholder   Questionable PDx   Manifestation   Unspecified   UPD Unacceptable PDx   H1 -H14 HAC   HCC CMS-HCC Dx   HIV HIV Dx

Chapter 8. Diseases of the Ear and Mastoid Process (H60–H95)

Chapter-specific Guidelines with Coding Examples
Reserved for future guideline expansion.

Chapter 8. Diseases of the Ear and Mastoid Process (H60-H95)

NOTE   Use an external cause code following the code for the ear condition, if applicable, to identify the cause of the ear condition

EXCLUDES 2   certain conditions originating in the perinatal period (P04-P96)
certain infectious and parasitic diseases (A00-B99)
complications of pregnancy, childbirth and the puerperium (O00-O9A)
congenital malformations, deformations and chromosomal abnormalities (Q00-Q99)
endocrine, nutritional and metabolic diseases (E00-E88)
injury, poisoning and certain other consequences of external causes (S00-T88)
neoplasms (C00-D49)
symptoms, signs and abnormal clinical and laboratory findings, not elsewhere classified (R00-R94)

This chapter contains the following blocks:
H60-H62   Diseases of external ear
H65-H75   Diseases of middle ear and mastoid
H80-H83   Diseases of inner ear
H90-H94   Other disorders of ear
H95   Intraoperative and postprocedural complications and disorders of ear and mastoid process, not elsewhere classified

Diseases of external ear (H60-H62)

✓4th **H60   Otitis externa**

✓5th **H60.0   Abscess of external ear**
Boil of external ear
Carbuncle of auricle or external auditory canal
Furuncle of external ear
   H60.00   Abscess of external ear, unspecified ear
   H60.01   Abscess of right external ear
   H60.02   Abscess of left external ear
   H60.03   Abscess of external ear, bilateral

✓5th **H60.1   Cellulitis of external ear**
Cellulitis of auricle
Cellulitis of external auditory canal
   H60.10   Cellulitis of external ear, unspecified ear
   H60.11   Cellulitis of right external ear
   H60.12   Cellulitis of left external ear
   H60.13   Cellulitis of external ear, bilateral

✓5th **H60.2   Malignant otitis externa**
   H60.20   Malignant otitis externa, unspecified ear   `CC` `UNS`
   H60.21   Malignant otitis externa, right ear   `CC`
   H60.22   Malignant otitis externa, left ear   `CC`
   H60.23   Malignant otitis externa, bilateral   `CC`

✓5th **H60.3   Other infective otitis externa**
  ✓6th **H60.31   Diffuse otitis externa**
   H60.311   Diffuse otitis externa, right ear
   H60.312   Diffuse otitis externa, left ear
   H60.313   Diffuse otitis externa, bilateral
   H60.319   Diffuse otitis externa, unspecified ear
  ✓6th **H60.32   Hemorrhagic otitis externa**
   H60.321   Hemorrhagic otitis externa, right ear
   H60.322   Hemorrhagic otitis externa, left ear
   H60.323   Hemorrhagic otitis externa, bilateral
   H60.329   Hemorrhagic otitis externa, unspecified ear
  ✓6th **H60.33   Swimmer's ear**
   DEF: Commonly occurs when water gets trapped in the ear after swimming.
   H60.331   Swimmer's ear, right ear
   H60.332   Swimmer's ear, left ear
   H60.333   Swimmer's ear, bilateral
   H60.339   Swimmer's ear, unspecified ear
  ✓6th **H60.39   Other infective otitis externa**
   H60.391   Other infective otitis externa, right ear
   H60.392   Other infective otitis externa, left ear
   H60.393   Other infective otitis externa, bilateral
   H60.399   Other infective otitis externa, unspecified ear

✓5th **H60.4   Cholesteatoma of external ear**
Keratosis obturans of external ear (canal)
EXCLUDES 2   cholesteatoma of middle ear (H71.-)
recurrent cholesteatoma of postmastoidectomy cavity (H95.0-)
DEF: Cholesteatoma: Noncancerous cyst-like mass of cell debris, including cholesterol and epithelial cells resulting from trauma, repeated or improperly healed infections, and congenital enclosure of epidermal cells.
   H60.40   Cholesteatoma of external ear, unspecified ear
   H60.41   Cholesteatoma of right external ear
   H60.42   Cholesteatoma of left external ear
   H60.43   Cholesteatoma of external ear, bilateral

✓5th **H60.5   Acute noninfective otitis externa**
  ✓6th **H60.50   Unspecified acute noninfective otitis externa**
   Acute otitis externa NOS
   H60.501   Unspecified acute noninfective otitis externa, right ear
   H60.502   Unspecified acute noninfective otitis externa, left ear
   H60.503   Unspecified acute noninfective otitis externa, bilateral
   H60.509   Unspecified acute noninfective otitis externa, unspecified ear
  ✓6th **H60.51   Acute actinic otitis externa**
   H60.511   Acute actinic otitis externa, right ear
   H60.512   Acute actinic otitis externa, left ear
   H60.513   Acute actinic otitis externa, bilateral
   H60.519   Acute actinic otitis externa, unspecified ear
  ✓6th **H60.52   Acute chemical otitis externa**
   H60.521   Acute chemical otitis externa, right ear
   H60.522   Acute chemical otitis externa, left ear
   H60.523   Acute chemical otitis externa, bilateral
   H60.529   Acute chemical otitis externa, unspecified ear
  ✓6th **H60.53   Acute contact otitis externa**
   H60.531   Acute contact otitis externa, right ear
   H60.532   Acute contact otitis externa, left ear
   H60.533   Acute contact otitis externa, bilateral
   H60.539   Acute contact otitis externa, unspecified ear
  ✓6th **H60.54   Acute eczematoid otitis externa**
   H60.541   Acute eczematoid otitis externa, right ear
   H60.542   Acute eczematoid otitis externa, left ear
   H60.543   Acute eczematoid otitis externa, bilateral
   H60.549   Acute eczematoid otitis externa, unspecified ear
  ✓6th **H60.55   Acute reactive otitis externa**
   H60.551   Acute reactive otitis externa, right ear
   H60.552   Acute reactive otitis externa, left ear
   H60.553   Acute reactive otitis externa, bilateral
   H60.559   Acute reactive otitis externa, unspecified ear
  ✓6th **H60.59   Other noninfective acute otitis externa**
   H60.591   Other noninfective acute otitis externa, right ear
   H60.592   Other noninfective acute otitis externa, left ear
   H60.593   Other noninfective acute otitis externa, bilateral
   H60.599   Other noninfective acute otitis externa, unspecified ear

✓5th **H60.6   Unspecified chronic otitis externa**
   H60.60   Unspecified chronic otitis externa, unspecified ear
   H60.61   Unspecified chronic otitis externa, right ear
   H60.62   Unspecified chronic otitis externa, left ear
   H60.63   Unspecified chronic otitis externa, bilateral

✓5th **H60.8   Other otitis externa**
  ✓6th **H60.8X   Other otitis externa**
   H60.8X1   Other otitis externa, right ear
   H60.8X2   Other otitis externa, left ear
   H60.8X3   Other otitis externa, bilateral
   H60.8X9   Other otitis externa, unspecified ear

✓5th **H60.9   Unspecified otitis externa**
   H60.90   Unspecified otitis externa, unspecified ear
   H60.91   Unspecified otitis externa, right ear

N Newborn: 0   **P** Pediatric: 0-17   **M** Maternity: 9-64   **A** Adult: 15-124   **UNS** Unspecified Site   **MCC** Major Complication/Comorbidity   **CC** Complication/Comorbidity   **PE** POA Exempt

646
ICD-10-CM 2025

H60.92   Unspecified otitis externa, **left** ear

H60.93   Unspecified otitis externa, **bilateral**

✓4ᵗʰ **H61**   **Other disorders of external ear**

   ✓5ᵗʰ **H61.0**   **Chondritis and perichondritis of external ear**

     Chondrodermatitis nodularis chronica helicis

     Perichondritis of auricle

     Perichondritis of pinna

     ✓6ᵗʰ **H61.00**   **Unspecified perichondritis of external ear**

       H61.001   Unspecified perichondritis of **right** external ear

       H61.002   Unspecified perichondritis of **left** external ear

       H61.003   Unspecified perichondritis of external ear, **bilateral**

       H61.009   Unspecified perichondritis of external ear, unspecified ear

     ✓6ᵗʰ **H61.01**   **Acute perichondritis of external ear**

       H61.011   Acute perichondritis of **right** external ear

       H61.012   Acute perichondritis of **left** external ear

       H61.013   Acute perichondritis of external ear, **bilateral**

       H61.019   Acute perichondritis of external ear, unspecified ear

     ✓6ᵗʰ **H61.02**   **Chronic perichondritis of external ear**

       H61.021   Chronic perichondritis of **right** external ear

       H61.022   Chronic perichondritis of **left** external ear

       H61.023   Chronic perichondritis of external ear, **bilateral**

       H61.029   Chronic perichondritis of external ear, unspecified ear

     ✓6ᵗʰ **H61.03**   **Chondritis of external ear**

       Chondritis of auricle

       Chondritis of pinna

       AHA: 2015,1Q,18

       DEF: Infection that has progressed into the cartilage and presents as indurated and edematous skin over the pinna. Vascular compromise occurs with tissue necrosis and deformity.

       H61.031   Chondritis of **right** external ear

       H61.032   Chondritis of **left** external ear

       H61.033   Chondritis of external ear, **bilateral**

       H61.039   Chondritis of external ear, unspecified ear

   ✓5ᵗʰ **H61.1**   **Noninfective disorders of pinna**

     EXCLUDES 2   cauliflower ear (M95.1-)

                 gouty tophi of ear (M1A.-)

     ✓6ᵗʰ **H61.10**   **Unspecified noninfective disorders of pinna**

       Disorder of pinna NOS

       H61.101   Unspecified noninfective disorders of pinna, **right** ear

       H61.102   Unspecified noninfective disorders of pinna, **left** ear

       H61.103   Unspecified noninfective disorders of pinna, **bilateral**

       H61.109   Unspecified noninfective disorders of pinna, unspecified ear

     ✓6ᵗʰ **H61.11**   **Acquired deformity of pinna**

       Acquired deformity of auricle

       EXCLUDES 2   cauliflower ear (M95.1-)

       H61.111   Acquired deformity of pinna, **right** ear

       H61.112   Acquired deformity of pinna, **left** ear

       H61.113   Acquired deformity of pinna, **bilateral**

       H61.119   Acquired deformity of pinna, unspecified ear

     ✓6ᵗʰ **H61.12**   **Hematoma of pinna**

       Hematoma of auricle

       H61.121   Hematoma of pinna, **right** ear

       H61.122   Hematoma of pinna, **left** ear

       H61.123   Hematoma of pinna, **bilateral**

       H61.129   Hematoma of pinna, unspecified ear

     ✓6ᵗʰ **H61.19**   **Other noninfective disorders of pinna**

       H61.191   Noninfective disorders of pinna, **right** ear

       H61.192   Noninfective disorders of pinna, **left** ear

       H61.193   Noninfective disorders of pinna, **bilateral**

       H61.199   Noninfective disorders of pinna, unspecified ear

   ✓5ᵗʰ **H61.2**   **Impacted cerumen**

     Wax in ear

     H61.20   **Impacted cerumen, unspecified ear**

H61.21   **Impacted cerumen, right ear**

H61.22   **Impacted cerumen, left ear**

H61.23   **Impacted cerumen, bilateral**

   ✓5ᵗʰ **H61.3**   **Acquired stenosis of external ear canal**

     Collapse of external ear canal

     EXCLUDES 1   postprocedural stenosis of external ear canal (H95.81-)

     ✓6ᵗʰ **H61.30**   **Acquired stenosis of external ear canal, unspecified**

       H61.301   Acquired stenosis of **right** external ear canal, unspecified

       H61.302   Acquired stenosis of **left** external ear canal, unspecified

       H61.303   Acquired stenosis of external ear canal, unspecified, **bilateral**

       H61.309   Acquired stenosis of external ear canal, unspecified, unspecified ear

     ✓6ᵗʰ **H61.31**   **Acquired stenosis of external ear canal secondary to trauma**

       H61.311   Acquired stenosis of **right** external ear canal secondary to trauma

       H61.312   Acquired stenosis of **left** external ear canal secondary to trauma

       H61.313   Acquired stenosis of external ear canal secondary to trauma, **bilateral**

       H61.319   Acquired stenosis of external ear canal secondary to trauma, unspecified ear

     ✓6ᵗʰ **H61.32**   **Acquired stenosis of external ear canal secondary to inflammation and infection**

       DEF: Narrowing of the external ear canal due to chronic inflammation or infection.

       H61.321   Acquired stenosis of **right** external ear canal secondary to inflammation and infection

       H61.322   Acquired stenosis of **left** external ear canal secondary to inflammation and infection

       H61.323   Acquired stenosis of external ear canal secondary to inflammation and infection, **bilateral**

       H61.329   Acquired stenosis of external ear canal secondary to inflammation and infection, unspecified ear

     ✓6ᵗʰ **H61.39**   **Other acquired stenosis of external ear canal**

       H61.391   Other acquired stenosis of **right** external ear canal

       H61.392   Other acquired stenosis of **left** external ear canal

       H61.393   Other acquired stenosis of external ear canal, **bilateral**

       H61.399   Other acquired stenosis of external ear canal, unspecified ear

   ✓5ᵗʰ **H61.8**   **Other specified disorders of external ear**

     ✓6ᵗʰ **H61.81**   **Exostosis of external canal**

       H61.811   Exostosis of **right** external canal

       H61.812   Exostosis of **left** external canal

       H61.813   Exostosis of external canal, **bilateral**

       H61.819   Exostosis of external canal, unspecified ear

     ✓6ᵗʰ **H61.89**   **Other specified disorders of external ear**

       H61.891   Other specified disorders of **right** external ear

       H61.892   Other specified disorders of **left** external ear

       H61.893   Other specified disorders of external ear, **bilateral**

       H61.899   Other specified disorders of external ear, unspecified ear

   ✓5ᵗʰ **H61.9**   **Disorder of external ear, unspecified**

     H61.90   Disorder of external ear, unspecified, unspecified ear

     H61.91   Disorder of **right** external ear, unspecified

     H61.92   Disorder of **left** external ear, unspecified

     H61.93   Disorder of external ear, unspecified, **bilateral**

✔ Additional Character Required   ✓x7ᵗʰ Placeholder   Questionable PDx   Manifestation   Unspecified   UPD Unacceptable PDx   H1–H14 HAC   HCC CMS-HCC Dx   HIV HIV Dx

✓4th H62 Disorders of external ear in diseases classified elsewhere

✓5th H62.4 Otitis externa in other diseases classified elsewhere

Code first underlying disease, such as:
erysipelas (A46)
impetigo (LØ1.Ø-)

EXCLUDES 1   *otitis externa (in):*
candidiasis (B37.84)
herpes viral [herpes simplex] (BØØ.1)
herpes zoster (BØ2.8)

H62.4Ø *Otitis externa in other diseases classified elsewhere, unspecified ear*

H62.41 *Otitis externa in other diseases classified elsewhere, right ear*

H62.42 *Otitis externa in other diseases classified elsewhere, left ear*

H62.43 *Otitis externa in other diseases classified elsewhere, bilateral*

✓5th H62.8 Other disorders of external ear in diseases classified elsewhere

Code first underlying disease, such as:
gout (M1A.-, M1Ø.-)

✓6th H62.8X Other disorders of external ear in diseases classified elsewhere

H62.8X1 *Other disorders of right external ear in diseases classified elsewhere*

H62.8X2 *Other disorders of left external ear in diseases classified elsewhere*

H62.8X3 *Other disorders of external ear in diseases classified elsewhere, bilateral*

H62.8X9 *Other disorders of external ear in diseases classified elsewhere, unspecified ear*

Diseases of middle ear and mastoid (H65-H75)

✓4th H65 Nonsuppurative otitis media

INCLUDES   nonsuppurative otitis media with myringitis

Use additional code for any associated perforated tympanic membrane (H72.-)
Use additional code, if applicable, to identify:
exposure to environmental tobacco smoke (Z77.22)
exposure to tobacco smoke in the perinatal period (P96.81)
history of tobacco dependence (Z87.891)
infectious agent (B95-B97)
occupational exposure to environmental tobacco smoke (Z57.31)
tobacco dependence (F17.-)
tobacco use (Z72.Ø)

✓5th H65.Ø Acute serous otitis media

Acute and subacute secretory otitis

H65.ØØ Acute serous otitis media, unspecified ear
H65.Ø1 Acute serous otitis media, right ear
H65.Ø2 Acute serous otitis media, left ear
H65.Ø3 Acute serous otitis media, bilateral
H65.Ø4 Acute serous otitis media, recurrent, right ear
H65.Ø5 Acute serous otitis media, recurrent, left ear
H65.Ø6 Acute serous otitis media, recurrent, bilateral
H65.Ø7 Acute serous otitis media, recurrent, unspecified ear

✓5th H65.1 Other acute nonsuppurative otitis media

EXCLUDES 1   *otitic barotrauma (T7Ø.Ø)*
otitis media (acute) NOS (H66.9)

✓6th H65.11 Acute and subacute allergic otitis media (mucoid) (sanguinous) (serous)

H65.111 Acute and subacute allergic otitis media (mucoid) (sanguinous) (serous), right ear
H65.112 Acute and subacute allergic otitis media (mucoid) (sanguinous) (serous), left ear
H65.113 Acute and subacute allergic otitis media (mucoid) (sanguinous) (serous), bilateral
H65.114 Acute and subacute allergic otitis media (mucoid) (sanguinous) (serous), recurrent, right ear
H65.115 Acute and subacute allergic otitis media (mucoid) (sanguinous) (serous), recurrent, left ear
H65.116 Acute and subacute allergic otitis media (mucoid) (sanguinous) (serous), recurrent, bilateral
H65.117 Acute and subacute allergic otitis media (mucoid) (sanguinous) (serous), recurrent, unspecified ear

H65.119 Acute and subacute allergic otitis media (mucoid) (sanguinous) (serous), unspecified ear

✓6th H65.19 Other acute nonsuppurative otitis media

Acute and subacute mucoid otitis media
Acute and subacute nonsuppurative otitis media NOS
Acute and subacute sanguinous otitis media
Acute and subacute seromucinous otitis media

H65.191 Other acute nonsuppurative otitis media, right ear
H65.192 Other acute nonsuppurative otitis media, left ear
H65.193 Other acute nonsuppurative otitis media, bilateral
H65.194 Other acute nonsuppurative otitis media, recurrent, right ear
H65.195 Other acute nonsuppurative otitis media, recurrent, left ear
H65.196 Other acute nonsuppurative otitis media, recurrent, bilateral
H65.197 Other acute nonsuppurative otitis media, recurrent, unspecified ear
H65.199 Other acute nonsuppurative otitis media, unspecified ear

✓5th H65.2 Chronic serous otitis media

Chronic tubotympanal catarrh

H65.2Ø Chronic serous otitis media, unspecified ear
H65.21 Chronic serous otitis media, right ear
H65.22 Chronic serous otitis media, left ear
H65.23 Chronic serous otitis media, bilateral

✓5th H65.3 Chronic mucoid otitis media

Chronic mucinous otitis media
Chronic secretory otitis media
Chronic transudative otitis media
Glue ear

EXCLUDES 1   *adhesive middle ear disease (H74.1)*

H65.3Ø Chronic mucoid otitis media, unspecified ear
H65.31 Chronic mucoid otitis media, right ear
H65.32 Chronic mucoid otitis media, left ear
H65.33 Chronic mucoid otitis media, bilateral

✓5th H65.4 Other chronic nonsuppurative otitis media

✓6th H65.41 Chronic allergic otitis media

H65.411 Chronic allergic otitis media, right ear
H65.412 Chronic allergic otitis media, left ear
H65.413 Chronic allergic otitis media, bilateral
H65.419 Chronic allergic otitis media, unspecified ear

✓6th H65.49 Other chronic nonsuppurative otitis media

Chronic exudative otitis media
Chronic nonsuppurative otitis media NOS
Chronic otitis media with effusion (nonpurulent)
Chronic seromucinous otitis media

H65.491 Other chronic nonsuppurative otitis media, right ear
H65.492 Other chronic nonsuppurative otitis media, left ear
H65.493 Other chronic nonsuppurative otitis media, bilateral
H65.499 Other chronic nonsuppurative otitis media, unspecified ear

✓5th H65.9 Unspecified nonsuppurative otitis media

Allergic otitis media NOS
Catarrhal otitis media NOS
Exudative otitis media NOS
Mucoid otitis media NOS
Otitis media with effusion (nonpurulent) NOS
Secretory otitis media NOS
Seromucinous otitis media NOS
Serous otitis media NOS
Transudative otitis media NOS

H65.9Ø Unspecified nonsuppurative otitis media, unspecified ear
H65.91 Unspecified nonsuppurative otitis media, right ear
H65.92 Unspecified nonsuppurative otitis media, left ear
H65.93 Unspecified nonsuppurative otitis media, bilateral

✓4ᵗʰ **H66 Suppurative and unspecified otitis media**

INCLUDES suppurative and unspecified otitis media with myringitis

Use additional code to identify:
exposure to environmental tobacco smoke (Z77.22)
exposure to tobacco smoke in the perinatal period (P96.81)
history of tobacco dependence (Z87.891)
occupational exposure to environmental tobacco smoke (Z57.31)
tobacco dependence (F17.-)
tobacco use (Z72.0)

AHA: 2016,1Q,34

✓5ᵗʰ **H66.0 Acute suppurative otitis media**

✓6ᵗʰ **H66.00 Acute suppurative otitis media without spontaneous rupture of ear drum**

H66.001 Acute suppurative otitis media without spontaneous rupture of ear drum, **right ear**

H66.002 Acute suppurative otitis media without spontaneous rupture of ear drum, **left ear**

H66.003 Acute suppurative otitis media without spontaneous rupture of ear drum, **bilateral**

H66.004 Acute suppurative otitis media without spontaneous rupture of ear drum, **recurrent, right ear**

H66.005 Acute suppurative otitis media without spontaneous rupture of ear drum, **recurrent, left ear**

H66.006 Acute suppurative otitis media without spontaneous rupture of ear drum, **recurrent, bilateral**

H66.007 Acute suppurative otitis media without spontaneous rupture of ear drum, **recurrent, unspecified ear**

H66.009 Acute suppurative otitis media without spontaneous rupture of ear drum, unspecified ear

✓6ᵗʰ **H66.01 Acute suppurative otitis media with spontaneous rupture of ear drum**

DEF: Sudden, severe inflammation of the middle ear, causing pressure that perforates the ear drum tissue.

H66.011 Acute suppurative otitis media with spontaneous rupture of ear drum, **right ear**

H66.012 Acute suppurative otitis media with spontaneous rupture of ear drum, **left ear**

H66.013 Acute suppurative otitis media with spontaneous rupture of ear drum, **bilateral**

H66.014 Acute suppurative otitis media with spontaneous rupture of ear drum, **recurrent, right ear**

H66.015 Acute suppurative otitis media with spontaneous rupture of ear drum, **recurrent, left ear**

H66.016 Acute suppurative otitis media with spontaneous rupture of ear drum, **recurrent, bilateral**

H66.017 Acute suppurative otitis media with spontaneous rupture of ear drum, **recurrent, unspecified ear**

H66.019 Acute suppurative otitis media with spontaneous rupture of ear drum, unspecified ear

✓5ᵗʰ **H66.1 Chronic tubotympanic suppurative otitis media**

Benign chronic suppurative otitis media
Chronic tubotympanic disease
Use additional code for any associated perforated tympanic membrane (H72.-)

H66.10 Chronic tubotympanic suppurative otitis media, unspecified

H66.11 Chronic tubotympanic suppurative otitis media, **right ear**

H66.12 Chronic tubotympanic suppurative otitis media, **left ear**

H66.13 Chronic tubotympanic suppurative otitis media, **bilateral**

✓5ᵗʰ **H66.2 Chronic atticoantral suppurative otitis media**

Chronic atticoantral disease
Use additional code for any associated perforated tympanic membrane (H72.-)

H66.20 Chronic atticoantral suppurative otitis media, unspecified ear

H66.21 Chronic atticoantral suppurative otitis media, **right ear**

H66.22 Chronic atticoantral suppurative otitis media, **left ear**

H66.23 Chronic atticoantral suppurative otitis media, **bilateral**

✓5ᵗʰ **H66.3 Other chronic suppurative otitis media**

Chronic suppurative otitis media NOS
Use additional code for any associated perforated tympanic membrane (H72.-)

EXCLUDES 1 tuberculous otitis media (A18.6)

✓6ᵗʰ **H66.3X Other chronic suppurative otitis media**

H66.3X1 Other chronic suppurative otitis media, **right ear**

H66.3X2 Other chronic suppurative otitis media, **left ear**

H66.3X3 Other chronic suppurative otitis media, **bilateral**

H66.3X9 Other chronic suppurative otitis media, unspecified ear

✓5ᵗʰ **H66.4 Suppurative otitis media, unspecified**

Purulent otitis media NOS
Use additional code for any associated perforated tympanic membrane (H72.-)

H66.40 Suppurative otitis media, unspecified, unspecified ear

H66.41 Suppurative otitis media, unspecified, **right ear**

H66.42 Suppurative otitis media, unspecified, **left ear**

H66.43 Suppurative otitis media, unspecified, **bilateral**

✓5ᵗʰ **H66.9 Otitis media, unspecified**

Otitis media NOS
Acute otitis media NOS
Chronic otitis media NOS
Use additional code for any associated perforated tympanic membrane (H72.-)

H66.90 Otitis media, unspecified, unspecified ear

H66.91 Otitis media, unspecified, **right ear**

H66.92 Otitis media, unspecified, **left ear**

H66.93 Otitis media, unspecified, **bilateral**

✓4ᵗʰ **H67 Otitis media in diseases classified elsewhere**

Code first underlying disease, such as:
plasminogen deficiency (E88.02)
viral disease NEC (B00-B34)
Use additional code for any associated perforated tympanic membrane (H72.-)

EXCLUDES 1 otitis media in:
     influenza (J09.X9, J10.83, J11.83)
     measles (B05.3)
     scarlet fever (A38.0)
     tuberculosis (A18.6)

H67.1 *Otitis media in diseases classified elsewhere, **right** ear*

H67.2 *Otitis media in diseases classified elsewhere, **left** ear*

H67.3 *Otitis media in diseases classified elsewhere, **bilateral***

H67.9 *Otitis media in diseases classified elsewhere, unspecified ear*

✓4ᵗʰ **H68 Eustachian salpingitis and obstruction**

DEF: Eustachian tube: Internal channel between the tympanic cavity and the nasopharynx that equalizes internal pressure to the outside pressure and drains mucous production from the middle ear.

✓5ᵗʰ **H68.0 Eustachian salpingitis**

✓6ᵗʰ **H68.00 Unspecified Eustachian salpingitis**

H68.001 Unspecified Eustachian salpingitis, **right ear**

H68.002 Unspecified Eustachian salpingitis, **left ear**

H68.003 Unspecified Eustachian salpingitis, **bilateral**

H68.009 Unspecified Eustachian salpingitis, unspecified ear

✓6ᵗʰ **H68.01 Acute Eustachian salpingitis**

H68.011 Acute Eustachian salpingitis, **right ear**

H68.012 Acute Eustachian salpingitis, **left ear**

H68.013 Acute Eustachian salpingitis, **bilateral**

H68.019 Acute Eustachian salpingitis, unspecified ear

✓6ᵗʰ **H68.02 Chronic Eustachian salpingitis**

H68.021 Chronic Eustachian salpingitis, **right ear**

H68.022 Chronic Eustachian salpingitis, **left ear**

H68.023 Chronic Eustachian salpingitis, **bilateral**

H68.029 Chronic Eustachian salpingitis, unspecified ear

✓ Additional Character Required   ✓x7ᵗʰ Placeholder   Questionable PDx   Manifestation   Unspecified   **UPD** Unacceptable PDx   **H1-H4** HAC   **HCC** CMS-HCC Dx   **HIV** HIV Dx

✓5ᵗʰ **H68.1**   **Obstruction** of Eustachian tube
> Stenosis of Eustachian tube
> Stricture of Eustachian tube

   ✓6ᵗʰ **H68.10**   **Unspecified obstruction of Eustachian tube**
- **H68.101**   Unspecified obstruction of Eustachian tube, **right** ear
- **H68.102**   Unspecified obstruction of Eustachian tube, **left** ear
- **H68.103**   Unspecified obstruction of Eustachian tube, **bilateral**
- **H68.109**   Unspecified obstruction of Eustachian tube, unspecified ear

   ✓6ᵗʰ **H68.11**   **Osseous** obstruction of Eustachian tube
- **H68.111**   Osseous obstruction of Eustachian tube, **right** ear
- **H68.112**   Osseous obstruction of Eustachian tube, **left** ear
- **H68.113**   Osseous obstruction of Eustachian tube, **bilateral**
- **H68.119**   Osseous obstruction of Eustachian tube, unspecified ear

   ✓6ᵗʰ **H68.12**   **Intrinsic cartilagenous** obstruction of Eustachian tube
- **H68.121**   Intrinsic cartilagenous obstruction of Eustachian tube, **right** ear
- **H68.122**   Intrinsic cartilagenous obstruction of Eustachian tube, **left** ear
- **H68.123**   Intrinsic cartilagenous obstruction of Eustachian tube, **bilateral**
- **H68.129**   Intrinsic cartilagenous obstruction of Eustachian tube, unspecified ear

   ✓6ᵗʰ **H68.13**   **Extrinsic cartilagenous** obstruction of Eustachian tube
> Compression of Eustachian tube
- **H68.131**   Extrinsic cartilagenous obstruction of Eustachian tube, **right** ear
- **H68.132**   Extrinsic cartilagenous obstruction of Eustachian tube, **left** ear
- **H68.133**   Extrinsic cartilagenous obstruction of Eustachian tube, **bilateral**
- **H68.139**   Extrinsic cartilagenous obstruction of Eustachian tube, unspecified ear

✓4ᵗʰ **H69**   **Other and unspecified disorders of Eustachian tube**
> **DEF:** Eustachian tube: Internal channel between the tympanic cavity and the nasopharynx that equalizes internal pressure to the outside pressure and drains mucous production from the middle ear.

   ✓5ᵗʰ **H69.0**   **Patulous** Eustachian tube
- **H69.00**   Patulous Eustachian tube, unspecified ear
- **H69.01**   Patulous Eustachian tube, **right** ear
- **H69.02**   Patulous Eustachian tube, **left** ear
- **H69.03**   Patulous Eustachian tube, **bilateral**

   ✓5ᵗʰ **H69.8**   **Other specified disorders of Eustachian tube**
- **H69.80**   Other specified disorders of Eustachian tube, unspecified ear
- **H69.81**   Other specified disorders of Eustachian tube, **right** ear
- **H69.82**   Other specified disorders of Eustachian tube, **left** ear
- **H69.83**   Other specified disorders of Eustachian tube, **bilateral**

   ✓5ᵗʰ **H69.9**   **Unspecified Eustachian tube disorder**
- **H69.90**   Unspecified Eustachian tube disorder, unspecified ear
- **H69.91**   Unspecified Eustachian tube disorder, **right** ear
- **H69.92**   Unspecified Eustachian tube disorder, **left** ear
- **H69.93**   Unspecified Eustachian tube disorder, **bilateral**

✓4ᵗʰ **H70**   **Mastoiditis and related conditions**

   ✓5ᵗʰ **H70.0**   **Acute** mastoiditis
> Abscess of mastoid
> Empyema of mastoid

    ✓6ᵗʰ **H70.00**   **Acute mastoiditis without complications**
- **H70.001**   Acute mastoiditis without complications, **right** ear   CC
- **H70.002**   Acute mastoiditis without complications, **left** ear   CC
- **H70.003**   Acute mastoiditis without complications, **bilateral**   CC
- **H70.009**   Acute mastoiditis without complications, unspecified ear   CC UNS

✓6ᵗʰ **H70.01**   **Subperiosteal abscess** of mastoid
- **H70.011**   Subperiosteal abscess of mastoid, **right** ear   CC
- **H70.012**   Subperiosteal abscess of mastoid, **left** ear   CC
- **H70.013**   Subperiosteal abscess of mastoid, **bilateral**   CC
- **H70.019**   Subperiosteal abscess of mastoid, unspecified ear   CC UNS

   ✓6ᵗʰ **H70.09**   **Acute mastoiditis with other complications**
- **H70.091**   Acute mastoiditis with other complications, **right** ear   CC
- **H70.092**   Acute mastoiditis with other complications, **left** ear   CC
- **H70.093**   Acute mastoiditis with other complications, **bilateral**   CC
- **H70.099**   Acute mastoiditis with other complications, unspecified ear   CC UNS

   ✓5ᵗʰ **H70.1**   **Chronic** mastoiditis
> Caries of mastoid
> Fistula of mastoid
> **EXCLUDES 1**   tuberculous mastoiditis (A18.03)
- **H70.10**   Chronic mastoiditis, unspecified ear
- **H70.11**   Chronic mastoiditis, **right** ear
- **H70.12**   Chronic mastoiditis, **left** ear
- **H70.13**   Chronic mastoiditis, **bilateral**

   ✓5ᵗʰ **H70.2**   **Petrositis**
> Inflammation of petrous bone

    ✓6ᵗʰ **H70.20**   **Unspecified petrositis**
- **H70.201**   Unspecified petrositis, **right** ear
- **H70.202**   Unspecified petrositis, **left** ear
- **H70.203**   Unspecified petrositis, **bilateral**
- **H70.209**   Unspecified petrositis, unspecified ear

    ✓6ᵗʰ **H70.21**   **Acute** petrositis
> **DEF:** Sudden, severe inflammation of the petrous temporal bone behind the ear, associated with a middle ear infection.
- **H70.211**   Acute petrositis, **right** ear
- **H70.212**   Acute petrositis, **left** ear
- **H70.213**   Acute petrositis, **bilateral**
- **H70.219**   Acute petrositis, unspecified ear

    ✓6ᵗʰ **H70.22**   **Chronic** petrositis
- **H70.221**   Chronic petrositis, **right** ear
- **H70.222**   Chronic petrositis, **left** ear
- **H70.223**   Chronic petrositis, **bilateral**
- **H70.229**   Chronic petrositis, unspecified ear

   ✓5ᵗʰ **H70.8**   **Other mastoiditis and related conditions**
> **EXCLUDES 1**   preauricular sinus and cyst (Q18.1)
> sinus, fistula, and cyst of branchial cleft (Q18.0)

    ✓6ᵗʰ **H70.81**   **Postauricular fistula**
- **H70.811**   Postauricular fistula, **right** ear
- **H70.812**   Postauricular fistula, **left** ear
- **H70.813**   Postauricular fistula, **bilateral**
- **H70.819**   Postauricular fistula, unspecified ear

    ✓6ᵗʰ **H70.89**   **Other mastoiditis and related conditions**
- **H70.891**   Other mastoiditis and related conditions, **right** ear
- **H70.892**   Other mastoiditis and related conditions, **left** ear
- **H70.893**   Other mastoiditis and related conditions, **bilateral**
- **H70.899**   Other mastoiditis and related conditions, unspecified ear

   ✓5ᵗʰ **H70.9**   **Unspecified mastoiditis**
- **H70.90**   Unspecified mastoiditis, unspecified ear
- **H70.91**   Unspecified mastoiditis, **right** ear
- **H70.92**   Unspecified mastoiditis, **left** ear
- **H70.93**   Unspecified mastoiditis, **bilateral**

N Newborn: 0   P Pediatric: 0-17   M Maternity: 9-64   A Adult: 15-124   UNS Unspecified Site   MCC Major Complication/Comorbidity   CC Complication/Comorbidity   PE POA Exempt

650

H68.1–H70.93

ICD-10-CM 2025

✓4ᵗʰ H71   Cholesteatoma of middle ear

EXCLUDES 2   *cholesteatoma of external ear (H60.4-)*
recurrent cholesteatoma of postmastoidectomy cavity (H95.0-)

AHA: 2021,3Q,8
DEF: Cholesteatoma: Noncancerous cyst-like mass of cell debris including cholesterol and epithelial cells resulting from trauma, repeated or improperly healed infections, and congenital enclosure of epidermal cells.

Cholesteatoma of Middle Ear

Middle ear chamber
Ear drum
Cholesteatoma sac

✓5ᵗʰ H71.0   Cholesteatoma of attic
- H71.00   Cholesteatoma of attic, unspecified ear
- H71.01   Cholesteatoma of attic, right ear
- H71.02   Cholesteatoma of attic, left ear
- H71.03   Cholesteatoma of attic, bilateral

✓5ᵗʰ H71.1   Cholesteatoma of tympanum
- H71.10   Cholesteatoma of tympanum, unspecified ear
- H71.11   Cholesteatoma of tympanum, right ear
- H71.12   Cholesteatoma of tympanum, left ear
- H71.13   Cholesteatoma of tympanum, bilateral

✓5ᵗʰ H71.2   Cholesteatoma of mastoid
- H71.20   Cholesteatoma of mastoid, unspecified ear
- H71.21   Cholesteatoma of mastoid, right ear
- H71.22   Cholesteatoma of mastoid, left ear
- H71.23   Cholesteatoma of mastoid, bilateral

✓5ᵗʰ H71.3   Diffuse cholesteatosis
AHA: 2021,3Q,8
- H71.30   Diffuse cholesteatosis, unspecified ear
- H71.31   Diffuse cholesteatosis, right ear
- H71.32   Diffuse cholesteatosis, left ear
- H71.33   Diffuse cholesteatosis, bilateral

✓5ᵗʰ H71.9   Unspecified cholesteatoma
- H71.90   Unspecified cholesteatoma, unspecified ear
- H71.91   Unspecified cholesteatoma, right ear
- H71.92   Unspecified cholesteatoma, left ear
- H71.93   Unspecified cholesteatoma, bilateral

✓4ᵗʰ H72   Perforation of tympanic membrane

INCLUDES   persistent post-traumatic perforation of ear drum
postinflammatory perforation of ear drum

Code first any associated otitis media (H65.-, H66.1-, H66.2-, H66.3-, H66.4-, H66.9-, H67.-)

EXCLUDES 1   *acute suppurative otitis media with rupture of the tympanic membrane (H66.01-)*
traumatic rupture of ear drum (S09.2-)

✓5ᵗʰ H72.0   Central perforation of tympanic membrane
- H72.00   Central perforation of tympanic membrane, unspecified ear
- H72.01   Central perforation of tympanic membrane, right ear
- H72.02   Central perforation of tympanic membrane, left ear
- H72.03   Central perforation of tympanic membrane, bilateral

✓5ᵗʰ H72.1   Attic perforation of tympanic membrane
Perforation of pars flaccida
- H72.10   Attic perforation of tympanic membrane, unspecified ear
- H72.11   Attic perforation of tympanic membrane, right ear
- H72.12   Attic perforation of tympanic membrane, left ear
- H72.13   Attic perforation of tympanic membrane, bilateral

✓5ᵗʰ H72.2   Other marginal perforations of tympanic membrane
- ✓6ᵗʰ H72.2X   Other marginal perforations of tympanic membrane
  - H72.2X1   Other marginal perforations of tympanic membrane, right ear
  - H72.2X2   Other marginal perforations of tympanic membrane, left ear
  - H72.2X3   Other marginal perforations of tympanic membrane, bilateral
  - H72.2X9   Other marginal perforations of tympanic membrane, unspecified ear

✓5ᵗʰ H72.8   Other perforations of tympanic membrane
- ✓6ᵗʰ H72.81   Multiple perforations of tympanic membrane
  - H72.811   Multiple perforations of tympanic membrane, right ear
  - H72.812   Multiple perforations of tympanic membrane, left ear
  - H72.813   Multiple perforations of tympanic membrane, bilateral
  - H72.819   Multiple perforations of tympanic membrane, unspecified ear
- ✓6ᵗʰ H72.82   Total perforations of tympanic membrane
  - H72.821   Total perforations of tympanic membrane, right ear
  - H72.822   Total perforations of tympanic membrane, left ear
  - H72.823   Total perforations of tympanic membrane, bilateral
  - H72.829   Total perforations of tympanic membrane, unspecified ear

✓5ᵗʰ H72.9   Unspecified perforation of tympanic membrane
- H72.90   Unspecified perforation of tympanic membrane, unspecified ear
- H72.91   Unspecified perforation of tympanic membrane, right ear
- H72.92   Unspecified perforation of tympanic membrane, left ear
- H72.93   Unspecified perforation of tympanic membrane, bilateral

✓4ᵗʰ H73   Other disorders of tympanic membrane

✓5ᵗʰ H73.0   Acute myringitis
EXCLUDES 1   *acute myringitis with otitis media (H65, H66)*
- ✓6ᵗʰ H73.00   Unspecified acute myringitis
  Acute tympanitis NOS
  - H73.001   Acute myringitis, right ear
  - H73.002   Acute myringitis, left ear
  - H73.003   Acute myringitis, bilateral
  - H73.009   Acute myringitis, unspecified ear
- ✓6ᵗʰ H73.01   Bullous myringitis
  DEF: Bacterial or viral otitis media that is characterized by the appearance of serous or hemorrhagic blebs on the ear drum and sudden onset of severe pain in ear.
  - H73.011   Bullous myringitis, right ear
  - H73.012   Bullous myringitis, left ear
  - H73.013   Bullous myringitis, bilateral
  - H73.019   Bullous myringitis, unspecified ear
- ✓6ᵗʰ H73.09   Other acute myringitis
  - H73.091   Other acute myringitis, right ear
  - H73.092   Other acute myringitis, left ear
  - H73.093   Other acute myringitis, bilateral
  - H73.099   Other acute myringitis, unspecified ear

✓5ᵗʰ H73.1   Chronic myringitis
Chronic tympanitis
EXCLUDES 1   *chronic myringitis with otitis media (H65, H66)*
- H73.10   Chronic myringitis, unspecified ear
- H73.11   Chronic myringitis, right ear
- H73.12   Chronic myringitis, left ear
- H73.13   Chronic myringitis, bilateral

✓5ᵗʰ H73.2   Unspecified myringitis
- H73.20   Unspecified myringitis, unspecified ear
- H73.21   Unspecified myringitis, right ear
- H73.22   Unspecified myringitis, left ear
- H73.23   Unspecified myringitis, bilateral

✓5ᵗʰ H73.8   Other specified disorders of tympanic membrane
- ✓6ᵗʰ H73.81   Atrophic flaccid tympanic membrane
  - H73.811   Atrophic flaccid tympanic membrane, right ear

☑ Additional Character Required   ✓x7ᵗʰ Placeholder   Questionable PDx   Manifestation   Unspecified   UPD Unacceptable PDx   H1-H14 HAC   HCC CMS-HCC Dx   HIV HIV Dx

Chapter 8. Diseases of the Ear and Mastoid Process

H73.812 Atrophic flaccid tympanic membrane, left ear

H73.813 Atrophic flaccid tympanic membrane, bilateral

H73.819 Atrophic flaccid tympanic membrane, unspecified ear

✓6th **H73.82** Atrophic nonflaccid tympanic membrane

H73.821 Atrophic nonflaccid tympanic membrane, right ear

H73.822 Atrophic nonflaccid tympanic membrane, left ear

H73.823 Atrophic nonflaccid tympanic membrane, bilateral

H73.829 Atrophic nonflaccid tympanic membrane, unspecified ear

✓6th **H73.89** Other specified disorders of tympanic membrane

H73.891 Other specified disorders of tympanic membrane, right ear

H73.892 Other specified disorders of tympanic membrane, left ear

H73.893 Other specified disorders of tympanic membrane, bilateral

H73.899 Other specified disorders of tympanic membrane, unspecified ear

✓5th **H73.9** Unspecified disorder of tympanic membrane

H73.90 Unspecified disorder of tympanic membrane, unspecified ear

H73.91 Unspecified disorder of tympanic membrane, right ear

H73.92 Unspecified disorder of tympanic membrane, left ear

H73.93 Unspecified disorder of tympanic membrane, bilateral

✓4th **H74** Other disorders of middle ear mastoid

EXCLUDES 2   mastoiditis (H70.-)

✓5th **H74.0** Tympanosclerosis

DEF: Calcification of tissue in the ear drum, middle ear bones, and middle ear canal.

H74.01 Tympanosclerosis, right ear

H74.02 Tympanosclerosis, left ear

H74.03 Tympanosclerosis, bilateral

H74.09 Tympanosclerosis, unspecified ear

✓5th **H74.1** Adhesive middle ear disease

Adhesive otitis

EXCLUDES 1   glue ear (H65.3-)

H74.11 Adhesive right middle ear disease

H74.12 Adhesive left middle ear disease

H74.13 Adhesive middle ear disease, bilateral

H74.19 Adhesive middle ear disease, unspecified ear

✓5th **H74.2** Discontinuity and dislocation of ear ossicles

H74.20 Discontinuity and dislocation of ear ossicles, unspecified ear

H74.21 Discontinuity and dislocation of right ear ossicles

H74.22 Discontinuity and dislocation of left ear ossicles

H74.23 Discontinuity and dislocation of ear ossicles, bilateral

✓5th **H74.3** Other acquired abnormalities of ear ossicles

✓6th **H74.31** Ankylosis of ear ossicles

H74.311 Ankylosis of ear ossicles, right ear

H74.312 Ankylosis of ear ossicles, left ear

H74.313 Ankylosis of ear ossicles, bilateral

H74.319 Ankylosis of ear ossicles, unspecified ear

✓6th **H74.32** Partial loss of ear ossicles

H74.321 Partial loss of ear ossicles, right ear

H74.322 Partial loss of ear ossicles, left ear

H74.323 Partial loss of ear ossicles, bilateral

H74.329 Partial loss of ear ossicles, unspecified ear

✓6th **H74.39** Other acquired abnormalities of ear ossicles

H74.391 Other acquired abnormalities of right ear ossicles

H74.392 Other acquired abnormalities of left ear ossicles

H74.393 Other acquired abnormalities of ear ossicles, bilateral

H74.399 Other acquired abnormalities of ear ossicles, unspecified ear

✓5th **H74.4** Polyp of middle ear

H74.40 Polyp of middle ear, unspecified ear

H74.41 Polyp of right middle ear

H74.42 Polyp of left middle ear

H74.43 Polyp of middle ear, bilateral

✓5th **H74.8** Other specified disorders of middle ear and mastoid

✓6th **H74.8X** Other specified disorders of middle ear and mastoid

H74.8X1 Other specified disorders of right middle ear and mastoid

H74.8X2 Other specified disorders of left middle ear and mastoid

H74.8X3 Other specified disorders of middle ear and mastoid, bilateral

H74.8X9 Other specified disorders of middle ear and mastoid, unspecified ear

✓5th **H74.9** Unspecified disorder of middle ear and mastoid

H74.90 Unspecified disorder of middle ear and mastoid, unspecified ear

H74.91 Unspecified disorder of right middle ear and mastoid

H74.92 Unspecified disorder of left middle ear and mastoid

H74.93 Unspecified disorder of middle ear and mastoid, bilateral

✓4th **H75** Other disorders of middle ear and mastoid in diseases classified elsewhere

Code first underlying disease

✓5th **H75.0** Mastoiditis in infectious and parasitic diseases classified elsewhere

EXCLUDES 1   mastoiditis (in):

    syphilis (A52.77)

    tuberculosis (A18.03)

H75.00 *Mastoiditis in infectious and parasitic diseases classified elsewhere, unspecified ear*

H75.01 *Mastoiditis in infectious and parasitic diseases classified elsewhere, right ear*

H75.02 *Mastoiditis in infectious and parasitic diseases classified elsewhere, left ear*

H75.03 *Mastoiditis in infectious and parasitic diseases classified elsewhere, bilateral*

✓5th **H75.8** Other specified disorders of middle ear and mastoid in diseases classified elsewhere

H75.80 *Other specified disorders of middle ear and mastoid in diseases classified elsewhere, unspecified ear*

H75.81 *Other specified disorders of right middle ear and mastoid in diseases classified elsewhere*

H75.82 *Other specified disorders of left middle ear and mastoid in diseases classified elsewhere*

H75.83 *Other specified disorders of middle ear and mastoid in diseases classified elsewhere, bilateral*

Diseases of inner ear (H80-H83)

✓4th **H80** Otosclerosis

INCLUDES   otospongiosis

✓5th **H80.0** Otosclerosis involving oval window, nonobliterative

H80.00 Otosclerosis involving oval window, nonobliterative, unspecified ear

H80.01 Otosclerosis involving oval window, nonobliterative, right ear

H80.02 Otosclerosis involving oval window, nonobliterative, left ear

H80.03 Otosclerosis involving oval window, nonobliterative, bilateral

✓5th **H80.1** Otosclerosis involving oval window, obliterative

H80.10 Otosclerosis involving oval window, obliterative, unspecified ear

H80.11 Otosclerosis involving oval window, obliterative, right ear

H80.12 Otosclerosis involving oval window, obliterative, left ear

H80.13 Otosclerosis involving oval window, obliterative, bilateral

✓5th **H80.2** Cochlear otosclerosis

Otosclerosis involving otic capsule

Otosclerosis involving round window

H80.20 Cochlear otosclerosis, unspecified ear

H80.21 Cochlear otosclerosis, right ear

H80.22 Cochlear otosclerosis, left ear

H80.23 Cochlear otosclerosis, bilateral

✓5th **H80.8** Other otosclerosis

H80.80 Other otosclerosis, unspecified ear

H80.81 Other otosclerosis, right ear

H80.82 Other otosclerosis, left ear

N Newborn: 0   P Pediatric: 0-17   M Maternity: 9-64   A Adult: 15-124   UNS Unspecified Site   MCC Major Complication/Comorbidity   CC Complication/Comorbidity   PE POA Exempt

652   ICD-10-CM 2025

H80.83   Other otosclerosis, **bilateral**

✓5ᵗʰ H80.9   **Unspecified otosclerosis**

    H80.90   Unspecified otosclerosis, unspecified ear
    H80.91   Unspecified otosclerosis, **right** ear
    H80.92   Unspecified otosclerosis, **left** ear
    H80.93   Unspecified otosclerosis, **bilateral**

✓4ᵗʰ H81   **Disorders of vestibular function**

    EXCLUDES 1   epidemic vertigo (A88.1)
       vertigo NOS (R42)

✓5ᵗʰ H81.0   **Meniere's disease**

    Labyrinthine hydrops
    Meniere's syndrome or vertigo
    DEF: Distended membranous labyrinth of the middle ear from fluctuating pressure of fluid (hydrops) that causes vertigo, tinnitus, pressure, and hearing loss that may last on and off for several hours. Episodes may occur in clusters or may subside for weeks, months, or even years.

    H81.01   Meniere's disease, **right** ear
    H81.02   Meniere's disease, **left** ear
    H81.03   Meniere's disease, **bilateral**
    H81.09   Meniere's disease, unspecified ear

✓5ᵗʰ H81.1   **Benign paroxysmal vertigo**

    H81.10   Benign paroxysmal vertigo, unspecified ear
    H81.11   Benign paroxysmal vertigo, **right** ear
    H81.12   Benign paroxysmal vertigo, **left** ear
    H81.13   Benign paroxysmal vertigo, **bilateral**

✓5ᵗʰ H81.2   **Vestibular neuronitis**

    DEF: Transient benign vertigo caused by inflammation of the vestibular nerve. It is characterized by response to caloric stimulation on one side and nystagmus with rhythmic movement of the eyes. Normal auditory function is present.

    H81.20   Vestibular neuronitis, unspecified ear
    H81.21   Vestibular neuronitis, **right** ear
    H81.22   Vestibular neuronitis, **left** ear
    H81.23   Vestibular neuronitis, **bilateral**

✓5ᵗʰ H81.3   **Other peripheral vertigo**

    ✓6ᵗʰ H81.31   **Aural** vertigo
       H81.311   Aural vertigo, **right** ear
       H81.312   Aural vertigo, **left** ear
       H81.313   Aural vertigo, **bilateral**
       H81.319   Aural vertigo, unspecified ear

    ✓6ᵗʰ H81.39   **Other peripheral vertigo**
       Lermoyez' syndrome
       Otogenic vertigo
       Peripheral vertigo NOS
       H81.391   Other peripheral vertigo, **right** ear
       H81.392   Other peripheral vertigo, **left** ear
       H81.393   Other peripheral vertigo, **bilateral**
       H81.399   Other peripheral vertigo, unspecified ear

H81.4   **Vertigo of central origin**
    Central positional nystagmus

✓5ᵗʰ H81.8   **Other disorders of vestibular function**

    ✓6ᵗʰ H81.8X   **Other disorders of vestibular function**
       H81.8X1   Other disorders of vestibular function, **right** ear
       H81.8X2   Other disorders of vestibular function, **left** ear
       H81.8X3   Other disorders of vestibular function, **bilateral**
       H81.8X9   Other disorders of vestibular function, unspecified ear
       AHA: 2022,2Q,12

✓5ᵗʰ H81.9   **Unspecified disorder of vestibular function**
    Vertiginous syndrome NOS
    H81.90   Unspecified disorder of vestibular function, unspecified ear
    H81.91   Unspecified disorder of vestibular function, **right** ear
    H81.92   Unspecified disorder of vestibular function, **left** ear
    H81.93   Unspecified disorder of vestibular function, **bilateral**

✓4ᵗʰ H82   **Vertiginous syndromes in diseases classified elsewhere**
    Code first underlying disease
    EXCLUDES 1   epidemic vertigo (A88.1)
    H82.1   *Vertiginous syndromes in diseases classified elsewhere, right ear*
    H82.2   *Vertiginous syndromes in diseases classified elsewhere, left ear*
    H82.3   *Vertiginous syndromes in diseases classified elsewhere, bilateral*

H82.9   *Vertiginous syndromes in diseases classified elsewhere, unspecified ear*

✓4ᵗʰ H83   **Other diseases of inner ear**

✓5ᵗʰ H83.0   **Labyrinthitis**
    DEF: Inflammation of the inner ear, or labyrinth, characterized by pus, vertigo, dizziness, nausea, and hearing loss.
    H83.01   Labyrinthitis, **right** ear
    H83.02   Labyrinthitis, **left** ear
    H83.03   Labyrinthitis, **bilateral**
    H83.09   Labyrinthitis, unspecified ear

✓5ᵗʰ H83.1   **Labyrinthine fistula**
    H83.11   Labyrinthine fistula, **right** ear
    H83.12   Labyrinthine fistula, **left** ear
    H83.13   Labyrinthine fistula, **bilateral**
    H83.19   Labyrinthine fistula, unspecified ear

✓5ᵗʰ H83.2   **Labyrinthine dysfunction**
    Labyrinthine hypersensitivity
    Labyrinthine hypofunction
    Labyrinthine loss of function
    DEF: Decreased function of the labyrinth sensors.
    ✓6ᵗʰ H83.2X   **Labyrinthine dysfunction**
       H83.2X1   Labyrinthine dysfunction, **right** ear
       H83.2X2   Labyrinthine dysfunction, **left** ear
       H83.2X3   Labyrinthine dysfunction, **bilateral**
       H83.2X9   Labyrinthine dysfunction, unspecified ear

✓5ᵗʰ H83.3   **Noise effects on inner ear**
    Acoustic trauma of inner ear
    Noise-induced hearing loss of inner ear
    ✓6ᵗʰ H83.3X   **Noise effects on inner ear**
       H83.3X1   Noise effects on **right** inner ear
       H83.3X2   Noise effects on **left** inner ear
       H83.3X3   Noise effects on inner ear, **bilateral**
       H83.3X9   Noise effects on inner ear, unspecified ear

✓5ᵗʰ H83.8   **Other specified diseases of inner ear**
    ✓6ᵗʰ H83.8X   **Other specified diseases of inner ear**
       H83.8X1   Other specified diseases of **right** inner ear
       H83.8X2   Other specified diseases of **left** inner ear
       H83.8X3   Other specified diseases of inner ear, **bilateral**
       H83.8X9   Other specified diseases of inner ear, unspecified ear

✓5ᵗʰ H83.9   **Unspecified disease of inner ear**
    H83.90   Unspecified disease of inner ear, unspecified ear
    H83.91   Unspecified disease of **right** inner ear
    H83.92   Unspecified disease of **left** inner ear
    H83.93   Unspecified disease of inner ear, **bilateral**

Other disorders of ear (H90-H94)

✓4ᵗʰ H90   **Conductive and sensorineural hearing loss**
    EXCLUDES 1   deaf nonspeaking NEC (H91.3)
       deafness NOS (H91.9-)
       hearing loss NOS (H91.9-)
       noise-induced hearing loss (H83.3-)
       ototoxic hearing loss (H91.0-)
       sudden (idiopathic) hearing loss (H91.2-)
    AHA: 2015,2Q,7
    DEF: Conductive hearing loss: Hearing loss due to the inability of soundwaves to move from the outer (external) ear to the inner ear.
    DEF: Sensorineural hearing loss: Hearing loss that occurs from damage to the hair cells of the inner ear or problems with the nerve pathways from the inner ear to the brain.
    H90.0   **Conductive** hearing loss, **bilateral**
    ✓5ᵗʰ H90.1   **Conductive** hearing loss, **unilateral** with unrestricted hearing on the contralateral side
       H90.11   Conductive hearing loss, unilateral, **right** ear, with unrestricted hearing on the contralateral side
       H90.12   Conductive hearing loss, unilateral, **left** ear, with unrestricted hearing on the contralateral side
    H90.2   **Conductive** hearing loss, unspecified
       Conductive deafness NOS
    H90.3   **Sensorineural** hearing loss, **bilateral**
    ✓5ᵗʰ H90.4   **Sensorineural** hearing loss, **unilateral** with unrestricted hearing on the contralateral side
       H90.41   Sensorineural hearing loss, unilateral, **right** ear, with unrestricted hearing on the contralateral side

Chapter 8. Diseases of the Ear and Mastoid Process

H90.42 Sensorineural hearing loss, unilateral, **left** ear, with unrestricted hearing on the contralateral side

H90.5 Unspecified **sensorineural** hearing loss
Central hearing loss NOS
Congenital deafness NOS
Neural hearing loss NOS
Perceptive hearing loss NOS
Sensorineural deafness NOS
Sensory hearing loss NOS
> **EXCLUDES 1**   *abnormal auditory perception (H93.2-)*
> *psychogenic deafness (F44.6)*

H90.6 **Mixed** conductive and sensorineural hearing loss, **bilateral**
AHA: 2015,2Q,7

✓5th **H90.7** **Mixed** conductive and sensorineural hearing loss, **unilateral** with unrestricted hearing on the contralateral side

    H90.71 Mixed conductive and sensorineural hearing loss, unilateral, **right** ear, with unrestricted hearing on the contralateral side

    H90.72 Mixed conductive and sensorineural hearing loss, unilateral, **left** ear, with unrestricted hearing on the contralateral side

H90.8 **Mixed** conductive and sensorineural hearing loss, unspecified

✓5th **H90.A** Conductive and sensorineural hearing loss with restricted hearing on the contralateral side
AHA: 2016,4Q,23-25

  ✓6th **H90.A1** Conductive hearing loss, unilateral, with restricted hearing on the contralateral side

    H90.A11 Conductive hearing loss, unilateral, **right** ear with restricted hearing on the contralateral side

    H90.A12 Conductive hearing loss, unilateral, **left** ear with restricted hearing on the contralateral side

  ✓6th **H90.A2** Sensorineural hearing loss, unilateral, with restricted hearing on the contralateral side

    H90.A21 Sensorineural hearing loss, unilateral, **right** ear, with restricted hearing on the contralateral side

    H90.A22 Sensorineural hearing loss, unilateral, **left** ear, with restricted hearing on the contralateral side

  ✓6th **H90.A3** Mixed conductive and sensorineural hearing loss, unilateral with restricted hearing on the contralateral side

    H90.A31 Mixed conductive and sensorineural hearing loss, unilateral, **right** ear with restricted hearing on the contralateral side

    H90.A32 Mixed conductive and sensorineural hearing, unilateral, **left** ear with restricted hearing on the contralateral side

✓4th **H91** Other and unspecified hearing loss
> **EXCLUDES 1**   *abnormal auditory perception (H93.2-)*
> *hearing loss as classified in H90.-*
> *impacted cerumen (H61.2-)*
> *noise-induced hearing loss (H83.3-)*
> *psychogenic deafness (F44.6)*
> *transient ischemic deafness (H93.01-)*

✓5th **H91.0** Ototoxic hearing loss
Code first poisoning due to drug or toxin, if applicable (T36-T65 with fifth or sixth character 1-4)
Use additional code for adverse effect, if applicable, to identify drug (T36-T50 with fifth or sixth character 5)

  H91.01 Ototoxic hearing loss, **right** ear
  H91.02 Ototoxic hearing loss, **left** ear
  H91.03 Ototoxic hearing loss, **bilateral**
  H91.09 Ototoxic hearing loss, unspecified ear

✓5th **H91.1** Presbycusis
Presbyacusia
  H91.10 Presbycusis, unspecified ear
  H91.11 Presbycusis, **right** ear
  H91.12 Presbycusis, **left** ear
  H91.13 Presbycusis, **bilateral**

✓5th **H91.2** Sudden idiopathic hearing loss
Sudden hearing loss NOS
  H91.20 Sudden idiopathic hearing loss, unspecified ear
  H91.21 Sudden idiopathic hearing loss, **right** ear
  H91.22 Sudden idiopathic hearing loss, **left** ear
  H91.23 Sudden idiopathic hearing loss, **bilateral**

H91.3 Deaf nonspeaking, not elsewhere classified

✓5th **H91.8** Other specified hearing loss
  ✓6th **H91.8X** Other specified hearing loss
    H91.8X1 Other specified hearing loss, **right** ear
    H91.8X2 Other specified hearing loss, **left** ear
    H91.8X3 Other specified hearing loss, **bilateral**
    H91.8X9 Other specified hearing loss, unspecified ear

✓5th **H91.9** Unspecified hearing loss
Deafness NOS
High frequency deafness
Low frequency deafness
  H91.90 Unspecified hearing loss, unspecified ear
  H91.91 Unspecified hearing loss, **right** ear
  H91.92 Unspecified hearing loss, **left** ear
  H91.93 Unspecified hearing loss, **bilateral**

✓4th **H92** Otalgia and effusion of ear

✓5th **H92.0** Otalgia
  H92.01 Otalgia, **right** ear
  H92.02 Otalgia, **left** ear
  H92.03 Otalgia, **bilateral**
  H92.09 Otalgia, unspecified ear

✓5th **H92.1** Otorrhea
> **EXCLUDES 1**   *leakage of cerebrospinal fluid through ear (G96.0)*

  H92.10 Otorrhea, unspecified ear
  H92.11 Otorrhea, **right** ear
  H92.12 Otorrhea, **left** ear
  H92.13 Otorrhea, **bilateral**

✓5th **H92.2** Otorrhagia
> **EXCLUDES 1**   *traumatic otorrhagia - code to injury*

  H92.20 Otorrhagia, unspecified ear
  H92.21 Otorrhagia, **right** ear
  H92.22 Otorrhagia, **left** ear
  H92.23 Otorrhagia, **bilateral**

✓4th **H93** Other disorders of ear, not elsewhere classified

✓5th **H93.0** Degenerative and vascular disorders of ear
> **EXCLUDES 1**   *presbycusis (H91.1)*

  ✓6th **H93.01** Transient ischemic deafness
    H93.011 Transient ischemic deafness, **right** ear
    H93.012 Transient ischemic deafness, **left** ear
    H93.013 Transient ischemic deafness, **bilateral**
    H93.019 Transient ischemic deafness, unspecified ear

  ✓6th **H93.09** Unspecified degenerative and vascular disorders of ear
    H93.091 Unspecified degenerative and vascular disorders of **right** ear
    H93.092 Unspecified degenerative and vascular disorders of **left** ear
    H93.093 Unspecified degenerative and vascular disorders of ear, **bilateral**
    H93.099 Unspecified degenerative and vascular disorders of unspecified ear

✓5th **H93.1** Tinnitus
  H93.11 Tinnitus, **right** ear
  H93.12 Tinnitus, **left** ear
  H93.13 Tinnitus, **bilateral**
  H93.19 Tinnitus, unspecified ear

✓5th **H93.A** Pulsatile tinnitus
AHA: 2023,2Q,18; 2016,4Q,25-26
  H93.A1 Pulsatile tinnitus, **right** ear
  H93.A2 Pulsatile tinnitus, **left** ear
  H93.A3 Pulsatile tinnitus, **bilateral**
  H93.A9 Pulsatile tinnitus, unspecified ear

✓5th **H93.2** Other abnormal auditory perceptions
> **EXCLUDES 2**   *auditory hallucinations (R44.0)*

  ✓6th **H93.21** Auditory recruitment
    H93.211 Auditory recruitment, **right** ear
    H93.212 Auditory recruitment, **left** ear
    H93.213 Auditory recruitment, **bilateral**
    H93.219 Auditory recruitment, unspecified ear

  ✓6th **H93.22** Diplacusis
    H93.221 Diplacusis, **right** ear
    H93.222 Diplacusis, **left** ear
    H93.223 Diplacusis, **bilateral**
    H93.229 Diplacusis, unspecified ear

N Newborn: 0   **P** Pediatric: 0-17   **M** Maternity: 9-64   **A** Adult: 15-124   **UNS** Unspecified Site   **MCC** Major Complication/Comorbidity   **CC** Complication/Comorbidity   **PE** POA Exempt

√6ᵗʰ **H93.23 Hyperacusis**

DEF: Exceptionally acute sense of hearing caused by such conditions as Bell's palsy. This term may also refer to painful sensitivity to sounds.

H93.231 Hyperacusis, **right** ear
H93.232 Hyperacusis, **left** ear
H93.233 Hyperacusis, **bilateral**
H93.239 Hyperacusis, unspecified ear

√6ᵗʰ **H93.24 Temporary auditory threshold shift**

H93.241 Temporary auditory threshold shift, **right** ear
H93.242 Temporary auditory threshold shift, **left** ear
H93.243 Temporary auditory threshold shift, **bilateral**
H93.249 Temporary auditory threshold shift, unspecified ear

H93.25 Central auditory processing disorder
Congenital auditory imperception
Word deafness
EXCLUDES 1   mixed receptive-expressive language disorder (F80.2)

√6ᵗʰ **H93.29 Other abnormal auditory perceptions**

H93.291 Other abnormal auditory perceptions, **right** ear
H93.292 Other abnormal auditory perceptions, **left** ear
H93.293 Other abnormal auditory perceptions, **bilateral**
H93.299 Other abnormal auditory perceptions, unspecified ear

√5ᵗʰ **H93.3 Disorders of acoustic nerve**
Disorder of 8th cranial nerve
EXCLUDES 1   acoustic neuroma (D33.3)
         syphilitic acoustic neuritis (A52.15)

√6ᵗʰ **H93.3X Disorders of acoustic nerve**

H93.3X1 Disorders of **right** acoustic nerve
H93.3X2 Disorders of **left** acoustic nerve
H93.3X3 Disorders of **bilateral** acoustic nerves
H93.3X9 Disorders of unspecified acoustic nerve

√5ᵗʰ **H93.8 Other specified disorders of ear**

√6ᵗʰ **H93.8X Other specified disorders of ear**

H93.8X1 Other specified disorders of **right** ear
H93.8X2 Other specified disorders of **left** ear
H93.8X3 Other specified disorders of ear, **bilateral**
H93.8X9 Other specified disorders of ear, unspecified ear

√5ᵗʰ **H93.9 Unspecified disorder of ear**

H93.90 Unspecified disorder of ear, unspecified ear   UPD
H93.91 Unspecified disorder of **right** ear   UPD
H93.92 Unspecified disorder of **left** ear   UPD
H93.93 Unspecified disorder of ear, **bilateral**   UPD

√4ᵗʰ **H94 Other disorders of ear in diseases classified elsewhere**

√5ᵗʰ **H94.0 Acoustic neuritis in infectious and parasitic diseases classified elsewhere**
Code first underlying disease, such as:
parasitic disease (B65-B89)
EXCLUDES 1   acoustic neuritis (in):
         herpes zoster (B02.29)
         syphilis (A52.15)

H94.00 *Acoustic neuritis in infectious and parasitic diseases classified elsewhere, unspecified ear*
H94.01 *Acoustic neuritis in infectious and parasitic diseases classified elsewhere, right ear*
H94.02 *Acoustic neuritis in infectious and parasitic diseases classified elsewhere, left ear*
H94.03 *Acoustic neuritis in infectious and parasitic diseases classified elsewhere, bilateral*

√5ᵗʰ **H94.8 Other specified disorders of ear in diseases classified elsewhere**
Code first underlying disease, such as:
congenital syphilis (A50.0)
EXCLUDES 1   aural myiasis (B87.4)
         syphilitic labyrinthitis (A52.79)

H94.80 *Other specified disorders of ear in diseases classified elsewhere, unspecified ear*
H94.81 *Other specified disorders of right ear in diseases classified elsewhere*

H94.82 *Other specified disorders of left ear in diseases classified elsewhere*
H94.83 *Other specified disorders of ear in diseases classified elsewhere, bilateral*

Intraoperative and postprocedural complications and disorders of ear and mastoid process, not elsewhere classified (H95)

√4ᵗʰ **H95 Intraoperative and postprocedural complications and disorders of ear and mastoid process, not elsewhere classified**
AHA: 2016,4Q,9-10

√5ᵗʰ **H95.0 Recurrent cholesteatoma of postmastoidectomy cavity**

H95.00 Recurrent cholesteatoma of postmastoidectomy cavity, unspecified ear
H95.01 Recurrent cholesteatoma of postmastoidectomy cavity, **right** ear
H95.02 Recurrent cholesteatoma of postmastoidectomy cavity, **left** ear
H95.03 Recurrent cholesteatoma of postmastoidectomy cavity, **bilateral** ears

√5ᵗʰ **H95.1 Other disorders of ear and mastoid process following mastoidectomy**

√6ᵗʰ **H95.11 Chronic inflammation of postmastoidectomy cavity**

H95.111 Chronic inflammation of postmastoidectomy cavity, **right** ear
H95.112 Chronic inflammation of postmastoidectomy cavity, **left** ear
H95.113 Chronic inflammation of postmastoidectomy cavity, **bilateral** ears
H95.119 Chronic inflammation of postmastoidectomy cavity, unspecified ear

√6ᵗʰ **H95.12 Granulation of postmastoidectomy cavity**

H95.121 Granulation of postmastoidectomy cavity, **right** ear
H95.122 Granulation of postmastoidectomy cavity, **left** ear
H95.123 Granulation of postmastoidectomy cavity, **bilateral** ears
H95.129 Granulation of postmastoidectomy cavity, unspecified ear

√6ᵗʰ **H95.13 Mucosal cyst of postmastoidectomy cavity**

H95.131 Mucosal cyst of postmastoidectomy cavity, **right** ear
H95.132 Mucosal cyst of postmastoidectomy cavity, **left** ear
H95.133 Mucosal cyst of postmastoidectomy cavity, **bilateral** ears
H95.139 Mucosal cyst of postmastoidectomy cavity, unspecified ear

√6ᵗʰ **H95.19 Other disorders following mastoidectomy**

H95.191 Other disorders following mastoidectomy, **right** ear
H95.192 Other disorders following mastoidectomy, **left** ear
H95.193 Other disorders following mastoidectomy, **bilateral** ears
H95.199 Other disorders following mastoidectomy, unspecified ear

√5ᵗʰ **H95.2 Intraoperative hemorrhage and hematoma of ear and mastoid process complicating a procedure**
EXCLUDES 1   intraoperative hemorrhage and hematoma of ear and mastoid process due to accidental puncture or laceration during a procedure (H95.3-)

H95.21 Intraoperative hemorrhage and hematoma of ear and mastoid process complicating a **procedure on the ear and mastoid process**   CC
H95.22 Intraoperative hemorrhage and hematoma of ear and mastoid process complicating **other procedure**   CC

√5ᵗʰ **H95.3 Accidental puncture and laceration of ear and mastoid process during a procedure**

H95.31 Accidental puncture and laceration of the ear and mastoid process during a **procedure on the ear and mastoid process**   CC
H95.32 Accidental puncture and laceration of the ear and mastoid process during **other procedure**   CC

✔ Additional Character Required   √x7ᵗʰ Placeholder   Questionable PDx   Manifestation   Unspecified   UPD Unacceptable PDx   H1-H14 HAC   HCC CMS-HCC Dx   HIV HIV Dx

✓5ᵗʰ **H95.4** **Postprocedural hemorrhage** of ear and mastoid process following a procedure

    H95.41 Postprocedural hemorrhage of ear and mastoid process following a **procedure on the ear and mastoid process** `CC`

    H95.42 Postprocedural hemorrhage of ear and mastoid process following **other procedure** `CC`

✓5ᵗʰ **H95.5** **Postprocedural hematoma and seroma** of ear and mastoid process following a procedure

    H95.51 Postprocedural **hematoma** of ear and mastoid process following a **procedure on the ear and mastoid process** `CC`

    H95.52 Postprocedural **hematoma** of ear and mastoid process following **other procedure** `CC`

    H95.53 Postprocedural **seroma** of ear and mastoid process following a **procedure on the ear and mastoid process** `CC`

    H95.54 Postprocedural **seroma** of ear and mastoid process following **other procedure** `CC`

✓5ᵗʰ **H95.8** Other intraoperative and postprocedural complications and disorders of the ear and mastoid process, not elsewhere classified

        EXCLUDES 2   *postprocedural complications and disorders following mastoidectomy (H95.0-, H95.1-)*

    ✓6ᵗʰ **H95.81** **Postprocedural stenosis** of external ear canal

        H95.811 Postprocedural stenosis of **right** external ear canal `CC`

        H95.812 Postprocedural stenosis of **left** external ear canal `CC`

        H95.813 Postprocedural stenosis of external ear canal, **bilateral** `CC`

        H95.819 Postprocedural stenosis of unspecified external ear canal `CC` `UNS`

    H95.88 Other intraoperative complications and disorders of the ear and mastoid process, not elsewhere classified `CC`

        Use additional code, if applicable, to further specify disorder

    H95.89 Other postprocedural complications and disorders of the ear and mastoid process, not elsewhere classified `CC`

        Use additional code, if applicable, to further specify disorder

Chapter 9. Diseases of the Circulatory System (I00–I99)

Chapter-specific Guidelines with Coding Examples

The chapter-specific guidelines from the ICD-10-CM Official Guidelines for Coding and Reporting have been provided below. Along with these guidelines are coding examples, contained in the shaded boxes, that have been developed to help illustrate the coding and/or sequencing guidance found in these guidelines.

a. Hypertension

The classification presumes a causal relationship between hypertension and heart involvement and between hypertension and kidney involvement, as the two conditions are linked by the term "with" in the Alphabetic Index. These conditions should be coded as related even in the absence of provider documentation explicitly linking them, unless the documentation clearly states the conditions are unrelated.

For hypertension and conditions not specifically linked by relational terms such as "with," "associated with" or "due to" in the classification, provider documentation must link the conditions in order to code them as related.

1) Hypertension with heart disease

Hypertension with heart conditions classified to I50.- or I51.4–I51.7, I51.89, I51.9, are assigned to a code from category I11, Hypertensive heart disease. Use additional code(s) from category I50, Heart failure, to identify the type(s) of heart failure in those patients with heart failure.

The same heart conditions (I50.-, I51.4–I51.7, I51.89, I51.9) with hypertension are coded separately if the provider has documented they are unrelated to the hypertension. Sequence according to the circumstances of the admission/encounter.

2) Hypertensive chronic kidney disease

Assign codes from category I12, Hypertensive chronic kidney disease, when both hypertension and a condition classifiable to category N18, Chronic kidney disease (CKD), are present. CKD should not be coded as hypertensive if the provider indicates the CKD is not related to the hypertension.

The appropriate code from category N18 should be used as a secondary code with a code from category I12 to identify the stage of chronic kidney disease.

See Section I.C.14. Chronic kidney disease.

If a patient has hypertensive chronic kidney disease and acute renal failure, the acute renal failure should also be coded. Sequence according to the circumstances of the admission/encounter.

> Patient is admitted with stage IV chronic kidney disease (CKD) due to polycystic kidney disease. Patient also is on lisinopril for hypertension.
>
> **N18.4**   **Chronic kidney disease, stage 4 (severe)**
>
> **Q61.3**   **Polycystic kidney, unspecified**
>
> **I10**   **Essential (primary) hypertension**
>
> *Explanation*: A combination code describing a relationship between hypertension and CKD is not used because the physician documentation identifies the polycystic kidney disease as the cause for the CKD.

3) Hypertensive heart and chronic kidney disease

Assign codes from combination category I13, Hypertensive heart and chronic kidney disease, when there is hypertension with both heart and kidney involvement. If heart failure is present, assign an additional code from category I50 to identify the type of heart failure.

The appropriate code from category N18, Chronic kidney disease, should be used as a secondary code with a code from category I13 to identify the stage of chronic kidney disease.

See Section I.C.14. Chronic kidney disease.

The codes in category I13, Hypertensive heart and chronic kidney disease, are combination codes that include hypertension, heart disease and chronic kidney disease. The Includes note at I13 specifies that the conditions included at I11 and I12 are included together in I13. If a patient has hypertension, heart disease and chronic kidney disease, then a code from I13 should be used, not individual codes for hypertension, heart disease and chronic kidney disease, or codes from I11 or I12.

For patients with both acute renal failure and chronic kidney disease, the acute renal failure should also be coded. Sequence according to the circumstances of the admission/encounter.

> Patient admitted with acute tubular necrosis, history of hypertensive heart and kidney disease with congestive heart failure and stage 3a chronic kidney disease
>
> **N17.0**   **Acute kidney failure with tubular necrosis**
>
> **I13.0**   **Hypertensive heart and chronic kidney disease with heart failure and stage 1 through stage 4 chronic kidney disease, or unspecified chronic kidney disease**
>
> **I50.9**   **Heart failure, unspecified**
>
> **N18.31**   **Chronic kidney disease, stage 3a**
>
> *Explanation*: It is appropriate to report an acute kidney failure code and a chronic kidney failure code when both conditions are treated during an encounter. In this instance, the acute renal failure was the focus of treatment and therefore sequenced as principal diagnosis. Combination codes in category I13 are used to report conditions classifiable to *both* categories I11 and I12. Do not report conditions classifiable to I11 and I12 separately. Use additional codes to report the type of heart failure and stage of CKD.

4) Hypertensive cerebrovascular disease

For hypertensive cerebrovascular disease, first assign the appropriate code from categories I60–I69, followed by the appropriate hypertension code.

> Rupture of cerebral aneurysm caused by malignant hypertension
>
> **I60.7**   **Nontraumatic subarachnoid hemorrhage from unspecified intracranial artery**
>
> **I10**   **Essential (primary) hypertension**
>
> *Explanation*: Hypertensive cerebrovascular disease requires two codes: the appropriate I60–I69 code followed by the appropriate hypertension code.

5) Hypertensive retinopathy

Subcategory H35.0, Background retinopathy and retinal vascular changes, should be used along with a code from categories I10–I15, in the Hypertensive diseases section, to include the systemic hypertension. The sequencing is based on the reason for the encounter.

6) Hypertension, secondary

Secondary hypertension is due to an underlying condition. Two codes are required: one to identify the underlying etiology and one from category I15 to identify the hypertension. Sequencing of codes is determined by the reason for admission/encounter.

> Renovascular hypertension due to renal artery atherosclerosis
>
> **I15.0**   **Renovascular hypertension**
>
> **I70.1**   **Atherosclerosis of renal artery**
>
> *Explanation*: Secondary hypertension requires two codes: a code to identify the etiology and the appropriate I15 code.

7) Hypertension, transient

Assign code R03.0, Elevated blood pressure reading without diagnosis of hypertension, unless patient has an established diagnosis of hypertension. Assign code O13.-, Gestational [pregnancy-induced] hypertension without significant proteinuria, or O14.-, Pre-eclampsia, for transient hypertension of pregnancy.

8) Hypertension, controlled

This diagnostic statement usually refers to an existing state of hypertension under control by therapy. Assign the appropriate code from categories I10–I15, Hypertensive diseases.

9) Hypertension, uncontrolled

Uncontrolled hypertension may refer to untreated hypertension or hypertension not responding to current therapeutic regimen. In either case, assign the appropriate code from categories I10–I15, Hypertensive diseases.

10) Hypertensive crisis

Assign a code from category I16, Hypertensive crisis, for documented hypertensive urgency, hypertensive emergency or unspecified hypertensive crisis. Code also any identified hypertensive disease (I10–I15). The sequencing is based on the reason for the encounter.

11) Pulmonary hypertension

Pulmonary hypertension is classified to category I27, Other pulmonary heart diseases. For secondary pulmonary hypertension (I27.1, I27.2-), code also any associated conditions or adverse effects of drugs or toxins. The sequencing is based on the reason for the encounter, except for adverse effects of drugs (See Section I.C.19.e.).

12) Hypertension, Resistant

Resistant hypertension refers to blood pressure of a patient with hypertension that remains above goal in spite of the use of antihypertensive medications. Assign code I1A.Ø, Resistant hypertension, as an additional code when apparent treatment resistant hypertension, treatment resistant hypertension, or true resistant hypertension is documented by the provider. A code for the specific type of existing hypertension is sequenced first, if known.

b. Atherosclerotic coronary artery disease and angina

ICD-10-CM has combination codes for atherosclerotic heart disease with angina pectoris. The subcategories for these codes are I25.11, Atherosclerotic heart disease of native coronary artery with angina pectoris and I25.7, Atherosclerosis of coronary artery bypass graft(s) and coronary artery of transplanted heart with angina pectoris.

When using one of these combination codes it is not necessary to use an additional code for angina pectoris. A causal relationship can be assumed in a patient with both atherosclerosis and angina pectoris, unless the documentation indicates the angina is due to something other than the atherosclerosis.

If a patient with coronary artery disease is admitted due to an acute myocardial infarction (AMI), the AMI should be sequenced before the coronary artery disease.

See Section I.C.9. Acute myocardial infarction (AMI)

c. Intraoperative and postprocedural cerebrovascular accident

Medical record documentation should clearly specify the cause- and- effect relationship between the medical intervention and the cerebrovascular accident in order to assign a code for intraoperative or postprocedural cerebrovascular accident.

Proper code assignment depends on whether it was an infarction or hemorrhage and whether it occurred intraoperatively or postoperatively. If it was a cerebral hemorrhage, code assignment depends on the type of procedure performed.

d. Sequelae of cerebrovascular disease

1) Category I69, Sequelae of cerebrovascular disease

Category I69 is used to indicate conditions classifiable to categories I6Ø–I67 as the causes of sequela (neurologic deficits), themselves classified elsewhere. These "late effects" include neurologic deficits that persist after initial onset of conditions classifiable to categories I6Ø–I67. The neurologic deficits caused by cerebrovascular disease may be present from the onset or may arise at any time after the onset of the condition classifiable to categories I6Ø–I67.

Codes from category I69, Sequelae of cerebrovascular disease, that specify hemiplegia, hemiparesis and monoplegia identify whether the dominant or nondominant side is affected. Should the affected side be documented, but not specified as dominant or nondominant, and the classification system does not indicate a default, code selection is as follows:

- For ambidextrous patients, the default should be dominant.
- If the left side is affected, the default is non-dominant.
- If the right side is affected, the default is dominant.

2) Codes from category I69 with codes from I6Ø–I67

Codes from category I69 may be assigned on a health care record with codes from I6Ø–I67, if the patient has a current cerebrovascular disease and deficits from an old cerebrovascular disease.

3) Codes from category I69 and personal history of transient ischemic attack (TIA) and cerebral infarction (Z86.73)

Codes from category I69 should not be assigned if the patient does not have neurologic deficits.

See Section I.C.21.4. History (of) for use of personal history codes

e. Acute myocardial infarction (AMI)

1) Type 1 ST elevation myocardial infarction (STEMI) and non ST elevation myocardial infarction (NSTEMI)

The ICD-10-CM codes for type 1 acute myocardial infarction (AMI) identify the site, such as anterolateral wall or true posterior wall. Subcategories I21.Ø-I21.2 and code I21.3 are used for type 1 ST elevation myocardial infarction (STEMI). Code I21.4, Non-ST elevation (NSTEMI) myocardial infarction, is used for type 1 non-ST elevation myocardial infarction (NSTEMI) and nontransmural MIs.

If a type 1 NSTEMI evolves to STEMI, assign the STEMI code. If a type 1 STEMI converts to NSTEMI due to thrombolytic therapy, it is still coded as STEMI.

For encounters occurring while the myocardial infarction is equal to, or less than, four weeks old, including transfers to another acute setting or a postacute setting, and the myocardial infarction meets the definition for "other diagnoses" (see Section III, Reporting Additional Diagnoses), codes from category I21 may continue to be reported. For encounters after the 4-week time frame and the patient is still receiving care related to the myocardial infarction, the appropriate aftercare code should be assigned, rather than a code from category I21. For old or healed myocardial infarctions not requiring further care, code I25.2, Old myocardial infarction, may be assigned.

2) Acute myocardial infarction, unspecified

Code I21.9, Acute myocardial infarction, unspecified, is the default for unspecified acute myocardial infarction or unspecified type. If only type 1 STEMI or transmural MI without the site is documented, assign code I21.3, ST elevation (STEMI) myocardial infarction of unspecified site.

3) AMI documented as nontransmural or subendocardial but site provided

If an AMI is documented as nontransmural or subendocardial, but the site is provided, it is still coded as a subendocardial AMI.

See Section I.C.21.3. for information on coding status post administration of tPA in a different facility within the last 24 hours.

4) Subsequent acute myocardial infarction

A code from category I22, Subsequent ST elevation (STEMI) and non-ST elevation (NSTEMI) myocardial infarction, is to be used when a patient who has suffered a type 1 or unspecified AMI has a new AMI within the 4-week time frame of the initial AMI. A code from category I22 must be used in conjunction with a code from category I21. The sequencing of the I22 and I21 codes depends on the circumstances of the encounter.

Do not assign code I22 for subsequent myocardial infarctions other than type 1 or unspecified. For subsequent type 2 AMI assign only code I21.A1. For subsequent type 4 or type 5 AMI, assign only code I21.A9.

If a subsequent myocardial infarction of one type occurs within 4 weeks of a myocardial infarction of a different type, assign the appropriate codes from category I21 to identify each type. Do not assign a code from I22. Codes from category I22 should only be assigned if both the initial and subsequent myocardial infarctions are type 1 or unspecified.

5) Other types of myocardial infarction

The ICD-10-CM provides codes for different types of myocardial infarction. Type 1 myocardial infarctions are assigned to codes I21.Ø–I21.4.

Type 2 myocardial infarction (myocardial infarction due to demand ischemia or secondary to ischemic imbalance) is assigned to code I21.A1, Myocardial infarction type 2 with the underlying cause coded first, **if applicable**. Do not assign code I24.89, Other forms of acute ischemic heart disease, for the demand ischemia. If a type 2 AMI is described as NSTEMI or STEMI, only assign code I21.A1. Codes I21.Ø1-I21.4 should only be assigned for type 1 AMIs.

Acute myocardial infarctions type 3, 4a, 4b, 4c and 5 are assigned to code I21.A9, Other myocardial infarction type.

The "Code also" and "Code first" notes should be followed related to complications, and for coding of postprocedural myocardial infarctions during or following cardiac surgery.

Myocardial infarction involving the left circumflex artery occurring during PTCA with stent insertion to treat coronary artery disease	
I25.1Ø	**Atherosclerotic heart disease of native coronary artery without angina pectoris**
I97.79Ø	**Other intraoperative cardiac functional disturbances during cardiac surgery**
I21.A9	**Other myocardial infarction type**

Explanation: A myocardial infarction occurring during a revascularization procedure is not considered a type 1 myocardial infarction (MI) and should not be coded to a type 1 MI code (I21.Ø-, I21.1-, I21.2-, I21.3) even when the specific site of the MI is documented. According to the code first instruction at I21.A9, the complication code (I97.79Ø) should be sequenced before code I21.A9.

6) Myocardial Infarction with Coronary Microvascular Dysfunction

Coronary microvascular dysfunction (CMD) is a condition that impacts the microvasculature by restricting microvascular flow and increasing microvascular resistance. Code I21.B, Myocardial infarction with coronary microvascular dysfunction, is assigned for myocardial infarction with coronary microvascular disease, myocardial infarction with coronary microvascular dysfunction, and myocardial infarction with non-obstructive coronary arteries (MINOCA) with microvascular disease.

Chapter 9. Diseases of the Circulatory System (I00-I99)

EXCLUDES 2   certain conditions originating in the perinatal period (P04-P96)
certain infectious and parasitic diseases (A00-B99)
complications of pregnancy, childbirth and the puerperium (O00-O9A)
congenital malformations, deformations, and chromosomal abnormalities (Q00-Q99)
endocrine, nutritional and metabolic diseases (E00-E88)
injury, poisoning and certain other consequences of external causes (S00-T88)
neoplasms (C00-D49)
symptoms, signs and abnormal clinical and laboratory findings, not elsewhere classified (R00-R94)
systemic connective tissue disorders (M30-M36)
transient cerebral ischemic attacks and related syndromes (G45.-)

This chapter contains the following blocks:

I00-I02	Acute rheumatic fever
I05-I09	Chronic rheumatic heart diseases
I10-I1A	Hypertensive diseases
I20-I25	Ischemic heart diseases
I26-I28	Pulmonary heart disease and diseases of pulmonary circulation
I30-I5A	Other forms of heart disease
I60-I69	Cerebrovascular diseases
I70-I79	Diseases of arteries, arterioles and capillaries
I80-I89	Diseases of veins, lymphatic vessels and lymph nodes, not elsewhere classified
I95-I99	Other and unspecified disorders of the circulatory system

Acute rheumatic fever (I00-I02)

DEF: Rheumatic fever: Inflammatory disease that can follow a throat infection by group A *streptococci*. Complications can involve the joints (arthritis), subcutaneous tissue (nodules), skin (erythema marginatum), heart (carditis), or brain (chorea).

I00 Rheumatic fever without heart involvement
     INCLUDES   arthritis, rheumatic, acute or subacute
     EXCLUDES 1   rheumatic fever with heart involvement (I01.0-I01.9)

✓4ᵗʰ **I01 Rheumatic fever with heart involvement**
     EXCLUDES 1   chronic diseases of rheumatic origin (I05-I09) unless rheumatic fever is also present or there is evidence of reactivation or activity of the rheumatic process

   I01.0 Acute rheumatic pericarditis   CC
     Any condition in I00 with pericarditis
     Rheumatic pericarditis (acute)
     EXCLUDES 1   acute pericarditis not specified as rheumatic (I30.-)

   I01.1 Acute rheumatic endocarditis   CC
     Any condition in I00 with endocarditis or valvulitis
     Acute rheumatic valvulitis

   I01.2 Acute rheumatic myocarditis   CC
     Any condition in I00 with myocarditis

   I01.8 Other acute rheumatic heart disease   CC
     Any condition in I00 with other or multiple types of heart involvement
     Acute rheumatic pancarditis

   I01.9 Acute rheumatic heart disease, unspecified   CC
     Any condition in I00 with unspecified type of heart involvement
     Rheumatic carditis, acute
     Rheumatic heart disease, active or acute

✓4ᵗʰ **I02 Rheumatic chorea**
     INCLUDES   Sydenham's chorea
     EXCLUDES 1   chorea NOS (G25.5)
         Huntington's chorea (G10)

   I02.0 Rheumatic chorea with heart involvement   CC
     Chorea NOS with heart involvement
     Rheumatic chorea with heart involvement of any type classifiable under I01.-

   I02.9 Rheumatic chorea without heart involvement   CC
     Rheumatic chorea NOS

Chronic rheumatic heart diseases (I05-I09)

✓4ᵗʰ **I05 Rheumatic mitral valve diseases**
     INCLUDES   conditions classifiable to both I05.0 and I05.2-I05.9, whether specified as rheumatic or not
     EXCLUDES 1   mitral valve disease specified as nonrheumatic (I34.-)
         mitral valve disease with aortic and/or tricuspid valve involvement (I08.-)

   I05.0 Rheumatic mitral stenosis
     Mitral (valve) obstruction (rheumatic)

   I05.1 Rheumatic mitral insufficiency
     Rheumatic mitral incompetence
     Rheumatic mitral regurgitation
     EXCLUDES 1   mitral insufficiency not specified as rheumatic (I34.0)

   I05.2 Rheumatic mitral stenosis with insufficiency
     Rheumatic mitral stenosis with incompetence or regurgitation

   I05.8 Other rheumatic mitral valve diseases
     Rheumatic mitral (valve) failure

   I05.9 Rheumatic mitral valve disease, unspecified
     Rheumatic mitral (valve) disorder (chronic) NOS

✓4ᵗʰ **I06 Rheumatic aortic valve diseases**
     EXCLUDES 1   aortic valve disease not specified as rheumatic (I35.-)
         aortic valve disease with mitral and/or tricuspid valve involvement (I08.-)

   I06.0 Rheumatic aortic stenosis
     Rheumatic aortic (valve) obstruction

   I06.1 Rheumatic aortic insufficiency
     Rheumatic aortic incompetence
     Rheumatic aortic regurgitation

   I06.2 Rheumatic aortic stenosis with insufficiency
     Rheumatic aortic stenosis with incompetence or regurgitation

   I06.8 Other rheumatic aortic valve diseases

   I06.9 Rheumatic aortic valve disease, unspecified
     Rheumatic aortic (valve) disease NOS

✓4ᵗʰ **I07 Rheumatic tricuspid valve diseases**
     INCLUDES   rheumatic tricuspid valve diseases specified as rheumatic or unspecified
     EXCLUDES 1   tricuspid valve disease specified as nonrheumatic (I36.-)
         tricuspid valve disease with aortic and/or mitral valve involvement (I08.-)

   I07.0 Rheumatic tricuspid stenosis
     Tricuspid (valve) stenosis (rheumatic)

   I07.1 Rheumatic tricuspid insufficiency
     Tricuspid (valve) insufficiency (rheumatic)

   I07.2 Rheumatic tricuspid stenosis and insufficiency

   I07.8 Other rheumatic tricuspid valve diseases

   I07.9 Rheumatic tricuspid valve disease, unspecified
     Rheumatic tricuspid valve disorder NOS

✓4ᵗʰ **I08 Multiple valve diseases**
     INCLUDES   multiple valve diseases specified as rheumatic or unspecified
     EXCLUDES 1   endocarditis, valve unspecified (I38)
         ~~multiple valve disease specified as nonrheumatic (I34.-, I35.-, I36.-, I37.-, I38.-, Q22.-, Q23.-,Q24.8-)~~
         rheumatic valve disease NOS (I09.1)
     EXCLUDES 2   ▶multiple valve disease specified as nonrheumatic (I34.-, I35.-, I36.-, I37.-, I38.-, Q22.-, Q23.-,Q24.8-)◀

   I08.0 Rheumatic disorders of both mitral and aortic valves
     Involvement of both mitral and aortic valves specified as rheumatic or unspecified
     AHA: 2019,2Q,5

   I08.1 Rheumatic disorders of both mitral and tricuspid valves

   I08.2 Rheumatic disorders of both aortic and tricuspid valves

   I08.3 Combined rheumatic disorders of mitral, aortic and tricuspid valves

   I08.8 Other rheumatic multiple valve diseases

   I08.9 Rheumatic multiple valve disease, unspecified

✓4ᵗʰ **I09 Other rheumatic heart diseases**

   I09.0 Rheumatic myocarditis   CC
     EXCLUDES 1   myocarditis not specified as rheumatic (I51.4)

   I09.1 Rheumatic diseases of endocardium, valve unspecified
     Rheumatic endocarditis (chronic)
     Rheumatic valvulitis (chronic)
     EXCLUDES 1   endocarditis, valve unspecified (I38)

   I09.2 Chronic rheumatic pericarditis   CC
     Adherent pericardium, rheumatic
     Chronic rheumatic mediastinopericarditis
     Chronic rheumatic myopericarditis
     EXCLUDES 1   chronic pericarditis not specified as rheumatic (I31.-)

✓5ᵗʰ   **I09.8 Other specified rheumatic heart diseases**

     I09.81 Rheumatic heart failure   CC HCC
       Use additional code to identify type of heart failure (I50.-)

     I09.89 Other specified rheumatic heart diseases
       Rheumatic disease of pulmonary valve

✔ Additional Character Required   ✓x7ᵗʰ Placeholder   Questionable PDx   Manifestation   Unspecified   UPD Unacceptable PDx   H1-H14 HAC   HCC CMS-HCC Dx   HIV HIV Dx

ICD-10-CM 2025   659

I09.9 Rheumatic heart disease, unspecified
Rheumatic carditis
EXCLUDES 1   *rheumatoid carditis (M05.31)*

Hypertensive diseases (I10-I1A)

Use additional code to identify:
exposure to environmental tobacco smoke (Z77.22)
history of tobacco dependence (Z87.891)
occupational exposure to environmental tobacco smoke (Z57.31)
tobacco dependence (F17.-)
tobacco use (Z72.0)
EXCLUDES 1   *neonatal hypertension (P29.2)*
primary pulmonary hypertension (I27.0)
EXCLUDES 2   *hypertensive disease complicating pregnancy, childbirth and the puerperium (O10-O11, O13-O16)*

I10 Essential (primary) hypertension
INCLUDES   high blood pressure
hypertension (arterial) (benign) (essential) (malignant) (primary) (systemic)
EXCLUDES 1   *hypertensive disease complicating pregnancy, childbirth and the puerperium (O10-O11, O13-O16)*
EXCLUDES 2   *essential (primary) hypertension involving vessels of brain (I60-I69)*
essential (primary) hypertension involving vessels of eye (H35.0-)
AHA: 2023,4Q,24; 2022,1Q,36; 2020,1Q,12; 2018,2Q,9; 2016,4Q,27

✓4ᵗʰ I11 Hypertensive heart disease
INCLUDES   any condition in I50.- or I51.4-I51.7, I51.89, I51.9 due to hypertension
AHA: 2018,2Q,9
TIP: Do not assign a code from this category when provider documentation indicates the heart disease is attributable to another cause.

I11.0 Hypertensive heart disease with heart failure   HCC
Hypertensive heart failure
Use additional code to identify type of heart failure (I50.-)
AHA: 2017,1Q,47

I11.9 Hypertensive heart disease without heart failure
Hypertensive heart disease NOS

✓4ᵗʰ I12 Hypertensive chronic kidney disease
INCLUDES   any condition in N18 and N26 — due to hypertension
arteriosclerosis of kidney
arteriosclerotic nephritis (chronic) (interstitial)
hypertensive nephropathy
nephrosclerosis
EXCLUDES 1   *hypertension due to kidney disease (I15.0, I15.1)*
renovascular hypertension (I15.0)
secondary hypertension (I15.-)
EXCLUDES 2   *acute kidney failure (N17.-)*
AHA: 2019,3Q,3; 2018,4Q,88; 2016,3Q,22
TIP: Do not assign a code from this category when provider documentation indicates the chronic kidney disease (CKD) is attributable to another cause.

I12.0 Hypertensive chronic kidney disease with stage 5 chronic kidney disease or end stage renal disease   CC HCC
Use additional code to identify the stage of chronic kidney disease (N18.5, N18.6)

I12.9 Hypertensive chronic kidney disease with stage 1 through stage 4 chronic kidney disease, or unspecified chronic kidney disease
Hypertensive chronic kidney disease NOS
Hypertensive renal disease NOS
Use additional code to identify the stage of chronic kidney disease (N18.1-N18.4, N18.9)

✓4ᵗʰ I13 Hypertensive heart and chronic kidney disease
INCLUDES   any condition in I11.- with any condition in I12.-
cardiorenal disease
cardiovascular renal disease
TIP: Do not assign a code from this category when provider documentation indicates the heart and/or chronic kidney disease is attributable to another cause.

I13.0 Hypertensive heart and chronic kidney disease with heart failure and stage 1 through stage 4 chronic kidney disease, or unspecified chronic kidney disease   CC HCC
Use additional code to identify type of heart failure (I50.-)
Use additional code to identify stage of chronic kidney disease (N18.1-N18.4, N18.9)

✓5ᵗʰ I13.1 Hypertensive heart and chronic kidney disease without heart failure

I13.10 Hypertensive heart and chronic kidney disease without heart failure, with stage 1 through stage 4 chronic kidney disease, or unspecified chronic kidney disease
Hypertensive heart disease and hypertensive chronic kidney disease NOS
Use additional code to identify the stage of chronic kidney disease (N18.1-N18.4, N18.9)

I13.11 Hypertensive heart and chronic kidney disease without heart failure, with stage 5 chronic kidney disease, or end stage renal disease   CC HCC
Use additional code to identify the stage of chronic kidney disease (N18.5, N18.6)

I13.2 Hypertensive heart and chronic kidney disease with heart failure and with stage 5 chronic kidney disease, or end stage renal disease   CC HCC
Use additional code to identify type of heart failure (I50.-)
Use additional code to identify the stage of chronic kidney disease (N18.5, N18.6)

✓4ᵗʰ I15 Secondary hypertension
Code also underlying condition
EXCLUDES 1   *postprocedural hypertension (I97.3)*
EXCLUDES 2   *secondary hypertension involving vessels of brain (I60-I69)*
secondary hypertension involving vessels of eye (H35.0-)

I15.0 Renovascular hypertension

I15.1 Hypertension secondary to other renal disorders
AHA: 2016,3Q,22

I15.2 Hypertension secondary to endocrine disorders
AHA: 2023,2Q,16

I15.8 Other secondary hypertension

I15.9 Secondary hypertension, unspecified

✓4ᵗʰ I16 Hypertensive crisis
Code also any identified hypertensive disease (I10-I15, I1A)
AHA: 2016,4Q,26-28

I16.0 Hypertensive urgency

I16.1 Hypertensive emergency   CC
▶Use additional code, if applicable, to identify specific organ dysfunction, such as:◀
▶acute kidney injury (N17.-)◀
▶acute myocardial infarction (I21.-)◀
▶acute pulmonary edema (left and/or right ventricular failure) (J81.0, I50.-)◀
▶aortic dissection (I71.0-)◀
▶cerebral hemorrhage (I60.-. I61.-, I62.-)◀
▶cerebral infarction (I63.-)◀
▶eclampsia (O15.-)◀
▶hypertensive encephalopathy (I67.4)◀
▶seizure (R56.9)◀
AHA: 2023,4Q,24

I16.9 Hypertensive crisis, unspecified   CC

✓4ᵗʰ I1A Other hypertension
AHA: 2023,4Q,23-25

I1A.0 Resistant hypertension
Apparent treatment resistant hypertension
Treatment resistant hypertension
True resistant hypertension
Code first specific type of existing hypertension, if known, such as:
essential hypertension (I10)
secondary hypertension (I15.-)

Ischemic heart diseases (I20-I25)

Code also the presence of hypertension (I10-I1A)

✓4th **I20 Angina pectoris**

Use additional code to identify:
exposure to environmental tobacco smoke (Z77.22)
history of tobacco dependence (Z87.891)
occupational exposure to environmental tobacco smoke (Z57.31)
tobacco dependence (F17.-)
tobacco use (Z72.0)

EXCLUDES 1   *angina pectoris with atherosclerotic heart disease of native coronary arteries (I25.1-)*
atherosclerosis of coronary artery bypass graft(s) and coronary artery of transplanted heart with angina pectoris (I25.7-)
postinfarction angina (I23.7)

DEF: Chest pain due to reduced blood flow resulting in a lack of oxygen to the heart muscles.

   I20.0 Unstable angina   CC HCC
     Accelerated angina
     Crescendo angina
     De novo effort angina
     Intermediate coronary syndrome
     Preinfarction syndrome
     Worsening effort angina

   I20.1 Angina pectoris with documented spasm   CC
     Angiospastic angina
     Prinzmetal angina
     Spasm-induced angina
     Variant angina

   I20.2 Refractory angina pectoris   CC
     AHA: 2022,4Q,20-21

✓5th **I20.8 Other forms of angina pectoris**
     Use additional code(s) for symptoms associated with angina equivalent
     AHA: 2023,4Q,25-26

     I20.81 Angina pectoris with coronary microvascular dysfunction
       Angina pectoris with coronary microvascular disease

     I20.89 Other forms of angina pectoris
       Angina equivalent
       Angina of effort
       Coronary slow flow syndrome
       Stable angina
       Stenocardia

   I20.9 Angina pectoris, unspecified
     Angina NOS
     Anginal syndrome
     Cardiac angina
     Ischemic chest pain

✓4th **I21 Acute myocardial infarction**

INCLUDES   cardiac infarction
coronary (artery) embolism
coronary (artery) occlusion
coronary (artery) rupture
coronary (artery) thrombosis
infarction of heart, myocardium, or ventricle
myocardial infarction specified as acute or with a stated duration of 4 weeks (28 days) or less from onset

Use additional code, if applicable, to identify:
exposure to environmental tobacco smoke (Z77.22)
history of tobacco dependence (Z87.891)
occupational exposure to environmental tobacco smoke (Z57.31)
status post administration of tPA (rtPA) in a different facility within the last 24 hours prior to admission to current facility (Z92.82)
tobacco dependence (F17.-)
tobacco use (Z72.0)

EXCLUDES 2   *old myocardial infarction (I25.2)*
postmyocardial infarction syndrome (I24.1)
subsequent type 1 myocardial infarction (I22.-)

AHA: 2019,2Q,5; 2018,4Q,68; 2018,3Q,5; 2017,4Q,12-14; 2017,1Q,44-45; 2016,4Q,140; 2015,2Q,16; 2013,1Q,25; 2012,4Q,96,102-103

TIP: When chronic total occlusion and myocardial infarction are documented as being in different vessels, assign code I25.82 Chronic total occlusion of coronary artery, in addition to the myocardial infarction code.

✓5th **I21.0 ST elevation (STEMI) myocardial infarction of anterior wall**
     Type 1 ST elevation myocardial infarction of anterior wall
     DEF: ST elevation myocardial infarction: Complete obstruction of one or more coronary arteries causing decreased blood flow (ischemia) and necrosis of myocardial muscle cells.

     I21.01 ST elevation (STEMI) myocardial infarction involving left main coronary artery   MCC HCC

     I21.02 ST elevation (STEMI) myocardial infarction involving left anterior descending coronary artery   MCC HCC
       ST elevation (STEMI) myocardial infarction involving diagonal coronary artery
       AHA: 2013,1Q,25

     I21.09 ST elevation (STEMI) myocardial infarction involving other coronary artery of anterior wall   MCC HCC
       Acute transmural myocardial infarction of anterior wall
       Anteroapical transmural (Q wave) infarction (acute)
       Anterolateral transmural (Q wave) infarction (acute)
       Anteroseptal transmural (Q wave) infarction (acute)
       Transmural (Q wave) infarction (acute) (of) anterior (wall) NOS
       AHA: 2012,4Q,102-103

✓5th **I21.1 ST elevation (STEMI) myocardial infarction of inferior wall**
     Type 1 ST elevation myocardial infarction of inferior wall
     DEF: ST elevation myocardial infarction: Complete obstruction of one or more coronary arteries causing decreased blood flow (ischemia) and necrosis of myocardial muscle cells.

     I21.11 ST elevation (STEMI) myocardial infarction involving right coronary artery   MCC HCC
       Inferoposterior transmural (Q wave) infarction (acute)

     I21.19 ST elevation (STEMI) myocardial infarction involving other coronary artery of inferior wall   MCC HCC
       Acute transmural myocardial infarction of inferior wall
       Inferolateral transmural (Q wave) infarction (acute)
       Transmural (Q wave) infarction (acute) (of) diaphragmatic wall
       Transmural (Q wave) infarction (acute) (of) inferior (wall) NOS

       EXCLUDES 2   *ST elevation (STEMI) myocardial infarction involving left circumflex coronary artery (I21.21)*

       AHA: 2012,4Q,96

✓5th **I21.2 ST elevation (STEMI) myocardial infarction of other sites**
     Type 1 ST elevation myocardial infarction of other sites
     DEF: ST elevation myocardial infarction: Complete obstruction of one or more coronary arteries causing decreased blood flow (ischemia) and necrosis of myocardial muscle cells.

     I21.21 ST elevation (STEMI) myocardial infarction involving left circumflex coronary artery   MCC HCC
       ST elevation (STEMI) myocardial infarction involving oblique marginal coronary artery

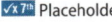 Additional Character Required   ✓x7th Placeholder   Questionable PDx   Manifestation   Unspecified   UPD Unacceptable PDx   H1-H14 HAC   HCC CMS-HCC Dx   HIV HIV Dx

ICD-10-CM 2025   661

Chapter 9. Diseases of the Circulatory System

I21.29   **ST elevation (STEMI) myocardial infarction involving other sites**   `MCC` `HCC`
Acute transmural myocardial infarction of other sites
Apical-lateral transmural (Q wave) infarction (acute)
Basal-lateral transmural (Q wave) infarction (acute)
High lateral transmural (Q wave) infarction (acute)
Lateral (wall) NOS transmural (Q wave) infarction (acute)
Posterior (true) transmural (Q wave) infarction (acute)
Posterobasal transmural (Q wave) infarction (acute)
Posterolateral transmural (Q wave) infarction (acute)
Posteroseptal transmural (Q wave) infarction (acute)
Septal transmural (Q wave) infarction (acute) NOS

I21.3   **ST elevation (STEMI) myocardial infarction of unspecified site**   `MCC` `HCC`
Acute transmural myocardial infarction of unspecified site
Transmural (Q wave) myocardial infarction NOS
Type 1 ST elevation myocardial infarction of unspecified site
DEF: ST elevation myocardial infarction: Complete obstruction of one or more coronary arteries causing decreased blood flow (ischemia) and necrosis of myocardial muscle cells.

I21.4   **Non-ST elevation (NSTEMI) myocardial infarction**   `MCC` `HCC`
Acute subendocardial myocardial infarction
Non-Q wave myocardial infarction NOS
Nontransmural myocardial infarction NOS
Type 1 non-ST elevation myocardial infarction
AHA: 2024,1Q,28; 2023,2Q,29; 2021,3Q,6; 2019,2Q,33; 2017,1Q,44-45
DEF: Partial obstruction of one or more coronary arteries that causes decreased blood flow (ischemia) and may cause partial thickness necrosis of myocardial muscle cells.

I21.9   **Acute myocardial infarction, unspecified**   `MCC` `HCC`
Myocardial infarction (acute) NOS

I21.A   **Other type of myocardial infarction**
AHA: 2019,2Q,5

I21.A1   **Myocardial infarction type 2**   `MCC` `HCC`
Myocardial infarction due to demand ischemia
Myocardial infarction secondary to ischemic imbalance
▶Code first, if applicable, the underlying cause, such as:◀
anemia (D50.0-D64.9)
chronic obstructive pulmonary disease (J44.-)
paroxysmal tachycardia (I47.0-I47.9)
shock (R57.0-R57.9)
AHA: 2019,4Q,53; 2017,4Q,13-14
DEF: Often referred to as due to demand ischemia, myocardial infarction (MI) type 2 refers to an MI due to ischemia and necrosis resulting from an oxygen imbalance to the heart. This mismatch between oxygen decreased supply and increased demand is caused by conditions other than coronary artery disease such as vasospasm, embolism, anemia, hypertension, hypotension, or arrhythmias.

I21.A9   **Other myocardial infarction type**   `MCC` `HCC`
Myocardial infarction associated with revascularization procedure
Myocardial infarction type 3
Myocardial infarction type 4a
Myocardial infarction type 4b
Myocardial infarction type 4c
Myocardial infarction type 5
Code first, if applicable, postprocedural myocardial infarction following cardiac surgery (I97.190), or postprocedural myocardial infarction during cardiac surgery (I97.790)
Code also complication, if known and applicable, such as:
(acute) stent occlusion (T82.897-)
(acute) stent stenosis (T82.855-)
(acute) stent thrombosis (T82.867-)
cardiac arrest due to underlying cardiac condition (I46.2)
complication of percutaneous coronary intervention (PCI) (I97.89)
occlusion of coronary artery bypass graft (T82.218-)
AHA: 2021,3Q,6; 2019,2Q,33

I21.B   **Myocardial infarction with coronary microvascular dysfunction**   `MCC` `HCC`
Myocardial infarction with coronary microvascular disease
Myocardial infarction with nonobstructive coronary arteries [MINOCA] with microvascular disease
AHA: 2023,4Q,25-26

I22   **Subsequent ST elevation (STEMI) and non-ST elevation (NSTEMI) myocardial infarction**
`INCLUDES`   acute myocardial infarction occurring within four weeks (28 days) of a previous acute myocardial infarction, regardless of site
cardiac infarction
coronary (artery) embolism
coronary (artery) occlusion
coronary (artery) rupture
coronary (artery) thrombosis
infarction of heart, myocardium, or ventricle
recurrent myocardial infarction
reinfarction of myocardium
rupture of heart, myocardium, or ventricle
subsequent type 1 myocardial infarction
Use additional code, if applicable, to identify:
exposure to environmental tobacco smoke (Z77.22)
history of tobacco dependence (Z87.891)
occupational exposure to environmental tobacco smoke (Z57.31)
status post administration of tPA (rtPA) in a different facility within the last 24 hours prior to admission to current facility (Z92.82)
tobacco dependence (F17.-)
tobacco use (Z72.0)
`EXCLUDES 1`   subsequent myocardial infarction, type 2 (I21.A1)
subsequent myocardial infarction of other type (type 3) (type 4) (type 5) (I21.A9)
AHA: 2018,4Q,68; 2018,3Q,5; 2017,4Q,12-13; 2017,2Q,11; 2013,1Q,25; 2012,4Q,97,102-103
DEF: Non-ST elevation myocardial infarction: Partial obstruction of one or more coronary arteries that causes decreased blood flow (ischemia) and may cause partial thickness necrosis of myocardial muscle cells.
DEF: ST elevation myocardial infarction: Complete obstruction of one or more coronary arteries causing decreased blood flow (ischemia) and necrosis of myocardial muscle cells.
TIP: When chronic total occlusion and myocardial infarction are documented as being in different vessels, assign code I25.82 Chronic total occlusion of coronary artery, in addition to the myocardial infarction code.

I22.0   **Subsequent ST elevation (STEMI) myocardial infarction of anterior wall**   `MCC` `HCC`
Subsequent acute transmural myocardial infarction of anterior wall
Subsequent transmural (Q wave) infarction (acute)(of) anterior (wall) NOS
Subsequent anteroapical transmural (Q wave) infarction (acute)
Subsequent anterolateral transmural (Q wave) infarction (acute)
Subsequent anteroseptal transmural (Q wave) infarction (acute)

I22.1   **Subsequent ST elevation (STEMI) myocardial infarction of inferior wall**   `MCC` `HCC`
Subsequent acute transmural myocardial infarction of inferior wall
Subsequent transmural (Q wave) infarction (acute)(of) diaphragmatic wall
Subsequent transmural (Q wave) infarction (acute)(of) inferior (wall) NOS
Subsequent inferolateral transmural (Q wave) infarction (acute)
Subsequent inferoposterior transmural (Q wave) infarction (acute)
AHA: 2012,4Q,102

I22.2   **Subsequent non-ST elevation (NSTEMI) myocardial infarction**   `MCC` `HCC`
Subsequent acute subendocardial myocardial infarction
Subsequent non-Q wave myocardial infarction NOS
Subsequent nontransmural myocardial infarction NOS

I22.8 **Subsequent ST elevation (STEMI) myocardial infarction of other sites** `MCC` `HCC`

Subsequent acute transmural myocardial infarction of other sites

Subsequent apical-lateral transmural (Q wave) myocardial infarction (acute)

Subsequent basal-lateral transmural (Q wave) myocardial infarction (acute)

Subsequent high lateral transmural (Q wave) myocardial infarction (acute)

Subsequent posterior (true) transmural (Q wave) myocardial infarction (acute)

Subsequent posterobasal transmural (Q wave) myocardial infarction (acute)

Subsequent posterolateral transmural (Q wave) myocardial infarction (acute)

Subsequent posteroseptal transmural (Q wave) myocardial infarction (acute)

Subsequent septal NOS transmural (Q wave) myocardial infarction (acute)

Subsequent transmural (Q wave) myocardial infarction (acute) (of) lateral (wall) NOS

I22.9 **Subsequent ST elevation (STEMI) myocardial infarction of unspecified site** `MCC` `HCC`

Subsequent acute myocardial infarction of unspecified site

Subsequent myocardial infarction (acute) NOS

✓4th **I23** **Certain current complications following ST elevation (STEMI) and non-ST elevation (NSTEMI) myocardial infarction (within the 28 day period)**

AHA: 2017,2Q,11

DEF: ST elevation myocardial infarction: Complete obstruction of one or more coronary arteries causing decreased blood flow (ischemia) and necrosis of myocardial muscle cells.

DEF: Non-ST elevation myocardial infarction: Partial obstruction of one or more coronary arteries that causes decreased blood flow (ischemia) and may cause partial thickness necrosis of myocardial muscle cells.

I23.0 **Hemopericardium as current complication following acute myocardial infarction** `CC` `HCC` `A`

EXCLUDES 1   *hemopericardium not specified as current complication following acute myocardial infarction (I31.2)*

I23.1 **Atrial septal defect as current complication following acute myocardial infarction** `CC` `HCC`

EXCLUDES 1   *acquired atrial septal defect not specified as current complication following acute myocardial infarction (I51.0)*

I23.2 **Ventricular septal defect as current complication following acute myocardial infarction** `CC` `HCC` `A`

EXCLUDES 1   *acquired ventricular septal defect not specified as current complication following acute myocardial infarction (I51.0)*

I23.3 **Rupture of cardiac wall without hemopericardium as current complication following acute myocardial infarction** `CC` `HCC` `A`

I23.4 **Rupture of chordae tendineae as current complication following acute myocardial infarction** `MCC` `HCC`

EXCLUDES 1   *rupture of chordae tendineae not specified as current complication following acute myocardial infarction (I51.1)*

I23.5 **Rupture of papillary muscle as current complication following acute myocardial infarction** `MCC` `HCC`

EXCLUDES 1   *rupture of papillary muscle not specified as current complication following acute myocardial infarction (I51.2)*

I23.6 **Thrombosis of atrium, auricular appendage, and ventricle as current complications following acute myocardial infarction** `CC` `HCC` `A`

EXCLUDES 1   *thrombosis of atrium, auricular appendage, and ventricle not specified as current complication following acute myocardial infarction (I51.3)*

I23.7 **Postinfarction angina** `CC` `HCC` `A`

AHA: 2015,2Q,16

TIP: When postinfarction angina occurs with atherosclerotic coronary artery disease, code both I23.7 and I25.118 for atherosclerotic disease with other forms of angina pectoris.

I23.8 **Other current complications following acute myocardial infarction** `CC` `HCC` `A`

✓4th **I24** **Other acute ischemic heart diseases**

EXCLUDES 1   *angina pectoris (I20.-)*

transient myocardial ischemia in newborn (P29.4)

EXCLUDES 2   *non-ischemic myocardial injury (I5A)*

I24.0 **Acute coronary thrombosis not resulting in myocardial infarction** `CC` `HCC`

Acute coronary (artery) (vein) embolism not resulting in myocardial infarction

Acute coronary (artery) (vein) occlusion not resulting in myocardial infarction

Acute coronary (artery) (vein) thromboembolism not resulting in myocardial infarction

EXCLUDES 1   *atherosclerotic heart disease (I25.1-)*

AHA: 2013,1Q,24

I24.1 **Dressler's syndrome** `CC` `HCC`

Postmyocardial infarction syndrome

EXCLUDES 1   *postinfarction angina (I23.7)*

DEF: Fever, leukocytosis, chest pain, evidence of pericarditis, pleurisy, and pneumonia occurring days or weeks after a myocardial infarction.

✓5th **I24.8** **Other forms of acute ischemic heart disease**

EXCLUDES 1   *myocardial infarction due to demand ischemia (I21.A1)*

AHA: 2023,4Q,25-26; 2019,4Q,53; 2017,4Q,13

I24.81 **Acute coronary microvascular dysfunction** `CC` `HCC`

Acute (presentation of) coronary microvascular disease

I24.89 **Other forms of acute ischemic heart disease** `CC` `HCC`

I24.9 **Acute ischemic heart disease, unspecified** `CC` `HCC`

EXCLUDES 1   *ischemic heart disease (chronic) NOS (I25.9)*

✓4th **I25** **Chronic ischemic heart disease**

Use additional code to identify:

chronic total occlusion of coronary artery (I25.82)

exposure to environmental tobacco smoke (Z77.22)

history of tobacco dependence (Z87.891)

occupational exposure to environmental tobacco smoke (Z57.31)

tobacco dependence (F17.-)

tobacco use (Z72.0)

EXCLUDES 2   *non-ischemic myocardial injury (I5A)*

AHA: 2022,4Q,20-21

✓5th **I25.1** **Atherosclerotic heart disease of native coronary artery**

Atherosclerotic cardiovascular disease

Coronary (artery) atheroma

Coronary (artery) atherosclerosis

Coronary (artery) disease

Coronary (artery) sclerosis

Use additional code, if applicable, to identify:

coronary atherosclerosis due to calcified coronary lesion (I25.84)

coronary atherosclerosis due to lipid rich plaque (I25.83)

EXCLUDES 2   *atheroembolism (I75.-)*

atherosclerosis of coronary artery bypass graft(s) and transplanted heart (I25.7-)

Atheromas

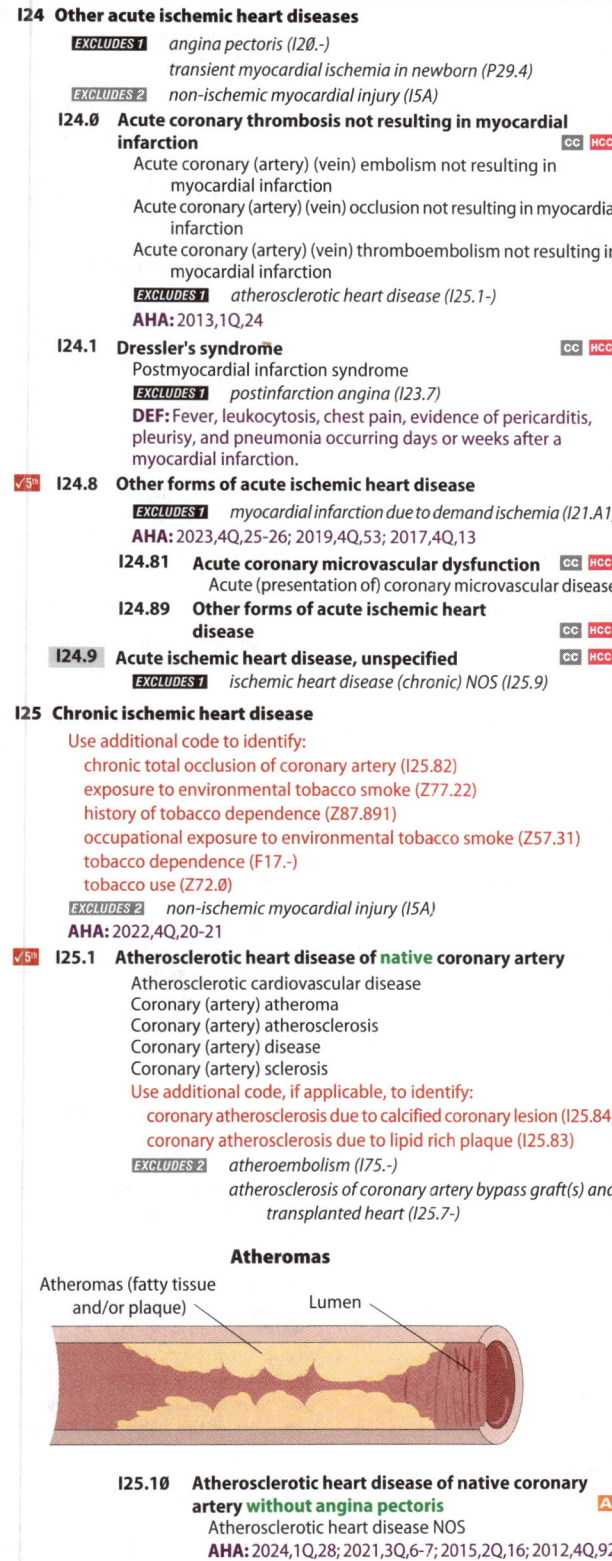

Atheromas (fatty tissue and/or plaque)   Lumen

I25.10 **Atherosclerotic heart disease of native coronary artery without angina pectoris** `A`

Atherosclerotic heart disease NOS

AHA: 2024,1Q,28; 2021,3Q,6-7; 2015,2Q,16; 2012,4Q,92

✓6th **I25.11** **Atherosclerotic heart disease of native coronary artery with angina pectoris**

AHA: 2024,1Q,28

I25.110 **Atherosclerotic heart disease of native coronary artery with unstable angina pectoris** `CC` `HCC` `A`

EXCLUDES 1   *unstable angina without atherosclerotic heart disease (I20.0)*

☑ Additional Character Required   ✓x7th Placeholder   Questionable PDx   Manifestation   Unspecified   `UPD` Unacceptable PDx   `H1`-`H14` HAC   `HCC` CMS-HCC Dx   `HIV` HIV Dx

ICD-10-CM 2025   663

I25.111 Atherosclerotic heart disease of native coronary artery with angina pectoris with documented spasm `A`
> *EXCLUDES 1*   *angina pectoris with documented spasm without atherosclerotic heart disease (I20.1)*

I25.112 Atherosclerotic heart disease of native coronary artery with refractory angina pectoris `CC` `A`

I25.118 Atherosclerotic heart disease of native coronary artery with other forms of angina pectoris `A`
> *EXCLUDES 1*   *other forms of angina pectoris without atherosclerotic heart disease (I20.8-)*

AHA: 2015,2Q,16
TIP: When postinfarction angina occurs with atherosclerotic coronary artery disease, code both I23.7 and I25.118 for atherosclerotic disease with other forms of angina pectoris.

I25.119 Atherosclerotic heart disease of native coronary artery with unspecified angina pectoris `A`
> Atherosclerotic heart disease with angina NOS
> Atherosclerotic heart disease with ischemic chest pain
> *EXCLUDES 1*   *unspecified angina pectoris without atherosclerotic heart disease (I20.9)*

I25.2 Old myocardial infarction `PE`
> Healed myocardial infarction
> Past myocardial infarction diagnosed by ECG or other investigation, but currently presenting no symptoms

I25.3 Aneurysm of heart `CC`
> Mural aneurysm
> Ventricular aneurysm

✓5th **I25.4 Coronary artery aneurysm and dissection**

I25.41 Coronary artery aneurysm
> Coronary arteriovenous fistula, acquired
> *EXCLUDES 1*   *congenital coronary (artery) aneurysm (Q24.5)*

I25.42 Coronary artery dissection `MCC`
> DEF: Tear in the intimal arterial wall of a coronary artery resulting in the sudden intrusion of blood within the layers of the wall.

I25.5 Ischemic cardiomyopathy
> *EXCLUDES 2*   *coronary atherosclerosis (I25.1-, I25.7-)*
> AHA: 2022,3Q,17

I25.6 Silent myocardial ischemia

✓5th **I25.7 Atherosclerosis of coronary artery bypass graft(s) and coronary artery of transplanted heart with angina pectoris**
> Use additional code, if applicable, to identify:
> coronary atherosclerosis due to calcified coronary lesion (I25.84)
> coronary atherosclerosis due to lipid rich plaque (I25.83)
> *EXCLUDES 1*   *atherosclerosis of bypass graft(s) of transplanted heart without angina pectoris (I25.812)*
> *atherosclerosis of coronary artery bypass graft(s) without angina pectoris (I25.810)*
> *atherosclerosis of native coronary artery of transplanted heart without angina pectoris (I25.811)*

✓6th **I25.70 Atherosclerosis of coronary artery bypass graft(s), unspecified, with angina pectoris**

I25.700 Atherosclerosis of coronary artery bypass graft(s), unspecified, with unstable angina pectoris `CC` `HCC` `A`
> *EXCLUDES 1*   *unstable angina pectoris without atherosclerosis of coronary artery bypass graft (I20.0)*

I25.701 Atherosclerosis of coronary artery bypass graft(s), unspecified, with angina pectoris with documented spasm `A`
> *EXCLUDES 1*   *angina pectoris with documented spasm without atherosclerosis of coronary artery bypass graft (I20.1)*

I25.702 Atherosclerosis of coronary artery bypass graft(s), unspecified, with refractory angina pectoris `CC` `A`
> AHA: 2022,4Q,21

I25.708 Atherosclerosis of coronary artery bypass graft(s), unspecified, with other forms of angina pectoris `A`
> *EXCLUDES 1*   *other forms of angina pectoris without atherosclerosis of coronary artery bypass graft (I20.8-)*

I25.709 Atherosclerosis of coronary artery bypass graft(s), unspecified, with unspecified angina pectoris `A`
> *EXCLUDES 1*   *unspecified angina pectoris without atherosclerosis of coronary artery bypass graft (I20.9)*

✓6th **I25.71 Atherosclerosis of autologous vein coronary artery bypass graft(s) with angina pectoris**

I25.710 Atherosclerosis of autologous vein coronary artery bypass graft(s) with unstable angina pectoris `CC` `HCC` `A`
> *EXCLUDES 1*   *unstable angina without atherosclerosis of autologous vein coronary artery bypass graft(s) (I20.0)*
> *EXCLUDES 2*   *embolism or thrombus of coronary artery bypass graft(s) (T82.8-)*

I25.711 Atherosclerosis of autologous vein coronary artery bypass graft(s) with angina pectoris with documented spasm `CC` `A`
> *EXCLUDES 1*   *angina pectoris with documented spasm without atherosclerosis of autologous vein coronary artery bypass graft(s) (I20.1)*

I25.712 Atherosclerosis of autologous vein coronary artery bypass graft(s) with refractory angina pectoris `CC` `A`

I25.718 Atherosclerosis of autologous vein coronary artery bypass graft(s) with other forms of angina pectoris `CC` `A`
> *EXCLUDES 1*   *other forms of angina pectoris without atherosclerosis of autologous vein coronary artery bypass graft(s) (I20.8-)*

I25.719 Atherosclerosis of autologous vein coronary artery bypass graft(s) with unspecified angina pectoris `CC` `A`
> *EXCLUDES 1*   *unspecified angina pectoris without atherosclerosis of autologous vein coronary artery bypass graft(s) (I20.9)*

`N` Newborn: 0   `P` Pediatric: 0-17   `M` Maternity: 9-64   `A` Adult: 15-124   `UNS` Unspecified Site   `MCC` Major Complication/Comorbidity   `CC` Complication/Comorbidity   `PE` POA Exempt

664   ICD-10-CM 2025

√6ᵗʰ **I25.72** **Atherosclerosis of autologous artery coronary artery bypass graft(s) with angina pectoris**
Atherosclerosis of internal mammary artery graft with angina pectoris

I25.720 **Atherosclerosis of autologous artery coronary artery bypass graft(s) with unstable angina pectoris** cc HCC A
EXCLUDES 1 unstable angina without atherosclerosis of autologous artery coronary artery bypass graft(s) (I20.0)

I25.721 **Atherosclerosis of autologous artery coronary artery bypass graft(s) with angina pectoris with documented spasm** cc A
EXCLUDES 1 angina pectoris with documented spasm without atherosclerosis of autologous artery coronary artery bypass graft(s) (I20.1)

I25.722 **Atherosclerosis of autologous artery coronary artery bypass graft(s) with refractory angina pectoris** cc A

I25.728 **Atherosclerosis of autologous artery coronary artery bypass graft(s) with other forms of angina pectoris** cc A
EXCLUDES 1 other forms of angina pectoris without atherosclerosis of autologous artery coronary artery bypass graft(s) (I20.8-)

I25.729 **Atherosclerosis of autologous artery coronary artery bypass graft(s) with unspecified angina pectoris** cc A
EXCLUDES 1 unspecified angina pectoris without atherosclerosis of autologous artery coronary artery bypass graft(s) (I20.9)

√6ᵗʰ **I25.73** **Atherosclerosis of nonautologous biological coronary artery bypass graft(s) with angina pectoris**

I25.730 **Atherosclerosis of nonautologous biological coronary artery bypass graft(s) with unstable angina pectoris** cc HCC A
EXCLUDES 1 unstable angina without atherosclerosis of nonautologous biological coronary artery bypass graft(s) (I20.0)

I25.731 **Atherosclerosis of nonautologous biological coronary artery bypass graft(s) with angina pectoris with documented spasm** cc A
EXCLUDES 1 angina pectoris with documented spasm without atherosclerosis of nonautologous biological coronary artery bypass graft(s) (I20.1)

I25.732 **Atherosclerosis of nonautologous biological coronary artery bypass graft(s) with refractory angina pectoris** cc A

I25.738 **Atherosclerosis of nonautologous biological coronary artery bypass graft(s) with other forms of angina pectoris** cc A
EXCLUDES 1 other forms of angina pectoris without atherosclerosis of nonautologous biological coronary artery bypass graft(s) (I20.8-)

I25.739 **Atherosclerosis of nonautologous biological coronary artery bypass graft(s) with unspecified angina pectoris** cc A
EXCLUDES 1 unspecified angina pectoris without atherosclerosis of nonautologous biological coronary artery bypass graft(s) (I20.9)

√6ᵗʰ **I25.75** **Atherosclerosis of native coronary artery of transplanted heart with angina pectoris**
EXCLUDES 1 atherosclerosis of native coronary artery of transplanted heart without angina pectoris (I25.811)

I25.750 **Atherosclerosis of native coronary artery of transplanted heart with unstable angina** cc HCC

I25.751 **Atherosclerosis of native coronary artery of transplanted heart with angina pectoris with documented spasm** cc

I25.752 **Atherosclerosis of native coronary artery of transplanted heart with refractory angina pectoris** cc A

I25.758 **Atherosclerosis of native coronary artery of transplanted heart with other forms of angina pectoris** cc

I25.759 **Atherosclerosis of native coronary artery of transplanted heart with unspecified angina pectoris** cc

√6ᵗʰ **I25.76** **Atherosclerosis of bypass graft of coronary artery of transplanted heart with angina pectoris**
EXCLUDES 1 atherosclerosis of bypass graft of coronary artery of transplanted heart without angina pectoris (I25.812)

I25.760 **Atherosclerosis of bypass graft of coronary artery of transplanted heart with unstable angina** cc HCC A

I25.761 **Atherosclerosis of bypass graft of coronary artery of transplanted heart with angina pectoris with documented spasm** cc A

I25.762 **Atherosclerosis of bypass graft of coronary artery of transplanted heart with refractory angina pectoris** cc A

I25.768 **Atherosclerosis of bypass graft of coronary artery of transplanted heart with other forms of angina pectoris** cc A

I25.769 **Atherosclerosis of bypass graft of coronary artery of transplanted heart with unspecified angina pectoris** cc A

√6ᵗʰ **I25.79** **Atherosclerosis of other coronary artery bypass graft(s) with angina pectoris**

I25.790 **Atherosclerosis of other coronary artery bypass graft(s) with unstable angina pectoris** cc HCC A
EXCLUDES 1 unstable angina without atherosclerosis of other coronary artery bypass graft(s) (I20.0)

I25.791 **Atherosclerosis of other coronary artery bypass graft(s) with angina pectoris with documented spasm** cc A
EXCLUDES 1 angina pectoris with documented spasm without atherosclerosis of other coronary artery bypass graft(s) (I20.1)

I25.792 **Atherosclerosis of other coronary artery bypass graft(s) with refractory angina pectoris** cc A

I25.798 **Atherosclerosis of other coronary artery bypass graft(s) with other forms of angina pectoris** cc A
EXCLUDES 1 other forms of angina pectoris without atherosclerosis of other coronary artery bypass graft(s) (I20.8-)

✔ Additional Character Required   √x7ᵗʰ Placeholder   Questionable PDx   Manifestation   Unspecified   UPD Unacceptable PDx   H1-H14 HAC   HCC CMS-HCC Dx   HIV HIV Dx

ICD-10-CM 2025   **665**

Chapter 9. Diseases of the Circulatory System

I25.799   **Atherosclerosis of other coronary artery bypass graft(s) with unspecified angina pectoris** `CC` `A`

> *EXCLUDES 1*   *unspecified angina pectoris without atherosclerosis of other coronary artery bypass graft(s) (I20.9)*

☑5ᵗʰ **I25.8**   **Other forms of chronic ischemic heart disease**

☑6ᵗʰ **I25.81**   **Atherosclerosis of other coronary vessels without angina pectoris**

Use additional code, if applicable, to identify:
> coronary atherosclerosis due to calcified coronary lesion (I25.84)
> coronary atherosclerosis due to lipid rich plaque (I25.83)

> *EXCLUDES 2*   *atherosclerotic heart disease of native coronary artery without angina pectoris (I25.10)*

I25.810   **Atherosclerosis of coronary artery bypass graft(s) without angina pectoris** `CC` `A`

Atherosclerosis of coronary artery bypass graft NOS

> *EXCLUDES 1*   *atherosclerosis of coronary bypass graft(s) with angina pectoris (I25.70-I25.73-, I25.79-)*

I25.811   **Atherosclerosis of native coronary artery of transplanted heart without angina pectoris** `CC`

Atherosclerosis of native coronary artery of transplanted heart NOS

> *EXCLUDES 1*   *atherosclerosis of native coronary artery of transplanted heart with angina pectoris (I25.75-)*

I25.812   **Atherosclerosis of bypass graft of coronary artery of transplanted heart without angina pectoris** `CC` `A`

Atherosclerosis of bypass graft of transplanted heart NOS

> *EXCLUDES 1*   *atherosclerosis of bypass graft of transplanted heart with angina pectoris (I25.76)*

I25.82   **Chronic total occlusion of coronary artery** `UPD`

Complete occlusion of coronary artery
Total occlusion of coronary artery
Code first coronary atherosclerosis (I25.1-, I25.7-, I25.81-)

> *EXCLUDES 1*   *acute coronary occlusion with myocardial infarction (I21.0-I21.B, I22.-)*
> *acute coronary occlusion without myocardial infarction (I24.0)*

AHA: 2018,3Q,5
DEF: Complete blockage of the coronary artery due to plaque accumulation over an extended period of time, resulting in substantial reduction of blood flow. Symptoms include angina or chest pain.
TIP: Report this code in addition to a code from category I21 or I22 when the chronic total occlusion and the myocardial infarction are documented as being in different vessels.

I25.83   **Coronary atherosclerosis due to lipid rich plaque** `UPD` `A`

Code first coronary atherosclerosis (I25.1-, I25.7-, I25.81-)

I25.84   **Coronary atherosclerosis due to calcified coronary lesion** `UPD`

Coronary atherosclerosis due to severely calcified coronary lesion
Code first coronary atherosclerosis (I25.1-, I25.7-, I25.81-)

I25.85   **Chronic coronary microvascular dysfunction**

Chronic (presentation of) coronary microvascular disease
Coronary microvascular dysfunction NOS
AHA: 2023,4Q,25-26

I25.89   **Other forms of chronic ischemic heart disease**

I25.9   **Chronic ischemic heart disease, unspecified**

Ischemic heart disease (chronic) NOS

Pulmonary heart disease and diseases of pulmonary circulation (I26-I28)

☑4ᵗʰ **I26**   **Pulmonary embolism**

INCLUDES   pulmonary (acute)(artery)(vein) infarction
pulmonary (acute) (artery)(vein) thromboembolism
pulmonary (acute)(artery)(vein) thrombosis

> *EXCLUDES 1*   *cor pulmonale without embolism (I27.81)*
> *EXCLUDES 2*   *chronic pulmonary embolism (I27.82)*
> *personal history of pulmonary embolism (Z86.711)*
> *pulmonary embolism complicating abortion, ectopic or molar pregnancy (O00-O07, O08.2)*
> *pulmonary embolism complicating pregnancy, childbirth and the puerperium (O88.-)*
> *pulmonary embolism due to trauma (T79.0, T79.1)*
> *pulmonary embolism due to complications of surgical and medical care (T80.0, T81.7-, T82.8-)*
> *septic (non-pulmonary) arterial embolism (I76)*

AHA: 2022,3Q,8

☑5ᵗʰ **I26.0**   **Pulmonary embolism with acute cor pulmonale**

DEF: Cor pulmonale: Heart-lung disease appearing in identifiable forms as chronic or acute. The chronic form of this heart-lung disease is marked by dilation, hypertrophy and failure of the right ventricle due to a disease that has affected the function of the lungs, excluding congenital or left heart diseases and is also called chronic cardiopulmonary disease. The acute form is an overload of the right ventricle from a rapid onset of pulmonary hypertension, usually arising from a pulmonary embolism.

I26.01   **Septic pulmonary embolism with acute cor pulmonale** `MCC` `UPD` `HCC`

Code first underlying infection

I26.02   **Saddle embolus of pulmonary artery with acute cor pulmonale** `MCC` `H10` `HCC`

I26.03   **Cement embolism of pulmonary artery with acute cor pulmonale** `MCC` `H10` `UPD`

Code first complication of other artery following a procedure (T81.718)

I26.04   **Fat embolism of pulmonary artery with acute cor pulmonale** `MCC` `H10`

Code first, if applicable:
> complication of other artery following a procedure (T81.718)
> traumatic fat embolism (T79.1)

I26.09   **Other pulmonary embolism with acute cor pulmonale** `MCC` `H10` `HCC`

Acute cor pulmonale NOS
▶Other thrombotic pulmonary embolism with acute cor pulmonale◀
AHA: 2014,4Q,21

☑5ᵗʰ **I26.9**   **Pulmonary embolism without acute cor pulmonale**

I26.90   **Septic pulmonary embolism without acute cor pulmonale** `MCC` `UPD` `HCC`

Code first underlying infection

I26.92   **Saddle embolus of pulmonary artery without acute cor pulmonale** `MCC` `H10` `HCC`

I26.93   **Single subsegmental thrombotic pulmonary embolism without acute cor pulmonale** `MCC` `H10` `HCC`

Subsegmental pulmonary embolism NOS
AHA: 2021,2Q,9; 2019,4Q,6-7

I26.94   **Multiple subsegmental thrombotic pulmonary emboli without acute cor pulmonale** `MCC` `H10` `HCC`

AHA: 2022,2Q,13; 2021,2Q,9; 2019,4Q,6-7

I26.95   **Cement embolism of pulmonary artery without acute cor pulmonale** `MCC` `H10` `UPD`

Code first complication of other artery following a procedure (T81.718)

I26.96   **Fat embolism of pulmonary artery without acute cor pulmonale** `MCC` `H10`

Code first, if applicable:
> complication of other artery following a procedure (T81.718)
> traumatic fat embolism (T79.1)

`N` Newborn: 0   `P` Pediatric: 0-17   `M` Maternity: 9-64   `A` Adult: 15-124   `UNS` Unspecified Site   `MCC` Major Complication/Comorbidity   `CC` Complication/Comorbidity   `PE` POA Exempt

666

ICD-10-CM 2025

I26.99   **Other pulmonary embolism without acute cor pulmonale**   `MCC` `H10` `HCC`
Acute pulmonary embolism NOS
▶Other thrombotic pulmonary embolism without acute cor pulmonale◀
Pulmonary embolism NOS
AHA: 2022,2Q,13; 2020,3Q,10-11; 2019,2Q,22

✓4th **I27**   **Other pulmonary heart diseases**

I27.0   **Primary pulmonary hypertension**   `CC` `HCC`
Heritable pulmonary arterial hypertension
Idiopathic pulmonary arterial hypertension
Primary group 1 pulmonary hypertension
Primary pulmonary arterial hypertension
EXCLUDES 1   *persistent pulmonary hypertension of newborn (P29.30)*
pulmonary hypertension NOS (I27.20)
secondary pulmonary arterial hypertension (I27.21)
secondary pulmonary hypertension (I27.25)
DEF: Condition that occurs when pressure within the pulmonary artery is elevated and vascular resistance is observed in the lungs.

I27.1   **Kyphoscoliotic heart disease**   `CC` `HCC`

✓5th **I27.2**   **Other secondary pulmonary hypertension**
Code also associated underlying condition
EXCLUDES 1   *Eisenmenger's syndrome (I27.83)*
AHA: 2017,4Q,14-15; 2014,4Q,21
DEF: Condition that occurs when pressure within the pulmonary artery is elevated and vascular resistance is observed in the lungs.

    I27.20   **Pulmonary hypertension, unspecified**   `HCC`
Pulmonary hypertension NOS

    I27.21   **Secondary pulmonary arterial hypertension**   `HCC`
(Associated) (drug-induced) (toxin-induced) pulmonary arterial hypertension NOS
(Associated) (drug-induced) (toxin-induced) (secondary) group 1 pulmonary hypertension
Code also associated conditions if applicable, or adverse effects of drugs or toxins, such as:
adverse effect of appetite depressants (T50.5X5)
congenital heart disease (Q20-Q28)
human immunodeficiency virus [HIV] disease (B20)
polymyositis (M33.2-)
portal hypertension (K76.6)
rheumatoid arthritis (M05.-)
schistosomiasis (B65.-)
Sjogren syndrome (M35.0-)
systemic sclerosis (M34.-)

    I27.22   **Pulmonary hypertension due to left heart disease**   `HCC`
Group 2 pulmonary hypertension
Code also associated left heart disease, if known, such as:
multiple valve disease (I08.-)
rheumatic aortic valve diseases (I06.-)
rheumatic mitral valve diseases (I05.-)

    I27.23   **Pulmonary hypertension due to lung diseases and hypoxia**   `HCC`
Group 3 pulmonary hypertension
Code also associated lung disease, if known, such as:
bronchiectasis (J47.-)
cystic fibrosis with pulmonary manifestations (E84.0)
interstitial lung disease (J84.-)
pleural effusion (J90)
sleep apnea (G47.3-)

    I27.24   **Chronic thromboembolic pulmonary hypertension**   `HCC`
Group 4 pulmonary hypertension
Code also associated pulmonary embolism, if applicable (I26.-, I27.82)

I27.29   **Other secondary pulmonary hypertension**   `HCC`
Group 5 pulmonary hypertension
Pulmonary hypertension with unclear multifactorial mechanisms
Pulmonary hypertension due to hematologic disorders
Pulmonary hypertension due to metabolic disorders
Pulmonary hypertension due to other systemic disorders
Code also other associated disorders, if known, such as:
chronic myeloid leukemia (C92.10-C92.22)
essential thrombocythemia (D47.3)
Gaucher disease (E75.22)
hypertensive chronic kidney disease with end stage renal disease (I12.0, I13.11, I13.2)
hyperthyroidism (E05.-)
hypothyroidism (E00-E03)
polycythemia vera (D45)
sarcoidosis (D86.-)
AHA: 2016,2Q,8

✓5th **I27.8**   **Other specified pulmonary heart diseases**

    I27.81   **Cor pulmonale (chronic)**   `HCC`
Cor pulmonale NOS
Code also, if applicable, right heart failure (I50.81-)
EXCLUDES 1   *acute cor pulmonale (I26.0-)*
AHA: 2014,4Q,21
DEF: Heart-lung disease appearing in identifiable forms as chronic or acute. The chronic form of this heart-lung disease is marked by dilation, hypertrophy and failure of the right ventricle due to a disease that has affected the function of the lungs, excluding congenital or left heart diseases and is also called chronic cardiopulmonary disease. The acute form is an overload of the right ventricle from a rapid onset of pulmonary hypertension, usually arising from a pulmonary embolism.

    I27.82   **Chronic pulmonary embolism**   `CC` `HCC`
Use additional code, if applicable, for associated long-term (current) use of anticoagulants (Z79.01)
EXCLUDES 1   *personal history of pulmonary embolism (Z86.711)*
AHA: 2021,2Q,9
DEF: Long-standing condition commonly associated with pulmonary hypertension in which small blood clots travel to the lungs repeatedly over many weeks, months, or years, requiring continuation of established anticoagulant or thrombolytic therapy.

    I27.83   **Eisenmenger's syndrome**   `HCC`
Eisenmenger's complex
(Irreversible) Eisenmenger's disease
Pulmonary hypertension with right to left shunt related to congenital heart disease
Code also underlying heart defect, if known, such as:
atrial septal defect (Q21.1-)
Eisenmenger's defect (Q21.8)
patent ductus arteriosus (Q25.0)
ventricular septal defect (Q21.0)
DEF: Pulmonary hypertension with congenital communication between two circulations resulting in a right to left shunt. This causes reduced oxygen saturation in the arterial blood, leading to cyanosis and organ damage. Once it develops, this life-threating condition is irreversible.

    I27.89   **Other specified pulmonary heart diseases**   `HCC`

    I27.9   **Pulmonary heart disease, unspecified**   `HCC`
Chronic cardiopulmonary disease

✓4th **I28**   **Other diseases of pulmonary vessels**

    I28.0   **Arteriovenous fistula of pulmonary vessels**   `CC` `HCC`
EXCLUDES 1   *congenital arteriovenous fistula (Q25.72)*

    I28.1   **Aneurysm of pulmonary artery**   `CC` `HCC`
EXCLUDES 1   *congenital aneurysm (Q25.79)*
congenital arteriovenous aneurysm (Q25.72)

    I28.8   **Other diseases of pulmonary vessels**   `HCC`
Pulmonary arteritis
Pulmonary endarteritis
Rupture of pulmonary vessels
Stenosis of pulmonary vessels
Stricture of pulmonary vessels

    I28.9   **Disease of pulmonary vessels, unspecified**   `HCC`

✔ Additional Character Required   ✓x7th Placeholder   Questionable PDx   Manifestation   Unspecified   `UPD` Unacceptable PDx   `H1`-`H14` HAC   `HCC` CMS-HCC Dx   `HIV` HIV Dx

Other forms of heart disease (I30–I5A)

✓4ᵗʰ I30 Acute pericarditis

INCLUDES
acute mediastinopericarditis
acute myopericarditis
acute pericardial effusion
acute pleuropericarditis
acute pneumopericarditis

EXCLUDES 1
Dressler's syndrome (I24.1)
rheumatic pericarditis (acute) (I01.0)
►*viral pericarditis due to Coxsackie virus*◄ *(B33.23)*

DEF: Pericarditis: Inflammation affecting the pericardium, the fibroserous membrane that surrounds the heart.

I30.0   Acute **nonspecific idiopathic** pericarditis   `CC`

I30.1   **Infective** pericarditis   `CC`
Pneumococcal pericarditis
Pneumopyopericardium
Purulent pericarditis
Pyopericarditis
Pyopericardium
Pyopneumopericardium
Staphylococcal pericarditis
Streptococcal pericarditis
Suppurative pericarditis
Viral pericarditis
Use additional code (B95-B97) to identify infectious agent

I30.8   Other forms of acute pericarditis   `CC`

I30.9   Acute pericarditis, unspecified   `CC`

✓4ᵗʰ I31 Other diseases of pericardium

EXCLUDES 1
diseases of pericardium specified as rheumatic (I09.2)
postcardiotomy syndrome (I97.0)
traumatic injury to pericardium (S26.-)

I31.0   Chronic **adhesive** pericarditis   `CC`
Accretio cordis
Adherent pericardium
Adhesive mediastinopericarditis

I31.1   Chronic **constrictive** pericarditis   `CC`
Concretio cordis
Pericardial calcification

I31.2   Hemopericardium, not elsewhere classified   `CC`
EXCLUDES 1 *hemopericardium as current complication following acute myocardial infarction (I23.0)*
malignant pericardial effusion (I31.31)
DEF: Presence of blood in the pericardial sac (pericardium). It can lead to potentially fatal cardiac tamponade if enough blood enters the pericardial cavity.

✓5ᵗʰ I31.3   Pericardial effusion (noninflammatory)
EXCLUDES 1 *acute pericardial effusion (I30.9)*
AHA: 2022,4Q,22; 2019,1Q,16

    I31.31   *Malignant* pericardial effusion in diseases classified elsewhere   `CC` `HCC`
Code first underlying neoplasm (C00-D49)
AHA: 2022,4Q,22

    I31.39   Other pericardial effusion (noninflammatory)   `CC`
Chylopericardium

I31.4   **Cardiac tamponade**   `CC` `UPD`
Code first underlying cause
DEF: Life-threatening condition in which fluid or blood accumulates in the space between the muscle of the heart (myocardium) and the outer sac that covers the heart (pericardium), resulting in compression of the heart.

Cardiac Tamponade

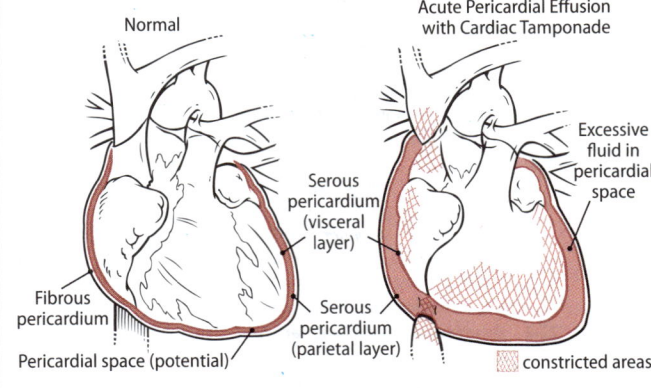

Normal   Acute Pericardial Effusion with Cardiac Tamponade

Serous pericardium (visceral layer) — Excessive fluid in pericardial space — Fibrous pericardium — Serous pericardium (parietal layer) — Pericardial space (potential) — constricted areas

I31.8   Other specified diseases of pericardium   `CC`
Epicardial plaques
Focal pericardial adhesions

I31.9   Disease of pericardium, unspecified   `CC`
Pericarditis (chronic) NOS

I32 Pericarditis in diseases classified elsewhere   `CC`
Code first underlying disease
EXCLUDES 1 *pericarditis (in):*
coxsackie (virus) (B33.23)
gonococcal (A54.83)
meningococcal (A39.53)
rheumatoid (arthritis) (M05.31)
syphilitic (A52.06)
systemic lupus erythematosus (M32.12)
tuberculosis (A18.84)
DEF: Pericarditis: Inflammation affecting the pericardium, the fibroserous membrane that surrounds the heart.

✓4ᵗʰ I33 Acute and subacute endocarditis
EXCLUDES 1 *acute rheumatic endocarditis (I01.1)*
endocarditis NOS (I38)
DEF: Endocarditis: Inflammatory disease of the interior lining of the heart chamber and heart valves.

I33.0   Acute and subacute **infective** endocarditis   `HIV` `MCC`
Bacterial endocarditis (acute) (subacute)
Infective endocarditis (acute) (subacute) NOS
Endocarditis lenta (acute) (subacute)
Malignant endocarditis (acute) (subacute)
Purulent endocarditis (acute) (subacute)
Septic endocarditis (acute) (subacute)
Ulcerative endocarditis (acute) (subacute)
Vegetative endocarditis (acute) (subacute)
Use additional code (B95-B97) to identify infectious agent

I33.9   Acute and subacute endocarditis, unspecified   `HIV` `MCC`
Acute endocarditis NOS
Acute myoendocarditis NOS
Acute periendocarditis NOS
Subacute endocarditis NOS
Subacute myoendocarditis NOS
Subacute periendocarditis NOS

✓4ᵗʰ **I34** **Nonrheumatic mitral valve disorders**

> **EXCLUDES 1**   mitral valve disease (I05.9)
> mitral valve failure (I05.8)
> mitral valve stenosis (I05.0)
> mitral valve disorder of unspecified cause with diseases of aortic and/or tricuspid valve(s) (I08.-)
> mitral valve disorder of unspecified cause with mitral stenosis or obstruction (I05.0)
> mitral valve disorder specified as congenital (Q23.2, Q23.9)
> mitral valve disorder specified as rheumatic (I05.-)

I34.0 **Nonrheumatic mitral (valve) insufficiency**
Nonrheumatic mitral (valve) incompetence NOS
Nonrheumatic mitral (valve) regurgitation NOS
Code also, if applicable:
nonrheumatic mitral (valve) annulus calcification (I34.81)

I34.1 **Nonrheumatic mitral (valve) prolapse**
Floppy nonrheumatic mitral valve syndrome
> **EXCLUDES 1**   Marfan's syndrome (Q87.4-)

I34.2 **Nonrheumatic mitral (valve) stenosis**
Code also, if applicable:
nonrheumatic mitral (valve) annulus calcification (I34.81)

✓5ᵗʰ **I34.8** **Other nonrheumatic mitral valve disorders**

> **AHA:** 2022,4Q,23

I34.81 **Nonrheumatic mitral (valve) annulus calcification**
Nonrheumatic mitral (valve) annular calcification
Mitral (valve) annulus calcification NOS
Code also, if applicable:
nonrheumatic mitral (valve) insufficiency (I34.0)
nonrheumatic mitral (valve) stenosis (I34.2)

I34.89 **Other nonrheumatic mitral valve disorders**

I34.9 **Nonrheumatic mitral valve disorder, unspecified**

✓4ᵗʰ **I35** **Nonrheumatic aortic valve disorders**

▶Code also, if applicable, bicuspid aortic valve (Q23.81)◀
> **EXCLUDES 1**   aortic valve disorder of unspecified cause but with diseases of mitral and/or tricuspid valve(s) (I08.-)
> aortic valve disorder specified as congenital (Q23.0, Q23.1)
> aortic valve disorder specified as rheumatic (I06.-)
> hypertrophic subaortic stenosis (I42.1)
> **EXCLUDES 2**   ▶aortic valve disorder of unspecified cause but with diseases of mitral and/or tricuspid valve(s) (I08.-)◀
> ▶aortic valve disorder specified as congenital (Q23.0, Q23.1)◀
> ▶aortic valve disorder specified as rheumatic (I06.-)◀
> ▶hypertrophic subaortic stenosis (I42.1)◀

I35.0 **Nonrheumatic aortic (valve) stenosis**

I35.1 **Nonrheumatic aortic (valve) insufficiency**
Nonrheumatic aortic (valve) incompetence NOS
Nonrheumatic aortic (valve) regurgitation NOS

I35.2 **Nonrheumatic aortic (valve) stenosis with insufficiency**

I35.8 **Other nonrheumatic aortic valve disorders**

I35.9 **Nonrheumatic aortic valve disorder, unspecified**

✓4ᵗʰ **I36** **Nonrheumatic tricuspid valve disorders**

> **EXCLUDES 1**   tricuspid valve disorders of unspecified cause (I07.-)
> tricuspid valve disorders specified as congenital (Q22.4, Q22.8, Q22.9)
> tricuspid valve disorders specified as rheumatic (I07.-)
> tricuspid valve disorders with aortic and/or mitral valve involvement (I08.-)

I36.0 **Nonrheumatic tricuspid (valve) stenosis**

I36.1 **Nonrheumatic tricuspid (valve) insufficiency**
Nonrheumatic tricuspid (valve) incompetence
Nonrheumatic tricuspid (valve) regurgitation

I36.2 **Nonrheumatic tricuspid (valve) stenosis with insufficiency**

I36.8 **Other nonrheumatic tricuspid valve disorders**

I36.9 **Nonrheumatic tricuspid valve disorder, unspecified**

✓4ᵗʰ **I37** **Nonrheumatic pulmonary valve disorders**

> **EXCLUDES 1**   pulmonary valve disorder specified as congenital (Q22.1, Q22.2, Q22.3)
> pulmonary valve disorder specified as rheumatic (I09.89)

I37.0 **Nonrheumatic pulmonary valve stenosis**

I37.1 **Nonrheumatic pulmonary valve insufficiency**
Nonrheumatic pulmonary valve incompetence
Nonrheumatic pulmonary valve regurgitation

I37.2 **Nonrheumatic pulmonary valve stenosis with insufficiency**

I37.8 **Other nonrheumatic pulmonary valve disorders**

I37.9 **Nonrheumatic pulmonary valve disorder, unspecified**

I38 **Endocarditis, valve unspecified**   **CC**

> **INCLUDES**   endocarditis (chronic) NOS
> valvular incompetence NOS
> valvular insufficiency NOS
> valvular regurgitation NOS
> valvular stenosis NOS
> valvulitis (chronic) NOS
> **EXCLUDES 1**   congenital insufficiency of cardiac valve NOS (Q24.8)
> congenital stenosis of cardiac valve NOS (Q24.8)
> endocardial fibroelastosis (I42.4)
> endocarditis specified as rheumatic (I09.1)

DEF: Endocarditis: Inflammatory disease of the interior lining of the heart chamber and heart valves.

I39 *Endocarditis and heart valve disorders in diseases classified elsewhere*   **CC**

Code first underlying disease, such as:
Q fever (A78)
> **EXCLUDES 1**   endocardial involvement in:
> candidiasis (B37.6)
> gonococcal infection (A54.83)
> Libman-Sacks disease (M32.11)
> listerosis (A32.82)
> meningococcal infection (A39.51)
> rheumatoid arthritis (M05.31)
> syphilis (A52.03)
> tuberculosis (A18.84)
> typhoid fever (A01.02)

DEF: Endocarditis: Inflammatory disease of the interior lining of the heart chamber and heart valves.

✓4ᵗʰ **I40** **Acute myocarditis**

> **INCLUDES**   subacute myocarditis
> **EXCLUDES 1**   acute rheumatic myocarditis (I01.2)

DEF: Myocarditis: Inflammation of the middle layer of the heart, which is composed of muscle tissue.

I40.0 **Infective myocarditis**   **HIV** **MCC**
Septic myocarditis
Use additional code (B95-B97) to identify infectious agent

I40.1 **Isolated myocarditis**   **HIV** **MCC**
Fiedler's myocarditis
Giant cell myocarditis
Idiopathic myocarditis

I40.8 **Other acute myocarditis**   **HIV** **MCC**

I40.9 **Acute myocarditis, unspecified**   **HIV** **MCC**

I41 *Myocarditis in diseases classified elsewhere*   **MCC**

Code first underlying disease, such as:
typhus (A75.0-A75.9)
> **EXCLUDES 1**   myocarditis (in):
> Chagas' disease (chronic) (B57.2)
> acute (B57.0)
> coxsackie (virus) infection (B33.22)
> diphtheritic (A36.81)
> gonococcal (A54.83)
> influenzal (J09.X9, J10.82, J11.82)
> meningococcal (A39.52)
> mumps (B26.82)
> rheumatoid arthritis (M05.31)
> sarcoid (D86.85)
> syphilis (A52.06)
> toxoplasmosis (B58.81)
> tuberculous (A18.84)

DEF: Myocarditis: Inflammation of the middle layer of the heart, which is composed of muscle tissue.

✓4ᵗʰ **I42** **Cardiomyopathy**

> **INCLUDES**   myocardiopathy

Code first pre-existing cardiomyopathy complicating pregnancy and puerperium (O99.4)
> **EXCLUDES 2**   ischemic cardiomyopathy (I25.5)
> peripartum cardiomyopathy (O90.3)
> ventricular hypertrophy (I51.7)

I42.0 **Dilated cardiomyopathy**   **CC** **HCC**
Congestive cardiomyopathy

✔ Additional Character Required   **✓x7ᵗʰ** Placeholder   **Questionable PDx**   **Manifestation**   **Unspecified**   **UPD** Unacceptable PDx   **H1 - H14** HAC   **HCC** CMS-HCC Dx   **HIV** HIV Dx

ICD-10-CM 2025   669

Chapter 9. Diseases of the Circulatory System

I42.1 **Obstructive hypertrophic cardiomyopathy** `CC` `HCC`
Hypertrophic subaortic stenosis (idiopathic)
DEF: Cardiomyopathy marked by left ventricle hypertrophy and an enlarged septum that result in obstructed blood flow, arrhythmias, mitral regurgitation, and sudden cardiac death.
TIP: When this condition is described as inherited, assign code Q24.8.

I42.2 **Other hypertrophic cardiomyopathy** `CC` `HCC`
Nonobstructive hypertrophic cardiomyopathy

I42.3 **Endomyocardial (eosinophilic) disease** `CC` `HCC`
Endomyocardial (tropical) fibrosis
Loffler's endocarditis

I42.4 **Endocardial fibroelastosis** `CC` `HCC`
Congenital cardiomyopathy
Elastomyofibrosis

I42.5 **Other restrictive cardiomyopathy** `CC` `HCC`
Constrictive cardiomyopathy NOS

I42.6 **Alcoholic cardiomyopathy** `CC` `HCC`
Code also presence of alcoholism (F10.-)

I42.7 **Cardiomyopathy due to drug and external agent** `CC`
Code first poisoning due to drug or toxin, if applicable (T36-T65 with fifth or sixth character 1-4)
Use additional code for adverse effect, if applicable, to identify drug (T36-T50 with fifth or sixth character 5)
AHA: 2021,3Q,8

I42.8 **Other cardiomyopathies** `CC` `HCC`

I42.9 **Cardiomyopathy, unspecified** `CC` `HCC`
Cardiomyopathy (primary) (secondary) NOS

I43 *Cardiomyopathy in diseases classified elsewhere* `CC` `HCC`
Code first underlying disease, such as:
  amyloidosis (E85.-)
  glycogen storage disease (E74.0-)
  gout (M10.0-)
  thyrotoxicosis (E05.0-E05.9-)
  EXCLUDES 1 cardiomyopathy (in):
    coxsackie (virus) (B33.24)
    diphtheria (A36.81)
    sarcoidosis (D86.85)
    tuberculosis (A18.84)
AHA: AHA:2024,2Q,9

I44 **Atrioventricular and left bundle-branch block** ✓4ᵗʰ

I44.0 **Atrioventricular block, first degree**

I44.1 **Atrioventricular block, second degree**
Atrioventricular block, type I and II
Möbitz block, type I and II
Second degree block, type I and II
Wenckebach's block

I44.2 **Atrioventricular block, complete** `CC` `HCC`
Complete heart block NOS
Third degree block
AHA: 2019,2Q,4

I44.3 ✓5ᵗʰ **Other and unspecified atrioventricular block**
Atrioventricular block NOS
     I44.30 **Unspecified atrioventricular block**
     I44.39 **Other atrioventricular block**

I44.4 **Left anterior fascicular block**

I44.5 **Left posterior fascicular block**

I44.6 ✓5ᵗʰ **Other and unspecified fascicular block**
     I44.60 **Unspecified fascicular block**
        Left bundle-branch hemiblock NOS
     I44.69 **Other fascicular block**

I44.7 **Left bundle-branch block, unspecified**

Conduction Disorders

Sinoatrial node (pacemaker)
Internodal tracts:
  Anterior
  Middle
  Posterior
Atrioventricular node
Atrioventricular bundle (of His)
Atrioventricular block
Accessory bundle (of Kent)
Right bundle branch
Right bundle branch block
Moderator band
Purkinje fibers
Bachmann's bundle
Left bundle branch block
Left bundle branch:
  Anterior fascicle
  Posterior fascicle
Left bundle branch hemiblock

I45 ✓4ᵗʰ **Other conduction disorders**

I45.0 **Right fascicular block**

I45.1 ✓5ᵗʰ **Other and unspecified right bundle-branch block**
     I45.10 **Unspecified right bundle-branch block**
        Right bundle-branch block NOS
     I45.19 **Other right bundle-branch block**

I45.2 **Bifascicular block** `CC`

I45.3 **Trifascicular block** `CC`

I45.4 **Nonspecific intraventricular block**
Bundle-branch block NOS

I45.5 **Other specified heart block**
Sinoatrial block
Sinoauricular block
EXCLUDES 1 heart block NOS (I45.9)

I45.6 **Pre-excitation syndrome**
Accelerated atrioventricular conduction
Accessory atrioventricular conduction
Anomalous atrioventricular excitation
Lown-Ganong-Levine syndrome
Pre-excitation atrioventricular conduction
Wolff-Parkinson-White syndrome

I45.8 ✓5ᵗʰ **Other specified conduction disorders**
     I45.81 **Long QT syndrome**
        DEF: Condition characterized by recurrent syncope, malignant arrhythmias, and sudden death. This syndrome has a characteristic prolonged Q-T interval on an electrocardiogram.
     I45.89 **Other specified conduction disorders** `CC`
        Atrioventricular [AV] dissociation
        Interference dissociation
        Isorhythmic dissociation
        Nonparoxysmal AV nodal tachycardia
        AHA: 2013,2Q,31

I45.9 **Conduction disorder, unspecified**
Heart block NOS
Stokes-Adams syndrome

I46 ✓4ᵗʰ **Cardiac arrest**
EXCLUDES 2 cardiogenic shock (R57.0)
AHA: 2019,2Q,4-5

I46.2 **Cardiac arrest due to underlying cardiac condition** `MCC` `UPD` `HCC`
Code first underlying cardiac condition
AHA: 2024,1Q,27
TIP: MCC only when patient is discharged alive.

I46.8 **Cardiac arrest due to other underlying condition** `MCC` `UPD` `HCC`
Code first underlying condition
TIP: MCC only when patient is discharged alive.

I46.9 **Cardiac arrest, cause unspecified** `MCC` `HCC`
    AHA: 2020,3Q,26
    TIP: MCC only when patient is discharged alive.

✓4ᵗʰ **I47** **Paroxysmal tachycardia**
    Code first tachycardia complicating:
        abortion or ectopic or molar pregnancy (O00-O07, O08.8)
        obstetric surgery and procedures (O75.4)
    EXCLUDES 1   *tachycardia NOS (R00.0)*
          sinoauricular tachycardia NOS (R00.0)
          sinus [sinusal] tachycardia NOS (R00.0)

    I47.0 **Re-entry ventricular arrhythmia** `CC` `HCC`
✓5ᵗʰ **I47.1** **Supraventricular tachycardia**
      AHA: 2023,4Q,26-27

        I47.10 **Supraventricular tachycardia, unspecified** `CC`
        I47.11 **Inappropriate sinus tachycardia, so stated** `CC`
            IST
        I47.19 **Other supraventricular tachycardia** `CC`
            Atrial (paroxysmal) tachycardia
            Atrioventricular [AV] (paroxysmal) tachycardia
            Atrioventricular re-entrant (nodal) tachycardia [AVNRT]
              [AVRT]
            Junctional (paroxysmal) tachycardia
            Nodal (paroxysmal) tachycardia

✓5ᵗʰ **I47.2** **Ventricular tachycardia**
      AHA: 2022,4Q,23-24; 2021,3Q,11; 2013,3Q,23

        I47.20 **Ventricular tachycardia, unspecified** `CC` `HCC`
        I47.21 **Torsades de pointes** `CC` `HCC`
            Code also, if applicable, long QT syndrome (I45.81)
            Use additional code for adverse effect, if applicable, to
              identify drug (T36-T50 with fifth or sixth character
              5)
            AHA: 2022,4Q,24
            DEF: Torsades de pointes (TdP): Accelerated heart
              rhythm, anywhere between 150 and 300 beats per
              minute, that initiates in the lower chambers of the heart
              (ventricles). Most commonly occurs in the setting of
              inherited or medication-induced long QT syndrome.

        I47.29 **Other ventricular tachycardia** `CC` `HCC`
    I47.9 **Paroxysmal tachycardia, unspecified** `HCC`
        Bouveret (-Hoffman) syndrome

✓4ᵗʰ **I48** **Atrial fibrillation and flutter**
    I48.0 **Paroxysmal atrial fibrillation** `HCC`
      AHA: 2021,2Q,8; 2018,3Q,6
✓5ᵗʰ **I48.1** **Persistent atrial fibrillation**
        EXCLUDES 1   *permanent atrial fibrillation (I48.21)*
      AHA: 2021,2Q,8; 2019,4Q,7; 2019,2Q,3; 2018,3Q,6

        I48.11 **Longstanding persistent atrial fibrillation** `CC` `HCC`
        I48.19 **Other persistent atrial fibrillation** `CC` `HCC`
            Chronic persistent atrial fibrillation
            Persistent atrial fibrillation, NOS
            AHA: 2019,4Q,7

✓5ᵗʰ **I48.2** **Chronic atrial fibrillation**
      AHA: 2021,2Q,8; 2019,4Q,7; 2019,2Q,3; 2018,3Q,6

        I48.20 **Chronic atrial fibrillation, unspecified** `CC` `HCC`
           EXCLUDES 1 *chronic persistent atrial fibrillation (I48.19)*
        I48.21 **Permanent atrial fibrillation** `CC` `HCC`
    I48.3 **Typical atrial flutter** `CC` `HCC`
        Type I atrial flutter
    I48.4 **Atypical atrial flutter** `CC` `HCC`
        Type II atrial flutter
✓5ᵗʰ **I48.9** **Unspecified atrial fibrillation and atrial flutter**

        I48.91 **Unspecified atrial fibrillation** `HCC`
        I48.92 **Unspecified atrial flutter** `CC` `HCC`

✓4ᵗʰ **I49** **Other cardiac arrhythmias**
    Code first cardiac arrhythmia complicating:
        abortion or ectopic or molar pregnancy (O00-O07, O08.8)
        obstetric surgery and procedures (O75.4)
    EXCLUDES 1   *neonatal dysrhythmia (P29.1-)*
          sinoatrial bradycardia (R00.1)
          sinus bradycardia (R00.1)
          vagal bradycardia (R00.1)
    EXCLUDES 2   *bradycardia NOS (R00.1)*
        ▶*neonatal dysrhythmia (P29.1-)*◀
        ▶*sinoatrial bradycardia (R00.1)*◀
        ▶*sinus bradycardia (R00.1)*◀
        ▶*vagal bradycardia (R00.1)*◀

✓5ᵗʰ **I49.0** **Ventricular fibrillation and flutter**
        I49.01 **Ventricular fibrillation** `MCC` `HCC`
            AHA: 2022,2Q,14
            TIP: MCC only when patient is discharged alive.
        I49.02 **Ventricular flutter** `MCC` `HCC`
    I49.1 **Atrial premature depolarization**
        Atrial premature beats
    I49.2 **Junctional premature depolarization** `CC` `HCC`
    I49.3 **Ventricular premature depolarization**
      AHA: 2020,2Q,23
✓5ᵗʰ **I49.4** **Other and unspecified premature depolarization**
        I49.40 **Unspecified premature depolarization**
            Premature beats NOS
        I49.49 **Other premature depolarization**
            Ectopic beats
            Extrasystoles
            Extrasystolic arrhythmias
            Premature contractions
    I49.5 **Sick sinus syndrome** `HCC`
        Tachycardia-bradycardia syndrome
      AHA: 2019,1Q,33
      TIP: The presence of a pacemaker controls but does not cure sick
      sinus syndrome and therefore is considered a reportable chronic
      condition. When a pacemaker is evaluated by a provider, this
      code and code Z95.0 Presence of cardiac pacemaker, should be
      reported, even in the absence of any notable changes or
      management.
    I49.8 **Other specified cardiac arrhythmias**
        Brugada syndrome
        Coronary sinus rhythm disorder
        Ectopic rhythm disorder
        Nodal rhythm disorder
    I49.9 **Cardiac arrhythmia, unspecified**
        Arrhythmia (cardiac) NOS

✓4ᵗʰ **I50** **Heart failure**
    Code first:
        heart failure complicating abortion or ectopic or molar pregnancy
          (O00-O07, O08.8)
        heart failure due to hypertension (I11.0)
        heart failure due to hypertension with chronic kidney disease (I13.-)
        heart failure following surgery (I97.13-)
        obstetric surgery and procedures (O75.4)
        rheumatic heart failure (I09.81)
    EXCLUDES 2   *cardiac arrest (I46.-)*
          neonatal cardiac failure (P29.0)
    AHA: 2018,4Q,67; 2018,2Q,9; 2017,1Q,47; 2014,1Q,25; 2013,2Q,33

    I50.1 **Left ventricular failure, unspecified** `CC` `HCC`
        Cardiac asthma
        Edema of lung with heart disease NOS
        Edema of lung with heart failure
        Left heart failure
        Pulmonary edema with heart disease NOS
        Pulmonary edema with heart failure
        EXCLUDES 1 *edema of lung without heart disease or heart failure*
            (J81.-)
            pulmonary edema without heart disease or failure
            (J81.-)

✓5ᵗʰ **I50.2　Systolic (congestive) heart failure**
Heart failure with reduced ejection fraction [HFrEF]
Systolic left ventricular heart failure
Code also end stage heart failure, if applicable (I50.84)
EXCLUDES 1　combined systolic (congestive) and diastolic (congestive) heart failure (I50.4-)
AHA: 2020,3Q,32; 2017,1Q,46; 2016,1Q,10

I50.20　Unspecified systolic (congestive) heart failure　CC HCC

I50.21　Acute systolic (congestive) heart failure　MCC HCC

I50.22　Chronic systolic (congestive) heart failure　CC HCC

I50.23　Acute on chronic systolic (congestive) heart failure　MCC HCC

✓5ᵗʰ **I50.3　Diastolic (congestive) heart failure**
Diastolic left ventricular heart failure
Heart failure with normal ejection fraction
Heart failure with preserved ejection fraction [HFpEF]
Code also end stage heart failure, if applicable (I50.84)
EXCLUDES 1　combined systolic (congestive) and diastolic (congestive) heart failure (I50.4-)
AHA: 2024,2Q,9; 2020,3Q,32; 2017,1Q,46; 2016,1Q,10

I50.30　Unspecified diastolic (congestive) heart failure　CC HCC

I50.31　Acute diastolic (congestive) heart failure　MCC HCC

I50.32　Chronic diastolic (congestive) heart failure　CC HCC
AHA: 2023,3Q,14
DEF: HFrecEF: Heart failure with recovered ejection fraction
DEF: HFimpEF: Heart failure with improved ejection fraction

I50.33　Acute on chronic diastolic (congestive) heart failure　MCC HCC

✓5ᵗʰ **I50.4　Combined systolic (congestive) and diastolic (congestive) heart failure**
Combined systolic and diastolic left ventricular heart failure
Heart failure with reduced ejection fraction and diastolic dysfunction
Code also end stage heart failure, if applicable (I50.84)
AHA: 2017,1Q,46; 2016,1Q,10

I50.40　Unspecified combined systolic (congestive) and diastolic (congestive) heart failure　CC HCC

I50.41　Acute combined systolic (congestive) and diastolic (congestive) heart failure　MCC HCC

I50.42　Chronic combined systolic (congestive) and diastolic (congestive) heart failure　CC HCC

I50.43　Acute on chronic combined systolic (congestive) and diastolic (congestive) heart failure　MCC HCC

✓5ᵗʰ **I50.8　Other heart failure**
AHA: 2022,3Q,16; 2017,4Q,15-16

✓6ᵗʰ **I50.81　Right heart failure**
Right ventricular failure
AHA: 2023,3Q,14

I50.810　Right heart failure, unspecified　HCC
Right heart failure without mention of left heart failure
Right ventricular failure NOS

I50.811　Acute right heart failure　HCC
Acute isolated right heart failure
Acute (isolated) right ventricular failure

I50.812　Chronic right heart failure　HCC
Chronic isolated right heart failure
Chronic (isolated) right ventricular failure

I50.813　Acute on chronic right heart failure　HCC
Acute on chronic isolated right heart failure
Acute on chronic (isolated) right ventricular failure
Acute decompensation of chronic (isolated) right ventricular failure
Acute exacerbation of chronic (isolated) right ventricular failure

I50.814　Right heart failure due to left heart failure　HCC
Right ventricular failure secondary to left ventricular failure
Code also the type of left ventricular failure, if known (I50.2-I50.43)
EXCLUDES 1　right heart failure with but not due to left heart failure (I50.82)

I50.82　Biventricular heart failure　HCC
Code also the type of left ventricular failure as systolic, diastolic, or combined, if known (I50.2-I50.43)

I50.83　High output heart failure　HCC
DEF: Occurs when the high demand for blood exceeds the capacity of a normally functioning heart to meet the demand.

I50.84　End stage heart failure　HCC
Stage D heart failure
Code also the type of heart failure as systolic, diastolic, or combined, if known (I50.2-I50.43)

I50.89　Other heart failure　HCC

I50.9　Heart failure, unspecified　HCC
Cardiac, heart or myocardial failure NOS
Congestive heart disease
Congestive heart failure NOS
EXCLUDES 2　fluid overload unrelated to congestive heart failure (E87.70)
AHA: 2017,4Q,15-16; 2017,1Q,45-46; 2014,4Q,21; 2012,4Q,92

✓4ᵗʰ **I51　Complications and ill-defined descriptions of heart disease**
EXCLUDES 1　any condition in I51.4-I51.9 due to hypertension (I11.-)
any condition in I51.4-I51.9 due to hypertension and chronic kidney disease (I13.-)
heart disease specified as rheumatic (I00-I09)

I51.0　Cardiac septal defect, acquired　CC A
Acquired septal atrial defect (old)
Acquired septal auricular defect (old)
Acquired septal ventricular defect (old)
EXCLUDES 1　cardiac septal defect as current complication following acute myocardial infarction (I23.1, I23.2)
DEF: Abnormal communication between opposite heart chambers due to a defect of the septum. It is not present at birth.

I51.1　Rupture of chordae tendineae, not elsewhere classified　MCC HCC
EXCLUDES 1　rupture of chordae tendineae as current complication following acute myocardial infarction (I23.4)

I51.2　Rupture of papillary muscle, not elsewhere classified　MCC HCC
EXCLUDES 1　rupture of papillary muscle as current complication following acute myocardial infarction (I23.5)

I51.3　Intracardiac thrombosis, not elsewhere classified
Apical thrombosis (old)
Atrial thrombosis (old)
Auricular thrombosis (old)
Mural thrombosis (old)
Ventricular thrombosis (old)
EXCLUDES 1　intracardiac thrombosis as current complication following acute myocardial infarction (I23.6)
AHA: 2013,1Q,24

I51.4　Myocarditis, unspecified　HCC
Chronic (interstitial) myocarditis
Myocardial fibrosis
Myocarditis NOS
EXCLUDES 1　acute or subacute myocarditis (I40.-)
AHA: 2018,4Q,67; 2018,2Q,9

I51.5　Myocardial degeneration　HCC
Fatty degeneration of heart or myocardium
Myocardial disease
Senile degeneration of heart or myocardium
AHA: 2018,4Q,67; 2018,2Q,9

I51.7　Cardiomegaly
Cardiac dilatation
Cardiac hypertrophy
Ventricular dilatation
AHA: 2018,4Q,67; 2018,2Q,9

✓5th **I51.8**   **Other ill-defined heart diseases**
    AHA: 2018,2Q,9

   I51.81   **Takotsubo syndrome**   CC
     Reversible left ventricular dysfunction following sudden emotional stress
     Stress induced cardiomyopathy
     Takotsubo cardiomyopathy
     Transient left ventricular apical ballooning syndrome
     DEF: Complex of symptoms mimicking myocardial infarct in absence of heart disease, with the majority of cases occurring in postmenopausal women. Heart muscles are temporarily weakened, and a sudden, massive surge of adrenalin stuns the heart, greatly reducing the ability to pump blood.

   I51.89   **Other ill-defined heart diseases**
     Carditis (acute)(chronic)
     Pancarditis (acute)(chronic)
     AHA: 2019,2Q,5; 2018,4Q,67

I51.9   **Heart disease, unspecified**
    AHA: 2018,4Q,67; 2018,2Q,9

I52   *Other heart disorders in diseases classified elsewhere*
   Code first underlying disease, such as:
    congenital syphilis (A50.5)
    mucopolysaccharidosis (E76.3)
    schistosomiasis (B65.0-B65.9)
   EXCLUDES 1   heart disease (in):
     gonococcal infection (A54.83)
     meningococcal infection (A39.50)
     rheumatoid arthritis (M05.31)
     syphilis (A52.06)

I5A   **Non-ischemic myocardial injury (non-traumatic)**   CC
   Acute (non-ischemic) myocardial injury
   Chronic (non-ischemic) myocardial injury
   Unspecified (non-ischemic) myocardial injury
   Code first the underlying cause, if known and applicable, such as:
    acute kidney failure (N17.-)
    acute myocarditis (I40.-)
    cardiomyopathy (I42.-)
    chronic kidney disease (CKD) (N18.-)
    heart failure (I50.-)
    hypertensive urgency (I16.0)
    nonrheumatic aortic valve disorders (I35.-)
    paroxysmal tachycardia (I47.-)
    pulmonary embolism (I26.-)
    pulmonary hypertension (I27.0, I27.2-)
    sepsis (A41.-)
    takotsubo syndrome (I51.81)
   EXCLUDES 1   acute myocardial infarction (I21.-)
     injury of heart (S26.-)
   EXCLUDES 2   other acute ischemic heart diseases (I24.-)
   AHA: 2021,4Q,14-15

Cerebrovascular diseases (I60-I69)

Use additional code to identify presence of:
   alcohol abuse and dependence (F10.-)
   exposure to environmental tobacco smoke (Z77.22)
   history of tobacco dependence (Z87.891)
   hypertension (I10-I1A)
   occupational exposure to environmental tobacco smoke (Z57.31)
   tobacco dependence (F17.-)
   tobacco use (Z72.0)
EXCLUDES 1   traumatic intracranial hemorrhage (S06.-)
AHA: 2014,3Q,5; 2012,4Q,91-92

✓4th **I60**   **Nontraumatic subarachnoid hemorrhage**
   Use additional code, if known, to indicate National Institutes of Health Stroke Scale (NIHSS) score (R29.7-)
   EXCLUDES 1   syphilitic ruptured cerebral aneurysm (A52.05)
   EXCLUDES 2   sequelae of subarachnoid hemorrhage (I69.0-)

✓5th **I60.0**   **Nontraumatic subarachnoid hemorrhage from carotid siphon and bifurcation**

   I60.00   **Nontraumatic subarachnoid hemorrhage from unspecified carotid siphon and bifurcation**   MCC HCC

   I60.01   **Nontraumatic subarachnoid hemorrhage from right carotid siphon and bifurcation**   MCC HCC

   I60.02   **Nontraumatic subarachnoid hemorrhage from left carotid siphon and bifurcation**   MCC HCC

✓5th **I60.1**   **Nontraumatic subarachnoid hemorrhage from middle cerebral artery**

   I60.10   **Nontraumatic subarachnoid hemorrhage from unspecified middle cerebral artery**   MCC HCC

   I60.11   **Nontraumatic subarachnoid hemorrhage from right middle cerebral artery**   MCC HCC

   I60.12   **Nontraumatic subarachnoid hemorrhage from left middle cerebral artery**   MCC HCC

I60.2   **Nontraumatic subarachnoid hemorrhage from anterior communicating artery**   MCC HCC

✓5th **I60.3**   **Nontraumatic subarachnoid hemorrhage from posterior communicating artery**

   I60.30   **Nontraumatic subarachnoid hemorrhage from unspecified posterior communicating artery**   MCC HCC

   I60.31   **Nontraumatic subarachnoid hemorrhage from right posterior communicating artery**   MCC HCC

   I60.32   **Nontraumatic subarachnoid hemorrhage from left posterior communicating artery**   MCC HCC

I60.4   **Nontraumatic subarachnoid hemorrhage from basilar artery**   MCC HCC

✓5th **I60.5**   **Nontraumatic subarachnoid hemorrhage from vertebral artery**

   I60.50   **Nontraumatic subarachnoid hemorrhage from unspecified vertebral artery**   MCC HCC

   I60.51   **Nontraumatic subarachnoid hemorrhage from right vertebral artery**   MCC HCC

   I60.52   **Nontraumatic subarachnoid hemorrhage from left vertebral artery**   MCC HCC

I60.6   **Nontraumatic subarachnoid hemorrhage from other intracranial arteries**   MCC HCC

I60.7   **Nontraumatic subarachnoid hemorrhage from unspecified intracranial artery**   MCC HCC
    Ruptured (congenital) berry aneurysm
    Ruptured (congenital) cerebral aneurysm
    Subarachnoid hemorrhage (nontraumatic) from cerebral artery NOS
    Subarachnoid hemorrhage (nontraumatic) from communicating artery NOS
   EXCLUDES 1   berry aneurysm, nonruptured (I67.1)

I60.8   **Other nontraumatic subarachnoid hemorrhage**   MCC HCC
    Meningeal hemorrhage
    Rupture of cerebral arteriovenous malformation

I60.9   **Nontraumatic subarachnoid hemorrhage, unspecified**   MCC HCC

✓4th **I61**   **Nontraumatic intracerebral hemorrhage**
   Use additional code, if known, to indicate National Institutes of Health Stroke Scale (NIHSS) score (R29.7-)
   EXCLUDES 2   sequelae of intracerebral hemorrhage (I69.1-)
   AHA: 2022,3Q,9-10; 2017,2Q,9-10

I61.0   **Nontraumatic intracerebral hemorrhage in hemisphere, subcortical**   MCC HCC
    Deep intracerebral hemorrhage (nontraumatic)
    AHA: 2016,4Q,27

I61.1   **Nontraumatic intracerebral hemorrhage in hemisphere, cortical**   MCC HCC
    Cerebral lobe hemorrhage (nontraumatic)
    Superficial intracerebral hemorrhage (nontraumatic)

I61.2   **Nontraumatic intracerebral hemorrhage in hemisphere, unspecified**   MCC HCC

I61.3   **Nontraumatic intracerebral hemorrhage in brain stem**   MCC HCC
    AHA: 2023,4Q,42

I61.4   **Nontraumatic intracerebral hemorrhage in cerebellum**   MCC HCC

I61.5   **Nontraumatic intracerebral hemorrhage, intraventricular**   MCC HCC

I61.6   **Nontraumatic intracerebral hemorrhage, multiple localized**   MCC HCC

I61.8   **Other nontraumatic intracerebral hemorrhage**   MCC HCC
    AHA: AHA:2024,2Q,25

I61.9   **Nontraumatic intracerebral hemorrhage, unspecified**   MCC HCC

✔ Additional Character Required   ✓x7th Placeholder   Questionable PDx   Manifestation   Unspecified   UPD Unacceptable PDx   H1-H14 HAC   HCC CMS-HCC Dx   HIV HIV Dx

ICD-10-CM 2025   673

✓4ʰ **I62　Other and unspecified nontraumatic intracranial hemorrhage**

Use additional code, if known, to indicate National Institutes of Health Stroke Scale (NIHSS) score (R29.7-)

EXCLUDES 2　sequelae of intracranial hemorrhage (I69.2)

✓5ʰ **I62.0　Nontraumatic subdural hemorrhage**

I62.00　Nontraumatic subdural hemorrhage, unspecified　MCC HCC

I62.01　Nontraumatic acute subdural hemorrhage　MCC HCC

I62.02　Nontraumatic subacute subdural hemorrhage　MCC HCC

I62.03　Nontraumatic chronic subdural hemorrhage　MCC HCC

I62.1　Nontraumatic extradural hemorrhage　MCC HCC
Nontraumatic epidural hemorrhage
AHA: 2023,3Q,21

I62.9　Nontraumatic intracranial hemorrhage, unspecified　CC HCC

✓4ʰ **I63　Cerebral infarction**

INCLUDES　occlusion and stenosis of cerebral and precerebral arteries, resulting in cerebral infarction

Use additional code, if applicable, to identify status post administration of tPA (rtPA) in a different facility within the last 24 hours prior to admission to current facility (Z92.82)

Use additional code, if known, to indicate National Institutes of Health Stroke Scale (NIHSS) score (R29.7-)

EXCLUDES 1　neonatal cerebral infarction (P91.82-)

EXCLUDES 2　chronic, without residual deficits (sequelae) (Z86.73)
sequelae of cerebral infarction (I69.3-)

AHA: 2024,1Q,26; 2017,2Q,9-10; 2016,4Q,28,61-62; 2015,1Q,25; 2014,1Q,23

TIP: Weakness on one side of the body documented as secondary to stroke is synonymous with hemiparesis/hemiplegia (G81.-). Weakness of one limb documented as secondary to stroke is synonymous with monoplegia (G83.1-, G83.2-, G83.3-).

✓5ʰ **I63.0　Cerebral infarction due to thrombosis of precerebral arteries**

I63.00　Cerebral infarction due to thrombosis of unspecified precerebral artery　MCC HCC

✓6ʰ **I63.01　Cerebral infarction due to thrombosis of vertebral artery**

I63.011　Cerebral infarction due to thrombosis of right vertebral artery　MCC HCC

I63.012　Cerebral infarction due to thrombosis of left vertebral artery　MCC HCC

I63.013　Cerebral infarction due to thrombosis of bilateral vertebral arteries　MCC HCC

I63.019　Cerebral infarction due to thrombosis of unspecified vertebral artery　MCC HCC

I63.02　Cerebral infarction due to thrombosis of basilar artery　MCC HCC

✓6ʰ **I63.03　Cerebral infarction due to thrombosis of carotid artery**

I63.031　Cerebral infarction due to thrombosis of right carotid artery　MCC HCC

I63.032　Cerebral infarction due to thrombosis of left carotid artery　MCC HCC

I63.033　Cerebral infarction due to thrombosis of bilateral carotid arteries　MCC HCC

I63.039　Cerebral infarction due to thrombosis of unspecified carotid artery　MCC HCC

I63.09　Cerebral infarction due to thrombosis of other precerebral artery　MCC HCC

✓5ʰ **I63.1　Cerebral infarction due to embolism of precerebral arteries**

I63.10　Cerebral infarction due to embolism of unspecified precerebral artery　MCC HCC

✓6ʰ **I63.11　Cerebral infarction due to embolism of vertebral artery**

I63.111　Cerebral infarction due to embolism of right vertebral artery　MCC HCC

I63.112　Cerebral infarction due to embolism of left vertebral artery　MCC HCC

I63.113　Cerebral infarction due to embolism of bilateral vertebral arteries　MCC HCC

I63.119　Cerebral infarction due to embolism of unspecified vertebral artery　MCC HCC

I63.12　Cerebral infarction due to embolism of basilar artery　MCC HCC

✓6ʰ **I63.13　Cerebral infarction due to embolism of carotid artery**

I63.131　Cerebral infarction due to embolism of right carotid artery　MCC HCC

I63.132　Cerebral infarction due to embolism of left carotid artery　MCC HCC

I63.133　Cerebral infarction due to embolism of bilateral carotid arteries　MCC HCC

I63.139　Cerebral infarction due to embolism of unspecified carotid artery　MCC HCC

I63.19　Cerebral infarction due to embolism of other precerebral artery　MCC HCC

✓5ʰ **I63.2　Cerebral infarction due to unspecified occlusion or stenosis of precerebral arteries**

AHA: 2020,3Q,27-28

I63.20　Cerebral infarction due to unspecified occlusion or stenosis of unspecified precerebral arteries　MCC HCC

✓6ʰ **I63.21　Cerebral infarction due to unspecified occlusion or stenosis of vertebral arteries**

I63.211　Cerebral infarction due to unspecified occlusion or stenosis of right vertebral artery　MCC HCC

I63.212　Cerebral infarction due to unspecified occlusion or stenosis of left vertebral artery　MCC HCC

I63.213　Cerebral infarction due to unspecified occlusion or stenosis of bilateral vertebral arteries　MCC HCC

I63.219　Cerebral infarction due to unspecified occlusion or stenosis of unspecified vertebral artery　MCC HCC

I63.22　Cerebral infarction due to unspecified occlusion or stenosis of basilar artery　MCC HCC

✓6ʰ **I63.23　Cerebral infarction due to unspecified occlusion or stenosis of carotid arteries**

I63.231　Cerebral infarction due to unspecified occlusion or stenosis of right carotid arteries　MCC HCC

I63.232　Cerebral infarction due to unspecified occlusion or stenosis of left carotid arteries　MCC HCC

I63.233　Cerebral infarction due to unspecified occlusion or stenosis of bilateral carotid arteries　MCC HCC

I63.239　Cerebral infarction due to unspecified occlusion or stenosis of unspecified carotid artery　MCC HCC

I63.29　Cerebral infarction due to unspecified occlusion or stenosis of other precerebral arteries　MCC HCC

✓5ʰ **I63.3　Cerebral infarction due to thrombosis of cerebral arteries**

I63.30　Cerebral infarction due to thrombosis of unspecified cerebral artery　MCC HCC

✓6ʰ **I63.31　Cerebral infarction due to thrombosis of middle cerebral artery**

I63.311　Cerebral infarction due to thrombosis of right middle cerebral artery　MCC HCC

I63.312　Cerebral infarction due to thrombosis of left middle cerebral artery　MCC HCC

I63.313　Cerebral infarction due to thrombosis of bilateral middle cerebral arteries　MCC HCC

I63.319　Cerebral infarction due to thrombosis of unspecified middle cerebral artery　MCC HCC

✓6ʰ **I63.32　Cerebral infarction due to thrombosis of anterior cerebral artery**

I63.321　Cerebral infarction due to thrombosis of right anterior cerebral artery　MCC HCC

I63.322　Cerebral infarction due to thrombosis of left anterior cerebral artery　MCC HCC

I63.323　Cerebral infarction due to thrombosis of bilateral anterior cerebral arteries　MCC HCC

I63.329　Cerebral infarction due to thrombosis of unspecified anterior cerebral artery　MCC HCC

✓6ʰ **I63.33　Cerebral infarction due to thrombosis of posterior cerebral artery**

I63.331　Cerebral infarction due to thrombosis of right posterior cerebral artery　MCC HCC

N Newborn: 0　P Pediatric: 0-17　M Maternity: 9-64　A Adult: 15-124　UNS Unspecified Site　MCC Major Complication/Comorbidity　CC Complication/Comorbidity　PE POA Exempt

674　　　ICD-10-CM 2025

I63.332   Cerebral infarction due to thrombosis of **left** posterior cerebral artery `MCC` `HCC`

I63.333   Cerebral infarction due to thrombosis of **bilateral** posterior cerebral arteries `MCC` `HCC`

I63.339   Cerebral infarction due to thrombosis of unspecified posterior cerebral artery `MCC` `HCC`

✓6ᵗʰ **I63.34**   Cerebral infarction due to thrombosis of **cerebellar** artery

I63.341   Cerebral infarction due to thrombosis of **right** cerebellar artery `MCC` `HCC`

I63.342   Cerebral infarction due to thrombosis of **left** cerebellar artery `MCC` `HCC`

I63.343   Cerebral infarction due to thrombosis of **bilateral** cerebellar arteries `MCC` `HCC`

I63.349   Cerebral infarction due to thrombosis of unspecified cerebellar artery `MCC` `HCC`

I63.39   Cerebral infarction due to thrombosis of other cerebral artery `MCC` `HCC`

✓5ᵗʰ **I63.4**   Cerebral infarction due to **embolism of cerebral** arteries

I63.40   Cerebral infarction due to embolism of unspecified cerebral artery `MCC` `HCC`

✓6ᵗʰ **I63.41**   Cerebral infarction due to embolism of **middle** cerebral artery

I63.411   Cerebral infarction due to embolism of **right** middle cerebral artery `MCC` `HCC`

I63.412   Cerebral infarction due to embolism of **left** middle cerebral artery `MCC` `HCC`

I63.413   Cerebral infarction due to embolism of **bilateral** middle cerebral arteries `MCC` `HCC`

I63.419   Cerebral infarction due to embolism of unspecified middle cerebral artery `MCC` `HCC`

✓6ᵗʰ **I63.42**   Cerebral infarction due to embolism of **anterior** cerebral artery

I63.421   Cerebral infarction due to embolism of **right** anterior cerebral artery `MCC` `HCC`

I63.422   Cerebral infarction due to embolism of **left** anterior cerebral artery `MCC` `HCC`

I63.423   Cerebral infarction due to embolism of **bilateral** anterior cerebral arteries `MCC` `HCC`

I63.429   Cerebral infarction due to embolism of unspecified anterior cerebral artery `MCC` `HCC`

✓6ᵗʰ **I63.43**   Cerebral infarction due to embolism of **posterior** cerebral artery

I63.431   Cerebral infarction due to embolism of **right** posterior cerebral artery `MCC` `HCC`

I63.432   Cerebral infarction due to embolism of **left** posterior cerebral artery `MCC` `HCC`

I63.433   Cerebral infarction due to embolism of **bilateral** posterior cerebral arteries `MCC` `HCC`

I63.439   Cerebral infarction due to embolism of unspecified posterior cerebral artery `MCC` `HCC`

✓6ᵗʰ **I63.44**   Cerebral infarction due to embolism of **cerebellar** artery

I63.441   Cerebral infarction due to embolism of **right** cerebellar artery `MCC` `HCC`

I63.442   Cerebral infarction due to embolism of **left** cerebellar artery `MCC` `HCC`

I63.443   Cerebral infarction due to embolism of **bilateral** cerebellar arteries `MCC` `HCC`

I63.449   Cerebral infarction due to embolism of unspecified cerebellar artery `MCC` `HCC`

I63.49   Cerebral infarction due to embolism of other cerebral artery `MCC` `HCC`

✓5ᵗʰ **I63.5**   Cerebral infarction due to unspecified **occlusion or stenosis of cerebral** arteries

I63.50   Cerebral infarction due to unspecified occlusion or stenosis of unspecified cerebral artery `MCC` `HCC`

✓6ᵗʰ **I63.51**   Cerebral infarction due to unspecified occlusion or stenosis of **middle** cerebral artery

I63.511   Cerebral infarction due to unspecified occlusion or stenosis of **right** middle cerebral artery `MCC` `HCC`

I63.512   Cerebral infarction due to unspecified occlusion or stenosis of **left** middle cerebral artery `MCC` `HCC`

I63.513   Cerebral infarction due to unspecified occlusion or stenosis of **bilateral** middle cerebral arteries `MCC` `HCC`

I63.519   Cerebral infarction due to unspecified occlusion or stenosis of unspecified middle cerebral artery `MCC` `HCC`

✓6ᵗʰ **I63.52**   Cerebral infarction due to unspecified occlusion or stenosis of **anterior** cerebral artery

I63.521   Cerebral infarction due to unspecified occlusion or stenosis of **right** anterior cerebral artery `MCC` `HCC`

I63.522   Cerebral infarction due to unspecified occlusion or stenosis of **left** anterior cerebral artery `MCC` `HCC`

I63.523   Cerebral infarction due to unspecified occlusion or stenosis of **bilateral** anterior cerebral arteries `MCC` `HCC`

I63.529   Cerebral infarction due to unspecified occlusion or stenosis of unspecified anterior cerebral artery `MCC` `HCC`

✓6ᵗʰ **I63.53**   Cerebral infarction due to unspecified occlusion or stenosis of **posterior** cerebral artery

I63.531   Cerebral infarction due to unspecified occlusion or stenosis of **right** posterior cerebral artery `MCC` `HCC`

I63.532   Cerebral infarction due to unspecified occlusion or stenosis of **left** posterior cerebral artery `MCC` `HCC`

I63.533   Cerebral infarction due to unspecified occlusion or stenosis of **bilateral** posterior cerebral arteries `MCC` `HCC`

I63.539   Cerebral infarction due to unspecified occlusion or stenosis of unspecified posterior cerebral artery `MCC` `HCC`

✓6ᵗʰ **I63.54**   Cerebral infarction due to unspecified occlusion or stenosis of **cerebellar** artery

I63.541   Cerebral infarction due to unspecified occlusion or stenosis of **right** cerebellar artery `MCC` `HCC`

I63.542   Cerebral infarction due to unspecified occlusion or stenosis of **left** cerebellar artery `MCC` `HCC`

I63.543   Cerebral infarction due to unspecified occlusion or stenosis of **bilateral** cerebellar arteries `MCC` `HCC`

I63.549   Cerebral infarction due to unspecified occlusion or stenosis of unspecified cerebellar artery `MCC` `HCC`

I63.59   Cerebral infarction due to unspecified occlusion or stenosis of other cerebral artery `MCC` `HCC`

I63.6   Cerebral infarction due to **cerebral venous thrombosis, nonpyogenic** `MCC` `HCC`

✓5ᵗʰ **I63.8**   Other cerebral infarction

   AHA: 2018,4Q,16

I63.81   Other cerebral infarction due to **occlusion or stenosis of small artery** `MCC` `HCC`
    Lacunar infarction
    AHA: 2020,3Q,27

I63.89   Other cerebral infarction `MCC` `HCC`
    AHA: 2024,1Q,32; 2022,1Q,25

I63.9   Cerebral infarction, unspecified `MCC` `HCC`
    Stroke NOS
    EXCLUDES 2   *transient cerebral ischemic attacks and related syndromes (G45.-)*
    AHA: 2020,2Q,29
    TIP: When provider documentation does not identify the location of an infarction, imaging reports can be used to pinpoint the location and lead to a more specific infarction code.

☑ Additional Character Required   ✓x7ᵗʰ Placeholder   **Questionable PDx**   Manifestation   Unspecified   **UPD** Unacceptable PDx   **H1**-**H14** HAC   **HCC** CMS-HCC Dx   **HIV** HIV Dx

ICD-10-CM 2025   675

✓4th I65 Occlusion and stenosis of precerebral arteries, not resulting in cerebral infarction

> INCLUDES   embolism of precerebral artery
> narrowing of precerebral artery
> obstruction (complete) (partial) of precerebral artery
> thrombosis of precerebral artery
>
> EXCLUDES 1   *insufficiency, NOS, of precerebral artery (G45.-)*
> *insufficiency of precerebral arteries causing cerebral infarction (I63.0-I63.2)*
>
> **AHA:** 2018,2Q,9

✓5th I65.0 Occlusion and stenosis of vertebral artery

    I65.01 Occlusion and stenosis of right vertebral artery
    I65.02 Occlusion and stenosis of left vertebral artery
    I65.03 Occlusion and stenosis of bilateral vertebral arteries
    I65.09 Occlusion and stenosis of unspecified vertebral artery

   I65.1 Occlusion and stenosis of basilar artery

✓5th I65.2 Occlusion and stenosis of carotid artery

> **AHA:** 2021,1Q,4; 2020,3Q,28

    I65.21 Occlusion and stenosis of right carotid artery
    I65.22 Occlusion and stenosis of left carotid artery
    I65.23 Occlusion and stenosis of bilateral carotid arteries
    I65.29 Occlusion and stenosis of unspecified carotid artery

   I65.8 Occlusion and stenosis of other precerebral arteries

   I65.9 Occlusion and stenosis of unspecified precerebral artery
     Occlusion and stenosis of precerebral artery NOS

✓4th I66 Occlusion and stenosis of cerebral arteries, not resulting in cerebral infarction

> INCLUDES   embolism of cerebral artery
> narrowing of cerebral artery
> obstruction (complete) (partial) of cerebral artery
> thrombosis of cerebral artery
>
> EXCLUDES 1   *occlusion and stenosis of cerebral artery causing cerebral infarction (I63.3-I63.5)*

✓5th I66.0 Occlusion and stenosis of middle cerebral artery

    I66.01 Occlusion and stenosis of right middle cerebral artery
    I66.02 Occlusion and stenosis of left middle cerebral artery
    I66.03 Occlusion and stenosis of bilateral middle cerebral arteries
    I66.09 Occlusion and stenosis of unspecified middle cerebral artery

✓5th I66.1 Occlusion and stenosis of anterior cerebral artery

    I66.11 Occlusion and stenosis of right anterior cerebral artery
    I66.12 Occlusion and stenosis of left anterior cerebral artery
    I66.13 Occlusion and stenosis of bilateral anterior cerebral arteries
    I66.19 Occlusion and stenosis of unspecified anterior cerebral artery

✓5th I66.2 Occlusion and stenosis of posterior cerebral artery

    I66.21 Occlusion and stenosis of right posterior cerebral artery
    I66.22 Occlusion and stenosis of left posterior cerebral artery
    I66.23 Occlusion and stenosis of bilateral posterior cerebral arteries
    I66.29 Occlusion and stenosis of unspecified posterior cerebral artery

   I66.3 Occlusion and stenosis of cerebellar arteries

   I66.8 Occlusion and stenosis of other cerebral arteries
     Occlusion and stenosis of perforating arteries

   I66.9 Occlusion and stenosis of unspecified cerebral artery

✓4th I67 Other cerebrovascular diseases

> EXCLUDES 1   *occlusion and stenosis of cerebral artery causing cerebral infarction (I63.3-I63.5-)*
> *occlusion and stenosis of precerebral artery causing cerebral infarction (I63.2-)*
>
> EXCLUDES 2   *sequelae of the listed conditions (I69.8)*

   I67.0 Dissection of cerebral arteries, nonruptured   MCC
> EXCLUDES 1   *ruptured cerebral arteries (I60.7)*
>
> **AHA:** 2021,3Q,5
> **DEF:** Dissecting aneurysm: Tear within an arterial wall that allows blood to accumulate between the outer and middle layers, creating a false lumen.

I67.1 Cerebral aneurysm, nonruptured
    Cerebral aneurysm NOS
    Cerebral arteriovenous fistula, acquired
    Internal carotid artery aneurysm, intracranial portion
    Internal carotid artery aneurysm, NOS

> EXCLUDES 1   *congenital cerebral aneurysm, nonruptured (Q28.-)*
> *ruptured cerebral aneurysm (I60.7)*
>
> **AHA:** 2021,3Q,5
> **TIP:** A diagnosis of dissecting aneurysm should be coded to the dissection code, I67.0. The bulging/aneurysm, although present, occurred secondary to the dissection. The dissection represents the most significant problem.

Berry Aneurysm

Berry aneurysms form at the site of a weakness in an arterial wall, often at a junction

Berry aneurysm

Anterior communicating artery

Anterior cerebral artery   40%

34%

Internal carotid   20%   Middle cerebral artery

Posterior cerebral artery   4%

Posterior communicating artery

Basilar artery

Common sites of berry aneurysms in the circle of Willis arteries

I67.2 Cerebral atherosclerosis   A
    Atheroma of cerebral and precerebral arteries

I67.3 Progressive vascular leukoencephalopathy   HIV CC MCC
    Binswanger's disease

I67.4 Hypertensive encephalopathy   CC
    Code also, if applicable, associated hypertensive conditions such as:
     essential (primary) hypertension (I10)
     hypertensive chronic kidney disease (I12.-)
     hypertensive heart and chronic kidney disease (I13.-)
     hypertensive heart disease (I11.-)

> EXCLUDES 2   *insufficiency, NOS, of precerebral arteries (G45.2)*
>
> **AHA:** 2023,4Q,24

I67.5 Moyamoya disease   CC
    DEF: Cerebrovascular ischemia. Vessels occlude and rupture, causing tiny hemorrhages at the base of brain. It affects predominantly Japanese people.

I67.6 Nonpyogenic thrombosis of intracranial venous system   CC
    Nonpyogenic thrombosis of cerebral vein
    Nonpyogenic thrombosis of intracranial venous sinus

> EXCLUDES 1   *nonpyogenic thrombosis of intracranial venous system causing infarction (I63.6)*

I67.7 Cerebral arteritis, not elsewhere classified   CC
    Granulomatous angiitis of the nervous system

> EXCLUDES 1   *allergic granulomatous angiitis (M30.1)*

✓5th I67.8 Other specified cerebrovascular diseases

   I67.81 Acute cerebrovascular insufficiency   CC
     Acute cerebrovascular insufficiency unspecified as to location or reversibility

   I67.82 Cerebral ischemia   CC
     Chronic cerebral ischemia

   I67.83 Posterior reversible encephalopathy syndrome   HIV MCC
     PRES

✓6ᵗʰ **I67.84 Cerebral vasospasm and vasoconstriction**

    I67.841 Reversible cerebrovascular vasoconstriction syndrome CC
        Call-Fleming syndrome
        Code first underlying condition, if applicable, such as eclampsia (O15.ØØ-O15.9)

    I67.848 Other cerebrovascular vasospasm and vasoconstriction CC

✓6ᵗʰ **I67.85 Hereditary cerebrovascular diseases**
    AHA: 2018,4Q,17

    I67.85Ø Cerebral autosomal dominant arteriopathy with subcortical infarcts and leukoencephalopathy CC
        CADASIL
        Code also any associated diagnoses, such as:
          epilepsy (G4Ø.-)
          stroke (I63.-)
          vascular dementia (FØ1.-)

    I67.858 Other hereditary cerebrovascular disease CC

  I67.89 Other cerebrovascular disease CC
    AHA: 2023,2Q,18

I67.9 Cerebrovascular disease, unspecified

✓4ᵗʰ **I68 Cerebrovascular disorders in diseases classified elsewhere**

  I68.Ø Cerebral amyloid angiopathy
    Code first underlying amyloidosis (E85.-)

  I68.2 Cerebral arteritis in other diseases classified elsewhere CC
    Code first underlying disease
    EXCLUDES 1 cerebral arteritis (in):
        listerosis (A32.89)
        syphilis (A52.Ø4)
        systemic lupus erythematosus (M32.19)
        tuberculosis (A18.89)

  I68.8 Other cerebrovascular disorders in diseases classified elsewhere
    Code first underlying disease
    EXCLUDES 1 syphilitic cerebral aneurysm (A52.Ø5)

✓4ᵗʰ **I69 Sequelae of cerebrovascular disease**

  NOTE Category I69 is to be used to indicate conditions in I6Ø-I67 as the cause of sequelae. The "sequelae" include conditions specified as such or as residuals which may occur at any time after the onset of the causal condition

  EXCLUDES 1 personal history of cerebral infarction without residual deficit (Z86.73)
    personal history of prolonged reversible ischemic neurologic deficit (PRIND) (Z86.73)
    personal history of reversible ischemic neurol*o*gcial deficit (RIND) (Z86.73)
    sequelae of traumatic intracranial injury (SØ6.-)

  AHA: 2023,1Q,37; 2020,2Q,29; 2017,1Q,47; 2016,4Q,28; 2015,1Q,25; 2012,4Q,106

  TIP: Weakness on one side of the body (unilateral weakness) documented as secondary to old cerebrovascular disease is synonymous with hemiparesis/hemiplegia. Weakness of one limb documented as secondary to old cerebrovascular disease is synonymous with monoplegia.

  TIP: For codes describing hemiplegia, hemiparesis, and monoplegia; if the documentation identifies the affected side but not whether it is the dominant or nondominant side, the default is as follows: for ambidextrous patients, the default is dominant; when the left side is affected, the default is nondominant; and when the right side is affected, the default is dominant.

✓5ᵗʰ **I69.Ø Sequelae of nontraumatic subarachnoid hemorrhage**

  I69.ØØ Unspecified sequelae of nontraumatic subarachnoid hemorrhage PE

✓6ᵗʰ **I69.Ø1 Cognitive deficits following nontraumatic subarachnoid hemorrhage**

    I69.Ø1Ø Attention and concentration deficit following nontraumatic subarachnoid hemorrhage PE

    I69.Ø11 Memory deficit following nontraumatic subarachnoid hemorrhage PE

    I69.Ø12 Visuospatial deficit and spatial neglect following nontraumatic subarachnoid hemorrhage PE

    I69.Ø13 Psychomotor deficit following nontraumatic subarachnoid hemorrhage PE

    I69.Ø14 Frontal lobe and executive function deficit following nontraumatic subarachnoid hemorrhage PE

    I69.Ø15 Cognitive social or emotional deficit following nontraumatic subarachnoid hemorrhage PE

    I69.Ø18 Other symptoms and signs involving cognitive functions following nontraumatic subarachnoid hemorrhage PE

    I69.Ø19 Unspecified symptoms and signs involving cognitive functions following nontraumatic subarachnoid hemorrhage PE

✓6ᵗʰ **I69.Ø2 Speech and language deficits following nontraumatic subarachnoid hemorrhage**

    I69.Ø2Ø Aphasia following nontraumatic subarachnoid hemorrhage PE

    I69.Ø21 Dysphasia following nontraumatic subarachnoid hemorrhage PE

    I69.Ø22 Dysarthria following nontraumatic subarachnoid hemorrhage PE

    I69.Ø23 Fluency disorder following nontraumatic subarachnoid hemorrhage PE
        Stuttering following nontraumatic subarachnoid hemorrhage

    I69.Ø28 Other speech and language deficits following nontraumatic subarachnoid hemorrhage PE

✓6ᵗʰ **I69.Ø3 Monoplegia of upper limb following nontraumatic subarachnoid hemorrhage**
    AHA: 2017,1Q,47

    I69.Ø31 Monoplegia of upper limb following nontraumatic subarachnoid hemorrhage affecting right dominant side HCC PE

    I69.Ø32 Monoplegia of upper limb following nontraumatic subarachnoid hemorrhage affecting left dominant side HCC PE

    I69.Ø33 Monoplegia of upper limb following nontraumatic subarachnoid hemorrhage affecting right non-dominant side HCC PE

    I69.Ø34 Monoplegia of upper limb following nontraumatic subarachnoid hemorrhage affecting left non-dominant side HCC PE

    I69.Ø39 Monoplegia of upper limb following nontraumatic subarachnoid hemorrhage affecting unspecified side HCC PE

✓6ᵗʰ **I69.Ø4 Monoplegia of lower limb following nontraumatic subarachnoid hemorrhage**
    AHA: 2017,1Q,47

    I69.Ø41 Monoplegia of lower limb following nontraumatic subarachnoid hemorrhage affecting right dominant side HCC PE

    I69.Ø42 Monoplegia of lower limb following nontraumatic subarachnoid hemorrhage affecting left dominant side HCC PE

    I69.Ø43 Monoplegia of lower limb following nontraumatic subarachnoid hemorrhage affecting right non-dominant side HCC PE

    I69.Ø44 Monoplegia of lower limb following nontraumatic subarachnoid hemorrhage affecting left non-dominant side HCC PE

    I69.Ø49 Monoplegia of lower limb following nontraumatic subarachnoid hemorrhage affecting unspecified side HCC PE

✓6ᵗʰ **I69.Ø5 Hemiplegia and hemiparesis following nontraumatic subarachnoid hemorrhage**
    AHA: 2015,1Q,25

    I69.Ø51 Hemiplegia and hemiparesis following nontraumatic subarachnoid hemorrhage affecting right dominant side CC HCC PE

    I69.Ø52 Hemiplegia and hemiparesis following nontraumatic subarachnoid hemorrhage affecting left dominant side CC HCC PE

Chapter 9. Diseases of the Circulatory System

I69.053 Hemiplegia and hemiparesis following nontraumatic subarachnoid hemorrhage affecting **right non-dominant** side `CC` `HCC` `PE`

I69.054 Hemiplegia and hemiparesis following nontraumatic subarachnoid hemorrhage affecting **left non-dominant** side `CC` `HCC` `PE`

I69.059 Hemiplegia and hemiparesis following nontraumatic subarachnoid hemorrhage affecting unspecified side `CC` `UNS` `HCC` `PE`

✓6ᵗʰ **I69.06** Other **paralytic syndrome** following nontraumatic subarachnoid hemorrhage

Use additional code to identify type of paralytic syndrome, such as:
locked-in state (G83.5)
quadriplegia (G82.5-)

EXCLUDES 1 hemiplegia/hemiparesis following nontraumatic subarachnoid hemorrhage (I69.05-)
monoplegia of lower limb following nontraumatic subarachnoid hemorrhage (I69.04-)
monoplegia of upper limb following nontraumatic subarachnoid hemorrhage (I69.03-)

I69.061 Other paralytic syndrome following nontraumatic subarachnoid hemorrhage affecting **right dominant** side `HCC` `PE`

I69.062 Other paralytic syndrome following nontraumatic subarachnoid hemorrhage affecting **left dominant** side `HCC` `PE`

I69.063 Other paralytic syndrome following nontraumatic subarachnoid hemorrhage affecting **right non-dominant** side `HCC` `PE`

I69.064 Other paralytic syndrome following nontraumatic subarachnoid hemorrhage affecting **left non-dominant** side `HCC` `PE`

I69.065 Other paralytic syndrome following nontraumatic subarachnoid hemorrhage, **bilateral** `HCC` `PE`

I69.069 Other paralytic syndrome following nontraumatic subarachnoid hemorrhage affecting unspecified side `HCC` `PE`

✓6ᵗʰ **I69.09** Other sequelae of nontraumatic subarachnoid hemorrhage

I69.090 **Apraxia** following nontraumatic subarachnoid hemorrhage `PE`

I69.091 **Dysphagia** following nontraumatic subarachnoid hemorrhage `PE`

Use additional code to identify the type of dysphagia, if known (R13.11-R13.19)

I69.092 **Facial weakness** following nontraumatic subarachnoid hemorrhage `PE`

Facial droop following nontraumatic subarachnoid hemorrhage

I69.093 **Ataxia** following nontraumatic subarachnoid hemorrhage `PE`

I69.098 Other sequelae following nontraumatic subarachnoid hemorrhage `PE`

Alterations of sensation following nontraumatic subarachnoid hemorrhage
Disturbance of vision following nontraumatic subarachnoid hemorrhage

Use additional code to identify the sequelae

✓5ᵗʰ **I69.1** Sequelae of nontraumatic **intracerebral** hemorrhage

I69.10 Unspecified sequelae of nontraumatic intracerebral hemorrhage `PE`

✓6ᵗʰ **I69.11** **Cognitive deficits** following nontraumatic intracerebral hemorrhage

I69.110 **Attention and concentration** deficit following nontraumatic intracerebral hemorrhage `PE`

I69.111 **Memory** deficit following nontraumatic intracerebral hemorrhage `PE`

I69.112 **Visuospatial** deficit and **spatial neglect** following nontraumatic intracerebral hemorrhage `PE`

I69.113 **Psychomotor** deficit following nontraumatic intracerebral hemorrhage `PE`

I69.114 **Frontal lobe and executive function** deficit following nontraumatic intracerebral hemorrhage `PE`

I69.115 **Cognitive social or emotional** deficit following nontraumatic intracerebral hemorrhage `PE`

I69.118 Other symptoms and signs involving cognitive functions following nontraumatic intracerebral hemorrhage `PE`

I69.119 Unspecified symptoms and signs involving cognitive functions following nontraumatic intracerebral hemorrhage `PE`

✓6ᵗʰ **I69.12** **Speech and language deficits** following nontraumatic intracerebral hemorrhage

I69.120 **Aphasia** following nontraumatic intracerebral hemorrhage `PE`

I69.121 **Dysphasia** following nontraumatic intracerebral hemorrhage `PE`

I69.122 **Dysarthria** following nontraumatic intracerebral hemorrhage `PE`

I69.123 **Fluency disorder** following nontraumatic intracerebral hemorrhage `PE`

Stuttering following nontraumatic intracerebral hemorrhage

I69.128 Other speech and language deficits following nontraumatic intracerebral hemorrhage `PE`

✓6ᵗʰ **I69.13** **Monoplegia of upper limb** following nontraumatic intracerebral hemorrhage

AHA: 2017,1Q,47

I69.131 Monoplegia of upper limb following nontraumatic intracerebral hemorrhage affecting **right dominant** side `HCC` `PE`

I69.132 Monoplegia of upper limb following nontraumatic intracerebral hemorrhage affecting **left dominant** side `HCC` `PE`

I69.133 Monoplegia of upper limb following nontraumatic intracerebral hemorrhage affecting **right non-dominant** side `HCC` `PE`

I69.134 Monoplegia of upper limb following nontraumatic intracerebral hemorrhage affecting **left non-dominant** side `HCC` `PE`

I69.139 Monoplegia of upper limb following nontraumatic intracerebral hemorrhage affecting unspecified side `HCC` `PE`

✓6ᵗʰ **I69.14** **Monoplegia of lower limb** following nontraumatic intracerebral hemorrhage

AHA: 2017,1Q,47

I69.141 Monoplegia of lower limb following nontraumatic intracerebral hemorrhage affecting **right dominant** side `HCC` `PE`

I69.142 Monoplegia of lower limb following nontraumatic intracerebral hemorrhage affecting **left dominant** side `HCC` `PE`

I69.143 Monoplegia of lower limb following nontraumatic intracerebral hemorrhage affecting **right non-dominant** side `HCC` `PE`

I69.144 Monoplegia of lower limb following nontraumatic intracerebral hemorrhage affecting **left non-dominant** side `HCC` `PE`

I69.149 Monoplegia of lower limb following nontraumatic intracerebral hemorrhage affecting unspecified side `HCC` `PE`

✓6ᵗʰ **I69.15** **Hemiplegia and hemiparesis** following nontraumatic intracerebral hemorrhage

AHA: 2015,1Q,25

I69.151 Hemiplegia and hemiparesis following nontraumatic intracerebral hemorrhage affecting **right dominant** side `CC` `HCC` `PE`

`N` Newborn: 0   `P` Pediatric: 0-17   `M` Maternity: 9-64   `A` Adult: 15-124   `UNS` Unspecified Site   `MCC` Major Complication/Comorbidity   `CC` Complication/Comorbidity   `PE` POA Exempt

678

ICD-10-CM 2025

I69.152   Hemiplegia and hemiparesis following nontraumatic intracerebral hemorrhage affecting **left dominant** side   `CC` `HCC` `PE`

I69.153   Hemiplegia and hemiparesis following nontraumatic intracerebral hemorrhage affecting **right non-dominant** side   `CC` `HCC` `PE`

I69.154   Hemiplegia and hemiparesis following nontraumatic intracerebral hemorrhage affecting **left non-dominant** side   `CC` `HCC` `PE`

I69.159   Hemiplegia and hemiparesis following nontraumatic intracerebral hemorrhage affecting unspecified side   `CC` `UnS` `HCC` `PE`

✓6th **I69.16**   Other **paralytic syndrome** following nontraumatic intracerebral hemorrhage

Use additional code to identify type of paralytic syndrome, such as:
locked-in state (G83.5)
quadriplegia (G82.5-)

EXCLUDES 1   hemiplegia/hemiparesis following nontraumatic intracerebral hemorrhage (I69.15-)
monoplegia of lower limb following nontraumatic intracerebral hemorrhage (I69.14-)
monoplegia of upper limb following nontraumatic intracerebral hemorrhage (I69.13-)

I69.161   Other paralytic syndrome following nontraumatic intracerebral hemorrhage affecting **right dominant** side   `HCC` `PE`

I69.162   Other paralytic syndrome following nontraumatic intracerebral hemorrhage affecting **left dominant** side   `HCC` `PE`

I69.163   Other paralytic syndrome following nontraumatic intracerebral hemorrhage affecting **right non-dominant** side   `HCC` `PE`

I69.164   Other paralytic syndrome following nontraumatic intracerebral hemorrhage affecting **left non-dominant** side   `HCC` `PE`

I69.165   Other paralytic syndrome following nontraumatic intracerebral hemorrhage, **bilateral**   `HCC` `PE`

I69.169   Other paralytic syndrome following nontraumatic intracerebral hemorrhage affecting unspecified side   `HCC` `PE`

✓6th **I69.19**   Other sequelae of nontraumatic intracerebral hemorrhage

I69.190   **Apraxia** following nontraumatic intracerebral hemorrhage   `PE`

I69.191   **Dysphagia** following nontraumatic intracerebral hemorrhage   `PE`

Use additional code to identify the type of dysphagia, if known (R13.11-R13.19)

I69.192   **Facial weakness** following nontraumatic intracerebral hemorrhage   `PE`

Facial droop following nontraumatic intracerebral hemorrhage

I69.193   **Ataxia** following nontraumatic intracerebral hemorrhage   `PE`

I69.198   Other sequelae of nontraumatic intracerebral hemorrhage   `PE`

Alteration of sensations following nontraumatic intracerebral hemorrhage
Disturbance of vision following nontraumatic intracerebral hemorrhage

Use additional code to identify the sequelae

✓5th **I69.2**   Sequelae of other nontraumatic **intracranial** hemorrhage

I69.20   Unspecified sequelae of other nontraumatic intracranial hemorrhage   `PE`

✓6th **I69.21**   **Cognitive deficits** following other nontraumatic intracranial hemorrhage

I69.210   **Attention and concentration** deficit following other nontraumatic intracranial hemorrhage   `PE`

I69.211   **Memory** deficit following other nontraumatic intracranial hemorrhage   `PE`

I69.212   **Visuospatial** deficit and **spatial neglect** following other nontraumatic intracranial hemorrhage   `PE`

I69.213   **Psychomotor** deficit following other nontraumatic intracranial hemorrhage   `PE`

I69.214   **Frontal lobe and executive function** deficit following other nontraumatic intracranial hemorrhage   `PE`

I69.215   **Cognitive social or emotional** deficit following other nontraumatic intracranial hemorrhage   `PE`

I69.218   Other symptoms and signs involving cognitive functions following other nontraumatic intracranial hemorrhage   `PE`

I69.219   Unspecified symptoms and signs involving cognitive functions following other nontraumatic intracranial hemorrhage   `PE`

✓6th **I69.22**   **Speech and language deficits** following other nontraumatic intracranial hemorrhage

I69.220   **Aphasia** following other nontraumatic intracranial hemorrhage   `PE`

I69.221   **Dysphasia** following other nontraumatic intracranial hemorrhage   `PE`

I69.222   **Dysarthria** following other nontraumatic intracranial hemorrhage   `PE`

I69.223   **Fluency** disorder following other nontraumatic intracranial hemorrhage   `PE`

Stuttering following other nontraumatic intracranial hemorrhage

I69.228   Other speech and language deficits following other nontraumatic intracranial hemorrhage   `PE`

✓6th **I69.23**   **Monoplegia of upper limb** following other nontraumatic intracranial hemorrhage

AHA: 2017,1Q,47

I69.231   Monoplegia of upper limb following other nontraumatic intracranial hemorrhage affecting **right dominant** side   `HCC` `PE`

I69.232   Monoplegia of upper limb following other nontraumatic intracranial hemorrhage affecting **left dominant** side   `HCC` `PE`

I69.233   Monoplegia of upper limb following other nontraumatic intracranial hemorrhage affecting **right non-dominant** side   `HCC` `PE`

I69.234   Monoplegia of upper limb following other nontraumatic intracranial hemorrhage affecting **left non-dominant** side   `HCC` `PE`

I69.239   Monoplegia of upper limb following other nontraumatic intracranial hemorrhage affecting unspecified side   `HCC` `PE`

✓6th **I69.24**   **Monoplegia of lower limb** following other nontraumatic intracranial hemorrhage

AHA: 2017,1Q,47

I69.241   Monoplegia of lower limb following other nontraumatic intracranial hemorrhage affecting **right dominant** side   `HCC` `PE`

I69.242   Monoplegia of lower limb following other nontraumatic intracranial hemorrhage affecting **left dominant** side   `HCC` `PE`

I69.243   Monoplegia of lower limb following other nontraumatic intracranial hemorrhage affecting **right non-dominant** side   `HCC` `PE`

I69.244   Monoplegia of lower limb following other nontraumatic intracranial hemorrhage affecting **left non-dominant** side   `HCC` `PE`

I69.249   Monoplegia of lower limb following other nontraumatic intracranial hemorrhage affecting unspecified side   `HCC` `PE`

✓ Additional Character Required   ✓x7th Placeholder   Questionable PDx   Manifestation   Unspecified   `UPD` Unacceptable PDx   `H1`-`H14` HAC   `HCC` CMS-HCC Dx   `HIV` HIV Dx

ICD-10-CM 2025   679

Chapter 9. Diseases of the Circulatory System

✓6th **I69.25** **Hemiplegia and hemiparesis** following other nontraumatic intracranial hemorrhage
AHA: 2015,1Q,25

I69.251 Hemiplegia and hemiparesis following other nontraumatic intracranial hemorrhage affecting **right dominant** side `CC` `HCC` `PE`

I69.252 Hemiplegia and hemiparesis following other nontraumatic intracranial hemorrhage affecting **left dominant** side `CC` `HCC` `PE`

I69.253 Hemiplegia and hemiparesis following other nontraumatic intracranial hemorrhage affecting **right non-dominant** side `CC` `HCC` `PE`

I69.254 Hemiplegia and hemiparesis following other nontraumatic intracranial hemorrhage affecting **left non-dominant** side `CC` `HCC` `PE`

I69.259 Hemiplegia and hemiparesis following other nontraumatic intracranial hemorrhage affecting unspecified side `CC` `UNS` `HCC` `PE`

✓6th **I69.26** Other **paralytic syndrome** following other nontraumatic intracranial hemorrhage
Use additional code to identify type of paralytic syndrome, such as:
  locked-in state (G83.5)
  quadriplegia (G82.5-)
EXCLUDES 1 hemiplegia/hemiparesis following other nontraumatic intracranial hemorrhage (I69.25-)
  monoplegia of lower limb following other nontraumatic intracranial hemorrhage (I69.24-)
  monoplegia of upper limb following other nontraumatic intracranial hemorrhage (I69.23-)

I69.261 Other paralytic syndrome following other nontraumatic intracranial hemorrhage affecting **right dominant** side `HCC` `PE`

I69.262 Other paralytic syndrome following other nontraumatic intracranial hemorrhage affecting **left dominant** side `HCC` `PE`

I69.263 Other paralytic syndrome following other nontraumatic intracranial hemorrhage affecting **right non-dominant** side `HCC` `PE`

I69.264 Other paralytic syndrome following other nontraumatic intracranial hemorrhage affecting **left non-dominant** side `HCC` `PE`

I69.265 Other paralytic syndrome following other nontraumatic intracranial hemorrhage, **bilateral** `HCC` `PE`

I69.269 Other paralytic syndrome following other nontraumatic intracranial hemorrhage affecting unspecified side `HCC` `PE`

✓6th **I69.29** Other sequelae of other nontraumatic intracranial hemorrhage

I69.290 **Apraxia** following other nontraumatic intracranial hemorrhage `PE`

I69.291 **Dysphagia** following other nontraumatic intracranial hemorrhage `PE`
Use additional code to identify the type of dysphagia, if known (R13.11-R13.19)

I69.292 **Facial weakness** following other nontraumatic intracranial hemorrhage `PE`
Facial droop following other nontraumatic intracranial hemorrhage

I69.293 **Ataxia** following other nontraumatic intracranial hemorrhage `PE`

I69.298 Other sequelae of other nontraumatic intracranial hemorrhage
Alteration of sensation following other nontraumatic intracranial hemorrhage
Disturbance of vision following other nontraumatic intracranial hemorrhage
Use additional code to identify the sequelae

✓5th **I69.3** Sequelae of **cerebral infarction**
Sequelae of stroke NOS
AHA: 2013,4Q,127-128; 2012,4Q,92,94

I69.30 Unspecified sequelae of cerebral infarction `PE`

✓6th **I69.31** **Cognitive** deficits following cerebral infarction

I69.310 **Attention and concentration** deficit following cerebral infarction `PE`

I69.311 **Memory** deficit following cerebral infarction `PE`

I69.312 **Visuospatial** deficit and **spatial neglect** following cerebral infarction `PE`

I69.313 **Psychomotor** deficit following cerebral infarction `PE`

I69.314 **Frontal lobe and executive function** deficit following cerebral infarction `PE`

I69.315 **Cognitive social or emotional** deficit following cerebral infarction `PE`

I69.318 Other symptoms and signs involving cognitive functions following cerebral infarction `PE`

I69.319 Unspecified symptoms and signs involving cognitive functions following cerebral infarction `PE`

✓6th **I69.32** **Speech and language deficits** following cerebral infarction

I69.320 **Aphasia** following cerebral infarction `PE`

I69.321 **Dysphasia** following cerebral infarction `PE`
AHA: 2012,4Q,91

I69.322 **Dysarthria** following cerebral infarction `PE`
EXCLUDES 2 transient ischemic attack (TIA) (G45.9)

I69.323 **Fluency disorder** following cerebral infarction `PE`
Stuttering following cerebral infarction

I69.328 Other speech and language deficits following cerebral infarction `PE`

✓6th **I69.33** **Monoplegia of upper limb** following cerebral infarction
AHA: 2017,1Q,47

I69.331 Monoplegia of upper limb following cerebral infarction affecting **right dominant** side `HCC` `PE`

I69.332 Monoplegia of upper limb following cerebral infarction affecting **left dominant** side `HCC` `PE`

I69.333 Monoplegia of upper limb following cerebral infarction affecting **right non-dominant** side `HCC` `PE`

I69.334 Monoplegia of upper limb following cerebral infarction affecting **left non-dominant** side `HCC` `PE`

I69.339 Monoplegia of upper limb following cerebral infarction affecting unspecified side `HCC` `PE`

✓6th **I69.34** **Monoplegia of lower limb** following cerebral infarction
AHA: 2017,1Q,47

I69.341 Monoplegia of lower limb following cerebral infarction affecting **right dominant** side `HCC` `PE`

I69.342 Monoplegia of lower limb following cerebral infarction affecting **left dominant** side `HCC` `PE`

I69.343 Monoplegia of lower limb following cerebral infarction affecting **right non-dominant** side `HCC` `PE`

I69.344 Monoplegia of lower limb following cerebral infarction affecting **left non-dominant** side `HCC` `PE`

I69.349 Monoplegia of lower limb following cerebral infarction affecting unspecified side `HCC` `PE`

✓6th **I69.35 Hemiplegia and hemiparesis** following cerebral infarction
AHA: 2015,1Q,25

I69.351 Hemiplegia and hemiparesis following cerebral infarction affecting right dominant side `CC` `HCC` `PE`
EXCLUDES 2   *transient ischemic attack (TIA) (G45.9)*

I69.352 Hemiplegia and hemiparesis following cerebral infarction affecting left dominant side `CC` `HCC` `PE`

I69.353 Hemiplegia and hemiparesis following cerebral infarction affecting right non-dominant side `CC` `HCC` `PE`

I69.354 Hemiplegia and hemiparesis following cerebral infarction affecting left non-dominant side `CC` `HCC` `PE`
AHA: 2012,4Q,91

I69.359 Hemiplegia and hemiparesis following cerebral infarction affecting unspecified side `CC` `UNS` `HCC` `PE`

✓6th **I69.36 Other paralytic syndrome** following cerebral infarction
Use additional code to identify type of paralytic syndrome, such as:
locked-in state (G83.5)
quadriplegia (G82.5-)
EXCLUDES 1   *hemiplegia/hemiparesis following cerebral infarction (I69.35-)*
monoplegia of lower limb following cerebral infarction (I69.34-)
monoplegia of upper limb following cerebral infarction (I69.33-)

I69.361 Other paralytic syndrome following cerebral infarction affecting right dominant side `HCC` `PE`

I69.362 Other paralytic syndrome following cerebral infarction affecting left dominant side `HCC` `PE`

I69.363 Other paralytic syndrome following cerebral infarction affecting right non-dominant side `HCC` `PE`

I69.364 Other paralytic syndrome following cerebral infarction affecting left non-dominant side `HCC` `PE`

I69.365 Other paralytic syndrome following cerebral infarction, bilateral `HCC` `PE`

I69.369 Other paralytic syndrome following cerebral infarction affecting unspecified side `HCC` `PE`

✓6th **I69.39 Other sequelae of cerebral infarction**

I69.390 Apraxia following cerebral infarction `PE`

I69.391 Dysphagia following cerebral infarction `PE`
Use additional code to identify the type of dysphagia, if known (R13.11-R13.19)

I69.392 Facial weakness following cerebral infarction `PE`
Facial droop following cerebral infarction
AHA: AHA:2024,2Q,13

I69.393 Ataxia following cerebral infarction `PE`

I69.398 Other sequelae of cerebral infarction `PE`
Alteration of sensation following cerebral infarction
Disturbance of vision following cerebral infarction
Use additional code to identify the sequelae
AHA: 2024,2Q,13; 2020,2Q,29

✓5th **I69.8 Sequelae of other cerebrovascular diseases**
EXCLUDES 1   *sequelae of traumatic intracranial injury (S06.-)*

I69.80 Unspecified sequelae of other cerebrovascular disease `PE`

✓6th **I69.81 Cognitive deficits** following other cerebrovascular disease

I69.810 Attention and concentration deficit following other cerebrovascular disease `PE`

I69.811 Memory deficit following other cerebrovascular disease `PE`

I69.812 Visuospatial deficit and spatial neglect following other cerebrovascular disease `PE`

I69.813 Psychomotor deficit following other cerebrovascular disease `PE`

I69.814 Frontal lobe and executive function deficit following other cerebrovascular disease `PE`

I69.815 Cognitive social or emotional deficit following other cerebrovascular disease `PE`

I69.818 Other symptoms and signs involving cognitive functions following other cerebrovascular disease `PE`

I69.819 Unspecified symptoms and signs involving cognitive functions following other cerebrovascular disease `PE`

✓6th **I69.82 Speech and language deficits** following other cerebrovascular disease

I69.820 Aphasia following other cerebrovascular disease `PE`

I69.821 Dysphasia following other cerebrovascular disease `PE`

I69.822 Dysarthria following other cerebrovascular disease `PE`

I69.823 Fluency disorder following other cerebrovascular disease `PE`
Stuttering following other cerebrovascular disease

I69.828 Other speech and language deficits following other cerebrovascular disease `PE`
AHA: 2019,3Q,8

✓6th **I69.83 Monoplegia of upper limb** following other cerebrovascular disease
AHA: 2017,1Q,47

I69.831 Monoplegia of upper limb following other cerebrovascular disease affecting right dominant side `HCC` `PE`

I69.832 Monoplegia of upper limb following other cerebrovascular disease affecting left dominant side `HCC` `PE`

I69.833 Monoplegia of upper limb following other cerebrovascular disease affecting right non-dominant side `HCC` `PE`

I69.834 Monoplegia of upper limb following other cerebrovascular disease affecting left non-dominant side `HCC` `PE`

I69.839 Monoplegia of upper limb following other cerebrovascular disease affecting unspecified side `HCC` `PE`

✓6th **I69.84 Monoplegia of lower limb** following other cerebrovascular disease
AHA: 2017,1Q,47

I69.841 Monoplegia of lower limb following other cerebrovascular disease affecting right dominant side `HCC` `PE`

I69.842 Monoplegia of lower limb following other cerebrovascular disease affecting left dominant side `HCC` `PE`

I69.843 Monoplegia of lower limb following other cerebrovascular disease affecting right non-dominant side `HCC` `PE`

I69.844 Monoplegia of lower limb following other cerebrovascular disease affecting left non-dominant side `HCC` `PE`

I69.849 Monoplegia of lower limb following other cerebrovascular disease affecting unspecified side `HCC` `PE`

✓6th **I69.85 Hemiplegia and hemiparesis** following other cerebrovascular disease
AHA: 2015,1Q,25

I69.851 Hemiplegia and hemiparesis following other cerebrovascular disease affecting right dominant side `CC` `HCC` `PE`

I69.852 Hemiplegia and hemiparesis following other cerebrovascular disease affecting left dominant side `CC` `HCC` `PE`

Chapter 9. Diseases of the Circulatory System

I69.853 Hemiplegia and hemiparesis following other cerebrovascular disease affecting **right non-dominant** side `CC` `HCC` `PE`

I69.854 Hemiplegia and hemiparesis following other cerebrovascular disease affecting **left non-dominant** side `CC` `HCC` `PE`

I69.859 Hemiplegia and hemiparesis following other cerebrovascular disease affecting unspecified side `CC` `UNS` `HCC` `PE`

✓6ᵗʰ **I69.86** Other **paralytic syndrome** following other cerebrovascular disease

Use additional code to identify type of paralytic syndrome, such as:
locked-in state (G83.5)
quadriplegia (G82.5-)

EXCLUDES 1   hemiplegia/hemiparesis following other cerebrovascular disease (I69.85-)
monoplegia of lower limb following other cerebrovascular disease (I69.84-)
monoplegia of upper limb following other cerebrovascular disease (I69.83-)

I69.861 Other paralytic syndrome following other cerebrovascular disease affecting **right dominant** side `HCC` `PE`

I69.862 Other paralytic syndrome following other cerebrovascular disease affecting **left dominant** side `HCC` `PE`

I69.863 Other paralytic syndrome following other cerebrovascular disease affecting **right non-dominant** side `HCC` `PE`

I69.864 Other paralytic syndrome following other cerebrovascular disease affecting **left non-dominant** side `HCC` `PE`

I69.865 Other paralytic syndrome following other cerebrovascular disease, **bilateral** `HCC` `PE`

I69.869 Other paralytic syndrome following other cerebrovascular disease affecting unspecified side `HCC` `PE`

✓6ᵗʰ **I69.89** Other sequelae of other cerebrovascular disease

I69.890 **Apraxia** following other cerebrovascular disease `PE`

I69.891 **Dysphagia** following other cerebrovascular disease `PE`
Use additional code to identify the type of dysphagia, if known (R13.11-R13.19)

I69.892 **Facial weakness** following other cerebrovascular disease `PE`
Facial droop following other cerebrovascular disease

I69.893 **Ataxia** following other cerebrovascular disease `PE`

I69.898 Other sequelae of other cerebrovascular disease `PE`
Alteration of sensation following other cerebrovascular disease
Disturbance of vision following other cerebrovascular disease
Use additional code to identify the sequelae

✓5ᵗʰ **I69.9** Sequelae of unspecified **cerebrovascular diseases**

EXCLUDES 1   sequelae of stroke (I69.3)
sequelae of traumatic intracranial injury (S06.-)

I69.90 Unspecified sequelae of unspecified cerebrovascular disease `PE`

✓6ᵗʰ **I69.91** **Cognitive deficits** following unspecified cerebrovascular disease

I69.910 **Attention and concentration** deficit following unspecified cerebrovascular disease

I69.911 **Memory** deficit following unspecified cerebrovascular disease

I69.912 **Visuospatial** deficit and **spatial neglect** following unspecified cerebrovascular disease

I69.913 **Psychomotor** deficit following unspecified cerebrovascular disease

I69.914 **Frontal lobe and executive function** deficit following unspecified cerebrovascular disease

I69.915 **Cognitive social or emotional deficit** following unspecified cerebrovascular disease

I69.918 Other symptoms and signs involving cognitive functions following unspecified cerebrovascular disease

I69.919 Unspecified symptoms and signs involving cognitive functions following unspecified cerebrovascular disease

✓6ᵗʰ **I69.92** **Speech and language deficits** following unspecified cerebrovascular disease

I69.920 **Aphasia** following unspecified cerebrovascular disease `PE`

I69.921 **Dysphasia** following unspecified cerebrovascular disease `PE`

I69.922 **Dysarthria** following unspecified cerebrovascular disease `PE`

I69.923 **Fluency disorder** following unspecified cerebrovascular disease `PE`
Stuttering following unspecified cerebrovascular disease

I69.928 Other speech and language deficits following unspecified cerebrovascular disease `PE`

✓6ᵗʰ **I69.93** **Monoplegia of upper limb** following unspecified cerebrovascular disease
AHA: 2017,1Q,47

I69.931 Monoplegia of upper limb following unspecified cerebrovascular disease affecting **right dominant** side `HCC` `PE`

I69.932 Monoplegia of upper limb following unspecified cerebrovascular disease affecting **left dominant** side `HCC` `PE`

I69.933 Monoplegia of upper limb following unspecified cerebrovascular disease affecting **right non-dominant** side `HCC` `PE`

I69.934 Monoplegia of upper limb following unspecified cerebrovascular disease affecting **left non-dominant** side `HCC` `PE`

I69.939 Monoplegia of upper limb following unspecified cerebrovascular disease affecting unspecified side `HCC` `PE`

✓6ᵗʰ **I69.94** **Monoplegia of lower limb** following unspecified cerebrovascular disease
AHA: 2017,1Q,47

I69.941 Monoplegia of lower limb following unspecified cerebrovascular disease affecting **right dominant** side `HCC` `PE`

I69.942 Monoplegia of lower limb following unspecified cerebrovascular disease affecting **left dominant** side `HCC` `PE`

I69.943 Monoplegia of lower limb following unspecified cerebrovascular disease affecting **right non-dominant** side `HCC` `PE`

I69.944 Monoplegia of lower limb following unspecified cerebrovascular disease affecting **left non-dominant** side `HCC` `PE`

I69.949 Monoplegia of lower limb following unspecified cerebrovascular disease affecting unspecified side `HCC` `PE`

✓6ᵗʰ **I69.95** **Hemiplegia and hemiparesis** following unspecified cerebrovascular disease
AHA: 2015,1Q,25

I69.951 Hemiplegia and hemiparesis following unspecified cerebrovascular disease affecting **right dominant** side `CC` `HCC` `PE`

I69.952 Hemiplegia and hemiparesis following unspecified cerebrovascular disease affecting **left dominant** side `CC` `HCC` `PE`

I69.953 Hemiplegia and hemiparesis following unspecified cerebrovascular disease affecting **right non-dominant** side `CC` `HCC` `PE`

I69.954 Hemiplegia and hemiparesis following unspecified cerebrovascular disease affecting **left non-dominant** side `CC` `HCC` `PE`

`N` Newborn: 0   `P` Pediatric: 0-17   `M` Maternity: 9-64   `A` Adult: 15-124   `UNS` Unspecified Site   `MCC` Major Complication/Comorbidity   `CC` Complication/Comorbidity   `PE` POA Exempt

682
ICD-10-CM 2025

I69.959 Hemiplegia and hemiparesis following unspecified cerebrovascular disease affecting unspecified side   `CC` `UNS` `HCC` `PE`

✓6ᵗʰ **I69.96** Other **paralytic syndrome** following unspecified cerebrovascular disease

Use additional code to identify type of paralytic syndrome, such as:
locked-in state (G83.5)
quadriplegia (G82.5-)

EXCLUDES 1   *hemiplegia/hemiparesis following unspecified cerebrovascular disease (I69.95-)*
monoplegia of lower limb following unspecified cerebrovascular disease (I69.94-)
monoplegia of upper limb following unspecified cerebrovascular disease (I69.93-)

I69.961 Other paralytic syndrome following unspecified cerebrovascular disease affecting **right dominant** side   `HCC` `PE`

I69.962 Other paralytic syndrome following unspecified cerebrovascular disease affecting **left dominant** side   `HCC` `PE`

I69.963 Other paralytic syndrome following unspecified cerebrovascular disease affecting **right non-dominant** side   `HCC` `PE`

I69.964 Other paralytic syndrome following unspecified cerebrovascular disease affecting **left non-dominant** side   `HCC` `PE`

I69.965 Other paralytic syndrome following unspecified cerebrovascular disease, **bilateral**   `HCC` `PE`

I69.969 Other paralytic syndrome following unspecified cerebrovascular disease affecting unspecified side   `HCC` `PE`

✓6ᵗʰ **I69.99** Other sequelae of unspecified cerebrovascular disease

I69.990 **Apraxia** following unspecified cerebrovascular disease   `PE`

I69.991 **Dysphagia** following unspecified cerebrovascular disease   `PE`
Use additional code to identify the type of dysphagia, if known (R13.11-R13.19)

I69.992 **Facial weakness** following unspecified cerebrovascular disease   `PE`
Facial droop following unspecified cerebrovascular disease

I69.993 **Ataxia** following unspecified cerebrovascular disease   `PE`

I69.998 Other sequelae following unspecified cerebrovascular disease   `PE`
Alteration in sensation following unspecified cerebrovascular disease
Disturbance of vision following unspecified cerebrovascular disease
Use additional code to identify the sequelae

Diseases of arteries, arterioles and capillaries (I70-I79)

✓4ᵗʰ **I70** **Atherosclerosis**

INCLUDES   arterial degeneration
arteriolosclerosis
arteriosclerosis
arteriosclerotic vascular disease
arteriovascular degeneration
atheroma
endarteritis deformans or obliterans
senile arteritis
senile endarteritis
vascular degeneration

Use additional code to identify:
exposure to environmental tobacco smoke (Z77.22)
history of tobacco dependence (Z87.891)
occupational exposure to environmental tobacco smoke (Z57.31)
tobacco dependence (F17.-)
tobacco use (Z72.0)

EXCLUDES 2   *arteriosclerotic cardiovascular disease (I25.1-)*
arteriosclerotic heart disease (I25.1-)
atheroembolism (I75.-)
cerebral atherosclerosis (I67.2)
coronary atherosclerosis (I25.1-)
mesenteric atherosclerosis (K55.1)
precerebral atherosclerosis (I67.2)
primary pulmonary atherosclerosis (I27.0)

I70.0 Atherosclerosis of **aorta**   `A`

I70.1 Atherosclerosis of **renal** artery   `A`
Goldblatt's kidney
EXCLUDES 2   *atherosclerosis of renal arterioles (I12.-)*

✓5ᵗʰ **I70.2** Atherosclerosis of **native** arteries of the **extremities**
Monckeberg's (medial) sclerosis
Use additional code, if applicable, to identify chronic total occlusion of artery of extremity (I70.92)
EXCLUDES 2   *atherosclerosis of bypass graft of extremities (I70.30-I70.79)*
AHA: 2020,4Q,98; 2018,3Q,4; 2018,2Q,7

✓6ᵗʰ **I70.20** Unspecified atherosclerosis of native arteries of extremities

I70.201 Unspecified atherosclerosis of native arteries of extremities, **right leg**   `A`

I70.202 Unspecified atherosclerosis of native arteries of extremities, **left leg**   `A`

I70.203 Unspecified atherosclerosis of native arteries of extremities, **bilateral legs**   `A`

I70.208 Unspecified atherosclerosis of native arteries of extremities, other extremity   `A`

I70.209 Unspecified atherosclerosis of native arteries of extremities, unspecified extremity   `A`

✓6ᵗʰ **I70.21** Atherosclerosis of native arteries of extremities with **intermittent claudication**

I70.211 Atherosclerosis of native arteries of extremities with intermittent claudication, **right leg**   `A`

I70.212 Atherosclerosis of native arteries of extremities with intermittent claudication, **left leg**   `A`

I70.213 Atherosclerosis of native arteries of extremities with intermittent claudication, **bilateral legs**   `A`

I70.218 Atherosclerosis of native arteries of extremities with intermittent claudication, other extremity   `A`

I70.219 Atherosclerosis of native arteries of extremities with intermittent claudication, unspecified extremity   `A`

✓6th **I70.22 Atherosclerosis of native arteries of extremities with rest pain**

INCLUDES   any condition classifiable to I70.21-
chronic limb-threatening ischemia NOS of native arteries of extremities
chronic limb-threatening ischemia of native arteries of extremities with rest pain
critical limb ischemia NOS of native arteries of extremities
critical limb ischemia of native arteries of extremities with rest pain

I70.221 Atherosclerosis of native arteries of extremities with rest pain, right leg HCC A

I70.222 Atherosclerosis of native arteries of extremities with rest pain, left leg HCC A

I70.223 Atherosclerosis of native arteries of extremities with rest pain, bilateral legs HCC A

I70.228 Atherosclerosis of native arteries of extremities with rest pain, other extremity HCC A

I70.229 Atherosclerosis of native arteries of extremities with rest pain, unspecified extremity HCC A

✓6th **I70.23 Atherosclerosis of native arteries of right leg with ulceration**

INCLUDES   any condition classifiable to I70.211 and I70.221
chronic limb-threatening ischemia of native arteries of right leg with ulceration
critical limb ischemia of native arteries of right leg with ulceration

Use additional code to identify severity of ulcer (L97.-)

I70.231 Atherosclerosis of native arteries of right leg with ulceration of thigh HCC A

I70.232 Atherosclerosis of native arteries of right leg with ulceration of calf HCC A

I70.233 Atherosclerosis of native arteries of right leg with ulceration of ankle HCC A

I70.234 Atherosclerosis of native arteries of right leg with ulceration of heel and midfoot HCC A

Atherosclerosis of native arteries of right leg with ulceration of plantar surface of midfoot

I70.235 Atherosclerosis of native arteries of right leg with ulceration of other part of foot HCC A

Atherosclerosis of native arteries of right leg extremities with ulceration of toe

I70.238 Atherosclerosis of native arteries of right leg with ulceration of other part of lower leg HCC A

I70.239 Atherosclerosis of native arteries of right leg with ulceration of unspecified site HCC A

✓6th **I70.24 Atherosclerosis of native arteries of left leg with ulceration**

INCLUDES   any condition classifiable to I70.212 and I70.222
chronic limb-threatening ischemia of native arteries of left leg with ulceration
critical limb ischemia of native arteries of left leg with ulceration

Use additional code to identify severity of ulcer (L97.-)

I70.241 Atherosclerosis of native arteries of left leg with ulceration of thigh HCC A

I70.242 Atherosclerosis of native arteries of left leg with ulceration of calf HCC A

I70.243 Atherosclerosis of native arteries of left leg with ulceration of ankle HCC A

I70.244 Atherosclerosis of native arteries of left leg with ulceration of heel and midfoot HCC A

Atherosclerosis of native arteries of left leg with ulceration of plantar surface of midfoot

I70.245 Atherosclerosis of native arteries of left leg with ulceration of other part of foot HCC A

Atherosclerosis of native arteries of left leg extremities with ulceration of toe

I70.248 Atherosclerosis of native arteries of left leg with ulceration of other part of lower leg HCC A

I70.249 Atherosclerosis of native arteries of left leg with ulceration of unspecified site HCC A

I70.25 Atherosclerosis of native arteries of other extremities with ulceration HCC A

INCLUDES   any condition classifiable to I70.218 and I70.228

Use additional code to identify the severity of the ulcer (L98.49-)

✓6th **I70.26 Atherosclerosis of native arteries of extremities with gangrene**

INCLUDES   any condition classifiable to I70.21-, I70.22-, I70.23-, I70.24-, and I70.25-
chronic limb-threatening ischemia of native arteries of extremities with gangrene
critical limb ischemia of native arteries of extremities with gangrene

Use additional code to identify the severity of any ulcer (L97.-, L98.49-), if applicable

I70.261 Atherosclerosis of native arteries of extremities with gangrene, right leg CC HCC A

I70.262 Atherosclerosis of native arteries of extremities with gangrene, left leg CC HCC A

I70.263 Atherosclerosis of native arteries of extremities with gangrene, bilateral legs CC HCC A

I70.268 Atherosclerosis of native arteries of extremities with gangrene, other extremity CC HCC A

I70.269 Atherosclerosis of native arteries of extremities with gangrene, unspecified extremity CC UNS HCC A

✓6th **I70.29 Other atherosclerosis of native arteries of extremities**

I70.291 Other atherosclerosis of native arteries of extremities, right leg A

I70.292 Other atherosclerosis of native arteries of extremities, left leg A

I70.293 Other atherosclerosis of native arteries of extremities, bilateral legs A

I70.298 Other atherosclerosis of native arteries of extremities, other extremity A

I70.299 Other atherosclerosis of native arteries of extremities, unspecified extremity A

✓5th **I70.3 Atherosclerosis of unspecified type of bypass graft(s) of the extremities**

Use additional code, if applicable, to identify chronic total occlusion of artery of extremity (I70.92)

EXCLUDES 1   embolism or thrombus of bypass graft(s) of extremities (T82.8-)

AHA: 2020,4Q,98

✓6th **I70.30 Unspecified atherosclerosis of unspecified type of bypass graft(s) of the extremities**

I70.301 Unspecified atherosclerosis of unspecified type of bypass graft(s) of the extremities, right leg A

I70.302 Unspecified atherosclerosis of unspecified type of bypass graft(s) of the extremities, left leg A

I70.303 Unspecified atherosclerosis of unspecified type of bypass graft(s) of the extremities, bilateral legs A

I70.308 Unspecified atherosclerosis of unspecified type of bypass graft(s) of the extremities, other extremity A

N Newborn: 0   P Pediatric: 0-17   M Maternity: 9-64   A Adult: 15-124   UNS Unspecified Site   MCC Major Complication/Comorbidity   CC Complication/Comorbidity   PE POA Exempt

684   ICD-10-CM 2025

I70.309 Unspecified atherosclerosis of unspecified type of bypass graft(s) of the extremities, unspecified extremity

✓6ᵗʰ **I70.31** Atherosclerosis of unspecified type of bypass graft(s) of the extremities with intermittent claudication

I70.311 Atherosclerosis of unspecified type of bypass graft(s) of the extremities with intermittent claudication, right leg   A

I70.312 Atherosclerosis of unspecified type of bypass graft(s) of the extremities with intermittent claudication, left leg   A

I70.313 Atherosclerosis of unspecified type of bypass graft(s) of the extremities with intermittent claudication, bilateral legs   A

I70.318 Atherosclerosis of unspecified type of bypass graft(s) of the extremities with intermittent claudication, other extremity   A

I70.319 Atherosclerosis of unspecified type of bypass graft(s) of the extremities with intermittent claudication, unspecified extremity   A

✓6ᵗʰ **I70.32** Atherosclerosis of unspecified type of bypass graft(s) of the extremities with rest pain

INCLUDES   any condition classifiable to I70.31-
chronic limb-threatening ischemia NOS of unspecified type of bypass graft(s) of the extremities
chronic limb-threatening ischemia of unspecified type of bypass graft(s) of the extremities with rest pain
critical limb ischemia NOS of unspecified type of bypass graft(s) of the extremities
critical limb ischemia of unspecified type of bypass graft(s) of the extremities with rest pain

I70.321 Atherosclerosis of unspecified type of bypass graft(s) of the extremities with rest pain, right leg   HCC A

I70.322 Atherosclerosis of unspecified type of bypass graft(s) of the extremities with rest pain, left leg   HCC A

I70.323 Atherosclerosis of unspecified type of bypass graft(s) of the extremities with rest pain, bilateral legs   HCC A

I70.328 Atherosclerosis of unspecified type of bypass graft(s) of the extremities with rest pain, other extremity   HCC A

I70.329 Atherosclerosis of unspecified type of bypass graft(s) of the extremities with rest pain, unspecified extremity   HCC A

✓6ᵗʰ **I70.33** Atherosclerosis of unspecified type of bypass graft(s) of the right leg with ulceration

INCLUDES   any condition classifiable to I70.311 and I70.321
chronic limb-threatening ischemia of unspecified type of bypass graft(s) of the right leg with ulceration
critical limb ischemia of unspecified type of bypass graft(s) of the right leg with ulceration

Use additional code to identify severity of ulcer (L97.-)

I70.331 Atherosclerosis of unspecified type of bypass graft(s) of the right leg with ulceration of thigh   CC HCC A

I70.332 Atherosclerosis of unspecified type of bypass graft(s) of the right leg with ulceration of calf   CC HCC A

I70.333 Atherosclerosis of unspecified type of bypass graft(s) of the right leg with ulceration of ankle   CC HCC A

I70.334 Atherosclerosis of unspecified type of bypass graft(s) of the right leg with ulceration of heel and midfoot   CC HCC A
Atherosclerosis of unspecified type of bypass graft(s) of right leg with ulceration of plantar surface of midfoot

I70.335 Atherosclerosis of unspecified type of bypass graft(s) of the right leg with ulceration of other part of foot   HCC A
Atherosclerosis of unspecified type of bypass graft(s) of the right leg with ulceration of toe

I70.338 Atherosclerosis of unspecified type of bypass graft(s) of the right leg with ulceration of other part of lower leg   CC HCC A

I70.339 Atherosclerosis of unspecified type of bypass graft(s) of the right leg with ulceration of unspecified site   CC HCC A

✓6ᵗʰ **I70.34** Atherosclerosis of unspecified type of bypass graft(s) of the left leg with ulceration

INCLUDES   any condition classifiable to I70.312 and I70.322
chronic limb-threatening ischemia of unspecified type of bypass graft(s) of the left leg with ulceration
critical limb ischemia of unspecified type of bypass graft(s) of the left leg with ulceration

Use additional code to identify severity of ulcer (L97.-)

I70.341 Atherosclerosis of unspecified type of bypass graft(s) of the left leg with ulceration of thigh   CC HCC A

I70.342 Atherosclerosis of unspecified type of bypass graft(s) of the left leg with ulceration of calf   CC HCC A

I70.343 Atherosclerosis of unspecified type of bypass graft(s) of the left leg with ulceration of ankle   CC HCC A

I70.344 Atherosclerosis of unspecified type of bypass graft(s) of the left leg with ulceration of heel and midfoot   CC HCC A
Atherosclerosis of unspecified type of bypass graft(s) of left leg with ulceration of plantar surface of midfoot

I70.345 Atherosclerosis of unspecified type of bypass graft(s) of the left leg with ulceration of other part of foot   HCC A
Atherosclerosis of unspecified type of bypass graft(s) of the left leg with ulceration of toe

I70.348 Atherosclerosis of unspecified type of bypass graft(s) of the left leg with ulceration of other part of lower leg   CC HCC A

I70.349 Atherosclerosis of unspecified type of bypass graft(s) of the left leg with ulceration of unspecified site   CC HCC A

I70.35 Atherosclerosis of unspecified type of bypass graft(s) of other extremity with ulceration   HCC A

INCLUDES   any condition classifiable to I70.318 and I70.328

Use additional code to identify severity of ulcer (L98.49-)

✓6ᵗʰ **I70.36** Atherosclerosis of unspecified type of bypass graft(s) of the extremities with gangrene

INCLUDES   any condition classifiable to I70.31-, I70.32-, I70.33-, I70.34-, I70.35
chronic limb-threatening ischemia of unspecified type of bypass graft(s) of the extremities with gangrene
critical limb ischemia of unspecified type of bypass graft(s) of the extremities with gangrene

Use additional code to identify the severity of any ulcer (L97.-, L98.49-), if applicable

I70.361 Atherosclerosis of unspecified type of bypass graft(s) of the extremities with gangrene, right leg   CC HCC

I70.362 Atherosclerosis of unspecified type of bypass graft(s) of the extremities with gangrene, left leg   CC HCC

I70.363 Atherosclerosis of unspecified type of bypass graft(s) of the extremities with gangrene, bilateral legs   CC HCC A

I70.368 Atherosclerosis of unspecified type of bypass graft(s) of the extremities with gangrene, other extremity   `CC` `HCC` `A`

I70.369 Atherosclerosis of unspecified type of bypass graft(s) of the extremities with gangrene, unspecified extremity   `CC` `UNS` `HCC` `A`

✓6ᵗʰ **I70.39** Other atherosclerosis of unspecified type of bypass graft(s) of the extremities

I70.391 Other atherosclerosis of unspecified type of bypass graft(s) of the extremities, right leg   `A`

I70.392 Other atherosclerosis of unspecified type of bypass graft(s) of the extremities, left leg   `A`

I70.393 Other atherosclerosis of unspecified type of bypass graft(s) of the extremities, bilateral legs   `A`

I70.398 Other atherosclerosis of unspecified type of bypass graft(s) of the extremities, other extremity   `A`

I70.399 Other atherosclerosis of unspecified type of bypass graft(s) of the extremities, unspecified extremity   `A`

✓5ᵗʰ **I70.4** Atherosclerosis of autologous vein bypass graft(s) of the extremities

Use additional code, if applicable, to identify chronic total occlusion of artery of extremity (I70.92)

AHA: 2020,4Q,98

✓6ᵗʰ **I70.40** Unspecified atherosclerosis of autologous vein bypass graft(s) of the extremities

I70.401 Unspecified atherosclerosis of autologous vein bypass graft(s) of the extremities, right leg   `A`

I70.402 Unspecified atherosclerosis of autologous vein bypass graft(s) of the extremities, left leg   `A`

I70.403 Unspecified atherosclerosis of autologous vein bypass graft(s) of the extremities, bilateral legs   `A`

I70.408 Unspecified atherosclerosis of autologous vein bypass graft(s) of the extremities, other extremity   `A`

I70.409 Unspecified atherosclerosis of autologous vein bypass graft(s) of the extremities, unspecified extremity   `A`

✓6ᵗʰ **I70.41** Atherosclerosis of autologous vein bypass graft(s) of the extremities with intermittent claudication

I70.411 Atherosclerosis of autologous vein bypass graft(s) of the extremities with intermittent claudication, right leg   `A`

I70.412 Atherosclerosis of autologous vein bypass graft(s) of the extremities with intermittent claudication, left leg   `A`

I70.413 Atherosclerosis of autologous vein bypass graft(s) of the extremities with intermittent claudication, bilateral legs   `A`

I70.418 Atherosclerosis of autologous vein bypass graft(s) of the extremities with intermittent claudication, other extremity   `A`

I70.419 Atherosclerosis of autologous vein bypass graft(s) of the extremities with intermittent claudication, unspecified extremity   `A`

✓6ᵗʰ **I70.42** Atherosclerosis of autologous vein bypass graft(s) of the extremities with rest pain

INCLUDES   any condition classifiable to I70.41-

chronic limb-threatening ischemia NOS of autologous vein bypass graft(s) of the extremities

chronic limb-threatening ischemia of autologous vein bypass graft(s) of the extremities with rest pain

critical limb ischemia NOS of autologous vein bypass graft(s) of the extremities

critical limb ischemia of autologous vein bypass graft(s) of the extremities with rest pain

I70.421 Atherosclerosis of autologous vein bypass graft(s) of the extremities with rest pain, right leg   `HCC` `A`

I70.422 Atherosclerosis of autologous vein bypass graft(s) of the extremities with rest pain, left leg   `HCC` `A`

I70.423 Atherosclerosis of autologous vein bypass graft(s) of the extremities with rest pain, bilateral legs   `HCC` `A`

I70.428 Atherosclerosis of autologous vein bypass graft(s) of the extremities with rest pain, other extremity   `HCC` `A`

I70.429 Atherosclerosis of autologous vein bypass graft(s) of the extremities with rest pain, unspecified extremity   `HCC` `A`

✓6ᵗʰ **I70.43** Atherosclerosis of autologous vein bypass graft(s) of the right leg with ulceration

INCLUDES   any condition classifiable to I70.411 and I70.421

chronic limb-threatening ischemia of autologous vein bypass graft(s) of the right leg with ulceration

critical limb ischemia of autologous vein bypass graft(s) of the right leg with ulceration

Use additional code to identify severity of ulcer (L97.-)

I70.431 Atherosclerosis of autologous vein bypass graft(s) of the right leg with ulceration of thigh   `CC` `HCC` `A`

I70.432 Atherosclerosis of autologous vein bypass graft(s) of the right leg with ulceration of calf   `CC` `HCC` `A`

I70.433 Atherosclerosis of autologous vein bypass graft(s) of the right leg with ulceration of ankle   `CC` `HCC` `A`

I70.434 Atherosclerosis of autologous vein bypass graft(s) of the right leg with ulceration of heel and midfoot   `CC` `HCC` `A`

Atherosclerosis of autologous vein bypass graft(s) of right leg with ulceration of plantar surface of midfoot

I70.435 Atherosclerosis of autologous vein bypass graft(s) of the right leg with ulceration of other part of foot   `HCC` `A`

Atherosclerosis of autologous vein bypass graft(s) of right leg with ulceration of toe

I70.438 Atherosclerosis of autologous vein bypass graft(s) of the right leg with ulceration of other part of lower leg   `CC` `HCC` `A`

I70.439 Atherosclerosis of autologous vein bypass graft(s) of the right leg with ulceration of unspecified site   `CC` `HCC` `A`

✓6ᵗʰ **I70.44** Atherosclerosis of autologous vein bypass graft(s) of the left leg with ulceration

INCLUDES   any condition classifiable to I70.412 and I70.422

chronic limb-threatening ischemia of autologous vein bypass graft(s) of the left leg with ulceration

critical limb ischemia of autologous vein bypass graft(s) of the left leg with ulceration

Use additional code to identify severity of ulcer (L97.-)

I70.441 Atherosclerosis of autologous vein bypass graft(s) of the left leg with ulceration of thigh   `CC` `HCC` `A`

`N` Newborn: 0   `P` Pediatric: 0-17   `M` Maternity: 9-64   `A` Adult: 15-124   `UNS` Unspecified Site   `MCC` Major Complication/Comorbidity   `CC` Complication/Comorbidity   `PE` POA Exempt

686   ICD-10-CM 2025

I70.442 **Atherosclerosis of autologous vein bypass graft(s) of the left leg with ulceration of calf** CC HCC A

I70.443 **Atherosclerosis of autologous vein bypass graft(s) of the left leg with ulceration of ankle** CC HCC A

I70.444 **Atherosclerosis of autologous vein bypass graft(s) of the left leg with ulceration of heel and midfoot** CC HCC A

Atherosclerosis of autologous vein bypass graft(s) of left leg with ulceration of plantar surface of midfoot

I70.445 **Atherosclerosis of autologous vein bypass graft(s) of the left leg with ulceration of other part of foot** HCC A

Atherosclerosis of autologous vein bypass graft(s) of left leg with ulceration of toe

I70.448 **Atherosclerosis of autologous vein bypass graft(s) of the left leg with ulceration of other part of lower leg** CC HCC A

I70.449 **Atherosclerosis of autologous vein bypass graft(s) of the left leg with ulceration of unspecified site** CC HCC A

I70.45 **Atherosclerosis of autologous vein bypass graft(s) of other extremity with ulceration** HCC A

INCLUDES any condition classifiable to I70.418, I70.428, and I70.438

Use additional code to identify severity of ulcer (L98.49)

✓6th **I70.46** **Atherosclerosis of autologous vein bypass graft(s) of the extremities with gangrene**

INCLUDES any condition classifiable to I70.41-, I70.42-, and I70.43-, I70.44-, I70.45

chronic limb-threatening ischemia of autologous vein bypass graft(s) of the extremities with gangrene

critical limb ischemia of autologous vein bypass graft(s) of the extremities with gangrene

Use additional code to identify the severity of any ulcer (L97.-, L98.49-), if applicable

I70.461 **Atherosclerosis of autologous vein bypass graft(s) of the extremities with gangrene, right leg** CC HCC A

I70.462 **Atherosclerosis of autologous vein bypass graft(s) of the extremities with gangrene, left leg** CC HCC A

I70.463 **Atherosclerosis of autologous vein bypass graft(s) of the extremities with gangrene, bilateral legs** CC HCC A

I70.468 **Atherosclerosis of autologous vein bypass graft(s) of the extremities with gangrene, other extremity** CC HCC A

I70.469 **Atherosclerosis of autologous vein bypass graft(s) of the extremities with gangrene, unspecified extremity** CC UMS HCC A

✓6th **I70.49** **Other atherosclerosis of autologous vein bypass graft(s) of the extremities**

I70.491 **Other atherosclerosis of autologous vein bypass graft(s) of the extremities, right leg** A

I70.492 **Other atherosclerosis of autologous vein bypass graft(s) of the extremities, left leg** A

I70.493 **Other atherosclerosis of autologous vein bypass graft(s) of the extremities, bilateral legs** A

I70.498 **Other atherosclerosis of autologous vein bypass graft(s) of the extremities, other extremity** A

I70.499 **Other atherosclerosis of autologous vein bypass graft(s) of the extremities, unspecified extremity** A

✓5th **I70.5** **Atherosclerosis of nonautologous biological bypass graft(s) of the extremities**

Use additional code, if applicable, to identify chronic total occlusion of artery of extremity (I70.92)

AHA: 2020,4Q,98

✓6th **I70.50** **Unspecified atherosclerosis of nonautologous biological bypass graft(s) of the extremities**

I70.501 **Unspecified atherosclerosis of nonautologous biological bypass graft(s) of the extremities, right leg** A

I70.502 **Unspecified atherosclerosis of nonautologous biological bypass graft(s) of the extremities, left leg** A

I70.503 **Unspecified atherosclerosis of nonautologous biological bypass graft(s) of the extremities, bilateral legs** A

I70.508 **Unspecified atherosclerosis of nonautologous biological bypass graft(s) of the extremities, other extremity** A

I70.509 **Unspecified atherosclerosis of nonautologous biological bypass graft(s) of the extremities, unspecified extremity** A

✓6th **I70.51** **Atherosclerosis of nonautologous biological bypass graft(s) of the extremities intermittent claudication**

I70.511 **Atherosclerosis of nonautologous biological bypass graft(s) of the extremities with intermittent claudication, right leg** A

I70.512 **Atherosclerosis of nonautologous biological bypass graft(s) of the extremities with intermittent claudication, left leg** A

I70.513 **Atherosclerosis of nonautologous biological bypass graft(s) of the extremities with intermittent claudication, bilateral legs** A

I70.518 **Atherosclerosis of nonautologous biological bypass graft(s) of the extremities with intermittent claudication, other extremity** A

I70.519 **Atherosclerosis of nonautologous biological bypass graft(s) of the extremities with intermittent claudication, unspecified extremity** A

✓6th **I70.52** **Atherosclerosis of nonautologous biological bypass graft(s) of the extremities with rest pain**

INCLUDES any condition classifiable to I70.51-

chronic limb-threatening ischemia NOS of nonautologous biological bypass graft(s) of the extremities

chronic limb-threatening ischemia of nonautologous biological bypass graft(s) of the extremities with rest pain

critical limb ischemia NOS of nonautologous biological bypass graft(s) of the extremities

critical limb ischemia of nonautologous biological bypass graft(s) of the extremities with rest pain

I70.521 **Atherosclerosis of nonautologous biological bypass graft(s) of the extremities with rest pain, right leg** HCC A

I70.522 **Atherosclerosis of nonautologous biological bypass graft(s) of the extremities with rest pain, left leg** HCC A

I70.523 **Atherosclerosis of nonautologous biological bypass graft(s) of the extremities with rest pain, bilateral legs** HCC A

I70.528 **Atherosclerosis of nonautologous biological bypass graft(s) of the extremities with rest pain, other extremity** HCC A

I70.529 **Atherosclerosis of nonautologous biological bypass graft(s) of the extremities with rest pain, unspecified extremity** HCC A

✓6th **I70.53** **Atherosclerosis of nonautologous biological bypass graft(s) of the right leg with ulceration**

INCLUDES any condition classifiable to I70.511 and I70.521

chronic limb-threatening ischemia of nonautologous biological bypass graft(s) of the right leg with ulceration

critical limb ischemia of nonautologous biological bypass graft(s) of the right leg with ulceration

Use additional code to identify severity of ulcer (L97.-)

I70.531 **Atherosclerosis of nonautologous biological bypass graft(s) of the right leg with ulceration of thigh** CC HCC A

✓ Additional Character Required   ✓x7th Placeholder   Questionable PDx   Manifestation   Unspecified   UPD Unacceptable PDx   H1-H14 HAC   HCC CMS-HCC Dx   HIV HIV Dx

ICD-10-CM 2025   687

I70.532   **Atherosclerosis of nonautologous biological bypass graft(s) of the right leg with ulceration of calf** `CC` `HCC` `A`

I70.533   **Atherosclerosis of nonautologous biological bypass graft(s) of the right leg with ulceration of ankle** `CC` `HCC` `A`

I70.534   **Atherosclerosis of nonautologous biological bypass graft(s) of the right leg with ulceration of heel and midfoot** `CC` `HCC` `A`
Atherosclerosis of nonautologous biological bypass graft(s) of right leg with ulceration of plantar surface of midfoot

I70.535   **Atherosclerosis of nonautologous biological bypass graft(s) of the right leg with ulceration of other part of foot** `HCC` `A`
Atherosclerosis of nonautologous biological bypass graft(s) of the right leg with ulceration of toe

I70.538   **Atherosclerosis of nonautologous biological bypass graft(s) of the right leg with ulceration of other part of lower leg** `CC` `HCC` `A`

I70.539   **Atherosclerosis of nonautologous biological bypass graft(s) of the right leg with ulceration of unspecified site** `CC` `HCC` `A`

✓6th   I70.54   **Atherosclerosis of nonautologous biological bypass graft(s) of the left leg with ulceration**
| INCLUDES | any condition classifiable to I70.512 and I70.522
chronic limb-threatening ischemia of nonautologous biological bypass graft(s) of the left leg with ulceration
critical limb ischemia of nonautologous biological bypass graft(s) of the left leg with ulceration

Use additional code to identify severity of ulcer (L97.-)

I70.541   **Atherosclerosis of nonautologous biological bypass graft(s) of the left leg with ulceration of thigh** `CC` `HCC` `A`

I70.542   **Atherosclerosis of nonautologous biological bypass graft(s) of the left leg with ulceration of calf** `CC` `HCC` `A`

I70.543   **Atherosclerosis of nonautologous biological bypass graft(s) of the left leg with ulceration of ankle** `CC` `HCC` `A`

I70.544   **Atherosclerosis of nonautologous biological bypass graft(s) of the left leg with ulceration of heel and midfoot** `CC` `HCC` `A`
Atherosclerosis of nonautologous biological bypass graft(s) of left leg with ulceration of plantar surface of midfoot

I70.545   **Atherosclerosis of nonautologous biological bypass graft(s) of the left leg with ulceration of other part of foot** `HCC` `A`
Atherosclerosis of nonautologous biological bypass graft(s) of the left leg with ulceration of toe

I70.548   **Atherosclerosis of nonautologous biological bypass graft(s) of the left leg with ulceration of other part of lower leg** `CC` `HCC` `A`

I70.549   **Atherosclerosis of nonautologous biological bypass graft(s) of the left leg with ulceration of unspecified site** `CC` `HCC` `A`

I70.55   **Atherosclerosis of nonautologous biological bypass graft(s) of other extremity with ulceration** `HCC` `A`
| INCLUDES | any condition classifiable to I70.518, I70.528, and I70.538
Use additional code to identify severity of ulcer (L98.49)

✓6th   I70.56   **Atherosclerosis of nonautologous biological bypass graft(s) of the extremities with gangrene**
| INCLUDES | any condition classifiable to I70.51-, I70.52-, and I70.53-, I70.54-, I70.55
chronic limb-threatening ischemia of nonautologous biological bypass graft(s) of the extremities with gangrene
critical limb ischemia of nonautologous biological bypass graft(s) of the extremities with gangrene

Use additional code to identify the severity of any ulcer (L97.-, L98.49-), if applicable

I70.561   **Atherosclerosis of nonautologous biological bypass graft(s) of the extremities with gangrene, right leg** `CC` `HCC` `A`

I70.562   **Atherosclerosis of nonautologous biological bypass graft(s) of the extremities with gangrene, left leg** `CC` `HCC` `A`

I70.563   **Atherosclerosis of nonautologous biological bypass graft(s) of the extremities with gangrene, bilateral legs** `CC` `HCC` `A`

I70.568   **Atherosclerosis of nonautologous biological bypass graft(s) of the extremities with gangrene, other extremity** `CC` `HCC` `A`

I70.569   **Atherosclerosis of nonautologous biological bypass graft(s) of the extremities with gangrene, unspecified extremity** `CC` `UNS` `HCC` `A`

✓6th   I70.59   **Other atherosclerosis of nonautologous biological bypass graft(s) of the extremities**

I70.591   **Other atherosclerosis of nonautologous biological bypass graft(s) of the extremities, right leg** `A`

I70.592   **Other atherosclerosis of nonautologous biological bypass graft(s) of the extremities, left leg** `A`

I70.593   **Other atherosclerosis of nonautologous biological bypass graft(s) of the extremities, bilateral legs** `A`

I70.598   **Other atherosclerosis of nonautologous biological bypass graft(s) of the extremities, other extremity** `A`

I70.599   **Other atherosclerosis of nonautologous biological bypass graft(s) of the extremities, unspecified extremity** `A`

✓5th   I70.6   **Atherosclerosis of nonbiological bypass graft(s) of the extremities**
Use additional code, if applicable, to identify chronic total occlusion of artery of extremity (I70.92)
AHA: 2020,4Q,98

✓6th   I70.60   **Unspecified atherosclerosis of nonbiological bypass graft(s) of the extremities**

I70.601   **Unspecified atherosclerosis of nonbiological bypass graft(s) of the extremities, right leg** `A`

I70.602   **Unspecified atherosclerosis of nonbiological bypass graft(s) of the extremities, left leg** `A`

I70.603   **Unspecified atherosclerosis of nonbiological bypass graft(s) of the extremities, bilateral legs** `A`

I70.608   **Unspecified atherosclerosis of nonbiological bypass graft(s) of the extremities, other extremity** `A`

I70.609   **Unspecified atherosclerosis of nonbiological bypass graft(s) of the extremities, unspecified extremity** `A`

✓6th   I70.61   **Atherosclerosis of nonbiological bypass graft(s) of the extremities with intermittent claudication**

I70.611   **Atherosclerosis of nonbiological bypass graft(s) of the extremities with intermittent claudication, right leg** `A`

I70.612   **Atherosclerosis of nonbiological bypass graft(s) of the extremities with intermittent claudication, left leg** `A`

I70.613   **Atherosclerosis of nonbiological bypass graft(s) of the extremities with intermittent claudication, bilateral legs** `A`

`N` Newborn: 0   `P` Pediatric: 0-17   `M` Maternity: 9-64   `A` Adult: 15-124   `UNS` Unspecified Site   `MCC` Major Complication/Comorbidity   `CC` Complication/Comorbidity   `PE` POA Exempt

688   ICD-10-CM 2025

I70.618 Atherosclerosis of nonbiological bypass graft(s) of the extremities with intermittent claudication, other extremity `A`

I70.619 Atherosclerosis of nonbiological bypass graft(s) of the extremities with intermittent claudication, unspecified extremity `A`

✓6ᵗʰ **I70.62 Atherosclerosis of nonbiological bypass graft(s) of the extremities with rest pain**

INCLUDES   any condition classifiable to I70.61-
chronic limb-threatening ischemia NOS of nonbiological bypass graft(s) of the extremities
chronic limb-threatening ischemia of nonbiological bypass graft(s) of the extremities with rest pain
critical limb ischemia NOS of nonbiological bypass graft(s) of the extremities
critical limb ischemia of nonbiological bypass graft(s) of the extremities with rest pain

I70.621 Atherosclerosis of nonbiological bypass graft(s) of the extremities with rest pain, right leg `HCC` `A`

I70.622 Atherosclerosis of nonbiological bypass graft(s) of the extremities with rest pain, left leg `HCC` `A`

I70.623 Atherosclerosis of nonbiological bypass graft(s) of the extremities with rest pain, bilateral legs `HCC` `A`

I70.628 Atherosclerosis of nonbiological bypass graft(s) of the extremities with rest pain, other extremity `HCC` `A`

I70.629 Atherosclerosis of nonbiological bypass graft(s) of the extremities with rest pain, unspecified extremity `HCC` `A`

✓6ᵗʰ **I70.63 Atherosclerosis of nonbiological bypass graft(s) of the right leg with ulceration**

INCLUDES   any condition classifiable to I70.611 and I70.621
chronic limb-threatening ischemia of nonbiological bypass graft(s) of the right leg with ulceration
critical limb ischemia of nonbiological bypass graft(s) of the right leg with ulceration

Use additional code to identify severity of ulcer (L97.-)

I70.631 Atherosclerosis of nonbiological bypass graft(s) of the right leg with ulceration of thigh `CC` `HCC` `A`

I70.632 Atherosclerosis of nonbiological bypass graft(s) of the right leg with ulceration of calf `CC` `HCC` `A`

I70.633 Atherosclerosis of nonbiological bypass graft(s) of the right leg with ulceration of ankle `CC` `HCC` `A`

I70.634 Atherosclerosis of nonbiological bypass graft(s) of the right leg with ulceration of heel and midfoot `CC` `HCC` `A`
Atherosclerosis of nonbiological bypass graft(s) of right leg with ulceration of plantar surface of midfoot

I70.635 Atherosclerosis of nonbiological bypass graft(s) of the right leg with ulceration of other part of foot `HCC` `A`
Atherosclerosis of nonbiological bypass graft(s) of the right leg with ulceration of toe

I70.638 Atherosclerosis of nonbiological bypass graft(s) of the right leg with ulceration of other part of lower leg `CC` `HCC` `A`

I70.639 Atherosclerosis of nonbiological bypass graft(s) of the right leg with ulceration of unspecified site `CC` `HCC` `A`

✓6ᵗʰ **I70.64 Atherosclerosis of nonbiological bypass graft(s) of the left leg with ulceration**

INCLUDES   any condition classifiable to I70.612 and I70.622
chronic limb-threatening ischemia of nonbiological bypass graft(s) of the left leg with ulceration
critical limb ischemia of nonbiological bypass graft(s) of the left leg with ulceration

Use additional code to identify severity of ulcer (L97.-)

I70.641 Atherosclerosis of nonbiological bypass graft(s) of the left leg with ulceration of thigh `CC` `HCC` `A`

I70.642 Atherosclerosis of nonbiological bypass graft(s) of the left leg with ulceration of calf `CC` `HCC` `A`

I70.643 Atherosclerosis of nonbiological bypass graft(s) of the left leg with ulceration of ankle `CC` `HCC` `A`

I70.644 Atherosclerosis of nonbiological bypass graft(s) of the left leg with ulceration of heel and midfoot `CC` `HCC` `A`
Atherosclerosis of nonbiological bypass graft(s) of left leg with ulceration of plantar surface of midfoot

I70.645 Atherosclerosis of nonbiological bypass graft(s) of the left leg with ulceration of other part of foot `HCC` `A`
Atherosclerosis of nonbiological bypass graft(s) of the left leg with ulceration of toe

I70.648 Atherosclerosis of nonbiological bypass graft(s) of the left leg with ulceration of other part of lower leg `CC` `HCC` `A`

I70.649 Atherosclerosis of nonbiological bypass graft(s) of the left leg with ulceration of unspecified site `CC` `HCC` `A`

I70.65 Atherosclerosis of nonbiological bypass graft(s) of other extremity with ulceration `HCC` `A`

INCLUDES   any condition classifiable to I70.618 and I70.628

Use additional code to identify severity of ulcer (L98.49)

✓6ᵗʰ **I70.66 Atherosclerosis of nonbiological bypass graft(s) of the extremities with gangrene**

INCLUDES   any condition classifiable to I70.61-, I70.62-, I70.63-, I70.64-, I70.65
chronic limb-threatening ischemia of nonbiological bypass graft(s) of the extremities with gangrene
critical limb ischemia of nonbiological bypass graft(s) of the extremities with gangrene

Use additional code to identify the severity of any ulcer (L97.-, L98.49-), if applicable

I70.661 Atherosclerosis of nonbiological bypass graft(s) of the extremities with gangrene, right leg `CC` `HCC` `A`

I70.662 Atherosclerosis of nonbiological bypass graft(s) of the extremities with gangrene, left leg `CC` `HCC` `A`

I70.663 Atherosclerosis of nonbiological bypass graft(s) of the extremities with gangrene, bilateral legs `CC` `HCC` `A`

I70.668 Atherosclerosis of nonbiological bypass graft(s) of the extremities with gangrene, other extremity `CC` `HCC` `A`

I70.669 Atherosclerosis of nonbiological bypass graft(s) of the extremities with gangrene, unspecified extremity `CC` `UNS` `HCC` `A`

✓6ᵗʰ **I70.69 Other atherosclerosis of nonbiological bypass graft(s) of the extremities**

I70.691 Other atherosclerosis of nonbiological bypass graft(s) of the extremities, right leg `A`

I70.692 Other atherosclerosis of nonbiological bypass graft(s) of the extremities, left leg `A`

I70.693 Other atherosclerosis of nonbiological bypass graft(s) of the extremities, bilateral legs `A`

 Additional Character Required   ✓x7ᵗʰ Placeholder   Questionable PDx   Manifestation   Unspecified   UPD Unacceptable PDx   H1-H14 HAC   HCC CMS-HCC Dx   HIV HIV Dx

ICD-10-CM 2025   689

      I70.698   **Other atherosclerosis of nonbiological bypass graft(s) of the extremities, other extremity** A

      I70.699   **Other atherosclerosis of nonbiological bypass graft(s) of the extremities, unspecified extremity** A

√5th   **I70.7**   **Atherosclerosis of other type of bypass graft(s) of the extremities**
     Use additional code, if applicable, to identify chronic total occlusion of artery of extremity (I70.92)
     AHA: 2020,4Q,98

√6th   **I70.70**   **Unspecified atherosclerosis of other type of bypass graft(s) of the extremities**

      I70.701   **Unspecified atherosclerosis of other type of bypass graft(s) of the extremities, right leg** A

      I70.702   **Unspecified atherosclerosis of other type of bypass graft(s) of the extremities, left leg** A

      I70.703   **Unspecified atherosclerosis of other type of bypass graft(s) of the extremities, bilateral legs** A

      I70.708   **Unspecified atherosclerosis of other type of bypass graft(s) of the extremities, other extremity** A

      I70.709   **Unspecified atherosclerosis of other type of bypass graft(s) of the extremities, unspecified extremity** A

√6th   **I70.71**   **Atherosclerosis of other type of bypass graft(s) of the extremities with intermittent claudication**

      I70.711   **Atherosclerosis of other type of bypass graft(s) of the extremities with intermittent claudication, right leg** A

      I70.712   **Atherosclerosis of other type of bypass graft(s) of the extremities with intermittent claudication, left leg** A

      I70.713   **Atherosclerosis of other type of bypass graft(s) of the extremities with intermittent claudication, bilateral legs** A

      I70.718   **Atherosclerosis of other type of bypass graft(s) of the extremities with intermittent claudication, other extremity** A

      I70.719   **Atherosclerosis of other type of bypass graft(s) of the extremities with intermittent claudication, unspecified extremity** A

√6th   **I70.72**   **Atherosclerosis of other type of bypass graft(s) of the extremities with rest pain**
     INCLUDES   any condition classifiable to I70.71-
       chronic limb-threatening ischemia NOS of other type of bypass graft(s) of the extremities
       chronic limb-threatening ischemia of other type of bypass graft(s) of the extremities with rest pain
       critical limb ischemia NOS of other type of bypass graft(s) of the extremities
       critical limb ischemia of other type of bypass graft(s) of the extremities with rest pain

      I70.721   **Atherosclerosis of other type of bypass graft(s) of the extremities with rest pain, right leg** HCC A

      I70.722   **Atherosclerosis of other type of bypass graft(s) of the extremities with rest pain, left leg** HCC A

      I70.723   **Atherosclerosis of other type of bypass graft(s) of the extremities with rest pain, bilateral legs** HCC A

      I70.728   **Atherosclerosis of other type of bypass graft(s) of the extremities with rest pain, other extremity** HCC A

      I70.729   **Atherosclerosis of other type of bypass graft(s) of the extremities with rest pain, unspecified extremity** HCC A

√6th   **I70.73**   **Atherosclerosis of other type of bypass graft(s) of the right leg with ulceration**
     INCLUDES   any condition classifiable to I70.711 and I70.721
       chronic limb-threatening ischemia of other type of bypass graft(s) of the right leg with ulceration
       critical limb ischemia of other type of bypass graft(s) of the right leg with ulceration
     Use additional code to identify severity of ulcer (L97.-)

      I70.731   **Atherosclerosis of other type of bypass graft(s) of the right leg with ulceration of thigh** CC HCC

      I70.732   **Atherosclerosis of other type of bypass graft(s) of the right leg with ulceration of calf** CC HCC A

      I70.733   **Atherosclerosis of other type of bypass graft(s) of the right leg with ulceration of ankle** CC HCC A

      I70.734   **Atherosclerosis of other type of bypass graft(s) of the right leg with ulceration of heel and midfoot** CC HCC A
       Atherosclerosis of other type of bypass graft(s) of right leg with ulceration of plantar surface of midfoot

      I70.735   **Atherosclerosis of other type of bypass graft(s) of the right leg with ulceration of other part of foot** HCC A
       Atherosclerosis of other type of bypass graft(s) of right leg with ulceration of toe

      I70.738   **Atherosclerosis of other type of bypass graft(s) of the right leg with ulceration of other part of lower leg** CC HCC A

      I70.739   **Atherosclerosis of other type of bypass graft(s) of the right leg with ulceration of unspecified site** CC HCC A

√6th   **I70.74**   **Atherosclerosis of other type of bypass graft(s) of the left leg with ulceration**
     INCLUDES   any condition classifiable to I70.712 and I70.722
       chronic limb-threatening ischemia of other type of bypass graft(s) of the left leg with ulceration
       critical limb ischemia of other type of bypass graft(s) of the left leg with ulceration
     Use additional code to identify severity of ulcer (L97.-)

      I70.741   **Atherosclerosis of other type of bypass graft(s) of the left leg with ulceration of thigh** CC HCC A

      I70.742   **Atherosclerosis of other type of bypass graft(s) of the left leg with ulceration of calf** CC HCC A

      I70.743   **Atherosclerosis of other type of bypass graft(s) of the left leg with ulceration of ankle** CC HCC A

      I70.744   **Atherosclerosis of other type of bypass graft(s) of the left leg with ulceration of heel and midfoot** CC HCC A
       Atherosclerosis of other type of bypass graft(s) of left leg with ulceration of plantar surface of midfoot

      I70.745   **Atherosclerosis of other type of bypass graft(s) of the left leg with ulceration of other part of foot** HCC A
       Atherosclerosis of other type of bypass graft(s) of left leg with ulceration of toe

      I70.748   **Atherosclerosis of other type of bypass graft(s) of the left leg with ulceration of other part of lower leg** CC HCC A

      I70.749   **Atherosclerosis of other type of bypass graft(s) of the left leg with ulceration of unspecified site** CC HCC A

     I70.75   **Atherosclerosis of other type of bypass graft(s) of other extremity with ulceration** HCC A
     INCLUDES   any condition classifiable to I70.718 and I70.728
     Use additional code to identify severity of ulcer (L98.49)

✓6th I70.76 Atherosclerosis of other type of bypass graft(s) of the extremities with **gangrene**

  INCLUDES any condition classifiable to I70.71-, I70.72-, I70.73-, I70.74-, I70.75 chronic limb-threatening ischemia of other type of bypass graft(s) of the extremities with gangrene critical limb ischemia of other type of bypass graft(s) of the extremities with gangrene

  Use additional code to identify the severity of any ulcer (L97.-, L98.49-), if applicable

  I70.761 Atherosclerosis of other type of bypass graft(s) of the extremities with gangrene, **right leg** CC HCC A

  I70.762 Atherosclerosis of other type of bypass graft(s) of the extremities with gangrene, **left leg** CC HCC A

  I70.763 Atherosclerosis of other type of bypass graft(s) of the extremities with gangrene, **bilateral legs** CC HCC A

  I70.768 Atherosclerosis of other type of bypass graft(s) of the extremities with gangrene, **other extremity** CC HCC A

  I70.769 Atherosclerosis of other type of bypass graft(s) of the extremities with gangrene, **unspecified extremity** CC UNS HCC A

✓6th I70.79 Other atherosclerosis of other type of bypass graft(s) of the extremities

  I70.791 Other atherosclerosis of other type of bypass graft(s) of the extremities, **right leg** A

  I70.792 Other atherosclerosis of other type of bypass graft(s) of the extremities, **left leg** A

  I70.793 Other atherosclerosis of other type of bypass graft(s) of the extremities, **bilateral legs** A

  I70.798 Other atherosclerosis of other type of bypass graft(s) of the extremities, **other extremity** A

  I70.799 Other atherosclerosis of other type of bypass graft(s) of the extremities, **unspecified extremity** A

I70.8 Atherosclerosis of other arteries A

  TIP: Arteriosclerosis of the iliac arteries is coded here.

✓5th I70.9 Other and unspecified atherosclerosis

  I70.90 Unspecified atherosclerosis A

  I70.91 **Generalized** atherosclerosis A

  I70.92 **Chronic total occlusion** of artery of the extremities CC UPD A

    Complete occlusion of artery of the extremities
    Total occlusion of artery of the extremities
    Code first atherosclerosis of arteries of the extremities (I70.2-, I70.3-, I70.4-, I70.5-, I70.6-, I70.7-)

✓4th I71 Aortic aneurysm and dissection

  Code first, if applicable:
    syphilitic aortic aneurysm (A52.01)
    traumatic aortic aneurysm (S25.09, S35.09)

  AHA: 2022,4Q,24-26

  TIP: A diagnosis of dissecting aneurysm should be coded to subcategory I71.0 only. The bulging/aneurysm, although present, occurred secondary to the dissection. The dissection represents the most significant problem.

✓5th I71.0 **Dissection of aorta**

  I71.00 Dissection of unspecified site of aorta MCC HCC

  ✓6th I71.01 Dissection of **thoracic** aorta

    AHA: AHA:2024,2Q,17

    I71.010 Dissection of **ascending** aorta MCC HCC

    I71.011 Dissection of **aortic arch** MCC HCC

    I71.012 Dissection of **descending** thoracic aorta MCC HCC

    I71.019 Dissection of thoracic aorta, unspecified MCC HCC

  I71.02 Dissection of **abdominal** aorta MCC HCC

  I71.03 Dissection of **thoracoabdominal** aorta MCC HCC

✓5th I71.1 **Thoracic** aortic aneurysm, **ruptured**

  I71.10 Thoracic aortic aneurysm, ruptured, unspecified MCC HCC

  I71.11 Aneurysm of the **ascending** aorta, ruptured MCC HCC

  I71.12 Aneurysm of the **aortic arch**, ruptured MCC HCC

  I71.13 Aneurysm of the **descending** thoracic aorta, ruptured MCC HCC

✓5th I71.2 **Thoracic** aortic aneurysm, **without rupture**

  I71.20 Thoracic aortic aneurysm, without rupture, unspecified

  I71.21 Aneurysm of the **ascending** aorta, without rupture

  I71.22 Aneurysm of the **aortic arch**, without rupture

  I71.23 Aneurysm of the **descending** thoracic aorta, without rupture

✓5th I71.3 **Abdominal** aortic aneurysm, **ruptured**

  I71.30 Abdominal aortic aneurysm, ruptured, unspecified MCC HCC

  I71.31 **Pararenal** abdominal aortic aneurysm, ruptured MCC HCC

  I71.32 **Juxtarenal** abdominal aortic aneurysm, ruptured MCC HCC

  I71.33 **Infrarenal** abdominal aortic aneurysm, ruptured MCC HCC

✓5th I71.4 **Abdominal** aortic aneurysm, **without rupture**

  I71.40 Abdominal aortic aneurysm, without rupture, unspecified

  I71.41 **Pararenal** abdominal aortic aneurysm, without rupture

    AHA: AHA:2024,2Q,16

  I71.42 **Juxtarenal** abdominal aortic aneurysm, without rupture

  I71.43 **Infrarenal** abdominal aortic aneurysm, without rupture

✓5th I71.5 **Thoracoabdominal** aortic aneurysm, **ruptured**

  I71.50 Thoracoabdominal aortic aneurysm, ruptured, unspecified MCC HCC

  I71.51 **Supraceliac** aneurysm of the thoracoabdominal aorta, ruptured MCC HCC

  I71.52 **Paravisceral** aneurysm of the thoracoabdominal aorta, ruptured MCC HCC

✓5th I71.6 **Thoracoabdominal** aortic aneurysm, **without rupture**

  I71.60 Thoracoabdominal aortic aneurysm, without rupture, unspecified

  I71.61 **Supraceliac** aneurysm of the thoracoabdominal aorta, without rupture

  I71.62 **Paravisceral** aneurysm of the thoracoabdominal aorta, without rupture

I71.8 Aortic aneurysm of unspecified site, **ruptured** MCC HCC

    Rupture of aorta NOS

I71.9 Aortic aneurysm of unspecified site, **without rupture**

    Aneurysm of aorta
    Dilatation of aorta
    Hyaline necrosis of aorta

✔ Additional Character Required   ✓x7th Placeholder   Questionable PDx   Manifestation   Unspecified   UPD Unacceptable PDx   H1-H14 HAC   HCC CMS-HCC Dx   HIV HIV Dx

✓4ᵗʰ I72   Other aneurysm

INCLUDES   aneurysm (cirsoid) (false) (ruptured)
EXCLUDES 2   *acquired aneurysm (I77.0)*
aneurysm (of) aorta (I71.-)
aneurysm (of) arteriovenous NOS (Q27.3-)
carotid artery dissection (I77.71)
cerebral (nonruptured) aneurysm (I67.1)
coronary aneurysm (I25.4)
coronary artery dissection (I25.42)
dissection of artery NEC (I77.79)
dissection of precerebral artery, congenital (nonruptured) (Q28.1)
heart aneurysm (I25.3)
iliac artery dissection (I77.72)
precerebral artery, congential (nonruptured) (Q28.1)
pulmonary artery aneurysm (I28.1)
renal artery dissection (I77.73)
retinal aneurysm (H35.0)
ruptured cerebral aneurysm (I60.7)
varicose aneurysm (I77.0)
vertebral artery dissection (I77.74)

AHA: 2016,4Q,28-29

I72.0   Aneurysm of carotid artery
Aneurysm of common carotid artery
Aneurysm of external carotid artery
Aneurysm of internal carotid artery, extracranial portion
EXCLUDES 1   *aneurysm of internal carotid artery, intracranial portion (I67.1)*
aneurysm of internal carotid artery NOS (I67.1)

I72.1   Aneurysm of artery of upper extremity

I72.2   Aneurysm of renal artery

I72.3   Aneurysm of iliac artery

I72.4   Aneurysm of artery of lower extremity
AHA: 2019,2Q,21

I72.5   Aneurysm of other precerebral arteries
Aneurysm of basilar artery (trunk)
EXCLUDES 2   *aneurysm of carotid artery (I72.0)*
aneurysm of vertebral artery (I72.6)
dissection of carotid artery (I77.71)
dissection of other precerebral arteries (I77.75)
dissection of vertebral artery (I77.74)

I72.6   Aneurysm of vertebral artery
EXCLUDES 2   *dissection of vertebral artery (I77.74)*

I72.8   Aneurysm of other specified arteries

I72.9   Aneurysm of unspecified site

Aneurysm

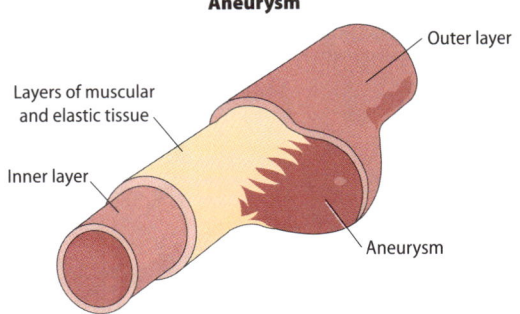

Outer layer

Layers of muscular and elastic tissue

Inner layer

Aneurysm

✓4ᵗʰ I73   Other peripheral vascular diseases

EXCLUDES 2   *chilblains (T69.1)*
frostbite (T33-T34)
immersion hand or foot (T69.0-)
spasm of cerebral artery (G45.9)

AHA: 2018,4Q,87

✓5ᵗʰ I73.0   Raynaud's syndrome
Raynaud's disease
Raynaud's phenomenon (secondary)
DEF: Constriction of the arteries of the digits caused by cold or by nerve or arterial damage and can be prompted by stress or emotion. Blood cannot reach the skin and soft tissues and the skin turns white with blue mottling.

I73.00   Raynaud's syndrome without gangrene

I73.01   Raynaud's syndrome with gangrene   CC HCC

I73.1   Thromboangiitis obliterans [Buerger's disease]
DEF: Inflammatory disease of the extremity blood vessels, mainly the lower blood vessels. This disease is associated with heavy tobacco use. The arteries are more affected than veins. It occurs primarily in young men and leads to tissue ischemia and gangrene.

✓5ᵗʰ I73.8   Other specified peripheral vascular diseases
EXCLUDES 1   *diabetic (peripheral) angiopathy (E08-E13 with .51-.52)*

I73.81   Erythromelalgia

I73.89   Other specified peripheral vascular diseases
Acrocyanosis
Erythrocyanosis
Simple acroparesthesia [Schultze's type]
Vasomotor acroparesthesia [Nothnagel's type]

I73.9   Peripheral vascular disease, unspecified
Intermittent claudication
Peripheral angiopathy NOS
Spasm of artery
EXCLUDES 1   *atherosclerosis of the extremities (I70.2-I70.7-)*
AHA: 2018,2Q,7

✓4ᵗʰ I74   Arterial embolism and thrombosis

INCLUDES   embolic infarction
embolic occlusion
thrombotic infarction
thrombotic occlusion

Code first:
  embolism and thrombosis complicating abortion or ectopic or molar pregnancy (O00-O07, O08.2)
  embolism and thrombosis complicating pregnancy, childbirth and the puerperium (O88.-)
EXCLUDES 2   *atheroembolism (I75.-)*
basilar embolism and thrombosis (I63.0-I63.2, I65.1)
carotid embolism and thrombosis (I63.0-I63.2, I65.2)
cerebral embolism and thrombosis (I63.3-I63.5, I66.-)
coronary embolism and thrombosis (I21-I25)
mesenteric embolism and thrombosis (K55.0-)
ophthalmic embolism and thrombosis (H34.-)
precerebral embolism and thrombosis NOS (I63.0-I63.2, I65.9)
pulmonary embolism and thrombosis (I26.-)
renal embolism and thrombosis (N28.0)
retinal embolism and thrombosis (H34.-)
septic embolism and thrombosis (I76)
vertebral embolism and thrombosis (I63.0-I63.2, I65.0)

AHA: 2023,2Q,7

✓5ᵗʰ I74.0   Embolism and thrombosis of abdominal aorta

I74.01   Saddle embolus of abdominal aorta   MCC HCC

I74.09   Other arterial embolism and thrombosis of abdominal aorta   CC HCC
Aortic bifurcation syndrome
Aortoiliac obstruction
Leriche's syndrome

✓5ᵗʰ I74.1   Embolism and thrombosis of other and unspecified parts of aorta

I74.10   Embolism and thrombosis of unspecified parts of aorta   CC HCC

I74.11   Embolism and thrombosis of thoracic aorta   CC HCC

I74.19   Embolism and thrombosis of other parts of aorta   CC HCC

I74.2   Embolism and thrombosis of arteries of the upper extremities   CC HCC

I74.3   Embolism and thrombosis of arteries of the lower extremities   CC HCC

I74.4   Embolism and thrombosis of arteries of extremities, unspecified   CC HCC
Peripheral arterial embolism NOS

I74.5   Embolism and thrombosis of iliac artery   CC HCC

I74.8   Embolism and thrombosis of other arteries   CC HCC

I74.9   Embolism and thrombosis of unspecified artery   CC HCC

✓4ᵗʰ I75   Atheroembolism

INCLUDES   atherothrombotic microembolism
cholesterol embolism

✓5ᵗʰ I75.0   Atheroembolism of extremities

✓6ᵗʰ I75.01   Atheroembolism of upper extremity

I75.011   Atheroembolism of right upper extremity   CC HCC

N Newborn: 0   P Pediatric: 0-17   M Maternity: 9-64   A Adult: 15-124   UNS Unspecified Site   MCC Major Complication/Comorbidity   CC Complication/Comorbidity   PE POA Exempt

692   ICD-10-CM 2025

I75.012 Atheroembolism of **left** upper extremity `CC` `HCC`

I75.013 Atheroembolism of **bilateral** upper extremities `CC` `HCC`

I75.019 Atheroembolism of unspecified upper extremity `CC` `UNS` `HCC`

✓6th **I75.02** Atheroembolism of **lower** extremity

I75.021 Atheroembolism of **right** lower extremity `CC` `HCC`

I75.022 Atheroembolism of **left** lower extremity `CC` `HCC`

I75.023 Atheroembolism of **bilateral** lower extremities `CC` `HCC`

I75.029 Atheroembolism of unspecified lower extremity `CC` `UNS` `HCC`

✓5th **I75.8** Atheroembolism of other sites

I75.81 Atheroembolism of **kidney** `CC` `HCC`

Use additional code for any associated acute kidney failure and chronic kidney disease (N17.-, N18.-)

I75.89 Atheroembolism of other site `CC` `HCC`

I76 Septic arterial embolism `CC` `UPD` `HCC`

Code first underlying infection, such as:
infective endocarditis (I33.0)
lung abscess (J85.-)
Use additional code to identify the site of the embolism (I74.-)

EXCLUDES 2   septic pulmonary embolism (I26.01, I26.90)

✓4th **I77 Other disorders of arteries and arterioles**

EXCLUDES 2   collagen (vascular) diseases (M30-M36)
hypersensitivity angiitis (M31.0)
pulmonary artery (I28.-)

I77.0 Arteriovenous fistula, acquired
Aneurysmal varix
Arteriovenous aneurysm, acquired

EXCLUDES 1   arteriovenous aneurysm NOS (Q27.3-)
presence of arteriovenous shunt (fistula) for dialysis (Z99.2)
traumatic - see injury of blood vessel by body region

EXCLUDES 2   cerebral (I67.1)
coronary (I25.4)

DEF: Communication between an artery and vein caused by trauma or invasive procedures.

I77.1 Stricture of artery
Narrowing of artery
AHA: 2021,3Q,12

I77.2 Rupture of artery `CC`
Erosion of artery
Fistula of artery
Ulcer of artery

EXCLUDES 1   traumatic rupture of artery - see injury of blood vessel by body region

I77.3 Arterial fibromuscular dysplasia
Fibromuscular hyperplasia (of) carotid artery
Fibromuscular hyperplasia (of) renal artery

I77.4 Celiac artery compression syndrome `CC`
AHA: 2021,3Q,12

I77.5 Necrosis of artery `CC`

I77.6 Arteritis, unspecified
Aortitis NOS
Endarteritis NOS

EXCLUDES 1   arteritis or endarteritis:
aortic arch (M31.4)
cerebral NEC (I67.7)
coronary (I25.89)
deformans (I70.-)
giant cell (M31.5, M31.6)
obliterans (I70.-)
senile (I70.-)

✓5th **I77.7 Other arterial dissection**

EXCLUDES 2   dissection of aorta (I71.0-)
dissection of coronary artery (I25.42)
AHA: 2016,4Q,28-29

I77.70 Dissection of unspecified artery `MCC`

I77.71 Dissection of **carotid** artery `MCC`

I77.72 Dissection of **iliac** artery `MCC`

I77.73 Dissection of **renal** artery `MCC`

I77.74 Dissection of **vertebral** artery `MCC`

EXCLUDES 2   aneurysm of vertebral artery (I72.6)
AHA: 2024,1Q,26

I77.75 Dissection of other precerebral arteries `MCC`
Dissection of basilar artery (trunk)

EXCLUDES 2   aneurysm of carotid artery (I72.0)
aneurysm of other precerebral arteries (I72.5)
aneurysm of vertebral artery (I72.6)
dissection of carotid artery (I77.71)
dissection of vertebral artery (I77.74)

I77.76 Dissection of artery of **upper extremity** `MCC`

I77.77 Dissection of artery of **lower extremity** `MCC`

I77.79 Dissection of other specified artery `MCC`

✓5th **I77.8 Other specified disorders of arteries and arterioles**

✓6th **I77.81 Aortic ectasia**
Ectasis aorta

EXCLUDES 1   aortic aneurysm and dissection (I71.-)

I77.810 **Thoracic** aortic ectasia

I77.811 **Abdominal** aortic ectasia

I77.812 **Thoracoabdominal** aortic ectasia

I77.819 Aortic ectasia, unspecified site

I77.82 Antineutrophilic cytoplasmic antibody [ANCA] vasculitis `HCC`
ANCA associated vasculitis
ANCA positive vasculitis

EXCLUDES 2   eosinophilic granulomatosis with polyangiitis (M30.1)
granulomatosis with polyangiitis (M31.3-)
microscopic polyangiitis (M31.7)

AHA: 2022,4Q,26-27

I77.89 Other specified disorders of arteries and arterioles
AHA: 2021,1Q,23

I77.9 Disorder of arteries and arterioles, unspecified
AHA: 2021,1Q,4; 2018,2Q,7

✓4th **I78 Diseases of capillaries**

I78.0 Hereditary hemorrhagic telangiectasia
Rendu-Osler-Weber disease

I78.1 Nevus, non-neoplastic
Araneus nevus
Senile nevus
Spider nevus
Stellar nevus

EXCLUDES 1   nevus NOS (D22.-)
vascular NOS (Q82.5)

EXCLUDES 2   blue nevus (D22.-)
flammeus nevus (Q82.5)
hairy nevus (D22.-)
melanocytic nevus (D22.-)
pigmented nevus (D22.-)
portwine nevus (Q82.5)
sanguineous nevus (Q82.5)
strawberry nevus (Q82.5)
verrucous nevus (Q82.5)

AHA: 2019,1Q,21

I78.8 Other diseases of capillaries

I78.9 Disease of capillaries, unspecified

✓4th **I79 Disorders of arteries, arterioles and capillaries in diseases classified elsewhere**

I79.0 *Aneurysm of aorta in diseases classified elsewhere*
Code first underlying disease

EXCLUDES 1   syphilitic aneurysm (A52.01)

I79.1 *Aortitis in diseases classified elsewhere*
Code first underlying disease

EXCLUDES 1   syphilitic aortitis (A52.02)

I79.8 *Other disorders of arteries, arterioles and capillaries in diseases classified elsewhere*
Code first underlying disease, such as:
amyloidosis (E85.-)

EXCLUDES 1   diabetic (peripheral) angiopathy (E08-E13 with .51-.52)
syphilitic endarteritis (A52.09)
tuberculous endarteritis (A18.89)

| ✓ Additional Character Required | ✓x 7th Placeholder | Questionable PDx | Manifestation | Unspecified | UPD Unacceptable PDx | H1-H4 HAC | HCC CMS-HCC Dx | HIV HIV Dx |

ICD-10-CM 2025

693

Diseases of veins, lymphatic vessels and lymph nodes, not elsewhere classified (I80-I89)

✓4th I80 Phlebitis and thrombophlebitis

INCLUDES   endophlebitis
inflammation, vein
periphlebitis
suppurative phlebitis

Code first:
phlebitis and thrombophlebitis complicating abortion, ectopic or molar pregnancy (O00-O07, O08.7)
phlebitis and thrombophlebitis complicating pregnancy, childbirth and the puerperium (O22.-, O87.-)

EXCLUDES 1   venous embolism and thrombosis of lower extremities (I82.4-, I82.5-, I82.81-)

✓5th I80.0 Phlebitis and thrombophlebitis of superficial vessels of lower extremities
Phlebitis and thrombophlebitis of femoropopliteal vein

I80.00   Phlebitis and thrombophlebitis of superficial vessels of unspecified lower extremity

I80.01   Phlebitis and thrombophlebitis of superficial vessels of right lower extremity

I80.02   Phlebitis and thrombophlebitis of superficial vessels of left lower extremity

I80.03   Phlebitis and thrombophlebitis of superficial vessels of lower extremities, bilateral

✓5th I80.1 Phlebitis and thrombophlebitis of femoral vein
Phlebitis and thrombophlebitis of common femoral vein
Phlebitis and thrombophlebitis of deep femoral vein

I80.10   Phlebitis and thrombophlebitis of unspecified femoral vein   CC UNS HCC

I80.11   Phlebitis and thrombophlebitis of right femoral vein   CC HCC

I80.12   Phlebitis and thrombophlebitis of left femoral vein   CC HCC

I80.13   Phlebitis and thrombophlebitis of femoral vein, bilateral   CC HCC

✓5th I80.2 Phlebitis and thrombophlebitis of other and unspecified deep vessels of lower extremities

✓6th I80.20 Phlebitis and thrombophlebitis of unspecified deep vessels of lower extremities

I80.201   Phlebitis and thrombophlebitis of unspecified deep vessels of right lower extremity   CC HCC

I80.202   Phlebitis and thrombophlebitis of unspecified deep vessels of left lower extremity   CC HCC

I80.203   Phlebitis and thrombophlebitis of unspecified deep vessels of lower extremities, bilateral   CC HCC

I80.209   Phlebitis and thrombophlebitis of unspecified deep vessels of unspecified lower extremity   CC UNS HCC

✓6th I80.21 Phlebitis and thrombophlebitis of iliac vein
Phlebitis and thrombophlebitis of common iliac vein
Phlebitis and thrombophlebitis of external iliac vein
Phlebitis and thrombophlebitis of internal iliac vein

I80.211   Phlebitis and thrombophlebitis of right iliac vein   CC HCC

I80.212   Phlebitis and thrombophlebitis of left iliac vein   CC HCC

I80.213   Phlebitis and thrombophlebitis of iliac vein, bilateral   CC HCC

I80.219   Phlebitis and thrombophlebitis of unspecified iliac vein   CC UNS HCC

✓6th I80.22 Phlebitis and thrombophlebitis of popliteal vein

I80.221   Phlebitis and thrombophlebitis of right popliteal vein   CC HCC

I80.222   Phlebitis and thrombophlebitis of left popliteal vein   CC HCC

I80.223   Phlebitis and thrombophlebitis of popliteal vein, bilateral   CC HCC

I80.229   Phlebitis and thrombophlebitis of unspecified popliteal vein   CC UNS HCC

✓6th I80.23 Phlebitis and thrombophlebitis of tibial vein
Phlebitis and thrombophlebitis of anterior tibial vein
Phlebitis and thrombophlebitis of posterior tibial vein

I80.231   Phlebitis and thrombophlebitis of right tibial vein   CC HCC

I80.232   Phlebitis and thrombophlebitis of left tibial vein   CC HCC

I80.233   Phlebitis and thrombophlebitis of tibial vein, bilateral   CC HCC

I80.239   Phlebitis and thrombophlebitis of unspecified tibial vein   CC UNS HCC

✓6th I80.24 Phlebitis and thrombophlebitis of peroneal vein
AHA: 2019,4Q,8

I80.241   Phlebitis and thrombophlebitis of right peroneal vein   CC HCC

I80.242   Phlebitis and thrombophlebitis of left peroneal vein   CC HCC

I80.243   Phlebitis and thrombophlebitis of peroneal vein, bilateral   CC HCC

I80.249   Phlebitis and thrombophlebitis of unspecified peroneal vein   CC UNS HCC

✓6th I80.25 Phlebitis and thrombophlebitis of calf muscular vein
Phlebitis and thrombophlebitis of calf muscular vein, NOS
Phlebitis and thrombophlebitis of gastrocnemial vein
Phlebitis and thrombophlebitis of soleal vein
AHA: 2019,4Q,8

I80.251   Phlebitis and thrombophlebitis of right calf muscular vein   HCC

I80.252   Phlebitis and thrombophlebitis of left calf muscular vein   HCC

I80.253   Phlebitis and thrombophlebitis of calf muscular vein, bilateral   HCC

I80.259   Phlebitis and thrombophlebitis of unspecified calf muscular vein   HCC

✓6th I80.29 Phlebitis and thrombophlebitis of other deep vessels of lower extremities

I80.291   Phlebitis and thrombophlebitis of other deep vessels of right lower extremity   CC HCC

I80.292   Phlebitis and thrombophlebitis of other deep vessels of left lower extremity   CC HCC

I80.293   Phlebitis and thrombophlebitis of other deep vessels of lower extremity, bilateral   CC HCC

I80.299   Phlebitis and thrombophlebitis of other deep vessels of unspecified lower extremity   CC UNS HCC

I80.3   Phlebitis and thrombophlebitis of lower extremities, unspecified

I80.8   Phlebitis and thrombophlebitis of other sites

I80.9   Phlebitis and thrombophlebitis of unspecified site

I81 Portal vein thrombosis   MCC
Portal (vein) obstruction

EXCLUDES 2   hepatic vein thrombosis (I82.0)
phlebitis of portal vein (K75.1)

AHA: 2019,4Q,68

✓4th I82 Other venous embolism and thrombosis

Code first venous embolism and thrombosis complicating:
abortion, ectopic or molar pregnancy (O00-O07, O08.7)
pregnancy, childbirth and the puerperium (O22.-, O87.-)

EXCLUDES 2   venous embolism and thrombosis (of):
cerebral (I63.6, I67.6)
coronary (I21-I25)
intracranial and intraspinal, septic or NOS (G08)
intracranial, nonpyogenic (I67.6)
intraspinal, nonpyogenic (G95.1)
mesenteric (K55.0-)
portal (I81)
pulmonary (I26.-)

I82.0   Budd-Chiari syndrome   MCC HCC
Hepatic vein thrombosis
DEF: Thrombosis or other obstruction of the hepatic veins. Symptoms include an enlarged liver, extensive collateral vessels, intractable ascites, and severe portal hypertension.

I82.1   Thrombophlebitis migrans   CC

N Newborn: 0   P Pediatric: 0-17   M Maternity: 9-64   A Adult: 15-124   UNS Unspecified Site   MCC Major Complication/Comorbidity   CC Complication/Comorbidity   PE POA Exempt

✓5ᵗʰ **I82.2** **Embolism and thrombosis of vena cava and other thoracic veins**

   ✓6ᵗʰ **I82.21** **Embolism and thrombosis of superior vena cava**

     I82.210 **Acute embolism and thrombosis of superior vena cava** `CC` `HCC`

       Embolism and thrombosis of superior vena cava NOS

     I82.211 **Chronic embolism and thrombosis of superior vena cava** `CC` `HCC`

   ✓6ᵗʰ **I82.22** **Embolism and thrombosis of inferior vena cava**

     I82.220 **Acute embolism and thrombosis of inferior vena cava** `MCC` `HCC`

       Embolism and thrombosis of inferior vena cava NOS

     I82.221 **Chronic embolism and thrombosis of inferior vena cava** `MCC` `HCC`

   ✓6ᵗʰ **I82.29** **Embolism and thrombosis of other thoracic veins**

       Embolism and thrombosis of brachiocephalic (innominate) vein

     I82.290 **Acute embolism and thrombosis of other thoracic veins** `CC` `HCC`

     I82.291 **Chronic embolism and thrombosis of other thoracic veins** `CC` `HCC`

I82.3 **Embolism and thrombosis of renal vein** `CC` `HCC`

✓5ᵗʰ **I82.4** **Acute embolism and thrombosis of deep veins of lower extremity**

   ✓6ᵗʰ **I82.40** **Acute embolism and thrombosis of unspecified deep veins of lower extremity**

       Deep vein thrombosis NOS
       DVT NOS

       EXCLUDES 1 *acute embolism and thrombosis of unspecified deep veins of distal lower extremity (I82.4Z-)*

         acute embolism and thrombosis of unspecified deep veins of proximal lower extremity (I82.4Y-)

     I82.401 **Acute embolism and thrombosis of unspecified deep veins of right lower extremity** `CC` `H10` `HCC`

     I82.402 **Acute embolism and thrombosis of unspecified deep veins of left lower extremity** `CC` `H10` `HCC`

     I82.403 **Acute embolism and thrombosis of unspecified deep veins of lower extremity, bilateral** `CC` `H10` `HCC`

     I82.409 **Acute embolism and thrombosis of unspecified deep veins of unspecified lower extremity** `CC` `H10` `UNS` `HCC`

   ✓6ᵗʰ **I82.41** **Acute embolism and thrombosis of femoral vein**

       Acute embolism and thrombosis of common femoral vein
       Acute embolism and thrombosis of deep femoral vein
       AHA: 2023,3Q,12

     I82.411 **Acute embolism and thrombosis of right femoral vein** `CC` `H10` `HCC`

     I82.412 **Acute embolism and thrombosis of left femoral vein** `CC` `H10` `HCC`

     I82.413 **Acute embolism and thrombosis of femoral vein, bilateral** `CC` `H10` `HCC`

     I82.419 **Acute embolism and thrombosis of unspecified femoral vein** `CC` `H10` `UNS` `HCC`

   ✓6ᵗʰ **I82.42** **Acute embolism and thrombosis of iliac vein**

       Acute embolism and thrombosis of common iliac vein
       Acute embolism and thrombosis of external iliac vein
       Acute embolism and thrombosis of internal iliac vein

     I82.421 **Acute embolism and thrombosis of right iliac vein** `CC` `H10` `HCC`

     I82.422 **Acute embolism and thrombosis of left iliac vein** `CC` `H10` `HCC`

     I82.423 **Acute embolism and thrombosis of iliac vein, bilateral** `CC` `H10` `HCC`

     I82.429 **Acute embolism and thrombosis of unspecified iliac vein** `CC` `H10` `UNS` `HCC`

   ✓6ᵗʰ **I82.43** **Acute embolism and thrombosis of popliteal vein**

     I82.431 **Acute embolism and thrombosis of right popliteal vein** `CC` `H10` `HCC`

     I82.432 **Acute embolism and thrombosis of left popliteal vein** `CC` `H10` `HCC`

     I82.433 **Acute embolism and thrombosis of popliteal vein, bilateral** `CC` `H10` `HCC`

     I82.439 **Acute embolism and thrombosis of unspecified popliteal vein** `CC` `H10` `UNS` `HCC`

   ✓6ᵗʰ **I82.44** **Acute embolism and thrombosis of tibial vein**

       Acute embolism and thrombosis of anterior tibial vein
       Acute embolism and thrombosis of posterior tibial vein

     I82.441 **Acute embolism and thrombosis of right tibial vein** `CC` `H10` `HCC`

     I82.442 **Acute embolism and thrombosis of left tibial vein** `CC` `H10` `HCC`

     I82.443 **Acute embolism and thrombosis of tibial vein, bilateral** `CC` `H10` `HCC`

     I82.449 **Acute embolism and thrombosis of unspecified tibial vein** `CC` `H10` `UNS` `HCC`

   ✓6ᵗʰ **I82.45** **Acute embolism and thrombosis of peroneal vein**

       AHA: 2019,4Q,8-10

     I82.451 **Acute embolism and thrombosis of right peroneal vein** `CC` `H10` `HCC`

     I82.452 **Acute embolism and thrombosis of left peroneal vein** `CC` `H10` `HCC`

     I82.453 **Acute embolism and thrombosis of peroneal vein, bilateral** `CC` `H10` `HCC`

     I82.459 **Acute embolism and thrombosis of unspecified peroneal vein** `CC` `H10` `UNS` `HCC`

   ✓6ᵗʰ **I82.46** **Acute embolism and thrombosis of calf muscular vein**

       Acute embolism and thrombosis of calf muscular vein, NOS
       Acute embolism and thrombosis of gastrocnemial vein
       Acute embolism and thrombosis of soleal vein
       AHA: 2019,4Q,8-10

     I82.461 **Acute embolism and thrombosis of right calf muscular vein** `HCC`

     I82.462 **Acute embolism and thrombosis of left calf muscular vein** `HCC`

     I82.463 **Acute embolism and thrombosis of calf muscular vein, bilateral** `HCC`

     I82.469 **Acute embolism and thrombosis of unspecified calf muscular vein** `HCC`

   ✓6ᵗʰ **I82.49** **Acute embolism and thrombosis of other specified deep vein of lower extremity**

     I82.491 **Acute embolism and thrombosis of other specified deep vein of right lower extremity** `CC` `H10` `HCC`

     I82.492 **Acute embolism and thrombosis of other specified deep vein of left lower extremity** `CC` `H10` `HCC`

     I82.493 **Acute embolism and thrombosis of other specified deep vein of lower extremity, bilateral** `CC` `H10` `HCC`

     I82.499 **Acute embolism and thrombosis of other specified deep vein of unspecified lower extremity** `CC` `H10` `UNS` `HCC`

   ✓6ᵗʰ **I82.4Y** **Acute embolism and thrombosis of unspecified deep veins of proximal lower extremity**

       Acute embolism and thrombosis of deep vein of thigh NOS
       Acute embolism and thrombosis of deep vein of upper leg NOS

     I82.4Y1 **Acute embolism and thrombosis of unspecified deep veins of right proximal lower extremity** `CC` `H10` `HCC`

     I82.4Y2 **Acute embolism and thrombosis of unspecified deep veins of left proximal lower extremity** `CC` `H10` `HCC`

     I82.4Y3 **Acute embolism and thrombosis of unspecified deep veins of proximal lower extremity, bilateral** `CC` `H10` `HCC`

     I82.4Y9 **Acute embolism and thrombosis of unspecified deep veins of unspecified proximal lower extremity** `CC` `H10` `UNS` `HCC`

✓ Additional Character Required   ✓x 7ᵗʰ Placeholder   `Questionable PDx`   `Manifestation`   `Unspecified`   `UPD` Unacceptable PDx   `H1`-`H14` HAC   `HCC` CMS-HCC Dx   `HIV` HIV Dx

ICD-10-CM 2025   **695**

✓6ᵗʰ I82.4Z Acute embolism and thrombosis of unspecified deep veins of distal lower extremity
Acute embolism and thrombosis of deep vein of calf NOS
Acute embolism and thrombosis of deep vein of lower leg NOS

    I82.4Z1 Acute embolism and thrombosis of unspecified deep veins of right distal lower extremity `CC` `H10` `HCC`

    I82.4Z2 Acute embolism and thrombosis of unspecified deep veins of left distal lower extremity `CC` `H10` `HCC`

    I82.4Z3 Acute embolism and thrombosis of unspecified deep veins of distal lower extremity, bilateral `CC` `H10` `HCC`

    I82.4Z9 Acute embolism and thrombosis of unspecified deep veins of unspecified distal lower extremity `CC` `H10` `UNS` `HCC`

✓5ᵗʰ I82.5 Chronic embolism and thrombosis of deep veins of lower extremity
Use additional code, if applicable, for associated long-term (current) use of anticoagulants (Z79.01)
    `EXCLUDES 1` *personal history of venous embolism and thrombosis (Z86.718)*
    AHA: 2020,2Q,20

✓6ᵗʰ I82.50 Chronic embolism and thrombosis of unspecified deep veins of lower extremity
    `EXCLUDES 1` *chronic embolism and thrombosis of unspecified deep veins of distal lower extremity (I82.5Z-)*
chronic embolism and thrombosis of unspecified deep veins of proximal lower extremity (I82.5Y-)

    I82.501 Chronic embolism and thrombosis of unspecified deep veins of right lower extremity `CC` `HCC`

    I82.502 Chronic embolism and thrombosis of unspecified deep veins of left lower extremity `CC` `HCC`

    I82.503 Chronic embolism and thrombosis of unspecified deep veins of lower extremity, bilateral `CC` `HCC`

    I82.509 Chronic embolism and thrombosis of unspecified deep veins of unspecified lower extremity `CC` `UNS` `HCC`

✓6ᵗʰ I82.51 Chronic embolism and thrombosis of femoral vein
Chronic embolism and thrombosis of common femoral vein
Chronic embolism and thrombosis of deep femoral vein

    I82.511 Chronic embolism and thrombosis of right femoral vein `CC` `HCC`

    I82.512 Chronic embolism and thrombosis of left femoral vein `CC` `HCC`

    I82.513 Chronic embolism and thrombosis of femoral vein, bilateral `CC` `HCC`

    I82.519 Chronic embolism and thrombosis of unspecified femoral vein `CC` `UNS` `HCC`

✓6ᵗʰ I82.52 Chronic embolism and thrombosis of iliac vein
Chronic embolism and thrombosis of common iliac vein
Chronic embolism and thrombosis of external iliac vein
Chronic embolism and thrombosis of internal iliac vein

    I82.521 Chronic embolism and thrombosis of right iliac vein `CC` `HCC`

    I82.522 Chronic embolism and thrombosis of left iliac vein `CC` `HCC`

    I82.523 Chronic embolism and thrombosis of iliac vein, bilateral `CC` `HCC`

    I82.529 Chronic embolism and thrombosis of unspecified iliac vein `CC` `UNS` `HCC`

✓6ᵗʰ I82.53 Chronic embolism and thrombosis of popliteal vein

    I82.531 Chronic embolism and thrombosis of right popliteal vein `CC` `HCC`

    I82.532 Chronic embolism and thrombosis of left popliteal vein `CC` `HCC`

    I82.533 Chronic embolism and thrombosis of popliteal vein, bilateral `CC` `HCC`

    I82.539 Chronic embolism and thrombosis of unspecified popliteal vein `CC` `UNS` `HCC`

✓6ᵗʰ I82.54 Chronic embolism and thrombosis of tibial vein
Chronic embolism and thrombosis of anterior tibial vein
Chronic embolism and thrombosis of posterior tibial vein

    I82.541 Chronic embolism and thrombosis of right tibial vein `CC` `HCC`

    I82.542 Chronic embolism and thrombosis of left tibial vein `CC` `HCC`

    I82.543 Chronic embolism and thrombosis of tibial vein, bilateral `CC` `HCC`

    I82.549 Chronic embolism and thrombosis of unspecified tibial vein `CC` `UNS` `HCC`

✓6ᵗʰ I82.55 Chronic embolism and thrombosis of peroneal vein
    AHA: 2019,4Q,8-10

    I82.551 Chronic embolism and thrombosis of right peroneal vein `CC` `HCC`

    I82.552 Chronic embolism and thrombosis of left peroneal vein `CC` `HCC`

    I82.553 Chronic embolism and thrombosis of peroneal vein, bilateral `CC` `HCC`

    I82.559 Chronic embolism and thrombosis of unspecified peroneal vein `CC` `UNS` `HCC`

✓6ᵗʰ I82.56 Chronic embolism and thrombosis of calf muscular vein
Chronic embolism and thrombosis of calf muscular vein NOS
Chronic embolism and thrombosis of gastrocnemial vein
Chronic embolism and thrombosis of soleal vein
    AHA: 2019,4Q,8-10

    I82.561 Chronic embolism and thrombosis of right calf muscular vein `HCC`

    I82.562 Chronic embolism and thrombosis of left calf muscular vein `HCC`

    I82.563 Chronic embolism and thrombosis of calf muscular vein, bilateral `HCC`

    I82.569 Chronic embolism and thrombosis of unspecified calf muscular vein `HCC`

✓6ᵗʰ I82.59 Chronic embolism and thrombosis of other specified deep vein of lower extremity

    I82.591 Chronic embolism and thrombosis of other specified deep vein of right lower extremity `CC` `HCC`

    I82.592 Chronic embolism and thrombosis of other specified deep vein of left lower extremity `CC` `HCC`

    I82.593 Chronic embolism and thrombosis of other specified deep vein of lower extremity, bilateral `CC` `HCC`

    I82.599 Chronic embolism and thrombosis of other specified deep vein of unspecified lower extremity `CC` `UNS` `HCC`

✓6ᵗʰ I82.5Y Chronic embolism and thrombosis of unspecified deep veins of proximal lower extremity
Chronic embolism and thrombosis of deep veins of thigh NOS
Chronic embolism and thrombosis of deep veins of upper leg NOS

    I82.5Y1 Chronic embolism and thrombosis of unspecified deep veins of right proximal lower extremity `CC` `HCC`

    I82.5Y2 Chronic embolism and thrombosis of unspecified deep veins of left proximal lower extremity `CC` `HCC`

    I82.5Y3 Chronic embolism and thrombosis of unspecified deep veins of proximal lower extremity, bilateral `CC` `HCC`

    I82.5Y9 Chronic embolism and thrombosis of unspecified deep veins of unspecified proximal lower extremity `CC` `UNS` `HCC`

✓6ᵗʰ I82.5Z Chronic embolism and thrombosis of unspecified deep veins of distal lower extremity
Chronic embolism and thrombosis of deep veins of calf NOS
Chronic embolism and thrombosis of deep veins of lower leg NOS

    I82.5Z1 Chronic embolism and thrombosis of unspecified deep veins of right distal lower extremity `CC` `HCC`

`N` Newborn: 0   `P` Pediatric: 0-17   `M` Maternity: 9-64   `A` Adult: 15-124   `UNS` Unspecified Site   `MCC` Major Complication/Comorbidity   `CC` Complication/Comorbidity   `PE` POA Exempt

696   ICD-10-CM 2025

I82.5Z2 Chronic embolism and thrombosis of unspecified deep veins of left distal lower extremity `CC` `HCC`

I82.5Z3 Chronic embolism and thrombosis of unspecified deep veins of distal lower extremity, bilateral `CC` `HCC`

I82.5Z9 Chronic embolism and thrombosis of unspecified deep veins of unspecified distal lower extremity `CC` `UNS` `HCC`

√5th **I82.6** Acute embolism and thrombosis of veins of upper extremity

√6th **I82.60** Acute embolism and thrombosis of unspecified veins of upper extremity

I82.601 Acute embolism and thrombosis of unspecified veins of right upper extremity `CC`

I82.602 Acute embolism and thrombosis of unspecified veins of left upper extremity `CC`

I82.603 Acute embolism and thrombosis of unspecified veins of upper extremity, bilateral `CC`

I82.609 Acute embolism and thrombosis of unspecified veins of unspecified upper extremity `CC` `UNS`

√6th **I82.61** Acute embolism and thrombosis of superficial veins of upper extremity

Acute embolism and thrombosis of antecubital vein
Acute embolism and thrombosis of basilic vein
Acute embolism and thrombosis of cephalic vein

I82.611 Acute embolism and thrombosis of superficial veins of right upper extremity `CC`

I82.612 Acute embolism and thrombosis of superficial veins of left upper extremity `CC`

I82.613 Acute embolism and thrombosis of superficial veins of upper extremity, bilateral `CC`

I82.619 Acute embolism and thrombosis of superficial veins of unspecified upper extremity `CC` `UNS`

√6th **I82.62** Acute embolism and thrombosis of deep veins of upper extremity

Acute embolism and thrombosis of brachial vein
Acute embolism and thrombosis of radial vein
Acute embolism and thrombosis of ulnar vein

I82.621 Acute embolism and thrombosis of deep veins of right upper extremity `CC` `HCC`

I82.622 Acute embolism and thrombosis of deep veins of left upper extremity `CC` `HCC`

I82.623 Acute embolism and thrombosis of deep veins of upper extremity, bilateral `CC` `HCC`

I82.629 Acute embolism and thrombosis of deep veins of unspecified upper extremity `CC` `UNS` `HCC`

√5th **I82.7** Chronic embolism and thrombosis of veins of upper extremity

Use additional code, if applicable, for associated long-term (current) use of anticoagulants (Z79.01)

EXCLUDES 1   *personal history of venous embolism and thrombosis (Z86.718)*

√6th **I82.70** Chronic embolism and thrombosis of unspecified veins of upper extremity

I82.701 Chronic embolism and thrombosis of unspecified veins of right upper extremity `CC`

I82.702 Chronic embolism and thrombosis of unspecified veins of left upper extremity `CC`

I82.703 Chronic embolism and thrombosis of unspecified veins of upper extremity, bilateral `CC`

I82.709 Chronic embolism and thrombosis of unspecified veins of unspecified upper extremity `CC` `UNS`

√6th **I82.71** Chronic embolism and thrombosis of superficial veins of upper extremity

Chronic embolism and thrombosis of antecubital vein
Chronic embolism and thrombosis of basilic vein
Chronic embolism and thrombosis of cephalic vein

I82.711 Chronic embolism and thrombosis of superficial veins of right upper extremity `CC`

I82.712 Chronic embolism and thrombosis of superficial veins of left upper extremity `CC`

I82.713 Chronic embolism and thrombosis of superficial veins of upper extremity, bilateral `CC`

I82.719 Chronic embolism and thrombosis of superficial veins of unspecified upper extremity `CC` `UNS`

√6th **I82.72** Chronic embolism and thrombosis of deep veins of upper extremity

Chronic embolism and thrombosis of brachial vein
Chronic embolism and thrombosis of radial vein
Chronic embolism and thrombosis of ulnar vein

I82.721 Chronic embolism and thrombosis of deep veins of right upper extremity `CC` `HCC`

I82.722 Chronic embolism and thrombosis of deep veins of left upper extremity `CC` `HCC`

I82.723 Chronic embolism and thrombosis of deep veins of upper extremity, bilateral `CC` `HCC`

I82.729 Chronic embolism and thrombosis of deep veins of unspecified upper extremity `CC` `UNS` `HCC`

√5th **I82.A** Embolism and thrombosis of axillary vein

√6th **I82.A1** Acute embolism and thrombosis of axillary vein

I82.A11 Acute embolism and thrombosis of right axillary vein `CC` `HCC`

I82.A12 Acute embolism and thrombosis of left axillary vein `CC` `HCC`

I82.A13 Acute embolism and thrombosis of axillary vein, bilateral `CC` `HCC`

I82.A19 Acute embolism and thrombosis of unspecified axillary vein `CC` `UNS` `HCC`

√6th **I82.A2** Chronic embolism and thrombosis of axillary vein

I82.A21 Chronic embolism and thrombosis of right axillary vein `CC` `HCC`

I82.A22 Chronic embolism and thrombosis of left axillary vein `CC` `HCC`

I82.A23 Chronic embolism and thrombosis of axillary vein, bilateral `CC` `HCC`

I82.A29 Chronic embolism and thrombosis of unspecified axillary vein `CC` `UNS` `HCC`

√5th **I82.B** Embolism and thrombosis of subclavian vein

√6th **I82.B1** Acute embolism and thrombosis of subclavian vein

I82.B11 Acute embolism and thrombosis of right subclavian vein `CC` `HCC`

I82.B12 Acute embolism and thrombosis of left subclavian vein `CC` `HCC`

I82.B13 Acute embolism and thrombosis of subclavian vein, bilateral `CC` `HCC`

I82.B19 Acute embolism and thrombosis of unspecified subclavian vein `CC` `UNS` `HCC`

√6th **I82.B2** Chronic embolism and thrombosis of subclavian vein

I82.B21 Chronic embolism and thrombosis of right subclavian vein `CC` `HCC`

I82.B22 Chronic embolism and thrombosis of left subclavian vein `CC` `HCC`

I82.B23 Chronic embolism and thrombosis of subclavian vein, bilateral `CC` `HCC`

I82.B29 Chronic embolism and thrombosis of unspecified subclavian vein `CC` `UNS` `HCC`

√5th **I82.C** Embolism and thrombosis of internal jugular vein

√6th **I82.C1** Acute embolism and thrombosis of internal jugular vein

I82.C11 Acute embolism and thrombosis of right internal jugular vein `CC` `HCC`

I82.C12 Acute embolism and thrombosis of left internal jugular vein `CC` `HCC`

I82.C13 Acute embolism and thrombosis of internal jugular vein, bilateral `CC` `HCC`

✔ Additional Character Required   √x7th Placeholder   `Questionable PDx`   Manifestation   Unspecified   `UPD` Unacceptable PDx   `H1`-`H14` HAC   `HCC` CMS-HCC Dx   `HIV` HIV Dx

ICD-10-CM 2025   697

I82.C19 Acute embolism and thrombosis of unspecified internal jugular vein `CC` `UNS` `HCC`

✓6th **I82.C2** Chronic embolism and thrombosis of internal jugular vein

    I82.C21 Chronic embolism and thrombosis of right internal jugular vein `CC` `HCC`

    I82.C22 Chronic embolism and thrombosis of left internal jugular vein `CC` `HCC`

    I82.C23 Chronic embolism and thrombosis of internal jugular vein, bilateral `CC` `HCC`

    I82.C29 Chronic embolism and thrombosis of unspecified internal jugular vein `CC` `UNS` `HCC`

✓5th **I82.8** Embolism and thrombosis of other specified veins

    Use additional code, if applicable, for associated long-term (current) use of anticoagulants (Z79.01)

  ✓6th **I82.81** Embolism and thrombosis of superficial veins of lower extremities

    Embolism and thrombosis of saphenous vein (greater) (lesser)

    I82.811 Embolism and thrombosis of superficial veins of right lower extremity `CC`

    I82.812 Embolism and thrombosis of superficial veins of left lower extremity `CC`

    I82.813 Embolism and thrombosis of superficial veins of lower extremities, bilateral `CC`

    I82.819 Embolism and thrombosis of superficial veins of unspecified lower extremity `CC` `UNS`

  ✓6th **I82.89** Embolism and thrombosis of other specified veins

    I82.890 Acute embolism and thrombosis of other specified veins `CC`

    I82.891 Chronic embolism and thrombosis of other specified veins `CC`

✓5th **I82.9** Embolism and thrombosis of unspecified vein

  I82.90 Acute embolism and thrombosis of unspecified vein `CC` `UNS`

    Embolism of vein NOS
    Thrombosis (vein) NOS

  I82.91 Chronic embolism and thrombosis of unspecified vein `CC` `UNS`

✓4th **I83** Varicose veins of lower extremities

  EXCLUDES 2 varicose veins complicating pregnancy (O22.0-)
    varicose veins complicating the puerperium (O87.4)

✓5th **I83.0** Varicose veins of lower extremities with ulcer

  Use additional code to identify severity of ulcer (L97.-)

  ✓6th **I83.00** Varicose veins of unspecified lower extremity with ulcer

    I83.001 Varicose veins of unspecified lower extremity with ulcer of thigh `HCC` `A`

    I83.002 Varicose veins of unspecified lower extremity with ulcer of calf `HCC` `A`

    I83.003 Varicose veins of unspecified lower extremity with ulcer of ankle `HCC` `A`

    I83.004 Varicose veins of unspecified lower extremity with ulcer of heel and midfoot `HCC` `A`
      Varicose veins of unspecified lower extremity with ulcer of plantar surface of midfoot

    I83.005 Varicose veins of unspecified lower extremity with ulcer other part of foot `HCC` `A`
      Varicose veins of unspecified lower extremity with ulcer of toe

    I83.008 Varicose veins of unspecified lower extremity with ulcer other part of lower leg `HCC` `A`

    I83.009 Varicose veins of unspecified lower extremity with ulcer of unspecified site `HCC` `A`

  ✓6th **I83.01** Varicose veins of right lower extremity with ulcer

    I83.011 Varicose veins of right lower extremity with ulcer of thigh `HCC` `A`

    I83.012 Varicose veins of right lower extremity with ulcer of calf `HCC` `A`

    I83.013 Varicose veins of right lower extremity with ulcer of ankle `HCC` `A`

    I83.014 Varicose veins of right lower extremity with ulcer of heel and midfoot `HCC` `A`
      Varicose veins of right lower extremity with ulcer of plantar surface of midfoot

    I83.015 Varicose veins of right lower extremity with ulcer other part of foot `HCC` `A`
      Varicose veins of right lower extremity with ulcer of toe

    I83.018 Varicose veins of right lower extremity with ulcer other part of lower leg `HCC` `A`

    I83.019 Varicose veins of right lower extremity with ulcer of unspecified site `HCC` `A`

  ✓6th **I83.02** Varicose veins of left lower extremity with ulcer

    I83.021 Varicose veins of left lower extremity with ulcer of thigh `HCC` `A`

    I83.022 Varicose veins of left lower extremity with ulcer of calf `HCC` `A`

    I83.023 Varicose veins of left lower extremity with ulcer of ankle `HCC` `A`

    I83.024 Varicose veins of left lower extremity with ulcer of heel and midfoot `HCC` `A`
      Varicose veins of left lower extremity with ulcer of plantar surface of midfoot

    I83.025 Varicose veins of left lower extremity with ulcer other part of foot `HCC` `A`
      Varicose veins of left lower extremity with ulcer of toe

    I83.028 Varicose veins of left lower extremity with ulcer other part of lower leg `HCC` `A`

    I83.029 Varicose veins of left lower extremity with ulcer of unspecified site `HCC` `A`

✓5th **I83.1** Varicose veins of lower extremities with inflammation

  I83.10 Varicose veins of unspecified lower extremity with inflammation `A`

  I83.11 Varicose veins of right lower extremity with inflammation `A`

  I83.12 Varicose veins of left lower extremity with inflammation `A`

✓5th **I83.2** Varicose veins of lower extremities with both ulcer and inflammation

  Use additional code to identify severity of ulcer (L97.-)

  ✓6th **I83.20** Varicose veins of unspecified lower extremity with both ulcer and inflammation

    I83.201 Varicose veins of unspecified lower extremity with both ulcer of thigh and inflammation `CC` `HCC`

    I83.202 Varicose veins of unspecified lower extremity with both ulcer of calf and inflammation `CC` `HCC`

    I83.203 Varicose veins of unspecified lower extremity with both ulcer of ankle and inflammation `CC` `HCC` `A`

    I83.204 Varicose veins of unspecified lower extremity with both ulcer of heel and midfoot and inflammation `CC` `HCC`
      Varicose veins of unspecified lower extremity with both ulcer of plantar surface of midfoot and inflammation

    I83.205 Varicose veins of unspecified lower extremity with both ulcer of other part of foot and inflammation `CC` `HCC` `A`
      Varicose veins of unspecified lower extremity with both ulcer of toe and inflammation

    I83.208 Varicose veins of unspecified lower extremity with both ulcer of other part of lower extremity and inflammation `CC` `HCC`

    I83.209 Varicose veins of unspecified lower extremity with both ulcer of unspecified site and inflammation `CC` `HCC`

  ✓6th **I83.21** Varicose veins of right lower extremity with both ulcer and inflammation

    I83.211 Varicose veins of right lower extremity with both ulcer of thigh and inflammation `CC` `HCC` `A`

    I83.212 Varicose veins of right lower extremity with both ulcer of calf and inflammation `CC` `HCC` `A`

    I83.213 Varicose veins of right lower extremity with both ulcer of ankle and inflammation `CC` `HCC` `A`

`N` Newborn: 0 `P` Pediatric: 0-17 `M` Maternity: 9-64 `A` Adult: 15-124 `UNS` Unspecified Site `MCC` Major Complication/Comorbidity `CC` Complication/Comorbidity `PE` POA Exempt

698   ICD-10-CM 2025

I83.214   Varicose veins of right lower extremity with both ulcer of heel and midfoot and inflammation `CC` `HCC` `A`
> Varicose veins of right lower extremity with both ulcer of plantar surface of midfoot and inflammation

I83.215   Varicose veins of right lower extremity with both ulcer other part of foot and inflammation `CC` `HCC` `A`
> Varicose veins of right lower extremity with both ulcer of toe and inflammation

I83.218   Varicose veins of right lower extremity with both ulcer of other part of lower extremity and inflammation `CC` `HCC` `A`

I83.219   Varicose veins of right lower extremity with both ulcer of unspecified site and inflammation `CC` `HCC` `A`

√6th **I83.22**   Varicose veins of left lower extremity with both ulcer and inflammation

I83.221   Varicose veins of left lower extremity with both ulcer of thigh and inflammation `CC` `HCC` `A`

I83.222   Varicose veins of left lower extremity with both ulcer of calf and inflammation `CC` `HCC` `A`

I83.223   Varicose veins of left lower extremity with both ulcer of ankle and inflammation `CC` `HCC` `A`

I83.224   Varicose veins of left lower extremity with both ulcer of heel and midfoot and inflammation `CC` `HCC` `A`
> Varicose veins of left lower extremity with both ulcer of plantar surface of midfoot and inflammation

I83.225   Varicose veins of left lower extremity with both ulcer other part of foot and inflammation `CC` `HCC` `A`
> Varicose veins of left lower extremity with both ulcer of toe and inflammation

I83.228   Varicose veins of left lower extremity with both ulcer of other part of lower extremity and inflammation `CC` `HCC` `A`

I83.229   Varicose veins of left lower extremity with both ulcer of unspecified site and inflammation `CC` `HCC` `A`

√5th **I83.8**   Varicose veins of lower extremities with other complications

√6th   **I83.81**   Varicose veins of lower extremities with pain

I83.811   Varicose veins of right lower extremity with pain `A`

I83.812   Varicose veins of left lower extremity with pain `A`

I83.813   Varicose veins of bilateral lower extremities with pain `A`

I83.819   Varicose veins of unspecified lower extremity with pain `A`

√6th   **I83.89**   Varicose veins of lower extremities with other complications
> Varicose veins of lower extremities with edema
> Varicose veins of lower extremities with swelling

I83.891   Varicose veins of right lower extremity with other complications `A`

I83.892   Varicose veins of left lower extremity with other complications `A`

I83.893   Varicose veins of bilateral lower extremities with other complications `A`

I83.899   Varicose veins of unspecified lower extremity with other complications `A`

√5th **I83.9**   Asymptomatic varicose veins of lower extremities
> Phlebectasia of lower extremities
> Varicose veins of lower extremities
> Varix of lower extremities

I83.90   Asymptomatic varicose veins of unspecified lower extremity `A`
> Varicose veins NOS

I83.91   Asymptomatic varicose veins of right lower extremity `A`

I83.92   Asymptomatic varicose veins of left lower extremity `A`

I83.93   Asymptomatic varicose veins of bilateral lower extremities `A`

√4th **I85**   **Esophageal varices**
> Use additional code to identify:
> alcohol abuse and dependence (F10.-)

√5th   **I85.0**   Esophageal varices
> Idiopathic esophageal varices
> Primary esophageal varices

I85.00   Esophageal varices without bleeding `CC` `HCC`
> Esophageal varices NOS

I85.01   Esophageal varices with bleeding `MCC` `HCC`

√5th   **I85.1**   Secondary esophageal varices
> Esophageal varices secondary to alcoholic liver disease
> Esophageal varices secondary to cirrhosis of liver
> Esophageal varices secondary to schistosomiasis
> Esophageal varices secondary to toxic liver disease
> Code first underlying disease

I85.10   Secondary esophageal varices without bleeding `CC` `HCC`

I85.11   Secondary esophageal varices with bleeding `MCC` `HCC`

√4th **I86**   **Varicose veins of other sites**
> *EXCLUDES 1*   varicose veins of unspecified site (I83.9-)
> *EXCLUDES 2*   retinal varices (H35.0-)

I86.0   Sublingual varices
> DEF: Distended, tortuous veins beneath the tongue.

I86.1   Scrotal varices
> Varicocele

I86.2   Pelvic varices

I86.3   Vulval varices
> *EXCLUDES 1*   vulval varices complicating childbirth and the puerperium (O87.8)
>   vulval varices complicating pregnancy (O22.1-)

I86.4   Gastric varices

I86.8   Varicose veins of other specified sites `A`
> Varicose ulcer of nasal septum

√4th **I87**   **Other disorders of veins**

√5th   **I87.0**   Postthrombotic syndrome
> Chronic venous hypertension due to deep vein thrombosis
> Postphlebitic syndrome
> *EXCLUDES 1*   chronic venous hypertension without deep vein thrombosis (I87.3-)

√6th   **I87.00**   Postthrombotic syndrome without complications
> Asymptomatic postthrombotic syndrome

I87.001   Postthrombotic syndrome without complications of right lower extremity

I87.002   Postthrombotic syndrome without complications of left lower extremity

I87.003   Postthrombotic syndrome without complications of bilateral lower extremity

I87.009   Postthrombotic syndrome without complications of unspecified extremity
> Postthrombotic syndrome NOS

√6th   **I87.01**   Postthrombotic syndrome with ulcer
> Use additional code to specify site and severity of ulcer (L97.-)

I87.011   Postthrombotic syndrome with ulcer of right lower extremity `CC` `HCC`

I87.012   Postthrombotic syndrome with ulcer of left lower extremity `CC` `HCC`

I87.013   Postthrombotic syndrome with ulcer of bilateral lower extremity `CC` `HCC`

I87.019   Postthrombotic syndrome with ulcer of unspecified lower extremity `CC` `UNS` `HCC`

√6th   **I87.02**   Postthrombotic syndrome with inflammation

I87.021   Postthrombotic syndrome with inflammation of right lower extremity

I87.022   Postthrombotic syndrome with inflammation of left lower extremity

I87.023   Postthrombotic syndrome with inflammation of bilateral lower extremity

I87.029   Postthrombotic syndrome with inflammation of unspecified lower extremity

✓ Additional Character Required   ✓x7th Placeholder   Questionable PDx   Manifestation   Unspecified   `UPD` Unacceptable PDx   `H1`-`H14` HAC   `HCC` CMS-HCC Dx   `HIV` HIV Dx

ICD-10-CM 2025   699

✓6th I87.Ø3   **Postthrombotic syndrome with ulcer and inflammation**

Use additional code to specify site and severity of ulcer (L97.-)

I87.Ø31   **Postthrombotic syndrome with ulcer and inflammation of right lower extremity** CC HCC

I87.Ø32   **Postthrombotic syndrome with ulcer and inflammation of left lower extremity** CC HCC

I87.Ø33   **Postthrombotic syndrome with ulcer and inflammation of bilateral lower extremity** CC HCC

I87.Ø39   **Postthrombotic syndrome with ulcer and inflammation of unspecified lower extremity** CC UNS HCC

✓6th I87.Ø9   **Postthrombotic syndrome with other complications**

I87.Ø91   **Postthrombotic syndrome with other complications of right lower extremity**

I87.Ø92   **Postthrombotic syndrome with other complications of left lower extremity**

I87.Ø93   **Postthrombotic syndrome with other complications of bilateral lower extremity**

I87.Ø99   **Postthrombotic syndrome with other complications of unspecified lower extremity**

I87.1   **Compression of vein**   CC

Stricture of vein

Vena cava syndrome (inferior) (superior)

EXCLUDES 2   compression of pulmonary vein (I28.8)

AHA: 2023,2Q,8

I87.2   **Venous insufficiency (chronic) (peripheral)**

Stasis dermatitis

Use additional code, if applicable, to specify site and severity of ulcer (L97.-)

Code also, if applicable, associated hypertensive conditions such as:

essential (primary) hypertension (I1Ø)

hypertensive chronic kidney disease (I12.-)

hypertensive heart and chronic kidney disease (I13.-)

hypertensive heart disease (I11.-)

EXCLUDES 1   stasis dermatitis with varicose veins of lower extremities (I83.1-, I83.2-)

AHA: 2024,1Q,16

DEF: Insufficient drainage of venous blood in any part of the body that results in edema or dermatosis.

✓5th I87.3   **Chronic venous hypertension (idiopathic)**

Stasis edema

EXCLUDES 1   chronic venous hypertension due to deep vein thrombosis (I87.Ø-)

varicose veins of lower extremities (I83.-)

✓6th I87.3Ø   **Chronic venous hypertension (idiopathic) without complications**

Asymptomatic chronic venous hypertension (idiopathic)

I87.3Ø1   **Chronic venous hypertension (idiopathic) without complications of right lower extremity**

I87.3Ø2   **Chronic venous hypertension (idiopathic) without complications of left lower extremity**

I87.3Ø3   **Chronic venous hypertension (idiopathic) without complications of bilateral lower extremity**

I87.3Ø9   **Chronic venous hypertension (idiopathic) without complications of unspecified lower extremity**

Chronic venous hypertension NOS

✓6th I87.31   **Chronic venous hypertension (idiopathic) with ulcer**

Use additional code to specify site and severity of ulcer (L97.-)

I87.311   **Chronic venous hypertension (idiopathic) with ulcer of right lower extremity** CC HCC

I87.312   **Chronic venous hypertension (idiopathic) with ulcer of left lower extremity** CC HCC

I87.313   **Chronic venous hypertension (idiopathic) with ulcer of bilateral lower extremity** CC HCC

I87.319   **Chronic venous hypertension (idiopathic) with ulcer of unspecified lower extremity** CC UNS HCC

✓6th I87.32   **Chronic venous hypertension (idiopathic) with inflammation**

I87.321   **Chronic venous hypertension (idiopathic) with inflammation of right lower extremity**

I87.322   **Chronic venous hypertension (idiopathic) with inflammation of left lower extremity**

I87.323   **Chronic venous hypertension (idiopathic) with inflammation of bilateral lower extremity**

I87.329   **Chronic venous hypertension (idiopathic) with inflammation of unspecified lower extremity**

✓6th I87.33   **Chronic venous hypertension (idiopathic) with ulcer and inflammation**

Use additional code to specify site and severity of ulcer (L97.-)

I87.331   **Chronic venous hypertension (idiopathic) with ulcer and inflammation of right lower extremity** CC HCC

I87.332   **Chronic venous hypertension (idiopathic) with ulcer and inflammation of left lower extremity** CC HCC

I87.333   **Chronic venous hypertension (idiopathic) with ulcer and inflammation of bilateral lower extremity** CC HCC

I87.339   **Chronic venous hypertension (idiopathic) with ulcer and inflammation of unspecified lower extremity** CC UNS HCC

✓6th I87.39   **Chronic venous hypertension (idiopathic) with other complications**

I87.391   **Chronic venous hypertension (idiopathic) with other complications of right lower extremity**

I87.392   **Chronic venous hypertension (idiopathic) with other complications of left lower extremity**

I87.393   **Chronic venous hypertension (idiopathic) with other complications of bilateral lower extremity**

I87.399   **Chronic venous hypertension (idiopathic) with other complications of unspecified lower extremity**

I87.8   **Other specified disorders of veins**

Phlebosclerosis

Venofibrosis

I87.9   **Disorder of vein, unspecified**

✓4th I88   **Nonspecific lymphadenitis**

EXCLUDES 1   acute lymphadenitis, except mesenteric (LØ4.-)

enlarged lymph nodes NOS (R59.-)

human immunodeficiency virus [HIV] disease resulting in generalized lymphadenopathy (B2Ø)

I88.Ø   **Nonspecific mesenteric lymphadenitis**

Mesenteric lymphadenitis (acute)(chronic)

I88.1   **Chronic lymphadenitis, except mesenteric**

Adenitis

Lymphadenitis

I88.8   **Other nonspecific lymphadenitis**

I88.9   **Nonspecific lymphadenitis, unspecified**

Lymphadenitis NOS

✓4th I89   **Other noninfective disorders of lymphatic vessels and lymph nodes**

EXCLUDES 1   chylocele, tunica vaginalis (nonfilarial) NOS (N5Ø.89)

enlarged lymph nodes NOS (R59.-)

filarial chylocele (B74.-)

hereditary lymphedema (Q82.Ø)

I89.Ø   **Lymphedema, not elsewhere classified**

Elephantiasis (nonfilarial) NOS

Lymphangiectasis

Obliteration, lymphatic vessel

Praecox lymphedema

Secondary lymphedema

EXCLUDES 1   postmastectomy lymphedema (I97.2)

AHA: 2024,1Q,16

N Newborn: 0   P Pediatric: 0-17   M Maternity: 9-64   A Adult: 15-124   UNS Unspecified Site   MCC Major Complication/Comorbidity   CC Complication/Comorbidity   PE POA Exempt

700   ICD-10-CM 2025

I89.1 Lymphangitis
    Chronic lymphangitis
    Lymphangitis NOS
    Subacute lymphangitis
    EXCLUDES 1   *acute lymphangitis (L03.-)*

I89.8 Other specified noninfective disorders of lymphatic vessels and lymph nodes
    Chylocele (nonfilarial)
    Chylous ascites
    Chylous cyst
    Lipomelanotic reticulosis
    Lymph node or vessel fistula
    Lymph node or vessel infarction
    Lymph node or vessel rupture

I89.9 Noninfective disorder of lymphatic vessels and lymph nodes, unspecified
    Disease of lymphatic vessels NOS

Other and unspecified disorders of the circulatory system (I95-I99)

☑4ᵗʰ I95 Hypotension
    EXCLUDES 1   *cardiovascular collapse (R57.9) (~R57.9)*
          maternal hypotension syndrome (O26.5-)
          nonspecific low blood pressure reading NOS (R03.1)

I95.0 Idiopathic hypotension

I95.1 Orthostatic hypotension
    Hypotension, postural
    EXCLUDES 1   *neurogenic orthostatic hypotension [Shy-Drager] (G90.3)*
          orthostatic hypotension due to drugs (I95.2)
    AHA: 2023,2Q,8

I95.2 Hypotension due to drugs
    Orthostatic hypotension due to drugs
    Use additional code for adverse effect, if applicable, to identify drug (T36-T50 with fifth or sixth character 5)

I95.3 Hypotension of hemodialysis
    Intra-dialytic hypotension

☑5ᵗʰ I95.8 Other hypotension
    I95.81 Postprocedural hypotension
    I95.89 Other hypotension
          Chronic hypotension

I95.9 Hypotension, unspecified

I96 Gangrene, not elsewhere classified   `CC` `HCC`
    Gangrenous cellulitis
    EXCLUDES 1   *gangrene in atherosclerosis of native arteries of the extremities (I70.26)*
          gangrene in hernia (K40.1, K40.4, K41.1, K41.4, K42.1, K43.1-, K44.1, K45.1, K46.1)
          gangrene in other peripheral vascular diseases (I73.-)
          gangrene of certain specified sites - see Alphabetical Index
          gas gangrene (A48.0)
          pyoderma gangrenosum (L88)
    EXCLUDES 2   *gangrene in diabetes mellitus (E08-E13 with .52)*
    AHA: 2022,3Q,13; 2018,4Q,87; 2018,3Q,3; 2017,3Q,6; 2013,2Q,34

☑4ᵗʰ I97 Intraoperative and postprocedural complications and disorders of circulatory system, not elsewhere classified
    EXCLUDES 2   *postprocedural shock (T81.1-)*
    AHA: 2021,1Q,13; 2019,2Q,21

I97.0 Postcardiotomy syndrome

☑5ᵗʰ I97.1 Other postprocedural cardiac functional disturbances
    EXCLUDES 2   *acute pulmonary insufficiency following thoracic surgery (J95.1)*
          intraoperative cardiac functional disturbances (I97.7-)

    ☑6ᵗʰ I97.11 Postprocedural cardiac insufficiency
        I97.110 Postprocedural cardiac insufficiency following cardiac surgery   `CC`
        I97.111 Postprocedural cardiac insufficiency following other surgery   `CC`

    ☑6ᵗʰ I97.12 Postprocedural cardiac arrest
        I97.120 Postprocedural cardiac arrest following cardiac surgery   `CC`
        I97.121 Postprocedural cardiac arrest following other surgery   `CC`

☑6ᵗʰ I97.13 Postprocedural heart failure
    Use additional code to identify the heart failure (I50.-)
    I97.130 Postprocedural heart failure following cardiac surgery   `CC`
    I97.131 Postprocedural heart failure following other surgery   `CC`

☑6ᵗʰ I97.19 Other postprocedural cardiac functional disturbances
    Use additional code, if applicable, to further specify disorder
    I97.190 Other postprocedural cardiac functional disturbances following cardiac surgery   `CC`
        Use additional code, if applicable, for type 4 or type 5 myocardial infarction, to further specify disorder
        AHA: 2019,2Q,33
    I97.191 Other postprocedural cardiac functional disturbances following other surgery   `CC`

I97.2 Postmastectomy lymphedema syndrome   `A`
    Elephantiasis due to mastectomy
    Obliteration of lymphatic vessels

I97.3 Postprocedural hypertension

☑5ᵗʰ I97.4 Intraoperative hemorrhage and hematoma of a circulatory system organ or structure complicating a procedure
    EXCLUDES 1   *intraoperative hemorrhage and hematoma of a circulatory system organ or structure due to accidental puncture and laceration during a procedure (I97.5-)*
    EXCLUDES 2   *intraoperative cerebrovascular hemorrhage complicating a procedure (G97.3-)*

    ☑6ᵗʰ I97.41 Intraoperative hemorrhage and hematoma of a circulatory system organ or structure complicating a circulatory system procedure
        I97.410 Intraoperative hemorrhage and hematoma of a circulatory system organ or structure complicating a cardiac catheterization   `CC`
        I97.411 Intraoperative hemorrhage and hematoma of a circulatory system organ or structure complicating a cardiac bypass   `CC`
        I97.418 Intraoperative hemorrhage and hematoma of a circulatory system organ or structure complicating other circulatory system procedure   `CC`

    I97.42 Intraoperative hemorrhage and hematoma of a circulatory system organ or structure complicating other procedure   `CC`
        AHA: 2020,1Q,19

☑5ᵗʰ I97.5 Accidental puncture and laceration of a circulatory system organ or structure during a procedure
    EXCLUDES 2   *accidental puncture and laceration of brain during a procedure (G97.4-)*

    I97.51 Accidental puncture and laceration of a circulatory system organ or structure during a circulatory system procedure   `CC`
        AHA: 2019,2Q,24

    I97.52 Accidental puncture and laceration of a circulatory system organ or structure during other procedure   `CC`

☑5ᵗʰ I97.6 Postprocedural hemorrhage, hematoma and seroma of a circulatory system organ or structure following a procedure
    EXCLUDES 2   *postprocedural cerebrovascular hemorrhage complicating a procedure (G97.5-)*
    AHA: 2016,4Q,9-10

    ☑6ᵗʰ I97.61 Postprocedural hemorrhage of a circulatory system organ or structure following a circulatory system procedure
        I97.610 Postprocedural hemorrhage of a circulatory system organ or structure following a cardiac catheterization   `CC`
        I97.611 Postprocedural hemorrhage of a circulatory system organ or structure following cardiac bypass   `CC`
        I97.618 Postprocedural hemorrhage of a circulatory system organ or structure following other circulatory system procedure   `CC`

√6ᵗʰ **I97.62 Postprocedural hemorrhage, hematoma and seroma** of a circulatory system organ or structure following other procedure

     I97.620 Postprocedural **hemorrhage** of a circulatory system organ or structure following other procedure `CC`

     I97.621 Postprocedural **hematoma** of a circulatory system organ or structure following other procedure `CC`

     I97.622 Postprocedural **seroma** of a circulatory system organ or structure following other procedure `CC`

√6ᵗʰ **I97.63 Postprocedural hematoma** of a circulatory system organ or structure following a **circulatory system procedure**

     I97.630 Postprocedural hematoma of a circulatory system organ or structure following a **cardiac catheterization** `CC`

     I97.631 Postprocedural hematoma of a circulatory system organ or structure following **cardiac bypass** `CC`

     I97.638 Postprocedural hematoma of a circulatory system organ or structure following **other circulatory system procedure** `CC`

√6ᵗʰ **I97.64 Postprocedural seroma** of a circulatory system organ or structure following a circulatory system procedure

     I97.640 Postprocedural seroma of a circulatory system organ or structure following a **cardiac catheterization** `CC`

     I97.641 Postprocedural seroma of a circulatory system organ or structure following **cardiac bypass** `CC`

     I97.648 Postprocedural seroma of a circulatory system organ or structure following other **circulatory system procedure** `CC`

√5ᵗʰ **I97.7 Intraoperative cardiac functional disturbances**

     EXCLUDES 2   *acute pulmonary insufficiency following thoracic surgery (J95.1)*

                postprocedural cardiac functional disturbances (I97.1-)

√6ᵗʰ **I97.71 Intraoperative cardiac arrest**

     I97.710 Intraoperative cardiac arrest during **cardiac surgery** `CC`

     I97.711 Intraoperative cardiac arrest during **other surgery** `CC`

√6ᵗʰ **I97.79 Other intraoperative cardiac functional disturbances**

     Use additional code, if applicable, to further specify disorder

     I97.790 Other intraoperative cardiac functional disturbances during **cardiac surgery** `CC`

     I97.791 Other intraoperative cardiac functional disturbances during **other surgery** `CC`

√5ᵗʰ **I97.8 Other intraoperative and postprocedural complications and disorders of the circulatory system, not elsewhere classified**

     Use additional code, if applicable, to further specify disorder

√6ᵗʰ **I97.81 Intraoperative cerebrovascular infarction**

     I97.810 Intraoperative cerebrovascular infarction during **cardiac surgery** `CC`

     I97.811 Intraoperative cerebrovascular infarction during **other surgery** `CC`

√6ᵗʰ **I97.82 Postprocedural cerebrovascular infarction**

     I97.820 Postprocedural cerebrovascular infarction following **cardiac surgery** `CC`

     I97.821 Postprocedural cerebrovascular infarction following **other surgery** `CC`

     I97.88 Other intraoperative complications of the circulatory system, not elsewhere classified `CC`

     I97.89 Other postprocedural complications and disorders of the circulatory system, not elsewhere classified `CC`

         AHA: 2024,1Q,26; 2021,3Q,33; 2020,3Q,3-8; 2019,2Q,33

√4ᵗʰ **I99 Other and unspecified disorders of circulatory system**

     I99.8 Other disorder of circulatory system

         AHA: 2020,4Q,98

     I99.9 Unspecified disorder of circulatory system

N Newborn: 0   **P** Pediatric: 0-17   **M** Maternity: 9-64   **A** Adult: 15-124   **UNS** Unspecified Site   **MCC** Major Complication/Comorbidity   **CC** Complication/Comorbidity   **PE** POA Exempt

702   ICD-10-CM 2025

Chapter 10. Diseases of the Respiratory System (J00–J99), U07.0

Chapter-specific Guidelines with Coding Examples

The chapter-specific guidelines from the ICD-10-CM Official Guidelines for Coding and Reporting have been provided below. Along with these guidelines are coding examples, contained in the shaded boxes, that have been developed to help illustrate the coding and/or sequencing guidance found in these guidelines.

a. Chronic obstructive pulmonary disease [COPD] and asthma

1) Acute exacerbation of chronic obstructive bronchitis and asthma

The codes in categories J44 and J45 distinguish between uncomplicated cases and those in acute exacerbation. An acute exacerbation is a worsening or a decompensation of a chronic condition. An acute exacerbation is not equivalent to an infection superimposed on a chronic condition, though an exacerbation may be triggered by an infection.

Vancomycin IV was started to treat a patient with acute pneumonia due to *Streptococcus pneumoniae*. Patient also with acute exacerbation of COPD continued on home meds.

J13	Pneumonia due to Streptococcus pneumoniae
J44.0	Chronic obstructive pulmonary disease with (acute) lower respiratory infection
J44.1	Chronic obstructive pulmonary disease with (acute) exacerbation

Explanation: ICD-10-CM uses combination codes to create organism-specific classifications for acute pneumonia. Category J44 codes include combination codes with severity components, which differentiate between COPD with acute lower respiratory infection (acute pneumonia), COPD with acute exacerbation, and COPD without mention of a complication (unspecified).

An acute exacerbation is a worsening or a decompensation of a chronic condition. An acute exacerbation is not equivalent to an infection superimposed on a chronic condition, though an exacerbation may be triggered by an infection, as in this example. Treatment of the pneumonia necessitated the inpatient admission. Instructional notes at J44.0 say to "code also to identify the infection," which informs the coder that another code must be assigned if applicable. Sequencing of the pneumonia and COPD exacerbation are governed by the Section II, "Selection of Principal Diagnosis," guidelines. In this case it was the pneumonia that was "chiefly responsible for occasioning the admission" with the IV vancomycin treatment.

Exacerbation of moderate persistent asthma with status asthmaticus

J45.42	Moderate persistent asthma with status asthmaticus

Explanation: Category J45 Asthma includes severity-specific subcategories and fifth-character codes to distinguish between uncomplicated cases, those in acute exacerbation, and those with status asthmaticus.

---

b. Acute respiratory failure

1) Acute respiratory failure as principal diagnosis

A code from subcategory J96.0, Acute respiratory failure, or subcategory J96.2, Acute and chronic respiratory failure, may be assigned as a principal diagnosis when it is the condition established after study to be chiefly responsible for occasioning the admission to the hospital, and the selection is supported by the Alphabetic Index and Tabular List. However, chapter-specific coding guidelines (such as obstetrics, poisoning, HIV, newborn) that provide sequencing direction take precedence.

Acute hypoxic respiratory failure due to COPD exacerbation

J96.01	Acute respiratory failure with hypoxia
J44.1	Chronic obstructive pulmonary disease with (acute) exacerbation

Explanation: Category J96 classifies respiratory failure with combination codes that designate the severity and the presence of hypoxia and hypercapnia. Code J96.01 is sequenced as the first-listed diagnosis, as the reason for the admission. Respiratory failure may be assigned as a principal diagnosis when it is the condition established after study to be chiefly responsible for occasioning the admission to the hospital and the selection is supported by the Alphabetic Index and Tabular List.

---

2) Acute respiratory failure as secondary diagnosis

Respiratory failure may be listed as a secondary diagnosis if it occurs after admission, or if it is present on admission, but does not meet the definition of principal diagnosis.

Acute respiratory failure due to accidental oxycodone overdose

T40.2X1A	Poisoning by other opioids, accidental (unintentional), initial encounter
J96.00	Acute respiratory failure, unspecified whether with hypoxia or hypercapnia

Explanation: Respiratory failure may be assigned as a principal diagnosis when it is the condition established after study to be chiefly responsible for occasioning the admission to the hospital, and the selection is supported by the Alphabetic Index and Tabular List. However, chapter-specific coding guidelines, such as poisoning, that provide sequencing direction take precedence. When coding a poisoning or reaction to the improper use of a medication (e.g., overdose, wrong substance given or taken in error, wrong route of administration), first assign the appropriate code from categories T36–T50. Use additional code(s) for all manifestations of the poisoning. In this instance, the respiratory failure is a manifestation of the poisoning and is sequenced as a secondary diagnosis.

Acute pneumococcal pneumonia with subsequent development of acute respiratory failure

J13	Pneumonia due to Streptococcus pneumoniae
J96.00	Acute respiratory failure, unspecified whether with hypoxia or hypercapnia

Explanation: Acute respiratory failure may be listed as a secondary diagnosis if it occurs after admission, or if it is present on admission but does not meet the definition of principal diagnosis.

---

3) Sequencing of acute respiratory failure and another acute condition

When a patient is admitted with respiratory failure and another acute condition, (e.g., myocardial infarction, cerebrovascular accident, aspiration pneumonia), the principal diagnosis will not be the same in every situation. This applies whether the other acute condition is a respiratory or nonrespiratory condition. Selection of the principal diagnosis will be dependent on the circumstances of admission. If both the respiratory failure and the other acute condition are equally responsible for occasioning the admission to the hospital, and there are no chapter-specific sequencing rules, the guideline regarding two or more diagnoses that equally meet the definition for principal diagnosis (*Section II, C.*) may be applied in these situations.

If the documentation is not clear as to whether acute respiratory failure and another condition are equally responsible for occasioning the admission, query the provider for clarification.

Acute pneumococcal pneumonia and acute respiratory failure, both present on admission

J96.00	Acute respiratory failure, unspecified whether with hypoxia or hypercapnia
J13	Pneumonia due to Streptococcus pneumoniae

Explanation: When a patient is admitted with respiratory failure and another acute condition, such as a bacterial pneumonia, the principal diagnosis is not the same in every situation. This applies whether the other acute condition is a respiratory or nonrespiratory condition. The principal diagnosis depends on the circumstances of admission.

---

c. Influenza due to certain identified influenza viruses

Code only confirmed cases of influenza due to certain identified influenza viruses (category J09), and due to other identified influenza virus (category J10). This is an exception to the hospital inpatient guideline Section II, H. (Uncertain Diagnosis).

In this context, "confirmation" does not require documentation of positive laboratory testing specific for avian or other novel influenza A or other identified influenza virus. However, coding should be based on the provider's diagnostic statement that the patient has avian influenza, or other novel influenza A, for category J09, or has another particular identified strain of influenza, such as H1N1 or H3N2, but not identified as novel or variant, for category J10.

If the provider records "suspected" or "possible" or "probable" avian influenza, or novel influenza, or other identified influenza, then the appropriate influenza code from category J11, Influenza due to unidentified influenza virus, should be assigned. A code from category J09, Influenza due to certain identified influenza viruses, should not be assigned nor should a code from category J10, Influenza due to other identified influenza virus.

Influenza due to avian influenza virus with pneumonia

J09.X1 Influenza due to identified novel influenza A virus with pneumonia

Explanation: Codes in category J09 Influenza due to certain identified influenza viruses should be assigned only for confirmed cases. "Confirmation" does not require positive laboratory testing of a specific influenza virus but does need to be based on the provider's diagnostic statement, which should not include terms such as "possible," "probable," or "suspected."

---

d. Ventilator associated pneumonia

1) Documentation of ventilator associated pneumonia

As with all procedural or postprocedural complications, code assignment is based on the provider's documentation of the relationship between the condition and the procedure.

Code J95.851, Ventilator associated pneumonia, should be assigned only when the provider has documented ventilator associated pneumonia (VAP). An additional code to identify the organism (e.g., Pseudomonas aeruginosa, code B96.5) should also be assigned. Do not assign an additional code from categories J12–J18 to identify the type of pneumonia.

Code J95.851 should not be assigned for cases where the patient has pneumonia and is on a mechanical ventilator and the provider has not specifically stated that the pneumonia is ventilator-associated pneumonia. If the documentation is unclear as to whether the patient has a pneumonia that is a complication attributable to the mechanical ventilator, query the provider.

2) Ventilator associated pneumonia develops after admission

A patient may be admitted with one type of pneumonia (e.g., code J13, Pneumonia due to Streptococcus pneumonia) and subsequently develop VAP. In this instance, the principal diagnosis would be the appropriate code from categories J12–J18 for the pneumonia diagnosed at the time of admission. Code J95.851, Ventilator associated pneumonia, would be assigned as an additional diagnosis when the provider has also documented the presence of ventilator associated pneumonia.

Patient with pneumonia due to *Klebsiella pneumoniae* develops superimposed MRSA ventilator-associated pneumonia

J15.0 Pneumonia due to Klebsiella pneumoniae

J95.851 Ventilator associated pneumonia

B95.62 Methicillin resistant Staphylococcus aureus infection as the cause of diseases classified elsewhere

Explanation: Code assignment for ventilator-associated pneumonia is based on the provider's documentation of the relationship between the condition and the procedure and is reported only when the provider has documented ventilator-associated pneumonia (VAP).

A patient may be admitted with one type of pneumonia and subsequently develop VAP. In this example, the principal diagnosis code describes the pneumonia diagnosed at the time of admission, with code J95.851 Ventilator associated pneumonia, assigned as secondary.

---

e. Vaping-related disorders

For patients presenting with condition(s) related to vaping, assign code U07.0, Vaping-related disorder, as the principal diagnosis. For lung injury due to vaping, assign only code U07.0. Assign additional codes for other manifestations, such as acute respiratory failure (subcategory J96.0-) or pneumonitis (code J68.0).

Associated respiratory signs and symptoms due to vaping, such as cough, shortness of breath, etc., are not coded separately, when a definitive diagnosis has been established. However, it would be appropriate to code separately any gastrointestinal symptoms, such as diarrhea and abdominal pain.

See Section I.C.1.g.1.c.i. for Pneumonia confirmed as due to COVID-19

23-year-old patient with history of anxiety disorder admitted with fever, dyspnea and nonproductive cough. Patient's respiratory function continued to clinically worsen, requiring intubation for suspected ARDS and required OGT suction for coffee ground hematemesis. Following extubating, patient confirmed the use of THC vaping cartridge preceding development of symptoms. Discharge diagnosis is ARDS due to EVALI and anxiety disorder.

U07.0 Vaping related disorder

J80 Acute respiratory distress syndrome

K92.0 Hematemesis

F41.9 Anxiety disorder, unspecified

Explanation: Codes U07.0 and J80 represent the vaping-related disorder and its associated manifestation, the acute respiratory distress syndrome (ARDS). The symptoms that brought the patient in are not coded separately because these are integral to the vaping disorder and the ARDS, unlike the hematemesis (vomiting blood) a gastrointestinal symptom that is not integral to either of these conditions.

Chapter 10. Diseases of the Respiratory System (J00-J99)

NOTE When a respiratory condition is described as occurring in more than one site and is not specifically indexed, it should be classified to the lower anatomic site (e.g., tracheobronchitis to bronchitis in J40).

Use additional code, where applicable, to identify:
exposure to environmental tobacco smoke (Z77.22)
exposure to tobacco smoke in the perinatal period (P96.81)
history of tobacco dependence (Z87.891)
occupational exposure to environmental tobacco smoke (Z57.31)
tobacco dependence (F17.-)
tobacco use (Z72.0)

EXCLUDES 2   certain conditions originating in the perinatal period (P04-P96)
certain infectious and parasitic diseases (A00-B99)
complications of pregnancy, childbirth and the puerperium (O00-O9A)
congenital malformations, deformations and chromosomal abnormalities (Q00-Q99)
endocrine, nutritional and metabolic diseases (E00-E88)
injury, poisoning and certain other consequences of external causes (S00-T88)
neoplasms (C00-D49)
smoke inhalation (T59.81-)
symptoms, signs and abnormal clinical and laboratory findings, not elsewhere classified (R00-R94)

This chapter contains the following blocks:

J00-J06	Acute upper respiratory infections
J09-J18	Influenza and pneumonia
J20-J22	Other acute lower respiratory infections
J30-J39	Other diseases of upper respiratory tract
J40-J4A	Chronic lower respiratory diseases
J60-J70	Lung diseases due to external agents
J80-J84	Other respiratory diseases principally affecting the interstitium
J85-J86	Suppurative and necrotic conditions of the lower respiratory tract
J90-J94	Other diseases of the pleura
J95	Intraoperative and postprocedural complications and disorders of respiratory system, not elsewhere classified
J96-J99	Other diseases of the respiratory system

Acute upper respiratory infections (J00-J06)

EXCLUDES 1   chronic obstructive pulmonary disease with acute lower respiratory infection (J44.0)

J00 Acute nasopharyngitis [common cold]
Acute rhinitis
Coryza (acute)
Infective nasopharyngitis NOS
Infective rhinitis
Nasal catarrh, acute
Nasopharyngitis NOS
> EXCLUDES 1   acute pharyngitis (J02.-)
> acute sore throat NOS (J02.9)
> influenza virus with other respiratory manifestations (J09.X2, J10.1, J11.1)
> pharyngitis NOS (J02.9)
> rhinitis NOS (J31.0)
> sore throat NOS (J02.9)
> EXCLUDES 2   allergic rhinitis (J30.1-J30.9)
> chronic pharyngitis (J31.2)
> chronic rhinitis (J31.0)
> chronic sore throat (J31.2)
> nasopharyngitis, chronic (J31.1)
> vasomotor rhinitis (J30.0)

✓4ᵗʰ J01 Acute sinusitis
INCLUDES   acute abscess of sinus
acute empyema of sinus
acute infection of sinus
acute inflammation of sinus
acute suppuration of sinus
Use additional code (B95-B97) to identify infectious agent
> EXCLUDES 1   sinusitis NOS (J32.9)
> EXCLUDES 2   chronic sinusitis (J32.0-J32.8)

✓5ᵗʰ J01.0 Acute maxillary sinusitis
Acute antritis
     J01.00   Acute maxillary sinusitis, unspecified
     J01.01   Acute recurrent maxillary sinusitis

✓5ᵗʰ J01.1 Acute frontal sinusitis
     J01.10   Acute frontal sinusitis, unspecified
     J01.11   Acute recurrent frontal sinusitis

✓5ᵗʰ J01.2 Acute ethmoidal sinusitis
     J01.20   Acute ethmoidal sinusitis, unspecified
     J01.21   Acute recurrent ethmoidal sinusitis

✓5ᵗʰ J01.3 Acute sphenoidal sinusitis
     J01.30   Acute sphenoidal sinusitis, unspecified
     J01.31   Acute recurrent sphenoidal sinusitis

✓5ᵗʰ J01.4 Acute pansinusitis
     J01.40   Acute pansinusitis, unspecified
     J01.41   Acute recurrent pansinusitis

✓5ᵗʰ J01.8 Other acute sinusitis
     J01.80   Other acute sinusitis
         Acute sinusitis involving more than one sinus but not pansinusitis
     J01.81   Other acute recurrent sinusitis
         Acute recurrent sinusitis involving more than one sinus but not pansinusitis

✓5ᵗʰ J01.9 Acute sinusitis, unspecified
     J01.90   Acute sinusitis, unspecified
     J01.91   Acute recurrent sinusitis, unspecified

✓4ᵗʰ J02 Acute pharyngitis
INCLUDES   acute sore throat
> EXCLUDES 1   acute laryngopharyngitis (J06.0)
> peritonsillar abscess (J36)
> pharyngeal abscess (J39.1)
> retropharyngeal abscess (J39.0)
> EXCLUDES 2   chronic pharyngitis (J31.2)

J02.0 Streptococcal pharyngitis
Septic pharyngitis
Streptococcal sore throat
> EXCLUDES 2   scarlet fever (A38.-)

J02.8 Acute pharyngitis due to other specified organisms
Use additional code (B95-B97) to identify infectious agent
> EXCLUDES 1   acute pharyngitis due to coxsackie virus (B08.5)
> acute pharyngitis due to gonococcus (A54.5)
> acute pharyngitis due to herpes [simplex] virus (B00.2)
> acute pharyngitis due to infectious mononucleosis (B27.-)
> enteroviral vesicular pharyngitis (B08.5)

J02.9 Acute pharyngitis, unspecified
Gangrenous pharyngitis (acute)
Infective pharyngitis (acute) NOS
Pharyngitis (acute) NOS
Sore throat (acute) NOS
Suppurative pharyngitis (acute)
Ulcerative pharyngitis (acute)
> EXCLUDES 1   influenza virus with other respiratory manifestations (J09.X2, J10.1, J11.1)

✓4ᵗʰ J03 Acute tonsillitis
> EXCLUDES 1   acute sore throat (J02.-)
> hypertrophy of tonsils (J35.1)
> peritonsillar abscess (J36)
> sore throat NOS (J02.9)
> streptococcal sore throat (J02.0)
> EXCLUDES 2   chronic tonsillitis (J35.0)

✓5ᵗʰ J03.0 Streptococcal tonsillitis
     J03.00   Acute streptococcal tonsillitis, unspecified
     J03.01   Acute recurrent streptococcal tonsillitis

✓5ᵗʰ J03.8 Acute tonsillitis due to other specified organisms
Use additional code (B95-B97) to identify infectious agent
> EXCLUDES 1   diphtheritic tonsillitis (A36.0)
> herpesviral pharyngotonsillitis (B00.2)
> streptococcal tonsillitis (J03.0)
> tuberculous tonsillitis (A15.8)
> Vincent's tonsillitis (A69.1)
     J03.80   Acute tonsillitis due to other specified organisms
     J03.81   Acute recurrent tonsillitis due to other specified organisms

☑ Additional Character Required   ✓x7ᵗʰ Placeholder   Questionable PDx   Manifestation   Unspecified   UPD Unacceptable PDx   H1-H14 HAC   HCC CMS-HCC Dx   HIV HIV Dx

ICD-10-CM 2025   705

Chapter 10. Diseases of the Respiratory System

J03.9–J09.X9

✓5ᵗʰ **J03.9 Acute tonsillitis, unspecified**
Follicular tonsillitis (acute)
Gangrenous tonsillitis (acute)
Infective tonsillitis (acute)
Tonsillitis (acute) NOS
Ulcerative tonsillitis (acute)
EXCLUDES 1   *influenza virus with other respiratory manifestations (J09.X2, J10.1, J11.1)*

J03.90 Acute tonsillitis, unspecified
J03.91 Acute recurrent tonsillitis, unspecified

✓4ᵗʰ **J04 Acute laryngitis and tracheitis**
Code also influenza, if present, such as:
influenza due to identified novel influenza A virus with other respiratory manifestations (J09.X2)
influenza due to other identified influenza virus with other respiratory manifestations (J10.1)
influenza due to unidentified influenza virus with other respiratory manifestations (J11.1)
Use additional code (B95-B97) to identify infectious agent
EXCLUDES 1   *acute obstructive laryngitis [croup] and epiglottitis (J05.-)*
EXCLUDES 2   *laryngismus (stridulus) (J38.5)*

J04.0 Acute laryngitis
Edematous laryngitis (acute)
Laryngitis (acute) NOS
Subglottic laryngitis (acute)
Suppurative laryngitis (acute)
Ulcerative laryngitis (acute)
EXCLUDES 1   *acute obstructive laryngitis (J05.0)*
EXCLUDES 2   *chronic laryngitis (J37.0)*

✓5ᵗʰ **J04.1 Acute tracheitis**
Acute viral tracheitis
Catarrhal tracheitis (acute)
Tracheitis (acute) NOS
EXCLUDES 2   *chronic tracheitis (J42)*

J04.10 Acute tracheitis without obstruction
J04.11 Acute tracheitis with obstruction   MCC

J04.2 Acute laryngotracheitis
Laryngotracheitis NOS
Tracheitis (acute) with laryngitis (acute)
EXCLUDES 1   *acute obstructive laryngotracheitis (J05.0)*
EXCLUDES 2   *chronic laryngotracheitis (J37.1)*

✓5ᵗʰ **J04.3 Supraglottitis, unspecified**
J04.30 Supraglottitis, unspecified, without obstruction
J04.31 Supraglottitis, unspecified, with obstruction   MCC

✓4ᵗʰ **J05 Acute obstructive laryngitis [croup] and epiglottitis**
Code also, influenza, if present, such as:
influenza due to identified novel influenza A virus with other respiratory manifestations (J09.X2)
influenza due to other identified influenza virus with other respiratory manifestations (J10.1)
influenza due to unidentified influenza virus with other respiratory manifestations (J11.1)
Use additional code (B95-B97) to identify infectious agent

J05.0 Acute obstructive laryngitis [croup]
Obstructive laryngitis (acute) NOS
Obstructive laryngotracheitis NOS
DEF: Acute laryngeal obstruction due to allergies, foreign bodies, or in the majority of cases a viral infection. Symptoms include a harsh, barking cough, hoarseness, and a persistent, high-pitched respiratory sound (stridor).

✓5ᵗʰ **J05.1 Acute epiglottitis**
EXCLUDES 2   *epiglottitis, chronic (J37.0)*
J05.10 Acute epiglottitis without obstruction   CC
Epiglottitis NOS
J05.11 Acute epiglottitis with obstruction   MCC

✓4ᵗʰ **J06 Acute upper respiratory infections of multiple and unspecified sites**
EXCLUDES 1   *acute respiratory infection NOS (J22)*
influenza virus with other respiratory manifestations (J09.X2, J10.1, J11.1)
streptococcal pharyngitis (J02.0)

J06.0 Acute laryngopharyngitis

J06.9 Acute upper respiratory infection, unspecified
Upper respiratory disease, acute
Upper respiratory infection NOS
Use additional code (B95-B97) to identify infectious agent, if known, such as:
respiratory syncytial virus (RSV) (B97.4)
AHA: 2020,1Q,22

Influenza and pneumonia (J09-J18)

Use additional code, if applicable, to identify resistance to antimicrobial drugs (Z16.-)
EXCLUDES 2   *allergic or eosinophilic pneumonia (J82)*
aspiration pneumonia NOS (J69.0)
meconium pneumonia (P24.01)
neonatal aspiration pneumonia (P24.-)
pneumonia due to solids and liquids (J69.-)
congenital pneumonia (P23.9)
lipid pneumonia (J69.1)
rheumatic pneumonia (I00)
ventilator associated pneumonia (J95.851)
AHA: 2017,4Q,96
TIP: Hemoptysis (R04.2) is not customarily associated with pneumonia and may be reported separately.

✓4ᵗʰ **J09 Influenza due to certain identified influenza viruses**
EXCLUDES 1   *influenza A/H1N1 (J10.-)*
influenza due to other identified influenza virus (J10.-)
influenza due to unidentified influenza virus (J11.-)
seasonal influenza due to other identified influenza virus (J10.-)
seasonal influenza due to unidentified influenza virus (J11.-)

✓5ᵗʰ **J09.X Influenza due to identified novel influenza A virus**
Avian influenza
Bird influenza
Influenza A/H5N1
Influenza of other animal origin, not bird or swine
Swine influenza virus (viruses that normally cause infections in pigs)
AHA: 2016,3Q,10

J09.X1 Influenza due to identified novel influenza A virus with pneumonia   HIV MCC
Code also, if applicable, associated:
lung abscess (J85.1)
other specified type of pneumonia

J09.X2 Influenza due to identified novel influenza A virus with other respiratory manifestations
Influenza due to identified novel influenza A virus NOS
Influenza due to identified novel influenza A virus with laryngitis
Influenza due to identified novel influenza A virus with pharyngitis
Influenza due to identified novel influenza A virus with upper respiratory symptoms
Use additional code, if applicable, for associated:
pleural effusion (J91.8)
sinusitis (J01.-)

J09.X3 Influenza due to identified novel influenza A virus with gastrointestinal manifestations
Influenza due to identified novel influenza A virus gastroenteritis
EXCLUDES 1   *'intestinal flu' [viral gastroenteritis] (A08.-)*

J09.X9 Influenza due to identified novel influenza A virus with other manifestations
Influenza due to identified novel influenza A virus with encephalopathy
Influenza due to identified novel influenza A virus with myocarditis
Influenza due to identified novel influenza A virus with otitis media
Use additional code to identify manifestation

N Newborn: 0   P Pediatric: 0-17   M Maternity: 9-64   A Adult: 15-124   UNS Unspecified Site   MCC Major Complication/Comorbidity   CC Complication/Comorbidity   PE POA Exempt

706   ICD-10-CM 2025

☑4ᵗʰ **J10** **Influenza due to other identified influenza virus**

     INCLUDES   influenza A (non-novel)
                 influenza B
                 influenza C
     EXCLUDES 1   *influenza due to avian influenza virus (J09.X-)*
                 influenza due to swine flu (J09.X-)
                 influenza due to unidentified influenza virus (J11.-)

✓5ᵗʰ **J10.0** **Influenza due to other identified influenza virus with pneumonia**
        Code also associated lung abscess, if applicable (J85.1)

    J10.00 **Influenza due to other identified influenza virus with unspecified type of pneumonia**   MCC

    J10.01 **Influenza due to other identified influenza virus with the same other identified influenza virus pneumonia**   MCC

    J10.08 **Influenza due to other identified influenza virus with other specified pneumonia**   HIV MCC
          Code also other specified type of pneumonia

   J10.1 **Influenza due to other identified influenza virus with other respiratory manifestations**
       Influenza due to other identified influenza virus NOS
       Influenza due to other identified influenza virus with laryngitis
       Influenza due to other identified influenza virus with pharyngitis
       Influenza due to other identified influenza virus with upper respiratory symptoms
       Use additional code for associated pleural effusion, if applicable (J91.8)
       Use additional code for associated sinusitis, if applicable (J01.-)
       AHA: 2016,3Q,10-11

   J10.2 **Influenza due to other identified influenza virus with gastrointestinal manifestations**
       Influenza due to other identified influenza virus gastroenteritis
       EXCLUDES 1   *"intestinal flu" [viral gastroenteritis] (A08.-)*

✓5ᵗʰ **J10.8** **Influenza due to other identified influenza virus with other manifestations**

    J10.81 **Influenza due to other identified influenza virus with encephalopathy**

    J10.82 **Influenza due to other identified influenza virus with myocarditis**

    J10.83 **Influenza due to other identified influenza virus with otitis media**
        Use additional code for any associated perforated tympanic membrane (H72.-)

    J10.89 **Influenza due to other identified influenza virus with other manifestations**
        Use additional codes to identify the manifestations

☑4ᵗʰ **J11** **Influenza due to unidentified influenza virus**

✓5ᵗʰ **J11.0** **Influenza due to unidentified influenza virus with pneumonia**
       Code also associated lung abscess, if applicable (J85.1)
       AHA: 2016,3Q,11

    J11.00 **Influenza due to unidentified influenza virus with unspecified type of pneumonia**   MCC
        Influenza with pneumonia NOS

    J11.08 **Influenza due to unidentified influenza virus with specified pneumonia**   MCC
        Code also other specified type of pneumonia

   J11.1 **Influenza due to unidentified influenza virus with other respiratory manifestations**
       Influenza NOS
       Influenzal laryngitis NOS
       Influenzal pharyngitis NOS
       Influenza with upper respiratory symptoms NOS
       Use additional code for associated pleural effusion, if applicable (J91.8)
       Use additional code for associated sinusitis, if applicable (J01.-)

   J11.2 **Influenza due to unidentified influenza virus with gastrointestinal manifestations**
       Influenza gastroenteritis NOS
       EXCLUDES 1   *"intestinal flu" [viral gastroenteritis] (A08.-)*

✓5ᵗʰ **J11.8** **Influenza due to unidentified influenza virus with other manifestations**

    J11.81 **Influenza due to unidentified influenza virus with encephalopathy**
        Influenzal encephalopathy NOS

    J11.82 **Influenza due to unidentified influenza virus with myocarditis**
        Influenzal myocarditis NOS

    J11.83 **Influenza due to unidentified influenza virus with otitis media**
        Influenzal otitis media NOS
        Use additional code for any associated perforated tympanic membrane (H72.-)

    J11.89 **Influenza due to unidentified influenza virus with other manifestations**
        Use additional codes to identify the manifestations

☑4ᵗʰ **J12** **Viral pneumonia, not elsewhere classified**

     INCLUDES   bronchopneumonia due to viruses other than influenza viruses
     Code first associated influenza, if applicable (J09.X1, J10.0-, J11.0-)
     Code also associated abscess, if applicable (J85.1)
     EXCLUDES 1   ~~aspiration pneumonia due to anesthesia during labor and delivery (O74.0)~~
               ~~aspiration pneumonia due to anesthesia during pregnancy (O29)~~
               ~~aspiration pneumonia due to anesthesia during puerperium (O89.0)~~
               ~~aspiration pneumonia due to solids and liquids (J69.-)~~
               ~~aspiration pneumonia NOS (J69.0)~~
               ~~congenital pneumonia (P23.0)~~
               ~~congenital rubella pneumonitis (P35.0)~~
               ~~interstitial pneumonia NOS (J84.9)~~
               ~~lipid pneumonia (J69.1)~~
               ~~neonatal aspiration pneumonia (P24.-)~~
     EXCLUDES 2   ▸*aspiration pneumonia due to anesthesia during delivery (O74.0)*◂
              ▸*aspiration pneumonia due to anesthesia during pregnancy (O29)*◂
              ▸*aspiration pneumonia due to anesthesia during puerperium (O89.0)*◂
              ▸*aspiration pneumonia due to solids and liquids (J69.-)*◂
              ▸*aspiration pneumonia NOS (J69.0)*◂
              ▸*congenital pneumonia (P23.0)*◂
              ▸*congenital rubella pneumonitis (P35.0)*◂
              ▸*interstitial pneumonia NOS (J84.9)*◂
              ▸*lipid pneumonia (J69.1)*◂
              ▸*neonatal aspiration pneumonia (P24.-)*◂
     AHA: 2020,2Q,28; 2019,1Q,35; 2018,3Q,24; 2016,3Q,15; 2013,4Q,118

   J12.0 **Adenoviral pneumonia**   MCC

   J12.1 **Respiratory syncytial virus pneumonia**   MCC
       RSV pneumonia

   J12.2 **Parainfluenza virus pneumonia**   MCC

   J12.3 **Human metapneumovirus pneumonia**   HIV MCC

✓5ᵗʰ **J12.8** **Other viral pneumonia**

    J12.81 **Pneumonia due to SARS-associated coronavirus**   HIV MCC
        Severe acute respiratory syndrome NOS
        DEF: Inflammation of the lungs with consolidation, caused by the severe adult respiratory syndrome (SARS)-associated coronavirus or SARS-CoV. This pneumonia should not be confused with that caused by SARS-CoV-2 (COVID-19).

    J12.82 **Pneumonia due to coronavirus disease 2019**   HIV MCC UPD
        Pneumonia due to 2019 novel coronavirus (SARS-CoV-2)
        Pneumonia due to COVID-19
        Code first COVID-19 (U07.1)
        AHA: 2021,1Q,25-30,31-49

    J12.89 **Other viral pneumonia**   HIV MCC
        AHA: 2021,1Q,33-34; 2020,2Q,8,11; 2020,1Q,34-36

   J12.9 **Viral pneumonia, unspecified**   HIV MCC

J13 **Pneumonia due to Streptococcus pneumoniae**   HIV MCC
       Bronchopneumonia due to S. pneumoniae
       ▸Code first, if applicable, associated influenza◂ (J09.X1, J10.0-, J11.0-)
       ▸Code also, if applicable, any associated condition such as:◂
       ▸abscess (J85.1)◂
       ▸aspiration pneumonia (J69.-)◂
       EXCLUDES 1   *congenital pneumonia due to S. pneumoniae (P23.6)*
              lobar pneumonia, unspecified organism (J18.1)
              pneumonia due to other streptococci (J15.3-J15.4)
       AHA: 2020,2Q,28; 2019,1Q,35; 2018,3Q,24; 2016,3Q,15; 2013,4Q,118

Chapter 10. Diseases of the Respiratory System

J14 Pneumonia due to Hemophilus influenzae `HIV` `MCC`
Bronchopneumonia due to H. influenzae
▶Code first, if applicable, associated influenza◀ (JØ9.X1, J1Ø.Ø-, J11.Ø-)
▶Code also, if applicable, any associated condition such as:◀
  ▶abscess (J85.1)◀
  ▶aspiration pneumonia (J69.-)◀
  EXCLUDES 1   congenital pneumonia due to H. influenzae (P23.6)
  AHA: 2020,2Q,28; 2019,1Q,35; 2018,3Q,24; 2016,3Q,15; 2013,4Q,118

✓4ᵗʰ J15 Bacterial pneumonia, not elsewhere classified
  INCLUDES   Bronchopneumonia due to bacteria other than S. pneumoniae and H. influenzae
▶Code first, if applicable, associated influenza◀ (JØ9.X1, J1Ø.Ø-, J11.Ø-)
▶Code also, if applicable, any associated condition such as:◀
  ▶abscess (J85.1)◀
  ▶aspiration pneumonia (J69.-)◀
  EXCLUDES 1   chlamydial pneumonia (J16.Ø)
                congenital pneumonia (P23.-)
                Legionnaires' disease (A48.1)
                spirochetal pneumonia (A69.8)
  AHA: 2020,2Q,28; 2019,1Q,35; 2018,3Q,24; 2016,3Q,15; 2013,4Q,118

J15.Ø Pneumonia due to Klebsiella pneumoniae `HIV` `MCC` `HCC`
J15.1 Pneumonia due to Pseudomonas `HIV` `MCC` `HCC`
✓5ᵗʰ J15.2 Pneumonia due to staphylococcus

  J15.2Ø Pneumonia due to staphylococcus, unspecified `HIV` `MCC` `HCC`
  ✓6ᵗʰ J15.21 Pneumonia due to Staphylococcus aureus
    J15.211 Pneumonia due to methicillin susceptible Staphylococcus aureus `HIV` `MCC` `HCC`
      MSSA pneumonia
      Pneumonia due to Staphylococcus aureus NOS
    J15.212 Pneumonia due to methicillin resistant Staphylococcus aureus `HIV` `MCC` `HCC`
  J15.29 Pneumonia due to other staphylococcus `HIV` `MCC` `HCC`

J15.3 Pneumonia due to streptococcus, group B `HIV` `MCC`
J15.4 Pneumonia due to other streptococci `HIV`
  EXCLUDES 1   pneumonia due to streptococcus, group B (J15.3)
                pneumonia due to Streptococcus pneumoniae (J13)
J15.5 Pneumonia due to Escherichia coli `HIV` `MCC` `HCC`
✓5ᵗʰ J15.6 Pneumonia due to other Gram-negative bacteria
  AHA: 2023,4Q,27; 2020,2Q,28
  J15.61 Pneumonia due to Acinetobacter baumannii `MCC` `HCC`
  J15.69 Pneumonia due to other Gram-negative bacteria `MCC` `HCC`
    Pneumonia due to other aerobic Gram-negative bacteria
    Pneumonia due to Serratia marcescens
J15.7 Pneumonia due to Mycoplasma pneumoniae `MCC`
J15.8 Pneumonia due to other specified bacteria `HIV` `MCC` `HCC`
J15.9 Unspecified bacterial pneumonia `HIV` `MCC`
  Pneumonia due to gram-positive bacteria

✓4ᵗʰ J16 Pneumonia due to other infectious organisms, not elsewhere classified
▶Code first, if applicable, associated influenza◀ (JØ9.X1, J1Ø.Ø-, J11.Ø-)
▶Code also, if applicable, any associated condition such as:◀
  ▶abscess (J85.1)◀
  ▶aspiration pneumonia (J69.-)◀
  EXCLUDES 1   congenital pneumonia (P23.-)
                ornithosis (A7Ø)
                pneumocystosis (B59)
                pneumonia NOS (J18.9)
  AHA: 2020,2Q,28; 2019,1Q,35; 2018,3Q,24; 2016,3Q,15; 2013,4Q,118
J16.Ø Chlamydial pneumonia `MCC`
J16.8 Pneumonia due to other specified infectious organisms `MCC`

J17 Pneumonia in diseases classified elsewhere `MCC`
Code first underlying disease, such as:
  Q fever (A78)
  rheumatic fever (IØØ)
  schistosomiasis (B65.Ø-B65.9)
▶Code also, if applicable, any associated condition such as:◀
  ▶abscess (J85.1)◀
  ▶aspiration pneumonia (J69.-)◀
  EXCLUDES 1   candidial pneumonia (B37.1)
                chlamydial pneumonia (J16.Ø)
                gonorrheal pneumonia (A54.84)
                histoplasmosis pneumonia (B39.Ø-B39.2)
                measles pneumonia (BØ5.2)
                nocardiosis pneumonia (A43.Ø)
                pneumocystosis (B59)
                pneumonia due to Pneumocystis carinii (B59)
                pneumonia due to Pneumocystis jiroveci (B59)
                pneumonia in actinomycosis (A42.Ø)
                pneumonia in anthrax (A22.1)
                pneumonia in ascariasis (B77.81)
                pneumonia in aspergillosis (B44.Ø-B44.1)
                pneumonia in coccidioidomycosis (B38.Ø-B38.2)
                pneumonia in cytomegalovirus disease (B25.Ø)
                pneumonia in toxoplasmosis (B58.3)
                rubella pneumonia (BØ6.81)
                salmonella pneumonia (AØ2.22)
                spirochetal infection NEC with pneumonia (A69.8)
                tularemia pneumonia (A21.2)
                typhoid fever with pneumonia (AØ1.Ø3)
                varicella pneumonia (BØ1.2)
                whooping cough with pneumonia (A37 with fifth character 1)
  AHA: 2020,2Q,28; 2019,1Q,35; 2016,3Q,15; 2013,4Q,118

✓4ᵗʰ J18 Pneumonia, unspecified organism
▶Code first, if applicable, associated influenza◀ (JØ9.X1, J1Ø.Ø-, J11.Ø-)
▶Code also, if applicable, any associated condition such as:◀
  ▶aspiration pneumonia (J69.-)◀
  EXCLUDES 1   abscess of lung with pneumonia (J85.1)
                aspiration pneumonia due to anesthesia during labor and delivery (O74.Ø)
                aspiration pneumonia due to anesthesia during pregnancy (O29)
                aspiration pneumonia due to anesthesia during puerperium (O89.Ø)
                aspiration pneumonia due to solids and liquids (J69.-)
                aspiration pneumonia NOS (J69.Ø)
                congenital pneumonia (P23.Ø)
                drug-induced interstitial lung disorder (J7Ø.2-J7Ø.4)
                interstitial pneumonia NOS (J84.9)
                lipid pneumonia (J69.1)
                neonatal aspiration pneumonia (P24.-)
                pneumonitis due to external agents (J67-J7Ø)
                pneumonitis due to fumes and vapors (J68.Ø)
                usual interstitial pneumonia (J84.178)
  EXCLUDES 2   ▶abscess of lung with pneumonia (J85.1)◀
                ▶aspiration pneumonia due to anesthesia during labor and delivery (O74.Ø)◀
                ▶aspiration pneumonia due to anesthesia during pregnancy (O29)◀
                ▶aspiration pneumonia due to anesthesia during puerperium (O89.Ø)◀
                ▶aspiration pneumonia due to solids and liquids (J69.-)◀
                ▶aspiration pneumonia NOS (J69.Ø)◀
                ▶lipid pneumonia (J69.1)◀
                ▶pneumonitis due to external agents (J67-J7Ø)◀
  AHA: 2020,2Q,28; 2019,1Q,35; 2016,3Q,15; 2013,4Q,118

J18.Ø Bronchopneumonia, unspecified organism `MCC`
  EXCLUDES 1   hypostatic bronchopneumonia (J18.2)
                lipid pneumonia (J69.1)
  EXCLUDES 2   acute bronchiolitis (J21.-)
                chronic bronchiolitis ▶(J44.89)◀
                ▶other specified chronic obstructive pulmonary disease (J44.89)◀

J18.1 **Lobar** pneumonia, unspecified organism   `HIV` `MCC`
AHA: 2019,3Q,37; 2018,3Q,24
DEF: Lobar pneumonia is characterized by consolidated inflammation confined or localized to only one or a few lobes of the lung. The consolidation affects primarily the alveolar air spaces, unlike bronchopneumonia, which arises from the bronchi or bronchioles and affects a wide area without any localization.
TIP: Documentation of right upper lobe, left upper lobe, right lower lobe, left lower lobe, or right middle lobe pneumonia alone is not synonymous with "lobar pneumonia," nor should a diagnosis of lobar pneumonia be assumed based on an imaging report that identifies pneumonia in a specific lobe. Assign J18.1 only when the provider specifically documents "lobar pneumonia" without specifying a causal organism.

J18.2 **Hypostatic** pneumonia, unspecified organism   `CC`
Hypostatic bronchopneumonia
Passive pneumonia

J18.8 Other pneumonia, unspecified organism   `HIV` `MCC`

J18.9 Pneumonia, unspecified organism   `HIV` `MCC`
AHA: 2020,2Q,28; 2019,3Q,15; 2019,2Q,28; 2014,3Q,4; 2013,4Q,119; 2012,4Q,94

Other acute lower respiratory infections (J20-J22)

> `EXCLUDES 2`   *chronic obstructive pulmonary disease with acute lower respiratory infection (J44.0)*

`✓4th` **J20** **Acute bronchitis**

`INCLUDES`   acute and subacute bronchitis (with) bronchospasm
acute and subacute bronchitis (with) tracheitis
acute and subacute bronchitis (with) tracheobronchitis, acute
acute and subacute fibrinous bronchitis
acute and subacute membranous bronchitis
acute and subacute purulent bronchitis
acute and subacute septic bronchitis

`EXCLUDES 1`   *bronchitis NOS (J40)*
tracheobronchitis NOS (J40)

`EXCLUDES 2`   *acute bronchitis with bronchiectasis (J47.0)*
acute bronchitis with chronic obstructive asthma (J44.0)
acute bronchitis with chronic obstructive pulmonary disease (J44.0)
allergic bronchitis NOS (J45.909-)
bronchitis due to chemicals, fumes and vapors (J68.0)
chronic bronchitis NOS (J42)
chronic mucopurulent bronchitis (J41.1)
chronic obstructive bronchitis (J44.-)
chronic obstructive tracheobronchitis (J44.-)
chronic simple bronchitis (J41.0)
chronic tracheobronchitis (J42)

AHA: 2019,1Q,35; 2016,3Q,10,16
DEF: Acute inflammation of the main branches of the bronchial tree due to infectious or irritant agents. Symptoms include cough with a varied production of sputum, fever, substernal soreness, and lung rales. Bronchitis usually lasts three to 10 days.

J20.0 Acute bronchitis due to **Mycoplasma pneumoniae**

J20.1 Acute bronchitis due to **Hemophilus influenzae**

J20.2 Acute bronchitis due to **streptococcus**

J20.3 Acute bronchitis due to **coxsackievirus**

J20.4 Acute bronchitis due to **parainfluenza virus**

J20.5 Acute bronchitis due to **respiratory syncytial virus**
Acute bronchitis due to RSV

J20.6 Acute bronchitis due to **rhinovirus**

J20.7 Acute bronchitis due to **echovirus**

J20.8 Acute bronchitis due to other specified organisms
AHA: 2020,1Q,34-36

J20.9 Acute bronchitis, unspecified

`✓4th` **J21** **Acute bronchiolitis**

`INCLUDES`   acute bronchiolitis with bronchospasm
`EXCLUDES 2`   *respiratory bronchiolitis interstitial lung disease (J84.115)*

J21.0 Acute bronchiolitis due to **respiratory syncytial virus**   `CC`
Acute bronchiolitis due to RSV

J21.1 Acute bronchiolitis due to **human metapneumovirus**   `CC`

J21.8 Acute bronchiolitis due to other specified organisms   `CC`

J21.9 Acute bronchiolitis, unspecified   `CC`
Bronchiolitis (acute)
`EXCLUDES 1`   *chronic bronchiolitis ▶(J44.89)◄*

J22 **Unspecified acute lower respiratory infection**
Acute (lower) respiratory (tract) infection NOS
`EXCLUDES 1`   *upper respiratory infection (acute) (J06.9)*
AHA: 2020,1Q,22,34-36

Other diseases of upper respiratory tract (J30-J39)

`✓4th` **J30** **Vasomotor and allergic rhinitis**

`INCLUDES`   spasmodic rhinorrhea
`EXCLUDES 1`   *allergic rhinitis with asthma (bronchial) (J45.909)*
rhinitis NOS (J31.0)

J30.0 **Vasomotor** rhinitis
DEF: Noninfectious and nonallergic type of rhinitis for which the cause is often unknown. Symptoms often mimic those of allergic rhinitis with a diagnosis of vasomotor rhinitis typically made after ruling out allergens as the cause.

J30.1 **Allergic** rhinitis **due to pollen**
Allergy NOS due to pollen
Hay fever
Pollinosis

J30.2 Other **seasonal allergic** rhinitis

J30.5 Allergic rhinitis **due to food**

`✓5th` **J30.8** Other allergic rhinitis

J30.81 Allergic rhinitis due to **animal** (cat) (dog) **hair and dander**

J30.89 Other allergic rhinitis
Perennial allergic rhinitis

J30.9 Allergic rhinitis, unspecified

`✓4th` **J31** **Chronic rhinitis, nasopharyngitis and pharyngitis**

J31.0 **Chronic rhinitis**
Atrophic rhinitis (chronic)
Granulomatous rhinitis (chronic)
Hypertrophic rhinitis (chronic)
Obstructive rhinitis (chronic)
Ozena
Purulent rhinitis (chronic)
Rhinitis (chronic) NOS
Ulcerative rhinitis (chronic)
`EXCLUDES 1`   *allergic rhinitis (J30.1-J30.9)*
vasomotor rhinitis (J30.0)
DEF: Persistent inflammation of the mucous membranes of the nose, characterized by a postnasal drip.

J31.1 **Chronic nasopharyngitis**
`EXCLUDES 2`   *acute nasopharyngitis (J00)*
DEF: Persistent inflammation of the mucous membranes extending from the nares to the pharynx. It is characterized by constant irritation in the nasopharynx and postnasal drip.

J31.2 **Chronic pharyngitis**
Atrophic pharyngitis (chronic)
Chronic sore throat
Granular pharyngitis (chronic)
Hypertrophic pharyngitis (chronic)
`EXCLUDES 2`   *acute pharyngitis (J02.9)*

`✓4th` **J32** **Chronic sinusitis**

`INCLUDES`   sinus abscess
sinus empyema
sinus infection
sinus suppuration

Use additional code to identify:
infectious agent (B95-B97)
`EXCLUDES 2`   *acute sinusitis (J01.-)*

J32.0 **Chronic maxillary sinusitis**
Antritis (chronic)
Maxillary sinusitis NOS

J32.1 **Chronic frontal sinusitis**
Frontal sinusitis NOS

J32.2 **Chronic ethmoidal sinusitis**
Ethmoidal sinusitis NOS
`EXCLUDES 1`   *Woakes' ethmoiditis (J33.1)*

J32.3 **Chronic sphenoidal sinusitis**
Sphenoidal sinusitis NOS

J32.4 **Chronic pansinusitis**
Pansinusitis NOS

J32.8 **Other chronic sinusitis**
Sinusitis (chronic) involving more than one sinus but not pansinusitis

J32.9 **Chronic sinusitis, unspecified**
Sinusitis (chronic) NOS

Chapter 10. Diseases of the Respiratory System

J33–J38.1

✅4ᵗʰ **J33** **Nasal polyp**
- EXCLUDES 1   adenomatous polyps (D14.0)

J33.0 **Polyp of nasal cavity**
- Choanal polyp
- Nasopharyngeal polyp

J33.1 **Polypoid sinus degeneration**
- Woakes' syndrome or ethmoiditis

J33.8 **Other polyp of sinus**
- Accessory polyp of sinus
- Ethmoidal polyp of sinus
- Maxillary polyp of sinus
- Sphenoidal polyp of sinus

J33.9 **Nasal polyp, unspecified**

✅4ᵗʰ **J34** **Other and unspecified disorders of nose and nasal sinuses**
- EXCLUDES 2   varicose ulcer of nasal septum (I86.8)

J34.0 **Abscess, furuncle and carbuncle of nose**
- Cellulitis of nose
- Necrosis of nose
- Ulceration of nose

J34.1 **Cyst and mucocele of nose and nasal sinus**

J34.2 **Deviated nasal septum**
- Deflection or deviation of septum (nasal) (acquired)
- EXCLUDES 1   congenital deviated nasal septum (Q67.4)
- **DEF:** Condition in which the nasal septum, a thin wall composed of cartilage and bone that separates the two nostrils, is crooked or displaced from the midline.

J34.3 **Hypertrophy of nasal turbinates**
- **DEF:** Overgrowth of bones within the nasal turbinate, which are ridges of bone and soft tissue that project from the sidewalls of the nasal passages. Hypertrophy can cause obstruction of the nasal passages.

✅5ᵗʰ **J34.8** **Other specified disorders of nose and nasal sinuses**

J34.81 **Nasal mucositis (ulcerative)**
- Code also type of associated therapy, such as:
  - antineoplastic and immunosuppressive drugs (T45.1X-)
  - radiological procedure and radiotherapy (Y84.2)
- EXCLUDES 2   gastrointestinal mucositis (ulcerative) (K92.81)
  - mucositis (ulcerative) of vagina and vulva (N76.81)
  - oral mucositis (ulcerative) (K12.3-)

● ✅6ᵗʰ **J34.82** **Nasal valve collapse**
- Nasal valve compromise
- Nasal valve stenosis
- Code first underlying cause, such as:
  - deviated nasal septum (J34.2)

● ✅7ᵗʰ **J34.820** **Internal nasal valve collapse**
●   **J34.8200** **Internal nasal valve collapse, unspecified** UPD
●   **J34.8201** **Internal nasal valve collapse, static** UPD
-      Narrowing of the septum, head of the inferior turbinate and the upper lateral cartilage
●   **J34.8202** **Internal nasal valve collapse, dynamic** UPD
-      Collapse or falling of the upper, middle sidewall of the nose on inspiration

● ✅7ᵗʰ **J34.821** **External nasal valve collapse**
●   **J34.8210** **External nasal valve collapse, unspecified** UPD
●   **J34.8211** **External nasal valve collapse, static** UPD
-      Fixed narrowing of the caudal septum, lower lateral cartilage, alar rim and nasal sill
●   **J34.8212** **External nasal valve collapse, dynamic** UPD
-      Collapse or falling of the lower sidewall or nostril of the nose on inspiration

●   **J34.829** **Nasal valve collapse, unspecified** UPD
- Nasal valve collapse, NOS

J34.89 **Other specified disorders of nose and nasal sinuses**
- Perforation of nasal septum NOS
- Rhinolith

J34.9 **Unspecified disorder of nose and nasal sinuses**

✅4ᵗʰ **J35** **Chronic diseases of tonsils and adenoids**

✅5ᵗʰ **J35.0** **Chronic tonsillitis and adenoiditis**
- EXCLUDES 2   acute tonsillitis (J03.-)

J35.01 **Chronic tonsillitis**

J35.02 **Chronic adenoiditis**

J35.03 **Chronic tonsillitis and adenoiditis**

J35.1 **Hypertrophy of tonsils**
- Enlargement of tonsils
- EXCLUDES 1   hypertrophy of tonsils with tonsillitis (J35.0-)

J35.2 **Hypertrophy of adenoids**
- Enlargement of adenoids
- EXCLUDES 1   hypertrophy of adenoids with adenoiditis (J35.0-)

J35.3 **Hypertrophy of tonsils with hypertrophy of adenoids**
- EXCLUDES 1   hypertrophy of tonsils and adenoids with tonsillitis and adenoiditis (J35.03)

J35.8 **Other chronic diseases of tonsils and adenoids**
- Adenoid vegetations
- Amygdalolith
- Calculus, tonsil
- Cicatrix of tonsil (and adenoid)
- Tonsillar tag
- Ulcer of tonsil

J35.9 **Chronic disease of tonsils and adenoids, unspecified**
- Disease (chronic) of tonsils and adenoids NOS

J36 **Peritonsillar abscess** CC
- INCLUDES   abscess of tonsil
  - peritonsillar cellulitis
  - quinsy
- Use additional code (B95-B97) to identify infectious agent
- EXCLUDES 1   acute tonsillitis (J03.-)
  - chronic tonsillitis (J35.0)
  - retropharyngeal abscess (J39.0)
  - tonsillitis NOS (J03.9-)

✅4ᵗʰ **J37** **Chronic laryngitis and laryngotracheitis**
- Use additional code to identify:
  - exposure to environmental tobacco smoke (Z77.22)
  - exposure to tobacco smoke in the perinatal period (P96.81)
  - history of tobacco dependence (Z87.891)
  - infectious agent (B95-B97)
  - occupational exposure to environmental tobacco smoke (Z57.31)
  - tobacco dependence (F17.-)
  - tobacco use (Z72.0)

J37.0 **Chronic laryngitis**
- Catarrhal laryngitis
- Hypertrophic laryngitis
- Sicca laryngitis
- EXCLUDES 2   acute laryngitis (J04.0)
  - obstructive (acute) laryngitis (J05.0)

J37.1 **Chronic laryngotracheitis**
- Laryngitis, chronic, with tracheitis (chronic)
- Tracheitis, chronic, with laryngitis
- EXCLUDES 1   chronic tracheitis (J42)
- EXCLUDES 2   acute laryngotracheitis (J04.2)
  - acute tracheitis (J04.1)

✅4ᵗʰ **J38** **Diseases of vocal cords and larynx, not elsewhere classified**
- EXCLUDES 1   congenital laryngeal stridor (P28.89)
  - obstructive laryngitis (acute) (J05.0)
  - postprocedural subglottic stenosis (J95.5)
  - stridor (R06.1)
  - ulcerative laryngitis (J04.0)

✅5ᵗʰ **J38.0** **Paralysis of vocal cords and larynx**
- Laryngoplegia
- Paralysis of glottis

J38.00 **Paralysis of vocal cords and larynx, unspecified**

J38.01 **Paralysis of vocal cords and larynx, unilateral**

J38.02 **Paralysis of vocal cords and larynx, bilateral**

J38.1 **Polyp of vocal cord and larynx**
- EXCLUDES 1   adenomatous polyps (D14.1)

N Newborn: 0   **P** Pediatric: 0-17   **M** Maternity: 9-64   **A** Adult: 15-124   **UNS** Unspecified Site   **MCC** Major Complication/Comorbidity   **CC** Complication/Comorbidity   **PE** POA Exempt

710   ICD-10-CM 2025

J38.2 **Nodules** of vocal cords
Chorditis (fibrinous)(nodosa)(tuberosa)
Singer's nodes
Teacher's nodes

J38.3 **Other diseases of vocal cords**
Abscess of vocal cords
Cellulitis of vocal cords
Granuloma of vocal cords
Leukokeratosis of vocal cords
Leukoplakia of vocal cords

J38.4 **Edema** of larynx
Edema (of) glottis
Subglottic edema
Supraglottic edema
> *EXCLUDES 1*   acute obstructive laryngitis [croup] (J05.0)
>   edematous laryngitis (J04.0)

J38.5 **Laryngeal** **spasm**
Laryngismus (stridulus)

J38.6 **Stenosis of larynx**

J38.7 **Other diseases of larynx**
Abscess of larynx
Cellulitis of larynx
Disease of larynx NOS
Necrosis of larynx
Pachyderma of larynx
Perichondritis of larynx
Ulcer of larynx

✓4ᵗʰ J39 **Other diseases of upper respiratory tract**
> *EXCLUDES 1*   acute respiratory infection NOS (J22)
>   acute upper respiratory infection (J06.9)
>   upper respiratory inflammation due to chemicals, gases, fumes or vapors (J68.2)

J39.0 **Retropharyngeal** and **parapharyngeal** **abscess**   `CC`
Peripharyngeal abscess
> *EXCLUDES 1*   peritonsillar abscess (J36)

DEF: Purulent infection behind the pharynx and the front of the precerebral fascia, characterized by neck stiffness, cervical lymphadenopathy, sore throat, fever, and stridor.

J39.1 **Other** **abscess** of pharynx   `CC`
Cellulitis of pharynx
Nasopharyngeal abscess

J39.2 **Other diseases of pharynx**
Cyst of pharynx
Edema of pharynx
> *EXCLUDES 2*   chronic pharyngitis (J31.2)
>   ulcerative pharyngitis (J02.9)

J39.3 **Upper respiratory tract hypersensitivity reaction, site unspecified**
> *EXCLUDES 1*   hypersensitivity reaction of upper respiratory tract, such as:
>   extrinsic allergic alveolitis (J67.9)
>   pneumoconiosis (J60-J67.9)

J39.8 **Other specified diseases of upper respiratory tract**
AHA: 2023,1Q,30

J39.9 **Disease of upper respiratory tract, unspecified**

Chronic lower respiratory diseases (J40-J4A)

> *EXCLUDES 1*   bronchitis due to chemicals, gases, fumes and vapors (J68.0)
> *EXCLUDES 2*   cystic fibrosis (E84.-)

J40 **Bronchitis, not specified as acute or chronic**
Bronchitis NOS
Bronchitis with tracheitis NOS
Catarrhal bronchitis
Tracheobronchitis NOS
Use additional code to identify:
exposure to environmental tobacco smoke (Z77.22)
exposure to tobacco smoke in the perinatal period (P96.81)
history of tobacco dependence (Z87.891)
occupational exposure to environmental tobacco smoke (Z57.31)
tobacco dependence (F17.-)
tobacco use (Z72.0)
> *EXCLUDES 1*   acute bronchitis (J20.-)
>   allergic bronchitis NOS (J45.909-)
>   asthmatic bronchitis NOS (J45.9-)
>   bronchitis due to chemicals, gases, fumes and vapors (J68.0)

AHA: 2020,1Q,34-36

✓4ᵗʰ J41 **Simple and mucopurulent chronic bronchitis**
Use additional code to identify:
exposure to environmental tobacco smoke (Z77.22)
exposure to tobacco smoke in the perinatal period (P96.81)
history of tobacco dependence (Z87.891)
occupational exposure to environmental tobacco smoke (Z57.31)
tobacco dependence (F17.-)
tobacco use (Z72.0)
> *EXCLUDES 2*   chronic bronchitis NOS (J42)
>   chronic obstructive bronchitis (J44.-)

J41.0 **Simple** chronic bronchitis   `HCC`

J41.1 **Mucopurulent** chronic bronchitis   `HCC`

J41.8 **Mixed** simple and mucopurulent chronic bronchitis   `HCC`

J42 **Unspecified** **chronic** bronchitis   `HCC`
Chronic bronchitis NOS
Chronic tracheitis
Chronic tracheobronchitis
Use additional code to identify:
exposure to environmental tobacco smoke (Z77.22)
exposure to tobacco smoke in the perinatal period (P96.81)
history of tobacco dependence (Z87.891)
occupational exposure to environmental tobacco smoke (Z57.31)
tobacco dependence (F17.-)
tobacco use (Z72.0)
> *EXCLUDES 1*   bronchiolitis obliterans and bronchiolitis obliterans syndrome (J44.81)
>   chronic asthmatic bronchitis (J44.-)
>   chronic bronchitis with airways obstruction (J44.-)
>   chronic emphysematous bronchitis (J44.-)
>   chronic obstructive pulmonary disease NOS (J44.9)
>   simple and mucopurulent chronic bronchitis (J41.-)

✓4ᵗʰ J43 **Emphysema**
> *EXCLUDES 1*   compensatory emphysema (J98.3)
>   emphysema due to inhalation of chemicals, gases, fumes or vapors (J68.4)
>   interstitial emphysema (J98.2)
>   mediastinal emphysema (J98.2)
>   neonatal interstitial emphysema (P25.0)
>   surgical (subcutaneous) emphysema (T81.82)
> *EXCLUDES 2*   emphysema with chronic (obstructive) bronchitis (J44.-)
>   emphysematous (obstructive) bronchitis (J44.-)
>   traumatic subcutaneous emphysema (T79.7)

Emphysema

Healthy alveoli   **Alveoli w/ Emphysema**
Patent bronchiole
Collapsed bronchiole
Well-vascularized
Broken/ fewer capillaries
Enlarged alveoli
Dilated alveoli
Alveolar membranes break down
Excess mucus

DEF: Pathological condition in which there is destructive enlargement of the air sacs in the lungs resulting in damage and lack of elasticity to the alveolar walls, commonly seen in long-term smokers.

J43.0 **Unilateral pulmonary** emphysema [MacLeod's syndrome]   `HCC`
Swyer-James syndrome
Unilateral emphysema
Unilateral hyperlucent lung
Unilateral pulmonary artery functional hypoplasia
Unilateral transparency of lung

J43.1 **Panlobular** emphysema   `HCC`
Panacinar emphysema

J43.2 **Centrilobular** emphysema   `HCC`

J43.8 **Other emphysema**   `HCC`

✔ Additional Character Required   ✔x7ᵗʰ Placeholder   Questionable PDx   Manifestation   Unspecified   **UPD** Unacceptable PDx   H1 - H14 HAC   HCC CMS-HCC Dx   HIV HIV Dx

ICD-10-CM 2025   711

J43.9 **Emphysema, unspecified** `HCC`
Bullous emphysema (lung)(pulmonary)
Emphysema (lung)(pulmonary) NOS
Emphysematous bleb
Vesicular emphysema (lung)(pulmonary)
AHA: 2024,2Q,4; 2019,1Q,34-36; 2017,4Q,97-98

✓4ᵗʰ **J44** **Other chronic obstructive pulmonary disease**
INCLUDES asthma with chronic obstructive pulmonary disease
chronic asthmatic (obstructive) bronchitis
chronic bronchitis with airway obstruction
chronic bronchitis with emphysema
chronic emphysematous bronchitis
chronic obstructive asthma
chronic obstructive bronchitis
chronic obstructive tracheobronchitis
Code also type of asthma, if applicable (J45.-)
EXCLUDES 1 *chronic bronchitis NOS (J42)*
chronic simple and mucopurulent bronchitis (J41.-)
chronic tracheitis (J42)
chronic tracheobronchitis (J42)
EXCLUDES 2 *bronchiectasis (J47.-)*
emphysema without chronic bronchitis (J43.-)
AHA: 2024,2Q,3–5; 2019,1Q,34-36; 2017,4Q,97-98; 2017,1Q,25-26; 2016,3Q,15-16; 2013,4Q,109

J44.0 **Chronic obstructive pulmonary disease with (acute) lower respiratory infection** `CC` `HCC`
Code also to identify the infection
AHA: 2019,1Q,35; 2017,4Q,96; 2017,1Q,24-25
TIP: Do not assign when only aspiration pneumonia is present. Aspiration pneumonia is not classified as a respiratory infection.

J44.1 **Chronic obstructive pulmonary disease with (acute) exacerbation** `CC` `HCC`
Decompensated COPD
Decompensated COPD with (acute) exacerbation
EXCLUDES 2 *chronic obstructive pulmonary disease [COPD] with acute bronchitis (J44.0)*
lung diseases due to external agents (J60-J70)
AHA: 2019,1Q,34; 2017,4Q,96; 2017,1Q,26; 2016,1Q,36
TIP: Exacerbation of COPD should not be assumed based upon worsening of a concomitant respiratory disease or when COPD is described as end-stage.

✓5ᵗʰ **J44.8** **Other specified chronic obstructive pulmonary disease**
AHA: 2023,4Q,27

J44.81 **Bronchiolitis obliterans and bronchiolitis obliterans syndrome** `HCC`
Obliterative bronchiolitis
Code first, if applicable:
complication of bone marrow transplant (T86.09)
complication of stem cell transplant (T86.5)
heart-lung transplant rejection (T86.31)
lung transplant rejection (T86.810)
other complications of heart-lung transplant (T86.39)
other complications of lung transplant (T86.818)
Code also, if applicable, associated conditions, such as:
chronic graft-versus-host disease (D89.811)
chronic lung allograft dysfunction (J4A.-)
chronic respiratory conditions due to chemicals, gases, fumes and vapors (J68.4)

J44.89 **Other specified chronic obstructive pulmonary disease** `HCC`
Chronic asthmatic (obstructive) bronchitis
Chronic emphysematous bronchitis

J44.9 **Chronic obstructive pulmonary disease, unspecified** `HCC`
Chronic obstructive airway disease NOS
Chronic obstructive lung disease NOS
EXCLUDES 2 *lung diseases due to external agents (J60-J70)*
AHA: 2019,1Q,36; 2017,4Q,96-97; 2016,1Q,36; 2014,4Q,21; 2013,4Q,109

✓4ᵗʰ **J4A** **Chronic lung allograft dysfunction**
Code first, if applicable:
heart-lung transplant rejection (T86.31)
lung transplant rejection (T86.810)
other complications of heart-lung transplant (T86.39)
other complications of lung transplant (T86.818)
Code also, if applicable, bronchiolitis obliterans syndrome (J44.81)
AHA: 2023,4Q,28

J4A.0 **Restrictive allograft syndrome** `HCC`
Code also, if applicable, for mixed chronic lung allograft dysfunction, bronchiolitis obliterans syndrome (J44.81)

J4A.8 **Other chronic lung allograft dysfunction** `HCC`

J4A.9 **Chronic lung allograft dysfunction, unspecified** `HCC`

✓4ᵗʰ **J45** **Asthma**
INCLUDES allergic (predominantly) asthma
allergic bronchitis NOS
allergic rhinitis with asthma
atopic asthma
extrinsic allergic asthma
hay fever with asthma
idiosyncratic asthma
intrinsic nonallergic asthma
nonallergic asthma
Use additional code to identify:
eosinophilic asthma (J82.83)
exposure to environmental tobacco smoke (Z77.22)
exposure to tobacco smoke in the perinatal period (P96.81)
history of tobacco dependence (Z87.891)
occupational exposure to environmental tobacco smoke (Z57.31)
tobacco dependence (F17.-)
tobacco use (Z72.0)
EXCLUDES 1 *detergent asthma (J69.8)*
miner's asthma (J60)
wheezing NOS (R06.2)
wood asthma (J67.8)
EXCLUDES 2 *asthma with chronic obstructive pulmonary disease ▶(J44.89)◄*
chronic asthmatic (obstructive) bronchitis ▶(J44.89)◄
chronic obstructive asthma ▶(J44.89)◄
▶other specified chronic obstructive pulmonary disease (J44.89)◄
AHA: 2024,2Q,3; 2023,1Q,17; 2019,1Q,36; 2017,1Q,25-26; 2012,4Q,99
DEF: Status asthmaticus: Severe, intractable episode of asthma that is unresponsive to normal therapeutic measures.

✓5ᵗʰ **J45.2** **Mild intermittent asthma**
J45.20 **Mild intermittent asthma, uncomplicated**
Mild intermittent asthma NOS
J45.21 **Mild intermittent asthma with (acute) exacerbation** `CC`
J45.22 **Mild intermittent asthma with status asthmaticus** `CC`

✓5ᵗʰ **J45.3** **Mild persistent asthma**
J45.30 **Mild persistent asthma, uncomplicated**
Mild persistent asthma NOS
J45.31 **Mild persistent asthma with (acute) exacerbation** `CC`
AHA: 2016,1Q,35
J45.32 **Mild persistent asthma with status asthmaticus** `CC`

✓5ᵗʰ **J45.4** **Moderate persistent asthma**
J45.40 **Moderate persistent asthma, uncomplicated**
Moderate persistent asthma NOS
J45.41 **Moderate persistent asthma with (acute) exacerbation** `CC`
AHA: 2017,1Q,26
J45.42 **Moderate persistent asthma with status asthmaticus** `CC`

✓5ᵗʰ **J45.5** **Severe persistent asthma**
J45.50 **Severe persistent asthma, uncomplicated** `HCC`
Severe persistent asthma NOS
J45.51 **Severe persistent asthma with (acute) exacerbation** `CC` `HCC`
J45.52 **Severe persistent asthma with status asthmaticus** `CC` `HCC`

N Newborn: 0   P Pediatric: 0-17   M Maternity: 9-64   A Adult: 15-124   UNS Unspecified Site   MCC Major Complication/Comorbidity   CC Complication/Comorbidity   PE POA Exempt

712   ICD-10-CM 2025

√5ᵗʰ **J45.9**   **Other and unspecified asthma**

  √6ᵗʰ **J45.90**   **Unspecified asthma**
       Asthmatic bronchitis NOS
       Childhood asthma NOS
       Late onset asthma
       AHA: 2017,4Q,96; 2017,1Q,25

     J45.901   **Unspecified asthma with (acute) exacerbation**   CC

     J45.902   **Unspecified asthma with status asthmaticus**   CC

     J45.909   **Unspecified asthma, uncomplicated**
         Asthma NOS
         EXCLUDES 2   lung diseases due to external agents (J60-J70)
         AHA: 2017,1Q,25

  √6ᵗʰ **J45.99**   **Other asthma**
     J45.990   **Exercise induced bronchospasm**
     J45.991   **Cough variant asthma**
     J45.998   **Other asthma**

√4ᵗʰ **J47**   **Bronchiectasis**
     INCLUDES   bronchiolectasis
     Use additional code to identify:
       exposure to environmental tobacco smoke (Z77.22)
       exposure to tobacco smoke in the perinatal period (P96.81)
       history of tobacco dependence (Z87.891)
       occupational exposure to environmental tobacco smoke (Z57.31)
       tobacco dependence (F17.-)
       tobacco use (Z72.0)
     EXCLUDES 1   congenital bronchiectasis (Q33.4)
         tuberculous bronchiectasis (current disease) (A15.0)
     DEF: Dilation of the bronchi with mucus production and persistent cough due to infection or chronic conditions that causes diminished lung capacity and frequent infections of the lung.

   J47.0   **Bronchiectasis with acute lower respiratory infection**   CC HCC
     Bronchiectasis with acute bronchitis
     Code also to identify infection, if applicable

   J47.1   **Bronchiectasis with (acute) exacerbation**   CC HCC
     AHA: 2021,1Q,23

   J47.9   **Bronchiectasis, uncomplicated**   HCC
     Bronchiectasis NOS
     AHA: AHA:2024,2Q,5

Lung diseases due to external agents (J60-J70)

     EXCLUDES 2   asthma (J45.-)
         malignant neoplasm of bronchus and lung (C34.-)
     DEF: Pneumoconiosis: Condition caused by inhaling inorganic dust particles, typically associated with occupations that require regular exposure to mineral dusts. A form of interstitial lung disease that contributes to the inflammation of the air sacs, causing the lung tissue to harden.

J60   **Coalworker's pneumoconiosis**   HCC A
   Anthracosilicosis
   Anthracosis
   Black lung disease
   Coalworker's lung
   EXCLUDES 1   coalworker pneumoconiosis with tuberculosis, any type in A15 (J65)

J61   **Pneumoconiosis due to asbestos and other mineral fibers**   HCC A
   Asbestosis
   EXCLUDES 1   pleural plaque with asbestosis (J92.0)
         pneumoconiosis with tuberculosis, any type in A15 (J65)

√4ᵗʰ **J62**   **Pneumoconiosis due to dust containing silica**
   INCLUDES   silicotic fibrosis (massive) of lung
   EXCLUDES 1   pneumoconiosis with tuberculosis, any type in A15 (J65)
   J62.0   **Pneumoconiosis due to talc dust**   HCC
   J62.8   **Pneumoconiosis due to other dust containing silica**   HCC
     Silicosis NOS

√4ᵗʰ **J63**   **Pneumoconiosis due to other inorganic dusts**
   EXCLUDES 1   pneumoconiosis with tuberculosis, any type in A15 (J65)
   J63.0   **Aluminosis (of lung)**   HCC
   J63.1   **Bauxite fibrosis (of lung)**   HCC
   J63.2   **Berylliosis**   HCC
   J63.3   **Graphite fibrosis (of lung)**   HCC

   J63.4   **Siderosis**   HCC
     AHA: 2019,3Q,8
   J63.5   **Stannosis**   HCC
   J63.6   **Pneumoconiosis due to other specified inorganic dusts**   HCC

J64   **Unspecified pneumoconiosis**   HCC
   EXCLUDES 1   pneumoconiosis with tuberculosis, any type in A15 (J65)

J65   **Pneumoconiosis associated with tuberculosis**   HCC
   Any condition in J60-J64 with tuberculosis, any type in A15
   Silicotuberculosis

√4ᵗʰ **J66**   **Airway disease due to specific organic dust**
   EXCLUDES 2   allergic alveolitis (J67.-)
         asbestosis (J61)
         bagassosis (J67.1)
         farmer's lung (J67.0)
         hypersensitivity pneumonitis due to organic dust (J67.-)
         reactive airways dysfunction syndrome (J68.3)
   J66.0   **Byssinosis**   HCC
     Airway disease due to cotton dust
   J66.1   **Flax-dressers' disease**   HCC
   J66.2   **Cannabinosis**   HCC
   J66.8   **Airway disease due to other specific organic dusts**   HCC

√4ᵗʰ **J67**   **Hypersensitivity pneumonitis due to organic dust**
   INCLUDES   allergic alveolitis and pneumonitis due to inhaled organic dust and particles of fungal, actinomycetic or other origin
   EXCLUDES 1   pneumonitis due to inhalation of chemicals, gases, fumes or vapors (J68.0)
   J67.0   **Farmer's lung**   HCC
     Harvester's lung
     Haymaker's lung
     Moldy hay disease
   J67.1   **Bagassosis**   HCC
     Bagasse disease
     Bagasse pneumonitis
   J67.2   **Bird fancier's lung**   HCC
     Budgerigar fancier's disease or lung
     Pigeon fancier's disease or lung
   J67.3   **Suberosis**   HCC
     Corkhandler's disease or lung
     Corkworker's disease or lung
   J67.4   **Maltworker's lung**   HCC
     Alveolitis due to Aspergillus clavatus
   J67.5   **Mushroom-worker's lung**   HCC
   J67.6   **Maple-bark-stripper's lung**   HCC
     Alveolitis due to Cryptostroma corticale
     Cryptostromosis
   J67.7   **Air conditioner and humidifier lung**   CC HCC
     Allergic alveolitis due to fungal, thermophilic actinomycetes and other organisms growing in ventilation [air conditioning] systems
   J67.8   **Hypersensitivity pneumonitis due to other organic dusts**   CC HCC
     Cheese-washer's lung
     Coffee-worker's lung
     Fish-meal worker's lung
     Furrier's lung
     Sequoiosis
   J67.9   **Hypersensitivity pneumonitis due to unspecified organic dust**   CC HCC
     Allergic alveolitis (extrinsic) NOS
     Hypersensitivity pneumonitis NOS

√4ᵗʰ **J68**   **Respiratory conditions due to inhalation of chemicals, gases, fumes and vapors**
   Code first (T51-T65) to identify cause
   Use additional code to identify associated respiratory conditions, such as:
     acute respiratory failure (J96.0-)
   J68.0   **Bronchitis and pneumonitis due to chemicals, gases, fumes and vapors**   CC HCC
     Chemical bronchitis (acute)
     AHA: 2019,2Q,31
   J68.1   **Pulmonary edema due to chemicals, gases, fumes and vapors**   MCC HCC
     Chemical pulmonary edema (acute) (chronic)
     EXCLUDES 1   pulmonary edema (acute) (chronic) NOS (J81.-)
   J68.2   **Upper respiratory inflammation due to chemicals, gases, fumes and vapors, not elsewhere classified**   HCC

Chapter 10. Diseases of the Respiratory System

J45.9–J68.2

J68.3 Other **acute and subacute respiratory conditions** due to chemicals, gases, fumes and vapors `HCC`
Reactive airways dysfunction syndrome

J68.4 **Chronic respiratory conditions** due to chemicals, gases, fumes and vapors `HCC`
Code also, if applicable, chronic conditions, such as:
emphysema (J43.-)
obliterative bronchiolitis (J44.81)
pulmonary fibrosis (J84.10)
EXCLUDES 1 *chronic pulmonary edema due to chemicals, gases, fumes and vapors (J68.1)*

J68.8 Other respiratory conditions due to chemicals, gases, fumes and vapors `HCC`

J68.9 Unspecified respiratory condition due to chemicals, fumes and vapors `HCC`

✓4ᵗʰ **J69** Pneumonitis due to solids and liquids
▶Codes also, if applicable, other types of pneumonias◀
EXCLUDES 1 *neonatal aspiration syndromes (P24.-)*
postprocedural pneumonitis (J95.4)
AHA: 2017,1Q,24
DEF: Pneumonitis: Noninfectious inflammation of the walls of the alveoli in the lung tissue due to inhalation of food, vomit, oils, essences, or other solids or liquids.

J69.0 Pneumonitis due to **inhalation of food and vomit** `MCC` `HCC`
Aspiration pneumonia NOS
Aspiration pneumonia (due to) food (regurgitated)
Aspiration pneumonia (due to) gastric secretions
Aspiration pneumonia (due to) milk
Aspiration pneumonia (due to) vomit
Code also any associated foreign body in respiratory tract (T17.-)
EXCLUDES 1 *chemical pneumonitis due to anesthesia (J95.4)*
obstetric aspiration pneumonitis (O74.0)
AHA: 2020,2Q,11,28; 2019,3Q,17; 2019,2Q,6,31

J69.1 Pneumonitis due to **inhalation of oils and essences** `MCC` `HCC`
Exogenous lipoid pneumonia
Lipid pneumonia NOS
Code first (T51-T65) to identify substance
EXCLUDES 1 *endogenous lipoid pneumonia (J84.89)*

J69.8 Pneumonitis due to inhalation of other solids and liquids `MCC` `HCC`
Pneumonitis due to aspiration of blood
Pneumonitis due to aspiration of detergent
Code first (T51-T65) to identify substance

✓4ᵗʰ **J70** Respiratory conditions due to other external agents

J70.0 **Acute** pulmonary manifestations due to **radiation** `CC`
Radiation pneumonitis
Use additional code (W88-W90, X39.0-) to identify the external cause

J70.1 **Chronic** and other pulmonary manifestations due to **radiation** `CC`
Fibrosis of lung following radiation
Use additional code (W88-W90, X39.0-) to identify the external cause

J70.2 **Acute drug-induced interstitial** lung disorders
Use additional code for adverse effect, if applicable, to identify drug (T36-T50 with fifth or sixth character 5)
EXCLUDES 1 *interstitial pneumonia NOS (J84.9)*
lymphoid interstitial pneumonia (J84.2)
AHA: 2019,2Q,28

J70.3 **Chronic drug-induced interstitial** lung disorders
Use additional code for adverse effect, if applicable, to identify drug (T36-T50 with fifth or sixth character 5)
EXCLUDES 1 *interstitial pneumonia NOS (J84.9)*
lymphoid interstitial pneumonia (J84.2)

J70.4 Drug-induced interstitial lung disorders, unspecified
Use additional code for adverse effect, if applicable, to identify drug (T36-T50 with fifth or sixth character 5)
EXCLUDES 1 *interstitial pneumonia NOS (J84.9)*
lymphoid interstitial pneumonia (J84.2)
AHA: 2019,2Q,28

J70.5 Respiratory conditions due to **smoke inhalation**
Code first smoke inhalation (T59.81-)
EXCLUDES 2 *smoke inhalation due to chemicals, gases, fumes and vapors (J68.9)*
AHA: 2013,4Q,121

J70.8 Respiratory conditions due to other specified external agents
Code first (T51-T65) to identify the external agent

J70.9 Respiratory conditions due to unspecified external agent
Code first (T51-T65) to identify the external agent

Other respiratory diseases principally affecting the interstitium (J80-J84)

J80 Acute respiratory distress syndrome `MCC` `HCC`
Acute respiratory distress syndrome in adult or child
Adult hyaline membrane disease
EXCLUDES 1 *respiratory distress syndrome in newborn (perinatal) (P22.0)*
AHA: 2021,1Q,23; 2020,4Q,96; 2020,1Q,34-36; 2017,1Q,26
DEF: Lung inflammation or injury resulting in a build-up of fluid in the air sacs, preventing the passage of oxygen from the air into the bloodstream.

✓4ᵗʰ **J81** Pulmonary edema
Use additional code to identify:
exposure to environmental tobacco smoke (Z77.22)
history of tobacco dependence (Z87.891)
occupational exposure to environmental tobacco smoke (Z57.31)
tobacco dependence (F17.-)
tobacco use (Z72.0)
EXCLUDES 1 *chemical (acute) pulmonary edema (J68.1)*
hypostatic pneumonia (J18.2)
passive pneumonia (J18.2)
pulmonary edema due to external agents (J60-J70)
pulmonary edema with heart disease NOS (I50.1)
pulmonary edema with heart failure (I50.1)
DEF: Accumulation of fluid in the air sacs of the lungs, making it difficult to breathe.

J81.0 **Acute** pulmonary edema `MCC` `HCC`
Acute edema of lung
AHA: 2023,1Q,25; 2020,3Q,27

J81.1 **Chronic** pulmonary edema `CC`
Pulmonary congestion (chronic) (passive)
Pulmonary edema NOS

✓4ᵗʰ **J82** Pulmonary eosinophilia, not elsewhere classified
EXCLUDES 2 *pulmonary eosinophilia due to aspergillosis (B44.-)*
pulmonary eosinophilia due to drugs (J70.2-J70.4)
pulmonary eosinophilia due to specified parasitic infection (B50-B83)
pulmonary eosinophilia due to systemic connective tissue disorders (M30-M36)
pulmonary infiltrate NOS (R91.8)
DEF: Infiltration of eosinophils (white blood cells of the immune system) into the parenchyma of the lungs, resulting in cough, fever, and dyspnea.

✓5ᵗʰ **J82.8** Pulmonary eosinophilia, not elsewhere classified
AHA: 2020,4Q,25-27

J82.81 **Chronic** eosinophilic pneumonia `CC` `HCC`
Eosinophilic pneumonia, NOS

J82.82 **Acute** eosinophilic pneumonia `CC`

J82.83 Eosinophilic **asthma** `CC`
Code first asthma, by type, such as:
mild intermittent asthma (J45.2-)
mild persistent asthma (J45.3-)
moderate persistent asthma (J45.4-)
severe persistent asthma (J45.5-)

J82.89 Other pulmonary eosinophilia, not elsewhere classified `CC`
Allergic pneumonia
Loffler's pneumonia
Tropical (pulmonary) eosinophilia NOS

✓4ᵗʰ **J84** Other **interstitial** pulmonary diseases
▶Code also, if applicable, associated condition◀
EXCLUDES 1 *drug-induced interstitial lung disorders (J70.2-J70.4)*
interstitial emphysema (J98.2)
EXCLUDES 2 *lung diseases due to external agents (J60-J70)*
DEF: Interstitial: Within the small spaces or gaps occurring in tissue or organs.

✓5ᵗʰ **J84.0** Alveolar and parieto-alveolar conditions

J84.01 Alveolar **proteinosis** `CC` `HCC`
DEF: Reduced ventilation due to proteinaceous deposits on alveoli. Symptoms include dyspnea, cough, chest pain, weakness, weight loss, and hemoptysis.

J84.02 Pulmonary alveolar **microlithiasis** `CC` `HCC`

J84.03   *Idiopathic pulmonary hemosiderosis* `CC` `HCC`
Essential brown induration of lung
Code first underlying disease, such as:
  disorders of iron metabolism (E83.1-)
  EXCLUDES 1   *acute idiopathic pulmonary hemorrhage in infants [AIPHI] (R04.81)*
DEF: Fibrosis of the alveolar walls marked by abnormal accumulation of iron as hemosiderin in the lungs. It primarily affects children and symptoms include anemia, fluid in the lungs, and blood in the sputum. Etiology is unknown.

J84.09   **Other alveolar and parieto-alveolar conditions** `CC` `HCC`

√5ᵗʰ J84.1   **Other interstitial pulmonary diseases with fibrosis**
  EXCLUDES 1   *pulmonary fibrosis (chronic) due to inhalation of chemicals, gases, fumes or vapors (J68.4)*
       pulmonary fibrosis (chronic) following radiation (J70.1)

  J84.10   **Pulmonary fibrosis, unspecified** `HCC`
    Capillary fibrosis of lung
    Cirrhosis of lung (chronic) NOS
    Fibrosis of lung (atrophic) (chronic) (confluent) (massive) (perialveolar) (peribronchial) NOS
    Induration of lung (chronic) NOS
    Postinflammatory pulmonary fibrosis
    AHA: AHA:2024,2Q,20

  √6ᵗʰ J84.11   **Idiopathic interstitial pneumonia**
    EXCLUDES 1   *lymphoid interstitial pneumonia (J84.2)*
       pneumocystis pneumonia (B59)

    J84.111   **Idiopathic interstitial pneumonia, not otherwise specified** `HCC`

    J84.112   **Idiopathic pulmonary fibrosis** `HCC`
      Cryptogenic fibrosing alveolitis
      Idiopathic fibrosing alveolitis

    J84.113   **Idiopathic non-specific interstitial pneumonitis** `HCC`
      EXCLUDES 1   *non-specific interstitial pneumonia NOS, or due to known underlying cause (J84.89)*

    J84.114   **Acute interstitial pneumonitis** `CC` `HCC`
      Hamman-Rich syndrome
      EXCLUDES 1   *pneumocystis pneumonia (B59)*

    J84.115   **Respiratory bronchiolitis interstitial lung disease** `HCC`

    J84.116   **Cryptogenic organizing pneumonia** `CC` `HCC`
      EXCLUDES 1   *organizing pneumonia NOS, or due to known underlying cause (J84.89)*

    J84.117   **Desquamative interstitial pneumonia** `CC` `HCC`

  √6ᵗʰ J84.17   **Other interstitial pulmonary diseases with fibrosis in diseases classified elsewhere**
    AHA: 2020,4Q,27-28

    J84.170   *Interstitial lung disease with progressive fibrotic phenotype in diseases classified elsewhere* `HCC`
      Progressive fibrotic interstitial lung disease
      Code first underlying disease, such as:
        lung diseases due to external agents (J60-J70)
        rheumatoid arthritis (M05.00-M06.9)
        sarcoidosis (D86.-)
        systemic connective tissue disorders (M30-M36)

J84.178   *Other interstitial pulmonary diseases with fibrosis in diseases classified elsewhere* `HCC`
  Interstitial pneumonia (nonspecific) (usual) due to collagen vascular disease
  Interstitial pneumonia (nonspecific) (usual) in diseases classified elsewhere
  Organizing pneumonia due to collagen vascular disease
  Organizing pneumonia in diseases classified elsewhere
  Code first underlying disease, such as:
    progressive systemic sclerosis (M34.0)
    rheumatoid arthritis (M05.00-M06.9)
    systemic lupus erythematosis (M32.0-M32.9)

J84.2   **Lymphoid interstitial pneumonia** `CC` `HCC`
  Lymphoid interstitial pneumonitis

√5ᵗʰ J84.8   **Other specified interstitial pulmonary diseases**
  EXCLUDES 1   *exogenous lipoid pneumonia (J69.1)*
     unspecified lipoid pneumonia (J69.1)

  J84.81   **Lymphangioleiomyomatosis** `MCC` `HCC`
    Lymphangiomyomatosis

  J84.82   **Adult pulmonary Langerhans cell histiocytosis** `CC` `HCC` `A`
    Adult PLCH

  J84.83   **Surfactant mutations of the lung** `MCC`
    DEF: Genetic disorder resulting in insufficient secretion of a complex mixture of phospholipids and proteins that reduce surface tension in the alveoli following the onset of breathing to facilitate lung expansion in the newborn. It is the leading indication for pediatric lung transplantation.

  √6ᵗʰ J84.84   **Other interstitial lung diseases of childhood**

    J84.841   **Neuroendocrine cell hyperplasia of infancy** `MCC`

    J84.842   **Pulmonary interstitial glycogenosis** `MCC`

    J84.843   **Alveolar capillary dysplasia with vein misalignment** `MCC`

    J84.848   **Other interstitial lung diseases of childhood** `MCC`

  J84.89   **Other specified interstitial pulmonary diseases** `HCC`
    Endogenous lipoid pneumonia
    Interstitial pneumonitis
    Non-specific interstitial pneumonitis NOS
    Organizing pneumonia NOS
    Code first, if applicable:
      poisoning due to drug or toxin (T51-T65 with fifth or sixth character to indicate intent), for toxic pneumonopathy
      underlying cause of pneumonopathy, if known
    Use additional code, for adverse effect, to identify drug (T36-T50 with fifth or sixth character 5), if drug-induced
    EXCLUDES 1   *cryptogenic organizing pneumonia (J84.116)*
       idiopathic non-specific interstitial pneumonitis (J84.113)
       lymphoid interstitial pneumonia (J84.2)
       lipoid pneumonia, exogenous or unspecified (J69.1)
    AHA: 2021,4Q,106; 2021,1Q,48; 2019,2Q,28

J84.9   **Interstitial pulmonary disease, unspecified** `CC` `HCC`
  Interstitial pneumonia NOS

Suppurative and necrotic conditions of the lower respiratory tract (J85-J86)

√4ᵗʰ J85   **Abscess of lung and mediastinum**
  Use additional code (B95-B97) to identify infectious agent

  J85.0   **Gangrene and necrosis of lung** `MCC` `HCC`

  J85.1   **Abscess of lung with pneumonia** `MCC` `HCC`
    Code also the type of pneumonia

  J85.2   **Abscess of lung without pneumonia** `MCC` `HCC`
    Abscess of lung NOS

  J85.3   **Abscess of mediastinum** `MCC` `HCC`

✓4ᵗʰ J86 Pyothorax

Use additional code (B95-B97) to identify infectious agent

EXCLUDES 1   abscess of lung (J85.-)

pyothorax due to tuberculosis (A15.6)

DEF: Collection of pus in the pleural space that is commonly caused by an infection that spreads from the lung, such as bacterial pneumonia or a lung abscess.

J86.0   Pyothorax with fistula   `MCC` `HCC`

Bronchocutaneous fistula

Bronchopleural fistula

Hepatopleural fistula

Mediastinal fistula

Pleural fistula

Thoracic fistula

Any condition classifiable to J86.9 with fistula

▶Code also, if applicable, disruption of internal operation (surgical) wound (T81.32-)◀

DEF: Purulent infection of the respiratory cavity, with communication from a cavity to another structure.

J86.9   Pyothorax without fistula   `MCC` `HCC`

Abscess of pleura

Abscess of thorax

Empyema (chest) (lung) (pleura)

Fibrinopurulent pleurisy

Purulent pleurisy

Pyopneumothorax

Septic pleurisy

Seropurulent pleurisy

Suppurative pleurisy

Other diseases of the pleura (J90-J94)

J90   Pleural effusion, not elsewhere classified   `CC`

Encysted pleurisy

Pleural effusion NOS

Pleurisy with effusion (exudative) (serous)

EXCLUDES 1   chylous (pleural) effusion (J94.0)

malignant pleural effusion (J91.0)

pleurisy NOS (R09.1)

tuberculous pleural effusion (A15.6)

DEF: Collection of lymph and other fluid within the pleural space.

✓4ᵗʰ J91   Pleural effusion in conditions classified elsewhere

EXCLUDES 2   pleural effusion in heart failure (I50.-)

pleural effusion in systemic lupus erythematosus (M32.13)

DEF: Collection of lymph and other fluid within the pleural space.

J91.0   _Malignant pleural effusion_   `CC` `HCC`

Code first underlying neoplasm (C00-D49)

AHA: 2024,2Q,11; 2022,3Q,14

J91.8   _Pleural effusion in other conditions classified elsewhere_   `CC`

Code first underlying disease, such as:

filariasis (B74.0-B74.9)

influenza (J09.X2, J10.1, J11.1)

AHA: 2015,2Q,15

TIP: Assign this code as a secondary diagnosis to congestive heart failure (I50.-) only if pleural effusion is specifically evaluated or treated.

Pleural Effusion

Right lung

Left lung

Pleura

Pleural space

Pleural effusion

✓4ᵗʰ J92   Pleural plaque

INCLUDES   pleural thickening

DEF: Areas of fibrous thickening that form on the parietal or visceral pleura, the membranes that line the ribs and lungs.

J92.0   Pleural plaque with presence of asbestos

J92.9   Pleural plaque without asbestos

Pleural plaque NOS

✓4ᵗʰ J93   Pneumothorax and air leak

EXCLUDES 1   congenital or perinatal pneumothorax (P25.1)

postprocedural air leak (J95.812)

postprocedural pneumothorax (J95.811)

pyopneumothorax (J86.-)

traumatic pneumothorax (S27.0)

tuberculous (current disease) pneumothorax (A15.-)

DEF: Pneumothorax: Lung displacement due to abnormal leakage of air or gas that is trapped in the pleural space formed by the membrane that encloses the lungs and lines the thoracic cavity.

J93.0   Spontaneous tension pneumothorax   `MCC`

DEF: Leaking air from the lung into the lining, causing collapse.

✓5ᵗʰ J93.1   Other spontaneous pneumothorax

J93.11   Primary spontaneous pneumothorax   `CC`

J93.12   Secondary spontaneous pneumothorax   `CC` `UPD`

Code first underlying condition, such as:

catamenial pneumothorax due to endometriosis (N80.B-)

cystic fibrosis (E84.-)

eosinophilic pneumonia (J82.81-J82.82)

lymphangioleiomyomatosis (J84.81)

malignant neoplasm of bronchus and lung (C34.-)

Marfan syndrome (Q87.4-)

pneumonia due to Pneumocystis carinii (B59)

secondary malignant neoplasm of lung (C78.0-)

spontaneous rupture of the esophagus (K22.3)

✓5ᵗʰ J93.8   Other pneumothorax and air leak

J93.81   Chronic pneumothorax   `CC`

J93.82   Other air leak   `CC`

Persistent air leak

J93.83   Other pneumothorax   `CC`

Acute pneumothorax

Spontaneous pneumothorax NOS

AHA: 2020,3Q,9-10

J93.9   Pneumothorax, unspecified   `CC`

Pneumothorax NOS

✓4ᵗʰ J94   Other pleural conditions

EXCLUDES 1   pleurisy NOS (R09.1)

traumatic hemopneumothorax (S27.2)

traumatic hemothorax (S27.1)

tuberculous pleural conditions (current disease) (A15.-)

J94.0   Chylous effusion   `CC`

Chyliform effusion

DEF: Fluid within the pleural space due to the leaking of lymph contents into the space, usually as a result of thoracic duct damage or injury or mediastinal lymphoma.

J94.1   Fibrothorax

DEF: Fibrosis within the pleural lining of the lungs commonly seen as a stiff layer surrounding the lung typically attributed to traumatic hemothorax or pleural effusion.

J94.2   Hemothorax   `CC`

Hemopneumothorax

J94.8   Other specified pleural conditions   `CC`

Hydropneumothorax

Hydrothorax

AHA: 2021,1Q,48

J94.9   Pleural condition, unspecified

N Newborn: 0   P Pediatric: 0-17   M Maternity: 9-64   A Adult: 15-124   UNS Unspecified Site   MCC Major Complication/Comorbidity   CC Complication/Comorbidity   PE POA Exempt

716   ICD-10-CM 2025

Intraoperative and postprocedural complications and disorders of respiratory system, not elsewhere classified (J95)

✓4th J95 Intraoperative and postprocedural complications and disorders of respiratory system, not elsewhere classified

    EXCLUDES 2   *aspiration pneumonia (J69.-)*
           emphysema (subcutaneous) resulting from a procedure (T81.82)
           hypostatic pneumonia (J18.2)
           pulmonary manifestations due to radiation (J70.0-J70.1)

✓5th J95.0 Tracheostomy complications

    DEF: Tracheostomy: Formation of a tracheal opening on the neck surface with tube insertion to allow for respiration in cases of obstruction or decreased patency. A tracheostomy may be planned or performed on an emergency basis for temporary or long-term use.

    J95.00 Unspecified tracheostomy complication `CC` `HCC`

    J95.01 Hemorrhage from tracheostomy stoma `CC` `HCC`

    J95.02 Infection of tracheostomy stoma `CC` `HCC`
       Use additional code to identify type of infection, such as:
         cellulitis of neck (L03.221)
         sepsis (A40, A41.-)

    J95.03 Malfunction of tracheostomy stoma `CC` `HCC`
       Mechanical complication of tracheostomy stoma
       Obstruction of tracheostomy airway
       Tracheal stenosis due to tracheostomy

    J95.04 Tracheo-esophageal fistula following tracheostomy `CC` `HCC`

    J95.09 Other tracheostomy complication `CC` `HCC`

J95.1 Acute pulmonary insufficiency following thoracic surgery `MCC`

    EXCLUDES 2   *functional disturbances following cardiac surgery (I97.0, I97.1-)*

J95.2 Acute pulmonary insufficiency following nonthoracic surgery `MCC`

    EXCLUDES 2   *functional disturbances following cardiac surgery (I97.0, I97.1-)*

J95.3 Chronic pulmonary insufficiency following surgery `MCC`

    EXCLUDES 2   *functional disturbances following cardiac surgery (I97.0, I97.1-)*

J95.4 Chemical pneumonitis due to anesthesia `CC`
    Mendelson's syndrome
    Postprocedural aspiration pneumonia
    Use additional code for adverse effect, if applicable, to identify drug (T41.- with fifth or sixth character 5)

    EXCLUDES 1   *aspiration pneumonitis due to anesthesia complicating labor and delivery (O74.0)*
           aspiration pneumonitis due to anesthesia complicating pregnancy (O29)
           aspiration pneumonitis due to anesthesia complicating the puerperium (O89.01)

J95.5 Postprocedural subglottic stenosis `CC`

✓5th J95.6 Intraoperative hemorrhage and hematoma of a respiratory system organ or structure complicating a procedure

    EXCLUDES 1   *intraoperative hemorrhage and hematoma of a respiratory system organ or structure due to accidental puncture and laceration during procedure (J95.7-)*

    J95.61 Intraoperative hemorrhage and hematoma of a respiratory system organ or structure complicating a respiratory system procedure `CC`

    J95.62 Intraoperative hemorrhage and hematoma of a respiratory system organ or structure complicating other procedure `CC`

✓5th J95.7 Accidental puncture and laceration of a respiratory system organ or structure during a procedure

    EXCLUDES 2   *postprocedural pneumothorax (J95.811)*

    J95.71 Accidental puncture and laceration of a respiratory system organ or structure during a respiratory system procedure `CC`

    J95.72 Accidental puncture and laceration of a respiratory system organ or structure during other procedure `CC`

✓5th J95.8 Other intraoperative and postprocedural complications and disorders of respiratory system, not elsewhere classified
    AHA: 2016,4Q,9-10

    ✓6th J95.81 Postprocedural pneumothorax and air leak

       J95.811 Postprocedural pneumothorax `CC` `H14`
          AHA: 2021,1Q,48

       J95.812 Postprocedural air leak `CC`

    ✓6th J95.82 Postprocedural respiratory failure

       EXCLUDES 1   *respiratory failure in other conditions (J96.-)*

       J95.821 Acute postprocedural respiratory failure `MCC`
          Postprocedural respiratory failure NOS

       J95.822 Acute and chronic postprocedural respiratory failure `MCC`

    ✓6th J95.83 Postprocedural hemorrhage of a respiratory system organ or structure following a procedure
       AHA: 2023,2Q,28

       J95.830 Postprocedural hemorrhage of a respiratory system organ or structure following a respiratory system procedure `CC`

       J95.831 Postprocedural hemorrhage of a respiratory system organ or structure following other procedure `CC`

    J95.84 Transfusion-related acute lung injury (TRALI) `CC`
       DEF: Relatively rare, but serious, pulmonary complication of blood transfusion, with acute respiratory distress, noncardiogenic pulmonary edema, cyanosis, hypoxemia, hypotension, fever, and chills.

    ✓6th J95.85 Complication of respirator [ventilator]

       J95.850 Mechanical complication of respirator `CC` `HCC`
         EXCLUDES 1   *encounter for respirator [ventilator] dependence during power failure (Z99.12)*

       J95.851 Ventilator associated pneumonia `CC` `HCC`
         Ventilator associated pneumonitis
         Use additional code to identify the organism, if known (B95.-, B96.-, B97.-)
         EXCLUDES 1   *ventilator lung in newborn (P27.8)*
         AHA: 2020,2Q,17; 2017,1Q,25

       J95.859 Other complication of respirator [ventilator] `CC` `HCC`
         AHA: 2021,1Q,48

    ✓6th J95.86 Postprocedural hematoma and seroma of a respiratory system organ or structure following a procedure

       J95.860 Postprocedural hematoma of a respiratory system organ or structure following a respiratory system procedure `CC`

       J95.861 Postprocedural hematoma of a respiratory system organ or structure following other procedure `CC`

       J95.862 Postprocedural seroma of a respiratory system organ or structure following a respiratory system procedure `CC`

       J95.863 Postprocedural seroma of a respiratory system organ or structure following other procedure `CC`

    J95.87 Transfusion-associated dyspnea (TAD) `CC`
       EXCLUDES 1   *transfusion associated circulatory overload (TACO) (E87.71)*
          transfusion-related acute lung injury (TRALI) (J95.84)
       AHA: 2022,4Q,27

    J95.88 Other intraoperative complications of respiratory system, not elsewhere classified `CC`

    J95.89 Other postprocedural complications and disorders of respiratory system, not elsewhere classified `CC`
       Use additional code to identify disorder, such as:
         aspiration pneumonia (J69.-)
         bacterial or viral pneumonia (J12-J18)
       EXCLUDES 2   *acute pulmonary insufficiency following thoracic surgery (J95.1)*
          postprocedural subglottic stenosis (J95.5)

Other diseases of the respiratory system (J96-J99)

✓4th J96   Respiratory failure, not elsewhere classified

     EXCLUDES 1   *acute respiratory distress syndrome (J80)*
           cardiorespiratory failure (R09.2)
           newborn respiratory distress syndrome (P22.0)
           postprocedural respiratory failure (J95.82-)
           respiratory arrest (R09.2)
           respiratory arrest of newborn (P28.81)
           respiratory failure of newborn (P28.5)

     AHA: 2021,1Q,27,44-45; 2020,4Q,96

✓5th J96.0   Acute respiratory failure

     J96.00   Acute respiratory failure, unspecified whether with hypoxia or hypercapnia `MCC` `HCC`
         AHA: 2016,3Q,14; 2013,4Q,121

     J96.01   Acute respiratory failure with hypoxia `MCC` `HCC`
         AHA: 2024,2Q,11; 2020,3Q,12

     J96.02   Acute respiratory failure with hypercapnia `MCC` `HCC`
         Acute respiratory acidosis

✓5th J96.1   Chronic respiratory failure

     J96.10   Chronic respiratory failure, unspecified whether with hypoxia or hypercapnia `CC` `HCC`
         AHA: 2016,1Q,38; 2015,1Q,21

     J96.11   Chronic respiratory failure with hypoxia `CC` `HCC`
         AHA: 2013,4Q,129

     J96.12   Chronic respiratory failure with hypercapnia `CC` `HCC`
         Chronic respiratory acidosis

✓5th J96.2   Acute and chronic respiratory failure

     Acute on chronic respiratory failure

     J96.20   Acute and chronic respiratory failure, unspecified whether with hypoxia or hypercapnia `MCC` `HCC`

     J96.21   Acute and chronic respiratory failure with hypoxia `MCC` `HCC`

     J96.22   Acute and chronic respiratory failure with hypercapnia `MCC` `HCC`

✓5th J96.9   Respiratory failure, unspecified

     J96.90   Respiratory failure, unspecified, unspecified whether with hypoxia or hypercapnia `MCC` `HCC`

     J96.91   Respiratory failure, unspecified with hypoxia `MCC` `HCC`

     J96.92   Respiratory failure, unspecified with hypercapnia `MCC` `HCC`

✓4th J98   Other respiratory disorders

     Use additional code to identify:
     exposure to environmental tobacco smoke (Z77.22)
     exposure to tobacco smoke in the perinatal period (P96.81)
     history of tobacco dependence (Z87.891)
     occupational exposure to environmental tobacco smoke (Z57.31)
     tobacco dependence (F17.-)
     tobacco use (Z72.0)

     EXCLUDES 1   *newborn apnea (P28.4-)*
           newborn sleep apnea (P28.3-)
     EXCLUDES 2   *apnea NOS (R06.81)*
           sleep apnea (G47.3-)

✓5th J98.0   Diseases of bronchus, not elsewhere classified

     J98.01   Acute bronchospasm
         EXCLUDES 1   *acute bronchiolitis with bronchospasm (J21.-)*
             acute bronchitis with bronchospasm (J20.-)
             asthma (J45.-)
             exercise induced bronchospasm (J45.990)

     J98.09   Other diseases of bronchus, not elsewhere classified
         Broncholithiasis
         Calcification of bronchus
         Stenosis of bronchus
         Tracheobronchial collapse
         Tracheobronchial dyskinesia
         Ulcer of bronchus
         AHA: 2022,3Q,8

✓5th J98.1   Pulmonary collapse

     EXCLUDES 1   *therapeutic collapse of lung status (Z98.3)*

     J98.11   Atelectasis `CC`
         EXCLUDES 1   *newborn atelectasis*
             tuberculous atelectasis (current disease) (A15)
         DEF: Collapse of lung tissue affecting part or all of one lung, preventing normal oxygen absorption to healthy tissues.

     J98.19   Other pulmonary collapse `CC`

J98.2   Interstitial emphysema `HCC`

     Mediastinal emphysema
     EXCLUDES 1   *emphysema NOS (J43.9)*
           emphysema in newborn (P25.0)
           surgical emphysema (subcutaneous) (T81.82)
           traumatic subcutaneous emphysema (T79.7)

J98.3   Compensatory emphysema `HCC`

     DEF: Distention of all or part of the lung caused by disease processes or surgical intervention that decreased volume in another part of the lung, causing an overcompensation reaction. Compensatory emphysema occurs in association with pneumonias, pleural effusions, atelectasis, empyema, and pneumothorax.

J98.4   Other disorders of lung

     Calcification of lung
     Cystic lung disease (acquired)
     Lung disease NOS
     Pulmolithiasis
     EXCLUDES 1   *acute interstitial pneumonitis (J84.114)*
           pulmonary insufficiency following surgery (J95.1-J95.2)
     AHA: AHA:2024,2Q,20

✓5th J98.5   Diseases of mediastinum, not elsewhere classified

     EXCLUDES 2   *abscess of mediastinum (J85.3)*
     AHA: 2016,4Q,29

     J98.51   Mediastinitis `MCC` `H8`
         Code first underlying condition, if applicable, such as postoperative mediastinitis (T81.-)

     J98.59   Other diseases of mediastinum, not elsewhere classified `MCC` `H8`
         Fibrosis of mediastinum
         Hernia of mediastinum
         Retraction of mediastinum

J98.6   Disorders of diaphragm

     Diaphragmatitis
     Paralysis of diaphragm
     Relaxation of diaphragm
     EXCLUDES 1   *congenital malformation of diaphragm NEC (Q79.1)*
           congenital diaphragmatic hernia (Q79.0)
     EXCLUDES 2   *diaphragmatic hernia (K44.-)*

J98.8   Other specified respiratory disorders
     AHA: 2020,1Q,34-36

J98.9   Respiratory disorder, unspecified
     Respiratory disease (chronic) NOS

`N` Newborn: 0   `P` Pediatric: 0-17   `M` Maternity: 9-64   `A` Adult: 15-124   `UNS` Unspecified Site   `MCC` Major Complication/Comorbidity   `CC` Complication/Comorbidity   `PE` POA Exempt

J99 Respiratory disorders in diseases classified elsewhere   `HCC`

Code first underlying disease, such as:

amyloidosis (E85.-)

ankylosing spondylitis (M45.-)

congenital syphilis (A50.-)

cryoglobulinemia (D89.1)

early congenital syphilis (A50.0-)

plasminogen deficiency (E88.02)

schistosomiasis (B65.0-B65.9)

`EXCLUDES 1`   *respiratory disorders in:*

amebiasis (A06.5)

blastomycosis (B40.0-B40.2)

candidiasis (B37.1)

coccidioidomycosis (B38.0-B38.2)

cystic fibrosis with pulmonary manifestations (E84.0)

dermatomyositis (M33.01, M33.11)

histoplasmosis (B39.0-B39.2)

late syphilis (A52.72, A52.73)

polymyositis (M33.21)

Sjogren syndrome (M35.02)

systemic lupus erythematosus (M32.13)

systemic sclerosis (M34.81)

Wegener's granulomatosis (M31.30-M31.31)

☑ Additional Character Required   √x7ᵗʰ Placeholder   Questionable PDx   Manifestation   Unspecified   `UPD` Unacceptable PDx   `H1`-`H14` HAC   `HCC` CMS-HCC Dx   `HIV` HIV Dx

ICD-10-CM 2025

719

Chapter 11. Diseases of the Digestive System (K00–K95)

Chapter-specific Guidelines with Coding Examples
Reserved for future guideline expansion.

Chapter 11. Diseases of the Digestive System (K00–K95)

> **EXCLUDES 2**   certain conditions originating in the perinatal period (P04-P96)
> certain infectious and parasitic diseases (A00-B99)
> complications of pregnancy, childbirth and the puerperium (O00-O9A)
> congenital malformations, deformations and chromosomal abnormalities (Q00-Q99)
> endocrine, nutritional and metabolic diseases (E00-E88)
> injury, poisoning and certain other consequences of external causes (S00-T88)
> neoplasms (C00-D49)
> symptoms, signs and abnormal clinical and laboratory findings, not elsewhere classified (R00-R94)

This chapter contains the following blocks:

K00-K14	Diseases of oral cavity and salivary glands
K20-K31	Diseases of esophagus, stomach and duodenum
K35-K38	Diseases of appendix
K40-K46	Hernia
K50-K52	Noninfective enteritis and colitis
K55-K64	Other diseases of intestines
K65-K68	Diseases of peritoneum and retroperitoneum
K70-K77	Diseases of liver
K80-K87	Disorders of gallbladder, biliary tract and pancreas
K90-K95	Other diseases of the digestive system

Diseases of oral cavity and salivary glands (K00-K14)

✓4ᵗʰ K00 Disorders of tooth development and eruption

> **EXCLUDES 2**   embedded and impacted teeth (K01.-)

K00.0 Anodontia
Hypodontia
Oligodontia
> **EXCLUDES 1**   acquired absence of teeth (K08.1-)

DEF: Partial or complete absence of teeth due to a congenital defect involving the tooth bud.

K00.1 Supernumerary teeth
Distomolar
Fourth molar
Mesiodens
Paramolar
Supplementary teeth
> **EXCLUDES 2**   supernumerary roots (K00.2)

K00.2 Abnormalities of size and form of teeth
Concrescence of teeth
Fusion of teeth
Gemination of teeth
Dens evaginatus
Dens in dente
Dens invaginatus
Enamel pearls
Macrodontia
Microdontia
Peg-shaped [conical] teeth
Supernumerary roots
Taurodontism
Tuberculum paramolare
> **EXCLUDES 1**   abnormalities of teeth due to congenital syphilis (A50.5)
> tuberculum Carabelli, which is regarded as a normal variation and should not be coded

K00.3 Mottled teeth
Dental fluorosis
Mottling of enamel
Nonfluoride enamel opacities
> **EXCLUDES 2**   deposits [accretions] on teeth (K03.6)

K00.4 Disturbances in tooth formation
Aplasia and hypoplasia of cementum
Dilaceration of tooth
Enamel hypoplasia (neonatal) (postnatal) (prenatal)
Regional odontodysplasia
Turner's tooth
> **EXCLUDES 1**   Hutchinson's teeth and mulberry molars in congenital syphilis (A50.5)
> **EXCLUDES 2**   mottled teeth (K00.3)

K00.5 Hereditary disturbances in tooth structure, not elsewhere classified
Amelogenesis imperfecta
Dentinogenesis imperfecta
Odontogenesis imperfecta
Dentinal dysplasia
Shell teeth

K00.6 Disturbances in tooth eruption
Dentia praecox
Natal tooth
Neonatal tooth
Premature eruption of tooth
Premature shedding of primary [deciduous] tooth
Prenatal teeth
Retained [persistent] primary tooth
> **EXCLUDES 2**   embedded and impacted teeth (K01.-)

K00.7 Teething syndrome

K00.8 Other disorders of tooth development
Color changes during tooth formation
Intrinsic staining of teeth NOS
> **EXCLUDES 2**   posteruptive color changes (K03.7)

K00.9 Disorder of tooth development, unspecified
Disorder of odontogenesis NOS

✓4ᵗʰ K01 Embedded and impacted teeth

> **EXCLUDES 1**   abnormal position of fully erupted teeth (M26.3-)

K01.0 Embedded teeth

K01.1 Impacted teeth

✓4ᵗʰ K02 Dental caries

> **INCLUDES**   caries of dentine
> dental cavities
> early childhood caries
> pre-eruptive caries
> recurrent caries (dentino enamel junction) (enamel) (to the pulp)
> tooth decay

Tooth Anatomy

Enamel
Dentin
Pulp chamber
Root canal
Cementum

K02.3 Arrested dental caries
Arrested coronal and root caries

✓5ᵗʰ K02.5 Dental caries on pit and fissure surface
Dental caries on chewing surface of tooth

K02.51 Dental caries on pit and fissure surface limited to enamel
White spot lesions [initial caries] on pit and fissure surface of tooth

K02.52 Dental caries on pit and fissure surface penetrating into dentin
Primary dental caries, cervical origin

K02.53 Dental caries on pit and fissure surface penetrating into pulp

✓5ᵗʰ K02.6 Dental caries on smooth surface

K02.61 Dental caries on smooth surface limited to enamel
White spot lesions [initial caries] on smooth surface of tooth

K02.62 Dental caries on smooth surface penetrating into dentin

K02.63 Dental caries on smooth surface penetrating into pulp

K02.7 Dental root caries

K02.9 Dental caries, unspecified

N Newborn: 0   P Pediatric: 0-17   M Maternity: 9-64   A Adult: 15-124   UNS Unspecified Site   MCC Major Complication/Comorbidity   CC Complication/Comorbidity   PE POA Exempt

722   ICD-10-CM 2025

✓4ᵗʰ **K03** **Other diseases of hard tissues of teeth**

> *EXCLUDES 2*   bruxism (F45.8)
> dental caries (K02.-)
> teeth-grinding NOS (F45.8)

K03.0 **Excessive attrition of teeth**
Approximal wear of teeth
Occlusal wear of teeth
DEF: Attrition: In dentistry, wearing away or erosion of tooth surface from abrasive food or grinding teeth.

K03.1 **Abrasion of teeth**
Dentifrice abrasion of teeth
Habitual abrasion of teeth
Occupational abrasion of teeth
Ritual abrasion of teeth
Traditional abrasion of teeth
Wedge defect NOS

K03.2 **Erosion of teeth**
Erosion of teeth due to diet
Erosion of teeth due to drugs and medicaments
Erosion of teeth due to persistent vomiting
Erosion of teeth NOS
Idiopathic erosion of teeth
Occupational erosion of teeth

K03.3 **Pathological resorption of teeth**
Internal granuloma of pulp
Resorption of teeth (external)

K03.4 **Hypercementosis**
Cementation hyperplasia

K03.5 **Ankylosis of teeth**

K03.6 **Deposits [accretions] on teeth**
Betel deposits [accretions] on teeth
Black deposits [accretions] on teeth
Extrinsic staining of teeth NOS
Green deposits [accretions] on teeth
Materia alba deposits [accretions] on teeth
Orange deposits [accretions] on teeth
Staining of teeth NOS
Subgingival dental calculus
Supragingival dental calculus
Tobacco deposits [accretions] on teeth

K03.7 **Posteruptive color changes of dental hard tissues**
> *EXCLUDES 2*   deposits [accretions] on teeth (K03.6)

✓5ᵗʰ **K03.8** **Other specified diseases of hard tissues of teeth**

K03.81 **Cracked tooth**
> *EXCLUDES 1*   asymptomatic craze lines in enamel - omit code
> broken or fractured tooth due to trauma (S02.5)

K03.89 **Other specified diseases of hard tissues of teeth**

K03.9 **Disease of hard tissues of teeth, unspecified**

✓4ᵗʰ **K04** **Diseases of pulp and periapical tissues**
AHA: 2016,4Q,29-30

✓5ᵗʰ **K04.0** **Pulpitis**
Acute pulpitis
Chronic (hyperplastic) (ulcerative) pulpitis

K04.01 **Reversible pulpitis**   CC

K04.02 **Irreversible pulpitis**   CC

K04.1 **Necrosis of pulp**
Pulpal gangrene

K04.2 **Pulp degeneration**
Denticles
Pulpal calcifications
Pulpal stones

K04.3 **Abnormal hard tissue formation in pulp**
Secondary or irregular dentine

K04.4 **Acute apical periodontitis of pulpal origin**   CC
Acute apical periodontitis NOS
> *EXCLUDES 1*   acute periodontitis (K05.2-)
> **DEF:** Severe inflammation of the area surrounding the tip of a tooth's root that is often secondary to infection or trauma.

K04.5 **Chronic apical periodontitis**
Apical or periapical granuloma
Apical periodontitis NOS
> *EXCLUDES 1*   chronic periodontitis (K05.3-)

K04.6 **Periapical abscess with sinus**
Dental abscess with sinus
Dentoalveolar abscess with sinus

K04.7 **Periapical abscess without sinus**
Dental abscess without sinus
Dentoalveolar abscess without sinus

K04.8 **Radicular cyst**
Apical (periodontal) cyst
Periapical cyst
Residual radicular cyst
> *EXCLUDES 2*   lateral periodontal cyst (K09.0)
> **DEF:** Most common odontogenic cyst in tissue around the tooth apex due to chronic inflammation of dental pulp.

✓5ᵗʰ **K04.9** **Other and unspecified diseases of pulp and periapical tissues**

K04.90 **Unspecified diseases of pulp and periapical tissues**

K04.99 **Other diseases of pulp and periapical tissues**

✓4ᵗʰ **K05** **Gingivitis and periodontal diseases**
Use additional code to identify:
alcohol abuse and dependence (F10.-)
exposure to environmental tobacco smoke (Z77.22)
exposure to tobacco smoke in the perinatal period (P96.81)
history of tobacco dependence (Z87.891)
occupational exposure to environmental tobacco smoke (Z57.31)
tobacco dependence (F17.-)
tobacco use (Z72.0)
AHA: 2016,4Q,29-30

✓5ᵗʰ **K05.0** **Acute gingivitis**
> *EXCLUDES 1*   acute necrotizing ulcerative gingivitis (A69.1)
> herpesviral [herpes simplex] gingivostomatitis (B00.2)

K05.00 **Acute gingivitis, plaque induced**
Acute gingivitis NOS
Plaque induced gingival disease

K05.01 **Acute gingivitis, non-plaque induced**

✓5ᵗʰ **K05.1** **Chronic gingivitis**
Desquamative gingivitis (chronic)
Gingivitis (chronic) NOS
Hyperplastic gingivitis (chronic)
Pregnancy associated gingivitis
Simple marginal gingivitis (chronic)
Ulcerative gingivitis (chronic)
Code first, if applicable, diseases of the digestive system complicating pregnacy (O99.61-)

K05.10 **Chronic gingivitis, plaque induced**
Chronic gingivitis NOS
Gingivitis NOS

K05.11 **Chronic gingivitis, non-plaque induced**

✓5ᵗʰ **K05.2** **Aggressive periodontitis**
Acute pericoronitis
> *EXCLUDES 1*   acute apical periodontitis (K04.4)
> periapical abscess (K04.7)
> periapical abscess with sinus (K04.6)

K05.20 **Aggressive periodontitis, unspecified**

✓6ᵗʰ **K05.21** **Aggressive periodontitis, localized**
Periodontal abscess

K05.211 **Aggressive periodontitis, localized, slight**

K05.212 **Aggressive periodontitis, localized, moderate**

K05.213 **Aggressive periodontitis, localized, severe**

K05.219 **Aggressive periodontitis, localized, unspecified severity**

✓6ᵗʰ **K05.22** **Aggressive periodontitis, generalized**

K05.221 **Aggressive periodontitis, generalized, slight**

K05.222 **Aggressive periodontitis, generalized, moderate**

K05.223 **Aggressive periodontitis, generalized, severe**

K05.229 **Aggressive periodontitis, generalized, unspecified severity**

✓5ᵗʰ **K05.3** **Chronic periodontitis**
Chronic pericoronitis
Complex periodontitis
Periodontitis NOS
Simplex periodontitis
> *EXCLUDES 1*   chronic apical periodontitis (K04.5)

K05.30 **Chronic periodontitis, unspecified**

✓6ᵗʰ **K05.31** **Chronic periodontitis, localized**

K05.311 **Chronic periodontitis, localized, slight**

K05.312 **Chronic periodontitis, localized, moderate**

K05.313 **Chronic periodontitis, localized, severe**

✓ Additional Character Required   ✓x7ᵗʰ Placeholder   Questionable PDx   Manifestation   Unspecified   UPD Unacceptable PDx   H1 - H14 HAC   HCC CMS-HCC Dx   HIV HIV Dx

         K05.319   **Chronic periodontitis, localized, unspecified severity**

     ✓6th   **K05.32**   **Chronic periodontitis, generalized**

         K05.321   **Chronic periodontitis, generalized, slight**

         K05.322   **Chronic periodontitis, generalized, moderate**

         K05.323   **Chronic periodontitis, generalized, severe**

         K05.329   **Chronic periodontitis, generalized, unspecified**

   K05.4   **Periodontosis**
       Juvenile periodontosis

   K05.5   **Other periodontal diseases**
       Combined periodontic-endodontic lesion
       Narrow gingival width (of periodontal soft tissue)
       EXCLUDES 2   *leukoplakia of gingiva (K13.21)*

   K05.6   **Periodontal disease, unspecified**

✓4th   **K06**   **Other disorders of gingiva and edentulous alveolar ridge**
     EXCLUDES 2   *acute gingivitis (K05.0)*
                atrophy of edentulous alveolar ridge (K08.2)
                chronic gingivitis (K05.1)
                gingivitis NOS (K05.1)
     AHA: 2016,4Q,29-30

✓5th   **K06.0**   **Gingival recession**
       Gingival recession (postinfective) (postprocedural)
     AHA: 2017,4Q,16

     ✓6th   **K06.01**   **Gingival recession, localized**

         K06.010   **Localized gingival recession, unspecified**
              Localized gingival recession, NOS

         K06.011   **Localized gingival recession, minimal**

         K06.012   **Localized gingival recession, moderate**

         K06.013   **Localized gingival recession, severe**

     ✓6th   **K06.02**   **Gingival recession, generalized**

         K06.020   **Generalized gingival recession, unspecified**
              Generalized gingival recession, NOS

         K06.021   **Generalized gingival recession, minimal**

         K06.022   **Generalized gingival recession, moderate**

         K06.023   **Generalized gingival recession, severe**

   K06.1   **Gingival enlargement**
       Gingival fibromatosis

   K06.2   **Gingival and edentulous alveolar ridge lesions associated with trauma**
       Irritative hyperplasia of edentulous ridge [denture hyperplasia]
       Use additional code (Chapter 20) to identify external cause or denture status (Z97.2)

   K06.3   **Horizontal alveolar bone loss**

   K06.8   **Other specified disorders of gingiva and edentulous alveolar ridge**
       Fibrous epulis
       Flabby alveolar ridge
       Giant cell epulis
       Peripheral giant cell granuloma of gingiva
       Pyogenic granuloma of gingiva
       Vertical ridge deficiency
       EXCLUDES 2   *gingival cyst (K09.0)*

   K06.9   **Disorder of gingiva and edentulous alveolar ridge, unspecified**

✓4th   **K08**   **Other disorders of teeth and supporting structures**
     EXCLUDES 2   *dentofacial anomalies [including malocclusion] (M26.-)*
                disorders of jaw (M27.-)
     AHA: 2016,4Q,29-30

   K08.0   **Exfoliation of teeth due to systemic causes**
       Code also underlying systemic condition

✓5th   **K08.1**   **Complete loss of teeth**
       Acquired loss of teeth, complete
       EXCLUDES 1   *congenital absence of teeth (K00.0)*
                exfoliation of teeth due to systemic causes (K08.0)
                partial loss of teeth (K08.4-)

     ✓6th   **K08.10**   **Complete loss of teeth, unspecified cause**

         K08.101   **Complete loss of teeth, unspecified cause, class I**

         K08.102   **Complete loss of teeth, unspecified cause, class II**

         K08.103   **Complete loss of teeth, unspecified cause, class III**

         K08.104   **Complete loss of teeth, unspecified cause, class IV**

         K08.109   **Complete loss of teeth, unspecified cause, unspecified class**
              Edentulism NOS

     ✓6th   **K08.11**   **Complete loss of teeth due to trauma**

         K08.111   **Complete loss of teeth due to trauma, class I**

         K08.112   **Complete loss of teeth due to trauma, class II**

         K08.113   **Complete loss of teeth due to trauma, class III**

         K08.114   **Complete loss of teeth due to trauma, class IV**

         K08.119   **Complete loss of teeth due to trauma, unspecified class**

     ✓6th   **K08.12**   **Complete loss of teeth due to periodontal diseases**

         K08.121   **Complete loss of teeth due to periodontal diseases, class I**

         K08.122   **Complete loss of teeth due to periodontal diseases, class II**

         K08.123   **Complete loss of teeth due to periodontal diseases, class III**

         K08.124   **Complete loss of teeth due to periodontal diseases, class IV**

         K08.129   **Complete loss of teeth due to periodontal diseases, unspecified class**

     ✓6th   **K08.13**   **Complete loss of teeth due to caries**

         K08.131   **Complete loss of teeth due to caries, class I**

         K08.132   **Complete loss of teeth due to caries, class II**

         K08.133   **Complete loss of teeth due to caries, class III**

         K08.134   **Complete loss of teeth due to caries, class IV**

         K08.139   **Complete loss of teeth due to caries, unspecified class**

     ✓6th   **K08.19**   **Complete loss of teeth due to other specified cause**

         K08.191   **Complete loss of teeth due to other specified cause, class I**

         K08.192   **Complete loss of teeth due to other specified cause, class II**

         K08.193   **Complete loss of teeth due to other specified cause, class III**

         K08.194   **Complete loss of teeth due to other specified cause, class IV**

         K08.199   **Complete loss of teeth due to other specified cause, unspecified class**

✓5th   **K08.2**   **Atrophy of edentulous alveolar ridge**

         K08.20   **Unspecified atrophy of edentulous alveolar ridge**
              Atrophy of the mandible NOS
              Atrophy of the maxilla NOS

       K08.21   **Minimal atrophy of the mandible**
            Minimal atrophy of the edentulous mandible

       K08.22   **Moderate atrophy of the mandible**
            Moderate atrophy of the edentulous mandible

       K08.23   **Severe atrophy of the mandible**
            Severe atrophy of the edentulous mandible

       K08.24   **Minimal atrophy of maxilla**
            Minimal atrophy of the edentulous maxilla

       K08.25   **Moderate atrophy of the maxilla**
            Moderate atrophy of the edentulous maxilla

       K08.26   **Severe atrophy of the maxilla**
            Severe atrophy of the edentulous maxilla

   K08.3   **Retained dental root**

✓5th   **K08.4**   **Partial loss of teeth**
       Acquired loss of teeth, partial
       EXCLUDES 1   *complete loss of teeth (K08.1-)*
                congenital absence of teeth (K00.0)
       EXCLUDES 2   *exfoliation of teeth due to systemic causes (K08.0)*

     ✓6th   **K08.40**   **Partial loss of teeth, unspecified cause**

         K08.401   **Partial loss of teeth, unspecified cause, class I**

         K08.402   **Partial loss of teeth, unspecified cause, class II**

         K08.403   **Partial loss of teeth, unspecified cause, class III**

         K08.404   **Partial loss of teeth, unspecified cause, class IV**

N Newborn: 0   P Pediatric: 0-17   M Maternity: 9-64   A Adult: 15-124   UNS Unspecified Site   MCC Major Complication/Comorbidity   CC Complication/Comorbidity   PE POA Exempt

724   ICD-10-CM 2025

K08.409   **Partial loss of teeth, unspecified cause, unspecified class**
    Tooth extraction status NOS

√6ᵗʰ **K08.41**   **Partial loss of teeth due to trauma**

K08.411   **Partial loss of teeth due to trauma, class I**
K08.412   **Partial loss of teeth due to trauma, class II**
K08.413   **Partial loss of teeth due to trauma, class III**
K08.414   **Partial loss of teeth due to trauma, class IV**
K08.419   **Partial loss of teeth due to trauma, unspecified class**

√6ᵗʰ **K08.42**   **Partial loss of teeth due to periodontal diseases**

K08.421   **Partial loss of teeth due to periodontal diseases, class I**
K08.422   **Partial loss of teeth due to periodontal diseases, class II**
K08.423   **Partial loss of teeth due to periodontal diseases, class III**
K08.424   **Partial loss of teeth due to periodontal diseases, class IV**
K08.429   **Partial loss of teeth due to periodontal diseases, unspecified class**

√6ᵗʰ **K08.43**   **Partial loss of teeth due to caries**

K08.431   **Partial loss of teeth due to caries, class I**
K08.432   **Partial loss of teeth due to caries, class II**
K08.433   **Partial loss of teeth due to caries, class III**
K08.434   **Partial loss of teeth due to caries, class IV**
K08.439   **Partial loss of teeth due to caries, unspecified class**

√6ᵗʰ **K08.49**   **Partial loss of teeth due to other specified cause**

K08.491   **Partial loss of teeth due to other specified cause, class I**
K08.492   **Partial loss of teeth due to other specified cause, class II**
K08.493   **Partial loss of teeth due to other specified cause, class III**
K08.494   **Partial loss of teeth due to other specified cause, class IV**
K08.499   **Partial loss of teeth due to other specified cause, unspecified class**

√5ᵗʰ **K08.5**   **Unsatisfactory restoration of tooth**
    Defective bridge, crown, filling
    Defective dental restoration
    EXCLUDES 1   *dental restoration status (Z98.811)*
    EXCLUDES 2   *endosseous dental implant failure (M27.6-)*
       unsatisfactory endodontic treatment (M27.5-)

K08.50   **Unsatisfactory restoration of tooth, unspecified**
    Defective dental restoration NOS

K08.51   **Open restoration margins of tooth**
    Dental restoration failure of marginal integrity
    Open margin on tooth restoration
    Poor gingival margin to tooth restoration

K08.52   **Unrepairable overhanging of dental restorative materials**
    Overhanging of tooth restoration

√6ᵗʰ **K08.53**   **Fractured dental restorative material**
    EXCLUDES 1   *cracked tooth (K03.81)*
       traumatic fracture of tooth (S02.5)

K08.530   **Fractured dental restorative material without loss of material**
K08.531   **Fractured dental restorative material with loss of material**
K08.539   **Fractured dental restorative material, unspecified**

K08.54   **Contour of existing restoration of tooth biologically incompatible with oral health**
    Dental restoration failure of periodontal anatomical integrity
    Unacceptable contours of existing restoration of tooth
    Unacceptable morphology of existing restoration of tooth

K08.55   **Allergy to existing dental restorative material**
    Use additional code to identify the specific type of allergy

K08.56   **Poor aesthetic of existing restoration of tooth**
    Dental restoration aesthetically inadequate or displeasing

K08.59   **Other unsatisfactory restoration of tooth**
    Other defective dental restoration

√5ᵗʰ **K08.8**   **Other specified disorders of teeth and supporting structures**

K08.81   **Primary occlusal trauma**

K08.82   **Secondary occlusal trauma**
K08.89   **Other specified disorders of teeth and supporting structures**
    Enlargement of alveolar ridge NOS
    Insufficient anatomic crown height
    Insufficient clinical crown length
    Irregular alveolar process
    Toothache NOS

K08.9   **Disorder of teeth and supporting structures, unspecified**

√4ᵗʰ **K09**   **Cysts of oral region, not elsewhere classified**
    INCLUDES   lesions showing histological features both of aneurysmal cyst and of another fibro-osseous lesion
    EXCLUDES 2   *cysts of jaw (M27.0-, M27.4-)*
       radicular cyst (K04.8)

K09.0   **Developmental odontogenic cysts**
    Dentigerous cyst
    Eruption cyst
    Follicular cyst
    Gingival cyst
    Lateral periodontal cyst
    Primordial cyst
    EXCLUDES 2   *keratocysts (D16.4, D16.5)*
       odontogenic keratocystic tumors (D16.4, D16.5)

K09.1   **Developmental (nonodontogenic) cysts of oral region**
    Cyst (of) incisive canal
    Cyst (of) palatine of papilla
    Globulomaxillary cyst
    Median palatal cyst
    Nasoalveolar cyst
    Nasolabial cyst
    Nasopalatine duct cyst

K09.8   **Other cysts of oral region, not elsewhere classified**
    Dermoid cyst
    Epidermoid cyst
    Epstein's pearl
    Lymphoepithelial cyst

K09.9   **Cyst of oral region, unspecified**

√4ᵗʰ **K11**   **Diseases of salivary glands**
    Use additional code to identify:
    alcohol abuse and dependence (F10.-)
    exposure to environmental tobacco smoke (Z77.22)
    exposure to tobacco smoke in the perinatal period (P96.81)
    history of tobacco dependence (Z87.891)
    occupational exposure to environmental tobacco smoke (Z57.31)
    tobacco dependence (F17.-)
    tobacco use (Z72.0)

K11.0   **Atrophy of salivary gland**
K11.1   **Hypertrophy of salivary gland**
    DEF: Overgrowth of or enlarged salivary gland tissue caused by infection, salivary duct blockage, autoimmune diseases, and benign and malignant tumors.

√5ᵗʰ **K11.2**   **Sialoadenitis**
    Parotitis
    EXCLUDES 1   *epidemic parotitis (B26.-)*
       mumps (B26.-)
       uveoparotid fever [Heerfordt] (D86.89)
    DEF: Inflammation of the salivary gland.

K11.20   **Sialoadenitis, unspecified**
K11.21   **Acute sialoadenitis**
    EXCLUDES 1   *acute recurrent sialoadenitis (K11.22)*

K11.22   **Acute recurrent sialoadenitis**
K11.23   **Chronic sialoadenitis**

K11.3   **Abscess of salivary gland**   CC
K11.4   **Fistula of salivary gland**   CC
    EXCLUDES 1   *congenital fistula of salivary gland (Q38.4)*

K11.5   **Sialolithiasis**
    Calculus of salivary gland or duct
    Stone of salivary gland or duct

K11.6   **Mucocele of salivary gland**
    Mucous extravasation cyst of salivary gland
    Mucous retention cyst of salivary gland
    Ranula

K11.7   **Disturbances of salivary secretion**
    Hypoptyalism
    Ptyalism
    Xerostomia
    EXCLUDES 2   *dry mouth NOS (R68.2)*

✔ Additional Character Required   √x7ᵗʰ Placeholder   Questionable PDx   Manifestation   Unspecified   UPD Unacceptable PDx   H1–H14 HAC   HCC CMS-HCC Dx   HIV HIV Dx

ICD-10-CM 2025   725

K11.8   Other diseases of salivary glands
Benign lymphoepithelial lesion of salivary gland
Mikulicz' disease
Necrotizing sialometaplasia
Sialectasia
Stenosis of salivary duct
Stricture of salivary duct
EXCLUDES 1   *Sjogren syndrome (M35.0-)*

K11.9   Disease of salivary gland, unspecified
Sialoadenopathy NOS

✓4ᵗʰ **K12   Stomatitis and related lesions**
Use additional code to identify:
alcohol abuse and dependence (F10.-)
exposure to environmental tobacco smoke (Z77.22)
exposure to tobacco smoke in the perinatal period (P96.81)
history of tobacco dependence (Z87.891)
occupational exposure to environmental tobacco smoke (Z57.31)
tobacco dependence (F17.-)
tobacco use (Z72.0)
EXCLUDES 1   *cancrum oris (A69.0)*
     cheilitis (K13.0)
     gangrenous stomatitis (A69.0)
     herpesviral [herpes simplex] gingivostomatitis (B00.2)
     noma (A69.0)

K12.0   Recurrent oral aphthae
Aphthous stomatitis (major) (minor)
Bednar's aphthae
Periadenitis mucosa necrotica recurrens
Recurrent aphthous ulcer
Stomatitis herpetiformis
DEF: Disorder of unknown etiology with small oval or round painful ulcers of the mouth marked by a grayish exudate and a red halo effect.

K12.1   Other forms of stomatitis
Stomatitis NOS
Denture stomatitis
Ulcerative stomatitis
Vesicular stomatitis
EXCLUDES 1   *acute necrotizing ulcerative stomatitis (A69.1)*
     Vincent's stomatitis (A69.1)

K12.2   Cellulitis and abscess of mouth   CC
Cellulitis of mouth (floor)
Submandibular abscess
EXCLUDES 2   *abscess of salivary gland (K11.3)*
     abscess of tongue (K14.0)
     periapical abscess (K04.6-K04.7)
     periodontal abscess (K05.21)
     peritonsillar abscess (J36)

✓5ᵗʰ **K12.3   Oral mucositis (ulcerative)**
Mucositis (oral) (oropharyneal)
EXCLUDES 2   *gastrointestinal mucositis (ulcerative) (K92.81)*
     mucositis (ulcerative) of vagina and vulva (N76.81)
     nasal mucositis (ulcerative) (J34.81)

K12.30   Oral mucositis (ulcerative), unspecified
K12.31   Oral mucositis (ulcerative) due to antineoplastic therapy
Use additional code for adverse effect, if applicable, to identify antineoplastic and immunosuppressive drugs (T45.1X5)
Use additional code for other antineoplastic therapy, such as:
radiological procedure and radiotherapy (Y84.2)
K12.32   Oral mucositis (ulcerative) due to other drugs
Use additional code for adverse effect, if applicable, to identify drug (T36-T50 with fifth or sixth character 5)
K12.33   Oral mucositis (ulcerative) due to radiation
Use additional external cause code (W88-W90, X39.0-) to identify cause
K12.39   Other oral mucositis (ulcerative)
Viral oral mucositis (ulcerative)

✓4ᵗʰ **K13   Other diseases of lip and oral mucosa**
INCLUDES   epithelial disturbances of tongue
Use additional code to identify:
alcohol abuse and dependence (F10.-)
exposure to environmental tobacco smoke (Z77.22)
exposure to tobacco smoke in the perinatal period (P96.81)
history of tobacco dependence (Z87.891)
occupational exposure to environmental tobacco smoke (Z57.31)
tobacco dependence (F17.-)
tobacco use (Z72.0)
EXCLUDES 2   *certain disorders of gingiva and edentulous alveolar ridge (K05-K06)*
     cysts of oral region (K09.-)
     diseases of tongue (K14.-)
     stomatitis and related lesions (K12.-)

K13.0   Diseases of lips
Abscess of lips
Angular cheilitis
Cellulitis of lips
Cheilitis NOS
Cheilodynia
Cheilosis
Exfoliative cheilitis
Fistula of lips
Glandular cheilitis
Hypertrophy of lips
Perlèche NEC
EXCLUDES 1   *ariboflavinosis (E53.0)*
     cheilitis due to radiation-related disorders (L55-L59)
     congenital fistula of lips (Q38.0)
     congenital hypertrophy of lips (Q18.6)
     perlèche due to candidiasis (B37.83)
     perlèche due to riboflavin deficiency (E53.0)

K13.1   Cheek and lip biting

✓5ᵗʰ **K13.2   Leukoplakia and other disturbances of oral epithelium, including tongue**
EXCLUDES 1   *carcinoma in situ of oral epithelium (D00.0-)*
     hairy leukoplakia (K13.3)
DEF: Leukoplakia: Thickened white patches or lesions appearing on a mucous membrane, such as oral mucosa or tongue.

K13.21   Leukoplakia of oral mucosa, including tongue
Leukokeratosis of oral mucosa
Leukoplakia of gingiva, lips, tongue
EXCLUDES 1   *hairy leukoplakia (K13.3)*
     leukokeratosis nicotina palati (K13.24)
K13.22   Minimal keratinized residual ridge mucosa
Minimal keratinization of alveolar ridge mucosa
K13.23   Excessive keratinized residual ridge mucosa
Excessive keratinization of alveolar ridge mucosa
K13.24   Leukokeratosis nicotina palati
Smoker's palate
K13.29   Other disturbances of oral epithelium, including tongue
Erythroplakia of mouth or tongue
Focal epithelial hyperplasia of mouth or tongue
Leukoedema of mouth or tongue
Other oral epithelium disturbances

K13.3   Hairy leukoplakia
K13.4   Granuloma and granuloma-like lesions of oral mucosa
Eosinophilic granuloma
Granuloma pyogenicum
Verrucous xanthoma
K13.5   Oral submucous fibrosis
Submucous fibrosis of tongue
K13.6   Irritative hyperplasia of oral mucosa
EXCLUDES 2   *irritative hyperplasia of edentulous ridge [denture hyperplasia] (K06.2)*

✓5ᵗʰ **K13.7   Other and unspecified lesions of oral mucosa**
K13.70   Unspecified lesions of oral mucosa
K13.79   Other lesions of oral mucosa
Focal oral mucinosis
AHA: 2022,2Q,7

☑4ᵗʰ K14 Diseases of tongue

Use additional code to identify:
alcohol abuse and dependence (F1Ø.-)
exposure to environmental tobacco smoke (Z77.22)
history of tobacco dependence (Z87.891)
occupational exposure to environmental tobacco smoke (Z57.31)
tobacco dependence (F17.-)
tobacco use (Z72.Ø)

EXCLUDES 2   erythroplakia (K13.29)
         focal epithelial hyperplasia (K13.29)
         ►leukoedema of tongue◄ (K13.29)
         leukoplakia of tongue (K13.21)
         hairy leukoplakia (K13.3)
         macroglossia (congenital) (Q38.2)
         submucous fibrosis of tongue (K13.5)

K14.Ø Glossitis
Abscess of tongue
Ulceration (traumatic) of tongue
EXCLUDES 1   atrophic glossitis (K14.4)
DEF: Inflammation and swelling of the tongue that may be associated with infection, adverse drug reactions, smoking, or injury.

K14.1 Geographic tongue
Benign migratory glossitis
Glossitis areata exfoliativa

K14.2 Median rhomboid glossitis

K14.3 Hypertrophy of tongue papillae
Black hairy tongue
Coated tongue
Hypertrophy of foliate papillae
Lingua villosa nigra

K14.4 Atrophy of tongue papillae
Atrophic glossitis

K14.5 Plicated tongue
Fissured tongue
Furrowed tongue
Scrotal tongue
EXCLUDES 1   fissured tongue, congenital (Q38.3)

K14.6 Glossodynia
Glossopyrosis
Painful tongue

K14.8 Other diseases of tongue
Atrophy of tongue
Crenated tongue
Enlargement of tongue
Glossocele
Glossoptosis
Hypertrophy of tongue

K14.9 Disease of tongue, unspecified
Glossopathy NOS

Diseases of esophagus, stomach and duodenum (K2Ø-K31)

EXCLUDES 2   hiatus hernia (K44.-)

☑4ᵗʰ K2Ø Esophagitis

Use additional code to identify:
alcohol abuse and dependence (F1Ø.-)
EXCLUDES 1   erosion of esophagus (K22.1-)
         esophagitis with gastro-esophageal reflux disease (K21.Ø-)
         reflux esophagitis (K21.Ø-)
         ulcerative esophagitis (K22.1-)
EXCLUDES 2   eosinophilic gastritis or gastroenteritis (K52.81)
AHA: 2023,1Q,20

K2Ø.Ø Eosinophilic esophagitis
AHA: 2020,4Q,9

☑5ᵗʰ K2Ø.8 Other esophagitis
AHA: 2020,4Q,28-29
K2Ø.8Ø Other esophagitis without bleeding
Abscess of esophagus
Other esophagitis NOS
K2Ø.81 Other esophagitis with bleeding   MCC

☑5ᵗʰ K2Ø.9 Esophagitis, unspecified
AHA: 2020,4Q,28-29
K2Ø.9Ø Esophagitis, unspecified without bleeding
Esophagitis NOS
K2Ø.91 Esophagitis, unspecified with bleeding   MCC

☑4ᵗʰ K21 Gastro-esophageal reflux disease

EXCLUDES 1   newborn esophageal reflux (P78.83)

☑5ᵗʰ K21.Ø Gastro-esophageal reflux disease with esophagitis
AHA: 2020,4Q,28-29
K21.ØØ Gastro-esophageal reflux disease with esophagitis, without bleeding
Reflux esophagitis
K21.Ø1 Gastro-esophageal reflux disease with esophagitis, with bleeding   MCC

K21.9 Gastro-esophageal reflux disease without esophagitis
Esophageal reflux NOS
AHA: 2016,1Q,18

☑4ᵗʰ K22 Other diseases of esophagus

EXCLUDES 2   esophageal varices (I85.-)

K22.Ø Achalasia of cardia
Achalasia NOS
Cardiospasm
EXCLUDES 1   congenital cardiospasm (Q39.5)
DEF: Esophageal motility disorder that is caused by absence of the esophageal peristalsis and impaired relaxation of the lower esophageal sphincter. It is characterized by dysphagia, regurgitation, and heartburn.

☑5ᵗʰ K22.1 Ulcer of esophagus
Barrett's ulcer
Erosion of esophagus
Fungal ulcer of esophagus
Peptic ulcer of esophagus
Ulcer of esophagus due to ingestion of chemicals
Ulcer of esophagus due to ingestion of drugs and medicaments
Ulcerative esophagitis
Code first poisoning due to drug or toxin, if applicable (T36-T65 with fifth or sixth character 1-4)
Use additional code for adverse effect, if applicable, to identify drug (T36-T5Ø with fifth or sixth character 5)
EXCLUDES 1   Barrett's esophagus (K22.7-)
AHA: 2018,3Q,22; 2017,3Q,27
TIP: Assign a code for "with bleeding" when an esophageal ulcer and bleeding (hematemesis) are documented. The ICD-10-CM classification assumes the two are related without the provider linking the two conditions. Evidence of bleeding during a procedure is not required.
K22.1Ø Ulcer of esophagus without bleeding   CC
Ulcer of esophagus NOS
K22.11 Ulcer of esophagus with bleeding   MCC
EXCLUDES 2   bleeding esophageal varices (I85.Ø1, I85.11)
AHA: 2023,1Q,20
TIP: For bleeding esophageal ulcers resulting from anticoagulant therapy, assign this code, code D68.32 Hemorrhagic disorder due to extrinsic circulating anticoagulant, and adverse effect code T45.515- with the appropriate seventh character. Either code K22.11 or D68.32 may be sequenced first, depending on the circumstances of admission.

K22.2 Esophageal obstruction
Compression of esophagus
Constriction of esophagus
Stenosis of esophagus
Stricture of esophagus
EXCLUDES 1   congenital stenosis or stricture of esophagus (Q39.3)

K22.3 Perforation of esophagus   MCC
Rupture of esophagus
EXCLUDES 1   traumatic perforation of (thoracic) esophagus (S27.8-)

K22.4 Dyskinesia of esophagus
Corkscrew esophagus
Diffuse esophageal spasm
Spasm of esophagus
EXCLUDES 1   cardiospasm (K22.Ø)

K22.5 Diverticulum of esophagus, acquired
Esophageal pouch, acquired
EXCLUDES 1   diverticulum of esophagus (congenital) (Q39.6)

K22.6 Gastro-esophageal laceration-hemorrhage syndrome   MCC
Mallory-Weiss syndrome

☑ Additional Character Required   ✓x7ᵗʰ Placeholder   Questionable PDx   Manifestation   Unspecified   UPD Unacceptable PDx   H1-H14 HAC   HCC CMS-HCC Dx   HIV HIV Dx

ICD-10-CM 2025   727

✓5th **K22.7** **Barrett's** esophagus

Barrett's disease
Barrett's syndrome

EXCLUDES 1   *Barrett's ulcer (K22.1)*

malignant neoplasm of esophagus (C15.-)

DEF: Metaplastic disorder in which specialized columnar epithelial cells replace the normal squamous epithelial cells. Secondary to chronic gastroesophageal reflux damage to the mucosa, this disorder increases the risk of developing adenocarcinoma.

K22.70   **Barrett's esophagus without dysplasia**

Barrett's esophagus NOS

✓6th **K22.71**   **Barrett's esophagus with dysplasia**

K22.710   Barrett's esophagus with **low grade dysplasia**

K22.711   Barrett's esophagus with **high grade dysplasia**

K22.719   Barrett's esophagus with dysplasia, unspecified

✓5th **K22.8** **Other specified diseases of esophagus**

EXCLUDES 2   *esophageal varices (I85.-)*

Paterson-Kelly syndrome (D50.1)

AHA: 2021,4Q,15; 2020,1Q,16

K22.81   **Esophageal polyp**

EXCLUDES 1   *benign neoplasm of esophagus (D13.0)*

K22.82   **Esophagogastric junction polyp**

EXCLUDES 1   *benign neoplasm of stomach (D13.1)*

K22.89   **Other specified disease of esophagus**

Hemorrhage of esophagus NOS

AHA: AHA:2024,2Q,26

K22.9 **Disease of esophagus, unspecified**

K23   ***Disorders of esophagus in diseases classified elsewhere***

Code first underlying disease, such as:
congenital syphilis (A50.5)

EXCLUDES 1   *late syphilis (A52.79)*

megaesophagus due to Chagas' disease (B57.31)

tuberculosis (A18.83)

✓4th **K25** **Gastric ulcer**

INCLUDES   erosion (acute) of stomach
pylorus ulcer (peptic)
stomach ulcer (peptic)

Use additional code to identify:
alcohol abuse and dependence (F10.-)

EXCLUDES 1   *acute gastritis (K29.0-)*

peptic ulcer NOS (K27.-)

AHA: 2021,1Q,9,11; 2017,3Q,27

TIP: Assign a code for "with hemorrhage" when a gastric ulcer and GI bleeding are documented. The ICD-10-CM classification assumes the two are related without the provider linking the two conditions. Evidence of bleeding during a procedure is not required.

TIP: For bleeding ulcers resulting from anticoagulant therapy, assign the appropriate "with hemorrhage" ulcer code from this category, code D68.32 Hemorrhagic disorder due to extrinsic circulating anticoagulant, and adverse effect code T45.515- with the appropriate seventh character. Either the bleeding ulcer code or code D68.32 may be sequenced first, depending on the circumstances of admission.

K25.0   **Acute gastric ulcer with hemorrhage** `MCC`

AHA: 2023,1Q,16

K25.1   **Acute gastric ulcer with perforation** `MCC` `HCC`

K25.2   **Acute gastric ulcer with both hemorrhage and perforation** `MCC` `HCC`

K25.3   **Acute gastric ulcer without hemorrhage or perforation** `CC`

K25.4   **Chronic or unspecified gastric ulcer with hemorrhage** `MCC`

K25.5   **Chronic or unspecified gastric ulcer with perforation** `MCC` `HCC`

K25.6   **Chronic or unspecified gastric ulcer with both hemorrhage and perforation** `MCC` `HCC`

K25.7   **Chronic gastric ulcer without hemorrhage or perforation**

K25.9   **Gastric ulcer, unspecified as acute or chronic, without hemorrhage or perforation**

Gastrointestinal Ulcers

Esophagus
Esophageal ulcer
Stomach
Duodenal ulcer
Gastric ulcer
Small intestine

✓4th **K26** **Duodenal ulcer**

INCLUDES   duodenum ulcer (peptic)
erosion (acute) of duodenum
postpyloric ulcer (peptic)

Use additional code to identify:
alcohol abuse and dependence (F10.-)

EXCLUDES 1   *peptic ulcer NOS (K27.-)*

AHA: 2023,2Q,11; 2017,3Q,27

TIP: Assign a code for "with hemorrhage" when a duodenal ulcer and GI bleeding are documented. The ICD-10-CM classification assumes the two are related without the provider linking the two conditions. Evidence of bleeding during a procedure is not required.

TIP: For bleeding ulcers resulting from anticoagulant therapy, assign the appropriate "with hemorrhage" ulcer code from this category, code D68.32 Hemorrhagic disorder due to extrinsic circulating anticoagulant, and adverse effect code T45.515- with the appropriate seventh character. Either the bleeding ulcer code or code D68.32 may be sequenced first, depending on the circumstances of admission.

K26.0   **Acute duodenal ulcer with hemorrhage** `MCC`

K26.1   **Acute duodenal ulcer with perforation** `MCC` `HCC`

K26.2   **Acute duodenal ulcer with both hemorrhage and perforation** `MCC` `HCC`

K26.3   **Acute duodenal ulcer without hemorrhage or perforation** `CC`

K26.4   **Chronic or unspecified duodenal ulcer with hemorrhage** `MCC`

AHA: 2016,1Q,14

K26.5   **Chronic or unspecified duodenal ulcer with perforation** `MCC` `HCC`

K26.6   **Chronic or unspecified duodenal ulcer with both hemorrhage and perforation** `MCC` `HCC`

K26.7   **Chronic duodenal ulcer without hemorrhage or perforation**

K26.9   **Duodenal ulcer, unspecified as acute or chronic, without hemorrhage or perforation**

✓4th **K27** **Peptic ulcer, site unspecified**

INCLUDES   gastroduodenal ulcer NOS
peptic ulcer NOS

Use additional code to identify:
alcohol abuse and dependence (F10.-)

EXCLUDES 1   *peptic ulcer of newborn (P78.82)*

AHA: 2017,3Q,27

TIP: Assign a code for "with hemorrhage" when a peptic ulcer and GI bleeding are documented. The ICD-10-CM classification assumes the two are related without the provider linking the two conditions. Evidence of bleeding during a procedure is not required.

TIP: For bleeding ulcers resulting from anticoagulant therapy, assign the appropriate "with hemorrhage" ulcer code from this category, code D68.32 Hemorrhagic disorder due to extrinsic circulating anticoagulant, and adverse effect code T45.515- with the appropriate seventh character. Either the bleeding ulcer code or code D68.32 may be sequenced first, depending on the circumstances of admission.

K27.0   **Acute peptic ulcer, site unspecified, with hemorrhage** `MCC`

K27.1   **Acute peptic ulcer, site unspecified, with perforation** `MCC` `HCC`

K27.2   **Acute peptic ulcer, site unspecified, with both hemorrhage and perforation** `MCC` `HCC`

K27.3   **Acute peptic ulcer, site unspecified, without hemorrhage or perforation** `CC`

N Newborn: 0   **P** Pediatric: 0-17   **M** Maternity: 9-64   **A** Adult: 15-124   **UNS** Unspecified Site   **MCC** Major Complication/Comorbidity   **CC** Complication/Comorbidity   **PE** POA Exempt

728   ICD-10-CM 2025

K27.4 **Chronic** or unspecified peptic ulcer, site unspecified, **with hemorrhage** `MCC`

K27.5 **Chronic** or unspecified peptic ulcer, site unspecified, **with perforation** `MCC` `HCC`

K27.6 **Chronic** or unspecified peptic ulcer, site unspecified, **with both hemorrhage and perforation** `MCC` `HCC`

K27.7 **Chronic** peptic ulcer, site unspecified, without hemorrhage or perforation

K27.9 Peptic ulcer, site unspecified, unspecified as acute or chronic, without hemorrhage or perforation

`√4th` **K28** **Gastrojejunal** ulcer

INCLUDES　　anastomotic ulcer (peptic) or erosion
gastrocolic ulcer (peptic) or erosion
gastrointestinal ulcer (peptic) or erosion
gastrojejunal ulcer (peptic) or erosion
jejunal ulcer (peptic) or erosion
marginal ulcer (peptic) or erosion
stomal ulcer (peptic) or erosion

Use additional code to identify:
alcohol abuse and dependence (F10.-)

EXCLUDES 1　　primary ulcer of small intestine (K63.3)

AHA: 2017,3Q,27

TIP: Assign a code for "with hemorrhage" when a gastrojejunal ulcer and GI bleeding are documented. The ICD-10-CM classification assumes the two are related without the provider linking the two conditions. Evidence of bleeding during a procedure is not required.

TIP: For bleeding ulcers resulting from anticoagulant therapy, assign the appropriate "with hemorrhage" ulcer code from this category, code D68.32 Hemorrhagic disorder due to extrinsic circulating anticoagulant, and adverse effect code T45.515- with the appropriate seventh character. Either the bleeding ulcer code or code D68.32 may be sequenced first, depending on the circumstances of admission.

K28.0 **Acute** gastrojejunal ulcer **with hemorrhage** `MCC`

K28.1 **Acute** gastrojejunal ulcer **with perforation** `MCC` `HCC`

K28.2 **Acute** gastrojejunal ulcer **with both hemorrhage and perforation** `MCC` `HCC`

K28.3 **Acute** gastrojejunal ulcer without hemorrhage or perforation `CC`

K28.4 **Chronic** or unspecified gastrojejunal ulcer **with hemorrhage** `MCC`
AHA: 2023,3Q,10

K28.5 **Chronic** or unspecified gastrojejunal ulcer **with perforation** `MCC` `HCC`

K28.6 **Chronic** or unspecified gastrojejunal ulcer **with both hemorrhage and perforation** `MCC` `HCC`

K28.7 **Chronic** gastrojejunal ulcer without hemorrhage or perforation

K28.9 Gastrojejunal ulcer, unspecified as acute or chronic, without hemorrhage or perforation

`√4th` **K29** **Gastritis and duodenitis**

EXCLUDES 1　　eosinophilic gastritis or gastroenteritis (K52.81)
Zollinger-Ellison syndrome (E16.4)

AHA: 2018,3Q,22

TIP: Assign a code for "with bleeding" when gastritis or duodenitis and GI bleeding are documented. The ICD-10-CM classification assumes the two are related without the provider linking the two conditions. Evidence of bleeding during a procedure is not required.

TIP: For bleeding ulcers resulting from anticoagulant therapy, assign the appropriate "with hemorrhage" ulcer code from this category, code D68.32 Hemorrhagic disorder due to extrinsic circulating anticoagulant, and adverse effect code T45.515- with the appropriate seventh character. Either the bleeding ulcer code or code D68.32 may be sequenced first, depending on the circumstances of admission.

`√5th` **K29.0** **Acute** gastritis

Use additional code to identify:
alcohol abuse and dependence (F10.-)

EXCLUDES 1　　erosion (acute) of stomach (K25.-)

K29.00 **Acute** gastritis **without bleeding**

K29.01 **Acute** gastritis **with bleeding** `MCC`

`√5th` **K29.2** **Alcoholic** gastritis

Use additional code to identify:
alcohol abuse and dependence (F10.-)

K29.20 **Alcoholic** gastritis **without bleeding**

K29.21 **Alcoholic** gastritis **with bleeding** `MCC`

`√5th` **K29.3** **Chronic superficial** gastritis

K29.30 **Chronic superficial** gastritis **without bleeding**

K29.31 **Chronic superficial** gastritis **with bleeding** `MCC`

`√5th` **K29.4** **Chronic atrophic** gastritis

Gastric atrophy

K29.40 **Chronic atrophic** gastritis **without bleeding**

K29.41 **Chronic atrophic** gastritis **with bleeding** `MCC`

`√5th` **K29.5** **Unspecified chronic** gastritis

Chronic antral gastritis
Chronic fundal gastritis

K29.50 **Unspecified chronic** gastritis **without bleeding**

K29.51 **Unspecified chronic** gastritis **with bleeding** `MCC`

`√5th` **K29.6** **Other** gastritis

Giant hypertrophic gastritis
Granulomatous gastritis
Menetrier's disease

K29.60 **Other** gastritis **without bleeding**

K29.61 **Other** gastritis **with bleeding** `MCC`

`√5th` **K29.7** **Gastritis, unspecified**

K29.70 **Gastritis, unspecified, without bleeding**

K29.71 **Gastritis, unspecified, with bleeding** `MCC`

`√5th` **K29.8** **Duodenitis**

K29.80 **Duodenitis without bleeding**

K29.81 **Duodenitis with bleeding** `MCC`

`√5th` **K29.9** **Gastroduodenitis, unspecified**

K29.90 **Gastroduodenitis, unspecified, without bleeding**

K29.91 **Gastroduodenitis, unspecified, with bleeding** `MCC`

K30 **Functional dyspepsia**

Indigestion

EXCLUDES 1　　dyspepsia NOS (R10.13)
heartburn (R12)
nervous dyspepsia (F45.8)
neurotic dyspepsia (F45.8)
psychogenic dyspepsia (F45.8)

`√4th` **K31** **Other diseases of stomach and duodenum**

INCLUDES　　functional disorders of stomach

EXCLUDES 2　　diabetic gastroparesis (E08.43, E09.43, E10.43, E11.43, E13.43)
diverticulum of duodenum (K57.00-K57.13)

K31.0 **Acute dilatation of stomach** `CC`

Acute distention of stomach

K31.1 **Adult hypertrophic pyloric stenosis** `CC` `A`

Pyloric stenosis NOS

EXCLUDES 1　　congenital or infantile pyloric stenosis (Q40.0)

AHA: 2023,3Q,11

K31.2 **Hourglass stricture and stenosis of stomach**

EXCLUDES 1　　congenital hourglass stomach (Q40.2)
hourglass contraction of stomach (K31.89)

K31.3 **Pylorospasm, not elsewhere classified**

EXCLUDES 1　　congenital or infantile pylorospasm (Q40.0)
neurotic pylorospasm (F45.8)
psychogenic pylorospasm (F45.8)

K31.4 **Gastric diverticulum**

EXCLUDES 1　　congenital diverticulum of stomach (Q40.2)

K31.5 **Obstruction of duodenum** `CC`

Constriction of duodenum
Duodenal ileus (chronic)
Stenosis of duodenum
Stricture of duodenum
Volvulus of duodenum

EXCLUDES 1　　congenital stenosis of duodenum (Q41.0)

K31.6 **Fistula of stomach and duodenum** `CC`

Gastrocolic fistula
Gastrojejunocolic fistula

▶Code also, if applicable, disruption of internal operation (surgical) wound (T81.32-)◀

K31.7 **Polyp of stomach and duodenum**

EXCLUDES 1　　adenomatous polyp of stomach (D13.1)

AHA: 2020,1Q,16

✔ Additional Character Required　`√x7th` Placeholder　Questionable PDx　Manifestation　Unspecified　`UPD` Unacceptable PDx　`H1`-`H14` HAC　`HCC` CMS-HCC Dx　`HIV` HIV Dx

ICD-10-CM 2025　　　　729

Chapter 11. Diseases of the Digestive System

✓5ᵗʰ **K31.8** **Other specified diseases of stomach and duodenum**

✓6ᵗʰ **K31.81** **Angiodysplasia of stomach and duodenum**

TIP: Assign a code for "with bleeding" when angiodysplasia of the stomach or the duodenum and GI bleeding are documented. The ICD-10-CM classification assumes the two are related without the provider linking the two conditions. Evidence of bleeding during a procedure is not required.

K31.811 **Angiodysplasia of stomach and duodenum with bleeding** MCC

AHA: 2023,1Q,16

K31.819 **Angiodysplasia of stomach and duodenum without bleeding**

Angiodysplasia of stomach and duodenum NOS

K31.82 **Dieulafoy lesion (hemorrhagic) of stomach and duodenum** MCC

EXCLUDES 2   *Dieulafoy lesion of intestine (K63.81)*

DEF: Abnormally large submucosal artery protruding through a defect in the stomach mucosa or intestines that can cause massive and life-threatening hemorrhaging.

K31.83 **Achlorhydria**

DEF: Absence of hydrochloric acid in gastric secretions due to gastric mucosa atrophy. Achlorhydria is unresponsive to histamines.

K31.84 **Gastroparesis**

Gastroparalysis

Code first underlying disease, if known, such as:
anorexia nervosa (F50.0-)
diabetes mellitus (E08.43, E09.43, E10.43, E11.43, E13.43)
scleroderma (M34.-)

AHA: 2013,4Q,114

K31.89 **Other diseases of stomach and duodenum**

AHA: 2024,2Q,26; 2020,1Q,15; 2017,1Q,28

K31.9 **Disease of stomach and duodenum, unspecified**

✓5ᵗʰ **K31.A** **Gastric intestinal metaplasia**

AHA: 2021,4Q,15-16

K31.A0 **Gastric intestinal metaplasia, unspecified**

Gastric intestinal metaplasia indefinite for dysplasia

Gastric intestinal metaplasia NOS

✓6ᵗʰ **K31.A1** **Gastric intestinal metaplasia without dysplasia**

K31.A11 **Gastric intestinal metaplasia without dysplasia, involving the antrum**

K31.A12 **Gastric intestinal metaplasia without dysplasia, involving the body (corpus)**

K31.A13 **Gastric intestinal metaplasia without dysplasia, involving the fundus**

K31.A14 **Gastric intestinal metaplasia without dysplasia, involving the cardia**

K31.A15 **Gastric intestinal metaplasia without dysplasia, involving multiple sites**

K31.A19 **Gastric intestinal metaplasia without dysplasia, unspecified site**

✓6ᵗʰ **K31.A2** **Gastric intestinal metaplasia with dysplasia**

K31.A21 **Gastric intestinal metaplasia with low grade dysplasia**

K31.A22 **Gastric intestinal metaplasia with high grade dysplasia**

K31.A29 **Gastric intestinal metaplasia with dysplasia, unspecified**

Diseases of appendix (K35-K38)

✓4ᵗʰ **K35** **Acute appendicitis**

AHA: 2018,4Q,17-18

✓5ᵗʰ **K35.2** **Acute appendicitis with generalized peritonitis**

AHA: 2023,4Q,28-29

✓6ᵗʰ **K35.20** **Acute appendicitis with generalized peritonitis, without abscess**

K35.200 **Acute appendicitis with generalized peritonitis, without perforation or abscess** CC

(Acute) appendicitis with generalized peritonitis without rupture or perforation of appendix NOS

K35.201 **Acute appendicitis with generalized peritonitis, with perforation, without abscess** CC

Appendicitis (acute) with generalized (diffuse) peritonitis following rupture or perforation of appendix NOS

K35.209 **Acute appendicitis with generalized peritonitis, without abscess, unspecified as to perforation** CC

(Acute) appendicitis with generalized peritonitis NOS

✓6ᵗʰ **K35.21** **Acute appendicitis with generalized peritonitis, with abscess**

K35.210 **Acute appendicitis with generalized peritonitis, without perforation, with abscess** MCC

(Acute) appendicitis with generalized peritonitis without rupture or perforation of appendix, with abscess

K35.211 **Acute appendicitis with generalized peritonitis, with perforation and abscess** MCC

Appendicitis (acute) with generalized (diffuse) peritonitis following rupture or perforation of appendix, with abscess

K35.219 **Acute appendicitis with generalized peritonitis, with abscess, unspecified as to perforation** MCC

(Acute) appendicitis with generalized peritonitis and abscess NOS

✓5ᵗʰ **K35.3** **Acute appendicitis with localized peritonitis**

K35.30 **Acute appendicitis with localized peritonitis, without perforation or gangrene** CC

Acute appendicitis with localized peritonitis NOS

K35.31 **Acute appendicitis with localized peritonitis and gangrene, without perforation** CC

K35.32 **Acute appendicitis with perforation, localized peritonitis, and gangrene, without abscess** MCC

(Acute) appendicitis with perforation NOS

Perforated appendix NOS

Ruptured appendix (with localized peritonitis) NOS

AHA: 2020,1Q,16

K35.33 **Acute appendicitis with perforation, localized peritonitis, and gangrene, with abscess** MCC

(Acute) appendicitis with (peritoneal) abscess NOS

Ruptured appendix with localized peritonitis and abscess

✓5ᵗʰ **K35.8** **Other and unspecified acute appendicitis**

K35.80 **Unspecified acute appendicitis** CC

Acute appendicitis NOS

Acute appendicitis without (localized) (generalized) peritonitis

✓6ᵗʰ **K35.89** **Other acute appendicitis**

AHA: 2020,1Q,16

K35.890 **Other acute appendicitis without perforation or gangrene** CC

K35.891 **Other acute appendicitis without perforation, with gangrene** CC

(Acute) appendicitis with gangrene NOS

K36 **Other appendicitis**

Chronic appendicitis

Recurrent appendicitis

K37 **Unspecified appendicitis**

EXCLUDES 1   *unspecified appendicitis with peritonitis (K35.2-, K35.3-)*

✓4ᵗʰ **K38** **Other diseases of appendix**

K38.0 **Hyperplasia of appendix**

K38.1 **Appendicular concretions**

Fecalith of appendix

Stercolith of appendix

K38.2 **Diverticulum of appendix**

K38.3 **Fistula of appendix**

K38.8 **Other specified diseases of appendix**

Intussusception of appendix

K38.9 **Disease of appendix, unspecified**

N Newborn: 0   P Pediatric: 0-17   M Maternity: 9-64   A Adult: 15-124   UNS Unspecified Site   MCC Major Complication/Comorbidity   CC Complication/Comorbidity   PE POA Exempt

730   ICD-10-CM 2025

Hernia (K40-K46)

NOTE   Hernia with both gangrene and obstruction is classified to hernia with gangrene.

INCLUDES   acquired hernia
congenital [except diaphragmatic or hiatus] hernia
recurrent hernia

AHA: 2021,3Q,30-31

TIP: Do not assign a code for bilateral hernia when the right and left sides have differing pathology. For example, two codes would be assigned for bilateral femoral hernia in which the left side is incarcerated (with obstruction) but the right side is not incarcerated; the code for bilateral would not apply in this case.

☑4ᵗʰ K40 Inguinal hernia

> **INCLUDES**   bubonocele
> direct inguinal hernia
> double inguinal hernia
> indirect inguinal hernia
> inguinal hernia NOS
> oblique inguinal hernia
> scrotal hernia.
>
> **DEF:** Within the groin region.

> **☑5ᵗʰ K40.0 Bilateral inguinal hernia, with obstruction, without gangrene**
> Inguinal hernia (bilateral) causing obstruction without gangrene
> Incarcerated inguinal hernia (bilateral) without gangrene
> Irreducible inguinal hernia (bilateral) without gangrene
> Strangulated inguinal hernia (bilateral) without gangrene
>
>> **K40.00 Bilateral inguinal hernia, with obstruction, without gangrene, not specified as recurrent** CC
>> Bilateral inguinal hernia, with obstruction, without gangrene NOS
>>
>> **K40.01 Bilateral inguinal hernia, with obstruction, without gangrene, recurrent** CC

> **☑5ᵗʰ K40.1 Bilateral inguinal hernia, with gangrene**
>> **K40.10 Bilateral inguinal hernia, with gangrene, not specified as recurrent** MCC
>> Bilateral inguinal hernia, with gangrene NOS
>>
>> **K40.11 Bilateral inguinal hernia, with gangrene, recurrent** MCC

> **☑5ᵗʰ K40.2 Bilateral inguinal hernia, without obstruction or gangrene**
>> **K40.20 Bilateral inguinal hernia, without obstruction or gangrene, not specified as recurrent**
>> Bilateral inguinal hernia NOS
>>
>> **K40.21 Bilateral inguinal hernia, without obstruction or gangrene, recurrent**

> **☑5ᵗʰ K40.3 Unilateral inguinal hernia, with obstruction, without gangrene**
> Inguinal hernia (unilateral) causing obstruction without gangrene
> Incarcerated inguinal hernia (unilateral) without gangrene
> Irreducible inguinal hernia (unilateral) without gangrene
> Strangulated inguinal hernia (unilateral) without gangrene
>
>> **K40.30 Unilateral inguinal hernia, with obstruction, without gangrene, not specified as recurrent** CC
>> Inguinal hernia, with obstruction NOS
>> Unilateral inguinal hernia, with obstruction, without gangrene NOS
>>
>> **K40.31 Unilateral inguinal hernia, with obstruction, without gangrene, recurrent** CC

> **☑5ᵗʰ K40.4 Unilateral inguinal hernia, with gangrene**
>> **K40.40 Unilateral inguinal hernia, with gangrene, not specified as recurrent** MCC
>> Inguinal hernia with gangrene NOS
>> Unilateral inguinal hernia with gangrene NOS
>>
>> **K40.41 Unilateral inguinal hernia, with gangrene, recurrent** MCC

> **☑5ᵗʰ K40.9 Unilateral inguinal hernia, without obstruction or gangrene**
>> **K40.90 Unilateral inguinal hernia, without obstruction or gangrene, not specified as recurrent**
>> Inguinal hernia NOS
>> Unilateral inguinal hernia NOS

>> **K40.91 Unilateral inguinal hernia, without obstruction or gangrene, recurrent**

Hernia Sites

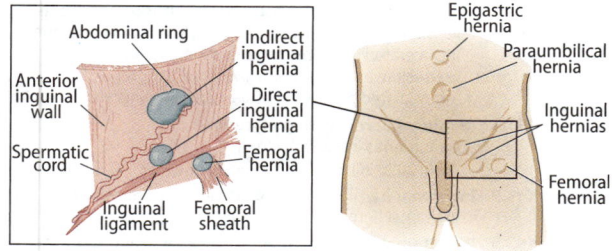

☑4ᵗʰ K41 Femoral hernia

> **☑5ᵗʰ K41.0 Bilateral femoral hernia, with obstruction, without gangrene**
> Femoral hernia (bilateral) causing obstruction, without gangrene
> Incarcerated femoral hernia (bilateral), without gangrene
> Irreducible femoral hernia (bilateral), without gangrene
> Strangulated femoral hernia (bilateral), without gangrene
>
>> **K41.00 Bilateral femoral hernia, with obstruction, without gangrene, not specified as recurrent** CC
>> Bilateral femoral hernia, with obstruction, without gangrene NOS
>>
>> **K41.01 Bilateral femoral hernia, with obstruction, without gangrene, recurrent** CC

> **☑5ᵗʰ K41.1 Bilateral femoral hernia, with gangrene**
>> **K41.10 Bilateral femoral hernia, with gangrene, not specified as recurrent** MCC
>> Bilateral femoral hernia, with gangrene NOS
>>
>> **K41.11 Bilateral femoral hernia, with gangrene, recurrent** MCC

> **☑5ᵗʰ K41.2 Bilateral femoral hernia, without obstruction or gangrene**
>> **K41.20 Bilateral femoral hernia, without obstruction or gangrene, not specified as recurrent**
>> Bilateral femoral hernia NOS
>>
>> **K41.21 Bilateral femoral hernia, without obstruction or gangrene, recurrent**

> **☑5ᵗʰ K41.3 Unilateral femoral hernia, with obstruction, without gangrene**
> Femoral hernia (unilateral) causing obstruction, without gangrene
> Incarcerated femoral hernia (unilateral), without gangrene
> Irreducible femoral hernia (unilateral), without gangrene
> Strangulated femoral hernia (unilateral), without gangrene
>
>> **K41.30 Unilateral femoral hernia, with obstruction, without gangrene, not specified as recurrent** CC
>> Femoral hernia, with obstruction NOS
>> Unilateral femoral hernia, with obstruction NOS
>>
>> **K41.31 Unilateral femoral hernia, with obstruction, without gangrene, recurrent** CC

> **☑5ᵗʰ K41.4 Unilateral femoral hernia, with gangrene**
>> **K41.40 Unilateral femoral hernia, with gangrene, not specified as recurrent** MCC
>> Femoral hernia, with gangrene NOS
>> Unilateral femoral hernia, with gangrene NOS
>>
>> **K41.41 Unilateral femoral hernia, with gangrene, recurrent** MCC

> **☑5ᵗʰ K41.9 Unilateral femoral hernia, without obstruction or gangrene**
>> **K41.90 Unilateral femoral hernia, without obstruction or gangrene, not specified as recurrent**
>> Femoral hernia NOS
>> Unilateral femoral hernia NOS
>>
>> **K41.91 Unilateral femoral hernia, without obstruction or gangrene, recurrent**

☑4ᵗʰ K42 Umbilical hernia

> **INCLUDES**   paraumbilical hernia
> **EXCLUDES 1**   *omphalocele (Q79.2)*

> **K42.0 Umbilical hernia with obstruction, without gangrene** CC
> Umbilical hernia causing obstruction, without gangrene
> Incarcerated umbilical hernia, without gangrene
> Irreducible umbilical hernia, without gangrene
> Strangulated umbilical hernia, without gangrene

> **K42.1 Umbilical hernia with gangrene** MCC
> Gangrenous umbilical hernia

> **K42.9 Umbilical hernia without obstruction or gangrene**
> Umbilical hernia NOS

☑ Additional Character Required   ☑x7ᵗʰ Placeholder   Questionable PDx   Manifestation   Unspecified   UPD Unacceptable PDx   H1-H14 HAC   HCC CMS-HCC Dx   HIV HIV Dx

ICD-10-CM 2025   **731**

✓4ᵗʰ K43 Ventral hernia

DEF: Condition in which a loop of bowel protrudes through a weakness in the abdominal wall muscles that may occur as a birth defect, past surgical site (incisional), or form at a stomal site (parastomal).

K43.0 Incisional hernia with obstruction, without gangrene `CC`
Incisional hernia causing obstruction, without gangrene
Incarcerated incisional hernia, without gangrene
Irreducible incisional hernia, without gangrene
Strangulated incisional hernia, without gangrene

K43.1 Incisional hernia with gangrene `MCC`
Gangrenous incisional hernia
AHA: 2020,2Q,22

K43.2 Incisional hernia without obstruction or gangrene
Incisional hernia NOS

K43.3 Parastomal hernia with obstruction, without gangrene `CC`
Incarcerated parastomal hernia, without gangrene
Irreducible parastomal hernia, without gangrene
Parastomal hernia causing obstruction, without gangrene
Strangulated parastomal hernia, without gangrene

K43.4 Parastomal hernia with gangrene `MCC`
Gangrenous parastomal hernia

K43.5 Parastomal hernia without obstruction or gangrene
Parastomal hernia NOS

K43.6 Other and unspecified ventral hernia with obstruction, without gangrene `CC`
Epigastric hernia causing obstruction, without gangrene
Hypogastric hernia causing obstruction, without gangrene
Incarcerated epigastric hernia without gangrene
Incarcerated hypogastric hernia without gangrene
Incarcerated midline hernia without gangrene
Incarcerated spigelian hernia without gangrene
Incarcerated subxiphoid hernia without gangrene
Irreducible epigastric hernia without gangrene
Irreducible hypogastric hernia without gangrene
Irreducible midline hernia without gangrene
Irreducible spigelian hernia without gangrene
Irreducible subxiphoid hernia without gangrene
Midline hernia causing obstruction, without gangrene
Spigelian hernia causing obstruction, without gangrene
Strangulated epigastric hernia without gangrene
Strangulated hypogastric hernia without gangrene
Strangulated midline hernia without gangrene
Strangulated spigelian hernia without gangrene
Strangulated subxiphoid hernia without gangrene
Subxiphoid hernia causing obstruction, without gangrene

K43.7 Other and unspecified ventral hernia with gangrene `MCC`
Any condition listed under K43.6 specified as gangrenous

K43.9 Ventral hernia without obstruction or gangrene
Epigastric hernia
Ventral hernia NOS

✓4ᵗʰ K44 Diaphragmatic hernia

`INCLUDES`   hiatus hernia (esophageal) (sliding)
         paraesophageal hernia
`EXCLUDES 1`   *congenital diaphragmatic hernia (Q79.0)*
         congenital hiatus hernia (Q40.1)

DEF: Protrusion of an abdominal organ, usually the stomach, through the esophageal opening within the diaphragm and occurring in two types: the sliding hiatal hernia and the paraesophageal hernia.

Hiatal Hernia

Gastroesophageal junction (slides up and down)

Sliding hiatal hernia

Gastroesophageal junction (remains in place)

Esophagus

Stomach

Diaphragm

Paraesophageal hiatal hernia

K44.0 Diaphragmatic hernia with obstruction, without gangrene `CC`
Diaphragmatic hernia causing obstruction
Incarcerated diaphragmatic hernia
Irreducible diaphragmatic hernia
Strangulated diaphragmatic hernia
AHA: 2022,2Q,13

K44.1 Diaphragmatic hernia with gangrene `MCC`
Gangrenous diaphragmatic hernia

K44.9 Diaphragmatic hernia without obstruction or gangrene
Diaphragmatic hernia NOS

✓4ᵗʰ K45 Other abdominal hernia

`INCLUDES`   abdominal hernia, specified site NEC
         lumbar hernia
         obturator hernia
         pudendal hernia
         retroperitoneal hernia
         sciatic hernia

K45.0 Other specified abdominal hernia with obstruction, without gangrene `CC`
Other specified abdominal hernia causing obstruction
Other specified incarcerated abdominal hernia
Other specified irreducible abdominal hernia
Other specified strangulated abdominal hernia

K45.1 Other specified abdominal hernia with gangrene `MCC`
Any condition listed under K45 specified as gangrenous
AHA: AHA:2024,2Q,22

K45.8 Other specified abdominal hernia without obstruction or gangrene

✓4ᵗʰ K46 Unspecified abdominal hernia

`INCLUDES`   enterocele
         epiplocele
         hernia NOS
         interstitial hernia
         intestinal hernia
         intra-abdominal hernia
`EXCLUDES 1`   *vaginal enterocele (N81.5)*

K46.0 Unspecified abdominal hernia with obstruction, without gangrene `CC`
Unspecified abdominal hernia causing obstruction
Unspecified incarcerated abdominal hernia
Unspecified irreducible abdominal hernia
Unspecified strangulated abdominal hernia

K46.1 Unspecified abdominal hernia with gangrene `MCC`
Any condition listed under K46 specified as gangrenous

`N` Newborn: 0   `P` Pediatric: 0-17   `M` Maternity: 9-64   `A` Adult: 15-124   `UNS` Unspecified Site   `MCC` Major Complication/Comorbidity   `CC` Complication/Comorbidity   `PE` POA Exempt

732   ICD-10-CM 2025

K46.9   **Unspecified abdominal hernia without obstruction or gangrene**
       Abdominal hernia NOS

Noninfective enteritis and colitis (K50-K52)

INCLUDES   noninfective inflammatory bowel disease
EXCLUDES 1   irritable bowel syndrome (K58.-)
         megacolon (K59.3-)

√4th **K50   Crohn's disease [regional enteritis]**

     INCLUDES   granulomatous enteritis
     ▶Use additional code to identify any associated fistulas, if applicable:◀
     ▶anal fistula (K60.3-)◀
     ▶anorectal fistula (K60.5-)◀
     ▶rectal fistula (K60.4-)◀
     Use additional code to identify manifestations, such as:
       pyoderma gangrenosum (L88)
     EXCLUDES 1   ulcerative colitis (K51.-)
     AHA: 2019,3Q,5; 2012,4Q,104
     DEF: Chronic inflammation of the gastrointestinal tract characterized by chronic granulomatous disease, most commonly affecting the intestines and the terminal ileum.

√5th **K50.0   Crohn's disease of small intestine**

     Crohn's disease [regional enteritis] of duodenum
     Crohn's disease [regional enteritis] of ileum
     Crohn's disease [regional enteritis] of jejunum
     Regional ileitis
     Terminal ileitis
     EXCLUDES 1   Crohn's disease of both small and large intestine (K50.8-)

     K50.00   **Crohn's disease of small intestine without complications**   CC HCC

     √6th **K50.01**   **Crohn's disease of small intestine with complications**

         K50.011   **Crohn's disease of small intestine with rectal bleeding**   CC HCC
         K50.012   **Crohn's disease of small intestine with intestinal obstruction**   CC HCC
         K50.013   **Crohn's disease of small intestine with fistula**   CC HCC
         K50.014   **Crohn's disease of small intestine with abscess**   CC HCC
           AHA: 2012,4Q,104
         K50.018   **Crohn's disease of small intestine with other complication**   CC HCC
         K50.019   **Crohn's disease of small intestine with unspecified complications**   CC HCC

√5th **K50.1   Crohn's disease of large intestine**

     Crohn's disease [regional enteritis] of colon
     Crohn's disease [regional enteritis] of large bowel
     Crohn's disease [regional enteritis] of rectum
     Granulomatous colitis
     Regional colitis
     EXCLUDES 1   Crohn's disease of both small and large intestine (K50.8)

     K50.10   **Crohn's disease of large intestine without complications**   CC HCC

     √6th **K50.11**   **Crohn's disease of large intestine with complications**

         K50.111   **Crohn's disease of large intestine with rectal bleeding**   CC HCC
         K50.112   **Crohn's disease of large intestine with intestinal obstruction**   CC HCC
         K50.113   **Crohn's disease of large intestine with fistula**   CC HCC
         K50.114   **Crohn's disease of large intestine with abscess**   CC HCC
         K50.118   **Crohn's disease of large intestine with other complication**   CC HCC
         K50.119   **Crohn's disease of large intestine with unspecified complications**   CC HCC

√5th **K50.8   Crohn's disease of both small and large intestine**

     K50.80   **Crohn's disease of both small and large intestine without complications**   CC HCC

     √6th **K50.81**   **Crohn's disease of both small and large intestine with complications**

         K50.811   **Crohn's disease of both small and large intestine with rectal bleeding**   CC HCC
         K50.812   **Crohn's disease of both small and large intestine with intestinal obstruction**   CC HCC

K50.813   **Crohn's disease of both small and large intestine with fistula**   CC HCC

K50.814   **Crohn's disease of both small and large intestine with abscess**   CC HCC

K50.818   **Crohn's disease of both small and large intestine with other complication**   CC HCC

K50.819   **Crohn's disease of both small and large intestine with unspecified complications**   CC HCC

√5th **K50.9   Crohn's disease, unspecified**

     K50.90   **Crohn's disease, unspecified, without complications**   CC HCC
       Crohn's disease NOS
       Regional enteritis NOS

     √6th **K50.91**   **Crohn's disease, unspecified, with complications**

         K50.911   **Crohn's disease, unspecified, with rectal bleeding**   CC HCC
         K50.912   **Crohn's disease, unspecified, with intestinal obstruction**   CC HCC
         K50.913   **Crohn's disease, unspecified, with fistula**   CC HCC
         K50.914   **Crohn's disease, unspecified, with abscess**   CC HCC
         K50.918   **Crohn's disease, unspecified, with other complication**   CC HCC
         K50.919   **Crohn's disease, unspecified, with unspecified complications**   CC HCC

√4th **K51   Ulcerative colitis**

     ▶Use additional code to identify any associated fistulas, if applicable:◀
     ▶anal fistula (K60.3-)◀
     ▶anorectal fistula (K60.5-)◀
     ▶rectal fistula (K60.4-)◀
     Use additional code to identify manifestations, such as:
       pyoderma gangrenosum (L88)
     EXCLUDES 1   Crohn's disease [regional enteritis] (K50.-)

√5th **K51.0   Ulcerative (chronic) pancolitis**

     Backwash ileitis

     K51.00   **Ulcerative (chronic) pancolitis without complications**   CC HCC
       Ulcerative (chronic) pancolitis NOS

     √6th **K51.01**   **Ulcerative (chronic) pancolitis with complications**

         K51.011   **Ulcerative (chronic) pancolitis with rectal bleeding**   CC HCC
         K51.012   **Ulcerative (chronic) pancolitis with intestinal obstruction**   CC HCC
         K51.013   **Ulcerative (chronic) pancolitis with fistula**   CC HCC
         K51.014   **Ulcerative (chronic) pancolitis with abscess**   CC HCC
         K51.018   **Ulcerative (chronic) pancolitis with other complication**   CC HCC
         K51.019   **Ulcerative (chronic) pancolitis with unspecified complications**   CC HCC

√5th **K51.2   Ulcerative (chronic) proctitis**

     K51.20   **Ulcerative (chronic) proctitis without complications**   CC HCC
       Ulcerative (chronic) proctitis NOS

     √6th **K51.21**   **Ulcerative (chronic) proctitis with complications**

         K51.211   **Ulcerative (chronic) proctitis with rectal bleeding**   CC HCC
         K51.212   **Ulcerative (chronic) proctitis with intestinal obstruction**   CC HCC
         K51.213   **Ulcerative (chronic) proctitis with fistula**   CC HCC
         K51.214   **Ulcerative (chronic) proctitis with abscess**   CC HCC
         K51.218   **Ulcerative (chronic) proctitis with other complication**   CC HCC
         K51.219   **Ulcerative (chronic) proctitis with unspecified complications**   CC HCC

√5th **K51.3   Ulcerative (chronic) rectosigmoiditis**

     K51.30   **Ulcerative (chronic) rectosigmoiditis without complications**   CC HCC
       Ulcerative (chronic) rectosigmoiditis NOS

✓6ᵗʰ **K51.31** **Ulcerative (chronic) rectosigmoiditis with complications**

K51.311 **Ulcerative (chronic) rectosigmoiditis with rectal bleeding** `CC` `HCC`

K51.312 **Ulcerative (chronic) rectosigmoiditis with intestinal obstruction** `CC` `HCC`

K51.313 **Ulcerative (chronic) rectosigmoiditis with fistula** `CC` `HCC`

K51.314 **Ulcerative (chronic) rectosigmoiditis with abscess** `CC` `HCC`

K51.318 **Ulcerative (chronic) rectosigmoiditis with other complication** `CC` `HCC`

K51.319 **Ulcerative (chronic) rectosigmoiditis with unspecified complications** `CC` `HCC`

✓5ᵗʰ **K51.4** **Inflammatory polyps of colon**

> EXCLUDES 2   adenomatous polyp of colon (D12.6)
> polyposis of colon (D12.6)
> polyps of colon NOS (K63.5)

K51.40 **Inflammatory polyps of colon without complications** `CC` `HCC`
Inflammatory polyps of colon NOS

✓6ᵗʰ **K51.41** **Inflammatory polyps of colon with complications**

K51.411 **Inflammatory polyps of colon with rectal bleeding** `CC` `HCC`

K51.412 **Inflammatory polyps of colon with intestinal obstruction** `CC` `HCC`

K51.413 **Inflammatory polyps of colon with fistula** `CC` `HCC`

K51.414 **Inflammatory polyps of colon with abscess** `CC` `HCC`

K51.418 **Inflammatory polyps of colon with other complication** `CC` `HCC`

K51.419 **Inflammatory polyps of colon with unspecified complications** `CC` `HCC`

✓5ᵗʰ **K51.5** **Left sided colitis**
Left hemicolitis

K51.50 **Left sided colitis without complications** `CC` `HCC`
Left sided colitis NOS

✓6ᵗʰ **K51.51** **Left sided colitis with complications**

K51.511 **Left sided colitis with rectal bleeding** `CC` `HCC`

K51.512 **Left sided colitis with intestinal obstruction** `CC` `HCC`

K51.513 **Left sided colitis with fistula** `CC` `HCC`

K51.514 **Left sided colitis with abscess** `CC` `HCC`

K51.518 **Left sided colitis with other complication** `CC` `HCC`

K51.519 **Left sided colitis with unspecified complications** `CC` `HCC`

✓5ᵗʰ **K51.8** **Other ulcerative colitis**

K51.80 **Other ulcerative colitis without complications** `CC` `HCC`

✓6ᵗʰ **K51.81** **Other ulcerative colitis with complications**

K51.811 **Other ulcerative colitis with rectal bleeding** `CC` `HCC`

K51.812 **Other ulcerative colitis with intestinal obstruction** `CC` `HCC`

K51.813 **Other ulcerative colitis with fistula** `CC` `HCC`

K51.814 **Other ulcerative colitis with abscess** `CC` `HCC`

K51.818 **Other ulcerative colitis with other complication** `CC` `HCC`

K51.819 **Other ulcerative colitis with unspecified complications** `CC` `HCC`

✓5ᵗʰ **K51.9** **Ulcerative colitis, unspecified**

K51.90 **Ulcerative colitis, unspecified, without complications** `CC` `HCC`

✓6ᵗʰ **K51.91** **Ulcerative colitis, unspecified, with complications**

K51.911 **Ulcerative colitis, unspecified with rectal bleeding** `CC` `HCC`

K51.912 **Ulcerative colitis, unspecified with intestinal obstruction** `CC` `HCC`

K51.913 **Ulcerative colitis, unspecified with fistula** `CC` `HCC`

K51.914 **Ulcerative colitis, unspecified with abscess** `CC` `HCC`

K51.918 **Ulcerative colitis, unspecified with other complication** `CC` `HCC`

K51.919 **Ulcerative colitis, unspecified with unspecified complications** `CC` `HCC`

✓4ᵗʰ **K52** **Other and unspecified noninfective gastroenteritis and colitis**
    AHA: 2016,4Q,30-31

K52.0 **Gastroenteritis and colitis due to radiation** `CC`

K52.1 **Toxic gastroenteritis and colitis** `CC`
Drug-induced gastroenteritis and colitis
Code first (T51-T65) to identify toxic agent
Use additional code for adverse effect, if applicable, to identify drug (T36-T50 with fifth or sixth character 5)
AHA: 2019,1Q,17

✓5ᵗʰ **K52.2** **Allergic and dietetic gastroenteritis and colitis**
Food hypersensitivity gastroenteritis or colitis
Use additional code to identify type of food allergy (Z91.01-, Z91.02-)

> EXCLUDES 2   allergic eosinophilic colitis (K52.82)
> allergic eosinophilic esophagitis (K20.0)
> allergic eosinophilic gastritis (K52.81)
> allergic eosinophilic gastroenteritis (K52.81)

DEF: True immunoglobulin E (IgE)-mediated allergic reaction of the lining of the stomach, intestines, or colon to food proteins. It causes nausea, vomiting, diarrhea, and abdominal cramping.

K52.21 **Food protein-induced enterocolitis syndrome**
FPIES
Use additional code for hypovolemic shock, if present (R57.1)

K52.22 **Food protein-induced enteropathy**

K52.29 **Other allergic and dietetic gastroenteritis and colitis**
Allergic proctocolitis
Food hypersensitivity gastroenteritis or colitis
Food-induced eosinophilic proctocolitis
Food protein-induced proctocolitis
Immediate gastrointestinal hypersensitivity
Milk protein-induced proctocolitis

K52.3 **Indeterminate colitis**
Colonic inflammatory bowel disease unclassified (IBDU)

> EXCLUDES 1   unspecified colitis (K52.9)

✓5ᵗʰ **K52.8** **Other specified noninfective gastroenteritis and colitis**

K52.81 **Eosinophilic gastritis or gastroenteritis**
Eosinophilic enteritis

> EXCLUDES 2   eosinophilic esophagitis (K20.0)

DEF: Disorder involving the accumulation of eosinophil in the lining of the stomach or multiple levels of the gastrointestinal tract, but without a known cause such as connective tissue disease, drug reaction, malignancy, or parasitic infection.

K52.82 **Eosinophilic colitis**

> EXCLUDES 2   allergic proctocolitis (K52.29)
> food-induced eosinophilic proctocolitis (K52.29)
> food protein-induced enterocolitis syndrome (FPIES) (K52.21)
> food protein-induced proctocolitis (K52.29)
> milk protein-induced proctocolitis (K52.29)

DEF: Disorder involving the accumulation of eosinophil in the tissues lining the colon, but without a known cause such as connective tissue disease, drug reaction, malignancy, or parasitic infection. The resultant inflammation may cause extreme abdominal pain, diarrhea, or bloody stool.

✓6ᵗʰ **K52.83** **Microscopic colitis**

K52.831 **Collagenous colitis**

K52.832 **Lymphocytic colitis**

K52.838 **Other microscopic colitis**

K52.839 **Microscopic colitis, unspecified**

K52.89 **Other specified noninfective gastroenteritis and colitis**
AHA: 2019,1Q,20

N Newborn: 0   **P** Pediatric: 0-17   **M** Maternity: 9-64   **A** Adult: 15-124   **UNS** Unspecified Site   **MCC** Major Complication/Comorbidity   **CC** Complication/Comorbidity   **PE** POA Exempt

734

ICD-10-CM 2025

K52.9 **Noninfective gastroenteritis and colitis, unspecified**
Colitis NOS
Enteritis NOS
Gastroenteritis NOS
Ileitis NOS
Jejunitis NOS
Sigmoiditis NOS

EXCLUDES 1   *diarrhea NOS (R19.7)*
functional diarrhea (K59.1)
infectious gastroenteritis and colitis NOS (A09)
neonatal diarrhea (noninfective) (P78.3)
psychogenic diarrhea (F45.8)

AHA: 2021,3Q,3

Other diseases of intestines (K55-K64)

K55 **Vascular disorders of intestine**

EXCLUDES 1   *necrotizing enterocolitis of newborn (P77.-)*
EXCLUDES 2   *angioectasia (angiodysplasia) duodenum (K31.81-)*
AHA: 2016,4Q,32

K55.0 **Acute vascular disorders of intestine**
Infarction of appendices epiploicae
Mesenteric (artery) (vein) embolism
Mesenteric (artery) (vein) infarction
Mesenteric (artery) (vein) thrombosis
AHA: 2019,4Q,68

K55.01 **Acute (reversible) ischemia of small intestine**

K55.011 **Focal** (segmental) acute (reversible) ischemia of small intestine   `MCC`

K55.012 **Diffuse** acute (reversible) ischemia of small intestine   `MCC`

K55.019 Acute (reversible) ischemia of small intestine, extent unspecified   `MCC`

K55.02 **Acute infarction of small intestine**
Gangrene of small intestine
Necrosis of small intestine

K55.021 **Focal** (segmental) acute infarction of small intestine   `MCC`

K55.022 **Diffuse** acute infarction of small intestine   `MCC`

K55.029 Acute infarction of small intestine, extent unspecified   `MCC`

K55.03 **Acute (reversible) ischemia of large intestine**
Acute fulminant ischemic colitis
Subacute ischemic colitis

K55.031 **Focal** (segmental) acute (reversible) ischemia of large intestine   `MCC`

K55.032 **Diffuse** acute (reversible) ischemia of large intestine   `MCC`

K55.039 Acute (reversible) ischemia of large intestine, extent unspecified   `MCC`
AHA: 2019,4Q,68

K55.04 **Acute infarction of large intestine**
Gangrene of large intestine
Necrosis of large intestine

K55.041 **Focal** (segmental) acute infarction of large intestine   `MCC`

K55.042 **Diffuse** acute infarction of large intestine   `MCC`

K55.049 Acute infarction of large intestine, extent unspecified   `MCC`

K55.05 **Acute (reversible) ischemia of intestine, part unspecified**

K55.051 **Focal** (segmental) acute (reversible) ischemia of intestine, part unspecified   `MCC`

K55.052 **Diffuse** acute (reversible) ischemia of intestine, part unspecified   `MCC`

K55.059 Acute (reversible) ischemia of intestine, part and extent unspecified   `MCC`

K55.06 **Acute infarction of intestine, part unspecified**
Acute intestinal infarction
Gangrene of intestine
Necrosis of intestine

K55.061 **Focal** (segmental) acute infarction of intestine, part unspecified   `MCC`

K55.062 **Diffuse** acute infarction of intestine, part unspecified   `MCC`

K55.069 **Acute infarction of intestine, part and extent unspecified**   `MCC`

K55.1 **Chronic vascular disorders of intestine**   `CC`
Chronic ischemic colitis
Chronic ischemic enteritis
Chronic ischemic enterocolitis
Ischemic stricture of intestine
Mesenteric atherosclerosis
Mesenteric vascular insufficiency

K55.2 **Angiodysplasia of colon**
AHA: 2018,3Q,21
TIP: Assign a code for "with hemorrhage" when angiodysplasia and GI bleeding are documented. The ICD-10-CM classification assumes the two are related without the provider linking the two conditions. Evidence of bleeding during a procedure is not required.

K55.20 **Angiodysplasia of colon without hemorrhage**

K55.21 **Angiodysplasia of colon with hemorrhage**   `MCC`
DEF: Small vascular abnormalities due to fragile blood vessels in the colon, resulting in blood loss from the gastrointestinal (GI) tract.

K55.3 **Necrotizing enterocolitis**
EXCLUDES 1   *necrotizing enterocolitis of newborn (P77.-)*
EXCLUDES 2   *necrotizing enterocolitis due to Clostridium difficile (A04.7-)*

K55.30 **Necrotizing enterocolitis, unspecified**   `MCC`
Necrotizing enterocolitis, NOS

K55.31 **Stage 1 necrotizing enterocolitis**   `MCC`
Necrotizing enterocolitis without pneumatosis, without perforation

K55.32 **Stage 2 necrotizing enterocolitis**   `MCC`
Necrotizing enterocolitis with pneumatosis, without perforation

K55.33 **Stage 3 necrotizing enterocolitis**   `MCC`
Necrotizing enterocolitis with perforation
Necrotizing enterocolitis with pneumatosis and perforation

K55.8 **Other vascular disorders of intestine**   `CC`

K55.9 **Vascular disorder of intestine, unspecified**   `CC`
Ischemic colitis
Ischemic enteritis
Ischemic enterocolitis

K56 **Paralytic ileus and intestinal obstruction without hernia**
EXCLUDES 1   *congenital stricture or stenosis of intestine (Q41-Q42)*
cystic fibrosis with meconium ileus (E84.11)
ischemic stricture of intestine (K55.1)
meconium ileus NOS (P76.0)
neonatal intestinal obstructions classifiable to P76.-
obstruction of duodenum (K31.5)
postprocedural intestinal obstruction (K91.3-)
EXCLUDES 2   *stenosis of anus or rectum (K62.4)*

K56.0 **Paralytic ileus**   `CC` `HCC`
Paralysis of bowel
Paralysis of colon
Paralysis of intestine
EXCLUDES 1   *gallstone ileus (K56.3)*
ileus NOS (K56.7)
obstructive ileus NOS (K56.69-)
DEF: Intestinal obstruction due to paralysis of bowel motility or peristalsis.

K56.1 **Intussusception**   `CC` `HCC`
Intussusception or invagination of bowel
Intussusception or invagination of colon
Intussusception or invagination of intestine
Intussusception or invagination of rectum
EXCLUDES 2   *intussusception of appendix (K38.8)*
AHA: 2023,3Q,11
DEF: Intestinal obstruction due to prolapse of a bowel section into an adjacent section. It occurs primarily in children and symptoms include acute abdominal pain, vomiting, and passage of blood and mucus from the rectum.

K56.2 Volvulus `MCC` `HCC`
Strangulation of colon or intestine
Torsion of colon or intestine
Twist of colon or intestine
EXCLUDES 2   *volvulus of duodenum (K31.5)*
AHA: AHA:2024,2Q,22
DEF: Twisting, knotting, or entanglement of the bowel on itself that may quickly compromise oxygen supply to the intestinal tissues. A volvulus usually occurs at the sigmoid and ileocecal areas of the intestines.

Volvulus

Knotted intestine (volvulus)

K56.3 Gallstone ileus `CC` `HCC`
Obstruction of intestine by gallstone

✓5ᵗʰ **K56.4 Other impaction of intestine**
    K56.41 Fecal impaction `HCC`
       EXCLUDES 1   *constipation (K59.0-)*
       EXCLUDES 2   *incomplete defecation (R15.0)*
       AHA: AHA:2024,2Q,6
    K56.49 Other impaction of intestine `CC` `HCC`

✓5ᵗʰ **K56.5 Intestinal adhesions [bands] with obstruction (postinfection)**
Abdominal hernia due to adhesions with obstruction
Peritoneal adhesions [bands] with intestinal obstruction (postinfection)
AHA: 2017,4Q,16-17
    K56.50 Intestinal adhesions [bands], unspecified as to partial versus complete obstruction `CC` `HCC`
       Intestinal adhesions with obstruction NOS
    K56.51 Intestinal adhesions [bands], with partial obstruction `CC` `HCC`
       Intestinal adhesions with incomplete obstruction
    K56.52 Intestinal adhesions [bands] with complete obstruction `CC` `HCC`

✓5ᵗʰ **K56.6 Other and unspecified intestinal obstruction**
    AHA: 2017,4Q,16-17; 2017,2Q,12
   ✓6ᵗʰ **K56.60 Unspecified intestinal obstruction**
       K56.600 Partial intestinal obstruction, unspecified as to cause `CC` `HCC`
          Incomplete intestinal obstruction, NOS
       K56.601 Complete intestinal obstruction, unspecified as to cause `CC` `HCC`
       K56.609 Unspecified intestinal obstruction, unspecified as to partial versus complete obstruction `CC` `HCC`
          Intestinal obstruction NOS
   ✓6ᵗʰ **K56.69 Other intestinal obstruction**
       Enterostenosis NOS
       Obstructive ileus NOS
       Occlusion of colon or intestine NOS
       Stenosis of colon or intestine NOS
       Stricture of colon or intestine NOS
       K56.690 Other partial intestinal obstruction `CC` `HCC`
          Other incomplete intestinal obstruction
       K56.691 Other complete intestinal obstruction `CC` `HCC`

K56.699 Other intestinal obstruction unspecified as to partial versus complete obstruction `CC` `HCC`
Other intestinal obstruction, NEC
AHA: 2023,3Q,10

K56.7 Ileus, unspecified `CC` `HCC`
EXCLUDES 1   *obstructive ileus (K56.69-)*
EXCLUDES 2   *intestinal obstruction with hernia (K40-K46)*
AHA: 2017,1Q,40

✓4ᵗʰ **K57 Diverticular disease of intestine**
Code also if applicable peritonitis K65.-
EXCLUDES 1   *congenital diverticulum of intestine (Q43.8)*
              Meckel's diverticulum (Q43.0)
EXCLUDES 2   *diverticulum of appendix (K38.2)*
AHA: 2022,1Q,26-27; 2021,1Q,9,11; 2018,3Q,21
TIP: Assign a code for "with bleeding" when diverticular disease of the intestine and GI bleeding are documented. The ICD-10-CM classification assumes the two are related without the provider linking the two conditions. Evidence of bleeding during a procedure is not required.

✓5ᵗʰ **K57.0 Diverticulitis of small intestine with perforation and abscess**
       EXCLUDES 1   *diverticulitis of both small and large intestine with perforation and abscess (K57.4-)*
    K57.00 Diverticulitis of small intestine with perforation and abscess without bleeding `CC`
    K57.01 Diverticulitis of small intestine with perforation and abscess with bleeding `MCC`

✓5ᵗʰ **K57.1 Diverticular disease of small intestine without perforation or abscess**
       EXCLUDES 1   *diverticular disease of both small and large intestine without perforation or abscess (K57.5-)*
    K57.10 Diverticulosis of small intestine without perforation or abscess without bleeding
       Diverticular disease of small intestine NOS
    K57.11 Diverticulosis of small intestine without perforation or abscess with bleeding `MCC`
    K57.12 Diverticulitis of small intestine without perforation or abscess without bleeding `CC`
    K57.13 Diverticulitis of small intestine without perforation or abscess with bleeding `MCC`

✓5ᵗʰ **K57.2 Diverticulitis of large intestine with perforation and abscess**
       EXCLUDES 1   *diverticulitis of both small and large intestine with perforation and abscess (K57.4-)*
    K57.20 Diverticulitis of large intestine with perforation and abscess without bleeding `CC`
    K57.21 Diverticulitis of large intestine with perforation and abscess with bleeding `MCC`

✓5ᵗʰ **K57.3 Diverticular disease of large intestine without perforation or abscess**
       EXCLUDES 1   *diverticular disease of both small and large intestine without perforation or abscess (K57.5-)*
    K57.30 Diverticulosis of large intestine without perforation or abscess without bleeding
       Diverticular disease of colon NOS
    K57.31 Diverticulosis of large intestine without perforation or abscess with bleeding `MCC`
    K57.32 Diverticulitis of large intestine without perforation or abscess without bleeding `CC`
    K57.33 Diverticulitis of large intestine without perforation or abscess with bleeding `MCC`

✓5ᵗʰ **K57.4 Diverticulitis of both small and large intestine with perforation and abscess**
    K57.40 Diverticulitis of both small and large intestine with perforation and abscess without bleeding `CC`
    K57.41 Diverticulitis of both small and large intestine with perforation and abscess with bleeding `MCC`

✓5ᵗʰ **K57.5 Diverticular disease of both small and large intestine without perforation or abscess**
    K57.50 Diverticulosis of both small and large intestine without perforation or abscess without bleeding
       Diverticular disease of both small and large intestine NOS
    K57.51 Diverticulosis of both small and large intestine without perforation or abscess with bleeding `MCC`
    K57.52 Diverticulitis of both small and large intestine without perforation or abscess without bleeding `CC`
    K57.53 Diverticulitis of both small and large intestine without perforation or abscess with bleeding `MCC`

√5ᵗʰ K57.8 Diverticulitis of intestine, part unspecified, with perforation and abscess

    K57.80 Diverticulitis of intestine, part unspecified, with perforation and abscess without bleeding `CC`

    K57.81 Diverticulitis of intestine, part unspecified, with perforation and abscess with bleeding `MCC`

√5ᵗʰ K57.9 Diverticular disease of intestine, part unspecified, without perforation or abscess

    K57.90 Diverticulosis of intestine, part unspecified, without perforation or abscess without bleeding
        Diverticular disease of intestine NOS

    K57.91 Diverticulosis of intestine, part unspecified, without perforation or abscess with bleeding `MCC`

    K57.92 Diverticulitis of intestine, part unspecified, without perforation or abscess without bleeding `CC`

    K57.93 Diverticulitis of intestine, part unspecified, without perforation or abscess with bleeding `MCC`

√4ᵗʰ K58 Irritable bowel syndrome

    `INCLUDES`   irritable colon
           spastic colon
    AHA: 2016,4Q,32-33

    K58.0 Irritable bowel syndrome with diarrhea

    K58.1 Irritable bowel syndrome with constipation

    K58.2 Mixed irritable bowel syndrome

    K58.8 Other irritable bowel syndrome

▲   **K58.9 Irritable bowel syndrome, unspecified**
        Irritable bowel syndrome NOS

√4ᵗʰ K59 Other functional intestinal disorders

    `EXCLUDES 1`   change in bowel habit NOS (R19.4)
             intestinal malabsorption (K90.-)
             psychogenic intestinal disorders (F45.8)
    `EXCLUDES 2`   functional disorders of stomach (K31.-)

    √5ᵗʰ K59.0 Constipation

        `EXCLUDES 1`   fecal impaction (K56.41)
        `EXCLUDES 2`   incomplete defecation (R15.0)
        AHA: 2024,2Q,6; 2016,4Q,33

        K59.00 Constipation, unspecified

        K59.01 Slow transit constipation
            DEF: Delay in the transit of fecal material through the colon secondary to smooth muscle dysfunction or decreased peristaltic contractions along the colon.

        K59.02 Outlet dysfunction constipation
            AHA: 2023,1Q,24
            TIP: Report this code for documented pelvic floor dyssynergia, outlet type constipation, or anismus.

        K59.03 Drug induced constipation
            Use additional code for adverse effect, if applicable, to identify drug (T36-T50 with fifth or sixth character 5)

        K59.04 Chronic idiopathic constipation
            Functional constipation

        K59.09 Other constipation
            Chronic constipation

    K59.1 Functional diarrhea
        `EXCLUDES 1`   diarrhea NOS (R19.7)
              irritable bowel syndrome with diarrhea (K58.0)

    K59.2 Neurogenic bowel, not elsewhere classified `CC`
        DEF: Disorder of bowel due to a spinal cord lesion because of injury or as a complication of conditions such as multiple sclerosis (MS) or spina bifida. Loss of bowel control is the primary symptom, manifested as constipation or bowel incontinence.

    √5ᵗʰ K59.3 Megacolon, not elsewhere classified
        Dilatation of colon
        Code first, if applicable (T51-T65) to identify toxic agent
        `EXCLUDES 1`   congenital megacolon (aganglionic) (Q43.1)
              megacolon (due to) (in) Chagas' disease (B57.32)
              megacolon (due to) (in) Clostridium difficile (A04.7-)
              megacolon (due to) (in) Hirschsprung's disease (Q43.1)
        AHA: 2016,4Q,33-34

        K59.31 Toxic megacolon `CC` `HCC`

        K59.39 Other megacolon `CC`
            Megacolon NOS

    K59.4 Anal spasm
        Proctalgia fugax

√5ᵗʰ K59.8 Other specified functional intestinal disorders
    AHA: 2020,4Q,29-30

    K59.81 Ogilvie syndrome
        Acute colonic pseudo-obstruction (ACPO)

    K59.89 Other specified functional intestinal disorders
        Atony of colon
        Pseudo-obstruction (acute) (chronic) of intestine

K59.9 Functional intestinal disorder, unspecified

√4ᵗʰ K60 Fissure and fistula of anal and rectal regions

    `EXCLUDES 1`   fissure and fistula of anal and rectal regions with abscess or cellulitis (K61.-)
    `EXCLUDES 2`   ►abscess or cellulitis of anal and rectal regions (K61.-)◄
              anal sphincter tear (healed) (nontraumatic) (old) (K62.81)

K60.0 Acute anal fissure

K60.1 Chronic anal fissure

K60.2 Anal fissure, unspecified

▲ **√5ᵗʰ K60.3 Anal fistula**

    ►Code first, if applicable:◄
    ►Crohn's disease (K50.-)◄
    ►ulcerative colitis (K51.-)◄
    `EXCLUDES 1`   ►congenital fistula (Q43.6)◄

    K60.30 Anal fistula, unspecified
        Anal fistula NOS

    √6ᵗʰ K60.31 Anal fistula, simple
        Low intersphincteric anal fistula
        Superficial anal fistula

        K60.311 Anal fistula, simple, initial
            Anal fistula, simple, new

        K60.312 Anal fistula, simple, persistent
            Anal fistula, simple, chronic

        K60.313 Anal fistula, simple, recurrent
            Anal fistula simple, occurring following complete healing

        K60.319 Anal fistula, simple, unspecified

    √6ᵗʰ K60.32 Anal fistula, complex
        Extrasphincteric anal fistula
        High intersphincteric anal fistula
        Suprasphincteric anal fistula
        Transsphincteric anal fistula
        Code also, if applicable:
            perianal abscess (K61.0)
            rectovaginal fistula (N82.3)
            stenosis of anus and rectum (K62.4)

        K60.321 Anal fistula, complex, initial
            Anal fistula, complex, new

        K60.322 Anal fistula, complex, persistent
            Anal fistula, complex, chronic

        K60.323 Anal fistula, complex, recurrent
            Anal fistula complex, occurring following complete healing

        K60.329 Anal fistula, complex, unspecified

▲ **√5ᵗʰ K60.4 Rectal fistula**
    Fistula of rectum to skin
    ►Code first, if applicable:◄
    ►Crohn's disease (K50.-)◄
    ►ulcerative colitis (K51.-)◄
    `EXCLUDES 1`   ►congenital fistula (Q43.6)◄
              rectovaginal fistula (N82.3)
              vesicorectal fistual (N32.1)

    K60.40 Rectal fistula, unspecified
        Rectal fistula NOS

    √6ᵗʰ K60.41 Rectal fistula, simple
        Low intersphincteric rectal fistula
        Superficial rectal fistula

        K60.411 Rectal fistula, simple, initial
            Rectal, fistula, simple, new

        K60.412 Rectal fistula, simple, persistent
            Rectal fistula, simple, chronic

        K60.413 Rectal fistula, simple, recurrent
            Rectal fistula simple, occurring following complete healing

        K60.419 Rectal fistula, simple, unspecified

☑ Additional Character Required   √x7ᵗʰ Placeholder   Questionable PDx   Manifestation   Unspecified   `UPD` Unacceptable PDx   H1-H14 HAC   `HCC` CMS-HCC Dx   HIV HIV Dx

Chapter 11. Diseases of the Digestive System

● ✓6ᵗʰ **K60.42** **Rectal fistula, complex**
  Extrasphincteric rectal fistula
  High intersphincteric rectal fistula
  Suprasphincteric rectal fistula
  Transsphincteric rectal fistula
  Code also, if applicable:
  perianal abscess (K61.0)
  rectovaginal fistula (N82.3)
  stenosis of anus and rectum (K62.4)

● **K60.421** **Rectal fistula, complex, initial**
  Rectal fistula, complex, new

● **K60.422** **Rectal fistula, complex, persistent**
  Rectal fistula, complex, chronic

● **K60.423** **Rectal fistula, complex, recurrent**
  Rectal fistula complex occurring following complete healing

● **K60.429** **Rectal fistula, complex, unspecified**

▲ ✓5ᵗʰ **K60.5** **Anorectal fistula**
  ▶Code first, if applicable:◀
  ▶Crohn's disease (K50.-)◀
  ▶ulcerative colitis (K51.-)◀
  EXCLUDES 1 ▶congenital fistula (Q43.6)◀

● **K60.50** **Anorectal fistula, unspecified**
  Anorectal fistula NOS

● ✓6ᵗʰ **K60.51** **Anorectal fistula, simple**
  Low intersphincteric anorectal fistula
  Superficial anorectal fistula

● **K60.511** **Anorectal fistula, simple, initial**
  Anorectal fistula, simple, new

● **K60.512** **Anorectal fistula, simple, persistent**
  Anorectal fistula, simple, chronic

● **K60.513** **Anorectal fistula, simple, recurrent**
  Anorectal fistula simple, occurring following complete healing

● **K60.519** **Anorectal fistula, simple, unspecified**

● ✓6ᵗʰ **K60.52** **Anorectal fistula, complex**
  Extrasphincteric anorectal fistula
  High intersphincteric anorectal fistula
  Suprasphincteric anorectal fistula
  Transsphincteric anorectal fistula
  Code also, if applicable:
  perianal abscess (K61.0)
  rectovaginal fistula (N82.3)
  stenosis of anus and rectum (K62.4)

● **K60.521** **Anorectal fistula, complex, initial**
  Anorectal fistula, complex, new

● **K60.522** **Anorectal fistula, complex, persistent**
  Anorectal fistula, complex, chronic

● **K60.523** **Anorectal fistula, complex, recurrent**
  Anorectal fistula complex, occurring following complete healing

● **K60.529** **Anorectal fistula, complex, unspecified**

✓4ᵗʰ **K61** **Abscess of anal and rectal regions**
  INCLUDES abscess of anal and rectal regions
  cellulitis of anal and rectal regions

K61.0 **Anal abscess** `CC`
  Perianal abscess
  EXCLUDES 2 intrasphincteric abscess (K61.4)

K61.1 **Rectal abscess** `CC`
  Perirectal abscess
  EXCLUDES 1 ischiorectal abscess (K61.39)
  AHA: 2012,4Q,104

K61.2 **Anorectal abscess** `CC`

✓5ᵗʰ **K61.3** **Ischiorectal abscess**
  AHA: 2018,4Q,19

K61.31 **Horseshoe abscess**

K61.39 **Other ischiorectal abscess**
  Abscess of ischiorectal fossa
  Ischiorectal abscess, NOS

K61.4 **Intrasphincteric abscess** `CC`
  Intersphincteric abscess

K61.5 **Supralevator abscess**
  AHA: 2018,4Q,19

✓4ᵗʰ **K62** **Other diseases of anus and rectum**
  INCLUDES anal canal
  EXCLUDES 2 colostomy and enterostomy malfunction (K94.0-, K94.1-)
  fecal incontinence (R15.-)
  hemorrhoids (K64.-)

K62.0 **Anal polyp**

K62.1 **Rectal polyp**
  EXCLUDES 1 adenomatous polyp (D12.8)
  AHA: 2018,1Q,6

K62.2 **Anal prolapse**
  Prolapse of anal canal

K62.3 **Rectal prolapse**
  Prolapse of rectal mucosa

K62.4 **Stenosis of anus and rectum**
  Stricture of anus (sphincter)
  AHA: 2019,2Q,13

K62.5 **Hemorrhage of anus and rectum** `CC`
  EXCLUDES 1 gastrointestinal bleeding NOS (K92.2)
  melena (K92.1)
  neonatal rectal hemorrhage (P54.2)
  AHA: 2019,1Q,21

K62.6 **Ulcer of anus and rectum** `CC`
  Solitary ulcer of anus and rectum
  Stercoral ulcer of anus and rectum
  EXCLUDES 1 fissure and fistula of anus and rectum (K60.-)
  ulcerative colitis (K51.-)

K62.7 **Radiation proctitis**
  Use additional code to identify the type of radiation (W88.-) or radiation therapy (Y84.2)
  AHA: 2019,1Q,21

✓5ᵗʰ **K62.8** **Other specified diseases of anus and rectum**
  EXCLUDES 2 ulcerative proctitis (K51.2)

K62.81 **Anal sphincter tear (healed) (nontraumatic) (old)**
  Tear of anus, nontraumatic
  Use additional code for any associated fecal incontinence (R15.-)
  EXCLUDES 2 anal fissure (K60.-)
  anal sphincter tear (healed) (old) complicating delivery (O34.7-)
  traumatic tear of anal sphincter (S31.831)

K62.82 **Dysplasia of anus**
  Anal intraepithelial neoplasia I and II (AIN I and II) (histologically confirmed)
  Dysplasia of anus NOS
  Mild and moderate dysplasia of anus (histologically confirmed)
  EXCLUDES 1 abnormal results from anal cytologic examination without histologic confirmation (R85.61-)
  anal intraepithelial neoplasia III (D01.3)
  carcinoma in situ of anus (D01.3)
  HGSIL of anus (R85.613)
  severe dysplasia of anus (D01.3)

K62.89 **Other specified diseases of anus and rectum**
  Proctitis NOS
  Use additional code for any associated fecal incontinence (R15.-)

K62.9 **Disease of anus and rectum, unspecified**

✓4ᵗʰ **K63** **Other diseases of intestine**

K63.0 **Abscess of intestine** `CC`
  EXCLUDES 1 abscess of intestine with Crohn's disease (K50.014, K50.114, K50.814, K50.914)
  abscess of intestine with diverticular disease (K57.0, K57.2, K57.4, K57.8)
  abscess of intestine with ulcerative colitis (K51.014, K51.214, K51.314, K51.414, K51.514, K51.814, K51.914)
  EXCLUDES 2 abscess of anal and rectal regions (K61.-)
  abscess of appendix (K35.3-)

N Newborn: 0   **P** Pediatric: 0-17   **M** Maternity: 9-64   **A** Adult: 15-124   **UNS** Unspecified Site   **MCC** Major Complication/Comorbidity   **CC** Complication/Comorbidity   **PE** POA Exempt

738

ICD-10-CM 2025

K63.1 **Perforation** of intestine (nontraumatic)   `MCC` `HCC`
     Perforation (nontraumatic) of rectum
     `EXCLUDES 1`   perforation (nontraumatic) of duodenum (K26.-)
               perforation (nontraumatic) of intestine with
                 diverticular disease (K57.0, K57.2, K57.4, K57.8)
     `EXCLUDES 2`   perforation (nontraumatic) of appendix (K35.2-, K35.3-)
     AHA: 2020,2Q,22

K63.2 **Fistula** of intestine   `CC`
     ▶Code also, if applicable, disruption of internal operation (surgical)
       wound (T81.32-)◀
     `EXCLUDES 1`   fistula of duodenum (K31.6)
                fistula of intestine with Crohn's disease (K50.013,
                 K50.113, K50.813, K50.913)
                fistula of intestine with ulcerative colitis (K51.013,
                 K51.213, K51.313, K51.413, K51.513, K51.813,
                 K51.913)
     `EXCLUDES 2`   fistula of anal and rectal regions (K60.-)
                fistula of appendix (K38.3)
                intestinal-genital fistula, female (N82.2-N82.4)
                vesicointestinal fistula (N32.1)
     AHA: 2017,3Q,4

K63.3 **Ulcer** of intestine   `CC`
     Primary ulcer of small intestine
     `EXCLUDES 1`   duodenal ulcer (K26.-)
                gastrointestinal ulcer (K28.-)
                gastrojejunal ulcer (K28.-)
                jejunal ulcer (K28.-)
                peptic ulcer, site unspecified (K27.-)
                ulcer of intestine with perforation (K63.1)
                ulcer of anus or rectum (K62.6)
                ulcerative colitis (K51.-)

K63.4 **Enteroptosis**

K63.5 **Polyp** of colon
     `EXCLUDES 2`   adenomatous polyp of colon (D12.-)
                inflammatory polyp of colon (K51.4-)
                polyposis of colon (D12.6)
     AHA: 2019,1Q,33; 2018,2Q,14; 2017,1Q,15; 2015,2Q,14
     TIP: Assign this code when documentation states hyperplastic
     colon polyp regardless of the site in the colon. Slow-growing,
     hyperplastic polyps are not precancerous and are classified
     differently from benign or adenomatous polyps.

`√5th` **K63.8** **Other specified diseases of intestine**

     K63.81 **Dieulafoy lesion of intestine**   `MCC`
           `EXCLUDES 2`   Dieulafoy lesion of stomach and duodenum
                   (K31.82)
           DEF: Abnormally large submucosal artery protruding
           through a defect in the stomach mucosa or intestines
           that can cause massive and life-threatening
           hemorrhaging.

     `√6th` **K63.82** **Intestinal microbial overgrowth**
           AHA: 2023,4Q,29-30

         `√7th` **K63.821** **Small intestinal bacterial overgrowth**

                K63.8211 **Small intestinal bacterial**
                        overgrowth, hydrogen-subtype

                K63.8212 **Small intestinal bacterial**
                        overgrowth, hydrogen
                        sulfide-subtype

                K63.8219 **Small intestinal bacterial**
                        overgrowth, unspecified

         K63.822 **Small intestinal fungal overgrowth**

         K63.829 **Intestinal methanogen overgrowth,**
                 unspecified

     K63.89 **Other specified diseases of intestine**
           AHA: 2013,2Q,31

K63.9 **Disease of intestine, unspecified**

`√4th` **K64** **Hemorrhoids and perianal venous thrombosis**
     `INCLUDES`   piles
     `EXCLUDES 1`   hemorrhoids complicating childbirth and the puerperium
                (O87.2)
                hemorrhoids complicating pregnancy (O22.4)

Hemorrhoids

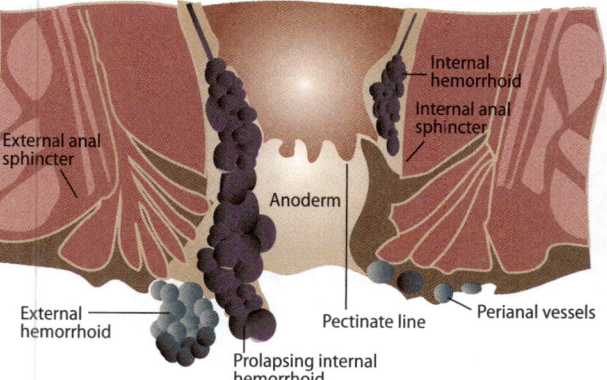

K64.0 **First degree** hemorrhoids
     Grade/stage I hemorrhoids
     Hemorrhoids (bleeding) without prolapse outside of anal canal

K64.1 **Second degree** hemorrhoids
     Grade/stage II hemorrhoids
     Hemorrhoids (bleeding) that prolapse with straining, but retract
       spontaneously

K64.2 **Third degree** hemorrhoids
     Grade/stage III hemorrhoids
     Hemorrhoids (bleeding) that prolapse with straining and require
       manual replacement back inside anal canal

K64.3 **Fourth degree** hemorrhoids
     Grade/stage IV hemorrhoids
     Hemorrhoids (bleeding) with prolapsed tissue that cannot be
       manually replaced

K64.4 **Residual** hemorrhoidal **skin tags**
     External hemorrhoids, NOS
     Skin tags of anus

K64.5 **Perianal venous thrombosis**
     External hemorrhoids with thrombosis
     Perianal hematoma
     Thrombosed hemorrhoids NOS

K64.8 **Other hemorrhoids**
     Internal hemorrhoids, without mention of degree
     Prolapsed hemorrhoids, degree not specified

K64.9 **Unspecified hemorrhoids**
     Hemorrhoids (bleeding) NOS
     Hemorrhoids (bleeding) without mention of degree

✔ Additional Character Required   `√x 7th` Placeholder   `Questionable PDx`   `Manifestation`   `Unspecified`   `UPD` Unacceptable PDx   `H1`-`H14` HAC   `HCC` CMS-HCC Dx   `HIV` HIV Dx

ICD-10-CM 2025   739

Diseases of peritoneum and retroperitoneum (K65-K68)

✓4ᵗʰ K65 Peritonitis

Use additional code (B95-B97), to identify infectious agent, if known
Code also if applicable diverticular disease of intestine (K57.-)

EXCLUDES 1   *acute appendicitis with generalized peritonitis (K35.2-)*
aseptic peritonitis (T81.6)
benign paroxysmal peritonitis (E85.0)
chemical peritonitis (T81.6)
gonococcal peritonitis (A54.85)
neonatal peritonitis (P78.0-P78.1)
pelvic peritonitis, female (N73.3-N73.5)
periodic familial peritonitis (E85.0)
peritonitis due to talc or other foreign substance (T81.6)
peritonitis in chlamydia (A74.81)
peritonitis in diphtheria (A36.89)
peritonitis in syphilis (late) (A52.74)
peritonitis in tuberculosis (A18.31)
peritonitis with or following abortion or ectopic or molar pregnancy (O00-O07, O08.0)
peritonitis with or following appendicitis (K35.-)
puerperal peritonitis (O85)
retroperitoneal infections (K68.-)

K65.0 Generalized (acute) peritonitis   MCC HCC
Pelvic peritonitis (acute), male
Subphrenic peritonitis (acute)
Suppurative peritonitis (acute)

K65.1 Peritoneal abscess   MCC HCC
Abdominopelvic abscess
Abscess (of) omentum
Abscess (of) peritoneum
Mesenteric abscess
Retrocecal abscess
Subdiaphragmatic abscess
Subhepatic abscess
Subphrenic abscess
AHA: 2024,1Q,20; 2022,1Q,26; 2019,1Q,15

K65.2 Spontaneous bacterial peritonitis   MCC HCC
EXCLUDES 1   *bacterial peritonitis NOS (K65.9)*

K65.3 Choleperitonitis   MCC HCC
Peritonitis due to bile
DEF: Inflammation of the peritoneum due to leakage of bile into the peritoneal cavity resulting from rupture of the bile passages or gallbladder.

K65.4 Sclerosing mesenteritis   CC HCC
Fat necrosis of peritoneum
(Idiopathic) sclerosing mesenteric fibrosis
Mesenteric lipodystrophy
Mesenteric panniculitis
Retractile mesenteritis

K65.8 Other peritonitis   MCC HCC
Chronic proliferative peritonitis
Peritonitis due to urine

K65.9 Peritonitis, unspecified   MCC HCC
Bacterial peritonitis NOS
AHA: 2022,1Q,27; 2013,2Q,31

✓4ᵗʰ K66 Other disorders of peritoneum

EXCLUDES 2   *ascites (R18.-)*
peritoneal effusion (chronic) (R18.8)

K66.0 Peritoneal adhesions (postprocedural) (postinfection)
Adhesions (of) abdominal (wall)
Adhesions (of) diaphragm
Adhesions (of) intestine
Adhesions (of) male pelvis
Adhesions (of) omentum
Adhesions (of) stomach
Adhesive bands
Mesenteric adhesions
EXCLUDES 1   *peritoneal adhesions with intestinal obstruction (K56.5-)*
female pelvic adhesions [bands] (N73.6)
EXCLUDES 2   ▶*female pelvic adhesions [bands] (N73.6)*◀
▶*female pelvic postprocedural adhesions (N99.4)*◀

K66.1 Hemoperitoneum   MCC
Peritoneal hematoma
Peritoneal hemorrhage
EXCLUDES 1   *traumatic hemoperitoneum (S36.8-)*
EXCLUDES 2   *retroperitoneal hematoma (K68.3)*
retroperitoneal hemorrhage (K68.3)
AHA: 2022,1Q,22-23

K66.8 Other specified disorders of peritoneum
K66.9 Disorder of peritoneum, unspecified

K67 Disorders of peritoneum in infectious diseases classified elsewhere   MCC HCC

Code first underlying disease, such as:
congenital syphilis (A50.0)
helminthiasis (B65.0-B83.9)

EXCLUDES 1   *peritonitis in chlamydia (A74.81)*
peritonitis in diphtheria (A36.89)
peritonitis in gonococcal (A54.85)
peritonitis in syphilis (late) (A52.74)
peritonitis in tuberculosis (A18.31)

✓4ᵗʰ K68 Disorders of retroperitoneum

✓5ᵗʰ K68.1 Retroperitoneal abscess

K68.11 Postprocedural retroperitoneal abscess   CC H11 H12 H13
EXCLUDES 2   *infection following procedure (T81.4-)*

K68.12 Psoas muscle abscess   MCC HCC

K68.19 Other retroperitoneal abscess   MCC HCC
AHA: 2023,2Q,27; 2019,1Q,15
TIP: This code should be used for a diagnosis of internal presacral abscess. If an intra-abdominal abscess is also present, code K65.1 can also be assigned; sequencing depends on the circumstances of admission.

K68.2 Retroperitoneal fibrosis   MCC
Code also, if applicable, associated obstruction of ureter (N13.5)
AHA: 2023,4Q,30-31

K68.3 Retroperitoneal hematoma   MCC
Retroperitoneal hemorrhage
AHA: 2023,4Q,30-31

K68.9 Other disorders of retroperitoneum   MCC

Diseases of liver (K70-K77)

EXCLUDES 1   *jaundice NOS (R17)*
EXCLUDES 2   *hemochromatosis (E83.11-)*
Reye's syndrome (G93.7)
viral hepatitis (B15-B19)
Wilson's disease (E83.01)

✓4ᵗʰ K70 Alcoholic liver disease

Use additional code to identify:
alcohol abuse and dependence (F10.-)

K70.0 Alcoholic fatty liver   A

✓5ᵗʰ K70.1 Alcoholic hepatitis
K70.10 Alcoholic hepatitis without ascites   HCC A
K70.11 Alcoholic hepatitis with ascites   HCC A

K70.2 Alcoholic fibrosis and sclerosis of liver   A

✓5ᵗʰ K70.3 Alcoholic cirrhosis of liver
Alcoholic cirrhosis NOS
K70.30 Alcoholic cirrhosis of liver without ascites   HCC A
K70.31 Alcoholic cirrhosis of liver with ascites   HCC A
AHA: 2018,1Q,4

✓5ᵗʰ K70.4 Alcoholic hepatic failure
Acute alcoholic hepatic failure
Alcoholic hepatic failure NOS
Chronic alcoholic hepatic failure
Subacute alcoholic hepatic failure
K70.40 Alcoholic hepatic failure without coma   HCC A
K70.41 Alcoholic hepatic failure with coma   MCC HCC A

K70.9 Alcoholic liver disease, unspecified   A

✓4th **K71　Toxic liver disease**

> INCLUDES　drug-induced idiosyncratic (unpredictable) liver disease
> drug-induced toxic (predictable) liver disease

> Code first poisoning due to drug or toxin, if applicable (T36-T65 with fifth or sixth character 1-4)
> Use additional code for adverse effect, if applicable, to identify drug (T36-T50 with fifth or sixth character 5)

> EXCLUDES 2　alcoholic liver disease (K70.-)
> Budd-Chiari syndrome (I82.0)

K71.0　Toxic liver disease with cholestasis
Cholestasis with hepatocyte injury
"Pure" cholestasis

✓5th **K71.1　Toxic liver disease with hepatic necrosis**
Hepatic failure (acute) (chronic) due to drugs

K71.10　Toxic liver disease with hepatic necrosis, without coma

K71.11　Toxic liver disease with hepatic necrosis, with coma　MCC

K71.2　Toxic liver disease with acute hepatitis

K71.3　Toxic liver disease with chronic persistent hepatitis　HCC

K71.4　Toxic liver disease with chronic lobular hepatitis　HCC

✓5th **K71.5　Toxic liver disease with chronic active hepatitis**
Toxic liver disease with lupoid hepatitis

K71.50　Toxic liver disease with chronic active hepatitis without ascites　HCC

K71.51　Toxic liver disease with chronic active hepatitis with ascites　HCC
AHA: 2018,1Q,4

K71.6　Toxic liver disease with hepatitis, not elsewhere classified

K71.7　Toxic liver disease with fibrosis and cirrhosis of liver　HCC

K71.8　Toxic liver disease with other disorders of liver
Toxic liver disease with focal nodular hyperplasia
Toxic liver disease with hepatic granulomas
Toxic liver disease with peliosis hepatis
Toxic liver disease with veno-occlusive disease of liver
AHA: 2024,1Q,25; 2015,2Q,17

K71.9　Toxic liver disease, unspecified

✓4th **K72　Hepatic failure, not elsewhere classified**

> INCLUDES　fulminant hepatitis NEC, with hepatic failure
> liver (cell) necrosis with hepatic failure
> malignant hepatitis NEC, with hepatic failure
> yellow liver atrophy or dystrophy

> EXCLUDES 1　alcoholic hepatic failure (K70.4)
> hepatic failure with toxic liver disease (K71.1-)
> icterus of newborn (P55-P59)
> postprocedural hepatic failure (K91.82)

> EXCLUDES 2　hepatic failure complicating abortion or ectopic or molar pregnancy (O00-O07, O08.8)
> hepatic failure complicating pregnancy, childbirth and the puerperium (O26.6-)
> viral hepatitis with hepatic coma (B15-B19)

AHA: 2017,1Q,41

✓5th **K72.0　Acute and subacute hepatic failure**
Acute non-viral hepatitis NOS
AHA: 2015,2Q,17; 2014,2Q,13

K72.00　Acute and subacute hepatic failure without coma　MCC
AHA: 2021,1Q,13

K72.01　Acute and subacute hepatic failure with coma　MCC

✓5th **K72.1　Chronic hepatic failure**
End stage liver disease

K72.10　Chronic hepatic failure without coma　HCC
AHA: 2021,1Q,13

K72.11　Chronic hepatic failure with coma　MCC　HCC

✓5th **K72.9　Hepatic failure, unspecified**

K72.90　Hepatic failure, unspecified without coma　HCC
AHA: 2022,1Q,52; 2018,4Q,20; 2016,2Q,35

K72.91　Hepatic failure, unspecified with coma　MCC　HCC
Hepatic coma NOS

✓4th **K73　Chronic hepatitis, not elsewhere classified**

> EXCLUDES 1　alcoholic hepatitis (chronic) (K70.1-)
> drug-induced hepatitis (chronic) (K71.-)
> granulomatous hepatitis (chronic) NEC (K75.3)
> reactive, nonspecific hepatitis (chronic) (K75.2)
> viral hepatitis (chronic) (B15-B19)

K73.0　Chronic persistent hepatitis, not elsewhere classified　HCC

K73.1　Chronic lobular hepatitis, not elsewhere classified　HCC

K73.2　Chronic active hepatitis, not elsewhere classified　HCC

K73.8　Other chronic hepatitis, not elsewhere classified　HCC

K73.9　Chronic hepatitis, unspecified　HCC

✓4th **K74　Fibrosis and cirrhosis of liver**

> Code also, if applicable, viral hepatitis (acute) (chronic) (B15-B19)

> EXCLUDES 1　alcoholic cirrhosis (of liver) (K70.3)
> alcoholic fibrosis of liver (K70.2)
> cardiac sclerosis of liver (K76.1)
> cirrhosis (of liver) with toxic liver disease (K71.7)
> congenital cirrhosis (of liver) (P78.81)
> pigmentary cirrhosis (of liver) (E83.110)

✓5th **K74.0　Hepatic fibrosis**

> Code first underlying liver disease, such as:
> nonalcoholic steatohepatitis (NASH) (K75.81)
> **AHA:** 2020,4Q,30-31

K74.00　Hepatic fibrosis, unspecified　UPD

K74.01　Hepatic fibrosis, early fibrosis　UPD
Hepatic fibrosis, stage F1 or stage F2

K74.02　Hepatic fibrosis, advanced fibrosis　UPD
Hepatic fibrosis, stage F3

> EXCLUDES 1　cirrhosis of liver (K74.6-)
> hepatic fibrosis, stage F4 (K74.6-)

K74.1　Hepatic sclerosis

K74.2　Hepatic fibrosis with hepatic sclerosis

K74.3　Primary biliary cirrhosis　HCC
Chronic nonsuppurative destructive cholangitis
Primary biliary cholangitis
> EXCLUDES 2　primary sclerosing cholangitis (K83.01)

K74.4　Secondary biliary cirrhosis　HCC

K74.5　Biliary cirrhosis, unspecified　HCC

✓5th **K74.6　Other and unspecified cirrhosis of liver**
AHA: 2020,4Q,30-31

K74.60　Unspecified cirrhosis of liver　HCC
Cirrhosis (of liver) NOS
AHA: 2018,1Q,4

K74.69　Other cirrhosis of liver　HCC
Cryptogenic cirrhosis (of liver)
Macronodular cirrhosis (of liver)
Micronodular cirrhosis (of liver)
Mixed type cirrhosis (of liver)
Portal cirrhosis (of liver)
Postnecrotic cirrhosis (of liver)

✓4th **K75　Other inflammatory liver diseases**

> EXCLUDES 2　toxic liver disease (K71.-)

K75.0　Abscess of liver　MCC
Cholangitic hepatic abscess
Hematogenic hepatic abscess
Hepatic abscess NOS
Lymphogenic hepatic abscess
Pylephlebitic hepatic abscess
> EXCLUDES 1　amebic liver abscess (A06.4)
> cholangitis without liver abscess (K83.09)
> pylephlebitis without liver abscess (K75.1)
> EXCLUDES 2　acute or subacute hepatitis NOS (B17.9)
> acute or subacute non-viral hepatitis (K72.0)
> chronic hepatitis NEC (K73.8)

K75.1　Phlebitis of portal vein　MCC
Pylephlebitis
> EXCLUDES 1　pylephlebitic liver abscess (K75.0)
> **DEF:** Inflammation of the portal vein or branches due to diverticulitis, perforated appendicitis, or peritonitis. Symptoms include fever, chills, jaundice, sweating, and abscess in various body parts.

✔ Additional Character Required　✓x7th Placeholder　Questionable PDx　Manifestation　Unspecified　UPD Unacceptable PDx　H1 - H14 HAC　HCC CMS-HCC Dx　HIV HIV Dx

Chapter 11. Diseases of the Digestive System

K75.2   Nonspecific reactive hepatitis
> EXCLUDES 1   *acute or subacute hepatitis (K72.0-)*
> *chronic hepatitis NEC (K73.-)*
> *viral hepatitis (B15-B19)*

K75.3   Granulomatous hepatitis, not elsewhere classified
> EXCLUDES 1   *acute or subacute hepatitis (K72.0-)*
> *chronic hepatitis NEC (K73.-)*
> *viral hepatitis (B15-B19)*

K75.4   Autoimmune hepatitis   `HCC`
> Lupoid hepatitis NEC

√5ᵗʰ **K75.8   Other specified inflammatory liver diseases**

     K75.81   Nonalcoholic steatohepatitis (NASH)
> Use additional code, if applicable, hepatic fibrosis (K74.0-)

     K75.89   Other specified inflammatory liver diseases

K75.9   Inflammatory liver disease, unspecified
> Hepatitis NOS
> EXCLUDES 1   *acute or subacute hepatitis (K72.0-)*
> *chronic hepatitis NEC (K73.-)*
> *viral hepatitis (B15-B19)*
>
> **AHA:** 2015,2Q,17

√4ᵗʰ **K76   Other diseases of liver**
> EXCLUDES 2   *alcoholic liver disease (K70.-)*
> *amyloid degeneration of liver (E85.-)*
> *cystic disease of liver (congenital) (Q44.6)*
> *hepatic vein thrombosis (I82.0)*
> *hepatomegaly NOS (R16.0)*
> *pigmentary cirrhosis (of liver) (E83.110)*
> *portal vein thrombosis (I81)*
> *toxic liver disease (K71.-)*

K76.0   Fatty (change of) liver, not elsewhere classified
> Nonalcoholic fatty liver disease (NAFLD)
> EXCLUDES 1   *nonalcoholic steatohepatitis (NASH) (K75.81)*

K76.1   Chronic passive congestion of liver
> Cardiac cirrhosis
> Cardiac sclerosis

K76.2   Central hemorrhagic necrosis of liver   `MCC`
> EXCLUDES 1   *liver necrosis with hepatic failure (K72.-)*

K76.3   Infarction of liver   `MCC`

K76.4   Peliosis hepatis
> Hepatic angiomatosis

K76.5   Hepatic veno-occlusive disease
> EXCLUDES 1   *Budd-Chiari syndrome (I82.0)*

K76.6   Portal hypertension   `CC` `HCC`
> Use additional code for any associated complications, such as:
> portal hypertensive gastropathy (K31.89)
> **AHA:** 2020,1Q,15

K76.7   Hepatorenal syndrome   `MCC` `HCC`
> EXCLUDES 1   *hepatorenal syndrome following labor and delivery (O90.41)*
> *postprocedural hepatorenal syndrome (K91.83)*

√5ᵗʰ **K76.8   Other specified diseases of liver**

     K76.81   Hepatopulmonary syndrome   `UPD` `HCC`
> Code first underlying liver disease, such as:
> alcoholic cirrhosis of liver (K70.3-)
> cirrhosis of liver without mention of alcohol (K74.6-)

K76.82   Hepatic encephalopathy   `HCC`
> Hepatic encephalopathy, NOS
> Hepatic encephalopathy without coma
> Hepatocerebral intoxication
> Portal-systemic encephalopathy
> Code also underlying liver disease, such as:
> acute and subacute hepatic failure without coma (K72.00)
> alcoholic hepatic failure without coma (K70.40)
> chronic hepatic failure without coma (K72.10)
> hepatic failure with toxic liver disease without coma (K71.10)
> hepatic failure without coma (K72.90)
> icterus of newborn (P55-P59)
> postprocedural hepatic failure (K91.82)
> viral hepatitis without hepatic coma (B15.9, B16.1, B16.9, B17.10, B19.10, B19.20, B19.9)
> EXCLUDES 1   *acute and subacute hepatic failure with coma (K72.01)*
> *alcoholic hepatic failure with coma (K70.41)*
> *chronic hepatic failure with coma (K72.11)*
> *hepatic failure with coma (K72.91)*
>
> **AHA:** 2022,4Q,27-28

K76.89   Other specified diseases of liver
> Cyst (simple) of liver
> Focal nodular hyperplasia of liver
> Hepatoptosis
> **AHA:** 2023,1Q,26; 2022,3Q,7
> **TIP:** Assign codes E80.6 and K76.89 to report benign recurrent intrahepatic cholestasis (BRIC) or progressive familial intrahepatic cholestasis (PFIC).

K76.9   Liver disease, unspecified

K77   *Liver disorders in diseases classified elsewhere*   `CC`
> Code first underlying disease, such as:
> amyloidosis (E85.-)
> congenital syphilis (A50.0, A50.5)
> congenital toxoplasmosis (P37.1)
> infectious mononucleosis with liver disease (B27.0-B27.9 with fifth character 9)
> schistosomiasis (B65.0-B65.9)
> EXCLUDES 1   *alcoholic hepatitis (K70.1-)*
> *alcoholic liver disease (K70.-)*
> *cytomegaloviral hepatitis (B25.1)*
> *herpesviral [herpes simplex] hepatitis (B00.81)*
> *mumps hepatitis (B26.81)*
> *sarcoidosis with liver disease (D86.89)*
> *secondary syphilis with liver disease (A51.45)*
> *syphilis (late) with liver disease (A52.74)*
> *toxoplasmosis (acquired) hepatitis (B58.1)*
> *tuberculosis with liver disease (A18.83)*

N Newborn: 0   **P** Pediatric: 0-17   **M** Maternity: 9-64   **A** Adult: 15-124   **UNS** Unspecified Site   **MCC** Major Complication/Comorbidity   **CC** Complication/Comorbidity   **PE** POA Exempt

742

ICD-10-CM 2025

Disorders of gallbladder, biliary tract and pancreas (K80-K87)

✓4ᵗʰ **K80 Cholelithiasis**

> **EXCLUDES 1** retained cholelithiasis following cholecystectomy (K91.86)
> **AHA:** 2018,4Q,20
> **DEF:** Presence or formation of concretions (calculi or "gallstones") in the gallbladder. The stones contain cholesterol, calcium carbonate, or calcium bilirubinate in pure forms or in various combinations.

Cholelithiasis

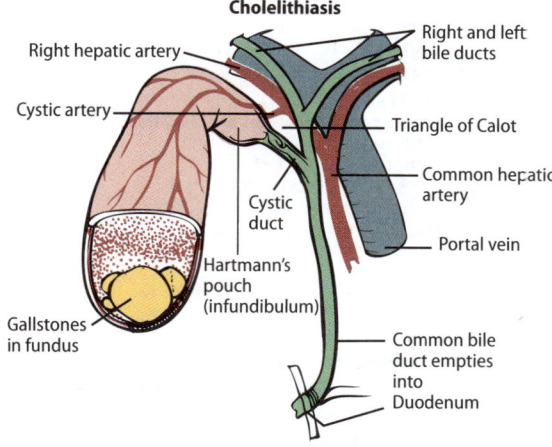

Right hepatic artery
Cystic artery
Cystic duct
Hartmann's pouch (infundibulum)
Gallstones in fundus
Right and left bile ducts
Triangle of Calot
Common hepatic artery
Portal vein
Common bile duct empties into Duodenum

✓5ᵗʰ **K80.0 Calculus of gallbladder with acute cholecystitis**
> Any condition listed in K80.2 with acute cholecystitis
> Use additional code if applicable for associated gangrene of gallbladder (K82.A1), or perforation of gallbladder (K82.A2)

K80.00 Calculus of gallbladder with acute cholecystitis without obstruction
> **AHA:** 2023,2Q,11   `CC`

K80.01 Calculus of gallbladder with acute cholecystitis with obstruction   `CC`

✓5ᵗʰ **K80.1 Calculus of gallbladder with other cholecystitis**
> Use additional code if applicable for associated gangrene of gallbladder (K82.A1), or perforation of gallbladder (K82.A2)

K80.10 Calculus of gallbladder with chronic cholecystitis without obstruction
> Cholelithiasis with cholecystitis NOS

K80.11 Calculus of gallbladder with chronic cholecystitis with obstruction   `CC`

K80.12 Calculus of gallbladder with acute and chronic cholecystitis without obstruction   `CC`

K80.13 Calculus of gallbladder with acute and chronic cholecystitis with obstruction   `CC`

K80.18 Calculus of gallbladder with other cholecystitis without obstruction   `CC`

K80.19 Calculus of gallbladder with other cholecystitis with obstruction   `CC`

✓5ᵗʰ **K80.2 Calculus of gallbladder without cholecystitis**
> Cholecystolithiasis without cholecystitis
> Cholelithiasis (without cholecystitis)
> Colic (recurrent) of gallbladder (without cholecystitis)
> Gallstone (impacted) of cystic duct (without cholecystitis)
> Gallstone (impacted) of gallbladder (without cholecystitis)

K80.20 Calculus of gallbladder without cholecystitis without obstruction

K80.21 Calculus of gallbladder without cholecystitis with obstruction   `CC`

✓5ᵗʰ **K80.3 Calculus of bile duct with cholangitis**
> Any condition listed in K80.5 with cholangitis
> **DEF:** Cholangitis: Inflammation of the bile ducts.

K80.30 Calculus of bile duct with cholangitis, unspecified, without obstruction   `CC`

K80.31 Calculus of bile duct with cholangitis, unspecified, with obstruction   `CC`

K80.32 Calculus of bile duct with acute cholangitis without obstruction   `CC`

K80.33 Calculus of bile duct with acute cholangitis with obstruction   `CC`

K80.34 Calculus of bile duct with chronic cholangitis without obstruction   `CC`

K80.35 Calculus of bile duct with chronic cholangitis with obstruction   `CC`

K80.36 Calculus of bile duct with acute and chronic cholangitis without obstruction   `CC`

K80.37 Calculus of bile duct with acute and chronic cholangitis with obstruction   `CC`

✓5ᵗʰ **K80.4 Calculus of bile duct with cholecystitis**
> Any condition listed in K80.5 with cholecystitis (with cholangitis)
> Code also, if applicable, fistula of bile duct (K83.3)
> Use additional code if applicable for associated gangrene of gallbladder (K82.A1), or perforation of gallbladder (K82.A2)
> **AHA:** 2019,1Q,17

K80.40 Calculus of bile duct with cholecystitis, unspecified, without obstruction   `CC`

K80.41 Calculus of bile duct with cholecystitis, unspecified, with obstruction   `CC`
> **AHA:** 2019,1Q,17

K80.42 Calculus of bile duct with acute cholecystitis without obstruction   `CC`

K80.43 Calculus of bile duct with acute cholecystitis with obstruction   `CC`

K80.44 Calculus of bile duct with chronic cholecystitis without obstruction   `CC`

K80.45 Calculus of bile duct with chronic cholecystitis with obstruction   `CC`

K80.46 Calculus of bile duct with acute and chronic cholecystitis without obstruction   `CC`

K80.47 Calculus of bile duct with acute and chronic cholecystitis with obstruction   `CC`

✓5ᵗʰ **K80.5 Calculus of bile duct without cholangitis or cholecystitis**
> Choledocholithiasis (without cholangitis or cholecystitis)
> Gallstone (impacted) of bile duct NOS (without cholangitis or cholecystitis)
> Gallstone (impacted) of common duct (without cholangitis or cholecystitis)
> Gallstone (impacted) of hepatic duct (without cholangitis or cholecystitis)
> Hepatic cholelithiasis (without cholangitis or cholecystitis)
> Hepatic colic (recurrent) (without cholangitis or cholecystitis)
> **DEF:** Cholangitis: Inflammation of the bile ducts.

K80.50 Calculus of bile duct without cholangitis or cholecystitis without obstruction

K80.51 Calculus of bile duct without cholangitis or cholecystitis with obstruction   `CC`

✓5ᵗʰ **K80.6 Calculus of gallbladder and bile duct with cholecystitis**
> Use additional code if applicable for associated gangrene of gallbladder (K82.A1), or perforation of gallbladder (K82.A2)

K80.60 Calculus of gallbladder and bile duct with cholecystitis, unspecified, without obstruction   `CC`

K80.61 Calculus of gallbladder and bile duct with cholecystitis, unspecified, with obstruction   `CC`

K80.62 Calculus of gallbladder and bile duct with acute cholecystitis without obstruction   `CC`

K80.63 Calculus of gallbladder and bile duct with acute cholecystitis with obstruction   `CC`

K80.64 Calculus of gallbladder and bile duct with chronic cholecystitis without obstruction   `CC`

K80.65 Calculus of gallbladder and bile duct with chronic cholecystitis with obstruction   `CC`

K80.66 Calculus of gallbladder and bile duct with acute and chronic cholecystitis without obstruction   `CC`

K80.67 Calculus of gallbladder and bile duct with acute and chronic cholecystitis with obstruction   `MCC`

✓5ᵗʰ **K80.7 Calculus of gallbladder and bile duct without cholecystitis**

K80.70 Calculus of gallbladder and bile duct without cholecystitis without obstruction

K80.71 Calculus of gallbladder and bile duct without cholecystitis with obstruction   `CC`

✓5ᵗʰ **K80.8 Other cholelithiasis**

K80.80 Other cholelithiasis without obstruction

K80.81 Other cholelithiasis with obstruction   `CC`

☑ Additional Character Required   ✓x7ᵗʰ Placeholder   Questionable PDx   Manifestation   Unspecified   UPD Unacceptable PDx   H1 - H14 HAC   HCC CMS-HCC Dx   HIV HIV Dx

ICD-10-CM 2025   743

√4ᵗʰ K81 Cholecystitis

Use additional code if applicable for associated gangrene of gallbladder (K82.A1), or perforation of gallbladder (K82.A2)

EXCLUDES 1   *cholecystitis with cholelithiasis (K80.-)*

AHA: 2018,4Q,20

K81.0 Acute cholecystitis   `CC`
Abscess of gallbladder
Angiocholecystitis
Emphysematous (acute) cholecystitis
Empyema of gallbladder
Gangrene of gallbladder
Gangrenous cholecystitis
Suppurative cholecystitis

K81.1 Chronic cholecystitis

K81.2 Acute cholecystitis with chronic cholecystitis   `CC`

K81.9 Cholecystitis, unspecified

√4ᵗʰ K82 Other diseases of gallbladder

EXCLUDES 1   *nonvisualization of gallbladder (R93.2)*
       postcholecystectomy syndrome (K91.5)

K82.0 Obstruction of gallbladder   `CC`
Occlusion of cystic duct or gallbladder without cholelithiasis
Stenosis of cystic duct or gallbladder without cholelithiasis
Stricture of cystic duct or gallbladder without cholelithiasis

EXCLUDES 1   *obstruction of gallbladder with cholelithiasis (K80.-)*

K82.1 Hydrops of gallbladder   `CC`
Mucocele of gallbladder

K82.2 Perforation of gallbladder   `MCC`
Rupture of cystic duct or gallbladder

EXCLUDES 1   *perforation of gallbladder in cholecystitis (K82.A2)*

K82.3 Fistula of gallbladder   `CC`
Cholecystocolic fistula
Cholecystoduodenal fistula

▶Code also, if applicable, disruption of internal operation (surgical) wound (T81.32-)◀

K82.4 Cholesterolosis of gallbladder
Strawberry gallbladder

EXCLUDES 1   *cholesterolosis of gallbladder with cholecystitis (K81.-)*
       cholesterolosis of gallbladder with cholelithiasis (K80.-)

K82.8 Other specified diseases of gallbladder
Adhesions of cystic duct or gallbladder
Atrophy of cystic duct or gallbladder
Cyst of cystic duct or gallbladder
Dyskinesia of cystic duct or gallbladder
Hypertrophy of cystic duct or gallbladder
Nonfunctioning of cystic duct or gallbladder
Ulcer of cystic duct or gallbladder

K82.9 Disease of gallbladder, unspecified

√5ᵗʰ K82.A Disorders of gallbladder in diseases classified elsewhere

Code first the type of cholecystitis (K81.-), or cholelithiasis with cholecystitis (K80.00-K80.19, K80.40-K80.47, K80.60-K80.67)

AHA: 2018,4Q,19-20

K82.A1 Gangrene of gallbladder in cholecystitis
K82.A2 Perforation of gallbladder in cholecystitis   `CC`

√4ᵗʰ K83 Other diseases of biliary tract

EXCLUDES 1   *postcholecystectomy syndrome (K91.5)*
EXCLUDES 2   *conditions involving the cystic duct (K81-K82)*
       conditions involving the gallbladder (K81-K82)

√5ᵗʰ K83.0 Cholangitis

EXCLUDES 1   *cholangitic liver abscess (K75.0)*
       cholangitis with choledocholithiasis (K80.3-, K80.4-)
EXCLUDES 2   *chronic nonsuppurative destructive cholangitis (K74.3)*
       primary biliary cholangitis (K74.3)
       primary biliary cirrhosis (K74.3)

AHA: 2018,4Q,20

K83.01 Primary sclerosing cholangitis   `CC` `HCC`
K83.09 Other cholangitis   `CC` `HCC`
Ascending cholangitis
Cholangitis NOS
Primary cholangitis
Recurrent cholangitis
Sclerosing cholangitis
Secondary cholangitis
Stenosing cholangitis
Suppurative cholangitis

K83.1 Obstruction of bile duct   `MCC` `HCC`
Occlusion of bile duct without cholelithiasis
Stenosis of bile duct without cholelithiasis
Stricture of bile duct without cholelithiasis

EXCLUDES 1   *congenital obstruction of bile duct (Q44.3)*
       obstruction of bile duct with cholelithiasis (K80.-)

AHA: 2023,1Q,26; 2016,1Q,18

K83.2 Perforation of bile duct   `MCC`
Rupture of bile duct

K83.3 Fistula of bile duct   `CC`
Choledochoduodenal fistula

AHA: 2019,1Q,17

K83.4 Spasm of sphincter of Oddi

K83.5 Biliary cyst

K83.8 Other specified diseases of biliary tract
Adhesions of biliary tract
Atrophy of biliary tract
Hypertrophy of biliary tract
Ulcer of biliary tract

K83.9 Disease of biliary tract, unspecified

√4ᵗʰ K85 Acute pancreatitis

INCLUDES   acute (recurrent) pancreatitis
       subacute pancreatitis

AHA: 2016,4Q,34

√5ᵗʰ K85.0 Idiopathic acute pancreatitis

K85.00 Idiopathic acute pancreatitis without necrosis or infection   `MCC`
K85.01 Idiopathic acute pancreatitis with uninfected necrosis   `MCC`
K85.02 Idiopathic acute pancreatitis with infected necrosis   `MCC`

√5ᵗʰ K85.1 Biliary acute pancreatitis
Gallstone pancreatitis

AHA: 2023,2Q,11

K85.10 Biliary acute pancreatitis without necrosis or infection   `MCC`
K85.11 Biliary acute pancreatitis with uninfected necrosis   `MCC`
K85.12 Biliary acute pancreatitis with infected necrosis   `MCC`

√5ᵗʰ K85.2 Alcohol induced acute pancreatitis

EXCLUDES 2   *alcohol induced chronic pancreatitis (K86.0)*

K85.20 Alcohol induced acute pancreatitis without necrosis or infection   `MCC`
     AHA: 2020,1Q,9
K85.21 Alcohol induced acute pancreatitis with uninfected necrosis   `MCC`
K85.22 Alcohol induced acute pancreatitis with infected necrosis   `MCC`

√5ᵗʰ K85.3 Drug induced acute pancreatitis

Use additional code for adverse effect, if applicable, to identify drug (T36-T50 with fifth or sixth character 5)
Use additional code to identify drug abuse and dependence (F11.-F17.-)

K85.30 Drug induced acute pancreatitis without necrosis or infection   `MCC`
K85.31 Drug induced acute pancreatitis with uninfected necrosis   `MCC`
K85.32 Drug induced acute pancreatitis with infected necrosis   `MCC`

√5ᵗʰ K85.8 Other acute pancreatitis

K85.80 Other acute pancreatitis without necrosis or infection   `MCC`
K85.81 Other acute pancreatitis with uninfected necrosis   `MCC`
K85.82 Other acute pancreatitis with infected necrosis   `MCC`

√5ᵗʰ K85.9 Acute pancreatitis, unspecified
Pancreatitis NOS

K85.90 Acute pancreatitis without necrosis or infection, unspecified   `MCC`
K85.91 Acute pancreatitis with uninfected necrosis, unspecified   `MCC`
K85.92 Acute pancreatitis with infected necrosis, unspecified   `MCC`

`N` Newborn: 0   `P` Pediatric: 0-17   `M` Maternity: 9-64   `A` Adult: 15-124   `UNS` Unspecified Site   `MCC` Major Complication/Comorbidity   `CC` Complication/Comorbidity   `PE` POA Exempt

744   ICD-10-CM 2025

✓4ᵗʰ **K86 Other diseases of pancreas**

> EXCLUDES 2   fibrocystic disease of pancreas (E84.-)
> islet cell tumor (of pancreas) (D13.7)
> pancreatic steatorrhea (K90.3)

K86.0 Alcohol-induced chronic pancreatitis CC ⊦CC
Use additional code to identify:
alcohol abuse and dependence (F10.-)
Code also exocrine pancreatic insufficiency (K86.81)
> EXCLUDES 2   alcohol induced acute pancreatitis (K85.2-)

K86.1 Other chronic pancreatitis CC ⊦CC
Chronic pancreatitis NOS
Infectious chronic pancreatitis
Recurrent chronic pancreatitis
Relapsing chronic pancreatitis
Code also exocrine pancreatic insufficiency (K86.81)

K86.2 Cyst of pancreas CC

K86.3 Pseudocyst of pancreas CC

✓5ᵗʰ **K86.8 Other specified diseases of pancreas**
AHA: 2016,4Q,34-35

     K86.81 Exocrine pancreatic insufficiency

     K86.89 Other specified diseases of pancreas
Aseptic pancreatic necrosis, unrelated to acute pancreatitis
Atrophy of pancreas
Calculus of pancreas
Cirrhosis of pancreas
Fibrosis of pancreas
Pancreatic fat necrosis, unrelated to acute pancreatitis
Pancreatic infantilism
Pancreatic necrosis NOS, unrelated to acute pancreatitis

K86.9 Disease of pancreas, unspecified

K87 Disorders of gallbladder, biliary tract and pancreas in diseases classified elsewhere
Code first underlying disease
> EXCLUDES 1   cytomegaloviral pancreatitis (B25.2)
> mumps pancreatitis (B26.3)
> syphilitic gallbladder (A52.74)
> syphilitic pancreas (A52.74)
> tuberculosis of gallbladder (A18.83)
> tuberculosis of pancreas (A18.83)

Other diseases of the digestive system (K90-K95)

✓4ᵗʰ **K90 Intestinal malabsorption**
> EXCLUDES 1   intestinal malabsorption following gastrointestinal surgery (K91.2)

AHA: 2017,4Q,108

K90.0 Celiac disease
Celiac disease with steatorrhea
Celiac gluten-sensitive enteropathy
Nontropical sprue
Use additional code for associated disorders including:
dermatitis herpetiformis (L13.0)
gluten ataxia (G32.81)
Code also exocrine pancreatic insufficiency (K86.81)
DEF: Malabsorption syndrome due to gluten consumption. Symptoms include fetid, bulky, frothy, oily stools; a distended abdomen; gas; asthenia; electrolyte depletion; and vitamin E, D, and K deficiency.

K90.1 Tropical sprue CC
Sprue NOS
Tropical steatorrhea

K90.2 Blind loop syndrome, not elsewhere classified CC
Blind loop syndrome NOS
> EXCLUDES 1   congenital blind loop syndrome (Q43.8)
> postsurgical blind loop syndrome (K91.2)

K90.3 Pancreatic steatorrhea CC

✓5ᵗʰ **K90.4 Other malabsorption due to intolerance**
> EXCLUDES 2   celiac gluten-sensitive enteropathy (K90.0)
> lactose intolerance (E73.-)

AHA: 2016,4Q,35-36

     K90.41 Non-celiac gluten sensitivity CC
Gluten sensitivity NOS
Non-celiac gluten sensitive enteropathy

     K90.49 Malabsorption due to intolerance, not elsewhere classified CC
Malabsorption due to intolerance to carbohydrate
Malabsorption due to intolerance to fat
Malabsorption due to intolerance to protein
Malabsorption due to intolerance to starch

✓5ᵗʰ **K90.8 Other intestinal malabsorption**
AHA: 2023,4Q,31-33

     K90.81 Whipple's disease CC

✓6ᵗʰ   **K90.82 Short bowel syndrome**
Short gut syndrome

       K90.821 Short bowel syndrome with colon in continuity CC
Short bowel syndrome with colonic continuity

       K90.822 Short bowel syndrome without colon in continuity CC
Short bowel syndrome without colonic continuity

       K90.829 Short bowel syndrome, unspecified CC

     K90.83 Intestinal failure CC

     K90.89 Other intestinal malabsorption CC

K90.9 Intestinal malabsorption, unspecified CC

✓4ᵗʰ **K91 Intraoperative and postprocedural complications and disorders of digestive system, not elsewhere classified**
> EXCLUDES 2   complications of artificial opening of digestive system (K94.-)
> complications of bariatric procedures (K95.-)
> gastrojejunal ulcer (K28.-)
> postprocedural (radiation) retroperitoneal abscess (K68.11)
> radiation colitis (K52.0)
> radiation gastroenteritis (K52.0)
> radiation proctitis (K62.7)

AHA: 2016,4Q,9-10

K91.0 Vomiting following gastrointestinal surgery

K91.1 Postgastric surgery syndromes
Dumping syndrome
Postgastrectomy syndrome
Postvagotomy syndrome

K91.2 Postsurgical malabsorption, not elsewhere classified CC
Postsurgical blind loop syndrome
> EXCLUDES 1   malabsorption osteomalacia in adults (M83.2)
> malabsorption osteoporosis, postsurgical (M80.8-, M81.8)

✓5ᵗʰ **K91.3 Postprocedural intestinal obstruction**
AHA: 2017,4Q,16-17; 2017,1Q,40

     K91.30 Postprocedural intestinal obstruction, unspecified as to partial versus complete CC
Postprocedural intestinal obstruction NOS

     K91.31 Postprocedural partial intestinal obstruction CC
Postprocedural incomplete intestinal obstruction

     K91.32 Postprocedural complete intestinal obstruction CC

K91.5 Postcholecystectomy syndrome

✓5ᵗʰ **K91.6 Intraoperative hemorrhage and hematoma of a digestive system organ or structure complicating a procedure**
> EXCLUDES 1   intraoperative hemorrhage and hematoma of a digestive system organ or structure due to accidental puncture and laceration during a procedure (K91.7-)

     K91.61 Intraoperative hemorrhage and hematoma of a digestive system organ or structure complicating a digestive system procedure CC
AHA: 2020,1Q,19

     K91.62 Intraoperative hemorrhage and hematoma of a digestive system organ or structure complicating other procedure CC

✓5ᵗʰ **K91.7 Accidental puncture and laceration of a digestive system organ or structure during a procedure**
AHA: 2022,1Q,51

     K91.71 Accidental puncture and laceration of a digestive system organ or structure during a digestive system procedure CC
AHA: 2021,2Q,11

     K91.72 Accidental puncture and laceration of a digestive system organ or structure during other procedure CC
AHA: 2019,2Q,23

✓5th K91.8 Other intraoperative and postprocedural complications and disorders of digestive system

K91.81 Other intraoperative complications of digestive system `CC`

K91.82 Postprocedural hepatic failure `CC`

K91.83 Postprocedural hepatorenal syndrome `CC`

✓6th K91.84 Postprocedural hemorrhage of a digestive system organ or structure following a procedure

K91.840 Postprocedural hemorrhage of a digestive system organ or structure following a digestive system procedure `CC`
AHA: 2016,1Q,15

K91.841 Postprocedural hemorrhage of a digestive system organ or structure following other procedure `CC`

✓6th K91.85 Complications of intestinal pouch

K91.850 Pouchitis `CC` `HCC`
Inflammation of internal ileoanal pouch
DEF: Inflammatory complication of an existing surgically created ileoanal pouch, resulting in multiple GI complaints, including diarrhea, abdominal pain, rectal bleeding, fecal urgency, or incontinence.

K91.858 Other complications of intestinal pouch `CC` `HCC`
AHA: 2019,2Q,13

K91.86 Retained cholelithiasis following cholecystectomy `CC`

✓6th K91.87 Postprocedural hematoma and seroma of a digestive system organ or structure following a procedure

K91.870 Postprocedural hematoma of a digestive system organ or structure following a digestive system procedure `CC`
AHA: 2022,1Q,24

K91.871 Postprocedural hematoma of a digestive system organ or structure following other procedure `CC`

K91.872 Postprocedural seroma of a digestive system organ or structure following a digestive system procedure `CC`

K91.873 Postprocedural seroma of a digestive system organ or structure following other procedure `CC`

K91.89 Other postprocedural complications and disorders of digestive system `CC`
Use additional code, if applicable, to further specify disorder
EXCLUDES 2   *postprocedural retroperitoneal abscess (K68.11)*
AHA: 2020,2Q,22; 2017,1Q,40

✓4th K92 Other diseases of digestive system
EXCLUDES 1   *neonatal gastrointestinal hemorrhage (P54.0-P54.3)*

K92.0 Hematemesis `CC`

K92.1 Melena `CC`
EXCLUDES 1   *occult blood in feces (R19.5)*

K92.2 Gastrointestinal hemorrhage, unspecified `CC`
Gastric hemorrhage NOS
Intestinal hemorrhage NOS
EXCLUDES 1   *acute hemorrhagic gastritis (K29.01)*
hemorrhage of anus and rectum (K62.5)
angiodysplasia of stomach with hemorrhage (K31.811)
diverticular disease with hemorrhage (K57.-)
gastritis and duodenitis with hemorrhage (K29.-)
peptic ulcer with hemorrhage (K25-K28)
AHA: 2021,1Q,11

✓5th K92.8 Other specified diseases of the digestive system

K92.81 Gastrointestinal mucositis (ulcerative) `CC`
Code also type of associated therapy, such as:
antineoplastic and immunosuppressive drugs (T45.1X-)
radiological procedure and radiotherapy (Y84.2)
EXCLUDES 2   *mucositis (ulcerative) of vagina and vulva (N76.81)*
nasal mucositis (ulcerative) (J34.81)
oral mucositis (ulcerative) (K12.3-)

K92.89 Other specified diseases of the digestive system

K92.9 Disease of digestive system, unspecified

✓4th K94 Complications of artificial openings of the digestive system

✓5th K94.0 Colostomy complications

K94.00 Colostomy complication, unspecified `HCC`

K94.01 Colostomy hemorrhage `CC` `HCC`

K94.02 Colostomy infection `CC` `HCC`
Use additional code to specify type of infection, such as:
cellulitis of abdominal wall (L03.311)
sepsis (A40.-, A41.-)

K94.03 Colostomy malfunction `CC` `HCC`
Mechanical complication of colostomy

K94.09 Other complications of colostomy `CC` `HCC`

✓5th K94.1 Enterostomy complications

K94.10 Enterostomy complication, unspecified `HCC`

K94.11 Enterostomy hemorrhage `CC` `HCC`

K94.12 Enterostomy infection `CC` `HCC`
Use additional code to specify type of infection, such as:
cellulitis of abdominal wall (L03.311)
sepsis (A40.-, A41.-)

K94.13 Enterostomy malfunction `CC` `HCC`
Mechanical complication of enterostomy

K94.19 Other complications of enterostomy `CC` `HCC`

✓5th K94.2 Gastrostomy complications

K94.20 Gastrostomy complication, unspecified `HCC`

K94.21 Gastrostomy hemorrhage `HCC`

K94.22 Gastrostomy infection `CC` `HCC`
Use additional code to specify type of infection, such as:
cellulitis of abdominal wall (L03.311)
sepsis (A40.-, A41.-)

K94.23 Gastrostomy malfunction `CC` `HCC`
Mechanical complication of gastrostomy
AHA: 2019,1Q,26

K94.29 Other complications of gastrostomy `HCC`

✓5th K94.3 Esophagostomy complications

K94.30 Esophagostomy complications, unspecified `CC` `HCC`

K94.31 Esophagostomy hemorrhage `CC` `HCC`

K94.32 Esophagostomy infection `CC` `HCC`
Use additional code to identify the infection

K94.33 Esophagostomy malfunction `CC` `HCC`
Mechanical complication of esophagostomy

K94.39 Other complications of esophagostomy `CC` `HCC`

✓4th K95 Complications of bariatric procedures

✓5th K95.0 Complications of gastric band procedure

K95.01 Infection due to gastric band procedure `CC` `H11`
Use additional code to specify type of infection or organism, such as:
bacterial and viral infectious agents (B95.-, B96.-)
cellulitis of abdominal wall (L03.311)
sepsis (A40.-, A41.-)

K95.09 Other complications of gastric band procedure `CC`
Use additional code, if applicable, to further specify complication

✓5th K95.8 Complications of other bariatric procedure
EXCLUDES 1   *complications of gastric band surgery (K95.0-)*

K95.81 Infection due to other bariatric procedure `CC` `H11`
Use additional code to specify type of infection or organism, such as:
bacterial and viral infectious agents (B95.-, B96.-)
cellulitis of abdominal wall (L03.311)
sepsis (A40.-, A41.-)

K95.89 Other complications of other bariatric procedure `CC`
Use additional code, if applicable, to further specify complication

---

`N` Newborn: 0   `P` Pediatric: 0-17   `M` Maternity: 9-64   `A` Adult: 15-124   `UNS` Unspecified Site   `MCC` Major Complication/Comorbidity   `CC` Complication/Comorbidity   `PE` POA Exempt

Chapter 12. Diseases of the Skin and Subcutaneous Tissue (L00–L99)

Chapter-specific Guidelines with Coding Examples

The chapter-specific guidelines from the ICD-10-CM Official Guidelines for Coding and Reporting have been provided below. Along with these guidelines are coding examples, contained in the shaded boxes, that have been developed to help illustrate the coding and/or sequencing guidance found in these guidelines.

a. Pressure ulcer stage codes

1) Pressure ulcer stages

Codes in category L89, Pressure ulcer, identify the site and stage of the pressure ulcer.

The ICD-10-CM classifies pressure ulcer stages based on severity, which is designated by stages 1-4, deep tissue pressure injury, unspecified stage, and unstageable.

Assign as many codes from category L89 as needed to identify all the pressure ulcers the patient has, if applicable.

See Section I.B.14. for pressure ulcer stage documentation by clinicians other than patient's provider

> Nursing notes: Dressings changed daily on stage 4 ulcer on heel and stage 2 ulcer on elbow
>
> Discharge summary: Pressure ulcers on right heel and left elbow
>
> **L89.614**   **Pressure ulcer of right heel, stage 4**
>
> **L89.022**   **Pressure ulcer of left elbow, stage 2**
>
> *Explanation:* Right heel and left elbow pressure ulcers were documented by the patient's provider in the discharge summary. Although the stage of these ulcers was not included in the provider's diagnostic statement, it is appropriate to code the stage from documentation from other clinicians involved in the patient's care, such as the nurse's notes, according to section I.B.14. Combination codes from category L89 Pressure ulcer, identify the site of the pressure ulcer as well as the stage. Assign as many codes from category L89 as needed to identify all the pressure ulcers the patient has.

2) Unstageable pressure ulcers

Assignment of the code for unstageable pressure ulcer (L89.--0) should be based on the clinical documentation. These codes are used for pressure ulcers whose stage cannot be clinically determined (e.g., the ulcer is covered by eschar or has been treated with a skin or muscle graft). This code should not be confused with the codes for unspecified stage (L89.--9). When there is no documentation regarding the stage of the pressure ulcer, assign the appropriate code for unspecified stage (L89.--9).

> Pressure ulcer of the right lower back documented as unstageable due to the presence of thick eschar covering the ulcer
>
> **L89.130**   **Pressure ulcer of right lower back, unstageable**
>
> *Explanation:* Codes for unstageable pressure ulcers are assigned when the stage cannot be clinically determined (e.g., the ulcer is covered by eschar or has been treated with a skin or muscle graft).

If during an encounter, the stage of an unstageable pressure ulcer is revealed after debridement, assign only the code for the stage revealed following debridement.

3) Documented pressure ulcer stage

Assignment of the pressure ulcer stage code should be guided by clinical documentation of the stage or documentation of the terms found in the Alphabetic Index. For clinical terms describing the stage that are not found in the Alphabetic Index, and there is no documentation of the stage, the provider should be queried.

> Left heel pressure ulcer with partial thickness skin loss involving the dermis
>
> **L89.622**   **Pressure ulcer of left heel, stage 2**
>
> *Explanation:* Code assignment for the pressure ulcer stage should be guided by either the clinical documentation of the stage or the documentation of terms found in the Alphabetic Index. The clinical documentation describing the left heel pressure ulcer "partial thickness skin loss involving the dermis" matches the ICD-10-CM index parenthetical description for stage 2 "(abrasion, blister, partial thickness skin loss involving epidermis and/or dermis)."

4) Patients admitted with pressure ulcers documented as healed

No code is assigned if the documentation states that the pressure ulcer is completely healed at the time of admission.

5) Pressure ulcers documented as healing

Pressure ulcers described as healing should be assigned the appropriate pressure ulcer stage code based on the documentation in the medical record. If the documentation does not provide information about the stage of the healing pressure ulcer, assign the appropriate code for unspecified stage.

If the documentation is unclear as to whether the patient has a current (new) pressure ulcer or if the patient is being treated for a healing pressure ulcer, query the provider.

For ulcers that were present on admission but healed at the time of discharge, assign the code for the site and stage of the pressure ulcer at the time of admission.

> H & P noted healing stage 2 sacral pressure ulcer. Resolved at time of discharge summary.
>
> **L89.152**   **Pressure ulcer of sacral region, stage 2**
>
> *Explanation:* Although completely healed upon discharge, the pressure ulcer required observation and/or treatment and should be coded based on the site and stage upon admission.

6) Patient admitted with pressure ulcer evolving into another stage during the admission

If a patient is admitted to an inpatient hospital with a pressure ulcer at one stage and it progresses to a higher stage, two separate codes should be assigned: one code for the site and stage of the ulcer on admission and a second code for the same ulcer site and the highest stage reported during the stay.

> Stage 3 right hip pressure ulcer worsened during admission to a stage 4
>
> **L89.213**   **Pressure ulcer of right hip, stage 3**
>
> **L89.214**   **Pressure ulcer of right hip, stage 4**
>
> *Explanation:* A pressure ulcer that progresses from a lower stage to a higher stage is assigned two codes, one for the documented stage upon admission and one for the documented stage at discharge.

7) Pressure-induced deep tissue damage

For pressure-induced deep tissue damage or deep tissue pressure injury, assign only the appropriate code for pressure-induced deep tissue damage (L89.--6).

b. Non-pressure chronic ulcers

1) Patients admitted with non-pressure ulcers documented as healed

No code is assigned if the documentation states that the non-pressure ulcer is completely healed at the time of admission.

2) Non-pressure ulcers documented as healing

Non-pressure ulcers described as healing should be assigned the appropriate non-pressure ulcer code based on the documentation in the medical record. If the documentation does not provide information about the severity of the healing non-pressure ulcer, assign the appropriate code for unspecified severity.

If the documentation is unclear as to whether the patient has a current (new) non-pressure ulcer or if the patient is being treated for a healing non-pressure ulcer, query the provider.

For ulcers that were present on admission but healed at the time of discharge, assign the code for the site and severity of the non-pressure ulcer at the time of admission.

> Admission diagnosis: Chronic ulcer, fat layer exposed, on left ankle
>
> Discharge diagnosis: Resolution of ulcer on the left ankle
>
> **L97.322**   **Non-pressure chronic ulcer of left ankle with fat layer exposed**
>
> *Explanation:* Although the ulcer was documented as resolved (healed) at discharge, a code representing the site and severity of the ulcer upon admission should be appended.

3) Patient admitted with non-pressure ulcer that progresses to another severity level during the admission

If a patient is admitted to an inpatient hospital with a non-pressure ulcer at one severity level and it progresses to a higher severity level, two separate codes should be assigned: one code for the site and severity level of the ulcer on admission and a second code for the same ulcer site and the highest severity level reported during the stay.

See Section I.B.14. for pressure ulcer stage documentation by clinicians other than patient's provider

Chapter 12. Diseases of the Skin and Subcutaneous Tissue (L00-L99)

EXCLUDES 2　certain conditions originating in the perinatal period (P04-P96)
certain infectious and parasitic diseases (A00-B99)
complications of pregnancy, childbirth and the puerperium (O00-O9A)
congenital malformations, deformations, and chromosomal abnormalities (Q00-Q99)
endocrine, nutritional and metabolic diseases (E00-E88)
lipomelanotic reticulosis (I89.8)
neoplasms (C00-D49)
symptoms, signs and abnormal clinical and laboratory findings, not elsewhere classified (R00-R94)
systemic connective tissue disorders (M30-M36)
viral warts (B07.-)

AHA: 2022,2Q,7

This chapter contains the following blocks:

L00-L08　Infections of the skin and subcutaneous tissue
L10-L14　Bullous disorders
L20-L30　Dermatitis and eczema
L40-L45　Papulosquamous disorders
L49-L54　Urticaria and erythema
L55-L59　Radiation-related disorders of the skin and subcutaneous tissue
L60-L75　Disorders of skin appendages
L76　　　Intraoperative and postprocedural complications of skin and subcutaneous tissue
L80-L99　Other disorders of the skin and subcutaneous tissue

Infections of the skin and subcutaneous tissue (L00-L08)

Use additional code (B95-B97) to identify infectious agent

EXCLUDES 2　hordeolum (H00.0)
infective dermatitis (L30.3)
local infections of skin classified in Chapter 1
lupus panniculitis (L93.2)
panniculitis NOS (M79.3)
panniculitis of neck and back (M54.0-)
perlèche NOS (K13.0)
perlèche due to candidiasis (B37.0)
perlèche due to riboflavin deficiency (E53.0)
pyogenic granuloma (L98.0)
relapsing panniculitis [Weber-Christian] (M35.6)
viral warts (B07.-)
zoster (B02.-)

L00　Staphylococcal scalded skin syndrome
Ritter's disease
Use additional code to identify percentage of skin exfoliation (L49.-)
EXCLUDES 1　bullous impetigo (L01.03)
pemphigus neonatorum (L01.03)
toxic epidermal necrolysis [Lyell] (L51.2)
DEF: Infectious skin disease of children younger than 5 years marked by eruptions ranging from a few localized blisters to widespread, easily ruptured, fine vesicles and bullae affecting almost the entire body. It results in exfoliation of large planes of skin and leaves raw areas.

L01　Impetigo
EXCLUDES 1　impetigo herpetiformis (L40.1)
DEF: Acute, superficial, highly contagious skin infection commonly occurring in children. Skin lesions usually appear on the face and consist of vesicles and bullae that burst and form yellow crusts.

L01.0　Impetigo
Impetigo contagiosa
Impetigo vulgaris
L01.00　Impetigo, unspecified
Impetigo NOS
L01.01　Non-bullous impetigo
L01.02　Bockhart's impetigo
Impetigo follicularis
Perifolliculitis NOS
Superficial pustular perifolliculitis
DEF: Superficial inflammation of the hair follicles commonly caused by *Staphylococcus aureus* that manifests as rounded, sphere-shaped, pustular eruptions in the areas of the scalp, beard, underarms, extremities, and buttocks.
L01.03　Bullous impetigo
Impetigo neonatorum
Pemphigus neonatorum
L01.09　Other impetigo
Ulcerative impetigo

L01.1　Impetiginization of other dermatoses

L02　Cutaneous abscess, furuncle and carbuncle
Use additional code to identify organism (B95-B96)
EXCLUDES 2　abscess of anus and rectal regions (K61.-)
abscess of female genital organs (external) (N76.4)
abscess of male genital organs (external) (N48.2, N49.-)
DEF: Carbuncle: Infection of the skin that arises from a collection of interconnected infected boils or furuncles, usually from hair follicles infected by *Staphylococcus*. This condition can produce pus and form drainage cavities.
DEF: Furuncle: Inflamed, painful abscess, cyst, or nodule on the skin caused by bacteria, often *Staphylococcus*, entering along the hair follicle.

L02.0　Cutaneous abscess, furuncle and carbuncle of face
EXCLUDES 2　abscess of ear, external (H60.0)
abscess of eyelid (H00.0)
abscess of head [any part, except face] (L02.8)
abscess of lacrimal gland (H04.0)
abscess of lacrimal passages (H04.3)
abscess of mouth (K12.2)
abscess of nose (J34.0)
abscess of orbit (H05.0)
submandibular abscess (K12.2)
L02.01　Cutaneous abscess of face　CC
L02.02　Furuncle of face
Boil of face
Folliculitis of face
L02.03　Carbuncle of face

L02.1　Cutaneous abscess, furuncle and carbuncle of neck
L02.11　Cutaneous abscess of neck　CC
L02.12　Furuncle of neck
Boil of neck
Folliculitis of neck
L02.13　Carbuncle of neck

L02.2　Cutaneous abscess, furuncle and carbuncle of trunk
EXCLUDES 1　non-newborn omphalitis (L08.82)
omphalitis of newborn (P38.-)
EXCLUDES 2　abscess of breast (N61.1)
abscess of buttocks (L02.3)
abscess of female external genital organs (N76.4)
abscess of hip (L02.4)
abscess of male external genital organs (N48.2, N49.-)

L02.21　Cutaneous abscess of trunk
L02.211　Cutaneous abscess of abdominal wall　CC
L02.212　Cutaneous abscess of back [any part, except buttock]　CC
L02.213　Cutaneous abscess of chest wall　CC
L02.214　Cutaneous abscess of groin　CC
L02.215　Cutaneous abscess of perineum　CC
L02.216　Cutaneous abscess of umbilicus　CC
L02.219　Cutaneous abscess of trunk, unspecified　CC

L02.22　Furuncle of trunk
Boil of trunk
Folliculitis of trunk
L02.221　Furuncle of abdominal wall
L02.222　Furuncle of back [any part, except buttock]
L02.223　Furuncle of chest wall
L02.224　Furuncle of groin
L02.225　Furuncle of perineum
L02.226　Furuncle of umbilicus
L02.229　Furuncle of trunk, unspecified

L02.23　Carbuncle of trunk
L02.231　Carbuncle of abdominal wall
L02.232　Carbuncle of back [any part, except buttock]
L02.233　Carbuncle of chest wall
L02.234　Carbuncle of groin
L02.235　Carbuncle of perineum
L02.236　Carbuncle of umbilicus
L02.239　Carbuncle of trunk, unspecified

L02.3　Cutaneous abscess, furuncle and carbuncle of buttock
EXCLUDES 1　pilonidal cyst with abscess (L05.01)
L02.31　Cutaneous abscess of buttock　CC
Cutaneous abscess of gluteal region

N Newborn: 0　**P** Pediatric: 0-17　**M** Maternity: 9-64　**A** Adult: 15-124　**UNS** Unspecified Site　**MCC** Major Complication/Comorbidity　**CC** Complication/Comorbidity　**PE** POA Exempt

748　　　　　　　　　　　　　　　　　　　　　　　　　　　　　　　　　　　　　　ICD-10-CM 2025

L02.32   **Furuncle** of buttock
     Boil of buttock
     Folliculitis of buttock
     Furuncle of gluteal region

L02.33   **Carbuncle** of buttock
     Carbuncle of gluteal region

☑5ᵗʰ **L02.4**   Cutaneous abscess, furuncle and carbuncle of **limb**
    EXCLUDES 2   cutaneous abscess, furuncle and carbuncle of foot (L02.6-)
           cutaneous abscess, furuncle and carbuncle of groin (L02.214, L02.224, L02.234)
           cutaneous abscess, furuncle and carbuncle of hand (L02.5-)

☑6ᵗʰ **L02.41**   **Cutaneous abscess** of limb
    L02.411   Cutaneous abscess of **right axilla**   CC
    L02.412   Cutaneous abscess of **left axilla**   CC
    L02.413   Cutaneous abscess of **right upper** limb   CC
    L02.414   Cutaneous abscess of **left upper** limb   CC
    L02.415   Cutaneous abscess of **right lower** limb   CC
    L02.416   Cutaneous abscess of **left lower** limb   CC
    L02.419   Cutaneous abscess of limb, unspecified   CC UNS

☑6ᵗʰ **L02.42**   **Furuncle** of limb
     Boil of limb
     Folliculitis of limb
    L02.421   Furuncle of **right axilla**
    L02.422   Furuncle of **left axilla**
    L02.423   Furuncle of **right upper** limb
    L02.424   Furuncle of **left upper** limb
    L02.425   Furuncle of **right lower** limb
    L02.426   Furuncle of **left lower** limb
    L02.429   Furuncle of limb, unspecified

☑6ᵗʰ **L02.43**   **Carbuncle** of limb
    L02.431   Carbuncle of **right axilla**
    L02.432   Carbuncle of **left axilla**
    L02.433   Carbuncle of **right upper** limb
    L02.434   Carbuncle of **left upper** limb
    L02.435   Carbuncle of **right lower** limb
    L02.436   Carbuncle of **left lower** limb
    L02.439   Carbuncle of limb, unspecified

☑5ᵗʰ **L02.5**   Cutaneous abscess, furuncle and carbuncle of **hand**
☑6ᵗʰ **L02.51**   **Cutaneous abscess** of hand
    L02.511   Cutaneous abscess of **right** hand   CC
    L02.512   Cutaneous abscess of **left** hand   CC
    L02.519   Cutaneous abscess of unspecified hand   CC UNS

☑6ᵗʰ **L02.52**   **Furuncle** hand
     Boil of hand
     Folliculitis of hand
    L02.521   Furuncle **right** hand
    L02.522   Furuncle **left** hand
    L02.529   Furuncle unspecified hand

☑6ᵗʰ **L02.53**   **Carbuncle** of hand
    L02.531   Carbuncle of **right** hand
    L02.532   Carbuncle of **left** hand
    L02.539   Carbuncle of unspecified hand

☑5ᵗʰ **L02.6**   Cutaneous abscess, furuncle and carbuncle of **foot**
☑6ᵗʰ **L02.61**   **Cutaneous abscess** of foot
    L02.611   Cutaneous abscess of **right** foot   CC
    L02.612   Cutaneous abscess of **left** foot   CC
    L02.619   Cutaneous abscess of unspecified foot   CC UNS

☑6ᵗʰ **L02.62**   **Furuncle** of foot
     Boil of foot
     Folliculitis of foot
    L02.621   Furuncle of **right** foot
    L02.622   Furuncle of **left** foot
    L02.629   Furuncle of unspecified foot

☑6ᵗʰ **L02.63**   **Carbuncle** of foot
    L02.631   Carbuncle of **right** foot
    L02.632   Carbuncle of **left** foot
    L02.639   Carbuncle of unspecified foot

☑5ᵗʰ **L02.8**   Cutaneous abscess, furuncle and carbuncle of other sites
☑6ᵗʰ **L02.81**   **Cutaneous abscess** of other sites
    L02.811   Cutaneous abscess of **head** [any part, except face]   CC
    L02.818   Cutaneous abscess of other sites   CC

☑6ᵗʰ **L02.82**   **Furuncle** of other sites
     Boil of other sites
     Folliculitis of other sites
    L02.821   Furuncle of **head** [any part, except face]
    L02.828   Furuncle of other sites

☑6ᵗʰ **L02.83**   **Carbuncle** of other sites
    L02.831   Carbuncle of **head** [any part, except face]
    L02.838   Carbuncle of other sites

☑5ᵗʰ **L02.9**   Cutaneous abscess, furuncle and carbuncle, unspecified
   L02.91   **Cutaneous abscess**, unspecified   CC
   L02.92   **Furuncle**, unspecified
     Boil NOS
     Furunculosis NOS
   L02.93   **Carbuncle**, unspecified

☑4ᵗʰ **L03**   **Cellulitis and acute lymphangitis**
    EXCLUDES 2   cellulitis of anal and rectal region (K61.-)
           cellulitis of external auditory canal (H60.1)
           cellulitis of eyelid (H00.0)
           cellulitis of female external genital organs (N76.4)
           cellulitis of lacrimal apparatus (H04.3)
           cellulitis of male external genital organs (N48.2, N49.-)
           cellulitis of mouth (K12.2)
           cellulitis of nose (J34.0)
           eosinophilic cellulitis [Wells] (L98.3)
           febrile neutrophilic dermatosis [Sweet] (L98.2)
           lymphangitis (chronic) (subacute) (I89.1)

AHA: 2017,4Q,100
DEF: Cellulitis: Infection of the skin and subcutaneous tissues, most often caused by *Staphylococcus* or *Streptococcus* bacteria secondary to a cutaneous lesion. Progression of the inflammation may lead to abscess and tissue death, or even systemic infection-like bacteremia.
DEF: Lymphangitis: Inflammation of the lymph channels most often caused by *Streptococcus*.

☑5ᵗʰ **L03.0**   Cellulitis and acute lymphangitis of **finger and toe**
     Infection of nail
     Onychia
     Paronychia
     Perionychia

☑6ᵗʰ **L03.01**   **Cellulitis** of **finger**
     Felon
     Whitlow
    EXCLUDES 1   herpetic whitlow (B00.89)
    DEF: Felon: Superficial bacterial skin infection at the tip of the finger.
    L03.011   Cellulitis of **right** finger
    L03.012   Cellulitis of **left** finger
    L03.019   Cellulitis of unspecified finger

☑6ᵗʰ **L03.02**   **Acute lymphangitis** of **finger**
     Hangnail with lymphangitis of finger
    L03.021   Acute lymphangitis of **right** finger
    L03.022   Acute lymphangitis of **left** finger
    L03.029   Acute lymphangitis of unspecified finger

☑6ᵗʰ **L03.03**   **Cellulitis** of **toe**
    L03.031   Cellulitis of **right** toe
    L03.032   Cellulitis of **left** toe
    L03.039   Cellulitis of unspecified toe

☑6ᵗʰ **L03.04**   **Acute lymphangitis** of **toe**
     Hangnail with lymphangitis of toe
    L03.041   Acute lymphangitis of **right** toe
    L03.042   Acute lymphangitis of **left** toe
    L03.049   Acute lymphangitis of unspecified toe

☑5ᵗʰ **L03.1**   Cellulitis and acute lymphangitis of other parts of limb
☑6ᵗʰ **L03.11**   **Cellulitis** of other parts of limb
    EXCLUDES 2   cellulitis of fingers (L03.01-)
           cellulitis of toes (L03.03-)
           groin (L03.314)
    L03.111   Cellulitis of **right axilla**   CC
    L03.112   Cellulitis of **left axilla**   CC
    L03.113   Cellulitis of **right upper** limb   CC
    L03.114   Cellulitis of **left upper** limb   CC

☑ Additional Character Required   ☑x7ᵗʰ Placeholder   Questionable PDx   Manifestation   Unspecified   UPD Unacceptable PDx   H1 - H4 HAC   HCC CMS-HCC Dx   HIV HIV Dx

ICD-10-CM 2025   749

L03.115 Cellulitis of **right lower** limb `CC`
L03.116 Cellulitis of **left lower** limb `CC`
L03.119 Cellulitis of unspecified part of limb `CC` `UNS`

√6th L03.12 **Acute lymphangitis** of other parts of limb
EXCLUDES 2   acute lymphangitis of fingers (L03.2-)
     acute lymphangitis of groin (L03.324)
     acute lymphangitis of toes (L03.04-)

L03.121 Acute lymphangitis of **right axilla** `CC`
L03.122 Acute lymphangitis of **left axilla** `CC`
L03.123 Acute lymphangitis of **right upper** limb `CC`
L03.124 Acute lymphangitis of **left upper** limb `CC`
L03.125 Acute lymphangitis of **right lower** limb `CC`
L03.126 Acute lymphangitis of **left lower** limb `CC`
L03.129 Acute lymphangitis of unspecified part of limb `CC` `UNS`

√5th L03.2 Cellulitis and acute lymphangitis of **face and neck**
√6th L03.21 Cellulitis and acute lymphangitis of **face**
L03.211 **Cellulitis** of face `CC`
EXCLUDES 2   abscess of orbit (H05.01-)
     cellulitis of ear (H60.1-)
     cellulitis of eyelid (H00.0-)
     cellulitis of head (L03.81)
     cellulitis of lacrimal apparatus (H04.3)
     cellulitis of lip (K13.0)
     cellulitis of mouth (K12.2)
     cellulitis of nose (internal) (J34.0)
     cellulitis of orbit (H05.01-)
     cellulitis of scalp (L03.81)
AHA: 2013,4Q,123

L03.212 **Acute lymphangitis** of face `CC`
L03.213 **Periorbital cellulitis** `CC`
Preseptal cellulitis
AHA: 2016,4Q,36

√6th L03.22 Cellulitis and acute lymphangitis of **neck**
L03.221 **Cellulitis** of neck `CC`
L03.222 **Acute lymphangitis** of neck `CC`

√5th L03.3 Cellulitis and acute lymphangitis of **trunk**
√6th L03.31 **Cellulitis** of trunk
EXCLUDES 2   cellulitis of anal and rectal regions (K61.-)
     cellulitis of breast NOS (N61.0)
     cellulitis of female external genital organs (N76.4)
     cellulitis of male external genital organs (N48.2, N49.-)
     omphalitis of newborn (P38.-)
     puerperal cellulitis of breast (O91.2)

L03.311 Cellulitis of **abdominal wall** `CC`
EXCLUDES 2   cellulitis of umbilicus (L03.316)
     cellulitis of groin (L03.314)
L03.312 Cellulitis of **back** [any part except buttock] `CC`
L03.313 Cellulitis of **chest wall** `CC`
L03.314 Cellulitis of **groin** `CC`
L03.315 Cellulitis of **perineum** `CC`
L03.316 Cellulitis of **umbilicus** `CC`
L03.317 Cellulitis of **buttock** `CC`
L03.319 Cellulitis of trunk, unspecified `CC`

√6th L03.32 **Acute lymphangitis** of trunk
L03.321 Acute lymphangitis of **abdominal wall** `CC`
L03.322 Acute lymphangitis of **back** [any part except buttock] `CC`
L03.323 Acute lymphangitis of **chest wall** `CC`
L03.324 Acute lymphangitis of **groin** `CC`
L03.325 Acute lymphangitis of **perineum** `CC`
L03.326 Acute lymphangitis of **umbilicus** `CC`
L03.327 Acute lymphangitis of **buttock** `CC`

L03.329 Acute lymphangitis of trunk, unspecified `CC`

√5th L03.8 Cellulitis and acute lymphangitis of other sites
√6th L03.81 **Cellulitis** of other sites
L03.811 Cellulitis of **head** [any part, except face] `CC`
Cellulitis of scalp
EXCLUDES 2   cellulitis of face (L03.211)
L03.818 Cellulitis of other sites `CC`

√6th L03.89 **Acute lymphangitis** of other sites
L03.891 Acute lymphangitis of **head** [any part, except face] `CC`
L03.898 Acute lymphangitis of other sites `CC`

√5th L03.9 Cellulitis and acute lymphangitis, unspecified
L03.90 **Cellulitis**, unspecified `CC`
L03.91 **Acute lymphangitis**, unspecified `CC`
EXCLUDES 1   lymphangitis NOS (I89.1)

√4th L04 **Acute lymphadenitis**
INCLUDES   abscess (acute) of lymph nodes, except mesenteric
     acute lymphadenitis, except mesenteric
EXCLUDES 1   chronic or subacute lymphadenitis, except mesenteric (I88.1)
     enlarged lymph nodes (R59.-)
     human immunodeficiency virus [HIV] disease resulting in generalized lymphadenopathy (B20)
     lymphadenitis NOS (I88.9)
     nonspecific mesenteric lymphadenitis (I88.0)
DEF: Inflammation or enlargement of the lymph nodes.

L04.0 Acute lymphadenitis of **face, head and neck**
L04.1 Acute lymphadenitis of **trunk**
L04.2 Acute lymphadenitis of **upper limb**
Acute lymphadenitis of axilla
Acute lymphadenitis of shoulder
L04.3 Acute lymphadenitis of **lower limb**
Acute lymphadenitis of hip
EXCLUDES 2   acute lymphadenitis of groin (L04.1)
L04.8 Acute lymphadenitis of other sites
L04.9 Acute lymphadenitis, unspecified

√4th L05 **Pilonidal cyst and sinus**
DEF: Pilonidal cyst: Sac or sinus cavity of trapped epithelial tissues in the sacrococcygeal region, usually associated with ingrown hair.
DEF: Pilonidal sinus: Fistula, tract, or channel that extends from an infected area of ingrown hair to another site within the skin or out to the skin surface.

Pilonidal Cyst

Skin
Fistula
Pilonidal cyst
Fat
Bone

√5th L05.0 Pilonidal cyst and sinus **with abscess**
L05.01 Pilonidal **cyst** with abscess `CC`
Pilonidal abscess
Pilonidal dimple with abscess
Postanal dimple with abscess
EXCLUDES 2   congenital sacral dimple (Q82.6)
     parasacral dimple (Q82.6)
L05.02 Pilonidal **sinus** with abscess `CC`
Coccygeal fistula with abscess
Coccygeal sinus with abscess
Pilonidal fistula with abscess

✓5ᵗʰ **L05.9**   **Pilonidal cyst and sinus without abscess**

     L05.91   **Pilonidal cyst without abscess**
         Pilonidal dimple
         Postanal dimple
         Pilonidal cyst NOS
         EXCLUDES 2   congenital sacral dimple (Q82.6)
                     parasacral dimple (Q82.6)

     L05.92   **Pilonidal sinus without abscess**
         Coccygeal fistula
         Coccygeal sinus without abscess
         Pilonidal fistula

✓4ᵗʰ **L08**   **Other local infections of skin and subcutaneous tissue**

     L08.0   **Pyoderma**
         Dermatitis gangrenosa
         Purulent dermatitis
         Septic dermatitis
         Suppurative dermatitis
         EXCLUDES 1   pyoderma gangrenosum (L88)
                     pyoderma vegetans (L08.81)
         DEF: Any superficial skin disease commonly characterized by the discharging of pus not attributed to another condition.

     L08.1   **Erythrasma**   HIV CC
         DEF: Chronic, superficial skin infection of brown scaly patches, commonly found in skin folds most prevalent in the overweight or diabetic population.

✓5ᵗʰ **L08.8**   **Other specified local infections of the skin and subcutaneous tissue**

     L08.81   **Pyoderma vegetans**
         EXCLUDES 1   pyoderma gangrenosum (L88)
                     pyoderma NOS (L08.0)

     L08.82   **Omphalitis not of newborn**
         EXCLUDES 1   omphalitis of newborn (P38.-)

     L08.89   **Other specified local infections of the skin and subcutaneous tissue**

     L08.9   **Local infection of the skin and subcutaneous tissue, unspecified**

Bullous disorders (L10-L14)

EXCLUDES 1   benign familial pemphigus [Hailey-Hailey] (Q82.8)
              staphylococcal scalded skin syndrome (L00)
              toxic epidermal necrolysis [Lyell] (L51.2)

✓4ᵗʰ **L10**   **Pemphigus**

     EXCLUDES 1   pemphigus neonatorum (L01.03)

     L10.0   **Pemphigus vulgaris**   CC HCC
     L10.1   **Pemphigus vegetans**   CC HCC
     L10.2   **Pemphigus foliaceous**   CC HCC
     L10.3   **Brazilian pemphigus [fogo selvagem]**   CC HCC
     L10.4   **Pemphigus erythematosus**   CC HCC
         Senear-Usher syndrome

     L10.5   **Drug-induced pemphigus**   CC
         Use additional code for adverse effect, if applicable, to identify drug (T36-T50 with fifth or sixth character 5)

✓5ᵗʰ **L10.8**   **Other pemphigus**

     L10.81   **Paraneoplastic pemphigus**   CC HCC
     L10.89   **Other pemphigus**   CC HCC

     L10.9   **Pemphigus, unspecified**   CC HCC

✓4ᵗʰ **L11**   **Other acantholytic disorders**

     L11.0   **Acquired keratosis follicularis**
         EXCLUDES 1   keratosis follicularis (congenital) [Darier-White] (Q82.8)
         AHA: 2021,3Q,10

     L11.1   **Transient acantholytic dermatosis [Grover]**
     L11.8   **Other specified acantholytic disorders**
     L11.9   **Acantholytic disorder, unspecified**

✓4ᵗʰ **L12**   **Pemphigoid**

     EXCLUDES 1   herpes gestationis (O26.4-)
                impetigo herpetiformis (L40.1)

     L12.0   **Bullous pemphigoid**   CC HCC
     L12.1   **Cicatricial pemphigoid**   HCC
         Benign mucous membrane pemphigoid
         DEF: Chronic autoimmune disease characterized by subepidermal blistering lesions of the mucosa, including the conjunctiva. It is seen predominantly in the elderly and produces adhesions and scarring.

     L12.2   **Chronic bullous disease of childhood**   P
         Juvenile dermatitis herpetiformis

✓5ᵗʰ **L12.3**   **Acquired epidermolysis bullosa**

     EXCLUDES 1   epidermolysis bullosa (congenital) (Q81.-)

     L12.30   **Acquired epidermolysis bullosa, unspecified**   CC
     L12.31   **Epidermolysis bullosa due to drug**   CC
         Use additional code for adverse effect, if applicable, to identify drug (T36-T50 with fifth or sixth character 5)

     L12.35   **Other acquired epidermolysis bullosa**   CC

     L12.8   **Other pemphigoid**   CC HCC
     L12.9   **Pemphigoid, unspecified**   CC HCC

✓4ᵗʰ **L13**   **Other bullous disorders**

     L13.0   **Dermatitis herpetiformis**
         Duhring's disease
         Hydroa herpetiformis
         EXCLUDES 1   juvenile dermatitis herpetiformis (L12.2)
                     senile dermatitis herpetiformis (L13.0)
         DEF: Skin disease to which people are genetically predisposed resulting from an immunological response to gluten. Dermatitis herpetiformis is an extremely pruritic eruption of various lesions that frequently heal, leaving hyperpigmentation or hypopigmentation and occasionally scarring. It is usually associated with asymptomatic gluten-sensitive enteropathy.

     L13.1   **Subcorneal pustular dermatitis**
         Sneddon-Wilkinson disease

     L13.8   **Other specified bullous disorders**
     L13.9   **Bullous disorder, unspecified**

L14   *Bullous disorders in diseases classified elsewhere*
     Code first underlying disease

Dermatitis and eczema (L20-L30)

NOTE   In this block the terms dermatitis and eczema are used synonymously and interchangeably.

EXCLUDES 2   chronic (childhood) granulomatous disease (D71)
              dermatitis gangrenosa (L08.0)
              dermatitis herpetiformis (L13.0)
              dry skin dermatitis (L85.3)
              factitial dermatitis (L98.1)
              perioral dermatitis (L71.0)
              radiation-related disorders of the skin and subcutaneous tissue (L55-L59)
              stasis dermatitis (I87.2)

✓4ᵗʰ **L20**   **Atopic dermatitis**

     L20.0   **Besnier's prurigo**

✓5ᵗʰ **L20.8**   **Other atopic dermatitis**

     EXCLUDES 2   circumscribed neurodermatitis (L28.0)

     L20.81   **Atopic neurodermatitis**
         Diffuse neurodermatitis

     L20.82   **Flexural eczema**
     L20.83   **Infantile (acute) (chronic) eczema**   P
     L20.84   **Intrinsic (allergic) eczema**
     L20.89   **Other atopic dermatitis**

     L20.9   **Atopic dermatitis, unspecified**

✓4ᵗʰ **L21**   **Seborrheic dermatitis**

     EXCLUDES 2   infective dermatitis (L30.3)
              seborrheic keratosis (L82.-)

     L21.0   **Seborrhea capitis**
         Cradle cap
         AHA: 2018,1Q,6
         TIP: Assign for dandruff in an adult patient.

     L21.1   **Seborrheic infantile dermatitis**   P
     L21.8   **Other seborrheic dermatitis**
     L21.9   **Seborrheic dermatitis, unspecified**
         Seborrhea NOS

L22   **Diaper dermatitis**
     Diaper erythema
     Diaper rash
     Psoriasiform diaper rash
     AHA: 2021,4Q,18

✓ Additional Character Required   ✓x 7ᵗʰ Placeholder   Questionable PDx   Manifestation   Unspecified   UPD Unacceptable PDx   H1-H14 HAC   HCC CMS-HCC Dx   HIV HIV Dx

✓4ᵗʰ L23 Allergic contact dermatitis

> **EXCLUDES 1**   allergy NOS (T78.40)
> contact dermatitis NOS (L25.9)
> dermatitis NOS (L30.9)
>
> **EXCLUDES 2**   dermatitis due to substances taken internally (L27.-)
> dermatitis of eyelid (H01.1-)
> diaper dermatitis (L22)
> eczema of external ear (H60.5-)
> irritant contact dermatitis (L24.-)
> perioral dermatitis (L71.0)
> radiation-related disorders of the skin and subcutaneous tissue
> (L55-L59)

L23.0 Allergic contact dermatitis due to metals
Allergic contact dermatitis due to chromium
Allergic contact dermatitis due to nickel

L23.1 Allergic contact dermatitis due to adhesives

L23.2 Allergic contact dermatitis due to cosmetics

L23.3 Allergic contact dermatitis due to drugs in contact with skin
Use additional code for adverse effect, if applicable, to identify
drug (T36-T50 with fifth or sixth character 5)
> **EXCLUDES 2**   dermatitis due to ingested drugs and medicaments
> (L27.0-L27.1)

L23.4 Allergic contact dermatitis due to dyes

L23.5 Allergic contact dermatitis due to other chemical products
Allergic contact dermatitis due to cement
Allergic contact dermatitis due to insecticide
Allergic contact dermatitis due to plastic
Allergic contact dermatitis due to rubber

L23.6 Allergic contact dermatitis due to food in contact with the skin
> **EXCLUDES 2**   dermatitis due to ingested food (L27.2)

L23.7 Allergic contact dermatitis due to plants, except food
> **EXCLUDES 2**   allergy NOS due to pollen (J30.1)

✓5ᵗʰ L23.8 Allergic contact dermatitis due to other agents

L23.81 Allergic contact dermatitis due to animal (cat) (dog) dander
Allergic contact dermatitis due to animal (cat) (dog) hair

L23.89 Allergic contact dermatitis due to other agents

L23.9 Allergic contact dermatitis, unspecified cause
Allergic contact eczema NOS

✓4ᵗʰ L24 Irritant contact dermatitis

> **EXCLUDES 1**   allergy NOS (T78.40)
> contact dermatitis NOS (L25.9)
> dermatitis NOS (L30.9)
>
> **EXCLUDES 2**   allergic contact dermatitis (L23.-)
> dermatitis due to substances taken internally (L27.-)
> dermatitis of eyelid (H01.1-)
> diaper dermatitis (L22)
> eczema of external ear (H60.5-)
> perioral dermatitis (L71.0)
> radiation-related disorders of the skin and subcutaneous tissue
> (L55-L59)

L24.0 Irritant contact dermatitis due to detergents

L24.1 Irritant contact dermatitis due to oils and greases

L24.2 Irritant contact dermatitis due to solvents
Irritant contact dermatitis due to chlorocompound
Irritant contact dermatitis due to cyclohexane
Irritant contact dermatitis due to ester
Irritant contact dermatitis due to glycol
Irritant contact dermatitis due to hydrocarbon
Irritant contact dermatitis due to ketone

L24.3 Irritant contact dermatitis due to cosmetics

L24.4 Irritant contact dermatitis due to drugs in contact with skin
Use additional code for adverse effect, if applicable, to identify
drug (T36-T50 with fifth or sixth character 5)

L24.5 Irritant contact dermatitis due to other chemical products
Irritant contact dermatitis due to cement
Irritant contact dermatitis due to insecticide
Irritant contact dermatitis due to plastic
Irritant contact dermatitis due to rubber

L24.6 Irritant contact dermatitis due to food in contact with skin
> **EXCLUDES 2**   dermatitis due to ingested food (L27.2)

L24.7 Irritant contact dermatitis due to plants, except food
> **EXCLUDES 2**   allergy NOS to pollen (J30.1)

✓5ᵗʰ L24.8 Irritant contact dermatitis due to other agents

L24.81 Irritant contact dermatitis due to metals
Irritant contact dermatitis due to chromium
Irritant contact dermatitis due to nickel

L24.89 Irritant contact dermatitis due to other agents
Irritant contact dermatitis due to dyes

L24.9 Irritant contact dermatitis, unspecified cause
Irritant contact eczema NOS

✓5ᵗʰ L24.A Irritant contact dermatitis due to friction or contact with body fluids
> **EXCLUDES 1**   irritant contact dermatitis related to stoma or fistula
> (L24.B-)
>
> **EXCLUDES 2**   erythema intertrigo (L30.4)
>
> **AHA:** 2021,4Q,16-18

L24.A0 Irritant contact dermatitis due to friction or contact with body fluids, unspecified

L24.A1 Irritant contact dermatitis due to saliva

L24.A2 Irritant contact dermatitis due to fecal, urinary or dual incontinence
> **EXCLUDES 1**   diaper dermatitis (L22)

L24.A9 Irritant contact dermatitis due friction or contact with other specified body fluids
Irritant contact dermatitis related to endotracheal tube
Wound fluids, exudate

✓5ᵗʰ L24.B Irritant contact dermatitis related to stoma or fistula
Use additional code to identify any artificial opening status (Z93.-),
if applicable, for contact dermatitis related to stoma
secretions
> **AHA:** 2021,4Q,16-18

L24.B0 Irritant contact dermatitis related to unspecified stoma or fistula
Irritant contact dermatitis related to fistula NOS
Irritant contact dermatitis related to stoma NOS

L24.B1 Irritant contact dermatitis related to digestive stoma or fistula
Irritant contact dermatitis related to gastrostomy
Irritant contact dermatitis related to jejunostomy
Irritant contact dermatitis related to saliva or spit fistula

L24.B2 Irritant contact dermatitis related to respiratory stoma or fistula
Irritant contact dermatitis related to tracheostomy

L24.B3 Irritant contact dermatitis related to fecal or urinary stoma or fistula
Irritant contact dermatitis related to colostomy
Irritant contact dermatitis related to enterocutaneous fistula
Irritant contact dermatitis related to ileostomy

✓4ᵗʰ L25 Unspecified contact dermatitis

> **EXCLUDES 1**   allergic contact dermatitis (L23.-)
> allergy NOS (T78.40)
> dermatitis NOS (L30.9)
> irritant contact dermatitis (L24.-)
>
> **EXCLUDES 2**   dermatitis due to ingested substances (L27.-)
> dermatitis of eyelid (H01.1-)
> eczema of external ear (H60.5-)
> perioral dermatitis (L71.0)
> radiation-related disorders of the skin and subcutaneous tissue
> (L55-L59)

L25.0 Unspecified contact dermatitis due to cosmetics

L25.1 Unspecified contact dermatitis due to drugs in contact with skin
Use additional code for adverse effect, if applicable, to identify
drug (T36-T50 with fifth or sixth character 5)
> **EXCLUDES 2**   dermatitis due to ingested drugs and medicaments
> (L27.0-L27.1)

L25.2 Unspecified contact dermatitis due to dyes

L25.3 Unspecified contact dermatitis due to other chemical products
Unspecified contact dermatitis due to cement
Unspecified contact dermatitis due to insecticide

L25.4 Unspecified contact dermatitis due to food in contact with skin
> **EXCLUDES 2**   dermatitis due to ingested food (L27.2)

L25.5 Unspecified contact dermatitis due to plants, except food
> **EXCLUDES 1**   nettle rash (L50.9)
>
> **EXCLUDES 2**   allergy NOS due to pollen (J30.1)

L25.8 Unspecified contact dermatitis due to other agents

L25.9   Unspecified contact dermatitis, unspecified cause
Contact dermatitis (occupational) NOS
Contact eczema (occupational) NOS

L26   **Exfoliative dermatitis**
Hebra's pityriasis
EXCLUDES 1   *Ritter's disease (L00)*

✓4ᵗʰ **L27**   **Dermatitis due to substances taken internally**
EXCLUDES 1   *allergy NOS (T78.40)*
EXCLUDES 2   *adverse food reaction, except dermatitis (T78.0-T78.1)*
contact dermatitis (L23-L25)
drug photoallergic response (L56.1)
drug phototoxic response (L56.0)
urticaria (L50.-)

L27.0   **Generalized skin eruption due to drugs and medicaments taken internally**
Use additional code for adverse effect, if applicable, to identify drug (T36-T50 with fifth or sixth character 5)

L27.1   **Localized skin eruption due to drugs and medicaments taken internally**
Use additional code for adverse effect, if applicable, to identify drug (T36-T50 with fifth or sixth character 5)

L27.2   **Dermatitis due to ingested food**
EXCLUDES 2   *dermatitis due to food in contact with skin (L23.6, L24.6, L25.4)*

L27.8   Dermatitis due to other substances taken internally
L27.9   Dermatitis due to unspecified substance taken internally

✓4ᵗʰ **L28**   **Lichen simplex chronicus and prurigo**
L28.0   **Lichen simplex chronicus**
Circumscribed neurodermatitis
Lichen NOS

L28.1   **Prurigo nodularis**
L28.2   **Other prurigo**
Prurigo NOS
Prurigo Hebra
Prurigo mitis
Urticaria papulosa

✓4ᵗʰ **L29**   **Pruritus**
EXCLUDES 1   *neurotic excoriation (L98.1)*
psychogenic pruritus (F45.8)

L29.0   **Pruritus ani**
L29.1   **Pruritus scroti**
L29.2   **Pruritus vulvae**
L29.3   **Anogenital pruritus, unspecified**

▲   ✓5ᵗʰ **L29.8**   **Other pruritus**
●   **L29.81**   **Cholestatic pruritus**
Code also, if applicable, type of liver disease
Use additional code for adverse effect, if applicable, to identify drug (T36-T50 with fifth or sixth character 5)

●   **L29.89**   **Other pruritus**
L29.9   **Pruritus, unspecified**
Itch NOS

✓4ᵗʰ **L30**   **Other and unspecified dermatitis**
EXCLUDES 2   *contact dermatitis (L23-L25)*
dry skin dermatitis (L85.3)
small plaque parapsoriasis (L41.3)
stasis dermatitis (I87.2)

L30.0   **Nummular dermatitis**
L30.1   **Dyshidrosis [pompholyx]**
L30.2   **Cutaneous autosensitization**
Candidid [levurid]
Dermatophytid
Eczematid

L30.3   **Infective dermatitis**
Infectious eczematoid dermatitis

L30.4   **Erythema intertrigo**
L30.5   **Pityriasis alba**
AHA: 2018,1Q,6

L30.8   **Other specified dermatitis**
L30.9   **Dermatitis, unspecified**
Eczema NOS

Papulosquamous disorders (L40-L45)

✓4ᵗʰ **L40**   **Psoriasis**
DEF: Chronic autoimmune condition that speeds up skin cell growth, causing excessive immature skin cells to form raised, rounded erythematous lesions covered by dry, silvery scaling patches. Most commonly found on the scalp, elbows, knees, hands, feet, and genitals, it can also affect the joints with stiffness and swelling.

L40.0   **Psoriasis vulgaris**
Nummular psoriasis
Plaque psoriasis

L40.1   **Generalized pustular psoriasis**
Impetigo herpetiformis
Von Zumbusch's disease

L40.2   **Acrodermatitis continua**
L40.3   **Pustulosis palmaris et plantaris**
L40.4   **Guttate psoriasis**

✓5ᵗʰ **L40.5**   **Arthropathic psoriasis**
L40.50   **Arthropathic psoriasis, unspecified**   HCC
L40.51   **Distal interphalangeal psoriatic arthropathy**   HCC
L40.52   **Psoriatic arthritis mutilans**   HCC
L40.53   **Psoriatic spondylitis**   HCC
L40.54   **Psoriatic juvenile arthropathy**   HCC
L40.59   **Other psoriatic arthropathy**   HCC

L40.8   **Other psoriasis**
Flexural psoriasis

L40.9   Psoriasis, unspecified

✓4ᵗʰ **L41**   **Parapsoriasis**
EXCLUDES 1   *poikiloderma vasculare atrophicans (L94.5)*

L41.0   **Pityriasis lichenoides et varioliformis acuta**
Mucha-Habermann disease

L41.1   **Pityriasis lichenoides chronica**
L41.3   **Small plaque parapsoriasis**
L41.4   **Large plaque parapsoriasis**
L41.5   **Retiform parapsoriasis**
L41.8   **Other parapsoriasis**
L41.9   **Parapsoriasis, unspecified**

L42   **Pityriasis rosea**

✓4ᵗʰ **L43**   **Lichen planus**
EXCLUDES 1   *lichen planopilaris ▶(L66.1-)◀*

L43.0   **Hypertrophic lichen planus**
L43.1   **Bullous lichen planus**
L43.2   **Lichenoid drug reaction**
Use additional code for adverse effect, if applicable, to identify drug (T36-T50 with fifth or sixth character 5)

L43.3   **Subacute (active) lichen planus**
Lichen planus tropicus

L43.8   **Other lichen planus**
L43.9   **Lichen planus, unspecified**

✓4ᵗʰ **L44**   **Other papulosquamous disorders**
L44.0   **Pityriasis rubra pilaris**
L44.1   **Lichen nitidus**
DEF: Chronic, inflammatory, asymptomatic skin disorder, characterized by numerous glistening, flat-topped, discrete, skin-colored micropapules, most often on the penis, lower abdomen, inner thighs, wrists, forearms, breasts, and buttocks.

L44.2   **Lichen striatus**
L44.3   **Lichen ruber moniliformis**
L44.4   **Infantile papular acrodermatitis [Gianotti-Crosti]**   P
L44.8   **Other specified papulosquamous disorders**
L44.9   **Papulosquamous disorder, unspecified**

L45   *Papulosquamous disorders in diseases classified elsewhere*
Code first underlying disease

✓ Additional Character Required   ✓x7ᵗʰ Placeholder   Questionable PDx   Manifestation   Unspecified   UPD Unacceptable PDx   H1 -H14 HAC   HCC CMS-HCC Dx   HIV HIV Dx

ICD-10-CM 2025   753

Chapter 12. Diseases of the Skin and Subcutaneous Tissue

L49–L55.9

Urticaria and erythema (L49-L54)

EXCLUDES 1   Lyme disease (A69.2-)
                    rosacea (L71.-)

✓4ᵗʰ **L49 Exfoliation due to erythematous conditions according to extent of body surface involved**

     Code first erythematous condition causing exfoliation, such as:
         Ritter's disease (L00)
         (Staphylococcal) scalded skin syndrome (L00)
         Stevens-Johnson syndrome (L51.1)
         Stevens-Johnson syndrome-toxic epidermal necrolysis overlap syndrome (L51.3)
         toxic epidermal necrolysis (L51.2)

     DEF: Exfoliation: Falling or sloughing off skin in layers.

L49.0 Exfoliation due to erythematous condition involving less than 10 percent of body surface UPD
     Exfoliation due to erythematous condition NOS

L49.1 Exfoliation due to erythematous condition involving 10-19 percent of body surface UPD

L49.2 Exfoliation due to erythematous condition involving 20-29 percent of body surface UPD

L49.3 Exfoliation due to erythematous condition involving 30-39 percent of body surface CC UPD

L49.4 Exfoliation due to erythematous condition involving 40-49 percent of body surface CC UPD

L49.5 Exfoliation due to erythematous condition involving 50-59 percent of body surface CC UPD

L49.6 Exfoliation due to erythematous condition involving 60-69 percent of body surface CC UPD

L49.7 Exfoliation due to erythematous condition involving 70-79 percent of body surface CC UPD

L49.8 Exfoliation due to erythematous condition involving 80-89 percent of body surface CC UPD

L49.9 Exfoliation due to erythematous condition involving 90 or more percent of body surface CC UPD

✓4ᵗʰ **L50 Urticaria**

     EXCLUDES 1   allergic contact dermatitis (L23.-)
                   angioneurotic edema (T78.3)
                   giant urticaria (T78.3)
                   hereditary angio-edema (D84.1)
                   Quincke's edema (T78.3)
                   serum urticaria (T80.6-)
                   solar urticaria (L56.3)
                   urticaria neonatorum (P83.8)
                   urticaria papulosa (L28.2)
                   urticaria pigmentosa (D47.01)

     DEF: Eruption of itching edema of the skin. **Synonym(s): hives.**

L50.0 Allergic urticaria

L50.1 Idiopathic urticaria

L50.2 Urticaria due to cold and heat
     EXCLUDES 2   familial cold urticaria (M04.2)

L50.3 Dermatographic urticaria

L50.4 Vibratory urticaria

L50.5 Cholinergic urticaria

L50.6 Contact urticaria

L50.8 Other urticaria
     Chronic urticaria
     Recurrent periodic urticaria

L50.9 Urticaria, unspecified

✓4ᵗʰ **L51 Erythema multiforme**

     Use additional code for adverse effect, if applicable, to identify drug (T36-T50 with fifth or sixth character 5)
     Use additional code to identify associated manifestations, such as:
         arthropathy associated with dermatological disorders (M14.8-)
         conjunctival edema (H11.42)
         conjunctivitis (H10.22-)
         corneal scars and opacities (H17.-)
         corneal ulcer (H16.0-)
         edema of eyelid (H02.84-)
         inflammation of eyelid (H01.8)
         keratoconjunctivitis sicca (H16.22-)
         mechanical lagophthalmos (H02.22-)
         stomatitis (K12.-)
         symblepharon (H11.23-)
     Use additional code to identify percentage of skin exfoliation (L49.-)

     EXCLUDES 1   staphylococcal scalded skin syndrome (L00)
                   Ritter's disease (L00)

     DEF: Acute complex of symptoms with a varied pattern of skin eruptions, such as macular, bullous, papular, nodose, or vesicular lesions on the neck, face, and legs. Erythema (redness of skin and mucous membranes) multiforme (multiple forms) is a hypersensitivity (allergic) reaction that can occur at any age but primarily affects children or young adults.

L51.0 Nonbullous erythema multiforme

L51.1 Stevens-Johnson syndrome CC

L51.2 Toxic epidermal necrolysis [Lyell] CC

L51.3 Stevens-Johnson syndrome-toxic epidermal necrolysis overlap syndrome CC
     SJS-TEN overlap syndrome

L51.8 Other erythema multiforme

L51.9 Erythema multiforme, unspecified
     Erythema iris
     Erythema multiforme major NOS
     Erythema multiforme minor NOS
     Herpes iris

L52 Erythema nodosum

     EXCLUDES 1   tuberculous erythema nodosum (A18.4)
     DEF: Form of panniculitis (inflammation of the fat layer beneath the skin) most often occurring in women. Commonly seen as a hypersensitivity reaction to infections, drugs, sarcoidosis, and specific enteropathies. The acute stage is associated with fever, malaise, and arthralgia. The lesions are pink to blue in color as tender nodules and are found on the front of the legs below the knees.

✓4ᵗʰ **L53 Other erythematous conditions**

     EXCLUDES 1   erythema ab igne (L59.0)
                   erythema due to external agents in contact with skin (L23-L25)
                   erythema intertrigo (L30.4)

L53.0 Toxic erythema CC
     Code first poisoning due to drug or toxin, if applicable (T36-T65 with fifth or sixth character 1-4)
     Use additional code for adverse effect, if applicable, to identify drug (T36-T50 with fifth or sixth character 5)
     EXCLUDES 1   neonatal erythema toxicum (P83.1)

L53.1 Erythema annulare centrifugum CC

L53.2 Erythema marginatum CC

L53.3 Other chronic figurate erythema CC

L53.8 Other specified erythematous conditions

L53.9 Erythematous condition, unspecified
     Erythema NOS
     Erythroderma NOS

L54 Erythema in diseases classified elsewhere
     Code first underlying disease

Radiation-related disorders of the skin and subcutaneous tissue (L55-L59)

✓4ᵗʰ **L55 Sunburn**

L55.0 Sunburn of first degree

L55.1 Sunburn of second degree

L55.2 Sunburn of third degree

L55.9 Sunburn, unspecified

✓4th **L56 Other acute skin changes due to ultraviolet radiation**

Use additional code to identify the source of the ultraviolet radiation (W89, X32)

L56.0 Drug phototoxic response

Use additional code for adverse effect, if applicable, to identify drug (T36-T50 with fifth or sixth character 5)

L56.1 Drug photoallergic response

Use additional code for adverse effect, if applicable, to identify drug (T36-T50 with fifth or sixth character 5)

L56.2 Photocontact dermatitis [berloque dermatitis]

L56.3 Solar urticaria

L56.4 Polymorphous light eruption

L56.5 Disseminated superficial actinic porokeratosis (DSAP)

DEF: Autosomal dominant skin condition occurring in sun-exposed areas of the skin (particularly the arms and legs), characterized by superficial annular, keratotic, brownish-red spots or thickenings with depressed centers and sharp, ridged borders. It may evolve into squamous cell carcinoma.

L56.8 Other specified acute skin changes due to ultraviolet radiation

L56.9 Acute skin change due to ultraviolet radiation, unspecified

✓4th **L57 Skin changes due to chronic exposure to nonionizing radiation**

Use additional code to identify the source of the ultraviolet radiation (W89), or other nonionizing radiation (W90)

L57.0 Actinic keratosis

Keratosis NOS
Senile keratosis
Solar keratosis

L57.1 Actinic reticuloid

L57.2 Cutis rhomboidalis nuchae

L57.3 Poikiloderma of Civatte

L57.4 Cutis laxa senilis

Elastosis senilis

L57.5 Actinic granuloma

L57.8 Other skin changes due to chronic exposure to nonionizing radiation

Farmer's skin
Sailor's skin
Solar dermatitis

L57.9 Skin changes due to chronic exposure to nonionizing radiation, unspecified

✓4th **L58 Radiodermatitis**

Use additional code to identify the source of the radiation (W88, W90)

L58.0 Acute radiodermatitis

L58.1 Chronic radiodermatitis

L58.9 Radiodermatitis, unspecified

✓4th **L59 Other disorders of skin and subcutaneous tissue related to radiation**

L59.0 Erythema ab igne [dermatitis ab igne]

L59.8 Other specified disorders of the skin and subcutaneous tissue related to radiation

AHA: 2017,1Q,33

L59.9 Disorder of the skin and subcutaneous tissue related to radiation, unspecified

Disorders of skin appendages (L60-L75)

EXCLUDES 1   congenital malformations of integument (Q84.-)

✓4th **L60 Nail disorders**

EXCLUDES 2   clubbing of nails (R68.3)
                onychia and paronychia (L03.0-)

Nail Disorders

Normal

Koilonychia

Beau's Lines

L60.0 Ingrowing nail

L60.1 Onycholysis

L60.2 Onychogryphosis

L60.3 Nail dystrophy

L60.4 Beau's lines

L60.5 Yellow nail syndrome

L60.8 Other nail disorders

L60.9 Nail disorder, unspecified

L62 Nail disorders in diseases classified elsewhere

Code first underlying disease, such as:
pachydermoperiostosis (M89.4-)

✓4th **L63 Alopecia areata**

L63.0 Alopecia (capitis) totalis

L63.1 Alopecia universalis

L63.2 Ophiasis

L63.8 Other alopecia areata

L63.9 Alopecia areata, unspecified

✓4th **L64 Androgenic alopecia**

INCLUDES   male-pattern baldness

L64.0 Drug-induced androgenic alopecia

Use additional code for adverse effect, if applicable, to identify drug (T36-T50 with fifth or sixth character 5)

L64.8 Other androgenic alopecia

L64.9 Androgenic alopecia, unspecified

✓4th **L65 Other nonscarring hair loss**

Use additional code for adverse effect, if applicable, to identify drug (T36-T50 with fifth or sixth character 5)

EXCLUDES 1   trichotillomania (F63.3)

L65.0 Telogen effluvium

DEF: Form of nonscarring alopecia characterized by shedding of hair from premature telogen development in follicles due to stress, including shock, childbirth, surgery, drugs, or weight loss.

L65.1 Anagen effluvium

L65.2 Alopecia mucinosa

L65.8 Other specified nonscarring hair loss

L65.9 Nonscarring hair loss, unspecified

Alopecia NOS

✓4th **L66 Cicatricial alopecia [scarring hair loss]**

L66.0 Pseudopelade

▲ ✓5th **L66.1 Lichen planopilaris**

~~Follicular lichen planus~~

●   **L66.10 Lichen planopilaris, unspecified**

●   **L66.11 Classic lichen planopilaris**

Follicular lichen planus

●   **L66.12 Frontal fibrosing alopecia**

FFA

Chapter 12. Diseases of the Skin and Subcutaneous Tissue

●   L66.19   **Other lichen planopilaris**
       Lassueur Graham-Little Piccardi syndrome

   L66.2   **Folliculitis decalvans**

   L66.3   **Perifolliculitis capitis abscedens**

   L66.4   **Folliculitis ulerythematosa reticulata**

▲   ✓5ᵗʰ   L66.8   **Other cicatricial alopecia**
       AHA: 2015,1Q,19

●   L66.81   **Central centrifugal** cicatricial alopecia
       CCCA

●   L66.89   **Other cicatricial alopecia**

   L66.9   **Cicatricial alopecia, unspecified**

✓4ᵗʰ   **L67   Hair color and hair shaft abnormalities**
     EXCLUDES 1   monilethrix (Q84.1)
          pili annulati (Q84.1)
          telogen effluvium (L65.0)

   L67.0   **Trichorrhexis nodosa**

   L67.1   **Variations in hair color**
       Canities
       Greyness, hair (premature)
       Heterochromia of hair
       Poliosis circumscripta, acquired
       Poliosis NOS

   L67.8   **Other hair color and hair shaft abnormalities**
       Fragilitas crinium

   L67.9   **Hair color and hair shaft abnormality, unspecified**

✓4ᵗʰ   **L68   Hypertrichosis**
     INCLUDES   excess hair
     EXCLUDES 1   congenital hypertrichosis (Q84.2)
          persistent lanugo (Q84.2)

   L68.0   **Hirsutism**

   L68.1   **Acquired hypertrichosis lanuginosa**

   L68.2   **Localized hypertrichosis**

   L68.3   **Polytrichia**

   L68.8   **Other hypertrichosis**

   L68.9   **Hypertrichosis, unspecified**

✓4ᵗʰ   **L70   Acne**
     EXCLUDES 2   acne keloid (L73.0)

   L70.0   **Acne vulgaris**

   L70.1   **Acne conglobata**

   L70.2   **Acne varioliformis**
       Acne necrotica miliaris
       DEF: Rare form of acne characterized by development of persistent brown papulopustules followed by scar formation. This type of acne usually presents on the brow and temporoparietal part of the scalp.

   L70.3   **Acne tropica**

   L70.4   **Infantile acne**   P

   L70.5   **Acné excoriée**
       Acné excoriée des jeunes filles
       Picker's acne

   L70.8   **Other acne**

   L70.9   **Acne, unspecified**

✓4ᵗʰ   **L71   Rosacea**
     Use additional code for adverse effect, if applicable, to identify drug (T36-T50 with fifth or sixth character 5)

   L71.0   **Perioral dermatitis**

   L71.1   **Rhinophyma**

   L71.8   **Other rosacea**
       AHA: 2018,4Q,15

   L71.9   **Rosacea, unspecified**

✓4ᵗʰ   **L72   Follicular cysts of skin and subcutaneous tissue**

   L72.0   **Epidermal cyst**

✓5ᵗʰ   L72.1   **Pilar and trichodermal cyst**

     L72.11   **Pilar cyst**

     L72.12   **Trichodermal cyst**
       Trichilemmal (proliferating) cyst

   L72.2   **Steatocystoma multiplex**

   L72.3   **Sebaceous cyst**
     EXCLUDES 2   pilar cyst (L72.11)
          trichilemmal (proliferating) cyst (L72.12)

   L72.8   **Other follicular cysts of the skin and subcutaneous tissue**

   L72.9   **Follicular cyst of the skin and subcutaneous tissue, unspecified**

✓4ᵗʰ   **L73   Other follicular disorders**

   L73.0   **Acne keloid**

   L73.1   **Pseudofolliculitis barbae**

   L73.2   **Hidradenitis suppurativa**

   L73.8   **Other specified follicular disorders**
       Sycosis barbae

   L73.9   **Follicular disorder, unspecified**

✓4ᵗʰ   **L74   Eccrine sweat disorders**
     EXCLUDES 2   generalized hyperhidrosis (R61)
     DEF: Eccrine sweat glands: Glands found in the dermal and hypodermal layer of the skin throughout the body, particularly on the forehead, scalp, axillae, palms, and soles. These glands produce watery and neutral or slightly acidic sweat.

   L74.0   **Miliaria rubra**

   L74.1   **Miliaria crystallina**

   L74.2   **Miliaria profunda**
       Miliaria tropicalis

   L74.3   **Miliaria, unspecified**

   L74.4   **Anhidrosis**
       Hypohidrosis
       DEF: Inability to sweat normally. When the body can't cool itself through perspiration it can lead to heatstroke, a life-threatening condition.

✓5ᵗʰ   L74.5   **Focal hyperhidrosis**

     ✓6ᵗʰ   L74.51   **Primary focal hyperhidrosis**

         L74.510   **Primary focal hyperhidrosis, axilla**

         L74.511   **Primary focal hyperhidrosis, face**

         L74.512   **Primary focal hyperhidrosis, palms**

         L74.513   **Primary focal hyperhidrosis, soles**

         L74.519   **Primary focal hyperhidrosis, unspecified**

     L74.52   **Secondary focal hyperhidrosis**
       Frey's syndrome

   L74.8   **Other eccrine sweat disorders**

   L74.9   **Eccrine sweat disorder, unspecified**
       Sweat gland disorder NOS

✓4ᵗʰ   **L75   Apocrine sweat disorders**
     EXCLUDES 1   dyshidrosis (L30.1)
          hidradenitis suppurativa (L73.2)
     DEF: Apocrine sweat glands: Found in the axilla, areola, and circumanal region, these glands begin to function in puberty and produce viscid milky secretions in response to external stimuli.

   L75.0   **Bromhidrosis**

   L75.1   **Chromhidrosis**

   L75.2   **Apocrine miliaria**
       Fox-Fordyce disease
       DEF: Chronic, usually pruritic disease evidenced by small follicular papular eruptions, especially in the axillary and pubic areas. Apocrine miliaria develops from the closure and rupture of the affected apocrine glands' intraepidermal portion of the ducts.

   L75.8   **Other apocrine sweat disorders**

   L75.9   **Apocrine sweat disorder, unspecified**

Intraoperative and postprocedural complications of skin and subcutaneous tissue (L76)

✓4ᵗʰ   **L76   Intraoperative and postprocedural complications of skin and subcutaneous tissue**
     AHA: 2016,4Q,9-10

✓5ᵗʰ   L76.0   **Intraoperative hemorrhage and hematoma of skin and subcutaneous tissue complicating a procedure**
     EXCLUDES 1   intraoperative hemorrhage and hematoma of skin and subcutaneous tissue due to accidental puncture and laceration during a procedure (L76.1-)

     L76.01   **Intraoperative hemorrhage and hematoma of skin and subcutaneous tissue complicating a dermatologic procedure**   CC

     L76.02   **Intraoperative hemorrhage and hematoma of skin and subcutaneous tissue complicating other procedure**   CC

✓5ᵗʰ   L76.1   **Accidental puncture and laceration of skin and subcutaneous tissue during a procedure**

     L76.11   **Accidental puncture and laceration of skin and subcutaneous tissue during a dermatologic procedure**   CC

     L76.12   **Accidental puncture and laceration of skin and subcutaneous tissue during other procedure**   CC

√5ᵗʰ **L76.2** Postprocedural hemorrhage of skin and subcutaneous tissue following a procedure

L76.21 Postprocedural hemorrhage of skin and subcutaneous tissue following a dermatologic procedure `CC`

L76.22 Postprocedural hemorrhage of skin and subcutaneous tissue following other procedure `CC`

√5ᵗʰ **L76.3** Postprocedural hematoma and seroma of skin and subcutaneous tissue following a procedure

L76.31 Postprocedural hematoma of skin and subcutaneous tissue following a dermatologic procedure `CC`

L76.32 Postprocedural hematoma of skin and subcutaneous tissue following other procedure `CC`

L76.33 Postprocedural seroma of skin and subcutaneous tissue following a dermatologic procedure `CC`

L76.34 Postprocedural seroma of skin and subcutaneous tissue following other procedure `CC`

√5ᵗʰ **L76.8** Other intraoperative and postprocedural complications of skin and subcutaneous tissue

Use additional code, if applicable, to further specify disorder

L76.81 Other intraoperative complications of skin and subcutaneous tissue

L76.82 Other postprocedural complications of skin and subcutaneous tissue

AHA: 2017,3Q,6

Other disorders of the skin and subcutaneous tissue (L80-L99)

L80 Vitiligo

EXCLUDES 2 vitiligo of eyelids (H02.73-)

vitiligo of vulva (N90.89)

DEF: Persistent, progressive development of nonpigmented white patches on otherwise normal skin.

√4ᵗʰ **L81** Other disorders of pigmentation

EXCLUDES 1 birthmark NOS (Q82.5)

Peutz-Jeghers syndrome (Q85.89)

EXCLUDES 2 nevus - see Alphabetical Index

L81.0 Postinflammatory hyperpigmentation

L81.1 Chloasma

L81.2 Freckles

L81.3 Cafe au lait spots

L81.4 Other melanin hyperpigmentation
Lentigo

L81.5 Leukoderma, not elsewhere classified

L81.6 Other disorders of diminished melanin formation

L81.7 Pigmented purpuric dermatosis
Angioma serpiginosum

L81.8 Other specified disorders of pigmentation
Iron pigmentation
Tattoo pigmentation

L81.9 Disorder of pigmentation, unspecified

√4ᵗʰ **L82** Seborrheic keratosis

INCLUDES basal cell papilloma
dermatosis papulosa nigra
Leser-Trélat disease

EXCLUDES 2 seborrheic dermatitis (L21.-)

DEF: Common, benign, noninvasive, lightly pigmented, warty growth composed of basaloid cells that usually appear at middle age as soft, easily crumbling plaques on the face, trunk, and extremities.

L82.0 Inflamed seborrheic keratosis
AHA: 2023,2Q,12; 2021,3Q,10

L82.1 Other seborrheic keratosis
Seborrheic keratosis NOS

L83 Acanthosis nigricans
Confluent and reticulated papillomatosis

DEF: Diffuse, velvety hyperplasia of the spinous skin layer of the axilla and other body folds marked by gray, brown, or black pigmentation. In adult form, it is often associated with malignant acanthosis nigricans in a benign, nevoid form relatively generalized.

L84 Corns and callosities
Callus
Clavus

√4ᵗʰ **L85** Other epidermal thickening

EXCLUDES 2 hypertrophic disorders of the skin (L91.-)

L85.0 Acquired ichthyosis
EXCLUDES 1 congenital ichthyosis (Q80.-)

L85.1 Acquired keratosis [keratoderma] palmaris et plantaris
EXCLUDES 1 inherited keratosis palmaris et plantaris (Q82.8)

L85.2 Keratosis punctata (palmaris et plantaris)

L85.3 Xerosis cutis
Dry skin dermatitis

L85.8 Other specified epidermal thickening
Cutaneous horn

L85.9 Epidermal thickening, unspecified

L86 *Keratoderma in diseases classified elsewhere*

Code first underlying disease, such as:
Reiter's disease (M02.3-)

EXCLUDES 1 gonococcal keratoderma (A54.89)
gonococcal keratosis (A54.89)
keratoderma due to vitamin A deficiency (E50.8)
keratosis due to vitamin A deficiency (E50.8)
xeroderma due to vitamin A deficiency (E50.8)

√4ᵗʰ **L87** Transepidermal elimination disorders

EXCLUDES 1 granuloma annulare (perforating) (L92.0)

L87.0 Keratosis follicularis et parafollicularis in cutem penetrans
Hyperkeratosis follicularis penetrans
Kyrle disease

L87.1 Reactive perforating collagenosis

L87.2 Elastosis perforans serpiginosa

L87.8 Other transepidermal elimination disorders

L87.9 Transepidermal elimination disorder, unspecified

L88 Pyoderma gangrenosum `CC` `HCC`
Phagedenic pyoderma

EXCLUDES 1 dermatitis gangrenosa (L08.0)

DEF: Persistent debilitating skin disease characterized by irregular, boggy, blue-red ulcerations, with central healing and undermined edges.

√4ᵗʰ **L89** Pressure ulcer

INCLUDES bed sore
decubitus ulcer
plaster ulcer
pressure area
pressure sore

Code first any associated gangrene (I96)

EXCLUDES 2 decubitus (trophic) ulcer of cervix (uteri) (N86)
diabetic ulcers (E08.621, E08.622, E09.621, E09.622, E10.621, E10.622, E11.621, E11.622, E13.621, E13.622)
non-pressure chronic ulcer of skin (L97.-)
skin infections (L00-L08)
varicose ulcer (I83.0, I83.2)

AHA: 2022,2Q,8; 2021,1Q,24; 2019,4Q,10-11,54; 2018,4Q,69; 2018,3Q,3; 2018,2Q,21; 2017,4Q,109; 2017,1Q,49; 2016,4Q,143

TIP: The stage of a diagnosed pressure ulcer can be based on documentation from clinicians who are not the patient's provider.

Four Stages of Pressure Ulcer

Stage 1
Persistent focal edema

Stage 2
Abrasion, blister, partial thickness skin loss involving epidermis and/or dermis

Stage 3
Full thickness skin loss involving damage or necrosis of subcutaneous tissue

Stage 4
Necrosis of soft tissues through to underlying muscle, tendon, or bone

√5ᵗʰ **L89.0** Pressure ulcer of elbow

√6ᵗʰ **L89.00** Pressure ulcer of unspecified elbow

L89.000 Pressure ulcer of unspecified elbow, unstageable `HCC`

☑ Additional Character Required √x7ᵗʰ Placeholder Questionable PDx Manifestation Unspecified UPD Unacceptable PDx H1-H14 HAC HCC CMS-HCC Dx HIV HIV Dx

ICD-10-CM 2025 757

L89.001 **Pressure ulcer of unspecified elbow, stage 1**

Healing pressure ulcer of unspecified elbow, stage 1

Pressure pre-ulcer skin changes limited to persistent focal edema, unspecified elbow

L89.002 **Pressure ulcer of unspecified elbow, stage 2** `HCC`

Healing pressure ulcer of unspecified elbow, stage 2

Pressure ulcer with abrasion, blister, partial thickness skin loss involving epidermis and/or dermis, unspecified elbow

L89.003 **Pressure ulcer of unspecified elbow, stage 3** `MCC` `H4` `UNS` `HCC`

Healing pressure ulcer of unspecified elbow, stage 3

Pressure ulcer with full thickness skin loss involving damage or necrosis of subcutaneous tissue, unspecified elbow

L89.004 **Pressure ulcer of unspecified elbow, stage 4** `MCC` `H4` `UNS` `HCC`

Healing pressure ulcer of unspecified elbow, stage 4

Pressure ulcer with necrosis of soft tissues through to underlying muscle, tendon, or bone, unspecified elbow

L89.006 **Pressure-induced deep tissue damage of unspecified elbow**

L89.009 **Pressure ulcer of unspecified elbow, unspecified stage**

Healing pressure ulcer of elbow NOS

Healing pressure ulcer of unspecified elbow, unspecified stage

✓6ᵗʰ **L89.01** **Pressure ulcer of right elbow**

L89.010 **Pressure ulcer of right elbow, unstageable** `HCC`

L89.011 **Pressure ulcer of right elbow, stage 1**

Healing pressure ulcer of right elbow, stage 1

Pressure pre-ulcer skin changes limited to persistent focal edema, right elbow

L89.012 **Pressure ulcer of right elbow, stage 2** `HCC`

Healing pressure ulcer of right elbow, stage 2

Pressure ulcer with abrasion, blister, partial thickness skin loss involving epidermis and/or dermis, right elbow

L89.013 **Pressure ulcer of right elbow, stage 3** `MCC` `H4` `HCC`

Healing pressure ulcer of right elbow, stage 3

Pressure ulcer with full thickness skin loss involving damage or necrosis of subcutaneous tissue, right elbow

L89.014 **Pressure ulcer of right elbow, stage 4** `MCC` `H4` `HCC`

Healing pressure ulcer of right elbow, stage 4

Pressure ulcer with necrosis of soft tissues through to underlying muscle, tendon, or bone, right elbow

L89.016 **Pressure-induced deep tissue damage of right elbow**

L89.019 **Pressure ulcer of right elbow, unspecified stage**

Healing pressure ulcer of right elbow NOS

✓6ᵗʰ **L89.02** **Pressure ulcer of left elbow**

L89.020 **Pressure ulcer of left elbow, unstageable** `HCC`

L89.021 **Pressure ulcer of left elbow, stage 1**

Healing pressure ulcer of left elbow, stage 1

Pressure pre-ulcer skin changes limited to persistent focal edema, left elbow

L89.022 **Pressure ulcer of left elbow, stage 2** `HCC`

Healing pressure ulcer of left elbow, stage 2

Pressure ulcer with abrasion, blister, partial thickness skin loss involving epidermis and/or dermis, left elbow

L89.023 **Pressure ulcer of left elbow, stage 3** `MCC` `H4` `HCC`

Healing pressure ulcer of left elbow, stage 3

Pressure ulcer with full thickness skin loss involving damage or necrosis of subcutaneous tissue, left elbow

L89.024 **Pressure ulcer of left elbow, stage 4** `MCC` `H4` `HCC`

Healing pressure ulcer of left elbow, stage 4

Pressure ulcer with necrosis of soft tissues through to underlying muscle, tendon, or bone, left elbow

L89.026 **Pressure-induced deep tissue damage of left elbow**

L89.029 **Pressure ulcer of left elbow, unspecified stage**

Healing pressure ulcer of left elbow NOS

✓5ᵗʰ **L89.1** **Pressure ulcer of back**

✓6ᵗʰ **L89.10** **Pressure ulcer of unspecified part of back**

L89.100 **Pressure ulcer of unspecified part of back, unstageable** `HCC`

L89.101 **Pressure ulcer of unspecified part of back, stage 1**

Healing pressure ulcer of unspecified part of back, stage 1

Pressure pre-ulcer skin changes limited to persistent focal edema, unspecified part of back

L89.102 **Pressure ulcer of unspecified part of back, stage 2** `HCC`

Healing pressure ulcer of unspecified part of back, stage 2

Pressure ulcer with abrasion, blister, partial thickness skin loss involving epidermis and/or dermis, unspecified part of back

L89.103 **Pressure ulcer of unspecified part of back, stage 3** `MCC` `H4` `UNS` `HCC`

Healing pressure ulcer of unspecified part of back, stage 3

Pressure ulcer with full thickness skin loss involving damage or necrosis of subcutaneous tissue, unspecified part of back

L89.104 **Pressure ulcer of unspecified part of back, stage 4** `MCC` `H4` `UNS` `HCC`

Healing pressure ulcer of unspecified part of back, stage 4

Pressure ulcer with necrosis of soft tissues through to underlying muscle, tendon, or bone, unspecified part of back

L89.106 **Pressure-induced deep tissue damage of unspecified part of back**

L89.109 **Pressure ulcer of unspecified part of back, unspecified stage**

Healing pressure ulcer of unspecified part of back NOS

Healing pressure ulcer of unspecified part of back, unspecified stage

✓6ᵗʰ **L89.11** **Pressure ulcer of right upper back**

Pressure ulcer of right shoulder blade

L89.110 **Pressure ulcer of right upper back, unstageable** `HCC`

L89.111 **Pressure ulcer of right upper back, stage 1**

Healing pressure ulcer of right upper back, stage 1

Pressure pre-ulcer skin changes limited to persistent focal edema, right upper back

L89.112 **Pressure ulcer of right upper back, stage 2** `HCC`

Healing pressure ulcer of right upper back, stage 2

Pressure ulcer with abrasion, blister, partial thickness skin loss involving epidermis and/or dermis, right upper back

L89.113 **Pressure ulcer of right upper back, stage 3** `MCC` `H4` `HCC`

Healing pressure ulcer of right upper back, stage 3

Pressure ulcer with full thickness skin loss involving damage or necrosis of subcutaneous tissue, right upper back

`N` Newborn: 0   `P` Pediatric: 0-17   `M` Maternity: 9-64   `A` Adult: 15-124   `UNS` Unspecified Site   `MCC` Major Complication/Comorbidity   `CC` Complication/Comorbidity   `PE` POA Exempt

758

ICD-10-CM 2025

L89.114 **Pressure ulcer of right upper back, stage 4** `MCC` `H4` `HCC`
Healing pressure ulcer of right upper back, stage 4
Pressure ulcer with necrosis of soft tissues through to underlying muscle, tendon, or bone, right upper back

L89.116 **Pressure-induced deep tissue damage of right upper back**

L89.119 **Pressure ulcer of right upper back, unspecified stage**
Healing pressure ulcer of right upper back NOS
Healing pressure ulcer of right upper back, unspecified stage

√6ᵗʰ **L89.12** **Pressure ulcer of left upper back**
Pressure ulcer of left shoulder blade

L89.120 **Pressure ulcer of left upper back, unstageable** `HCC`

L89.121 **Pressure ulcer of left upper back, stage 1**
Healing pressure ulcer of left upper back, stage 1
Pressure pre-ulcer skin changes limited to persistent focal edema, left upper back

L89.122 **Pressure ulcer of left upper back, stage 2** `HCC`
Healing pressure ulcer of left upper back, stage 2
Pressure ulcer with abrasion, blister, partial thickness skin loss involving epidermis and/or dermis, left upper back

L89.123 **Pressure ulcer of left upper back, stage 3** `MCC` `H4` `HCC`
Healing pressure ulcer of left upper back, stage 3
Pressure ulcer with full thickness skin loss involving damage or necrosis of subcutaneous tissue, left upper back

L89.124 **Pressure ulcer of left upper back, stage 4** `MCC` `H4` `HCC`
Healing pressure ulcer of left upper back, stage 4
Pressure ulcer with necrosis of soft tissues through to underlying muscle, tendon, or bone, left upper back

L89.126 **Pressure-induced deep tissue damage of left upper back**

L89.129 **Pressure ulcer of left upper back, unspecified stage**
Healing pressure ulcer of left upper back NOS
Healing pressure ulcer of left upper back, unspecified stage

√6ᵗʰ **L89.13** **Pressure ulcer of right lower back**

L89.130 **Pressure ulcer of right lower back, unstageable** `HCC`

L89.131 **Pressure ulcer of right lower back, stage 1**
Healing pressure ulcer of right lower back, stage 1
Pressure pre-ulcer skin changes limited to persistent focal edema, right lower back

L89.132 **Pressure ulcer of right lower back, stage 2** `HCC`
Healing pressure ulcer of right lower back, stage 2
Pressure ulcer with abrasion, blister, partial thickness skin loss involving epidermis and/or dermis, right lower back

L89.133 **Pressure ulcer of right lower back, stage 3** `MCC` `H4` `HCC`
Healing pressure ulcer of right lower back, stage 3
Pressure ulcer with full thickness skin loss involving damage or necrosis of subcutaneous tissue, right lower back

L89.134 **Pressure ulcer of right lower back, stage 4** `MCC` `H4` `HCC`
Healing pressure ulcer of right lower back, stage 4
Pressure ulcer with necrosis of soft tissues through to underlying muscle, tendon, or bone, right lower back

L89.136 **Pressure-induced deep tissue damage of right lower back**

L89.139 **Pressure ulcer of right lower back, unspecified stage**
Healing pressure ulcer of right lower back NOS
Healing pressure ulcer of right lower back, unspecified stage

√6ᵗʰ **L89.14** **Pressure ulcer of left lower back**

L89.140 **Pressure ulcer of left lower back, unstageable** `HCC`

L89.141 **Pressure ulcer of left lower back, stage 1**
Healing pressure ulcer of left lower back, stage 1
Pressure pre-ulcer skin changes limited to persistent focal edema, left lower back

L89.142 **Pressure ulcer of left lower back, stage 2** `HCC`
Healing pressure ulcer of left lower back, stage 2
Pressure ulcer with abrasion, blister, partial thickness skin loss involving epidermis and/or dermis, left lower back

L89.143 **Pressure ulcer of left lower back, stage 3** `MCC` `H4` `HCC`
Healing pressure ulcer of left lower back, stage 3
Pressure ulcer with full thickness skin loss involving damage or necrosis of subcutaneous tissue, left lower back

L89.144 **Pressure ulcer of left lower back, stage 4** `MCC` `H4` `HCC`
Healing pressure ulcer of left lower back, stage 4
Pressure ulcer with necrosis of soft tissues through to underlying muscle, tendon, or bone, left lower back

L89.146 **Pressure-induced deep tissue damage of left lower back**

L89.149 **Pressure ulcer of left lower back, unspecified stage**
Healing pressure ulcer of left lower back NOS
Healing pressure ulcer of left lower back, unspecified stage

√6ᵗʰ **L89.15** **Pressure ulcer of sacral region**
Pressure ulcer of coccyx
Pressure ulcer of tailbone
AHA: 2021,3Q,10

L89.150 **Pressure ulcer of sacral region, unstageable** `HCC`

L89.151 **Pressure ulcer of sacral region, stage 1**
Healing pressure ulcer of sacral region, stage 1
Pressure pre-ulcer skin changes limited to persistent focal edema, sacral region

L89.152 **Pressure ulcer of sacral region, stage 2** `HCC`
Healing pressure ulcer of sacral region, stage 2
Pressure ulcer with abrasion, blister, partial thickness skin loss involving epidermis and/or dermis, sacral region

L89.153 **Pressure ulcer of sacral region, stage 3** `MCC` `H4` `HCC`
Healing pressure ulcer of sacral region, stage 3
Pressure ulcer with full thickness skin loss involving damage or necrosis of subcutaneous tissue, sacral region

L89.154 **Pressure ulcer of sacral region, stage 4** `MCC` `H4` `HCC`
Healing pressure ulcer of sacral region, stage 4
Pressure ulcer with necrosis of soft tissues through to underlying muscle, tendon, or bone, sacral region
AHA: 2022,2Q,8

L89.156 **Pressure-induced deep tissue damage of sacral region**

L89.159 **Pressure ulcer of sacral region, unspecified stage**
Healing pressure ulcer of sacral region NOS
Healing pressure ulcer of sacral region, unspecified stage

✓5th **L89.2** **Pressure ulcer of hip**

✓6th **L89.20** **Pressure ulcer of unspecified hip**

L89.200 **Pressure ulcer of unspecified hip, unstageable** `HCC`

L89.201 **Pressure ulcer of unspecified hip, stage 1**
Healing pressure ulcer of unspecified hip back, stage 1
Pressure pre-ulcer skin changes limited to persistent focal edema, unspecified hip

L89.202 **Pressure ulcer of unspecified hip, stage 2** `HCC`
Healing pressure ulcer of unspecified hip, stage 2
Pressure ulcer with abrasion, blister, partial thickness skin loss involving epidermis and/or dermis, unspecified hip

L89.203 **Pressure ulcer of unspecified hip, stage 3** `MCC` `H4` `UNS` `HCC`
Healing pressure ulcer of unspecified hip, stage 3
Pressure ulcer with full thickness skin loss involving damage or necrosis of subcutaneous tissue, unspecified hip

L89.204 **Pressure ulcer of unspecified hip, stage 4** `MCC` `H4` `UNS` `HCC`
Healing pressure ulcer of unspecified hip, stage 4
Pressure ulcer with necrosis of soft tissues through to underlying muscle, tendon, or bone, unspecified hip

L89.206 **Pressure-induced deep tissue damage of unspecified hip**

L89.209 **Pressure ulcer of unspecified hip, unspecified stage**
Healing pressure ulcer of unspecified hip NOS
Healing pressure ulcer of unspecified hip, unspecified stage

✓6th **L89.21** **Pressure ulcer of right hip**

L89.210 **Pressure ulcer of right hip, unstageable** `HCC`

L89.211 **Pressure ulcer of right hip, stage 1**
Healing pressure ulcer of right hip back, stage 1
Pressure pre-ulcer skin changes limited to persistent focal edema, right hip

L89.212 **Pressure ulcer of right hip, stage 2** `HCC`
Healing pressure ulcer of right hip, stage 2
Pressure ulcer with abrasion, blister, partial thickness skin loss involving epidermis and/or dermis, right hip

L89.213 **Pressure ulcer of right hip, stage 3** `MCC` `H4` `HCC`
Healing pressure ulcer of right hip, stage 3
Pressure ulcer with full thickness skin loss involving damage or necrosis of subcutaneous tissue, right hip

L89.214 **Pressure ulcer of right hip, stage 4** `MCC` `H4` `HCC`
Healing pressure ulcer of right hip, stage 4
Pressure ulcer with necrosis of soft tissues through to underlying muscle, tendon, or bone, right hip

L89.216 **Pressure-induced deep tissue damage of right hip**

L89.219 **Pressure ulcer of right hip, unspecified stage**
Healing pressure ulcer of right hip NOS
Healing pressure ulcer of right hip, unspecified stage

✓6th **L89.22** **Pressure ulcer of left hip**

L89.220 **Pressure ulcer of left hip, unstageable** `HCC`

L89.221 **Pressure ulcer of left hip, stage 1**
Healing pressure ulcer of left hip back, stage 1
Pressure pre-ulcer skin changes limited to persistent focal edema, left hip

L89.222 **Pressure ulcer of left hip, stage 2** `HCC`
Healing pressure ulcer of left hip, stage 2
Pressure ulcer with abrasion, blister, partial thickness skin loss involving epidermis and/or dermis, left hip

L89.223 **Pressure ulcer of left hip, stage 3** `MCC` `H4` `HCC`
Healing pressure ulcer of left hip, stage 3
Pressure ulcer with full thickness skin loss involving damage or necrosis of subcutaneous tissue, left hip

L89.224 **Pressure ulcer of left hip, stage 4** `MCC` `H4` `HCC`
Healing pressure ulcer of left hip, stage 4
Pressure ulcer with necrosis of soft tissues through to underlying muscle, tendon, or bone, left hip

L89.226 **Pressure-induced deep tissue damage of left hip**

L89.229 **Pressure ulcer of left hip, unspecified stage**
Healing pressure ulcer of left hip NOS
Healing pressure ulcer of left hip, unspecified stage

✓5th **L89.3** **Pressure ulcer of buttock**
AHA: 2021,3Q,10

✓6th **L89.30** **Pressure ulcer of unspecified buttock**

L89.300 **Pressure ulcer of unspecified buttock, unstageable** `HCC`

L89.301 **Pressure ulcer of unspecified buttock, stage 1**
Healing pressure ulcer of unspecified buttock, stage 1
Pressure pre-ulcer skin changes limited to persistent focal edema, unspecified buttock

L89.302 **Pressure ulcer of unspecified buttock, stage 2** `HCC`
Healing pressure ulcer of unspecified buttock, stage 2
Pressure ulcer with abrasion, blister, partial thickness skin loss involving epidermis and/or dermis, unspecified buttock

L89.303 **Pressure ulcer of unspecified buttock, stage 3** `MCC` `H4` `UNS` `HCC`
Healing pressure ulcer of unspecified buttock, stage 3
Pressure ulcer with full thickness skin loss involving damage or necrosis of subcutaneous tissue, unspecified buttock

L89.304 **Pressure ulcer of unspecified buttock, stage 4** `MCC` `H4` `UNS` `HCC`
Healing pressure ulcer of unspecified buttock, stage 4
Pressure ulcer with necrosis of soft tissues through to underlying muscle, tendon, or bone, unspecified buttock

L89.306 **Pressure-induced deep tissue damage of unspecified buttock**

L89.309 **Pressure ulcer of unspecified buttock, unspecified stage**
Healing pressure ulcer of unspecified buttock NOS
Healing pressure ulcer of unspecified buttock, unspecified stage

✓6th **L89.31** **Pressure ulcer of right buttock**

L89.310 **Pressure ulcer of right buttock, unstageable** `HCC`

L89.311 Pressure ulcer of right buttock, stage 1
Healing pressure ulcer of right buttock, stage 1
Pressure pre-ulcer skin changes limited to persistent focal edema, right buttock

L89.312 Pressure ulcer of right buttock, stage 2 `HCC`
Healing pressure ulcer of right buttock, stage 2
Pressure ulcer with abrasion, blister, partial thickness skin loss involving epidermis and/or dermis, right buttock

L89.313 Pressure ulcer of right buttock, stage 3 `MCC` `H4` `HCC`
Healing pressure ulcer of right buttock, stage 3
Pressure ulcer with full thickness skin loss involving damage or necrosis of subcutaneous tissue, right buttock

L89.314 Pressure ulcer of right buttock, stage 4 `MCC` `H4` `HCC`
Healing pressure ulcer of right buttock, stage 4
Pressure ulcer with necrosis of soft tissues through to underlying muscle, tendon, or bone, right buttock

L89.316 Pressure-induced deep tissue damage of right buttock

L89.319 Pressure ulcer of right buttock, unspecified stage
Healing pressure ulcer of right buttock NOS
Healing pressure ulcer of right buttock, unspecified stage

√6ᵗʰ **L89.32 Pressure ulcer of left buttock**

L89.320 Pressure ulcer of left buttock, unstageable `HCC`

L89.321 Pressure ulcer of left buttock, stage 1
Healing pressure ulcer of left buttock, stage 1
Pressure pre-ulcer skin changes limited to persistent focal edema, left buttock

L89.322 Pressure ulcer of left buttock, stage 2 `HCC`
Healing pressure ulcer of left buttock, stage 2
Pressure ulcer with abrasion, blister, partial thickness skin loss involving epidermis and/or dermis, left buttock

L89.323 Pressure ulcer of left buttock, stage 3 `MCC` `H4` `HCC`
Healing pressure ulcer of left buttock, stage 3
Pressure ulcer with full thickness skin loss involving damage or necrosis of subcutaneous tissue, left buttock

L89.324 Pressure ulcer of left buttock, stage 4 `MCC` `H4` `HCC`
Healing pressure ulcer of left buttock, stage 4
Pressure ulcer with necrosis of soft tissues through to underlying muscle, tendon, or bone, left buttock

L89.326 Pressure-induced deep tissue damage of left buttock

L89.329 Pressure ulcer of left buttock, unspecified stage
Healing pressure ulcer of left buttock NOS
Healing pressure ulcer of left buttock, unspecified stage

√5ᵗʰ **L89.4 Pressure ulcer of contiguous site of back, buttock and hip**

L89.40 Pressure ulcer of contiguous site of back, buttock and hip, unspecified stage
Healing pressure ulcer of contiguous site of back, buttock and hip NOS
Healing pressure ulcer of contiguous site of back, buttock and hip, unspecified stage

L89.41 Pressure ulcer of contiguous site of back, buttock and hip, stage 1
Healing pressure ulcer of contiguous site of back, buttock and hip, stage 1
Pressure pre-ulcer skin changes limited to persistent focal edema, contiguous site of back, buttock and hip

L89.42 Pressure ulcer of contiguous site of back, buttock and hip, stage 2 `HCC`
Healing pressure ulcer of contiguous site of back, buttock and hip, stage 2
Pressure ulcer with abrasion, blister, partial thickness skin loss involving epidermis and/or dermis, contiguous site of back, buttock and hip

L89.43 Pressure ulcer of contiguous site of back, buttock and hip, stage 3 `MCC` `H4` `HCC`
Healing pressure ulcer of contiguous site of back, buttock and hip, stage 3
Pressure ulcer with full thickness skin loss involving damage or necrosis of subcutaneous tissue, contiguous site of back, buttock and hip

L89.44 Pressure ulcer of contiguous site of back, buttock and hip, stage 4 `MCC` `H4` `HCC`
Healing pressure ulcer of contiguous site of back, buttock and hip, stage 4
Pressure ulcer with necrosis of soft tissues through to underlying muscle, tendon, or bone, contiguous site of back, buttock and hip

L89.45 Pressure ulcer of contiguous site of back, buttock and hip, unstageable `HCC`

L89.46 Pressure-induced deep tissue damage of contiguous site of back, buttock and hip

√5ᵗʰ **L89.5 Pressure ulcer of ankle**

√6ᵗʰ **L89.50 Pressure ulcer of unspecified ankle**

L89.500 Pressure ulcer of unspecified ankle, unstageable `HCC`

L89.501 Pressure ulcer of unspecified ankle, stage 1
Healing pressure ulcer of unspecified ankle, stage 1
Pressure pre-ulcer skin changes limited to persistent focal edema, unspecified ankle

L89.502 Pressure ulcer of unspecified ankle, stage 2 `HCC`
Healing pressure ulcer of unspecified ankle, stage 2
Pressure ulcer with abrasion, blister, partial thickness skin loss involving epidermis and/or dermis, unspecified ankle

L89.503 Pressure ulcer of unspecified ankle, stage 3 `MCC` `H4` `IJNS` `HCC`
Healing pressure ulcer of unspecified ankle, stage 3
Pressure ulcer with full thickness skin loss involving damage or necrosis of subcutaneous tissue, unspecified ankle

L89.504 Pressure ulcer of unspecified ankle, stage 4 `MCC` `H4` `IJNS` `HCC`
Healing pressure ulcer of unspecified ankle, stage 4
Pressure ulcer with necrosis of soft tissues through to underlying muscle, tendon, or bone, unspecified ankle

L89.506 Pressure-induced deep tissue damage of unspecified ankle

L89.509 Pressure ulcer of unspecified ankle, unspecified stage
Healing pressure ulcer of unspecified ankle NOS
Healing pressure ulcer of unspecified ankle, unspecified stage

√6ᵗʰ **L89.51 Pressure ulcer of right ankle**

L89.510 Pressure ulcer of right ankle, unstageable `HCC`

L89.511 Pressure ulcer of right ankle, stage 1
Healing pressure ulcer of right ankle, stage 1
Pressure pre-ulcer skin changes limited to persistent focal edema, right ankle

✔ Additional Character Required   √x7ᵗʰ Placeholder   Questionable PDx   Manifestation   Unspecified   `UPD` Unacceptable PDx   `H1`-`H14` HAC   `HCC` CMS-HCC Dx   `HIV` HIV Dx

ICD-10-CM 2025   761

Chapter 12. Diseases of the Skin and Subcutaneous Tissue

L89.512–L89.810

L89.512 Pressure ulcer of right ankle, stage 2 `HCC`
Healing pressure ulcer of right ankle, stage 2
Pressure ulcer with abrasion, blister, partial thickness skin loss involving epidermis and/or dermis, right ankle

L89.513 Pressure ulcer of right ankle, stage 3 `MCC` `H4` `HCC`
Healing pressure ulcer of right ankle, stage 3
Pressure ulcer with full thickness skin loss involving damage or necrosis of subcutaneous tissue, right ankle

L89.514 Pressure ulcer of right ankle, stage 4 `MCC` `H4` `HCC`
Healing pressure ulcer of right ankle, stage 4
Pressure ulcer with necrosis of soft tissues through to underlying muscle, tendon, or bone, right ankle

L89.516 Pressure-induced deep tissue damage of right ankle

L89.519 Pressure ulcer of right ankle, unspecified stage
Healing pressure ulcer of right ankle NOS
Healing pressure ulcer of right ankle, unspecified stage

✓6th **L89.52 Pressure ulcer of left ankle**

L89.520 Pressure ulcer of left ankle, unstageable `HCC`

L89.521 Pressure ulcer of left ankle, stage 1
Healing pressure ulcer of left ankle, stage 1
Pressure pre-ulcer skin changes limited to persistent focal edema, left ankle

L89.522 Pressure ulcer of left ankle, stage 2 `HCC`
Healing pressure ulcer of left ankle, stage 2
Pressure ulcer with abrasion, blister, partial thickness skin loss involving epidermis and/or dermis, left ankle

L89.523 Pressure ulcer of left ankle, stage 3 `MCC` `H4` `HCC`
Healing pressure ulcer of left ankle, stage 3
Pressure ulcer with full thickness skin loss involving damage or necrosis of subcutaneous tissue, left ankle

L89.524 Pressure ulcer of left ankle, stage 4 `MCC` `H4` `HCC`
Healing pressure ulcer of left ankle, stage 4
Pressure ulcer with necrosis of soft tissues through to underlying muscle, tendon, or bone, left ankle

L89.526 Pressure-induced deep tissue damage of left ankle

L89.529 Pressure ulcer of left ankle, unspecified stage
Healing pressure ulcer of left ankle NOS
Healing pressure ulcer of left ankle, unspecified stage

✓5th **L89.6 Pressure ulcer of heel**

✓6th **L89.60 Pressure ulcer of unspecified heel**

L89.600 Pressure ulcer of unspecified heel, unstageable `HCC`

L89.601 Pressure ulcer of unspecified heel, stage 1
Healing pressure ulcer of unspecified heel, stage 1
Pressure pre-ulcer skin changes limited to persistent focal edema, unspecified heel

L89.602 Pressure ulcer of unspecified heel, stage 2 `HCC`
Healing pressure ulcer of unspecified heel, stage 2
Pressure ulcer with abrasion, blister, partial thickness skin loss involving epidermis and/or dermis, unspecified heel

L89.603 Pressure ulcer of unspecified heel, stage 3 `MCC` `H4` `UNS` `HCC`
Healing pressure ulcer of unspecified heel, stage 3
Pressure ulcer with full thickness skin loss involving damage or necrosis of subcutaneous tissue, unspecified heel

L89.604 Pressure ulcer of unspecified heel, stage 4 `MCC` `H4` `UNS` `HCC`
Healing pressure ulcer of unspecified heel, stage 4
Pressure ulcer with necrosis of soft tissues through to underlying muscle, tendon, or bone, unspecified heel

L89.606 Pressure-induced deep tissue damage of unspecified heel

L89.609 Pressure ulcer of unspecified heel, unspecified stage
Healing pressure ulcer of unspecified heel NOS
Healing pressure ulcer of unspecified heel, unspecified stage

✓6th **L89.61 Pressure ulcer of right heel**

L89.610 Pressure ulcer of right heel, unstageable `HCC`

L89.611 Pressure ulcer of right heel, stage 1
Healing pressure ulcer of right heel, stage 1
Pressure pre-ulcer skin changes limited to persistent focal edema, right heel

L89.612 Pressure ulcer of right heel, stage 2 `HCC`
Healing pressure ulcer of right heel, stage 2
Pressure ulcer with abrasion, blister, partial thickness skin loss involving epidermis and/or dermis, right heel

L89.613 Pressure ulcer of right heel, stage 3 `MCC` `H4` `HCC`
Healing pressure ulcer of right heel, stage 3
Pressure ulcer with full thickness skin loss involving damage or necrosis of subcutaneous tissue, right heel

L89.614 Pressure ulcer of right heel, stage 4 `MCC` `H4` `HCC`
Healing pressure ulcer of right heel, stage 4
Pressure ulcer with necrosis of soft tissues through to underlying muscle, tendon, or bone, right heel

L89.616 Pressure-induced deep tissue damage of right heel

L89.619 Pressure ulcer of right heel, unspecified stage
Healing pressure ulcer of right heel NOS
Healing pressure ulcer of right heel, unspecified stage

✓6th **L89.62 Pressure ulcer of left heel**

L89.620 Pressure ulcer of left heel, unstageable `HCC`

L89.621 Pressure ulcer of left heel, stage 1
Healing pressure ulcer of left heel, stage 1
Pressure pre-ulcer skin changes limited to persistent focal edema, left heel

L89.622 Pressure ulcer of left heel, stage 2 `HCC`
Healing pressure ulcer of left heel, stage 2
Pressure ulcer with abrasion, blister, partial thickness skin loss involving epidermis and/or dermis, left heel

L89.623 Pressure ulcer of left heel, stage 3 `MCC` `H4` `HCC`
Healing pressure ulcer of left heel, stage 3
Pressure ulcer with full thickness skin loss involving damage or necrosis of subcutaneous tissue, left heel

L89.624 Pressure ulcer of left heel, stage 4 `MCC` `H4` `HCC`
Healing pressure ulcer of left heel, stage 4
Pressure ulcer with necrosis of soft tissues through to underlying muscle, tendon, or bone, left heel

L89.626 Pressure-induced deep tissue damage of left heel

L89.629 Pressure ulcer of left heel, unspecified stage
Healing pressure ulcer of left heel NOS
Healing pressure ulcer of left heel, unspecified stage

✓5th **L89.8 Pressure ulcer of other site**

✓6th **L89.81 Pressure ulcer of head**
Pressure ulcer of face

L89.810 Pressure ulcer of head, unstageable `HCC`

L89.811 Pressure ulcer of head, stage 1
Healing pressure ulcer of head, stage 1
Pressure pre-ulcer skin changes limited to persistent focal edema, head

L89.812 Pressure ulcer of head, stage 2 `HCC`
Healing pressure ulcer of head, stage 2
Pressure ulcer with abrasion, blister, partial thickness skin loss involving epidermis and/or dermis, head

L89.813 Pressure ulcer of head, stage 3 `MCC` `H4` `HCC`
Healing pressure ulcer of head, stage 3
Pressure ulcer with full thickness skin loss involving damage or necrosis of subcutaneous tissue, head

L89.814 Pressure ulcer of head, stage 4 `MCC` `H4` `HCC`
Healing pressure ulcer of head, stage 4
Pressure ulcer with necrosis of soft tissues through to underlying muscle, tendon, or bone, head

L89.816 Pressure-induced deep tissue damage of head

L89.819 Pressure ulcer of head, unspecified stage
Healing pressure ulcer of head NOS
Healing pressure ulcer of head, unspecified stage

✓6th **L89.89 Pressure ulcer of other site**

L89.890 Pressure ulcer of other site, unstageable `HCC`

L89.891 Pressure ulcer of other site, stage 1
Healing pressure ulcer of other site, stage 1
Pressure pre-ulcer skin changes limited to persistent focal edema, other site

L89.892 Pressure ulcer of other site, stage 2 `HCC`
Healing pressure ulcer of other site, stage 2
Pressure ulcer with abrasion, blister, partial thickness skin loss involving epidermis and/or dermis, other site

L89.893 Pressure ulcer of other site, stage 3 `MCC` `H4` `HCC`
Healing pressure ulcer of other site, stage 3
Pressure ulcer with full thickness skin loss involving damage or necrosis of subcutaneous tissue, other site

L89.894 Pressure ulcer of other site, stage 4 `MCC` `H4` `HCC`
Healing pressure ulcer of other site, stage 4
Pressure ulcer with necrosis of soft tissues through to underlying muscle, tendon, or bone, other site

L89.896 Pressure-induced deep tissue damage of other site

L89.899 Pressure ulcer of other site, unspecified stage
Healing pressure ulcer of other site NOS
Healing pressure ulcer of other site, unspecified stage

✓5th **L89.9 Pressure ulcer of unspecified site**

L89.90 Pressure ulcer of unspecified site, unspecified stage
Healing pressure ulcer of unspecified site NOS
Healing pressure ulcer of unspecified site, unspecified stage

L89.91 Pressure ulcer of unspecified site, stage 1
Healing pressure ulcer of unspecified site, stage 1
Pressure pre-ulcer skin changes limited to persistent focal edema, unspecified site

L89.92 Pressure ulcer of unspecified site, stage 2 `HCC`
Healing pressure ulcer of unspecified site, stage 2
Pressure ulcer with abrasion, blister, partial thickness skin loss involving epidermis and/or dermis, unspecified site

L89.93 Pressure ulcer of unspecified site, stage 3 `MCC` `H4` `UNS` `HCC`
Healing pressure ulcer of unspecified site, stage 3
Pressure ulcer with full thickness skin loss involving damage or necrosis of subcutaneous tissue, unspecified site

L89.94 Pressure ulcer of unspecified site, stage 4 `MCC` `H4` `UNS` `HCC`
Healing pressure ulcer of unspecified site, stage 4
Pressure ulcer with necrosis of soft tissues through to underlying muscle, tendon, or bone, unspecified site

L89.95 Pressure ulcer of unspecified site, unstageable `HCC`

L89.96 Pressure-induced deep tissue damage of unspecified site

✓4th **L90 Atrophic disorders of skin**

L90.0 Lichen sclerosus et atrophicus
EXCLUDES 2   *lichen sclerosus of external female genital organs (N90.4)*
lichen sclerosus of external male genital organs (N48.0)

L90.1 Anetoderma of Schweninger-Buzzi

L90.2 Anetoderma of Jadassohn-Pellizzari

L90.3 Atrophoderma of Pasini and Pierini

L90.4 Acrodermatitis chronica atrophicans

L90.5 Scar conditions and fibrosis of skin
Adherent scar (skin)
Cicatrix
Disfigurement of skin due to scar
Fibrosis of skin NOS
Scar NOS
EXCLUDES 2   *hypertrophic scar (L91.0)*
keloid scar (L91.0)
AHA: 2016,2Q,5; 2015,1Q,19

L90.6 Striae atrophicae

L90.8 Other atrophic disorders of skin

L90.9 Atrophic disorder of skin, unspecified

✓4th **L91 Hypertrophic disorders of skin**

L91.0 Hypertrophic scar
Keloid
Keloid scar
EXCLUDES 2   *acne keloid (L73.0)*
scar NOS (L90.5)
DEF: Overgrowth of scar tissue due to excess amounts of collagen during connective tissue repair, occurring mainly on the upper trunk and face.

L91.8 Other hypertrophic disorders of the skin

L91.9 Hypertrophic disorder of the skin, unspecified

✓4th **L92 Granulomatous disorders of skin and subcutaneous tissue**
EXCLUDES 2   *actinic granuloma (L57.5)*

L92.0 Granuloma annulare
Perforating granuloma annulare

L92.1 Necrobiosis lipoidica, not elsewhere classified
EXCLUDES 1   *necrobiosis lipoidica associated with diabetes mellitus (E08-E13 with .620)*

L92.2 Granuloma faciale [eosinophilic granuloma of skin]

L92.3 Foreign body granuloma of the skin and subcutaneous tissue
Use additional code to identify the type of retained foreign body (Z18.-)

L92.8 Other granulomatous disorders of the skin and subcutaneous tissue

L92.9 Granulomatous disorder of the skin and subcutaneous tissue, unspecified
EXCLUDES 2   *umbilical granuloma (P83.81)*
AHA: 2017,4Q,21-22

✓4th **L93 Lupus erythematosus**
Use additional code for adverse effect, if applicable, to identify drug (T36-T50 with fifth or sixth character 5)
EXCLUDES 1   *lupus exedens (A18.4)*
lupus vulgaris (A18.4)
scleroderma (M34.-)
systemic lupus erythematosus (M32.-)
DEF: Inflammatory, autoimmune skin condition in which the body's autoimmune system attacks healthy tissue of the integumentary system.

L93.0 Discoid lupus erythematosus
Lupus erythematosus NOS

L93.1 Subacute cutaneous lupus erythematosus

L93.2 Other local lupus erythematosus
Lupus erythematosus profundus
Lupus panniculitis

L94 Other localized connective tissue disorders

EXCLUDES 1   systemic connective tissue disorders (M30-M36)

L94.0 Localized scleroderma [morphea]
Circumscribed scleroderma

L94.1 Linear scleroderma
En coup de sabre lesion

L94.2 Calcinosis cutis

L94.3 Sclerodactyly

L94.4 Gottron's papules

L94.5 Poikiloderma vasculare atrophicans

L94.6 Ainhum

L94.8 Other specified localized connective tissue disorders

L94.9 Localized connective tissue disorder, unspecified

L95 Vasculitis limited to skin, not elsewhere classified

EXCLUDES 1   angioma serpiginosum (L81.7)
Henoch(-Schonlein) purpura (D69.0)
hypersensitivity angiitis (M31.0)
lupus panniculitis (L93.2)
panniculitis NOS (M79.3)
panniculitis of neck and back (M54.0-)
polyarteritis nodosa (M30.0)
relapsing panniculitis (M35.6)
rheumatoid vasculitis (M05.2)
serum sickness (T80.6-)
urticaria (L50.-)
Wegener's granulomatosis (M31.3-)

L95.0 Livedoid vasculitis
Atrophie blanche (en plaque)

L95.1 Erythema elevatum diutinum

L95.8 Other vasculitis limited to the skin

L95.9 Vasculitis limited to the skin, unspecified

L97 Non-pressure chronic ulcer of lower limb, not elsewhere classified

INCLUDES   chronic ulcer of skin of lower limb NOS
non-healing ulcer of skin
non-infected sinus of skin
trophic ulcer NOS
tropical ulcer NOS
ulcer of skin of lower limb NOS

Code first any associated underlying condition, such as:
any associated gangrene (I96)
atherosclerosis of the lower extremities (I70.23-, I70.24-, I70.33-, I70.34-, I70.43-, I70.44-, I70.53-, I70.54-, I70.63-, I70.64-, I70.74-)
chronic venous hypertension (I87.31-, I87.33-)
diabetic ulcers (E08.621, E08.622, E09.621, E09.622, E10.621, E10.622, E11.621, E11.622, E13.621, E13.622)
postphlebitic syndrome (I87.01-, I87.03-)
postthrombotic syndrome (I87.01-, I87.03-)
varicose ulcer (I83.0-, I83.2-)

EXCLUDES 2   pressure ulcer (pressure area) (L89.-)
skin infections (L00-L08)
specific infections classified to A00-B99

AHA: 2021,1Q,7; 2020,2Q,19; 2018,4Q,69; 2017,4Q,17

TIP: The depth and/or severity of a diagnosed nonpressure ulcer can be determined based on medical record documentation from clinicians who are not the patient's provider.

L97.1 Non-pressure chronic ulcer of thigh

L97.10 Non-pressure chronic ulcer of unspecified thigh

L97.101 Non-pressure chronic ulcer of unspecified thigh limited to breakdown of skin `CC` `UNS` `HCC`

L97.102 Non-pressure chronic ulcer of unspecified thigh with fat layer exposed `CC` `UNS` `HCC`

L97.103 Non-pressure chronic ulcer of unspecified thigh with necrosis of muscle `CC` `UNS` `HCC`

L97.104 Non-pressure chronic ulcer of unspecified thigh with necrosis of bone `CC` `UNS` `HCC`

L97.105 Non-pressure chronic ulcer of unspecified thigh with muscle involvement without evidence of necrosis `CC` `UNS` `HCC`

L97.106 Non-pressure chronic ulcer of unspecified thigh with bone involvement without evidence of necrosis `CC` `UNS` `HCC`

L97.108 Non-pressure chronic ulcer of unspecified thigh with other specified severity `CC` `UNS` `HCC`

L97.109 Non-pressure chronic ulcer of unspecified thigh with unspecified severity `CC` `UNS` `HCC`

L97.11 Non-pressure chronic ulcer of right thigh

L97.111 Non-pressure chronic ulcer of right thigh limited to breakdown of skin `CC` `HCC`

L97.112 Non-pressure chronic ulcer of right thigh with fat layer exposed `CC` `HCC`

L97.113 Non-pressure chronic ulcer of right thigh with necrosis of muscle `CC` `HCC`

L97.114 Non-pressure chronic ulcer of right thigh with necrosis of bone `CC` `HCC`

L97.115 Non-pressure chronic ulcer of right thigh with muscle involvement without evidence of necrosis `CC` `HCC`

L97.116 Non-pressure chronic ulcer of right thigh with bone involvement without evidence of necrosis `CC` `HCC`

L97.118 Non-pressure chronic ulcer of right thigh with other specified severity `CC` `HCC`

L97.119 Non-pressure chronic ulcer of right thigh with unspecified severity `CC` `HCC`

L97.12 Non-pressure chronic ulcer of left thigh

L97.121 Non-pressure chronic ulcer of left thigh limited to breakdown of skin `CC` `HCC`

L97.122 Non-pressure chronic ulcer of left thigh with fat layer exposed `CC` `HCC`

L97.123 Non-pressure chronic ulcer of left thigh with necrosis of muscle `CC` `HCC`

L97.124 Non-pressure chronic ulcer of left thigh with necrosis of bone `CC` `HCC`

L97.125 Non-pressure chronic ulcer of left thigh with muscle involvement without evidence of necrosis `CC` `HCC`

L97.126 Non-pressure chronic ulcer of left thigh with bone involvement without evidence of necrosis `CC` `HCC`

L97.128 Non-pressure chronic ulcer of left thigh with other specified severity `CC` `HCC`

L97.129 Non-pressure chronic ulcer of left thigh with unspecified severity `CC` `HCC`

L97.2 Non-pressure chronic ulcer of calf

AHA: 2024,1Q,16

L97.20 Non-pressure chronic ulcer of unspecified calf

L97.201 Non-pressure chronic ulcer of unspecified calf limited to breakdown of skin `CC` `UNS` `HCC`

L97.202 Non-pressure chronic ulcer of unspecified calf with fat layer exposed `CC` `UNS` `HCC`

L97.203 Non-pressure chronic ulcer of unspecified calf with necrosis of muscle `CC` `UNS` `HCC`

L97.204 Non-pressure chronic ulcer of unspecified calf with necrosis of bone `CC` `UNS` `HCC`

L97.205 Non-pressure chronic ulcer of unspecified calf with muscle involvement without evidence of necrosis `CC` `UNS` `HCC`

L97.206 Non-pressure chronic ulcer of unspecified calf with bone involvement without evidence of necrosis `CC` `UNS` `HCC`

L97.208 Non-pressure chronic ulcer of unspecified calf with other specified severity `CC` `UNS` `HCC`

L97.209 Non-pressure chronic ulcer of unspecified calf with unspecified severity `CC` `UNS` `HCC`

L97.21 Non-pressure chronic ulcer of right calf

L97.211 Non-pressure chronic ulcer of right calf limited to breakdown of skin `CC` `HCC`

L97.212 Non-pressure chronic ulcer of right calf with fat layer exposed `CC` `HCC`

L97.213 Non-pressure chronic ulcer of right calf with necrosis of muscle `CC` `HCC`

L97.214 Non-pressure chronic ulcer of right calf with necrosis of bone `CC` `HCC`

L97.215 Non-pressure chronic ulcer of right calf with muscle involvement without evidence of necrosis `CC` `HCC`

L97.216 Non-pressure chronic ulcer of right calf with bone involvement without evidence of necrosis `CC` `HCC`

N Newborn: 0   **P** Pediatric: 0-17   **M** Maternity: 9-64   **A** Adult: 15-124   **UNS** Unspecified Site   **MCC** Major Complication/Comorbidity   **CC** Complication/Comorbidity   **PE** POA Exempt

764

ICD-10-CM 2025

L97.218   Non-pressure chronic ulcer of right calf with other specified severity `CC` `HCC`

L97.219   Non-pressure chronic ulcer of right calf with unspecified severity `CC` `HCC`

✓6ᵗʰ   **L97.22**   **Non-pressure chronic ulcer of left calf**

L97.221   Non-pressure chronic ulcer of left calf limited to breakdown of skin `CC` `HCC`

L97.222   Non-pressure chronic ulcer of left calf with fat layer exposed `CC` `HCC`

L97.223   Non-pressure chronic ulcer of left calf with necrosis of muscle `CC` `HCC`

L97.224   Non-pressure chronic ulcer of left calf with necrosis of bone `CC` `HCC`

L97.225   Non-pressure chronic ulcer of left calf with muscle involvement without evidence of necrosis `CC` `HCC`

L97.226   Non-pressure chronic ulcer of left calf with bone involvement without evidence of necrosis `CC` `HCC`

L97.228   Non-pressure chronic ulcer of left calf with other specified severity `CC` `HCC`

L97.229   Non-pressure chronic ulcer of left calf with unspecified severity `CC` `HCC`

✓5ᵗʰ   **L97.3**   **Non-pressure chronic ulcer of ankle**

✓6ᵗʰ   **L97.30**   **Non-pressure chronic ulcer of unspecified ankle**

L97.301   Non-pressure chronic ulcer of unspecified ankle limited to breakdown of skin `CC` `UNS` `HCC`

L97.302   Non-pressure chronic ulcer of unspecified ankle with fat layer exposed `CC` `UNS` `HCC`

L97.303   Non-pressure chronic ulcer of unspecified ankle with necrosis of muscle `CC` `UNS` `HCC`

L97.304   Non-pressure chronic ulcer of unspecified ankle with necrosis of bone `CC` `UNS` `HCC`

L97.305   Non-pressure chronic ulcer of unspecified ankle with muscle involvement without evidence of necrosis `CC` `UNS` `HCC`

L97.306   Non-pressure chronic ulcer of unspecified ankle with bone involvement without evidence of necrosis `CC` `UNS` `HCC`

L97.308   Non-pressure chronic ulcer of unspecified ankle with other specified severity `CC` `UNS` `HCC`

L97.309   Non-pressure chronic ulcer of unspecified ankle with unspecified severity `CC` `UNS` `HCC`

✓6ᵗʰ   **L97.31**   **Non-pressure chronic ulcer of right ankle**

L97.311   Non-pressure chronic ulcer of right ankle limited to breakdown of skin `CC` `HCC`

L97.312   Non-pressure chronic ulcer of right ankle with fat layer exposed `CC` `HCC`

L97.313   Non-pressure chronic ulcer of right ankle with necrosis of muscle `CC` `HCC`

L97.314   Non-pressure chronic ulcer of right ankle with necrosis of bone `CC` `HCC`

L97.315   Non-pressure chronic ulcer of right ankle with muscle involvement without evidence of necrosis `CC` `HCC`

L97.316   Non-pressure chronic ulcer of right ankle with bone involvement without evidence of necrosis `CC` `HCC`

L97.318   Non-pressure chronic ulcer of right ankle with other specified severity `CC` `HCC`

L97.319   Non-pressure chronic ulcer of right ankle with unspecified severity `CC` `HCC`

✓6ᵗʰ   **L97.32**   **Non-pressure chronic ulcer of left ankle**

L97.321   Non-pressure chronic ulcer of left ankle limited to breakdown of skin `CC` `HCC`

L97.322   Non-pressure chronic ulcer of left ankle with fat layer exposed `CC` `HCC`

L97.323   Non-pressure chronic ulcer of left ankle with necrosis of muscle `CC` `HCC`

L97.324   Non-pressure chronic ulcer of left ankle with necrosis of bone `CC` `HCC`

L97.325   Non-pressure chronic ulcer of left ankle with muscle involvement without evidence of necrosis `CC` `HCC`

L97.326   Non-pressure chronic ulcer of left ankle with bone involvement without evidence of necrosis `CC` `HCC`

L97.328   Non-pressure chronic ulcer of left ankle with other specified severity `CC` `HCC`

L97.329   Non-pressure chronic ulcer of left ankle with unspecified severity `CC` `HCC`

✓5ᵗʰ   **L97.4**   **Non-pressure chronic ulcer of heel and midfoot**

    Non-pressure chronic ulcer of plantar surface of midfoot

✓6ᵗʰ   **L97.40**   **Non-pressure chronic ulcer of unspecified heel and midfoot**

L97.401   Non-pressure chronic ulcer of unspecified heel and midfoot limited to breakdown of skin `CC` `UNS` `HCC`

L97.402   Non-pressure chronic ulcer of unspecified heel and midfoot with fat layer exposed `CC` `UNS` `HCC`

L97.403   Non-pressure chronic ulcer of unspecified heel and midfoot with necrosis of muscle `CC` `UNS` `HCC`

L97.404   Non-pressure chronic ulcer of unspecified heel and midfoot with necrosis of bone `CC` `UNS` `HCC`

L97.405   Non-pressure chronic ulcer of unspecified heel and midfoot with muscle involvement without evidence of necrosis `CC` `UNS` `HCC`

L97.406   Non-pressure chronic ulcer of unspecified heel and midfoot with bone involvement without evidence of necrosis `CC` `UNS` `HCC`

L97.408   Non-pressure chronic ulcer of unspecified heel and midfoot with other specified severity `CC` `UNS` `HCC`

L97.409   Non-pressure chronic ulcer of unspecified heel and midfoot with unspecified severity `CC` `UNS` `HCC`

✓6ᵗʰ   **L97.41**   **Non-pressure chronic ulcer of right heel and midfoot**

L97.411   Non-pressure chronic ulcer of right heel and midfoot limited to breakdown of skin `CC` `HCC`

L97.412   Non-pressure chronic ulcer of right heel and midfoot with fat layer exposed `CC` `HCC`
    AHA: 2020,2Q,19

L97.413   Non-pressure chronic ulcer of right heel and midfoot with necrosis of muscle `CC` `HCC`

L97.414   Non-pressure chronic ulcer of right heel and midfoot with necrosis of bone `CC` `HCC`

L97.415   Non-pressure chronic ulcer of right heel and midfoot with muscle involvement without evidence of necrosis `CC` `HCC`

L97.416   Non-pressure chronic ulcer of right heel and midfoot with bone involvement without evidence of necrosis `CC` `HCC`

L97.418   Non-pressure chronic ulcer of right heel and midfoot with other specified severity `CC` `HCC`

L97.419   Non-pressure chronic ulcer of right heel and midfoot with unspecified severity `CC` `HCC`

✓6ᵗʰ   **L97.42**   **Non-pressure chronic ulcer of left heel and midfoot**

L97.421   Non-pressure chronic ulcer of left heel and midfoot limited to breakdown of skin `CC` `HCC`
    AHA: 2016,1Q,12

L97.422   Non-pressure chronic ulcer of left heel and midfoot with fat layer exposed `CC` `HCC`
    AHA: 2020,2Q,19

L97.423   Non-pressure chronic ulcer of left heel and midfoot with necrosis of muscle `CC` `HCC`

L97.424   Non-pressure chronic ulcer of left heel and midfoot with necrosis of bone `CC` `HCC`

L97.425   Non-pressure chronic ulcer of left heel and midfoot with muscle involvement without evidence of necrosis `CC` `HCC`

L97.426   Non-pressure chronic ulcer of left heel and midfoot with bone involvement without evidence of necrosis `CC` `HCC`

✔ Additional Character Required   ✓x7ᵗʰ Placeholder   Questionable PDx   Manifestation   Unspecified   `UPD` Unacceptable PDx   `H1`-`H14` HAC   `HCC` CMS-HCC Dx   `HIV` HIV Dx

ICD-10-CM 2025   765

Chapter 12. Diseases of the Skin and Subcutaneous Tissue

L97.428–L97.828

L97.428 Non-pressure chronic ulcer of left heel and midfoot with other specified severity `CC` `HCC`

L97.429 Non-pressure chronic ulcer of left heel and midfoot with unspecified severity `CC` `HCC`

✓5ᵗʰ **L97.5** Non-pressure chronic ulcer of other part of foot
Non-pressure chronic ulcer of toe

✓6ᵗʰ **L97.50** Non-pressure chronic ulcer of other part of unspecified foot

L97.501 Non-pressure chronic ulcer of other part of unspecified foot limited to breakdown of skin `HCC`

L97.502 Non-pressure chronic ulcer of other part of unspecified foot with fat layer exposed `HCC`

L97.503 Non-pressure chronic ulcer of other part of unspecified foot with necrosis of muscle `HCC`

L97.504 Non-pressure chronic ulcer of other part of unspecified foot with necrosis of bone `HCC`

L97.505 Non-pressure chronic ulcer of other part of unspecified foot with muscle involvement without evidence of necrosis `CC` `HCC`

L97.506 Non-pressure chronic ulcer of other part of unspecified foot with bone involvement without evidence of necrosis `CC` `HCC`

L97.508 Non-pressure chronic ulcer of other part of unspecified foot with other specified severity `CC` `HCC`

L97.509 Non-pressure chronic ulcer of other part of unspecified foot with unspecified severity `HCC`

✓6ᵗʰ **L97.51** Non-pressure chronic ulcer of other part of right foot
AHA: 2020,1Q,12

L97.511 Non-pressure chronic ulcer of other part of right foot limited to breakdown of skin `HCC`

L97.512 Non-pressure chronic ulcer of other part of right foot with fat layer exposed `HCC`
AHA: 2020,2Q,19

L97.513 Non-pressure chronic ulcer of other part of right foot with necrosis of muscle `HCC`

L97.514 Non-pressure chronic ulcer of other part of right foot with necrosis of bone `HCC`

L97.515 Non-pressure chronic ulcer of other part of right foot with muscle involvement without evidence of necrosis `CC` `HCC`

L97.516 Non-pressure chronic ulcer of other part of right foot with bone involvement without evidence of necrosis `CC` `HCC`

L97.518 Non-pressure chronic ulcer of other part of right foot with other specified severity `CC` `HCC`

L97.519 Non-pressure chronic ulcer of other part of right foot with unspecified severity `HCC`

✓6ᵗʰ **L97.52** Non-pressure chronic ulcer of other part of left foot
AHA: 2020,1Q,12

L97.521 Non-pressure chronic ulcer of other part of left foot limited to breakdown of skin `HCC`

L97.522 Non-pressure chronic ulcer of other part of left foot with fat layer exposed `HCC`
AHA: 2020,2Q,19

L97.523 Non-pressure chronic ulcer of other part of left foot with necrosis of muscle `HCC`

L97.524 Non-pressure chronic ulcer of other part of left foot with necrosis of bone `HCC`

L97.525 Non-pressure chronic ulcer of other part of left foot with muscle involvement without evidence of necrosis `CC` `HCC`

L97.526 Non-pressure chronic ulcer of other part of left foot with bone involvement without evidence of necrosis `CC` `HCC`

L97.528 Non-pressure chronic ulcer of other part of left foot with other specified severity `CC` `HCC`

L97.529 Non-pressure chronic ulcer of other part of left foot with unspecified severity `HCC`

✓5ᵗʰ **L97.8** Non-pressure chronic ulcer of other part of lower leg

✓6ᵗʰ **L97.80** Non-pressure chronic ulcer of other part of unspecified lower leg

L97.801 Non-pressure chronic ulcer of other part of unspecified lower leg limited to breakdown of skin `CC` `HCC`

L97.802 Non-pressure chronic ulcer of other part of unspecified lower leg with fat layer exposed `CC` `HCC`

L97.803 Non-pressure chronic ulcer of other part of unspecified lower leg with necrosis of muscle `CC` `HCC`

L97.804 Non-pressure chronic ulcer of other part of unspecified lower leg with necrosis of bone `CC` `HCC`

L97.805 Non-pressure chronic ulcer of other part of unspecified lower leg with muscle involvement without evidence of necrosis `CC` `HCC`

L97.806 Non-pressure chronic ulcer of other part of unspecified lower leg with bone involvement without evidence of necrosis `CC` `HCC`

L97.808 Non-pressure chronic ulcer of other part of unspecified lower leg with other specified severity `CC` `HCC`

L97.809 Non-pressure chronic ulcer of other part of unspecified lower leg with unspecified severity `CC` `HCC`

✓6ᵗʰ **L97.81** Non-pressure chronic ulcer of other part of right lower leg

L97.811 Non-pressure chronic ulcer of other part of right lower leg limited to breakdown of skin `HCC`

L97.812 Non-pressure chronic ulcer of other part of right lower leg with fat layer exposed `CC` `HCC`

L97.813 Non-pressure chronic ulcer of other part of right lower leg with necrosis of muscle `CC` `HCC`

L97.814 Non-pressure chronic ulcer of other part of right lower leg with necrosis of bone `CC` `HCC`

L97.815 Non-pressure chronic ulcer of other part of right lower leg with muscle involvement without evidence of necrosis `CC` `HCC`

L97.816 Non-pressure chronic ulcer of other part of right lower leg with bone involvement without evidence of necrosis `CC` `HCC`

L97.818 Non-pressure chronic ulcer of other part of right lower leg with other specified severity `CC` `HCC`

L97.819 Non-pressure chronic ulcer of other part of right lower leg with unspecified severity `CC` `HCC`

✓6ᵗʰ **L97.82** Non-pressure chronic ulcer of other part of left lower leg

L97.821 Non-pressure chronic ulcer of other part of left lower leg limited to breakdown of skin `CC` `HCC`

L97.822 Non-pressure chronic ulcer of other part of left lower leg with fat layer exposed `CC` `HCC`

L97.823 Non-pressure chronic ulcer of other part of left lower leg with necrosis of muscle `CC` `HCC`

L97.824 Non-pressure chronic ulcer of other part of left lower leg with necrosis of bone `CC` `HCC`

L97.825 Non-pressure chronic ulcer of other part of left lower leg with muscle involvement without evidence of necrosis `CC` `HCC`

L97.826 Non-pressure chronic ulcer of other part of left lower leg with bone involvement without evidence of necrosis `CC` `HCC`

L97.828 Non-pressure chronic ulcer of other part of left lower leg with other specified severity `CC` `HCC`

L97.829 Non-pressure chronic ulcer of other part of left lower leg with unspecified severity `CC` `HCC`

☑5th **L97.9** Non-pressure chronic ulcer of unspecified part of lower leg

  ☑6th **L97.90** Non-pressure chronic ulcer of unspecified part of unspecified lower leg

L97.901 Non-pressure chronic ulcer of unspecified part of unspecified lower leg limited to breakdown of skin `CC` `UNS` `HCC`

L97.902 Non-pressure chronic ulcer of unspecified part of unspecified lower leg with fat layer exposed `CC` `UNS` `HCC`

L97.903 Non-pressure chronic ulcer of unspecified part of unspecified lower leg with necrosis of muscle `CC` `UNS` `HCC`

L97.904 Non-pressure chronic ulcer of unspecified part of unspecified lower leg with necrosis of bone `CC` `UNS` `HCC`

L97.905 Non-pressure chronic ulcer of unspecified part of unspecified lower leg with muscle involvement without evidence of necrosis `CC` `UNS` `HCC`

L97.906 Non-pressure chronic ulcer of unspecified part of unspecified lower leg with bone involvement without evidence of necrosis `CC` `UNS` `HCC`

L97.908 Non-pressure chronic ulcer of unspecified part of unspecified lower leg with other specified severity `CC` `UNS` `HCC`

L97.909 Non-pressure chronic ulcer of unspecified part of unspecified lower leg with unspecified severity `CC` `UNS` `HCC`

  ☑6th **L97.91** Non-pressure chronic ulcer of unspecified part of right lower leg

L97.911 Non-pressure chronic ulcer of unspecified part of right lower leg limited to breakdown of skin `CC` `HCC`

L97.912 Non-pressure chronic ulcer of unspecified part of right lower leg with fat layer exposed `CC` `HCC`

L97.913 Non-pressure chronic ulcer of unspecified part of right lower leg with necrosis of muscle `CC` `HCC`

L97.914 Non-pressure chronic ulcer of unspecified part of right lower leg with necrosis of bone `CC` `HCC`

L97.915 Non-pressure chronic ulcer of unspecified part of right lower leg with muscle involvement without evidence of necrosis `CC` `HCC`

L97.916 Non-pressure chronic ulcer of unspecified part of right lower leg with bone involvement without evidence of necrosis `CC` `HCC`

L97.918 Non-pressure chronic ulcer of unspecified part of right lower leg with other specified severity `CC` `HCC`

L97.919 Non-pressure chronic ulcer of unspecified part of right lower leg with unspecified severity `CC` `HCC`

  ☑6th **L97.92** Non-pressure chronic ulcer of unspecified part of left lower leg

L97.921 Non-pressure chronic ulcer of unspecified part of left lower leg limited to breakdown of skin `CC` `HCC`

L97.922 Non-pressure chronic ulcer of unspecified part of left lower leg with fat layer exposed `CC` `HCC`

L97.923 Non-pressure chronic ulcer of unspecified part of left lower leg with necrosis of muscle `CC` `HCC`

L97.924 Non-pressure chronic ulcer of unspecified part of left lower leg with necrosis of bone `CC` `HCC`

L97.925 Non-pressure chronic ulcer of unspecified part of left lower leg with muscle involvement without evidence of necrosis `CC` `HCC`

L97.926 Non-pressure chronic ulcer of unspecified part of left lower leg with bone involvement without evidence of necrosis `CC` `HCC`

L97.928 Non-pressure chronic ulcer of unspecified part of left lower leg with other specified severity `CC` `HCC`

L97.929 Non-pressure chronic ulcer of unspecified part of left lower leg with unspecified severity `CC` `HCC`

☑4th **L98** Other disorders of skin and subcutaneous tissue, not elsewhere classified

L98.0 Pyogenic granuloma

EXCLUDES 2   pyogenic granuloma of gingiva (K06.8)
pyogenic granuloma of maxillary alveolar ridge (K04.5)
pyogenic granuloma of oral mucosa (K13.4)

DEF: Solitary polypoid capillary hemangioma often associated with local irritation, trauma, and superimposed inflammation. Located on the skin and gingival or oral mucosa, they bleed easily and may ulcerate and form crusted sores.

L98.1 Factitial dermatitis

Neurotic excoriation

EXCLUDES 1   excoriation (skin-picking) disorder (F42.4)

AHA: 2016,4Q,15

DEF: Self-inflicted skin lesions to satisfy an unconscious psychological or emotional need. Methods used to injure the skin include deep excoriations with a sharp instrument, scarification with a knife, or the application of caustic chemicals and burning, sometimes with a cigarette.

L98.2 Febrile neutrophilic dermatosis [Sweet]

L98.3 Eosinophilic cellulitis [Wells] `CC`

☑5th **L98.4** Non-pressure chronic ulcer of skin, not elsewhere classified

Chronic ulcer of skin NOS
Tropical ulcer NOS
Ulcer of skin NOS

EXCLUDES 2   gangrene (I96)
pressure ulcer (pressure area) (L89.-)
skin infections (L00-L08)
specific infections classified to A00-B99
ulcer of lower limb NEC (L97.-)
varicose ulcer (I83.0-I83.93)

AHA: 2017,4Q,17

TIP: The depth and/or severity of a diagnosed nonpressure ulcer can be determined based on medical record documentation from clinicians who are not the patient's provider.

  ☑6th **L98.41** Non-pressure chronic ulcer of buttock

L98.411 Non-pressure chronic ulcer of buttock limited to breakdown of skin `HCC`

L98.412 Non-pressure chronic ulcer of buttock with fat layer exposed `HCC`

L98.413 Non-pressure chronic ulcer of buttock with necrosis of muscle `HCC`

L98.414 Non-pressure chronic ulcer of buttock with necrosis of bone `HCC`

L98.415 Non-pressure chronic ulcer of buttock with muscle involvement without evidence of necrosis `CC` `HCC`

L98.416 Non-pressure chronic ulcer of buttock with bone involvement without evidence of necrosis `CC` `HCC`

L98.418 Non-pressure chronic ulcer of buttock with other specified severity `CC` `HCC`

L98.419 Non-pressure chronic ulcer of buttock with unspecified severity `HCC`

  ☑6th **L98.42** Non-pressure chronic ulcer of back

L98.421 Non-pressure chronic ulcer of back limited to breakdown of skin `HCC`

L98.422 Non-pressure chronic ulcer of back with fat layer exposed `HCC`

L98.423 Non-pressure chronic ulcer of back with necrosis of muscle `HCC`

L98.424 Non-pressure chronic ulcer of back with necrosis of bone `HCC`

L98.425 Non-pressure chronic ulcer of back with muscle involvement without evidence of necrosis `CC` `HCC`

L98.426 Non-pressure chronic ulcer of back with bone involvement without evidence of necrosis `CC` `HCC`

L98.428 Non-pressure chronic ulcer of back with other specified severity `CC` `HCC`

L98.429 Non-pressure chronic ulcer of back with unspecified severity `HCC`

☑ Additional Character Required   ☑x7th Placeholder   Questionable PDx   Manifestation   Unspecified   `UPD` Unacceptable PDx   `H1`-`H14` HAC   `HCC` CMS-HCC Dx   `HIV` HIV Dx

ICD-10-CM 2025   767

√6ᵗʰ **L98.49   Non-pressure chronic ulcer of skin of other sites**
   Non-pressure chronic ulcer of skin NOS
  L98.491   Non-pressure chronic ulcer of skin of other sites limited to breakdown of skin HCC
  L98.492   Non-pressure chronic ulcer of skin of other sites with fat layer exposed HCC
  L98.493   Non-pressure chronic ulcer of skin of other sites with necrosis of muscle HCC
  L98.494   Non-pressure chronic ulcer of skin of other sites with necrosis of bone HCC
  L98.495   Non-pressure chronic ulcer of skin of other sites with muscle involvement without evidence of necrosis CC HCC
  L98.496   Non-pressure chronic ulcer of skin of other sites with bone involvement without evidence of necrosis CC HCC
  L98.498   Non-pressure chronic ulcer of skin of other sites with other specified severity CC HCC
  L98.499   Non-pressure chronic ulcer of skin of other sites with unspecified severity HCC

L98.5   Mucinosis of the skin
  Focal mucinosis
  Lichen myxedematosus
  Reticular erythematous mucinosis
  EXCLUDES 1 *focal oral mucinosis (K13.79)*
      myxedema (E03.9)

L98.6   Other infiltrative disorders of the skin and subcutaneous tissue
  EXCLUDES 1 *hyalinosis cutis et mucosae (E78.89)*

L98.7   Excessive and redundant skin and subcutaneous tissue
  Loose or sagging skin, following bariatric surgery weight loss
  Loose or sagging skin following dietary weight loss
  Loose or sagging skin, NOS
  EXCLUDES 2 *acquired excess or redundant skin of eyelid (H02.3-)*
      congenital excess or redundant skin of eyelid (Q10.3)
      skin changes due to chronic exposure to nonionizing radiation (L57.-)
  AHA: 2022,3Q,11; 2016,4Q,36

L98.8   Other specified disorders of the skin and subcutaneous tissue
  AHA: 2013,2Q,32

L98.9   Disorder of the skin and subcutaneous tissue, unspecified

L99   *Other disorders of skin and subcutaneous tissue in diseases classified elsewhere*
  Code first underlying disease, such as:
  amyloidosis (E85.-)
  EXCLUDES 1 *skin disorders in diabetes (E08-E13 with .62-)*
      skin disorders in gonorrhea (A54.89)
      skin disorders in syphilis (A51.31, A52.79)
  AHA: 2021,1Q,39

N Newborn: 0 P Pediatric: 0-17 M Maternity: 9-64 A Adult: 15-124 UNS Unspecified Site MCC Major Complication/Comorbidity CC Complication/Comorbidity PE POA Exempt

768 ICD-10-CM 2025

Chapter 13. Diseases of the Musculoskeletal System and Connective Tissue (M00–M99)

Chapter-specific Guidelines with Coding Examples

The chapter-specific guidelines from the ICD-10-CM Official Guidelines for Coding and Reporting have been provided below. Along with these guidelines are coding examples, contained in the shaded boxes, that have been developed to help illustrate the coding and/or sequencing guidance found in these guidelines.

a. Site and laterality

Most of the codes within Chapter 13 have site and laterality designations. The site represents the bone, joint or the muscle involved. For some conditions where more than one bone, joint or muscle is usually involved, such as osteoarthritis, there is a "multiple sites" code available. For categories where no multiple site code is provided and more than one bone, joint or muscle is involved, multiple codes should be used to indicate the different sites involved.

> Rheumatoid arthritis of multiple sites without rheumatoid factor
>
> **M06.09   Rheumatoid arthritis without rheumatoid factor, multiple sites**
>
> *Explanation:* For some conditions where more than one bone, joint or muscle is usually involved, such as rheumatoid arthritis, there is a "multiple sites" code available.

> Osteomyelitis of the fourth thoracic and second lumbar vertebrae
>
> **M46.24   Osteomyelitis of vertebra, thoracic region**
>
> **M46.26   Osteomyelitis of vertebra, lumbar region**
>
> *Explanation:* For categories without a multiple site code and more than one bone, joint, or muscle is involved, multiple codes should be used to indicate the different sites involved.

1) Bone versus joint

For certain conditions, the bone may be affected at the upper or lower end, (e.g., avascular necrosis of bone, M87, Osteoporosis, M80, M81). Though the portion of the bone affected may be at the joint, the site designation will be the bone, not the joint.

> Idiopathic avascular necrosis of the femoral head of the left hip joint
>
> **M87.052   Idiopathic aseptic necrosis of left femur**
>
> *Explanation:* For certain conditions such as avascular necrosis, the bone may be affected at the joint, but the site designation is the bone, not the joint.

b. Acute traumatic versus chronic or recurrent musculoskeletal conditions

Many musculoskeletal conditions are a result of previous injury or trauma to a site, or are recurrent conditions. Bone, joint or muscle conditions that are the result of a healed injury are usually found in chapter 13. Recurrent bone, joint or muscle conditions are also usually found in chapter 13. Any current, acute injury should be coded to the appropriate injury code from chapter 19. Chronic or recurrent conditions should generally be coded with a code from chapter 13. If it is difficult to determine from the documentation in the record which code is best to describe a condition, query the provider.

> Acute traumatic bucket-handle tear of right medial meniscus
>
> **S83.211A   Bucket-handle tear of medial meniscus, current injury, right knee, initial encounter**
>
> *Explanation:* Any current, acute injury is not coded in chapter 13. It should instead be coded to the appropriate injury code from chapter 19.

> Old bucket-handle tear of right medial meniscus
>
> **M23.203   Derangement of unspecified medial meniscus due to old tear or injury, right knee**
>
> *Explanation:* Chronic or recurrent conditions should generally be coded with a code from chapter 13.

c. Coding of pathologic fractures

7th character A is for use as long as the patient is receiving active treatment for the fracture. Examples of active treatment are: surgical treatment, emergency department encounter, evaluation and continuing treatment by the same or a different physician. While the patient may be seen by a new or different provider over the course of treatment for a pathological fracture, assignment of the 7th character is based on whether the patient is undergoing active treatment and not whether the provider is seeing the patient for the first time.

> Patient admitted for repair of pathologic fracture of left foot, unknown cause. The surgery will be performed by his orthopedic specialist who he has been seeing for this fracture for the past month.
>
> **M84.475A   Pathological fracture, left foot, initial encounter for fracture**
>
> *Explanation:* Seventh character A is for use as long as the patient is receiving active treatment for a pathologic fracture. Examples of active treatment are surgical treatment, emergency department encounter, evaluation, and continuing treatment by the same or a different physician.
>
> The seventh character is based on whether the patient is undergoing active treatment such as surgery, and not whether the provider is seeing the patient for the first time.

7th character D is to be used for encounters after the patient has completed active treatment for the fracture and is receiving routine care for the fracture during the healing or recovery phase. The other 7th characters, listed under each subcategory in the Tabular List, are to be used for subsequent encounters for treatment of problems associated with the healing, such as malunions, nonunions, and sequelae.

Care for complications of surgical treatment for fracture repairs during the healing or recovery phase should be coded with the appropriate complication codes.

See Section I.C.19. Coding of traumatic fractures.

d. Osteoporosis

Osteoporosis is a systemic condition, meaning that all bones of the musculoskeletal system are affected. Therefore, site is not a component of the codes under category M81, Osteoporosis without current pathological fracture. The site codes under category M80, Osteoporosis with current pathological fracture, identify the site of the fracture, not the osteoporosis.

1) Osteoporosis without pathological fracture

Category M81, Osteoporosis without current pathological fracture, is for use for patients with osteoporosis who do not currently have a pathologic fracture due to the osteoporosis, even if they have had a fracture in the past. For patients with a history of osteoporosis fractures, status code Z87.310, Personal history of (healed) osteoporosis fracture, should follow the code from M81.

> Age-related osteoporosis with healed osteoporotic fracture of the lumbar vertebra
>
> **M81.0   Age-related osteoporosis without current pathological fracture**
>
> **Z87.310   Personal history of (healed) osteoporosis fracture**
>
> *Explanation:* Category M81 is used for patients with osteoporosis who do not currently have a pathologic fracture due to the osteoporosis. To report a previous (healed) fracture, status code Z87.310 Personal history of (healed) osteoporosis fracture, should follow the code from M81.

2) Osteoporosis with current pathological fracture

Category M80, Osteoporosis with current pathological fracture, is for patients who have a current pathologic fracture at the time of an encounter. The codes under M80 identify the site of the fracture. A code from category M80, not a traumatic fracture code, should be used for any patient with known osteoporosis who suffers a fracture, even if the patient had a minor fall or trauma, if that fall or trauma would not usually break a normal, healthy bone.

> Disuse osteoporosis with current fracture of right shoulder sustained lifting a grocery bag, initial encounter
>
> **M80.811A   Other osteoporosis with current pathological fracture, right shoulder, initial encounter for fracture**
>
> *Explanation:* A code from category M80, not a traumatic fracture code, should be used for any patient with known osteoporosis who suffers a fracture, even if the patient had a minor fall or trauma, if that fall or trauma would not usually break a normal, healthy bone.

e. Multisystem inflammatory syndrome

See Section I.C.1.g.1.l. for Multisystem Inflammatory Syndrome

Muscle/Tendon Table

ICD-10-CM categorizes certain muscles and tendons in the upper and lower extremities by their action (e.g., extension, flexion), their anatomical location (e.g., posterior, anterior), and/or whether they are intrinsic or extrinsic to a certain anatomical area. The Muscle/Tendon Table is provided at the beginning of chapters 13 and 19 as a resource to help users when code selection depends on one or more of these characteristics. Please note that this table is not all-inclusive, and proper code assignment should be based on the provider's documentation.

Body Region	Muscle	Extensor Tendon	Flexor Tendon	Other Tendon
Shoulder				
	Deltoid	Posterior deltoid	Anterior deltoid	
	Rotator cuff			
	Infraspinatus			Infraspinatus
	Subscapularis			Subscapularis
	Supraspinatus			Supraspinatus
	Teres minor			Teres minor
	Teres major	Teres major		
Upper arm				
	Anterior muscles			
	Biceps brachii — long head		Biceps brachii — long head	
	Biceps brachii — short head		Biceps brachii — short head	
	Brachialis		Brachialis	
	Coracobrachialis		Coracobrachialis	
	Posterior muscles			
	Triceps brachii	Triceps brachii		
Forearm				
	Anterior muscles			
	Flexors			
	Deep			
	Flexor digitorum profundus		Flexor digitorum profundus	
	Flexor pollicis longus		Flexor pollicis longus	
	Intermediate			
	Flexor digitorum superficialis		Flexor digitorum superficialis	
	Superficial			
	Flexor carpi radialis		Flexor carpi radialis	
	Flexor carpi ulnaris		Flexor carpi ulnaris	
	Palmaris longus		Palmaris longus	
	Pronators			
	Pronator quadratus			Pronator quadratus
	Pronator teres			Pronator teres
	Posterior muscles			
	Extensors			
	Deep			
	Abductor pollicis longus			Abductor pollicis longus
	Extensor indicis	Extensor indicis		
	Extensor pollicis brevis	Extensor pollicis brevis		
	Extensor pollicis longus	Extensor pollicis longus		
	Superficial			
	Brachioradialis			Brachioradialis
	Extensor carpi radialis brevis	Extensor carpi radialis brevis		
	Extensor carpi radialis longus	Extensor carpi radialis longus		
	Extensor carpi ulnaris	Extensor carpi ulnaris		
	Extensor digiti minimi	Extensor digiti minimi		
	Extensor digitorum	Extensor digitorum		
	Anconeus	Anconeus		
	Supinator			Supinator

Body Region	Muscle	Extensor Tendon	Flexor Tendon	Other Tendon
Hand				
Extrinsic — attach to a site in the forearm as well as a site in the hand with action related to hand movement at the wrist				
	Extensor carpi radialis brevis	Extensor carpi radialis brevis		
	Extensor carpi radialis longus	Extensor carpi radialis longus		
	Extensor carpi ulnaris	Extensor carpi ulnaris		
	Flexor carpi radialis		Flexor carpi radialis	
	Flexor carpi ulnaris		Flexor carpi ulnaris	
	Flexor digitorum superficialis		Flexor digitorum superficialis	
	Palmaris longus		Palmaris longus	
Extrinsic — attach to a site in the forearm as well as a site in the hand with action in the hand related to finger movement				
	Adductor pollicis longus			Adductor pollicis longus
	Extensor digiti minimi	Extensor digiti minimi		
	Extensor digitorum	Extensor digitorum		
	Extensor indicis	Extensor indicis		
	Flexor digitorum profundus		Flexor digitorum profundus	
	Flexor digitorum superficialis		Flexor digitorum superficialis	
Extrinsic — attach to a site in the forearm as well as a site in the hand with action in the hand related to thumb movement				
	Extensor pollicis brevis	Extensor pollicis brevis		
	Extensor pollicis longus	Extensor pollicis longus		
	Flexor pollicis longus		Flexor pollicis longus	
Intrinsic — found within the hand only				
	Adductor pollicis			Adductor pollicis
	Dorsal interossei	Dorsal interossei	Dorsal interossei	
	Lumbricals	Lumbricals	Lumbricals	
	Palmaris brevis			Palmaris brevis
	Palmar interossei	Palmar interossei	Palmar interossei	
	Hypothenar muscles			
	Abductor digiti minimi			Abductor digiti minimi
	Flexor digiti minimi brevis		Flexor digiti minimi brevis	
	Opponens digiti minimi		Opponens digiti minimi	
	Thenar muscles			
	Abductor pollicis brevis			Abductor pollicis brevis
	Flexor pollicis brevis		Flexor pollicis brevis	
	Opponens pollicis		Opponens pollicis	
Thigh				
	Anterior muscles			
	Iliopsoas		Iliopsoas	
	Pectineus		Pectineus	
	Quadriceps	Quadriceps		
	Rectus femoris	Rectus femoris — Extends knee	Rectus femoris — Flexes hip	
	Vastus intermedius	Vastus intermedius		
	Vastus lateralis	Vastus lateralis		
	Vastus medialis	Vastus medialis		
	Sartorius		Sartorius	
	Medial muscles			
	Adductor brevis			Adductor brevis
	Adductor longus			Adductor longus
	Adductor magnus			Adductor magnus
	Gracilis			Gracilis
	Obturator externus			Obturator externus
	Posterior muscles			
	Hamstring	Hamstring — Extends hip	Hamstring — Flexes knee	
	Biceps femoris	Biceps femoris	Biceps femoris	
	Semimembranosus	Semimembranosus	Semimembranosus	
	Semitendinosus	Semitendinosus	Semitendinosus	

Chapter 13. Diseases of the Musculoskeletal System and Connective Tissue

Body Region	Muscle	Extensor Tendon	Flexor Tendon	Other Tendon
Lower leg				
	Anterior muscles			
	Extensor digitorum longus	Extensor digitorum longus		
	Extensor hallucis longus	Extensor hallucis longus		
	Fibularis (peroneus) tertius	Fibularis (peroneus) tertius		
	Tibialis anterior	Tibialis anterior		Tibialis anterior
	Lateral muscles			
	Fibularis (peroneus) brevis		Fibularis (peroneus) brevis	
	Fibularis (peroneus) longus		Fibularis (peroneus) longus	
	Posterior muscles			
	Deep			
	Flexor digitorum longus		Flexor digitorum longus	
	Flexor hallucis longus		Flexor hallucis longus	
	Popliteus		Popliteus	
	Tibialis posterior		Tibialis posterior	
	Superficial			
	Gastrocnemius		Gastrocnemius	
	Plantaris		Plantaris	
	Soleus		Soleus	
				Calcaneal (Achilles)
Ankle/Foot				
Extrinsic — attach to a site in the lower leg as well as a site in the foot with action related to foot movement at the ankle				
	Plantaris		Plantaris	
	Soleus		Soleus	
	Tibialis anterior	Tibialis anterior		
	Tibialis posterior		Tibialis posterior	
Extrinsic — attach to a site in the lower leg as well as a site in the foot with action in the foot related to toe movement				
	Extensor digitorum longus	Extensor digitorum longus		
	Extensor hallucis longus	Extensor hallucis longus		
	Flexor digitorum longus		Flexor digitorum longus	
	Flexor hallucis longus		Flexor hallucis longus	
Intrinsic — found within the ankle/foot only				
	Dorsal muscles			
	Extensor digitorum brevis	Extensor digitorum brevis		
	Extensor hallucis brevis	Extensor hallucis brevis		
	Plantar muscles			
	Abductor digiti minimi		Abductor digiti minimi	
	Abductor hallucis		Abductor hallucis	
	Dorsal interossei	Dorsal interossei	Dorsal interossei	
	Flexor digiti minimi brevis		Flexor digiti minimi brevis	
	Flexor digitorum brevis		Flexor digitorum brevis	
	Flexor hallucis brevis		Flexor hallucis brevis	
	Lumbricals	Lumbricals	Lumbricals	
	Quadratus plantae		Quadratus plantae	
	Plantar interossei	Plantar interossei	Plantar interossei	

Chapter 13. Diseases of the Musculoskeletal System and Connective Tissue (M00-M99)

NOTE   Use an external cause code following the code for the musculoskeletal condition, if applicable, to identify the cause of the musculoskeletal condition

EXCLUDES 2   arthropathic psoriasis (L40.5-)
certain conditions originating in the perinatal period (P04-P96)
certain infectious and parasitic diseases (A00-B99)
compartment syndrome (traumatic) (T79.A-)
complications of pregnancy, childbirth and the puerperium (O00-O9A)
congenital malformations, deformations, and chromosomal abnormalities (Q00-Q99)
endocrine, nutritional and metabolic diseases (E00-E88)
injury, poisoning and certain other consequences of external causes (S00-T88)
neoplasms (C00-D49)
symptoms, signs and abnormal clinical and laboratory findings, not elsewhere classified (R00-R94)

This chapter contains the following blocks:

M00-M02	Infectious arthropathies
M04	Autoinflammatory syndromes
M05-M14	Inflammatory polyarthropathies
M15-M19	Osteoarthritis
M20-M25	Other joint disorders
M26-M27	Dentofacial anomalies [including malocclusion] and other disorders of jaw
M30-M36	Systemic connective tissue disorders
M40-M43	Deforming dorsopathies
M45-M49	Spondylopathies
M50-M54	Other dorsopathies
M60-M63	Disorders of muscles
M65-M67	Disorders of synovium and tendon
M70-M79	Other soft tissue disorders
M80-M85	Disorders of bone density and structure
M86-M90	Other osteopathies
M91-M94	Chondropathies
M95	Other disorders of the musculoskeletal system and connective tissue
M96	Intraoperative and postprocedural complications and disorders of musculoskeletal system, not elsewhere classified
M97	Periprosthetic fracture around internal prosthetic joint
M99	Biomechanical lesions, not elsewhere classified

ARTHROPATHIES (M00-M25)

INCLUDES   disorders affecting predominantly peripheral (limb) joints

Infectious arthropathies (M00-M02)

NOTE   This block comprises arthropathies due to microbiological agents. Distinction is made between the following types of etiological relationship:

a) direct infection of joint, where organisms invade synovia tissue and microbial antigen is present in the joint;

b) indirect infection, which may be of two types: a reactive arthropathy, where microbial infection of the body is established but neither organisms nor antigens can be identified in the joint, and a postinfective arthropathy, where microbial antigen is present but recovery of an organism is inconstant and evidence of local multiplication is lacking.

AHA: 2019,3Q,16

✓4ᵗʰ **M00 Pyogenic arthritis**

EXCLUDES 2   infection and inflammatory reaction due to internal joint prosthesis (T84.5-)

AHA: 2022,1Q,31
DEF: Pyogenic: Relating to or involving pus production, often referred to as suppurative or purulent.

✓5ᵗʰ **M00.0 Staphylococcal arthritis and polyarthritis**

Use additional code (B95.61-B95.8) to identify bacterial agent

M00.00 **Staphylococcal arthritis, unspecified joint**   CC UNS HCC

✓6ᵗʰ M00.01 **Staphylococcal arthritis, shoulder**
M00.011 **Staphylococcal arthritis, right shoulder**   CC HCC
M00.012 **Staphylococcal arthritis, left shoulder**   CC HCC
M00.019 **Staphylococcal arthritis, unspecified shoulder**   CC UNS HCC

✓6ᵗʰ M00.02 **Staphylococcal arthritis, elbow**
M00.021 **Staphylococcal arthritis, right elbow**   CC HCC
M00.022 **Staphylococcal arthritis, left elbow**   CC HCC
M00.029 **Staphylococcal arthritis, unspecified elbow**   CC UNS HCC

✓6ᵗʰ M00.03 **Staphylococcal arthritis, wrist**
Staphylococcal arthritis of carpal bones
M00.031 **Staphylococcal arthritis, right wrist**   CC HCC
M00.032 **Staphylococcal arthritis, left wrist**   CC HCC
M00.039 **Staphylococcal arthritis, unspecified wrist**   CC UNS HCC

✓6ᵗʰ M00.04 **Staphylococcal arthritis, hand**
Staphylococcal arthritis of metacarpus and phalanges
M00.041 **Staphylococcal arthritis, right hand**   CC HCC
M00.042 **Staphylococcal arthritis, left hand**   CC HCC
M00.049 **Staphylococcal arthritis, unspecified hand**   CC UNS HCC

✓6ᵗʰ M00.05 **Staphylococcal arthritis, hip**
M00.051 **Staphylococcal arthritis, right hip**   CC HCC
M00.052 **Staphylococcal arthritis, left hip**   CC HCC
M00.059 **Staphylococcal arthritis, unspecified hip**   CC UNS HCC

✓6ᵗʰ M00.06 **Staphylococcal arthritis, knee**
M00.061 **Staphylococcal arthritis, right knee**   CC HCC
M00.062 **Staphylococcal arthritis, left knee**   CC HCC
M00.069 **Staphylococcal arthritis, unspecified knee**   CC UNS HCC

✓6ᵗʰ M00.07 **Staphylococcal arthritis, ankle and foot**
Staphylococcal arthritis, tarsus, metatarsus and phalanges
M00.071 **Staphylococcal arthritis, right ankle and foot**   CC HCC
M00.072 **Staphylococcal arthritis, left ankle and foot**   CC HCC
M00.079 **Staphylococcal arthritis, unspecified ankle and foot**   CC UNS HCC

M00.08 **Staphylococcal arthritis, vertebrae**   CC HCC
M00.09 **Staphylococcal polyarthritis**   CC HCC

✓5ᵗʰ **M00.1 Pneumococcal arthritis and polyarthritis**

M00.10 **Pneumococcal arthritis, unspecified joint**   CC UNS HCC

✓6ᵗʰ M00.11 **Pneumococcal arthritis, shoulder**
M00.111 **Pneumococcal arthritis, right shoulder**   CC HCC
M00.112 **Pneumococcal arthritis, left shoulder**   CC HCC
M00.119 **Pneumococcal arthritis, unspecified shoulder**   CC UNS HCC

✓6ᵗʰ M00.12 **Pneumococcal arthritis, elbow**
M00.121 **Pneumococcal arthritis, right elbow**   CC HCC
M00.122 **Pneumococcal arthritis, left elbow**   CC HCC
M00.129 **Pneumococcal arthritis, unspecified elbow**   CC UNS HCC

✓6ᵗʰ M00.13 **Pneumococcal arthritis, wrist**
Pneumococcal arthritis of carpal bones
M00.131 **Pneumococcal arthritis, right wrist**   CC HCC
M00.132 **Pneumococcal arthritis, left wrist**   CC HCC
M00.139 **Pneumococcal arthritis, unspecified wrist**   CC UNS HCC

✓6ᵗʰ M00.14 **Pneumococcal arthritis, hand**
Pneumococcal arthritis of metacarpus and phalanges
M00.141 **Pneumococcal arthritis, right hand**   CC HCC
M00.142 **Pneumococcal arthritis, left hand**   CC HCC
M00.149 **Pneumococcal arthritis, unspecified hand**   CC UNS HCC

√6th **M00.15** Pneumococcal arthritis, **hip**

    M00.151 Pneumococcal arthritis, **right** hip `CC` `HCC`

    M00.152 Pneumococcal arthritis, **left** hip `CC` `HCC`

    M00.159 Pneumococcal arthritis, unspecified hip `CC` `UNS` `HCC`

√6th **M00.16** Pneumococcal arthritis, **knee**

    M00.161 Pneumococcal arthritis, **right** knee `CC` `HCC`

    M00.162 Pneumococcal arthritis, **left** knee `CC` `HCC`

    M00.169 Pneumococcal arthritis, unspecified knee `CC` `UNS` `HCC`

√6th **M00.17** Pneumococcal arthritis, **ankle and foot**

    Pneumococcal arthritis, tarsus, metatarsus and phalanges

    M00.171 Pneumococcal arthritis, **right** ankle and foot `CC` `HCC`

    M00.172 Pneumococcal arthritis, **left** ankle and foot `CC` `HCC`

    M00.179 Pneumococcal arthritis, unspecified ankle and foot `CC` `UNS` `HCC`

M00.18 Pneumococcal arthritis, **vertebrae** `CC` `HCC`

M00.19 Pneumococcal **polyarthritis** `CC` `HCC`

√5th **M00.2** Other streptococcal arthritis and polyarthritis

    Use additional code (B95.0-B95.2, B95.4-B95.5) to identify bacterial agent

    M00.20 Other streptococcal arthritis, unspecified **joint** `CC` `UNS` `HCC`

√6th **M00.21** Other streptococcal arthritis, **shoulder**

    M00.211 Other streptococcal arthritis, **right** shoulder `CC` `HCC`

    M00.212 Other streptococcal arthritis, **left** shoulder `CC` `HCC`

    M00.219 Other streptococcal arthritis, unspecified shoulder `CC` `UNS` `HCC`

√6th **M00.22** Other streptococcal arthritis, **elbow**

    M00.221 Other streptococcal arthritis, **right** elbow `CC` `HCC`

    M00.222 Other streptococcal arthritis, **left** elbow `CC` `HCC`

    M00.229 Other streptococcal arthritis, unspecified elbow `CC` `UNS` `HCC`

√6th **M00.23** Other streptococcal arthritis, **wrist**

    Other streptococcal arthritis of carpal bones

    M00.231 Other streptococcal arthritis, **right** wrist `CC` `HCC`

    M00.232 Other streptococcal arthritis, **left** wrist `CC` `HCC`

    M00.239 Other streptococcal arthritis, unspecified wrist `CC` `UNS` `HCC`

√6th **M00.24** Other streptococcal arthritis, **hand**

    Other streptococcal arthritis metacarpus and phalanges

    M00.241 Other streptococcal arthritis, **right** hand `CC` `HCC`

    M00.242 Other streptococcal arthritis, **left** hand `CC` `HCC`

    M00.249 Other streptococcal arthritis, unspecified hand `CC` `UNS` `HCC`

√6th **M00.25** Other streptococcal arthritis, **hip**

    M00.251 Other streptococcal arthritis, **right** hip `CC` `HCC`

    M00.252 Other streptococcal arthritis, **left** hip `CC` `HCC`

    M00.259 Other streptococcal arthritis, unspecified hip `CC` `UNS` `HCC`

√6th **M00.26** Other streptococcal arthritis, **knee**

    M00.261 Other streptococcal arthritis, **right** knee `CC` `HCC`

    M00.262 Other streptococcal arthritis, **left** knee `CC` `HCC`

    M00.269 Other streptococcal arthritis, unspecified knee `CC` `UNS` `HCC`

√6th **M00.27** Other streptococcal arthritis, **ankle and foot**

    Other streptococcal arthritis, tarsus, metatarsus and phalanges

    M00.271 Other streptococcal arthritis, **right** ankle and foot `CC` `HCC`

    M00.272 Other streptococcal arthritis, **left** ankle and foot `CC` `HCC`

    M00.279 Other streptococcal arthritis, unspecified ankle and foot `CC` `UNS` `HCC`

M00.28 Other streptococcal arthritis, **vertebrae** `CC` `HCC`

M00.29 Other streptococcal **polyarthritis** `CC` `HCC`

√5th **M00.8** Arthritis and polyarthritis due to other bacteria

    Use additional code (B96) to identify bacteria

    M00.80 Arthritis due to other bacteria, unspecified joint `CC` `UNS` `HCC`

√6th **M00.81** Arthritis due to other bacteria, **shoulder**

    M00.811 Arthritis due to other bacteria, **right** shoulder `CC` `HCC`

    M00.812 Arthritis due to other bacteria, **left** shoulder `CC` `HCC`

    M00.819 Arthritis due to other bacteria, unspecified shoulder `CC` `UNS` `HCC`

√6th **M00.82** Arthritis due to other bacteria, **elbow**

    M00.821 Arthritis due to other bacteria, **right** elbow `CC` `HCC`

    M00.822 Arthritis due to other bacteria, **left** elbow `CC` `HCC`

    M00.829 Arthritis due to other bacteria, unspecified elbow `CC` `UNS` `HCC`

√6th **M00.83** Arthritis due to other bacteria, **wrist**

    Arthritis due to other bacteria, carpal bones

    M00.831 Arthritis due to other bacteria, **right** wrist `CC` `HCC`

    M00.832 Arthritis due to other bacteria, **left** wrist `CC` `HCC`

    M00.839 Arthritis due to other bacteria, unspecified wrist `CC` `UNS` `HCC`

√6th **M00.84** Arthritis due to other bacteria, **hand**

    Arthritis due to other bacteria, metacarpus and phalanges

    M00.841 Arthritis due to other bacteria, **right** hand `CC` `HCC`

    M00.842 Arthritis due to other bacteria, **left** hand `CC` `HCC`

    M00.849 Arthritis due to other bacteria, unspecified hand `CC` `UNS` `HCC`

√6th **M00.85** Arthritis due to other bacteria, **hip**

    M00.851 Arthritis due to other bacteria, **right** hip `CC` `HCC`

    M00.852 Arthritis due to other bacteria, **left** hip `CC` `HCC`

    M00.859 Arthritis due to other bacteria, unspecified hip `CC` `UNS` `HCC`

√6th **M00.86** Arthritis due to other bacteria, **knee**

    AHA: 2019,3Q,16

    M00.861 Arthritis due to other bacteria, **right** knee `CC` `HCC`

    M00.862 Arthritis due to other bacteria, **left** knee `CC` `HCC`

    M00.869 Arthritis due to other bacteria, unspecified knee `CC` `UNS` `HCC`

√6th **M00.87** Arthritis due to other bacteria, **ankle and foot**

    Arthritis due to other bacteria, tarsus, metatarsus, and phalanges

    M00.871 Arthritis due to other bacteria, **right** ankle and foot `CC` `HCC`

    M00.872 Arthritis due to other bacteria, **left** ankle and foot `CC` `HCC`

    M00.879 Arthritis due to other bacteria, unspecified ankle and foot `CC` `UNS` `HCC`

M00.88 Arthritis due to other bacteria, **vertebrae** `CC` `HCC`

M00.89 **Polyarthritis** due to other bacteria `CC` `HCC`

M00.9 Pyogenic arthritis, unspecified `CC` `HCC`

    Infective arthritis NOS

`N` Newborn: 0   `P` Pediatric: 0-17   `M` Maternity: 9-64   `A` Adult: 15-124   `UNS` Unspecified Site   `MCC` Major Complication/Comorbidity   `CC` Complication/Comorbidity   `PE` POA Exempt

774   ICD-10-CM 2025

✓4th M01   Direct infections of joint in infectious and parasitic diseases classified elsewhere

Code first underlying disease, such as:
leprosy [Hansen's disease] (A30.-)
mycoses (B35-B49)
O'nyong-nyong fever (A92.1)
paratyphoid fever (A01.1-A01.4)

EXCLUDES 1   arthropathy in Lyme disease (A69.23)
gonococcal arthritis (A54.42)
meningococcal arthritis (A39.83)
mumps arthritis (B26.85)
postinfective arthropathy (M02.-)
postmeningococcal arthritis (A39.84)
reactive arthritis (M02.3)
rubella arthritis (B06.82)
sarcoidosis arthritis (D86.86)
tuberculosis arthritis (A18.01-A18.02)
typhoid fever arthritis (A01.04)

✓5th M01.X   Direct infection of joint in infectious and parasitic diseases classified elsewhere

    M01.X0   *Direct infection of unspecified joint in infectious and parasitic diseases classified elsewhere*   CC UNS HCC

✓6th M01.X1   Direct infection of shoulder joint in infectious and parasitic diseases classified elsewhere

    M01.X11   *Direct infection of right shoulder in infectious and parasitic diseases classified elsewhere*   CC HCC

    M01.X12   *Direct infection of left shoulder in infectious and parasitic diseases classified elsewhere*   CC HCC

    M01.X19   *Direct infection of unspecified shoulder in infectious and parasitic diseases classified elsewhere*   CC UNS HCC

✓6th M01.X2   Direct infection of elbow in infectious and parasitic diseases classified elsewhere

    M01.X21   *Direct infection of right elbow in infectious and parasitic diseases classified elsewhere*   CC HCC

    M01.X22   *Direct infection of left elbow in infectious and parasitic diseases classified elsewhere*   CC HCC

    M01.X29   *Direct infection of unspecified elbow in infectious and parasitic diseases classified elsewhere*   CC UNS HCC

✓6th M01.X3   Direct infection of wrist in infectious and parasitic diseases classified elsewhere

Direct infection of carpal bones in infectious and parasitic diseases classified elsewhere

    M01.X31   *Direct infection of right wrist in infectious and parasitic diseases classified elsewhere*   CC HCC

    M01.X32   *Direct infection of left wrist in infectious and parasitic diseases classified elsewhere*   CC HCC

    M01.X39   *Direct infection of unspecified wrist in infectious and parasitic diseases classified elsewhere*   CC UNS HCC

✓6th M01.X4   Direct infection of hand in infectious and parasitic diseases classified elsewhere

Direct infection of metacarpus and phalanges in infectious and parasitic diseases classified elsewhere

    M01.X41   *Direct infection of right hand in infectious and parasitic diseases classified elsewhere*   CC HCC

    M01.X42   *Direct infection of left hand in infectious and parasitic diseases classified elsewhere*   CC HCC

    M01.X49   *Direct infection of unspecified hand in infectious and parasitic diseases classified elsewhere*   CC UNS HCC

✓6th M01.X5   Direct infection of hip in infectious and parasitic diseases classified elsewhere

    M01.X51   *Direct infection of right hip in infectious and parasitic diseases classified elsewhere*   CC HCC

    M01.X52   *Direct infection of left hip in infectious and parasitic diseases classified elsewhere*   CC HCC

    M01.X59   *Direct infection of unspecified hip in infectious and parasitic diseases classified elsewhere*   CC UNS HCC

✓6th M01.X6   Direct infection of knee in infectious and parasitic diseases classified elsewhere

    M01.X61   *Direct infection of right knee in infectious and parasitic diseases classified elsewhere*   CC HCC

    M01.X62   *Direct infection of left knee in infectious and parasitic diseases classified elsewhere*   CC HCC

    M01.X69   *Direct infection of unspecified knee in infectious and parasitic diseases classified elsewhere*   CC UNS HCC

✓6th M01.X7   Direct infection of ankle and foot in infectious and parasitic diseases classified elsewhere

Direct infection of tarsus, metatarsus and phalanges in infectious and parasitic diseases classified elsewhere

    M01.X71   *Direct infection of right ankle and foot in infectious and parasitic diseases classified elsewhere*   CC HCC

    M01.X72   *Direct infection of left ankle and foot in infectious and parasitic diseases classified elsewhere*   CC HCC

    M01.X79   *Direct infection of unspecified ankle and foot in infectious and parasitic diseases classified elsewhere*   CC UNS HCC

    M01.X8   *Direct infection of vertebrae in infectious and parasitic diseases classified elsewhere*   CC HCC

    M01.X9   *Direct infection of multiple joints in infectious and parasitic diseases classified elsewhere*   CC HCC

✓4th M02   Postinfective and reactive arthropathies

Code first underlying disease, such as:
congenital syphilis [Clutton's joints] (A50.5)
enteritis due to Yersinia enterocolitica (A04.6)
infective endocarditis (I33.0)
viral hepatitis (B15-B19)

EXCLUDES 1   Behcet's disease (M35.2)
direct infections of joint in infectious and parasitic diseases classified elsewhere (M01.-)
mumps arthritis (B26.85)
postmeningococcal arthritis (A39.84)
rheumatic fever (I00)
rubella arthritis (B06.82)
syphilis arthritis (late) (A52.77)
tabetic arthropathy [Charcôt's] (A52.16)

✓5th M02.0   Arthropathy following intestinal bypass

    M02.00   Arthropathy following intestinal bypass, unspecified site

✓6th M02.01   Arthropathy following intestinal bypass, shoulder

    M02.011   Arthropathy following intestinal bypass, right shoulder

    M02.012   Arthropathy following intestinal bypass, left shoulder

    M02.019   Arthropathy following intestinal bypass, unspecified shoulder

✓6th M02.02   Arthropathy following intestinal bypass, elbow

    M02.021   Arthropathy following intestinal bypass, right elbow

    M02.022   Arthropathy following intestinal bypass, left elbow

    M02.029   Arthropathy following intestinal bypass, unspecified elbow

✓6th M02.03   Arthropathy following intestinal bypass, wrist

Arthropathy following intestinal bypass, carpal bones

    M02.031   Arthropathy following intestinal bypass, right wrist

    M02.032   Arthropathy following intestinal bypass, left wrist

    M02.039   Arthropathy following intestinal bypass, unspecified wrist

✓6th M02.04   Arthropathy following intestinal bypass, hand

Arthropathy following intestinal bypass, metacarpals and phalanges

    M02.041   Arthropathy following intestinal bypass, right hand

    M02.042   Arthropathy following intestinal bypass, left hand

✔ Additional Character Required   ✓x7th Placeholder   Questionable PDx   Manifestation   Unspecified   UPD Unacceptable PDx   H1 - H14 HAC   HCC CMS-HCC Dx   HIV HIV Dx

ICD-10-CM 2025   775

Chapter 13. Diseases of the Musculoskeletal System and Connective Tissue

        M02.049 Arthropathy following intestinal bypass, unspecified hand

√6ᵗʰ **M02.05** Arthropathy following intestinal bypass, **hip**

        M02.051 Arthropathy following intestinal bypass, **right** hip

        M02.052 Arthropathy following intestinal bypass, **left** hip

        M02.059 Arthropathy following intestinal bypass, unspecified hip

√6ᵗʰ **M02.06** Arthropathy following intestinal bypass, **knee**

        M02.061 Arthropathy following intestinal bypass, **right** knee

        M02.062 Arthropathy following intestinal bypass, **left** knee

        M02.069 Arthropathy following intestinal bypass, unspecified knee

√6ᵗʰ **M02.07** Arthropathy following intestinal bypass, **ankle and foot**

     Arthropathy following intestinal bypass, tarsus, metatarsus and phalanges

        M02.071 Arthropathy following intestinal bypass, **right** ankle and foot

        M02.072 Arthropathy following intestinal bypass, **left** ankle and foot

        M02.079 Arthropathy following intestinal bypass, unspecified ankle and foot

     M02.08 Arthropathy following intestinal bypass, **vertebrae**

     M02.09 Arthropathy following intestinal bypass, **multiple sites**

√5ᵗʰ **M02.1** **Postdysenteric** arthropathy

     M02.10 Postdysenteric arthropathy, unspecified site   CC UNS HCC

√6ᵗʰ **M02.11** Postdysenteric arthropathy, **shoulder**

        M02.111 Postdysenteric arthropathy, **right** shoulder   CC HCC

        M02.112 Postdysenteric arthropathy, **left** shoulder   CC HCC

        M02.119 Postdysenteric arthropathy, unspecified shoulder   CC UNS HCC

√6ᵗʰ **M02.12** Postdysenteric arthropathy, **elbow**

        M02.121 Postdysenteric arthropathy, **right** elbow   CC HCC

        M02.122 Postdysenteric arthropathy, **left** elbow   CC HCC

        M02.129 Postdysenteric arthropathy, unspecified elbow   CC UNS HCC

√6ᵗʰ **M02.13** Postdysenteric arthropathy, **wrist**

     Postdysenteric arthropathy, carpal bones

        M02.131 Postdysenteric arthropathy, **right** wrist   CC HCC

        M02.132 Postdysenteric arthropathy, **left** wrist   CC HCC

        M02.139 Postdysenteric arthropathy, unspecified wrist   CC UNS HCC

√6ᵗʰ **M02.14** Postdysenteric arthropathy, **hand**

     Postdysenteric arthropathy, metacarpus and phalanges

        M02.141 Postdysenteric arthropathy, **right** hand   CC HCC

        M02.142 Postdysenteric arthropathy, **left** hand   CC HCC

        M02.149 Postdysenteric arthropathy, unspecified hand   CC UNS HCC

√6ᵗʰ **M02.15** Postdysenteric arthropathy, **hip**

        M02.151 Postdysenteric arthropathy, **right** hip   CC HCC

        M02.152 Postdysenteric arthropathy, **left** hip   CC HCC

        M02.159 Postdysenteric arthropathy, unspecified hip   CC UNS HCC

√6ᵗʰ **M02.16** Postdysenteric arthropathy, **knee**

        M02.161 Postdysenteric arthropathy, **right** knee   CC HCC

        M02.162 Postdysenteric arthropathy, **left** knee   CC HCC

        M02.169 Postdysenteric arthropathy, unspecified knee   CC UNS HCC

√6ᵗʰ **M02.17** Postdysenteric arthropathy, **ankle and foot**

     Postdysenteric arthropathy, tarsus, metatarsus and phalanges

        M02.171 Postdysenteric arthropathy, **right** ankle and foot   CC HCC

        M02.172 Postdysenteric arthropathy, **left** ankle and foot   CC HCC

        M02.179 Postdysenteric arthropathy, unspecified ankle and foot   CC UNS HCC

     M02.18 Postdysenteric arthropathy, **vertebrae**   CC HCC

     M02.19 Postdysenteric arthropathy, **multiple sites**   CC HCC

√5ᵗʰ **M02.2** **Postimmunization** arthropathy

     M02.20 Postimmunization arthropathy, unspecified site

√6ᵗʰ **M02.21** Postimmunization arthropathy, **shoulder**

        M02.211 Postimmunization arthropathy, **right** shoulder

        M02.212 Postimmunization arthropathy, **left** shoulder

        M02.219 Postimmunization arthropathy, unspecified shoulder

√6ᵗʰ **M02.22** Postimmunization arthropathy, **elbow**

        M02.221 Postimmunization arthropathy, **right** elbow

        M02.222 Postimmunization arthropathy, **left** elbow

        M02.229 Postimmunization arthropathy, unspecified elbow

√6ᵗʰ **M02.23** Postimmunization arthropathy, **wrist**

     Postimmunization arthropathy, carpal bones

        M02.231 Postimmunization arthropathy, **right** wrist

        M02.232 Postimmunization arthropathy, **left** wrist

        M02.239 Postimmunization arthropathy, unspecified wrist

√6ᵗʰ **M02.24** Postimmunization arthropathy, **hand**

     Postimmunization arthropathy, metacarpus and phalanges

        M02.241 Postimmunization arthropathy, **right** hand

        M02.242 Postimmunization arthropathy, **left** hand

        M02.249 Postimmunization arthropathy, unspecified hand

√6ᵗʰ **M02.25** Postimmunization arthropathy, **hip**

        M02.251 Postimmunization arthropathy, **right** hip

        M02.252 Postimmunization arthropathy, **left** hip

        M02.259 Postimmunization arthropathy, unspecified hip

√6ᵗʰ **M02.26** Postimmunization arthropathy, **knee**

        M02.261 Postimmunization arthropathy, **right** knee

        M02.262 Postimmunization arthropathy, **left** knee

        M02.269 Postimmunization arthropathy, unspecified knee

√6ᵗʰ **M02.27** Postimmunization arthropathy, **ankle and foot**

     Postimmunization arthropathy, tarsus, metatarsus and phalanges

        M02.271 Postimmunization arthropathy, **right** ankle and foot

        M02.272 Postimmunization arthropathy, **left** ankle and foot

        M02.279 Postimmunization arthropathy, unspecified ankle and foot

     M02.28 Postimmunization arthropathy, **vertebrae**

     M02.29 Postimmunization arthropathy, **multiple sites**

√5ᵗʰ **M02.3** **Reiter's disease**

     Reactive arthritis

     DEF: Arthritis, iridocyclitis, and urethritis, sometimes with diarrhea. While symptoms may recur, arthritis is constant.

     M02.30 Reiter's disease, unspecified site   CC UNS HCC

√6ᵗʰ **M02.31** Reiter's disease, **shoulder**

        M02.311 Reiter's disease, **right** shoulder   CC HCC

        M02.312 Reiter's disease, **left** shoulder   CC HCC

        M02.319 Reiter's disease, unspecified shoulder   CC UNS HCC

√6ᵗʰ **M02.32** Reiter's disease, **elbow**

        M02.321 Reiter's disease, **right** elbow   CC HCC

        M02.322 Reiter's disease, **left** elbow   CC HCC

        M02.329 Reiter's disease, unspecified elbow   CC UNS HCC

N Newborn: 0   P Pediatric: 0-17   M Maternity: 9-64   A Adult: 15-124   UNS Unspecified Site   MCC Major Complication/Comorbidity   CC Complication/Comorbidity   PE POA Exempt

776   ICD-10-CM 2025

√6ᵗʰ **M02.33** Reiter's disease, **wrist**
Reiter's disease, carpal bones
     M02.331 Reiter's disease, **right** wrist   `CC` `HCC`
     M02.332 Reiter's disease, **left** wrist   `CC` `HCC`
     M02.339 Reiter's disease, **unspecified** wrist   `CC` `UNS` `HCC`

√6ᵗʰ **M02.34** Reiter's disease, **hand**
Reiter's disease, metacarpus and phalanges
     M02.341 Reiter's disease, **right** hand   `CC` `HCC`
     M02.342 Reiter's disease, **left** hand   `CC` `HCC`
     M02.349 Reiter's disease, **unspecified** hand   `CC` `UNS` `HCC`

√6ᵗʰ **M02.35** Reiter's disease, **hip**
     M02.351 Reiter's disease, **right** hip   `CC` `HCC`
     M02.352 Reiter's disease, **left** hip   `CC` `HCC`
     M02.359 Reiter's disease, **unspecified** hip   `CC` `UNS` `HCC`

√6ᵗʰ **M02.36** Reiter's disease, **knee**
     M02.361 Reiter's disease, **right** knee   `CC` `HCC`
     M02.362 Reiter's disease, **left** knee   `CC` `HCC`
     M02.369 Reiter's disease, **unspecified** knee   `CC` `UNS` `HCC`

√6ᵗʰ **M02.37** Reiter's disease, **ankle and foot**
Reiter's disease, tarsus, metatarsus and phalanges
     M02.371 Reiter's disease, **right** ankle and foot   `CC` `HCC`
     M02.372 Reiter's disease, **left** ankle and foot   `CC` `HCC`
     M02.379 Reiter's disease, **unspecified** ankle and foot   `CC` `UNS` `HCC`

     M02.38 Reiter's disease, **vertebrae**   `CC` `HCC`
     M02.39 Reiter's disease, **multiple sites**   `CC` `HCC`

√5ᵗʰ **M02.8** Other **reactive** arthropathies
     M02.80 Other reactive arthropathies, **unspecified site**   `CC` `UNS` `HCC`

√6ᵗʰ **M02.81** Other reactive arthropathies, **shoulder**
     M02.811 Other reactive arthropathies, right shoulder   `CC` `HCC`
     M02.812 Other reactive arthropathies, left shoulder   `CC` `HCC`
     M02.819 Other reactive arthropathies, unspecified shoulder   `CC` `UNS` `HCC`

√6ᵗʰ **M02.82** Other reactive arthropathies, **elbow**
     M02.821 Other reactive arthropathies, right elbow   `CC` `HCC`
     M02.822 Other reactive arthropathies, left elbow   `CC` `HCC`
     M02.829 Other reactive arthropathies, unspecified elbow   `CC` `UNS` `HCC`

√6ᵗʰ **M02.83** Other reactive arthropathies, **wrist**
Other reactive arthropathies, carpal bones
     M02.831 Other reactive arthropathies, right wrist   `CC` `HCC`
     M02.832 Other reactive arthropathies, left wrist   `CC` `HCC`
     M02.839 Other reactive arthropathies, unspecified wrist   `CC` `UNS` `HCC`

√6ᵗʰ **M02.84** Other reactive arthropathies, **hand**
Other reactive arthropathies, metacarpus and phalanges
     M02.841 Other reactive arthropathies, right hand   `CC` `HCC`
     M02.842 Other reactive arthropathies, left hand   `CC` `HCC`
     M02.849 Other reactive arthropathies, unspecified hand   `CC` `UNS` `HCC`

√6ᵗʰ **M02.85** Other reactive arthropathies, **hip**
     M02.851 Other reactive arthropathies, right hip   `CC` `HCC`
     M02.852 Other reactive arthropathies, left hip   `CC` `HCC`
     M02.859 Other reactive arthropathies, unspecified hip   `CC` `UNS` `HCC`

√6ᵗʰ **M02.86** Other reactive arthropathies, **knee**
     M02.861 Other reactive arthropathies, right knee   `CC` `HCC`

     M02.862 Other reactive arthropathies, left knee   `CC` `HCC`
     M02.869 Other reactive arthropathies, unspecified knee   `CC` `UNS` `HCC`

√6ᵗʰ **M02.87** Other reactive arthropathies, **ankle and foot**
Other reactive arthropathies, tarsus, metatarsus and phalanges
     M02.871 Other reactive arthropathies, right ankle and foot   `CC` `HCC`
     M02.872 Other reactive arthropathies, left ankle and foot   `CC` `HCC`
     M02.879 Other reactive arthropathies, unspecified ankle and foot   `CC` `UNS` `HCC`

     M02.88 Other reactive arthropathies, vertebrae   `CC` `HCC`
     M02.89 Other reactive arthropathies, multiple sites   `CC` `HCC`

M02.9 Reactive arthropathy, unspecified   `HCC`

Autoinflammatory syndromes (M04)

√4ᵗʰ **M04** Autoinflammatory syndromes
     EXCLUDES 2   Crohn's disease (K50.-)
     AHA: 2016,4Q,37

     M04.1 Periodic fever syndromes   `HCC`
       Familial Mediterranean fever
       Hyperimmunoglobin D syndrome
       Mevalonate kinase deficiency
       Tumor necrosis factor receptor associated periodic syndrome [TRAPS]

     M04.2 Cryopyrin-associated periodic syndromes   `HCC`
       Chronic infantile neurological, cutaneous and articular syndrome [CINCA]
       Familial cold autoinflammatory syndrome
       Familial cold urticaria
       Muckle-Wells syndrome
       Neonatal onset multisystemic inflammatory disorder [NOMID]

     M04.8 Other autoinflammatory syndromes   `HCC`
       Blau syndrome
       Deficiency of interleukin 1 receptor antagonist [DIRA]
       Majeed syndrome
       Periodic fever, aphthous stomatitis, pharyngitis, and adenopathy syndrome [PFAPA]
       Pyogenic arthritis, pyoderma gangrenosum, and acne syndrome [PAPA]

     M04.9 Autoinflammatory syndrome, unspecified   `HCC`

Inflammatory polyarthropathies (M05-M14)

√4ᵗʰ **M05** Rheumatoid arthritis with rheumatoid factor
     EXCLUDES 1   juvenile rheumatoid arthritis (M08.-)
         rheumatic fever (I00)
         rheumatoid arthritis of spine (M45.-)
     AHA: 2020,4Q,31-32
     DEF: Rheumatoid arthritis: Autoimmune systemic disease that causes chronic inflammation of the joints and other areas of the body, manifested by inflammatory changes in articular structures and synovial membranes, atrophy, and loss in bone density.

√5ᵗʰ **M05.0** Felty's syndrome
     Rheumatoid arthritis with splenoadenomegaly and leukopenia
     M05.00 Felty's syndrome, unspecified site   `HCC`

√6ᵗʰ **M05.01** Felty's syndrome, **shoulder**
     M05.011 Felty's syndrome, **right** shoulder   `HCC`
     M05.012 Felty's syndrome, **left** shoulder   `HCC`
     M05.019 Felty's syndrome, **unspecified** shoulder   `HCC`

√6ᵗʰ **M05.02** Felty's syndrome, **elbow**
     M05.021 Felty's syndrome, **right** elbow   `HCC`
     M05.022 Felty's syndrome, **left** elbow   `HCC`
     M05.029 Felty's syndrome, **unspecified** elbow   `HCC`

√6ᵗʰ **M05.03** Felty's syndrome, **wrist**
     Felty's syndrome, carpal bones
     M05.031 Felty's syndrome, **right** wrist   `HCC`
     M05.032 Felty's syndrome, **left** wrist   `HCC`
     M05.039 Felty's syndrome, unspecified wrist   `HCC`

√6ᵗʰ **M05.04** Felty's syndrome, **hand**
     Felty's syndrome, metacarpus and phalanges
     M05.041 Felty's syndrome, **right** hand   `HCC`
     M05.042 Felty's syndrome, **left** hand   `HCC`

M05.049 **Felty's syndrome, unspecified hand** `HCC`

✓6ᵗʰ M05.05 **Felty's syndrome, hip**

M05.051 **Felty's syndrome, right hip** `HCC`

M05.052 **Felty's syndrome, left hip** `HCC`

M05.059 **Felty's syndrome, unspecified hip** `HCC`

✓6ᵗʰ M05.06 **Felty's syndrome, knee**

M05.061 **Felty's syndrome, right knee** `HCC`

M05.062 **Felty's syndrome, left knee** `HCC`

M05.069 **Felty's syndrome, unspecified knee** `HCC`

✓6ᵗʰ M05.07 **Felty's syndrome, ankle and foot**

Felty's syndrome, tarsus, metatarsus and phalanges

M05.071 **Felty's syndrome, right ankle and foot** `HCC`

M05.072 **Felty's syndrome, left ankle and foot** `HCC`

M05.079 **Felty's syndrome, unspecified ankle and foot** `HCC`

M05.09 **Felty's syndrome, multiple sites** `HCC`

✓5ᵗʰ M05.1 **Rheumatoid lung disease with rheumatoid arthritis**

M05.10 **Rheumatoid lung disease with rheumatoid arthritis of unspecified site** `HCC`

✓6ᵗʰ M05.11 **Rheumatoid lung disease with rheumatoid arthritis of shoulder**

M05.111 **Rheumatoid lung disease with rheumatoid arthritis of right shoulder** `HCC`

M05.112 **Rheumatoid lung disease with rheumatoid arthritis of left shoulder** `HCC`

M05.119 **Rheumatoid lung disease with rheumatoid arthritis of unspecified shoulder** `HCC`

✓6ᵗʰ M05.12 **Rheumatoid lung disease with rheumatoid arthritis of elbow**

M05.121 **Rheumatoid lung disease with rheumatoid arthritis of right elbow** `HCC`

M05.122 **Rheumatoid lung disease with rheumatoid arthritis of left elbow** `HCC`

M05.129 **Rheumatoid lung disease with rheumatoid arthritis of unspecified elbow** `HCC`

✓6ᵗʰ M05.13 **Rheumatoid lung disease with rheumatoid arthritis of wrist**

Rheumatoid lung disease with rheumatoid arthritis, carpal bones

M05.131 **Rheumatoid lung disease with rheumatoid arthritis of right wrist** `HCC`

M05.132 **Rheumatoid lung disease with rheumatoid arthritis of left wrist** `HCC`

M05.139 **Rheumatoid lung disease with rheumatoid arthritis of unspecified wrist** `HCC`

✓6ᵗʰ M05.14 **Rheumatoid lung disease with rheumatoid arthritis of hand**

Rheumatoid lung disease with rheumatoid arthritis, metacarpus and phalanges

M05.141 **Rheumatoid lung disease with rheumatoid arthritis of right hand** `HCC`

M05.142 **Rheumatoid lung disease with rheumatoid arthritis of left hand** `HCC`

M05.149 **Rheumatoid lung disease with rheumatoid arthritis of unspecified hand** `HCC`

✓6ᵗʰ M05.15 **Rheumatoid lung disease with rheumatoid arthritis of hip**

M05.151 **Rheumatoid lung disease with rheumatoid arthritis of right hip** `HCC`

M05.152 **Rheumatoid lung disease with rheumatoid arthritis of left hip** `HCC`

M05.159 **Rheumatoid lung disease with rheumatoid arthritis of unspecified hip** `HCC`

✓6ᵗʰ M05.16 **Rheumatoid lung disease with rheumatoid arthritis of knee**

M05.161 **Rheumatoid lung disease with rheumatoid arthritis of right knee** `HCC`

M05.162 **Rheumatoid lung disease with rheumatoid arthritis of left knee** `HCC`

M05.169 **Rheumatoid lung disease with rheumatoid arthritis of unspecified knee** `HCC`

✓6ᵗʰ M05.17 **Rheumatoid lung disease with rheumatoid arthritis of ankle and foot**

Rheumatoid lung disease with rheumatoid arthritis, tarsus, metatarsus and phalanges

M05.171 **Rheumatoid lung disease with rheumatoid arthritis of right ankle and foot** `HCC`

M05.172 **Rheumatoid lung disease with rheumatoid arthritis of left ankle and foot** `HCC`

M05.179 **Rheumatoid lung disease with rheumatoid arthritis of unspecified ankle and foot** `HCC`

M05.19 **Rheumatoid lung disease with rheumatoid arthritis of multiple sites** `HCC`

✓5ᵗʰ M05.2 **Rheumatoid vasculitis with rheumatoid arthritis**

M05.20 **Rheumatoid vasculitis with rheumatoid arthritis of unspecified site** `HCC`

✓6ᵗʰ M05.21 **Rheumatoid vasculitis with rheumatoid arthritis of shoulder**

M05.211 **Rheumatoid vasculitis with rheumatoid arthritis of right shoulder** `HCC`

M05.212 **Rheumatoid vasculitis with rheumatoid arthritis of left shoulder** `HCC`

M05.219 **Rheumatoid vasculitis with rheumatoid arthritis of unspecified shoulder** `HCC`

✓6ᵗʰ M05.22 **Rheumatoid vasculitis with rheumatoid arthritis of elbow**

M05.221 **Rheumatoid vasculitis with rheumatoid arthritis of right elbow** `HCC`

M05.222 **Rheumatoid vasculitis with rheumatoid arthritis of left elbow** `HCC`

M05.229 **Rheumatoid vasculitis with rheumatoid arthritis of unspecified elbow** `HCC`

✓6ᵗʰ M05.23 **Rheumatoid vasculitis with rheumatoid arthritis of wrist**

Rheumatoid vasculitis with rheumatoid arthritis, carpal bones

M05.231 **Rheumatoid vasculitis with rheumatoid arthritis of right wrist** `HCC`

M05.232 **Rheumatoid vasculitis with rheumatoid arthritis of left wrist** `HCC`

M05.239 **Rheumatoid vasculitis with rheumatoid arthritis of unspecified wrist** `HCC`

✓6ᵗʰ M05.24 **Rheumatoid vasculitis with rheumatoid arthritis of hand**

Rheumatoid vasculitis with rheumatoid arthritis, metacarpus and phalanges

M05.241 **Rheumatoid vasculitis with rheumatoid arthritis of right hand** `HCC`

M05.242 **Rheumatoid vasculitis with rheumatoid arthritis of left hand** `HCC`

M05.249 **Rheumatoid vasculitis with rheumatoid arthritis of unspecified hand** `HCC`

✓6ᵗʰ M05.25 **Rheumatoid vasculitis with rheumatoid arthritis of hip**

M05.251 **Rheumatoid vasculitis with rheumatoid arthritis of right hip** `HCC`

M05.252 **Rheumatoid vasculitis with rheumatoid arthritis of left hip** `HCC`

M05.259 **Rheumatoid vasculitis with rheumatoid arthritis of unspecified hip** `HCC`

✓6ᵗʰ M05.26 **Rheumatoid vasculitis with rheumatoid arthritis of knee**

M05.261 **Rheumatoid vasculitis with rheumatoid arthritis of right knee** `HCC`

M05.262 **Rheumatoid vasculitis with rheumatoid arthritis of left knee** `HCC`

M05.269 **Rheumatoid vasculitis with rheumatoid arthritis of unspecified knee** `HCC`

✓6ᵗʰ M05.27 **Rheumatoid vasculitis with rheumatoid arthritis of ankle and foot**

Rheumatoid vasculitis with rheumatoid arthritis, tarsus, metatarsus and phalanges

M05.271 **Rheumatoid vasculitis with rheumatoid arthritis of right ankle and foot** `HCC`

M05.272 **Rheumatoid vasculitis with rheumatoid arthritis of left ankle and foot** `HCC`

M05.279 **Rheumatoid vasculitis with rheumatoid arthritis of unspecified ankle and foot** `HCC`

M05.29 **Rheumatoid vasculitis with rheumatoid arthritis of multiple sites** `HCC`

N Newborn: 0   **P** Pediatric: 0-17   **M** Maternity: 9-64   **A** Adult: 15-124   **UNS** Unspecified Site   **MCC** Major Complication/Comorbidity   **CC** Complication/Comorbidity   **PE** POA Exempt

778   ICD-10-CM 2025

✓5ᵗʰ **M05.3** Rheumatoid **heart disease with rheumatoid arthritis**

Rheumatoid carditis
Rheumatoid endocarditis
Rheumatoid myocarditis
Rheumatoid pericarditis

M05.30 Rheumatoid heart disease with rheumatoid arthritis of unspecified site `HCC`

✓6ᵗʰ **M05.31** Rheumatoid heart disease with rheumatoid arthritis of **shoulder**

M05.311 Rheumatoid heart disease with rheumatoid arthritis of **right** shoulder `HCC`

M05.312 Rheumatoid heart disease with rheumatoid arthritis of **left** shoulder `HCC`

M05.319 Rheumatoid heart disease with rheumatoid arthritis of unspecified shoulder

✓6ᵗʰ **M05.32** Rheumatoid heart disease with rheumatoid arthritis of **elbow**

M05.321 Rheumatoid heart disease with rheumatoid arthritis of **right** elbow `HCC`

M05.322 Rheumatoid heart disease with rheumatoid arthritis of **left** elbow `HCC`

M05.329 Rheumatoid heart disease with rheumatoid arthritis of unspecified elbow `HCC`

✓6ᵗʰ **M05.33** Rheumatoid heart disease with rheumatoid arthritis of **wrist**

Rheumatoid heart disease with rheumatoid arthritis, carpal bones

M05.331 Rheumatoid heart disease with rheumatoid arthritis of **right** wrist `HCC`

M05.332 Rheumatoid heart disease with rheumatoid arthritis of **left** wrist `HCC`

M05.339 Rheumatoid heart disease with rheumatoid arthritis of unspecified wrist `HCC`

✓6ᵗʰ **M05.34** Rheumatoid heart disease with rheumatoid arthritis of **hand**

Rheumatoid heart disease with rheumatoid arthritis, metacarpus and phalanges

M05.341 Rheumatoid heart disease with rheumatoid arthritis of **right** hand `HCC`

M05.342 Rheumatoid heart disease with rheumatoid arthritis of **left** hand `HCC`

M05.349 Rheumatoid heart disease with rheumatoid arthritis of unspecified hand `HCC`

✓6ᵗʰ **M05.35** Rheumatoid heart disease with rheumatoid arthritis of **hip**

M05.351 Rheumatoid heart disease with rheumatoid arthritis of **right** hip `HCC`

M05.352 Rheumatoid heart disease with rheumatoid arthritis of **left** hip `HCC`

M05.359 Rheumatoid heart disease with rheumatoid arthritis of unspecified hip `HCC`

✓6ᵗʰ **M05.36** Rheumatoid heart disease with rheumatoid arthritis of **knee**

M05.361 Rheumatoid heart disease with rheumatoid arthritis of **right** knee `HCC`

M05.362 Rheumatoid heart disease with rheumatoid arthritis of **left** knee `HCC`

M05.369 Rheumatoid heart disease with rheumatoid arthritis of unspecified knee `HCC`

✓6ᵗʰ **M05.37** Rheumatoid heart disease with rheumatoid arthritis of **ankle and foot**

Rheumatoid heart disease with rheumatoid arthritis, tarsus, metatarsus and phalanges

M05.371 Rheumatoid heart disease with rheumatoid arthritis of **right** ankle and foot `HCC`

M05.372 Rheumatoid heart disease with rheumatoid arthritis of **left** ankle and foot `HCC`

M05.379 Rheumatoid heart disease with rheumatoid arthritis of unspecified ankle and foot `HCC`

M05.39 Rheumatoid heart disease with rheumatoid arthritis of **multiple sites** `HCC`

✓5ᵗʰ **M05.4** Rheumatoid **myopathy with rheumatoid arthritis**

M05.40 Rheumatoid myopathy with rheumatoid arthritis of unspecified site `CC` `UNS` `HCC`

✓6ᵗʰ **M05.41** Rheumatoid myopathy with rheumatoid arthritis of **shoulder**

M05.411 Rheumatoid myopathy with rheumatoid arthritis of **right** shoulder `CC` `HCC`

M05.412 Rheumatoid myopathy with rheumatoid arthritis of **left** shoulder `CC` `HCC`

M05.419 Rheumatoid myopathy with rheumatoid arthritis of unspecified shoulder `CC` `UNS` `HCC`

✓6ᵗʰ **M05.42** Rheumatoid myopathy with rheumatoid arthritis of **elbow**

M05.421 Rheumatoid myopathy with rheumatoid arthritis of **right** elbow `CC` `HCC`

M05.422 Rheumatoid myopathy with rheumatoid arthritis of **left** elbow `CC` `HCC`

M05.429 Rheumatoid myopathy with rheumatoid arthritis of unspecified elbow `CC` `UNS` `HCC`

✓6ᵗʰ **M05.43** Rheumatoid myopathy with rheumatoid arthritis of **wrist**

Rheumatoid myopathy with rheumatoid arthritis, carpal bones

M05.431 Rheumatoid myopathy with rheumatoid arthritis of **right** wrist `CC` `HCC`

M05.432 Rheumatoid myopathy with rheumatoid arthritis of **left** wrist `CC` `HCC`

M05.439 Rheumatoid myopathy with rheumatoid arthritis of unspecified wrist `CC` `UNS` `HCC`

✓6ᵗʰ **M05.44** Rheumatoid myopathy with rheumatoid arthritis of **hand**

Rheumatoid myopathy with rheumatoid arthritis, metacarpus and phalanges

M05.441 Rheumatoid myopathy with rheumatoid arthritis of **right** hand `CC` `HCC`

M05.442 Rheumatoid myopathy with rheumatoid arthritis of **left** hand `CC` `HCC`

M05.449 Rheumatoid myopathy with rheumatoid arthritis of unspecified hand `CC` `UNS` `HCC`

✓6ᵗʰ **M05.45** Rheumatoid myopathy with rheumatoid arthritis of **hip**

M05.451 Rheumatoid myopathy with rheumatoid arthritis of **right** hip `CC` `HCC`

M05.452 Rheumatoid myopathy with rheumatoid arthritis of **left** hip `CC` `HCC`

M05.459 Rheumatoid myopathy with rheumatoid arthritis of unspecified hip `CC` `UNS` `HCC`

✓6ᵗʰ **M05.46** Rheumatoid myopathy with rheumatoid arthritis of **knee**

M05.461 Rheumatoid myopathy with rheumatoid arthritis of **right** knee `CC` `HCC`

M05.462 Rheumatoid myopathy with rheumatoid arthritis of **left** knee `CC` `HCC`

M05.469 Rheumatoid myopathy with rheumatoid arthritis of unspecified knee `CC` `UNS` `HCC`

✓6ᵗʰ **M05.47** Rheumatoid myopathy with rheumatoid arthritis of **ankle and foot**

Rheumatoid myopathy with rheumatoid arthritis, tarsus, metatarsus and phalanges

M05.471 Rheumatoid myopathy with rheumatoid arthritis of **right** ankle and foot `CC` `HCC`

M05.472 Rheumatoid myopathy with rheumatoid arthritis of **left** ankle and foot `CC` `HCC`

M05.479 Rheumatoid myopathy with rheumatoid arthritis of unspecified ankle and foot `CC` `UNS` `HCC`

M05.49 Rheumatoid myopathy with rheumatoid arthritis of **multiple sites** `CC` `HCC`

✓5ᵗʰ **M05.5** Rheumatoid **polyneuropathy with rheumatoid arthritis**

M05.50 Rheumatoid polyneuropathy with rheumatoid arthritis of unspecified site `HCC`

✓6ᵗʰ **M05.51** Rheumatoid polyneuropathy with rheumatoid arthritis of **shoulder**

M05.511 Rheumatoid polyneuropathy with rheumatoid arthritis of **right** shoulder `HCC`

☑ Additional Character Required   ✓x7ᵗʰ Placeholder   **Questionable PDx**   Manifestation   Unspecified   `UPD` Unacceptable PDx   `H1`-`H14` HAC   `HCC` CMS-HCC Dx   `HIV` HIV Dx

ICD-10-CM 2025   **779**

M05.512 Rheumatoid polyneuropathy with rheumatoid arthritis of left shoulder `HCC`

M05.519 Rheumatoid polyneuropathy with rheumatoid arthritis of unspecified shoulder `HCC`

✓6ᵗʰ **M05.52** Rheumatoid polyneuropathy with rheumatoid arthritis of elbow

M05.521 Rheumatoid polyneuropathy with rheumatoid arthritis of right elbow `HCC`

M05.522 Rheumatoid polyneuropathy with rheumatoid arthritis of left elbow `HCC`

M05.529 Rheumatoid polyneuropathy with rheumatoid arthritis of unspecified elbow `HCC`

✓6ᵗʰ **M05.53** Rheumatoid polyneuropathy with rheumatoid arthritis of wrist

Rheumatoid polyneuropathy with rheumatoid arthritis, carpal bones

M05.531 Rheumatoid polyneuropathy with rheumatoid arthritis of right wrist `HCC`

M05.532 Rheumatoid polyneuropathy with rheumatoid arthritis of left wrist `HCC`

M05.539 Rheumatoid polyneuropathy with rheumatoid arthritis of unspecified wrist `HCC`

✓6ᵗʰ **M05.54** Rheumatoid polyneuropathy with rheumatoid arthritis of hand

Rheumatoid polyneuropathy with rheumatoid arthritis, metacarpus and phalanges

M05.541 Rheumatoid polyneuropathy with rheumatoid arthritis of right hand `HCC`

M05.542 Rheumatoid polyneuropathy with rheumatoid arthritis of left hand `HCC`

M05.549 Rheumatoid polyneuropathy with rheumatoid arthritis of unspecified hand `HCC`

✓6ᵗʰ **M05.55** Rheumatoid polyneuropathy with rheumatoid arthritis of hip

M05.551 Rheumatoid polyneuropathy with rheumatoid arthritis of right hip `HCC`

M05.552 Rheumatoid polyneuropathy with rheumatoid arthritis of left hip `HCC`

M05.559 Rheumatoid polyneuropathy with rheumatoid arthritis of unspecified hip `HCC`

✓6ᵗʰ **M05.56** Rheumatoid polyneuropathy with rheumatoid arthritis of knee

M05.561 Rheumatoid polyneuropathy with rheumatoid arthritis of right knee `HCC`

M05.562 Rheumatoid polyneuropathy with rheumatoid arthritis of left knee `HCC`

M05.569 Rheumatoid polyneuropathy with rheumatoid arthritis of unspecified knee `HCC`

✓6ᵗʰ **M05.57** Rheumatoid polyneuropathy with rheumatoid arthritis of ankle and foot

Rheumatoid polyneuropathy with rheumatoid arthritis, tarsus, metatarsus and phalanges

M05.571 Rheumatoid polyneuropathy with rheumatoid arthritis of right ankle and foot `HCC`

M05.572 Rheumatoid polyneuropathy with rheumatoid arthritis of left ankle and foot `HCC`

M05.579 Rheumatoid polyneuropathy with rheumatoid arthritis of unspecified ankle and foot `HCC`

M05.59 Rheumatoid polyneuropathy with rheumatoid arthritis of multiple sites `HCC`

✓5ᵗʰ **M05.6** Rheumatoid arthritis with involvement of other organs and systems

M05.60 Rheumatoid arthritis of unspecified site with involvement of other organs and systems `HCC`

✓6ᵗʰ **M05.61** Rheumatoid arthritis of shoulder with involvement of other organs and systems

M05.611 Rheumatoid arthritis of right shoulder with involvement of other organs and systems `HCC`

M05.612 Rheumatoid arthritis of left shoulder with involvement of other organs and systems `HCC`

M05.619 Rheumatoid arthritis of unspecified shoulder with involvement of other organs and systems `HCC`

✓6ᵗʰ **M05.62** Rheumatoid arthritis of elbow with involvement of other organs and systems

M05.621 Rheumatoid arthritis of right elbow with involvement of other organs and systems `HCC`

M05.622 Rheumatoid arthritis of left elbow with involvement of other organs and systems `HCC`

M05.629 Rheumatoid arthritis of unspecified elbow with involvement of other organs and systems `HCC`

✓6ᵗʰ **M05.63** Rheumatoid arthritis of wrist with involvement of other organs and systems

Rheumatoid arthritis of carpal bones with involvement of other organs and systems

M05.631 Rheumatoid arthritis of right wrist with involvement of other organs and systems `HCC`

M05.632 Rheumatoid arthritis of left wrist with involvement of other organs and systems `HCC`

M05.639 Rheumatoid arthritis of unspecified wrist with involvement of other organs and systems `HCC`

✓6ᵗʰ **M05.64** Rheumatoid arthritis of hand with involvement of other organs and systems

Rheumatoid arthritis of metacarpus and phalanges with involvement of other organs and systems

M05.641 Rheumatoid arthritis of right hand with involvement of other organs and systems `HCC`

M05.642 Rheumatoid arthritis of left hand with involvement of other organs and systems `HCC`

M05.649 Rheumatoid arthritis of unspecified hand with involvement of other organs and systems `HCC`

✓6ᵗʰ **M05.65** Rheumatoid arthritis of hip with involvement of other organs and systems

M05.651 Rheumatoid arthritis of right hip with involvement of other organs and systems `HCC`

M05.652 Rheumatoid arthritis of left hip with involvement of other organs and systems `HCC`

M05.659 Rheumatoid arthritis of unspecified hip with involvement of other organs and systems `HCC`

✓6ᵗʰ **M05.66** Rheumatoid arthritis of knee with involvement of other organs and systems

M05.661 Rheumatoid arthritis of right knee with involvement of other organs and systems `HCC`

M05.662 Rheumatoid arthritis of left knee with involvement of other organs and systems `HCC`

M05.669 Rheumatoid arthritis of unspecified knee with involvement of other organs and systems `HCC`

✓6ᵗʰ **M05.67** Rheumatoid arthritis of ankle and foot with involvement of other organs and systems

Rheumatoid arthritis of tarsus, metatarsus and phalanges with involvement of other organs and systems

M05.671 Rheumatoid arthritis of right ankle and foot with involvement of other organs and systems `HCC`

M05.672 Rheumatoid arthritis of left ankle and foot with involvement of other organs and systems `HCC`

M05.679 Rheumatoid arthritis of unspecified ankle and foot with involvement of other organs and systems `HCC`

M05.69 Rheumatoid arthritis of multiple sites with involvement of other organs and systems `HCC`

✓5ᵗʰ **M05.7** Rheumatoid arthritis with rheumatoid factor without organ or systems involvement

M05.70 Rheumatoid arthritis with rheumatoid factor of unspecified site without organ or systems involvement `HCC`

Ⓝ Newborn: 0   Ⓟ Pediatric: 0-17   Ⓜ Maternity: 9-64   Ⓐ Adult: 15-124   ⓊⓃⓈ Unspecified Site   ⓂⒸⒸ Major Complication/Comorbidity   ⒸⒸ Complication/Comorbidity   ⓅⒺ POA Exempt

780

ICD-10-CM 2025

√6ᵗʰ **M05.71** Rheumatoid arthritis with rheumatoid factor of shoulder without organ or systems involvement

　　M05.711 Rheumatoid arthritis with rheumatoid factor of right shoulder without organ or systems involvement `HCC`

　　M05.712 Rheumatoid arthritis with rheumatoid factor of left shoulder without organ or systems involvement `HCC`

　　M05.719 Rheumatoid arthritis with rheumatoid factor of unspecified shoulder without organ or systems involvement `HCC`

√6ᵗʰ **M05.72** Rheumatoid arthritis with rheumatoid factor of elbow without organ or systems involvement

　　M05.721 Rheumatoid arthritis with rheumatoid factor of right elbow without organ or systems involvement `HCC`

　　M05.722 Rheumatoid arthritis with rheumatoid factor of left elbow without organ or systems involvement `HCC`

　　M05.729 Rheumatoid arthritis with rheumatoid factor of unspecified elbow without organ or systems involvement `HCC`

√6ᵗʰ **M05.73** Rheumatoid arthritis with rheumatoid factor of wrist without organ or systems involvement

　　M05.731 Rheumatoid arthritis with rheumatoid factor of right wrist without organ or systems involvement `HCC`

　　M05.732 Rheumatoid arthritis with rheumatoid factor of left wrist without organ or systems involvement `HCC`

　　M05.739 Rheumatoid arthritis with rheumatoid factor of unspecified wrist without organ or systems involvement `HCC`

√6ᵗʰ **M05.74** Rheumatoid arthritis with rheumatoid factor of hand without organ or systems involvement

　　M05.741 Rheumatoid arthritis with rheumatoid factor of right hand without organ or systems involvement `HCC`

　　M05.742 Rheumatoid arthritis with rheumatoid factor of left hand without organ or systems involvement `HCC`

　　M05.749 Rheumatoid arthritis with rheumatoid factor of unspecified hand without organ or systems involvement `HCC`

√6ᵗʰ **M05.75** Rheumatoid arthritis with rheumatoid factor of hip without organ or systems involvement

　　M05.751 Rheumatoid arthritis with rheumatoid factor of right hip without organ or systems involvement `HCC`

　　M05.752 Rheumatoid arthritis with rheumatoid factor of left hip without organ or systems involvement `HCC`

　　M05.759 Rheumatoid arthritis with rheumatoid factor of unspecified hip without organ or systems involvement `HCC`

√6ᵗʰ **M05.76** Rheumatoid arthritis with rheumatoid factor of knee without organ or systems involvement

　　M05.761 Rheumatoid arthritis with rheumatoid factor of right knee without organ or systems involvement `HCC`

　　M05.762 Rheumatoid arthritis with rheumatoid factor of left knee without organ or systems involvement `HCC`

　　M05.769 Rheumatoid arthritis with rheumatoid factor of unspecified knee without organ or systems involvement `HCC`

√6ᵗʰ **M05.77** Rheumatoid arthritis with rheumatoid factor of ankle and foot without organ or systems involvement

　　M05.771 Rheumatoid arthritis with rheumatoid factor of right ankle and foot without organ or systems involvement `HCC`

　　M05.772 Rheumatoid arthritis with rheumatoid factor of left ankle and foot without organ or systems involvement `HCC`

　　M05.779 Rheumatoid arthritis with rheumatoid factor of unspecified ankle and foot without organ or systems involvement `HCC`

　M05.79 Rheumatoid arthritis with rheumatoid factor of multiple sites without organ or systems involvement `HCC`

M05.7A Rheumatoid arthritis with rheumatoid factor of other specified site without organ or systems involvement `HCC`

√5ᵗʰ **M05.8** Other rheumatoid arthritis with rheumatoid factor

　M05.80 Other rheumatoid arthritis with rheumatoid factor of unspecified site `HCC`

√6ᵗʰ **M05.81** Other rheumatoid arthritis with rheumatoid factor of shoulder

　　M05.811 Other rheumatoid arthritis with rheumatoid factor of right shoulder `HCC`

　　M05.812 Other rheumatoid arthritis with rheumatoid factor of left shoulder `HCC`

　　M05.819 Other rheumatoid arthritis with rheumatoid factor of unspecified shoulder `HCC`

√6ᵗʰ **M05.82** Other rheumatoid arthritis with rheumatoid factor of elbow

　　M05.821 Other rheumatoid arthritis with rheumatoid factor of right elbow `HCC`

　　M05.822 Other rheumatoid arthritis with rheumatoid factor of left elbow `HCC`

　　M05.829 Other rheumatoid arthritis with rheumatoid factor of unspecified elbow `HCC`

√6ᵗʰ **M05.83** Other rheumatoid arthritis with rheumatoid factor of wrist

　　M05.831 Other rheumatoid arthritis with rheumatoid factor of right wrist `HCC`

　　M05.832 Other rheumatoid arthritis with rheumatoid factor of left wrist `HCC`

　　M05.839 Other rheumatoid arthritis with rheumatoid factor of unspecified wrist `HCC`

√6ᵗʰ **M05.84** Other rheumatoid arthritis with rheumatoid factor of hand

　　M05.841 Other rheumatoid arthritis with rheumatoid factor of right hand `HCC`

　　M05.842 Other rheumatoid arthritis with rheumatoid factor of left hand `HCC`

　　M05.849 Other rheumatoid arthritis with rheumatoid factor of unspecified hand `HCC`

√6ᵗʰ **M05.85** Other rheumatoid arthritis with rheumatoid factor of hip

　　M05.851 Other rheumatoid arthritis with rheumatoid factor of right hip `HCC`

　　M05.852 Other rheumatoid arthritis with rheumatoid factor of left hip `HCC`

　　M05.859 Other rheumatoid arthritis with rheumatoid factor of unspecified hip `HCC`

√6ᵗʰ **M05.86** Other rheumatoid arthritis with rheumatoid factor of knee

　　M05.861 Other rheumatoid arthritis with rheumatoid factor of right knee `HCC`

　　M05.862 Other rheumatoid arthritis with rheumatoid factor of left knee `HCC`

　　M05.869 Other rheumatoid arthritis with rheumatoid factor of unspecified knee `HCC`

√6ᵗʰ **M05.87** Other rheumatoid arthritis with rheumatoid factor of ankle and foot

　　M05.871 Other rheumatoid arthritis with rheumatoid factor of right ankle and foot `HCC`

　　M05.872 Other rheumatoid arthritis with rheumatoid factor of left ankle and foot `HCC`

　　M05.879 Other rheumatoid arthritis with rheumatoid factor of unspecified ankle and foot `HCC`

　M05.89 Other rheumatoid arthritis with rheumatoid factor of multiple sites `HCC`

　M05.8A Other rheumatoid arthritis with rheumatoid factor of other specified site `HCC`

M05.9 Rheumatoid arthritis with rheumatoid factor, unspecified `HCC`

✔ Additional Character Required　　√x7ᵗʰ Placeholder　　Questionable PDx　　Manifestation　　Unspecified　　`UPD` Unacceptable PDx　　`H1`-`H14` HAC　　`HCC` CMS-HCC Dx　　`HIV` HIV Dx

ICD-10-CM 2025

781

Chapter 13. Diseases of the Musculoskeletal System and Connective Tissue

M05.71–M05.9

✓4ᵗʰ M06 Other rheumatoid arthritis

AHA: 2020,4Q,31-32

DEF: Rheumatoid arthritis: Autoimmune systemic disease that causes chronic inflammation of the joints and other areas of the body, manifested by inflammatory changes in articular structures and synovial membranes, atrophy, and loss in bone density.

✓5ᵗʰ M06.0 Rheumatoid arthritis without rheumatoid factor

  M06.00 Rheumatoid arthritis without rheumatoid factor, unspecified site   HCC

  ✓6ᵗʰ M06.01 Rheumatoid arthritis without rheumatoid factor, shoulder

    M06.011 Rheumatoid arthritis without rheumatoid factor, right shoulder   HCC

    M06.012 Rheumatoid arthritis without rheumatoid factor, left shoulder   HCC

    M06.019 Rheumatoid arthritis without rheumatoid factor, unspecified shoulder   HCC

  ✓6ᵗʰ M06.02 Rheumatoid arthritis without rheumatoid factor, elbow

    M06.021 Rheumatoid arthritis without rheumatoid factor, right elbow   HCC

    M06.022 Rheumatoid arthritis without rheumatoid factor, left elbow   HCC

    M06.029 Rheumatoid arthritis without rheumatoid factor, unspecified elbow   HCC

  ✓6ᵗʰ M06.03 Rheumatoid arthritis without rheumatoid factor, wrist

    M06.031 Rheumatoid arthritis without rheumatoid factor, right wrist   HCC

    M06.032 Rheumatoid arthritis without rheumatoid factor, left wrist   HCC

    M06.039 Rheumatoid arthritis without rheumatoid factor, unspecified wrist   HCC

  ✓6ᵗʰ M06.04 Rheumatoid arthritis without rheumatoid factor, hand

    M06.041 Rheumatoid arthritis without rheumatoid factor, right hand   HCC

    M06.042 Rheumatoid arthritis without rheumatoid factor, left hand   HCC

    M06.049 Rheumatoid arthritis without rheumatoid factor, unspecified hand   HCC

  ✓6ᵗʰ M06.05 Rheumatoid arthritis without rheumatoid factor, hip

    M06.051 Rheumatoid arthritis without rheumatoid factor, right hip   HCC

    M06.052 Rheumatoid arthritis without rheumatoid factor, left hip   HCC

    M06.059 Rheumatoid arthritis without rheumatoid factor, unspecified hip   HCC

  ✓6ᵗʰ M06.06 Rheumatoid arthritis without rheumatoid factor, knee

    M06.061 Rheumatoid arthritis without rheumatoid factor, right knee   HCC

    M06.062 Rheumatoid arthritis without rheumatoid factor, left knee   HCC

    M06.069 Rheumatoid arthritis without rheumatoid factor, unspecified knee   HCC

  ✓6ᵗʰ M06.07 Rheumatoid arthritis without rheumatoid factor, ankle and foot

    M06.071 Rheumatoid arthritis without rheumatoid factor, right ankle and foot   HCC

    M06.072 Rheumatoid arthritis without rheumatoid factor, left ankle and foot   HCC

    M06.079 Rheumatoid arthritis without rheumatoid factor, unspecified ankle and foot   HCC

  M06.08 Rheumatoid arthritis without rheumatoid factor, vertebrae   HCC

  M06.09 Rheumatoid arthritis without rheumatoid factor, multiple sites   HCC

  M06.0A Rheumatoid arthritis without rheumatoid factor, other specified site   HCC

M06.1 Adult-onset Still's disease   HCC A

  EXCLUDES 1   Still's disease NOS (M08.2-)

  DEF: Type of systemic arthritis characterized by a transient rash and spiking fevers. This condition may resolve or develop into a chronic condition and may affect internal organs, as well as joints.

  Synonym(s): *AOSD*

✓5ᵗʰ M06.2 Rheumatoid bursitis

  M06.20 Rheumatoid bursitis, unspecified site   HCC

✓6ᵗʰ M06.21 Rheumatoid bursitis, shoulder

  M06.211 Rheumatoid bursitis, right shoulder   HCC

  M06.212 Rheumatoid bursitis, left shoulder   HCC

  M06.219 Rheumatoid bursitis, unspecified shoulder   HCC

✓6ᵗʰ M06.22 Rheumatoid bursitis, elbow

  M06.221 Rheumatoid bursitis, right elbow   HCC

  M06.222 Rheumatoid bursitis, left elbow   HCC

  M06.229 Rheumatoid bursitis, unspecified elbow   HCC

✓6ᵗʰ M06.23 Rheumatoid bursitis, wrist

  M06.231 Rheumatoid bursitis, right wrist   HCC

  M06.232 Rheumatoid bursitis, left wrist   HCC

  M06.239 Rheumatoid bursitis, unspecified wrist   HCC

✓6ᵗʰ M06.24 Rheumatoid bursitis, hand

  M06.241 Rheumatoid bursitis, right hand   HCC

  M06.242 Rheumatoid bursitis, left hand   HCC

  M06.249 Rheumatoid bursitis, unspecified hand   HCC

✓6ᵗʰ M06.25 Rheumatoid bursitis, hip

  M06.251 Rheumatoid bursitis, right hip   HCC

  M06.252 Rheumatoid bursitis, left hip   HCC

  M06.259 Rheumatoid bursitis, unspecified hip   HCC

✓6ᵗʰ M06.26 Rheumatoid bursitis, knee

  M06.261 Rheumatoid bursitis, right knee   HCC

  M06.262 Rheumatoid bursitis, left knee   HCC

  M06.269 Rheumatoid bursitis, unspecified knee   HCC

✓6ᵗʰ M06.27 Rheumatoid bursitis, ankle and foot

  M06.271 Rheumatoid bursitis, right ankle and foot   HCC

  M06.272 Rheumatoid bursitis, left ankle and foot   HCC

  M06.279 Rheumatoid bursitis, unspecified ankle and foot   HCC

M06.28 Rheumatoid bursitis, vertebrae   HCC

M06.29 Rheumatoid bursitis, multiple sites   HCC

✓5ᵗʰ M06.3 Rheumatoid nodule

  M06.30 Rheumatoid nodule, unspecified site   HCC

  ✓6ᵗʰ M06.31 Rheumatoid nodule, shoulder

    M06.311 Rheumatoid nodule, right shoulder   HCC

    M06.312 Rheumatoid nodule, left shoulder   HCC

    M06.319 Rheumatoid nodule, unspecified shoulder   HCC

  ✓6ᵗʰ M06.32 Rheumatoid nodule, elbow

    M06.321 Rheumatoid nodule, right elbow   HCC

    M06.322 Rheumatoid nodule, left elbow   HCC

    M06.329 Rheumatoid nodule, unspecified elbow   HCC

  ✓6ᵗʰ M06.33 Rheumatoid nodule, wrist

    M06.331 Rheumatoid nodule, right wrist   HCC

    M06.332 Rheumatoid nodule, left wrist   HCC

    M06.339 Rheumatoid nodule, unspecified wrist   HCC

  ✓6ᵗʰ M06.34 Rheumatoid nodule, hand

    M06.341 Rheumatoid nodule, right hand   HCC

    M06.342 Rheumatoid nodule, left hand   HCC

    M06.349 Rheumatoid nodule, unspecified hand   HCC

  ✓6ᵗʰ M06.35 Rheumatoid nodule, hip

    M06.351 Rheumatoid nodule, right hip   HCC

    M06.352 Rheumatoid nodule, left hip   HCC

    M06.359 Rheumatoid nodule, unspecified hip   HCC

  ✓6ᵗʰ M06.36 Rheumatoid nodule, knee

    M06.361 Rheumatoid nodule, right knee   HCC

    M06.362 Rheumatoid nodule, left knee   HCC

    M06.369 Rheumatoid nodule, unspecified knee   HCC

M06-M06.369

N Newborn: 0   P Pediatric: 0-17   M Maternity: 9-64   A Adult: 15-124   UNS Unspecified Site   MCC Major Complication/Comorbidity   CC Complication/Comorbidity   PE POA Exempt

782   ICD-10-CM 2025

√6ᵗʰ **M06.37** Rheumatoid nodule, ankle and foot

     M06.371 Rheumatoid nodule, right ankle and foot `HCC`

     M06.372 Rheumatoid nodule, left ankle and foot `HCC`

     M06.379 Rheumatoid nodule, unspecified ankle and foot `HCC`

   M06.38 Rheumatoid nodule, vertebrae `HCC`

   M06.39 Rheumatoid nodule, multiple sites `HCC`

M06.4 Inflammatory polyarthropathy

   EXCLUDES 1   polyarthritis NOS (M13.0)

   AHA: 2024,1Q,17

√5ᵗʰ **M06.8** Other specified rheumatoid arthritis

   M06.80 Other specified rheumatoid arthritis, unspecified site `HCC`

   √6ᵗʰ **M06.81** Other specified rheumatoid arthritis, shoulder

     M06.811 Other specified rheumatoid arthritis, right shoulder `HCC`

     M06.812 Other specified rheumatoid arthritis, left shoulder `HCC`

     M06.819 Other specified rheumatoid arthritis, unspecified shoulder `HCC`

   √6ᵗʰ **M06.82** Other specified rheumatoid arthritis, elbow

     M06.821 Other specified rheumatoid arthritis, right elbow `HCC`

     M06.822 Other specified rheumatoid arthritis, left elbow `HCC`

     M06.829 Other specified rheumatoid arthritis, unspecified elbow `HCC`

   √6ᵗʰ **M06.83** Other specified rheumatoid arthritis, wrist

     M06.831 Other specified rheumatoid arthritis, right wrist `HCC`

     M06.832 Other specified rheumatoid arthritis, left wrist `HCC`

     M06.839 Other specified rheumatoid arthritis, unspecified wrist `HCC`

   √6ᵗʰ **M06.84** Other specified rheumatoid arthritis, hand

     M06.841 Other specified rheumatoid arthritis, right hand `HCC`

     M06.842 Other specified rheumatoid arthritis, left hand `HCC`

     M06.849 Other specified rheumatoid arthritis, unspecified hand `HCC`

   √6ᵗʰ **M06.85** Other specified rheumatoid arthritis, hip

     M06.851 Other specified rheumatoid arthritis, right hip `HCC`

     M06.852 Other specified rheumatoid arthritis, left hip `HCC`

     M06.859 Other specified rheumatoid arthritis, unspecified hip `HCC`

   √6ᵗʰ **M06.86** Other specified rheumatoid arthritis, knee

     M06.861 Other specified rheumatoid arthritis, right knee `HCC`

     M06.862 Other specified rheumatoid arthritis, left knee `HCC`

     M06.869 Other specified rheumatoid arthritis, unspecified knee `HCC`

   √6ᵗʰ **M06.87** Other specified rheumatoid arthritis, ankle and foot

     M06.871 Other specified rheumatoid arthritis, right ankle and foot `HCC`

     M06.872 Other specified rheumatoid arthritis, left ankle and foot `HCC`

     M06.879 Other specified rheumatoid arthritis, unspecified ankle and foot `HCC`

   M06.88 Other specified rheumatoid arthritis, vertebrae `HCC`

   M06.89 Other specified rheumatoid arthritis, multiple sites `HCC`

   M06.8A Other specified rheumatoid arthritis, other specified site `HCC`

M06.9 Rheumatoid arthritis, unspecified `HCC`

   AHA: 2024,1Q,17

√4ᵗʰ **M07 Enteropathic arthropathies**

Code also associated enteropathy, such as:
regional enteritis [Crohn's disease] (K50.-)
ulcerative colitis (K51.-)

   EXCLUDES 1   psoriatic arthropathies (L40.5-)

√5ᵗʰ **M07.6** Enteropathic arthropathies

   M07.60 Enteropathic arthropathies, unspecified site

   √6ᵗʰ **M07.61** Enteropathic arthropathies, shoulder

     M07.611 Enteropathic arthropathies, right shoulder

     M07.612 Enteropathic arthropathies, left shoulder

     M07.619 Enteropathic arthropathies, unspecified shoulder

   √6ᵗʰ **M07.62** Enteropathic arthropathies, elbow

     M07.621 Enteropathic arthropathies, right elbow

     M07.622 Enteropathic arthropathies, left elbow

     M07.629 Enteropathic arthropathies, unspecified elbow

   √6ᵗʰ **M07.63** Enteropathic arthropathies, wrist

     M07.631 Enteropathic arthropathies, right wrist

     M07.632 Enteropathic arthropathies, left wrist

     M07.639 Enteropathic arthropathies, unspecified wrist

   √6ᵗʰ **M07.64** Enteropathic arthropathies, hand

     M07.641 Enteropathic arthropathies, right hand

     M07.642 Enteropathic arthropathies, left hand

     M07.649 Enteropathic arthropathies, unspecified hand

   √6ᵗʰ **M07.65** Enteropathic arthropathies, hip

     M07.651 Enteropathic arthropathies, right hip

     M07.652 Enteropathic arthropathies, left hip

     M07.659 Enteropathic arthropathies, unspecified hip

   √6ᵗʰ **M07.66** Enteropathic arthropathies, knee

     M07.661 Enteropathic arthropathies, right knee

     M07.662 Enteropathic arthropathies, left knee

     M07.669 Enteropathic arthropathies, unspecified knee

   √6ᵗʰ **M07.67** Enteropathic arthropathies, ankle and foot

     M07.671 Enteropathic arthropathies, right ankle and foot

     M07.672 Enteropathic arthropathies, left ankle and foot

     M07.679 Enteropathic arthropathies, unspecified ankle and foot

   M07.68 Enteropathic arthropathies, vertebrae

   M07.69 Enteropathic arthropathies, multiple sites

√4ᵗʰ **M08 Juvenile arthritis**

Code also any associated underlying condition, such as:
regional enteritis [Crohn's disease] (K50.-)
ulcerative colitis (K51.-)

   EXCLUDES 1   arthropathy in Whipple's disease (M14.8)

        Felty's syndrome (M05.0)

        juvenile dermatomyositis (M33.0-)

        psoriatic juvenile arthropathy (L40.54)

   AHA: 2020,4Q,31-32

√5ᵗʰ **M08.0** Unspecified juvenile rheumatoid arthritis

   Juvenile rheumatoid arthritis with or without rheumatoid factor

   M08.00 Unspecified juvenile rheumatoid arthritis of unspecified site `HCC`

   √6ᵗʰ **M08.01** Unspecified juvenile rheumatoid arthritis, shoulder

     M08.011 Unspecified juvenile rheumatoid arthritis, right shoulder `HCC`

     M08.012 Unspecified juvenile rheumatoid arthritis, left shoulder `HCC`

     M08.019 Unspecified juvenile rheumatoid arthritis, unspecified shoulder `HCC`

   √6ᵗʰ **M08.02** Unspecified juvenile rheumatoid arthritis of elbow

     M08.021 Unspecified juvenile rheumatoid arthritis, right elbow `HCC`

     M08.022 Unspecified juvenile rheumatoid arthritis, left elbow `HCC`

     M08.029 Unspecified juvenile rheumatoid arthritis, unspecified elbow `HCC`

   √6ᵗʰ **M08.03** Unspecified juvenile rheumatoid arthritis, wrist

     M08.031 Unspecified juvenile rheumatoid arthritis, right wrist `HCC`

✔ Additional Character Required	√x7ᵗʰ Placeholder	Questionable PDx	Manifestation	Unspecified	UPD Unacceptable PDx	H1-H14 HAC	HCC CMS-HCC Dx	HIV HIV Dx

ICD-10-CM 2025

Chapter 13. Diseases of the Musculoskeletal System and Connective Tissue

M06.37–M08.031

783

M08.032   **Unspecified juvenile rheumatoid arthritis, left wrist**   `HCC`

M08.039   **Unspecified juvenile rheumatoid arthritis, unspecified wrist**   `HCC`

✓6ᵗʰ   **M08.04**   **Unspecified juvenile rheumatoid arthritis, hand**

M08.041   **Unspecified juvenile rheumatoid arthritis, right hand**   `HCC`

M08.042   **Unspecified juvenile rheumatoid arthritis, left hand**   `HCC`

M08.049   **Unspecified juvenile rheumatoid arthritis, unspecified hand**   `HCC`

✓6ᵗʰ   **M08.05**   **Unspecified juvenile rheumatoid arthritis, hip**

M08.051   **Unspecified juvenile rheumatoid arthritis, right hip**   `HCC`

M08.052   **Unspecified juvenile rheumatoid arthritis, left hip**   `HCC`

M08.059   **Unspecified juvenile rheumatoid arthritis, unspecified hip**   `HCC`

✓6ᵗʰ   **M08.06**   **Unspecified juvenile rheumatoid arthritis, knee**

M08.061   **Unspecified juvenile rheumatoid arthritis, right knee**   `HCC`

M08.062   **Unspecified juvenile rheumatoid arthritis, left knee**   `HCC`

M08.069   **Unspecified juvenile rheumatoid arthritis, unspecified knee**   `HCC`

✓6ᵗʰ   **M08.07**   **Unspecified juvenile rheumatoid arthritis, ankle and foot**

M08.071   **Unspecified juvenile rheumatoid arthritis, right ankle and foot**   `HCC`

M08.072   **Unspecified juvenile rheumatoid arthritis, left ankle and foot**   `HCC`

M08.079   **Unspecified juvenile rheumatoid arthritis, unspecified ankle and foot**   `HCC`

M08.08   **Unspecified juvenile rheumatoid arthritis, vertebrae**   `HCC`

M08.09   **Unspecified juvenile rheumatoid arthritis, multiple sites**   `HCC`

M08.0A   **Unspecified juvenile rheumatoid arthritis, other specified site**   `HCC`

M08.1   **Juvenile ankylosing spondylitis**   `HCC`

> **EXCLUDES 1**   *ankylosing spondylitis in adults (M45.0-)*

✓5ᵗʰ   **M08.2**   **Juvenile rheumatoid arthritis with systemic onset**

Still's disease NOS

> **EXCLUDES 1**   *adult-onset Still's disease (M06.1-)*

DEF: Systemic juvenile rheumatoid arthritis characterized by a transient rash and spiking fevers that may affect internal organs, as well as joints.

M08.20   **Juvenile rheumatoid arthritis with systemic onset, unspecified site**   `HCC`

✓6ᵗʰ   **M08.21**   **Juvenile rheumatoid arthritis with systemic onset, shoulder**

M08.211   **Juvenile rheumatoid arthritis with systemic onset, right shoulder**   `HCC`

M08.212   **Juvenile rheumatoid arthritis with systemic onset, left shoulder**   `HCC`

M08.219   **Juvenile rheumatoid arthritis with systemic onset, unspecified shoulder**   `HCC`

✓6ᵗʰ   **M08.22**   **Juvenile rheumatoid arthritis with systemic onset, elbow**

M08.221   **Juvenile rheumatoid arthritis with systemic onset, right elbow**   `HCC`

M08.222   **Juvenile rheumatoid arthritis with systemic onset, left elbow**   `HCC`

M08.229   **Juvenile rheumatoid arthritis with systemic onset, unspecified elbow**   `HCC`

✓6ᵗʰ   **M08.23**   **Juvenile rheumatoid arthritis with systemic onset, wrist**

M08.231   **Juvenile rheumatoid arthritis with systemic onset, right wrist**   `HCC`

M08.232   **Juvenile rheumatoid arthritis with systemic onset, left wrist**   `HCC`

M08.239   **Juvenile rheumatoid arthritis with systemic onset, unspecified wrist**   `HCC`

✓6ᵗʰ   **M08.24**   **Juvenile rheumatoid arthritis with systemic onset, hand**

M08.241   **Juvenile rheumatoid arthritis with systemic onset, right hand**   `HCC`

M08.242   **Juvenile rheumatoid arthritis with systemic onset, left hand**   `HCC`

M08.249   **Juvenile rheumatoid arthritis with systemic onset, unspecified hand**   `HCC`

✓6ᵗʰ   **M08.25**   **Juvenile rheumatoid arthritis with systemic onset, hip**

M08.251   **Juvenile rheumatoid arthritis with systemic onset, right hip**   `HCC`

M08.252   **Juvenile rheumatoid arthritis with systemic onset, left hip**   `HCC`

M08.259   **Juvenile rheumatoid arthritis with systemic onset, unspecified hip**   `HCC`

✓6ᵗʰ   **M08.26**   **Juvenile rheumatoid arthritis with systemic onset, knee**

M08.261   **Juvenile rheumatoid arthritis with systemic onset, right knee**   `HCC`

M08.262   **Juvenile rheumatoid arthritis with systemic onset, left knee**   `HCC`

M08.269   **Juvenile rheumatoid arthritis with systemic onset, unspecified knee**   `HCC`

✓6ᵗʰ   **M08.27**   **Juvenile rheumatoid arthritis with systemic onset, ankle and foot**

M08.271   **Juvenile rheumatoid arthritis with systemic onset, right ankle and foot**   `HCC`

M08.272   **Juvenile rheumatoid arthritis with systemic onset, left ankle and foot**   `HCC`

M08.279   **Juvenile rheumatoid arthritis with systemic onset, unspecified ankle and foot**   `HCC`

M08.28   **Juvenile rheumatoid arthritis with systemic onset, vertebrae**   `HCC`

M08.29   **Juvenile rheumatoid arthritis with systemic onset, multiple sites**   `HCC`

M08.2A   **Juvenile rheumatoid arthritis with systemic onset, other specified site**   `HCC`

M08.3   **Juvenile rheumatoid polyarthritis (seronegative)**   `HCC`

✓5ᵗʰ   **M08.4**   **Pauciarticular juvenile rheumatoid arthritis**

M08.40   **Pauciarticular juvenile rheumatoid arthritis, unspecified site**   `HCC`

✓6ᵗʰ   **M08.41**   **Pauciarticular juvenile rheumatoid arthritis, shoulder**

M08.411   **Pauciarticular juvenile rheumatoid arthritis, right shoulder**   `HCC`

M08.412   **Pauciarticular juvenile rheumatoid arthritis, left shoulder**   `HCC`

M08.419   **Pauciarticular juvenile rheumatoid arthritis, unspecified shoulder**   `HCC`

✓6ᵗʰ   **M08.42**   **Pauciarticular juvenile rheumatoid arthritis, elbow**

M08.421   **Pauciarticular juvenile rheumatoid arthritis, right elbow**   `HCC`

M08.422   **Pauciarticular juvenile rheumatoid arthritis, left elbow**   `HCC`

M08.429   **Pauciarticular juvenile rheumatoid arthritis, unspecified elbow**   `HCC`

✓6ᵗʰ   **M08.43**   **Pauciarticular juvenile rheumatoid arthritis, wrist**

M08.431   **Pauciarticular juvenile rheumatoid arthritis, right wrist**   `HCC`

M08.432   **Pauciarticular juvenile rheumatoid arthritis, left wrist**   `HCC`

M08.439   **Pauciarticular juvenile rheumatoid arthritis, unspecified wrist**   `HCC`

✓6ᵗʰ   **M08.44**   **Pauciarticular juvenile rheumatoid arthritis, hand**

M08.441   **Pauciarticular juvenile rheumatoid arthritis, right hand**   `HCC`

M08.442   **Pauciarticular juvenile rheumatoid arthritis, left hand**   `HCC`

M08.449   **Pauciarticular juvenile rheumatoid arthritis, unspecified hand**   `HCC`

✓6ᵗʰ   **M08.45**   **Pauciarticular juvenile rheumatoid arthritis, hip**

M08.451   **Pauciarticular juvenile rheumatoid arthritis, right hip**   `HCC`

M08.452   **Pauciarticular juvenile rheumatoid arthritis, left hip**   `HCC`

M08.459   **Pauciarticular juvenile rheumatoid arthritis, unspecified hip**   `HCC`

✓6ᵗʰ   **M08.46**   **Pauciarticular juvenile rheumatoid arthritis, knee**

M08.461   **Pauciarticular juvenile rheumatoid arthritis, right knee**   `HCC`

`N` Newborn: 0   `P` Pediatric: 0-17   `M` Maternity: 9-64   `A` Adult: 15-124   `UNS` Unspecified Site   `MCC` Major Complication/Comorbidity   `CC` Complication/Comorbidity   `PE` POA Exempt

784   ICD-10-CM 2025

M08.462   Pauciarticular juvenile rheumatoid arthritis, **left** knee   `HCC`

M08.469   Pauciarticular juvenile rheumatoid arthritis, unspecified knee   `HCC`

√6th   **M08.47**   Pauciarticular juvenile rheumatoid arthritis, **ankle and foot**

    M08.471   Pauciarticular juvenile rheumatoid arthritis, **right** ankle and foot   `HCC`

    M08.472   Pauciarticular juvenile rheumatoid arthritis, **left** ankle and foot   `HCC`

    M08.479   Pauciarticular juvenile rheumatoid arthritis, unspecified ankle and foot   `HCC`

   M08.48   Pauciarticular juvenile rheumatoid arthritis, **vertebrae**   `HCC`

   M08.4A   Pauciarticular juvenile rheumatoid arthritis, other specified site   `HCC`

√5th   **M08.8**   **Other juvenile arthritis**

   M08.80   Other juvenile arthritis, unspecified site   `HCC`

√6th   **M08.81**   Other juvenile arthritis, **shoulder**

    M08.811   Other juvenile arthritis, **right** shoulder

    M08.812   Other juvenile arthritis, **left** shoulder   `HCC`

    M08.819   Other juvenile arthritis, unspecified shoulder   `HCC`

√6th   **M08.82**   Other juvenile arthritis, **elbow**

    M08.821   Other juvenile arthritis, **right** elbow   `HCC`

    M08.822   Other juvenile arthritis, **left** elbow   `HCC`

    M08.829   Other juvenile arthritis, unspecified elbow   `HCC`

√6th   **M08.83**   Other juvenile arthritis, **wrist**

    M08.831   Other juvenile arthritis, **right** wrist   `HCC`

    M08.832   Other juvenile arthritis, **left** wrist   `HCC`

    M08.839   Other juvenile arthritis, unspecified wrist   `HCC`

√6th   **M08.84**   Other juvenile arthritis, **hand**

    M08.841   Other juvenile arthritis, **right** hand   `HCC`

    M08.842   Other juvenile arthritis, **left** hand   `HCC`

    M08.849   Other juvenile arthritis, unspecified hand   `HCC`

√6th   **M08.85**   Other juvenile arthritis, **hip**

    M08.851   Other juvenile arthritis, **right** hip   `HCC`

    M08.852   Other juvenile arthritis, **left** hip   `HCC`

    M08.859   Other juvenile arthritis, unspecified hip   `HCC`

√6th   **M08.86**   Other juvenile arthritis, **knee**

    M08.861   Other juvenile arthritis, **right** knee   `HCC`

    M08.862   Other juvenile arthritis, **left** knee   `HCC`

    M08.869   Other juvenile arthritis, unspecified knee   `HCC`

√6th   **M08.87**   Other juvenile arthritis, **ankle and foot**

    M08.871   Other juvenile arthritis, **right** ankle and foot   `HCC`

    M08.872   Other juvenile arthritis, **left** ankle and foot   `HCC`

    M08.879   Other juvenile arthritis, unspecified ankle and foot   `HCC`

   M08.88   Other juvenile arthritis, other specified site   `HCC`

     Other juvenile arthritis, vertebrae

   M08.89   Other juvenile arthritis, **multiple sites**   `HCC`

√5th   **M08.9**   **Juvenile arthritis, unspecified**

    EXCLUDES 1   *juvenile rheumatoid arthritis, unspecified (M08.0-)*

   M08.90   Juvenile arthritis, unspecified, unspecified site   `HCC`

√6th   **M08.91**   Juvenile arthritis, unspecified, **shoulder**

    M08.911   Juvenile arthritis, unspecified, **right** shoulder   `HCC`

    M08.912   Juvenile arthritis, unspecified, **left** shoulder   `HCC`

    M08.919   Juvenile arthritis, unspecified, unspecified shoulder   `HCC`

√6th   **M08.92**   Juvenile arthritis, unspecified, **elbow**

    M08.921   Juvenile arthritis, unspecified, **right** elbow   `HCC`

    M08.922   Juvenile arthritis, unspecified, **left** elbow   `HCC`

    M08.929   Juvenile arthritis, unspecified, unspecified elbow   `HCC`

√6th   **M08.93**   Juvenile arthritis, unspecified, **wrist**

    M08.931   Juvenile arthritis, unspecified, **right** wrist   `HCC`

    M08.932   Juvenile arthritis, unspecified, **left** wrist   `HCC`

    M08.939   Juvenile arthritis, unspecified, unspecified wrist   `HCC`

√6th   **M08.94**   Juvenile arthritis, unspecified, **hand**

    M08.941   Juvenile arthritis, unspecified, **right** hand   `HCC`

    M08.942   Juvenile arthritis, unspecified, **left** hand   `HCC`

    M08.949   Juvenile arthritis, unspecified, unspecified hand   `HCC`

√6th   **M08.95**   Juvenile arthritis, unspecified, **hip**

    M08.951   Juvenile arthritis, unspecified, **right** hip   `HCC`

    M08.952   Juvenile arthritis, unspecified, **left** hip   `HCC`

    M08.959   Juvenile arthritis, unspecified, unspecified hip   `HCC`

√6th   **M08.96**   Juvenile arthritis, unspecified, **knee**

    M08.961   Juvenile arthritis, unspecified, **right** knee   `HCC`

    M08.962   Juvenile arthritis, unspecified, **left** knee   `HCC`

    M08.969   Juvenile arthritis, unspecified, unspecified knee   `HCC`

√6th   **M08.97**   Juvenile arthritis, unspecified, **ankle and foot**

    M08.971   Juvenile arthritis, unspecified, **right** ankle and foot   `HCC`

    M08.972   Juvenile arthritis, unspecified, **left** ankle and foot   `HCC`

    M08.979   Juvenile arthritis, unspecified, unspecified ankle and foot   `HCC`

   M08.98   Juvenile arthritis, unspecified, **vertebrae**   `HCC`

   M08.99   Juvenile arthritis, unspecified, **multiple sites**   `HCC`

   M08.9A   Juvenile arthritis, unspecified, other specified site   `HCC`

√4th   **M1A   Chronic gout**

   Use additional code to identify:

    autonomic neuropathy in diseases classified elsewhere (G99.0)

    calculus of urinary tract in diseases classified elsewhere (N22)

    cardiomyopathy in diseases classified elsewhere (I43)

    disorders of external ear in diseases classified elsewhere (H61.1-, H62.8-)

    disorders of iris and ciliary body in diseases classified elsewhere (H22)

    glomerular disorders in diseases classified elsewhere (N08)

   EXCLUDES 1   *gout NOS (M10.-)*

   EXCLUDES 2   *acute gout (M10.-)*

   The appropriate 7th character is to be added to each code from category M1A.

   0   without tophus (tophi)

   1   with tophus (tophi)

√5th   **M1A.0**   **Idiopathic** chronic gout

    Chronic gouty bursitis

    Primary chronic gout

√x7th   **M1A.00**   Idiopathic chronic gout, unspecified site

√6th   **M1A.01**   Idiopathic chronic gout, **shoulder**

    √7th   M1A.011   Idiopathic chronic gout, **right** shoulder

    √7th   M1A.012   Idiopathic chronic gout, **left** shoulder

    √7th   M1A.019   Idiopathic chronic gout, unspecified shoulder

√6th   **M1A.02**   Idiopathic chronic gout, **elbow**

    √7th   M1A.021   Idiopathic chronic gout, **right** elbow

    √7th   M1A.022   Idiopathic chronic gout, **left** elbow

    √7th   M1A.029   Idiopathic chronic gout, unspecified elbow

√6th   **M1A.03**   Idiopathic chronic gout, **wrist**

    √7th   M1A.031   Idiopathic chronic gout, **right** wrist

    √7th   M1A.032   Idiopathic chronic gout, **left** wrist

    √7th   M1A.039   Idiopathic chronic gout, unspecified wrist

✔ Additional Character Required   ✓x7th Placeholder   Questionable PDx   Manifestation   Unspecified   `UPD` Unacceptable PDx   `H1`-`H14` HAC   `HCC` CMS-HCC Dx   `HIV` HIV Dx

ICD-10-CM 2025

785

✓6ᵗʰ **M1A.04**   Idiopathic chronic gout, **hand**
- ✓7ᵗʰ **M1A.041**   Idiopathic chronic gout, **right** hand
- ✓7ᵗʰ **M1A.042**   Idiopathic chronic gout, **left** hand
- ✓7ᵗʰ **M1A.049**   Idiopathic chronic gout, unspecified hand

✓6ᵗʰ **M1A.05**   Idiopathic chronic gout, **hip**
- ✓7ᵗʰ **M1A.051**   Idiopathic chronic gout, **right** hip
- ✓7ᵗʰ **M1A.052**   Idiopathic chronic gout, **left** hip
- ✓7ᵗʰ **M1A.059**   Idiopathic chronic gout, unspecified hip

✓6ᵗʰ **M1A.06**   Idiopathic chronic gout, **knee**
- ✓7ᵗʰ **M1A.061**   Idiopathic chronic gout, **right** knee
- ✓7ᵗʰ **M1A.062**   Idiopathic chronic gout, **left** knee
- ✓7ᵗʰ **M1A.069**   Idiopathic chronic gout, unspecified knee

✓6ᵗʰ **M1A.07**   Idiopathic chronic gout, **ankle and foot**
- ✓7ᵗʰ **M1A.071**   Idiopathic chronic gout, **right** ankle and foot
- ✓7ᵗʰ **M1A.072**   Idiopathic chronic gout, **left** ankle and foot
- ✓7ᵗʰ **M1A.079**   Idiopathic chronic gout, unspecified ankle and foot

✓x7ᵗʰ **M1A.08**   Idiopathic chronic gout, **vertebrae**

✓x7ᵗʰ **M1A.09**   Idiopathic chronic gout, **multiple sites**

✓5ᵗʰ **M1A.1**   **Lead-induced** chronic gout

Code first toxic effects of lead and its compounds (T56.0-)

✓x7ᵗʰ **M1A.10**   Lead-induced chronic gout, unspecified site

✓6ᵗʰ **M1A.11**   Lead-induced chronic gout, **shoulder**
- ✓7ᵗʰ **M1A.111**   Lead-induced chronic gout, **right** shoulder
- ✓7ᵗʰ **M1A.112**   Lead-induced chronic gout, **left** shoulder
- ✓7ᵗʰ **M1A.119**   Lead-induced chronic gout, unspecified shoulder

✓6ᵗʰ **M1A.12**   Lead-induced chronic gout, **elbow**
- ✓7ᵗʰ **M1A.121**   Lead-induced chronic gout, **right** elbow
- ✓7ᵗʰ **M1A.122**   Lead-induced chronic gout, **left** elbow
- ✓7ᵗʰ **M1A.129**   Lead-induced chronic gout, unspecified elbow

✓6ᵗʰ **M1A.13**   Lead-induced chronic gout, **wrist**
- ✓7ᵗʰ **M1A.131**   Lead-induced chronic gout, **right** wrist
- ✓7ᵗʰ **M1A.132**   Lead-induced chronic gout, **left** wrist
- ✓7ᵗʰ **M1A.139**   Lead-induced chronic gout, unspecified wrist

✓6ᵗʰ **M1A.14**   Lead-induced chronic gout, **hand**
- ✓7ᵗʰ **M1A.141**   Lead-induced chronic gout, **right** hand
- ✓7ᵗʰ **M1A.142**   Lead-induced chronic gout, **left** hand
- ✓7ᵗʰ **M1A.149**   Lead-induced chronic gout, unspecified hand

✓6ᵗʰ **M1A.15**   Lead-induced chronic gout, **hip**
- ✓7ᵗʰ **M1A.151**   Lead-induced chronic gout, **right** hip
- ✓7ᵗʰ **M1A.152**   Lead-induced chronic gout, **left** hip
- ✓7ᵗʰ **M1A.159**   Lead-induced chronic gout, unspecified hip

✓6ᵗʰ **M1A.16**   Lead-induced chronic gout, **knee**
- ✓7ᵗʰ **M1A.161**   Lead-induced chronic gout, **right** knee
- ✓7ᵗʰ **M1A.162**   Lead-induced chronic gout, **left** knee
- ✓7ᵗʰ **M1A.169**   Lead-induced chronic gout, unspecified knee

✓6ᵗʰ **M1A.17**   Lead-induced chronic gout, **ankle and foot**
- ✓7ᵗʰ **M1A.171**   Lead-induced chronic gout, **right** ankle and foot
- ✓7ᵗʰ **M1A.172**   Lead-induced chronic gout, **left** ankle and foot
- ✓7ᵗʰ **M1A.179**   Lead-induced chronic gout, unspecified ankle and foot

✓x7ᵗʰ **M1A.18**   Lead-induced chronic gout, **vertebrae**

✓x7ᵗʰ **M1A.19**   Lead-induced chronic gout, **multiple sites**

✓5ᵗʰ **M1A.2**   **Drug-induced** chronic gout

Use additional code for adverse effect, if applicable, to identify drug (T36-T50 with fifth or sixth character 5)

✓x7ᵗʰ **M1A.20**   Drug-induced chronic gout, unspecified site

✓6ᵗʰ **M1A.21**   Drug-induced chronic gout, **shoulder**
- ✓7ᵗʰ **M1A.211**   Drug-induced chronic gout, **right** shoulder
- ✓7ᵗʰ **M1A.212**   Drug-induced chronic gout, **left** shoulder
- ✓7ᵗʰ **M1A.219**   Drug-induced chronic gout, unspecified shoulder

✓6ᵗʰ **M1A.22**   Drug-induced chronic gout, **elbow**
- ✓7ᵗʰ **M1A.221**   Drug-induced chronic gout, **right** elbow
- ✓7ᵗʰ **M1A.222**   Drug-induced chronic gout, **left** elbow
- ✓7ᵗʰ **M1A.229**   Drug-induced chronic gout, unspecified elbow

✓6ᵗʰ **M1A.23**   Drug-induced chronic gout, **wrist**
- ✓7ᵗʰ **M1A.231**   Drug-induced chronic gout, **right** wrist
- ✓7ᵗʰ **M1A.232**   Drug-induced chronic gout, **left** wrist
- ✓7ᵗʰ **M1A.239**   Drug-induced chronic gout, unspecified wrist

✓6ᵗʰ **M1A.24**   Drug-induced chronic gout, **hand**
- ✓7ᵗʰ **M1A.241**   Drug-induced chronic gout, **right** hand
- ✓7ᵗʰ **M1A.242**   Drug-induced chronic gout, **left** hand
- ✓7ᵗʰ **M1A.249**   Drug-induced chronic gout, unspecified hand

✓6ᵗʰ **M1A.25**   Drug-induced chronic gout, **hip**
- ✓7ᵗʰ **M1A.251**   Drug-induced chronic gout, **right** hip
- ✓7ᵗʰ **M1A.252**   Drug-induced chronic gout, **left** hip
- ✓7ᵗʰ **M1A.259**   Drug-induced chronic gout, unspecified hip

✓6ᵗʰ **M1A.26**   Drug-induced chronic gout, **knee**
- ✓7ᵗʰ **M1A.261**   Drug-induced chronic gout, **right** knee
- ✓7ᵗʰ **M1A.262**   Drug-induced chronic gout, **left** knee
- ✓7ᵗʰ **M1A.269**   Drug-induced chronic gout, unspecified knee

✓6ᵗʰ **M1A.27**   Drug-induced chronic gout, **ankle and foot**
- ✓7ᵗʰ **M1A.271**   Drug-induced chronic gout, **right** ankle and foot
- ✓7ᵗʰ **M1A.272**   Drug-induced chronic gout, **left** ankle and foot
- ✓7ᵗʰ **M1A.279**   Drug-induced chronic gout, unspecified ankle and foot

✓x7ᵗʰ **M1A.28**   Drug-induced chronic gout, **vertebrae**

✓x7ᵗʰ **M1A.29**   Drug-induced chronic gout, **multiple sites**

✓5ᵗʰ **M1A.3**   Chronic gout **due to renal impairment**

Code first associated renal disease

✓x7ᵗʰ **M1A.30**   Chronic gout due to renal impairment, unspecified site

✓6ᵗʰ **M1A.31**   Chronic gout due to renal impairment, **shoulder**
- ✓7ᵗʰ **M1A.311**   Chronic gout due to renal impairment, **right** shoulder
- ✓7ᵗʰ **M1A.312**   Chronic gout due to renal impairment, **left** shoulder
- ✓7ᵗʰ **M1A.319**   Chronic gout due to renal impairment, unspecified shoulder

✓6ᵗʰ **M1A.32**   Chronic gout due to renal impairment, **elbow**
- ✓7ᵗʰ **M1A.321**   Chronic gout due to renal impairment, **right** elbow
- ✓7ᵗʰ **M1A.322**   Chronic gout due to renal impairment, **left** elbow
- ✓7ᵗʰ **M1A.329**   Chronic gout due to renal impairment, unspecified elbow

✓6ᵗʰ **M1A.33**   Chronic gout due to renal impairment, **wrist**
- ✓7ᵗʰ **M1A.331**   Chronic gout due to renal impairment, **right** wrist
- ✓7ᵗʰ **M1A.332**   Chronic gout due to renal impairment, **left** wrist
- ✓7ᵗʰ **M1A.339**   Chronic gout due to renal impairment, unspecified wrist

✓6ᵗʰ **M1A.34**   Chronic gout due to renal impairment, **hand**
- ✓7ᵗʰ **M1A.341**   Chronic gout due to renal impairment, **right** hand
- ✓7ᵗʰ **M1A.342**   Chronic gout due to renal impairment, **left** hand
- ✓7ᵗʰ **M1A.349**   Chronic gout due to renal impairment, unspecified hand

✓6ᵗʰ **M1A.35**   Chronic gout due to renal impairment, **hip**
- ✓7ᵗʰ **M1A.351**   Chronic gout due to renal impairment, **right** hip
- ✓7ᵗʰ **M1A.352**   Chronic gout due to renal impairment, **left** hip
- ✓7ᵗʰ **M1A.359**   Chronic gout due to renal impairment, unspecified hip

✓6ᵗʰ **M1A.36**   Chronic gout due to renal impairment, **knee**
- ✓7ᵗʰ **M1A.361**   Chronic gout due to renal impairment, **right** knee

N Newborn: 0   **P** Pediatric: 0-17   **M** Maternity: 9-64   **A** Adult: 15-124   **UNS** Unspecified Site   **MCC** Major Complication/Comorbidity   **CC** Complication/Comorbidity   **PE** POA Exempt

786

ICD-10-CM 2025

√7ᵗʰ **M1A.362** Chronic gout due to renal impairment, left knee

√7ᵗʰ **M1A.369** Chronic gout due to renal impairment, unspecified knee

√6ᵗʰ **M1A.37** Chronic gout due to renal impairment, ankle and foot

√7ᵗʰ **M1A.371** Chronic gout due to renal impairment, right ankle and foot

√7ᵗʰ **M1A.372** Chronic gout due to renal impairment, left ankle and foot

√7ᵗʰ **M1A.379** Chronic gout due to renal impairment, unspecified ankle and foot

√x7ᵗʰ **M1A.38** Chronic gout due to renal impairment, vertebrae

√x7ᵗʰ **M1A.39** Chronic gout due to renal impairment, multiple sites

√5ᵗʰ **M1A.4** Other secondary chronic gout

Code first associated condition

√x7ᵗʰ **M1A.40** Other secondary chronic gout, unspecified site

√6ᵗʰ **M1A.41** Other secondary chronic gout, shoulder

√7ᵗʰ **M1A.411** Other secondary chronic gout, right shoulder

√7ᵗʰ **M1A.412** Other secondary chronic gout, left shoulder

√7ᵗʰ **M1A.419** Other secondary chronic gout, unspecified shoulder

√6ᵗʰ **M1A.42** Other secondary chronic gout, elbow

√7ᵗʰ **M1A.421** Other secondary chronic gout, right elbow

√7ᵗʰ **M1A.422** Other secondary chronic gout, left elbow

√7ᵗʰ **M1A.429** Other secondary chronic gout, unspecified elbow

√6ᵗʰ **M1A.43** Other secondary chronic gout, wrist

√7ᵗʰ **M1A.431** Other secondary chronic gout, right wrist

√7ᵗʰ **M1A.432** Other secondary chronic gout, left wrist

√7ᵗʰ **M1A.439** Other secondary chronic gout, unspecified wrist

√6ᵗʰ **M1A.44** Other secondary chronic gout, hand

√7ᵗʰ **M1A.441** Other secondary chronic gout, right hand

√7ᵗʰ **M1A.442** Other secondary chronic gout, left hand

√7ᵗʰ **M1A.449** Other secondary chronic gout, unspecified hand

√6ᵗʰ **M1A.45** Other secondary chronic gout, hip

√7ᵗʰ **M1A.451** Other secondary chronic gout, right hip

√7ᵗʰ **M1A.452** Other secondary chronic gout, left hip

√7ᵗʰ **M1A.459** Other secondary chronic gout, unspecified hip

√6ᵗʰ **M1A.46** Other secondary chronic gout, knee

√7ᵗʰ **M1A.461** Other secondary chronic gout, right knee

√7ᵗʰ **M1A.462** Other secondary chronic gout, left knee

√7ᵗʰ **M1A.469** Other secondary chronic gout, unspecified knee

√6ᵗʰ **M1A.47** Other secondary chronic gout, ankle and foot

√7ᵗʰ **M1A.471** Other secondary chronic gout, right ankle and foot

√7ᵗʰ **M1A.472** Other secondary chronic gout, left ankle and foot

√7ᵗʰ **M1A.479** Other secondary chronic gout, unspecified ankle and foot

√x7ᵗʰ **M1A.48** Other secondary chronic gout, vertebrae

√x7ᵗʰ **M1A.49** Other secondary chronic gout, multiple sites

√x7ᵗʰ **M1A.9** Chronic gout, unspecified

√4ᵗʰ **M10** **Gout**

Acute gout
Gout attack
Gout flare
Podagra

Use additional code to identify:

autonomic neuropathy in diseases classified elsewhere (G99.0)

calculus of urinary tract in diseases classified elsewhere (N22)

cardiomyopathy in diseases classified elsewhere (I43)

disorders of external ear in diseases classified elsewhere (H61.1-, H62.8-)

disorders of iris and ciliary body in diseases classified elsewhere (H22)

glomerular disorders in diseases classified elsewhere (N08)

EXCLUDES 2   chronic gout (M1A.-)

DEF: Purine and pyrimidine metabolic disorders, manifested by hyperuricemia and recurrent acute inflammatory arthritis. Monosodium urate or monohydrate crystals may be deposited in and around the joints, leading to joint destruction and severe crippling.

√5ᵗʰ **M10.0** **Idiopathic gout**

Gouty bursitis
Primary gout

M10.00 Idiopathic gout, unspecified site

√6ᵗʰ **M10.01** Idiopathic gout, shoulder

M10.011 Idiopathic gout, right shoulder

M10.012 Idiopathic gout, left shoulder

M10.019 Idiopathic gout, unspecified shoulder

√6ᵗʰ **M10.02** Idiopathic gout, elbow

M10.021 Idiopathic gout, right elbow

M10.022 Idiopathic gout, left elbow

M10.029 Idiopathic gout, unspecified elbow

√6ᵗʰ **M10.03** Idiopathic gout, wrist

M10.031 Idiopathic gout, right wrist

M10.032 Idiopathic gout, left wrist

M10.039 Idiopathic gout, unspecified wrist

√6ᵗʰ **M10.04** Idiopathic gout, hand

M10.041 Idiopathic gout, right hand

M10.042 Idiopathic gout, left hand

M10.049 Idiopathic gout, unspecified hand

√6ᵗʰ **M10.05** Idiopathic gout, hip

M10.051 Idiopathic gout, right hip

M10.052 Idiopathic gout, left hip

M10.059 Idiopathic gout, unspecified hip

√6ᵗʰ **M10.06** Idiopathic gout, knee

M10.061 Idiopathic gout, right knee

M10.062 Idiopathic gout, left knee

M10.069 Idiopathic gout, unspecified knee

√6ᵗʰ **M10.07** Idiopathic gout, ankle and foot

M10.071 Idiopathic gout, right ankle and foot

M10.072 Idiopathic gout, left ankle and foot

M10.079 Idiopathic gout, unspecified ankle and foot

M10.08 Idiopathic gout, vertebrae

M10.09 Idiopathic gout, multiple sites

√5ᵗʰ **M10.1** **Lead-induced gout**

Code first toxic effects of lead and its compounds (T56.0-)

M10.10 Lead-induced gout, unspecified site

√6ᵗʰ **M10.11** Lead-induced gout, shoulder

M10.111 Lead-induced gout, right shoulder

M10.112 Lead-induced gout, left shoulder

M10.119 Lead-induced gout, unspecified shoulder

√6ᵗʰ **M10.12** Lead-induced gout, elbow

M10.121 Lead-induced gout, right elbow

M10.122 Lead-induced gout, left elbow

M10.129 Lead-induced gout, unspecified elbow

√6ᵗʰ **M10.13** Lead-induced gout, wrist

M10.131 Lead-induced gout, right wrist

M10.132 Lead-induced gout, left wrist

M10.139 Lead-induced gout, unspecified wrist

√6ᵗʰ **M10.14** Lead-induced gout, hand

M10.141 Lead-induced gout, right hand

M10.142 Lead-induced gout, left hand

M10.149 Lead-induced gout, unspecified hand

√6ᵗʰ **M10.15** Lead-induced gout, hip

M10.151 Lead-induced gout, right hip

M10.152 Lead-induced gout, left hip

M10.159 Lead-induced gout, unspecified hip

√6ᵗʰ **M10.16** Lead-induced gout, knee

M10.161 Lead-induced gout, right knee

✔ Additional Character Required   √x7ᵗʰ Placeholder   Questionable PDx   Manifestation   Unspecified   **UPD** Unacceptable PDx   **H1**-**H14** HAC   **HCC** CMS-HCC Dx   **HIV** HIV Dx

ICD-10-CM 2025   **787**

    M10.162   Lead-induced gout, **left** knee
    M10.169   Lead-induced gout, unspecified knee

✓6th   M10.17   Lead-induced gout, **ankle and foot**

    M10.171   Lead-induced gout, **right** ankle and foot
    M10.172   Lead-induced gout, **left** ankle and foot
    M10.179   Lead-induced gout, unspecified ankle and foot

  M10.18   Lead-induced gout, **vertebrae**
  M10.19   Lead-induced gout, **multiple sites**

✓5th   **M10.2**   **Drug-induced** gout

Use additional code for adverse effect, if applicable, to identify drug (T36-T50 with fifth or sixth character 5)

  M10.20   Drug-induced gout, unspecified site

✓6th   M10.21   Drug-induced gout, **shoulder**

    M10.211   Drug-induced gout, **right** shoulder
    M10.212   Drug-induced gout, **left** shoulder
    M10.219   Drug-induced gout, unspecified shoulder

✓6th   M10.22   Drug-induced gout, **elbow**

    M10.221   Drug-induced gout, **right** elbow
    M10.222   Drug-induced gout, **left** elbow
    M10.229   Drug-induced gout, unspecified elbow

✓6th   M10.23   Drug-induced gout, **wrist**

    M10.231   Drug-induced gout, **right** wrist
    M10.232   Drug-induced gout, **left** wrist
    M10.239   Drug-induced gout, unspecified wrist

✓6th   M10.24   Drug-induced gout, **hand**

    M10.241   Drug-induced gout, **right** hand
    M10.242   Drug-induced gout, **left** hand
    M10.249   Drug-induced gout, unspecified hand

✓6th   M10.25   Drug-induced gout, **hip**

    M10.251   Drug-induced gout, **right** hip
    M10.252   Drug-induced gout, **left** hip
    M10.259   Drug-induced gout, unspecified hip

✓6th   M10.26   Drug-induced gout, **knee**

    M10.261   Drug-induced gout, **right** knee
    M10.262   Drug-induced gout, **left** knee
    M10.269   Drug-induced gout, unspecified knee

✓6th   M10.27   Drug-induced gout, **ankle and foot**

    M10.271   Drug-induced gout, **right** ankle and foot
    M10.272   Drug-induced gout, **left** ankle and foot
    M10.279   Drug-induced gout, unspecified ankle and foot

  M10.28   Drug-induced gout, **vertebrae**
  M10.29   Drug-induced gout, **multiple sites**

✓5th   **M10.3**   **Gout due to renal impairment**

Code first associated renal disease

  M10.30   Gout due to renal impairment, unspecified site

✓6th   M10.31   Gout due to renal impairment, **shoulder**

    M10.311   Gout due to renal impairment, **right** shoulder
    M10.312   Gout due to renal impairment, **left** shoulder
    M10.319   Gout due to renal impairment, unspecified shoulder

✓6th   M10.32   Gout due to renal impairment, **elbow**

    M10.321   Gout due to renal impairment, **right** elbow
    M10.322   Gout due to renal impairment, **left** elbow
    M10.329   Gout due to renal impairment, unspecified elbow

✓6th   M10.33   Gout due to renal impairment, **wrist**

    M10.331   Gout due to renal impairment, **right** wrist
    M10.332   Gout due to renal impairment, **left** wrist
    M10.339   Gout due to renal impairment, unspecified wrist

✓6th   M10.34   Gout due to renal impairment, **hand**

    M10.341   Gout due to renal impairment, **right** hand
    M10.342   Gout due to renal impairment, **left** hand
    M10.349   Gout due to renal impairment, unspecified hand

✓6th   M10.35   Gout due to renal impairment, **hip**

    M10.351   Gout due to renal impairment, **right** hip
    M10.352   Gout due to renal impairment, **left** hip
    M10.359   Gout due to renal impairment, unspecified hip

✓6th   M10.36   Gout due to renal impairment, **knee**

    M10.361   Gout due to renal impairment, **right** knee

    M10.362   Gout due to renal impairment, **left** knee
    M10.369   Gout due to renal impairment, unspecified knee

✓6th   M10.37   Gout due to renal impairment, **ankle and foot**

    M10.371   Gout due to renal impairment, **right** ankle and foot
    M10.372   Gout due to renal impairment, **left** ankle and foot
    M10.379   Gout due to renal impairment, unspecified ankle and foot

  M10.38   Gout due to renal impairment, **vertebrae**
  M10.39   Gout due to renal impairment, **multiple sites**

✓5th   **M10.4**   **Other secondary gout**

Code first associated condition

  M10.40   Other secondary gout, unspecified site

✓6th   M10.41   Other secondary gout, **shoulder**

    M10.411   Other secondary gout, **right** shoulder
    M10.412   Other secondary gout, **left** shoulder
    M10.419   Other secondary gout, unspecified shoulder

✓6th   M10.42   Other secondary gout, **elbow**

    M10.421   Other secondary gout, **right** elbow
    M10.422   Other secondary gout, **left** elbow
    M10.429   Other secondary gout, unspecified elbow

✓6th   M10.43   Other secondary gout, **wrist**

    M10.431   Other secondary gout, **right** wrist
    M10.432   Other secondary gout, **left** wrist
    M10.439   Other secondary gout, unspecified wrist

✓6th   M10.44   Other secondary gout, **hand**

    M10.441   Other secondary gout, **right** hand
    M10.442   Other secondary gout, **left** hand
    M10.449   Other secondary gout, unspecified hand

✓6th   M10.45   Other secondary gout, **hip**

    M10.451   Other secondary gout, **right** hip
    M10.452   Other secondary gout, **left** hip
    M10.459   Other secondary gout, unspecified hip

✓6th   M10.46   Other secondary gout, **knee**

    M10.461   Other secondary gout, **right** knee
    M10.462   Other secondary gout, **left** knee
    M10.469   Other secondary gout, unspecified knee

✓6th   M10.47   Other secondary gout, **ankle and foot**

    M10.471   Other secondary gout, **right** ankle and foot
    M10.472   Other secondary gout, **left** ankle and foot
    M10.479   Other secondary gout, unspecified ankle and foot

  M10.48   Other secondary gout, **vertebrae**
  M10.49   Other secondary gout, **multiple sites**

  M10.9   Gout, unspecified

    Gout NOS

✓4th   **M11**   **Other crystal arthropathies**

✓5th   **M11.0**   **Hydroxyapatite deposition disease**

DEF: Disease caused by deposits of calcium phosphate crystals in the soft tissues close to the joint (especially tendons) or in the joints. These calcifications can be mono or polyarticular and can cause destruction of the joint involved.

  M11.00   Hydroxyapatite deposition disease, unspecified site

✓6th   M11.01   Hydroxyapatite deposition disease, **shoulder**

    M11.011   Hydroxyapatite deposition disease, **right** shoulder
    M11.012   Hydroxyapatite deposition disease, **left** shoulder
    M11.019   Hydroxyapatite deposition disease, unspecified shoulder

✓6th   M11.02   Hydroxyapatite deposition disease, **elbow**

    M11.021   Hydroxyapatite deposition disease, **right** elbow
    M11.022   Hydroxyapatite deposition disease, **left** elbow
    M11.029   Hydroxyapatite deposition disease, unspecified elbow

✓6th   M11.03   Hydroxyapatite deposition disease, **wrist**

    M11.031   Hydroxyapatite deposition disease, **right** wrist
    M11.032   Hydroxyapatite deposition disease, **left** wrist
    M11.039   Hydroxyapatite deposition disease, unspecified wrist

N Newborn: 0   **P** Pediatric: 0-17   **M** Maternity: 9-64   **A** Adult: 15-124   **UNS** Unspecified Site   **MCC** Major Complication/Comorbidity   **CC** Complication/Comorbidity   **PE** POA Exempt

788   ICD-10-CM 2025

✓6th **M11.04** **Hydroxyapatite deposition disease, hand**

     M11.041 **Hydroxyapatite deposition disease, right hand**

     M11.042 **Hydroxyapatite deposition disease, left hand**

     M11.049 **Hydroxyapatite deposition disease, unspecified hand**

✓6th **M11.05** **Hydroxyapatite deposition disease, hip**

     M11.051 **Hydroxyapatite deposition disease, right hip**

     M11.052 **Hydroxyapatite deposition disease, left hip**

     M11.059 **Hydroxyapatite deposition disease, unspecified hip**

✓6th **M11.06** **Hydroxyapatite deposition disease, knee**

     M11.061 **Hydroxyapatite deposition disease, right knee**

     M11.062 **Hydroxyapatite deposition disease, left knee**

     M11.069 **Hydroxyapatite deposition disease, unspecified knee**

✓6th **M11.07** **Hydroxyapatite deposition disease, ankle and foot**

     M11.071 **Hydroxyapatite deposition disease, right ankle and foot**

     M11.072 **Hydroxyapatite deposition disease, left ankle and foot**

     M11.079 **Hydroxyapatite deposition disease, unspecified ankle and foot**

   M11.08 **Hydroxyapatite deposition disease, vertebrae**

   M11.09 **Hydroxyapatite deposition disease, multiple sites**

✓5th **M11.1** **Familial chondrocalcinosis**

   M11.10 **Familial chondrocalcinosis, unspecified site**

✓6th **M11.11** **Familial chondrocalcinosis, shoulder**

     M11.111 **Familial chondrocalcinosis, right shoulder**

     M11.112 **Familial chondrocalcinosis, left shoulder**

     M11.119 **Familial chondrocalcinosis, unspecified shoulder**

✓6th **M11.12** **Familial chondrocalcinosis, elbow**

     M11.121 **Familial chondrocalcinosis, right elbow**

     M11.122 **Familial chondrocalcinosis, left elbow**

     M11.129 **Familial chondrocalcinosis, unspecified elbow**

✓6th **M11.13** **Familial chondrocalcinosis, wrist**

     M11.131 **Familial chondrocalcinosis, right wrist**

     M11.132 **Familial chondrocalcinosis, left wrist**

     M11.139 **Familial chondrocalcinosis, unspecified wrist**

✓6th **M11.14** **Familial chondrocalcinosis, hand**

     M11.141 **Familial chondrocalcinosis, right hand**

     M11.142 **Familial chondrocalcinosis, left hand**

     M11.149 **Familial chondrocalcinosis, unspecified hand**

✓6th **M11.15** **Familial chondrocalcinosis, hip**

     M11.151 **Familial chondrocalcinosis, right hip**

     M11.152 **Familial chondrocalcinosis, left hip**

     M11.159 **Familial chondrocalcinosis, unspecified hip**

✓6th **M11.16** **Familial chondrocalcinosis, knee**

     M11.161 **Familial chondrocalcinosis, right knee**

     M11.162 **Familial chondrocalcinosis, left knee**

     M11.169 **Familial chondrocalcinosis, unspecified knee**

✓6th **M11.17** **Familial chondrocalcinosis, ankle and foot**

     M11.171 **Familial chondrocalcinosis, right ankle and foot**

     M11.172 **Familial chondrocalcinosis, left ankle and foot**

     M11.179 **Familial chondrocalcinosis, unspecified ankle and foot**

   M11.18 **Familial chondrocalcinosis, vertebrae**

   M11.19 **Familial chondrocalcinosis, multiple sites**

✓5th **M11.2** **Other chondrocalcinosis**

   Chondrocalcinosis NOS

   AHA: 2018,3Q,20

   TIP: Pseudogout is captured with codes in this subcategory.

   M11.20 **Other chondrocalcinosis, unspecified site**

✓6th **M11.21** **Other chondrocalcinosis, shoulder**

     M11.211 **Other chondrocalcinosis, right shoulder**

     M11.212 **Other chondrocalcinosis, left shoulder**

     M11.219 **Other chondrocalcinosis, unspecified shoulder**

✓6th **M11.22** **Other chondrocalcinosis, elbow**

     M11.221 **Other chondrocalcinosis, right elbow**

     M11.222 **Other chondrocalcinosis, left elbow**

     M11.229 **Other chondrocalcinosis, unspecified elbow**

✓6th **M11.23** **Other chondrocalcinosis, wrist**

     M11.231 **Other chondrocalcinosis, right wrist**

     M11.232 **Other chondrocalcinosis, left wrist**

     M11.239 **Other chondrocalcinosis, unspecified wrist**

✓6th **M11.24** **Other chondrocalcinosis, hand**

     M11.241 **Other chondrocalcinosis, right hand**

     M11.242 **Other chondrocalcinosis, left hand**

     M11.249 **Other chondrocalcinosis, unspecified hand**

✓6th **M11.25** **Other chondrocalcinosis, hip**

     M11.251 **Other chondrocalcinosis, right hip**

     M11.252 **Other chondrocalcinosis, left hip**

     M11.259 **Other chondrocalcinosis, unspecified hip**

✓6th **M11.26** **Other chondrocalcinosis, knee**

     M11.261 **Other chondrocalcinosis, right knee**

     M11.262 **Other chondrocalcinosis, left knee**

     M11.269 **Other chondrocalcinosis, unspecified knee**

✓6th **M11.27** **Other chondrocalcinosis, ankle and foot**

     M11.271 **Other chondrocalcinosis, right ankle and foot**

     M11.272 **Other chondrocalcinosis, left ankle and foot**

     M11.279 **Other chondrocalcinosis, unspecified ankle and foot**

   M11.28 **Other chondrocalcinosis, vertebrae**

   M11.29 **Other chondrocalcinosis, multiple sites**

✓5th **M11.8** **Other specified crystal arthropathies**

   M11.80 **Other specified crystal arthropathies, unspecified site**

✓6th **M11.81** **Other specified crystal arthropathies, shoulder**

     M11.811 **Other specified crystal arthropathies, right shoulder**

     M11.812 **Other specified crystal arthropathies, left shoulder**

     M11.819 **Other specified crystal arthropathies, unspecified shoulder**

✓6th **M11.82** **Other specified crystal arthropathies, elbow**

     M11.821 **Other specified crystal arthropathies, right elbow**

     M11.822 **Other specified crystal arthropathies, left elbow**

     M11.829 **Other specified crystal arthropathies, unspecified elbow**

✓6th **M11.83** **Other specified crystal arthropathies, wrist**

     M11.831 **Other specified crystal arthropathies, right wrist**

     M11.832 **Other specified crystal arthropathies, left wrist**

     M11.839 **Other specified crystal arthropathies, unspecified wrist**

✓6th **M11.84** **Other specified crystal arthropathies, hand**

     M11.841 **Other specified crystal arthropathies, right hand**

     M11.842 **Other specified crystal arthropathies, left hand**

     M11.849 **Other specified crystal arthropathies, unspecified hand**

✓6th **M11.85** **Other specified crystal arthropathies, hip**

     M11.851 **Other specified crystal arthropathies, right hip**

     M11.852 **Other specified crystal arthropathies, left hip**

     M11.859 **Other specified crystal arthropathies, unspecified hip**

✓6th **M11.86** **Other specified crystal arthropathies, knee**

     M11.861 **Other specified crystal arthropathies, right knee**

     M11.862 **Other specified crystal arthropathies, left knee**

     M11.869 **Other specified crystal arthropathies, unspecified knee**

✓ Additional Character Required   ✓x7th Placeholder   **Questionable PDx**   Manifestation   Unspecified   **UPD** Unacceptable PDx   **H1-H14** HAC   **HCC** CMS-HCC Dx   **HIV** HIV Dx

ICD-10-CM 2025   789

✓6th **M11.87** **Other specified crystal arthropathies, ankle and foot**

M11.871 Other specified crystal arthropathies, right ankle and foot

M11.872 Other specified crystal arthropathies, left ankle and foot

M11.879 Other specified crystal arthropathies, unspecified ankle and foot

M11.88 Other specified crystal arthropathies, vertebrae

M11.89 Other specified crystal arthropathies, multiple sites

M11.9 **Crystal arthropathy, unspecified**

✓4th **M12** **Other and unspecified arthropathy**

EXCLUDES 1   arthrosis (M15-M19)

cricoarytenoid arthropathy (J38.7)

✓5th **M12.0** **Chronic postrheumatic arthropathy [Jaccoud]**

M12.00 Chronic postrheumatic arthropathy [Jaccoud], unspecified site   HCC

✓6th **M12.01** Chronic postrheumatic arthropathy [Jaccoud], shoulder

M12.011 Chronic postrheumatic arthropathy [Jaccoud], right shoulder   HCC

M12.012 Chronic postrheumatic arthropathy [Jaccoud], left shoulder   HCC

M12.019 Chronic postrheumatic arthropathy [Jaccoud], unspecified shoulder   HCC

✓6th **M12.02** Chronic postrheumatic arthropathy [Jaccoud], elbow

M12.021 Chronic postrheumatic arthropathy [Jaccoud], right elbow   HCC

M12.022 Chronic postrheumatic arthropathy [Jaccoud], left elbow   HCC

M12.029 Chronic postrheumatic arthropathy [Jaccoud], unspecified elbow   HCC

✓6th **M12.03** Chronic postrheumatic arthropathy [Jaccoud], wrist

M12.031 Chronic postrheumatic arthropathy [Jaccoud], right wrist   HCC

M12.032 Chronic postrheumatic arthropathy [Jaccoud], left wrist   HCC

M12.039 Chronic postrheumatic arthropathy [Jaccoud], unspecified wrist   HCC

✓6th **M12.04** Chronic postrheumatic arthropathy [Jaccoud], hand

M12.041 Chronic postrheumatic arthropathy [Jaccoud], right hand   HCC

M12.042 Chronic postrheumatic arthropathy [Jaccoud], left hand   HCC

M12.049 Chronic postrheumatic arthropathy [Jaccoud], unspecified hand   HCC

✓6th **M12.05** Chronic postrheumatic arthropathy [Jaccoud], hip

M12.051 Chronic postrheumatic arthropathy [Jaccoud], right hip   HCC

M12.052 Chronic postrheumatic arthropathy [Jaccoud], left hip   HCC

M12.059 Chronic postrheumatic arthropathy [Jaccoud], unspecified hip   HCC

✓6th **M12.06** Chronic postrheumatic arthropathy [Jaccoud], knee

M12.061 Chronic postrheumatic arthropathy [Jaccoud], right knee   HCC

M12.062 Chronic postrheumatic arthropathy [Jaccoud], left knee   HCC

M12.069 Chronic postrheumatic arthropathy [Jaccoud], unspecified knee   HCC

✓6th **M12.07** Chronic postrheumatic arthropathy [Jaccoud], ankle and foot

M12.071 Chronic postrheumatic arthropathy [Jaccoud], right ankle and foot   HCC

M12.072 Chronic postrheumatic arthropathy [Jaccoud], left ankle and foot   HCC

M12.079 Chronic postrheumatic arthropathy [Jaccoud], unspecified ankle and foot   HCC

M12.08 Chronic postrheumatic arthropathy [Jaccoud], other specified site   HCC

Chronic postrheumatic arthropathy [Jaccoud], vertebrae

M12.09 Chronic postrheumatic arthropathy [Jaccoud], multiple sites   HCC

✓5th **M12.1** **Kaschin-Beck disease**

Osteochondroarthrosis deformans endemica

M12.10 Kaschin-Beck disease, unspecified site

✓6th **M12.11** Kaschin-Beck disease, shoulder

M12.111 Kaschin-Beck disease, right shoulder

M12.112 Kaschin-Beck disease, left shoulder

M12.119 Kaschin-Beck disease, unspecified shoulder

✓6th **M12.12** Kaschin-Beck disease, elbow

M12.121 Kaschin-Beck disease, right elbow

M12.122 Kaschin-Beck disease, left elbow

M12.129 Kaschin-Beck disease, unspecified elbow

✓6th **M12.13** Kaschin-Beck disease, wrist

M12.131 Kaschin-Beck disease, right wrist

M12.132 Kaschin-Beck disease, left wrist

M12.139 Kaschin-Beck disease, unspecified wrist

✓6th **M12.14** Kaschin-Beck disease, hand

M12.141 Kaschin-Beck disease, right hand

M12.142 Kaschin-Beck disease, left hand

M12.149 Kaschin-Beck disease, unspecified hand

✓6th **M12.15** Kaschin-Beck disease, hip

M12.151 Kaschin-Beck disease, right hip

M12.152 Kaschin-Beck disease, left hip

M12.159 Kaschin-Beck disease, unspecified hip

✓6th **M12.16** Kaschin-Beck disease, knee

M12.161 Kaschin-Beck disease, right knee

M12.162 Kaschin-Beck disease, left knee

M12.169 Kaschin-Beck disease, unspecified knee

✓6th **M12.17** Kaschin-Beck disease, ankle and foot

M12.171 Kaschin-Beck disease, right ankle and foot

M12.172 Kaschin-Beck disease, left ankle and foot

M12.179 Kaschin-Beck disease, unspecified ankle and foot

M12.18 Kaschin-Beck disease, vertebrae

M12.19 Kaschin-Beck disease, multiple sites

✓5th **M12.2** **Villonodular synovitis (pigmented)**

M12.20 Villonodular synovitis (pigmented), unspecified site

✓6th **M12.21** Villonodular synovitis (pigmented), shoulder

M12.211 Villonodular synovitis (pigmented), right shoulder

M12.212 Villonodular synovitis (pigmented), left shoulder

M12.219 Villonodular synovitis (pigmented), unspecified shoulder

✓6th **M12.22** Villonodular synovitis (pigmented), elbow

M12.221 Villonodular synovitis (pigmented), right elbow

M12.222 Villonodular synovitis (pigmented), left elbow

M12.229 Villonodular synovitis (pigmented), unspecified elbow

✓6th **M12.23** Villonodular synovitis (pigmented), wrist

M12.231 Villonodular synovitis (pigmented), right wrist

M12.232 Villonodular synovitis (pigmented), left wrist

M12.239 Villonodular synovitis (pigmented), unspecified wrist

✓6th **M12.24** Villonodular synovitis (pigmented), hand

M12.241 Villonodular synovitis (pigmented), right hand

M12.242 Villonodular synovitis (pigmented), left hand

M12.249 Villonodular synovitis (pigmented), unspecified hand

✓6th **M12.25** Villonodular synovitis (pigmented), hip

M12.251 Villonodular synovitis (pigmented), right hip

M12.252 Villonodular synovitis (pigmented), left hip

M12.259 Villonodular synovitis (pigmented), unspecified hip

✓6th **M12.26** Villonodular synovitis (pigmented), knee

M12.261 Villonodular synovitis (pigmented), right knee

M12.262 Villonodular synovitis (pigmented), left knee

M12.269 Villonodular synovitis (pigmented), unspecified knee

✓6th **M12.27** Villonodular synovitis (pigmented), ankle and foot

M12.271 Villonodular synovitis (pigmented), right ankle and foot

N Newborn: 0   P Pediatric: 0-17   M Maternity: 9-64   A Adult: 15-124   UNS Unspecified Site   MCC Major Complication/Comorbidity   CC Complication/Comorbidity   PE POA Exempt

790

ICD-10-CM 2025

M12.272 Villonodular synovitis (pigmented), **left ankle and foot**

M12.279 Villonodular synovitis (pigmented), unspecified ankle and foot

M12.28 Villonodular synovitis (pigmented), other specified site
Villonodular synovitis (pigmented), vertebrae

M12.29 Villonodular synovitis (pigmented), **multiple sites**

✓5th **M12.3 Palindromic rheumatism**

DEF: Sudden and recurring attacks of moderate to severe joint pain and swelling generally occurring in the hands or feet of unknown etiology. After the attack subsides, the joints appear normal again.

M12.30 Palindromic rheumatism, unspecified site

✓6th M12.31 Palindromic rheumatism, **shoulder**

M12.311 Palindromic rheumatism, **right** shoulder
M12.312 Palindromic rheumatism, **left** shoulder
M12.319 Palindromic rheumatism, unspecified shoulder

✓6th M12.32 Palindromic rheumatism, **elbow**

M12.321 Palindromic rheumatism, **right** elbow
M12.322 Palindromic rheumatism, **left** elbow
M12.329 Palindromic rheumatism, unspecified elbow

✓6th M12.33 Palindromic rheumatism, **wrist**

M12.331 Palindromic rheumatism, **right** wrist
M12.332 Palindromic rheumatism, **left** wrist
M12.339 Palindromic rheumatism, unspecified wrist

✓6th M12.34 Palindromic rheumatism, **hand**

M12.341 Palindromic rheumatism, **right** hand
M12.342 Palindromic rheumatism, **left** hand
M12.349 Palindromic rheumatism, unspecified hand

✓6th M12.35 Palindromic rheumatism, **hip**

M12.351 Palindromic rheumatism, **right** hip
M12.352 Palindromic rheumatism, **left** hip
M12.359 Palindromic rheumatism, unspecified hip

✓6th M12.36 Palindromic rheumatism, **knee**

M12.361 Palindromic rheumatism, **right** knee
M12.362 Palindromic rheumatism, **left** knee
M12.369 Palindromic rheumatism, unspecified knee

✓6th M12.37 Palindromic rheumatism, **ankle and foot**

M12.371 Palindromic rheumatism, **right** ankle and foot
M12.372 Palindromic rheumatism, **left** ankle and foot
M12.379 Palindromic rheumatism, unspecified ankle and foot

M12.38 Palindromic rheumatism, other specified site
Palindromic rheumatism, vertebrae

M12.39 Palindromic rheumatism, **multiple sites**

✓5th **M12.4 Intermittent hydrarthrosis**

M12.40 Intermittent hydrarthrosis, unspecified site

✓6th M12.41 Intermittent hydrarthrosis, **shoulder**

M12.411 Intermittent hydrarthrosis, **right** shoulder
M12.412 Intermittent hydrarthrosis, **left** shoulder
M12.419 Intermittent hydrarthrosis, unspecified shoulder

✓6th M12.42 Intermittent hydrarthrosis, **elbow**

M12.421 Intermittent hydrarthrosis, **right** elbow
M12.422 Intermittent hydrarthrosis, **left** elbow
M12.429 Intermittent hydrarthrosis, unspecified elbow

✓6th M12.43 Intermittent hydrarthrosis, **wrist**

M12.431 Intermittent hydrarthrosis, **right** wrist
M12.432 Intermittent hydrarthrosis, **left** wrist
M12.439 Intermittent hydrarthrosis, unspecified wrist

✓6th M12.44 Intermittent hydrarthrosis, **hand**

M12.441 Intermittent hydrarthrosis, **right** hand
M12.442 Intermittent hydrarthrosis, **left** hand
M12.449 Intermittent hydrarthrosis, unspecified hand

✓6th M12.45 Intermittent hydrarthrosis, **hip**

M12.451 Intermittent hydrarthrosis, **right** hip
M12.452 Intermittent hydrarthrosis, **left** hip
M12.459 Intermittent hydrarthrosis, unspecified hip

✓6th M12.46 Intermittent hydrarthrosis, **knee**

M12.461 Intermittent hydrarthrosis, **right** knee
M12.462 Intermittent hydrarthrosis, **left** knee
M12.469 Intermittent hydrarthrosis, unspecified knee

✓6th M12.47 Intermittent hydrarthrosis, **ankle and foot**

M12.471 Intermittent hydrarthrosis, **right** ankle and foot
M12.472 Intermittent hydrarthrosis, **left** ankle and foot
M12.479 Intermittent hydrarthrosis, unspecified ankle and foot

M12.48 Intermittent hydrarthrosis, other site

M12.49 Intermittent hydrarthrosis, **multiple sites**

✓5th **M12.5 Traumatic arthropathy**

EXCLUDES 1 current injury–see Alphabetic Index
post-traumatic osteoarthritis of first carpometacarpal joint (M18.2-M18.3)
post-traumatic osteoarthritis of hip (M16.4-M16.5)
post-traumatic osteoarthritis of knee (M17.2-M17.3)
post-traumatic osteoarthritis NOS (M19.1-)
post-traumatic osteoarthritis of other single joints (M19.1-)

AHA: 2015,1Q,17

M12.50 Traumatic arthropathy, unspecified site

✓6th M12.51 Traumatic arthropathy, **shoulder**

M12.511 Traumatic arthropathy, **right** shoulder
M12.512 Traumatic arthropathy, **left** shoulder
M12.519 Traumatic arthropathy, unspecified shoulder

✓6th M12.52 Traumatic arthropathy, **elbow**

M12.521 Traumatic arthropathy, **right** elbow
M12.522 Traumatic arthropathy, **left** elbow
M12.529 Traumatic arthropathy, unspecified elbow

✓6th M12.53 Traumatic arthropathy, **wrist**

M12.531 Traumatic arthropathy, **right** wrist
M12.532 Traumatic arthropathy, **left** wrist
M12.539 Traumatic arthropathy, unspecified wrist

✓6th M12.54 Traumatic arthropathy, **hand**

M12.541 Traumatic arthropathy, **right** hand
M12.542 Traumatic arthropathy, **left** hand
M12.549 Traumatic arthropathy, unspecified hand

✓6th M12.55 Traumatic arthropathy, **hip**

M12.551 Traumatic arthropathy, **right** hip
M12.552 Traumatic arthropathy, **left** hip
M12.559 Traumatic arthropathy, unspecified hip

✓6th M12.56 Traumatic arthropathy, **knee**

M12.561 Traumatic arthropathy, **right** knee
M12.562 Traumatic arthropathy, **left** knee
M12.569 Traumatic arthropathy, unspecified knee

✓6th M12.57 Traumatic arthropathy, **ankle and foot**

M12.571 Traumatic arthropathy, **right** ankle and foot
M12.572 Traumatic arthropathy, **left** ankle and foot
M12.579 Traumatic arthropathy, unspecified ankle and foot

M12.58 Traumatic arthropathy, other specified site
Traumatic arthropathy, vertebrae

M12.59 Traumatic arthropathy, **multiple sites**

✓5th **M12.8 Other specific arthropathies, not elsewhere classified**
Transient arthropathy

M12.80 Other specific arthropathies, not elsewhere classified, unspecified site

✓6th M12.81 Other specific arthropathies, not elsewhere classified, **shoulder**

M12.811 Other specific arthropathies, not elsewhere classified, **right** shoulder
M12.812 Other specific arthropathies, not elsewhere classified, **left** shoulder
M12.819 Other specific arthropathies, not elsewhere classified, unspecified shoulder

✓6th M12.82 Other specific arthropathies, not elsewhere classified, **elbow**

M12.821 Other specific arthropathies, not elsewhere classified, **right** elbow
M12.822 Other specific arthropathies, not elsewhere classified, **left** elbow

M12.829 Other specific arthropathies, not elsewhere classified, unspecified elbow

✓6th **M12.83** Other specific arthropathies, not elsewhere classified, **wrist**

    M12.831 Other specific arthropathies, not elsewhere classified, **right** wrist

    M12.832 Other specific arthropathies, not elsewhere classified, **left** wrist

    M12.839 Other specific arthropathies, not elsewhere classified, unspecified wrist

✓6th **M12.84** Other specific arthropathies, not elsewhere classified, **hand**

    M12.841 Other specific arthropathies, not elsewhere classified, **right** hand

    M12.842 Other specific arthropathies, not elsewhere classified, **left** hand

    M12.849 Other specific arthropathies, not elsewhere classified, unspecified hand

✓6th **M12.85** Other specific arthropathies, not elsewhere classified, **hip**

    M12.851 Other specific arthropathies, not elsewhere classified, **right** hip

    M12.852 Other specific arthropathies, not elsewhere classified, **left** hip

    M12.859 Other specific arthropathies, not elsewhere classified, unspecified hip

✓6th **M12.86** Other specific arthropathies, not elsewhere classified, **knee**

    M12.861 Other specific arthropathies, not elsewhere classified, **right** knee

    M12.862 Other specific arthropathies, not elsewhere classified, **left** knee

    M12.869 Other specific arthropathies, not elsewhere classified, unspecified knee

✓6th **M12.87** Other specific arthropathies, not elsewhere classified, **ankle and foot**

    M12.871 Other specific arthropathies, not elsewhere classified, **right** ankle and foot

    M12.872 Other specific arthropathies, not elsewhere classified, **left** ankle and foot

    M12.879 Other specific arthropathies, not elsewhere classified, unspecified ankle and foot

M12.88 Other specific arthropathies, not elsewhere classified, other specified site

    Other specific arthropathies, not elsewhere classified, vertebrae

M12.89 Other specific arthropathies, not elsewhere classified, **multiple sites**

M12.9 Arthropathy, unspecified

✓4th **M13** Other arthritis

    EXCLUDES 1   arthrosis (M15-M19)

                   osteoarthritis (M15-M19)

M13.0 Polyarthritis, unspecified

✓5th **M13.1** Monoarthritis, not elsewhere classified

    M13.10 Monoarthritis, not elsewhere classified, unspecified site

✓6th **M13.11** Monoarthritis, not elsewhere classified, **shoulder**

    M13.111 Monoarthritis, not elsewhere classified, **right** shoulder

    M13.112 Monoarthritis, not elsewhere classified, **left** shoulder

    M13.119 Monoarthritis, not elsewhere classified, unspecified shoulder

✓6th **M13.12** Monoarthritis, not elsewhere classified, **elbow**

    M13.121 Monoarthritis, not elsewhere classified, **right** elbow

    M13.122 Monoarthritis, not elsewhere classified, **left** elbow

    M13.129 Monoarthritis, not elsewhere classified, unspecified elbow

✓6th **M13.13** Monoarthritis, not elsewhere classified, **wrist**

    M13.131 Monoarthritis, not elsewhere classified, **right** wrist

    M13.132 Monoarthritis, not elsewhere classified, **left** wrist

    M13.139 Monoarthritis, not elsewhere classified, unspecified wrist

✓6th **M13.14** Monoarthritis, not elsewhere classified, **hand**

    M13.141 Monoarthritis, not elsewhere classified, **right** hand

M13.142 Monoarthritis, not elsewhere classified, **left** hand

M13.149 Monoarthritis, not elsewhere classified, unspecified hand

✓6th **M13.15** Monoarthritis, not elsewhere classified, **hip**

    M13.151 Monoarthritis, not elsewhere classified, **right** hip

    M13.152 Monoarthritis, not elsewhere classified, **left** hip

    M13.159 Monoarthritis, not elsewhere classified, unspecified hip

✓6th **M13.16** Monoarthritis, not elsewhere classified, **knee**

    M13.161 Monoarthritis, not elsewhere classified, **right** knee

    M13.162 Monoarthritis, not elsewhere classified, **left** knee

    M13.169 Monoarthritis, not elsewhere classified, unspecified knee

✓6th **M13.17** Monoarthritis, not elsewhere classified, **ankle and foot**

    M13.171 Monoarthritis, not elsewhere classified, **right** ankle and foot

    M13.172 Monoarthritis, not elsewhere classified, **left** ankle and foot

    M13.179 Monoarthritis, not elsewhere classified, unspecified ankle and foot

✓5th **M13.8** Other specified arthritis

    Allergic arthritis

    EXCLUDES 1   osteoarthritis (M15-M19)

    M13.80 Other specified arthritis, unspecified site

✓6th **M13.81** Other specified arthritis, **shoulder**

    M13.811 Other specified arthritis, **right** shoulder

    M13.812 Other specified arthritis, **left** shoulder

    M13.819 Other specified arthritis, unspecified shoulder

✓6th **M13.82** Other specified arthritis, **elbow**

    M13.821 Other specified arthritis, **right** elbow

    M13.822 Other specified arthritis, **left** elbow

    M13.829 Other specified arthritis, unspecified elbow

✓6th **M13.83** Other specified arthritis, **wrist**

    M13.831 Other specified arthritis, **right** wrist

    M13.832 Other specified arthritis, **left** wrist

    M13.839 Other specified arthritis, unspecified wrist

✓6th **M13.84** Other specified arthritis, **hand**

    M13.841 Other specified arthritis, **right** hand

    M13.842 Other specified arthritis, **left** hand

    M13.849 Other specified arthritis, unspecified hand

✓6th **M13.85** Other specified arthritis, **hip**

    M13.851 Other specified arthritis, **right** hip

    M13.852 Other specified arthritis, **left** hip

    M13.859 Other specified arthritis, unspecified hip

✓6th **M13.86** Other specified arthritis, **knee**

    M13.861 Other specified arthritis, **right** knee

    M13.862 Other specified arthritis, **left** knee

    M13.869 Other specified arthritis, unspecified knee

✓6th **M13.87** Other specified arthritis, **ankle and foot**

    M13.871 Other specified arthritis, **right** ankle and foot

    M13.872 Other specified arthritis, **left** ankle and foot

    M13.879 Other specified arthritis, unspecified ankle and foot

M13.88 Other specified arthritis, other site

M13.89 Other specified arthritis, **multiple sites**

N Newborn: 0   **P** Pediatric: 0-17   **M** Maternity: 9-64   **A** Adult: 15-124   **UNS** Unspecified Site   **MCC** Major Complication/Comorbidity   **CC** Complication/Comorbidity   **PE** POA Exempt

792

ICD-10-CM 2025

✓4ᵗʰ **M14 Arthropathies in other diseases classified elsewhere**

     EXCLUDES 1   *arthropathy in:*
          diabetes mellitus (E08-E13 with .61-)
          hematological disorders (M36.2-M36.3)
          hypersensitivity reactions (M36.4)
          neoplastic disease (M36.1)
          neurosyphillis (A52.16)
          sarcoidosis (D86.86)
       enteropathic arthropathies (M07.-)
       juvenile psoriatic arthropathy (L40.54)
       lipoid dermatoarthritis (E78.81)

✓5ᵗʰ **M14.6 Charcôt's joint**

     Neuropathic arthropathy
     EXCLUDES 1   *Charcôt's joint in diabetes mellitus (E08-E13 with .610)*
          Charcôt's joint in tabes dorsalis (A52.16)

     DEF: Progressive neurologic arthropathy in which chronic degeneration of joints in the weight-bearing areas with peripheral hypertrophy occurs as a complication of a neuropathy disorder. Supporting structures relax from a loss of sensation resulting in chronic joint instability.

     M14.60   Charcôt's joint, unspecified site

   ✓6ᵗʰ M14.61   Charcôt's joint, shoulder
       M14.611   Charcôt's joint, right shoulder
       M14.612   Charcôt's joint, left shoulder
       M14.619   Charcôt's joint, unspecified shoulder

   ✓6ᵗʰ M14.62   Charcôt's joint, elbow
       M14.621   Charcôt's joint, right elbow
       M14.622   Charcôt's joint, left elbow
       M14.629   Charcôt's joint, unspecified elbow

   ✓6ᵗʰ M14.63   Charcôt's joint, wrist
       M14.631   Charcôt's joint, right wrist
       M14.632   Charcôt's joint, left wrist
       M14.639   Charcôt's joint, unspecified wrist

   ✓6ᵗʰ M14.64   Charcôt's joint, hand
       M14.641   Charcôt's joint, right hand
       M14.642   Charcôt's joint, left hand
       M14.649   Charcôt's joint, unspecified hand

   ✓6ᵗʰ M14.65   Charcôt's joint, hip
       M14.651   Charcôt's joint, right hip
       M14.652   Charcôt's joint, left hip
       M14.659   Charcôt's joint, unspecified hip

   ✓6ᵗʰ M14.66   Charcôt's joint, knee
       M14.661   Charcôt's joint, right knee
       M14.662   Charcôt's joint, left knee
       M14.669   Charcôt's joint, unspecified knee

   ✓6ᵗʰ M14.67   Charcôt's joint, ankle and foot
       M14.671   Charcôt's joint, right ankle and foot
       M14.672   Charcôt's joint, left ankle and foot
       M14.679   Charcôt's joint, unspecified ankle and foot

     M14.68   Charcôt's joint, vertebrae
     M14.69   Charcôt's joint, multiple sites

✓5ᵗʰ **M14.8 Arthropathies in other specified diseases classified elsewhere**

     Code first underlying disease, such as:
       amyloidosis (E85.-)
       erythema multiforme (L51.-)
       erythema nodosum (L52)
       hemochromatosis (E83.11-)
       hyperparathyroidism (E21.-)
       hypothyroidism (E00-E03)
       sickle-cell disorders (D57.-)
       thyrotoxicosis [hyperthyroidism] (E05.-)
       Whipple's disease (K90.81)

     M14.80   *Arthropathies in other specified diseases classified elsewhere, unspecified site*

   ✓6ᵗʰ M14.81   Arthropathies in other specified diseases classified elsewhere, shoulder
       M14.811   *Arthropathies in other specified diseases classified elsewhere, right shoulder*
       M14.812   *Arthropathies in other specified diseases classified elsewhere, left shoulder*
       M14.819   *Arthropathies in other specified diseases classified elsewhere, unspecified shoulder*

   ✓6ᵗʰ M14.82   Arthropathies in other specified diseases classified elsewhere, elbow
       M14.821   *Arthropathies in other specified diseases classified elsewhere, right elbow*

       M14.822   *Arthropathies in other specified diseases classified elsewhere, left elbow*
       M14.829   *Arthropathies in other specified diseases classified elsewhere, unspecified elbow*

   ✓6ᵗʰ M14.83   Arthropathies in other specified diseases classified elsewhere, wrist
       M14.831   *Arthropathies in other specified diseases classified elsewhere, right wrist*
       M14.832   *Arthropathies in other specified diseases classified elsewhere, left wrist*
       M14.839   *Arthropathies in other specified diseases classified elsewhere, unspecified wrist*

   ✓6ᵗʰ M14.84   Arthropathies in other specified diseases classified elsewhere, hand
       M14.841   *Arthropathies in other specified diseases classified elsewhere, right hand*
       M14.842   *Arthropathies in other specified diseases classified elsewhere, left hand*
       M14.849   *Arthropathies in other specified diseases classified elsewhere, unspecified hand*

   ✓6ᵗʰ M14.85   Arthropathies in other specified diseases classified elsewhere, hip
       M14.851   *Arthropathies in other specified diseases classified elsewhere, right hip*
       M14.852   *Arthropathies in other specified diseases classified elsewhere, left hip*
       M14.859   *Arthropathies in other specified diseases classified elsewhere, unspecified hip*

   ✓6ᵗʰ M14.86   Arthropathies in other specified diseases classified elsewhere, knee
       M14.861   *Arthropathies in other specified diseases classified elsewhere, right knee*
       M14.862   *Arthropathies in other specified diseases classified elsewhere, left knee*
       M14.869   *Arthropathies in other specified diseases classified elsewhere, unspecified knee*

   ✓6ᵗʰ M14.87   Arthropathies in other specified diseases classified elsewhere, ankle and foot
       M14.871   *Arthropathies in other specified diseases classified elsewhere, right ankle and foot*
       M14.872   *Arthropathies in other specified diseases classified elsewhere, left ankle and foot*
       M14.879   *Arthropathies in other specified diseases classified elsewhere, unspecified ankle and foot*

     M14.88   *Arthropathies in other specified diseases classified elsewhere, vertebrae*
     M14.89   *Arthropathies in other specified diseases classified elsewhere, multiple sites*

Osteoarthritis (M15-M19)

     EXCLUDES 2   *osteoarthritis of spine (M47.-)*
     AHA: 2020,2Q,14; 2016,4Q,147
     TIP: Assign a primary osteoarthritis code when the site of the osteoarthritis is documented but the type of osteoarthritis — primary, secondary, generalized, or post-traumatic — is not documented. Primary is considered the default.

✓4ᵗʰ **M15 Polyosteoarthritis**

     INCLUDES   arthritis of multiple sites
     EXCLUDES 1   *bilateral involvement of single joint (M16-M19)*

     M15.0 Primary generalized (osteo)arthritis
     M15.1 Heberden's nodes (with arthropathy)
       Interphalangeal distal osteoarthritis
     M15.2 Bouchard's nodes (with arthropathy)
       Juxtaphalangeal distal osteoarthritis
     M15.3 Secondary multiple arthritis
       Post-traumatic polyosteoarthritis
     M15.4 Erosive (osteo)arthritis
     M15.8 Other polyosteoarthritis
     M15.9 Polyosteoarthritis, unspecified
       Generalized osteoarthritis NOS

✓4ᵗʰ **M16 Osteoarthritis of hip**

     AHA: 2016,4Q,146

     M16.0 Bilateral primary osteoarthritis of hip
       AHA: 2018,2Q,15

   ✓5ᵗʰ **M16.1 Unilateral primary osteoarthritis of hip**
       Primary osteoarthritis of hip NOS
       AHA: 2018,2Q,15

     M16.10   Unilateral primary osteoarthritis, unspecified hip
     M16.11   Unilateral primary osteoarthritis, right hip
     M16.12   Unilateral primary osteoarthritis, left hip

✔ Additional Character Required   ✔x7ᵗʰ Placeholder   Questionable PDx   Manifestation   Unspecified   UPD Unacceptable PDx   H1 -H14 HAC   HCC CMS-HCC Dx   HIV HIV Dx

Chapter 13. Diseases of the Musculoskeletal System and Connective Tissue

M16.2 **Bilateral** osteoarthritis resulting from **hip dysplasia**

✓5ᵗʰ M16.3 **Unilateral** osteoarthritis resulting from **hip dysplasia**

Dysplastic osteoarthritis of hip NOS

     M16.30 Unilateral osteoarthritis resulting from hip dysplasia, unspecified hip

     M16.31 Unilateral osteoarthritis resulting from hip dysplasia, **right** hip

     M16.32 Unilateral osteoarthritis resulting from hip dysplasia, **left** hip

M16.4 **Bilateral post-traumatic** osteoarthritis of hip

✓5ᵗʰ M16.5 **Unilateral post-traumatic** osteoarthritis of hip

Post-traumatic osteoarthritis of hip NOS

     M16.50 Unilateral post-traumatic osteoarthritis, unspecified hip

     M16.51 Unilateral post-traumatic osteoarthritis, **right** hip

     M16.52 Unilateral post-traumatic osteoarthritis, **left** hip

M16.6 Other bilateral secondary osteoarthritis of hip

M16.7 Other unilateral secondary osteoarthritis of hip

Secondary osteoarthritis of hip NOS

     M16.9 Osteoarthritis of hip, unspecified

✓4ᵗʰ **M17 Osteoarthritis of knee**

     AHA: 2016,4Q,146-147

M17.0 **Bilateral primary** osteoarthritis of knee

     AHA: 2018,2Q,15

✓5ᵗʰ M17.1 **Unilateral primary** osteoarthritis of knee

Primary osteoarthritis of knee NOS

     AHA: 2018,2Q,15

     M17.10 Unilateral primary osteoarthritis, unspecified knee

     M17.11 Unilateral primary osteoarthritis, **right** knee

     M17.12 Unilateral primary osteoarthritis, **left** knee

M17.2 **Bilateral post-traumatic** osteoarthritis of knee

✓5ᵗʰ M17.3 **Unilateral post-traumatic** osteoarthritis of knee

Post-traumatic osteoarthritis of knee NOS

     M17.30 Unilateral post-traumatic osteoarthritis, unspecified knee

     M17.31 Unilateral post-traumatic osteoarthritis, **right** knee

     M17.32 Unilateral post-traumatic osteoarthritis, **left** knee

M17.4 **Other bilateral secondary** osteoarthritis of knee

M17.5 **Other unilateral secondary** osteoarthritis of knee

Secondary osteoarthritis of knee NOS

     M17.9 Osteoarthritis of knee, unspecified

✓4ᵗʰ **M18 Osteoarthritis of first carpometacarpal joint**

M18.0 **Bilateral primary** osteoarthritis of first carpometacarpal joints

✓5ᵗʰ M18.1 **Unilateral primary** osteoarthritis of first carpometacarpal joint

Primary osteoarthritis of first carpometacarpal joint NOS

     M18.10 Unilateral primary osteoarthritis of first carpometacarpal joint, unspecified hand

     M18.11 Unilateral primary osteoarthritis of first carpometacarpal joint, **right** hand

     M18.12 Unilateral primary osteoarthritis of first carpometacarpal joint, **left** hand

M18.2 **Bilateral post-traumatic** osteoarthritis of first carpometacarpal joints

✓5ᵗʰ M18.3 **Unilateral post-traumatic** osteoarthritis of first carpometacarpal joint

Post-traumatic osteoarthritis of first carpometacarpal joint NOS

     M18.30 Unilateral post-traumatic osteoarthritis of first carpometacarpal joint, unspecified hand

     M18.31 Unilateral post-traumatic osteoarthritis of first carpometacarpal joint, **right** hand

     M18.32 Unilateral post-traumatic osteoarthritis of first carpometacarpal joint, **left** hand

M18.4 Other **bilateral secondary** osteoarthritis of first carpometacarpal joints

✓5ᵗʰ M18.5 Other **unilateral secondary** osteoarthritis of first carpometacarpal joint

Secondary osteoarthritis of first carpometacarpal joint NOS

     M18.50 Other unilateral secondary osteoarthritis of first carpometacarpal joint, unspecified hand

     M18.51 Other unilateral secondary osteoarthritis of first carpometacarpal joint, **right** hand

     M18.52 Other unilateral secondary osteoarthritis of first carpometacarpal joint, **left** hand

     M18.9 Osteoarthritis of first carpometacarpal joint, unspecified

✓4ᵗʰ **M19 Other and unspecified osteoarthritis**

     EXCLUDES 1   polyarthritis (M15.-)

     EXCLUDES 2   arthrosis of spine (M47.-)

           hallux rigidus (M20.2)

           osteoarthritis of spine (M47.-)

     AHA: 2020,4Q,31-32

✓5ᵗʰ M19.0 **Primary** osteoarthritis of other joints

     AHA: 2018,2Q,15; 2016,4Q,145

✓6ᵗʰ M19.01 Primary osteoarthritis, **shoulder**

     M19.011 Primary osteoarthritis, **right** shoulder

     M19.012 Primary osteoarthritis, **left** shoulder

     M19.019 Primary osteoarthritis, unspecified shoulder

✓6ᵗʰ M19.02 Primary osteoarthritis, **elbow**

     M19.021 Primary osteoarthritis, **right** elbow

     M19.022 Primary osteoarthritis, **left** elbow

     M19.029 Primary osteoarthritis, unspecified elbow

✓6ᵗʰ M19.03 Primary osteoarthritis, **wrist**

     M19.031 Primary osteoarthritis, **right** wrist

     M19.032 Primary osteoarthritis, **left** wrist

     M19.039 Primary osteoarthritis, unspecified wrist

✓6ᵗʰ M19.04 Primary osteoarthritis, **hand**

     EXCLUDES 2   primary osteoarthritis of first carpometacarpal joint (M18.0-, M18.1-)

     M19.041 Primary osteoarthritis, **right** hand

     M19.042 Primary osteoarthritis, **left** hand

     M19.049 Primary osteoarthritis, unspecified hand

✓6ᵗʰ M19.07 Primary osteoarthritis **ankle and foot**

     M19.071 Primary osteoarthritis, **right** ankle and foot

     M19.072 Primary osteoarthritis, **left** ankle and foot

     M19.079 Primary osteoarthritis, unspecified ankle and foot

     M19.09 Primary osteoarthritis, other specified site

✓5ᵗʰ M19.1 **Post-traumatic** osteoarthritis of other joints

✓6ᵗʰ M19.11 Post-traumatic osteoarthritis, **shoulder**

     M19.111 Post-traumatic osteoarthritis, **right** shoulder

     M19.112 Post-traumatic osteoarthritis, **left** shoulder

     M19.119 Post-traumatic osteoarthritis, unspecified shoulder

✓6ᵗʰ M19.12 Post-traumatic osteoarthritis, **elbow**

     M19.121 Post-traumatic osteoarthritis, **right** elbow

     M19.122 Post-traumatic osteoarthritis, **left** elbow

     M19.129 Post-traumatic osteoarthritis, unspecified elbow

✓6ᵗʰ M19.13 Post-traumatic osteoarthritis, **wrist**

     M19.131 Post-traumatic osteoarthritis, **right** wrist

     M19.132 Post-traumatic osteoarthritis, **left** wrist

     M19.139 Post-traumatic osteoarthritis, unspecified wrist

✓6ᵗʰ M19.14 Post-traumatic osteoarthritis, **hand**

     EXCLUDES 2   post-traumatic osteoarthritis of first carpometacarpal joint (M18.2-, M18.3-)

     M19.141 Post-traumatic osteoarthritis, **right** hand

     M19.142 Post-traumatic osteoarthritis, **left** hand

     M19.149 Post-traumatic osteoarthritis, unspecified hand

✓6ᵗʰ M19.17 Post-traumatic osteoarthritis, **ankle and foot**

     M19.171 Post-traumatic osteoarthritis, **right** ankle and foot

     M19.172 Post-traumatic osteoarthritis, **left** ankle and foot

     M19.179 Post-traumatic osteoarthritis, unspecified ankle and foot

     M19.19 Post-traumatic osteoarthritis, other specified site

✓5ᵗʰ M19.2 **Secondary** osteoarthritis of other joints

✓6ᵗʰ M19.21 Secondary osteoarthritis, **shoulder**

     M19.211 Secondary osteoarthritis, **right** shoulder

     M19.212 Secondary osteoarthritis, **left** shoulder

     M19.219 Secondary osteoarthritis, unspecified shoulder

✓6ᵗʰ M19.22 Secondary osteoarthritis, **elbow**

     M19.221 Secondary osteoarthritis, **right** elbow

     M19.222 Secondary osteoarthritis, **left** elbow

N Newborn: 0   P Pediatric: 0-17   M Maternity: 9-64   A Adult: 15-124   UNS Unspecified Site   MCC Major Complication/Comorbidity   CC Complication/Comorbidity   PE POA Exempt

794   ICD-10-CM 2025

M19.229   **Secondary osteoarthritis, unspecified elbow**

√6ᵗʰ   M19.23   **Secondary osteoarthritis, wrist**

   M19.231   **Secondary osteoarthritis, right wrist**

   M19.232   **Secondary osteoarthritis, left wrist**

   M19.239   **Secondary osteoarthritis, unspecified wrist**

√6ᵗʰ   M19.24   **Secondary osteoarthritis, hand**

   M19.241   **Secondary osteoarthritis, right hand**

   M19.242   **Secondary osteoarthritis, left hand**

   M19.249   **Secondary osteoarthritis, unspecified hand**

√6ᵗʰ   M19.27   **Secondary osteoarthritis, ankle and foot**

   M19.271   **Secondary osteoarthritis, right ankle and foot**

   M19.272   **Secondary osteoarthritis, left ankle and foot**

   M19.279   **Secondary osteoarthritis, unspecified ankle and foot**

   M19.29   **Secondary osteoarthritis, other specified site**

√5ᵗʰ   M19.9   **Osteoarthritis, unspecified site**

   TIP: Assign M19.90 when neither the site nor the type of osteoarthritis — primary, secondary, or post-traumatic — is documented.

   M19.90   **Unspecified osteoarthritis, unspecified site**
     Arthritis NOS
     Arthrosis NOS
     Osteoarthritis NOS
     AHA: 2016,4Q,145-147

   M19.91   **Primary osteoarthritis, unspecified site**
     Primary osteoarthritis NOS

   M19.92   **Post-traumatic osteoarthritis, unspecified site**
     Post-traumatic osteoarthritis NOS

   M19.93   **Secondary osteoarthritis, unspecified site**
     Secondary osteoarthritis NOS

Other joint disorders (M20-M25)

EXCLUDES 2   *joints of the spine (M40-M54)*

√4ᵗʰ   **M20   Acquired deformities of fingers and toes**

   EXCLUDES 1   *acquired absence of fingers and toes (Z89.-)*
     congenital absence of fingers and toes (Q71.3-, Q72.3-)
     congenital deformities and malformations of fingers and toes (Q66.-, Q68-Q70, Q74.-)

√5ᵗʰ   M20.0   **Deformity of finger(s)**

   EXCLUDES 1   *clubbing of fingers (R68.3)*
     palmar fascial fibromatosis [Dupuytren] (M72.0)
     trigger finger (M65.3)

   √6ᵗʰ   M20.00   **Unspecified deformity of finger(s)**

     M20.001   **Unspecified deformity of right finger(s)**

     M20.002   **Unspecified deformity of left finger(s)**

     M20.009   **Unspecified deformity of unspecified finger(s)**

   √6ᵗʰ   M20.01   **Mallet finger**

     M20.011   **Mallet finger of right finger(s)**

     M20.012   **Mallet finger of left finger(s)**

     M20.019   **Mallet finger of unspecified finger(s)**

   √6ᵗʰ   M20.02   **Boutonnière deformity**

     DEF: Deformity of the finger caused by flexion of the proximal interphalangeal joint and hyperextension of the distal joint. The deformity results from rheumatoid arthritis, osteoarthritis, or injury.

     M20.021   **Boutonnière deformity of right finger(s)**

     M20.022   **Boutonnière deformity of left finger(s)**

     M20.029   **Boutonnière deformity of unspecified finger(s)**

   √6ᵗʰ   M20.03   **Swan-neck deformity**

     DEF: Flexed distal and hyperextended proximal interphalangeal joint most commonly caused by rheumatoid arthritis.

     M20.031   **Swan-neck deformity of right finger(s)**

     M20.032   **Swan-neck deformity of left finger(s)**

     M20.039   **Swan-neck deformity of unspecified finger(s)**

   √6ᵗʰ   M20.09   **Other deformity of finger(s)**

     M20.091   **Other deformity of right finger(s)**

     M20.092   **Other deformity of left finger(s)**

     M20.099   **Other deformity of finger(s), unspecified finger(s)**

√5ᵗʰ   M20.1   **Hallux valgus (acquired)**

   EXCLUDES 2   *bunion (M21.6-)*

   AHA: 2016,4Q,38

   DEF: Deformity in which the great toe deviates toward the other toes and may even be positioned over or under the second toe.

Hallux Valgus

Hallux valgus

Medial eminence of metatarsal bone

Right foot

   M20.10   **Hallux valgus (acquired), unspecified foot**

   M20.11   **Hallux valgus (acquired), right foot**

   M20.12   **Hallux valgus (acquired), left foot**

√5ᵗʰ   M20.2   **Hallux rigidus**

   M20.20   **Hallux rigidus, unspecified foot**

   M20.21   **Hallux rigidus, right foot**

   M20.22   **Hallux rigidus, left foot**

√5ᵗʰ   M20.3   **Hallux varus (acquired)**

   DEF: Deformity in which the great toe deviates away from the other toes.

   M20.30   **Hallux varus (acquired), unspecified foot**

   M20.31   **Hallux varus (acquired), right foot**

   M20.32   **Hallux varus (acquired), left foot**

√5ᵗʰ   M20.4   **Other hammer toe(s) (acquired)**

   M20.40   **Other hammer toe(s) (acquired), unspecified foot**

   M20.41   **Other hammer toe(s) (acquired), right foot**

   M20.42   **Other hammer toe(s) (acquired), left foot**

√5ᵗʰ   M20.5   **Other deformities of toe(s) (acquired)**

   √6ᵗʰ   M20.5X   **Other deformities of toe(s) (acquired)**

     M20.5X1   **Other deformities of toe(s) (acquired), right foot**

     M20.5X2   **Other deformities of toe(s) (acquired), left foot**

     M20.5X9   **Other deformities of toe(s) (acquired), unspecified foot**

√5ᵗʰ   M20.6   **Acquired deformities of toe(s), unspecified**

   M20.60   **Acquired deformities of toe(s), unspecified, unspecified foot**

   M20.61   **Acquired deformities of toe(s), unspecified, right foot**

   M20.62   **Acquired deformities of toe(s), unspecified, left foot**

√4ᵗʰ   **M21   Other acquired deformities of limbs**

   EXCLUDES 1   *acquired absence of limb (Z89.-)*
     congenital absence of limbs (Q71-Q73)
     congenital deformities and malformations of limbs (Q65-Q66, Q68-Q74)

   EXCLUDES 2   *acquired deformities of fingers or toes (M20.-)*
     coxa plana (M91.2)

√5ᵗʰ   M21.0   **Valgus deformity, not elsewhere classified**

   EXCLUDES 1   *metatarsus valgus (Q66.6)*
     talipes calcaneovalgus (Q66.4-)

   M21.00   **Valgus deformity, not elsewhere classified, unspecified site**

   √6ᵗʰ   M21.02   **Valgus deformity, not elsewhere classified, elbow**
     Cubitus valgus

     M21.021   **Valgus deformity, not elsewhere classified, right elbow**

☑ Additional Character Required   ✓x7ᵗʰ Placeholder   Questionable PDx   Manifestation   Unspecified   UPD Unacceptable PDx   H1 -H14 HAC   HCC CMS-HCC Dx   HIV HIV Dx

ICD-10-CM 2025   795

    M21.022 Valgus deformity, not elsewhere classified, **left** elbow

    M21.029 Valgus deformity, not elsewhere classified, unspecified elbow

✓6th **M21.05** Valgus deformity, not elsewhere classified, **hip**

    M21.051 Valgus deformity, not elsewhere classified, **right** hip

    M21.052 Valgus deformity, not elsewhere classified, **left** hip

    M21.059 Valgus deformity, not elsewhere classified, unspecified hip

✓6th **M21.06** Valgus deformity, not elsewhere classified, **knee**

    Genu valgum
    Knock knee
    DEF: Genu valga/valgum: Condition in which the thighs slant inward, causing the knees to be angled abnormally close together, leaving the space between the ankles wider than normal.

Genu Valga (knock-knee)

    M21.061 Valgus deformity, not elsewhere classified, **right** knee

    M21.062 Valgus deformity, not elsewhere classified, **left** knee

    M21.069 Valgus deformity, not elsewhere classified, unspecified knee

✓6th **M21.07** Valgus deformity, not elsewhere classified, **ankle**

    M21.071 Valgus deformity, not elsewhere classified, **right** ankle

    M21.072 Valgus deformity, not elsewhere classified, **left** ankle

    M21.079 Valgus deformity, not elsewhere classified, unspecified ankle

✓5th **M21.1** **Varus** deformity, not elsewhere classified

    EXCLUDES 1   metatarsus varus (Q66.22-)
               tibia vara (M92.51-)

    M21.10 Varus deformity, not elsewhere classified, unspecified site

✓6th **M21.12** Varus deformity, not elsewhere classified, **elbow**

    Cubitus varus, elbow

    M21.121 Varus deformity, not elsewhere classified, **right** elbow

    M21.122 Varus deformity, not elsewhere classified, **left** elbow

    M21.129 Varus deformity, not elsewhere classified, unspecified elbow

✓6th **M21.15** Varus deformity, not elsewhere classified, **hip**

    M21.151 Varus deformity, not elsewhere classified, **right** hip

    M21.152 Varus deformity, not elsewhere classified, **left** hip

    M21.159 Varus deformity, not elsewhere classified, unspecified

✓6th **M21.16** Varus deformity, not elsewhere classified, **knee**

    Bow leg
    Genu varum
    DEF: Genu varus/varum: Condition in which the thighs and/or legs are bowed in an outward curve with an abnormally increased space between the knees.

Genu Varus (bowleg)

    M21.161 Varus deformity, not elsewhere classified, **right** knee

    M21.162 Varus deformity, not elsewhere classified, **left** knee

    M21.169 Varus deformity, not elsewhere classified, unspecified knee

✓6th **M21.17** Varus deformity, not elsewhere classified, **ankle**

    M21.171 Varus deformity, not elsewhere classified, **right** ankle

    M21.172 Varus deformity, not elsewhere classified, **left** ankle

    M21.179 Varus deformity, not elsewhere classified, unspecified ankle

✓5th **M21.2** **Flexion** deformity

    M21.20 Flexion deformity, unspecified site

✓6th **M21.21** Flexion deformity, **shoulder**

    M21.211 Flexion deformity, **right** shoulder
    M21.212 Flexion deformity, **left** shoulder
    M21.219 Flexion deformity, unspecified shoulder

✓6th **M21.22** Flexion deformity, **elbow**

    M21.221 Flexion deformity, **right** elbow
    M21.222 Flexion deformity, **left** elbow
    M21.229 Flexion deformity, unspecified elbow

✓6th **M21.23** Flexion deformity, **wrist**

    M21.231 Flexion deformity, **right** wrist
    M21.232 Flexion deformity, **left** wrist
    M21.239 Flexion deformity, unspecified wrist

✓6th **M21.24** Flexion deformity, **finger joints**

    M21.241 Flexion deformity, **right** finger joints
    M21.242 Flexion deformity, **left** finger joints
    M21.249 Flexion deformity, unspecified finger joints

✓6th **M21.25** Flexion deformity, **hip**

    M21.251 Flexion deformity, **right** hip
    M21.252 Flexion deformity, **left** hip
    M21.259 Flexion deformity, unspecified hip

✓6th **M21.26** Flexion deformity, **knee**

    M21.261 Flexion deformity, **right** knee
    M21.262 Flexion deformity, **left** knee
    M21.269 Flexion deformity, unspecified knee

✓6th **M21.27** Flexion deformity, **ankle and toes**

    M21.271 Flexion deformity, **right** ankle and toes
    M21.272 Flexion deformity, **left** ankle and toes
    M21.279 Flexion deformity, unspecified ankle and toes

N Newborn: 0   P Pediatric: 0-17   M Maternity: 9-64   A Adult: 15-124   UNS Unspecified Site   MCC Major Complication/Comorbidity   CC Complication/Comorbidity   PE POA Exempt

796   ICD-10-CM 2025

✓5ᵗʰ M21.3 Wrist or foot drop (acquired)

   ✓6ᵗʰ M21.33 Wrist drop (acquired)

      M21.331 Wrist drop, **right** wrist
      M21.332 Wrist drop, **left** wrist
      M21.339 Wrist drop, unspecified wrist

   ✓6ᵗʰ M21.37 Foot drop (acquired)

      M21.371 Foot drop, **right** foot
      M21.372 Foot drop, **left** foot
      M21.379 Foot drop, unspecified foot

✓5ᵗʰ M21.4 Flat foot [pes planus] (acquired)

   EXCLUDES 1   congenital pes planus (Q66.5-)

   M21.40 Flat foot [pes planus] (acquired), unspecified foot
   M21.41 Flat foot [pes planus] (acquired), **left** foot
   M21.42 Flat foot [pes planus] (acquired), **right** foot

✓5ᵗʰ M21.5 Acquired clawhand, clubhand, clawfoot and clubfoot

   EXCLUDES 1   clubfoot, not specified as acquired (Q66.89)

   ✓6ᵗʰ M21.51 Acquired clawhand

      M21.511 Acquired clawhand, **right** hand
      M21.512 Acquired clawhand, **left** hand
      M21.519 Acquired clawhand, unspecified hand

   ✓6ᵗʰ M21.52 Acquired clubhand

      M21.521 Acquired clubhand, **right** hand
      M21.522 Acquired clubhand, **left** hand
      M21.529 Acquired clubhand, unspecified hand

   ✓6ᵗʰ M21.53 Acquired clawfoot

      DEF: High foot arch with hyperextended toes at the metatarsophalangeal joint and flexed toes at the distal joints.

      M21.531 Acquired clawfoot, **right** foot
      M21.532 Acquired clawfoot, **left** foot
      M21.539 Acquired clawfoot, unspecified foot

   ✓6ᵗʰ M21.54 Acquired clubfoot

      DEF: Acquired anomaly of the foot with the heel elevated and rotated outward and the toes pointing inward.

      M21.541 Acquired clubfoot, **right** foot
      M21.542 Acquired clubfoot, **left** foot
      M21.549 Acquired clubfoot, unspecified foot

✓5ᵗʰ M21.6 Other acquired deformities of foot

   EXCLUDES 2   deformities of toe (acquired) (M20.1-M20.6-)
   AHA: 2016,4Q,38

   ✓6ᵗʰ M21.61 Bunion

      M21.611 Bunion of **right** foot
      M21.612 Bunion of **left** foot
      M21.619 Bunion of unspecified foot

   ✓6ᵗʰ M21.62 Bunionette

      M21.621 Bunionette of **right** foot
      M21.622 Bunionette of **left** foot
      M21.629 Bunionette of unspecified foot

   ✓6ᵗʰ M21.6X Other acquired deformities of foot

      AHA: 2023,3Q,20

      M21.6X1 Other acquired deformities of **right** foot
      M21.6X2 Other acquired deformities of **left** foot
      M21.6X9 Other acquired deformities of unspecified foot

✓5ᵗʰ M21.7 Unequal limb length (acquired)

   NOTE   The site used should correspond to the shorter limb

   M21.70 Unequal limb length (acquired), unspecified site

   ✓6ᵗʰ M21.72 Unequal limb length (acquired), humerus

      M21.721 Unequal limb length (acquired), **right** humerus
      M21.722 Unequal limb length (acquired), **left** humerus
      M21.729 Unequal limb length (acquired), unspecified humerus

   ✓6ᵗʰ M21.73 Unequal limb length (acquired), ulna and radius

      M21.731 Unequal limb length (acquired), **right** ulna
      M21.732 Unequal limb length (acquired), **left** ulna
      M21.733 Unequal limb length (acquired), **right** radius
      M21.734 Unequal limb length (acquired), **left** radius
      M21.739 Unequal limb length (acquired), unspecified ulna and radius

✓6ᵗʰ M21.75 Unequal limb length (acquired), femur

   M21.751 Unequal limb length (acquired), **right** femur
   M21.752 Unequal limb length (acquired), **left** femur
   M21.759 Unequal limb length (acquired), unspecified femur

✓6ᵗʰ M21.76 Unequal limb length (acquired), tibia and fibula

   M21.761 Unequal limb length (acquired), **right tibia**
   M21.762 Unequal limb length (acquired), **left tibia**
   M21.763 Unequal limb length (acquired), **right fibula**
   M21.764 Unequal limb length (acquired), **left fibula**
   M21.769 Unequal limb length (acquired), unspecified tibia and fibula

✓5ᵗʰ M21.8 Other specified acquired deformities of limbs

   EXCLUDES 2   coxa plana (M91.2)

   M21.80 Other specified acquired deformities of unspecified limb

   ✓6ᵗʰ M21.82 Other specified acquired deformities of upper arm

      M21.821 Other specified acquired deformities of **right** upper arm
      M21.822 Other specified acquired deformities of **left** upper arm
      M21.829 Other specified acquired deformities of unspecified upper arm

   ✓6ᵗʰ M21.83 Other specified acquired deformities of forearm

      M21.831 Other specified acquired deformities of **right** forearm
      M21.832 Other specified acquired deformities of **left** forearm
      M21.839 Other specified acquired deformities of unspecified forearm

   ✓6ᵗʰ M21.85 Other specified acquired deformities of thigh

      M21.851 Other specified acquired deformities of **right** thigh
      M21.852 Other specified acquired deformities of **left** thigh
      M21.859 Other specified acquired deformities of unspecified thigh

   ✓6ᵗʰ M21.86 Other specified acquired deformities of lower leg

      M21.861 Other specified acquired deformities of **right** lower leg
      M21.862 Other specified acquired deformities of **left** lower leg
      M21.869 Other specified acquired deformities of unspecified lower leg

✓5ᵗʰ M21.9 Unspecified acquired deformity of limb and hand

   M21.90 Unspecified acquired deformity of unspecified limb

   ✓6ᵗʰ M21.92 Unspecified acquired deformity of upper arm

      M21.921 Unspecified acquired deformity of **right** upper arm
      M21.922 Unspecified acquired deformity of **left** upper arm
      M21.929 Unspecified acquired deformity of unspecified upper arm

   ✓6ᵗʰ M21.93 Unspecified acquired deformity of forearm

      M21.931 Unspecified acquired deformity of **right** forearm
      M21.932 Unspecified acquired deformity of **left** forearm
      M21.939 Unspecified acquired deformity of unspecified forearm

   ✓6ᵗʰ M21.94 Unspecified acquired deformity of hand

      M21.941 Unspecified acquired deformity of hand, **right** hand
      M21.942 Unspecified acquired deformity of hand, **left** hand
      M21.949 Unspecified acquired deformity of hand, unspecified hand

   ✓6ᵗʰ M21.95 Unspecified acquired deformity of thigh

      M21.951 Unspecified acquired deformity of **right** thigh
      M21.952 Unspecified acquired deformity of **left** thigh
      M21.959 Unspecified acquired deformity of unspecified thigh

   ✓6ᵗʰ M21.96 Unspecified acquired deformity of lower leg

      M21.961 Unspecified acquired deformity of **right** lower leg

---

✓ Additional Character Required ✓x7ᵗʰ Placeholder <mark>Questionable PDx</mark> Manifestation Unspecified **UPD** Unacceptable PDx **H1–H14** HAC **HCC** CMS-HCC Dx **HIV** HIV Dx

Chapter 13. Diseases of the Musculoskeletal System and Connective Tissue

M21.962   **Unspecified acquired deformity of** left **lower leg**

M21.969   **Unspecified acquired deformity of unspecified lower leg**

✓4ᵗʰ **M22   Disorder of patella**

   EXCLUDES 2   *traumatic dislocation of patella (S83.0-)*

✓5ᵗʰ **M22.0   Recurrent dislocation of patella**

   M22.00   Recurrent dislocation of patella, unspecified knee

   M22.01   Recurrent dislocation of patella, right knee

   M22.02   Recurrent dislocation of patella, left knee

✓5ᵗʰ **M22.1   Recurrent subluxation of patella**

   Incomplete dislocation of patella

   M22.10   Recurrent subluxation of patella, unspecified knee

   M22.11   Recurrent subluxation of patella, right knee

   M22.12   Recurrent subluxation of patella, left knee

✓5ᵗʰ **M22.2   Patellofemoral disorders**

   ✓6ᵗʰ **M22.2X   Patellofemoral disorders**

     M22.2X1   Patellofemoral disorders, right knee

     M22.2X2   Patellofemoral disorders, left knee

     M22.2X9   Patellofemoral disorders, unspecified knee

✓5ᵗʰ **M22.3   Other derangements of patella**

   ✓6ᵗʰ **M22.3X   Other derangements of patella**

     M22.3X1   Other derangements of patella, right knee

     M22.3X2   Other derangements of patella, left knee

     M22.3X9   Other derangements of patella, unspecified knee

✓5ᵗʰ **M22.4   Chondromalacia patellae**

   M22.40   Chondromalacia patellae, unspecified knee

   M22.41   Chondromalacia patellae, right knee

   M22.42   Chondromalacia patellae, left knee

✓5ᵗʰ **M22.8   Other disorders of patella**

   ✓6ᵗʰ **M22.8X   Other disorders of patella**

     M22.8X1   Other disorders of patella, right knee

     M22.8X2   Other disorders of patella, left knee

     M22.8X9   Other disorders of patella, unspecified knee

✓5ᵗʰ **M22.9   Unspecified disorder of patella**

   M22.90   Unspecified disorder of patella, unspecified knee

   M22.91   Unspecified disorder of patella, right knee

   M22.92   Unspecified disorder of patella, left knee

✓4ᵗʰ **M23   Internal derangement of knee**

   EXCLUDES 1   *ankylosis (M24.66)*

     deformity of knee (M21.-)

     osteochondritis dissecans (M93.2)

   EXCLUDES 2   *current injury - see injury of knee and lower leg (S80-S89)*

     recurrent dislocation or subluxation of joints (M24.4)

     recurrent dislocation or subluxation of patella (M22.0-M22.1)

   ✓5ᵗʰ **M23.0   Cystic meniscus**

     ✓6ᵗʰ **M23.00   Cystic meniscus, unspecified meniscus**

      Cystic meniscus, unspecified lateral meniscus

      Cystic meniscus, unspecified medial meniscus

      M23.000   Cystic meniscus, unspecified lateral meniscus, right knee

      M23.001   Cystic meniscus, unspecified lateral meniscus, left knee

      M23.002   Cystic meniscus, unspecified lateral meniscus, unspecified knee

      M23.003   Cystic meniscus, unspecified medial meniscus, right knee

      M23.004   Cystic meniscus, unspecified medial meniscus, left knee

      M23.005   Cystic meniscus, unspecified medial meniscus, unspecified knee

      M23.006   Cystic meniscus, unspecified meniscus, right knee

      M23.007   Cystic meniscus, unspecified meniscus, left knee

      M23.009   Cystic meniscus, unspecified meniscus, unspecified knee

     ✓6ᵗʰ **M23.01   Cystic meniscus, anterior horn of medial meniscus**

      M23.011   Cystic meniscus, anterior horn of medial meniscus, right knee

      M23.012   Cystic meniscus, anterior horn of medial meniscus, left knee

      M23.019   Cystic meniscus, anterior horn of medial meniscus, unspecified knee

✓6ᵗʰ **M23.02   Cystic meniscus, posterior horn of medial meniscus**

   M23.021   Cystic meniscus, posterior horn of medial meniscus, right knee

   M23.022   Cystic meniscus, posterior horn of medial meniscus, left knee

   M23.029   Cystic meniscus, posterior horn of medial meniscus, unspecified knee

✓6ᵗʰ **M23.03   Cystic meniscus, other medial meniscus**

   M23.031   Cystic meniscus, other medial meniscus, right knee

   M23.032   Cystic meniscus, other medial meniscus, left knee

   M23.039   Cystic meniscus, other medial meniscus, unspecified knee

✓6ᵗʰ **M23.04   Cystic meniscus, anterior horn of lateral meniscus**

   M23.041   Cystic meniscus, anterior horn of lateral meniscus, right knee

   M23.042   Cystic meniscus, anterior horn of lateral meniscus, left knee

   M23.049   Cystic meniscus, anterior horn of lateral meniscus, unspecified knee

✓6ᵗʰ **M23.05   Cystic meniscus, posterior horn of lateral meniscus**

   M23.051   Cystic meniscus, posterior horn of lateral meniscus, right knee

   M23.052   Cystic meniscus, posterior horn of lateral meniscus, left knee

   M23.059   Cystic meniscus, posterior horn of lateral meniscus, unspecified knee

✓6ᵗʰ **M23.06   Cystic meniscus, other lateral meniscus**

   M23.061   Cystic meniscus, other lateral meniscus, right knee

   M23.062   Cystic meniscus, other lateral meniscus, left knee

   M23.069   Cystic meniscus, other lateral meniscus, unspecified knee

✓5ᵗʰ **M23.2   Derangement of meniscus due to old tear or injury**

   Old bucket-handle tear

   AHA: 2019,2Q,26

Derangement of Meniscus

Lateral meniscus

Posterior cruciate ligament

Medial meniscus

Anterior horns

Patellar ligament

Posterior horns

Anterior cruciate ligament

Bucket handle tear

Radial tear

Meniscus

Overhead view of right knee

✓6ᵗʰ **M23.20   Derangement of unspecified meniscus due to old tear or injury**

   Derangement of unspecified lateral meniscus due to old tear or injury

   Derangement of unspecified medial meniscus due to old tear or injury

   M23.200   Derangement of unspecified lateral meniscus due to old tear or injury, right knee

   M23.201   Derangement of unspecified lateral meniscus due to old tear or injury, left knee

   M23.202   Derangement of unspecified lateral meniscus due to old tear or injury, unspecified knee

   M23.203   Derangement of unspecified medial meniscus due to old tear or injury, right knee

   M23.204   Derangement of unspecified medial meniscus due to old tear or injury, left knee

N Newborn: 0   **P** Pediatric: 0-17   **M** Maternity: 9-64   **A** Adult: 15-124   **UNS** Unspecified Site   **MCC** Major Complication/Comorbidity   **CC** Complication/Comorbidity   **PE** POA Exempt

798   ICD-10-CM 2025

M23.205 Derangement of unspecified medial meniscus due to old tear or injury, unspecified knee

M23.206 Derangement of unspecified meniscus due to old tear or injury, right knee

M23.207 Derangement of unspecified meniscus due to old tear or injury, left knee

M23.209 Derangement of unspecified meniscus due to old tear or injury, unspecified knee

√6th **M23.21** Derangement of anterior horn of medial meniscus due to old tear or injury

M23.211 Derangement of anterior horn of medial meniscus due to old tear or injury, right knee

M23.212 Derangement of anterior horn of medial meniscus due to old tear or injury, left knee

M23.219 Derangement of anterior horn of medial meniscus due to old tear or injury, unspecified knee

√6th **M23.22** Derangement of posterior horn of medial meniscus due to old tear or injury

M23.221 Derangement of posterior horn of medial meniscus due to old tear or injury, right knee

M23.222 Derangement of posterior horn of medial meniscus due to old tear or injury, left knee

M23.229 Derangement of posterior horn of medial meniscus due to old tear or injury, unspecified knee

√6th **M23.23** Derangement of other medial meniscus due to old tear or injury

M23.231 Derangement of other medial meniscus due to old tear or injury, right knee

M23.232 Derangement of other medial meniscus due to old tear or injury, left knee

M23.239 Derangement of other medial meniscus due to old tear or injury, unspecified knee

√6th **M23.24** Derangement of anterior horn of lateral meniscus due to old tear or injury

M23.241 Derangement of anterior horn of lateral meniscus due to old tear or injury, right knee

M23.242 Derangement of anterior horn of lateral meniscus due to old tear or injury, left knee

M23.249 Derangement of anterior horn of lateral meniscus due to old tear or injury, unspecified knee

√6th **M23.25** Derangement of posterior horn of lateral meniscus due to old tear or injury

M23.251 Derangement of posterior horn of lateral meniscus due to old tear or injury, right knee

M23.252 Derangement of posterior horn of lateral meniscus due to old tear or injury, left knee

M23.259 Derangement of posterior horn of lateral meniscus due to old tear or injury, unspecified knee

√6th **M23.26** Derangement of other lateral meniscus due to old tear or injury

M23.261 Derangement of other lateral meniscus due to old tear or injury, right knee

M23.262 Derangement of other lateral meniscus due to old tear or injury, left knee

M23.269 Derangement of other lateral meniscus due to old tear or injury, unspecified knee

√5th **M23.3** Other meniscus derangements

Degenerate meniscus
Detached meniscus
Retained meniscus

√6th **M23.30** Other meniscus derangements, unspecified meniscus

Other meniscus derangements, unspecified lateral meniscus
Other meniscus derangements, unspecified medial meniscus

M23.300 Other meniscus derangements, unspecified lateral meniscus, right knee

M23.301 Other meniscus derangements, unspecified lateral meniscus, left knee

M23.302 Other meniscus derangements, unspecified lateral meniscus, unspecified knee

M23.303 Other meniscus derangements, unspecified medial meniscus, right knee

M23.304 Other meniscus derangements, unspecified medial meniscus, left knee

M23.305 Other meniscus derangements, unspecified medial meniscus, unspecified knee

M23.306 Other meniscus derangements, unspecified meniscus, right knee

M23.307 Other meniscus derangements, unspecified meniscus, left knee

M23.309 Other meniscus derangements, unspecified meniscus, unspecified knee

√6th **M23.31** Other meniscus derangements, anterior horn of medial meniscus

M23.311 Other meniscus derangements, anterior horn of medial meniscus, right knee

M23.312 Other meniscus derangements, anterior horn of medial meniscus, left knee

M23.319 Other meniscus derangements, anterior horn of medial meniscus, unspecified knee

√6th **M23.32** Other meniscus derangements, posterior horn of medial meniscus

M23.321 Other meniscus derangements, posterior horn of medial meniscus, right knee

M23.322 Other meniscus derangements, posterior horn of medial meniscus, left knee

M23.329 Other meniscus derangements, posterior horn of medial meniscus, unspecified knee

√6th **M23.33** Other meniscus derangements, other medial meniscus

M23.331 Other meniscus derangements, other medial meniscus, right knee

M23.332 Other meniscus derangements, other medial meniscus, left knee

M23.339 Other meniscus derangements, other medial meniscus, unspecified knee

√6th **M23.34** Other meniscus derangements, anterior horn of lateral meniscus

M23.341 Other meniscus derangements, anterior horn of lateral meniscus, right knee

M23.342 Other meniscus derangements, anterior horn of lateral meniscus, left knee

M23.349 Other meniscus derangements, anterior horn of lateral meniscus, unspecified knee

√6th **M23.35** Other meniscus derangements, posterior horn of lateral meniscus

M23.351 Other meniscus derangements, posterior horn of lateral meniscus, right knee

M23.352 Other meniscus derangements, posterior horn of lateral meniscus, left knee

M23.359 Other meniscus derangements, posterior horn of lateral meniscus, unspecified knee

√6th **M23.36** Other meniscus derangements, other lateral meniscus

M23.361 Other meniscus derangements, other lateral meniscus, right knee

M23.362 Other meniscus derangements, other lateral meniscus, left knee

M23.369 Other meniscus derangements, other lateral meniscus, unspecified knee

√5th **M23.4** Loose body in knee

M23.40 Loose body in knee, unspecified knee

M23.41 Loose body in knee, right knee

M23.42 Loose body in knee, left knee

√5th **M23.5** Chronic instability of knee

M23.50 Chronic instability of knee, unspecified knee

M23.51 Chronic instability of knee, right knee

M23.52 Chronic instability of knee, left knee

√5th **M23.6** Other spontaneous disruption of ligament(s) of knee

√6th **M23.60** Other spontaneous disruption of unspecified ligament of knee

M23.601 Other spontaneous disruption of unspecified ligament of right knee

M23.602 Other spontaneous disruption of unspecified ligament of left knee

M23.609 Other spontaneous disruption of unspecified ligament of unspecified knee

√6th **M23.61** Other spontaneous disruption of anterior cruciate ligament of knee

M23.611 Other spontaneous disruption of anterior cruciate ligament of right knee

M23.612 Other spontaneous disruption of anterior cruciate ligament of left knee

M23.619 Other spontaneous disruption of anterior cruciate ligament of unspecified knee

✓6th **M23.62** Other spontaneous disruption of **posterior cruciate** ligament of knee
- **M23.621** Other spontaneous disruption of posterior cruciate ligament of **right** knee
- **M23.622** Other spontaneous disruption of posterior cruciate ligament of **left** knee
- **M23.629** Other spontaneous disruption of posterior cruciate ligament of unspecified knee

✓6th **M23.63** Other spontaneous disruption of **medial collateral** ligament of knee
- **M23.631** Other spontaneous disruption of medial collateral ligament of **right** knee
- **M23.632** Other spontaneous disruption of medial collateral ligament of **left** knee
- **M23.639** Other spontaneous disruption of medial collateral ligament of unspecified knee

✓6th **M23.64** Other spontaneous disruption of **lateral collateral** ligament of knee
- **M23.641** Other spontaneous disruption of lateral collateral ligament of **right** knee
- **M23.642** Other spontaneous disruption of lateral collateral ligament of **left** knee
- **M23.649** Other spontaneous disruption of lateral collateral ligament of unspecified knee

✓6th **M23.67** Other spontaneous disruption of **capsular** ligament of knee
- **M23.671** Other spontaneous disruption of capsular ligament of **right** knee
- **M23.672** Other spontaneous disruption of capsular ligament of **left** knee
- **M23.679** Other spontaneous disruption of capsular ligament of unspecified knee

✓5th **M23.8** Other internal derangements of knee
  Laxity of ligament of knee
  Snapping knee

✓6th **M23.8X** Other internal derangements of knee
- **M23.8X1** Other internal derangements of **right** knee
- **M23.8X2** Other internal derangements of **left** knee
- **M23.8X9** Other internal derangements of unspecified knee

✓5th **M23.9** Unspecified internal derangement of knee
- **M23.90** Unspecified internal derangement of unspecified knee
- **M23.91** Unspecified internal derangement of **right** knee
- **M23.92** Unspecified internal derangement of **left** knee

✓4th **M24** Other specific joint derangements
  EXCLUDES 1 current injury - see injury of joint by body region
  EXCLUDES 2 ganglion (M67.4)
  snapping knee (M23.8-)
  temporomandibular joint disorders (M26.6-)
  AHA: 2020,4Q,31-32

✓5th **M24.0** Loose body in joint
  EXCLUDES 2 loose body in knee (M23.4)
- **M24.00** Loose body in unspecified joint

✓6th **M24.01** Loose body in **shoulder**
- **M24.011** Loose body in **right** shoulder
- **M24.012** Loose body in **left** shoulder
- **M24.019** Loose body in unspecified shoulder

✓6th **M24.02** Loose body in **elbow**
- **M24.021** Loose body in **right** elbow
- **M24.022** Loose body in **left** elbow
- **M24.029** Loose body in unspecified elbow

✓6th **M24.03** Loose body in **wrist**
- **M24.031** Loose body in **right** wrist
- **M24.032** Loose body in **left** wrist
- **M24.039** Loose body in unspecified wrist

✓6th **M24.04** Loose body in **finger joints**
- **M24.041** Loose body in **right** finger joint(s)
- **M24.042** Loose body in **left** finger joint(s)
- **M24.049** Loose body in unspecified finger joint(s)

✓6th **M24.05** Loose body in **hip**
- **M24.051** Loose body in **right** hip
- **M24.052** Loose body in **left** hip
- **M24.059** Loose body in unspecified hip

✓6th **M24.07** Loose body in **ankle and toe joints**
- **M24.071** Loose body in **right ankle**

- **M24.072** Loose body in **left ankle**
- **M24.073** Loose body in unspecified ankle
- **M24.074** Loose body in **right toe joint(s)**
- **M24.075** Loose body in **left toe joint(s)**
- **M24.076** Loose body in unspecified toe joints

M24.08 Loose body, other site

✓5th **M24.1** Other articular cartilage disorders
  EXCLUDES 2 chondrocalcinosis (M11.1-, M11.2-)
  internal derangement of knee (M23.-)
  metastatic calcification (E83.59)
  ochronosis (E70.29)

- **M24.10** Other articular cartilage disorders, unspecified site

✓6th **M24.11** Other articular cartilage disorders, **shoulder**
- **M24.111** Other articular cartilage disorders, **right** shoulder
- **M24.112** Other articular cartilage disorders, **left** shoulder
- **M24.119** Other articular cartilage disorders, unspecified shoulder

✓6th **M24.12** Other articular cartilage disorders, **elbow**
- **M24.121** Other articular cartilage disorders, **right** elbow
- **M24.122** Other articular cartilage disorders, **left** elbow
- **M24.129** Other articular cartilage disorders, unspecified elbow

✓6th **M24.13** Other articular cartilage disorders, **wrist**
- **M24.131** Other articular cartilage disorders, **right** wrist
- **M24.132** Other articular cartilage disorders, **left** wrist
- **M24.139** Other articular cartilage disorders, unspecified wrist

✓6th **M24.14** Other articular cartilage disorders, **hand**
- **M24.141** Other articular cartilage disorders, **right** hand
- **M24.142** Other articular cartilage disorders, **left** hand
- **M24.149** Other articular cartilage disorders, unspecified hand

✓6th **M24.15** Other articular cartilage disorders, **hip**
- **M24.151** Other articular cartilage disorders, **right** hip
- **M24.152** Other articular cartilage disorders, **left** hip
- **M24.159** Other articular cartilage disorders, unspecified hip

✓6th **M24.17** Other articular cartilage disorders, **ankle and foot**
- **M24.171** Other articular cartilage disorders, **right ankle**
- **M24.172** Other articular cartilage disorders, **left ankle**
- **M24.173** Other articular cartilage disorders, unspecified ankle
- **M24.174** Other articular cartilage disorders, **right foot**
- **M24.175** Other articular cartilage disorders, **left foot**
- **M24.176** Other articular cartilage disorders, unspecified foot

M24.19 Other articular cartilage disorders, other specified site

✓5th **M24.2** Disorder of ligament
  Instability secondary to old ligament injury
  Ligamentous laxity NOS
  EXCLUDES 1 familial ligamentous laxity (M35.7)
  EXCLUDES 2 internal derangement of knee (M23.5-M23.8X9)

- **M24.20** Disorder of ligament, unspecified site

✓6th **M24.21** Disorder of ligament, **shoulder**
- **M24.211** Disorder of ligament, **right** shoulder
- **M24.212** Disorder of ligament, **left** shoulder
- **M24.219** Disorder of ligament, unspecified shoulder

✓6th **M24.22** Disorder of ligament, **elbow**
- **M24.221** Disorder of ligament, **right** elbow
- **M24.222** Disorder of ligament, **left** elbow
- **M24.229** Disorder of ligament, unspecified elbow

✓6th **M24.23** Disorder of ligament, **wrist**
- **M24.231** Disorder of ligament, **right** wrist
- **M24.232** Disorder of ligament, **left** wrist
- **M24.239** Disorder of ligament, unspecified wrist

✓6th **M24.24** Disorder of ligament, **hand**

     M24.241 Disorder of ligament, **right** hand
     M24.242 Disorder of ligament, **left** hand
     M24.249 Disorder of ligament, unspecified hand

✓6th **M24.25** Disorder of ligament, **hip**

     M24.251 Disorder of ligament, **right** hip
     M24.252 Disorder of ligament, **left** hip
     M24.259 Disorder of ligament, unspecified hip

✓6th **M24.27** Disorder of ligament, **ankle and foot**

     M24.271 Disorder of ligament, **right** ankle
     M24.272 Disorder of ligament, **left** ankle
     M24.273 Disorder of ligament, unspecified ankle
     M24.274 Disorder of ligament, **right** foot
     M24.275 Disorder of ligament, **left** foot
     M24.276 Disorder of ligament, unspecified foot

M24.28 Disorder of ligament, **vertebrae**
     AHA: 2023,2Q,13

M24.29 Disorder of ligament, other specified site

✓5th **M24.3** Pathological dislocation of joint, not elsewhere classified

     EXCLUDES 1   *congenital dislocation or displacement of joint - see congenital malformations and deformations of the musculoskeletal system (Q65-Q79)*

         current injury - see injury of joints and ligaments by body region

         recurrent dislocation of joint (M24.4-)

M24.30 Pathological dislocation of unspecified joint, not elsewhere classified

✓6th **M24.31** Pathological dislocation of **shoulder,** not elsewhere classified

     M24.311 Pathological dislocation of **right** shoulder, not elsewhere classified
     M24.312 Pathological dislocation of **left** shoulder, not elsewhere classified
     M24.319 Pathological dislocation of unspecified shoulder, not elsewhere classified

✓6th **M24.32** Pathological dislocation of **elbow,** not elsewhere classified

     M24.321 Pathological dislocation of **right** elbow, not elsewhere classified
     M24.322 Pathological dislocation of **left** elbow, not elsewhere classified
     M24.329 Pathological dislocation of unspecified elbow, not elsewhere classified

✓6th **M24.33** Pathological dislocation of **wrist,** not elsewhere classified

     M24.331 Pathological dislocation of **right** wrist, not elsewhere classified
     M24.332 Pathological dislocation of **left** wrist, not elsewhere classified
     M24.339 Pathological dislocation of unspecified wrist, not elsewhere classified

✓6th **M24.34** Pathological dislocation of **hand,** not elsewhere classified

     M24.341 Pathological dislocation of **right** hand, not elsewhere classified
     M24.342 Pathological dislocation of **left** hand, not elsewhere classified
     M24.349 Pathological dislocation of unspecified hand, not elsewhere classified

✓6th **M24.35** Pathological dislocation of **hip,** not elsewhere classified
     AHA: 2022,1Q,32

     M24.351 Pathological dislocation of **right** hip, not elsewhere classified
     M24.352 Pathological dislocation of **left** hip, not elsewhere classified
     M24.359 Pathological dislocation of unspecified hip, not elsewhere classified

✓6th **M24.36** Pathological dislocation of **knee,** not elsewhere classified

     M24.361 Pathological dislocation of **right** knee, not elsewhere classified
     M24.362 Pathological dislocation of **left** knee, not elsewhere classified
     M24.369 Pathological dislocation of unspecified knee, not elsewhere classified

✓6th **M24.37** Pathological dislocation of **ankle and foot,** not elsewhere classified

     M24.371 Pathological dislocation of **right** ankle, not elsewhere classified

     M24.372 Pathological dislocation of **left** ankle, not elsewhere classified
     M24.373 Pathological dislocation of unspecified ankle, not elsewhere classified
     M24.374 Pathological dislocation of **right** foot, not elsewhere classified
     M24.375 Pathological dislocation of **left** foot, not elsewhere classified
     M24.376 Pathological dislocation of unspecified foot, not elsewhere classified

M24.39 Pathological dislocation of other specified joint, not elsewhere classified

✓5th **M24.4** Recurrent dislocation of joint

     Recurrent subluxation of joint
     EXCLUDES 2   *recurrent dislocation of patella (M22.0-M22.1)*
         recurrent vertebral dislocation (M43.3-, M43.4, M43.5-)

M24.40 Recurrent dislocation, unspecified joint

✓6th **M24.41** Recurrent dislocation, **shoulder**

     M24.411 Recurrent dislocation, **right** shoulder
     M24.412 Recurrent dislocation, **left** shoulder
     M24.419 Recurrent dislocation, unspecified shoulder

✓6th **M24.42** Recurrent dislocation, **elbow**

     M24.421 Recurrent dislocation, **right** elbow
     M24.422 Recurrent dislocation, **left** elbow
     M24.429 Recurrent dislocation, unspecified elbow

✓6th **M24.43** Recurrent dislocation, **wrist**

     M24.431 Recurrent dislocation, **right** wrist
     M24.432 Recurrent dislocation, **left** wrist
     M24.439 Recurrent dislocation, unspecified wrist

✓6th **M24.44** Recurrent dislocation, **hand and finger(s)**

     M24.441 Recurrent dislocation, **right** hand
     M24.442 Recurrent dislocation, **left** hand
     M24.443 Recurrent dislocation, unspecified hand
     M24.444 Recurrent dislocation, **right** finger
     M24.445 Recurrent dislocation, **left** finger
     M24.446 Recurrent dislocation, unspecified finger

✓6th **M24.45** Recurrent dislocation, **hip**

     M24.451 Recurrent dislocation, **right** hip
     M24.452 Recurrent dislocation, **left** hip
     M24.459 Recurrent dislocation, unspecified hip

✓6th **M24.46** Recurrent dislocation, **knee**

     M24.461 Recurrent dislocation, **right** knee
     M24.462 Recurrent dislocation, **left** knee
     M24.469 Recurrent dislocation, unspecified knee

✓6th **M24.47** Recurrent dislocation, **ankle, foot and toes**

     M24.471 Recurrent dislocation, **right** ankle
     M24.472 Recurrent dislocation, **left** ankle
     M24.473 Recurrent dislocation, unspecified ankle
     M24.474 Recurrent dislocation, **right** foot
     M24.475 Recurrent dislocation, **left** foot
     M24.476 Recurrent dislocation, unspecified foot
     M24.477 Recurrent dislocation, **right** toe(s)
     M24.478 Recurrent dislocation, **left** toe(s)
     M24.479 Recurrent dislocation, unspecified toe(s)

M24.49 Recurrent dislocation, other specified joint

✓5th **M24.5** Contracture of joint

     EXCLUDES 1   *contracture of muscle without contracture of joint (M62.4-)*
         contracture of tendon (sheath) without contracture of joint (M62.4-)
         Dupuytren's contracture (M72.0)
     EXCLUDES 2   *acquired deformities of limbs (M20-M21)*
     AHA: 2016,2Q,6

M24.50 Contracture, unspecified joint

✓6th **M24.51** Contracture, **shoulder**

     M24.511 Contracture, **right** shoulder
     M24.512 Contracture, **left** shoulder
     M24.519 Contracture, unspecified shoulder

✓6th **M24.52** Contracture, **elbow**

     M24.521 Contracture, **right** elbow
     M24.522 Contracture, **left** elbow
     M24.529 Contracture, unspecified elbow

✓6th **M24.53** Contracture, **wrist**

     M24.531 Contracture, **right** wrist
     M24.532 Contracture, **left** wrist

☑ Additional Character Required   ✓x7th Placeholder   Questionable PDx   Manifestation   Unspecified   UPD Unacceptable PDx   H1-H14 HAC   HCC CMS-HCC Dx   HIV HIV Dx

ICD-10-CM 2025   **801**

M24.539 Contracture, unspecified wrist

✓6ᵗʰ **M24.54** **Contracture, hand**

M24.541 Contracture, **right** hand
M24.542 Contracture, **left** hand
M24.549 Contracture, unspecified hand

✓6ᵗʰ **M24.55** **Contracture, hip**

M24.551 Contracture, **right** hip
M24.552 Contracture, **left** hip
M24.559 Contracture, unspecified hip

✓6ᵗʰ **M24.56** **Contracture, knee**

M24.561 Contracture, **right** knee
M24.562 Contracture, **left** knee
M24.569 Contracture, unspecified knee

✓6ᵗʰ **M24.57** **Contracture, ankle and foot**

M24.571 Contracture, **right** ankle
M24.572 Contracture, **left** ankle
M24.573 Contracture, unspecified ankle
M24.574 Contracture, **right** foot
M24.575 Contracture, **left** foot
M24.576 Contracture, unspecified foot

M24.59 Contracture, other specified joint

✓5ᵗʰ **M24.6** **Ankylosis of joint**

EXCLUDES 1 *stiffness of joint without ankylosis (M25.6-)*
EXCLUDES 2 *spine (M43.2-)*
DEF: Ankylosis: Abnormal union or fusion of bones in a joint, which is normally moveable.

M24.60 **Ankylosis, unspecified joint**

✓6ᵗʰ **M24.61** **Ankylosis, shoulder**

M24.611 Ankylosis, **right** shoulder
M24.612 Ankylosis, **left** shoulder
M24.619 Ankylosis, unspecified shoulder

✓6ᵗʰ **M24.62** **Ankylosis, elbow**

M24.621 Ankylosis, **right** elbow
M24.622 Ankylosis, **left** elbow
M24.629 Ankylosis, unspecified elbow

✓6ᵗʰ **M24.63** **Ankylosis, wrist**

M24.631 Ankylosis, **right** wrist
M24.632 Ankylosis, **left** wrist
M24.639 Ankylosis, unspecified wrist

✓6ᵗʰ **M24.64** **Ankylosis, hand**

M24.641 Ankylosis, **right** hand
M24.642 Ankylosis, **left** hand
M24.649 Ankylosis, unspecified hand

✓6ᵗʰ **M24.65** **Ankylosis, hip**

M24.651 Ankylosis, **right** hip
M24.652 Ankylosis, **left** hip
M24.659 Ankylosis, unspecified hip

✓6ᵗʰ **M24.66** **Ankylosis, knee**

M24.661 Ankylosis, **right** knee
M24.662 Ankylosis, **left** knee
M24.669 Ankylosis, unspecified knee

✓6ᵗʰ **M24.67** **Ankylosis, ankle and foot**

M24.671 Ankylosis, **right** ankle
M24.672 Ankylosis, **left** ankle
M24.673 Ankylosis, unspecified ankle
M24.674 Ankylosis, **right** foot
M24.675 Ankylosis, **left** foot
M24.676 Ankylosis, unspecified foot

M24.69 Ankylosis, other specified joint

M24.7 **Protrusio acetabuli**

DEF: Intrapelvic protrusion of the acetabulum characterized by the sinking of the floor of the acetabulum, causing the femoral head to protrude. It limits hip movement and is of unknown etiology. **Synonym(s):** *Otto's pelvis.*

✓5ᵗʰ **M24.8** **Other specific joint derangements, not elsewhere classified**

EXCLUDES 2 *iliotibial band syndrome (M76.3)*

M24.80 **Other specific joint derangements of unspecified joint, not elsewhere classified**

✓6ᵗʰ **M24.81** **Other specific joint derangements of shoulder, not elsewhere classified**

M24.811 Other specific joint derangements of **right** shoulder, not elsewhere classified
M24.812 Other specific joint derangements of **left** shoulder, not elsewhere classified
M24.819 Other specific joint derangements of unspecified shoulder, not elsewhere classified

✓6ᵗʰ **M24.82** **Other specific joint derangements of elbow, not elsewhere classified**

M24.821 Other specific joint derangements of **right** elbow, not elsewhere classified
M24.822 Other specific joint derangements of **left** elbow, not elsewhere classified
M24.829 Other specific joint derangements of unspecified elbow, not elsewhere classified

✓6ᵗʰ **M24.83** **Other specific joint derangements of wrist, not elsewhere classified**

M24.831 Other specific joint derangements of **right** wrist, not elsewhere classified
M24.832 Other specific joint derangements of **left** wrist, not elsewhere classified
M24.839 Other specific joint derangements of unspecified wrist, not elsewhere classified

✓6ᵗʰ **M24.84** **Other specific joint derangements of hand, not elsewhere classified**

M24.841 Other specific joint derangements of **right** hand, not elsewhere classified
M24.842 Other specific joint derangements of **left** hand, not elsewhere classified
M24.849 Other specific joint derangements of unspecified hand, not elsewhere classified

✓6ᵗʰ **M24.85** **Other specific joint derangements of hip, not elsewhere classified**

Irritable hip

M24.851 Other specific joint derangements of **right** hip, not elsewhere classified
M24.852 Other specific joint derangements of **left** hip, not elsewhere classified
M24.859 Other specific joint derangements of unspecified hip, not elsewhere classified

✓6ᵗʰ **M24.87** **Other specific joint derangements of ankle and foot, not elsewhere classified**

M24.871 Other specific joint derangements of **right** ankle, not elsewhere classified
M24.872 Other specific joint derangements of **left** ankle, not elsewhere classified
M24.873 Other specific joint derangements of unspecified ankle, not elsewhere classified
M24.874 Other specific joint derangements of **right** foot, not elsewhere classified
M24.875 Other specific joint derangements **left** foot, not elsewhere classified
M24.876 Other specific joint derangements of unspecified foot, not elsewhere classified

M24.89 Other specific joint derangement of other specified joint, not elsewhere classified

M24.9 **Joint derangement, unspecified**

✓4ᵗʰ **M25** **Other joint disorder, not elsewhere classified**

EXCLUDES 2 *abnormality of gait and mobility (R26.-)*
acquired deformities of limb (M20-M21)
calcification of bursa (M71.4-)
calcification of shoulder (joint) (M75.3)
calcification of tendon (M65.2-)
difficulty in walking (R26.2)
temporomandibular joint disorder (M26.6-)

AHA: 2020,4Q,31-32

✓5ᵗʰ **M25.0** **Hemarthrosis**

EXCLUDES 1 *current injury - see injury of joint by body region*
hemophilic arthropathy (M36.2)

M25.00 **Hemarthrosis, unspecified joint** CC UNS

✓6ᵗʰ **M25.01** **Hemarthrosis, shoulder**

M25.011 Hemarthrosis, **right** shoulder CC
M25.012 Hemarthrosis, **left** shoulder CC
M25.019 Hemarthrosis, unspecified shoulder CC UNS

✓6ᵗʰ **M25.02** **Hemarthrosis, elbow**

M25.021 Hemarthrosis, **right** elbow CC
M25.022 Hemarthrosis, **left** elbow CC
M25.029 Hemarthrosis, unspecified elbow CC UNS

✓6ᵗʰ **M25.03** **Hemarthrosis, wrist**

M25.031 Hemarthrosis, **right** wrist CC
M25.032 Hemarthrosis, **left** wrist CC
M25.039 Hemarthrosis, unspecified wrist CC UNS

√6ᵗʰ M25.04 Hemarthrosis, hand

    M25.041 Hemarthrosis, **right** hand   `CC`
    M25.042 Hemarthrosis, **left** hand   `CC`
    M25.049 Hemarthrosis, unspecified hand   `CC` `UNS`

√6ᵗʰ M25.05 Hemarthrosis, hip

    M25.051 Hemarthrosis, **right** hip   `CC`
    M25.052 Hemarthrosis, **left** hip   `CC`
    M25.059 Hemarthrosis, unspecified hip   `CC` `UNS`

√6ᵗʰ M25.06 Hemarthrosis, knee

    M25.061 Hemarthrosis, **right** knee   `CC`
    M25.062 Hemarthrosis, **left** knee   `CC`
    M25.069 Hemarthrosis, unspecified knee   `CC` `UNS`

√6ᵗʰ M25.07 Hemarthrosis, ankle and foot

    M25.071 Hemarthrosis, **right** ankle   `CC`
    M25.072 Hemarthrosis, **left** ankle   `CC`
    M25.073 Hemarthrosis, unspecified ankle   `CC` `UNS`
    M25.074 Hemarthrosis, **right** foot   `CC`
    M25.075 Hemarthrosis, **left** foot   `CC`
    M25.076 Hemarthrosis, unspecified foot   `CC` `UNS`

    M25.08 Hemarthrosis, other specified site   `CC`
      Hemarthrosis, vertebrae

√5ᵗʰ M25.1 Fistula of joint

    M25.10 Fistula, unspecified joint

√6ᵗʰ M25.11 Fistula, shoulder

    M25.111 Fistula, **right** shoulder
    M25.112 Fistula, **left** shoulder
    M25.119 Fistula, unspecified shoulder

√6ᵗʰ M25.12 Fistula, elbow

    M25.121 Fistula, **right** elbow
    M25.122 Fistula, **left** elbow
    M25.129 Fistula, unspecified elbow

√6ᵗʰ M25.13 Fistula, wrist

    M25.131 Fistula, **right** wrist
    M25.132 Fistula, **left** wrist
    M25.139 Fistula, unspecified wrist

√6ᵗʰ M25.14 Fistula, hand

    M25.141 Fistula, **right** hand
    M25.142 Fistula, **left** hand
    M25.149 Fistula, unspecified hand

√6ᵗʰ M25.15 Fistula, hip

    M25.151 Fistula, **right** hip
    M25.152 Fistula, **left** hip
    M25.159 Fistula, unspecified hip

√6ᵗʰ M25.16 Fistula, knee

    M25.161 Fistula, **right** knee
    M25.162 Fistula, **left** knee
    M25.169 Fistula, unspecified knee

√6ᵗʰ M25.17 Fistula, ankle and foot

    M25.171 Fistula, **right** ankle
    M25.172 Fistula, **left** ankle
    M25.173 Fistula, unspecified ankle
    M25.174 Fistula, **right** foot
    M25.175 Fistula, **left** foot
    M25.176 Fistula, unspecified foot

    M25.18 Fistula, other specified site
      Fistula, vertebrae

√5ᵗʰ M25.2 Flail joint

    DEF: Hinged joint that exhibits an abnormal or excessive degree of range and mobility.

    M25.20 Flail joint, unspecified joint

√6ᵗʰ M25.21 Flail joint, shoulder

    M25.211 Flail joint, **right** shoulder
    M25.212 Flail joint, **left** shoulder
    M25.219 Flail joint, unspecified shoulder

√6ᵗʰ M25.22 Flail joint, elbow

    M25.221 Flail joint, **right** elbow
    M25.222 Flail joint, **left** elbow
    M25.229 Flail joint, unspecified elbow

√6ᵗʰ M25.23 Flail joint, wrist

    M25.231 Flail joint, **right** wrist
    M25.232 Flail joint, **left** wrist
    M25.239 Flail joint, unspecified wrist

√6ᵗʰ M25.24 Flail joint, hand

    M25.241 Flail joint, **right** hand
    M25.242 Flail joint, **left** hand
    M25.249 Flail joint, unspecified hand

√6ᵗʰ M25.25 Flail joint, hip

    M25.251 Flail joint, **right** hip
    M25.252 Flail joint, **left** hip
    M25.259 Flail joint, unspecified hip

√6ᵗʰ M25.26 Flail joint, knee

    M25.261 Flail joint, **right** knee
    M25.262 Flail joint, **left** knee
    M25.269 Flail joint, unspecified knee

√6ᵗʰ M25.27 Flail joint, ankle and foot

    M25.271 Flail joint, **right** ankle and foot
    M25.272 Flail joint, **left** ankle and foot
    M25.279 Flail joint, unspecified ankle and foot

    M25.28 Flail joint, other site

√5ᵗʰ M25.3 Other instability of joint

    `EXCLUDES 1`   *instability of joint secondary to old ligament injury (M24.2-)*
                 instability of joint secondary to removal of joint prosthesis (M96.8-)
    `EXCLUDES 2`   *spinal instabilities (M53.2-)*

    M25.30 Other instability, unspecified joint

√6ᵗʰ M25.31 Other instability, shoulder

    M25.311 Other instability, **right** shoulder
    M25.312 Other instability, **left** shoulder
    M25.319 Other instability, unspecified shoulder

√6ᵗʰ M25.32 Other instability, elbow

    M25.321 Other instability, **right** elbow
    M25.322 Other instability, **left** elbow
    M25.329 Other instability, unspecified elbow

√6ᵗʰ M25.33 Other instability, wrist

    M25.331 Other instability, **right** wrist
    M25.332 Other instability, **left** wrist
    M25.339 Other instability, unspecified wrist

√6ᵗʰ M25.34 Other instability, hand

    M25.341 Other instability, **right** hand
    M25.342 Other instability, **left** hand
    M25.349 Other instability, unspecified hand

√6ᵗʰ M25.35 Other instability, hip

    M25.351 Other instability, **right** hip
    M25.352 Other instability, **left** hip
    M25.359 Other instability, unspecified hip

√6ᵗʰ M25.36 Other instability, knee

    M25.361 Other instability, **right** knee
    M25.362 Other instability, **left** knee
    M25.369 Other instability, unspecified knee

√6ᵗʰ M25.37 Other instability, ankle and foot

    M25.371 Other instability, **right** ankle
    M25.372 Other instability, **left** ankle
    M25.373 Other instability, unspecified ankle
    M25.374 Other instability, **right** foot
    M25.375 Other instability, **left** foot
    M25.376 Other instability, unspecified foot

    M25.39 Other instability, other specified joint

√5ᵗʰ M25.4 Effusion of joint

    `EXCLUDES 1`   *hydrarthrosis in yaws (A66.6)*
                 intermittent hydrarthrosis (M12.4-)
                 other infective (teno)synovitis (M65.1-)

    M25.40 Effusion, unspecified joint

√6ᵗʰ M25.41 Effusion, shoulder

    M25.411 Effusion, **right** shoulder
    M25.412 Effusion, **left** shoulder
    M25.419 Effusion, unspecified shoulder

√6ᵗʰ M25.42 Effusion, elbow

    M25.421 Effusion, **right** elbow
    M25.422 Effusion, **left** elbow
    M25.429 Effusion, unspecified elbow

√6ᵗʰ M25.43 Effusion, wrist

    M25.431 Effusion, **right** wrist
    M25.432 Effusion, **left** wrist
    M25.439 Effusion, unspecified wrist

Chapter 13. Diseases of the Musculoskeletal System and Connective Tissue

✓6ᵗʰ **M25.44 Effusion, hand**

     M25.441 Effusion, **right** hand
     M25.442 Effusion, **left** hand
     M25.449 Effusion, unspecified hand

✓6ᵗʰ **M25.45 Effusion, hip**

     M25.451 Effusion, **right** hip
     M25.452 Effusion, **left** hip
     M25.459 Effusion, unspecified hip

✓6ᵗʰ **M25.46 Effusion, knee**

     M25.461 Effusion, **right** knee
     M25.462 Effusion, **left** knee
     M25.469 Effusion, unspecified knee

✓6ᵗʰ **M25.47 Effusion, ankle and foot**

     M25.471 Effusion, **right** ankle
     M25.472 Effusion, **left** ankle
     M25.473 Effusion, unspecified ankle
     M25.474 Effusion, **right** foot
     M25.475 Effusion, **left** foot
     M25.476 Effusion, unspecified foot

     M25.48 Effusion, other site

✓5ᵗʰ **M25.5 Pain in joint**

     EXCLUDES 2   *pain in fingers (M79.64-)*
                      pain in foot (M79.67-)
                      pain in hand (M79.64-)
                      pain in limb (M79.6-)
                      pain in toes (M79.67-)

     M25.50 Pain in unspecified joint

✓6ᵗʰ **M25.51 Pain in shoulder**

     M25.511 Pain in **right** shoulder
     M25.512 Pain in **left** shoulder
     M25.519 Pain in unspecified shoulder

✓6ᵗʰ **M25.52 Pain in elbow**

     M25.521 Pain in **right** elbow
     M25.522 Pain in **left** elbow
     M25.529 Pain in unspecified elbow

✓6ᵗʰ **M25.53 Pain in wrist**

     M25.531 Pain in **right** wrist
     M25.532 Pain in **left** wrist
     M25.539 Pain in unspecified wrist

✓6ᵗʰ **M25.54 Pain in joints of hand**

     AHA: 2016,4Q,38
     M25.541 Pain in joints of **right** hand
     M25.542 Pain in joints of **left** hand
     M25.549 Pain in joints of unspecified hand
                 Pain in joints of hand NOS

✓6ᵗʰ **M25.55 Pain in hip**

     M25.551 Pain in **right** hip
     M25.552 Pain in **left** hip
     M25.559 Pain in unspecified hip

✓6ᵗʰ **M25.56 Pain in knee**

     M25.561 Pain in **right** knee
     M25.562 Pain in **left** knee
     M25.569 Pain in unspecified knee

✓6ᵗʰ **M25.57 Pain in ankle and joints of foot**

     M25.571 Pain in **right** ankle and joints of right foot
     M25.572 Pain in **left** ankle and joints of left foot
     M25.579 Pain in unspecified ankle and joints of unspecified foot

     M25.59 Pain in other specified joint

✓5ᵗʰ **M25.6 Stiffness of joint, not elsewhere classified**

     EXCLUDES 1   *ankylosis of joint (M24.6-)*
                      contracture of joint (M24.5-)

     M25.60 Stiffness of unspecified joint, not elsewhere classified

✓6ᵗʰ **M25.61 Stiffness of shoulder, not elsewhere classified**

     M25.611 Stiffness of **right** shoulder, not elsewhere classified
     M25.612 Stiffness of **left** shoulder, not elsewhere classified
     M25.619 Stiffness of unspecified shoulder, not elsewhere classified

✓6ᵗʰ **M25.62 Stiffness of elbow, not elsewhere classified**

     M25.621 Stiffness of **right** elbow, not elsewhere classified
     M25.622 Stiffness of **left** elbow, not elsewhere classified

     M25.629 Stiffness of unspecified elbow, not elsewhere classified

✓6ᵗʰ **M25.63 Stiffness of wrist, not elsewhere classified**

     M25.631 Stiffness of **right** wrist, not elsewhere classified
     M25.632 Stiffness of **left** wrist, not elsewhere classified
     M25.639 Stiffness of unspecified wrist, not elsewhere classified

✓6ᵗʰ **M25.64 Stiffness of hand, not elsewhere classified**

     M25.641 Stiffness of **right** hand, not elsewhere classified
     M25.642 Stiffness of **left** hand, not elsewhere classified
     M25.649 Stiffness of unspecified hand, not elsewhere classified

✓6ᵗʰ **M25.65 Stiffness of hip, not elsewhere classified**

     M25.651 Stiffness of **right** hip, not elsewhere classified
     M25.652 Stiffness of **left** hip, not elsewhere classified
     M25.659 Stiffness of unspecified hip, not elsewhere classified

✓6ᵗʰ **M25.66 Stiffness of knee, not elsewhere classified**

     M25.661 Stiffness of **right** knee, not elsewhere classified
     M25.662 Stiffness of **left** knee, not elsewhere classified
     M25.669 Stiffness of unspecified knee, not elsewhere classified

✓6ᵗʰ **M25.67 Stiffness of ankle and foot, not elsewhere classified**

     M25.671 Stiffness of **right** ankle, not elsewhere classified
     M25.672 Stiffness of **left** ankle, not elsewhere classified
     M25.673 Stiffness of unspecified ankle, not elsewhere classified
     M25.674 Stiffness of **right** foot, not elsewhere classified
     M25.675 Stiffness of **left** foot, not elsewhere classified
     M25.676 Stiffness of unspecified foot, not elsewhere classified

     M25.69 Stiffness of other specified joint, not elsewhere classified

✓5ᵗʰ **M25.7 Osteophyte**

     M25.70 Osteophyte, unspecified joint

✓6ᵗʰ **M25.71 Osteophyte, shoulder**

     M25.711 Osteophyte, **right** shoulder
     M25.712 Osteophyte, **left** shoulder
     M25.719 Osteophyte, unspecified shoulder

✓6ᵗʰ **M25.72 Osteophyte, elbow**

     M25.721 Osteophyte, **right** elbow
     M25.722 Osteophyte, **left** elbow
     M25.729 Osteophyte, unspecified elbow

✓6ᵗʰ **M25.73 Osteophyte, wrist**

     M25.731 Osteophyte, **right** wrist
     M25.732 Osteophyte, **left** wrist
     M25.739 Osteophyte, unspecified wrist

✓6ᵗʰ **M25.74 Osteophyte, hand**

     M25.741 Osteophyte, **right** hand
     M25.742 Osteophyte, **left** hand
     M25.749 Osteophyte, unspecified hand

✓6ᵗʰ **M25.75 Osteophyte, hip**

     M25.751 Osteophyte, **right** hip
     M25.752 Osteophyte, **left** hip
     M25.759 Osteophyte, unspecified hip

✓6ᵗʰ **M25.76 Osteophyte, knee**

     M25.761 Osteophyte, **right** knee
     M25.762 Osteophyte, **left** knee
     M25.769 Osteophyte, unspecified knee

✓6ᵗʰ **M25.77 Osteophyte, ankle and foot**

     M25.771 Osteophyte, **right** ankle
     M25.772 Osteophyte, **left** ankle
     M25.773 Osteophyte, unspecified ankle
     M25.774 Osteophyte, **right** foot
     M25.775 Osteophyte, **left** foot
     M25.776 Osteophyte, unspecified foot

N Newborn: 0   **P** Pediatric: 0-17   **M** Maternity: 9-64   **A** Adult: 15-124   **UNS** Unspecified Site   **MCC** Major Complication/Comorbidity   **CC** Complication/Comorbidity   **PE** POA Exempt

804   ICD-10-CM 2025

M25.78   Osteophyte, **vertebrae**

√5ᵗʰ **M25.8**   **Other specified joint disorders**

    M25.80   Other specified joint disorders, unspecified joint

√6ᵗʰ **M25.81**   **Other specified joint disorders, shoulder**

     AHA: 2022,3Q,18

     M25.811   Other specified joint disorders, **right** shoulder

     M25.812   Other specified joint disorders, **left** shoulder

     M25.819   Other specified joint disorders, unspecified shoulder

√6ᵗʰ **M25.82**   **Other specified joint disorders, elbow**

     M25.821   Other specified joint disorders, **right** elbow

     M25.822   Other specified joint disorders, **left** elbow

     M25.829   Other specified joint disorders, unspecified elbow

√6ᵗʰ **M25.83**   **Other specified joint disorders, wrist**

     M25.831   Other specified joint disorders, **right** wrist

     M25.832   Other specified joint disorders, **left** wrist

     M25.839   Other specified joint disorders, unspecified wrist

√6ᵗʰ **M25.84**   **Other specified joint disorders, hand**

     M25.841   Other specified joint disorders, **right** hand

     M25.842   Other specified joint disorders, **left** hand

     M25.849   Other specified joint disorders, unspecified hand

√6ᵗʰ **M25.85**   **Other specified joint disorders, hip**

     AHA: 2014,4Q,25

     M25.851   Other specified joint disorders, **right** hip

     M25.852   Other specified joint disorders, **left** hip

     M25.859   Other specified joint disorders, unspecified hip

√6ᵗʰ **M25.86**   **Other specified joint disorders, knee**

     M25.861   Other specified joint disorders, **right** knee

     M25.862   Other specified joint disorders, **left** knee

     M25.869   Other specified joint disorders, unspecified knee

√6ᵗʰ **M25.87**   **Other specified joint disorders, ankle and foot**

     M25.871   Other specified joint disorders, **right** ankle and foot

     M25.872   Other specified joint disorders, **left** ankle and foot

     M25.879   Other specified joint disorders, unspecified ankle and foot

    M25.9   Joint disorder, unspecified

Dentofacial anomalies [including malocclusion] and other disorders of jaw (M26-M27)

EXCLUDES 1   hemifacial atrophy or hypertrophy (Q67.4)
       unilateral condylar hyperplasia or hypoplasia (M27.8)

√4ᵗʰ **M26**   **Dentofacial anomalies [including malocclusion]**

√5ᵗʰ **M26.0**   **Major anomalies of jaw size**

     EXCLUDES 1   acromegaly (E22.0)
           Robin's syndrome (Q87.0)

    M26.00   Unspecified anomaly of jaw size

    M26.01   Maxillary hyperplasia

    M26.02   Maxillary hypoplasia

     AHA: 2014,3Q,23

    M26.03   Mandibular hyperplasia

    M26.04   Mandibular hypoplasia

    M26.05   Macrogenia

    M26.06   Microgenia

    M26.07   Excessive tuberosity of jaw
        Entire maxillary tuberosity

    M26.09   Other specified anomalies of jaw size

√5ᵗʰ **M26.1**   **Anomalies of jaw-cranial base relationship**

    M26.10   Unspecified anomaly of jaw-cranial base relationship

    M26.11   Maxillary asymmetry

    M26.12   Other jaw asymmetry

    M26.19   Other specified anomalies of jaw-cranial base relationship

     AHA: 2020,1Q,21

√5ᵗʰ **M26.2**   **Anomalies of dental arch relationship**

    M26.20   Unspecified anomaly of dental arch relationship

√6ᵗʰ **M26.21**   **Malocclusion, Angle's class**

     M26.211   **Malocclusion, Angle's class I**
         Neutro-occlusion

     M26.212   **Malocclusion, Angle's class II**
         Disto-occlusion Division I
         Disto-occlusion Division II

     M26.213   **Malocclusion, Angle's class III**
         Mesio-occlusion

     M26.219   Malocclusion, Angle's class, unspecified

√6ᵗʰ **M26.22**   **Open occlusal relationship**

     M26.220   **Open anterior occlusal relationship**
         Anterior open bite

     M26.221   **Open posterior occlusal relationship**
         Posterior open bite

    M26.23   **Excessive horizontal overlap**
       Excessive horizontal overjet

    M26.24   **Reverse articulation**
       Crossbite (anterior) (posterior)

    M26.25   **Anomalies of interarch distance**

    M26.29   **Other anomalies of dental arch relationship**
       Midline deviation of dental arch
       Overbite (excessive) deep
       Overbite (excessive) horizontal
       Overbite (excessive) vertical
       Posterior lingual occlusion of mandibular teeth

√5ᵗʰ **M26.3**   **Anomalies of tooth position of fully erupted tooth or teeth**

     EXCLUDES 2   embedded and impacted teeth (K01.-)

    M26.30   **Unspecified anomaly of tooth position of fully erupted tooth or teeth**
       Abnormal spacing of fully erupted tooth or teeth NOS
       Displacement of fully erupted tooth or teeth NOS
       Transposition of fully erupted tooth or teeth NOS

    M26.31   **Crowding of fully erupted teeth**

    M26.32   **Excessive spacing of fully erupted teeth**
       Diastema of fully erupted tooth or teeth NOS

    M26.33   **Horizontal displacement of fully erupted tooth or teeth**
       Tipped tooth or teeth
       Tipping of fully erupted tooth

    M26.34   **Vertical displacement of fully erupted tooth or teeth**
       Extruded tooth
       Infraeruption of tooth or teeth
       Supraeruption of tooth or teeth

    M26.35   **Rotation of fully erupted tooth or teeth**

    M26.36   **Insufficient interocclusal distance of fully erupted teeth (ridge)**
       Lack of adequate intermaxillary vertical dimension of fully erupted teeth

    M26.37   **Excessive interocclusal distance of fully erupted teeth**
       Excessive intermaxillary vertical dimension of fully erupted teeth
       Loss of occlusal vertical dimension of fully erupted teeth

    M26.39   **Other anomalies of tooth position of fully erupted tooth or teeth**

    M26.4   **Malocclusion, unspecified**

√5ᵗʰ **M26.5**   **Dentofacial functional abnormalities**

     EXCLUDES 1   bruxism (F45.8)
           teeth-grinding NOS (F45.8)

    M26.50   Dentofacial functional abnormalities, unspecified

    M26.51   Abnormal jaw closure

    M26.52   Limited mandibular range of motion

    M26.53   Deviation in opening and closing of the mandible

    M26.54   Insufficient anterior guidance
       Insufficient anterior occlusal guidance

    M26.55   Centric occlusion maximum intercuspation discrepancy
      EXCLUDES 1   centric occlusion NOS (M26.59)

    M26.56   Non-working side interference
       Balancing side interference

    M26.57   Lack of posterior occlusal support

    M26.59   Other dentofacial functional abnormalities
       Centric occlusion (of teeth) NOS
       Malocclusion due to abnormal swallowing
       Malocclusion due to mouth breathing
       Malocclusion due to tongue, lip or finger habits

☑ Additional Character Required   √x7ᵗʰ Placeholder   Questionable PDx   Manifestation   Unspecified   UPD Unacceptable PDx   H1-H14 HAC   HCC CMS-HCC Dx   HIV HIV Dx

ICD-10-CM 2025   805

✓5ᵗʰ **M26.6 Temporomandibular joint disorders**

EXCLUDES 2 current temporomandibular joint dislocation (S03.0)

current temporomandibular joint sprain (S03.4)

AHA: 2016,4Q,38-39

Temporomandibular Joint

Cutaway detail

Upper joint space

Articular disc (meniscus)

Lower joint space

Condyle

Mandible

Cutaway view of temporomandibular joint (TMJ)

✓6ᵗʰ **M26.60 Temporomandibular joint disorder, unspecified**

M26.601 Right temporomandibular joint disorder, unspecified

M26.602 Left temporomandibular joint disorder, unspecified

M26.603 Bilateral temporomandibular joint disorder, unspecified

M26.609 Unspecified temporomandibular joint disorder, unspecified side

Temporomandibular joint disorder NOS

✓6ᵗʰ **M26.61 Adhesions and ankylosis of temporomandibular joint**

M26.611 Adhesions and ankylosis of right temporomandibular joint

M26.612 Adhesions and ankylosis of left temporomandibular joint

M26.613 Adhesions and ankylosis of bilateral temporomandibular joint

M26.619 Adhesions and ankylosis of temporomandibular joint, unspecified side

✓6ᵗʰ **M26.62 Arthralgia of temporomandibular joint**

M26.621 Arthralgia of right temporomandibular joint

M26.622 Arthralgia of left temporomandibular joint

M26.623 Arthralgia of bilateral temporomandibular joint

M26.629 Arthralgia of temporomandibular joint, unspecified side

✓6ᵗʰ **M26.63 Articular disc disorder of temporomandibular joint**

M26.631 Articular disc disorder of right temporomandibular joint

M26.632 Articular disc disorder of left temporomandibular joint

M26.633 Articular disc disorder of bilateral temporomandibular joint

M26.639 Articular disc disorder of temporomandibular joint, unspecified side

✓6ᵗʰ **M26.64 Arthritis of temporomandibular joint**

AHA: 2020,4Q,32

M26.641 Arthritis of right temporomandibular joint

M26.642 Arthritis of left temporomandibular joint

M26.643 Arthritis of bilateral temporomandibular joint

M26.649 Arthritis of unspecified temporomandibular joint

✓6ᵗʰ **M26.65 Arthropathy of temporomandibular joint**

AHA: 2020,4Q,32

M26.651 Arthropathy of right temporomandibular joint

M26.652 Arthropathy of left temporomandibular joint

M26.653 Arthropathy of bilateral temporomandibular joint

M26.659 Arthropathy of unspecified temporomandibular joint

M26.69 Other specified disorders of temporomandibular joint

✓5ᵗʰ **M26.7 Dental alveolar anomalies**

M26.70 Unspecified alveolar anomaly

M26.71 Alveolar maxillary hyperplasia

M26.72 Alveolar mandibular hyperplasia

M26.73 Alveolar maxillary hypoplasia

M26.74 Alveolar mandibular hypoplasia

M26.79 Other specified alveolar anomalies

✓5ᵗʰ **M26.8 Other dentofacial anomalies**

M26.81 Anterior soft tissue impingement

Anterior soft tissue impingement on teeth

M26.82 Posterior soft tissue impingement

Posterior soft tissue impingement on teeth

M26.89 Other dentofacial anomalies

M26.9 Dentofacial anomaly, unspecified

✓4ᵗʰ **M27 Other diseases of jaws**

M27.0 Developmental disorders of jaws

Latent bone cyst of jaw

Stafne's cyst

Torus mandibularis

Torus palatinus

M27.1 Giant cell granuloma, central

Giant cell granuloma NOS

EXCLUDES 1 peripheral giant cell granuloma (K06.8)

M27.2 Inflammatory conditions of jaws

Osteitis of jaw(s)

Osteomyelitis (neonatal) jaw(s)

Osteoradionecrosis jaw(s)

Periostitis jaw(s)

Sequestrum of jaw bone

Use additional code (W88-W90, X39.0) to identify radiation, if radiation-induced

EXCLUDES 2 osteonecrosis of jaw due to drug (M87.180)

M27.3 Alveolitis of jaws

Alveolar osteitis

Dry socket

✓5ᵗʰ **M27.4 Other and unspecified cysts of jaw**

EXCLUDES 1 cysts of oral region (K09.-)

latent bone cyst of jaw (M27.0)

Stafne's cyst (M27.0)

M27.40 Unspecified cyst of jaw

Cyst of jaw NOS

M27.49 Other cysts of jaw

Aneurysmal cyst of jaw

Hemorrhagic cyst of jaw

Traumatic cyst of jaw

✓5ᵗʰ **M27.5 Periradicular pathology associated with previous endodontic treatment**

M27.51 Perforation of root canal space due to endodontic treatment

M27.52 Endodontic overfill

M27.53 Endodontic underfill

M27.59 Other periradicular pathology associated with previous endodontic treatment

✓5ᵗʰ **M27.6 Endosseous dental implant failure**

M27.61 Osseointegration failure of dental implant

Hemorrhagic complications of dental implant placement

Iatrogenic osseointegration failure of dental implant

Osseointegration failure of dental implant due to complications of systemic disease

Osseointegration failure of dental implant due to poor bone quality

Pre-integration failure of dental implant NOS

Pre-osseointegration failure of dental implant

M27.62 Post-osseointegration biological failure of dental implant

Failure of dental implant due to lack of attached gingiva

Failure of dental implant due to occlusal trauma (caused by poor prosthetic design)

Failure of dental implant due to parafunctional habits

Failure of dental implant due to periodontal infection (peri-implantitis)

Failure of dental implant due to poor oral hygiene

Iatrogenic post-osseointegration failure of dental implant

Post-osseointegration failure of dental implant due to complications of systemic disease

N Newborn: 0 P Pediatric: 0-17 M Maternity: 9-64 A Adult: 15-124 UNS Unspecified Site MCC Major Complication/Comorbidity CC Complication/Comorbidity PE POA Exempt

806 ICD-10-CM 2025

M27.63 **Post-osseointegration mechanical** failure of dental implant

Failure of dental prosthesis causing loss of dental implant

Fracture of dental implant

EXCLUDES 2 *cracked tooth (KØ3.81)*

fractured dental restorative material with loss of material (KØ8.531)

fractured dental restorative material without loss of material (KØ8.530)

fractured tooth (SØ2.5)

M27.69 **Other endosseous dental implant failure**
Dental implant failure NOS

M27.8 **Other specified diseases of jaws**
Cherubism
Exostosis
Fibrous dysplasia
Unilateral condylar hyperplasia
Unilateral condylar hypoplasia

EXCLUDES 1 *jaw pain (R68.84)*

M27.9 **Disease of jaws, unspecified**

Systemic connective tissue disorders (M3Ø-M36)

INCLUDES   autoimmune disease NOS
collagen (vascular) disease NOS
systemic autoimmune disease
systemic collagen (vascular) disease

EXCLUDES 1 *autoimmune disease, single organ or single cell-type -code to relevant condition category*

✓4th **M3Ø Polyarteritis nodosa and related conditions**

EXCLUDES 1 *microscopic polyarteritis (M31.7)*

M3Ø.Ø **Polyarteritis nodosa** `CC` `HCC`

M3Ø.1 **Polyarteritis with lung involvement [Churg-Strauss]** `CC` `HCC`
Allergic granulomatous angiitis
Eosinophilic granulomatosis with polyangiitis [EGPA]
AHA: 2021,1Q,23

M3Ø.2 **Juvenile polyarteritis** `CC` `HCC`

M3Ø.3 **Mucocutaneous lymph node syndrome [Kawasaki]** `CC` `HCC`

M3Ø.8 **Other conditions related to polyarteritis nodosa** `CC` `HCC`
Polyangiitis overlap syndrome

✓4th **M31 Other necrotizing vasculopathies**

M31.Ø **Hypersensitivity angiitis** `CC` `HCC`
Goodpasture's syndrome

✓5th M31.1 **Thrombotic microangiopathy**
AHA: 2021,4Q,19

M31.1Ø **Thrombotic microangiopathy, unspecified** `MCC` `HCC`

M31.11 **Hematopoietic stem cell transplantation-associated thrombotic microangiopathy [HSCT-TMA]** `MCC` `HCC`
Transplant-associated thrombotic microangiopathy [TA-TMA]
Code first if applicable:
complications of bone marrow transplant (T86.Ø-)
complications of stem cell transplant (T86.5)
Use additional code to identify specific organ dysfunction, such as:
acute kidney failure (N17.-)
acute respiratory distress syndrome (J8Ø)
capillary leak syndrome (I78.8)
diffuse alveolar hemorrhage (RØ4.89)
encephalopathy (metabolic) (septic) (G93.41)
fluid overload, unspecified (E87.7Ø)
graft versus host disease (D89.81-)
hemolytic uremic syndrome (D59.3-)
hepatic failure (K72.-)
hepatic veno-occlusive disease (K76.5)
idiopathic interstitial pneumonia (J84.11-)
sinusoidal obstruction syndrome (K76.5)

M31.19 **Other thrombotic microangiopathy** `MCC` `HCC`
Thrombotic thrombocytopenic purpura

M31.2 **Lethal midline granuloma** `CC` `HCC`

✓5th **M31.3 Wegener's granulomatosis**
Granulomatosis with polyangiitis
Necrotizing respiratory granulomatosis
AHA: 2021,1Q,23

M31.3Ø **Wegener's granulomatosis without renal involvement** `CC` `HCC`
Wegener's granulomatosis NOS
AHA: 2021,2Q,10

M31.31 **Wegener's granulomatosis with renal involvement** `CC` `HCC`

M31.4 **Aortic arch syndrome [Takayasu]** `CC` `HCC`

M31.5 **Giant cell arteritis with polymyalgia rheumatica** `HCC`

M31.6 **Other giant cell arteritis** `HCC`

M31.7 **Microscopic polyangiitis** `CC` `HCC`
Microscopic polyarteritis
EXCLUDES 1 *polyarteritis nodosa (M3Ø.Ø)*
AHA: 2021,1Q,23

M31.8 **Other specified necrotizing vasculopathies** `CC` `HCC`
Hypocomplementemic vasculitis
Septic vasculitis

M31.9 **Necrotizing vasculopathy, unspecified** `CC` `HCC`

✓4th **M32 Systemic lupus erythematosus (SLE)**

EXCLUDES 1 *lupus erythematosus (discoid) (NOS) (L93.Ø)*

AHA: 2020,4Q,11; 2018,3Q,14

TIP: There is no default code for "lupus NOS." Query the provider for the specific type of lupus in order to assign the appropriate code.

M32.Ø **Drug-induced systemic lupus erythematosus**
Use additional code for adverse effect, if applicable, to identify drug (T36-T5Ø with fifth or sixth character 5)

✓5th M32.1 **Systemic lupus erythematosus with organ or system involvement**

M32.1Ø **Systemic lupus erythematosus, organ or system involvement unspecified** `HCC`

M32.11 **Endocarditis in systemic lupus erythematosus** `CC` `HCC`
Libman-Sacks disease

M32.12 **Pericarditis in systemic lupus erythematosus** `CC` `HCC`
Lupus pericarditis

M32.13 **Lung involvement in systemic lupus erythematosus** `HCC`
Pleural effusion due to systemic lupus erythematosus

M32.14 **Glomerular disease in systemic lupus erythematosus** `HCC`
Lupus renal disease NOS
AHA: 2013,4Q,125

M32.15 **Tubulo-interstitial nephropathy in systemic lupus erythematosus** `HCC`

M32.19 **Other organ or system involvement in systemic lupus erythematosus**
Use additional code(s) to identify organ or system involvement, such as encephalitis (GØ5.3)

M32.8 **Other forms of systemic lupus erythematosus** `HCC`

M32.9 **Systemic lupus erythematosus, unspecified** `HCC`
SLE NOS
Systemic lupus erythematosus NOS
Systemic lupus erythematosus without organ involvement

✓4th **M33 Dermatopolymyositis**
AHA: 2017,4Q,18

✓5th M33.Ø **Juvenile dermatomyositis**

M33.ØØ **Juvenile dermatomyositis, organ involvement unspecified** `CC` `HCC`

M33.Ø1 **Juvenile dermatomyositis with respiratory involvement** `CC` `HCC`

M33.Ø2 **Juvenile dermatomyositis with myopathy** `CC` `HCC`

M33.Ø3 **Juvenile dermatomyositis without myopathy** `CC` `HCC`

M33.Ø9 **Juvenile dermatomyositis with other organ involvement** `CC` `HCC`

✓5th M33.1 **Other dermatomyositis**
Adult dermatomyositis

M33.1Ø **Other dermatomyositis, organ involvement unspecified** `CC` `HCC`

M33.11 **Other dermatomyositis with respiratory involvement** `CC` `HCC`

M33.12 **Other dermatomyositis with myopathy** `CC` `HCC`

M33.13 **Other dermatomyositis without myopathy** `CC` `HCC`
Dermatomyositis NOS

M33.19 **Other dermatomyositis with other organ involvement** `CC` `HCC`

√5th **M33.2** **Polymyositis**

M33.20 **Polymyositis, organ involvement unspecified** `CC` `HCC`

M33.21 **Polymyositis with respiratory involvement** `CC` `HCC`

M33.22 **Polymyositis with myopathy** `CC` `HCC`

M33.29 **Polymyositis with other organ involvement** `CC` `HCC`

√5th **M33.9** **Dermatopolymyositis, unspecified**

M33.90 **Dermatopolymyositis, unspecified, organ involvement unspecified** `CC` `HCC`

M33.91 **Dermatopolymyositis, unspecified with respiratory involvement** `CC` `HCC`

M33.92 **Dermatopolymyositis, unspecified with myopathy** `CC` `HCC`

M33.93 **Dermatopolymyositis, unspecified without myopathy** `CC` `HCC`

M33.99 **Dermatopolymyositis, unspecified with other organ involvement** `CC` `HCC`

√4th **M34** **Systemic sclerosis [scleroderma]**
EXCLUDES 1   circumscribed scleroderma (L94.0)
neonatal scleroderma (P83.88)

M34.0 **Progressive systemic sclerosis** `HCC`

M34.1 **CR(E)ST syndrome** `HCC`
Combination of calcinosis, Raynaud's phenomenon, esophageal dysfunction, sclerodactyly, telangiectasia

M34.2 **Systemic sclerosis induced by drug and chemical**
Code first poisoning due to drug or toxin, if applicable (T36-T65 with fifth or sixth character 1-4)
Use additional code for adverse effect, if applicable, to identify drug (T36-T50 with fifth or sixth character 5)

√5th **M34.8** **Other forms of systemic sclerosis**

M34.81 **Systemic sclerosis with lung involvement** `CC` `HCC`
Code also if applicable:
other interstitial pulmonary diseases (J84.89)
secondary pulmonary arterial hypertension (I27.21)

M34.82 **Systemic sclerosis with myopathy** `CC` `HCC`

M34.83 **Systemic sclerosis with polyneuropathy** `HCC`

M34.89 **Other systemic sclerosis** `HCC`

M34.9 **Systemic sclerosis, unspecified** `HCC`

√4th **M35** **Other systemic involvement of connective tissue**
EXCLUDES 1   reactive perforating collagenosis (L87.1)

√5th **M35.0** **Sjogren syndrome**
Sicca syndrome
Use additional code to identify associated manifestations
EXCLUDES 1   dry mouth, unspecified (R68.2)
AHA: 2021,4Q,20
DEF: Autoimmune disease associated with keratoconjunctivitis, laryngopharyngitis, rhinitis, dry mouth, enlarged parotid gland, and chronic polyarthritis.

M35.00 **Sjogren syndrome, unspecified**

M35.01 **Sjogren syndrome with keratoconjunctivitis**

M35.02 **Sjogren syndrome with lung involvement** `HCC`

M35.03 **Sjogren syndrome with myopathy** `CC`

M35.04 **Sjogren syndrome with tubulo-interstitial nephropathy**
Renal tubular acidosis in sicca syndrome

M35.05 **Sjogren syndrome with inflammatory arthritis**

M35.06 **Sjogren syndrome with peripheral nervous system involvement**

M35.07 **Sjogren syndrome with central nervous system involvement** `CC`

M35.08 **Sjogren syndrome with gastrointestinal involvement**

M35.0A **Sjogren syndrome with glomerular disease**

M35.0B **Sjogren syndrome with vasculitis**

M35.0C **Sjogren syndrome with dental involvement**

M35.09 **Sjogren syndrome with other organ involvement**

M35.1 **Other overlap syndromes** `CC`
Mixed connective tissue disease
EXCLUDES 1   polyangiitis overlap syndrome (M30.8)

M35.2 **Behcet's disease** `CC` `HCC`

M35.3 **Polymyalgia rheumatica**
EXCLUDES 1   polymyalgia rheumatica with giant cell arteritis (M31.5)

M35.4 **Diffuse (eosinophilic) fasciitis**

M35.5 **Multifocal fibrosclerosis** `CC`

M35.6 **Relapsing panniculitis [Weber-Christian]**
EXCLUDES 1   lupus panniculitis (L93.2)
panniculitis NOS (M79.3-)

M35.7 **Hypermobility syndrome**
Familial ligamentous laxity
EXCLUDES 1   ligamentous laxity, NOS (M24.2-)
EXCLUDES 2   Ehlers-Danlos syndromes (Q79.6-)

√5th **M35.8** **Other specified systemic involvement of connective tissue**
AHA: 2021,1Q,36; 2020,3Q,13-14

M35.81 **Multisystem inflammatory syndrome** `CC` `HCC`
MIS-A
MIS-C
Multisystem inflammatory syndrome in adults
Multisystem inflammatory syndrome in children
Pediatric inflammatory multisystem syndrome
PIMS
Code first, if applicable, COVID-19 (U07.1)
Code also any associated complications such as:
acute hepatic failure (K72.0-)
acute kidney failure (N17.-)
acute myocarditis (I40.-)
acute respiratory distress syndrome (J80)
cardiac arrhythmia (I47-I49.-)
pneumonia due to COVID-19 (J12.82)
severe sepsis (R65.2-)
viral cardiomyopathy (B33.24)
viral pericarditis (B33.23)
Use additional code, if applicable, for:
exposure to COVID-19 or SARS-CoV-2 infection (Z20.822)
personal history of COVID-19 (Z86.16)
post COVID-19 condition (U09.9)
AHA: 2021,4Q,102; 2021,1Q,29,36,41
DEF: Hyperinflammatory condition that seems to be largely associated with past or present coronavirus disease 2019 (COVID-19) infection. Predominantly occurring in children, with less frequent occurrences in adults, symptoms often include fever, laboratory evidence of inflammation, and evidence of clinically severe illness requiring hospitalization with multisystem (two or more) organ involvement. *Synonym(s): MIS, MIS-C.*

M35.89 **Other specified systemic involvement of connective tissue** `CC`

M35.9 **Systemic involvement of connective tissue, unspecified**
Autoimmune disease (systemic) NOS
Collagen (vascular) disease NOS

√4th **M36** **Systemic disorders of connective tissue in diseases classified elsewhere**
EXCLUDES 2   arthropathies in diseases classified elsewhere (M14.-)

M36.0 *Dermato(poly)myositis in neoplastic disease* `CC` `HCC`
Code first underlying neoplasm (C00-D49)

M36.1 *Arthropathy in neoplastic disease*
Code first underlying neoplasm, such as:
leukemia (C91-C95)
malignant histiocytosis (C96.A)
multiple myeloma (C90.0)

M36.2 *Hemophilic arthropathy*
Hemarthrosis in hemophilic arthropathy
Code first underlying disease, such as:
factor VIII deficiency (D66)
with vascular defect (D68.0-)
factor IX deficiency (D67)
hemophilia (classical) (D66)
hemophilia B (D67)
hemophilia C (D68.1)

M36.3 *Arthropathy in other blood disorders*

M36.4 *Arthropathy in hypersensitivity reactions classified elsewhere*
Code first underlying disease, such as:
Henoch (-Schonlein) purpura (D69.0)
serum sickness (T80.6-)

M36.8 *Systemic disorders of connective tissue in other diseases classified elsewhere*

Code first underlying disease, such as:
  alkaptonuria (E70.29)
  hypogammaglobulinemia (D80.-)
  ochronosis (E70.29)

DORSOPATHIES (M40-M54)

Deforming dorsopathies (M40-M43)

√4ᵗʰ **M40** **Kyphosis and lordosis**

Code first underlying disease

EXCLUDES 1   *congenital kyphosis and lordosis (Q76.4)*
  kyphoscoliosis (M41.-)
  postprocedural kyphosis and lordosis (M96.-)

Kyphosis and Lordosis

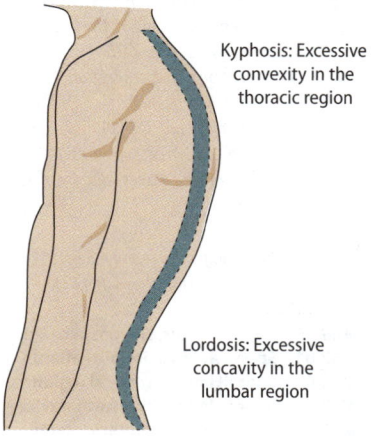

Kyphosis: Excessive convexity in the thoracic region

Lordosis: Excessive concavity in the lumbar region

√5ᵗʰ **M40.0** **Postural kyphosis**

  EXCLUDES 1   *osteochondrosis of spine (M42.-)*

  M40.00 Postural kyphosis, site unspecified
  M40.03 Postural kyphosis, cervicothoracic region
  M40.04 Postural kyphosis, thoracic region
  M40.05 Postural kyphosis, thoracolumbar region

√5ᵗʰ **M40.1** **Other secondary kyphosis**

  M40.10 Other secondary kyphosis, site unspecified **UPD**
  M40.12 Other secondary kyphosis, cervical region **UPD**
  M40.13 Other secondary kyphosis, cervicothoracic region **UPD**
  M40.14 Other secondary kyphosis, thoracic region **UPD**
  M40.15 Other secondary kyphosis, thoracolumbar region **UPD**

√5ᵗʰ **M40.2** **Other and unspecified kyphosis**

  √6ᵗʰ **M40.20** **Unspecified kyphosis**

    M40.202 Unspecified kyphosis, cervical region
    M40.203 Unspecified kyphosis, cervicothoracic region
    M40.204 Unspecified kyphosis, thoracic region
    M40.205 Unspecified kyphosis, thoracolumbar region
    M40.209 Unspecified kyphosis, site unspecified

  √6ᵗʰ **M40.29** **Other kyphosis**

    M40.292 Other kyphosis, cervical region
    M40.293 Other kyphosis, cervicothoracic region
    M40.294 Other kyphosis, thoracic region
    M40.295 Other kyphosis, thoracolumbar region
    M40.299 Other kyphosis, site unspecified

√5ᵗʰ **M40.3** **Flatback syndrome**

  M40.30 Flatback syndrome, site unspecified
  M40.35 Flatback syndrome, thoracolumbar region
  M40.36 Flatback syndrome, lumbar region
  M40.37 Flatback syndrome, lumbosacral region

√5ᵗʰ **M40.4** **Postural lordosis**

  Acquired lordosis

  M40.40 Postural lordosis, site unspecified
  M40.45 Postural lordosis, thoracolumbar region
  M40.46 Postural lordosis, lumbar region

  M40.47 Postural lordosis, lumbosacral region

√5ᵗʰ **M40.5** **Lordosis, unspecified**

  M40.50 Lordosis, unspecified, site unspecified
  M40.55 Lordosis, unspecified, thoracolumbar region
  M40.56 Lordosis, unspecified, lumbar region
  M40.57 Lordosis, unspecified, lumbosacral region

√4ᵗʰ **M41** **Scoliosis**

  INCLUDES   kyphoscoliosis
  EXCLUDES 1   *congenital scoliosis due to bony malformation (Q76.3)*
    congenital scoliosis NOS (Q67.5)
    kyphoscoliotic heart disease (I27.1)
    postural congenital scoliosis (Q67.5)
  EXCLUDES 2   *postprocedural scoliosis (M96.89)*
    postradiation scoliosis (M96.5)

Scoliosis

Lateral curvature of spine

AHA: 2022,1Q,30

√5ᵗʰ **M41.0** **Infantile idiopathic scoliosis**

  AHA: 2014,4Q,26

  M41.00 Infantile idiopathic scoliosis, site unspecified
  M41.02 Infantile idiopathic scoliosis, cervical region
  M41.03 Infantile idiopathic scoliosis, cervicothoracic region
  M41.04 Infantile idiopathic scoliosis, thoracic region
  M41.05 Infantile idiopathic scoliosis, thoracolumbar region
  M41.06 Infantile idiopathic scoliosis, lumbar region
  M41.07 Infantile idiopathic scoliosis, lumbosacral region
  M41.08 Infantile idiopathic scoliosis, sacral and sacrococcygeal region

√5ᵗʰ **M41.1** **Juvenile and adolescent idiopathic scoliosis**

  √6ᵗʰ **M41.11** **Juvenile idiopathic scoliosis**

    AHA: 2014,4Q,28

    M41.112 Juvenile idiopathic scoliosis, cervical region
    M41.113 Juvenile idiopathic scoliosis, cervicothoracic region
    M41.114 Juvenile idiopathic scoliosis, thoracic region
    M41.115 Juvenile idiopathic scoliosis, thoracolumbar region
    M41.116 Juvenile idiopathic scoliosis, lumbar region
    M41.117 Juvenile idiopathic scoliosis, lumbosacral region
    M41.119 Juvenile idiopathic scoliosis, site unspecified

  √6ᵗʰ **M41.12** **Adolescent idiopathic scoliosis**

    AHA: 2024,1Q,23

    M41.122 Adolescent idiopathic scoliosis, cervical region
    M41.123 Adolescent idiopathic scoliosis, cervicothoracic region
    M41.124 Adolescent idiopathic scoliosis, thoracic region
    M41.125 Adolescent idiopathic scoliosis, thoracolumbar region
    M41.126 Adolescent idiopathic scoliosis, lumbar region

✔ Additional Character Required   √x7ᵗʰ Placeholder   **Questionable PDx**   Manifestation   Unspecified   **UPD** Unacceptable PDx   **H1 - H14** HAC   **HCC** CMS-HCC Dx   **HIV** HIV Dx

ICD-10-CM 2025   **809**

M41.127 Adolescent idiopathic scoliosis, **lumbosacral** region

M41.129 Adolescent idiopathic scoliosis, site unspecified

✓5ᵗʰ **M41.2** Other idiopathic scoliosis

     M41.20 Other idiopathic scoliosis, site unspecified

     M41.22 Other idiopathic scoliosis, **cervical** region

     M41.23 Other idiopathic scoliosis, **cervicothoracic** region

     M41.24 Other idiopathic scoliosis, **thoracic** region

     M41.25 Other idiopathic scoliosis, **thoracolumbar** region

     M41.26 Other idiopathic scoliosis, **lumbar** region

     M41.27 Other idiopathic scoliosis, **lumbosacral** region

✓5ᵗʰ **M41.3** **Thoracogenic** scoliosis

     M41.30 Thoracogenic scoliosis, site unspecified

     M41.34 Thoracogenic scoliosis, **thoracic** region

     M41.35 Thoracogenic scoliosis, **thoracolumbar** region

✓5ᵗʰ **M41.4** **Neuromuscular** scoliosis

Scoliosis secondary to cerebral palsy, Friedreich's ataxia, poliomyelitis and other neuromuscular disorders

Code also underlying condition

AHA: 2014,4Q,27

     M41.40 Neuromuscular scoliosis, site unspecified

     M41.41 Neuromuscular scoliosis, **occipito-atlanto-axial** region

     M41.42 Neuromuscular scoliosis, **cervical** region

     M41.43 Neuromuscular scoliosis, **cervicothoracic** region

     M41.44 Neuromuscular scoliosis, **thoracic** region

     M41.45 Neuromuscular scoliosis, **thoracolumbar** region

     M41.46 Neuromuscular scoliosis, **lumbar** region

     M41.47 Neuromuscular scoliosis, **lumbosacral** region

✓5ᵗʰ **M41.5** Other **secondary** scoliosis

Code first underlying disease

AHA: 2019,1Q,19

     M41.50 Other secondary scoliosis, site unspecified   `UPD`

     M41.52 Other secondary scoliosis, **cervical** region   `UPD`

     M41.53 Other secondary scoliosis, **cervicothoracic** region   `UPD`

     M41.54 Other secondary scoliosis, **thoracic** region   `UPD`

     M41.55 Other secondary scoliosis, **thoracolumbar** region   `UPD`

     M41.56 Other secondary scoliosis, **lumbar** region   `UPD`

     M41.57 Other secondary scoliosis, **lumbosacral** region   `UPD`

✓5ᵗʰ **M41.8** Other forms of scoliosis

AHA: 2022,1Q,30

     M41.80 Other forms of scoliosis, site unspecified

     M41.82 Other forms of scoliosis, **cervical** region

     M41.83 Other forms of scoliosis, **cervicothoracic** region

     M41.84 Other forms of scoliosis, **thoracic** region

     M41.85 Other forms of scoliosis, **thoracolumbar** region

     M41.86 Other forms of scoliosis, **lumbar** region

     M41.87 Other forms of scoliosis, **lumbosacral** region

M41.9 Scoliosis, unspecified

AHA: 2022,1Q,30

✓4ᵗʰ **M42** Spinal osteochondrosis

✓5ᵗʰ **M42.0** **Juvenile** osteochondrosis of spine

Calve's disease

Scheuermann's disease

EXCLUDES 1 *postural kyphosis (M40.0)*

     M42.00 Juvenile osteochondrosis of spine, site unspecified

     M42.01 Juvenile osteochondrosis of spine, **occipito-atlanto-axial** region

     M42.02 Juvenile osteochondrosis of spine, **cervical** region

     M42.03 Juvenile osteochondrosis of spine, **cervicothoracic** region

     M42.04 Juvenile osteochondrosis of spine, **thoracic** region

     M42.05 Juvenile osteochondrosis of spine, **thoracolumbar** region

     M42.06 Juvenile osteochondrosis of spine, **lumbar** region

     M42.07 Juvenile osteochondrosis of spine, **lumbosacral** region

     M42.08 Juvenile osteochondrosis of spine, **sacral and sacrococcygeal** region

     M42.09 Juvenile osteochondrosis of spine, **multiple sites** in spine

✓5ᵗʰ **M42.1** **Adult** osteochondrosis of spine

     M42.10 Adult osteochondrosis of spine, site unspecified   `A`

M42.11 Adult osteochondrosis of spine, **occipito-atlanto-axial** region   `A`

M42.12 Adult osteochondrosis of spine, **cervical** region   `A`

M42.13 Adult osteochondrosis of spine, **cervicothoracic** region   `A`

M42.14 Adult osteochondrosis of spine, **thoracic** region   `A`

M42.15 Adult osteochondrosis of spine, **thoracolumbar** region   `A`

M42.16 Adult osteochondrosis of spine, **lumbar** region   `A`

M42.17 Adult osteochondrosis of spine, **lumbosacral** region   `A`

M42.18 Adult osteochondrosis of **spine, sacral and sacrococcygeal** region   `A`

M42.19 Adult osteochondrosis of spine, **multiple sites** in spine   `A`

M42.9 Spinal osteochondrosis, unspecified

✓4ᵗʰ **M43** **Other deforming dorsopathies**

EXCLUDES 1 *congenital spondylolysis and spondylolisthesis (Q76.2)*

hemivertebra (Q76.3-Q76.4)

Klippel-Feil syndrome (Q76.1)

lumbarization and sacralization (Q76.4)

platyspondylisis (Q76.4)

spina bifida occulta (Q76.0)

spinal curvature in osteoporosis (M80.-)

spinal curvature in Paget's disease of bone [osteitis deformans] (M88.-)

✓5ᵗʰ **M43.0** Spondylolysis

EXCLUDES 1 *congenital spondylolysis (Q76.2)*

spondylolisthesis (M43.1)

AHA: 2023,3Q,20

     M43.00 Spondylolysis, site unspecified

     M43.01 Spondylolysis, **occipito-atlanto-axial** region

     M43.02 Spondylolysis, **cervical** region

     M43.03 Spondylolysis, **cervicothoracic** region

     M43.04 Spondylolysis, **thoracic** region

     M43.05 Spondylolysis, **thoracolumbar** region

     M43.06 Spondylolysis, **lumbar** region

     M43.07 Spondylolysis, **lumbosacral** region

     M43.08 Spondylolysis, **sacral and sacrococcygeal** region

     M43.09 Spondylolysis, **multiple sites** in spine

✓5ᵗʰ **M43.1** Spondylolisthesis

EXCLUDES 1 *acute traumatic of lumbosacral region (S33.1)*

acute traumatic of sites other than lumbosacral - code to Fracture, vertebra, by region

congenital spondylolisthesis (Q76.2)

AHA: 2023,3Q,20; 2020,2Q,21; 2018,3Q,18

DEF: anterolisthesis: Forward displacement of one vertebra slipping over another. This condition can cause compression of the nerve roots exiting the spine.

DEF: retrolisthesis: Backward displacement of one vertebra slipping over another. This condition can cause compression of the nerve roots exiting the spine.

TIP: Code also any associated radiculopathy (M54.1-) and/or myelopathy (G99.2).

     M43.10 Spondylolisthesis, site unspecified

     M43.11 Spondylolisthesis, **occipito-atlanto-axial** region

     M43.12 Spondylolisthesis, **cervical** region

     M43.13 Spondylolisthesis, **cervicothoracic** region

     M43.14 Spondylolisthesis, **thoracic** region

     M43.15 Spondylolisthesis, **thoracolumbar** region

     M43.16 Spondylolisthesis, **lumbar** region

       AHA: 2024,1Q,17

     M43.17 Spondylolisthesis, **lumbosacral** region

     M43.18 Spondylolisthesis, **sacral and sacrococcygeal** region

     M43.19 Spondylolisthesis, **multiple sites** in spine

✓5ᵗʰ **M43.2** Fusion of spine

Ankylosis of spinal joint

EXCLUDES 1 *ankylosing spondylitis (M45.0-)*

congenital fusion of spine (Q76.4)

EXCLUDES 2 *arthrodesis status (Z98.1)*

pseudoarthrosis after fusion or arthrodesis (M96.0)

     M43.20 Fusion of spine, site unspecified

     M43.21 Fusion of spine, **occipito-atlanto-axial** region

     M43.22 Fusion of spine, **cervical** region

     M43.23 Fusion of spine, **cervicothoracic** region

     M43.24 Fusion of spine, **thoracic** region

`N` Newborn: 0   `P` Pediatric: 0-17   `M` Maternity: 9-64   `A` Adult: 15-124   `UNS` Unspecified Site   `MCC` Major Complication/Comorbidity   `CC` Complication/Comorbidity   `PE` POA Exempt

810

ICD-10-CM 2025

M43.25   Fusion of spine, **thoracolumbar** region
M43.26   Fusion of spine, **lumbar** region
M43.27   Fusion of spine, **lumbosacral** region
M43.28   Fusion of spine, **sacral and sacrococcygeal** region
M43.3   Recurrent atlantoaxial dislocation with myelopathy
M43.4   Other recurrent atlantoaxial dislocation
✓5th M43.5   Other recurrent vertebral dislocation
     EXCLUDES 1   biomechanical lesions NEC (M99.-)

✓6th M43.5X   Other recurrent vertebral dislocation
     M43.5X2   Other recurrent vertebral dislocation, **cervical** region
     M43.5X3   Other recurrent vertebral dislocation, **cervicothoracic** region
     M43.5X4   Other recurrent vertebral dislocation, **thoracic** region
     M43.5X5   Other recurrent vertebral dislocation, **thoracolumbar** region
     M43.5X6   Other recurrent vertebral dislocation, **lumbar** region
     M43.5X7   Other recurrent vertebral dislocation, **lumbosacral** region
     M43.5X8   Other recurrent vertebral dislocation, **sacral and sacrococcygeal** region
     M43.5X9   Other recurrent vertebral dislocation, site unspecified

M43.6   Torticollis
     EXCLUDES 1   congenital (sternomastoid) torticollis (Q68.0)
          current injury - see Injury, of spine, by body region
          ocular torticollis (R29.891)
          psychogenic torticollis (F45.8)
          spasmodic torticollis (G24.3)
          torticollis due to birth injury (P15.2)
     DEF: Twisted, unnatural position of the neck due to contracted cervical muscles that pull the head to one side.

✓5th M43.8   Other specified deforming dorsopathies
     EXCLUDES 2   kyphosis and lordosis (M40.-)
          scoliosis (M41.-)

✓6th M43.8X   Other specified deforming dorsopathies
     M43.8X1   Other specified deforming dorsopathies, **occipito-atlanto-axial** region
     M43.8X2   Other specified deforming dorsopathies, **cervical** region
     M43.8X3   Other specified deforming dorsopathies, **cervicothoracic** region
     M43.8X4   Other specified deforming dorsopathies, **thoracic** region
     M43.8X5   Other specified deforming dorsopathies, **thoracolumbar** region
     M43.8X6   Other specified deforming dorsopathies, **lumbar** region
     M43.8X7   Other specified deforming dorsopathies, **lumbosacral** region
     M43.8X8   Other specified deforming dorsopathies, **sacral and sacrococcygeal** region
     M43.8X9   Other specified deforming dorsopathies, site unspecified

M43.9   Deforming dorsopathy, unspecified
     Curvature of spine NOS

Spondylopathies (M45-M49)

✓4th M45   Ankylosing spondylitis
     Rheumatoid arthritis of spine
     EXCLUDES 1   arthropathy in Reiter's disease (M02.3-)
          juvenile (ankylosing) spondylitis (M08.1)
     EXCLUDES 2   Behcet's disease (M35.2)

M45.0   Ankylosing spondylitis of **multiple sites** in spine   HCC
M45.1   Ankylosing spondylitis of **occipito-atlanto-axial** region   HCC
M45.2   Ankylosing spondylitis of **cervical** region   HCC
M45.3   Ankylosing spondylitis of **cervicothoracic** region   HCC
M45.4   Ankylosing spondylitis of **thoracic** region   HCC
M45.5   Ankylosing spondylitis of **thoracolumbar** region   HCC
M45.6   Ankylosing spondylitis **lumbar** region   HCC
M45.7   Ankylosing spondylitis of **lumbosacral** region   HCC
M45.8   Ankylosing spondylitis **sacral and sacrococcygeal** region   HCC
M45.9   Ankylosing spondylitis of unspecified sites in spine   HCC

✓5th M45.A   Non-radiographic axial spondyloarthritis
     AHA: 2021,4Q,21-22
     M45.A0   Non-radiographic axial spondyloarthritis of unspecified sites in spine   HCC
     M45.A1   Non-radiographic axial spondyloarthritis of **occipito-atlanto-axial** region   HCC
     M45.A2   Non-radiographic axial spondyloarthritis of **cervical** region   HCC
     M45.A3   Non-radiographic axial spondyloarthritis of **cervicothoracic** region   HCC
     M45.A4   Non-radiographic axial spondyloarthritis of **thoracic** region   HCC
     M45.A5   Non-radiographic axial spondyloarthritis of **thoracolumbar** region   HCC
     M45.A6   Non-radiographic axial spondyloarthritis of **lumbar** region   HCC
     M45.A7   Non-radiographic axial spondyloarthritis of **lumbosacral** region   HCC
     M45.A8   Non-radiographic axial spondyloarthritis of **sacral and sacrococcygeal** region   HCC
     M45.AB   Non-radiographic axial spondyloarthritis of **multiple sites** in spine   HCC

✓4th M46   Other inflammatory spondylopathies
✓5th M46.0   Spinal enthesopathy
     Disorder of ligamentous or muscular attachments of spine
     M46.00   Spinal enthesopathy, site unspecified
     M46.01   Spinal enthesopathy, **occipito-atlanto-axial** region
     M46.02   Spinal enthesopathy, **cervical** region
     M46.03   Spinal enthesopathy, **cervicothoracic** region
     M46.04   Spinal enthesopathy, **thoracic** region
     M46.05   Spinal enthesopathy, **thoracolumbar** region
     M46.06   Spinal enthesopathy, **lumbar** region
     M46.07   Spinal enthesopathy, **lumbosacral** region
     M46.08   Spinal enthesopathy, **sacral and sacrococcygeal** region
     M46.09   Spinal enthesopathy, **multiple sites** in spine

M46.1   Sacroiliitis, not elsewhere classified
     AHA: 2020,2Q,14
     DEF: Inflammation of the sacroiliac joint (situated at the juncture of the sacrum and hip). Symptoms include pain in the buttocks or lower back that can extend down one or both legs.

✓5th M46.2   Osteomyelitis of vertebra
     M46.20   Osteomyelitis of vertebra, site unspecified   CC UNS HCC
     M46.21   Osteomyelitis of vertebra, **occipito-atlanto-axial** region   CC HCC
     M46.22   Osteomyelitis of vertebra, **cervical** region   CC HCC
     M46.23   Osteomyelitis of vertebra, **cervicothoracic** region   CC HCC
     M46.24   Osteomyelitis of vertebra, **thoracic** region   CC HCC
     M46.25   Osteomyelitis of vertebra, **thoracolumbar** region   CC HCC
     M46.26   Osteomyelitis of vertebra, **lumbar** region   CC HCC
     M46.27   Osteomyelitis of vertebra, **lumbosacral** region   CC HCC
     M46.28   Osteomyelitis of vertebra, **sacral and sacrococcygeal** region   CC HCC

✓5th M46.3   Infection of intervertebral disc (pyogenic)
     Use additional code (B95-B97) to identify infectious agent
     M46.30   Infection of intervertebral disc (pyogenic), site unspecified   CC UNS HCC
     M46.31   Infection of intervertebral disc (pyogenic), **occipito-atlanto-axial** region   CC HCC
     M46.32   Infection of intervertebral disc (pyogenic), **cervical** region   CC HCC
     M46.33   Infection of intervertebral disc (pyogenic), **cervicothoracic** region   CC HCC
     M46.34   Infection of intervertebral disc (pyogenic), **thoracic** region   CC HCC
     M46.35   Infection of intervertebral disc (pyogenic), **thoracolumbar** region   CC HCC
     M46.36   Infection of intervertebral disc (pyogenic), **lumbar** region   CC HCC
     M46.37   Infection of intervertebral disc (pyogenic), **lumbosacral** region   CC HCC
     M46.38   Infection of intervertebral disc (pyogenic), **sacral and sacrococcygeal** region   CC HCC

Chapter 13. Diseases of the Musculoskeletal System and Connective Tissue

M46.39 Infection of intervertebral disc (pyogenic), multiple sites in spine   CC HCC

√5th **M46.4 Discitis, unspecified**

M46.40 Discitis, unspecified, site unspecified

M46.41 Discitis, unspecified, occipito-atlanto-axial region

M46.42 Discitis, unspecified, cervical region

M46.43 Discitis, unspecified, cervicothoracic region

M46.44 Discitis, unspecified, thoracic region

M46.45 Discitis, unspecified, thoracolumbar region

M46.46 Discitis, unspecified, lumbar region

M46.47 Discitis, unspecified, lumbosacral region

M46.48 Discitis, unspecified, sacral and sacrococcygeal region

M46.49 Discitis, unspecified, multiple sites in spine

√5th **M46.5 Other infective spondylopathies**

M46.50 Other infective spondylopathies, site unspecified

M46.51 Other infective spondylopathies, occipito-atlanto-axial region

M46.52 Other infective spondylopathies, cervical region

M46.53 Other infective spondylopathies, cervicothoracic region

M46.54 Other infective spondylopathies, thoracic region

M46.55 Other infective spondylopathies, thoracolumbar region

M46.56 Other infective spondylopathies, lumbar region

M46.57 Other infective spondylopathies, lumbosacral region

M46.58 Other infective spondylopathies, sacral and sacrococcygeal region

M46.59 Other infective spondylopathies, multiple sites in spine

√5th **M46.8 Other specified inflammatory spondylopathies**

M46.80 Other specified inflammatory spondylopathies, site unspecified

M46.81 Other specified inflammatory spondylopathies, occipito-atlanto-axial region

M46.82 Other specified inflammatory spondylopathies, cervical region

M46.83 Other specified inflammatory spondylopathies, cervicothoracic region

M46.84 Other specified inflammatory spondylopathies, thoracic region

M46.85 Other specified inflammatory spondylopathies, thoracolumbar region

M46.86 Other specified inflammatory spondylopathies, lumbar region

M46.87 Other specified inflammatory spondylopathies, lumbosacral region

M46.88 Other specified inflammatory spondylopathies, sacral and sacrococcygeal region

M46.89 Other specified inflammatory spondylopathies, multiple sites in spine

√5th **M46.9 Unspecified inflammatory spondylopathy**

M46.90 Unspecified inflammatory spondylopathy, site unspecified

M46.91 Unspecified inflammatory spondylopathy, occipito-atlanto-axial region

M46.92 Unspecified inflammatory spondylopathy, cervical region
AHA: 2019,3Q,10

M46.93 Unspecified inflammatory spondylopathy, cervicothoracic region

M46.94 Unspecified inflammatory spondylopathy, thoracic region

M46.95 Unspecified inflammatory spondylopathy, thoracolumbar region

M46.96 Unspecified inflammatory spondylopathy, lumbar region

M46.97 Unspecified inflammatory spondylopathy, lumbosacral region

M46.98 Unspecified inflammatory spondylopathy, sacral and sacrococcygeal region

M46.99 Unspecified inflammatory spondylopathy, multiple sites in spine

√4th **M47 Spondylosis**

INCLUDES arthrosis or osteoarthritis of spine
degeneration of facet joints
AHA: 2020,1Q,17; 2019,3Q,10-11; 2016,4Q,147

√5th **M47.0 Anterior spinal and vertebral artery compression syndromes**

√6th **M47.01 Anterior spinal artery compression syndromes**

M47.011 Anterior spinal artery compression syndromes, occipito-atlanto-axial region   CC

M47.012 Anterior spinal artery compression syndromes, cervical region   CC
AHA: 2023,1Q,37

M47.013 Anterior spinal artery compression syndromes, cervicothoracic region   CC

M47.014 Anterior spinal artery compression syndromes, thoracic region   CC

M47.015 Anterior spinal artery compression syndromes, thoracolumbar region   CC

M47.016 Anterior spinal artery compression syndromes, lumbar region   CC

M47.019 Anterior spinal artery compression syndromes, site unspecified   CC UNS

√6th **M47.02 Vertebral artery compression syndromes**

M47.021 Vertebral artery compression syndromes, occipito-atlanto-axial region   CC

M47.022 Vertebral artery compression syndromes, cervical region   CC
AHA: 2023,1Q,37

M47.029 Vertebral artery compression syndromes, site unspecified   CC UNS

√5th **M47.1 Other spondylosis with myelopathy**

Spondylogenic compression of spinal cord
EXCLUDES 1 vertebral subluxation (M43.3-M43.5X9)
AHA: 2020,1Q,17

M47.10 Other spondylosis with myelopathy, site unspecified   CC UNS

M47.11 Other spondylosis with myelopathy, occipito-atlanto-axial region   CC

M47.12 Other spondylosis with myelopathy, cervical region   CC

M47.13 Other spondylosis with myelopathy, cervicothoracic region   CC

M47.14 Other spondylosis with myelopathy, thoracic region   CC

M47.15 Other spondylosis with myelopathy, thoracolumbar region   CC

M47.16 Other spondylosis with myelopathy, lumbar region   CC

√5th **M47.2 Other spondylosis with radiculopathy**
AHA: 2020,1Q,17

M47.20 Other spondylosis with radiculopathy, site unspecified

M47.21 Other spondylosis with radiculopathy, occipito-atlanto-axial region

M47.22 Other spondylosis with radiculopathy, cervical region

M47.23 Other spondylosis with radiculopathy, cervicothoracic region

M47.24 Other spondylosis with radiculopathy, thoracic region

M47.25 Other spondylosis with radiculopathy, thoracolumbar region

M47.26 Other spondylosis with radiculopathy, lumbar region

M47.27 Other spondylosis with radiculopathy, lumbosacral region

M47.28 Other spondylosis with radiculopathy, sacral and sacrococcygeal region

√5th **M47.8 Other spondylosis**

√6th **M47.81 Spondylosis without myelopathy or radiculopathy**
AHA: 2019,3Q,10-11; 2018,2Q,14

M47.811 Spondylosis without myelopathy or radiculopathy, occipito-atlanto-axial region

M47.812 Spondylosis without myelopathy or radiculopathy, cervical region

M47.813 Spondylosis without myelopathy or radiculopathy, cervicothoracic region

M47.814 Spondylosis without myelopathy or radiculopathy, thoracic region

M47.815 Spondylosis without myelopathy or radiculopathy, **thoracolumbar** region
M47.816 Spondylosis without myelopathy or radiculopathy, **lumbar** region
M47.817 Spondylosis without myelopathy or radiculopathy, **lumbosacral** region
M47.818 Spondylosis without myelopathy or radiculopathy, **sacral and sacrococcygeal** region
M47.819 Spondylosis without myelopathy or radiculopathy, site unspecified

✓6th **M47.89 Other spondylosis**
M47.891 Other spondylosis, **occipito-atlanto-axial** region
M47.892 Other spondylosis, **cervical** region
M47.893 Other spondylosis, **cervicothoracic** region
M47.894 Other spondylosis, **thoracic** region
M47.895 Other spondylosis, **thoracolumbar** region
M47.896 Other spondylosis, **lumbar** region
M47.897 Other spondylosis, **lumbosacral** region
M47.898 Other spondylosis, **sacral and sacrococcygeal** region
M47.899 Other spondylosis, site unspecified

M47.9 Spondylosis, unspecified

✓4th **M48 Other spondylopathies**

✓5th **M48.0 Spinal stenosis**
Caudal stenosis
AHA: 2020,1Q,17; 2018,3Q,18-19
TIP: Code also any associated radiculopathy (M54.1-) and/or myelopathy (G99.2).
M48.00 Spinal stenosis, site unspecified
M48.01 Spinal stenosis, **occipito-atlanto-axial** region
M48.02 Spinal stenosis, **cervical** region
M48.03 Spinal stenosis, **cervicothoracic** region
M48.04 Spinal stenosis, **thoracic** region
M48.05 Spinal stenosis, **thoracolumbar** region
✓6th **M48.06 Spinal stenosis, lumbar** region
AHA: 2018,3Q,19; 2017,4Q,18-19
M48.061 Spinal stenosis, lumbar region **without neurogenic claudication**
Spinal stenosis, lumbar region NOS
M48.062 Spinal stenosis, lumbar region **with neurogenic claudication**
M48.07 Spinal stenosis, **lumbosacral** region
M48.08 Spinal stenosis, **sacral and sacrococcygeal** region

✓5th **M48.1 Ankylosing hyperostosis [Forestier]**
Diffuse idiopathic skeletal hyperostosis [DISH]
M48.10 Ankylosing hyperostosis [Forestier], site unspecified
M48.11 Ankylosing hyperostosis [Forestier], **occipito-atlanto-axial** region
M48.12 Ankylosing hyperostosis [Forestier], **cervical** region
M48.13 Ankylosing hyperostosis [Forestier], **cervicothoracic** region
M48.14 Ankylosing hyperostosis [Forestier], **thoracic** region
M48.15 Ankylosing hyperostosis [Forestier], **thoracolumbar** region
M48.16 Ankylosing hyperostosis [Forestier], **lumbar** region
M48.17 Ankylosing hyperostosis [Forestier], **lumbosacral** region
M48.18 Ankylosing hyperostosis [Forestier], **sacral and sacrococcygeal** region
M48.19 Ankylosing hyperostosis [Forestier], **multiple sites** in spine

✓5th **M48.2 Kissing spine**
M48.20 Kissing spine, site unspecified
M48.21 Kissing spine, **occipito-atlanto-axial** region
M48.22 Kissing spine, **cervical** region
M48.23 Kissing spine, **cervicothoracic** region
M48.24 Kissing spine, **thoracic** region
M48.25 Kissing spine, **thoracolumbar** region
M48.26 Kissing spine, **lumbar** region
M48.27 Kissing spine, **lumbosacral** region

✓5th **M48.3 Traumatic spondylopathy**
M48.30 Traumatic spondylopathy, site unspecified `CC` `U-S`
M48.31 Traumatic spondylopathy, **occipito-atlanto-axial** region `CC`
M48.32 Traumatic spondylopathy, **cervical** region `CC`

M48.33 Traumatic spondylopathy, **cervicothoracic** region `CC`
M48.34 Traumatic spondylopathy, **thoracic** region `CC`
M48.35 Traumatic spondylopathy, **thoracolumbar** region `CC`
M48.36 Traumatic spondylopathy, **lumbar** region `CC`
M48.37 Traumatic spondylopathy, **lumbosacral** region `CC`
M48.38 Traumatic spondylopathy, **sacral and sacrococcygeal** region `CC`

✓5th **M48.4 Fatigue fracture of vertebra**
Stress fracture of vertebra
EXCLUDES 1 *pathological fracture NOS (M84.4-)*
pathological fracture of vertebra due to neoplasm (M84.58)
pathological fracture of vertebra due to osteoporosis (M80.-)
pathological fracture of vertebra due to other diagnosis (M84.68)
traumatic fracture of vertebrae (S12.0-S12.3-, S22.0-, S32.0-)

The appropriate 7th character is to be added to each code from subcategory M48.4.
A   initial encounter for fracture
D   subsequent encounter for fracture with routine healing
G   subsequent encounter for fracture with delayed healing
S   sequela of fracture

✓x7th **M48.40 Fatigue fracture of vertebra, site unspecified**
✓x7th **M48.41 Fatigue fracture of vertebra, occipito-atlanto-axial** region
✓x7th **M48.42 Fatigue fracture of vertebra, cervical** region
✓x7th **M48.43 Fatigue fracture of vertebra, cervicothoracic** region
✓x7th **M48.44 Fatigue fracture of vertebra, thoracic** region
✓x7th **M48.45 Fatigue fracture of vertebra, thoracolumbar** region
✓x7th **M48.46 Fatigue fracture of vertebra, lumbar** region
✓x7th **M48.47 Fatigue fracture of vertebra, lumbosacral** region
✓x7th **M48.48 Fatigue fracture of vertebra, sacral and sacrococcygeal** region

✓5th **M48.5 Collapsed vertebra, not elsewhere classified**
Collapsed vertebra NOS
Compression fracture of vertebra NOS
Wedging of vertebra NOS
EXCLUDES 1 *current injury - see Injury of spine, by body region*
fatigue fracture of vertebra (M48.4)
pathological fracture NOS (M84.4-)
pathological fracture of vertebra due to neoplasm (M84.58)
pathological fracture of vertebra due to osteoporosis (M80.-)
pathological fracture of vertebra due to other diagnosis (M84.68)
stress fracture of vertebra (M48.4-)
traumatic fracture of vertebra (S12.-, S22.-, S32.-)

The appropriate 7th character is to be added to each code from subcategory M48.5.
A   initial encounter for fracture
D   subsequent encounter for fracture with routine healing
G   subsequent encounter for fracture with delayed healing
S   sequela of fracture

✓x7th **M48.50 Collapsed vertebra, not elsewhere classified, site unspecified** `CC` `UNS` `HCC`
✓x7th **M48.51 Collapsed vertebra, not elsewhere classified, occipito-atlanto-axial** region `CC` `HCC`
✓x7th **M48.52 Collapsed vertebra, not elsewhere classified, cervical** region `CC` `HCC`
✓x7th **M48.53 Collapsed vertebra, not elsewhere classified, cervicothoracic** region `CC` `HCC`
✓x7th **M48.54 Collapsed vertebra, not elsewhere classified, thoracic** region `CC` `HCC`
✓x7th **M48.55 Collapsed vertebra, not elsewhere classified, thoracolumbar** region `CC` `HCC`
✓x7th **M48.56 Collapsed vertebra, not elsewhere classified, lumbar** region `CC` `HCC`
✓x7th **M48.57 Collapsed vertebra, not elsewhere classified, lumbosacral** region `CC` `HCC`

√x7ᵗʰ M48.58 Collapsed vertebra, not elsewhere classified, sacral and sacrococcygeal region `CC` `HCC`

√5ᵗʰ M48.8 Other specified spondylopathies
Ossification of posterior longitudinal ligament

√6ᵗʰ M48.8X Other specified spondylopathies
M48.8X1 Other specified spondylopathies, occipito-atlanto-axial region `HCC`
M48.8X2 Other specified spondylopathies, cervical region `HCC`
M48.8X3 Other specified spondylopathies, cervicothoracic region `HCC`
M48.8X4 Other specified spondylopathies, thoracic region `HCC`
M48.8X5 Other specified spondylopathies, thoracolumbar region `HCC`
M48.8X6 Other specified spondylopathies, lumbar region `HCC`
M48.8X7 Other specified spondylopathies, lumbosacral region `HCC`
M48.8X8 Other specified spondylopathies, sacral and sacrococcygeal region `HCC`
M48.8X9 Other specified spondylopathies, site unspecified `HCC`

M48.9 Spondylopathy, unspecified

√4ᵗʰ M49 Spondylopathies in diseases classified elsewhere
[INCLUDES] curvature of spine in diseases classified elsewhere
deformity of spine in diseases classified elsewhere
kyphosis in diseases classified elsewhere
scoliosis in diseases classified elsewhere
spondylopathy in diseases classified elsewhere

Code first underlying disease, such as:
brucellosis (A23.-)
Charcôt-Marie-Tooth disease (G60.0)
enterobacterial infections (A01-A04)
osteitis fibrosa cystica (E21.0)

[EXCLUDES 1] curvature of spine in tuberculosis [Pott's] (A18.01)
enteropathic arthropathies (M07.-)
gonococcal spondylitis (A54.41)
neuropathic spondylopathy in syringomyelia (G95.0)
neuropathic spondylopathy in tabes dorsalis (A52.11)
neuropathic [tabes dorsalis] spondylitis (A52.11)
nonsyphilitic neuropathic spondylopathy NEC (G98.0)
spondylitis in syphilis (acquired) (A52.77)
tuberculous spondylitis (A18.01)
typhoid fever spondylitis (A01.05)

√5ᵗʰ M49.8 Spondylopathy in diseases classified elsewhere
M49.80 *Spondylopathy in diseases classified elsewhere, site unspecified*
M49.81 *Spondylopathy in diseases classified elsewhere, occipito-atlanto-axial region*
M49.82 *Spondylopathy in diseases classified elsewhere, cervical region*
M49.83 *Spondylopathy in diseases classified elsewhere, cervicothoracic region*
M49.84 *Spondylopathy in diseases classified elsewhere, thoracic region*
M49.85 *Spondylopathy in diseases classified elsewhere, thoracolumbar region*
M49.86 *Spondylopathy in diseases classified elsewhere, lumbar region*
M49.87 *Spondylopathy in diseases classified elsewhere, lumbosacral region*
M49.88 *Spondylopathy in diseases classified elsewhere, sacral and sacrococcygeal region*
M49.89 *Spondylopathy in diseases classified elsewhere, multiple sites in spine*

Other dorsopathies (M50-M54)

[EXCLUDES 1] current injury - see injury of spine by body region
discitis NOS (M46.4-)

√4ᵗʰ M50 Cervical disc disorders
[INCLUDES] cervicothoracic disc disorders
cervicothoracic disc disorders with cervicalgia
AHA: 2016,4Q,39-40; 2016,1Q,17

√5ᵗʰ M50.0 Cervical disc disorder with myelopathy
AHA: 2018,3Q,19
M50.00 Cervical disc disorder with myelopathy, unspecified cervical region `CC` `UNS`
M50.01 Cervical disc disorder with myelopathy, high cervical region `CC`
C2-C3 disc disorder with myelopathy
C3-C4 disc disorder with myelopathy
√6ᵗʰ M50.02 Cervical disc disorder with myelopathy, mid-cervical region
M50.020 Cervical disc disorder with myelopathy, mid-cervical region, unspecified level `CC` `UNS`
M50.021 Cervical disc disorder at C4-C5 level with myelopathy `CC`
C4-C5 disc disorder with myelopathy
M50.022 Cervical disc disorder at C5-C6 level with myelopathy `CC`
C5-C6 disc disorder with myelopathy
M50.023 Cervical disc disorder at C6-C7 level with myelopathy `CC`
C6-C7 disc disorder with myelopathy
M50.03 Cervical disc disorder with myelopathy, cervicothoracic region `CC`
C7-T1 disc disorder with myelopathy

√5ᵗʰ M50.1 Cervical disc disorder with radiculopathy
[EXCLUDES 2] brachial radiculitis NOS (M54.13)
AHA: 2018,3Q,19
M50.10 Cervical disc disorder with radiculopathy, unspecified cervical region
M50.11 Cervical disc disorder with radiculopathy, high cervical region
C2-C3 disc disorder with radiculopathy
C3 radiculopathy due to disc disorder
C3-C4 disc disorder with radiculopathy
C4 radiculopathy due to disc disorder
√6ᵗʰ M50.12 Cervical disc disorder with radiculopathy, mid-cervical region
M50.120 Mid-cervical disc disorder, unspecified level
M50.121 Cervical disc disorder at C4-C5 level with radiculopathy
C4-C5 disc disorder with radiculopathy
C5 radiculopathy due to disc disorder
M50.122 Cervical disc disorder at C5-C6 level with radiculopathy
C5-C6 disc disorder with radiculopathy
C6 radiculopathy due to disc disorder
M50.123 Cervical disc disorder at C6-C7 level with radiculopathy
C6-C7 disc disorder with radiculopathy
C7 radiculopathy due to disc disorder
M50.13 Cervical disc disorder with radiculopathy, cervicothoracic region
C7-T1 disc disorder with radiculopathy
C8 radiculopathy due to disc disorder

√5ᵗʰ M50.2 Other cervical disc displacement
M50.20 Other cervical disc displacement, unspecified cervical region
M50.21 Other cervical disc displacement, high cervical region
Other C2-C3 cervical disc displacement
Other C3-C4 cervical disc displacement
√6ᵗʰ M50.22 Other cervical disc displacement, mid-cervical region
M50.220 Other cervical disc displacement, mid-cervical region, unspecified level
M50.221 Other cervical disc displacement at C4-C5 level
Other C4-C5 cervical disc displacement
M50.222 Other cervical disc displacement at C5-C6 level
Other C5-C6 cervical disc displacement

N Newborn: 0   **P** Pediatric: 0-17   **M** Maternity: 9-64   **A** Adult: 15-124   **UNS** Unspecified Site   **MCC** Major Complication/Comorbidity   **CC** Complication/Comorbidity   **PE** POA Exempt

814   **ICD-10-CM 2025**

M50.223 Other cervical disc displacement at C6-C7 level
Other C6-C7 cervical disc displacement

– **M50.23 Other cervical disc displacement, cervicothoracic region**
Other C7-T1 cervical disc displacement

✓5th **M50.3 Other cervical disc degeneration**

M50.30 Other cervical disc degeneration, unspecified cervical region

M50.31 Other cervical disc degeneration, high cervical region
Other C2-C3 cervical disc degeneration
Other C3-C4 cervical disc degeneration

✓6th **M50.32 Other cervical disc degeneration, mid-cervical region**

M50.320 Other cervical disc degeneration, mid-cervical region, unspecified level

M50.321 Other cervical disc degeneration at C4-C5 level
Other C4-C5 cervical disc degeneration

M50.322 Other cervical disc degeneration at C5-C6 level
Other C5-C6 cervical disc degeneration

M50.323 Other cervical disc degeneration at C6-C7 level
Other C6-C7 cervical disc degeneration

M50.33 Other cervical disc degeneration, cervicothoracic region
Other C7-T1 cervical disc degeneration

✓5th **M50.8 Other cervical disc disorders**

M50.80 Other cervical disc disorders, unspecified cervical region

M50.81 Other cervical disc disorders, high cervical region
Other C2-C3 cervical disc disorders
Other C3-C4 cervical disc disorders

✓6th **M50.82 Other cervical disc disorders, mid-cervical region**

M50.820 Other cervical disc disorders, mid-cervical region, unspecified level

M50.821 Other cervical disc disorders at C4-C5 level
Other C4-C5 cervical disc disorders

M50.822 Other cervical disc disorders at C5-C6 level
Other C5-C6 cervical disc disorders

M50.823 Other cervical disc disorders at C6-C7 level
Other C6-C7 cervical disc disorders

M50.83 Other cervical disc disorders, cervicothoracic region
Other C7-T1 cervical disc disorders

✓5th **M50.9 Cervical disc disorder, unspecified**

M50.90 Cervical disc disorder, unspecified, unspecified cervical region

M50.91 Cervical disc disorder, unspecified, high cervical region
C2-C3 cervical disc disorder, unspecified
C3-C4 cervical disc disorder, unspecified

✓6th **M50.92 Cervical disc disorder, unspecified, mid-cervical region**

M50.920 Unspecified cervical disc disorder, mid-cervical region, unspecified level

M50.921 Unspecified cervical disc disorder at C4-C5 level
Unspecified C4-C5 cervical disc disorder

M50.922 Unspecified cervical disc disorder at C5-C6 level
Unspecified C5-C6 cervical disc disorder

M50.923 Unspecified cervical disc disorder at C6-C7 level
Unspecified C6-C7 cervical disc disorder

M50.93 Cervical disc disorder, unspecified, cervicothoracic region
C7-T1 cervical disc disorder, unspecified

✓4th **M51 Thoracic, thoracolumbar, and lumbosacral intervertebral disc disorders**
EXCLUDES 2   cervical and cervicothoracic disc disorders (M50.-)
sacral and sacrococcygeal disorders (M53.3)

✓5th **M51.0 Thoracic, thoracolumbar and lumbosacral intervertebral disc disorders with myelopathy**

M51.04 Intervertebral disc disorders with myelopathy, thoracic region   CC

M51.05 Intervertebral disc disorders with myelopathy, thoracolumbar region   CC

M51.06 Intervertebral disc disorders with myelopathy, lumbar region   CC

✓5th **M51.1 Thoracic, thoracolumbar and lumbosacral intervertebral disc disorders with radiculopathy**
Sciatica due to intervertebral disc disorder
EXCLUDES 1   lumbar radiculitis NOS (M54.16)
sciatica NOS (M54.3)
AHA: 2018,3Q,18

M51.14 Intervertebral disc disorders with radiculopathy, thoracic region

M51.15 Intervertebral disc disorders with radiculopathy, thoracolumbar region

M51.16 Intervertebral disc disorders with radiculopathy, lumbar region

M51.17 Intervertebral disc disorders with radiculopathy, lumbosacral region

✓5th **M51.2 Other thoracic, thoracolumbar and lumbosacral intervertebral disc displacement**
Lumbago due to displacement of intervertebral disc
AHA: 2022,1Q,26

Displacement Intervertebral Disc

Nucleus pulposus · Lamina · Ligamentum flavum · Spinal cord · Herniates through annulus · Spinal nerve · Disc annulus · Nucleus pulposus

Normal Top View   Herniated Top View

M51.24 Other intervertebral disc displacement, thoracic region

M51.25 Other intervertebral disc displacement, thoracolumbar region

M51.26 Other intervertebral disc displacement, lumbar region

M51.27 Other intervertebral disc displacement, lumbosacral region

✓5th **M51.3 Other thoracic, thoracolumbar and lumbosacral intervertebral disc degeneration**
AHA: 2022,1Q,26; 2018,2Q,15; 2013,3Q,22

M51.34 Other intervertebral disc degeneration, thoracic region

M51.35 Other intervertebral disc degeneration, thoracolumbar region

✓6th **M51.36 Other intervertebral disc degeneration, lumbar region**

M51.360 Other intervertebral disc degeneration, lumbar region with discogenic back pain only
Other intervertebral disc degeneration, lumbar region with axial back pain only

M51.361 Other intervertebral disc degeneration, lumbar region with lower extremity pain only
Other intervertebral disc degeneration, lumbar region with leg pain only
Other intervertebral disc degeneration, lumbar region with referred sclerotomal pain only

M51.362 Other intervertebral disc degeneration, lumbar region with discogenic back pain and lower extremity pain
Other intervertebral disc degeneration, lumbar region with discogenic back pain and leg pain
Other intervertebral disc degeneration, lumbar region with axial back pain and referred sclerotomal pain

Chapter 13. Diseases of the Musculoskeletal System and Connective Tissue

M50.223–M51.362

Chapter 13. Diseases of the Musculoskeletal System and Connective Tissue

●   **M51.369 Other intervertebral disc degeneration, lumbar region without mention of lumbar back pain or lower extremity pain**
Other intervertebral disc degeneration, lumbar region without mention of lumbar back pain or leg pain
Other intervertebral disc degeneration, lumbar region, NOS

▲   √6ᵗʰ **M51.37 Other intervertebral disc degeneration, lumbosacral region**

●   **M51.370 Other intervertebral disc degeneration, lumbosacral region with discogenic back pain only**
Other intervertebral disc degeneration, lumbosacral region with axial back pain only

●   **M51.371 Other intervertebral disc degeneration, lumbosacral region with lower extremity pain only**
Other intervertebral disc degeneration, lumbosacral region with leg pain only
Other intervertebral disc degeneration, lumbosacral region with referred sclerotomal pain only

●   **M51.372 Other intervertebral disc degeneration, lumbosacral region with discogenic back pain and lower extremity pain**
Other intervertebral disc degeneration, lumbosacral region with discogenic back pain and leg pain
Other intervertebral disc degeneration, lumbosacral region with axial back pain and referred sclerotomal pain

●   **M51.379 Other intervertebral disc degeneration, lumbosacral region without mention of lumbar back pain or lower extremity pain**
Other intervertebral disc degeneration, lumbosacral region without mention of lumbar back pain or leg pain
Other intervertebral disc degeneration, lumbosacral region, NOS

√5ᵗʰ **M51.4 Schmorl's nodes**
DEF: Irregular bone defect in the margin of the vertebral body that causes herniation into the end plate of the vertebral body.
M51.44 Schmorl's nodes, thoracic region
M51.45 Schmorl's nodes, thoracolumbar region
M51.46 Schmorl's nodes, lumbar region
M51.47 Schmorl's nodes, lumbosacral region

√5ᵗʰ **M51.8 Other thoracic, thoracolumbar and lumbosacral intervertebral disc disorders**
M51.84 Other intervertebral disc disorders, thoracic region
M51.85 Other intervertebral disc disorders, thoracolumbar region
M51.86 Other intervertebral disc disorders, lumbar region
M51.87 Other intervertebral disc disorders, lumbosacral region

M51.9 Unspecified thoracic, thoracolumbar and lumbosacral intervertebral disc disorder

√5ᵗʰ **M51.A Other lumbar and lumbosacral annulus fibrosus disc defects**
AHA: 2022,4Q,28-29
M51.A0 Intervertebral annulus fibrosus defect, lumbar region, unspecified size
Code first, if applicable, lumbar disc herniation (M51.06, M51.16, M51.26)
M51.A1 Intervertebral annulus fibrosus defect, small, lumbar region
Code first, if applicable, lumbar disc herniation (M51.06, M51.16, M51.26)
M51.A2 Intervertebral annulus fibrosus defect, large, lumbar region
Code first, if applicable, lumbar disc herniation (M51.06, M51.16, M51.26)
M51.A3 Intervertebral annulus fibrosus defect, lumbosacral region, unspecified size
Code first, if applicable, lumbosacral disc herniation (M51.17, M51.27)
M51.A4 Intervertebral annulus fibrosus defect, small, lumbosacral region
Code first, if applicable, lumbosacral disc herniation (M51.17, M51.27)

M51.A5 Intervertebral annulus fibrosus defect, large, lumbosacral region
Code first, if applicable, lumbosacral disc herniation (M51.17, M51.27)

√4ᵗʰ **M53 Other and unspecified dorsopathies, not elsewhere classified**

M53.0 Cervicocranial syndrome
Posterior cervical sympathetic syndrome

M53.1 Cervicobrachial syndrome
EXCLUDES 2   cervical disc disorder (M50.-)
thoracic outlet syndrome (G54.0)

√5ᵗʰ **M53.2 Spinal instabilities**
√6ᵗʰ **M53.2X Spinal instabilities**
M53.2X1 Spinal instabilities, occipito-atlanto-axial region
M53.2X2 Spinal instabilities, cervical region
M53.2X3 Spinal instabilities, cervicothoracic region
M53.2X4 Spinal instabilities, thoracic region
M53.2X5 Spinal instabilities, thoracolumbar region
M53.2X6 Spinal instabilities, lumbar region
M53.2X7 Spinal instabilities, lumbosacral region
M53.2X8 Spinal instabilities, sacral and sacrococcygeal region
M53.2X9 Spinal instabilities, site unspecified

M53.3 Sacrococcygeal disorders, not elsewhere classified
Coccygodynia

√5ᵗʰ **M53.8 Other specified dorsopathies**
M53.80 Other specified dorsopathies, site unspecified
M53.81 Other specified dorsopathies, occipito-atlanto-axial region
M53.82 Other specified dorsopathies, cervical region
M53.83 Other specified dorsopathies, cervicothoracic region
M53.84 Other specified dorsopathies, thoracic region
M53.85 Other specified dorsopathies, thoracolumbar region
M53.86 Other specified dorsopathies, lumbar region
M53.87 Other specified dorsopathies, lumbosacral region
M53.88 Other specified dorsopathies, sacral and sacrococcygeal region
M53.9 Dorsopathy, unspecified

√4ᵗʰ **M54 Dorsalgia**
EXCLUDES 1   psychogenic dorsalgia (F45.41)

√5ᵗʰ **M54.0 Panniculitis affecting regions of neck and back**
EXCLUDES 1   lupus panniculitis (L93.2)
panniculitis NOS (M79.3)
relapsing [Weber-Christian] panniculitis (M35.6)
M54.00 Panniculitis affecting regions of neck and back, site unspecified
M54.01 Panniculitis affecting regions of neck and back, occipito-atlanto-axial region
M54.02 Panniculitis affecting regions of neck and back, cervical region
M54.03 Panniculitis affecting regions of neck and back, cervicothoracic region
M54.04 Panniculitis affecting regions of neck and back, thoracic region
M54.05 Panniculitis affecting regions of neck and back, thoracolumbar region
M54.06 Panniculitis affecting regions of neck and back, lumbar region
M54.07 Panniculitis affecting regions of neck and back, lumbosacral region
M54.08 Panniculitis affecting regions of neck and back, sacral and sacrococcygeal region
M54.09 Panniculitis affecting regions, neck and back, multiple sites in spine

✓5ᵗʰ **M54.1 Radiculopathy**

Brachial neuritis or radiculitis NOS
Lumbar neuritis or radiculitis NOS
Lumbosacral neuritis or radiculitis NOS
Radiculitis NOS
Thoracic neuritis or radiculitis NOS

EXCLUDES 1   *neuralgia and neuritis NOS (M79.2)*
radiculopathy with cervical disc disorder (M50.1)
radiculopathy with lumbar and other intervertebral disc disorder (M51.1-)
radiculopathy with spondylosis (M47.2-)

AHA: 2018,3Q,18

TIP: A code from this subcategory can be used in addition to a spondylolisthesis code (M43.1-) or a spinal stenosis code (M48.0-) when either condition is documented as the cause of the radiculopathy.

M54.10 **Radiculopathy, site unspecified**
M54.11 **Radiculopathy, occipito-atlanto-axial region**
M54.12 **Radiculopathy, cervical region**
M54.13 **Radiculopathy, cervicothoracic region**
M54.14 **Radiculopathy, thoracic region**
M54.15 **Radiculopathy, thoracolumbar region**
M54.16 **Radiculopathy, lumbar region**
M54.17 **Radiculopathy, lumbosacral region**
M54.18 **Radiculopathy, sacral and sacrococcygeal region**

M54.2 Cervicalgia

EXCLUDES 1   *cervicalgia due to intervertebral cervical disc disorder (M50.-)*

✓5ᵗʰ **M54.3 Sciatica**

EXCLUDES 1   ▶*intervertebral disc degeneration, lumbar region with lower extremity pain only (M51.361)*◀
▶*intervertebral disc degeneration, lumbosacral region with lower extremity pain only (M51.371)*◀
lesion of sciatic nerve (G57.0)
sciatica due to intervertebral disc disorder (M51.1-)
sciatica with lumbago (M54.4-)

M54.30 **Sciatica, unspecified side**
M54.31 **Sciatica, right side**
M54.32 **Sciatica, left side**

✓5ᵗʰ **M54.4 Lumbago with sciatica**

EXCLUDES 1   ▶*intervertebral disc degeneration, lumbar region with discogenic back pain and lower extremity pain (M51.362)*◀
▶*intervertebral disc degeneration, lumbosacral region with discogenic back pain and lower extremity pain (M51.372)*◀
lumbago with sciatica due to intervertebral disc disorder (M51.1-)

AHA: 2016,2Q,7

M54.40 **Lumbago with sciatica, unspecified side**
M54.41 **Lumbago with sciatica, right side**
M54.42 **Lumbago with sciatica, left side**

✓5ᵗʰ **M54.5 Low back pain**

EXCLUDES 1   ▶*intervertebral disc degeneration, lumbar region with discogenic back pain only (M51.360)*◀
▶*intervertebral disc degeneration, lumbosacral region with discogenic back pain only (M51.370)*◀
low back strain (S39.012)
lumbago due to intervertebral disc displacement (M51.2-)
lumbago with sciatica (M54.4-)

AHA: 2021,4Q,22

M54.50 **Low back pain, unspecified**
Loin pain
Lumbago NOS
M54.51 **Vertebrogenic low back pain**
Low back vertebral endplate pain
M54.59 **Other low back pain**

M54.6 Pain in thoracic spine

EXCLUDES 1   *pain in thoracic spine due to intervertebral disc disorder (M51.-)*

✓5ᵗʰ **M54.8 Other dorsalgia**

EXCLUDES 1   *dorsalgia in thoracic region (M54.6)*
low back pain (M54.5-)

M54.81 **Occipital neuralgia**
M54.89 **Other dorsalgia**

M54.9 **Dorsalgia, unspecified**
Backache NOS
Back pain NOS

SOFT TISSUE DISORDERS (M60-M79)

Disorders of muscles (M60-M63)

EXCLUDES 1   *dermatopolymyositis (M33.-)*
myopathy in amyloidosis (E85.-)
myopathy in polyarteritis nodosa (M30.0)
myopathy in rheumatoid arthritis (M05.32)
myopathy in scleroderma (M34.-)
myopathy in Sjögren's syndrome (M35.03)
myopathy in systemic lupus erythematosus (M32.-)

EXCLUDES 2   *muscular dystrophies and myopathies (G71-G72)*

✓4ᵗʰ **M60 Myositis**

EXCLUDES 2   *inclusion body myositis [IBM] (G72.41)*

✓5ᵗʰ **M60.0 Infective myositis**
Tropical pyomyositis
Use additional code (B95-B97) to identify infectious agent

✓6ᵗʰ M60.00 **Infective myositis, unspecified site**

M60.000 **Infective myositis, unspecified right arm** CC
Infective myositis, right upper limb NOS
M60.001 **Infective myositis, unspecified left arm** CC
Infective myositis, left upper limb NOS
M60.002 **Infective myositis, unspecified arm** CC UNS
Infective myositis, upper limb NOS
M60.003 **Infective myositis, unspecified right leg** CC
Infective myositis, right lower limb NOS
M60.004 **Infective myositis, unspecified left leg** CC
Infective myositis, left lower limb NOS
M60.005 **Infective myositis, unspecified leg** CC UNS
Infective myositis, lower limb NOS
M60.009 **Infective myositis, unspecified site** CC UNS

✓6ᵗʰ M60.01 **Infective myositis, shoulder**

M60.011 **Infective myositis, right shoulder** CC
M60.012 **Infective myositis, left shoulder** CC
M60.019 **Infective myositis, unspecified shoulder** CC UNS

✓6ᵗʰ M60.02 **Infective myositis, upper arm**

M60.021 **Infective myositis, right upper arm** CC
M60.022 **Infective myositis, left upper arm** CC
M60.029 **Infective myositis, unspecified upper arm** CC UNS

✓6ᵗʰ M60.03 **Infective myositis, forearm**

M60.031 **Infective myositis, right forearm** CC
M60.032 **Infective myositis, left forearm** CC
M60.039 **Infective myositis, unspecified forearm** CC UNS

✓6ᵗʰ M60.04 **Infective myositis, hand and fingers**

M60.041 **Infective myositis, right hand** CC
M60.042 **Infective myositis, left hand** CC
M60.043 **Infective myositis, unspecified hand** CC UNS
M60.044 **Infective myositis, right finger(s)** CC
M60.045 **Infective myositis, left finger(s)** CC
M60.046 **Infective myositis, unspecified finger(s)** CC UNS

✓6ᵗʰ M60.05 **Infective myositis, thigh**

M60.051 **Infective myositis, right thigh** CC
M60.052 **Infective myositis, left thigh** CC
M60.059 **Infective myositis, unspecified thigh** CC UNS

✓6ᵗʰ M60.06 **Infective myositis, lower leg**

M60.061 **Infective myositis, right lower leg** CC
M60.062 **Infective myositis, left lower leg** CC
M60.069 **Infective myositis, unspecified lower leg** CC UNS

√6ᵗʰ **M60.07** Infective myositis, **ankle, foot and toes**
     M60.070 Infective myositis, **right ankle** `CC`
     M60.071 Infective myositis, **left ankle** `CC`
     M60.072 Infective myositis, unspecified ankle `CC` `UNS`
     M60.073 Infective myositis, **right foot** `CC`
     M60.074 Infective myositis, **left foot** `CC`
     M60.075 Infective myositis, unspecified foot `CC` `UNS`
     M60.076 Infective myositis, **right toe(s)** `CC`
     M60.077 Infective myositis, **left toe(s)** `CC`
     M60.078 Infective myositis, unspecified toe(s) `CC` `UNS`
M60.08 Infective myositis, other site `CC`
M60.09 Infective myositis, **multiple sites** `CC`

√5ᵗʰ **M60.1** Interstitial myositis
     M60.10 Interstitial myositis of unspecified site
√6ᵗʰ **M60.11** Interstitial myositis, **shoulder**
     M60.111 Interstitial myositis, **right** shoulder
     M60.112 Interstitial myositis, **left** shoulder
     M60.119 Interstitial myositis, unspecified shoulder
√6ᵗʰ **M60.12** Interstitial myositis, **upper arm**
     M60.121 Interstitial myositis, **right** upper arm
     M60.122 Interstitial myositis, **left** upper arm
     M60.129 Interstitial myositis, unspecified upper arm
√6ᵗʰ **M60.13** Interstitial myositis, **forearm**
     M60.131 Interstitial myositis, **right** forearm
     M60.132 Interstitial myositis, **left** forearm
     M60.139 Interstitial myositis, unspecified forearm
√6ᵗʰ **M60.14** Interstitial myositis, **hand**
     M60.141 Interstitial myositis, **right** hand
     M60.142 Interstitial myositis, **left** hand
     M60.149 Interstitial myositis, unspecified hand
√6ᵗʰ **M60.15** Interstitial myositis, **thigh**
     M60.151 Interstitial myositis, **right** thigh
     M60.152 Interstitial myositis, **left** thigh
     M60.159 Interstitial myositis, unspecified thigh
√6ᵗʰ **M60.16** Interstitial myositis, **lower leg**
     M60.161 Interstitial myositis, **right** lower leg
     M60.162 Interstitial myositis, **left** lower leg
     M60.169 Interstitial myositis, unspecified lower leg
√6ᵗʰ **M60.17** Interstitial myositis, **ankle and foot**
     M60.171 Interstitial myositis, **right** ankle and foot
     M60.172 Interstitial myositis, **left** ankle and foot
     M60.179 Interstitial myositis, unspecified ankle and foot
M60.18 Interstitial myositis, other site
M60.19 Interstitial myositis, **multiple sites**

√5ᵗʰ **M60.2** Foreign body granuloma of soft tissue, not elsewhere classified
Use additional code to identify the type of retained foreign body (Z18.-)
> **EXCLUDES 1** *foreign body granuloma of skin and subcutaneous tissue (L92.3)*

     M60.20 Foreign body granuloma of soft tissue, not elsewhere classified, unspecified site
√6ᵗʰ **M60.21** Foreign body granuloma of soft tissue, not elsewhere classified, **shoulder**
     M60.211 Foreign body granuloma of soft tissue, not elsewhere classified, **right** shoulder
     M60.212 Foreign body granuloma of soft tissue, not elsewhere classified, **left** shoulder
     M60.219 Foreign body granuloma of soft tissue, not elsewhere classified, unspecified shoulder
√6ᵗʰ **M60.22** Foreign body granuloma of soft tissue, not elsewhere classified, **upper arm**
     M60.221 Foreign body granuloma of soft tissue, not elsewhere classified, **right** upper arm
     M60.222 Foreign body granuloma of soft tissue, not elsewhere classified, **left** upper arm
     M60.229 Foreign body granuloma of soft tissue, not elsewhere classified, unspecified upper arm
√6ᵗʰ **M60.23** Foreign body granuloma of soft tissue, not elsewhere classified, **forearm**
     M60.231 Foreign body granuloma of soft tissue, not elsewhere classified, **right** forearm
     M60.232 Foreign body granuloma of soft tissue, not elsewhere classified, **left** forearm
     M60.239 Foreign body granuloma of soft tissue, not elsewhere classified, unspecified forearm
√6ᵗʰ **M60.24** Foreign body granuloma of soft tissue, not elsewhere classified, **hand**
     M60.241 Foreign body granuloma of soft tissue, not elsewhere classified, **right** hand
     M60.242 Foreign body granuloma of soft tissue, not elsewhere classified, **left** hand
     M60.249 Foreign body granuloma of soft tissue, not elsewhere classified, unspecified hand
√6ᵗʰ **M60.25** Foreign body granuloma of soft tissue, not elsewhere classified, **thigh**
     M60.251 Foreign body granuloma of soft tissue, not elsewhere classified, **right** thigh
     M60.252 Foreign body granuloma of soft tissue, not elsewhere classified, **left** thigh
     M60.259 Foreign body granuloma of soft tissue, not elsewhere classified, unspecified thigh
√6ᵗʰ **M60.26** Foreign body granuloma of soft tissue, not elsewhere classified, **lower leg**
     M60.261 Foreign body granuloma of soft tissue, not elsewhere classified, **right** lower leg
     M60.262 Foreign body granuloma of soft tissue, not elsewhere classified, **left** lower leg
     M60.269 Foreign body granuloma of soft tissue, not elsewhere classified, unspecified lower leg
√6ᵗʰ **M60.27** Foreign body granuloma of soft tissue, not elsewhere classified, **ankle and foot**
     M60.271 Foreign body granuloma of soft tissue, not elsewhere classified, **right** ankle and foot
     M60.272 Foreign body granuloma of soft tissue, not elsewhere classified, **left** ankle and foot
     M60.279 Foreign body granuloma of soft tissue, not elsewhere classified, unspecified ankle and foot
M60.28 Foreign body granuloma of soft tissue, not elsewhere classified, other site

√5ᵗʰ **M60.8** Other myositis
     M60.80 Other myositis, unspecified site
√6ᵗʰ **M60.81** Other myositis **shoulder**
     M60.811 Other myositis, **right** shoulder
     M60.812 Other myositis, **left** shoulder
     M60.819 Other myositis, unspecified shoulder
√6ᵗʰ **M60.82** Other myositis, **upper arm**
     M60.821 Other myositis, **right** upper arm
     M60.822 Other myositis, **left** upper arm
     M60.829 Other myositis, unspecified upper arm
√6ᵗʰ **M60.83** Other myositis, **forearm**
     M60.831 Other myositis, **right** forearm
     M60.832 Other myositis, **left** forearm
     M60.839 Other myositis, unspecified forearm
√6ᵗʰ **M60.84** Other myositis, **hand**
     M60.841 Other myositis, **right** hand
     M60.842 Other myositis, **left** hand
     M60.849 Other myositis, unspecified hand
√6ᵗʰ **M60.85** Other myositis, **thigh**
     M60.851 Other myositis, **right** thigh
     M60.852 Other myositis, **left** thigh
     M60.859 Other myositis, unspecified thigh
√6ᵗʰ **M60.86** Other myositis, **lower leg**
     M60.861 Other myositis, **right** lower leg
     M60.862 Other myositis, **left** lower leg
     M60.869 Other myositis, unspecified lower leg
√6ᵗʰ **M60.87** Other myositis, **ankle and foot**
     M60.871 Other myositis, **right** ankle and foot
     M60.872 Other myositis, **left** ankle and foot
     M60.879 Other myositis, unspecified ankle and foot
M60.88 Other myositis, other site
M60.89 Other myositis, **multiple sites**
M60.9 Myositis, unspecified

√4ᵗʰ **M61** Calcification and ossification of muscle
√5ᵗʰ **M61.0** Myositis ossificans **traumatica**
     M61.00 Myositis ossificans traumatica, unspecified site
√6ᵗʰ **M61.01** Myositis ossificans traumatica, **shoulder**
     M61.011 Myositis ossificans traumatica, **right** shoulder

     M61.012 Myositis ossificans traumatica, left shoulder

     M61.019 Myositis ossificans traumatica, unspecified shoulder

✓6ᵗʰ M61.02 Myositis ossificans traumatica, upper arm

     M61.021 Myositis ossificans traumatica, right upper arm

     M61.022 Myositis ossificans traumatica, left upper arm

     M61.029 Myositis ossificans traumatica, unspecified upper arm

✓6ᵗʰ M61.03 Myositis ossificans traumatica, forearm

     M61.031 Myositis ossificans traumatica, right forearm

     M61.032 Myositis ossificans traumatica, left forearm

     M61.039 Myositis ossificans traumatica, unspecified forearm

✓6ᵗʰ M61.04 Myositis ossificans traumatica, hand

     M61.041 Myositis ossificans traumatica, right hand

     M61.042 Myositis ossificans traumatica, left hand

     M61.049 Myositis ossificans traumatica, unspecified hand

✓6ᵗʰ M61.05 Myositis ossificans traumatica, thigh

     M61.051 Myositis ossificans traumatica, right thigh

     M61.052 Myositis ossificans traumatica, left thigh

     M61.059 Myositis ossificans traumatica, unspecified thigh

✓6ᵗʰ M61.06 Myositis ossificans traumatica, lower leg

     M61.061 Myositis ossificans traumatica, right lower leg

     M61.062 Myositis ossificans traumatica, left lower leg

     M61.069 Myositis ossificans traumatica, unspecified lower leg

✓6ᵗʰ M61.07 Myositis ossificans traumatica, ankle and foot

     M61.071 Myositis ossificans traumatica, right ankle and foot

     M61.072 Myositis ossificans traumatica, left ankle and foot

     M61.079 Myositis ossificans traumatica, unspecified ankle and foot

M61.08 Myositis ossificans traumatica, other site

M61.09 Myositis ossificans traumatica, multiple sites

✓5ᵗʰ M61.1 Myositis ossificans progressiva

     Fibrodysplasia ossificans progressiva

     M61.10 Myositis ossificans progressiva, unspecified site

✓6ᵗʰ M61.11 Myositis ossificans progressiva, shoulder

     M61.111 Myositis ossificans progressiva, right shoulder

     M61.112 Myositis ossificans progressiva, left shoulder

     M61.119 Myositis ossificans progressiva, unspecified shoulder

✓6ᵗʰ M61.12 Myositis ossificans progressiva, upper arm

     M61.121 Myositis ossificans progressiva, right upper arm

     M61.122 Myositis ossificans progressiva, left upper arm

     M61.129 Myositis ossificans progressiva, unspecified arm

✓6ᵗʰ M61.13 Myositis ossificans progressiva, forearm

     M61.131 Myositis ossificans progressiva, right forearm

     M61.132 Myositis ossificans progressiva, left forearm

     M61.139 Myositis ossificans progressiva, unspecified forearm

✓6ᵗʰ M61.14 Myositis ossificans progressiva, hand and finger(s)

     M61.141 Myositis ossificans progressiva, right hand

     M61.142 Myositis ossificans progressiva, left hand

     M61.143 Myositis ossificans progressiva, unspecified hand

     M61.144 Myositis ossificans progressiva, right finger(s)

     M61.145 Myositis ossificans progressiva, left finger(s)

     M61.146 Myositis ossificans progressiva, unspecified finger(s)

✓6ᵗʰ M61.15 Myositis ossificans progressiva, thigh

     M61.151 Myositis ossificans progressiva, right thigh

     M61.152 Myositis ossificans progressiva, left thigh

     M61.159 Myositis ossificans progressiva, unspecified thigh

✓6ᵗʰ M61.16 Myositis ossificans progressiva, lower leg

     M61.161 Myositis ossificans progressiva, right lower leg

     M61.162 Myositis ossificans progressiva, left lower leg

     M61.169 Myositis ossificans progressiva, unspecified lower leg

✓6ᵗʰ M61.17 Myositis ossificans progressiva, ankle, foot and toe(s)

     M61.171 Myositis ossificans progressiva, right ankle

     M61.172 Myositis ossificans progressiva, left ankle

     M61.173 Myositis ossificans progressiva, unspecified ankle

     M61.174 Myositis ossificans progressiva, right foot

     M61.175 Myositis ossificans progressiva, left foot

     M61.176 Myositis ossificans progressiva, unspecified foot

     M61.177 Myositis ossificans progressiva, right toe(s)

     M61.178 Myositis ossificans progressiva, left toe(s)

     M61.179 Myositis ossificans progressiva, unspecified toe(s)

M61.18 Myositis ossificans progressiva, other site

M61.19 Myositis ossificans progressiva, multiple sites

✓5ᵗʰ M61.2 Paralytic calcification and ossification of muscle

     Myositis ossificans associated with quadriplegia or paraplegia

     M61.20 Paralytic calcification and ossification of muscle, unspecified site

✓6ᵗʰ M61.21 Paralytic calcification and ossification of muscle, shoulder

     M61.211 Paralytic calcification and ossification of muscle, right shoulder

     M61.212 Paralytic calcification and ossification of muscle, left shoulder

     M61.219 Paralytic calcification and ossification of muscle, unspecified shoulder

✓6ᵗʰ M61.22 Paralytic calcification and ossification of muscle, upper arm

     M61.221 Paralytic calcification and ossification of muscle, right upper arm

     M61.222 Paralytic calcification and ossification of muscle, left upper arm

     M61.229 Paralytic calcification and ossification of muscle, unspecified upper arm

✓6ᵗʰ M61.23 Paralytic calcification and ossification of muscle, forearm

     M61.231 Paralytic calcification and ossification of muscle, right forearm

     M61.232 Paralytic calcification and ossification of muscle, left forearm

     M61.239 Paralytic calcification and ossification of muscle, unspecified forearm

✓6ᵗʰ M61.24 Paralytic calcification and ossification of muscle, hand

     M61.241 Paralytic calcification and ossification of muscle, right hand

     M61.242 Paralytic calcification and ossification of muscle, left hand

     M61.249 Paralytic calcification and ossification of muscle, unspecified hand

✓6ᵗʰ M61.25 Paralytic calcification and ossification of muscle, thigh

     M61.251 Paralytic calcification and ossification of muscle, right thigh

     M61.252 Paralytic calcification and ossification of muscle, left thigh

     M61.259 Paralytic calcification and ossification of muscle, unspecified thigh

✓6ᵗʰ M61.26 Paralytic calcification and ossification of muscle, lower leg

     M61.261 Paralytic calcification and ossification of muscle, right lower leg

     M61.262 Paralytic calcification and ossification of muscle, left lower leg

     M61.269 Paralytic calcification and ossification of muscle, unspecified lower leg

✔ Additional Character Required   ✓x7ᵗʰ Placeholder   Questionable PDx   Manifestation   Unspecified   UPD Unacceptable PDx   H1 - H14 HAC   HCC CMS-HCC Dx   HIV HIV Dx

ICD-10-CM 2025   819

✓6ᵗʰ **M61.27 Paralytic calcification and ossification of muscle, ankle and foot**

    M61.271 Paralytic calcification and ossification of muscle, right ankle and foot

    M61.272 Paralytic calcification and ossification of muscle, left ankle and foot

    M61.279 Paralytic calcification and ossification of muscle, unspecified ankle and foot

M61.28 Paralytic calcification and ossification of muscle, other site

M61.29 Paralytic calcification and ossification of muscle, multiple sites

✓5ᵗʰ **M61.3 Calcification and ossification of muscles associated with burns**

    Myositis ossificans associated with burns

    M61.30 Calcification and ossification of muscles associated with burns, unspecified site

✓6ᵗʰ   **M61.31 Calcification and ossification of muscles associated with burns, shoulder**

    M61.311 Calcification and ossification of muscles associated with burns, right shoulder

    M61.312 Calcification and ossification of muscles associated with burns, left shoulder

    M61.319 Calcification and ossification of muscles associated with burns, unspecified shoulder

✓6ᵗʰ   **M61.32 Calcification and ossification of muscles associated with burns, upper arm**

    M61.321 Calcification and ossification of muscles associated with burns, right upper arm

    M61.322 Calcification and ossification of muscles associated with burns, left upper arm

    M61.329 Calcification and ossification of muscles associated with burns, unspecified upper arm

✓6ᵗʰ   **M61.33 Calcification and ossification of muscles associated with burns, forearm**

    M61.331 Calcification and ossification of muscles associated with burns, right forearm

    M61.332 Calcification and ossification of muscles associated with burns, left forearm

    M61.339 Calcification and ossification of muscles associated with burns, unspecified forearm

✓6ᵗʰ   **M61.34 Calcification and ossification of muscles associated with burns, hand**

    M61.341 Calcification and ossification of muscles associated with burns, right hand

    M61.342 Calcification and ossification of muscles associated with burns, left hand

    M61.349 Calcification and ossification of muscles associated with burns, unspecified hand

✓6ᵗʰ   **M61.35 Calcification and ossification of muscles associated with burns, thigh**

    M61.351 Calcification and ossification of muscles associated with burns, right thigh

    M61.352 Calcification and ossification of muscles associated with burns, left thigh

    M61.359 Calcification and ossification of muscles associated with burns, unspecified thigh

✓6ᵗʰ   **M61.36 Calcification and ossification of muscles associated with burns, lower leg**

    M61.361 Calcification and ossification of muscles associated with burns, right lower leg

    M61.362 Calcification and ossification of muscles associated with burns, left lower leg

    M61.369 Calcification and ossification of muscles associated with burns, unspecified lower leg

✓6ᵗʰ   **M61.37 Calcification and ossification of muscles associated with burns, ankle and foot**

    M61.371 Calcification and ossification of muscles associated with burns, right ankle and foot

    M61.372 Calcification and ossification of muscles associated with burns, left ankle and foot

    M61.379 Calcification and ossification of muscles associated with burns, unspecified ankle and foot

M61.38 Calcification and ossification of muscles associated with burns, other site

M61.39 Calcification and ossification of muscles associated with burns, multiple sites

✓5ᵗʰ **M61.4 Other calcification of muscle**

    EXCLUDES 1   *calcific tendinitis NOS (M65.2-)*

                  calcific tendinitis of shoulder (M75.3)

    M61.40 Other calcification of muscle, unspecified site

✓6ᵗʰ   **M61.41 Other calcification of muscle, shoulder**

    M61.411 Other calcification of muscle, right shoulder

    M61.412 Other calcification of muscle, left shoulder

    M61.419 Other calcification of muscle, unspecified shoulder

✓6ᵗʰ   **M61.42 Other calcification of muscle, upper arm**

    M61.421 Other calcification of muscle, right upper arm

    M61.422 Other calcification of muscle, left upper arm

    M61.429 Other calcification of muscle, unspecified upper arm

✓6ᵗʰ   **M61.43 Other calcification of muscle, forearm**

    M61.431 Other calcification of muscle, right forearm

    M61.432 Other calcification of muscle, left forearm

    M61.439 Other calcification of muscle, unspecified forearm

✓6ᵗʰ   **M61.44 Other calcification of muscle, hand**

    M61.441 Other calcification of muscle, right hand

    M61.442 Other calcification of muscle, left hand

    M61.449 Other calcification of muscle, unspecified hand

✓6ᵗʰ   **M61.45 Other calcification of muscle, thigh**

    M61.451 Other calcification of muscle, right thigh

    M61.452 Other calcification of muscle, left thigh

    M61.459 Other calcification of muscle, unspecified thigh

✓6ᵗʰ   **M61.46 Other calcification of muscle, lower leg**

    M61.461 Other calcification of muscle, right lower leg

    M61.462 Other calcification of muscle, left lower leg

    M61.469 Other calcification of muscle, unspecified lower leg

✓6ᵗʰ   **M61.47 Other calcification of muscle, ankle and foot**

    M61.471 Other calcification of muscle, right ankle and foot

    M61.472 Other calcification of muscle, left ankle and foot

    M61.479 Other calcification of muscle, unspecified ankle and foot

M61.48 Other calcification of muscle, other site

M61.49 Other calcification of muscle, multiple sites

✓5ᵗʰ **M61.5 Other ossification of muscle**

    M61.50 Other ossification of muscle, unspecified site

✓6ᵗʰ   **M61.51 Other ossification of muscle, shoulder**

    M61.511 Other ossification of muscle, right shoulder

    M61.512 Other ossification of muscle, left shoulder

    M61.519 Other ossification of muscle, unspecified shoulder

✓6ᵗʰ   **M61.52 Other ossification of muscle, upper arm**

    M61.521 Other ossification of muscle, right upper arm

    M61.522 Other ossification of muscle, left upper arm

    M61.529 Other ossification of muscle, unspecified upper arm

✓6ᵗʰ   **M61.53 Other ossification of muscle, forearm**

    M61.531 Other ossification of muscle, right forearm

    M61.532 Other ossification of muscle, left forearm

    M61.539 Other ossification of muscle, unspecified forearm

✓6ᵗʰ   **M61.54 Other ossification of muscle, hand**

    M61.541 Other ossification of muscle, right hand

    M61.542 Other ossification of muscle, left hand

    M61.549 Other ossification of muscle, unspecified hand

✓6ᵗʰ   **M61.55 Other ossification of muscle, thigh**

    M61.551 Other ossification of muscle, right thigh

    M61.552 Other ossification of muscle, left thigh

    M61.559 Other ossification of muscle, unspecified thigh

N Newborn: 0   **P** Pediatric: 0-17   **M** Maternity: 9-64   **A** Adult: 15-124   **UNS** Unspecified Site   **MCC** Major Complication/Comorbidity   **CC** Complication/Comorbidity   **PE** POA Exempt

820   ICD-10-CM 2025

✓6th **M61.56** Other ossification of muscle, lower leg

     M61.561 Other ossification of muscle, right lower leg

     M61.562 Other ossification of muscle, left lower leg

     M61.569 Other ossification of muscle, unspecified lower leg

✓6th **M61.57** Other ossification of muscle, ankle and foot

     M61.571 Other ossification of muscle, right ankle and foot

     M61.572 Other ossification of muscle, left ankle and foot

     M61.579 Other ossification of muscle, unspecified ankle and foot

M61.58 Other ossification of muscle, other site

M61.59 Other ossification of muscle, multiple sites

M61.9 Calcification and ossification of muscle, unspecified

✓4th **M62** **Other disorders of muscle**

     EXCLUDES 1   *alcoholic myopathy (G72.1)*

               cramp and spasm (R25.2)

               drug-induced myopathy (G72.0)

               myalgia (M79.1-)

               stiff-man syndrome (G25.82)

     EXCLUDES 2   *nontraumatic hematoma of muscle (M79.81)*

✓5th **M62.0** **Separation of muscle (nontraumatic)**

     Diastasis of muscle

     EXCLUDES 1   *diastasis recti complicating pregnancy, labor and delivery (O71.8)*

               traumatic separation of muscle - see strain of muscle by body region

     M62.00 Separation of muscle (nontraumatic), unspecified site

✓6th **M62.01** Separation of muscle (nontraumatic), shoulder

     M62.011 Separation of muscle (nontraumatic), right shoulder

     M62.012 Separation of muscle (nontraumatic), left shoulder

     M62.019 Separation of muscle (nontraumatic), unspecified shoulder

✓6th **M62.02** Separation of muscle (nontraumatic), upper arm

     M62.021 Separation of muscle (nontraumatic), right upper arm

     M62.022 Separation of muscle (nontraumatic), left upper arm

     M62.029 Separation of muscle (nontraumatic), unspecified upper arm

✓6th **M62.03** Separation of muscle (nontraumatic), forearm

     M62.031 Separation of muscle (nontraumatic), right forearm

     M62.032 Separation of muscle (nontraumatic), left forearm

     M62.039 Separation of muscle (nontraumatic), unspecified forearm

✓6th **M62.04** Separation of muscle (nontraumatic), hand

     M62.041 Separation of muscle (nontraumatic), right hand

     M62.042 Separation of muscle (nontraumatic), left hand

     M62.049 Separation of muscle (nontraumatic), unspecified hand

✓6th **M62.05** Separation of muscle (nontraumatic), thigh

     M62.051 Separation of muscle (nontraumatic), right thigh

     M62.052 Separation of muscle (nontraumatic), left thigh

     M62.059 Separation of muscle (nontraumatic), unspecified thigh

✓6th **M62.06** Separation of muscle (nontraumatic), lower leg

     M62.061 Separation of muscle (nontraumatic), right lower leg

     M62.062 Separation of muscle (nontraumatic), left lower leg

     M62.069 Separation of muscle (nontraumatic), unspecified lower leg

✓6th **M62.07** Separation of muscle (nontraumatic), ankle and foot

     M62.071 Separation of muscle (nontraumatic), right ankle and foot

     M62.072 Separation of muscle (nontraumatic), left ankle and foot

     M62.079 Separation of muscle (nontraumatic), unspecified ankle and foot

M62.08 Separation of muscle (nontraumatic), other site

✓5th **M62.1** **Other rupture of muscle (nontraumatic)**

     EXCLUDES 1   *traumatic rupture of muscle - see strain of muscle by body region*

     EXCLUDES 2   *rupture of tendon (M66.-)*

     M62.10 Other rupture of muscle (nontraumatic), unspecified site

✓6th **M62.11** Other rupture of muscle (nontraumatic), shoulder

     M62.111 Other rupture of muscle (nontraumatic), right shoulder

     M62.112 Other rupture of muscle (nontraumatic), left shoulder

     M62.119 Other rupture of muscle (nontraumatic), unspecified shoulder

✓6th **M62.12** Other rupture of muscle (nontraumatic), upper arm

     M62.121 Other rupture of muscle (nontraumatic), right upper arm

     M62.122 Other rupture of muscle (nontraumatic), left upper arm

     M62.129 Other rupture of muscle (nontraumatic), unspecified upper arm

✓6th **M62.13** Other rupture of muscle (nontraumatic), forearm

     M62.131 Other rupture of muscle (nontraumatic), right forearm

     M62.132 Other rupture of muscle (nontraumatic), left forearm

     M62.139 Other rupture of muscle (nontraumatic), unspecified forearm

✓6th **M62.14** Other rupture of muscle (nontraumatic), hand

     M62.141 Other rupture of muscle (nontraumatic), right hand

     M62.142 Other rupture of muscle (nontraumatic), left hand

     M62.149 Other rupture of muscle (nontraumatic), unspecified hand

✓6th **M62.15** Other rupture of muscle (nontraumatic), thigh

     M62.151 Other rupture of muscle (nontraumatic), right thigh

     M62.152 Other rupture of muscle (nontraumatic), left thigh

     M62.159 Other rupture of muscle (nontraumatic), unspecified thigh

✓6th **M62.16** Other rupture of muscle (nontraumatic), lower leg

     M62.161 Other rupture of muscle (nontraumatic), right lower leg

     M62.162 Other rupture of muscle (nontraumatic), left lower leg

     M62.169 Other rupture of muscle (nontraumatic), unspecified lower leg

✓6th **M62.17** Other rupture of muscle (nontraumatic), ankle and foot

     M62.171 Other rupture of muscle (nontraumatic), right ankle and foot

     M62.172 Other rupture of muscle (nontraumatic), left ankle and foot

     M62.179 Other rupture of muscle (nontraumatic), unspecified ankle and foot

M62.18 Other rupture of muscle (nontraumatic), other site

✓5th **M62.2** **Nontraumatic ischemic infarction of muscle**

     EXCLUDES 1   *compartment syndrome (traumatic) (T79.A-)*

               nontraumatic compartment syndrome (M79.A-)

               rhabdomyolysis (M62.82)

               traumatic ischemia of muscle (T79.6)

               Volkmann's ischemic contracture (T79.6)

     M62.20 Nontraumatic ischemic infarction of muscle, unspecified site

✓6th **M62.21** Nontraumatic ischemic infarction of muscle, shoulder

     M62.211 Nontraumatic ischemic infarction of muscle, right shoulder

     M62.212 Nontraumatic ischemic infarction of muscle, left shoulder

     M62.219 Nontraumatic ischemic infarction of muscle, unspecified shoulder

✓6th **M62.22** Nontraumatic ischemic infarction of muscle, upper arm

     M62.221 Nontraumatic ischemic infarction of muscle, right upper arm

✔ Additional Character Required   ✓x7th Placeholder   Questionable PDx   Manifestation   Unspecified   UPD Unacceptable PDx   H1-H4 HAC   HCC CMS-HCC Dx   HIV HIV Dx

ICD-10-CM 2025   821

        M62.222 Nontraumatic ischemic infarction of muscle, left upper arm

        M62.229 Nontraumatic ischemic infarction of muscle, unspecified upper arm

✓6ᵗʰ M62.23 Nontraumatic ischemic infarction of muscle, forearm

        M62.231 Nontraumatic ischemic infarction of muscle, right forearm

        M62.232 Nontraumatic ischemic infarction of muscle, left forearm

        M62.239 Nontraumatic ischemic infarction of muscle, unspecified forearm

✓6ᵗʰ M62.24 Nontraumatic ischemic infarction of muscle, hand

        M62.241 Nontraumatic ischemic infarction of muscle, right hand

        M62.242 Nontraumatic ischemic infarction of muscle, left hand

        M62.249 Nontraumatic ischemic infarction of muscle, unspecified hand

✓6ᵗʰ M62.25 Nontraumatic ischemic infarction of muscle, thigh

        M62.251 Nontraumatic ischemic infarction of muscle, right thigh

        M62.252 Nontraumatic ischemic infarction of muscle, left thigh

        M62.259 Nontraumatic ischemic infarction of muscle, unspecified thigh

✓6ᵗʰ M62.26 Nontraumatic ischemic infarction of muscle, lower leg

        M62.261 Nontraumatic ischemic infarction of muscle, right lower leg

        M62.262 Nontraumatic ischemic infarction of muscle, left lower leg

        M62.269 Nontraumatic ischemic infarction of muscle, unspecified lower leg

✓6ᵗʰ M62.27 Nontraumatic ischemic infarction of muscle, ankle and foot

        M62.271 Nontraumatic ischemic infarction of muscle, right ankle and foot

        M62.272 Nontraumatic ischemic infarction of muscle, left ankle and foot

        M62.279 Nontraumatic ischemic infarction of muscle, unspecified ankle and foot

    M62.28 Nontraumatic ischemic infarction of muscle, other site

  M62.3 Immobility syndrome (paraplegic)

✓5ᵗʰ M62.4 Contracture of muscle

    Contracture of tendon (sheath)

    EXCLUDES 1   contracture of joint (M24.5-)

    M62.40 Contracture of muscle, unspecified site

✓6ᵗʰ M62.41 Contracture of muscle, shoulder

        M62.411 Contracture of muscle, right shoulder

        M62.412 Contracture of muscle, left shoulder

        M62.419 Contracture of muscle, unspecified shoulder

✓6ᵗʰ M62.42 Contracture of muscle, upper arm

        M62.421 Contracture of muscle, right upper arm

        M62.422 Contracture of muscle, left upper arm

        M62.429 Contracture of muscle, unspecified upper arm

✓6ᵗʰ M62.43 Contracture of muscle, forearm

        M62.431 Contracture of muscle, right forearm

        M62.432 Contracture of muscle, left forearm

        M62.439 Contracture of muscle, unspecified forearm

✓6ᵗʰ M62.44 Contracture of muscle, hand

        M62.441 Contracture of muscle, right hand

        M62.442 Contracture of muscle, left hand

        M62.449 Contracture of muscle, unspecified hand

✓6ᵗʰ M62.45 Contracture of muscle, thigh

        M62.451 Contracture of muscle, right thigh

        M62.452 Contracture of muscle, left thigh

        M62.459 Contracture of muscle, unspecified thigh

✓6ᵗʰ M62.46 Contracture of muscle, lower leg

    AHA: 2023,2Q,14

        M62.461 Contracture of muscle, right lower leg

        M62.462 Contracture of muscle, left lower leg

        M62.469 Contracture of muscle, unspecified lower leg

✓6ᵗʰ M62.47 Contracture of muscle, ankle and foot

        M62.471 Contracture of muscle, right ankle and foot

        M62.472 Contracture of muscle, left ankle and foot

        M62.479 Contracture of muscle, unspecified ankle and foot

  M62.48 Contracture of muscle, other site

  M62.49 Contracture of muscle, multiple sites

✓5ᵗʰ M62.5 Muscle wasting and atrophy, not elsewhere classified

    Disuse atrophy NEC

    EXCLUDES 1   neuralgic amyotrophy (G54.5)

        progressive muscular atrophy (G12.21)

        sarcopenia (M62.84)

    EXCLUDES 2   pelvic muscle wasting (N81.84)

    M62.50 Muscle wasting and atrophy, not elsewhere classified, unspecified site

✓6ᵗʰ M62.51 Muscle wasting and atrophy, not elsewhere classified, shoulder

        M62.511 Muscle wasting and atrophy, not elsewhere classified, right shoulder

        M62.512 Muscle wasting and atrophy, not elsewhere classified, left shoulder

        M62.519 Muscle wasting and atrophy, not elsewhere classified, unspecified shoulder

✓6ᵗʰ M62.52 Muscle wasting and atrophy, not elsewhere classified, upper arm

        M62.521 Muscle wasting and atrophy, not elsewhere classified, right upper arm

        M62.522 Muscle wasting and atrophy, not elsewhere classified, left upper arm

        M62.529 Muscle wasting and atrophy, not elsewhere classified, unspecified upper arm

✓6ᵗʰ M62.53 Muscle wasting and atrophy, not elsewhere classified, forearm

        M62.531 Muscle wasting and atrophy, not elsewhere classified, right forearm

        M62.532 Muscle wasting and atrophy, not elsewhere classified, left forearm

        M62.539 Muscle wasting and atrophy, not elsewhere classified, unspecified forearm

✓6ᵗʰ M62.54 Muscle wasting and atrophy, not elsewhere classified, hand

        M62.541 Muscle wasting and atrophy, not elsewhere classified, right hand

        M62.542 Muscle wasting and atrophy, not elsewhere classified, left hand

        M62.549 Muscle wasting and atrophy, not elsewhere classified, unspecified hand

✓6ᵗʰ M62.55 Muscle wasting and atrophy, not elsewhere classified, thigh

        M62.551 Muscle wasting and atrophy, not elsewhere classified, right thigh

        M62.552 Muscle wasting and atrophy, not elsewhere classified, left thigh

        M62.559 Muscle wasting and atrophy, not elsewhere classified, unspecified thigh

✓6ᵗʰ M62.56 Muscle wasting and atrophy, not elsewhere classified, lower leg

        M62.561 Muscle wasting and atrophy, not elsewhere classified, right lower leg

        M62.562 Muscle wasting and atrophy, not elsewhere classified, left lower leg

        M62.569 Muscle wasting and atrophy, not elsewhere classified, unspecified lower leg

✓6ᵗʰ M62.57 Muscle wasting and atrophy, not elsewhere classified, ankle and foot

        M62.571 Muscle wasting and atrophy, not elsewhere classified, right ankle and foot

        M62.572 Muscle wasting and atrophy, not elsewhere classified, left ankle and foot

        M62.579 Muscle wasting and atrophy, not elsewhere classified, unspecified ankle and foot

  M62.58 Muscle wasting and atrophy, not elsewhere classified, other site

  M62.59 Muscle wasting and atrophy, not elsewhere classified, multiple sites

✓6ᵗʰ M62.5A Muscle wasting and atrophy, not elsewhere classified, back

    AHA: 2022,4Q,29

        M62.5A0 Muscle wasting and atrophy, not elsewhere classified, back, cervical

        M62.5A1 Muscle wasting and atrophy, not elsewhere classified, back, thoracic

        M62.5A2 Muscle wasting and atrophy, not elsewhere classified, back, lumbosacral

N Newborn: 0   P Pediatric: 0-17   M Maternity: 9-64   A Adult: 15-124   UNS Unspecified Site   MCC Major Complication/Comorbidity   CC Complication/Comorbidity   PE POA Exempt

822   ICD-10-CM 2025

M62.5A9   Muscle wasting and atrophy, not elsewhere classified, back, unspecified level

√5ᵗʰ **M62.8**   **Other specified disorders of muscle**

EXCLUDES 2   nontraumatic hematoma of muscle (M79.81)

M62.81   **Muscle weakness (generalized)**

EXCLUDES 1   muscle weakness in sarcopenia (M62.84)

M62.82   **Rhabdomyolysis**   ▭▷

EXCLUDES 1   traumatic rhabdomyolysis (T79.6)

AHA: 2019,2Q,12

DEF: Rapid disintegration or destruction of skeletal muscle caused by direct or indirect injury, resulting in the excretion of muscle protein myoglobin into the urine.

√6ᵗʰ **M62.83**   **Muscle spasm**

M62.830   **Muscle spasm of back**

M62.831   **Muscle spasm of calf**

Charley-horse

M62.838   **Other muscle spasm**

M62.84   **Sarcopenia**

Age-related sarcopenia

Code first underlying disease, if applicable, such as:

disorders of myoneural junction and muscle disease in diseases classified elsewhere (G73.-)

other and unspecified myopathies (G72.-)

primary disorders of muscles (G71.-)

AHA: 2016,4Q,41

● **M62.85**   **Dysfunction of the multifidus muscles, lumbar region**

M62.89   **Other specified disorders of muscle**

Muscle (sheath) hernia

M62.9   **Disorder of muscle, unspecified**

√4ᵗʰ **M63**   **Disorders of muscle in diseases classified elsewhere**

Code first underlying disease, such as:

leprosy (A30.-)

neoplasm (C49.-, C79.89, D21.-, D48.1-)

schistosomiasis (B65.-)

trichinellosis (B75)

EXCLUDES 1   myopathy in cysticercosis (B69.81)

myopathy in endocrine diseases (G73.7)

myopathy in metabolic diseases (G73.7)

myopathy in sarcoidosis (D86.87)

myopathy in secondary syphilis (A51.49)

myopathy in syphilis (late) (A52.78)

myopathy in toxoplasmosis (B58.82)

myopathy in tuberculosis (A18.09)

√5ᵗʰ **M63.8**   **Disorders of muscle in diseases classified elsewhere**

M63.80   *Disorders of muscle in diseases classified elsewhere, unspecified site*

√6ᵗʰ **M63.81**   **Disorders of muscle in diseases classified elsewhere, shoulder**

M63.811   *Disorders of muscle in diseases classified elsewhere, right shoulder*

M63.812   *Disorders of muscle in diseases classified elsewhere, left shoulder*

M63.819   *Disorders of muscle in diseases classified elsewhere, unspecified shoulder*

√6ᵗʰ **M63.82**   **Disorders of muscle in diseases classified elsewhere, upper arm**

M63.821   *Disorders of muscle in diseases classified elsewhere, right upper arm*

M63.822   *Disorders of muscle in diseases classified elsewhere, left upper arm*

M63.829   *Disorders of muscle in diseases classified elsewhere, unspecified upper arm*

√6ᵗʰ **M63.83**   **Disorders of muscle in diseases classified elsewhere, forearm**

M63.831   *Disorders of muscle in diseases classified elsewhere, right forearm*

M63.832   *Disorders of muscle in diseases classified elsewhere, left forearm*

M63.839   *Disorders of muscle in diseases classified elsewhere, unspecified forearm*

√6ᵗʰ **M63.84**   **Disorders of muscle in diseases classified elsewhere, hand**

M63.841   *Disorders of muscle in diseases classified elsewhere, right hand*

M63.842   *Disorders of muscle in diseases classified elsewhere, left hand*

M63.849   *Disorders of muscle in diseases classified elsewhere, unspecified hand*

√6ᵗʰ **M63.85**   **Disorders of muscle in diseases classified elsewhere, thigh**

M63.851   *Disorders of muscle in diseases classified elsewhere, right thigh*

M63.852   *Disorders of muscle in diseases classified elsewhere, left thigh*

M63.859   *Disorders of muscle in diseases classified elsewhere, unspecified thigh*

√6ᵗʰ **M63.86**   **Disorders of muscle in diseases classified elsewhere, lower leg**

M63.861   *Disorders of muscle in diseases classified elsewhere, right lower leg*

M63.862   *Disorders of muscle in diseases classified elsewhere, left lower leg*

M63.869   *Disorders of muscle in diseases classified elsewhere, unspecified lower leg*

√6ᵗʰ **M63.87**   **Disorders of muscle in diseases classified elsewhere, ankle and foot**

M63.871   *Disorders of muscle in diseases classified elsewhere, right ankle and foot*

M63.872   *Disorders of muscle in diseases classified elsewhere, left ankle and foot*

M63.879   *Disorders of muscle in diseases classified elsewhere, unspecified ankle and foot*

M63.88   *Disorders of muscle in diseases classified elsewhere, other site*

M63.89   *Disorders of muscle in diseases classified elsewhere, multiple sites*

Disorders of synovium and tendon (M65-M67)

√4ᵗʰ **M65**   **Synovitis and tenosynovitis**

EXCLUDES 1   chronic crepitant synovitis of hand and wrist (M70.0-)

current injury - see injury of ligament or tendon by body region

soft tissue disorders related to use, overuse and pressure (M70.-)

√5ᵗʰ **M65.0**   **Abscess of tendon sheath**

Use additional code (B95-B96) to identify bacterial agent.

M65.00   **Abscess of tendon sheath, unspecified site**

√6ᵗʰ **M65.01**   **Abscess of tendon sheath, shoulder**

M65.011   **Abscess of tendon sheath, right shoulder**

M65.012   **Abscess of tendon sheath, left shoulder**

M65.019   **Abscess of tendon sheath, unspecified shoulder**

√6ᵗʰ **M65.02**   **Abscess of tendon sheath, upper arm**

M65.021   **Abscess of tendon sheath, right upper arm**

M65.022   **Abscess of tendon sheath, left upper arm**

M65.029   **Abscess of tendon sheath, unspecified upper arm**

√6ᵗʰ **M65.03**   **Abscess of tendon sheath, forearm**

M65.031   **Abscess of tendon sheath, right forearm**

M65.032   **Abscess of tendon sheath, left forearm**

M65.039   **Abscess of tendon sheath, unspecified forearm**

√6ᵗʰ **M65.04**   **Abscess of tendon sheath, hand**

M65.041   **Abscess of tendon sheath, right hand**

M65.042   **Abscess of tendon sheath, left hand**

M65.049   **Abscess of tendon sheath, unspecified hand**

√6ᵗʰ **M65.05**   **Abscess of tendon sheath, thigh**

M65.051   **Abscess of tendon sheath, right thigh**

M65.052   **Abscess of tendon sheath, left thigh**

M65.059   **Abscess of tendon sheath, unspecified thigh**

√6ᵗʰ **M65.06**   **Abscess of tendon sheath, lower leg**

M65.061   **Abscess of tendon sheath, right lower leg**

M65.062   **Abscess of tendon sheath, left lower leg**

M65.069   **Abscess of tendon sheath, unspecified lower leg**

√6ᵗʰ **M65.07**   **Abscess of tendon sheath, ankle and foot**

M65.071   **Abscess of tendon sheath, right ankle and foot**

M65.072   **Abscess of tendon sheath, left ankle and foot**

M65.079   **Abscess of tendon sheath, unspecified ankle and foot**

M65.08   **Abscess of tendon sheath, other site**

☑ Additional Character Required   √x7ᵗʰ Placeholder   Questionable PDx   Manifestation   Unspecified   UPD Unacceptable PDx   H1-H14 HAC   HCC CMS-HCC Dx   HIV HIV Dx

ICD-10-CM 2025   823

✓5ᵗʰ **M65.1** **Other infective (teno)synovitis**

    M65.10 Other infective (teno)synovitis, unspecified site

    ✓6ᵗʰ **M65.11** Other infective (teno)synovitis, **shoulder**

        M65.111 Other infective (teno)synovitis, **right** shoulder

        M65.112 Other infective (teno)synovitis, **left** shoulder

        M65.119 Other infective (teno)synovitis, unspecified shoulder

    ✓6ᵗʰ **M65.12** Other infective (teno)synovitis, **elbow**

        M65.121 Other infective (teno)synovitis, **right** elbow

        M65.122 Other infective (teno)synovitis, **left** elbow

        M65.129 Other infective (teno)synovitis, unspecified elbow

    ✓6ᵗʰ **M65.13** Other infective (teno)synovitis, **wrist**

        M65.131 Other infective (teno)synovitis, **right** wrist

        M65.132 Other infective (teno)synovitis, **left** wrist

        M65.139 Other infective (teno)synovitis, unspecified wrist

    ✓6ᵗʰ **M65.14** Other infective (teno)synovitis, **hand**

        M65.141 Other infective (teno)synovitis, **right** hand

        M65.142 Other infective (teno)synovitis, **left** hand

        M65.149 Other infective (teno)synovitis, unspecified hand

    ✓6ᵗʰ **M65.15** Other infective (teno)synovitis, **hip**

        M65.151 Other infective (teno)synovitis, **right** hip

        M65.152 Other infective (teno)synovitis, **left** hip

        M65.159 Other infective (teno)synovitis, unspecified hip

    ✓6ᵗʰ **M65.16** Other infective (teno)synovitis, **knee**

        M65.161 Other infective (teno)synovitis, **right** knee

        M65.162 Other infective (teno)synovitis, **left** knee

        M65.169 Other infective (teno)synovitis, unspecified knee

    ✓6ᵗʰ **M65.17** Other infective (teno)synovitis, **ankle and foot**

        M65.171 Other infective (teno)synovitis, **right** ankle and foot

        M65.172 Other infective (teno)synovitis, **left** ankle and foot

        M65.179 Other infective (teno)synovitis, unspecified ankle and foot

    M65.18 Other infective (teno)synovitis, other site

    M65.19 Other infective (teno)synovitis, **multiple sites**

✓5ᵗʰ **M65.2** **Calcific tendinitis**

    EXCLUDES 1 *tendinitis as classified in M75-M77*
        calcified tendinitis of shoulder (M75.3)

    M65.20 Calcific tendinitis, unspecified site

    ✓6ᵗʰ **M65.22** Calcific tendinitis, **upper arm**

        M65.221 Calcific tendinitis, **right** upper arm

        M65.222 Calcific tendinitis, **left** upper arm

        M65.229 Calcific tendinitis, unspecified upper arm

    ✓6ᵗʰ **M65.23** Calcific tendinitis, **forearm**

        M65.231 Calcific tendinitis, **right** forearm

        M65.232 Calcific tendinitis, **left** forearm

        M65.239 Calcific tendinitis, unspecified forearm

    ✓6ᵗʰ **M65.24** Calcific tendinitis, **hand**

        M65.241 Calcific tendinitis, **right** hand

        M65.242 Calcific tendinitis, **left** hand

        M65.249 Calcific tendinitis, unspecified hand

    ✓6ᵗʰ **M65.25** Calcific tendinitis, **thigh**

        M65.251 Calcific tendinitis, **right** thigh

        M65.252 Calcific tendinitis, **left** thigh

        M65.259 Calcific tendinitis, unspecified thigh

    ✓6ᵗʰ **M65.26** Calcific tendinitis, **lower** leg

        M65.261 Calcific tendinitis, **right** lower leg

        M65.262 Calcific tendinitis, **left** lower leg

        M65.269 Calcific tendinitis, unspecified lower leg

    ✓6ᵗʰ **M65.27** Calcific tendinitis, **ankle and foot**

        M65.271 Calcific tendinitis, **right** ankle and foot

        M65.272 Calcific tendinitis, **left** ankle and foot

        M65.279 Calcific tendinitis, unspecified ankle and foot

    M65.28 Calcific tendinitis, other site

    M65.29 Calcific tendinitis, **multiple sites**

✓5ᵗʰ **M65.3** **Trigger finger**

    Nodular tendinous disease

    M65.30 Trigger finger, unspecified finger

    ✓6ᵗʰ **M65.31** Trigger **thumb**

        M65.311 Trigger thumb, **right** thumb

        M65.312 Trigger thumb, **left** thumb

        M65.319 Trigger thumb, unspecified thumb

    ✓6ᵗʰ **M65.32** Trigger finger, **index finger**

        M65.321 Trigger finger, **right** index finger

        M65.322 Trigger finger, **left** index finger

        M65.329 Trigger finger, unspecified index finger

    ✓6ᵗʰ **M65.33** Trigger finger, **middle finger**

        M65.331 Trigger finger, **right** middle finger

        M65.332 Trigger finger, **left** middle finger

        M65.339 Trigger finger, unspecified middle finger

    ✓6ᵗʰ **M65.34** Trigger finger, **ring finger**

        M65.341 Trigger finger, **right** ring finger

        M65.342 Trigger finger, **left** ring finger

        M65.349 Trigger finger, unspecified ring finger

    ✓6ᵗʰ **M65.35** Trigger finger, **little finger**

        M65.351 Trigger finger, **right** little finger

        M65.352 Trigger finger, **left** little finger

        M65.359 Trigger finger, unspecified little finger

M65.4 Radial styloid tenosynovitis [de Quervain]

✓5ᵗʰ **M65.8** **Other synovitis and tenosynovitis**

    M65.80 Other synovitis and tenosynovitis, unspecified site

    ✓6ᵗʰ **M65.81** Other synovitis and tenosynovitis, **shoulder**

        M65.811 Other synovitis and tenosynovitis, **right** shoulder

        M65.812 Other synovitis and tenosynovitis, **left** shoulder

        M65.819 Other synovitis and tenosynovitis, unspecified shoulder

    ✓6ᵗʰ **M65.82** Other synovitis and tenosynovitis, **upper arm**

        M65.821 Other synovitis and tenosynovitis, **right** upper arm

        M65.822 Other synovitis and tenosynovitis, **left** upper arm

        M65.829 Other synovitis and tenosynovitis, unspecified upper arm

    ✓6ᵗʰ **M65.83** Other synovitis and tenosynovitis, **forearm**

        M65.831 Other synovitis and tenosynovitis, **right** forearm

        M65.832 Other synovitis and tenosynovitis, **left** forearm

        M65.839 Other synovitis and tenosynovitis, unspecified forearm

    ✓6ᵗʰ **M65.84** Other synovitis and tenosynovitis, **hand**

        M65.841 Other synovitis and tenosynovitis, **right** hand

        M65.842 Other synovitis and tenosynovitis, **left** hand

        M65.849 Other synovitis and tenosynovitis, unspecified hand

    ✓6ᵗʰ **M65.85** Other synovitis and tenosynovitis, **thigh**

        M65.851 Other synovitis and tenosynovitis, **right** thigh

        M65.852 Other synovitis and tenosynovitis, **left** thigh

        M65.859 Other synovitis and tenosynovitis, unspecified thigh

    ✓6ᵗʰ **M65.86** Other synovitis and tenosynovitis, **lower leg**

        M65.861 Other synovitis and tenosynovitis, **right** lower leg

        M65.862 Other synovitis and tenosynovitis, **left** lower leg

        M65.869 Other synovitis and tenosynovitis, unspecified lower leg

    ✓6ᵗʰ **M65.87** Other synovitis and tenosynovitis, **ankle and foot**

        M65.871 Other synovitis and tenosynovitis, **right** ankle and foot

        M65.872 Other synovitis and tenosynovitis, **left** ankle and foot

        M65.879 Other synovitis and tenosynovitis, unspecified ankle and foot

    M65.88 Other synovitis and tenosynovitis, other site

    M65.89 Other synovitis and tenosynovitis, **multiple sites**

N Newborn: 0   **P** Pediatric: 0-17   **M** Maternity: 9-64   **A** Adult: 15-124   **UNS** Unspecified Site   **MCC** Major Complication/Comorbidity   **CC** Complication/Comorbidity   **PE** POA Exempt

824

ICD-10-CM 2025

▲ ✓5ᵗʰ **M65.9** **Synovitis and tenosynovitis, unspecified**

● **M65.90** Unspecified synovitis and tenosynovitis, unspecified site

● ✓6ᵗʰ **M65.91** Unspecified synovitis and tenosynovitis, **shoulder**

● **M65.911** Unspecified synovitis and tenosynovitis, **right** shoulder

● **M65.912** Unspecified synovitis and tenosynovitis, **left** shoulder

● **M65.919** Unspecified synovitis and tenosynovitis, unspecified shoulder

● ✓6ᵗʰ **M65.92** Unspecified synovitis and tenosynovitis, **upper arm**

● **M65.921** Unspecified synovitis and tenosynovitis, **right** upper arm

● **M65.922** Unspecified synovitis and tenosynovitis, **left** upper arm

● **M65.929** Unspecified synovitis and tenosynovitis, unspecified upper arm

● ✓6ᵗʰ **M65.93** Unspecified synovitis and tenosynovitis, **forearm**

● **M65.931** Unspecified synovitis and tenosynovitis, **right** forearm

● **M65.932** Unspecified synovitis and tenosynovitis, **left** forearm

● **M65.939** Unspecified synovitis and tenosynovitis, unspecified forearm

● ✓6ᵗʰ **M65.94** Unspecified synovitis and tenosynovitis, **hand**

● **M65.941** Unspecified synovitis and tenosynovitis, **right** hand

● **M65.942** Unspecified synovitis and tenosynovitis, **left** hand

● **M65.949** Unspecified synovitis and tenosynovitis, unspecified hand

● ✓6ᵗʰ **M65.95** Unspecified synovitis and tenosynovitis, **thigh**

● **M65.951** Unspecified synovitis and tenosynovitis, **right** thigh

● **M65.952** Unspecified synovitis and tenosynovitis, **left** thigh

● **M65.959** Unspecified synovitis and tenosynovitis, unspecified thigh

● ✓6ᵗʰ **M65.96** Unspecified synovitis and tenosynovitis, **lower leg**

● **M65.961** Unspecified synovitis and tenosynovitis, **right** lower leg

● **M65.962** Unspecified synovitis and tenosynovitis, **left** lower leg

● **M65.969** Unspecified synovitis and tenosynovitis, unspecified lower leg

● ✓6ᵗʰ **M65.97** Unspecified synovitis and tenosynovitis, **ankle and foot**

● **M65.971** Unspecified synovitis and tenosynovitis, **right** ankle and foot

● **M65.972** Unspecified synovitis and tenosynovitis, **left** ankle and foot

● **M65.979** Unspecified synovitis and tenosynovitis, unspecified ankle and foot

● **M65.98** Unspecified synovitis and tenosynovitis, **other site**

● **M65.99** Unspecified synovitis and tenosynovitis, **multiple sites**

✓4ᵗʰ **M66** **Spontaneous rupture of synovium and tendon**

INCLUDES   rupture that occurs when a normal force is applied to tissues that are inferred to have less than normal strength

EXCLUDES 2   rotator cuff syndrome (M75.1-)

rupture where an abnormal force is applied to normal tissue - see injury of tendon by body region

M66.0 **Rupture of popliteal cyst**

✓5ᵗʰ **M66.1** **Rupture of synovium**

Rupture of synovial cyst

EXCLUDES 2   rupture of popliteal cyst (M66.0)

M66.10 Rupture of synovium, unspecified joint

✓6ᵗʰ **M66.11** Rupture of synovium, **shoulder**

M66.111 Rupture of synovium, **right** shoulder
M66.112 Rupture of synovium, **left** shoulder
M66.119 Rupture of synovium, unspecified shoulder

✓6ᵗʰ **M66.12** Rupture of synovium, **elbow**

M66.121 Rupture of synovium, **right** elbow
M66.122 Rupture of synovium, **left** elbow
M66.129 Rupture of synovium, unspecified elbow

✓6ᵗʰ **M66.13** Rupture of synovium, **wrist**

M66.131 Rupture of synovium, **right** wrist
M66.132 Rupture of synovium, **left** wrist

M66.139 Rupture of synovium, unspecified wrist

✓6ᵗʰ **M66.14** Rupture of synovium, **hand and fingers**

M66.141 Rupture of synovium, **right** hand
M66.142 Rupture of synovium, **left** hand
M66.143 Rupture of synovium, unspecified hand
M66.144 Rupture of synovium, **right** finger(s)
M66.145 Rupture of synovium, **left** finger(s)
M66.146 Rupture of synovium, unspecified finger(s)

✓6ᵗʰ **M66.15** Rupture of synovium, **hip**

M66.151 Rupture of synovium, **right** hip
M66.152 Rupture of synovium, **left** hip
M66.159 Rupture of synovium, unspecified hip

✓6ᵗʰ **M66.17** Rupture of synovium, **ankle, foot and toes**

M66.171 Rupture of synovium, **right** ankle
M66.172 Rupture of synovium, **left** ankle
M66.173 Rupture of synovium, unspecified ankle
M66.174 Rupture of synovium, **right** foot
M66.175 Rupture of synovium, **left** foot
M66.176 Rupture of synovium, unspecified foot
M66.177 Rupture of synovium, **right** toe(s)
M66.178 Rupture of synovium, **left** toe(s)
M66.179 Rupture of synovium, unspecified toe(s)

M66.18 Rupture of synovium, other site

✓5ᵗʰ **M66.2** **Spontaneous rupture of extensor tendons**

TIP: Refer to the Muscle/Tendon table at the beginning of this chapter.

M66.20 Spontaneous rupture of extensor tendons, unspecified site

✓6ᵗʰ **M66.21** Spontaneous rupture of extensor tendons, **shoulder**

M66.211 Spontaneous rupture of extensor tendons, **right** shoulder
M66.212 Spontaneous rupture of extensor tendons, **left** shoulder
M66.219 Spontaneous rupture of extensor tendons, unspecified shoulder

✓6ᵗʰ **M66.22** Spontaneous rupture of extensor tendons, **upper arm**

M66.221 Spontaneous rupture of extensor tendons, **right** upper arm
M66.222 Spontaneous rupture of extensor tendons, **left** upper arm
M66.229 Spontaneous rupture of extensor tendons, unspecified upper arm

✓6ᵗʰ **M66.23** Spontaneous rupture of extensor tendons, **forearm**

M66.231 Spontaneous rupture of extensor tendons, **right** forearm
M66.232 Spontaneous rupture of extensor tendons, **left** forearm
M66.239 Spontaneous rupture of extensor tendons, unspecified forearm

✓6ᵗʰ **M66.24** Spontaneous rupture of extensor tendons, **hand**

M66.241 Spontaneous rupture of extensor tendons, **right** hand
M66.242 Spontaneous rupture of extensor tendons, **left** hand
M66.249 Spontaneous rupture of extensor tendons, unspecified hand

✓6ᵗʰ **M66.25** Spontaneous rupture of extensor tendons, **thigh**

M66.251 Spontaneous rupture of extensor tendons, **right** thigh
M66.252 Spontaneous rupture of extensor tendons, **left** thigh
M66.259 Spontaneous rupture of extensor tendons, unspecified thigh

✓6ᵗʰ **M66.26** Spontaneous rupture of extensor tendons, **lower leg**

M66.261 Spontaneous rupture of extensor tendons, **right** lower leg
M66.262 Spontaneous rupture of extensor tendons, **left** lower leg
M66.269 Spontaneous rupture of extensor tendons, unspecified lower leg

✓6ᵗʰ **M66.27** Spontaneous rupture of extensor tendons, **ankle and foot**

M66.271 Spontaneous rupture of extensor tendons, **right** ankle and foot
M66.272 Spontaneous rupture of extensor tendons, **left** ankle and foot
M66.279 Spontaneous rupture of extensor tendons, unspecified ankle and foot

M66.28 Spontaneous rupture of extensor tendons, other site

✓ Additional Character Required   ✓x7ᵗʰ Placeholder   Questionable PDx   Manifestation   Unspecified   UPD Unacceptable PDx   H1-H4 HAC   HCC CMS-HCC Dx   HIV HIV Dx

ICD-10-CM 2025   825

Chapter 13. Diseases of the Musculoskeletal System and Connective Tissue

      M66.29   Spontaneous rupture of extensor tendons, multiple sites

✓5th M66.3   **Spontaneous rupture of flexor tendons**

> **TIP:** Refer to the Muscle/Tendon table at the beginning of this chapter.

     M66.30   Spontaneous rupture of flexor tendons, unspecified site

✓6th M66.31   Spontaneous rupture of flexor tendons, shoulder

     M66.311   Spontaneous rupture of flexor tendons, right shoulder

     M66.312   Spontaneous rupture of flexor tendons, left shoulder

     M66.319   Spontaneous rupture of flexor tendons, unspecified shoulder

✓6th M66.32   Spontaneous rupture of flexor tendons, upper arm

     M66.321   Spontaneous rupture of flexor tendons, right upper arm

     M66.322   Spontaneous rupture of flexor tendons, left upper arm

     M66.329   Spontaneous rupture of flexor tendons, unspecified upper arm

✓6th M66.33   Spontaneous rupture of flexor tendons, forearm

     M66.331   Spontaneous rupture of flexor tendons, right forearm

     M66.332   Spontaneous rupture of flexor tendons, left forearm

     M66.339   Spontaneous rupture of flexor tendons, unspecified forearm

✓6th M66.34   Spontaneous rupture of flexor tendons, hand

     M66.341   Spontaneous rupture of flexor tendons, right hand

     M66.342   Spontaneous rupture of flexor tendons, left hand

     M66.349   Spontaneous rupture of flexor tendons, unspecified hand

✓6th M66.35   Spontaneous rupture of flexor tendons, thigh

     M66.351   Spontaneous rupture of flexor tendons, right thigh

     M66.352   Spontaneous rupture of flexor tendons, left thigh

     M66.359   Spontaneous rupture of flexor tendons, unspecified thigh

✓6th M66.36   Spontaneous rupture of flexor tendons, lower leg

     M66.361   Spontaneous rupture of flexor tendons, right lower leg

     M66.362   Spontaneous rupture of flexor tendons, left lower leg

     M66.369   Spontaneous rupture of flexor tendons, unspecified lower leg

✓6th M66.37   Spontaneous rupture of flexor tendons, ankle and foot

     M66.371   Spontaneous rupture of flexor tendons, right ankle and foot

     M66.372   Spontaneous rupture of flexor tendons, left ankle and foot

     M66.379   Spontaneous rupture of flexor tendons, unspecified ankle and foot

     M66.38   Spontaneous rupture of flexor tendons, other site

     M66.39   Spontaneous rupture of flexor tendons, multiple sites

✓5th M66.8   **Spontaneous rupture of other tendons**

> **TIP:** Refer to the Muscle/Tendon table at the beginning of this chapter.

     M66.80   Spontaneous rupture of other tendons, unspecified site

✓6th M66.81   Spontaneous rupture of other tendons, shoulder

     M66.811   Spontaneous rupture of other tendons, right shoulder

     M66.812   Spontaneous rupture of other tendons, left shoulder

     M66.819   Spontaneous rupture of other tendons, unspecified shoulder

✓6th M66.82   Spontaneous rupture of other tendons, upper arm

     M66.821   Spontaneous rupture of other tendons, right upper arm

     M66.822   Spontaneous rupture of other tendons, left upper arm

     M66.829   Spontaneous rupture of other tendons, unspecified upper arm

✓6th M66.83   Spontaneous rupture of other tendons, forearm

     M66.831   Spontaneous rupture of other tendons, right forearm

     M66.832   Spontaneous rupture of other tendons, left forearm

     M66.839   Spontaneous rupture of other tendons, unspecified forearm

✓6th M66.84   Spontaneous rupture of other tendons, hand

     M66.841   Spontaneous rupture of other tendons, right hand

     M66.842   Spontaneous rupture of other tendons, left hand

     M66.849   Spontaneous rupture of other tendons, unspecified hand

✓6th M66.85   Spontaneous rupture of other tendons, thigh

     M66.851   Spontaneous rupture of other tendons, right thigh

     M66.852   Spontaneous rupture of other tendons, left thigh

     M66.859   Spontaneous rupture of other tendons, unspecified thigh

✓6th M66.86   Spontaneous rupture of other tendons, lower leg

     M66.861   Spontaneous rupture of other tendons, right lower leg

     M66.862   Spontaneous rupture of other tendons, left lower leg

     M66.869   Spontaneous rupture of other tendons, unspecified lower leg

✓6th M66.87   Spontaneous rupture of other tendons, ankle and foot

     M66.871   Spontaneous rupture of other tendons, right ankle and foot

     M66.872   Spontaneous rupture of other tendons, left ankle and foot

     M66.879   Spontaneous rupture of other tendons, unspecified ankle and foot

     M66.88   Spontaneous rupture of other tendons, other sites

     M66.89   Spontaneous rupture of other tendons, multiple sites

M66.9   **Spontaneous rupture of unspecified tendon**

> Rupture at musculotendinous junction, nontraumatic

✓4th **M67   Other disorders of synovium and tendon**

> **EXCLUDES 1**   palmar fascial fibromatosis [Dupuytren] (M72.0)
> tendinitis NOS (M77.9-)
> xanthomatosis localized to tendons (E78.2)

✓5th M67.0   **Short Achilles tendon (acquired)**

     M67.00   Short Achilles tendon (acquired), unspecified ankle

     M67.01   Short Achilles tendon (acquired), right ankle

     M67.02   Short Achilles tendon (acquired), left ankle

✓5th M67.2   **Synovial hypertrophy, not elsewhere classified**

> **EXCLUDES 1**   villonodular synovitis (pigmented) (M12.2-)

     M67.20   Synovial hypertrophy, not elsewhere classified, unspecified site

✓6th M67.21   Synovial hypertrophy, not elsewhere classified, shoulder

     M67.211   Synovial hypertrophy, not elsewhere classified, right shoulder

     M67.212   Synovial hypertrophy, not elsewhere classified, left shoulder

     M67.219   Synovial hypertrophy, not elsewhere classified, unspecified shoulder

✓6th M67.22   Synovial hypertrophy, not elsewhere classified, upper arm

     M67.221   Synovial hypertrophy, not elsewhere classified, right upper arm

     M67.222   Synovial hypertrophy, not elsewhere classified, left upper arm

     M67.229   Synovial hypertrophy, not elsewhere classified, unspecified upper arm

✓6th M67.23   Synovial hypertrophy, not elsewhere classified, forearm

     M67.231   Synovial hypertrophy, not elsewhere classified, right forearm

     M67.232   Synovial hypertrophy, not elsewhere classified, left forearm

     M67.239   Synovial hypertrophy, not elsewhere classified, unspecified forearm

✓6th M67.24   Synovial hypertrophy, not elsewhere classified, hand

     M67.241   Synovial hypertrophy, not elsewhere classified, right hand

N Newborn: 0   P Pediatric: 0-17   M Maternity: 9-64   A Adult: 15-124   UNS Unspecified Site   MCC Major Complication/Comorbidity   CC Complication/Comorbidity   PE POA Exempt

826

ICD-10-CM 2025

M67.242   Synovial hypertrophy, not elsewhere classified, **left** hand

M67.249   Synovial hypertrophy, not elsewhere classified, unspecified hand

✓6th   M67.25   Synovial hypertrophy, not elsewhere classified, **thigh**

    M67.251   Synovial hypertrophy, not elsewhere classified, **right** thigh

    M67.252   Synovial hypertrophy, not elsewhere classified, **left** thigh

    M67.259   Synovial hypertrophy, not elsewhere classified, unspecified thigh

✓6th   M67.26   Synovial hypertrophy, not elsewhere classified, **lower leg**

    M67.261   Synovial hypertrophy, not elsewhere classified, **right** lower leg

    M67.262   Synovial hypertrophy, not elsewhere classified, **left** lower leg

    M67.269   Synovial hypertrophy, not elsewhere classified, unspecified lower leg

✓6th   M67.27   Synovial hypertrophy, not elsewhere classified, **ankle and foot**

    M67.271   Synovial hypertrophy, not elsewhere classified, **right** ankle and foot

    M67.272   Synovial hypertrophy, not elsewhere classified, **left** ankle and foot

    M67.279   Synovial hypertrophy, not elsewhere classified, unspecified ankle and foot

M67.28   Synovial hypertrophy, not elsewhere classified, other site

M67.29   Synovial hypertrophy, not elsewhere classified, **multiple sites**

✓5th   **M67.3   Transient synovitis**

    Toxic synovitis

    EXCLUDES 1   palindromic rheumatism (M12.3-)

M67.30   Transient synovitis, unspecified site

✓6th   M67.31   Transient synovitis, **shoulder**

    M67.311   Transient synovitis, **right** shoulder

    M67.312   Transient synovitis, **left** shoulder

    M67.319   Transient synovitis, unspecified shoulder

✓6th   M67.32   Transient synovitis, **elbow**

    M67.321   Transient synovitis, **right** elbow

    M67.322   Transient synovitis, **left** elbow

    M67.329   Transient synovitis, unspecified elbow

✓6th   M67.33   Transient synovitis, **wrist**

    M67.331   Transient synovitis, **right** wrist

    M67.332   Transient synovitis, **left** wrist

    M67.339   Transient synovitis, unspecified wrist

✓6th   M67.34   Transient synovitis, **hand**

    M67.341   Transient synovitis, **right** hand

    M67.342   Transient synovitis, **left** hand

    M67.349   Transient synovitis, unspecified hand

✓6th   M67.35   Transient synovitis, **hip**

    M67.351   Transient synovitis, **right** hip

    M67.352   Transient synovitis, **left** hip

    M67.359   Transient synovitis, unspecified hip

✓6th   M67.36   Transient synovitis, **knee**

    M67.361   Transient synovitis, **right** knee

    M67.362   Transient synovitis, **left** knee

    M67.369   Transient synovitis, unspecified knee

✓6th   M67.37   Transient synovitis, **ankle and foot**

    M67.371   Transient synovitis, **right** ankle and foot

    M67.372   Transient synovitis, **left** ankle and foot

    M67.379   Transient synovitis, unspecified ankle and foot

M67.38   Transient synovitis, other site

M67.39   Transient synovitis, **multiple sites**

✓5th   **M67.4   Ganglion**

    Ganglion of joint or tendon (sheath)

    EXCLUDES 1   ganglion in yaws (A66.6)

    EXCLUDES 2   cyst of bursa (M71.2-M71.3)

           cyst of synovium (M71.2-M71.3)

    DEF: Fluid-filled, benign cyst appearing on a tendon sheath or aponeurosis, frequently connecting to an underlying joint.

M67.40   Ganglion, unspecified site

✓6th   M67.41   Ganglion, **shoulder**

    M67.411   Ganglion, **right** shoulder

    M67.412   Ganglion, **left** shoulder

    M67.419   Ganglion, unspecified shoulder

✓6th   M67.42   Ganglion, **elbow**

    M67.421   Ganglion, **right** elbow

    M67.422   Ganglion, **left** elbow

    M67.429   Ganglion, unspecified elbow

✓6th   M67.43   Ganglion, **wrist**

Ganglion of Wrist

Extensor tendon sheaths

Ganglion of wrist (fluid-filled sac)

    M67.431   Ganglion, **right** wrist

    M67.432   Ganglion, **left** wrist

    M67.439   Ganglion, unspecified wrist

✓6th   M67.44   Ganglion, **hand**

    M67.441   Ganglion, **right** hand

    M67.442   Ganglion, **left** hand

    M67.449   Ganglion, unspecified hand

✓6th   M67.45   Ganglion, **hip**

    M67.451   Ganglion, **right** hip

    M67.452   Ganglion, **left** hip

    M67.459   Ganglion, unspecified hip

✓6th   M67.46   Ganglion, **knee**

    M67.461   Ganglion, **right** knee

    M67.462   Ganglion, **left** knee

    M67.469   Ganglion, unspecified knee

✓6th   M67.47   Ganglion, **ankle and foot**

    M67.471   Ganglion, **right** ankle and foot

    M67.472   Ganglion, **left** ankle and foot

    M67.479   Ganglion, unspecified ankle and foot

M67.48   Ganglion, other site

M67.49   Ganglion, **multiple sites**

✓5th   **M67.5   Plica syndrome**

    Plica knee

M67.50   Plica syndrome, unspecified knee

M67.51   Plica syndrome, **right** knee

M67.52   Plica syndrome, **left** knee

✓5th   **M67.8   Other specified disorders of synovium and tendon**

M67.80   Other specified disorders of synovium and tendon, unspecified site

✓6th   M67.81   Other specified disorders of synovium and tendon, **shoulder**

    M67.811   Other specified disorders of synovium, **right** shoulder

    M67.812   Other specified disorders of synovium, **left** shoulder

    M67.813   Other specified disorders of tendon, **right** shoulder

    M67.814   Other specified disorders of tendon, **left** shoulder

    M67.819   Other specified disorders of synovium and tendon, unspecified shoulder

✓6th   M67.82   Other specified disorders of synovium and tendon, **elbow**

    M67.821   Other specified disorders of synovium, **right** elbow

    M67.822   Other specified disorders of synovium, **left** elbow

    M67.823   Other specified disorders of tendon, **right** elbow

✓ Additional Character Required   ✓x7th Placeholder   Questionable PDx   Manifestation   Unspecified   UPD Unacceptable PDx   H1-H14 HAC   HCC CMS-HCC Dx   HIV HIV Dx

ICD-10-CM 2025   827

M67.824 Other specified disorders of tendon, **left** elbow

M67.829 Other specified disorders of synovium and tendon, unspecified elbow

√6ᵗʰ **M67.83** Other specified disorders of synovium and tendon, **wrist**

M67.831 Other specified disorders of synovium, **right** wrist

M67.832 Other specified disorders of synovium, **left** wrist

M67.833 Other specified disorders of tendon, **right** wrist

M67.834 Other specified disorders of tendon, **left** wrist

M67.839 Other specified disorders of synovium and tendon, unspecified wrist

√6ᵗʰ **M67.84** Other specified disorders of synovium and tendon, **hand**

M67.841 Other specified disorders of synovium, **right** hand

M67.842 Other specified disorders of synovium, **left** hand

M67.843 Other specified disorders of tendon, **right** hand

M67.844 Other specified disorders of tendon, **left** hand

M67.849 Other specified disorders of synovium and tendon, unspecified hand

√6ᵗʰ **M67.85** Other specified disorders of synovium and tendon, **hip**

M67.851 Other specified disorders of synovium, **right** hip

M67.852 Other specified disorders of synovium, **left** hip

M67.853 Other specified disorders of tendon, **right** hip

M67.854 Other specified disorders of tendon, **left** hip

M67.859 Other specified disorders of synovium and tendon, unspecified hip

√6ᵗʰ **M67.86** Other specified disorders of synovium and tendon, **knee**

M67.861 Other specified disorders of synovium, **right** knee

M67.862 Other specified disorders of synovium, **left** knee

M67.863 Other specified disorders of tendon, **right** knee

M67.864 Other specified disorders of tendon, **left** knee

M67.869 Other specified disorders of synovium and tendon, unspecified knee

√6ᵗʰ **M67.87** Other specified disorders of synovium and tendon, **ankle and foot**

M67.871 Other specified disorders of synovium, **right** ankle and foot

M67.872 Other specified disorders of synovium, **left** ankle and foot

M67.873 Other specified disorders of tendon, **right** ankle and foot

M67.874 Other specified disorders of tendon, **left** ankle and foot

M67.879 Other specified disorders of synovium and tendon, unspecified ankle and foot

M67.88 Other specified disorders of synovium and tendon, other site

M67.89 Other specified disorders of synovium and tendon, multiple sites

√5ᵗʰ **M67.9** Unspecified disorder of synovium and tendon

M67.90 Unspecified disorder of synovium and tendon, unspecified site

√6ᵗʰ **M67.91** Unspecified disorder of synovium and tendon, **shoulder**

M67.911 Unspecified disorder of synovium and tendon, **right** shoulder

M67.912 Unspecified disorder of synovium and tendon, **left** shoulder

M67.919 Unspecified disorder of synovium and tendon, unspecified shoulder

√6ᵗʰ **M67.92** Unspecified disorder of synovium and tendon, upper **arm**

M67.921 Unspecified disorder of synovium and tendon, **right** upper arm

M67.922 Unspecified disorder of synovium and tendon, **left** upper arm

M67.929 Unspecified disorder of synovium and tendon, unspecified upper arm

√6ᵗʰ **M67.93** Unspecified disorder of synovium and tendon, **forearm**

M67.931 Unspecified disorder of synovium and tendon, **right** forearm

M67.932 Unspecified disorder of synovium and tendon, **left** forearm

M67.939 Unspecified disorder of synovium and tendon, unspecified forearm

√6ᵗʰ **M67.94** Unspecified disorder of synovium and tendon, **hand**

M67.941 Unspecified disorder of synovium and tendon, **right** hand

M67.942 Unspecified disorder of synovium and tendon, **left** hand

M67.949 Unspecified disorder of synovium and tendon, unspecified hand

√6ᵗʰ **M67.95** Unspecified disorder of synovium and tendon, **thigh**

M67.951 Unspecified disorder of synovium and tendon, **right** thigh

M67.952 Unspecified disorder of synovium and tendon, **left** thigh

M67.959 Unspecified disorder of synovium and tendon, unspecified thigh

√6ᵗʰ **M67.96** Unspecified disorder of synovium and tendon, **lower leg**

M67.961 Unspecified disorder of synovium and tendon, **right** lower leg

M67.962 Unspecified disorder of synovium and tendon, **left** lower leg

M67.969 Unspecified disorder of synovium and tendon, unspecified lower leg

√6ᵗʰ **M67.97** Unspecified disorder of synovium and tendon, **ankle and foot**

M67.971 Unspecified disorder of synovium and tendon, **right** ankle and foot

M67.972 Unspecified disorder of synovium and tendon, **left** ankle and foot

M67.979 Unspecified disorder of synovium and tendon, unspecified ankle and foot

M67.98 Unspecified disorder of synovium and tendon, other site

M67.99 Unspecified disorder of synovium and tendon, **multiple sites**

Other soft tissue disorders (M70-M79)

√4ᵗʰ **M70** **Soft tissue disorders related to use, overuse and pressure**

INCLUDES   soft tissue disorders of occupational origin

Use additional external cause code to identify activity causing disorder (Y93.-)

EXCLUDES 1   bursitis NOS (M71.9-)

EXCLUDES 2   bursitis of shoulder (M75.5)

enthesopathies (M76-M77)

pressure ulcer (pressure area) (L89.-)

√5ᵗʰ **M70.0** **Crepitant synovitis (acute) (chronic) of hand and wrist**

√6ᵗʰ **M70.03** Crepitant synovitis (acute) (chronic), **wrist**

M70.031 Crepitant synovitis (acute) (chronic), **right** wrist

M70.032 Crepitant synovitis (acute) (chronic), **left** wrist

M70.039 Crepitant synovitis (acute) (chronic), unspecified wrist

√6ᵗʰ **M70.04** Crepitant synovitis (acute) (chronic), **hand**

M70.041 Crepitant synovitis (acute) (chronic), **right** hand

M70.042 Crepitant synovitis (acute) (chronic), **left** hand

M70.049 Crepitant synovitis (acute) (chronic), unspecified hand

√5ᵗʰ **M70.1** **Bursitis of hand**

M70.10 Bursitis, unspecified hand

M70.11 Bursitis, **right** hand

M70.12 Bursitis, **left** hand

√5ᵗʰ **M70.2** **Olecranon bursitis**

M70.20 Olecranon bursitis, unspecified elbow

M70.21 Olecranon bursitis, **right** elbow

M70.22 Olecranon bursitis, **left** elbow

✓5ᵗʰ **M70.3** Other bursitis of **elbow**

    M70.30 Other bursitis of elbow, unspecified elbow

    M70.31 Other bursitis of elbow, **right** elbow

    M70.32 Other bursitis of elbow, **left** elbow

✓5ᵗʰ **M70.4** **Prepatellar** bursitis

    M70.40 Prepatellar bursitis, unspecified knee

    M70.41 Prepatellar bursitis, **right** knee

    M70.42 Prepatellar bursitis, **left** knee

Knee Bursae

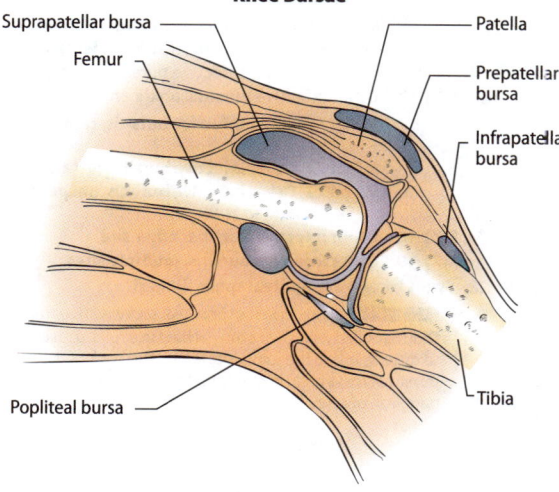

Suprapatellar bursa

Femur

Patella

Prepatellar bursa

Infrapatellar bursa

Popliteal bursa

Tibia

✓5ᵗʰ **M70.5** Other bursitis of **knee**

    M70.50 Other bursitis of knee, unspecified knee

    M70.51 Other bursitis of knee, **right** knee

    M70.52 Other bursitis of knee, **left** knee

✓5ᵗʰ **M70.6** **Trochanteric** bursitis

    Trochanteric tendinitis

    M70.60 Trochanteric bursitis, unspecified hip

    M70.61 Trochanteric bursitis, **right** hip

    M70.62 Trochanteric bursitis, **left** hip

✓5ᵗʰ **M70.7** Other bursitis of **hip**

    Ischial bursitis

    M70.70 Other bursitis of hip, unspecified hip

    M70.71 Other bursitis of hip, **right** hip

    M70.72 Other bursitis of hip, **left** hip

✓5ᵗʰ **M70.8** Other soft tissue disorders related to use, overuse and pressure

    M70.80 Other soft tissue disorders related to use, overuse and pressure of unspecified site

  ✓6ᵗʰ M70.81 Other soft tissue disorders related to use, overuse and pressure of **shoulder**

    M70.811 Other soft tissue disorders related to use, overuse and pressure, **right** shoulder

    M70.812 Other soft tissue disorders related to use, overuse and pressure, **left** shoulder

    M70.819 Other soft tissue disorders related to use, overuse and pressure, unspecified shoulder

  ✓6ᵗʰ M70.82 Other soft tissue disorders related to use, overuse and pressure of **upper arm**

    M70.821 Other soft tissue disorders related to use, overuse and pressure, **right** upper arm

    M70.822 Other soft tissue disorders related to use, overuse and pressure, **left** upper arm

    M70.829 Other soft tissue disorders related to use, overuse and pressure, unspecified upper arms

  ✓6ᵗʰ M70.83 Other soft tissue disorders related to use, overuse and pressure of **forearm**

    M70.831 Other soft tissue disorders related to use, overuse and pressure, **right** forearm

    M70.832 Other soft tissue disorders related to use, overuse and pressure, **left** forearm

    M70.839 Other soft tissue disorders related to use, overuse and pressure, unspecified forearm

  ✓6ᵗʰ M70.84 Other soft tissue disorders related to use, overuse and pressure of **hand**

    M70.841 Other soft tissue disorders related to use, overuse and pressure, **right** hand

    M70.842 Other soft tissue disorders related to use, overuse and pressure, **left** hand

    M70.849 Other soft tissue disorders related to use, overuse and pressure, unspecified hand

  ✓6ᵗʰ M70.85 Other soft tissue disorders related to use, overuse and pressure of **thigh**

    M70.851 Other soft tissue disorders related to use, overuse and pressure, **right** thigh

    M70.852 Other soft tissue disorders related to use, overuse and pressure, **left** thigh

    M70.859 Other soft tissue disorders related to use, overuse and pressure, unspecified thigh

  ✓6ᵗʰ M70.86 Other soft tissue disorders related to use, overuse and pressure **lower leg**

    M70.861 Other soft tissue disorders related to use, overuse and pressure, **right** lower leg

    M70.862 Other soft tissue disorders related to use, overuse and pressure, **left** lower leg

    M70.869 Other soft tissue disorders related to use, overuse and pressure, unspecified leg

  ✓6ᵗʰ M70.87 Other soft tissue disorders related to use, overuse and pressure of **ankle and foot**

    M70.871 Other soft tissue disorders related to use, overuse and pressure, **right** ankle and foot

    M70.872 Other soft tissue disorders related to use, overuse and pressure, **left** ankle and foot

    M70.879 Other soft tissue disorders related to use, overuse and pressure, unspecified ankle and foot

    M70.88 Other soft tissue disorders related to use and pressure other site

    M70.89 Other soft tissue disorders related to use, overuse and pressure **multiple sites**

✓5ᵗʰ **M70.9** Unspecified soft tissue disorder related to use, overuse and pressure

    M70.90 Unspecified soft tissue disorder related to use, overuse and pressure of unspecified site

  ✓6ᵗʰ M70.91 Unspecified soft tissue disorder related to use, overuse and pressure of **shoulder**

    M70.911 Unspecified soft tissue disorder related to use, overuse and pressure, **right** shoulder

    M70.912 Unspecified soft tissue disorder related to use, overuse and pressure, **left** shoulder

    M70.919 Unspecified soft tissue disorder related to use, overuse and pressure, unspecified shoulder

  ✓6ᵗʰ M70.92 Unspecified soft tissue disorder related to use, overuse and pressure of **upper arm**

    M70.921 Unspecified soft tissue disorder related to use, overuse and pressure, **right** upper arm

    M70.922 Unspecified soft tissue disorder related to use, overuse and pressure, **left** upper arm

    M70.929 Unspecified soft tissue disorder related to use, overuse and pressure, unspecified upper arm

  ✓6ᵗʰ M70.93 Unspecified soft tissue disorder related to use, overuse and pressure of **forearm**

    M70.931 Unspecified soft tissue disorder related to use, overuse and pressure, **right** forearm

    M70.932 Unspecified soft tissue disorder related to use, overuse and pressure, **left** forearm

    M70.939 Unspecified soft tissue disorder related to use, overuse and pressure, unspecified forearm

  ✓6ᵗʰ M70.94 Unspecified soft tissue disorder related to use, overuse and pressure of **hand**

    M70.941 Unspecified soft tissue disorder related to use, overuse and pressure, **right** hand

    M70.942 Unspecified soft tissue disorder related to use, overuse and pressure, **left** hand

    M70.949 Unspecified soft tissue disorder related to use, overuse and pressure, unspecified hand

  ✓6ᵗʰ M70.95 Unspecified soft tissue disorder related to use, overuse and pressure of **thigh**

    M70.951 Unspecified soft tissue disorder related to use, overuse and pressure, **right** thigh

    M70.952 Unspecified soft tissue disorder related to use, overuse and pressure, **left** thigh

    M70.959 Unspecified soft tissue disorder related to use, overuse and pressure, unspecified thigh

✔ Additional Character Required ✓x7ᵗʰ Placeholder Questionable PDx Manifestation Unspecified UPD Unacceptable PDx H1 - H14 HAC HCC CMS-HCC Dx HIV HIV Dx

ICD-10-CM 2025   829

✓6ᵗʰ **M70.96** Unspecified soft tissue disorder related to use, overuse and pressure **lower leg**

   M70.961 Unspecified soft tissue disorder related to use, overuse and pressure, **right** lower leg

   M70.962 Unspecified soft tissue disorder related to use, overuse and pressure, **left** lower leg

   M70.969 Unspecified soft tissue disorder related to use, overuse and pressure, unspecified lower leg

✓6ᵗʰ **M70.97** Unspecified soft tissue disorder related to use, overuse and pressure of **ankle and foot**

   M70.971 Unspecified soft tissue disorder related to use, overuse and pressure, **right** ankle and foot

   M70.972 Unspecified soft tissue disorder related to use, overuse and pressure, **left** ankle and foot

   M70.979 Unspecified soft tissue disorder related to use, overuse and pressure, unspecified ankle and foot

   M70.98 Unspecified soft tissue disorder related to use, overuse and pressure other

   M70.99 Unspecified soft tissue disorder related to use, overuse and pressure **multiple sites**

✓4ᵗʰ **M71 Other bursopathies**

   EXCLUDES 1   bunion (M20.1)

        bursitis related to use, overuse or pressure (M70.-)

        enthesopathies (M76-M77)

✓5ᵗʰ **M71.0 Abscess of bursa**

   Use additional code (B95.-, B96.-) to identify causative organism

   M71.00   Abscess of bursa, unspecified site

✓6ᵗʰ   **M71.01**   Abscess of bursa, **shoulder**

   M71.011 Abscess of bursa, **right** shoulder
   M71.012 Abscess of bursa, **left** shoulder
   M71.019 Abscess of bursa, unspecified shoulder

✓6ᵗʰ   **M71.02**   Abscess of bursa, **elbow**

   M71.021 Abscess of bursa, **right** elbow
   M71.022 Abscess of bursa, **left** elbow
   M71.029 Abscess of bursa, unspecified elbow

✓6ᵗʰ   **M71.03**   Abscess of bursa, **wrist**

   M71.031 Abscess of bursa, **right** wrist
   M71.032 Abscess of bursa, **left** wrist
   M71.039 Abscess of bursa, unspecified wrist

✓6ᵗʰ   **M71.04**   Abscess of bursa, **hand**

   M71.041 Abscess of bursa, **right** hand
   M71.042 Abscess of bursa, **left** hand
   M71.049 Abscess of bursa, unspecified hand

✓6ᵗʰ   **M71.05**   Abscess of bursa, **hip**

   M71.051 Abscess of bursa, **right** hip
   M71.052 Abscess of bursa, **left** hip
   M71.059 Abscess of bursa, unspecified hip

✓6ᵗʰ   **M71.06**   Abscess of bursa, **knee**

   M71.061 Abscess of bursa, **right** knee
   M71.062 Abscess of bursa, **left** knee
   M71.069 Abscess of bursa, unspecified knee

✓6ᵗʰ   **M71.07**   Abscess of bursa, **ankle and foot**

   M71.071 Abscess of bursa, **right** ankle and foot
   M71.072 Abscess of bursa, **left** ankle and foot
   M71.079 Abscess of bursa, unspecified ankle and foot

   M71.08   Abscess of bursa, other site
   M71.09   Abscess of bursa, **multiple sites**

✓5ᵗʰ **M71.1 Other infective bursitis**

   Use additional code (B95.-, B96.-) to identify causative organism

   M71.10   Other infective bursitis, unspecified site

✓6ᵗʰ   **M71.11**   Other infective bursitis, **shoulder**

   M71.111 Other infective bursitis, **right** shoulder
   M71.112 Other infective bursitis, **left** shoulder
   M71.119 Other infective bursitis, unspecified shoulder

✓6ᵗʰ   **M71.12**   Other infective bursitis, **elbow**

   M71.121 Other infective bursitis, **right** elbow
   M71.122 Other infective bursitis, **left** elbow
   M71.129 Other infective bursitis, unspecified elbow

✓6ᵗʰ   **M71.13**   Other infective bursitis, **wrist**

   M71.131 Other infective bursitis, **right** wrist
   M71.132 Other infective bursitis, **left** wrist

   M71.139 Other infective bursitis, unspecified wrist

✓6ᵗʰ   **M71.14**   Other infective bursitis, **hand**

   M71.141 Other infective bursitis, **right** hand
   M71.142 Other infective bursitis, **left** hand
   M71.149 Other infective bursitis, unspecified hand

✓6ᵗʰ   **M71.15**   Other infective bursitis, **hip**

   M71.151 Other infective bursitis, **right** hip
   M71.152 Other infective bursitis, **left** hip
   M71.159 Other infective bursitis, unspecified hip

✓6ᵗʰ   **M71.16**   Other infective bursitis, **knee**

   M71.161 Other infective bursitis, **right** knee
   M71.162 Other infective bursitis, **left** knee
   M71.169 Other infective bursitis, unspecified knee

✓6ᵗʰ   **M71.17**   Other infective bursitis, **ankle and foot**

   M71.171 Other infective bursitis, **right** ankle and foot
   M71.172 Other infective bursitis, **left** ankle and foot
   M71.179 Other infective bursitis, unspecified ankle and foot

   M71.18   Other infective bursitis, other site
   M71.19   Other infective bursitis, **multiple sites**

✓5ᵗʰ **M71.2 Synovial cyst of popliteal space [Baker]**

   EXCLUDES 1   synovial cyst of popliteal space with rupture (M66.0)

   DEF: Sac filled with clear synovial fluid in adults, usually secondary to disease inside the joint, located on the back of the knee in the popliteal fossa area. In children, the cyst usually represents a ganglion of one of the tendons in the knee.

Baker's Cyst

Baker's cyst connected to knee joint synovial cavity

   M71.20   Synovial cyst of popliteal space [Baker], unspecified knee
   M71.21   Synovial cyst of popliteal space [Baker], **right** knee
   M71.22   Synovial cyst of popliteal space [Baker], **left** knee

✓5ᵗʰ **M71.3 Other bursal cyst**

   Synovial cyst NOS

   EXCLUDES 1   synovial cyst with rupture (M66.1-)

   M71.30   Other bursal cyst, unspecified site

✓6ᵗʰ   **M71.31**   Other bursal cyst, **shoulder**

   M71.311 Other bursal cyst, **right** shoulder
   M71.312 Other bursal cyst, **left** shoulder
   M71.319 Other bursal cyst, unspecified shoulder

✓6ᵗʰ   **M71.32**   Other bursal cyst, **elbow**

   M71.321 Other bursal cyst, **right** elbow
   M71.322 Other bursal cyst, **left** elbow
   M71.329 Other bursal cyst, unspecified elbow

✓6ᵗʰ   **M71.33**   Other bursal cyst, **wrist**

   M71.331 Other bursal cyst, **right** wrist
   M71.332 Other bursal cyst, **left** wrist
   M71.339 Other bursal cyst, unspecified wrist

✓6ᵗʰ   **M71.34**   Other bursal cyst, **hand**

   M71.341 Other bursal cyst, **right** hand
   M71.342 Other bursal cyst, **left** hand
   M71.349 Other bursal cyst, unspecified hand

✓6ᵗʰ   **M71.35**   Other bursal cyst, **hip**

   M71.351 Other bursal cyst, **right** hip

M71.352 Other bursal cyst, **left** hip

M71.359 Other bursal cyst, unspecified hip

✓6th M71.37 Other bursal cyst, **ankle and foot**

M71.371 Other bursal cyst, **right** ankle and foot

M71.372 Other bursal cyst, **left** ankle and foot

M71.379 Other bursal cyst, unspecified ankle and foot

M71.38 Other bursal cyst, other site

M71.39 Other bursal cyst, **multiple sites**

✓5th **M71.4 Calcium deposit in bursa**

> EXCLUDES 2   calcium deposit in bursa of shoulder (M75.3)

M71.40 Calcium deposit in bursa, unspecified site

✓6th M71.42 Calcium deposit in bursa, **elbow**

M71.421 Calcium deposit in bursa, **right** elbow

M71.422 Calcium deposit in bursa, **left** elbow

M71.429 Calcium deposit in bursa, unspecified elbow

✓6th M71.43 Calcium deposit in bursa, **wrist**

M71.431 Calcium deposit in bursa, **right** wrist

M71.432 Calcium deposit in bursa, **left** wrist

M71.439 Calcium deposit in bursa, unspecified wrist

✓6th M71.44 Calcium deposit in bursa, **hand**

M71.441 Calcium deposit in bursa, **right** hand

M71.442 Calcium deposit in bursa, **left** hand

M71.449 Calcium deposit in bursa, unspecified hand

✓6th M71.45 Calcium deposit in bursa, **hip**

M71.451 Calcium deposit in bursa, **right** hip

M71.452 Calcium deposit in bursa, **left** hip

M71.459 Calcium deposit in bursa, unspecified hip

✓6th M71.46 Calcium deposit in bursa, **knee**

M71.461 Calcium deposit in bursa, **right** knee

M71.462 Calcium deposit in bursa, **left** knee

M71.469 Calcium deposit in bursa, unspecified knee

✓6th M71.47 Calcium deposit in bursa, **ankle and foot**

M71.471 Calcium deposit in bursa, **right** ankle and foot

M71.472 Calcium deposit in bursa, **left** ankle and foot

M71.479 Calcium deposit in bursa, unspecified ankle and foot

M71.48 Calcium deposit in bursa, other site

M71.49 Calcium deposit in bursa, **multiple sites**

✓5th **M71.5 Other bursitis, not elsewhere classified**

> EXCLUDES 1   bursitis NOS (M71.9-)
>
> EXCLUDES 2   bursitis of shoulder (M75.5)
>
>   bursitis of tibial collateral [Pellegrini-Stieda] (M76.4-)

M71.50 Other bursitis, not elsewhere classified, unspecified site

✓6th M71.52 Other bursitis, not elsewhere classified, **elbow**

M71.521 Other bursitis, not elsewhere classified, **right** elbow

M71.522 Other bursitis, not elsewhere classified, **left** elbow

M71.529 Other bursitis, not elsewhere classified, unspecified elbow

✓6th M71.53 Other bursitis, not elsewhere classified, **wrist**

M71.531 Other bursitis, not elsewhere classified, **right** wrist

M71.532 Other bursitis, not elsewhere classified, **left** wrist

M71.539 Other bursitis, not elsewhere classified, unspecified wrist

✓6th M71.54 Other bursitis, not elsewhere classified, **hand**

M71.541 Other bursitis, not elsewhere classified, **right** hand

M71.542 Other bursitis, not elsewhere classified, **left** hand

M71.549 Other bursitis, not elsewhere classified, unspecified hand

✓6th M71.55 Other bursitis, not elsewhere classified, **hip**

M71.551 Other bursitis, not elsewhere classified, **right** hip

M71.552 Other bursitis, not elsewhere classified, **left** hip

M71.559 Other bursitis, not elsewhere classified, unspecified hip

✓6th M71.56 Other bursitis, not elsewhere classified, **knee**

M71.561 Other bursitis, not elsewhere classified, **right** knee

M71.562 Other bursitis, not elsewhere classified, **left** knee

M71.569 Other bursitis, not elsewhere classified, unspecified knee

✓6th M71.57 Other bursitis, not elsewhere classified, **ankle and foot**

M71.571 Other bursitis, not elsewhere classified, **right** ankle and foot

M71.572 Other bursitis, not elsewhere classified, **left** ankle and foot

M71.579 Other bursitis, not elsewhere classified, unspecified ankle and foot

M71.58 Other bursitis, not elsewhere classified, other site

✓5th **M71.8 Other specified bursopathies**

M71.80 Other specified bursopathies, unspecified site

✓6th M71.81 Other specified bursopathies, **shoulder**

M71.811 Other specified bursopathies, **right** shoulder

M71.812 Other specified bursopathies, **left** shoulder

M71.819 Other specified bursopathies, unspecified shoulder

✓6th M71.82 Other specified bursopathies, **elbow**

M71.821 Other specified bursopathies, **right** elbow

M71.822 Other specified bursopathies, **left** elbow

M71.829 Other specified bursopathies, unspecified elbow

✓6th M71.83 Other specified bursopathies, **wrist**

M71.831 Other specified bursopathies, **right** wrist

M71.832 Other specified bursopathies, **left** wrist

M71.839 Other specified bursopathies, unspecified wrist

✓6th M71.84 Other specified bursopathies, **hand**

M71.841 Other specified bursopathies, **right** hand

M71.842 Other specified bursopathies, **left** hand

M71.849 Other specified bursopathies, unspecified hand

✓6th M71.85 Other specified bursopathies, **hip**

M71.851 Other specified bursopathies, **right** hip

M71.852 Other specified bursopathies, **left** hip

M71.859 Other specified bursopathies, unspecified hip

✓6th M71.86 Other specified bursopathies, **knee**

M71.861 Other specified bursopathies, **right** knee

M71.862 Other specified bursopathies, **left** knee

M71.869 Other specified bursopathies, unspecified knee

✓6th M71.87 Other specified bursopathies, **ankle and foot**

M71.871 Other specified bursopathies, **right** ankle and foot

M71.872 Other specified bursopathies, **left** ankle and foot

M71.879 Other specified bursopathies, unspecified ankle and foot

M71.88 Other specified bursopathies, other site

M71.89 Other specified bursopathies, **multiple sites**

M71.9 **Bursopathy, unspecified**
    Bursitis NOS

✓4th **M72 Fibroblastic disorders**

> EXCLUDES 2   retroperitoneal fibromatosis (D48.3)

M72.0 **Palmar fascial fibromatosis [Dupuytren]**   A

    DEF: Dupuytren's contracture: Flexion deformity of a finger, due to shortened, thickened fibrosing of palmar fascia. The cause is unknown, but it is associated with long-standing epilepsy.

M72.1 **Knuckle pads**

M72.2 **Plantar fascial fibromatosis**
    Plantar fasciitis
    DEF: Rapid-growing and multiplanar nodular swellings and pain in the foot that is not associated with contractures.

M72.4 **Pseudosarcomatous fibromatosis**
    Nodular fasciitis

M72.6 **Necrotizing fasciitis**   MCC HCC
    Use additional code (B95.-, B96.-) to identify causative organism

☑ Additional Character Required   ✓x7th Placeholder   Questionable PDx   Manifestation   Unspecified   UPD Unacceptable PDx   H1-H14 HAC   HCC CMS-HCC Dx   HIV HIV Dx

ICD-10-CM 2025   831

M72.8 Other fibroblastic disorders
Abscess of fascia
Fasciitis NEC
Other infective fasciitis
Use additional code to (B95.-, B96.-) identify causative organism
> EXCLUDES 1   *diffuse (eosinophilic) fasciitis (M35.4)*
> *necrotizing fasciitis (M72.6)*
> *nodular fasciitis (M72.4)*
> *perirenal fasciitis NOS (N13.5)*
> *perirenal fasciitis with infection (N13.6)*
> *plantar fasciitis (M72.2)*

M72.9 Fibroblastic disorder, unspecified
Fasciitis NOS
Fibromatosis NOS

✓4th M75 Shoulder lesions
> EXCLUDES 2   *shoulder-hand syndrome (M89.0-)*

✓5th M75.0 Adhesive capsulitis of shoulder
Frozen shoulder
Periarthritis of shoulder
AHA: 2015,2Q,23
   M75.00 Adhesive capsulitis of unspecified shoulder
   M75.01 Adhesive capsulitis of right shoulder
   M75.02 Adhesive capsulitis of left shoulder

✓5th M75.1 Rotator cuff tear or rupture, not specified as traumatic
Rotator cuff syndrome
Supraspinatus syndrome
Supraspinatus tear or rupture, not specified as traumatic
> EXCLUDES 1   *tear of rotator cuff, traumatic (S46.01-)*

   ✓6th M75.10 Unspecified rotator cuff tear or rupture, not specified as traumatic
     M75.100 Unspecified rotator cuff tear or rupture of unspecified shoulder, not specified as traumatic
     M75.101 Unspecified rotator cuff tear or rupture of right shoulder, not specified as traumatic
     M75.102 Unspecified rotator cuff tear or rupture of left shoulder, not specified as traumatic

   ✓6th M75.11 Incomplete rotator cuff tear or rupture not specified as traumatic
     M75.110 Incomplete rotator cuff tear or rupture of unspecified shoulder, not specified as traumatic
     M75.111 Incomplete rotator cuff tear or rupture of right shoulder, not specified as traumatic
     M75.112 Incomplete rotator cuff tear or rupture of left shoulder, not specified as traumatic

   ✓6th M75.12 Complete rotator cuff tear or rupture not specified as traumatic
     M75.120 Complete rotator cuff tear or rupture of unspecified shoulder, not specified as traumatic
     M75.121 Complete rotator cuff tear or rupture of right shoulder, not specified as traumatic
     M75.122 Complete rotator cuff tear or rupture of left shoulder, not specified as traumatic

✓5th M75.2 Bicipital tendinitis
   M75.20 Bicipital tendinitis, unspecified shoulder
   M75.21 Bicipital tendinitis, right shoulder
   M75.22 Bicipital tendinitis, left shoulder

✓5th M75.3 Calcific tendinitis of shoulder
Calcified bursa of shoulder
   M75.30 Calcific tendinitis of unspecified shoulder
   M75.31 Calcific tendinitis of right shoulder
   M75.32 Calcific tendinitis of left shoulder

✓5th M75.4 Impingement syndrome of shoulder
AHA: 2022,3Q,18
   M75.40 Impingement syndrome of unspecified shoulder
   M75.41 Impingement syndrome of right shoulder
   M75.42 Impingement syndrome of left shoulder

✓5th M75.5 Bursitis of shoulder
   M75.50 Bursitis of unspecified shoulder
   M75.51 Bursitis of right shoulder
   M75.52 Bursitis of left shoulder

✓5th M75.8 Other shoulder lesions
   M75.80 Other shoulder lesions, unspecified shoulder
   M75.81 Other shoulder lesions, right shoulder
   M75.82 Other shoulder lesions, left shoulder

✓5th M75.9 Shoulder lesion, unspecified
   M75.90 Shoulder lesion, unspecified, unspecified shoulder
   M75.91 Shoulder lesion, unspecified, right shoulder
   M75.92 Shoulder lesion, unspecified, left shoulder

✓4th M76 Enthesopathies, lower limb, excluding foot
> EXCLUDES 2   *bursitis due to use, overuse and pressure (M70.-)*
> *enthesopathies of ankle and foot (M77.5-)*

✓5th M76.0 Gluteal tendinitis
   M76.00 Gluteal tendinitis, unspecified hip
   M76.01 Gluteal tendinitis, right hip
   M76.02 Gluteal tendinitis, left hip

✓5th M76.1 Psoas tendinitis
   M76.10 Psoas tendinitis, unspecified hip
   M76.11 Psoas tendinitis, right hip
   M76.12 Psoas tendinitis, left hip

✓5th M76.2 Iliac crest spur
   M76.20 Iliac crest spur, unspecified hip
   M76.21 Iliac crest spur, right hip
   M76.22 Iliac crest spur, left hip

✓5th M76.3 Iliotibial band syndrome
   M76.30 Iliotibial band syndrome, unspecified leg
   M76.31 Iliotibial band syndrome, right leg
   M76.32 Iliotibial band syndrome, left leg

✓5th M76.4 Tibial collateral bursitis [Pellegrini-Stieda]
   M76.40 Tibial collateral bursitis [Pellegrini-Stieda], unspecified leg
   M76.41 Tibial collateral bursitis [Pellegrini-Stieda], right leg
   M76.42 Tibial collateral bursitis [Pellegrini-Stieda], left leg

✓5th M76.5 Patellar tendinitis
   M76.50 Patellar tendinitis, unspecified knee
   M76.51 Patellar tendinitis, right knee
   M76.52 Patellar tendinitis, left knee

✓5th M76.6 Achilles tendinitis
Achilles bursitis
   M76.60 Achilles tendinitis, unspecified leg
   M76.61 Achilles tendinitis, right leg
   M76.62 Achilles tendinitis, left leg

✓5th M76.7 Peroneal tendinitis
   M76.70 Peroneal tendinitis, unspecified leg
   M76.71 Peroneal tendinitis, right leg
   M76.72 Peroneal tendinitis, left leg

✓5th M76.8 Other specified enthesopathies of lower limb, excluding foot
   ✓6th M76.81 Anterior tibial syndrome
     M76.811 Anterior tibial syndrome, right leg
     M76.812 Anterior tibial syndrome, left leg
     M76.819 Anterior tibial syndrome, unspecified leg

   ✓6th M76.82 Posterior tibial tendinitis
     M76.821 Posterior tibial tendinitis, right leg
     M76.822 Posterior tibial tendinitis, left leg
     M76.829 Posterior tibial tendinitis, unspecified leg

   ✓6th M76.89 Other specified enthesopathies of lower limb, excluding foot
     M76.891 Other specified enthesopathies of right lower limb, excluding foot
     M76.892 Other specified enthesopathies of left lower limb, excluding foot
     M76.899 Other specified enthesopathies of unspecified lower limb, excluding foot

M76.9 Unspecified enthesopathy, lower limb, excluding foot

✓4th M77 Other enthesopathies
> EXCLUDES 1   *bursitis NOS (M71.9-)*
> EXCLUDES 2   *bursitis due to use, overuse and pressure (M70.-)*
> *osteophyte (M25.7)*
> *spinal enthesopathy (M46.0-)*

✓5th M77.0 Medial epicondylitis
   M77.00 Medial epicondylitis, unspecified elbow
   M77.01 Medial epicondylitis, right elbow
   M77.02 Medial epicondylitis, left elbow

✓5th M77.1 Lateral epicondylitis
Tennis elbow
   M77.10 Lateral epicondylitis, unspecified elbow
   M77.11 Lateral epicondylitis, right elbow
   M77.12 Lateral epicondylitis, left elbow

N Newborn: 0   **P** Pediatric: 0-17   **M** Maternity: 9-64   **A** Adult: 15-124   **UNS** Unspecified Site   **MCC** Major Complication/Comorbidity   **CC** Complication/Comorbidity   **PE** POA Exempt

832   ICD-10-CM 2025

✓5th **M77.2** **Periarthritis of wrist**

     M77.20 Periarthritis, unspecified wrist

     M77.21 Periarthritis, **right** wrist

     M77.22 Periarthritis, **left** wrist

✓5th **M77.3** **Calcaneal spur**

     DEF: Overgrowth of calcaneus bone on the underside of the heel that causes pain on walking. Calcaneal spur is due to a chronic avulsion injury of the plantar fascia from the calcaneus.

     M77.30 Calcaneal spur, unspecified foot

     M77.31 Calcaneal spur, **right** foot

     M77.32 Calcaneal spur, **left** foot

✓5th **M77.4** **Metatarsalgia**

     EXCLUDES 1   *Morton's metatarsalgia (G57.6)*

     M77.40 Metatarsalgia, unspecified foot

     M77.41 Metatarsalgia, **right** foot

     M77.42 Metatarsalgia, **left** foot

✓5th **M77.5** Other enthesopathy of **foot and ankle**

     M77.50 Other enthesopathy of unspecified foot and ankle

     M77.51 Other enthesopathy of **right** foot and ankle

     M77.52 Other enthesopathy of **left** foot and ankle

M77.8 Other enthesopathies, not elsewhere classified

M77.9 Enthesopathy, unspecified

     Bone spur NOS

     Capsulitis NOS

     Periarthritis NOS

     Tendinitis NOS

✓4th **M79** **Other and unspecified soft tissue disorders, not elsewhere classified**

     EXCLUDES 1   *psychogenic rheumatism (F45.8)*

         soft tissue pain, psychogenic (F45.41)

M79.0 Rheumatism, unspecified

     EXCLUDES 1   *fibromyalgia (M79.7)*

         palindromic rheumatism (M12.3-)

✓5th **M79.1** **Myalgia**

     Myofascial pain syndrome

     EXCLUDES 1   *fibromyalgia (M79.7)*

         myositis (M60.-)

     AHA: 2018,4Q,21

     M79.10 Myalgia, unspecified site

     M79.11 Myalgia of **mastication muscle**

     M79.12 Myalgia of **auxiliary muscles, head and neck**

     M79.18 Myalgia, other site

M79.2 Neuralgia and neuritis, unspecified

     EXCLUDES 1   *brachial radiculitis NOS (M54.1)*

         lumbosacral radiculitis NOS (M54.1)

         mononeuropathies (G56-G58)

         radiculitis NOS (M54.1)

         sciatica (M54.3-M54.4)

     TIP: Assign for documented neuropathic pain.

M79.3 Panniculitis, unspecified

     EXCLUDES 1   *lupus panniculitis (L93.2)*

         neck and back panniculitis (M54.0-)

         relapsing [Weber-Christian] panniculitis (M35.6)

     AHA: 2024,1Q,16

M79.4 Hypertrophy of (infrapatellar) fat pad

M79.5 Residual foreign body in soft tissue

     EXCLUDES 1   *foreign body granuloma of skin and subcutaneous tissue (L92.3)*

         foreign body granuloma of soft tissue (M60.2-)

     AHA: 2023,2Q,27

✓5th **M79.6** Pain in limb, hand, foot, fingers and toes

     EXCLUDES 2   *pain in joint (M25.5-)*

     ✓6th **M79.60** Pain in limb, unspecified

         M79.601 Pain in **right** arm

             Pain in right upper limb NOS

         M79.602 Pain in **left** arm

             Pain in left upper limb NOS

         M79.603 Pain in arm, unspecified

             Pain in upper limb NOS

         M79.604 Pain in **right** leg

             Pain in right lower limb NOS

         M79.605 Pain in **left** leg

             Pain in left lower limb NOS

         M79.606 Pain in leg, unspecified

             Pain in lower limb NOS

         M79.609 Pain in unspecified limb

             Pain in limb NOS

     ✓6th **M79.62** Pain in **upper arm**

         Pain in axillary region

         M79.621 Pain in **right** upper arm

         M79.622 Pain in **left** upper arm

         M79.629 Pain in unspecified upper arm

     ✓6th **M79.63** Pain in **forearm**

         M79.631 Pain in **right** forearm

         M79.632 Pain in **left** forearm

         M79.639 Pain in unspecified forearm

     ✓6th **M79.64** Pain in **hand and fingers**

         M79.641 Pain in **right** hand

         M79.642 Pain in **left** hand

         M79.643 Pain in unspecified hand

         M79.644 Pain in **right** finger(s)

         M79.645 Pain in **left** finger(s)

         M79.646 Pain in unspecified finger(s)

     ✓6th **M79.65** Pain in **thigh**

         M79.651 Pain in **right** thigh

         M79.652 Pain in **left** thigh

         M79.659 Pain in unspecified thigh

     ✓6th **M79.66** Pain in **lower leg**

         M79.661 Pain in **right** lower leg

         M79.662 Pain in **left** lower leg

         M79.669 Pain in unspecified lower leg

     ✓6th **M79.67** Pain in **foot and toes**

         M79.671 Pain in **right** foot

         M79.672 Pain in **left** foot

         M79.673 Pain in unspecified foot

         M79.674 Pain in **right** toe(s)

         M79.675 Pain in **left** toe(s)

         M79.676 Pain in unspecified toe(s)

M79.7 **Fibromyalgia**

     Fibromyositis

     Fibrositis

     Myofibrositis

✓5th **M79.A** **Nontraumatic compartment syndrome**

     Code first, if applicable, associated postprocedural complication

     EXCLUDES 1   *compartment syndrome NOS (T79.A-)*

         fibromyalgia (M79.7)

         nontraumatic ischemic infarction of muscle (M62.2-)

         traumatic compartment syndrome (T79.A-)

     ✓6th **M79.A1** Nontraumatic compartment syndrome of **upper extremity**

         Nontraumatic compartment syndrome of shoulder, arm, forearm, wrist, hand, and fingers

         M79.A11 Nontraumatic compartment syndrome of **right** upper extremity   CC

         M79.A12 Nontraumatic compartment syndrome of **left** upper extremity   CC

         M79.A19 Nontraumatic compartment syndrome of unspecified upper extremity   CC UNS

     ✓6th **M79.A2** Nontraumatic compartment syndrome of **lower extremity**

         Nontraumatic compartment syndrome of hip, buttock, thigh, leg, foot, and toes

         M79.A21 Nontraumatic compartment syndrome of **right** lower extremity   CC

         M79.A22 Nontraumatic compartment syndrome of **left** lower extremity   CC

         M79.A29 Nontraumatic compartment syndrome of unspecified lower extremity   CC UNS

     M79.A3 Nontraumatic compartment syndrome of **abdomen**   CC

     M79.A9 Nontraumatic compartment syndrome of other sites   CC

✓5th **M79.8** Other specified soft tissue disorders

     M79.81 Nontraumatic hematoma of soft tissue

         Nontraumatic hematoma of muscle

         Nontraumatic seroma of muscle and soft tissue

     M79.89 Other specified soft tissue disorders

         Polyalgia

M79.9 Soft tissue disorder, unspecified

✔ Additional Character Required   ✔x7th Placeholder   Questionable PDx   Manifestation   Unspecified   UPD Unacceptable PDx   H1-H14 HAC   HCC CMS-HCC Dx   HIV HIV Dx

ICD-10-CM 2025   833

Chapter 13. Diseases of the Musculoskeletal System and Connective Tissue

OSTEOPATHIES AND CHONDROPATHIES (M80–M94)

Disorders of bone density and structure (M80–M85)

√4ᵗʰ **M80**   Osteoporosis **with current pathological fracture**

INCLUDES   osteoporosis with current fragility fracture

Use additional code to identify major osseous defect, if applicable (M89.7-)

EXCLUDES 1   collapsed vertebra NOS (M48.5)
pathological fracture NOS (M84.4)
wedging of vertebra NOS (M48.5)

EXCLUDES 2   personal history of (healed) osteoporosis fracture (Z87.310)

AHA: 2018,2Q,12

TIP: The site codes in this category identify the site of the fracture, not the site of the osteoporosis.

> The appropriate 7th character is to be added to each code from category M80:
>
> A   initial encounter for fracture
> D   subsequent encounter for fracture with routine healing
> G   subsequent encounter for fracture with delayed healing
> K   subsequent encounter for fracture with nonunion
> P   subsequent encounter for fracture with malunion
> S   sequela

√5ᵗʰ **M80.0**   **Age-related** osteoporosis with current pathological fracture

Involutional osteoporosis with current pathological fracture
Osteoporosis NOS with current pathological fracture
Postmenopausal osteoporosis with current pathological fracture
Senile osteoporosis with current pathological fracture

√x 7ᵗʰ **M80.00**   Age-related osteoporosis with current pathological fracture, unspecified site   CC UNS A PE

√6ᵗʰ **M80.01**   Age-related osteoporosis with current pathological fracture, **shoulder**

√7ᵗʰ **M80.011**   Age-related osteoporosis with current pathological fracture, **right** shoulder   CC A PE

√7ᵗʰ **M80.012**   Age-related osteoporosis with current pathological fracture, **left** shoulder   CC A PE

√7ᵗʰ **M80.019**   Age-related osteoporosis with current pathological fracture, unspecified shoulder   CC UNS A PE

√6ᵗʰ **M80.02**   Age-related osteoporosis with current pathological fracture, **humerus**

√7ᵗʰ **M80.021**   Age-related osteoporosis with current pathological fracture, **right** humerus   CC A PE

√7ᵗʰ **M80.022**   Age-related osteoporosis with current pathological fracture, **left** humerus   CC A PE

√7ᵗʰ **M80.029**   Age-related osteoporosis with current pathological fracture, unspecified humerus   CC UNS A PE

√6ᵗʰ **M80.03**   Age-related osteoporosis with current pathological fracture, **forearm**

Age-related osteoporosis with current pathological fracture of wrist

√7ᵗʰ **M80.031**   Age-related osteoporosis with current pathological fracture, **right** forearm   CC A PE

√7ᵗʰ **M80.032**   Age-related osteoporosis with current pathological fracture, **left** forearm   CC A PE

√7ᵗʰ **M80.039**   Age-related osteoporosis with current pathological fracture, unspecified forearm   CC UNS A PE

√6ᵗʰ **M80.04**   Age-related osteoporosis with current pathological fracture, **hand**

√7ᵗʰ **M80.041**   Age-related osteoporosis with current pathological fracture, **right** hand   CC A PE

√7ᵗʰ **M80.042**   Age-related osteoporosis with current pathological fracture, **left** hand   CC A PE

√7ᵗʰ **M80.049**   Age-related osteoporosis with current pathological fracture, unspecified hand   CC UNS A PE

√6ᵗʰ **M80.05**   Age-related osteoporosis with current pathological fracture, **femur**

Age-related osteoporosis with current pathological fracture of hip

√7ᵗʰ **M80.051**   Age-related osteoporosis with current pathological fracture, **right** femur   CC HCC A PE

√7ᵗʰ **M80.052**   Age-related osteoporosis with current pathological fracture, **left** femur   CC HCC A PE

√7ᵗʰ **M80.059**   Age-related osteoporosis with current pathological fracture, unspecified femur   CC UNS HCC A PE

√6ᵗʰ **M80.06**   Age-related osteoporosis with current pathological fracture, **lower leg**

√7ᵗʰ **M80.061**   Age-related osteoporosis with current pathological fracture, **right** lower leg   CC A PE

√7ᵗʰ **M80.062**   Age-related osteoporosis with current pathological fracture, **left** lower leg   CC A PE

√7ᵗʰ **M80.069**   Age-related osteoporosis with current pathological fracture, unspecified lower leg   CC UNS A PE

√6ᵗʰ **M80.07**   Age-related osteoporosis with current pathological fracture, **ankle and foot**

√7ᵗʰ **M80.071**   Age-related osteoporosis with current pathological fracture, **right** ankle and foot   CC A PE

√7ᵗʰ **M80.072**   Age-related osteoporosis with current pathological fracture, **left** ankle and foot   CC A PE

√7ᵗʰ **M80.079**   Age-related osteoporosis with current pathological fracture, unspecified ankle and foot   CC UNS A PE

√x 7ᵗʰ **M80.08**   Age-related osteoporosis with current pathological fracture, **vertebra(e)**   CC HCC A PE

√x 7ᵗʰ **M80.0A**   Age-related osteoporosis with current pathological fracture, other site   CC A PE

AHA: 2020,4Q,32-33

√6ᵗʰ **M80.0B**   Age-related osteoporosis with current pathological fracture, **pelvis**

AHA: 2023,4Q,33-34

√7ᵗʰ **M80.0B1**   Age-related osteoporosis with current pathological fracture, **right** pelvis   CC A PE

√7ᵗʰ **M80.0B2**   Age-related osteoporosis with current pathological fracture, **left** pelvis   CC A PE

√7ᵗʰ **M80.0B9**   Age-related osteoporosis with current pathological fracture, unspecified pelvis   CC UNS A PE

√5ᵗʰ **M80.8**   **Other osteoporosis with current pathological fracture**

Drug-induced osteoporosis with current pathological fracture
Idiopathic osteoporosis with current pathological fracture
Osteoporosis of disuse with current pathological fracture
Postoophorectomy osteoporosis with current pathological fracture
Postsurgical malabsorption osteoporosis with current pathological fracture
Post-traumatic osteoporosis with current pathological fracture

Use additional code for adverse effect, if applicable, to identify drug (T36-T50 with fifth or sixth character 5)

√x 7ᵗʰ **M80.80**   Other osteoporosis with current pathological fracture, unspecified site   CC UNS PE

√6ᵗʰ **M80.81**   Other osteoporosis with pathological fracture, **shoulder**

√7ᵗʰ **M80.811**   Other osteoporosis with current pathological fracture, **right** shoulder   CC PE

√7ᵗʰ **M80.812**   Other osteoporosis with current pathological fracture, **left** shoulder   CC PE

√7ᵗʰ **M80.819**   Other osteoporosis with current pathological fracture, unspecified shoulder   CC UNS PE

√6ᵗʰ **M80.82**   Other osteoporosis with current pathological fracture, **humerus**

√7ᵗʰ **M80.821**   Other osteoporosis with current pathological fracture, **right** humerus   CC PE

N Newborn: 0   P Pediatric: 0-17   M Maternity: 9-64   A Adult: 15-124   UNS Unspecified Site   MCC Major Complication/Comorbidity   CC Complication/Comorbidity   PE POA Exempt

834   ICD-10-CM 2025

√7ᵗʰ **M80.822** Other osteoporosis with current pathological fracture, **left** humerus   `CC` `PE`

√7ᵗʰ **M80.829** Other osteoporosis with current pathological fracture, unspecified humerus   `CC` `UNS` `PE`

√6ᵗʰ **M80.83** Other osteoporosis with current pathological fracture, **forearm**

Other osteoporosis with current pathological fracture of wrist

√7ᵗʰ **M80.831** Other osteoporosis with current pathological fracture, **right** forearm   `CC` `PE`

√7ᵗʰ **M80.832** Other osteoporosis with current pathological fracture, **left** forearm   `CC` `PE`

√7ᵗʰ **M80.839** Other osteoporosis with current pathological fracture, unspecified forearm   `CC` `UNS` `PE`

√6ᵗʰ **M80.84** Other osteoporosis with current pathological fracture, **hand**

√7ᵗʰ **M80.841** Other osteoporosis with current pathological fracture, **right** hand   `CC` `PE`

√7ᵗʰ **M80.842** Other osteoporosis with current pathological fracture, **left** hand   `CC` `PE`

√7ᵗʰ **M80.849** Other osteoporosis with current pathological fracture, unspecified hand   `CC` `UNS` `PE`

√6ᵗʰ **M80.85** Other osteoporosis with current pathological fracture, **femur**

Other osteoporosis with current pathological fracture of hip

√7ᵗʰ **M80.851** Other osteoporosis with current pathological fracture, **right** femur   `CC` `HCC` `PE`

√7ᵗʰ **M80.852** Other osteoporosis with current pathological fracture, **left** femur   `CC` `HCC` `PE`

√7ᵗʰ **M80.859** Other osteoporosis with current pathological fracture, unspecified femur   `CC` `UNS` `HCC` `PE`

√6ᵗʰ **M80.86** Other osteoporosis with current pathological fracture, **lower leg**

√7ᵗʰ **M80.861** Other osteoporosis with current pathological fracture, **right** lower leg   `CC` `PE`

√7ᵗʰ **M80.862** Other osteoporosis with current pathological fracture, **left** lower leg   `CC` `PE`

√7ᵗʰ **M80.869** Other osteoporosis with current pathological fracture, unspecified lower leg   `CC` `UNS` `PE`

√6ᵗʰ **M80.87** Other osteoporosis with current pathological fracture, **ankle and foot**

√7ᵗʰ **M80.871** Other osteoporosis with current pathological fracture, **right** ankle and foot   `CC` `PE`

√7ᵗʰ **M80.872** Other osteoporosis with current pathological fracture, **left** ankle and foot   `CC` `PE`

√7ᵗʰ **M80.879** Other osteoporosis with current pathological fracture, unspecified ankle and foot   `CC` `UNS` `PE`

√x7ᵗʰ **M80.88** Other osteoporosis with current pathological fracture, **vertebra(e)**   `CC` `HCC` `PE`

√x7ᵗʰ **M80.8A** Other osteoporosis with current pathological fracture, **other site**   `CC` `PE`

AHA: 2020,4Q,32

√6ᵗʰ **M80.8B** Other osteoporosis with current pathological fracture, **pelvis**

AHA: 2023,4Q,33-34

√7ᵗʰ **M80.8B1** Other osteoporosis with current pathological fracture, **right** pelvis   `CC` `PE`

√7ᵗʰ **M80.8B2** Other osteoporosis with current pathological fracture, **left** pelvis   `CC` `PE`

√7ᵗʰ **M80.8B9** Other osteoporosis with current pathological fracture, unspecified pelvis   `CC` `UNS` `PE`

√4ᵗʰ **M81** **Osteoporosis** **without current pathological fracture**

Use additional code to identify:

major osseous defect, if applicable (M89.7-)

personal history of (healed) osteoporosis fracture, if applicable (Z87.310)

EXCLUDES 1   *osteoporosis with current pathological fracture (M80.-)*

Sudeck's atrophy (M89.0)

M81.0 **Age-related** osteoporosis without current pathological fracture   `A`

Involutional osteoporosis without current pathological fracture

Osteoporosis NOS

Postmenopausal osteoporosis without current pathological fracture

Senile osteoporosis without current pathological fracture

M81.6 **Localized** osteoporosis [Lequesne]

EXCLUDES 1   *Sudeck's atrophy (M89.0)*

M81.8 **Other** osteoporosis without current pathological fracture

Drug-induced osteoporosis without current pathological fracture

Idiopathic osteoporosis without current pathological fracture

Osteoporosis of disuse without current pathological fracture

Postoophorectomy osteoporosis without current pathological fracture

Postsurgical malabsorption osteoporosis without current pathological fracture

Post-traumatic osteoporosis without current pathological fracture

Use additional code for adverse effect, if applicable, to identify drug (T36-T50 with fifth or sixth character 5)

√4ᵗʰ **M83** **Adult osteomalacia**

EXCLUDES 1   *infantile and juvenile osteomalacia (E55.0)*

renal osteodystrophy (N25.0)

rickets (active) (E55.0)

rickets (active) sequelae (E64.3)

vitamin D-resistant osteomalacia (E83.31)

vitamin D-resistant rickets (active) (E83.31)

M83.0 **Puerperal** osteomalacia   `M`

M83.1 **Senile** osteomalacia   `M` `A`

M83.2 Adult osteomalacia **due to malabsorption**   `A`

Postsurgical malabsorption osteomalacia in adults

M83.3 Adult osteomalacia **due to malnutrition**   `A`

M83.4 **Aluminum bone disease**

M83.5 Other **drug-induced** osteomalacia in adults   `A`

Use additional code for adverse effect, if applicable, to identify drug (T36-T50 with fifth or sixth character 5)

M83.8 **Other** adult osteomalacia   `A`

M83.9 Adult osteomalacia, unspecified   `A`

√4ᵗʰ **M84** **Disorder of continuity of bone**

EXCLUDES 2   *traumatic fracture of bone-see fracture, by site*

√5ᵗʰ **M84.3** **Stress fracture**

Fatigue fracture

March fracture

Stress fracture NOS

Stress reaction

Use additional external cause code(s) to identify the cause of the stress fracture

EXCLUDES 1   *pathological fracture due to osteoporosis (M80.-)*

pathological fracture NOS (M84.4.-)

traumatic fracture (S12.-, S22.-, S32.-, S42.-, S52.-, S62.-, S72.-, S82.-, S92.-)

EXCLUDES 2   *personal history of (healed) stress (fatigue) fracture (Z87.312)*

stress fracture of vertebra (M48.4-)

> The appropriate 7th character is to be added to each code from subcategory M84.3.
>
> A   initial encounter for fracture
>
> D   subsequent encounter for fracture with routine healing
>
> G   subsequent encounter for fracture with delayed healing
>
> K   subsequent encounter for fracture with nonunion
>
> P   subsequent encounter for fracture with malunion
>
> S   sequela

√x7ᵗʰ **M84.30** Stress fracture, unspecified site   `CC` `UNS`

√6ᵗʰ **M84.31** Stress fracture, **shoulder**

√7ᵗʰ **M84.311** Stress fracture, **right** shoulder   `CC`

√7ᵗʰ **M84.312** Stress fracture, **left** shoulder   `CC`

√7ᵗʰ **M84.319** Stress fracture, unspecified shoulder   `CC` `UNS`

✅ Additional Character Required   √x7ᵗʰ Placeholder   Questionable PDx   Manifestation   Unspecified   `UPD` Unacceptable PDx   `H1`-`H4` HAC   `HCC` CMS-HCC Dx   `HIV` HIV Dx

ICD-10-CM 2025   835

Chapter 13. Diseases of the Musculoskeletal System and Connective Tissue (side tab)

√6th **M84.32** Stress fracture, **humerus**
- √7th **M84.321** Stress fracture, **right** humerus `CC`
- √7th **M84.322** Stress fracture, **left** humerus `CC`
- √7th **M84.329** Stress fracture, unspecified humerus `CC` `UNS`

√6th **M84.33** Stress fracture, **ulna and radius**
- √7th **M84.331** Stress fracture, **right** ulna `CC`
- √7th **M84.332** Stress fracture, **left** ulna `CC`
- √7th **M84.333** Stress fracture, **right** radius `CC`
- √7th **M84.334** Stress fracture, **left** radius `CC`
- √7th **M84.339** Stress fracture, unspecified ulna and radius `UNS`

√6th **M84.34** Stress fracture, **hand and fingers**
- √7th **M84.341** Stress fracture, **right** hand `CC`
- √7th **M84.342** Stress fracture, **left** hand `CC`
- √7th **M84.343** Stress fracture, unspecified hand `CC` `UNS`
- √7th **M84.344** Stress fracture, **right** finger(s) `CC`
- √7th **M84.345** Stress fracture, **left** finger(s) `CC`
- √7th **M84.346** Stress fracture, unspecified finger(s) `CC` `UNS`

√6th **M84.35** Stress fracture, **pelvis and femur**
    Stress fracture, hip
- √7th **M84.35Ø** Stress fracture, **pelvis** `CC`
- √7th **M84.351** Stress fracture, **right** femur `CC`
- √7th **M84.352** Stress fracture, **left** femur `CC`
- √7th **M84.353** Stress fracture, unspecified femur `CC` `UNS`
- √7th **M84.359** Stress fracture, hip, unspecified `CC`

√6th **M84.36** Stress fracture, **tibia and fibula**
- √7th **M84.361** Stress fracture, **right** tibia `CC`
- √7th **M84.362** Stress fracture, **left** tibia `CC`
- √7th **M84.363** Stress fracture, **right** fibula `CC`
- √7th **M84.364** Stress fracture, **left** fibula `CC`
- √7th **M84.369** Stress fracture, unspecified tibia and fibula `CC` `UNS`

√6th **M84.37** Stress fracture, **ankle, foot and toes**
- √7th **M84.371** Stress fracture, **right** ankle `CC`
- √7th **M84.372** Stress fracture, **left** ankle `CC`
- √7th **M84.373** Stress fracture, unspecified ankle `CC` `UNS`
- √7th **M84.374** Stress fracture, **right** foot `CC`
- √7th **M84.375** Stress fracture, **left** foot `CC`
- √7th **M84.376** Stress fracture, unspecified foot `CC` `UNS`
- √7th **M84.377** Stress fracture, **right** toe(s) `CC`
- √7th **M84.378** Stress fracture, **left** toe(s) `CC`
- √7th **M84.379** Stress fracture, unspecified toe(s) `CC` `UNS`

√x7th **M84.38** Stress fracture, other site `CC`
    EXCLUDES 2   stress fracture of vertebra (M48.4-)

√5th **M84.4** Pathological fracture, not elsewhere classified
    Chronic fracture
    Pathological fracture NOS
    EXCLUDES 1   collapsed vertebra NEC (M48.5)
           pathological fracture in neoplastic disease (M84.5-)
           pathological fracture in osteoporosis (M8Ø.-)
           pathological fracture in other disease (M84.6-)
           stress fracture (M84.3-)
           traumatic fracture (S12.-, S22.-, S32.-, S42.-, S52.-, S62.-, S72.-, S82.-, S92.-)
    EXCLUDES 2   personal history of (healed) pathological fracture (Z87.311)

The appropriate 7th character is to be added to each code from subcategory M84.4.
A   initial encounter for fracture
D   subsequent encounter for fracture with routine healing
G   subsequent encounter for fracture with delayed healing
K   subsequent encounter for fracture with nonunion
P   subsequent encounter for fracture with malunion
S   sequela

√x7th **M84.4Ø** Pathological fracture, unspecified site `CC` `UNS`

√6th **M84.41** Pathological fracture, **shoulder**
- √7th **M84.411** Pathological fracture, **right** shoulder `CC`
- √7th **M84.412** Pathological fracture, **left** shoulder `CC`
- √7th **M84.419** Pathological fracture, unspecified shoulder `CC` `UNS`

√6th **M84.42** Pathological fracture, **humerus**
- √7th **M84.421** Pathological fracture, **right** humerus `CC`
- √7th **M84.422** Pathological fracture, **left** humerus `CC`
- √7th **M84.429** Pathological fracture, unspecified humerus `CC` `UNS`

√6th **M84.43** Pathological fracture, **ulna and radius**
- √7th **M84.431** Pathological fracture, **right** ulna `CC`
- √7th **M84.432** Pathological fracture, **left** ulna `CC`
- √7th **M84.433** Pathological fracture, **right** radius `CC`
- √7th **M84.434** Pathological fracture, **left** radius `CC`
- √7th **M84.439** Pathological fracture, unspecified ulna and radius `CC` `UNS`

√6th **M84.44** Pathological fracture, **hand and fingers**
- √7th **M84.441** Pathological fracture, **right** hand `CC`
- √7th **M84.442** Pathological fracture, **left** hand `CC`
- √7th **M84.443** Pathological fracture, unspecified hand `CC` `UNS`
- √7th **M84.444** Pathological fracture, **right** finger(s) `CC`
- √7th **M84.445** Pathological fracture, **left** finger(s) `CC`
- √7th **M84.446** Pathological fracture, unspecified finger(s) `CC` `UNS`

√6th **M84.45** Pathological fracture, **femur and pelvis**
    AHA: 2016,4Q,43
- √7th **M84.451** Pathological fracture, **right** femur `CC` `HCC`
- √7th **M84.452** Pathological fracture, **left** femur `CC` `HCC`
- √7th **M84.453** Pathological fracture, unspecified femur `CC` `UNS` `HCC`
- √7th **M84.454** Pathological fracture, **pelvis** `CC`
- √7th **M84.459** Pathological fracture, hip, unspecified `CC` `HCC`

√6th **M84.46** Pathological fracture, **tibia and fibula**
- √7th **M84.461** Pathological fracture, **right** tibia `CC`
- √7th **M84.462** Pathological fracture, **left** tibia `CC`
- √7th **M84.463** Pathological fracture, **right** fibula `CC`
- √7th **M84.464** Pathological fracture, **left** fibula `CC`
- √7th **M84.469** Pathological fracture, unspecified tibia and fibula `CC` `UNS`

√6th **M84.47** Pathological fracture, **ankle, foot and toes**
- √7th **M84.471** Pathological fracture, **right** ankle `CC`
- √7th **M84.472** Pathological fracture, **left** ankle `CC`
- √7th **M84.473** Pathological fracture, unspecified ankle `CC` `UNS`
- √7th **M84.474** Pathological fracture, **right** foot `CC`
- √7th **M84.475** Pathological fracture, **left** foot `CC`
- √7th **M84.476** Pathological fracture, unspecified foot `CC` `UNS`
- √7th **M84.477** Pathological fracture, **right** toe(s) `CC`
- √7th **M84.478** Pathological fracture, **left** toe(s) `CC`
- √7th **M84.479** Pathological fracture, unspecified toe(s) `CC` `UNS`

√x7th **M84.48** Pathological fracture, other site `CC`

√5th **M84.5** Pathological fracture in **neoplastic disease**
    Code also underlying neoplasm

The appropriate 7th character is to be added to each code from subcategory M84.5.
A   initial encounter for fracture
D   subsequent encounter for fracture with routine healing
G   subsequent encounter for fracture with delayed healing
K   subsequent encounter for fracture with nonunion
P   subsequent encounter for fracture with malunion
S   sequela

√x7th **M84.5Ø** Pathological fracture in neoplastic disease, unspecified site `CC` `UNS`

N Newborn: 0   P Pediatric: 0-17   M Maternity: 9-64   A Adult: 15-124   `UNS` Unspecified Site   `MCC` Major Complication/Comorbidity   `CC` Complication/Comorbidity   `PE` POA Exempt

836   ICD-10-CM 2025

√6th **M84.51** Pathological fracture in neoplastic disease, shoulder

√7th **M84.511** Pathological fracture in neoplastic disease, right shoulder `CC`

√7th **M84.512** Pathological fracture in neoplastic disease, left shoulder `CC`

√7th **M84.519** Pathological fracture in neoplastic disease, unspecified shoulder `CC` `UNS`

√6th **M84.52** Pathological fracture in neoplastic disease, humerus

√7th **M84.521** Pathological fracture in neoplastic disease, right humerus `CC`

√7th **M84.522** Pathological fracture in neoplastic disease, left humerus `CC`

√7th **M84.529** Pathological fracture in neoplastic disease, unspecified humerus `CC` `UNS`

√6th **M84.53** Pathological fracture in neoplastic disease, ulna and radius

√7th **M84.531** Pathological fracture in neoplastic disease, right ulna `CC`

√7th **M84.532** Pathological fracture in neoplastic disease, left ulna `CC`

√7th **M84.533** Pathological fracture in neoplastic disease, right radius `CC`

√7th **M84.534** Pathological fracture in neoplastic disease, left radius `CC`

√7th **M84.539** Pathological fracture in neoplastic disease, unspecified ulna and radius `CC` `UNS`

√6th **M84.54** Pathological fracture in neoplastic disease, hand

√7th **M84.541** Pathological fracture in neoplastic disease, right hand `CC`

√7th **M84.542** Pathological fracture in neoplastic disease, left hand `CC`

√7th **M84.549** Pathological fracture in neoplastic disease, unspecified hand `CC` `UNS`

√6th **M84.55** Pathological fracture in neoplastic disease, pelvis and femur

√7th **M84.550** Pathological fracture in neoplastic disease, pelvis `CC`

√7th **M84.551** Pathological fracture in neoplastic disease, right femur `CC` `HCC`

√7th **M84.552** Pathological fracture in neoplastic disease, left femur `CC` `HCC`

√7th **M84.553** Pathological fracture in neoplastic disease, unspecified femur `CC` `UNS` `HCC`

√7th **M84.559** Pathological fracture in neoplastic disease, hip, unspecified `CC` `UNS` `HCC`

√6th **M84.56** Pathological fracture in neoplastic disease, tibia and fibula

√7th **M84.561** Pathological fracture in neoplastic disease, right tibia `CC`

√7th **M84.562** Pathological fracture in neoplastic disease, left tibia `CC`

√7th **M84.563** Pathological fracture in neoplastic disease, right fibula `CC`

√7th **M84.564** Pathological fracture in neoplastic disease, left fibula `CC`

√7th **M84.569** Pathological fracture in neoplastic disease, unspecified tibia and fibula `CC` `UNS`

√6th **M84.57** Pathological fracture in neoplastic disease, ankle and foot

√7th **M84.571** Pathological fracture in neoplastic disease, right ankle `CC`

√7th **M84.572** Pathological fracture in neoplastic disease, left ankle `CC`

√7th **M84.573** Pathological fracture in neoplastic disease, unspecified ankle `CC` `UNS`

√7th **M84.574** Pathological fracture in neoplastic disease, right foot `CC`

√7th **M84.575** Pathological fracture in neoplastic disease, left foot `CC`

√7th **M84.576** Pathological fracture in neoplastic disease, unspecified foot `CC` `UNS`

√x7th **M84.58** Pathological fracture in neoplastic disease, other specified site `CC`

Pathological fracture in neoplastic disease, vertebrae

√5th **M84.6** Pathological fracture in other disease

Code also underlying condition

EXCLUDES 1   *pathological fracture in osteoporosis (M80.-)*

The appropriate 7th character is to be added to each code from subcategory M84.6.
A   initial encounter for fracture
D   subsequent encounter for fracture with routine healing
G   subsequent encounter for fracture with delayed healing
K   subsequent encounter for fracture with nonunion
P   subsequent encounter for fracture with malunion
S   sequela

√x7th **M84.60** Pathological fracture in other disease, unspecified site `CC` `UNS`

√6th **M84.61** Pathological fracture in other disease, shoulder

√7th **M84.611** Pathological fracture in other disease, right shoulder `CC`

√7th **M84.612** Pathological fracture in other disease, left shoulder `CC`

√7th **M84.619** Pathological fracture in other disease, unspecified shoulder `CC` `UNS`

√6th **M84.62** Pathological fracture in other disease, humerus

√7th **M84.621** Pathological fracture in other disease, right humerus `CC`

√7th **M84.622** Pathological fracture in other disease, left humerus `CC`

√7th **M84.629** Pathological fracture in other disease, unspecified humerus `CC` `UNS`

√6th **M84.63** Pathological fracture in other disease, ulna and radius

√7th **M84.631** Pathological fracture in other disease, right ulna `CC`

√7th **M84.632** Pathological fracture in other disease, left ulna `CC`

√7th **M84.633** Pathological fracture in other disease, right radius `CC`

√7th **M84.634** Pathological fracture in other disease, left radius `CC`

√7th **M84.639** Pathological fracture in other disease, unspecified ulna and radius `CC` `UNS`

√6th **M84.64** Pathological fracture in other disease, hand

√7th **M84.641** Pathological fracture in other disease, right hand `CC`

√7th **M84.642** Pathological fracture in other disease, left hand `CC`

√7th **M84.649** Pathological fracture in other disease, unspecified hand `CC` `UNS`

√6th **M84.65** Pathological fracture in other disease, pelvis and femur

√7th **M84.650** Pathological fracture in other disease, pelvis `CC`

√7th **M84.651** Pathological fracture in other disease, right femur `CC` `HCC`

√7th **M84.652** Pathological fracture in other disease, left femur `CC` `HCC`

√7th **M84.653** Pathological fracture in other disease, unspecified femur `CC` `UNS` `HCC`

√7th **M84.659** Pathological fracture in other disease, hip, unspecified `CC` `HCC`

√6th **M84.66** Pathological fracture in other disease, tibia and fibula

√7th **M84.661** Pathological fracture in other disease, right tibia `CC`

√7th **M84.662** Pathological fracture in other disease, left tibia `CC`

√7th **M84.663** Pathological fracture in other disease, right fibula `CC`

√7th **M84.664** Pathological fracture in other disease, left fibula `CC`

√7th **M84.669** Pathological fracture in other disease, unspecified tibia and fibula `CC` `UNS`

√6th **M84.67** Pathological fracture in other disease, ankle and foot

√7th **M84.671** Pathological fracture in other disease, right ankle `CC`

√7th **M84.672** Pathological fracture in other disease, left ankle `CC`

√7th **M84.673** Pathological fracture in other disease, unspecified ankle `CC` `UNS`

√7th **M84.674** Pathological fracture in other disease, right foot `CC`

✔ Additional Character Required   √x7th Placeholder   Questionable PDx   Manifestation   Unspecified   UPD Unacceptable PDx   H1 - H14 HAC   HCC CMS-HCC Dx   HIV HIV Dx

ICD-10-CM 2025   **837**

√7ᵗʰ **M84.675** Pathological fracture in other disease, **left foot** `CC`

√7ᵗʰ **M84.676** Pathological fracture in other disease, **unspecified foot** `CC` `UNS`

√x7ᵗʰ **M84.68** Pathological fracture in other disease, other site `CC`

√5ᵗʰ **M84.7** Nontraumatic fracture, not elsewhere classified

√6ᵗʰ **M84.75** **Atypical** femoral fracture

     AHA: 2016,4Q,41-42

> The appropriate 7th character is to be added to each code from M84.75.
> A   initial encounter for fracture
> D   subsequent encounter for fracture with routine healing
> G   subsequent encounter for fracture with delayed healing
> K   subsequent encounter for fracture with nonunion
> P   subsequent encounter for fracture with malunion
> S   sequela

√7ᵗʰ **M84.75Ø** Atypical femoral fracture, **unspecified** `CC` `PE`

√7ᵗʰ **M84.751** **Incomplete** atypical femoral fracture, **right leg** `CC` `PE`

√7ᵗʰ **M84.752** **Incomplete** atypical femoral fracture, **left leg** `CC` `PE`

√7ᵗʰ **M84.753** **Incomplete** atypical femoral fracture, **unspecified leg** `CC` `UNS` `PE`

√7ᵗʰ **M84.754** **Complete transverse** atypical femoral fracture, **right leg** `CC` `HCC` `PE`

√7ᵗʰ **M84.755** **Complete transverse** atypical femoral fracture, **left leg** `CC` `HCC` `PE`

√7ᵗʰ **M84.756** **Complete transverse** atypical femoral fracture, **unspecified leg** `CC` `UNS` `HCC` `PE`

√7ᵗʰ **M84.757** **Complete oblique** atypical femoral fracture, **right leg** `CC` `HCC` `PE`

√7ᵗʰ **M84.758** **Complete oblique** atypical femoral fracture, **left leg** `CC` `HCC` `PE`

√7ᵗʰ **M84.759** **Complete oblique** atypical femoral fracture, **unspecified leg** `CC` `UNS` `HCC` `PE`

√5ᵗʰ **M84.8** Other disorders of continuity of bone

M84.8Ø Other disorders of continuity of bone, unspecified site

√6ᵗʰ **M84.81** Other disorders of continuity of bone, **shoulder**

M84.811 Other disorders of continuity of bone, **right shoulder**

M84.812 Other disorders of continuity of bone, **left shoulder**

M84.819 Other disorders of continuity of bone, **unspecified shoulder**

√6ᵗʰ **M84.82** Other disorders of continuity of bone, **humerus**

M84.821 Other disorders of continuity of bone, **right humerus**

M84.822 Other disorders of continuity of bone, **left humerus**

M84.829 Other disorders of continuity of bone, **unspecified humerus**

√6ᵗʰ **M84.83** Other disorders of continuity of bone, **ulna and radius**

M84.831 Other disorders of continuity of bone, **right ulna**

M84.832 Other disorders of continuity of bone, **left ulna**

M84.833 Other disorders of continuity of bone, **right radius**

M84.834 Other disorders of continuity of bone, **left radius**

M84.839 Other disorders of continuity of bone, **unspecified ulna and radius**

√6ᵗʰ **M84.84** Other disorders of continuity of bone, **hand**

M84.841 Other disorders of continuity of bone, **right hand**

M84.842 Other disorders of continuity of bone, **left hand**

M84.849 Other disorders of continuity of bone, **unspecified hand**

√6ᵗʰ **M84.85** Other disorders of continuity of bone, **pelvic region and thigh**

M84.851 Other disorders of continuity of bone, **right pelvic region and thigh**

M84.852 Other disorders of continuity of bone, **left pelvic region and thigh**

M84.859 Other disorders of continuity of bone, **unspecified pelvic region and thigh**

√6ᵗʰ **M84.86** Other disorders of continuity of bone, **tibia and fibula**

M84.861 Other disorders of continuity of bone, **right tibia**

M84.862 Other disorders of continuity of bone, **left tibia**

M84.863 Other disorders of continuity of bone, **right fibula**

M84.864 Other disorders of continuity of bone, **left fibula**

M84.869 Other disorders of continuity of bone, **unspecified tibia and fibula**

√6ᵗʰ **M84.87** Other disorders of continuity of bone, **ankle and foot**

M84.871 Other disorders of continuity of bone, **right ankle and foot**

M84.872 Other disorders of continuity of bone, **left ankle and foot**

M84.879 Other disorders of continuity of bone, **unspecified ankle and foot**

M84.88 Other disorders of continuity of bone, other site

M84.9 Disorder of continuity of bone, unspecified

√4ᵗʰ **M85** **Other disorders of bone density and structure**

   `EXCLUDES 1`   *osteogenesis imperfecta (Q78.Ø)*
               osteopetrosis (Q78.2)
               osteopoikilosis (Q78.8)
               polyostotic fibrous dysplasia (Q78.1)

√5ᵗʰ **M85.Ø** Fibrous dysplasia (monostotic)

   `EXCLUDES 2`   *fibrous dysplasia of jaw (M27.8)*

M85.ØØ Fibrous dysplasia (monostotic), unspecified site

√6ᵗʰ **M85.Ø1** Fibrous dysplasia (monostotic), **shoulder**

M85.Ø11 Fibrous dysplasia (monostotic), **right shoulder**

M85.Ø12 Fibrous dysplasia (monostotic), **left shoulder**

M85.Ø19 Fibrous dysplasia (monostotic), **unspecified shoulder**

√6ᵗʰ **M85.Ø2** Fibrous dysplasia (monostotic), **upper arm**

M85.Ø21 Fibrous dysplasia (monostotic), **right** upper arm

M85.Ø22 Fibrous dysplasia (monostotic), **left** upper arm

M85.Ø29 Fibrous dysplasia (monostotic), **unspecified upper arm**

√6ᵗʰ **M85.Ø3** Fibrous dysplasia (monostotic), **forearm**

M85.Ø31 Fibrous dysplasia (monostotic), **right forearm**

M85.Ø32 Fibrous dysplasia (monostotic), **left forearm**

M85.Ø39 Fibrous dysplasia (monostotic), **unspecified forearm**

√6ᵗʰ **M85.Ø4** Fibrous dysplasia (monostotic), **hand**

M85.Ø41 Fibrous dysplasia (monostotic), **right** hand

M85.Ø42 Fibrous dysplasia (monostotic), **left** hand

M85.Ø49 Fibrous dysplasia (monostotic), **unspecified hand**

√6ᵗʰ **M85.Ø5** Fibrous dysplasia (monostotic), **thigh**

M85.Ø51 Fibrous dysplasia (monostotic), **right** thigh

M85.Ø52 Fibrous dysplasia (monostotic), **left** thigh

M85.Ø59 Fibrous dysplasia (monostotic), **unspecified thigh**

√6ᵗʰ **M85.Ø6** Fibrous dysplasia (monostotic), **lower leg**

M85.Ø61 Fibrous dysplasia (monostotic), **right** lower leg

M85.Ø62 Fibrous dysplasia (monostotic), **left** lower leg

M85.Ø69 Fibrous dysplasia (monostotic), **unspecified lower leg**

√6ᵗʰ **M85.Ø7** Fibrous dysplasia (monostotic), **ankle and foot**

M85.Ø71 Fibrous dysplasia (monostotic), **right** ankle and foot

M85.Ø72 Fibrous dysplasia (monostotic), **left** ankle and foot

M85.Ø79 Fibrous dysplasia (monostotic), **unspecified ankle and foot**

M85.Ø8 Fibrous dysplasia (monostotic), other site

M85.Ø9 Fibrous dysplasia (monostotic), **multiple sites**

✓5ᵗʰ **M85.1**   **Skeletal fluorosis**

    M85.10   Skeletal fluorosis, unspecified site

✓6ᵗʰ   M85.11   Skeletal fluorosis, shoulder

    M85.111   Skeletal fluorosis, right shoulder
    M85.112   Skeletal fluorosis, left shoulder
    M85.119   Skeletal fluorosis, unspecified shoulder

✓6ᵗʰ   M85.12   Skeletal fluorosis, upper arm

    M85.121   Skeletal fluorosis, right upper arm
    M85.122   Skeletal fluorosis, left upper arm
    M85.129   Skeletal fluorosis, unspecified upper arm

✓6ᵗʰ   M85.13   Skeletal fluorosis, forearm

    M85.131   Skeletal fluorosis, right forearm
    M85.132   Skeletal fluorosis, left forearm
    M85.139   Skeletal fluorosis, unspecified forearm

✓6ᵗʰ   M85.14   Skeletal fluorosis, hand

    M85.141   Skeletal fluorosis, right hand
    M85.142   Skeletal fluorosis, left hand
    M85.149   Skeletal fluorosis, unspecified hand

✓6ᵗʰ   M85.15   Skeletal fluorosis, thigh

    M85.151   Skeletal fluorosis, right thigh
    M85.152   Skeletal fluorosis, left thigh
    M85.159   Skeletal fluorosis, unspecified thigh

✓6ᵗʰ   M85.16   Skeletal fluorosis, lower leg

    M85.161   Skeletal fluorosis, right lower leg
    M85.162   Skeletal fluorosis, left lower leg
    M85.169   Skeletal fluorosis, unspecified lower leg

✓6ᵗʰ   M85.17   Skeletal fluorosis, ankle and foot

    M85.171   Skeletal fluorosis, right ankle and foot
    M85.172   Skeletal fluorosis, left ankle and foot
    M85.179   Skeletal fluorosis, unspecified ankle and foot

    M85.18   Skeletal fluorosis, other site
    M85.19   Skeletal fluorosis, multiple sites

M85.2   **Hyperostosis of skull**

    DEF: Abnormal bone growth on the inner aspect of the cranial bones.

✓5ᵗʰ **M85.3**   **Osteitis condensans**

    M85.30   Osteitis condensans, unspecified site

✓6ᵗʰ   M85.31   Osteitis condensans, shoulder

    M85.311   Osteitis condensans, right shoulder
    M85.312   Osteitis condensans, left shoulder
    M85.319   Osteitis condensans, unspecified shoulder

✓6ᵗʰ   M85.32   Osteitis condensans, upper arm

    M85.321   Osteitis condensans, right upper arm
    M85.322   Osteitis condensans, left upper arm
    M85.329   Osteitis condensans, unspecified upper arm

✓6ᵗʰ   M85.33   Osteitis condensans, forearm

    M85.331   Osteitis condensans, right forearm
    M85.332   Osteitis condensans, left forearm
    M85.339   Osteitis condensans, unspecified forearm

✓6ᵗʰ   M85.34   Osteitis condensans, hand

    M85.341   Osteitis condensans, right hand
    M85.342   Osteitis condensans, left hand
    M85.349   Osteitis condensans, unspecified hand

✓6ᵗʰ   M85.35   Osteitis condensans, thigh

    M85.351   Osteitis condensans, right thigh
    M85.352   Osteitis condensans, left thigh
    M85.359   Osteitis condensans, unspecified thigh

✓6ᵗʰ   M85.36   Osteitis condensans, lower leg

    M85.361   Osteitis condensans, right lower leg
    M85.362   Osteitis condensans, left lower leg
    M85.369   Osteitis condensans, unspecified lower leg

✓6ᵗʰ   M85.37   Osteitis condensans, ankle and foot

    M85.371   Osteitis condensans, right ankle and foot
    M85.372   Osteitis condensans, left ankle and foot
    M85.379   Osteitis condensans, unspecified ankle and foot

    M85.38   Osteitis condensans, other site
    M85.39   Osteitis condensans, multiple sites

✓5ᵗʰ **M85.4**   **Solitary bone cyst**

    EXCLUDES 2   solitary cyst of jaw (M27.4)

    M85.40   Solitary bone cyst, unspecified site

✓6ᵗʰ   M85.41   Solitary bone cyst, shoulder

    M85.411   Solitary bone cyst, right shoulder

    M85.412   Solitary bone cyst, left shoulder
    M85.419   Solitary bone cyst, unspecified shoulder

✓6ᵗʰ   M85.42   Solitary bone cyst, humerus

    M85.421   Solitary bone cyst, right humerus
    M85.422   Solitary bone cyst, left humerus
    M85.429   Solitary bone cyst, unspecified humerus

✓6ᵗʰ   M85.43   Solitary bone cyst, ulna and radius

    M85.431   Solitary bone cyst, right ulna and radius
    M85.432   Solitary bone cyst, left ulna and radius
    M85.439   Solitary bone cyst, unspecified ulna and radius

✓6ᵗʰ   M85.44   Solitary bone cyst, hand

    M85.441   Solitary bone cyst, right hand
    M85.442   Solitary bone cyst, left hand
    M85.449   Solitary bone cyst, unspecified hand

✓6ᵗʰ   M85.45   Solitary bone cyst, pelvis

    M85.451   Solitary bone cyst, right pelvis
    M85.452   Solitary bone cyst, left pelvis
    M85.459   Solitary bone cyst, unspecified pelvis

✓6ᵗʰ   M85.46   Solitary bone cyst, tibia and fibula

    M85.461   Solitary bone cyst, right tibia and fibula
    M85.462   Solitary bone cyst, left tibia and fibula
    M85.469   Solitary bone cyst, unspecified tibia and fibula

✓6ᵗʰ   M85.47   Solitary bone cyst, ankle and foot

    M85.471   Solitary bone cyst, right ankle and foot
    M85.472   Solitary bone cyst, left ankle and foot
    M85.479   Solitary bone cyst, unspecified ankle and foot

    M85.48   Solitary bone cyst, other site

✓5ᵗʰ **M85.5**   **Aneurysmal bone cyst**

    EXCLUDES 2   aneurysmal cyst of jaw (M27.4)

    DEF: Solitary bone lesion that bulges into the periosteum and is marked by a calcified rim.

    M85.50   Aneurysmal bone cyst, unspecified site

✓6ᵗʰ   M85.51   Aneurysmal bone cyst, shoulder

    M85.511   Aneurysmal bone cyst, right shoulder
    M85.512   Aneurysmal bone cyst, left shoulder
    M85.519   Aneurysmal bone cyst, unspecified shoulder

✓6ᵗʰ   M85.52   Aneurysmal bone cyst, upper arm

    M85.521   Aneurysmal bone cyst, right upper arm
    M85.522   Aneurysmal bone cyst, left upper arm
    M85.529   Aneurysmal bone cyst, unspecified upper arm

✓6ᵗʰ   M85.53   Aneurysmal bone cyst, forearm

    M85.531   Aneurysmal bone cyst, right forearm
    M85.532   Aneurysmal bone cyst, left forearm
    M85.539   Aneurysmal bone cyst, unspecified forearm

✓6ᵗʰ   M85.54   Aneurysmal bone cyst, hand

    M85.541   Aneurysmal bone cyst, right hand
    M85.542   Aneurysmal bone cyst, left hand
    M85.549   Aneurysmal bone cyst, unspecified hand

✓6ᵗʰ   M85.55   Aneurysmal bone cyst, thigh

    M85.551   Aneurysmal bone cyst, right thigh
    M85.552   Aneurysmal bone cyst, left thigh
    M85.559   Aneurysmal bone cyst, unspecified thigh

✓6ᵗʰ   M85.56   Aneurysmal bone cyst, lower leg

    M85.561   Aneurysmal bone cyst, right lower leg
    M85.562   Aneurysmal bone cyst, left lower leg
    M85.569   Aneurysmal bone cyst, unspecified lower leg

✓6ᵗʰ   M85.57   Aneurysmal bone cyst, ankle and foot

    M85.571   Aneurysmal bone cyst, right ankle and foot
    M85.572   Aneurysmal bone cyst, left ankle and foot
    M85.579   Aneurysmal bone cyst, unspecified ankle and foot

    M85.58   Aneurysmal bone cyst, other site
    M85.59   Aneurysmal bone cyst, multiple sites

✓5ᵗʰ **M85.6**   **Other cyst of bone**

    EXCLUDES 1   cyst of jaw NEC (M27.4)
             osteitis fibrosa cystica generalisata [von Recklinghausen's disease of bone] (E21.0)

    M85.60   Other cyst of bone, unspecified site

✓6ᵗʰ   M85.61   Other cyst of bone, shoulder

    M85.611   Other cyst of bone, right shoulder

✔ Additional Character Required   ✓x7ᵗʰ Placeholder   Questionable PDx   Manifestation   Unspecified   UPD Unacceptable PDx   H1-H14 HAC   HCC CMS-HCC Dx   HIV HIV Dx

ICD-10-CM 2025   839

Chapter 13. Diseases of the Musculoskeletal System and Connective Tissue

M85.612   Other cyst of bone, **left** shoulder
M85.619   Other cyst of bone, unspecified shoulder

✓6th   **M85.62**   Other cyst of bone, **upper arm**

M85.621   Other cyst of bone, **right** upper arm
M85.622   Other cyst of bone, **left** upper arm
M85.629   Other cyst of bone, unspecified upper arm

✓6th   **M85.63**   Other cyst of bone, **forearm**

M85.631   Other cyst of bone, **right** forearm
M85.632   Other cyst of bone, **left** forearm
M85.639   Other cyst of bone, unspecified forearm

✓6th   **M85.64**   Other cyst of bone, **hand**

M85.641   Other cyst of bone, **right** hand
M85.642   Other cyst of bone, **left** hand
M85.649   Other cyst of bone, unspecified hand

✓6th   **M85.65**   Other cyst of bone, **thigh**

M85.651   Other cyst of bone, **right** thigh
M85.652   Other cyst of bone, **left** thigh
M85.659   Other cyst of bone, unspecified thigh

✓6th   **M85.66**   Other cyst of bone, **lower leg**

M85.661   Other cyst of bone, **right** lower leg
M85.662   Other cyst of bone, **left** lower leg
M85.669   Other cyst of bone, unspecified lower leg

✓6th   **M85.67**   Other cyst of bone, **ankle and foot**

M85.671   Other cyst of bone, **right** ankle and foot
M85.672   Other cyst of bone, **left** ankle and foot
M85.679   Other cyst of bone, unspecified ankle and foot

M85.68   Other cyst of bone, other site
M85.69   Other cyst of bone, **multiple sites**

✓5th   **M85.8**   **Other specified disorders of bone density and structure**

Hyperostosis of bones, except skull
Osteosclerosis, acquired

EXCLUDES 1   *diffuse idiopathic skeletal hyperostosis [DISH] (M48.1)*
osteosclerosis congenita (Q77.4)
osteosclerosis fragilitas (generalista) (Q78.2)
osteosclerosis myelofibrosis (D75.81)

M85.80   Other specified disorders of bone density and structure, unspecified site

✓6th   **M85.81**   Other specified disorders of bone density and structure, **shoulder**

M85.811   Other specified disorders of bone density and structure, **right** shoulder
M85.812   Other specified disorders of bone density and structure, **left** shoulder
M85.819   Other specified disorders of bone density and structure, unspecified shoulder

✓6th   **M85.82**   Other specified disorders of bone density and structure, **upper arm**

M85.821   Other specified disorders of bone density and structure, **right** upper arm
M85.822   Other specified disorders of bone density and structure, **left** upper arm
M85.829   Other specified disorders of bone density and structure, unspecified upper arm

✓6th   **M85.83**   Other specified disorders of bone density and structure, **forearm**

M85.831   Other specified disorders of bone density and structure, **right** forearm
M85.832   Other specified disorders of bone density and structure, **left** forearm
M85.839   Other specified disorders of bone density and structure, unspecified forearm

✓6th   **M85.84**   Other specified disorders of bone density and structure, **hand**

M85.841   Other specified disorders of bone density and structure, **right** hand
M85.842   Other specified disorders of bone density and structure, **left** hand
M85.849   Other specified disorders of bone density and structure, unspecified hand

✓6th   **M85.85**   Other specified disorders of bone density and structure, **thigh**

M85.851   Other specified disorders of bone density and structure, **right** thigh
M85.852   Other specified disorders of bone density and structure, **left** thigh
M85.859   Other specified disorders of bone density and structure, unspecified thigh

✓6th   **M85.86**   Other specified disorders of bone density and structure, **lower leg**

M85.861   Other specified disorders of bone density and structure, **right** lower leg
M85.862   Other specified disorders of bone density and structure, **left** lower leg
M85.869   Other specified disorders of bone density and structure, unspecified lower leg

✓6th   **M85.87**   Other specified disorders of bone density and structure, **ankle and foot**

M85.871   Other specified disorders of bone density and structure, **right** ankle and foot
M85.872   Other specified disorders of bone density and structure, **left** ankle and foot
M85.879   Other specified disorders of bone density and structure, unspecified ankle and foot

M85.88   Other specified disorders of bone density and structure, other site
M85.89   Other specified disorders of bone density and structure, **multiple sites**

M85.9   **Disorder of bone density and structure, unspecified**
AHA: 2021,3Q,11

Other osteopathies (M86-M90)

EXCLUDES 1   *postprocedural osteopathies (M96.-)*

✓4th   **M86 Osteomyelitis**

Use additional code (B95-B97) to identify infectious agent
Use additional code to identify major osseous defect, if applicable (M89.7-)

EXCLUDES 1   *osteomyelitis due to:*
echinococcus (B67.2)
gonococcus (A54.43)
salmonella (A02.24)

EXCLUDES 2   *ostemyelitis of:*
orbit (H05.0-)
petrous bone (H70.2-)
vertebra (M46.2-)

✓5th   **M86.0**   **Acute hematogenous osteomyelitis**

M86.00   Acute hematogenous osteomyelitis, unspecified site   CC UNS HCC

✓6th   **M86.01**   Acute hematogenous osteomyelitis, **shoulder**

M86.011   Acute hematogenous osteomyelitis, **right** shoulder   CC HCC
M86.012   Acute hematogenous osteomyelitis, **left** shoulder   CC HCC
M86.019   Acute hematogenous osteomyelitis, unspecified shoulder   CC UNS HCC

✓6th   **M86.02**   Acute hematogenous osteomyelitis, **humerus**

M86.021   Acute hematogenous osteomyelitis, **right** humerus   CC HCC
M86.022   Acute hematogenous osteomyelitis, **left** humerus   CC HCC
M86.029   Acute hematogenous osteomyelitis, unspecified humerus   CC UNS HCC

✓6th   **M86.03**   Acute hematogenous osteomyelitis, **radius and ulna**

M86.031   Acute hematogenous osteomyelitis, **right** radius and ulna   CC HCC
M86.032   Acute hematogenous osteomyelitis, **left** radius and ulna   CC HCC
M86.039   Acute hematogenous osteomyelitis, unspecified radius and ulna   CC UNS HCC

✓6th   **M86.04**   Acute hematogenous osteomyelitis, **hand**

M86.041   Acute hematogenous osteomyelitis, **right** hand   CC HCC
M86.042   Acute hematogenous osteomyelitis, **left** hand   CC HCC
M86.049   Acute hematogenous osteomyelitis, unspecified hand   CC UNS HCC

✓6th   **M86.05**   Acute hematogenous osteomyelitis, **femur**

M86.051   Acute hematogenous osteomyelitis, **right** femur   CC HCC
M86.052   Acute hematogenous osteomyelitis, **left** femur   CC HCC
M86.059   Acute hematogenous osteomyelitis, unspecified femur   CC UNS HCC

✓6th   **M86.06**   Acute hematogenous osteomyelitis, **tibia and fibula**

M86.061   Acute hematogenous osteomyelitis, **right** tibia and fibula   CC HCC

M86.062 Acute hematogenous osteomyelitis, **left** tibia and fibula `CC` `HCC`

M86.069 Acute hematogenous osteomyelitis, unspecified tibia and fibula `CC` `UNS` `HCC`

✓6ᵗʰ M86.07 Acute hematogenous osteomyelitis, **ankle and foot**

M86.071 Acute hematogenous osteomyelitis, **right** ankle and foot `CC` `HCC`

M86.072 Acute hematogenous osteomyelitis, **left** ankle and foot `CC` `HCC`

M86.079 Acute hematogenous osteomyelitis, unspecified ankle and foot `CC` `UNS` `HCC`

M86.08 Acute hematogenous osteomyelitis, other sites `CC` `HCC`

M86.09 Acute hematogenous osteomyelitis, **multiple sites** `CC` `HCC`

✓5ᵗʰ M86.1 **Other acute** osteomyelitis

M86.10 Other acute osteomyelitis, unspecified site `CC` `UNS` `HCC`

✓6ᵗʰ M86.11 Other acute osteomyelitis, **shoulder**

M86.111 Other acute osteomyelitis, **right** shoulder `CC` `HCC`

M86.112 Other acute osteomyelitis, **left** shoulder `CC` `HCC`

M86.119 Other acute osteomyelitis, unspecified shoulder `CC` `UNS` `HCC`

✓6ᵗʰ M86.12 Other acute osteomyelitis, **humerus**

M86.121 Other acute osteomyelitis, **right** humerus `CC` `HCC`

M86.122 Other acute osteomyelitis, **left** humerus `CC` `HCC`

M86.129 Other acute osteomyelitis, unspecified humerus `CC` `UNS` `HCC`

✓6ᵗʰ M86.13 Other acute osteomyelitis, **radius and ulna**

M86.131 Other acute osteomyelitis, **right** radius and ulna `CC` `HCC`

M86.132 Other acute osteomyelitis, **left** radius and ulna `CC` `HCC`

M86.139 Other acute osteomyelitis, unspecified radius and ulna `CC` `UNS` `HCC`

✓6ᵗʰ M86.14 Other acute osteomyelitis, **hand**

M86.141 Other acute osteomyelitis, **right** hand `CC` `HCC`

M86.142 Other acute osteomyelitis, **left** hand `CC` `HCC`

M86.149 Other acute osteomyelitis, unspecified hand `CC` `UNS` `HCC`

✓6ᵗʰ M86.15 Other acute osteomyelitis, **femur**

M86.151 Other acute osteomyelitis, **right** femur `CC` `HCC`

M86.152 Other acute osteomyelitis, **left** femur `CC` `HCC`

M86.159 Other acute osteomyelitis, unspecified femur `CC` `UNS` `HCC`

✓6ᵗʰ M86.16 Other acute osteomyelitis, **tibia and fibula**

M86.161 Other acute osteomyelitis, **right** tibia and fibula `CC` `HCC`

M86.162 Other acute osteomyelitis, **left** tibia and fibula `CC` `HCC`

M86.169 Other acute osteomyelitis, unspecified tibia and fibula `CC` `UNS` `HCC`

✓6ᵗʰ M86.17 Other acute osteomyelitis, **ankle and foot**

AHA: 2020,1Q,12

M86.171 Other acute osteomyelitis, **right** ankle and foot `CC` `HCC`

M86.172 Other acute osteomyelitis, **left** ankle and foot `CC` `HCC`

M86.179 Other acute osteomyelitis, unspecified ankle and foot `CC` `UNS` `HCC`

M86.18 Other acute osteomyelitis, other site `CC` `HCC`

M86.19 Other acute osteomyelitis, **multiple sites** `CC` `HCC`

✓5ᵗʰ M86.2 **Subacute** osteomyelitis

M86.20 Subacute osteomyelitis, unspecified site `CC` `UNS` `HCC`

✓6ᵗʰ M86.21 Subacute osteomyelitis, **shoulder**

M86.211 Subacute osteomyelitis, **right** shoulder `CC` `HCC`

M86.212 Subacute osteomyelitis, **left** shoulder `CC` `HCC`

M86.219 Subacute osteomyelitis, unspecified shoulder `CC` `UNS` `HCC`

✓6ᵗʰ M86.22 Subacute osteomyelitis, **humerus**

M86.221 Subacute osteomyelitis, **right** humerus `CC` `HCC`

M86.222 Subacute osteomyelitis, **left** humerus `CC` `HCC`

M86.229 Subacute osteomyelitis, unspecified humerus `CC` `UNS` `HCC`

✓6ᵗʰ M86.23 Subacute osteomyelitis, **radius and ulna**

M86.231 Subacute osteomyelitis, **right** radius and ulna `CC` `HCC`

M86.232 Subacute osteomyelitis, **left** radius and ulna `CC` `HCC`

M86.239 Subacute osteomyelitis, unspecified radius and ulna `CC` `UNS` `HCC`

✓6ᵗʰ M86.24 Subacute osteomyelitis, **hand**

M86.241 Subacute osteomyelitis, **right** hand `CC` `HCC`

M86.242 Subacute osteomyelitis, **left** hand `CC` `HCC`

M86.249 Subacute osteomyelitis, unspecified hand `CC` `UNS` `HCC`

✓6ᵗʰ M86.25 Subacute osteomyelitis, **femur**

M86.251 Subacute osteomyelitis, **right** femur `CC` `HCC`

M86.252 Subacute osteomyelitis, **left** femur `CC` `HCC`

M86.259 Subacute osteomyelitis, unspecified femur `CC` `UNS` `HCC`

✓6ᵗʰ M86.26 Subacute osteomyelitis, **tibia and fibula**

M86.261 Subacute osteomyelitis, **right** tibia and fibula `CC` `HCC`

M86.262 Subacute osteomyelitis, **left** tibia and fibula `CC` `HCC`

M86.269 Subacute osteomyelitis, unspecified tibia and fibula `CC` `UNS` `HCC`

✓6ᵗʰ M86.27 Subacute osteomyelitis, **ankle and foot**

M86.271 Subacute osteomyelitis, **right** ankle and foot `CC` `HCC`

M86.272 Subacute osteomyelitis, **left** ankle and foot `CC` `HCC`

M86.279 Subacute osteomyelitis, unspecified ankle and foot `CC` `UNS` `HCC`

M86.28 Subacute osteomyelitis, other site `CC` `HCC`

M86.29 Subacute osteomyelitis, **multiple sites** `CC` `HCC`

✓5ᵗʰ M86.3 **Chronic multifocal** osteomyelitis

M86.30 Chronic multifocal osteomyelitis, unspecified site `CC` `UNS` `HCC`

✓6ᵗʰ M86.31 Chronic multifocal osteomyelitis, **shoulder**

M86.311 Chronic multifocal osteomyelitis, **right** shoulder `CC` `HCC`

M86.312 Chronic multifocal osteomyelitis, **left** shoulder `CC` `HCC`

M86.319 Chronic multifocal osteomyelitis, unspecified shoulder `CC` `UNS` `HCC`

✓6ᵗʰ M86.32 Chronic multifocal osteomyelitis, **humerus**

M86.321 Chronic multifocal osteomyelitis, **right** humerus `CC` `HCC`

M86.322 Chronic multifocal osteomyelitis, **left** humerus `CC` `HCC`

M86.329 Chronic multifocal osteomyelitis, unspecified humerus `CC` `UNS` `HCC`

✓6ᵗʰ M86.33 Chronic multifocal osteomyelitis, **radius and ulna**

M86.331 Chronic multifocal osteomyelitis, **right** radius and ulna `CC` `HCC`

M86.332 Chronic multifocal osteomyelitis, **left** radius and ulna `CC` `HCC`

M86.339 Chronic multifocal osteomyelitis, unspecified radius and ulna `CC` `UNS` `HCC`

✓6ᵗʰ M86.34 Chronic multifocal osteomyelitis, **hand**

M86.341 Chronic multifocal osteomyelitis, **right** hand `CC` `HCC`

M86.342 Chronic multifocal osteomyelitis, **left** hand `CC` `HCC`

☑ Additional Character Required   ✓x7ᵗʰ Placeholder   **Questionable PDx**   Manifestation   Unspecified   `UPD` Unacceptable PDx   `H1`-`H14` HAC   `HCC` CMS-HCC Dx   `HIV` HIV Dx

ICD-10-CM 2025

841

M86.349   Chronic multifocal osteomyelitis, unspecified hand   `CC` `UNS` `HCC`

√6ᵗʰ   **M86.35**   Chronic multifocal osteomyelitis, **femur**

M86.351   Chronic multifocal osteomyelitis, **right** femur   `CC` `HCC`

M86.352   Chronic multifocal osteomyelitis, **left** femur   `CC` `HCC`

M86.359   Chronic multifocal osteomyelitis, unspecified femur   `CC` `UNS` `HCC`

√6ᵗʰ   **M86.36**   Chronic multifocal osteomyelitis, **tibia and fibula**

M86.361   Chronic multifocal osteomyelitis, **right** tibia and fibula   `CC` `HCC`

M86.362   Chronic multifocal osteomyelitis, **left** tibia and fibula   `CC` `HCC`

M86.369   Chronic multifocal osteomyelitis, unspecified tibia and fibula   `CC` `UNS` `HCC`

√6ᵗʰ   **M86.37**   Chronic multifocal osteomyelitis, **ankle and foot**

M86.371   Chronic multifocal osteomyelitis, **right** ankle and foot   `CC` `HCC`

M86.372   Chronic multifocal osteomyelitis, **left** ankle and foot   `CC` `HCC`

M86.379   Chronic multifocal osteomyelitis, unspecified ankle and foot   `CC` `UNS` `HCC`

M86.38   Chronic multifocal osteomyelitis, other site   `CC` `HCC`

M86.39   Chronic multifocal osteomyelitis, **multiple sites**   `CC` `HCC`

√5ᵗʰ   **M86.4**   **Chronic** osteomyelitis **with draining sinus**

M86.40   Chronic osteomyelitis with draining sinus, unspecified site   `CC` `UNS` `HCC`

√6ᵗʰ   **M86.41**   Chronic osteomyelitis with draining sinus, **shoulder**

M86.411   Chronic osteomyelitis with draining sinus, **right** shoulder   `CC` `HCC`

M86.412   Chronic osteomyelitis with draining sinus, **left** shoulder   `CC` `HCC`

M86.419   Chronic osteomyelitis with draining sinus, unspecified shoulder   `CC` `UNS` `HCC`

√6ᵗʰ   **M86.42**   Chronic osteomyelitis with draining sinus, **humerus**

M86.421   Chronic osteomyelitis with draining sinus, **right** humerus   `CC` `HCC`

M86.422   Chronic osteomyelitis with draining sinus, **left** humerus   `CC` `HCC`

M86.429   Chronic osteomyelitis with draining sinus, unspecified humerus   `CC` `UNS` `HCC`

√6ᵗʰ   **M86.43**   Chronic osteomyelitis with draining sinus, **radius and ulna**

M86.431   Chronic osteomyelitis with draining sinus, **right** radius and ulna   `CC` `HCC`

M86.432   Chronic osteomyelitis with draining sinus, **left** radius and ulna   `CC` `HCC`

M86.439   Chronic osteomyelitis with draining sinus, unspecified radius and ulna   `CC` `UNS` `HCC`

√6ᵗʰ   **M86.44**   Chronic osteomyelitis with draining sinus, **hand**

M86.441   Chronic osteomyelitis with draining sinus, **right** hand   `CC` `HCC`

M86.442   Chronic osteomyelitis with draining sinus, **left** hand   `CC` `HCC`

M86.449   Chronic osteomyelitis with draining sinus, unspecified hand   `CC` `UNS` `HCC`

√6ᵗʰ   **M86.45**   Chronic osteomyelitis with draining sinus, **femur**

M86.451   Chronic osteomyelitis with draining sinus, **right** femur   `CC` `HCC`

M86.452   Chronic osteomyelitis with draining sinus, **left** femur   `CC` `HCC`

M86.459   Chronic osteomyelitis with draining sinus, unspecified femur   `CC` `UNS` `HCC`

√6ᵗʰ   **M86.46**   Chronic osteomyelitis with draining sinus, **tibia and fibula**

M86.461   Chronic osteomyelitis with draining sinus, **right** tibia and fibula   `CC` `HCC`

M86.462   Chronic osteomyelitis with draining sinus, **left** tibia and fibula   `CC` `HCC`

M86.469   Chronic osteomyelitis with draining sinus, unspecified tibia and fibula   `CC` `UNS` `HCC`

√6ᵗʰ   **M86.47**   Chronic osteomyelitis with draining sinus, **ankle and foot**

M86.471   Chronic osteomyelitis with draining sinus, **right** ankle and foot   `CC` `HCC`

M86.472   Chronic osteomyelitis with draining sinus, **left** ankle and foot   `CC` `HCC`

M86.479   Chronic osteomyelitis with draining sinus, unspecified ankle and foot   `CC` `HCC`

M86.48   Chronic osteomyelitis with draining sinus, other site   `CC` `HCC`

M86.49   Chronic osteomyelitis with draining sinus, **multiple sites**   `CC` `HCC`

√5ᵗʰ   **M86.5**   **Other chronic hematogenous** osteomyelitis

M86.50   Other chronic hematogenous osteomyelitis, unspecified site   `CC` `UNS` `HCC`

√6ᵗʰ   **M86.51**   Other chronic hematogenous osteomyelitis, **shoulder**

M86.511   Other chronic hematogenous osteomyelitis, **right** shoulder   `CC` `HCC`

M86.512   Other chronic hematogenous osteomyelitis, **left** shoulder   `CC` `HCC`

M86.519   Other chronic hematogenous osteomyelitis, unspecified shoulder   `CC` `UNS` `HCC`

√6ᵗʰ   **M86.52**   Other chronic hematogenous osteomyelitis, **humerus**

M86.521   Other chronic hematogenous osteomyelitis, **right** humerus   `CC` `HCC`

M86.522   Other chronic hematogenous osteomyelitis, **left** humerus   `CC` `HCC`

M86.529   Other chronic hematogenous osteomyelitis, unspecified humerus   `CC` `UNS` `HCC`

√6ᵗʰ   **M86.53**   Other chronic hematogenous osteomyelitis, **radius and ulna**

M86.531   Other chronic hematogenous osteomyelitis, **right** radius and ulna   `CC` `HCC`

M86.532   Other chronic hematogenous osteomyelitis, **left** radius and ulna   `CC` `HCC`

M86.539   Other chronic hematogenous osteomyelitis, unspecified radius and ulna   `CC` `UNS` `HCC`

√6ᵗʰ   **M86.54**   Other chronic hematogenous osteomyelitis, **hand**

M86.541   Other chronic hematogenous osteomyelitis, **right** hand   `CC` `HCC`

M86.542   Other chronic hematogenous osteomyelitis, **left** hand   `CC` `HCC`

M86.549   Other chronic hematogenous osteomyelitis, unspecified hand   `CC` `UNS` `HCC`

√6ᵗʰ   **M86.55**   Other chronic hematogenous osteomyelitis, **femur**

M86.551   Other chronic hematogenous osteomyelitis, **right** femur   `CC` `HCC`

M86.552   Other chronic hematogenous osteomyelitis, **left** femur   `CC` `HCC`

M86.559   Other chronic hematogenous osteomyelitis, unspecified femur   `CC` `UNS` `HCC`

√6ᵗʰ   **M86.56**   Other chronic hematogenous osteomyelitis, **tibia and fibula**

M86.561   Other chronic hematogenous osteomyelitis, **right** tibia and fibula   `CC` `HCC`

M86.562   Other chronic hematogenous osteomyelitis, **left** tibia and fibula   `CC` `HCC`

M86.569   Other chronic hematogenous osteomyelitis, unspecified tibia and fibula   `CC` `UNS` `HCC`

√6ᵗʰ   **M86.57**   Other chronic hematogenous osteomyelitis, **ankle and foot**

M86.571   Other chronic hematogenous osteomyelitis, **right** ankle and foot   `CC` `HCC`

M86.572   Other chronic hematogenous osteomyelitis, **left** ankle and foot   `CC` `HCC`

M86.579   Other chronic hematogenous osteomyelitis, unspecified ankle and foot   `CC` `UNS` `HCC`

M86.58   Other chronic hematogenous osteomyelitis, other site   `CC` `HCC`

M86.59   Other chronic hematogenous osteomyelitis, **multiple sites**   `CC` `HCC`

N Newborn: 0   **P** Pediatric: 0-17   **M** Maternity: 9-64   **A** Adult: 15-124   `UNS` Unspecified Site   `MCC` Major Complication/Comorbidity   `CC` Complication/Comorbidity   `PE` POA Exempt

842   ICD-10-CM 2025

√5th M86.6 Other chronic osteomyelitis

> **M86.60 Other chronic osteomyelitis, unspecified site** `CC` `UNS` `HCC`

> **√6th M86.61 Other chronic osteomyelitis, shoulder**
>> **M86.611 Other chronic osteomyelitis, right shoulder** `CC` `HCC`
>> **M86.612 Other chronic osteomyelitis, left shoulder** `CC` `HCC`
>> **M86.619 Other chronic osteomyelitis, unspecified shoulder** `CC` `UNS` `HCC`

> **√6th M86.62 Other chronic osteomyelitis, humerus**
>> **M86.621 Other chronic osteomyelitis, right humerus** `CC` `HCC`
>> **M86.622 Other chronic osteomyelitis, left humerus** `CC` `HCC`
>> **M86.629 Other chronic osteomyelitis, unspecified humerus** `CC` `UNS` `HCC`

> **√6th M86.63 Other chronic osteomyelitis, radius and ulna**
>> **M86.631 Other chronic osteomyelitis, right radius and ulna** `CC` `HCC`
>> **M86.632 Other chronic osteomyelitis, left radius and ulna** `CC` `HCC`
>> **M86.639 Other chronic osteomyelitis, unspecified radius and ulna** `CC` `UNS` `HCC`

> **√6th M86.64 Other chronic osteomyelitis, hand**
>> **M86.641 Other chronic osteomyelitis, right hand** `CC` `HCC`
>> **M86.642 Other chronic osteomyelitis, left hand** `CC` `HCC`
>> **M86.649 Other chronic osteomyelitis, unspecified hand** `CC` `UNS` `HCC`

> **√6th M86.65 Other chronic osteomyelitis, thigh**
>> **M86.651 Other chronic osteomyelitis, right thigh** `CC` `HCC`
>> **M86.652 Other chronic osteomyelitis, left thigh** `CC` `HCC`
>> **M86.659 Other chronic osteomyelitis, unspecified thigh** `CC` `UNS` `HCC`

> **√6th M86.66 Other chronic osteomyelitis, tibia and fibula**
>> **M86.661 Other chronic osteomyelitis, right tibia and fibula** `CC` `HCC`
>> **M86.662 Other chronic osteomyelitis, left tibia and fibula** `CC` `HCC`
>> **M86.669 Other chronic osteomyelitis, unspecified tibia and fibula** `CC` `UNS` `HCC`

> **√6th M86.67 Other chronic osteomyelitis, ankle and foot**
>> **M86.671 Other chronic osteomyelitis, right ankle and foot** `CC` `HCC`
>>> **AHA:** 2016,1Q,13
>> **M86.672 Other chronic osteomyelitis, left ankle and foot** `CC` `HCC`
>> **M86.679 Other chronic osteomyelitis, unspecified ankle and foot** `CC` `UNS` `HCC`

> **M86.68 Other chronic osteomyelitis, other site** `CC` `HCC`
> **M86.69 Other chronic osteomyelitis, multiple sites** `CC` `HCC`

√5th M86.8 Other osteomyelitis
> Brodie's abscess
> **AHA:** 2022,1Q,31

> **√6th M86.8X Other osteomyelitis**
>> **M86.8X0 Other osteomyelitis, multiple sites** `CC` `HCC`
>> **M86.8X1 Other osteomyelitis, shoulder** `CC` `HCC`
>> **M86.8X2 Other osteomyelitis, upper arm** `CC` `HCC`
>> **M86.8X3 Other osteomyelitis, forearm** `CC` `HCC`
>> **M86.8X4 Other osteomyelitis, hand** `CC` `HCC`
>> **M86.8X5 Other osteomyelitis, thigh** `CC` `HCC`
>> **M86.8X6 Other osteomyelitis, lower leg** `CC` `HCC`
>> **M86.8X7 Other osteomyelitis, ankle and foot** `CC` `HCC`
>> **M86.8X8 Other osteomyelitis, other site** `CC` `HCC`
>> **M86.8X9 Other osteomyelitis, unspecified sites** `CC` `UNS` `HCC`

> **M86.9 Osteomyelitis, unspecified** `CC` `HCC`
>> Infection of bone NOS
>> Periostitis without osteomyelitis

√4th M87 Osteonecrosis

> `INCLUDES` avascular necrosis of bone
> Use additional code to identify major osseous defect, if applicable (M89.7-)
> `EXCLUDES 1` juvenile osteonecrosis (M91-M92)
> osteochondropathies (M90-M93)

> **√5th M87.0 Idiopathic aseptic necrosis of bone**

>> **M87.00 Idiopathic aseptic necrosis of unspecified bone** `CC` `UNS` `HCC`

>> **√6th M87.01 Idiopathic aseptic necrosis of shoulder**
>>> Idiopathic aseptic necrosis of clavicle and scapula
>>> **M87.011 Idiopathic aseptic necrosis of right shoulder** `CC` `HCC`
>>> **M87.012 Idiopathic aseptic necrosis of left shoulder** `CC` `HCC`
>>> **M87.019 Idiopathic aseptic necrosis of unspecified shoulder** `CC` `UNS` `HCC`

>> **√6th M87.02 Idiopathic aseptic necrosis of humerus**
>>> **M87.021 Idiopathic aseptic necrosis of right humerus** `CC` `HCC`
>>> **M87.022 Idiopathic aseptic necrosis of left humerus** `CC` `HCC`
>>> **M87.029 Idiopathic aseptic necrosis of unspecified humerus** `CC` `UNS` `HCC`

>> **√6th M87.03 Idiopathic aseptic necrosis of radius, ulna and carpus**
>>> **M87.031 Idiopathic aseptic necrosis of right radius** `CC` `HCC`
>>> **M87.032 Idiopathic aseptic necrosis of left radius** `CC` `HCC`
>>> **M87.033 Idiopathic aseptic necrosis of unspecified radius** `CC` `UNS` `HCC`
>>> **M87.034 Idiopathic aseptic necrosis of right ulna** `CC` `HCC`
>>> **M87.035 Idiopathic aseptic necrosis of left ulna** `CC` `HCC`
>>> **M87.036 Idiopathic aseptic necrosis of unspecified ulna** `CC` `UNS` `HCC`
>>> **M87.037 Idiopathic aseptic necrosis of right carpus** `CC` `HCC`
>>> **M87.038 Idiopathic aseptic necrosis of left carpus** `CC` `HCC`
>>> **M87.039 Idiopathic aseptic necrosis of unspecified carpus** `CC` `UNS` `HCC`

>> **√6th M87.04 Idiopathic aseptic necrosis of hand and fingers**
>>> Idiopathic aseptic necrosis of metacarpals and phalanges of hands
>>> **M87.041 Idiopathic aseptic necrosis of right hand** `CC` `HCC`
>>> **M87.042 Idiopathic aseptic necrosis of left hand** `CC` `HCC`
>>> **M87.043 Idiopathic aseptic necrosis of unspecified hand** `CC` `UNS` `HCC`
>>> **M87.044 Idiopathic aseptic necrosis of right finger(s)** `CC` `HCC`
>>> **M87.045 Idiopathic aseptic necrosis of left finger(s)** `CC` `HCC`
>>> **M87.046 Idiopathic aseptic necrosis of unspecified finger(s)** `CC` `UNS` `HCC`

>> **√6th M87.05 Idiopathic aseptic necrosis of pelvis and femur**
>>> **M87.050 Idiopathic aseptic necrosis of pelvis** `CC` `HCC`
>>> **M87.051 Idiopathic aseptic necrosis of right femur** `CC` `HCC`
>>> **M87.052 Idiopathic aseptic necrosis of left femur** `CC` `HCC`
>>> **M87.059 Idiopathic aseptic necrosis of unspecified femur** `CC` `UNS` `HCC`

>> **√6th M87.06 Idiopathic aseptic necrosis of tibia and fibula**
>>> **M87.061 Idiopathic aseptic necrosis of right tibia** `CC` `HCC`
>>> **M87.062 Idiopathic aseptic necrosis of left tibia** `CC` `HCC`
>>> **M87.063 Idiopathic aseptic necrosis of unspecified tibia** `CC` `UNS` `HCC`
>>> **M87.064 Idiopathic aseptic necrosis of right fibula** `CC` `HCC`
>>> **M87.065 Idiopathic aseptic necrosis of left fibula** `CC` `HCC`

☑ Additional Character Required   √x7th Placeholder   Questionable PDx   Manifestation   Unspecified   `UPD` Unacceptable PDx   H1-H14 HAC   `HCC` CMS-HCC Dx   `HIV` HIV Dx

ICD-10-CM 2025   **843**

M87.066 Idiopathic aseptic necrosis of unspecified fibula `CC` `UNS` `HCC`

✓6ᵗʰ **M87.07** Idiopathic aseptic necrosis of **ankle, foot and toes**

Idiopathic aseptic necrosis of metatarsus, tarsus, and phalanges of toes

M87.071 Idiopathic aseptic necrosis of **right ankle** `CC` `HCC`

M87.072 Idiopathic aseptic necrosis of **left ankle** `CC` `HCC`

M87.073 Idiopathic aseptic necrosis of unspecified ankle `CC` `UNS` `HCC`

M87.074 Idiopathic aseptic necrosis of **right foot** `CC` `HCC`

M87.075 Idiopathic aseptic necrosis of **left foot** `CC` `HCC`

M87.076 Idiopathic aseptic necrosis of unspecified foot `CC` `UNS` `HCC`

M87.077 Idiopathic aseptic necrosis of **right toe(s)** `CC` `HCC`

M87.078 Idiopathic aseptic necrosis of **left toe(s)** `CC` `HCC`

M87.079 Idiopathic aseptic necrosis of unspecified toe(s) `CC` `UNS` `HCC`

M87.08 Idiopathic aseptic necrosis of bone, other site `CC` `HCC`

M87.09 Idiopathic aseptic necrosis of bone, **multiple sites** `CC` `HCC`

✓5ᵗʰ **M87.1** Osteonecrosis **due to drugs**

Use additional code for adverse effect, if applicable, to identify drug (T36-T50 with fifth or sixth character 5)

M87.10 Osteonecrosis due to drugs, unspecified bone `CC` `UNS`

✓6ᵗʰ **M87.11** Osteonecrosis due to drugs, **shoulder**

M87.111 Osteonecrosis due to drugs, **right shoulder** `CC`

M87.112 Osteonecrosis due to drugs, **left shoulder** `CC`

M87.119 Osteonecrosis due to drugs, unspecified shoulder `CC` `UNS`

✓6ᵗʰ **M87.12** Osteonecrosis due to drugs, **humerus**

M87.121 Osteonecrosis due to drugs, **right humerus** `CC`

M87.122 Osteonecrosis due to drugs, **left humerus** `CC`

M87.129 Osteonecrosis due to drugs, unspecified humerus `CC` `UNS`

✓6ᵗʰ **M87.13** Osteonecrosis due to drugs of **radius, ulna and carpus**

M87.131 Osteonecrosis due to drugs of **right radius** `CC`

M87.132 Osteonecrosis due to drugs of **left radius** `CC`

M87.133 Osteonecrosis due to drugs of unspecified radius `CC` `UNS`

M87.134 Osteonecrosis due to drugs of **right ulna** `CC`

M87.135 Osteonecrosis due to drugs of **left ulna** `CC`

M87.136 Osteonecrosis due to drugs of unspecified ulna `CC` `UNS`

M87.137 Osteonecrosis due to drugs of **right carpus** `CC`

M87.138 Osteonecrosis due to drugs of **left carpus** `CC`

M87.139 Osteonecrosis due to drugs of unspecified carpus `CC` `UNS`

✓6ᵗʰ **M87.14** Osteonecrosis due to drugs, **hand and fingers**

M87.141 Osteonecrosis due to drugs, **right hand** `CC`

M87.142 Osteonecrosis due to drugs, **left hand** `CC`

M87.143 Osteonecrosis due to drugs, unspecified hand `CC` `UNS`

M87.144 Osteonecrosis due to drugs, **right finger(s)** `CC`

M87.145 Osteonecrosis due to drugs, **left finger(s)** `CC`

M87.146 Osteonecrosis due to drugs, unspecified finger(s) `CC` `UNS`

✓6ᵗʰ **M87.15** Osteonecrosis due to drugs, **pelvis and femur**

M87.150 Osteonecrosis due to drugs, **pelvis** `CC`

M87.151 Osteonecrosis due to drugs, **right femur** `CC`

M87.152 Osteonecrosis due to drugs, **left femur** `CC`

M87.159 Osteonecrosis due to drugs, unspecified femur `CC` `UNS`

✓6ᵗʰ **M87.16** Osteonecrosis due to drugs, **tibia and fibula**

M87.161 Osteonecrosis due to drugs, **right tibia** `CC`

M87.162 Osteonecrosis due to drugs, **left tibia** `CC`

M87.163 Osteonecrosis due to drugs, unspecified tibia `CC` `UNS`

M87.164 Osteonecrosis due to drugs, **right fibula** `CC`

M87.165 Osteonecrosis due to drugs, **left fibula** `CC`

M87.166 Osteonecrosis due to drugs, unspecified fibula `CC` `UNS`

✓6ᵗʰ **M87.17** Osteonecrosis due to drugs, **ankle, foot and toes**

M87.171 Osteonecrosis due to drugs, **right ankle** `CC`

M87.172 Osteonecrosis due to drugs, **left ankle** `CC`

M87.173 Osteonecrosis due to drugs, unspecified ankle `CC` `UNS`

M87.174 Osteonecrosis due to drugs, **right foot** `CC`

M87.175 Osteonecrosis due to drugs, **left foot** `CC`

M87.176 Osteonecrosis due to drugs, unspecified foot `CC` `UNS`

M87.177 Osteonecrosis due to drugs, **right toe(s)** `CC`

M87.178 Osteonecrosis due to drugs, **left toe(s)** `CC`

M87.179 Osteonecrosis due to drugs, unspecified toe(s) `CC` `UNS`

✓6ᵗʰ **M87.18** Osteonecrosis due to drugs, other site

M87.180 Osteonecrosis due to drugs, **jaw** `CC`

M87.188 Osteonecrosis due to drugs, other site `CC`

M87.19 Osteonecrosis due to drugs, **multiple sites** `CC`

✓5ᵗʰ **M87.2** Osteonecrosis **due to previous trauma**

M87.20 Osteonecrosis due to previous trauma, unspecified bone `CC` `UNS` `HCC`

✓6ᵗʰ **M87.21** Osteonecrosis due to previous trauma, **shoulder**

M87.211 Osteonecrosis due to previous trauma, **right** shoulder `CC` `HCC`

M87.212 Osteonecrosis due to previous trauma, **left** shoulder `CC` `HCC`

M87.219 Osteonecrosis due to previous trauma, unspecified shoulder `CC` `UNS` `HCC`

✓6ᵗʰ **M87.22** Osteonecrosis due to previous trauma, **humerus**

M87.221 Osteonecrosis due to previous trauma, **right** humerus `CC` `HCC`

M87.222 Osteonecrosis due to previous trauma, **left** humerus `CC` `HCC`

M87.229 Osteonecrosis due to previous trauma, unspecified humerus `CC` `UNS` `HCC`

✓6ᵗʰ **M87.23** Osteonecrosis due to previous trauma of **radius, ulna and carpus**

M87.231 Osteonecrosis due to previous trauma of **right radius** `CC` `HCC`

M87.232 Osteonecrosis due to previous trauma of **left radius** `CC` `HCC`

M87.233 Osteonecrosis due to previous trauma of unspecified radius `CC` `UNS` `HCC`

M87.234 Osteonecrosis due to previous trauma of **right ulna** `CC` `HCC`

M87.235 Osteonecrosis due to previous trauma of **left ulna** `CC` `HCC`

M87.236 Osteonecrosis due to previous trauma of unspecified ulna `CC` `UNS` `HCC`

M87.237 Osteonecrosis due to previous trauma of **right carpus** `CC` `HCC`

`N` Newborn: 0   `P` Pediatric: 0-17   `M` Maternity: 9-64   `A` Adult: 15-124   `UNS` Unspecified Site   `MCC` Major Complication/Comorbidity   `CC` Complication/Comorbidity   `PE` POA Exempt

844

ICD-10-CM 2025

M87.238 Osteonecrosis due to previous trauma of left carpus `CC` `HCC`

M87.239 Osteonecrosis due to previous trauma of unspecified carpus `CC` `UNS` `HCC`

√6ᵗʰ **M87.24** Osteonecrosis due to previous trauma, hand and fingers

M87.241 Osteonecrosis due to previous trauma, right hand `CC` `HCC`

M87.242 Osteonecrosis due to previous trauma, left hand `CC` `HCC`

M87.243 Osteonecrosis due to previous trauma, unspecified hand `CC` `UNS` `HCC`

M87.244 Osteonecrosis due to previous trauma, right finger(s) `CC` `HCC`

M87.245 Osteonecrosis due to previous trauma, left finger(s) `CC` `HCC`

M87.246 Osteonecrosis due to previous trauma, unspecified finger(s) `CC` `UNS` `HCC`

√6ᵗʰ **M87.25** Osteonecrosis due to previous trauma, pelvis and femur

M87.250 Osteonecrosis due to previous trauma, pelvis `CC` `HCC`

M87.251 Osteonecrosis due to previous trauma, right femur `CC` `HCC`

M87.252 Osteonecrosis due to previous trauma, left femur `CC` `HCC`

M87.256 Osteonecrosis due to previous trauma, unspecified femur `CC` `UNS` `HCC`

√6ᵗʰ **M87.26** Osteonecrosis due to previous trauma, tibia and fibula

M87.261 Osteonecrosis due to previous trauma, right tibia `CC` `HCC`

M87.262 Osteonecrosis due to previous trauma, left tibia `CC` `HCC`

M87.263 Osteonecrosis due to previous trauma, unspecified tibia `CC` `UNS` `HCC`

M87.264 Osteonecrosis due to previous trauma, right fibula `CC` `HCC`

M87.265 Osteonecrosis due to previous trauma, left fibula `CC` `HCC`

M87.266 Osteonecrosis due to previous trauma, unspecified fibula `CC` `UNS` `HCC`

√6ᵗʰ **M87.27** Osteonecrosis due to previous trauma, ankle, foot and toes

M87.271 Osteonecrosis due to previous trauma, right ankle `CC` `HCC`

M87.272 Osteonecrosis due to previous trauma, left ankle `CC` `HCC`

M87.273 Osteonecrosis due to previous trauma, unspecified ankle `CC` `UNS` `HCC`

M87.274 Osteonecrosis due to previous trauma, right foot `CC` `HCC`

M87.275 Osteonecrosis due to previous trauma, left foot `CC` `HCC`

M87.276 Osteonecrosis due to previous trauma, unspecified foot `CC` `UNS` `HCC`

M87.277 Osteonecrosis due to previous trauma, right toe(s) `CC` `HCC`

M87.278 Osteonecrosis due to previous trauma, left toe(s) `CC` `HCC`

M87.279 Osteonecrosis due to previous trauma, unspecified toe(s) `CC` `UNS` `HCC`

M87.28 Osteonecrosis due to previous trauma, other site `CC` `HCC`

M87.29 Osteonecrosis due to previous trauma, multiple sites `CC` `HCC`

√5ᵗʰ **M87.3** Other secondary osteonecrosis

M87.30 Other secondary osteonecrosis, unspecified bone `CC` `UNS` `HCC`

√6ᵗʰ **M87.31** Other secondary osteonecrosis, shoulder

M87.311 Other secondary osteonecrosis, right shoulder `CC` `HCC`

M87.312 Other secondary osteonecrosis, left shoulder `CC` `HCC`

M87.319 Other secondary osteonecrosis, unspecified shoulder `CC` `UNS` `HCC`

√6ᵗʰ **M87.32** Other secondary osteonecrosis, humerus

M87.321 Other secondary osteonecrosis, right humerus `CC` `HCC`

M87.322 Other secondary osteonecrosis, left humerus `CC` `HCC`

M87.329 Other secondary osteonecrosis, unspecified humerus `CC` `UNS` `HCC`

√6ᵗʰ **M87.33** Other secondary osteonecrosis of radius, ulna and carpus

M87.331 Other secondary osteonecrosis of right radius `CC` `HCC`

M87.332 Other secondary osteonecrosis of left radius `CC` `HCC`

M87.333 Other secondary osteonecrosis of unspecified radius `CC` `UNS` `HCC`

M87.334 Other secondary osteonecrosis of right ulna `CC` `HCC`

M87.335 Other secondary osteonecrosis of left ulna `CC` `HCC`

M87.336 Other secondary osteonecrosis of unspecified ulna `CC` `UNS` `HCC`

M87.337 Other secondary osteonecrosis of right carpus `CC` `HCC`

M87.338 Other secondary osteonecrosis of left carpus `CC` `HCC`

M87.339 Other secondary osteonecrosis of unspecified carpus `CC` `UNS` `HCC`

√6ᵗʰ **M87.34** Other secondary osteonecrosis, hand and fingers

M87.341 Other secondary osteonecrosis, right hand `CC` `HCC`

M87.342 Other secondary osteonecrosis, left hand `CC` `HCC`

M87.343 Other secondary osteonecrosis, unspecified hand `CC` `UNS` `HCC`

M87.344 Other secondary osteonecrosis, right finger(s) `CC` `HCC`

M87.345 Other secondary osteonecrosis, left finger(s) `CC` `HCC`

M87.346 Other secondary osteonecrosis, unspecified finger(s) `CC` `UNS` `HCC`

√6ᵗʰ **M87.35** Other secondary osteonecrosis, pelvis and femur

M87.350 Other secondary osteonecrosis, pelvis `CC` `HCC`

M87.351 Other secondary osteonecrosis, right femur `CC` `HCC`

M87.352 Other secondary osteonecrosis, left femur `CC` `HCC`

M87.353 Other secondary osteonecrosis, unspecified femur `CC` `UNS` `HCC`

√6ᵗʰ **M87.36** Other secondary osteonecrosis, tibia and fibula

M87.361 Other secondary osteonecrosis, right tibia `CC` `HCC`

M87.362 Other secondary osteonecrosis, left tibia `CC` `HCC`

M87.363 Other secondary osteonecrosis, unspecified tibia `CC` `UNS` `HCC`

M87.364 Other secondary osteonecrosis, right fibula `CC` `HCC`

M87.365 Other secondary osteonecrosis, left fibula `CC` `HCC`

M87.366 Other secondary osteonecrosis, unspecified fibula `CC` `UNS` `HCC`

√6ᵗʰ **M87.37** Other secondary osteonecrosis, ankle and foot

M87.371 Other secondary osteonecrosis, right ankle `CC` `HCC`

M87.372 Other secondary osteonecrosis, left ankle `CC` `HCC`

M87.373 Other secondary osteonecrosis, unspecified ankle `CC` `UNS` `HCC`

M87.374 Other secondary osteonecrosis, right foot `CC` `HCC`

M87.375 Other secondary osteonecrosis, left foot `CC` `HCC`

M87.376 Other secondary osteonecrosis, unspecified foot `CC` `UNS` `HCC`

M87.377 Other secondary osteonecrosis, right toe(s) `CC` `HCC`

M87.378 Other secondary osteonecrosis, left toe(s) `CC` `HCC`

M87.379 Other secondary osteonecrosis, unspecified toe(s) `CC` `UNS` `HCC`

M87.38 Other secondary osteonecrosis, other site `CC` `HCC`

✔ Additional Character Required   √x7ᵗʰ Placeholder   Questionable PDx   Manifestation   Unspecified   `UPD` Unacceptable PDx   `H1`-`H14` HAC   `HCC` CMS-HCC Dx   `HIV` HIV Dx

ICD-10-CM 2025   845

Chapter 13. Diseases of the Musculoskeletal System and Connective Tissue

M87.39–M89.041

M87.39   Other secondary osteonecrosis, **multiple sites** `CC` `HCC`

√5ᵗʰ **M87.8   Other osteonecrosis**

    M87.80   Other osteonecrosis, unspecified bone `CC` `UNS` `HCC`

    √6ᵗʰ M87.81   Other osteonecrosis, **shoulder**

        M87.811   Other osteonecrosis, **right** shoulder `CC` `HCC`

        M87.812   Other osteonecrosis, **left** shoulder `CC` `HCC`

        M87.819   Other osteonecrosis, unspecified shoulder `CC` `UNS` `HCC`

    √6ᵗʰ M87.82   Other osteonecrosis, **humerus**

        M87.821   Other osteonecrosis, **right** humerus `CC` `HCC`

        M87.822   Other osteonecrosis, **left** humerus `CC` `HCC`

        M87.829   Other osteonecrosis, unspecified humerus `CC` `UNS` `HCC`

    √6ᵗʰ M87.83   Other osteonecrosis of **radius, ulna and carpus**

        M87.831   Other osteonecrosis of **right** radius `CC` `HCC`

        M87.832   Other osteonecrosis of **left** radius `CC` `HCC`

        M87.833   Other osteonecrosis of unspecified radius `CC` `UNS` `HCC`

        M87.834   Other osteonecrosis of **right** ulna `CC` `HCC`

        M87.835   Other osteonecrosis of **left** ulna `CC` `HCC`

        M87.836   Other osteonecrosis of unspecified ulna `CC` `UNS` `HCC`

        M87.837   Other osteonecrosis of **right** carpus `CC` `HCC`

        M87.838   Other osteonecrosis of **left** carpus `CC` `HCC`

        M87.839   Other osteonecrosis of unspecified carpus `CC` `UNS` `HCC`

    √6ᵗʰ M87.84   Other osteonecrosis, **hand and fingers**

        M87.841   Other osteonecrosis, **right hand** `CC` `HCC`

        M87.842   Other osteonecrosis, **left hand** `CC` `HCC`

        M87.843   Other osteonecrosis, unspecified hand `CC` `UNS` `HCC`

        M87.844   Other osteonecrosis, **right finger(s)** `CC` `HCC`

        M87.845   Other osteonecrosis, **left finger(s)** `CC` `HCC`

        M87.849   Other osteonecrosis, unspecified finger(s) `CC` `UNS` `HCC`

    √6ᵗʰ M87.85   Other osteonecrosis, **pelvis and femur**

        M87.850   Other osteonecrosis, **pelvis** `CC` `HCC`

        M87.851   Other osteonecrosis, **right** femur `CC` `HCC`

        M87.852   Other osteonecrosis, **left** femur `CC` `HCC`

        M87.859   Other osteonecrosis, unspecified femur `CC` `UNS` `HCC`

    √6ᵗʰ M87.86   Other osteonecrosis, **tibia and fibula**

        M87.861   Other osteonecrosis, **right tibia** `CC` `HCC`

        M87.862   Other osteonecrosis, **left tibia** `CC` `HCC`

        M87.863   Other osteonecrosis, unspecified tibia `CC` `UNS` `HCC`

        M87.864   Other osteonecrosis, **right fibula** `CC` `HCC`

        M87.865   Other osteonecrosis, **left fibula** `CC` `HCC`

        M87.869   Other osteonecrosis, unspecified fibula `CC` `UNS` `HCC`

    √6ᵗʰ M87.87   Other osteonecrosis, **ankle, foot and toes**

        M87.871   Other osteonecrosis, **right ankle** `CC` `HCC`

        M87.872   Other osteonecrosis, **left ankle** `CC` `HCC`

        M87.873   Other osteonecrosis, unspecified ankle `CC` `UNS` `HCC`

        M87.874   Other osteonecrosis, **right foot** `CC` `HCC`

        M87.875   Other osteonecrosis, **left foot** `CC` `HCC`

        M87.876   Other osteonecrosis, unspecified foot `CC` `UNS` `HCC`

        M87.877   Other osteonecrosis, **right toe(s)** `CC` `HCC`

        M87.878   Other osteonecrosis, **left toe(s)** `CC` `HCC`

        M87.879   Other osteonecrosis, unspecified toe(s) `CC` `UNS` `HCC`

    M87.88   Other osteonecrosis, other site `CC` `HCC`

    M87.89   Other osteonecrosis, **multiple sites** `CC` `HCC`

M87.9   Osteonecrosis, unspecified `CC` `HCC`
    Necrosis of bone NOS

√4ᵗʰ **M88   Osteitis deformans [Paget's disease of bone]**

    EXCLUDES 1   osteitis deformans in neoplastic disease (M90.6)

    DEF: Bone disease characterized by numerous cycles of bone resorption by the body. Resorption is followed by accelerated repair attempts, causing bone deformities and bowing, with associated fractures and pain.

    M88.0   Osteitis deformans of skull

    M88.1   Osteitis deformans of vertebrae

    √5ᵗʰ **M88.8   Osteitis deformans of other bones**

        √6ᵗʰ M88.81   Osteitis deformans of **shoulder**

            M88.811   Osteitis deformans of **right** shoulder

            M88.812   Osteitis deformans of **left** shoulder

            M88.819   Osteitis deformans of unspecified shoulder

        √6ᵗʰ M88.82   Osteitis deformans of **upper arm**

            M88.821   Osteitis deformans of **right** upper arm

            M88.822   Osteitis deformans of **left** upper arm

            M88.829   Osteitis deformans of unspecified upper arm

        √6ᵗʰ M88.83   Osteitis deformans of **forearm**

            M88.831   Osteitis deformans of **right** forearm

            M88.832   Osteitis deformans of **left** forearm

            M88.839   Osteitis deformans of unspecified forearm

        √6ᵗʰ M88.84   Osteitis deformans of **hand**

            M88.841   Osteitis deformans of **right** hand

            M88.842   Osteitis deformans of **left** hand

            M88.849   Osteitis deformans of unspecified hand

        √6ᵗʰ M88.85   Osteitis deformans of **thigh**

            M88.851   Osteitis deformans of **right** thigh

            M88.852   Osteitis deformans of **left** thigh

            M88.859   Osteitis deformans of unspecified thigh

        √6ᵗʰ M88.86   Osteitis deformans of **lower leg**

            M88.861   Osteitis deformans of **right** lower leg

            M88.862   Osteitis deformans of **left** lower leg

            M88.869   Osteitis deformans of unspecified lower leg

        √6ᵗʰ M88.87   Osteitis deformans of **ankle and foot**

            M88.871   Osteitis deformans of **right** ankle and foot

            M88.872   Osteitis deformans of **left** ankle and foot

            M88.879   Osteitis deformans of unspecified ankle and foot

        M88.88   Osteitis deformans of other bones

            EXCLUDES 2   osteitis deformans of skull (M88.0)
                      osteitis deformans of vertebrae (M88.1)

        M88.89   Osteitis deformans of **multiple sites**

    M88.9   Osteitis deformans of unspecified bone

√4ᵗʰ **M89   Other disorders of bone**

    √5ᵗʰ **M89.0   Algoneurodystrophy**
        Shoulder-hand syndrome
        Sudeck's atrophy

        EXCLUDES 1   causalgia, lower limb (G57.7-)
                causalgia, upper limb (G56.4-)
                complex regional pain syndrome II, lower limb (G57.7-)
                complex regional pain syndrome II, upper limb (G56.4-)
                reflex sympathetic dystrophy (G90.5-)

        M89.00   Algoneurodystrophy, unspecified site

        √6ᵗʰ M89.01   Algoneurodystrophy, **shoulder**

            M89.011   Algoneurodystrophy, **right** shoulder

            M89.012   Algoneurodystrophy, **left** shoulder

            M89.019   Algoneurodystrophy, unspecified shoulder

        √6ᵗʰ M89.02   Algoneurodystrophy, **upper arm**

            M89.021   Algoneurodystrophy, **right** upper arm

            M89.022   Algoneurodystrophy, **left** upper arm

            M89.029   Algoneurodystrophy, unspecified upper arm

        √6ᵗʰ M89.03   Algoneurodystrophy, **forearm**

            M89.031   Algoneurodystrophy, **right** forearm

            M89.032   Algoneurodystrophy, **left** forearm

            M89.039   Algoneurodystrophy, unspecified forearm

        √6ᵗʰ M89.04   Algoneurodystrophy, **hand**

            M89.041   Algoneurodystrophy, **right** hand

`N` Newborn: 0   `P` Pediatric: 0-17   `M` Maternity: 9-64   `A` Adult: 15-124   `UNS` Unspecified Site   `MCC` Major Complication/Comorbidity   `CC` Complication/Comorbidity   `PE` POA Exempt

846

ICD-10-CM 2025

M89.042   Algoneurodystrophy, **left** hand
M89.049   Algoneurodystrophy, unspecified hand

√6ᵗʰ   M89.05   Algoneurodystrophy, **thigh**

M89.051   Algoneurodystrophy, **right** thigh
M89.052   Algoneurodystrophy, **left** thigh
M89.059   Algoneurodystrophy, unspecified thigh

√6ᵗʰ   M89.06   Algoneurodystrophy, **lower leg**

M89.061   Algoneurodystrophy, **right** lower leg
M89.062   Algoneurodystrophy, **left** lower leg
M89.069   Algoneurodystrophy, unspecified lower leg

√6ᵗʰ   M89.07   Algoneurodystrophy, **ankle and foot**

M89.071   Algoneurodystrophy, **right** ankle and foot
M89.072   Algoneurodystrophy, **left** ankle and foot
M89.079   Algoneurodystrophy, unspecified ankle and foot

M89.08   Algoneurodystrophy, other site
M89.09   Algoneurodystrophy, **multiple sites**

√5ᵗʰ   M89.1   **Physeal arrest**

Arrest of growth plate
Epiphyseal arrest
Growth plate arrest

√6ᵗʰ   M89.12   Physeal arrest, **humerus**

M89.121   **Complete** physeal arrest, **right proximal** humerus
M89.122   **Complete** physeal arrest, **left proximal** humerus
M89.123   **Partial** physeal arrest, **right proximal** humerus
M89.124   **Partial** physeal arrest, **left proximal** humerus
M89.125   **Complete** physeal arrest, **right distal** humerus
M89.126   **Complete** physeal arrest, **left distal** humerus
M89.127   **Partial** physeal arrest, **right distal** humerus
M89.128   **Partial** physeal arrest, **left distal** humerus
M89.129   Physeal arrest, humerus, unspecified

√6ᵗʰ   M89.13   Physeal arrest, **forearm**

M89.131   **Complete** physeal arrest, **right** distal radius
M89.132   **Complete** physeal arrest, **left** distal radius
M89.133   **Partial** physeal arrest, **right** distal radius
M89.134   **Partial** physeal arrest, **left** distal radius
M89.138   Other physeal arrest of forearm
M89.139   Physeal arrest, forearm, unspecified

√6ᵗʰ   M89.15   Physeal arrest, **femur**

M89.151   **Complete** physeal arrest, **right proximal** femur
M89.152   **Complete** physeal arrest, **left proximal** femur
M89.153   **Partial** physeal arrest, **right proximal** femur
M89.154   **Partial** physeal arrest, **left proximal** femur
M89.155   **Complete** physeal arrest, **right distal** femur
M89.156   **Complete** physeal arrest, **left distal** femur
M89.157   **Partial** physeal arrest, **right distal** femur
M89.158   **Partial** physeal arrest, **left distal** femur
M89.159   Physeal arrest, femur, unspecified

√6ᵗʰ   M89.16   Physeal arrest, **lower leg**

M89.160   **Complete** physeal arrest, **right proximal** tibia
M89.161   **Complete** physeal arrest, **left proximal** tibia
M89.162   **Partial** physeal arrest, **right proximal** tibia
M89.163   **Partial** physeal arrest, **left proximal** tibia
M89.164   **Complete** physeal arrest, **right distal** tibia
M89.165   **Complete** physeal arrest, **left distal** tibia
M89.166   **Partial** physeal arrest, **right distal** tibia
M89.167   **Partial** physeal arrest, **left distal** tibia
M89.168   Other physeal arrest of lower leg
M89.169   Physeal arrest, lower leg, unspecified

M89.18   Physeal arrest, other site

√5ᵗʰ   M89.2   **Other disorders of bone development and growth**

M89.20   Other disorders of bone development and growth, unspecified site

√6ᵗʰ   M89.21   Other disorders of bone development and growth, **shoulder**

M89.211   Other disorders of bone development and growth, **right** shoulder
M89.212   Other disorders of bone development and growth, **left** shoulder

M89.219   Other disorders of bone development and growth, unspecified shoulder

√6ᵗʰ   M89.22   Other disorders of bone development and growth, **humerus**

M89.221   Other disorders of bone development and growth, **right** humerus
M89.222   Other disorders of bone development and growth, **left** humerus
M89.229   Other disorders of bone development and growth, unspecified humerus

√6ᵗʰ   M89.23   Other disorders of bone development and growth, **ulna and radius**

M89.231   Other disorders of bone development and growth, **right ulna**
M89.232   Other disorders of bone development and growth, **left ulna**
M89.233   Other disorders of bone development and growth, **right radius**
M89.234   Other disorders of bone development and growth, **left radius**
M89.239   Other disorders of bone development and growth, unspecified ulna and radius

√6ᵗʰ   M89.24   Other disorders of bone development and growth, **hand**

M89.241   Other disorders of bone development and growth, **right** hand
M89.242   Other disorders of bone development and growth, **left** hand
M89.249   Other disorders of bone development and growth, unspecified hand

√6ᵗʰ   M89.25   Other disorders of bone development and growth, **femur**

M89.251   Other disorders of bone development and growth, **right** femur
M89.252   Other disorders of bone development and growth, **left** femur
M89.259   Other disorders of bone development and growth, unspecified femur

√6ᵗʰ   M89.26   Other disorders of bone development and growth, **tibia and fibula**

M89.261   Other disorders of bone development and growth, **right tibia**
M89.262   Other disorders of bone development and growth, **left tibia**
M89.263   Other disorders of bone development and growth, **right fibula**
M89.264   Other disorders of bone development and growth, **left fibula**
M89.269   Other disorders of bone development and growth, unspecified lower leg

√6ᵗʰ   M89.27   Other disorders of bone development and growth, **ankle and foot**

M89.271   Other disorders of bone development and growth, **right** ankle and foot
M89.272   Other disorders of bone development and growth, **left** ankle and foot
M89.279   Other disorders of bone development and growth, unspecified ankle and foot

M89.28   Other disorders of bone development and growth, other site
M89.29   Other disorders of bone development and growth, **multiple sites**

√5ᵗʰ   M89.3   **Hypertrophy of bone**

M89.30   Hypertrophy of bone, unspecified site

√6ᵗʰ   M89.31   Hypertrophy of bone, **shoulder**

M89.311   Hypertrophy of bone, **right** shoulder
M89.312   Hypertrophy of bone, **left** shoulder
M89.319   Hypertrophy of bone, unspecified shoulder

√6ᵗʰ   M89.32   Hypertrophy of bone, **humerus**

M89.321   Hypertrophy of bone, **right** humerus
M89.322   Hypertrophy of bone, **left** humerus
M89.329   Hypertrophy of bone, unspecified humerus

√6ᵗʰ   M89.33   Hypertrophy of bone, **ulna and radius**

M89.331   Hypertrophy of bone, **right ulna**
M89.332   Hypertrophy of bone, **left ulna**
M89.333   Hypertrophy of bone, **right radius**
M89.334   Hypertrophy of bone, **left radius**
M89.339   Hypertrophy of bone, unspecified ulna and radius

√6ᵗʰ   M89.34   Hypertrophy of bone, **hand**

M89.341   Hypertrophy of bone, **right** hand

Chapter 13. Diseases of the Musculoskeletal System and Connective Tissue

M89.342 Hypertrophy of bone, **left** hand
M89.349 Hypertrophy of bone, unspecified hand

√6ᵗʰ M89.35 Hypertrophy of bone, **femur**

M89.351 Hypertrophy of bone, **right** femur
M89.352 Hypertrophy of bone, **left** femur
M89.359 Hypertrophy of bone, unspecified femur

√6ᵗʰ M89.36 Hypertrophy of bone, **tibia and fibula**

M89.361 Hypertrophy of bone, **right** tibia
M89.362 Hypertrophy of bone, **left** tibia
M89.363 Hypertrophy of bone, **right** fibula
M89.364 Hypertrophy of bone, **left** fibula
M89.369 Hypertrophy of bone, unspecified tibia and fibula

√6ᵗʰ M89.37 Hypertrophy of bone, **ankle and foot**

M89.371 Hypertrophy of bone, **right** ankle and foot
M89.372 Hypertrophy of bone, **left** ankle and foot
M89.379 Hypertrophy of bone, unspecified ankle and foot

M89.38 Hypertrophy of bone, other site
M89.39 Hypertrophy of bone, **multiple sites**

√5ᵗʰ M89.4 **Other hypertrophic osteoarthropathy**

Marie-Bamberger disease
Pachydermoperiostosis

M89.40 Other hypertrophic osteoarthropathy, unspecified site

√6ᵗʰ M89.41 Other hypertrophic osteoarthropathy, **shoulder**

M89.411 Other hypertrophic osteoarthropathy, **right** shoulder
M89.412 Other hypertrophic osteoarthropathy, **left** shoulder
M89.419 Other hypertrophic osteoarthropathy, unspecified shoulder

√6ᵗʰ M89.42 Other hypertrophic osteoarthropathy, **upper arm**

M89.421 Other hypertrophic osteoarthropathy, **right** upper arm
M89.422 Other hypertrophic osteoarthropathy, **left** upper arm
M89.429 Other hypertrophic osteoarthropathy, unspecified upper arm

√6ᵗʰ M89.43 Other hypertrophic osteoarthropathy, **forearm**

M89.431 Other hypertrophic osteoarthropathy, **right** forearm
M89.432 Other hypertrophic osteoarthropathy, **left** forearm
M89.439 Other hypertrophic osteoarthropathy, unspecified forearm

√6ᵗʰ M89.44 Other hypertrophic osteoarthropathy, **hand**

M89.441 Other hypertrophic osteoarthropathy, **right** hand
M89.442 Other hypertrophic osteoarthropathy, **left** hand
M89.449 Other hypertrophic osteoarthropathy, unspecified hand

√6ᵗʰ M89.45 Other hypertrophic osteoarthropathy, **thigh**

M89.451 Other hypertrophic osteoarthropathy, **right** thigh
M89.452 Other hypertrophic osteoarthropathy, **left** thigh
M89.459 Other hypertrophic osteoarthropathy, unspecified thigh

√6ᵗʰ M89.46 Other hypertrophic osteoarthropathy, **lower leg**

M89.461 Other hypertrophic osteoarthropathy, **right** lower leg
M89.462 Other hypertrophic osteoarthropathy, **left** lower leg
M89.469 Other hypertrophic osteoarthropathy, unspecified lower leg

√6ᵗʰ M89.47 Other hypertrophic osteoarthropathy, **ankle and foot**

M89.471 Other hypertrophic osteoarthropathy, **right** ankle and foot
M89.472 Other hypertrophic osteoarthropathy, **left** ankle and foot
M89.479 Other hypertrophic osteoarthropathy, unspecified ankle and foot

M89.48 Other hypertrophic osteoarthropathy, other site
M89.49 Other hypertrophic osteoarthropathy, **multiple sites**

√5ᵗʰ M89.5 **Osteolysis**

Use additional code to identify major osseous defect, if applicable (M89.7-)

EXCLUDES 2   periprosthetic osteolysis of internal prosthetic joint (T84.05-)

M89.50 Osteolysis, unspecified site

√6ᵗʰ M89.51 Osteolysis, **shoulder**

M89.511 Osteolysis, **right** shoulder
M89.512 Osteolysis, **left** shoulder
M89.519 Osteolysis, unspecified shoulder

√6ᵗʰ M89.52 Osteolysis, **upper arm**

M89.521 Osteolysis, **right** upper arm
M89.522 Osteolysis, **left** upper arm
M89.529 Osteolysis, unspecified upper arm

√6ᵗʰ M89.53 Osteolysis, **forearm**

M89.531 Osteolysis, **right** forearm
M89.532 Osteolysis, **left** forearm
M89.539 Osteolysis, unspecified forearm

√6ᵗʰ M89.54 Osteolysis, **hand**

M89.541 Osteolysis, **right** hand
M89.542 Osteolysis, **left** hand
M89.549 Osteolysis, unspecified hand

√6ᵗʰ M89.55 Osteolysis, **thigh**

M89.551 Osteolysis, **right** thigh
M89.552 Osteolysis, **left** thigh
M89.559 Osteolysis, unspecified thigh

√6ᵗʰ M89.56 Osteolysis, **lower leg**

M89.561 Osteolysis, **right** lower leg
M89.562 Osteolysis, **left** lower leg
M89.569 Osteolysis, unspecified lower leg

√6ᵗʰ M89.57 Osteolysis, **ankle and foot**

M89.571 Osteolysis, **right** ankle and foot
M89.572 Osteolysis, **left** ankle and foot
M89.579 Osteolysis, unspecified ankle and foot

M89.58 Osteolysis, other site
M89.59 Osteolysis, **multiple sites**

√5ᵗʰ M89.6 **Osteopathy after poliomyelitis**

Use additional code (B91) to identify previous poliomyelitis

EXCLUDES 1   postpolio syndrome (G14)

M89.60 Osteopathy after poliomyelitis, unspecified site   **HCC**

√6ᵗʰ M89.61 Osteopathy after poliomyelitis, **shoulder**

M89.611 Osteopathy after poliomyelitis, **right** shoulder   **HCC**
M89.612 Osteopathy after poliomyelitis, **left** shoulder   **HCC**
M89.619 Osteopathy after poliomyelitis, unspecified shoulder   **HCC**

√6ᵗʰ M89.62 Osteopathy after poliomyelitis, **upper arm**

M89.621 Osteopathy after poliomyelitis, **right** upper arm   **HCC**
M89.622 Osteopathy after poliomyelitis, **left** upper arm   **HCC**
M89.629 Osteopathy after poliomyelitis, unspecified upper arm   **HCC**

√6ᵗʰ M89.63 Osteopathy after poliomyelitis, **forearm**

M89.631 Osteopathy after poliomyelitis, **right** forearm   **HCC**
M89.632 Osteopathy after poliomyelitis, **left** forearm   **HCC**
M89.639 Osteopathy after poliomyelitis, unspecified forearm   **HCC**

√6ᵗʰ M89.64 Osteopathy after poliomyelitis, **hand**

M89.641 Osteopathy after poliomyelitis, **right** hand   **HCC**
M89.642 Osteopathy after poliomyelitis, **left** hand   **HCC**
M89.649 Osteopathy after poliomyelitis, unspecified hand   **HCC**

√6ᵗʰ M89.65 Osteopathy after poliomyelitis, **thigh**

M89.651 Osteopathy after poliomyelitis, **right** thigh   **HCC**
M89.652 Osteopathy after poliomyelitis, **left** thigh   **HCC**
M89.659 Osteopathy after poliomyelitis, unspecified thigh   **HCC**

N Newborn: 0   **P** Pediatric: 0-17   **M** Maternity: 9-64   **A** Adult: 15-124   **UNS** Unspecified Site   **MCC** Major Complication/Comorbidity   **CC** Complication/Comorbidity   **PE** POA Exempt

848   ICD-10-CM 2025

✓6ᵗʰ **M89.66** **Osteopathy after poliomyelitis, lower leg**

    M89.661 Osteopathy after poliomyelitis, right lower leg   HCC

    M89.662 Osteopathy after poliomyelitis, left lower leg   HCC

    M89.669 Osteopathy after poliomyelitis, unspecified lower leg   HCC

✓6ᵗʰ **M89.67** **Osteopathy after poliomyelitis, ankle and foot**

    M89.671 Osteopathy after poliomyelitis, right ankle and foot

    M89.672 Osteopathy after poliomyelitis, left ankle and foot   HCC

    M89.679 Osteopathy after poliomyelitis, unspecified ankle and foot   HCC

M89.68 **Osteopathy after poliomyelitis, other site**   HCC

M89.69 **Osteopathy after poliomyelitis, multiple sites**   HCC

✓5ᵗʰ **M89.7** **Major osseous defect**

Code first underlying disease, if known, such as:
   aseptic necrosis of bone (M87.-)
   malignant neoplasm of bone (C40.-)
   osteolysis (M89.5-)
   osteomyelitis (M86.-)
   osteonecrosis (M87.-)
   osteoporosis (M80.-, M81.-)
   periprosthetic osteolysis (T84.05-)

M89.70 **Major osseous defect, unspecified site**

✓6ᵗʰ **M89.71** **Major osseous defect, shoulder region**

   Major osseous defect clavicle or scapula

    M89.711 Major osseous defect, right shoulder region

    M89.712 Major osseous defect, left shoulder region

    M89.719 Major osseous defect, unspecified shoulder region

✓6ᵗʰ **M89.72** **Major osseous defect, humerus**

    M89.721 Major osseous defect, right humerus

    M89.722 Major osseous defect, left humerus

    M89.729 Major osseous defect, unspecified humerus

✓6ᵗʰ **M89.73** **Major osseous defect, forearm**

   Major osseous defect of radius and ulna

    M89.731 Major osseous defect, right forearm

    M89.732 Major osseous defect, left forearm

    M89.739 Major osseous defect, unspecified forearm

✓6ᵗʰ **M89.74** **Major osseous defect, hand**

   Major osseous defect of carpus, fingers, metacarpus

    M89.741 Major osseous defect, right hand

    M89.742 Major osseous defect, left hand

    M89.749 Major osseous defect, unspecified hand

✓6ᵗʰ **M89.75** **Major osseous defect, pelvic region and thigh**

   Major osseous defect of femur and pelvis

    M89.751 Major osseous defect, right pelvic region and thigh

    M89.752 Major osseous defect, left pelvic region and thigh

    M89.759 Major osseous defect, unspecified pelvic region and thigh

✓6ᵗʰ **M89.76** **Major osseous defect, lower leg**

   Major osseous defect of fibula and tibia

    M89.761 Major osseous defect, right lower leg

    M89.762 Major osseous defect, left lower leg

    M89.769 Major osseous defect, unspecified lower leg

✓6ᵗʰ **M89.77** **Major osseous defect, ankle and foot**

   Major osseous defect of metatarsus, tarsus, toes

    M89.771 Major osseous defect, right ankle and foot

    M89.772 Major osseous defect, left ankle and foot

    M89.779 Major osseous defect, unspecified ankle and foot

M89.78 **Major osseous defect, other site**

M89.79 **Major osseous defect, multiple sites**

✓5ᵗʰ **M89.8** **Other specified disorders of bone**

   Infantile cortical hyperostoses
   Post-traumatic subperiosteal ossification
   AHA: 2022,2Q,10

✓6ᵗʰ **M89.8X** **Other specified disorders of bone**

    M89.8X0 Other specified disorders of bone, multiple sites

    M89.8X1 Other specified disorders of bone, shoulder

    M89.8X2 Other specified disorders of bone, upper arm

    M89.8X3 Other specified disorders of bone, forearm
     AHA: 2019,3Q,9

    M89.8X4 Other specified disorders of bone, hand

    M89.8X5 Other specified disorders of bone, thigh

    M89.8X6 Other specified disorders of bone, lower leg

    M89.8X7 Other specified disorders of bone, ankle and foot

    M89.8X8 Other specified disorders of bone, other site
     AHA: 2023,2Q,18

    M89.8X9 Other specified disorders of bone, unspecified site

M89.9 **Disorder of bone, unspecified**

✓4ᵗʰ **M90** **Osteopathies in diseases classified elsewhere**

   EXCLUDES 1   osteochondritis, osteomyelitis, and osteopathy (in):
     cryptococcosis (B45.3)
     diabetes mellitus (E08-E13 with .69-)
     gonococcal (A54.43)
     neurogenic syphilis (A52.11)
     renal osteodystrophy (N25.0)
     salmonellosis (A02.24)
     secondary syphilis (A51.46)
     syphilis (late) (A52.77)

✓5ᵗʰ **M90.5** **Osteonecrosis in diseases classified elsewhere**

   Code first underlying disease, such as:
    caisson disease (T70.3)
    hemoglobinopathy (D50-D64)

    M90.50 *Osteonecrosis in diseases classified elsewhere, unspecified site*   CC UNS HCC

✓6ᵗʰ **M90.51** **Osteonecrosis in diseases classified elsewhere, shoulder**

    M90.511 *Osteonecrosis in diseases classified elsewhere, right shoulder*   CC HCC

    M90.512 *Osteonecrosis in diseases classified elsewhere, left shoulder*   CC HCC

    M90.519 *Osteonecrosis in diseases classified elsewhere, unspecified shoulder*   CC UNS HCC

✓6ᵗʰ **M90.52** **Osteonecrosis in diseases classified elsewhere, upper arm**

    M90.521 *Osteonecrosis in diseases classified elsewhere, right upper arm*   CC HCC

    M90.522 *Osteonecrosis in diseases classified elsewhere, left upper arm*   CC HCC

    M90.529 *Osteonecrosis in diseases classified elsewhere, unspecified upper arm*   CC UNS HCC

✓6ᵗʰ **M90.53** **Osteonecrosis in diseases classified elsewhere, forearm**

    M90.531 *Osteonecrosis in diseases classified elsewhere, right forearm*   CC HCC

    M90.532 *Osteonecrosis in diseases classified elsewhere, left forearm*   CC HCC

    M90.539 *Osteonecrosis in diseases classified elsewhere, unspecified forearm*   CC UNS HCC

✓6ᵗʰ **M90.54** **Osteonecrosis in diseases classified elsewhere, hand**

    M90.541 *Osteonecrosis in diseases classified elsewhere, right hand*   CC HCC

    M90.542 *Osteonecrosis in diseases classified elsewhere, left hand*   CC HCC

    M90.549 *Osteonecrosis in diseases classified elsewhere, unspecified hand*   CC UNS HCC

✓6ᵗʰ **M90.55** **Osteonecrosis in diseases classified elsewhere, thigh**

    M90.551 *Osteonecrosis in diseases classified elsewhere, right thigh*   CC HCC

    M90.552 *Osteonecrosis in diseases classified elsewhere, left thigh*   CC HCC

    M90.559 *Osteonecrosis in diseases classified elsewhere, unspecified thigh*   CC UNS HCC

✓6ᵗʰ **M90.56** **Osteonecrosis in diseases classified elsewhere, lower leg**

    M90.561 *Osteonecrosis in diseases classified elsewhere, right lower leg*   CC HCC

Chapter 13. Diseases of the Musculoskeletal System and Connective Tissue

M89.66–M90.561

✅ Additional Character Required   ✓x7ᵗʰ Placeholder   Questionable PDx   Manifestation   Unspecified   UPD Unacceptable PDx   H1-H14 HAC   HCC CMS-HCC Dx   HIV HIV Dx

ICD-10-CM 2025   **849**

Chapter 13. Diseases of the Musculoskeletal System and Connective Tissue

      M90.562 *Osteonecrosis in diseases classified elsewhere, left lower leg* CC HCC

      M90.569 *Osteonecrosis in diseases classified elsewhere, unspecified lower leg* CC UNS HCC

✓6th M90.57 Osteonecrosis in diseases classified elsewhere, ankle and foot

      M90.571 *Osteonecrosis in diseases classified elsewhere, right ankle and foot* CC HCC

      M90.572 *Osteonecrosis in diseases classified elsewhere, left ankle and foot* CC HCC

      M90.579 *Osteonecrosis in diseases classified elsewhere, unspecified ankle and foot* CC UNS HCC

    M90.58 Osteonecrosis in diseases classified elsewhere, other site CC HCC

    M90.59 Osteonecrosis in diseases classified elsewhere, multiple sites CC HCC

✓5th M90.6 Osteitis deformans in neoplastic diseases

    Osteitis deformans in malignant neoplasm of bone

    Code first the neoplasm (C40.-, C41.-)

    EXCLUDES 1   osteitis deformans [Paget's disease of bone] (M88.-)

    M90.60 *Osteitis deformans in neoplastic diseases, unspecified site*

    ✓6th M90.61 Osteitis deformans in neoplastic diseases, shoulder

      M90.611 *Osteitis deformans in neoplastic diseases, right shoulder*

      M90.612 *Osteitis deformans in neoplastic diseases, left shoulder*

      M90.619 *Osteitis deformans in neoplastic diseases, unspecified shoulder*

    ✓6th M90.62 Osteitis deformans in neoplastic diseases, upper arm

      M90.621 *Osteitis deformans in neoplastic diseases, right upper arm*

      M90.622 *Osteitis deformans in neoplastic diseases, left upper arm*

      M90.629 *Osteitis deformans in neoplastic diseases, unspecified upper arm*

    ✓6th M90.63 Osteitis deformans in neoplastic diseases, forearm

      M90.631 *Osteitis deformans in neoplastic diseases, right forearm*

      M90.632 *Osteitis deformans in neoplastic diseases, left forearm*

      M90.639 *Osteitis deformans in neoplastic diseases, unspecified forearm*

    ✓6th M90.64 Osteitis deformans in neoplastic diseases, hand

      M90.641 *Osteitis deformans in neoplastic diseases, right hand*

      M90.642 *Osteitis deformans in neoplastic diseases, left hand*

      M90.649 *Osteitis deformans in neoplastic diseases, unspecified hand*

    ✓6th M90.65 Osteitis deformans in neoplastic diseases, thigh

      M90.651 *Osteitis deformans in neoplastic diseases, right thigh*

      M90.652 *Osteitis deformans in neoplastic diseases, left thigh*

      M90.659 *Osteitis deformans in neoplastic diseases, unspecified thigh*

    ✓6th M90.66 Osteitis deformans in neoplastic diseases, lower leg

      M90.661 *Osteitis deformans in neoplastic diseases, right lower leg*

      M90.662 *Osteitis deformans in neoplastic diseases, left lower leg*

      M90.669 *Osteitis deformans in neoplastic diseases, unspecified lower leg*

    ✓6th M90.67 Osteitis deformans in neoplastic diseases, ankle and foot

      M90.671 *Osteitis deformans in neoplastic diseases, right ankle and foot*

      M90.672 *Osteitis deformans in neoplastic diseases, left ankle and foot*

      M90.679 *Osteitis deformans in neoplastic diseases, unspecified ankle and foot*

    M90.68 *Osteitis deformans in neoplastic diseases, other site*

    M90.69 *Osteitis deformans in neoplastic diseases, multiple sites*

✓5th M90.8 Osteopathy in diseases classified elsewhere

    Code first underlying disease, such as:

      rickets (E55.0)

      vitamin-D-resistant rickets (E83.31)

    M90.80 *Osteopathy in diseases classified elsewhere, unspecified site*

    ✓6th M90.81 Osteopathy in diseases classified elsewhere, shoulder

      M90.811 *Osteopathy in diseases classified elsewhere, right shoulder*

      M90.812 *Osteopathy in diseases classified elsewhere, left shoulder*

      M90.819 *Osteopathy in diseases classified elsewhere, unspecified shoulder*

    ✓6th M90.82 Osteopathy in diseases classified elsewhere, upper arm

      M90.821 *Osteopathy in diseases classified elsewhere, right upper arm*

      M90.822 *Osteopathy in diseases classified elsewhere, left upper arm*

      M90.829 *Osteopathy in diseases classified elsewhere, unspecified upper arm*

    ✓6th M90.83 Osteopathy in diseases classified elsewhere, forearm

      M90.831 *Osteopathy in diseases classified elsewhere, right forearm*

      M90.832 *Osteopathy in diseases classified elsewhere, left forearm*

      M90.839 *Osteopathy in diseases classified elsewhere, unspecified forearm*

    ✓6th M90.84 Osteopathy in diseases classified elsewhere, hand

      M90.841 *Osteopathy in diseases classified elsewhere, right hand*

      M90.842 *Osteopathy in diseases classified elsewhere, left hand*

      M90.849 *Osteopathy in diseases classified elsewhere, unspecified hand*

    ✓6th M90.85 Osteopathy in diseases classified elsewhere, thigh

      M90.851 *Osteopathy in diseases classified elsewhere, right thigh*

      M90.852 *Osteopathy in diseases classified elsewhere, left thigh*

      M90.859 *Osteopathy in diseases classified elsewhere, unspecified thigh*

    ✓6th M90.86 Osteopathy in diseases classified elsewhere, lower leg

      M90.861 *Osteopathy in diseases classified elsewhere, right lower leg*

      M90.862 *Osteopathy in diseases classified elsewhere, left lower leg*

      M90.869 *Osteopathy in diseases classified elsewhere, unspecified lower leg*

    ✓6th M90.87 Osteopathy in diseases classified elsewhere, ankle and foot

      M90.871 *Osteopathy in diseases classified elsewhere, right ankle and foot*

      M90.872 *Osteopathy in diseases classified elsewhere, left ankle and foot*

      M90.879 *Osteopathy in diseases classified elsewhere, unspecified ankle and foot*

    M90.88 *Osteopathy in diseases classified elsewhere, other site*

    M90.89 *Osteopathy in diseases classified elsewhere, multiple sites*

Chondropathies (M91-M94)

EXCLUDES 1   postprocedural chondropathies (M96.-)

✓4th M91 Juvenile osteochondrosis of hip and pelvis

    EXCLUDES 1   slipped upper femoral epiphysis (nontraumatic) (M93.0-)

    M91.0 Juvenile osteochondrosis of pelvis

      Osteochondrosis (juvenile) of acetabulum

      Osteochondrosis (juvenile) of iliac crest [Buchanan]

      Osteochondrosis (juvenile) of ischiopubic synchondrosis [van Neck]

      Osteochondrosis (juvenile) of symphysis pubis [Pierson]

    ✓5th M91.1 Juvenile osteochondrosis of head of femur [Legg-Calve-Perthes]

      M91.10 Juvenile osteochondrosis of head of femur [Legg-Calve-Perthes], unspecified leg

      M91.11 Juvenile osteochondrosis of head of femur [Legg-Calve-Perthes], right leg

      M91.12 Juvenile osteochondrosis of head of femur [Legg-Calve-Perthes], left leg

N Newborn: 0   **P** Pediatric: 0-17   **M** Maternity: 9-64   **A** Adult: 15-124   UNS Unspecified Site   MCC Major Complication/Comorbidity   CC Complication/Comorbidity   PE POA Exempt

850   ICD-10-CM 2025

√5th **M91.2 Coxa plana**

Hip deformity due to previous juvenile osteochondrosis

    M91.20   Coxa plana, unspecified hip
    M91.21   Coxa plana, right hip
    M91.22   Coxa plana, left hip

√5th **M91.3 Pseudocoxalgia**

    M91.30   Pseudocoxalgia, unspecified hip
    M91.31   Pseudocoxalgia, right hip
    M91.32   Pseudocoxalgia, left hip

√5th **M91.4 Coxa magna**

    M91.40   Coxa magna, unspecified hip
    M91.41   Coxa magna, right hip
    M91.42   Coxa magna, left hip

√5th **M91.8 Other juvenile osteochondrosis of hip and pelvis**

Juvenile osteochondrosis after reduction of congenital dislocation of hip

    M91.80   Other juvenile osteochondrosis of hip and pelvis, unspecified leg
    M91.81   Other juvenile osteochondrosis of hip and pelvis, right leg
    M91.82   Other juvenile osteochondrosis of hip and pelvis, left leg

√5th **M91.9 Juvenile osteochondrosis of hip and pelvis, unspecified**

    M91.90   Juvenile osteochondrosis of hip and pelvis, unspecified, unspecified leg
    M91.91   Juvenile osteochondrosis of hip and pelvis, unspecified, right leg
    M91.92   Juvenile osteochondrosis of hip and pelvis, unspecified, left leg

√4th **M92 Other juvenile osteochondrosis**

√5th **M92.0 Juvenile osteochondrosis of humerus**

Osteochondrosis (juvenile) of capitulum of humerus [Panner]
Osteochondrosis (juvenile) of head of humerus [Haas]

    M92.00   Juvenile osteochondrosis of humerus, unspecified arm
    M92.01   Juvenile osteochondrosis of humerus, right arm
    M92.02   Juvenile osteochondrosis of humerus, left arm

√5th **M92.1 Juvenile osteochondrosis of radius and ulna**

Osteochondrosis (juvenile) of lower ulna [Burns]
Osteochondrosis (juvenile) of radial head [Brailsford]

    M92.10   Juvenile osteochondrosis of radius and ulna, unspecified arm
    M92.11   Juvenile osteochondrosis of radius and ulna, right arm
    M92.12   Juvenile osteochondrosis of radius and ulna, left arm

√5th **M92.2 Juvenile osteochondrosis, hand**

√6th   **M92.20 Unspecified juvenile osteochondrosis, hand**

    M92.201   Unspecified juvenile osteochondrosis, right hand
    M92.202   Unspecified juvenile osteochondrosis, left hand
    M92.209   Unspecified juvenile osteochondrosis, unspecified hand

√6th   **M92.21 Osteochondrosis (juvenile) of carpal lunate [Kienbock]**

    M92.211   Osteochondrosis (juvenile) of carpal lunate [Kienbock], right hand
    M92.212   Osteochondrosis (juvenile) of carpal lunate [Kienbock], left hand
    M92.219   Osteochondrosis (juvenile) of carpal lunate [Kienbock], unspecified hand

√6th   **M92.22 Osteochondrosis (juvenile) of metacarpal heads [Mauclaire]**

    M92.221   Osteochondrosis (juvenile) of metacarpal heads [Mauclaire], right hand
    M92.222   Osteochondrosis (juvenile) of metacarpal heads [Mauclaire], left hand
    M92.229   Osteochondrosis (juvenile) of metacarpal heads [Mauclaire], unspecified hand

√6th   **M92.29 Other juvenile osteochondrosis, hand**

    M92.291   Other juvenile osteochondrosis, right hand
    M92.292   Other juvenile osteochondrosis, left hand
    M92.299   Other juvenile osteochondrosis, unspecified hand

√5th **M92.3 Other juvenile osteochondrosis, upper limb**

    M92.30   Other juvenile osteochondrosis, unspecified upper limb
    M92.31   Other juvenile osteochondrosis, right upper limb

    M92.32   Other juvenile osteochondrosis, left upper limb

√5th **M92.4 Juvenile osteochondrosis of patella**

Osteochondrosis (juvenile) of primary patellar center [Kohler]
Osteochondrosis (juvenile) of secondary patellar centre [Sinding Larsen]

    M92.40   Juvenile osteochondrosis of patella, unspecified knee
    M92.41   Juvenile osteochondrosis of patella, right knee
    M92.42   Juvenile osteochondrosis of patella, left knee

√5th **M92.5 Juvenile osteochondrosis of tibia and fibula**

    AHA: 2020,4Q,33-34

√6th   **M92.50 Unspecified juvenile osteochondrosis of tibia and fibula**

    M92.501   Unspecified juvenile osteochondrosis, right leg
    M92.502   Unspecified juvenile osteochondrosis, left leg
    M92.503   Unspecified juvenile osteochondrosis, bilateral leg
    M92.509   Unspecified juvenile osteochondrosis, unspecified leg

√6th   **M92.51 Juvenile osteochondrosis of proximal tibia**

Blount disease
Tibia vara

    M92.511   Juvenile osteochondrosis of proximal tibia, right leg
    M92.512   Juvenile osteochondrosis of proximal tibia, left leg
    M92.513   Juvenile osteochondrosis of proximal tibia, bilateral
    M92.519   Juvenile osteochondrosis of proximal tibia, unspecified leg

√6th   **M92.52 Juvenile osteochondrosis of tibia tubercle**

Osgood-Schlatter disease

    M92.521   Juvenile osteochondrosis of tibia tubercle, right leg
    M92.522   Juvenile osteochondrosis of tibia tubercle, left leg
    M92.523   Juvenile osteochondrosis of tibia tubercle, bilateral
    M92.529   Juvenile osteochondrosis of tibia tubercle, unspecified leg

√6th   **M92.59 Other juvenile osteochondrosis of tibia and fibula**

    M92.591   Other juvenile osteochondrosis of tibia and fibula, right leg
    M92.592   Other juvenile osteochondrosis of tibia and fibula, left leg
    M92.593   Other juvenile osteochondrosis of tibia and fibula, bilateral
    M92.599   Other juvenile osteochondrosis of tibia and fibula, unspecified leg

√5th **M92.6 Juvenile osteochondrosis of tarsus**

Osteochondrosis (juvenile) of calcaneum [Sever]
Osteochondrosis (juvenile) of os tibiale externum [Haglund]
Osteochondrosis (juvenile) of talus [Diaz]
Osteochondrosis (juvenile) of tarsal navicular [Kohler]

    M92.60   Juvenile osteochondrosis of tarsus, unspecified ankle
    M92.61   Juvenile osteochondrosis of tarsus, right ankle
    M92.62   Juvenile osteochondrosis of tarsus, left ankle

√5th **M92.7 Juvenile osteochondrosis of metatarsus**

Osteochondrosis (juvenile) of fifth metatarsus [Iselin]
Osteochondrosis (juvenile) of second metatarsus [Freiberg]

    M92.70   Juvenile osteochondrosis of metatarsus, unspecified foot
    M92.71   Juvenile osteochondrosis of metatarsus, right foot
    M92.72   Juvenile osteochondrosis of metatarsus, left foot

M92.8 Other specified juvenile osteochondrosis

~~Calcaneal apophysitis~~
DEF: Calcaneal apophysitis: Inflammation of the calcaneus at the point of Achilles tendon insertion usually occurring in boys ages 8 to 14. Pain, tenderness, and localized swelling are present.

M92.9 Juvenile osteochondrosis, unspecified

Juvenile apophysitis NOS
Juvenile epiphysitis NOS
Juvenile osteochondritis NOS
Juvenile osteochondrosis NOS

✔ Additional Character Required   √x7th Placeholder   Questionable PDx   Manifestation   Unspecified   UPD Unacceptable PDx   H1-H14 HAC   HCC CMS-HCC Dx   HIV HIV Dx

ICD-10-CM 2025   851

Chapter 13. Diseases of the Musculoskeletal System and Connective Tissue

√4ᵗʰ **M93** **Other osteochondropathies**

EXCLUDES 2   osteochondrosis of spine (M42.-)

√5ᵗʰ **M93.0** **Slipped upper femoral epiphysis (nontraumatic)**

Slipped capital femoral epiphysis (SCFE)
Slipped upper femoral epiphysis (SUFE)
Use additional code for associated chondrolysis (M94.3)
AHA: 2022,4Q,30-31

√6ᵗʰ **M93.00** **Unspecified slipped upper femoral epiphysis (nontraumatic)**

M93.001 Unspecified slipped upper femoral epiphysis (nontraumatic), **right** hip

M93.002 Unspecified slipped upper femoral epiphysis (nontraumatic), **left** hip

M93.003 Unspecified slipped upper femoral epiphysis (nontraumatic), unspecified hip

M93.004 Unspecified slipped upper femoral epiphysis (nontraumatic), **bilateral** hips

√6ᵗʰ **M93.01** **Acute** slipped upper femoral epiphysis, **stable** (nontraumatic)

M93.011 Acute slipped upper femoral epiphysis, stable (nontraumatic), **right** hip

M93.012 Acute slipped upper femoral epiphysis, stable (nontraumatic), **left** hip

M93.013 Acute slipped upper femoral epiphysis, stable (nontraumatic), unspecified hip

M93.014 Acute slipped upper femoral epiphysis, stable (nontraumatic), **bilateral** hips

√6ᵗʰ **M93.02** **Chronic** slipped upper femoral epiphysis, **stable** (nontraumatic)

M93.021 Chronic slipped upper femoral epiphysis, stable (nontraumatic), **right** hip

M93.022 Chronic slipped upper femoral epiphysis, stable (nontraumatic), **left** hip

M93.023 Chronic slipped upper femoral epiphysis, stable (nontraumatic), unspecified hip

M93.024 Chronic slipped upper femoral epiphysis, stable (nontraumatic), **bilateral** hips

√6ᵗʰ **M93.03** **Acute on chronic** slipped upper femoral epiphysis, **stable** (nontraumatic)

M93.031 Acute on chronic slipped upper femoral epiphysis, stable (nontraumatic), **right** hip

M93.032 Acute on chronic slipped upper femoral epiphysis, stable (nontraumatic), **left** hip

M93.033 Acute on chronic slipped upper femoral epiphysis, stable (nontraumatic), unspecified hip

M93.034 Acute on chronic slipped upper femoral epiphysis, stable (nontraumatic), **bilateral** hips

√6ᵗʰ **M93.04** **Acute** slipped upper femoral epiphysis, **unstable** (nontraumatic)

M93.041 Acute slipped upper femoral epiphysis, unstable (nontraumatic), **right** hip

M93.042 Acute slipped upper femoral epiphysis, unstable (nontraumatic), **left** hip

M93.043 Acute slipped upper femoral epiphysis, unstable (nontraumatic), unspecified hip

M93.044 Acute slipped upper femoral epiphysis, unstable (nontraumatic), **bilateral** hips

√6ᵗʰ **M93.05** **Acute on chronic** slipped upper femoral epiphysis, **unstable** (nontraumatic)

M93.051 Acute on chronic slipped upper femoral epiphysis, unstable (nontraumatic), **right** hip

M93.052 Acute on chronic slipped upper femoral epiphysis, unstable (nontraumatic), **left** hip

M93.053 Acute on chronic slipped upper femoral epiphysis, unstable (nontraumatic), unspecified hip

M93.054 Acute on chronic slipped upper femoral epiphysis, unstable (nontraumatic), **bilateral** hips

√6ᵗʰ **M93.06** **Acute** slipped upper femoral epiphysis, unspecified stability (nontraumatic)

M93.061 Acute slipped upper femoral epiphysis, unspecified stability (nontraumatic), **right** hip

M93.062 Acute slipped upper femoral epiphysis, unspecified stability (nontraumatic), **left** hip

M93.063 Acute slipped upper femoral epiphysis, unspecified stability (nontraumatic), unspecified hip

M93.064 Acute slipped upper femoral epiphysis, unspecified stability (nontraumatic), **bilateral** hips

√6ᵗʰ **M93.07** **Acute on chronic** slipped upper femoral epiphysis, unspecified stability (nontraumatic)

M93.071 Acute on chronic slipped upper femoral epiphysis, unspecified stability (nontraumatic), **right** hip

M93.072 Acute on chronic slipped upper femoral epiphysis, unspecified stability (nontraumatic), **left** hip

M93.073 Acute on chronic slipped upper femoral epiphysis, unspecified stability (nontraumatic), unspecified hip

M93.074 Acute on chronic slipped upper femoral epiphysis, unspecified stability (nontraumatic), **bilateral** hips

M93.1 **Kienbock's disease of adults**   A

Adult osteochondrosis of carpal lunates

√5ᵗʰ **M93.2** **Osteochondritis dissecans**

DEF: Avascular necrosis caused by lack of blood flow to the bone and cartilage of a joint causing the bone to die. This can result in splinters or pieces of cartilage breaking off in the joint.

M93.20 Osteochondritis dissecans of unspecified site

√6ᵗʰ **M93.21** Osteochondritis dissecans of **shoulder**

M93.211 Osteochondritis dissecans, **right** shoulder
M93.212 Osteochondritis dissecans, **left** shoulder
M93.219 Osteochondritis dissecans, unspecified shoulder

√6ᵗʰ **M93.22** Osteochondritis dissecans of **elbow**

M93.221 Osteochondritis dissecans, **right** elbow
M93.222 Osteochondritis dissecans, **left** elbow
M93.229 Osteochondritis dissecans, unspecified elbow

√6ᵗʰ **M93.23** Osteochondritis dissecans of **wrist**

M93.231 Osteochondritis dissecans, **right** wrist
M93.232 Osteochondritis dissecans, **left** wrist
M93.239 Osteochondritis dissecans, unspecified wrist

√6ᵗʰ **M93.24** Osteochondritis dissecans of joints of **hand**

M93.241 Osteochondritis dissecans, joints of **right** hand

M93.242 Osteochondritis dissecans, joints of **left** hand

M93.249 Osteochondritis dissecans, joints of unspecified hand

√6ᵗʰ **M93.25** Osteochondritis dissecans of **hip**

M93.251 Osteochondritis dissecans, **right** hip
M93.252 Osteochondritis dissecans, **left** hip
M93.259 Osteochondritis dissecans, unspecified hip

√6ᵗʰ **M93.26** Osteochondritis dissecans **knee**

M93.261 Osteochondritis dissecans, **right** knee
M93.262 Osteochondritis dissecans, **left** knee
M93.269 Osteochondritis dissecans, unspecified knee

√6ᵗʰ **M93.27** Osteochondritis dissecans of **ankle and joints of foot**

M93.271 Osteochondritis dissecans, **right** ankle and joints of **right** foot

M93.272 Osteochondritis dissecans, **left** ankle and joints of **left** foot

M93.279 Osteochondritis dissecans, unspecified ankle and joints of foot

M93.28 Osteochondritis dissecans other site
M93.29 Osteochondritis dissecans **multiple sites**

√5ᵗʰ **M93.8** **Other specified osteochondropathies**

M93.80 Other specified osteochondropathies of unspecified site

√6ᵗʰ **M93.81** Other specified osteochondropathies of **shoulder**

M93.811 Other specified osteochondropathies, **right** shoulder

M93.812 Other specified osteochondropathies, **left** shoulder

M93.819 Other specified osteochondropathies, unspecified shoulder

√6ᵗʰ **M93.82** Other specified osteochondropathies of **upper arm**

M93.821 Other specified osteochondropathies, **right** upper arm

N Newborn: 0   P Pediatric: 0-17   M Maternity: 9-64   A Adult: 15-124   UNS Unspecified Site   MCC Major Complication/Comorbidity   CC Complication/Comorbidity   PE POA Exempt

852

ICD-10-CM 2025

M93.822 Other specified osteochondropathies, left upper arm

M93.829 Other specified osteochondropathies, unspecified upper arm

✓6ᵗʰ **M93.83** Other specified osteochondropathies of forearm

M93.831 Other specified osteochondropathies, right forearm

M93.832 Other specified osteochondropathies, left forearm

M93.839 Other specified osteochondropathies, unspecified forearm

✓6ᵗʰ **M93.84** Other specified osteochondropathies of hand

M93.841 Other specified osteochondropathies, right hand

M93.842 Other specified osteochondropathies, left hand

M93.849 Other specified osteochondropathies, unspecified hand

✓6ᵗʰ **M93.85** Other specified osteochondropathies of thigh

M93.851 Other specified osteochondropathies, right thigh

M93.852 Other specified osteochondropathies, left thigh

M93.859 Other specified osteochondropathies, unspecified thigh

✓6ᵗʰ **M93.86** Other specified osteochondropathies lower leg

M93.861 Other specified osteochondropathies, right lower leg

M93.862 Other specified osteochondropathies, left lower leg

M93.869 Other specified osteochondropathies, unspecified lower leg

✓6ᵗʰ **M93.87** Other specified osteochondropathies of ankle and foot

M93.871 Other specified osteochondropathies, right ankle and foot

M93.872 Other specified osteochondropathies, left ankle and foot

M93.879 Other specified osteochondropathies, unspecified ankle and foot

M93.88 Other specified osteochondropathies other site

M93.89 Other specified osteochondropathies multiple sites

✓5ᵗʰ **M93.9** Osteochondropathy, unspecified

Apophysitis NOS
Epiphysitis NOS
Osteochondritis NOS
Osteochondrosis NOS

M93.90 Osteochondropathy, unspecified of unspecified site

✓6ᵗʰ **M93.91** Osteochondropathy, unspecified of shoulder

M93.911 Osteochondropathy, unspecified, right shoulder

M93.912 Osteochondropathy, unspecified, left shoulder

M93.919 Osteochondropathy, unspecified, unspecified shoulder

✓6ᵗʰ **M93.92** Osteochondropathy, unspecified of upper arm

M93.921 Osteochondropathy, unspecified, right upper arm

M93.922 Osteochondropathy, unspecified, left upper arm

M93.929 Osteochondropathy, unspecified, unspecified upper arm

✓6ᵗʰ **M93.93** Osteochondropathy, unspecified of forearm

M93.931 Osteochondropathy, unspecified, right forearm

M93.932 Osteochondropathy, unspecified, left forearm

M93.939 Osteochondropathy, unspecified, unspecified forearm

✓6ᵗʰ **M93.94** Osteochondropathy, unspecified of hand

M93.941 Osteochondropathy, unspecified, right hand

M93.942 Osteochondropathy, unspecified, left hand

M93.949 Osteochondropathy, unspecified, unspecified hand

✓6ᵗʰ **M93.95** Osteochondropathy, unspecified of thigh

M93.951 Osteochondropathy, unspecified, right thigh

M93.952 Osteochondropathy, unspecified, left thigh

M93.959 Osteochondropathy, unspecified, unspecified thigh

✓6ᵗʰ **M93.96** Osteochondropathy, unspecified lower leg

M93.961 Osteochondropathy, unspecified, right lower leg

M93.962 Osteochondropathy, unspecified, left lower leg

M93.969 Osteochondropathy, unspecified, unspecified lower leg

✓6ᵗʰ **M93.97** Osteochondropathy, unspecified of ankle and foot

M93.971 Osteochondropathy, unspecified, right ankle and foot

M93.972 Osteochondropathy, unspecified, left ankle and foot

M93.979 Osteochondropathy, unspecified, unspecified ankle and foot

M93.98 Osteochondropathy, unspecified other site

M93.99 Osteochondropathy, unspecified multiple sites

✓4ᵗʰ **M94** Other disorders of cartilage

M94.0 Chondrocostal junction syndrome [Tietze]
Costochondritis

M94.1 Relapsing polychondritis

✓5ᵗʰ **M94.2** Chondromalacia

EXCLUDES 1   chondromalacia patellae (M22.4)

M94.20 Chondromalacia, unspecified site

✓6ᵗʰ **M94.21** Chondromalacia, shoulder

M94.211 Chondromalacia, right shoulder
M94.212 Chondromalacia, left shoulder
M94.219 Chondromalacia, unspecified shoulder

✓6ᵗʰ **M94.22** Chondromalacia, elbow

M94.221 Chondromalacia, right elbow
M94.222 Chondromalacia, left elbow
M94.229 Chondromalacia, unspecified elbow

✓6ᵗʰ **M94.23** Chondromalacia, wrist

M94.231 Chondromalacia, right wrist
M94.232 Chondromalacia, left wrist
M94.239 Chondromalacia, unspecified wrist

✓6ᵗʰ **M94.24** Chondromalacia, joints of hand

M94.241 Chondromalacia, joints of right hand
M94.242 Chondromalacia, joints of left hand
M94.249 Chondromalacia, joints of unspecified hand

✓6ᵗʰ **M94.25** Chondromalacia, hip

M94.251 Chondromalacia, right hip
M94.252 Chondromalacia, left hip
M94.259 Chondromalacia, unspecified hip

✓6ᵗʰ **M94.26** Chondromalacia, knee

M94.261 Chondromalacia, right knee
M94.262 Chondromalacia, left knee
M94.269 Chondromalacia, unspecified knee

✓6ᵗʰ **M94.27** Chondromalacia, ankle and joints of foot

M94.271 Chondromalacia, right ankle and joints of right foot

M94.272 Chondromalacia, left ankle and joints of left foot

M94.279 Chondromalacia, unspecified ankle and joints of foot

M94.28 Chondromalacia, other site

M94.29 Chondromalacia, multiple sites

✓5ᵗʰ **M94.3** Chondrolysis

Code first any associated slipped upper femoral epiphysis (nontraumatic) (M93.0-)

✓6ᵗʰ **M94.35** Chondrolysis, hip

M94.351 Chondrolysis, right hip
M94.352 Chondrolysis, left hip
M94.359 Chondrolysis, unspecified hip

✓5ᵗʰ **M94.8** Other specified disorders of cartilage

✓6ᵗʰ **M94.8X** Other specified disorders of cartilage

M94.8X0 Other specified disorders of cartilage, multiple sites

M94.8X1 Other specified disorders of cartilage, shoulder

M94.8X2 Other specified disorders of cartilage, upper arm

M94.8X3 Other specified disorders of cartilage, forearm

M94.8X4 Other specified disorders of cartilage, hand

✓ Additional Character Required   ✓x7ᵗʰ Placeholder   Questionable PDx   Manifestation   Unspecified   UPD Unacceptable PDx   H1–H14 HAC   HCC CMS-HCC Dx   HIV HIV Dx

ICD-10-CM 2025

853

M94.8X5   Other specified disorders of cartilage, **thigh**

M94.8X6   Other specified disorders of cartilage, **lower leg**

M94.8X7   Other specified disorders of cartilage, **ankle and foot**

M94.8X8   Other specified disorders of cartilage, **other site**

M94.8X9   Other specified disorders of cartilage, **unspecified sites**

M94.9   Disorder of cartilage, unspecified

Other disorders of the musculoskeletal system and connective tissue (M95)

✓4th **M95**   **Other acquired deformities of musculoskeletal system and connective tissue**

> EXCLUDES 2   acquired absence of limbs and organs (Z89-Z90)
> acquired deformities of limbs (M20-M21)
> congenital malformations and deformations of the musculoskeletal system (Q65-Q79)
> deforming dorsopathies (M40-M43)
> dentofacial anomalies [including malocclusion] (M26.-)
> postprocedural musculoskeletal disorders (M96.-)

M95.0   **Acquired deformity of nose**
> EXCLUDES 2   deviated nasal septum (J34.2)

✓5th **M95.1**   **Cauliflower ear**
> EXCLUDES 2   other acquired deformities of ear (H61.1)
> **DEF:** Acquired deformity of the external ear due to injury or subsequent perichondritis.

  M95.10   **Cauliflower ear, unspecified ear**

  M95.11   **Cauliflower ear, right ear**

  M95.12   **Cauliflower ear, left ear**

M95.2   **Other acquired deformity of head**
> **AHA:** 2023,1Q,30; 2022,1Q,34

M95.3   **Acquired deformity of neck**

M95.4   **Acquired deformity of chest and rib**
> **AHA:** 2022,2Q,14; 2014,4Q,26-27

M95.5   **Acquired deformity of pelvis**
> EXCLUDES 1   maternal care for known or suspected disproportion (O33.-)

M95.8   **Other specified acquired deformities of musculoskeletal system**

M95.9   **Acquired deformity of musculoskeletal system, unspecified**

Intraoperative and postprocedural complications and disorders of musculoskeletal system, not elsewhere classified (M96)

✓4th **M96**   **Intraoperative and postprocedural complications and disorders of musculoskeletal system, not elsewhere classified**

> EXCLUDES 2   arthropathy following intestinal bypass (M02.0-)
> complications of internal orthopedic prosthetic devices, implants and grafts (T84.-)
> disorders associated with osteoporosis (M80)
> periprosthetic fracture around internal prosthetic joint (M97.-)
> presence of functional implants and other devices (Z96-Z97)

M96.0   **Pseudarthrosis after fusion or arthrodesis** `CC`

M96.1   **Postlaminectomy syndrome, not elsewhere classified**
> **AHA:** 2024,1Q,17

M96.2   **Postradiation kyphosis**

M96.3   **Postlaminectomy kyphosis**

M96.4   **Postsurgical lordosis**

M96.5   **Postradiation scoliosis**

✓5th **M96.6**   **Fracture of bone following insertion of orthopedic implant, joint prosthesis, or bone plate**
> Intraoperative fracture of bone during insertion of orthopedic implant, joint prosthesis, or bone plate
> EXCLUDES 2   complication of internal orthopedic devices, implants or grafts (T84.-)

  ✓6th **M96.62**   **Fracture of humerus following insertion of orthopedic implant, joint prosthesis, or bone plate**

    M96.621   Fracture of humerus following insertion of orthopedic implant, joint prosthesis, or bone plate, **right arm** `CC`

    M96.622   Fracture of humerus following insertion of orthopedic implant, joint prosthesis, or bone plate, **left arm**

    M96.629   Fracture of humerus following insertion of orthopedic implant, joint prosthesis, or bone plate, unspecified arm `CC` `UNS`

  ✓6th **M96.63**   **Fracture of radius or ulna following insertion of orthopedic implant, joint prosthesis, or bone plate**

    M96.631   Fracture of radius or ulna following insertion of orthopedic implant, joint prosthesis, or bone plate, **right arm** `CC`

    M96.632   Fracture of radius or ulna following insertion of orthopedic implant, joint prosthesis, or bone plate, **left arm** `CC`

    M96.639   Fracture of radius or ulna following insertion of orthopedic implant, joint prosthesis, or bone plate, unspecified arm `CC` `UNS`

  M96.65   **Fracture of pelvis following insertion of orthopedic implant, joint prosthesis, or bone plate** `CC`

  ✓6th **M96.66**   **Fracture of femur following insertion of orthopedic implant, joint prosthesis, or bone plate**

    M96.661   Fracture of femur following insertion of orthopedic implant, joint prosthesis, or bone plate, **right leg** `CC`

    M96.662   Fracture of femur following insertion of orthopedic implant, joint prosthesis, or bone plate, **left leg** `CC`

    M96.669   Fracture of femur following insertion of orthopedic implant, joint prosthesis, or bone plate, unspecified leg `CC` `UNS`

  ✓6th **M96.67**   **Fracture of tibia or fibula following insertion of orthopedic implant, joint prosthesis, or bone plate**

    M96.671   Fracture of tibia or fibula following insertion of orthopedic implant, joint prosthesis, or bone plate, **right leg** `CC`

    M96.672   Fracture of tibia or fibula following insertion of orthopedic implant, joint prosthesis, or bone plate, **left leg** `CC`

    M96.679   Fracture of tibia or fibula following insertion of orthopedic implant, joint prosthesis, or bone plate, unspecified leg `CC` `UNS`

  M96.69   **Fracture of other bone following insertion of orthopedic implant, joint prosthesis, or bone plate** `CC`

✓5th **M96.8**   **Other intraoperative and postprocedural complications and disorders of musculoskeletal system, not elsewhere classified**
> **AHA:** 2016,4Q,9-10

  ✓6th **M96.81**   **Intraoperative hemorrhage and hematoma of a musculoskeletal structure complicating a procedure**
> EXCLUDES 1   intraoperative hemorrhage and hematoma of a musculoskeletal structure due to accidental puncture and laceration during a procedure (M96.82-)

    M96.810   Intraoperative hemorrhage and hematoma of a musculoskeletal structure complicating a **musculoskeletal system procedure** `CC`

    M96.811   Intraoperative hemorrhage and hematoma of a musculoskeletal structure complicating **other procedure** `CC`

  ✓6th **M96.82**   **Accidental puncture and laceration of a musculoskeletal structure during a procedure**

    M96.820   Accidental puncture and laceration of a musculoskeletal structure during a **musculoskeletal system procedure** `CC`

    M96.821   Accidental puncture and laceration of a musculoskeletal structure during **other procedure** `CC`

  ✓6th **M96.83**   **Postprocedural hemorrhage of a musculoskeletal structure following a procedure**

    M96.830   Postprocedural hemorrhage of a musculoskeletal structure following a **musculoskeletal system procedure** `CC`

    M96.831   Postprocedural hemorrhage of a musculoskeletal structure following **other procedure** `CC`

  ✓6th **M96.84**   **Postprocedural hematoma and seroma of a musculoskeletal structure following a procedure**

    M96.840   Postprocedural **hematoma** of a musculoskeletal structure following a **musculoskeletal system procedure** `CC`

N Newborn: 0   P Pediatric: 0-17   M Maternity: 9-64   A Adult: 15-124   UNS Unspecified Site   MCC Major Complication/Comorbidity   CC Complication/Comorbidity   PE POA Exempt

854   ICD-10-CM 2025

M96.841 Postprocedural hematoma of a musculoskeletal structure following other procedure `CC`
AHA: 2016,4Q,10

M96.842 Postprocedural seroma of a musculoskeletal structure following a musculoskeletal system procedure `CC`

M96.843 Postprocedural seroma of a musculoskeletal structure following other procedure `CC`
AHA: 2023,2Q,13; 2018,3Q,6

M96.89 Other intraoperative and postprocedural complications and disorders of the musculoskeletal system `CC`
Instability of joint secondary to removal of joint prosthesis
Use additional code, if applicable, to further specify disorder
AHA: 2024,1Q,17,23; 2023,2Q,14; 2022,2Q,14; 2021,1Q,5

√5th **M96.A** Fracture of ribs, sternum and thorax associated with compression of the chest and cardiopulmonary resuscitation
AHA: 2022,4Q,31-33

M96.A1 Fracture of sternum associated with chest compression and cardiopulmonary resuscitation `CC`
Fracture of xiphoid process associated with chest compression and cardiopulmonary resuscitation

M96.A2 Fracture of one rib associated with chest compression and cardiopulmonary resuscitation `CC`

M96.A3 Multiple fractures of ribs associated with chest compression and cardiopulmonary resuscitation `CC`
AHA: 2022,4Q,32

M96.A4 Flail chest associated with chest compression and cardiopulmonary resuscitation `MCC`

M96.A9 Other fracture associated with chest compression and cardiopulmonary resuscitation `CC`

Periprosthetic fractures around internal prosthetic joint (M97)

√4th **M97** Periprosthetic fracture around internal prosthetic joint
Code first, if known, the specific type and cause of fracture, such as traumatic or pathological
EXCLUDES 2   fracture of bone following insertion of orthopedic implant, joint prosthesis or bone plate (M96.6-)
breakage (fracture) of prosthetic joint (T84.01-)
AHA: 2016,4Q,42-43

> The appropriate 7th character is to be added to each code from category M97.
> A   initial encounter
> D   subsequent encounter
> S   sequela

√5th **M97.0** Periprosthetic fracture around internal prosthetic hip joint
AHA: 2018,1Q,21; 2016,4Q,42

√x7th **M97.01** Periprosthetic fracture around internal prosthetic right hip joint `CC` `HCC` `PE`

√x7th **M97.02** Periprosthetic fracture around internal prosthetic left hip joint `CC` `HCC` `PE`

√5th **M97.1** Periprosthetic fracture around internal prosthetic knee joint

√x7th **M97.11** Periprosthetic fracture around internal prosthetic right knee joint `CC` `FE`

√x7th **M97.12** Periprosthetic fracture around internal prosthetic left knee joint `CC` `FE`

√5th **M97.2** Periprosthetic fracture around internal prosthetic ankle joint

√x7th **M97.21** Periprosthetic fracture around internal prosthetic right ankle joint `CC` `PE`

√x7th **M97.22** Periprosthetic fracture around internal prosthetic left ankle joint `CC` `PE`

√5th **M97.3** Periprosthetic fracture around internal prosthetic shoulder joint

√x7th **M97.31** Periprosthetic fracture around internal prosthetic right shoulder joint `CC` `PE`

√x7th **M97.32** Periprosthetic fracture around internal prosthetic left shoulder joint `CC` `PE`

√5th **M97.4** Periprosthetic fracture around internal prosthetic elbow joint

√x7th **M97.41** Periprosthetic fracture around internal prosthetic right elbow joint `CC` `PE`

√x7th **M97.42** Periprosthetic fracture around internal prosthetic left elbow joint `CC` `PE`

√x7th **M97.8** Periprosthetic fracture around other internal prosthetic joint `CC` `PE`
Periprosthetic fracture around internal prosthetic finger joint
Periprosthetic fracture around internal prosthetic spinal joint
Periprosthetic fracture around internal prosthetic toe joint
Periprosthetic fracture around internal prosthetic wrist joint
Use additional code to identify the joint (Z96.6-)

√x7th **M97.9** Periprosthetic fracture around unspecified internal prosthetic joint `CC` `PE`

Biomechanical lesions, not elsewhere classified (M99)

√4th **M99** Biomechanical lesions, not elsewhere classified
NOTE   This category should not be used if the condition can be classified elsewhere.
DEF: Biomechanical lesion: Term used by osteopathic and chiropractic physicians to describe musculoskeletal conditions treated that are not more appropriately classified elsewhere.

√5th **M99.0** Segmental and somatic dysfunction

M99.00 Segmental and somatic dysfunction of head region
M99.01 Segmental and somatic dysfunction of cervical region
M99.02 Segmental and somatic dysfunction of thoracic region
M99.03 Segmental and somatic dysfunction of lumbar region
M99.04 Segmental and somatic dysfunction of sacral region
M99.05 Segmental and somatic dysfunction of pelvic region
M99.06 Segmental and somatic dysfunction of lower extremity
M99.07 Segmental and somatic dysfunction of upper extremity
M99.08 Segmental and somatic dysfunction of rib cage
M99.09 Segmental and somatic dysfunction of abdomen and other regions

√5th **M99.1** Subluxation complex (vertebral)

M99.10 Subluxation complex (vertebral) of head region `CC` `H5`
M99.11 Subluxation complex (vertebral) of cervical region `CC` `H5`
M99.12 Subluxation complex (vertebral) of thoracic region
M99.13 Subluxation complex (vertebral) of lumbar region
M99.14 Subluxation complex (vertebral) of sacral region
M99.15 Subluxation complex (vertebral) of pelvic region
M99.16 Subluxation complex (vertebral) of lower extremity
M99.17 Subluxation complex (vertebral) of upper extremity
M99.18 Subluxation complex (vertebral) of rib cage `CC` `H5`
M99.19 Subluxation complex (vertebral) of abdomen and other regions

√5th **M99.2** Subluxation stenosis of neural canal

M99.20 Subluxation stenosis of neural canal of head region
M99.21 Subluxation stenosis of neural canal of cervical region
M99.22 Subluxation stenosis of neural canal of thoracic region
M99.23 Subluxation stenosis of neural canal of lumbar region
M99.24 Subluxation stenosis of neural canal of sacral region
M99.25 Subluxation stenosis of neural canal of pelvic region
M99.26 Subluxation stenosis of neural canal of lower extremity
M99.27 Subluxation stenosis of neural canal of upper extremity
M99.28 Subluxation stenosis of neural canal of rib cage
M99.29 Subluxation stenosis of neural canal of abdomen and other regions

√5th **M99.3** Osseous stenosis of neural canal

M99.30 Osseous stenosis of neural canal of head region
M99.31 Osseous stenosis of neural canal of cervical region
M99.32 Osseous stenosis of neural canal of thoracic region
M99.33 Osseous stenosis of neural canal of lumbar region
M99.34 Osseous stenosis of neural canal of sacral region
M99.35 Osseous stenosis of neural canal of pelvic region
M99.36 Osseous stenosis of neural canal of lower extremity
M99.37 Osseous stenosis of neural canal of upper extremity
M99.38 Osseous stenosis of neural canal of rib cage
M99.39 Osseous stenosis of neural canal of abdomen and other regions

✓5ᵗʰ **M99.4 Connective tissue stenosis of neural canal**

M99.40 Connective tissue stenosis of neural canal of **head** region

M99.41 Connective tissue stenosis of neural canal of **cervical** region

M99.42 Connective tissue stenosis of neural canal of **thoracic** region

M99.43 Connective tissue stenosis of neural canal of **lumbar** region

M99.44 Connective tissue stenosis of neural canal of **sacral** region

M99.45 Connective tissue stenosis of neural canal of **pelvic** region

M99.46 Connective tissue stenosis of neural canal of **lower extremity**

M99.47 Connective tissue stenosis of neural canal of **upper extremity**

M99.48 Connective tissue stenosis of neural canal of **rib cage**

M99.49 Connective tissue stenosis of neural canal of **abdomen and other** regions

✓5ᵗʰ **M99.5 Intervertebral disc stenosis of neural canal**

M99.50 Intervertebral disc stenosis of neural canal of **head** region

M99.51 Intervertebral disc stenosis of neural canal of **cervical** region

M99.52 Intervertebral disc stenosis of neural canal of **thoracic** region

M99.53 Intervertebral disc stenosis of neural canal of **lumbar** region

M99.54 Intervertebral disc stenosis of neural canal of **sacral** region

M99.55 Intervertebral disc stenosis of neural canal of **pelvic** region

M99.56 Intervertebral disc stenosis of neural canal of **lower extremity**

M99.57 Intervertebral disc stenosis of neural canal of **upper extremity**

M99.58 Intervertebral disc stenosis of neural canal of **rib cage**

M99.59 Intervertebral disc stenosis of neural canal of **abdomen and other** regions

✓5ᵗʰ **M99.6 Osseous and subluxation stenosis of intervertebral foramina**

M99.60 Osseous and subluxation stenosis of intervertebral foramina of **head** region

M99.61 Osseous and subluxation stenosis of intervertebral foramina of **cervical** region

M99.62 Osseous and subluxation stenosis of intervertebral foramina of **thoracic** region

M99.63 Osseous and subluxation stenosis of intervertebral foramina of **lumbar** region

M99.64 Osseous and subluxation stenosis of intervertebral foramina of **sacral** region

M99.65 Osseous and subluxation stenosis of intervertebral foramina of **pelvic** region

M99.66 Osseous and subluxation stenosis of intervertebral foramina of **lower extremity**

M99.67 Osseous and subluxation stenosis of intervertebral foramina of **upper extremity**

M99.68 Osseous and subluxation stenosis of intervertebral foramina of **rib cage**

M99.69 Osseous and subluxation stenosis of intervertebral foramina of **abdomen and other** regions

✓5ᵗʰ **M99.7 Connective tissue and disc stenosis of intervertebral foramina**

M99.70 Connective tissue and disc stenosis of intervertebral foramina of **head** region

M99.71 Connective tissue and disc stenosis of intervertebral foramina of **cervical** region

M99.72 Connective tissue and disc stenosis of intervertebral foramina of **thoracic** region

M99.73 Connective tissue and disc stenosis of intervertebral foramina of **lumbar** region

M99.74 Connective tissue and disc stenosis of intervertebral foramina of **sacral** region

M99.75 Connective tissue and disc stenosis of intervertebral foramina of **pelvic** region

M99.76 Connective tissue and disc stenosis of intervertebral foramina of **lower extremity**

M99.77 Connective tissue and disc stenosis of intervertebral foramina of **upper extremity**

M99.78 Connective tissue and disc stenosis of intervertebral foramina of **rib cage**

M99.79 Connective tissue and disc stenosis of intervertebral foramina of **abdomen and other** regions

✓5ᵗʰ **M99.8 Other biomechanical lesions**

M99.80 Other biomechanical lesions of **head** region

M99.81 Other biomechanical lesions of **cervical** region

M99.82 Other biomechanical lesions of **thoracic** region

M99.83 Other biomechanical lesions of **lumbar** region

M99.84 Other biomechanical lesions of **sacral** region

M99.85 Other biomechanical lesions of **pelvic** region

M99.86 Other biomechanical lesions of **lower extremity**

M99.87 Other biomechanical lesions of **upper extremity**

M99.88 Other biomechanical lesions of **rib cage**

M99.89 Other biomechanical lesions of **abdomen and other** regions

M99.9 Biomechanical lesion, unspecified

Chapter 14. Diseases of Genitourinary System (N00–N99)

Chapter-specific Guidelines with Coding Examples

The chapter-specific guidelines from the ICD-10-CM Official Guidelines for Coding and Reporting have been provided below. Along with these guidelines are coding examples, contained in the shaded boxes, that have been developed to help illustrate the coding and/or sequencing guidance found in these guidelines.

a. Chronic kidney disease

1) Stages of chronic kidney disease (CKD)

The ICD-10-CM classifies CKD based on severity. The severity of CKD is designated by stages 1-5. Stage 2, code N18.2, equates to mild CKD; stage 3, codes N18.30-N18.32, equate to moderate CKD; and stage 4, code N18.4, equates to severe CKD. Code N18.6, End stage renal disease (ESRD), is assigned when the provider has documented end-stage renal disease (ESRD).

If both a stage of CKD and ESRD are documented, assign code N18.6 only.

> Stage 5 chronic kidney disease with ESRD requiring chronic dialysis
>
> **N18.6**   **End stage renal disease**
>
> **Z99.2**   **Dependence on renal dialysis**
>
> *Explanation:* The diagnostic statement indicates the patient has chronic kidney disease, documented both as stage 5 and as ESRD requiring chronic dialysis. Code N18.6 End stage renal disease (ESRD), is assigned when the provider has documented end-stage-renal disease (ESRD). If both a stage of CKD and ESRD are documented, assign code N18.6 only.

2) Chronic kidney disease and kidney transplant status

Patients who have undergone kidney transplant may still have some form of chronic kidney disease (CKD) because the kidney transplant may not fully restore kidney function. Therefore, the presence of CKD alone does not constitute a transplant complication. Assign the appropriate N18 code for the patient's stage of CKD and code Z94.0, Kidney transplant status. If a transplant complication such as failure or rejection or other transplant complication is documented, see section I.C.19.g for information on coding complications of a kidney transplant. If the documentation is unclear as to whether the patient has a complication of the transplant, query the provider.

> Patient with residual chronic kidney disease stage 1 after kidney transplant
>
> **N18.1**   **Chronic kidney disease, stage 1**
>
> **Z94.0**   **Kidney transplant status**
>
> *Explanation:* Patients who have undergone kidney transplant may still have some form of chronic kidney disease (CKD) because the kidney transplant may not fully restore kidney function. The presence of CKD alone does not constitute a transplant complication. Assign the appropriate N18 code for the patient's stage of CKD and code Z94.0 Kidney transplant status.

3) Chronic kidney disease with other conditions

Patients with CKD may also suffer from other serious conditions, most commonly diabetes mellitus and hypertension. The sequencing of the CKD code in relationship to codes for other contributing conditions is based on the conventions in the Tabular List.

See I.C.9. Hypertensive chronic kidney disease.

See I.C.19. Chronic kidney disease and kidney transplant complications.

> Type 1 diabetic chronic kidney disease, stage 2
>
> **E10.22**   **Type 1 diabetes mellitus with diabetic chronic kidney disease**
>
> **N18.2**   **Chronic kidney disease, stage 2 (mild)**
>
> *Explanation:* Patients with CKD may also suffer from other serious conditions such as diabetes mellitus. The sequencing of the CKD code in relationship to codes for other contributing conditions is based on the conventions in the Tabular List. Diabetic CKD code E10.22 includes an instructional note to "Use additional code to identify stage of chronic kidney disease (N18.1–N18.6)," thus providing sequencing direction.

Chapter 14. Diseases of the Genitourinary System (N00-N99)

EXCLUDES 2
certain conditions originating in the perinatal period (P04-P96)
certain infectious and parasitic diseases (A00-B99)
complications of pregnancy, childbirth and the puerperium (O00-O9A)
congenital malformations, deformations and chromosomal abnormalities (Q00-Q99)
endocrine, nutritional and metabolic diseases (E00-E88)
injury, poisoning and certain other consequences of external causes (S00-T88)
neoplasms (C00-D49)
symptoms, signs and abnormal clinical and laboratory findings, not elsewhere classified (R00-R94)

This chapter contains the following blocks:

N00-N08   Glomerular diseases
N10-N16   Renal tubulo-interstitial diseases
N17-N19   Acute kidney failure and chronic kidney disease
N20-N23   Urolithiasis
N25-N29   Other disorders of kidney and ureter
N30-N39   Other diseases of the urinary system
N40-N53   Diseases of male genital organs
N60-N65   Disorders of breast
N70-N77   Inflammatory diseases of female pelvic organs
N80-N98   Noninflammatory disorders of female genital tract
N99   Intraoperative and postprocedural complications and disorders of genitourinary system, not elsewhere classified

Glomerular diseases (N00-N08)

Code also any associated kidney failure (N17-N19).

EXCLUDES 1   *hypertensive chronic kidney disease (I12.-)*

AHA: 2020,4Q,34-35

DEF: Glomeruli: Clusters of microscopic blood vessels located within the kidneys containing small pores through which waste products are filtered from the blood and urine is formed.

DEF: Glomerulonephritis: Disease of the kidney with diffuse inflammation of the capillary loops of the glomeruli.

✓4ᵗʰ N00   Acute nephritic syndrome

INCLUDES   acute glomerular disease
       acute glomerulonephritis
       acute nephritis

EXCLUDES 1   *acute tubulo-interstitial nephritis (N10)*
       nephritic syndrome NOS (N05.-)

AHA: 2021,1Q,23

N00.0   **Acute nephritic syndrome with minor glomerular abnormality**   MCC
Acute nephritic syndrome with minimal change lesion

N00.1   **Acute nephritic syndrome with focal and segmental glomerular lesions**   MCC
Acute nephritic syndrome with focal and segmental hyalinosis
Acute nephritic syndrome with focal and segmental sclerosis
Acute nephritic syndrome with focal glomerulonephritis

N00.2   **Acute nephritic syndrome with diffuse membranous glomerulonephritis**   MCC

N00.3   **Acute nephritic syndrome with diffuse mesangial proliferative glomerulonephritis**   MCC

N00.4   **Acute nephritic syndrome with diffuse endocapillary proliferative glomerulonephritis**   MCC

N00.5   **Acute nephritic syndrome with diffuse mesangiocapillary glomerulonephritis**   MCC
Acute nephritic syndrome with membranoproliferative glomerulonephritis, types 1 and 3, or NOS
EXCLUDES 1   *acute nephritic syndrome with C3 glomerulonephritis (N00.A)*
       acute nephritic syndrome with C3 glomerulopathy (N00.A)

N00.6   **Acute nephritic syndrome with dense deposit disease**   MCC
Acute nephritic syndrome with C3 glomerulopathy with dense deposit disease
Acute nephritic syndrome with membranoproliferative glomerulonephritis, type 2

N00.7   **Acute nephritic syndrome with diffuse crescentic glomerulonephritis**   MCC
Acute nephritic syndrome with extracapillary glomerulonephritis

N00.8   **Acute nephritic syndrome with other morphologic changes**   MCC
Acute nephritic syndrome with proliferative glomerulonephritis NOS

N00.9   **Acute nephritic syndrome with unspecified morphologic changes**   MCC

N00.A   **Acute nephritic syndrome with C3 glomerulonephritis**   MCC
Acute nephritic syndrome with C3 glomerulopathy, NOS
EXCLUDES 1   *acute nephritic syndrome (with C3 glomerulopathy) with dense deposit disease (N00.6)*

✓4ᵗʰ N01   Rapidly progressive nephritic syndrome

INCLUDES   rapidly progressive glomerular disease
       rapidly progressive glomerulonephritis
       rapidly progressive nephritis

EXCLUDES 1   *nephritic syndrome NOS (N05.-)*

AHA: 2021,1Q,23

N01.0   **Rapidly progressive nephritic syndrome with minor glomerular abnormality**   MCC
Rapidly progressive nephritic syndrome with minimal change lesion

N01.1   **Rapidly progressive nephritic syndrome with focal and segmental glomerular lesions**   MCC
Rapidly progressive nephritic syndrome with focal and segmental hyalinosis
Rapidly progressive nephritic syndrome with focal and segmental sclerosis
Rapidly progressive nephritic syndrome with focal glomerulonephritis

N01.2   **Rapidly progressive nephritic syndrome with diffuse membranous glomerulonephritis**   MCC

N01.3   **Rapidly progressive nephritic syndrome with diffuse mesangial proliferative glomerulonephritis**   MCC

N01.4   **Rapidly progressive nephritic syndrome with diffuse endocapillary proliferative glomerulonephritis**   MCC

N01.5   **Rapidly progressive nephritic syndrome with diffuse mesangiocapillary glomerulonephritis**   MCC
Rapidly progressive nephritic syndrome with membranoproliferative glomerulonephritis, types 1 and 3, or NOS
EXCLUDES 1   *rapidly progressive nephritic syndrome with C3 glomerulonephritis (N01.A)*
       rapidly progressive nephritic syndrome with C3 glomerulopathy (N01.A)

N01.6   **Rapidly progressive nephritic syndrome with dense deposit disease**   MCC
Rapidly progressive nephritic syndrome with C3 glomerulopathy with dense deposit disease
Rapidly progressive nephritic syndrome with membranoproliferative glomerulonephritis, type 2

N01.7   **Rapidly progressive nephritic syndrome with diffuse crescentic glomerulonephritis**   MCC
Rapidly progressive nephritic syndrome with extracapillary glomerulonephritis

N01.8   **Rapidly progressive nephritic syndrome with other morphologic changes**   MCC
Rapidly progressive nephritic syndrome with proliferative glomerulonephritis NOS

N01.9   **Rapidly progressive nephritic syndrome with unspecified morphologic changes**   MCC

N01.A   **Rapidly progressive nephritic syndrome with C3 glomerulonephritis**   MCC
Rapidly progressive nephritic syndrome with C3 glomerulopathy, NOS
EXCLUDES 1   *rapidly progressive nephritic syndrome (with C3 glomerulopathy) with dense deposit disease (N01.6)*

✓4ᵗʰ N02   Recurrent and persistent hematuria

EXCLUDES 1   *acute cystitis with hematuria (N30.01)*
       hematuria NOS (R31.9)
       hematuria not associated with specified morphologic lesions (R31.-)

N02.0   **Recurrent and persistent hematuria with minor glomerular abnormality**   CC
Recurrent and persistent hematuria with minimal change lesion

N02.1   **Recurrent and persistent hematuria with focal and segmental glomerular lesions**   CC
Recurrent and persistent hematuria with focal and segmental hyalinosis
Recurrent and persistent hematuria with focal and segmental sclerosis
Recurrent and persistent hematuria with focal glomerulonephritis

N02.2   **Recurrent and persistent hematuria with diffuse membranous glomerulonephritis**   CC

N02.3   **Recurrent and persistent hematuria with diffuse mesangial proliferative glomerulonephritis**   CC

N02.4   **Recurrent and persistent hematuria with diffuse endocapillary proliferative glomerulonephritis**   `CC`

N02.5   **Recurrent and persistent hematuria with diffuse mesangiocapillary glomerulonephritis**   `CC`

Recurrent and persistent hematuria with membranoproliferative glomerulonephritis, types 1 and 3, or NOS

> *EXCLUDES 1*   *recurrent and persistent hematuria with C3 glomerulonephritis (N02.A)*
>
> *recurrent and persistent hematuria with C3 glomerulopathy (N02.A)*

N02.6   **Recurrent and persistent hematuria with dense deposit disease**   `CC`

Recurrent and persistent hematuria with C3 glomerulopathy with dense deposit disease

Recurrent and persistent hematuria with membranoproliferative glomerulonephritis, type 2

N02.7   **Recurrent and persistent hematuria with diffuse crescentic glomerulonephritis**   `CC`

Recurrent and persistent hematuria with extracapillary glomerulonephritis

N02.8   **Recurrent and persistent hematuria with other morphologic changes**   `CC`

Recurrent and persistent hematuria with proliferative glomerulonephritis NOS

N02.9   **Recurrent and persistent hematuria with unspecified morphologic changes**   `CC`

AHA: 2017,2Q,5

N02.A   **Recurrent and persistent hematuria with C3 glomerulonephritis**   `CC`

Recurrent and persistent hematuria with C3 glomerulopathy

> *EXCLUDES 1*   *recurrent and persistent hematuria (with C3 glomerulopathy) with dense deposit disease (N02.6)*

√5th **N02.B**   **Recurrent and persistent immunoglobulin A nephropathy**

AHA: 2023,4Q,34-35

N02.B1   **Recurrent and persistent immunoglobulin A nephropathy with glomerular lesion**   `CC`

N02.B2   **Recurrent and persistent immunoglobulin A nephropathy with focal and segmental glomerular lesion**   `CC`

Recurrent and persistent immunoglobulin A nephropathy with focal and segmental hyalinosis or sclerosis

N02.B3   **Recurrent and persistent immunoglobulin A nephropathy with diffuse membranoproliferative glomerulonephritis**   `CC`

N02.B4   **Recurrent and persistent immunoglobulin A nephropathy with diffuse membranous glomerulonephritis**   `CC`

N02.B5   **Recurrent and persistent immunoglobulin A nephropathy with diffuse mesangial proliferative glomerulonephritis**   `CC`

N02.B6   **Recurrent and persistent immunoglobulin A nephropathy with diffuse mesangiocapillary glomerulonephritis**   `CC`

N02.B9   **Other recurrent and persistent immunoglobulin A nephropathy**   `CC`

√4th **N03**   **Chronic nephritic syndrome**

> *INCLUDES*   chronic glomerular disease
> chronic glomerulonephritis
> chronic nephritis
>
> *EXCLUDES 1*   *chronic tubulo-interstitial nephritis (N11.-)*
> *diffuse sclerosing glomerulonephritis (N05.8-)*
> *nephritic syndrome NOS (N05.-)*

AHA: 2021,1Q,23

DEF: Slow, progressive type of nephritis characterized by inflammation of the capillary loops in the glomeruli of the kidney, which leads to renal failure.

N03.0   **Chronic nephritic syndrome with minor glomerular abnormality**   `CC`

Chronic nephritic syndrome with minimal change lesion

N03.1   **Chronic nephritic syndrome with focal and segmental glomerular lesions**   `CC`

Chronic nephritic syndrome with focal and segmental hyalinosis
Chronic nephritic syndrome with focal and segmental sclerosis
Chronic nephritic syndrome with focal glomerulonephritis

N03.2   **Chronic nephritic syndrome with diffuse membranous glomerulonephritis**   `CC`

N03.3   **Chronic nephritic syndrome with diffuse mesangial proliferative glomerulonephritis**   `CC`

N03.4   **Chronic nephritic syndrome with diffuse endocapillary proliferative glomerulonephritis**   `CC`

N03.5   **Chronic nephritic syndrome with diffuse mesangiocapillary glomerulonephritis**   `CC`

Chronic nephritic syndrome with membranoproliferative glomerulonephritis, types 1 and 3, or NOS

> *EXCLUDES 1*   *chronic nephritic syndrome with C3 glomerulonephritis (N03.A)*
>
> *chronic nephritic syndrome with C3 glomerulopathy (N03.A)*

N03.6   **Chronic nephritic syndrome with dense deposit disease**   `CC`

Chronic nephritic syndrome with C3 glomerulopathy with dense deposit disease

Chronic nephritic syndrome with membranoproliferative glomerulonephritis, type 2

N03.7   **Chronic nephritic syndrome with diffuse crescentic glomerulonephritis**   `CC`

Chronic nephritic syndrome with extracapillary glomerulonephritis

N03.8   **Chronic nephritic syndrome with other morphologic changes**   `CC`

Chronic nephritic syndrome with proliferative glomerulonephritis NOS

N03.9   **Chronic nephritic syndrome with unspecified morphologic changes**   `CC`

N03.A   **Chronic nephritic syndrome with C3 glomerulonephritis**   `CC`

Chronic nephritic syndrome with C3 glomerulopathy

> *EXCLUDES 1*   *chronic nephritic syndrome (with C3 glomerulopathy) with dense deposit disease (N03.6)*

√4th **N04**   **Nephrotic syndrome**

> *INCLUDES*   congenital nephrotic syndrome
> lipoid nephrosis

N04.0   **Nephrotic syndrome with minor glomerular abnormality**   `CC`

Nephrotic syndrome with minimal change lesion

N04.1   **Nephrotic syndrome with focal and segmental glomerular lesions**   `CC`

Nephrotic syndrome with focal and segmental hyalinosis
Nephrotic syndrome with focal and segmental sclerosis
Nephrotic syndrome with focal glomerulonephritis

√5th **N04.2**   **Nephrotic syndrome with diffuse membranous glomerulonephritis**

AHA: 2023,4Q,35-36

N04.20   **Nephrotic syndrome with diffuse membranous glomerulonephritis, unspecified**

Membranous nephropathy NOS with nephrotic syndrome

N04.21   **Primary membranous nephropathy with nephrotic syndrome**   `CC`

Idiopathic membranous nephropathy with nephrotic syndrome

N04.22   **Secondary membranous nephropathy with nephrotic syndrome**   `CC`

Code first, if applicable, other disease or disorder or poisoning causing membranous nephropathy

Use additional code, if applicable, for adverse effect of drug causing membranous nephropathy

N04.29   **Other nephrotic syndrome with diffuse membranous glomerulonephritis**   `CC`

N04.3   **Nephrotic syndrome with diffuse mesangial proliferative glomerulonephritis**

N04.4   **Nephrotic syndrome with diffuse endocapillary proliferative glomerulonephritis**

N04.5   **Nephrotic syndrome with diffuse mesangiocapillary glomerulonephritis**   `CC`

Nephrotic syndrome with membranoproliferative glomerulonephritis, types 1 and 3, or NOS

> *EXCLUDES 1*   *nephrotic syndrome with C3 glomerulonephritis (N04.A)*
>
> *nephrotic syndrome with C3 glomerulopathy (N04.A)*

N04.6   **Nephrotic syndrome with dense deposit disease**   `CC`

Nephrotic syndrome with C3 glomerulopathy with dense deposit disease

Nephrotic syndrome with membranoproliferative glomerulonephritis, type 2

N04.7   **Nephrotic syndrome with diffuse crescentic glomerulonephritis**   `CC`

Nephrotic syndrome with extracapillary glomerulonephritis

✔ Additional Character Required   √7th Placeholder   Questionable PDx   Manifestation   Unspecified   UPD Unacceptable PDx   H1-H14 HAC   HCC CMS-HCC Dx   HIV HIV Dx

N04.8 **Nephrotic syndrome with other morphologic changes** `CC`
Nephrotic syndrome with proliferative glomerulonephritis NOS

N04.9 **Nephrotic syndrome with unspecified morphologic changes** `CC`

N04.A **Nephrotic syndrome with C3 glomerulonephritis** `CC`
Nephrotic syndrome with C3 glomerulopathy
EXCLUDES 1 *nephrotic syndrome (with C3 glomerulopathy) with dense deposit disease (N04.6)*

✓4th **N05** **Unspecified nephritic syndrome**
INCLUDES glomerular disease NOS
glomerulonephritis NOS
nephritis NOS
nephropathy NOS and renal disease NOS with morphological lesion specified in .0-.8
EXCLUDES 1 *nephropathy NOS with no stated morphological lesion (N28.9)*
renal disease NOS with no stated morphological lesion (N28.9)
tubulo-interstitial nephritis NOS (N12)

N05.0 **Unspecified nephritic syndrome with minor glomerular abnormality**
Unspecified nephritic syndrome with minimal change lesion

N05.1 **Unspecified nephritic syndrome with focal and segmental glomerular lesions**
Unspecified nephritic syndrome with focal and segmental hyalinosis
Unspecified nephritic syndrome with focal and segmental sclerosis
Unspecified nephritic syndrome with focal glomerulonephritis

N05.2 **Unspecified nephritic syndrome with diffuse membranous glomerulonephritis** `CC`

N05.3 **Unspecified nephritic syndrome with diffuse mesangial proliferative glomerulonephritis** `CC`

N05.4 **Unspecified nephritic syndrome with diffuse endocapillary proliferative glomerulonephritis** `CC`

N05.5 **Unspecified nephritic syndrome with diffuse mesangiocapillary glomerulonephritis** `CC`
Unspecified nephritic syndrome with membranoproliferative glomerulonephritis, types 1 and 3, or NOS
EXCLUDES 1 *unspecified nephritic syndrome with C3 glomerulonephritis (N05.A)*
unspecified nephritic syndrome with C3 glomerulopathy (N05.A)

N05.6 **Unspecified nephritic syndrome with dense deposit disease**
Unspecified nephritic syndrome with C3 glomerulopathy with dense deposit disease
Unspecified nephritic syndrome with membranoproliferative glomerulonephritis, type 2

N05.7 **Unspecified nephritic syndrome with diffuse crescentic glomerulonephritis**
Unspecified nephritic syndrome with extracapillary glomerulonephritis

N05.8 **Unspecified nephritic syndrome with other morphologic changes**
Unspecified nephritic syndrome with proliferative glomerulonephritis NOS

N05.9 **Unspecified nephritic syndrome with unspecified morphologic changes**

N05.A **Unspecified nephritic syndrome with C3 glomerulonephritis** `CC`
Unspecified nephritic syndrome with C3 glomerulopathy
EXCLUDES 1 *unspecified nephritic syndrome (with C3 glomerulopathy) with dense deposit disease (N05.6)*

✓4th **N06** **Isolated proteinuria with specified morphological lesion**
EXCLUDES 1 *proteinuria not associated with specific morphologic lesions (R80.0)*

N06.0 **Isolated proteinuria with minor glomerular abnormality**
Isolated proteinuria with minimal change lesion

N06.1 **Isolated proteinuria with focal and segmental glomerular lesions**
Isolated proteinuria with focal and segmental hyalinosis
Isolated proteinuria with focal and segmental sclerosis
Isolated proteinuria with focal glomerulonephritis

✓5th **N06.2** **Isolated proteinuria with diffuse membranous glomerulonephritis**
AHA: 2023,4Q,35-36

N06.20 **Isolated proteinuria with diffuse membranous glomerulonephritis, unspecified** `CC`
Membranous nephropathy, NOS
EXCLUDES 1 *membranous nephropathy NOS with nephrotic syndrome (N04.20)*

N06.21 **Primary membranous nephropathy with isolated proteinuria** `CC`
Idiopathic membranous nephropathy (with isolated proteinuria)
Primary membranous nephropathy, NOS
EXCLUDES 1 *primary membranous nephropathy with nephrotic syndrome (N04.21)*

N06.22 **Secondary membranous nephropathy with isolated proteinuria** `CC`
Secondary membranous nephropathy, NOS
Code first, if applicable, other disease or disorder or poisoning causing membranous nephropathy
Use additional code, if applicable, for adverse effect of drug causing membranous nephropathy
EXCLUDES 1 *secondary membranous nephropathy with nephrotic syndrome (N04.22)*

N06.29 **Other isolated proteinuria with diffuse membranous glomerulonephritis** `CC`

N06.3 **Isolated proteinuria with diffuse mesangial proliferative glomerulonephritis** `CC`

N06.4 **Isolated proteinuria with diffuse endocapillary proliferative glomerulonephritis** `CC`

N06.5 **Isolated proteinuria with diffuse mesangiocapillary glomerulonephritis** `CC`
Isolated proteinuria with membranoproliferative glomerulonephritis, types 1 and 3, or NOS
EXCLUDES 1 *isolated proteinuria with C3 glomerulonephritis (N06.A)*
isolated proteinuria with C3 glomerulopathy (N06.A)

N06.6 **Isolated proteinuria with dense deposit disease**
Isolated proteinuria with C3 glomerulopathy with dense deposit disease
Isolated proteinuria with membranoproliferative glomerulonephritis, type 2

N06.7 **Isolated proteinuria with diffuse crescentic glomerulonephritis**
Isolated proteinuria with extracapillary glomerulonephritis

N06.8 **Isolated proteinuria with other morphologic lesion**
Isolated proteinuria with proliferative glomerulonephritis NOS

N06.9 **Isolated proteinuria with unspecified morphologic lesion**

N06.A **Isolated proteinuria with C3 glomerulonephritis** `CC`
Isolated proteinuria with C3 glomerulopathy
EXCLUDES 1 *isolated proteinuria (with C3 glomerulopathy) with dense deposit disease (N06.6)*

✓4th **N07** **Hereditary nephropathy, not elsewhere classified**
EXCLUDES 2 *Alport's syndrome (Q87.81-)*
hereditary amyloid nephropathy (E85.-)
nail patella syndrome (Q87.2)
non-neuropathic heredofamilial amyloidosis (E85.-)

N07.0 **Hereditary nephropathy, not elsewhere classified with minor glomerular abnormality**
Hereditary nephropathy, not elsewhere classified with minimal change lesion

N07.1 **Hereditary nephropathy, not elsewhere classified with focal and segmental glomerular lesions**
Hereditary nephropathy, not elsewhere classified with focal and segmental hyalinosis
Hereditary nephropathy, not elsewhere classified with focal and segmental sclerosis
Hereditary nephropathy, not elsewhere classified with focal glomerulonephritis

N07.2 **Hereditary nephropathy, not elsewhere classified with diffuse membranous glomerulonephritis** `CC`

N07.3 **Hereditary nephropathy, not elsewhere classified with diffuse mesangial proliferative glomerulonephritis** `CC`

N07.4 **Hereditary nephropathy, not elsewhere classified with diffuse endocapillary proliferative glomerulonephritis** `CC`

N07.5   **Hereditary nephropathy, not elsewhere classified with diffuse mesangiocapillary glomerulonephritis**   `CC`
Hereditary nephropathy, not elsewhere classified with membranoproliferative glomerulonephritis, types 1 and 3, or NOS
> EXCLUDES 1   *hereditary nephropathy, not elsewhere classified with C3 glomerulonephritis (N07.A)*
> *hereditary nephropathy, not elsewhere classified with C3 glomerulopathy (N07.A)*

N07.6   **Hereditary nephropathy, not elsewhere classified with dense deposit disease**
Hereditary nephropathy, not elsewhere classified with C3 glomerulopathy with dense deposit disease
Hereditary nephropathy, not elsewhere classified with membranoproliferative glomerulonephritis, type 2

N07.7   **Hereditary nephropathy, not elsewhere classified with diffuse crescentic glomerulonephritis**
Hereditary nephropathy, not elsewhere classified with extracapillary glomerulonephritis

N07.8   **Hereditary nephropathy, not elsewhere classified with other morphologic lesions**
Hereditary nephropathy, not elsewhere classified with proliferative glomerulonephritis NOS

N07.9   **Hereditary nephropathy, not elsewhere classified with unspecified morphologic lesions**

N07.A   **Hereditary nephropathy, not elsewhere classified with C3 glomerulonephritis**   `CC`
Hereditary nephropathy, not elsewhere classified with C3 glomerulopathy
> EXCLUDES 1   *hereditary nephropathy, not elsewhere classified (with C3 glomerulopathy) with dense deposit disease (N07.6)*

N08   ***Glomerular disorders in diseases classified elsewhere***
Glomerulonephritis
Nephritis
Nephropathy
Code first underlying disease, such as:
   amyloidosis (E85.-)
   congenital syphilis (A50.5)
   cryoglobulinemia (D89.1)
   disseminated intravascular coagulation (D65)
   gout (M1A.-, M10.-)
   microscopic polyangiitis (M31.7)
   multiple myeloma (C90.0-)
   sepsis (A40.0-A41.9)
   sickle-cell disease (D57.0-D57.8)
> EXCLUDES 1   *glomerulonephritis, nephritis and nephropathy (in):*
> *antiglomerular basement membrane disease (M31.0)*
> *diabetes (E08-E13 with .21)*
> *gonococcal (A54.21)*
> *Goodpasture's syndrome (M31.0)*
> *hemolytic-uremic syndrome (D59.3-)*
> *lupus (M32.14)*
> *mumps (B26.83)*
> *syphilis (A52.75)*
> *systemic lupus erythematosus (M32.14)*
> *Wegener's granulomatosis (M31.31)*
> *pyelonephritis in diseases classified elsewhere (N16)*
> *renal tubulo-interstitial disorders classified elsewhere (N16)*

Renal tubulo-interstitial diseases (N10-N16)

INCLUDES   pyelonephritis
EXCLUDES 1   *pyeloureteritis cystica (N28.85)*

N10   **Acute pyelonephritis**   `CC` `H6`
Acute infectious interstitial nephritis
Acute pyelitis
Acute tubulo-interstitial nephritis
Hemoglobin nephrosis
Myoglobin nephrosis
Use additional code (B95-B97), to identify infectious agent
AHA: 2020,3Q,25; 2019,3Q,13

N11   **Chronic tubulo-interstitial nephritis**   ✓4ᵗʰ
INCLUDES   chronic infectious interstitial nephritis
          chronic pyelitis
          chronic pyelonephritis
Use additional code (B95-B97), to identify infectious agent

N11.0   **Nonobstructive reflux-associated chronic pyelonephritis**
Pyelonephritis (chronic) associated with (vesicoureteral) reflux
> EXCLUDES 1   *vesicoureteral reflux NOS (N13.70)*

N11.1   **Chronic obstructive pyelonephritis**   `CC`
Pyelonephritis (chronic) associated with anomaly of pelviureteric junction
Pyelonephritis (chronic) associated with anomaly of pyeloureteric junction
Pyelonephritis (chronic) associated with crossing of vessel
Pyelonephritis (chronic) associated with kinking of ureter
Pyelonephritis (chronic) associated with obstruction of ureter
Pyelonephritis (chronic) associated with stricture of pelviureteric junction
Pyelonephritis (chronic) associated with stricture of ureter
> EXCLUDES 1   *calculous pyelonephritis (N20.9)*
> *obstructive uropathy (N13.-)*

N11.8   **Other chronic tubulo-interstitial nephritis**   `CC`
Nonobstructive chronic pyelonephritis NOS

N11.9   **Chronic tubulo-interstitial nephritis, unspecified**   `CC` `H6`
Chronic interstitial nephritis NOS
Chronic pyelitis NOS
Chronic pyelonephritis NOS

N12   **Tubulo-interstitial nephritis, not specified as acute or chronic**   `CC` `H6`
Interstitial nephritis NOS
Pyelitis NOS
Pyelonephritis NOS
> EXCLUDES 1   *calculous pyelonephritis (N20.9)*

N13   **Obstructive and reflux uropathy**   ✓4ᵗʰ
> EXCLUDES 2   *calculus of kidney and ureter without hydronephrosis (N20.-)*
> *congenital obstructive defects of renal pelvis and ureter (Q62.0-Q62.3)*
> *hydronephrosis with ureteropelvic junction obstruction (Q62.11)*
> *obstructive pyelonephritis (N11.1)*

DEF: Hydronephrosis: Distension of the kidney caused by an accumulation of urine that cannot flow out due to an obstruction that may be caused by conditions such as kidney stones or vesicoureteral reflux.

N13.0   **Hydronephrosis with ureteropelvic junction obstruction**   `CC`
Hydronephrosis due to acquired occlusion of ureteropelvic junction
> EXCLUDES 2   *hydronephrosis with ureteropelvic junction obstruction due to calculus (N13.2)*

AHA: 2016,4Q,43

Hydronephrosis/UPJ Obstruction

Hydronephrosis

Ureteropelvic junction obstruction

Kidney

Ureters

Bladder

Chapter 14. Diseases of the Genitourinary System

N13.1 **Hydronephrosis with ureteral stricture, not elsewhere classified** `CC`
  EXCLUDES 1   hydronephrosis with ureteral stricture with infection (N13.6)

N13.2 **Hydronephrosis with renal and ureteral calculous obstruction** `CC`
  EXCLUDES 1   hydronephrosis with renal and ureteral calculous obstruction with infection (N13.6)

✓5ᵗʰ **N13.3** **Other and unspecified hydronephrosis**
  EXCLUDES 1   hydronephrosis with infection (N13.6)

     N13.30 **Unspecified hydronephrosis** `CC`

     N13.39 **Other hydronephrosis** `CC`

N13.4 **Hydroureter** `CC`
  EXCLUDES 1   congenital hydroureter (Q62.3-)
       hydroureter with infection (N13.6)
       vesicoureteral-reflux with hydroureter (N13.73-)
  DEF: Abnormal enlargement or distension of the ureter with water or urine caused by an obstruction.

N13.5 **Crossing vessel and stricture of ureter without hydronephrosis**
  Kinking and stricture of ureter without hydronephrosis
  EXCLUDES 1   crossing vessel and stricture of ureter without hydronephrosis with infection (N13.6)

N13.6 **Pyonephrosis** `CC` `H6`
  Conditions in N13.0-N13.5 with infection
  Obstructive uropathy with infection
  Use additional code (B95-B97), to identify infectious agent
  AHA: 2018,2Q,21

✓5ᵗʰ **N13.7** **Vesicoureteral-reflux**
  EXCLUDES 1   reflux-associated pyelonephritis (N11.0)
  DEF: Urine passage from the bladder flows backward up into the ureter and kidneys that can lead to bacterial infection and an increase in hydrostatic pressure, causing kidney damage.

Vesicoureteral Reflux

Kidneys

Ureters

Bladder

Normal flow of urine   Urine flowing the wrong way (VUR)

     N13.70 **Vesicoureteral-reflux, unspecified**
       Vesicoureteral-reflux NOS

     N13.71 **Vesicoureteral-reflux without reflux nephropathy**

✓6ᵗʰ **N13.72** **Vesicoureteral-reflux with reflux nephropathy without hydroureter**
       N13.721 **Vesicoureteral-reflux with reflux nephropathy without hydroureter, unilateral**
       N13.722 **Vesicoureteral-reflux with reflux nephropathy without hydroureter, bilateral**
       N13.729 **Vesicoureteral-reflux with reflux nephropathy without hydroureter, unspecified**

✓6ᵗʰ **N13.73** **Vesicoureteral-reflux with reflux nephropathy with hydroureter**
       N13.731 **Vesicoureteral-reflux with reflux nephropathy with hydroureter, unilateral**
       N13.732 **Vesicoureteral-reflux with reflux nephropathy with hydroureter, bilateral**
       N13.739 **Vesicoureteral-reflux with reflux nephropathy with hydroureter, unspecified**

N13.8 **Other obstructive and reflux uropathy** `CC`
  Urinary tract obstruction due to specified cause
  Code first, if applicable, any causal condition, such as:
       enlarged prostate (N40.1)

N13.9 **Obstructive and reflux uropathy, unspecified**
  Urinary tract obstruction NOS

✓4ᵗʰ **N14** **Drug- and heavy-metal-induced tubulo-interstitial and tubular conditions**
  Code first poisoning due to drug or toxin, if applicable (T36-T65 with fifth or sixth character 1-4)
  Use additional code for adverse effect, if applicable, to identify drug (T36-T50 with fifth or sixth character 5)

N14.0 **Analgesic nephropathy**

✓5ᵗʰ **N14.1** **Nephropathy induced by other drugs, medicaments and biological substances**
  AHA: 2022,4Q,33; 2021,3Q,9-10

     N14.11 **Contrast-induced nephropathy**
       Contrast medium, radiography nephropathy
       EXCLUDES 2   acute kidney failure (N17.-)

     N14.19 **Nephropathy induced by other drugs, medicaments and biological substances**

N14.2 **Nephropathy induced by unspecified drug, medicament or biological substance**

N14.3 **Nephropathy induced by heavy metals**

N14.4 **Toxic nephropathy, not elsewhere classified**

✓4ᵗʰ **N15** **Other renal tubulo-interstitial diseases**

N15.0 **Balkan nephropathy**
  Balkan endemic nephropathy

N15.1 **Renal and perinephric abscess** `MCC` `H6`

N15.8 **Other specified renal tubulo-interstitial diseases**

N15.9 **Renal tubulo-interstitial disease, unspecified**
  Infection of kidney NOS
  EXCLUDES 1   urinary tract infection NOS (N39.0)

N16 ***Renal tubulo-interstitial disorders in diseases classified elsewhere***
  Pyelonephritis
  Tubulo-interstitial nephritis
  Code first underlying disease, such as:
       brucellosis (A23.0-A23.9)
       cryoglobulinemia (D89.1)
       glycogen storage disease (E74.0-)
       leukemia (C91-C95)
       lymphoma (C81.0-C85.9, C96.0-C96.9)
       multiple myeloma (C90.0-)
       sepsis (A40.0-A41.9)
       Wilson's disease (E83.01)
  EXCLUDES 1   diphtheritic pyelonephritis and tubulo-interstitial nephritis (A36.84)
       pyelonephritis and tubulo-interstitial nephritis in candidiasis (B37.49)
       pyelonephritis and tubulo-interstitial nephritis in cystinosis (E72.04)
       pyelonephritis and tubulo-interstitial nephritis in salmonella infection (A02.25)
       pyelonephritis and tubulo-interstitial nephritis in sarcoidosis (D86.84)
       pyelonephritis and tubulo-interstitial nephritis in Sjogren syndrome (M35.04)
       pyelonephritis and tubulo-interstitial nephritis in systemic lupus erythematosus (M32.15)
       pyelonephritis and tubulo-interstitial nephritis in toxoplasmosis (B58.83)
       renal tubular degeneration in diabetes (E08-E13 with .29)
       syphilitic pyelonephritis and tubulo-interstitial nephritis (A52.75)

N Newborn: 0   **P** Pediatric: 0-17   **M** Maternity: 9-64   **A** Adult: 15-124   **UMS** Unspecified Site   **MCC** Major Complication/Comorbidity   **CC** Complication/Comorbidity   **PE** POA Exempt

862   ICD-10-CM 2025

Acute kidney failure and chronic kidney disease (N17-N19)

EXCLUDES 2   congenital renal failure (P96.0)
drug- and heavy-metal-induced tubulo-interstitial and tubular conditions (N14.-)
extrarenal uremia (R39.2)
hemolytic-uremic syndrome (D59.3-)
hepatorenal syndrome (K76.7)
postpartum hepatorenal syndrome (O90.41)
posttraumatic renal failure (T79.5)
prerenal uremia (R39.2)
renal failure complicating abortion or ectopic or molar pregnancy (O00-O07, O08.4)
renal failure following labor and delivery (O90.41)
renal failure postprocedural (N99.0)

✓4ᵗʰ **N17**   **Acute** kidney failure
Code also associated underlying condition
EXCLUDES 1   posttraumatic renal failure (T79.5)
AHA: 2020,3Q,22; 2019,2Q,7; 2019,1Q,12; 2013,4Q,124

    N17.0   **Acute kidney failure with tubular necrosis**   `MCC`
        Acute tubular necrosis
        Renal tubular necrosis
        Tubular necrosis NOS
        AHA: 2022,4Q,33; 2021,3Q,10

    N17.1   **Acute kidney failure with acute cortical necrosis**   `MCC`
        Acute cortical necrosis
        Cortical necrosis NOS
        Renal cortical necrosis

    N17.2   **Acute kidney failure with medullary necrosis**   `MCC`
        Medullary [papillary] necrosis NOS
        Acute medullary [papillary] necrosis
        Renal medullary [papillary] necrosis

    N17.8   **Other acute kidney failure**   `CC`

    N17.9   **Acute kidney failure, unspecified**   `CC`
        Acute kidney injury (nontraumatic)
        EXCLUDES 2   traumatic kidney injury (S37.0-)

✓4ᵗʰ **N18**   **Chronic** kidney disease (CKD)
Code first any associated:
   diabetic chronic kidney disease (E08.22, E09.22, E10.22, E11.22, E13.22)
   hypertensive chronic kidney disease (I12.-, I13.-)
Use additional code to identify kidney transplant status, if applicable, (Z94.0)
AHA: 2023,1Q,17; 2022,4Q,14; 2019,3Q,3; 2018,4Q,88; 2013,1Q,24

    N18.1   **Chronic kidney disease, stage 1**

    N18.2   **Chronic kidney disease, stage 2 (mild)**

✓5ᵗʰ   **N18.3**   **Chronic kidney disease, stage 3 (moderate)**
        AHA: 2020,4Q,35

      N18.30   **Chronic kidney disease, stage 3 unspecified**   `I-CC`
      N18.31   **Chronic kidney disease, stage 3a**   `I-CC`
      N18.32   **Chronic kidney disease, stage 3b**   `I-CC`

    N18.4   **Chronic kidney disease, stage 4 (severe)**   `CC` `I-CC`

    N18.5   **Chronic kidney disease, stage 5**   `CC` `I-CC`
        EXCLUDES 1   chronic kidney disease, stage 5 requiring chronic dialysis (N18.6)
        DEF: End-stage renal disease (ESRD) with a GFR value of 15 ml/min or less not yet requiring chronic dialysis.
        TIP: When both ESRD and CKD 5 are documented, code only for ESRD.

    N18.6   **End stage renal disease**   `MCC` `I-CC`
        Chronic kidney disease requiring chronic dialysis
        Use additional code to identify dialysis status (Z99.2)
        AHA: 2023,1Q,19; 2022,3Q,15; 2016,3Q,22; 2016,1Q,12; 2013,4Q,124-125
        TIP: When both ESRD and CKD 5 are documented, code only for ESRD.

    N18.9   **Chronic kidney disease, unspecified**
        Chronic renal disease
        Chronic renal failure NOS
        Chronic renal insufficiency
        Chronic uremia NOS
        Diffuse sclerosing glomerulonephritis NOS

N19   **Unspecified kidney failure**
Uremia NOS
EXCLUDES 1   acute kidney failure (N17.-)
            chronic kidney disease (N18.-)
            chronic uremia (N18.9)
            extrarenal uremia (R39.2)
            prerenal uremia (R39.2)
            renal insufficiency (acute) (N28.9)
            uremia of newborn (P96.0)

Urolithiasis (N20-N23)

AHA: 2017,1Q,5; 2015,2Q,8

✓4ᵗʰ **N20**   **Calculus of kidney and ureter**
Calculous pyelonephritis
EXCLUDES 1   nephrocalcinosis (E83.59)
            that with hydronephrosis (N13.2)
AHA: 2019,3Q,13

    N20.0   **Calculus of kidney**
        Nephrolithiasis NOS
        Renal calculus
        Renal stone
        Staghorn calculus
        Stone in kidney
        AHA: 2019,3Q,13

    N20.1   **Calculus of ureter**   `CC`
        Calculus of the ureteropelvic junction
        Ureteric stone
        AHA: 2016,3Q,22

    N20.2   **Calculus of kidney with calculus of ureter**   `CC`

    N20.9   **Urinary calculus, unspecified**

✓4ᵗʰ **N21**   **Calculus of lower urinary tract**
INCLUDES   calculus of lower urinary tract with cystitis and urethritis

    N21.0   **Calculus in bladder**
        Calculus in diverticulum of bladder
        Urinary bladder stone
        EXCLUDES 2   staghorn calculus (N20.0)

    N21.1   **Calculus in urethra**
        EXCLUDES 2   calculus of prostate (N42.0)

    N21.8   **Other lower urinary tract calculus**

    N21.9   **Calculus of lower urinary tract, unspecified**
        EXCLUDES 1   calculus of urinary tract NOS (N20.9)

N22   *Calculus of urinary tract in diseases classified elsewhere*
Code first underlying disease, such as:
   gout (M1A.-, M10.-)
   schistosomiasis (B65.0-B65.9)

N23   **Unspecified renal colic**

Other disorders of kidney and ureter (N25-N29)

EXCLUDES 2   disorders of kidney and ureter with urolithiasis (N20-N23)

✓4ᵗʰ **N25**   **Disorders resulting from impaired renal tubular function**

    N25.0   **Renal osteodystrophy**
        Azotemic osteodystrophy
        Phosphate-losing tubular disorders
        Renal rickets
        Renal short stature
        EXCLUDES 2   metabolic disorders classifiable to E70-E88
        DEF: Various bone diseases occurring when kidney function is impaired or fails. Abnormal levels of phosphorous and calcium can lead to osteomalacia, osteoporosis, or osteosclerosis.

    N25.1   **Nephrogenic diabetes insipidus**   `CC`
        EXCLUDES 1   diabetes insipidus NOS (E23.2)
        DEF: Type of diabetes due to the inability of renal tubules to reabsorb water back into the body. It is not responsive to vasopressin (antidiuretic hormone) and it is characterized by excessive thirst and excessive urine production. It may develop into chronic renal insufficiency.

✅ Additional Character Required   ✓x7ᵗʰ Placeholder   <mark>Questionable PDx</mark>   Manifestation   Unspecified   `UPD` Unacceptable PDx   `H1`-`H14` HAC   `HCC` CMS-HCC Dx   `HIV` HIV Dx

ICD-10-CM 2025

863

N25.8   Other disorders resulting from impaired renal tubular function

     N25.81   Secondary hyperparathyroidism of renal origin   CC

        EXCLUDES 1   secondary hyperparathyroidism, non-renal (E21.1)

        EXCLUDES 2   metabolic disorders classifiable to E70-E88

        DEF: Parathyroid dysfunction caused by chronic renal failure. Phosphate clearance and vitamin D production is impaired resulting in lowered calcium blood levels and an excessive production of parathyroid hormone.

     N25.89   Other disorders resulting from impaired renal tubular function

        Hypokalemic nephropathy

        Lightwood-Albright syndrome

        Renal tubular acidosis NOS

N25.9   Disorder resulting from impaired renal tubular function, unspecified

N26   Unspecified contracted kidney

        EXCLUDES 1   contracted kidney due to hypertension (I12.-)

                    diffuse sclerosing glomerulonephritis (N05.8-)

                    hypertensive nephrosclerosis (arteriolar) (arteriosclerotic) (I12.-)

                    small kidney of unknown cause (N27.-)

     N26.1   Atrophy of kidney (terminal)

     N26.2   Page kidney

     N26.9   Renal sclerosis, unspecified

N27   Small kidney of unknown cause

        INCLUDES   oligonephronia

     N27.0   Small kidney, unilateral

     N27.1   Small kidney, bilateral

     N27.9   Small kidney, unspecified

N28   Other disorders of kidney and ureter, not elsewhere classified

     N28.0   Ischemia and infarction of kidney   CC

        Renal artery embolism

        Renal artery obstruction

        Renal artery occlusion

        Renal artery thrombosis

        Renal infarct

        EXCLUDES 1   atherosclerosis of renal artery (extrarenal part) (I70.1)

                    congenital stenosis of renal artery (Q27.1)

                    Goldblatt's kidney (I70.1)

     N28.1   Cyst of kidney, acquired

        Cyst (multiple) (solitary) of kidney (acquired)

        EXCLUDES 1   cystic kidney disease (congenital) (Q61.-)

     N28.8   Other specified disorders of kidney and ureter

        EXCLUDES 1   hydroureter (N13.4)

                    ureteric stricture with hydronephrosis (N13.1)

                    ureteric stricture without hydronephrosis (N13.5)

        N28.81   Hypertrophy of kidney

        N28.82   Megaloureter

        N28.83   Nephroptosis

        N28.84   Pyelitis cystica   CC   H6

        N28.85   Pyeloureteritis cystica   CC   H6

        N28.86   Ureteritis cystica   CC   H6

        N28.89   Other specified disorders of kidney and ureter

             AHA: 2023,3Q,5

     N28.9   Disorder of kidney and ureter, unspecified

        Nephropathy NOS

        Renal disease (acute) NOS

        Renal insufficiency (acute)

        EXCLUDES 1   chronic renal insufficiency (N18.9)

                    unspecified nephritic syndrome (N05.-)

        AHA: 2016,1Q,13

N29   *Other disorders of kidney and ureter in diseases classified elsewhere*

     Code first underlying disease, such as:

     amyloidosis (E85.-)

     nephrocalcinosis (E83.59)

     schistosomiasis (B65.0-B65.9)

        EXCLUDES 1   disorders of kidney and ureter in:

                    cystinosis (E72.0)

                    gonorrhea (A54.21)

                    syphilis (A52.75)

                    tuberculosis (A18.11)

Other diseases of the urinary system (N30-N39)

     EXCLUDES 2   urinary infection (complicating):

            abortion or ectopic or molar pregnancy (O00-O07, O08.8)

            pregnancy, childbirth and the puerperium (O23.-, O75.3, O86.2-)

N30   Cystitis

     Use additional code to identify infectious agent (B95-B97)

        EXCLUDES 1   prostatocystitis (N41.3)

     AHA: 2017,1Q,6

     DEF: Inflammation of the urinary bladder. Symptoms include dysuria, frequency of urination, urgency, and hematuria.

     N30.0   Acute cystitis

        EXCLUDES 1   irradiation cystitis (N30.4-)

                    trigonitis (N30.3-)

        N30.00   Acute cystitis without hematuria   CC   H6

        N30.01   Acute cystitis with hematuria   CC   H6

     N30.1   Interstitial cystitis (chronic)

        N30.10   Interstitial cystitis (chronic) without hematuria

        N30.11   Interstitial cystitis (chronic) with hematuria

     N30.2   Other chronic cystitis

        N30.20   Other chronic cystitis without hematuria

        N30.21   Other chronic cystitis with hematuria

     N30.3   Trigonitis

        Urethrotrigonitis

        N30.30   Trigonitis without hematuria

        N30.31   Trigonitis with hematuria

     N30.4   Irradiation cystitis

        N30.40   Irradiation cystitis without hematuria   CC

        N30.41   Irradiation cystitis with hematuria   CC

     N30.8   Other cystitis

        Abscess of bladder

        N30.80   Other cystitis without hematuria

        N30.81   Other cystitis with hematuria

     N30.9   Cystitis, unspecified

        N30.90   Cystitis, unspecified without hematuria

        N30.91   Cystitis, unspecified with hematuria

N31   Neuromuscular dysfunction of bladder, not elsewhere classified

     Use additional code to identify any associated urinary incontinence (N39.3-N39.4-)

        EXCLUDES 1   cord bladder NOS (G95.89)

                    neurogenic bladder due to cauda equina syndrome (G83.4)

                    neuromuscular dysfunction due to spinal cord lesion (G95.89)

     N31.0   Uninhibited neuropathic bladder, not elsewhere classified

     N31.1   Reflex neuropathic bladder, not elsewhere classified

     N31.2   Flaccid neuropathic bladder, not elsewhere classified

        Atonic (motor) (sensory) neuropathic bladder

        Autonomous neuropathic bladder

        Nonreflex neuropathic bladder

     N31.8   Other neuromuscular dysfunction of bladder

     N31.9   Neuromuscular dysfunction of bladder, unspecified

        Neurogenic bladder dysfunction NOS

N32   Other disorders of bladder

        EXCLUDES 2   calculus of bladder (N21.0)

                    cystocele (N81.1-)

                    hernia or prolapse of bladder, female (N81.1-)

     N32.0   Bladder-neck obstruction

        Bladder-neck stenosis (acquired)

        EXCLUDES 1   congenital bladder-neck obstruction (Q64.3-)

        DEF: Bladder outlet and vesicourethral obstruction that occurs as a consequence of benign prostatic hypertrophy or prostatic cancer. It may also occur in either sex due to strictures, radiation, cystoscopy, catheterization, injury, infection, blood clots, bladder cancer, impaction, or other disease that compresses the bladder neck.

     N32.1   Vesicointestinal fistula   CC

        Vesicorectal fistula

     N32.2   Vesical fistula, not elsewhere classified   CC

        EXCLUDES 1   fistula between bladder and female genital tract (N82.0-N82.1)

     N32.3   Diverticulum of bladder

        EXCLUDES 1   congenital diverticulum of bladder (Q64.6)

                    diverticulitis of bladder (N30.8-)

N Newborn: 0   **P** Pediatric: 0-17   **M** Maternity: 9-64   **A** Adult: 15-124   **UNS** Unspecified Site   **MCC** Major Complication/Comorbidity   **CC** Complication/Comorbidity   **PE** POA Exempt

864   ICD-10-CM 2025

√5ᵗʰ **N32.8 Other specified disorders of bladder**

N32.81 Overactive bladder
Detrusor muscle hyperactivity
EXCLUDES 1   *frequent urination due to specified bladder condition — code to condition*
DEF: Sudden involuntary contractions of the muscular wall of the bladder that results in a sudden, strong urge to urinate.

N32.89 Other specified disorders of bladder
Bladder hemorrhage
Bladder hypertrophy
Calcified bladder
Contracted bladder

N32.9 Bladder disorder, unspecified

N33 Bladder disorders in diseases classified elsewhere
Code first underlying disease, such as:
schistosomiasis (B65.0-B65.9)
EXCLUDES 1   *bladder disorder in syphilis (A52.76)*
bladder disorder in tuberculosis (A18.12)
candidal cystitis (B37.41)
chlamydial cystitis (A56.01)
cystitis in gonorrhea (A54.01)
cystitis in neurogenic bladder (N31.-)
diphtheritic cystitis (A36.85)
neurogenic bladder (N31.-)
syphilitic cystitis (A52.76)
trichomonal cystitis (A59.03)

√4ᵗʰ **N34 Urethritis and urethral syndrome**
Use additional code (B95-B97), to identify infectious agent
EXCLUDES 2   *Reiter's disease (M02.3-)*
urethritis in diseases with a predominantly sexual mode of transmission (A50-A64)
urethrotrigonitis (N30.3-)
AHA: 2017,1Q,6

N34.0 Urethral abscess   `CC` `H6`
Abscess (of) Cowper's gland
Abscess (of) Littre's gland
Abscess (of) urethral (gland)
Periurethral abscess
EXCLUDES 1   *urethral caruncle (N36.2)*

N34.1 Nonspecific urethritis
Nongonococcal urethritis
Nonvenereal urethritis

N34.2 Other urethritis
Meatitis, urethral
Postmenopausal urethritis
Ulcer of urethra (meatus)
Urethritis NOS

N34.3 Urethral syndrome, unspecified

√4ᵗʰ **N35 Urethral stricture**
EXCLUDES 1   *congenital urethral stricture (Q64.3-)*
postprocedural urethral stricture (N99.1-)
AHA: 2018,4Q,21-22

√5ᵗʰ **N35.0 Post-traumatic urethral stricture**
Urethral stricture due to injury
EXCLUDES 1   *postprocedural urethral stricture (N99.1-)*

√6ᵗʰ **N35.01 Post-traumatic urethral stricture, male**
N35.010 Post-traumatic urethral stricture, male, meatal
N35.011 Post-traumatic bulbous urethral stricture
N35.012 Post-traumatic membranous urethral stricture
N35.013 Post-traumatic anterior urethral stricture
N35.014 Post-traumatic urethral stricture, male, unspecified
N35.016 Post-traumatic urethral stricture, male, overlapping sites

√6ᵗʰ **N35.02 Post-traumatic urethral stricture, female**
N35.021 Urethral stricture due to childbirth
N35.028 Other post-traumatic urethral stricture, female

√5ᵗʰ **N35.1 Postinfective urethral stricture, not elsewhere classified**
EXCLUDES 1   *gonococcal urethral stricture (A54.01)*
syphilitic urethral stricture (A52.76)
urethral stricture associated with schistosomiasis (B65.-, N29)

√6ᵗʰ **N35.11 Postinfective urethral stricture, not elsewhere classified, male**
N35.111 Postinfective urethral stricture, not elsewhere classified, male, meatal
N35.112 Postinfective bulbous urethral stricture, not elsewhere classified, male
N35.113 Postinfective membranous urethral stricture, not elsewhere classified, male
N35.114 Postinfective anterior urethral stricture, not elsewhere classified, male
N35.116 Postinfective urethral stricture, not elsewhere classified, male, overlapping sites
N35.119 Postinfective urethral stricture, not elsewhere classified, male, unspecified

N35.12 Postinfective urethral stricture, not elsewhere classified, female

√5ᵗʰ **N35.8 Other urethral stricture**
EXCLUDES 1   *postprocedural urethral stricture (N99.1-)*

√6ᵗʰ **N35.81 Other urethral stricture, male**
N35.811 Other urethral stricture, male, meatal
N35.812 Other bulbous urethral stricture, male
N35.813 Other membranous urethral stricture, male
N35.814 Other anterior urethral stricture, male
N35.816 Other urethral stricture, male, overlapping sites
N35.819 Other urethral stricture, male, unspecified site

N35.82 Other urethral stricture, female

√5ᵗʰ **N35.9 Urethral stricture, unspecified**

√6ᵗʰ **N35.91 Urethral stricture, unspecified, male**
N35.911 Unspecified urethral stricture, male, meatal
N35.912 Unspecified bulbous urethral stricture, male
N35.913 Unspecified membranous urethral stricture, male
N35.914 Unspecified anterior urethral stricture, male
N35.916 Unspecified urethral stricture, male, overlapping sites
N35.919 Unspecified urethral stricture, male, unspecified site
Pinhole meatus NOS
Urethral stricture NOS

N35.92 Unspecified urethral stricture, female

√4ᵗʰ **N36 Other disorders of urethra**

N36.0 Urethral fistula   `CC`
Urethroperineal fistula
Urethrorectal fistula
Urinary fistula NOS
EXCLUDES 1   *urethroscrotal fistula (N50.89)*
urethrovaginal fistula (N82.1)
urethrovesicovaginal fistula (N82.1)

N36.1 Urethral diverticulum

N36.2 Urethral caruncle

√5ᵗʰ **N36.4 Urethral functional and muscular disorders**
Use additional code to identify associated urinary stress incontinence (N39.3)
N36.41 Hypermobility of urethra
N36.42 Intrinsic sphincter deficiency (ISD)
N36.43 Combined hypermobility of urethra and intrinsic sphincter deficiency
N36.44 Muscular disorders of urethra
Bladder sphincter dyssynergy

N36.5 Urethral false passage

N36.8 Other specified disorders of urethra
EXCLUDES 1   *congenital urethrocele (Q64.7)*
female urethrocele (N81.0)
AHA: 2022,2Q,7

N36.9 Urethral disorder, unspecified

Chapter 14. Diseases of the Genitourinary System

N37 **Urethral disorders in diseases classified elsewhere**
     Code first underlying disease
      EXCLUDES 1   urethritis (in):
           candidal infection (B37.41)
           chlamydial (A56.Ø1)
           gonorrhea (A54.Ø1)
           syphilis (A52.76)
           trichomonal infection (A59.Ø3)
           tuberculosis (A18.13)

√4ᵗʰ N39 **Other disorders of urinary system**
      EXCLUDES 2   hematuria NOS (R31.-)
           proteinuria NOS (R8Ø.-)
           recurrent or persistent hematuria (NØ2.-)
           recurrent or persistent hematuria with specified morphological
             lesion (NØ2.-)

    N39.Ø   **Urinary tract infection, site not specified**   CC   H6
       Use additional code (B95-B97), to identify infectious agent
       EXCLUDES 1   candidiasis of urinary tract (B37.4-)
           neonatal urinary tract infection (P39.3)
           pyuria (R82.81)
           urinary tract infection of specified site, such as:
             cystitis (N3Ø.-)
             ▶pyonephrosis (N13.6)◀
             urethritis (N34.-)
       AHA: 2019,3Q,17; 2018,2Q,21,22; 2018,1Q,16; 2017,1Q,6;
       2012,4Q,94

    N39.3   **Stress incontinence (female) (male)**
       Code also any associated overactive bladder (N32.81)
       EXCLUDES 1   mixed incontinence (N39.46)

   √5ᵗʰ N39.4   **Other specified urinary incontinence**
       Code also any associated overactive bladder (N32.81)
       EXCLUDES 1   enuresis NOS (R32)
           functional urinary incontinence (R39.81)
           urinary incontinence associated with cognitive
             impairment (R39.81)
           urinary incontinence NOS (R32)
           urinary incontinence of nonorganic origin (F98.Ø)

     N39.41   **Urge incontinence**
        EXCLUDES 1   mixed incontinence (N39.46)

     N39.42   **Incontinence without sensory awareness**
        Insensible (urinary) incontinence

     N39.43   **Post-void dribbling**

     N39.44   **Nocturnal enuresis**
        EXCLUDES 2   nocturnal polyuria (R35.81)

     N39.45   **Continuous leakage**

     N39.46   **Mixed incontinence**
        Urge and stress incontinence

   √6ᵗʰ N39.49   **Other specified urinary incontinence**
        AHA: 2016,4Q,44

       N39.49Ø   **Overflow incontinence**
       N39.491   **Coital incontinence**
       N39.492   **Postural (urinary) incontinence**
       N39.498   **Other specified urinary incontinence**
           Reflex incontinence
           Total incontinence

   N39.8   **Other specified disorders of urinary system**
   N39.9   **Disorder of urinary system, unspecified**

Diseases of male genital organs (N4Ø-N53)

√4ᵗʰ N4Ø **Benign prostatic hyperplasia**
     INCLUDES   adenofibromatous hypertrophy of prostate
           benign hypertrophy of the prostate
           benign prostatic hypertrophy
           BPH
           enlarged prostate
           nodular prostate
           polyp of prostate
     EXCLUDES 1   benign neoplasms of prostate (adenoma, benign)
             (fibroadenoma) (fibroma) (myoma) (D29.1)
     EXCLUDES 2   malignant neoplasm of prostate (C61)
     DEF: Enlargement of the prostate gland due to an abnormal proliferation
     of fibrostromal tissue in the paraurethral glands. This condition causes
     impingement of the urethra resulting in obstructed urinary flow.

   N4Ø.Ø   **Benign prostatic hyperplasia without lower urinary tract**
      symptoms   A
       Enlarged prostate NOS
       Enlarged prostate without LUTS

   N4Ø.1   **Benign prostatic hyperplasia with lower urinary tract**
      symptoms   A
       Enlarged prostate with LUTS
       Use additional code for associated symptoms, when specified:
           incomplete bladder emptying (R39.14)
           nocturia (R35.1)
           straining on urination (R39.16)
           urinary frequency (R35.Ø)
           urinary hesitancy (R39.11)
           urinary incontinence (N39.4-)
           urinary obstruction (N13.8)
           urinary retention (R33.8)
           urinary urgency (R39.15)
           weak urinary stream (R39.12)
       AHA: 2018,4Q,55

   N4Ø.2   **Nodular prostate without lower urinary tract symptoms**   A
       Nodular prostate without LUTS

   N4Ø.3   **Nodular prostate with lower urinary tract symptoms**   A
       Use additional code for associated symptoms, when specified:
           incomplete bladder emptying (R39.14)
           nocturia (R35.1)
           straining on urination (R39.16)
           urinary frequency (R35.Ø)
           urinary hesitancy (R39.11)
           urinary incontinence (N39.4-)
           urinary obstruction (N13.8)
           urinary retention (R33.8)
           urinary urgency (R39.15)
           weak urinary stream (R39.12)

√4ᵗʰ N41 **Inflammatory diseases of prostate**
     Use additional code (B95-B97), to identify infectious agent

   N41.Ø   **Acute prostatitis**   CC   A
       AHA: 2024,1Q,16

   N41.1   **Chronic prostatitis**   A

   N41.2   **Abscess of prostate**   CC   A

   N41.3   **Prostatocystitis**   A
       AHA: 2024,1Q,16

   N41.4   **Granulomatous prostatitis**   A

   N41.8   **Other inflammatory diseases of prostate**   A

   N41.9   **Inflammatory disease of prostate, unspecified**   A
       Prostatitis NOS

√4ᵗʰ N42 **Other and unspecified disorders of prostate**

   N42.Ø   **Calculus of prostate**   A
       Prostatic stone
       DEF: Formation of a small, solid stone often composed of calcium
       carbonate or calcium phosphate in the prostate gland.

   N42.1   **Congestion and hemorrhage of prostate**   A
       EXCLUDES 1   enlarged prostate (N4Ø.-)
           hematuria (R31.-)
           hyperplasia of prostate (N4Ø.-)
           inflammatory diseases of prostate (N41.-)

   √5ᵗʰ N42.3   **Dysplasia of prostate**
       AHA: 2016,4Q,44

     N42.3Ø   **Unspecified dysplasia of prostate**

N42.31 **Prostatic intraepithelial neoplasia**
PIN
Prostatic intraepithelial neoplasia I (PIN I)
Prostatic intraepithelial neoplasia II (PIN II)
EXCLUDES 1 *prostatic intraepithelial neoplasia III (PIN III) (D07.5)*
DEF: Abnormality of shape and size of the intraepithelial tissues of the prostate. It is a premalignant condition characterized by stalks and absence of a basilar cell layer.

N42.32 **Atypical small acinar proliferation of prostate**
N42.39 **Other dysplasia of prostate**

✓5th N42.8 **Other specified disorders of prostate**
N42.81 **Prostatodynia syndrome**   A
Painful prostate syndrome
N42.82 **Prostatosis syndrome**   A
N42.83 **Cyst of prostate**   A
N42.89 **Other specified disorders of prostate**   A
N42.9 **Disorder of prostate, unspecified**   A

✓4th **N43 Hydrocele and spermatocele**
INCLUDES hydrocele of spermatic cord, testis or tunica vaginalis
EXCLUDES 1 *congenital hydrocele (P83.5)*
DEF: Hydrocele: Serous fluid that collects in the tunica vaginalis of the scrotum along the spermatic cord in males.
N43.0 **Encysted hydrocele**
N43.1 **Infected hydrocele**   CC
Use additional code (B95-B97), to identify infectious agent
N43.2 **Other hydrocele**

Hydrocele

Normal   Noncommunicating hydrocele   Communicating hydrocele   Hydrocele of the cord

Testicle
Scrotum

N43.3 **Hydrocele, unspecified**
✓5th N43.4 **Spermatocele of epididymis**
Spermatic cyst
DEF: Spermatocele: Noncancerous accumulation of fluid and dead sperm cells normally located at the head of the epididymis that exhibits itself as a hard, smooth scrotal mass and do not normally require treatment unless they become enlarged or cause pain.
N43.40 **Spermatocele of epididymis, unspecified**
N43.41 **Spermatocele of epididymis, single**
N43.42 **Spermatocele of epididymis, multiple**

✓4th **N44 Noninflammatory disorders of testis**
✓5th N44.0 **Torsion of testis**
N44.00 **Torsion of testis, unspecified**   CC
N44.01 **Extravaginal torsion of spermatic cord**   CC
DEF: Torsion of the spermatic cord just below the tunica vaginalis attachments.
N44.02 **Intravaginal torsion of spermatic cord**   CC
Torsion of spermatic cord NOS
N44.03 **Torsion of appendix testis**   CC
N44.04 **Torsion of appendix epididymis**   CC
N44.1 **Cyst of tunica albuginea testis**
N44.2 **Benign cyst of testis**
N44.8 **Other noninflammatory disorders of the testis**

✓4th **N45 Orchitis and epididymitis**
Use additional code (B95-B97), to identify infectious agent
N45.1 **Epididymitis**
N45.2 **Orchitis**
N45.3 **Epididymo-orchitis**
N45.4 **Abscess of epididymis or testis**   CC

✓4th **N46 Male infertility**
EXCLUDES 1 *vasectomy status (Z98.52)*
✓5th N46.0 **Azoospermia**
Absolute male infertility
Male infertility due to germinal (cell) aplasia
Male infertility due to spermatogenic arrest (complete)
DEF: Failure of the development of sperm or the absence of sperm in semen.
N46.01 **Organic azoospermia**   A
Azoospermia NOS
✓6th N46.02 **Azoospermia due to extratesticular causes**
Code also associated cause
N46.021 **Azoospermia due to drug therapy**   A
N46.022 **Azoospermia due to infection**   A
N46.023 **Azoospermia due to obstruction of efferent ducts**   A
N46.024 **Azoospermia due to radiation**
N46.025 **Azoospermia due to systemic disease**   A
N46.029 **Azoospermia due to other extratesticular causes**   A

✓5th N46.1 **Oligospermia**
Male infertility due to germinal cell desquamation
Male infertility due to hypospermatogenesis
Male infertility due to incomplete spermatogenic arrest
DEF: Insufficient production of sperm in semen.
N46.11 **Organic oligospermia**   A
Oligospermia NOS
✓6th N46.12 **Oligospermia due to extratesticular causes**
Code also associated cause
N46.121 **Oligospermia due to drug therapy**   A
N46.122 **Oligospermia due to infection**   A
N46.123 **Oligospermia due to obstruction of efferent ducts**   A
N46.124 **Oligospermia due to radiation**   A
N46.125 **Oligospermia due to systemic disease**   A
N46.129 **Oligospermia due to other extratesticular causes**

N46.8 **Other male infertility**   A
N46.9 **Male infertility, unspecified**   A

✓4th **N47 Disorders of prepuce**
N47.0 **Adherent prepuce, newborn**   N
N47.1 **Phimosis**
DEF: Condition in which the foreskin is contracted and cannot be drawn back behind the glans penis.
N47.2 **Paraphimosis**
N47.3 **Deficient foreskin**
N47.4 **Benign cyst of prepuce**
N47.5 **Adhesions of prepuce and glans penis**
N47.6 **Balanoposthitis**
Use additional code (B95-B97), to identify infectious agent
EXCLUDES 1 *balanitis (N48.1)*
N47.7 **Other inflammatory diseases of prepuce**
Use additional code (B95-B97), to identify infectious agent
N47.8 **Other disorders of prepuce**

✓4th **N48 Other disorders of penis**
N48.0 **Leukoplakia of penis**
Balanitis xerotica obliterans
Kraurosis of penis
Lichen sclerosus of external male genital organs
EXCLUDES 1 *carcinoma in situ of penis (D07.4)*
N48.1 **Balanitis**
Use additional code (B95-B97), to identify infectious agent
EXCLUDES 1 *amebic balanitis (A06.8)*
balanitis xerotica obliterans (N48.0)
candidal balanitis (B37.42)
gonococcal balanitis (A54.23)
herpesviral [herpes simplex] balanitis (A60.01)
DEF: Inflammation of the glans penis, most often affecting uncircumcised males.

√5ᵗʰ N48.2 Other inflammatory disorders of penis
Use additional code (B95-B97), to identify infectious agent
EXCLUDES 1   *balanitis (N48.1)*
          balanitis xerotica obliterans (N48.0)
          balanoposthitis (N47.6)
   N48.21 Abscess of corpus cavernosum and penis
   N48.22 Cellulitis of corpus cavernosum and penis
   N48.29 Other inflammatory disorders of penis

√5ᵗʰ N48.3 Priapism
Painful erection
Code first underlying cause
   N48.30 Priapism, unspecified   CC
   N48.31 Priapism due to trauma   CC
   N48.32 Priapism due to disease classified elsewhere   CC
   N48.33 Priapism, drug-induced   CC
   N48.39 Other priapism   CC

N48.5 Ulcer of penis

N48.6 Induration penis plastica
Peyronie's disease
Plastic induration of penis

√5ᵗʰ N48.8 Other specified disorders of penis
   N48.81 Thrombosis of superficial vein of penis
   N48.82 Acquired torsion of penis
     Acquired torsion of penis NOS
     EXCLUDES 1   *congenital torsion of penis (Q55.63)*
   N48.83 Acquired buried penis
     EXCLUDES 1   *congenital hidden penis (Q55.64)*
   N48.89 Other specified disorders of penis

N48.9 Disorder of penis, unspecified

√4ᵗʰ N49 Inflammatory disorders of male genital organs, not elsewhere classified
Use additional code (B95-B97), to identify infectious agent
EXCLUDES 1   *inflammation of penis (N48.1, N48.2-)*
          orchitis and epididymitis (N45.-)

N49.0 Inflammatory disorders of seminal vesicle
Vesiculitis NOS

N49.1 Inflammatory disorders of spermatic cord, tunica vaginalis and vas deferens
Vasitis

N49.2 Inflammatory disorders of scrotum

N49.3 Fournier gangrene   HCC
AHA: 2020,2Q,18

N49.8 Inflammatory disorders of other specified male genital organs
Inflammation of multiple sites in male genital organs

N49.9 Inflammatory disorder of unspecified male genital organ
Abscess of unspecified male genital organ
Boil of unspecified male genital organ
Carbuncle of unspecified male genital organ
Cellulitis of unspecified male genital organ

√4ᵗʰ N50 Other and unspecified disorders of male genital organs
EXCLUDES 2   *torsion of testis (N44.0-)*

N50.0 Atrophy of testis

N50.1 Vascular disorders of male genital organs
Hematocele, NOS, of male genital organs
Hemorrhage of male genital organs
Thrombosis of male genital organs

N50.3 Cyst of epididymis

√5ᵗʰ N50.8 Other specified disorders of male genital organs
AHA: 2016,4Q,45
   √6ᵗʰ N50.81 Testicular pain
     N50.811 Right testicular pain
     N50.812 Left testicular pain
     N50.819 Testicular pain, unspecified
   N50.82 Scrotal pain

N50.89 Other specified disorders of the male genital organs
Atrophy of scrotum, seminal vesicle, spermatic cord, tunica vaginalis and vas deferens
Chylocele, tunica vaginalis (nonfilarial) NOS
Edema of scrotum, seminal vesicle, spermatic cord, tunica vaginalis and vas deferens
Hypertrophy of scrotum, seminal vesicle, spermatic cord, tunica vaginalis and vas deferens
Stricture of spermatic cord, tunica vaginalis, and vas deferens
Ulcer of scrotum, seminal vesicle, spermatic cord, testis, tunica vaginalis and vas deferens
Urethroscrotal fistula

N50.9 Disorder of male genital organs, unspecified

N51 Disorders of male genital organs in diseases classified elsewhere
Code first underlying disease, such as:
filariasis (B74.0-B74.9)
EXCLUDES 1   *amebic balanitis (A06.8)*
          candidal balanitis (B37.42)
          gonococcal balanitis (A54.23)
          gonococcal prostatitis (A54.22)
          herpesviral [herpes simplex] balanitis (A60.01)
          trichomonal prostatitis (A59.02)
          tuberculous prostatitis (A18.14)

√4ᵗʰ N52 Male erectile dysfunction
EXCLUDES 1   *psychogenic impotence (F52.21)*

√5ᵗʰ N52.0 Vasculogenic erectile dysfunction
   N52.01 Erectile dysfunction due to arterial insufficiency   A
   N52.02 Corporo-venous occlusive erectile dysfunction   A
   N52.03 Combined arterial insufficiency and corporo-venous occlusive erectile dysfunction   A

√5ᵗʰ N52.1 *Erectile dysfunction due to diseases classified elsewhere*   A
Code first underlying disease

N52.2 Drug-induced erectile dysfunction   A

√5ᵗʰ N52.3 Postprocedural erectile dysfunction
AHA: 2016,4Q,45
   N52.31 Erectile dysfunction following radical prostatectomy   A
   N52.32 Erectile dysfunction following radical cystectomy   A
   N52.33 Erectile dysfunction following urethral surgery   A
   N52.34 Erectile dysfunction following simple prostatectomy   A
   N52.35 Erectile dysfunction following radiation therapy   A
   N52.36 Erectile dysfunction following interstitial seed therapy   A
   N52.37 Erectile dysfunction following prostate ablative therapy   A
     Erectile dysfunction following cryotherapy
     Erectile dysfunction following other prostate ablative therapies
     Erectile dysfunction following ultrasound ablative therapies
   N52.39 Other and unspecified postprocedural erectile dysfunction   A

N52.8 Other male erectile dysfunction   A

N52.9 Male erectile dysfunction, unspecified   A
Impotence NOS

√4ᵗʰ N53 Other male sexual dysfunction
EXCLUDES 1   *psychogenic sexual dysfunction (F52.-)*

√5ᵗʰ N53.1 Ejaculatory dysfunction
EXCLUDES 1   *premature ejaculation (F52.4)*
   N53.11 Retarded ejaculation
   N53.12 Painful ejaculation
   N53.13 Anejaculatory orgasm
   N53.14 Retrograde ejaculation
     DEF: Form of male sexual dysfunction in which the semen enters the bladder instead of going out through the urethra during ejaculation.
   N53.19 Other ejaculatory dysfunction
     Ejaculatory dysfunction NOS

N53.8 Other male sexual dysfunction

N53.9 Unspecified male sexual dysfunction

Disorders of breast (N60-N65)

EXCLUDES 1   *disorders of breast associated with childbirth (O91-O92)*

☑4th **N60** **Benign mammary dysplasia**

     INCLUDES   fibrocystic mastopathy

    ☑5th **N60.0** **Solitary cyst of breast**

      Cyst of breast

      N60.01   Solitary cyst of **right** breast

      N60.02   Solitary cyst of **left** breast

      N60.09   Solitary cyst of unspecified breast

    ☑5th **N60.1** **Diffuse cystic mastopathy**

      Cystic breast

      Fibrocystic disease of breast

       EXCLUDES 1   *diffuse cystic mastopathy with epithelial proliferation (N60.3-)*

      N60.11   Diffuse cystic mastopathy of **right** breast   🅰

      N60.12   Diffuse cystic mastopathy of **left** breast   🅰

      N60.19   Diffuse cystic mastopathy of unspecified breast   🅰

    ☑5th **N60.2** **Fibroadenosis of breast**

      Adenofibrosis of breast

       EXCLUDES 2   *fibroadenoma of breast (D24.-)*

      N60.21   Fibroadenosis of **right** breast

      N60.22   Fibroadenosis of **left** breast

      N60.29   Fibroadenosis of unspecified breast

    ☑5th **N60.3** **Fibrosclerosis of breast**

      Cystic mastopathy with epithelial proliferation

      N60.31   Fibrosclerosis of **right** breast

      N60.32   Fibrosclerosis of **left** breast

      N60.39   Fibrosclerosis of unspecified breast

    ☑5th **N60.4** **Mammary duct ectasia**

      N60.41   Mammary duct ectasia of **right** breast

      N60.42   Mammary duct ectasia of **left** breast

      N60.49   Mammary duct ectasia of unspecified breast

    ☑5th **N60.8** **Other benign mammary dysplasias**

      N60.81   Other benign mammary dysplasias of **right** breast

      N60.82   Other benign mammary dysplasias of **left** breast

      N60.89   Other benign mammary dysplasias of unspecified breast

    ☑5th **N60.9** **Unspecified benign mammary dysplasia**

      N60.91   Unspecified benign mammary dysplasia of **right** breast

      N60.92   Unspecified benign mammary dysplasia of **left** breast

      N60.99   Unspecified benign mammary dysplasia of unspecified breast

☑4th **N61** **Inflammatory disorders of breast**

     EXCLUDES 1   *inflammatory carcinoma of breast (C50.9)*

         inflammatory disorder of breast associated with childbirth (O91.-)

         neonatal infective mastitis (P39.0)

         thrombophlebitis of breast [Mondor's disease] (I80.8)

    N61.0 **Mastitis without abscess**

      Infective mastitis (acute) (nonpuerperal) (subacute)

      Mastitis (acute) (nonpuerperal) (subacute) NOS

      Cellulitis (acute) (nonpuerperal) (subacute) of breast NOS

      Cellulitis (acute) (nonpuerperal) (subacute) of nipple NOS

    N61.1 **Abscess of the breast and nipple**

      Abscess (acute) (chronic) (nonpuerperal) of areola

      Abscess (acute) (chronic) (nonpuerperal) of breast

      Carbuncle of breast

      Mastitis with abscess

    ☑5th **N61.2** **Granulomatous mastitis**

      AHA: 2020,4Q,35

      N61.20   Granulomatous mastitis, unspecified breast

      N61.21   Granulomatous mastitis, **right** breast

      N61.22   Granulomatous mastitis, **left** breast

      N61.23   Granulomatous mastitis, **bilateral** breast

N62 **Hypertrophy of breast**

     Gynecomastia

     Hypertrophy of breast NOS

     Massive pubertal hypertrophy of breast

      EXCLUDES 1   *breast engorgement of newborn (P83.4)*

         disproportion of reconstructed breast (N65.1)

     AHA: 2023,3Q,22

☑4th **N63** **Unspecified lump in breast**

     Nodule(s) NOS in breast

     AHA: 2022,3Q,8; 2019,4Q,12; 2017,4Q,19

    N63.0 **Unspecified lump in unspecified breast**

    ☑5th **N63.1** **Unspecified lump in the right breast**

      N63.10   Unspecified lump in the right breast, unspecified quadrant

      N63.11   Unspecified lump in the right breast, **upper outer quadrant**

      N63.12   Unspecified lump in the right breast, **upper inner quadrant**

      N63.13   Unspecified lump in the right breast, **lower outer quadrant**

      N63.14   Unspecified lump in the right breast, **lower inner quadrant**

      N63.15   Unspecified lump in the right breast, **overlapping quadrants**

    ☑5th **N63.2** **Unspecified lump in the left breast**

      N63.20   Unspecified lump in the left breast, unspecified quadrant

      N63.21   Unspecified lump in the left breast, **upper outer quadrant**

      N63.22   Unspecified lump in the left breast, **upper inner quadrant**

      N63.23   Unspecified lump in the left breast, **lower outer quadrant**

      N63.24   Unspecified lump in the left breast, **lower inner quadrant**

      N63.25   Unspecified lump in the left breast, **overlapping quadrants**

    ☑5th **N63.3** **Unspecified lump in axillary tail**

      N63.31   Unspecified lump in axillary tail of the **right** breast

      N63.32   Unspecified lump in axillary tail of the **left** breast

    ☑5th **N63.4** **Unspecified lump in breast, subareolar**

      N63.41   Unspecified lump in **right** breast, subareolar

      N63.42   Unspecified lump in **left** breast, subareolar

☑4th **N64** **Other disorders of breast**

     EXCLUDES 2   *mechanical complication of breast prosthesis and implant (T85.4-)*

    N64.0 **Fissure and fistula of nipple**

    N64.1 **Fat necrosis of breast**   UPD

      Fat necrosis (segmental) of breast

      Code first breast fat necrosis due to breast graft (T85.898)

    N64.2 **Atrophy of breast**

    N64.3 **Galactorrhea not associated with childbirth**

    N64.4 **Mastodynia**

    ☑5th **N64.5** **Other signs and symptoms in breast**

      EXCLUDES 2   *abnormal findings on diagnostic imaging of breast (R92.-)*

      N64.51   Induration of breast

      N64.52   Nipple discharge

        EXCLUDES 1   *abnormal findings in nipple discharge (R89.-)*

      N64.53   Retraction of nipple

      N64.59   Other signs and symptoms in breast

    ☑5th **N64.8** **Other specified disorders of breast**

      N64.81   Ptosis of breast   🅰

        EXCLUDES 1   *ptosis of native breast in relation to reconstructed breast (N65.1)*

      N64.82   Hypoplasia of breast   🅰

        Micromastia

        EXCLUDES 1   *congenital absence of breast (Q83.0)*

           hypoplasia of native breast in relation to reconstructed breast (N65.1)

      N64.89   Other specified disorders of breast

        Galactocele

        Subinvolution of breast (postlactational)

        AHA: 2019,1Q,32; 2018,1Q,3

    N64.9 **Disorder of breast, unspecified**

☑4th **N65** **Deformity and disproportion of reconstructed breast**

    N65.0 **Deformity of reconstructed breast**   🅰

      Contour irregularity in reconstructed breast

      Excess tissue in reconstructed breast

      Misshapen reconstructed breast

☑ Additional Character Required   ☑x7th Placeholder   Questionable PDx   Manifestation   Unspecified   UPD Unacceptable PDx   H1-H14 HAC   HCC CMS-HCC Dx   HIV HIV Dx

Chapter 14. Diseases of the Genitourinary System

N65.1   **Disproportion of reconstructed breast**   <kbd>A</kbd>
Breast asymmetry between native breast and reconstructed breast
Disproportion between native breast and reconstructed breast

Inflammatory diseases of female pelvic organs (N70-N77)

EXCLUDES 1   inflammatory diseases of female pelvic organs complicating:
abortion or ectopic or molar pregnancy (O00-O07, O08.0)
pregnancy, childbirth and the puerperium (O23.-, O75.3, O85, O86.-)

✓4th **N70**   **Salpingitis and oophoritis**
    INCLUDES   abscess (of) fallopian tube
               abscess (of) ovary
               pyosalpinx
               salpingo-oophoritis
               tubo-ovarian abscess
               tubo-ovarian inflammatory disease
    Use additional code (B95-B97), to identify infectious agent
    EXCLUDES 1   gonococcal infection (A54.24)
                   tuberculous infection (A18.17)

✓5th **N70.0**   **Acute salpingitis and oophoritis**
    N70.01   **Acute salpingitis**   <kbd>CC</kbd>
    N70.02   **Acute oophoritis**   <kbd>CC</kbd>
    N70.03   **Acute salpingitis and oophoritis**   <kbd>CC</kbd>

✓5th **N70.1**   **Chronic salpingitis and oophoritis**
    Hydrosalpinx
    N70.11   **Chronic salpingitis**
    N70.12   **Chronic oophoritis**
    N70.13   **Chronic salpingitis and oophoritis**

✓5th **N70.9**   **Salpingitis and oophoritis, unspecified**
    N70.91   **Salpingitis, unspecified**
    N70.92   **Oophoritis, unspecified**
    N70.93   **Salpingitis and oophoritis, unspecified**

✓4th **N71**   **Inflammatory disease of uterus, except cervix**
    INCLUDES   endo (myo) metritis
               metritis
               myometritis
               pyometra
               uterine abscess
    Use additional code (B95-B97), to identify infectious agent
    EXCLUDES 1   hyperplastic endometritis (N85.0-)
                   infection of uterus following delivery (O85, O86.-)

N71.0   **Acute inflammatory disease of uterus**   <kbd>CC</kbd>
N71.1   **Chronic inflammatory disease of uterus**
N71.9   **Inflammatory disease of uterus, unspecified**

N72   **Inflammatory disease of cervix uteri**
    INCLUDES   cervicitis (with or without erosion or ectropion)
               endocervicitis (with or without erosion or ectropion)
               exocervicitis (with or without erosion or ectropion)
    Use additional code (B95-B97), to identify infectious agent
    EXCLUDES 1   erosion and ectropion of cervix without cervicitis (N86)

✓4th **N73**   **Other female pelvic inflammatory diseases**
    Use additional code (B95-B97), to identify infectious agent

N73.0   **Acute parametritis and pelvic cellulitis**   <kbd>CC</kbd>
    Abscess of broad ligament
    Abscess of parametrium
    Pelvic cellulitis, female
    DEF: Parametritis: Inflammation of the parametrium.

N73.1   **Chronic parametritis and pelvic cellulitis**
    Any condition in N73.0 specified as chronic
    EXCLUDES 1   tuberculous parametritis and pelvic cellultis (A18.17)

N73.2   **Unspecified parametritis and pelvic cellulitis**
    Any condition in N73.0 unspecified whether acute or chronic

N73.3   **Female acute pelvic peritonitis**   <kbd>MCC</kbd>
N73.4   **Female chronic pelvic peritonitis**   <kbd>CC</kbd>
    EXCLUDES 1   tuberculous pelvic (female) peritonitis (A18.17)

N73.5   **Female pelvic peritonitis, unspecified**
N73.6   **Female pelvic peritoneal adhesions (postinfective)**
    EXCLUDES 2   postprocedural pelvic peritoneal adhesions (N99.4)
    AHA: 2014,1Q,6

N73.8   **Other specified female pelvic inflammatory diseases**
N73.9   **Female pelvic inflammatory disease, unspecified**
    Female pelvic infection or inflammation NOS

N74   *Female pelvic inflammatory disorders in diseases classified elsewhere*
    Code first underlying disease
    EXCLUDES 1   chlamydial cervicitis (A56.02)
                   chlamydial pelvic inflammatory disease (A56.11)
                   gonococcal cervicitis (A54.03)
                   gonococcal pelvic inflammatory disease (A54.24)
                   herpesviral [herpes simplex] cervicitis (A60.03)
                   herpesviral [herpes simplex] pelvic inflammatory disease (A60.09)
                   syphilitic cervicitis (A52.76)
                   syphilitic pelvic inflammatory disease (A52.76)
                   trichomonal cervicitis (A59.09)
                   tuberculous cervicitis (A18.16)
                   tuberculous pelvic inflammatory disease (A18.17)

✓4th **N75**   **Diseases of Bartholin's gland**
    DEF: Bartholin's gland: Mucous-producing gland found in the vestibular bulbs on either side of the vaginal orifice and connected to the mucosal membrane at the opening by a duct.

N75.0   **Cyst of Bartholin's gland**
N75.1   **Abscess of Bartholin's gland**   <kbd>CC</kbd>
N75.8   **Other diseases of Bartholin's gland**
    Bartholinitis
N75.9   **Disease of Bartholin's gland, unspecified**

✓4th **N76**   **Other inflammation of vagina and vulva**
    Use additional code (B95-B97), to identify infectious agent
    EXCLUDES 2   senile (atrophic) vaginitis (N95.2)
                   vulvar vestibulitis (N94.810)

N76.0   **Acute vaginitis**
    Acute vulvovaginitis
    Vaginitis NOS
    Vulvovaginitis NOS

N76.1   **Subacute and chronic vaginitis**
    Chronic vulvovaginitis
    Subacute vulvovaginitis

N76.2   **Acute vulvitis**
    Vulvitis NOS

N76.3   **Subacute and chronic vulvitis**
N76.4   **Abscess of vulva**   <kbd>CC</kbd>
    Furuncle of vulva
N76.5   **Ulceration of vagina**
N76.6   **Ulceration of vulva**

✓5th **N76.8**   **Other specified inflammation of vagina and vulva**
    N76.81   **Mucositis (ulcerative) of vagina and vulva**   <kbd>CC</kbd>
        Code also type of associated therapy, such as:
            antineoplastic and immunosuppressive drugs (T45.1X-)
            radiological procedure and radiotherapy (Y84.2)
        EXCLUDES 2   gastrointestinal mucositis (ulcerative) (K92.81)
                       nasal mucositis (ulcerative) (J34.81)
                       oral mucositis (ulcerative) (K12.3-)

    N76.82   **Fournier disease of vagina and vulva**   <kbd>HCC</kbd>
        Fournier gangrene of vagina and vulva
        Code also, if applicable, diabetes mellitus (E08-E13 with .9)
        EXCLUDES 1   gangrene in diabetes mellitus (E08-E13 with .52)
        AHA: 2022,4Q,34

    N76.89   **Other specified inflammation of vagina and vulva**

✓4th **N77**   **Vulvovaginal ulceration and inflammation in diseases classified elsewhere**
    N77.0   *Ulceration of vulva in diseases classified elsewhere*
        Code first underlying disease, such as:
        Behcet's disease (M35.2)
        EXCLUDES 1   ulceration of vulva in gonococcal infection (A54.02)
                       ulceration of vulva in herpesviral [herpes simplex] infection (A60.04)
                       ulceration of vulva in syphilis (A51.0)
                       ulceration of vulva in tuberculosis (A18.18)

<kbd>N</kbd> Newborn: 0   <kbd>P</kbd> Pediatric: 0-17   <kbd>M</kbd> Maternity: 9-64   <kbd>A</kbd> Adult: 15-124   <kbd>UNS</kbd> Unspecified Site   <kbd>MCC</kbd> Major Complication/Comorbidity   <kbd>CC</kbd> Complication/Comorbidity   <kbd>PE</kbd> POA Exempt

870   ICD-10-CM 2025

N77.1   *Vaginitis, vulvitis and vulvovaginitis in diseases classified elsewhere*

Code first underlying disease, such as:
pinworm (B80)

EXCLUDES 1   candidal vulvovaginitis (B37.3-)
chlamydial vulvovaginitis (A56.02)
gonococcal vulvovaginitis (A54.02)
herpesviral [herpes simplex] vulvovaginitis (A60.04)
trichomonal vulvovaginitis (A59.01)
tuberculous vulvovaginitis (A18.18)
vulvovaginitis in early syphilis (A51.0)
vulvovaginitis in late syphilis (A52.76)

Noninflammatory disorders of female genital tract (N80-N98)

N80   **Endometriosis**

AHA: 2022,4Q,34-36
DEF: Aberrant uterine mucosal tissue appearing in areas of the pelvic cavity outside of its normal location, lining the uterus, and inflaming surrounding tissues often resulting in infertility or spontaneous abortion.

N80.0   **Endometriosis of uterus**

Endometriosis of the cervix
EXCLUDES 1   stromal endometriosis (D39.0)

N80.00   Endometriosis of the uterus, unspecified
N80.01   **Superficial** endometriosis of the uterus
N80.02   **Deep** endometriosis of the uterus
Deep retrocervical endometriosis
N80.03   **Adenomyosis** of the uterus
Adenomyosis NOS

N80.1   **Endometriosis of ovary**

N80.10   Endometriosis of ovary, unspecified depth
    N80.101   Endometriosis of **right** ovary, unspecified depth
    N80.102   Endometriosis of **left** ovary, unspecified depth
    N80.103   Endometriosis of **bilateral** ovaries, unspecified depth
    N80.109   Endometriosis of ovary, unspecified side, unspecified depth
       Endometriosis of ovary NOS

N80.11   **Superficial** endometriosis of the ovary
    N80.111   Superficial endometriosis of **right** ovary
       AHA: 2022,4Q,35
    N80.112   Superficial endometriosis of **left** ovary
    N80.113   Superficial endometriosis of **bilateral** ovaries
    N80.119   Superficial endometriosis of ovary, unspecified ovary

N80.12   **Deep** endometriosis of ovary
Deep ovarian endometriosis
Endometrioma
    N80.121   Deep endometriosis of **right** ovary
    N80.122   Deep endometriosis of **left** ovary
    N80.123   Deep endometriosis of **bilateral** ovaries
    N80.129   Deep endometriosis of ovary, unspecified ovary

N80.2   **Endometriosis of fallopian tube**

N80.20   Endometriosis of fallopian tube, unspecified depth
    N80.201   Endometriosis of **right** fallopian tube, unspecified depth
    N80.202   Endometriosis of **left** fallopian tube, unspecified depth
    N80.203   Endometriosis of **bilateral** fallopian tubes, unspecified depth
    N80.209   Endometriosis of unspecified fallopian tube, unspecified depth
       Endometriosis fallopian tube NOS

N80.21   **Superficial** endometriosis of fallopian tube
    N80.211   Superficial endometriosis of **right** fallopian tube
    N80.212   Superficial endometriosis of **left** fallopian tube
    N80.213   Superficial endometriosis of **bilateral** fallopian tubes
    N80.219   Superficial endometriosis of unspecified fallopian tube

N80.22   **Deep** endometriosis of the fallopian tube
Deep endometriosis involving muscular wall of fallopian tube
    N80.221   Deep endometriosis of **right** fallopian tube
    N80.222   Deep endometriosis of **left** fallopian tube
    N80.223   Deep endometriosis of **bilateral** fallopian tubes
    N80.229   Deep endometriosis of unspecified fallopian tube

N80.3   **Endometriosis of pelvic peritoneum**

N80.30   Endometriosis of pelvic peritoneum, unspecified
Endometriosis of the retroperitoneum NOS

N80.31   Endometriosis of the **anterior cul-de-sac**
    N80.311   **Superficial** endometriosis of the anterior cul-de-sac
    N80.312   **Deep** endometriosis of the anterior cul-de-sac
    N80.319   Endometriosis of the anterior cul-de-sac, unspecified depth
       Endometriosis of the anterior cul-de-sac NOS

N80.32   Endometriosis of the **posterior cul-de-sac**
    N80.321   **Superficial** endometriosis of the posterior cul-de-sac
    N80.322   **Deep** endometriosis of the posterior cul-de-sac
    N80.329   Endometriosis of the posterior cul-de-sac, unspecified depth
       Endometriosis of the posterior cul-de-sac NOS

N80.33   **Superficial** endometriosis of the **pelvic sidewall**
    N80.331   Superficial endometriosis of the **right** pelvic sidewall
    N80.332   Superficial endometriosis of the **left** pelvic sidewall
    N80.333   Superficial endometriosis of **bilateral** pelvic sidewall
    N80.339   Superficial endometriosis of pelvic sidewall, unspecified side

N80.34   **Deep** endometriosis of the **pelvic sidewall**
    N80.341   Deep endometriosis of the **right** pelvic sidewall
    N80.342   Deep endometriosis of the **left** pelvic sidewall
    N80.343   Deep endometriosis of the **bilateral** pelvic sidewall
    N80.349   Deep endometriosis of the pelvic sidewall, unspecified side
       AHA: 2022,4Q,36

N80.35   Endometriosis of the pelvic sidewall, unspecified depth
    N80.351   Endometriosis of the **right** pelvic sidewall, unspecified depth
    N80.352   Endometriosis of the **left** pelvic sidewall, unspecified depth
    N80.353   Endometriosis of **bilateral** pelvic sidewall, unspecified depth
    N80.359   Endometriosis of pelvic sidewall, unspecified side, unspecified depth
       Endometriosis of the pelvic sidewall NOS

N80.36   **Superficial** endometriosis of the **pelvic brim**
    N80.361   Superficial endometriosis of the **right** pelvic brim
    N80.362   Superficial endometriosis of the **left** pelvic brim
    N80.363   Superficial endometriosis of **bilateral** pelvic brim
    N80.369   Superficial endometriosis of the pelvic brim, unspecified side

N80.37   **Deep** endometriosis of the **pelvic brim**
    N80.371   Deep endometriosis of the **right** pelvic brim
    N80.372   Deep endometriosis of the **left** pelvic brim
    N80.373   Deep endometriosis of **bilateral** pelvic brim
    N80.379   Deep endometriosis of the pelvic brim, unspecified side

N80.38   Endometriosis of the pelvic brim, unspecified depth
    N80.381   Endometriosis of the **right** pelvic brim, unspecified depth
    N80.382   Endometriosis of the **left** pelvic brim, unspecified depth

Chapter 14. Diseases of the Genitourinary System *(side tab)*

N80.383   Endometriosis of **bilateral** pelvic brim, unspecified depth

N80.389   Endometriosis of the pelvic brim, unspecified side, unspecified depth
     Endometriosis of the pelvic brim NOS

✓6ᵗʰ   **N80.3A**   **Superficial** endometriosis of the **uterosacral ligament(s)**

     N80.3A1   Superficial endometriosis of the **right** uterosacral ligament

     N80.3A2   Superficial endometriosis of the **left** uterosacral ligament

     N80.3A3   Superficial endometriosis of the **bilateral** uterosacral ligament(s)

     N80.3A9   Superficial endometriosis of the uterosacral ligament(s), unspecified side

✓6ᵗʰ   **N80.3B**   **Deep** endometriosis of the **uterosacral ligament(s)**

     N80.3B1   Deep endometriosis of the **right** uterosacral ligament

     N80.3B2   Deep endometriosis of the **left** uterosacral ligament

     N80.3B3   Deep endometriosis of **bilateral** uterosacral ligament(s)

     N80.3B9   Deep endometriosis of the uterosacral ligament(s), unspecified side

✓6ᵗʰ   **N80.3C**   Endometriosis of the **uterosacral ligament(s)**, unspecified depth

     N80.3C1   Endometriosis of the **right** uterosacral ligament, unspecified depth

     N80.3C2   Endometriosis of the **left** uterosacral ligament, unspecified depth

     N80.3C3   Endometriosis of **bilateral** uterosacral ligament(s), unspecified depth

     N80.3C9   Endometriosis of the uterosacral ligament(s), unspecified side, unspecified depth
       Endometriosis of the uterosacral ligament(s) NOS

✓6ᵗʰ   **N80.39**   Endometriosis of other pelvic peritoneum

     N80.391   **Superficial** endometriosis of the pelvic peritoneum, other specified sites

     N80.392   **Deep** endometriosis of the pelvic peritoneum, other specified sites

     N80.399   Endometriosis of the pelvic peritoneum, other specified sites, unspecified depth

✓5ᵗʰ   **N80.4**   Endometriosis of **rectovaginal septum and vagina**

     N80.40   Endometriosis of rectovaginal septum, unspecified involvement of vagina
       Endometriosis of the rectovaginal septum, NOS

     N80.41   Endometriosis of rectovaginal septum **without involvement of vagina**

     N80.42   Endometriosis of rectovaginal septum **with involvement of vagina**

✓5ᵗʰ   **N80.5**   Endometriosis of **intestine**

     N80.50   Endometriosis of intestine, unspecified

✓6ᵗʰ   **N80.51**   Endometriosis of the **rectum**

     N80.511   **Superficial** endometriosis of the rectum

     N80.512   **Deep** endometriosis of the rectum
       Deep endometriosis of the rectum, multifocal

     N80.519   Endometriosis of the rectum, unspecified depth
       Endometriosis of the rectum NOS

✓6ᵗʰ   **N80.52**   Endometriosis of the **sigmoid colon**

     N80.521   **Superficial** endometriosis of the sigmoid colon

     N80.522   **Deep** endometriosis of the sigmoid colon

     N80.529   Endometriosis of the sigmoid colon, unspecified depth
       Endometriosis of the sigmoid colon NOS

✓6ᵗʰ   **N80.53**   Endometriosis of the **cecum**

     N80.531   **Superficial** endometriosis of the cecum

     N80.532   **Deep** endometriosis of the cecum

     N80.539   Endometriosis of the cecum, unspecified depth
       Endometriosis of the cecum NOS

✓6ᵗʰ   **N80.54**   Endometriosis of the **appendix**

     N80.541   **Superficial** endometriosis of the appendix

     N80.542   **Deep** endometriosis of the appendix

N80.549   Endometriosis of the appendix, unspecified depth
     Endometriosis of the appendix NOS

✓6ᵗʰ   **N80.55**   Endometriosis of other parts of the **colon**
     Endometriosis of descending colon
     Endometriosis of transverse colon

     N80.551   **Superficial** endometriosis of other parts of the colon

     N80.552   **Deep** endometriosis of other parts of the colon

     N80.559   Endometriosis of other parts of the colon, unspecified depth
       Endometriosis of colon NOS

✓6ᵗʰ   **N80.56**   Endometriosis of the **small intestine**

     N80.561   **Superficial** endometriosis of the small intestine

     N80.562   **Deep** endometriosis of the small intestine
       Deep endometriosis of the small intestine, multifocal

     N80.569   Endometriosis of the small intestine, unspecified depth
       Endometriosis of the small intestine NOS

N80.6   Endometriosis in **cutaneous scar**

✓5ᵗʰ   **N80.A**   Endometriosis of bladder and ureters

     N80.A0   Endometriosis of **bladder**, unspecified depth
       Endometriosis of bladder NOS

     N80.A1   **Superficial** endometriosis of **bladder**

     N80.A2   **Deep** endometriosis of **bladder**

✓6ᵗʰ   **N80.A4**   **Superficial** endometriosis of **ureter**
     Extrinsic endometriosis of ureter
     Code also, if applicable, obstructive and reflux uropathy (N13.-)

     N80.A41   Superficial endometriosis of **right** ureter

     N80.A42   Superficial endometriosis of **left** ureter

     N80.A43   Superficial endometriosis of **bilateral** ureters

     N80.A49   Superficial endometriosis of unspecified ureter

✓6ᵗʰ   **N80.A5**   **Deep** endometriosis of **ureter**
     Intrinsic endometriosis of ureter
     Code also, if applicable, obstructive and reflux uropathy (N13.-)

     N80.A51   Deep endometriosis of **right** ureter

     N80.A52   Deep endometriosis of **left** ureter

     N80.A53   Deep endometriosis of **bilateral** ureters

     N80.A59   Deep endometriosis of unspecified ureter

✓6ᵗʰ   **N80.A6**   Endometriosis of **ureter**, unspecified depth
     Code also, if applicable, obstructive and reflux uropathy (N13.-)

     N80.A61   Endometriosis of **right** ureter, unspecified depth

     N80.A62   Endometriosis of **left** ureter, unspecified depth

     N80.A63   Endometriosis of **bilateral** ureters, unspecified depth

     N80.A69   Endometriosis of unspecified ureter, unspecified depth

✓5ᵗʰ   **N80.B**   Endometriosis of **cardiothoracic space**
     Endometriosis of thorax
     Code also, if applicable:
       catamenial hemothorax (J94.2)
       catamenial pneumothorax (J93.12)

     N80.B1   Endometriosis of **pleura**

     N80.B2   Endometriosis of **lung**

✓6ᵗʰ   **N80.B3**   Endometriosis of **diaphragm**

     N80.B31   **Superficial** endometriosis of diaphragm

     N80.B32   **Deep** endometriosis of diaphragm

     N80.B39   Endometriosis of diaphragm, unspecified depth
       Endometriosis of the diaphragm NOS

     N80.B4   Endometriosis of the **pericardial space**

     N80.B5   Endometriosis of the **mediastinal space**

     N80.B6   Endometriosis of **cardiothoracic space**

✓5ᵗʰ   **N80.C**   Endometriosis of the **abdomen**

     N80.C0   Endometriosis of the abdomen, unspecified
       Endometriosis of the abdomen NOS

✓6ᵗʰ   **N80.C1**   Endometriosis of the **anterior** abdominal wall

     N80.C10   Endometriosis of the anterior abdominal wall, **subcutaneous tissue**

N Newborn: 0   **P** Pediatric: 0-17   **M** Maternity: 9-64   **A** Adult: 15-124   **UNS** Unspecified Site   **MCC** Major Complication/Comorbidity   **CC** Complication/Comorbidity   **PE** POA Exempt

872   ICD-10-CM 2025

N80.C11   **Endometriosis of the anterior abdominal wall, fascia and muscular layers**

N80.C19   **Endometriosis of the anterior abdominal wall, unspecified depth**
Endometriosis of the anterior abdominal wall NOS

N80.C2   **Endometriosis of the umbilicus**

N80.C3   **Endometriosis of the inguinal canal**

N80.C4   **Endometriosis of extra-pelvic abdominal peritoneum**

N80.C9   **Endometriosis of other site of abdomen**

✓5th **N80.D**   **Endometriosis of the pelvic nerves**
Endometriosis of the nerves of the retroperitoneum

N80.D0   **Endometriosis of the pelvic nerves, unspecified**
Endometriosis of nerve of the retroperitoneum, NOS

N80.D1   **Endometriosis of the sacral splanchnic nerves**
Endometriosis of the pelvic splanchnic nerves

N80.D2   **Endometriosis of the sacral nerve roots**

N80.D3   **Endometriosis of the obturator nerve**

N80.D4   **Endometriosis of the sciatic nerve**

N80.D5   **Endometriosis of the pudendal nerve**

N80.D6   **Endometriosis of the femoral nerve**

N80.D9   **Endometriosis of other pelvic nerve**
Endometriosis of the other nerves of the retroperitoneum

N80.8   **Other endometriosis**
Endometriosis of other site

N80.9   **Endometriosis, unspecified**

✓4th **N81**   **Female genital prolapse**
     EXCLUDES 1   genital prolapse complicating pregnancy, labor or delivery (O34.5-)
           prolapse and hernia of ovary and fallopian tube (N83.4-)
           prolapse of vaginal vault after hysterectomy (N99.3)

Types of Pelvic Organ Prolapse

Urethrocele   Cystocele

Rectocele   Enterocele

N81.0   **Urethrocele**
     EXCLUDES 1   urethrocele with cystocele (N81.1-)
           urethrocele with prolapse of uterus (N81.2-N81.4)

✓5th **N81.1**   **Cystocele**
Cystocele with urethrocele
Cystourethrocele
     EXCLUDES 1   cystocele with prolapse of uterus (N81.2-N81.4)

N81.10   **Cystocele, unspecified**
Prolapse of (anterior) vaginal wall NOS

N81.11   **Cystocele, midline**

N81.12   **Cystocele, lateral**
Paravaginal cystocele
DEF: Detachment of the lateral support connections of the vagina at the arcus tendineus fasciae pelvis (ATFP) that results in bladder drop. The bladder herniates into the vagina laterally.

N81.2   **Incomplete uterovaginal prolapse**
First degree uterine prolapse
Prolapse of cervix NOS
Second degree uterine prolapse
     EXCLUDES 1   cervical stump prolapse (N81.85)

N81.3   **Complete uterovaginal prolapse**
Procidentia (uteri) NOS
Third degree uterine prolapse

N81.4   **Uterovaginal prolapse, unspecified**
Prolapse of uterus NOS

N81.5   **Vaginal enterocele**
     EXCLUDES 1   enterocele with prolapse of uterus (N81.2-N81.4)

N81.6   **Rectocele**
Prolapse of posterior vaginal wall
Use additional code for any associated fecal incontinence, if applicable (R15.-)
     EXCLUDES 1   rectocele with prolapse of uterus (N81.2-N81.4)
     EXCLUDES 2   perineocele (N81.81)
           rectal prolapse (K62.3)

✓5th **N81.8**   **Other female genital prolapse**

N81.81   **Perineocele**

N81.82   **Incompetence or weakening of pubocervical tissue**

N81.83   **Incompetence or weakening of rectovaginal tissue**

N81.84   **Pelvic muscle wasting**
Disuse atrophy of pelvic muscles and anal sphincter

N81.85   **Cervical stump prolapse**

N81.89   **Other female genital prolapse**
Deficient perineum
Old laceration of muscles of pelvic floor

N81.9   **Female genital prolapse, unspecified**

✓4th **N82**   **Fistulae involving female genital tract**
     EXCLUDES 1   vesicointestinal fistulae (N32.1)

N82.0   **Vesicovaginal fistula**   `cc`

N82.1   **Other female urinary-genital tract fistulae**   `cc`
Cervicovesical fistula
Ureterovaginal fistula
Urethrovaginal fistula
Uteroureteric fistula
Uterovesical fistula
AHA: 2017,3Q,3

N82.2   **Fistula of vagina to small intestine**   `cc`

N82.3   **Fistula of vagina to large intestine**   `cc`
Rectovaginal fistula

N82.4   **Other female intestinal-genital tract fistulae**   `cc`
Intestinouterine fistula

N82.5   **Female genital tract-skin fistulae**   `cc`
Uterus to abdominal wall fistula
Vaginoperineal fistula

N82.8   **Other female genital tract fistulae**   `cc`

N82.9   **Female genital tract fistula, unspecified**   `cc`

✓4th **N83**   **Noninflammatory disorders of ovary, fallopian tube and broad ligament**
     EXCLUDES 2   hydrosalpinx (N70.1-)
AHA: 2016,4Q,46

✓5th **N83.0**   **Follicular cyst of ovary**
Cyst of graafian follicle
Hemorrhagic follicular cyst (of ovary)

N83.00   **Follicular cyst of ovary, unspecified side**

N83.01   **Follicular cyst of right ovary**

N83.02   **Follicular cyst of left ovary**

✓5th **N83.1**   **Corpus luteum cyst**
Hemorrhagic corpus luteum cyst
AHA: 2022,1Q,23

N83.10   **Corpus luteum cyst of ovary, unspecified side**

N83.11   **Corpus luteum cyst of right ovary**

N83.12   **Corpus luteum cyst of left ovary**

✓5th **N83.2**   **Other and unspecified ovarian cysts**
     EXCLUDES 1   developmental ovarian cyst (Q50.1)
           neoplastic ovarian cyst (D27.-)
           polycystic ovarian syndrome (E28.2)
           Stein-Leventhal syndrome (E28.2)
AHA: 2022,1Q,23

✓6th **N83.20**   **Unspecified ovarian cysts**

N83.201   **Unspecified ovarian cyst, right side**

N83.202   **Unspecified ovarian cyst, left side**

N83.209   **Unspecified ovarian cyst, unspecified side**
Ovarian cyst, NOS

✓6th **N83.29**   **Other ovarian cysts**
Retention cyst of ovary
Simple cyst of ovary

N83.291   **Other ovarian cyst, right side**

✓ Additional Character Required   ✓x7th Placeholder   Questionable PDx   Manifestation   Unspecified   UPD Unacceptable PDx   H1 - H14 HAC   HCC CMS-HCC Dx   HIV HIV Dx

ICD-10-CM 2025   873

N83.292 Other ovarian cyst, **left** side

N83.299 Other ovarian cyst, unspecified side

✓5th **N83.3** **Acquired atrophy** of ovary and fallopian tube

  ✓6th **N83.31** Acquired atrophy of **ovary**

N83.311 Acquired atrophy of **right** ovary

N83.312 Acquired atrophy of **left** ovary

N83.319 Acquired atrophy of ovary, unspecified side
    Acquired atrophy of ovary, NOS

  ✓6th **N83.32** Acquired atrophy of **fallopian tube**

N83.321 Acquired atrophy of **right** fallopian tube

N83.322 Acquired atrophy of **left** fallopian tube

N83.329 Acquired atrophy of fallopian tube, unspecified side
    Acquired atrophy of fallopian tube, NOS

  ✓6th **N83.33** Acquired atrophy of **ovary and fallopian tube**

N83.331 Acquired atrophy of **right** ovary and fallopian tube

N83.332 Acquired atrophy of **left** ovary and fallopian tube

N83.339 Acquired atrophy of ovary and fallopian tube, unspecified side
    Acquired atrophy of ovary and fallopian tube, NOS

✓5th **N83.4** **Prolapse and hernia** of ovary and fallopian tube

N83.40 Prolapse and hernia of ovary and fallopian tube, unspecified side
    Prolapse and hernia of ovary and fallopian tube, NOS

N83.41 Prolapse and hernia of **right** ovary and fallopian tube

N83.42 Prolapse and hernia of **left** ovary and fallopian tube

✓5th **N83.5** **Torsion** of ovary, ovarian pedicle and fallopian tube
  Torsion of accessory tube

  ✓6th **N83.51** Torsion of **ovary and ovarian pedicle**

N83.511 Torsion of **right** ovary and ovarian pedicle `CC`

N83.512 Torsion of **left** ovary and ovarian pedicle `CC`

N83.519 Torsion of ovary and ovarian pedicle, unspecified side `CC` `UNS`
    Torsion of ovary and ovarian pedicle, NOS

  ✓6th **N83.52** Torsion of **fallopian tube**
    Torsion of hydatid of Morgagni

N83.521 Torsion of **right** fallopian tube `CC`

N83.522 Torsion of **left** fallopian tube `CC`

N83.529 Torsion of fallopian tube, unspecified side `CC` `UNS`
    Torsion of fallopian tube, NOS

  N83.53 Torsion of **ovary, ovarian pedicle and fallopian tube** `CC`

N83.6 **Hematosalpinx**
  EXCLUDES 1 *hematosalpinx (with) (in):*
      hematocolpos (N89.7)
      hematometra (N85.7)
      tubal pregnancy (O00.1-)

N83.7 **Hematoma of broad ligament**

N83.8 **Other noninflammatory disorders of ovary, fallopian tube and broad ligament**
  Broad ligament laceration syndrome [Allen-Masters]

N83.9 **Noninflammatory disorder of ovary, fallopian tube and broad ligament, unspecified**

✓4th **N84** **Polyp of female genital tract**
  EXCLUDES 1 *adenomatous polyp (D28.-)*
      ▾ *placental polyp (O90.89)*

N84.0 Polyp of **corpus uteri**
  Polyp of endometrium
  Polyp of uterus NOS
  EXCLUDES 1 *polypoid endometrial hyperplasia (N85.0-)*

N84.1 Polyp of **cervix uteri**
  Mucous polyp of cervix

N84.2 Polyp of **vagina**

N84.3 Polyp of **vulva**
  Polyp of labia

N84.8 Polyp of other parts of female genital tract

N84.9 Polyp of female genital tract, unspecified

✓4th **N85** **Other noninflammatory disorders of uterus, except cervix**
  EXCLUDES 1 *endometriosis (N80.-)*
      inflammatory diseases of uterus (N71.-)
      noninflammatory disorders of cervix, except malposition (N86-N88)
      polyp of corpus uteri (N84.0)
      uterine prolapse (N81.-)

✓5th **N85.0** **Endometrial hyperplasia**

  N85.00 **Endometrial hyperplasia, unspecified**
    Hyperplasia (adenomatous) (cystic) (glandular) of endometrium
    Hyperplastic endometritis

  N85.01 **Benign** endometrial hyperplasia
    Endometrial hyperplasia (complex) (simple) without atypia

  N85.02 **Endometrial intraepithelial neoplasia [EIN]**
    Endometrial hyperplasia with atypia
    EXCLUDES 1 *malignant neoplasm of endometrium (with endometrial intraepithelial neoplasia [EIN]) (C54.1)*

N85.2 **Hypertrophy of uterus**
  Bulky or enlarged uterus
  EXCLUDES 1 *puerperal hypertrophy of uterus (O90.89)*

N85.3 **Subinvolution of uterus**
  EXCLUDES 1 *puerperal subinvolution of uterus (O90.89)*

N85.4 **Malposition of uterus**
  Anteversion of uterus
  Retroflexion of uterus
  Retroversion of uterus
  EXCLUDES 1 *malposition of uterus complicating pregnancy, labor or delivery (O34.5-, O65.5)*

N85.5 **Inversion of uterus**
  EXCLUDES 1 *current obstetric trauma (O71.2)*
      postpartum inversion of uterus (O71.2)
  DEF: Abnormality in which the uterus turns inside out.

Inversion of Uterus

Uterus

N85.6 **Intrauterine synechiae**

N85.7 **Hematometra**
  Hematosalpinx with hematometra
  EXCLUDES 1 *hematometra with hematocolpos (N89.7)*
  DEF: Accumulation of blood within the uterus.

N85.8 **Other specified noninflammatory disorders of uterus**
  Atrophy of uterus, acquired
  Fibrosis of uterus NOS

N85.9 **Noninflammatory disorder of uterus, unspecified**
  Disorder of uterus NOS

N85.A **Isthmocele**
  Isthmocele (non-pregnant state)
  Code also any associated conditions such as:
    abnormal uterine and vaginal bleeding, unspecified (N93.9)
    female infertility of uterine origin (N97.2)
    pelvic and perineal pain (R10.2)
  EXCLUDES 1 *maternal care for cesarean scar defect (isthmocele) (O34.22)*
  AHA: 2022,4Q,36-37

N86 **Erosion and ectropion of cervix uteri**
  Decubitus (trophic) ulcer of cervix
  Eversion of cervix
  EXCLUDES 1 *erosion and ectropion of cervix with cervicitis (N72)*

`N` Newborn: 0   `P` Pediatric: 0-17   `M` Maternity: 9-64   `A` Adult: 15-124   `UNS` Unspecified Site   `MCC` Major Complication/Comorbidity   `CC` Complication/Comorbidity   `PE` POA Exempt

874

ICD-10-CM 2025

✓4ᵗʰ **N87 Dysplasia of cervix uteri**

EXCLUDES 1   *abnormal results from cervical cytologic examination without*
     histologic confirmation (R87.61-)
carcinoma in situ of cervix uteri (D06.-)
cervical intraepithelial neoplasia III [CIN III] (D06.-)
HGSIL of cervix (R87.613)
severe dysplasia of cervix uteri (D06.-)

N87.0 Mild cervical dysplasia
Cervical intraepithelial neoplasia I [CIN I]

N87.1 Moderate cervical dysplasia
Cervical intraepithelial neoplasia II [CIN II]

N87.9 Dysplasia of cervix uteri, unspecified
Anaplasia of cervix
Cervical atypism
Cervical dysplasia NOS

✓4ᵗʰ **N88 Other noninflammatory disorders of cervix uteri**

EXCLUDES 2   *inflammatory disease of cervix (N72)*
polyp of cervix (N84.1)

N88.0 Leukoplakia of cervix uteri
N88.1 Old laceration of cervix uteri
Adhesions of cervix
EXCLUDES 1   *current obstetric trauma (O71.3)*

N88.2 Stricture and stenosis of cervix uteri
EXCLUDES 1   *stricture and stenosis of cervix uteri complicating labor*
     (O65.5)

N88.3 Incompetence of cervix uteri
Investigation and management of (suspected) cervical
incompetence in a nonpregnant woman
EXCLUDES 1   *cervical incompetence complicating pregnancy*
     (O34.3-)

DEF: Inadequate functioning of the cervix marked by abnormal
widening during pregnancy and causing premature birth or
miscarriage.

N88.4 Hypertrophic elongation of cervix uteri
N88.8 Other specified noninflammatory disorders of cervix uteri
EXCLUDES 1   *current obstetric trauma (O71.3)*
N88.9 Noninflammatory disorder of cervix uteri, unspecified

✓4ᵗʰ **N89 Other noninflammatory disorders of vagina**

EXCLUDES 1   *abnormal results from vaginal cytologic examination without*
     histologic confirmation (R87.62-)
carcinoma in situ of vagina (D07.2)
HGSIL of vagina (R87.623)
inflammation of vagina (N76.-)
senile (atrophic) vaginitis (N95.2)
severe dysplasia of vagina (D07.2)
trichomonal leukorrhea (A59.00)
vaginal intraepithelial neoplasia [VAIN], grade III (D07.2)

N89.0 Mild vaginal dysplasia
Vaginal intraepithelial neoplasia [VAIN], grade I

N89.1 Moderate vaginal dysplasia
Vaginal intraepithelial neoplasia [VAIN], grade II

N89.3 Dysplasia of vagina, unspecified
N89.4 Leukoplakia of vagina
N89.5 Stricture and atresia of vagina
Vaginal adhesions
Vaginal stenosis
EXCLUDES 1   *congenital atresia or stricture (Q52.4)*
     postprocedural adhesions of vagina (N99.2)

N89.6 Tight hymenal ring
Rigid hymen
Tight introitus
EXCLUDES 1   *imperforate hymen (Q52.3)*

N89.7 Hematocolpos
Hematocolpos with hematometra or hematosalpinx
AHA: 2016,4Q,58

N89.8 Other specified noninflammatory disorders of vagina
Leukorrhea NOS
Old vaginal laceration
Pessary ulcer of vagina
EXCLUDES 1   *current obstetric trauma (O70.-, O71.4, O71.7-O71.8)*
     old laceration involving muscles of pelvic floor (N81.8)

N89.9 Noninflammatory disorder of vagina, unspecified

✓4ᵗʰ **N90 Other noninflammatory disorders of vulva and perineum**

EXCLUDES 1   *anogenital (venereal) warts (A63.0)*
carcinoma in situ of vulva (D07.1)
condyloma acuminatum (A63.0)
current obstetric trauma (O70.-, O71.7-O71.8)
inflammation of vulva (N76.-)
severe dysplasia of vulva (D07.1)
vulvar intraepithelial neoplasm III [VIN III] (D07.1)

N90.0 Mild vulvar dysplasia
Vulvar intraepithelial neoplasia [VIN], grade I

N90.1 Moderate vulvar dysplasia
Vulvar intraepithelial neoplasia [VIN], grade II

N90.3 Dysplasia of vulva, unspecified
N90.4 Leukoplakia of vulva
Dystrophy of vulva
Kraurosis of vulva
Lichen sclerosus of external female genital organs

N90.5 Atrophy of vulva
Stenosis of vulva

✓5ᵗʰ **N90.6 Hypertrophy of vulva**
AHA: 2016,4Q,46

N90.60 Unspecified hypertrophy of vulva
Unspecified hypertrophy of labia

N90.61 Childhood asymmetric labium majus enlargement
CALME

N90.69 Other specified hypertrophy of vulva
Other specified hypertrophy of labia

N90.7 Vulvar cyst

✓5ᵗʰ **N90.8 Other specified noninflammatory disorders of vulva and perineum**

✓6ᵗʰ **N90.81 Female genital mutilation status**
Female genital cutting status

N90.810 Female genital mutilation status, unspecified
Female genital cutting status, unspecified
Female genital mutilation status NOS

N90.811 Female genital mutilation Type I status
Clitorectomy status
Female genital cutting Type I status

N90.812 Female genital mutilation Type II status
Clitorectomy with excision of labia minora status
Female genital cutting Type II status

N90.813 Female genital mutilation Type III status
Female genital cutting Type III status
Infibulation status

N90.818 Other female genital mutilation status
Female genital cutting Type IV status
Female genital mutilation Type IV status
Other female genital cutting status

N90.89 Other specified noninflammatory disorders of vulva and perineum
Adhesions of vulva
Hypertrophy of clitoris

N90.9 Noninflammatory disorder of vulva and perineum, unspecified

✓4ᵗʰ **N91 Absent, scanty and rare menstruation**

EXCLUDES 1   *ovarian dysfunction (E28.-)*

N91.0 Primary amenorrhea
N91.1 Secondary amenorrhea
N91.2 Amenorrhea, unspecified
N91.3 Primary oligomenorrhea
N91.4 Secondary oligomenorrhea
N91.5 Oligomenorrhea, unspecified
Hypomenorrhea NOS

✓4ᵗʰ **N92 Excessive, frequent and irregular menstruation**

EXCLUDES 1   *postmenopausal bleeding (N95.0)*
precocious puberty (menstruation) (E30.1)

N92.0 Excessive and frequent menstruation with regular cycle
Heavy periods NOS
Menorrhagia NOS
Polymenorrhea

N92.1 Excessive and frequent menstruation with irregular cycle
Irregular intermenstrual bleeding
Irregular, shortened intervals between menstrual bleeding
Menometrorrhagia
Metrorrhagia

N92.2 Excessive menstruation at puberty   P
Excessive bleeding associated with onset of menstrual periods
Pubertal menorrhagia
Puberty bleeding

N92.3 Ovulation bleeding
Regular intermenstrual bleeding

N92.4 Excessive bleeding in the premenopausal period
Climacteric menorrhagia or metrorrhagia
Menopausal menorrhagia or metrorrhagia
Perimenopausal bleeding
Perimenopausal menorrhagia or metrorrhagia
Preclimacteric menorrhagia or metrorrhagia
Premenopausal menorrhagia or metrorrhagia

N92.5 Other specified irregular menstruation

N92.6 Irregular menstruation, unspecified
Irregular bleeding NOS
Irregular periods NOS
    EXCLUDES 1   *irregular menstruation with:*
        lengthened intervals or scanty bleeding
         (N91.3-N91.5)
        shortened intervals or excessive bleeding (N92.1)

✓4th **N93 Other abnormal uterine and vaginal bleeding**
    EXCLUDES 1   *neonatal vaginal hemorrhage (P54.6)*
        precocious puberty (menstruation) (E30.1)
        pseudomenses (P54.6)

N93.0 Postcoital and contact bleeding

N93.1 Pre-pubertal vaginal bleeding
    AHA: 2016,4Q,47

N93.8 Other specified abnormal uterine and vaginal bleeding
Dysfunctional or functional uterine or vaginal bleeding NOS

N93.9 Abnormal uterine and vaginal bleeding, unspecified

✓4th **N94 Pain and other conditions associated with female genital organs and menstrual cycle**

N94.0 Mittelschmerz
    DEF: One-sided, lower abdominal pain occurring between menstrual periods that is associated with ovulation.

✓5th **N94.1 Dyspareunia**
    EXCLUDES 1   *psychogenic dyspareunia (F52.6)*
    AHA: 2016,4Q,47
     N94.10 Unspecified dyspareunia
     N94.11 Superficial (introital) dyspareunia
     N94.12 Deep dyspareunia
     N94.19 Other specified dyspareunia

N94.2 Vaginismus
    EXCLUDES 1   *psychogenic vaginismus (F52.5)*
    DEF: Spontaneous contractions of the muscles surrounding the vagina, causing it to constrict or close.

N94.3 Premenstrual tension syndrome
    Code also associated menstrual migraine (G43.82-, G43.83-)
    EXCLUDES 1   *premenstrual dysphoric disorder (F32.81)*

N94.4 Primary dysmenorrhea

N94.5 Secondary dysmenorrhea

N94.6 Dysmenorrhea, unspecified
    EXCLUDES 1   *psychogenic dysmenorrhea (F45.8)*

✓5th **N94.8 Other specified conditions associated with female genital organs and menstrual cycle**
   ✓6th **N94.81 Vulvodynia**
     N94.810 Vulvar vestibulitis
     N94.818 Other vulvodynia
     N94.819 Vulvodynia, unspecified
       Vulvodynia NOS
     N94.89 Other specified conditions associated with female genital organs and menstrual cycle
       DEF: Hydrocele: Serous fluid that collects in the canal of Nuck in females.

N94.9 Unspecified condition associated with female genital organs and menstrual cycle

✓4th **N95 Menopausal and other perimenopausal disorders**
Menopausal and other perimenopausal disorders due to naturally occurring (age-related) menopause and perimenopause
    EXCLUDES 1   *excessive bleeding in the premenopausal period (N92.4)*
        menopausal and perimenopausal disorders due to artificial or premature menopause (E89.4-, E28.31-)
        premature menopause (E28.31-)
    EXCLUDES 2   *postmenopausal osteoporosis (M81.0-)*
        postmenopausal osteoporosis with current pathological fracture (M80.0-)
        postmenopausal urethritis (N34.2)

N95.0 Postmenopausal bleeding

N95.1 Menopausal and female climacteric states
Symptoms such as flushing, sleeplessness, headache, lack of concentration, associated with natural (age-related) menopause
Use additional code for associated symptoms
    EXCLUDES 1   *asymptomatic menopausal state (Z78.0)*
        symptoms associated with artificial menopause (E89.41)
        symptoms associated with premature menopause (E28.310)

N95.2 Postmenopausal atrophic vaginitis
Senile (atrophic) vaginitis

N95.8 Other specified menopausal and perimenopausal disorders

N95.9 Unspecified menopausal and perimenopausal disorder

N96 Recurrent pregnancy loss
Investigation or care in a nonpregnant woman with history of recurrent pregnancy loss
    EXCLUDES 1   *recurrent pregnancy loss with current pregnancy (O26.2-)*

✓4th **N97 Female infertility**
    INCLUDES   inability to achieve a pregnancy
        sterility, female NOS
    EXCLUDES 2   *female infertility associated with:*
        hypopituitarism (E23.0)
        incompetence of cervix uteri (N88.3)
        Stein-Leventhal syndrome (E28.2)
    DEF: Infertility: Inability to conceive for at least one year with regular intercourse.
    DEF: Primary infertility: Infertility occurring in patients who have never conceived.
    DEF: Secondary infertility: Infertility occurring in patients who have previously conceived.

N97.0 Female infertility associated with anovulation
    AHA: 2022,2Q,16

N97.1 Female infertility of tubal origin
Female infertility associated with congenital anomaly of tube
Female infertility due to tubal block
Female infertility due to tubal occlusion
Female infertility due to tubal stenosis

N97.2 Female infertility of uterine origin
Female infertility associated with congenital anomaly of uterus
Female infertility due to nonimplantation of ovum

N97.8 Female infertility of other origin
    AHA: 2022,2Q,15

N97.9 Female infertility, unspecified

✓4th **N98 Complications associated with artificial fertilization**

N98.0 Infection associated with artificial insemination   CC

N98.1 Hyperstimulation of ovaries   CC
Hyperstimulation of ovaries NOS
Hyperstimulation of ovaries associated with induced ovulation

N98.2 Complications of attempted introduction of fertilized ovum following in vitro fertilization   CC

N98.3 Complications of attempted introduction of embryo in embryo transfer   CC

N98.8 Other complications associated with artificial fertilization   CC

N98.9 Complication associated with artificial fertilization, unspecified   CC

Intraoperative and postprocedural complications and disorders of genitourinary system, not elsewhere classified (N99)

✓4ᵗʰ **N99** **Intraoperative and postprocedural complications and disorders of genitourinary system, not elsewhere classified**

> EXCLUDES 2   irradiation cystitis (N30.4-)
> postoophorectomy osteoporosis with current pathological fracture (M80.8-)
> postoophorectomy osteoporosis without current pathological fracture (M81.8)

N99.0 **Postprocedural (acute) (chronic) kidney failure**
Use additional code to type of kidney disease

✓5ᵗʰ **N99.1** **Postprocedural urethral stricture**
Postcatheterization urethral stricture

  ✓6ᵗʰ **N99.11** **Postprocedural urethral stricture, male**
AHA: 2016,4Q,47-48

    N99.110 **Postprocedural urethral stricture, male, meatal**

    N99.111 **Postprocedural bulbous urethral stricture, male**

    N99.112 **Postprocedural membranous urethral stricture, male**

    N99.113 **Postprocedural anterior bulbous urethral stricture, male**

    N99.114 **Postprocedural urethral stricture, male, unspecified**

    N99.115 **Postprocedural fossa navicularis urethral stricture**

    N99.116 **Postprocedural urethral stricture, male, overlapping sites**

  N99.12 **Postprocedural urethral stricture, female**

N99.2 **Postprocedural adhesions of vagina**

N99.3 **Prolapse of vaginal vault after hysterectomy**

N99.4 **Postprocedural pelvic peritoneal adhesions**

> EXCLUDES 2   pelvic peritoneal adhesions NOS (N73.6)
> postinfective pelvic peritoneal adhesions (N73.6)

✓5ᵗʰ **N99.5** **Complications of stoma of urinary tract**

> EXCLUDES 2   mechanical complication of urinary catheter (T83.0–)

AHA: 2016,4Q,48

  ✓6ᵗʰ **N99.51** **Complication of cystostomy**

    N99.510 **Cystostomy hemorrhage** `CC`

    N99.511 **Cystostomy infection** `CC`

    N99.512 **Cystostomy malfunction** `CC`

    N99.518 **Other cystostomy complication** `CC`

  ✓6ᵗʰ **N99.52** **Complication of incontinent external stoma of urinary tract**

    N99.520 **Hemorrhage of incontinent external stoma of urinary tract**

    N99.521 **Infection of incontinent external stoma of urinary tract**

    N99.522 **Malfunction of incontinent external stoma of urinary tract**

    N99.523 **Herniation of incontinent stoma of urinary tract**

    N99.524 **Stenosis of incontinent stoma of urinary tract**

    N99.528 **Other complication of incontinent external stoma of urinary tract**

  ✓6ᵗʰ **N99.53** **Complication of continent stoma of urinary tract**

    N99.530 **Hemorrhage of continent stoma of urinary tract**

    N99.531 **Infection of continent stoma of urinary tract**

    N99.532 **Malfunction of continent stoma of urinary tract**

    N99.533 **Herniation of continent stoma of urinary tract**

    N99.534 **Stenosis of continent stoma of urinary tract**

    N99.538 **Other complication of continent stoma of urinary tract**

✓5ᵗʰ **N99.6** **Intraoperative hemorrhage and hematoma of a genitourinary system organ or structure complicating a procedure**

> EXCLUDES 1   intraoperative hemorrhage and hematoma of a genitourinary system organ or structure due to accidental puncture or laceration during a procedure (N99.7-)

  N99.61 **Intraoperative hemorrhage and hematoma of a genitourinary system organ or structure complicating a genitourinary system procedure** `CC`

  N99.62 **Intraoperative hemorrhage and hematoma of a genitourinary system organ or structure complicating other procedure** `CC`

✓5ᵗʰ **N99.7** **Accidental puncture and laceration of a genitourinary system organ or structure during a procedure**

  N99.71 **Accidental puncture and laceration of a genitourinary system organ or structure during a genitourinary system procedure** `CC`

  N99.72 **Accidental puncture and laceration of a genitourinary system organ or structure during other procedure** `CC`

✓5ᵗʰ **N99.8** **Other intraoperative and postprocedural complications and disorders of genitourinary system**
AHA: 2016,4Q,9-10

  N99.81 **Other intraoperative complications of genitourinary system**

  ✓6ᵗʰ **N99.82** **Postprocedural hemorrhage of a genitourinary system organ or structure following a procedure**

    N99.820 **Postprocedural hemorrhage of a genitourinary system organ or structure following a genitourinary system procedure** `CC`

    N99.821 **Postprocedural hemorrhage of a genitourinary system organ or structure following other procedure** `CC`

  N99.83 **Residual ovary syndrome**

  ✓6ᵗʰ **N99.84** **Postprocedural hematoma and seroma of a genitourinary system organ or structure following a procedure**

    N99.840 **Postprocedural hematoma of a genitourinary system organ or structure following a genitourinary system procedure** `CC`

    N99.841 **Postprocedural hematoma of a genitourinary system organ or structure following other procedure** `CC`

    N99.842 **Postprocedural seroma of a genitourinary system organ or structure following a genitourinary system procedure** `CC`

    N99.843 **Postprocedural seroma of a genitourinary system organ or structure following other procedure** `CC`

  N99.85 **Post endometrial ablation syndrome**
AHA: 2019,4Q,12

  N99.89 **Other postprocedural complications and disorders of genitourinary system**

✔ Additional Character Required   ✓x7ᵗʰ Placeholder   Questionable PDx   Manifestation   Unspecified   UPD Unacceptable PDx   H1-H14 HAC   HCC CMS-HCC Dx   HIV HIV Dx

ICD-10-CM 2025   877

Chapter 15. Pregnancy, Childbirth, and the Puerperium (O00–O9A)

Chapter-specific Guidelines with Coding Examples

The chapter-specific guidelines from the ICD-10-CM Official Guidelines for Coding and Reporting have been provided below. Along with these guidelines are coding examples, contained in the shaded boxes, that have been developed to help illustrate the coding and/or sequencing guidance found in these guidelines.

a. General rules for obstetric cases

1) Codes from Chapter 15 and sequencing priority

Obstetric cases require codes from chapter 15, codes in the range O00–O9A, Pregnancy, Childbirth, and the Puerperium. Chapter 15 codes have sequencing priority over codes from other chapters. Additional codes from other chapters may be used in conjunction with chapter 15 codes to further specify conditions. Should the provider document that the pregnancy is incidental to the encounter, then code Z33.1, Pregnant state, incidental, should be used in place of any chapter 15 codes. It is the provider's responsibility to state that the condition being treated is not affecting the pregnancy.

Pregnant patient at 25 weeks' gestation admitted for bladder abscess	
O23.12	Infections of bladder in pregnancy, second trimester
N30.80	Other cystitis without hematuria
Z3A.25	25 weeks gestation of pregnancy

Explanation: The documentation does not indicate that the pregnancy is incidental or in any way unaffected by the bladder abscess; therefore, an obstetrics code should be sequenced first. An additional code was provided to identify the specific bladder condition as this information is not called out specifically in the obstetrics code.

2) Chapter 15 codes used only on the maternal record

Chapter 15 codes are to be used only on the maternal record, never on the record of the newborn.

3) Final character for trimester

The majority of codes in Chapter 15 have a final character indicating the trimester of pregnancy. The timeframes for the trimesters are indicated at the beginning of the chapter. If trimester is not a component of a code, it is because the condition always occurs in a specific trimester, or the concept of trimester of pregnancy is not applicable. Certain codes have characters for only certain trimesters because the condition does not occur in all trimesters, but it may occur in more than just one.

Assignment of the final character for trimester should be based on the provider's documentation of the trimester (or number of weeks) for the current admission/encounter. This applies to the assignment of trimester for pre-existing conditions as well as those that develop during or are due to the pregnancy. The provider's documentation of the number of weeks may be used to assign the appropriate code identifying the trimester.

Whenever delivery occurs during the current admission, and there is an "in childbirth" option for the obstetric complication being coded, the "in childbirth" code should be assigned. When the classification does not provide an obstetric code with an "in childbirth" option, it is appropriate to assign a code describing the current trimester.

Pregnant patient at 21 weeks' gestation admitted with excessive vomiting	
O21.2	Late vomiting of pregnancy
Z3A.21	21 weeks gestation of pregnancy

Explanation: Category O21 classifies vomiting in pregnancy. Although code selection is based on whether the vomiting is before or after 20 completed weeks, these codes are not further classified by trimester. If vomiting only in the second trimester was documented, the provider should be queried for the specific week of gestation, as this will affect code selection.

4) Selection of trimester for inpatient admissions that encompass more than one trimester

In instances when a patient is admitted to a hospital for complications of pregnancy during one trimester and remains in the hospital into a subsequent trimester, the trimester character for the antepartum complication code should be assigned on the basis of the trimester when the complication developed, not the trimester of the discharge. If the condition developed prior to the current admission/encounter or represents a pre-existing condition, the trimester character for the trimester at the time of the admission/encounter should be assigned.

Patient admitted at 27 6/7 weeks' gestation for hemorrhaging from partial placenta previa; three days after admission at 28 1/7 weeks' gestation, she developed gestational hypertension	
O44.32	Partial placenta previa with hemorrhage, second trimester
O13.3	Gestational [pregnancy-induced] hypertension without significant proteinuria, third trimester
Z3A.27	27 weeks gestation of pregnancy

Explanation: The patient presented with hemorrhaging from partial placenta previa while still in her 27th week, which falls within the second trimester. The gestational hypertension did not occur until three days after admission, putting the patient in her 28th week of pregnancy or what is considered to be the third trimester. The weeks of gestation captured by a code from category Z3A should represent only the gestational weeks upon admission.

5) Unspecified trimester

Each category that includes codes for trimester has a code for "unspecified trimester." The "unspecified trimester" code should rarely be used, such as when the documentation in the record is insufficient to determine the trimester and it is not possible to obtain clarification.

6) 7th character for fetus identification

Where applicable, a 7th character is to be assigned for certain categories (O31, O32, O33.3–O33.6, O35, O36, O40, O41, O60.1, O60.2, O64, and O69) to identify the fetus for which the complication code applies.

Assign 7th character "0":

- For single gestations
- When the documentation in the record is insufficient to determine the fetus affected and it is not possible to obtain clarification.
- When it is not possible to clinically determine which fetus is affected.

7) Completed weeks of gestation

In ICD-10-CM, "completed" weeks of gestation refers to full weeks. For example, if the provider documents gestation at 39 weeks and 6 days, the code for 39 weeks of gestation should be assigned, as the patient has not yet reached 40 completed weeks.

b. Selection of OB principal or first-listed diagnosis

1) Routine outpatient prenatal visits

For routine outpatient prenatal visits when no complications are present, a code from category Z34, Encounter for supervision of normal pregnancy, should be used as the first-listed diagnosis. These codes should not be used in conjunction with chapter 15 codes.

2) Supervision of high-risk pregnancy

Codes from category O09, Supervision of high-risk pregnancy, are intended for use only during the prenatal period. For complications during the labor or delivery episode as a result of a high-risk pregnancy, assign the applicable complication codes from Chapter 15. If there are no complications during the labor or delivery episode, assign code O80, Encounter for full-term uncomplicated delivery.

For routine prenatal outpatient visits for patients with high-risk pregnancies, a code from category O09, Supervision of high-risk pregnancy, should be used as the first-listed diagnosis. Secondary chapter 15 codes may be used in conjunction with these codes if appropriate.

36-year-old with history of preterm labor admitted in labor with second child at 39 weeks' gestation, delivered healthy baby without complications	
O80	Encounter for full-term uncomplicated delivery
Z3A.39	39 weeks gestation of pregnancy
Z37.0	Single live birth

Explanation: Although this patient is over 35 and having her second child (elderly multigravida) and has a history of preterm labor with her first child, no codes from category O09.- should be appended. In the absence of any other complications noted during the encounter, code O80 is the most appropriate code to describe the principal diagnosis.

3) Episodes when no delivery occurs

In episodes when no delivery occurs, the principal diagnosis should correspond to the principal complication of the pregnancy which necessitated the encounter. Should more than one complication exist, all

Chapter 15. Pregnancy, Childbirth, and the Puerperium

of which are treated or monitored, any of the complication codes may be sequenced first.

4) When a delivery occurs

When an obstetric patient is admitted and delivers during that admission, the condition that prompted the admission should be sequenced as the principal diagnosis. If multiple conditions prompted the admission, sequence the one most related to the delivery as the principal diagnosis. A code for any complication of the delivery should be assigned as an additional diagnosis. In cases of cesarean delivery, if the patient was admitted with a condition that resulted in the performance of a cesarean procedure, that condition should be selected as the principal diagnosis. If the reason for the admission was unrelated to the condition resulting in the cesarean delivery, the condition related to the reason for the admission should be selected as the principal diagnosis.

> Maternal patient with diet-controlled gestational diabetes was admitted at 38 weeks' gestation in obstructed labor due to footling presentation; cesarean performed for the malpresentation
>
> | O64.8XXØ | Obstructed labor due to other malposition and malpresentation, not applicable or unspecified |
> | O24.42Ø | Gestational diabetes mellitus in childbirth, diet controlled |
> | Z3A.38 | 38 weeks gestation of pregnancy |
> | Z37.Ø | Single live birth |
>
> *Explanation:* The obstructed labor necessitated the cesarean procedure.

> At 39 weeks' gestation, a maternal patient presents with hemorrhage with coagulation defect; the next day the patient goes into labor and eventually delivers via cesarean section due to arrested active phase of labor
>
> | O46.003 | Antepartum hemorrhage with coagulation defect, unspecified, third trimester |
> | O62.1 | Secondary uterine inertia |
> | Z3A.39 | 39 weeks gestation of pregnancy |
> | Z37.Ø | Single live birth |
>
> *Explanation:* The patient was admitted because of the antepartum hemorrhage with coagulation defect. The arrested active phase, although the reason for the cesarean delivery, did not develop until later into the stay.

5) Outcome of delivery

A code from category Z37, Outcome of delivery, should be included on every maternal record when a delivery has occurred. These codes are not to be used on subsequent records or on the newborn record.

c. Pre-existing conditions versus conditions due to the pregnancy

Certain categories in Chapter 15 distinguish between conditions of the mother that existed prior to pregnancy (pre-existing) and those that are a direct result of pregnancy. When assigning codes from Chapter 15, it is important to assess if a condition was pre-existing prior to pregnancy or developed during or due to the pregnancy in order to assign the correct code.

Categories that do not distinguish between pre-existing and pregnancy-related conditions may be used for either. It is acceptable to use codes specifically for the puerperium with codes complicating pregnancy and childbirth if a condition arises postpartum during the delivery encounter.

d. Pre-existing hypertension in pregnancy

Category O1Ø, Pre-existing hypertension complicating pregnancy, childbirth and the puerperium, includes codes for hypertensive heart and hypertensive chronic kidney disease. When assigning one of the O1Ø codes that includes hypertensive heart disease or hypertensive chronic kidney disease, it is necessary to add a secondary code from the appropriate hypertension category to specify the type of heart failure or chronic kidney disease.

See Section I.C.9. Hypertension.

e. Fetal conditions affecting the management of the mother

1) Codes from categories O35 and O36

Codes from categories O35, Maternal care for known or suspected fetal abnormality and damage, and O36, Maternal care for other fetal problems, are assigned only when the fetal condition is actually responsible for modifying the management of the mother, i.e., by requiring diagnostic studies, additional observation, special care, or

termination of pregnancy. The fact that the fetal condition exists does not justify assigning a code from this series to the mother's record.

> A patient is seen in ED for spotting 15 weeks into her pregnancy; the doctors also suspect fetal hydrocephalus.
>
> | O26.852 | Spotting complicating pregnancy, second trimester |
> | Z3A.15 | 15 weeks gestation of pregnancy |
>
> *Explanation:* Whether the fetal hydrocephalus was suspected or confirmed, an additional code is not warranted for this condition as the documentation does not indicate that this fetal condition is in any way altering the management of the mother or complicating her pregnancy.

2) In utero surgery

In cases when surgery is performed on the fetus, a diagnosis code from category O35, Maternal care for known or suspected fetal abnormality and damage, should be assigned identifying the fetal condition. Assign the appropriate procedure code for the procedure performed.

No code from Chapter 16, the perinatal codes, should be used on the mother's record to identify fetal conditions. Surgery performed in utero on a fetus is still to be coded as an obstetric encounter.

f. HIV infection in pregnancy, childbirth and the puerperium

During pregnancy, childbirth or the puerperium, a patient admitted because of an HIV-related illness should receive a principal diagnosis from subcategory O98.7-, Human immunodeficiency [HIV] disease complicating pregnancy, childbirth and the puerperium, followed by the code(s) for the HIV-related illness(es).

Patients with asymptomatic HIV infection status admitted during pregnancy, childbirth, or the puerperium should receive codes of O98.7- and Z21, Asymptomatic human immunodeficiency virus [HIV] infection status.

> A previously asymptomatic HIV patient who is 13 weeks pregnant is admitted with oral thrush.
>
> | O98.711 | Human immunodeficiency virus [HIV] disease complicating pregnancy, first trimester |
> | B2Ø | Human immunodeficiency virus [HIV] disease |
> | B37.Ø | Candidal stomatitis |
> | Z3A.13 | 13 weeks gestation of pregnancy |
>
> *Explanation:* Because oral thrush is an HIV-related condition, this patient is now considered to have HIV disease. An obstetrics code indicating that HIV is complicating the pregnancy is coded first, followed by B2Ø for HIV disease as well as a code for the oral thrush.

g. Diabetes mellitus in pregnancy

Diabetes mellitus is a significant complicating factor in pregnancy. Pregnant patients who are diabetic should be assigned a code from category O24, Diabetes mellitus in pregnancy, childbirth, and the puerperium, first, followed by the appropriate diabetes code(s) (EØ8–E13) from Chapter 4.

h. Long term use of insulin and oral hypoglycemics

See section I.C.4.a.3 for information on the long-term use of insulin and oral hypoglycemics.

i. Gestational (pregnancy induced) diabetes

Gestational (pregnancy induced) diabetes can occur during the second and third trimester of pregnancy in patients who were not diabetic prior to pregnancy. Gestational diabetes can cause complications in the pregnancy similar to those of pre-existing diabetes mellitus. It also puts the patient at greater risk of developing diabetes after the pregnancy.

Codes for gestational diabetes are in subcategory O24.4, Gestational diabetes mellitus. No other code from category O24, Diabetes mellitus in pregnancy, childbirth, and the puerperium, should be used with a code from O24.4.

The codes under subcategory O24.4 include diet controlled, insulin controlled, and controlled by oral hypoglycemic drugs. If a patient with gestational diabetes is treated with both diet and insulin, only the code for insulin-controlled is required. If a patient with gestational diabetes is treated with both diet and oral hypoglycemic medications, only the code for "controlled by oral hypoglycemic drugs" is required. Codes Z79.4, Long-term (current) use of insulin, Z79.84, Long-term (current) use of oral hypoglycemic drugs, and Z79.85, Long-term (current) use of injectable non-insulin antidiabetic drugs, should not be assigned with codes from subcategory O24.4.

An abnormal glucose tolerance in pregnancy is assigned a code from subcategory O99.81, Abnormal glucose complicating pregnancy, childbirth, and the puerperium.

> Patient at 39 weeks term pregnancy with gestational diabetes was admitted in labor and delivered a healthy newborn. Patient is on a diabetic diet with daily metformin.
>
> **O24.425**   **Gestational diabetes mellitus in childbirth, controlled by oral hypoglycemic drugs**
>
> **Z3A.39**   **39 weeks gestation of pregnancy**
>
> **Z37.0**   **Single live birth**
>
> *Explanation:* When the patient is admitted for delivery and the patient's gestational diabetes is controlled by both diet and oral hypoglycemic medications, only the combination code in subcategory O24.4- Gestational diabetes mellitus, is reported. No code is added for diet controlled diabetes, and no Z code for long-term use of oral hypoglycemics is reported with the O24.4 combination codes.

j. Sepsis and septic shock complicating abortion, pregnancy, childbirth and the puerperium

When assigning a chapter 15 code for sepsis complicating abortion, pregnancy, childbirth, and the puerperium, a code for the specific type of infection should be assigned as an additional diagnosis. If severe sepsis is present, a code from subcategory R65.2, Severe sepsis, and code(s) for associated organ dysfunction(s) should also be assigned as additional diagnoses.

> Patient is seen several days after a miscarriage with sepsis; cultures return MSSA
>
> **O03.87**   **Sepsis following complete or unspecified spontaneous abortion**
>
> **B95.61**   **Methicillin susceptible Staphylococcus aureus infection as the cause of diseases classified elsewhere**
>
> *Explanation:* The type of infection that caused this patient to become septic was methicillin susceptible *Staphylococcus aureus* (MSSA), which as a secondary code helps capture all aspects related to this patient's septic condition.

k. Puerperal sepsis

Code O85, Puerperal sepsis, should be assigned with a secondary code to identify the causal organism (e.g., for a bacterial infection, assign a code from category B95–B96, Bacterial infections in conditions classified elsewhere). A code from category A40, Streptococcal sepsis, or A41, Other sepsis, should not be used for puerperal sepsis. If applicable, use additional codes to identify severe sepsis (R65.2-) and any associated acute organ dysfunction.

Code O85 should not be assigned for sepsis following an obstetrical procedure (See Section I.C.1.d.5.b., Sepsis due to a postprocedural infection).

l. Alcohol, tobacco and drug use during pregnancy, childbirth and the puerperium

   1) Alcohol use during pregnancy, childbirth and the puerperium

Codes under subcategory O99.31, Alcohol use complicating pregnancy, childbirth, and the puerperium, should be assigned for any pregnancy case when a patient uses alcohol during the pregnancy or postpartum. A secondary code from category F10, Alcohol related disorders, should also be assigned to identify manifestations of the alcohol use.

   2) Tobacco use during pregnancy, childbirth and the puerperium

Codes under subcategory O99.33, Smoking (tobacco) complicating pregnancy, childbirth, and the puerperium, should be assigned for any pregnancy case when a patient uses any type of tobacco product during the pregnancy or postpartum.

A secondary code from category F17, Nicotine dependence, should also be assigned to identify the type of nicotine dependence.

   3) Drug use during pregnancy, childbirth and the puerperium

Codes under subcategory O99.32, Drug use complicating pregnancy, childbirth, and the puerperium, should be assigned for any pregnancy case when a patient uses drugs during the pregnancy or postpartum. This can involve illegal drugs, or inappropriate use or abuse of prescription drugs. Secondary code(s) from categories F11–F16 and F18–F19 should also be assigned to identify manifestations of the drug use.

m. Poisoning, toxic effects, adverse effects and underdosing in a pregnant patient

A code from subcategory O9A.2, Injury, poisoning and certain other consequences of external causes complicating pregnancy, childbirth, and the puerperium, should be sequenced first, followed by the appropriate injury, poisoning, toxic effect, adverse effect or underdosing code, and then the additional code(s) that specifies the condition caused by the poisoning, toxic effect, adverse effect or underdosing.

See Section I.C.19. Adverse effects, poisoning, underdosing and toxic effects.

> Patient admitted with accidental carbon monoxide poisoning from a gas heating implement; the patient is 18 weeks pregnant
>
> **O9A.212**   **Injury, poisoning and certain other consequences of external causes complicating pregnancy, second trimester**
>
> **T58.11XA**   **Toxic effect of carbon monoxide from utility gas, accidental (unintentional), initial encounter**
>
> **Z3A.18**   **18 weeks gestation of pregnancy**
>
> *Explanation:* Although the carbon monoxide poisoning is the reason the patient was admitted, a code from the obstetrics chapter must be sequenced first. Chapter 15 codes have sequencing priority over codes from other chapters.

n. Normal delivery, code O80

   1) Encounter for full term uncomplicated delivery

Code O80 should be assigned when a patient is admitted for a full-term normal delivery and delivers a single, healthy infant without any complications antepartum, during the delivery, or postpartum during the delivery episode. Code O80 is always a principal diagnosis. It is not to be used if any other code from chapter 15 is needed to describe a current complication of the antenatal, delivery, or postnatal period. Additional codes from other chapters may be used with code O80 if they are not related to or are in any way complicating the pregnancy.

   2) Uncomplicated delivery with resolved antepartum complication

Code O80 may be used if the patient had a complication at some point during the pregnancy, but the complication is not present at the time of the admission for delivery.

> Patient presents in labor at 39 weeks' gestation and delivers a healthy newborn; patient had abnormal glucose levels in her first trimester, which have since resolved
>
> **O80**   **Encounter for full-term uncomplicated delivery**
>
> **Z37.0**   **Single live birth**
>
> *Explanation:* The abnormal glucose levels during the first trimester cannot be coded if they are not affecting the patient's current trimester. Without additional complications associated with the pregnancy, fetus, or mother, code O80 is appropriate.

   3) Outcome of delivery for O80

Z37.0, Single live birth, is the only outcome of delivery code appropriate for use with O80.

o. The peripartum and postpartum periods

   1) Peripartum and postpartum periods

The postpartum period begins immediately after delivery and continues for six weeks following delivery. The peripartum period is defined as the last month of pregnancy to five months postpartum.

   2) Peripartum and postpartum complication

A postpartum complication is any complication occurring within the six-week period.

   3) Pregnancy-related complications after 6-week period

Chapter 15 codes may also be used to describe pregnancy-related complications after the peripartum or postpartum period if the provider documents that a condition is pregnancy related.

> Patient admitted for varicose veins. She had a baby boy three months ago; the varicose veins started to appear one month ago. The doctor attributes the patient's pregnancy as the cause of the varicose veins, which continue to be painful and bother the patient. She is seeking surgical relief.
>
> **O87.4**   **Varicose veins of the lower extremity in the puerperium**
>
> *Explanation:* Although the varicose veins occurred several months after the delivery of the newborn, the doctor attributed the varicose veins to pregnancy and therefore a code from chapter 15 is appropriate.

4) Admission for routine postpartum care following delivery outside hospital

When the mother delivers outside the hospital prior to admission and is admitted for routine postpartum care and no complications are noted, code Z39.0, Encounter for care and examination of mother immediately after delivery, should be assigned as the principal diagnosis.

5) Pregnancy associated cardiomyopathy

Pregnancy associated cardiomyopathy, code O90.3, is unique in that it may be diagnosed in the third trimester of pregnancy but may continue to progress months after delivery. For this reason, it is referred to as peripartum cardiomyopathy. Code O90.3 is only for use when the cardiomyopathy develops as a result of pregnancy in a patient who did not have pre-existing heart disease.

p. Code O94, Sequelae of complication of pregnancy, childbirth, and the puerperium

1) Code O94

Code O94, Sequelae of complication of pregnancy, childbirth, and the puerperium, is for use in those cases when an initial complication of a pregnancy develops a sequela or sequelae requiring care or treatment at a future date.

2) After the initial postpartum period

This code may be used at any time after the initial postpartum period.

3) Sequencing of code O94

This code, like all sequela codes, is to be sequenced following the code describing the sequelae of the complication.

q. Termination of pregnancy and spontaneous abortions

1) Abortion with liveborn fetus

When an attempted termination of pregnancy results in a liveborn fetus, assign code Z33.2, Encounter for elective termination of pregnancy and a code from category Z37, Outcome of Delivery.

2) Retained products of conception following an abortion

Subsequent encounters for retained products of conception following a spontaneous abortion or elective termination of pregnancy, without complications are assigned O03.4, Incomplete spontaneous, abortion without complication, or code O07.4, Failed attempted termination of pregnancy without complication. This advice is appropriate even when the patient was discharged previously with a discharge diagnosis of complete abortion. If the patient has a specific complication associated with the spontaneous abortion or elective termination of pregnancy in addition to retained products of conception, assign the appropriate complication code (e.g., O03.-, O04.-, O07.-) instead of code O03.4 or O07.4.

> Patient was seen two days ago for complete spontaneous abortion but returns today for urinary tract infection (UTI) with ultrasound showing retained products of conception
>
> **O03.38   Urinary tract infection following incomplete spontaneous abortion**
>
> *Explanation:* Although the diagnosis from the patient's previous stay indicated that the patient had a complete abortion, it is now determined that there were actually retained products of conception (POC). An abortion with retained POC is considered incomplete and in this case resulted in the patient developing a UTI.

3) Complications leading to abortion

Codes from Chapter 15 may be used as additional codes to identify any documented complications of the pregnancy in conjunction with codes in categories in O04, O07 and O08.

4) Hemorrhage following elective abortion

For hemorrhage post elective abortion, assign code O04.6, Delayed or excessive hemorrhage following (induced) termination of pregnancy. Do not assign code O72.1, Other immediate postpartum hemorrhage, as this code should not be assigned for post abortion conditions.

r. Abuse in a pregnant patient

For suspected or confirmed cases of abuse of a pregnant patient, a code(s) from subcategories O9A.3, Physical abuse complicating pregnancy, childbirth, and the puerperium, O9A.4, Sexual abuse complicating pregnancy, childbirth, and the puerperium, and O9A.5, Psychological abuse complicating pregnancy, childbirth, and the puerperium, should be sequenced first, followed by the appropriate codes (if applicable) to identify any associated current injury due to physical abuse, sexual abuse, and the perpetrator of abuse.

See Section I.C.19. Adult and child abuse, neglect and other maltreatment.

s. COVID-19 infection in pregnancy, childbirth, and the puerperium

During pregnancy, childbirth or the puerperium, when COVID-19 is the reason for admission/encounter , code O98.5-, Other viral diseases complicating pregnancy, childbirth and the puerperium, should be sequenced as the principal/first-listed diagnosis, and code U07.1, COVID-19, and the appropriate codes for associated manifestation(s) should be assigned as additional diagnoses. Codes from Chapter 15 always take sequencing priority.

If the reason for admission/encounter is unrelated to COVID-19 but the patient tests positive for COVID-19 during the admission/encounter, the appropriate code for the reason for admission/encounter should be sequenced as the principal/first-listed diagnosis, and codes O98.5- and U07.1, as well as the appropriate codes for associated COVID-19 manifestations, should be assigned as additional diagnoses.

> Patient admitted in labor at 39 weeks' gestation and delivered a healthy newborn. Prenatal care consisted of some hyperemesis early in the pregnancy that has since resolved. No complications encountered during or following delivery. As per hospital protocol, during the pandemic, all patients are to be screened for COVID-19, and the patient tested positive. She remains asymptomatic, will be sent home to quarantine for 14 days.
>
> | O98.52 | Other viral diseases complicating childbirth |
> |---|---|
> | U07.1 | COVID-19 |
> | Z3A.39 | 39 weeks gestation of pregnancy |
> | Z37.0 | Single live birth |
>
> *Explanation:* No code is assigned for the hyperemesis as it resolved prior to this admission. Per guideline I.C.1.g.1.f, a screening code is generally not appropriate during the pandemic phase of COVID-19. Most hospitals screen their patients upon admission to the hospital to ensure proper protocols are in place for monitoring and treating those patients who do test positive for the disease. A positive test result alone is confirmation of the disease, according to guideline I.C.1.g.1.a, and code U07.1 should be assigned. A claim for any patient admitted during pregnancy, childbirth, or the puerperium and who tests positive or is treated for COVID-19 should have a code from subcategory O98.5- sequenced first, followed by code U07.1. As the patient was asymptomatic, no additional codes are assigned to represent any manifestation of the COVID-19 infection.

Chapter 15. Pregnancy, Childbirth and the Puerperium (O00-O9A)

NOTE CODES FROM THIS CHAPTER ARE FOR USE ONLY ON MATERNAL RECORDS, NEVER ON NEWBORN RECORDS

Codes from this chapter are for use for conditions related to or aggravated by the pregnancy, childbirth, or by the puerperium (maternal causes or obstetric causes)

NOTE Trimesters are counted from the first day of the last menstrual period. They are defined as follows:

1st trimester- less than 14 weeks 0 days

2nd trimester- 14 weeks 0 days to less than 28 weeks 0 days

3rd trimester- 28 weeks 0 days until delivery

Use additional code, if applicable, from category Z3A, Weeks of gestation, to identify the specific week of the pregnancy, if known.

EXCLUDES 1 *supervision of normal pregnancy (Z34.-)*

EXCLUDES 2 *mental and behavioral disorders associated with the puerperium (F53.-)*
obstetrical tetanus (A34)
postpartum necrosis of pituitary gland (E23.0)
puerperal osteomalacia (M83.0)

AHA: 2016,1Q,3-5; 2014,3Q,17

This chapter contains the following blocks:

O00-O08   Pregnancy with abortive outcome
O09   Supervision of high risk pregnancy
O10-O16   Edema, proteinuria and hypertensive disorders in pregnancy, childbirth and the puerperium
O20-O29   Other maternal disorders predominantly related to pregnancy
O30-O48   Maternal care related to the fetus and amniotic cavity and possible delivery problems
O60-O77   Complications of labor and delivery
O80-O82   Encounter for delivery
O85-O92   Complications predominantly related to the puerperium
O94-O9A   Other obstetric conditions, not elsewhere classified

Pregnancy with abortive outcome (O00-O08)

EXCLUDES 1 *continuing pregnancy in multiple gestation after abortion of one fetus or more (O31.1-, O31.3-)*

TIP: Do not assign a code from category Z3A with codes in this code block.

✓4ᵗʰ O00   Ectopic pregnancy

INCLUDES ruptured ectopic pregnancy

Use additional code from category O08 to identify any associated complication

AHA: 2016,4Q,48-50; 2014,3Q,17

DEF: Implantation of a fertilized egg outside the uterus, usually in the fallopian tube or abdomen that requires emergency treatment.

✓5ᵗʰ **O00.0   Abdominal pregnancy**

EXCLUDES 1 *maternal care for viable fetus in abdominal pregnancy (O36.7-)*

O00.00   Abdominal pregnancy without intrauterine pregnancy CC M
Abdominal pregnancy NOS

O00.01   Abdominal pregnancy with intrauterine pregnancy CC M

✓5ᵗʰ **O00.1   Tubal pregnancy**
Fallopian pregnancy
Rupture of (fallopian) tube due to pregnancy
Tubal abortion
AHA: 2017,4Q,20

✓6ᵗʰ **O00.10   Tubal pregnancy without intrauterine pregnancy**
Tubal pregnancy NOS

O00.101   Right tubal pregnancy without intrauterine pregnancy CC M

O00.102   Left tubal pregnancy without intrauterine pregnancy CC M

O00.109   Unspecified tubal pregnancy without intrauterine pregnancy CC UNS M

✓6ᵗʰ **O00.11   Tubal pregnancy with intrauterine pregnancy**

O00.111   Right tubal pregnancy with intrauterine pregnancy CC M

O00.112   Left tubal pregnancy with intrauterine pregnancy CC M

O00.119   Unspecified tubal pregnancy with intrauterine pregnancy CC UNS M

✓5ᵗʰ **O00.2   Ovarian pregnancy**
AHA: 2017,4Q,20

✓6ᵗʰ **O00.20   Ovarian pregnancy without intrauterine pregnancy**
Ovarian pregnancy NOS

O00.201   Right ovarian pregnancy without intrauterine pregnancy CC M

O00.202   Left ovarian pregnancy without intrauterine pregnancy CC M

O00.209   Unspecified ovarian pregnancy without intrauterine pregnancy CC UNS M

✓6ᵗʰ **O00.21   Ovarian pregnancy with intrauterine pregnancy**

O00.211   Right ovarian pregnancy with intrauterine pregnancy CC M

O00.212   Left ovarian pregnancy with intrauterine pregnancy CC M

O00.219   Unspecified ovarian pregnancy with intrauterine pregnancy CC UNS M

✓5ᵗʰ **O00.8   Other ectopic pregnancy**
Cervical pregnancy
Cornual pregnancy
Intraligamentous pregnancy
Mural pregnancy

O00.80   Other ectopic pregnancy without intrauterine pregnancy CC M
Other ectopic pregnancy NOS

O00.81   Other ectopic pregnancy with intrauterine pregnancy CC M

✓5ᵗʰ **O00.9   Ectopic pregnancy, unspecified**

O00.90   Unspecified ectopic pregnancy without intrauterine pregnancy CC M
Ectopic pregnancy NOS

O00.91   Unspecified ectopic pregnancy with intrauterine pregnancy CC M

✓4ᵗʰ O01   Hydatidiform mole

Use additional code from category O08 to identify any associated complication

EXCLUDES 1 *chorioadenoma (destruens) (D39.2)*
malignant hydatidiform mole (D39.2)

AHA: 2014,3Q,17

DEF: Abnormal product of pregnancy, marked by a mass of cysts resembling a bunch of grapes due to chorionic villi proliferation and dissolution. It must be surgically removed.

O01.0   Classical hydatidiform mole M
Complete hydatidiform mole

O01.1   Incomplete and partial hydatidiform mole M

O01.9   Hydatidiform mole, unspecified M
Trophoblastic disease NOS
Vesicular mole NOS

✓4ᵗʰ O02   Other abnormal products of conception

Use additional code from category O08 to identify any associated complication

EXCLUDES 1 *papyraceous fetus (O31.0-)*

AHA: 2014,3Q,17

O02.0   Blighted ovum and nonhydatidiform mole M
Carneous mole
Fleshy mole
Intrauterine mole NOS
Molar pregnancy NEC
Pathological ovum

O02.1   Missed abortion M
Early fetal death, before completion of 20 weeks of gestation, with retention of dead fetus

EXCLUDES 1 *failed induced abortion (O07.-)*
fetal death (intrauterine) (late) (O36.4)
missed abortion with blighted ovum (O02.0)
missed abortion with hydatidiform mole (O01.-)
missed abortion with nonhydatidiform (O02.0)
missed abortion with other abnormal products of conception (O02.8-)
missed delivery (O36.4)
stillbirth (P95)

AHA: 2022,2Q,3; 2019,3Q,11

✔ Additional Character Required   ✔x7ᵗʰ Placeholder   Questionable PDx   Manifestation   Unspecified   UPD Unacceptable PDx   H1-H14 HAC   HCC CMS-HCC Dx   HIV HIV Dx

ICD-10-CM 2025   883

✓5ᵗʰ **O02.8 Other specified abnormal products of conception**

EXCLUDES 1 *abnormal products of conception with blighted ovum (O02.0)*

abnormal products of conception with hydatidiform mole (O01.-)

abnormal products of conception with nonhydatidiform mole (O02.0)

O02.81 Inappropriate change in quantitative human chorionic gonadotropin (hCG) in early pregnancy M

Biochemical pregnancy

Chemical pregnancy

Inappropriate level of quantitative human chorionic gonadotropin (hCG) for gestational age in early pregnancy

O02.89 Other abnormal products of conception M

O02.9 Abnormal product of conception, unspecified M

✓4ᵗʰ **O03 Spontaneous abortion**

NOTE Incomplete abortion includes retained products of conception following spontaneous abortion

INCLUDES miscarriage

AHA: 2023,1Q,17

O03.0 Genital tract and pelvic infection following incomplete spontaneous abortion CC M

Endometritis following incomplete spontaneous abortion

Oophoritis following incomplete spontaneous abortion

Parametritis following incomplete spontaneous abortion

Pelvic peritonitis following incomplete spontaneous abortion

Salpingitis following incomplete spontaneous abortion

Salpingo-oophoritis following incomplete spontaneous abortion

EXCLUDES 1 *sepsis following incomplete spontaneous abortion (O03.37)*

urinary tract infection following incomplete spontaneous abortion (O03.38)

O03.1 Delayed or excessive hemorrhage following incomplete spontaneous abortion M

Afibrinogenemia following incomplete spontaneous abortion

Defibrination syndrome following incomplete spontaneous abortion

Hemolysis following incomplete spontaneous abortion

Intravascular coagulation following incomplete spontaneous abortion

AHA: 2022,1Q,19

O03.2 Embolism following incomplete spontaneous abortion MCC M

Air embolism following incomplete spontaneous abortion

Amniotic fluid embolism following incomplete spontaneous abortion

Blood-clot embolism following incomplete spontaneous abortion

Embolism NOS following incomplete spontaneous abortion

Fat embolism following incomplete spontaneous abortion

Pulmonary embolism following incomplete spontaneous abortion

Pyemic embolism following incomplete spontaneous abortion

Septic or septicopyemic embolism following incomplete spontaneous abortion

Soap embolism following incomplete spontaneous abortion

✓5ᵗʰ **O03.3 Other and unspecified complications following incomplete spontaneous abortion**

O03.30 Unspecified complication following incomplete spontaneous abortion CC M

O03.31 Shock following incomplete spontaneous abortion MCC M

Circulatory collapse following incomplete spontaneous abortion

Shock (postprocedural) following incomplete spontaneous abortion

EXCLUDES 1 *shock due to infection following incomplete spontaneous abortion (O03.37)*

O03.32 Renal failure following incomplete spontaneous abortion MCC M

Kidney failure (acute) following incomplete spontaneous abortion

Oliguria following incomplete spontaneous abortion

Renal shutdown following incomplete spontaneous abortion

Renal tubular necrosis following incomplete spontaneous abortion

Uremia following incomplete spontaneous abortion

O03.33 Metabolic disorder following incomplete spontaneous abortion CC M

O03.34 Damage to pelvic organs following incomplete spontaneous abortion CC M

Laceration, perforation, tear or chemical damage of bladder following incomplete spontaneous abortion

Laceration, perforation, tear or chemical damage of bowel following incomplete spontaneous abortion

Laceration, perforation, tear or chemical damage of broad ligament following incomplete spontaneous abortion

Laceration, perforation, tear or chemical damage of cervix following incomplete spontaneous abortion

Laceration, perforation, tear or chemical damage of periurethral tissue following incomplete spontaneous abortion

Laceration, perforation, tear or chemical damage of uterus following incomplete spontaneous abortion

Laceration, perforation, tear or chemical damage of vagina following incomplete spontaneous abortion

O03.35 Other venous complications following incomplete spontaneous abortion CC M

O03.36 Cardiac arrest following incomplete spontaneous abortion CC M

O03.37 Sepsis following incomplete spontaneous abortion CC M

Use additional code to identify infectious agent (B95-B97)

Use additional code to identify severe sepsis, if applicable (R65.2-)

EXCLUDES 1 *septic or septicopyemic embolism following incomplete spontaneous abortion (O03.2)*

O03.38 Urinary tract infection following incomplete spontaneous abortion CC M

Cystitis following incomplete spontaneous abortion

O03.39 Incomplete spontaneous abortion with other complications CC M

O03.4 Incomplete spontaneous abortion without complication M

O03.5 Genital tract and pelvic infection following complete or unspecified spontaneous abortion CC M

Endometritis following complete or unspecified spontaneous abortion

Oophoritis following complete or unspecified spontaneous abortion

Parametritis following complete or unspecified spontaneous abortion

Pelvic peritonitis following complete or unspecified spontaneous abortion

Salpingitis following complete or unspecified spontaneous abortion

Salpingo-oophoritis following complete or unspecified spontaneous abortion

EXCLUDES 1 *sepsis following complete or unspecified spontaneous abortion (O03.87)*

urinary tract infection following complete or unspecified spontaneous abortion (O03.88)

O03.6 Delayed or excessive hemorrhage following complete or unspecified spontaneous abortion M

Afibrinogenemia following complete or unspecified spontaneous abortion

Defibrination syndrome following complete or unspecified spontaneous abortion

Hemolysis following complete or unspecified spontaneous abortion

Intravascular coagulation following complete or unspecified spontaneous abortion

AHA: 2022,1Q,19

N Newborn: 0   P Pediatric: 0-17   M Maternity: 9-64   A Adult: 15-124   UNS Unspecified Site   MCC Major Complication/Comorbidity   CC Complication/Comorbidity   PE POA Exempt

O03.7 **Embolism** following **complete or unspecified** spontaneous abortion   `CC` `M`

Air embolism following complete or unspecified spontaneous abortion

Amniotic fluid embolism following complete or unspecified spontaneous abortion

Blood-clot embolism following complete or unspecified spontaneous abortion

Embolism NOS following complete or unspecified spontaneous abortion

Fat embolism following complete or unspecified spontaneous abortion

Pulmonary embolism following complete or unspecified spontaneous abortion

Pyemic embolism following complete or unspecified spontaneous abortion

Septic or septicopyemic embolism following complete or unspecified spontaneous abortion

Soap embolism following complete or unspecified spontaneous abortion

☑5ᵗʰ **O03.8** **Other and unspecified complications following complete or unspecified spontaneous abortion**

  O03.80 **Unspecified complication following complete or unspecified** spontaneous abortion   `CC` `M`

  O03.81 **Shock following complete or unspecified spontaneous abortion**   `MCC` `M`

Circulatory collapse following complete or unspecified spontaneous abortion

Shock (postprocedural) following complete or unspecified spontaneous abortion

> **EXCLUDES 1**   *shock due to infection following complete or unspecified spontaneous abortion (O03.87)*

  O03.82 **Renal failure following complete or unspecified spontaneous abortion**   `MCC` `M`

Kidney failure (acute) following complete or unspecified spontaneous abortion

Oliguria following complete or unspecified spontaneous abortion

Renal shutdown following complete or unspecified spontaneous abortion

Renal tubular necrosis following complete or unspecified spontaneous abortion

Uremia following complete or unspecified spontaneous abortion

  O03.83 **Metabolic disorder following complete or unspecified spontaneous abortion**   `CC` `M`

  O03.84 **Damage to pelvic organs following complete or unspecified spontaneous abortion**

Laceration, perforation, tear or chemical damage of bladder following complete or unspecified spontaneous abortion

Laceration, perforation, tear or chemical damage of bowel following complete or unspecified spontaneous abortion

Laceration, perforation, tear or chemical damage of broad ligament following complete or unspecified spontaneous abortion

Laceration, perforation, tear or chemical damage of cervix following complete or unspecified spontaneous abortion

Laceration, perforation, tear or chemical damage of periurethral tissue following complete or unspecified spontaneous abortion

Laceration, perforation, tear or chemical damage of uterus following complete or unspecified spontaneous abortion

Laceration, perforation, tear or chemical damage of vagina following complete or unspecified spontaneous abortion

  O03.85 **Other venous complications following complete or unspecified spontaneous abortion**   `CC` `M`

  O03.86 **Cardiac arrest following complete or unspecified spontaneous abortion**   `CC` `M`

  O03.87 **Sepsis following complete or unspecified spontaneous abortion**   `CC` `M`

Use additional code to identify infectious agent (B95-B97)

Use additional code to identify severe sepsis, if applicable (R65.2-)

> **EXCLUDES 1**   *septic or septicopyemic embolism following complete or unspecified spontaneous abortion (O03.7)*

  O03.88 **Urinary tract infection following complete or unspecified** spontaneous abortion   `CC` `M`

Cystitis following complete or unspecified spontaneous abortion

  O03.89 **Complete or unspecified** spontaneous abortion with **other complications**   `CC` `M`

O03.9 **Complete or unspecified** spontaneous abortion without **complication**   `M`

Miscarriage NOS

Spontaneous abortion NOS

☑4ᵗʰ **O04** **Complications** following (induced) **termination of pregnancy**

> **INCLUDES**   complications following (induced) termination of pregnancy
>
> **EXCLUDES 2**   *encounter for elective termination of pregnancy, uncomplicated (Z33.2)*
>
>   *failed attempted termination of pregnancy (O07.-)*

O04.5 **Genital tract and pelvic infection following (induced) termination of pregnancy**   `CC` `M`

Endometritis following (induced) termination of pregnancy

Oophoritis following (induced) termination of pregnancy

Parametritis following (induced) termination of pregnancy

Pelvic peritonitis following (induced) termination of pregnancy

Salpingitis following (induced) termination of pregnancy

Salpingo-oophoritis following (induced) termination of pregnancy

> **EXCLUDES 1**   *sepsis following (induced) termination of pregnancy (O04.87)*
>
>   *urinary tract infection following (induced) termination of pregnancy (O04.88)*

O04.6 **Delayed or excessive hemorrhage following (induced) termination of pregnancy**   `M`

Afibrinogenemia following (induced) termination of pregnancy

Defibrination syndrome following (induced) termination of pregnancy

Hemolysis following (induced) termination of pregnancy

Intravascular coagulation following (induced) termination of pregnancy

AHA: 2023,2Q,15; 2019,3Q,11

O04.7 **Embolism following (induced) termination of pregnancy**   `MCC` `M`

Air embolism following (induced) termination of pregnancy

Amniotic fluid embolism following (induced) termination of pregnancy

Blood-clot embolism following (induced) termination of pregnancy

Embolism NOS following (induced) termination of pregnancy

Fat embolism following (induced) termination of pregnancy

Pulmonary embolism following (induced) termination of pregnancy

Pyemic embolism following (induced) termination of pregnancy

Septic or septicopyemic embolism following (induced) termination of pregnancy

Soap embolism following (induced) termination of pregnancy

☑5ᵗʰ **O04.8** **(Induced) termination of pregnancy with other and unspecified complications**

  O04.80 **(Induced) termination of pregnancy with unspecified complications**   `CC` `M`

  O04.81 **Shock following (induced) termination of pregnancy**   `MCC` `M`

Circulatory collapse following (induced) termination of pregnancy

Shock (postprocedural) following (induced) termination of pregnancy

> **EXCLUDES 1**   *shock due to infection following (induced) termination of pregnancy (O04.87)*

 Additional Character Required   ☑x7ᵗʰ Placeholder   Questionable PDx   Manifestation   Unspecified   `UPD` Unacceptable PDx   `H1`-`H14` HAC   `HCC` CMS-HCC Dx   `HIV` HIV Dx

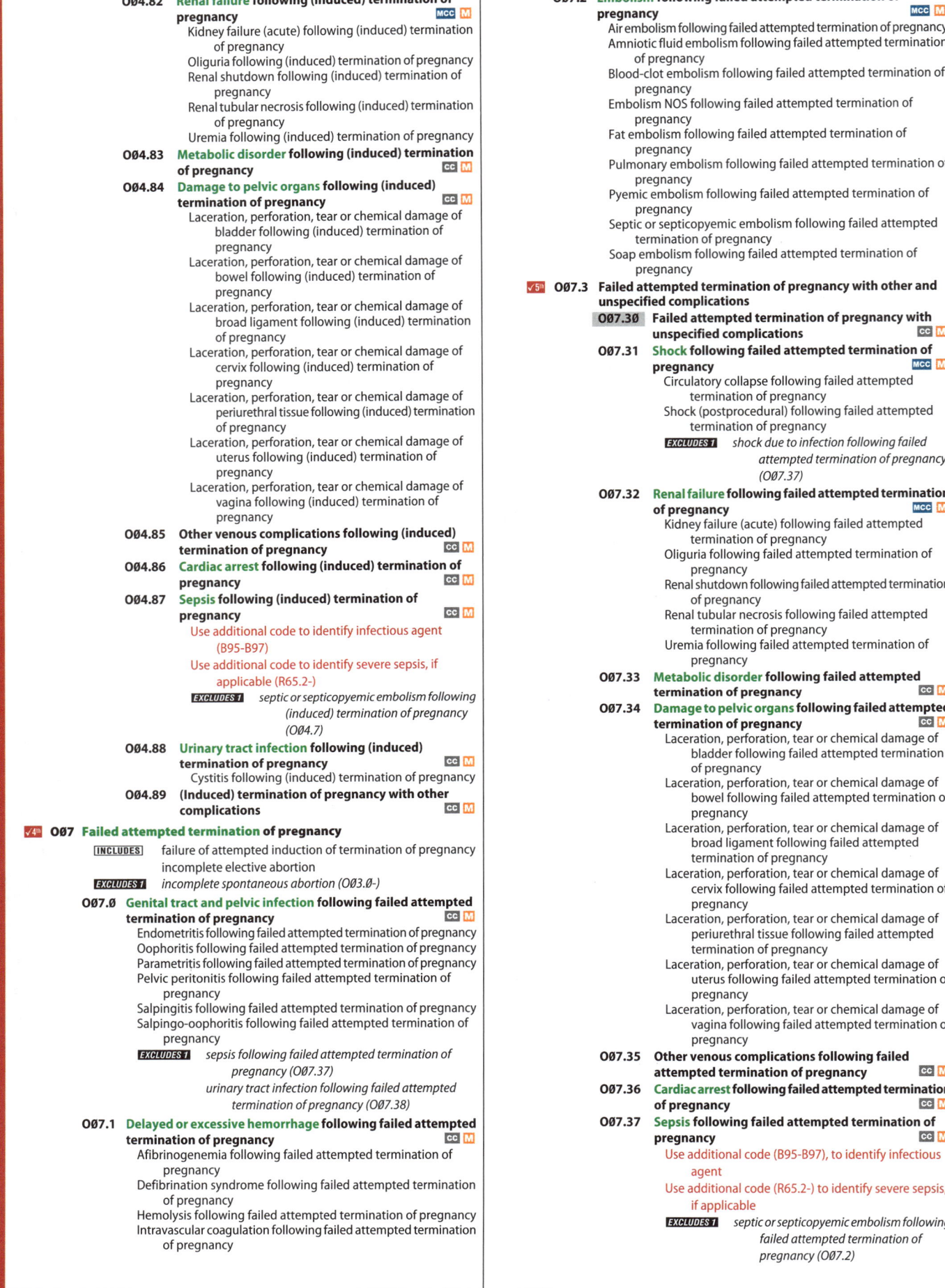

O04.82 **Renal failure** following (induced) termination of pregnancy   MCC M
- Kidney failure (acute) following (induced) termination of pregnancy
- Oliguria following (induced) termination of pregnancy
- Renal shutdown following (induced) termination of pregnancy
- Renal tubular necrosis following (induced) termination of pregnancy
- Uremia following (induced) termination of pregnancy

O04.83 **Metabolic disorder** following (induced) termination of pregnancy   CC M

O04.84 **Damage to pelvic organs** following (induced) termination of pregnancy   CC M
- Laceration, perforation, tear or chemical damage of bladder following (induced) termination of pregnancy
- Laceration, perforation, tear or chemical damage of bowel following (induced) termination of pregnancy
- Laceration, perforation, tear or chemical damage of broad ligament following (induced) termination of pregnancy
- Laceration, perforation, tear or chemical damage of cervix following (induced) termination of pregnancy
- Laceration, perforation, tear or chemical damage of periurethral tissue following (induced) termination of pregnancy
- Laceration, perforation, tear or chemical damage of uterus following (induced) termination of pregnancy
- Laceration, perforation, tear or chemical damage of vagina following (induced) termination of pregnancy

O04.85 **Other venous complications following (induced) termination of pregnancy**   CC M

O04.86 **Cardiac arrest** following (induced) termination of pregnancy   CC M

O04.87 **Sepsis** following (induced) termination of pregnancy   CC M

Use additional code to identify infectious agent (B95-B97)

Use additional code to identify severe sepsis, if applicable (R65.2-)

    EXCLUDES 1   *septic or septicopyemic embolism following (induced) termination of pregnancy (O04.7)*

O04.88 **Urinary tract infection** following (induced) termination of pregnancy   CC M
- Cystitis following (induced) termination of pregnancy

O04.89 **(Induced) termination of pregnancy with other complications**   CC M

✓4th **O07** **Failed attempted termination** of pregnancy

    INCLUDES   failure of attempted induction of termination of pregnancy
incomplete elective abortion

    EXCLUDES 1   *incomplete spontaneous abortion (O03.0-)*

O07.0 **Genital tract and pelvic infection** following failed attempted termination of pregnancy   CC M
- Endometritis following failed attempted termination of pregnancy
- Oophoritis following failed attempted termination of pregnancy
- Parametritis following failed attempted termination of pregnancy
- Pelvic peritonitis following failed attempted termination of pregnancy
- Salpingitis following failed attempted termination of pregnancy
- Salpingo-oophoritis following failed attempted termination of pregnancy

    EXCLUDES 1   *sepsis following failed attempted termination of pregnancy (O07.37)*
urinary tract infection following failed attempted termination of pregnancy (O07.38)

O07.1 **Delayed or excessive hemorrhage** following failed attempted termination of pregnancy   CC M
- Afibrinogenemia following failed attempted termination of pregnancy
- Defibrination syndrome following failed attempted termination of pregnancy
- Hemolysis following failed attempted termination of pregnancy
- Intravascular coagulation following failed attempted termination of pregnancy

O07.2 **Embolism** following failed attempted termination of pregnancy   MCC M
- Air embolism following failed attempted termination of pregnancy
- Amniotic fluid embolism following failed attempted termination of pregnancy
- Blood-clot embolism following failed attempted termination of pregnancy
- Embolism NOS following failed attempted termination of pregnancy
- Fat embolism following failed attempted termination of pregnancy
- Pulmonary embolism following failed attempted termination of pregnancy
- Pyemic embolism following failed attempted termination of pregnancy
- Septic or septicopyemic embolism following failed attempted termination of pregnancy
- Soap embolism following failed attempted termination of pregnancy

✓5th **O07.3** **Failed attempted termination of pregnancy with other and unspecified complications**

    O07.30 **Failed attempted termination of pregnancy with unspecified complications**   CC M

    O07.31 **Shock** following failed attempted termination of pregnancy   MCC M
- Circulatory collapse following failed attempted termination of pregnancy
- Shock (postprocedural) following failed attempted termination of pregnancy

      EXCLUDES 1   *shock due to infection following failed attempted termination of pregnancy (O07.37)*

    O07.32 **Renal failure** following failed attempted termination of pregnancy   MCC M
- Kidney failure (acute) following failed attempted termination of pregnancy
- Oliguria following failed attempted termination of pregnancy
- Renal shutdown following failed attempted termination of pregnancy
- Renal tubular necrosis following failed attempted termination of pregnancy
- Uremia following failed attempted termination of pregnancy

    O07.33 **Metabolic disorder** following failed attempted termination of pregnancy   CC M

    O07.34 **Damage to pelvic organs** following failed attempted termination of pregnancy   CC M
- Laceration, perforation, tear or chemical damage of bladder following failed attempted termination of pregnancy
- Laceration, perforation, tear or chemical damage of bowel following failed attempted termination of pregnancy
- Laceration, perforation, tear or chemical damage of broad ligament following failed attempted termination of pregnancy
- Laceration, perforation, tear or chemical damage of cervix following failed attempted termination of pregnancy
- Laceration, perforation, tear or chemical damage of periurethral tissue following failed attempted termination of pregnancy
- Laceration, perforation, tear or chemical damage of uterus following failed attempted termination of pregnancy
- Laceration, perforation, tear or chemical damage of vagina following failed attempted termination of pregnancy

    O07.35 **Other venous complications following failed attempted termination of pregnancy**   CC M

    O07.36 **Cardiac arrest** following failed attempted termination of pregnancy   CC M

    O07.37 **Sepsis** following failed attempted termination of pregnancy   CC M

Use additional code (B95-B97), to identify infectious agent

Use additional code (R65.2-) to identify severe sepsis, if applicable

      EXCLUDES 1   *septic or septicopyemic embolism following failed attempted termination of pregnancy (O07.2)*

N Newborn: 0   P Pediatric: 0-17   M Maternity: 9-64   A Adult: 15-124   UNS Unspecified Site   MCC Major Complication/Comorbidity   CC Complication/Comorbidity   PE POA Exempt

886   ICD-10-CM 2025

O07.38 **Urinary tract infection** following failed attempted termination of pregnancy `CC` `M`
  Cystitis following failed attempted termination of pregnancy

O07.39 Failed attempted termination of pregnancy with other complications `CC` `M`

O07.4 Failed attempted termination of pregnancy **without complication** `M`

✓4ᵗʰ **O08** **Complications following ectopic and molar** pregnancy
  This category is for use with categories O00-O02 to identify any associated complications

O08.0 **Genital tract and pelvic infection** following ectopic and molar pregnancy `CC` `M`
  Endometritis following ectopic and molar pregnancy
  Oophoritis following ectopic and molar pregnancy
  Parametritis following ectopic and molar pregnancy
  Pelvic peritonitis following ectopic and molar pregnancy
  Salpingitis following ectopic and molar pregnancy
  Salpingo-oophoritis following ectopic and molar pregnancy
  EXCLUDES 1 *sepsis following ectopic and molar pregnancy (O08.82)*
    urinary tract infection (O08.83)

O08.1 **Delayed or excessive hemorrhage** following ectopic and molar pregnancy `CC` `M`
  Afibrinogenemia following ectopic and molar pregnancy
  Defibrination syndrome following ectopic and molar pregnancy
  Hemolysis following ectopic and molar pregnancy
  Intravascular coagulation following ectopic and molar pregnancy
  EXCLUDES 1 *delayed or excessive hemorrhage due to incomplete abortion (O03.1)*

O08.2 **Embolism following ectopic and molar pregnancy** `MCC` `M`
  Air embolism following ectopic and molar pregnancy
  Amniotic fluid embolism following ectopic and molar pregnancy
  Blood-clot embolism following ectopic and molar pregnancy
  Embolism NOS following ectopic and molar pregnancy
  Fat embolism following ectopic and molar pregnancy
  Pulmonary embolism following ectopic and molar pregnancy
  Pyemic embolism following ectopic and molar pregnancy
  Septic or septicopyemic embolism following ectopic and molar pregnancy
  Soap embolism following ectopic and molar pregnancy

O08.3 **Shock** following ectopic and molar pregnancy `MCC` `M`
  Circulatory collapse following ectopic and molar pregnancy
  Shock (postprocedural) following ectopic and molar pregnancy
  EXCLUDES 1 *shock due to infection following ectopic and molar pregnancy (O08.82)*

O08.4 **Renal failure** following ectopic and molar pregnancy `MCC` `M`
  Kidney failure (acute) following ectopic and molar pregnancy
  Oliguria following ectopic and molar pregnancy
  Renal shutdown following ectopic and molar pregnancy
  Renal tubular necrosis following ectopic and molar pregnancy
  Uremia following ectopic and molar pregnancy

O08.5 **Metabolic disorders** following an ectopic and molar pregnancy `CC` `M`

O08.6 **Damage to pelvic organs and tissues** following an ectopic and molar pregnancy `CC` `M`
  Laceration, perforation, tear or chemical damage of bladder following an ectopic and molar pregnancy
  Laceration, perforation, tear or chemical damage of bowel following an ectopic and molar pregnancy
  Laceration, perforation, tear or chemical damage of broad ligament following an ectopic and molar pregnancy
  Laceration, perforation, tear or chemical damage of cervix following an ectopic and molar pregnancy
  Laceration, perforation, tear or chemical damage of periurethral tissue following an ectopic and molar pregnancy
  Laceration, perforation, tear or chemical damage of uterus following an ectopic and molar pregnancy
  Laceration, perforation, tear or chemical damage of vagina following an ectopic and molar pregnancy

O08.7 Other venous complications following an ectopic and molar pregnancy `CC` `M`

✓5ᵗʰ O08.8 **Other complications following an ectopic and molar pregnancy**

O08.81 **Cardiac arrest** following an ectopic and molar pregnancy `CC` `M`

O08.82 **Sepsis** following ectopic and molar pregnancy `CC` `M`
  Use additional code (B95-B97), to identify infectious agent
  Use additional code (R65.2-) to identify severe sepsis, if applicable
  EXCLUDES 1 *septic or septicopyemic embolism following ectopic and molar pregnancy (O08.2)*

O08.83 **Urinary tract infection** following an ectopic and molar pregnancy `CC` `M`
  Cystitis following an ectopic and molar pregnancy

O08.89 **Other complications** following an ectopic and molar pregnancy `CC` `M`

O08.9 Unspecified complication following an ectopic and molar pregnancy `CC` `M`

Supervision of high risk pregnancy (O09)

✓4ᵗʰ **O09** **Supervision of high risk** pregnancy
  AHA: 2019,3Q,5; 2016,4Q,48-50,150

✓5ᵗʰ O09.0 **Supervision of pregnancy with history of infertility**

O09.00 **Supervision of pregnancy with history of infertility, unspecified trimester** `UPD` `M` `PE`

O09.01 **Supervision of pregnancy with history of infertility, first trimester** `UPD` `M` `PE`

O09.02 **Supervision of pregnancy with history of infertility, second trimester** `UPD` `M` `PE`

O09.03 **Supervision of pregnancy with history of infertility, third trimester** `UPD` `M` `PE`

✓5ᵗʰ O09.1 **Supervision of pregnancy with history of ectopic** pregnancy

O09.10 **Supervision of pregnancy with history of ectopic pregnancy, unspecified trimester** `UPD` `M` `PE`

O09.11 **Supervision of pregnancy with history of ectopic pregnancy, first trimester** `UPD` `M` `PE`

O09.12 **Supervision of pregnancy with history of ectopic pregnancy, second trimester** `UPD` `M` `PE`

O09.13 **Supervision of pregnancy with history of ectopic pregnancy, third trimester** `UPD` `M` `PE`

✓5ᵗʰ O09.A **Supervision of pregnancy with history of molar** pregnancy
  DEF: Molar pregnancy: Trophoblastic neoplasm that mimics pregnancy by proliferating from a pathologic ovum and resulting only in a mass of cysts resembling grapes, 80 percent of which are benign, but require surgical removal.

O09.A0 **Supervision of pregnancy with history of molar pregnancy, unspecified trimester** `UPD` `M` `PE`

O09.A1 **Supervision of pregnancy with history of molar pregnancy, first trimester** `UPD` `M` `PE`

O09.A2 **Supervision of pregnancy with history of molar pregnancy, second trimester** `UPD` `M` `PE`

O09.A3 **Supervision of pregnancy with history of molar pregnancy, third trimester** `UPD` `M` `PE`

✓5ᵗʰ O09.2 **Supervision of pregnancy with other poor reproductive or obstetric history**
  EXCLUDES 2 *pregnancy care for patient with history of recurrent pregnancy loss (O26.2-)*

✓6ᵗʰ O09.21 **Supervision of pregnancy with history of pre-term labor**

O09.211 **Supervision of pregnancy with history of pre-term labor, first trimester** `UPD` `M` `PE`

O09.212 **Supervision of pregnancy with history of pre-term labor, second trimester** `UPD` `M` `PE`

O09.213 **Supervision of pregnancy with history of pre-term labor, third trimester** `UPD` `M` `PE`

O09.219 **Supervision of pregnancy with history of pre-term labor, unspecified trimester** `UPD` `M` `PE`

✓6ᵗʰ O09.29 **Supervision of pregnancy with other poor reproductive or obstetric history**
  Supervision of pregnancy with history of neonatal death
  Supervision of pregnancy with history of stillbirth

O09.291 **Supervision of pregnancy with other poor reproductive or obstetric history, first trimester** `UPD` `M` `PE`

O09.292 **Supervision of pregnancy with other poor reproductive or obstetric history, second trimester** `UPD` `M` `PE`

O09.293 Supervision of pregnancy with other poor reproductive or obstetric history, third trimester **UPD M**

O09.299 Supervision of pregnancy with other poor reproductive or obstetric history, unspecified trimester **UPD M PE**

√5th **O09.3** Supervision of pregnancy with insufficient antenatal care

Supervision of concealed pregnancy
Supervision of hidden pregnancy

O09.30 Supervision of pregnancy with insufficient antenatal care, unspecified trimester **UPD M PE**

O09.31 Supervision of pregnancy with insufficient antenatal care, first trimester

O09.32 Supervision of pregnancy with insufficient antenatal care, second trimester

O09.33 Supervision of pregnancy with insufficient antenatal care, third trimester **UPD M PE**

√5th **O09.4** Supervision of pregnancy with grand multiparity

O09.40 Supervision of pregnancy with grand multiparity, unspecified trimester **UPD M PE**

O09.41 Supervision of pregnancy with grand multiparity, first trimester

O09.42 Supervision of pregnancy with grand multiparity, second trimester

O09.43 Supervision of pregnancy with grand multiparity, third trimester **UPD M PE**

√5th **O09.5** Supervision of elderly primigravida and multigravida

Pregnancy for a female 35 years and older at expected date of delivery

√6th **O09.51** Supervision of elderly primigravida

O09.511 Supervision of elderly primigravida, first trimester **UPD M PE**

O09.512 Supervision of elderly primigravida, second trimester **UPD M PE**

O09.513 Supervision of elderly primigravida, third trimester **UPD M PE**

O09.519 Supervision of elderly primigravida, unspecified trimester **UPD M PE**

√6th **O09.52** Supervision of elderly multigravida

O09.521 Supervision of elderly multigravida, first trimester **UPD M PE**

O09.522 Supervision of elderly multigravida, second trimester **UPD M PE**

O09.523 Supervision of elderly multigravida, third trimester **UPD M PE**

O09.529 Supervision of elderly multigravida, unspecified trimester **UPD M PE**

√5th **O09.6** Supervision of young primigravida and multigravida

Supervision of pregnancy for a female less than 16 years old at expected date of delivery

√6th **O09.61** Supervision of young primigravida

O09.611 Supervision of young primigravida, first trimester **UPD M PE**

O09.612 Supervision of young primigravida, second trimester **UPD M PE**

O09.613 Supervision of young primigravida, third trimester **UPD M PE**

O09.619 Supervision of young primigravida, unspecified trimester **UPD M PE**

√6th **O09.62** Supervision of young multigravida

O09.621 Supervision of young multigravida, first trimester **UPD M PE**

O09.622 Supervision of young multigravida, second trimester **UPD M PE**

O09.623 Supervision of young multigravida, third trimester **UPD M PE**

O09.629 Supervision of young multigravida, unspecified trimester **UPD M PE**

√5th **O09.7** Supervision of high risk pregnancy due to social problems

O09.70 Supervision of high risk pregnancy due to social problems, unspecified trimester **UPD M PE**

O09.71 Supervision of high risk pregnancy due to social problems, first trimester **UPD M PE**

O09.72 Supervision of high risk pregnancy due to social problems, second trimester **UPD M PE**

O09.73 Supervision of high risk pregnancy due to social problems, third trimester **UPD M PE**

√5th **O09.8** Supervision of other high risk pregnancies

√6th **O09.81** Supervision of pregnancy resulting from assisted reproductive technology

Supervision of pregnancy resulting from in-vitro fertilization

EXCLUDES 2 gestational carrier status (Z33.3)

O09.811 Supervision of pregnancy resulting from assisted reproductive technology, first trimester **UPD M PE**

O09.812 Supervision of pregnancy resulting from assisted reproductive technology, second trimester **UPD M PE**

O09.813 Supervision of pregnancy resulting from assisted reproductive technology, third trimester **UPD M PE**

O09.819 Supervision of pregnancy resulting from assisted reproductive technology, unspecified trimester **UPD M PE**

√6th **O09.82** Supervision of pregnancy with history of in utero procedure during previous pregnancy

O09.821 Supervision of pregnancy with history of in utero procedure during previous pregnancy, first trimester **UPD M PE**

O09.822 Supervision of pregnancy with history of in utero procedure during previous pregnancy, second trimester **UPD M PE**

O09.823 Supervision of pregnancy with history of in utero procedure during previous pregnancy, third trimester **UPD M PE**

O09.829 Supervision of pregnancy with history of in utero procedure during previous pregnancy, unspecified trimester **UPD M PE**

EXCLUDES 1 supervision of pregnancy affected by in utero procedure during current pregnancy (O35.7)

√6th **O09.89** Supervision of other high risk pregnancies

O09.891 Supervision of other high risk pregnancies, first trimester **UPD M**

O09.892 Supervision of other high risk pregnancies, second trimester **UPD M**

O09.893 Supervision of other high risk pregnancies, third trimester **UPD M**

O09.899 Supervision of other high risk pregnancies, unspecified trimester **UPD M**

√5th **O09.9** Supervision of high risk pregnancy, unspecified

O09.90 Supervision of high risk pregnancy, unspecified, unspecified trimester **UPD M PE**

O09.91 Supervision of high risk pregnancy, unspecified, first trimester **UPD M PE**

O09.92 Supervision of high risk pregnancy, unspecified, second trimester **UPD M PE**

O09.93 Supervision of high risk pregnancy, unspecified, third trimester **UPD M PE**

Edema, proteinuria and hypertensive disorders in pregnancy, childbirth and the puerperium (O10-O16)

AHA: 2016,4Q,50

√4th **O10** Pre-existing hypertension complicating pregnancy, childbirth and the puerperium

INCLUDES pre-existing hypertension with pre-existing proteinuria complicating pregnancy, childbirth and the puerperium

EXCLUDES 2 pre-existing hypertension with superimposed pre-eclampsia complicating pregnancy, childbirth and the puerperium (O11.-)

√5th **O10.0** Pre-existing essential hypertension complicating pregnancy, childbirth and the puerperium

Any condition in I10 specified as a reason for obstetric care during pregnancy, childbirth or the puerperium

√6th **O10.01** Pre-existing essential hypertension complicating pregnancy

O10.011 Pre-existing essential hypertension complicating pregnancy, first trimester **CC M**

O10.012 Pre-existing essential hypertension complicating pregnancy, second trimester **CC M**

N Newborn: 0 | P Pediatric: 0-17 | M Maternity: 9-64 | A Adult: 15-124 | UNS Unspecified Site | MCC Major Complication/Comorbidity | CC Complication/Comorbidity | PE POA Exempt

888

ICD-10-CM 2025

O10.013   Pre-existing essential hypertension complicating pregnancy, **third trimester**   `cc` `M`

O10.019   Pre-existing essential hypertension complicating pregnancy, unspecified trimester   `M`

O10.02   Pre-existing essential hypertension complicating **childbirth**   `cc` `M`

O10.03   Pre-existing essential hypertension complicating the **puerperium**   `M`

√5ᵗʰ   **O10.1**   Pre-existing hypertensive **heart disease** complicating pregnancy, childbirth and the puerperium

Any condition in I11 specified as a reason for obstetric care during pregnancy, childbirth or the puerperium

Use additional code from I11 to identify the type of hypertensive heart disease

√6ᵗʰ   **O10.11**   Pre-existing hypertensive heart disease complicating **pregnancy**

O10.111   Pre-existing hypertensive heart disease complicating pregnancy, **first trimester**   `M`

O10.112   Pre-existing hypertensive heart disease complicating pregnancy, **second trimester**   `M`

O10.113   Pre-existing hypertensive heart disease complicating pregnancy, **third trimester**   `M`

O10.119   Pre-existing hypertensive heart disease complicating pregnancy, unspecified trimester   `M`

O10.12   Pre-existing hypertensive heart disease complicating **childbirth**   `M`

O10.13   Pre-existing hypertensive heart disease complicating the **puerperium**   `M`

√5ᵗʰ   **O10.2**   Pre-existing hypertensive **chronic kidney disease** complicating pregnancy, childbirth and the puerperium

Any condition in I12 specified as a reason for obstetric care during pregnancy, childbirth or the puerperium

Use additional code from I12 to identify the type of hypertensive chronic kidney disease

√6ᵗʰ   **O10.21**   Pre-existing hypertensive chronic kidney disease complicating **pregnancy**

O10.211   Pre-existing hypertensive chronic kidney disease complicating pregnancy, **first trimester**   `M`

O10.212   Pre-existing hypertensive chronic kidney disease complicating pregnancy, **second trimester**   `M`

O10.213   Pre-existing hypertensive chronic kidney disease complicating pregnancy, **third trimester**   `M`

O10.219   Pre-existing hypertensive chronic kidney disease complicating pregnancy, unspecified trimester   `M`

O10.22   Pre-existing hypertensive chronic kidney disease complicating **childbirth**   `M`

O10.23   Pre-existing hypertensive chronic kidney disease complicating the **puerperium**   `M`

√5ᵗʰ   **O10.3**   Pre-existing hypertensive **heart and chronic kidney disease** complicating pregnancy, childbirth and the puerperium

Any condition in I13 specified as a reason for obstetric care during pregnancy, childbirth or the puerperium

Use additional code from I13 to identify the type of hypertensive heart and chronic kidney disease

√6ᵗʰ   **O10.31**   Pre-existing hypertensive heart and chronic kidney disease complicating **pregnancy**

O10.311   Pre-existing hypertensive heart and chronic kidney disease complicating pregnancy, **first trimester**   `M`

O10.312   Pre-existing hypertensive heart and chronic kidney disease complicating pregnancy, **second trimester**   `M`

O10.313   Pre-existing hypertensive heart and chronic kidney disease complicating pregnancy, **third trimester**   `M`

O10.319   Pre-existing hypertensive heart and chronic kidney disease complicating pregnancy, unspecified trimester   `M`

O10.32   Pre-existing hypertensive heart and chronic kidney disease complicating **childbirth**   `M`

O10.33   Pre-existing hypertensive heart and chronic kidney disease complicating the **puerperium**   `M`

√5ᵗʰ   **O10.4**   Pre-existing **secondary** hypertension complicating pregnancy, childbirth and the puerperium

Any condition in I15 specified as a reason for obstetric care during pregnancy, childbirth or the puerperium

Use additional code from I15 to identify the type of secondary hypertension

√6ᵗʰ   **O10.41**   Pre-existing secondary hypertension complicating **pregnancy**

O10.411   Pre-existing secondary hypertension complicating pregnancy, **first trimester**   `cc` `M`

O10.412   Pre-existing secondary hypertension complicating pregnancy, **second trimester**   `cc` `M`

O10.413   Pre-existing secondary hypertension complicating pregnancy, **third trimester**   `cc` `M`

O10.419   Pre-existing secondary hypertension complicating pregnancy, unspecified trimester   `M`

O10.42   Pre-existing secondary hypertension complicating **childbirth**   `MCC` `M`

O10.43   Pre-existing secondary hypertension complicating the **puerperium**   `cc` `M`

√5ᵗʰ   **O10.9**   Unspecified pre-existing hypertension complicating pregnancy, childbirth and the puerperium

√6ᵗʰ   **O10.91**   Unspecified pre-existing hypertension complicating **pregnancy**

O10.911   Unspecified pre-existing hypertension complicating pregnancy, **first trimester**   `cc` `M`

O10.912   Unspecified pre-existing hypertension complicating pregnancy, **second trimester**   `cc` `M`

O10.913   Unspecified pre-existing hypertension complicating pregnancy, **third trimester**   `cc` `M`

O10.919   Unspecified pre-existing hypertension complicating pregnancy, unspecified trimester   `M`

O10.92   Unspecified pre-existing hypertension complicating **childbirth**   `cc` `M`

O10.93   Unspecified pre-existing hypertension complicating the **puerperium**   `M`

√4ᵗʰ   **O11**   **Pre-existing hypertension with pre-eclampsia**

`INCLUDES`   conditions in O10 complicated by pre-eclampsia
pre-eclampsia superimposed pre-existing in hypertension

Use additional code from O10 to identify the type of hypertension

DEF: Complication of pregnancy manifesting in the development of borderline hypertension, protein in the urine, and unresponsive swelling between the 20th week of pregnancy and the end of the first week following birth in mild to moderate cases. Severe preeclampsia presents with hypertension, associated with marked swelling, proteinuria, abdominal pain, and/or visual changes.

O11.1   Pre-existing hypertension with pre-eclampsia, **first trimester**   `MCC` `M`

O11.2   Pre-existing hypertension with pre-eclampsia, **second trimester**   `MCC` `M`

O11.3   Pre-existing hypertension with pre-eclampsia, **third trimester**   `MCC` `M`

O11.4   Pre-existing hypertension with pre-eclampsia, complicating **childbirth**   `M`

O11.5   Pre-existing hypertension with pre-eclampsia, complicating the **puerperium**   `M`

O11.9   Pre-existing hypertension with pre-eclampsia, unspecified trimester   `M`

√4ᵗʰ   **O12**   **Gestational [pregnancy-induced] edema and proteinuria without hypertension**

√5ᵗʰ   **O12.0**   Gestational **edema**

O12.00   Gestational edema, unspecified trimester   `M`

O12.01   Gestational edema, **first trimester**   `M`

O12.02   Gestational edema, **second trimester**   `M`

O12.03   Gestational edema, **third trimester**   `M`

O12.04   Gestational edema, complicating **childbirth**   `M`

O12.05   Gestational edema, complicating the **puerperium**   `M`

√5ᵗʰ   **O12.1**   Gestational **proteinuria**

O12.10   Gestational proteinuria, unspecified trimester   `M`

O12.11   Gestational proteinuria, **first trimester**   `cc` `M`

✔ Additional Character Required   √x7ᵗʰ Placeholder   Questionable PDx   Manifestation   Unspecified   `UPD` Unacceptable PDx   H1-H14 HAC   HCC CMS-HCC Dx   HIV HIV Dx

ICD-10-CM 2025   889

Chapter 15. Pregnancy, Childbirth and the Puerperium (side tab)

O12.12–O21.9 (side tab)

O12.12   Gestational proteinuria, **second trimester** `CC` `M`

O12.13   Gestational proteinuria, **third trimester** `CC` `M`

O12.14   Gestational proteinuria, complicating **childbirth** `M`

O12.15   Gestational proteinuria, complicating the **puerperium** `M`

✓5th O12.2   Gestational **edema with proteinuria**

   O12.20   Gestational edema with proteinuria, unspecified trimester `M`

   O12.21   Gestational edema with proteinuria, **first trimester** `CC` `M`

   O12.22   Gestational edema with proteinuria, **second trimester** `CC` `M`

   O12.23   Gestational edema with proteinuria, **third trimester** `CC` `M`

   O12.24   Gestational edema with proteinuria, complicating **childbirth**

   O12.25   Gestational edema with proteinuria, complicating the **puerperium** `M`

✓4th **O13**   Gestational **[pregnancy-induced] hypertension without significant proteinuria**

> `INCLUDES`   gestational hypertension NOS
> transient hypertension of pregnancy
> **AHA:** 2016,1Q,5

O13.1   Gestational [pregnancy-induced] hypertension without significant proteinuria, **first trimester** `M`

O13.2   Gestational [pregnancy-induced] hypertension without significant proteinuria, **second trimester** `M`

O13.3   Gestational [pregnancy-induced] hypertension without significant proteinuria, **third trimester** `M`

O13.4   Gestational [pregnancy-induced] hypertension without significant proteinuria, complicating **childbirth** `M`

O13.5   Gestational [pregnancy-induced] hypertension without significant proteinuria, complicating the **puerperium** `M`

O13.9   Gestational [pregnancy-induced] hypertension without significant proteinuria, unspecified trimester `M`

✓4th **O14**   **Pre-eclampsia**

> `EXCLUDES 1`   pre-existing hypertension with pre-eclampsia (O11)
> **DEF:** Complication of pregnancy manifesting in the development of borderline hypertension, protein in the urine, and unresponsive swelling between the 20th week of pregnancy and the end of the first week following birth in mild to moderate cases. Severe preeclampsia presents with hypertension, associated with marked swelling, proteinuria, abdominal pain, and/or visual changes.

✓5th O14.0   **Mild to moderate** pre-eclampsia

> **AHA:** 2019,3Q,12; 2019,2Q,8

   O14.00   Mild to moderate pre-eclampsia, unspecified trimester `M`

   O14.02   Mild to moderate pre-eclampsia, **second trimester** `CC` `M`

   O14.03   Mild to moderate pre-eclampsia, **third trimester** `CC` `M`

   O14.04   Mild to moderate pre-eclampsia, complicating **childbirth** `M`

> **AHA:** 2019,2Q,8

   O14.05   Mild to moderate pre-eclampsia, complicating the **puerperium** `M`

✓5th O14.1   **Severe** pre-eclampsia

> `EXCLUDES 1`   HELLP syndrome (O14.2-)
> **AHA:** 2019,3Q,12

   O14.10   Severe pre-eclampsia, unspecified trimester `M`

   O14.12   Severe pre-eclampsia, **second trimester** `MCC` `M`

   O14.13   Severe pre-eclampsia, **third trimester** `MCC` `M`

   O14.14   Severe pre-eclampsia complicating **childbirth** `M`

   O14.15   Severe pre-eclampsia, complicating the **puerperium** `M`

✓5th O14.2   **HELLP syndrome**

> Severe pre-eclampsia with hemolysis, elevated liver enzymes and low platelet count (HELLP)
> **AHA:** 2019,3Q,12

   O14.20   HELLP syndrome (HELLP), unspecified trimester `M`

   O14.22   HELLP syndrome (HELLP), **second trimester** `MCC` `M`

   O14.23   HELLP syndrome (HELLP), **third trimester** `MCC` `M`

   O14.24   HELLP syndrome, complicating **childbirth** `M`

   O14.25   HELLP syndrome, complicating the **puerperium** `M`

✓5th O14.9   Unspecified pre-eclampsia

   O14.90   Unspecified pre-eclampsia, unspecified trimester `M`

   O14.92   Unspecified pre-eclampsia, **second trimester** `CC` `M`

   O14.93   Unspecified pre-eclampsia, **third trimester** `CC` `M`

   O14.94   Unspecified pre-eclampsia, complicating **childbirth** `M`

   O14.95   Unspecified pre-eclampsia, complicating the **puerperium** `M`

✓4th **O15**   **Eclampsia**

> `INCLUDES`   convulsions following conditions in O10-O14 and O16
> **DEF:** Tetany and toxemia producing seizure activity or coma in a pregnant patient who most often has presented with prior preeclampsia (i.e., hypertension, albuminuria, and edema).

✓5th O15.0   Eclampsia **complicating pregnancy**

   O15.00   Eclampsia complicating pregnancy, unspecified trimester `M`

   O15.02   Eclampsia complicating pregnancy, **second trimester** `MCC` `M`

   O15.03   Eclampsia complicating pregnancy, **third trimester** `MCC` `M`

O15.1   Eclampsia complicating **labor** `MCC` `M`

O15.2   Eclampsia complicating the **puerperium** `MCC` `M`

O15.9   Eclampsia, unspecified as to time period `M`
> Eclampsia NOS

✓4th **O16**   Unspecified maternal hypertension

O16.1   Unspecified maternal hypertension, **first trimester** `CC` `M`

O16.2   Unspecified maternal hypertension, **second trimester** `CC` `M`

O16.3   Unspecified maternal hypertension, **third trimester** `CC` `M`

O16.4   Unspecified maternal hypertension, complicating **childbirth** `M`

O16.5   Unspecified maternal hypertension, complicating the **puerperium** `M`

O16.9   Unspecified maternal hypertension, unspecified trimester `M`

Other maternal disorders predominantly related to pregnancy (O20–O29)

> `EXCLUDES 2`   maternal care related to the fetus and amniotic cavity and possible delivery problems (O30-O48)
> maternal diseases classifiable elsewhere but complicating pregnancy, labor and delivery, and the puerperium (O98-O99)

✓4th **O20**   Hemorrhage in early pregnancy

> `INCLUDES`   hemorrhage before completion of 20 weeks gestation
> `EXCLUDES 1`   pregnancy with abortive outcome (O00-O08)

O20.0   Threatened abortion `CC` `M`
> Hemorrhage specified as due to threatened abortion
> **DEF:** Bloody discharge during pregnancy. The cervix may be dilated and pregnancy threatened, but the pregnancy is not terminated.

O20.8   Other hemorrhage in early pregnancy `M`
> **AHA:** 2023,3Q,18

O20.9   Hemorrhage in early pregnancy, unspecified `CC` `M`

✓4th **O21**   Excessive vomiting in pregnancy

O21.0   Mild **hyperemesis gravidarum** `M`
> Hyperemesis gravidarum, mild or unspecified, starting before the end of the 20th week of gestation

O21.1   Hyperemesis gravidarum with **metabolic disturbance** `M`
> Hyperemesis gravidarum, starting before the end of the 20th week of gestation, with metabolic disturbance such as carbohydrate depletion
> Hyperemesis gravidarum, starting before the end of the 20th week of gestation, with metabolic disturbance such as dehydration
> Hyperemesis gravidarum, starting before the end of the 20th week of gestation, with metabolic disturbance such as electrolyte imbalance

O21.2   **Late** vomiting of pregnancy `M`
> Excessive vomiting starting after 20 completed weeks of gestation

O21.8   Other vomiting complicating pregnancy `M`
> Vomiting due to diseases classified elsewhere, complicating pregnancy
> Use additional code, to identify cause

O21.9   Vomiting of pregnancy, unspecified `M`

√4th **O22**   **Venous complications and hemorrhoids in pregnancy**

> EXCLUDES 1   venous complications of:
> abortion NOS (O03.9)
> ectopic or molar pregnancy (O08.7)
> failed attempted abortion (O07.35)
> induced abortion (O04.85)
> spontaneous abortion (O03.89)
>
> EXCLUDES 2   obstetric pulmonary embolism (O88.-)
> venous complications and hemorrhoids of childbirth and the puerperium (O87.-)

√5th **O22.0**   **Varicose veins of lower extremity in pregnancy**

> Varicose veins NOS in pregnancy
> **DEF:** Distended, tortuous veins of the lower extremities associated with pregnancy.

   O22.00   **Varicose veins of lower extremity in pregnancy, unspecified trimester**   M

   O22.01   **Varicose veins of lower extremity in pregnancy, first trimester**   M

   O22.02   **Varicose veins of lower extremity in pregnancy, second trimester**   M

   O22.03   **Varicose veins of lower extremity in pregnancy, third trimester**   M

√5th **O22.1**   **Genital varices in pregnancy**

> Perineal varices in pregnancy
> Vaginal varices in pregnancy
> Vulval varices in pregnancy

   O22.10   **Genital varices in pregnancy, unspecified trimester**   M

   O22.11   **Genital varices in pregnancy, first trimester**   M

   O22.12   **Genital varices in pregnancy, second trimester**   M

   O22.13   **Genital varices in pregnancy, third trimester**   M

√5th **O22.2**   **Superficial thrombophlebitis in pregnancy**

> Phlebitis in pregnancy NOS
> Thrombophlebitis of legs in pregnancy
> Thrombosis in pregnancy NOS
> Use additional code to identify the superficial thrombophlebitis (I80.0-)

   O22.20   **Superficial thrombophlebitis in pregnancy, unspecified trimester**   CC M

   O22.21   **Superficial thrombophlebitis in pregnancy, first trimester**   CC M

   O22.22   **Superficial thrombophlebitis in pregnancy, second trimester**   CC M

   O22.23   **Superficial thrombophlebitis in pregnancy, third trimester**   CC M

√5th **O22.3**   **Deep phlebothrombosis in pregnancy**

> Deep vein thrombosis, antepartum
> Use additional code to identify the deep vein thrombosis (I82.4-, I82.5-, I82.62-, I82.72-)
> Use additional code, if applicable, for associated long-term (current) use of anticoagulants (Z79.01)

   O22.30   **Deep phlebothrombosis in pregnancy, unspecified trimester**   CC M

   O22.31   **Deep phlebothrombosis in pregnancy, first trimester**   MCC M

   O22.32   **Deep phlebothrombosis in pregnancy, second trimester**   MCC M

   O22.33   **Deep phlebothrombosis in pregnancy, third trimester**   MCC M

√5th **O22.4**   **Hemorrhoids in pregnancy**

   O22.40   **Hemorrhoids in pregnancy, unspecified trimester**   CC M

   O22.41   **Hemorrhoids in pregnancy, first trimester**   CC M

   O22.42   **Hemorrhoids in pregnancy, second trimester**   CC M

   O22.43   **Hemorrhoids in pregnancy, third trimester**   CC M

√5th **O22.5**   **Cerebral venous thrombosis in pregnancy**

> Cerebrovenous sinus thrombosis in pregnancy

   O22.50   **Cerebral venous thrombosis in pregnancy, unspecified trimester**   CC M

   O22.51   **Cerebral venous thrombosis in pregnancy, first trimester**   CC M

   O22.52   **Cerebral venous thrombosis in pregnancy, second trimester**   CC M

   O22.53   **Cerebral venous thrombosis in pregnancy, third trimester**   CC M

√5th **O22.8**   **Other venous complications in pregnancy**

√6th   **O22.8X**   **Other venous complications in pregnancy**

   O22.8X1   **Other venous complications in pregnancy, first trimester**   CC M

   O22.8X2   **Other venous complications in pregnancy, second trimester**   CC M

   O22.8X3   **Other venous complications in pregnancy, third trimester**   CC M

   O22.8X9   **Other venous complications in pregnancy, unspecified trimester**   M

√5th **O22.9**   **Venous complication in pregnancy, unspecified**

> Gestational phlebitis NOS
> Gestational phlebopathy NOS
> Gestational thrombosis NOS

   O22.90   **Venous complication in pregnancy, unspecified, unspecified trimester**   CC M

   O22.91   **Venous complication in pregnancy, unspecified, first trimester**   M

   O22.92   **Venous complication in pregnancy, unspecified, second trimester**   M

   O22.93   **Venous complication in pregnancy, unspecified, third trimester**   M

√4th **O23**   **Infections of genitourinary tract in pregnancy**

> Use additional code to identify organism (B95.-, B96.-)
>
> EXCLUDES 2   gonococcal infections complicating pregnancy, childbirth and the puerperium (O98.2)
> infections with a predominantly sexual mode of transmission NOS complicating pregnancy, childbirth and the puerperium (O98.3)
> syphilis complicating pregnancy, childbirth and the puerperium (O98.1)
> tuberculosis of genitourinary system complicating pregnancy, childbirth and the puerperium (O98.0)
> venereal disease NOS complicating pregnancy, childbirth and the puerperium (O98.3)
>
> AHA: 2018,2Q,20

√5th **O23.0**   **Infections of kidney in pregnancy**

> Pyelonephritis in pregnancy

   O23.00   **Infections of kidney in pregnancy, unspecified trimester**   M

   O23.01   **Infections of kidney in pregnancy, first trimester**   CC M

   O23.02   **Infections of kidney in pregnancy, second trimester**   CC M

   O23.03   **Infections of kidney in pregnancy, third trimester**   CC M

√5th **O23.1**   **Infections of bladder in pregnancy**

   O23.10   **Infections of bladder in pregnancy, unspecified trimester**   M

   O23.11   **Infections of bladder in pregnancy, first trimester**   CC M

   O23.12   **Infections of bladder in pregnancy, second trimester**   CC M

   O23.13   **Infections of bladder in pregnancy, third trimester**   CC M

√5th **O23.2**   **Infections of urethra in pregnancy**

   O23.20   **Infections of urethra in pregnancy, unspecified trimester**   M

   O23.21   **Infections of urethra in pregnancy, first trimester**   CC M

   O23.22   **Infections of urethra in pregnancy, second trimester**   CC M

   O23.23   **Infections of urethra in pregnancy, third trimester**   CC M

√5th **O23.3**   **Infections of other parts of urinary tract in pregnancy**

   O23.30   **Infections of other parts of urinary tract in pregnancy, unspecified trimester**   M

   O23.31   **Infections of other parts of urinary tract in pregnancy, first trimester**   CC M

   O23.32   **Infections of other parts of urinary tract in pregnancy, second trimester**   CC M

   O23.33   **Infections of other parts of urinary tract in pregnancy, third trimester**   CC M

√5th **O23.4**   **Unspecified infection of urinary tract in pregnancy**

   O23.40   **Unspecified infection of urinary tract in pregnancy, unspecified trimester**   M

√ Additional Character Required   √x7th Placeholder   Questionable PDx   Manifestation   Unspecified   UPD Unacceptable PDx   H1 - H14 HAC   HCC CMS-HCC Dx   HIV HIV Dx

O23.41 **Unspecified infection of urinary tract in pregnancy, first trimester** CC M

O23.42 **Unspecified infection of urinary tract in pregnancy, second trimester** CC M

O23.43 **Unspecified infection of urinary tract in pregnancy, third trimester** CC M

√5ᵗʰ O23.5 **Infections of the genital tract in pregnancy**

  √6ᵗʰ O23.51 **Infection of cervix in pregnancy**

    O23.511 **Infections of cervix in pregnancy, first trimester** CC M

    O23.512 **Infections of cervix in pregnancy, second trimester** CC M

    O23.513 **Infections of cervix in pregnancy, third trimester** CC M

    O23.519 **Infections of cervix in pregnancy, unspecified trimester** M

  √6ᵗʰ O23.52 **Salpingo-oophoritis in pregnancy**

    Oophoritis in pregnancy
    Salpingitis in pregnancy

    O23.521 **Salpingo-oophoritis in pregnancy, first trimester** CC M

    O23.522 **Salpingo-oophoritis in pregnancy, second trimester** CC M

    O23.523 **Salpingo-oophoritis in pregnancy, third trimester** CC M

    O23.529 **Salpingo-oophoritis in pregnancy, unspecified trimester** M

  √6ᵗʰ O23.59 **Infection of other part of genital tract in pregnancy**

    AHA: 2022,1Q,20

    O23.591 **Infection of other part of genital tract in pregnancy, first trimester** CC M

    O23.592 **Infection of other part of genital tract in pregnancy, second trimester** CC M

    O23.593 **Infection of other part of genital tract in pregnancy, third trimester** CC M

    O23.599 **Infection of other part of genital tract in pregnancy, unspecified trimester** M

√5ᵗʰ O23.9 **Unspecified genitourinary tract infection in pregnancy**

  Genitourinary tract infection in pregnancy NOS

  O23.90 **Unspecified genitourinary tract infection in pregnancy, unspecified trimester** M

  O23.91 **Unspecified genitourinary tract infection in pregnancy, first trimester** CC M

  O23.92 **Unspecified genitourinary tract infection in pregnancy, second trimester** CC M

  O23.93 **Unspecified genitourinary tract infection in pregnancy, third trimester** CC M

√4ᵗʰ O24 **Diabetes mellitus in pregnancy, childbirth and the puerperium**

  √5ᵗʰ O24.0 **Pre-existing type 1 diabetes mellitus, in pregnancy, childbirth and the puerperium**

    Juvenile onset diabetes mellitus, in pregnancy, childbirth and the puerperium
    Ketosis-prone diabetes mellitus in pregnancy, childbirth and the puerperium

    Use additional code from category E10 to further identify any manifestations

    √6ᵗʰ O24.01 **Pre-existing type 1 diabetes mellitus, in pregnancy**

      O24.011 **Pre-existing type 1 diabetes mellitus, in pregnancy, first trimester** CC M

      O24.012 **Pre-existing type 1 diabetes mellitus, in pregnancy, second trimester** CC M

      O24.013 **Pre-existing type 1 diabetes mellitus, in pregnancy, third trimester** CC M

      O24.019 **Pre-existing type 1 diabetes mellitus, in pregnancy, unspecified trimester** CC M

    O24.02 **Pre-existing type 1 diabetes mellitus, in childbirth** MCC M

    O24.03 **Pre-existing type 1 diabetes mellitus, in the puerperium** CC M

√5ᵗʰ O24.1 **Pre-existing type 2 diabetes mellitus, in pregnancy, childbirth and the puerperium**

  Insulin-resistant diabetes mellitus in pregnancy, childbirth and the puerperium

  Use additional code (for):
    from category E11 to further identify any manifestations
    ►injectable non-insulin antidiabetic drugs (Z79.85)◄
    long-term (current) use of insulin (Z79.4)

  √6ᵗʰ O24.11 **Pre-existing type 2 diabetes mellitus, in pregnancy**

    O24.111 **Pre-existing type 2 diabetes mellitus, in pregnancy, first trimester** CC M

    O24.112 **Pre-existing type 2 diabetes mellitus, in pregnancy, second trimester** CC M

    O24.113 **Pre-existing type 2 diabetes mellitus, in pregnancy, third trimester** CC M

    O24.119 **Pre-existing type 2 diabetes mellitus, in pregnancy, unspecified trimester** CC M

  O24.12 **Pre-existing type 2 diabetes mellitus, in childbirth** MCC M

  O24.13 **Pre-existing type 2 diabetes mellitus, in the puerperium** CC M

√5ᵗʰ O24.3 **Unspecified pre-existing diabetes mellitus in pregnancy, childbirth and the puerperium**

  Use additional code (for):
    from category E11 to further identify any manifestation
    ►injectable non-insulin antidiabetic drugs (Z79.85)◄
    long-term (current) use of insulin (Z79.4)

  √6ᵗʰ O24.31 **Unspecified pre-existing diabetes mellitus in pregnancy**

    O24.311 **Unspecified pre-existing diabetes mellitus in pregnancy, first trimester** CC M

    O24.312 **Unspecified pre-existing diabetes mellitus in pregnancy, second trimester** CC M

    O24.313 **Unspecified pre-existing diabetes mellitus in pregnancy, third trimester** CC M

    O24.319 **Unspecified pre-existing diabetes mellitus in pregnancy, unspecified trimester** CC M

  O24.32 **Unspecified pre-existing diabetes mellitus in childbirth** MCC M

  O24.33 **Unspecified pre-existing diabetes mellitus in the puerperium** CC M

√5ᵗʰ O24.4 **Gestational diabetes mellitus**

  Diabetes mellitus arising in pregnancy
  Gestational diabetes mellitus NOS
  AHA: 2020,3Q,30; 2016,4Q,50; 2015,4Q,34

  √6ᵗʰ O24.41 **Gestational diabetes mellitus in pregnancy**

    O24.410 **Gestational diabetes mellitus in pregnancy, diet controlled** M

    O24.414 **Gestational diabetes mellitus in pregnancy, insulin controlled** M

    O24.415 **Gestational diabetes mellitus in pregnancy, controlled by oral hypoglycemic drugs** M

      Gestational diabetes mellitus in pregnancy, controlled by oral antidiabetic drugs

    O24.419 **Gestational diabetes mellitus in pregnancy, unspecified control** M

  √6ᵗʰ O24.42 **Gestational diabetes mellitus in childbirth**

    AHA: 2016,1Q,5

    O24.420 **Gestational diabetes mellitus in childbirth, diet controlled** M

    O24.424 **Gestational diabetes mellitus in childbirth, insulin controlled** M

    O24.425 **Gestational diabetes mellitus in childbirth, controlled by oral hypoglycemic drugs** M

      Gestational diabetes mellitus in childbirth, controlled by oral antidiabetic drugs

    O24.429 **Gestational diabetes mellitus in childbirth, unspecified control** M

  √6ᵗʰ O24.43 **Gestational diabetes mellitus in the puerperium**

    O24.430 **Gestational diabetes mellitus in the puerperium, diet controlled** M

    O24.434 **Gestational diabetes mellitus in the puerperium, insulin controlled** M

N Newborn: 0   P Pediatric: 0-17   M Maternity: 9-64   A Adult: 15-124   UNS Unspecified Site   MCC Major Complication/Comorbidity   CC Complication/Comorbidity   PE POA Exempt

892
ICD-10-CM 2025

O24.435   **Gestational diabetes mellitus in puerperium, controlled by oral hypoglycemic drugs**   M

     Gestational diabetes mellitus in puerperium, controlled by oral antidiabetic drugs

O24.439   **Gestational diabetes mellitus in the puerperium, unspecified control**   M

✓5th **O24.8**   **Other pre-existing diabetes mellitus in pregnancy, childbirth, and the puerperium**

Use additional code (for):

from categories E08, E09 and E13 to further identify any manifestation

►injectable non-insulin antidiabetic drugs (Z79.85)◄

long-term (current) use of insulin (Z79.4)

✓6th **O24.81**   **Other pre-existing diabetes mellitus in pregnancy**

O24.811   **Other pre-existing diabetes mellitus in pregnancy, first trimester**   CC M

O24.812   **Other pre-existing diabetes mellitus in pregnancy, second trimester**   CC M

O24.813   **Other pre-existing diabetes mellitus in pregnancy, third trimester**   CC M

O24.819   **Other pre-existing diabetes mellitus in pregnancy, unspecified trimester**   CC M

O24.82   **Other pre-existing diabetes mellitus in childbirth**   MCC M

O24.83   **Other pre-existing diabetes mellitus in the puerperium**   CC M

✓5th **O24.9**   **Unspecified diabetes mellitus in pregnancy, childbirth and the puerperium**

►Use additional code (for):◄

►from categories E08, E09 and E13 to further identify any manifestation◄

►injectable non-insulin antidiabetic drugs (Z79.85)◄

►long-term (current) use of insulin (Z79.4)◄

✓6th **O24.91**   **Unspecified diabetes mellitus in pregnancy**

O24.911   **Unspecified diabetes mellitus in pregnancy, first trimester**   CC M

O24.912   **Unspecified diabetes mellitus in pregnancy, second trimester**   CC M

O24.913   **Unspecified diabetes mellitus in pregnancy, third trimester**   CC M

O24.919   **Unspecified diabetes mellitus in pregnancy, unspecified trimester**   CC M

O24.92   **Unspecified diabetes mellitus in childbirth**   M

O24.93   **Unspecified diabetes mellitus in the puerperium**   CC M

✓4th **O25**   **Malnutrition in pregnancy, childbirth and the puerperium**

✓5th **O25.1**   **Malnutrition in pregnancy**

O25.10   **Malnutrition in pregnancy, unspecified trimester**   M

O25.11   **Malnutrition in pregnancy, first trimester**   M

O25.12   **Malnutrition in pregnancy, second trimester**   M

O25.13   **Malnutrition in pregnancy, third trimester**   M

O25.2   **Malnutrition in childbirth**   M

O25.3   **Malnutrition in the puerperium**   M

✓4th **O26**   **Maternal care for other conditions predominantly related to pregnancy**

✓5th **O26.0**   **Excessive weight gain in pregnancy**

EXCLUDES 2   gestational edema (O12.0, O12.2)

O26.00   **Excessive weight gain in pregnancy, unspecified trimester**   M

O26.01   **Excessive weight gain in pregnancy, first trimester**   M

O26.02   **Excessive weight gain in pregnancy, second trimester**   M

O26.03   **Excessive weight gain in pregnancy, third trimester**   M

✓5th **O26.1**   **Low weight gain in pregnancy**

O26.10   **Low weight gain in pregnancy, unspecified trimester**   M

O26.11   **Low weight gain in pregnancy, first trimester**   M

O26.12   **Low weight gain in pregnancy, second trimester**   M

O26.13   **Low weight gain in pregnancy, third trimester**   M

✓5th **O26.2**   **Pregnancy care for patient with recurrent pregnancy loss**

O26.20   **Pregnancy care for patient with recurrent pregnancy loss, unspecified trimester**   M

O26.21   **Pregnancy care for patient with recurrent pregnancy loss, first trimester**   M

O26.22   **Pregnancy care for patient with recurrent pregnancy loss, second trimester**   M

O26.23   **Pregnancy care for patient with recurrent pregnancy loss, third trimester**   M

✓5th **O26.3**   **Retained intrauterine contraceptive device in pregnancy**

O26.30   **Retained intrauterine contraceptive device in pregnancy, unspecified trimester**   M

O26.31   **Retained intrauterine contraceptive device in pregnancy, first trimester**   M

O26.32   **Retained intrauterine contraceptive device in pregnancy, second trimester**   M

O26.33   **Retained intrauterine contraceptive device in pregnancy, third trimester**   M

✓5th **O26.4**   **Herpes gestationis**

DEF: Rare skin disorder of unknown origin that appears on the abdomen in the second and third trimester as intensely itchy blisters that spread to other sites.

O26.40   **Herpes gestationis, unspecified trimester**   M

O26.41   **Herpes gestationis, first trimester**   M

O26.42   **Herpes gestationis, second trimester**   M

O26.43   **Herpes gestationis, third trimester**   M

✓5th **O26.5**   **Maternal hypotension syndrome**

Supine hypotensive syndrome

O26.50   **Maternal hypotension syndrome, unspecified trimester**   M

O26.51   **Maternal hypotension syndrome, first trimester**   M

O26.52   **Maternal hypotension syndrome, second trimester**   M

O26.53   **Maternal hypotension syndrome, third trimester**   M

✓5th **O26.6**   **Liver and biliary tract disorders in pregnancy, childbirth and the puerperium**

Use additional code to identify the specific disorder

EXCLUDES 2   hepatorenal syndrome following labor and delivery (O90.41)

✓6th **O26.61**   **Liver and biliary tract disorders in pregnancy**

O26.611   **Liver and biliary tract disorders in pregnancy, first trimester**   CC M

O26.612   **Liver and biliary tract disorders in pregnancy, second trimester**   CC M

O26.613   **Liver and biliary tract disorders in pregnancy, third trimester**   CC M

O26.619   **Liver and biliary tract disorders in pregnancy, unspecified trimester**   M

O26.62   **Liver and biliary tract disorders in childbirth**   CC M
   AHA: 2023,1Q,26

O26.63   **Liver and biliary tract disorders in the puerperium**   M

✓6th **O26.64**   **Intrahepatic cholestasis of pregnancy**
   AHA: 2023,4Q,36-37

O26.641   **Intrahepatic cholestasis of pregnancy, first trimester**   CC M

O26.642   **Intrahepatic cholestasis of pregnancy, second trimester**   CC M

O26.643   **Intrahepatic cholestasis of pregnancy, third trimester**   CC M

O26.649   **Intrahepatic cholestasis of pregnancy, unspecified trimester**

✓5th **O26.7**   **Subluxation of symphysis (pubis) in pregnancy, childbirth and the puerperium**

EXCLUDES 1   traumatic separation of symphysis (pubis) during childbirth (O71.6)

✓6th **O26.71**   **Subluxation of symphysis (pubis) in pregnancy**

O26.711   **Subluxation of symphysis (pubis) in pregnancy, first trimester**   M

O26.712   **Subluxation of symphysis (pubis) in pregnancy, second trimester**   M

O26.713   **Subluxation of symphysis (pubis) in pregnancy, third trimester**   M

O26.719   **Subluxation of symphysis (pubis) in pregnancy, unspecified trimester**   M

✓ Additional Character Required   ✓x7th Placeholder   Questionable PDx   Manifestation   Unspecified   UPD Unacceptable PDx   H1-H14 HAC   HCC CMS-HCC Dx   HIV HIV Dx

ICD-10-CM 2025   893

O26.72 **Subluxation of symphysis (pubis) in** childbirth **M**

O26.73 **Subluxation of symphysis (pubis) in the** puerperium **M**

√5th O26.8 **Other specified pregnancy related conditions**

√6th O26.81 **Pregnancy related exhaustion and fatigue**

O26.811 **Pregnancy related exhaustion and fatigue,** first trimester **M**

O26.812 **Pregnancy related exhaustion and fatigue,** second trimester **M**

O26.813 **Pregnancy related exhaustion and fatigue,** third trimester **M**

O26.819 **Pregnancy related exhaustion and fatigue, unspecified trimester** **M**

√6th O26.82 **Pregnancy related peripheral neuritis**

O26.821 **Pregnancy related peripheral neuritis,** first trimester **M**

O26.822 **Pregnancy related peripheral neuritis,** second trimester **M**

O26.823 **Pregnancy related peripheral neuritis,** third trimester **M**

O26.829 **Pregnancy related peripheral neuritis, unspecified trimester** **M**

√6th O26.83 **Pregnancy related renal disease**

Use additional code to identify the specific disorder

O26.831 **Pregnancy related renal disease,** first trimester **CC M**

O26.832 **Pregnancy related renal disease,** second trimester **CC M**

O26.833 **Pregnancy related renal disease,** third trimester **CC M**

O26.839 **Pregnancy related renal disease, unspecified trimester** **M**

√6th O26.84 **Uterine size-date discrepancy complicating pregnancy**

EXCLUDES 1 *encounter for suspected problem with fetal growth ruled out (Z03.74)*

O26.841 **Uterine size-date discrepancy,** first trimester **M**

O26.842 **Uterine size-date discrepancy,** second trimester **M**

O26.843 **Uterine size-date discrepancy,** third trimester **M**

O26.849 **Uterine size-date discrepancy, unspecified trimester** **M**

√6th O26.85 **Spotting complicating pregnancy**

O26.851 **Spotting complicating pregnancy,** first trimester **M**

O26.852 **Spotting complicating pregnancy,** second trimester **M**

O26.853 **Spotting complicating pregnancy,** third trimester **M**

O26.859 **Spotting complicating pregnancy, unspecified trimester** **M**

O26.86 **Pruritic urticarial papules and plaques of pregnancy (PUPPP)** **M**

Polymorphic eruption of pregnancy

√6th O26.87 **Cervical shortening**

EXCLUDES 1 *encounter for suspected cervical shortening ruled out (Z03.75)*

DEF: Cervix that has shortened to less than 25 mm before the 24th week of pregnancy. A shortened cervix is a warning sign for impending premature delivery and is treated by cervical cerclage placement or progesterone.

O26.872 **Cervical shortening,** second trimester **CC M**

O26.873 **Cervical shortening,** third trimester **CC M**

O26.879 **Cervical shortening, unspecified trimester** **CC M**

√6th O26.89 **Other specified pregnancy related conditions**

Use additional code, if applicable, to identify specific condition such as insulin resistance (E88.81-)

AHA: 2015,3Q,40

O26.891 **Other specified pregnancy related conditions,** first trimester **M**

O26.892 **Other specified pregnancy related conditions,** second trimester **M**

O26.893 **Other specified pregnancy related conditions,** third trimester **M**

O26.899 **Other specified pregnancy related conditions, unspecified trimester** **M**

√5th O26.9 **Pregnancy related conditions, unspecified**

O26.90 **Pregnancy related conditions, unspecified, unspecified trimester** **M**

O26.91 **Pregnancy related conditions, unspecified,** first trimester **M**

O26.92 **Pregnancy related conditions, unspecified,** second trimester **M**

O26.93 **Pregnancy related conditions, unspecified,** third trimester **M**

√4th O28 **Abnormal findings on antenatal screening of mother**

EXCLUDES 1 *diagnostic findings classified elsewhere - see Alphabetical Index*

O28.0 **Abnormal** hematological **finding on antenatal screening of mother** **M**

O28.1 **Abnormal** biochemical **finding on antenatal screening of mother** **M**

O28.2 **Abnormal** cytological **finding on antenatal screening of mother** **M**

O28.3 **Abnormal** ultrasonic **finding on antenatal screening of mother** **M**

O28.4 **Abnormal** radiological **finding on antenatal screening of mother** **M**

O28.5 **Abnormal** chromosomal and genetic **finding on antenatal screening of mother** **M**

O28.8 **Other abnormal findings on antenatal screening of mother** **M**

O28.9 **Unspecified abnormal findings on antenatal screening of mother** **M**

√4th O29 **Complications of anesthesia during pregnancy**

INCLUDES maternal complications arising from the administration of a general, regional or local anesthetic, analgesic or other sedation during pregnancy

Use additional code, if necessary, to identify the complication

EXCLUDES 2 *complications of anesthesia during labor and delivery (O74.-)*
complications of anesthesia during the puerperium (O89.-)

√5th O29.0 **Pulmonary complications of anesthesia during pregnancy**

√6th O29.01 **Aspiration pneumonitis due to anesthesia during pregnancy**

Inhalation of stomach contents or secretions NOS due to anesthesia during pregnancy

Mendelson's syndrome due to anesthesia during pregnancy

O29.011 **Aspiration pneumonitis due to anesthesia during pregnancy,** first trimester **M**

O29.012 **Aspiration pneumonitis due to anesthesia during pregnancy,** second trimester **M**

O29.013 **Aspiration pneumonitis due to anesthesia during pregnancy,** third trimester **M**

O29.019 **Aspiration pneumonitis due to anesthesia during pregnancy, unspecified trimester** **M**

√6th O29.02 **Pressure collapse of lung due to anesthesia during pregnancy**

O29.021 **Pressure collapse of lung due to anesthesia during pregnancy,** first trimester **M**

O29.022 **Pressure collapse of lung due to anesthesia during pregnancy,** second trimester **M**

O29.023 **Pressure collapse of lung due to anesthesia during pregnancy,** third trimester **M**

O29.029 **Pressure collapse of lung due to anesthesia during pregnancy, unspecified trimester** **M**

√6th O29.09 **Other pulmonary complications of anesthesia during pregnancy**

O29.091 **Other pulmonary complications of anesthesia during pregnancy,** first trimester **M**

O29.092 **Other pulmonary complications of anesthesia during pregnancy,** second trimester **M**

O29.093 **Other pulmonary complications of anesthesia during pregnancy,** third trimester **M**

O29.099 **Other pulmonary complications of anesthesia during pregnancy, unspecified trimester** **M**

N Newborn: 0   **P** Pediatric: 0-17   **M** Maternity: 9-64   **A** Adult: 15-124   **UNS** Unspecified Site   **MCC** Major Complication/Comorbidity   **CC** Complication/Comorbidity   **PE** POA Exempt

894   ICD-10-CM 2025

✓5ᵗʰ O29.1 Cardiac complications of anesthesia during pregnancy

    ✓6ᵗʰ O29.11 Cardiac arrest due to anesthesia during pregnancy

        O29.111 Cardiac arrest due to anesthesia during pregnancy, first trimester Ⓜ

        O29.112 Cardiac arrest due to anesthesia during pregnancy, second trimester Ⓜ

        O29.113 Cardiac arrest due to anesthesia during pregnancy, third trimester Ⓜ

        O29.119 Cardiac arrest due to anesthesia during pregnancy, unspecified trimester Ⓜ

    ✓6ᵗʰ O29.12 Cardiac failure due to anesthesia during pregnancy

        O29.121 Cardiac failure due to anesthesia during pregnancy, first trimester Ⓜ

        O29.122 Cardiac failure due to anesthesia during pregnancy, second trimester Ⓜ

        O29.123 Cardiac failure due to anesthesia during pregnancy, third trimester Ⓜ

        O29.129 Cardiac failure due to anesthesia during pregnancy, unspecified trimester Ⓜ

    ✓6ᵗʰ O29.19 Other cardiac complications of anesthesia during pregnancy

        O29.191 Other cardiac complications of anesthesia during pregnancy, first trimester Ⓜ

        O29.192 Other cardiac complications of anesthesia during pregnancy, second trimester Ⓜ

        O29.193 Other cardiac complications of anesthesia during pregnancy, third trimester Ⓜ

        O29.199 Other cardiac complications of anesthesia during pregnancy, unspecified trimester Ⓜ

✓5ᵗʰ O29.2 Central nervous system complications of anesthesia during pregnancy

    ✓6ᵗʰ O29.21 Cerebral anoxia due to anesthesia during pregnancy

        O29.211 Cerebral anoxia due to anesthesia during pregnancy, first trimester Ⓜ

        O29.212 Cerebral anoxia due to anesthesia during pregnancy, second trimester Ⓜ

        O29.213 Cerebral anoxia due to anesthesia during pregnancy, third trimester Ⓜ

        O29.219 Cerebral anoxia due to anesthesia during pregnancy, unspecified trimester Ⓜ

    ✓6ᵗʰ O29.29 Other central nervous system complications of anesthesia during pregnancy

        O29.291 Other central nervous system complications of anesthesia during pregnancy, first trimester Ⓜ

        O29.292 Other central nervous system complications of anesthesia during pregnancy, second trimester Ⓜ

        O29.293 Other central nervous system complications of anesthesia during pregnancy, third trimester Ⓜ

        O29.299 Other central nervous system complications of anesthesia during pregnancy, unspecified trimester Ⓜ

✓5ᵗʰ O29.3 Toxic reaction to local anesthesia during pregnancy

    ✓6ᵗʰ O29.3X Toxic reaction to local anesthesia during pregnancy

        O29.3X1 Toxic reaction to local anesthesia during pregnancy, first trimester Ⓜ

        O29.3X2 Toxic reaction to local anesthesia during pregnancy, second trimester Ⓜ

        O29.3X3 Toxic reaction to local anesthesia during pregnancy, third trimester Ⓜ

        O29.3X9 Toxic reaction to local anesthesia during pregnancy, unspecified trimester Ⓜ

✓5ᵗʰ O29.4 Spinal and epidural anesthesia induced headache during pregnancy

    O29.40 Spinal and epidural anesthesia induced headache during pregnancy, unspecified trimester Ⓜ

    O29.41 Spinal and epidural anesthesia induced headache during pregnancy, first trimester Ⓜ

    O29.42 Spinal and epidural anesthesia induced headache during pregnancy, second trimester Ⓜ

    O29.43 Spinal and epidural anesthesia induced headache during pregnancy, third trimester Ⓜ

✓5ᵗʰ O29.5 Other complications of spinal and epidural anesthesia during pregnancy

    ✓6ᵗʰ O29.5X Other complications of spinal and epidural anesthesia during pregnancy

        O29.5X1 Other complications of spinal and epidural anesthesia during pregnancy, first trimester Ⓜ

        O29.5X2 Other complications of spinal and epidural anesthesia during pregnancy, second trimester Ⓜ

        O29.5X3 Other complications of spinal and epidural anesthesia during pregnancy, third trimester Ⓜ

        O29.5X9 Other complications of spinal and epidural anesthesia during pregnancy, unspecified trimester Ⓜ

✓5ᵗʰ O29.6 Failed or difficult intubation for anesthesia during pregnancy

    O29.60 Failed or difficult intubation for anesthesia during pregnancy, unspecified trimester Ⓜ

    O29.61 Failed or difficult intubation for anesthesia during pregnancy, first trimester Ⓜ

    O29.62 Failed or difficult intubation for anesthesia during pregnancy, second trimester Ⓜ

    O29.63 Failed or difficult intubation for anesthesia during pregnancy, third trimester Ⓜ

✓5ᵗʰ O29.8 Other complications of anesthesia during pregnancy

    ✓6ᵗʰ O29.8X Other complications of anesthesia during pregnancy

        O29.8X1 Other complications of anesthesia during pregnancy, first trimester Ⓜ

        O29.8X2 Other complications of anesthesia during pregnancy, second trimester Ⓜ

        O29.8X3 Other complications of anesthesia during pregnancy, third trimester Ⓜ

        O29.8X9 Other complications of anesthesia during pregnancy, unspecified trimester Ⓜ

✓5ᵗʰ O29.9 Unspecified complication of anesthesia during pregnancy

    O29.90 Unspecified complication of anesthesia during pregnancy, unspecified trimester Ⓜ

    O29.91 Unspecified complication of anesthesia during pregnancy, first trimester Ⓜ

    O29.92 Unspecified complication of anesthesia during pregnancy, second trimester Ⓜ

    O29.93 Unspecified complication of anesthesia during pregnancy, third trimester Ⓜ

Maternal care related to the fetus and amniotic cavity and possible delivery problems (O30-O48)

✓4ᵗʰ O30 Multiple gestation

    Code also any complications specific to multiple gestation
    AHA: 2016,4Q,51

    ✓5ᵗʰ O30.0 Twin pregnancy

        ✓6ᵗʰ O30.00 Twin pregnancy, unspecified number of placenta and unspecified number of amniotic sacs

            O30.001 Twin pregnancy, unspecified number of placenta and unspecified number of amniotic sacs, first trimester Ⓜ

            O30.002 Twin pregnancy, unspecified number of placenta and unspecified number of amniotic sacs, second trimester Ⓜ

            O30.003 Twin pregnancy, unspecified number of placenta and unspecified number of amniotic sacs, third trimester Ⓜ

            O30.009 Twin pregnancy, unspecified number of placenta and unspecified number of amniotic sacs, unspecified trimester Ⓜ

        ✓6ᵗʰ O30.01 Twin pregnancy, monochorionic/monoamniotic

            Twin pregnancy, one placenta, one amniotic sac
            EXCLUDES 1   *conjoined twins (O30.02-)*

            O30.011 Twin pregnancy, monochorionic/monoamniotic, first trimester Ⓜ

            O30.012 Twin pregnancy, monochorionic/monoamniotic, second trimester Ⓜ

            O30.013 Twin pregnancy, monochorionic/monoamniotic, third trimester Ⓜ

✔ Additional Character Required   ✔7ᵗʰ Placeholder   Questionable PDx   Manifestation   Unspecified   UPD Unacceptable PDx   H1-H14 HAC   HCC CMS-HCC Dx   HIV HIV Dx

ICD-10-CM 2025   895

O30.019 Twin pregnancy, monochorionic/monoamniotic, unspecified trimester **M**

√6ᵗʰ **O30.02** Conjoined twin pregnancy

 O30.021 Conjoined twin pregnancy, first trimester **M**

 O30.022 Conjoined twin pregnancy, second trimester **M**

 O30.023 Conjoined twin pregnancy, third trimester **M**

 O30.029 Conjoined twin pregnancy, unspecified trimester **M**

√6ᵗʰ **O30.03** Twin pregnancy, monochorionic/diamniotic

 Twin pregnancy, one placenta, two amniotic sacs

 O30.031 Twin pregnancy, monochorionic/diamniotic, first trimester **M**

 O30.032 Twin pregnancy, monochorionic/diamniotic, second trimester **M**

 O30.033 Twin pregnancy, monochorionic/diamniotic, third trimester **M**

 O30.039 Twin pregnancy, monochorionic/diamniotic, unspecified trimester **M**

√6ᵗʰ **O30.04** Twin pregnancy, dichorionic/diamniotic

 Twin pregnancy, two placentae, two amniotic sacs

 O30.041 Twin pregnancy, dichorionic/diamniotic, first trimester **M**

 O30.042 Twin pregnancy, dichorionic/diamniotic, second trimester **M**

 O30.043 Twin pregnancy, dichorionic/diamniotic, third trimester **M**

 O30.049 Twin pregnancy, dichorionic/diamniotic, unspecified trimester **M**

√6ᵗʰ **O30.09** Twin pregnancy, unable to determine number of placenta and number of amniotic sacs

 O30.091 Twin pregnancy, unable to determine number of placenta and number of amniotic sacs, first trimester **M**

 O30.092 Twin pregnancy, unable to determine number of placenta and number of amniotic sacs, second trimester **M**

 O30.093 Twin pregnancy, unable to determine number of placenta and number of amniotic sacs, third trimester **M**

 O30.099 Twin pregnancy, unable to determine number of placenta and number of amniotic sacs, unspecified trimester **M**

√5ᵗʰ **O30.1** Triplet pregnancy

√6ᵗʰ **O30.10** Triplet pregnancy, unspecified number of placenta and unspecified number of amniotic sacs

 AHA: 2016,2Q,8

 O30.101 Triplet pregnancy, unspecified number of placenta and unspecified number of amniotic sacs, first trimester **CC M**

 O30.102 Triplet pregnancy, unspecified number of placenta and unspecified number of amniotic sacs, second trimester **CC M**

 O30.103 Triplet pregnancy, unspecified number of placenta and unspecified number of amniotic sacs, third trimester **CC M**

 O30.109 Triplet pregnancy, unspecified number of placenta and unspecified number of amniotic sacs, unspecified trimester **M**

√6ᵗʰ **O30.11** Triplet pregnancy with two or more monochorionic fetuses

 O30.111 Triplet pregnancy with two or more monochorionic fetuses, first trimester **CC M**

 O30.112 Triplet pregnancy with two or more monochorionic fetuses, second trimester **CC M**

 O30.113 Triplet pregnancy with two or more monochorionic fetuses, third trimester **CC M**

 O30.119 Triplet pregnancy with two or more monochorionic fetuses, unspecified trimester **M**

√6ᵗʰ **O30.12** Triplet pregnancy with two or more monoamniotic fetuses

 O30.121 Triplet pregnancy with two or more monoamniotic fetuses, first trimester **CC M**

 O30.122 Triplet pregnancy with two or more monoamniotic fetuses, second trimester **CC M**

 O30.123 Triplet pregnancy with two or more monoamniotic fetuses, third trimester **CC M**

 O30.129 Triplet pregnancy with two or more monoamniotic fetuses, unspecified trimester **M**

√6ᵗʰ **O30.13** Triplet pregnancy, trichorionic/triamniotic

 AHA: 2018,4Q,22

 O30.131 Triplet pregnancy, trichorionic/triamniotic, first trimester **CC M**

 O30.132 Triplet pregnancy, trichorionic/triamniotic, second trimester **CC M**

 O30.133 Triplet pregnancy, trichorionic/triamniotic, third trimester **CC M**

 O30.139 Triplet pregnancy, trichorionic/triamniotic, unspecified trimester **M**

√6ᵗʰ **O30.19** Triplet pregnancy, unable to determine number of placenta and number of amniotic sacs

 O30.191 Triplet pregnancy, unable to determine number of placenta and number of amniotic sacs, first trimester **CC M**

 O30.192 Triplet pregnancy, unable to determine number of placenta and number of amniotic sacs, second trimester **CC M**

 O30.193 Triplet pregnancy, unable to determine number of placenta and number of amniotic sacs, third trimester **CC M**

 O30.199 Triplet pregnancy, unable to determine number of placenta and number of amniotic sacs, unspecified trimester **M**

√5ᵗʰ **O30.2** Quadruplet pregnancy

√6ᵗʰ **O30.20** Quadruplet pregnancy, unspecified number of placenta and unspecified number of amniotic sacs

 O30.201 Quadruplet pregnancy, unspecified number of placenta and unspecified number of amniotic sacs, first trimester **CC M**

 O30.202 Quadruplet pregnancy, unspecified number of placenta and unspecified number of amniotic sacs, second trimester **CC M**

 O30.203 Quadruplet pregnancy, unspecified number of placenta and unspecified number of amniotic sacs, third trimester **CC M**

 O30.209 Quadruplet pregnancy, unspecified number of placenta and unspecified number of amniotic sacs, unspecified trimester **M**

√6ᵗʰ **O30.21** Quadruplet pregnancy with two or more monochorionic fetuses

 O30.211 Quadruplet pregnancy with two or more monochorionic fetuses, first trimester **CC M**

 O30.212 Quadruplet pregnancy with two or more monochorionic fetuses, second trimester **CC M**

 O30.213 Quadruplet pregnancy with two or more monochorionic fetuses, third trimester **CC M**

 O30.219 Quadruplet pregnancy with two or more monochorionic fetuses, unspecified trimester **M**

√6ᵗʰ **O30.22** Quadruplet pregnancy with two or more monoamniotic fetuses

 O30.221 Quadruplet pregnancy with two or more monoamniotic fetuses, first trimester **CC M**

 O30.222 Quadruplet pregnancy with two or more monoamniotic fetuses, second trimester **CC M**

 O30.223 Quadruplet pregnancy with two or more monoamniotic fetuses, third trimester **CC M**

N Newborn: 0 **P** Pediatric: 0-17 **M** Maternity: 9-64 **A** Adult: 15-124 **UNS** Unspecified Site **MCC** Major Complication/Comorbidity **CC** Complication/Comorbidity **PE** POA Exempt

896 ICD-10-CM 2025

O30.229 Quadruplet pregnancy with two or more monoamniotic fetuses, unspecified trimester M

√6th O30.23 Quadruplet pregnancy, quadrachorionic/quadra-amniotic
AHA: 2018,4Q,22

O30.231 Quadruplet pregnancy, quadrachorionic/quadra-amniotic, first trimester CC M

O30.232 Quadruplet pregnancy, quadrachorionic/quadra-amniotic, second trimester CC M

O30.233 Quadruplet pregnancy, quadrachorionic/quadra-amniotic, third trimester CC M

O30.239 Quadruplet pregnancy, quadrachorionic/quadra-amniotic, unspecified trimester M

√6th O30.29 Quadruplet pregnancy, unable to determine number of placenta and number of amniotic sacs

O30.291 Quadruplet pregnancy, unable to determine number of placenta and number of amniotic sacs, first trimester CC M

O30.292 Quadruplet pregnancy, unable to determine number of placenta and number of amniotic sacs, second trimester CC M

O30.293 Quadruplet pregnancy, unable to determine number of placenta and number of amniotic sacs, third trimester CC M

O30.299 Quadruplet pregnancy, unable to determine number of placenta and number of amniotic sacs, unspecified trimester M

√5th O30.8 Other specified multiple gestation
Multiple gestation pregnancy greater then quadruplets

√6th O30.80 Other specified multiple gestation, unspecified number of placenta and unspecified number of amniotic sacs

O30.801 Other specified multiple gestation, unspecified number of placenta and unspecified number of amniotic sacs, first trimester CC M

O30.802 Other specified multiple gestation, unspecified number of placenta and unspecified number of amniotic sacs, second trimester CC M

O30.803 Other specified multiple gestation, unspecified number of placenta and unspecified number of amniotic sacs, third trimester CC M

O30.809 Other specified multiple gestation, unspecified number of placenta and unspecified number of amniotic sacs, unspecified trimester M

√6th O30.81 Other specified multiple gestation with two or more monochorionic fetuses

O30.811 Other specified multiple gestation with two or more monochorionic fetuses, first trimester CC M

O30.812 Other specified multiple gestation with two or more monochorionic fetuses, second trimester CC M

O30.813 Other specified multiple gestation with two or more monochorionic fetuses, third trimester CC M

O30.819 Other specified multiple gestation with two or more monochorionic fetuses, unspecified trimester M

√6th O30.82 Other specified multiple gestation with two or more monoamniotic fetuses

O30.821 Other specified multiple gestation with two or more monoamniotic fetuses, first trimester CC M

O30.822 Other specified multiple gestation with two or more monoamniotic fetuses, second trimester CC M

O30.823 Other specified multiple gestation with two or more monoamniotic fetuses, third trimester CC M

O30.829 Other specified multiple gestation with two or more monoamniotic fetuses, unspecified trimester M

√6th O30.83 Other specified multiple gestation, number of chorions and amnions are both equal to the number of fetuses
Pentachorionic, penta-amniotic pregnancy (quintuplets)
Hexachorionic, hexa-amniotic pregnancy (sextuplets)
Heptachorionic, hepta-amniotic pregnancy (septuplets)
AHA: 2018,4Q,22

O30.831 Other specified multiple gestation, number of chorions and amnions are both equal to the number of fetuses, first trimester CC M

O30.832 Other specified multiple gestation, number of chorions and amnions are both equal to the number of fetuses, second trimester CC M

O30.833 Other specified multiple gestation, number of chorions and amnions are both equal to the number of fetuses, third trimester CC M

O30.839 Other specified multiple gestation, number of chorions and amnions are both equal to the number of fetuses, unspecified trimester M

√6th O30.89 Other specified multiple gestation, unable to determine number of placenta and number of amniotic sacs

O30.891 Other specified multiple gestation, unable to determine number of placenta and number of amniotic sacs, first trimester CC M

O30.892 Other specified multiple gestation, unable to determine number of placenta and number of amniotic sacs, second trimester CC M

O30.893 Other specified multiple gestation, unable to determine number of placenta and number of amniotic sacs, third trimester CC M

O30.899 Other specified multiple gestation, unable to determine number of placenta and number of amniotic sacs, unspecified trimester M

√5th O30.9 Multiple gestation, unspecified
Multiple pregnancy NOS

O30.90 Multiple gestation, unspecified, unspecified trimester M

O30.91 Multiple gestation, unspecified, first trimester M

O30.92 Multiple gestation, unspecified, second trimester M

O30.93 Multiple gestation, unspecified, third trimester M

√4th O31 Complications specific to multiple gestation
EXCLUDES 2   delayed delivery of second twin, triplet, etc. (O63.2)
malpresentation of one fetus or more (O32.9)
placental transfusion syndromes (O43.0-)
AHA: 2012,4Q,107

One of the following 7th characters is to be assigned to each code under category O31. 7th character 0 is for single gestations and multiple gestations where the fetus is unspecified. 7th characters 1 through 9 are for cases of multiple gestations to identify the fetus for which the code applies. The appropriate code from category O30, Multiple gestation, must also be assigned when assigning a code from category O31 that has a 7th character of 1 through 9.
0   not applicable or unspecified
1   fetus 1
2   fetus 2
3   fetus 3
4   fetus 4
5   fetus 5
9   other fetus

√5th O31.0 Papyraceous fetus
Fetus compressus
DEF: Fetus that has died, but remains in utero for weeks before delivery, becoming compacted and mummified in appearance, with skin resembling parchment. Occurs most commonly in multigestational pregnancies. Synonym(s): paper doll fetus.

√x7th O31.00 Papyraceous fetus, unspecified trimester M

√x7th O31.01 Papyraceous fetus, first trimester M

√x7th O31.02 Papyraceous fetus, second trimester M

√x 7ᵗʰ **O31.Ø3** **Papyraceous fetus, third trimester**   M

√ 5ᵗʰ **O31.1** **Continuing pregnancy after spontaneous abortion of one fetus or more**

√x 7ᵗʰ **O31.10** **Continuing pregnancy after spontaneous abortion of one fetus or more, unspecified trimester**   M

√x 7ᵗʰ **O31.11** **Continuing pregnancy after spontaneous abortion of one fetus or more, first trimester**   M

√x 7ᵗʰ **O31.12** **Continuing pregnancy after spontaneous abortion of one fetus or more, second trimester**   M

√x 7ᵗʰ **O31.13** **Continuing pregnancy after spontaneous abortion of one fetus or more, third trimester**   M

√ 5ᵗʰ **O31.2** **Continuing pregnancy after intrauterine death of one fetus or more**

√x 7ᵗʰ **O31.20** **Continuing pregnancy after intrauterine death of one fetus or more, unspecified trimester**   M

√x 7ᵗʰ **O31.21** **Continuing pregnancy after intrauterine death of one fetus or more, first trimester**   M

√x 7ᵗʰ **O31.22** **Continuing pregnancy after intrauterine death of one fetus or more, second trimester**   M

√x 7ᵗʰ **O31.23** **Continuing pregnancy after intrauterine death of one fetus or more, third trimester**   M

√ 5ᵗʰ **O31.3** **Continuing pregnancy after elective fetal reduction of one fetus or more**

Continuing pregnancy after selective termination of one fetus or more

√x 7ᵗʰ **O31.30** **Continuing pregnancy after elective fetal reduction of one fetus or more, unspecified trimester**   M

√x 7ᵗʰ **O31.31** **Continuing pregnancy after elective fetal reduction of one fetus or more, first trimester**   M

√x 7ᵗʰ **O31.32** **Continuing pregnancy after elective fetal reduction of one fetus or more, second trimester**   M

√x 7ᵗʰ **O31.33** **Continuing pregnancy after elective fetal reduction of one fetus or more, third trimester**   M

√ 5ᵗʰ **O31.8** **Other complications specific to multiple gestation**

√ 6ᵗʰ **O31.8X** **Other complications specific to multiple gestation**

√ 7ᵗʰ **O31.8X1** **Other complications specific to multiple gestation, first trimester**   CC M

√ 7ᵗʰ **O31.8X2** **Other complications specific to multiple gestation, second trimester**   CC M

√ 7ᵗʰ **O31.8X3** **Other complications specific to multiple gestation, third trimester**   CC M

√ 7ᵗʰ **O31.8X9** **Other complications specific to multiple gestation, unspecified trimester**   CC M

√ 4ᵗʰ **O32** **Maternal care for malpresentation of fetus**

INCLUDES   the listed conditions as a reason for observation, hospitalization or other obstetric care of the mother, or for cesarean delivery before onset of labor

EXCLUDES 1   *malpresentation of fetus with obstructed labor (O64.-)*

AHA: 2012,4Q,107

One of the following 7th characters is to be assigned to each code under category O32. 7th character Ø is for single gestations and multiple gestations where the fetus is unspecified. 7th characters 1 through 9 are for cases of multiple gestations to identify the fetus for which the code applies. The appropriate code from category O30, Multiple gestation, must also be assigned when assigning a code from category O32 that has a 7th character of 1 through 9.

Ø   not applicable or unspecified
1   fetus 1
2   fetus 2
3   fetus 3
4   fetus 4
5   fetus 5
9   other fetus

Fetal Malpresentation

Breech — Mother's pelvis
Shoulder (arm prolapse)
Compound (extremity together with head)
Face (mentum)
Oblique

√x 7ᵗʰ **O32.0** **Maternal care for unstable lie**   M

√x 7ᵗʰ **O32.1** **Maternal care for breech presentation**   M

Maternal care for buttocks presentation
Maternal care for complete breech
Maternal care for frank breech

EXCLUDES 1   *footling presentation (O32.8)*
incomplete breech (O32.8)

DEF: Fetus presentation in a longitudinal lie with the buttocks or feet closest to birth canal that may require external cephalic version or cesarean delivery.

√x 7ᵗʰ **O32.2** **Maternal care for transverse and oblique lie**   M

Maternal care for oblique presentation
Maternal care for transverse presentation

√x 7ᵗʰ **O32.3** **Maternal care for face, brow and chin presentation**   M

√x 7ᵗʰ **O32.4** **Maternal care for high head at term**   M

Maternal care for failure of head to enter pelvic brim

√x 7ᵗʰ **O32.6** **Maternal care for compound presentation**   M

√x 7ᵗʰ **O32.8** **Maternal care for other malpresentation of fetus**   M

Maternal care for footling presentation
Maternal care for incomplete breech

√x 7ᵗʰ **O32.9** **Maternal care for malpresentation of fetus, unspecified**   M

√ 4ᵗʰ **O33** **Maternal care for disproportion**

INCLUDES   the listed conditions as a reason for observation, hospitalization or other obstetric care of the mother, or for cesarean delivery before onset of labor

EXCLUDES 1   *disproportion with obstructed labor (O65-O66)*

O33.0 **Maternal care for disproportion due to deformity of maternal pelvic bones**   CC M

Maternal care for disproportion due to pelvic deformity causing disproportion NOS

O33.1 **Maternal care for disproportion due to generally contracted pelvis**   M

Maternal care for disproportion due to contracted pelvis NOS causing disproportion

N Newborn: 0   P Pediatric: 0-17   M Maternity: 9-64   A Adult: 15-124   UNS Unspecified Site   MCC Major Complication/Comorbidity   CC Complication/Comorbidity   PE POA Exempt

898   ICD-10-CM 2025

O33.2 Maternal care for disproportion due to inlet contraction of pelvis M

Maternal care for disproportion due to inlet contraction (pelvis) causing disproportion

√x7ᵗʰ **O33.3 Maternal care for disproportion due to outlet contraction of pelvis** M

Maternal care for disproportion due to mid-cavity contraction (pelvis)

Maternal care for disproportion due to outlet contraction (pelvis)

One of the following 7th characters is to be assigned to code O33.3. 7th character Ø is for single gestations and multiple gestations where the fetus is unspecified. 7th characters 1 through 9 are for cases of multiple gestations to identify the fetus for which the code applies. The appropriate code from category O3Ø, Multiple gestation, must also be assigned when assigning code O33.3 with a 7th character of 1 through 9.

Ø   not applicable or unspecified
1   fetus 1
2   fetus 2
3   fetus 3
4   fetus 4
5   fetus 5
9   other fetus

√x7ᵗʰ **O33.4 Maternal care for disproportion of mixed maternal and fetal origin** M

One of the following 7th characters is to be assigned to code O33.4. 7th character Ø is for single gestations and multiple gestations where the fetus is unspecified. 7th characters 1 through 9 are for cases of multiple gestations to identify the fetus for which the code applies. The appropriate code from category O3Ø, Multiple gestation, must also be assigned when assigning code O33.4 with a 7th character of 1 through 9.

Ø   not applicable or unspecified
1   fetus 1
2   fetus 2
3   fetus 3
4   fetus 4
5   fetus 5
9   other fetus

√x7ᵗʰ **O33.5 Maternal care for disproportion due to unusually large fetus** M

Maternal care for disproportion due to disproportion of fetal origin with normally formed fetus

Maternal care for disproportion due to fetal disproportion NOS

One of the following 7th characters is to be assigned to code O33.5. 7th character Ø is for single gestations and multiple gestations where the fetus is unspecified. 7th characters 1 through 9 are for cases of multiple gestations to identify the fetus for which the code applies. The appropriate code from category O3Ø, Multiple gestation, must also be assigned when assigning code O33.5 with a 7th character of 1 through 9.

Ø   not applicable or unspecified
1   fetus 1
2   fetus 2
3   fetus 3
4   fetus 4
5   fetus 5
9   other fetus

√x7ᵗʰ **O33.6 Maternal care for disproportion due to hydrocephalic fetus** M

One of the following 7th characters is to be assigned to code O33.6. 7th character Ø is for single gestations and multiple gestations where the fetus is unspecified. 7th characters 1 through 9 are for cases of multiple gestations to identify the fetus for which the code applies. The appropriate code from category O3Ø, Multiple gestation, must also be assigned when assigning code O33.6 with a 7th character of 1 through 9.

Ø   not applicable or unspecified
1   fetus 1
2   fetus 2
3   fetus 3
4   fetus 4
5   fetus 5
9   other fetus

√x7ᵗʰ **O33.7 Maternal care for disproportion due to other fetal deformities** M

Maternal care for disproportion due to fetal ascites
Maternal care for disproportion due to fetal hydrops
Maternal care for disproportion due to fetal meningomyelocele
Maternal care for disproportion due to fetal sacral teratoma
Maternal care for disproportion due to fetal tumor

EXCLUDES 1   obstructed labor due to other fetal deformities (O66.3)

AHA: 2016,4Q,51

One of the following 7th characters is to be assigned to code O33.7. 7th character Ø is for single gestations and multiple gestations where the fetus is unspecified. 7th characters 1 through 9 are for cases of multiple gestations to identify the fetus for which the code applies. The appropriate code from category O3Ø, Multiple gestation, must also be assigned when assigning code O33.7 with a 7th character of 1 through 9.

Ø   not applicable or unspecified
1   fetus 1
2   fetus 2
3   fetus 3
4   fetus 4
5   fetus 5
9   other fetus

O33.8 Maternal care for disproportion of other origin M

O33.9 Maternal care for disproportion, unspecified M

Maternal care for disproportion due to cephalopelvic disproportion NOS

Maternal care for disproportion due to fetopelvic disproportion NOS

√4ᵗʰ **O34 Maternal care for abnormality of pelvic organs**

INCLUDES   the listed conditions as a reason for hospitalization or other obstetric care of the mother, or for cesarean delivery before onset of labor

Code first any associated obstructed labor (O65.5)

Use additional code for specific condition

√5ᵗʰ **O34.Ø Maternal care for congenital malformation of uterus**

Maternal care for double uterus
Maternal care for uterus bicornis

O34.ØØ Maternal care for unspecified congenital malformation of uterus, unspecified trimester M

O34.Ø1 Maternal care for unspecified congenital malformation of uterus, first trimester M

O34.Ø2 Maternal care for unspecified congenital malformation of uterus, second trimester M

O34.Ø3 Maternal care for unspecified congenital malformation of uterus, third trimester M

√5ᵗʰ **O34.1 Maternal care for benign tumor of corpus uteri**

EXCLUDES 2   maternal care for benign tumor of cervix (O34.4-)
maternal care for malignant neoplasm of uterus (O9A.1-)

O34.1Ø Maternal care for benign tumor of corpus uteri, unspecified trimester M

O34.11 Maternal care for benign tumor of corpus uteri, first trimester M

O34.12 Maternal care for benign tumor of corpus uteri, second trimester M

O34.13 Maternal care for benign tumor of corpus uteri, third trimester M

√5ᵗʰ **O34.2 Maternal care due to uterine scar from previous surgery**

AHA: 2020,4Q,36; 2016,4Q,76

√6ᵗʰ **O34.21 Maternal care for scar from previous cesarean delivery**

AHA: 2018,3Q,23; 2016,4Q,51-52

O34.211 Maternal care for low transverse scar from previous cesarean delivery M

O34.212 Maternal care for vertical scar from previous cesarean delivery M

Maternal care for classical scar from previous cesarean delivery

O34.218 Maternal care for other type scar from previous cesarean delivery M

Mid-transverse T incision

O34.219 Maternal care for unspecified type scar from previous cesarean delivery M

O34.22 Maternal care for cesarean scar defect (isthmocele) M

☑ Additional Character Required   √x7ᵗʰ Placeholder   Questionable PDx   Manifestation   Unspecified   UPD Unacceptable PDx   H1–H14 HAC   HCC CMS-HCC Dx   HIV HIV Dx

ICD-10-CM 2025   899

O34.29   **Maternal care due to uterine scar from other previous surgery**   M

Maternal care due to uterine scar from other transmural uterine incision

✓5ᵗʰ **O34.3**   **Maternal care for cervical incompetence**

Maternal care for cerclage with or without cervical incompetence

Maternal care for Shirodkar suture with or without cervical incompetence

DEF: Inadequate functioning of the cervix marked by abnormal widening during pregnancy and causing premature birth or miscarriage.

O34.30   **Maternal care for cervical incompetence, unspecified trimester**   M

O34.31   **Maternal care for cervical incompetence, first trimester**   MCC M

O34.32   **Maternal care for cervical incompetence, second trimester**   MCC M

O34.33   **Maternal care for cervical incompetence, third trimester**   MCC M

✓5ᵗʰ **O34.4**   **Maternal care for other abnormalities of cervix**

O34.40   **Maternal care for other abnormalities of cervix, unspecified trimester**   M

O34.41   **Maternal care for other abnormalities of cervix, first trimester**   M

O34.42   **Maternal care for other abnormalities of cervix, second trimester**   M

O34.43   **Maternal care for other abnormalities of cervix, third trimester**   M

✓5ᵗʰ **O34.5**   **Maternal care for other abnormalities of gravid uterus**

✓6ᵗʰ **O34.51**   **Maternal care for incarceration of gravid uterus**

O34.511   **Maternal care for incarceration of gravid uterus, first trimester**   M

O34.512   **Maternal care for incarceration of gravid uterus, second trimester**   M

O34.513   **Maternal care for incarceration of gravid uterus, third trimester**   M

O34.519   **Maternal care for incarceration of gravid uterus, unspecified trimester**   M

✓6ᵗʰ **O34.52**   **Maternal care for prolapse of gravid uterus**

O34.521   **Maternal care for prolapse of gravid uterus, first trimester**   M

O34.522   **Maternal care for prolapse of gravid uterus, second trimester**   M

O34.523   **Maternal care for prolapse of gravid uterus, third trimester**   M

O34.529   **Maternal care for prolapse of gravid uterus, unspecified trimester**   M

✓6ᵗʰ **O34.53**   **Maternal care for retroversion of gravid uterus**

O34.531   **Maternal care for retroversion of gravid uterus, first trimester**   M

O34.532   **Maternal care for retroversion of gravid uterus, second trimester**   M

O34.533   **Maternal care for retroversion of gravid uterus, third trimester**   M

O34.539   **Maternal care for retroversion of gravid uterus, unspecified trimester**   M

✓6ᵗʰ **O34.59**   **Maternal care for other abnormalities of gravid uterus**

O34.591   **Maternal care for other abnormalities of gravid uterus, first trimester**   M

O34.592   **Maternal care for other abnormalities of gravid uterus, second trimester**   M

O34.593   **Maternal care for other abnormalities of gravid uterus, third trimester**   M

O34.599   **Maternal care for other abnormalities of gravid uterus, unspecified trimester**   M

✓5ᵗʰ **O34.6**   **Maternal care for abnormality of vagina**

EXCLUDES 2   *maternal care for vaginal varices in pregnancy (O22.1-)*

O34.60   **Maternal care for abnormality of vagina, unspecified trimester**   M

O34.61   **Maternal care for abnormality of vagina, first trimester**   M

O34.62   **Maternal care for abnormality of vagina, second trimester**   M

O34.63   **Maternal care for abnormality of vagina, third trimester**   M

✓5ᵗʰ **O34.7**   **Maternal care for abnormality of vulva and perineum**

EXCLUDES 2   *maternal care for perineal and vulval varices in pregnancy (O22.1-)*

O34.70   **Maternal care for abnormality of vulva and perineum, unspecified trimester**   M

O34.71   **Maternal care for abnormality of vulva and perineum, first trimester**   M

O34.72   **Maternal care for abnormality of vulva and perineum, second trimester**   M

O34.73   **Maternal care for abnormality of vulva and perineum, third trimester**   M

✓5ᵗʰ **O34.8**   **Maternal care for other abnormalities of pelvic organs**

O34.80   **Maternal care for other abnormalities of pelvic organs, unspecified trimester**   M

O34.81   **Maternal care for other abnormalities of pelvic organs, first trimester**   M

O34.82   **Maternal care for other abnormalities of pelvic organs, second trimester**   M

O34.83   **Maternal care for other abnormalities of pelvic organs, third trimester**   M

✓5ᵗʰ **O34.9**   **Maternal care for abnormality of pelvic organ, unspecified**

O34.90   **Maternal care for abnormality of pelvic organ, unspecified, unspecified trimester**   M

O34.91   **Maternal care for abnormality of pelvic organ, unspecified, first trimester**   M

O34.92   **Maternal care for abnormality of pelvic organ, unspecified, second trimester**   M

O34.93   **Maternal care for abnormality of pelvic organ, unspecified, third trimester**   M

✓4ᵗʰ **O35**   **Maternal care for known or suspected fetal abnormality and damage**

INCLUDES   the listed conditions in the fetus as a reason for hospitalization or other obstetric care to the mother, or for termination of pregnancy

Code also any associated maternal condition

EXCLUDES 1   *encounter for suspected maternal and fetal conditions ruled out (Z03.7-)*

AHA: 2022,4Q,37

One of the following 7th characters is to be assigned to each code under category O35. 7th character 0 is for single gestations and multiple gestations where the fetus is unspecified. 7th characters 1 through 9 are for cases of multiple gestations to identify the fetus for which the code applies. The appropriate code from category O30, Multiple gestation, must also be assigned when assigning a code from category O35 that has a 7th character of 1 through 9.

0   not applicable or unspecified
1   fetus 1
2   fetus 2
3   fetus 3
4   fetus 4
5   fetus 5
9   other fetus

✓5ᵗʰ **O35.0**   **Maternal care for (suspected) central nervous system malformation in fetus**

EXCLUDES 2   *chromosomal abnormality in fetus (O35.1-)*

✓x7ᵗʰ **O35.00**   **Maternal care for (suspected) central nervous system malformation or damage in fetus, unspecified**   M

✓x7ᵗʰ **O35.01**   **Maternal care for (suspected) central nervous system malformation or damage in fetus, agenesis of the corpus callosum**   M

✓x7ᵗʰ **O35.02**   **Maternal care for (suspected) central nervous system malformation or damage in fetus, anencephaly**   M

✓x7ᵗʰ **O35.03**   **Maternal care for (suspected) central nervous system malformation or damage in fetus, choroid plexus cysts**   M

✓x7ᵗʰ **O35.04**   **Maternal care for (suspected) central nervous system malformation or damage in fetus, encephalocele**   M

✓x7ᵗʰ **O35.05**   **Maternal care for (suspected) central nervous system malformation or damage in fetus, holoprosencephaly**   M

✓x7ᵗʰ **O35.06**   **Maternal care for (suspected) central nervous system malformation or damage in fetus, hydrocephaly**   M

Maternal care for fetal hydrocephalus

✓x7ᵗʰ **O35.07**   **Maternal care for (suspected) central nervous system malformation or damage in fetus, microcephaly**   M

N Newborn: 0   P Pediatric: 0-17   M Maternity: 9-64   A Adult: 15-124   UNS Unspecified Site   MCC Major Complication/Comorbidity   CC Complication/Comorbidity   PE POA Exempt

900   ICD-10-CM 2025

√x 7th **O35.Ø8** **Maternal care for (suspected) central nervous system malformation or damage in fetus, spina bifida** M

√x 7th **O35.Ø9** **Maternal care for (suspected) other central nervous system malformation or damage in fetus** M

√5th **O35.1** **Maternal care for (suspected) chromosomal abnormality in fetus**
AHA: 2023,2Q,15

√x 7th **O35.1Ø** **Maternal care for (suspected) chromosomal abnormality in fetus, unspecified** M

√x 7th **O35.11** **Maternal care for (suspected) chromosomal abnormality in fetus, Trisomy 13** M

√x 7th **O35.12** **Maternal care for (suspected) chromosomal abnormality in fetus, Trisomy 18** M

√x 7th **O35.13** **Maternal care for (suspected) chromosomal abnormality in fetus, Trisomy 21** M

√x 7th **O35.14** **Maternal care for (suspected) chromosomal abnormality in fetus, Turner Syndrome** M

√x 7th **O35.15** **Maternal care for (suspected) chromosomal abnormality in fetus, sex chromosome abnormality** M

√x 7th **O35.19** **Maternal care for (suspected) chromosomal abnormality in fetus, other chromosomal abnormality** M

√x 7th **O35.A** **Maternal care for other (suspected) fetal abnormality and damage, fetal facial anomalies** M

√x 7th **O35.B** **Maternal care for other (suspected) fetal abnormality and damage, fetal cardiac anomalies** M

√x 7th **O35.C** **Maternal care for other (suspected) fetal abnormality and damage, fetal pulmonary anomalies** M

√x 7th **O35.D** **Maternal care for other (suspected) fetal abnormality and damage, fetal gastrointestinal anomalies** M

√x 7th **O35.E** **Maternal care for other (suspected) fetal abnormality and damage, fetal genitourinary anomalies** M

√x 7th **O35.F** **Maternal care for other (suspected) fetal abnormality and damage, fetal musculoskeletal anomalies of trunk** M

> EXCLUDES 2   *maternal care for other (suspected) fetal abnormality and damage, fetal lower extremities anomalies (O35.H)*
> *maternal care for other (suspected) fetal abnormality and damage, fetal upper extremities anomalies (O35.G)*

√x 7th **O35.G** **Maternal care for other (suspected) fetal abnormality and damage, fetal upper extremities anomalies** M

√x 7th **O35.H** **Maternal care for other (suspected) fetal abnormality and damage, fetal lower extremities anomalies** M

√x 7th **O35.2** **Maternal care for (suspected) hereditary disease in fetus** M

> EXCLUDES 2   *chromosomal abnormality in fetus (O35.1-)*

√x 7th **O35.3** **Maternal care for (suspected) damage to fetus from viral disease in mother** M
Maternal care for damage to fetus from maternal cytomegalovirus infection
Maternal care for damage to fetus from maternal rubella

√x 7th **O35.4** **Maternal care for (suspected) damage to fetus from alcohol** M

√x 7th **O35.5** **Maternal care for (suspected) damage to fetus by drugs** M
Maternal care for damage to fetus from drug addiction

√x 7th **O35.6** **Maternal care for (suspected) damage to fetus by radiation** M

√x 7th **O35.7** **Maternal care for (suspected) damage to fetus by other medical procedures** M
Maternal care for damage to fetus by amniocentesis
Maternal care for damage to fetus by biopsy procedures
Maternal care for damage to fetus by hematological investigation
Maternal care for damage to fetus by intrauterine contraceptive device
Maternal care for damage to fetus by intrauterine surgery

√x 7th **O35.8** **Maternal care for other (suspected) fetal abnormality and damage** M
Maternal care for damage to fetus from maternal listeriosis
Maternal care for damage to fetus from maternal toxoplasmosis

√x 7th **O35.9** **Maternal care for (suspected) fetal abnormality and damage, unspecified** M

√4th **O36** **Maternal care for other fetal problems**

> INCLUDES   the listed conditions in the fetus as a reason for hospitalization or other obstetric care of the mother, or for termination of pregnancy
> EXCLUDES 1   *encounter for suspected maternal and fetal conditions ruled out (Z03.7-)*
> *placental transfusion syndromes (O43.Ø-)*
> EXCLUDES 2   *labor and delivery complicated by fetal stress (O77.-)*

AHA: 2015,3Q,40

> One of the following 7th characters is to be assigned to each code under category O36. 7th character Ø is for single gestations and multiple gestations where the fetus is unspecified. 7th characters 1 through 9 are for cases of multiple gestations to identify the fetus for which the code applies. The appropriate code from category O30, Multiple gestation, must also be assigned when assigning a code from category O36 that has a 7th character of 1 through 9.
> Ø   not applicable or unspecified
> 1   fetus 1
> 2   fetus 2
> 3   fetus 3
> 4   fetus 4
> 5   fetus 5
> 9   other fetus

√5th **O36.Ø** **Maternal care for rhesus isoimmunization**
Maternal care for Rh incompatibility (with hydrops fetalis)

√6th **O36.Ø1** **Maternal care for anti-D [Rh] antibodies**
AHA: 2014,4Q,17

√7th **O36.Ø11** **Maternal care for anti-D [Rh] antibodies, first trimester** CC M

√7th **O36.Ø12** **Maternal care for anti-D [Rh] antibodies, second trimester** CC M

√7th **O36.Ø13** **Maternal care for anti-D [Rh] antibodies, third trimester** CC M

√7th **O36.Ø19** **Maternal care for anti-D [Rh] antibodies, unspecified trimester** M

√6th **O36.Ø9** **Maternal care for other rhesus isoimmunization**

√7th **O36.Ø91** **Maternal care for other rhesus isoimmunization, first trimester** CC M

√7th **O36.Ø92** **Maternal care for other rhesus isoimmunization, second trimester** CC M

√7th **O36.Ø93** **Maternal care for other rhesus isoimmunization, third trimester** CC M

√7th **O36.Ø99** **Maternal care for other rhesus isoimmunization, unspecified trimester** M

√5th **O36.1** **Maternal care for other isoimmunization**
Maternal care for ABO isoimmunization

√6th **O36.11** **Maternal care for Anti-A sensitization**
Maternal care for isoimmunization NOS (with hydrops fetalis)

√7th **O36.111** **Maternal care for Anti-A sensitization, first trimester** M

√7th **O36.112** **Maternal care for Anti-A sensitization, second trimester** M

√7th **O36.113** **Maternal care for Anti-A sensitization, third trimester** M

√7th **O36.119** **Maternal care for Anti-A sensitization, unspecified trimester** M

√6th **O36.19** **Maternal care for other isoimmunization**
Maternal care for Anti-B sensitization

√7th **O36.191** **Maternal care for other isoimmunization, first trimester** M

√7th **O36.192** **Maternal care for other isoimmunization, second trimester** M

√7th **O36.193** **Maternal care for other isoimmunization, third trimester** M

√7th **O36.199** **Maternal care for other isoimmunization, unspecified trimester** M

✔ Additional Character Required   √x 7th Placeholder   Questionable PDx   Manifestation   Unspecified   UPD Unacceptable PDx   H1-H14 HAC   HCC CMS-HCC Dx   HIV HIV Dx

ICD-10-CM 2025   901

√5th **O36.2 Maternal care for hydrops fetalis**

Maternal care for hydrops fetalis NOS

Maternal care for hydrops fetalis not associated with isoimmunization

> EXCLUDES 1   *hydrops fetalis associated with ABO isoimmunization (O36.1-)*
>
> *hydrops fetalis associated with rhesus isoimmunization (O36.0-)*

DEF: Hydrops fetalis: Abnormal fluid buildup in at least two of the following fetal organ spaces: the skin (edema), abdomen (ascites), around the heart (pericardia effusion), and around the lung (pleural effusion). Fluid accumulation may also occur in the mother as polyhydramnios and edema of the placenta.

√x7th **O36.20 Maternal care for hydrops fetalis, unspecified trimester** M

√x7th **O36.21 Maternal care for hydrops fetalis, first trimester** M

√x7th **O36.22 Maternal care for hydrops fetalis, second trimester** M

√x7th **O36.23 Maternal care for hydrops fetalis, third trimester** M

√x7th **O36.4 Maternal care for intrauterine death** CC M

Maternal care for intrauterine fetal death NOS

Maternal care for intrauterine fetal death after completion of 20 weeks of gestation

Maternal care for late fetal death

Maternal care for missed delivery

> EXCLUDES 1   *missed abortion (O02.1)*
>
> *stillbirth (P95)*

AHA: 2022,2Q,3

√5th **O36.5 Maternal care for known or suspected poor fetal growth**

√6th **O36.51 Maternal care for known or suspected placental insufficiency**

√7th **O36.511 Maternal care for known or suspected placental insufficiency, first trimester** M

√7th **O36.512 Maternal care for known or suspected placental insufficiency, second trimester** M

√7th **O36.513 Maternal care for known or suspected placental insufficiency, third trimester** M

√7th **O36.519 Maternal care for known or suspected placental insufficiency, unspecified trimester** M

√6th **O36.59 Maternal care for other known or suspected poor fetal growth**

Maternal care for known or suspected light-for-dates NOS

Maternal care for known or suspected small-for-dates NOS

√7th **O36.591 Maternal care for other known or suspected poor fetal growth, first trimester** M

√7th **O36.592 Maternal care for other known or suspected poor fetal growth, second trimester** M

√7th **O36.593 Maternal care for other known or suspected poor fetal growth, third trimester** M

√7th **O36.599 Maternal care for other known or suspected poor fetal growth, unspecified trimester** M

√5th **O36.6 Maternal care for excessive fetal growth**

Maternal care for known or suspected large-for-dates

√x7th **O36.60 Maternal care for excessive fetal growth, unspecified trimester** M

√x7th **O36.61 Maternal care for excessive fetal growth, first trimester** M

√x7th **O36.62 Maternal care for excessive fetal growth, second trimester** M

√x7th **O36.63 Maternal care for excessive fetal growth, third trimester** M

√5th **O36.7 Maternal care for viable fetus in abdominal pregnancy**

√x7th **O36.70 Maternal care for viable fetus in abdominal pregnancy, unspecified trimester** M

√x7th **O36.71 Maternal care for viable fetus in abdominal pregnancy, first trimester** M

√x7th **O36.72 Maternal care for viable fetus in abdominal pregnancy, second trimester** M

√x7th **O36.73 Maternal care for viable fetus in abdominal pregnancy, third trimester** M

√5th **O36.8 Maternal care for other specified fetal problems**

√x7th **O36.80 Pregnancy with inconclusive fetal viability** UPD M

Encounter to determine fetal viability of pregnancy

AHA: 2019,2Q,29

√6th **O36.81 Decreased fetal movements**

√7th **O36.812 Decreased fetal movements, second trimester** M

√7th **O36.813 Decreased fetal movements, third trimester** M

√7th **O36.819 Decreased fetal movements, unspecified trimester** M

√6th **O36.82 Fetal anemia and thrombocytopenia**

√7th **O36.821 Fetal anemia and thrombocytopenia, first trimester** M

√7th **O36.822 Fetal anemia and thrombocytopenia, second trimester** M

√7th **O36.823 Fetal anemia and thrombocytopenia, third trimester** M

√7th **O36.829 Fetal anemia and thrombocytopenia, unspecified trimester** M

√6th **O36.83 Maternal care for abnormalities of the fetal heart rate or rhythm**

Maternal care for depressed fetal heart rate tones

Maternal care for fetal bradycardia

Maternal care for fetal heart rate abnormal variability

Maternal care for fetal heart rate decelerations

Maternal care for fetal heart rate irregularity

Maternal care for fetal tachycardia

Maternal care for non-reassuring fetal heart rate or rhythm

AHA: 2017,4Q,20

TIP: Assign for documented fetal tachycardia, bradycardia, decelerations, or loss of variability detected during antenatal testing.

√7th **O36.831 Maternal care for abnormalities of the fetal heart rate or rhythm, first trimester** M

√7th **O36.832 Maternal care for abnormalities of the fetal heart rate or rhythm, second trimester** M

√7th **O36.833 Maternal care for abnormalities of the fetal heart rate or rhythm, third trimester** M

√7th **O36.839 Maternal care for abnormalities of the fetal heart rate or rhythm, unspecified trimester** M

√6th **O36.89 Maternal care for other specified fetal problems**

√7th **O36.891 Maternal care for other specified fetal problems, first trimester** M

√7th **O36.892 Maternal care for other specified fetal problems, second trimester** M

√7th **O36.893 Maternal care for other specified fetal problems, third trimester** M

√7th **O36.899 Maternal care for other specified fetal problems, unspecified trimester** M

√5th **O36.9 Maternal care for fetal problem, unspecified**

√x7th **O36.90 Maternal care for fetal problem, unspecified, unspecified trimester** M

√x7th **O36.91 Maternal care for fetal problem, unspecified, first trimester** M

√x7th **O36.92 Maternal care for fetal problem, unspecified, second trimester** M

√x7th **O36.93 Maternal care for fetal problem, unspecified, third trimester** M

N Newborn: 0   P Pediatric: 0-17   M Maternity: 9-64   A Adult: 15-124   UNS Unspecified Site   MCC Major Complication/Comorbidity   CC Complication/Comorbidity   PE POA Exempt

902   ICD-10-CM 2025

✓4th O40 Polyhydramnios

> INCLUDES   hydramnios
> EXCLUDES 1   encounter for suspected maternal and fetal conditions ruled out (Z03.7-)

AHA: 2016,1Q,4
DEF: Excess amniotic fluid surrounding the fetus, typically defined as a total fluid volume of greater than 24 cm.

> One of the following 7th characters is to be assigned to each code under category O40. 7th character 0 is for single gestations and multiple gestations where the fetus is unspecified. 7th characters 1 through 9 are for cases of multiple gestations to identify the fetus for which the code applies. The appropriate code from category O30, Multiple gestation, must also be assigned when assigning a code from category O40 that has a 7th character of 1 through 9.
> 0   not applicable or unspecified
> 1   fetus 1
> 2   fetus 2
> 3   fetus 3
> 4   fetus 4
> 5   fetus 5
> 9   other fetus

✓x7th O40.1 Polyhydramnios, first trimester   M
✓x7th O40.2 Polyhydramnios, second trimester   M
✓x7th O40.3 Polyhydramnios, third trimester   M
✓x7th O40.9 Polyhydramnios, unspecified trimester   M

✓4th O41 Other disorders of amniotic fluid and membranes

> EXCLUDES 1   encounter for suspected maternal and fetal conditions ruled out (Z03.7-)

> One of the following 7th characters is to be assigned to each code under category O41. 7th character 0 is for single gestations and multiple gestations where the fetus is unspecified. 7th characters 1 through 9 are for cases of multiple gestations to identify the fetus for which the code applies. The appropriate code from category O30, Multiple gestation, must also be assigned when assigning a code from category O41 that has a 7th character of 1 through 9.
> 0   not applicable or unspecified
> 1   fetus 1
> 2   fetus 2
> 3   fetus 3
> 4   fetus 4
> 5   fetus 5
> 9   other fetus

✓5th O41.0 Oligohydramnios

> Oligohydramnios without rupture of membranes
> **DEF:** Low amniotic fluid, occurring most frequently in the last trimester.

   ✓x7th O41.00 Oligohydramnios, unspecified trimester   M
   ✓x7th O41.01 Oligohydramnios, first trimester   CC M
   ✓x7th O41.02 Oligohydramnios, second trimester   CC M
   ✓x7th O41.03 Oligohydramnios, third trimester   CC M

✓5th O41.1 Infection of amniotic sac and membranes

   ✓6th O41.10 Infection of amniotic sac and membranes, unspecified

     ✓7th O41.101 Infection of amniotic sac and membranes, unspecified, first trimester   MCC M
     ✓7th O41.102 Infection of amniotic sac and membranes, unspecified, second trimester   MCC M
     ✓7th O41.103 Infection of amniotic sac and membranes, unspecified, third trimester   MCC M
     ✓7th O41.109 Infection of amniotic sac and membranes, unspecified, unspecified trimester   M

   ✓6th O41.12 Chorioamnionitis

     AHA: 2019,2Q,34

     ✓7th O41.121 Chorioamnionitis, first trimester   MCC M
     ✓7th O41.122 Chorioamnionitis, second trimester   MCC M
     ✓7th O41.123 Chorioamnionitis, third trimester   MCC M
     ✓7th O41.129 Chorioamnionitis, unspecified trimester   M

   ✓6th O41.14 Placentitis

     ✓7th O41.141 Placentitis, first trimester   MCC M
     ✓7th O41.142 Placentitis, second trimester   MCC M
     ✓7th O41.143 Placentitis, third trimester   MCC M

     ✓7th O41.149 Placentitis, unspecified trimester   M

✓5th O41.8 Other specified disorders of amniotic fluid and membranes

   ✓6th O41.8X Other specified disorders of amniotic fluid and membranes

     AHA: 2024,1Q,13

     ✓7th O41.8X1 Other specified disorders of amniotic fluid and membranes, first trimester   M
     ✓7th O41.8X2 Other specified disorders of amniotic fluid and membranes, second trimester   M
     ✓7th O41.8X3 Other specified disorders of amniotic fluid and membranes, third trimester   M
     ✓7th O41.8X9 Other specified disorders of amniotic fluid and membranes, unspecified trimester   M

✓5th O41.9 Disorder of amniotic fluid and membranes, unspecified

   ✓x7th O41.90 Disorder of amniotic fluid and membranes, unspecified, unspecified trimester   M
   ✓x7th O41.91 Disorder of amniotic fluid and membranes, unspecified, first trimester   M
   ✓x7th O41.92 Disorder of amniotic fluid and membranes, unspecified, second trimester   M
   ✓x7th O41.93 Disorder of amniotic fluid and membranes, unspecified, third trimester   M

✓4th O42 Premature rupture of membranes

> **AHA:** 2023,3Q,17; 2016,1Q,3

✓5th O42.0 Premature rupture of membranes, onset of labor within 24 hours of rupture

   O42.00 Premature rupture of membranes, onset of labor within 24 hours of rupture, unspecified weeks of gestation   M

   ✓6th O42.01 Preterm premature rupture of membranes, onset of labor within 24 hours of rupture

> Premature rupture of membranes before 37 completed weeks of gestation

     O42.011 Preterm premature rupture of membranes, onset of labor within 24 hours of rupture, first trimester   M
     O42.012 Preterm premature rupture of membranes, onset of labor within 24 hours of rupture, second trimester   M
     O42.013 Preterm premature rupture of membranes, onset of labor within 24 hours of rupture, third trimester   M
     O42.019 Preterm premature rupture of membranes, onset of labor within 24 hours of rupture, unspecified trimester   M

   O42.02 Full-term premature rupture of membranes, onset of labor within 24 hours of rupture

> Premature rupture of membranes at or after 37 completed weeks of gestation, onset of labor within 24 hours of rupture

✓5th O42.1 Premature rupture of membranes, onset of labor more than 24 hours following rupture

> **AHA:** 2016,1Q,5

   O42.10 Premature rupture of membranes, onset of labor more than 24 hours following rupture, unspecified weeks of gestation

   ✓6th O42.11 Preterm premature rupture of membranes, onset of labor more than 24 hours following rupture

> Premature rupture of membranes before 37 completed weeks of gestation

     O42.111 Preterm premature rupture of membranes, onset of labor more than 24 hours following rupture, first trimester   M
     O42.112 Preterm premature rupture of membranes, onset of labor more than 24 hours following rupture, second trimester   M
     O42.113 Preterm premature rupture of membranes, onset of labor more than 24 hours following rupture, third trimester   M
     O42.119 Preterm premature rupture of membranes, onset of labor more than 24 hours following rupture, unspecified trimester   M

   O42.12 Full-term premature rupture of membranes, onset of labor more than 24 hours following rupture   M

> Premature rupture of membranes at or after 37 completed weeks of gestation, onset of labor more than 24 hours following rupture

✔ Additional Character Required   ✓x7th Placeholder   Questionable PDx   Manifestation   Unspecified   UPD Unacceptable PDx   H1-H14 HAC   HCC CMS-HCC Dx   HIV HIV Dx

ICD-10-CM 2025   903

✓5ᵗʰ **O42.9 Premature rupture of membranes, unspecified as to length of time between rupture and onset of labor**

    O42.90 Premature rupture of membranes, unspecified as to length of time between rupture and onset of labor, unspecified weeks of gestation M

    ✓6ᵗʰ **O42.91 Preterm premature rupture of membranes, unspecified as to length of time between rupture and onset of labor**

        Premature rupture of membranes before 37 completed weeks of gestation

        O42.911 Preterm premature rupture of membranes, unspecified as to length of time between rupture and onset of labor, first trimester M

        O42.912 Preterm premature rupture of membranes, unspecified as to length of time between rupture and onset of labor, second trimester M

        O42.913 Preterm premature rupture of membranes, unspecified as to length of time between rupture and onset of labor, third trimester M

        O42.919 Preterm premature rupture of membranes, unspecified as to length of time between rupture and onset of labor, unspecified trimester M

    O42.92 Full-term premature rupture of membranes, unspecified as to length of time between rupture and onset of labor

        Premature rupture of membranes at or after 37 completed weeks of gestation, unspecified as to length of time between rupture and onset of labor

✓4ᵗʰ **O43 Placental disorders**

    EXCLUDES 2 *maternal care for poor fetal growth due to placental insufficiency (O36.5-)*
        placenta previa (O44.-)
        placental polyp (O90.89)
        placentitis (O41.14-)
        premature separation of placenta [abruptio placentae] (O45.-)

    ✓5ᵗʰ **O43.0 Placental transfusion syndromes**

        ✓6ᵗʰ **O43.01 Fetomaternal placental transfusion syndrome**

            Maternofetal placental transfusion syndrome

            O43.011 Fetomaternal placental transfusion syndrome, first trimester M

            O43.012 Fetomaternal placental transfusion syndrome, second trimester M

            O43.013 Fetomaternal placental transfusion syndrome, third trimester M

            O43.019 Fetomaternal placental transfusion syndrome, unspecified trimester M

        ✓6ᵗʰ **O43.02 Fetus-to-fetus placental transfusion syndrome**

            DEF: Condition in which an imbalance in amniotic fluid occurs due to uneven blood flow between twins sharing a placenta.

Twin to Twin Transfusion Syndrome (TTTS)

Healthy twins   Twins with TTTS

            O43.021 Fetus-to-fetus placental transfusion syndrome, first trimester M

            O43.022 Fetus-to-fetus placental transfusion syndrome, second trimester M

            O43.023 Fetus-to-fetus placental transfusion syndrome, third trimester M

            O43.029 Fetus-to-fetus placental transfusion syndrome, unspecified trimester M

    ✓5ᵗʰ **O43.1 Malformation of placenta**

        ✓6ᵗʰ **O43.10 Malformation of placenta, unspecified**

            Abnormal placenta NOS

            O43.101 Malformation of placenta, unspecified, first trimester M

            O43.102 Malformation of placenta, unspecified, second trimester M

            O43.103 Malformation of placenta, unspecified, third trimester M

            O43.109 Malformation of placenta, unspecified, unspecified trimester M

        ✓6ᵗʰ **O43.11 Circumvallate placenta**

            O43.111 Circumvallate placenta, first trimester M

            O43.112 Circumvallate placenta, second trimester M

            O43.113 Circumvallate placenta, third trimester M

            O43.119 Circumvallate placenta, unspecified trimester M

        ✓6ᵗʰ **O43.12 Velamentous insertion of umbilical cord**

            O43.121 Velamentous insertion of umbilical cord, first trimester M

            O43.122 Velamentous insertion of umbilical cord, second trimester M

            O43.123 Velamentous insertion of umbilical cord, third trimester M

            O43.129 Velamentous insertion of umbilical cord, unspecified trimester M

        ✓6ᵗʰ **O43.19 Other malformation of placenta**

            O43.191 Other malformation of placenta, first trimester M

            O43.192 Other malformation of placenta, second trimester M

            O43.193 Other malformation of placenta, third trimester M

            O43.199 Other malformation of placenta, unspecified trimester M

    ✓5ᵗʰ **O43.2 Morbidly adherent placenta**

        Code also associated third stage postpartum hemorrhage, if applicable (O72.0)

        EXCLUDES 1 *retained placenta (O73.-)*

        ✓6ᵗʰ **O43.21 Placenta accreta**

            DEF: Condition where the placenta adheres too deeply to the uterine wall; often associated with placenta previa.

            O43.211 Placenta accreta, first trimester M

            O43.212 Placenta accreta, second trimester M

            O43.213 Placenta accreta, third trimester M

            O43.219 Placenta accreta, unspecified trimester M

        ✓6ᵗʰ **O43.22 Placenta increta**

            AHA: 2022,1Q,20
            DEF: Condition where the placenta adheres too deeply to the uterine wall and penetrates the muscle; often associated with placenta previa.

            O43.221 Placenta increta, first trimester M

            O43.222 Placenta increta, second trimester M

            O43.223 Placenta increta, third trimester M

            O43.229 Placenta increta, unspecified trimester M

        ✓6ᵗʰ **O43.23 Placenta percreta**

            DEF: Condition where the placenta attaches through the uterine muscle and may invade other organs, resulting in antenatal complications, premature delivery, retention of all or a portion of the placenta, or postpartum bleeding.

            O43.231 Placenta percreta, first trimester M

            O43.232 Placenta percreta, second trimester M

            O43.233 Placenta percreta, third trimester M

            O43.239 Placenta percreta, unspecified trimester M

    ✓5ᵗʰ **O43.8 Other placental disorders**

        ✓6ᵗʰ **O43.81 Placental infarction**

            O43.811 Placental infarction, first trimester M

O43.812 **Placental infarction, second trimester** M

O43.813 **Placental infarction, third trimester** M

O43.819 **Placental infarction, unspecified trimester** M

√6th O43.89 **Other placental disorders**
Placental dysfunction

O43.891 **Other placental disorders, first trimester** M

O43.892 **Other placental disorders, second trimester** M

O43.893 **Other placental disorders, third trimester** M

O43.899 **Other placental disorders, unspecified trimester** M

√5th O43.9 **Unspecified placental disorder**

O43.90 **Unspecified placental disorder, unspecified trimester** M

O43.91 **Unspecified placental disorder, first trimester** M

O43.92 **Unspecified placental disorder, second trimester** M

O43.93 **Unspecified placental disorder, third trimester** M

√4th O44 **Placenta previa**
AHA: 2016,4Q,52-53
DEF: Placenta implanted in the lower segment of the uterus, which commonly causes hemorrhage in the last trimester of pregnancy.

√5th O44.0 **Complete placenta previa NOS or without hemorrhage**
Placenta previa NOS

O44.00 **Complete placenta previa NOS or without hemorrhage, unspecified trimester** M

O44.01 **Complete placenta previa NOS or without hemorrhage, first trimester** CC M

O44.02 **Complete placenta previa NOS or without hemorrhage, second trimester** CC M

O44.03 **Complete placenta previa NOS or without hemorrhage, third trimester** CC M

√5th O44.1 **Complete placenta previa with hemorrhage**
EXCLUDES 1   labor and delivery complicated by hemorrhage from vasa previa (O69.4)

O44.10 **Complete placenta previa with hemorrhage, unspecified trimester** M

O44.11 **Complete placenta previa with hemorrhage, first trimester** MCC M

O44.12 **Complete placenta previa with hemorrhage, second trimester** MCC M

O44.13 **Complete placenta previa with hemorrhage, third trimester** MCC M

√5th O44.2 **Partial placenta previa without hemorrhage**
Marginal placenta previa, NOS or without hemorrhage

O44.20 **Partial placenta previa NOS or without hemorrhage, unspecified trimester** M

O44.21 **Partial placenta previa NOS or without hemorrhage, first trimester** CC M

O44.22 **Partial placenta previa NOS or without hemorrhage, second trimester** CC M

O44.23 **Partial placenta previa NOS or without hemorrhage, third trimester** CC M

√5th O44.3 **Partial placenta previa with hemorrhage**
Marginal placenta previa with hemorrhage

O44.30 **Partial placenta previa with hemorrhage, unspecified trimester** M

O44.31 **Partial placenta previa with hemorrhage, first trimester** MCC M

O44.32 **Partial placenta previa with hemorrhage, second trimester** MCC M

O44.33 **Partial placenta previa with hemorrhage, third trimester** MCC M

√5th O44.4 **Low lying placenta NOS or without hemorrhage**
Low implantation of placenta NOS or without hemorrhage

O44.40 **Low lying placenta NOS or without hemorrhage, unspecified trimester** M

O44.41 **Low lying placenta NOS or without hemorrhage, first trimester** CC M

O44.42 **Low lying placenta NOS or without hemorrhage, second trimester** CC M

O44.43 **Low lying placenta NOS or without hemorrhage, third trimester** CC M

√5th O44.5 **Low lying placenta with hemorrhage**
Low implantation of placenta with hemorrhage

O44.50 **Low lying placenta with hemorrhage, unspecified trimester** M

O44.51 **Low lying placenta with hemorrhage, first trimester** MCC M

O44.52 **Low lying placenta with hemorrhage, second trimester** MCC M

O44.53 **Low lying placenta with hemorrhage, third trimester** MCC M

√4th O45 **Premature separation of placenta [abruptio placentae]**

√5th O45.0 **Premature separation of placenta with coagulation defect**

√6th O45.00 **Premature separation of placenta with coagulation defect, unspecified**

O45.001 **Premature separation of placenta with coagulation defect, unspecified, first trimester** MCC M

O45.002 **Premature separation of placenta with coagulation defect, unspecified, second trimester** MCC M

O45.003 **Premature separation of placenta with coagulation defect, unspecified, third trimester** MCC M

O45.009 **Premature separation of placenta with coagulation defect, unspecified, unspecified trimester** M

√6th O45.01 **Premature separation of placenta with afibrinogenemia**
Premature separation of placenta with hypofibrinogenemia

O45.011 **Premature separation of placenta with afibrinogenemia, first trimester** MCC M

O45.012 **Premature separation of placenta with afibrinogenemia, second trimester** MCC M

O45.013 **Premature separation of placenta with afibrinogenemia, third trimester** MCC M

O45.019 **Premature separation of placenta with afibrinogenemia, unspecified trimester** M

√6th O45.02 **Premature separation of placenta with disseminated intravascular coagulation**

O45.021 **Premature separation of placenta with disseminated intravascular coagulation, first trimester** MCC M

O45.022 **Premature separation of placenta with disseminated intravascular coagulation, second trimester** MCC M

O45.023 **Premature separation of placenta with disseminated intravascular coagulation, third trimester** MCC M

O45.029 **Premature separation of placenta with disseminated intravascular coagulation, unspecified trimester** M

√6th O45.09 **Premature separation of placenta with other coagulation defect**

O45.091 **Premature separation of placenta with other coagulation defect, first trimester** MCC M

O45.092 **Premature separation of placenta with other coagulation defect, second trimester** MCC M

O45.093 **Premature separation of placenta with other coagulation defect, third trimester** MCC M

O45.099 **Premature separation of placenta with other coagulation defect, unspecified trimester** M

√5th O45.8 **Other premature separation of placenta**

√6th O45.8X **Other premature separation of placenta**

O45.8X1 **Other premature separation of placenta, first trimester** MCC M

O45.8X2 **Other premature separation of placenta, second trimester** MCC M

O45.8X3 **Other premature separation of placenta, third trimester** MCC M

O45.8X9 **Other premature separation of placenta, unspecified trimester** M

☑ Additional Character Required   √x7th Placeholder   Questionable PDx   Manifestation   Unspecified   UPD Unacceptable PDx   H1-H14 HAC   HCC CMS-HCC Dx   HIV HIV Dx

√5ᵗʰ **O45.9　Premature separation of placenta, unspecified**
　　　Abruptio placentae NOS
　　　O45.90　Premature separation of placenta, unspecified, unspecified trimester　M
　　　O45.91　Premature separation of placenta, unspecified, first trimester　MCC M
　　　O45.92　Premature separation of placenta, unspecified, second trimester　MCC M
　　　O45.93　Premature separation of placenta, unspecified, third trimester　MCC M

√4ᵗʰ **O46　Antepartum hemorrhage, not elsewhere classified**
　　EXCLUDES 1　hemorrhage in early pregnancy (O20.-)
　　　　　　　intrapartum hemorrhage NEC (O67.-)
　　　　　　　placenta previa (O44.-)
　　　　　　　premature separation of placenta [abruptio placentae] (O45.-)
　　DEF: Uterine hemorrhage prior to delivery that is not related to placenta previa or abruptio placentae.

√5ᵗʰ **O46.0　Antepartum hemorrhage with coagulation defect**
　　√6ᵗʰ **O46.00　Antepartum hemorrhage with coagulation defect, unspecified**
　　　　O46.001　Antepartum hemorrhage with coagulation defect, unspecified, first trimester　MCC M
　　　　O46.002　Antepartum hemorrhage with coagulation defect, unspecified, second trimester　MCC M
　　　　O46.003　Antepartum hemorrhage with coagulation defect, unspecified, third trimester　MCC M
　　　　O46.009　Antepartum hemorrhage with coagulation defect, unspecified, unspecified trimester　M
　　√6ᵗʰ **O46.01　Antepartum hemorrhage with afibrinogenemia**
　　　　Antepartum hemorrhage with hypofibrinogenemia
　　　　O46.011　Antepartum hemorrhage with afibrinogenemia, first trimester　MCC M
　　　　O46.012　Antepartum hemorrhage with afibrinogenemia, second trimester　MCC M
　　　　O46.013　Antepartum hemorrhage with afibrinogenemia, third trimester　MCC M
　　　　O46.019　Antepartum hemorrhage with afibrinogenemia, unspecified trimester　M
　　√6ᵗʰ **O46.02　Antepartum hemorrhage with disseminated intravascular coagulation**
　　　　O46.021　Antepartum hemorrhage with disseminated intravascular coagulation, first trimester　MCC M
　　　　O46.022　Antepartum hemorrhage with disseminated intravascular coagulation, second trimester　MCC M
　　　　O46.023　Antepartum hemorrhage with disseminated intravascular coagulation, third trimester　MCC M
　　　　O46.029　Antepartum hemorrhage with disseminated intravascular coagulation, unspecified trimester　M
　　√6ᵗʰ **O46.09　Antepartum hemorrhage with other coagulation defect**
　　　　O46.091　Antepartum hemorrhage with other coagulation defect, first trimester　MCC M
　　　　O46.092　Antepartum hemorrhage with other coagulation defect, second trimester　MCC M
　　　　O46.093　Antepartum hemorrhage with other coagulation defect, third trimester　MCC M
　　　　O46.099　Antepartum hemorrhage with other coagulation defect, unspecified trimester　M

√5ᵗʰ **O46.8　Other antepartum hemorrhage**
　　√6ᵗʰ **O46.8X　Other antepartum hemorrhage**
　　　　O46.8X1　Other antepartum hemorrhage, first trimester　M
　　　　O46.8X2　Other antepartum hemorrhage, second trimester　M
　　　　O46.8X3　Other antepartum hemorrhage, third trimester　M

　　　　O46.8X9　Other antepartum hemorrhage, unspecified trimester　M
√5ᵗʰ **O46.9　Antepartum hemorrhage, unspecified**
　　　O46.90　Antepartum hemorrhage, unspecified, unspecified trimester　M
　　　O46.91　Antepartum hemorrhage, unspecified, first trimester　M
　　　O46.92　Antepartum hemorrhage, unspecified, second trimester　M
　　　O46.93　Antepartum hemorrhage, unspecified, third trimester　M

√4ᵗʰ **O47　False labor**
　　INCLUDES　Braxton Hicks contractions
　　　　　　　threatened labor
　　EXCLUDES 1　preterm labor (O60.-)
　　AHA: 2021,1Q,10
√5ᵗʰ **O47.0　False labor before 37 completed weeks of gestation**
　　　O47.00　False labor before 37 completed weeks of gestation, unspecified trimester　M
　　　O47.02　False labor before 37 completed weeks of gestation, second trimester　CC M
　　　O47.03　False labor before 37 completed weeks of gestation, third trimester　CC M
　　O47.1　False labor at or after 37 completed weeks of gestation　CC M
　　O47.9　False labor, unspecified　M

√4ᵗʰ **O48　Late pregnancy**
　　AHA: 2022,2Q,3
　　O48.0　Post-term pregnancy　M
　　　　Pregnancy over 40 completed weeks to 42 completed weeks gestation
　　O48.1　Prolonged pregnancy　M
　　　　Pregnancy which has advanced beyond 42 completed weeks gestation
　　AHA: 2016,1Q,5

Complications of labor and delivery (O60-O77)

√4ᵗʰ **O60　Preterm labor**
　　INCLUDES　onset (spontaneous) of labor before 37 completed weeks of gestation
　　EXCLUDES 1　false labor (O47.0-)
　　　　　　　threatened labor NOS (O47.0-)
√5ᵗʰ **O60.0　Preterm labor without delivery**
　　　O60.00　Preterm labor without delivery, unspecified trimester　M
　　　O60.02　Preterm labor without delivery, second trimester　MCC M
　　　O60.03　Preterm labor without delivery, third trimester　MCC M
√5ᵗʰ **O60.1　Preterm labor with preterm delivery**
　　AHA: 2016,2Q,10

> One of the following 7th characters is to be assigned to each code under subcategory O60.1. 7th character 0 is for single gestations and multiple gestations where the fetus is unspecified. 7th characters 1 through 9 are for cases of multiple gestations to identify the fetus for which the code applies. The appropriate code from category O30, Multiple gestation, must also be assigned when assigning a code from subcategory O60.1 that has a 7th character of 1 through 9.
> 0　not applicable or unspecified
> 1　fetus 1
> 2　fetus 2
> 3　fetus 3
> 4　fetus 4
> 5　fetus 5
> 9　other fetus

　√x 7ᵗʰ **O60.10**　Preterm labor with preterm delivery, unspecified trimester　CC M
　　　　Preterm labor with delivery NOS
　√x 7ᵗʰ **O60.12**　Preterm labor second trimester with preterm delivery second trimester　MCC M
　√x 7ᵗʰ **O60.13**　Preterm labor second trimester with preterm delivery third trimester　MCC M
　√x 7ᵗʰ **O60.14**　Preterm labor third trimester with preterm delivery third trimester　MCC M

☑5ᵗʰ O60.2 Term delivery with preterm labor

One of the following 7th characters is to be assigned to each code under subcategory O60.2. 7th character Ø is for single gestations and multiple gestations where the fetus is unspecified. 7th characters 1 through 9 are for cases of multiple gestations to identify the fetus for which the code applies. The appropriate code from category O30, Multiple gestation, must also be assigned when assigning a code from subcategory O60.2 that has a 7th character of 1 through 9.

Ø   not applicable or unspecified
1   fetus 1
2   fetus 2
3   fetus 3
4   fetus 4
5   fetus 5
9   other fetus

- **☑x7ᵗʰ O60.20 Term delivery with preterm labor, unspecified trimester** `CC` `M`
- **☑x7ᵗʰ O60.22 Term delivery with preterm labor, second trimester** `MCC` `M`
- **☑x7ᵗʰ O60.23 Term delivery with preterm labor, third trimester** `MCC` `M`

☑4ᵗʰ O61 Failed induction of labor

- **O61.Ø Failed medical induction of labor** `M`
  Failed induction (of labor) by oxytocin
  Failed induction (of labor) by prostaglandins

- **O61.1 Failed instrumental induction of labor** `M`
  Failed mechanical induction (of labor)
  Failed surgical induction (of labor)

- **O61.8 Other failed induction of labor** `M`
- **O61.9 Failed induction of labor, unspecified** `M`

☑4ᵗʰ O62 Abnormalities of forces of labor

DEF: Uterine inertia: Weak or poorly coordinated contractions of the uterus during labor.

- **O62.Ø Primary inadequate contractions** `M`
  Failure of cervical dilatation
  Primary hypotonic uterine dysfunction
  Uterine inertia during latent phase of labor
  AHA: 2024,1Q,13

- **O62.1 Secondary uterine inertia** `M`
  Arrested active phase of labor
  Secondary hypotonic uterine dysfunction

- **O62.2 Other uterine inertia** `M`
  Atony of uterus without hemorrhage
  Atony of uterus NOS
  Desultory labor
  Hypotonic uterine dysfunction NOS
  Irregular labor
  Poor contractions
  Slow slope active phase of labor
  Uterine inertia NOS
  > **EXCLUDES 1**   atony of uterus with hemorrhage (postpartum) (O72.1)
  > postpartum atony of uterus without hemorrhage (O75.89)

  DEF: Uterine atony: Failure of the uterine muscles to contract after the fetus and placenta are delivered.

- **O62.3 Precipitate labor** `M`
  DEF: Rapid labor with delivery occurring in three hours or less from the onset of contractions.

- **O62.4 Hypertonic, incoordinate, and prolonged uterine contractions** `M`
  Cervical spasm
  Contraction ring dystocia
  Dyscoordinate labor
  Hour-glass contraction of uterus
  Hypertonic uterine dysfunction
  Incoordinate uterine action
  Tetanic contractions
  Uterine dystocia NOS
  Uterine spasm
  > **EXCLUDES 1**   dystocia (fetal) (maternal) NOS (O66.9)

- **O62.8 Other abnormalities of forces of labor** `M`
- **O62.9 Abnormality of forces of labor, unspecified** `M`

☑4ᵗʰ O63 Long labor

- **O63.Ø Prolonged first stage (of labor)** `M`
- **O63.1 Prolonged second stage (of labor)** `M`
- **O63.2 Delayed delivery of second twin, triplet, etc.** `M`

O63.9 Long labor, unspecified `CC` `M`
Prolonged labor NOS

☑4ᵗʰ O64 Obstructed labor due to malposition and malpresentation of fetus

One of the following 7th characters is to be assigned to each code under category O64. 7th character Ø is for single gestations and multiple gestations where the fetus is unspecified. 7th characters 1 through 9 are for cases of multiple gestations to identify the fetus for which the code applies. The appropriate code from category O30, Multiple gestation, must also be assigned when assigning a code from category O64 that has a 7th character of 1 through 9.

Ø   not applicable or unspecified
1   fetus 1
2   fetus 2
3   fetus 3
4   fetus 4
5   fetus 5
9   other fetus

Fetal Malposition

Breech
Mother's pelvis

Shoulder (arm prolapse)

Compound (extremity together with head)

Face (mentum)

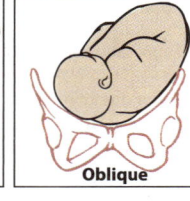
Oblique

- **☑x7ᵗʰ O64.Ø Obstructed labor due to incomplete rotation of fetal head** `M`
  Deep transverse arrest
  Obstructed labor due to persistent occipitoiliac (position)
  Obstructed labor due to persistent occipitoposterior (position)
  Obstructed labor due to persistent occipitosacral (position)
  Obstructed labor due to persistent occipitotransverse (position)

- **☑x7ᵗʰ O64.1 Obstructed labor due to breech presentation**
  Obstructed labor due to buttocks presentation
  Obstructed labor due to complete breech presentation
  Obstructed labor due to frank breech presentation

- **☑x7ᵗʰ O64.2 Obstructed labor due to face presentation** `M`
  Obstructed labor due to chin presentation

- **☑x7ᵗʰ O64.3 Obstructed labor due to brow presentation** `M`

- **☑x7ᵗʰ O64.4 Obstructed labor due to shoulder presentation** `M`
  Prolapsed arm
  > **EXCLUDES 1**   impacted shoulders (O66.Ø)
  > shoulder dystocia (O66.Ø)

- **☑x7ᵗʰ O64.5 Obstructed labor due to compound presentation** `M`

- **☑x7ᵗʰ O64.8 Obstructed labor due to other malposition and malpresentation** `M`
  Obstructed labor due to footling presentation
  Obstructed labor due to incomplete breech presentation

- **☑x7ᵗʰ O64.9 Obstructed labor due to malposition and malpresentation, unspecified** `M`

☑4ᵗʰ O65 Obstructed labor due to maternal pelvic abnormality

- **O65.Ø Obstructed labor due to deformed pelvis** `M`
- **O65.1 Obstructed labor due to generally contracted pelvis** `M`
- **O65.2 Obstructed labor due to pelvic inlet contraction** `M`
- **O65.3 Obstructed labor due to pelvic outlet and mid-cavity contraction** `M`
- **O65.4 Obstructed labor due to fetopelvic disproportion, unspecified** `M`
  > **EXCLUDES 1**   dystocia due to abnormality of fetus (O66.2-O66.3)

☑ Additional Character Required   ☑x7ᵗʰ Placeholder   `Questionable PDx`   Manifestation   Unspecified   `UPD` Unacceptable PDx   `H1`-`H14` HAC   `HCC` CMS-HCC Dx   `HIV` HIV Dx

ICD-10-CM 2025   907

O65.5   **Obstructed labor due to abnormality of maternal pelvic organs**   **M**
Obstructed labor due to conditions listed in O34.-
Use additional code to identify abnormality of pelvic organs O34.-

O65.8   **Obstructed labor due to other maternal pelvic abnormalities**   **M**

O65.9   **Obstructed labor due to maternal pelvic abnormality, unspecified**   **M**

✓4ᵗʰ **O66**   **Other obstructed labor**

O66.0   **Obstructed labor due to shoulder dystocia**   **M**
Impacted shoulders
DEF: Obstructed labor due to impacted fetal shoulders. It is an emergency condition that may require cesarean section, forceps delivery, vacuum extraction, or symphysiotomy.

O66.1   **Obstructed labor due to locked twins**   **M**

O66.2   **Obstructed labor due to unusually large fetus**   **M**

O66.3   **Obstructed labor due to other abnormalities of fetus**   **M**
Dystocia due to fetal ascites
Dystocia due to fetal hydrops
Dystocia due to fetal meningomyelocele
Dystocia due to fetal sacral teratoma
Dystocia due to fetal tumor
Dystocia due to hydrocephalic fetus
Use additional code to identify cause of obstruction

✓5ᵗʰ **O66.4**   **Failed trial of labor**

O66.40   **Failed trial of labor, unspecified**   **M**

O66.41   **Failed attempted vaginal birth after previous cesarean delivery**   **M**
Code first rupture of uterus, if applicable (O71.0-, O71.1)

O66.5   **Attempted application of vacuum extractor and forceps**   **M** **PE**
Attempted application of vacuum or forceps, with subsequent delivery by forceps or cesarean delivery

O66.6   **Obstructed labor due to other multiple fetuses**   **M**

O66.8   **Other specified obstructed labor**   **M**
Use additional code to identify cause of obstruction

O66.9   **Obstructed labor, unspecified**   **M**
Dystocia NOS
Fetal dystocia NOS
Maternal dystocia NOS

✓4ᵗʰ **O67**   **Labor and delivery complicated by intrapartum hemorrhage, not elsewhere classified**
EXCLUDES 1   antepartum hemorrhage NEC (O46.-)
    placenta previa (O44.-)
    premature separation of placenta [abruptio placentae] (O45.-)
EXCLUDES 2   postpartum hemorrhage (O72.-)

O67.0   **Intrapartum hemorrhage with coagulation defect**   **MCC** **M**
Intrapartum hemorrhage (excessive) associated with afibrinogenemia
Intrapartum hemorrhage (excessive) associated with disseminated intravascular coagulation
Intrapartum hemorrhage (excessive) associated with hyperfibrinolysis
Intrapartum hemorrhage (excessive) associated with hypofibrinogenemia

O67.8   **Other intrapartum hemorrhage**   **M**
Excessive intrapartum hemorrhage

O67.9   **Intrapartum hemorrhage, unspecified**   **M**

O68   **Labor and delivery complicated by abnormality of fetal acid-base balance**   **CC** **M**
Fetal acidemia complicating labor and delivery
Fetal acidosis complicating labor and delivery
Fetal alkalosis complicating labor and delivery
Fetal metabolic acidemia complicating labor and delivery
EXCLUDES 1   fetal stress NOS (O77.9)
    labor and delivery complicated by electrocardiographic evidence of fetal stress (O77.8)
    labor and delivery complicated by ultrasonic evidence of fetal stress (O77.8)
EXCLUDES 2   abnormality in fetal heart rate or rhythm (O76)
    labor and delivery complicated by meconium in amniotic fluid (O77.0)

✓4ᵗʰ **O69**   **Labor and delivery complicated by umbilical cord complications**
AHA: 2016,1Q,5

One of the following 7th characters is to be assigned to each code under category O69. 7th character 0 is for single gestations and multiple gestations where the fetus is unspecified. 7th characters 1 through 9 are for cases of multiple gestations to identify the fetus for which the code applies. The appropriate code from category O30, Multiple gestation, must also be assigned when assigning a code from category O69 that has a 7th character of 1 through 9.
0   not applicable or unspecified
1   fetus 1
2   fetus 2
3   fetus 3
4   fetus 4
5   fetus 5
9   other fetus

✓x7ᵗʰ **O69.0**   **Labor and delivery complicated by prolapse of cord**   **M**
DEF: Abnormal presentation of the fetus marked by a protruding umbilical cord during labor. It can cause fetal death.

✓x7ᵗʰ **O69.1**   **Labor and delivery complicated by cord around neck, with compression**   **M**
EXCLUDES 1   labor and delivery complicated by cord around neck, without compression (O69.81)

✓x7ᵗʰ **O69.2**   **Labor and delivery complicated by other cord entanglement, with compression**   **M**
Labor and delivery complicated by compression of cord NOS
Labor and delivery complicated by entanglement of cords of twins in monoamniotic sac
Labor and delivery complicated by knot in cord
EXCLUDES 1   labor and delivery complicated by other cord entanglement, without compression (O69.82)

✓x7ᵗʰ **O69.3**   **Labor and delivery complicated by short cord**   **M**

✓x7ᵗʰ **O69.4**   **Labor and delivery complicated by vasa previa**   **M**
Labor and delivery complicated by hemorrhage from vasa previa

✓x7ᵗʰ **O69.5**   **Labor and delivery complicated by vascular lesion of cord**   **M**
Labor and delivery complicated by cord bruising
Labor and delivery complicated by cord hematoma
Labor and delivery complicated by thrombosis of umbilical vessels

✓5ᵗʰ **O69.8**   **Labor and delivery complicated by other cord complications**

✓x7ᵗʰ **O69.81**   **Labor and delivery complicated by cord around neck, without compression**   **M**
AHA: 2016,1Q,5

✓x7ᵗʰ **O69.82**   **Labor and delivery complicated by other cord entanglement, without compression**   **M**

✓x7ᵗʰ **O69.89**   **Labor and delivery complicated by other cord complications**   **M**
AHA: 2023,2Q,29

✓x7ᵗʰ **O69.9**   **Labor and delivery complicated by cord complication, unspecified**   **M**

✓4ᵗʰ **O70**   **Perineal laceration during delivery**
INCLUDES   episiotomy extended by laceration
EXCLUDES 1   obstetric high vaginal laceration alone (O71.4)
AHA: 2016,2Q,34; 2016,1Q,3-4,5

O70.0   **First degree perineal laceration during delivery**   **M**
Perineal laceration, rupture or tear involving fourchette during delivery
Perineal laceration, rupture or tear involving labia during delivery
Perineal laceration, rupture or tear involving skin during delivery
Perineal laceration, rupture or tear involving vagina during delivery
Perineal laceration, rupture or tear involving vulva during delivery
Slight perineal laceration, rupture or tear during delivery

O70.1   **Second degree perineal laceration during delivery**   **M**
Perineal laceration, rupture or tear during delivery as in O70.0, also involving pelvic floor
Perineal laceration, rupture or tear during delivery as in O70.0, also involving perineal muscles
Perineal laceration, rupture or tear during delivery as in O70.0, also involving vaginal muscles
EXCLUDES 1   perineal laceration involving anal sphincter (O70.2)

N Newborn: 0   **P** Pediatric: 0-17   **M** Maternity: 9-64   **A** Adult: 15-124   **UNS** Unspecified Site   **MCC** Major Complication/Comorbidity   **CC** Complication/Comorbidity   **PE** POA Exempt

908

ICD-10-CM 2025

✓5ᵗʰ **O70.2** **Third degree** perineal laceration during delivery

Perineal laceration, rupture or tear during delivery as in O70.1, also involving anal sphincter

Perineal laceration, rupture or tear during delivery as in O70.1, also involving rectovaginal septum

Perineal laceration, rupture or tear during delivery as in O70.1, also involving sphincter NOS

EXCLUDES 1 *anal sphincter tear during delivery without third degree perineal laceration (O70.4)*

perineal laceration involving anal or rectal mucosa (O70.3)

AHA: 2016,4Q,53-54

O70.20 **Third degree perineal laceration during delivery, unspecified** CC M

O70.21 **Third degree perineal laceration during delivery, IIIa** CC M

Third degree perineal laceration during delivery with less than 50% of external anal sphincter (EAS) thickness torn

O70.22 **Third degree perineal laceration during delivery, IIIb** CC M

Third degree perineal laceration during delivery with more than 50% external anal sphincter (EAS) thickness torn

O70.23 **Third degree perineal laceration during delivery, IIIc** CC M

Third degree perineal laceration during delivery with both external anal sphincter (EAS) and internal anal sphincter (IAS) torn

O70.3 **Fourth degree** perineal laceration during delivery CC M

Perineal laceration, rupture or tear during delivery as in O70.2, also involving anal mucosa

Perineal laceration, rupture or tear during delivery as in O70.2, also involving rectal mucosa

O70.4 **Anal sphincter tear** complicating delivery, not associated with third degree laceration CC M

EXCLUDES 1 *anal sphincter tear with third degree perineal laceration (O70.2)*

O70.9 **Perineal laceration during delivery, unspecified** M

✓4ᵗʰ **O71** **Other obstetric trauma**

INCLUDES obstetric damage from instruments

✓5ᵗʰ **O71.0** **Rupture of uterus (spontaneous)** before onset of labor

EXCLUDES 1 *disruption of (current) cesarean delivery wound (O90.0)*

laceration of uterus, NEC (O71.81)

O71.00 **Rupture of uterus before onset of labor, unspecified trimester**

O71.02 **Rupture of uterus before onset of labor, second trimester** MCC M

O71.03 **Rupture of uterus before onset of labor, third trimester** MCC M

O71.1 **Rupture of uterus during labor** MCC M

Rupture of uterus not stated as occurring before onset of labor

EXCLUDES 1 *disruption of cesarean delivery wound (O90.0)*

laceration of uterus, NEC (O71.81)

O71.2 **Postpartum inversion of uterus** CC M

O71.3 **Obstetric laceration of cervix** CC M

Annular detachment of cervix

O71.4 **Obstetric high vaginal laceration alone** CC M

Laceration of vaginal wall without perineal laceration

EXCLUDES 1 *obstetric high vaginal laceration with perineal laceration (O70.-)*

AHA: 2016,1Q,5

O71.5 **Other obstetric injury to pelvic organs** CC M

Obstetric injury to bladder

Obstetric injury to urethra

EXCLUDES 2 *obstetric periurethral trauma (O71.82)*

AHA: 2014,4Q,18

O71.6 **Obstetric damage to pelvic joints and ligaments** CC M

Obstetric avulsion of inner symphyseal cartilage

Obstetric damage to coccyx

Obstetric traumatic separation of symphysis (pubis)

O71.7 **Obstetric hematoma of pelvis** CC M

Obstetric hematoma of perineum

Obstetric hematoma of vagina

Obstetric hematoma of vulva

✓5ᵗʰ **O71.8** **Other specified obstetric trauma**

O71.81 **Laceration of uterus, not elsewhere classified** M

O71.82 **Other specified trauma to perineum and vulva** M

Obstetric periurethral trauma

AHA: 2016,1Q,4; 2014,4Q,18

O71.89 **Other specified obstetric trauma** M

O71.9 **Obstetric trauma, unspecified** M

✓4ᵗʰ **O72** **Postpartum hemorrhage**

INCLUDES hemorrhage after delivery of fetus or infant

O72.0 **Third-stage** hemorrhage CC M

Hemorrhage associated with retained, trapped or adherent placenta

Retained placenta NOS

Code also type of adherent placenta (O43.2-)

AHA: 2019,3Q,11

O72.1 **Other immediate postpartum hemorrhage** CC M

Hemorrhage following delivery of placenta

Postpartum hemorrhage (atonic) NOS

Uterine atony with hemorrhage

EXCLUDES 1 *uterine atony NOS (O62.2)*

uterine atony without hemorrhage (O62.2)

postpartum atony of uterus without hemorrhage (O75.89)

AHA: 2023,2Q,15; 2016,1Q,4

DEF: Uterine atony: Failure of the uterine muscles to contract after the fetus and placenta are delivered.

O72.2 **Delayed and secondary** postpartum hemorrhage CC M

Hemorrhage associated with retained portions of placenta or membranes after the first 24 hours following delivery of placenta

Retained products of conception NOS, following delivery

O72.3 **Postpartum coagulation defects** M

Postpartum afibrinogenemia

Postpartum fibrinolysis

✓4ᵗʰ **O73** **Retained placenta and membranes, without hemorrhage**

EXCLUDES 1 *placenta accreta (O43.21-)*

placenta increta (O43.22-)

placenta percreta (O43.23-)

DEF: Postpartum condition resulting from failure to expel placental membrane tissues due to failed contractions of the uterine wall.

O73.0 **Retained placenta without hemorrhage** M

Adherent placenta, without hemorrhage

Trapped placenta without hemorrhage

O73.1 **Retained portions of placenta and membranes, without hemorrhage** M

Retained products of conception following delivery, without hemorrhage

✓4ᵗʰ **O74** **Complications of anesthesia during labor and delivery**

INCLUDES maternal complications arising from the administration of a general, regional or local anesthetic, analgesic or other sedation during labor and delivery

Use additional code, if applicable, to identify specific complication

O74.0 **Aspiration pneumonitis** due to anesthesia during labor and delivery M

Inhalation of stomach contents or secretions NOS due to anesthesia during labor and delivery

Mendelson's syndrome due to anesthesia during labor and delivery

O74.1 **Other pulmonary complications of anesthesia during labor and delivery** M

O74.2 **Cardiac complications of anesthesia during labor and delivery** M

O74.3 **Central nervous system complications of anesthesia during labor and delivery** M

O74.4 **Toxic reaction to local anesthesia during labor and delivery** M

O74.5 **Spinal and epidural anesthesia-induced headache during labor and delivery** M

O74.6 **Other complications of spinal and epidural anesthesia during labor and delivery** M

O74.7 **Failed or difficult intubation for anesthesia during labor and delivery** M

O74.8 **Other complications of anesthesia during labor and delivery** M

O74.9 **Complication of anesthesia during labor and delivery, unspecified** M

☑4ᵗʰ O75 Other complications of labor and delivery, not elsewhere classified
- EXCLUDES 2   *puerperal (postpartum) infection (O86.-)*
- *puerperal (postpartum) sepsis (O85)*

O75.0 Maternal distress during labor and delivery M

O75.1 Shock during or following labor and delivery MCC M
- Obstetric shock following labor and delivery

O75.2 Pyrexia during labor, not elsewhere classified CC M

O75.3 Other infection during labor MCC M
- Sepsis during labor
- Use additional code (B95-B97), to identify infectious agent

O75.4 Other complications of obstetric surgery and procedures M
- Cardiac arrest following obstetric surgery or procedures
- Cardiac failure following obstetric surgery or procedures
- Cerebral anoxia following obstetric surgery or procedures
- Pulmonary edema following obstetric surgery or procedures
- Use additional code to identify specific complication
  - EXCLUDES 2   *complications of anesthesia during labor and delivery (O74.-)*
  - *disruption of obstetrical (surgical) wound (O90.0-O90.1)*
  - *hematoma of obstetrical (surgical) wound (O90.2)*
  - *infection of obstetrical (surgical) wound (O86.0-)*

O75.5 Delayed delivery after artificial rupture of membranes M

☑5ᵗʰ O75.8 Other specified complications of labor and delivery

O75.81 Maternal exhaustion complicating labor and delivery M

O75.82 Onset (spontaneous) of labor after 37 completed weeks of gestation but before 39 completed weeks gestation, with delivery by (planned) cesarean section UPD M
- Delivery by (planned) cesarean section occurring after 37 completed weeks of gestation but before 39 completed weeks gestation due to (spontaneous) onset of labor
- Code first to specify reason for planned cesarean section such as:
  - cephalopelvic disproportion (normally formed fetus) (O33.9)
  - previous cesarean delivery (O34.21-)
- AHA: 2022,2Q,3

O75.89 Other specified complications of labor and delivery M

O75.9 Complication of labor and delivery, unspecified M

O76 Abnormality in fetal heart rate and rhythm complicating labor and delivery M
- Depressed fetal heart rate tones complicating labor and delivery
- Fetal bradycardia complicating labor and delivery
- Fetal heart rate decelerations complicating labor and delivery
- Fetal heart rate irregularity complicating labor and delivery
- Fetal heart rate abnormal variability complicating labor and delivery
- Fetal tachycardia complicating labor and delivery
- Non-reassuring fetal heart rate or rhythm complicating labor and delivery
  - EXCLUDES 1   *fetal stress NOS (O77.9)*
  - *labor and delivery complicated by electrocardiographic evidence of fetal stress (O77.8)*
  - *labor and delivery complicated by ultrasonic evidence of fetal stress (O77.8)*
  - EXCLUDES 2   *fetal metabolic acidemia (O68)*
  - *other fetal stress (O77.0-O77.1)*
- AHA: 2013,4Q,118

☑4ᵗʰ O77 Other fetal stress complicating labor and delivery

O77.0 Labor and delivery complicated by meconium in amniotic fluid M
- AHA: 2022,2Q,16; 2013,4Q,117-118

O77.1 Fetal stress in labor or delivery due to drug administration M

O77.8 Labor and delivery complicated by other evidence of fetal stress M
- Labor and delivery complicated by electrocardiographic evidence of fetal stress
- Labor and delivery complicated by ultrasonic evidence of fetal stress
  - EXCLUDES 1   *abnormality of fetal acid-base balance (O68)*
  - *abnormality in fetal heart rate or rhythm (O76)*
  - *fetal metabolic acidemia (O68)*

O77.9 Labor and delivery complicated by fetal stress, unspecified M
- EXCLUDES 1   *abnormality of fetal acid-base balance (O68)*
- *abnormality in fetal heart rate or rhythm (O76)*
- *fetal metabolic acidemia (O68)*

Encounter for delivery (O80-O82)

O80 Encounter for full-term uncomplicated delivery M PE
- NOTE   Delivery requiring minimal or no assistance, with or without episiotomy, without fetal manipulation [e.g., rotation version] or instrumentation [forceps] of a spontaneous, cephalic, vaginal, full-term, single, live-born infant. This code is for use as a single diagnosis code and is not to be used with any other code from chapter 15.
- Use additional code to indicate outcome of delivery (Z37.0)
- AHA: 2016,4Q,150; 2014,2Q,9

O82 Encounter for cesarean delivery without indication M
- Use additional code to indicate outcome of delivery (Z37.0)

Complications predominantly related to the puerperium (O85-O92)

- EXCLUDES 2   *mental and behavioral disorders associated with the puerperium (F53.-)*
- *obstetrical tetanus (A34)*
- *puerperal osteomalacia (M83.0)*

O85 Puerperal sepsis MCC M
- Postpartum sepsis
- Puerperal peritonitis
- Puerperal pyemia
- Use additional code (B95-B97), to identify infectious agent
- Use additional code (R65.2-) to identify severe sepsis, if applicable
  - EXCLUDES 1   *fever of unknown origin following delivery (O86.4)*
  - ~~*genital tract infection following delivery (O86.1-)*~~
  - *obstetric pyemic and septic embolism (O88.3-)*
  - *puerperal septic thrombophlebitis (O86.81)*
  - ~~*urinary tract infection following delivery (O86.2-)*~~
  - EXCLUDES 2   ▶*genital tract infection following delivery (O86.1-)*◄
  - *sepsis during labor (O75.3)*
  - ▶*urinary tract infection following delivery (O86.2-)*◄
- AHA: 2022,2Q,5; 2020,2Q,32; 2019,2Q,39; 2018,4Q,23

☑4ᵗʰ O86 Other puerperal infections
- Use additional code (B95-B97), to identify infectious agent
  - EXCLUDES 2   *infection during labor (O75.3)*
  - *obstetrical tetanus (A34)*

☑5ᵗʰ O86.0 Infection of obstetric surgical wound
- Infected cesarean delivery wound following delivery
- Infected perineal repair following delivery
  - EXCLUDES 1   *complications of procedures, not elsewhere classified (T81.4-)*
  - *postprocedural fever NOS (R50.82)*
  - *postprocedural retroperitoneal abscess (K68.11)*
- AHA: 2020,2Q,32; 2018,4Q,22-23,62

O86.00 Infection of obstetric surgical wound, unspecified M

O86.01 Infection of obstetric surgical wound, superficial incisional site M
- Subcutaneous abscess following an obstetrical procedure
- Stitch abscess following an obstetrical procedure

O86.02 Infection of obstetric surgical wound, deep incisional site M
- Intramuscular abscess following an obstetrical procedure
- Sub-fascial abscess following an obstetrical procedure
- AHA: 2020,2Q,32

O86.03 Infection of obstetric surgical wound, organ and space site M
- Intraabdominal abscess following an obstetrical procedure
- Subphrenic abscess following an obstetrical procedure

O86.04 Sepsis following an obstetrical procedure MCC M
- Use additional code to identify the sepsis
- AHA: 2020,2Q,32; 2019,2Q,39

O86.09 Infection of obstetric surgical wound, other surgical site M

N Newborn: 0   P Pediatric: 0-17   M Maternity: 9-64   A Adult: 15-124   UNS Unspecified Site   MCC Major Complication/Comorbidity   CC Complication/Comorbidity   PE POA Exempt

✓5ᵗʰ O86.1 Other infection of genital tract following delivery

     O86.11 **Cervicitis following delivery** `CC` `M`

     O86.12 **Endometritis following delivery** `CC` `M`

     O86.13 **Vaginitis following delivery** `CC` `M`

     O86.19 **Other infection of genital tract following delivery** `CC` `M`

✓5ᵗʰ O86.2 Urinary tract infection following delivery

     O86.20 **Urinary tract infection following delivery, unspecified** `CC` `M`
         Puerperal urinary tract infection NOS
         AHA: 2022,2Q,5

     O86.21 **Infection of kidney following delivery** `CC` `M`

     O86.22 **Infection of bladder following delivery** `CC` `M`
         Infection of urethra following delivery

     O86.29 **Other urinary tract infection following delivery** `CC` `M`

O86.4 Pyrexia of unknown origin following delivery `CC` `M`
     Puerperal infection NOS following delivery
     Puerperal pyrexia NOS following delivery
     EXCLUDES 2   *pyrexia during labor (O75.2)*
     DEF: Fever of unknown origin experienced by the mother after childbirth.

✓5ᵗʰ O86.8 Other specified puerperal infections

     O86.81 **Puerperal septic thrombophlebitis** `MCC` `M`

     O86.89 **Other specified puerperal infections** `MCC` `M`

✓4ᵗʰ O87 Venous complications and hemorrhoids in the puerperium

     `INCLUDES`   venous complications in labor, delivery and the puerperium
     EXCLUDES 2   *obstetric embolism (O88.-)*
         puerperal septic thrombophlebitis (O86.81)
         venous complications in pregnancy (O22.-)

O87.0 Superficial thrombophlebitis in the puerperium `CC` `M`
     Puerperal phlebitis NOS
     Puerperal thrombosis NOS
     Use additional code, if applicable, to identify the superficial vein thrombosis, such as thrombosis of superficial vessels of lower extremities (I80.0-)

O87.1 Deep phlebothrombosis in the puerperium `MCC` `M`
     Deep vein thrombosis, postpartum
     Pelvic thrombophlebitis, postpartum
     Use additional code to identify the deep vein thrombosis (I82.4-, I82.5-, I82.62-, I82.72-)
     Use additional code, if applicable, for associated long-term (current) use of anticoagulants (Z79.01)

O87.2 Hemorrhoids in the puerperium `CC` `M`

O87.3 Cerebral venous thrombosis in the puerperium `CC` `M`
     Cerebrovenous sinus thrombosis in the puerperium

O87.4 Varicose veins of lower extremity in the puerperium `M`

O87.8 Other venous complications in the puerperium `CC` `M`
     Genital varices in the puerperium

O87.9 Venous complication in the puerperium, unspecified `M`
     Puerperal phlebopathy NOS

✓4ᵗʰ O88 Obstetric embolism

     EXCLUDES 1   *embolism complicating abortion NOS (O03.2)*
         embolism complicating ectopic or molar pregnancy (O08.2)
         embolism complicating failed attempted abortion (O07.2)
         embolism complicating induced abortion (O04.7)
         embolism complicating spontaneous abortion (O03.2, O03.7)

✓5ᵗʰ O88.0 Obstetric air embolism
     DEF: Sudden blocking of the pulmonary artery or right ventricle with air or nitrogen bubbles.

     ✓6ᵗʰ O88.01 Obstetric air embolism in pregnancy

         O88.011 **Air embolism in pregnancy, first trimester** `MCC` `M`

         O88.012 **Air embolism in pregnancy, second trimester** `MCC` `M`

         O88.013 **Air embolism in pregnancy, third trimester** `MCC` `M`

         O88.019 **Air embolism in pregnancy, unspecified trimester** `M`

     O88.02 **Air embolism in childbirth** `MCC` `M`

     O88.03 **Air embolism in the puerperium** `MCC` `M`

✓5ᵗʰ O88.1 Amniotic fluid embolism
     Anaphylactoid syndrome in pregnancy

     ✓6ᵗʰ O88.11 Amniotic fluid embolism in pregnancy

         O88.111 **Amniotic fluid embolism in pregnancy, first trimester** `MCC` `M`

         O88.112 **Amniotic fluid embolism in pregnancy, second trimester** `MCC` `M`

         O88.113 **Amniotic fluid embolism in pregnancy, third trimester** `MCC` `M`

         O88.119 **Amniotic fluid embolism in pregnancy, unspecified trimester** `M`

     O88.12 **Amniotic fluid embolism in childbirth** `MCC` `M`

     O88.13 **Amniotic fluid embolism in the puerperium** `MCC` `M`

✓5ᵗʰ O88.2 Obstetric thromboembolism

     ✓6ᵗʰ O88.21 Thromboembolism in pregnancy
         Obstetric (pulmonary) embolism NOS

         O88.211 **Thromboembolism in pregnancy, first trimester** `MCC` `M`

         O88.212 **Thromboembolism in pregnancy, second trimester** `MCC` `M`

         O88.213 **Thromboembolism in pregnancy, third trimester** `MCC` `M`

         O88.219 **Thromboembolism in pregnancy, unspecified trimester** `M`

     O88.22 **Thromboembolism in childbirth** `MCC` `M`

     O88.23 **Thromboembolism in the puerperium** `MCC` `M`
         Puerperal (pulmonary) embolism NOS

✓5ᵗʰ O88.3 Obstetric pyemic and septic embolism

     ✓6ᵗʰ O88.31 Pyemic and septic embolism in pregnancy

         O88.311 **Pyemic and septic embolism in pregnancy, first trimester** `MCC` `M`

         O88.312 **Pyemic and septic embolism in pregnancy, second trimester** `MCC` `M`

         O88.313 **Pyemic and septic embolism in pregnancy, third trimester** `MCC` `M`

         O88.319 **Pyemic and septic embolism in pregnancy, unspecified trimester** `CC` `M`

     O88.32 **Pyemic and septic embolism in childbirth** `MCC` `M`

     O88.33 **Pyemic and septic embolism in the puerperium** `MCC` `M`

✓5ᵗʰ O88.8 Other obstetric embolism
     Obstetric fat embolism

     ✓6ᵗʰ O88.81 Other embolism in pregnancy

         O88.811 **Other embolism in pregnancy, first trimester** `MCC` `M`

         O88.812 **Other embolism in pregnancy, second trimester** `MCC` `M`

         O88.813 **Other embolism in pregnancy, third trimester** `MCC` `M`

         O88.819 **Other embolism in pregnancy, unspecified trimester** `M`

     O88.82 **Other embolism in childbirth** `MCC` `M`

     O88.83 **Other embolism in the puerperium** `MCC` `M`

✓4ᵗʰ O89 Complications of anesthesia during the puerperium

     `INCLUDES`   maternal complications arising from the administration of a general, regional or local anesthetic, analgesic or other sedation during the puerperium
     Use additional code, if applicable, to identify specific complication

✓5ᵗʰ O89.0 Pulmonary complications of anesthesia during the puerperium

     O89.01 **Aspiration pneumonitis due to anesthesia during the puerperium** `M`
         Inhalation of stomach contents or secretions NOS due to anesthesia during the puerperium
         Mendelson's syndrome due to anesthesia during the puerperium

     O89.09 **Other pulmonary complications of anesthesia during the puerperium** `M`

O89.1 Cardiac complications of anesthesia during the puerperium `M`

O89.2 Central nervous system complications of anesthesia during the puerperium `M`

O89.3 Toxic reaction to local anesthesia during the puerperium `M`

O89.4 Spinal and epidural anesthesia-induced headache during the puerperium `M`

✔ Additional Character Required   `✓x7ᵗʰ` Placeholder   `Questionable PDx`   `Manifestation`   `Unspecified`   `UPD` Unacceptable PDx   `H1`-`H14` HAC   `HCC` CMS-HCC Dx   `HIV` HIV Dx

ICD-10-CM 2025   911

O89.5 Other complications of spinal and epidural anesthesia during the puerperium   M

O89.6 Failed or difficult intubation for anesthesia during the puerperium   M

O89.8 Other complications of anesthesia during the puerperium   M

O89.9 Complication of anesthesia during the puerperium, unspecified   M

√4ᵗʰ **O90 Complications of the puerperium, not elsewhere classified**

O90.0 Disruption of cesarean delivery wound   M
Dehiscence of cesarean delivery wound
EXCLUDES 1   *rupture of uterus (spontaneous) before onset of labor (O71.0-)*
rupture of uterus during labor (O71.1)

O90.1 Disruption of perineal obstetric wound   M
Disruption of wound of episiotomy
Disruption of wound of perineal laceration
Secondary perineal tear

O90.2 Hematoma of obstetric wound   M

O90.3 Peripartum cardiomyopathy   MCC M
Conditions in I42- arising during pregnancy and the puerperium
EXCLUDES 1   *pre-existing heart disease complicating pregnancy and the puerperium (O99.4-)*
AHA: 2022,3Q,16-17
DEF: Any structural or functional abnormality of the ventricular myocardium. It is a noninflammatory disease of obscure or unknown etiology with onset during the postpartum period.

√5ᵗʰ **O90.4** Postpartum acute kidney failure
EXCLUDES 1   *non-anuria and oliguria (R34)*
AHA: 2023,4Q,37

O90.41 Hepatorenal syndrome following labor and delivery   MCC M

O90.49 Other postpartum acute kidney failure   MCC M
Postpartum acute kidney failure
Puerperal anuria
Puerperal oliguria

O90.5 Postpartum thyroiditis   M

O90.6 Postpartum mood disturbance   M
Postpartum blues
Postpartum dysphoria
Postpartum sadness
EXCLUDES 1   *postpartum depression (F53.0)*
puerperal psychosis (F53.1)

√5ᵗʰ **O90.8** Other complications of the puerperium, not elsewhere classified

O90.81 Anemia of the puerperium   M
Postpartum anemia NOS
EXCLUDES 1   *pre-existing anemia complicating the puerperium (O99.03)*
AHA: 2019,3Q,11

O90.89 Other complications of the puerperium, not elsewhere classified   M
Placental polyp

O90.9 Complication of the puerperium, unspecified   M

√4ᵗʰ **O91 Infections of breast associated with pregnancy, the puerperium and lactation**
Use additional code to identify infection

√5ᵗʰ **O91.0** Infection of nipple associated with pregnancy, the puerperium and lactation

√6ᵗʰ **O91.01** Infection of nipple associated with pregnancy
Gestational abscess of nipple

O91.011 Infection of nipple associated with pregnancy, first trimester   M

O91.012 Infection of nipple associated with pregnancy, second trimester   M

O91.013 Infection of nipple associated with pregnancy, third trimester   M

O91.019 Infection of nipple associated with pregnancy, unspecified trimester   M

O91.02 Infection of nipple associated with the puerperium   M
Puerperal abscess of nipple

O91.03 Infection of nipple associated with lactation   M
Abscess of nipple associated with lactation

√5ᵗʰ **O91.1** Abscess of breast associated with pregnancy, the puerperium and lactation

√6ᵗʰ **O91.11** Abscess of breast associated with pregnancy
Gestational mammary abscess
Gestational purulent mastitis
Gestational subareolar abscess

O91.111 Abscess of breast associated with pregnancy, first trimester   M

O91.112 Abscess of breast associated with pregnancy, second trimester   M

O91.113 Abscess of breast associated with pregnancy, third trimester   M

O91.119 Abscess of breast associated with pregnancy, unspecified trimester   M

O91.12 Abscess of breast associated with the puerperium   M
Puerperal mammary abscess
Puerperal purulent mastitis
Puerperal subareolar abscess

O91.13 Abscess of breast associated with lactation   M
Mammary abscess associated with lactation
Purulent mastitis associated with lactation
Subareolar abscess associated with lactation

√5ᵗʰ **O91.2** Nonpurulent mastitis associated with pregnancy, the puerperium and lactation

√6ᵗʰ **O91.21** Nonpurulent mastitis associated with pregnancy
Gestational interstitial mastitis
Gestational lymphangitis of breast
Gestational mastitis NOS
Gestational parenchymatous mastitis

O91.211 Nonpurulent mastitis associated with pregnancy, first trimester   M

O91.212 Nonpurulent mastitis associated with pregnancy, second trimester   M

O91.213 Nonpurulent mastitis associated with pregnancy, third trimester   M

O91.219 Nonpurulent mastitis associated with pregnancy, unspecified trimester   M

O91.22 Nonpurulent mastitis associated with the puerperium   M
Puerperal interstitial mastitis
Puerperal lymphangitis of breast
Puerperal mastitis NOS
Puerperal parenchymatous mastitis

O91.23 Nonpurulent mastitis associated with lactation   M
Interstitial mastitis associated with lactation
Lymphangitis of breast associated with lactation
Mastitis NOS associated with lactation
Parenchymatous mastitis associated with lactation

√4ᵗʰ **O92 Other disorders of breast and disorders of lactation associated with pregnancy and the puerperium**

√5ᵗʰ **O92.0** Retracted nipple associated with pregnancy, the puerperium, and lactation

√6ᵗʰ **O92.01** Retracted nipple associated with pregnancy

O92.011 Retracted nipple associated with pregnancy, first trimester   M

O92.012 Retracted nipple associated with pregnancy, second trimester   M

O92.013 Retracted nipple associated with pregnancy, third trimester   M

O92.019 Retracted nipple associated with pregnancy, unspecified trimester   M

O92.02 Retracted nipple associated with the puerperium   M

O92.03 Retracted nipple associated with lactation   M

√5ᵗʰ **O92.1** Cracked nipple associated with pregnancy, the puerperium, and lactation
Fissure of nipple, gestational or puerperal

√6ᵗʰ **O92.11** Cracked nipple associated with pregnancy

O92.111 Cracked nipple associated with pregnancy, first trimester   M

O92.112 Cracked nipple associated with pregnancy, second trimester   M

O92.113 Cracked nipple associated with pregnancy, third trimester   M

O92.119 Cracked nipple associated with pregnancy, unspecified trimester   M

O92.12 Cracked nipple associated with the puerperium   M

O92.13 Cracked nipple associated with lactation   M

✓5ᵗʰ O92.2 Other and unspecified disorders of breast associated with pregnancy and the puerperium

    O92.20 Unspecified disorder of breast associated with pregnancy and the puerperium M

    O92.29 Other disorders of breast associated with pregnancy and the puerperium M

O92.3 Agalactia M
    Primary agalactia
    EXCLUDES 1   elective agalactia (O92.5)
                secondary agalactia (O92.5)
                therapeutic agalactia (O92.5)
    DEF: Absence of milk secretion in a female after delivery.

O92.4 Hypogalactia M

O92.5 Suppressed lactation M
    Elective agalactia
    Secondary agalactia
    Therapeutic agalactia
    EXCLUDES 1   primary agalactia (O92.3)

O92.6 Galactorrhea M
    DEF: Excessive or persistent milk secretion by the breast that may occur in the absence of nursing.

✓5ᵗʰ O92.7 Other and unspecified disorders of lactation

    O92.70 Unspecified disorders of lactation M

    O92.79 Other disorders of lactation M
        Puerperal galactocele

Other obstetric conditions, not elsewhere classified (O94-O9A)

O94 Sequelae of complication of pregnancy, childbirth, and the puerperium UPD M PE

    NOTE   This category is to be used to indicate conditions in O00-O77.-, O85-O94 and O98-O9A.- as the cause of late effects. The sequelae include conditions specified as such, or as late effects, which may occur at any time after the puerperium

    Code first condition resulting from (sequela) of complication of pregnancy, childbirth, and the puerperium
    AHA: 2022,3Q,16-17

✓4ᵗʰ O98 Maternal infectious and parasitic diseases classifiable elsewhere but complicating pregnancy, childbirth and the puerperium

    INCLUDES   the listed conditions when complicating the pregnant state, when aggravated by the pregnancy, or as a reason for obstetric care

    Use additional code (Chapter 1), to identify specific infectious or parasitic disease

    EXCLUDES 2   herpes gestationis (O26.4-)
                infectious carrier state (O99.82-, O99.83-)
                obstetrical tetanus (A34)
                puerperal infection (O86.-)
                puerperal sepsis (O85)
                when the reason for maternal care is that the disease is known or suspected to have affected the fetus (O35-O36)

✓5ᵗʰ O98.0 Tuberculosis complicating pregnancy, childbirth and the puerperium
    Conditions in A15-A19

    ✓6ᵗʰ O98.01 Tuberculosis complicating pregnancy

        O98.011 Tuberculosis complicating pregnancy, first trimester CC M

        O98.012 Tuberculosis complicating pregnancy, second trimester CC M

        O98.013 Tuberculosis complicating pregnancy, third trimester CC M

        O98.019 Tuberculosis complicating pregnancy, unspecified trimester M

    O98.02 Tuberculosis complicating childbirth CC M

    O98.03 Tuberculosis complicating the puerperium CC M

✓5ᵗʰ O98.1 Syphilis complicating pregnancy, childbirth and the puerperium
    Conditions in A50-A53

    ✓6ᵗʰ O98.11 Syphilis complicating pregnancy

        O98.111 Syphilis complicating pregnancy, first trimester CC M

        O98.112 Syphilis complicating pregnancy, second trimester CC M

        O98.113 Syphilis complicating pregnancy, third trimester CC M

        O98.119 Syphilis complicating pregnancy, unspecified trimester M

    O98.12 Syphilis complicating childbirth CC M

    O98.13 Syphilis complicating the puerperium CC M

✓5ᵗʰ O98.2 Gonorrhea complicating pregnancy, childbirth and the puerperium
    Conditions in A54.-

    ✓6ᵗʰ O98.21 Gonorrhea complicating pregnancy

        O98.211 Gonorrhea complicating pregnancy, first trimester CC M

        O98.212 Gonorrhea complicating pregnancy, second trimester CC M

        O98.213 Gonorrhea complicating pregnancy, third trimester CC M

        O98.219 Gonorrhea complicating pregnancy, unspecified trimester M

    O98.22 Gonorrhea complicating childbirth CC M

    O98.23 Gonorrhea complicating the puerperium CC M

✓5ᵗʰ O98.3 Other infections with a predominantly sexual mode of transmission complicating pregnancy, childbirth and the puerperium
    Conditions in A55-A64
    AHA: 2020,1Q,20

    ✓6ᵗʰ O98.31 Other infections with a predominantly sexual mode of transmission complicating pregnancy

        O98.311 Other infections with a predominantly sexual mode of transmission complicating pregnancy, first trimester CC M

        O98.312 Other infections with a predominantly sexual mode of transmission complicating pregnancy, second trimester CC M

        O98.313 Other infections with a predominantly sexual mode of transmission complicating pregnancy, third trimester CC M

        O98.319 Other infections with a predominantly sexual mode of transmission complicating pregnancy, unspecified trimester M

    O98.32 Other infections with a predominantly sexual mode of transmission complicating childbirth CC M

    O98.33 Other infections with a predominantly sexual mode of transmission complicating the puerperium CC M

✓5ᵗʰ O98.4 Viral hepatitis complicating pregnancy, childbirth and the puerperium
    Conditions in B15-B19

    ✓6ᵗʰ O98.41 Viral hepatitis complicating pregnancy

        O98.411 Viral hepatitis complicating pregnancy, first trimester CC M

        O98.412 Viral hepatitis complicating pregnancy, second trimester CC M

        O98.413 Viral hepatitis complicating pregnancy, third trimester CC M

        O98.419 Viral hepatitis complicating pregnancy, unspecified trimester M

    O98.42 Viral hepatitis complicating childbirth CC M

    O98.43 Viral hepatitis complicating the puerperium CC M

✓5ᵗʰ O98.5 Other viral diseases complicating pregnancy, childbirth and the puerperium
    Conditions in A80-B09, B25-B34, R87.81-, R87.82-
    EXCLUDES 1   human immunodeficiency virus [HIV] disease complicating pregnancy, childbirth and the puerperium (O98.7-)

    TIP: Assign a code from this subcategory as the principal or first-listed diagnosis for a patient admitted/presenting during pregnancy, childbirth, or the puerperium because of COVID-19; assign U07.1 and codes for associated manifestations as secondary codes.

    ✓6ᵗʰ O98.51 Other viral diseases complicating pregnancy

        O98.511 Other viral diseases complicating pregnancy, first trimester CC M

        O98.512 Other viral diseases complicating pregnancy, second trimester CC M

        O98.513 Other viral diseases complicating pregnancy, third trimester CC M

        O98.519 Other viral diseases complicating pregnancy, unspecified trimester M

    O98.52 Other viral diseases complicating childbirth CC M

    O98.53 Other viral diseases complicating the puerperium CC M

✓ Additional Character Required   ✓x7ᵗʰ Placeholder   Questionable PDx   Manifestation   Unspecified   UPD Unacceptable PDx   H1-H14 HAC   HCC CMS-HCC Dx   HIV HIV Dx

√5ᵗʰ **O98.6** **Protozoal diseases** complicating pregnancy, childbirth and the puerperium
Conditions in B5Ø-B64

√6ᵗʰ **O98.61** **Protozoal diseases complicating pregnancy**

O98.611 **Protozoal diseases complicating pregnancy, first trimester** CC M

O98.612 **Protozoal diseases complicating pregnancy, second trimester** CC M

O98.613 **Protozoal diseases complicating pregnancy, third trimester** CC M

O98.619 **Protozoal diseases complicating pregnancy, unspecified trimester** M

O98.62 **Protozoal diseases complicating childbirth** CC M

O98.63 **Protozoal diseases complicating the puerperium** CC M

√5ᵗʰ **O98.7** **Human immunodeficiency virus [HIV] disease** complicating pregnancy, childbirth and the puerperium
Use additional code to identify the type of HIV disease:
acquired immune deficiency syndrome (AIDS) (B2Ø)
asymptomatic HIV status (Z21)
HIV positive NOS (Z21)
symptomatic HIV disease (B2Ø)

√6ᵗʰ **O98.71** **Human immunodeficiency virus [HIV] disease complicating pregnancy**

O98.711 **Human immunodeficiency virus [HIV] disease complicating pregnancy, first trimester** CC M

O98.712 **Human immunodeficiency virus [HIV] disease complicating pregnancy, second trimester** CC M

O98.713 **Human immunodeficiency virus [HIV] disease complicating pregnancy, third trimester** CC M

O98.719 **Human immunodeficiency virus [HIV] disease complicating pregnancy, unspecified trimester** M

O98.72 **Human immunodeficiency virus [HIV] disease complicating childbirth** CC M

O98.73 **Human immunodeficiency virus [HIV] disease complicating the puerperium** CC M

√5ᵗʰ **O98.8** **Other maternal infectious and parasitic diseases complicating pregnancy, childbirth and the puerperium**
AHA: 2020,1Q,10

√6ᵗʰ **O98.81** **Other maternal infectious and parasitic diseases complicating pregnancy**

O98.811 **Other maternal infectious and parasitic diseases complicating pregnancy, first trimester** CC M

O98.812 **Other maternal infectious and parasitic diseases complicating pregnancy, second trimester** CC M

O98.813 **Other maternal infectious and parasitic diseases complicating pregnancy, third trimester** CC M

O98.819 **Other maternal infectious and parasitic diseases complicating pregnancy, unspecified trimester** M

O98.82 **Other maternal infectious and parasitic diseases complicating childbirth** CC M

O98.83 **Other maternal infectious and parasitic diseases complicating the puerperium** CC M
AHA: 2022,2Q,5

√5ᵗʰ **O98.9** **Unspecified maternal infectious and parasitic disease complicating pregnancy, childbirth and the puerperium**

√6ᵗʰ **O98.91** **Unspecified maternal infectious and parasitic disease complicating pregnancy**

O98.911 **Unspecified maternal infectious and parasitic disease complicating pregnancy, first trimester** CC M

O98.912 **Unspecified maternal infectious and parasitic disease complicating pregnancy, second trimester** CC M

O98.913 **Unspecified maternal infectious and parasitic disease complicating pregnancy, third trimester** CC M

O98.919 **Unspecified maternal infectious and parasitic disease complicating pregnancy, unspecified trimester** M

O98.92 **Unspecified maternal infectious and parasitic disease complicating childbirth** CC M

O98.93 **Unspecified maternal infectious and parasitic disease complicating the puerperium** CC M

√4ᵗʰ **O99** **Other maternal diseases classifiable elsewhere but complicating pregnancy, childbirth and the puerperium**
INCLUDES conditions which complicate the pregnant state, are aggravated by the pregnancy or are a main reason for obstetric care
Use additional code to identify specific condition
EXCLUDES 2 when the reason for maternal care is that the condition is known or suspected to have affected the fetus (O35-O36)

√5ᵗʰ **O99.Ø** **Anemia** complicating pregnancy, childbirth and the puerperium
Conditions in D5Ø-D64
EXCLUDES 1 anemia arising in the puerperium (O9Ø.81)
postpartum anemia NOS (O9Ø.81)
AHA: 2019,3Q,11

√6ᵗʰ **O99.Ø1** **Anemia complicating pregnancy**
AHA: 2016,1Q,4

O99.Ø11 **Anemia complicating pregnancy, first trimester** M

O99.Ø12 **Anemia complicating pregnancy, second trimester** M

O99.Ø13 **Anemia complicating pregnancy, third trimester** M

O99.Ø19 **Anemia complicating pregnancy, unspecified trimester** M

O99.Ø2 **Anemia complicating childbirth** M

O99.Ø3 **Anemia complicating the puerperium** M
EXCLUDES 1 postpartum anemia not pre-existing prior to delivery (O9Ø.81)

√5ᵗʰ **O99.1** **Other diseases of the blood and blood-forming organs** and certain disorders **involving the immune mechanism** complicating pregnancy, childbirth and the puerperium
Conditions in D65-D89
EXCLUDES 1 hemorrhage with coagulation defects (O45.-, O46.Ø-, O67.Ø, O72.3)

√6ᵗʰ **O99.11** **Other diseases of the blood and blood-forming organs and certain disorders involving the immune mechanism complicating pregnancy**

O99.111 **Other diseases of the blood and blood-forming organs and certain disorders involving the immune mechanism complicating pregnancy, first trimester** CC M

O99.112 **Other diseases of the blood and blood-forming organs and certain disorders involving the immune mechanism complicating pregnancy, second trimester** CC M

O99.113 **Other diseases of the blood and blood-forming organs and certain disorders involving the immune mechanism complicating pregnancy, third trimester** CC M

O99.119 **Other diseases of the blood and blood-forming organs and certain disorders involving the immune mechanism complicating pregnancy, unspecified trimester** CC M

O99.12 **Other diseases of the blood and blood-forming organs and certain disorders involving the immune mechanism complicating childbirth** CC M

O99.13 **Other diseases of the blood and blood-forming organs and certain disorders involving the immune mechanism complicating the puerperium** CC M

√5ᵗʰ **O99.2** **Endocrine, nutritional and metabolic diseases** complicating pregnancy, childbirth and the puerperium
Conditions in EØØ-E89
EXCLUDES 2 diabetes mellitus (O24.-)
malnutrition (O25.-)
postpartum thyroiditis (O9Ø.5)

√6ᵗʰ **O99.21** **Obesity** complicating pregnancy, childbirth, and the puerperium
Use additional code to identify the type of obesity (E66.-)
AHA: 2021,2Q,10; 2018,4Q,80
TIP: Do not assign a BMI code (Z68.-) for obese or overweight patients who are pregnant.

O99.21Ø **Obesity complicating pregnancy, unspecified trimester** M

O99.211 **Obesity complicating pregnancy, first trimester** M

O99.212 **Obesity complicating pregnancy, second trimester** M

O99.213 **Obesity complicating pregnancy, third trimester** M

O99.214 **Obesity complicating childbirth** M

O99.215 **Obesity complicating the puerperium** M

✓6ᵗʰ O99.28 **Other endocrine, nutritional and metabolic diseases complicating pregnancy, childbirth and the puerperium**
AHA: 2021,1Q,8

O99.280 **Endocrine, nutritional and metabolic diseases complicating pregnancy, unspecified trimester** M

O99.281 **Endocrine, nutritional and metabolic diseases complicating pregnancy, first trimester** M

O99.282 **Endocrine, nutritional and metabolic diseases complicating pregnancy, second trimester** M

O99.283 **Endocrine, nutritional and metabolic diseases complicating pregnancy, third trimester** M

O99.284 **Endocrine, nutritional and metabolic diseases complicating childbirth** M

O99.285 **Endocrine, nutritional and metabolic diseases complicating the puerperium** M

✓5ᵗʰ O99.3 **Mental disorders and diseases of the nervous system complicating pregnancy, childbirth and the puerperium**

✓6ᵗʰ O99.31 **Alcohol use complicating pregnancy, childbirth, and the puerperium**
Use additional code(s) from F10 to identify manifestations of the alcohol use

O99.310 **Alcohol use complicating pregnancy, unspecified trimester** M

O99.311 **Alcohol use complicating pregnancy, first trimester** M

O99.312 **Alcohol use complicating pregnancy, second trimester** M

O99.313 **Alcohol use complicating pregnancy, third trimester** M

O99.314 **Alcohol use complicating childbirth** M

O99.315 **Alcohol use complicating the puerperium** M

✓6ᵗʰ O99.32 **Drug use complicating pregnancy, childbirth, and the puerperium**
Use additional code(s) from F11-F16 and F18-F19 to identify manifestations of the drug use
AHA: 2018,4Q,69-70; 2018,2Q,10
TIP: When drug use is documented during pregnancy, assign first a code from this subcategory followed by an additional code from F11-F16 and F18-F19 identifying the specific drug use even if not documented as associated with a physical, mental, or behavioral disorder. According to chapter 15 guidelines, it is the provider's responsibility to state that the condition being treated is *not* affecting the pregnancy.

O99.320 **Drug use complicating pregnancy, unspecified trimester** M

O99.321 **Drug use complicating pregnancy, first trimester** CC M

O99.322 **Drug use complicating pregnancy, second trimester** CC M

O99.323 **Drug use complicating pregnancy, third trimester** CC M

O99.324 **Drug use complicating childbirth** CC M

O99.325 **Drug use complicating the puerperium** CC M

✓6ᵗʰ O99.33 **Tobacco use disorder complicating pregnancy, childbirth, and the puerperium**
Smoking complicating pregnancy, childbirth, and the puerperium
Use additional code from category F17 to identify type of tobacco nicotine dependence

O99.330 **Smoking (tobacco) complicating pregnancy, unspecified trimester** M

O99.331 **Smoking (tobacco) complicating pregnancy, first trimester** M

O99.332 **Smoking (tobacco) complicating pregnancy, second trimester** M

O99.333 **Smoking (tobacco) complicating pregnancy, third trimester** M

O99.334 **Smoking (tobacco) complicating childbirth** M

O99.335 **Smoking (tobacco) complicating the puerperium** M

✓6ᵗʰ O99.34 **Other mental disorders complicating pregnancy, childbirth, and the puerperium**
Conditions in F01-F09, F20-F52 and F54-F99
EXCLUDES 2   *postpartum mood disturbance (O90.6)*
postnatal psychosis (F53.1)
puerperal psychosis (F53.1)

O99.340 **Other mental disorders complicating pregnancy, unspecified trimester** M

O99.341 **Other mental disorders complicating pregnancy, first trimester** M

O99.342 **Other mental disorders complicating pregnancy, second trimester** M

O99.343 **Other mental disorders complicating pregnancy, third trimester** M

O99.344 **Other mental disorders complicating childbirth** M

O99.345 **Other mental disorders complicating the puerperium** M
AHA: 2018,4Q,8

✓6ᵗʰ O99.35 **Diseases of the nervous system complicating pregnancy, childbirth, and the puerperium**
Conditions in G00-G99
EXCLUDES 2   *pregnancy related peripheral neuritis (O26.8-)*

O99.350 **Diseases of the nervous system complicating pregnancy, unspecified trimester** M

O99.351 **Diseases of the nervous system complicating pregnancy, first trimester** M

O99.352 **Diseases of the nervous system complicating pregnancy, second trimester** M

O99.353 **Diseases of the nervous system complicating pregnancy, third trimester** M

O99.354 **Diseases of the nervous system complicating childbirth** CC M

O99.355 **Diseases of the nervous system complicating the puerperium** CC M

✓5ᵗʰ O99.4 **Diseases of the circulatory system complicating pregnancy, childbirth and the puerperium**
Conditions in I00-I99
EXCLUDES 1   *peripartum cardiomyopathy (O90.3)*
EXCLUDES 2   *hypertensive disorders (O10-O16)*
obstetric embolism (O88.-)
venous complications and cerebrovenous sinus thrombosis in labor, childbirth and the puerperium (O87.-)
venous complications and cerebrovenous sinus thrombosis in pregnancy (O22.-)
AHA: 2016,2Q,8

✓6ᵗʰ O99.41 **Diseases of the circulatory system complicating pregnancy**

O99.411 **Diseases of the circulatory system complicating pregnancy, first trimester** CC M

O99.412 **Diseases of the circulatory system complicating pregnancy, second trimester** CC M

O99.413 **Diseases of the circulatory system complicating pregnancy, third trimester** CC M

O99.419 **Diseases of the circulatory system complicating pregnancy, unspecified trimester** M

O99.42 **Diseases of the circulatory system complicating childbirth** MCC M

O99.43 **Diseases of the circulatory system complicating the puerperium** CC M

✓5ᵗʰ **O99.5** **Diseases of the respiratory system complicating pregnancy, childbirth and the puerperium**
Conditions in J00–J99

   ✓6ᵗʰ **O99.51** **Diseases of the respiratory system complicating pregnancy**

     O99.511 **Diseases of the respiratory system complicating pregnancy, first trimester** M

     O99.512 **Diseases of the respiratory system complicating pregnancy, second trimester** M

     O99.513 **Diseases of the respiratory system complicating pregnancy, third trimester** M

     O99.519 **Diseases of the respiratory system complicating pregnancy, unspecified trimester** M

   O99.52 **Diseases of the respiratory system complicating childbirth** M

   O99.53 **Diseases of the respiratory system complicating the puerperium** M

✓5ᵗʰ **O99.6** **Diseases of the digestive system complicating pregnancy, childbirth and the puerperium**
Conditions in K00–K93

   EXCLUDES 2   hemorrhoids in pregnancy (O22.4-)
       liver and biliary tract disorders in pregnancy, childbirth and the puerperium (O26.6-)

   ✓6ᵗʰ **O99.61** **Diseases of the digestive system complicating pregnancy**
     AHA: 2016,1Q,4

     O99.611 **Diseases of the digestive system complicating pregnancy, first trimester** M

     O99.612 **Diseases of the digestive system complicating pregnancy, second trimester** M

     O99.613 **Diseases of the digestive system complicating pregnancy, third trimester** M

     O99.619 **Diseases of the digestive system complicating pregnancy, unspecified trimester** M

   O99.62 **Diseases of the digestive system complicating childbirth** M

   O99.63 **Diseases of the digestive system complicating the puerperium** M

✓5ᵗʰ **O99.7** **Diseases of the skin and subcutaneous tissue complicating pregnancy, childbirth and the puerperium**
Conditions in L00–L99

   EXCLUDES 2   herpes gestationis (O26.4)
       pruritic urticarial papules and plaques of pregnancy (PUPPP) (O26.86)

   ✓6ᵗʰ **O99.71** **Diseases of the skin and subcutaneous tissue complicating pregnancy**

     O99.711 **Diseases of the skin and subcutaneous tissue complicating pregnancy, first trimester** M

     O99.712 **Diseases of the skin and subcutaneous tissue complicating pregnancy, second trimester** M

     O99.713 **Diseases of the skin and subcutaneous tissue complicating pregnancy, third trimester** M

     O99.719 **Diseases of the skin and subcutaneous tissue complicating pregnancy, unspecified trimester**

   O99.72 **Diseases of the skin and subcutaneous tissue complicating childbirth** M

   O99.73 **Diseases of the skin and subcutaneous tissue complicating the puerperium** M

✓5ᵗʰ **O99.8** **Other specified diseases and conditions complicating pregnancy, childbirth and the puerperium**
Conditions in D00-D48, H00-H95, M00-N99, and Q00-Q99
Use additional code to identify condition

   EXCLUDES 2   genitourinary infections in pregnancy (O23.-)
       infection of genitourinary tract following delivery (O86.1-O86.4)
       malignant neoplasm complicating pregnancy, childbirth and the puerperium (O9A.1-)
       maternal care for known or suspected abnormality of maternal pelvic organs (O34.-)
       postpartum acute kidney failure (O90.49)
       traumatic injuries in pregnancy (O9A.2-)

   ✓6ᵗʰ **O99.81** **Abnormal glucose complicating pregnancy, childbirth and the puerperium**
     EXCLUDES 1   gestational diabetes (O24.4-)

     O99.810 **Abnormal glucose complicating pregnancy** M

     O99.814 **Abnormal glucose complicating childbirth** M

     O99.815 **Abnormal glucose complicating the puerperium** M

   ✓6ᵗʰ **O99.82** **Streptococcus B carrier state complicating pregnancy, childbirth and the puerperium**
     EXCLUDES 1   carrier of streptococcus group B (GBS) in a nonpregnant woman (Z22.330)
     DEF: *Streptococcus* group B colonization: Bacteria normally found in the vagina or lower intestine of many healthy adult women that may infect the fetus during childbirth, causing mental or physical handicaps or death. Women who test positive for *Streptococcus* group B during pregnancy are considered a "colonized" status and are treated with IV antibiotics at the time of delivery and may also be treated with oral antibiotics during the pregnancy.

     O99.820 **Streptococcus B carrier state complicating pregnancy** UPD M

     O99.824 **Streptococcus B carrier state complicating childbirth** M
       AHA: 2019,2Q,8

     O99.825 **Streptococcus B carrier state complicating the puerperium** UPD M

   ✓6ᵗʰ **O99.83** **Other infection carrier state complicating pregnancy, childbirth and the puerperium**
Use additional code to identify the carrier state (Z22.-)

     O99.830 **Other infection carrier state complicating pregnancy** CC M

     O99.834 **Other infection carrier state complicating childbirth** CC M

     O99.835 **Other infection carrier state complicating the puerperium** CC M

   ✓6ᵗʰ **O99.84** **Bariatric surgery status complicating pregnancy, childbirth and the puerperium**
Gastric banding status complicating pregnancy, childbirth and the puerperium
Gastric bypass status for obesity complicating pregnancy, childbirth and the puerperium
Obesity surgery status complicating pregnancy, childbirth and the puerperium

     O99.840 **Bariatric surgery status complicating pregnancy, unspecified trimester** M

     O99.841 **Bariatric surgery status complicating pregnancy, first trimester** M

     O99.842 **Bariatric surgery status complicating pregnancy, second trimester** M

     O99.843 **Bariatric surgery status complicating pregnancy, third trimester** M

     O99.844 **Bariatric surgery status complicating childbirth** M

     O99.845 **Bariatric surgery status complicating the puerperium** M

   ✓6ᵗʰ **O99.89** **Other specified diseases and conditions complicating pregnancy, childbirth and the puerperium**
     AHA: 2023,3Q,17; 2020,4Q,36-37

     O99.891 **Other specified diseases and conditions complicating pregnancy** M

     O99.892 **Other specified diseases and conditions complicating childbirth** M

     O99.893 **Other specified diseases and conditions complicating puerperium** M

N Newborn: 0   P Pediatric: 0-17   M Maternity: 9-64   A Adult: 15-124   UNS Unspecified Site   MCC Major Complication/Comorbidity   CC Complication/Comorbidity   PE POA Exempt

✓4ᵗʰ O9A **Maternal malignant neoplasms, traumatic injuries and abuse classifiable elsewhere but complicating pregnancy, childbirth and the puerperium**

✓5ᵗʰ O9A.1 **Malignant neoplasm complicating pregnancy, childbirth and the puerperium**
Conditions in C00-C96
Use additional code to identify neoplasm
EXCLUDES 2   *maternal care for benign tumor of corpus uteri (O34.1-)*
maternal care for benign tumor of cervix (C34.4-)
AHA: 2015,3Q,19

   ✓6ᵗʰ O9A.11 **Malignant neoplasm complicating pregnancy**
     O9A.111 **Malignant neoplasm complicating pregnancy, first trimester** Ⓜ
     O9A.112 **Malignant neoplasm complicating pregnancy, second trimester** Ⓜ
     O9A.113 **Malignant neoplasm complicating pregnancy, third trimester** Ⓜ
     O9A.119 **Malignant neoplasm complicating pregnancy, unspecified trimester** Ⓜ
   O9A.12 **Malignant neoplasm complicating childbirth** Ⓜ
   O9A.13 **Malignant neoplasm complicating the puerperium** Ⓜ

✓5ᵗʰ O9A.2 **Injury, poisoning and certain other consequences of external causes complicating pregnancy, childbirth and the puerperium**
Conditions in S00-T88, except T74 and T76
Use additional code(s) to identify the injury or poisoning
EXCLUDES 2   *physical, sexual and psychological abuse complicating pregnancy, childbirth and the puerperium (O9A.3-, O9A.4-, O9A.5-)*

   ✓6ᵗʰ O9A.21 **Injury, poisoning and certain other consequences of external causes complicating pregnancy**
     O9A.211 **Injury, poisoning and certain other consequences of external causes complicating pregnancy, first trimester** Ⓜ
     O9A.212 **Injury, poisoning and certain other consequences of external causes complicating pregnancy, second trimester** Ⓜ
     O9A.213 **Injury, poisoning and certain other consequences of external causes complicating pregnancy, third trimester** Ⓜ
     O9A.219 **Injury, poisoning and certain other consequences of external causes complicating pregnancy, unspecified trimester** Ⓜ
   O9A.22 **Injury, poisoning and certain other consequences of external causes complicating childbirth** Ⓜ
   O9A.23 **Injury, poisoning and certain other consequences of external causes complicating the puerperium** Ⓜ

✓5ᵗʰ O9A.3 **Physical abuse complicating pregnancy, childbirth and the puerperium**
Conditions in T74.11 or T76.11
Use additional code (if applicable):
to identify any associated current injury due to physical abuse
to identify the perpetrator of abuse (Y07.-)
EXCLUDES 2   *sexual abuse complicating pregnancy, childbirth and the puerperium (O9A.4)*

   ✓6ᵗʰ O9A.31 **Physical abuse complicating pregnancy**
     O9A.311 **Physical abuse complicating pregnancy, first trimester** Ⓜ
     O9A.312 **Physical abuse complicating pregnancy, second trimester** Ⓜ
     O9A.313 **Physical abuse complicating pregnancy, third trimester** Ⓜ
     O9A.319 **Physical abuse complicating pregnancy, unspecified trimester** Ⓜ
   O9A.32 **Physical abuse complicating childbirth** Ⓜ
   O9A.33 **Physical abuse complicating the puerperium** Ⓜ

✓5ᵗʰ O9A.4 **Sexual abuse complicating pregnancy, childbirth and the puerperium**
Conditions in T74.21 or T76.21
Use additional code (if applicable):
to identify any associated current injury due to sexual abuse
to identify the perpetrator of abuse (Y07.-)

   ✓6ᵗʰ O9A.41 **Sexual abuse complicating pregnancy**
     O9A.411 **Sexual abuse complicating pregnancy, first trimester** Ⓜ
     O9A.412 **Sexual abuse complicating pregnancy, second trimester** Ⓜ
     O9A.413 **Sexual abuse complicating pregnancy, third trimester** Ⓜ
     O9A.419 **Sexual abuse complicating pregnancy, unspecified trimester** Ⓜ
   O9A.42 **Sexual abuse complicating childbirth** Ⓜ
   O9A.43 **Sexual abuse complicating the puerperium** Ⓜ

✓5ᵗʰ O9A.5 **Psychological abuse complicating pregnancy, childbirth and the puerperium**
Conditions in T74.31 or T76.31
Use additional code to identify the perpetrator of abuse (Y07.-)

   ✓6ᵗʰ O9A.51 **Psychological abuse complicating pregnancy**
     O9A.511 **Psychological abuse complicating pregnancy, first trimester** Ⓜ
     O9A.512 **Psychological abuse complicating pregnancy, second trimester** Ⓜ
     O9A.513 **Psychological abuse complicating pregnancy, third trimester** Ⓜ
     O9A.519 **Psychological abuse complicating pregnancy, unspecified trimester** Ⓜ
   O9A.52 **Psychological abuse complicating childbirth** Ⓜ
   O9A.53 **Psychological abuse complicating the puerperium** Ⓜ

✓ Additional Character Required   ✓x7ᵗʰ Placeholder   Questionable PDx   Manifestation   Unspecified   UPD Unacceptable PDx   H1 - H14 HAC   HCC CMS-HCC Dx   HIV HIV Dx

Chapter 16. Certain Conditions Originating in the Perinatal Period (PØØ–P96)

Chapter-specific Guidelines with Coding Examples

The chapter-specific guidelines from the ICD-10-CM Official Guidelines for Coding and Reporting have been provided below. Along with these guidelines are coding examples, contained in the shaded boxes, that have been developed to help illustrate the coding and/or sequencing guidance found in these guidelines.

For coding and reporting purposes the perinatal period is defined as before birth through the 28th day following birth. The following guidelines are provided for reporting purposes

a. General perinatal rules

1) Use of Chapter 16 codes

Codes in this chapter are <u>never</u> for use on the maternal record. Codes from Chapter 15, the obstetric chapter, are never permitted on the newborn record. Chapter 16 codes may be used throughout the life of the patient if the condition is still present.

2) Principal diagnosis for birth record

When coding the birth episode in a newborn record, assign a code from category Z38, Liveborn infants according to place of birth and type of delivery, as the principal diagnosis. A code from category Z38 is assigned only once, to a newborn at the time of birth. If a newborn is transferred to another institution, a code from category Z38 should not be used at the receiving hospital.

A code from category Z38 is used only on the newborn record, not on the mother's record.

> Newborn delivered via vaginal delivery in Rural Hospital A, experienced meconium aspiration resulting in pneumonia. Rural Hospital A is not equipped to handle the extensive respiratory therapy this baby needs and transfers the patient to Metropolis Hospital B, where the pneumonia resolves and the newborn is eventually discharged.
>
> *Rural Hospital A*
>
> **Z38.ØØ**   **Single liveborn infant, delivered vaginally**
>
> **P24.Ø1**   **Meconium aspiration with respiratory symptoms**
>
> Metropolis Hospital B
>
> **P24.Ø1**   **Meconium aspiration with respiratory symptoms**
>
> *Explanation:* A code from category Z38 is a one-time use only code. The hospital that actually delivered the newborn, in this case Rural Hospital A, can append a code from category Z38 but for the delivery admission only. Once the patient is transferred or discharged, the Z38 category no longer applies for that patient.
>
> The reason for the transfer to Metropolis Hospital B was for the respiratory symptoms (pneumonia) the newborn was exhibiting secondary to aspirating meconium.

3) Use of codes from other chapters with codes from Chapter 16

Codes from other chapters may be used with codes from chapter 16 if the codes from the other chapters provide more specific detail. Codes for signs and symptoms may be assigned when a definitive diagnosis has not been established. If the reason for the encounter is a perinatal condition, the code from chapter 16 should be sequenced first.

4) Use of Chapter 16 codes after the perinatal period

Should a condition originate in the perinatal period, and continue throughout the life of the patient, the perinatal code should continue to be used regardless of the patient's age.

> A 7-year-old patient with history of birth injury that resulted in Erb's palsy is seen for subscapularis release
>
> **P14.Ø**   **Erb's paralysis due to birth injury**
>
> *Explanation:* Although in this instance Erb's palsy is specifically related to a birth injury, it has not resolved and continues to be a health concern. A perinatal code is appropriate even though this patient is beyond the perinatal period.

5) Birth process or community acquired conditions

If a newborn has a condition that may be either due to the birth process or community acquired and the documentation does not indicate which it is, the default is due to the birth process and the code from Chapter 16 should be used. If the condition is community-acquired, a code from Chapter 16 should not be assigned.

For COVID-19 infection in a newborn, see guideline I.C.16.h.

6) Code all clinically significant conditions

All clinically significant conditions noted on routine newborn examination should be coded. A condition is clinically significant if it requires:

clinical evaluation; or

therapeutic treatment; or

diagnostic procedures; or

extended length of hospital stay; or

increased nursing care and/or monitoring; or

has implications for future health care needs

Note: The perinatal guidelines listed above are the same as the general coding guidelines for "additional diagnoses", except for the final point regarding implications for future health care needs. Codes should be assigned for conditions that have been specified by the provider as having implications for future health care needs.

b. Observation and evaluation of newborns for suspected conditions not found

1) Use of ZØ5 codes

Assign a code from category ZØ5, Observation and evaluation of newborn for suspected diseases and conditions ruled out, to identify those instances when a healthy newborn is evaluated for a suspected condition/disease that is determined after study not to be present. Do not use a code from category ZØ5 when the patient is documented to have signs or symptoms of a suspected problem; in such cases code the sign or symptom.

2) ZØ5 on other than the birth record

A code from category ZØ5 may also be assigned as a principal or first-listed code for readmissions or encounters when the code from category Z38 code no longer applies. Codes from category ZØ5 are for use only for healthy newborns and infants for which no condition after study is found to be present.

3) ZØ5 on a birth record

A code from category ZØ5 is to be used as a secondary code after the code from category Z38, Liveborn infants according to place of birth and type of delivery.

> Newborn delivered via vaginal delivery; previous ultrasounds showed what appeared to be an abnormality of the right kidney. Kidney function tests were performed and ultrasounds taken and any genitourinary conditions ruled out.
>
> **Z38.ØØ**   **Single liveborn infant, delivered vaginally**
>
> **ZØ5.6**   **Observation and evaluation of newborn for suspected genitourinary condition ruled out**
>
> Explanation: The newborn had no signs or symptoms of kidney or other genitourinary condition but was evaluated after delivery due to the abnormal prenatal ultrasound findings. A Z code describing the type and place of birth should be coded first, followed by a ZØ5 category code for the work performed to rule out a suspected genitourinary condition.

c. Coding additional perinatal diagnoses

1) Assigning codes for conditions that require treatment

Assign codes for conditions that require treatment or further investigation, prolong the length of stay, or require resource utilization.

Chapter 16. Certain Conditions Originating in the Perinatal Period

2) Codes for conditions specified as having implications for future health care needs

Assign codes for conditions that have been specified by the provider as having implications for future health care needs.

Note: This guideline should not be used for adult patients.

An abnormal noise was heard in the left hip of a post-term newborn during a physical examination. The pediatrician would like to follow the patient after discharge as a hip click can be an early sign of hip dysplasia. The newborn was delivered via cesarean at 41 weeks.

Z38.Ø1	Single liveborn infant, delivered by cesarean
P08.21	Post-term newborn
R29.4	Clicking hip

Explanation: The abnormal hip noise or click is appended as a secondary diagnosis not only because it is an abnormal finding upon examination, but also due to its potential to be part of a bigger health issue. The hip dysplasia has not yet been diagnosed and does not warrant a code at this time.

d. Prematurity and fetal growth retardation

Providers utilize different criteria in determining prematurity. A code for prematurity should not be assigned unless it is documented. Assignment of codes in categories P05, Disorders of newborn related to slow fetal growth and fetal malnutrition, and P07, Disorders of newborn related to short gestation and low birth weight, not elsewhere classified, should be based on the recorded birth weight and estimated gestational age.

When both birth weight and gestational age are available, two codes from category P07 should be assigned, with the code for birth weight sequenced before the code for gestational age.

e. Low birth weight and immaturity status

Codes from category P07, Disorders of newborn related to short gestation and low birth weight, not elsewhere classified, are for use for a child or adult who was premature or had a low birth weight as a newborn and this is affecting the patient's current health status.

See Section I.C.21. Factors influencing health status and contact with health services, Status.

A 35-year-old patient, who weighed 659 grams at birth, is seen for heart disease documented as being a consequence of the low birth weight

| I51.9 | Heart disease, unspecified |
| P07.02 | Extremely low birth weight newborn, 500–749 grams |

Explanation: A code from subcategories P07.0- and P07.1- is appropriate, regardless of the age of the patient, as long as the documentation provides a clear link between the patient's current illness and the low birth weight.

f. Bacterial sepsis of newborn

Category P36, Bacterial sepsis of newborn, includes congenital sepsis. If a perinate is documented as having sepsis without documentation of congenital or community acquired, the default is congenital and a code from category P36 should be assigned. If the P36 code includes the causal organism, an additional code from category B95, Streptococcus, Staphylococcus, and Enterococcus as the cause of diseases classified elsewhere, or B96, Other bacterial agents as the cause of diseases classified elsewhere, should not be assigned. If the P36 code does not include the causal organism, assign an additional code from category B96. If applicable, use additional codes to identify severe sepsis (R65.2-) and any associated acute organ dysfunction.

A full-term infant develops severe sepsis 24 hours after discharge from the hospital and is readmitted; cultures identified *E. coli* as the infective agent

| P36.4 | Sepsis of newborn due to Escherichia coli |
| R65.2Ø | Severe sepsis without septic shock |

Explanation: Even though this newborn was discharged and could have acquired *E. coli* from his/her external environment, due to the lack of documentation specifying specifically how this pathogen was acquired, the default is to code the *E. coli* sepsis as congenital. A code from chapter 1, "Certain Infectious and Parasitic Diseases," is not required because the perinatal sepsis code identifies both the sepsis and the bacteria causing the sepsis.

g. Stillbirth

Code P95, Stillbirth, is only for use in institutions that maintain separate records for stillbirths. No other code should be used with P95. Code P95 should not be used on the mother's record.

h. COVID-19 infection in newborn

For a newborn that tests positive for COVID-19, assign code U07.1, COVID-19, and the appropriate codes for associated manifestation(s) in neonates/newborns in the absence of documentation indicating a specific type of transmission. For a newborn that tests positive for COVID-19 and the provider documents the condition was contracted in utero or during the birth process, assign codes P35.8, Other congenital viral diseases, and U07.1, COVID-19. When coding the birth episode in a newborn record, the appropriate code from category Z38, Liveborn infants according to place of birth and type of delivery, should be assigned as the principal diagnosis.

Chapter 16. Certain Conditions Originating in the Perinatal Period (P00-P96)

NOTE   Codes from this chapter are for use on newborn records only, never on maternal records

INCLUDES   conditions that have their origin in the fetal or perinatal period (before birth through the first 28 days after birth) even if morbidity occurs later

EXCLUDES 2   congenital malformations, deformations and chromosomal abnormalities (Q00-Q99)
endocrine, nutritional and metabolic diseases (E00-E88)
injury, poisoning and certain other consequences of external causes (S00-T88)
neoplasms (C00-D49)
tetanus neonatorum (A33)

This chapter contains the following blocks:

P00-P04	Newborn affected by maternal factors and by complications of pregnancy, labor, and delivery
P05-P08	Disorders of newborn related to length of gestation and fetal growth
P09	Abnormal findings on neonatal screening
P10-P15	Birth trauma
P19-P29	Respiratory and cardiovascular disorders specific to the perinatal period
P35-P39	Infections specific to the perinatal period
P50-P61	Hemorrhagic and hematological disorders of newborn
P70-P74	Transitory endocrine and metabolic disorders specific to newborn
P76-P78	Digestive system disorders of newborn
P80-P83	Conditions involving the integument and temperature regulation of newborn
P84	Other problems with newborn
P90-P96	Other disorders originating in the perinatal period

Newborn affected by maternal factors and by complications of pregnancy, labor, and delivery (P00-P04)

NOTE   These codes are for use when the listed maternal conditions are specified as the cause of confirmed morbidity or potential morbidity which have their origin in the perinatal period (before birth through the first 28 days after birth).

AHA: 2016,4Q,54-55

☑4ᵗʰ P00 Newborn affected by maternal conditions that may be unrelated to present pregnancy

Code first any current condition in newborn

EXCLUDES 2   encounter for observation of newborn for suspected diseases and conditions ruled out (Z05.-)
newborn affected by maternal complications of pregnancy (P01.-)
newborn affected by maternal endocrine and metabolic disorders (P70-P74)
newborn affected by noxious substances transmitted via placenta or breast milk (P04.-)

P00.0 Newborn affected by maternal hypertensive disorders **PE**
Newborn affected by maternal conditions classifiable to O10-O11, O13-O16

P00.1 Newborn affected by maternal renal and urinary tract diseases **PE**
Newborn affected by maternal conditions classifiable to N00-N39

P00.2 Newborn affected by maternal infectious and parasitic diseases **PE**
Newborn affected by maternal infectious disease classifiable to A00-B99, J09 and J10

EXCLUDES 1   maternal genital tract or other localized infections (P00.8)

EXCLUDES 2   infections specific to the perinatal period (P35-P39)
newborn affected by (positive) maternal group B streptococcus (GBS) colonization (P00.82)

AHA: 2019,2Q,10; 2015,3Q,20

P00.3 Newborn affected by other maternal circulatory and respiratory diseases **PE**
Newborn affected by maternal conditions classifiable to I00-I99, J00-J99, Q20-Q34 and not included in P00.0, P00.2

P00.4 Newborn affected by maternal nutritional disorders **PE**
Newborn affected by maternal disorders classifiable to E40-E64
Maternal malnutrition NOS

P00.5 Newborn affected by maternal injury **PE**
Newborn affected by maternal conditions classifiable to O9A.2-

P00.6 Newborn affected by surgical procedure on mother **PE**
Newborn affected by amniocentesis

EXCLUDES 1   Cesarean delivery for present delivery (P03.4)
damage to placenta from amniocentesis, Cesarean delivery or surgical induction (P02.1)
previous surgery to uterus or pelvic organs (P03.89)

EXCLUDES 2   newborn affected by complication of (fetal) intrauterine procedure (P96.5)

P00.7 Newborn affected by other medical procedures on mother, not elsewhere classified **PE**
Newborn affected by radiation to mother

EXCLUDES 1   damage to placenta from amniocentesis, cesarean delivery or surgical induction (P02.1)
newborn affected by other complications of labor and delivery (P03.-)

☑5ᵗʰ P00.8 Newborn affected by other maternal conditions

P00.81 Newborn affected by periodontal disease in mother **PE**

P00.82 Newborn affected by (positive) maternal group B streptococcus (GBS) colonization **PE**
Contact with positive maternal group B streptococcus
AHA: 2021,4Q,23

P00.89 Newborn affected by other maternal conditions **PE**
Newborn affected by conditions classifiable to T80-T88
Newborn affected by maternal genital tract or other localized infections
Newborn affected by maternal systemic lupus erythematosus
Use additional code to identify infectious agent, if known

EXCLUDES 2   newborn affected by positive maternal group B streptococcus (GBS) colonization (P00.82)

AHA: 2019,2Q,9

P00.9 Newborn affected by unspecified maternal condition **PE**

☑4ᵗʰ P01 Newborn affected by maternal complications of pregnancy

Code first any current condition in newborn

EXCLUDES 2   encounter for observation of newborn for suspected diseases and conditions ruled out (Z05.-)

P01.0 Newborn affected by incompetent cervix

P01.1 Newborn affected by premature rupture of membranes

P01.2 Newborn affected by oligohydramnios

EXCLUDES 1   oligohydramnios due to premature rupture of membranes (P01.1)
DEF: Low amniotic fluid level, resulting in underdeveloped organs in the fetus.

P01.3 Newborn affected by polyhydramnios
Newborn affected by hydramnios
DEF: Excess amniotic fluid surrounding the fetus, typically defined as a total fluid volume of greater than 24 cm.

P01.4 Newborn affected by ectopic pregnancy
Newborn affected by abdominal pregnancy

P01.5 Newborn affected by multiple pregnancy
Newborn affected by triplet (pregnancy)
Newborn affected by twin (pregnancy)

P01.6 Newborn affected by maternal death

P01.7 Newborn affected by malpresentation before labor
Newborn affected by breech presentation before labor
Newborn affected by external version before labor
Newborn affected by face presentation before labor
Newborn affected by transverse lie before labor
Newborn affected by unstable lie before labor

P01.8 Newborn affected by other maternal complications of pregnancy

P01.9 Newborn affected by maternal complication of pregnancy, unspecified

☑4ᵗʰ P02 Newborn affected by complications of placenta, cord and membranes

Code first any current condition in newborn

EXCLUDES 2   encounter for observation of newborn for suspected diseases and conditions ruled out (Z05.-)

P02.0 Newborn affected by placenta previa
DEF: Placenta developed in the lower segment of the uterus that can cause hemorrhaging leading to preterm delivery.

☑ Additional Character Required   ☑x7ᵗʰ Placeholder   Questionable PDx   Manifestation   Unspecified   **UPD** Unacceptable PDx   **H1-H14** HAC   **HCC** CMS-HCC Dx   **HIV** HIV Dx

ICD-10-CM 2025   **921**

Chapter 16. Certain Conditions Originating in the Perinatal Period

P02.1   **Newborn affected by other forms of placental separation and hemorrhage**
Newborn affected by abruptio placenta
Newborn affected by accidental hemorrhage
Newborn affected by antepartum hemorrhage
Newborn affected by damage to placenta from amniocentesis, cesarean delivery or surgical induction
Newborn affected by maternal blood loss
Newborn affected by premature separation of placenta

✓5th **P02.2**   **Newborn affected by other and unspecified morphological and functional abnormalities of placenta**

   P02.20   **Newborn affected by unspecified morphological and functional abnormalities of placenta**

   P02.29   **Newborn affected by other morphological and functional abnormalities of placenta**
Newborn affected by placental dysfunction
Newborn affected by placental infarction
Newborn affected by placental insufficiency

P02.3   **Newborn affected by placental transfusion syndromes**
Newborn affected by placental and cord abnormalities resulting in twin-to-twin or other transplacental transfusion

P02.4   **Newborn affected by prolapsed cord**

P02.5   **Newborn affected by other compression of umbilical cord**
Newborn affected by entanglement of umbilical cord
Newborn affected by knot in umbilical cord
Newborn affected by umbilical cord (tightly) around neck
AHA: 2022,1Q,22

✓5th **P02.6**   **Newborn affected by other and unspecified conditions of umbilical cord**

   P02.60   **Newborn affected by unspecified conditions of umbilical cord**

   P02.69   **Newborn affected by other conditions of umbilical cord**
Newborn affected by short umbilical cord
Newborn affected by vasa previa
EXCLUDES 1   *newborn affected by single umbilical artery (Q27.0)*

✓5th **P02.7**   **Newborn affected by chorioamnionitis**
AHA: 2018,4Q,23-24
DEF: Inflammation of the fetal membranes due to maternal infection characterized by fetal tachycardia, respiratory distress, apnea, weak cries, and poor sucking.

   P02.70   **Newborn affected by fetal inflammatory response syndrome** **HCC**
Newborn affected by FIRS

   P02.78   **Newborn affected by other conditions from chorioamnionitis**
Newborn affected by amnionitis
Newborn affected by membranitis
Newborn affected by placentitis

P02.8   **Newborn affected by other abnormalities of membranes**

P02.9   **Newborn affected by abnormality of membranes, unspecified**

✓4th **P03**   **Newborn affected by other complications of labor and delivery**
Code first any current condition in newborn
EXCLUDES 2   *encounter for observation of newborn for suspected diseases and conditions ruled out (Z05.-)*

P03.0   **Newborn affected by breech delivery and extraction**

P03.1   **Newborn affected by other malpresentation, malposition and disproportion during labor and delivery**
Newborn affected by contracted pelvis
Newborn affected by conditions classifiable to O64-O66
Newborn affected by persistent occipitoposterior
Newborn affected by transverse lie

P03.2   **Newborn affected by forceps delivery**

Forceps Assisted Birth

Forceps extractor

P03.3   **Newborn affected by delivery by vacuum extractor [ventouse]**

Vacuum Assisted Birth

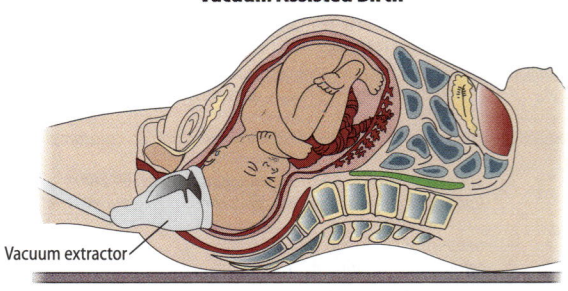

Vacuum extractor

P03.4   **Newborn affected by Cesarean delivery**

P03.5   **Newborn affected by precipitate delivery**
Newborn affected by rapid second stage

P03.6   **Newborn affected by abnormal uterine contractions**
Newborn affected by conditions classifiable to O62.-, except O62.3
Newborn affected by hypertonic labor
Newborn affected by uterine inertia

✓5th **P03.8**   **Newborn affected by other specified complications of labor and delivery**

   ✓6th **P03.81**   **Newborn affected by abnormality in fetal (intrauterine) heart rate or rhythm**
EXCLUDES 1   *neonatal cardiac dysrhythmia (P29.1-)*

     P03.810   **Newborn affected by abnormality in fetal (intrauterine) heart rate or rhythm before the onset of labor**

     P03.811   **Newborn affected by abnormality in fetal (intrauterine) heart rate or rhythm during labor**

     P03.819   **Newborn affected by abnormality in fetal (intrauterine) heart rate or rhythm, unspecified as to time of onset**

   P03.82   **Meconium passage during delivery**
EXCLUDES 1   *meconium aspiration (P24.00, P24.01)*
meconium staining (P96.83)
DEF: Fetal intestinal activity that increases in response to a fetomaternal distressed state during delivery. The anal sphincter relaxes and meconium is passed into the amniotic fluid.

   P03.89   **Newborn affected by other specified complications of labor and delivery**
Newborn affected by abnormality of maternal soft tissues
Newborn affected by conditions classifiable to O60-O75 and by procedures used in labor and delivery not included in P02.- and P03.0-P03.6
Newborn affected by induction of labor

P03.9   **Newborn affected by complication of labor and delivery, unspecified**

✓4th **P04**   **Newborn affected by noxious substances transmitted via placenta or breast milk**
INCLUDES   nonteratogenic effects of substances transmitted via placenta
Code first any current condition in newborn, if applicable
EXCLUDES 2   *congenital malformations (Q00-Q99)*
encounter for observation of newborn for suspected diseases and conditions ruled out (Z05.-)
neonatal jaundice from excessive hemolysis due to drugs or toxins transmitted from mother (P58.4)
newborn in contact with and (suspected) exposures hazardous to health not transmitted via placenta or breast milk (Z77.-)

P04.0   **Newborn affected by maternal anesthesia and analgesia in pregnancy, labor and delivery** **HCC**
Newborn affected by reactions and intoxications from maternal opiates and tranquilizers administered for procedures during pregnancy or labor and delivery
EXCLUDES 2   *newborn affected by other maternal medication (P04.1-)*

N Newborn: 0   **P** Pediatric: 0-17   **M** Maternity: 9-64   **A** Adult: 15-124   **UNS** Unspecified Site   **MCC** Major Complication/Comorbidity   **CC** Complication/Comorbidity   **PE** POA Exempt

922

ICD-10-CM 2025

✓5ᵗʰ P04.1 Newborn affected by other maternal medication

Code first, if applicable, withdrawal symptoms from maternal use of drugs of addiction (P96.1)

withdrawal symptoms from therapeutic use of drugs in newborn (P96.2)

EXCLUDES 1   dysmorphism due to warfarin (Q86.2)

      fetal hydantoin syndrome (Q86.1)

EXCLUDES 2   maternal anesthesia and analgesia in pregnancy, labor and delivery (P04.0)

      maternal use of drugs of addiction (P04.4-)

AHA: 2018,4Q,24-25

   P04.11   **Newborn affected by maternal antineoplastic chemotherapy**   HCC

   P04.12   **Newborn affected by maternal cytotoxic drugs**   HCC

   P04.13   **Newborn affected by maternal use of anticonvulsants**   HCC

   P04.14   **Newborn affected by maternal use of opiates**   HCC

   P04.15   **Newborn affected by maternal use of antidepressants**   HCC

   P04.16   **Newborn affected by maternal use of amphetamines**   HCC

   P04.17   **Newborn affected by maternal use of sedative-hypnotics**   HCC

   P04.1A   **Newborn affected by maternal use of anxiolytics**   HCC

   P04.18   **Newborn affected by other maternal medication**   HCC

   P04.19   **Newborn affected by maternal use of unspecified medication**   HCC

P04.2 Newborn affected by maternal use of tobacco   HCC

Newborn affected by exposure in utero to tobacco smoke

EXCLUDES 2   newborn exposure to environmental tobacco smoke (P96.81)

P04.3 Newborn affected by maternal use of alcohol   HCC

EXCLUDES 1   fetal alcohol syndrome (Q86.0)

✓5ᵗʰ P04.4 Newborn affected by maternal use of drugs of addiction

AHA: 2018,4Q,25

   P04.40   **Newborn affected by maternal use of unspecified drugs of addiction**   HCC

   P04.41   **Newborn affected by maternal use of cocaine**   HCC

   P04.42   **Newborn affected by maternal use of hallucinogens**   HCC

     EXCLUDES 2   newborn affected by other maternal medication (P04.1-)

   P04.49   **Newborn affected by maternal use of other drugs of addiction**   HCC

     EXCLUDES 2   newborn affected by maternal anesthesia and analgesia (P04.0)

       withdrawal symptoms from maternal use of drugs of addiction (P96.1)

P04.5 Newborn affected by maternal use of nutritional chemical substances   HCC

P04.6 Newborn affected by maternal exposure to environmental chemical substances   HCC

✓5ᵗʰ P04.8 Newborn affected by other maternal noxious substances

AHA: 2018,4Q,25

   P04.81   **Newborn affected by maternal use of cannabis**   HCC

   P04.89   **Newborn affected by other maternal noxious substances**   HCC

   P04.9   **Newborn affected by maternal noxious substance, unspecified**   HCC

Disorders of newborn related to length of gestation and fetal growth (P05-P08)

✓4ᵗʰ P05 Disorders of newborn related to slow fetal growth and fetal malnutrition

AHA: 2016,4Q,55-56

✓5ᵗʰ P05.0 Newborn light for gestational age

Newborn light-for-dates

Weight below but length above 10th percentile for gestational age

   P05.00   **Newborn light for gestational age, unspecified weight**

   P05.01   **Newborn light for gestational age, less than 500 grams**

   P05.02   **Newborn light for gestational age, 500-749 grams**

   P05.03   **Newborn light for gestational age, 750-999 grams**

   P05.04   **Newborn light for gestational age, 1000-1249 grams**

   P05.05   **Newborn light for gestational age, 1250-1499 grams**

   P05.06   **Newborn light for gestational age, 1500-1749 grams**

   P05.07   **Newborn light for gestational age, 1750-1999 grams**

   P05.08   **Newborn light for gestational age, 2000-2499 grams**

   P05.09   **Newborn light for gestational age, 2500 grams and over**

     Newborn light for gestational age, other

✓5ᵗʰ P05.1 Newborn small for gestational age

Newborn small-and-light-for-dates

Newborn small-for-dates

Weight and length below 10th percentile for gestational age

   P05.10   **Newborn small for gestational age, unspecified weight**

   P05.11   **Newborn small for gestational age, less than 500 grams**

   P05.12   **Newborn small for gestational age, 500-749 grams**

   P05.13   **Newborn small for gestational age, 750-999 grams**

   P05.14   **Newborn small for gestational age, 1000-1249 grams**

   P05.15   **Newborn small for gestational age, 1250-1499 grams**

   P05.16   **Newborn small for gestational age, 1500-1749 grams**

   P05.17   **Newborn small for gestational age, 1750-1999 grams**

   P05.18   **Newborn small for gestational age, 2000-2499 grams**

   P05.19   **Newborn small for gestational age, other**

     Newborn small for gestational age, 2500 grams and over

P05.2 Newborn affected by fetal (intrauterine) malnutrition not light or small for gestational age

Infant, not light or small for gestational age, showing signs of fetal malnutrition, such as dry, peeling skin and loss of subcutaneous tissue

EXCLUDES 1   newborn affected by fetal malnutrition with light for gestational age (P05.0-)

      newborn affected by fetal malnutrition with small for gestational age (P05.1-)

P05.9 Newborn affected by slow intrauterine growth, unspecified

Newborn affected by fetal growth retardation NOS

✓4ᵗʰ P07 Disorders of newborn related to short gestation and low birth weight, not elsewhere classified

NOTE   When both birth weight and gestational age of the newborn are available, both should be coded with birth weight sequenced before gestational age

INCLUDES   the listed conditions, without further specification, as the cause of morbidity or additional care, in newborn

✓5ᵗʰ P07.0 Extremely low birth weight newborn

Newborn birth weight 999 g. or less

EXCLUDES 1   low birth weight due to slow fetal growth and fetal malnutrition (P05.-)

   P07.00   **Extremely low birth weight newborn, unspecified weight**

   P07.01   **Extremely low birth weight newborn, less than 500 grams**

   P07.02   **Extremely low birth weight newborn, 500-749 grams**

   P07.03   **Extremely low birth weight newborn, 750-999 grams**

✓5ᵗʰ P07.1 Other low birth weight newborn

Newborn birth weight 1000-2499 g.

EXCLUDES 1   low birth weight due to slow fetal growth and fetal malnutrition (P05.-)

   P07.10   **Other low birth weight newborn, unspecified weight**

   P07.14   **Other low birth weight newborn, 1000-1249 grams**

   P07.15   **Other low birth weight newborn, 1250-1499 grams**

   P07.16   **Other low birth weight newborn, 1500-1749 grams**

   P07.17   **Other low birth weight newborn, 1750-1999 grams**

   P07.18   **Other low birth weight newborn, 2000-2499 grams**

✓5ᵗʰ P07.2 Extreme immaturity of newborn

Less than 28 completed weeks (less than 196 completed days) of gestation.

   P07.20   **Extreme immaturity of newborn, unspecified weeks of gestation**

     Gestational age less than 28 completed weeks NOS

   P07.21   **Extreme immaturity of newborn, gestational age less than 23 completed weeks**

     Extreme immaturity of newborn, gestational age less than 23 weeks, 0 days

✔ Additional Character Required   ✓x7ᵗʰ Placeholder   Questionable PDx   Manifestation   Unspecified   UPD Unacceptable PDx   H1-H14 HAC   HCC CMS-HCC Dx   HIV HIV Dx

ICD-10-CM 2025   923

P07.22   **Extreme immaturity of newborn, gestational age 23 completed weeks**
Extreme immaturity of newborn, gestational age 23 weeks, 0 days through 23 weeks, 6 days

P07.23   **Extreme immaturity of newborn, gestational age 24 completed weeks**
Extreme immaturity of newborn, gestational age 24 weeks, 0 days through 24 weeks, 6 days

P07.24   **Extreme immaturity of newborn, gestational age 25 completed weeks**
Extreme immaturity of newborn, gestational age 25 weeks, 0 days through 25 weeks, 6 days

P07.25   **Extreme immaturity of newborn, gestational age 26 completed weeks**
Extreme immaturity of newborn, gestational age 26 weeks, 0 days through 26 weeks, 6 days

P07.26   **Extreme immaturity of newborn, gestational age 27 completed weeks**
Extreme immaturity of newborn, gestational age 27 weeks, 0 days through 27 weeks, 6 days

✓5ᵗʰ **P07.3**   **Preterm [premature] newborn [other]**
28 completed weeks or more but less than 37 completed weeks (196 completed days but less than 259 completed days) of gestation
Prematurity NOS
AHA: 2017,3Q,26

    P07.30   Preterm newborn, unspecified weeks of gestation

    P07.31   **Preterm newborn, gestational age 28 completed weeks**
Preterm newborn, gestational age 28 weeks, 0 days through 28 weeks, 6 days

    P07.32   **Preterm newborn, gestational age 29 completed weeks**
Preterm newborn, gestational age 29 weeks, 0 days through 29 weeks, 6 days

    P07.33   **Preterm newborn, gestational age 30 completed weeks**
Preterm newborn, gestational age 30 weeks, 0 days through 30 weeks, 6 days

    P07.34   **Preterm newborn, gestational age 31 completed weeks**
Preterm newborn, gestational age 31 weeks, 0 days through 31 weeks, 6 days

    P07.35   **Preterm newborn, gestational age 32 completed weeks**
Preterm newborn, gestational age 32 weeks, 0 days through 32 weeks, 6 days

    P07.36   **Preterm newborn, gestational age 33 completed weeks**
Preterm newborn, gestational age 33 weeks, 0 days through 33 weeks, 6 days

    P07.37   **Preterm newborn, gestational age 34 completed weeks**
Preterm newborn, gestational age 34 weeks, 0 days through 34 weeks, 6 days

    P07.38   **Preterm newborn, gestational age 35 completed weeks**
Preterm newborn, gestational age 35 weeks, 0 days through 35 weeks, 6 days

    P07.39   **Preterm newborn, gestational age 36 completed weeks**
Preterm newborn, gestational age 36 weeks, 0 days through 36 weeks, 6 days

✓4ᵗʰ **P08**   **Disorders of newborn related to long gestation and high birth weight**

    NOTE   When both birth weight and gestational age of the newborn are available, priority of assignment should be given to birth weight

    INCLUDES   the listed conditions, without further specification, as causes of morbidity or additional care, in newborn

    P08.0   **Exceptionally large newborn baby**
Usually implies a birth weight of 4500 g. or more
    EXCLUDES 1   *syndrome of infant of diabetic mother (P70.1)*
syndrome of infant of mother with gestational diabetes (P70.0)

P08.1   **Other heavy for gestational age newborn**
Other newborn heavy- or large-for-dates regardless of period of gestation
Usually implies a birth weight of 4000 g. to 4499 g.
    EXCLUDES 1   *newborn with a birth weight of 4500 or more (P08.0)*
syndrome of infant of diabetic mother (P70.1)
syndrome of infant of mother with gestational diabetes (P70.0)

✓5ᵗʰ **P08.2**   **Late newborn, not heavy for gestational age**
AHA: 2014,1Q,14

    P08.21   **Post-term newborn**
Newborn with gestation period over 40 completed weeks to 42 completed weeks

    P08.22   **Prolonged gestation of newborn**
Newborn with gestation period over 42 completed weeks (294 days or more), not heavy- or large-for-dates.
Postmaturity NOS

Abnormal findings on neonatal screening (P09)

✓4ᵗʰ **P09**   **Abnormal findings on neonatal screening**

    INCLUDES   abnormal findings on state mandated newborn screens
failed newborn screening

    EXCLUDES 2   *nonspecific serologic evidence of human immunodeficiency virus [HIV] (R75)*

    AHA: 2021,4Q,24

    P09.1   **Abnormal findings on neonatal screening for inborn errors of metabolism**

    P09.2   **Abnormal findings on neonatal screening for congenital endocrine disease**
Abnormal findings on neonatal screening for congenital adrenal hyperplasia
Abnormal findings on neonatal screening for hypothyroidism screen

    P09.3   **Abnormal findings on neonatal screening for congenital hematologic disorders**
Abnormal findings for hemoglobinopathy screening
Abnormal findings on red cell membrane defects screen
Abnormal findings on sickle cell screen

    P09.4   **Abnormal findings on neonatal screening for cystic fibrosis**

    P09.5   **Abnormal findings on neonatal screening for critical congenital heart disease**
Neonatal congenital heart disease screening failure

    P09.6   **Abnormal findings on neonatal screening for neonatal hearing loss**
    EXCLUDES 2   *encounter for hearing examination following failed hearing screening (Z01.110)*

    P09.8   **Other abnormal findings on neonatal screening**
    P09.9   **Abnormal findings on neonatal screening, unspecified**

Birth trauma (P10-P15)

✓4ᵗʰ **P10**   **Intracranial laceration and hemorrhage due to birth injury**
    EXCLUDES 1   *intracranial hemorrhage of newborn NOS (P52.9)*
intracranial hemorrhage of newborn due to anoxia or hypoxia (P52.-)
nontraumatic intracranial hemorrhage of newborn (P52.-)

    P10.0   **Subdural hemorrhage due to birth injury**   MCC HCC
Subdural hematoma (localized) due to birth injury
    EXCLUDES 1   *subdural hemorrhage accompanying tentorial tear (P10.4)*

    P10.1   **Cerebral hemorrhage due to birth injury**   MCC HCC
    P10.2   **Intraventricular hemorrhage due to birth injury**   CC HCC
    P10.3   **Subarachnoid hemorrhage due to birth injury**   MCC HCC
    P10.4   **Tentorial tear due to birth injury**   MCC HCC
    P10.8   **Other intracranial lacerations and hemorrhages due to birth injury**   MCC HCC
    P10.9   **Unspecified intracranial laceration and hemorrhage due to birth injury**   MCC HCC

✓4ᵗʰ **P11**   **Other birth injuries to central nervous system**
    P11.0   **Cerebral edema due to birth injury**   MCC HCC
    P11.1   **Other specified brain damage due to birth injury**   HCC
    P11.2   **Unspecified brain damage due to birth injury**   MCC HCC
    P11.3   **Birth injury to facial nerve**
Facial palsy due to birth injury
    P11.4   **Birth injury to other cranial nerves**

P11.5   Birth injury to **spine and spinal cord**   HCC
     Fracture of spine due to birth injury

P11.9   Birth injury to **central nervous system, unspecified**   MCC

✓4th **P12**   Birth injury to **scalp**

Birth Injuries to Scalp

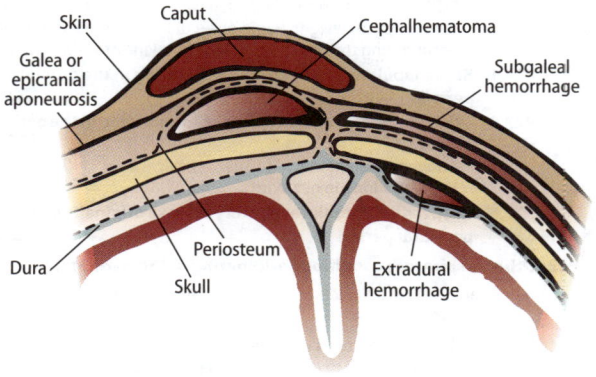

Skin · Caput · Cephalhematoma · Galea or epicranial aponeurosis · Subgaleal hemorrhage · Dura · Periosteum · Skull · Extradural hemorrhage

P12.0   **Cephalhematoma** due to birth injury
     DEF: Condition that occurs in a neonate when blood vessels between the skull and periosteum rupture and blood collects in the subperiosteal space (below the periosteum). It is typically caused by prolonged labor or trauma due to instrument-assisted delivery (e.g., forceps, vacuum extraction), although in rare circumstances, it may indicate a linear skull fracture with intracranial hemorrhage.

P12.1   **Chignon (from vacuum extraction)** due to birth injury
     DEF: Artificial swelling of the scalp that occurs when a collection of interstitial fluid and blood forms in the area of the scalp where the suction cup was applied during a vacuum-assisted delivery.

P12.2   **Epicranial subaponeurotic hemorrhage** due to birth injury   CC HCC
     Subgaleal hemorrhage

P12.3   **Bruising of scalp** due to birth injury

P12.4   Injury of scalp of newborn due to **monitoring equipment**
     Sampling incision of scalp of newborn
     Scalp clip (electrode) injury of newborn

✓5th **P12.8**   Other birth injuries to scalp

     P12.81   **Caput succedaneum**
         DEF: Swelling of the scalp as a result of pressure being exerted on the head from the vaginal walls, uterus, or instrumentation used in assisting a delivery (e.g., vacuum).

     P12.89   Other birth injuries to scalp

P12.9   Birth injury to scalp, unspecified

✓4th **P13**   Birth injury to **skeleton**

     EXCLUDES 2   birth injury to spine (P11.5)

P13.0   **Fracture of skull** due to birth injury

P13.1   Other birth injuries to skull
     EXCLUDES 1   cephalhematoma (P12.0)

P13.2   Birth injury to **femur**

P13.3   Birth injury to other long bones

P13.4   **Fracture of clavicle** due to birth injury

P13.8   Birth injuries to other parts of skeleton

P13.9   Birth injury to skeleton, unspecified

✓4th **P14**   Birth injury to **peripheral nervous system**

     P14.0   **Erb's paralysis** due to birth injury
         DEF: Erb's paralysis: Most common type of brachial plexus (peripheral nerve) injury in a neonate that involves nerve damage at the level of C5-C6. **Synonym(s):** Erb's palsy

     P14.1   **Klumpke's paralysis** due to birth injury

     P14.2   **Phrenic nerve paralysis** due to birth injury

     P14.3   Other brachial plexus birth injuries

     P14.8   Birth injuries to other parts of peripheral nervous system

     P14.9   Birth injury to peripheral nervous system, unspecified

✓4th **P15**   Other birth injuries

     P15.0   Birth injury to **liver**
         Rupture of liver due to birth injury

     P15.1   Birth injury to **spleen**
         Rupture of spleen due to birth injury

     P15.2   **Sternomastoid** injury due to birth injury

     P15.3   Birth injury to **eye**
         Subconjunctival hemorrhage due to birth injury
         Traumatic glaucoma due to birth injury

     P15.4   Birth injury to **face**
         Facial congestion due to birth injury

     P15.5   Birth injury to **external genitalia**

     P15.6   **Subcutaneous fat necrosis** due to birth injury

     P15.8   **Other specified birth injuries**

     P15.9   **Birth injury, unspecified**

Respiratory and cardiovascular disorders specific to the perinatal period (P19-P29)

✓4th **P19**   Metabolic acidemia in newborn

     INCLUDES   metabolic acidemia in newborn

     P19.0   Metabolic acidemia in newborn first noted **before onset of labor**

     P19.1   Metabolic acidemia in newborn first noted **during labor**

     P19.2   Metabolic acidemia noted **at birth**

     P19.9   Metabolic acidemia in newborn, unspecified

✓4th **P22**   Respiratory distress of newborn

     AHA: 2019,2Q,29

     P22.0   Respiratory distress syndrome of newborn   MCC HCC
         Cardiorespiratory distress syndrome of newborn
         Hyaline membrane disease
         Idiopathic respiratory distress syndrome [IRDS or RDS] of newborn
         Pulmonary hypoperfusion syndrome
         Respiratory distress syndrome, type I
         EXCLUDES 2   respiratory arrest of newborn (P28.81)
                    respiratory failure of newborn NOS (P28.5)

         AHA: 2019,2Q,29
         DEF: Severe chest contractions upon air intake and expiratory grunting. The infant appears blue due to oxygen deficiency and has a rapid respiratory rate, formerly called hyaline membrane disease.

     P22.1   Transient tachypnea of newborn
         Idiopathic tachypnea of newborn
         Respiratory distress syndrome, type II
         Wet lung syndrome
         DEF: Rapid, labored breathing of a newborn. It is a short-term problem that begins after birth and lasts about three days.

     P22.8   Other respiratory distress of newborn
         EXCLUDES 1   respiratory arrest of newborn (P28.81)
                    respiratory failure of newborn NOS (P28.5)

     P22.9   Respiratory distress of newborn, unspecified
         EXCLUDES 1   respiratory arrest of newborn (P28.81)
                    respiratory failure of newborn NOS (P28.5)

✓4th **P23**   Congenital pneumonia

     INCLUDES   infective pneumonia acquired in utero or during birth
     EXCLUDES 1   neonatal pneumonia resulting from aspiration (P24.-)

     P23.0   Congenital pneumonia due to **viral agent**   MCC
         Use additional code (B97) to identify organism
         EXCLUDES 1   congenital rubella pneumonitis (P35.0)

     P23.1   Congenital pneumonia due to **Chlamydia**   MCC

     P23.2   Congenital pneumonia due to **staphylococcus**   MCC

     P23.3   Congenital pneumonia due to **streptococcus, group B**   MCC

     P23.4   Congenital pneumonia due to **Escherichia coli**   MCC

     P23.5   Congenital pneumonia due to **Pseudomonas**   MCC

     P23.6   Congenital pneumonia due to other bacterial agents   MCC
         Congenital pneumonia due to Hemophilus influenzae
         Congenital pneumonia due to Klebsiella pneumoniae
         Congenital pneumonia due to Mycoplasma
         Congenital pneumonia due to Streptococcus, except group B
         Use additional code (B95-B96) to identify organism

     P23.8   Congenital pneumonia due to other organisms   MCC

     P23.9   Congenital pneumonia, unspecified   MCC

✓4th **P24**   Neonatal aspiration

     INCLUDES   aspiration in utero and during delivery

✓5th   **P24.0**   **Meconium** aspiration
         EXCLUDES 1   meconium passage (without aspiration) during delivery (P03.82)
                    meconium staining (P96.83)
         DEF: Meconium in the trachea or seen on chest x-ray after birth.

         P24.00   Meconium aspiration **without respiratory symptoms**
                 Meconium aspiration NOS

✓ Additional Character Required   ✓x7th Placeholder   Questionable PDx   Manifestation   Unspecified   UPD Unacceptable PDx   H1 - H4 HAC   HCC CMS-HCC Dx   HIV HIV Dx

ICD-10-CM 2025   925

P24.01 Meconium aspiration with respiratory symptoms `MCC`
Meconium aspiration pneumonia
Meconium aspiration pneumonitis
Meconium aspiration syndrome NOS
Use additional code to identify any secondary pulmonary hypertension, if applicable (I27.2-)
DEF: Aspiration of fetal intestinal material during or prior to delivery. It is usually a complication of placental insufficiency, causing pneumonitis and bronchial obstruction (inflammatory reaction of lungs).

√5th **P24.1 Neonatal aspiration of (clear) amniotic fluid and mucus**
Neonatal aspiration of liquor (amnii)

P24.10 Neonatal aspiration of (clear) amniotic fluid and mucus without respiratory symptoms
Neonatal aspiration of amniotic fluid and mucus NOS

P24.11 Neonatal aspiration of (clear) amniotic fluid and mucus with respiratory symptoms `MCC`
Neonatal aspiration of amniotic fluid and mucus with pneumonia
Neonatal aspiration of amniotic fluid and mucus with pneumonitis
Use additional code to identify any secondary pulmonary hypertension, if applicable (I27.2-)

√5th **P24.2 Neonatal aspiration of blood**

P24.20 Neonatal aspiration of blood without respiratory symptoms
Neonatal aspiration of blood NOS

P24.21 Neonatal aspiration of blood with respiratory symptoms `MCC`
Neonatal aspiration of blood with pneumonia
Neonatal aspiration of blood with pneumonitis
Use additional code to identify any secondary pulmonary hypertension, if applicable (I27.2-)

√5th **P24.3 Neonatal aspiration of milk and regurgitated food**
Neonatal aspiration of stomach contents

P24.30 Neonatal aspiration of milk and regurgitated food without respiratory symptoms
Neonatal aspiration of milk and regurgitated food NOS

P24.31 Neonatal aspiration of milk and regurgitated food with respiratory symptoms `MCC`
Neonatal aspiration of milk and regurgitated food with pneumonia
Neonatal aspiration of milk and regurgitated food with pneumonitis
Use additional code to identify any secondary pulmonary hypertension, if applicable (I27.2-)

√5th **P24.8 Other neonatal aspiration**

P24.80 Other neonatal aspiration without respiratory symptoms
Neonatal aspiration NEC

P24.81 Other neonatal aspiration with respiratory symptoms `MCC`
Neonatal aspiration pneumonia NEC
Neonatal aspiration with pneumonitis NEC
Neonatal aspiration with pneumonia NOS
Neonatal aspiration with pneumonitis NOS
Use additional code to identify any secondary pulmonary hypertension, if applicable (I27.2-)

P24.9 Neonatal aspiration, unspecified

√4th **P25 Interstitial emphysema and related conditions originating in the perinatal period**

P25.0 Interstitial emphysema originating in the perinatal period `MCC`

P25.1 Pneumothorax originating in the perinatal period `MCC`

P25.2 Pneumomediastinum originating in the perinatal period `MCC`

P25.3 Pneumopericardium originating in the perinatal period `MCC`

P25.8 Other conditions related to interstitial emphysema originating in the perinatal period `MCC`

√4th **P26 Pulmonary hemorrhage originating in the perinatal period**
EXCLUDES 1 acute idiopathic hemorrhage in infants over 28 days old (R04.81)

P26.0 Tracheobronchial hemorrhage originating in the perinatal period `MCC` `HCC`

P26.1 Massive pulmonary hemorrhage originating in the perinatal period `MCC` `HCC`

P26.8 Other pulmonary hemorrhages originating in the perinatal period `MCC` `HCC`

P26.9 Unspecified pulmonary hemorrhage originating in the perinatal period `MCC` `HCC`

√4th **P27 Chronic respiratory disease originating in the perinatal period**
EXCLUDES 2 respiratory distress of newborn (P22.0-P22.9)

P27.0 Wilson-Mikity syndrome `MCC` `HCC`
Pulmonary dysmaturity
DEF: Pulmonary insufficiency in newborn babies, especially those with low birth weight. Rapid onset of hypercapnia and cyanosis occur during the first month of life frequently resulting in death.

P27.1 Bronchopulmonary dysplasia originating in the perinatal period `MCC` `HCC`

P27.8 Other chronic respiratory diseases originating in the perinatal period `MCC` `HCC`
Congenital pulmonary fibrosis
Ventilator lung in newborn

P27.9 Unspecified chronic respiratory disease originating in the perinatal period `MCC` `HCC`

√4th **P28 Other respiratory conditions originating in the perinatal period**
Code also, if applicable, congenital malformations of the respiratory system (Q30-Q34)

P28.0 Primary atelectasis of newborn `CC` `HCC`
Primary failure to expand terminal respiratory units
Pulmonary hypoplasia associated with short gestation
Pulmonary immaturity NOS

√5th **P28.1 Other and unspecified atelectasis of newborn**

P28.10 Unspecified atelectasis of newborn `CC` `HCC`
Atelectasis of newborn NOS

P28.11 Resorption atelectasis without respiratory distress syndrome `CC` `HCC`
EXCLUDES 1 resorption atelectasis with respiratory distress syndrome (P22.0)

P28.19 Other atelectasis of newborn `CC` `HCC`
Partial atelectasis of newborn
Secondary atelectasis of newborn

P28.2 Cyanotic attacks of newborn `CC`
EXCLUDES 1 apnea of newborn (P28.3- - P28.4-)

√5th **P28.3 Primary sleep apnea of newborn**
Sleep apnea of newborn NOS
EXCLUDES 2 other apnea of newborn (P28.4-)
AHA: 2022,4Q,38-39
DEF: Unexplained cessation of breathing when a neonate makes no respiratory effort for 20 seconds or longer or when a neonate's breathing cessation is accompanied by cyanosis, bradycardia, or hypotonia.

P28.30 Primary sleep apnea of newborn, unspecified `CC`
Transient oxygen desaturation spells of newborn during sleep

P28.31 Primary central sleep apnea of newborn `CC`

P28.32 Primary obstructive sleep apnea of newborn `CC`

P28.33 Primary mixed sleep apnea of newborn `CC`

P28.39 Other primary sleep apnea of newborn `CC`

√5th **P28.4 Other apnea of newborn**
EXCLUDES 2 primary sleep apnea of newborn (P28.3-)
AHA: 2022,4Q,38-39

P28.40 Unspecified apnea of newborn `CC`
Apnea of newborn, NOS
Transient oxygen desaturation spells of newborn

P28.41 Central neonatal apnea of newborn `CC`

P28.42 Obstructive apnea of newborn `CC`

P28.43 Mixed neonatal apnea of newborn `CC`

P28.49 Other apnea of newborn `CC`
Apnea of prematurity

P28.5 Respiratory failure of newborn `MCC` `HCC`
EXCLUDES 2 respiratory arrest of newborn (P28.81)
respiratory distress of newborn ▶(P22.0)◀
AHA: 2019,2Q,29

√5th **P28.8 Other specified respiratory conditions of newborn**

P28.81 Respiratory arrest of newborn `MCC` `HCC`

P28.89 Other specified respiratory conditions of newborn
Congenital laryngeal stridor
Sniffles in newborn
Snuffles in newborn
EXCLUDES 1 early congenital syphilitic rhinitis (A50.05)

P28.9 Respiratory condition of newborn, unspecified
Respiratory depression in newborn

✓4ᵗʰ P29 Cardiovascular disorders originating in the perinatal period

> *EXCLUDES 2*   *congenital malformations of the circulatory system (Q20–Q28)*

P29.0 Neonatal cardiac failure   `HCC`
Code also associated underlying condition

✓5ᵗʰ P29.1 Neonatal cardiac dysrhythmia

P29.11 Neonatal tachycardia

P29.12 Neonatal bradycardia

P29.2 Neonatal hypertension

✓5ᵗʰ P29.3 Persistent fetal circulation
AHA: 2017,4Q,20-21

P29.30 Pulmonary hypertension of newborn   `MCC` `PE`
Persistent pulmonary hypertension of newborn
DEF: Condition that occurs when pressure within the pulmonary artery is elevated and vascular resistance is observed in the lungs.

P29.38 Other persistent fetal circulation   `MCC` `PE`
Delayed closure of ductus arteriosus

P29.4 Transient myocardial ischemia in newborn

✓5ᵗʰ P29.8 Other cardiovascular disorders originating in the perinatal period

P29.81 Cardiac arrest of newborn   `MCC` `HCC`

P29.89 Other cardiovascular disorders originating in the perinatal period
AHA: 2014,4Q,23

P29.9 Cardiovascular disorder originating in the perinatal period, unspecified

Infections specific to the perinatal period (P35-P39)

Infections acquired in utero, during birth via the umbilicus, or during the first 28 days after birth

> *EXCLUDES 2*   *asymptomatic human immunodeficiency virus [HIV] infection status (Z21)*
> *congenital gonococcal infection (A54.-)*
> *congenital pneumonia (P23.-)*
> *congenital syphilis (A50.-)*
> *human immunodeficiency virus [HIV] disease (B20)*
> *infant botulism (A48.51)*
> *infectious diseases not specific to the perinatal period (A00–B99, J09, J10.-)*
> *intestinal infectious disease (A00–A09)*
> *laboratory evidence of human immunodeficiency virus [HIV] (R75)*
> *tetanus neonatorum (A33)*

✓4ᵗʰ P35 Congenital viral diseases

> *INCLUDES*   infections acquired in utero or during birth

P35.0 Congenital rubella syndrome   `CC`
Congenital rubella pneumonitis

P35.1 Congenital cytomegalovirus infection   `MCC`

P35.2 Congenital herpesviral [herpes simplex] infection   `MCC`

P35.3 Congenital viral hepatitis   `MCC`

P35.4 Congenital Zika virus disease   `MCC`
Use additional code to identify manifestations of congenital Zika virus disease
AHA: 2018,4Q,25-26

P35.8 Other congenital viral diseases   `MCC`
Congenital varicella [chickenpox]
AHA: 2020,2Q,13

P35.9 Congenital viral disease, unspecified   `MCC`

✓4ᵗʰ P36 Bacterial sepsis of newborn

> *INCLUDES*   congenital sepsis

Use additional code(s), if applicable, to identify severe sepsis (R65.2-) and associated acute organ dysfunction(s)

P36.0 Sepsis of newborn due to streptococcus, group B   `MCC` `HCC`

✓5ᵗʰ P36.1 Sepsis of newborn due to other and unspecified streptococci

P36.10 Sepsis of newborn due to unspecified streptococci   `MCC` `HCC`

P36.19 Sepsis of newborn due to other streptococci   `MCC` `HCC`

P36.2 Sepsis of newborn due to Staphylococcus aureus   `MCC` `HCC`

✓5ᵗʰ P36.3 Sepsis of newborn due to other and unspecified staphylococci

P36.30 Sepsis of newborn due to unspecified staphylococci   `MCC` `HCC`

P36.39 Sepsis of newborn due to other staphylococci   `MCC` `HCC`

P36.4 Sepsis of newborn due to Escherichia coli   `MCC` `HCC`

P36.5 Sepsis of newborn due to anaerobes   `MCC` `HCC`

P36.8 Other bacterial sepsis of newborn   `MCC` `HCC`
Use additional code from category B96 to identify organism

P36.9 Bacterial sepsis of newborn, unspecified   `MCC` `HCC`

✓4ᵗʰ P37 Other congenital infectious and parasitic diseases

> *EXCLUDES 2*   *congenital syphilis (A50.-)*
> *infectious neonatal diarrhea (A00–A09)*
> *necrotizing enterocolitis in newborn (P77.-)*
> *noninfectious neonatal diarrhea (P78.3)*
> *ophthalmia neonatorum due to gonococcus (A54.31)*
> *tetanus neonatorum (A33)*

P37.0 Congenital tuberculosis   `MCC`

P37.1 Congenital toxoplasmosis   `MCC`
Hydrocephalus due to congenital toxoplasmosis

P37.2 Neonatal (disseminated) listeriosis   `MCC`

P37.3 Congenital falciparum malaria   `MCC`

P37.4 Other congenital malaria   `MCC`

P37.5 Neonatal candidiasis

P37.8 Other specified congenital infectious and parasitic diseases   `MCC`

P37.9 Congenital infectious or parasitic disease, unspecified   `MCC`

✓4ᵗʰ P38 Omphalitis of newborn

> *EXCLUDES 1*   *omphalitis not of newborn (L08.82)*
> *tetanus omphalitis (A33)*
> *umbilical hemorrhage of newborn (P51.-)*

DEF: Omphalitis: Infection and inflammation of the umbilical stump, often due to bacteria that can spread beyond the umbilical stump to the fascia, muscle, or even the umbilical vessels.

P38.1 Omphalitis with mild hemorrhage   `CC`

P38.9 Omphalitis without hemorrhage   `CC`
Omphalitis of newborn NOS

✓4ᵗʰ P39 Other infections specific to the perinatal period
Use additional code to identify organism or specific infection

P39.0 Neonatal infective mastitis   `CC`

> *EXCLUDES 1*   *breast engorgement of newborn (P83.4)*
> *noninfective mastitis of newborn (P83.4)*

P39.1 Neonatal conjunctivitis and dacryocystitis
Neonatal chlamydial conjunctivitis
Ophthalmia neonatorum NOS

> *EXCLUDES 1*   *gonococcal conjunctivitis (A54.31)*

P39.2 Intra-amniotic infection affecting newborn, not elsewhere classified   `CC`

P39.3 Neonatal urinary tract infection   `CC`

P39.4 Neonatal skin infection   `CC`
Neonatal pyoderma

> *EXCLUDES 1*   *pemphigus neonatorum (L00)*
> *staphylococcal scalded skin syndrome (L00)*

P39.8 Other specified infections specific to the perinatal period   `CC`

P39.9 Infection specific to the perinatal period, unspecified   `CC`

Hemorrhagic and hematological disorders of newborn (P50-P61)

> *EXCLUDES 1*   *congenital stenosis and stricture of bile ducts (Q44.3)*
> *Crigler-Najjar syndrome (E80.5)*
> *Dubin-Johnson syndrome (E80.6)*
> *Gilbert syndrome (E80.4)*
> *hereditary hemolytic anemias (D55-D58)*

✓4ᵗʰ P50 Newborn affected by intrauterine (fetal) blood loss

> *EXCLUDES 1*   *congenital anemia from intrauterine (fetal) blood loss (P61.3)*

P50.0 Newborn affected by intrauterine (fetal) blood loss from vasa previa

P50.1 Newborn affected by intrauterine (fetal) blood loss from ruptured cord

P50.2 Newborn affected by intrauterine (fetal) blood loss from placenta

P50.3 Newborn affected by hemorrhage into co-twin

P50.4 Newborn affected by hemorrhage into maternal circulation

P50.5 Newborn affected by intrauterine (fetal) blood loss from cut end of co-twin's cord

P50.8 Newborn affected by other intrauterine (fetal) blood loss

P50.9 Newborn affected by intrauterine (fetal) blood loss, unspecified
Newborn affected by fetal hemorrhage NOS

Chapter 16. Certain Conditions Originating in the Perinatal Period

P51–P59.9

√4ᵗʰ **P51** **Umbilical** hemorrhage of newborn
- EXCLUDES 1   *omphalitis with mild hemorrhage (P38.1)*
- *umbilical hemorrhage from cut end of co-twins cord (P50.5)*

P51.0 **Massive** umbilical hemorrhage of newborn

P51.8 **Other umbilical hemorrhages of newborn**
- Slipped umbilical ligature NOS

P51.9 Umbilical hemorrhage of newborn, unspecified

√4ᵗʰ **P52** **Intracranial nontraumatic hemorrhage** of newborn
- INCLUDES   intracranial hemorrhage due to anoxia or hypoxia
- EXCLUDES 1   *intracranial hemorrhage due to birth injury (P10.-)*
- *intracranial hemorrhage due to other injury (S06.-)*

P52.0 **Intraventricular (nontraumatic) hemorrhage, grade 1, of newborn** CC HCC
- Bleeding into germinal matrix
- Subependymal hemorrhage (without intraventricular extension)

P52.1 **Intraventricular (nontraumatic) hemorrhage, grade 2, of newborn** CC HCC
- Bleeding into ventricle
- Subependymal hemorrhage with intraventricular extension

√5ᵗʰ **P52.2** **Intraventricular (nontraumatic) hemorrhage, grade 3 and grade 4, of newborn**

     P52.21 **Intraventricular (nontraumatic) hemorrhage, grade 3, of newborn** MCC HCC
       Subependymal hemorrhage with intraventricular extension with enlargement of ventricle

     P52.22 **Intraventricular (nontraumatic) hemorrhage, grade 4, of newborn** MCC HCC
       Bleeding into cerebral cortex
       Subependymal hemorrhage with intracerebral extension

P52.3 **Unspecified intraventricular (nontraumatic) hemorrhage of newborn** CC HCC

P52.4 **Intracerebral** (nontraumatic) hemorrhage of newborn MCC HCC

P52.5 **Subarachnoid** (nontraumatic) hemorrhage of newborn MCC HCC

P52.6 **Cerebellar** (nontraumatic) and posterior fossa hemorrhage of newborn MCC HCC

P52.8 **Other intracranial (nontraumatic) hemorrhages of newborn** MCC HCC

P52.9 Intracranial (nontraumatic) hemorrhage of newborn, unspecified MCC HCC

P53 **Hemorrhagic disease** of newborn CC
- Vitamin K deficiency of newborn

√4ᵗʰ **P54** **Other neonatal hemorrhages**
- EXCLUDES 1   *newborn affected by (intrauterine) blood loss (P50.-)*
- *pulmonary hemorrhage originating in the perinatal period (P26.-)*

P54.0 **Neonatal hematemesis**
- EXCLUDES 1   *neonatal hematemesis due to swallowed maternal blood (P78.2)*

P54.1 **Neonatal melena** MCC
- EXCLUDES 1   *neonatal melena due to swallowed maternal blood (P78.2)*

P54.2 **Neonatal rectal hemorrhage** MCC

P54.3 **Other neonatal gastrointestinal hemorrhage** MCC

P54.4 **Neonatal adrenal hemorrhage** CC

P54.5 **Neonatal cutaneous hemorrhage**
- Neonatal bruising
- Neonatal ecchymoses
- Neonatal petechiae
- Neonatal superficial hematomata
- EXCLUDES 2   *bruising of scalp due to birth injury (P12.3)*
- *cephalhematoma due to birth injury (P12.0)*

P54.6 **Neonatal vaginal hemorrhage**
- Neonatal pseudomenses

P54.8 **Other specified neonatal hemorrhages**

P54.9 Neonatal hemorrhage, unspecified

√4ᵗʰ **P55** **Hemolytic disease of newborn**

P55.0 **Rh** isoimmunization of newborn HCC
- **DEF:** Incompatible Rh fetal-maternal blood grouping that prematurely destroys red blood cells. Symptoms include jaundice, asphyxia, pulmonary hypertension, edema, respiratory distress, kernicterus, and coagulopathies. It is detected by a Coombs test.
- **TIP:** A positive Coombs test without documentation of associated Rh isoimmunization should be coded to R79.89 Other specified abnormal findings of blood chemistry.

P55.1 **ABO** isoimmunization of newborn HCC
- **AHA:** 2015,3Q,20

P55.8 **Other hemolytic diseases of newborn** HCC
- **AHA:** 2018,3Q,24

P55.9 Hemolytic disease of newborn, unspecified HCC

√4ᵗʰ **P56** **Hydrops fetalis due to hemolytic disease**
- EXCLUDES 1   *hydrops fetalis NOS (P83.2)*

P56.0 **Hydrops fetalis due to isoimmunization** MCC HCC

√5ᵗʰ **P56.9** **Hydrops fetalis due to other and unspecified hemolytic disease**

     P56.90 **Hydrops fetalis due to unspecified hemolytic disease** MCC HCC

     P56.99 **Hydrops fetalis due to other hemolytic disease** MCC HCC

√4ᵗʰ **P57** **Kernicterus**

P57.0 **Kernicterus due to isoimmunization** MCC HCC
- **DEF:** Complication of erythroblastosis fetalis associated with severe neural symptoms, high blood bilirubin levels, and nerve cell destruction. It results in bilirubin-pigmented gray matter of the central nervous system.

P57.8 **Other specified kernicterus** MCC HCC
- EXCLUDES 1   *Crigler-Najjar syndrome (E80.5)*

P57.9 **Kernicterus, unspecified** MCC HCC

√4ᵗʰ **P58** **Neonatal jaundice due to other excessive hemolysis**
- EXCLUDES 1   *jaundice due to isoimmunization (P55-P57)*

P58.0 **Neonatal jaundice due to bruising**

P58.1 **Neonatal jaundice due to bleeding**

P58.2 **Neonatal jaundice due to infection**

P58.3 **Neonatal jaundice due to polycythemia**

√5ᵗʰ **P58.4** **Neonatal jaundice due to drugs or toxins transmitted from mother or given to newborn**
- Code first poisoning due to drug or toxin, if applicable (T36-T65 with fifth or sixth character 1-4)
- Use additional code for adverse effect, if applicable, to identify drug (T36-T50 with fifth or sixth character 5)

     P58.41 **Neonatal jaundice due to drugs or toxins transmitted from mother**

     P58.42 **Neonatal jaundice due to drugs or toxins given to newborn**

P58.5 **Neonatal jaundice due to swallowed maternal blood**

P58.8 **Neonatal jaundice due to other specified excessive hemolysis**

P58.9 Neonatal jaundice due to excessive hemolysis, unspecified

√4ᵗʰ **P59** **Neonatal jaundice from other and unspecified causes**
- EXCLUDES 1   *jaundice due to inborn errors of metabolism (E70-E88)*
- *kernicterus (P57.-)*

P59.0 **Neonatal jaundice associated with preterm delivery**
- Hyperbilirubinemia of prematurity
- Jaundice due to delayed conjugation associated with preterm delivery

P59.1 **Inspissated bile syndrome** MCC
- **DEF:** Biliary obstruction in newborn resulting from obstruction of outflow tract.

√5ᵗʰ **P59.2** **Neonatal jaundice from other and unspecified hepatocellular damage**
- EXCLUDES 1   *congenital viral hepatitis (P35.3)*

     P59.20 **Neonatal jaundice from unspecified hepatocellular damage** MCC

     P59.29 **Neonatal jaundice from other hepatocellular damage** MCC
       Neonatal giant cell hepatitis
       Neonatal (idiopathic) hepatitis

P59.3 **Neonatal jaundice from breast milk inhibitor**

P59.8 **Neonatal jaundice from other specified causes**

P59.9 Neonatal jaundice, unspecified
- Neonatal physiological jaundice (intense)(prolonged) NOS
- **AHA:** 2015,3Q,20

N Newborn: 0   P Pediatric: 0-17   M Maternity: 9-64   A Adult: 15-124   UNS Unspecified Site   MCC Major Complication/Comorbidity   CC Complication/Comorbidity   PE POA Exempt

928   ICD-10-CM 2025

P60 **Disseminated intravascular coagulation of newborn** `MCC`
    Defibrination syndrome of newborn

√4ᵗʰ **P61** **Other perinatal hematological disorders**
    EXCLUDES 1   *transient hypogammaglobulinemia of infancy (D80.7)*

    P61.0 **Transient neonatal thrombocytopenia** `MCC`
        Neonatal thrombocytopenia due to exchange transfusion
        Neonatal thrombocytopenia due to idiopathic maternal thrombocytopenia
        Neonatal thrombocytopenia due to isoimmunization
        DEF: Temporary decrease in blood platelets of a newborn that is secondary to placental insufficiency.

    P61.1 **Polycythemia neonatorum**
        DEF: Abnormal increase of total red blood cells of a newborn that results in hyperviscosity, which slows the flow of blood through small blood vessels.

    P61.2 **Anemia of prematurity** `CC`

    P61.3 **Congenital anemia from fetal blood loss** `CC`

    P61.4 **Other congenital anemias, not elsewhere classified** `CC`
        Congenital anemia NOS

    P61.5 **Transient neonatal neutropenia** `MCC`
        EXCLUDES 1   *congenital neutropenia (nontransient) (D70.0)*
        DEF: Low blood neutrophil counts of newborn that occurs due to maternal hypertension, sepsis, twin-twin transfusion, alloimmunization, and hemolytic disease.

    P61.6 **Other transient neonatal disorders of coagulation** `CC`

    P61.8 **Other specified perinatal hematological disorders**

    P61.9 **Perinatal hematological disorder, unspecified**

Transitory endocrine and metabolic disorders specific to newborn (P70-P74)

    `INCLUDES`   transitory endocrine and metabolic disturbances caused by the infant's response to maternal endocrine and metabolic factors, or its adjustment to extrauterine environment

    AHA: 2018,2Q,6

√4ᵗʰ **P70** **Transitory disorders of carbohydrate metabolism specific to newborn**

    P70.0 **Syndrome of infant of mother with gestational diabetes**
        Newborn (with hypoglycemia) affected by maternal gestational diabetes
        EXCLUDES 1   *newborn (with hypoglycemia) affected by maternal (pre-existing) diabetes mellitus (P70.1)*
                   syndrome of infant of a diabetic mother (P70.1)

    P70.1 **Syndrome of infant of a diabetic mother**
        Newborn (with hypoglycemia) affected by maternal (pre-existing) diabetes mellitus
        EXCLUDES 1   *newborn (with hypoglycemia) affected by maternal gestational diabetes (P70.0)*
                   syndrome of infant of mother with gestational diabetes (P70.0)

    P70.2 **Neonatal diabetes mellitus** `CC`

    P70.3 **Iatrogenic neonatal hypoglycemia**

    P70.4 **Other neonatal hypoglycemia**
        Transitory neonatal hypoglycemia

    P70.8 **Other transitory disorders of carbohydrate metabolism of newborn** `CC`

    P70.9 **Transitory disorder of carbohydrate metabolism of newborn, unspecified**

√4ᵗʰ **P71** **Transitory neonatal disorders of calcium and magnesium metabolism**

    P71.0 **Cow's milk hypocalcemia in newborn** `CC`

    P71.1 **Other neonatal hypocalcemia** `CC`
        EXCLUDES 1   *neonatal hypoparathyroidism (P71.4)*

    P71.2 **Neonatal hypomagnesemia** `CC`

    P71.3 **Neonatal tetany without calcium or magnesium deficiency** `CC`
        Neonatal tetany NOS

    P71.4 **Transitory neonatal hypoparathyroidism** `CC`

    P71.8 **Other transitory neonatal disorders of calcium and magnesium metabolism** `CC`
        AHA: 2016,4Q,54

    P71.9 **Transitory neonatal disorder of calcium and magnesium metabolism, unspecified** `CC`

√4ᵗʰ **P72** **Other transitory neonatal endocrine disorders**
    EXCLUDES 1   *congenital hypothyroidism with or without goiter (E03.0-E03.1)*
               dyshormogenetic goiter (E07.1)
               ▶*dyshormonogenetic goiter (E07.1)*◀
               Pendred's syndrome (E07.1)

    P72.0 **Neonatal goiter, not elsewhere classified** `CC`
        Transitory congenital goiter with normal functioning

    P72.1 **Transitory neonatal hyperthyroidism** `CC`
        Neonatal thyrotoxicosis

    P72.2 **Other transitory neonatal disorders of thyroid function, not elsewhere classified** `CC`
        Transitory neonatal hypothyroidism

    P72.8 **Other specified transitory neonatal endocrine disorders** `CC`

    P72.9 **Transitory neonatal endocrine disorder, unspecified**

√4ᵗʰ **P74** **Other transitory neonatal electrolyte and metabolic disturbances**
    AHA: 2018,4Q,26-27

    P74.0 **Late metabolic acidosis of newborn** `MCC`
        EXCLUDES 1   *(fetal) metabolic acidosis of newborn (P19)*

    P74.1 **Dehydration of newborn**

√5ᵗʰ   **P74.2** **Disturbances of sodium balance of newborn**
        P74.21 **Hypernatremia of newborn**
        P74.22 **Hyponatremia of newborn**

√5ᵗʰ   **P74.3** **Disturbances of potassium balance of newborn**
        P74.31 **Hyperkalemia of newborn**
        P74.32 **Hypokalemia of newborn**

√5ᵗʰ   **P74.4** **Other transitory electrolyte disturbances of newborn**
        P74.41 **Alkalosis of newborn** `CC`
            Hyperbicarbonatemia
        √6ᵗʰ   **P74.42** **Disturbances of chlorine balance of newborn**
            P74.421 **Hyperchloremia of newborn**
               Hyperchloremic metabolic acidosis
               EXCLUDES 2   *late metabolic acidosis of the newborn (P74.0)*
            P74.422 **Hypochloremia of newborn**
            P74.49 **Other transitory electrolyte disturbance of newborn**

    P74.5 **Transitory tyrosinemia of newborn** `CC`

    P74.6 **Transitory hyperammonemia of newborn** `CC`

    P74.8 **Other transitory metabolic disturbances of newborn** `CC`
        Amino-acid metabolic disorders described as transitory

    P74.9 **Transitory metabolic disturbance of newborn, unspecified**

Digestive system disorders of newborn (P76-P78)

√4ᵗʰ **P76** **Other intestinal obstruction of newborn**

    P76.0 **Meconium plug syndrome**
        Meconium ileus NOS
        EXCLUDES 1   *meconium ileus in cystic fibrosis (E84.11)*
        DEF: Meconium obstruction of a newborn's intestines, resulting from unusually thick or hard meconium.

    P76.1 **Transitory ileus of newborn** `CC`
        EXCLUDES 1   *Hirschsprung's disease (Q43.1)*

    P76.2 **Intestinal obstruction due to inspissated milk**

    P76.8 **Other specified intestinal obstruction of newborn**
        EXCLUDES 1   *intestinal obstruction classifiable to K56.-*

    P76.9 **Intestinal obstruction of newborn, unspecified**

√4ᵗʰ **P77** **Necrotizing enterocolitis of newborn**
    DEF: Serious intestinal infection and inflammation in preterm infants. Severity is measured by stages and may progress to life-threatening perforation or peritonitis. Resection surgical treatment may be necessary.

    P77.1 **Stage 1 necrotizing enterocolitis in newborn** `MCC` `HCC`
        Necrotizing enterocolitis without pneumatosis, without perforation
        DEF: Broad-spectrum symptoms with nonspecific signs, including feeding intolerance, abdominal distention, bradycardia, and metabolic abnormalities.

    P77.2 **Stage 2 necrotizing enterocolitis in newborn** `MCC` `HCC`
        Necrotizing enterocolitis with pneumatosis, without perforation
        DEF: Radiographic confirmation of necrotizing enterocolitis showing intestinal dilatation, fixed loops of bowels, pneumatosis intestinalis, metabolic acidosis, and thrombocytopenia.

P77.3 **Stage 3** necrotizing enterocolitis in newborn   MCC HCC
Necrotizing enterocolitis with perforation
Necrotizing enterocolitis with pneumatosis and perforation
DEF: Advanced stage in which an infant demonstrates signs of bowel perforation, septic shock, metabolic acidosis, ascites, disseminated intravascular coagulopathy, and neutropenia.

P77.9 Necrotizing enterocolitis in newborn, unspecified   MCC HCC
Necrotizing enterocolitis in newborn, NOS

√4th **P78** **Other perinatal digestive system disorders**
EXCLUDES 1   cystic fibrosis (E84.0-E84.9)
                  neonatal gastrointestinal hemorrhages (P54.0-P54.3)

P78.0 Perinatal intestinal perforation   MCC HCC
Meconium peritonitis

P78.1 Other neonatal peritonitis
Neonatal peritonitis NOS

P78.2 Neonatal hematemesis and melena due to swallowed maternal blood

P78.3 Noninfective neonatal diarrhea
Neonatal diarrhea NOS

√5th **P78.8** Other specified perinatal digestive system disorders

P78.81 Congenital cirrhosis (of liver)

P78.82 Peptic ulcer of newborn

P78.83 Newborn esophageal reflux
Neonatal esophageal reflux

P78.84 Gestational alloimmune liver disease   PE
GALD
Neonatal hemochromatosis
EXCLUDES 1   hemochromatosis (E83.11-)
AHA: 2017,4Q,21
DEF: Severe hepatic injury with onset during fetal development with manifestations beginning during fetal life. It is due to maternal antibodies to fetal hepatic cells (hepatocytes) that cross the placenta into the fetal circulation, causing hepatic cell necrosis.

P78.89 Other specified perinatal digestive system disorders

P78.9 Perinatal digestive system disorder, unspecified

Conditions involving the integument and temperature regulation of newborn (P80-P83)

√4th **P80** **Hypothermia of newborn**
DEF: Decrease in newborn body temperature due to their larger ratio of surface area to body weight, thin skin with blood vessels close to the surface, and a limited amount of subcutaneous fat.

P80.0 Cold injury syndrome
Severe and usually chronic hypothermia associated with a pink flushed appearance, edema and neurological and biochemical abnormalities.
EXCLUDES 1   mild hypothermia of newborn (P80.8)

P80.8 Other hypothermia of newborn
Mild hypothermia of newborn

P80.9 Hypothermia of newborn, unspecified

√4th **P81** **Other disturbances of temperature regulation of newborn**

P81.0 Environmental hyperthermia of newborn

P81.8 Other specified disturbances of temperature regulation of newborn

P81.9 Disturbance of temperature regulation of newborn, unspecified
Fever of newborn NOS

√4th **P83** **Other conditions of integument specific to newborn**
EXCLUDES 1   congenital malformations of skin and integument (Q80-Q84)
                  hydrops fetalis due to hemolytic disease (P56.-)
                  neonatal skin infection (P39.4)
                  staphylococcal scalded skin syndrome (L00)
EXCLUDES 2   cradle cap (L21.0)
                  diaper [napkin] dermatitis (L22)

P83.0 Sclerema neonatorum   CC
DEF: Diffuse, rapidly progressing white, waxy, nonpitting hardening of tissue, usually of legs and feet that is life-threatening. It is found in preterm or debilitated infants. Etiology is unknown.

P83.1 Neonatal erythema toxicum

P83.2 Hydrops fetalis not due to hemolytic disease   MCC
Hydrops fetalis NOS
DEF: Severe, life-threatening problem of a newborn characterized by severe edema of the entire body. It is unrelated to immune response.

√5th **P83.3** Other and unspecified edema specific to newborn

P83.30 Unspecified edema specific to newborn   CC

P83.39 Other edema specific to newborn   CC

P83.4 Breast engorgement of newborn
Noninfective mastitis of newborn

P83.5 Congenital hydrocele
DEF: Hydrocele: Serous fluid that collects in the tunica vaginalis of the scrotum along the spermatic cord in males.

P83.6 Umbilical polyp of newborn

√5th **P83.8** Other specified conditions of integument specific to newborn
AHA: 2017,4Q,21-22

P83.81 Umbilical granuloma   PE
EXCLUDES 2   granulomatous disorder of the skin and subcutaneous tissue, unspecified (L92.9)

P83.88 Other specified conditions of integument specific to newborn   PE
Bronze baby syndrome
Neonatal scleroderma
Urticaria neonatorum

P83.9 Condition of the integument specific to newborn, unspecified

Other problems with newborn (P84)

P84 **Other problems with newborn**
Acidemia of newborn
Acidosis of newborn
Anoxia of newborn NOS
Asphyxia of newborn NOS
Hypercapnia of newborn
Hypoxemia of newborn
Hypoxia of newborn NOS
Mixed metabolic and respiratory acidosis of newborn
EXCLUDES 1   intracranial hemorrhage due to anoxia or hypoxia (P52.-)
                  hypoxic ischemic encephalopathy [HIE] (P91.6-)
                  late metabolic acidosis of newborn (P74.0)

Other disorders originating in the perinatal period (P90-P96)

P90 **Convulsions of newborn**   MCC HCC
EXCLUDES 1   benign myoclonic epilepsy in infancy (G40.3-)
                  benign neonatal convulsions (familial) (G40.3-)

√4th **P91** **Other disturbances of cerebral status of newborn**

P91.0 Neonatal cerebral ischemia   MCC HCC
EXCLUDES 1   neonatal cerebral infarction (P91.82-)

P91.1 Acquired periventricular cysts of newborn   MCC HCC

P91.2 Neonatal cerebral leukomalacia   MCC HCC
Periventricular leukomalacia

P91.3 Neonatal cerebral irritability   MCC HCC

P91.4 Neonatal cerebral depression   MCC HCC

P91.5 Neonatal coma   MCC HCC

√5th **P91.6** Hypoxic ischemic encephalopathy [HIE]
EXCLUDES 1   neonatal cerebral depression (P91.4)
                  neonatal cerebral irritability (P91.3)
                  neonatal coma (P91.5)
AHA: 2017,4Q,22

P91.60 Hypoxic ischemic encephalopathy [HIE], unspecified   CC HCC

P91.61 Mild hypoxic ischemic encephalopathy [HIE]   CC HCC

P91.62 Moderate hypoxic ischemic encephalopathy [HIE]   CC HCC

P91.63 Severe hypoxic ischemic encephalopathy [HIE]   MCC HCC

√5th **P91.8** Other specified disturbances of cerebral status of newborn
AHA: 2017,4Q,22

√6th **P91.81** Neonatal encephalopathy

P91.811 Neonatal encephalopathy in diseases classified elsewhere   HCC PE
Code first underlying condition, if known, such as:
congenital cirrhosis (of liver) (P78.81)
intracranial nontraumatic hemorrhage of newborn (P52.-)
kernicterus (P57.-)

P91.819 Neonatal encephalopathy, unspecified   HCC PE

√6ᵗʰ   **P91.82**   **Neonatal cerebral infarction**
Neonatal stroke
Perinatal arterial ischemic stroke
Perinatal cerebral infarction
EXCLUDES 1   *cerebral infarction (I63.-)*
EXCLUDES 2   *intracranial hemorrhage of newborn (P52.-)*
AHA: 2020,4Q,37-38

     P91.821   **Neonatal cerebral infarction, right side of brain**   `MCC` `HCC` `PE`

     P91.822   **Neonatal cerebral infarction, left side of brain**   `MCC` `HCC` `PE`

     P91.823   **Neonatal cerebral infarction, bilateral**   `MCC` `HCC` `PE`

     P91.829   **Neonatal cerebral infarction, unspecified side**   `MCC` `HCC`

   P91.88   **Other specified disturbances of cerebral status of newborn**   `HCC` `PE`

P91.9   **Disturbance of cerebral status of newborn, unspecified**   `HCC`

√4ᵗʰ   **P92**   **Feeding problems of newborn**
EXCLUDES 1   *eating disorders (F50.-)*
EXCLUDES 2   *feeding problems in child over 28 days old (R63.3-)*
AHA: 2016,3Q,19

  √5ᵗʰ   **P92.0**   **Vomiting of newborn**
EXCLUDES 1   *vomiting of child over 28 days old (R11.-)*

     P92.01   **Bilious vomiting of newborn**   `MCC`
EXCLUDES 1   *bilious vomiting in child over 28 days old (R11.14)*

     P92.09   **Other vomiting of newborn**
EXCLUDES 1   *regurgitation of food in newborn (P92.1)*

  P92.1   **Regurgitation and rumination of newborn**

  P92.2   **Slow feeding of newborn**

  P92.3   **Underfeeding of newborn**

  P92.4   **Overfeeding of newborn**

  P92.5   **Neonatal difficulty in feeding at breast**
AHA: 2017,1Q,28

  P92.6   **Failure to thrive in newborn**
EXCLUDES 1   *failure to thrive in child over 28 days old (R62.51)*

  P92.8   **Other feeding problems of newborn**

  P92.9   **Feeding problem of newborn, unspecified**

√4ᵗʰ   **P93**   **Reactions and intoxications due to drugs administered to newborn**
INCLUDES   reactions and intoxications due to drugs administered to fetus affecting newborn
EXCLUDES 1   *jaundice due to drugs or toxins transmitted from mother or given to newborn (P58.4-)*
reactions and intoxications from maternal opiates, tranquilizers and other medication (P04.0-P04.1, P04.4-)
withdrawal symptoms from maternal use of drugs of addiction (P96.1)
withdrawal symptoms from therapeutic use of drugs in newborn (P96.2)

  P93.0   **Grey baby syndrome**   `CC` `HCC`
Grey syndrome from chloramphenicol administration in newborn

  P93.8   **Other reactions and intoxications due to drugs administered to newborn**   `CC` `HCC`
Use additional code for adverse effect, if applicable, to identify drug (T36-T50 with fifth or sixth character 5)

√4ᵗʰ   **P94**   **Disorders of muscle tone of newborn**

  P94.0   **Transient neonatal myasthenia gravis**   `CC`
EXCLUDES 1   *myasthenia gravis (G70.0)*

  P94.1   **Congenital hypertonia**

  P94.2   **Congenital hypotonia**
Floppy baby syndrome, unspecified

  P94.8   **Other disorders of muscle tone of newborn**

  P94.9   **Disorder of muscle tone of newborn, unspecified**

P95   **Stillbirth**
Deadborn fetus NOS
Fetal death of unspecified cause
Stillbirth NOS
EXCLUDES 1   *maternal care for intrauterine death (O36.4)*
missed abortion (O02.1)
outcome of delivery, stillbirth (Z37.1, Z37.3, Z37.4, Z37.7)

√4ᵗʰ   **P96**   **Other conditions originating in the perinatal period**

  P96.0   **Congenital renal failure**
Uremia of newborn

  P96.1   **Neonatal withdrawal symptoms from maternal use of drugs of addiction**   `CC` `HCC`
Drug withdrawal syndrome in infant of dependent mother
Neonatal abstinence syndrome
EXCLUDES 1   *reactions and intoxications from maternal opiates and tranquilizers administered during labor and delivery (P04.0)*
AHA: 2018,4Q,24-25

  P96.2   **Withdrawal symptoms from therapeutic use of drugs in newborn**   `CC` `HCC`

  P96.3   **Wide cranial sutures of newborn**
Neonatal craniotabes

  P96.5   **Complication to newborn due to (fetal) intrauterine procedure**
EXCLUDES 2   *newborn affected by amniocentesis (P00.6)*

  √5ᵗʰ   **P96.8**   **Other specified conditions originating in the perinatal period**

     P96.81   **Exposure to (parental) (environmental) tobacco smoke in the perinatal period**
EXCLUDES 2   *exposure to environmental tobacco smoke after the perinatal period (Z77.22)*
newborn affected by in utero exposure to tobacco (P04.2)

     P96.82   **Delayed separation of umbilical cord**

     P96.83   **Meconium staining**
EXCLUDES 1   *meconium aspiration (P24.00, P24.01)*
meconium passage during delivery (P03.82)
DEF: Meconium passed in utero causing discoloration on the fetal skin and nails or on the umbilicus. This staining may be incidental or may be an indicator of significant fetal stress that could affect outcomes.

     P96.89   **Other specified conditions originating in the perinatal period**
Use additional code to specify condition
AHA: 2023,3Q,3

  P96.9   **Condition originating in the perinatal period, unspecified**
Congenital debility NOS

Chapter 17. Congenital Malformations, Deformations, and Chromosomal Abnormalities (Q00–Q99)

Chapter-specific Guidelines with Coding Examples

The chapter-specific guidelines from the ICD-10-CM Official Guidelines for Coding and Reporting have been provided below. Along with these guidelines are coding examples, contained in the shaded boxes, that have been developed to help illustrate the coding and/or sequencing guidance found in these guidelines.

Assign an appropriate code(s) from categories Q00–Q99, Congenital malformations, deformations, and chromosomal abnormalities when a malformation/deformation or chromosomal abnormality is documented. A malformation/deformation/or chromosomal abnormality may be the principal/first-listed diagnosis on a record or a secondary diagnosis.

When a malformation/deformation/or chromosomal abnormality does not have a unique code assignment, assign additional code(s) for any manifestations that may be present.

When the code assignment specifically identifies the malformation/deformation/or chromosomal abnormality, manifestations that are an inherent component of the anomaly should not be coded separately. Additional codes should be assigned for manifestations that are not an inherent component.

> **8-day-old infant with tetralogy of Fallot and pulmonary stenosis**
>
> **Q21.3** **Tetralogy of Fallot**
>
> *Explanation:* Pulmonary stenosis is inherent in the disease process of tetralogy of Fallot. When the code assignment specifically identifies the malformation/deformation/or chromosomal abnormality, manifestations that are inherent components of the anomaly should not be coded separately.

> **7-month-old infant with Down syndrome and common atrioventricular canal**
>
> **Q90.9** **Down syndrome, unspecified**
>
> **Q21.23** **Complete atrioventricular septal defect**
>
> *Explanation:* While a common atrioventricular canal is often associated with patients with Down syndrome, this manifestation is not an inherent component and may be reported separately. When the code assignment specifically identifies the anomaly, manifestations that are inherent components of the condition should not be coded separately. Additional codes should be assigned for manifestations that are not inherent components.

Codes from Chapter 17 may be used throughout the life of the patient. If a congenital malformation or deformity has been corrected, a personal history code should be used to identify the history of the malformation or deformity. Although present at birth, a malformation/deformation/or chromosomal abnormality may not be identified until later in life. Whenever the condition is diagnosed by the provider, it is appropriate to assign a code from codes Q00–Q99. For the birth admission, the appropriate code from category Z38, Liveborn infants, according to place of birth and type of delivery, should be sequenced as the principal diagnosis, followed by any congenital anomaly codes, Q00–Q99.

> **Three-year-old with history of corrected ventricular septal defect**
>
> **Z87.74** **Personal history of (corrected) congenital malformations of heart and circulatory system**
>
> *Explanation:* If a congenital malformation or deformity has been corrected, a personal history code should be used to identify the history of the malformation or deformity.

> **Forty-year-old man with headaches diagnosed with congenital arteriovenous malformation of cerebral vessels by brain scan**
>
> **Q28.2** **Arteriovenous malformation of cerebral vessels**
>
> *Explanation:* Although present at birth, malformations may not be identified until later in life. Whenever a congenital condition is diagnosed by the physician, it is appropriate to assign a code from the range Q00–Q99.

> **Newborn with anencephaly delivered vaginally in hospital**
>
> **Z38.00** **Single liveborn infant, delivered vaginally**
>
> **Q00.0** **Anencephaly**
>
> *Explanation:* For the birth admission, the appropriate code from category Z38 Liveborn infants, according to place of birth and type of delivery, should be sequenced as the principal diagnosis, followed by any congenital anomaly codes, Q00–Q99.

Chapter 17. Congenital Malformations, Deformations and Chromosomal Abnormalities (Q00-Q99)

NOTE Codes from this chapter are not for use on maternal records

EXCLUDES 2 *inborn errors of metabolism (E70-E88)*

This chapter contains the following blocks:

Q00-Q07 Congenital malformations of the nervous system
Q10-Q18 Congenital malformations of eye, ear, face and neck
Q20-Q28 Congenital malformations of the circulatory system
Q30-Q34 Congenital malformations of the respiratory system
Q35-Q37 Cleft lip and cleft palate
Q38-Q45 Other congenital malformations of the digestive system
Q50-Q56 Congenital malformations of genital organs
Q60-Q64 Congenital malformations of the urinary system
Q65-Q79 Congenital malformations and deformations of the musculoskeletal system
Q80-Q89 Other congenital malformations
Q90-Q99 Chromosomal abnormalities, not elsewhere classified

Congenital malformations of the nervous system (Q00-Q07)

Q00 ✓4th **Anencephaly and similar malformations**

Q00.0 Anencephaly `MCC` `HCC` `PE`
Acephaly
Acrania
Amyelencephaly
Hemianencephaly
Hemicephaly

Q00.1 Craniorachischisis `MCC` `HCC` `PE`

Q00.2 Iniencephaly `MCC` `HCC` `PE`

Q01 ✓4th **Encephalocele**

INCLUDES Arnold-Chiari syndrome, type III
encephalocystocele
encephalomyelocele
hydroencephalocele
hydromeningocele, cranial
meningocele, cerebral
meningoencephalocele

EXCLUDES 1 *Meckel-Gruber syndrome (Q61.9)*

DEF: Congenital protrusion of brain tissue through a defect in the skull.

Q01.0 Frontal encephalocele `CC` `HCC` `PE`

Q01.1 Nasofrontal encephalocele `CC` `HCC` `PE`

Q01.2 Occipital encephalocele `CC` `HCC` `PE`

Q01.8 Encephalocele of other sites `CC` `HCC` `PE`

Q01.9 Encephalocele, unspecified `CC` `HCC` `PE`

Q02 Microcephaly `HCC` `PE`

INCLUDES hydromicrocephaly
micrencephalon

Code first, if applicable, congenital Zika virus disease

EXCLUDES 1 *Meckel-Gruber syndrome (Q61.9)*

AHA: 2018,4Q,26

DEF: Congenital disorder in which the head circumference is more than two standard deviations below the mean for age, sex, race, and gestation and associated with a decreased life expectancy.

Q03 ✓4th **Congenital hydrocephalus**

INCLUDES hydrocephalus in newborn

EXCLUDES 1 *acquired hydrocephalus (G91.-)*
Arnold-Chiari syndrome, type II (Q07.0-)
hydrocephalus due to congenital toxoplasmosis (P37.1)
hydrocephalus with spina bifida (Q05.0-Q05.4)

DEF: Hydrocephalus: Abnormal buildup of cerebrospinal fluid in the brain causing dilation of the ventricles.

Congenital Hydrocephalus

Normal ventricles   Hydrocephalic ventricles

Pressure

Q03.0 Malformations of aqueduct of Sylvius `HCC` `PE`
Anomaly of aqueduct of Sylvius
Obstruction of aqueduct of Sylvius, congenital
Stenosis of aqueduct of Sylvius

Q03.1 Atresia of foramina of Magendie and Luschka `HCC` `PE`
Dandy-Walker syndrome

Q03.8 Other congenital hydrocephalus `HCC` `PE`

Q03.9 Congenital hydrocephalus, unspecified `HCC` `PE`

Q04 ✓4th **Other congenital malformations of brain**

EXCLUDES 1 *cyclopia (Q87.0)*
macrocephaly (Q75.3)

Q04.0 Congenital malformations of corpus callosum `MCC` `HCC` `PE`
Agenesis of corpus callosum

Q04.1 Arhinencephaly `MCC` `HCC` `PE`

Q04.2 Holoprosencephaly `MCC` `HCC` `PE`

Q04.3 Other reduction deformities of brain `MCC` `HCC` `PE`
Absence of part of brain
Agenesis of part of brain
Agyria
Aplasia of part of brain
Hydranencephaly
Hypoplasia of part of brain
Lissencephaly
Microgyria
Pachygyria

EXCLUDES 1 *congenital malformations of corpus callosum (Q04.0)*

Q04.4 Septo-optic dysplasia of brain `CC` `HCC` `PE`

Q04.5 Megalencephaly `CC` `HCC` `PE`

Q04.6 Congenital cerebral cysts `CC` `HCC` `PE`
Porencephaly
Schizencephaly

EXCLUDES 1 *acquired porencephalic cyst (G93.0)*

Q04.8 Other specified congenital malformations of brain `CC` `HCC` `PE`
Arnold-Chiari syndrome, type IV
Macrogyria

Q04.9 Congenital malformation of brain, unspecified `HCC` `PE`
Congenital anomaly NOS of brain
Congenital deformity NOS of brain
Congenital disease or lesion NOS of brain
Multiple anomalies NOS of brain, congenital

✓4th **Q05 Spina bifida**

INCLUDES   hydromeningocele (spinal)
meningocele (spinal)
meningomyelocele
myelocele
myelomeningocele
rachischisis
spina bifida (aperta)(cystica)
syringomyelocele

Use additional code for any associated paraplegia (paraparesis) (G82.2-)

EXCLUDES 1   Arnold-Chiari syndrome, type II (Q07.0-)
spina bifida occulta (Q76.0)

DEF: Lack of closure in the vertebral column with protrusion of the spinal cord through the defect, often in the lumbosacral area. This condition can be recognized by the presence of alpha-fetoproteins in the amniotic fluid.

Spina Bifida

Spina bifida occulta   Meningocele   Myelomeningocele

Q05.0	**Cervical spina bifida with hydrocephalus**	CC HCC PE
Q05.1	**Thoracic spina bifida with hydrocephalus** Dorsal spina bifida with hydrocephalus Thoracolumbar spina bifida with hydrocephalus	CC HCC PE
Q05.2	**Lumbar spina bifida with hydrocephalus** Lumbosacral spina bifida with hydrocephalus	CC HCC PE
Q05.3	**Sacral spina bifida with hydrocephalus**	CC HCC PE
Q05.4	**Unspecified spina bifida with hydrocephalus**	CC HCC PE
Q05.5	**Cervical spina bifida without hydrocephalus**	HCC PE
Q05.6	**Thoracic spina bifida without hydrocephalus** Dorsal spina bifida NOS Thoracolumbar spina bifida NOS	HCC PE
Q05.7	**Lumbar spina bifida without hydrocephalus** Lumbosacral spina bifida NOS	HCC PE
Q05.8	**Sacral spina bifida without hydrocephalus**	HCC PE
Q05.9	**Spina bifida, unspecified**	HCC PE

✓4th **Q06 Other congenital malformations of spinal cord**

Q06.0	**Amyelia**	HCC PE
Q06.1	**Hypoplasia and dysplasia of spinal cord** Atelomyelia Myelatelia Myelodysplasia of spinal cord	HCC PE
Q06.2	**Diastematomyelia** **DEF:** Rare congenital anomaly often associated with spina bifida. The spinal cord is separated into longitudinal halves by a bony, cartilaginous or fibrous septum, each half surrounded by a dural sac.	HCC PE
Q06.3	**Other congenital cauda equina malformations**	HCC PE
Q06.4	**Hydromyelia** Hydrorachis	HCC PE
Q06.8	**Other specified congenital malformations of spinal cord**	HCC PE
Q06.9	**Congenital malformation of spinal cord, unspecified** Congenital anomaly NOS of spinal cord Congenital deformity NOS of spinal cord Congenital disease or lesion NOS of spinal cord	HCC PE

✓4th **Q07 Other congenital malformations of nervous system**

EXCLUDES 2   congenital central alveolar hypoventilation syndrome (G47.35)
familial dysautonomia [Riley-Day] (G90.1)
neurofibromatosis (nonmalignant) (Q85.0-)

✓5th **Q07.0 Arnold-Chiari syndrome**
Arnold-Chiari syndrome, type II

EXCLUDES 1   Arnold-Chiari syndrome, type III (Q01.-)
Arnold-Chiari syndrome, type IV (Q04.8)

DEF: Congenital malformation of the brain in which the cerebellum protrudes through the foramen magnum into the spinal canal.

Q07.00	**Arnold-Chiari syndrome without spina bifida or hydrocephalus**	HCC PE
Q07.01	**Arnold-Chiari syndrome with spina bifida**	HCC PE
Q07.02	**Arnold-Chiari syndrome with hydrocephalus**	CC HCC PE
Q07.03	**Arnold-Chiari syndrome with spina bifida and hydrocephalus**	CC HCC PE

Q07.8	**Other specified congenital malformations of nervous system** Agenesis of nerve Displacement of brachial plexus Jaw-winking syndrome Marcus Gunn's syndrome	HCC PE
Q07.9	**Congenital malformation of nervous system, unspecified** Congenital anomaly NOS of nervous system Congenital deformity NOS of nervous system Congenital disease or lesion NOS of nervous system	HCC PE

Congenital malformations of eye, ear, face and neck (Q10-Q18)

EXCLUDES 2   cleft lip and cleft palate (Q35-Q37)
congenital malformation of cervical spine (Q05.0, Q05.5, Q67.5, Q76.0-Q76.4)
congenital malformation of larynx (Q31.-)
congenital malformation of lip NEC (Q38.0)
congenital malformation of nose (Q30.-)
congenital malformation of parathyroid gland (Q89.2)
congenital malformation of thyroid gland (Q89.2)

✓4th **Q10 Congenital malformations of eyelid, lacrimal apparatus and orbit**

EXCLUDES 1   cryptophthalmos NOS (Q11.2)
cryptophthalmos syndrome (Q87.0)

Q10.0	**Congenital ptosis** **DEF:** Congenital drooping of the eyelid. Ptosis is mostly idiopathic, but may occur genetically.	PE
Q10.1	**Congenital ectropion**	PE
Q10.2	**Congenital entropion**	PE
Q10.3	**Other congenital malformations of eyelid** Ablepharon Blepharophimosis, congenital Coloboma of eyelid Congenital absence or agenesis of cilia Congenital absence or agenesis of eyelid Congenital accessory eyelid Congenital accessory eye muscle Congenital malformation of eyelid NOS	PE
Q10.4	**Absence and agenesis of lacrimal apparatus** Congenital absence of punctum lacrimale	PE
Q10.5	**Congenital stenosis and stricture of lacrimal duct**	PE
Q10.6	**Other congenital malformations of lacrimal apparatus** Congenital malformation of lacrimal apparatus NOS	PE
Q10.7	**Congenital malformation of orbit**	PE

✓4th **Q11 Anophthalmos, microphthalmos and macrophthalmos**

Q11.0	**Cystic eyeball**	PE
Q11.1	**Other anophthalmos** Anophthalmos NOS Agenesis of eye Aplasia of eye	PE
Q11.2	**Microphthalmos** Cryptophthalmos NOS Dysplasia of eye Hypoplasia of eye Rudimentary eye EXCLUDES 1 cryptophthalmos syndrome (Q87.0)	PE
Q11.3	**Macrophthalmos** EXCLUDES 1 macrophthalmos in congenital glaucoma (Q15.0)	PE

✓ Additional Character Required   ✓x7th Placeholder   Questionable PDx   Manifestation   Unspecified   UPD Unacceptable PDx   H1 -H14 HAC   HCC CMS-HCC Dx   HIV HIV Dx

ICD-10-CM 2025   **935**

Chapter 17. Congenital Malformations, Deformations and Chromosomal Abnormalities

Q12–Q18.1

✓4th **Q12** Congenital **lens** malformations

Q12.0 Congenital **cataract**   PE

Q12.1 Congenital **displaced lens**   PE

Q12.2 **Coloboma of lens**

Coloboma of Lens

Coloboma of Lens illustration

Coloboma

Q12.3 Congenital **aphakia**   PE

Q12.4 **Spherophakia**   PE

Q12.8 Other congenital lens malformations   PE
Microphakia

Q12.9 Congenital lens malformation, unspecified   PE

✓4th **Q13** Congenital malformations of **anterior segment of eye**

Q13.0 **Coloboma** of **iris**   PE
Coloboma NOS
DEF: Defective or absent section of ocular tissue that may present as mild cupping or a small pit in the ocular disc due to extensive defects in the iris, ciliary body, choroids, and retina.

Q13.1 **Absence** of **iris**   PE
Aniridia
Use additional code for associated glaucoma (H42)
DEF: Incompletely formed or absent iris. It affects both eyes and is a dominant trait.

Q13.2 Other congenital malformations of iris   PE
Anisocoria, congenital
Atresia of pupil
Congenital malformation of iris NOS
Corectopia

Q13.3 Congenital **corneal opacity**   PE

Q13.4 Other congenital corneal malformations   PE
Congenital malformation of cornea NOS
Microcornea
Peter's anomaly

Q13.5 **Blue sclera**   PE

✓5th Q13.8 Other congenital malformations of anterior segment of eye

▲ Q13.81 Rieger anomaly   PE
▶Axenfeld-Rieger syndrome◀
▶Code also any other associated congenital malformations such as cardiac defects◀
Use additional code for associated glaucoma (H42)

Q13.89 Other congenital malformations of anterior segment of eye   PE

Q13.9 Congenital malformation of anterior segment of eye, unspecified   PE

✓4th **Q14** Congenital malformations of **posterior segment of eye**

EXCLUDES 2   optic nerve hypoplasia (H47.03-)

Q14.0 Congenital malformation of **vitreous humor**   PE
Congenital vitreous opacity

Q14.1 Congenital malformation of **retina**   PE
Congenital retinal aneurysm

Q14.2 Congenital malformation of **optic disc**   PE
Coloboma of optic disc

Q14.3 Congenital malformation of **choroid**   PE

Q14.8 Other congenital malformations of posterior segment of eye   PE
Coloboma of the fundus

Q14.9 Congenital malformation of posterior segment of eye, unspecified   PE

✓4th **Q15** Other congenital malformations of **eye**

EXCLUDES 1   congenital nystagmus (H55.01)
ocular albinism (E70.31-)
optic nerve hypoplasia (H47.03-)
retinitis pigmentosa (H35.52)

Q15.0 Congenital **glaucoma**   PE
Axenfeld's anomaly
Buphthalmos
Glaucoma of childhood
Glaucoma of newborn
Hydrophthalmos
Keratoglobus, congenital, with glaucoma
Macrocornea with glaucoma
Macrophthalmos in congenital glaucoma
Megalocornea with glaucoma

Q15.8 Other specified congenital malformations of eye   PE

Q15.9 Congenital malformation of eye, unspecified   PE
Congenital anomaly of eye
Congenital deformity of eye

✓4th **Q16** Congenital malformations of **ear causing impairment of hearing**

EXCLUDES 1   congenital deafness (H90.-)

Q16.0 Congenital absence of (ear) **auricle**   PE

Q16.1 Congenital absence, **atresia and stricture of auditory canal (external)**   PE
Congenital atresia or stricture of osseous meatus

Q16.2 Absence of **eustachian tube**   PE

Q16.3 Congenital malformation of **ear ossicles**   PE
Congenital fusion of ear ossicles

Q16.4 Other congenital malformations of middle ear   PE
Congenital malformation of middle ear NOS

Q16.5 Congenital malformation of **inner ear**   PE
Congenital anomaly of membranous labyrinth
Congenital anomaly of organ of Corti

Q16.9 Congenital malformation of ear causing impairment of hearing, unspecified   PE
Congenital absence of ear NOS

✓4th **Q17** Other congenital malformations of **ear**

EXCLUDES 1   congenital malformations of ear with impairment of hearing (Q16.0-Q16.9)
preauricular sinus (Q18.1)

Q17.0 **Accessory auricle**   PE
Accessory tragus
Polyotia
Preauricular appendage or tag
Supernumerary ear
Supernumerary lobule

Q17.1 **Macrotia**   PE
DEF: Birth defect characterized by abnormal enlargement of the pinna of the ear.

Q17.2 **Microtia**   PE

Q17.3 **Other misshapen ear**   PE
Pointed ear

Q17.4 **Misplaced ear**   PE
Low-set ears
EXCLUDES 1   cervical auricle (Q18.2)

Q17.5 **Prominent ear**   PE
Bat ear

Q17.8 Other specified congenital malformations of ear   PE
Congenital absence of lobe of ear

Q17.9 Congenital malformation of ear, unspecified   PE
Congenital anomaly of ear NOS

✓4th **Q18** Other congenital malformations of **face and neck**

EXCLUDES 1   cleft lip and cleft palate (Q35-Q37)
conditions classified to Q67.0-Q67.4
congenital malformations of skull and face bones (Q75.-)
cyclopia (Q87.0)
dentofacial anomalies [including malocclusion] (M26.-)
malformation syndromes affecting facial appearance (Q87.0)
persistent thyroglossal duct (Q89.2)

Q18.0 Sinus, fistula and cyst of branchial cleft   PE
Branchial vestige

Q18.1 Preauricular sinus and cyst   PE
Cervicoaural fistula
Fistula of auricle, congenital

Q18.2 Other branchial cleft malformations `PE`
Branchial cleft malformation NOS
Cervical auricle
Otocephaly

Q18.3 Webbing of neck `PE`
Pterygium colli
DEF: Congenital malformation characterized by a thick, triangular skinfold that stretches from the lateral side of the neck across the shoulder. It is associated with genetic conditions such as Turner's and Noonan's syndromes.

Q18.4 Macrostomia `PE`
DEF: Rare congenital craniofacial bilateral or unilateral anomaly of the mouth due to malformed maxillary and mandibular processes. It results in an abnormally large mouth extending toward the ear.

Q18.5 Microstomia `PE`

Q18.6 Macrocheilia `PE`
Hypertrophy of lip, congenital

Q18.7 Microcheilia `PE`

Q18.8 Other specified congenital malformations of face and neck `PE`
Medial cyst of face and neck
Medial fistula of face and neck
Medial sinus of face and neck

Q18.9 Congenital malformation of face and neck, unspecified `PE`
Congenital anomaly NOS of face and neck

Congenital malformations of the circulatory system (Q20-Q28)

`✓4ᵗʰ` **Q20 Congenital malformations of cardiac chambers and connections**
  `EXCLUDES 1` *dextrocardia with situs inversus (Q89.3)*
              mirror-image atrial arrangement with situs inversus (Q89.3)

Q20.0 Common arterial trunk `MCC` `PE`
Persistent truncus arteriosus
  `EXCLUDES 1` *aortic septal defect (Q21.4)*

Q20.1 Double outlet right ventricle `MCC` `PE`
Taussig-Bing syndrome

Q20.2 Double outlet left ventricle `MCC` `PE`

Q20.3 Discordant ventriculoarterial connection `MCC` `PE`
Dextrotransposition of aorta
Transposition of great vessels (complete)

Q20.4 Double inlet ventricle `MCC` `PE`
Common ventricle
Cor triloculare biatriatum
Single ventricle

Q20.5 Discordant atrioventricular connection `CC` `PE`
Corrected transposition
Levotransposition
Ventricular inversion

Q20.6 Isomerism of atrial appendages `PE`
Isomerism of atrial appendages with asplenia or polysplenia

Q20.8 Other congenital malformations of cardiac chambers and connections `PE`
Cor binoculare

Q20.9 Congenital malformation of cardiac chambers and connections, unspecified `PE`

`✓4ᵗʰ` **Q21 Congenital malformations of cardiac septa**
  `EXCLUDES 1` *acquired cardiac septal defect (I51.0)*

Q21.0 Ventricular septal defect `CC` `PE`
Roger's disease

Ventricular Septal Defect

`✓5ᵗʰ` **Q21.1 Atrial septal defect**
  `EXCLUDES 2` *ostium primum atrial septal defect (type I) (Q21.20)*
  AHA: 2022,4Q,39-40

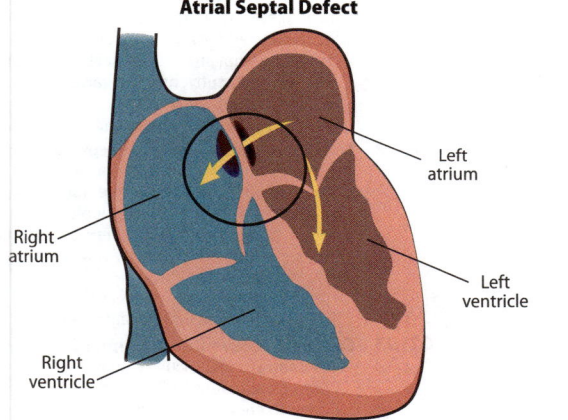

Atrial Septal Defect

Left atrium

Right atrium

Left ventricle

Right ventricle

Q21.10 Atrial septal defect, unspecified `CC` `PE`

Q21.11 Secundum atrial septal defect `CC` `PE`
Fenestrated atrial septum
Patent or persistent ostium secundum defect (type II)

Q21.12 Patent foramen ovale `CC` `PE`
Persistent foramen ovale

Q21.13 Coronary sinus atrial septal defect `CC` `PE`
Coronary sinus defect
Unroofed coronary sinus

Q21.14 Superior sinus venosus atrial septal defect `CC` `PE`
Superior vena cava type atrial septal defect

Q21.15 Inferior sinus venosus atrial septal defect `CC` `PE`
Inferior vena cava type atrial septal defect

Q21.16 Sinus venosus atrial septal defect, unspecified `CC` `PE`
Sinus venosus defect, NOS

Q21.19 Other specified atrial septal defect `CC` `PE`
Common atrium
Other specified atrial septal abnormality

☑ Additional Character Required   ✓x 7ᵗʰ Placeholder   Questionable PDx   Manifestation   Unspecified   UPD Unacceptable PDx   H1-H14 HAC   HCC CMS-HCC Dx   HIV HIV Dx

ICD-10-CM 2025   937

√5ᵗʰ **Q21.2** **Atrioventricular** septal defect
Atrioventricular canal defect
Endocardial cushion defect
Ostium primum atrial septal defect (type I)
AHA: 2022,4Q,39-40

Atrioventricular Septal Defect

Q21.20 **Atrioventricular septal defect, unspecified as to partial or complete** CC PE
Atrioventricular canal, NOS
Endocardial cushion defect NOS
Ostium primum atrial septal defect (type I) NOS

Q21.21 **Partial** atrioventricular septal defect CC PE
Incomplete atrioventricular canal
Incomplete atrioventricular septal defect
Incomplete endocardial cushion defect
Ostium primum atrial septal defect (type I) with separate atrioventricular valves
Partial atrioventricular canal
Partial endocardial cushion defect

Q21.22 **Transitional** atrioventricular septal defect CC PE
Intermediate atrioventricular canal
Intermediate atrioventricular septal defect
Intermediate endocardial cushion defect
Ostium primum atrial septal defect (type I) with separate atrioventricular valves and a small or restrictive inlet VSD
Transitional atrioventricular canal
Transitional endocardial cushion defect

Q21.23 **Complete** atrioventricular septal defect CC PE
Common atrioventricular canal
Common atrioventricular septal defect
Common endocardial cushion defect
Ostium primum atrial septal defect (type I) with common atrioventricular valve and a moderate or larger inlet VSD

Q21.3 **Tetralogy of Fallot** MCC PE
Ventricular septal defect with pulmonary stenosis or atresia, dextroposition of aorta and hypertrophy of right ventricle.
AHA: 2014,3Q,16

Q21.4 **Aortopulmonary** septal defect PE
Aortic septal defect
Aortopulmonary window

Q21.8 **Other congenital malformations of cardiac septa** PE
Eisenmenger's defect
Pentalogy of Fallot
Code also, if applicable:
Eisenmenger's complex (I27.83)
Eisenmenger's syndrome (I27.83)

Q21.9 **Congenital malformation of cardiac septum, unspecified** PE
Septal (heart) defect NOS

√4ᵗʰ **Q22** **Congenital malformations of pulmonary and tricuspid valves**

Q22.0 **Pulmonary** valve atresia MCC PE

Q22.1 **Congenital pulmonary valve stenosis** CC PE

Q22.2 **Congenital pulmonary valve insufficiency** CC PE
Congenital pulmonary valve regurgitation
AHA: 2022,4Q,39-40

Q22.3 **Other congenital malformations of pulmonary valve** CC PE
Congenital malformation of pulmonary valve NOS
Supernumerary cusps of pulmonary valve

Q22.4 **Congenital tricuspid stenosis** MCC PE
Congenital tricuspid atresia

Q22.5 **Ebstein's anomaly** MCC PE
DEF: Malformation of the tricuspid valve characterized by septal and posterior leaflets attaching to the wall of the right ventricle. Ebstein's anomaly causes the right ventricle to fuse with the atrium into a large right atrium and a small ventricle and leads to heart failure and abnormal cardiac rhythm.

Q22.6 **Hypoplastic right heart syndrome** MCC PE

Q22.8 **Other congenital malformations of tricuspid valve** MCC PE

Q22.9 **Congenital malformation of tricuspid valve, unspecified** MCC PE

√4ᵗʰ **Q23** **Congenital malformations of aortic and mitral valves**

Q23.0 **Congenital stenosis of aortic valve** CC PE
Congenital aortic atresia
Congenital aortic stenosis NOS
EXCLUDES 1 congenital stenosis of aortic valve in hypoplastic left heart syndrome (Q23.4)
congenital subaortic stenosis (Q24.4)
supravalvular aortic stenosis (congenital) (Q25.3)

Q23.1 **Congenital insufficiency of aortic valve** CC PE
~~Bicuspid aortic valve~~
Congenital aortic insufficiency

Q23.2 **Congenital mitral stenosis** CC PE
Congenital mitral atresia

Q23.3 **Congenital mitral insufficiency** CC PE

Q23.4 **Hypoplastic left heart syndrome** MCC PE

▲ √5ᵗʰ **Q23.8** **Other congenital malformations of aortic and mitral valves**

● **Q23.81** **Bicuspid aortic valve** PE
Congenital bicuspid aortic valve
Unicuspid (congenital) aortic valve (at birth)
Code also, if applicable, acquired aortic valve disorders, such as:
aortic (valve) insufficiency (nonrheumatic) (I35.1)
aortic (valve) stenosis (nonrheumatic) (I35.0)
aortic (valve) stenosis with insufficiency (nonrheumatic) (I35.2)

● **Q23.82** **Congenital mitral valve cleft leaflet** PE
Cleft mitral valve leaflet at birth

● **Q23.88** **Other congenital malformations of aortic and mitral valves** PE

Q23.9 **Congenital malformation of aortic and mitral valves, unspecified** PE

√4ᵗʰ **Q24** **Other congenital malformations of heart**
EXCLUDES 1 endocardial fibroelastosis (I42.4)

Q24.0 **Dextrocardia** CC PE
EXCLUDES 1 dextrocardia with situs inversus (Q89.3)
isomerism of atrial appendages (with asplenia or polysplenia) (Q20.6)
mirror-image atrial arrangement with situs inversus (Q89.3)
DEF: Congenital condition in which the heart is located on the right side of the chest rather than in its normal position on the left.

Q24.1 **Levocardia** CC PE

Q24.2 **Cor triatriatum** MCC PE

Q24.3 **Pulmonary infundibular stenosis** CC PE
Subvalvular pulmonic stenosis

Q24.4 **Congenital subaortic stenosis** MCC PE
DEF: Congenital heart defect characterized by stenosis of the left ventricular outflow tract due to a fibrous tissue ring or septal hypertrophy below the aortic valve.

Q24.5 **Malformation of coronary vessels** CC PE
Congenital coronary (artery) aneurysm

Q24.6 **Congenital heart block** MCC PE

Q24.8 **Other specified congenital malformations of heart** PE
Congenital diverticulum of left ventricle
Congenital malformation of myocardium
Congenital malformation of pericardium
Malposition of heart
Uhl's disease

Q24.9 **Congenital malformation of heart, unspecified** PE
Congenital anomaly of heart
Congenital disease of heart

☑4th **Q25 Congenital malformations of great arteries**

Q25.0 Patent ductus arteriosus `CC` `PE`
Patent ductus Botallo
Persistent ductus arteriosus
DEF: Condition in which the normal channel between the pulmonary artery and the aorta fails to close at birth, causing arterial blood to recirculate in the lungs and inhibiting the blood supply to the aorta. **Synonym(s):** PDA.

Q25.1 Coarctation of aorta `CC` `PE`
Coarctation of aorta (preductal) (postductal)
Stenosis of aorta
AHA: 2016,4Q,56-57

☑5th **Q25.2 Atresia of aorta**
AHA: 2016,4Q,56-57

Q25.21 Interruption of aortic arch `CC` `PE`
Atresia of aortic arch

Q25.29 Other atresia of aorta `CC` `PE`
Atresia of aorta

Q25.3 Supravalvular aortic stenosis `CC` `PE`
EXCLUDES 1   congenital aortic stenosis NOS (Q23.0)
congenital stenosis of aortic valve (Q23.0)

☑5th **Q25.4 Other congenital malformations of aorta**
EXCLUDES 1   hypoplasia of aorta in hypoplastic left heart syndrome (Q23.4)
AHA: 2016,4Q,57

Q25.40 Congenital malformation of aorta unspecified `CC` `PE`

Q25.41 Absence and aplasia of aorta `CC` `PE`

Q25.42 Hypoplasia of aorta `CC` `PE`

Q25.43 Congenital aneurysm of aorta `CC` `PE`
Congenital aneurysm of aortic root
Congenital aneurysm of aortic sinus

Q25.44 Congenital dilation of aorta `CC` `PE`

Q25.45 Double aortic arch
Vascular ring of aorta

Aortic Arch Anomalies

Normal aortic arch

Double aortic arch   Right aortic arch

Q25.46 Tortuous aortic arch `CC` `PE`
Persistent convolutions of aortic arch

Q25.47 Right aortic arch `CC` `PE`
Persistent right aortic arch

Q25.48 Anomalous origin of subclavian artery `CC` `PE`

Q25.49 Other congenital malformations of aorta `CC` `PE`
Aortic arch
Bovine arch

Q25.5 Atresia of pulmonary artery `MCC` `PE`

Q25.6 Stenosis of pulmonary artery `MCC` `PE`
Supravalvular pulmonary stenosis

☑5th **Q25.7 Other congenital malformations of pulmonary artery**

Q25.71 Coarctation of pulmonary artery `MCC` `PE`

Q25.72 Congenital pulmonary arteriovenous malformation `MCC` `PE`
Congenital pulmonary arteriovenous aneurysm

Q25.79 Other congenital malformations of pulmonary artery `MCC` `PE`
Aberrant pulmonary artery
Agenesis of pulmonary artery
Congenital aneurysm of pulmonary artery
Congenital anomaly of pulmonary artery
Hypoplasia of pulmonary artery

Q25.8 Other congenital malformations of other great arteries `CC` `PE`

Q25.9 Congenital malformation of great arteries, unspecified `CC` `PE`

☑4th **Q26 Congenital malformations of great veins**

Q26.0 Congenital stenosis of vena cava `CC` `PE`
Congenital stenosis of vena cava (inferior)(superior)

Q26.1 Persistent left superior vena cava `CC` `PE`

Q26.2 Total anomalous pulmonary venous connection `CC` `PE`
Total anomalous pulmonary venous return [TAPVR], subdiaphragmatic
Total anomalous pulmonary venous return [TAPVR], supradiaphragmatic

Q26.3 Partial anomalous pulmonary venous connection `CC` `PE`
Partial anomalous pulmonary venous return

Q26.4 Anomalous pulmonary venous connection, unspecified `CC` `PE`

Q26.5 Anomalous portal venous connection `PE`

Q26.6 Portal vein-hepatic artery fistula `PE`

Q26.8 Other congenital malformations of great veins `CC` `PE`
Absence of vena cava (inferior) (superior)
Azygos continuation of inferior vena cava
Persistent left posterior cardinal vein
Scimitar syndrome

Q26.9 Congenital malformation of great vein, unspecified `CC` `PE`
Congenital anomaly of vena cava (inferior) (superior) NOS

☑4th **Q27 Other congenital malformations of peripheral vascular system**
EXCLUDES 2   anomalies of cerebral and precerebral vessels (Q28.0-Q28.3)
anomalies of coronary vessels (Q24.5)
anomalies of pulmonary artery (Q25.5-Q25.7)
congenital retinal aneurysm (Q14.1)
hemangioma and lymphangioma (D18.-)

Q27.0 Congenital absence and hypoplasia of umbilical artery `PE`
Single umbilical artery

Q27.1 Congenital renal artery stenosis `PE`

Q27.2 Other congenital malformations of renal artery `PE`
Congenital malformation of renal artery NOS
Multiple renal arteries

☑5th **Q27.3 Arteriovenous malformation (peripheral)**
Arteriovenous aneurysm
EXCLUDES 1   acquired arteriovenous aneurysm (I77.0)
EXCLUDES 2   arteriovenous malformation of cerebral vessels (Q28.2)
arteriovenous malformation of precerebral vessels (Q28.0)
DEF: Arteriovenous malformation: Connecting passage between an artery and a vein.

Q27.30 Arteriovenous malformation, site unspecified `CC` `PE`

Q27.31 Arteriovenous malformation of vessel of upper limb `PE`

Q27.32 Arteriovenous malformation of vessel of lower limb `PE`

Q27.33 Arteriovenous malformation of digestive system vessel `PE`
AHA: 2018,3Q,21

Q27.34 Arteriovenous malformation of renal vessel `PE`

Q27.39 Arteriovenous malformation, other site `PE`

Q27.4 Congenital phlebectasia `CC` `PE`

Q27.8 Other specified congenital malformations of peripheral vascular system `PE`
Absence of peripheral vascular system
Atresia of peripheral vascular system
Congenital aneurysm (peripheral)
Congenital stricture, artery
Congenital varix
EXCLUDES 1   arteriovenous malformation (Q27.3-)

✓ Additional Character Required   ✓x7th Placeholder   Questionable PDx   Manifestation   Unspecified   `UPD` Unacceptable PDx   `H1`-`H14` HAC   `HCC` CMS-HCC Dx   `HIV` HIV Dx

ICD-10-CM 2025   **939**

Q27.9 Congenital malformation of peripheral vascular system, unspecified `PE`
Anomaly of artery or vein NOS

✓4th Q28 Other congenital malformations of circulatory system

EXCLUDES 1   congenital aneurysm NOS (Q27.8)
congenital coronary aneurysm (Q24.5)
ruptured cerebral arteriovenous malformation (I60.8)
ruptured malformation of precerebral vessels (I72.0)

EXCLUDES 2   congenital peripheral aneurysm (Q27.8)
congenital pulmonary aneurysm (Q25.79)
congenital retinal aneurysm (Q14.1)

Q28.0 Arteriovenous malformation of precerebral vessels `CC` `PE`
Congenital arteriovenous precerebral aneurysm (nonruptured)

Q28.1 Other malformations of precerebral vessels `CC` `PE`
Congenital malformation of precerebral vessels NOS
Congenital precerebral aneurysm (nonruptured)

Q28.2 Arteriovenous malformation of cerebral vessels `MCC` `PE`
Arteriovenous malformation of brain NOS
Congenital arteriovenous cerebral aneurysm (nonruptured)

Q28.3 Other malformations of cerebral vessels `MCC` `PE`
Congenital cerebral aneurysm (nonruptured)
Congenital malformation of cerebral vessels NOS
Developmental venous anomaly

Q28.8 Other specified congenital malformations of circulatory system `CC` `PE`
Congenital aneurysm, specified site NEC
Spinal vessel anomaly

Q28.9 Congenital malformation of circulatory system, unspecified `CC` `PE`

Congenital malformations of the respiratory system (Q30-Q34)

✓4th Q30 Congenital malformations of nose

EXCLUDES 1   congenital deviation of nasal septum (Q67.4)

Q30.0 Choanal atresia `PE`
Atresia of nares (anterior) (posterior)
Congenital stenosis of nares (anterior) (posterior)

Q30.1 Agenesis and underdevelopment of nose `PE`
Congenital absent of nose

Q30.2 Fissured, notched and cleft nose `PE`

Q30.3 Congenital perforated nasal septum `PE`

Q30.8 Other congenital malformations of nose `PE`
Accessory nose
Congenital anomaly of nasal sinus wall
AHA: 2022,2Q,17

Q30.9 Congenital malformation of nose, unspecified `PE`

✓4th Q31 Congenital malformations of larynx

EXCLUDES 1   congenital laryngeal stridor NOS (P28.89)

Q31.0 Web of larynx `PE`
Glottic web of larynx
Subglottic web of larynx
Web of larynx NOS
DEF: Congenital malformation of the larynx marked by thin, translucent, or thick fibrotic membrane-like structure between the vocal folds. It is characterized by shortness of breath and stridor.

Q31.1 Congenital subglottic stenosis `CC` `PE`

Q31.2 Laryngeal hypoplasia `CC` `PE`

Q31.3 Laryngocele `CC` `PE`

Q31.5 Congenital laryngomalacia `CC` `PE`

Q31.8 Other congenital malformations of larynx `CC` `PE`
Absence of larynx
Agenesis of larynx
Atresia of larynx
Congenital cleft thyroid cartilage
Congenital fissure of epiglottis
Congenital stenosis of larynx NEC
Posterior cleft of cricoid cartilage

Q31.9 Congenital malformation of larynx, unspecified `CC` `PE`

✓4th Q32 Congenital malformations of trachea and bronchus

EXCLUDES 1   congenital bronchiectasis (Q33.4)

Q32.0 Congenital tracheomalacia `CC` `PE`

Q32.1 Other congenital malformations of trachea `CC` `PE`
Atresia of trachea
Congenital anomaly of tracheal cartilage
Congenital dilatation of trachea
Congenital malformation of trachea
Congenital stenosis of trachea
Congenital tracheocele

Q32.2 Congenital bronchomalacia `CC` `PE`

Q32.3 Congenital stenosis of bronchus `CC` `PE`

Q32.4 Other congenital malformations of bronchus `CC` `PE`
Absence of bronchus
Agenesis of bronchus
Atresia of bronchus
Congenital diverticulum of bronchus
Congenital malformation of bronchus NOS

✓4th Q33 Congenital malformations of lung

Q33.0 Congenital cystic lung `CC` `PE`
Congenital cystic lung disease
Congenital honeycomb lung
Congenital polycystic lung disease
EXCLUDES 1   cystic fibrosis (E84.0)
cystic lung disease, acquired or unspecified (J98.4)

Q33.1 Accessory lobe of lung `PE`
Azygos lobe (fissured), lung

Q33.2 Sequestration of lung `MCC` `PE`

Q33.3 Agenesis of lung `MCC` `PE`
Congenital absence of lung (lobe)

Q33.4 Congenital bronchiectasis `CC` `PE`

Q33.5 Ectopic tissue in lung `PE`

Q33.6 Congenital hypoplasia and dysplasia of lung `MCC` `PE`
EXCLUDES 1   pulmonary hypoplasia associated with short gestation (P28.0)

Q33.8 Other congenital malformations of lung `PE`

Q33.9 Congenital malformation of lung, unspecified `PE`

✓4th Q34 Other congenital malformations of respiratory system

EXCLUDES 2   congenital central alveolar hypoventilation syndrome (G47.35)

Q34.0 Anomaly of pleura `PE`

Q34.1 Congenital cyst of mediastinum `PE`

Q34.8 Other specified congenital malformations of respiratory system `PE`
Atresia of nasopharynx

Q34.9 Congenital malformation of respiratory system, unspecified `PE`
Congenital absence of respiratory system
Congenital anomaly of respiratory system NOS

Cleft lip and cleft palate (Q35-Q37)

Use additional code to identify associated malformation of the nose (Q30.2)
EXCLUDES 2   Robin's syndrome (Q87.0)

✓4th Q35 Cleft palate

INCLUDES   fissure of palate
palatoschisis
EXCLUDES 1   cleft palate with cleft lip (Q37.-)
DEF: Congenital fissure or defect of the roof of the mouth opening to the nasal cavity due to failure of embryonic cells to fuse completely.

Cleft Palate

Cleft in soft palate   Cleft in hard and soft palate

Hard palate
Soft palate
Cleft

Q35.1 Cleft hard palate `PE`

Q35.3 Cleft soft palate `PE`

Q35.5 Cleft hard palate with cleft soft palate `PE`

Q35.7 Cleft uvula `PE`

Q35.9 Cleft palate, unspecified `PE`
Cleft palate NOS

✓4ᵗʰ Q36 Cleft lip

INCLUDES cheiloschisis
congenital fissure of lip
harelip
labium leporinum

EXCLUDES 1 cleft lip with cleft palate (Q37.-)

DEF: Congenital fissure or opening in the upper lip due to failure of embryonic cells to fuse completely.

Cleft Lip

Unilateral incomplete

Unilateral complete

Bilateral complete

Q36.Ø **Cleft lip, bilateral**   PE
Q36.1 **Cleft lip, median**   PE
Q36.9 **Cleft lip, unilateral**   PE
          Cleft lip NOS

✓4ᵗʰ Q37 Cleft palate with cleft lip

INCLUDES cheilopalatoschisis

Q37.Ø **Cleft hard palate with bilateral cleft lip**   PE
Q37.1 **Cleft hard palate with unilateral cleft lip** PE
          Cleft hard palate with cleft lip NOS
Q37.2 **Cleft soft palate with bilateral cleft lip**   PE
Q37.3 **Cleft soft palate with unilateral cleft lip** PE
          Cleft soft palate with cleft lip NOS
Q37.4 **Cleft hard and soft palate with bilateral cleft lip**   PE
Q37.5 **Cleft hard and soft palate with unilateral cleft lip** PE
          Cleft hard and soft palate with cleft lip NOS
Q37.8 **Unspecified cleft palate with bilateral cleft lip**   PE
Q37.9 **Unspecified cleft palate with unilateral cleft lip**   PE
          Cleft palate with cleft lip NOS

Other congenital malformations of the digestive system (Q38-Q45)

✓4ᵗʰ Q38 Other congenital malformations of tongue, mouth and pharynx

EXCLUDES 1 dentofacial anomalies (M26.-)
macrostomia (Q18.4)
microstomia (Q18.5)

Q38.Ø **Congenital malformations of lips, not elsewhere classified**   PE
          Congenital fistula of lip
          Congenital malformation of lip NOS
          Van der Woude's syndrome
          EXCLUDES 1 cleft lip (Q36.-)
                      cleft lip with cleft palate (Q37.-)
                      macrocheilia (Q18.6)
                      microcheilia (Q18.7)

Q38.1 **Ankyloglossia**   PE
          Tongue tie
Q38.2 **Macroglossia**   PE
          Congenital hypertrophy of tongue
Q38.3 **Other congenital malformations of tongue**   PE
          Aglossia
          Bifid tongue
          Congenital adhesion of tongue
          Congenital fissure of tongue
          Congenital malformation of tongue NOS
          Double tongue
          Hypoglossia
          Hypoplasia of tongue
          Microglossia
Q38.4 **Congenital malformations of salivary glands and ducts**   PE
          Atresia of salivary glands and ducts
          Congenital absence of salivary glands and ducts
          Congenital accessory salivary glands and ducts
          Congenital fistula of salivary gland

Q38.5 **Congenital malformations of palate, not elsewhere classified**   PE
          Congenital absence of uvula
          Congenital high arched palate
          Congenital malformation of palate NOS
          EXCLUDES 1 cleft palate (Q35.-)
                      cleft palate with cleft lip (Q37.-)
Q38.6 **Other congenital malformations of mouth**   PE
          Congenital malformation of mouth NOS
Q38.7 **Congenital pharyngeal pouch**   PE
          Congenital diverticulum of pharynx
          EXCLUDES 1 pharyngeal pouch syndrome (D82.1)
Q38.8 **Other congenital malformations of pharynx**   PE
          Congenital malformation of pharynx NOS
          Imperforate pharynx

✓4ᵗʰ Q39 Congenital malformations of esophagus

Q39.Ø **Atresia of esophagus without fistula**   MCC PE
          Atresia of esophagus NOS
Q39.1 **Atresia of esophagus with tracheo-esophageal fistula**   MCC PE
          Atresia of esophagus with broncho-esophageal fistula
Q39.2 **Congenital tracheo-esophageal fistula without atresia**   MCC PE
          Congenital tracheo-esophageal fistula NOS
Q39.3 **Congenital stenosis and stricture of esophagus**   MCC PE
Q39.4 **Esophageal web**   MCC PE
Q39.5 **Congenital dilatation of esophagus**   CC PE
          Congenital cardiospasm
Q39.6 **Congenital diverticulum of esophagus**   CC PE
          Congenital esophageal pouch
Q39.8 **Other congenital malformations of esophagus**   CC PE
          Congenital absence of esophagus
          Congenital displacement of esophagus
          Congenital duplication of esophagus
Q39.9 **Congenital malformation of esophagus, unspecified**   CC PE

✓4ᵗʰ Q4Ø Other congenital malformations of upper alimentary tract

Q4Ø.Ø **Congenital hypertrophic pyloric stenosis**   HCC PE
          Congenital or infantile constriction
          Congenital or infantile hypertrophy
          Congenital or infantile spasm
          Congenital or infantile stenosis
          Congenital or infantile stricture
Q4Ø.1 **Congenital hiatus hernia**   PE
          Congenital displacement of cardia through esophageal hiatus
          EXCLUDES 1 congenital diaphragmatic hernia (Q79.Ø)
Q4Ø.2 **Other specified congenital malformations of stomach**   PE
          Congenital displacement of stomach
          Congenital diverticulum of stomach
          Congenital hourglass stomach
          Congenital duplication of stomach
          Megalogastria
          Microgastria
Q4Ø.3 **Congenital malformation of stomach, unspecified**   PE
Q4Ø.8 **Other specified congenital malformations of upper alimentary tract**   PE
Q4Ø.9 **Congenital malformation of upper alimentary tract, unspecified**   PE
          Congenital anomaly of upper alimentary tract
          Congenital deformity of upper alimentary tract

✓4ᵗʰ Q41 Congenital absence, atresia and stenosis of small intestine

INCLUDES congenital obstruction, occlusion or stricture of small intestine or intestine NOS

EXCLUDES 1 cystic fibrosis with intestinal manifestation (E84.11)
meconium ileus NOS (without cystic fibrosis) (P76.Ø)

Q41.Ø **Congenital absence, atresia and stenosis of duodenum**   CC HCC PE
Q41.1 **Congenital absence, atresia and stenosis of jejunum**   CC HCC PE
          Apple peel syndrome
          Imperforate jejunum
Q41.2 **Congenital absence, atresia and stenosis of ileum**   CC HCC PE
Q41.8 **Congenital absence, atresia and stenosis of other specified parts of small intestine**   CC HCC PE

✔ Additional Character Required   ✓x7ᵗʰ Placeholder   Questionable PDx   Manifestation   Unspecified   UPD Unacceptable PDx   H1-H14 HAC   HCC CMS-HCC Dx   HIV HIV Dx

ICD-10-CM 2025   941

Q41.9 **Congenital absence, atresia and stenosis of small intestine, part unspecified** `CC` `HCC` `PE`
Congenital absence, atresia and stenosis of intestine NOS

✓4th **Q42** **Congenital absence, atresia and stenosis of large intestine**

INCLUDES   congenital obstruction, occlusion and stricture of large intestine

Q42.0 **Congenital absence, atresia and stenosis of rectum with fistula** `CC` `HCC` `PE`

Q42.1 **Congenital absence, atresia and stenosis of rectum without fistula** `CC` `HCC` `PE`
Imperforate rectum

Q42.2 **Congenital absence, atresia and stenosis of anus with fistula** `CC` `HCC` `PE`

Q42.3 **Congenital absence, atresia and stenosis of anus without fistula** `CC` `HCC` `PE`
Imperforate anus

Q42.8 **Congenital absence, atresia and stenosis of other parts of large intestine** `CC` `HCC` `PE`

Q42.9 **Congenital absence, atresia and stenosis of large intestine, part unspecified** `CC` `HCC` `PE`

✓4th **Q43** **Other congenital malformations of intestine**

Q43.0 **Meckel's diverticulum (displaced) (hypertrophic)** `PE`
Persistent omphalomesenteric duct
Persistent vitelline duct
DEF: Congenital, abnormal remnant of embryonic digestive system development that leaves a sacculation or outpouching from the wall of the small intestine near the terminal part of the ileum made of acid-secreting tissue as in the stomach.

Q43.1 **Hirschsprung's disease** `CC` `HCC` `PE`
Aganglionosis
Congenital (aganglionic) megacolon
DEF: Congenital enlargement or dilation of the colon, with the absence of nerve cells in a segment of colon distally that causes the inability to defecate.

Q43.2 **Other congenital functional disorders of colon** `CC` `HCC` `PE`
Congenital dilatation of colon

Q43.3 **Congenital malformations of intestinal fixation** `CC` `HCC` `PE`
Congenital omental, anomalous adhesions [bands]
Congenital peritoneal adhesions [bands]
Incomplete rotation of cecum and colon
Insufficient rotation of cecum and colon
Jackson's membrane
Malrotation of colon
Rotation failure of cecum and colon
Universal mesentery

Q43.4 **Duplication of intestine** `CC` `PE`

Q43.5 **Ectopic anus** `CC` `PE`

Q43.6 **Congenital fistula of rectum and anus** `CC` `PE`
EXCLUDES 1   congenital fistula of anus with absence, atresia and stenosis (Q42.2)
congenital fistula of rectum with absence, atresia and stenosis (Q42.0)
congenital rectovaginal fistula (Q52.2)
congenital urethrorectal fistula (Q64.73)
pilonidal fistula or sinus (L05.-)

Q43.7 **Persistent cloaca** `CC` `PE`
Cloaca NOS

Q43.8 **Other specified congenital malformations of intestine** `CC` `PE`
Congenital blind loop syndrome
Congenital diverticulitis, colon
Congenital diverticulum, intestine
Dolichocolon
Megaloappendix
Megaloduodenum
Microcolon
Transposition of appendix
Transposition of colon
Transposition of intestine
AHA: 2013,2Q,31

Q43.9 **Congenital malformation of intestine, unspecified** `CC` `PE`

✓4th **Q44** **Congenital malformations of gallbladder, bile ducts and liver**

Q44.0 **Agenesis, aplasia and hypoplasia of gallbladder** `CC` `PE`
Congenital absence of gallbladder

Q44.1 **Other congenital malformations of gallbladder** `CC` `PE`
Congenital malformation of gallbladder NOS
Intrahepatic gallbladder

Q44.2 **Atresia of bile ducts** `MCC` `HCC` `PE`

Q44.3 **Congenital stenosis and stricture of bile ducts** `MCC` `HCC` `PE`

Q44.4 **Choledochal cyst** `CC` `PE`

Q44.5 **Other congenital malformations of bile ducts** `CC` `PE`
Accessory hepatic duct
Biliary duct duplication
Congenital malformation of bile duct NOS
Cystic duct duplication

Q44.6 **Cystic disease of liver** `CC` `PE`
Fibrocystic disease of liver

✓5th **Q44.7** **Other congenital malformations of liver**
Code also, if applicable, associated malformations affecting other systems
AHA: 2023,4Q,37-38

Q44.70 **Other congenital malformation of liver, unspecified** `CC` `PE`
Congenital malformation of liver, NOS

Q44.71 **Alagille syndrome** `CC` `HCC` `PE`
Alagille-Watson syndrome

Q44.79 **Other congenital malformations of liver** `CC` `PE`
Accessory liver
Congenital absence of liver
Congenital hepatomegaly

✓4th **Q45** **Other congenital malformations of digestive system**
EXCLUDES 2   congenital diaphragmatic hernia (Q79.0)
congenital hiatus hernia (Q40.1)

Q45.0 **Agenesis, aplasia and hypoplasia of pancreas** `CC` `PE`
Congenital absence of pancreas

Q45.1 **Annular pancreas** `CC` `PE`

Q45.2 **Congenital pancreatic cyst** `CC` `PE`

Q45.3 **Other congenital malformations of pancreas and pancreatic duct** `CC` `PE`
Accessory pancreas
Congenital malformation of pancreas or pancreatic duct NOS
EXCLUDES 1   congenital diabetes mellitus (E10.-)
cystic fibrosis (E84.0-E84.9)
fibrocystic disease of pancreas (E84.-)
neonatal diabetes mellitus (P70.2)

Q45.8 **Other specified congenital malformations of digestive system** `PE`
Absence (complete) (partial) of alimentary tract NOS
Duplication of digestive system
Malposition, congenital of digestive system

Q45.9 **Congenital malformation of digestive system, unspecified** `PE`
Congenital anomaly of digestive system
Congenital deformity of digestive system

Congenital malformations of genital organs (Q50-Q56)

EXCLUDES 1   androgen insensitivity syndrome (E34.5-)
syndromes associated with anomalies in the number and form of chromosomes (Q90-Q99)

✓4th **Q50** **Congenital malformations of ovaries, fallopian tubes and broad ligaments**

✓5th **Q50.0** **Congenital absence of ovary**
EXCLUDES 1   Turner's syndrome (Q96.-)

Q50.01 **Congenital absence of ovary, unilateral** `PE`

Q50.02 **Congenital absence of ovary, bilateral** `PE`

Q50.1 **Developmental ovarian cyst** `PE`

Q50.2 **Congenital torsion of ovary** `PE`

✓5th **Q50.3** **Other congenital malformations of ovary**

Q50.31 **Accessory ovary** `PE`

Q50.32 **Ovarian streak** `PE`
46, XX with streak gonads

Q50.39 **Other congenital malformation of ovary** `PE`
Congenital malformation of ovary NOS

Q50.4 **Embryonic cyst of fallopian tube** `PE`
Fimbrial cyst

Q50.5 **Embryonic cyst of broad ligament** `PE`
Epoophoron cyst
Parovarian cyst

`N` Newborn: 0   `P` Pediatric: 0-17   `M` Maternity: 9-64   `A` Adult: 15-124   `UNS` Unspecified Site   `MCC` Major Complication/Comorbidity   `CC` Complication/Comorbidity   `PE` POA Exempt

942   ICD-10-CM 2025

Q50.6 **Other congenital malformations of fallopian tube and broad ligament** `PE`
  Absence of fallopian tube and broad ligament
  Accessory fallopian tube and broad ligament
  Atresia of fallopian tube and broad ligament
  Congenital malformation of fallopian tube or broad ligament NOS

`✓4th` **Q51** **Congenital malformations of uterus and cervix**

Q51.0 **Agenesis and aplasia of uterus** `PE`
  Congenital absence of uterus

`✓5th` **Q51.1** **Doubling of uterus with doubling of cervix and vagina**

  Q51.10 **Doubling of uterus with doubling of cervix and vagina without obstruction** `PE`
    Doubling of uterus with doubling of cervix and vagina NOS

  Q51.11 **Doubling of uterus with doubling of cervix and vagina with obstruction** `PE`

`✓5th` **Q51.2** **Other doubling of uterus**
  Doubling of uterus NOS
  Septate uterus
  AHA: 2018,4Q,27

  Q51.21 **Complete doubling of uterus** `PE`
    Complete septate uterus

  Q51.22 **Partial doubling of uterus** `PE`
    Partial septate uterus

  Q51.28 **Other and unspecified doubling of uterus** `PE`
    Septate uterus NOS

Q51.3 **Bicornate uterus** `PE`
  Bicornate uterus, complete or partial

Q51.4 **Unicornate uterus** `PE`
  Unicornate uterus with or without a separate uterine horn
  Uterus with only one functioning horn

Q51.5 **Agenesis and aplasia of cervix** `PE`
  Congenital absence of cervix

Q51.6 **Embryonic cyst of cervix** `PE`

Q51.7 **Congenital fistulae between uterus and digestive and urinary tracts** `PE`

`✓5th` **Q51.8** **Other congenital malformations of uterus and cervix**

  `✓6th` **Q51.81** **Other congenital malformations of uterus**

    Q51.810 **Arcuate uterus** `PE`
      Arcuatus uterus

    Q51.811 **Hypoplasia of uterus** `PE`

    Q51.818 **Other congenital malformations of uterus** `PE`
      Mullerian anomaly of uterus NEC

  `✓6th` **Q51.82** **Other congenital malformations of cervix**

    Q51.820 **Cervical duplication** `PE`

    Q51.821 **Hypoplasia of cervix** `PE`

    Q51.828 **Other congenital malformations of cervix** `PE`

Q51.9 **Congenital malformation of uterus and cervix, unspecified** `PE`

`✓4th` **Q52** **Other congenital malformations of female genitalia**

Q52.0 **Congenital absence of vagina** `PE`
  Vaginal agenesis, total or partial

`✓5th` **Q52.1** **Doubling of vagina**
  EXCLUDES 1 *doubling of vagina with doubling of uterus and cervix (Q51.1-)*

  Q52.10 **Doubling of vagina, unspecified** `PE`
    Septate vagina NOS

  Q52.11 **Transverse vaginal septum** `PE`

  `✓6th` **Q52.12** **Longitudinal vaginal septum**
    AHA: 2016,4Q,58-59

    Q52.120 **Longitudinal vaginal septum, nonobstructing** `PE`

    Q52.121 **Longitudinal vaginal septum, obstructing, right side** `PE`

    Q52.122 **Longitudinal vaginal septum, obstructing, left side** `PE`

    Q52.123 **Longitudinal vaginal septum, microperforate, right side** `PE`

    Q52.124 **Longitudinal vaginal septum, microperforate, left side** `PE`

    Q52.129 **Other and unspecified longitudinal vaginal septum** `PE`

Q52.2 **Congenital rectovaginal fistula** `PE`
  EXCLUDES 1 *cloaca (Q43.7)*

Q52.3 **Imperforate hymen** `PE`
  DEF: Obstructive anomaly of vagina, characterized by complete closure of the membranous fold around the external opening of the vagina, obstructing the vaginal introitus.

Q52.4 **Other congenital malformations of vagina** `PE`
  Canal of Nuck cyst, congenital
  Congenital malformation of vagina NOS
  Embryonic vaginal cyst
  Gartner's duct cyst
  AHA: 2022,2Q,15

Q52.5 **Fusion of labia** `PE`

Q52.6 **Congenital malformation of clitoris** `PE`

`✓5th` **Q52.7** **Other and unspecified congenital malformations of vulva**

  Q52.70 **Unspecified congenital malformations of vulva** `PE`
    Congenital malformation of vulva NOS

  Q52.71 **Congenital absence of vulva** `PE`

  Q52.79 **Other congenital malformations of vulva** `PE`
    Congenital cyst of vulva

Q52.8 **Other specified congenital malformations of female genitalia** `PE`

Q52.9 **Congenital malformation of female genitalia, unspecified** `PE`

`✓4th` **Q53** **Undescended and ectopic testicle**

`✓5th` **Q53.0** **Ectopic testis**

  Q53.00 **Ectopic testis, unspecified** `PE`
  Q53.01 **Ectopic testis, unilateral** `PE`
  Q53.02 **Ectopic testes, bilateral** `PE`

`✓5th` **Q53.1** **Undescended testicle, unilateral**
  AHA: 2017,4Q,22-23

  Q53.10 **Unspecified undescended testicle, unilateral** `PE`

  `✓6th` **Q53.11** **Abdominal testis, unilateral**
    Q53.111 **Unilateral intraabdominal testis** `PE`
    Q53.112 **Unilateral inguinal testis** `PE`

  Q53.12 **Ectopic perineal testis, unilateral** `PE`
  Q53.13 **Unilateral high scrotal testis** `PE`

`✓5th` **Q53.2** **Undescended testicle, bilateral**
  AHA: 2017,4Q,22-23

  Q53.20 **Undescended testicle, unspecified, bilateral** `PE`

  `✓6th` **Q53.21** **Abdominal testis, bilateral**
    Q53.211 **Bilateral intraabdominal testes** `PE`
    Q53.212 **Bilateral inguinal testes** `PE`

  Q53.22 **Ectopic perineal testis, bilateral** `PE`
  Q53.23 **Bilateral high scrotal testes** `PE`

Q53.9 **Undescended testicle, unspecified** `PE`
  Cryptorchism NOS

`✓4th` **Q54** **Hypospadias**
  EXCLUDES 1 *epispadias (Q64.0)*
  DEF: Abnormal opening of the urethra on the ventral (underside) surface of the penis.

Hypospadias

Balanic (glanular, coronal) hypospadias
Subcoronal hypospadias
Penile hypospadias
Penile raphe
Scrotal hypospadias
Penoscrotal hypospadias
Scrotum
Scrotal raphe
Perineal hypospadias
Hypospadias (ventral view)

Q54.0 **Hypospadias, balanic** `PE`
  Hypospadias, coronal
  Hypospadias, glandular

Q54.1 **Hypospadias, penile** `PE`

Q54.2 **Hypospadias, penoscrotal** `PE`

Q54.3 **Hypospadias, perineal** `PE`

✓ Additional Character Required · `✓x7th` Placeholder · Questionable PDx · Manifestation · Unspecified · `UPD` Unacceptable PDx · `H1`-`H14` HAC · `HCC` CMS-HCC Dx · `HIV` HIV Dx

ICD-10-CM 2025

943

Q54.4 Congenital chordee `PE`
  Chordee without hypospadias

Q54.8 Other hypospadias `PE`
  Hypospadias with intersex state

Q54.9 Hypospadias, unspecified `PE`

`✓4th` **Q55 Other congenital malformations of male genital organs**
  EXCLUDES 1 congenital hydrocele (P83.5)
    hypospadias (Q54.-)

Q55.0 Absence and aplasia of testis `PE`
  Monorchism

Q55.1 Hypoplasia of testis and scrotum `PE`
  Fusion of testes

`✓5th` **Q55.2 Other and unspecified congenital malformations of testis and scrotum**

  Q55.20 Unspecified congenital malformations of testis and scrotum
    Congenital malformation of testis or scrotum NOS

  Q55.21 Polyorchism `PE`
    DEF: Congenital anomaly in which there are more than two testes.

  Q55.22 Retractile testis `PE`

  Q55.23 Scrotal transposition `PE`

  Q55.29 Other congenital malformations of testis and scrotum `PE`

Q55.3 Atresia of vas deferens `PE`
  Code first any associated cystic fibrosis (E84.-)

Q55.4 Other congenital malformations of vas deferens, epididymis, seminal vesicles and prostate `PE`
  Absence or aplasia of prostate
  Absence or aplasia of spermatic cord
  Congenital malformation of vas deferens, epididymis, seminal vesicles or prostate NOS

Q55.5 Congenital absence and aplasia of penis `PE`

`✓5th` **Q55.6 Other congenital malformations of penis**

  Q55.61 Curvature of penis (lateral) `PE`

  Q55.62 Hypoplasia of penis `PE`
    Micropenis

  Q55.63 Congenital torsion of penis `PE`
    EXCLUDES 1 acquired torsion of penis (N48.82)

  Q55.64 Hidden penis `PE`
    Buried penis
    Concealed penis
    EXCLUDES 1 acquired buried penis (N48.83)

  Q55.69 Other congenital malformation of penis `PE`
    Congenital malformation of penis NOS

Q55.7 Congenital vasocutaneous fistula `PE`

Q55.8 Other specified congenital malformations of male genital organs `PE`

Q55.9 Congenital malformation of male genital organ, unspecified `PE`
  Congenital anomaly of male genital organ
  Congenital deformity of male genital organ

`✓4th` **Q56 Indeterminate sex and pseudohermaphroditism**
  EXCLUDES 1 46, XX true hermaphrodite (Q99.1)
    androgen insensitivity syndrome (E34.5-)
    chimera 46, XX/46, XY true hermaphrodite (Q99.0)
    female pseudohermaphroditism with adrenocortical disorder (E25.-)
    pseudohermaphroditism with specified chromosomal anomaly (Q96-Q99)
    pure gonadal dysgenesis (Q99.1)
  DEF: Indeterminate sex: External genitalia that is nondescript, lacking the physical appearance specific to either sex.
  DEF: Pseudohermaphroditism: Presence of gonads of one sex and external genitalia of another sex.

Q56.0 Hermaphroditism, not elsewhere classified `PE`
  Ovotestis

Q56.1 Male pseudohermaphroditism, not elsewhere classified `PE`
  46, XY with streak gonads
  Male pseudohermaphroditism NOS

Q56.2 Female pseudohermaphroditism, not elsewhere classified `PE`
  Female pseudohermaphroditism NOS

Q56.3 Pseudohermaphroditism, unspecified

Q56.4 Indeterminate sex, unspecified `PE`
  Ambiguous genitalia

Congenital malformations of the urinary system (Q60-Q64)

`✓4th` **Q60 Renal agenesis and other reduction defects of kidney**
  INCLUDES congenital absence of kidney
    congenital atrophy of kidney
    infantile atrophy of kidney

Q60.0 Renal agenesis, unilateral `CC` `PE`

Q60.1 Renal agenesis, bilateral `CC` `PE`

Q60.2 Renal agenesis, unspecified `CC` `PE`

Q60.3 Renal hypoplasia, unilateral `CC` `PE`

Q60.4 Renal hypoplasia, bilateral `CC` `PE`

Q60.5 Renal hypoplasia, unspecified `CC` `PE`

Q60.6 Potter's syndrome `CC` `PE`

`✓4th` **Q61 Cystic kidney disease**
  EXCLUDES 1 acquired cyst of kidney (N28.1)
    Potter's syndrome (Q60.6)

`✓5th` **Q61.0 Congenital renal cyst**

  Q61.00 Congenital renal cyst, unspecified `CC` `PE`
    Cyst of kidney NOS (congenital)

  Q61.01 Congenital single renal cyst `CC` `PE`

  Q61.02 Congenital multiple renal cysts `CC` `PE`

`✓5th` **Q61.1 Polycystic kidney, infantile type**
  Polycystic kidney, autosomal recessive

  Q61.11 Cystic dilatation of collecting ducts `CC` `PE`

  Q61.19 Other polycystic kidney, infantile type `CC` `PE`

Q61.2 Polycystic kidney, adult type `CC` `PE`
  Polycystic kidney, autosomal dominant

Q61.3 Polycystic kidney, unspecified `CC` `PE`
  AHA: 2016,3Q,22

Q61.4 Renal dysplasia `CC` `PE`
  Multicystic dysplastic kidney
  Multicystic kidney (development)
  Multicystic kidney disease
  Multicystic renal dysplasia
  EXCLUDES 1 polycystic kidney disease (Q61.11-Q61.3)

Q61.5 Medullary cystic kidney `CC` `PE`
  Nephronophthisis
  Sponge kidney NOS
  DEF: Sponge kidney: Dilated collecting tubules that are usually asymptomatic. Calcinosis in tubules may cause renal insufficiency.

Q61.8 Other cystic kidney diseases `CC` `PE`
  Fibrocystic kidney
  Fibrocystic renal degeneration or disease

Q61.9 Cystic kidney disease, unspecified `CC` `PE`
  Meckel-Gruber syndrome

`✓4th` **Q62 Congenital obstructive defects of renal pelvis and congenital malformations of ureter**

Q62.0 Congenital hydronephrosis `CC` `PE`

`✓5th` **Q62.1 Congenital occlusion of ureter**
  Atresia and stenosis of ureter

  Q62.10 Congenital occlusion of ureter, unspecified `CC` `PE`

  Q62.11 Congenital occlusion of ureteropelvic junction `CC` `PE`

  Q62.12 Congenital occlusion of ureterovesical orifice `CC` `PE`

Q62.2 Congenital megaureter `CC` `PE`
  Congenital dilatation of ureter

`✓5th` **Q62.3 Other obstructive defects of renal pelvis and ureter**

  Q62.31 Congenital ureterocele, orthotopic `CC` `PE`

  Q62.32 Cecoureterocele `CC` `PE`
    Ectopic ureterocele

  Q62.39 Other obstructive defects of renal pelvis and ureter `CC` `PE`
    Ureteropelvic junction obstruction NOS

Q62.4 Agenesis of ureter `PE`
  Congenital absence ureter

Q62.5 Duplication of ureter `PE`
  Accessory ureter
  Double ureter

`✓5th` **Q62.6 Malposition of ureter**

  Q62.60 Malposition of ureter, unspecified `PE`

  Q62.61 Deviation of ureter `PE`

Q62.62   **Displacement** of ureter   `PE`

Q62.63   **Anomalous implantation** of ureter   `PE`
     Ectopia of ureter
     Ectopic ureter

Q62.69   **Other malposition** of ureter   `PE`

Q62.7   Congenital **vesico-uretero-renal reflux**   `PE`

Q62.8   Other congenital malformations of ureter   `PE`
     Anomaly of ureter NOS

√4th **Q63**   Other congenital malformations of **kidney**

     EXCLUDES 1   congenital nephrotic syndrome (N04.-)

Q63.0   **Accessory** kidney   `PE`

Q63.1   **Lobulated, fused and horseshoe** kidney   `PE`

Q63.2   **Ectopic** kidney   `PE`
     Congenital displaced kidney
     Malrotation of kidney

Q63.3   **Hyperplastic and giant** kidney   `PE`
     Compensatory hypertrophy of kidney

Q63.8   Other specified congenital malformations of kidney   `PE`
     Congenital renal calculi

Q63.9   Congenital malformation of kidney, unspecified   `PE`

√4th **Q64**   Other congenital malformations of **urinary system**

Q64.0   **Epispadias**   `PE`

     EXCLUDES 1   hypospadias (Q54.-)

Epispadias

Normal external urethral orifice

Glans penis

Foreskin (retracted)

Epispadias

Epispadias (dorsal view)

√5th Q64.1   **Exstrophy of urinary bladder**

Q64.10   Exstrophy of urinary bladder, unspecified   `CC` `PE`
     Ectopia vesicae

Q64.11   **Supravesical fissure** of urinary bladder   `CC` `PE`

Q64.12   **Cloacal exstrophy** of urinary bladder   `CC` `PE`

Q64.19   Other exstrophy of urinary bladder   `CC` `PE`
     Extroversion of bladder

Q64.2   Congenital **posterior urethral valves**   `CC` `PE`

√5th Q64.3   Other atresia and stenosis of **urethra and bladder neck**

Q64.31   Congenital **bladder neck obstruction**   `CC` `PE`
     Congenital obstruction of vesicourethral orifice

Q64.32   Congenital **stricture of urethra**   `CC` `PE`

Q64.33   Congenital **stricture of urinary meatus**   `CC` `PE`

Q64.39   Other atresia and stenosis of urethra and bladder neck   `CC` `PE`
     Atresia and stenosis of urethra and bladder neck NOS

Q64.4   Malformation of **urachus**   `PE`
     Cyst of urachus
     Patent urachus
     Prolapse of urachus

Q64.5   Congenital **absence of bladder and urethra**   `PE`

Q64.6   Congenital **diverticulum of bladder**   `PE`

√5th Q64.7   Other and unspecified congenital malformations of bladder and urethra

     EXCLUDES 1   congenital prolapse of bladder (mucosa) (Q79.4)

Q64.70   Unspecified congenital malformation of bladder and urethra   `PE`
     Malformation of bladder or urethra NOS

Q64.71   Congenital **prolapse** of **urethra**   `PE`

Q64.72   Congenital **prolapse** of **urinary meatus**   `PE`

Q64.73   Congenital **urethrorectal fistula**   `PE`

Q64.74   **Double urethra**   `PE`

Q64.75   **Double urinary meatus**   `PE`

Q64.79   Other congenital malformations of bladder and urethra   `PE`

Q64.8   Other specified congenital malformations of urinary system   `PE`

Q64.9   Congenital malformation of urinary system, unspecified   `PE`
     Congenital anomaly NOS of urinary system
     Congenital deformity NOS of urinary system

Congenital malformations and deformations of the musculoskeletal system (Q65-Q79)

√4th **Q65**   Congenital deformities of **hip**

     EXCLUDES 1   clicking hip (R29.4)

√5th Q65.0   Congenital **dislocation** of hip, **unilateral**

Q65.00   Congenital dislocation of unspecified hip, unilateral   `PE`

Q65.01   Congenital dislocation of **right** hip, unilateral   `PE`

Q65.02   Congenital dislocation of **left** hip, unilateral   `PE`

Q65.1   Congenital **dislocation** of hip, **bilateral**   `PE`

Q65.2   Congenital dislocation of hip, unspecified   `PE`

√5th Q65.3   Congenital **partial dislocation** of hip, **unilateral**

Q65.30   Congenital partial dislocation of unspecified hip, unilateral   `PE`

Q65.31   Congenital partial dislocation of **right** hip, unilateral   `PE`

Q65.32   Congenital partial dislocation of **left** hip, unilateral   `PE`

Q65.4   Congenital **partial dislocation** of hip, **bilateral**   `PE`

Q65.5   Congenital partial dislocation of hip, unspecified   `PE`

Q65.6   Congenital **unstable** hip   `PE`
     Congenital dislocatable hip

√5th Q65.8   Other congenital deformities of hip

Q65.81   Congenital **coxa valga**   `PE`

Q65.82   Congenital **coxa vara**   `PE`

Q65.89   Other specified congenital deformities of hip
     Anteversion of femoral neck
     Congenital acetabular dysplasia

Q65.9   Congenital deformity of hip, unspecified   `PE`

√4th **Q66**   Congenital deformities of **feet**

     EXCLUDES 1   reduction defects of feet (Q72.-)
                valgus deformities (acquired) (M21.0-)
                varus deformities (acquired) (M21.1-)

     AHA: 2019,4Q,13

√5th Q66.0   Congenital **talipes equinovarus**

Q66.00   Congenital talipes equinovarus, unspecified foot   `PE`

Q66.01   Congenital talipes equinovarus, **right** foot   `PE`

Q66.02   Congenital talipes equinovarus, **left** foot   `PE`

√5th Q66.1   Congenital **talipes calcaneovarus**

Q66.10   Congenital talipes calcaneovarus, unspecified foot   `PE`

Q66.11   Congenital talipes calcaneovarus, **right** foot   `PE`

Q66.12   Congenital talipes calcaneovarus, **left** foot   `PE`

√5th Q66.2   Congenital metatarsus (primus) varus

     AHA: 2016,4Q,59

√6th Q66.21   Congenital **metatarsus primus varus**

Q66.211   Congenital metatarsus primus varus, **right** foot   `PE`

Q66.212   Congenital metatarsus primus varus, **left** foot   `PE`

Q66.219   Congenital metatarsus primus varus, unspecified foot   `PE`

√6th Q66.22   Congenital **metatarsus adductus**
     Congenital metatarsus varus

Q66.221   Congenital metatarsus adductus, **right** foot   `PE`

Q66.222   Congenital metatarsus adductus, **left** foot   `PE`

Q66.229   Congenital metatarsus adductus, unspecified foot   `PE`

√5th Q66.3   Other congenital varus deformities of feet
     Hallux varus, congenital
     AHA: 2023,3Q,20

Q66.30   Other congenital varus deformities of feet, unspecified foot   `PE`

Q66.31   Other congenital varus deformities of feet, **right** foot   `PE`

Q66.32   Other congenital varus deformities of feet, **left** foot   `PE`

✓5ᵗʰ Q66.4   Congenital talipes calcaneovalgus

    Q66.40   Congenital talipes calcaneovalgus, unspecified foot   **PE**

    Q66.41   Congenital talipes calcaneovalgus, right foot   **PE**

    Q66.42   Congenital talipes calcaneovalgus, left foot   **PE**

✓5ᵗʰ Q66.5   Congenital pes planus

    Congenital flat foot
    Congenital rigid flat foot
    Congenital spastic (everted) flat foot

    EXCLUDES 1   pes planus, acquired (M21.4)

    Q66.50   Congenital pes planus, unspecified foot   **PE**

    Q66.51   Congenital pes planus, right foot   **PE**

    Q66.52   Congenital pes planus, left foot   **PE**

Q66.6   Other congenital valgus deformities of feet   **PE**

    Congenital metatarsus valgus

✓5ᵗʰ Q66.7   Congenital pes cavus

    Q66.70   Congenital pes cavus, unspecified foot   **PE**

    Q66.71   Congenital pes cavus, right foot   **PE**

    Q66.72   Congenital pes cavus, left foot   **PE**

✓5ᵗʰ Q66.8   Other congenital deformities of feet

    Q66.80   Congenital vertical talus deformity, unspecified foot   **PE**

    Q66.81   Congenital vertical talus deformity, right foot   **PE**

    Q66.82   Congenital vertical talus deformity, left foot   **PE**

    Q66.89   Other specified congenital deformities of feet   **PE**

    Congenital asymmetric talipes
    Congenital clubfoot NOS
    Congenital talipes NOS
    Congenital tarsal coalition
    Hammer toe, congenital

    DEF: Clubfoot: Congenital anomaly of the foot with the heel elevated and rotated outward and the toes pointing inward.

✓5ᵗʰ Q66.9   Congenital deformity of feet, unspecified

    Q66.90   Congenital deformity of feet, unspecified, unspecified foot   **PE**

    Q66.91   Congenital deformity of feet, unspecified, right foot   **PE**

    Q66.92   Congenital deformity of feet, unspecified, left foot   **PE**

✓4ᵗʰ Q67   Congenital musculoskeletal deformities of head, face, spine and chest

    EXCLUDES 1   congenital malformation syndromes classified to Q87.- Potter's syndrome (Q60.6)

Q67.0   Congenital facial asymmetry   **PE**

Q67.1   Congenital compression facies   **PE**

Q67.2   Dolichocephaly

    EXCLUDES 1   sagittal craniosynostosis (Q75.01)

Q67.3   Plagiocephaly

    EXCLUDES 1   coronal craniosynostosis (Q75.02-)
                lambdoid craniosynostosis (Q75.04-)

Q67.4   Other congenital deformities of skull, face and jaw   **PE**

    Congenital depressions in skull
    Congenital hemifacial atrophy or hypertrophy
    Deviation of nasal septum, congenital
    Squashed or bent nose, congenital

    EXCLUDES 1   dentofacial anomalies [including malocclusion] (M26.-)
                syphilitic saddle nose (A50.5)

    DEF: Deviated septum: Condition in which the nasal septum, a thin wall composed of cartilage and bone that separates the two nostrils, is crooked or displaced from the midline.

Q67.5   Congenital deformity of spine   **CC**   **PE**

    Congenital postural scoliosis
    Congenital scoliosis NOS

    EXCLUDES 1   infantile idiopathic scoliosis (M41.0)
                scoliosis due to congenital bony malformation (Q76.3)

    AHA: 2014,4Q,26

Q67.6   Pectus excavatum   **PE**

    Congenital funnel chest

Q67.7   Pectus carinatum   **PE**

    Congenital pigeon chest

Q67.8   Other congenital deformities of chest   **CC**   **PE**

    Congenital deformity of chest wall NOS

✓4ᵗʰ Q68   Other congenital musculoskeletal deformities

    EXCLUDES 1   reduction defects of limb(s) (Q71-Q73)
    EXCLUDES 2   congenital myotonic chondrodystrophy (G71.13)

Q68.0   Congenital deformity of sternocleidomastoid muscle   **PE**

    Congenital contracture of sternocleidomastoid (muscle)
    Congenital (sternomastoid) torticollis
    Sternomastoid tumor (congenital)

Q68.1   Congenital deformity of finger(s) and hand   **CC**   **PE**

    Congenital clubfinger
    Spade-like hand (congenital)

Q68.2   Congenital deformity of knee

    Congenital dislocation of knee
    Congenital genu recurvatum

Q68.3   Congenital bowing of femur   **PE**

    EXCLUDES 1   anteversion of femur (neck) (Q65.89)

Q68.4   Congenital bowing of tibia and fibula   **PE**

Q68.5   Congenital bowing of long bones of leg, unspecified   **PE**

Q68.6   Discoid meniscus   **PE**

Q68.8   Other specified congenital musculoskeletal deformities   **PE**

    Congenital deformity of clavicle
    Congenital deformity of elbow
    Congenital deformity of forearm
    Congenital deformity of scapula
    Congenital deformity of wrist
    Congenital dislocation of elbow
    Congenital dislocation of shoulder
    Congenital dislocation of wrist

✓4ᵗʰ Q69   Polydactyly

Q69.0   Accessory finger(s)   **PE**

Q69.1   Accessory thumb(s)   **PE**

Q69.2   Accessory toe(s)   **PE**

    Accessory hallux

Q69.9   Polydactyly, unspecified   **PE**

    Supernumerary digit(s) NOS

✓4ᵗʰ Q70   Syndactyly

✓5ᵗʰ Q70.0   Fused fingers

    Complex syndactyly of fingers with synostosis

    Q70.00   Fused fingers, unspecified hand   **PE**

    Q70.01   Fused fingers, right hand   **PE**

    Q70.02   Fused fingers, left hand   **PE**

    Q70.03   Fused fingers, bilateral   **PE**

✓5ᵗʰ Q70.1   Webbed fingers

    Simple syndactyly of fingers without synostosis

    Q70.10   Webbed fingers, unspecified hand   **PE**

    Q70.11   Webbed fingers, right hand   **PE**

    Q70.12   Webbed fingers, left hand   **PE**

    Q70.13   Webbed fingers, bilateral   **PE**

✓5ᵗʰ Q70.2   Fused toes

    Complex syndactyly of toes with synostosis

    Q70.20   Fused toes, unspecified foot   **PE**

    Q70.21   Fused toes, right foot   **PE**

    Q70.22   Fused toes, left foot   **PE**

    Q70.23   Fused toes, bilateral   **PE**

✓5ᵗʰ Q70.3   Webbed toes

    Simple syndactyly of toes without synostosis

    Q70.30   Webbed toes, unspecified foot   **PE**

    Q70.31   Webbed toes, right foot   **PE**

    Q70.32   Webbed toes, left foot   **PE**

    Q70.33   Webbed toes, bilateral   **PE**

Q70.4   Polysyndactyly, unspecified   **PE**

    EXCLUDES 1   specified syndactyly of hand and feet - code to specified conditions (Q70.0-Q70.3-)

Q70.9   Syndactyly, unspecified   **PE**

    Symphalangy NOS

✓4ᵗʰ Q71   Reduction defects of upper limb

✓5ᵗʰ Q71.0   Congenital complete absence of upper limb

    Q71.00   Congenital complete absence of unspecified upper limb   **PE**

    Q71.01   Congenital complete absence of right upper limb   **PE**

    Q71.02   Congenital complete absence of left upper limb   **PE**

    Q71.03   Congenital complete absence of upper limb, bilateral   **PE**

N Newborn: 0   **P** Pediatric: 0-17   **M** Maternity: 9-64   **A** Adult: 15-124   **UNS** Unspecified Site   **MCC** Major Complication/Comorbidity   **CC** Complication/Comorbidity   **PE** POA Exempt

946   ICD-10-CM 2025

✓5ᵗʰ **Q71.1** Congenital absence of upper arm and forearm with hand present

     Q71.10 Congenital absence of unspecified upper arm and forearm with hand present `PE`

     Q71.11 Congenital absence of right upper arm and forearm with hand present `PE`

     Q71.12 Congenital absence of left upper arm and forearm with hand present `PE`

     Q71.13 Congenital absence of upper arm and forearm with hand present, bilateral `PE`

✓5ᵗʰ **Q71.2** Congenital absence of both forearm and hand

     Q71.20 Congenital absence of both forearm and hand, unspecified upper limb `PE`

     Q71.21 Congenital absence of both forearm and hand, right upper limb `PE`

     Q71.22 Congenital absence of both forearm and hand, left upper limb `PE`

     Q71.23 Congenital absence of both forearm and hand, bilateral `PE`

✓5ᵗʰ **Q71.3** Congenital absence of hand and finger

     Q71.30 Congenital absence of unspecified hand and finger `PE`

     Q71.31 Congenital absence of right hand and finger `PE`

     Q71.32 Congenital absence of left hand and finger `PE`

     Q71.33 Congenital absence of hand and finger, bilateral `PE`

✓5ᵗʰ **Q71.4** Longitudinal reduction defect of radius
     Clubhand (congenital)
     Radial clubhand

     Q71.40 Longitudinal reduction defect of unspecified radius `PE`

     Q71.41 Longitudinal reduction defect of right radius `PE`

     Q71.42 Longitudinal reduction defect of left radius `PE`

     Q71.43 Longitudinal reduction defect of radius, bilateral `PE`

✓5ᵗʰ **Q71.5** Longitudinal reduction defect of ulna

     Q71.50 Longitudinal reduction defect of unspecified ulna `PE`

     Q71.51 Longitudinal reduction defect of right ulna `PE`

     Q71.52 Longitudinal reduction defect of left ulna `PE`

     Q71.53 Longitudinal reduction defect of ulna, bilateral `PE`

✓5ᵗʰ **Q71.6** Lobster-claw hand

     Q71.60 Lobster-claw hand, unspecified hand `PE`

     Q71.61 Lobster-claw right hand `PE`

     Q71.62 Lobster-claw left hand `PE`

     Q71.63 Lobster-claw hand, bilateral `PE`

✓5ᵗʰ **Q71.8** Other reduction defects of upper limb

     ✓6ᵗʰ **Q71.81** Congenital shortening of upper limb

         Q71.811 Congenital shortening of right upper limb `PE`

         Q71.812 Congenital shortening of left upper limb `PE`

         Q71.813 Congenital shortening of upper limb, bilateral `PE`

         Q71.819 Congenital shortening of unspecified upper limb `PE`

     ✓6ᵗʰ **Q71.89** Other reduction defects of upper limb

         Q71.891 Other reduction defects of right upper limb `PE`

         Q71.892 Other reduction defects of left upper limb `PE`

         Q71.893 Other reduction defects of upper limb, bilateral `PE`

         Q71.899 Other reduction defects of unspecified upper limb `PE`

✓5ᵗʰ **Q71.9** Unspecified reduction defect of upper limb

     Q71.90 Unspecified reduction defect of unspecified upper limb `PE`

     Q71.91 Unspecified reduction defect of right upper limb `PE`

     Q71.92 Unspecified reduction defect of left upper limb `PE`

     Q71.93 Unspecified reduction defect of upper limb, bilateral `PE`

✓4ᵗʰ **Q72** Reduction defects of lower limb

✓5ᵗʰ **Q72.0** Congenital complete absence of lower limb

     Q72.00 Congenital complete absence of unspecified lower limb `PE`

     Q72.01 Congenital complete absence of right lower limb `PE`

     Q72.02 Congenital complete absence of left lower limb `PE`

     Q72.03 Congenital complete absence of lower limb, bilateral `PE`

✓5ᵗʰ **Q72.1** Congenital absence of thigh and lower leg with foot present

     Q72.10 Congenital absence of unspecified thigh and lower leg with foot present `PE`

     Q72.11 Congenital absence of right thigh and lower leg with foot present `PE`

     Q72.12 Congenital absence of left thigh and lower leg with foot present `PE`

     Q72.13 Congenital absence of thigh and lower leg with foot present, bilateral `PE`

✓5ᵗʰ **Q72.2** Congenital absence of both lower leg and foot

     Q72.20 Congenital absence of both lower leg and foot, unspecified lower limb `PE`

     Q72.21 Congenital absence of both lower leg and foot, right lower limb `PE`

     Q72.22 Congenital absence of both lower leg and foot, left lower limb `PE`

     Q72.23 Congenital absence of both lower leg and foot, bilateral `PE`

✓5ᵗʰ **Q72.3** Congenital absence of foot and toe(s)

     Q72.30 Congenital absence of unspecified foot and toe(s) `PE`

     Q72.31 Congenital absence of right foot and toe(s) `PE`

     Q72.32 Congenital absence of left foot and toe(s) `PE`

     Q72.33 Congenital absence of foot and toe(s), bilateral `PE`

✓5ᵗʰ **Q72.4** Longitudinal reduction defect of femur
     Proximal femoral focal deficiency

     Q72.40 Longitudinal reduction defect of unspecified femur `PE`

     Q72.41 Longitudinal reduction defect of right femur `PE`

     Q72.42 Longitudinal reduction defect of left femur `PE`

     Q72.43 Longitudinal reduction defect of femur, bilateral `PE`

✓5ᵗʰ **Q72.5** Longitudinal reduction defect of tibia

     Q72.50 Longitudinal reduction defect of unspecified tibia `PE`

     Q72.51 Longitudinal reduction defect of right tibia `PE`

     Q72.52 Longitudinal reduction defect of left tibia `PE`

     Q72.53 Longitudinal reduction defect of tibia, bilateral `PE`

✓5ᵗʰ **Q72.6** Longitudinal reduction defect of fibula

     Q72.60 Longitudinal reduction defect of unspecified fibula `PE`

     Q72.61 Longitudinal reduction defect of right fibula `PE`

     Q72.62 Longitudinal reduction defect of left fibula `PE`

     Q72.63 Longitudinal reduction defect of fibula, bilateral `PE`

✓5ᵗʰ **Q72.7** Split foot

     Q72.70 Split foot, unspecified lower limb `PE`

     Q72.71 Split foot, right lower limb `PE`

     Q72.72 Split foot, left lower limb `PE`

     Q72.73 Split foot, bilateral `PE`

✓5ᵗʰ **Q72.8** Other reduction defects of lower limb

     ✓6ᵗʰ **Q72.81** Congenital shortening of lower limb

         Q72.811 Congenital shortening of right lower limb `PE`

         Q72.812 Congenital shortening of left lower limb `PE`

         Q72.813 Congenital shortening of lower limb, bilateral `PE`

         Q72.819 Congenital shortening of unspecified lower limb `PE`

     ✓6ᵗʰ **Q72.89** Other reduction defects of lower limb

         Q72.891 Other reduction defects of right lower limb `PE`

✔ Additional Character Required   ✓x7ᵗʰ Placeholder   Questionable PDx   Manifestation   Unspecified   `UPD` Unacceptable PDx   `H1`-`H4` HAC   `HCC` CMS-HCC Dx   `HIV` HIV Dx

ICD-10-CM 2025   **947**

Q72.892 Other reduction defects of left lower limb `PE`

Q72.893 Other reduction defects of lower limb, bilateral `PE`

Q72.899 Other reduction defects of unspecified lower limb `PE`

✓5ᵗʰ **Q72.9 Unspecified reduction defect of lower limb**

Q72.90 Unspecified reduction defect of unspecified lower limb `PE`

Q72.91 Unspecified reduction defect of right lower limb `PE`

Q72.92 Unspecified reduction defect of left lower limb `PE`

Q72.93 Unspecified reduction defect of lower limb, bilateral `PE`

✓4ᵗʰ **Q73 Reduction defects of unspecified limb**

Q73.0 Congenital absence of unspecified limb(s) `PE`
Amelia NOS

Q73.1 Phocomelia, unspecified limb(s) `PE`
Phocomelia NOS

Q73.8 Other reduction defects of unspecified limb(s) `PE`
Longitudinal reduction deformity of unspecified limb(s)
Ectromelia of limb NOS
Hemimelia of limb NOS
Reduction defect of limb NOS

✓4ᵗʰ **Q74 Other congenital malformations of limb(s)**

EXCLUDES 1   *polydactyly (Q69.-)*
reduction defect of limb (Q71-Q73)
syndactyly (Q70.-)

Q74.0 Other congenital malformations of upper limb(s), including shoulder girdle `PE`
Accessory carpal bones
Cleidocranial dysostosis
Congenital pseudarthrosis of clavicle
Macrodactylia (fingers)
Madelung's deformity
Radioulnar synostosis
Sprengel's deformity
Triphalangeal thumb

Q74.1 Congenital malformation of knee `PE`
Congenital absence of patella
Congenital dislocation of patella
Congenital genu valgum
Congenital genu varum
Rudimentary patella
EXCLUDES 1   *congenital dislocation of knee (Q68.2)*
congenital genu recurvatum (Q68.2)
nail patella syndrome (Q87.2)

Q74.2 Other congenital malformations of lower limb(s), including pelvic girdle `PE`
Congenital fusion of sacroiliac joint
Congenital malformation of ankle joint
Congenital malformation of sacroiliac joint
EXCLUDES 1   *anteversion of femur (neck) (Q65.89)*

Q74.3 Arthrogryposis multiplex congenita `CC` `PE`

Q74.8 Other specified congenital malformations of limb(s) `PE`

Q74.9 Unspecified congenital malformation of limb(s) `PE`
Congenital anomaly of limb(s) NOS

✓4ᵗʰ **Q75 Other congenital malformations of skull and face bones**

EXCLUDES 1   *congenital malformation of face NOS (Q18.-)*
congenital malformation syndromes classified to Q87.-
dentofacial anomalies [including malocclusion] (M26.-)
musculoskeletal deformities of head and face (Q67.0-Q67.4)
skull defects associated with congenital anomalies of brain such as:
anencephaly (Q00.0)
encephalocele (Q01.-)
hydrocephalus (Q03.-)
microcephaly (Q02)

✓5ᵗʰ **Q75.0 Craniosynostosis**
AHA: 2023,4Q,38-39
DEF: Congenital condition in which one or more of the cranial sutures fuse prematurely, creating a deformed or aberrant head shape.

✓6ᵗʰ **Q75.00 Craniosynostosis unspecified**
Craniosynostosis NOS

Q75.001 Craniosynostosis unspecified, unilateral

Q75.002 Craniosynostosis unspecified, bilateral `PE`

Q75.009 Craniosynostosis unspecified `PE`
Imperfect fusion of skull

Q75.01 Sagittal craniosynostosis `PE`
Non-deformational dolichocephaly
Non-deformational scaphocephaly
EXCLUDES 1   *plagiocephaly (Q67.3)*

✓6ᵗʰ **Q75.02 Coronal craniosynostosis**
Non-deformational anterior plagiocephaly
EXCLUDES 1   *dolichocephaly (Q67.2)*

Q75.021 Coronal craniosynostosis unilateral `PE`
Non-deformational anterior plagiocephaly

Q75.022 Coronal craniosynostosis bilateral `PE`
Non-deformational brachycephaly

Q75.029 Coronal craniosynostosis unspecified `PE`

Q75.03 Metopic craniosynostosis `PE`
Trigonocephaly

✓6ᵗʰ **Q75.04 Lambdoid craniosynostosis**
Non-deformational posterior plagiocephaly
EXCLUDES 1   *dolichocephaly (Q67.2)*

Q75.041 Lambdoid craniosynostosis, unilateral `PE`

Q75.042 Lambdoid craniosynostosis, bilateral `PE`

Q75.049 Lambdoid craniosynostosis, unspecified `PE`

✓6ᵗʰ **Q75.05 Multi-suture craniosynostosis**

Q75.051 Cloverleaf skull `PE`
Kleeblattschaedel skull

Q75.052 Pansynostosis `PE`

Q75.058 Other multi-suture craniosynostosis `PE`
EXCLUDES 1   *coronal craniosynostosis, bilateral (Q75.022)*
lambdoid craniosynostosis, bilateral (Q75.042)

Q75.08 Other single-suture craniosynostosis `PE`

Q75.1 Craniofacial dysostosis `PE`
Crouzon's disease

Q75.2 Hypertelorism `PE`

Q75.3 Macrocephaly `PE`

Q75.4 Mandibulofacial dysostosis `PE`
Franceschetti syndrome
Treacher Collins syndrome

Q75.5 Oculomandibular dysostosis `PE`

Q75.8 Other specified congenital malformations of skull and face bones `PE`
Absence of skull bone, congenital
Congenital deformity of forehead
Platybasia

Q75.9 Congenital malformation of skull and face bones, unspecified `PE`
Congenital anomaly of face bones NOS
Congenital anomaly of skull NOS

☑️4th **Q76 Congenital malformations of spine and bony thorax**

> EXCLUDES 1   congenital musculoskeletal deformities of spine and chest (Q67.5-Q67.8)

Q76.Ø Spina bifida occulta   `PE`
> EXCLUDES 1   meningocele (spinal) (QØ5.-)
> spina bifida (aperta) (cystica) (QØ5.-)

Q76.1 Klippel-Feil syndrome   `PE`
Cervical fusion syndrome

Q76.2 Congenital spondylolisthesis   `PE`
Congenital spondylolysis
> EXCLUDES 1   spondylolisthesis (acquired) (M43.1-)
> spondylolysis (acquired) (M43.Ø-)

Q76.3 Congenital scoliosis due to congenital bony malformation   `CC` `PE`
Hemivertebra fusion or failure of segmentation with scoliosis

☑️5th **Q76.4 Other congenital malformations of spine, not associated with scoliosis**

> ☑️6th **Q76.41 Congenital kyphosis**
>
> **Q76.411 Congenital kyphosis, occipito-atlanto-axial region**   `PE`
>
> **Q76.412 Congenital kyphosis, cervical region**   `PE`
>
> **Q76.413 Congenital kyphosis, cervicothoracic region**   `PE`
>
> **Q76.414 Congenital kyphosis, thoracic region**   `PE`
>
> **Q76.415 Congenital kyphosis, thoracolumbar region**   `PE`
>
> **Q76.419 Congenital kyphosis, unspecified region**   `PE`
>
> ☑️6th **Q76.42 Congenital lordosis**
>
> **Q76.425 Congenital lordosis, thoracolumbar region**   `CC` `PE`
>
> **Q76.426 Congenital lordosis, lumbar region**   `CC` `PE`
>
> **Q76.427 Congenital lordosis, lumbosacral region**   `CC` `PE`
>
> **Q76.428 Congenital lordosis, sacral and sacrococcygeal region**   `CC` `PE`
>
> **Q76.429 Congenital lordosis, unspecified region**   `CC` `PE`
>
> **Q76.49 Other congenital malformations of spine, not associated with scoliosis**   `PE`
> Congenital absence of vertebra NOS
> Congenital fusion of spine NOS
> Congenital malformation of lumbosacral (joint) (region) NOS
> Congenital malformation of spine NOS
> Hemivertebra NOS
> Malformation of spine NOS
> Platyspondylisis NOS
> Supernumerary vertebra NOS

Q76.5 Cervical rib   `PE`
Supernumerary rib in cervical region

Q76.6 Other congenital malformations of ribs   `CC` `PE`
Accessory rib
Congenital absence of rib
Congenital fusion of ribs
Congenital malformation of ribs NOS
> EXCLUDES 1   short rib syndrome (Q77.2)

Q76.7 Congenital malformation of sternum   `CC` `PE`
Congenital absence of sternum
Sternum bifidum

Q76.8 Other congenital malformations of bony thorax   `CC` `PE`

Q76.9 Congenital malformation of bony thorax, unspecified   `CC` `PE`

☑️4th **Q77 Osteochondrodysplasia with defects of growth of tubular bones and spine**

> EXCLUDES 1   mucopolysaccharidosis (E76.Ø-E76.3)
> EXCLUDES 2   congenital myotonic chondrodystrophy (G71.13)

Q77.Ø Achondrogenesis   `PE`
Hypochondrogenesis

Q77.1 Thanatophoric short stature   `PE`

Q77.2 Short rib syndrome   `CC` `PE`
Asphyxiating thoracic dysplasia [Jeune]

Q77.3 Chondrodysplasia punctata   `PE`
> EXCLUDES 1   Rhizomelic chondrodysplasia punctata (E71.43)

Q77.4 Achondroplasia   `PE`
Hypochondroplasia
Osteosclerosis congenita

Q77.5 Diastrophic dysplasia   `PE`

Q77.6 Chondroectodermal dysplasia   `PE`
Ellis-van Creveld syndrome

Q77.7 Spondyloepiphyseal dysplasia   `PE`

Q77.8 Other osteochondrodysplasia with defects of growth of tubular bones and spine   `PE`

Q77.9 Osteochondrodysplasia with defects of growth of tubular bones and spine, unspecified   `PE`

☑️4th **Q78 Other osteochondrodysplasias**

> EXCLUDES 2   congenital myotonic chondrodystrophy (G71.13)

Q78.Ø Osteogenesis imperfecta   `CC` `PE`
Fragilitas ossium
Osteopsathyrosis

Q78.1 Polyostotic fibrous dysplasia   `PE`
Albright(-McCune)(-Sternberg) syndrome

Q78.2 Osteopetrosis   `CC` `PE`
Albers-Schonberg syndrome
Osteosclerosis NOS
DEF: Rare congenital condition in which the bones are excessively dense, resulting from a discrepancy in the formation and breakdown of bone.

Q78.3 Progressive diaphyseal dysplasia   `PE`
Camurati-Engelmann syndrome

Q78.4 Enchondromatosis   `PE`
Maffucci's syndrome
Ollier's disease

Q78.5 Metaphyseal dysplasia   `PE`
Pyle's syndrome

Q78.6 Multiple congenital exostoses   `PE`
Diaphyseal aclasis

Q78.8 Other specified osteochondrodysplasias   `PE`
Osteopoikilosis

Q78.9 Osteochondrodysplasia, unspecified   `PE`
Chondrodystrophy NOS
Osteodystrophy NOS

☑️4th **Q79 Congenital malformations of musculoskeletal system, not elsewhere classified**

> EXCLUDES 2   congenital (sternomastoid) torticollis (Q68.Ø)

Q79.Ø Congenital diaphragmatic hernia   `MCC` `PE`
> EXCLUDES 1   congenital hiatus hernia (Q4Ø.1)

Q79.1 Other congenital malformations of diaphragm   `MCC` `PE`
Absence of diaphragm
Congenital malformation of diaphragm NOS
Eventration of diaphragm

Q79.2 Exomphalos   `MCC` `PE`
Omphalocele
> EXCLUDES 1   umbilical hernia (K42.-)

Q79.3 Gastroschisis   `MCC` `PE`

Gastroschisis

Herniated small bowel (gastroschisis)

Rectus abdominus m.

Umbilicus

distal   proximal

skin

Defect

Q79.4 Prune belly syndrome   `MCC` `PE`
Congenital prolapse of bladder mucosa
Eagle-Barrett syndrome

☑️5th **Q79.5 Other congenital malformations of abdominal wall**
> EXCLUDES 1   umbilical hernia (K42.-)

> **Q79.51 Congenital hernia of bladder**   `MCC` `PE`
>
> **Q79.59 Other congenital malformations of abdominal wall**   `MCC` `PE`

✅ Additional Character Required   ✓x7th Placeholder   Questionable PDx   Manifestation   Unspecified   `UPD` Unacceptable PDx   H1 - H14 HAC   HCC CMS-HCC Dx   HIV HIV Dx

ICD-10-CM 2025   **949**

Chapter 17. Congenital Malformations, Deformations and Chromosomal Abnormalities

Q79.6–Q84.9

√5th **Q79.6** **Ehlers-Danlos syndromes**

AHA: 2019,4Q,13-14

DEF: Connective tissue disorder that causes hyperextended skin and joints and results in fragile blood vessels with bleeding, poor wound healing, and subcutaneous pseudotumors.

    Q79.60 **Ehlers-Danlos syndrome, unspecified** `CC` `PE`

    Q79.61 **Classical** **Ehlers-Danlos syndrome** `CC` `PE`
       Classical EDS (cEDS)

    Q79.62 **Hypermobile** **Ehlers-Danlos syndrome** `CC` `PE`
       Hypermobile EDS (hEDS)

    Q79.63 **Vascular** **Ehlers-Danlos syndrome** `CC` `PE`
       Vascular EDS (vEDS)

    Q79.69 **Other Ehlers-Danlos syndromes** `CC` `PE`

Q79.8 **Other congenital malformations of musculoskeletal system** `PE`
    Absence of muscle
    Absence of tendon
    Accessory muscle
    Amyotrophia congenita
    Congenital constricting bands
    Congenital shortening of tendon
    Poland syndrome

Q79.9 **Congenital malformation of musculoskeletal system, unspecified** `PE`
    Congenital anomaly of musculoskeletal system NOS
    Congenital deformity of musculoskeletal system NOS

Other congenital malformations (Q80-Q89)

√4th **Q80** **Congenital ichthyosis**

EXCLUDES 1   *Refsum's disease (G60.1)*

DEF: Excessive production of skin cells resulting in red, dry, scaly skin.

Q80.0 **Ichthyosis vulgaris** `PE`

Q80.1 **X-linked ichthyosis** `PE`

Q80.2 **Lamellar ichthyosis** `PE`
    Collodion baby

Q80.3 **Congenital bullous ichthyosiform erythroderma** `PE`

Q80.4 **Harlequin fetus** `PE`

Q80.8 **Other congenital ichthyosis** `PE`

Q80.9 **Congenital ichthyosis, unspecified** `PE`

√4th **Q81** **Epidermolysis bullosa**

Q81.0 **Epidermolysis bullosa simplex** `PE`
    EXCLUDES 1   *Cockayne's syndrome (Q87.19)*

Q81.1 **Epidermolysis bullosa letalis** `PE`
    Herlitz' syndrome

Q81.2 **Epidermolysis bullosa dystrophica** `PE`

Q81.8 **Other epidermolysis bullosa** `PE`

Q81.9 **Epidermolysis bullosa, unspecified** `PE`

√4th **Q82** **Other congenital malformations of skin**

EXCLUDES 1   *acrodermatitis enteropathica (E83.2)*
       congenital erythropoietic porphyria (E80.0)
       pilonidal cyst or sinus (L05.-)
       Sturge-Weber (-Dimitri) syndrome (Q85.89)

Q82.0 **Hereditary lymphedema** `PE`

Q82.1 **Xeroderma pigmentosum** `PE`

Q82.2 **Congenital cutaneous mastocytosis** `PE`
    Congenital diffuse cutaneous mastocytosis
    Congenital maculopapular cutaneous mastocytosis
    Congenital urticaria pigmentosa
    EXCLUDES 1   *cutaneous mastocytosis NOS (D47.01)*
       diffuse cutaneous mastocytosis (with onset after newborn period) (D47.01)
       malignant mastocytosis (C96.2-)
       systemic mastocytosis (D47.02)
       urticaria pigmentosa (non-congenital) (with onset after newborn period) (D47.01)

    AHA: 2017,4Q,5

Q82.3 **Incontinentia pigmenti** `PE`

Q82.4 **Ectodermal dysplasia (anhidrotic)** `PE`
    EXCLUDES 1   *Ellis-van Creveld syndrome (Q77.6)*

Q82.5 **Congenital non-neoplastic nevus** `PE`
    Birthmark NOS
    Flammeus Nevus
    Portwine Nevus
    Sanguineous Nevus
    Strawberry Nevus
    Vascular Nevus NOS
    Verrucous Nevus
    EXCLUDES 2   *araneus nevus (I78.1)*
       Cafe au lait spots (L81.3)
       lentigo (L81.4)
       melanocytic nevus (D22.-)
       nevus NOS (D22.-)
       pigmented nevus (D22.-)
       spider nevus (I78.1)
       stellar nevus (I78.1)

Q82.6 **Congenital sacral dimple** `PE`
    Parasacral dimple
    EXCLUDES 2   *pilonidal cyst with abscess (L05.01)*
       pilonidal cyst without abscess (L05.91)
    AHA: 2016,4Q,60

Q82.8 **Other specified congenital malformations of skin** `PE`
    Abnormal palmar creases
    Accessory skin tags
    Benign familial pemphigus [Hailey-Hailey]
    Congenital poikiloderma
    Cutis laxa (hyperelastica)
    Dermatoglyphic anomalies
    Inherited keratosis palmaris et plantaris
    Keratosis follicularis [Darier-White]
    EXCLUDES 1   *Ehlers-Danlos syndromes (Q79.6-)*
    AHA: 2021,3Q,10; 2016,1Q,17

Q82.9 **Congenital malformation of skin, unspecified** `PE`

√4th **Q83** **Congenital malformations of breast**

EXCLUDES 2   *absence of pectoral muscle (Q79.8)*
       hypoplasia of breast (N64.82)
       micromastia (N64.82)

Q83.0 **Congenital absence of breast with absent nipple** `PE`

Q83.1 **Accessory breast** `PE`
    Supernumerary breast

Q83.2 **Absent nipple** `PE`

Q83.3 **Accessory nipple** `PE`
    Supernumerary nipple

Q83.8 **Other congenital malformations of breast** `PE`

Q83.9 **Congenital malformation of breast, unspecified** `PE`

√4th **Q84** **Other congenital malformations of integument**

Q84.0 **Congenital alopecia** `PE`
    Congenital atrichosis

Q84.1 **Congenital morphological disturbances of hair, not elsewhere classified** `PE`
    Beaded hair
    Monilethrix
    Pili annulati
    EXCLUDES 1   *Menkes' kinky hair syndrome (E83.09)*

Q84.2 **Other congenital malformations of hair** `PE`
    Congenital hypertrichosis
    Congenital malformation of hair NOS
    Persistent lanugo

Q84.3 **Anonychia** `PE`
    EXCLUDES 1   *nail patella syndrome (Q87.2)*

Q84.4 **Congenital leukonychia** `PE`

Q84.5 **Enlarged and hypertrophic nails** `PE`
    Congenital onychauxis
    Pachyonychia

Q84.6 **Other congenital malformations of nails** `PE`
    Congenital clubnail
    Congenital koilonychia
    Congenital malformation of nail NOS

Q84.8 **Other specified congenital malformations of integument** `PE`
    Aplasia cutis congenita

Q84.9 **Congenital malformation of integument, unspecified** `PE`
    Congenital anomaly of integument NOS
    Congenital deformity of integument NOS

`N` Newborn: 0   `P` Pediatric: 0-17   `M` Maternity: 9-64   `A` Adult: 15-124   `UNS` Unspecified Site   `MCC` Major Complication/Comorbidity   `CC` Complication/Comorbidity   `PE` POA Exempt

950   ICD-10-CM 2025

✓4th Q85 Phakomatoses, not elsewhere classified

> EXCLUDES 1   *ataxia telangiectasia [Louis-Bar] (G11.3)*
> *familial dysautonomia [Riley-Day] (G90.1)*

✓5th Q85.0 Neurofibromatosis (nonmalignant)

Q85.00 Neurofibromatosis, unspecified   HCC PE

Q85.01 Neurofibromatosis, type 1   HCC PE
Von Recklinghausen disease

Q85.02 Neurofibromatosis, type 2   HCC PE
Acoustic neurofibromatosis
DEF: Inherited condition with cutaneous lesions, benign tumors of peripheral nerves, and bilateral 8th nerve masses.

Q85.03 Schwannomatosis   HCC PE
DEF: Genetic mutation (SMARCB1/INI1) causing multiple benign tumors along the nerve pathways, except on the 8th cranial (vestibular) nerve.

Q85.09 Other neurofibromatosis   HCC PE

Q85.1 Tuberous sclerosis   CC HCC PE
Bourneville's disease
Epiloia

✓5th Q85.8 Other phakomatoses, not elsewhere classified

> EXCLUDES 1   *Meckel-Gruber syndrome (Q61.9)*
AHA: 2022,4Q,40-41; 2021,3Q,12

Q85.81 PTEN hamartoma tumor syndrome   CC HCC PE
PHTS
PTEN related Cowden syndrome
Code also, if applicable, genetic susceptibility to malignant neoplasm (Z15.0-)
AHA: 2022,4Q,41
TIP: PTEN hamartoma tumor syndrome (PHTS) manifests differently in each patient. Separate codes should be assigned in addition to code Q85.81 for any manifestations of PHTS, such as macrocephaly, autism, or learning delays.

Q85.82 Other Cowden syndrome   CC HCC PE

Q85.83 Von Hippel-Lindau syndrome   CC HCC PE
Code also manifestations
AHA: 2023,2Q,16

Q85.89 Other phakomatoses, not elsewhere classified   CC HCC PE
Peutz-Jeghers syndrome
Sturge-Weber(-Dimitri) syndrome

Q85.9 Phakomatosis, unspecified   CC HCC PE
Hamartosis NOS

✓4th Q86 Congenital malformation syndromes due to known exogenous causes, not elsewhere classified

> EXCLUDES 2   *iodine-deficiency-related hypothyroidism (E00-E02)*
> *nonteratogenic effects of substances transmitted via placenta or breast milk (P04.-)*

Q86.0 Fetal alcohol syndrome (dysmorphic)   PE

Q86.1 Fetal hydantoin syndrome   PE
Meadow's syndrome

Q86.2 Dysmorphism due to warfarin   PE

Q86.8 Other congenital malformation syndromes due to known exogenous causes   PE

✓4th Q87 Other specified congenital malformation syndromes affecting multiple systems
Use additional code(s) to identify all associated manifestations

Q87.0 Congenital malformation syndromes predominantly affecting facial appearance   PE
Acrocephalopolysyndactyly
Acrocephalosyndactyly [Apert]
Cryptophthalmos syndrome
Cyclopia
Goldenhar syndrome
Moebius syndrome
Oro-facial-digital syndrome
Robin syndrome
Whistling face

✓5th Q87.1 Congenital malformation syndromes predominantly associated with short stature

> EXCLUDES 1   *Ellis-van Creveld syndrome (Q77.6)*
> *Smith-Lemli-Opitz syndrome (E78.72)*
AHA: 2019,4Q,14-15

Q87.11 Prader-Willi syndrome   CC PE

Q87.19 Other congenital malformation syndromes predominantly associated with short stature   CC PE
Aarskog syndrome
Cockayne syndrome
De Lange syndrome
Dubowitz syndrome
Noonan syndrome
Robinow-Silverman-Smith syndrome
Russell-Silver syndrome
Seckel syndrome

Q87.2 Congenital malformation syndromes predominantly involving limbs   CC PE
Holt-Oram syndrome
Klippel-Trenaunay-Weber syndrome
Nail patella syndrome
Rubinstein-Taybi syndrome
Sirenomelia syndrome
Thrombocytopenia with absent radius [TAR] syndrome
VATER syndrome

Q87.3 Congenital malformation syndromes involving early overgrowth   CC PE
Beckwith-Wiedemann syndrome
Sotos syndrome
Weaver syndrome

✓5th Q87.4 Marfan syndrome
DEF: Disorder that affects the connective tissue of multiple systems, including disproportionally long or abnormal bone structure and eye and cardiovascular complications.

Q87.40 Marfan syndrome, unspecified   CC PE

✓6th Q87.41 Marfan syndrome with cardiovascular manifestations

Q87.410 Marfan syndrome with aortic dilation   CC PE

Q87.418 Marfan syndrome with other cardiovascular manifestations   CC PE

Q87.42 Marfan syndrome with ocular manifestations   CC PE

Q87.43 Marfan syndrome with skeletal manifestation   CC PE

Q87.5 Other congenital malformation syndromes with other skeletal changes   CC PE

✓5th Q87.8 Other specified congenital malformation syndromes, not elsewhere classified

> EXCLUDES 1   *Zellweger syndrome (E71.510)*
AHA: 2023,4Q,39-40

Q87.81 Alport syndrome   CC PE
Use additional code to identify stage of chronic kidney disease (N18.1-N18.6)

Q87.82 Arterial tortuosity syndrome   CC PE
AHA: 2016,4Q,60-61

Q87.83 Bardet-Biedl syndrome   CC PE

Q87.84 Laurence-Moon syndrome   CC PE

Q87.85 MED13L syndrome   CC PE
Asadollahi-Rauch syndrome
Mediator complex subunit 13L syndrome
Code also, if applicable, any associated manifestations such as:
autism spectrum disorder (F84.0-)
congenital malformations of cardiac septa ▶(Q21.-)◀
epilepsy and recurrent seizures (G40.-)
intellectual disability (F70-F79)

Q87.86 Kleefstra syndrome   CC PE

Q87.89 Other specified congenital malformation syndromes, not elsewhere classified   CC PE

✓4th Q89 Other congenital malformations, not elsewhere classified

✓5th Q89.0 Congenital absence and malformations of spleen

> EXCLUDES 1   *isomerism of atrial appendages (with asplenia or polysplenia) (Q20.6)*

Q89.01 Asplenia (congenital)   CC PE

Q89.09 Congenital malformations of spleen   CC PE
Congenital splenomegaly

Q89.1 Congenital malformations of adrenal gland   PE

> EXCLUDES 1   *adrenogenital disorders (E25.-)*
> *congenital adrenal hyperplasia (E25.0)*

☑ Additional Character Required   ✓x7th Placeholder   Questionable PDx   Manifestation   Unspecified   UPD Unacceptable PDx   H1-H14 HAC   HCC CMS-HCC Dx   HIV HIV Dx

ICD-10-CM 2025   951

Q89.2   Congenital malformations of other endocrine glands   PE
Congenital malformation of parathyroid or thyroid gland
Persistent thyroglossal duct
Thyroglossal cyst
EXCLUDES 1   *congenital goiter (E03.0)*
                 congenital hypothyroidism (E03.1)

Q89.3   Situs inversus   CC PE
Dextrocardia with situs inversus
Mirror-image atrial arrangement with situs inversus
Situs inversus or transversus abdominalis
Situs inversus or transversus thoracis
Transposition of abdominal viscera
Transposition of thoracic viscera
EXCLUDES 1   *dextrocardia NOS (Q24.0)*
DEF: Congenital anomaly in which the internal thoracic and abdominal organs are transposed laterally and found on the opposite side from the normal position.

Q89.4   Conjoined twins   MCC PE
Craniopagus
Dicephaly
Pygopagus
Thoracopagus

Q89.7   Multiple congenital malformations, not elsewhere classified   CC PE
Multiple congenital anomalies NOS
Multiple congenital deformities NOS
EXCLUDES 1   *congenital malformation syndromes affecting multiple systems (Q87.-)*

Q89.8   Other specified congenital malformations   CC PE
Use additional code(s) to identify all associated manifestations
AHA: 2021,3Q,12

Q89.9   Congenital malformation, unspecified   PE
Congenital anomaly NOS
Congenital deformity NOS

Chromosomal abnormalities, not elsewhere classified (Q90-Q99)

EXCLUDES 2   *mitochondrial metabolic disorders (E88.4-)*

✓4th **Q90   Down syndrome**
Code also associated physical condition(s), such as atrioventricular septal defect (Q21.2-)
Use additional code(s) to identify any associated degree of intellectual disabilities (F70-F79)

Q90.0   Trisomy 21, nonmosaicism (meiotic nondisjunction)   PE

Q90.1   Trisomy 21, mosaicism (mitotic nondisjunction)   PE

Q90.2   Trisomy 21, translocation   PE

Q90.9   Down syndrome, unspecified   PE
Trisomy 21 NOS

✓4th **Q91   Trisomy 18 and Trisomy 13**

Q91.0   Trisomy 18, nonmosaicism (meiotic nondisjunction)   CC PE

Q91.1   Trisomy 18, mosaicism (mitotic nondisjunction)   CC PE

Q91.2   Trisomy 18, translocation   CC PE

Q91.3   Trisomy 18, unspecified   CC PE

Q91.4   Trisomy 13, nonmosaicism (meiotic nondisjunction)   CC PE

Q91.5   Trisomy 13, mosaicism (mitotic nondisjunction)   CC PE

Q91.6   Trisomy 13, translocation   CC PE

Q91.7   Trisomy 13, unspecified   CC PE

✓4th **Q92   Other trisomies and partial trisomies of the autosomes, not elsewhere classified**
INCLUDES   unbalanced translocations and insertions
EXCLUDES 1   *trisomies of chromosomes 13, 18, 21 (Q90-Q91)*

Q92.0   Whole chromosome trisomy, nonmosaicism (meiotic nondisjunction)   PE

Q92.1   Whole chromosome trisomy, mosaicism (mitotic nondisjunction)   PE

Q92.2   Partial trisomy   PE
Less than whole arm duplicated
Whole arm or more duplicated
EXCLUDES 1   *partial trisomy due to unbalanced translocation (Q92.5)*

Q92.5   Duplications with other complex rearrangements   PE
Partial trisomy due to unbalanced translocations
Code also any associated deletions due to unbalanced translocations, inversions and insertions (Q93.7)

✓5th **Q92.6   Marker chromosomes**
Trisomies due to dicentrics
Trisomies due to extra rings
Trisomies due to isochromosomes
Individual with marker heterochromatin

Q92.61   Marker chromosomes in normal individual   PE

Q92.62   Marker chromosomes in abnormal individual   PE

Q92.7   Triploidy and polyploidy   PE

Q92.8   Other specified trisomies and partial trisomies of autosomes   PE
Duplications identified by fluorescence in situ hybridization (FISH)
Duplications identified by in situ hybridization (ISH)
Duplications seen only at prometaphase

Q92.9   Trisomy and partial trisomy of autosomes, unspecified   PE

✓4th **Q93   Monosomies and deletions from the autosomes, not elsewhere classified**

Q93.0   Whole chromosome monosomy, nonmosaicism (meiotic nondisjunction)   PE

Q93.1   Whole chromosome monosomy, mosaicism (mitotic nondisjunction)   PE

Q93.2   Chromosome replaced with ring, dicentric or isochromosome   PE

Q93.3   Deletion of short arm of chromosome 4   CC PE
Wolff-Hirschorn syndrome

Q93.4   Deletion of short arm of chromosome 5   CC PE
Cri-du-chat syndrome

✓5th **Q93.5   Other deletions of part of a chromosome**
AHA: 2018,4Q,28

Q93.51   Angelman syndrome   CC PE

Q93.52   Phelan-McDermid syndrome   CC PE
22q13.3 deletion syndrome
Use additional code(s) to identify any associated conditions, such as:
autism spectrum disorder (F84.0)
degree of intellectual disabilities (F70-F79)
epilepsy and recurrent seizures (G40.-)
lymphedema (I89.0)
AHA: 2023,4Q,40-41

Q93.59   Other deletions of part of a chromosome   CC PE

Q93.7   Deletions with other complex rearrangements   CC PE
Deletions due to unbalanced translocations, inversions and insertions
Code also any associated duplications due to unbalanced translocations, inversions and insertions (Q92.5)

✓5th **Q93.8   Other deletions from the autosomes**

Q93.81   Velo-cardio-facial syndrome   MCC PE
Deletion 22q11.2
AHA: 2019,3Q,14
DEF: Microdeletion syndrome affecting multiple organs characterized by a cleft palate, heart defects, an elongated face with almond-shaped eyes, wide nose, small ears, weak immune system, weak musculature, hypothyroidism, short stature, and scoliosis. The deletion occurs at q11.2 on the long arm of the chromosome 22.

Q93.82   Williams syndrome   CC PE
AHA: 2018,4Q,28-29

Q93.88   Other microdeletions   CC PE
Miller-Dieker syndrome
Smith-Magenis syndrome

Q93.89   Other deletions from the autosomes   CC PE
Deletions identified by fluorescence in situ hybridization (FISH)
Deletions identified by in situ hybridization (ISH)
Deletions seen only at prometaphase

Q93.9   Deletion from autosomes, unspecified   CC PE

✓4th **Q95   Balanced rearrangements and structural markers, not elsewhere classified**
INCLUDES   Robertsonian and balanced reciprocal translocations and insertions

Q95.0   Balanced translocation and insertion in normal individual   PE

Q95.1   Chromosome inversion in normal individual   PE

Q95.2   Balanced autosomal rearrangement in abnormal individual   PE

Q95.3   Balanced sex/autosomal rearrangement in abnormal individual   PE

Q89.2–Q95.3
Chapter 17. Congenital Malformations, Deformations and Chromosomal Abnormalities

Q95.5   Individual with autosomal fragile site   PE

Q95.8   Other balanced rearrangements and structural markers   PE

Q95.9   Balanced rearrangement and structural marker, unspecified   PE

☑4ᵗʰ **Q96**   **Turner's syndrome**

    EXCLUDES 1   Noonan syndrome (Q87.19)

Q96.0   Karyotype 45, X   PE

Q96.1   Karyotype 46, X iso (Xq)   PE

     Karyotype 46, isochromosome Xq

Q96.2   Karyotype 46, X with abnormal sex chromosome, except iso (Xq)   PE

     Karyotype 46, X with abnormal sex chromosome, except isochromosome Xq

Q96.3   Mosaicism, 45, X/46, XX or XY   PE

Q96.4   Mosaicism, 45, X/other cell line(s) with abnormal sex chromosome   PE

Q96.8   Other variants of Turner's syndrome   PE

Q96.9   Turner's syndrome, unspecified   PE

☑4ᵗʰ **Q97**   **Other sex chromosome abnormalities, female phenotype, not elsewhere classified**

    EXCLUDES 1   Turner's syndrome (Q96.-)

Q97.0   Karyotype 47, XXX   PE

Q97.1   Female with more than three X chromosomes   PE

Q97.2   Mosaicism, lines with various numbers of X chromosomes   PE

Q97.3   Female with 46, XY karyotype   PE

Q97.8   Other specified sex chromosome abnormalities, female phenotype   PE

Q97.9   Sex chromosome abnormality, female phenotype, unspecified   PE

☑4ᵗʰ **Q98**   **Other sex chromosome abnormalities, male phenotype, not elsewhere classified**

Q98.0   Klinefelter syndrome karyotype 47, XXY   PE

Q98.1   Klinefelter syndrome, male with more than two X chromosomes   PE

Q98.3   Other male with 46, XX karyotype   PE

Q98.4   Klinefelter syndrome, unspecified   PE

Q98.5   Karyotype 47, XYY   PE

Q98.6   Male with structurally abnormal sex chromosome   PE

Q98.7   Male with sex chromosome mosaicism   PE

Q98.8   Other specified sex chromosome abnormalities, male phenotype   PE

Q98.9   Sex chromosome abnormality, male phenotype, unspecified   PE

☑4ᵗʰ **Q99**   **Other chromosome abnormalities, not elsewhere classified**

Q99.0   Chimera 46, XX/46, XY   PE

     Chimera 46, XX/46, XY true hermaphrodite

Q99.1   46, XX true hermaphrodite   PE

     46, XX with streak gonads

     46, XY with streak gonads

     Pure gonadal dysgenesis

Q99.2   Fragile X chromosome   PE

     Fragile X syndrome

Q99.8   Other specified chromosome abnormalities   PE

Q99.9   Chromosomal abnormality, unspecified   PE

☑ Additional Character Required   ☑x7ᵗʰ Placeholder   Questionable PDx   Manifestation   Unspecified   UPD Unacceptable PDx   H1 - H14 HAC   HCC CMS-HCC Dx   HIV HIV Dx

ICD-10-CM 2025   **953**

Chapter 18. Symptoms, Signs, and Abnormal Clinical and Laboratory Findings, Not Elsewhere Classified (RØØ–R99)

Chapter-specific Guidelines with Coding Examples

The chapter-specific guidelines from the ICD-10-CM Official Guidelines for Coding and Reporting have been provided below. Along with these guidelines are coding examples, contained in the shaded boxes, that have been developed to help illustrate the coding and/or sequencing guidance found in these guidelines.

Chapter 18 includes symptoms, signs, abnormal results of clinical or other investigative procedures, and ill-defined conditions regarding which no diagnosis classifiable elsewhere is recorded. Signs and symptoms that point to a specific diagnosis have been assigned to a category in other chapters of the classification.

a. Use of symptom codes

Codes that describe symptoms and signs are acceptable for reporting purposes when a related definitive diagnosis has not been established (confirmed) by the provider.

> Chest pain of unknown origin
>
> **R07.9**   **Chest pain, unspecified**
>
> *Explanation:* Codes that describe symptoms such as chest pain are acceptable for reporting purposes when the provider has not established (confirmed) a related definitive diagnosis.

b. Use of a symptom code with a definitive diagnosis code

Codes for signs and symptoms may be reported in addition to a related definitive diagnosis when the sign or symptom is not routinely associated with that diagnosis, such as the various signs and symptoms associated with complex syndromes. The definitive diagnosis code should be sequenced before the symptom code.

Signs or symptoms that are associated routinely with a disease process should not be assigned as additional codes, unless otherwise instructed by the classification.

> Pneumonia with hemoptysis
>
> **J18.9**   **Pneumonia, unspecified organism**
>
> **R04.2**   **Hemoptysis**
>
> *Explanation:* Codes for signs and symptoms may be reported in addition to a related definitive diagnosis when the sign or symptom is not routinely associated with that diagnosis.

> Abdominal pain due to acute appendicitis
>
> **K35.80**   **Unspecified acute appendicitis**
>
> *Explanation:* Codes for signs or symptoms routinely associated with a disease process should not be assigned unless the classification instructs otherwise.

c. Combination codes that include symptoms

ICD-10-CM contains a number of combination codes that identify both the definitive diagnosis and common symptoms of that diagnosis. When using one of these combination codes, an additional code should not be assigned for the symptom.

> Acute gastritis with hemorrhage
>
> **K29.01**   **Acute gastritis with bleeding**
>
> *Explanation:* When a combination code identifies both the definitive diagnosis and the symptom, an additional code should not be assigned for the symptom.

d. Repeated falls

Code R29.6, Repeated falls, is for use for encounters when a patient has recently fallen and the reason for the fall is being investigated.

Code Z91.81, History of falling, is for use when a patient has fallen in the past and is at risk for future falls. When appropriate, both codes R29.6 and Z91.81 may be assigned together.

e. Coma

Code R40.20, Unspecified coma, should be assigned when the underlying cause of the coma is not known, or the cause is a traumatic brain injury and the coma scale is not documented in the medical record.

Do not report codes for unspecified coma, individual or total Glasgow coma scale scores for a patient with a medically induced coma or a sedated patient.

1) Coma scale

The coma scale codes (R40.21- to R40.24-) can be used in conjunction with traumatic brain injury codes. These codes cannot be used with R40.2A, Nontraumatic coma due to underlying condition. They are primarily for use by trauma registries, but they may be used in any setting where this information is collected. The coma scale codes should be sequenced after the diagnosis code(s).

These codes, one from each subcategory, are needed to complete the scale. The 7th character indicates when the scale was recorded. The 7th character should match for all three codes.

At a minimum, report the initial score documented on presentation at your facility. This may be a score from the emergency medicine technician (EMT) or in the emergency department. If desired, a facility may choose to capture multiple coma scale scores.

Assign code R40.24-, Glasgow coma scale, total score, when only the total score is documented in the medical record and not the individual score(s).

If multiple coma scores are captured within the first 24 hours after hospital admission, assign only the code for the score at the time of admission. ICD-10-CM does not classify coma scores that are reported after admission but less than 24 hours later.

See Section I.B.14. for coma scale documentation by clinicians other than patient's provider

> 23-year-old man found down after unknown injury with skull fracture and with concussion and loss of consciousness of unknown duration. EMS evaluated the patient in the field and reported the individual Glasgow coma scores:
>
> Eye opening response—3: eyes open to speech
>
> Verbal response—4: confused but coherent speech
>
> Motor response—6: obeys commands fully
>
> **S02.0XXA**   **Fracture of vault of skull, initial encounter for closed fracture**
>
> **S06.0X9A**   **Concussion with loss of consciousness of unspecified duration, initial encounter**
>
> **R40.2131**   **Coma scale, eyes open, to sound, in the field [EMT or ambulance]**
>
> **R40.2241**   **Coma scale, best verbal response, confused conversation, in the field [EMT or ambulance]**
>
> **R40.2361**   **Coma scale, best motor response, obeys commands, in the field [EMT or ambulance]**
>
> *Explanation:* When individual scores for the Glasgow coma scale are documented, one code from each category is needed to complete the scale. The seventh character indicates when the scale was recorded and should match for all three codes. Assign a code from subcategory R40.24- Glasgow coma scale, total score, when only the total and not the individual score(s) is documented.

f. Functional quadriplegia

GUIDELINE HAS BEEN DELETED EFFECTIVE OCTOBER 1, 2017

g. SIRS due to non-infectious process

The systemic inflammatory response syndrome (SIRS) can develop as a result of certain non-infectious disease processes, such as trauma, malignant neoplasm, or pancreatitis. When SIRS is documented with a noninfectious condition, and no subsequent infection is documented, the code for the underlying condition, such as an injury, should be assigned, followed by code R65.10, Systemic inflammatory response syndrome (SIRS) of non-infectious origin without acute organ dysfunction, or code R65.11, Systemic inflammatory response syndrome (SIRS) of non-infectious origin with acute organ dysfunction. If an associated acute organ dysfunction is documented, the appropriate code(s) for the specific type of organ dysfunction(s) should be assigned in addition to code R65.11. If acute organ dysfunction is documented, but it cannot be determined if the acute organ dysfunction is associated with SIRS or due to another condition (e.g., directly due to the trauma), the provider should be queried.

Systemic inflammatory response syndrome (SIRS) due to acute gallstone pancreatitis

K85.1Ø   **Biliary acute pancreatitis without necrosis or infection**

R65.1Ø   **Systemic inflammatory response syndrome [SIRS] of non-infectious origin without acute organ dysfunction**

Explanation: When SIRS is documented with a non-infectious condition without subsequent infection documented, the code for the underlying condition such as pancreatitis should be assigned followed by the appropriate code for SIRS of noninfectious origin, either with or without associated organ dysfunction.

h. Death NOS

Code R99, Ill-defined and unknown cause of mortality, is only for use in the very limited circumstance when a patient who has already died is brought into an emergency department or other healthcare facility and is pronounced dead upon arrival. It does not represent the discharge disposition of death.

i. NIHSS stroke scale

The NIH stroke scale (NIHSS) codes (R29.7- -) can be used in conjunction with acute stroke codes (I6Ø-I63) to identify the patient's neurological status and the severity of the stroke. The stroke scale codes should be sequenced after the acute stroke diagnosis code(s).

At a minimum, report the initial score documented. If desired, a facility may choose to capture multiple stroke scale scores.

See Section I.B.14. for NIHSS stroke scale documentation by clinicians other than patient's provider

Patient admitted with CVA seen by neurology consult who documents moderate to severe stroke, 17 on NIHSS stroke scale.

I63.9   **Cerebral infarction, unspecified**

R29.717   **NIHSS score 17**

Explanation: Unspecified cerebral vascular accident (CVA) is sequenced before the NIHSS stroke scale score code. The stroke scale is an assessment tool to help measure stroke-related neurological deficits. Fifteen items are evaluated by trained observers and include such conditions as levels of consciousness, language, dysarthria, ataxia, and sensory loss. A facility may report multiple stroke scale scores if it wants to.

Chapter 18. Symptoms, Signs and Abnormal Clinical and Laboratory Findings, Not Elsewhere Classified (R00-R99)

NOTE This chapter includes symptoms, signs, abnormal results of clinical or other investigative procedures, and ill-defined conditions regarding which no diagnosis classifiable elsewhere is recorded.

Signs and symptoms that point rather definitely to a given diagnosis have been assigned to a category in other chapters of the classification. In general, categories in this chapter include the less well-defined conditions and symptoms that, without the necessary study of the case to establish a final diagnosis, point perhaps equally to two or more diseases or to two or more systems of the body. Practically all categories in the chapter could be designated 'not otherwise specified', 'unknown etiology' or 'transient'. The Alphabetical Index should be consulted to determine which symptoms and signs are to be allocated here and which to other chapters. The residual subcategories, numbered .8, are generally provided for other relevant symptoms that cannot be allocated elsewhere in the classification.

The conditions and signs or symptoms included in categories R00-R94 consist of:

(a) cases for which no more specific diagnosis can be made even after all the facts bearing on the case have been investigated;

(b) signs or symptoms existing at the time of initial encounter that proved to be transient and whose causes could not be determined;

(c) provisional diagnosis in a patient who failed to return for further investigation or care;

(d) cases referred elsewhere for investigation or treatment before the diagnosis was made;

(e) cases in which a more precise diagnosis was not available for any other reason;

(f) certain symptoms, for which supplementary information is provided, that represent important problems in medical care in their own right.

> **EXCLUDES 2**   abnormal findings on antenatal screening of mother (O28.-)
> certain conditions originating in the perinatal period (P04-P96)
> signs and symptoms classified in the body system chapters
> signs and symptoms of breast (N63, N64.5)

AHA: 2017,1Q,6,7

This chapter contains the following blocks:

R00-R09 Symptoms and signs involving the circulatory and respiratory systems
R10-R19 Symptoms and signs involving the digestive system and abdomen
R20-R23 Symptoms and signs involving the skin and subcutaneous tissue
R25-R29 Symptoms and signs involving the nervous and musculoskeletal systems
R30-R39 Symptoms and signs involving the genitourinary system
R40-R46 Symptoms and signs involving cognition, perception, emotional state and behavior
R47-R49 Symptoms and signs involving speech and voice
R50-R69 General symptoms and signs
R70-R79 Abnormal findings on examination of blood, without diagnosis
R80-R82 Abnormal findings on examination of urine, without diagnosis
R83-R89 Abnormal findings on examination of other body fluids, substances and tissues, without diagnosis
R90-R94 Abnormal findings on diagnostic imaging and in function studies, without diagnosis
R97 Abnormal tumor markers
R99 Ill-defined and unknown cause of mortality

Symptoms and signs involving the circulatory and respiratory systems (R00-R09)

✓4ᵗʰ R00 Abnormalities of heart beat
> **EXCLUDES 1**   abnormalities originating in the perinatal period (P29.1-)
> **EXCLUDES 2**   specified arrhythmias (I47-I49)

R00.0 Tachycardia, unspecified
Rapid heart beat
Sinoauricular tachycardia NOS
Sinus [sinusal] tachycardia NOS
> **EXCLUDES 1**   inappropriate sinus tachycardia, so stated (I47.11)
> neonatal tachycardia (P29.11)
> paroxysmal tachycardia (I47.-)

AHA: 2022,4Q,46
DEF: Excessively rapid heart rate of more than 100 beats per minute.

R00.1 Bradycardia, unspecified
Sinoatrial bradycardia
Sinus bradycardia
Slow heart beat
Vagal bradycardia
Use additional code for adverse effect, if applicable, to identify drug (T36-T50 with fifth or sixth character 5)
> **EXCLUDES 1**   neonatal bradycardia (P29.12)

AHA: 2020,2Q,23
DEF: Slowed heartbeat, usually defined as a rate fewer than 60 beats per minute. Heart rhythm may be slow as a result of a congenital defect or an acquired problem.

R00.2 Palpitations
Awareness of heart beat

R00.8 Other abnormalities of heart beat

R00.9 Unspecified abnormalities of heart beat

✓4ᵗʰ R01 Cardiac murmurs and other cardiac sounds
> **EXCLUDES 1**   cardiac murmurs and sounds originating in the perinatal period (P29.8)

R01.0 Benign and innocent cardiac murmurs
Functional cardiac murmur

R01.1 Cardiac murmur, unspecified
Cardiac bruit NOS
Heart murmur NOS
Systolic murmur NOS

R01.2 Other cardiac sounds
Cardiac dullness, increased or decreased
Precordial friction

✓4ᵗʰ R03 Abnormal blood-pressure reading, without diagnosis

R03.0 Elevated blood-pressure reading, without diagnosis of hypertension
> **NOTE** This category is to be used to record an episode of elevated blood pressure in a patient in whom no formal diagnosis of hypertension has been made, or as an isolated incidental finding.

R03.1 Nonspecific low blood-pressure reading
> **EXCLUDES 1**   hypotension (I95.-)
> maternal hypotension syndrome (O26.5-)
> neurogenic orthostatic hypotension (G90.3)

✓4ᵗʰ R04 Hemorrhage from respiratory passages

R04.0 Epistaxis
Hemorrhage from nose
Nosebleed
AHA: 2023,2Q,28

R04.1 Hemorrhage from throat
> **EXCLUDES 2**   hemoptysis (R04.2)

R04.2 Hemoptysis   CC
Blood-stained sputum
Cough with hemorrhage
AHA: 2013,4Q,118

✓5ᵗʰ R04.8 Hemorrhage from other sites in respiratory passages

R04.81 Acute idiopathic pulmonary hemorrhage in infants   CC P
AIPHI
Acute idiopathic hemorrhage in infants over 28 days old
> **EXCLUDES 1**   perinatal pulmonary hemorrhage (P26.-)
> von Willebrand disease (D68.0-)

R04.89 Hemorrhage from other sites in respiratory passages   CC
Pulmonary hemorrhage NOS

R04.9 Hemorrhage from respiratory passages, unspecified   CC

✓4ᵗʰ R05 Cough
> **EXCLUDES 1**   paroxysmal cough due to Bordetella pertussis (A37.0-)
> smoker's cough (J41.0)
> **EXCLUDES 2**   cough with hemorrhage (R04.2)

AHA: 2021,4Q,24-25; 2016,2Q,33

R05.1 Acute cough

R05.2 Subacute cough

R05.3 Chronic cough
Persistent cough
Refractory cough
Unexplained cough

R05.4 Cough syncope   UPD
Code first syncope and collapse (R55)

R05.8 Other specified cough

☑ Additional Character Required   ✓x7ᵗʰ Placeholder   Questionable PDx   Manifestation   Unspecified   UPD Unacceptable PDx   H1 - H14 HAC   HCC CMS-HCC Dx   HIV HIV Dx

ICD-10-CM 2025   **957**

Chapter 18. Symptoms, Signs and Abnormal Clinical and Laboratory Findings

R00–R05.8

Chapter 18. Symptoms, Signs and Abnormal Clinical and Laboratory Findings

R05.9	**Cough, unspecified**

✓4ᵗʰ R06 Abnormalities of breathing

> *EXCLUDES 1*   *acute respiratory distress syndrome (J80)*
> *respiratory arrest (R09.2)*
> *respiratory arrest of newborn (P28.81)*
> *respiratory distress syndrome of newborn (P22.-)*
> *respiratory failure (J96.-)*
> *respiratory failure of newborn (P28.5)*

✓5ᵗʰ R06.0 Dyspnea

> *EXCLUDES 1*   *tachypnea NOS (R06.82)*
> *transient tachypnea of newborn (P22.1)*

   R06.00 Dyspnea, unspecified
     AHA: 2017,1Q,26
   R06.01 Orthopnea
   R06.02 Shortness of breath
   R06.03 Acute respiratory distress
     AHA: 2017,4Q,23
   R06.09 Other forms of dyspnea

R06.1 Stridor

> *EXCLUDES 1*   *congenital laryngeal stridor (P28.89)*
> *laryngismus (stridulus) (J38.5)*

   DEF: Certain type of wheezing described as a loud, constant, musical sound produced when breathing with an obstructed airway, like the inspiratory sound heard when laryngeal or esophageal obstruction is present.

R06.2 Wheezing

> *EXCLUDES 1*   *asthma (J45.-)*

   AHA: 2016,2Q,33
   DEF: High-pitched whistling sound during breathing due to stenosis of the respiratory passageway. Wheezing is associated with asthma, sleep apnea, bronchiectasis, bronchiolitis, COPD, and pleural effusion.

R06.3 Periodic breathing   `CC`
   Cheyne-Stokes breathing

R06.4 Hyperventilation

> *EXCLUDES 1*   *psychogenic hyperventilation (F45.8)*

R06.5 Mouth breathing

> *EXCLUDES 2*   *dry mouth NOS (R68.2)*

R06.6 Hiccough

> *EXCLUDES 1*   *psychogenic hiccough (F45.8)*

R06.7 Sneezing

✓5ᵗʰ R06.8 Other abnormalities of breathing

   R06.81 Apnea, not elsewhere classified
     Apnea NOS

> *EXCLUDES 1*   *apnea (of) newborn (P28.4-)*
> *sleep apnea (G47.3-)*
> *sleep apnea of newborn (primary) (P28.3-)*

   R06.82 Tachypnea, not elsewhere classified
     Tachypnea NOS

> *EXCLUDES 1*   *transitory tachypnea of newborn (P22.1)*

   R06.83 Snoring
   R06.89 Other abnormalities of breathing
     Breath-holding (spells)
     Sighing

R06.9	**Unspecified abnormalities of breathing**

✓4ᵗʰ R07 Pain in throat and chest

> *EXCLUDES 1*   *epidemic myalgia (B33.0)*
> *EXCLUDES 2*   *jaw pain R68.84*
> *pain in breast (N64.4)*

R07.0 Pain in throat

> *EXCLUDES 1*   *chronic sore throat (J31.2)*
> *sore throat (acute) NOS (J02.9)*
> *EXCLUDES 2*   *dysphagia (R13.1-)*
> *pain in neck (M54.2)*

R07.1 Chest pain on breathing
   Painful respiration

R07.2 Precordial pain
   DEF: Pain felt in the anterior (front) chest wall over the region of the heart. This type of pain is generally felt slightly to the left of the sternum, but may also extend into the surrounding chest wall region.

✓5ᵗʰ R07.8 Other chest pain

   R07.81 Pleurodynia
     Pleurodynia NOS

> *EXCLUDES 1*   *epidemic pleurodynia (B33.0)*

   R07.82 Intercostal pain
   R07.89 Other chest pain
     Anterior chest-wall pain NOS
     AHA: 2021,1Q,42

R07.9	**Chest pain, unspecified**

✓4ᵗʰ R09 Other symptoms and signs involving the circulatory and respiratory system

> *EXCLUDES 1*   *acute respiratory distress syndrome (J80)*
> *respiratory arrest of newborn (P28.81)*
> *respiratory distress syndrome of newborn (P22.0)*
> *respiratory failure (J96.-)*
> *respiratory failure of newborn (P28.5)*

✓5ᵗʰ R09.0 Asphyxia and hypoxemia

> *EXCLUDES 1*   *asphyxia due to carbon monoxide (T58.-)*
> *asphyxia due to foreign body in respiratory tract (T17.-)*
> *birth (intrauterine) asphyxia (P84)*
> *hyperventilation (R06.4)*
> *traumatic asphyxia (T71.-)*
> *EXCLUDES 2*   *hypercapnia (R06.89)*

   R09.01 Asphyxia   `CC`
     DEF: Interference of oxygen intake due to obstruction or injury of airways resulting in a lack of oxygen perfusion to the tissues or excessive carbon dioxide in the blood. Can cause unconsciousness or death.

   R09.02 Hypoxemia
     AHA: 2019,3Q,15
     DEF: Insufficient oxygen in the arterial blood resulting in inadequate delivery of oxygen to the body tissues.

R09.1 Pleurisy

> *EXCLUDES 1*   *pleurisy with effusion (J90)*

R09.2 Respiratory arrest   `MCC` `HCC`
   Cardiorespiratory failure

> *EXCLUDES 1*   *cardiac arrest (I46.-)*
> *respiratory arrest of newborn (P28.81)*
> *respiratory distress of newborn (P22.0)*
> *respiratory failure (J96.-)*
> *respiratory failure of newborn (P28.5)*
> *respiratory insufficiency (R06.89)*
> *respiratory insufficiency of newborn (P28.5)*

   TIP: MCC only when patient is discharged alive.

R09.3 Abnormal sputum
   Abnormal amount of sputum
   Abnormal color of sputum
   Abnormal odor of sputum
   Excessive sputum

> *EXCLUDES 1*   *blood-stained sputum (R04.2)*

✓5ᵗʰ R09.8 Other specified symptoms and signs involving the circulatory and respiratory systems

   R09.81 Nasal congestion
   R09.82 Postnasal drip
   R09.89 Other specified symptoms and signs involving the circulatory and respiratory systems
     Abnormal chest percussion
     Bruit (arterial)
     Chest tympany
     Choking sensation
     Friction sounds in chest
     Rales
     Weak pulse

> *EXCLUDES 2*   *foreign body in throat (T17.2-)*
> *wheezing (R06.2)*

     AHA: 2021,1Q,42

✓5ᵗʰ R09.A Foreign body sensation of the circulatory and respiratory system
   AHA: 2023,4Q,41-42

R09.A0	**Foreign body sensation, unspecified**

   R09.A1 Foreign body sensation, nose
   R09.A2 Foreign body sensation, throat
     Foreign body sensation globus
   R09.A9 Foreign body sensation, other site

R05.9–R09.A9

`N` Newborn: 0   `P` Pediatric: 0-17   `M` Maternity: 9-64   `A` Adult: 15-124   `UNS` Unspecified Site   `MCC` Major Complication/Comorbidity   `CC` Complication/Comorbidity   `PE` POA Exempt

958   ICD-10-CM 2025

Symptoms and signs involving the digestive system and abdomen (R10-R19)

> **EXCLUDES 2**   congenital or infantile pylorospasm (Q40.0)
> gastrointestinal hemorrhage (K92.0-K92.2)
> intestinal obstruction (K56.-)
> newborn gastrointestinal hemorrhage (P54.0-P54.3)
> newborn intestinal obstruction (P76.-)
> pylorospasm (K31.3)
> signs and symptoms involving the urinary system (R30-R39)
> symptoms referable to female genital organs (N94.-)
> symptoms referable to male genital organs (N48-N50)

✓4th R10   Abdominal and pelvic pain

> **EXCLUDES 1**   renal colic (N23)
> **EXCLUDES 2**   dorsalgia (M54.-)
> flatulence and related conditions (R14.-)

    R10.0   Acute abdomen
        Severe abdominal pain (generalized) (with abdominal rigidity)
> **EXCLUDES 1**   abdominal rigidity NOS (R19.3)
> generalized abdominal pain NOS (R10.84)
> localized abdominal pain (R10.1-R10.3-)

    ✓5th R10.1   Pain localized to upper abdomen

        R10.10   Upper abdominal pain, unspecified
        R10.11   Right upper quadrant pain
        R10.12   Left upper quadrant pain
        R10.13   Epigastric pain
            Dyspepsia
> **EXCLUDES 1**   functional dyspepsia (K30)

Abdominal Pain

Right upper quadrant (RUQ)   Left upper quadrant (LUQ)
Epigastric
Periumbilical
Right lower quadrant (RLQ)   Left lower quadrant (LLQ)

    R10.2   Pelvic and perineal pain
> **EXCLUDES 1**   vulvodynia (N94.81)

    ✓5th R10.3   Pain localized to other parts of lower abdomen

        R10.30   Lower abdominal pain, unspecified
        R10.31   Right lower quadrant pain
        R10.32   Left lower quadrant pain
        R10.33   Periumbilical pain

    ✓5th R10.8   Other abdominal pain

      ✓6th R10.81   Abdominal tenderness
        Abdominal tenderness NOS
        R10.811   Right upper quadrant abdominal tenderness
        R10.812   Left upper quadrant abdominal tenderness
        R10.813   Right lower quadrant abdominal tenderness
        R10.814   Left lower quadrant abdominal tenderness
        R10.815   Periumbilic abdominal tenderness
        R10.816   Epigastric abdominal tenderness
        R10.817   Generalized abdominal tenderness
        R10.819   Abdominal tenderness, unspecified site

      ✓6th R10.82   Rebound abdominal tenderness
        R10.821   Right upper quadrant rebound abdominal tenderness
        R10.822   Left upper quadrant rebound abdominal tenderness
        R10.823   Right lower quadrant rebound abdominal tenderness
        R10.824   Left lower quadrant rebound abdominal tenderness

        R10.825   Periumbilic rebound abdominal tenderness
        R10.826   Epigastric rebound abdominal tenderness
        R10.827   Generalized rebound abdominal tenderness
        R10.829   Rebound abdominal tenderness, unspecified site

      R10.83   Colic   🅿
        Colic NOS
        Infantile colic
> **EXCLUDES 1**   colic in adult and child over 12 months old (R10.84)

        DEF: Inconsolable crying in an otherwise well-fed and healthy infant for more than three hours a day, three days a week, for more than three weeks.

      R10.84   Generalized abdominal pain
> **EXCLUDES 1**   generalized abdominal pain associated with acute abdomen (R10.0)

    R10.9   Unspecified abdominal pain

✓4th R11   Nausea and vomiting

> **EXCLUDES 1**   cyclical vomiting associated with migraine (G43.A-)
> excessive vomiting in pregnancy (O21.-)
> hematemesis (K92.0)
> neonatal hematemesis (P54.0)
> newborn vomiting (P92.0-)
> psychogenic vomiting (F50.89)
> vomiting associated with bulimia nervosa ▶(F50.2-)◀
> vomiting following gastrointestinal surgery (K91.0)

    AHA: 2017,1Q,28

    R11.0   Nausea
        Nausea NOS
        Nausea without vomiting

    ✓5th R11.1   Vomiting

        R11.10   Vomiting, unspecified
            Vomiting NOS
        R11.11   Vomiting without nausea
        R11.12   Projectile vomiting
        R11.13   Vomiting of fecal matter
        R11.14   Bilious vomiting
            Bilious emesis
        R11.15   Cyclical vomiting syndrome unrelated to migraine
            Cyclic vomiting syndrome NOS
            Persistent vomiting
> **EXCLUDES 1**   cyclical vomiting in migraine (G43.A-)
> **EXCLUDES 2**   bulimia nervosa ▶(F50.20)◀
> diabetes mellitus due to underlying condition (E08.-)

        AHA: 2019,4Q,15

    R11.2   Nausea with vomiting, unspecified
        Persistent nausea with vomiting NOS
        AHA: 2020,1Q,8

R12   Heartburn
> **EXCLUDES 1**   dyspepsia NOS (R10.13)
> functional dyspepsia (K30)

✓4th R13   Aphagia and dysphagia

    R13.0   Aphagia
        Inability to swallow
> **EXCLUDES 1**   psychogenic aphagia (F50.9)

✓ Additional Character Required   ✓x7th Placeholder   Questionable PDx   Manifestation   Unspecified   UPD Unacceptable PDx   H1-H14 HAC   HCC CMS-HCC Dx   HIV HIV Dx

ICD-10-CM 2025   959

✓5ᵗʰ R13.1 Dysphagia

Code first, if applicable, dysphagia following cerebrovascular disease (I69. with final characters -91)

EXCLUDES 1 *psychogenic dysphagia (F45.8)*

Swallowing Function

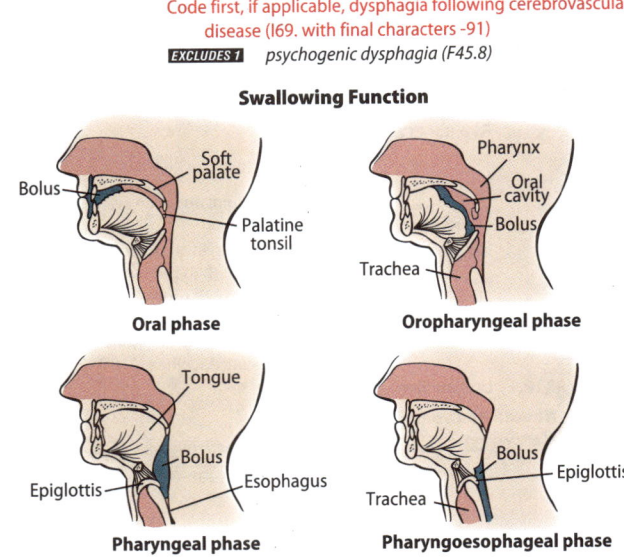

Oral phase — Bolus, Soft palate, Palatine tonsil

Oropharyngeal phase — Pharynx, Oral cavity, Bolus, Trachea

Pharyngeal phase — Tongue, Bolus, Epiglottis, Esophagus

Pharyngoesophageal phase — Bolus, Trachea, Epiglottis

R13.10	**Dysphagia, unspecified**	
	Difficulty in swallowing NOS	
R13.11	**Dysphagia, oral phase**	
R13.12	**Dysphagia, oropharyngeal phase**	
R13.13	**Dysphagia, pharyngeal phase**	
R13.14	**Dysphagia, pharyngoesophageal phase**	
R13.19	**Other dysphagia**	
	Cervical dysphagia	
	Neurogenic dysphagia	

✓4ᵗʰ R14 Flatulence and related conditions

    EXCLUDES 1 *psychogenic aerophagy (F45.8)*

R14.0 Abdominal distension (gaseous)
    Bloating
    Tympanites (abdominal) (intestinal)

R14.1 Gas pain

R14.2 Eructation

R14.3 Flatulence

✓4ᵗʰ R15 Fecal incontinence

    INCLUDES encopresis NOS
    EXCLUDES 1 *fecal incontinence of nonorganic origin (F98.1)*

R15.0 Incomplete defecation
    EXCLUDES 1 *constipation (K59.0-)*
         fecal impaction (K56.41)

R15.1 Fecal smearing
    Fecal soiling

R15.2 Fecal urgency

R15.9 Full incontinence of feces
    Fecal incontinence NOS

✓4ᵗʰ R16 Hepatomegaly and splenomegaly, not elsewhere classified

R16.0 Hepatomegaly, not elsewhere classified
    Hepatomegaly NOS

R16.1 Splenomegaly, not elsewhere classified
    Splenomegaly NOS

R16.2 Hepatomegaly with splenomegaly, not elsewhere classified
    Hepatosplenomegaly NOS

R17 Unspecified jaundice   `CC`
    EXCLUDES 1 *neonatal jaundice (P55, P57-P59)*

✓4ᵗʰ R18 Ascites

    INCLUDES fluid in peritoneal cavity
    EXCLUDES 1 *ascites in alcoholic cirrhosis (K70.31)*
         ascites in alcoholic hepatitis (K70.11)
         ascites in toxic liver disease with chronic active hepatitis (K71.51)

DEF: Abnormal accumulation of free fluid in the abdominal cavity, causing distention and tightness in addition to shortness of breath as the fluid accumulates. Ascites is usually an underlying disorder and can be a manifestation of any number of diseases.

R18.0 Malignant ascites   `CC` `UPD` `HCC`
    Code first malignancy, such as:
        malignant neoplasm of ovary (C56.-)
        secondary malignant neoplasm of retroperitoneum and peritoneum (C78.6)

R18.8 Other ascites   `CC`
    Ascites NOS
    Peritoneal effusion (chronic)
    AHA: 2018,1Q,4

✓4ᵗʰ R19 Other symptoms and signs involving the digestive system and abdomen

    EXCLUDES 1 *acute abdomen (R10.0)*

✓5ᵗʰ R19.0 Intra-abdominal and pelvic swelling, mass and lump

    EXCLUDES 1 *abdominal distension (gaseous) (R14.-)*
         ascites (R18.-)

R19.00	**Intra-abdominal and pelvic swelling, mass and lump, unspecified site**	
R19.01	**Right upper quadrant abdominal swelling, mass and lump**	
R19.02	**Left upper quadrant abdominal swelling, mass and lump**	
R19.03	**Right lower quadrant abdominal swelling, mass and lump**	
R19.04	**Left lower quadrant abdominal swelling, mass and lump**	
R19.05	**Periumbilic swelling, mass or lump**	
	Diffuse or generalized umbilical swelling or mass	
R19.06	**Epigastric swelling, mass or lump**	
R19.07	**Generalized intra-abdominal and pelvic swelling, mass and lump**	
	Diffuse or generalized intra-abdominal swelling or mass NOS	
	Diffuse or generalized pelvic swelling or mass NOS	
R19.09	**Other intra-abdominal and pelvic swelling, mass and lump**	

✓5ᵗʰ R19.1 Abnormal bowel sounds

    R19.11 **Absent bowel sounds**
    R19.12 **Hyperactive bowel sounds**
    R19.15 **Other abnormal bowel sounds**
        Abnormal bowel sounds NOS

R19.2 Visible peristalsis
    Hyperperistalsis
    DEF: Visible movements of muscular attempts to move food through the digestive tract due to pyloric obstruction, stomach obstruction, or intestinal obstruction.

✓5ᵗʰ R19.3 Abdominal rigidity

    EXCLUDES 1 *abdominal rigidity with severe abdominal pain (R10.0)*

R19.30	**Abdominal rigidity, unspecified site**	
R19.31	**Right upper quadrant abdominal rigidity**	
R19.32	**Left upper quadrant abdominal rigidity**	
R19.33	**Right lower quadrant abdominal rigidity**	
R19.34	**Left lower quadrant abdominal rigidity**	
R19.35	**Periumbilic abdominal rigidity**	
R19.36	**Epigastric abdominal rigidity**	
R19.37	**Generalized abdominal rigidity**	

R19.4 Change in bowel habit
    EXCLUDES 1 *constipation (K59.0-)*
         functional diarrhea (K59.1)

R19.5 Other fecal abnormalities
    Abnormal stool color
    Bulky stools
    Mucus in stools
    Occult blood in feces
    Occult blood in stools
    EXCLUDES 1 *melena (K92.1)*
         neonatal melena (P54.1)
    AHA: 2021,1Q,9; 2019,1Q,32

R19.6 Halitosis

N Newborn: 0   **P** Pediatric: 0-17   **M** Maternity: 9-64   **A** Adult: 15-124   **UNS** Unspecified Site   **MCC** Major Complication/Comorbidity   **CC** Complication/Comorbidity   **PE** POA Exempt

960   ICD-10-CM 2025

R19.7　Diarrhea, unspecified
Diarrhea NOS
EXCLUDES 1　functional diarrhea (K59.1)
　　　　　　　neonatal diarrhea (P78.3)
　　　　　　　psychogenic diarrhea (F45.8)
AHA: 2021,3Q,3

R19.8　Other specified symptoms and signs involving the digestive system and abdomen

Symptoms and signs involving the skin and subcutaneous tissue (R20-R23)

EXCLUDES 2　symptoms relating to breast (N64.4-N64.5)

√4th　**R20　Disturbances of skin sensation**
EXCLUDES 1　dissociative anesthesia and sensory loss (F44.6)
　　　　　　　psychogenic disturbances (F45.8)

R20.0　Anesthesia of skin
R20.1　Hypoesthesia of skin
R20.2　Paresthesia of skin
Formication
Pins and needles
Tingling skin
EXCLUDES 1　acroparesthesia (I73.8)

R20.3　Hyperesthesia
R20.8　Other disturbances of skin sensation
R20.9　Unspecified disturbances of skin sensation

R21　Rash and other nonspecific skin eruption
INCLUDES　rash NOS
EXCLUDES 1　specified type of rash - code to condition
　　　　　　　vesicular eruption (R23.8)

√4th　**R22　Localized swelling, mass and lump of skin and subcutaneous tissue**
INCLUDES　subcutaneous nodules (localized)(superficial)
EXCLUDES 1　abnormal findings on diagnostic imaging (R90-R93)
　　　　　　　edema (R60.-)
　　　　　　　enlarged lymph nodes (R59.-)
　　　　　　　localized adiposity (E65)
　　　　　　　swelling of joint (M25.4-)

R22.0　Localized swelling, mass and lump, head
R22.1　Localized swelling, mass and lump, neck
R22.2　Localized swelling, mass and lump, trunk
EXCLUDES 1　intra-abdominal or pelvic mass and lump (R19.0-)
　　　　　　　intra-abdominal or pelvic swelling (R19.0-)
EXCLUDES 2　breast mass and lump (N63)
AHA: 2022,3Q,8

√5th　**R22.3　Localized swelling, mass and lump, upper limb**
　R22.30　Localized swelling, mass and lump, unspecified upper limb
　R22.31　Localized swelling, mass and lump, right upper limb
　R22.32　Localized swelling, mass and lump, left upper limb
　R22.33　Localized swelling, mass and lump, upper limb, bilateral

√5th　**R22.4　Localized swelling, mass and lump, lower limb**
　R22.40　Localized swelling, mass and lump, unspecified lower limb
　R22.41　Localized swelling, mass and lump, right lower limb
　R22.42　Localized swelling, mass and lump, left lower limb
　R22.43　Localized swelling, mass and lump, lower limb, bilateral

R22.9　Localized swelling, mass and lump, unspecified

√4th　**R23　Other skin changes**
R23.0　Cyanosis
EXCLUDES 1　acrocyanosis (I73.8)
　　　　　　　cyanotic attacks of newborn (P28.2)
DEF: Bluish or purplish discoloration of the skin due to an inadequate oxygen blood level.

R23.1　Pallor
Clammy skin
R23.2　Flushing
Excessive blushing
Code first, if applicable, menopausal and female climacteric states (N95.1)
R23.3　Spontaneous ecchymoses
Petechiae
EXCLUDES 1　ecchymoses of newborn (P54.5)
　　　　　　　purpura (D69.-)

R23.4　Changes in skin texture
Desquamation of skin
Induration of skin
Scaling of skin
EXCLUDES 1　epidermal thickening NOS (L85.9)

R23.8　Other skin changes
R23.9　Unspecified skin changes

Symptoms and signs involving the nervous and musculoskeletal systems (R25-R29)

√4th　**R25　Abnormal involuntary movements**
EXCLUDES 1　specific movement disorders (G20-G26)
　　　　　　　stereotyped movement disorders (F98.4)
　　　　　　　tic disorders (F95.-)

R25.0　Abnormal head movements
R25.1　Tremor, unspecified
EXCLUDES 1　chorea NOS (G25.5)
　　　　　　　essential tremor (G25.0)
　　　　　　　hysterical tremor (F44.4)
　　　　　　　intention tremor (G25.2)

R25.2　Cramp and spasm
EXCLUDES 2　carpopedal spasm (R29.0)
　　　　　　　charley-horse (M62.831)
　　　　　　　infantile spasms (G40.4-)
　　　　　　　muscle spasm of back (M62.830)
　　　　　　　muscle spasm of calf (M62.831)

R25.3　Fasciculation
Twitching NOS
R25.8　Other abnormal involuntary movements
R25.9　Unspecified abnormal involuntary movements

√4th　**R26　Abnormalities of gait and mobility**
EXCLUDES 1　ataxia NOS (R27.0)
　　　　　　　hereditary ataxia (G11.-)
　　　　　　　locomotor (syphilitic) ataxia (A52.11)
　　　　　　　immobility syndrome (paraplegic) (M62.3)

R26.0　Ataxic gait
Staggering gait
AHA: 2022,2Q,12
R26.1　Paralytic gait
Spastic gait
R26.2　Difficulty in walking, not elsewhere classified
EXCLUDES 1　falling (R29.6)
　　　　　　　unsteadiness on feet (R26.81)
AHA: 2016,2Q,7

√5th　**R26.8　Other abnormalities of gait and mobility**
　R26.81　Unsteadiness on feet
　R26.89　Other abnormalities of gait and mobility
　　AHA: 2020,2Q,29

R26.9　Unspecified abnormalities of gait and mobility

√4th　**R27　Other lack of coordination**
EXCLUDES 1　ataxic gait (R26.0)
　　　　　　　hereditary ataxia (G11.-)
　　　　　　　vertigo NOS (R42)

R27.0　Ataxia, unspecified
EXCLUDES 1　ataxia following cerebrovascular disease (I69. with final characters -93)

R27.8　Other lack of coordination
R27.9　Unspecified lack of coordination

√4th　**R29　Other symptoms and signs involving the nervous and musculoskeletal systems**
R29.0　Tetany　　　　　　　　　　　　　　　CC
Carpopedal spasm
EXCLUDES 1　hysterical tetany (F44.5)
　　　　　　　neonatal tetany (P71.3)
　　　　　　　parathyroid tetany (E20.9)
　　　　　　　post-thyroidectomy tetany (E89.2)
DEF: Calcium or other mineral imbalance causing voluntary muscles such as hands, feet, or larynx to spasm rhythmically.

R29.1　Meningismus　　　　　　　　　　　　CC
R29.2　Abnormal reflex
EXCLUDES 2　abnormal pupillary reflex (H57.0)
　　　　　　　hyperactive gag reflex (J39.2)
　　　　　　　vasovagal reaction or syncope (R55)

R29.3　Abnormal posture

R29.4 Clicking hip
> EXCLUDES 1 *congenital deformities of hip (Q65.-)*

R29.5 Transient paralysis `CC`
> Code first any associated spinal cord injury (S14.Ø, S14.1-, S24.Ø, S24.1-, S34.Ø-, S34.1-)
> EXCLUDES 1 *transient ischemic attack (G45.9)*

R29.6 Repeated falls
Falling
Tendency to fall
> EXCLUDES 2 *at risk for falling (Z91.81)*
> *history of falling (Z91.81)*
> **AHA:** 2016,2Q,6

✓5th **R29.7 National Institutes of Health Stroke Scale (NIHSS) score**
> Code first the type of cerebral infarction (I63.-)
> **AHA:** 2016,4Q,61-62
> **TIP:** Codes from this subcategory may be assigned based on medical record documentation from clinicians who are not the patient's provider.

✓6th **R29.70 NIHSS score Ø-9**
R29.70Ø	NIHSS score Ø	`UPD`
R29.7Ø1	NIHSS score 1	`UPD`
R29.7Ø2	NIHSS score 2	`UPD`
R29.7Ø3	NIHSS score 3	`UPD`
R29.7Ø4	NIHSS score 4	`UPD`
R29.7Ø5	NIHSS score 5	`UPD`
R29.7Ø6	NIHSS score 6	`UPD`
R29.7Ø7	NIHSS score 7	`UPD`
R29.7Ø8	NIHSS score 8	`UPD`
R29.7Ø9	NIHSS score 9	`UPD`

✓6th **R29.71 NIHSS score 1Ø-19**
R29.71Ø	NIHSS score 1Ø	`UPD`
R29.711	NIHSS score 11	`UPD`
R29.712	NIHSS score 12	`UPD`
R29.713	NIHSS score 13	`UPD`
R29.714	NIHSS score 14	`UPD`
R29.715	NIHSS score 15	`UPD`
R29.716	NIHSS score 16	`UPD`
R29.717	NIHSS score 17	`UPD`
R29.718	NIHSS score 18	`UPD`
R29.719	NIHSS score 19	`UPD`

✓6th **R29.72 NIHSS score 2Ø-29**
R29.72Ø	NIHSS score 2Ø	`UPD`
R29.721	NIHSS score 21	`UPD`
R29.722	NIHSS score 22	`UPD`
R29.723	NIHSS score 23	`UPD`
R29.724	NIHSS score 24	`UPD`
R29.725	NIHSS score 25	`UPD`
R29.726	NIHSS score 26	`UPD`
R29.727	NIHSS score 27	`UPD`
R29.728	NIHSS score 28	`UPD`
R29.729	NIHSS score 29	`UPD`

✓6th **R29.73 NIHSS score 3Ø-39**
R29.73Ø	NIHSS score 3Ø	`UPD`
R29.731	NIHSS score 31	`UPD`
R29.732	NIHSS score 32	`UPD`
R29.733	NIHSS score 33	`UPD`
R29.734	NIHSS score 34	`UPD`
R29.735	NIHSS score 35	`UPD`
R29.736	NIHSS score 36	`UPD`
R29.737	NIHSS score 37	`UPD`
R29.738	NIHSS score 38	`UPD`
R29.739	NIHSS score 39	`UPD`

✓6th **R29.74 NIHSS score 4Ø-42**
R29.74Ø	NIHSS score 4Ø	`UPD`
R29.741	NIHSS score 41	`UPD`
R29.742	NIHSS score 42	`UPD`

✓5th **R29.8 Other symptoms and signs involving the nervous and musculoskeletal systems**

✓6th **R29.81 Other symptoms and signs involving the nervous system**

R29.81Ø Facial weakness
Facial droop
> EXCLUDES 1 *Bell's palsy (G51.Ø)*
> *facial weakness following cerebrovascular disease (I69. with final characters -92)*

R29.818 Other symptoms and signs involving the nervous system

✓6th **R29.89 Other symptoms and signs involving the musculoskeletal system**
> EXCLUDES 2 *pain in limb (M79.6-)*

R29.89Ø Loss of height
> EXCLUDES 1 *osteoporosis (M8Ø-M81)*

R29.891 Ocular torticollis
> EXCLUDES 1 *congenital (sternomastoid) torticollis Q68.Ø*
> *psychogenic torticollis (F45.8)*
> *spasmodic torticollis (G24.3)*
> *torticollis due to birth injury (P15.8)*
> *torticollis NOS M43.6*
> **DEF:** Abnormal head posture as a result of a contracted state of cervical muscles to correct a visual disturbance, either double vision or a visual field defect.

R29.898 Other symptoms and signs involving the musculoskeletal system

✓5th **R29.9 Unspecified symptoms and signs involving the nervous and musculoskeletal systems**

R29.9Ø Unspecified symptoms and signs involving the nervous system

R29.91 Unspecified symptoms and signs involving the musculoskeletal system

Symptoms and signs involving the genitourinary system (R3Ø-R39)

✓4th **R3Ø Pain associated with micturition**
> EXCLUDES 1 *psychogenic pain associated with micturition (F45.8)*

R3Ø.Ø Dysuria
Strangury

R3Ø.1 Vesical tenesmus
> **DEF:** Feeling of a full bladder even when there is little or no urine in the bladder.

R3Ø.9 Painful micturition, unspecified
Painful urination NOS

✓4th **R31 Hematuria**
> EXCLUDES 1 *hematuria included with underlying conditions, such as:*
> *acute cystitis with hematuria (N3Ø.Ø1)*
> *recurrent and persistent hematuria in glomerular diseases (NØ2.-)*
> **AHA:** 2017,1Q,17

R31.Ø Gross hematuria

R31.1 Benign essential microscopic hematuria

✓5th **R31.2 Other microscopic hematuria**
> **AHA:** 2016,4Q,62

R31.21 Asymptomatic microscopic hematuria
AMH

R31.29 Other microscopic hematuria

R31.9 Hematuria, unspecified

✓4th **R32 Unspecified urinary incontinence**
Enuresis NOS
> EXCLUDES 1 *functional urinary incontinence (R39.81)*
> *nonorganic enuresis (F98.Ø)*
> *stress incontinence and other specified urinary incontinence (N39.3-N39.4-)*
> *urinary incontinence associated with cognitive impairment (R39.81)*

☑4th **R33** **Retention of urine**

> EXCLUDES 1   *psychogenic retention of urine (F45.8)*

R33.0 **Drug induced** retention of urine

> Use additional code for adverse effect, if applicable, to identify drug (T36-T50 with fifth or sixth character 5)

R33.8 **Other retention of urine**

> Code first, if applicable, any causal condition, such as:
> enlarged prostate (N40.1)
> **AHA:** 2018,4Q,55

R33.9 **Retention of urine, unspecified**

R34 **Anuria and oliguria**

> EXCLUDES 1   *anuria and oliguria complicating abortion or ectopic or molar pregnancy (O00-O07, O08.4)*
> *anuria and oliguria complicating pregnancy (O26.83-)*
> *anuria and oliguria complicating the puerperium (O90.49)*

☑4th **R35** **Polyuria**

> Code first, if applicable, any causal condition, such as:
> enlarged prostate (N40.1)
> EXCLUDES 1   *psychogenic polyuria (F45.8)*

R35.0 **Frequency of micturition**

R35.1 **Nocturia**

☑5th **R35.8** **Other polyuria**

> **AHA:** 2021,4Q,26

     R35.81 **Nocturnal** polyuria

> > EXCLUDES 2   *nocturnal enuresis (N39.44)*

     R35.89 **Other polyuria**
> > Polyuria NOS

☑4th **R36** **Urethral discharge**

R36.0 **Urethral discharge without blood**

R36.1 **Hematospermia**

R36.9 **Urethral discharge, unspecified**
> Penile discharge NOS
> Urethrorrhea

R37 **Sexual dysfunction, unspecified**

☑4th **R39** **Other and unspecified symptoms and signs involving the genitourinary system**

R39.0 **Extravasation of urine**   CC

☑5th **R39.1** **Other difficulties with micturition**

> Code first, if applicable, any causal condition, such as:
> enlarged prostate (N40.1)

     R39.11 **Hesitancy of micturition**

     R39.12 **Poor urinary stream**
> > Weak urinary stream

     R39.13 **Splitting of urinary stream**

     R39.14 **Feeling of incomplete bladder emptying**

     R39.15 **Urgency of urination**
> > EXCLUDES 1   *urge incontinence (N39.41, N39.46)*

     R39.16 **Straining to void**

     ☑6th **R39.19** **Other difficulties with micturition**
> > **AHA:** 2016,4Q,63
> > > **R39.191** **Need to immediately re-void**
> > > **R39.192** **Position dependent micturition**
> > > **R39.198** **Other difficulties with micturition**

R39.2 **Extrarenal uremia**
> Prerenal uremia
> EXCLUDES 1   *uremia NOS (N19)*

☑5th **R39.8** **Other symptoms and signs involving the genitourinary system**

> **AHA:** 2017,4Q,22-23

     R39.81 **Functional urinary incontinence**
> > Urinary incontinence due to cognitive impairment, or severe physical disability or immobility
> > EXCLUDES 1   *stress incontinence and other specified urinary incontinence (N39.3-N39.4-)*
> > *urinary incontinence NOS (R32)*

     R39.82 **Chronic bladder pain**
> > **AHA:** 2016,4Q,64

     R39.83 **Unilateral non-palpable testicle**

     R39.84 **Bilateral non-palpable testicles**

     R39.89 **Other symptoms and signs involving the genitourinary system**

R39.9 **Unspecified symptoms and signs involving the genitourinary system**

Symptoms and signs involving cognition, perception, emotional state and behavior (R40-R46)

> EXCLUDES 2   *symptoms and signs constituting part of a pattern of mental disorder (F01-F99)*

☑4th **R40** **Somnolence, stupor and coma**

> EXCLUDES 1   *neonatal coma (P91.5)*
> *somnolence, stupor and coma in diabetes (E08-E13)*
> *somnolence, stupor and coma in hepatic failure (K72.-)*
> *somnolence, stupor and coma in hypoglycemia (nondiabetic) (E15)*

R40.0 **Somnolence**
> Drowsiness
> EXCLUDES 1   *coma (R40.2-)*

R40.1 **Stupor**
> Catatonic stupor
> Semicoma
> EXCLUDES 1   *catatonic schizophrenia (F20.2)*
> *coma (R40.2-)*
> *depressive stupor (F31-F33)*
> *dissociative stupor (F44.2)*
> *manic stupor (F30.2)*

☑5th **R40.2** **Coma**

> Code first any associated:
> fracture of skull (S02.-)
> intracranial injury (S06.-)

> NOTE   One code from each subcategory, R40.21-R40.23, is required to complete the coma scale

> **AHA:** 2020,3Q,46; 2019,2Q,12; 2018,4Q,70; 2017,4Q,23-25,95; 2015,2Q,17; 2014,1Q,19

> **TIP:** The codes for individual (R40.21-, R40.22-, R40.23-) or total (R40.24-) coma scale scores are only assigned as secondary diagnoses with traumatic brain injury (TBI) codes (S06.2X-, S06.30-, S06.9X-). While individual or total coma scale scores may be useful to providers in their clinical decision making when trying to establish a diagnosis, the codes reflecting these scores may not be assigned in conjunction with conditions other than TBIs.

> **TIP:** Codes for individual (R40.21-, R40.22-, R40.23-) or total (R40.24-) coma scale scores may be assigned based on medical record documentation from clinicians who are not the patient's provider.

> **TIP:** It is not appropriate to assign individual (R40.21-, R40.22-, R40.23-) or total (R40.24-) coma scale score codes for patients who are sedated or in medically induced comas, nor in conjunction with code R40.2A.

     R40.20 **Unspecified coma**   MCC HCC
> > Coma NOS
> > Unconsciousness NOS
> > **AHA:** 2021,4Q,112-113; 2021,2Q,5

     ☑6th **R40.21** **Coma scale, eyes open**

> > The following appropriate 7th character is to be added to subcategory R40.21-, R40.22-, R40.23-, and R40.24-.
> > 0   unspecified time
> > 1   in the field [EMT or ambulance]
> > 2   at arrival to emergency department
> > 3   at hospital admission
> > 4   24 hours or more after hospital admission

> > ☑7th **R40.211** **Coma scale, eyes open, never**   MCC UPD HCC
> > > Coma scale eye opening score of 1

> > ☑7th **R40.212** **Coma scale, eyes open, to pain**   MCC UPD HCC
> > > Coma scale eye opening score of 2

> > ☑7th **R40.213** **Coma scale, eyes open, to sound**   UPD
> > > Coma scale eye opening score of 3

> > ☑7th **R40.214** **Coma scale, eyes open, spontaneous**   UPD
> > > Coma scale eye opening score of 4

     ☑6th **R40.22** **Coma scale, best verbal response**

> > ☑7th **R40.221** **Coma scale, best verbal response, none**   MCC UPD HCC
> > > Coma scale verbal score of 1

☑ Additional Character Required   ☑x7th Placeholder   Questionable PDx   Manifestation   Unspecified   UPD Unacceptable PDx   H1-H14 HAC   HCC CMS-HCC Dx   HIV HIV Dx

✓7th **R40.222** **Coma scale, best verbal response, incomprehensible words** `MCC` `UPD` `HCC`
Coma scale verbal score of 2
Incomprehensible sounds (2-5 years of age)
Moans/grunts to pain; restless (< 2 years old)

✓7th **R40.223** **Coma scale, best verbal response, inappropriate words** `UPD`
Coma scale verbal score of 3
Inappropriate crying or screaming (< 2 years of age)
Screaming (2-5 years of age)

✓7th **R40.224** **Coma scale, best verbal response, confused conversation** `UPD`
Coma scale verbal score of 4
Inappropriate words (2-5 years of age)
Irritable cries (< 2 years of age)

✓7th **R40.225** **Coma scale, best verbal response, oriented** `UPD`
Coma scale verbal score of 5
Cooing or babbling or crying appropriately (< 2 years of age)
Uses appropriate words (2-5 years of age)

✓6th **R40.23** **Coma scale, best motor response**

✓7th **R40.231** **Coma scale, best motor response, none** `MCC` `UPD` `HCC`
Coma scale motor score of 1

✓7th **R40.232** **Coma scale, best motor response, extension** `MCC` `UPD` `HCC`
Abnormal extensor posturing to pain or noxious stimuli (< 2 years of age)
Coma scale motor score of 2
Extensor posturing to pain or noxious stimuli (2-5 years of age)

✓7th **R40.233** **Coma scale, best motor response, abnormal flexion** `UPD`
Abnormal flexure posturing to pain or noxious stimuli (2-5 years of age)
Coma scale motor score of 3
Flexion/decorticate posturing (< 2 years of age)

✓7th **R40.234** **Coma scale, best motor response, flexion withdrawal** `MCC` `UPD`
Coma scale motor score of 4
Withdraws from pain or noxious stimuli (2-5 years of age)

✓7th **R40.235** **Coma scale, best motor response, localizes pain** `UPD`
Coma scale motor score of 5
Localizes pain (2-5 years of age)
Withdraws to touch (< 2 years of age)

✓7th **R40.236** **Coma scale, best motor response, obeys commands** `UPD`
Coma scale motor score of 6
Normal or spontaneous movement (< 2 years of age)
Obeys commands (2-5 years of age)

✓6th **R40.24** **Glasgow coma scale, total score**

> `NOTE` Assign a code from subcategory R40.24, when only the total coma score is documented

AHA: 2021,2Q,4; 2016,4Q,64-65

✓7th **R40.241** **Glasgow coma scale score 13-15** `UPD`
✓7th **R40.242** **Glasgow coma scale score 9-12** `UPD`
✓7th **R40.243** **Glasgow coma scale score 3-8** `UPD` `HCC`
✓7th **R40.244** **Other coma, without documented Glasgow coma scale score, or with partial score reported** `UPD` `HCC`

R40.2A **Nontraumatic coma due to underlying condition** `MCC` `UPD` `HCC`
Secondary coma
Code first underlying condition
AHA: 2023,4Q,42

R40.3 **Persistent vegetative state** `CC` `HCC`
DEF: Persistent wakefulness without consciousness due to a nonfunctioning cerebral cortex.

R40.4 **Transient alteration of awareness**
AHA: 2020,2Q,24

✓4th **R41** **Other symptoms and signs involving cognitive functions and awareness**
> `EXCLUDES 1` dissociative [conversion] disorders (F44.-)
> mild cognitive impairment of uncertain or unknown etiology) (G31.84)

R41.0 **Disorientation, unspecified**
Confusion NOS
Delirium NOS
> `EXCLUDES 1` ►delirium due to known physiological condition (F05)◄
AHA: 2022,2Q,11; 2019,2Q,34

R41.1 **Anterograde amnesia**

R41.2 **Retrograde amnesia**

R41.3 **Other amnesia**
Amnesia NOS
Memory loss NOS
> `EXCLUDES 1` amnestic disorder due to known physiologic condition (F04)
> amnestic syndrome due to psychoactive substance use (F10-F19 with 5th character .6)
> mild memory disturbance due to known physiological condition (F06.8)
> transient global amnesia (G45.4)

R41.4 **Neurologic neglect syndrome** `CC`
Asomatognosia
Hemi-akinesia
Hemi-inattention
Hemispatial neglect
Left-sided neglect
Sensory neglect
Visuospatial neglect
> `EXCLUDES 1` visuospatial deficit (R41.842)

✓5th **R41.8** **Other symptoms and signs involving cognitive functions and awareness**

R41.81 **Age-related cognitive decline** `A`
Senility NOS

R41.82 **Altered mental status, unspecified**
Change in mental status NOS
> `EXCLUDES 1` altered level of consciousness (R40.-)
> altered mental status due to known condition - code to condition
> delirium NOS (R41.0)
AHA: 2012,4Q,97

R41.83 **Borderline intellectual functioning** `UPD`
IQ level 71 to 84
> `EXCLUDES 1` intellectual disabilities (F70-F79)

✓6th **R41.84** **Other specified cognitive deficit**
> ►Code first the underlying condition, if known, such as:◄
> ►schizophrenia (F20.-)◄
> `EXCLUDES 1` cognitive deficits as sequelae of cerebrovascular disease (I69.01-, I69.11-, I69.21-, I69.31-, I69.81-, I69.91-)

R41.840 **Attention and concentration deficit**
> `EXCLUDES 1` attention-deficit hyperactivity disorders (F90.-)

R41.841 **Cognitive communication deficit**
R41.842 **Visuospatial deficit**
R41.843 **Psychomotor deficit**
R41.844 **Frontal lobe and executive function deficit**

● **R41.85** **Anosognosia**

R41.89 **Other symptoms and signs involving cognitive functions and awareness**
~~Anosognosia~~

R41.9 **Unspecified symptoms and signs involving cognitive functions and awareness**
Unspecified neurocognitive disorder

R42 **Dizziness and giddiness**
Light-headedness
Vertigo NOS
> `EXCLUDES 1` vertiginous syndromes (H81.-)
> vertigo from infrasound (T75.23)

✓4th **R43** **Disturbances of smell and taste**

R43.0 **Anosmia**
DEF: Permanent or transient absence of smell that may be congenital or acquired.

`N` Newborn: 0   `P` Pediatric: 0-17   `M` Maternity: 9-64   `A` Adult: 15-124   `UNS` Unspecified Site   `MCC` Major Complication/Comorbidity   `CC` Complication/Comorbidity   `PE` POA Exempt

964

ICD-10-CM 2025

R43.1   **Parosmia**
    DEF: Abnormal perception of smell usually triggered by environmental odors.

R43.2   **Parageusia**
    DEF: Abnormal perception of taste.

R43.8   **Other disturbances of smell and taste**
    Mixed disturbance of smell and taste

R43.9   **Unspecified disturbances of smell and taste**

☑4ᵗʰ **R44**   **Other symptoms and signs involving general sensations and perceptions**
    EXCLUDES 1   *alcoholic hallucinations (F10.151, F10.251, F10.951)*
      hallucinations in drug psychosis (F11-F19 with fifth to sixth characters 51)
      hallucinations in mood disorders with psychotic symptoms (F30.2, F31.5, F32.3, F33.3)
      hallucinations in schizophrenia, schizotypal and delusional disorders (F20-F29)
    EXCLUDES 2   *disturbances of skin sensation (R20.-)*

R44.0   **Auditory hallucinations**   `CC`

R44.1   **Visual hallucinations**

R44.2   **Other hallucinations**   `CC`

R44.3   **Hallucinations, unspecified**   `CC`
    AHA: 2022,2Q,11

R44.8   **Other symptoms and signs involving general sensations and perceptions**

R44.9   **Unspecified symptoms and signs involving general sensations and perceptions**

☑4ᵗʰ **R45**   **Symptoms and signs involving emotional state**

R45.0   **Nervousness**
    Nervous tension

R45.1   **Restlessness and agitation**

R45.2   **Unhappiness**

R45.3   **Demoralization and apathy**
    EXCLUDES 1   *anhedonia (R45.84)*

R45.4   **Irritability and anger**

R45.5   **Hostility**

R45.6   **Violent behavior**

R45.7   **State of emotional shock and stress, unspecified**

☑5ᵗʰ **R45.8**   **Other symptoms and signs involving emotional state**

    R45.81   **Low self-esteem**
    R45.82   **Worries**
    R45.83   **Excessive crying of child, adolescent or adult**
      EXCLUDES 1   *excessive crying of infant (baby) R68.11*
    R45.84   **Anhedonia**
    ☑6ᵗʰ **R45.85**   **Homicidal and suicidal ideations**
      EXCLUDES 1   *suicide attempt (T14.91)*
      R45.850   **Homicidal ideations**   `UPD`
      R45.851   **Suicidal ideations**   `CC`
        AHA: 2022,1Q,29
        DEF: Thoughts of committing suicide but no actual attempt of suicide has been made.
    R45.86   **Emotional lability**
    R45.87   **Impulsiveness**
    R45.88   **Nonsuicidal self-harm**   `HCC`
      Nonsuicidal self-injury
      Nonsuicidal self-mutilation
      Self-inflicted injury without suicidal intent
      Code also injury, if known
      AHA: 2021,4Q,26-27
    R45.89   **Other symptoms and signs involving emotional state**
      Flat affect
      Loneliness

☑4ᵗʰ **R46**   **Symptoms and signs involving appearance and behavior**
    EXCLUDES 1   *appearance and behavior in schizophrenia, schizotypal and delusional disorders (F20-F29)*
      mental and behavioral disorders (F01-F99)

R46.0   **Very low level of personal hygiene**

R46.1   **Bizarre personal appearance**

R46.2   **Strange and inexplicable behavior**

R46.3   **Overactivity**

R46.4   **Slowness and poor responsiveness**
    EXCLUDES 1   *stupor (R40.1)*

R46.5   **Suspiciousness and marked evasiveness**

R46.6   **Undue concern and preoccupation with stressful events**

R46.7   **Verbosity and circumstantial detail obscuring reason for contact**

☑5ᵗʰ **R46.8**   **Other symptoms and signs involving appearance and behavior**

    R46.81   **Obsessive-compulsive behavior**   `UPD`
      EXCLUDES 1   *obsessive-compulsive disorder (F42.-)*
    R46.89   **Other symptoms and signs involving appearance and behavior**   `UPD`

Symptoms and signs involving speech and voice (R47-R49)

☑4ᵗʰ **R47**   **Speech disturbances, not elsewhere classified**
    EXCLUDES 1   *autism (F84.0)*
      cluttering (F80.81)
      specific developmental disorders of speech and language (F80.-)
      stuttering (F80.81)

☑5ᵗʰ **R47.0**   **Dysphasia and aphasia**

    R47.01   **Aphasia**   `CC`
      EXCLUDES 1   *aphasia following cerebrovascular disease (I69. with final characters -20)*
        progressive isolated aphasia (G31.01)
    R47.02   **Dysphasia**
      EXCLUDES 1   *dysphasia following cerebrovascular disease (I69. with final characters -21)*

R47.1   **Dysarthria and anarthria**
    EXCLUDES 1   *dysarthria following cerebrovascular disease (I69. with final characters -22)*

☑5ᵗʰ **R47.8**   **Other speech disturbances**
    EXCLUDES 1   *dysarthria following cerebrovascular disease (I69. with final characters -28)*

    R47.81   **Slurred speech**
    R47.82   ***Fluency disorder in conditions classified elsewhere***
      Stuttering in conditions classified elsewhere
      Code first underlying disease or condition, such as:
      Parkinson's disease (G20.-)
      EXCLUDES 1   *adult onset fluency disorder (F98.5)*
        childhood onset fluency disorder (F80.81)
        fluency disorder (stuttering) following cerebrovascular disease (I69. with final characters -23)
    R47.89   **Other speech disturbances**

R47.9   **Unspecified speech disturbances**

☑4ᵗʰ **R48**   **Dyslexia and other symbolic dysfunctions, not elsewhere classified**
    EXCLUDES 1   *specific developmental disorders of scholastic skills (F81.-)*

R48.0   **Dyslexia and alexia**

R48.1   **Agnosia**
    Astereognosia (astereognosis)
    Autotopagnosia
    EXCLUDES 1   *visual object agnosia (R48.3)*
    DEF: Inability to recognize common things such as faces, objects, smells, or voices.

R48.2   **Apraxia**
    EXCLUDES 1   *apraxia following cerebrovascular disease (I69. with final characters -90)*

R48.3   **Visual agnosia**
    Prosopagnosia
    Simultanagnosia (asimultagnosia)

R48.8   **Other symbolic dysfunctions**
    Acalculia
    Agraphia
    AHA: 2017,1Q,27

R48.9   **Unspecified symbolic dysfunctions**

☑4ᵗʰ **R49**   **Voice and resonance disorders**
    EXCLUDES 1   *psychogenic voice and resonance disorders (F44.4)*

R49.0   **Dysphonia**
    Hoarseness

R49.1   **Aphonia**
    Loss of voice

☑5ᵗʰ **R49.2**   **Hypernasality and hyponasality**

    R49.21   **Hypernasality**
    R49.22   **Hyponasality**

R49.8   **Other voice and resonance disorders**

R49.9   **Unspecified voice and resonance disorder**
    Change in voice NOS
    Resonance disorder NOS

☑ Additional Character Required   ☑x7ᵗʰ Placeholder   Questionable PDx   Manifestation   Unspecified   `UPD` Unacceptable PDx   `H1`-`H14` HAC   `HCC` CMS-HCC Dx   `HIV` HIV Dx

ICD-10-CM 2025   **965**

Chapter 18. Symptoms, Signs and Abnormal Clinical and Laboratory Findings

General symptoms and signs (R5Ø-R69)

✓4ᵗʰ R5Ø   Fever of other and unknown origin

> EXCLUDES 1   *chills without fever (R68.83)*
> *febrile convulsions (R56.Ø-)*
> *fever of unknown origin during labor (O75.2)*
> *fever of unknown origin in newborn (P81.9)*
> *hypothermia due to illness (R68.Ø)*
> *malignant hyperthermia due to anesthesia (T88.3)*
> *puerperal pyrexia NOS (O86.4)*

R5Ø.2   **Drug induced** fever
Use additional code for adverse effect, if applicable, to identify drug (T36-T5Ø with fifth or sixth character 5)
> EXCLUDES 1   *postvaccination (postimmunization) fever (R5Ø.83)*

✓5ᵗʰ R5Ø.8   **Other specified fever**

R5Ø.81   *Fever presenting with conditions classified elsewhere*
Code first underlying condition when associated fever is present, such as with:
leukemia (C91-C95)
neutropenia (D7Ø.-)
sickle-cell disease (D57.-)
AHA: 2020,3Q,22; 2014,4Q,22

R5Ø.82   **Postprocedural** fever
> EXCLUDES 1   *postprocedural infection (T81.4-)*
> *posttransfusion fever (R5Ø.84)*
> *postvaccination (postimmunization) fever (R5Ø.83)*

R5Ø.83   **Postvaccination** fever
Postimmunization fever

R5Ø.84   **Febrile nonhemolytic transfusion reaction**
FNHTR
Posttransfusion fever

R5Ø.9   **Fever, unspecified**
Fever NOS
Fever of unknown origin [FUO]
Fever with chills
Fever with rigors
Hyperpyrexia NOS
Persistent fever
Pyrexia NOS

✓4ᵗʰ R51   Headache

> EXCLUDES 2   *atypical face pain (G5Ø.1)*
> *migraine and other headache syndromes (G43-G44)*
> *trigeminal neuralgia (G5Ø.Ø)*

AHA: 2020,4Q,38-39

R51.Ø   **Headache with orthostatic component, not elsewhere classified**
Headache with positional component, not elsewhere classified

R51.9   **Headache, unspecified**
Facial pain NOS

R52   Pain, unspecified
Acute pain NOS
Generalized pain NOS
Pain NOS
> EXCLUDES 1   *acute and chronic pain, not elsewhere classified (G89.-)*
> *localized pain, unspecified type - code to pain by site, such as:*
> *abdomen pain (R1Ø.-)*
> *back pain (M54.9)*
> *breast pain (N64.4)*
> *chest pain (RØ7.1-RØ7.9)*
> *ear pain (H92.Ø-)*
> *eye pain (H57.1)*
> *headache (R51.9)*
> *joint pain (M25.5-)*
> *limb pain (M79.6-)*
> *lumbar region pain (M54.5-)*
> *pelvic and perineal pain (R1Ø.2)*
> *renal colic (N23)*
> *shoulder pain (M25.51-)*
> *spine pain (M54.-)*
> *throat pain (RØ7.Ø)*
> *tongue pain (K14.6)*
> *tooth pain (KØ8.8)*
> *pain disorders exclusively related to psychological factors (F45.41)*

✓4ᵗʰ R53   Malaise and fatigue

R53.Ø   **Neoplastic (malignant) related fatigue**
Code first associated neoplasm

R53.1   **Weakness**
Asthenia NOS
> EXCLUDES 1   *age-related weakness (R54)*
> *muscle weakness (generalized) (M62.81)*
> *sarcopenia (M62.84)*
> *senile asthenia (R54)*

AHA: 2017,1Q,7; 2015,1Q,25

R53.2   **Functional quadriplegia**   MCC   HCC
Complete immobility due to severe physical disability or frailty
> EXCLUDES 1   *frailty NOS (R54)*
> *hysterical paralysis (F44.4)*
> *immobility syndrome (M62.3)*
> *neurologic quadriplegia (G82.5-)*
> *quadriplegia (G82.5Ø)*

AHA: 2022,4Q,15; 2016,2Q,6
DEF: Inability to move due to a nonphysiological condition, such as dementia. The patient has no mental ability to move independently.

✓5ᵗʰ R53.8   **Other malaise and fatigue**
> EXCLUDES 1   *combat exhaustion and fatigue (F43.Ø)*
> *congenital debility (P96.9)*
> *exhaustion and fatigue due to excessive exertion (T73.3)*
> *exhaustion and fatigue due to exposure (T73.2)*
> *exhaustion and fatigue due to heat (T67.-)*
> *exhaustion and fatigue due to pregnancy (O26.8-)*
> *exhaustion and fatigue due to recurrent depressive episode (F33)*
> *exhaustion and fatigue due to senile debility (R54)*

R53.81   **Other malaise**
Chronic debility
Debility NOS
General physical deterioration
Malaise NOS
Nervous debility
> EXCLUDES 1   *age-related physical debility (R54)*

AHA: 2021,1Q,43

R53.82   **Chronic fatigue, unspecified**
> EXCLUDES 1   *chronic fatigue syndrome (G93.32)*
> *myalgic encephalomyelitis (G93.32)*
> *other post infection and related fatigue syndromes (G93.39)*
> *postviral fatigue syndrome (G93.31)*

N Newborn: 0   P Pediatric: 0-17   M Maternity: 9-64   A Adult: 15-124   UNS Unspecified Site   MCC Major Complication/Comorbidity   CC Complication/Comorbidity   PE POA Exempt

966   ICD-10-CM 2025

R53.83   **Other fatigue**
Fatigue NOS
Lack of energy
Lethargy
Tiredness
EXCLUDES 2   exhaustion and fatigue due to depressive episode (F32.-)

R54   **Age-related physical debility**   A
Frailty
Old age
Senescence
Senile asthenia
Senile debility
EXCLUDES 1   age-related cognitive decline (R41.81)
sarcopenia (M62.84)
senile psychosis ▶(F03.-)◀
senility NOS (R41.81)

R55   **Syncope and collapse**
Blackout
Fainting
Vasovagal attack
EXCLUDES 1   cardiogenic shock (R57.0)
carotid sinus syncope (G90.01)
heat syncope (T67.1)
neurocirculatory asthenia (F45.8)
neurogenic orthostatic hypotension (G90.3)
orthostatic hypotension (I95.1)
postprocedural shock (T81.1-)
psychogenic syncope (F48.8)
shock NOS (R57.9)
shock complicating or following abortion or ectopic or molar pregnancy (O00-O07, O08.3)
shock complicating or following labor and delivery (O75.1)
Stokes-Adams attack (I45.9)
unconsciousness NOS (R40.2-)

✓4ᵗʰ   **R56**   **Convulsions, not elsewhere classified**
EXCLUDES 1   dissociative convulsions and seizures (F44.5)
epileptic convulsions and seizures (G40.-)
newborn convulsions and seizures (P90)

✓5ᵗʰ   **R56.0**   **Febrile convulsions**

R56.00   **Simple febrile convulsions**   CC HCC
Febrile convulsion NOS
Febrile seizure NOS

R56.01   **Complex febrile convulsions**   CC HCC
Atypical febrile seizure
Complex febrile seizure
Complicated febrile seizure
EXCLUDES 1   status epilepticus (G40.901)

R56.1   **Post traumatic seizures**   CC HCC
EXCLUDES 1   post traumatic epilepsy (G40.-)

R56.9   **Unspecified convulsions**   HCC
Convulsion disorder
Fit NOS
Recurrent convulsions
Seizure(s) (convulsive) NOS
AHA: 2022,4Q,46; 2021,1Q,3; 2019,1Q,19

✓4ᵗʰ   **R57**   **Shock, not elsewhere classified**
EXCLUDES 1   anaphylactic shock NOS (T78.2)
anaphylactic reaction or shock due to adverse food reaction (T78.0-)
anaphylactic shock due to adverse effect of correct drug or medicament properly administered (T88.6)
anaphylactic shock due to serum (T80.5-)
electric shock (T75.4)
obstetric shock (O75.1)
postprocedural shock (T81.1-)
psychic shock (F43.0)
shock complicating or following ectopic or molar pregnancy (O00-O07, O08.3)
shock due to anesthesia (T88.2)
shock due to lightning (T75.01)
toxic shock syndrome (A48.3)
traumatic shock (T79.4)

R57.0   **Cardiogenic shock**   MCC HCC
EXCLUDES 2   septic shock (R65.21)
AHA: 2020,3Q,26
DEF: Associated with myocardial infarction, cardiac tamponade, and massive pulmonary embolism. Symptoms include mental confusion, reduced blood pressure, tachycardia, pallor, and cold, clammy skin.
TIP: MCC only when patient is discharged alive.

R57.1   **Hypovolemic shock**   MCC HCC
AHA: 2019,2Q,7
TIP: MCC only when patient is discharged alive.

R57.8   **Other shock**   MCC HCC
TIP: MCC only when patient is discharged alive.

R57.9   **Shock, unspecified**   CC HCC
Failure of peripheral circulation NOS

R58   **Hemorrhage, not elsewhere classified**
Hemorrhage NOS
EXCLUDES 1   hemorrhage included with underlying conditions, such as:
   acute duodenal ulcer with hemorrhage (K26.0)
   acute gastritis with bleeding (K29.01)
   ulcerative enterocolitis with rectal bleeding (K51.01)

✓4ᵗʰ   **R59**   **Enlarged lymph nodes**
INCLUDES   swollen glands
EXCLUDES 1   acute lymphadenitis (L04.-)
chronic lymphadenitis (I88.1)
lymphadenitis NOS (I88.9)
mesenteric (acute) (chronic) lymphadenitis (I88.0)

R59.0   **Localized enlarged lymph nodes**

R59.1   **Generalized enlarged lymph nodes**
Lymphadenopathy NOS

R59.9   **Enlarged lymph nodes, unspecified**

✓4ᵗʰ   **R60**   **Edema, not elsewhere classified**
EXCLUDES 1   angioneurotic edema (T78.3)
ascites (R18.-)
cerebral edema (G93.6)
cerebral edema due to birth injury (P11.0)
edema of larynx (J38.4)
edema of nasopharynx (J39.2)
edema of pharynx (J39.2)
gestational edema (O12.0-)
hereditary edema (Q82.0)
hydrops fetalis NOS (P83.2)
hydrothorax (J94.8)
newborn edema (P83.3)
pulmonary edema (J81.-)

R60.0   **Localized edema**

R60.1   **Generalized edema**
EXCLUDES 2   nutritional edema (E40-E46)

R60.9   **Edema, unspecified**
Fluid retention NOS

Chapter 18. Symptoms, Signs and Abnormal Clinical and Laboratory Findings

R61   Generalized hyperhidrosis
Excessive sweating
Night sweats
Secondary hyperhidrosis
Code first, if applicable, menopausal and female climacteric states (N95.1)
EXCLUDES 1   *focal (primary) (secondary) hyperhidrosis (L74.5-)*
Frey's syndrome (L74.52)
localized (primary) (secondary) hyperhidrosis (L74.5-)

✓4ᵗʰ R62   Lack of expected normal physiological development in childhood and adults
EXCLUDES 1   *delayed puberty (E30.0)*
gonadal dysgenesis (Q99.1)
hypopituitarism (E23.0)

R62.0   Delayed milestone in childhood   P
Delayed attainment of expected physiological developmental stage
Late talker
Late walker

✓5ᵗʰ R62.5   Other and unspecified lack of expected normal physiological development in childhood
EXCLUDES 1   *HIV disease resulting in failure to thrive (B20)*
physical retardation due to malnutrition (E45)

R62.50   Unspecified lack of expected normal physiological development in childhood
Infantilism NOS

R62.51   Failure to thrive (child)   P
Failure to gain weight
EXCLUDES 1   *failure to thrive in child under 28 days old (P92.6)*

AHA: 2018,4Q,82
DEF: Organic failure to thrive (FTT): Acute or chronic illness that interferes with nutritional intake, absorption, metabolism excretion, and energy requirements.
DEF: Nonorganic failure to thrive (FTT): Symptom of neglect or abuse.

R62.52   Short stature (child)
Lack of growth
Physical retardation
Short stature NOS
EXCLUDES 1   *short stature due to endocrine disorder (E34.3-)*

R62.59   Other lack of expected normal physiological development in childhood

R62.7   Adult failure to thrive   A

✓4ᵗʰ R63   Symptoms and signs concerning food and fluid intake
EXCLUDES 1   *bulimia NOS ▶(F50.2-)◀*

R63.0   Anorexia
Loss of appetite
EXCLUDES 1   *anorexia nervosa (F50.0-)*
loss of appetite of nonorganic origin (F50.89)

AHA: 2018,4Q,82
TIP: Assign an additional code from category Z68 when BMI is documented. BMI can be based on documentation from clinicians who are not the patient's provider.

R63.1   Polydipsia
Excessive thirst

R63.2   Polyphagia
Excessive eating
Hyperalimentation NOS

✓5ᵗʰ R63.3   Feeding difficulties
EXCLUDES 2   *eating disorders (F50.-)*
feeding problems of newborn (P92.-)
infant feeding disorder of nonorganic origin (F98.2-)

AHA: 2021,4Q,27-28; 2017,1Q,28; 2016,3Q,19

R63.30   Feeding difficulties, unspecified

R63.31   Pediatric feeding disorder, acute   P
Pediatric feeding dysfunction, acute
Code also, if applicable, associated conditions such as:
aspiration pneumonia (J69.0)
dysphagia (R13.1-)
gastro-esophageal reflux disease (K21.-)
malnutrition (E40-E46)

R63.32   Pediatric feeding disorder, chronic   P
Pediatric feeding dysfunction, chronic
Code also, if applicable, associated conditions such as:
aspiration pneumonia (J69.0)
dysphagia (R13.1-)
gastro-esophageal reflux disease (K21.-)
malnutrition (E40-E46)

R63.39   Other feeding difficulties
Feeding problem (elderly) (infant) NOS
Picky eater

R63.4   Abnormal weight loss
AHA: 2018,4Q,82
TIP: Assign an additional code from category Z68 when BMI is documented. BMI can be based on documentation from clinicians who are not the patient's provider.

R63.5   Abnormal weight gain
EXCLUDES 1   *excessive weight gain in pregnancy (O26.0-)*
obesity (E66.-)
AHA: 2018,4Q,82
TIP: Assign an additional code from category Z68 when BMI is documented. BMI can be based on documentation from clinicians who are not the patient's provider.

R63.6   Underweight
Use additional code to identify body mass index (BMI), if known (Z68.-)
EXCLUDES 1   *abnormal weight loss (R63.4)*
anorexia nervosa (F50.0-)
malnutrition (E40-E46)
AHA: 2018,4Q,82

R63.8   Other symptoms and signs concerning food and fluid intake

R64   Cachexia   CC
EXCLUDES 1   *abnormal weight loss (R63.4)*
cachexia due to underlying condition (E88.A)
nutritional marasmus (E41)
AHA: 2018,4Q,82; 2017,3Q,24

✓4ᵗʰ R65   Symptoms and signs specifically associated with systemic inflammation and infection
AHA: 2019,2Q,38
TIP: When documentation states SIRS with an infection, assign only a code for the infection. ICD-10-CM does not offer a code for SIRS due to infectious process. If sepsis is suspected, query the provider.

✓5ᵗʰ R65.1   Systemic inflammatory response syndrome [SIRS] of non-infectious origin
Code first underlying condition, such as:
heatstroke (T67.0-)
injury and trauma (S00-T88)
EXCLUDES 1   *sepsis - code to infection*
severe sepsis (R65.2)

R65.10   Systemic inflammatory response syndrome [SIRS] of non-infectious origin without acute organ dysfunction   CC   IJPD   HCC
Systemic inflammatory response syndrome (SIRS) NOS
AHA: 2019,2Q,24

R65.11   Systemic inflammatory response syndrome [SIRS] of non-infectious origin with acute organ dysfunction   MCC   IJPD   HCC
Use additional code to identify specific acute organ dysfunction, such as:
acute kidney failure (N17.-)
acute respiratory failure (J96.0-)
critical illness myopathy (G72.81)
critical illness polyneuropathy (G62.81)
disseminated intravascular coagulopathy [DIC] (D65)
encephalopathy (metabolic) (septic) (G93.41)
hepatic failure (K72.0-)

✓5ᵗʰ R65.2 Severe sepsis

Infection with associated acute organ dysfunction

Sepsis with acute organ dysfunction

Sepsis with multiple organ dysfunction

Systemic inflammatory response syndrome due to infectious process with acute organ dysfunction

Code first underlying infection, such as:

infection following a procedure (T81.4-)

infections following infusion, transfusion and therapeutic injection (T80.2-)

puerperal sepsis (O85)

sepsis following complete or unspecified spontaneous abortion (O03.87)

sepsis following ectopic and molar pregnancy (O08.82)

sepsis following incomplete spontaneous abortion (O03.37)

sepsis following (induced) termination of pregnancy (O04.87)

sepsis NOS (A41.9)

Use additional code to identify specific acute organ dysfunction, such as:

acute kidney failure (N17.-)

acute respiratory failure (J96.0-)

critical illness myopathy (G72.81)

critical illness polyneuropathy (G62.81)

disseminated intravascular coagulopathy [DIC] (D65)

encephalopathy (metabolic) (septic) (G93.41)

hepatic failure (K72.0-)

AHA: 2020,2Q,17; 2018,4Q,62-63; 2017,4Q,98-99; 2016,3Q,8

R65.20 Severe sepsis without septic shock `MCC` `UPD` `HCC`

Severe sepsis NOS

AHA: 2020,2Q,17; 2016,3Q,14; 2013,4Q,119

R65.21 Severe sepsis with septic shock `MCC` `UPD` `HCC`

AHA: 2018,4Q,63

✓4ᵗʰ R68 Other general symptoms and signs

R68.0 Hypothermia, not associated with low environmental temperature

`EXCLUDES 1` *hypothermia NOS (accidental) (T68)*

hypothermia due to anesthesia (T88.51)

hypothermia due to low environmental temperature (T68)

newborn hypothermia (P80.-)

✓5ᵗʰ R68.1 Nonspecific symptoms peculiar to infancy

`EXCLUDES 1` *colic, infantile (R10.83)*

neonatal cerebral irritability (P91.3)

teething syndrome (K00.7)

R68.11 Excessive crying of infant (baby) `P`

`EXCLUDES 1` *excessive crying of child, adolescent, or adult (R45.83)*

R68.12 Fussy infant (baby) `P`

Irritable infant

R68.13 Apparent life threatening event in infant (ALTE) `P`

Apparent life threatening event in newborn

Brief resolved unexplained event (BRUE)

Code first confirmed diagnosis, if known

Use additional code(s) for associated signs and symptoms if no confirmed diagnosis established, or if signs and symptoms are not associated routinely with confirmed diagnosis, or provide additional information for cause of ALTE

R68.19 Other nonspecific symptoms peculiar to infancy `P`

R68.2 Dry mouth, unspecified

`EXCLUDES 1` *dry mouth due to dehydration (E86.0)*

dry mouth due to Sjogren syndrome (M35.0-)

~~*salivary gland hyposecretion (K11.7)*~~

`EXCLUDES 2` ▶*salivary gland hyposecretion (K11.7)*◀

R68.3 Clubbing of fingers

Clubbing of nails

`EXCLUDES 1` *congenital clubfinger (Q68.1)*

DEF: Enlarged soft tissue of the distal fingers that usually occurs in heart and lung diseases.

✓5ᵗʰ R68.8 Other general symptoms and signs

R68.81 Early satiety

DEF: Premature feeling of being full after eating only a small amount of food. The mechanism of satiety is multifactorial.

R68.82 Decreased libido `A`

Decreased sexual desire

R68.83 Chills (without fever)

Chills NOS

`EXCLUDES 1` *chills with fever (R50.9)*

R68.84 Jaw pain

Mandibular pain

Maxilla pain

`EXCLUDES 1` *temporomandibular joint arthralgia (M26.62-)*

R68.89 Other general symptoms and signs

R69 Illness, unspecified

Unknown and unspecified cases of morbidity

Abnormal findings on examination of blood, without diagnosis (R70-R79)

`EXCLUDES 2` *abnormal findings on antenatal screening of mother (O28.-)*

abnormalities of lipids (E78.-)

abnormalities of platelets and thrombocytes (D69.-)

abnormalities of white blood cells classified elsewhere (D70-D72)

coagulation hemorrhagic disorders (D65-D68)

diagnostic abnormal findings classified elsewhere - see Alphabetical Index

hemorrhagic and hematological disorders of newborn (P50-P61)

✓4ᵗʰ R70 Elevated erythrocyte sedimentation rate and abnormality of plasma viscosity

R70.0 Elevated erythrocyte sedimentation rate

R70.1 Abnormal plasma viscosity

✓4ᵗʰ R71 Abnormality of red blood cells

`EXCLUDES 1` *anemias (D50-D64)*

anemia of premature infant (P61.2)

benign (familial) polycythemia (D75.0)

congenital anemias (P61.2-P61.4)

newborn anemia due to isoimmunization (P55.-)

polycythemia neonatorum (P61.1)

polycythemia NOS (D75.1)

polycythemia vera (D45)

secondary polycythemia (D75.1)

R71.0 Precipitous drop in hematocrit `CC`

Drop (precipitous) in hemoglobin

Drop in hematocrit

R71.8 Other abnormality of red blood cells

Abnormal red-cell morphology NOS

Abnormal red-cell volume NOS

Anisocytosis

Poikilocytosis

✓4ᵗʰ R73 Elevated blood glucose level

`EXCLUDES 1` *diabetes mellitus (E08-E13)*

diabetes mellitus in pregnancy, childbirth and the puerperium (O24.-)

neonatal disorders (P70.0-P70.2)

postsurgical hypoinsulinemia (E89.1)

✓5ᵗʰ R73.0 Abnormal glucose

`EXCLUDES 1` *abnormal glucose in pregnancy (O99.81-)*

diabetes mellitus (E08-E13)

dysmetabolic syndrome X (E88.81-)

gestational diabetes (O24.4-)

glycosuria (R81)

hypoglycemia (E16.2)

▶*type 1 diabetes mellitus, presymptomatic (E10.A-)*◀

R73.01 Impaired fasting glucose

Elevated fasting glucose

R73.02 Impaired glucose tolerance (oral)

Elevated glucose tolerance

R73.03 Prediabetes

Latent diabetes

AHA: 2016,4Q,65

R73.09 Other abnormal glucose

Abnormal glucose NOS

Abnormal non-fasting glucose tolerance

R73.9 Hyperglycemia, unspecified

✔ Additional Character Required   `✓x7ᵗʰ` Placeholder   Questionable PDx   Manifestation   Unspecified   `UPD` Unacceptable PDx   `H1`-`H14` HAC   `HCC` CMS-HCC Dx   `HIV` HIV Dx

ICD-10-CM 2025

969

✓4th R74 Abnormal serum enzyme levels

✓5th R74.0 Nonspecific elevation of levels of transaminase and lactic acid dehydrogenase [LDH]
AHA: 2020,4Q,39

R74.01 **Elevation of levels of liver transaminase levels**
Elevation of levels of alanine transaminase (ALT)
Elevation of levels of aspartate transaminase (AST)

R74.02 **Elevation of levels of lactic acid dehydrogenase [LDH]**

R74.8 **Abnormal levels of other serum enzymes**
Abnormal level of acid phosphatase
Abnormal level of alkaline phosphatase
Abnormal level of amylase
Abnormal level of lipase [triacylglycerol lipase]
AHA: 2019,2Q,6

R74.9 **Abnormal serum enzyme level, unspecified**

R75 **Inconclusive laboratory evidence of human immunodeficiency virus [HIV]**
Nonconclusive HIV-test finding in infants
EXCLUDES 1 *asymptomatic human immunodeficiency virus [HIV] infection status (Z21)*
human immunodeficiency virus [HIV] disease (B20)

✓4th R76 Other abnormal immunological findings in serum

R76.0 **Raised antibody titer**
EXCLUDES 1 *isoimmunization in pregnancy (O36.0-O36.1)*
isoimmunization affecting newborn (P55.-)
AHA: 2021,1Q,6

✓5th R76.1 Nonspecific reaction to test for tuberculosis

R76.11 **Nonspecific reaction to tuberculin skin test without active tuberculosis**
Abnormal result of Mantoux test
PPD positive
Tuberculin (skin test) positive
Tuberculin (skin test) reactor
EXCLUDES 1 *nonspecific reaction to cell mediated immunity measurement of gamma interferon antigen response without active tuberculosis (R76.12)*

R76.12 **Nonspecific reaction to cell mediated immunity measurement of gamma interferon antigen response without active tuberculosis**
Nonspecific reaction to QuantiFERON-TB test (QFT) without active tuberculosis
EXCLUDES 1 *nonspecific reaction to tuberculin skin test without active tuberculosis (R76.11)*
positive tuberculin skin test (R76.11)

R76.8 **Other specified abnormal immunological findings in serum**
Raised level of immunoglobulins NOS
AHA: 2021,1Q,6

R76.9 **Abnormal immunological finding in serum, unspecified**

✓4th R77 Other abnormalities of plasma proteins
EXCLUDES 1 *disorders of plasma-protein metabolism (E88.0-)*

R77.0 **Abnormality of albumin**

R77.1 **Abnormality of globulin**
Hyperglobulinemia NOS

R77.2 **Abnormality of alphafetoprotein**

R77.8 **Other specified abnormalities of plasma proteins**

R77.9 **Abnormality of plasma protein, unspecified**
AHA: 2019,2Q,6

✓4th R78 Findings of drugs and other substances, not normally found in blood
Use additional code to identify the any retained foreign body, if applicable (Z18.-)
EXCLUDES 2 *mental or behavioral disorders due to psychoactive substance use (F10-F19)*

R78.0 **Finding of alcohol in blood**
Use additional external cause code (Y90.-), for detail regarding alcohol level

R78.1 **Finding of opiate drug in blood**

R78.2 **Finding of cocaine in blood**

R78.3 **Finding of hallucinogen in blood**

R78.4 **Finding of other drugs of addictive potential in blood**

R78.5 **Finding of other psychotropic drug in blood**

R78.6 **Finding of steroid agent in blood**

✓5th R78.7 Finding of abnormal level of heavy metals in blood

R78.71 **Abnormal lead level in blood**
EXCLUDES 1 *lead poisoning (T56.0-)*

R78.79 **Finding of abnormal level of heavy metals in blood**

✓5th R78.8 Finding of other specified substances, not normally found in blood

R78.81 **Bacteremia** CC
EXCLUDES 1 *sepsis — code to specified infection*
DEF: Laboratory finding of bacteria in the blood in the absence of two or more signs of sepsis. Transient in nature, it can progress to septicemia with a severe infectious process.

R78.89 **Finding of other specified substances, not normally found in blood**
Finding of abnormal level of lithium in blood

R78.9 **Finding of unspecified substance, not normally found in blood**

✓4th R79 Other abnormal findings of blood chemistry
Use additional code to identify any retained foreign body, if applicable (Z18.-)
EXCLUDES 1 *asymptomatic hyperuricemia (E79.0)*
hyperglycemia NOS (R73.9)
hypoglycemia NOS (E16.2)
neonatal hypoglycemia (P70.3-P70.4)
specific findings indicating disorder of amino-acid metabolism (E70-E72)
specific findings indicating disorder of carbohydrate metabolism (E73-E74)
specific findings indicating disorder of lipid metabolism (E75.-)

R79.0 **Abnormal level of blood mineral**
Abnormal blood level of cobalt
Abnormal blood level of copper
Abnormal blood level of iron
Abnormal blood level of magnesium
Abnormal blood level of mineral NEC
Abnormal blood level of zinc
EXCLUDES 1 *abnormal level of lithium (R78.89)*
disorders of mineral metabolism (E83.-)
neonatal hypomagnesemia (P71.2)
nutritional mineral deficiency (E58-E61)

R79.1 **Abnormal coagulation profile**
Abnormal or prolonged bleeding time
Abnormal or prolonged coagulation time
Abnormal or prolonged partial thromboplastin time [PTT]
Abnormal or prolonged prothrombin time [PT]
Low von Willebrand factor
EXCLUDES 1 *coagulation defects (D68.-)*
EXCLUDES 2 *abnormality of fluid, electrolyte or acid-base balance (E86-E87)*

✓5th R79.8 Other specified abnormal findings of blood chemistry

R79.81 **Abnormal blood-gas level**

R79.82 **Elevated C-reactive protein [CRP]**

R79.83 **Abnormal findings of blood amino-acid level**
Homocysteinemia
EXCLUDES 1 *disorders of amino-acid metabolism (E70-E72)*
AHA: 2021,4Q,28

R79.89 **Other specified abnormal findings of blood chemistry**
AHA: 2019,2Q,6
TIP: Assign for positive Coombs test when not further clarified in the documentation.

R79.9 **Abnormal finding of blood chemistry, unspecified**

Abnormal findings on examination of urine, without diagnosis (R80-R82)

EXCLUDES 1 *abnormal findings on antenatal screening of mother (O28.-)*
diagnostic abnormal findings classified elsewhere - see Alphabetical Index
specific findings indicating disorder of amino-acid metabolism (E70-E72)
specific findings indicating disorder of carbohydrate metabolism (E73-E74)

✓4th R80 Proteinuria
EXCLUDES 1 *gestational proteinuria (O12.1-)*

R80.0 **Isolated proteinuria**
Idiopathic proteinuria
EXCLUDES 1 *isolated proteinuria with specific morphological lesion (N06.-)*

R80.1 **Persistent proteinuria, unspecified**

R80.2 **Orthostatic proteinuria, unspecified**
Postural proteinuria

R80.3 **Bence Jones proteinuria**

R80.8 **Other proteinuria**

R80.9   **Proteinuria, unspecified**
Albuminuria NOS

R81   **Glycosuria**
    EXCLUDES 1   *renal glycosuria (E74.818)*

☑4th **R82**   **Other and unspecified abnormal findings in urine**
    INCLUDES   chromoabnormalities in urine
    Use additional code to identify any retained foreign body, if applicable (Z18.-)
    EXCLUDES 2   *hematuria (R31.-)*

   R82.0   **Chyluria**   CC
       EXCLUDES 1   *filarial chyluria (B74.-)*

   R82.1   **Myoglobinuria**   CC
   R82.2   **Biliuria**
   R82.3   **Hemoglobinuria**
       EXCLUDES 1   *hemoglobinuria due to hemolysis from external causes NEC (D59.6)*
             hemoglobinuria due to paroxysmal nocturnal [Marchiafava-Micheli] (D59.5)
       DEF: Free hemoglobin in blood due to rapid hemolysis of red blood cells. Causes include burns, crushed injury, sickle cell anemia, thalassemia, parasitic infections, or kidney infections.

   R82.4   **Acetonuria**
       Ketonuria
       DEF: Excessive excretion of acetone in urine that commonly occurs in diabetic acidosis.

   R82.5   **Elevated urine levels of drugs, medicaments and biological substances**
       Elevated urine levels of catecholamines
       Elevated urine levels of indoleacetic acid
       Elevated urine levels of 17-ketosteroids
       Elevated urine levels of steroids

   R82.6   **Abnormal urine levels of substances chiefly nonmedicinal as to source**
       Abnormal urine level of heavy metals

☑5th **R82.7**   **Abnormal findings on microbiological examination of urine**
       EXCLUDES 1   *colonization status (Z22.-)*
       AHA: 2016,4Q,65

     R82.71   **Bacteriuria**
     R82.79   **Other abnormal findings on microbiological examination of urine**
         Positive culture findings of urine

☑5th **R82.8**   **Abnormal findings on cytological and histological examination of urine**
       AHA: 2019,4Q,16

     R82.81   **Pyuria**
         Sterile pyuria
     R82.89   **Other abnormal findings on cytological and histological examination of urine**

☑5th **R82.9**   **Other and unspecified abnormal findings in urine**

     R82.90   **Unspecified abnormal findings in urine**
     R82.91   **Other chromoabnormalities of urine**
         Chromoconversion (dipstick)
         Idiopathic dipstick converts positive for blood with no cellular forms in sediment
         EXCLUDES 1   *hemoglobinuria (R82.3)*
                 myoglobinuria (R82.1)

     ☑6th **R82.99**   **Other abnormal findings in urine**
         AHA: 2018,4Q,29-30

       R82.991   **Hypocitraturia**
       R82.992   **Hyperoxaluria**
           EXCLUDES 1   *primary hyperoxaluria (E72.53)*
       R82.993   **Hyperuricosuria**
       R82.994   **Hypercalciuria**
           Idiopathic hypercalciuria
       R82.998   **Other abnormal findings in urine**
           Cells and casts in urine
           Crystalluria
           Melanuria

Abnormal findings on examination of other body fluids, substances and tissues, without diagnosis (R83-R89)

   EXCLUDES 1   *abnormal findings on antenatal screening of mother (O28.-)*
           diagnostic abnormal findings classified elsewhere - see Alphabetical Index
   EXCLUDES 2   *abnormal findings on examination of blood, without diagnosis (R70-R79)*
           abnormal findings on examination of urine, without diagnosis (R80-R82)
           abnormal tumor markers (R97.-)

☑4th **R83**   **Abnormal findings in cerebrospinal fluid**

   R83.0   **Abnormal level of enzymes in cerebrospinal fluid**
   R83.1   **Abnormal level of hormones in cerebrospinal fluid**
   R83.2   **Abnormal level of other drugs, medicaments and biological substances in cerebrospinal fluid**
   R83.3   **Abnormal level of substances chiefly nonmedicinal as to source in cerebrospinal fluid**
   R83.4   **Abnormal immunological findings in cerebrospinal fluid**
   R83.5   **Abnormal microbiological findings in cerebrospinal fluid**
       Positive culture findings in cerebrospinal fluid
       EXCLUDES 1   *colonization status (Z22.-)*
   R83.6   **Abnormal cytological findings in cerebrospinal fluid**
   R83.8   **Other abnormal findings in cerebrospinal fluid**
       Abnormal chromosomal findings in cerebrospinal fluid
   R83.9   **Unspecified abnormal finding in cerebrospinal fluid**

☑4th **R84**   **Abnormal findings in specimens from respiratory organs and thorax**
       INCLUDES   abnormal findings in bronchial washings
              abnormal findings in nasal secretions
              abnormal findings in pleural fluid
              abnormal findings in sputum
              abnormal findings in throat scrapings
       EXCLUDES 1   *blood-stained sputum (R04.2)*

   R84.0   **Abnormal level of enzymes in specimens from respiratory organs and thorax**
   R84.1   **Abnormal level of hormones in specimens from respiratory organs and thorax**
   R84.2   **Abnormal level of other drugs, medicaments and biological substances in specimens from respiratory organs and thorax**
   R84.3   **Abnormal level of substances chiefly nonmedicinal as to source in specimens from respiratory organs and thorax**
   R84.4   **Abnormal immunological findings in specimens from respiratory organs and thorax**
   R84.5   **Abnormal microbiological findings in specimens from respiratory organs and thorax**
       Positive culture findings in specimens from respiratory organs and thorax
       EXCLUDES 1   *colonization status (Z22.-)*
   R84.6   **Abnormal cytological findings in specimens from respiratory organs and thorax**
   R84.7   **Abnormal histological findings in specimens from respiratory organs and thorax**
   R84.8   **Other abnormal findings in specimens from respiratory organs and thorax**
       Abnormal chromosomal findings in specimens from respiratory organs and thorax
   R84.9   **Unspecified abnormal finding in specimens from respiratory organs and thorax**

☑4th **R85**   **Abnormal findings in specimens from digestive organs and abdominal cavity**
       INCLUDES   abnormal findings in peritoneal fluid
              abnormal findings in saliva
       EXCLUDES 1   *cloudy peritoneal dialysis effluent (R88.0)*
           fecal abnormalities (R19.5)

   R85.0   **Abnormal level of enzymes in specimens from digestive organs and abdominal cavity**
   R85.1   **Abnormal level of hormones in specimens from digestive organs and abdominal cavity**
   R85.2   **Abnormal level of other drugs, medicaments and biological substances in specimens from digestive organs and abdominal cavity**
   R85.3   **Abnormal level of substances chiefly nonmedicinal as to source in specimens from digestive organs and abdominal cavity**
   R85.4   **Abnormal immunological findings in specimens from digestive organs and abdominal cavity**

R85.5   **Abnormal microbiological findings in specimens from digestive organs and abdominal cavity**
Positive culture findings in specimens from digestive organs and abdominal cavity
EXCLUDES 1   colonization status (Z22.-)

✓5ᵗʰ **R85.6**   **Abnormal cytological findings in specimens from digestive organs and abdominal cavity**

    ✓6ᵗʰ **R85.61**   **Abnormal cytologic smear of anus**
      EXCLUDES 1   abnormal cytological findings in specimens from other digestive organs and abdominal cavity (R85.69)
       anal intraepithelial neoplasia I [AIN I] (K62.82)
       anal intraepithelial neoplasia II [AIN II] (K62.82)
       anal intraepithelial neoplasia III [AIN III] (D01.3)
       carcinoma in situ of anus (histologically confirmed) (D01.3)
       dysplasia (mild) (moderate) of anus (histologically confirmed) (K62.82)
       severe dysplasia of anus (histologically confirmed) (D01.3)
      EXCLUDES 2   anal high risk human papillomavirus (HPV) DNA test positive (R85.81)
       anal low risk human papillomavirus (HPV) DNA test positive (R85.82)

      R85.610   **Atypical squamous cells of undetermined significance on cytologic smear of anus [ASC-US]**

      R85.611   **Atypical squamous cells cannot exclude high grade squamous intraepithelial lesion on cytologic smear of anus [ASC-H]**

      R85.612   **Low grade squamous intraepithelial lesion on cytologic smear of anus [LGSIL]**

      R85.613   **High grade squamous intraepithelial lesion on cytologic smear of anus [HGSIL]**

      R85.614   **Cytologic evidence of malignancy on smear of anus**

      R85.615   **Unsatisfactory cytologic smear of anus**
       Inadequate sample of cytologic smear of anus

      R85.616   **Satisfactory anal smear but lacking transformation zone**

      R85.618   **Other abnormal cytological findings on specimens from anus**

      R85.619   **Unspecified abnormal cytological findings in specimens from anus**
       Abnormal anal cytology NOS
       Atypical glandular cells of anus NOS

    R85.69   **Abnormal cytological findings in specimens from other digestive organs and abdominal cavity**

R85.7   **Abnormal histological findings in specimens from digestive organs and abdominal cavity**

✓5ᵗʰ **R85.8**   **Other abnormal findings in specimens from digestive organs and abdominal cavity**

    R85.81   **Anal high risk human papillomavirus [HPV] DNA test positive**
      EXCLUDES 1   anogenital warts due to human papillomavirus (HPV) (A63.0)
       condyloma acuminatum (A63.0)

    R85.82   **Anal low risk human papillomavirus [HPV] DNA test positive**
      Use additional code for associated human papillomavirus (B97.7)

    R85.89   **Other abnormal findings in specimens from digestive organs and abdominal cavity**
      Abnormal chromosomal findings in specimens from digestive organs and abdominal cavity

R85.9   **Unspecified abnormal finding in specimens from digestive organs and abdominal cavity**

✓4ᵗʰ **R86**   **Abnormal findings in specimens from male genital organs**
    INCLUDES   abnormal findings in prostatic secretions
      abnormal findings in semen, seminal fluid
      abnormal spermatozoa
    EXCLUDES 1   azoospermia (N46.0-)
      oligospermia (N46.1-)

    R86.0   **Abnormal level of enzymes in specimens from male genital organs**

R86.1   **Abnormal level of hormones in specimens from male genital organs**

R86.2   **Abnormal level of other drugs, medicaments and biological substances in specimens from male genital organs**

R86.3   **Abnormal level of substances chiefly nonmedicinal as to source in specimens from male genital organs**

R86.4   **Abnormal immunological findings in specimens from male genital organs**

R86.5   **Abnormal microbiological findings in specimens from male genital organs**
Positive culture findings in specimens from male genital organs
EXCLUDES 1   colonization status (Z22.-)

R86.6   **Abnormal cytological findings in specimens from male genital organs**

R86.7   **Abnormal histological findings in specimens from male genital organs**

R86.8   **Other abnormal findings in specimens from male genital organs**
Abnormal chromosomal findings in specimens from male genital organs

R86.9   **Unspecified abnormal finding in specimens from male genital organs**

✓4ᵗʰ **R87**   **Abnormal findings in specimens from female genital organs**
    INCLUDES   abnormal findings in secretion and smears from cervix uteri
      abnormal findings in secretion and smears from vagina
      abnormal findings in secretion and smears from vulva

R87.0   **Abnormal level of enzymes in specimens from female genital organs**

R87.1   **Abnormal level of hormones in specimens from female genital organs**

R87.2   **Abnormal level of other drugs, medicaments and biological substances in specimens from female genital organs**

R87.3   **Abnormal level of substances chiefly nonmedicinal as to source in specimens from female genital organs**

R87.4   **Abnormal immunological findings in specimens from female genital organs**

R87.5   **Abnormal microbiological findings in specimens from female genital organs**
Positive culture findings in specimens from female genital organs
EXCLUDES 1   colonization status (Z22.-)

✓5ᵗʰ **R87.6**   **Abnormal cytological findings in specimens from female genital organs**

    ✓6ᵗʰ **R87.61**   **Abnormal cytological findings in specimens from cervix uteri**
      EXCLUDES 1   abnormal cytological findings in specimens from other female genital organs (R87.69)
       abnormal cytological findings in specimens from vagina (R87.62-)
       carcinoma in situ of cervix uteri (histologically confirmed) (D06.-)
       cervical intraepithelial neoplasia I [CIN I] (N87.0)
       cervical intraepithelial neoplasia II [CIN II] (N87.1)
       cervical intraepithelial neoplasia III [CIN III] (D06.-)
       dysplasia (mild) (moderate) of cervix uteri (histologically confirmed) (N87.-)
       severe dysplasia of cervix uteri (histologically confirmed) (D06.-)
      EXCLUDES 2   cervical high risk human papillomavirus (HPV) DNA test positive (R87.810)
       cervical low risk human papillomavirus (HPV) DNA test positive (R87.820)

      R87.610   **Atypical squamous cells of undetermined significance on cytologic smear of cervix [ASC-US]**

      R87.611   **Atypical squamous cells cannot exclude high grade squamous intraepithelial lesion on cytologic smear of cervix [ASC-H]**

      R87.612   **Low grade squamous intraepithelial lesion on cytologic smear of cervix [LGSIL]**

      R87.613   **High grade squamous intraepithelial lesion on cytologic smear of cervix [HGSIL]**

      R87.614   **Cytologic evidence of malignancy on smear of cervix**

R87.615 **Unsatisfactory** cytologic smear of cervix
Inadequate sample of cytologic smear of cervix

R87.616 **Satisfactory** cervical smear but **lacking transformation zone**

R87.618 **Other abnormal cytological findings on specimens from cervix uteri**

R87.619 **Unspecified abnormal cytological findings in specimens from cervix uteri**
Abnormal cervical cytology NOS
Abnormal Papanicolaou smear of cervix NOS
Abnormal thin preparation smear of cervix NOS
Atypical endocervial cells of cervix NOS
Atypical endometrial cells of cervix NOS
Atypical glandular cells of cervix NOS

✓6ᵗʰ **R87.62** **Abnormal cytological findings in specimens from vagina**
Use additional code to identify acquired absence of uterus and cervix, if applicable (Z90.71-)

EXCLUDES 1   *abnormal cytological findings in specimens from cervix uteri (R87.61-)*
abnormal cytological findings in specimens from other female genital organs (R87.69)
carcinoma in situ of vagina (histologically confirmed) (D07.2)
dysplasia (mild) (moderate) of vagina (histologically confirmed) (N89.-)
severe dysplasia of vagina (histologically confirmed) (D07.2)
vaginal intraepithelial neoplasia I [VAIN I] (N89.0)
vaginal intraepithelial neoplasia II [VAIN II] (N89.1)
vaginal intraepithelial neoplasia III [VAIN III] (D07.2)

EXCLUDES 2   *vaginal high risk human papillomavirus (HPV) DNA test positive (R87.811)*
vaginal low risk human papillomavirus (HPV) DNA test positive (R87.821)

R87.620 **Atypical** squamous cells of **undetermined significance** on cytologic smear of vagina **[ASC-US]**

R87.621 **Atypical** squamous cells cannot exclude **high grade** squamous intraepithelial lesion on cytologic smear of vagina **[ASC-H]**

R87.622 **Low grade** squamous intraepithelial lesion on cytologic smear of vagina **[LGSIL]**

R87.623 **High grade** squamous intraepithelial lesion on cytologic smear of vagina **[HGSIL]**

R87.624 **Cytologic evidence of malignancy** on smear of vagina

R87.625 **Unsatisfactory** cytologic smear of vagina
Inadequate sample of cytologic smear of vagina

R87.628 **Other abnormal cytological findings on specimens from vagina**

R87.629 **Unspecified abnormal cytological findings in specimens from vagina**
Abnormal Papanicolaou smear of vagina NOS
Abnormal thin preparation smear of vagina NOS
Abnormal vaginal cytology NOS
Atypical endocervial cells of vagina NOS
Atypical endometrial cells of vagina NOS
Atypical glandular cells of vagina NOS

R87.69 **Abnormal cytological findings in specimens from other female genital organs**
Abnormal cytological findings in specimens from female genital organs NOS
EXCLUDES 1   *dysplasia of vulva (histologically confirmed) (N90.0-N90.3)*

R87.7 **Abnormal histological findings in specimens from female genital organs**
EXCLUDES 1   *carcinoma in situ (histologically confirmed) of female genital organs (D06-D07.3)*
cervical intraepithelial neoplasia I [CIN I] (N87.0)
cervical intraepithelial neoplasia II [CIN II] (N87.1)
cervical intraepithelial neoplasia III [CIN III] (D06.-)
dysplasia (mild) (moderate) of cervix uteri (histologically confirmed) (N87.-)
dysplasia (mild) (moderate) of vagina (histologically confirmed) (N89.-)
severe dysplasia of cervix uteri (histologically confirmed) (D06.-)
severe dysplasia of vagina (histologically confirmed) (D07.2)
vaginal intraepithelial neoplasia I [VAIN I] (N89.0)
vaginal intraepithelial neoplasia II [VAIN II] (N89.1)
vaginal intraepithelial neoplasia III [VAIN III] (D07.2)

✓5ᵗʰ **R87.8** **Other abnormal findings in specimens from female genital organs**

✓6ᵗʰ **R87.81** **High risk human papillomavirus [HPV] DNA test positive from female genital organs**
EXCLUDES 1   *anogenital warts due to human papillomavirus (HPV) (A63.0)*
condyloma acuminatum (A63.0)

R87.810 **Cervical** high risk human papillomavirus **[HPV] DNA test positive**

R87.811 **Vaginal** high risk human papillomavirus **[HPV] DNA test positive**

✓6ᵗʰ **R87.82** **Low risk human papillomavirus [HPV] DNA test positive from female genital organs**
Use additional code for associated human papillomavirus (B97.7)

R87.820 **Cervical** low risk human papillomavirus **[HPV] DNA test positive**

R87.821 **Vaginal** low risk human papillomavirus **[HPV] DNA test positive**

R87.89 **Other abnormal findings in specimens from female genital organs**
Abnormal chromosomal findings in specimens from female genital organs

R87.9 **Unspecified abnormal finding in specimens from female genital organs**

✓4ᵗʰ **R88** **Abnormal findings in other body fluids and substances**

R88.0 **Cloudy (hemodialysis) (peritoneal) dialysis effluent**

R88.8 **Abnormal findings in other body fluids and substances**

✓4ᵗʰ **R89** **Abnormal findings in specimens from other organs, systems and tissues**
INCLUDES   abnormal findings in nipple discharge
abnormal findings in synovial fluid
abnormal findings in wound secretions

R89.0 **Abnormal level of enzymes in specimens from other organs, systems and tissues**

R89.1 **Abnormal level of hormones in specimens from other organs, systems and tissues**

R89.2 **Abnormal level of other drugs, medicaments and biological substances in specimens from other organs, systems and tissues**

R89.3 **Abnormal level of substances chiefly nonmedicinal as to source in specimens from other organs, systems and tissues**

R89.4 **Abnormal immunological findings in specimens from other organs, systems and tissues**

R89.5 **Abnormal microbiological findings in specimens from other organs, systems and tissues**
Positive culture findings in specimens from other organs, systems and tissues
EXCLUDES 1   *colonization status (Z22.-)*

R89.6 **Abnormal cytological findings in specimens from other organs, systems and tissues**

R89.7 **Abnormal histological findings in specimens from other organs, systems and tissues**

R89.8 **Other abnormal findings in specimens from other organs, systems and tissues**
Abnormal chromosomal findings in specimens from other organs, systems and tissues

R89.9 **Unspecified abnormal finding in specimens from other organs, systems and tissues**

✓ Additional Character Required   ✓x7ᵗʰ Placeholder   Questionable PDx   Manifestation   Unspecified   UPD Unacceptable PDx   H1-H14 HAC   HCC CMS-HCC Dx   HIV HIV Dx

ICD-10-CM 2025   973

Chapter 18. Symptoms, Signs and Abnormal Clinical and Laboratory Findings   R87.615–R89.9

Chapter 18. Symptoms, Signs and Abnormal Clinical and Laboratory Findings

Abnormal findings on diagnostic imaging and in function studies, without diagnosis (R90-R94)

INCLUDES nonspecific abnormal findings on diagnostic imaging by computerized axial tomography [CAT scan]
nonspecific abnormal findings on diagnostic imaging by magnetic resonance imaging [MRI][NMR]
nonspecific abnormal findings on diagnostic imaging by positron emission tomography [PET scan]
nonspecific abnormal findings on diagnostic imaging by thermography
nonspecific abnormal findings on diagnostic imaging by ultrasound [echogram]
nonspecific abnormal findings on diagnostic imaging by X-ray examination

EXCLUDES 1 *abnormal findings on antenatal screening of mother (O28.-)*
diagnostic abnormal findings classified elsewhere - see Alphabetical Index

√4th **R90** **Abnormal findings on diagnostic imaging of central nervous system**

  R90.0 **Intracranial space-occupying lesion found on diagnostic imaging of central nervous system**

  √5th **R90.8** **Other abnormal findings on diagnostic imaging of central nervous system**

    R90.81 **Abnormal echoencephalogram**

    R90.82 **White matter disease, unspecified**

    R90.89 **Other abnormal findings on diagnostic imaging of central nervous system**
Other cerebrovascular abnormality found on diagnostic imaging of central nervous system

√4th **R91** **Abnormal findings on diagnostic imaging of lung**

  R91.1 **Solitary pulmonary nodule**
Coin lesion lung
Solitary pulmonary nodule, subsegmental branch of the bronchial tree

  R91.8 **Other nonspecific abnormal finding of lung field**
Lung mass NOS found on diagnostic imaging of lung
Pulmonary infiltrate NOS
Shadow, lung

√4th **R92** **Abnormal and inconclusive findings on diagnostic imaging of breast**

  R92.0 **Mammographic microcalcification found on diagnostic imaging of breast**

    EXCLUDES 2 *mammographic calcification (calculus) found on diagnostic imaging of breast (R92.1)*

    DEF: Calcium and cellular debris deposits in the breast that cannot be felt but can be detected on a mammogram. The deposits can be a sign of cancer, benign conditions, or changes in the breast tissue as a result of inflammation, injury, or an obstructed duct.

  R92.1 **Mammographic calcification found on diagnostic imaging of breast**
Mammographic calculus found on diagnostic imaging of breast

  R92.2 **Inconclusive mammogram**
Inconclusive mammogram NEC
Inconclusive mammography NEC
AHA: 2015,1Q,24

  √5th **R92.3** **Mammographic density found on imaging of breast**
Code also, if applicable, inconclusive mammogram (R92.2)
AHA: 2023,4Q,42-44

    R92.30 **Dense breasts, unspecified**
Dense breasts NOS
Low density

  √6th **R92.31** **Mammographic fatty tissue density of breast**
Breast Imaging Reporting and Data System (BI-RADS): A
Breast Imaging Reporting and Data System (BI-RADS): 1

    R92.311 **Mammographic fatty tissue density, right breast**

    R92.312 **Mammographic fatty tissue density, left breast**

    R92.313 **Mammographic fatty tissue density, bilateral breasts**

  √6th **R92.32** **Mammographic fibroglandular density of breast**
Breast Imaging Reporting and Data System (BI-RADS): B
Breast Imaging Reporting and Data System (BI-RADS): 2

    R92.321 **Mammographic fibroglandular density, right breast**

    R92.322 **Mammographic fibroglandular density, left breast**

    R92.323 **Mammographic fibroglandular density, bilateral breasts**

  √6th **R92.33** **Mammographic heterogeneous density of breast**
Breast Imaging Reporting and Data System (BI-RADS): C
Breast Imaging Reporting and Data System (BI-RADS): 3

    R92.331 **Mammographic heterogeneous density, right breast**

    R92.332 **Mammographic heterogeneous density, left breast**

    R92.333 **Mammographic heterogeneous density, bilateral breasts**

  √6th **R92.34** **Mammographic extreme density of breast**
Breast Imaging Reporting and Data System (BI-RADS): D
Breast Imaging Reporting and Data System (BI-RADS): 4

    R92.341 **Mammographic extreme density, right breast**

    R92.342 **Mammographic extreme density, left breast**

    R92.343 **Mammographic extreme density, bilateral breasts**

  R92.8 **Other abnormal and inconclusive findings on diagnostic imaging of breast**

√4th **R93** **Abnormal findings on diagnostic imaging of other body structures**

  R93.0 **Abnormal findings on diagnostic imaging of skull and head, not elsewhere classified**

    EXCLUDES 1 *intracranial space-occupying lesion found on diagnostic imaging (R90.0)*

  R93.1 **Abnormal findings on diagnostic imaging of heart and coronary circulation**
Abnormal echocardiogram NOS
Abnormal heart shadow

  R93.2 **Abnormal findings on diagnostic imaging of liver and biliary tract**
Nonvisualization of gallbladder

  R93.3 **Abnormal findings on diagnostic imaging of other parts of digestive tract**

  √5th **R93.4** **Abnormal findings on diagnostic imaging of urinary organs**

    EXCLUDES 2 *hypertrophy of kidney (N28.81)*

    AHA: 2016,4Q,66

    R93.41 **Abnormal radiologic findings on diagnostic imaging of renal pelvis, ureter, or bladder**
Filling defect of bladder found on diagnostic imaging
Filling defect of renal pelvis found on diagnostic imaging
Filling defect of ureter found on diagnostic imaging

  √6th **R93.42** **Abnormal radiologic findings on diagnostic imaging of kidney**

    R93.421 **Abnormal radiologic findings on diagnostic imaging of right kidney**

    R93.422 **Abnormal radiologic findings on diagnostic imaging of left kidney**

    R93.429 **Abnormal radiologic findings on diagnostic imaging of unspecified kidney**

    R93.49 **Abnormal radiologic findings on diagnostic imaging of other urinary organs**

  R93.5 **Abnormal findings on diagnostic imaging of other abdominal regions, including retroperitoneum**

  R93.6 **Abnormal findings on diagnostic imaging of limbs**

    EXCLUDES 2 *abnormal finding in skin and subcutaneous tissue (R93.8-)*

    AHA: 2020,1Q,14

  R93.7 **Abnormal findings on diagnostic imaging of other parts of musculoskeletal system**

    EXCLUDES 2 *abnormal findings on diagnostic imaging of skull (R93.0)*

  √5th **R93.8** **Abnormal findings on diagnostic imaging of other specified body structures**

    AHA: 2018,4Q,30

  √6th **R93.81** **Abnormal radiologic findings on diagnostic imaging of testis**

    R93.811 **Abnormal radiologic findings on diagnostic imaging of right testicle**

    R93.812 **Abnormal radiologic findings on diagnostic imaging of left testicle**

    R93.813 **Abnormal radiologic findings on diagnostic imaging of testicles, bilateral**

N Newborn: 0   P Pediatric: 0-17   M Maternity: 9-64   A Adult: 15-124   UNS Unspecified Site   MCC Major Complication/Comorbidity   CC Complication/Comorbidity   PE POA Exempt

974   ICD-10-CM 2025

R93.819   Abnormal radiologic findings on diagnostic imaging of unspecified testicle

R93.89   Abnormal findings on diagnostic imaging of other specified body structures
  Abnormal finding by radioisotope localization of placenta
  Abnormal radiological finding in skin and subcutaneous tissue
  Mediastinal shift

R93.9   Diagnostic imaging inconclusive due to **excess body fat** of patient

✓4th **R94**   **Abnormal results of function studies**

INCLUDES   abnormal results of radionuclide [radioisotope] uptake studies
  abnormal results of scintigraphy

✓5th **R94.0**   **Abnormal results of function studies of central nervous system**

R94.01   Abnormal **electroencephalogram** [EEG]

R94.02   Abnormal **brain scan**

R94.09   Abnormal results of other function studies of central nervous system

✓5th **R94.1**   **Abnormal results of function studies of peripheral nervous system and special senses**

✓6th **R94.11**   Abnormal results of function studies of **eye**

R94.110   Abnormal **electro-oculogram** [EOG]

R94.111   Abnormal **electroretinogram** [ERG]
  Abnormal retinal function study

R94.112   Abnormal **visually evoked potential** [VEP]

R94.113   Abnormal **oculomotor** study

R94.118   Abnormal results of other function studies of eye

✓6th **R94.12**   Abnormal results of function studies of **ear and other special senses**
  AHA: 2016,3Q,17

R94.120   Abnormal **auditory** function study

R94.121   Abnormal **vestibular** function study

R94.128   Abnormal results of other function studies of ear and other special senses

✓6th **R94.13**   Abnormal results of function studies of **peripheral nervous system**

R94.130   Abnormal response to nerve stimulation, unspecified

R94.131   Abnormal **electromyogram** [EMG]
  EXCLUDES 1   electromyogram of eye (R94.113)

R94.138   Abnormal results of other function studies of peripheral nervous system

R94.2   **Abnormal results of pulmonary function studies**
  Reduced ventilatory capacity
  Reduced vital capacity

✓5th **R94.3**   **Abnormal results of cardiovascular function studies**

R94.30   Abnormal result of cardiovascular function study, unspecified

R94.31   Abnormal **electrocardiogram** [ECG] [EKG]
  EXCLUDES 1   long QT syndrome (I45.81)

R94.39   Abnormal result of other cardiovascular function study
  Abnormal electrophysiological intracardiac studies
  Abnormal phonocardiogram
  Abnormal vectorcardiogram
  AHA: 2023,1Q,25

R94.4   **Abnormal results of kidney function studies**
  Abnormal renal function test

R94.5   **Abnormal results of liver function studies**

R94.6   **Abnormal results of thyroid function studies**

R94.7   **Abnormal results of other endocrine function studies**
  EXCLUDES 2   abnormal glucose (R73.0-)

R94.8   **Abnormal results of function studies of other organs and systems**
  Abnormal basal metabolic rate [BMR]
  Abnormal bladder function test
  Abnormal splenic function test

Abnormal tumor markers (R97)

✓4th **R97**   **Abnormal tumor markers**
  Elevated tumor associated antigens [TAA]
  Elevated tumor specific antigens [TSA]

R97.0   **Elevated carcinoembryonic antigen [CEA]**

R97.1   **Elevated cancer antigen 125 [CA 125]**

✓5th **R97.2**   **Elevated prostate specific antigen [PSA]**
  AHA: 2016,4Q,66

R97.20   Elevated prostate specific antigen [PSA]   A

R97.21   Rising PSA following treatment for malignant neoplasm of prostate   A
  AHA: 2023,2Q,5

R97.8   **Other abnormal tumor markers**

Ill-defined and unknown cause of mortality (R99)

R99   **Ill-defined and unknown cause of mortality**
  Death (unexplained) NOS
  Unspecified cause of mortality

✓ Additional Character Required   ✓x7th Placeholder   Questionable PDx   Manifestation   Unspecified   UPD Unacceptable PDx   H1-H14 HAC   HCC CMS-HCC Dx   HIV HIV Dx

ICD-10-CM 2025   975

Chapter 19. Injury, Poisoning, and Certain Other Consequences of External Causes (S00–T88)

Chapter-specific Guidelines with Coding Examples

The chapter-specific guidelines from the ICD-10-CM Official Guidelines for Coding and Reporting have been provided below. Along with these guidelines are coding examples, contained in the shaded boxes, that have been developed to help illustrate the coding and/or sequencing guidance found in these guidelines.

a. Application of 7th characters in Chapter 19

Most categories in chapter 19 have a 7th character requirement for each applicable code. Most categories in this chapter have three 7th character values (with the exception of fractures): A, initial encounter, D, subsequent encounter and S, sequela. Categories for traumatic fractures have additional 7th character values. While the patient may be seen by a new or different provider over the course of treatment for an injury, assignment of the 7th character is based on whether the patient is undergoing active treatment and not whether the provider is seeing the patient for the first time.

For complication codes, active treatment refers to treatment for the condition described by the code, even though it may be related to an earlier precipitating problem. For example, code T84.50XA, Infection and inflammatory reaction due to unspecified internal joint prosthesis, initial encounter, is used when active treatment is provided for the infection, even though the condition relates to the prosthetic device, implant or graft that was placed at a previous encounter.

7th character "A", initial encounter is used for each encounter where the patient is receiving active treatment for the condition.

> Patient admitted after fall from a skateboard onto the sidewalk, x-rays identify a nondisplaced fracture to the distal pole of the right scaphoid bone. The patient is placed in a cast.
>
> **S62.014A**   **Nondisplaced fracture of distal pole of navicular [scaphoid] bone of right wrist, initial encounter for closed fracture**
>
> **V00.131A**   **Fall from skateboard, initial encounter**
>
> **Y92.480**   **Sidewalk as the place of occurrence of the external cause**
>
> **Y93.51**   **Activity, roller skating (inline) and skateboarding**
>
> **Y99.8**   **Other external cause status**
>
> *Explanation:* This fracture would be coded with a seventh character A for initial encounter because the patient received x-rays to identify the site of the fracture and treatment was rendered; this would be considered active treatment.

7th character "D" subsequent encounter is used for encounters after the patient has completed active treatment of the condition and is receiving routine care for the condition during the healing or recovery phase.

> Patient admitted after fall from a skateboard onto the sidewalk resulted in casting of the right arm. X-rays are taken to evaluate how well the nondisplaced fracture to the distal pole of the right scaphoid bone is healing. The physician feels the fracture is healing appropriately; no adjustments to the cast are made.
>
> **S62.014D**   **Nondisplaced fracture of distal pole of navicular [scaphoid] bone of right wrist, subsequent encounter for fracture with routine healing**
>
> **V00.131D**   **Fall from skateboard, subsequent encounter**
>
> *Explanation:* This fracture would be coded with a seventh character D for subsequent encounter, whether the same physician who provided the initial cast application or a different physician is now seeing the patient. Although the patient received x-rays, the intent of the x-rays was to assess how the fracture was healing. There was no active treatment rendered and the visit is therefore considered a subsequent encounter.

The aftercare Z codes should not be used for aftercare for conditions such as injuries or poisonings, where 7th characters are provided to identify subsequent care. For example, for aftercare of an injury, assign the acute injury code with the 7th character "D" (subsequent encounter).

7th character "S", sequela, is for use for complications or conditions that arise as a direct result of a condition, such as scar formation after a burn. The scars are sequelae of the burn. When using 7th character "S", it is necessary to use both the injury code that precipitated the sequela and the code for the sequela itself. The "S" is added only to the injury code, not the sequela code. The 7th character "S" identifies the injury responsible for the sequela. The specific type of sequela (e.g. scar) is sequenced first, followed by the injury code.

See Section I.B.10. Sequelae, (Late Effects)

> Patient with a history of a nondisplaced fracture to the distal pole of the right scaphoid bone due to a fall from a skateboard is admitted for evaluation of arthritis to the right wrist that has developed as a consequence of the traumatic fracture.
>
> **M12.531**   **Traumatic arthropathy, right wrist**
>
> **S62.014S**   **Nondisplaced fracture of distal pole of navicular [scaphoid] bone of right wrist, sequela**
>
> **V00.131S**   **Fall from skateboard, sequela**
>
> *Explanation:* The code identifying the specific sequela condition (traumatic arthritis) should be coded first followed by the injury that instigated the development of the sequela (fracture). The scaphoid fracture injury code is given a 7th character S for sequela to represent its role as the inciting injury. The fracture has healed and is not being managed or treated on this admit and therefore is not applicable as a first listed or principal diagnosis. However, it is directly related to the development of the arthritis and should be appended as a secondary code to signify this cause and effect relationship.

b. Coding of injuries

When coding injuries, assign separate codes for each injury unless a combination code is provided, in which case the combination code is assigned. Codes from category T07, Unspecified multiple injuries should not be assigned in the inpatient setting unless information for a more specific code is not available. Traumatic injury codes (S00–T14.9) are not to be used for normal, healing surgical wounds or to identify complications of surgical wounds.

The code for the most serious injury, as determined by the provider and the focus of treatment, is sequenced first.

1) Superficial injuries

Superficial injuries such as abrasions or contusions are not coded when associated with more severe injuries of the same site.

2) Primary injury with damage to nerves/blood vessels

When a primary injury results in minor damage to peripheral nerves or blood vessels, the primary injury is sequenced first with additional code(s) for injuries to nerves and spinal cord (such as category S04), and/or injury to blood vessels (such as category S15). When the primary injury is to the blood vessels or nerves, that injury should be sequenced first.

3) Iatrogenic injuries

Injury codes from Chapter 19 should not be assigned for injuries that occur during, or as a result of, a medical intervention. Assign the appropriate complication code(s).

c. Coding of traumatic fractures

The principles of multiple coding of injuries should be followed in coding fractures. Fractures of specified sites are coded individually by site in accordance with both the provisions within categories S02, S12, S22, S32, S42, S49, S52, S59, S62, S72, S79, S82, S89, S92 and the level of detail furnished by medical record content.

A fracture not indicated as open or closed should be coded to closed. A fracture not indicated whether displaced or not displaced should be coded to displaced.

More specific guidelines are as follows:

1) Initial vs. subsequent encounter for fractures

Traumatic fractures are coded using the appropriate 7th character for initial encounter (A, B, C) for each encounter where the patient is receiving active treatment for the fracture. The appropriate 7th character for initial encounter should also be assigned for a patient who delayed seeking treatment for the fracture or nonunion.

Fractures are coded using the appropriate 7th character for subsequent care for encounters after the patient has completed active treatment of the fracture and is receiving routine care for the fracture during the healing or recovery phase.

Care for complications of surgical treatment for fracture repairs during the healing or recovery phase should be coded with the appropriate complication codes.

Care of complications of fractures, such as malunion and nonunion, should be reported with the appropriate 7th character for subsequent care with nonunion (K, M, N,) or subsequent care with malunion (P, Q, R).

Malunion/nonunion: The appropriate 7th character for initial encounter should also be assigned for a patient who delayed seeking treatment for the fracture or nonunion.

	Female patient fell during a forest hiking excursion almost six months ago and until recently did not feel she needed to seek medical attention for her left ankle pain; x-rays show nonunion of lateral malleolus and surgery has been scheduled
S82.62XA	**Displaced fracture of lateral malleolus of left fibula, initial encounter for closed fracture**
W01.0XXA	**Fall on same level from slipping, tripping and stumbling without subsequent striking against object, initial encounter**
Y92.821	**Forest as place of occurrence of the external cause**
Y93.01	**Activity, walking, marching and hiking**
Y99.8	**Other external cause status**

Explanation: A seventh character of A is used for the lateral malleolus nonunion fracture to signify that the fracture is receiving active treatment. The delayed care for the fracture has resulted in a nonunion, but capturing the nonunion in the seventh character is trumped by the provision of active care.

The open fracture designations in the assignment of the 7th character for fractures of the forearm, femur and lower leg, including ankle are based on the Gustilo open fracture classification. When the Gustilo classification type is not specified for an open fracture, the 7th character for open fracture type I or II should be assigned (B, E, H, M, Q).

	A 17-year-old arrives at the trauma center with open, displaced right forearm fracture with extensive soft tissue damage. He fell while being tackled playing football for his high school team. On-call orthopaedic specialist documents segmental type IIIA fracture of radial shaft with no need for plastic consult.
S52.361C	**Displaced segmental fracture of shaft of radius, right arm, initial encounter for open fracture type IIIA, IIIB, or IIIC**
W03.XXXA	**Other fall on same level due to collision with another person, initial encounter**
Y92.321	**Football field as the place of occurrence of the external cause**
Y93.61	**Activity, American tackle football**

Explanation: The seventh character for forearm fractures capture the type of encounter and whether the fracture is open or closed; open fractures are broken down further by the type of fracture based on the Gustilo classification. The Gustilo classification describes the severity of open fracture and soft tissue injury. Type IIIA describes an open fracture with extensive soft tissue injury but adequate soft tissue remaining for wound coverage. A segmental fracture means that the bone is broken in two places, leaving at least one segment unattached to the bone. There is no need to report an additional code for the soft tissue injury as it is captured in the fracture code.

A code from category M80, not a traumatic fracture code, should be used for any patient with known osteoporosis who suffers a fracture, even if the patient had a minor fall or trauma, if that fall or trauma would not usually break a normal, healthy bone.

See Section I.C.13. Osteoporosis.

The aftercare Z codes should not be used for aftercare for traumatic fractures. For aftercare of a traumatic fracture, assign the acute fracture code with the appropriate 7th character.

2) Multiple fractures sequencing

Multiple fractures are sequenced in accordance with the severity of the fracture.

3) Physeal fractures

For physeal fractures, assign only the code identifying the type of physeal fracture. Do not assign a separate code to identify the specific bone that is fractured.

d. Coding of burns and corrosions

The ICD-10-CM makes a distinction between burns and corrosions. The burn codes are for thermal burns, except sunburns, that come from a heat source, such as a fire or hot appliance. The burn codes are also for burns resulting from electricity and radiation. Corrosions are burns due to chemicals. The guidelines are the same for burns and corrosions.

Current burns (T20–T25) are classified by depth, extent and by agent (X code). Burns are classified by depth as first degree (erythema), second degree (blistering), and third degree (full-thickness involvement). Burns of the eye and internal organs (T26–T28) are classified by site, but not by degree.

1) Sequencing of burn and related condition codes

Sequence first the code that reflects the highest degree of burn when more than one burn is present.

a. When the reason for the admission or encounter is for treatment of external multiple burns, sequence first the code that reflects the burn of the highest degree.

b. When a patient has both internal and external burns, the circumstances of admission govern the selection of the principal diagnosis or first-listed diagnosis.

c. When a patient is admitted for burn injuries and other related conditions such as smoke inhalation and/or respiratory failure, the circumstances of admission govern the selection of the principal or first-listed diagnosis.

	Patient admitted with minor first-degree burns to multiple sites of her right and left hands as well as severe smoke inhalation. While she was sleeping at home, a candle on her dresser lit the bedroom curtains on fire.
T59.811A	**Toxic effect of smoke, accidental (unintentional), initial encounter**
J70.5	**Respiratory conditions due to smoke inhalation**
T23.191A	**Burn of first degree of multiple sites of right wrist and hand, initial encounter**
T23.192A	**Burn of first degree of multiple sites of left wrist and hand, initial encounter**
X08.8XXA	**Exposure to other specified smoke, fire and flames, initial encounter**
Y92.003	**Bedroom of unspecified non-institutional (private) residence as the place of occurrence of the external cause**
Y93.84	**Activity, sleeping**

Explanation: Based on the documentation, the inhalation injury is more severe than the first-degree burns and is sequenced first. The burns to the hands are appended as secondary diagnoses.

2) Burns of the same anatomic site

Classify burns of the same anatomic site and on the same side but of different degrees to the subcategory identifying the highest degree recorded in the diagnosis (e.g., for second and third degree burns of right thigh, assign only code T24.311-).

3) Non-healing burns

Non-healing burns are coded as acute burns.

Necrosis of burned skin should be coded as a non-healed burn.

4) Infected burn

For any documented infected burn site, use an additional code for the infection.

5) Assign separate codes for each burn site

When coding burns, assign separate codes for each burn site. Category T30, Burn and corrosion, body region unspecified is extremely vague and should rarely be used.

Codes for burns of "multiple sites" should only be assigned when the medical record documentation does not specify the individual sites.

	Patient is admitted with third-degree burns of the scalp as well as second-degree burns to the back of the right hand
T20.35XA	**Burn of third degree of scalp [any part], initial encounter**
T23.261A	**Burn of second degree of back of right hand, initial encounter**

Explanation: Two codes may be reported as the hand and face represent distinct burn sites.

6) Burns and corrosions classified according to extent of body surface involved

Assign codes from category T31, Burns classified according to extent of body surface involved, or T32, Corrosions classified according to extent of body surface involved, for acute burns or corrosions when the site of the burn or corrosion is not specified or when there is a need for additional data. It is advisable to use category T31 as additional coding when needed to provide data for evaluating burn mortality, such as that needed by burn units. It is also advisable to use category T31 as an additional code for reporting purposes when there is mention of a third-degree burn involving 20 percent or more of the body surface. Codes from categories T31 and T32 should not be used for sequelae of burns or corrosions.

Categories T31 and T32 are based on the classic "rule of nines" in estimating body surface involved: head and neck are assigned nine percent, each arm nine percent, each leg 18 percent, the anterior trunk 18 percent, posterior trunk 18 percent, and genitalia one percent. Providers may change these percentage assignments where necessary to accommodate infants and children who have proportionately larger heads than adults, and patients who have large buttocks, thighs, or abdomen that involve burns.

> Patient seen in burn unit for dressing change after he accidentally spilled acetic acid on himself two days ago. The second-degree burns to his right thigh, covering about 3 percent of his body surface, are healing appropriately.
>
> **T54.2X1D**   **Toxic effect of corrosive acids and acid-like substances, accidental (unintentional), subsequent encounter**
>
> **T24.611D**   **Corrosion of second degree of right thigh, subsequent encounter**
>
> **T32.0**   **Corrosions involving less than 10% of body surface**
>
> *Explanation:* Code T32.0 provides additional information as to how much of the patient's body was affected by the corrosive substance.

7) Encounters for treatment of sequela of burns

Encounters for the treatment of the late effects of burns or corrosions (i.e., scars or joint contractures) should be coded with a burn or corrosion code with the 7th character "S" for sequela.

8) Sequelae with a late effect code and current burn

When appropriate, both a code for a current burn or corrosion with 7th character "A" or "D" and a burn or corrosion code with 7th character "S" may be assigned on the same record (when both a current burn and sequelae of an old burn exist). Burns and corrosions do not heal at the same rate and a current healing wound may still exist with sequela of a healed burn or corrosion.

See Section I.B.10. Sequela (Late Effects)

> Female patient seen in ED for second-degree burn to the left ear; she also has significant scarring on her left elbow from a third-degree burn from childhood
>
> **T20.212A**   **Burn of second degree of left ear [any part, except ear drum], initial encounter**
>
> **L90.5**   **Scar conditions and fibrosis of skin**
>
> **T22.322S**   **Burn of third degree of left elbow, sequela**
>
> *Explanation:* The patient is being seen for management of a current second-degree burn, which is reflected in the code by appending the seventh character of A, indicating active treatment or management of this burn. The elbow scarring is a sequela of a previous third-degree burn. The sequela condition precedes the original burn injury, which is appended with a seventh character of S.

9) Use of an external cause code with burns and corrosions

An external cause code should be used with burns and corrosions to identify the source and intent of the burn, as well as the place where it occurred.

e. Adverse effects, poisoning, and toxic effects

Codes in categories T36–T65 are combination codes that include the substance that was taken as well as the intent. No additional external cause code is required for poisonings, toxic effects, adverse effects and underdosing codes.

1) Do not code directly from the Table of Drugs

Do not code directly from the Table of Drugs and Chemicals. Always refer back to the Tabular List.

2) Use as many codes as necessary to describe

Use as many codes as necessary to describe completely all drugs, medicinal or biological substances.

3) If the same code would describe the causative agent

If the same code would describe the causative agent for more than one adverse reaction, poisoning, toxic effect or underdosing, assign the code only once.

4) If two or more drugs, medicinal or biological substances

If two or more drugs, medicinal or biological substances are taken, code each individually unless a combination code is listed in the Table of Drugs and Chemicals.

If multiple unspecified drugs, medicinal or biological substances were taken, assign the appropriate code from subcategory T50.91, Poisoning by, adverse effect of and underdosing of multiple unspecified drugs, medicaments and biological substances.

5) The occurrence of drug toxicity is classified in ICD-10-CM as follows:

(a) Adverse effect

When coding an adverse effect of a drug that has been correctly prescribed and properly administered, assign the appropriate code for the nature of the adverse effect followed by the appropriate code for

the adverse effect of the drug (T36–T50). The code for the drug should have a 5th or 6th character "5" (for example T36.0X5-) Examples of the nature of an adverse effect are tachycardia, delirium, gastrointestinal hemorrhaging, vomiting, hypokalemia, hepatitis, renal failure, or respiratory failure.

> Patient admitted for stomach pain and jaundice, indicated by physician as possible side-effects of Inderal, recently started for hypertension. Inderal was discontinued and the patient switched to Atenolol instead.
>
> **R10.9**   **Unspecified abdominal pain**
>
> **R17**   **Unspecified jaundice**
>
> **T44.7X5A**   **Adverse effect of beta-adrenoreceptor antagonists, initial encounter**
>
> **I10**   **Essential (primary) hypertension**
>
> *Explanation:* The side-effects caused by the drug are listed first, followed by the code for the adverse effect of the drug to capture the specific drug that was used.

(b) Poisoning

When coding a poisoning or reaction to the improper use of a medication (e.g., overdose, wrong substance given or taken in error, wrong route of administration), first assign the appropriate code from categories T36–T50. The poisoning codes have an associated intent as their 5th or 6th character (accidental, intentional self-harm, assault and undetermined). If the intent of the poisoning is unknown or unspecified, code the intent as accidental intent. The undetermined intent is only for use if the documentation in the record specifies that the intent cannot be determined. Use additional code(s) for all manifestations of poisonings.

> A 55-year-old female status post recent left knee replacement is admitted due to confusion, dizziness, and nausea. Her spouse brought in her prescribed Xanax, Ambien, and Percocet bottles but has no idea how many she took. It is suspected that her symptoms are due to an overdose of these medications.
>
> **T42.4X1A**   **Poisoning by benzodiazepines, accidental (unintentional), initial encounter**
>
> **T42.6X1A**   **Poisoning by other antiepileptic and sedative-hypnotic drugs, accidental (unintentional), initial encounter**
>
> **T40.2X1A**   **Poisoning by other opioids, accidental (unintentional), initial encounter**
>
> **R41.0**   **Disorientation, unspecified**
>
> **R42**   **Dizziness and giddiness**
>
> **R11.0**   **Nausea**
>
> *Explanation:* It was not documented whether the overdose of the drugs was accidental or intentional; therefore the correct reporting of the poisoning codes is accidental intent. The poisoning codes are sequenced first, followed by manifestations of the poisoning.

If there is also a diagnosis of abuse or dependence of the substance, the abuse or dependence is assigned as an additional code.

Examples of poisoning include:

(i)   Error was made in drug prescription
Errors made in drug prescription or in the administration of the drug by provider, nurse, patient, or other person.

(ii)   Overdose of a drug intentionally taken
If an overdose of a drug was intentionally taken or administered and resulted in drug toxicity, it would be coded as a poisoning.

(iii)   Nonprescribed drug taken with correctly prescribed and properly administered drug
If a nonprescribed drug or medicinal agent was taken in combination with a correctly prescribed and properly administered drug, any drug toxicity or other reaction resulting from the interaction of the two drugs would be classified as a poisoning.

(iv)   Interaction of drug(s) and alcohol
When a reaction results from the interaction of a drug(s) and alcohol, this would be classified as poisoning.
See Section I.C.4. if poisoning is the result of insulin pump malfunctions.
For Sequela (Late Effects) see Section I.B.10.

(c) Underdosing

Underdosing refers to taking less of a medication than is prescribed by a provider or a manufacturer's instruction. Discontinuing the use of a prescribed medication on the patient's own initiative (not directed by the patient's provider) is also classified as an underdosing. For

Chapter 19. Injury, Poisoning, and Certain Other Consequences of External Causes

underdosing, assign the code from categories T36–T5Ø (fifth or sixth character "6"). Documentation of a change in the patient's condition is not required in order to assign an underdosing code. Documentation that the patient is taking less of a medication than is prescribed or discontinued the prescribed medication is sufficient for code assignment.

Codes for underdosing should never be assigned as principal or first-listed codes. If a patient has a relapse or exacerbation of the medical condition for which the drug is prescribed because of the reduction in dose, then the medical condition itself should be coded.

Noncompliance (Z91.12-, Z91.13-, Z91.14- and Z91.A4-) or complication of care (Y63.6-Y63.9) codes are to be used with an underdosing code to indicate intent, if known.

> Patient admitted for atrial fibrillation with history of chronic atrial fibrillation for which she is prescribed amiodarone. Financial concerns have left the patient unable to pay for her prescriptions and she has been skipping her amiodarone dose every other day to offset the cost.
>
> **I48.2Ø**   **Chronic atrial fibrillation, unspecified**
>
> **T46.2X6A**   **Underdosing of other antidysrhythmic drugs, initial encounter**
>
> **Z91.12Ø**   **Patient's intentional underdosing of medication regimen due to financial hardship**
>
> *Explanation:* By skipping her amiodarone pill every other day, the patient's atrial fibrillation returned. The condition for which the drug was being taken is reported first, followed by an underdosing code to show that the patient was not adhering to her prescription regimen. The Z code helps elaborate on the patient's social and/or economic circumstances that led to the patient taking less then what she was prescribed.

(d) Toxic effects

When a harmful substance is ingested or comes in contact with a person, this is classified as a toxic effect. The toxic effect codes are in categories T51–T65. When coding a toxic effect, assign the toxic effect code first, followed by codes for all associated manifestations of the toxic effect.

Toxic effect codes have an associated intent: accidental, intentional self-harm, assault and undetermined.

For Sequela (Late Effects) see Section I.B.1Ø. Sequela

f. Adult and child abuse, neglect and other maltreatment

Sequence first the appropriate code from categories T74.- (Adult and child abuse, neglect and other maltreatment, confirmed) or T76.- (Adult and child abuse, neglect and other maltreatment, suspected) for abuse, neglect and other maltreatment, followed by any accompanying mental health or injury code(s).

If the documentation in the medical record states abuse or neglect it is coded as confirmed (T74.-). It is coded as suspected if it is documented as suspected (T76.-).

For cases of confirmed abuse or neglect an external cause code from the assault section (X92–Y09) should be added to identify the cause of any physical injuries. A perpetrator code (YØ7) should be added when the perpetrator of the abuse is known. For suspected cases of abuse or neglect, do not report external cause or perpetrator code.

If a suspected case of abuse, neglect or mistreatment is ruled out during an encounter code ZØ4.71, Encounter for examination and observation following alleged physical adult abuse, ruled out, or code ZØ4.72, Encounter for examination and observation following alleged child physical abuse, ruled out, should be used, not a code from T76.

If a suspected case of alleged rape or sexual abuse is ruled out during an encounter code ZØ4.41, Encounter for examination and observation following alleged adult rape or code ZØ4.42, Encounter for examination and observation following alleged child rape, should be used, not a code from T76.

If a suspected case of forced sexual exploitation or forced labor exploitation is ruled out during an encounter, code ZØ4.81, Encounter for examination and observation of victim following forced sexual exploitation, or code ZØ4.82, Encounter for examination and observation of victim following forced labor exploitation, should be used, not a code from T76.

See Section I.C.15. Abuse in a pregnant patient.

g. Complications of care

1) General guidelines for complications of care

(a) Documentation of complications of care

See Section I.B.16. for information on documentation of complications of care.

2) Pain due to medical devices

Pain associated with devices, implants or grafts left in a surgical site (for example painful hip prosthesis) is assigned to the appropriate code(s) found in Chapter 19, Injury, poisoning, and certain other consequences of external causes. Specific codes for pain due to medical devices are found in the T code section of the ICD-10-CM. Use additional code(s) from category G89 to identify acute or chronic pain due to presence of the device, implant or graft (G89.18 or G89.28).

3) Transplant complications

(a) Transplant complications other than kidney

Codes under category T86, Complications of transplanted organs and tissues, are for use for both complications and rejection of transplanted organs. A transplant complication code is only assigned if the complication affects the function of the transplanted organ. Two codes are required to fully describe a transplant complication: the appropriate code from category T86 and a secondary code that identifies the complication.

Pre-existing conditions or conditions that develop after the transplant are not coded as complications unless they affect the function of the transplanted organs.

See I.C.21. for transplant organ removal status

See I.C.2. for malignant neoplasm associated with transplanted organ.

See I.C.1.d.4. for sequencing of sepsis due to infection in transplanted organ

(b) Kidney transplant complications

Patients who have undergone kidney transplant may still have some form of chronic kidney disease (CKD) because the kidney transplant may not fully restore kidney function. Code T86.1- should be assigned for documented complications of a kidney transplant, such as transplant failure or rejection or other transplant complication. Code T86.1- should not be assigned for post kidney transplant patients who have chronic kidney (CKD) unless a transplant complication such as transplant failure or rejection is documented. If the documentation is unclear as to whether the patient has a complication of the transplant, query the provider.

Conditions that affect the function of the transplanted kidney, other than CKD, should be assigned a code from subcategory T86.1, Complications of transplanted organ, Kidney, and a secondary code that identifies the complication.

For patients with CKD following a kidney transplant, but who do not have a complication such as failure or rejection, *see section I.C.14. Chronic kidney disease and kidney transplant status.*

See I.C.1.d.4. for sequencing of sepsis due to infection in transplanted organ

> Patient with chronic kidney disease stage 2; history of successful kidney transplant with no complications identified
>
> **N18.2**   **Chronic kidney disease, stage 2 (mild)**
>
> **Z94.Ø**   **Kidney transplant status**
>
> *Explanation:* This patient's stage 2 CKD is not indicated as being due to the transplanted kidney but instead is just the residual disease the patient had prior to the transplant.

4) Complication codes that include the external cause

As with certain other T codes, some of the complications of care codes have the external cause included in the code. The code includes the nature of the complication as well as the type of procedure that caused the complication. No external cause code indicating the type of procedure is necessary for these codes.

5) Complications of care codes within the body system chapters

Intraoperative and postprocedural complication codes are found within the body system chapters with codes specific to the organs and structures of that body system. These codes should be sequenced first, followed by a code(s) for the specific complication, if applicable.

Complication codes from the body system chapters should be assigned for intraoperative and postprocedural complications (e.g., the appropriate complication code from chapter 9 would be assigned for a vascular intraoperative or postprocedural complication) unless the complication is specifically indexed to a T code in chapter 19.

> During a spinal fusion procedure, the surgeon inadvertently punctured the dura. The midline durotomy was repaired, and the fusion procedure was completed.
>
> **G97.41**   **Accidental puncture or laceration of dura during a procedure**
>
> *Explanation:* The accidental durotomy is not coded to an injury code in chapter 19 but instead is categorized to the nervous system chapter.

Muscle/Tendon Table

ICD-10-CM categorizes certain muscles and tendons in the upper and lower extremities by their action (e.g., extension, flexion), their anatomical location (e.g., posterior, anterior), and/or whether they are intrinsic or extrinsic to a certain anatomical area. The Muscle/Tendon Table is provided at the beginning of chapters 13 and 19 as a resource to help users when code selection depends on one or more of these characteristics. Please note that this table is not all-inclusive, and proper code assignment should be based on the provider's documentation.

Body Region	Muscle	Extensor Tendon	Flexor Tendon	Other Tendon
Shoulder				
	Deltoid	Posterior deltoid	Anterior deltoid	
	Rotator cuff			
	Infraspinatus			Infraspinatus
	Subscapularis			Subscapularis
	Supraspinatus			Supraspinatus
	Teres minor			Teres minor
	Teres major	Teres major		
Upper arm				
	Anterior muscles			
	Biceps brachii — long head		Biceps brachii — long head	
	Biceps brachii — short head		Biceps brachii — short head	
	Brachialis		Brachialis	
	Coracobrachialis		Coracobrachialis	
	Posterior muscles			
	Triceps brachii	Triceps brachii		
Forearm				
	Anterior muscles			
	Flexors			
	Deep			
	Flexor digitorum profundus		Flexor digitorum profundus	
	Flexor pollicis longus		Flexor pollicis longus	
	Intermediate			
	Flexor digitorum superficialis		Flexor digitorum superficialis	
	Superficial			
	Flexor carpi radialis		Flexor carpi radialis	
	Flexor carpi ulnaris		Flexor carpi ulnaris	
	Palmaris longus		Palmaris longus	
	Pronators			
	Pronator quadratus			Pronator quadratus
	Pronator teres			Pronator teres
	Posterior muscles			
	Extensors			
	Deep			
	Abductor pollicis longus			Abductor pollicis longus
	Extensor indicis	Extensor indicis		
	Extensor pollicis brevis	Extensor pollicis brevis		
	Extensor pollicis longus	Extensor pollicis longus		
	Superficial			
	Brachioradialis			Brachioradialis
	Extensor carpi radialis brevis	Extensor carpi radialis brevis		
	Extensor carpi radialis longus	Extensor carpi radialis longus		
	Extensor carpi ulnaris	Extensor carpi ulnaris		
	Extensor digiti minimi	Extensor digiti minimi		
	Extensor digitorum	Extensor digitorum		
	Anconeus	Anconeus		
	Supinator			Supinator

Chapter 19. Injury, Poisoning, and Certain Other Consequences of External Causes

Body Region	Muscle	Extensor Tendon	Flexor Tendon	Other Tendon
Hand				
Extrinsic — attach to a site in the forearm as well as a site in the hand with action related to hand movement at the wrist				
	Extensor carpi radialis brevis	Extensor carpi radialis brevis		
	Extensor carpi radialis longus	Extensor carpi radialis longus		
	Extensor carpi ulnaris	Extensor carpi ulnaris		
	Flexor carpi radialis		Flexor carpi radialis	
	Flexor carpi ulnaris		Flexor carpi ulnaris	
	Flexor digitorum superficialis		Flexor digitorum superficialis	
	Palmaris longus		Palmaris longus	
Extrinsic — attach to a site in the forearm as well as a site in the hand with action in the hand related to finger movement				
	Adductor pollicis longus			Adductor pollicis longus
	Extensor digiti minimi	Extensor digiti minimi		
	Extensor digitorum	Extensor digitorum		
	Extensor indicis	Extensor indicis		
	Flexor digitorum profundus		Flexor digitorum profundus	
	Flexor digitorum superficialis		Flexor digitorum superficialis	
Extrinsic — attach to a site in the forearm as well as a site in the hand with action in the hand related to thumb movement				
	Extensor pollicis brevis	Extensor pollicis brevis		
	Extensor pollicis longus	Extensor pollicis longus		
	Flexor pollicis longus		Flexor pollicis longus	
Intrinsic — found within the hand only				
	Adductor pollicis			Adductor pollicis
	Dorsal interossei	Dorsal interossei	Dorsal interossei	
	Lumbricals	Lumbricals	Lumbricals	
	Palmaris brevis			Palmaris brevis
	Palmar interossei	Palmar interossei	Palmar interossei	
	Hypothenar muscles			
	Abductor digiti minimi			Abductor digiti minimi
	Flexor digiti minimi brevis		Flexor digiti minimi brevis	
	Opponens digiti minimi		Opponens digiti minimi	
	Thenar muscles			
	Abductor pollicis brevis			Abductor pollicis brevis
	Flexor pollicis brevis		Flexor pollicis brevis	
	Opponens pollicis		Opponens pollicis	
Thigh				
	Anterior muscles			
	Iliopsoas		Iliopsoas	
	Pectineus		Pectineus	
	Quadriceps	Quadriceps		
	Rectus femoris	Rectus femoris — Extends knee	Rectus femoris — Flexes hip	
	Vastus intermedius	Vastus intermedius		
	Vastus lateralis	Vastus lateralis		
	Vastus medialis	Vastus medialis		
	Sartorius		Sartorius	
	Medial muscles			
	Adductor brevis			Adductor brevis
	Adductor longus			Adductor longus
	Adductor magnus			Adductor magnus
	Gracilis			Gracilis
	Obturator externus			Obturator externus
	Posterior muscles			
	Hamstring	Hamstring — Extends hip	Hamstring — Flexes knee	
	Biceps femoris	Biceps femoris	Biceps femoris	
	Semimembranosus	Semimembranosus	Semimembranosus	
	Semitendinosus	Semitendinosus	Semitendinosus	

Body Region	Muscle	Extensor Tendon	Flexor Tendon	Other Tendon
Lower leg				
	Anterior muscles			
	Extensor digitorum longus	Extensor digitorum longus		
	Extensor hallucis longus	Extensor hallucis longus		
	Fibularis (peroneus) tertius	Fibularis (peroneus) tertius		
	Tibialis anterior	Tibialis anterior		Tibialis anterior
	Lateral muscles			
	Fibularis (peroneus) brevis		Fibularis (peroneus) brevis	
	Fibularis (peroneus) longus		Fibularis (peroneus) longus	
	Posterior muscles			
	Deep			
	Flexor digitorum longus		Flexor digitorum longus	
	Flexor hallucis longus		Flexor hallucis longus	
	Popliteus		Popliteus	
	Tibialis posterior		Tibialis posterior	
	Superficial			
	Gastrocnemius		Gastrocnemius	
	Plantaris		Plantaris	
	Soleus		Soleus	
				Calcaneal (Achilles)
Ankle/Foot				
Extrinsic — attach to a site in the lower leg as well as a site in the foot with action related to foot movement at the ankle				
	Plantaris		Plantaris	
	Soleus		Soleus	
	Tibialis anterior	Tibialis anterior		
	Tibialis posterior		Tibialis posterior	
Extrinsic — attach to a site in the lower leg as well as a site in the foot with action in the foot related to toe movement				
	Extensor digitorum longus	Extensor digitorum longus		
	Extensor hallucis longus	Extensor hallucis longus		
	Flexor digitorum longus		Flexor digitorum longus	
	Flexor hallucis longus		Flexor hallucis longus	
Intrinsic — found within the ankle/foot only				
	Dorsal muscles			
	Extensor digitorum brevis	Extensor digitorum brevis		
	Extensor hallucis brevis	Extensor hallucis brevis		
	Plantar muscles			
	Abductor digiti minimi		Abductor digiti minimi	
	Abductor hallucis		Abductor hallucis	
	Dorsal interossei	Dorsal interossei	Dorsal interossei	
	Flexor digiti minimi brevis		Flexor digiti minimi brevis	
	Flexor digitorum brevis		Flexor digitorum brevis	
	Flexor hallucis brevis		Flexor hallucis brevis	
	Lumbricals	Lumbricals	Lumbricals	
	Quadratus plantae		Quadratus plantae	
	Plantar interossei	Plantar interossei	Plantar interossei	

Chapter 19. Injury, Poisoning and Certain Other Consequences of External Causes (S00-T88)

NOTE Use secondary code(s) from Chapter 20, External causes of morbidity, to indicate cause of injury. Codes within the T section that include the external cause do not require an additional external cause code.

Use additional code to identify any retained foreign body, if applicable (Z18.-)

EXCLUDES 1 birth trauma (P10-P15)
obstetric trauma (O70-O71)

NOTE The chapter uses the S-section for coding different types of injuries related to single body regions and the T-section to cover injuries to unspecified body regions as well as poisoning and certain other consequences of external causes.

AHA: 2016,2Q,3-7; 2015,4Q,35-38; 2015,3Q,37-39,40; 2015,2Q,6; 2015,1Q,3-21
TIP: The specific site of an injury can be determined from the radiology report when authenticated by a radiologist and available at the time of code assignment.

This chapter contains the following blocks:

S00-S09	Injuries to the head
S10-S19	Injuries to the neck
S20-S29	Injuries to the thorax
S30-S39	Injuries to the abdomen, lower back, lumbar spine, pelvis and external genitals
S40-S49	Injuries to the shoulder and upper arm
S50-S59	Injuries to the elbow and forearm
S60-S69	Injuries to the wrist, hand and fingers
S70-S79	Injuries to the hip and thigh
S80-S89	Injuries to the knee and lower leg
S90-S99	Injuries to the ankle and foot
T07	Injuries involving multiple body regions
T14	Injury of unspecified body region
T15-T19	Effects of foreign body entering through natural orifice
T20-T25	Burns and corrosions of external body surface, specified by site
T26-T28	Burns and corrosions confined to eye and internal organs
T30-T32	Burns and corrosions of multiple and unspecified body regions
T33-T34	Frostbite
T36-T50	Poisoning by, adverse effect of and underdosing of drugs, medicaments and biological substances
T51-T65	Toxic effects of substances chiefly nonmedicinal as to source
T66-T78	Other and unspecified effects of external causes
T79	Certain early complications of trauma
T80-T88	Complications of surgical and medical care, not elsewhere classified

Injuries to the head (S00-S09)

INCLUDES injuries of ear
injuries of eye
injuries of face [any part]
injuries of gum
injuries of jaw
injuries of oral cavity
injuries of palate
injuries of periocular area
injuries of scalp
injuries of temporomandibular joint area
injuries of tongue
injuries of tooth

Code also for any associated infection

EXCLUDES 2 burns and corrosions (T20-T32)
effects of foreign body in ear (T16)
effects of foreign body in larynx (T17.3)
effects of foreign body in mouth NOS (T18.0)
effects of foreign body in nose (T17.0-T17.1)
effects of foreign body in pharynx (T17.2)
effects of foreign body on external eye (T15.-)
frostbite (T33-T34)
insect bite or sting, venomous (T63.4)

√4th S00 **Superficial injury of head**

EXCLUDES 1 diffuse cerebral contusion (S06.2-)
focal cerebral contusion (S06.3-)
injury of eye and orbit (S05.-)
open wound of head (S01.-)

The appropriate 7th character is to be added to each code from category S00.
A initial encounter
D subsequent encounter
S sequela

√5th S00.0 **Superficial injury of scalp**

√x 7th S00.00 Unspecified superficial injury of scalp **PE**

√x 7th S00.01 **Abrasion** of scalp **PE**

√x 7th S00.02 **Blister** (nonthermal) of scalp **PE**

√x 7th S00.03 **Contusion** of scalp **PE**
Bruise of scalp
Hematoma of scalp

√x 7th S00.04 **External constriction** of part of scalp **PE**

√x 7th S00.05 **Superficial foreign body** of scalp **PE**
Splinter in the scalp

√x 7th S00.06 **Insect bite** (nonvenomous) of scalp **PE**

√x 7th S00.07 Other superficial **bite** of scalp **PE**
EXCLUDES 1 open bite of scalp (S01.05)

√5th S00.1 **Contusion** of **eyelid and periocular area**
Black eye
EXCLUDES 2 contusion of eyeball and orbital tissues (S05.1-)

√x 7th S00.10 Contusion of unspecified eyelid and periocular area **PE**

√x 7th S00.11 Contusion of **right** eyelid and periocular area **PE**

√x 7th S00.12 Contusion of **left** eyelid and periocular area **PE**

√5th S00.2 **Other and unspecified superficial injuries of eyelid and periocular area**
EXCLUDES 2 superficial injury of conjunctiva and cornea (S05.0-)

√6th S00.20 Unspecified superficial injury of eyelid and periocular area

7th S00.201 Unspecified superficial injury of **right** eyelid and periocular area **PE**

7th S00.202 Unspecified superficial injury of **left** eyelid and periocular area **PE**

7th S00.209 Unspecified superficial injury of unspecified eyelid and periocular area **PE**

√6th S00.21 **Abrasion** of eyelid and periocular area

7th S00.211 Abrasion of **right** eyelid and periocular area **PE**

7th S00.212 Abrasion of **left** eyelid and periocular area **PE**

7th S00.219 Abrasion of unspecified eyelid and periocular area **PE**

√6th S00.22 **Blister** (nonthermal) of eyelid and periocular area

7th S00.221 Blister (nonthermal) of **right** eyelid and periocular area **PE**

7th S00.222 Blister (nonthermal) of **left** eyelid and periocular area **PE**

7th S00.229 Blister (nonthermal) of unspecified eyelid and periocular area **PE**

√6th S00.24 **External constriction** of eyelid and periocular area

7th S00.241 External constriction of **right** eyelid and periocular area **PE**

7th S00.242 External constriction of **left** eyelid and periocular area **PE**

7th S00.249 External constriction of unspecified eyelid and periocular area **PE**

√6th S00.25 Superficial **foreign body** of eyelid and periocular area
Splinter of eyelid and periocular area
EXCLUDES 2 retained foreign body in eyelid (H02.81-)

7th S00.251 Superficial foreign body of **right** eyelid and periocular area **PE**

7th S00.252 Superficial foreign body of **left** eyelid and periocular area **PE**

7th S00.259 Superficial foreign body of unspecified eyelid and periocular area **PE**

√6th S00.26 **Insect bite** (nonvenomous) of eyelid and periocular area

7th S00.261 Insect bite (nonvenomous) of **right** eyelid and periocular area **PE**

7th S00.262 Insect bite (nonvenomous) of **left** eyelid and periocular area **PE**

7th S00.269 Insect bite (nonvenomous) of unspecified eyelid and periocular area **PE**

√6th S00.27 Other superficial **bite** of eyelid and periocular area
EXCLUDES 1 open bite of eyelid and periocular area (S01.15)

7th S00.271 Other superficial bite of **right** eyelid and periocular area **PE**

7th S00.272 Other superficial bite of **left** eyelid and periocular area **PE**

7th S00.279 Other superficial bite of unspecified eyelid and periocular area **PE**

√5th S00.3 Superficial injury of **nose**

√x 7th S00.30 Unspecified superficial injury of nose **PE**

N Newborn: 0   P Pediatric: 0-17   M Maternity: 9-64   A Adult: 15-124   UNS Unspecified Site   MCC Major Complication/Comorbidity   CC Complication/Comorbidity   PE POA Exempt

984   ICD-10-CM 2025

√x 7th **S00.31** **Abrasion** of nose `PE`

√x 7th **S00.32** **Blister** (nonthermal) of nose `PE`

√x 7th **S00.33** **Contusion** of nose `PE`
Bruise of nose
Hematoma of nose

√x 7th **S00.34** **External constriction** of nose `PE`

√x 7th **S00.35** Superficial **foreign body** of nose `PE`
Splinter in the nose

√x 7th **S00.36** **Insect bite** (nonvenomous) of nose `PE`

√x 7th **S00.37** Other superficial **bite** of nose `PE`
EXCLUDES 1 *open bite of nose (S01.25)*

√5th **S00.4** Superficial injury of **ear**

√6th **S00.40** Unspecified superficial injury of ear

√7th **S00.401** Unspecified superficial injury of **right** ear `PE`

√7th **S00.402** Unspecified superficial injury of **left** ear `PE`

√7th **S00.409** Unspecified superficial injury of unspecified ear `PE`

√6th **S00.41** **Abrasion** of ear

√7th **S00.411** Abrasion of **right** ear `PE`

√7th **S00.412** Abrasion of **left** ear `PE`

√7th **S00.419** Abrasion of unspecified ear `PE`

√6th **S00.42** **Blister** (nonthermal) of ear

√7th **S00.421** Blister (nonthermal) of **right** ear `PE`

√7th **S00.422** Blister (nonthermal) of **left** ear `PE`

√7th **S00.429** Blister (nonthermal) of unspecified ear `PE`

√6th **S00.43** **Contusion** of ear
Bruise of ear
Hematoma of ear

√7th **S00.431** Contusion of **right** ear `PE`

√7th **S00.432** Contusion of **left** ear `PE`

√7th **S00.439** Contusion of unspecified ear `PE`

√6th **S00.44** **External constriction** of ear

√7th **S00.441** External constriction of **right** ear `PE`

√7th **S00.442** External constriction of **left** ear `PE`

√7th **S00.449** External constriction of unspecified ear `PE`

√6th **S00.45** Superficial **foreign body** of ear
Splinter in the ear

√7th **S00.451** Superficial foreign body of **right** ear `PE`

√7th **S00.452** Superficial foreign body of **left** ear `PE`

√7th **S00.459** Superficial foreign body of unspecified ear `PE`

√6th **S00.46** **Insect bite** (nonvenomous) of ear

√7th **S00.461** Insect bite (nonvenomous) of **right** ear `PE`

√7th **S00.462** Insect bite (nonvenomous) of **left** ear `PE`

√7th **S00.469** Insect bite (nonvenomous) of unspecified ear `PE`

√6th **S00.47** Other superficial **bite** of ear
EXCLUDES 1 *open bite of ear (S01.35)*

√7th **S00.471** Other superficial bite of **right** ear `PE`

√7th **S00.472** Other superficial bite of **left** ear `PE`

√7th **S00.479** Other superficial bite of unspecified ear `PE`

√5th **S00.5** Superficial injury of **lip and oral cavity**

√6th **S00.50** Unspecified superficial injury of lip and oral cavity

√7th **S00.501** Unspecified superficial injury of **lip** `PE`

√7th **S00.502** Unspecified superficial injury of **oral cavity** `PE`

√6th **S00.51** **Abrasion** of lip and oral cavity

√7th **S00.511** Abrasion of **lip** `PE`

√7th **S00.512** Abrasion of **oral cavity** `PE`

√6th **S00.52** **Blister** (nonthermal) of lip and oral cavity

√7th **S00.521** Blister (nonthermal) of **lip** `PE`

√7th **S00.522** Blister (nonthermal) of **oral cavity** `PE`

√6th **S00.53** **Contusion** of lip and oral cavity

√7th **S00.531** Contusion of **lip** `PE`
Bruise of lip
Hematoma of lip

√7th **S00.532** Contusion of **oral cavity** `PE`
Bruise of oral cavity
Hematoma of oral cavity

√6th **S00.54** **External constriction** of lip and oral cavity

√7th **S00.541** External constriction of **lip** `PE`

√7th **S00.542** External constriction of **oral cavity** `PE`

√6th **S00.55** Superficial **foreign body** of lip and oral cavity

√7th **S00.551** Superficial foreign body of **lip** `PE`
Splinter of lip and oral cavity

√7th **S00.552** Superficial foreign body of **oral cavity** `PE`
Splinter of lip and oral cavity

√6th **S00.56** **Insect bite** (nonvenomous) of lip and oral cavity

√7th **S00.561** Insect bite (nonvenomous) of **lip** `PE`

√7th **S00.562** Insect bite (nonvenomous) of **oral cavity** `PE`

√6th **S00.57** Other superficial **bite** of lip and oral cavity

√7th **S00.571** Other superficial bite of **lip** `PE`
EXCLUDES 1 *open bite of lip (S01.551)*

√7th **S00.572** Other superficial bite of **oral cavity** `PE`
EXCLUDES 1 *open bite of oral cavity (S01.552)*

√5th **S00.8** Superficial injury of other parts of head
Superficial injuries of face [any part]

√x 7th **S00.80** Unspecified superficial injury of other part of head `PE`

√x 7th **S00.81** **Abrasion** of other part of head `PE`

√x 7th **S00.82** **Blister** (nonthermal) of other part of head `PE`

√x 7th **S00.83** **Contusion** of other part of head `PE`
Bruise of other part of head
Hematoma of other part of head

√x 7th **S00.84** **External constriction** of other part of head `PE`

√x 7th **S00.85** Superficial **foreign body** of other part of head `PE`
Splinter in other part of head

√x 7th **S00.86** **Insect bite** (nonvenomous) of other part of head `PE`

√x 7th **S00.87** Other superficial **bite** of other part of head `PE`
EXCLUDES 1 *open bite of other part of head (S01.85)*

√5th **S00.9** Superficial injury of unspecified part of head

√x 7th **S00.90** Unspecified superficial injury of unspecified part of head `PE`

√x 7th **S00.91** **Abrasion** of unspecified part of head `PE`

√x 7th **S00.92** **Blister** (nonthermal) of unspecified part of head `PE`

√x 7th **S00.93** **Contusion** of unspecified part of head `PE`
Bruise of head
Hematoma of head

√x 7th **S00.94** **External constriction** of unspecified part of head `PE`

√x 7th **S00.95** Superficial **foreign body** of unspecified part of head `PE`
Splinter of head

√x 7th **S00.96** **Insect bite** (nonvenomous) of unspecified part of head `PE`

√x 7th **S00.97** Other superficial **bite** of unspecified part of head `PE`
EXCLUDES 1 *open bite of head (S01.95)*

✔ Additional Character Required | √x 7th Placeholder | Questionable PDx | Manifestation | Unspecified | UPD Unacceptable PDx | H1-H14 HAC | HCC CMS-HCC Dx | HIV HIV Dx

✓4ᵗʰ S01 Open wound of head

Code also any associated:
 injury of cranial nerve (S04.-)
 injury of muscle and tendon of head (S09.1-)
 intracranial injury (S06.-)
 wound infection

EXCLUDES 1   open skull fracture (S02.- with 7th character B)
EXCLUDES 2   injury of eye and orbit (S05.-)
 traumatic amputation of part of head (S08.-)

The appropriate 7th character is to be added to each code from category S01.
A   initial encounter
D   subsequent encounter
S   sequela

✓5ᵗʰ S01.0 Open wound of scalp

EXCLUDES 1   avulsion of scalp (S08.0-)

✓x7ᵗʰ **S01.00 Unspecified open wound of scalp** PE
✓x7ᵗʰ **S01.01 Laceration without foreign body of scalp** PE
✓x7ᵗʰ **S01.02 Laceration with foreign body of scalp** PE
✓x7ᵗʰ **S01.03 Puncture wound without foreign body of scalp** PE
✓x7ᵗʰ **S01.04 Puncture wound with foreign body of scalp** PE
✓x7ᵗʰ **S01.05 Open bite of scalp** PE
 Bite of scalp NOS
 EXCLUDES 1   superficial bite of scalp (S00.06, S00.07-)

✓5ᵗʰ S01.1 Open wound of eyelid and periocular area

Open wound of eyelid and periocular area with or without involvement of lacrimal passages

✓6ᵗʰ **S01.10 Unspecified open wound of eyelid and periocular area**
 ✓7ᵗʰ **S01.101 Unspecified open wound of right eyelid and periocular area** CC PE
 ✓7ᵗʰ **S01.102 Unspecified open wound of left eyelid and periocular area** CC PE
 ✓7ᵗʰ **S01.109 Unspecified open wound of unspecified eyelid and periocular area** CC UNS PE

✓6ᵗʰ **S01.11 Laceration without foreign body of eyelid and periocular area**
 ✓7ᵗʰ **S01.111 Laceration without foreign body of right eyelid and periocular area** PE
 ✓7ᵗʰ **S01.112 Laceration without foreign body of left eyelid and periocular area** PE
 ✓7ᵗʰ **S01.119 Laceration without foreign body of unspecified eyelid and periocular area** PE

✓6ᵗʰ **S01.12 Laceration with foreign body of eyelid and periocular area**
 ✓7ᵗʰ **S01.121 Laceration with foreign body of right eyelid and periocular area** PE
 ✓7ᵗʰ **S01.122 Laceration with foreign body of left eyelid and periocular area** PE
 ✓7ᵗʰ **S01.129 Laceration with foreign body of unspecified eyelid and periocular area** PE

✓6ᵗʰ **S01.13 Puncture wound without foreign body of eyelid and periocular area**
 ✓7ᵗʰ **S01.131 Puncture wound without foreign body of right eyelid and periocular area** PE
 ✓7ᵗʰ **S01.132 Puncture wound without foreign body of left eyelid and periocular area** PE
 ✓7ᵗʰ **S01.139 Puncture wound without foreign body of unspecified eyelid and periocular area** PE

✓6ᵗʰ **S01.14 Puncture wound with foreign body of eyelid and periocular area**
 ✓7ᵗʰ **S01.141 Puncture wound with foreign body of right eyelid and periocular area** PE
 ✓7ᵗʰ **S01.142 Puncture wound with foreign body of left eyelid and periocular area** PE
 ✓7ᵗʰ **S01.149 Puncture wound with foreign body of unspecified eyelid and periocular area** PE

✓6ᵗʰ **S01.15 Open bite of eyelid and periocular area**
 Bite of eyelid and periocular area NOS
 EXCLUDES 1   superficial bite of eyelid and periocular area (S00.26, S00.27)
 ✓7ᵗʰ **S01.151 Open bite of right eyelid and periocular area** PE

 ✓7ᵗʰ **S01.152 Open bite of left eyelid and periocular area** PE
 ✓7ᵗʰ **S01.159 Open bite of unspecified eyelid and periocular area** PE

✓5ᵗʰ S01.2 Open wound of nose

✓x7ᵗʰ **S01.20 Unspecified open wound of nose** PE
✓x7ᵗʰ **S01.21 Laceration without foreign body of nose** PE
✓x7ᵗʰ **S01.22 Laceration with foreign body of nose** PE
✓x7ᵗʰ **S01.23 Puncture wound without foreign body of nose** PE
✓x7ᵗʰ **S01.24 Puncture wound with foreign body of nose** PE
✓x7ᵗʰ **S01.25 Open bite of nose** PE
 Bite of nose NOS
 EXCLUDES 1   superficial bite of nose (S00.36, S00.37)

✓5ᵗʰ S01.3 Open wound of ear

✓6ᵗʰ **S01.30 Unspecified open wound of ear**
 ✓7ᵗʰ **S01.301 Unspecified open wound of right ear** PE
 ✓7ᵗʰ **S01.302 Unspecified open wound of left ear** PE
 ✓7ᵗʰ **S01.309 Unspecified open wound of unspecified ear** PE

✓6ᵗʰ **S01.31 Laceration without foreign body of ear**
 ✓7ᵗʰ **S01.311 Laceration without foreign body of right ear** PE
 ✓7ᵗʰ **S01.312 Laceration without foreign body of left ear** PE
 ✓7ᵗʰ **S01.319 Laceration without foreign body of unspecified ear** PE

✓6ᵗʰ **S01.32 Laceration with foreign body of ear**
 ✓7ᵗʰ **S01.321 Laceration with foreign body of right ear** PE
 ✓7ᵗʰ **S01.322 Laceration with foreign body of left ear** PE
 ✓7ᵗʰ **S01.329 Laceration with foreign body of unspecified ear** PE

✓6ᵗʰ **S01.33 Puncture wound without foreign body of ear**
 ✓7ᵗʰ **S01.331 Puncture wound without foreign body of right ear** PE
 ✓7ᵗʰ **S01.332 Puncture wound without foreign body of left ear** PE
 ✓7ᵗʰ **S01.339 Puncture wound without foreign body of unspecified ear** PE

✓6ᵗʰ **S01.34 Puncture wound with foreign body of ear**
 ✓7ᵗʰ **S01.341 Puncture wound with foreign body of right ear** PE
 ✓7ᵗʰ **S01.342 Puncture wound with foreign body of left ear** PE
 ✓7ᵗʰ **S01.349 Puncture wound with foreign body of unspecified ear** PE

✓6ᵗʰ **S01.35 Open bite of ear**
 Bite of ear NOS
 EXCLUDES 1   superficial bite of ear (S00.46, S00.47)
 ✓7ᵗʰ **S01.351 Open bite of right ear** PE
 ✓7ᵗʰ **S01.352 Open bite of left ear** PE
 ✓7ᵗʰ **S01.359 Open bite of unspecified ear** PE

✓5ᵗʰ S01.4 Open wound of cheek and temporomandibular area

✓6ᵗʰ **S01.40 Unspecified open wound of cheek and temporomandibular area**
 ✓7ᵗʰ **S01.401 Unspecified open wound of right cheek and temporomandibular area** PE
 ✓7ᵗʰ **S01.402 Unspecified open wound of left cheek and temporomandibular area** PE
 ✓7ᵗʰ **S01.409 Unspecified open wound of unspecified cheek and temporomandibular area** PE

✓6ᵗʰ **S01.41 Laceration without foreign body of cheek and temporomandibular area**
 ✓7ᵗʰ **S01.411 Laceration without foreign body of right cheek and temporomandibular area** PE
 ✓7ᵗʰ **S01.412 Laceration without foreign body of left cheek and temporomandibular area** PE
 ✓7ᵗʰ **S01.419 Laceration without foreign body of unspecified cheek and temporomandibular area** PE

N Newborn: 0   P Pediatric: 0-17   M Maternity: 9-64   A Adult: 15-124   UNS Unspecified Site   MCC Major Complication/Comorbidity   CC Complication/Comorbidity   PE POA Exempt

✓6ᵗʰ **S01.42** **Laceration with foreign body** of cheek and temporomandibular area

   ✓7ᵗʰ **S01.421** Laceration with foreign body of **right** cheek and temporomandibular area   **PE**

   ✓7ᵗʰ **S01.422** Laceration with foreign body of **left** cheek and temporomandibular area   **PE**

   ✓7ᵗʰ **S01.429** Laceration with foreign body of unspecified cheek and temporomandibular area   **PE**

✓6ᵗʰ **S01.43** **Puncture wound without foreign body** of cheek and temporomandibular area

   ✓7ᵗʰ **S01.431** Puncture wound without foreign body of **right** cheek and temporomandibular area   **PE**

   ✓7ᵗʰ **S01.432** Puncture wound without foreign body of **left** cheek and temporomandibular area   **PE**

   ✓7ᵗʰ **S01.439** Puncture wound without foreign body of unspecified cheek and temporomandibular area   **PE**

✓6ᵗʰ **S01.44** **Puncture wound with foreign body** of cheek and temporomandibular area

   ✓7ᵗʰ **S01.441** Puncture wound with foreign body of **right** cheek and temporomandibular area   **PE**

   ✓7ᵗʰ **S01.442** Puncture wound with foreign body of **left** cheek and temporomandibular area   **PE**

   ✓7ᵗʰ **S01.449** Puncture wound with foreign body of unspecified cheek and temporomandibular area   **PE**

✓6ᵗʰ **S01.45** **Open bite** of cheek and temporomandibular area

   Bite of cheek and temporomandibular area NOS

   EXCLUDES 2   *superficial bite of cheek and temporomandibular area (S00.86, S00.87)*

   ✓7ᵗʰ **S01.451** Open bite of **right** cheek and temporomandibular area   **PE**

   ✓7ᵗʰ **S01.452** Open bite of **left** cheek and temporomandibular area   **PE**

   ✓7ᵗʰ **S01.459** Open bite of unspecified cheek and temporomandibular area   **PE**

✓5ᵗʰ **S01.5** **Open wound of lip and oral cavity**

   EXCLUDES 2   *tooth dislocation (S03.2)*
                  tooth fracture (S02.5)

✓6ᵗʰ **S01.50** Unspecified open wound of lip and oral cavity

   ✓7ᵗʰ **S01.501** Unspecified open wound of **lip**   **PE**

   ✓7ᵗʰ **S01.502** Unspecified open wound of **oral cavity**   **PE**

✓6ᵗʰ **S01.51** **Laceration** of lip and oral cavity **without foreign body**

   ✓7ᵗʰ **S01.511** Laceration without foreign body of **lip**   **PE**

   ✓7ᵗʰ **S01.512** Laceration without foreign body of **oral cavity**   **PE**

✓6ᵗʰ **S01.52** **Laceration** of lip and oral cavity **with foreign body**

   ✓7ᵗʰ **S01.521** Laceration with foreign body of **lip**   **PE**

   ✓7ᵗʰ **S01.522** Laceration with foreign body of **oral cavity**   **PE**

✓6ᵗʰ **S01.53** **Puncture wound** of lip and oral cavity **without foreign body**

   ✓7ᵗʰ **S01.531** Puncture wound without foreign body of **lip**   **PE**

   ✓7ᵗʰ **S01.532** Puncture wound without foreign body of **oral cavity**   **PE**

✓6ᵗʰ **S01.54** **Puncture wound** of lip and oral cavity **with foreign body**

   ✓7ᵗʰ **S01.541** Puncture wound with foreign body of **lip**   **PE**

   ✓7ᵗʰ **S01.542** Puncture wound with foreign body of **oral cavity**   **PE**

✓6ᵗʰ **S01.55** **Open bite** of lip and oral cavity

   ✓7ᵗʰ **S01.551** Open bite of **lip**   **PE**

   Bite of lip NOS

   EXCLUDES 1   *superficial bite of lip (S00.571)*

   ✓7ᵗʰ **S01.552** Open bite of **oral cavity**   **PE**

   Bite of oral cavity NOS

   EXCLUDES 1   *superficial bite of oral cavity (S00.572)*

✓5ᵗʰ **S01.8** **Open wound of other parts of head**

   ✓x7ᵗʰ **S01.80** Unspecified open wound of other part of head   **PE**

   ✓x7ᵗʰ **S01.81** **Laceration without foreign body** of other part of head   **PE**

   ✓x7ᵗʰ **S01.82** **Laceration with foreign body** of other part of head   **PE**

   ✓x7ᵗʰ **S01.83** **Puncture wound without foreign body** of other part of head   **PE**

   ✓x7ᵗʰ **S01.84** **Puncture wound with foreign body** of other part of head   **PE**

   ✓x7ᵗʰ **S01.85** **Open bite** of other part of head   **PE**

   Bite of other part of head NOS

   EXCLUDES 1   *superficial bite of other part of head (S00.87)*

✓5ᵗʰ **S01.9** **Open wound of unspecified part of head**

   ✓x7ᵗʰ **S01.90** Unspecified open wound of unspecified part of head   **PE**

   ✓x7ᵗʰ **S01.91** **Laceration without foreign body** of unspecified part of head   **PE**

   ✓x7ᵗʰ **S01.92** **Laceration with foreign body** of unspecified part of head   **PE**

   ✓x7ᵗʰ **S01.93** **Puncture wound without foreign body** of unspecified part of head   **PE**

   ✓x7ᵗʰ **S01.94** **Puncture wound with foreign body** of unspecified part of head   **PE**

   ✓x7ᵗʰ **S01.95** **Open bite** of unspecified part of head   **PE**

   Bite of head NOS

   EXCLUDES 1   *superficial bite of head NOS (S00.97)*

✓4ᵗʰ **S02** **Fracture of skull and facial bones**

   NOTE   A fracture not indicated as open or closed should be coded to closed.

   Code also any associated intracranial injury (S06.-)

   AHA: 2021,1Q,6; 2017,1Q,42; 2016,4Q,66-67

   The appropriate 7th character is to be added to each code from category S02.
   A   initial encounter for closed fracture
   B   initial encounter for open fracture
   D   subsequent encounter for fracture with routine healing
   G   subsequent encounter for fracture with delayed healing
   K   subsequent encounter for fracture with nonunion
   S   sequela

   ✓x7ᵗʰ **S02.0** **Fracture of vault of skull**   **MCC CC H5 HCC PE**

   Fracture of frontal bone
   Fracture of parietal bone

   ✓5ᵗʰ **S02.1** **Fracture of base of skull**

   EXCLUDES 2   *lateral orbital wall (S02.84-)*
                  medial orbital wall (S02.83-)
                  orbital floor (S02.3-)

   AHA: 2019,4Q,16-17

   ✓6ᵗʰ **S02.10** Unspecified fracture of base of skull

      ✓7ᵗʰ **S02.101** Fracture of base of skull, **right** side   **MCC CC H5 HCC PE**

      ✓7ᵗʰ **S02.102** Fracture of base of skull, **left** side   **MCC CC H5 HCC PE**

      ✓7ᵗʰ **S02.109** Fracture of base of skull, unspecified side   **MCC CC H5 UNS HCC PE**

   ✓6ᵗʰ **S02.11** Fracture of **occiput**

      ✓7ᵗʰ **S02.110** **Type I** occipital condyle fracture, unspecified side   **MCC CC H5 UNS HCC PE**

      ✓7ᵗʰ **S02.111** **Type II** occipital condyle fracture, unspecified side   **MCC CC H5 UNS HCC PE**

      ✓7ᵗʰ **S02.112** **Type III** occipital condyle fracture, unspecified side   **MCC CC H5 UNS HCC PE**

      ✓7ᵗʰ **S02.113** **Unspecified** occipital condyle fracture   **MCC CC H5 HCC PE**

      ✓7ᵗʰ **S02.118** **Other** fracture of occiput, unspecified side   **MCC CC H5 HCC PE**

      ✓7ᵗʰ **S02.119** **Unspecified** fracture of occiput   **MCC CC H5 HCC PE**

      ✓7ᵗʰ **S02.11A** **Type I** occipital condyle fracture, **right** side   **MCC CC H5 HCC PE**

✓ Additional Character Required   ✓x7ᵗʰ Placeholder   Questionable PDx   Manifestation   Unspecified   **UPD** Unacceptable PDx   **H1-H14** HAC   **HCC** CMS-HCC Dx   **HIV** HIV Dx

ICD-10-CM 2025   987

√7ᵗʰ **S02.11B** **Type I** occipital condyle fracture, **left** side `MCC` `CC` `H5` `HCC` `PE`

√7ᵗʰ **S02.11C** **Type II** occipital condyle fracture, **right** side `MCC` `CC` `H5` `HCC` `PE`

√7ᵗʰ **S02.11D** **Type II** occipital condyle fracture, **left** side `MCC` `CC` `H5` `HCC` `PE`

√7ᵗʰ **S02.11E** **Type III** occipital condyle fracture, **right** side `MCC` `CC` `H5` `HCC` `PE`

√7ᵗʰ **S02.11F** **Type III** occipital condyle fracture, **left** side `MCC` `CC` `H5` `HCC` `PE`

√7ᵗʰ **S02.11G** **Other** fracture of occiput, **right** side `MCC` `CC` `H5` `HCC` `PE`

√7ᵗʰ **S02.11H** **Other** fracture of occiput, **left** side `MCC` `CC` `H5` `HCC` `PE`

√6ᵗʰ **S02.12** **Fracture of orbital roof**

　　AHA: 2019,4Q,16-17

√7ᵗʰ **S02.121** Fracture of orbital roof, **right** side `MCC` `CC` `H5` `HCC` `PE`

√7ᵗʰ **S02.122** Fracture of orbital roof, **left** side `MCC` `CC` `H5` `HCC` `PE`

√7ᵗʰ **S02.129** Fracture of orbital roof, **unspecified** `MCC` `CC` `UNS` `HCC` `PE`

√x7ᵗʰ **S02.19** **Other fracture of base of skull** `MCC` `CC` `H5` `HCC` `PE`

　　Fracture of anterior fossa of base of skull
　　Fracture of ethmoid sinus
　　Fracture of frontal sinus
　　Fracture of middle fossa of base of skull
　　Fracture of posterior fossa of base of skull
　　Fracture of sphenoid
　　Fracture of temporal bone

√x7ᵗʰ **S02.2** **Fracture of nasal bones** `CC` `H5` `PE`

√5ᵗʰ **S02.3** **Fracture of orbital floor**

　　Fracture of inferior orbital wall
　　EXCLUDES 1　orbit NOS (S02.85)
　　EXCLUDES 2　lateral orbital wall (S02.84-)
　　　　　　　medial orbital wall (S02.83-)
　　　　　　　orbital roof (S02.1-)

√x7ᵗʰ **S02.30** Fracture of orbital floor, **unspecified** side `CC` `H5` `UNS` `HCC` `PE`

√x7ᵗʰ **S02.31** Fracture of orbital floor, **right** side `CC` `H5` `HCC` `PE`

√x7ᵗʰ **S02.32** Fracture of orbital floor, **left** side `CC` `H5` `HCC` `PE`

√5ᵗʰ **S02.4** **Fracture of malar, maxillary and zygoma bones**

　　Fracture of superior maxilla
　　Fracture of upper jaw (bone)
　　Fracture of zygomatic process of temporal bone

√6ᵗʰ **S02.40** **Fracture of malar, maxillary and zygoma bones, unspecified**

√7ᵗʰ **S02.400** **Malar** fracture, unspecified side `CC` `H5` `UNS` `HCC` `PE`

√7ᵗʰ **S02.401** **Maxillary** fracture, unspecified side `CC` `H5` `UNS` `HCC` `PE`

√7ᵗʰ **S02.402** **Zygomatic** fracture, unspecified side `CC` `H5` `UNS` `HCC` `PE`

√7ᵗʰ **S02.40A** **Malar** fracture, **right** side `CC` `H5` `HCC` `PE`

√7ᵗʰ **S02.40B** **Malar** fracture, **left** side `CC` `H5` `HCC` `PE`

√7ᵗʰ **S02.40C** **Maxillary** fracture, **right** side `CC` `H5` `HCC` `PE`

√7ᵗʰ **S02.40D** **Maxillary** fracture, **left** side `CC` `H5` `HCC` `PE`

√7ᵗʰ **S02.40E** **Zygomatic** fracture, **right** side `CC` `H5` `HCC` `PE`

√7ᵗʰ **S02.40F** **Zygomatic** fracture, **left** side `CC` `H5` `HCC` `PE`

√6ᵗʰ **S02.41** **LeFort fracture**

　　DEF: Named for Rene Le Fort, these fractures describe different combinations of multiple fractures that occur from significant force to the midface. A common denominator in all three types of LeFort fractures is fracture of the pterygoid processes, which are two bony plates resembling wings that extend downward from the sphenoid bone.

LeFort Fracture Types

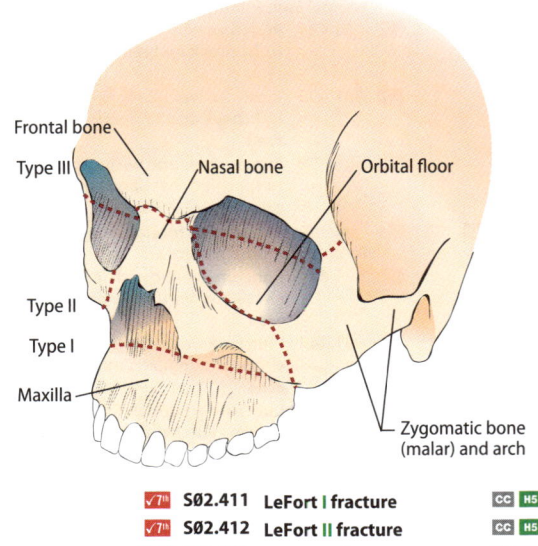

√7ᵗʰ **S02.411** **LeFort I** fracture `CC` `H5` `HCC` `PE`

√7ᵗʰ **S02.412** **LeFort II** fracture `CC` `H5` `HCC` `PE`

√7ᵗʰ **S02.413** **LeFort III** fracture `CC` `H5` `HCC` `PE`

√x7ᵗʰ **S02.42** **Fracture of alveolus of maxilla** `CC` `H5` `HCC` `PE`

√x7ᵗʰ **S02.5** **Fracture of tooth (traumatic)** `CC` `PE`

　　Broken tooth
　　EXCLUDES 1　cracked tooth (nontraumatic) (K03.81)

√5ᵗʰ **S02.6** **Fracture of mandible**

　　Fracture of lower jaw (bone)

√6ᵗʰ **S02.60** **Fracture of mandible, unspecified**

√7ᵗʰ **S02.600** Fracture of unspecified part of body of mandible, unspecified side `CC` `H5` `UNS` `HCC` `PE`

√7ᵗʰ **S02.601** Fracture of unspecified part of body of **right** mandible `CC` `H5` `HCC` `PE`

√7ᵗʰ **S02.602** Fracture of unspecified part of body of **left** mandible `CC` `H5` `HCC` `PE`

√7ᵗʰ **S02.609** Fracture of mandible, unspecified `CC` `H5` `HCC` `PE`

√6ᵗʰ **S02.61** **Fracture of condylar process of mandible**

√7ᵗʰ **S02.610** Fracture of condylar process of mandible, unspecified side `CC` `H5` `UNS` `HCC` `PE`

√7ᵗʰ **S02.611** Fracture of condylar process of **right** mandible `CC` `H5` `HCC` `PE`

√7ᵗʰ **S02.612** Fracture of condylar process of **left** mandible `CC` `H5` `HCC` `PE`

√6ᵗʰ **S02.62** **Fracture of subcondylar process of mandible**

√7ᵗʰ **S02.620** Fracture of subcondylar process of mandible, unspecified side `CC` `H5` `UNS` `HCC` `PE`

√7ᵗʰ **S02.621** Fracture of subcondylar process of **right** mandible `CC` `H5` `HCC` `PE`

√7ᵗʰ **S02.622** Fracture of subcondylar process of **left** mandible `CC` `H5` `HCC` `PE`

√6ᵗʰ **S02.63** **Fracture of coronoid process of mandible**

√7ᵗʰ **S02.630** Fracture of coronoid process of mandible, unspecified side `CC` `H5` `UNS` `HCC` `PE`

√7ᵗʰ **S02.631** Fracture of coronoid process of **right** mandible `CC` `H5` `HCC` `PE`

√7ᵗʰ **S02.632** Fracture of coronoid process of **left** mandible `CC` `H5` `PE`

√6ᵗʰ **S02.64** **Fracture of ramus of mandible**

√7ᵗʰ **S02.640** Fracture of ramus of mandible, unspecified side `CC` `H5` `UNS` `HCC` `PE`

√7ᵗʰ **S02.641** Fracture of ramus of **right** mandible `CC` `H5` `HCC` `PE`

`N` Newborn: 0　`P` Pediatric: 0-17　`M` Maternity: 9-64　`A` Adult: 15-124　`UNS` Unspecified Site　`MCC` Major Complication/Comorbidity　`CC` Complication/Comorbidity　`PE` POA Exempt

988

ICD-10-CM 2025

√7th **S02.642** Fracture of ramus of **left** mandible `CC` `H5` `HCC` `PE`

√6th **S02.65** Fracture of **angle** of mandible

   √7th **S02.650** Fracture of angle of mandible, **unspecified** side `CC` `H5` `UNS` `HCC` `PE`

   √7th **S02.651** Fracture of angle of **right** mandible `CC` `H5` `HCC` `PE`

   √7th **S02.652** Fracture of angle of **left** mandible `CC` `H5` `HCC` `PE`

√x7th **S02.66** Fracture of **symphysis** of mandible `CC` `H5` `HCC` `PE`

√6th **S02.67** Fracture of **alveolus** of mandible

   √7th **S02.670** Fracture of alveolus of mandible, **unspecified** side `CC` `H5` `UNS` `HCC` `PE`

   √7th **S02.671** Fracture of alveolus of **right** mandible `CC` `H5` `HCC` `PE`

   √7th **S02.672** Fracture of alveolus of **left** mandible `CC` `H5` `HCC` `PE`

√x7th **S02.69** Fracture of mandible of other specified site `CC` `H5` `HCC` `PE`

√5th **S02.8** Fractures of other specified skull and facial bones

Fracture of palate

   EXCLUDES 2   fracture of orbital floor (S02.3-)
               fracture of orbital roof (S02.12-)

√x7th **S02.80** Fracture of other specified skull and facial bones, **unspecified** side `CC` `H5` `UNS` `HCC` `PE`

√x7th **S02.81** Fracture of other specified skull and facial bones, **right** side `CC` `H5` `HCC` `PE`

√x7th **S02.82** Fracture of other specified skull and facial bones, **left** side `CC` `H5` `HCC` `PE`

√6th **S02.83** Fracture of **medial orbital wall**

   EXCLUDES 2   orbital floor (S02.3-)
               orbital roof (S02.12-)

   AHA: 2019,4Q,16-17

   √7th **S02.831** Fracture of medial orbital wall, **right** side `CC` `H5` `HCC` `PE`

   √7th **S02.832** Fracture of medial orbital wall, **left** side `CC` `H5` `HCC` `PE`

   √7th **S02.839** Fracture of medial orbital wall, unspecified side `CC` `H5` `HCC` `PE`

√6th **S02.84** Fracture of **lateral orbital wall**

   EXCLUDES 2   orbital floor (S02.3-)
               orbital roof (S02.12-)

   AHA: 2019,4Q,16-17

   √7th **S02.841** Fracture of lateral orbital wall, **right** side `CC` `H5` `HCC` `PE`

   √7th **S02.842** Fracture of lateral orbital wall, **left** side `CC` `H5` `HCC` `PE`

   √7th **S02.849** Fracture of lateral orbital wall, unspecified side `CC` `H5` `HCC` `PE`

√x7th **S02.85** Fracture of orbit, unspecified `CC` `H5` `HCC` `PE`

Fracture of orbit NOS
Fracture of orbit wall NOS

   EXCLUDES 1   lateral orbital wall (S02.84-)
               medial orbital wall (S02.83-)
               orbital floor (S02.3-)
               orbital roof (S02.12-)

√5th **S02.9** Fracture of unspecified skull and facial bones

√x7th **S02.91** Unspecified fracture of **skull** `MCC` `CC` `I-5` `HCC` `PE`

   AHA: 2020,2Q,24

√x7th **S02.92** Unspecified fracture of **facial bones** `CC` `I-5` `HCC` `PE`

√4th **S03** Dislocation and sprain of joints and ligaments of head

   `INCLUDES`   avulsion of joint (capsule) or ligament of head
                     laceration of cartilage, joint (capsule) or ligament of head
                     sprain of cartilage, joint (capsule) or ligament of head
                     traumatic hemarthrosis of joint or ligament of head
                     traumatic rupture of joint or ligament of head
                     traumatic subluxation of joint or ligament of head
                     traumatic tear of joint or ligament of head

Code also any associated open wound

   EXCLUDES 2   strain of muscle or tendon of head (S09.1)

> The appropriate 7th character is to be added to each code from category S03.
> A   initial encounter
> D   subsequent encounter
> S   sequela

√5th **S03.0** Dislocation of jaw

Dislocation of jaw (cartilage) (meniscus)
Dislocation of mandible
Dislocation of temporomandibular (joint)

   AHA: 2016,4Q,67

   √x7th **S03.00** Dislocation of jaw, unspecified side `PE`

   √x7th **S03.01** Dislocation of jaw, **right** side `PE`

   √x7th **S03.02** Dislocation of jaw, **left** side `PE`

   √x7th **S03.03** Dislocation of jaw, **bilateral** `PE`

√x7th **S03.1** Dislocation of septal cartilage of nose `PE`

√x7th **S03.2** Dislocation of tooth `PE`

√5th **S03.4** Sprain of jaw

Sprain of temporomandibular (joint) (ligament)

   AHA: 2016,4Q,67

   √x7th **S03.40** Sprain of jaw, unspecified side `PE`

   √x7th **S03.41** Sprain of jaw, **right** side `PE`

   √x7th **S03.42** Sprain of jaw, **left** side `PE`

   √x7th **S03.43** Sprain of jaw, **bilateral** `PE`

√x7th **S03.8** Sprain of joints and ligaments of other parts of head `PE`

√x7th **S03.9** Sprain of joints and ligaments of unspecified parts of head `PE`

√4th **S04** Injury of cranial nerve

The selection of side should be based on the side of the body being affected

Code first any associated intracranial injury (S06.-)
Code also any associated:
    open wound of head (S01.-)
    skull fracture (S02.-)

> The appropriate 7th character is to be added to each code from category S04.
> A   initial encounter
> D   subsequent encounter
> S   sequela

√5th **S04.0** Injury of optic nerve and pathways

Use additional code to identify any visual field defect or blindness (H53.4-, H54.-)

   √6th **S04.01** Injury of **optic nerve**

Injury of 2nd cranial nerve

      √7th **S04.011** Injury of optic nerve, **right** eye `CC` `PE`

      √7th **S04.012** Injury of optic nerve, **left** eye `CC` `PE`

      √7th **S04.019** Injury of optic nerve, unspecified eye `CC` `UNS` `PE`

Injury of optic nerve NOS

   √x7th **S04.02** Injury of optic **chiasm** `CC` `PE`

   √6th **S04.03** Injury of optic **tract and pathways**

Injury of optic radiation

      √7th **S04.031** Injury of optic tract and pathways, **right** side `CC` `PE`

      √7th **S04.032** Injury of optic tract and pathways, **left** side `CC` `PE`

      √7th **S04.039** Injury of optic tract and pathways, unspecified side `CC` `UNS` `PE`

Injury of optic tract and pathways NOS

   √6th **S04.04** Injury of **visual cortex**

      √7th **S04.041** Injury of visual cortex, **right** side `CC` `PE`

      √7th **S04.042** Injury of visual cortex, **left** side `CC` `PE`

✔ Additional Character Required   √x7th Placeholder   Questionable PDx   Manifestation   Unspecified   `UPD` Unacceptable PDx   `H1`-`H14` HAC   `HCC` CMS-HCC Dx   `HIV` HIV Dx

ICD-10-CM 2025   **989**

√7th **S04.049** **Injury of visual cortex, unspecified side** `CC` `UNS` `PE`
Injury of visual cortex NOS

√5th **S04.1** **Injury of oculomotor nerve**
Injury of 3rd cranial nerve
√x7th **S04.10** **Injury of oculomotor nerve, unspecified side** `CC` `UNS` `PE`
√x7th **S04.11** **Injury of oculomotor nerve, right side** `CC` `PE`
√x7th **S04.12** **Injury of oculomotor nerve, left side** `CC` `PE`

√5th **S04.2** **Injury of trochlear nerve**
Injury of 4th cranial nerve
√x7th **S04.20** **Injury of trochlear nerve, unspecified side** `CC` `UNS` `PE`
√x7th **S04.21** **Injury of trochlear nerve, right side** `CC` `PE`
√x7th **S04.22** **Injury of trochlear nerve, left side** `CC` `PE`

√5th **S04.3** **Injury of trigeminal nerve**
Injury of 5th cranial nerve
√x7th **S04.30** **Injury of trigeminal nerve, unspecified side** `CC` `UNS` `PE`
√x7th **S04.31** **Injury of trigeminal nerve, right side** `CC` `PE`
√x7th **S04.32** **Injury of trigeminal nerve, left side** `CC` `PE`

√5th **S04.4** **Injury of abducent nerve**
Injury of 6th cranial nerve
√x7th **S04.40** **Injury of abducent nerve, unspecified side** `CC` `UNS` `PE`
√x7th **S04.41** **Injury of abducent nerve, right side** `CC` `PE`
√x7th **S04.42** **Injury of abducent nerve, left side** `CC` `PE`

√5th **S04.5** **Injury of facial nerve**
Injury of 7th cranial nerve
√x7th **S04.50** **Injury of facial nerve, unspecified side** `CC` `UNS` `PE`
√x7th **S04.51** **Injury of facial nerve, right side** `CC` `PE`
√x7th **S04.52** **Injury of facial nerve, left side** `CC` `PE`

√5th **S04.6** **Injury of acoustic nerve**
Injury of auditory nerve
Injury of 8th cranial nerve
√x7th **S04.60** **Injury of acoustic nerve, unspecified side** `CC` `UNS` `PE`
√x7th **S04.61** **Injury of acoustic nerve, right side** `CC` `PE`
√x7th **S04.62** **Injury of acoustic nerve, left side** `CC` `PE`

√5th **S04.7** **Injury of accessory nerve**
Injury of 11th cranial nerve
√x7th **S04.70** **Injury of accessory nerve, unspecified side** `CC` `UNS` `PE`
√x7th **S04.71** **Injury of accessory nerve, right side** `CC` `PE`
√x7th **S04.72** **Injury of accessory nerve, left side** `CC` `PE`

√5th **S04.8** **Injury of other cranial nerves**
√6th **S04.81** **Injury of olfactory [1st] nerve**
√7th **S04.811** **Injury of olfactory [1st] nerve, right side** `CC` `PE`
√7th **S04.812** **Injury of olfactory [1st] nerve, left side** `CC` `PE`
√7th **S04.819** **Injury of olfactory [1st] nerve, unspecified side** `CC` `PE`
√6th **S04.89** **Injury of other cranial nerves**
Injury of vagus [10th] nerve
√7th **S04.891** **Injury of other cranial nerves, right side** `CC` `PE`
√7th **S04.892** **Injury of other cranial nerves, left side** `CC` `PE`
√7th **S04.899** **Injury of other cranial nerves, unspecified side** `CC` `UNS` `PE`

√x7th **S04.9** **Injury of unspecified cranial nerve** `CC` `PE`

√4th **S05** **Injury of eye and orbit**
`INCLUDES`   open wound of eye and orbit
`EXCLUDES 2`   2nd cranial [optic] nerve injury (S04.0-)
    3rd cranial [oculomotor] nerve injury (S04.1-)
    open wound of eyelid and periocular area (S01.1-)
    orbital bone fracture (S02.1-, S02.3-, S02.8-)
    superficial injury of eyelid (S00.1-S00.2)

> The appropriate 7th character is to be added to each code from category S05.
> A   initial encounter
> D   subsequent encounter
> S   sequela

√5th **S05.0** **Injury of conjunctiva and corneal abrasion without foreign body**
`EXCLUDES 1`   foreign body in conjunctival sac (T15.1)
    foreign body in cornea (T15.0)
√x7th **S05.00** **Injury of conjunctiva and corneal abrasion without foreign body, unspecified eye** `PE`
√x7th **S05.01** **Injury of conjunctiva and corneal abrasion without foreign body, right eye** `PE`
√x7th **S05.02** **Injury of conjunctiva and corneal abrasion without foreign body, left eye** `PE`

√5th **S05.1** **Contusion of eyeball and orbital tissues**
Traumatic hyphema
`EXCLUDES 2`   black eye NOS (S00.1)
    contusion of eyelid and periocular area (S00.1)
√x7th **S05.10** **Contusion of eyeball and orbital tissues, unspecified eye** `PE`
√x7th **S05.11** **Contusion of eyeball and orbital tissues, right eye** `PE`
√x7th **S05.12** **Contusion of eyeball and orbital tissues, left eye** `PE`

√5th **S05.2** **Ocular laceration and rupture with prolapse or loss of intraocular tissue**
√x7th **S05.20** **Ocular laceration and rupture with prolapse or loss of intraocular tissue, unspecified eye** `CC` `UNS` `PE`
√x7th **S05.21** **Ocular laceration and rupture with prolapse or loss of intraocular tissue, right eye** `CC` `PE`
√x7th **S05.22** **Ocular laceration and rupture with prolapse or loss of intraocular tissue, left eye** `CC` `PE`

√5th **S05.3** **Ocular laceration without prolapse or loss of intraocular tissue**
Laceration of eye NOS
AHA: 2022,1Q,33
DEF: Tear in ocular tissue without displacing structures that is due to blunt trauma. It is characterized by pain, redness, and decreased vision.
√x7th **S05.30** **Ocular laceration without prolapse or loss of intraocular tissue, unspecified eye** `CC` `UNS` `PE`
√x7th **S05.31** **Ocular laceration without prolapse or loss of intraocular tissue, right eye** `CC` `PE`
√x7th **S05.32** **Ocular laceration without prolapse or loss of intraocular tissue, left eye** `CC` `PE`

√5th **S05.4** **Penetrating wound of orbit with or without foreign body**
`EXCLUDES 2`   retained (old) foreign body following penetrating wound in orbit (H05.5-)
√x7th **S05.40** **Penetrating wound of orbit with or without foreign body, unspecified eye** `CC` `UNS` `PE`
√x7th **S05.41** **Penetrating wound of orbit with or without foreign body, right eye** `CC` `PE`
√x7th **S05.42** **Penetrating wound of orbit with or without foreign body, left eye** `CC` `PE`

√5th **S05.5** **Penetrating wound with foreign body of eyeball**
`EXCLUDES 2`   retained (old) intraocular foreign body (H44.6-, H44.7)
√x7th **S05.50** **Penetrating wound with foreign body of unspecified eyeball** `CC` `UNS` `PE`
√x7th **S05.51** **Penetrating wound with foreign body of right eyeball** `CC` `PE`
√x7th **S05.52** **Penetrating wound with foreign body of left eyeball** `CC` `PE`

√5th **S05.6** **Penetrating wound without foreign body of eyeball**
Ocular penetration NOS
√x7th **S05.60** **Penetrating wound without foreign body of unspecified eyeball** `PE`
√x7th **S05.61** **Penetrating wound without foreign body of right eyeball** `PE`
√x7th **S05.62** **Penetrating wound without foreign body of left eyeball** `PE`

`N` Newborn: 0   `P` Pediatric: 0-17   `M` Maternity: 9-64   `A` Adult: 15-124   `UNS` Unspecified Site   `MCC` Major Complication/Comorbidity   `CC` Complication/Comorbidity   `PE` POA Exempt

990   ICD-10-CM 2025

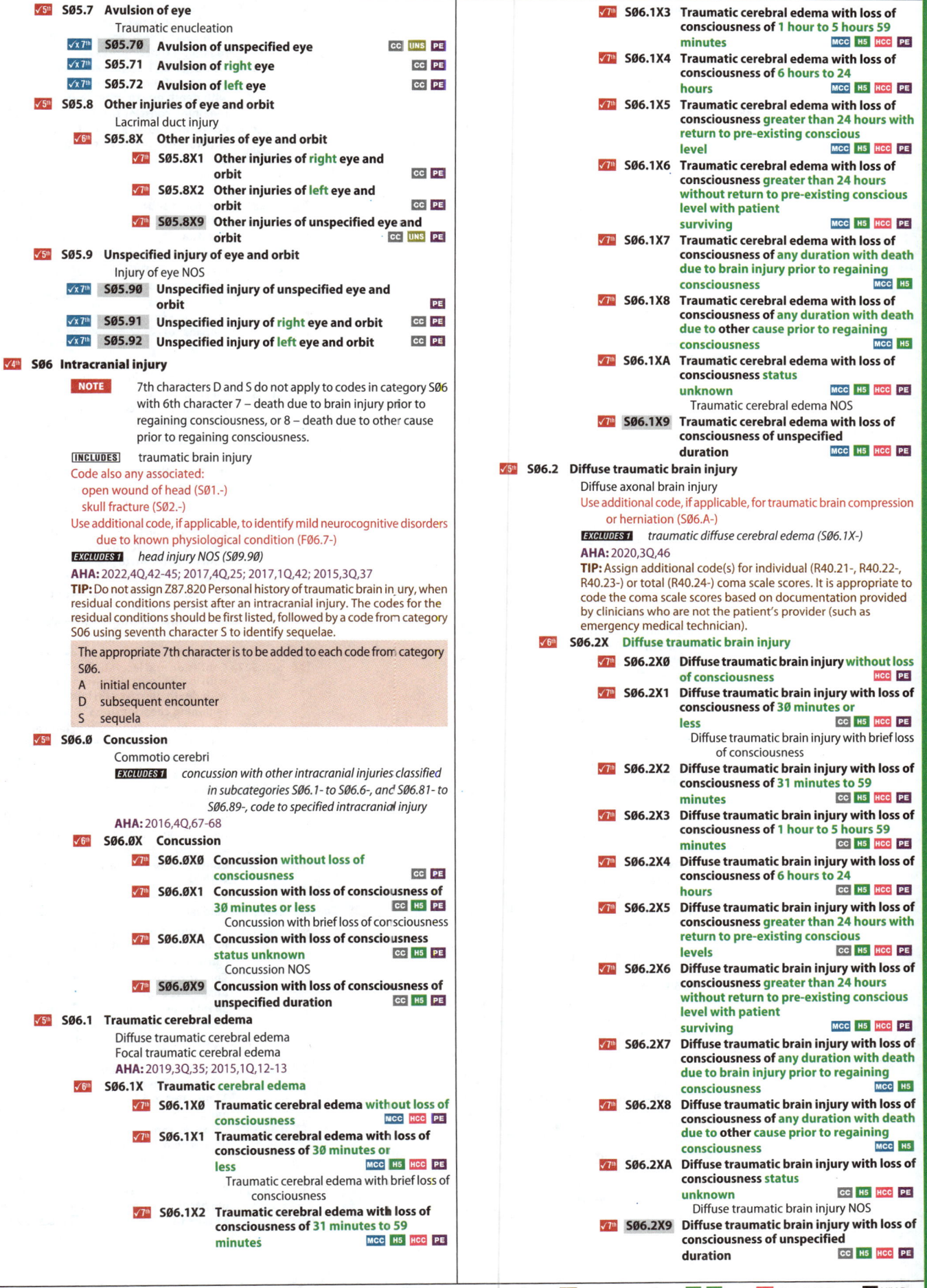

✓5ᵗʰ **S05.7 Avulsion of eye**
Traumatic enucleation

    ✓x7ᵗʰ **S05.70 Avulsion of unspecified eye** `CC` `UNS` `PE`

    ✓x7ᵗʰ **S05.71 Avulsion of right eye** `CC` `PE`

    ✓x7ᵗʰ **S05.72 Avulsion of left eye** `CC` `PE`

✓5ᵗʰ **S05.8 Other injuries of eye and orbit**
Lacrimal duct injury

    ✓6ᵗʰ **S05.8X Other injuries of eye and orbit**

        ✓7ᵗʰ **S05.8X1 Other injuries of right eye and orbit** `CC` `PE`

        ✓7ᵗʰ **S05.8X2 Other injuries of left eye and orbit** `CC` `PE`

        ✓7ᵗʰ **S05.8X9 Other injuries of unspecified eye and orbit** `CC` `UNS` `PE`

✓5ᵗʰ **S05.9 Unspecified injury of eye and orbit**
Injury of eye NOS

    ✓x7ᵗʰ **S05.90 Unspecified injury of unspecified eye and orbit** `PE`

    ✓x7ᵗʰ **S05.91 Unspecified injury of right eye and orbit** `CC` `PE`

    ✓x7ᵗʰ **S05.92 Unspecified injury of left eye and orbit** `CC` `PE`

✓4ᵗʰ **S06 Intracranial injury**

> **NOTE** 7th characters D and S do not apply to codes in category S06 with 6th character 7 – death due to brain injury prior to regaining consciousness, or 8 – death due to other cause prior to regaining consciousness.

INCLUDES traumatic brain injury

Code also any associated:
    open wound of head (S01.-)
    skull fracture (S02.-)
Use additional code, if applicable, to identify mild neurocognitive disorders due to known physiological condition (F06.7-)

EXCLUDES 1 head injury NOS (S09.90)

AHA: 2022,4Q,42-45; 2017,4Q,25; 2017,1Q,42; 2015,3Q,37

TIP: Do not assign Z87.820 Personal history of traumatic brain injury, when residual conditions persist after an intracranial injury. The codes for the residual conditions should be first listed, followed by a code from category S06 using seventh character S to identify sequelae.

> The appropriate 7th character is to be added to each code from category S06.
> A   initial encounter
> D   subsequent encounter
> S   sequela

✓5ᵗʰ **S06.0 Concussion**
Commotio cerebri

EXCLUDES 1 concussion with other intracranial injuries classified in subcategories S06.1- to S06.6-, and S06.81- to S06.89-, code to specified intracranial injury

AHA: 2016,4Q,67-68

    ✓6ᵗʰ **S06.0X Concussion**

        ✓7ᵗʰ **S06.0X0 Concussion without loss of consciousness** `CC` `PE`

        ✓7ᵗʰ **S06.0X1 Concussion with loss of consciousness 30 minutes or less** `CC` `H5` `PE`
            Concussion with brief loss of consciousness

        ✓7ᵗʰ **S06.0XA Concussion with loss of consciousness status unknown** `CC` `H5` `PE`
            Concussion NOS

        ✓7ᵗʰ **S06.0X9 Concussion with loss of consciousness of unspecified duration** `CC` `H5` `PE`

✓5ᵗʰ **S06.1 Traumatic cerebral edema**
Diffuse traumatic cerebral edema
Focal traumatic cerebral edema

AHA: 2019,3Q,35; 2015,1Q,12-13

    ✓6ᵗʰ **S06.1X Traumatic cerebral edema**

        ✓7ᵗʰ **S06.1X0 Traumatic cerebral edema without loss of consciousness** `NCC` `HCC` `PE`

        ✓7ᵗʰ **S06.1X1 Traumatic cerebral edema with loss of consciousness of 30 minutes or less** `MCC` `H5` `HCC` `PE`
            Traumatic cerebral edema with brief loss of consciousness

        ✓7ᵗʰ **S06.1X2 Traumatic cerebral edema with loss of consciousness of 31 minutes to 59 minutes** `MCC` `H5` `HCC` `PE`

        ✓7ᵗʰ **S06.1X3 Traumatic cerebral edema with loss of consciousness of 1 hour to 5 hours 59 minutes** `MCC` `H5` `PE`

        ✓7ᵗʰ **S06.1X4 Traumatic cerebral edema with loss of consciousness of 6 hours to 24 hours** `MCC` `H5` `HCC` `PE`

        ✓7ᵗʰ **S06.1X5 Traumatic cerebral edema with loss of consciousness greater than 24 hours with return to pre-existing conscious level** `MCC` `H5` `HCC` `PE`

        ✓7ᵗʰ **S06.1X6 Traumatic cerebral edema with loss of consciousness greater than 24 hours without return to pre-existing conscious level with patient surviving** `MCC` `H5` `HCC` `PE`

        ✓7ᵗʰ **S06.1X7 Traumatic cerebral edema with loss of consciousness of any duration with death due to brain injury prior to regaining consciousness** `MCC` `H5`

        ✓7ᵗʰ **S06.1X8 Traumatic cerebral edema with loss of consciousness of any duration with death due to other cause prior to regaining consciousness** `MCC` `H5`

        ✓7ᵗʰ **S06.1XA Traumatic cerebral edema with loss of consciousness status unknown** `MCC` `H5` `HCC` `PE`
            Traumatic cerebral edema NOS

        ✓7ᵗʰ **S06.1X9 Traumatic cerebral edema with loss of consciousness of unspecified duration** `MCC` `H5` `HCC` `PE`

✓5ᵗʰ **S06.2 Diffuse traumatic brain injury**
Diffuse axonal brain injury
Use additional code, if applicable, for traumatic brain compression or herniation (S06.A-)

EXCLUDES 1 traumatic diffuse cerebral edema (S06.1X-)

AHA: 2020,3Q,46

TIP: Assign additional code(s) for individual (R40.21-, R40.22-, R40.23-) or total (R40.24-) coma scale scores. It is appropriate to code the coma scale scores based on documentation provided by clinicians who are not the patient's provider (such as emergency medical technician).

    ✓6ᵗʰ **S06.2X Diffuse traumatic brain injury**

        ✓7ᵗʰ **S06.2X0 Diffuse traumatic brain injury without loss of consciousness** `HCC` `PE`

        ✓7ᵗʰ **S06.2X1 Diffuse traumatic brain injury with loss of consciousness of 30 minutes or less** `CC` `H5` `HCC` `PE`
            Diffuse traumatic brain injury with brief loss of consciousness

        ✓7ᵗʰ **S06.2X2 Diffuse traumatic brain injury with loss of consciousness of 31 minutes to 59 minutes** `CC` `H5` `HCC` `PE`

        ✓7ᵗʰ **S06.2X3 Diffuse traumatic brain injury with loss of consciousness of 1 hour to 5 hours 59 minutes** `CC` `H5` `HCC` `PE`

        ✓7ᵗʰ **S06.2X4 Diffuse traumatic brain injury with loss of consciousness of 6 hours to 24 hours** `CC` `H5` `HCC` `PE`

        ✓7ᵗʰ **S06.2X5 Diffuse traumatic brain injury with loss of consciousness greater than 24 hours with return to pre-existing conscious levels** `CC` `H5` `HCC` `PE`

        ✓7ᵗʰ **S06.2X6 Diffuse traumatic brain injury with loss of consciousness greater than 24 hours without return to pre-existing conscious level with patient surviving** `MCC` `H5` `HCC` `PE`

        ✓7ᵗʰ **S06.2X7 Diffuse traumatic brain injury with loss of consciousness of any duration with death due to brain injury prior to regaining consciousness** `MCC` `H5`

        ✓7ᵗʰ **S06.2X8 Diffuse traumatic brain injury with loss of consciousness of any duration with death due to other cause prior to regaining consciousness** `MCC` `H5`

        ✓7ᵗʰ **S06.2XA Diffuse traumatic brain injury with loss of consciousness status unknown** `CC` `H5` `HCC` `PE`
            Diffuse traumatic brain injury NOS

        ✓7ᵗʰ **S06.2X9 Diffuse traumatic brain injury with loss of consciousness of unspecified duration** `CC` `H5` `HCC` `PE`

✓ Additional Character Required   ✓x7ᵗʰ Placeholder   `Questionable PDx`   Manifestation   Unspecified   `UPD` Unacceptable PDx   `H1`-`H14` HAC   `HCC` CMS-HCC Dx   `HIV` HIV Dx

Chapter 19. Injury, Poisoning and Certain Other Consequences of External Causes

√5th **S06.3 Focal traumatic brain injury**

Use additional code, if applicable, for traumatic brain compression or herniation (S06.A-)

EXCLUDES 2   any condition classifiable to S06.4-S06.6 focal cerebral edema (S06.1)

AHA: 2020,3Q,46; 2019,3Q,35; 2015,1Q,12-13

TIP: Assign additional code(s) for individual (R40.21-, R40.22-, R40.23-) or total (R40.24-) coma scale scores. It is appropriate to code the coma scale scores based on documentation provided by clinicians who are not the patient's provider (such as emergency medical technician).

√6th **S06.30 Unspecified focal traumatic brain injury**

√7th **S06.300 Unspecified focal traumatic brain injury without loss of consciousness** HCC PE

√7th **S06.301 Unspecified focal traumatic brain injury with loss of consciousness of 30 minutes or less** CC H5 HCC PE
Unspecified focal traumatic brain injury with brief loss of consciousness

√7th **S06.302 Unspecified focal traumatic brain injury with loss of consciousness of 31 minutes to 59 minutes** CC H5 HCC PE

√7th **S06.303 Unspecified focal traumatic brain injury with loss of consciousness of 1 hour to 5 hours 59 minutes** CC H5 HCC PE

√7th **S06.304 Unspecified focal traumatic brain injury with loss of consciousness of 6 hours to 24 hours** CC H5 HCC PE

√7th **S06.305 Unspecified focal traumatic brain injury with loss of consciousness greater than 24 hours with return to pre-existing conscious level** CC H5 HCC PE

√7th **S06.306 Unspecified focal traumatic brain injury with loss of consciousness greater than 24 hours without return to pre-existing conscious level with patient surviving** MCC H5 HCC PE

√7th **S06.307 Unspecified focal traumatic brain injury with loss of consciousness of any duration with death due to brain injury prior to regaining consciousness** MCC H5

√7th **S06.308 Unspecified focal traumatic brain injury with loss of consciousness of any duration with death due to other cause prior to regaining consciousness** MCC H5

√7th **S06.30A Unspecified focal traumatic brain injury with loss of consciousness status unknown** CC H5 HCC PE
Unspecified focal traumatic brain injury NOS

√7th **S06.309 Unspecified focal traumatic brain injury with loss of consciousness of unspecified duration** CC H5 HCC PE

√6th **S06.31 Contusion and laceration of right cerebrum**

√7th **S06.310 Contusion and laceration of right cerebrum without loss of consciousness** MCC H5 HCC PE

√7th **S06.311 Contusion and laceration of right cerebrum with loss of consciousness of 30 minutes or less** MCC H5 HCC PE
Contusion and laceration of right cerebrum with brief loss of consciousness

√7th **S06.312 Contusion and laceration of right cerebrum with loss of consciousness of 31 minutes to 59 minutes** MCC H5 HCC PE

√7th **S06.313 Contusion and laceration of right cerebrum with loss of consciousness of 1 hour to 5 hours 59 minutes** MCC H5 HCC PE

√7th **S06.314 Contusion and laceration of right cerebrum with loss of consciousness of 6 hours to 24 hours** MCC H5 HCC PE

√7th **S06.315 Contusion and laceration of right cerebrum with loss of consciousness greater than 24 hours with return to pre-existing conscious level** MCC H5 HCC PE

√7th **S06.316 Contusion and laceration of right cerebrum with loss of consciousness greater than 24 hours without return to pre-existing conscious level with patient surviving** MCC H5 HCC PE

√7th **S06.317 Contusion and laceration of right cerebrum with loss of consciousness of any duration with death due to brain injury prior to regaining consciousness** MCC H5

√7th **S06.318 Contusion and laceration of right cerebrum with loss of consciousness of any duration with death due to other cause prior to regaining consciousness** MCC H5

√7th **S06.31A Contusion and laceration of right cerebrum with loss of consciousness status unknown** MCC H5 HCC PE
Contusion and laceration of right cerebrum NOS

√7th **S06.319 Contusion and laceration of right cerebrum with loss of consciousness of unspecified duration** MCC H5 HCC PE

√6th **S06.32 Contusion and laceration of left cerebrum**

√7th **S06.320 Contusion and laceration of left cerebrum without loss of consciousness** MCC H5 HCC PE

√7th **S06.321 Contusion and laceration of left cerebrum with loss of consciousness of 30 minutes or less** MCC H5 HCC PE
Contusion and laceration of left cerebrum with brief loss of consciousness

√7th **S06.322 Contusion and laceration of left cerebrum with loss of consciousness of 31 minutes to 59 minutes** MCC H5 HCC PE

√7th **S06.323 Contusion and laceration of left cerebrum with loss of consciousness of 1 hour to 5 hours 59 minutes** MCC H5 HCC PE

√7th **S06.324 Contusion and laceration of left cerebrum with loss of consciousness of 6 hours to 24 hours** MCC H5 HCC PE

√7th **S06.325 Contusion and laceration of left cerebrum with loss of consciousness greater than 24 hours with return to pre-existing conscious level** MCC H5 HCC PE

√7th **S06.326 Contusion and laceration of left cerebrum with loss of consciousness greater than 24 hours without return to pre-existing conscious level with patient surviving** MCC H5 HCC PE

√7th **S06.327 Contusion and laceration of left cerebrum with loss of consciousness of any duration with death due to brain injury prior to regaining consciousness** MCC H5

√7th **S06.328 Contusion and laceration of left cerebrum with loss of consciousness of any duration with death due to other cause prior to regaining consciousness** MCC H5

√7th **S06.32A Contusion and laceration of left cerebrum with loss of consciousness status unknown** MCC H5 HCC PE
Contusion and laceration of left cerebrum NOS

√7th **S06.329 Contusion and laceration of left cerebrum with loss of consciousness of unspecified duration** MCC H5 HCC PE

√6th **S06.33 Contusion and laceration of cerebrum, unspecified**

√7th **S06.330 Contusion and laceration of cerebrum, unspecified, without loss of consciousness** MCC H5 HCC PE

√7th **S06.331 Contusion and laceration of cerebrum, unspecified, with loss of consciousness of 30 minutes or less** MCC H5 HCC PE
Contusion and laceration of cerebrum, unspecified, with brief loss of consciousness

√7th **S06.332 Contusion and laceration of cerebrum, unspecified, with loss of consciousness of 31 minutes to 59 minutes** MCC H5 HCC PE

√7th **S06.333 Contusion and laceration of cerebrum, unspecified, with loss of consciousness of 1 hour to 5 hours 59 minutes** MCC H5 HCC PE

√7th **S06.334 Contusion and laceration of cerebrum, unspecified, with loss of consciousness of 6 hours to 24 hours** MCC H5 HCC PE

N Newborn: 0   P Pediatric: 0-17   M Maternity: 9-64   A Adult: 15-124   UNS Unspecified Site   MCC Major Complication/Comorbidity   CC Complication/Comorbidity   PE POA Exempt

992   ICD-10-CM 2025

√7ᵗʰ **S06.335** **Contusion and laceration of cerebrum, unspecified, with loss of consciousness greater than 24 hours with return to pre-existing conscious level** `MCC` `H5` `HCC` `PE`

√7ᵗʰ **S06.336** **Contusion and laceration of cerebrum, unspecified, with loss of consciousness greater than 24 hours without return to pre-existing conscious level with patient surviving** `MCC` `H5` `HCC` `PE`

√7ᵗʰ **S06.337** **Contusion and laceration of cerebrum, unspecified, with loss of consciousness of any duration with death due to brain injury prior to regaining consciousness** `MCC` `H5`

√7ᵗʰ **S06.338** **Contusion and laceration of cerebrum, unspecified, with loss of consciousness of any duration with death due to other cause prior to regaining consciousness** `MCC` `H5`

√7ᵗʰ **S06.33A** **Contusion and laceration of cerebrum, unspecified, with loss of consciousness status unknown** `MCC` `H5` `UNS` `HCC` `PE`
Contusion and laceration of cerebrum NOS

√7ᵗʰ **S06.339** **Contusion and laceration of cerebrum, unspecified, with loss of consciousness of unspecified duration** `MCC` `H5` `HCC` `PE`

√6ᵗʰ **S06.34** **Traumatic hemorrhage of right cerebrum**
Traumatic intracerebral hemorrhage and hematoma of right cerebrum

√7ᵗʰ **S06.340** **Traumatic hemorrhage of right cerebrum without loss of consciousness** `MCC` `H5` `HCC` `PE`

√7ᵗʰ **S06.341** **Traumatic hemorrhage of right cerebrum with loss of consciousness of 30 minutes or less** `MCC` `H5` `HCC` `PE`
▶Traumatic hemorrhage of right cerebrum with brief loss of consciousness◀

√7ᵗʰ **S06.342** **Traumatic hemorrhage of right cerebrum with loss of consciousness of 31 minutes to 59 minutes** `MCC` `H5` `HCC` `PE`

√7ᵗʰ **S06.343** **Traumatic hemorrhage of right cerebrum with loss of consciousness of 1 hours to 5 hours 59 minutes** `MCC` `H5` `HCC` `PE`

√7ᵗʰ **S06.344** **Traumatic hemorrhage of right cerebrum with loss of consciousness of 6 hours to 24 hours** `MCC` `H5` `HCC` `PE`

√7ᵗʰ **S06.345** **Traumatic hemorrhage of right cerebrum with loss of consciousness greater than 24 hours with return to pre-existing conscious level** `MCC` `H5` `HCC` `PE`

√7ᵗʰ **S06.346** **Traumatic hemorrhage of right cerebrum with loss of consciousness greater than 24 hours without return to pre-existing conscious level with patient surviving** `MCC` `H5` `HCC` `PE`

√7ᵗʰ **S06.347** **Traumatic hemorrhage of right cerebrum with loss of consciousness of any duration with death due to brain injury prior to regaining consciousness** `MCC` `H5`

√7ᵗʰ **S06.348** **Traumatic hemorrhage of right cerebrum with loss of consciousness of any duration with death due to other cause prior to regaining consciousness** `MCC` `H5`

√7ᵗʰ **S06.34A** **Traumatic hemorrhage of right cerebrum with loss of consciousness status unknown** `MCC` `H5` `HCC` `PE`
Traumatic hemorrhage of right cerebrum NOS

√7ᵗʰ **S06.349** **Traumatic hemorrhage of right cerebrum with loss of consciousness of unspecified duration** `MCC` `H5` `HCC` `PE`

√6ᵗʰ **S06.35** **Traumatic hemorrhage of left cerebrum**
Traumatic intracerebral hemorrhage and hematoma of left cerebrum

√7ᵗʰ **S06.350** **Traumatic hemorrhage of left cerebrum without loss of consciousness** `MCC` `H5` `HCC` `PE`

√7ᵗʰ **S06.351** **Traumatic hemorrhage of left cerebrum with loss of consciousness of 30 minutes or less** `MCC` `H5` `HCC` `PE`
Traumatic hemorrhage of left cerebrum with brief loss of consciousness

√7ᵗʰ **S06.352** **Traumatic hemorrhage of left cerebrum with loss of consciousness of 31 minutes to 59 minutes** `MCC` `H5` `HCC` `PE`

√7ᵗʰ **S06.353** **Traumatic hemorrhage of left cerebrum with loss of consciousness of 1 hours to 5 hours 59 minutes** `MCC` `H5` `HCC` `PE`

√7ᵗʰ **S06.354** **Traumatic hemorrhage of left cerebrum with loss of consciousness of 6 hours to 24 hours** `MCC` `H5` `HCC` `PE`

√7ᵗʰ **S06.355** **Traumatic hemorrhage of left cerebrum with loss of consciousness greater than 24 hours with return to pre-existing conscious level** `MCC` `H5` `HCC` `PE`

√7ᵗʰ **S06.356** **Traumatic hemorrhage of left cerebrum with loss of consciousness greater than 24 hours without return to pre-existing conscious level with patient surviving** `MCC` `H5` `HCC` `PE`

√7ᵗʰ **S06.357** **Traumatic hemorrhage of left cerebrum with loss of consciousness of any duration with death due to brain injury prior to regaining consciousness** `MCC` `H5`

√7ᵗʰ **S06.358** **Traumatic hemorrhage of left cerebrum with loss of consciousness of any duration with death due to other cause prior to regaining consciousness** `MCC` `H5`

√7ᵗʰ **S06.35A** **Traumatic hemorrhage of left cerebrum with loss of consciousness status unknown** `MCC` `H5` `HCC` `PE`
Traumatic hemorrhage of left cerebrum NOS

√7ᵗʰ **S06.359** **Traumatic hemorrhage of left cerebrum with loss of consciousness of unspecified duration** `MCC` `H5` `HCC` `PE`

√6ᵗʰ **S06.36** **Traumatic hemorrhage of cerebrum, unspecified**
Traumatic intracerebral hemorrhage and hematoma, unspecified

√7ᵗʰ **S06.360** **Traumatic hemorrhage of cerebrum, unspecified, without loss of consciousness** `MCC` `H5` `HCC` `PE`

√7ᵗʰ **S06.361** **Traumatic hemorrhage of cerebrum, unspecified, with loss of consciousness of 30 minutes or less** `MCC` `H5` `HCC` `PE`
Traumatic hemorrhage of cerebrum, unspecified, with brief loss of consciousness

√7ᵗʰ **S06.362** **Traumatic hemorrhage of cerebrum, unspecified, with loss of consciousness of 31 minutes to 59 minutes** `MCC` `H5` `HCC` `PE`

√7ᵗʰ **S06.363** **Traumatic hemorrhage of cerebrum, unspecified, with loss of consciousness of 1 hours to 5 hours 59 minutes** `MCC` `H5` `HCC` `PE`

√7ᵗʰ **S06.364** **Traumatic hemorrhage of cerebrum, unspecified, with loss of consciousness of 6 hours to 24 hours** `MCC` `H5` `HCC` `PE`

√7ᵗʰ **S06.365** **Traumatic hemorrhage of cerebrum, unspecified, with loss of consciousness greater than 24 hours with return to pre-existing conscious level** `MCC` `H5` `HCC` `PE`

√7ᵗʰ **S06.366** **Traumatic hemorrhage of cerebrum, unspecified, with loss of consciousness greater than 24 hours without return to pre-existing conscious level with patient surviving** `MCC` `H5` `HCC` `PE`

√7ᵗʰ **S06.367** **Traumatic hemorrhage of cerebrum, unspecified, with loss of consciousness of any duration with death due to brain injury prior to regaining consciousness** `MCC` `H5`

√7ᵗʰ **S06.368** **Traumatic hemorrhage of cerebrum, unspecified, with loss of consciousness of any duration with death due to other cause prior to regaining consciousness** `MCC` `H5`

√7ᵗʰ **S06.36A** **Traumatic hemorrhage of cerebrum, unspecified, with loss of consciousness status unknown** `MCC` `H5` `UNS` `HCC`
Traumatic hemorrhage of cerebrum NOS

√7ᵗʰ **S06.369** **Traumatic hemorrhage of cerebrum, unspecified, with loss of consciousness of unspecified duration** `MCC` `H5` `HCC` `PE`

√6ᵗʰ **S06.37** **Contusion, laceration, and hemorrhage of cerebellum**

√7ᵗʰ **S06.370** **Contusion, laceration, and hemorrhage of cerebellum without loss of consciousness** `MCC` `H5` `HCC` `PE`

√7ᵗʰ **S06.371** **Contusion, laceration, and hemorrhage of cerebellum with loss of consciousness of 30 minutes or less** `CC` `H5` `HCC` `PE`
Contusion, laceration, and hemorrhage of cerebellum with brief loss of consciousness

√7ᵗʰ **S06.372** **Contusion, laceration, and hemorrhage of cerebellum with loss of consciousness of 31 minutes to 59 minutes** `CC` `H5` `HCC` `PE`

√7ᵗʰ **S06.373** **Contusion, laceration, and hemorrhage of cerebellum with loss of consciousness of 1 hour to 5 hours 59 minutes** `CC` `H5` `HCC` `PE`

√7ᵗʰ **S06.374** **Contusion, laceration, and hemorrhage of cerebellum with loss of consciousness of 6 hours to 24 hours** `CC` `H5` `HCC` `PE`

√7ᵗʰ **S06.375** **Contusion, laceration, and hemorrhage of cerebellum with loss of consciousness greater than 24 hours with return to pre-existing conscious level** `CC` `H5` `HCC` `PE`

√7ᵗʰ **S06.376** **Contusion, laceration, and hemorrhage of cerebellum with loss of consciousness greater than 24 hours without return to pre-existing conscious level with patient surviving** `CC` `H5` `HCC` `PE`

√7ᵗʰ **S06.377** **Contusion, laceration, and hemorrhage of cerebellum with loss of consciousness of any duration with death due to brain injury prior to regaining consciousness** `MCC` `H5`

√7ᵗʰ **S06.378** **Contusion, laceration, and hemorrhage of cerebellum with loss of consciousness of any duration with death due to other cause prior to regaining consciousness** `MCC` `H5`

√7ᵗʰ **S06.37A** **Contusion, laceration, and hemorrhage of cerebellum with loss of consciousness status unknown** `CC` `H5` `HCC` `PE`
Contusion, laceration, and hemorrhage of cerebellum NOS

√7ᵗʰ **S06.379** **Contusion, laceration, and hemorrhage of cerebellum with loss of consciousness of unspecified duration** `CC` `H5` `HCC` `PE`

√6ᵗʰ **S06.38** **Contusion, laceration, and hemorrhage of brainstem**

√7ᵗʰ **S06.380** **Contusion, laceration, and hemorrhage of brainstem without loss of consciousness** `MCC` `H5` `HCC` `PE`

√7ᵗʰ **S06.381** **Contusion, laceration, and hemorrhage of brainstem with loss of consciousness of 30 minutes or less** `CC` `H5` `HCC` `PE`
Contusion, laceration, and hemorrhage of brainstem with brief loss of consciousness

√7ᵗʰ **S06.382** **Contusion, laceration, and hemorrhage of brainstem with loss of consciousness of 31 minutes to 59 minutes** `CC` `H5` `HCC` `PE`

√7ᵗʰ **S06.383** **Contusion, laceration, and hemorrhage of brainstem with loss of consciousness of 1 hour to 5 hours 59 minutes** `CC` `H5` `HCC` `PE`

√7ᵗʰ **S06.384** **Contusion, laceration, and hemorrhage of brainstem with loss of consciousness of 6 hours to 24 hours** `CC` `H5` `HCC` `PE`

√7ᵗʰ **S06.385** **Contusion, laceration, and hemorrhage of brainstem with loss of consciousness greater than 24 hours with return to pre-existing conscious level** `CC` `H5` `HCC` `PE`

√7ᵗʰ **S06.386** **Contusion, laceration, and hemorrhage of brainstem with loss of consciousness greater than 24 hours without return to pre-existing conscious level with patient surviving** `MCC` `H5` `HCC` `PE`

√7ᵗʰ **S06.387** **Contusion, laceration, and hemorrhage of brainstem with loss of consciousness of any duration with death due to brain injury prior to regaining consciousness** `MCC` `H5`

√7ᵗʰ **S06.388** **Contusion, laceration, and hemorrhage of brainstem with loss of consciousness of any duration with death due to other cause prior to regaining consciousness** `MCC` `H5`

√7ᵗʰ **S06.38A** **Contusion, laceration, and hemorrhage of brainstem with loss of consciousness status unknown** `MCC` `H5` `HCC` `PE`
Contusion, laceration, and hemorrhage of brainstem NOS

√7ᵗʰ **S06.389** **Contusion, laceration, and hemorrhage of brainstem with loss of consciousness of unspecified duration** `CC` `H5` `HCC` `PE`

√5ᵗʰ **S06.4** **Epidural hemorrhage**
Extradural hemorrhage NOS
Extradural hemorrhage (traumatic)
DEF: Epidural space: Space between the endosteum of the cranium (skull) and the dura mater, the outermost layer of a three-layer membrane that covers the brain.

√6ᵗʰ **S06.4X** **Epidural hemorrhage**

√7ᵗʰ **S06.4X0** **Epidural hemorrhage without loss of consciousness** `MCC` `H5` `HCC` `PE`

√7ᵗʰ **S06.4X1** **Epidural hemorrhage with loss of consciousness of 30 minutes or less** `MCC` `H5` `HCC` `PE`
Epidural hemorrhage with brief loss of consciousness

√7ᵗʰ **S06.4X2** **Epidural hemorrhage with loss of consciousness of 31 minutes to 59 minutes** `MCC` `H5` `HCC` `PE`

√7ᵗʰ **S06.4X3** **Epidural hemorrhage with loss of consciousness of 1 hour to 5 hours 59 minutes** `MCC` `H5` `HCC` `PE`

√7ᵗʰ **S06.4X4** **Epidural hemorrhage with loss of consciousness of 6 hours to 24 hours** `MCC` `H5` `HCC` `PE`

√7ᵗʰ **S06.4X5** **Epidural hemorrhage with loss of consciousness greater than 24 hours with return to pre-existing conscious level** `MCC` `H5` `HCC` `PE`

√7ᵗʰ **S06.4X6** **Epidural hemorrhage with loss of consciousness greater than 24 hours without return to pre-existing conscious level with patient surviving** `MCC` `H5` `HCC` `PE`

√7ᵗʰ **S06.4X7** **Epidural hemorrhage with loss of consciousness of any duration with death due to brain injury prior to regaining consciousness** `MCC` `H5`

√7ᵗʰ **S06.4X8** **Epidural hemorrhage with loss of consciousness of any duration with death due to other causes prior to regaining consciousness** `MCC` `H5`

√7ᵗʰ **S06.4XA** **Epidural hemorrhage with loss of consciousness status unknown** `MCC` `H5` `HCC` `PE`
Epidural hemorrhage NOS

√7ᵗʰ **S06.4X9** **Epidural hemorrhage with loss of consciousness of unspecified duration** `MCC` `H5` `HCC` `PE`

√5ᵗʰ **S06.5** **Traumatic subdural hemorrhage**
Use additional code, if applicable, for traumatic brain compression or herniation (S06.A-)
AHA: 2021,2Q,5; 2021,1Q,4
DEF: Subdural: Potential space between the dura mater and arachnoid membrane around the brain.

√6ᵗʰ **S06.5X** **Traumatic subdural hemorrhage**

√7ᵗʰ **S06.5X0** **Traumatic subdural hemorrhage without loss of consciousness** `MCC` `H5` `HCC` `PE`

`N` Newborn: 0   `P` Pediatric: 0-17   `M` Maternity: 9-64   `A` Adult: 15-124   `UNS` Unspecified Site   `MCC` Major Complication/Comorbidity   `CC` Complication/Comorbidity   `PE` POA Exempt

994

ICD-10-CM 2025

✓7ᵗʰ **S06.5X1 Traumatic subdural hemorrhage with loss of consciousness of 30 minutes or less** `MCC` `H5` `HCC` `PE`
> Traumatic subdural hemorrhage with brief loss of consciousness

✓7ᵗʰ **S06.5X2 Traumatic subdural hemorrhage with loss of consciousness of 31 minutes to 59 minutes** `MCC` `H5` `HCC` `PE`

✓7ᵗʰ **S06.5X3 Traumatic subdural hemorrhage with loss of consciousness of 1 hour to 5 hours 59 minutes** `MCC` `H5` `HCC` `PE`

✓7ᵗʰ **S06.5X4 Traumatic subdural hemorrhage with loss of consciousness of 6 hours to 24 hours** `MCC` `H5` `HCC` `PE`

✓7ᵗʰ **S06.5X5 Traumatic subdural hemorrhage with loss of consciousness greater than 24 hours with return to pre-existing conscious level** `MCC` `H5` `HCC` `PE`

✓7ᵗʰ **S06.5X6 Traumatic subdural hemorrhage with loss of consciousness greater than 24 hours without return to pre-existing conscious level with patient surviving** `MCC` `H5` `HCC` `PE`

✓7ᵗʰ **S06.5X7 Traumatic subdural hemorrhage with loss of consciousness of any duration with death due to brain injury before regaining consciousness** `MCC` `H5`

✓7ᵗʰ **S06.5X8 Traumatic subdural hemorrhage with loss of consciousness of any duration with death due to other cause before regaining consciousness** `MCC` `H5`

✓7ᵗʰ **S06.5XA Traumatic subdural hemorrhage with loss of consciousness status unknown** `MCC` `H5` `HCC` `PE`
> Traumatic subdural hemorrhage NOS
> **AHA:** 2022,4Q,44

✓7ᵗʰ **S06.5X9 Traumatic subdural hemorrhage with loss of consciousness of unspecified duration** `MCC` `H5` `HCC` `PE`

✓5ᵗʰ **S06.6 Traumatic subarachnoid hemorrhage**
> Use additional code, if applicable, for traumatic brain compression or herniation (S06.A-)
> **AHA:** 2021,2Q,5; 2021,1Q,4
> **DEF:** Subarachnoid: Space located between the arachnoid membrane and the pia mater that contains cerebrospinal fluid.

✓6ᵗʰ **S06.6X Traumatic subarachnoid hemorrhage**

✓7ᵗʰ **S06.6X0 Traumatic subarachnoid hemorrhage without loss of consciousness** `MCC` `H5` `HCC` `PE`

✓7ᵗʰ **S06.6X1 Traumatic subarachnoid hemorrhage with loss of consciousness of 30 minutes or less** `MCC` `H5` `HCC` `PE`
> Traumatic subarachnoid hemorrhage with brief loss of consciousness

✓7ᵗʰ **S06.6X2 Traumatic subarachnoid hemorrhage with loss of consciousness of 31 minutes to 59 minutes** `MCC` `H5` `HCC` `PE`

✓7ᵗʰ **S06.6X3 Traumatic subarachnoid hemorrhage with loss of consciousness of 1 hour to 5 hours 59 minutes** `MCC` `H5` `HCC` `PE`

✓7ᵗʰ **S06.6X4 Traumatic subarachnoid hemorrhage with loss of consciousness of 6 hours to 24 hours** `MCC` `H5` `HCC` `PE`

✓7ᵗʰ **S06.6X5 Traumatic subarachnoid hemorrhage with loss of consciousness greater than 24 hours with return to pre-existing conscious level** `MCC` `H5` `HCC` `PE`

✓7ᵗʰ **S06.6X6 Traumatic subarachnoid hemorrhage with loss of consciousness greater than 24 hours without return to pre-existing conscious level with patient surviving** `MCC` `H5` `HCC` `PE`

✓7ᵗʰ **S06.6X7 Traumatic subarachnoid hemorrhage with loss of consciousness of any duration with death due to brain injury prior to regaining consciousness** `MCC` `H5`

✓7ᵗʰ **S06.6X8 Traumatic subarachnoid hemorrhage with loss of consciousness of any duration with death due to other cause prior to regaining consciousness** `MCC` `H5`

✓7ᵗʰ **S06.6XA Traumatic subarachnoid hemorrhage with loss of consciousness status unknown** `MCC` `H5` `HCC` `PE`
> Traumatic subarachnoid hemorrhage NOS
> **AHA:** 2022,4Q,44

✓7ᵗʰ **S06.6X9 Traumatic subarachnoid hemorrhage with loss of consciousness of unspecified duration** `MCC` `H5` `HCC` `PE`

✓5ᵗʰ **S06.8 Other specified intracranial injuries**

✓6ᵗʰ **S06.81 Injury of right internal carotid artery, intracranial portion, not elsewhere classified**

✓7ᵗʰ **S06.810 Injury of right internal carotid artery, intracranial portion, not elsewhere classified without loss of consciousness** `HCC` `PE`

✓7ᵗʰ **S06.811 Injury of right internal carotid artery, intracranial portion, not elsewhere classified with loss of consciousness of 30 minutes or less** `CC` `H5` `HCC` `PE`
> Injury of right internal carotid artery, intracranial portion, not elsewhere classified with brief loss of consciousness

✓7ᵗʰ **S06.812 Injury of right internal carotid artery, intracranial portion, not elsewhere classified with loss of consciousness of 31 minutes to 59 minutes** `CC` `H5` `HCC` `PE`

✓7ᵗʰ **S06.813 Injury of right internal carotid artery, intracranial portion, not elsewhere classified with loss of consciousness of 1 hour to 5 hours 59 minutes** `CC` `H5` `HCC` `PE`

✓7ᵗʰ **S06.814 Injury of right internal carotid artery, intracranial portion, not elsewhere classified with loss of consciousness of 6 hours to 24 hours** `CC` `H5` `HCC` `PE`

✓7ᵗʰ **S06.815 Injury of right internal carotid artery, intracranial portion, not elsewhere classified with loss of consciousness greater than 24 hours with return to pre-existing conscious level** `CC` `H5` `HCC` `PE`

✓7ᵗʰ **S06.816 Injury of right internal carotid artery, intracranial portion, not elsewhere classified with loss of consciousness greater than 24 hours without return to pre-existing conscious level with patient surviving** `MCC` `H5` `HCC` `PE`

✓7ᵗʰ **S06.817 Injury of right internal carotid artery, intracranial portion, not elsewhere classified with loss of consciousness of any duration with death due to brain injury prior to regaining consciousness** `MCC` `H5`

✓7ᵗʰ **S06.818 Injury of right internal carotid artery, intracranial portion, not elsewhere classified with loss of consciousness of any duration with death due to other cause prior to regaining consciousness** `MCC` `H5`

✓7ᵗʰ **S06.81A Injury of right internal carotid artery, intracranial portion, not elsewhere classified with loss of consciousness status unknown** `CC` `H5` `HCC` `PE`
> Injury of right internal carotid artery, intracranial portion, not elsewhere classified NOS

✓7ᵗʰ **S06.819 Injury of right internal carotid artery, intracranial portion, not elsewhere classified with loss of consciousness of unspecified duration** `CC` `H5` `HCC` `PE`

✓6ᵗʰ **S06.82 Injury of left internal carotid artery, intracranial portion, not elsewhere classified**

✓7ᵗʰ **S06.820 Injury of left internal carotid artery, intracranial portion, not elsewhere classified without loss of consciousness** `HCC` `PE`

✓7th **S06.821** Injury of left internal carotid artery, intracranial portion, not elsewhere classified with loss of consciousness of **30 minutes or less** `CC` `H5` `HCC` `PE`

Injury of left internal carotid artery, intracranial portion, not elsewhere classified with brief loss of consciousness

✓7th **S06.822** Injury of left internal carotid artery, intracranial portion, not elsewhere classified with loss of consciousness of **31 minutes to 59 minutes** `CC` `H5` `HCC` `PE`

✓7th **S06.823** Injury of left internal carotid artery, intracranial portion, not elsewhere classified with loss of consciousness of **1 hour to 5 hours 59 minutes** `CC` `H5` `HCC` `PE`

✓7th **S06.824** Injury of left internal carotid artery, intracranial portion, not elsewhere classified with loss of consciousness of **6 hours to 24 hours** `CC` `H5` `HCC` `PE`

✓7th **S06.825** Injury of left internal carotid artery, intracranial portion, not elsewhere classified with loss of consciousness **greater than 24 hours with return to pre-existing conscious level** `CC` `H5` `HCC` `PE`

✓7th **S06.826** Injury of left internal carotid artery, intracranial portion, not elsewhere classified with loss of consciousness **greater than 24 hours without return to pre-existing conscious level with patient surviving** `MCC` `H5` `HCC` `PE`

✓7th **S06.827** Injury of left internal carotid artery, intracranial portion, not elsewhere classified with loss of consciousness of **any duration with death due to brain injury prior to regaining consciousness** `MCC` `H5`

✓7th **S06.828** Injury of left internal carotid artery, intracranial portion, not elsewhere classified with loss of consciousness of **any duration with death due to other cause prior to regaining consciousness** `MCC` `H5`

✓7th **S06.82A** Injury of left internal carotid artery, intracranial portion, not elsewhere classified with loss of consciousness **status unknown** `CC` `H5` `HCC` `PE`

Injury of left internal carotid artery, intracranial portion, not elsewhere classified NOS

✓7th **S06.829** Injury of left internal carotid artery, intracranial portion, not elsewhere classified with loss of consciousness of **unspecified duration** `CC` `H5` `HCC` `PE`

✓6th **S06.8A** Primary blast injury of brain, not elsewhere classified

Code also, if applicable, focal traumatic brain injury (S06.3-)

EXCLUDES 2   traumatic cerebral edema (S06.1)

✓7th **S06.8A0** Primary blast injury of brain, not elsewhere classified **without loss of consciousness** `CC` `H5` `HCC` `PE`

✓7th **S06.8A1** Primary blast injury of brain, not elsewhere classified with loss of consciousness of **30 minutes or less** `CC` `H5` `HCC` `PE`

Primary blast injury of brain, not elsewhere classified with brief loss of consciousness

✓7th **S06.8A2** Primary blast injury of brain, not elsewhere classified with loss of consciousness of **31 minutes to 59 minutes** `CC` `H5` `HCC` `PE`

✓7th **S06.8A3** Primary blast injury of brain, not elsewhere classified with loss of consciousness of **1 hour to 5 hours 59 minutes** `CC` `H5` `HCC` `PE`

✓7th **S06.8A4** Primary blast injury of brain, not elsewhere classified with loss of consciousness of **6 hours to 24 hours** `CC` `H5` `HCC` `PE`

✓7th **S06.8A5** Primary blast injury of brain, not elsewhere classified with loss of consciousness **greater than 24 hours with return to pre-existing conscious level** `CC` `H5` `HCC` `PE`

✓7th **S06.8A6** Primary blast injury of brain, not elsewhere classified with loss of consciousness **greater than 24 hours without return to pre-existing conscious level with patient surviving** `MCC` `H5` `HCC` `PE`

✓7th **S06.8A7** Primary blast injury of brain, not elsewhere classified with loss of consciousness of **any duration with death due to brain injury prior to regaining consciousness** `MCC` `H5`

✓7th **S06.8A8** Primary blast injury of brain, not elsewhere classified with loss of consciousness of **any duration with death due to other cause prior to regaining consciousness** `MCC` `H5`

✓7th **S06.8AA** Primary blast injury of brain, not elsewhere classified with loss of consciousness **status unknown** `CC` `H5` `HCC` `PE`

Primary blast injury of brain NOS

✓7th **S06.8A9** Primary blast injury of brain, not elsewhere classified with loss of consciousness of **unspecified duration** `CC` `H5` `HCC` `PE`

✓6th **S06.89** Other specified intracranial injury

EXCLUDES 1   concussion (S06.0X-)

AHA: AHA:2024,2Q,15

✓7th **S06.890** Other specified intracranial injury **without loss of consciousness** `HCC` `PE`

✓7th **S06.891** Other specified intracranial injury with loss of consciousness of **30 minutes or less** `CC` `H5` `HCC` `PE`

Other specified intracranial injury with brief loss of consciousness

✓7th **S06.892** Other specified intracranial injury with loss of consciousness of **31 minutes to 59 minutes** `CC` `H5` `HCC` `PE`

✓7th **S06.893** Other specified intracranial injury with loss of consciousness of **1 hour to 5 hours 59 minutes** `CC` `H5` `HCC` `PE`

✓7th **S06.894** Other specified intracranial injury with loss of consciousness of **6 hours to 24 hours** `CC` `H5` `HCC` `PE`

✓7th **S06.895** Other specified intracranial injury with loss of consciousness **greater than 24 hours with return to pre-existing conscious level** `CC` `H5` `HCC` `PE`

✓7th **S06.896** Other specified intracranial injury with loss of consciousness **greater than 24 hours without return to pre-existing conscious level with patient surviving** `MCC` `H5` `HCC` `PE`

✓7th **S06.897** Other specified intracranial injury with loss of consciousness of **any duration with death due to brain injury prior to regaining consciousness** `MCC` `H5`

✓7th **S06.898** Other specified intracranial injury with loss of consciousness of **any duration with death due to other cause prior to regaining consciousness** `MCC` `H5`

✓7th **S06.89A** Other specified intracranial injury with loss of consciousness **status unknown** `CC` `H5` `HCC` `PE`

✓7th **S06.899** Other specified intracranial injury with loss of consciousness of **unspecified duration** `CC` `H5` `HCC` `PE`

✓5th **S06.9** Unspecified intracranial injury

Brain injury NOS
Head injury NOS with loss of consciousness
Traumatic brain injury NOS

EXCLUDES 1   conditions classifiable to S06.0- to S06.8- code to specified intracranial injury
head injury NOS (S09.90)

AHA: 2020,3Q,46; 2020,2Q,31

TIP: Assign additional code(s) for individual (R40.21-, R40.22-, R40.23-) or total (R40.24-) coma scale scores. It is appropriate to code the coma scale scores based on documentation provided by clinicians who are not the patient's provider (such as emergency medical technician).

✓6th **S06.9X** Unspecified intracranial injury

✓7th **S06.9X0** Unspecified intracranial injury **without loss of consciousness** `HCC` `PE`

`N` Newborn: 0   `P` Pediatric: 0-17   `M` Maternity: 9-64   `A` Adult: 15-124   `UNS` Unspecified Site   `MCC` Major Complication/Comorbidity   `CC` Complication/Comorbidity   `PE` POA Exempt

996

ICD-10-CM 2025

√7ᵗʰ **S06.9X1** **Unspecified intracranial injury with loss of consciousness of 30 minutes or less** `CC` `H5` `HCC` `PE`
Unspecified intracranial injury with brief loss of consciousness

√7ᵗʰ **S06.9X2** **Unspecified intracranial injury with loss of consciousness of 31 minutes to 59 minutes** `CC` `H5` `HCC` `PE`

√7ᵗʰ **S06.9X3** **Unspecified intracranial injury with loss of consciousness of 1 hour to 5 hours 59 minutes** `CC` `H5` `HCC` `PE`

√7ᵗʰ **S06.9X4** **Unspecified intracranial injury with loss of consciousness of 6 hours to 24 hours** `CC` `H5` `HCC` `PE`

√7ᵗʰ **S06.9X5** **Unspecified intracranial injury with loss of consciousness greater than 24 hours with return to pre-existing conscious level** `CC` `H5` `HCC` `PE`

√7ᵗʰ **S06.9X6** **Unspecified intracranial injury with loss of consciousness greater than 24 hours without return to pre-existing conscious level with patient surviving** `MCC` `H5` `HCC` `FE`

√7ᵗʰ **S06.9X7** **Unspecified intracranial injury with loss of consciousness of any duration with death due to brain injury prior to regaining consciousness** `MCC` `H5`

√7ᵗʰ **S06.9X8** **Unspecified intracranial injury with loss of consciousness of any duration with death due to other cause prior to regaining consciousness** `MCC` `H5`

√7ᵗʰ **S06.9XA** **Unspecified intracranial injury with loss of consciousness status unknown** `CC` `H5` `HCC` `PE`

√7ᵗʰ **S06.9X9** **Unspecified intracranial injury with loss of consciousness of unspecified duration** `CC` `H5` `HCC` `PE`

√5ᵗʰ **S06.A** **Traumatic brain compression and herniation**
Traumatic cerebral compression
Code first the underlying traumatic brain injury, such as:
diffuse traumatic brain injury (S06.2-)
focal traumatic brain injury (S06.3-)
traumatic subarachnoid hemorrhage (S06.6-)
traumatic subdural hemorrhage (S06.5-)
AHA: 2021,4Q,29

√x7ᵗʰ **S06.A0** **Traumatic brain compression without herniation** `MCC` `UPD` `HCC` `PE`
Traumatic brain compression NOS
Traumatic cerebral compression NOS

√x7ᵗʰ **S06.A1** **Traumatic brain compression with herniation** `MCC` `UPD` `HCC` `PE`
Traumatic brain herniation
Traumatic brainstem compression with herniation
Traumatic cerebellar compression with herniation
Traumatic cerebral compression with herniation

√4ᵗʰ **S07** **Crushing injury of head**
Use additional code for all associated injuries, such as:
intracranial injuries (S06.-)
skull fractures (S02.-)

The appropriate 7th character is to be added to each code from category S07.
A   initial encounter
D   subsequent encounter
S   sequela

√x7ᵗʰ **S07.0** **Crushing injury of face** `CC` `H5` `PE`

√x7ᵗʰ **S07.1** **Crushing injury of skull** `CC` `H5` `PE`

√x7ᵗʰ **S07.8** **Crushing injury of other parts of head** `CC` `H5` `PE`

√x7ᵗʰ **S07.9** **Crushing injury of head, part unspecified** `CC` `H5` `PE`

√4ᵗʰ **S08** **Avulsion and traumatic amputation of part of head**
An amputation not identified as partial or complete should be coded to complete

The appropriate 7th character is to be added to each code from category S08.
A   initial encounter
D   subsequent encounter
S   sequela

√x7ᵗʰ **S08.0** **Avulsion of scalp** `PE`

√5ᵗʰ **S08.1** **Traumatic amputation of ear**

√6ᵗʰ **S08.11** **Complete traumatic amputation of ear**

√7ᵗʰ **S08.111** **Complete traumatic amputation of right ear** `PE`

√7ᵗʰ **S08.112** **Complete traumatic amputation of left ear** `PE`

√7ᵗʰ **S08.119** **Complete traumatic amputation of unspecified ear** `PE`

√6ᵗʰ **S08.12** **Partial traumatic amputation of ear**

√7ᵗʰ **S08.121** **Partial traumatic amputation of right ear** `PE`

√7ᵗʰ **S08.122** **Partial traumatic amputation of left ear** `PE`

√7ᵗʰ **S08.129** **Partial traumatic amputation of unspecified ear** `PE`

√5ᵗʰ **S08.8** **Traumatic amputation of other parts of head**

√6ᵗʰ **S08.81** **Traumatic amputation of nose**

√7ᵗʰ **S08.811** **Complete traumatic amputation of nose**

√7ᵗʰ **S08.812** **Partial traumatic amputation of nose** `PE`

√x7ᵗʰ **S08.89** **Traumatic amputation of other parts of head** `PE`

√4ᵗʰ **S09** **Other and unspecified injuries of head**

The appropriate 7th character is to be added to each code from category S09.
A   initial encounter
D   subsequent encounter
S   sequela

√x7ᵗʰ **S09.0** **Injury of blood vessels of head, not elsewhere classified** `CC` `PE`
EXCLUDES 1   injury of cerebral blood vessels (S06.-)
injury of precerebral blood vessels (S15.-)

√5ᵗʰ **S09.1** **Injury of muscle and tendon of head**
Code also any associated open wound (S01.-)
EXCLUDES 2   sprain to joints and ligament of head (S03.9)

√x7ᵗʰ **S09.10** **Unspecified injury of muscle and tendon of head** `PE`
Injury of muscle and tendon of head NOS

√x7ᵗʰ **S09.11** **Strain of muscle and tendon of head** `PE`

√x7ᵗʰ **S09.12** **Laceration of muscle and tendon of head** `PE`

√x7ᵗʰ **S09.19** **Other specified injury of muscle and tendon of head** `PE`

√5ᵗʰ **S09.2** **Traumatic rupture of ear drum**
EXCLUDES 1   traumatic rupture of ear drum due to blast injury (S09.31-)

√x7ᵗʰ **S09.20** **Traumatic rupture of unspecified ear drum** `CC` `UNS` `PE`

√x7ᵗʰ **S09.21** **Traumatic rupture of right ear drum** `CC` `PE`

√x7ᵗʰ **S09.22** **Traumatic rupture of left ear drum** `CC` `PE`

√5ᵗʰ **S09.3** **Other specified and unspecified injury of middle and inner ear**
EXCLUDES 1   injury to ear NOS (S09.91-)
EXCLUDES 2   injury to external ear (S00.4-, S01.3-, S08.1-)

√6ᵗʰ **S09.30** **Unspecified injury of middle and inner ear**

√7ᵗʰ **S09.301** **Unspecified injury of right middle and inner ear**

√7ᵗʰ **S09.302** **Unspecified injury of left middle and inner ear** `CC` `PE`

√7ᵗʰ **S09.309** **Unspecified injury of unspecified middle and inner ear** `CC` `UNS` `PE`

√6ᵗʰ **S09.31** **Primary blast injury of ear**
Blast injury of ear NOS

√7ᵗʰ **S09.311** **Primary blast injury of right ear** `CC` `PE`

√7ᵗʰ **S09.312** **Primary blast injury of left ear** `CC` `PE`

√7ᵗʰ **S09.313** **Primary blast injury of ear, bilateral** `CC` `PE`

√7ᵗʰ **S09.319** **Primary blast injury of unspecified ear** `CC` `UNS` `PE`

√6ᵗʰ **S09.39** **Other specified injury of middle and inner ear**
Secondary blast injury to ear

√7ᵗʰ **S09.391** **Other specified injury of right middle and inner ear** `CC` `PE`

√7ᵗʰ **S09.392** **Other specified injury of left middle and inner ear** `CC` `PE`

√7ᵗʰ **S09.399** Other specified injury of unspecified middle and inner ear   `CC` `UNS` `PE`

√7ᵗʰ **S09.8** Other specified injuries of head   `PE`

√5ᵗʰ **S09.9** Unspecified injury of face and head

   √x7ᵗʰ **S09.90** Unspecified injury of **head**   `PE`
Head injury NOS

     EXCLUDES 1   *brain injury NOS (S06.9-)*
head injury NOS with loss of consciousness (S06.9-)
intracranial injury NOS (S06.9-)

   √x7ᵗʰ **S09.91** Unspecified injury of **ear**   `PE`
Injury of ear NOS

   √x7ᵗʰ **S09.92** Unspecified injury of **nose**   `PE`
Injury of nose NOS

   √x7ᵗʰ **S09.93** Unspecified injury of **face**   `PE`
Injury of face NOS
AHA: 2019,2Q,23

Injuries to the neck (S10-S19)

INCLUDES   injuries of nape
injuries of supraclavicular region
injuries of throat

EXCLUDES 2   *burns and corrosions (T20-T32)*
effects of foreign body in esophagus (T18.1)
effects of foreign body in larynx (T17.3)
effects of foreign body in pharynx (T17.2)
effects of foreign body in trachea (T17.4)
frostbite (T33-T34)
insect bite or sting, venomous (T63.4)

√4ᵗʰ **S10 Superficial injury of neck**

> The appropriate 7th character is to be added to each code from category S10.
> A   initial encounter
> D   subsequent encounter
> S   sequela

√x7ᵗʰ **S10.0** Contusion of throat   `PE`
Contusion of cervical esophagus
Contusion of larynx
Contusion of pharynx
Contusion of trachea

√5ᵗʰ **S10.1** Other and unspecified superficial injuries of throat

   √x7ᵗʰ **S10.10** Unspecified superficial injuries of throat   `PE`

   √x7ᵗʰ **S10.11** **Abrasion** of throat   `PE`

   √x7ᵗʰ **S10.12** **Blister** (nonthermal) of throat   `PE`

   √x7ᵗʰ **S10.14** **External constriction** of part of throat   `PE`

   √x7ᵗʰ **S10.15** Superficial **foreign body** of throat   `PE`
Splinter in the throat

   √x7ᵗʰ **S10.16** **Insect bite** (nonvenomous) of throat   `PE`

   √x7ᵗʰ **S10.17** Other superficial **bite** of throat   `PE`
     EXCLUDES 1   *open bite of throat (S11.85)*

√5ᵗʰ **S10.8** Superficial injury of other specified parts of neck

   √x7ᵗʰ **S10.80** Unspecified superficial injury of other specified part of neck   `PE`

   √x7ᵗʰ **S10.81** **Abrasion** of other specified part of neck   `PE`

   √x7ᵗʰ **S10.82** **Blister** (nonthermal) of other specified part of neck   `PE`

   √x7ᵗʰ **S10.83** **Contusion** of other specified part of neck   `PE`

   √x7ᵗʰ **S10.84** **External constriction** of other specified part of neck   `PE`

   √x7ᵗʰ **S10.85** Superficial **foreign body** of other specified part of neck   `PE`
Splinter in other specified part of neck

   √x7ᵗʰ **S10.86** **Insect bite** of other specified part of neck   `PE`

   √x7ᵗʰ **S10.87** Other superficial **bite** of other specified part of neck   `PE`
     EXCLUDES 1   *open bite of other specified parts of neck (S11.85)*

√5ᵗʰ **S10.9** Superficial injury of unspecified part of neck

   √x7ᵗʰ **S10.90** Unspecified superficial injury of unspecified part of neck   `PE`

   √x7ᵗʰ **S10.91** **Abrasion** of unspecified part of neck   `PE`

   √x7ᵗʰ **S10.92** **Blister** (nonthermal) of unspecified part of neck   `PE`

   √x7ᵗʰ **S10.93** **Contusion** of unspecified part of neck   `PE`

   √x7ᵗʰ **S10.94** **External constriction** of unspecified part of neck   `PE`

   √x7ᵗʰ **S10.95** Superficial **foreign body** of unspecified part of neck   `PE`

   √x7ᵗʰ **S10.96** **Insect bite** of unspecified part of neck   `PE`

   √x7ᵗʰ **S10.97** Other superficial **bite** of unspecified part of neck   `PE`

√4ᵗʰ **S11 Open wound of neck**

Code also any associated:
   spinal cord injury (S14.0, S14.1-)
   wound infection
   EXCLUDES 2   *open fracture of vertebra (S12.- with 7th character B)*

> The appropriate 7th character is to be added to each code from category S11.
> A   initial encounter
> D   subsequent encounter
> S   sequela

√5ᵗʰ **S11.0** Open wound of larynx and trachea

   √6ᵗʰ **S11.01** Open wound of **larynx**
     EXCLUDES 2   *open wound of vocal cord (S11.03)*

     √7ᵗʰ **S11.011** **Laceration without foreign body** of larynx   `MCC` `PE`

     √7ᵗʰ **S11.012** **Laceration with foreign body** of larynx   `MCC` `PE`

     √7ᵗʰ **S11.013** **Puncture wound without foreign body** of larynx   `MCC` `PE`

     √7ᵗʰ **S11.014** **Puncture wound with foreign body** of larynx   `MCC` `PE`

     √7ᵗʰ **S11.015** **Open bite** of larynx   `MCC` `PE`
Bite of larynx NOS

     √7ᵗʰ **S11.019** **Unspecified open wound of larynx**   `MCC` `PE`

   √6ᵗʰ **S11.02** Open wound of **trachea**
Open wound of cervical trachea
Open wound of trachea NOS
     EXCLUDES 2   *open wound of thoracic trachea (S27.5-)*

     √7ᵗʰ **S11.021** **Laceration without foreign body** of trachea   `MCC` `PE`

     √7ᵗʰ **S11.022** **Laceration with foreign body** of trachea   `MCC` `PE`

     √7ᵗʰ **S11.023** **Puncture wound without foreign body** of trachea   `MCC` `PE`

     √7ᵗʰ **S11.024** **Puncture wound with foreign body** of trachea   `MCC` `PE`

     √7ᵗʰ **S11.025** **Open bite** of trachea   `MCC` `PE`
Bite of trachea NOS

     √7ᵗʰ **S11.029** **Unspecified open wound of trachea**   `MCC` `PE`

   √6ᵗʰ **S11.03** Open wound of **vocal cord**

     √7ᵗʰ **S11.031** **Laceration without foreign body** of vocal cord   `MCC` `PE`

     √7ᵗʰ **S11.032** **Laceration with foreign body** of vocal cord   `MCC` `PE`

     √7ᵗʰ **S11.033** **Puncture wound without foreign body** of vocal cord   `MCC` `PE`

     √7ᵗʰ **S11.034** **Puncture wound with foreign body** of vocal cord   `MCC` `PE`

     √7ᵗʰ **S11.035** **Open bite** of vocal cord   `MCC` `PE`
Bite of vocal cord NOS

     √7ᵗʰ **S11.039** **Unspecified open wound of vocal cord**   `MCC` `PE`

√5ᵗʰ **S11.1** Open wound of **thyroid gland**

   √x7ᵗʰ **S11.10** Unspecified open wound of thyroid gland   `CC` `PE`

   √x7ᵗʰ **S11.11** **Laceration without foreign body** of thyroid gland   `CC` `PE`

   √x7ᵗʰ **S11.12** **Laceration with foreign body** of thyroid gland   `CC` `PE`

   √x7ᵗʰ **S11.13** **Puncture wound without foreign body** of thyroid gland   `CC` `PE`

   √x7ᵗʰ **S11.14** **Puncture wound with foreign body** of thyroid gland   `CC` `PE`

   √x7ᵗʰ **S11.15** **Open bite** of thyroid gland   `CC` `PE`
Bite of thyroid gland NOS

`N` Newborn: 0   `P` Pediatric: 0-17   `M` Maternity: 9-64   `A` Adult: 15-124   `UNS` Unspecified Site   `MCC` Major Complication/Comorbidity   `CC` Complication/Comorbidity   `PE` POA Exempt

998   ICD-10-CM 2025

√5ᵗʰ **S11.2 Open wound of pharynx and cervical esophagus**

> EXCLUDES 1   *open wound of esophagus NOS (S27.8-)*

  √x7ᵗʰ **S11.20 Unspecified open wound of pharynx and cervical esophagus** `CC` `PE`

  √x7ᵗʰ **S11.21 Laceration without foreign body of pharynx and cervical esophagus** `CC` `PE`

  √x7ᵗʰ **S11.22 Laceration with foreign body of pharynx and cervical esophagus** `CC` `PE`

  √x7ᵗʰ **S11.23 Puncture wound without foreign body of pharynx and cervical esophagus** `CC` `PE`

  √x7ᵗʰ **S11.24 Puncture wound with foreign body of pharynx and cervical esophagus** `CC` `PE`

  √x7ᵗʰ **S11.25 Open bite of pharynx and cervical esophagus** `CC` `PE`
> Bite of pharynx and cervical esophagus NOS

√5ᵗʰ **S11.8 Open wound of other specified parts of neck**

  √x7ᵗʰ **S11.80 Unspecified open wound of other specified part of neck** `PE`

  √x7ᵗʰ **S11.81 Laceration without foreign body of other specified part of neck** `PE`

  √x7ᵗʰ **S11.82 Laceration with foreign body of other specified part of neck** `PE`

  √x7ᵗʰ **S11.83 Puncture wound without foreign body of other specified part of neck** `PE`

  √x7ᵗʰ **S11.84 Puncture wound with foreign body of other specified part of neck** `PE`

  √x7ᵗʰ **S11.85 Open bite of other specified part of neck** `PE`
> Bite of other specified part of neck NOS
>> EXCLUDES 1   *superficial bite of other specified part of neck (S10.87)*

  √x7ᵗʰ **S11.89 Other open wound of other specified part of neck** `PE`

√5ᵗʰ **S11.9 Open wound of unspecified part of neck**

  √x7ᵗʰ **S11.90 Unspecified open wound of unspecified part of neck** `PE`

  √x7ᵗʰ **S11.91 Laceration without foreign body of unspecified part of neck** `PE`

  √x7ᵗʰ **S11.92 Laceration with foreign body of unspecified part of neck** `PE`

  √x7ᵗʰ **S11.93 Puncture wound without foreign body of unspecified part of neck** `PE`

  √x7ᵗʰ **S11.94 Puncture wound with foreign body of unspecified part of neck** `PE`

  √x7ᵗʰ **S11.95 Open bite of unspecified part of neck** `PE`
> Bite of neck NOS
>> EXCLUDES 1   *superficial bite of neck (S10.97)*

√4ᵗʰ **S12 Fracture of cervical vertebra and other parts of neck**

> **NOTE**   A fracture not indicated as displaced or nondisplaced should be coded to displaced.
>
> A fracture not indicated as open or closed should be coded to closed.

> **INCLUDES**   fracture of cervical neural arch
> fracture of cervical spine
> fracture of cervical spinous process
> fracture of cervical transverse process
> fracture of cervical vertebral arch
> fracture of neck

Code first any associated cervical spinal cord injury (S14.0, S14.1-)

AHA: 2024,2Q,23; 2021,1Q,6; 2018,2Q,12; 2015,3Q,37-39

> The appropriate 7th character is to be added to all codes from subcategories S12.0-S12.6.
> A   initial encounter for closed fracture
> B   initial encounter for open fracture
> D   subsequent encounter for fracture with routine healing
> G   subsequent encounter for fracture with delayed healing
> K   subsequent encounter for fracture with nonunion
> S   sequela

√5ᵗʰ **S12.0 Fracture of first cervical vertebra**
> Atlas

  √6ᵗʰ **S12.00 Unspecified fracture of first cervical vertebra**

    √7ᵗʰ **S12.000 Unspecified displaced fracture of first cervical vertebra** `MCC` `CC` `H5` `HCC` `PE`

    √7ᵗʰ **S12.001 Unspecified nondisplaced fracture of first cervical vertebra** `MCC` `CC` `H5` `HCC` `PE`

    √7ᵗʰ **S12.01 Stable burst fracture of first cervical vertebra** `MCC` `CC` `H5` `HCC` `PE`

    √7ᵗʰ **S12.02 Unstable burst fracture of first cervical vertebra** `MCC` `CC` `H5` `HCC` `PE`

  √6ᵗʰ **S12.03 Posterior arch fracture of first cervical vertebra**

    √7ᵗʰ **S12.030 Displaced posterior arch fracture of first cervical vertebra** `MCC` `CC` `H5` `HCC` `PE`

    √7ᵗʰ **S12.031 Nondisplaced posterior arch fracture of first cervical vertebra** `MCC` `CC` `H5` `HCC` `PE`

  √6ᵗʰ **S12.04 Lateral mass fracture of first cervical vertebra**

    √7ᵗʰ **S12.040 Displaced lateral mass fracture of first cervical vertebra** `MCC` `CC` `H5` `HCC` `PE`

    √7ᵗʰ **S12.041 Nondisplaced lateral mass fracture of first cervical vertebra** `MCC` `CC` `H5` `HCC` `PE`

  √6ᵗʰ **S12.09 Other fracture of first cervical vertebra**

    √7ᵗʰ **S12.090 Other displaced fracture of first cervical vertebra** `MCC` `CC` `H5` `HCC` `PE`

    √7ᵗʰ **S12.091 Other nondisplaced fracture of first cervical vertebra** `MCC` `CC` `H5` `HCC` `PE`

√5ᵗʰ **S12.1 Fracture of second cervical vertebra**
> Axis

  √6ᵗʰ **S12.10 Unspecified fracture of second cervical vertebra**

    √7ᵗʰ **S12.100 Unspecified displaced fracture of second cervical vertebra** `MCC` `CC` `H5` `HCC` `PE`

    √7ᵗʰ **S12.101 Unspecified nondisplaced fracture of second cervical vertebra** `MCC` `CC` `H5` `HCC` `PE`

  √6ᵗʰ **S12.11 Type II dens fracture**

    √7ᵗʰ **S12.110 Anterior displaced Type II dens fracture** `MCC` `CC` `H5` `HCC` `PE`

    √7ᵗʰ **S12.111 Posterior displaced Type II dens fracture** `MCC` `CC` `H5` `HCC` `PE`

    √7ᵗʰ **S12.112 Nondisplaced Type II dens fracture** `MCC` `CC` `H5` `HCC` `PE`

  √6ᵗʰ **S12.12 Other dens fracture**

    √7ᵗʰ **S12.120 Other displaced dens fracture** `MCC` `CC` `H5` `HCC` `PE`

    √7ᵗʰ **S12.121 Other nondisplaced dens fracture** `MCC` `CC` `H5` `HCC` `PE`

  √6ᵗʰ **S12.13 Unspecified traumatic spondylolisthesis of second cervical vertebra**

    √7ᵗʰ **S12.130 Unspecified traumatic displaced spondylolisthesis of second cervical vertebra** `MCC` `CC` `H5` `HCC` `PE`

    √7ᵗʰ **S12.131 Unspecified traumatic nondisplaced spondylolisthesis of second cervical vertebra** `MCC` `CC` `H5` `HCC` `PE`

  √x7ᵗʰ **S12.14 Type III traumatic spondylolisthesis of second cervical vertebra** `MCC` `CC` `H5` `HCC` `PE`

  √6ᵗʰ **S12.15 Other traumatic spondylolisthesis of second cervical vertebra**

    √7ᵗʰ **S12.150 Other traumatic displaced spondylolisthesis of second cervical vertebra** `MCC` `CC` `H5` `HCC` `PE`

    √7ᵗʰ **S12.151 Other traumatic nondisplaced spondylolisthesis of second cervical vertebra** `MCC` `CC` `H5` `HCC` `PE`

  √6ᵗʰ **S12.19 Other fracture of second cervical vertebra**

    √7ᵗʰ **S12.190 Other displaced fracture of second cervical vertebra** `MCC` `CC` `H5` `HCC` `PE`

    √7ᵗʰ **S12.191 Other nondisplaced fracture of second cervical vertebra** `MCC` `CC` `H5` `HCC` `PE`

√5ᵗʰ **S12.2 Fracture of third cervical vertebra**

  √6ᵗʰ **S12.20 Unspecified fracture of third cervical vertebra**

    √7ᵗʰ **S12.200 Unspecified displaced fracture of third cervical vertebra** `MCC` `CC` `H5` `HCC` `PE`

    √7ᵗʰ **S12.201 Unspecified nondisplaced fracture of third cervical vertebra** `MCC` `CC` `H5` `HCC` `PE`

  √6ᵗʰ **S12.23 Unspecified traumatic spondylolisthesis of third cervical vertebra**

    √7ᵗʰ **S12.230 Unspecified traumatic displaced spondylolisthesis of third cervical vertebra** `MCC` `CC` `H5` `HCC` `PE`

    √7ᵗʰ **S12.231 Unspecified traumatic nondisplaced spondylolisthesis of third cervical vertebra** `MCC` `CC` `H5` `HCC` `PE`

☑ Additional Character Required   √x7ᵗʰ Placeholder   Questionable PDx   Manifestation   Unspecified   UPD Unacceptable PDx   H1–H14 HAC   HCC CMS-HCC Dx   HIV HIV Dx

ICD-10-CM 2025   999

√x 7th **S12.24** **Type III** traumatic **spondylolisthesis** of third cervical vertebra   MCC CC H5 HCC PE

√6th **S12.25** Other traumatic spondylolisthesis of third cervical vertebra

    √7th **S12.250** Other traumatic **displaced** spondylolisthesis of third cervical vertebra

    √7th **S12.251** Other traumatic **nondisplaced** spondylolisthesis of third cervical vertebra   MCC CC H5 HCC PE

√6th **S12.29** Other fracture of third cervical vertebra

    √7th **S12.290** Other **displaced** fracture of third cervical vertebra   MCC CC H5 HCC PE

    √7th **S12.291** Other **nondisplaced** fracture of third cervical vertebra   MCC CC H5 HCC PE

√5th **S12.3** Fracture of **fourth** cervical vertebra

   √6th **S12.30** Unspecified fracture of fourth cervical vertebra

     √7th **S12.300** Unspecified **displaced** fracture of fourth cervical vertebra   MCC CC H5 HCC PE

     √7th **S12.301** Unspecified **nondisplaced** fracture of fourth cervical vertebra

   √6th **S12.33** Unspecified traumatic **spondylolisthesis** of fourth cervical vertebra

     √7th **S12.330** Unspecified traumatic **displaced** spondylolisthesis of fourth cervical vertebra   MCC CC H5 HCC PE

     √7th **S12.331** Unspecified traumatic **nondisplaced** spondylolisthesis of fourth cervical vertebra   MCC CC H5 HCC PE

   √x 7th **S12.34** **Type III** traumatic **spondylolisthesis** of fourth cervical vertebra   MCC CC H5 HCC PE

   √6th **S12.35** Other traumatic **spondylolisthesis** of fourth cervical vertebra

     √7th **S12.350** Other traumatic **displaced** spondylolisthesis of fourth cervical vertebra

     √7th **S12.351** Other traumatic **nondisplaced** spondylolisthesis of fourth cervical vertebra   MCC CC H5 HCC PE

   √6th **S12.39** Other fracture of fourth cervical vertebra

     √7th **S12.390** Other **displaced** fracture of fourth cervical vertebra   MCC CC H5 HCC PE

     √7th **S12.391** Other **nondisplaced** fracture of fourth cervical vertebra   MCC CC H5 HCC PE

√5th **S12.4** Fracture of **fifth** cervical vertebra

   √6th **S12.40** Unspecified fracture of fifth cervical vertebra

     √7th **S12.400** Unspecified **displaced** fracture of fifth cervical vertebra   MCC CC H5 HCC PE

     √7th **S12.401** Unspecified **nondisplaced** fracture of fifth cervical vertebra   MCC CC H5 HCC PE

   √6th **S12.43** Unspecified traumatic **spondylolisthesis** of fifth cervical vertebra

     √7th **S12.430** Unspecified traumatic **displaced** spondylolisthesis of fifth cervical vertebra   MCC CC H5 HCC PE

     √7th **S12.431** Unspecified traumatic **nondisplaced** spondylolisthesis of fifth cervical vertebra   MCC CC H5 HCC PE

   √x 7th **S12.44** **Type III** traumatic **spondylolisthesis** of fifth cervical vertebra   MCC CC H5 HCC PE

   √6th **S12.45** Other traumatic **spondylolisthesis** of fifth cervical vertebra

     √7th **S12.450** Other traumatic **displaced** spondylolisthesis of fifth cervical vertebra   MCC CC H5 HCC PE

     √7th **S12.451** Other traumatic **nondisplaced** spondylolisthesis of fifth cervical vertebra   MCC CC H5 HCC PE

   √6th **S12.49** Other fracture of fifth cervical vertebra

     √7th **S12.490** Other **displaced** fracture of fifth cervical vertebra   MCC CC H5 HCC PE

     √7th **S12.491** Other **nondisplaced** fracture of fifth cervical vertebra   MCC CC H5 HCC PE

√5th **S12.5** Fracture of **sixth** cervical vertebra

   √6th **S12.50** Unspecified fracture of sixth cervical vertebra

     √7th **S12.500** Unspecified **displaced** fracture of sixth cervical vertebra   MCC CC H5 HCC

     √7th **S12.501** Unspecified **nondisplaced** fracture of sixth cervical vertebra   MCC CC H5 HCC PE

   √6th **S12.53** Unspecified traumatic **spondylolisthesis** of sixth cervical vertebra

     √7th **S12.530** Unspecified traumatic **displaced** spondylolisthesis of sixth cervical vertebra   MCC CC H5 HCC PE

     √7th **S12.531** Unspecified traumatic **nondisplaced** spondylolisthesis of sixth cervical vertebra   MCC CC H5 HCC PE

   √x 7th **S12.54** **Type III** traumatic **spondylolisthesis** of sixth cervical vertebra   MCC CC H5 HCC PE

   √6th **S12.55** Other traumatic **spondylolisthesis** of sixth cervical vertebra

     √7th **S12.550** Other traumatic **displaced** spondylolisthesis of sixth cervical vertebra   MCC CC H5 HCC PE

     √7th **S12.551** Other traumatic **nondisplaced** spondylolisthesis of sixth cervical vertebra   MCC CC H5 HCC PE

   √6th **S12.59** Other fracture of sixth cervical vertebra

     √7th **S12.590** Other **displaced** fracture of sixth cervical vertebra   MCC CC H5 HCC PE

     √7th **S12.591** Other **nondisplaced** fracture of sixth cervical vertebra   MCC CC H5 HCC PE

√5th **S12.6** Fracture of **seventh** cervical vertebra

   √6th **S12.60** Unspecified fracture of seventh cervical vertebra

     √7th **S12.600** Unspecified **displaced** fracture of seventh cervical vertebra   MCC CC H5 HCC PE

     √7th **S12.601** Unspecified **nondisplaced** fracture of seventh cervical vertebra   MCC CC H5 HCC PE

   √6th **S12.63** Unspecified traumatic **spondylolisthesis** of seventh cervical vertebra

     √7th **S12.630** Unspecified traumatic **displaced** spondylolisthesis of seventh cervical vertebra   MCC CC H5 HCC PE

     √7th **S12.631** Unspecified traumatic **nondisplaced** spondylolisthesis of seventh cervical vertebra   MCC CC H5 HCC PE

   √x 7th **S12.64** **Type III** traumatic **spondylolisthesis** of seventh cervical vertebra   MCC CC H5 HCC PE

   √6th **S12.65** Other traumatic **spondylolisthesis** of seventh cervical vertebra

     √7th **S12.650** Other traumatic **displaced** spondylolisthesis of seventh cervical vertebra   MCC CC H5 HCC PE

     √7th **S12.651** Other traumatic **nondisplaced** spondylolisthesis of seventh cervical vertebra   MCC CC H5 HCC PE

   √6th **S12.69** Other fracture of seventh cervical vertebra

     √7th **S12.690** Other **displaced** fracture of seventh cervical vertebra   MCC CC H5 HCC PE

     √7th **S12.691** Other **nondisplaced** fracture of seventh cervical vertebra   MCC CC H5 HCC PE

√x 7th **S12.8** **Fracture of other parts of neck**   MCC H5 HCC PE

   Hyoid bone
   Larynx
   Thyroid cartilage
   Trachea

> The appropriate 7th character is to be added to code S12.8.
> A   initial encounter
> D   subsequent encounter
> S   sequela

√x 7th **S12.9** **Fracture of neck, unspecified**   CC H5 HCC PE

   Fracture of neck NOS
   Fracture of cervical spine NOS
   Fracture of cervical vertebra NOS

> The appropriate 7th character is to be added to code S12.9.
> A   initial encounter
> D   subsequent encounter
> S   sequela

N Newborn: 0   P Pediatric: 0-17   M Maternity: 9-64   A Adult: 15-124   UNS Unspecified Site   MCC Major Complication/Comorbidity   CC Complication/Comorbidity   PE POA Exempt

1000

ICD-10-CM 2025

✔4ᵗʰ **S13** **Dislocation and sprain of joints and ligaments at neck level**

INCLUDES avulsion of joint or ligament at neck level
laceration of cartilage, joint or ligament at neck level
sprain of cartilage, joint or ligament at neck level
traumatic hemarthrosis of joint or ligament at neck level
traumatic rupture of joint or ligament at neck level
traumatic subluxation of joint or ligament at neck level
traumatic tear of joint or ligament at neck level

Code also any associated open wound

EXCLUDES 2 strain of muscle or tendon at neck level (S16.1)

The appropriate 7th character is to be added to each code from category S13.
A   initial encounter
D   subsequent encounter
S   sequela

✔x7ᵗʰ **S13.0** **Traumatic rupture of cervical intervertebral disc** CC H5 PE

EXCLUDES 1 rupture or displacement (nontraumatic) of cervical intervertebral disc NOS (M50.-)

✔6ᵗʰ **S13.1** **Subluxation and dislocation of cervical vertebrae**

Code also any associated:
open wound of neck (S11.-)
spinal cord injury (S14.1-)

EXCLUDES 2 fracture of cervical vertebrae (S12.0-S12.3-)

✔6ᵗʰ **S13.10** **Subluxation and dislocation of unspecified cervical vertebrae**

✔7ᵗʰ **S13.100** **Subluxation** of unspecified cervical vertebrae CC H5 PE

✔7ᵗʰ **S13.101** **Dislocation** of unspecified cervical vertebrae CC H5 PE

✔6ᵗʰ **S13.11** **Subluxation and dislocation of C0/C1 cervical vertebrae**
Subluxation and dislocation of atlantooccipital joint
Subluxation and dislocation of atloidooccipital joint
Subluxation and dislocation of occipitoatloid joint

✔7ᵗʰ **S13.110** **Subluxation** of C0/C1 cervical vertebrae CC H5 PE

✔7ᵗʰ **S13.111** **Dislocation** of C0/C1 cervical vertebrae CC H5 PE

✔6ᵗʰ **S13.12** **Subluxation and dislocation of C1/C2 cervical vertebrae**
Subluxation and dislocation of atlantoaxial joint

✔7ᵗʰ **S13.120** **Subluxation** of C1/C2 cervical vertebrae CC H5 PE

✔7ᵗʰ **S13.121** **Dislocation** of C1/C2 cervical vertebrae CC H5 PE

✔6ᵗʰ **S13.13** **Subluxation and dislocation of C2/C3 cervical vertebrae**

✔7ᵗʰ **S13.130** **Subluxation** of C2/C3 cervical vertebrae CC H5 PE

✔7ᵗʰ **S13.131** **Dislocation** of C2/C3 cervical vertebrae CC H5 PE

✔6ᵗʰ **S13.14** **Subluxation and dislocation of C3/C4 cervical vertebrae**

✔7ᵗʰ **S13.140** **Subluxation** of C3/C4 cervical vertebrae CC H5 PE

✔7ᵗʰ **S13.141** **Dislocation** of C3/C4 cervical vertebrae CC H5 PE

✔6ᵗʰ **S13.15** **Subluxation and dislocation of C4/C5 cervical vertebrae**

✔7ᵗʰ **S13.150** **Subluxation** of C4/C5 cervical vertebrae CC H5 PE

✔7ᵗʰ **S13.151** **Dislocation** of C4/C5 cervical vertebrae CC H5 PE

✔6ᵗʰ **S13.16** **Subluxation and dislocation of C5/C6 cervical vertebrae**

✔7ᵗʰ **S13.160** **Subluxation** of C5/C6 cervical vertebrae CC H5 PE

✔7ᵗʰ **S13.161** **Dislocation** of C5/C6 cervical vertebrae CC H5 PE

✔6ᵗʰ **S13.17** **Subluxation and dislocation of C6/C7 cervical vertebrae**

✔7ᵗʰ **S13.170** **Subluxation** of C6/C7 cervical vertebrae CC H5 PE

✔7ᵗʰ **S13.171** **Dislocation** of C6/C7 cervical vertebrae CC H5 PE

✔6ᵗʰ **S13.18** **Subluxation and dislocation of C7/T1 cervical vertebrae**

✔7ᵗʰ **S13.180** **Subluxation** of C7/T1 cervical vertebrae CC H5 PE

✔7ᵗʰ **S13.181** **Dislocation** of C7/T1 cervical vertebrae CC H5 PE

✔5ᵗʰ **S13.2** **Dislocation of other and unspecified parts of neck**

✔x7ᵗʰ **S13.20** **Dislocation of unspecified parts of neck** CC H5 PE

✔x7ᵗʰ **S13.29** **Dislocation of other parts of neck** CC H5 PE

✔x7ᵗʰ **S13.4** **Sprain of ligaments of cervical spine** PE
Sprain of anterior longitudinal (ligament), cervical
Sprain of atlanto-axial (joints)
Sprain of atlanto-occipital (joints)
Whiplash injury of cervical spine

✔x7ᵗʰ **S13.5** **Sprain of thyroid region** PE
Sprain of cricoarytenoid (joint) (ligament)
Sprain of cricothyroid (joint) (ligament)
Sprain of thyroid cartilage

✔x7ᵗʰ **S13.8** **Sprain of joints and ligaments of other parts of neck** PE

✔x7ᵗʰ **S13.9** **Sprain of joints and ligaments of unspecified parts of neck** PE

✔4ᵗʰ **S14** **Injury of nerves and spinal cord at neck level**

NOTE   Code to highest level of cervical cord injury

Code also any associated:
fracture of cervical vertebra (S12.0- — S12.6.-)
open wound of neck (S11.-)
transient paralysis (R29.5)

The appropriate 7th character is to be added to each code from category S14.
AHA: AHA:2024,2Q,23
A   initial encounter
D   subsequent encounter
S   sequela

✔x7ᵗʰ **S14.0** **Concussion and edema of cervical spinal cord** MCC HCC PE

✔5ᵗʰ **S14.1** **Other and unspecified injuries of cervical spinal cord**

✔6ᵗʰ **S14.10** **Unspecified injury of cervical spinal cord**

✔7ᵗʰ **S14.101** **Unspecified injury at C1 level** of cervical spinal cord MCC H5 HCC PE

✔7ᵗʰ **S14.102** **Unspecified injury at C2 level** of cervical spinal cord MCC H5 HCC PE

✔7ᵗʰ **S14.103** **Unspecified injury at C3 level** of cervical spinal cord MCC H5 HCC PE

✔7ᵗʰ **S14.104** **Unspecified injury at C4 level** of cervical spinal cord MCC H5 HCC PE

✔7ᵗʰ **S14.105** **Unspecified injury at C5 level** of cervical spinal cord MCC H5 HCC PE

✔7ᵗʰ **S14.106** **Unspecified injury at C6 level** of cervical spinal cord MCC H5 HCC PE

✔7ᵗʰ **S14.107** **Unspecified injury at C7 level** of cervical spinal cord MCC H5 HCC PE

✔7ᵗʰ **S14.108** **Unspecified injury at C8 level** of cervical spinal cord MCC HCC PE

✔7ᵗʰ **S14.109** **Unspecified injury at unspecified level** of cervical spinal cord MCC PE
Injury of cervical spinal cord NOS

✔6ᵗʰ **S14.11** **Complete lesion of cervical spinal cord**

✔7ᵗʰ **S14.111** **Complete lesion at C1 level** of cervical spinal cord MCC H5 HCC PE

✔7ᵗʰ **S14.112** **Complete lesion at C2 level** of cervical spinal cord MCC H5 HCC PE

✔7ᵗʰ **S14.113** **Complete lesion at C3 level** of cervical spinal cord MCC H5 HCC PE

✔7ᵗʰ **S14.114** **Complete lesion at C4 level** of cervical spinal cord MCC H5 HCC PE

✔7ᵗʰ **S14.115** **Complete lesion at C5 level** of cervical spinal cord MCC H5 HCC PE

✔7ᵗʰ **S14.116** **Complete lesion at C6 level** of cervical spinal cord MCC H5 HCC PE

✔7ᵗʰ **S14.117** **Complete lesion at C7 level** of cervical spinal cord MCC H5 HCC PE

✔7ᵗʰ **S14.118** **Complete lesion at C8 level** of cervical spinal cord MCC HCC PE

✔7ᵗʰ **S14.119** **Complete lesion at unspecified level** of cervical spinal cord HCC PE

✔6ᵗʰ **S14.12** **Central cord syndrome of cervical spinal cord**

✔7ᵗʰ **S14.121** **Central cord syndrome at C1 level** of cervical spinal cord MCC H5 HCC PE

✔7ᵗʰ **S14.122** **Central cord syndrome at C2 level** of cervical spinal cord MCC H5 HCC PE

Chapter 19. Injury, Poisoning and Certain Other Consequences of External Causes

S14.123–S15.191

✓7ᵗʰ **S14.123** Central cord syndrome at C3 level of cervical spinal cord `MCC` `H5` `HCC` `PE`

✓7ᵗʰ **S14.124** Central cord syndrome at C4 level of cervical spinal cord `MCC` `H5` `HCC` `PE`

✓7ᵗʰ **S14.125** Central cord syndrome at C5 level of cervical spinal cord `MCC` `H5` `HCC` `PE`

✓7ᵗʰ **S14.126** Central cord syndrome at C6 level of cervical spinal cord `MCC` `H5` `HCC` `PE`

✓7ᵗʰ **S14.127** Central cord syndrome at C7 level of cervical spinal cord `MCC` `H5` `HCC` `PE`

✓7ᵗʰ **S14.128** Central cord syndrome at C8 level of cervical spinal cord `MCC` `HCC` `PE`

✓7ᵗʰ **S14.129** Central cord syndrome at unspecified level of cervical spinal cord `HCC` `PE`

✓6ᵗʰ **S14.13** Anterior cord syndrome of cervical spinal cord

✓7ᵗʰ **S14.131** Anterior cord syndrome at C1 level of cervical spinal cord `MCC` `H5` `HCC` `PE`

✓7ᵗʰ **S14.132** Anterior cord syndrome at C2 level of cervical spinal cord `MCC` `H5` `HCC` `PE`

✓7ᵗʰ **S14.133** Anterior cord syndrome at C3 level of cervical spinal cord `MCC` `H5` `HCC` `PE`

✓7ᵗʰ **S14.134** Anterior cord syndrome at C4 level of cervical spinal cord `MCC` `H5` `HCC` `PE`

✓7ᵗʰ **S14.135** Anterior cord syndrome at C5 level of cervical spinal cord `MCC` `H5` `HCC` `PE`

✓7ᵗʰ **S14.136** Anterior cord syndrome at C6 level of cervical spinal cord `MCC` `H5` `HCC` `PE`

✓7ᵗʰ **S14.137** Anterior cord syndrome at C7 level of cervical spinal cord `MCC` `H5` `HCC` `PE`

✓7ᵗʰ **S14.138** Anterior cord syndrome at C8 level of cervical spinal cord `MCC` `HCC` `PE`

✓7ᵗʰ **S14.139** Anterior cord syndrome at unspecified level of cervical spinal cord `HCC` `PE`

✓6ᵗʰ **S14.14** Brown-Sequard syndrome of cervical spinal cord

✓7ᵗʰ **S14.141** Brown-Sequard syndrome at C1 level of cervical spinal cord `MCC` `HCC` `PE`

✓7ᵗʰ **S14.142** Brown-Sequard syndrome at C2 level of cervical spinal cord `MCC` `HCC` `PE`

✓7ᵗʰ **S14.143** Brown-Sequard syndrome at C3 level of cervical spinal cord `MCC` `HCC` `PE`

✓7ᵗʰ **S14.144** Brown-Sequard syndrome at C4 level of cervical spinal cord `MCC` `HCC` `PE`

✓7ᵗʰ **S14.145** Brown-Sequard syndrome at C5 level of cervical spinal cord `MCC` `HCC` `PE`

✓7ᵗʰ **S14.146** Brown-Sequard syndrome at C6 level of cervical spinal cord `MCC` `HCC` `PE`

✓7ᵗʰ **S14.147** Brown-Sequard syndrome at C7 level of cervical spinal cord `MCC` `HCC` `PE`

✓7ᵗʰ **S14.148** Brown-Sequard syndrome at C8 level of cervical spinal cord `MCC` `HCC` `PE`

✓7ᵗʰ **S14.149** Brown-Sequard syndrome at unspecified level of cervical spinal cord `HCC` `PE`

✓6ᵗʰ **S14.15** Other incomplete lesions of cervical spinal cord

Incomplete lesion of cervical spinal cord NOS
Posterior cord syndrome of cervical spinal cord

✓7ᵗʰ **S14.151** Other incomplete lesion at C1 level of cervical spinal cord `MCC` `H5` `HCC` `PE`

✓7ᵗʰ **S14.152** Other incomplete lesion at C2 level of cervical spinal cord `MCC` `H5` `HCC` `PE`

✓7ᵗʰ **S14.153** Other incomplete lesion at C3 level of cervical spinal cord `MCC` `H5` `HCC` `PE`

✓7ᵗʰ **S14.154** Other incomplete lesion at C4 level of cervical spinal cord `MCC` `H5` `HCC` `PE`

✓7ᵗʰ **S14.155** Other incomplete lesion at C5 level of cervical spinal cord `MCC` `H5` `HCC` `PE`

✓7ᵗʰ **S14.156** Other incomplete lesion at C6 level of cervical spinal cord `MCC` `H5` `HCC` `PE`

✓7ᵗʰ **S14.157** Other incomplete lesion at C7 level of cervical spinal cord `MCC` `H5` `HCC` `PE`

✓7ᵗʰ **S14.158** Other incomplete lesion at C8 level of cervical spinal cord `MCC` `HCC` `PE`

✓7ᵗʰ **S14.159** Other incomplete lesion at unspecified level of cervical spinal cord `HCC` `PE`

✓x7ᵗʰ **S14.2** Injury of nerve root of cervical spine `PE`

✓x7ᵗʰ **S14.3** Injury of brachial plexus `PE`

✓x7ᵗʰ **S14.4** Injury of peripheral nerves of neck `PE`

✓x7ᵗʰ **S14.5** Injury of cervical sympathetic nerves `PE`

✓x7ᵗʰ **S14.8** Injury of other specified nerves of neck `PE`

✓x7ᵗʰ **S14.9** Injury of unspecified nerves of neck `PE`

✓4ᵗʰ **S15** Injury of blood vessels at neck level

Code also any associated open wound (S11.-)

The appropriate 7th character is to be added to each code from category S15.
A   initial encounter
D   subsequent encounter
S   sequela

✓5ᵗʰ **S15.0** Injury of carotid artery of neck

Injury of carotid artery (common) (external) (internal, extracranial portion)
Injury of carotid artery NOS

EXCLUDES 1   injury of internal carotid artery, intracranial portion (S06.8)

✓6ᵗʰ **S15.00** Unspecified injury of carotid artery

✓7ᵗʰ **S15.001** Unspecified injury of right carotid artery `CC` `PE`

✓7ᵗʰ **S15.002** Unspecified injury of left carotid artery `CC` `PE`

✓7ᵗʰ **S15.009** Unspecified injury of unspecified carotid artery `CC` `UNS` `PE`

✓6ᵗʰ **S15.01** Minor laceration of carotid artery

Incomplete transection of carotid artery
Laceration of carotid artery NOS
Superficial laceration of carotid artery

✓7ᵗʰ **S15.011** Minor laceration of right carotid artery `CC` `PE`

✓7ᵗʰ **S15.012** Minor laceration of left carotid artery `CC` `PE`

✓7ᵗʰ **S15.019** Minor laceration of unspecified carotid artery `CC` `UNS` `PE`

✓6ᵗʰ **S15.02** Major laceration of carotid artery

Complete transection of carotid artery
Traumatic rupture of carotid artery

✓7ᵗʰ **S15.021** Major laceration of right carotid artery `CC` `PE`

✓7ᵗʰ **S15.022** Major laceration of left carotid artery `CC` `PE`

✓7ᵗʰ **S15.029** Major laceration of unspecified carotid artery `CC` `UNS` `PE`

✓6ᵗʰ **S15.09** Other specified injury of carotid artery

✓7ᵗʰ **S15.091** Other specified injury of right carotid artery `CC` `PE`

✓7ᵗʰ **S15.092** Other specified injury of left carotid artery `CC` `PE`

✓7ᵗʰ **S15.099** Other specified injury of unspecified carotid artery `CC` `UNS` `PE`

✓5ᵗʰ **S15.1** Injury of vertebral artery

✓6ᵗʰ **S15.10** Unspecified injury of vertebral artery

✓7ᵗʰ **S15.101** Unspecified injury of right vertebral artery `CC` `PE`

✓7ᵗʰ **S15.102** Unspecified injury of left vertebral artery `CC` `PE`

✓7ᵗʰ **S15.109** Unspecified injury of unspecified vertebral artery `CC` `UNS` `PE`

✓6ᵗʰ **S15.11** Minor laceration of vertebral artery

Incomplete transection of vertebral artery
Laceration of vertebral artery NOS
Superficial laceration of vertebral artery

✓7ᵗʰ **S15.111** Minor laceration of right vertebral artery `CC` `PE`

✓7ᵗʰ **S15.112** Minor laceration of left vertebral artery `CC` `PE`

✓7ᵗʰ **S15.119** Minor laceration of unspecified vertebral artery `CC` `UNS` `PE`

✓6ᵗʰ **S15.12** Major laceration of vertebral artery

Complete transection of vertebral artery
Traumatic rupture of vertebral artery

✓7ᵗʰ **S15.121** Major laceration of right vertebral artery `CC` `PE`

✓7ᵗʰ **S15.122** Major laceration of left vertebral artery `CC` `PE`

✓7ᵗʰ **S15.129** Major laceration of unspecified vertebral artery `CC` `UNS` `PE`

✓6ᵗʰ **S15.19** Other specified injury of vertebral artery

✓7ᵗʰ **S15.191** Other specified injury of right vertebral artery `CC` `PE`

√7ᵗʰ **S15.192** Other specified injury of left vertebral artery   CC PE

√7ᵗʰ **S15.199** Other specified injury of unspecified vertebral artery   CC UNS PE

√5ᵗʰ **S15.2** Injury of external jugular vein

  √6ᵗʰ **S15.20** Unspecified injury of external jugular vein

    √7ᵗʰ **S15.201** Unspecified injury of right external jugular vein   CC PE

    √7ᵗʰ **S15.202** Unspecified injury of left external jugular vein   CC PE

    √7ᵗʰ **S15.209** Unspecified injury of unspecified external jugular vein   CC UNS PE

  √6ᵗʰ **S15.21** Minor laceration of external jugular vein

    Incomplete transection of external jugular vein
    Laceration of external jugular vein NOS
    Superficial laceration of external jugular vein

    √7ᵗʰ **S15.211** Minor laceration of right external jugular vein   CC PE

    √7ᵗʰ **S15.212** Minor laceration of left external jugular vein   CC PE

    √7ᵗʰ **S15.219** Minor laceration of unspecified external jugular vein   CC UNS PE

  √6ᵗʰ **S15.22** Major laceration of external jugular vein

    Complete transection of external jugular vein
    Traumatic rupture of external jugular vein

    √7ᵗʰ **S15.221** Major laceration of right external jugular vein   CC PE

    √7ᵗʰ **S15.222** Major laceration of left external jugular vein   CC PE

    √7ᵗʰ **S15.229** Major laceration of unspecified external jugular vein   CC UNS PE

  √6ᵗʰ **S15.29** Other specified injury of external jugular vein

    √7ᵗʰ **S15.291** Other specified injury of right external jugular vein   CC PE

    √7ᵗʰ **S15.292** Other specified injury of left external jugular vein   CC PE

    √7ᵗʰ **S15.299** Other specified injury of unspecified external jugular vein   CC UNS PE

√5ᵗʰ **S15.3** Injury of internal jugular vein

  √6ᵗʰ **S15.30** Unspecified injury of internal jugular vein

    √7ᵗʰ **S15.301** Unspecified injury of right internal jugular vein   CC PE

    √7ᵗʰ **S15.302** Unspecified injury of left internal jugular vein   CC PE

    √7ᵗʰ **S15.309** Unspecified injury of unspecified internal jugular vein   CC UNS PE

  √6ᵗʰ **S15.31** Minor laceration of internal jugular vein

    Incomplete transection of internal jugular vein
    Laceration of internal jugular vein NOS
    Superficial laceration of internal jugular vein

    √7ᵗʰ **S15.311** Minor laceration of right internal jugular vein   CC PE

    √7ᵗʰ **S15.312** Minor laceration of left internal jugular vein   CC PE

    √7ᵗʰ **S15.319** Minor laceration of unspecified internal jugular vein   CC UNS PE

  √6ᵗʰ **S15.32** Major laceration of internal jugular vein

    Complete transection of internal jugular vein
    Traumatic rupture of internal jugular vein

    √7ᵗʰ **S15.321** Major laceration of right internal jugular vein   CC PE

    √7ᵗʰ **S15.322** Major laceration of left internal jugular vein   CC PE

    √7ᵗʰ **S15.329** Major laceration of unspecified internal jugular vein   CC UNS PE

  √6ᵗʰ **S15.39** Other specified injury of internal jugular vein

    √7ᵗʰ **S15.391** Other specified injury of right internal jugular vein   CC PE

    √7ᵗʰ **S15.392** Other specified injury of left internal jugular vein   CC PE

    √7ᵗʰ **S15.399** Other specified injury of unspecified internal jugular vein   CC UNS PE

√x7ᵗʰ **S15.8** Injury of other specified blood vessels at neck level   CC PE

√x7ᵗʰ **S15.9** Injury of unspecified blood vessel at neck level   CC PE

√4ᵗʰ **S16** Injury of muscle, fascia and tendon at neck level

  Code also any associated open wound (S11.-)

  EXCLUDES 2   *sprain of joint or ligament at neck level (S13.9)*

  The appropriate 7th character is to be added to each code from category S16.
  A   initial encounter
  D   subsequent encounter
  S   sequela

√x7ᵗʰ **S16.1** Strain of muscle, fascia and tendon at neck level   PE

√x7ᵗʰ **S16.2** Laceration of muscle, fascia and tendon at neck level   PE

√x7ᵗʰ **S16.8** Other specified injury of muscle, fascia and tendon at neck level   PE

√x7ᵗʰ **S16.9** Unspecified injury of muscle, fascia and tendon at neck level   PE

√4ᵗʰ **S17** Crushing injury of neck

  Use additional code for all associated injuries, such as:
    injury of blood vessels (S15.-)
    open wound of neck (S11.-)
    spinal cord injury (S14.0, S14.1-)
    vertebral fracture (S12.0- — S12.3-)

  The appropriate 7th character is to be added to each code from category S17.
  A   initial encounter
  D   subsequent encounter
  S   sequela

√x7ᵗʰ **S17.0** Crushing injury of larynx and trachea   CC H5 PE

√x7ᵗʰ **S17.8** Crushing injury of other specified parts of neck   CC H5 PE

√x7ᵗʰ **S17.9** Crushing injury of neck, part unspecified   CC H5 PE

√4ᵗʰ **S19** Other specified and unspecified injuries of neck

  The appropriate 7th character is to be added to each code from category S19.
  A   initial encounter
  D   subsequent encounter
  S   sequela

√5ᵗʰ **S19.8** Other specified injuries of neck

  √x7ᵗʰ **S19.80** Other specified injuries of unspecified part of neck   PE

  √x7ᵗʰ **S19.81** Other specified injuries of larynx   PE

  √x7ᵗʰ **S19.82** Other specified injuries of cervical trachea   PE

    EXCLUDES 2   *other specified injury of thoracic trachea (S27.5-)*

  √x7ᵗʰ **S19.83** Other specified injuries of vocal cord   PE

  √x7ᵗʰ **S19.84** Other specified injuries of thyroid gland   PE

  √x7ᵗʰ **S19.85** Other specified injuries of pharynx and cervical esophagus   PE
    AHA: 2022,1Q,27

  √x7ᵗʰ **S19.89** Other specified injuries of other specified part of neck   PE

√x7ᵗʰ **S19.9** Unspecified injury of neck   PE

Additional Character Required   √x7ᵗʰ Placeholder   Questionable PDx   Manifestation   Unspecified   UPD Unacceptable PDx   H1 - H14 HAC   HCC CMS-HCC Dx   HIV HIV Dx

ICD-10-CM 2025   1003

Injuries to the thorax (S20-S29)

INCLUDES
injuries of breast
injuries of chest (wall)
injuries of interscapular area

EXCLUDES 2
burns and corrosions (T20-T32)
effects of foreign body in bronchus (T17.5)
effects of foreign body in esophagus (T18.1)
effects of foreign body in lung (T17.8)
effects of foreign body in trachea (T17.4)
frostbite (T33-T34)
injuries of axilla
injuries of clavicle
injuries of scapular region
injuries of shoulder
insect bite or sting, venomous (T63.4)

√4ᵗʰ **S20   Superficial injury of thorax**

AHA: 2020,4Q,39

The appropriate 7th character is to be added to each code from category S20.
A   initial encounter
D   subsequent encounter
S   sequela

√5ᵗʰ **S20.0   Contusion of breast**

√x7ᵗʰ **S20.00   Contusion of breast, unspecified breast**   PE

√x7ᵗʰ **S20.01   Contusion of right breast**   PE

√x7ᵗʰ **S20.02   Contusion of left breast**   PE

√5ᵗʰ **S20.1   Other and unspecified superficial injuries of breast**

√6ᵗʰ **S20.10   Unspecified superficial injuries of breast**

√7ᵗʰ **S20.101   Unspecified superficial injuries of breast, right breast**   PE

√7ᵗʰ **S20.102   Unspecified superficial injuries of breast, left breast**   PE

√7ᵗʰ **S20.109   Unspecified superficial injuries of breast, unspecified breast**   PE

√6ᵗʰ **S20.11   Abrasion of breast**

√7ᵗʰ **S20.111   Abrasion of breast, right breast**   PE

√7ᵗʰ **S20.112   Abrasion of breast, left breast**   PE

√7ᵗʰ **S20.119   Abrasion of breast, unspecified breast**   PE

√6ᵗʰ **S20.12   Blister (nonthermal) of breast**

√7ᵗʰ **S20.121   Blister (nonthermal) of breast, right breast**   PE

√7ᵗʰ **S20.122   Blister (nonthermal) of breast, left breast**   PE

√7ᵗʰ **S20.129   Blister (nonthermal) of breast, unspecified breast**   PE

√6ᵗʰ **S20.14   External constriction of part of breast**

√7ᵗʰ **S20.141   External constriction of part of breast, right breast**   PE

√7ᵗʰ **S20.142   External constriction of part of breast, left breast**   PE

√7ᵗʰ **S20.149   External constriction of part of breast, unspecified breast**   PE

√6ᵗʰ **S20.15   Superficial foreign body of breast**
Splinter in the breast

√7ᵗʰ **S20.151   Superficial foreign body of breast, right breast**   PE

√7ᵗʰ **S20.152   Superficial foreign body of breast, left breast**   PE

√7ᵗʰ **S20.159   Superficial foreign body of breast, unspecified breast**   PE

√6ᵗʰ **S20.16   Insect bite (nonvenomous) of breast**

√7ᵗʰ **S20.161   Insect bite (nonvenomous) of breast, right breast**   PE

√7ᵗʰ **S20.162   Insect bite (nonvenomous) of breast, left breast**   PE

√7ᵗʰ **S20.169   Insect bite (nonvenomous) of breast, unspecified breast**   PE

√6ᵗʰ **S20.17   Other superficial bite of breast**

EXCLUDES 1   *open bite of breast (S21.05-)*

√7ᵗʰ **S20.171   Other superficial bite of breast, right breast**   PE

√7ᵗʰ **S20.172   Other superficial bite of breast, left breast**   PE

√7ᵗʰ **S20.179   Other superficial bite of breast, unspecified breast**   PE

√5ᵗʰ **S20.2   Contusion of thorax**

√x7ᵗʰ **S20.20   Contusion of thorax, unspecified**   PE

√6ᵗʰ **S20.21   Contusion of front wall of thorax**

√7ᵗʰ **S20.211   Contusion of right front wall of thorax**   PE

√7ᵗʰ **S20.212   Contusion of left front wall of thorax**   PE

√7ᵗʰ **S20.213   Contusion of bilateral front wall of thorax**   PE

√7ᵗʰ **S20.214   Contusion of middle front wall of thorax**   PE

√7ᵗʰ **S20.219   Contusion of unspecified front wall of thorax**   PE

√6ᵗʰ **S20.22   Contusion of back wall of thorax**

√7ᵗʰ **S20.221   Contusion of right back wall of thorax**   PE

√7ᵗʰ **S20.222   Contusion of left back wall of thorax**   PE

√7ᵗʰ **S20.223   Contusion of bilateral back wall of thorax**   PE

√7ᵗʰ **S20.224   Contusion of middle back wall of thorax**   PE

√7ᵗʰ **S20.229   Contusion of unspecified back wall of thorax**   PE

√5ᵗʰ **S20.3   Other and unspecified superficial injuries of front wall of thorax**

√6ᵗʰ **S20.30   Unspecified superficial injuries of front wall of thorax**

√7ᵗʰ **S20.301   Unspecified superficial injuries of right front wall of thorax**   PE

√7ᵗʰ **S20.302   Unspecified superficial injuries of left front wall of thorax**   PE

√7ᵗʰ **S20.303   Unspecified superficial injuries of bilateral front wall of thorax**   PE

√7ᵗʰ **S20.304   Unspecified superficial injuries of middle front wall of thorax**   PE

√7ᵗʰ **S20.309   Unspecified superficial injuries of unspecified front wall of thorax**   PE

√6ᵗʰ **S20.31   Abrasion of front wall of thorax**

√7ᵗʰ **S20.311   Abrasion of right front wall of thorax**   PE

√7ᵗʰ **S20.312   Abrasion of left front wall of thorax**   PE

√7ᵗʰ **S20.313   Abrasion of bilateral front wall of thorax**   PE

√7ᵗʰ **S20.314   Abrasion of middle front wall of thorax**   PE

√7ᵗʰ **S20.319   Abrasion of unspecified front wall of thorax**   PE

√6ᵗʰ **S20.32   Blister (nonthermal) of front wall of thorax**

√7ᵗʰ **S20.321   Blister (nonthermal) of right front wall of thorax**   PE

√7ᵗʰ **S20.322   Blister (nonthermal) of left front wall of thorax**   PE

√7ᵗʰ **S20.323   Blister (nonthermal) of bilateral front wall of thorax**   PE

√7ᵗʰ **S20.324   Blister (nonthermal) of middle front wall of thorax**   PE

√7ᵗʰ **S20.329   Blister (nonthermal) of unspecified front wall of thorax**   PE

√6ᵗʰ **S20.34   External constriction of front wall of thorax**

√7ᵗʰ **S20.341   External constriction of right front wall of thorax**   PE

√7ᵗʰ **S20.342   External constriction of left front wall of thorax**   PE

√7ᵗʰ **S20.343   External constriction of bilateral front wall of thorax**   PE

√7ᵗʰ **S20.344   External constriction of middle front wall of thorax**   PE

√7ᵗʰ **S20.349   External constriction of unspecified front wall of thorax**   PE

√6ᵗʰ **S20.35   Superficial foreign body of front wall of thorax**
Splinter in front wall of thorax

√7ᵗʰ **S20.351   Superficial foreign body of right front wall of thorax**   PE

√7ᵗʰ **S20.352   Superficial foreign body of left front wall of thorax**   PE

N Newborn: 0   P Pediatric: 0-17   M Maternity: 9-64   A Adult: 15-124   UNS Unspecified Site   MCC Major Complication/Comorbidity   CC Complication/Comorbidity   PE POA Exempt

1004   ICD-10-CM 2025

☑7ᵗʰ **S20.353** Superficial foreign body of **bilateral** front wall of thorax   PE

☑7ᵗʰ **S20.354** Superficial foreign body of **middle** front wall of thorax   PE

☑7ᵗʰ **S20.359** Superficial foreign body of unspecified front wall of thorax   PE

✓6ᵗʰ **S20.36** Insect bite (nonvenomous) of front wall of thorax

☑7ᵗʰ **S20.361** Insect bite (nonvenomous) of **right** front wall of thorax   PE

☑7ᵗʰ **S20.362** Insect bite (nonvenomous) of **left** front wall of thorax   PE

☑7ᵗʰ **S20.363** Insect bite (nonvenomous) of **bilateral** front wall of thorax   PE

☑7ᵗʰ **S20.364** Insect bite (nonvenomous) of **middle** front wall of thorax   PE

☑7ᵗʰ **S20.369** Insect bite (nonvenomous) of unspecified front wall of thorax   PE

✓6ᵗʰ **S20.37** Other superficial **bite** of front wall of thorax

EXCLUDES 1   *open bite of front wall of thorax (S21.15)*

☑7ᵗʰ **S20.371** Other superficial bite of **right** front wall of thorax   PE

☑7ᵗʰ **S20.372** Other superficial bite of **left** front wall of thorax   PE

☑7ᵗʰ **S20.373** Other superficial bite of **bilateral** front wall of thorax   PE

☑7ᵗʰ **S20.374** Other superficial bite of **middle** front wall of thorax   PE

☑7ᵗʰ **S20.379** Other superficial bite of unspecified front wall of thorax   PE

✓5ᵗʰ **S20.4** Other and unspecified superficial injuries of **back wall of thorax**

✓6ᵗʰ **S20.40** Unspecified superficial injuries of back wall of thorax

☑7ᵗʰ **S20.401** Unspecified superficial injuries of **right** back wall of thorax   PE

☑7ᵗʰ **S20.402** Unspecified superficial injuries of **left** back wall of thorax   PE

☑7ᵗʰ **S20.409** Unspecified superficial injuries of unspecified back wall of thorax   PE

✓6ᵗʰ **S20.41** **Abrasion** of back wall of thorax

☑7ᵗʰ **S20.411** Abrasion of **right** back wall of thorax   PE

☑7ᵗʰ **S20.412** Abrasion of **left** back wall of thorax   PE

☑7ᵗʰ **S20.419** Abrasion of unspecified back wall of thorax   PE

✓6ᵗʰ **S20.42** **Blister** (nonthermal) of back wall of thorax

☑7ᵗʰ **S20.421** Blister (nonthermal) of **right** back wall of thorax   PE

☑7ᵗʰ **S20.422** Blister (nonthermal) of **left** back wall of thorax   PE

☑7ᵗʰ **S20.429** Blister (nonthermal) of unspecified back wall of thorax   PE

✓6ᵗʰ **S20.44** **External constriction** of back wall of thorax

☑7ᵗʰ **S20.441** External constriction of **right** back wall of thorax   PE

☑7ᵗʰ **S20.442** External constriction of **left** back wall of thorax   PE

☑7ᵗʰ **S20.449** External constriction of unspecified back wall of thorax   PE

✓6ᵗʰ **S20.45** Superficial **foreign body** of back wall of thorax

Splinter of back wall of thorax

☑7ᵗʰ **S20.451** Superficial foreign body of **right** back wall of thorax   PE

☑7ᵗʰ **S20.452** Superficial foreign body of **left** back wall of thorax   PE

☑7ᵗʰ **S20.459** Superficial foreign body of unspecified back wall of thorax   PE

✓6ᵗʰ **S20.46** **Insect bite** (nonvenomous) of back wall of thorax

☑7ᵗʰ **S20.461** Insect bite (nonvenomous) of **right** back wall of thorax   PE

☑7ᵗʰ **S20.462** Insect bite (nonvenomous) of **left** back wall of thorax   PE

☑7ᵗʰ **S20.469** Insect bite (nonvenomous) of unspecified back wall of thorax   PE

✓6ᵗʰ **S20.47** Other superficial **bite** of back wall of thorax

EXCLUDES 1   *open bite of back wall of thorax (S21.25)*

☑7ᵗʰ **S20.471** Other superficial bite of **right** back wall of thorax

---

☑7ᵗʰ **S20.472** Other superficial bite of **left** back wall of thorax   PE

☑7ᵗʰ **S20.479** Other superficial bite of unspecified back wall of thorax   PE

✓5ᵗʰ **S20.9** **Superficial injury** of unspecified parts of thorax

EXCLUDES 1   *contusion of thorax NOS (S20.20)*

✓×7ᵗʰ **S20.90** Unspecified superficial injury of unspecified parts of thorax   PE

Superficial injury of thoracic wall NOS

✓×7ᵗʰ **S20.91** **Abrasion** of unspecified parts of thorax   PE

✓×7ᵗʰ **S20.92** **Blister** (nonthermal) of unspecified parts of thorax   PE

✓×7ᵗʰ **S20.94** **External constriction** of unspecified parts of thorax   PE

✓×7ᵗʰ **S20.95** Superficial **foreign body** of unspecified parts of thorax   PE

Splinter in thorax NOS

✓×7ᵗʰ **S20.96** **Insect bite** (nonvenomous) of unspecified parts of thorax   PE

✓×7ᵗʰ **S20.97** Other superficial **bite** of unspecified parts of thorax   PE

EXCLUDES 1   *open bite of thorax NOS (S21.95)*

✓4ᵗʰ **S21** **Open wound of thorax**

Code also any associated injury, such as:

injury of heart (S26.-)
injury of intrathoracic organs (S27.-)
rib fracture (S22.3-, S22.4-)
spinal cord injury (S24.0-, S24.1-)
traumatic hemopneumothorax (S27.3)
traumatic hemothorax (S27.1)
traumatic pneumothorax (S27.0)
wound infection

EXCLUDES 1   *traumatic amputation (partial) of thorax (S28.1)*

> The appropriate 7th character is to be added to each code from category S21.
> A   initial encounter
> D   subsequent encounter
> S   sequela

✓5ᵗʰ **S21.0** **Open wound of breast**

✓6ᵗʰ **S21.00** Unspecified open wound of breast

☑7ᵗʰ **S21.001** Unspecified open wound of **right** breast   PE

☑7ᵗʰ **S21.002** Unspecified open wound of **left** breast   PE

☑7ᵗʰ **S21.009** Unspecified open wound of unspecified breast   PE

✓6ᵗʰ **S21.01** **Laceration without foreign body** of breast

☑7ᵗʰ **S21.011** Laceration without foreign body of **right** breast   PE

☑7ᵗʰ **S21.012** Laceration without foreign body of **left** breast   PE

☑7ᵗʰ **S21.019** Laceration without foreign body of unspecified breast   PE

✓6ᵗʰ **S21.02** **Laceration with foreign body** of breast

☑7ᵗʰ **S21.021** Laceration with foreign body of **right** breast   PE

☑7ᵗʰ **S21.022** Laceration with foreign body of **left** breast   PE

☑7ᵗʰ **S21.029** Laceration with foreign body of unspecified breast   PE

✓6ᵗʰ **S21.03** **Puncture wound without foreign body** of breast

☑7ᵗʰ **S21.031** Puncture wound without foreign body of **right** breast   PE

☑7ᵗʰ **S21.032** Puncture wound without foreign body of **left** breast   PE

☑7ᵗʰ **S21.039** Puncture wound without foreign body of unspecified breast   PE

✓6ᵗʰ **S21.04** **Puncture wound with foreign body** of breast

☑7ᵗʰ **S21.041** Puncture wound with foreign body of **right** breast   PE

☑7ᵗʰ **S21.042** Puncture wound with foreign body of **left** breast   PE

☑7ᵗʰ **S21.049** Puncture wound with foreign body of unspecified breast

☑ Additional Character Required   ✓×7ᵗʰ Placeholder   Questionable PDx   Manifestation   Unspecified   UPD Unacceptable PDx   H1-H14 HAC   HCC CMS-HCC Dx   HIV HIV Dx

ICD-10-CM 2025   **1005**

√6ᵗʰ **S21.05** Open bite of breast
Bite of breast NOS
EXCLUDES 1   superficial bite of breast (S20.17)

√7ᵗʰ **S21.051** Open bite of right breast   PE

√7ᵗʰ **S21.052** Open bite of left breast   PE

√7ᵗʰ **S21.059** Open bite of unspecified breast   PE

√5ᵗʰ **S21.1** Open wound of front wall of thorax without penetration into thoracic cavity
Open wound of chest without penetration into thoracic cavity

√6ᵗʰ **S21.10** Unspecified open wound of front wall of thorax without penetration into thoracic cavity

√7ᵗʰ **S21.101** Unspecified open wound of right front wall of thorax without penetration into thoracic cavity   CC PE

√7ᵗʰ **S21.102** Unspecified open wound of left front wall of thorax without penetration into thoracic cavity   CC PE

√7ᵗʰ **S21.109** Unspecified open wound of unspecified front wall of thorax without penetration into thoracic cavity   CC UNS PE

√6ᵗʰ **S21.11** Laceration without foreign body of front wall of thorax without penetration into thoracic cavity

√7ᵗʰ **S21.111** Laceration without foreign body of right front wall of thorax without penetration into thoracic cavity   CC PE

√7ᵗʰ **S21.112** Laceration without foreign body of left front wall of thorax without penetration into thoracic cavity   CC PE

√7ᵗʰ **S21.119** Laceration without foreign body of unspecified front wall of thorax without penetration into thoracic cavity   CC UNS PE

√6ᵗʰ **S21.12** Laceration with foreign body of front wall of thorax without penetration into thoracic cavity

√7ᵗʰ **S21.121** Laceration with foreign body of right front wall of thorax without penetration into thoracic cavity   CC PE

√7ᵗʰ **S21.122** Laceration with foreign body of left front wall of thorax without penetration into thoracic cavity   CC PE

√7ᵗʰ **S21.129** Laceration with foreign body of unspecified front wall of thorax without penetration into thoracic cavity   CC UNS PE

√6ᵗʰ **S21.13** Puncture wound without foreign body of front wall of thorax without penetration into thoracic cavity

√7ᵗʰ **S21.131** Puncture wound without foreign body of right front wall of thorax without penetration into thoracic cavity   CC PE

√7ᵗʰ **S21.132** Puncture wound without foreign body of left front wall of thorax without penetration into thoracic cavity   CC PE

√7ᵗʰ **S21.139** Puncture wound without foreign body of unspecified front wall of thorax without penetration into thoracic cavity   CC UNS PE

√6ᵗʰ **S21.14** Puncture wound with foreign body of front wall of thorax without penetration into thoracic cavity

√7ᵗʰ **S21.141** Puncture wound with foreign body of right front wall of thorax without penetration into thoracic cavity   CC PE

√7ᵗʰ **S21.142** Puncture wound with foreign body of left front wall of thorax without penetration into thoracic cavity   CC PE

√7ᵗʰ **S21.149** Puncture wound with foreign body of unspecified front wall of thorax without penetration into thoracic cavity   CC UNS PE

√6ᵗʰ **S21.15** Open bite of front wall of thorax without penetration into thoracic cavity
Bite of front wall of thorax NOS
EXCLUDES 1   superficial bite of front wall of thorax (S20.37)

√7ᵗʰ **S21.151** Open bite of right front wall of thorax without penetration into thoracic cavity   CC PE

√7ᵗʰ **S21.152** Open bite of left front wall of thorax without penetration into thoracic cavity   CC PE

√7ᵗʰ **S21.159** Open bite of unspecified front wall of thorax without penetration into thoracic cavity   CC UNS PE

√5ᵗʰ **S21.2** Open wound of back wall of thorax without penetration into thoracic cavity

√6ᵗʰ **S21.20** Unspecified open wound of back wall of thorax without penetration into thoracic cavity

√7ᵗʰ **S21.201** Unspecified open wound of right back wall of thorax without penetration into thoracic cavity   PE

√7ᵗʰ **S21.202** Unspecified open wound of left back wall of thorax without penetration into thoracic cavity   PE

√7ᵗʰ **S21.209** Unspecified open wound of unspecified back wall of thorax without penetration into thoracic cavity   PE

√6ᵗʰ **S21.21** Laceration without foreign body of back wall of thorax without penetration into thoracic cavity

√7ᵗʰ **S21.211** Laceration without foreign body of right back wall of thorax without penetration into thoracic cavity   PE

√7ᵗʰ **S21.212** Laceration without foreign body of left back wall of thorax without penetration into thoracic cavity   PE

√7ᵗʰ **S21.219** Laceration without foreign body of unspecified back wall of thorax without penetration into thoracic cavity   PE

√6ᵗʰ **S21.22** Laceration with foreign body of back wall of thorax without penetration into thoracic cavity

√7ᵗʰ **S21.221** Laceration with foreign body of right back wall of thorax without penetration into thoracic cavity   PE

√7ᵗʰ **S21.222** Laceration with foreign body of left back wall of thorax without penetration into thoracic cavity   PE

√7ᵗʰ **S21.229** Laceration with foreign body of unspecified back wall of thorax without penetration into thoracic cavity   PE

√6ᵗʰ **S21.23** Puncture wound without foreign body of back wall of thorax without penetration into thoracic cavity

√7ᵗʰ **S21.231** Puncture wound without foreign body of right back wall of thorax without penetration into thoracic cavity   PE

√7ᵗʰ **S21.232** Puncture wound without foreign body of left back wall of thorax without penetration into thoracic cavity   PE

√7ᵗʰ **S21.239** Puncture wound without foreign body of unspecified back wall of thorax without penetration into thoracic cavity   PE

√6ᵗʰ **S21.24** Puncture wound with foreign body of back wall of thorax without penetration into thoracic cavity

√7ᵗʰ **S21.241** Puncture wound with foreign body of right back wall of thorax without penetration into thoracic cavity   PE

√7ᵗʰ **S21.242** Puncture wound with foreign body of left back wall of thorax without penetration into thoracic cavity   PE

√7ᵗʰ **S21.249** Puncture wound with foreign body of unspecified back wall of thorax without penetration into thoracic cavity   PE

√6ᵗʰ **S21.25** Open bite of back wall of thorax without penetration into thoracic cavity
Bite of back wall of thorax NOS
EXCLUDES 1   superficial bite of back wall of thorax (S20.47)

√7ᵗʰ **S21.251** Open bite of right back wall of thorax without penetration into thoracic cavity   PE

√7ᵗʰ **S21.252** Open bite of left back wall of thorax without penetration into thoracic cavity   PE

√7ᵗʰ **S21.259** Open bite of unspecified back wall of thorax without penetration into thoracic cavity   PE

√5ᵗʰ **S21.3** Open wound of front wall of thorax with penetration into thoracic cavity
Open wound of chest with penetration into thoracic cavity

√6ᵗʰ **S21.30** Unspecified open wound of front wall of thorax with penetration into thoracic cavity

√7ᵗʰ **S21.301** Unspecified open wound of right front wall of thorax with penetration into thoracic cavity   MCC PE

√7ᵗʰ **S21.302** Unspecified open wound of left front wall of thorax with penetration into thoracic cavity   MCC PE

√7ᵗʰ **S21.309** Unspecified open wound of unspecified front wall of thorax with penetration into thoracic cavity `MCC` `UNS` `PE`

√6ᵗʰ **S21.31** Laceration without foreign body of front wall of thorax with penetration into thoracic cavity

√7ᵗʰ **S21.311** Laceration without foreign body of right front wall of thorax with penetration into thoracic cavity `MCC` `PE`

√7ᵗʰ **S21.312** Laceration without foreign body of left front wall of thorax with penetration into thoracic cavity `MCC` `PE`

√7ᵗʰ **S21.319** Laceration without foreign body of unspecified front wall of thorax with penetration into thoracic cavity `MCC` `UNS` `PE`

√6ᵗʰ **S21.32** Laceration with foreign body of front wall of thorax with penetration into thoracic cavity

√7ᵗʰ **S21.321** Laceration with foreign body of right front wall of thorax with penetration into thoracic cavity `MCC` `PE`

√7ᵗʰ **S21.322** Laceration with foreign body of left front wall of thorax with penetration into thoracic cavity `MCC` `PE`

√7ᵗʰ **S21.329** Laceration with foreign body of unspecified front wall of thorax with penetration into thoracic cavity `MCC` `UNS` `PE`

√6ᵗʰ **S21.33** Puncture wound without foreign body of front wall of thorax with penetration into thoracic cavity

√7ᵗʰ **S21.331** Puncture wound without foreign body of right front wall of thorax with penetration into thoracic cavity `MCC` `PE`

√7ᵗʰ **S21.332** Puncture wound without foreign body of left front wall of thorax with penetration into thoracic cavity `MCC` `PE`

√7ᵗʰ **S21.339** Puncture wound without foreign body of unspecified front wall of thorax with penetration into thoracic cavity `MCC` `UNS` `PE`

√6ᵗʰ **S21.34** Puncture wound with foreign body of front wall of thorax with penetration into thoracic cavity

√7ᵗʰ **S21.341** Puncture wound with foreign body of right front wall of thorax with penetration into thoracic cavity `MCC` `FE`

√7ᵗʰ **S21.342** Puncture wound with foreign body of left front wall of thorax with penetration into thoracic cavity `MCC` `FE`

√7ᵗʰ **S21.349** Puncture wound with foreign body of unspecified front wall of thorax with penetration into thoracic cavity `MCC` `UNS` `FE`

√6ᵗʰ **S21.35** Open bite of front wall of thorax with penetration into thoracic cavity

> **EXCLUDES 1**   superficial bite of front wall of thorax (S20.37)

√7ᵗʰ **S21.351** Open bite of right front wall of thorax with penetration into thoracic cavity `MCC` `PE`

√7ᵗʰ **S21.352** Open bite of left front wall of thorax with penetration into thoracic cavity `MCC` `PE`

√7ᵗʰ **S21.359** Open bite of unspecified front wall of thorax with penetration into thoracic cavity `MCC` `UNS` `PE`

√5ᵗʰ **S21.4** Open wound of back wall of thorax with penetration into thoracic cavity

√6ᵗʰ **S21.40** Unspecified open wound of back wall of thorax with penetration into thoracic cavity

√7ᵗʰ **S21.401** Unspecified open wound of right back wall of thorax with penetration into thoracic cavity `MCC` `PE`

√7ᵗʰ **S21.402** Unspecified open wound of left back wall of thorax with penetration into thoracic cavity `MCC` `PE`

√7ᵗʰ **S21.409** Unspecified open wound of unspecified back wall of thorax with penetration into thoracic cavity `MCC` `UNS` `PE`

√6ᵗʰ **S21.41** Laceration without foreign body of back wall of thorax with penetration into thoracic cavity

√7ᵗʰ **S21.411** Laceration without foreign body of right back wall of thorax with penetration into thoracic cavity `MCC` `PE`

√7ᵗʰ **S21.412** Laceration without foreign body of left back wall of thorax with penetration into thoracic cavity `MCC` `PE`

√7ᵗʰ **S21.419** Laceration without foreign body of unspecified back wall of thorax with penetration into thoracic cavity `MCC` `UNS` `PE`

√6ᵗʰ **S21.42** Laceration with foreign body of back wall of thorax with penetration into thoracic cavity

√7ᵗʰ **S21.421** Laceration with foreign body of right back wall of thorax with penetration into thoracic cavity `MCC` `PE`

√7ᵗʰ **S21.422** Laceration with foreign body of left back wall of thorax with penetration into thoracic cavity `MCC` `PE`

√7ᵗʰ **S21.429** Laceration with foreign body of unspecified back wall of thorax with penetration into thoracic cavity `MCC` `UNS` `PE`

√6ᵗʰ **S21.43** Puncture wound without foreign body of back wall of thorax with penetration into thoracic cavity

√7ᵗʰ **S21.431** Puncture wound without foreign body of right back wall of thorax with penetration into thoracic cavity `MCC` `PE`

√7ᵗʰ **S21.432** Puncture wound without foreign body of left back wall of thorax with penetration into thoracic cavity `MCC` `PE`

√7ᵗʰ **S21.439** Puncture wound without foreign body of unspecified back wall of thorax with penetration into thoracic cavity `MCC` `UNS` `PE`

√6ᵗʰ **S21.44** Puncture wound with foreign body of back wall of thorax with penetration into thoracic cavity

√7ᵗʰ **S21.441** Puncture wound with foreign body of right back wall of thorax with penetration into thoracic cavity `MCC` `PE`

√7ᵗʰ **S21.442** Puncture wound with foreign body of left back wall of thorax with penetration into thoracic cavity `MCC` `PE`

√7ᵗʰ **S21.449** Puncture wound with foreign body of unspecified back wall of thorax with penetration into thoracic cavity `MCC` `UNS` `PE`

√6ᵗʰ **S21.45** Open bite of back wall of thorax with penetration into thoracic cavity

Bite of back wall of thorax NOS

> **EXCLUDES 1**   superficial bite of back wall of thorax (S20.47)

√7ᵗʰ **S21.451** Open bite of right back wall of thorax with penetration into thoracic cavity `MCC` `PE`

√7ᵗʰ **S21.452** Open bite of left back wall of thorax with penetration into thoracic cavity `MCC` `PE`

√7ᵗʰ **S21.459** Open bite of unspecified back wall of thorax with penetration into thoracic cavity `MCC` `UNS` `PE`

√5ᵗʰ **S21.9** Open wound of unspecified part of thorax

Open wound of thoracic wall NOS

√x7ᵗʰ **S21.90** Unspecified open wound of unspecified part of thorax `CC` `UNS` `PE`

√x7ᵗʰ **S21.91** Laceration without foreign body of unspecified part of thorax `CC` `UNS` `PE`

√x7ᵗʰ **S21.92** Laceration with foreign body of unspecified part of thorax `CC` `UNS` `PE`

√x7ᵗʰ **S21.93** Puncture wound without foreign body of unspecified part of thorax `CC` `UNS` `PE`

√x7ᵗʰ **S21.94** Puncture wound with foreign body of unspecified part of thorax `CC` `UNS` `PE`

√x7ᵗʰ **S21.95** Open bite of unspecified part of thorax `CC` `UNS` `PE`

> **EXCLUDES 1**   superficial bite of thorax (S20.97)

☑ Additional Character Required   √x7ᵗʰ Placeholder   Questionable PDx   Manifestation   Unspecified   **UPD** Unacceptable PDx   H1-H14 HAC   HCC CMS-HCC Dx   HIV HIV Dx

ICD-10-CM 2025   **1007**

✓4th **S22 Fracture of rib(s), sternum and thoracic spine**

NOTE A fracture not indicated as displaced or nondisplaced should be coded to displaced

A fracture not indicated as open or closed should be coded to closed

INCLUDES fracture of thoracic neural arch
fracture of thoracic spinous process
fracture of thoracic transverse process
fracture of thoracic vertebra
fracture of thoracic vertebral arch

►Code also, if applicable, any associated condition such as:◄
injury of intrathoracic organ (S27.-)
spinal cord injury (S24.0-, S24.1-)
►traumatic hemopneumothorax (S27.2)◄
►traumatic hemothorax (S27.1-)◄
►traumatic pneumothorax (S27.0)◄
EXCLUDES 1 transection of thorax (S28.1)
EXCLUDES 2 fracture of clavicle (S42.0-)
fracture of scapula (S42.1-)
AHA: 2021,1Q,6; 2018,2Q,12; 2015,3Q,37-39

The appropriate 7th character is to be added to each code from category S22.
A initial encounter for closed fracture
B initial encounter for open fracture
D subsequent encounter for fracture with routine healing
G subsequent encounter for fracture with delayed healing
K subsequent encounter for fracture with nonunion
S sequela

✓5th **S22.0 Fracture of thoracic vertebra**

✓6th **S22.00 Fracture of unspecified thoracic vertebra**

✓7th **S22.000 Wedge compression fracture of unspecified thoracic vertebra** `MCC` `CC` `H5` `HCC` `PE`

✓7th **S22.001 Stable burst fracture of unspecified thoracic vertebra** `MCC` `CC` `H5` `HCC` `PE`

✓7th **S22.002 Unstable burst fracture of unspecified thoracic vertebra** `MCC` `CC` `H5` `HCC` `PE`

✓7th **S22.008 Other fracture of unspecified thoracic vertebra** `MCC` `CC` `H5` `HCC` `PE`

✓7th **S22.009 Unspecified fracture of unspecified thoracic vertebra** `MCC` `CC` `H5` `HCC` `PE`

✓6th **S22.01 Fracture of first thoracic vertebra**

✓7th **S22.010 Wedge compression fracture of first thoracic vertebra** `MCC` `CC` `H5` `HCC` `PE`

✓7th **S22.011 Stable burst fracture of first thoracic vertebra** `MCC` `CC` `H5` `HCC` `PE`

✓7th **S22.012 Unstable burst fracture of first thoracic vertebra** `MCC` `CC` `H5` `HCC` `PE`

✓7th **S22.018 Other fracture of first thoracic vertebra** `MCC` `CC` `H5` `HCC` `PE`

✓7th **S22.019 Unspecified fracture of first thoracic vertebra** `MCC` `CC` `H5` `HCC` `PE`

✓6th **S22.02 Fracture of second thoracic vertebra**

✓7th **S22.020 Wedge compression fracture of second thoracic vertebra** `MCC` `CC` `H5` `HCC` `PE`

✓7th **S22.021 Stable burst fracture of second thoracic vertebra** `MCC` `CC` `H5` `HCC` `PE`

✓7th **S22.022 Unstable burst fracture of second thoracic vertebra** `MCC` `CC` `H5` `HCC` `PE`

✓7th **S22.028 Other fracture of second thoracic vertebra** `MCC` `CC` `H5` `HCC` `PE`

✓7th **S22.029 Unspecified fracture of second thoracic vertebra** `MCC` `CC` `H5` `HCC` `PE`

✓6th **S22.03 Fracture of third thoracic vertebra**

✓7th **S22.030 Wedge compression fracture of third thoracic vertebra** `MCC` `CC` `H5` `HCC` `PE`

✓7th **S22.031 Stable burst fracture of third thoracic vertebra** `MCC` `CC` `H5` `HCC` `PE`

✓7th **S22.032 Unstable burst fracture of third thoracic vertebra** `MCC` `CC` `H5` `HCC` `PE`

✓7th **S22.038 Other fracture of third thoracic vertebra** `MCC` `CC` `H5` `HCC` `PE`

✓7th **S22.039 Unspecified fracture of third thoracic vertebra** `MCC` `CC` `H5` `HCC` `PE`

✓6th **S22.04 Fracture of fourth thoracic vertebra**

✓7th **S22.040 Wedge compression fracture of fourth thoracic vertebra** `MCC` `CC` `H5` `HCC` `PE`

✓7th **S22.041 Stable burst fracture of fourth thoracic vertebra** `MCC` `CC` `H5` `HCC` `PE`

✓7th **S22.042 Unstable burst fracture of fourth thoracic vertebra** `MCC` `CC` `H5` `HCC` `PE`

✓7th **S22.048 Other fracture of fourth thoracic vertebra** `MCC` `CC` `H5` `HCC` `PE`

✓7th **S22.049 Unspecified fracture of fourth thoracic vertebra** `MCC` `CC` `H5` `HCC` `PE`

✓6th **S22.05 Fracture of T5-T6 vertebra**

✓7th **S22.050 Wedge compression fracture of T5-T6 vertebra** `MCC` `CC` `H5` `HCC` `PE`

✓7th **S22.051 Stable burst fracture of T5-T6 vertebra** `MCC` `CC` `H5` `HCC` `PE`

✓7th **S22.052 Unstable burst fracture of T5-T6 vertebra** `MCC` `CC` `H5` `HCC` `PE`

✓7th **S22.058 Other fracture of T5-T6 vertebra** `MCC` `CC` `H5` `HCC` `PE`

✓7th **S22.059 Unspecified fracture of T5-T6 vertebra** `MCC` `CC` `H5` `HCC` `PE`

✓6th **S22.06 Fracture of T7-T8 vertebra**

✓7th **S22.060 Wedge compression fracture of T7-T8 vertebra** `MCC` `CC` `H5` `HCC` `PE`

✓7th **S22.061 Stable burst fracture of T7-T8 vertebra** `MCC` `CC` `H5` `HCC` `PE`

✓7th **S22.062 Unstable burst fracture of T7-T8 vertebra** `MCC` `CC` `H5` `HCC` `PE`

✓7th **S22.068 Other fracture of T7-T8 thoracic vertebra** `MCC` `CC` `H5` `HCC` `PE`

✓7th **S22.069 Unspecified fracture of T7-T8 vertebra** `MCC` `CC` `H5` `HCC` `PE`

✓6th **S22.07 Fracture of T9-T10 vertebra**

✓7th **S22.070 Wedge compression fracture of T9-T10 vertebra** `MCC` `CC` `H5` `HCC` `PE`

✓7th **S22.071 Stable burst fracture of T9-T10 vertebra** `MCC` `CC` `H5` `HCC` `PE`

✓7th **S22.072 Unstable burst fracture of T9-T10 vertebra** `MCC` `CC` `H5` `HCC` `PE`

✓7th **S22.078 Other fracture of T9-T10 vertebra** `MCC` `CC` `H5` `HCC` `PE`

✓7th **S22.079 Unspecified fracture of T9-T10 vertebra** `MCC` `CC` `H5` `HCC` `PE`

✓6th **S22.08 Fracture of T11-T12 vertebra**

✓7th **S22.080 Wedge compression fracture of T11-T12 vertebra** `MCC` `CC` `H5` `HCC` `PE`

✓7th **S22.081 Stable burst fracture of T11-T12 vertebra** `MCC` `CC` `H5` `HCC` `PE`

✓7th **S22.082 Unstable burst fracture of T11-T12 vertebra** `MCC` `CC` `H5` `HCC` `PE`

✓7th **S22.088 Other fracture of T11-T12 vertebra** `MCC` `CC` `H5` `HCC` `PE`

✓7th **S22.089 Unspecified fracture of T11-T12 vertebra** `MCC` `CC` `H5` `HCC` `PE`

✓5th **S22.2 Fracture of sternum**

DEF: Break in flat bone (breast bone) in the anterior thorax caused by blunt trauma to the anterior chest.

✓x7th **S22.20 Unspecified fracture of sternum** `MCC` `CC` `H5` `PE`

✓x7th **S22.21 Fracture of manubrium** `MCC` `CC` `H5` `PE`

✓x7th **S22.22 Fracture of body of sternum** `MCC` `CC` `H5` `PE`

✓x7th **S22.23 Sternal manubrial dissociation** `MCC` `CC` `H5` `PE`

✓x7th **S22.24 Fracture of xiphoid process** `MCC` `CC` `H5` `PE`

✓5th **S22.3 Fracture of one rib**

AHA: 2021,1Q,5

✓x7th **S22.31 Fracture of one rib, right side** `MCC` `CC` `H5` `PE`

✓x7th **S22.32 Fracture of one rib, left side** `MCC` `CC` `H5` `PE`

✓x7th **S22.39 Fracture of one rib, unspecified side** `MCC` `CC` `H5` `UNS` `PE`

✓5th **S22.4 Multiple fractures of ribs**

Fractures of two or more ribs
EXCLUDES 1 flail chest (S22.5-)
AHA: 2021,1Q,5

✓x7th **S22.41 Multiple fractures of ribs, right side** `MCC` `CC` `H5` `PE`

✓x7th **S22.42 Multiple fractures of ribs, left side** `MCC` `CC` `H5` `PE`

√x7ᵗʰ **S22.43** **Multiple fractures of ribs, bilateral** `MCC` `CC` `H5` `PE`

√x7ᵗʰ **S22.49** **Multiple fractures of ribs, unspecified side** `MCC` `CC` `H5` `UNS` `PE`

√x7ᵗʰ **S22.5** **Flail chest** `MCC` `CC` `H5` `PE`

√x7ᵗʰ **S22.9** **Fracture of bony thorax, part unspecified** `MCC` `CC` `H5` `PE`

√4ᵗʰ **S23** **Dislocation and sprain of joints and ligaments of thorax**

> **INCLUDES** avulsion of joint or ligament of thorax
> laceration of cartilage, joint or ligament of thorax
> sprain of cartilage, joint or ligament of thorax
> traumatic hemarthrosis of joint or ligament of thorax
> traumatic rupture of joint or ligament of thorax
> traumatic subluxation of joint or ligament of thorax
> traumatic tear of joint or ligament of thorax

> Code also any associated open wound
> **EXCLUDES 2** dislocation, sprain of sternoclavicular joint (S43.2, S43.6)
> strain of muscle or tendon of thorax (S29.01-)

> The appropriate 7th character is to be added to each code from category S23.
> A   initial encounter
> D   subsequent encounter
> S   sequela

√x7ᵗʰ **S23.0** **Traumatic rupture of thoracic intervertebral disc** `PE`

> **EXCLUDES 1** rupture or displacement (nontraumatic) of thoracic intervertebral disc NOS (M51.- with fifth character 4)

√5ᵗʰ **S23.1** **Subluxation and dislocation of thoracic vertebra**

> Code also any associated:
> open wound of thorax (S21.-)
> spinal cord injury (S24.0-, S24.1-)
> **EXCLUDES 2** fracture of thoracic vertebrae (S22.0-)

√6ᵗʰ **S23.10** **Subluxation and dislocation of unspecified thoracic vertebra**

√7ᵗʰ **S23.100** **Subluxation of unspecified thoracic vertebra** `PE`

√7ᵗʰ **S23.101** **Dislocation of unspecified thoracic vertebra** `PE`

√6ᵗʰ **S23.11** **Subluxation and dislocation of T1/T2 thoracic vertebra**

√7ᵗʰ **S23.110** **Subluxation of T1/T2 thoracic vertebra** `PE`

√7ᵗʰ **S23.111** **Dislocation of T1/T2 thoracic vertebra** `PE`

√6ᵗʰ **S23.12** **Subluxation and dislocation of T2/T3-T3/T4 thoracic vertebra**

√7ᵗʰ **S23.120** **Subluxation of T2/T3 thoracic vertebra** `PE`

√7ᵗʰ **S23.121** **Dislocation of T2/T3 thoracic vertebra** `PE`

√7ᵗʰ **S23.122** **Subluxation of T3/T4 thoracic vertebra** `PE`

√7ᵗʰ **S23.123** **Dislocation of T3/T4 thoracic vertebra** `PE`

√6ᵗʰ **S23.13** **Subluxation and dislocation of T4/T5-T5/T6 thoracic vertebra**

√7ᵗʰ **S23.130** **Subluxation of T4/T5 thoracic vertebra** `PE`

√7ᵗʰ **S23.131** **Dislocation of T4/T5 thoracic vertebra** `PE`

√7ᵗʰ **S23.132** **Subluxation of T5/T6 thoracic vertebra** `PE`

√7ᵗʰ **S23.133** **Dislocation of T5/T6 thoracic vertebra** `PE`

√6ᵗʰ **S23.14** **Subluxation and dislocation of T6/T7-T7/T8 thoracic vertebra**

√7ᵗʰ **S23.140** **Subluxation of T6/T7 thoracic vertebra** `PE`

√7ᵗʰ **S23.141** **Dislocation of T6/T7 thoracic vertebra** `PE`

√7ᵗʰ **S23.142** **Subluxation of T7/T8 thoracic vertebra** `PE`

√7ᵗʰ **S23.143** **Dislocation of T7/T8 thoracic vertebra** `PE`

√6ᵗʰ **S23.15** **Subluxation and dislocation of T8/T9-T9/T10 thoracic vertebra**

√7ᵗʰ **S23.150** **Subluxation of T8/T9 thoracic vertebra** `PE`

√7ᵗʰ **S23.151** **Dislocation of T8/T9 thoracic vertebra** `PE`

√7ᵗʰ **S23.152** **Subluxation of T9/T10 thoracic vertebra** `PE`

√7ᵗʰ **S23.153** **Dislocation of T9/T10 thoracic vertebra** `PE`

√6ᵗʰ **S23.16** **Subluxation and dislocation of T10/T11-T11/T12 thoracic vertebra**

√7ᵗʰ **S23.160** **Subluxation of T10/T11 thoracic vertebra** `PE`

√7ᵗʰ **S23.161** **Dislocation of T10/T11 thoracic vertebra** `PE`

√7ᵗʰ **S23.162** **Subluxation of T11/T12 thoracic vertebra** `PE`

√7ᵗʰ **S23.163** **Dislocation of T11/T12 thoracic vertebra** `PE`

√6ᵗʰ **S23.17** **Subluxation and dislocation of T12/L1 thoracic vertebra**

√7ᵗʰ **S23.170** **Subluxation of T12/L1 thoracic vertebra** `PE`

√7ᵗʰ **S23.171** **Dislocation of T12/L1 thoracic vertebra** `PE`

√5ᵗʰ **S23.2** **Dislocation of other and unspecified parts of thorax**

√x7ᵗʰ **S23.20** **Dislocation of unspecified part of thorax** `PE`

√x7ᵗʰ **S23.29** **Dislocation of other parts of thorax** `PE`

√x7ᵗʰ **S23.3** **Sprain of ligaments of thoracic spine** `PE`

√5ᵗʰ **S23.4** **Sprain of ribs and sternum**

√x7ᵗʰ **S23.41** **Sprain of ribs** `PE`

√6ᵗʰ **S23.42** **Sprain of sternum**

√7ᵗʰ **S23.420** **Sprain of sternoclavicular (joint) (ligament)** `PE`

√7ᵗʰ **S23.421** **Sprain of chondrosternal joint** `PE`

√7ᵗʰ **S23.428** **Other sprain of sternum** `PE`

√7ᵗʰ **S23.429** **Unspecified sprain of sternum** `PE`

√x7ᵗʰ **S23.8** **Sprain of other specified parts of thorax** `PE`

√x7ᵗʰ **S23.9** **Sprain of unspecified parts of thorax** `PE`

√4ᵗʰ **S24** **Injury of nerves and spinal cord at thorax level**

> **NOTE** Code to highest level of thoracic spinal cord injury.
> Injuries to the spinal cord (S24.0 and S24.1) refer to the cord level and not bone level injury, and can affect nerve roots at and below the level given.

> Code also any associated:
> fracture of thoracic vertebra (S22.0-)
> open wound of thorax (S21.-)
> transient paralysis (R29.5)
> **EXCLUDES 2** injury of brachial plexus (S14.3)

> The appropriate 7th character is to be added to each code from category S24.
> A   initial encounter
> D   subsequent encounter
> S   sequela

√x7ᵗʰ **S24.0** **Concussion and edema of thoracic spinal cord** `MCC` `HCC` `PE`

√5ᵗʰ **S24.1** **Other and unspecified injuries of thoracic spinal cord**

√6ᵗʰ **S24.10** **Unspecified injury of thoracic spinal cord**

√7ᵗʰ **S24.101** **Unspecified injury at T1 level of thoracic spinal cord** `MCC` `H5` `HCC` `PE`

√7ᵗʰ **S24.102** **Unspecified injury at T2-T6 level of thoracic spinal cord** `MCC` `H5` `HCC` `PE`

√7ᵗʰ **S24.103** **Unspecified injury at T7-T10 level of thoracic spinal cord** `MCC` `H5` `HCC` `PE`

√7ᵗʰ **S24.104** **Unspecified injury at T11-T12 level of thoracic spinal cord** `MCC` `H5` `HCC` `PE`

√7ᵗʰ **S24.109** **Unspecified injury at unspecified level of thoracic spinal cord** `HCC` `PE`
Injury of thoracic spinal cord NOS

√6ᵗʰ **S24.11** **Complete lesion of thoracic spinal cord**

√7ᵗʰ **S24.111** **Complete lesion at T1 level of thoracic spinal cord** `MCC` `H5` `HCC` `PE`

√7ᵗʰ **S24.112** **Complete lesion at T2-T6 level of thoracic spinal cord** `MCC` `H5` `HCC` `PE`

√7ᵗʰ **S24.113** **Complete lesion at T7-T10 level of thoracic spinal cord** `MCC` `H5` `HCC` `PE`

√7ᵗʰ **S24.114** **Complete lesion at T11-T12 level of thoracic spinal cord** `MCC` `H5` `HCC` `PE`

Chapter 19. Injury, Poisoning and Certain Other Consequences of External Causes

✓7th **S24.119** Complete lesion at unspecified level of thoracic spinal cord `HCC` `PE`

✓6th **S24.13** Anterior cord syndrome of thoracic spinal cord

✓7th **S24.131** Anterior cord syndrome at T1 level of thoracic spinal cord `MCC` `H5` `HCC` `PE`

✓7th **S24.132** Anterior cord syndrome at T2-T6 level of thoracic spinal cord `MCC` `H5` `HCC` `PE`

✓7th **S24.133** Anterior cord syndrome at T7-T10 level of thoracic spinal cord `MCC` `H5` `HCC` `PE`

✓7th **S24.134** Anterior cord syndrome at T11-T12 level of thoracic spinal cord `MCC` `H5` `HCC` `PE`

✓7th **S24.139** Anterior cord syndrome at unspecified level of thoracic spinal cord `HCC` `PE`

✓6th **S24.14** Brown-Sequard syndrome of thoracic spinal cord

✓7th **S24.141** Brown-Sequard syndrome at T1 level of thoracic spinal cord `MCC` `HCC` `PE`

✓7th **S24.142** Brown-Sequard syndrome at T2-T6 level of thoracic spinal cord `MCC` `HCC` `PE`

✓7th **S24.143** Brown-Sequard syndrome at T7-T10 level of thoracic spinal cord `MCC` `HCC` `PE`

✓7th **S24.144** Brown-Sequard syndrome at T11-T12 level of thoracic spinal cord `MCC` `HCC` `PE`

✓7th **S24.149** Brown-Sequard syndrome at unspecified level of thoracic spinal cord `HCC` `PE`

✓6th **S24.15** Other incomplete lesions of thoracic spinal cord

Incomplete lesion of thoracic spinal cord NOS
Posterior cord syndrome of thoracic spinal cord

✓7th **S24.151** Other incomplete lesion at T1 level of thoracic spinal cord `MCC` `H5` `HCC` `PE`

✓7th **S24.152** Other incomplete lesion at T2-T6 level of thoracic spinal cord `MCC` `H5` `HCC` `PE`

✓7th **S24.153** Other incomplete lesion at T7-T10 level of thoracic spinal cord `MCC` `H5` `HCC` `PE`

✓7th **S24.154** Other incomplete lesion at T11-T12 level of thoracic spinal cord `MCC` `H5` `HCC` `PE`

✓7th **S24.159** Other incomplete lesion at unspecified level of thoracic spinal cord `HCC` `PE`

✓x7th **S24.2** Injury of nerve root of thoracic spine `PE`

✓x7th **S24.3** Injury of peripheral nerves of thorax `PE`

✓x7th **S24.4** Injury of thoracic sympathetic nervous system `PE`

Injury of cardiac plexus
Injury of esophageal plexus
Injury of pulmonary plexus
Injury of stellate ganglion
Injury of thoracic sympathetic ganglion

✓x7th **S24.8** Injury of other specified nerves of thorax `PE`

✓x7th **S24.9** Injury of unspecified nerve of thorax `PE`

✓4th **S25** Injury of blood vessels of thorax

Code also any associated open wound (S21.-)

The appropriate 7th character is to be added to each code from category S25.
A   initial encounter
D   subsequent encounter
S   sequela

✓5th **S25.0** Injury of thoracic aorta

Injury of aorta NOS

✓x7th **S25.00** Unspecified injury of thoracic aorta `MCC` `PE`

✓x7th **S25.01** Minor laceration of thoracic aorta `MCC` `PE`

Incomplete transection of thoracic aorta
Laceration of thoracic aorta NOS
Superficial laceration of thoracic aorta

✓x7th **S25.02** Major laceration of thoracic aorta `MCC` `PE`

Complete transection of thoracic aorta
Traumatic rupture of thoracic aorta

✓x7th **S25.09** Other specified injury of thoracic aorta `MCC` `PE`

✓5th **S25.1** Injury of innominate or subclavian artery

✓6th **S25.10** Unspecified injury of innominate or subclavian artery

✓7th **S25.101** Unspecified injury of right innominate or subclavian artery `MCC` `PE`

✓7th **S25.102** Unspecified injury of left innominate or subclavian artery `MCC` `PE`

✓7th **S25.109** Unspecified injury of unspecified innominate or subclavian artery `MCC` `UNS` `PE`

✓6th **S25.11** Minor laceration of innominate or subclavian artery

Incomplete transection of innominate or subclavian artery
Laceration of innominate or subclavian artery NOS
Superficial laceration of innominate or subclavian artery

✓7th **S25.111** Minor laceration of right innominate or subclavian artery `MCC` `PE`

✓7th **S25.112** Minor laceration of left innominate or subclavian artery `MCC` `PE`

✓7th **S25.119** Minor laceration of unspecified innominate or subclavian artery `MCC` `UNS` `PE`

✓6th **S25.12** Major laceration of innominate or subclavian artery

Complete transection of innominate or subclavian artery
Traumatic rupture of innominate or subclavian artery

✓7th **S25.121** Major laceration of right innominate or subclavian artery `MCC` `PE`

✓7th **S25.122** Major laceration of left innominate or subclavian artery `MCC` `PE`

✓7th **S25.129** Major laceration of unspecified innominate or subclavian artery `MCC` `UNS` `PE`

✓6th **S25.19** Other specified injury of innominate or subclavian artery

✓7th **S25.191** Other specified injury of right innominate or subclavian artery `MCC` `PE`

✓7th **S25.192** Other specified injury of left innominate or subclavian artery `MCC` `PE`

✓7th **S25.199** Other specified injury of unspecified innominate or subclavian artery `MCC` `UNS` `PE`

✓5th **S25.2** Injury of superior vena cava

Injury of vena cava NOS

✓x7th **S25.20** Unspecified injury of superior vena cava `MCC` `PE`

✓x7th **S25.21** Minor laceration of superior vena cava `MCC` `PE`

Incomplete transection of superior vena cava
Laceration of superior vena cava NOS
Superficial laceration of superior vena cava

✓x7th **S25.22** Major laceration of superior vena cava `MCC` `PE`

Complete transection of superior vena cava
Traumatic rupture of superior vena cava

✓x7th **S25.29** Other specified injury of superior vena cava `MCC` `PE`

✓5th **S25.3** Injury of innominate or subclavian vein

✓6th **S25.30** Unspecified injury of innominate or subclavian vein

✓7th **S25.301** Unspecified injury of right innominate or subclavian vein `MCC` `PE`

✓7th **S25.302** Unspecified injury of left innominate or subclavian vein `MCC` `PE`

✓7th **S25.309** Unspecified injury of unspecified innominate or subclavian vein `MCC` `UNS` `PE`

✓6th **S25.31** Minor laceration of innominate or subclavian vein

Incomplete transection of innominate or subclavian vein
Laceration of innominate or subclavian vein NOS
Superficial laceration of innominate or subclavian vein

✓7th **S25.311** Minor laceration of right innominate or subclavian vein `MCC` `PE`

✓7th **S25.312** Minor laceration of left innominate or subclavian vein `MCC` `PE`

✓7th **S25.319** Minor laceration of unspecified innominate or subclavian vein `MCC` `UNS` `PE`

✓6th **S25.32** Major laceration of innominate or subclavian vein

Complete transection of innominate or subclavian vein
Traumatic rupture of innominate or subclavian vein

✓7th **S25.321** Major laceration of right innominate or subclavian vein `MCC` `PE`

✓7th **S25.322** Major laceration of left innominate or subclavian vein `MCC` `PE`

✓7th **S25.329** Major laceration of unspecified innominate or subclavian vein `MCC` `UNS` `PE`

✓6th **S25.39** Other specified injury of innominate or subclavian vein

✓7th **S25.391** Other specified injury of right innominate or subclavian vein `MCC` `PE`

✓7th **S25.392** Other specified injury of left innominate or subclavian vein `MCC` `PE`

✓7th **S25.399** Other specified injury of unspecified innominate or subclavian vein `MCC` `UNS` `PE`

✓5th **S25.4** Injury of **pulmonary blood vessels**

✓6th **S25.40** Unspecified injury of pulmonary blood vessels

✓7th **S25.401** Unspecified injury of **right** pulmonary blood vessels `MCC` `PE`

✓7th **S25.402** Unspecified injury of **left** pulmonary blood vessels `MCC` `PE`

✓7th **S25.409** Unspecified injury of unspecified pulmonary blood vessels `MCC` `UNS` `PE`

✓6th **S25.41** **Minor laceration** of pulmonary blood vessels

Incomplete transection of pulmonary blood vessels
Laceration of pulmonary blood vessels NOS
Superficial laceration of pulmonary blood vessels

✓7th **S25.411** Minor laceration of **right** pulmonary blood vessels `MCC` `PE`

✓7th **S25.412** Minor laceration of **left** pulmonary blood vessels `MCC` `PE`

✓7th **S25.419** Minor laceration of unspecified pulmonary blood vessels `MCC` `UNS` `PE`

✓6th **S25.42** **Major laceration** of pulmonary blood vessels

Complete transection of pulmonary blood vessels
Traumatic rupture of pulmonary blood vessels

✓7th **S25.421** Major laceration of **right** pulmonary blood vessels `MCC` `PE`

✓7th **S25.422** Major laceration of **left** pulmonary blood vessels `MCC` `PE`

✓7th **S25.429** Major laceration of unspecified pulmonary blood vessels `MCC` `UNS` `PE`

✓6th **S25.49** Other specified injury of pulmonary blood vessels

✓7th **S25.491** Other specified injury of **right** pulmonary blood vessels `MCC` `PE`

✓7th **S25.492** Other specified injury of **left** pulmonary blood vessels `MCC` `PE`

✓7th **S25.499** Other specified injury of unspecified pulmonary blood vessels `MCC` `UNS` `PE`

✓5th **S25.5** Injury of **intercostal blood vessels**

✓6th **S25.50** Unspecified injury of intercostal blood vessels

✓7th **S25.501** Unspecified injury of intercostal blood vessels, **right** side `CC` `PE`

✓7th **S25.502** Unspecified injury of intercostal blood vessels, **left** side `CC` `PE`

✓7th **S25.509** Unspecified injury of intercostal blood vessels, unspecified side `CC` `UNS` `PE`

✓6th **S25.51** **Laceration** of intercostal blood vessels

✓7th **S25.511** Laceration of intercostal blood vessels, **right** side `CC` `PE`

✓7th **S25.512** Laceration of intercostal blood vessels, **left** side `CC` `PE`

✓7th **S25.519** Laceration of intercostal blood vessels, unspecified side `CC` `UNS` `PE`

✓6th **S25.59** Other specified injury of intercostal blood vessels

✓7th **S25.591** Other specified injury of intercostal blood vessels, **right** side `CC` `PE`

✓7th **S25.592** Other specified injury of intercostal blood vessels, **left** side `CC` `PE`

✓7th **S25.599** Other specified injury of intercostal blood vessels, unspecified side `CC` `UNS` `PE`

✓5th **S25.8** Injury of other blood vessels of thorax

Injury of azygos vein
Injury of mammary artery or vein

✓6th **S25.80** Unspecified injury of other blood vessels of thorax

✓7th **S25.801** Unspecified injury of other blood vessels of thorax, **right** side `CC` `PE`

✓7th **S25.802** Unspecified injury of other blood vessels of thorax, **left** side `CC` `PE`

✓7th **S25.809** Unspecified injury of other blood vessels of thorax, unspecified side `CC` `UNS` `PE`

✓6th **S25.81** **Laceration** of other blood vessels of thorax

✓7th **S25.811** Laceration of other blood vessels of thorax, **right** side `CC` `PE`

✓7th **S25.812** Laceration of other blood vessels of thorax, **left** side `CC` `PE`

✓7th **S25.819** Laceration of other blood vessels of thorax, unspecified side `CC` `UNS` `PE`

✓6th **S25.89** Other specified injury of other blood vessels of thorax

✓7th **S25.891** Other specified injury of other blood vessels of thorax, **right** side `CC` `PE`

✓7th **S25.892** Other specified injury of other blood vessels of thorax, **left** side `CC` `PE`

✓7th **S25.899** Other specified injury of other blood vessels of thorax, unspecified side `CC` `UNS` `PE`

✓5th **S25.9** Injury of unspecified blood vessel of thorax

✓x7th **S25.90** Unspecified injury of unspecified blood vessel of thorax `CC` `UNS` `PE`

✓x7th **S25.91** **Laceration** of unspecified blood vessel of thorax `CC` `UNS` `PE`

✓x7th **S25.99** Other specified injury of unspecified blood vessel of thorax `CC` `UNS` `PE`

✓4th **S26** **Injury of heart**

Code also any associated:
open wound of thorax (S21.-)
traumatic hemopneumothorax (S27.2)
traumatic hemothorax (S27.1)
traumatic pneumothorax (S27.0)

The appropriate 7th character is to be added to each code from category S26.
A   initial encounter
D   subsequent encounter
S   sequela

✓5th **S26.0** Injury of heart **with hemopericardium**

✓x7th **S26.00** Unspecified injury of heart with hemopericardium `CC` `PE`

✓x7th **S26.01** **Contusion** of heart with hemopericardium `CC` `PE`

✓6th **S26.02** **Laceration** of heart with hemopericardium

✓7th **S26.020** **Mild** laceration of heart with hemopericardium `MCC` `PE`

Laceration of heart without penetration of heart chamber

✓7th **S26.021** **Moderate** laceration of heart with hemopericardium `MCC` `PE`

Laceration of heart with penetration of heart chamber

✓7th **S26.022** **Major** laceration of heart with hemopericardium `MCC` `PE`

Laceration of heart with penetration of multiple heart chambers

✓x7th **S26.09** Other injury of heart with hemopericardium `CC` `PE`

✓5th **S26.1** Injury of heart **without hemopericardium**

✓x7th **S26.10** Unspecified injury of heart without hemopericardium `CC` `PE`

✓x7th **S26.11** **Contusion** of heart without hemopericardium `CC` `PE`

✓x7th **S26.12** **Laceration** of heart without hemopericardium `MCC` `PE`

✓x7th **S26.19** Other injury of heart without hemopericardium `CC` `PE`

✓5th **S26.9** Injury of heart, unspecified with or without hemopericardium

✓x7th **S26.90** Unspecified injury of heart, unspecified with or without hemopericardium `CC` `PE`

✓x7th **S26.91** **Contusion** of heart, unspecified with or without hemopericardium `CC` `PE`

DEF: Bruising within the heart muscle, with no mention of an open wound, usually caused by blunt chest trauma in motor vehicle accidents, falling from great heights, or receiving CPR.

✓x7th **S26.92** **Laceration** of heart, unspecified with or without hemopericardium `MCC` `PE`

Laceration of heart NOS
AHA: 2019,2Q,24

✓x7th **S26.99** Other injury of heart, unspecified with or without hemopericardium `CC` `PE`

☑ Additional Character Required
ICD-10-CM 2025

✓x7th Placeholder   **Questionable PDx**   Manifestation   Unspecified   `UPD` Unacceptable PDx   `H1`-`H14` HAC   `HCC` CMS-HCC Dx   `HIV` HIV Dx

1011

Chapter 19. Injury, Poisoning and Certain Other Consequences of External Causes

S27–S28.219

√4th S27 Injury of other and unspecified intrathoracic organs

Code also any associated open wound of thorax (S21.-)

EXCLUDES 2   injury of cervical esophagus (S1Ø-S19)
             injury of trachea (cervical) (S1Ø-S19)

> The appropriate 7th character is to be added to each code from category S27.
> A   initial encounter
> D   subsequent encounter
> S   sequela

√x 7th **S27.Ø**   **Traumatic pneumothorax**   CC PE
       EXCLUDES 1   spontaneous pneumothorax (J93.-)

√x 7th **S27.1**   **Traumatic hemothorax**   MCC PE

√x 7th **S27.2**   **Traumatic hemopneumothorax**   MCC PE

√5th **S27.3**   **Other and unspecified injuries of lung**

    √6th **S27.3Ø**   **Unspecified injury of lung**

       √7th **S27.3Ø1**   **Unspecified injury of lung, unilateral**   CC PE

       √7th **S27.3Ø2**   **Unspecified injury of lung, bilateral**   CC PE

       √7th **S27.3Ø9**   **Unspecified injury of lung, unspecified**   CC UNS PE

    √6th **S27.31**   **Primary blast injury of lung**
             Blast injury of lung NOS

       √7th **S27.311**   **Primary blast injury of lung, unilateral**   CC PE

       √7th **S27.312**   **Primary blast injury of lung, bilateral**   CC PE

       √7th **S27.319**   **Primary blast injury of lung, unspecified**   CC UNS PE

    √6th **S27.32**   **Contusion of lung**
             DEF: Bruising of the lung without mention of an open wound.

       √7th **S27.321**   **Contusion of lung, unilateral**   CC PE

       √7th **S27.322**   **Contusion of lung, bilateral**   CC PE

       √7th **S27.329**   **Contusion of lung, unspecified**   CC UNS PE

    √6th **S27.33**   **Laceration of lung**

       √7th **S27.331**   **Laceration of lung, unilateral**   MCC PE

       √7th **S27.332**   **Laceration of lung, bilateral**   MCC PE

       √7th **S27.339**   **Laceration of lung, unspecified**   MCC UNS PE

    √6th **S27.39**   **Other injuries of lung**
             Secondary blast injury of lung

       √7th **S27.391**   **Other injuries of lung, unilateral**   CC PE

       √7th **S27.392**   **Other injuries of lung, bilateral**   CC PE

       √7th **S27.399**   **Other injuries of lung, unspecified**   CC UNS PE

√5th **S27.4**   **Injury of bronchus**

    √6th **S27.4Ø**   **Unspecified injury of bronchus**

       √7th **S27.4Ø1**   **Unspecified injury of bronchus, unilateral**   MCC PE

       √7th **S27.4Ø2**   **Unspecified injury of bronchus, bilateral**   MCC PE

       √7th **S27.4Ø9**   **Unspecified injury of bronchus, unspecified**   MCC UNS PE

    √6th **S27.41**   **Primary blast injury of bronchus**
             Blast injury of bronchus NOS

       √7th **S27.411**   **Primary blast injury of bronchus, unilateral**   MCC PE

       √7th **S27.412**   **Primary blast injury of bronchus, bilateral**   MCC PE

       √7th **S27.419**   **Primary blast injury of bronchus, unspecified**   MCC UNS PE

    √6th **S27.42**   **Contusion of bronchus**

       √7th **S27.421**   **Contusion of bronchus, unilateral**   MCC PE

       √7th **S27.422**   **Contusion of bronchus, bilateral**   MCC PE

       √7th **S27.429**   **Contusion of bronchus, unspecified**   MCC UNS PE

    √6th **S27.43**   **Laceration of bronchus**

       √7th **S27.431**   **Laceration of bronchus, unilateral**   MCC PE

       √7th **S27.432**   **Laceration of bronchus, bilateral**   MCC PE

       √7th **S27.439**   **Laceration of bronchus, unspecified**   MCC UNS PE

    √6th **S27.49**   **Other injury of bronchus**
             Secondary blast injury of bronchus

       √7th **S27.491**   **Other injury of bronchus, unilateral**   MCC PE

       √7th **S27.492**   **Other injury of bronchus, bilateral**   MCC PE

       √7th **S27.499**   **Other injury of bronchus, unspecified**   MCC UNS PE

√5th **S27.5**   **Injury of thoracic trachea**

    √x 7th **S27.5Ø**   **Unspecified injury of thoracic trachea**   CC PE

    √x 7th **S27.51**   **Primary blast injury of thoracic trachea**   CC PE
             Blast injury of thoracic trachea NOS

    √x 7th **S27.52**   **Contusion of thoracic trachea**   CC PE

    √x 7th **S27.53**   **Laceration of thoracic trachea**   CC PE

    √x 7th **S27.59**   **Other injury of thoracic trachea**   CC PE
             Secondary blast injury of thoracic trachea

√5th **S27.6**   **Injury of pleura**

    √x 7th **S27.6Ø**   **Unspecified injury of pleura**   CC PE

    √x 7th **S27.63**   **Laceration of pleura**   CC PE

    √x 7th **S27.69**   **Other injury of pleura**   CC PE

√5th **S27.8**   **Injury of other specified intrathoracic organs**

    √6th **S27.8Ø**   **Injury of diaphragm**

       √7th **S27.8Ø2**   **Contusion of diaphragm**   CC PE

       √7th **S27.8Ø3**   **Laceration of diaphragm**   CC PE

       √7th **S27.8Ø8**   **Other injury of diaphragm**   CC PE

       √7th **S27.8Ø9**   **Unspecified injury of diaphragm**   CC PE

    √6th **S27.81**   **Injury of esophagus (thoracic part)**

       √7th **S27.812**   **Contusion of esophagus (thoracic part)**   MCC PE

       √7th **S27.813**   **Laceration of esophagus (thoracic part)**   MCC PE

       √7th **S27.818**   **Other injury of esophagus (thoracic part)**   MCC PE

       √7th **S27.819**   **Unspecified injury of esophagus (thoracic part)**   MCC PE

    √6th **S27.89**   **Injury of other specified intrathoracic organs**
             Injury of lymphatic thoracic duct
             Injury of thymus gland

       √7th **S27.892**   **Contusion of other specified intrathoracic organs**   CC PE

       √7th **S27.893**   **Laceration of other specified intrathoracic organs**   CC PE

       √7th **S27.898**   **Other injury of other specified intrathoracic organs**   CC PE

       √7th **S27.899**   **Unspecified injury of other specified intrathoracic organs**   CC PE

√x 7th **S27.9**   **Injury of unspecified intrathoracic organ**   CC PE

√4th S28 Crushing injury of thorax, and traumatic amputation of part of thorax

> The appropriate 7th character is to be added to each code from category S28.
> A   initial encounter
> D   subsequent encounter
> S   sequela

√x 7th **S28.Ø**   **Crushed chest**   PE
         Use additional code for all associated injuries
       EXCLUDES 1   flail chest (S22.5)

√x 7th **S28.1**   **Traumatic amputation (partial) of part of thorax, except breast**   CC PE

√5th **S28.2**   **Traumatic amputation of breast**

    √6th **S28.21**   **Complete traumatic amputation of breast**
             Traumatic amputation of breast NOS

       √7th **S28.211**   **Complete traumatic amputation of right breast**   PE

       √7th **S28.212**   **Complete traumatic amputation of left breast**   PE

       √7th **S28.219**   **Complete traumatic amputation of unspecified breast**   PE

N Newborn: 0   P Pediatric: 0-17   M Maternity: 9-64   A Adult: 15-124   UNS Unspecified Site   MCC Major Complication/Comorbidity   CC Complication/Comorbidity   PE POA Exempt

1012   ICD-10-CM 2025

√6ᵗʰ **S28.22** Partial traumatic amputation of breast

    √7ᵗʰ **S28.221** Partial traumatic amputation of right breast   PE

    √7ᵗʰ **S28.222** Partial traumatic amputation of left breast   PE

    √7ᵗʰ **S28.229** Partial traumatic amputation of unspecified breast   PE

√4ᵗʰ **S29** Other and unspecified injuries of thorax

Code also any associated open wound (S21.-)

The appropriate 7th character is to be added to each code from category S29.
A   initial encounter
D   subsequent encounter
S   sequela

√5ᵗʰ **S29.0** Injury of muscle and tendon at thorax level

    √6ᵗʰ **S29.00** Unspecified injury of muscle and tendon of thorax

      √7ᵗʰ **S29.001** Unspecified injury of muscle and tendon of front wall of thorax   PE

      √7ᵗʰ **S29.002** Unspecified injury of muscle and tendon of back wall of thorax   PE

      √7ᵗʰ **S29.009** Unspecified injury of muscle and tendon of unspecified wall of thorax   PE

    √6ᵗʰ **S29.01** Strain of muscle and tendon of thorax

      √7ᵗʰ **S29.011** Strain of muscle and tendon of front wall of thorax   PE

      √7ᵗʰ **S29.012** Strain of muscle and tendon of back wall of thorax   PE

      √7ᵗʰ **S29.019** Strain of muscle and tendon of unspecified wall of thorax   PE

    √6ᵗʰ **S29.02** Laceration of muscle and tendon of thorax

      √7ᵗʰ **S29.021** Laceration of muscle and tendon of front wall of thorax   CC PE

      √7ᵗʰ **S29.022** Laceration of muscle and tendon of back wall of thorax   PE

      √7ᵗʰ **S29.029** Laceration of muscle and tendon of unspecified wall of thorax   CC UNS PE

    √6ᵗʰ **S29.09** Other injury of muscle and tendon of thorax

      √7ᵗʰ **S29.091** Other injury of muscle and tendon of front wall of thorax   PE

      √7ᵗʰ **S29.092** Other injury of muscle and tendon of back wall of thorax   PE

      √7ᵗʰ **S29.099** Other injury of muscle and tendon of unspecified wall of thorax   PE

√x7ᵗʰ **S29.8** Other specified injuries of thorax   PE

√x7ᵗʰ **S29.9** Unspecified injury of thorax   PE

Injuries to the abdomen, lower back, lumbar spine, pelvis and external genitals (S30-S39)

INCLUDES
injuries to the abdominal wall
injuries to the anus
injuries to the buttock
injuries to the external genitalia
injuries to the flank
injuries to the groin

EXCLUDES 2
burns and corrosions (T20-T32)
effects of foreign body in anus and rectum (T18.5)
effects of foreign body in genitourinary tract (T19.-)
effects of foreign body in stomach, small intestine and colon (T18.2-T18.4)
frostbite (T33-T34)
insect bite or sting, venomous (T63.4)

√4ᵗʰ **S30** Superficial injury of abdomen, lower back, pelvis and external genitals

    EXCLUDES 2   *superficial injury of hip (S70.-)*

The appropriate 7th character is to be added to each code from category S30.
A   initial encounter
D   subsequent encounter
S   sequela

√x7ᵗʰ **S30.0** Contusion of lower back and pelvis   PE
Contusion of buttock

√x7ᵗʰ **S30.1** Contusion of abdominal wall   PE
Contusion of flank
Contusion of groin

√5ᵗʰ **S30.2** Contusion of external genital organs

    √6ᵗʰ **S30.20** Contusion of unspecified external genital organ

      √7ᵗʰ **S30.201** Contusion of unspecified external genital organ, male   PE

      √7ᵗʰ **S30.202** Contusion of unspecified external genital organ, female   PE

    √x7ᵗʰ **S30.21** Contusion of penis   PE

    √x7ᵗʰ **S30.22** Contusion of scrotum and testes   PE

    √x7ᵗʰ **S30.23** Contusion of vagina and vulva   PE

√x7ᵗʰ **S30.3** Contusion of anus   PE

√5ᵗʰ **S30.8** Other superficial injuries of abdomen, lower back, pelvis and external genitals

    √6ᵗʰ **S30.81** Abrasion of abdomen, lower back, pelvis and external genitals

      √7ᵗʰ **S30.810** Abrasion of lower back and pelvis   PE

      √7ᵗʰ **S30.811** Abrasion of abdominal wall   PE

      √7ᵗʰ **S30.812** Abrasion of penis   PE

      √7ᵗʰ **S30.813** Abrasion of scrotum and testes   PE

      √7ᵗʰ **S30.814** Abrasion of vagina and vulva   PE

      √7ᵗʰ **S30.815** Abrasion of unspecified external genital organs, male   PE

      √7ᵗʰ **S30.816** Abrasion of unspecified external genital organs, female   PE

      √7ᵗʰ **S30.817** Abrasion of anus   PE

    √6ᵗʰ **S30.82** Blister (nonthermal) of abdomen, lower back, pelvis and external genitals

      √7ᵗʰ **S30.820** Blister (nonthermal) of lower back and pelvis   PE

      √7ᵗʰ **S30.821** Blister (nonthermal) of abdominal wall   PE

      √7ᵗʰ **S30.822** Blister (nonthermal) of penis   PE

      √7ᵗʰ **S30.823** Blister (nonthermal) of scrotum and testes   PE

      √7ᵗʰ **S30.824** Blister (nonthermal) of vagina and vulva   PE

      √7ᵗʰ **S30.825** Blister (nonthermal) of unspecified external genital organs, male   PE

      √7ᵗʰ **S30.826** Blister (nonthermal) of unspecified external genital organs, female   PE

      √7ᵗʰ **S30.827** Blister (nonthermal) of anus   PE

    √6ᵗʰ **S30.84** External constriction of abdomen, lower back, pelvis and external genitals

      √7ᵗʰ **S30.840** External constriction of lower back and pelvis   PE

      √7ᵗʰ **S30.841** External constriction of abdominal wall   PE

      √7ᵗʰ **S30.842** External constriction of penis   PE
       Hair tourniquet syndrome of penis
       Use additional cause code to identify the constricting item (W49.0-)

      √7ᵗʰ **S30.843** External constriction of scrotum and testes   PE

      √7ᵗʰ **S30.844** External constriction of vagina and vulva   PE

      √7ᵗʰ **S30.845** External constriction of unspecified external genital organs, male   PE

      √7ᵗʰ **S30.846** External constriction of unspecified external genital organs, female   PE

    √6ᵗʰ **S30.85** Superficial foreign body of abdomen, lower back, pelvis and external genitals
      Splinter in the abdomen, lower back, pelvis and external genitals

      √7ᵗʰ **S30.850** Superficial foreign body of lower back and pelvis   PE

      √7ᵗʰ **S30.851** Superficial foreign body of abdominal wall   PE

      √7ᵗʰ **S30.852** Superficial foreign body of penis   PE

      √7ᵗʰ **S30.853** Superficial foreign body of scrotum and testes   PE

      √7ᵗʰ **S30.854** Superficial foreign body of vagina and vulva   PE

      √7ᵗʰ **S30.855** Superficial foreign body of unspecified external genital organs, male   PE

      √7ᵗʰ **S30.856** Superficial foreign body of unspecified external genital organs, female   PE

      √7ᵗʰ **S30.857** Superficial foreign body of anus   PE

✔ Additional Character Required   √x7ᵗʰ Placeholder   Questionable PDx   Manifestation   Unspecified   UPD Unacceptable PDx   H1-H14 HAC   HCC CMS-HCC Dx   HIV HIV Dx

ICD-10-CM 2025   1013

√6ᵗʰ **S30.86** Insect bite (nonvenomous) of abdomen, lower back, pelvis and external genitals

  √7ᵗʰ **S30.860** Insect bite (nonvenomous) of lower back and pelvis   PE

  √7ᵗʰ **S30.861** Insect bite (nonvenomous) of abdominal wall   PE

  √7ᵗʰ **S30.862** Insect bite (nonvenomous) of penis   PE

  √7ᵗʰ **S30.863** Insect bite (nonvenomous) of scrotum and testes   PE

  √7ᵗʰ **S30.864** Insect bite (nonvenomous) of vagina and vulva   PE

  √7ᵗʰ **S30.865** Insect bite (nonvenomous) of unspecified external genital organs, male   PE

  √7ᵗʰ **S30.866** Insect bite (nonvenomous) of unspecified external genital organs, female   PE

  √7ᵗʰ **S30.867** Insect bite (nonvenomous) of anus   PE

√6ᵗʰ **S30.87** Other superficial bite of abdomen, lower back, pelvis and external genitals

  EXCLUDES 1   open bite of abdomen, lower back, pelvis and external genitals (S31.05, S31.15, S31.25, S31.35, S31.45, S31.55)

  √7ᵗʰ **S30.870** Other superficial bite of lower back and pelvis   PE

  √7ᵗʰ **S30.871** Other superficial bite of abdominal wall   PE

  √7ᵗʰ **S30.872** Other superficial bite of penis   PE

  √7ᵗʰ **S30.873** Other superficial bite of scrotum and testes   PE

  √7ᵗʰ **S30.874** Other superficial bite of vagina and vulva   PE

  √7ᵗʰ **S30.875** Other superficial bite of unspecified external genital organs, male   PE

  √7ᵗʰ **S30.876** Other superficial bite of unspecified external genital organs, female   PE

  √7ᵗʰ **S30.877** Other superficial bite of anus   PE

√5ᵗʰ **S30.9** Unspecified superficial injury of abdomen, lower back, pelvis and external genitals

  √x7ᵗʰ **S30.91** Unspecified superficial injury of lower back and pelvis   PE

  √x7ᵗʰ **S30.92** Unspecified superficial injury of abdominal wall   PE

  √x7ᵗʰ **S30.93** Unspecified superficial injury of penis   PE

  √x7ᵗʰ **S30.94** Unspecified superficial injury of scrotum and testes   PE

  √x7ᵗʰ **S30.95** Unspecified superficial injury of vagina and vulva   PE

  √x7ᵗʰ **S30.96** Unspecified superficial injury of unspecified external genital organs, male   PE

  √x7ᵗʰ **S30.97** Unspecified superficial injury of unspecified external genital organs, female   PE

  √x7ᵗʰ **S30.98** Unspecified superficial injury of anus   PE

√4ᵗʰ **S31** Open wound of abdomen, lower back, pelvis and external genitals

Code also any associated:
  spinal cord injury (S24.0, S24.1-, S34.0-, S34.1-)
  wound infection

EXCLUDES 1   traumatic amputation of part of abdomen, lower back and pelvis (S38.2-, S38.3)

EXCLUDES 2   open fracture of pelvis (S32.1-- S32.9 with 7th character B)
  open wound of hip (S71.00-S71.02)

The appropriate 7th character is to be added to each code from category S31.
  A   initial encounter
  D   subsequent encounter
  S   sequela

√5ᵗʰ **S31.0** Open wound of lower back and pelvis

  √6ᵗʰ **S31.00** Unspecified open wound of lower back and pelvis

    √7ᵗʰ **S31.000** Unspecified open wound of lower back and pelvis without penetration into retroperitoneum   PE
     Unspecified open wound of lower back and pelvis NOS

    √7ᵗʰ **S31.001** Unspecified open wound of lower back and pelvis with penetration into retroperitoneum   MCC PE

√6ᵗʰ **S31.01** Laceration without foreign body of lower back and pelvis

  √7ᵗʰ **S31.010** Laceration without foreign body of lower back and pelvis without penetration into retroperitoneum   PE
    Laceration without foreign body of lower back and pelvis NOS

  √7ᵗʰ **S31.011** Laceration without foreign body of lower back and pelvis with penetration into retroperitoneum   MCC PE

√6ᵗʰ **S31.02** Laceration with foreign body of lower back and pelvis

  √7ᵗʰ **S31.020** Laceration with foreign body of lower back and pelvis without penetration into retroperitoneum   PE
    Laceration with foreign body of lower back and pelvis NOS

  √7ᵗʰ **S31.021** Laceration with foreign body of lower back and pelvis with penetration into retroperitoneum   MCC PE

√6ᵗʰ **S31.03** Puncture wound without foreign body of lower back and pelvis

  √7ᵗʰ **S31.030** Puncture wound without foreign body of lower back and pelvis without penetration into retroperitoneum   PE
    Puncture wound without foreign body of lower back and pelvis NOS

  √7ᵗʰ **S31.031** Puncture wound without foreign body of lower back and pelvis with penetration into retroperitoneum   MCC PE

√6ᵗʰ **S31.04** Puncture wound with foreign body of lower back and pelvis

  √7ᵗʰ **S31.040** Puncture wound with foreign body of lower back and pelvis without penetration into retroperitoneum   PE
    Puncture wound with foreign body of lower back and pelvis NOS

  √7ᵗʰ **S31.041** Puncture wound with foreign body of lower back and pelvis with penetration into retroperitoneum   MCC PE

√6ᵗʰ **S31.05** Open bite of lower back and pelvis

  Bite of lower back and pelvis NOS

  EXCLUDES 1   superficial bite of lower back and pelvis (S30.860, S30.870)

  √7ᵗʰ **S31.050** Open bite of lower back and pelvis without penetration into retroperitoneum   PE
    Open bite of lower back and pelvis NOS

  √7ᵗʰ **S31.051** Open bite of lower back and pelvis with penetration into retroperitoneum   MCC PE

√5ᵗʰ **S31.1** Open wound of abdominal wall without penetration into peritoneal cavity

  Open wound of abdominal wall NOS

  EXCLUDES 2   open wound of abdominal wall with penetration into peritoneal cavity (S31.6-)

√6ᵗʰ **S31.10** Unspecified open wound of abdominal wall without penetration into peritoneal cavity

  √7ᵗʰ **S31.100** Unspecified open wound of abdominal wall, right upper quadrant without penetration into peritoneal cavity   PE

  √7ᵗʰ **S31.101** Unspecified open wound of abdominal wall, left upper quadrant without penetration into peritoneal cavity   PE

  √7ᵗʰ **S31.102** Unspecified open wound of abdominal wall, epigastric region without penetration into peritoneal cavity   PE

  √7ᵗʰ **S31.103** Unspecified open wound of abdominal wall, right lower quadrant without penetration into peritoneal cavity   PE

  √7ᵗʰ **S31.104** Unspecified open wound of abdominal wall, left lower quadrant without penetration into peritoneal cavity   PE

  √7ᵗʰ **S31.105** Unspecified open wound of abdominal wall, periumbilic region without penetration into peritoneal cavity   PE

  √7ᵗʰ **S31.109** Unspecified open wound of abdominal wall, unspecified quadrant without penetration into peritoneal cavity   PE
    Unspecified open wound of abdominal wall NOS

N Newborn: 0   P Pediatric: 0-17   M Maternity: 9-64   A Adult: 15-124   UNS Unspecified Site   MCC Major Complication/Comorbidity   CC Complication/Comorbidity   PE POA Exempt

1014   ICD-10-CM 2025

☑6ᵗʰ S31.11 **Laceration without foreign body** of abdominal wall without penetration into peritoneal cavity

- **☑7ᵗʰ S31.110** Laceration without foreign body of abdominal wall, **right upper quadrant** without penetration into peritoneal cavity   PE
- **☑7ᵗʰ S31.111** Laceration without foreign body of abdominal wall, **left upper quadrant** without penetration into peritoneal cavity   PE
- **☑7ᵗʰ S31.112** Laceration without foreign body of abdominal wall, **epigastric region** without penetration into peritoneal cavity   PE
- **☑7ᵗʰ S31.113** Laceration without foreign body of abdominal wall, **right lower quadrant** without penetration into peritoneal cavity   PE
- **☑7ᵗʰ S31.114** Laceration without foreign body of abdominal wall, **left lower quadrant** without penetration into peritoneal cavity   PE
- **☑7ᵗʰ S31.115** Laceration without foreign body of abdominal wall, **periumbilic region** without penetration into peritoneal cavity   PE
- **☑7ᵗʰ S31.119** Laceration without foreign body of abdominal wall, unspecified quadrant without penetration into peritoneal cavity   PE

☑6ᵗʰ S31.12 **Laceration with foreign body** of abdominal wall without penetration into peritoneal cavity

- **☑7ᵗʰ S31.120** Laceration of abdominal wall with foreign body, **right upper quadrant** without penetration into peritoneal cavity   PE
- **☑7ᵗʰ S31.121** Laceration of abdominal wall with foreign body, **left upper quadrant** without penetration into peritoneal cavity   PE
- **☑7ᵗʰ S31.122** Laceration of abdominal wall with foreign body, **epigastric region** without penetration into peritoneal cavity   PE
- **☑7ᵗʰ S31.123** Laceration of abdominal wall with foreign body, **right lower quadrant** without penetration into peritoneal cavity   PE
- **☑7ᵗʰ S31.124** Laceration of abdominal wall with foreign body, **left lower quadrant** without penetration into peritoneal cavity   PE
- **☑7ᵗʰ S31.125** Laceration of abdominal wall with foreign body, **periumbilic region** without penetration into peritoneal cavity   PE
- **☑7ᵗʰ S31.129** Laceration of abdominal wall with foreign body, unspecified quadrant without penetration into peritoneal cavity   PE

☑6ᵗʰ S31.13 **Puncture wound** of abdominal wall **without foreign body** without penetration into peritoneal cavity

- **☑7ᵗʰ S31.130** Puncture wound of abdominal wall without foreign body, **right upper quadrant** without penetration into peritoneal cavity   PE
- **☑7ᵗʰ S31.131** Puncture wound of abdominal wall without foreign body, **left upper quadrant** without penetration into peritoneal cavity   PE
- **☑7ᵗʰ S31.132** Puncture wound of abdominal wall without foreign body, **epigastric region** without penetration into peritoneal cavity   PE
- **☑7ᵗʰ S31.133** Puncture wound of abdominal wall without foreign body, **right lower quadrant** without penetration into peritoneal cavity   PE
- **☑7ᵗʰ S31.134** Puncture wound of abdominal wall without foreign body, **left lower quadrant** without penetration into peritoneal cavity   PE
- **☑7ᵗʰ S31.135** Puncture wound of abdominal wall without foreign body, **periumbilic region** without penetration into peritoneal cavity   PE
- **☑7ᵗʰ S31.139** Puncture wound of abdominal wall without foreign body, unspecified quadrant without penetration into peritoneal cavity   PE

☑6ᵗʰ S31.14 **Puncture wound** of abdominal wall **with foreign body** without penetration into peritoneal cavity

- **☑7ᵗʰ S31.140** Puncture wound of abdominal wall with foreign body, **right upper quadrant** without penetration into peritoneal cavity   PE
- **☑7ᵗʰ S31.141** Puncture wound of abdominal wall with foreign body, **left upper quadrant** without penetration into peritoneal cavity   PE
- **☑7ᵗʰ S31.142** Puncture wound of abdominal wall with foreign body, **epigastric region** without penetration into peritoneal cavity   PE
- **☑7ᵗʰ S31.143** Puncture wound of abdominal wall with foreign body, **right lower quadrant** without penetration into peritoneal cavity   PE
- **☑7ᵗʰ S31.144** Puncture wound of abdominal wall with foreign body, **left lower quadrant** without penetration into peritoneal cavity   PE
- **☑7ᵗʰ S31.145** Puncture wound of abdominal wall with foreign body, **periumbilic region** without penetration into peritoneal cavity   PE
- **☑7ᵗʰ S31.149** Puncture wound of abdominal wall with foreign body, unspecified quadrant without penetration into peritoneal cavity   PE

☑6ᵗʰ S31.15 **Open bite** of abdominal wall without penetration into peritoneal cavity

    Bite of abdominal wall NOS

    EXCLUDES 1   *superficial bite of abdominal wall (S30.871)*

- **☑7ᵗʰ S31.150** Open bite of abdominal wall, **right upper quadrant** without penetration into peritoneal cavity   PE
- **☑7ᵗʰ S31.151** Open bite of abdominal wall, **left upper quadrant** without penetration into peritoneal cavity   PE
- **☑7ᵗʰ S31.152** Open bite of abdominal wall, **epigastric region** without penetration into peritoneal cavity   PE
- **☑7ᵗʰ S31.153** Open bite of abdominal wall, **right lower quadrant** without penetration into peritoneal cavity   PE
- **☑7ᵗʰ S31.154** Open bite of abdominal wall, **left lower quadrant** without penetration into peritoneal cavity   PE
- **☑7ᵗʰ S31.155** Open bite of abdominal wall, **periumbilic region** without penetration into peritoneal cavity   PE
- **☑7ᵗʰ S31.159** Open bite of abdominal wall, unspecified quadrant without penetration into peritoneal cavity   PE

☑5ᵗʰ S31.2 **Open wound of penis**

- **☑✕7ᵗʰ S31.20** Unspecified open wound of penis   PE
- **☑✕7ᵗʰ S31.21** **Laceration without foreign body** of penis   PE
- **☑✕7ᵗʰ S31.22** **Laceration with foreign body** of penis   PE
- **☑✕7ᵗʰ S31.23** **Puncture wound without foreign body** of penis   PE
- **☑✕7ᵗʰ S31.24** **Puncture wound with foreign body** of penis   PE
- **☑✕7ᵗʰ S31.25** **Open bite** of penis   PE

    Bite of penis NOS

    EXCLUDES 1   *superficial bite of penis (S30.862, S30.872)*

☑5ᵗʰ S31.3 **Open wound of scrotum and testes**

- **☑✕7ᵗʰ S31.30** Unspecified open wound of scrotum and testes   PE
- **☑✕7ᵗʰ S31.31** **Laceration without foreign body** of scrotum and testes   PE
- **☑✕7ᵗʰ S31.32** **Laceration with foreign body** of scrotum and testes   PE
- **☑✕7ᵗʰ S31.33** **Puncture wound without foreign body** of scrotum and testes   PE
- **☑✕7ᵗʰ S31.34** **Puncture wound with foreign body** of scrotum and testes   PE
- **☑✕7ᵗʰ S31.35** **Open bite** of scrotum and testes   PE

    Bite of scrotum and testes NOS

    EXCLUDES 1   *superficial bite of scrotum and testes (S30.863, S30.873)*

☑5ᵗʰ S31.4 **Open wound of vagina and vulva**

    EXCLUDES 1   *injury to vagina and vulva during delivery (O70.-, O71.4)*

- **☑✕7ᵗʰ S31.40** Unspecified open wound of vagina and vulva   PE

✔ Additional Character Required   ☑✕7ᵗʰ Placeholder   Questionable PDx   Manifestation   Unspecified   UPD Unacceptable PDx   H1-H14 HAC   HCC CMS-HCC Dx   HIV HIV Dx

ICD-10-CM 2025   1015

Chapter 19. Injury, Poisoning and Certain Other Consequences of External Causes

S31.41–S31.633

√x 7th **S31.41** **Laceration without foreign body** of vagina and vulva [PE]

√x 7th **S31.42** **Laceration with foreign body** of vagina and vulva [PE]

√x 7th **S31.43** **Puncture wound without foreign body** of vagina and vulva [PE]

√x 7th **S31.44** **Puncture wound with foreign body** of vagina and vulva [PE]

√x 7th **S31.45** **Open bite** of vagina and vulva
Bite of vagina and vulva NOS
EXCLUDES 1   superficial bite of vagina and vulva (S30.864, S30.874)

√5th **S31.5** **Open wound of unspecified external genital organs**
EXCLUDES 1   traumatic amputation of external genital organs (S38.21, S38.22)

√6th **S31.50** **Unspecified open wound** of unspecified external genital organs

√7th **S31.501** Unspecified open wound of unspecified external genital organs, **male** [PE]

√7th **S31.502** Unspecified open wound of unspecified external genital organs, **female** [PE]

√6th **S31.51** **Laceration without foreign body** of unspecified external genital organs

√7th **S31.511** Laceration without foreign body of unspecified external genital organs, **male** [PE]

√7th **S31.512** Laceration without foreign body of unspecified external genital organs, **female** [PE]

√6th **S31.52** **Laceration with foreign body** of unspecified external genital organs

√7th **S31.521** Laceration with foreign body of unspecified external genital organs, **male** [PE]

√7th **S31.522** Laceration with foreign body of unspecified external genital organs, **female** [PE]

√6th **S31.53** **Puncture wound without foreign body** of unspecified external genital organs

√7th **S31.531** Puncture wound without foreign body of unspecified external genital organs, **male** [PE]

√7th **S31.532** Puncture wound without foreign body of unspecified external genital organs, **female** [PE]

√6th **S31.54** **Puncture wound with foreign body** of unspecified external genital organs

√7th **S31.541** Puncture wound with foreign body of unspecified external genital organs, **male** [PE]

√7th **S31.542** Puncture wound with foreign body of unspecified external genital organs, **female** [PE]

√6th **S31.55** **Open bite** of unspecified external genital organs
Bite of unspecified external genital organs NOS
EXCLUDES 1   superficial bite of unspecified external genital organs (S30.865, S30.866, S30.875, S30.876)

√7th **S31.551** Open bite of unspecified external genital organs, **male** [PE]

√7th **S31.552** Open bite of unspecified external genital organs, **female** [PE]

√5th **S31.6** **Open wound of abdominal wall with penetration into peritoneal cavity**
AHA: 2023,3Q,8

√6th **S31.60** **Unspecified open wound** of abdominal wall with penetration into peritoneal cavity

√7th **S31.600** Unspecified open wound of abdominal wall, **right upper quadrant** with penetration into peritoneal cavity [MCC] [PE]

√7th **S31.601** Unspecified open wound of abdominal wall, **left upper quadrant** with penetration into peritoneal cavity [MCC] [PE]

√7th **S31.602** Unspecified open wound of abdominal wall, **epigastric region** with penetration into peritoneal cavity [MCC] [PE]

√7th **S31.603** Unspecified open wound of abdominal wall, **right lower quadrant** with penetration into peritoneal cavity [MCC] [PE]

√7th **S31.604** Unspecified open wound of abdominal wall, **left lower quadrant** with penetration into peritoneal cavity [MCC] [PE]

√7th **S31.605** Unspecified open wound of abdominal wall, **periumbilic region** with penetration into peritoneal cavity [MCC] [PE]

√7th **S31.609** Unspecified open wound of abdominal wall, unspecified quadrant with penetration into peritoneal cavity [MCC] [UNS] [PE]

√6th **S31.61** **Laceration without foreign body** of abdominal wall with penetration into peritoneal cavity

√7th **S31.610** Laceration without foreign body of abdominal wall, **right upper quadrant** with penetration into peritoneal cavity [MCC] [PE]

√7th **S31.611** Laceration without foreign body of abdominal wall, **left upper quadrant** with penetration into peritoneal cavity [MCC] [PE]

√7th **S31.612** Laceration without foreign body of abdominal wall, **epigastric region** with penetration into peritoneal cavity [MCC] [PE]

√7th **S31.613** Laceration without foreign body of abdominal wall, **right lower quadrant** with penetration into peritoneal cavity [MCC] [PE]

√7th **S31.614** Laceration without foreign body of abdominal wall, **left lower quadrant** with penetration into peritoneal cavity [MCC] [PE]

√7th **S31.615** Laceration without foreign body of abdominal wall, **periumbilic region** with penetration into peritoneal cavity [MCC] [PE]

√7th **S31.619** Laceration without foreign body of abdominal wall, unspecified quadrant with penetration into peritoneal cavity [MCC] [UNS] [PE]

√6th **S31.62** **Laceration with foreign body** of abdominal wall with penetration into peritoneal cavity

√7th **S31.620** Laceration with foreign body of abdominal wall, **right upper quadrant** with penetration into peritoneal cavity [MCC] [PE]

√7th **S31.621** Laceration with foreign body of abdominal wall, **left upper quadrant** with penetration into peritoneal cavity [MCC] [PE]

√7th **S31.622** Laceration with foreign body of abdominal wall, **epigastric region** with penetration into peritoneal cavity [MCC] [PE]

√7th **S31.623** Laceration with foreign body of abdominal wall, **right lower quadrant** with penetration into peritoneal cavity [MCC] [PE]

√7th **S31.624** Laceration with foreign body of abdominal wall, **left lower quadrant** with penetration into peritoneal cavity [MCC] [PE]

√7th **S31.625** Laceration with foreign body of abdominal wall, **periumbilic region** with penetration into peritoneal cavity [MCC] [PE]

√7th **S31.629** Laceration with foreign body of abdominal wall, unspecified quadrant with penetration into peritoneal cavity [MCC] [UNS] [PE]

√6th **S31.63** **Puncture wound without foreign body** of abdominal wall with penetration into peritoneal cavity

√7th **S31.630** Puncture wound without foreign body of abdominal wall, **right upper quadrant** with penetration into peritoneal cavity [MCC] [PE]

√7th **S31.631** Puncture wound without foreign body of abdominal wall, **left upper quadrant** with penetration into peritoneal cavity [MCC] [PE]

√7th **S31.632** Puncture wound without foreign body of abdominal wall, **epigastric region** with penetration into peritoneal cavity [MCC] [PE]

√7th **S31.633** Puncture wound without foreign body of abdominal wall, **right lower quadrant** with penetration into peritoneal cavity [MCC] [PE]

✓7ᵗʰ **S31.634** Puncture wound without foreign body of abdominal wall, **left lower quadrant** with penetration into peritoneal cavity   `MCC` `PE`

✓7ᵗʰ **S31.635** Puncture wound without foreign body of abdominal wall, **periumbilic region** with penetration into peritoneal cavity   `MCC` `PE`

✓7ᵗʰ **S31.639** Puncture wound without foreign body of abdominal wall, unspecified quadrant with penetration into peritoneal cavity   `MCC` `UNS` `PE`

✓6ᵗʰ **S31.64** **Puncture wound with foreign body** of abdominal wall with penetration into peritoneal cavity

✓7ᵗʰ **S31.640** Puncture wound with foreign body of abdominal wall, **right upper quadrant** with penetration into peritoneal cavity   `MCC` `PE`

✓7ᵗʰ **S31.641** Puncture wound with foreign body of abdominal wall, **left upper quadrant** with penetration into peritoneal cavity   `MCC` `PE`

✓7ᵗʰ **S31.642** Puncture wound with foreign body of abdominal wall, **epigastric region** with penetration into peritoneal cavity   `MCC` `PE`

✓7ᵗʰ **S31.643** Puncture wound with foreign body of abdominal wall, **right lower quadrant** with penetration into peritoneal cavity   `MCC` `PE`

✓7ᵗʰ **S31.644** Puncture wound with foreign body of abdominal wall, **left lower quadrant** with penetration into peritoneal cavity   `MCC` `PE`

✓7ᵗʰ **S31.645** Puncture wound with foreign body of abdominal wall, **periumbilic region** with penetration into peritoneal cavity   `MCC` `PE`

✓7ᵗʰ **S31.649** Puncture wound with foreign body of abdominal wall, unspecified quadrant with penetration into peritoneal cavity   `MCC` `UNS` `PE`

✓6ᵗʰ **S31.65** **Open bite** of abdominal wall with penetration into peritoneal cavity

    EXCLUDES 1   superficial bite of abdominal wall (S30.861, S30.871)

✓7ᵗʰ **S31.650** Open bite of abdominal wall, **right upper quadrant** with penetration into peritoneal cavity   `MCC` `PE`

✓7ᵗʰ **S31.651** Open bite of abdominal wall, **left upper quadrant** with penetration into peritoneal cavity   `MCC` `PE`

✓7ᵗʰ **S31.652** Open bite of abdominal wall, **epigastric region** with penetration into peritoneal cavity   `MCC` `PE`

✓7ᵗʰ **S31.653** Open bite of abdominal wall, **right lower quadrant** with penetration into peritoneal cavity   `MCC` `PE`

✓7ᵗʰ **S31.654** Open bite of abdominal wall, **left lower quadrant** with penetration into peritoneal cavity   `MCC` `PE`

✓7ᵗʰ **S31.655** Open bite of abdominal wall, **periumbilic region** with penetration into peritoneal cavity   `MCC` `PE`

✓7ᵗʰ **S31.659** Open bite of abdominal wall, unspecified quadrant with penetration into peritoneal cavity   `MCC` `UNS` `PE`

✓5ᵗʰ **S31.8** **Open wound of other parts of abdomen, lower back and pelvis**

✓6ᵗʰ **S31.80** **Open wound of unspecified buttock**

✓7ᵗʰ **S31.801** **Laceration without foreign body** of unspecified buttock   `PE`

✓7ᵗʰ **S31.802** **Laceration with foreign body** of unspecified buttock   `PE`

✓7ᵗʰ **S31.803** **Puncture wound without foreign body** of unspecified buttock   `PE`

✓7ᵗʰ **S31.804** **Puncture wound with foreign body** of unspecified buttock   `PE`

✓7ᵗʰ **S31.805** **Open bite** of unspecified buttock   `PE`

    Bite of buttock NOS

      EXCLUDES 1   superficial bite of buttock (S30.870)

✓7ᵗʰ **S31.809** Unspecified open wound of unspecified buttock   `PE`

✓6ᵗʰ **S31.81** **Open wound of right buttock**

✓7ᵗʰ **S31.811** **Laceration without foreign body** of right buttock   `PE`

✓7ᵗʰ **S31.812** **Laceration with foreign body** of right buttock   `PE`

✓7ᵗʰ **S31.813** **Puncture wound without foreign body** of right buttock   `PE`

✓7ᵗʰ **S31.814** **Puncture wound with foreign body** of right buttock   `PE`

✓7ᵗʰ **S31.815** **Open bite** of right buttock   `PE`

    Bite of right buttock NOS

      EXCLUDES 1   superficial bite of buttock (S30.870)

✓7ᵗʰ **S31.819** Unspecified open wound of right buttock   `PE`

✓6ᵗʰ **S31.82** **Open wound of left buttock**

✓7ᵗʰ **S31.821** **Laceration without foreign body** of left buttock   `PE`

✓7ᵗʰ **S31.822** **Laceration with foreign body** of left buttock   `PE`

✓7ᵗʰ **S31.823** **Puncture wound without foreign body** of left buttock   `PE`

✓7ᵗʰ **S31.824** **Puncture wound with foreign body** of left buttock   `PE`

✓7ᵗʰ **S31.825** **Open bite** of left buttock   `PE`

    Bite of left buttock NOS

      EXCLUDES 1   superficial bite of buttock (S30.870)

✓7ᵗʰ **S31.829** Unspecified open wound of left buttock   `PE`

✓6ᵗʰ **S31.83** **Open wound of anus**

✓7ᵗʰ **S31.831** **Laceration without foreign body** of anus   `PE`

✓7ᵗʰ **S31.832** **Laceration with foreign body** of anus   `PE`

✓7ᵗʰ **S31.833** **Puncture wound without foreign body** of anus   `PE`

✓7ᵗʰ **S31.834** **Puncture wound with foreign body** of anus   `PE`

✓7ᵗʰ **S31.835** **Open bite** of anus   `PE`

    Bite of anus NOS

      EXCLUDES 1   superficial bite of anus (S30.877)

✓7ᵗʰ **S31.839** Unspecified open wound of anus   `PE`

✓4ᵗʰ **S32** **Fracture of lumbar spine and pelvis**

    `NOTE`   A fracture not indicated as displaced or nondisplaced should be coded to displaced.

       A fracture not indicated as opened or closed should be coded to closed.

    `INCLUDES`   fracture of lumbosacral neural arch
       fracture of lumbosacral spinous process
       fracture of lumbosacral transverse process
       fracture of lumbosacral vertebra
       fracture of lumbosacral vertebral arch

Code first any associated spinal cord and spinal nerve injury (S34.-)

    EXCLUDES 1   transection of abdomen (S38.3)

    EXCLUDES 2   fracture of hip NOS (S72.0-)

AHA: 2021,1Q,6; 2018,2Q,12; 2015,3Q,37-39; 2012,4Q,93

The appropriate 7th character is to be added to each code from category S32.

A   initial encounter for closed fracture

B   initial encounter for open fracture

D   subsequent encounter for fracture with routine healing

G   subsequent encounter for fracture with delayed healing

K   subsequent encounter for fracture with nonunion

S   sequela

✓5ᵗʰ **S32.0** **Fracture of lumbar vertebra**

    Fracture of lumbar spine NOS

✓6ᵗʰ **S32.00** **Fracture of unspecified lumbar vertebra**

✓7ᵗʰ **S32.000** **Wedge compression** fracture of unspecified lumbar vertebra   `MCC` `CC` `H5` `HCC` `PE`

✓7ᵗʰ **S32.001** **Stable burst** fracture of unspecified lumbar vertebra   `MCC` `CC` `H5` `HCC` `PE`

✓ Additional Character Required   ✓7ᵗʰ Placeholder   Questionable PDx   Manifestation   Unspecified   `UPD` Unacceptable PDx   `H1`-`H14` HAC   `HCC` CMS-HCC Dx   `HIV` HIV Dx

ICD-10-CM 2025   1017

Chapter 19. Injury, Poisoning and Certain Other Consequences of External Causes

S32.002–S32.2

✓7th **S32.002** **Unstable burst** fracture of unspecified lumbar vertebra   MCC CC H5 HCC PE

✓7th **S32.008** Other fracture of unspecified lumbar vertebra   MCC CC H5 HCC PE

✓7th **S32.009** Unspecified fracture of unspecified lumbar vertebra   MCC CC H5 HCC PE

✓6th **S32.01** Fracture of **first** lumbar vertebra

✓7th **S32.010** **Wedge compression** fracture of first lumbar vertebra   MCC CC H5 HCC PE

✓7th **S32.011** **Stable burst** fracture of first lumbar vertebra   MCC CC H5 HCC PE

✓7th **S32.012** **Unstable burst** fracture of first lumbar vertebra   MCC CC H5 HCC PE

✓7th **S32.018** Other fracture of first lumbar vertebra   MCC CC H5 HCC PE

✓7th **S32.019** Unspecified fracture of first lumbar vertebra   MCC CC H5 HCC PE

✓6th **S32.02** Fracture of **second** lumbar vertebra

✓7th **S32.020** **Wedge compression** fracture of second lumbar vertebra   MCC CC H5 HCC PE

✓7th **S32.021** **Stable burst** fracture of second lumbar vertebra   MCC CC H5 HCC PE

✓7th **S32.022** **Unstable burst** fracture of second lumbar vertebra   MCC CC H5 HCC PE

✓7th **S32.028** Other fracture of second lumbar vertebra   MCC CC H5 HCC PE

✓7th **S32.029** Unspecified fracture of second lumbar vertebra   MCC CC H5 HCC PE

✓6th **S32.03** Fracture of **third** lumbar vertebra

✓7th **S32.030** **Wedge compression** fracture of third lumbar vertebra   MCC CC H5 HCC PE

✓7th **S32.031** **Stable burst** fracture of third lumbar vertebra   MCC CC H5 HCC PE

✓7th **S32.032** **Unstable burst** fracture of third lumbar vertebra   MCC CC H5 HCC PE

✓7th **S32.038** Other fracture of third lumbar vertebra   MCC CC H5 HCC PE

✓7th **S32.039** Unspecified fracture of third lumbar vertebra   MCC CC H5 HCC PE

✓6th **S32.04** Fracture of **fourth** lumbar vertebra

✓7th **S32.040** **Wedge compression** fracture of fourth lumbar vertebra   MCC CC H5 HCC PE

✓7th **S32.041** **Stable burst** fracture of fourth lumbar vertebra   MCC CC H5 HCC PE

✓7th **S32.042** **Unstable burst** fracture of fourth lumbar vertebra   MCC CC H5 HCC PE

✓7th **S32.048** Other fracture of fourth lumbar vertebra   MCC CC H5 HCC PE

✓7th **S32.049** Unspecified fracture of fourth lumbar vertebra   MCC CC H5 HCC PE

✓6th **S32.05** Fracture of **fifth** lumbar vertebra

✓7th **S32.050** **Wedge compression** fracture of fifth lumbar vertebra   MCC CC H5 HCC PE

✓7th **S32.051** **Stable burst** fracture of fifth lumbar vertebra   MCC CC H5 HCC PE

✓7th **S32.052** **Unstable burst** fracture of fifth lumbar vertebra   MCC CC H5 HCC PE

✓7th **S32.058** Other fracture of fifth lumbar vertebra   MCC CC H5 HCC PE

✓7th **S32.059** Unspecified fracture of fifth lumbar vertebra   MCC CC H5 HCC PE

✓5th **S32.1** Fracture of **sacrum**

NOTE For vertical fractures, code to most medial fracture extension

Use two codes if both a vertical and transverse fracture are present

Code also any associated fracture of pelvic ring (S32.8-)

✓x7th **S32.10** Unspecified fracture of sacrum   MCC CC H5 HCC PE

✓6th **S32.11** **Zone I** fracture of sacrum

Vertical sacral ala fracture of sacrum

Vertical Sacral Fracture Zones

Zones: ① ② ③

✓7th **S32.110** **Nondisplaced** Zone I fracture of sacrum   MCC CC H5 HCC PE

✓7th **S32.111** **Minimally displaced** Zone I fracture of sacrum   MCC CC H5 HCC PE

✓7th **S32.112** **Severely displaced** Zone I fracture of sacrum   MCC CC H5 HCC PE

✓7th **S32.119** Unspecified Zone I fracture of sacrum   MCC CC H5 HCC PE

✓6th **S32.12** **Zone II** fracture of sacrum

Vertical foraminal region fracture of sacrum

✓7th **S32.120** **Nondisplaced** Zone II fracture of sacrum   MCC CC H5 HCC PE

✓7th **S32.121** **Minimally displaced** Zone II fracture of sacrum   MCC CC H5 HCC PE

✓7th **S32.122** **Severely displaced** Zone II fracture of sacrum   MCC CC H5 HCC PE

✓7th **S32.129** Unspecified Zone II fracture of sacrum   MCC CC H5 HCC PE

✓6th **S32.13** **Zone III** fracture of sacrum

Vertical fracture into spinal canal region of sacrum

✓7th **S32.130** **Nondisplaced** Zone III fracture of sacrum   MCC CC H5 HCC PE

✓7th **S32.131** **Minimally displaced** Zone III fracture of sacrum   MCC CC H5 HCC PE

✓7th **S32.132** **Severely displaced** Zone III fracture of sacrum   MCC CC H5 HCC PE

✓7th **S32.139** Unspecified Zone III fracture of sacrum   MCC CC H5 HCC PE

Transverse Sacral Fracture Types

Type 1   Type 2   Type 3   Type 4

✓x7th **S32.14** **Type 1 fracture of sacrum**   MCC CC H5 HCC PE

Transverse flexion fracture of sacrum without displacement

✓x7th **S32.15** **Type 2 fracture of sacrum**   MCC CC H5 HCC PE

Transverse flexion fracture of sacrum with posterior displacement

✓x7th **S32.16** **Type 3 fracture of sacrum**   MCC CC H5 HCC PE

Transverse extension fracture of sacrum with anterior displacement

✓x7th **S32.17** **Type 4 fracture of sacrum**   MCC CC H5 HCC PE

Transverse segmental comminution of upper sacrum

✓x7th **S32.19** Other fracture of sacrum   MCC CC H5 HCC PE

✓x7th **S32.2** Fracture of **coccyx**   MCC CC H5 HCC PE

N Newborn: 0   P Pediatric: 0-17   M Maternity: 9-64   A Adult: 15-124   UHS Unspecified Site   MCC Major Complication/Comorbidity   CC Complication/Comorbidity   PE POA Exempt

1018   ICD-10-CM 2025

√5ᵗʰ S32.3 Fracture of ilium

> **EXCLUDES 1**   *fracture of ilium with associated disruption of pelvic ring (S32.8-)*

  √6ᵗʰ S32.30 Unspecified fracture of ilium

    √7ᵗʰ S32.301 Unspecified fracture of right ilium `MCC` `CC` `H5` `HCC` `PE`

    √7ᵗʰ S32.302 Unspecified fracture of left ilium `MCC` `CC` `H5` `HCC` `PE`

    √7ᵗʰ S32.309 Unspecified fracture of unspecified ilium `MCC` `CC` `H5` `UNS` `HCC` `PE`

  √6ᵗʰ S32.31 Avulsion fracture of ilium

    √7ᵗʰ S32.311 Displaced avulsion fracture of right ilium `MCC` `CC` `H5` `HCC` `PE`

    √7ᵗʰ S32.312 Displaced avulsion fracture of left ilium `MCC` `CC` `H5` `HCC` `PE`

    √7ᵗʰ S32.313 Displaced avulsion fracture of unspecified ilium `MCC` `CC` `H5` `UNS` `HCC` `PE`

    √7ᵗʰ S32.314 Nondisplaced avulsion fracture of right ilium `MCC` `CC` `H5` `HCC` `PE`

    √7ᵗʰ S32.315 Nondisplaced avulsion fracture of left ilium `MCC` `CC` `H5` `HCC` `PE`

    √7ᵗʰ S32.316 Nondisplaced avulsion fracture of unspecified ilium `MCC` `CC` `H5` `UNS` `HCC` `PE`

  √6ᵗʰ S32.39 Other fracture of ilium

    √7ᵗʰ S32.391 Other fracture of right ilium `MCC` `CC` `H5` `HCC` `PE`

    √7ᵗʰ S32.392 Other fracture of left ilium `MCC` `CC` `H5` `HCC` `PE`

    √7ᵗʰ S32.399 Other fracture of unspecified ilium `MCC` `CC` `H5` `UNS` `HCC` `PE`

√5ᵗʰ S32.4 Fracture of acetabulum

> Code also any associated fracture of pelvic ring (S32.8-)
> **AHA:** 2016,3Q,16

  √6ᵗʰ S32.40 Unspecified fracture of acetabulum

    √7ᵗʰ S32.401 Unspecified fracture of right acetabulum `MCC` `CC` `H5` `HCC` `PE`

    √7ᵗʰ S32.402 Unspecified fracture of left acetabulum `MCC` `CC` `H5` `HCC` `PE`

    √7ᵗʰ S32.409 Unspecified fracture of unspecified acetabulum `MCC` `CC` `H5` `UNS` `HCC` `PE`

  √6ᵗʰ S32.41 Fracture of anterior wall of acetabulum

    √7ᵗʰ S32.411 Displaced fracture of anterior wall of right acetabulum `MCC` `CC` `H5` `HCC` `PE`

    √7ᵗʰ S32.412 Displaced fracture of anterior wall of left acetabulum `MCC` `CC` `H5` `HCC` `PE`

    √7ᵗʰ S32.413 Displaced fracture of anterior wall of unspecified acetabulum `MCC` `CC` `H5` `UNS` `HCC` `PE`

    √7ᵗʰ S32.414 Nondisplaced fracture of anterior wall of right acetabulum `MCC` `CC` `H5` `HCC` `PE`

    √7ᵗʰ S32.415 Nondisplaced fracture of anterior wall of left acetabulum `MCC` `CC` `H5` `HCC` `PE`

    √7ᵗʰ S32.416 Nondisplaced fracture of anterior wall of unspecified acetabulum `MCC` `CC` `H5` `UNS` `HCC` `PE`

  √6ᵗʰ S32.42 Fracture of posterior wall of acetabulum

    √7ᵗʰ S32.421 Displaced fracture of posterior wall of right acetabulum `MCC` `CC` `H5` `HCC` `PE`

    √7ᵗʰ S32.422 Displaced fracture of posterior wall of left acetabulum `MCC` `CC` `H5` `HCC` `PE`

    √7ᵗʰ S32.423 Displaced fracture of posterior wall of unspecified acetabulum `MCC` `CC` `H5` `UNS` `HCC` `PE`

    √7ᵗʰ S32.424 Nondisplaced fracture of posterior wall of right acetabulum `MCC` `CC` `H5` `HCC` `PE`

    √7ᵗʰ S32.425 Nondisplaced fracture of posterior wall of left acetabulum `MCC` `CC` `H5` `HCC` `PE`

    √7ᵗʰ S32.426 Nondisplaced fracture of posterior wall of unspecified acetabulum `MCC` `CC` `H5` `UNS` `HCC` `PE`

  √6ᵗʰ S32.43 Fracture of anterior column [iliopubic] of acetabulum

    √7ᵗʰ S32.431 Displaced fracture of anterior column [iliopubic] of right acetabulum `MCC` `CC` `H5` `HCC` `PE`

    √7ᵗʰ S32.432 Displaced fracture of anterior column [iliopubic] of left acetabulum `MCC` `CC` `H5` `HCC` `PE`

    √7ᵗʰ S32.433 Displaced fracture of anterior column [iliopubic] of unspecified acetabulum `MCC` `CC` `H5` `UNS` `HCC` `PE`

    √7ᵗʰ S32.434 Nondisplaced fracture of anterior column [iliopubic] of right acetabulum `MCC` `CC` `H5` `HCC` `PE`

    √7ᵗʰ S32.435 Nondisplaced fracture of anterior column [iliopubic] of left acetabulum `MCC` `CC` `H5` `HCC` `PE`

    √7ᵗʰ S32.436 Nondisplaced fracture of anterior column [iliopubic] of unspecified acetabulum `MCC` `CC` `H5` `UNS` `HCC` `PE`

  √6ᵗʰ S32.44 Fracture of posterior column [ilioischial] of acetabulum

    √7ᵗʰ S32.441 Displaced fracture of posterior column [ilioischial] of right acetabulum `MCC` `CC` `H5` `HCC` `PE`

    √7ᵗʰ S32.442 Displaced fracture of posterior column [ilioischial] of left acetabulum `MCC` `CC` `H5` `HCC` `PE`

    √7ᵗʰ S32.443 Displaced fracture of posterior column [ilioischial] of unspecified acetabulum `MCC` `CC` `H5` `UNS` `HCC` `PE`

    √7ᵗʰ S32.444 Nondisplaced fracture of posterior column [ilioischial] of right acetabulum `MCC` `CC` `H5` `HCC` `PE`

    √7ᵗʰ S32.445 Nondisplaced fracture of posterior column [ilioischial] of left acetabulum `MCC` `CC` `H5` `HCC` `PE`

    √7ᵗʰ S32.446 Nondisplaced fracture of posterior column [ilioischial] of unspecified acetabulum `MCC` `CC` `H5` `UNS` `HCC` `PE`

  √6ᵗʰ S32.45 Transverse fracture of acetabulum

    √7ᵗʰ S32.451 Displaced transverse fracture of right acetabulum `MCC` `CC` `H5` `HCC` `PE`

    √7ᵗʰ S32.452 Displaced transverse fracture of left acetabulum `MCC` `CC` `H5` `HCC` `PE`

    √7ᵗʰ S32.453 Displaced transverse fracture of unspecified acetabulum `MCC` `CC` `H5` `UNS` `HCC` `PE`

    √7ᵗʰ S32.454 Nondisplaced transverse fracture of right acetabulum `MCC` `CC` `H5` `HCC` `PE`

    √7ᵗʰ S32.455 Nondisplaced transverse fracture of left acetabulum `MCC` `CC` `H5` `HCC` `PE`

    √7ᵗʰ S32.456 Nondisplaced transverse fracture of unspecified acetabulum `MCC` `CC` `H5` `UNS` `HCC` `PE`

  √6ᵗʰ S32.46 Associated transverse-posterior fracture of acetabulum

    √7ᵗʰ S32.461 Displaced associated transverse-posterior fracture of right acetabulum `MCC` `CC` `H5` `HCC` `PE`

    √7ᵗʰ S32.462 Displaced associated transverse-posterior fracture of left acetabulum `MCC` `CC` `H5` `HCC` `PE`

    √7ᵗʰ S32.463 Displaced associated transverse-posterior fracture of unspecified acetabulum `MCC` `CC` `H5` `UNS` `HCC` `PE`

    √7ᵗʰ S32.464 Nondisplaced associated transverse-posterior fracture of right acetabulum `MCC` `CC` `H5` `HCC` `PE`

    √7ᵗʰ S32.465 Nondisplaced associated transverse-posterior fracture of left acetabulum `MCC` `CC` `H5` `HCC` `PE`

    √7ᵗʰ S32.466 Nondisplaced associated transverse-posterior fracture of unspecified acetabulum `MCC` `CC` `H5` `UNS` `HCC` `PE`

  √6ᵗʰ S32.47 Fracture of medial wall of acetabulum

    √7ᵗʰ S32.471 Displaced fracture of medial wall of right acetabulum `MCC` `CC` `H5` `HCC` `PE`

    √7ᵗʰ S32.472 Displaced fracture of medial wall of left acetabulum `MCC` `CC` `H5` `HCC` `PE`

    √7ᵗʰ S32.473 Displaced fracture of medial wall of unspecified acetabulum `MCC` `CC` `H5` `UNS` `HCC` `PE`

    √7ᵗʰ S32.474 Nondisplaced fracture of medial wall of right acetabulum `MCC` `CC` `H5` `HCC` `PE`

    √7ᵗʰ S32.475 Nondisplaced fracture of medial wall of left acetabulum `MCC` `CC` `H5` `HCC` `PE`

✔ Additional Character Required   √x7ᵗʰ Placeholder   `Questionable PDx`   Manifestation   Unspecified   `UPD` Unacceptable PDx   `H1`-`H14` HAC   `HCC` CMS-HCC Dx   `HIV` HIV Dx

ICD-10-CM 2025   1019

√7ᵗʰ **S32.476** **Nondisplaced** fracture of medial wall of unspecified acetabulum   MCC CC H5 UNS HCC PE

√6ᵗʰ **S32.48** **Dome fracture** of acetabulum

   √7ᵗʰ **S32.481** **Displaced** dome fracture of **right** acetabulum   MCC CC H5 HCC PE

   √7ᵗʰ **S32.482** **Displaced** dome fracture of **left** acetabulum   MCC CC H5 HCC PE

   √7ᵗʰ **S32.483** **Displaced** dome fracture of **unspecified** acetabulum   MCC CC H5 UNS HCC PE

   √7ᵗʰ **S32.484** **Nondisplaced** dome fracture of **right** acetabulum   MCC CC H5 HCC PE

   √7ᵗʰ **S32.485** **Nondisplaced** dome fracture of **left** acetabulum   MCC CC H5 HCC PE

   √7ᵗʰ **S32.486** **Nondisplaced** dome fracture of **unspecified** acetabulum   MCC CC H5 UNS HCC PE

√6ᵗʰ **S32.49** **Other specified fracture of acetabulum**

   √7ᵗʰ **S32.491** **Other specified fracture of right** acetabulum   MCC CC H5 HCC PE

   √7ᵗʰ **S32.492** **Other specified fracture of left** acetabulum   MCC CC H5 HCC PE

   √7ᵗʰ **S32.499** **Other specified fracture of unspecified** acetabulum   MCC CC H5 UNS HCC PE

√5ᵗʰ **S32.5** **Fracture of pubis**

   EXCLUDES 1   *fracture of pubis with associated disruption of pelvic ring (S32.8-)*

   √6ᵗʰ **S32.50** **Unspecified fracture of pubis**

     √7ᵗʰ **S32.501** **Unspecified fracture of right** pubis   MCC CC H5 HCC PE

     √7ᵗʰ **S32.502** **Unspecified fracture of left** pubis   MCC CC H5 HCC PE

     √7ᵗʰ **S32.509** **Unspecified fracture of unspecified** pubis   MCC CC H5 UNS HCC PE

   √6ᵗʰ **S32.51** **Fracture of superior rim of pubis**

     √7ᵗʰ **S32.511** **Fracture of superior rim of right** pubis   MCC CC H5 HCC PE

     √7ᵗʰ **S32.512** **Fracture of superior rim of left** pubis   MCC CC H5 HCC PE

     √7ᵗʰ **S32.519** **Fracture of superior rim of unspecified** pubis   MCC CC H5 UNS HCC PE

   √6ᵗʰ **S32.59** **Other specified fracture of pubis**

     √7ᵗʰ **S32.591** **Other specified fracture of right** pubis   MCC CC H5 HCC PE

     √7ᵗʰ **S32.592** **Other specified fracture of left** pubis   MCC CC H5 HCC PE

     √7ᵗʰ **S32.599** **Other specified fracture of unspecified** pubis   MCC CC H5 UNS HCC PE

√5ᵗʰ **S32.6** **Fracture of ischium**

   EXCLUDES 1   *fracture of ischium with associated disruption of pelvic ring (S32.8-)*

   √6ᵗʰ **S32.60** **Unspecified fracture of ischium**

     √7ᵗʰ **S32.601** **Unspecified fracture of right** ischium   MCC CC H5 HCC PE

     √7ᵗʰ **S32.602** **Unspecified fracture of left** ischium   MCC CC H5 HCC PE

     √7ᵗʰ **S32.609** **Unspecified fracture of unspecified** ischium   MCC CC H5 UNS HCC PE

   √6ᵗʰ **S32.61** **Avulsion fracture of ischium**

     √7ᵗʰ **S32.611** **Displaced** avulsion fracture of **right** ischium   MCC CC H5 HCC PE

     √7ᵗʰ **S32.612** **Displaced** avulsion fracture of **left** ischium   MCC CC H5 HCC PE

     √7ᵗʰ **S32.613** **Displaced** avulsion fracture of **unspecified** ischium   MCC CC H5 UNS HCC PE

     √7ᵗʰ **S32.614** **Nondisplaced** avulsion fracture of **right** ischium   MCC CC H5 HCC PE

     √7ᵗʰ **S32.615** **Nondisplaced** avulsion fracture of **left** ischium   MCC CC H5 HCC PE

     √7ᵗʰ **S32.616** **Nondisplaced** avulsion fracture of **unspecified** ischium   MCC CC H5 UNS HCC PE

   √6ᵗʰ **S32.69** **Other specified fracture of ischium**

     √7ᵗʰ **S32.691** **Other specified fracture of right** ischium   MCC CC H5 HCC PE

     √7ᵗʰ **S32.692** **Other specified fracture of left** ischium   MCC CC H5 HCC PE

√7ᵗʰ **S32.699** **Other specified fracture of unspecified** ischium   MCC CC H5 UNS HCC PE

√5ᵗʰ **S32.8** **Fracture of other parts of pelvis**

   Code also any associated:
    fracture of acetabulum (S32.4-)
    sacral fracture (S32.1-)

Fractures Disrupting Pelvic Circle

Pelvic circle — **Stable**

Unstable (two-place fracture)

Iliac crest — Anterior superior iliac spine — Ischial spine — Acetabulum — Femur — Ischium — Ilium — L5 — **Pelvic Bones** — Sacrum — Coccyx — Pubis — Pubic symphysis

   √6ᵗʰ **S32.81** **Multiple fractures of pelvis with disruption of pelvic ring**
    Multiple pelvic fractures with disruption of pelvic circle

     √7ᵗʰ **S32.810** **Multiple fractures of pelvis with stable disruption of pelvic ring**   MCC CC H5 HCC PE

     √7ᵗʰ **S32.811** **Multiple fractures of pelvis with unstable disruption of pelvic ring**   MCC CC H5 HCC PE

   √x7ᵗʰ **S32.82** **Multiple fractures of pelvis without disruption of pelvic ring**   MCC CC H5 HCC PE
    Multiple pelvic fractures without disruption of pelvic circle

   √x7ᵗʰ **S32.89** **Fracture of other parts of pelvis**   MCC CC H5 HCC PE

√x7ᵗʰ **S32.9** **Fracture of unspecified parts of lumbosacral spine and pelvis**   MCC CC H5 HCC PE
   Fracture of lumbosacral spine NOS
   Fracture of pelvis NOS
   AHA: 2012,4Q,93

√4ᵗʰ **S33** **Dislocation and sprain of joints and ligaments of lumbar spine and pelvis**

   INCLUDES   avulsion of joint or ligament of lumbar spine and pelvis
      laceration of cartilage, joint or ligament of lumbar spine and pelvis
      sprain of cartilage, joint or ligament of lumbar spine and pelvis
      traumatic hemarthrosis of joint or ligament of lumbar spine and pelvis
      traumatic rupture of joint or ligament of lumbar spine and pelvis
      traumatic subluxation of joint or ligament of lumbar spine and pelvis
      traumatic tear of joint or ligament of lumbar spine and pelvis

   Code also any associated open wound

   EXCLUDES 1   *nontraumatic rupture or displacement of lumbar intervertebral disc NOS (M51.-)*
      obstetric damage to pelvic joints and ligaments (O71.6)

   EXCLUDES 2   *dislocation and sprain of joints and ligaments of hip (S73.-)*
      strain of muscle of lower back and pelvis (S39.01-)

> The appropriate 7th character is to be added to each code from category S33.
> A   initial encounter
> D   subsequent encounter
> S   sequela

√x7ᵗʰ **S33.0** **Traumatic rupture of lumbar intervertebral disc**   PE

   EXCLUDES 1   *rupture or displacement (nontraumatic) of lumbar intervertebral disc NOS (M51.- with fifth character 6)*

✓5th **S33.1** Subluxation and dislocation of lumbar vertebra

Code also any associated:
open wound of abdomen, lower back and pelvis (S31)
spinal cord injury (S24.0, S24.1-, S34.0-, S34.1-)

EXCLUDES 2   fracture of lumbar vertebrae (S32.0-)

✓6th **S33.10** Subluxation and dislocation of unspecified lumbar vertebra

✓7th **S33.100** **Subluxation** of unspecified lumbar vertebra   PE

✓7th **S33.101** **Dislocation** of unspecified lumbar vertebra   PE

✓6th **S33.11** Subluxation and dislocation of L1/L2 lumbar vertebra

✓7th **S33.110** **Subluxation** of L1/L2 lumbar vertebra   PE

✓7th **S33.111** **Dislocation** of L1/L2 lumbar vertebra   PE

✓6th **S33.12** Subluxation and dislocation of L2/L3 lumbar vertebra

✓7th **S33.120** **Subluxation** of L2/L3 lumbar vertebra   PE

✓7th **S33.121** **Dislocation** of L2/L3 lumbar vertebra   PE

✓6th **S33.13** Subluxation and dislocation of L3/L4 lumbar vertebra

✓7th **S33.130** **Subluxation** of L3/L4 lumbar vertebra   PE

✓7th **S33.131** **Dislocation** of L3/L4 lumbar vertebra   PE

✓6th **S33.14** Subluxation and dislocation of L4/L5 lumbar vertebra

✓7th **S33.140** **Subluxation** of L4/L5 lumbar vertebra   PE

✓7th **S33.141** **Dislocation** of L4/L5 lumbar vertebra   PE

✓x7th **S33.2** Dislocation of sacroiliac and sacrococcygeal joint   PE

✓5th **S33.3** Dislocation of other and unspecified parts of lumbar spine and pelvis

✓x7th **S33.30** Dislocation of unspecified parts of lumbar spine and pelvis   PE

✓x7th **S33.39** Dislocation of other parts of lumbar spine and pelvis   PE

✓x7th **S33.4** Traumatic rupture of symphysis pubis   PE

✓x7th **S33.5** Sprain of ligaments of lumbar spine   PE

✓x7th **S33.6** Sprain of sacroiliac joint   PE

✓x7th **S33.8** Sprain of other parts of lumbar spine and pelvis   PE

✓x7th **S33.9** Sprain of unspecified parts of lumbar spine and pelvis   PE

✓4th **S34** Injury of lumbar and sacral spinal cord and nerves at abdomen, lower back and pelvis level

NOTE   Code to highest level of lumbar cord injury.

Injuries to the spinal cord (S34.0 and S34.1) refer to the cord level and not bone level injury, and can affect nerve roots at and below the level given.

Code also any associated:
fracture of vertebra (S22.0-, S32.0-)
open wound of abdomen, lower back and pelvis (S31.-)
transient paralysis (R29.5)

The appropriate 7th character is to be added to each code from category S34.
A   initial encounter
D   subsequent encounter
S   sequela

✓5th **S34.0** Concussion and edema of lumbar and sacral spinal cord

✓x7th **S34.01** Concussion and edema of lumbar spinal cord   MCC HCC PE

✓x7th **S34.02** Concussion and edema of sacral spinal cord   MCC HCC PE
Concussion and edema of conus medullaris

✓5th **S34.1** Other and unspecified injury of lumbar and sacral spinal cord

✓6th **S34.10** Unspecified injury to lumbar spinal cord

✓7th **S34.101** Unspecified injury to L1 level of lumbar spinal cord   MCC H5 HCC PE
Unspecified injury to lumbar spinal cord level 1

✓7th **S34.102** Unspecified injury to L2 level of lumbar spinal cord   MCC H5 HCC PE
Unspecified injury to lumbar spinal cord level 2

✓7th **S34.103** Unspecified injury to L3 level of lumbar spinal cord   MCC H5 HCC PE
Unspecified injury to lumbar spinal cord level 3

✓7th **S34.104** Unspecified injury to L4 level of lumbar spinal cord   MCC H5 HCC PE
Unspecified injury to lumbar spinal cord level 4

✓7th **S34.105** Unspecified injury to L5 level of lumbar spinal cord   MCC H5 HCC PE
Unspecified injury to lumbar spinal cord level 5

✓7th **S34.109** Unspecified injury to unspecified level of lumbar spinal cord   MCC H5 HCC PE

✓6th **S34.11** Complete lesion of lumbar spinal cord

✓7th **S34.111** Complete lesion of L1 level of lumbar spinal cord   MCC H5 HCC PE
Complete lesion of lumbar spinal cord level 1

✓7th **S34.112** Complete lesion of L2 level of lumbar spinal cord   MCC H5 HCC PE
Complete lesion of lumbar spinal cord level 2

✓7th **S34.113** Complete lesion of L3 level of lumbar spinal cord   MCC H5 HCC PE
Complete lesion of lumbar spinal cord level 3

✓7th **S34.114** Complete lesion of L4 level of lumbar spinal cord   MCC H5 HCC PE
Complete lesion of lumbar spinal cord level 4

✓7th **S34.115** Complete lesion of L5 level of lumbar spinal cord   MCC H5 HCC PE
Complete lesion of lumbar spinal cord level 5

✓7th **S34.119** Complete lesion of unspecified level of lumbar spinal cord   MCC H5 HCC PE

✓6th **S34.12** Incomplete lesion of lumbar spinal cord

✓7th **S34.121** Incomplete lesion of L1 level of lumbar spinal cord   MCC H5 HCC PE
Incomplete lesion of lumbar spinal cord level 1

✓7th **S34.122** Incomplete lesion of L2 level of lumbar spinal cord   MCC H5 HCC PE
Incomplete lesion of lumbar spinal cord level 2

✓7th **S34.123** Incomplete lesion of L3 level of lumbar spinal cord   MCC H5 HCC PE
Incomplete lesion of lumbar spinal cord level 3

✓7th **S34.124** Incomplete lesion of L4 level of lumbar spinal cord   MCC H5 HCC PE
Incomplete lesion of lumbar spinal cord level 4

✓7th **S34.125** Incomplete lesion of L5 level of lumbar spinal cord   MCC H5 HCC PE
Incomplete lesion of lumbar spinal cord level 5

✓7th **S34.129** Incomplete lesion of unspecified level of lumbar spinal cord   MCC H5 HCC PE

✓6th **S34.13** Other and unspecified injury to sacral spinal cord
Other injury to conus medullaris

✓7th **S34.131** Complete lesion of sacral spinal cord   MCC H5 HCC PE
Complete lesion of conus medullaris

✓7th **S34.132** Incomplete lesion of sacral spinal cord   MCC H5 HCC PE
Incomplete lesion of conus medullaris

✓7th **S34.139** Unspecified injury to sacral spinal cord   MCC H5 HCC PE
Unspecified injury of conus medullaris

✓5th **S34.2** Injury of nerve root of lumbar and sacral spine

✓x7th **S34.21** Injury of nerve root of lumbar spine   PE

✓x7th **S34.22** Injury of nerve root of sacral spine   PE

✓x7th **S34.3** Injury of cauda equina   MCC H5 HCC PE

✓x7th **S34.4** Injury of lumbosacral plexus   PE

√x7th **S34.5** **Injury of lumbar, sacral and pelvic sympathetic nerves** PE
    Injury of celiac ganglion or plexus
    Injury of hypogastric plexus
    Injury of mesenteric plexus (inferior) (superior)
    Injury of splanchnic nerve

√x7th **S34.6** **Injury of peripheral nerve(s) at abdomen, lower back and pelvis level** PE

√x7th **S34.8** **Injury of other nerves at abdomen, lower back and pelvis level** PE

√x7th **S34.9** **Injury of unspecified nerves at abdomen, lower back and pelvis level** PE

√4th **S35** **Injury of blood vessels at abdomen, lower back and pelvis level**
    Code also any associated open wound (S31.-)

> The appropriate 7th character is to be added to each code from category S35.
> A   initial encounter
> D   subsequent encounter
> S   sequela

√5th **S35.0** **Injury of abdominal aorta**
    EXCLUDES 1   injury of aorta NOS (S25.0)

    √x7th **S35.00** **Unspecified injury of abdominal aorta** MCC PE

    √x7th **S35.01** **Minor laceration of abdominal aorta** MCC PE
       Incomplete transection of abdominal aorta
       Laceration of abdominal aorta NOS
       Superficial laceration of abdominal aorta

    √x7th **S35.02** **Major laceration of abdominal aorta** MCC PE
       Complete transection of abdominal aorta
       Traumatic rupture of abdominal aorta

    √x7th **S35.09** **Other injury of abdominal aorta** MCC PE

√5th **S35.1** **Injury of inferior vena cava**
    Injury of hepatic vein
    EXCLUDES 1   injury of vena cava NOS (S25.2)

    √x7th **S35.10** **Unspecified injury of inferior vena cava** MCC PE

    √x7th **S35.11** **Minor laceration of inferior vena cava** MCC PE
       Incomplete transection of inferior vena cava
       Laceration of inferior vena cava NOS
       Superficial laceration of inferior vena cava

    √x7th **S35.12** **Major laceration of inferior vena cava** MCC PE
       Complete transection of inferior vena cava
       Traumatic rupture of inferior vena cava

    √x7th **S35.19** **Other injury of inferior vena cava** MCC PE

√5th **S35.2** **Injury of celiac or mesenteric artery and branches**

    √6th **S35.21** **Injury of celiac artery**

       √7th **S35.211** **Minor laceration of celiac artery** MCC PE
          Incomplete transection of celiac artery
          Laceration of celiac artery NOS
          Superficial laceration of celiac artery

       √7th **S35.212** **Major laceration of celiac artery** MCC PE
          Complete transection of celiac artery
          Traumatic rupture of celiac artery

       √7th **S35.218** **Other injury of celiac artery** MCC PE

       √7th **S35.219** **Unspecified injury of celiac artery** MCC PE

    √6th **S35.22** **Injury of superior mesenteric artery**

       √7th **S35.221** **Minor laceration of superior mesenteric artery** MCC PE
          Incomplete transection of superior mesenteric artery
          Laceration of superior mesenteric artery NOS
          Superficial laceration of superior mesenteric artery

       √7th **S35.222** **Major laceration of superior mesenteric artery** MCC PE
          Complete transection of superior mesenteric artery
          Traumatic rupture of superior mesenteric artery

       √7th **S35.228** **Other injury of superior mesenteric artery** MCC PE

       √7th **S35.229** **Unspecified injury of superior mesenteric artery** MCC PE

√6th **S35.23** **Injury of inferior mesenteric artery**

    √7th **S35.231** **Minor laceration of inferior mesenteric artery** MCC PE
       Incomplete transection of inferior mesenteric artery
       Laceration of inferior mesenteric artery NOS
       Superficial laceration of inferior mesenteric artery

    √7th **S35.232** **Major laceration of inferior mesenteric artery** MCC PE
       Complete transection of inferior mesenteric artery
       Traumatic rupture of inferior mesenteric artery

    √7th **S35.238** **Other injury of inferior mesenteric artery** MCC PE

    √7th **S35.239** **Unspecified injury of inferior mesenteric artery** MCC PE

√6th **S35.29** **Injury of branches of celiac and mesenteric artery**
    Injury of gastric artery
    Injury of gastroduodenal artery
    Injury of hepatic artery
    Injury of splenic artery

    √7th **S35.291** **Minor laceration of branches of celiac and mesenteric artery** MCC PE
       Incomplete transection of branches of celiac and mesenteric artery
       Laceration of branches of celiac and mesenteric artery NOS
       Superficial laceration of branches of celiac and mesenteric artery

    √7th **S35.292** **Major laceration of branches of celiac and mesenteric artery** MCC PE
       Complete transection of branches of celiac and mesenteric artery
       Traumatic rupture of branches of celiac and mesenteric artery

    √7th **S35.298** **Other injury of branches of celiac and mesenteric artery** MCC PE

    √7th **S35.299** **Unspecified injury of branches of celiac and mesenteric artery** MCC PE

√5th **S35.3** **Injury of portal or splenic vein and branches**

    √6th **S35.31** **Injury of portal vein**

       √7th **S35.311** **Laceration of portal vein** MCC PE

       √7th **S35.318** **Other specified injury of portal vein** MCC PE

       √7th **S35.319** **Unspecified injury of portal vein** MCC PE

    √6th **S35.32** **Injury of splenic vein**

       √7th **S35.321** **Laceration of splenic vein** MCC PE

       √7th **S35.328** **Other specified injury of splenic vein** MCC PE

       √7th **S35.329** **Unspecified injury of splenic vein** MCC PE

    √6th **S35.33** **Injury of superior mesenteric vein**

       √7th **S35.331** **Laceration of superior mesenteric vein** MCC PE

       √7th **S35.338** **Other specified injury of superior mesenteric vein** MCC PE

       √7th **S35.339** **Unspecified injury of superior mesenteric vein** MCC PE

    √6th **S35.34** **Injury of inferior mesenteric vein**

       √7th **S35.341** **Laceration of inferior mesenteric vein** MCC PE

       √7th **S35.348** **Other specified injury of inferior mesenteric vein** MCC PE

       √7th **S35.349** **Unspecified injury of inferior mesenteric vein** MCC PE

√5th **S35.4** **Injury of renal blood vessels**

    √6th **S35.40** **Unspecified injury of renal blood vessel**

       √7th **S35.401** **Unspecified injury of right renal artery** MCC PE

       √7th **S35.402** **Unspecified injury of left renal artery** MCC PE

       √7th **S35.403** **Unspecified injury of unspecified renal artery** MCC UNS PE

       √7th **S35.404** **Unspecified injury of right renal vein** MCC PE

√7th **S35.405** Unspecified injury of left renal vein **MCC PE**

√7th **S35.406** Unspecified injury of unspecified renal vein **MCC UNS PE**

√6th **S35.41** Laceration of renal blood vessel

√7th **S35.411** Laceration of right renal artery **MCC PE**

√7th **S35.412** Laceration of left renal artery **MCC PE**

√7th **S35.413** Laceration of unspecified renal artery **MCC UNS PE**

√7th **S35.414** Laceration of right renal vein **MCC PE**

√7th **S35.415** Laceration of left renal vein **MCC PE**

√7th **S35.416** Laceration of unspecified renal vein **MCC UNS PE**

√6th **S35.49** Other specified injury of renal blood vessel

√7th **S35.491** Other specified injury of right renal artery **MCC PE**

√7th **S35.492** Other specified injury of left renal artery **MCC PE**

√7th **S35.493** Other specified injury of unspecified renal artery **MCC UNS PE**

√7th **S35.494** Other specified injury of right renal vein **MCC PE**

√7th **S35.495** Other specified injury of left renal vein **MCC PE**

√7th **S35.496** Other specified injury of unspecified renal vein **MCC UNS PE**

√5th **S35.5** Injury of iliac blood vessels

√x7th **S35.50** Injury of unspecified iliac blood vessel(s) **MCC PE**

√6th **S35.51** Injury of iliac artery or vein

Injury of hypogastric artery or vein

√7th **S35.511** Injury of right iliac artery **MCC PE**

√7th **S35.512** Injury of left iliac artery **MCC PE**

√7th **S35.513** Injury of unspecified iliac artery **MCC UNS PE**

√7th **S35.514** Injury of right iliac vein **MCC PE**

√7th **S35.515** Injury of left iliac vein **MCC PE**

√7th **S35.516** Injury of unspecified iliac vein **MCC UNS PE**

√6th **S35.53** Injury of uterine artery or vein

√7th **S35.531** Injury of right uterine artery **CC PE**

√7th **S35.532** Injury of left uterine artery **CC PE**

√7th **S35.533** Injury of unspecified uterine artery **CC UNS PE**

√7th **S35.534** Injury of right uterine vein **CC PE**

√7th **S35.535** Injury of left uterine vein **CC PE**

√7th **S35.536** Injury of unspecified uterine vein **CC UNS PE**

√x7th **S35.59** Injury of other iliac blood vessels **MCC PE**

√5th **S35.8** Injury of other blood vessels at abdomen, lower back and pelvis level

Injury of ovarian artery or vein

√6th **S35.8X** Injury of other blood vessels at abdomen, lower back and pelvis level

√7th **S35.8X1** Laceration of other blood vessels at abdomen, lower back and pelvis level **CC PE**

√7th **S35.8X8** Other specified injury of other blood vessels at abdomen, lower back and pelvis level **CC PE**

√7th **S35.8X9** Unspecified injury of other blood vessels at abdomen, lower back and pelvis level **CC PE**

√5th **S35.9** Injury of unspecified blood vessel at abdomen, lower back and pelvis level

√x7th **S35.90** Unspecified injury of unspecified blood vessel at abdomen, lower back and pelvis level **CC PE**

√x7th **S35.91** Laceration of unspecified blood vessel at abdomen, lower back and pelvis level **CC PE**

√x7th **S35.99** Other specified injury of unspecified blood vessel at abdomen, lower back and pelvis level **CC PE**

√4th **S36** Injury of intra-abdominal organs

Code also any associated open wound (S31.-)

TIP: Code only the most severe injury documented for each intra-abdominal organ injured; a laceration is more severe than a contusion.

The appropriate 7th character is to be added to each code from category S36.

A   initial encounter

D   subsequent encounter

S   sequela

√5th **S36.0** Injury of spleen

AHA: 2015,2Q,36; 2015,1Q,10

√x7th **S36.00** Unspecified injury of spleen **CC PE**

√6th **S36.02** Contusion of spleen

√7th **S36.020** Minor contusion of spleen **CC PE**

Contusion of spleen less than 2 cm

√7th **S36.021** Major contusion of spleen

Contusion of spleen greater than 2 cm

√7th **S36.029** Unspecified contusion of spleen **CC PE**

√6th **S36.03** Laceration of spleen

√7th **S36.030** Superficial (capsular) laceration of spleen **CC PE**

Laceration of spleen less than 1 cm

Minor laceration of spleen

√7th **S36.031** Moderate laceration of spleen **MCC PE**

Laceration of spleen 1 to 3 cm

√7th **S36.032** Major laceration of spleen **MCC PE**

Avulsion of spleen

Laceration of spleen greater than 3 cm

Massive laceration of spleen

Multiple moderate lacerations of spleen

Stellate laceration of spleen

√7th **S36.039** Unspecified laceration of spleen **CC PE**

√x7th **S36.09** Other injury of spleen **CC PE**

√5th **S36.1** Injury of liver and gallbladder and bile duct

√6th **S36.11** Injury of liver

AHA: 2024,1Q,25

√7th **S36.112** Contusion of liver **CC PE**

√7th **S36.113** Laceration of liver, unspecified degree **CC PE**

√7th **S36.114** Minor laceration of liver **CC PE**

Laceration involving capsule only, or, without significant involvement of hepatic parenchyma [i.e., less than 1 cm deep]

√7th **S36.115** Moderate laceration of liver **MCC PE**

Laceration involving parenchyma but without major disruption of parenchyma [i.e., less than 10 cm long and less than 3 cm deep]

√7th **S36.116** Major laceration of liver **MCC PE**

Laceration with significant disruption of hepatic parenchyma [i.e., greater than 10 cm long and 3 cm deep]

Multiple moderate lacerations, with or without hematoma

Stellate laceration of liver

√7th **S36.118** Other injury of liver **CC PE**

√7th **S36.119** Unspecified injury of liver **CC PE**

√6th **S36.12** Injury of gallbladder

√7th **S36.122** Contusion of gallbladder **CC PE**

√7th **S36.123** Laceration of gallbladder **CC PE**

√7th **S36.128** Other injury of gallbladder **CC PE**

√7th **S36.129** Unspecified injury of gallbladder **CC PE**

√x7th **S36.13** Injury of bile duct **CC PE**

√5th **S36.2** Injury of pancreas

√6th **S36.20** Unspecified injury of pancreas

√7th **S36.200** Unspecified injury of head of pancreas **CC PE**

√7th **S36.201** Unspecified injury of body of pancreas **CC PE**

√7th **S36.202** Unspecified injury of tail of pancreas **CC PE**

√7ᵗʰ **S36.209** Unspecified injury of unspecified part of pancreas `CC` `PE`

√6ᵗʰ **S36.22** Contusion of pancreas

√7ᵗʰ **S36.220** Contusion of head of pancreas `CC` `PE`

√7ᵗʰ **S36.221** Contusion of body of pancreas `CC` `PE`

√7ᵗʰ **S36.222** Contusion of tail of pancreas `CC` `PE`

√7ᵗʰ **S36.229** Contusion of unspecified part of pancreas `CC` `PE`

√6ᵗʰ **S36.23** Laceration of pancreas, unspecified degree

√7ᵗʰ **S36.230** Laceration of head of pancreas, unspecified degree `CC` `PE`

√7ᵗʰ **S36.231** Laceration of body of pancreas, unspecified degree `CC` `PE`

√7ᵗʰ **S36.232** Laceration of tail of pancreas, unspecified degree `CC` `PE`

√7ᵗʰ **S36.239** Laceration of unspecified part of pancreas, unspecified degree `CC` `PE`

√6ᵗʰ **S36.24** Minor laceration of pancreas

√7ᵗʰ **S36.240** Minor laceration of head of pancreas `CC` `PE`

√7ᵗʰ **S36.241** Minor laceration of body of pancreas `CC` `PE`

√7ᵗʰ **S36.242** Minor laceration of tail of pancreas `CC` `PE`

√7ᵗʰ **S36.249** Minor laceration of unspecified part of pancreas `CC` `PE`

√6ᵗʰ **S36.25** Moderate laceration of pancreas

√7ᵗʰ **S36.250** Moderate laceration of head of pancreas `CC` `PE`

√7ᵗʰ **S36.251** Moderate laceration of body of pancreas `CC` `PE`

√7ᵗʰ **S36.252** Moderate laceration of tail of pancreas `CC` `PE`

√7ᵗʰ **S36.259** Moderate laceration of unspecified part of pancreas `CC` `PE`

√6ᵗʰ **S36.26** Major laceration of pancreas

√7ᵗʰ **S36.260** Major laceration of head of pancreas `CC` `PE`

√7ᵗʰ **S36.261** Major laceration of body of pancreas `CC` `PE`

√7ᵗʰ **S36.262** Major laceration of tail of pancreas `CC` `PE`

√7ᵗʰ **S36.269** Major laceration of unspecified part of pancreas `CC` `PE`

√6ᵗʰ **S36.29** Other injury of pancreas

√7ᵗʰ **S36.290** Other injury of head of pancreas `CC` `PE`

√7ᵗʰ **S36.291** Other injury of body of pancreas `CC` `PE`

√7ᵗʰ **S36.292** Other injury of tail of pancreas `CC` `PE`

√7ᵗʰ **S36.299** Other injury of unspecified part of pancreas `CC` `PE`

√5ᵗʰ **S36.3** Injury of stomach

√x7ᵗʰ **S36.30** Unspecified injury of stomach `CC` `PE`

√x7ᵗʰ **S36.32** Contusion of stomach `CC` `PE`

√x7ᵗʰ **S36.33** Laceration of stomach `CC` `PE`

√x7ᵗʰ **S36.39** Other injury of stomach `CC` `PE`

√5ᵗʰ **S36.4** Injury of small intestine

√6ᵗʰ **S36.40** Unspecified injury of small intestine

√7ᵗʰ **S36.400** Unspecified injury of duodenum `CC` `PE`

√7ᵗʰ **S36.408** Unspecified injury of other part of small intestine `CC` `PE`

√7ᵗʰ **S36.409** Unspecified injury of unspecified part of small intestine `CC` `PE`

√6ᵗʰ **S36.41** Primary blast injury of small intestine

Blast injury of small intestine NOS

√7ᵗʰ **S36.410** Primary blast injury of duodenum `CC` `PE`

√7ᵗʰ **S36.418** Primary blast injury of other part of small intestine `CC` `PE`

√7ᵗʰ **S36.419** Primary blast injury of unspecified part of small intestine `CC` `PE`

√6ᵗʰ **S36.42** Contusion of small intestine

√7ᵗʰ **S36.420** Contusion of duodenum `CC` `PE`

√7ᵗʰ **S36.428** Contusion of other part of small intestine `CC` `PE`

√7ᵗʰ **S36.429** Contusion of unspecified part of small intestine `CC` `PE`

√6ᵗʰ **S36.43** Laceration of small intestine

√7ᵗʰ **S36.430** Laceration of duodenum `CC` `PE`

√7ᵗʰ **S36.438** Laceration of other part of small intestine `CC` `PE`

√7ᵗʰ **S36.439** Laceration of unspecified part of small intestine `CC` `PE`

√6ᵗʰ **S36.49** Other injury of small intestine

√7ᵗʰ **S36.490** Other injury of duodenum `CC` `PE`

√7ᵗʰ **S36.498** Other injury of other part of small intestine `CC` `PE`

    AHA: 2023,3Q,8

√7ᵗʰ **S36.499** Other injury of unspecified part of small intestine `CC` `PE`

√5ᵗʰ **S36.5** Injury of colon

EXCLUDES 2   injury of rectum (S36.6-)

√6ᵗʰ **S36.50** Unspecified injury of colon

√7ᵗʰ **S36.500** Unspecified injury of ascending [right] colon `CC` `PE`

√7ᵗʰ **S36.501** Unspecified injury of transverse colon `CC` `PE`

√7ᵗʰ **S36.502** Unspecified injury of descending [left] colon `CC` `PE`

√7ᵗʰ **S36.503** Unspecified injury of sigmoid colon `CC` `PE`

√7ᵗʰ **S36.508** Unspecified injury of other part of colon `CC` `PE`

√7ᵗʰ **S36.509** Unspecified injury of unspecified part of colon `CC` `PE`

√6ᵗʰ **S36.51** Primary blast injury of colon

Blast injury of colon NOS

√7ᵗʰ **S36.510** Primary blast injury of ascending [right] colon `CC` `PE`

√7ᵗʰ **S36.511** Primary blast injury of transverse colon `CC` `PE`

√7ᵗʰ **S36.512** Primary blast injury of descending [left] colon `CC` `PE`

√7ᵗʰ **S36.513** Primary blast injury of sigmoid colon `CC` `PE`

√7ᵗʰ **S36.518** Primary blast injury of other part of colon `CC` `PE`

√7ᵗʰ **S36.519** Primary blast injury of unspecified part of colon `CC` `PE`

√6ᵗʰ **S36.52** Contusion of colon

√7ᵗʰ **S36.520** Contusion of ascending [right] colon `CC` `PE`

√7ᵗʰ **S36.521** Contusion of transverse colon `CC` `PE`

√7ᵗʰ **S36.522** Contusion of descending [left] colon `CC` `PE`

√7ᵗʰ **S36.523** Contusion of sigmoid colon `CC` `PE`

√7ᵗʰ **S36.528** Contusion of other part of colon `CC` `PE`

√7ᵗʰ **S36.529** Contusion of unspecified part of colon `CC` `PE`

√6ᵗʰ **S36.53** Laceration of colon

√7ᵗʰ **S36.530** Laceration of ascending [right] colon `CC` `PE`

√7ᵗʰ **S36.531** Laceration of transverse colon `CC` `PE`

√7ᵗʰ **S36.532** Laceration of descending [left] colon `CC` `PE`

√7ᵗʰ **S36.533** Laceration of sigmoid colon `CC` `PE`

√7ᵗʰ **S36.538** Laceration of other part of colon `CC` `PE`

√7ᵗʰ **S36.539** Laceration of unspecified part of colon `CC` `PE`

√6ᵗʰ **S36.59** Other injury of colon

Secondary blast injury of colon

AHA: 2023,3Q,8

√7ᵗʰ **S36.590** Other injury of ascending [right] colon `CC` `PE`

√7ᵗʰ **S36.591** Other injury of transverse colon `CC` `PE`

√7ᵗʰ **S36.592** Other injury of descending [left] colon `CC` `PE`

√7ᵗʰ **S36.593** Other injury of sigmoid colon `CC` `PE`

√7ᵗʰ **S36.598** Other injury of other part of colon `CC` `PE`

`N` Newborn: 0   `P` Pediatric: 0-17   `M` Maternity: 9-64   `A` Adult: 15-124   `UNS` Unspecified Site   `MCC` Major Complication/Comorbidity   `CC` Complication/Comorbidity   `PE` POA Exempt

1024   ICD-10-CM 2025

√7ᵗʰ **S36.599** Other injury of unspecified part of colon   CC PE

√5ᵗʰ **S36.6** **Injury of rectum**

    √x7ᵗʰ **S36.60** Unspecified injury of rectum   CC PE

    √x7ᵗʰ **S36.61** **Primary blast** injury of rectum   CC PE
      Blast injury of rectum NOS

    √x7ᵗʰ **S36.62** **Contusion** of rectum   CC PE

    √x7ᵗʰ **S36.63** **Laceration** of rectum   CC PE

    √x7ᵗʰ **S36.69** Other injury of rectum   CC PE
      Secondary blast injury of rectum

√5ᵗʰ **S36.8** **Injury of other intra-abdominal organs**

    √x7ᵗʰ **S36.81** **Injury of peritoneum**   CC PE

    √6ᵗʰ **S36.89** Injury of other intra-abdominal organs
      Injury of retroperitoneum

      √7ᵗʰ **S36.892** **Contusion** of other intra-abdominal organs   CC PE

      √7ᵗʰ **S36.893** **Laceration** of other intra-abdominal organs   CC PE

      √7ᵗʰ **S36.898** Other injury of other intra-abdominal organs   CC PE

      √7ᵗʰ **S36.899** Unspecified injury of other intra-abdominal organs   CC PE

√5ᵗʰ **S36.9** **Injury of unspecified intra-abdominal organ**

    √x7ᵗʰ **S36.90** Unspecified injury of unspecified intra-abdominal organ   CC PE

    √x7ᵗʰ **S36.92** **Contusion** of unspecified intra-abdominal organ   CC PE

    √x7ᵗʰ **S36.93** **Laceration** of unspecified intra-abdominal organ   CC PE

    √x7ᵗʰ **S36.99** Other injury of unspecified intra-abdominal organ   CC PE

√4ᵗʰ **S37** **Injury of urinary and pelvic organs**

    Code also any associated open wound (S31.-)

    EXCLUDES 1   obstetric trauma to pelvic organs (O71.-)
    EXCLUDES 2   injury of peritoneum (S36.81)
            injury of retroperitoneum (S36.89-)

    The appropriate 7th character is to be added to each code from category S37.
    A   initial encounter
    D   subsequent encounter
    S   sequela

√5ᵗʰ **S37.0** **Injury of kidney**

    EXCLUDES 2   acute kidney injury (nontraumatic) (N17.9)

    √6ᵗʰ **S37.00** Unspecified injury of kidney

      √7ᵗʰ **S37.001** Unspecified injury of **right** kidney   CC PE

      √7ᵗʰ **S37.002** Unspecified injury of **left** kidney   CC PE

      √7ᵗʰ **S37.009** Unspecified injury of unspecified kidney   CC UNS PE

    √6ᵗʰ **S37.01** **Minor contusion** of kidney
      Contusion of kidney less than 2 cm
      Contusion of kidney NOS

      √7ᵗʰ **S37.011** Minor contusion of **right** kidney   CC PE

      √7ᵗʰ **S37.012** Minor contusion of **left** kidney   CC PE

      √7ᵗʰ **S37.019** Minor contusion of unspecified kidney   CC UNS PE

    √6ᵗʰ **S37.02** **Major contusion** of kidney
      Contusion of kidney greater than 2 cm

      √7ᵗʰ **S37.021** Major contusion of **right** kidney   CC PE

      √7ᵗʰ **S37.022** Major contusion of **left** kidney   CC PE

      √7ᵗʰ **S37.029** Major contusion of unspecified kidney   CC UNS PE

    √6ᵗʰ **S37.03** **Laceration** of kidney, unspecified degree

      √7ᵗʰ **S37.031** Laceration of **right** kidney, unspecified degree   CC PE

      √7ᵗʰ **S37.032** Laceration of **left** kidney, unspecified degree   CC PE

      √7ᵗʰ **S37.039** Laceration of unspecified kidney, unspecified degree   CC UNS PE

    √6ᵗʰ **S37.04** **Minor laceration** of kidney
      Laceration of kidney less than 1 cm

      √7ᵗʰ **S37.041** Minor laceration of **right** kidney   CC PE

      √7ᵗʰ **S37.042** Minor laceration of **left** kidney   CC PE

√7ᵗʰ **S37.049** Minor laceration of unspecified kidney   CC UNS PE

√6ᵗʰ **S37.05** **Moderate laceration** of kidney
    Laceration of kidney 1 to 3 cm

    √7ᵗʰ **S37.051** Moderate laceration of **right** kidney   CC PE

    √7ᵗʰ **S37.052** Moderate laceration of **left** kidney   CC PE

    √7ᵗʰ **S37.059** **Moderate laceration** of unspecified kidney   CC UNS PE

√6ᵗʰ **S37.06** **Major laceration** of kidney
    Avulsion of kidney
    Laceration of kidney greater than 3 cm
    Massive laceration of kidney
    Multiple moderate lacerations of kidney
    Stellate laceration of kidney

    √7ᵗʰ **S37.061** Major laceration of **right** kidney   MCC PE

    √7ᵗʰ **S37.062** Major laceration of **left** kidney   MCC PE

    √7ᵗʰ **S37.069** Major laceration of unspecified kidney   MCC UNS PE

√6ᵗʰ **S37.09** Other injury of kidney

    √7ᵗʰ **S37.091** Other injury of **right** kidney   MCC PE

    √7ᵗʰ **S37.092** Other injury of **left** kidney   MCC PE

    √7ᵗʰ **S37.099** Other injury of unspecified kidney   MCC UNS PE

√5ᵗʰ **S37.1** **Injury of ureter**

    √x7ᵗʰ **S37.10** Unspecified injury of ureter   CC PE

    √x7ᵗʰ **S37.12** **Contusion** of ureter   CC PE

    √x7ᵗʰ **S37.13** **Laceration** of ureter   CC PE

    √x7ᵗʰ **S37.19** Other injury of ureter   CC PE

√5ᵗʰ **S37.2** **Injury of bladder**

    √x7ᵗʰ **S37.20** Unspecified injury of bladder   CC PE

    √x7ᵗʰ **S37.22** **Contusion** of bladder   CC PE

    √x7ᵗʰ **S37.23** **Laceration** of bladder   CC PE

    √x7ᵗʰ **S37.29** Other injury of bladder   CC PE

√5ᵗʰ **S37.3** **Injury of urethra**

    √x7ᵗʰ **S37.30** Unspecified injury of urethra   CC PE

    √x7ᵗʰ **S37.32** **Contusion** of urethra   CC PE

    √x7ᵗʰ **S37.33** **Laceration** of urethra   CC PE

    √x7ᵗʰ **S37.39** Other injury of urethra   CC PE

√5ᵗʰ **S37.4** **Injury of ovary**

    √6ᵗʰ **S37.40** Unspecified injury of ovary

      √7ᵗʰ **S37.401** Unspecified injury of ovary, **unilateral**   PE

      √7ᵗʰ **S37.402** Unspecified injury of ovary, **bilateral**   PE

      √7ᵗʰ **S37.409** Unspecified injury of ovary, unspecified   PE

    √6ᵗʰ **S37.42** **Contusion** of ovary

      √7ᵗʰ **S37.421** Contusion of ovary, **unilateral**   PE

      √7ᵗʰ **S37.422** Contusion of ovary, **bilateral**   PE

      √7ᵗʰ **S37.429** Contusion of ovary, unspecified   PE

    √6ᵗʰ **S37.43** **Laceration** of ovary

      √7ᵗʰ **S37.431** Laceration of ovary, **unilateral**   PE

      √7ᵗʰ **S37.432** Laceration of ovary, **bilateral**   PE

      √7ᵗʰ **S37.439** Laceration of ovary, unspecified   PE

    √6ᵗʰ **S37.49** Other injury of ovary

      √7ᵗʰ **S37.491** Other injury of ovary, **unilateral**   PE

      √7ᵗʰ **S37.492** Other injury of ovary, **bilateral**   PE

      √7ᵗʰ **S37.499** Other injury of ovary, unspecified   PE

√5ᵗʰ **S37.5** **Injury of fallopian tube**

    √6ᵗʰ **S37.50** Unspecified injury of fallopian tube

      √7ᵗʰ **S37.501** Unspecified injury of fallopian tube, **unilateral**   PE

      √7ᵗʰ **S37.502** Unspecified injury of fallopian tube, **bilateral**   PE

      √7ᵗʰ **S37.509** Unspecified injury of fallopian tube, unspecified   PE

☑ Additional Character Required   √x7ᵗʰ Placeholder   Questionable PDx   Manifestation   Unspecified   UPD Unacceptable PDx   H1-H14 HAC   HCC CMS-HCC Dx   HIV HIV Dx

ICD-10-CM 2025   1025

√6ᵗʰ **S37.51**   **Primary blast** injury of fallopian tube
Blast injury of fallopian tube NOS

- √7ᵗʰ   **S37.511**   Primary blast injury of fallopian tube, **unilateral**   `PE`
- √7ᵗʰ   **S37.512**   Primary blast injury of fallopian tube, **bilateral**   `PE`
- √7ᵗʰ   **S37.519**   Primary blast injury of fallopian tube, unspecified   `PE`

√6ᵗʰ **S37.52**   **Contusion** of fallopian tube

- √7ᵗʰ   **S37.521**   Contusion of fallopian tube, **unilateral**   `PE`
- √7ᵗʰ   **S37.522**   Contusion of fallopian tube, **bilateral**   `PE`
- √7ᵗʰ   **S37.529**   Contusion of fallopian tube, unspecified   `PE`

√6ᵗʰ **S37.53**   **Laceration** of fallopian tube

- √7ᵗʰ   **S37.531**   Laceration of fallopian tube, **unilateral**   `PE`
- √7ᵗʰ   **S37.532**   Laceration of fallopian tube, **bilateral**   `PE`
- √7ᵗʰ   **S37.539**   Laceration of fallopian tube, unspecified   `PE`

√6ᵗʰ **S37.59**   **Other injury** of fallopian tube
Secondary blast injury of fallopian tube

- √7ᵗʰ   **S37.591**   Other injury of fallopian tube, **unilateral**   `PE`
- √7ᵗʰ   **S37.592**   Other injury of fallopian tube, **bilateral**   `PE`
- √7ᵗʰ   **S37.599**   Other injury of fallopian tube, unspecified   `PE`

√5ᵗʰ **S37.6**   **Injury of uterus**

> `EXCLUDES 1`   injury to gravid uterus (O9A.2-)
> injury to uterus during delivery (O71.-)

- √x7ᵗʰ   **S37.60**   Unspecified injury of uterus   `CC` `PE`
- √x7ᵗʰ   **S37.62**   **Contusion** of uterus   `CC` `PE`
- √x7ᵗʰ   **S37.63**   **Laceration** of uterus   `CC` `PE`
- √x7ᵗʰ   **S37.69**   Other injury of uterus   `CC` `PE`

√5ᵗʰ **S37.8**   **Injury of other urinary and pelvic organs**

√6ᵗʰ **S37.81**   Injury of **adrenal gland**

- √7ᵗʰ   **S37.812**   **Contusion** of adrenal gland   `CC` `PE`
- √7ᵗʰ   **S37.813**   **Laceration** of adrenal gland   `CC` `PE`
- √7ᵗʰ   **S37.818**   Other injury of adrenal gland   `CC` `PE`
- √7ᵗʰ   **S37.819**   Unspecified injury of adrenal gland   `CC` `PE`

√6ᵗʰ **S37.82**   Injury of **prostate**

- √7ᵗʰ   **S37.822**   **Contusion** of prostate   `PE`
- √7ᵗʰ   **S37.823**   **Laceration** of prostate   `PE`
- √7ᵗʰ   **S37.828**   Other injury of prostate   `PE`
- √7ᵗʰ   **S37.829**   Unspecified injury of prostate   `PE`

√6ᵗʰ **S37.89**   Injury of other urinary and pelvic organ

- √7ᵗʰ   **S37.892**   **Contusion** of other urinary and pelvic organ   `CC` `PE`
- √7ᵗʰ   **S37.893**   **Laceration** of other urinary and pelvic organ   `CC` `PE`
- √7ᵗʰ   **S37.898**   Other injury of other urinary and pelvic organ   `CC` `PE`
- √7ᵗʰ   **S37.899**   Unspecified injury of other urinary and pelvic organ   `CC` `PE`

√5ᵗʰ **S37.9**   **Injury of unspecified urinary and pelvic organ**

- √x7ᵗʰ   **S37.90**   Unspecified injury of unspecified urinary and pelvic organ   `CC` `PE`
- √x7ᵗʰ   **S37.92**   **Contusion** of unspecified urinary and pelvic organ   `CC` `PE`
- √x7ᵗʰ   **S37.93**   **Laceration** of unspecified urinary and pelvic organ   `CC` `PE`
- √x7ᵗʰ   **S37.99**   Other injury of unspecified urinary and pelvic organ   `CC` `PE`

√4ᵗʰ **S38**   **Crushing injury and traumatic amputation of abdomen, lower back, pelvis and external genitals**

> `NOTE`   An amputation not identified as partial or complete should be coded to complete

> The appropriate 7th character is to be added to each code from category S38.
> A   initial encounter
> D   subsequent encounter
> S   sequela

√5ᵗʰ **S38.0**   **Crushing injury** of **external genital organs**
Use additional code for any associated injuries

√6ᵗʰ **S38.00**   **Crushing injury of unspecified external genital organs**

- √7ᵗʰ   **S38.001**   **Crushing injury of unspecified external genital organs, male**   `PE`
- √7ᵗʰ   **S38.002**   **Crushing injury of unspecified external genital organs, female**   `PE`
- √x7ᵗʰ   **S38.01**   **Crushing injury of penis**   `PE`
- √x7ᵗʰ   **S38.02**   **Crushing injury of scrotum and testis**   `PE`
- √x7ᵗʰ   **S38.03**   **Crushing injury of vulva**   `PE`

√x7ᵗʰ **S38.1**   **Crushing injury of abdomen, lower back, and pelvis**   `PE`
Use additional code for all associated injuries, such as:
fracture of thoracic or lumbar spine and pelvis (S22.0-, S32.-)
injury to intra-abdominal organs (S36.-)
injury to urinary and pelvic organs (S37.-)
open wound of abdominal wall (S31.-)
spinal cord injury (S34.0, S34.1-)

> `EXCLUDES 2`   crushing injury of external genital organs (S38.0-)

√5ᵗʰ **S38.2**   **Traumatic amputation** of external genital organs

√6ᵗʰ **S38.21**   **Traumatic amputation of female external genital organs**
Traumatic amputation of clitoris
Traumatic amputation of labium (majus) (minus)
Traumatic amputation of vulva

- √7ᵗʰ   **S38.211**   **Complete** traumatic amputation of female external genital organs   `PE`
- √7ᵗʰ   **S38.212**   **Partial** traumatic amputation of female external genital organs   `PE`

√6ᵗʰ **S38.22**   Traumatic amputation of **penis**

- √7ᵗʰ   **S38.221**   **Complete** traumatic amputation of penis   `PE`
- √7ᵗʰ   **S38.222**   **Partial** traumatic amputation of penis   `PE`

√6ᵗʰ **S38.23**   Traumatic amputation of **scrotum and testis**

- √7ᵗʰ   **S38.231**   **Complete** traumatic amputation of scrotum and testis   `PE`
- √7ᵗʰ   **S38.232**   **Partial** traumatic amputation of scrotum and testis   `PE`

√x7ᵗʰ **S38.3**   **Transection (partial) of abdomen**   `PE`

√4ᵗʰ **S39**   **Other and unspecified injuries of abdomen, lower back, pelvis and external genitals**
Code also any associated open wound (S31.-)

> `EXCLUDES 2`   sprain of joints and ligaments of lumbar spine and pelvis (S33.-)

> The appropriate 7th character is to be added to each code from category S39.
> A   initial encounter
> D   subsequent encounter
> S   sequela

√5ᵗʰ **S39.0**   **Injury of muscle, fascia and tendon of abdomen, lower back and pelvis**

√6ᵗʰ **S39.00**   **Unspecified injury of muscle, fascia and tendon of abdomen, lower back and pelvis**

- √7ᵗʰ   **S39.001**   Unspecified injury of muscle, fascia and tendon of **abdomen**   `PE`
- √7ᵗʰ   **S39.002**   Unspecified injury of muscle, fascia and tendon of **lower back**   `PE`
- √7ᵗʰ   **S39.003**   Unspecified injury of muscle, fascia and tendon of **pelvis**   `PE`

√6ᵗʰ **S39.01**   **Strain** of muscle, fascia and tendon of abdomen, lower back and pelvis

- √7ᵗʰ   **S39.011**   Strain of muscle, fascia and tendon of **abdomen**   `PE`
- √7ᵗʰ   **S39.012**   Strain of muscle, fascia and tendon of **lower back**   `PE`
- √7ᵗʰ   **S39.013**   Strain of muscle, fascia and tendon of **pelvis**   `PE`

√6ᵗʰ **S39.02** **Laceration** of muscle, fascia and tendon of abdomen, lower back and pelvis

　　　√7ᵗʰ **S39.021** **Laceration of muscle, fascia and tendon of abdomen** PE

　　　√7ᵗʰ **S39.022** **Laceration of muscle, fascia and tendon of lower back** PE

　　　√7ᵗʰ **S39.023** **Laceration of muscle, fascia and tendon of pelvis** PE

√6ᵗʰ **S39.09** **Other injury of muscle, fascia and tendon of abdomen, lower back and pelvis**

　　　√7ᵗʰ **S39.091** **Other injury of muscle, fascia and tendon of abdomen** PE

　　　√7ᵗʰ **S39.092** **Other injury of muscle, fascia and tendon of lower back** PE

　　　√7ᵗʰ **S39.093** **Other injury of muscle, fascia and tendon of pelvis** PE

√5ᵗʰ **S39.8** **Other specified injuries of abdomen, lower back, pelvis and external genitals**

　　√x7ᵗʰ **S39.81** **Other specified injuries of abdomen** PE

　　√x7ᵗʰ **S39.82** **Other specified injuries of lower back** PE

　　√x7ᵗʰ **S39.83** **Other specified injuries of pelvis** PE

　　√6ᵗʰ **S39.84** **Other specified injuries of external genitals**

　　　√7ᵗʰ **S39.840** **Fracture of corpus cavernosum penis** PE

　　　√7ᵗʰ **S39.848** **Other specified injuries of external genitals** PE

√5ᵗʰ **S39.9** **Unspecified injury of abdomen, lower back, pelvis and external genitals**

　　√x7ᵗʰ **S39.91** **Unspecified injury of abdomen** PE

　　√x7ᵗʰ **S39.92** **Unspecified injury of lower back** PE

　　√x7ᵗʰ **S39.93** **Unspecified injury of pelvis** PE

　　√x7ᵗʰ **S39.94** **Unspecified injury of external genitals** PE

Injuries to the shoulder and upper arm (S40-S49)

INCLUDES　injuries of axilla
　　　　　injuries of scapular region
EXCLUDES 2　*burns and corrosions (T20-T32)*
　　　　　frostbite (T33-T34)
　　　　　injuries of elbow (S50-S59)
　　　　　insect bite or sting, venomous (T63.4)

√4ᵗʰ **S40** **Superficial injury of shoulder and upper arm**

The appropriate 7th character is to be added to each code from category S40.
A　initial encounter
D　subsequent encounter
S　sequela

√5ᵗʰ **S40.0** **Contusion** of shoulder and upper arm

　　√6ᵗʰ **S40.01** **Contusion of shoulder**

　　　√7ᵗʰ **S40.011** **Contusion of right shoulder** PE

　　　√7ᵗʰ **S40.012** **Contusion of left shoulder** PE

　　　√7ᵗʰ **S40.019** **Contusion of unspecified shoulder** PE

　　√6ᵗʰ **S40.02** **Contusion of upper arm**

　　　√7ᵗʰ **S40.021** **Contusion of right upper arm** PE

　　　√7ᵗʰ **S40.022** **Contusion of left upper arm** PE

　　　√7ᵗʰ **S40.029** **Contusion of unspecified upper arm** PE

√5ᵗʰ **S40.2** **Other superficial injuries of shoulder**

　　√6ᵗʰ **S40.21** **Abrasion of shoulder**

　　　√7ᵗʰ **S40.211** **Abrasion of right shoulder** PE

　　　√7ᵗʰ **S40.212** **Abrasion of left shoulder** PE

　　　√7ᵗʰ **S40.219** **Abrasion of unspecified shoulder** PE

　　√6ᵗʰ **S40.22** **Blister (nonthermal) of shoulder**

　　　√7ᵗʰ **S40.221** **Blister (nonthermal) of right shoulder** PE

　　　√7ᵗʰ **S40.222** **Blister (nonthermal) of left shoulder** PE

　　　√7ᵗʰ **S40.229** **Blister (nonthermal) of unspecified shoulder** PE

　　√6ᵗʰ **S40.24** **External constriction of shoulder**

　　　√7ᵗʰ **S40.241** **External constriction of right shoulder** PE

　　　√7ᵗʰ **S40.242** **External constriction of left shoulder** PE

　　　√7ᵗʰ **S40.249** **External constriction of unspecified shoulder** PE

　　√6ᵗʰ **S40.25** **Superficial foreign body of shoulder**

　　　　Splinter in the shoulder

　　　√7ᵗʰ **S40.251** **Superficial foreign body of right shoulder** PE

　　　√7ᵗʰ **S40.252** **Superficial foreign body of left shoulder** PE

　　　√7ᵗʰ **S40.259** **Superficial foreign body of unspecified shoulder** PE

　　√6ᵗʰ **S40.26** **Insect bite (nonvenomous) of shoulder**

　　　√7ᵗʰ **S40.261** **Insect bite (nonvenomous) of right shoulder** PE

　　　√7ᵗʰ **S40.262** **Insect bite (nonvenomous) of left shoulder** PE

　　　√7ᵗʰ **S40.269** **Insect bite (nonvenomous) of unspecified shoulder** PE

　　√6ᵗʰ **S40.27** **Other superficial bite of shoulder**

　　　　EXCLUDES 1　*open bite of shoulder (S41.05)*

　　　√7ᵗʰ **S40.271** **Other superficial bite of right shoulder** PE

　　　√7ᵗʰ **S40.272** **Other superficial bite of left shoulder** PE

　　　√7ᵗʰ **S40.279** **Other superficial bite of unspecified shoulder** PE

√5ᵗʰ **S40.8** **Other superficial injuries of upper arm**

　　√6ᵗʰ **S40.81** **Abrasion of upper arm**

　　　√7ᵗʰ **S40.811** **Abrasion of right upper arm** PE

　　　√7ᵗʰ **S40.812** **Abrasion of left upper arm** PE

　　　√7ᵗʰ **S40.819** **Abrasion of unspecified upper arm** PE

　　√6ᵗʰ **S40.82** **Blister (nonthermal) of upper arm**

　　　√7ᵗʰ **S40.821** **Blister (nonthermal) of right upper arm** PE

　　　√7ᵗʰ **S40.822** **Blister (nonthermal) of left upper arm** PE

　　　√7ᵗʰ **S40.829** **Blister (nonthermal) of unspecified upper arm** PE

　　√6ᵗʰ **S40.84** **External constriction of upper arm**

　　　√7ᵗʰ **S40.841** **External constriction of right upper arm** PE

　　　√7ᵗʰ **S40.842** **External constriction of left upper arm** PE

　　　√7ᵗʰ **S40.849** **External constriction of unspecified upper arm** PE

　　√6ᵗʰ **S40.85** **Superficial foreign body of upper arm**

　　　　Splinter in the upper arm

　　　√7ᵗʰ **S40.851** **Superficial foreign body of right upper arm** PE

　　　√7ᵗʰ **S40.852** **Superficial foreign body of left upper arm** PE

　　　√7ᵗʰ **S40.859** **Superficial foreign body of unspecified upper arm** PE

　　√6ᵗʰ **S40.86** **Insect bite (nonvenomous) of upper arm**

　　　√7ᵗʰ **S40.861** **Insect bite (nonvenomous) of right upper arm** PE

　　　√7ᵗʰ **S40.862** **Insect bite (nonvenomous) of left upper arm** PE

　　　√7ᵗʰ **S40.869** **Insect bite (nonvenomous) of unspecified upper arm** PE

　　√6ᵗʰ **S40.87** **Other superficial bite of upper arm**

　　　　EXCLUDES 1　*open bite of upper arm (S41.14)*
　　　　EXCLUDES 2　*other superficial bite of shoulder (S40.27-)*

　　　√7ᵗʰ **S40.871** **Other superficial bite of right upper arm** PE

　　　√7ᵗʰ **S40.872** **Other superficial bite of left upper arm** PE

　　　√7ᵗʰ **S40.879** **Other superficial bite of unspecified upper arm** PE

√5ᵗʰ **S40.9** **Unspecified superficial injury of shoulder and upper arm**

　　√6ᵗʰ **S40.91** **Unspecified superficial injury of shoulder**

　　　√7ᵗʰ **S40.911** **Unspecified superficial injury of right shoulder** PE

　　　√7ᵗʰ **S40.912** **Unspecified superficial injury of left shoulder** PE

　　　√7ᵗʰ **S40.919** **Unspecified superficial injury of unspecified shoulder** PE

✔ Additional Character Required　　√x7ᵗʰ Placeholder　　Questionable PDx　　Manifestation　　Unspecified　　UPD Unacceptable PDx　　H1-H14 HAC　　HCC CMS-HCC Dx　　HIV HIV Dx

ICD-10-CM 2025　　　1027

✓6th **S40.92** **Unspecified superficial injury of upper arm**

    ✓7th **S40.921** **Unspecified superficial injury of right upper arm** PE

    ✓7th **S40.922** **Unspecified superficial injury of left upper arm** PE

    ✓7th **S40.929** **Unspecified superficial injury of unspecified upper arm** PE

✓4th **S41** **Open wound of shoulder and upper arm**

Code also any associated wound infection

EXCLUDES 1   *traumatic amputation of shoulder and upper arm (S48.-)*

EXCLUDES 2   *open fracture of shoulder and upper arm (S42.- with 7th character B or C)*

The appropriate 7th character is to be added to each code from category S41.
A   initial encounter
D   subsequent encounter
S   sequela

✓5th **S41.0** **Open wound of shoulder**

  ✓6th **S41.00** **Unspecified open wound of shoulder**

    ✓7th **S41.001** **Unspecified open wound of right shoulder** PE

    ✓7th **S41.002** **Unspecified open wound of left shoulder** PE

    ✓7th **S41.009** **Unspecified open wound of unspecified shoulder** PE

  ✓6th **S41.01** **Laceration without foreign body of shoulder**

    ✓7th **S41.011** **Laceration without foreign body of right shoulder** PE

    ✓7th **S41.012** **Laceration without foreign body of left shoulder** PE

    ✓7th **S41.019** **Laceration without foreign body of unspecified shoulder** PE

  ✓6th **S41.02** **Laceration with foreign body of shoulder**

    ✓7th **S41.021** **Laceration with foreign body of right shoulder** PE

    ✓7th **S41.022** **Laceration with foreign body of left shoulder** PE

    ✓7th **S41.029** **Laceration with foreign body of unspecified shoulder** PE

  ✓6th **S41.03** **Puncture wound without foreign body of shoulder**

    ✓7th **S41.031** **Puncture wound without foreign body of right shoulder** PE

    ✓7th **S41.032** **Puncture wound without foreign body of left shoulder** PE

    ✓7th **S41.039** **Puncture wound without foreign body of unspecified shoulder** PE

  ✓6th **S41.04** **Puncture wound with foreign body of shoulder**

    ✓7th **S41.041** **Puncture wound with foreign body of right shoulder** PE

    ✓7th **S41.042** **Puncture wound with foreign body of left shoulder** PE

    ✓7th **S41.049** **Puncture wound with foreign body of unspecified shoulder** PE

  ✓6th **S41.05** **Open bite of shoulder**

Bite of shoulder NOS

EXCLUDES 1   *superficial bite of shoulder (S40.27)*

    ✓7th **S41.051** **Open bite of right shoulder** PE

    ✓7th **S41.052** **Open bite of left shoulder** PE

    ✓7th **S41.059** **Open bite of unspecified shoulder** PE

✓5th **S41.1** **Open wound of upper arm**

  ✓6th **S41.10** **Unspecified open wound of upper arm**

AHA: 2016,3Q,24

    ✓7th **S41.101** **Unspecified open wound of right upper arm** PE

    ✓7th **S41.102** **Unspecified open wound of left upper arm** PE

    ✓7th **S41.109** **Unspecified open wound of unspecified upper arm** PE

  ✓6th **S41.11** **Laceration without foreign body of upper arm**

    ✓7th **S41.111** **Laceration without foreign body of right upper arm** PE

    ✓7th **S41.112** **Laceration without foreign body of left upper arm** PE

    ✓7th **S41.119** **Laceration without foreign body of unspecified upper arm** PE

  ✓6th **S41.12** **Laceration with foreign body of upper arm**

    ✓7th **S41.121** **Laceration with foreign body of right upper arm** PE

    ✓7th **S41.122** **Laceration with foreign body of left upper arm** PE

    ✓7th **S41.129** **Laceration with foreign body of unspecified upper arm** PE

  ✓6th **S41.13** **Puncture wound without foreign body of upper arm**

AHA: 2016,3Q,24

    ✓7th **S41.131** **Puncture wound without foreign body of right upper arm** PE

    ✓7th **S41.132** **Puncture wound without foreign body of left upper arm** PE

    ✓7th **S41.139** **Puncture wound without foreign body of unspecified upper arm** PE

  ✓6th **S41.14** **Puncture wound with foreign body of upper arm**

AHA: 2016,3Q,24

    ✓7th **S41.141** **Puncture wound with foreign body of right upper arm** PE

    ✓7th **S41.142** **Puncture wound with foreign body of left upper arm** PE

    ✓7th **S41.149** **Puncture wound with foreign body of unspecified upper arm** PE

  ✓6th **S41.15** **Open bite of upper arm**

Bite of upper arm NOS

EXCLUDES 1   *superficial bite of upper arm (S40.87)*

    ✓7th **S41.151** **Open bite of right upper arm** PE

    ✓7th **S41.152** **Open bite of left upper arm** PE

    ✓7th **S41.159** **Open bite of unspecified upper arm** PE

✓4th **S42** **Fracture of shoulder and upper arm**

NOTE   A fracture not indicated as displaced or nondisplaced should be coded to displaced

A fracture not indicated as open or closed should be coded to closed

EXCLUDES 1   *traumatic amputation of shoulder and upper arm (S48.-)*

EXCLUDES 2   *periprosthetic fracture around internal prosthetic shoulder joint (M97.3)*

AHA: 2018,2Q,12; 2015,3Q,37-39

DEF: Diaphysis: Central shaft of a long bone.

DEF: Epiphysis: Proximal and distal rounded ends of a long bone, communicates with the joint.

DEF: Metaphysis: Section of a long bone located between the epiphysis and diaphysis at the proximal and distal ends.

DEF: Physis (growth plate): Narrow zone of cartilaginous tissue between the epiphysis and metaphysis at each end of a long bone. In childhood, proliferation of cells in this zone lengthens the bone. As the bone matures, this area thins, ossification eventually fusing into solid bone and growth stops. **Synonym(s):** Epiphyseal plate.

The appropriate 7th character is to be added to all codes from category S42 [unless otherwise indicated].
A   initial encounter for closed fracture
B   initial encounter for open fracture
D   subsequent encounter for fracture with routine healing
G   subsequent encounter for fracture with delayed healing
K   subsequent encounter for fracture with nonunion
P   subsequent encounter for fracture with malunion
S   sequela

✓5th **S42.0** **Fracture of clavicle**

  ✓6th **S42.00** **Fracture of unspecified part of clavicle**

    ✓7th **S42.001** **Fracture of unspecified part of right clavicle** CC H5 PE

    ✓7th **S42.002** **Fracture of unspecified part of left clavicle** CC H5 PE

    ✓7th **S42.009** **Fracture of unspecified part of unspecified clavicle** CC H5 UNS PE

AHA: 2012,4Q,93

  ✓6th **S42.01** **Fracture of sternal end of clavicle**

    ✓7th **S42.011** **Anterior displaced fracture of sternal end of right clavicle** CC H5 PE

    ✓7th **S42.012** **Anterior displaced fracture of sternal end of left clavicle** CC H5 PE

    ✓7th **S42.013** **Anterior displaced fracture of sternal end of unspecified clavicle** CC H5 UNS PE

Displaced fracture of sternal end of clavicle NOS

√7th **S42.014** **Posterior** displaced fracture of sternal end of **right** clavicle   `CC` `H5` `PE`

√7th **S42.015** **Posterior** displaced fracture of sternal end of **left** clavicle   `CC` `H5` `PE`

√7th **S42.016** **Posterior** displaced fracture of sternal end of unspecified clavicle   `CC` `H5` `UNS` `PE`

√7th **S42.017** **Nondisplaced** fracture of sternal end of **right** clavicle   `CC` `H5` `PE`

√7th **S42.018** **Nondisplaced** fracture of sternal end of **left** clavicle   `CC` `H5` `PE`

√7th **S42.019** **Nondisplaced** fracture of sternal end of unspecified clavicle   `CC` `H5` `UNS` `PE`

√6th **S42.02** Fracture of **shaft** of clavicle

√7th **S42.021** **Displaced** fracture of shaft of **right** clavicle   `CC` `H5` `PE`

√7th **S42.022** **Displaced** fracture of shaft of **left** clavicle   `CC` `H5` `PE`

√7th **S42.023** **Displaced** fracture of shaft of unspecified clavicle   `CC` `H5` `UNS` `PE`

√7th **S42.024** **Nondisplaced** fracture of shaft of **right** clavicle   `CC` `H5` `PE`

√7th **S42.025** **Nondisplaced** fracture of shaft of **left** clavicle   `CC` `H5` `PE`

√7th **S42.026** **Nondisplaced** fracture of shaft of unspecified clavicle   `CC` `H5` `UNS` `PE`

√6th **S42.03** Fracture of **lateral end** of clavicle

    Fracture of acromial end of clavicle

√7th **S42.031** **Displaced** fracture of lateral end of **right** clavicle   `CC` `H5` `PE`

√7th **S42.032** **Displaced** fracture of lateral end of **left** clavicle   `CC` `H5` `PE`

√7th **S42.033** **Displaced** fracture of lateral end of unspecified clavicle   `CC` `H5` `UNS` `PE`

√7th **S42.034** **Nondisplaced** fracture of lateral end of **right** clavicle   `CC` `H5` `PE`

√7th **S42.035** **Nondisplaced** fracture of lateral end of **left** clavicle   `CC` `H5` `PE`

√7th **S42.036** **Nondisplaced** fracture of lateral end of unspecified clavicle   `CC` `H5` `UNS` `PE`

√5th **S42.1** Fracture of **scapula**

√6th **S42.10** Fracture of unspecified part of scapula

√7th **S42.101** Fracture of unspecified part of scapula, **right** shoulder   `CC` `H5` `PE`

√7th **S42.102** Fracture of unspecified part of scapula, **left** shoulder   `CC` `H5` `PE`

√7th **S42.109** Fracture of unspecified part of scapula, unspecified shoulder   `CC` `H5` `UNS` `PE`

√6th **S42.11** Fracture of **body** of scapula

√7th **S42.111** **Displaced** fracture of body of scapula, **right** shoulder   `CC` `H5` `PE`

√7th **S42.112** **Displaced** fracture of body of scapula, **left** shoulder   `CC` `H5` `PE`

√7th **S42.113** **Displaced** fracture of body of scapula, unspecified shoulder   `CC` `H5` `UNS` `PE`

√7th **S42.114** **Nondisplaced** fracture of body of scapula, **right** shoulder   `CC` `H5` `PE`

√7th **S42.115** **Nondisplaced** fracture of body of scapula, **left** shoulder   `CC` `H5` `PE`

√7th **S42.116** **Nondisplaced** fracture of body of scapula, unspecified shoulder   `CC` `H5` `UNS` `PE`

√6th **S42.12** Fracture of **acromial process**

√7th **S42.121** **Displaced** fracture of acromial process, **right** shoulder   `CC` `H5` `PE`

√7th **S42.122** **Displaced** fracture of acromial process, **left** shoulder   `CC` `H5` `PE`

√7th **S42.123** **Displaced** fracture of acromial process, unspecified shoulder   `CC` `H5` `UNS` `PE`

√7th **S42.124** **Nondisplaced** fracture of acromial process, **right** shoulder   `CC` `H5` `PE`

√7th **S42.125** **Nondisplaced** fracture of acromial process, **left** shoulder   `CC` `H5` `PE`

√7th **S42.126** **Nondisplaced** fracture of acromial process, unspecified shoulder   `CC` `H5` `UNS` `PE`

√6th **S42.13** Fracture of **coracoid process**

√7th **S42.131** **Displaced** fracture of coracoid process, **right** shoulder   `CC` `H5` `PE`

√7th **S42.132** **Displaced** fracture of coracoid process, **left** shoulder   `CC` `H5` `PE`

√7th **S42.133** **Displaced** fracture of coracoid process, unspecified shoulder   `CC` `H5` `UNS` `PE`

√7th **S42.134** **Nondisplaced** fracture of coracoid process, **right** shoulder   `CC` `H5` `PE`

√7th **S42.135** **Nondisplaced** fracture of coracoid process, **left** shoulder   `CC` `H5` `PE`

√7th **S42.136** **Nondisplaced** fracture of coracoid process, unspecified shoulder   `CC` `H5` `UNS` `PE`

√6th **S42.14** Fracture of **glenoid cavity** of scapula

√7th **S42.141** **Displaced** fracture of glenoid cavity of scapula, **right** shoulder   `CC` `H5` `PE`

√7th **S42.142** **Displaced** fracture of glenoid cavity of scapula, **left** shoulder   `CC` `H5` `PE`

√7th **S42.143** **Displaced** fracture of glenoid cavity of scapula, unspecified shoulder   `CC` `H5` `UNS` `PE`

√7th **S42.144** **Nondisplaced** fracture of glenoid cavity of scapula, **right** shoulder   `CC` `H5` `PE`

√7th **S42.145** **Nondisplaced** fracture of glenoid cavity of scapula, **left** shoulder   `CC` `H5` `PE`

√7th **S42.146** **Nondisplaced** fracture of glenoid cavity of scapula, unspecified shoulder   `CC` `H5` `UNS` `PE`

√6th **S42.15** Fracture of **neck** of scapula

√7th **S42.151** **Displaced** fracture of neck of scapula, **right** shoulder   `CC` `H5` `PE`

√7th **S42.152** **Displaced** fracture of neck of scapula, **left** shoulder   `CC` `H5` `PE`

√7th **S42.153** **Displaced** fracture of neck of scapula, unspecified shoulder   `CC` `H5` `UNS` `PE`

√7th **S42.154** **Nondisplaced** fracture of neck of scapula, **right** shoulder   `CC` `H5` `PE`

√7th **S42.155** **Nondisplaced** fracture of neck of scapula, **left** shoulder   `CC` `H5` `PE`

√7th **S42.156** **Nondisplaced** fracture of neck of scapula, unspecified shoulder   `CC` `H5` `UNS` `PE`

√6th **S42.19** Fracture of other part of scapula

√7th **S42.191** Fracture of other part of scapula, **right** shoulder   `CC` `H5` `PE`

√7th **S42.192** Fracture of other part of scapula, **left** shoulder   `CC` `H5` `PE`

√7th **S42.199** Fracture of other part of scapula, unspecified shoulder   `CC` `H5` `UNS` `PE`

√5th **S42.2** Fracture of **upper end of humerus**

    Fracture of proximal end of humerus

    EXCLUDES 2   fracture of shaft of humerus (S42.3-)

              physeal fracture of upper end of humerus (S49.0-)

√6th **S42.20** Unspecified fracture of upper end of humerus

√7th **S42.201** Unspecified fracture of upper end of **right** humerus   `MCC` `CC` `H5` `PE`

√7th **S42.202** Unspecified fracture of upper end of **left** humerus   `MCC` `CC` `H5` `PE`

√7th **S42.209** Unspecified fracture of upper end of unspecified humerus   `MCC` `CC` `H5` `UNS` `PE`

√6th **S42.21** Unspecified fracture of **surgical neck** of humerus

    Fracture of neck of humerus NOS

√7th **S42.211** Unspecified **displaced** fracture of surgical neck of **right** humerus   `MCC` `CC` `H5` `PE`

√7th **S42.212** Unspecified **displaced** fracture of surgical neck of **left** humerus   `MCC` `CC` `H5` `PE`

√7th **S42.213** Unspecified **displaced** fracture of surgical neck of unspecified humerus   `MCC` `CC` `H5` `UNS` `PE`

√7th **S42.214** Unspecified **nondisplaced** fracture of surgical neck of **right** humerus   `MCC` `CC` `H5` `PE`

√7th **S42.215** Unspecified **nondisplaced** fracture of surgical neck of **left** humerus   `MCC` `CC` `H5` `PE`

√7th **S42.216** Unspecified **nondisplaced** fracture of surgical neck of unspecified humerus   `MCC` `CC` `H5` `UNS` `PE`

√6th **S42.22** **2-part** fracture of **surgical neck** of humerus

√7th **S42.221** 2-part **displaced** fracture of surgical neck of **right** humerus   `MCC` `CC` `H5` `PE`

✔ Additional Character Required   √x 7th Placeholder   Questionable PDx   Manifestation   Unspecified   `UPD` Unacceptable PDx   `H1`-`H14` HAC   `HCC` CMS-HCC Dx   `HIV` HIV Dx

ICD-10-CM 2025   **1029**

√7th **S42.222** 2-part **displaced** fracture of surgical neck of **left** humerus `MCC` `CC` `H5` `PE`

√7th **S42.223** 2-part **displaced** fracture of surgical neck of unspecified humerus `MCC` `CC` `H5` `UNS` `PE`

√7th **S42.224** 2-part **nondisplaced** fracture of surgical neck of **right** humerus `MCC` `CC` `H5` `PE`

√7th **S42.225** 2-part **nondisplaced** fracture of surgical neck of **left** humerus `MCC` `CC` `H5` `PE`

√7th **S42.226** 2-part **nondisplaced** fracture of surgical neck of unspecified humerus `MCC` `CC` `H5` `UNS` `PE`

√6th **S42.23** **3-part** fracture of **surgical neck** of humerus

√7th **S42.231** 3-part fracture of surgical neck of **right** humerus `MCC` `CC` `H5` `PE`

√7th **S42.232** 3-part fracture of surgical neck of **left** humerus `MCC` `CC` `H5` `PE`

√7th **S42.239** 3-part fracture of surgical neck of unspecified humerus `MCC` `CC` `H5` `UNS` `PE`

√6th **S42.24** **4-part** fracture of **surgical neck** of humerus

√7th **S42.241** 4-part fracture of surgical neck of **right** humerus `MCC` `CC` `H5` `PE`

√7th **S42.242** 4-part fracture of surgical neck of **left** humerus `MCC` `CC` `H5` `PE`

√7th **S42.249** 4-part fracture of surgical neck of unspecified humerus `MCC` `CC` `H5` `UNS` `PE`

√6th **S42.25** Fracture of **greater tuberosity** of humerus

√7th **S42.251** **Displaced** fracture of greater tuberosity of **right** humerus `MCC` `CC` `H5` `PE`

√7th **S42.252** **Displaced** fracture of greater tuberosity of **left** humerus `MCC` `CC` `H5` `PE`

√7th **S42.253** **Displaced** fracture of greater tuberosity of unspecified humerus `MCC` `CC` `H5` `UNS` `PE`

√7th **S42.254** **Nondisplaced** fracture of greater tuberosity of **right** humerus `MCC` `CC` `H5` `PE`

√7th **S42.255** **Nondisplaced** fracture of greater tuberosity of **left** humerus `MCC` `CC` `H5` `PE`

√7th **S42.256** **Nondisplaced** fracture of greater tuberosity of unspecified humerus `MCC` `CC` `H5` `UNS` `PE`

√6th **S42.26** Fracture of **lesser tuberosity** of humerus

√7th **S42.261** **Displaced** fracture of lesser tuberosity of **right** humerus `MCC` `CC` `H5` `PE`

√7th **S42.262** **Displaced** fracture of lesser tuberosity of **left** humerus `MCC` `CC` `H5` `PE`

√7th **S42.263** **Displaced** fracture of lesser tuberosity of unspecified humerus `MCC` `CC` `H5` `UNS` `PE`

√7th **S42.264** **Nondisplaced** fracture of lesser tuberosity of **right** humerus `MCC` `CC` `H5` `PE`

√7th **S42.265** **Nondisplaced** fracture of lesser tuberosity of **left** humerus `MCC` `CC` `H5` `PE`

√7th **S42.266** **Nondisplaced** fracture of lesser tuberosity of unspecified humerus `MCC` `CC` `H5` `UNS` `PE`

√6th **S42.27** **Torus** fracture of upper end of humerus

> The appropriate 7th character is to be added to all codes in subcategory S42.27
> A   initial encounter for closed fracture
> D   subsequent encounter for fracture with routine healing
> G   subsequent encounter for fracture with delayed healing
> K   subsequent encounter for fracture with nonunion
> P   subsequent encounter for fracture with malunion
> S   sequela

√7th **S42.271** Torus fracture of upper end of **right** humerus `CC` `H5` `PE`

√7th **S42.272** Torus fracture of upper end of **left** humerus `CC` `H5` `PE`

√7th **S42.279** Torus fracture of upper end of unspecified humerus `CC` `H5` `UNS` `PE`

√6th **S42.29** **Other fracture of upper end of humerus**

Fracture of anatomical neck of humerus
Fracture of articular head of humerus
AHA: 2024,2Q,24; 2019,1Q,18

√7th **S42.291** Other **displaced** fracture of upper end of **right** humerus `MCC` `CC` `H5` `PE`

√7th **S42.292** Other **displaced** fracture of upper end of **left** humerus `MCC` `CC` `H5` `PE`

√7th **S42.293** Other **displaced** fracture of upper end of unspecified humerus `MCC` `CC` `H5` `UNS` `PE`

√7th **S42.294** Other **nondisplaced** fracture of upper end of **right** humerus `MCC` `CC` `H5` `PE`

√7th **S42.295** Other **nondisplaced** fracture of upper end of **left** humerus `MCC` `CC` `H5` `PE`

√7th **S42.296** Other **nondisplaced** fracture of upper end of unspecified humerus `MCC` `CC` `H5` `UNS` `PE`

√5th **S42.3** Fracture of **shaft** of humerus

Fracture of humerus NOS
Fracture of upper arm NOS
EXCLUDES 2   physeal fractures of upper end of humerus (S49.0-)
    physeal fractures of lower end of humerus (S49.1-)

√6th **S42.30** Unspecified fracture of shaft of humerus

√7th **S42.301** Unspecified fracture of shaft of humerus, **right arm** `MCC` `CC` `H5` `PE`

√7th **S42.302** Unspecified fracture of shaft of humerus, **left arm** `MCC` `CC` `H5` `PE`

√7th **S42.309** Unspecified fracture of shaft of humerus, unspecified arm `MCC` `CC` `H5` `UNS` `PE`

√6th **S42.31** **Greenstick** fracture of shaft of humerus

> The appropriate 7th character is to be added to all codes in subcategory S42.31
> A   initial encounter for closed fracture
> D   subsequent encounter for fracture with routine healing
> G   subsequent encounter for fracture with delayed healing
> K   subsequent encounter for fracture with nonunion
> P   subsequent encounter for fracture with malunion
> S   sequela

√7th **S42.311** Greenstick fracture of shaft of humerus, **right arm** `CC` `H5` `PE`

√7th **S42.312** Greenstick fracture of shaft of humerus, **left arm** `CC` `H5` `PE`

√7th **S42.319** Greenstick fracture of shaft of humerus, unspecified arm `CC` `H5` `UNS` `PE`

√6th **S42.32** **Transverse** fracture of shaft of humerus

√7th **S42.321** **Displaced** transverse fracture of shaft of humerus, **right arm** `MCC` `CC` `H5` `PE`

√7th **S42.322** **Displaced** transverse fracture of shaft of humerus, **left arm** `MCC` `CC` `H5` `PE`

√7th **S42.323** **Displaced** transverse fracture of shaft of humerus, unspecified arm `MCC` `CC` `H5` `UNS` `PE`

√7th **S42.324** **Nondisplaced** transverse fracture of shaft of humerus, **right arm** `MCC` `CC` `H5` `PE`

√7th **S42.325** **Nondisplaced** transverse fracture of shaft of humerus, **left arm** `MCC` `CC` `H5` `PE`

√7th **S42.326** **Nondisplaced** transverse fracture of shaft of humerus, unspecified arm `MCC` `CC` `H5` `UNS` `PE`

√6th **S42.33** **Oblique** fracture of shaft of humerus

√7th **S42.331** **Displaced** oblique fracture of shaft of humerus, **right arm** `MCC` `CC` `H5` `PE`

√7th **S42.332** **Displaced** oblique fracture of shaft of humerus, **left arm** `MCC` `CC` `H5` `PE`

√7th **S42.333** **Displaced** oblique fracture of shaft of humerus, unspecified arm `MCC` `CC` `H5` `UNS` `PE`

√7th **S42.334** **Nondisplaced** oblique fracture of shaft of humerus, **right arm** `MCC` `CC` `H5` `PE`

√7th **S42.335** **Nondisplaced** oblique fracture of shaft of humerus, **left arm** `MCC` `CC` `H5` `PE`

√7th **S42.336** **Nondisplaced** oblique fracture of shaft of humerus, unspecified arm `MCC` `CC` `H5` `UNS` `PE`

`N` Newborn: 0   `P` Pediatric: 0-17   `M` Maternity: 9-64   `A` Adult: 15-124   `UNS` Unspecified Site   `MCC` Major Complication/Comorbidity   `CC` Complication/Comorbidity   `PE` POA Exempt

1030   ICD-10-CM 2025

S42.34 ✓6ᵗʰ **Spiral** fracture of shaft of humerus

  ✓7ᵗʰ **S42.341** **Displaced** spiral fracture of shaft of humerus, **right** arm `MCC` `CC` `H5` `PE`

  ✓7ᵗʰ **S42.342** **Displaced** spiral fracture of shaft of humerus, **left** arm `MCC` `CC` `H5` `PE`

  ✓7ᵗʰ **S42.343** **Displaced** spiral fracture of shaft of humerus, unspecified arm `MCC` `CC` `H5` `UNS` `PE`

  ✓7ᵗʰ **S42.344** **Nondisplaced** spiral fracture of shaft of humerus, **right** arm `MCC` `CC` `H5` `PE`

  ✓7ᵗʰ **S42.345** **Nondisplaced** spiral fracture of shaft of humerus, **left** arm `MCC` `CC` `H5` `PE`

  ✓7ᵗʰ **S42.346** **Nondisplaced** spiral fracture of shaft of humerus, unspecified arm `MCC` `CC` `H5` `UNS` `PE`

S42.35 ✓6ᵗʰ **Comminuted** fracture of shaft of humerus

  ✓7ᵗʰ **S42.351** **Displaced** comminuted fracture of shaft of humerus, **right** arm `MCC` `CC` `H5` `PE`

  ✓7ᵗʰ **S42.352** **Displaced** comminuted fracture of shaft of humerus, **left** arm `MCC` `CC` `H5` `PE`

  ✓7ᵗʰ **S42.353** **Displaced** comminuted fracture of shaft of humerus, unspecified arm `MCC` `CC` `H5` `UNS` `PE`

  ✓7ᵗʰ **S42.354** **Nondisplaced** comminuted fracture of shaft of humerus, **right** arm `MCC` `CC` `H5` `PE`

  ✓7ᵗʰ **S42.355** **Nondisplaced** comminuted fracture of shaft of humerus, **left** arm `MCC` `CC` `H5` `PE`

  ✓7ᵗʰ **S42.356** **Nondisplaced** comminuted fracture of shaft of humerus, unspecified arm `MCC` `CC` `H5` `UNS` `PE`

S42.36 ✓6ᵗʰ **Segmental** fracture of shaft of humerus

  ✓7ᵗʰ **S42.361** **Displaced** segmental fracture of shaft of humerus, **right** arm `MCC` `CC` `H5` `PE`

  ✓7ᵗʰ **S42.362** **Displaced** segmental fracture of shaft of humerus, **left** arm `MCC` `CC` `H5` `PE`

  ✓7ᵗʰ **S42.363** **Displaced** segmental fracture of shaft of humerus, unspecified arm `MCC` `CC` `H5` `UNS` `PE`

  ✓7ᵗʰ **S42.364** **Nondisplaced** segmental fracture of shaft of humerus, **right** arm `MCC` `CC` `H5` `PE`

  ✓7ᵗʰ **S42.365** **Nondisplaced** segmental fracture of shaft of humerus, **left** arm `MCC` `CC` `H5` `PE`

  ✓7ᵗʰ **S42.366** **Nondisplaced** segmental fracture of shaft of humerus, unspecified arm `MCC` `CC` `H5` `UNS` `PE`

S42.39 ✓6ᵗʰ **Other** fracture of shaft of humerus

  ✓7ᵗʰ **S42.391** Other fracture of shaft of **right** humerus `MCC` `CC` `H5` `PE`

  ✓7ᵗʰ **S42.392** Other fracture of shaft of **left** humerus `MCC` `CC` `H5` `PE`

  ✓7ᵗʰ **S42.399** Other fracture of shaft of unspecified humerus `MCC` `CC` `H5` `UNS` `PE`

S42.4 ✓5ᵗʰ Fracture of **lower end** of humerus

  Fracture of distal end of humerus

  EXCLUDES 2 *fracture of shaft of humerus (S42.3-)*
        physeal fracture of lower end of humerus (S49.1-)

S42.40 ✓6ᵗʰ Unspecified fracture of lower end of humerus

  Fracture of elbow NOS

  ✓7ᵗʰ **S42.401** Unspecified fracture of lower end of **right** humerus `MCC` `CC` `H5` `PE`

  ✓7ᵗʰ **S42.402** Unspecified fracture of lower end of **left** humerus `MCC` `CC` `H5` `PE`

  ✓7ᵗʰ **S42.409** Unspecified fracture of lower end of unspecified humerus `MCC` `CC` `H5` `UNS` `PE`

S42.41 ✓6ᵗʰ **Simple supracondylar** fracture **without intercondylar** fracture of humerus

  ✓7ᵗʰ **S42.411** **Displaced** simple supracondylar fracture without intercondylar fracture of **right** humerus `MCC` `CC` `H5` `PE`

  ✓7ᵗʰ **S42.412** **Displaced** simple supracondylar fracture without intercondylar fracture of **left** humerus `MCC` `CC` `H5` `PE`

  ✓7ᵗʰ **S42.413** **Displaced** simple supracondylar fracture without intercondylar fracture of unspecified humerus `MCC` `CC` `H5` `UNS` `PE`

  ✓7ᵗʰ **S42.414** **Nondisplaced** simple supracondylar fracture without intercondylar fracture of **right** humerus `MCC` `CC` `H5` `PE`

  ✓7ᵗʰ **S42.415** **Nondisplaced** simple supracondylar fracture without intercondylar fracture of **left** humerus `MCC` `CC` `H5` `PE`

  ✓7ᵗʰ **S42.416** **Nondisplaced** simple supracondylar fracture without intercondylar fracture of unspecified humerus `MCC` `CC` `H5` `UNS` `PE`

S42.42 ✓6ᵗʰ **Comminuted supracondylar** fracture **without intercondylar** fracture of humerus

  ✓7ᵗʰ **S42.421** **Displaced** comminuted supracondylar fracture without intercondylar fracture of **right** humerus `MCC` `CC` `H5` `PE`

  ✓7ᵗʰ **S42.422** **Displaced** comminuted supracondylar fracture without intercondylar fracture of **left** humerus `MCC` `CC` `H5` `PE`

  ✓7ᵗʰ **S42.423** **Displaced** comminuted supracondylar fracture without intercondylar fracture of unspecified humerus `MCC` `CC` `H5` `UNS` `PE`

  ✓7ᵗʰ **S42.424** **Nondisplaced** comminuted supracondylar fracture without intercondylar fracture of **right** humerus `MCC` `CC` `H5` `PE`

  ✓7ᵗʰ **S42.425** **Nondisplaced** comminuted supracondylar fracture without intercondylar fracture of **left** humerus `MCC` `CC` `H5` `PE`

  ✓7ᵗʰ **S42.426** **Nondisplaced** comminuted supracondylar fracture without intercondylar fracture of unspecified humerus `MCC` `CC` `H5` `UNS` `PE`

S42.43 ✓6ᵗʰ Fracture (avulsion) of **lateral epicondyle** of humerus

  ✓7ᵗʰ **S42.431** **Displaced** fracture (avulsion) of lateral epicondyle of **right** humerus `MCC` `CC` `H5` `PE`

  ✓7ᵗʰ **S42.432** **Displaced** fracture (avulsion) of lateral epicondyle of **left** humerus `MCC` `CC` `H5` `PE`

  ✓7ᵗʰ **S42.433** **Displaced** fracture (avulsion) of lateral epicondyle of unspecified humerus `MCC` `CC` `H5` `UNS` `PE`

  ✓7ᵗʰ **S42.434** **Nondisplaced** fracture (avulsion) of lateral epicondyle of **right** humerus `MCC` `CC` `H5` `PE`

  ✓7ᵗʰ **S42.435** **Nondisplaced** fracture (avulsion) of lateral epicondyle of **left** humerus `MCC` `CC` `H5` `PE`

  ✓7ᵗʰ **S42.436** **Nondisplaced** fracture (avulsion) of lateral epicondyle of unspecified humerus `MCC` `CC` `H5` `UNS` `PE`

S42.44 ✓6ᵗʰ Fracture (avulsion) of **medial epicondyle** of humerus

  ✓7ᵗʰ **S42.441** **Displaced** fracture (avulsion) of medial epicondyle of **right** humerus `MCC` `CC` `H5` `PE`

  ✓7ᵗʰ **S42.442** **Displaced** fracture (avulsion) of medial epicondyle of **left** humerus `MCC` `CC` `H5` `PE`

  ✓7ᵗʰ **S42.443** **Displaced** fracture (avulsion) of medial epicondyle of unspecified humerus `MCC` `CC` `H5` `UNS` `PE`

  ✓7ᵗʰ **S42.444** **Nondisplaced** fracture (avulsion) of medial epicondyle of **right** humerus `MCC` `CC` `H5` `PE`

  ✓7ᵗʰ **S42.445** **Nondisplaced** fracture (avulsion) of medial epicondyle of **left** humerus `MCC` `CC` `H5` `PE`

  ✓7ᵗʰ **S42.446** **Nondisplaced** fracture (avulsion) of medial epicondyle of unspecified humerus `MCC` `CC` `H5` `UNS` `PE`

  ✓7ᵗʰ **S42.447** **Incarcerated** fracture (avulsion) of medial epicondyle of **right** humerus `MCC` `CC` `H5` `PE`

  ✓7ᵗʰ **S42.448** **Incarcerated** fracture (avulsion) of medial epicondyle of **left** humerus `MCC` `CC` `H5` `PE`

  ✓7ᵗʰ **S42.449** **Incarcerated** fracture (avulsion) of medial epicondyle of unspecified humerus `MCC` `CC` `H5` `UNS` `PE`

✓ Additional Character Required   ✓x7ᵗʰ Placeholder   Questionable PDx   Manifestation   Unspecified   `UPD` Unacceptable PDx   `H1`-`H14` HAC   `HCC` CMS-HCC Dx   `HIV` HIV Dx

√6ᵗʰ **S42.45** **Fracture of lateral condyle of humerus**
Fracture of capitellum of humerus

√7ᵗʰ **S42.451** **Displaced fracture of lateral condyle of right humerus** MCC CC H5 PE

√7ᵗʰ **S42.452** **Displaced fracture of lateral condyle of left humerus** MCC CC H5 PE

√7ᵗʰ **S42.453** **Displaced fracture of lateral condyle of unspecified humerus** MCC CC H5 UNS PE

√7ᵗʰ **S42.454** **Nondisplaced fracture of lateral condyle of right humerus** MCC CC H5 PE

√7ᵗʰ **S42.455** **Nondisplaced fracture of lateral condyle of left humerus** MCC CC H5 PE

√7ᵗʰ **S42.456** **Nondisplaced fracture of lateral condyle of unspecified humerus** MCC CC H5 UNS PE

√6ᵗʰ **S42.46** **Fracture of medial condyle of humerus**
Trochlea fracture of humerus

√7ᵗʰ **S42.461** **Displaced fracture of medial condyle of right humerus** MCC CC H5 PE

√7ᵗʰ **S42.462** **Displaced fracture of medial condyle of left humerus** MCC CC H5 PE

√7ᵗʰ **S42.463** **Displaced fracture of medial condyle of unspecified humerus** MCC CC H5 UNS PE

√7ᵗʰ **S42.464** **Nondisplaced fracture of medial condyle of right humerus** MCC CC H5 PE

√7ᵗʰ **S42.465** **Nondisplaced fracture of medial condyle of left humerus** MCC CC H5 PE

√7ᵗʰ **S42.466** **Nondisplaced fracture of medial condyle of unspecified humerus** MCC CC H5 UNS PE

√6ᵗʰ **S42.47** **Transcondylar fracture of humerus**

√7ᵗʰ **S42.471** **Displaced transcondylar fracture of right humerus** MCC CC H5 PE

√7ᵗʰ **S42.472** **Displaced transcondylar fracture of left humerus** MCC CC H5 PE

√7ᵗʰ **S42.473** **Displaced transcondylar fracture of unspecified humerus** MCC CC H5 UNS PE

√7ᵗʰ **S42.474** **Nondisplaced transcondylar fracture of right humerus** MCC CC H5 PE

√7ᵗʰ **S42.475** **Nondisplaced transcondylar fracture of left humerus** MCC CC H5 PE

√7ᵗʰ **S42.476** **Nondisplaced transcondylar fracture of unspecified humerus** MCC CC H5 UNS PE

√6ᵗʰ **S42.48** **Torus fracture of lower end of humerus**

> The appropriate 7th character is to be added to all codes in subcategory S42.48.
> A   initial encounter for closed fracture
> D   subsequent encounter for fracture with routine healing
> G   subsequent encounter for fracture with delayed healing
> K   subsequent encounter for fracture with nonunion
> P   subsequent encounter for fracture with malunion
> S   sequela

√7ᵗʰ **S42.481** **Torus fracture of lower end of right humerus** CC H5 PE

√7ᵗʰ **S42.482** **Torus fracture of lower end of left humerus** CC H5 PE

√7ᵗʰ **S42.489** **Torus fracture of lower end of unspecified humerus** CC H5 UNS PE

√6ᵗʰ **S42.49** **Other fracture of lower end of humerus**

√7ᵗʰ **S42.491** **Other displaced fracture of lower end of right humerus** MCC CC H5 PE

√7ᵗʰ **S42.492** **Other displaced fracture of lower end of left humerus** MCC CC H5 PE

√7ᵗʰ **S42.493** **Other displaced fracture of lower end of unspecified humerus** MCC CC H5 UNS PE

√7ᵗʰ **S42.494** **Other nondisplaced fracture of lower end of right humerus** MCC CC H5 PE

√7ᵗʰ **S42.495** **Other nondisplaced fracture of lower end of left humerus** MCC CC H5 PE

√7ᵗʰ **S42.496** **Other nondisplaced fracture of lower end of unspecified humerus** MCC CC H5 UNS PE

√5ᵗʰ **S42.9** **Fracture of shoulder girdle, part unspecified**
Fracture of shoulder NOS

√x7ᵗʰ **S42.90** **Fracture of unspecified shoulder girdle, part unspecified** MCC CC H5 UNS PE

√x7ᵗʰ **S42.91** **Fracture of right shoulder girdle, part unspecified** MCC CC H5 PE

√x7ᵗʰ **S42.92** **Fracture of left shoulder girdle, part unspecified** MCC CC H5 PE

√4ᵗʰ **S43** **Dislocation and sprain of joints and ligaments of shoulder girdle**

INCLUDES | avulsion of joint or ligament of shoulder girdle
laceration of cartilage, joint or ligament of shoulder girdle
sprain of cartilage, joint or ligament of shoulder girdle
traumatic hemarthrosis of joint or ligament of shoulder girdle
traumatic rupture of joint or ligament of shoulder girdle
traumatic subluxation of joint or ligament of shoulder girdle
traumatic tear of joint or ligament of shoulder girdle

Code also any associated open wound

EXCLUDES 2 | strain of muscle, fascia and tendon of shoulder and upper arm (S46.-)

> The appropriate 7th character is to be added to each code from category S43.
> A   initial encounter
> D   subsequent encounter
> S   sequela

√5ᵗʰ **S43.0** **Subluxation and dislocation of shoulder joint**
Dislocation of glenohumeral joint
Subluxation of glenohumeral joint

√6ᵗʰ **S43.00** **Unspecified subluxation and dislocation of shoulder joint**
Dislocation of humerus NOS
Subluxation of humerus NOS

√7ᵗʰ **S43.001** **Unspecified subluxation of right shoulder joint** PE

√7ᵗʰ **S43.002** **Unspecified subluxation of left shoulder joint** PE

√7ᵗʰ **S43.003** **Unspecified subluxation of unspecified shoulder joint** PE

√7ᵗʰ **S43.004** **Unspecified dislocation of right shoulder joint** PE

√7ᵗʰ **S43.005** **Unspecified dislocation of left shoulder joint** PE

√7ᵗʰ **S43.006** **Unspecified dislocation of unspecified shoulder joint** PE

√6ᵗʰ **S43.01** **Anterior subluxation and dislocation of humerus**

√7ᵗʰ **S43.011** **Anterior subluxation of right humerus** PE

√7ᵗʰ **S43.012** **Anterior subluxation of left humerus** PE

√7ᵗʰ **S43.013** **Anterior subluxation of unspecified humerus** PE

√7ᵗʰ **S43.014** **Anterior dislocation of right humerus** PE

√7ᵗʰ **S43.015** **Anterior dislocation of left humerus** PE

√7ᵗʰ **S43.016** **Anterior dislocation of unspecified humerus** PE

√6ᵗʰ **S43.02** **Posterior subluxation and dislocation of humerus**

√7ᵗʰ **S43.021** **Posterior subluxation of right humerus** PE

√7ᵗʰ **S43.022** **Posterior subluxation of left humerus** PE

√7ᵗʰ **S43.023** **Posterior subluxation of unspecified humerus** PE

√7ᵗʰ **S43.024** **Posterior dislocation of right humerus** PE

√7ᵗʰ **S43.025** **Posterior dislocation of left humerus** PE

√7ᵗʰ **S43.026** **Posterior dislocation of unspecified humerus** PE

√6ᵗʰ **S43.03** **Inferior subluxation and dislocation of humerus**

√7ᵗʰ **S43.031** **Inferior subluxation of right humerus** PE

√7ᵗʰ **S43.032** **Inferior subluxation of left humerus** PE

√7ᵗʰ **S43.033** **Inferior subluxation of unspecified humerus** PE

√7ᵗʰ **S43.034** Inferior dislocation of right humerus `PE`

√7ᵗʰ **S43.035** Inferior dislocation of left humerus `PE`

√7ᵗʰ **S43.036** Inferior dislocation of unspecified humerus `PE`

✓6ᵗʰ **S43.08** Other subluxation and dislocation of shoulder joint

√7ᵗʰ **S43.081** Other subluxation of right shoulder joint `PE`

√7ᵗʰ **S43.082** Other subluxation of left shoulder joint `PE`

√7ᵗʰ **S43.083** Other subluxation of unspecified shoulder joint `PE`

√7ᵗʰ **S43.084** Other dislocation of right shoulder joint `PE`

√7ᵗʰ **S43.085** Other dislocation of left shoulder joint `PE`

√7ᵗʰ **S43.086** Other dislocation of unspecified shoulder joint `PE`

✓5ᵗʰ **S43.1** Subluxation and dislocation of acromioclavicular joint

✓6ᵗʰ **S43.10** Unspecified dislocation of acromioclavicular joint

√7ᵗʰ **S43.101** Unspecified dislocation of right acromioclavicular joint `PE`

√7ᵗʰ **S43.102** Unspecified dislocation of left acromioclavicular joint `PE`

√7ᵗʰ **S43.109** Unspecified dislocation of unspecified acromioclavicular joint `PE`

✓6ᵗʰ **S43.11** Subluxation of acromioclavicular joint

√7ᵗʰ **S43.111** Subluxation of right acromioclavicular joint `PE`

√7ᵗʰ **S43.112** Subluxation of left acromioclavicular joint `PE`

√7ᵗʰ **S43.119** Subluxation of unspecified acromioclavicular joint `PE`

✓6ᵗʰ **S43.12** Dislocation of acromioclavicular joint, 100%-200% displacement

√7ᵗʰ **S43.121** Dislocation of right acromioclavicular joint, 100%-200% displacement `PE`

√7ᵗʰ **S43.122** Dislocation of left acromioclavicular joint, 100%-200% displacement `PE`

√7ᵗʰ **S43.129** Dislocation of unspecified acromioclavicular joint, 100%-200% displacement `PE`

✓6ᵗʰ **S43.13** Dislocation of acromioclavicular joint, greater than 200% displacement

√7ᵗʰ **S43.131** Dislocation of right acromioclavicular joint, greater than 200% displacement `PE`

√7ᵗʰ **S43.132** Dislocation of left acromioclavicular joint, greater than 200% displacement `PE`

√7ᵗʰ **S43.139** Dislocation of unspecified acromioclavicular joint, greater than 200% displacement `PE`

✓6ᵗʰ **S43.14** Inferior dislocation of acromioclavicular joint

√7ᵗʰ **S43.141** Inferior dislocation of right acromioclavicular joint `PE`

√7ᵗʰ **S43.142** Inferior dislocation of left acromioclavicular joint `PE`

√7ᵗʰ **S43.149** Inferior dislocation of unspecified acromioclavicular joint `PE`

✓6ᵗʰ **S43.15** Posterior dislocation of acromioclavicular joint

√7ᵗʰ **S43.151** Posterior dislocation of right acromioclavicular joint `PE`

√7ᵗʰ **S43.152** Posterior dislocation of left acromioclavicular joint `PE`

√7ᵗʰ **S43.159** Posterior dislocation of unspecified acromioclavicular joint `PE`

✓5ᵗʰ **S43.2** Subluxation and dislocation of sternoclavicular joint

✓6ᵗʰ **S43.20** Unspecified subluxation and dislocation of sternoclavicular joint

√7ᵗʰ **S43.201** Unspecified subluxation of right sternoclavicular joint `CC` `H5` `PE`

√7ᵗʰ **S43.202** Unspecified subluxation of left sternoclavicular joint `CC` `H5` `PE`

√7ᵗʰ **S43.203** Unspecified subluxation of unspecified sternoclavicular joint `CC` `H5` `UNS` `PE`

√7ᵗʰ **S43.204** Unspecified dislocation of right sternoclavicular joint `CC` `H5` `PE`

√7ᵗʰ **S43.205** Unspecified dislocation of left sternoclavicular joint `CC` `H5` `PE`

√7ᵗʰ **S43.206** Unspecified dislocation of unspecified sternoclavicular joint `CC` `H5` `UNS` `PE`

✓6ᵗʰ **S43.21** Anterior subluxation and dislocation of sternoclavicular joint

√7ᵗʰ **S43.211** Anterior subluxation of right sternoclavicular joint `CC` `H5` `PE`

√7ᵗʰ **S43.212** Anterior subluxation of left sternoclavicular joint `CC` `H5` `PE`

√7ᵗʰ **S43.213** Anterior subluxation of unspecified sternoclavicular joint `CC` `H5` `UNS` `PE`

√7ᵗʰ **S43.214** Anterior dislocation of right sternoclavicular joint `CC` `H5` `PE`

√7ᵗʰ **S43.215** Anterior dislocation of left sternoclavicular joint `CC` `H5` `PE`

√7ᵗʰ **S43.216** Anterior dislocation of unspecified sternoclavicular joint `CC` `H5` `UNS` `PE`

✓6ᵗʰ **S43.22** Posterior subluxation and dislocation of sternoclavicular joint

√7ᵗʰ **S43.221** Posterior subluxation of right sternoclavicular joint `CC` `H5` `PE`

√7ᵗʰ **S43.222** Posterior subluxation of left sternoclavicular joint `CC` `H5` `PE`

√7ᵗʰ **S43.223** Posterior subluxation of unspecified sternoclavicular joint `CC` `H5` `UNS` `PE`

√7ᵗʰ **S43.224** Posterior dislocation of right sternoclavicular joint `CC` `H5` `PE`

√7ᵗʰ **S43.225** Posterior dislocation of left sternoclavicular joint `CC` `H5` `PE`

√7ᵗʰ **S43.226** Posterior dislocation of unspecified sternoclavicular joint `CC` `H5` `UNS` `PE`

✓5ᵗʰ **S43.3** Subluxation and dislocation of other and unspecified parts of shoulder girdle

✓6ᵗʰ **S43.30** Subluxation and dislocation of unspecified parts of shoulder girdle

Dislocation of shoulder girdle NOS
Subluxation of shoulder girdle NOS

√7ᵗʰ **S43.301** Subluxation of unspecified parts of right shoulder girdle `PE`

√7ᵗʰ **S43.302** Subluxation of unspecified parts of left shoulder girdle `PE`

√7ᵗʰ **S43.303** Subluxation of unspecified parts of unspecified shoulder girdle `PE`

√7ᵗʰ **S43.304** Dislocation of unspecified parts of right shoulder girdle `PE`

√7ᵗʰ **S43.305** Dislocation of unspecified parts of left shoulder girdle `PE`

√7ᵗʰ **S43.306** Dislocation of unspecified parts of unspecified shoulder girdle `PE`

✓6ᵗʰ **S43.31** Subluxation and dislocation of scapula

√7ᵗʰ **S43.311** Subluxation of right scapula `PE`

√7ᵗʰ **S43.312** Subluxation of left scapula `PE`

√7ᵗʰ **S43.313** Subluxation of unspecified scapula `PE`

√7ᵗʰ **S43.314** Dislocation of right scapula `PE`

√7ᵗʰ **S43.315** Dislocation of left scapula `PE`

√7ᵗʰ **S43.316** Dislocation of unspecified scapula `PE`

✓6ᵗʰ **S43.39** Subluxation and dislocation of other parts of shoulder girdle

√7ᵗʰ **S43.391** Subluxation of other parts of right shoulder girdle `PE`

√7ᵗʰ **S43.392** Subluxation of other parts of left shoulder girdle `PE`

√7ᵗʰ **S43.393** Subluxation of other parts of unspecified shoulder girdle `PE`

√7ᵗʰ **S43.394** Dislocation of other parts of right shoulder girdle `PE`

√7ᵗʰ **S43.395** Dislocation of other parts of left shoulder girdle `PE`

√7ᵗʰ **S43.396** Dislocation of other parts of unspecified shoulder girdle `PE`

✓5ᵗʰ **S43.4** Sprain of shoulder joint

✓6ᵗʰ **S43.40** Unspecified sprain of shoulder joint

√7ᵗʰ **S43.401** Unspecified sprain of right shoulder joint `PE`

√7ᵗʰ **S43.402** Unspecified sprain of left shoulder joint `PE`

√7ᵗʰ **S43.409** Unspecified sprain of unspecified shoulder joint `PE`

✓ Additional Character Required   ✓x7ᵗʰ Placeholder   Questionable PDx   Manifestation   Unspecified   `UPD` Unacceptable PDx   `H1`-`H14` HAC   `HCC` CMS-HCC Dx   `HIV` HIV Dx

√6ᵗʰ **S43.41** Sprain of **coracohumeral** (ligament)
    √7ᵗʰ **S43.411** Sprain of **right** coracohumeral (ligament)   PE
    √7ᵗʰ **S43.412** Sprain of **left** coracohumeral (ligament)   PE
    √7ᵗʰ **S43.419** Sprain of unspecified coracohumeral (ligament)   PE

√6ᵗʰ **S43.42** Sprain of **rotator cuff capsule**
    EXCLUDES 1   rotator cuff syndrome (complete) (incomplete), not specified as traumatic (M75.1-)
    EXCLUDES 2   injury of tendon of rotator cuff (S46.Ø-)
    √7ᵗʰ **S43.421** Sprain of **right** rotator cuff capsule   PE
    √7ᵗʰ **S43.422** Sprain of **left** rotator cuff capsule   PE
    √7ᵗʰ **S43.429** Sprain of unspecified rotator cuff capsule   PE

√6ᵗʰ **S43.43** **Superior glenoid labrum** lesion
    SLAP lesion
    AHA: 2024,2Q,24; 2019,2Q,26
    DEF: Detachment injury of the superior aspect of the glenoid labrum, which is the ring of fibrocartilage attached to the rim of the glenoid cavity of the scapula.
    √7ᵗʰ **S43.431** Superior glenoid labrum lesion of **right** shoulder   PE
    √7ᵗʰ **S43.432** Superior glenoid labrum lesion of **left** shoulder   PE
    √7ᵗʰ **S43.439** Superior glenoid labrum lesion of unspecified shoulder   PE

√6ᵗʰ **S43.49** Other sprain of shoulder joint
    √7ᵗʰ **S43.491** Other sprain of **right** shoulder joint   PE
    √7ᵗʰ **S43.492** Other sprain of **left** shoulder joint   PE
    √7ᵗʰ **S43.499** Other sprain of unspecified shoulder joint   PE

√5ᵗʰ **S43.5** Sprain of **acromioclavicular** joint
    Sprain of acromioclavicular ligament
    √x7ᵗʰ **S43.50** Sprain of unspecified acromioclavicular joint   PE
    √x7ᵗʰ **S43.51** Sprain of **right** acromioclavicular joint   PE
    √x7ᵗʰ **S43.52** Sprain of **left** acromioclavicular joint   PE

√5ᵗʰ **S43.6** Sprain of **sternoclavicular** joint
    √x7ᵗʰ **S43.60** Sprain of unspecified sternoclavicular joint   PE
    √x7ᵗʰ **S43.61** Sprain of **right** sternoclavicular joint   PE
    √x7ᵗʰ **S43.62** Sprain of **left** sternoclavicular joint   PE

√5ᵗʰ **S43.8** Sprain of other specified parts of shoulder girdle
    √x7ᵗʰ **S43.80** Sprain of other specified parts of unspecified shoulder girdle   PE
    √x7ᵗʰ **S43.81** Sprain of other specified parts of **right** shoulder girdle   PE
    √x7ᵗʰ **S43.82** Sprain of other specified parts of **left** shoulder girdle   PE

√5ᵗʰ **S43.9** Sprain of unspecified parts of shoulder girdle
    √x7ᵗʰ **S43.90** Sprain of unspecified parts of unspecified shoulder girdle   PE
    Sprain of shoulder girdle NOS
    √x7ᵗʰ **S43.91** Sprain of unspecified parts of **right** shoulder girdle   PE
    √x7ᵗʰ **S43.92** Sprain of unspecified parts of **left** shoulder girdle   PE

√4ᵗʰ **S44** Injury of nerves at shoulder and upper arm level
    Code also any associated open wound (S41.-)
    EXCLUDES 2   injury of brachial plexus (S14.3-)
    The appropriate 7th character is to be added to each code from category S44.
    A   initial encounter
    D   subsequent encounter
    S   sequela

√5ᵗʰ **S44.Ø** Injury of **ulnar nerve** at upper arm level
    EXCLUDES 1   ulnar nerve NOS (S54.Ø)
    √x7ᵗʰ **S44.00** Injury of ulnar nerve at upper arm level, unspecified arm   PE
    √x7ᵗʰ **S44.01** Injury of ulnar nerve at upper arm level, **right** arm   PE
    √x7ᵗʰ **S44.02** Injury of ulnar nerve at upper arm level, **left** arm   PE

√5ᵗʰ **S44.1** Injury of **median nerve** at upper arm level
    EXCLUDES 1   median nerve NOS (S54.1)
    √x7ᵗʰ **S44.10** Injury of median nerve at upper arm level, unspecified arm   PE
    √x7ᵗʰ **S44.11** Injury of median nerve at upper arm level, **right** arm   PE
    √x7ᵗʰ **S44.12** Injury of median nerve at upper arm level, **left** arm   PE

√5ᵗʰ **S44.2** Injury of **radial nerve** at upper arm level
    EXCLUDES 1   radial nerve NOS (S54.2)
    √x7ᵗʰ **S44.20** Injury of radial nerve at upper arm level, unspecified arm   PE
    √x7ᵗʰ **S44.21** Injury of radial nerve at upper arm level, **right** arm   PE
    √x7ᵗʰ **S44.22** Injury of radial nerve at upper arm level, **left** arm   PE

√5ᵗʰ **S44.3** Injury of **axillary nerve**
    √x7ᵗʰ **S44.30** Injury of axillary nerve, unspecified arm   PE
    √x7ᵗʰ **S44.31** Injury of axillary nerve, **right** arm   PE
    √x7ᵗʰ **S44.32** Injury of axillary nerve, **left** arm   PE

√5ᵗʰ **S44.4** Injury of **musculocutaneous nerve**
    √x7ᵗʰ **S44.40** Injury of musculocutaneous nerve, unspecified arm   PE
    √x7ᵗʰ **S44.41** Injury of musculocutaneous nerve, **right** arm   PE
    √x7ᵗʰ **S44.42** Injury of musculocutaneous nerve, **left** arm   PE

√5ᵗʰ **S44.5** Injury of **cutaneous sensory nerve** at shoulder and upper arm level
    √x7ᵗʰ **S44.50** Injury of cutaneous sensory nerve at shoulder and upper arm level, unspecified arm   PE
    √x7ᵗʰ **S44.51** Injury of cutaneous sensory nerve at shoulder and upper arm level, **right** arm   PE
    √x7ᵗʰ **S44.52** Injury of cutaneous sensory nerve at shoulder and upper arm level, **left** arm   PE

√5ᵗʰ **S44.8** Injury of other nerves at shoulder and upper arm level
    √6ᵗʰ **S44.8X** Injury of other nerves at shoulder and upper arm level
      √7ᵗʰ **S44.8X1** Injury of other nerves at shoulder and upper arm level, **right** arm   PE
      √7ᵗʰ **S44.8X2** Injury of other nerves at shoulder and upper arm level, **left** arm   PE
      √7ᵗʰ **S44.8X9** Injury of other nerves at shoulder and upper arm level, unspecified arm   PE

√5ᵗʰ **S44.9** Injury of unspecified nerve at shoulder and upper arm level
    √x7ᵗʰ **S44.90** Injury of unspecified nerve at shoulder and upper arm level, unspecified arm   PE
    √x7ᵗʰ **S44.91** Injury of unspecified nerve at shoulder and upper arm level, **right** arm   PE
    √x7ᵗʰ **S44.92** Injury of unspecified nerve at shoulder and upper arm level, **left** arm   PE

√4ᵗʰ **S45** Injury of blood vessels at shoulder and upper arm level
    Code also any associated open wound (S41.-)
    EXCLUDES 2   injury of subclavian artery (S25.1)
           injury of subclavian vein (S25.3)
    The appropriate 7th character is to be added to each code from category S45.
    A   initial encounter
    D   subsequent encounter
    S   sequela

√5ᵗʰ **S45.Ø** Injury of **axillary artery**
    √6ᵗʰ **S45.00** Unspecified injury of axillary artery
      √7ᵗʰ **S45.001** Unspecified injury of axillary artery, **right** side   MCC   PE
      √7ᵗʰ **S45.002** Unspecified injury of axillary artery, **left** side   MCC   PE
      √7ᵗʰ **S45.009** Unspecified injury of axillary artery, unspecified side   MCC   UNS   PE
    √6ᵗʰ **S45.01** **Laceration** of axillary artery
      √7ᵗʰ **S45.011** Laceration of axillary artery, **right** side   MCC   PE
      √7ᵗʰ **S45.012** Laceration of axillary artery, **left** side   MCC   PE
      √7ᵗʰ **S45.019** Laceration of axillary artery, unspecified side   MCC   UNS   PE

✓6ᵗʰ **S45.09** Other specified injury of axillary artery

   ✓7ᵗʰ **S45.091** Other specified injury of axillary artery, **right** side `MCC` `PE`

   ✓7ᵗʰ **S45.092** Other specified injury of axillary artery, **left** side `MCC` `PE`

   ✓7ᵗʰ **S45.099** Other specified injury of axillary artery, unspecified side `MCC` `UNS` `PE`

✓5ᵗʰ **S45.1** Injury of **brachial artery**

  ✓6ᵗʰ **S45.10** Unspecified injury of brachial artery

   ✓7ᵗʰ **S45.101** Unspecified injury of brachial artery, **right** side `CC` `PE`

   ✓7ᵗʰ **S45.102** Unspecified injury of brachial artery, **left** side `CC` `PE`

   ✓7ᵗʰ **S45.109** Unspecified injury of brachial artery, unspecified side `CC` `UNS` `PE`

  ✓6ᵗʰ **S45.11** **Laceration** of brachial artery

   ✓7ᵗʰ **S45.111** Laceration of brachial artery, **right** side `CC` `PE`

   ✓7ᵗʰ **S45.112** Laceration of brachial artery, **left** side `CC` `PE`

   ✓7ᵗʰ **S45.119** Laceration of brachial artery, unspecified side `CC` `UNS` `PE`

  ✓6ᵗʰ **S45.19** Other specified injury of brachial artery

   ✓7ᵗʰ **S45.191** Other specified injury of brachial artery, **right** side `CC` `PE`

   ✓7ᵗʰ **S45.192** Other specified injury of brachial artery, **left** side `CC` `PE`

   ✓7ᵗʰ **S45.199** Other specified injury of brachial artery, unspecified side `CC` `UNS` `PE`

✓5ᵗʰ **S45.2** Injury of **axillary or brachial vein**

  ✓6ᵗʰ **S45.20** Unspecified injury of axillary or brachial vein

   ✓7ᵗʰ **S45.201** Unspecified injury of axillary or brachial vein, **right** side `CC` `PE`

   ✓7ᵗʰ **S45.202** Unspecified injury of axillary or brachial vein, **left** side `CC` `PE`

   ✓7ᵗʰ **S45.209** Unspecified injury of axillary or brachial vein, unspecified side `CC` `UNS` `PE`

  ✓6ᵗʰ **S45.21** **Laceration** of axillary or brachial vein

   ✓7ᵗʰ **S45.211** Laceration of axillary or brachial vein, **right** side `CC` `PE`

   ✓7ᵗʰ **S45.212** Laceration of axillary or brachial vein, **left** side `CC` `PE`

   ✓7ᵗʰ **S45.219** Laceration of axillary or brachial vein, unspecified side `CC` `UNS` `PE`

  ✓6ᵗʰ **S45.29** Other specified injury of axillary or brachial vein

   ✓7ᵗʰ **S45.291** Other specified injury of axillary or brachial vein, **right** side `CC` `PE`

   ✓7ᵗʰ **S45.292** Other specified injury of axillary or brachial vein, **left** side `CC` `PE`

   ✓7ᵗʰ **S45.299** Other specified injury of axillary or brachial vein, unspecified side `CC` `UNS` `PE`

✓5ᵗʰ **S45.3** Injury of **superficial vein** at shoulder and upper arm level

  ✓6ᵗʰ **S45.30** Unspecified injury of superficial vein at shoulder and upper arm level

   ✓7ᵗʰ **S45.301** Unspecified injury of superficial vein at shoulder and upper arm level, **right** arm `CC` `PE`

   ✓7ᵗʰ **S45.302** Unspecified injury of superficial vein at shoulder and upper arm level, **left** arm `CC` `PE`

   ✓7ᵗʰ **S45.309** Unspecified injury of superficial vein at shoulder and upper arm level, unspecified arm `CC` `UNS` `PE`

  ✓6ᵗʰ **S45.31** **Laceration** of superficial vein at shoulder and upper arm level

   ✓7ᵗʰ **S45.311** Laceration of superficial vein at shoulder and upper arm level, **right** arm `CC` `PE`

   ✓7ᵗʰ **S45.312** Laceration of superficial vein at shoulder and upper arm level, **left** arm `CC` `PE`

   ✓7ᵗʰ **S45.319** Laceration of superficial vein at shoulder and upper arm level, unspecified arm `CC` `UNS` `PE`

  ✓6ᵗʰ **S45.39** Other specified injury of superficial vein at shoulder and upper arm level

   ✓7ᵗʰ **S45.391** Other specified injury of superficial vein at shoulder and upper arm level, **right** arm `CC` `PE`

   ✓7ᵗʰ **S45.392** Other specified injury of superficial vein at shoulder and upper arm level, **left** arm `CC` `PE`

   ✓7ᵗʰ **S45.399** Other specified injury of superficial vein at shoulder and upper arm level, unspecified arm `CC` `UNS` `PE`

✓5ᵗʰ **S45.8** Injury of other specified blood vessels at shoulder and upper arm level

  ✓6ᵗʰ **S45.80** Unspecified injury of other specified blood vessels at shoulder and upper arm level

   ✓7ᵗʰ **S45.801** Unspecified injury of other specified blood vessels at shoulder and upper arm level, **right** arm `CC` `PE`

   ✓7ᵗʰ **S45.802** Unspecified injury of other specified blood vessels at shoulder and upper arm level, **left** arm `CC` `PE`

   ✓7ᵗʰ **S45.809** Unspecified injury of other specified blood vessels at shoulder and upper arm level, unspecified arm `CC` `UNS` `PE`

  ✓6ᵗʰ **S45.81** **Laceration** of other specified blood vessels at shoulder and upper arm level

   ✓7ᵗʰ **S45.811** Laceration of other specified blood vessels at shoulder and upper arm level, **right** arm `CC` `PE`

   ✓7ᵗʰ **S45.812** Laceration of other specified blood vessels at shoulder and upper arm level, **left** arm `CC` `PE`

   ✓7ᵗʰ **S45.819** Laceration of other specified blood vessels at shoulder and upper arm level, unspecified arm `CC` `UNS` `PE`

  ✓6ᵗʰ **S45.89** Other specified injury of other specified blood vessels at shoulder and upper arm level

   ✓7ᵗʰ **S45.891** Other specified injury of other specified blood vessels at shoulder and upper arm level, **right** arm `CC` `PE`

   ✓7ᵗʰ **S45.892** Other specified injury of other specified blood vessels at shoulder and upper arm level, **left** arm `CC` `PE`

   ✓7ᵗʰ **S45.899** Other specified injury of other specified blood vessels at shoulder and upper arm level, unspecified arm `CC` `UNS` `PE`

✓5ᵗʰ **S45.9** Injury of unspecified blood vessel at shoulder and upper arm level

  ✓6ᵗʰ **S45.90** Unspecified injury of unspecified blood vessel at shoulder and upper arm level

   ✓7ᵗʰ **S45.901** Unspecified injury of unspecified blood vessel at shoulder and upper arm level, **right** arm `CC` `PE`

   ✓7ᵗʰ **S45.902** Unspecified injury of unspecified blood vessel at shoulder and upper arm level, **left** arm `CC` `PE`

   ✓7ᵗʰ **S45.909** Unspecified injury of unspecified blood vessel at shoulder and upper arm level, unspecified arm `CC` `UNS` `PE`

  ✓6ᵗʰ **S45.91** **Laceration** of unspecified blood vessel at shoulder and upper arm level

   ✓7ᵗʰ **S45.911** Laceration of unspecified blood vessel at shoulder and upper arm level, **right** arm `CC` `PE`

   ✓7ᵗʰ **S45.912** Laceration of unspecified blood vessel at shoulder and upper arm level, **left** arm `CC` `PE`

   ✓7ᵗʰ **S45.919** Laceration of unspecified blood vessel at shoulder and upper arm level, unspecified arm `CC` `UNS` `PE`

  ✓6ᵗʰ **S45.99** Other specified injury of unspecified blood vessel at shoulder and upper arm level

   ✓7ᵗʰ **S45.991** Other specified injury of unspecified blood vessel at shoulder and upper arm level, **right** arm `CC` `PE`

   ✓7ᵗʰ **S45.992** Other specified injury of unspecified blood vessel at shoulder and upper arm level, **left** arm `CC` `PE`

   ✓7ᵗʰ **S45.999** Other specified injury of unspecified blood vessel at shoulder and upper arm level, unspecified arm `CC` `UNS` `PE`

✔ Additional Character Required   ✔x7ᵗʰ Placeholder   **Questionable PDx**   Manifestation   Unspecified   `UPD` Unacceptable PDx   `H1`-`H14` HAC   `HCC` CMS-HCC Dx   `HIV` HIV Dx

√4th S46 Injury of muscle, fascia and tendon at shoulder and upper arm level

Code also any associated open wound (S41.-)

EXCLUDES 2 *injury of muscle, fascia and tendon at elbow (S56.-)*
sprain of joints and ligaments of shoulder girdle (S43.9)

TIP: Refer to the Muscle/Tendon table at the beginning of this chapter.

The appropriate 7th character is to be added to each code from category S46.
A   initial encounter
D   subsequent encounter
S   sequela

√5th S46.0 Injury of muscle(s) and tendon(s) of the rotator cuff of shoulder

√6th S46.00 Unspecified injury of muscle(s) and tendon(s) of the rotator cuff of shoulder

√7th S46.001 Unspecified injury of muscle(s) and tendon(s) of the rotator cuff of right shoulder `PE`

√7th S46.002 Unspecified injury of muscle(s) and tendon(s) of the rotator cuff of left shoulder `PE`

√7th S46.009 Unspecified injury of muscle(s) and tendon(s) of the rotator cuff of unspecified shoulder `PE`

√6th S46.01 Strain of muscle(s) and tendon(s) of the rotator cuff of shoulder

√7th S46.011 Strain of muscle(s) and tendon(s) of the rotator cuff of right shoulder `PE`

√7th S46.012 Strain of muscle(s) and tendon(s) of the rotator cuff of left shoulder `PE`

√7th S46.019 Strain of muscle(s) and tendon(s) of the rotator cuff of unspecified shoulder `PE`

√6th S46.02 Laceration of muscle(s) and tendon(s) of the rotator cuff of shoulder

√7th S46.021 Laceration of muscle(s) and tendon(s) of the rotator cuff of right shoulder `CC` `PE`

√7th S46.022 Laceration of muscle(s) and tendon(s) of the rotator cuff of left shoulder `CC` `PE`

√7th S46.029 Laceration of muscle(s) and tendon(s) of the rotator cuff of unspecified shoulder `CC` `UNS` `PE`

√6th S46.09 Other injury of muscle(s) and tendon(s) of the rotator cuff of shoulder

√7th S46.091 Other injury of muscle(s) and tendon(s) of the rotator cuff of right shoulder `PE`

√7th S46.092 Other injury of muscle(s) and tendon(s) of the rotator cuff of left shoulder `PE`

√7th S46.099 Other injury of muscle(s) and tendon(s) of the rotator cuff of unspecified shoulder `PE`

√5th S46.1 Injury of muscle, fascia and tendon of long head of biceps

√6th S46.10 Unspecified injury of muscle, fascia and tendon of long head of biceps

√7th S46.101 Unspecified injury of muscle, fascia and tendon of long head of biceps, right arm `PE`

√7th S46.102 Unspecified injury of muscle, fascia and tendon of long head of biceps, left arm `PE`

√7th S46.109 Unspecified injury of muscle, fascia and tendon of long head of biceps, unspecified arm `PE`

√6th S46.11 Strain of muscle, fascia and tendon of long head of biceps

AHA: 2020,1Q,38; 2019,2Q,27

√7th S46.111 Strain of muscle, fascia and tendon of long head of biceps, right arm `PE`

√7th S46.112 Strain of muscle, fascia and tendon of long head of biceps, left arm `PE`

√7th S46.119 Strain of muscle, fascia and tendon of long head of biceps, unspecified arm `PE`

√6th S46.12 Laceration of muscle, fascia and tendon of long head of biceps

√7th S46.121 Laceration of muscle, fascia and tendon of long head of biceps, right arm `CC` `PE`

√7th S46.122 Laceration of muscle, fascia and tendon of long head of biceps, left arm `CC` `PE`

√7th S46.129 Laceration of muscle, fascia and tendon of long head of biceps, unspecified arm `CC` `UNS` `PE`

√6th S46.19 Other injury of muscle, fascia and tendon of long head of biceps

√7th S46.191 Other injury of muscle, fascia and tendon of long head of biceps, right arm `PE`

√7th S46.192 Other injury of muscle, fascia and tendon of long head of biceps, left arm `PE`

√7th S46.199 Other injury of muscle, fascia and tendon of long head of biceps, unspecified arm `PE`

√5th S46.2 Injury of muscle, fascia and tendon of other parts of biceps

√6th S46.20 Unspecified injury of muscle, fascia and tendon of other parts of biceps

√7th S46.201 Unspecified injury of muscle, fascia and tendon of other parts of biceps, right arm `PE`

√7th S46.202 Unspecified injury of muscle, fascia and tendon of other parts of biceps, left arm `PE`

√7th S46.209 Unspecified injury of muscle, fascia and tendon of other parts of biceps, unspecified arm `PE`

√6th S46.21 Strain of muscle, fascia and tendon of other parts of biceps

√7th S46.211 Strain of muscle, fascia and tendon of other parts of biceps, right arm `PE`

√7th S46.212 Strain of muscle, fascia and tendon of other parts of biceps, left arm `PE`

√7th S46.219 Strain of muscle, fascia and tendon of other parts of biceps, unspecified arm `PE`

√6th S46.22 Laceration of muscle, fascia and tendon of other parts of biceps

√7th S46.221 Laceration of muscle, fascia and tendon of other parts of biceps, right arm `CC` `PE`

√7th S46.222 Laceration of muscle, fascia and tendon of other parts of biceps, left arm `CC` `PE`

√7th S46.229 Laceration of muscle, fascia and tendon of other parts of biceps, unspecified arm `CC` `UNS` `PE`

√6th S46.29 Other injury of muscle, fascia and tendon of other parts of biceps

√7th S46.291 Other injury of muscle, fascia and tendon of other parts of biceps, right arm `PE`

√7th S46.292 Other injury of muscle, fascia and tendon of other parts of biceps, left arm `PE`

√7th S46.299 Other injury of muscle, fascia and tendon of other parts of biceps, unspecified arm `PE`

√5th S46.3 Injury of muscle, fascia and tendon of triceps

√6th S46.30 Unspecified injury of muscle, fascia and tendon of triceps

√7th S46.301 Unspecified injury of muscle, fascia and tendon of triceps, right arm `PE`

√7th S46.302 Unspecified injury of muscle, fascia and tendon of triceps, left arm `PE`

√7th S46.309 Unspecified injury of muscle, fascia and tendon of triceps, unspecified arm `PE`

√6th S46.31 Strain of muscle, fascia and tendon of triceps

√7th S46.311 Strain of muscle, fascia and tendon of triceps, right arm `PE`

√7th S46.312 Strain of muscle, fascia and tendon of triceps, left arm `PE`

√7th S46.319 Strain of muscle, fascia and tendon of triceps, unspecified arm `PE`

√6th S46.32 Laceration of muscle, fascia and tendon of triceps

√7th S46.321 Laceration of muscle, fascia and tendon of triceps, right arm `CC` `PE`

√7th S46.322 Laceration of muscle, fascia and tendon of triceps, left arm `CC` `PE`

√7th S46.329 Laceration of muscle, fascia and tendon of triceps, unspecified arm `CC` `UNS` `PE`

√6th S46.39 Other injury of muscle, fascia and tendon of triceps

√7th S46.391 Other injury of muscle, fascia and tendon of triceps, right arm `PE`

√7th S46.392 Other injury of muscle, fascia and tendon of triceps, left arm `PE`

√7th S46.399 Other injury of muscle, fascia and tendon of triceps, unspecified arm `PE`

`N` Newborn: 0   `P` Pediatric: 0-17   `M` Maternity: 9-64   `A` Adult: 15-124   `UNS` Unspecified Site   `MCC` Major Complication/Comorbidity   `CC` Complication/Comorbidity   `PE` POA Exempt

1036

ICD-10-CM 2025

✓5ᵗʰ **S46.8 Injury of other muscles, fascia and tendons at shoulder and upper arm level**

  ✓6ᵗʰ **S46.80 Unspecified injury of other muscles, fascia and tendons at shoulder and upper arm level**

    ✓7ᵗʰ **S46.801** Unspecified injury of other muscles, fascia and tendons at shoulder and upper arm level, **right** arm   PE

    ✓7ᵗʰ **S46.802** Unspecified injury of other muscles, fascia and tendons at shoulder and upper arm level, **left** arm   PE

    ✓7ᵗʰ **S46.809** Unspecified injury of other muscles, fascia and tendons at shoulder and upper arm level, unspecified arm   PE

  ✓6ᵗʰ **S46.81 Strain of other muscles, fascia and tendons at shoulder and upper arm level**

    ✓7ᵗʰ **S46.811** Strain of other muscles, fascia and tendons at shoulder and upper arm level, **right** arm

    ✓7ᵗʰ **S46.812** Strain of other muscles, fascia and tendons at shoulder and upper arm level, **left** arm

    ✓7ᵗʰ **S46.819** Strain of other muscles, fascia and tendons at shoulder and upper arm level, unspecified arm   PE

  ✓6ᵗʰ **S46.82 Laceration of other muscles, fascia and tendons at shoulder and upper arm level**

    ✓7ᵗʰ **S46.821** Laceration of other muscles, fascia and tendons at shoulder and upper arm level, **right** arm   CC PE

    ✓7ᵗʰ **S46.822** Laceration of other muscles, fascia and tendons at shoulder and upper arm level, **left** arm   CC PE

    ✓7ᵗʰ **S46.829** Laceration of other muscles, fascia and tendons at shoulder and upper arm level, unspecified arm   CC UNS PE

  ✓6ᵗʰ **S46.89 Other injury of other muscles, fascia and tendons at shoulder and upper arm level**

    ✓7ᵗʰ **S46.891** Other injury of other muscles, fascia and tendons at shoulder and upper arm level, **right** arm   PE

    ✓7ᵗʰ **S46.892** Other injury of other muscles, fascia and tendons at shoulder and upper arm level, **left** arm   PE

    ✓7ᵗʰ **S46.899** Other injury of other muscles, fascia and tendons at shoulder and upper arm level, unspecified arm   PE

✓5ᵗʰ **S46.9 Injury of unspecified muscle, fascia and tendon at shoulder and upper arm level**

  ✓6ᵗʰ **S46.90 Unspecified injury of unspecified muscle, fascia and tendon at shoulder and upper arm level**

    ✓7ᵗʰ **S46.901** Unspecified injury of unspecified muscle, fascia and tendon at shoulder and upper arm level, **right** arm   PE

    ✓7ᵗʰ **S46.902** Unspecified injury of unspecified muscle, fascia and tendon at shoulder and upper arm level, **left** arm   PE

    ✓7ᵗʰ **S46.909** Unspecified injury of unspecified muscle, fascia and tendon at shoulder and upper arm level, unspecified arm   PE

  ✓6ᵗʰ **S46.91 Strain of unspecified muscle, fascia and tendon at shoulder and upper arm level**

    ✓7ᵗʰ **S46.911** Strain of unspecified muscle, fascia and tendon at shoulder and upper arm level, **right** arm   PE

    ✓7ᵗʰ **S46.912** Strain of unspecified muscle, fascia and tendon at shoulder and upper arm level, **left** arm   PE

    ✓7ᵗʰ **S46.919** Strain of unspecified muscle, fascia and tendon at shoulder and upper arm level, unspecified arm   PE

  ✓6ᵗʰ **S46.92 Laceration of unspecified muscle, fascia and tendon at shoulder and upper arm level**

    ✓7ᵗʰ **S46.921** Laceration of unspecified muscle, fascia and tendon at shoulder and upper arm level, **right** arm   CC PE

    ✓7ᵗʰ **S46.922** Laceration of unspecified muscle, fascia and tendon at shoulder and upper arm level, **left** arm   CC PE

    ✓7ᵗʰ **S46.929** Laceration of unspecified muscle, fascia and tendon at shoulder and upper arm level, unspecified arm   CC UNS PE

  ✓6ᵗʰ **S46.99 Other injury of unspecified muscle, fascia and tendon at shoulder and upper arm level**

    ✓7ᵗʰ **S46.991** Other injury of unspecified muscle, fascia and tendon at shoulder and upper arm level, **right** arm   PE

    ✓7ᵗʰ **S46.992** Other injury of unspecified muscle, fascia and tendon at shoulder and upper arm level, **left** arm   PE

    ✓7ᵗʰ **S46.999** Other injury of unspecified muscle, fascia and tendon at shoulder and upper arm level, unspecified arm   PE

✓4ᵗʰ **S47 Crushing injury of shoulder and upper arm**

Use additional code for all associated injuries

EXCLUDES 2   *crushing injury of elbow (S57.0-)*

> The appropriate 7th character is to be added to each code from category S47.
> A   initial encounter
> D   subsequent encounter
> S   sequela

✓x7ᵗʰ **S47.1 Crushing injury of right shoulder and upper arm**   PE

✓x7ᵗʰ **S47.2 Crushing injury of left shoulder and upper arm**   PE

✓x7ᵗʰ **S47.9 Crushing injury of shoulder and upper arm, unspecified arm**   PE

✓4ᵗʰ **S48 Traumatic amputation of shoulder and upper arm**

An amputation not identified as partial or complete should be coded to complete

EXCLUDES 1   *traumatic amputation at elbow level (S58.0)*

> The appropriate 7th character is to be added to each code from category S48.
> A   initial encounter
> D   subsequent encounter
> S   sequela

✓5ᵗʰ **S48.0 Traumatic amputation at shoulder joint**

  ✓6ᵗʰ **S48.01 Complete traumatic amputation at shoulder joint**

    ✓7ᵗʰ **S48.011** Complete traumatic amputation at **right** shoulder joint   CC HCC PE

    ✓7ᵗʰ **S48.012** Complete traumatic amputation at **left** shoulder joint   CC HCC PE

    ✓7ᵗʰ **S48.019** Complete traumatic amputation at unspecified shoulder joint   CC UNS HCC PE

  ✓6ᵗʰ **S48.02 Partial traumatic amputation at shoulder joint**

    ✓7ᵗʰ **S48.021** Partial traumatic amputation at **right** shoulder joint   CC HCC PE

    ✓7ᵗʰ **S48.022** Partial traumatic amputation at **left** shoulder joint   CC HCC PE

    ✓7ᵗʰ **S48.029** Partial traumatic amputation at unspecified shoulder joint   CC UNS HCC PE

✓5ᵗʰ **S48.1 Traumatic amputation at level between shoulder and elbow**

  ✓6ᵗʰ **S48.11 Complete traumatic amputation at level between shoulder and elbow**

    ✓7ᵗʰ **S48.111** Complete traumatic amputation at level between **right** shoulder and elbow   CC HCC PE

    ✓7ᵗʰ **S48.112** Complete traumatic amputation at level between **left** shoulder and elbow   CC HCC PE

    ✓7ᵗʰ **S48.119** Complete traumatic amputation at level between unspecified shoulder and elbow   CC UNS HCC PE

  ✓6ᵗʰ **S48.12 Partial traumatic amputation at level between shoulder and elbow**

    ✓7ᵗʰ **S48.121** Partial traumatic amputation at level between **right** shoulder and elbow   CC HCC PE

    ✓7ᵗʰ **S48.122** Partial traumatic amputation at level between **left** shoulder and elbow   CC HCC PE

    ✓7ᵗʰ **S48.129** Partial traumatic amputation at level between unspecified shoulder and elbow   CC UNS HCC PE

✓ Additional Character Required   ✓x7ᵗʰ Placeholder   Questionable PDx   Manifestation   Unspecified   UPD Unacceptable PDx   H1-H14 HAC   HCC CMS-HCC Dx   HIV HIV Dx

√5ᵗʰ **S48.9 Traumatic amputation of shoulder and upper arm, level unspecified**

√6ᵗʰ **S48.91 Complete** traumatic amputation of shoulder and upper arm, level unspecified

√7ᵗʰ **S48.911** Complete traumatic amputation of **right** shoulder and upper arm, level unspecified `CC` `HCC` `PE`

√7ᵗʰ **S48.912** Complete traumatic amputation of **left** shoulder and upper arm, level unspecified `CC` `HCC` `PE`

√7ᵗʰ **S48.919** Complete traumatic amputation of unspecified shoulder and upper arm, level unspecified `CC` `UNS` `HCC` `PE`

√6ᵗʰ **S48.92 Partial** traumatic amputation of shoulder and upper arm, level unspecified

√7ᵗʰ **S48.921** Partial traumatic amputation of **right** shoulder and upper arm, level unspecified `CC` `HCC` `PE`

√7ᵗʰ **S48.922** Partial traumatic amputation of **left** shoulder and upper arm, level unspecified `CC` `HCC` `PE`

√7ᵗʰ **S48.929** Partial traumatic amputation of unspecified shoulder and upper arm, level unspecified `CC` `UNS` `HCC` `PE`

√4ᵗʰ **S49 Other and unspecified injuries of shoulder and upper arm**

AHA: 2018,2Q,12; 2018,1Q,3

> The appropriate 7th character is to be added to each code from subcategories S49.0 and S49.1.
> A   initial encounter for closed fracture
> D   subsequent encounter for fracture with routine healing
> G   subsequent encounter for fracture with delayed healing
> K   subsequent encounter for fracture with nonunion
> P   subsequent encounter for fracture with malunion
> S   sequela

√5ᵗʰ **S49.0 Physeal fracture of upper end of humerus**

AHA: 2019,4Q,56

√6ᵗʰ **S49.00** Unspecified physeal fracture of upper end of humerus

√7ᵗʰ **S49.001** Unspecified physeal fracture of upper end of humerus, **right** arm `CC` `H5` `PE`

√7ᵗʰ **S49.002** Unspecified physeal fracture of upper end of humerus, **left** arm `CC` `H5` `PE`

√7ᵗʰ **S49.009** Unspecified physeal fracture of upper end of humerus, unspecified arm `CC` `H5` `UNS` `PE`

√6ᵗʰ **S49.01 Salter-Harris Type I** physeal fracture of upper end of humerus

√7ᵗʰ **S49.011** Salter-Harris Type I physeal fracture of upper end of humerus, **right** arm `CC` `H5` `PE`

√7ᵗʰ **S49.012** Salter-Harris Type I physeal fracture of upper end of humerus, **left** arm `CC` `H5` `PE`

√7ᵗʰ **S49.019** Salter-Harris Type I physeal fracture of upper end of humerus, unspecified arm `CC` `H5` `UNS` `PE`

√6ᵗʰ **S49.02 Salter-Harris Type II** physeal fracture of upper end of humerus

√7ᵗʰ **S49.021** Salter-Harris Type II physeal fracture of upper end of humerus, **right** arm `CC` `H5` `PE`

√7ᵗʰ **S49.022** Salter-Harris Type II physeal fracture of upper end of humerus, **left** arm `CC` `H5` `PE`

√7ᵗʰ **S49.029** Salter-Harris Type II physeal fracture of upper end of humerus, unspecified arm `CC` `H5` `UNS` `PE`

√6ᵗʰ **S49.03 Salter-Harris Type III** physeal fracture of upper end of humerus

√7ᵗʰ **S49.031** Salter-Harris Type III physeal fracture of upper end of humerus, **right** arm `CC` `H5` `PE`

√7ᵗʰ **S49.032** Salter-Harris Type III physeal fracture of upper end of humerus, **left** arm `CC` `H5` `PE`

√7ᵗʰ **S49.039** Salter-Harris Type III physeal fracture of upper end of humerus, unspecified arm `CC` `H5` `UNS` `PE`

√6ᵗʰ **S49.04 Salter-Harris Type IV** physeal fracture of upper end of humerus

√7ᵗʰ **S49.041** Salter-Harris Type IV physeal fracture of upper end of humerus, **right** arm `CC` `H5` `PE`

√7ᵗʰ **S49.042** Salter-Harris Type IV physeal fracture of upper end of humerus, **left** arm `CC` `H5` `PE`

√7ᵗʰ **S49.049** Salter-Harris Type IV physeal fracture of upper end of humerus, unspecified arm `CC` `H5` `UNS` `PE`

√6ᵗʰ **S49.09** Other physeal fracture of upper end of humerus

√7ᵗʰ **S49.091** Other physeal fracture of upper end of humerus, **right** arm `CC` `H5` `PE`

√7ᵗʰ **S49.092** Other physeal fracture of upper end of humerus, **left** arm `CC` `H5` `PE`

√7ᵗʰ **S49.099** Other physeal fracture of upper end of humerus, unspecified arm `CC` `H5` `UNS` `PE`

√5ᵗʰ **S49.1 Physeal fracture of lower end of humerus**

AHA: 2019,4Q,56

√6ᵗʰ **S49.10** Unspecified physeal fracture of lower end of humerus

√7ᵗʰ **S49.101** Unspecified physeal fracture of lower end of humerus, **right** arm `CC` `H5` `PE`

√7ᵗʰ **S49.102** Unspecified physeal fracture of lower end of humerus, **left** arm `CC` `H5` `PE`

√7ᵗʰ **S49.109** Unspecified physeal fracture of lower end of humerus, unspecified arm `CC` `H5` `UNS` `PE`

√6ᵗʰ **S49.11 Salter-Harris Type I** physeal fracture of lower end of humerus

√7ᵗʰ **S49.111** Salter-Harris Type I physeal fracture of lower end of humerus, **right** arm `CC` `H5` `PE`

√7ᵗʰ **S49.112** Salter-Harris Type I physeal fracture of lower end of humerus, **left** arm `CC` `H5` `PE`

√7ᵗʰ **S49.119** Salter-Harris Type I physeal fracture of lower end of humerus, unspecified arm `CC` `H5` `UNS` `PE`

√6ᵗʰ **S49.12 Salter-Harris Type II** physeal fracture of lower end of humerus

√7ᵗʰ **S49.121** Salter-Harris Type II physeal fracture of lower end of humerus, **right** arm `CC` `H5` `PE`

√7ᵗʰ **S49.122** Salter-Harris Type II physeal fracture of lower end of humerus, **left** arm `CC` `H5` `PE`

√7ᵗʰ **S49.129** Salter-Harris Type II physeal fracture of lower end of humerus, unspecified arm `CC` `H5` `UNS` `PE`

√6ᵗʰ **S49.13 Salter-Harris Type III** physeal fracture of lower end of humerus

√7ᵗʰ **S49.131** Salter-Harris Type III physeal fracture of lower end of humerus, **right** arm `CC` `H5` `PE`

√7ᵗʰ **S49.132** Salter-Harris Type III physeal fracture of lower end of humerus, **left** arm `CC` `H5` `PE`

√7ᵗʰ **S49.139** Salter-Harris Type III physeal fracture of lower end of humerus, unspecified arm `CC` `H5` `UNS` `PE`

√6ᵗʰ **S49.14 Salter-Harris Type IV** physeal fracture of lower end of humerus

√7ᵗʰ **S49.141** Salter-Harris Type IV physeal fracture of lower end of humerus, **right** arm `CC` `H5` `PE`

√7ᵗʰ **S49.142** Salter-Harris Type IV physeal fracture of lower end of humerus, **left** arm `CC` `H5` `PE`

√7ᵗʰ **S49.149** Salter-Harris Type IV physeal fracture of lower end of humerus, unspecified arm `CC` `H5` `UNS` `PE`

√6ᵗʰ **S49.19** Other physeal fracture of lower end of humerus

√7ᵗʰ **S49.191** Other physeal fracture of lower end of humerus, **right** arm `CC` `H5` `PE`

√7ᵗʰ **S49.192** Other physeal fracture of lower end of humerus, **left** arm `CC` `H5` `PE`

`N` Newborn: 0   `P` Pediatric: 0-17   `M` Maternity: 9-64   `A` Adult: 15-124   `UNS` Unspecified Site   `MCC` Major Complication/Comorbidity   `CC` Complication/Comorbidity   `PE` POA Exempt

1038

ICD-10-CM 2025

√7ᵗʰ **S49.199** Other physeal fracture of lower end of humerus, unspecified arm   CC HE UNS PE

√5ᵗʰ **S49.8** Other specified injuries of shoulder and upper arm

> The appropriate 7th character is to be added to each code in subcategory S49.8.
> A   initial encounter
> D   subsequent encounter
> S   sequela

√x7ᵗʰ **S49.80** Other specified injuries of shoulder and upper arm, unspecified arm   PE

√x7ᵗʰ **S49.81** Other specified injuries of right shoulder and upper arm   PE

√x7ᵗʰ **S49.82** Other specified injuries of left shoulder and upper arm   PE

√5ᵗʰ **S49.9** Unspecified injury of shoulder and upper arm

> The appropriate 7th character is to be added to each code in subcategory S49.9.
> A   initial encounter
> D   subsequent encounter
> S   sequela

√x7ᵗʰ **S49.90** Unspecified injury of shoulder and upper arm, unspecified arm   PE

√x7ᵗʰ **S49.91** Unspecified injury of right shoulder and upper arm   PE

√x7ᵗʰ **S49.92** Unspecified injury of left shoulder and upper arm   PE

Injuries to the elbow and forearm (S50-S59)

EXCLUDES 2   burns and corrosions (T20-T32)
frostbite (T33-T34)
injuries of wrist and hand (S60-S69)
insect bite or sting, venomous (T63.4)

√4ᵗʰ **S50** Superficial injury of elbow and forearm

EXCLUDES 2   superficial injury of wrist and hand (S60.-)

> The appropriate 7th character is to be added to each code from category S50.
> A   initial encounter
> D   subsequent encounter
> S   sequela

√5ᵗʰ **S50.0** Contusion of elbow

√x7ᵗʰ **S50.00** Contusion of unspecified elbow   PE

√x7ᵗʰ **S50.01** Contusion of right elbow   PE

√x7ᵗʰ **S50.02** Contusion of left elbow   PE

√5ᵗʰ **S50.1** Contusion of forearm

√x7ᵗʰ **S50.10** Contusion of unspecified forearm   PE

√x7ᵗʰ **S50.11** Contusion of right forearm   PE

√x7ᵗʰ **S50.12** Contusion of left forearm   PE

√5ᵗʰ **S50.3** Other superficial injuries of elbow

√6ᵗʰ **S50.31** Abrasion of elbow

√7ᵗʰ **S50.311** Abrasion of right elbow   PE

√7ᵗʰ **S50.312** Abrasion of left elbow   PE

√7ᵗʰ **S50.319** Abrasion of unspecified elbow   PE

√6ᵗʰ **S50.32** Blister (nonthermal) of elbow

√7ᵗʰ **S50.321** Blister (nonthermal) of right elbow   PE

√7ᵗʰ **S50.322** Blister (nonthermal) of left elbow   PE

√7ᵗʰ **S50.329** Blister (nonthermal) of unspecified elbow   PE

√6ᵗʰ **S50.34** External constriction of elbow

√7ᵗʰ **S50.341** External constriction of right elbow   PE

√7ᵗʰ **S50.342** External constriction of left elbow   PE

√7ᵗʰ **S50.349** External constriction of unspecified elbow   PE

√6ᵗʰ **S50.35** Superficial foreign body of elbow

> Splinter in the elbow

√7ᵗʰ **S50.351** Superficial foreign body of right elbow   PE

√7ᵗʰ **S50.352** Superficial foreign body of left elbow   PE

√7ᵗʰ **S50.359** Superficial foreign body of unspecified elbow   PE

√6ᵗʰ **S50.36** Insect bite (nonvenomous) of elbow

√7ᵗʰ **S50.361** Insect bite (nonvenomous) of right elbow   PE

√7ᵗʰ **S50.362** Insect bite (nonvenomous) of left elbow   PE

√7ᵗʰ **S50.369** Insect bite (nonvenomous) of unspecified elbow   PE

√6ᵗʰ **S50.37** Other superficial bite of elbow

EXCLUDES 1   open bite of elbow (S51.05)

√7ᵗʰ **S50.371** Other superficial bite of right elbow   PE

√7ᵗʰ **S50.372** Other superficial bite of left elbow   PE

√7ᵗʰ **S50.379** Other superficial bite of unspecified elbow   PE

√5ᵗʰ **S50.8** Other superficial injuries of forearm

√6ᵗʰ **S50.81** Abrasion of forearm

√7ᵗʰ **S50.811** Abrasion of right forearm   PE

√7ᵗʰ **S50.812** Abrasion of left forearm   PE

√7ᵗʰ **S50.819** Abrasion of unspecified forearm   PE

√6ᵗʰ **S50.82** Blister (nonthermal) of forearm

√7ᵗʰ **S50.821** Blister (nonthermal) of right forearm   PE

√7ᵗʰ **S50.822** Blister (nonthermal) of left forearm   PE

√7ᵗʰ **S50.829** Blister (nonthermal) of unspecified forearm   PE

√6ᵗʰ **S50.84** External constriction of forearm

√7ᵗʰ **S50.841** External constriction of right forearm   PE

√7ᵗʰ **S50.842** External constriction of left forearm   PE

√7ᵗʰ **S50.849** External constriction of unspecified forearm   PE

√6ᵗʰ **S50.85** Superficial foreign body of forearm

> Splinter in the forearm

√7ᵗʰ **S50.851** Superficial foreign body of right forearm   PE

√7ᵗʰ **S50.852** Superficial foreign body of left forearm   PE

√7ᵗʰ **S50.859** Superficial foreign body of unspecified forearm   PE

√6ᵗʰ **S50.86** Insect bite (nonvenomous) of forearm

√7ᵗʰ **S50.861** Insect bite (nonvenomous) of right forearm   PE

√7ᵗʰ **S50.862** Insect bite (nonvenomous) of left forearm   PE

√7ᵗʰ **S50.869** Insect bite (nonvenomous) of unspecified forearm   PE

√6ᵗʰ **S50.87** Other superficial bite of forearm

EXCLUDES 1   open bite of forearm (S51.85)

√7ᵗʰ **S50.871** Other superficial bite of right forearm   PE

√7ᵗʰ **S50.872** Other superficial bite of left forearm   PE

√7ᵗʰ **S50.879** Other superficial bite of unspecified forearm   PE

√5ᵗʰ **S50.9** Unspecified superficial injury of elbow and forearm

√6ᵗʰ **S50.90** Unspecified superficial injury of elbow

√7ᵗʰ **S50.901** Unspecified superficial injury of right elbow   PE

√7ᵗʰ **S50.902** Unspecified superficial injury of left elbow   PE

√7ᵗʰ **S50.909** Unspecified superficial injury of unspecified elbow   PE

√6ᵗʰ **S50.91** Unspecified superficial injury of forearm

√7ᵗʰ **S50.911** Unspecified superficial injury of right forearm   PE

√7ᵗʰ **S50.912** Unspecified superficial injury of left forearm   PE

√7ᵗʰ **S50.919** Unspecified superficial injury of unspecified forearm   PE

✔ Additional Character Required   √x7ᵗʰ Placeholder   Questionable PDx   Manifestation   Unspecified   UPD Unacceptable PDx   H1-H14 HAC   HCC CMS-HCC Dx   HIV HIV Dx

ICD-10-CM 2025   **1039**

√4th S51 Open wound of elbow and forearm

Code also any associated wound infection

> EXCLUDES 1   open fracture of elbow and forearm (S52.- with open fracture 7th character)
>
> traumatic amputation of elbow and forearm (S58.-)

> EXCLUDES 2   open wound of wrist and hand (S61.-)

The appropriate 7th character is to be added to each code from category S51.
A   initial encounter
D   subsequent encounter
S   sequela

√5th S51.0 Open wound of elbow

    √6th S51.00 Unspecified open wound of elbow

       √7th S51.001 Unspecified open wound of right elbow PE
          AHA: 2012,4Q,108

       √7th S51.002 Unspecified open wound of left elbow PE

       √7th S51.009 Unspecified open wound of unspecified elbow PE
          Open wound of elbow NOS

    √6th S51.01 Laceration without foreign body of elbow

       √7th S51.011 Laceration without foreign body of right elbow PE

       √7th S51.012 Laceration without foreign body of left elbow PE

       √7th S51.019 Laceration without foreign body of unspecified elbow PE

    √6th S51.02 Laceration with foreign body of elbow

       √7th S51.021 Laceration with foreign body of right elbow PE

       √7th S51.022 Laceration with foreign body of left elbow PE

       √7th S51.029 Laceration with foreign body of unspecified elbow PE

    √6th S51.03 Puncture wound without foreign body of elbow

       √7th S51.031 Puncture wound without foreign body of right elbow PE

       √7th S51.032 Puncture wound without foreign body of left elbow PE

       √7th S51.039 Puncture wound without foreign body of unspecified elbow PE

    √6th S51.04 Puncture wound with foreign body of elbow

       √7th S51.041 Puncture wound with foreign body of right elbow PE

       √7th S51.042 Puncture wound with foreign body of left elbow PE

       √7th S51.049 Puncture wound with foreign body of unspecified elbow PE

    √6th S51.05 Open bite of elbow
       Bite of elbow NOS
> EXCLUDES 1   superficial bite of elbow (S50.36, S50.37)

       √7th S51.051 Open bite, right elbow PE

       √7th S51.052 Open bite, left elbow PE

       √7th S51.059 Open bite, unspecified elbow PE

√5th S51.8 Open wound of forearm

> EXCLUDES 2   open wound of elbow (S51.0-)

    √6th S51.80 Unspecified open wound of forearm

       AHA: 2016,3Q,24

       √7th S51.801 Unspecified open wound of right forearm PE

       √7th S51.802 Unspecified open wound of left forearm PE

       √7th S51.809 Unspecified open wound of unspecified forearm PE
          Open wound of forearm NOS

    √6th S51.81 Laceration without foreign body of forearm

       √7th S51.811 Laceration without foreign body of right forearm PE

       √7th S51.812 Laceration without foreign body of left forearm PE

       √7th S51.819 Laceration without foreign body of unspecified forearm PE

    √6th S51.82 Laceration with foreign body of forearm

       √7th S51.821 Laceration with foreign body of right forearm PE

       √7th S51.822 Laceration with foreign body of left forearm PE

       √7th S51.829 Laceration with foreign body of unspecified forearm PE

    √6th S51.83 Puncture wound without foreign body of forearm

       AHA: 2016,3Q,24

       √7th S51.831 Puncture wound without foreign body of right forearm PE

       √7th S51.832 Puncture wound without foreign body of left forearm PE

       √7th S51.839 Puncture wound without foreign body of unspecified forearm PE

    √6th S51.84 Puncture wound with foreign body of forearm

       AHA: 2016,3Q,24

       √7th S51.841 Puncture wound with foreign body of right forearm PE

       √7th S51.842 Puncture wound with foreign body of left forearm PE

       √7th S51.849 Puncture wound with foreign body of unspecified forearm PE

    √6th S51.85 Open bite of forearm
       Bite of forearm NOS
> EXCLUDES 1   superficial bite of forearm (S50.86, S50.87)

       √7th S51.851 Open bite of right forearm PE

       √7th S51.852 Open bite of left forearm PE

       √7th S51.859 Open bite of unspecified forearm PE

N Newborn: 0   P Pediatric: 0-17   M Maternity: 9-64   A Adult: 15-124   UNS Unspecified Site   MCC Major Complication/Comorbidity   CC Complication/Comorbidity   PE POA Exempt

1040   ICD-10-CM 2025

✓4ᵗʰ **S52 Fracture of forearm**

NOTE A fracture not indicated as displaced or nondisplaced should be coded to displaced.

A fracture not indicated as open or closed should be coded to closed.

The open fracture designations are based on the Gustilo open fracture classification.

EXCLUDES 1   traumatic amputation of forearm (S58.-)

EXCLUDES 2   fracture at wrist and hand level (S62.-)

periprosthetic fracture around internal prosthetic elbow joint (M97.4)

AHA: 2018,2Q,12; 2016,1Q,33; 2015,3Q,37-39

DEF: Diaphysis: Central shaft of a long bone.

DEF: Epiphysis: Proximal and distal rounded ends of a long bone, communicates with the joint.

DEF: Metaphysis: Section of a long bone located between the epiphysis and diaphysis at the proximal and distal ends.

DEF: Physis (growth plate): Narrow zone of cartilaginous tissue between the epiphysis and metaphysis at each end of a long bone. In childhood, proliferation of cells in this zone lengthens the bone. As the bone matures, this area thins, ossification eventually fusing into solid bone and growth stops. *Synonym(s): Epiphyseal plate.*

The appropriate 7th character is to be added to all codes from category S52 [unless otherwise indicated].

A   initial encounter for closed fracture

B   initial encounter for open fracture type I or II
    initial encounter for open fracture NOS

C   initial encounter for open fracture type IIIA, IIIB, or IIIC

D   subsequent encounter for closed fracture with routine healing

E   subsequent encounter for open fracture type I or II with routine healing

F   subsequent encounter for open fracture type IIIA, IIIB, or IIIC with routine healing

G   subsequent encounter for closed fracture with delayed healing

H   subsequent encounter for open fracture type I or II with delayed healing

J   subsequent encounter for open fracture type IIIA, IIIB, or IIIC with delayed healing

K   subsequent encounter for closed fracture with nonunion

M   subsequent encounter for open fracture type I or II with nonunion

N   subsequent encounter for open fracture type IIIA, IIIB, or IIIC with nonunion

P   subsequent encounter for closed fracture with malunion

Q   subsequent encounter for open fracture type I or II with malunion

R   subsequent encounter for open fracture type IIIA, IIIB, or IIIC with malunion

S   sequela

✓5ᵗʰ **S52.0 Fracture of upper end of ulna**

Fracture of proximal end of ulna

EXCLUDES 2   fracture of elbow NOS (S42.40-)

fractures of shaft of ulna (S52.2-)

✓6ᵗʰ **S52.00 Unspecified fracture of upper end of ulna**

✓7ᵗʰ **S52.001 Unspecified fracture of upper end of right ulna** `MCC` `CC` `H5` `PE`

✓7ᵗʰ **S52.002 Unspecified fracture of upper end of left ulna** `MCC` `CC` `H5` `PE`

✓7ᵗʰ **S52.009 Unspecified fracture of upper end of unspecified ulna** `MCC` `CC` `H5` `UNS` `PE`

✓6ᵗʰ **S52.01 Torus fracture of upper end of ulna**

The appropriate 7th character is to be added to all codes in subcategory S52.01

A   initial encounter for closed fracture

D   subsequent encounter for fracture with routine healing

G   subsequent encounter for fracture with delayed healing

K   subsequent encounter for fracture with nonunion

P   subsequent encounter for fracture with malunion

S   sequela

✓7ᵗʰ **S52.011 Torus fracture of upper end of right ulna** `CC` `H5` `PE`

✓7ᵗʰ **S52.012 Torus fracture of upper end of left ulna** `CC` `H5` `PE`

✓7ᵗʰ **S52.019 Torus fracture of upper end of unspecified ulna** `CC` `H5` `UNS` `PE`

✓6ᵗʰ **S52.02 Fracture of olecranon process without intraarticular extension of ulna**

✓7ᵗʰ **S52.021 Displaced fracture of olecranon process without intraarticular extension of right ulna** `MCC` `CC` `H5` `PE`

✓7ᵗʰ **S52.022 Displaced fracture of olecranon process without intraarticular extension of left ulna** `MCC` `CC` `H5` `PE`

✓7ᵗʰ **S52.023 Displaced fracture of olecranon process without intraarticular extension of unspecified ulna** `MCC` `CC` `H5` `UNS` `PE`

✓7ᵗʰ **S52.024 Nondisplaced fracture of olecranon process without intraarticular extension of right ulna** `MCC` `CC` `H5` `PE`

✓7ᵗʰ **S52.025 Nondisplaced fracture of olecranon process without intraarticular extension of left ulna** `MCC` `CC` `H5` `PE`

✓7ᵗʰ **S52.026 Nondisplaced fracture of olecranon process without intraarticular extension of unspecified ulna** `MCC` `CC` `H5` `UNS` `PE`

✓6ᵗʰ **S52.03 Fracture of olecranon process with intraarticular extension of ulna**

✓7ᵗʰ **S52.031 Displaced fracture of olecranon process with intraarticular extension of right ulna** `MCC` `CC` `H5` `PE`

✓7ᵗʰ **S52.032 Displaced fracture of olecranon process with intraarticular extension of left ulna** `MCC` `CC` `H5` `PE`

✓7ᵗʰ **S52.033 Displaced fracture of olecranon process with intraarticular extension of unspecified ulna** `MCC` `CC` `H5` `UNS` `PE`

✓7ᵗʰ **S52.034 Nondisplaced fracture of olecranon process with intraarticular extension of right ulna** `MCC` `CC` `H5` `PE`

✓7ᵗʰ **S52.035 Nondisplaced fracture of olecranon process with intraarticular extension of left ulna** `MCC` `CC` `H5` `PE`

✓7ᵗʰ **S52.036 Nondisplaced fracture of olecranon process with intraarticular extension of unspecified ulna** `MCC` `CC` `H5` `PE`

✓6ᵗʰ **S52.04 Fracture of coronoid process of ulna**

✓7ᵗʰ **S52.041 Displaced fracture of coronoid process of right ulna** `MCC` `CC` `H5` `PE`

✓7ᵗʰ **S52.042 Displaced fracture of coronoid process of left ulna** `MCC` `CC` `H5` `PE`

✓7ᵗʰ **S52.043 Displaced fracture of coronoid process of unspecified ulna** `MCC` `CC` `H5` `UNS` `PE`

✓7ᵗʰ **S52.044 Nondisplaced fracture of coronoid process of right ulna** `MCC` `CC` `H5` `PE`

✓7ᵗʰ **S52.045 Nondisplaced fracture of coronoid process of left ulna** `MCC` `CC` `H5` `PE`

✓7ᵗʰ **S52.046 Nondisplaced fracture of coronoid process of unspecified ulna** `MCC` `CC` `H5` `UNS` `PE`

✓6ᵗʰ **S52.09 Other fracture of upper end of ulna**

✓7ᵗʰ **S52.091 Other fracture of upper end of right ulna** `MCC` `CC` `H5` `PE`

✓7ᵗʰ **S52.092 Other fracture of upper end of left ulna** `MCC` `CC` `H5` `PE`

✓7ᵗʰ **S52.099 Other fracture of upper end of unspecified ulna** `MCC` `CC` `H5` `UNS` `PE`

✓5ᵗʰ **S52.1 Fracture of upper end of radius**

Fracture of proximal end of radius

EXCLUDES 2   fracture of shaft of radius (S52.3-)

physeal fractures of upper end of radius (S59.2-)

✓6ᵗʰ **S52.10 Unspecified fracture of upper end of radius**

✓7ᵗʰ **S52.101 Unspecified fracture of upper end of right radius** `MCC` `CC` `H5` `PE`

✓7ᵗʰ **S52.102 Unspecified fracture of upper end of left radius** `MCC` `CC` `H5` `PE`

✓7ᵗʰ **S52.109 Unspecified fracture of upper end of unspecified radius** `MCC` `CC` `H5` `UNS` `PE`

✔ Additional Character Required   ✓x7ᵗʰ Placeholder   Questionable PDx   Manifestation   Unspecified   `UPD` Unacceptable PDx   `H1`-`H14` HAC   `HCC` CMS-HCC Dx   `HIV` HIV Dx

ICD-10-CM 2025   **1041**

√6ᵗʰ **S52.11** **Torus** fracture of upper end of radius

> The appropriate 7th character is to be added to all codes in subcategory S52.11
> A   initial encounter for closed fracture
> D   subsequent encounter for fracture with routine healing
> G   subsequent encounter for fracture with delayed healing
> K   subsequent encounter for fracture with nonunion
> P   subsequent encounter for fracture with malunion
> S   sequela

√7ᵗʰ **S52.111** Torus fracture of upper end of **right** radius   CC H5 PE

√7ᵗʰ **S52.112** Torus fracture of upper end of **left** radius   CC H5 PE

√7ᵗʰ **S52.119** Torus fracture of upper end of unspecified radius   CC H5 UNS PE

√6ᵗʰ **S52.12** Fracture of **head** of radius

√7ᵗʰ **S52.121** **Displaced** fracture of head of **right** radius   MCC CC H5 PE

√7ᵗʰ **S52.122** **Displaced** fracture of head of **left** radius   MCC CC H5 PE

√7ᵗʰ **S52.123** **Displaced** fracture of head of unspecified radius   MCC CC H5 UNS PE

√7ᵗʰ **S52.124** **Nondisplaced** fracture of head of **right** radius   MCC CC H5 PE

√7ᵗʰ **S52.125** **Nondisplaced** fracture of head of **left** radius   MCC CC H5 PE

√7ᵗʰ **S52.126** **Nondisplaced** fracture of head of unspecified radius   MCC CC H5 UNS PE

√6ᵗʰ **S52.13** Fracture of **neck** of radius

√7ᵗʰ **S52.131** **Displaced** fracture of neck of **right** radius   MCC CC H5 PE

√7ᵗʰ **S52.132** **Displaced** fracture of neck of **left** radius   MCC CC H5 PE

√7ᵗʰ **S52.133** **Displaced** fracture of neck of unspecified radius   MCC CC H5 UNS PE

√7ᵗʰ **S52.134** **Nondisplaced** fracture of neck of **right** radius   MCC CC H5 PE

√7ᵗʰ **S52.135** **Nondisplaced** fracture of neck of **left** radius   MCC CC H5 PE

√7ᵗʰ **S52.136** **Nondisplaced** fracture of neck of unspecified radius   MCC CC H5 UNS PE

√6ᵗʰ **S52.18** Other fracture of upper end of radius

√7ᵗʰ **S52.181** Other fracture of upper end of **right** radius   MCC CC H5 PE

√7ᵗʰ **S52.182** Other fracture of upper end of **left** radius   MCC CC H5 PE

√7ᵗʰ **S52.189** Other fracture of upper end of unspecified radius   MCC CC H5 UNS PE

√5ᵗʰ **S52.2** Fracture of **shaft of ulna**

√6ᵗʰ **S52.20** Unspecified fracture of shaft of ulna

> Fracture of ulna NOS

√7ᵗʰ **S52.201** Unspecified fracture of shaft of **right** ulna   MCC CC H5 PE

√7ᵗʰ **S52.202** Unspecified fracture of shaft of **left** ulna   MCC CC H5 PE

√7ᵗʰ **S52.209** Unspecified fracture of shaft of unspecified ulna   MCC CC H5 UNS PE

√6ᵗʰ **S52.21** **Greenstick** fracture of shaft of ulna

> The appropriate 7th character is to be added to all codes in subcategory S52.21
> A   initial encounter for closed fracture
> D   subsequent encounter for fracture with routine healing
> G   subsequent encounter for fracture with delayed healing
> K   subsequent encounter for fracture with nonunion
> P   subsequent encounter for fracture with malunion
> S   sequela

√7ᵗʰ **S52.211** Greenstick fracture of shaft of **right** ulna   CC H5 PE

√7ᵗʰ **S52.212** Greenstick fracture of shaft of **left** ulna   CC H5 PE

√7ᵗʰ **S52.219** Greenstick fracture of shaft of unspecified ulna   CC H5 UNS PE

√6ᵗʰ **S52.22** **Transverse** fracture of shaft of ulna

√7ᵗʰ **S52.221** **Displaced** transverse fracture of shaft of **right** ulna   MCC CC H5 PE

√7ᵗʰ **S52.222** **Displaced** transverse fracture of shaft of **left** ulna   MCC CC H5 PE

√7ᵗʰ **S52.223** **Displaced** transverse fracture of shaft of unspecified ulna   MCC CC H5 UNS PE

√7ᵗʰ **S52.224** **Nondisplaced** transverse fracture of shaft of **right** ulna   MCC CC H5 PE

√7ᵗʰ **S52.225** **Nondisplaced** transverse fracture of shaft of **left** ulna   MCC CC H5 PE

√7ᵗʰ **S52.226** **Nondisplaced** transverse fracture of shaft of unspecified ulna   MCC CC H5 UNS PE

√6ᵗʰ **S52.23** **Oblique** fracture of shaft of ulna

√7ᵗʰ **S52.231** **Displaced** oblique fracture of shaft of **right** ulna   MCC CC H5 PE

√7ᵗʰ **S52.232** **Displaced** oblique fracture of shaft of **left** ulna   MCC CC H5 PE

√7ᵗʰ **S52.233** **Displaced** oblique fracture of shaft of unspecified ulna   MCC CC H5 UNS PE

√7ᵗʰ **S52.234** **Nondisplaced** oblique fracture of shaft of **right** ulna   MCC CC H5 PE

√7ᵗʰ **S52.235** **Nondisplaced** oblique fracture of shaft of **left** ulna   MCC CC H5 PE

√7ᵗʰ **S52.236** **Nondisplaced** oblique fracture of shaft of unspecified ulna   MCC CC H5 UNS PE

√6ᵗʰ **S52.24** **Spiral** fracture of shaft of ulna

√7ᵗʰ **S52.241** **Displaced** spiral fracture of shaft of ulna, **right arm**   MCC CC H5 PE

√7ᵗʰ **S52.242** **Displaced** spiral fracture of shaft of ulna, **left arm**   MCC CC H5 PE

√7ᵗʰ **S52.243** **Displaced** spiral fracture of shaft of ulna, unspecified arm   MCC CC H5 UNS PE

√7ᵗʰ **S52.244** **Nondisplaced** spiral fracture of shaft of ulna, **right arm**   MCC CC H5 PE

√7ᵗʰ **S52.245** **Nondisplaced** spiral fracture of shaft of ulna, **left arm**   MCC CC H5 PE

√7ᵗʰ **S52.246** **Nondisplaced** spiral fracture of shaft of ulna, unspecified arm   MCC CC H5 UNS PE

√6ᵗʰ **S52.25** **Comminuted** fracture of shaft of ulna

√7ᵗʰ **S52.251** **Displaced** comminuted fracture of shaft of ulna, **right arm**   MCC CC H5 PE

√7ᵗʰ **S52.252** **Displaced** comminuted fracture of shaft of ulna, **left arm**   MCC CC H5 PE

√7ᵗʰ **S52.253** **Displaced** comminuted fracture of shaft of ulna, unspecified arm   MCC CC H5 UNS PE

√7ᵗʰ **S52.254** **Nondisplaced** comminuted fracture of shaft of ulna, **right arm**   MCC CC H5 PE

√7ᵗʰ **S52.255** **Nondisplaced** comminuted fracture of shaft of ulna, **left arm**   MCC CC H5 PE

√7ᵗʰ **S52.256** **Nondisplaced** comminuted fracture of shaft of ulna, unspecified arm   MCC CC H5 UNS PE

√6ᵗʰ **S52.26** **Segmental** fracture of shaft of ulna

√7ᵗʰ **S52.261** **Displaced** segmental fracture of shaft of ulna, **right arm**   MCC CC H5 PE

√7ᵗʰ **S52.262** **Displaced** segmental fracture of shaft of ulna, **left arm**   MCC CC H5 PE

√7ᵗʰ **S52.263** **Displaced** segmental fracture of shaft of ulna, unspecified arm   MCC CC H5 UNS PE

√7ᵗʰ **S52.264** **Nondisplaced** segmental fracture of shaft of ulna, **right arm**   MCC CC H5 PE

√7ᵗʰ **S52.265** **Nondisplaced** segmental fracture of shaft of ulna, **left arm**   MCC CC H5 PE

√7ᵗʰ **S52.266** **Nondisplaced** segmental fracture of shaft of ulna, unspecified arm   MCC CC H5 UNS PE

√6ᵗʰ **S52.27** **Monteggia's** fracture of ulna

> Fracture of upper shaft of ulna with dislocation of radial head

√7ᵗʰ **S52.271** Monteggia's fracture of **right** ulna   MCC CC H5 PE

√7ᵗʰ **S52.272** Monteggia's fracture of **left** ulna   MCC CC H5 PE

√7ᵗʰ **S52.279** Monteggia's fracture of unspecified ulna `MCC` `CC` `H5` `UNS` `PE`

√6ᵗʰ **S52.28** **Bent bone** of ulna

√7ᵗʰ **S52.281** Bent bone of **right** ulna `MCC` `CC` `H5` `PE`

√7ᵗʰ **S52.282** Bent bone of **left** ulna `MCC` `CC` `H5` `PE`

√7ᵗʰ **S52.283** Bent bone of unspecified ulna `MCC` `CC` `H5` `UNS` `PE`

√6ᵗʰ **S52.29** Other fracture of shaft of ulna

√7ᵗʰ **S52.291** Other fracture of shaft of **right** ulna `MCC` `CC` `H5` `PE`

√7ᵗʰ **S52.292** Other fracture of shaft of **left** ulna `MCC` `CC` `H5` `PE`

√7ᵗʰ **S52.299** Other fracture of shaft of unspecified ulna `MCC` `CC` `H5` `UNS` `PE`

√5ᵗʰ **S52.3** Fracture of **shaft of radius**

√6ᵗʰ **S52.30** **Unspecified** fracture of shaft of radius

√7ᵗʰ **S52.301** Unspecified fracture of shaft of **right** radius `MCC` `CC` `H5` `PE`

√7ᵗʰ **S52.302** Unspecified fracture of shaft of **left** radius `MCC` `CC` `H5` `PE`

√7ᵗʰ **S52.309** Unspecified fracture of shaft of unspecified radius `MCC` `CC` `H5` `UNS` `PE`

√6ᵗʰ **S52.31** **Greenstick** fracture of shaft of radius `MCC` `CC` `HE` `UNS` `PE`

> The appropriate 7th character is to be added to all codes in subcategory S52.31.
> A   initial encounter for closed fracture
> D   subsequent encounter for fracture with routine healing
> G   subsequent encounter for fracture with delayed healing
> K   subsequent encounter for fracture with nonunion
> P   subsequent encounter for fracture with malunion
> S   sequela

√7ᵗʰ **S52.311** Greenstick fracture of shaft of radius, **right** arm `CC` `H5` `PE`

√7ᵗʰ **S52.312** Greenstick fracture of shaft of radius, **left** arm `CC` `H5` `PE`

√7ᵗʰ **S52.319** Greenstick fracture of shaft of radius, unspecified arm `CC` `H5` `UNS` `PE`

√6ᵗʰ **S52.32** **Transverse** fracture of shaft of radius

√7ᵗʰ **S52.321** **Displaced** transverse fracture of shaft of **right** radius `MCC` `CC` `H5` `PE`

√7ᵗʰ **S52.322** **Displaced** transverse fracture of shaft of **left** radius `MCC` `CC` `H5` `PE`

√7ᵗʰ **S52.323** **Displaced** transverse fracture of shaft of unspecified radius `MCC` `CC` `H5` `UNS` `PE`

√7ᵗʰ **S52.324** **Nondisplaced** transverse fracture of shaft of **right** radius `MCC` `CC` `H5` `PE`

√7ᵗʰ **S52.325** **Nondisplaced** transverse fracture of shaft of **left** radius `MCC` `CC` `H5` `PE`

√7ᵗʰ **S52.326** **Nondisplaced** transverse fracture of shaft of unspecified radius `MCC` `CC` `H5` `UNS` `PE`

√6ᵗʰ **S52.33** **Oblique** fracture of shaft of radius

√7ᵗʰ **S52.331** **Displaced** oblique fracture of shaft of **right** radius `MCC` `CC` `H5` `PE`

√7ᵗʰ **S52.332** **Displaced** oblique fracture of shaft of **left** radius `MCC` `CC` `H5` `PE`

√7ᵗʰ **S52.333** **Displaced** oblique fracture of shaft of unspecified radius `MCC` `CC` `H5` `UNS` `PE`

√7ᵗʰ **S52.334** **Nondisplaced** oblique fracture of shaft of **right** radius `MCC` `CC` `H5` `PE`

√7ᵗʰ **S52.335** **Nondisplaced** oblique fracture of shaft of **left** radius `MCC` `CC` `H5` `PE`

√7ᵗʰ **S52.336** **Nondisplaced** oblique fracture of shaft of unspecified radius `MCC` `CC` `H5` `UNS` `PE`

√6ᵗʰ **S52.34** **Spiral** fracture of shaft of radius

√7ᵗʰ **S52.341** **Displaced** spiral fracture of shaft of radius, **right** arm `MCC` `CC` `H5` `PE`

√7ᵗʰ **S52.342** **Displaced** spiral fracture of shaft of radius, **left** arm `MCC` `CC` `H5` `PE`

√7ᵗʰ **S52.343** **Displaced** spiral fracture of shaft of radius, unspecified arm `MCC` `CC` `H5` `UNS` `PE`

√7ᵗʰ **S52.344** **Nondisplaced** spiral fracture of shaft of radius, **right** arm `MCC` `CC` `H5` `PE`

√7ᵗʰ **S52.345** **Nondisplaced** spiral fracture of shaft of radius, **left** arm `MCC` `CC` `H5` `PE`

√7ᵗʰ **S52.346** **Nondisplaced** spiral fracture of shaft of radius, unspecified arm `MCC` `CC` `H5` `UNS` `PE`

√6ᵗʰ **S52.35** **Comminuted** fracture of shaft of radius

√7ᵗʰ **S52.351** **Displaced** comminuted fracture of shaft of radius, **right** arm `MCC` `CC` `H5` `PE`

√7ᵗʰ **S52.352** **Displaced** comminuted fracture of shaft of radius, **left** arm `MCC` `CC` `H5` `PE`

√7ᵗʰ **S52.353** **Displaced** comminuted fracture of shaft of radius, unspecified arm `MCC` `CC` `H5` `UNS` `PE`

√7ᵗʰ **S52.354** **Nondisplaced** comminuted fracture of shaft of radius, **right** arm `MCC` `CC` `H5` `PE`

√7ᵗʰ **S52.355** **Nondisplaced** comminuted fracture of shaft of radius, **left** arm `MCC` `CC` `H5` `PE`

√7ᵗʰ **S52.356** **Nondisplaced** comminuted fracture of shaft of radius, unspecified arm `MCC` `CC` `H5` `PE`

√6ᵗʰ **S52.36** **Segmental** fracture of shaft of radius

√7ᵗʰ **S52.361** **Displaced** segmental fracture of shaft of radius, **right** arm `MCC` `CC` `H5` `PE`

√7ᵗʰ **S52.362** **Displaced** segmental fracture of shaft of radius, **left** arm `MCC` `CC` `H5` `PE`

√7ᵗʰ **S52.363** **Displaced** segmental fracture of shaft of radius, unspecified arm `MCC` `CC` `H5` `UNS` `PE`

√7ᵗʰ **S52.364** **Nondisplaced** segmental fracture of shaft of radius, **right** arm `MCC` `CC` `H5` `PE`

√7ᵗʰ **S52.365** **Nondisplaced** segmental fracture of shaft of radius, **left** arm `MCC` `CC` `H5` `PE`

√7ᵗʰ **S52.366** **Nondisplaced** segmental fracture of shaft of radius, unspecified arm `MCC` `CC` `H5` `UNS` `PE`

√6ᵗʰ **S52.37** **Galeazzi's** fracture

Fracture of lower shaft of radius with radioulnar joint dislocation

√7ᵗʰ **S52.371** Galeazzi's fracture of **right** radius `MCC` `CC` `H5` `PE`

√7ᵗʰ **S52.372** Galeazzi's fracture of **left** radius `MCC` `CC` `H5` `PE`

√7ᵗʰ **S52.379** Galeazzi's fracture of unspecified radius `MCC` `CC` `H5` `UNS` `PE`

√6ᵗʰ **S52.38** **Bent bone** of radius

√7ᵗʰ **S52.381** Bent bone of **right** radius `MCC` `CC` `H5` `PE`

√7ᵗʰ **S52.382** Bent bone of **left** radius `MCC` `CC` `H5` `PE`

√7ᵗʰ **S52.389** Bent bone of unspecified radius `MCC` `CC` `H5` `UNS` `PE`

√6ᵗʰ **S52.39** Other fracture of shaft of radius

√7ᵗʰ **S52.391** Other fracture of shaft of radius, **right** arm `MCC` `CC` `H5` `PE`

√7ᵗʰ **S52.392** Other fracture of shaft of radius, **left** arm `MCC` `CC` `H5` `PE`

√7ᵗʰ **S52.399** Other fracture of shaft of radius, unspecified arm `MCC` `CC` `H5` `UNS` `PE`

√5ᵗʰ **S52.5** Fracture of **lower end of radius**

Fracture of distal end of radius

EXCLUDES 2   physeal fractures of lower end of radius (S59.2-)

DEF: Fracture of the distal end of the radius above the wrist, most commonly caused by a fall onto an outstretched hand.

√6ᵗʰ **S52.50** **Unspecified** fracture of the lower end of radius

√7ᵗʰ **S52.501** Unspecified fracture of the lower end of **right** radius `MCC` `CC` `H5` `PE`

√7ᵗʰ **S52.502** Unspecified fracture of the lower end of **left** radius `MCC` `CC` `H5` `PE`

√7ᵗʰ **S52.509** Unspecified fracture of the lower end of unspecified radius `MCC` `CC` `H5` `UNS` `PE`

√6ᵗʰ **S52.51** Fracture of **radial styloid process**

√7ᵗʰ **S52.511** **Displaced** fracture of **right** radial styloid process `MCC` `CC` `H5` `PE`

√7ᵗʰ **S52.512** **Displaced** fracture of **left** radial styloid process `MCC` `CC` `H5` `PE`

√7ᵗʰ **S52.513** **Displaced** fracture of unspecified radial styloid process `MCC` `CC` `H5` `UNS` `PE`

√7ᵗʰ **S52.514** **Nondisplaced** fracture of **right** radial styloid process `MCC` `CC` `H5` `PE`

√7ᵗʰ **S52.515** **Nondisplaced** fracture of **left** radial styloid process `MCC` `CC` `H5` `PE`

✔ Additional Character Required   √x7ᵗʰ Placeholder   Questionable PDx   Manifestation   Unspecified   UPD Unacceptable PDx   H1-H14 HAC   HCC CMS-HCC Dx   HIV HIV Dx

ICD-10-CM 2025   1043

✓7ᵗʰ **S52.516** **Nondisplaced** fracture of unspecified radial styloid process   MCC CC H5 UNS PE

✓6ᵗʰ **S52.52** **Torus** fracture of lower end of radius

> The appropriate 7th character is to be added to all codes in subcategory S52.52.
> A   initial encounter for closed fracture
> D   subsequent encounter for fracture with routine healing
> G   subsequent encounter for fracture with delayed healing
> K   subsequent encounter for fracture with nonunion
> P   subsequent encounter for fracture with malunion
> S   sequela

✓7ᵗʰ **S52.521** **Torus** fracture of lower end of **right** radius   CC H5 PE

✓7ᵗʰ **S52.522** **Torus** fracture of lower end of **left** radius   CC H5 PE

✓7ᵗʰ **S52.529** **Torus** fracture of lower end of unspecified radius   CC H5 UNS PE

✓6ᵗʰ **S52.53** **Colles' fracture**
> **AHA:** 2016,2Q,4
> **DEF:** Fracture of the radius at the wrist in which the distal fragment is pushed posteriorly. The dorsal angulation of the fragment results in the wrist cocking up.

✓7ᵗʰ **S52.531** **Colles' fracture of right** radius   MCC CC H5 PE

✓7ᵗʰ **S52.532** **Colles' fracture of left** radius   MCC CC H5 PE

✓7ᵗʰ **S52.539** **Colles' fracture of unspecified** radius   MCC CC H5 UNS PE

✓6ᵗʰ **S52.54** **Smith's** fracture

✓7ᵗʰ **S52.541** **Smith's fracture of right** radius   MCC CC H5 PE

✓7ᵗʰ **S52.542** **Smith's fracture of left** radius   MCC CC H5 PE

✓7ᵗʰ **S52.549** **Smith's fracture of unspecified** radius   MCC CC H5 UNS PE

✓6ᵗʰ **S52.55** **Other extraarticular** fracture of lower end of radius

✓7ᵗʰ **S52.551** **Other extraarticular** fracture of lower end of **right** radius   MCC CC H5 PE

✓7ᵗʰ **S52.552** **Other extraarticular** fracture of lower end of **left** radius   MCC CC H5 PE

✓7ᵗʰ **S52.559** **Other extraarticular** fracture of lower end of unspecified radius   MCC CC H5 UNS PE

✓6ᵗʰ **S52.56** **Barton's** fracture

✓7ᵗʰ **S52.561** **Barton's fracture of right** radius   MCC CC H5 PE

✓7ᵗʰ **S52.562** **Barton's fracture of left** radius   MCC CC H5 PE

✓7ᵗʰ **S52.569** **Barton's fracture of unspecified** radius   MCC CC H5 UNS PE

✓6ᵗʰ **S52.57** **Other intraarticular** fracture of lower end of radius

✓7ᵗʰ **S52.571** **Other intraarticular** fracture of lower end of **right** radius   MCC CC H5 PE

✓7ᵗʰ **S52.572** **Other intraarticular** fracture of lower end of **left** radius   MCC CC H5 PE

✓7ᵗʰ **S52.579** **Other intraarticular** fracture of lower end of unspecified radius   MCC CC H5 UNS PE

✓6ᵗʰ **S52.59** **Other fractures of lower end of radius**
> **AHA:** 2019,3Q,9

✓7ᵗʰ **S52.591** **Other fractures of lower end of right** radius   MCC CC H5 PE

✓7ᵗʰ **S52.592** **Other fractures of lower end of left** radius   MCC CC H5 PE

✓7ᵗʰ **S52.599** **Other fractures of lower end of unspecified** radius   MCC CC H5 UNS PE

✓5ᵗʰ **S52.6** **Fracture of lower end of ulna**

✓6ᵗʰ **S52.60** **Unspecified fracture of lower end of ulna**

✓7ᵗʰ **S52.601** **Unspecified fracture of lower end of right** ulna   MCC CC H5 PE

✓7ᵗʰ **S52.602** **Unspecified fracture of lower end of left** ulna   MCC CC H5 PE

✓7ᵗʰ **S52.609** **Unspecified fracture of lower end of unspecified ulna**   MCC CC H5 UNS PE

✓6ᵗʰ **S52.61** **Fracture of ulna styloid process**

✓7ᵗʰ **S52.611** **Displaced** fracture of **right** ulna styloid process   MCC CC H5 PE

✓7ᵗʰ **S52.612** **Displaced** fracture of **left** ulna styloid process   MCC CC H5 PE

✓7ᵗʰ **S52.613** **Displaced** fracture of unspecified ulna styloid process   MCC CC H5 UNS PE

✓7ᵗʰ **S52.614** **Nondisplaced** fracture of **right** ulna styloid process   MCC CC H5 PE

✓7ᵗʰ **S52.615** **Nondisplaced** fracture of **left** ulna styloid process   MCC CC H5 PE

✓7ᵗʰ **S52.616** **Nondisplaced** fracture of unspecified ulna styloid process   MCC CC H5 UNS PE

✓6ᵗʰ **S52.62** **Torus** fracture of lower end of ulna

> The appropriate 7th character is to be added to all codes in subcategory S52.62.
> A   initial encounter for closed fracture
> D   subsequent encounter for fracture with routine healing
> G   subsequent encounter for fracture with delayed healing
> K   subsequent encounter for fracture with nonunion
> P   subsequent encounter for fracture with malunion
> S   sequela

✓7ᵗʰ **S52.621** **Torus** fracture of lower end of **right** ulna   CC H5 PE

✓7ᵗʰ **S52.622** **Torus** fracture of lower end of **left** ulna   CC H5 PE

✓7ᵗʰ **S52.629** **Torus** fracture of lower end of unspecified ulna   CC H5 UNS PE

✓6ᵗʰ **S52.69** **Other fracture of lower end of ulna**
> **AHA:** 2019,3Q,9

✓7ᵗʰ **S52.691** **Other fracture of lower end of right** ulna   MCC CC H5 PE

✓7ᵗʰ **S52.692** **Other fracture of lower end of left** ulna   MCC CC H5 PE

✓7ᵗʰ **S52.699** **Other fracture of lower end of unspecified** ulna   MCC CC H5 UNS PE

✓5ᵗʰ **S52.9** **Unspecified fracture of forearm**

✓x7ᵗʰ **S52.90** **Unspecified fracture of unspecified forearm**   MCC CC H5 UNS PE

✓x7ᵗʰ **S52.91** **Unspecified fracture of right forearm**   MCC CC H5 PE

✓x7ᵗʰ **S52.92** **Unspecified fracture of left forearm**   MCC CC H5 PE

✓4ᵗʰ **S53** **Dislocation and sprain of joints and ligaments of elbow**

> **INCLUDES**   avulsion of joint or ligament of elbow
> laceration of cartilage, joint or ligament of elbow
> sprain of cartilage, joint or ligament of elbow
> traumatic hemarthrosis of joint or ligament of elbow
> traumatic rupture of joint or ligament of elbow
> traumatic subluxation of joint or ligament of elbow
> traumatic tear of joint or ligament of elbow

Code also any associated open wound

> **EXCLUDES 2**   strain of muscle, fascia and tendon at forearm level (S56.-)

> The appropriate 7th character is to be added to each code from category S53.
> A   initial encounter
> D   subsequent encounter
> S   sequela

✓5ᵗʰ **S53.0** **Subluxation and dislocation of radial head**
> Dislocation of radiohumeral joint
> Subluxation of radiohumeral joint
> **EXCLUDES 1**   Monteggia's fracture-dislocation (S52.27-)

✓6ᵗʰ **S53.00** **Unspecified subluxation and dislocation of radial head**

✓7ᵗʰ **S53.001** **Unspecified subluxation of right radial head**   PE

✓7ᵗʰ **S53.002** **Unspecified subluxation of left radial head**   PE

✓7ᵗʰ **S53.003** **Unspecified subluxation of unspecified radial head**   PE

✓7ᵗʰ **S53.004** **Unspecified dislocation of right radial head**   PE

✓7ᵗʰ **S53.005** **Unspecified dislocation of left radial head**   PE

√7ᵗʰ **S53.006** Unspecified dislocation of unspecified radial head

√6ᵗʰ **S53.01** Anterior subluxation and dislocation of radial head

Anteriomedial subluxation and dislocation of radial head

√7ᵗʰ **S53.011** Anterior subluxation of right radial head   PE

√7ᵗʰ **S53.012** Anterior subluxation of left radial head   PE

√7ᵗʰ **S53.013** Anterior subluxation of unspecified radial head   PE

√7ᵗʰ **S53.014** Anterior dislocation of right radial head   PE

√7ᵗʰ **S53.015** Anterior dislocation of left radial head   PE

√7ᵗʰ **S53.016** Anterior dislocation of unspecified radial head   PE

√6ᵗʰ **S53.02** Posterior subluxation and dislocation of radial head

Posteriolateral subluxation and dislocation of radial head

√7ᵗʰ **S53.021** Posterior subluxation of right radial head   PE

√7ᵗʰ **S53.022** Posterior subluxation of left radial head   PE

√7ᵗʰ **S53.023** Posterior subluxation of unspecified radial head   PE

√7ᵗʰ **S53.024** Posterior dislocation of right radial head   PE

√7ᵗʰ **S53.025** Posterior dislocation of left radial head   PE

√7ᵗʰ **S53.026** Posterior dislocation of unspecified radial head   PE

√6ᵗʰ **S53.03** Nursemaid's elbow

√7ᵗʰ **S53.031** Nursemaid's elbow, right elbow   PE

√7ᵗʰ **S53.032** Nursemaid's elbow, left elbow   PE

√7ᵗʰ **S53.033** Nursemaid's elbow, unspecified elbow   PE

√6ᵗʰ **S53.09** Other subluxation and dislocation of radial head

√7ᵗʰ **S53.091** Other subluxation of right radial head   PE

√7ᵗʰ **S53.092** Other subluxation of left radial head   PE

√7ᵗʰ **S53.093** Other subluxation of unspecified radial head   PE

√7ᵗʰ **S53.094** Other dislocation of right radial head   PE

√7ᵗʰ **S53.095** Other dislocation of left radial head   PE

√7ᵗʰ **S53.096** Other dislocation of unspecified radial head   PE

√5ᵗʰ **S53.1** Subluxation and dislocation of ulnohumeral joint

Subluxation and dislocation of elbow NOS

EXCLUDES 1   dislocation of radial head alone (S53.0-)

√6ᵗʰ **S53.10** Unspecified subluxation and dislocation of ulnohumeral joint

√7ᵗʰ **S53.101** Unspecified subluxation of right ulnohumeral joint   PE

√7ᵗʰ **S53.102** Unspecified subluxation of left ulnohumeral joint   PE

√7ᵗʰ **S53.103** Unspecified subluxation of unspecified ulnohumeral joint   PE

√7ᵗʰ **S53.104** Unspecified dislocation of right ulnohumeral joint   PE

√7ᵗʰ **S53.105** Unspecified dislocation of left ulnohumeral joint   PE

√7ᵗʰ **S53.106** Unspecified dislocation of unspecified ulnohumeral joint   PE

√6ᵗʰ **S53.11** Anterior subluxation and dislocation of ulnohumeral joint

√7ᵗʰ **S53.111** Anterior subluxation of right ulnohumeral joint   PE

√7ᵗʰ **S53.112** Anterior subluxation of left ulnohumeral joint   PE

√7ᵗʰ **S53.113** Anterior subluxation of unspecified ulnohumeral joint   PE

√7ᵗʰ **S53.114** Anterior dislocation of right ulnohumeral joint   PE

AHA: 2012,4Q,108

√7ᵗʰ **S53.115** Anterior dislocation of left ulnohumeral joint   PE

√7ᵗʰ **S53.116** Anterior dislocation of unspecified ulnohumeral joint   PE

√6ᵗʰ **S53.12** Posterior subluxation and dislocation of ulnohumeral joint

√7ᵗʰ **S53.121** Posterior subluxation of right ulnohumeral joint   PE

√7ᵗʰ **S53.122** Posterior subluxation of left ulnohumeral joint   PE

√7ᵗʰ **S53.123** Posterior subluxation of unspecified ulnohumeral joint   PE

√7ᵗʰ **S53.124** Posterior dislocation of right ulnohumeral joint   PE

√7ᵗʰ **S53.125** Posterior dislocation of left ulnohumeral joint   PE

√7ᵗʰ **S53.126** Posterior dislocation of unspecified ulnohumeral joint   PE

√6ᵗʰ **S53.13** Medial subluxation and dislocation of ulnohumeral joint

√7ᵗʰ **S53.131** Medial subluxation of right ulnohumeral joint   PE

√7ᵗʰ **S53.132** Medial subluxation of left ulnohumeral joint   PE

√7ᵗʰ **S53.133** Medial subluxation of unspecified ulnohumeral joint   PE

√7ᵗʰ **S53.134** Medial dislocation of right ulnohumeral joint   PE

√7ᵗʰ **S53.135** Medial dislocation of left ulnohumeral joint   PE

√7ᵗʰ **S53.136** Medial dislocation of unspecified ulnohumeral joint   PE

√6ᵗʰ **S53.14** Lateral subluxation and dislocation of ulnohumeral joint

√7ᵗʰ **S53.141** Lateral subluxation of right ulnohumeral joint   PE

√7ᵗʰ **S53.142** Lateral subluxation of left ulnohumeral joint   PE

√7ᵗʰ **S53.143** Lateral subluxation of unspecified ulnohumeral joint   PE

√7ᵗʰ **S53.144** Lateral dislocation of right ulnohumeral joint   PE

√7ᵗʰ **S53.145** Lateral dislocation of left ulnohumeral joint   PE

√7ᵗʰ **S53.146** Lateral dislocation of unspecified ulnohumeral joint   PE

√6ᵗʰ **S53.19** Other subluxation and dislocation of ulnohumeral joint

√7ᵗʰ **S53.191** Other subluxation of right ulnohumeral joint   PE

√7ᵗʰ **S53.192** Other subluxation of left ulnohumeral joint   PE

√7ᵗʰ **S53.193** Other subluxation of unspecified ulnohumeral joint   PE

√7ᵗʰ **S53.194** Other dislocation of right ulnohumeral joint   PE

√7ᵗʰ **S53.195** Other dislocation of left ulnohumeral joint   PE

√7ᵗʰ **S53.196** Other dislocation of unspecified ulnohumeral joint   PE

√5ᵗʰ **S53.2** Traumatic rupture of radial collateral ligament

EXCLUDES 1   sprain of radial collateral ligament NOS (S53.43-)

√x7ᵗʰ **S53.20** Traumatic rupture of unspecified radial collateral ligament   PE

√x7ᵗʰ **S53.21** Traumatic rupture of right radial collateral ligament   PE

√x7ᵗʰ **S53.22** Traumatic rupture of left radial collateral ligament   PE

√5ᵗʰ **S53.3** Traumatic rupture of ulnar collateral ligament

EXCLUDES 1   sprain of ulnar collateral ligament (S53.44-)

√x7ᵗʰ **S53.30** Traumatic rupture of unspecified ulnar collateral ligament   PE

√x7ᵗʰ **S53.31** Traumatic rupture of right ulnar collateral ligament   PE

√x7ᵗʰ **S53.32** Traumatic rupture of left ulnar collateral ligament   PE

✔ Additional Character Required   √x7ᵗʰ Placeholder   Questionable PDx   Manifestation   Unspecified   UPD Unacceptable PDx   H1-H4 HAC   HCC CMS-HCC Dx   HIV HIV Dx

ICD-10-CM 2025   1045

√5th **S53.4 Sprain of elbow**

> EXCLUDES 2   traumatic rupture of radial collateral ligament (S53.2-)
> traumatic rupture of ulnar collateral ligament (S53.3-)

√6th   **S53.40 Unspecified sprain of elbow**

√7th   S53.401 **Unspecified sprain of right elbow** PE

√7th   S53.402 **Unspecified sprain of left elbow** PE

√7th   S53.409 **Unspecified sprain of unspecified elbow** PE
Sprain of elbow NOS

√6th   **S53.41 Radiohumeral (joint) sprain**

√7th   S53.411 **Radiohumeral (joint) sprain of right elbow** PE

√7th   S53.412 **Radiohumeral (joint) sprain of left elbow** PE

√7th   S53.419 **Radiohumeral (joint) sprain of unspecified elbow** PE

√6th   **S53.42 Ulnohumeral (joint) sprain**

√7th   S53.421 **Ulnohumeral (joint) sprain of right elbow** PE

√7th   S53.422 **Ulnohumeral (joint) sprain of left elbow** PE

√7th   S53.429 **Ulnohumeral (joint) sprain of unspecified elbow** PE

√6th   **S53.43 Radial collateral ligament sprain**

√7th   S53.431 **Radial collateral ligament sprain of right elbow** PE

√7th   S53.432 **Radial collateral ligament sprain of left elbow** PE

√7th   S53.439 **Radial collateral ligament sprain of unspecified elbow** PE

√6th   **S53.44 Ulnar collateral ligament sprain**

√7th   S53.441 **Ulnar collateral ligament sprain of right elbow** PE

√7th   S53.442 **Ulnar collateral ligament sprain of left elbow** PE

√7th   S53.449 **Ulnar collateral ligament sprain of unspecified elbow** PE

√6th   **S53.49 Other sprain of elbow**

√7th   S53.491 **Other sprain of right elbow** PE

√7th   S53.492 **Other sprain of left elbow** PE

√7th   S53.499 **Other sprain of unspecified elbow** PE

√4th **S54 Injury of nerves at forearm level**

> Code also any associated open wound (S51.-)
>
> EXCLUDES 2   injury of nerves at wrist and hand level (S64.-)

> The appropriate 7th character is to be added to each code from category S54.
> A   initial encounter
> D   subsequent encounter
> S   sequela

√5th   **S54.0 Injury of ulnar nerve at forearm level**
Injury of ulnar nerve NOS

√x7th   S54.00 **Injury of ulnar nerve at forearm level, unspecified arm** PE

√x7th   S54.01 **Injury of ulnar nerve at forearm level, right arm** PE

√x7th   S54.02 **Injury of ulnar nerve at forearm level, left arm** PE

√5th   **S54.1 Injury of median nerve at forearm level**
Injury of median nerve NOS

√x7th   S54.10 **Injury of median nerve at forearm level, unspecified arm** PE

√x7th   S54.11 **Injury of median nerve at forearm level, right arm** PE

√x7th   S54.12 **Injury of median nerve at forearm level, left arm** PE

√5th   **S54.2 Injury of radial nerve at forearm level**
Injury of radial nerve NOS

√x7th   S54.20 **Injury of radial nerve at forearm level, unspecified arm** PE

√x7th   S54.21 **Injury of radial nerve at forearm level, right arm** PE

√x7th   S54.22 **Injury of radial nerve at forearm level, left arm** PE

√5th   **S54.3 Injury of cutaneous sensory nerve at forearm level**

√x7th   S54.30 **Injury of cutaneous sensory nerve at forearm level, unspecified arm** PE

√x7th   S54.31 **Injury of cutaneous sensory nerve at forearm level, right arm** PE

√x7th   S54.32 **Injury of cutaneous sensory nerve at forearm level, left arm** PE

√5th   **S54.8 Injury of other nerves at forearm level**

√6th   **S54.8X Injury of other nerves at forearm level**

√7th   S54.8X1 **Injury of other nerves at forearm level, right arm** PE

√7th   S54.8X2 **Injury of other nerves at forearm level, left arm** PE

√7th   S54.8X9 **Injury of other nerves at forearm level, unspecified arm** PE

√5th   **S54.9 Injury of unspecified nerve at forearm level**

√x7th   S54.90 **Injury of unspecified nerve at forearm level, unspecified arm** PE

√x7th   S54.91 **Injury of unspecified nerve at forearm level, right arm** PE

√x7th   S54.92 **Injury of unspecified nerve at forearm level, left arm** PE

√4th **S55 Injury of blood vessels at forearm level**

> Code also any associated open wound (S51.-)
>
> EXCLUDES 2   injury of blood vessels at wrist and hand level (S65.-)
> injury of brachial vessels (S45.1-S45.2)

> The appropriate 7th character is to be added to each code from category S55.
> A   initial encounter
> D   subsequent encounter
> S   sequela

√5th   **S55.0 Injury of ulnar artery at forearm level**

√6th   **S55.00 Unspecified injury of ulnar artery at forearm level**

√7th   S55.001 **Unspecified injury of ulnar artery at forearm level, right arm** CC PE

√7th   S55.002 **Unspecified injury of ulnar artery at forearm level, left arm** CC PE

√7th   S55.009 **Unspecified injury of ulnar artery at forearm level, unspecified arm** CC UNS PE

√6th   **S55.01 Laceration of ulnar artery at forearm level**

√7th   S55.011 **Laceration of ulnar artery at forearm level, right arm** CC PE

√7th   S55.012 **Laceration of ulnar artery at forearm level, left arm** CC PE

√7th   S55.019 **Laceration of ulnar artery at forearm level, unspecified arm** CC UNS PE

√6th   **S55.09 Other specified injury of ulnar artery at forearm level**

√7th   S55.091 **Other specified injury of ulnar artery at forearm level, right arm** CC PE

√7th   S55.092 **Other specified injury of ulnar artery at forearm level, left arm** CC PE

√7th   S55.099 **Other specified injury of ulnar artery at forearm level, unspecified arm** CC UNS PE

√5th   **S55.1 Injury of radial artery at forearm level**

√6th   **S55.10 Unspecified injury of radial artery at forearm level**

√7th   S55.101 **Unspecified injury of radial artery at forearm level, right arm** CC PE

√7th   S55.102 **Unspecified injury of radial artery at forearm level, left arm** CC PE

√7th   S55.109 **Unspecified injury of radial artery at forearm level, unspecified arm** CC UNS PE

√6th   **S55.11 Laceration of radial artery at forearm level**

√7th   S55.111 **Laceration of radial artery at forearm level, right arm** CC PE

√7th   S55.112 **Laceration of radial artery at forearm level, left arm** CC PE

√7th   S55.119 **Laceration of radial artery at forearm level, unspecified arm** CC UNS PE

√6th   **S55.19 Other specified injury of radial artery at forearm level**

√7th   S55.191 **Other specified injury of radial artery at forearm level, right arm** CC PE

√7th   S55.192 **Other specified injury of radial artery at forearm level, left arm** CC PE

√7th   S55.199 **Other specified injury of radial artery at forearm level, unspecified arm** CC UNS PE

☑5ᵗʰ **S55.2 Injury of vein at forearm level**

  ☑6ᵗʰ **S55.20 Unspecified injury of vein at forearm level**

    ☑7ᵗʰ **S55.201 Unspecified injury of vein at forearm level, right arm** `CC` `PE`

    ☑7ᵗʰ **S55.202 Unspecified injury of vein at forearm level, left arm** `CC` `PE`

    ☑7ᵗʰ **S55.209 Unspecified injury of vein at forearm level, unspecified arm** `CC` `UNS` `PE`

  ☑6ᵗʰ **S55.21 Laceration of vein at forearm level**

    ☑7ᵗʰ **S55.211 Laceration of vein at forearm level, right arm** `CC` `PE`

    ☑7ᵗʰ **S55.212 Laceration of vein at forearm level, left arm** `CC` `PE`

    ☑7ᵗʰ **S55.219 Laceration of vein at forearm level, unspecified arm** `CC` `UNS` `PE`

  ☑6ᵗʰ **S55.29 Other specified injury of vein at forearm level**

    ☑7ᵗʰ **S55.291 Other specified injury of vein at forearm level, right arm** `CC` `PE`

    ☑7ᵗʰ **S55.292 Other specified injury of vein at forearm level, left arm** `CC` `PE`

    ☑7ᵗʰ **S55.299 Other specified injury of vein at forearm level, unspecified arm** `CC` `UNS` `PE`

☑5ᵗʰ **S55.8 Injury of other blood vessels at forearm level**

  ☑6ᵗʰ **S55.80 Unspecified injury of other blood vessels at forearm level**

    ☑7ᵗʰ **S55.801 Unspecified injury of other blood vessels at forearm level, right arm** `CC` `PE`

    ☑7ᵗʰ **S55.802 Unspecified injury of other blood vessels at forearm level, left arm** `CC` `PE`

    ☑7ᵗʰ **S55.809 Unspecified injury of other blood vessels at forearm level, unspecified arm** `CC` `UNS` `PE`

  ☑6ᵗʰ **S55.81 Laceration of other blood vessels at forearm level**

    ☑7ᵗʰ **S55.811 Laceration of other blood vessels at forearm level, right arm** `CC` `PE`

    ☑7ᵗʰ **S55.812 Laceration of other blood vessels at forearm level, left arm** `CC` `PE`

    ☑7ᵗʰ **S55.819 Laceration of other blood vessels at forearm level, unspecified arm** `CC` `UNS` `PE`

  ☑6ᵗʰ **S55.89 Other specified injury of other blood vessels at forearm level**

    ☑7ᵗʰ **S55.891 Other specified injury of other blood vessels at forearm level, right arm** `CC` `PE`

    ☑7ᵗʰ **S55.892 Other specified injury of other blood vessels at forearm level, left arm** `CC` `PE`

    ☑7ᵗʰ **S55.899 Other specified injury of other blood vessels at forearm level, unspecified arm** `CC` `UNS` `PE`

☑5ᵗʰ **S55.9 Injury of unspecified blood vessel at forearm level**

  ☑6ᵗʰ **S55.90 Unspecified injury of unspecified blood vessel at forearm level**

    ☑7ᵗʰ **S55.901 Unspecified injury of unspecified blood vessel at forearm level, right arm** `CC` `PE`

    ☑7ᵗʰ **S55.902 Unspecified injury of unspecified blood vessel at forearm level, left arm** `CC` `FE`

    ☑7ᵗʰ **S55.909 Unspecified injury of unspecified blood vessel at forearm level, unspecified arm** `CC` `UNS` `FE`

  ☑6ᵗʰ **S55.91 Laceration of unspecified blood vessel at forearm level**

    ☑7ᵗʰ **S55.911 Laceration of unspecified blood vessel at forearm level, right arm** `CC` `PE`

    ☑7ᵗʰ **S55.912 Laceration of unspecified blood vessel at forearm level, left arm** `CC` `PE`

    ☑7ᵗʰ **S55.919 Laceration of unspecified blood vessel at forearm level, unspecified arm** `CC` `UNS` `PE`

  ☑6ᵗʰ **S55.99 Other specified injury of unspecified blood vessel at forearm level**

    ☑7ᵗʰ **S55.991 Other specified injury of unspecified blood vessel at forearm level, right arm** `CC` `PE`

    ☑7ᵗʰ **S55.992 Other specified injury of unspecified blood vessel at forearm level, left arm** `CC` `PE`

    ☑7ᵗʰ **S55.999 Other specified injury of unspecified blood vessel at forearm level, unspecified arm** `CC` `UNS` `PE`

☑4ᵗʰ **S56 Injury of muscle, fascia and tendon at forearm level**

Code also any associated open wound (S51.-)

EXCLUDES 2 injury of muscle, fascia and tendon at or below wrist (S66.-)
sprain of joints and ligaments of elbow (S53.4-)

TIP: Refer to the Muscle/Tendon table at the beginning of this chapter

The appropriate 7th character is to be added to each code from category S56.
A initial encounter
D subsequent encounter
S sequela

☑5ᵗʰ **S56.0 Injury of flexor muscle, fascia and tendon of thumb at forearm level**

  ☑6ᵗʰ **S56.00 Unspecified injury of flexor muscle, fascia and tendon of thumb at forearm level**

    ☑7ᵗʰ **S56.001 Unspecified injury of flexor muscle, fascia and tendon of right thumb at forearm level** `PE`

    ☑7ᵗʰ **S56.002 Unspecified injury of flexor muscle, fascia and tendon of left thumb at forearm level** `PE`

    ☑7ᵗʰ **S56.009 Unspecified injury of flexor muscle, fascia and tendon of unspecified thumb at forearm level** `PE`

  ☑6ᵗʰ **S56.01 Strain of flexor muscle, fascia and tendon of thumb at forearm level**

    ☑7ᵗʰ **S56.011 Strain of flexor muscle, fascia and tendon of right thumb at forearm level** `PE`

    ☑7ᵗʰ **S56.012 Strain of flexor muscle, fascia and tendon of left thumb at forearm level** `PE`

    ☑7ᵗʰ **S56.019 Strain of flexor muscle, fascia and tendon of unspecified thumb at forearm level** `PE`

  ☑6ᵗʰ **S56.02 Laceration of flexor muscle, fascia and tendon of thumb at forearm level**

    ☑7ᵗʰ **S56.021 Laceration of flexor muscle, fascia and tendon of right thumb at forearm level** `CC` `PE`

    ☑7ᵗʰ **S56.022 Laceration of flexor muscle, fascia and tendon of left thumb at forearm level** `CC` `PE`

    ☑7ᵗʰ **S56.029 Laceration of flexor muscle, fascia and tendon of unspecified thumb at forearm level** `CC` `PE`

  ☑6ᵗʰ **S56.09 Other injury of flexor muscle, fascia and tendon of thumb at forearm level**

    ☑7ᵗʰ **S56.091 Other injury of flexor muscle, fascia and tendon of right thumb at forearm level** `PE`

    ☑7ᵗʰ **S56.092 Other injury of flexor muscle, fascia and tendon of left thumb at forearm level** `PE`

    ☑7ᵗʰ **S56.099 Other injury of flexor muscle, fascia and tendon of unspecified thumb at forearm level** `PE`

☑5ᵗʰ **S56.1 Injury of flexor muscle, fascia and tendon of other and unspecified finger at forearm level**

  ☑6ᵗʰ **S56.10 Unspecified injury of flexor muscle, fascia and tendon of other and unspecified finger at forearm level**

    ☑7ᵗʰ **S56.101 Unspecified injury of flexor muscle, fascia and tendon of right index finger at forearm level** `PE`

    ☑7ᵗʰ **S56.102 Unspecified injury of flexor muscle, fascia and tendon of left index finger at forearm level** `PE`

    ☑7ᵗʰ **S56.103 Unspecified injury of flexor muscle, fascia and tendon of right middle finger at forearm level** `PE`

    ☑7ᵗʰ **S56.104 Unspecified injury of flexor muscle, fascia and tendon of left middle finger at forearm level** `PE`

    ☑7ᵗʰ **S56.105 Unspecified injury of flexor muscle, fascia and tendon of right ring finger at forearm level** `PE`

    ☑7ᵗʰ **S56.106 Unspecified injury of flexor muscle, fascia and tendon of left ring finger at forearm level** `PE`

✓ Additional Character Required ✓x7ᵗʰ Placeholder **Questionable PDx** Manifestation Unspecified `UPD` Unacceptable PDx `H1`-`H14` HAC `HCC` CMS-HCC Dx `HIV` HIV Dx

ICD-10-CM 2025 **1047**

√7ᵗʰ **S56.107** Unspecified injury of flexor muscle, fascia and tendon of **right little finger** at forearm level `PE`

√7ᵗʰ **S56.108** Unspecified injury of flexor muscle, fascia and tendon of **left little finger** at forearm level `PE`

√7ᵗʰ **S56.109** Unspecified injury of flexor muscle, fascia and tendon of unspecified finger at forearm level `PE`

√6ᵗʰ **S56.11** **Strain** of flexor muscle, fascia and tendon of other and unspecified finger at forearm level

√7ᵗʰ **S56.111** Strain of flexor muscle, fascia and tendon of **right index finger** at forearm level `PE`

√7ᵗʰ **S56.112** Strain of flexor muscle, fascia and tendon of **left index finger** at forearm level `PE`

√7ᵗʰ **S56.113** Strain of flexor muscle, fascia and tendon of **right middle finger** at forearm level `PE`

√7ᵗʰ **S56.114** Strain of flexor muscle, fascia and tendon of **left middle finger** at forearm level `PE`

√7ᵗʰ **S56.115** Strain of flexor muscle, fascia and tendon of **right ring finger** at forearm level `PE`

√7ᵗʰ **S56.116** Strain of flexor muscle, fascia and tendon of **left ring finger** at forearm level `PE`

√7ᵗʰ **S56.117** Strain of flexor muscle, fascia and tendon of **right little finger** at forearm level `PE`

√7ᵗʰ **S56.118** Strain of flexor muscle, fascia and tendon of **left little finger** at forearm level `PE`

√7ᵗʰ **S56.119** Strain of flexor muscle, fascia and tendon of finger of unspecified finger at forearm level `PE`

√6ᵗʰ **S56.12** **Laceration** of flexor muscle, fascia and tendon of other and unspecified finger at forearm level

√7ᵗʰ **S56.121** Laceration of flexor muscle, fascia and tendon of **right index finger** at forearm level `CC` `PE`

√7ᵗʰ **S56.122** Laceration of flexor muscle, fascia and tendon of **left index finger** at forearm level `CC` `PE`

√7ᵗʰ **S56.123** Laceration of flexor muscle, fascia and tendon of **right middle finger** at forearm level `CC` `PE`

√7ᵗʰ **S56.124** Laceration of flexor muscle, fascia and tendon of **left middle finger** at forearm level `CC` `PE`

√7ᵗʰ **S56.125** Laceration of flexor muscle, fascia and tendon of **right ring finger** at forearm level `CC` `PE`

√7ᵗʰ **S56.126** Laceration of flexor muscle, fascia and tendon of **left ring finger** at forearm level `CC` `PE`

√7ᵗʰ **S56.127** Laceration of flexor muscle, fascia and tendon of **right little finger** at forearm level `CC` `PE`

√7ᵗʰ **S56.128** Laceration of flexor muscle, fascia and tendon of **left little finger** at forearm level `CC` `PE`

√7ᵗʰ **S56.129** Laceration of flexor muscle, fascia and tendon of unspecified finger at forearm level `CC` `UNS` `PE`

√6ᵗʰ **S56.19** **Other injury** of flexor muscle, fascia and tendon of other and unspecified finger at forearm level

√7ᵗʰ **S56.191** Other injury of flexor muscle, fascia and tendon of **right index finger** at forearm level `PE`

√7ᵗʰ **S56.192** Other injury of flexor muscle, fascia and tendon of **left index finger** at forearm level `PE`

√7ᵗʰ **S56.193** Other injury of flexor muscle, fascia and tendon of **right middle finger** at forearm level `PE`

√7ᵗʰ **S56.194** Other injury of flexor muscle, fascia and tendon of **left middle finger** at forearm level `PE`

√7ᵗʰ **S56.195** Other injury of flexor muscle, fascia and tendon of **right ring finger** at forearm level `PE`

√7ᵗʰ **S56.196** Other injury of flexor muscle, fascia and tendon of **left ring finger** at forearm level `PE`

√7ᵗʰ **S56.197** Other injury of flexor muscle, fascia and tendon of **right little finger** at forearm level `PE`

√7ᵗʰ **S56.198** Other injury of flexor muscle, fascia and tendon of **left little finger** at forearm level `PE`

√7ᵗʰ **S56.199** Other injury of flexor muscle, fascia and tendon of unspecified finger at forearm level `PE`

√5ᵗʰ **S56.2** Injury of other flexor muscle, fascia and tendon at forearm level

√6ᵗʰ **S56.20** Unspecified injury of other flexor muscle, fascia and tendon at forearm level

√7ᵗʰ **S56.201** Unspecified injury of other flexor muscle, fascia and tendon at forearm level, **right arm** `PE`

√7ᵗʰ **S56.202** Unspecified injury of other flexor muscle, fascia and tendon at forearm level, **left arm** `PE`

√7ᵗʰ **S56.209** Unspecified injury of other flexor muscle, fascia and tendon at forearm level, unspecified arm `PE`

√6ᵗʰ **S56.21** **Strain** of other flexor muscle, fascia and tendon at forearm level

√7ᵗʰ **S56.211** Strain of other flexor muscle, fascia and tendon at forearm level, **right arm** `PE`

√7ᵗʰ **S56.212** Strain of other flexor muscle, fascia and tendon at forearm level, **left arm** `PE`

√7ᵗʰ **S56.219** Strain of other flexor muscle, fascia and tendon at forearm level, unspecified arm `PE`

√6ᵗʰ **S56.22** **Laceration** of other flexor muscle, fascia and tendon at forearm level

√7ᵗʰ **S56.221** Laceration of other flexor muscle, fascia and tendon at forearm level, **right arm** `CC` `PE`

√7ᵗʰ **S56.222** Laceration of other flexor muscle, fascia and tendon at forearm level, **left arm** `CC` `PE`

√7ᵗʰ **S56.229** Laceration of other flexor muscle, fascia and tendon at forearm level, unspecified arm `CC` `UNS` `PE`

√6ᵗʰ **S56.29** **Other injury** of other flexor muscle, fascia and tendon at forearm level

√7ᵗʰ **S56.291** Other injury of other flexor muscle, fascia and tendon at forearm level, **right arm** `PE`

√7ᵗʰ **S56.292** Other injury of other flexor muscle, fascia and tendon at forearm level, **left arm** `PE`

√7ᵗʰ **S56.299** Other injury of other flexor muscle, fascia and tendon at forearm level, unspecified arm `PE`

√5ᵗʰ **S56.3** Injury of **extensor or abductor** muscles, fascia and tendons of **thumb** at forearm level

√6ᵗʰ **S56.30** Unspecified injury of extensor or abductor muscles, fascia and tendons of thumb at forearm level

√7ᵗʰ **S56.301** Unspecified injury of extensor or abductor muscles, fascia and tendons of **right thumb** at forearm level `PE`

√7ᵗʰ **S56.302** Unspecified injury of extensor or abductor muscles, fascia and tendons of **left thumb** at forearm level `PE`

√7ᵗʰ **S56.309** Unspecified injury of extensor or abductor muscles, fascia and tendons of unspecified thumb at forearm level `PE`

√6ᵗʰ **S56.31** **Strain** of extensor or abductor muscles, fascia and tendons of thumb at forearm level

√7ᵗʰ **S56.311** Strain of extensor or abductor muscles, fascia and tendons of **right thumb** at forearm level `PE`

√7ᵗʰ **S56.312** Strain of extensor or abductor muscles, fascia and tendons of **left thumb** at forearm level `PE`

√7ᵗʰ **S56.319** Strain of extensor or abductor muscles, fascia and tendons of unspecified thumb at forearm level `PE`

√6ᵗʰ **S56.32** **Laceration** of extensor or abductor muscles, fascia and tendons of thumb at forearm level

√7ᵗʰ **S56.321** Laceration of extensor or abductor muscles, fascia and tendons of **right thumb** at forearm level `CC` `PE`

`N` Newborn: 0   `P` Pediatric: 0-17   `M` Maternity: 9-64   `A` Adult: 15-124   `UNS` Unspecified Site   `MCC` Major Complication/Comorbidity   `CC` Complication/Comorbidity   `PE` POA Exempt

1048   ICD-10-CM 2025

✓7th **S56.322** Laceration of extensor or abductor muscles, fascia and tendons of left thumb at forearm level `CC` `PE`

✓7th **S56.329** Laceration of extensor or abductor muscles, fascia and tendons of unspecified thumb at forearm level `CC` `PE`

✓6th **S56.39** Other injury of extensor or abductor muscles, fascia and tendons of thumb at forearm level

✓7th **S56.391** Other injury of extensor or abductor muscles, fascia and tendons of right thumb at forearm level `PE`

✓7th **S56.392** Other injury of extensor or abductor muscles, fascia and tendons of left thumb at forearm level `PE`

✓7th **S56.399** Other injury of extensor or abductor muscles, fascia and tendons of unspecified thumb at forearm level `PE`

✓5th **S56.4** Injury of extensor muscle, fascia and tendon of other and unspecified finger at forearm level

✓6th **S56.40** Unspecified injury of extensor muscle, fascia and tendon of other and unspecified finger at forearm level

✓7th **S56.401** Unspecified injury of extensor muscle, fascia and tendon of right index finger at forearm level

✓7th **S56.402** Unspecified injury of extensor muscle, fascia and tendon of left index finger at forearm level `PE`

✓7th **S56.403** Unspecified injury of extensor muscle, fascia and tendon of right middle finger at forearm level `PE`

✓7th **S56.404** Unspecified injury of extensor muscle, fascia and tendon of left middle finger at forearm level `PE`

✓7th **S56.405** Unspecified injury of extensor muscle, fascia and tendon of right ring finger at forearm level `PE`

✓7th **S56.406** Unspecified injury of extensor muscle, fascia and tendon of left ring finger at forearm level `PE`

✓7th **S56.407** Unspecified injury of extensor muscle, fascia and tendon of right little finger at forearm level `PE`

✓7th **S56.408** Unspecified injury of extensor muscle, fascia and tendon of left little finger at forearm level `PE`

✓7th **S56.409** Unspecified injury of extensor muscle, fascia and tendon of unspecified finger at forearm level

✓6th **S56.41** Strain of extensor muscle, fascia and tendon of other and unspecified finger at forearm level

✓7th **S56.411** Strain of extensor muscle, fascia and tendon of right index finger at forearm level

✓7th **S56.412** Strain of extensor muscle, fascia and tendon of left index finger at forearm level `PE`

✓7th **S56.413** Strain of extensor muscle, fascia and tendon of right middle finger at forearm level

✓7th **S56.414** Strain of extensor muscle, fascia and tendon of left middle finger at forearm level

✓7th **S56.415** Strain of extensor muscle, fascia and tendon of right ring finger at forearm level `PE`

✓7th **S56.416** Strain of extensor muscle, fascia and tendon of left ring finger at forearm level `PE`

✓7th **S56.417** Strain of extensor muscle, fascia and tendon of right little finger at forearm level `PE`

✓7th **S56.418** Strain of extensor muscle, fascia and tendon of left little finger at forearm level `PE`

✓7th **S56.419** Strain of extensor muscle, fascia and tendon of finger, unspecified finger at forearm level `PE`

✓6th **S56.42** Laceration of extensor muscle, fascia and tendon of other and unspecified finger at forearm level

✓7th **S56.421** Laceration of extensor muscle, fascia and tendon of right index finger at forearm level `CC` `PE`

✓7th **S56.422** Laceration of extensor muscle, fascia and tendon of left index finger at forearm level `CC` `PE`

✓7th **S56.423** Laceration of extensor muscle, fascia and tendon of right middle finger at forearm level

✓7th **S56.424** Laceration of extensor muscle, fascia and tendon of left middle finger at forearm level `CC` `PE`

✓7th **S56.425** Laceration of extensor muscle, fascia and tendon of right ring finger at forearm level

✓7th **S56.426** Laceration of extensor muscle, fascia and tendon of left ring finger at forearm level `CC` `PE`

✓7th **S56.427** Laceration of extensor muscle, fascia and tendon of right little finger at forearm level `CC` `PE`

✓7th **S56.428** Laceration of extensor muscle, fascia and tendon of left little finger at forearm level `CC` `PE`

✓7th **S56.429** Laceration of extensor muscle, fascia and tendon of unspecified finger at forearm level `CC` `UNS` `PE`

✓6th **S56.49** Other injury of extensor muscle, fascia and tendon of other and unspecified finger at forearm level

✓7th **S56.491** Other injury of extensor muscle, fascia and tendon of right index finger at forearm level `PE`

✓7th **S56.492** Other injury of extensor muscle, fascia and tendon of left index finger at forearm level `PE`

✓7th **S56.493** Other injury of extensor muscle, fascia and tendon of right middle finger at forearm level `PE`

✓7th **S56.494** Other injury of extensor muscle, fascia and tendon of left middle finger at forearm level `PE`

✓7th **S56.495** Other injury of extensor muscle, fascia and tendon of right ring finger at forearm level `PE`

✓7th **S56.496** Other injury of extensor muscle, fascia and tendon of left ring finger at forearm level `PE`

✓7th **S56.497** Other injury of extensor muscle, fascia and tendon of right little finger at forearm level `PE`

✓7th **S56.498** Other injury of extensor muscle, fascia and tendon of left little finger at forearm level `PE`

✓7th **S56.499** Other injury of extensor muscle, fascia and tendon of unspecified finger at forearm level `PE`

✓5th **S56.5** Injury of other extensor muscle, fascia and tendon at forearm level

✓6th **S56.50** Unspecified injury of other extensor muscle, fascia and tendon at forearm level

✓7th **S56.501** Unspecified injury of other extensor muscle, fascia and tendon at forearm level, right arm `PE`

✓7th **S56.502** Unspecified injury of other extensor muscle, fascia and tendon at forearm level, left arm `PE`

✓7th **S56.509** Unspecified injury of other extensor muscle, fascia and tendon at forearm level, unspecified arm `PE`

✓6th **S56.51** Strain of other extensor muscle, fascia and tendon at forearm level

✓7th **S56.511** Strain of other extensor muscle, fascia and tendon at forearm level, right arm `PE`

✓7th **S56.512** Strain of other extensor muscle, fascia and tendon at forearm level, left arm `PE`

✓7th **S56.519** Strain of other extensor muscle, fascia and tendon at forearm level, unspecified arm `PE`

✓6th **S56.52** Laceration of other extensor muscle, fascia and tendon at forearm level

✓7th **S56.521** Laceration of other extensor muscle, fascia and tendon at forearm level, right arm `CC` `PE`

✓7th **S56.522** Laceration of other extensor muscle, fascia and tendon at forearm level, left arm `CC` `PE`

Chapter 19. Injury, Poisoning and Certain Other Consequences of External Causes

S56.529–S58.121

√7ᵗʰ **S56.529** Laceration of other extensor muscle, fascia and tendon at forearm level, unspecified arm `CC` `UNS` `PE`

√6ᵗʰ **S56.59** Other injury of other extensor muscle, fascia and tendon at forearm level

    √7ᵗʰ **S56.591** Other injury of other extensor muscle, fascia and tendon at forearm level, right arm `PE`

    √7ᵗʰ **S56.592** Other injury of other extensor muscle, fascia and tendon at forearm level, left arm `PE`

    √7ᵗʰ **S56.599** Other injury of other extensor muscle, fascia and tendon at forearm level, unspecified arm `PE`

√5ᵗʰ **S56.8** Injury of other muscles, fascia and tendons at forearm level

  √6ᵗʰ **S56.80** Unspecified injury of other muscles, fascia and tendons at forearm level

    √7ᵗʰ **S56.801** Unspecified injury of other muscles, fascia and tendons at forearm level, right arm `PE`

    √7ᵗʰ **S56.802** Unspecified injury of other muscles, fascia and tendons at forearm level, left arm `PE`

    √7ᵗʰ **S56.809** Unspecified injury of other muscles, fascia and tendons at forearm level, unspecified arm `PE`

  √6ᵗʰ **S56.81** Strain of other muscles, fascia and tendons at forearm level

    √7ᵗʰ **S56.811** Strain of other muscles, fascia and tendons at forearm level, right arm `PE`

    √7ᵗʰ **S56.812** Strain of other muscles, fascia and tendons at forearm level, left arm `PE`

    √7ᵗʰ **S56.819** Strain of other muscles, fascia and tendons at forearm level, unspecified arm `PE`

  √6ᵗʰ **S56.82** Laceration of other muscles, fascia and tendons at forearm level

    √7ᵗʰ **S56.821** Laceration of other muscles, fascia and tendons at forearm level, right arm `CC` `PE`

    √7ᵗʰ **S56.822** Laceration of other muscles, fascia and tendons at forearm level, left arm `CC` `PE`

    √7ᵗʰ **S56.829** Laceration of other muscles, fascia and tendons at forearm level, unspecified arm `CC` `UNS` `PE`

  √6ᵗʰ **S56.89** Other injury of other muscles, fascia and tendons at forearm level

    √7ᵗʰ **S56.891** Other injury of other muscles, fascia and tendons at forearm level, right arm `PE`

    √7ᵗʰ **S56.892** Other injury of other muscles, fascia and tendons at forearm level, left arm `PE`

    √7ᵗʰ **S56.899** Other injury of other muscles, fascia and tendons at forearm level, unspecified arm `PE`

√5ᵗʰ **S56.9** Injury of unspecified muscles, fascia and tendons at forearm level

  √6ᵗʰ **S56.90** Unspecified injury of unspecified muscles, fascia and tendons at forearm level

    √7ᵗʰ **S56.901** Unspecified injury of unspecified muscles, fascia and tendons at forearm level, right arm `PE`

    √7ᵗʰ **S56.902** Unspecified injury of unspecified muscles, fascia and tendons at forearm level, left arm `PE`

    √7ᵗʰ **S56.909** Unspecified injury of unspecified muscles, fascia and tendons at forearm level, unspecified arm `PE`

  √6ᵗʰ **S56.91** Strain of unspecified muscles, fascia and tendons at forearm level

    √7ᵗʰ **S56.911** Strain of unspecified muscles, fascia and tendons at forearm level, right arm `PE`

    √7ᵗʰ **S56.912** Strain of unspecified muscles, fascia and tendons at forearm level, left arm `PE`

    √7ᵗʰ **S56.919** Strain of unspecified muscles, fascia and tendons at forearm level, unspecified arm `PE`

  √6ᵗʰ **S56.92** Laceration of unspecified muscles, fascia and tendons at forearm level

    √7ᵗʰ **S56.921** Laceration of unspecified muscles, fascia and tendons at forearm level, right arm `CC` `PE`

√7ᵗʰ **S56.922** Laceration of unspecified muscles, fascia and tendons at forearm level, left arm `CC` `PE`

√7ᵗʰ **S56.929** Laceration of unspecified muscles, fascia and tendons at forearm level, unspecified arm `CC` `UNS` `PE`

√6ᵗʰ **S56.99** Other injury of unspecified muscles, fascia and tendons at forearm level

    √7ᵗʰ **S56.991** Other injury of unspecified muscles, fascia and tendons at forearm level, right arm `PE`

    √7ᵗʰ **S56.992** Other injury of unspecified muscles, fascia and tendons at forearm level, left arm `PE`

    √7ᵗʰ **S56.999** Other injury of unspecified muscles, fascia and tendons at forearm level, unspecified arm `PE`

√4ᵗʰ **S57** **Crushing injury** of elbow and forearm

Use additional code(s) for all associated injuries

EXCLUDES 2   crushing injury of wrist and hand (S67.-)

The appropriate 7th character is to be added to each code from category S57.
A   initial encounter
D   subsequent encounter
S   sequela

√5ᵗʰ **S57.0** Crushing injury of **elbow**

  √x7ᵗʰ **S57.00** Crushing injury of unspecified elbow `PE`

  √x7ᵗʰ **S57.01** Crushing injury of **right** elbow `PE`

  √x7ᵗʰ **S57.02** Crushing injury of **left** elbow `PE`

√5ᵗʰ **S57.8** Crushing injury of **forearm**

  √x7ᵗʰ **S57.80** Crushing injury of unspecified forearm `PE`

  √x7ᵗʰ **S57.81** Crushing injury of **right** forearm `PE`

  √x7ᵗʰ **S57.82** Crushing injury of **left** forearm `PE`

√4ᵗʰ **S58** **Traumatic amputation** of elbow and forearm

An amputation not identified as partial or complete should be coded to complete

EXCLUDES 1   traumatic amputation of wrist and hand (S68.-)

The appropriate 7th character is to be added to each code from category S58.
A   initial encounter
D   subsequent encounter
S   sequela

√5ᵗʰ **S58.0** Traumatic amputation at **elbow** level

  √6ᵗʰ **S58.01** **Complete** traumatic amputation at elbow level

    √7ᵗʰ **S58.011** Complete traumatic amputation at elbow level, **right** arm `CC` `HCC` `PE`

    √7ᵗʰ **S58.012** Complete traumatic amputation at elbow level, **left** arm `CC` `HCC` `PE`

    √7ᵗʰ **S58.019** Complete traumatic amputation at elbow level, unspecified arm `CC` `UNS` `HCC` `PE`

  √6ᵗʰ **S58.02** **Partial** traumatic amputation at elbow level

    √7ᵗʰ **S58.021** Partial traumatic amputation at elbow level, **right** arm `CC` `HCC` `PE`

    √7ᵗʰ **S58.022** Partial traumatic amputation at elbow level, **left** arm `CC` `HCC` `PE`

    √7ᵗʰ **S58.029** Partial traumatic amputation at elbow level, unspecified arm `CC` `UNS` `HCC` `PE`

√5ᵗʰ **S58.1** Traumatic amputation at level **between elbow and wrist**

  √6ᵗʰ **S58.11** **Complete** traumatic amputation at level between elbow and wrist

    √7ᵗʰ **S58.111** Complete traumatic amputation at level between elbow and wrist, **right** arm `CC` `HCC` `PE`

    √7ᵗʰ **S58.112** Complete traumatic amputation at level between elbow and wrist, **left** arm `CC` `HCC` `PE`

    √7ᵗʰ **S58.119** Complete traumatic amputation at level between elbow and wrist, unspecified arm `CC` `UNS` `HCC` `PE`

  √6ᵗʰ **S58.12** **Partial** traumatic amputation at level between elbow and wrist

    √7ᵗʰ **S58.121** Partial traumatic amputation at level between elbow and wrist, **right** arm `CC` `HCC` `PE`

N Newborn: 0   **P** Pediatric: 0-17   **M** Maternity: 9-64   **A** Adult: 15-124   **UNS** Unspecified Site   **MCC** Major Complication/Comorbidity   **CC** Complication/Comorbidity   **PE** POA Exempt

1050

ICD-10-CM 2025

√7ᵗʰ **S58.122** Partial traumatic amputation at level between elbow and wrist, **left** arm `CC` `HCC` `PE`

√7ᵗʰ **S58.129** Partial traumatic amputation at level between elbow and wrist, unspecified arm `CC` `UNS` `HCC` `PE`

√5ᵗʰ **S58.9** Traumatic amputation of **forearm, level unspecified**

> *EXCLUDES 1*   traumatic amputation of wrist (S68.-)

√6ᵗʰ **S58.91** **Complete** traumatic amputation of forearm, level unspecified

√7ᵗʰ **S58.911** Complete traumatic amputation of **right** forearm, level unspecified `CC` `HCC` `PE`

√7ᵗʰ **S58.912** Complete traumatic amputation of **left** forearm, level unspecified `CC` `HCC` `PE`

√7ᵗʰ **S58.919** Complete traumatic amputation of unspecified forearm, level unspecified `CC` `UNS` `HCC` `PE`

√6ᵗʰ **S58.92** **Partial** traumatic amputation of forearm, level unspecified

√7ᵗʰ **S58.921** Partial traumatic amputation of **right** forearm, level unspecified `CC` `HCC` `PE`

√7ᵗʰ **S58.922** Partial traumatic amputation of **left** forearm, level unspecified `CC` `HCC` `PE`

√7ᵗʰ **S58.929** Partial traumatic amputation of unspecified forearm, level unspecified `CC` `UNS` `HCC` `PE`

√4ᵗʰ **S59** Other and unspecified injuries of elbow and forearm

> *EXCLUDES 2*   other and unspecified injuries of wrist and hand (S69.-)
>
> AHA: 2018,2Q,12; 2018,1Q,3; 2015,3Q,37-39

> The appropriate 7th character is to be added to each code from subcategories S59.0, S59.1, and S59.2.
> A   initial encounter for closed fracture
> D   subsequent encounter for fracture with routine healing
> G   subsequent encounter for fracture with delayed healing
> K   subsequent encounter for fracture with nonunion
> P   subsequent encounter for fracture with malunion
> S   sequela

√5ᵗʰ **S59.0** Physeal fracture of **lower end of ulna**

> AHA: 2019,4Q,56

√6ᵗʰ **S59.00** Unspecified physeal fracture of lower end of ulna

√7ᵗʰ **S59.001** Unspecified physeal fracture of lower end of ulna, **right** arm `CC` `H5` `PE`

√7ᵗʰ **S59.002** Unspecified physeal fracture of lower end of ulna, **left** arm `CC` `H5` `PE`

√7ᵗʰ **S59.009** Unspecified physeal fracture of lower end of ulna, unspecified arm `CC` `H5` `UNS` `PE`

√6ᵗʰ **S59.01** **Salter-Harris Type I** physeal fracture of lower end of ulna

√7ᵗʰ **S59.011** Salter-Harris Type I physeal fracture of lower end of ulna, **right** arm `CC` `H5` `PE`

√7ᵗʰ **S59.012** Salter-Harris Type I physeal fracture of lower end of ulna, **left** arm `CC` `H5` `PE`

√7ᵗʰ **S59.019** Salter-Harris Type I physeal fracture of lower end of ulna, unspecified arm `CC` `H5` `UNS` `PE`

√6ᵗʰ **S59.02** **Salter-Harris Type II** physeal fracture of lower end of ulna

√7ᵗʰ **S59.021** Salter-Harris Type II physeal fracture of lower end of ulna, **right** arm `CC` `H5` `PE`

√7ᵗʰ **S59.022** Salter-Harris Type II physeal fracture of lower end of ulna, **left** arm `CC` `H5` `PE`

√7ᵗʰ **S59.029** Salter-Harris Type II physeal fracture of lower end of ulna, unspecified arm `CC` `H5` `UNS` `PE`

√6ᵗʰ **S59.03** **Salter-Harris Type III** physeal fracture of lower end of ulna

√7ᵗʰ **S59.031** Salter-Harris Type III physeal fracture of lower end of ulna, **right** arm `CC` `H5` `PE`

√7ᵗʰ **S59.032** Salter-Harris Type III physeal fracture of lower end of ulna, **left** arm `CC` `H5` `PE`

√7ᵗʰ **S59.039** Salter-Harris Type III physeal fracture of lower end of ulna, unspecified arm `CC` `H5` `UNS` `PE`

√6ᵗʰ **S59.04** **Salter-Harris Type IV** physeal fracture of lower end of ulna

√7ᵗʰ **S59.041** Salter-Harris Type IV physeal fracture of lower end of ulna, **right** arm

√7ᵗʰ **S59.042** Salter-Harris Type IV physeal fracture of lower end of ulna, **left** arm `CC` `H5` `PE`

√7ᵗʰ **S59.049** Salter-Harris Type IV physeal fracture of lower end of ulna, unspecified arm `CC` `H5` `UNS` `PE`

√6ᵗʰ **S59.09** Other physeal fracture of lower end of ulna

√7ᵗʰ **S59.091** Other physeal fracture of lower end of ulna, **right** arm `CC` `H5` `PE`

√7ᵗʰ **S59.092** Other physeal fracture of lower end of ulna, **left** arm `CC` `H5` `PE`

√7ᵗʰ **S59.099** Other physeal fracture of lower end of ulna, unspecified arm `CC` `H5` `UNS` `PE`

√5ᵗʰ **S59.1** Physeal fracture of **upper end of radius**

> AHA: 2019,4Q,56

√6ᵗʰ **S59.10** Unspecified physeal fracture of upper end of radius

√7ᵗʰ **S59.101** Unspecified physeal fracture of upper end of radius, **right** arm `CC` `PE`

√7ᵗʰ **S59.102** Unspecified physeal fracture of upper end of radius, **left** arm `CC` `PE`

√7ᵗʰ **S59.109** Unspecified physeal fracture of upper end of radius, unspecified arm `CC` `UNS` `PE`

√6ᵗʰ **S59.11** **Salter-Harris Type I** physeal fracture of upper end of radius

√7ᵗʰ **S59.111** Salter-Harris Type I physeal fracture of upper end of radius, **right** arm `CC` `PE`

√7ᵗʰ **S59.112** Salter-Harris Type I physeal fracture of upper end of radius, **left** arm `CC` `PE`

√7ᵗʰ **S59.119** Salter-Harris Type I physeal fracture of upper end of radius, unspecified arm `CC` `UNS` `PE`

√6ᵗʰ **S59.12** **Salter-Harris Type II** physeal fracture of upper end of radius

√7ᵗʰ **S59.121** Salter-Harris Type II physeal fracture of upper end of radius, **right** arm `CC` `PE`

√7ᵗʰ **S59.122** Salter-Harris Type II physeal fracture of upper end of radius, **left** arm `CC` `PE`

√7ᵗʰ **S59.129** Salter-Harris Type II physeal fracture of upper end of radius, unspecified arm `CC` `UNS` `PE`

√6ᵗʰ **S59.13** **Salter-Harris Type III** physeal fracture of upper end of radius

√7ᵗʰ **S59.131** Salter-Harris Type III physeal fracture of upper end of radius, **right** arm `CC` `PE`

√7ᵗʰ **S59.132** Salter-Harris Type III physeal fracture of upper end of radius, **left** arm `CC` `PE`

√7ᵗʰ **S59.139** Salter-Harris Type III physeal fracture of upper end of radius, unspecified arm `CC` `UNS` `PE`

√6ᵗʰ **S59.14** **Salter-Harris Type IV** physeal fracture of upper end of radius

√7ᵗʰ **S59.141** Salter-Harris Type IV physeal fracture of upper end of radius, **right** arm `CC` `PE`

√7ᵗʰ **S59.142** Salter-Harris Type IV physeal fracture of upper end of radius, **left** arm `CC` `PE`

√7ᵗʰ **S59.149** Salter-Harris Type IV physeal fracture of upper end of radius, unspecified arm `CC` `UNS` `PE`

√6ᵗʰ **S59.19** Other physeal fracture of upper end of radius

√7ᵗʰ **S59.191** Other physeal fracture of upper end of radius, **right** arm `CC` `PE`

√7ᵗʰ **S59.192** Other physeal fracture of upper end of radius, **left** arm `CC` `PE`

√7ᵗʰ **S59.199** Other physeal fracture of upper end of radius, unspecified arm `CC` `UNS` `PE`

√5ᵗʰ **S59.2** Physeal fracture of **lower end of radius**

> AHA: 2019,4Q,56

√6ᵗʰ **S59.20** Unspecified physeal fracture of lower end of radius

√7ᵗʰ **S59.201** Unspecified physeal fracture of lower end of radius, **right** arm `CC` `H5` `PE`

√7ᵗʰ **S59.202** Unspecified physeal fracture of lower end of radius, **left** arm `CC` `H5` `PE`

√7ᵗʰ **S59.209** Unspecified physeal fracture of lower end of radius, unspecified arm `CC` `H5` `UNS` `PE`

√6ᵗʰ **S59.21** **Salter-Harris Type I** physeal fracture of lower end of radius

√7ᵗʰ **S59.211** Salter-Harris Type I physeal fracture of lower end of radius, **right** arm `CC` `H5` `PE`

☑ Additional Character Required   √x7ᵗʰ Placeholder   Questionable PDx   Manifestation   Unspecified   `UPD` Unacceptable PDx   `H1`-`H14` HAC   `HCC` CMS-HCC Dx   `HIV` HIV Dx

ICD-10-CM 2025   1051

√7ᵗʰ **S59.212** Salter-Harris Type I physeal fracture of lower end of radius, **left** arm `CC` `H5` `PE`

√7ᵗʰ **S59.219** Salter-Harris Type I physeal fracture of lower end of radius, unspecified arm `CC` `H5` `UNS` `PE`

√6ᵗʰ **S59.22** **Salter-Harris Type II** physeal fracture of lower end of radius

√7ᵗʰ **S59.221** Salter-Harris Type II physeal fracture of lower end of radius, **right** arm `CC` `H5` `PE`

√7ᵗʰ **S59.222** Salter-Harris Type II physeal fracture of lower end of radius, **left** arm `CC` `H5` `PE`

√7ᵗʰ **S59.229** Salter-Harris Type II physeal fracture of lower end of radius, unspecified arm `CC` `H5` `UNS` `PE`

√6ᵗʰ **S59.23** **Salter-Harris Type III** physeal fracture of lower end of radius

√7ᵗʰ **S59.231** Salter-Harris Type III physeal fracture of lower end of radius, **right** arm `CC` `H5` `PE`

√7ᵗʰ **S59.232** Salter-Harris Type III physeal fracture of lower end of radius, **left** arm `CC` `H5` `PE`

√7ᵗʰ **S59.239** Salter-Harris Type III physeal fracture of lower end of radius, unspecified arm `CC` `H5` `UNS` `PE`

√6ᵗʰ **S59.24** **Salter-Harris Type IV** physeal fracture of lower end of radius

√7ᵗʰ **S59.241** Salter-Harris Type IV physeal fracture of lower end of radius, **right** arm `CC` `H5` `PE`

√7ᵗʰ **S59.242** Salter-Harris Type IV physeal fracture of lower end of radius, **left** arm `CC` `H5` `PE`

√7ᵗʰ **S59.249** Salter-Harris Type IV physeal fracture of lower end of radius, unspecified arm `CC` `H5` `UNS` `PE`

√6ᵗʰ **S59.29** Other physeal fracture of lower end of radius

√7ᵗʰ **S59.291** Other physeal fracture of lower end of radius, **right** arm `CC` `H5` `PE`

√7ᵗʰ **S59.292** Other physeal fracture of lower end of radius, **left** arm `CC` `H5` `PE`

√7ᵗʰ **S59.299** Other physeal fracture of lower end of radius, unspecified arm `CC` `H5` `UNS` `PE`

√5ᵗʰ **S59.8** Other specified injuries of elbow and forearm

> The appropriate 7th character is to be added to each code in subcategory S59.8.
> A   initial encounter
> D   subsequent encounter
> S   sequela

√6ᵗʰ **S59.80** Other specified injuries of **elbow**

√7ᵗʰ **S59.801** Other specified injuries of **right** elbow `PE`

√7ᵗʰ **S59.802** Other specified injuries of **left** elbow `PE`

√7ᵗʰ **S59.809** Other specified injuries of unspecified elbow `PE`

√6ᵗʰ **S59.81** Other specified injuries of **forearm**

√7ᵗʰ **S59.811** Other specified injuries **right** forearm `PE`

√7ᵗʰ **S59.812** Other specified injuries **left** forearm `PE`

√7ᵗʰ **S59.819** Other specified injuries unspecified forearm `PE`

√5ᵗʰ **S59.9** Unspecified injury of elbow and forearm

> The appropriate 7th character is to be added to each code in subcategory S59.9.
> A   initial encounter
> D   subsequent encounter
> S   sequela

√6ᵗʰ **S59.90** Unspecified injury of **elbow**

√7ᵗʰ **S59.901** Unspecified injury of **right** elbow `PE`

√7ᵗʰ **S59.902** Unspecified injury of **left** elbow `PE`

√7ᵗʰ **S59.909** Unspecified injury of unspecified elbow `PE`

√6ᵗʰ **S59.91** Unspecified injury of **forearm**

√7ᵗʰ **S59.911** Unspecified injury of **right** forearm `PE`

√7ᵗʰ **S59.912** Unspecified injury of **left** forearm `PE`

√7ᵗʰ **S59.919** Unspecified injury of unspecified forearm `PE`

Injuries to the wrist, hand and fingers (S60-S69)

EXCLUDES 2   burns and corrosions (T20-T32)
frostbite (T33-T34)
insect bite or sting, venomous (T63.4)

√4ᵗʰ **S60** Superficial injury of wrist, hand and fingers

> The appropriate 7th character is to be added to each code from category S60.
> A   initial encounter
> D   subsequent encounter
> S   sequela

√5ᵗʰ **S60.0** Contusion of **finger without damage to nail**

EXCLUDES 1   contusion involving nail (matrix) (S60.1)

√×7ᵗʰ **S60.00** Contusion of unspecified finger without damage to nail `PE`
Contusion of finger(s) NOS

√6ᵗʰ **S60.01** Contusion of **thumb** without damage to nail

√7ᵗʰ **S60.011** Contusion of **right** thumb without damage to nail `PE`

√7ᵗʰ **S60.012** Contusion of **left** thumb without damage to nail `PE`

√7ᵗʰ **S60.019** Contusion of unspecified thumb without damage to nail `PE`

√6ᵗʰ **S60.02** Contusion of **index finger** without damage to nail

√7ᵗʰ **S60.021** Contusion of **right** index finger without damage to nail `PE`

√7ᵗʰ **S60.022** Contusion of **left** index finger without damage to nail `PE`

√7ᵗʰ **S60.029** Contusion of unspecified index finger without damage to nail `PE`

√6ᵗʰ **S60.03** Contusion of **middle finger** without damage to nail

√7ᵗʰ **S60.031** Contusion of **right** middle finger without damage to nail `PE`

√7ᵗʰ **S60.032** Contusion of **left** middle finger without damage to nail `PE`

√7ᵗʰ **S60.039** Contusion of unspecified middle finger without damage to nail `PE`

√6ᵗʰ **S60.04** Contusion of **ring finger** without damage to nail

√7ᵗʰ **S60.041** Contusion of **right** ring finger without damage to nail `PE`

√7ᵗʰ **S60.042** Contusion of **left** ring finger without damage to nail `PE`

√7ᵗʰ **S60.049** Contusion of unspecified ring finger without damage to nail `PE`

√6ᵗʰ **S60.05** Contusion of **little finger** without damage to nail

√7ᵗʰ **S60.051** Contusion of **right** little finger without damage to nail `PE`

√7ᵗʰ **S60.052** Contusion of **left** little finger without damage to nail `PE`

√7ᵗʰ **S60.059** Contusion of unspecified little finger without damage to nail `PE`

√5ᵗʰ **S60.1** Contusion of **finger with damage to nail**

√×7ᵗʰ **S60.10** Contusion of unspecified finger with damage to nail `PE`

√6ᵗʰ **S60.11** Contusion of **thumb** with damage to nail

√7ᵗʰ **S60.111** Contusion of **right** thumb with damage to nail `PE`

√7ᵗʰ **S60.112** Contusion of **left** thumb with damage to nail `PE`

√7ᵗʰ **S60.119** Contusion of unspecified thumb with damage to nail `PE`

√6ᵗʰ **S60.12** Contusion of **index finger** with damage to nail

√7ᵗʰ **S60.121** Contusion of **right** index finger with damage to nail `PE`

√7ᵗʰ **S60.122** Contusion of **left** index finger with damage to nail `PE`

√7ᵗʰ **S60.129** Contusion of unspecified index finger with damage to nail `PE`

√6ᵗʰ **S60.13** Contusion of **middle finger** with damage to nail

√7ᵗʰ **S60.131** Contusion of **right** middle finger with damage to nail `PE`

√7ᵗʰ **S60.132** Contusion of **left** middle finger with damage to nail `PE`

√7th **S60.139** Contusion of unspecified middle finger with damage to nail   PE

√6th **S60.14** Contusion of ring finger with damage to nail

  √7th **S60.141** Contusion of right ring finger with damage to nail   PE

  √7th **S60.142** Contusion of left ring finger with damage to nail   PE

  √7th **S60.149** Contusion of unspecified ring finger with damage to nail   PE

√6th **S60.15** Contusion of little finger with damage to nail

  √7th **S60.151** Contusion of right little finger with damage to nail   PE

  √7th **S60.152** Contusion of left little finger with damage to nail   PE

  √7th **S60.159** Contusion of unspecified little finger with damage to nail   PE

√5th **S60.2** Contusion of wrist and hand

  EXCLUDES 2   contusion of fingers (S60.0-, S60.1-)

√6th **S60.21** Contusion of wrist

  √7th **S60.211** Contusion of right wrist   PE

  √7th **S60.212** Contusion of left wrist   PE

  √7th **S60.219** Contusion of unspecified wrist   PE

√6th **S60.22** Contusion of hand

  √7th **S60.221** Contusion of right hand   PE

  √7th **S60.222** Contusion of left hand   PE

  √7th **S60.229** Contusion of unspecified hand   PE

√5th **S60.3** Other superficial injuries of thumb

√6th **S60.31** Abrasion of thumb

  √7th **S60.311** Abrasion of right thumb   PE

  √7th **S60.312** Abrasion of left thumb   PE

  √7th **S60.319** Abrasion of unspecified thumb   PE

√6th **S60.32** Blister (nonthermal) of thumb

  √7th **S60.321** Blister (nonthermal) of right thumb   PE

  √7th **S60.322** Blister (nonthermal) of left thumb   PE

  √7th **S60.329** Blister (nonthermal) of unspecified thumb   PE

√6th **S60.34** External constriction of thumb

  Hair tourniquet syndrome of thumb

  Use additional cause code to identify the constricting item (W49.0-)

  √7th **S60.341** External constriction of right thumb   PE

  √7th **S60.342** External constriction of left thumb   PE

  √7th **S60.349** External constriction of unspecified thumb   PE

√6th **S60.35** Superficial foreign body of thumb

  Splinter in the thumb

  √7th **S60.351** Superficial foreign body of right thumb   PE

  √7th **S60.352** Superficial foreign body of left thumb   PE

  √7th **S60.359** Superficial foreign body of unspecified thumb   PE

√6th **S60.36** Insect bite (nonvenomous) of thumb

  √7th **S60.361** Insect bite (nonvenomous) of right thumb   PE

  √7th **S60.362** Insect bite (nonvenomous) of left thumb   PE

  √7th **S60.369** Insect bite (nonvenomous) of unspecified thumb   PE

√6th **S60.37** Other superficial bite of thumb

  EXCLUDES 1   open bite of thumb (S61.05-, S61.15-)

  √7th **S60.371** Other superficial bite of right thumb   PE

  √7th **S60.372** Other superficial bite of left thumb   PE

  √7th **S60.379** Other superficial bite of unspecified thumb   PE

√6th **S60.39** Other superficial injuries of thumb

  √7th **S60.391** Other superficial injuries of right thumb   PE

  √7th **S60.392** Other superficial injuries of left thumb   PE

  √7th **S60.399** Other superficial injuries of unspecified thumb   PE

√5th **S60.4** Other superficial injuries of other fingers

√6th **S60.41** Abrasion of fingers

  √7th **S60.410** Abrasion of right index finger   PE

  √7th **S60.411** Abrasion of left index finger   PE

  √7th **S60.412** Abrasion of right middle finger   PE

  √7th **S60.413** Abrasion of left middle finger   PE

  √7th **S60.414** Abrasion of right ring finger   PE

  √7th **S60.415** Abrasion of left ring finger   PE

  √7th **S60.416** Abrasion of right little finger   PE

  √7th **S60.417** Abrasion of left little finger   PE

  √7th **S60.418** Abrasion of other finger   PE

    Abrasion of specified finger with unspecified laterality

  √7th **S60.419** Abrasion of unspecified finger   PE

√6th **S60.42** Blister (nonthermal) of fingers

  √7th **S60.420** Blister (nonthermal) of right index finger   PE

  √7th **S60.421** Blister (nonthermal) of left index finger   PE

  √7th **S60.422** Blister (nonthermal) of right middle finger   PE

  √7th **S60.423** Blister (nonthermal) of left middle finger   PE

  √7th **S60.424** Blister (nonthermal) of right ring finger   PE

  √7th **S60.425** Blister (nonthermal) of left ring finger   PE

  √7th **S60.426** Blister (nonthermal) of right little finger   PE

  √7th **S60.427** Blister (nonthermal) of left little finger   PE

  √7th **S60.428** Blister (nonthermal) of other finger   PE

    Blister (nonthermal) of specified finger with unspecified laterality

  √7th **S60.429** Blister (nonthermal) of unspecified finger   PE

√6th **S60.44** External constriction of fingers

  Hair tourniquet syndrome of finger

  Use additional cause code to identify the constricting item (W49.0-)

  √7th **S60.440** External constriction of right index finger   PE

  √7th **S60.441** External constriction of left index finger   PE

  √7th **S60.442** External constriction of right middle finger   PE

  √7th **S60.443** External constriction of left middle finger   PE

  √7th **S60.444** External constriction of right ring finger   PE

  √7th **S60.445** External constriction of left ring finger   PE

  √7th **S60.446** External constriction of right little finger   PE

  √7th **S60.447** External constriction of left little finger   PE

  √7th **S60.448** External constriction of other finger   PE

    External constriction of specified finger with unspecified laterality

  √7th **S60.449** External constriction of unspecified finger   PE

√6th **S60.45** Superficial foreign body of fingers

  Splinter in the finger(s)

  √7th **S60.450** Superficial foreign body of right index finger   PE

  √7th **S60.451** Superficial foreign body of left index finger   PE

  √7th **S60.452** Superficial foreign body of right middle finger   PE

  √7th **S60.453** Superficial foreign body of left middle finger   PE

  √7th **S60.454** Superficial foreign body of right ring finger   PE

  √7th **S60.455** Superficial foreign body of left ring finger   PE

  √7th **S60.456** Superficial foreign body of right little finger   PE

✔ Additional Character Required   √x7th Placeholder   Questionable PDx   Manifestation   Unspecified   UPD Unacceptable PDx   H1-H14 HAC   HCC CMS-HCC Dx   HIV HIV Dx

ICD-10-CM 2025   1053

✓7ᵗʰ **S60.457** **Superficial foreign body of** left little **finger** PE

✓7ᵗʰ **S60.458** **Superficial foreign body of other finger** PE

Superficial foreign body of specified finger with unspecified laterality

✓7ᵗʰ **S60.459** **Superficial foreign body of unspecified finger** PE

✓6ᵗʰ **S60.46** **Insect bite** (nonvenomous) **of fingers**

✓7ᵗʰ **S60.460** **Insect bite (nonvenomous) of** right index **finger** PE

✓7ᵗʰ **S60.461** **Insect bite (nonvenomous) of** left index **finger** PE

✓7ᵗʰ **S60.462** **Insect bite (nonvenomous) of** right middle **finger** PE

✓7ᵗʰ **S60.463** **Insect bite (nonvenomous) of** left middle **finger** PE

✓7ᵗʰ **S60.464** **Insect bite (nonvenomous) of** right ring **finger** PE

✓7ᵗʰ **S60.465** **Insect bite (nonvenomous) of** left ring **finger** PE

✓7ᵗʰ **S60.466** **Insect bite (nonvenomous) of** right little **finger** PE

✓7ᵗʰ **S60.467** **Insect bite (nonvenomous) of** left little **finger** PE

✓7ᵗʰ **S60.468** **Insect bite (nonvenomous) of other finger** PE

Insect bite (nonvenomous) of specified finger with unspecified laterality

✓7ᵗʰ **S60.469** **Insect bite (nonvenomous) of unspecified finger** PE

✓6ᵗʰ **S60.47** **Other superficial** bite **of fingers**

EXCLUDES 1   open bite of fingers (S61.25-, S61.35-)

✓7ᵗʰ **S60.470** **Other superficial bite of** right index **finger** PE

✓7ᵗʰ **S60.471** **Other superficial bite of** left index **finger** PE

✓7ᵗʰ **S60.472** **Other superficial bite of** right middle **finger** PE

✓7ᵗʰ **S60.473** **Other superficial bite of** left middle **finger** PE

✓7ᵗʰ **S60.474** **Other superficial bite of** right ring **finger** PE

✓7ᵗʰ **S60.475** **Other superficial bite of** left ring **finger** PE

✓7ᵗʰ **S60.476** **Other superficial bite of** right little **finger** PE

✓7ᵗʰ **S60.477** **Other superficial bite of** left little **finger** PE

✓7ᵗʰ **S60.478** **Other superficial bite of other finger** PE

Other superficial bite of specified finger with unspecified laterality

✓7ᵗʰ **S60.479** **Other superficial bite of unspecified finger** PE

✓5ᵗʰ **S60.5** **Other superficial injuries of** hand

EXCLUDES 2   superficial injuries of fingers (S60.3-, S60.4-)

✓6ᵗʰ **S60.51** **Abrasion of hand**

✓7ᵗʰ **S60.511** **Abrasion of** right **hand** PE

✓7ᵗʰ **S60.512** **Abrasion of** left **hand** PE

✓7ᵗʰ **S60.519** **Abrasion of unspecified hand** PE

✓6ᵗʰ **S60.52** **Blister** (nonthermal) **of hand**

✓7ᵗʰ **S60.521** **Blister (nonthermal) of** right **hand** PE

✓7ᵗʰ **S60.522** **Blister (nonthermal) of** left **hand** PE

✓7ᵗʰ **S60.529** **Blister (nonthermal) of unspecified hand** PE

✓6ᵗʰ **S60.54** **External constriction of hand**

✓7ᵗʰ **S60.541** **External constriction of** right **hand** PE

✓7ᵗʰ **S60.542** **External constriction of** left **hand** PE

✓7ᵗʰ **S60.549** **External constriction of unspecified hand** PE

✓6ᵗʰ **S60.55** **Superficial** foreign body **of hand**

Splinter in the hand

✓7ᵗʰ **S60.551** **Superficial foreign body of** right **hand** PE

✓7ᵗʰ **S60.552** **Superficial foreign body of** left **hand** PE

✓7ᵗʰ **S60.559** **Superficial foreign body of unspecified hand** PE

✓6ᵗʰ **S60.56** **Insect bite** (nonvenomous) **of hand**

✓7ᵗʰ **S60.561** **Insect bite (nonvenomous) of** right **hand** PE

✓7ᵗʰ **S60.562** **Insect bite (nonvenomous) of** left **hand** PE

✓7ᵗʰ **S60.569** **Insect bite (nonvenomous) of unspecified hand** PE

✓6ᵗʰ **S60.57** **Other superficial** bite **of hand**

EXCLUDES 1   open bite of hand (S61.45-)

✓7ᵗʰ **S60.571** **Other superficial bite of hand of** right **hand** PE

✓7ᵗʰ **S60.572** **Other superficial bite of hand of** left **hand** PE

✓7ᵗʰ **S60.579** **Other superficial bite of hand of unspecified hand** PE

✓5ᵗʰ **S60.8** **Other superficial injuries of** wrist

✓6ᵗʰ **S60.81** **Abrasion** of wrist

✓7ᵗʰ **S60.811** **Abrasion of** right **wrist** PE

✓7ᵗʰ **S60.812** **Abrasion of** left **wrist** PE

✓7ᵗʰ **S60.819** **Abrasion of unspecified wrist** PE

✓6ᵗʰ **S60.82** **Blister** (nonthermal) **of wrist**

✓7ᵗʰ **S60.821** **Blister (nonthermal) of** right **wrist** PE

✓7ᵗʰ **S60.822** **Blister (nonthermal) of** left **wrist** PE

✓7ᵗʰ **S60.829** **Blister (nonthermal) of unspecified wrist** PE

✓6ᵗʰ **S60.84** **External constriction** of wrist

✓7ᵗʰ **S60.841** **External constriction of** right **wrist** PE

✓7ᵗʰ **S60.842** **External constriction of** left **wrist** PE

✓7ᵗʰ **S60.849** **External constriction of unspecified wrist** PE

✓6ᵗʰ **S60.85** **Superficial** foreign body **of wrist**

Splinter in the wrist

✓7ᵗʰ **S60.851** **Superficial foreign body of** right **wrist** PE

✓7ᵗʰ **S60.852** **Superficial foreign body of** left **wrist** PE

✓7ᵗʰ **S60.859** **Superficial foreign body of unspecified wrist** PE

✓6ᵗʰ **S60.86** **Insect bite** (nonvenomous) **of wrist**

✓7ᵗʰ **S60.861** **Insect bite (nonvenomous) of** right **wrist** PE

✓7ᵗʰ **S60.862** **Insect bite (nonvenomous) of** left **wrist** PE

✓7ᵗʰ **S60.869** **Insect bite (nonvenomous) of unspecified wrist** PE

✓6ᵗʰ **S60.87** **Other superficial** bite **of wrist**

EXCLUDES 1   open bite of wrist (S61.55)

✓7ᵗʰ **S60.871** **Other superficial bite of** right **wrist** PE

✓7ᵗʰ **S60.872** **Other superficial bite of** left **wrist** PE

✓7ᵗʰ **S60.879** **Other superficial bite of unspecified wrist** PE

✓5ᵗʰ **S60.9** **Unspecified superficial injury of wrist, hand and fingers**

✓6ᵗʰ **S60.91** **Unspecified superficial injury of** wrist

✓7ᵗʰ **S60.911** **Unspecified superficial injury of** right **wrist** PE

✓7ᵗʰ **S60.912** **Unspecified superficial injury of** left **wrist** PE

✓7ᵗʰ **S60.919** **Unspecified superficial injury of unspecified wrist** PE

✓6ᵗʰ **S60.92** **Unspecified superficial injury of** hand

✓7ᵗʰ **S60.921** **Unspecified superficial injury of** right **hand** PE

✓7ᵗʰ **S60.922** **Unspecified superficial injury of** left **hand** PE

✓7ᵗʰ **S60.929** **Unspecified superficial injury of unspecified hand** PE

✓6ᵗʰ **S60.93** **Unspecified superficial injury of** thumb

✓7ᵗʰ **S60.931** **Unspecified superficial injury of** right **thumb** PE

✓7ᵗʰ **S60.932** **Unspecified superficial injury of** left **thumb** PE

✓7ᵗʰ **S60.939** **Unspecified superficial injury of unspecified thumb** PE

√6th **S60.94 Unspecified superficial injury of other fingers**

√7th S60.940 Unspecified superficial injury of **right index** finger PE

√7th S60.941 Unspecified superficial injury of **left index** finger PE

√7th S60.942 Unspecified superficial injury of **right middle** finger PE

√7th S60.943 Unspecified superficial injury of **left middle** finger PE

√7th S60.944 Unspecified superficial injury of **right ring** finger PE

√7th S60.945 Unspecified superficial injury of **left ring** finger PE

√7th S60.946 Unspecified superficial injury of **right little** finger PE

√7th S60.947 Unspecified superficial injury of **left little** finger PE

√7th S60.948 Unspecified superficial injury of other finger PE
> Unspecified superficial injury of specified finger with unspecified laterality

√7th S60.949 Unspecified superficial injury of unspecified finger PE

√4th **S61 Open wound of wrist, hand and fingers**

Code also any associated wound infection

EXCLUDES 1   *open fracture of wrist, hand and finger (S62.- with 7th character B)*

    traumatic amputation of wrist and hand (S68.-)

> The appropriate 7th character is to be added to each code from category S61.
> A   initial encounter
> D   subsequent encounter
> S   sequela

√5th **S61.0 Open wound of thumb without damage to nail**

EXCLUDES 1   *open wound of thumb with damage to nail (S61.1-)*

√6th **S61.00 Unspecified open wound of thumb without damage to nail**

√7th S61.001 Unspecified open wound of **right** thumb without damage to nail PE

√7th S61.002 Unspecified open wound of **left** thumb without damage to nail PE

√7th S61.009 Unspecified open wound of unspecified thumb without damage to nail PE

√6th **S61.01 Laceration without foreign body of thumb without damage to nail**

√7th S61.011 Laceration without foreign body of **right** thumb without damage to nail PE

√7th S61.012 Laceration without foreign body of **left** thumb without damage to nail PE

√7th S61.019 Laceration without foreign body of unspecified thumb without damage to nail PE

√6th **S61.02 Laceration with foreign body of thumb without damage to nail**

√7th S61.021 Laceration with foreign body of **right** thumb without damage to nail PE

√7th S61.022 Laceration with foreign body of **left** thumb without damage to nail PE

√7th S61.029 Laceration with foreign body of unspecified thumb without damage to nail PE

√6th **S61.03 Puncture wound without foreign body of thumb without damage to nail**

√7th S61.031 Puncture wound without foreign body of **right** thumb without damage to nail PE

√7th S61.032 Puncture wound without foreign body of **left** thumb without damage to nail PE

√7th S61.039 Puncture wound without foreign body of unspecified thumb without damage to nail PE

√6th **S61.04 Puncture wound with foreign body of thumb without damage to nail**

√7th S61.041 Puncture wound with foreign body of **right** thumb without damage to nail PE

√7th S61.042 Puncture wound with foreign body of **left** thumb without damage to nail PE

√7th S61.049 Puncture wound with foreign body of unspecified thumb without damage to nail PE

√6th **S61.05 Open bite of thumb without damage to nail**
> Bite of thumb NOS

EXCLUDES 1   *superficial bite of thumb (S60.36-, S60.37-)*

√7th S61.051 Open bite of **right** thumb without damage to nail PE

√7th S61.052 Open bite of **left** thumb without damage to nail PE

√7th S61.059 Open bite of unspecified thumb without damage to nail PE

√5th **S61.1 Open wound of thumb with damage to nail**

√6th **S61.10 Unspecified open wound of thumb with damage to nail**

√7th S61.101 Unspecified open wound of **right** thumb with damage to nail PE

√7th S61.102 Unspecified open wound of **left** thumb with damage to nail PE

√7th S61.109 Unspecified open wound of unspecified thumb with damage to nail PE

√6th **S61.11 Laceration without foreign body of thumb with damage to nail**

√7th S61.111 Laceration without foreign body of **right** thumb with damage to nail PE

√7th S61.112 Laceration without foreign body of **left** thumb with damage to nail PE

√7th S61.119 Laceration without foreign body of unspecified thumb with damage to nail PE

√6th **S61.12 Laceration with foreign body of thumb with damage to nail**

√7th S61.121 Laceration with foreign body of **right** thumb with damage to nail PE

√7th S61.122 Laceration with foreign body of **left** thumb with damage to nail PE

√7th S61.129 Laceration with foreign body of unspecified thumb with damage to nail PE

√6th **S61.13 Puncture wound without foreign body of thumb with damage to nail**

√7th S61.131 Puncture wound without foreign body of **right** thumb with damage to nail PE

√7th S61.132 Puncture wound without foreign body of **left** thumb with damage to nail PE

√7th S61.139 Puncture wound without foreign body of unspecified thumb with damage to nail PE

√6th **S61.14 Puncture wound with foreign body of thumb with damage to nail**

√7th S61.141 Puncture wound with foreign body of **right** thumb with damage to nail PE

√7th S61.142 Puncture wound with foreign body of **left** thumb with damage to nail PE

√7th S61.149 Puncture wound with foreign body of unspecified thumb with damage to nail PE

√6th **S61.15 Open bite of thumb with damage to nail**
> Bite of thumb with damage to nail NOS

EXCLUDES 1   *superficial bite of thumb (S60.36-, S60.37-)*

√7th S61.151 Open bite of **right** thumb with damage to nail PE

√7th S61.152 Open bite of **left** thumb with damage to nail PE

√7th S61.159 Open bite of unspecified thumb with damage to nail PE

√5th **S61.2 Open wound of other finger without damage to nail**

EXCLUDES 1   *open wound of finger involving nail (matrix) (S61.3-)*

EXCLUDES 2   *open wound of thumb without damage to nail (S61.0-)*

√6th **S61.20 Unspecified open wound of other finger without damage to nail**

√7th S61.200 Unspecified open wound of **right index** finger without damage to nail PE

√7th S61.201 Unspecified open wound of **left index** finger without damage to nail PE

√7th S61.202 Unspecified open wound of **right middle** finger without damage to nail PE

√7th S61.203 Unspecified open wound of **left middle** finger without damage to nail PE

√7th S61.204 Unspecified open wound of **right ring** finger without damage to nail PE

√7th S61.205 Unspecified open wound of **left ring** finger without damage to nail

✔ Additional Character Required   √x7th Placeholder   Questionable PDx   Manifestation   Unspecified   UPD Unacceptable PDx   H1-H14 HAC   HCC CMS-HCC Dx   HIV HIV Dx

ICD-10-CM 2025   1055

✓7th **S61.206** **Unspecified open wound of** right little finger **without damage to nail** PE

✓7th **S61.207** **Unspecified open wound of** left little finger **without damage to nail** PE

✓7th **S61.208** **Unspecified open wound of other finger without damage to nail** PE

     Unspecified open wound of specified finger with unspecified laterality without damage to nail

✓7th **S61.209** **Unspecified open wound of unspecified finger without damage to nail** PE

✓6th **S61.21** **Laceration without foreign body of finger without damage to nail**

✓7th **S61.210** **Laceration without foreign body of** right index **finger without damage to nail** PE

✓7th **S61.211** **Laceration without foreign body of** left index **finger without damage to nail** PE

✓7th **S61.212** **Laceration without foreign body of** right middle **finger without damage to nail** PE

✓7th **S61.213** **Laceration without foreign body of** left middle **finger without damage to nail** PE

✓7th **S61.214** **Laceration without foreign body of** right ring **finger without damage to nail** PE

✓7th **S61.215** **Laceration without foreign body of** left ring **finger without damage to nail** PE

✓7th **S61.216** **Laceration without foreign body of** right little **finger without damage to nail** PE

✓7th **S61.217** **Laceration without foreign body of** left little **finger without damage to nail** PE

✓7th **S61.218** **Laceration without foreign body of other finger without damage to nail** PE

     Laceration without foreign body of specified finger with unspecified laterality without damage to nail

✓7th **S61.219** **Laceration without foreign body of unspecified finger without damage to nail** PE

✓6th **S61.22** **Laceration with foreign body of finger without damage to nail**

✓7th **S61.220** **Laceration with foreign body of** right index **finger without damage to nail** PE

✓7th **S61.221** **Laceration with foreign body of** left index **finger without damage to nail** PE

✓7th **S61.222** **Laceration with foreign body of** right middle **finger without damage to nail** PE

✓7th **S61.223** **Laceration with foreign body of** left middle **finger without damage to nail** PE

✓7th **S61.224** **Laceration with foreign body of** right ring **finger without damage to nail** PE

✓7th **S61.225** **Laceration with foreign body of** left ring **finger without damage to nail** PE

✓7th **S61.226** **Laceration with foreign body of** right little **finger without damage to nail** PE

✓7th **S61.227** **Laceration with foreign body of** left little **finger without damage to nail** PE

✓7th **S61.228** **Laceration with foreign body of other finger without damage to nail** PE

     Laceration with foreign body of specified finger with unspecified laterality without damage to nail

✓7th **S61.229** **Laceration with foreign body of unspecified finger without damage to nail** PE

✓6th **S61.23** **Puncture wound without foreign body of finger without damage to nail**

✓7th **S61.230** **Puncture wound without foreign body of** right index **finger without damage to nail** PE

✓7th **S61.231** **Puncture wound without foreign body of** left index **finger without damage to nail** PE

✓7th **S61.232** **Puncture wound without foreign body of** right middle **finger without damage to nail** PE

✓7th **S61.233** **Puncture wound without foreign body of** left middle **finger without damage to nail** PE

✓7th **S61.234** **Puncture wound without foreign body of** right ring **finger without damage to nail** PE

✓7th **S61.235** **Puncture wound without foreign body of** left ring **finger without damage to nail** PE

✓7th **S61.236** **Puncture wound without foreign body of** right little **finger without damage to nail** PE

✓7th **S61.237** **Puncture wound without foreign body of** left little **finger without damage to nail** PE

✓7th **S61.238** **Puncture wound without foreign body of other finger without damage to nail** PE

     Puncture wound without foreign body of specified finger with unspecified laterality without damage to nail

✓7th **S61.239** **Puncture wound without foreign body of unspecified finger without damage to nail** PE

✓6th **S61.24** **Puncture wound with foreign body of finger without damage to nail**

✓7th **S61.240** **Puncture wound with foreign body of** right index **finger without damage to nail** PE

✓7th **S61.241** **Puncture wound with foreign body of** left index **finger without damage to nail** PE

✓7th **S61.242** **Puncture wound with foreign body of** right middle **finger without damage to nail** PE

✓7th **S61.243** **Puncture wound with foreign body of** left middle **finger without damage to nail** PE

✓7th **S61.244** **Puncture wound with foreign body of** right ring **finger without damage to nail** PE

✓7th **S61.245** **Puncture wound with foreign body of** left ring **finger without damage to nail** PE

✓7th **S61.246** **Puncture wound with foreign body of** right little **finger without damage to nail** PE

✓7th **S61.247** **Puncture wound with foreign body of** left little **finger without damage to nail** PE

✓7th **S61.248** **Puncture wound with foreign body of other finger without damage to nail** PE

     Puncture wound with foreign body of specified finger with unspecified laterality without damage to nail

✓7th **S61.249** **Puncture wound with foreign body of unspecified finger without damage to nail** PE

✓6th **S61.25** **Open bite of finger without damage to nail**

     Bite of finger without damage to nail NOS

     EXCLUDES 1   *superficial bite of finger (S60.46-, S60.47-)*

✓7th **S61.250** **Open bite of** right index **finger without damage to nail** PE

✓7th **S61.251** **Open bite of** left index **finger without damage to nail** PE

✓7th **S61.252** **Open bite of** right middle **finger without damage to nail** PE

✓7th **S61.253** **Open bite of** left middle **finger without damage to nail** PE

✓7th **S61.254** **Open bite of** right ring **finger without damage to nail** PE

✓7th **S61.255** **Open bite of** left ring **finger without damage to nail** PE

✓7th **S61.256** **Open bite of** right little **finger without damage to nail** PE

✓7th **S61.257** **Open bite of** left little **finger without damage to nail** PE

✓7th **S61.258** **Open bite of other finger without damage to nail** PE

     Open bite of specified finger with unspecified laterality without damage to nail

✓7th **S61.259** **Open bite of unspecified finger without damage to nail** PE

✓5th **S61.3** **Open wound of other** finger with damage to nail

✓6th **S61.30** **Unspecified open wound of finger with damage to nail**

✓7th **S61.300** **Unspecified open wound of** right index **finger with damage to nail** PE

N Newborn: 0   P Pediatric: 0-17   M Maternity: 9-64   A Adult: 15-124   UNS Unspecified Site   MCC Major Complication/Comorbidity   CC Complication/Comorbidity   PE POA Exempt

1056   ICD-10-CM 2025

✓7ᵗʰ **S61.301** Unspecified open wound of left index finger with damage to nail **PE**

✓7ᵗʰ **S61.302** Unspecified open wound of right middle finger with damage to nail

✓7ᵗʰ **S61.303** Unspecified open wound of left middle finger with damage to nail **PE**

✓7ᵗʰ **S61.304** Unspecified open wound of right ring finger with damage to nail

✓7ᵗʰ **S61.305** Unspecified open wound of left ring finger with damage to nail **PE**

✓7ᵗʰ **S61.306** Unspecified open wound of right little finger with damage to nail

✓7ᵗʰ **S61.307** Unspecified open wound of left little finger with damage to nail

✓7ᵗʰ **S61.308** Unspecified open wound of other finger with damage to nail **PE**

Unspecified open wound of specified finger with unspecified laterality with damage to nail

✓7ᵗʰ **S61.309** Unspecified open wound of unspecified finger with damage to nail **PE**

✓6ᵗʰ **S61.31** Laceration without foreign body of finger with damage to nail

✓7ᵗʰ **S61.310** Laceration without foreign body of right index finger with damage to nail **PE**

✓7ᵗʰ **S61.311** Laceration without foreign body of left index finger with damage to nail **PE**

✓7ᵗʰ **S61.312** Laceration without foreign body of right middle finger with damage to nail **PE**

✓7ᵗʰ **S61.313** Laceration without foreign body of left middle finger with damage to nail **PE**

✓7ᵗʰ **S61.314** Laceration without foreign body of right ring finger with damage to nail **PE**

✓7ᵗʰ **S61.315** Laceration without foreign body of left ring finger with damage to nail **PE**

✓7ᵗʰ **S61.316** Laceration without foreign body of right little finger with damage to nail **PE**

✓7ᵗʰ **S61.317** Laceration without foreign body of left little finger with damage to nail **PE**

✓7ᵗʰ **S61.318** Laceration without foreign body of other finger with damage to nail **PE**

Laceration without foreign body of specified finger with unspecified laterality with damage to nail

✓7ᵗʰ **S61.319** Laceration without foreign body of unspecified finger with damage to nail **PE**

✓6ᵗʰ **S61.32** Laceration with foreign body of finger with damage to nail

✓7ᵗʰ **S61.320** Laceration with foreign body of right index finger with damage to nail **PE**

✓7ᵗʰ **S61.321** Laceration with foreign body of left index finger with damage to nail **PE**

✓7ᵗʰ **S61.322** Laceration with foreign body of right middle finger with damage to nail **PE**

✓7ᵗʰ **S61.323** Laceration with foreign body of left middle finger with damage to nail **PE**

✓7ᵗʰ **S61.324** Laceration with foreign body of right ring finger with damage to nail **PE**

✓7ᵗʰ **S61.325** Laceration with foreign body of left ring finger with damage to nail **PE**

✓7ᵗʰ **S61.326** Laceration with foreign body of right little finger with damage to nail **PE**

✓7ᵗʰ **S61.327** Laceration with foreign body of left little finger with damage to nail **PE**

✓7ᵗʰ **S61.328** Laceration with foreign body of other finger with damage to nail **PE**

Laceration with foreign body of specified finger with unspecified laterality with damage to nail

✓7ᵗʰ **S61.329** Laceration with foreign body of unspecified finger with damage to nail **PE**

✓6ᵗʰ **S61.33** Puncture wound without foreign body of finger with damage to nail

✓7ᵗʰ **S61.330** Puncture wound without foreign body of right index finger with damage to nail **PE**

✓7ᵗʰ **S61.331** Puncture wound without foreign body of left index finger with damage to nail **PE**

✓7ᵗʰ **S61.332** Puncture wound without foreign body of right middle finger with damage to nail

✓7ᵗʰ **S61.333** Puncture wound without foreign body of left middle finger with damage to nail **PE**

✓7ᵗʰ **S61.334** Puncture wound without foreign body of right ring finger with damage to nail

✓7ᵗʰ **S61.335** Puncture wound without foreign body of left ring finger with damage to nail **PE**

✓7ᵗʰ **S61.336** Puncture wound without foreign body of right little finger with damage to nail

✓7ᵗʰ **S61.337** Puncture wound without foreign body of left little finger with damage to nail **PE**

✓7ᵗʰ **S61.338** Puncture wound without foreign body of other finger with damage to nail **PE**

Puncture wound without foreign body of specified finger with unspecified laterality with damage to nail

✓7ᵗʰ **S61.339** Puncture wound without foreign body of unspecified finger with damage to nail **PE**

✓6ᵗʰ **S61.34** Puncture wound with foreign body of finger with damage to nail

✓7ᵗʰ **S61.340** Puncture wound with foreign body of right index finger with damage to nail **PE**

✓7ᵗʰ **S61.341** Puncture wound with foreign body of left index finger with damage to nail **PE**

✓7ᵗʰ **S61.342** Puncture wound with foreign body of right middle finger with damage to nail **PE**

✓7ᵗʰ **S61.343** Puncture wound with foreign body of left middle finger with damage to nail **PE**

✓7ᵗʰ **S61.344** Puncture wound with foreign body of right ring finger with damage to nail **PE**

✓7ᵗʰ **S61.345** Puncture wound with foreign body of left ring finger with damage to nail **PE**

✓7ᵗʰ **S61.346** Puncture wound with foreign body of right little finger with damage to nail **PE**

✓7ᵗʰ **S61.347** Puncture wound with foreign body of left little finger with damage to nail **PE**

✓7ᵗʰ **S61.348** Puncture wound with foreign body of other finger with damage to nail **PE**

Puncture wound with foreign body of specified finger with unspecified laterality with damage to nail

✓7ᵗʰ **S61.349** Puncture wound with foreign body of unspecified finger with damage to nail **PE**

✓6ᵗʰ **S61.35** Open bite of finger with damage to nail

Bite of finger with damage to nail NOS

EXCLUDES 1   superficial bite of finger (S60.46-, S60.47-)

✓7ᵗʰ **S61.350** Open bite of right index finger with damage to nail **PE**

✓7ᵗʰ **S61.351** Open bite of left index finger with damage to nail **PE**

✓7ᵗʰ **S61.352** Open bite of right middle finger with damage to nail **PE**

✓7ᵗʰ **S61.353** Open bite of left middle finger with damage to nail **PE**

✓7ᵗʰ **S61.354** Open bite of right ring finger with damage to nail **PE**

✓7ᵗʰ **S61.355** Open bite of left ring finger with damage to nail **PE**

✓7ᵗʰ **S61.356** Open bite of right little finger with damage to nail **PE**

✓7ᵗʰ **S61.357** Open bite of left little finger with damage to nail **PE**

✓7ᵗʰ **S61.358** Open bite of other finger with damage to nail **PE**

Open bite of specified finger with unspecified laterality with damage to nail

✓7ᵗʰ **S61.359** Open bite of unspecified finger with damage to nail **PE**

✓5ᵗʰ **S61.4** Open wound of hand

✓6ᵗʰ **S61.40** Unspecified open wound of hand

✓7ᵗʰ **S61.401** Unspecified open wound of right hand **PE**

✔ Additional Character Required   ✓x7ᵗʰ Placeholder   Questionable PDx   Manifestation   Unspecified   **UPD** Unacceptable PDx   **H1-H14** HAC   **HCC** CMS-HCC Dx   **HIV** HIV Dx

ICD-10-CM 2025   **1057**

√7ᵗʰ **S61.402** Unspecified open wound of left hand   PE

√7ᵗʰ **S61.409** Unspecified open wound of unspecified hand   PE

√6ᵗʰ **S61.41** Laceration without foreign body of hand

   √7ᵗʰ **S61.411** Laceration without foreign body of right hand   PE

   √7ᵗʰ **S61.412** Laceration without foreign body of left hand   PE

   √7ᵗʰ **S61.419** Laceration without foreign body of unspecified hand   PE

√6ᵗʰ **S61.42** Laceration with foreign body of hand

   √7ᵗʰ **S61.421** Laceration with foreign body of right hand   PE

   √7ᵗʰ **S61.422** Laceration with foreign body of left hand   PE

   √7ᵗʰ **S61.429** Laceration with foreign body of unspecified hand   PE

√6ᵗʰ **S61.43** Puncture wound without foreign body of hand

   √7ᵗʰ **S61.431** Puncture wound without foreign body of right hand   PE

   √7ᵗʰ **S61.432** Puncture wound without foreign body of left hand   PE

   √7ᵗʰ **S61.439** Puncture wound without foreign body of unspecified hand   PE

√6ᵗʰ **S61.44** Puncture wound with foreign body of hand

   √7ᵗʰ **S61.441** Puncture wound with foreign body of right hand   PE

   √7ᵗʰ **S61.442** Puncture wound with foreign body of left hand   PE

   √7ᵗʰ **S61.449** Puncture wound with foreign body of unspecified hand   PE

√6ᵗʰ **S61.45** Open bite of hand

   Bite of hand NOS

   EXCLUDES 1   *superficial bite of hand (S60.56-, S60.57-)*

   √7ᵗʰ **S61.451** Open bite of right hand   PE

   √7ᵗʰ **S61.452** Open bite of left hand   PE

   √7ᵗʰ **S61.459** Open bite of unspecified hand   PE

√5ᵗʰ **S61.5** Open wound of wrist

√6ᵗʰ **S61.50** Unspecified open wound of wrist

   √7ᵗʰ **S61.501** Unspecified open wound of right wrist   PE

   √7ᵗʰ **S61.502** Unspecified open wound of left wrist   PE

   √7ᵗʰ **S61.509** Unspecified open wound of unspecified wrist   PE

√6ᵗʰ **S61.51** Laceration without foreign body of wrist

   √7ᵗʰ **S61.511** Laceration without foreign body of right wrist   PE

   √7ᵗʰ **S61.512** Laceration without foreign body of left wrist   PE

   √7ᵗʰ **S61.519** Laceration without foreign body of unspecified wrist   PE

√6ᵗʰ **S61.52** Laceration with foreign body of wrist

   √7ᵗʰ **S61.521** Laceration with foreign body of right wrist   PE

   √7ᵗʰ **S61.522** Laceration with foreign body of left wrist   PE

   √7ᵗʰ **S61.529** Laceration with foreign body of unspecified wrist   PE

√6ᵗʰ **S61.53** Puncture wound without foreign body of wrist

   √7ᵗʰ **S61.531** Puncture wound without foreign body of right wrist   PE

   √7ᵗʰ **S61.532** Puncture wound without foreign body of left wrist   PE

   √7ᵗʰ **S61.539** Puncture wound without foreign body of unspecified wrist   PE

√6ᵗʰ **S61.54** Puncture wound with foreign body of wrist

   √7ᵗʰ **S61.541** Puncture wound with foreign body of right wrist   PE

   √7ᵗʰ **S61.542** Puncture wound with foreign body of left wrist   PE

   √7ᵗʰ **S61.549** Puncture wound with foreign body of unspecified wrist   PE

√6ᵗʰ **S61.55** Open bite of wrist

   Bite of wrist NOS

   EXCLUDES 1   *superficial bite of wrist (S60.86-, S60.87-)*

   √7ᵗʰ **S61.551** Open bite of right wrist   PE

   √7ᵗʰ **S61.552** Open bite of left wrist   PE

   √7ᵗʰ **S61.559** Open bite of unspecified wrist   PE

√4ᵗʰ **S62** Fracture at wrist and hand level

NOTE   A fracture not indicated as displaced or nondisplaced should be coded to displaced

     A fracture not indicated as open or closed should be coded to closed

EXCLUDES 1   *traumatic amputation of wrist and hand (S68.-)*

EXCLUDES 2   *fracture of distal parts of ulna and radius (S52.-)*

AHA: 2018,2Q,12; 2015,3Q,37-39

The appropriate 7th character is to be added to each code from category S62.

   A   initial encounter for closed fracture
   B   initial encounter for open fracture
   D   subsequent encounter for fracture with routine healing
   G   subsequent encounter for fracture with delayed healing
   K   subsequent encounter for fracture with nonunion
   P   subsequent encounter for fracture with malunion
   S   sequela

√5ᵗʰ **S62.0** Fracture of navicular [scaphoid] bone of wrist

√6ᵗʰ **S62.00** Unspecified fracture of navicular [scaphoid] bone of wrist

   √7ᵗʰ **S62.001** Unspecified fracture of navicular [scaphoid] bone of right wrist   CC H5 PE

   √7ᵗʰ **S62.002** Unspecified fracture of navicular [scaphoid] bone of left wrist   CC H5 PE

     AHA: 2012,4Q,106

   √7ᵗʰ **S62.009** Unspecified fracture of navicular [scaphoid] bone of unspecified wrist   CC H5 UNS PE

√6ᵗʰ **S62.01** Fracture of distal pole of navicular [scaphoid] bone of wrist

   Fracture of volar tuberosity of navicular [scaphoid] bone of wrist

   √7ᵗʰ **S62.011** Displaced fracture of distal pole of navicular [scaphoid] bone of right wrist   CC H5 PE

   √7ᵗʰ **S62.012** Displaced fracture of distal pole of navicular [scaphoid] bone of left wrist   CC H5 PE

   √7ᵗʰ **S62.013** Displaced fracture of distal pole of navicular [scaphoid] bone of unspecified wrist   CC H5 UNS PE

   √7ᵗʰ **S62.014** Nondisplaced fracture of distal pole of navicular [scaphoid] bone of right wrist   CC H5 PE

   √7ᵗʰ **S62.015** Nondisplaced fracture of distal pole of navicular [scaphoid] bone of left wrist   CC H5 PE

   √7ᵗʰ **S62.016** Nondisplaced fracture of distal pole of navicular [scaphoid] bone of unspecified wrist   CC H5 UNS PE

√6ᵗʰ **S62.02** Fracture of middle third of navicular [scaphoid] bone of wrist

   √7ᵗʰ **S62.021** Displaced fracture of middle third of navicular [scaphoid] bone of right wrist   CC H5 PE

   √7ᵗʰ **S62.022** Displaced fracture of middle third of navicular [scaphoid] bone of left wrist   CC H5 PE

   √7ᵗʰ **S62.023** Displaced fracture of middle third of navicular [scaphoid] bone of unspecified wrist   CC H5 UNS PE

   √7ᵗʰ **S62.024** Nondisplaced fracture of middle third of navicular [scaphoid] bone of right wrist   CC H5 PE

   √7ᵗʰ **S62.025** Nondisplaced fracture of middle third of navicular [scaphoid] bone of left wrist   CC H5 PE

   √7ᵗʰ **S62.026** Nondisplaced fracture of middle third of navicular [scaphoid] bone of unspecified wrist   CC H5 UNS PE

N Newborn: 0   **P** Pediatric: 0-17   **M** Maternity: 9-64   **A** Adult: 15-124   **UNS** Unspecified Site   **MCC** Major Complication/Comorbidity   **CC** Complication/Comorbidity   **PE** POA Exempt

1058   ICD-10-CM 2025

√6ᵗʰ **S62.03** Fracture of proximal third of navicular [scaphoid] bone of wrist

   √7ᵗʰ **S62.031** **Displaced** fracture of proximal third of navicular [scaphoid] bone of **right** wrist   CC H5 PE

   √7ᵗʰ **S62.032** **Displaced** fracture of proximal third of navicular [scaphoid] bone of **left** wrist   CC H5 PE

   √7ᵗʰ **S62.033** **Displaced** fracture of proximal third of navicular [scaphoid] bone of unspecified wrist   CC H5 UNS PE

   √7ᵗʰ **S62.034** **Nondisplaced** fracture of proximal third of navicular [scaphoid] bone of **right** wrist   CC H5 PE

   √7ᵗʰ **S62.035** **Nondisplaced** fracture of proximal third of navicular [scaphoid] bone of **left** wrist   CC H5 PE

   √7ᵗʰ **S62.036** **Nondisplaced** fracture of proximal third of navicular [scaphoid] bone of unspecified wrist   CC H5 UNS PE

√5ᵗʰ **S62.1** Fracture of other and unspecified **carpal** bone(s)

   EXCLUDES 2   *fracture of scaphoid of wrist (S62.0-)*

  √6ᵗʰ **S62.10** Fracture of unspecified carpal bone

   Fracture of wrist NOS

   √7ᵗʰ **S62.101** Fracture of unspecified carpal bone, **right** wrist   CC H5 PE

   √7ᵗʰ **S62.102** Fracture of unspecified carpal bone, **left** wrist   CC H5 PE

     AHA: 2012,4Q,95

   √7ᵗʰ **S62.109** Fracture of unspecified carpal bone, unspecified wrist   CC H5 UNS PE

  √6ᵗʰ **S62.11** Fracture of **triquetrum** [cuneiform] bone of wrist

   √7ᵗʰ **S62.111** **Displaced** fracture of triquetrum [cuneiform] bone, **right** wrist   CC H5 PE

   √7ᵗʰ **S62.112** **Displaced** fracture of triquetrum [cuneiform] bone, **left** wrist   CC H5 PE

   √7ᵗʰ **S62.113** **Displaced** fracture of triquetrum [cuneiform] bone, unspecified wrist   CC H5 UNS PE

   √7ᵗʰ **S62.114** **Nondisplaced** fracture of triquetrum [cuneiform] bone, **right** wrist   CC H5 PE

   √7ᵗʰ **S62.115** **Nondisplaced** fracture of triquetrum [cuneiform] bone, **left** wrist   CC H5 PE

   √7ᵗʰ **S62.116** **Nondisplaced** fracture of triquetrum [cuneiform] bone, unspecified wrist   CC H5 UNS PE

  √6ᵗʰ **S62.12** Fracture of **lunate** [semilunar]

   √7ᵗʰ **S62.121** **Displaced** fracture of lunate [semilunar], **right** wrist   CC H5 PE

   √7ᵗʰ **S62.122** **Displaced** fracture of lunate [semilunar], **left** wrist   CC H5 PE

   √7ᵗʰ **S62.123** **Displaced** fracture of lunate [semilunar], unspecified wrist   CC H5 UNS PE

   √7ᵗʰ **S62.124** **Nondisplaced** fracture of lunate [semilunar], **right** wrist   CC H5 PE

   √7ᵗʰ **S62.125** **Nondisplaced** fracture of lunate [semilunar], **left** wrist   CC H5 PE

   √7ᵗʰ **S62.126** **Nondisplaced** fracture of lunate [semilunar], unspecified wrist   CC H5 UNS PE

  √6ᵗʰ **S62.13** Fracture of **capitate** [os magnum] bone

   √7ᵗʰ **S62.131** **Displaced** fracture of capitate [os magnum] bone, **right** wrist   CC H5 PE

   √7ᵗʰ **S62.132** **Displaced** fracture of capitate [os magnum] bone, **left** wrist   CC H5 PE

   √7ᵗʰ **S62.133** **Displaced** fracture of capitate [os magnum] bone, unspecified wrist   CC H5 UNS PE

   √7ᵗʰ **S62.134** **Nondisplaced** fracture of capitate [os magnum] bone, **right** wrist   CC H5 PE

   √7ᵗʰ **S62.135** **Nondisplaced** fracture of capitate [os magnum] bone, **left** wrist   CC H5 PE

   √7ᵗʰ **S62.136** **Nondisplaced** fracture of capitate [os magnum] bone, unspecified wrist   CC H5 UNS PE

  √6ᵗʰ **S62.14** Fracture of **body of hamate** [unciform] bone

   Fracture of hamate [unciform] bone NOS

   √7ᵗʰ **S62.141** **Displaced** fracture of body of hamate [unciform] bone, **right** wrist   CC H5 PE

   √7ᵗʰ **S62.142** **Displaced** fracture of body of hamate [unciform] bone, **left** wrist   CC H5 PE

   √7ᵗʰ **S62.143** **Displaced** fracture of body of hamate [unciform] bone, unspecified wrist   CC H5 UNS PE

   √7ᵗʰ **S62.144** **Nondisplaced** fracture of body of hamate [unciform] bone, **right** wrist   CC H5 PE

   √7ᵗʰ **S62.145** **Nondisplaced** fracture of body of hamate [unciform] bone, **left** wrist   CC H5 PE

   √7ᵗʰ **S62.146** **Nondisplaced** fracture of body of hamate [unciform] bone, unspecified wrist   CC H5 UNS PE

  √6ᵗʰ **S62.15** Fracture of **hook process of hamate** [unciform] bone

   Fracture of unciform process of hamate [unciform] bone

   √7ᵗʰ **S62.151** **Displaced** fracture of hook process of hamate [unciform] bone, **right** wrist   CC H5 PE

   √7ᵗʰ **S62.152** **Displaced** fracture of hook process of hamate [unciform] bone, **left** wrist   CC H5 PE

   √7ᵗʰ **S62.153** **Displaced** fracture of hook process of hamate [unciform] bone, unspecified wrist   CC H5 UNS PE

   √7ᵗʰ **S62.154** **Nondisplaced** fracture of hook process of hamate [unciform] bone, **right** wrist   CC H5 PE

   √7ᵗʰ **S62.155** **Nondisplaced** fracture of hook process of hamate [unciform] bone, **left** wrist   CC H5 PE

   √7ᵗʰ **S62.156** **Nondisplaced** fracture of hook process of hamate [unciform] bone, unspecified wrist   CC H5 UNS PE

  √6ᵗʰ **S62.16** Fracture of **pisiform**

   √7ᵗʰ **S62.161** **Displaced** fracture of pisiform, **right** wrist   CC H5 PE

   √7ᵗʰ **S62.162** **Displaced** fracture of pisiform, **left** wrist   CC H5 PE

   √7ᵗʰ **S62.163** **Displaced** fracture of pisiform, unspecified wrist   CC H5 UNS PE

   √7ᵗʰ **S62.164** **Nondisplaced** fracture of pisiform, **right** wrist   CC H5 PE

   √7ᵗʰ **S62.165** **Nondisplaced** fracture of pisiform, **left** wrist   CC H5 PE

   √7ᵗʰ **S62.166** **Nondisplaced** fracture of pisiform, unspecified wrist   CC H5 UNS PE

  √6ᵗʰ **S62.17** Fracture of **trapezium** [larger multangular]

   √7ᵗʰ **S62.171** **Displaced** fracture of trapezium [larger multangular], **right** wrist   CC H5 PE

   √7ᵗʰ **S62.172** **Displaced** fracture of trapezium [larger multangular], **left** wrist   CC H5 PE

   √7ᵗʰ **S62.173** **Displaced** fracture of trapezium [larger multangular], unspecified wrist   CC H5 UNS PE

   √7ᵗʰ **S62.174** **Nondisplaced** fracture of trapezium [larger multangular], **right** wrist   CC H5 PE

   √7ᵗʰ **S62.175** **Nondisplaced** fracture of trapezium [larger multangular], **left** wrist   CC H5 PE

   √7ᵗʰ **S62.176** **Nondisplaced** fracture of trapezium [larger multangular], unspecified wrist   CC H5 UNS PE

  √6ᵗʰ **S62.18** Fracture of **trapezoid** [smaller multangular]

   √7ᵗʰ **S62.181** **Displaced** fracture of trapezoid [smaller multangular], **right** wrist   CC H5 PE

   √7ᵗʰ **S62.182** **Displaced** fracture of trapezoid [smaller multangular], **left** wrist   CC H5 PE

   √7ᵗʰ **S62.183** **Displaced** fracture of trapezoid [smaller multangular], unspecified wrist   CC H5 UNS PE

   √7ᵗʰ **S62.184** **Nondisplaced** fracture of trapezoid [smaller multangular], **right** wrist   CC H5 PE

   √7ᵗʰ **S62.185** **Nondisplaced** fracture of trapezoid [smaller multangular], **left** wrist   CC H5 PE

   √7ᵗʰ **S62.186** **Nondisplaced** fracture of trapezoid [smaller multangular], unspecified wrist   CC H5 UNS PE

✓ Additional Character Required   √x7ᵗʰ Placeholder   Questionable PDx   Manifestation   Unspecified   UPD Unacceptable PDx   H1-H14 HAC   HCC CMS-HCC Dx   HIV HIV Dx

ICD-10-CM 2025   1059

√5ᵗʰ **S62.2** **Fracture of first metacarpal bone**

    √6ᵗʰ **S62.20** **Unspecified fracture of first metacarpal bone**

        √7ᵗʰ **S62.201** **Unspecified fracture of first metacarpal bone, right hand** `CC` `H5` `PE`

        √7ᵗʰ **S62.202** **Unspecified fracture of first metacarpal bone, left hand** `CC` `H5` `PE`

        √7ᵗʰ **S62.209** **Unspecified fracture of first metacarpal bone, unspecified hand** `CC` `H5` `UNS` `PE`

    √6ᵗʰ **S62.21** **Bennett's fracture**

        DEF: Intra-articular, two-part fracture at the base of the first metacarpal bone (thumb) on the ulnar side at the carpometacarpal (CMC) joint.

        √7ᵗʰ **S62.211** **Bennett's fracture, right hand** `CC` `H5` `PE`

        √7ᵗʰ **S62.212** **Bennett's fracture, left hand** `CC` `H5` `PE`

        √7ᵗʰ **S62.213** **Bennett's fracture, unspecified hand** `CC` `H5` `UNS` `PE`

    √6ᵗʰ **S62.22** **Rolando's fracture**

        DEF: Comminuted, three part intra-articular fracture at the base of the thumb metacarpal.

        √7ᵗʰ **S62.221** **Displaced Rolando's fracture, right hand** `CC` `H5` `PE`

        √7ᵗʰ **S62.222** **Displaced Rolando's fracture, left hand** `CC` `H5` `PE`

        √7ᵗʰ **S62.223** **Displaced Rolando's fracture, unspecified hand** `CC` `H5` `UNS` `PE`

        √7ᵗʰ **S62.224** **Nondisplaced Rolando's fracture, right hand** `CC` `H5` `PE`

        √7ᵗʰ **S62.225** **Nondisplaced Rolando's fracture, left hand** `CC` `H5` `PE`

        √7ᵗʰ **S62.226** **Nondisplaced Rolando's fracture, unspecified hand** `CC` `H5` `UNS` `PE`

    √6ᵗʰ **S62.23** **Other fracture of base of first metacarpal bone**

        √7ᵗʰ **S62.231** **Other displaced fracture of base of first metacarpal bone, right hand** `CC` `H5` `PE`

        √7ᵗʰ **S62.232** **Other displaced fracture of base of first metacarpal bone, left hand** `CC` `H5` `PE`

        √7ᵗʰ **S62.233** **Other displaced fracture of base of first metacarpal bone, unspecified hand** `CC` `H5` `UNS` `PE`

        √7ᵗʰ **S62.234** **Other nondisplaced fracture of base of first metacarpal bone, right hand** `CC` `H5` `PE`

        √7ᵗʰ **S62.235** **Other nondisplaced fracture of base of first metacarpal bone, left hand** `CC` `H5` `PE`

        √7ᵗʰ **S62.236** **Other nondisplaced fracture of base of first metacarpal bone, unspecified hand** `CC` `H5` `UNS` `PE`

    √6ᵗʰ **S62.24** **Fracture of shaft of first metacarpal bone**

        √7ᵗʰ **S62.241** **Displaced fracture of shaft of first metacarpal bone, right hand** `CC` `H5` `PE`

        √7ᵗʰ **S62.242** **Displaced fracture of shaft of first metacarpal bone, left hand** `CC` `H5` `PE`

        √7ᵗʰ **S62.243** **Displaced fracture of shaft of first metacarpal bone, unspecified hand** `CC` `H5` `UNS` `PE`

        √7ᵗʰ **S62.244** **Nondisplaced fracture of shaft of first metacarpal bone, right hand** `CC` `H5` `PE`

        √7ᵗʰ **S62.245** **Nondisplaced fracture of shaft of first metacarpal bone, left hand** `CC` `H5` `PE`

        √7ᵗʰ **S62.246** **Nondisplaced fracture of shaft of first metacarpal bone, unspecified hand** `CC` `H5` `UNS` `PE`

    √6ᵗʰ **S62.25** **Fracture of neck of first metacarpal bone**

        √7ᵗʰ **S62.251** **Displaced fracture of neck of first metacarpal bone, right hand** `CC` `H5` `PE`

        √7ᵗʰ **S62.252** **Displaced fracture of neck of first metacarpal bone, left hand** `CC` `H5` `PE`

        √7ᵗʰ **S62.253** **Displaced fracture of neck of first metacarpal bone, unspecified hand** `CC` `H5` `UNS` `PE`

        √7ᵗʰ **S62.254** **Nondisplaced fracture of neck of first metacarpal bone, right hand** `CC` `H5` `PE`

        √7ᵗʰ **S62.255** **Nondisplaced fracture of neck of first metacarpal bone, left hand** `CC` `H5` `PE`

        √7ᵗʰ **S62.256** **Nondisplaced fracture of neck of first metacarpal bone, unspecified hand** `CC` `H5` `UNS` `PE`

√6ᵗʰ **S62.29** **Other fracture of first metacarpal bone**

    √7ᵗʰ **S62.291** **Other fracture of first metacarpal bone, right hand** `CC` `H5` `PE`

    √7ᵗʰ **S62.292** **Other fracture of first metacarpal bone, left hand** `CC` `H5` `PE`

    √7ᵗʰ **S62.299** **Other fracture of first metacarpal bone, unspecified hand** `CC` `H5` `UNS` `PE`

√5ᵗʰ **S62.3** **Fracture of other and unspecified metacarpal bone**

    EXCLUDES 2   fracture of first metacarpal bone (S62.2-)

    √6ᵗʰ **S62.30** **Unspecified fracture of other metacarpal bone**

        √7ᵗʰ **S62.300** **Unspecified fracture of second metacarpal bone, right hand** `CC` `H5` `PE`

        √7ᵗʰ **S62.301** **Unspecified fracture of second metacarpal bone, left hand** `CC` `H5` `PE`

        √7ᵗʰ **S62.302** **Unspecified fracture of third metacarpal bone, right hand** `CC` `H5` `PE`

        √7ᵗʰ **S62.303** **Unspecified fracture of third metacarpal bone, left hand** `CC` `H5` `PE`

        √7ᵗʰ **S62.304** **Unspecified fracture of fourth metacarpal bone, right hand** `CC` `H5` `PE`

        √7ᵗʰ **S62.305** **Unspecified fracture of fourth metacarpal bone, left hand** `CC` `H5` `PE`

        √7ᵗʰ **S62.306** **Unspecified fracture of fifth metacarpal bone, right hand** `CC` `H5` `PE`

        √7ᵗʰ **S62.307** **Unspecified fracture of fifth metacarpal bone, left hand** `CC` `H5` `PE`

        √7ᵗʰ **S62.308** **Unspecified fracture of other metacarpal bone** `CC` `H5` `PE`

            Unspecified fracture of specified metacarpal bone with unspecified laterality

        √7ᵗʰ **S62.309** **Unspecified fracture of unspecified metacarpal bone** `CC` `H5` `UNS` `PE`

    √6ᵗʰ **S62.31** **Displaced fracture of base of other metacarpal bone**

        √7ᵗʰ **S62.310** **Displaced fracture of base of second metacarpal bone, right hand** `CC` `H5` `PE`

        √7ᵗʰ **S62.311** **Displaced fracture of base of second metacarpal bone, left hand** `CC` `H5` `PE`

        √7ᵗʰ **S62.312** **Displaced fracture of base of third metacarpal bone, right hand** `CC` `H5` `PE`

        √7ᵗʰ **S62.313** **Displaced fracture of base of third metacarpal bone, left hand** `CC` `H5` `PE`

        √7ᵗʰ **S62.314** **Displaced fracture of base of fourth metacarpal bone, right hand** `CC` `H5` `PE`

        √7ᵗʰ **S62.315** **Displaced fracture of base of fourth metacarpal bone, left hand** `CC` `H5` `PE`

        √7ᵗʰ **S62.316** **Displaced fracture of base of fifth metacarpal bone, right hand** `CC` `H5` `PE`

        √7ᵗʰ **S62.317** **Displaced fracture of base of fifth metacarpal bone, left hand** `CC` `H5` `PE`

        √7ᵗʰ **S62.318** **Displaced fracture of base of other metacarpal bone** `CC` `H5` `PE`

            Displaced fracture of base of specified metacarpal bone with unspecified laterality

        √7ᵗʰ **S62.319** **Displaced fracture of base of unspecified metacarpal bone** `CC` `H5` `UNS` `PE`

    √6ᵗʰ **S62.32** **Displaced fracture of shaft of other metacarpal bone**

        √7ᵗʰ **S62.320** **Displaced fracture of shaft of second metacarpal bone, right hand** `CC` `H5` `PE`

        √7ᵗʰ **S62.321** **Displaced fracture of shaft of second metacarpal bone, left hand** `CC` `H5` `PE`

        √7ᵗʰ **S62.322** **Displaced fracture of shaft of third metacarpal bone, right hand** `CC` `H5` `PE`

        √7ᵗʰ **S62.323** **Displaced fracture of shaft of third metacarpal bone, left hand** `CC` `H5` `PE`

        √7ᵗʰ **S62.324** **Displaced fracture of shaft of fourth metacarpal bone, right hand** `CC` `H5` `PE`

        √7ᵗʰ **S62.325** **Displaced fracture of shaft of fourth metacarpal bone, left hand** `CC` `H5` `PE`

        √7ᵗʰ **S62.326** **Displaced fracture of shaft of fifth metacarpal bone, right hand** `CC` `H5` `PE`

        √7ᵗʰ **S62.327** **Displaced fracture of shaft of fifth metacarpal bone, left hand** `CC` `H5` `PE`

`N` Newborn: 0   `P` Pediatric: 0-17   `M` Maternity: 9-64   `A` Adult: 15-124   `UNS` Unspecified Site   `MCC` Major Complication/Comorbidity   `CC` Complication/Comorbidity   `PE` POA Exempt

1060   ICD-10-CM 2025

√7ᵗʰ **S62.328** **Displaced fracture of shaft of other metacarpal bone** `CC` `H5` `PE`
    Displaced fracture of shaft of specified metacarpal bone with unspecified laterality

√7ᵗʰ **S62.329** **Displaced fracture of shaft of unspecified metacarpal bone** `CC` `H5` `UNS` `PE`

√6ᵗʰ **S62.33** **Displaced fracture of neck of other metacarpal bone**

√7ᵗʰ **S62.330** **Displaced fracture of neck of second metacarpal bone, right hand** `CC` `H5` `PE`

√7ᵗʰ **S62.331** **Displaced fracture of neck of second metacarpal bone, left hand** `CC` `H5` `PE`

√7ᵗʰ **S62.332** **Displaced fracture of neck of third metacarpal bone, right hand** `CC` `H5` `PE`

√7ᵗʰ **S62.333** **Displaced fracture of neck of third metacarpal bone, left hand** `CC` `H5` `PE`

√7ᵗʰ **S62.334** **Displaced fracture of neck of fourth metacarpal bone, right hand** `CC` `H5` `PE`

√7ᵗʰ **S62.335** **Displaced fracture of neck of fourth metacarpal bone, left hand** `CC` `H5` `PE`

√7ᵗʰ **S62.336** **Displaced fracture of neck of fifth metacarpal bone, right hand** `CC` `H5` `PE`

√7ᵗʰ **S62.337** **Displaced fracture of neck of fifth metacarpal bone, left hand** `CC` `H5` `PE`

√7ᵗʰ **S62.338** **Displaced fracture of neck of other metacarpal bone** `CC` `H5` `PE`
    Displaced fracture of neck of specified metacarpal bone with unspecified laterality

√7ᵗʰ **S62.339** **Displaced fracture of neck of unspecified metacarpal bone** `CC` `H5` `UNS` `PE`

√6ᵗʰ **S62.34** **Nondisplaced fracture of base of other metacarpal bone**

√7ᵗʰ **S62.340** **Nondisplaced fracture of base of second metacarpal bone, right hand** `CC` `H5` `PE`

√7ᵗʰ **S62.341** **Nondisplaced fracture of base of second metacarpal bone, left hand** `CC` `H5` `PE`

√7ᵗʰ **S62.342** **Nondisplaced fracture of base of third metacarpal bone, right hand** `CC` `H5` `PE`

√7ᵗʰ **S62.343** **Nondisplaced fracture of base of third metacarpal bone, left hand** `CC` `H5` `PE`

√7ᵗʰ **S62.344** **Nondisplaced fracture of base of fourth metacarpal bone, right hand** `CC` `H5` `PE`

√7ᵗʰ **S62.345** **Nondisplaced fracture of base of fourth metacarpal bone, left hand** `CC` `H5` `PE`

√7ᵗʰ **S62.346** **Nondisplaced fracture of base of fifth metacarpal bone, right hand** `CC` `H5` `PE`

√7ᵗʰ **S62.347** **Nondisplaced fracture of base of fifth metacarpal bone, left hand** `CC` `H5` `PE`

√7ᵗʰ **S62.348** **Nondisplaced fracture of base of other metacarpal bone** `CC` `H5` `PE`
    Nondisplaced fracture of base of specified metacarpal bone with unspecified laterality

√7ᵗʰ **S62.349** **Nondisplaced fracture of base of unspecified metacarpal bone** `CC` `H5` `UNS` `PE`

√6ᵗʰ **S62.35** **Nondisplaced fracture of shaft of other metacarpal bone**

√7ᵗʰ **S62.350** **Nondisplaced fracture of shaft of second metacarpal bone, right hand** `CC` `H5` `PE`

√7ᵗʰ **S62.351** **Nondisplaced fracture of shaft of second metacarpal bone, left hand** `CC` `H5` `PE`

√7ᵗʰ **S62.352** **Nondisplaced fracture of shaft of third metacarpal bone, right hand** `CC` `H5` `PE`

√7ᵗʰ **S62.353** **Nondisplaced fracture of shaft of third metacarpal bone, left hand** `CC` `H5` `PE`

√7ᵗʰ **S62.354** **Nondisplaced fracture of shaft of fourth metacarpal bone, right hand** `CC` `H5` `PE`

√7ᵗʰ **S62.355** **Nondisplaced fracture of shaft of fourth metacarpal bone, left hand** `CC` `H5` `PE`

√7ᵗʰ **S62.356** **Nondisplaced fracture of shaft of fifth metacarpal bone, right hand** `CC` `H5` `PE`

√7ᵗʰ **S62.357** **Nondisplaced fracture of shaft of fifth metacarpal bone, left hand** `CC` `H5` `PE`

√7ᵗʰ **S62.358** **Nondisplaced fracture of shaft of other metacarpal bone** `CC` `H5` `PE`
    Nondisplaced fracture of shaft of specified metacarpal bone with unspecified laterality

√7ᵗʰ **S62.359** **Nondisplaced fracture of shaft of unspecified metacarpal bone** `CC` `H5` `UNS` `PE`

√6ᵗʰ **S62.36** **Nondisplaced fracture of neck of other metacarpal bone**

√7ᵗʰ **S62.360** **Nondisplaced fracture of neck of second metacarpal bone, right hand** `CC` `H5` `PE`

√7ᵗʰ **S62.361** **Nondisplaced fracture of neck of second metacarpal bone, left hand** `CC` `H5` `PE`

√7ᵗʰ **S62.362** **Nondisplaced fracture of neck of third metacarpal bone, right hand** `CC` `H5` `PE`

√7ᵗʰ **S62.363** **Nondisplaced fracture of neck of third metacarpal bone, left hand** `CC` `H5` `PE`

√7ᵗʰ **S62.364** **Nondisplaced fracture of neck of fourth metacarpal bone, right hand** `CC` `H5` `PE`

√7ᵗʰ **S62.365** **Nondisplaced fracture of neck of fourth metacarpal bone, left hand** `CC` `H5` `PE`

√7ᵗʰ **S62.366** **Nondisplaced fracture of neck of fifth metacarpal bone, right hand** `CC` `H5` `PE`

√7ᵗʰ **S62.367** **Nondisplaced fracture of neck of fifth metacarpal bone, left hand** `CC` `H5` `PE`

√7ᵗʰ **S62.368** **Nondisplaced fracture of neck of other metacarpal bone** `CC` `H5` `PE`
    Nondisplaced fracture of neck of specified metacarpal bone with unspecified laterality

√7ᵗʰ **S62.369** **Nondisplaced fracture of neck of unspecified metacarpal bone** `CC` `H5` `UNS` `PE`

√6ᵗʰ **S62.39** **Other fracture of other metacarpal bone**

√7ᵗʰ **S62.390** **Other fracture of second metacarpal bone, right hand** `CC` `H5` `PE`

√7ᵗʰ **S62.391** **Other fracture of second metacarpal bone, left hand** `CC` `H5` `PE`

√7ᵗʰ **S62.392** **Other fracture of third metacarpal bone, right hand** `CC` `H5` `PE`

√7ᵗʰ **S62.393** **Other fracture of third metacarpal bone, left hand** `CC` `H5` `PE`

√7ᵗʰ **S62.394** **Other fracture of fourth metacarpal bone, right hand** `CC` `H5` `PE`

√7ᵗʰ **S62.395** **Other fracture of fourth metacarpal bone, left hand** `CC` `H5` `PE`

√7ᵗʰ **S62.396** **Other fracture of fifth metacarpal bone, right hand** `CC` `H5` `PE`

√7ᵗʰ **S62.397** **Other fracture of fifth metacarpal bone, left hand** `CC` `H5` `PE`

√7ᵗʰ **S62.398** **Other fracture of other metacarpal bone** `CC` `H5` `PE`
    Other fracture of specified metacarpal bone with unspecified laterality

√7ᵗʰ **S62.399** **Other fracture of unspecified metacarpal bone** `CC` `H5` `UNS` `PE`

√5ᵗʰ **S62.5** **Fracture of thumb**

√6ᵗʰ **S62.50** **Fracture of unspecified phalanx of thumb**

√7ᵗʰ **S62.501** **Fracture of unspecified phalanx of right thumb** `CC` `H5` `PE`

√7ᵗʰ **S62.502** **Fracture of unspecified phalanx of left thumb** `CC` `H5` `PE`

√7ᵗʰ **S62.509** **Fracture of unspecified phalanx of unspecified thumb** `CC` `H5` `UNS` `PE`

√6ᵗʰ **S62.51** **Fracture of proximal phalanx of thumb**

√7ᵗʰ **S62.511** **Displaced fracture of proximal phalanx of right thumb** `CC` `H5` `PE`

√7ᵗʰ **S62.512** **Displaced fracture of proximal phalanx of left thumb** `CC` `H5` `PE`

√7ᵗʰ **S62.513** **Displaced fracture of proximal phalanx of unspecified thumb** `CC` `H5` `UNS` `PE`

√7ᵗʰ **S62.514** **Nondisplaced fracture of proximal phalanx of right thumb** `CC` `H5` `PE`

√7ᵗʰ **S62.515** **Nondisplaced fracture of proximal phalanx of left thumb** `CC` `H5` `PE`

√7ᵗʰ **S62.516** **Nondisplaced fracture of proximal phalanx of unspecified thumb** `CC` `H5` `PE`

✔ Additional Character Required   √x7ᵗʰ Placeholder   Questionable PDx   Manifestation   Unspecified   `UPD` Unacceptable PDx   `H1`-`H14` HAC   `HCC` CMS-HCC Dx   `HIV` HIV Dx

Chapter 19. Injury, Poisoning and Certain Other Consequences of External Causes

S62.52–S62.657

✓6ᵗʰ **S62.52** **Fracture of distal phalanx of thumb**
- ✓7ᵗʰ **S62.521** Displaced fracture of distal phalanx of right thumb   `CC` `H5` `PE`
- ✓7ᵗʰ **S62.522** Displaced fracture of distal phalanx of left thumb   `CC` `PE`
- ✓7ᵗʰ **S62.523** Displaced fracture of distal phalanx of unspecified thumb   `CC` `H5` `UNS` `PE`
- ✓7ᵗʰ **S62.524** Nondisplaced fracture of distal phalanx of right thumb   `CC` `H5` `PE`
- ✓7ᵗʰ **S62.525** Nondisplaced fracture of distal phalanx of left thumb   `CC` `H5` `PE`
- ✓7ᵗʰ **S62.526** Nondisplaced fracture of distal phalanx of unspecified thumb   `CC` `H5` `UNS` `PE`

✓5ᵗʰ **S62.6** **Fracture of other and unspecified finger(s)**

     EXCLUDES 2   *fracture of thumb (S62.5-)*

✓6ᵗʰ **S62.60** **Fracture of unspecified phalanx of finger**
- ✓7ᵗʰ **S62.600** Fracture of unspecified phalanx of right index finger   `CC` `H5` `PE`
- ✓7ᵗʰ **S62.601** Fracture of unspecified phalanx of left index finger   `CC` `H5` `PE`
- ✓7ᵗʰ **S62.602** Fracture of unspecified phalanx of right middle finger   `CC` `H5` `PE`
- ✓7ᵗʰ **S62.603** Fracture of unspecified phalanx of left middle finger   `CC` `H5` `PE`
- ✓7ᵗʰ **S62.604** Fracture of unspecified phalanx of right ring finger   `CC` `H5` `PE`
- ✓7ᵗʰ **S62.605** Fracture of unspecified phalanx of left ring finger   `CC` `H5` `PE`
- ✓7ᵗʰ **S62.606** Fracture of unspecified phalanx of right little finger   `CC` `H5` `PE`
- ✓7ᵗʰ **S62.607** Fracture of unspecified phalanx of left little finger   `CC` `H5` `PE`
- ✓7ᵗʰ **S62.608** Fracture of unspecified phalanx of other finger   `CC` `H5` `PE`
  Fracture of unspecified phalanx of specified finger with unspecified laterality
- ✓7ᵗʰ **S62.609** Fracture of unspecified phalanx of unspecified finger   `CC` `H5` `UNS` `PE`

✓6ᵗʰ **S62.61** **Displaced fracture of proximal phalanx of finger**
- ✓7ᵗʰ **S62.610** Displaced fracture of proximal phalanx of right index finger   `CC` `H5` `PE`
- ✓7ᵗʰ **S62.611** Displaced fracture of proximal phalanx of left index finger   `CC` `H5` `PE`
- ✓7ᵗʰ **S62.612** Displaced fracture of proximal phalanx of right middle finger   `CC` `H5` `PE`
- ✓7ᵗʰ **S62.613** Displaced fracture of proximal phalanx of left middle finger   `CC` `H5` `PE`
- ✓7ᵗʰ **S62.614** Displaced fracture of proximal phalanx of right ring finger   `CC` `H5` `PE`
- ✓7ᵗʰ **S62.615** Displaced fracture of proximal phalanx of left ring finger   `CC` `H5` `PE`
- ✓7ᵗʰ **S62.616** Displaced fracture of proximal phalanx of right little finger   `CC` `H5` `PE`
- ✓7ᵗʰ **S62.617** Displaced fracture of proximal phalanx of left little finger   `CC` `H5` `PE`
- ✓7ᵗʰ **S62.618** Displaced fracture of proximal phalanx of other finger   `CC` `H5` `PE`
  Displaced fracture of proximal phalanx of specified finger with unspecified laterality
- ✓7ᵗʰ **S62.619** Displaced fracture of proximal phalanx of unspecified finger   `CC` `H5` `UNS` `PE`

✓6ᵗʰ **S62.62** **Displaced fracture of middle phalanx of finger**
- ✓7ᵗʰ **S62.620** Displaced fracture of middle phalanx of right index finger   `CC` `H5` `PE`
- ✓7ᵗʰ **S62.621** Displaced fracture of middle phalanx of left index finger   `CC` `H5` `PE`
- ✓7ᵗʰ **S62.622** Displaced fracture of middle phalanx of right middle finger   `CC` `H5` `PE`
- ✓7ᵗʰ **S62.623** Displaced fracture of middle phalanx of left middle finger   `CC` `H5` `PE`
- ✓7ᵗʰ **S62.624** Displaced fracture of middle phalanx of right ring finger   `CC` `H5` `PE`
- ✓7ᵗʰ **S62.625** Displaced fracture of middle phalanx of left ring finger   `CC` `H5` `PE`
- ✓7ᵗʰ **S62.626** Displaced fracture of middle phalanx of right little finger   `CC` `H5` `PE`
- ✓7ᵗʰ **S62.627** Displaced fracture of middle phalanx of left little finger   `CC` `H5` `PE`
- ✓7ᵗʰ **S62.628** Displaced fracture of middle phalanx of other finger   `CC` `H5` `PE`
  Displaced fracture of middle phalanx of specified finger with unspecified laterality
- ✓7ᵗʰ **S62.629** Displaced fracture of middle phalanx of unspecified finger   `CC` `H5` `UNS` `PE`

✓6ᵗʰ **S62.63** **Displaced fracture of distal phalanx of finger**
- ✓7ᵗʰ **S62.630** Displaced fracture of distal phalanx of right index finger   `CC` `H5` `PE`
- ✓7ᵗʰ **S62.631** Displaced fracture of distal phalanx of left index finger   `CC` `H5` `PE`
- ✓7ᵗʰ **S62.632** Displaced fracture of distal phalanx of right middle finger   `CC` `H5` `PE`
- ✓7ᵗʰ **S62.633** Displaced fracture of distal phalanx of left middle finger   `CC` `H5` `PE`
- ✓7ᵗʰ **S62.634** Displaced fracture of distal phalanx of right ring finger   `CC` `H5` `PE`
- ✓7ᵗʰ **S62.635** Displaced fracture of distal phalanx of left ring finger   `CC` `H5` `PE`
- ✓7ᵗʰ **S62.636** Displaced fracture of distal phalanx of right little finger   `CC` `H5` `PE`
- ✓7ᵗʰ **S62.637** Displaced fracture of distal phalanx of left little finger   `CC` `H5` `PE`
- ✓7ᵗʰ **S62.638** Displaced fracture of distal phalanx of other finger   `CC` `H5` `PE`
  Displaced fracture of distal phalanx of specified finger with unspecified laterality
- ✓7ᵗʰ **S62.639** Displaced fracture of distal phalanx of unspecified finger   `CC` `H5` `UNS` `PE`

✓6ᵗʰ **S62.64** **Nondisplaced fracture of proximal phalanx of finger**
- ✓7ᵗʰ **S62.640** Nondisplaced fracture of proximal phalanx of right index finger   `CC` `H5` `PE`
- ✓7ᵗʰ **S62.641** Nondisplaced fracture of proximal phalanx of left index finger   `CC` `H5` `PE`
- ✓7ᵗʰ **S62.642** Nondisplaced fracture of proximal phalanx of right middle finger   `CC` `H5` `PE`
- ✓7ᵗʰ **S62.643** Nondisplaced fracture of proximal phalanx of left middle finger   `CC` `H5` `PE`
- ✓7ᵗʰ **S62.644** Nondisplaced fracture of proximal phalanx of right ring finger   `CC` `H5` `PE`
- ✓7ᵗʰ **S62.645** Nondisplaced fracture of proximal phalanx of left ring finger   `CC` `H5` `PE`
- ✓7ᵗʰ **S62.646** Nondisplaced fracture of proximal phalanx of right little finger   `CC` `H5` `PE`
- ✓7ᵗʰ **S62.647** Nondisplaced fracture of proximal phalanx of left little finger   `CC` `H5` `PE`
- ✓7ᵗʰ **S62.648** Nondisplaced fracture of proximal phalanx of other finger   `CC` `H5` `PE`
  Nondisplaced fracture of proximal phalanx of specified finger with unspecified laterality
- ✓7ᵗʰ **S62.649** Nondisplaced fracture of proximal phalanx of unspecified finger   `CC` `H5` `UNS` `PE`

✓6ᵗʰ **S62.65** **Nondisplaced fracture of middle phalanx of finger**
- ✓7ᵗʰ **S62.650** Nondisplaced fracture of middle phalanx of right index finger   `CC` `H5` `PE`
- ✓7ᵗʰ **S62.651** Nondisplaced fracture of middle phalanx of left index finger   `CC` `H5` `PE`
- ✓7ᵗʰ **S62.652** Nondisplaced fracture of middle phalanx of right middle finger   `CC` `H5` `PE`
- ✓7ᵗʰ **S62.653** Nondisplaced fracture of middle phalanx of left middle finger   `CC` `H5` `PE`
- ✓7ᵗʰ **S62.654** Nondisplaced fracture of middle phalanx of right ring finger   `CC` `H5` `PE`
- ✓7ᵗʰ **S62.655** Nondisplaced fracture of middle phalanx of left ring finger   `CC` `H5` `PE`
- ✓7ᵗʰ **S62.656** Nondisplaced fracture of middle phalanx of right little finger   `CC` `H5` `PE`
- ✓7ᵗʰ **S62.657** Nondisplaced fracture of middle phalanx of left little finger   `CC` `H5` `PE`

`N` Newborn: 0   `P` Pediatric: 0-17   `M` Maternity: 9-64   `A` Adult: 15-124   `UNS` Unspecified Site   `MCC` Major Complication/Comorbidity   `CC` Complication/Comorbidity   `PE` POA Exempt

1062   ICD-10-CM 2025

√7ᵗʰ **S62.658 Nondisplaced fracture of middle phalanx of other finger** `CC` `H5` `PE`
    Nondisplaced fracture of middle phalanx of specified finger with unspecified laterality

√7ᵗʰ **S62.659 Nondisplaced fracture of middle phalanx of unspecified finger** `CC` `H5` `UNS` `PE`

√6ᵗʰ **S62.66 Nondisplaced fracture of distal phalanx of finger**

√7ᵗʰ **S62.660 Nondisplaced fracture of distal phalanx of right index finger** `CC` `H5` `PE`

√7ᵗʰ **S62.661 Nondisplaced fracture of distal phalanx of left index finger** `CC` `H5` `PE`

√7ᵗʰ **S62.662 Nondisplaced fracture of distal phalanx of right middle finger** `CC` `H5` `PE`

√7ᵗʰ **S62.663 Nondisplaced fracture of distal phalanx of left middle finger** `CC` `H5` `PE`

√7ᵗʰ **S62.664 Nondisplaced fracture of distal phalanx of right ring finger** `CC` `H5` `PE`

√7ᵗʰ **S62.665 Nondisplaced fracture of distal phalanx of left ring finger** `CC` `H5` `PE`

√7ᵗʰ **S62.666 Nondisplaced fracture of distal phalanx of right little finger** `CC` `H5` `PE`

√7ᵗʰ **S62.667 Nondisplaced fracture of distal phalanx of left little finger** `CC` `H5` `PE`

√7ᵗʰ **S62.668 Nondisplaced fracture of distal phalanx of other finger** `CC` `H5` `PE`
    Nondisplaced fracture of distal phalanx of specified finger with unspecified laterality

√7ᵗʰ **S62.669 Nondisplaced fracture of distal phalanx of unspecified finger** `CC` `H5` `UNS` `PE`

√5ᵗʰ **S62.9 Unspecified fracture of wrist and hand**

√x7ᵗʰ **S62.90 Unspecified fracture of unspecified wrist and hand** `CC` `H5` `UNS` `PE`

√x7ᵗʰ **S62.91 Unspecified fracture of right wrist and hand** `CC` `H5` `PE`

√x7ᵗʰ **S62.92 Unspecified fracture of left wrist and hand** `CC` `H5` `PE`

√4ᵗʰ **S63 Dislocation and sprain of joints and ligaments at wrist and hand level**

`INCLUDES`   avulsion of joint or ligament at wrist and hand level
    laceration of cartilage, joint or ligament at wrist and hand level
    sprain of cartilage, joint or ligament at wrist and hand level
    traumatic hemarthrosis of joint or ligament at wrist and hand level
    traumatic rupture of joint or ligament at wrist and hand level
    traumatic subluxation of joint or ligament at wrist and hand level
    traumatic tear of joint or ligament at wrist and hand level

Code also any associated open wound

`EXCLUDES 2`   strain of muscle, fascia and tendon of wrist and hand (S66.-)

The appropriate 7th character is to be added to each code from category S63.
A   initial encounter
D   subsequent encounter
S   sequela

√5ᵗʰ **S63.0 Subluxation and dislocation of wrist and hand joints**

√6ᵗʰ **S63.00 Unspecified subluxation and dislocation of wrist and hand**
    Dislocation of carpal bone NOS
    Dislocation of distal end of radius NOS
    Subluxation of carpal bone NOS
    Subluxation of distal end of radius NOS

√7ᵗʰ **S63.001 Unspecified subluxation of right wrist and hand** `PE`

√7ᵗʰ **S63.002 Unspecified subluxation of left wrist and hand** `PE`

√7ᵗʰ **S63.003 Unspecified subluxation of unspecified wrist and hand** `PE`

√7ᵗʰ **S63.004 Unspecified dislocation of right wrist and hand** `PE`

√7ᵗʰ **S63.005 Unspecified dislocation of left wrist and hand** `PE`

√7ᵗʰ **S63.006 Unspecified dislocation of unspecified wrist and hand** `PE`

√6ᵗʰ **S63.01 Subluxation and dislocation of distal radioulnar joint**

√7ᵗʰ **S63.011 Subluxation of distal radioulnar joint of right wrist** `PE`

√7ᵗʰ **S63.012 Subluxation of distal radioulnar joint of left wrist** `PE`

√7ᵗʰ **S63.013 Subluxation of distal radioulnar joint of unspecified wrist** `PE`

√7ᵗʰ **S63.014 Dislocation of distal radioulnar joint of right wrist** `PE`

√7ᵗʰ **S63.015 Dislocation of distal radioulnar joint of left wrist** `PE`

√7ᵗʰ **S63.016 Dislocation of distal radioulnar joint of unspecified wrist** `PE`

√6ᵗʰ **S63.02 Subluxation and dislocation of radiocarpal joint**

√7ᵗʰ **S63.021 Subluxation of radiocarpal joint of right wrist** `PE`

√7ᵗʰ **S63.022 Subluxation of radiocarpal joint of left wrist** `PE`

√7ᵗʰ **S63.023 Subluxation of radiocarpal joint of unspecified wrist** `PE`

√7ᵗʰ **S63.024 Dislocation of radiocarpal joint of right wrist** `PE`

√7ᵗʰ **S63.025 Dislocation of radiocarpal joint of left wrist** `PE`

√7ᵗʰ **S63.026 Dislocation of radiocarpal joint of unspecified wrist** `PE`

√6ᵗʰ **S63.03 Subluxation and dislocation of midcarpal joint**

√7ᵗʰ **S63.031 Subluxation of midcarpal joint of right wrist** `PE`

√7ᵗʰ **S63.032 Subluxation of midcarpal joint of left wrist** `PE`

√7ᵗʰ **S63.033 Subluxation of midcarpal joint of unspecified wrist** `PE`

√7ᵗʰ **S63.034 Dislocation of midcarpal joint of right wrist** `PE`

√7ᵗʰ **S63.035 Dislocation of midcarpal joint of left wrist** `PE`

√7ᵗʰ **S63.036 Dislocation of midcarpal joint of unspecified wrist** `PE`

√6ᵗʰ **S63.04 Subluxation and dislocation of carpometacarpal joint of thumb**

`EXCLUDES 2`   interphalangeal subluxation and dislocation of thumb (S63.1-)

√7ᵗʰ **S63.041 Subluxation of carpometacarpal joint of right thumb** `PE`

√7ᵗʰ **S63.042 Subluxation of carpometacarpal joint of left thumb** `PE`

√7ᵗʰ **S63.043 Subluxation of carpometacarpal joint of unspecified thumb** `PE`

√7ᵗʰ **S63.044 Dislocation of carpometacarpal joint of right thumb** `PE`

√7ᵗʰ **S63.045 Dislocation of carpometacarpal joint of left thumb** `PE`

√7ᵗʰ **S63.046 Dislocation of carpometacarpal joint of unspecified thumb** `PE`

√6ᵗʰ **S63.05 Subluxation and dislocation of other carpometacarpal joint**

`EXCLUDES 2`   subluxation and dislocation of carpometacarpal joint of thumb (S63.04-)

√7ᵗʰ **S63.051 Subluxation of other carpometacarpal joint of right hand** `PE`

√7ᵗʰ **S63.052 Subluxation of other carpometacarpal joint of left hand** `PE`

√7ᵗʰ **S63.053 Subluxation of other carpometacarpal joint of unspecified hand** `PE`

√7ᵗʰ **S63.054 Dislocation of other carpometacarpal joint of right hand** `PE`

√7ᵗʰ **S63.055 Dislocation of other carpometacarpal joint of left hand** `PE`

√7ᵗʰ **S63.056 Dislocation of other carpometacarpal joint of unspecified hand** `PE`

√6ᵗʰ **S63.06 Subluxation and dislocation of metacarpal (bone), proximal end**

√7ᵗʰ **S63.061 Subluxation of metacarpal (bone), proximal end of right hand** `PE`

√7ᵗʰ **S63.062 Subluxation of metacarpal (bone), proximal end of left hand** `PE`

Chapter 19. Injury, Poisoning and Certain Other Consequences of External Causes

S62.658–S63.062

√7ᵗʰ **S63.063** Subluxation of metacarpal (bone), proximal end of unspecified hand PE

√7ᵗʰ S63.064 Dislocation of metacarpal (bone), proximal end of right hand

√7ᵗʰ S63.065 Dislocation of metacarpal (bone), proximal end of left hand

√7ᵗʰ S63.066 Dislocation of metacarpal (bone), proximal end of unspecified hand PE

√6ᵗʰ **S63.07** Subluxation and dislocation of distal end of ulna

√7ᵗʰ S63.071 Subluxation of distal end of right ulna PE

√7ᵗʰ S63.072 Subluxation of distal end of left ulna PE

√7ᵗʰ S63.073 Subluxation of distal end of unspecified ulna PE

√7ᵗʰ S63.074 Dislocation of distal end of right ulna PE

√7ᵗʰ S63.075 Dislocation of distal end of left ulna PE

√7ᵗʰ S63.076 Dislocation of distal end of unspecified ulna PE

√6ᵗʰ **S63.09** Other subluxation and dislocation of wrist and hand

√7ᵗʰ S63.091 Other subluxation of right wrist and hand

√7ᵗʰ S63.092 Other subluxation of left wrist and hand PE

√7ᵗʰ S63.093 Other subluxation of unspecified wrist and hand PE

√7ᵗʰ S63.094 Other dislocation of right wrist and hand

√7ᵗʰ S63.095 Other dislocation of left wrist and hand PE

√7ᵗʰ S63.096 Other dislocation of unspecified wrist and hand PE

√5ᵗʰ **S63.1** Subluxation and dislocation of thumb

√6ᵗʰ **S63.10** Unspecified subluxation and dislocation of thumb

√7ᵗʰ S63.101 Unspecified subluxation of right thumb

√7ᵗʰ S63.102 Unspecified subluxation of left thumb PE

√7ᵗʰ S63.103 Unspecified subluxation of unspecified thumb PE

√7ᵗʰ S63.104 Unspecified dislocation of right thumb

√7ᵗʰ S63.105 Unspecified dislocation of left thumb PE

√7ᵗʰ S63.106 Unspecified dislocation of unspecified thumb PE

√6ᵗʰ **S63.11** Subluxation and dislocation of metacarpophalangeal joint of thumb

√7ᵗʰ S63.111 Subluxation of metacarpophalangeal joint of right thumb PE

√7ᵗʰ S63.112 Subluxation of metacarpophalangeal joint of left thumb PE

√7ᵗʰ S63.113 Subluxation of metacarpophalangeal joint of unspecified thumb PE

√7ᵗʰ S63.114 Dislocation of metacarpophalangeal joint of right thumb PE

√7ᵗʰ S63.115 Dislocation of metacarpophalangeal joint of left thumb PE

√7ᵗʰ S63.116 Dislocation of metacarpophalangeal joint of unspecified thumb PE

√6ᵗʰ **S63.12** Subluxation and dislocation of interphalangeal joint of thumb

√7ᵗʰ S63.121 Subluxation of interphalangeal joint of right thumb PE

√7ᵗʰ S63.122 Subluxation of interphalangeal joint of left thumb PE

√7ᵗʰ S63.123 Subluxation of interphalangeal joint of unspecified thumb PE

√7ᵗʰ S63.124 Dislocation of interphalangeal joint of right thumb PE

√7ᵗʰ S63.125 Dislocation of interphalangeal joint of left thumb PE

√7ᵗʰ S63.126 Dislocation of interphalangeal joint of unspecified thumb PE

√5ᵗʰ **S63.2** Subluxation and dislocation of other finger(s)

EXCLUDES 2 subluxation and dislocation of thumb (S63.1-)

√6ᵗʰ **S63.20** Unspecified subluxation of other finger

√7ᵗʰ S63.200 Unspecified subluxation of right index finger PE

√7ᵗʰ S63.201 Unspecified subluxation of left index finger PE

√7ᵗʰ S63.202 Unspecified subluxation of right middle finger PE

√7ᵗʰ S63.203 Unspecified subluxation of left middle finger PE

√7ᵗʰ S63.204 Unspecified subluxation of right ring finger PE

√7ᵗʰ S63.205 Unspecified subluxation of left ring finger PE

√7ᵗʰ S63.206 Unspecified subluxation of right little finger PE

√7ᵗʰ S63.207 Unspecified subluxation of left little finger PE

√7ᵗʰ S63.208 Unspecified subluxation of other finger PE
Unspecified subluxation of specified finger with unspecified laterality

√7ᵗʰ S63.209 Unspecified subluxation of unspecified finger PE

√6ᵗʰ **S63.21** Subluxation of metacarpophalangeal joint of finger

√7ᵗʰ S63.210 Subluxation of metacarpophalangeal joint of right index finger PE

√7ᵗʰ S63.211 Subluxation of metacarpophalangeal joint of left index finger PE

√7ᵗʰ S63.212 Subluxation of metacarpophalangeal joint of right middle finger PE

√7ᵗʰ S63.213 Subluxation of metacarpophalangeal joint of left middle finger PE

√7ᵗʰ S63.214 Subluxation of metacarpophalangeal joint of right ring finger PE

√7ᵗʰ S63.215 Subluxation of metacarpophalangeal joint of left ring finger PE

√7ᵗʰ S63.216 Subluxation of metacarpophalangeal joint of right little finger PE

√7ᵗʰ S63.217 Subluxation of metacarpophalangeal joint of left little finger PE

√7ᵗʰ S63.218 Subluxation of metacarpophalangeal joint of other finger PE
Subluxation of metacarpophalangeal joint of specified finger with unspecified laterality

√7ᵗʰ S63.219 Subluxation of metacarpophalangeal joint of unspecified finger PE

√6ᵗʰ **S63.22** Subluxation of unspecified interphalangeal joint of finger

√7ᵗʰ S63.220 Subluxation of unspecified interphalangeal joint of right index finger PE

√7ᵗʰ S63.221 Subluxation of unspecified interphalangeal joint of left index finger PE

√7ᵗʰ S63.222 Subluxation of unspecified interphalangeal joint of right middle finger PE

√7ᵗʰ S63.223 Subluxation of unspecified interphalangeal joint of left middle finger PE

√7ᵗʰ S63.224 Subluxation of unspecified interphalangeal joint of right ring finger PE

√7ᵗʰ S63.225 Subluxation of unspecified interphalangeal joint of left ring finger PE

√7ᵗʰ S63.226 Subluxation of unspecified interphalangeal joint of right little finger PE

√7ᵗʰ S63.227 Subluxation of unspecified interphalangeal joint of left little finger PE

√7ᵗʰ **S63.228** **Subluxation of unspecified interphalangeal joint of other finger** **PE**
  Subluxation of unspecified interphalangeal joint of specified finger with unspecified laterality

√7ᵗʰ **S63.229** **Subluxation of unspecified interphalangeal joint of unspecified finger** **PE**

√6ᵗʰ **S63.23** **Subluxation of proximal interphalangeal joint of finger**

√7ᵗʰ **S63.230** **Subluxation of proximal interphalangeal joint of right index finger** **PE**

√7ᵗʰ **S63.231** **Subluxation of proximal interphalangeal joint of left index finger** **PE**

√7ᵗʰ **S63.232** **Subluxation of proximal interphalangeal joint of right middle finger** **PE**

√7ᵗʰ **S63.233** **Subluxation of proximal interphalangeal joint of left middle finger** **PE**

√7ᵗʰ **S63.234** **Subluxation of proximal interphalangeal joint of right ring finger** **PE**

√7ᵗʰ **S63.235** **Subluxation of proximal interphalangeal joint of left ring finger** **PE**

√7ᵗʰ **S63.236** **Subluxation of proximal interphalangeal joint of right little finger** **PE**

√7ᵗʰ **S63.237** **Subluxation of proximal interphalangeal joint of left little finger** **PE**

√7ᵗʰ **S63.238** **Subluxation of proximal interphalangeal joint of other finger** **PE**
  Subluxation of proximal interphalangeal joint of specified finger with unspecified laterality

√7ᵗʰ **S63.239** **Subluxation of proximal interphalangeal joint of unspecified finger** **PE**

√6ᵗʰ **S63.24** **Subluxation of distal interphalangeal joint of finger**

√7ᵗʰ **S63.240** **Subluxation of distal interphalangeal joint of right index finger** **PE**

√7ᵗʰ **S63.241** **Subluxation of distal interphalangeal joint of left index finger** **PE**

√7ᵗʰ **S63.242** **Subluxation of distal interphalangeal joint of right middle finger** **PE**

√7ᵗʰ **S63.243** **Subluxation of distal interphalangeal joint of left middle finger** **PE**

√7ᵗʰ **S63.244** **Subluxation of distal interphalangeal joint of right ring finger** **PE**

√7ᵗʰ **S63.245** **Subluxation of distal interphalangeal joint of left ring finger** **PE**

√7ᵗʰ **S63.246** **Subluxation of distal interphalangeal joint of right little finger** **PE**

√7ᵗʰ **S63.247** **Subluxation of distal interphalangeal joint of left little finger** **PE**

√7ᵗʰ **S63.248** **Subluxation of distal interphalangeal joint of other finger** **PE**
  Subluxation of distal interphalangeal joint of specified finger with unspecified laterality

√7ᵗʰ **S63.249** **Subluxation of distal interphalangeal joint of unspecified finger** **PE**

√6ᵗʰ **S63.25** **Unspecified dislocation of other finger**

√7ᵗʰ **S63.250** **Unspecified dislocation of right index finger** **PE**

√7ᵗʰ **S63.251** **Unspecified dislocation of left index finger** **PE**

√7ᵗʰ **S63.252** **Unspecified dislocation of right middle finger** **PE**

√7ᵗʰ **S63.253** **Unspecified dislocation of left middle finger** **PE**

√7ᵗʰ **S63.254** **Unspecified dislocation of right ring finger** **PE**

√7ᵗʰ **S63.255** **Unspecified dislocation of left ring finger** **PE**

√7ᵗʰ **S63.256** **Unspecified dislocation of right little finger** **PE**

√7ᵗʰ **S63.257** **Unspecified dislocation of left little finger** **PE**

√7ᵗʰ **S63.258** **Unspecified dislocation of other finger** **PE**
  Unspecified dislocation of specified finger with unspecified laterality

√7ᵗʰ **S63.259** **Unspecified dislocation of unspecified finger** **PE**
  Unspecified dislocation of unspecified finger with unspecified laterality

√6ᵗʰ **S63.26** **Dislocation of metacarpophalangeal joint of finger**

√7ᵗʰ **S63.260** **Dislocation of metacarpophalangeal joint of right index finger** **PE**

√7ᵗʰ **S63.261** **Dislocation of metacarpophalangeal joint of left index finger** **PE**

√7ᵗʰ **S63.262** **Dislocation of metacarpophalangeal joint of right middle finger** **PE**

√7ᵗʰ **S63.263** **Dislocation of metacarpophalangeal joint of left middle finger** **PE**

√7ᵗʰ **S63.264** **Dislocation of metacarpophalangeal joint of right ring finger** **PE**

√7ᵗʰ **S63.265** **Dislocation of metacarpophalangeal joint of left ring finger** **PE**

√7ᵗʰ **S63.266** **Dislocation of metacarpophalangeal joint of right little finger** **PE**

√7ᵗʰ **S63.267** **Dislocation of metacarpophalangeal joint of left little finger** **PE**

√7ᵗʰ **S63.268** **Dislocation of metacarpophalangeal joint of other finger** **PE**
  Dislocation of metacarpophalangeal joint of specified finger with unspecified laterality

√7ᵗʰ **S63.269** **Dislocation of metacarpophalangeal joint of unspecified finger** **PE**

√6ᵗʰ **S63.27** **Dislocation of unspecified interphalangeal joint of finger**

√7ᵗʰ **S63.270** **Dislocation of unspecified interphalangeal joint of right index finger** **PE**

√7ᵗʰ **S63.271** **Dislocation of unspecified interphalangeal joint of left index finger** **PE**

√7ᵗʰ **S63.272** **Dislocation of unspecified interphalangeal joint of right middle finger** **PE**

√7ᵗʰ **S63.273** **Dislocation of unspecified interphalangeal joint of left middle finger** **PE**

√7ᵗʰ **S63.274** **Dislocation of unspecified interphalangeal joint of right ring finger** **PE**

√7ᵗʰ **S63.275** **Dislocation of unspecified interphalangeal joint of left ring finger** **PE**

√7ᵗʰ **S63.276** **Dislocation of unspecified interphalangeal joint of right little finger** **PE**

√7ᵗʰ **S63.277** **Dislocation of unspecified interphalangeal joint of left little finger** **PE**

√7ᵗʰ **S63.278** **Dislocation of unspecified interphalangeal joint of other finger** **PE**
  Dislocation of unspecified interphalangeal joint of specified finger with unspecified laterality

√7ᵗʰ **S63.279** **Dislocation of unspecified interphalangeal joint of unspecified finger** **PE**
  Dislocation of unspecified interphalangeal joint of unspecified finger without specified laterality

√6ᵗʰ **S63.28** **Dislocation of proximal interphalangeal joint of finger**

√7ᵗʰ **S63.280** **Dislocation of proximal interphalangeal joint of right index finger** **PE**

√7ᵗʰ **S63.281** **Dislocation of proximal interphalangeal joint of left index finger** **PE**

√7ᵗʰ **S63.282** **Dislocation of proximal interphalangeal joint of right middle finger** **PE**

√7ᵗʰ **S63.283** **Dislocation of proximal interphalangeal joint of left middle finger** **PE**

√7ᵗʰ **S63.284** **Dislocation of proximal interphalangeal joint of right ring finger** **PE**

√7ᵗʰ **S63.285** **Dislocation of proximal interphalangeal joint of left ring finger** **PE**

√7ᵗʰ **S63.286** **Dislocation of proximal interphalangeal joint of right little finger** **PE**

√7ᵗʰ **S63.287** **Dislocation of proximal interphalangeal joint of left little finger** **PE**

√7ᵗʰ **S63.288** **Dislocation of proximal interphalangeal joint of other finger** **PE**
  Dislocation of proximal interphalangeal joint of specified finger with unspecified laterality

√7ᵗʰ **S63.289** **Dislocation of proximal interphalangeal joint of unspecified finger** **PE**

√6th **S63.29**   **Dislocation of distal interphalangeal joint** of finger

√7th **S63.290**   Dislocation of distal interphalangeal joint of **right index** finger   PE

√7th **S63.291**   Dislocation of distal interphalangeal joint of **left index** finger   PE

√7th **S63.292**   Dislocation of distal interphalangeal joint of **right middle** finger   PE

√7th **S63.293**   Dislocation of distal interphalangeal joint of **left middle** finger   PE

√7th **S63.294**   Dislocation of distal interphalangeal joint of **right ring** finger   PE

√7th **S63.295**   Dislocation of distal interphalangeal joint of **left ring** finger   PE

√7th **S63.296**   Dislocation of distal interphalangeal joint of **right little** finger   PE

√7th **S63.297**   Dislocation of distal interphalangeal joint of **left little** finger   PE

√7th **S63.298**   Dislocation of distal interphalangeal joint of **other finger**   PE

Dislocation of distal interphalangeal joint of specified finger with unspecified laterality

√7th **S63.299**   Dislocation of distal interphalangeal joint of **unspecified finger**   PE

√5th **S63.3**   **Traumatic rupture of ligament of wrist**

√6th **S63.30**   Traumatic rupture of unspecified ligament of wrist

√7th **S63.301**   Traumatic rupture of unspecified ligament of **right** wrist   PE

√7th **S63.302**   Traumatic rupture of unspecified ligament of **left** wrist   PE

√7th **S63.309**   Traumatic rupture of unspecified ligament of **unspecified wrist**   PE

√6th **S63.31**   Traumatic rupture of **collateral** ligament of wrist

√7th **S63.311**   Traumatic rupture of collateral ligament of **right** wrist   PE

√7th **S63.312**   Traumatic rupture of collateral ligament of **left** wrist   PE

√7th **S63.319**   Traumatic rupture of collateral ligament of **unspecified wrist**   PE

√6th **S63.32**   Traumatic rupture of **radiocarpal ligament**

√7th **S63.321**   Traumatic rupture of **right** radiocarpal ligament   PE

√7th **S63.322**   Traumatic rupture of **left** radiocarpal ligament   PE

√7th **S63.329**   Traumatic rupture of unspecified radiocarpal ligament   PE

√6th **S63.33**   Traumatic rupture of **ulnocarpal (palmar) ligament**

√7th **S63.331**   Traumatic rupture of **right** ulnocarpal (palmar) ligament   PE

√7th **S63.332**   Traumatic rupture of **left** ulnocarpal (palmar) ligament   PE

√7th **S63.339**   Traumatic rupture of unspecified ulnocarpal (palmar) ligament   PE

√6th **S63.39**   Traumatic rupture of other ligament of wrist

√7th **S63.391**   Traumatic rupture of other ligament of **right** wrist   PE

√7th **S63.392**   Traumatic rupture of other ligament of **left** wrist   PE

√7th **S63.399**   Traumatic rupture of other ligament of **unspecified** wrist   PE

√5th **S63.4**   **Traumatic rupture of ligament of finger at metacarpophalangeal and interphalangeal joint(s)**

√6th **S63.40**   Traumatic rupture of unspecified ligament of finger at metacarpophalangeal and interphalangeal joint

√7th **S63.400**   Traumatic rupture of unspecified ligament of **right index** finger at metacarpophalangeal and interphalangeal joint   PE

√7th **S63.401**   Traumatic rupture of unspecified ligament of **left index** finger at metacarpophalangeal and interphalangeal joint   PE

√7th **S63.402**   Traumatic rupture of unspecified ligament of **right middle** finger at metacarpophalangeal and interphalangeal joint   PE

√7th **S63.403**   Traumatic rupture of unspecified ligament of **left middle** finger at metacarpophalangeal and interphalangeal joint   PE

√7th **S63.404**   Traumatic rupture of unspecified ligament of **right ring** finger at metacarpophalangeal and interphalangeal joint   PE

√7th **S63.405**   Traumatic rupture of unspecified ligament of **left ring** finger at metacarpophalangeal and interphalangeal joint   PE

√7th **S63.406**   Traumatic rupture of unspecified ligament of **right little** finger at metacarpophalangeal and interphalangeal joint   PE

√7th **S63.407**   Traumatic rupture of unspecified ligament of **left little** finger at metacarpophalangeal and interphalangeal joint   PE

√7th **S63.408**   Traumatic rupture of unspecified ligament of **other finger** at metacarpophalangeal and interphalangeal joint   PE

Traumatic rupture of unspecified ligament of specified finger with unspecified laterality at metacarpophalangeal and interphalangeal joint

√7th **S63.409**   Traumatic rupture of unspecified ligament of **unspecified finger** at metacarpophalangeal and interphalangeal joint   PE

√6th **S63.41**   Traumatic rupture of **collateral ligament** of finger at metacarpophalangeal and interphalangeal joint

√7th **S63.410**   Traumatic rupture of collateral ligament of **right index** finger at metacarpophalangeal and interphalangeal joint   PE

√7th **S63.411**   Traumatic rupture of collateral ligament of **left index** finger at metacarpophalangeal and interphalangeal joint   PE

√7th **S63.412**   Traumatic rupture of collateral ligament of **right middle** finger at metacarpophalangeal and interphalangeal joint   PE

√7th **S63.413**   Traumatic rupture of collateral ligament of **left middle** finger at metacarpophalangeal and interphalangeal joint   PE

√7th **S63.414**   Traumatic rupture of collateral ligament of **right ring** finger at metacarpophalangeal and interphalangeal joint   PE

√7th **S63.415**   Traumatic rupture of collateral ligament of **left ring** finger at metacarpophalangeal and interphalangeal joint   PE

√7th **S63.416**   Traumatic rupture of collateral ligament of **right little** finger at metacarpophalangeal and interphalangeal joint   PE

√7th **S63.417**   Traumatic rupture of collateral ligament of **left little** finger at metacarpophalangeal and interphalangeal joint   PE

√7th **S63.418**   Traumatic rupture of collateral ligament of **other finger** at metacarpophalangeal and interphalangeal joint   PE

Traumatic rupture of collateral ligament of specified finger with unspecified laterality at metacarpophalangeal and interphalangeal joint

√7th **S63.419**   Traumatic rupture of collateral ligament of **unspecified finger** at metacarpophalangeal and interphalangeal joint   PE

√6th **S63.42**   Traumatic rupture of **palmar ligament** of finger at metacarpophalangeal and interphalangeal joint

√7th **S63.420**   Traumatic rupture of palmar ligament of **right index** finger at metacarpophalangeal and interphalangeal joint   PE

√7th **S63.421**   Traumatic rupture of palmar ligament of **left index** finger at metacarpophalangeal and interphalangeal joint   PE

√7th **S63.422**   Traumatic rupture of palmar ligament of **right middle** finger at metacarpophalangeal and interphalangeal joint   PE

✓7ᵗʰ **S63.423** Traumatic rupture of palmar ligament of **left middle** finger at metacarpophalangeal and interphalangeal joint   PE

✓7ᵗʰ **S63.424** Traumatic rupture of palmar ligament of **right ring** finger at metacarpophalangeal and interphalangeal joint   PE

✓7ᵗʰ **S63.425** Traumatic rupture of palmar ligament of **left ring** finger at metacarpophalangeal and interphalangeal joint   PE

✓7ᵗʰ **S63.426** Traumatic rupture of palmar ligament of **right little** finger at metacarpophalangeal and interphalangeal joint   PE

✓7ᵗʰ **S63.427** Traumatic rupture of palmar ligament of **left little** finger at metacarpophalangeal and interphalangeal joint   PE

✓7ᵗʰ **S63.428** Traumatic rupture of palmar ligament of other finger at metacarpophalangeal and interphalangeal joint

     Traumatic rupture of palmar ligament of specified finger with unspecified laterality at metacarpophalangeal and interphalangeal joint

✓7ᵗʰ **S63.429** Traumatic rupture of palmar ligament of unspecified finger at metacarpophalangeal and interphalangeal joint   PE

✓6ᵗʰ **S63.43** **Traumatic rupture of volar plate of finger at metacarpophalangeal and interphalangeal joint**

✓7ᵗʰ **S63.430** Traumatic rupture of volar plate of **right index** finger at metacarpophalangeal and interphalangeal joint   PE

✓7ᵗʰ **S63.431** Traumatic rupture of volar plate of **left index** finger at metacarpophalangeal and interphalangeal joint   PE

✓7ᵗʰ **S63.432** Traumatic rupture of volar plate of **right middle** finger at metacarpophalangeal and interphalangeal joint   PE

✓7ᵗʰ **S63.433** Traumatic rupture of volar plate of **left middle** finger at metacarpophalangeal and interphalangeal joint   PE

✓7ᵗʰ **S63.434** Traumatic rupture of volar plate of **right ring** finger at metacarpophalangeal and interphalangeal joint   PE

✓7ᵗʰ **S63.435** Traumatic rupture of volar plate of **left ring** finger at metacarpophalangeal and interphalangeal joint   PE

✓7ᵗʰ **S63.436** Traumatic rupture of volar plate of **right little** finger at metacarpophalangeal and interphalangeal joint   PE

✓7ᵗʰ **S63.437** Traumatic rupture of volar plate of **left little** finger at metacarpophalangeal and interphalangeal joint   PE

✓7ᵗʰ **S63.438** Traumatic rupture of volar plate of other finger at metacarpophalangeal and interphalangeal joint   PE

     Traumatic rupture of volar plate of specified finger with unspecified laterality at metacarpophalangeal and interphalangeal joint

✓7ᵗʰ **S63.439** Traumatic rupture of volar plate of unspecified finger at metacarpophalangeal and interphalangeal joint   PE

✓6ᵗʰ **S63.49** **Traumatic rupture of other ligament of finger at metacarpophalangeal and interphalangeal joint**

✓7ᵗʰ **S63.490** Traumatic rupture of other ligament of **right index** finger at metacarpophalangeal and interphalangeal joint   PE

✓7ᵗʰ **S63.491** Traumatic rupture of other ligament of **left index** finger at metacarpophalangeal and interphalangeal joint   PE

✓7ᵗʰ **S63.492** Traumatic rupture of other ligament of **right middle** finger at metacarpophalangeal and interphalangeal joint   PE

✓7ᵗʰ **S63.493** Traumatic rupture of other ligament of **left middle** finger at metacarpophalangeal and interphalangeal joint   PE

✓7ᵗʰ **S63.494** Traumatic rupture of other ligament of **right ring** finger at metacarpophalangeal and interphalangeal joint   PE

✓7ᵗʰ **S63.495** Traumatic rupture of other ligament of **left ring** finger at metacarpophalangeal and interphalangeal joint   PE

✓7ᵗʰ **S63.496** Traumatic rupture of other ligament of **right little** finger at metacarpophalangeal and interphalangeal joint   PE

✓7ᵗʰ **S63.497** Traumatic rupture of other ligament of **left little** finger at metacarpophalangeal and interphalangeal joint   PE

✓7ᵗʰ **S63.498** Traumatic rupture of other ligament of other finger at metacarpophalangeal and interphalangeal joint

     Traumatic rupture of ligament of specified finger with unspecified laterality at metacarpophalangeal and interphalangeal joint

✓7ᵗʰ **S63.499** Traumatic rupture of other ligament of unspecified finger at metacarpophalangeal and interphalangeal joint   PE

✓5ᵗʰ **S63.5** **Other and unspecified sprain of wrist**

✓6ᵗʰ **S63.50** **Unspecified sprain of wrist**

✓7ᵗʰ **S63.501** Unspecified sprain of **right** wrist   PE

✓7ᵗʰ **S63.502** Unspecified sprain of **left** wrist   PE

✓7ᵗʰ **S63.509** Unspecified sprain of unspecified wrist   PE

✓6ᵗʰ **S63.51** **Sprain of carpal (joint)**

✓7ᵗʰ **S63.511** Sprain of carpal joint of **right** wrist   PE

✓7ᵗʰ **S63.512** Sprain of carpal joint of **left** wrist   PE

✓7ᵗʰ **S63.519** Sprain of carpal joint of unspecified wrist   PE

✓6ᵗʰ **S63.52** **Sprain of radiocarpal joint**

     EXCLUDES 1   *traumatic rupture of radiocarpal ligament (S63.32-)*

✓7ᵗʰ **S63.521** Sprain of radiocarpal joint of **right** wrist   PE

✓7ᵗʰ **S63.522** Sprain of radiocarpal joint of **left** wrist   PE

✓7ᵗʰ **S63.529** Sprain of radiocarpal joint of unspecified wrist   PE

✓6ᵗʰ **S63.59** **Other specified sprain of wrist**

✓7ᵗʰ **S63.591** Other specified sprain of **right** wrist   PE

✓7ᵗʰ **S63.592** Other specified sprain of **left** wrist   PE

✓7ᵗʰ **S63.599** Other specified sprain of unspecified wrist   PE

✓5ᵗʰ **S63.6** **Other and unspecified sprain of finger(s)**

     EXCLUDES 1   *traumatic rupture of ligament of finger at metacarpophalangeal and interphalangeal joint(s) (S63.4-)*

✓6ᵗʰ **S63.60** **Unspecified sprain of thumb**

✓7ᵗʰ **S63.601** Unspecified sprain of **right** thumb   PE

✓7ᵗʰ **S63.602** Unspecified sprain of **left** thumb   PE

✓7ᵗʰ **S63.609** Unspecified sprain of unspecified thumb   PE

✓6ᵗʰ **S63.61** **Unspecified sprain of other and unspecified finger(s)**

✓7ᵗʰ **S63.610** Unspecified sprain of **right index** finger   PE

✓7ᵗʰ **S63.611** Unspecified sprain of **left index** finger   PE

✓7ᵗʰ **S63.612** Unspecified sprain of **right middle** finger   PE

✓7ᵗʰ **S63.613** Unspecified sprain of **left middle** finger   PE

✓7ᵗʰ **S63.614** Unspecified sprain of **right ring** finger   PE

✓7ᵗʰ **S63.615** Unspecified sprain of **left ring** finger   PE

✓7ᵗʰ **S63.616** Unspecified sprain of **right little** finger   PE

✓7ᵗʰ **S63.617** Unspecified sprain of **left little** finger   PE

✓7ᵗʰ **S63.618** Unspecified sprain of other finger   PE

     Unspecified sprain of specified finger with unspecified laterality

✓7ᵗʰ **S63.619** Unspecified sprain of unspecified finger   PE

✓6ᵗʰ **S63.62** **Sprain of interphalangeal joint of thumb**

✓7ᵗʰ **S63.621** Sprain of interphalangeal joint of **right** thumb   PE

✓ Additional Character Required   ✓x7ᵗʰ Placeholder   Questionable PDx   Manifestation   Unspecified   UPD Unacceptable PDx   H1-H14 HAC   HCC CMS-HCC Dx   HIV HIV Dx

ICD-10-CM 2025   1067

√7ᵗʰ **S63.622** Sprain of interphalangeal joint of left thumb   PE

√7ᵗʰ **S63.629** Sprain of interphalangeal joint of unspecified thumb   PE

√6ᵗʰ **S63.63** Sprain of interphalangeal joint of other and unspecified finger(s)

√7ᵗʰ **S63.630** Sprain of interphalangeal joint of right index finger

√7ᵗʰ **S63.631** Sprain of interphalangeal joint of left index finger

√7ᵗʰ **S63.632** Sprain of interphalangeal joint of right middle finger

√7ᵗʰ **S63.633** Sprain of interphalangeal joint of left middle finger

√7ᵗʰ **S63.634** Sprain of interphalangeal joint of right ring finger   PE

√7ᵗʰ **S63.635** Sprain of interphalangeal joint of left ring finger   PE

√7ᵗʰ **S63.636** Sprain of interphalangeal joint of right little finger

√7ᵗʰ **S63.637** Sprain of interphalangeal joint of left little finger   PE

√7ᵗʰ **S63.638** Sprain of interphalangeal joint of other finger

√7ᵗʰ **S63.639** Sprain of interphalangeal joint of unspecified finger   PE

√6ᵗʰ **S63.64** Sprain of metacarpophalangeal joint of thumb

√7ᵗʰ **S63.641** Sprain of metacarpophalangeal joint of right thumb   PE

√7ᵗʰ **S63.642** Sprain of metacarpophalangeal joint of left thumb   PE

√7ᵗʰ **S63.649** Sprain of metacarpophalangeal joint of unspecified thumb   PE

√6ᵗʰ **S63.65** Sprain of metacarpophalangeal joint of other and unspecified finger(s)

√7ᵗʰ **S63.650** Sprain of metacarpophalangeal joint of right index finger   PE

√7ᵗʰ **S63.651** Sprain of metacarpophalangeal joint of left index finger   PE

√7ᵗʰ **S63.652** Sprain of metacarpophalangeal joint of right middle finger   PE

√7ᵗʰ **S63.653** Sprain of metacarpophalangeal joint of left middle finger   PE

√7ᵗʰ **S63.654** Sprain of metacarpophalangeal joint of right ring finger   PE

√7ᵗʰ **S63.655** Sprain of metacarpophalangeal joint of left ring finger   PE

√7ᵗʰ **S63.656** Sprain of metacarpophalangeal joint of right little finger   PE

√7ᵗʰ **S63.657** Sprain of metacarpophalangeal joint of left little finger   PE

√7ᵗʰ **S63.658** Sprain of metacarpophalangeal joint of other finger

    Sprain of metacarpophalangeal joint of specified finger with unspecified laterality

√7ᵗʰ **S63.659** Sprain of metacarpophalangeal joint of unspecified finger   PE

√6ᵗʰ **S63.68** Other sprain of thumb

√7ᵗʰ **S63.681** Other sprain of right thumb   PE

√7ᵗʰ **S63.682** Other sprain of left thumb   PE

√7ᵗʰ **S63.689** Other sprain of unspecified thumb   PE

√6ᵗʰ **S63.69** Other sprain of other and unspecified finger(s)

√7ᵗʰ **S63.690** Other sprain of right index finger   PE

√7ᵗʰ **S63.691** Other sprain of left index finger   PE

√7ᵗʰ **S63.692** Other sprain of right middle finger   PE

√7ᵗʰ **S63.693** Other sprain of left middle finger   PE

√7ᵗʰ **S63.694** Other sprain of right ring finger   PE

√7ᵗʰ **S63.695** Other sprain of left ring finger   PE

√7ᵗʰ **S63.696** Other sprain of right little finger   PE

√7ᵗʰ **S63.697** Other sprain of left little finger   PE

√7ᵗʰ **S63.698** Other sprain of other finger   PE

    Other sprain of specified finger with unspecified laterality

√7ᵗʰ **S63.699** Other sprain of unspecified finger   PE

√5ᵗʰ **S63.8** Sprain of other part of wrist and hand

√6ᵗʰ **S63.8X** Sprain of other part of wrist and hand

√7ᵗʰ **S63.8X1** Sprain of other part of right wrist and hand   PE

√7ᵗʰ **S63.8X2** Sprain of other part of left wrist and hand   PE

√7ᵗʰ **S63.8X9** Sprain of other part of unspecified wrist and hand   PE

√5ᵗʰ **S63.9** Sprain of unspecified part of wrist and hand

√x7ᵗʰ **S63.90** Sprain of unspecified part of unspecified wrist and hand

√x7ᵗʰ **S63.91** Sprain of unspecified part of right wrist and hand   PE

√x7ᵗʰ **S63.92** Sprain of unspecified part of left wrist and hand   PE

√4ᵗʰ **S64** Injury of nerves at wrist and hand level

Code also any associated open wound (S61.-)

> The appropriate 7th character is to be added to each code from category S64.
> A   initial encounter
> D   subsequent encounter
> S   sequela

√5ᵗʰ **S64.0** Injury of ulnar nerve at wrist and hand level

√x7ᵗʰ **S64.00** Injury of ulnar nerve at wrist and hand level of unspecified arm   PE

√x7ᵗʰ **S64.01** Injury of ulnar nerve at wrist and hand level of right arm   PE

√x7ᵗʰ **S64.02** Injury of ulnar nerve at wrist and hand level of left arm   PE

√5ᵗʰ **S64.1** Injury of median nerve at wrist and hand level

√x7ᵗʰ **S64.10** Injury of median nerve at wrist and hand level of unspecified arm   PE

√x7ᵗʰ **S64.11** Injury of median nerve at wrist and hand level of right arm   PE

√x7ᵗʰ **S64.12** Injury of median nerve at wrist and hand level of left arm   PE

√5ᵗʰ **S64.2** Injury of radial nerve at wrist and hand level

√x7ᵗʰ **S64.20** Injury of radial nerve at wrist and hand level of unspecified arm   PE

√x7ᵗʰ **S64.21** Injury of radial nerve at wrist and hand level of right arm   PE

√x7ᵗʰ **S64.22** Injury of radial nerve at wrist and hand level of left arm   PE

√5ᵗʰ **S64.3** Injury of digital nerve of thumb

√x7ᵗʰ **S64.30** Injury of digital nerve of unspecified thumb   PE

√x7ᵗʰ **S64.31** Injury of digital nerve of right thumb   PE

√x7ᵗʰ **S64.32** Injury of digital nerve of left thumb   PE

√5ᵗʰ **S64.4** Injury of digital nerve of other and unspecified finger

√x7ᵗʰ **S64.40** Injury of digital nerve of unspecified finger   PE

√6ᵗʰ **S64.49** Injury of digital nerve of other finger

√7ᵗʰ **S64.490** Injury of digital nerve of right index finger   PE

√7ᵗʰ **S64.491** Injury of digital nerve of left index finger   PE

√7ᵗʰ **S64.492** Injury of digital nerve of right middle finger   PE

√7ᵗʰ **S64.493** Injury of digital nerve of left middle finger   PE

√7ᵗʰ **S64.494** Injury of digital nerve of right ring finger   PE

√7ᵗʰ **S64.495** Injury of digital nerve of left ring finger   PE

√7ᵗʰ **S64.496** Injury of digital nerve of right little finger   PE

√7ᵗʰ **S64.497** Injury of digital nerve of left little finger   PE

√7ᵗʰ **S64.498** Injury of digital nerve of other finger   PE

    Injury of digital nerve of specified finger with unspecified laterality

√5ᵗʰ **S64.8** Injury of other nerves at wrist and hand level

√6ᵗʰ **S64.8X** Injury of other nerves at wrist and hand level

√7ᵗʰ **S64.8X1** Injury of other nerves at wrist and hand level of right arm   PE

N Newborn: 0   **P** Pediatric: 0-17   **M** Maternity: 9-64   **A** Adult: 15-124   **UNS** Unspecified Site   **MCC** Major Complication/Comorbidity   **CC** Complication/Comorbidity   **PE** POA Exempt

1068   ICD-10-CM 2025

√7ᵗʰ **S64.8X2** Injury of other nerves at wrist and hand level of left arm   PE

√7ᵗʰ **S64.8X9** Injury of other nerves at wrist and hand level of unspecified arm   PE

√5ᵗʰ **S64.9** Injury of unspecified nerve at wrist and hand level

√x7ᵗʰ **S64.9Ø** Injury of unspecified nerve at wrist and hand level of unspecified arm   PE

√x7ᵗʰ **S64.91** Injury of unspecified nerve at wrist and hand level of right arm   PE

√x7ᵗʰ **S64.92** Injury of unspecified nerve at wrist and hand level of left arm   PE

√4ᵗʰ **S65 Injury of blood vessels at wrist and hand level**

Code also any associated open wound (S61.-)

The appropriate 7th character is to be added to each code from category S65.
A   initial encounter
D   subsequent encounter
S   sequela

√5ᵗʰ **S65.Ø** Injury of ulnar artery at wrist and hand level

√6ᵗʰ **S65.ØØ** Unspecified injury of ulnar artery at wrist and hand level

√7ᵗʰ **S65.ØØ1** Unspecified injury of ulnar artery at wrist and hand level of right arm   CC PE

√7ᵗʰ **S65.ØØ2** Unspecified injury of ulnar artery at wrist and hand level of left arm   CC PE

√7ᵗʰ **S65.ØØ9** Unspecified injury of ulnar artery at wrist and hand level of unspecified arm   CC UNS PE

√6ᵗʰ **S65.Ø1** Laceration of ulnar artery at wrist and hand level

√7ᵗʰ **S65.Ø11** Laceration of ulnar artery at wrist and hand level of right arm   CC PE

√7ᵗʰ **S65.Ø12** Laceration of ulnar artery at wrist and hand level of left arm   CC PE

√7ᵗʰ **S65.Ø19** Laceration of ulnar artery at wrist and hand level of unspecified arm   CC UNS PE

√6ᵗʰ **S65.Ø9** Other specified injury of ulnar artery at wrist and hand level

√7ᵗʰ **S65.Ø91** Other specified injury of ulnar artery at wrist and hand level of right arm   CC PE

√7ᵗʰ **S65.Ø92** Other specified injury of ulnar artery at wrist and hand level of left arm   CC PE

√7ᵗʰ **S65.Ø99** Other specified injury of ulnar artery at wrist and hand level of unspecified arm   CC UNS PE

√5ᵗʰ **S65.1** Injury of radial artery at wrist and hand level

√6ᵗʰ **S65.1Ø** Unspecified injury of radial artery at wrist and hand level

√7ᵗʰ **S65.1Ø1** Unspecified injury of radial artery at wrist and hand level of right arm   CC PE

√7ᵗʰ **S65.1Ø2** Unspecified injury of radial artery at wrist and hand level of left arm   CC PE

√7ᵗʰ **S65.1Ø9** Unspecified injury of radial artery at wrist and hand level of unspecified arm   CC UNS PE

√6ᵗʰ **S65.11** Laceration of radial artery at wrist and hand level

√7ᵗʰ **S65.111** Laceration of radial artery at wrist and hand level of right arm   CC PE

√7ᵗʰ **S65.112** Laceration of radial artery at wrist and hand level of left arm   CC PE

√7ᵗʰ **S65.119** Laceration of radial artery at wrist and hand level of unspecified arm   CC UNS PE

√6ᵗʰ **S65.19** Other specified injury of radial artery at wrist and hand level

√7ᵗʰ **S65.191** Other specified injury of radial artery at wrist and hand level of right arm   CC PE

√7ᵗʰ **S65.192** Other specified injury of radial artery at wrist and hand level of left arm   CC PE

√7ᵗʰ **S65.199** Other specified injury of radial artery at wrist and hand level of unspecified arm   CC UNS PE

√5ᵗʰ **S65.2** Injury of superficial palmar arch

√6ᵗʰ **S65.2Ø** Unspecified injury of superficial palmar arch

√7ᵗʰ **S65.2Ø1** Unspecified injury of superficial palmar arch of right hand   CC PE

√7ᵗʰ **S65.2Ø2** Unspecified injury of superficial palmar arch of left hand   CC PE

√7ᵗʰ **S65.2Ø9** Unspecified injury of superficial palmar arch of unspecified hand   CC UNS PE

√6ᵗʰ **S65.21** Laceration of superficial palmar arch

√7ᵗʰ **S65.211** Laceration of superficial palmar arch of right hand   CC PE

√7ᵗʰ **S65.212** Laceration of superficial palmar arch of left hand   CC PE

√7ᵗʰ **S65.219** Laceration of superficial palmar arch of unspecified hand   CC UNS PE

√6ᵗʰ **S65.29** Other specified injury of superficial palmar arch

√7ᵗʰ **S65.291** Other specified injury of superficial palmar arch of right hand   CC PE

√7ᵗʰ **S65.292** Other specified injury of superficial palmar arch of left hand   CC PE

√7ᵗʰ **S65.299** Other specified injury of superficial palmar arch of unspecified hand   CC UNS PE

√5ᵗʰ **S65.3** Injury of deep palmar arch

√6ᵗʰ **S65.3Ø** Unspecified injury of deep palmar arch

√7ᵗʰ **S65.3Ø1** Unspecified injury of deep palmar arch of right hand   CC PE

√7ᵗʰ **S65.3Ø2** Unspecified injury of deep palmar arch of left hand   CC PE

√7ᵗʰ **S65.3Ø9** Unspecified injury of deep palmar arch of unspecified hand   CC UNS PE

√6ᵗʰ **S65.31** Laceration of deep palmar arch

√7ᵗʰ **S65.311** Laceration of deep palmar arch of right hand   CC PE

√7ᵗʰ **S65.312** Laceration of deep palmar arch of left hand   CC PE

√7ᵗʰ **S65.319** Laceration of deep palmar arch of unspecified hand   CC UNS PE

√6ᵗʰ **S65.39** Other specified injury of deep palmar arch

√7ᵗʰ **S65.391** Other specified injury of deep palmar arch of right hand   CC PE

√7ᵗʰ **S65.392** Other specified injury of deep palmar arch of left hand   CC PE

√7ᵗʰ **S65.399** Other specified injury of deep palmar arch of unspecified hand   CC UNS PE

√5ᵗʰ **S65.4** Injury of blood vessel of thumb

√6ᵗʰ **S65.4Ø** Unspecified injury of blood vessel of thumb

√7ᵗʰ **S65.4Ø1** Unspecified injury of blood vessel of right thumb   CC PE

√7ᵗʰ **S65.4Ø2** Unspecified injury of blood vessel of left thumb   CC PE

√7ᵗʰ **S65.4Ø9** Unspecified injury of blood vessel of unspecified thumb   CC UNS PE

√6ᵗʰ **S65.41** Laceration of blood vessel of thumb

√7ᵗʰ **S65.411** Laceration of blood vessel of right thumb   CC PE

√7ᵗʰ **S65.412** Laceration of blood vessel of left thumb   CC PE

√7ᵗʰ **S65.419** Laceration of blood vessel of unspecified thumb   CC UNS PE

√6ᵗʰ **S65.49** Other specified injury of blood vessel of thumb

√7ᵗʰ **S65.491** Other specified injury of blood vessel of right thumb   CC PE

√7ᵗʰ **S65.492** Other specified injury of blood vessel of left thumb   CC PE

√7ᵗʰ **S65.499** Other specified injury of blood vessel of unspecified thumb   CC UNS PE

√5ᵗʰ **S65.5** Injury of blood vessel of other and unspecified finger

√6ᵗʰ **S65.5Ø** Unspecified injury of blood vessel of other and unspecified finger

√7ᵗʰ **S65.5ØØ** Unspecified injury of blood vessel of right index finger   CC PE

√7ᵗʰ **S65.5Ø1** Unspecified injury of blood vessel of left index finger   CC PE

√7ᵗʰ **S65.5Ø2** Unspecified injury of blood vessel of right middle finger   CC PE

√7ᵗʰ **S65.5Ø3** Unspecified injury of blood vessel of left middle finger   CC PE

√7ᵗʰ **S65.5Ø4** Unspecified injury of blood vessel of right ring finger   CC PE

√7ᵗʰ **S65.5Ø5** Unspecified injury of blood vessel of left ring finger   CC PE

√7ᵗʰ **S65.5Ø6** Unspecified injury of blood vessel of right little finger   CC PE

✔ Additional Character Required   √x7ᵗʰ Placeholder   Questionable PDx   Manifestation   Unspecified   UPD Unacceptable PDx   H1-H4 HAC   HCC CMS-HCC Dx   HIV HIV Dx

ICD-10-CM 2025

1069

√7ᵗʰ **S65.507** Unspecified injury of blood vessel of **left little** finger `CC` `PE`

√7ᵗʰ **S65.508** Unspecified injury of blood vessel of other finger `CC` `UNS` `PE`
> Unspecified injury of blood vessel of specified finger with unspecified laterality

√7ᵗʰ **S65.509** Unspecified injury of blood vessel of unspecified finger `CC` `UNS` `PE`

√6ᵗʰ **S65.51** **Laceration** of blood vessel of other and unspecified finger

√7ᵗʰ **S65.510** Laceration of blood vessel of **right index** finger `CC` `PE`

√7ᵗʰ **S65.511** Laceration of blood vessel of **left index** finger `CC` `PE`

√7ᵗʰ **S65.512** Laceration of blood vessel of **right middle** finger `CC` `PE`

√7ᵗʰ **S65.513** Laceration of blood vessel of **left middle** finger `CC` `PE`

√7ᵗʰ **S65.514** Laceration of blood vessel of **right ring** finger `CC` `PE`

√7ᵗʰ **S65.515** Laceration of blood vessel of **left ring** finger `CC` `PE`

√7ᵗʰ **S65.516** Laceration of blood vessel of **right little** finger `CC` `PE`

√7ᵗʰ **S65.517** Laceration of blood vessel of **left little** finger `CC` `PE`

√7ᵗʰ **S65.518** Laceration of blood vessel of other finger `CC` `PE`
> Laceration of blood vessel of specified finger with unspecified laterality

√7ᵗʰ **S65.519** Laceration of blood vessel of unspecified finger `CC` `UNS` `PE`

√6ᵗʰ **S65.59** **Other specified injury** of blood vessel of other and unspecified finger

√7ᵗʰ **S65.590** Other specified injury of blood vessel of **right index** finger `CC` `PE`

√7ᵗʰ **S65.591** Other specified injury of blood vessel of **left index** finger `CC` `PE`

√7ᵗʰ **S65.592** Other specified injury of blood vessel of **right middle** finger `CC` `PE`

√7ᵗʰ **S65.593** Other specified injury of blood vessel of **left middle** finger `CC` `PE`

√7ᵗʰ **S65.594** Other specified injury of blood vessel of **right ring** finger `CC` `PE`

√7ᵗʰ **S65.595** Other specified injury of blood vessel of **left ring** finger `CC` `PE`

√7ᵗʰ **S65.596** Other specified injury of blood vessel of **right little** finger `CC` `PE`

√7ᵗʰ **S65.597** Other specified injury of blood vessel of **left little** finger `CC` `PE`

√7ᵗʰ **S65.598** Other specified injury of blood vessel of other finger `CC` `PE`
> Other specified injury of blood vessel of specified finger with unspecified laterality

√7ᵗʰ **S65.599** Other specified injury of blood vessel of unspecified finger `CC` `UNS` `PE`

√5ᵗʰ **S65.8** **Injury of other blood vessels at wrist and hand level**

√6ᵗʰ **S65.80** **Unspecified injury** of other blood vessels at wrist and hand level

√7ᵗʰ **S65.801** Unspecified injury of other blood vessels at wrist and hand level of right arm `CC` `PE`

√7ᵗʰ **S65.802** Unspecified injury of other blood vessels at wrist and hand level of left arm `CC` `PE`

√7ᵗʰ **S65.809** Unspecified injury of other blood vessels at wrist and hand level of unspecified arm `CC` `UNS` `PE`

√6ᵗʰ **S65.81** **Laceration** of other blood vessels at wrist and hand level

√7ᵗʰ **S65.811** Laceration of other blood vessels at wrist and hand level of **right** arm `CC` `PE`

√7ᵗʰ **S65.812** Laceration of other blood vessels at wrist and hand level of **left** arm `CC` `PE`

√7ᵗʰ **S65.819** Laceration of other blood vessels at wrist and hand level of unspecified arm `CC` `UNS` `PE`

√6ᵗʰ **S65.89** **Other specified injury** of other blood vessels at wrist and hand level

√7ᵗʰ **S65.891** Other specified injury of other blood vessels at wrist and hand level of **right** arm `CC` `PE`

√7ᵗʰ **S65.892** Other specified injury of other blood vessels at wrist and hand level of **left** arm `CC` `PE`

√7ᵗʰ **S65.899** Other specified injury of other blood vessels at wrist and hand level of unspecified arm `CC` `UNS` `PE`

√5ᵗʰ **S65.9** **Injury of unspecified blood vessel at wrist and hand level**

√6ᵗʰ **S65.90** **Unspecified injury** of unspecified blood vessel at wrist and hand level

√7ᵗʰ **S65.901** Unspecified injury of unspecified blood vessel at wrist and hand level of **right** arm `CC` `PE`

√7ᵗʰ **S65.902** Unspecified injury of unspecified blood vessel at wrist and hand level of **left** arm `CC` `PE`

√7ᵗʰ **S65.909** Unspecified injury of unspecified blood vessel at wrist and hand level of unspecified arm `CC` `UNS` `PE`

√6ᵗʰ **S65.91** **Laceration** of unspecified blood vessel at wrist and hand level

√7ᵗʰ **S65.911** Laceration of unspecified blood vessel at wrist and hand level of **right** arm `CC` `PE`

√7ᵗʰ **S65.912** Laceration of unspecified blood vessel at wrist and hand level of **left** arm `CC` `PE`

√7ᵗʰ **S65.919** Laceration of unspecified blood vessel at wrist and hand level of unspecified arm `CC` `UNS` `PE`

√6ᵗʰ **S65.99** **Other specified injury** of unspecified blood vessel at wrist and hand level

√7ᵗʰ **S65.991** Other specified injury of unspecified blood vessel at wrist and hand of **right** arm `CC` `PE`

√7ᵗʰ **S65.992** Other specified injury of unspecified blood vessel at wrist and hand of **left** arm `CC` `PE`

√7ᵗʰ **S65.999** Other specified injury of unspecified blood vessel at wrist and hand of unspecified arm `CC` `UNS` `PE`

√4ᵗʰ **S66** **Injury of muscle, fascia and tendon at wrist and hand level**

Code also any associated open wound (S61.-)

EXCLUDES 2   *sprain of joints and ligaments of wrist and hand (S63.-)*

TIP: Refer to the Muscle/Tendon table at the beginning of this chapter.

> The appropriate 7th character is to be added to each code from category S66.
> A   initial encounter
> D   subsequent encounter
> S   sequela

√5ᵗʰ **S66.0** **Injury of long flexor muscle, fascia and tendon of thumb at wrist and hand level**

√6ᵗʰ **S66.00** **Unspecified injury** of long flexor muscle, fascia and tendon of thumb at wrist and hand level

√7ᵗʰ **S66.001** Unspecified injury of long flexor muscle, fascia and tendon of **right** thumb at wrist and hand level `PE`

√7ᵗʰ **S66.002** Unspecified injury of long flexor muscle, fascia and tendon of **left** thumb at wrist and hand level `PE`

√7ᵗʰ **S66.009** Unspecified injury of long flexor muscle, fascia and tendon of unspecified thumb at wrist and hand level `PE`

√6ᵗʰ **S66.01** **Strain** of long flexor muscle, fascia and tendon of thumb at wrist and hand level

√7ᵗʰ **S66.011** Strain of long flexor muscle, fascia and tendon of **right** thumb at wrist and hand level `PE`

√7ᵗʰ **S66.012** Strain of long flexor muscle, fascia and tendon of **left** thumb at wrist and hand level `PE`

√7ᵗʰ **S66.019** Strain of long flexor muscle, fascia and tendon of unspecified thumb at wrist and hand level `PE`

√6ᵗʰ **S66.02** **Laceration** of long flexor muscle, fascia and tendon of thumb at wrist and hand level

√7ᵗʰ **S66.021** Laceration of long flexor muscle, fascia and tendon of **right** thumb at wrist and hand level `CC` `PE`

√7th **S66.022** Laceration of long flexor muscle, fascia and tendon of **left** thumb at wrist and hand level   `CC` `PE`

√7th **S66.029** Laceration of long flexor muscle, fascia and tendon of unspecified thumb at wrist and hand level   `CC` `PE`

√6th **S66.09** Other specified injury of long flexor muscle, fascia and tendon of thumb at wrist and hand level

√7th **S66.091** Other specified injury of long flexor muscle, fascia and tendon of **right** thumb at wrist and hand level   `PE`

√7th **S66.092** Other specified injury of long flexor muscle, fascia and tendon of **left** thumb at wrist and hand level   `PE`

√7th **S66.099** Other specified injury of long flexor muscle, fascia and tendon of unspecified thumb at wrist and hand level   `PE`

√5th **S66.1** Injury of **flexor** muscle, fascia and tendon of other and unspecified **finger** at wrist and hand level

> EXCLUDES 2   injury of long flexor muscle, fascia and tendon of thumb at wrist and hand level (S66.0-)

√6th **S66.10** Unspecified injury of flexor muscle, fascia and tendon of other and unspecified finger at wrist and hand level

√7th **S66.100** Unspecified injury of flexor muscle, fascia and tendon of **right index** finger at wrist and hand level   `PE`

√7th **S66.101** Unspecified injury of flexor muscle, fascia and tendon of **left index** finger at wrist and hand level   `PE`

√7th **S66.102** Unspecified injury of flexor muscle, fascia and tendon of **right middle** finger at wrist and hand level   `PE`

√7th **S66.103** Unspecified injury of flexor muscle, fascia and tendon of **left middle** finger at wrist and hand level   `PE`

√7th **S66.104** Unspecified injury of flexor muscle, fascia and tendon of **right ring** finger at wrist and hand level   `PE`

√7th **S66.105** Unspecified injury of flexor muscle, fascia and tendon of **left ring** finger at wrist and hand level   `PE`

√7th **S66.106** Unspecified injury of flexor muscle, fascia and tendon of **right little** finger at wrist and hand level   `PE`

√7th **S66.107** Unspecified injury of flexor muscle, fascia and tendon of **left little** finger at wrist and hand level   `PE`

√7th **S66.108** Unspecified injury of flexor muscle, fascia and tendon of other finger at wrist and hand level   `PE`

> Unspecified injury of flexor muscle, fascia and tendon of specified finger with unspecified laterality at wrist and hand level

√7th **S66.109** Unspecified injury of flexor muscle, fascia and tendon of unspecified finger at wrist and hand level   `PE`

√6th **S66.11** Strain of flexor muscle, fascia and tendon of other and unspecified finger at wrist and hand level

√7th **S66.110** Strain of flexor muscle, fascia and tendon of **right index** finger at wrist and hand level   `PE`

√7th **S66.111** Strain of flexor muscle, fascia and tendon of **left index** finger at wrist and hand level   `PE`

√7th **S66.112** Strain of flexor muscle, fascia and tendon of **right middle** finger at wrist and hand level   `PE`

√7th **S66.113** Strain of flexor muscle, fascia and tendon of **left middle** finger at wrist and hand level   `PE`

√7th **S66.114** Strain of flexor muscle, fascia and tendon of **right ring** finger at wrist and hand level   `PE`

√7th **S66.115** Strain of flexor muscle, fascia and tendon of **left ring** finger at wrist and hand level   `PE`

√7th **S66.116** Strain of flexor muscle, fascia and tendon of **right little** finger at wrist and hand level   `PE`

√7th **S66.117** Strain of flexor muscle, fascia and tendon of **left little** finger at wrist and hand level   `PE`

√7th **S66.118** Strain of flexor muscle, fascia and tendon of other finger at wrist and hand level   `PE`

> Strain of flexor muscle, fascia and tendon of specified finger with unspecified laterality at wrist and hand level

√7th **S66.119** Strain of flexor muscle, fascia and tendon of unspecified finger at wrist and hand level   `PE`

√6th **S66.12** **Laceration** of flexor muscle, fascia and tendon of other and unspecified finger at wrist and hand level

√7th **S66.120** Laceration of flexor muscle, fascia and tendon of **right index** finger at wrist and hand level   `CC` `PE`

√7th **S66.121** Laceration of flexor muscle, fascia and tendon of **left index** finger at wrist and hand level   `CC` `PE`

√7th **S66.122** Laceration of flexor muscle, fascia and tendon of **right middle** finger at wrist and hand level   `CC` `PE`

√7th **S66.123** Laceration of flexor muscle, fascia and tendon of **left middle** finger at wrist and hand level   `CC` `PE`

√7th **S66.124** Laceration of flexor muscle, fascia and tendon of **right ring** finger at wrist and hand level   `CC` `PE`

√7th **S66.125** Laceration of flexor muscle, fascia and tendon of **left ring** finger at wrist and hand level   `CC` `PE`

√7th **S66.126** Laceration of flexor muscle, fascia and tendon of **right little** finger at wrist and hand level   `CC` `PE`

√7th **S66.127** Laceration of flexor muscle, fascia and tendon of **left little** finger at wrist and hand level   `CC` `PE`

√7th **S66.128** Laceration of flexor muscle, fascia and tendon of other finger at wrist and hand level   `CC` `PE`

> Laceration of flexor muscle, fascia and tendon of specified finger with unspecified laterality at wrist and hand level

√7th **S66.129** Laceration of flexor muscle, fascia and tendon of unspecified finger at wrist and hand level   `CC` `UNS` `PE`

√6th **S66.19** Other injury of flexor muscle, fascia and tendon of other and unspecified finger at wrist and hand level

√7th **S66.190** Other injury of flexor muscle, fascia and tendon of **right index** finger at wrist and hand level   `PE`

√7th **S66.191** Other injury of flexor muscle, fascia and tendon of **left index** finger at wrist and hand level   `PE`

√7th **S66.192** Other injury of flexor muscle, fascia and tendon of **right middle** finger at wrist and hand level   `PE`

√7th **S66.193** Other injury of flexor muscle, fascia and tendon of **left middle** finger at wrist and hand level   `PE`

√7th **S66.194** Other injury of flexor muscle, fascia and tendon of **right ring** finger at wrist and hand level   `PE`

√7th **S66.195** Other injury of flexor muscle, fascia and tendon of **left ring** finger at wrist and hand level   `PE`

√7th **S66.196** Other injury of flexor muscle, fascia and tendon of **right little** finger at wrist and hand level   `PE`

√7th **S66.197** Other injury of flexor muscle, fascia and tendon of **left little** finger at wrist and hand level   `PE`

√7th **S66.198** Other injury of flexor muscle, fascia and tendon of other finger at wrist and hand level   `PE`

> Other injury of flexor muscle, fascia and tendon of specified finger with unspecified laterality at wrist and hand level

☑ Additional Character Required   √x7th Placeholder   Questionable PDx   Manifestation   Unspecified   `UPD` Unacceptable PDx   `H1`-`H14` HAC   `HCC` CMS-HCC Dx   `HIV` HIV Dx

ICD-10-CM 2025   1071

√7ᵗʰ **S66.199** Other injury of flexor muscle, fascia and tendon of unspecified finger at wrist and hand level

√5ᵗʰ **S66.2** Injury of extensor muscle, fascia and tendon of thumb at wrist and hand level

  √6ᵗʰ **S66.20** Unspecified injury of extensor muscle, fascia and tendon of thumb at wrist and hand level

    √7ᵗʰ **S66.201** Unspecified injury of extensor muscle, fascia and tendon of right thumb at wrist and hand level **PE**

    √7ᵗʰ **S66.202** Unspecified injury of extensor muscle, fascia and tendon of left thumb at wrist and hand level **PE**

    √7ᵗʰ **S66.209** Unspecified injury of extensor muscle, fascia and tendon of unspecified thumb at wrist and hand level **PE**

  √6ᵗʰ **S66.21** Strain of extensor muscle, fascia and tendon of thumb at wrist and hand level

    √7ᵗʰ **S66.211** Strain of extensor muscle, fascia and tendon of right thumb at wrist and hand level **PE**

    √7ᵗʰ **S66.212** Strain of extensor muscle, fascia and tendon of left thumb at wrist and hand level **PE**

    √7ᵗʰ **S66.219** Strain of extensor muscle, fascia and tendon of unspecified thumb at wrist and hand level **PE**

  √6ᵗʰ **S66.22** Laceration of extensor muscle, fascia and tendon of thumb at wrist and hand level

    √7ᵗʰ **S66.221** Laceration of extensor muscle, fascia and tendon of right thumb at wrist and hand level **CC** **PE**

    √7ᵗʰ **S66.222** Laceration of extensor muscle, fascia and tendon of left thumb at wrist and hand level **CC** **PE**

    √7ᵗʰ **S66.229** Laceration of extensor muscle, fascia and tendon of unspecified thumb at wrist and hand level **CC** **PE**

  √6ᵗʰ **S66.29** Other specified injury of extensor muscle, fascia and tendon of thumb at wrist and hand level

    √7ᵗʰ **S66.291** Other specified injury of extensor muscle, fascia and tendon of right thumb at wrist and hand level **PE**

    √7ᵗʰ **S66.292** Other specified injury of extensor muscle, fascia and tendon of left thumb at wrist and hand level **PE**

    √7ᵗʰ **S66.299** Other specified injury of extensor muscle, fascia and tendon of unspecified thumb at wrist and hand level **PE**

√5ᵗʰ **S66.3** Injury of extensor muscle, fascia and tendon of other and unspecified finger at wrist and hand level

    EXCLUDES 2   injury of extensor muscle, fascia and tendon of thumb at wrist and hand level (S66.2-)

  √6ᵗʰ **S66.30** Unspecified injury of extensor muscle, fascia and tendon of other and unspecified finger at wrist and hand level

    √7ᵗʰ **S66.300** Unspecified injury of extensor muscle, fascia and tendon of right index finger at wrist and hand level **PE**

    √7ᵗʰ **S66.301** Unspecified injury of extensor muscle, fascia and tendon of left index finger at wrist and hand level **PE**

    √7ᵗʰ **S66.302** Unspecified injury of extensor muscle, fascia and tendon of right middle finger at wrist and hand level **PE**

    √7ᵗʰ **S66.303** Unspecified injury of extensor muscle, fascia and tendon of left middle finger at wrist and hand level **PE**

    √7ᵗʰ **S66.304** Unspecified injury of extensor muscle, fascia and tendon of right ring finger at wrist and hand level **PE**

    √7ᵗʰ **S66.305** Unspecified injury of extensor muscle, fascia and tendon of left ring finger at wrist and hand level **PE**

    √7ᵗʰ **S66.306** Unspecified injury of extensor muscle, fascia and tendon of right little finger at wrist and hand level **PE**

    √7ᵗʰ **S66.307** Unspecified injury of extensor muscle, fascia and tendon of left little finger at wrist and hand level **PE**

√7ᵗʰ **S66.308** Unspecified injury of extensor muscle, fascia and tendon of other finger at wrist and hand level **PE**

    Unspecified injury of extensor muscle, fascia and tendon of specified finger with unspecified laterality at wrist and hand level

√7ᵗʰ **S66.309** Unspecified injury of extensor muscle, fascia and tendon of unspecified finger at wrist and hand level **PE**

√6ᵗʰ **S66.31** Strain of extensor muscle, fascia and tendon of other and unspecified finger at wrist and hand level

    √7ᵗʰ **S66.310** Strain of extensor muscle, fascia and tendon of right index finger at wrist and hand level **PE**

    √7ᵗʰ **S66.311** Strain of extensor muscle, fascia and tendon of left index finger at wrist and hand level **PE**

    √7ᵗʰ **S66.312** Strain of extensor muscle, fascia and tendon of right middle finger at wrist and hand level **PE**

    √7ᵗʰ **S66.313** Strain of extensor muscle, fascia and tendon of left middle finger at wrist and hand level **PE**

    √7ᵗʰ **S66.314** Strain of extensor muscle, fascia and tendon of right ring finger at wrist and hand level **PE**

    √7ᵗʰ **S66.315** Strain of extensor muscle, fascia and tendon of left ring finger at wrist and hand level **PE**

    √7ᵗʰ **S66.316** Strain of extensor muscle, fascia and tendon of right little finger at wrist and hand level **PE**

    √7ᵗʰ **S66.317** Strain of extensor muscle, fascia and tendon of left little finger at wrist and hand level **PE**

    √7ᵗʰ **S66.318** Strain of extensor muscle, fascia and tendon of other finger at wrist and hand level **PE**

    Strain of extensor muscle, fascia and tendon of specified finger with unspecified laterality at wrist and hand level

    √7ᵗʰ **S66.319** Strain of extensor muscle, fascia and tendon of unspecified finger at wrist and hand level **PE**

√6ᵗʰ **S66.32** Laceration of extensor muscle, fascia and tendon of other and unspecified finger at wrist and hand level

    √7ᵗʰ **S66.320** Laceration of extensor muscle, fascia and tendon of right index finger at wrist and hand level **CC** **PE**

    √7ᵗʰ **S66.321** Laceration of extensor muscle, fascia and tendon of left index finger at wrist and hand level **CC** **PE**

    √7ᵗʰ **S66.322** Laceration of extensor muscle, fascia and tendon of right middle finger at wrist and hand level **CC** **PE**

    √7ᵗʰ **S66.323** Laceration of extensor muscle, fascia and tendon of left middle finger at wrist and hand level **CC** **PE**

    √7ᵗʰ **S66.324** Laceration of extensor muscle, fascia and tendon of right ring finger at wrist and hand level **CC** **PE**

    √7ᵗʰ **S66.325** Laceration of extensor muscle, fascia and tendon of left ring finger at wrist and hand level **CC** **PE**

    √7ᵗʰ **S66.326** Laceration of extensor muscle, fascia and tendon of right little finger at wrist and hand level **CC** **PE**

    √7ᵗʰ **S66.327** Laceration of extensor muscle, fascia and tendon of left little finger at wrist and hand level **CC** **PE**

    √7ᵗʰ **S66.328** Laceration of extensor muscle, fascia and tendon of other finger at wrist and hand level **CC** **PE**

    Laceration of extensor muscle, fascia and tendon of specified finger with unspecified laterality at wrist and hand level

    √7ᵗʰ **S66.329** Laceration of extensor muscle, fascia and tendon of unspecified finger at wrist and hand level **CC** **UNS** **PE**

N Newborn: 0   **P** Pediatric: 0-17   **M** Maternity: 9-64   **A** Adult: 15-124   **UNS** Unspecified Site   **MCC** Major Complication/Comorbidity   **CC** Complication/Comorbidity   **PE** POA Exempt

1072

ICD-10-CM 2025

✓6ᵗʰ **S66.39** **Other injury of extensor muscle, fascia and tendon of other and unspecified finger at wrist and hand level**

   ✓7ᵗʰ **S66.390** Other injury of extensor muscle, fascia and tendon of **right index** finger at wrist and hand level   PE

   ✓7ᵗʰ **S66.391** Other injury of extensor muscle, fascia and tendon of **left index** finger at wrist and hand level   PE

   ✓7ᵗʰ **S66.392** Other injury of extensor muscle, fascia and tendon of **right middle** finger at wrist and hand level   PE

   ✓7ᵗʰ **S66.393** Other injury of extensor muscle, fascia and tendon of **left middle** finger at wrist and hand level   PE

   ✓7ᵗʰ **S66.394** Other injury of extensor muscle, fascia and tendon of **right ring** finger at wrist and hand level   PE

   ✓7ᵗʰ **S66.395** Other injury of extensor muscle, fascia and tendon of **left ring** finger at wrist and hand level   PE

   ✓7ᵗʰ **S66.396** Other injury of extensor muscle, fascia and tendon of **right little** finger at wrist and hand level   PE

   ✓7ᵗʰ **S66.397** Other injury of extensor muscle, fascia and tendon of **left little** finger at wrist and hand level   PE

   ✓7ᵗʰ **S66.398** Other injury of extensor muscle, fascia and tendon of other finger at wrist and hand level   PE

        Other injury of extensor muscle, fascia and tendon of specified finger with unspecified laterality at wrist and hand level

   ✓7ᵗʰ **S66.399** Other injury of extensor muscle, fascia and tendon of unspecified finger at wrist and hand level   PE

✓5ᵗʰ **S66.4** **Injury of intrinsic muscle, fascia and tendon of thumb at wrist and hand level**

  ✓6ᵗʰ **S66.40** **Unspecified injury of intrinsic muscle, fascia and tendon of thumb at wrist and hand level**

   ✓7ᵗʰ **S66.401** Unspecified injury of intrinsic muscle, fascia and tendon of **right** thumb at wrist and hand level   PE

   ✓7ᵗʰ **S66.402** Unspecified injury of intrinsic muscle, fascia and tendon of **left** thumb at wrist and hand level   PE

   ✓7ᵗʰ **S66.409** Unspecified injury of intrinsic muscle, fascia and tendon of unspecified thumb at wrist and hand level

  ✓6ᵗʰ **S66.41** **Strain of intrinsic muscle, fascia and tendon of thumb at wrist and hand level**

   ✓7ᵗʰ **S66.411** Strain of intrinsic muscle, fascia and tendon of **right** thumb at wrist and hand level   PE

   ✓7ᵗʰ **S66.412** Strain of intrinsic muscle, fascia and tendon of **left** thumb at wrist and hand level   PE

   ✓7ᵗʰ **S66.419** Strain of intrinsic muscle, fascia and tendon of unspecified thumb at wrist and hand level   PE

  ✓6ᵗʰ **S66.42** **Laceration of intrinsic muscle, fascia and tendon of thumb at wrist and hand level**

   ✓7ᵗʰ **S66.421** Laceration of intrinsic muscle, fascia and tendon of **right** thumb at wrist and hand level   CC PE

   ✓7ᵗʰ **S66.422** Laceration of intrinsic muscle, fascia and tendon of **left** thumb at wrist and hand level   CC PE

   ✓7ᵗʰ **S66.429** Laceration of intrinsic muscle, fascia and tendon of unspecified thumb at wrist and hand level   CC PE

  ✓6ᵗʰ **S66.49** **Other specified injury of intrinsic muscle, fascia and tendon of thumb at wrist and hand level**

   ✓7ᵗʰ **S66.491** Other specified injury of intrinsic muscle, fascia and tendon of **right** thumb at wrist and hand level   PE

   ✓7ᵗʰ **S66.492** Other specified injury of intrinsic muscle, fascia and tendon of **left** thumb at wrist and hand level   PE

   ✓7ᵗʰ **S66.499** Other specified injury of intrinsic muscle, fascia and tendon of unspecified thumb at wrist and hand level   PE

✓5ᵗʰ **S66.5** **Injury of intrinsic muscle, fascia and tendon of other and unspecified finger at wrist and hand level**

   EXCLUDES 2   injury of intrinsic muscle, fascia and tendon of thumb at wrist and hand level (S66.4-)

  ✓6ᵗʰ **S66.50** **Unspecified injury of intrinsic muscle, fascia and tendon of other and unspecified finger at wrist and hand level**

   ✓7ᵗʰ **S66.500** Unspecified injury of intrinsic muscle, fascia and tendon of **right index** finger at wrist and hand level   PE

   ✓7ᵗʰ **S66.501** Unspecified injury of intrinsic muscle, fascia and tendon of **left index** finger at wrist and hand level   PE

   ✓7ᵗʰ **S66.502** Unspecified injury of intrinsic muscle, fascia and tendon of **right middle** finger at wrist and hand level   PE

   ✓7ᵗʰ **S66.503** Unspecified injury of intrinsic muscle, fascia and tendon of **left middle** finger at wrist and hand level   PE

   ✓7ᵗʰ **S66.504** Unspecified injury of intrinsic muscle, fascia and tendon of **right ring** finger at wrist and hand level   PE

   ✓7ᵗʰ **S66.505** Unspecified injury of intrinsic muscle, fascia and tendon of **left ring** finger at wrist and hand level   PE

   ✓7ᵗʰ **S66.506** Unspecified injury of intrinsic muscle, fascia and tendon of **right little** finger at wrist and hand level   PE

   ✓7ᵗʰ **S66.507** Unspecified injury of intrinsic muscle, fascia and tendon of **left little** finger at wrist and hand level   PE

   ✓7ᵗʰ **S66.508** Unspecified injury of intrinsic muscle, fascia and tendon of other finger at wrist and hand level   PE

        Unspecified injury of intrinsic muscle, fascia and tendon of specified finger with unspecified laterality at wrist and hand level

   ✓7ᵗʰ **S66.509** Unspecified injury of intrinsic muscle, fascia and tendon of unspecified finger at wrist and hand level   PE

  ✓6ᵗʰ **S66.51** **Strain of intrinsic muscle, fascia and tendon of other and unspecified finger at wrist and hand level**

   ✓7ᵗʰ **S66.510** Strain of intrinsic muscle, fascia and tendon of **right index** finger at wrist and hand level   PE

   ✓7ᵗʰ **S66.511** Strain of intrinsic muscle, fascia and tendon of **left index** finger at wrist and hand level   PE

   ✓7ᵗʰ **S66.512** Strain of intrinsic muscle, fascia and tendon of **right middle** finger at wrist and hand level   PE

   ✓7ᵗʰ **S66.513** Strain of intrinsic muscle, fascia and tendon of **left middle** finger at wrist and hand level   PE

   ✓7ᵗʰ **S66.514** Strain of intrinsic muscle, fascia and tendon of **right ring** finger at wrist and hand level   PE

   ✓7ᵗʰ **S66.515** Strain of intrinsic muscle, fascia and tendon of **left ring** finger at wrist and hand level   PE

   ✓7ᵗʰ **S66.516** Strain of intrinsic muscle, fascia and tendon of **right little** finger at wrist and hand level   PE

   ✓7ᵗʰ **S66.517** Strain of intrinsic muscle, fascia and tendon of **left little** finger at wrist and hand level   PE

   ✓7ᵗʰ **S66.518** Strain of intrinsic muscle, fascia and tendon of other finger at wrist and hand level   PE

        Strain of intrinsic muscle, fascia and tendon of specified finger with unspecified laterality at wrist and hand level

   ✓7ᵗʰ **S66.519** Strain of intrinsic muscle, fascia and tendon of unspecified finger at wrist and hand level   PE

  ✓6ᵗʰ **S66.52** **Laceration of intrinsic muscle, fascia and tendon of other and unspecified finger at wrist and hand level**

   ✓7ᵗʰ **S66.520** Laceration of intrinsic muscle, fascia and tendon of **right index** finger at wrist and hand level   CC PE

✓ Additional Character Required   ✓x7ᵗʰ Placeholder   Questionable PDx   Manifestation   Unspecified   UPD Unacceptable PDx   H1-H4 HAC   HCC CMS-HCC Dx   HIV HIV Dx

ICD-10-CM 2025   1073

Chapter 19. Injury, Poisoning and Certain Other Consequences of External Causes

S66.39–S66.520

√7ᵗʰ **S66.521 Laceration of intrinsic muscle, fascia and tendon of left index finger at wrist and hand level** CC PE

√7ᵗʰ **S66.522 Laceration of intrinsic muscle, fascia and tendon of right middle finger at wrist and hand level** CC PE

√7ᵗʰ **S66.523 Laceration of intrinsic muscle, fascia and tendon of left middle finger at wrist and hand level** CC PE

√7ᵗʰ **S66.524 Laceration of intrinsic muscle, fascia and tendon of right ring finger at wrist and hand level** CC PE

√7ᵗʰ **S66.525 Laceration of intrinsic muscle, fascia and tendon of left ring finger at wrist and hand level** CC PE

√7ᵗʰ **S66.526 Laceration of intrinsic muscle, fascia and tendon of right little finger at wrist and hand level** CC PE

√7ᵗʰ **S66.527 Laceration of intrinsic muscle, fascia and tendon of left little finger at wrist and hand level** CC PE

√7ᵗʰ **S66.528 Laceration of intrinsic muscle, fascia and tendon of other finger at wrist and hand level** CC PE
Laceration of intrinsic muscle, fascia and tendon of specified finger with unspecified laterality at wrist and hand level

√7ᵗʰ **S66.529 Laceration of intrinsic muscle, fascia and tendon of unspecified finger at wrist and hand level** CC UNS PE

√6ᵗʰ **S66.59 Other injury of intrinsic muscle, fascia and tendon of other and unspecified finger at wrist and hand level**

√7ᵗʰ **S66.590 Other injury of intrinsic muscle, fascia and tendon of right index finger at wrist and hand level** PE

√7ᵗʰ **S66.591 Other injury of intrinsic muscle, fascia and tendon of left index finger at wrist and hand level** PE

√7ᵗʰ **S66.592 Other injury of intrinsic muscle, fascia and tendon of right middle finger at wrist and hand level** PE

√7ᵗʰ **S66.593 Other injury of intrinsic muscle, fascia and tendon of left middle finger at wrist and hand level** PE

√7ᵗʰ **S66.594 Other injury of intrinsic muscle, fascia and tendon of right ring finger at wrist and hand level** PE

√7ᵗʰ **S66.595 Other injury of intrinsic muscle, fascia and tendon of left ring finger at wrist and hand level** PE

√7ᵗʰ **S66.596 Other injury of intrinsic muscle, fascia and tendon of right little finger at wrist and hand level** PE

√7ᵗʰ **S66.597 Other injury of intrinsic muscle, fascia and tendon of left little finger at wrist and hand level** PE

√7ᵗʰ **S66.598 Other injury of intrinsic muscle, fascia and tendon of other finger at wrist and hand level** PE
Other injury of intrinsic muscle, fascia and tendon of specified finger with unspecified laterality at wrist and hand level

√7ᵗʰ **S66.599 Other injury of intrinsic muscle, fascia and tendon of unspecified finger at wrist and hand level** PE

√5ᵗʰ **S66.8 Injury of other specified muscles, fascia and tendons at wrist and hand level**

√6ᵗʰ **S66.80 Unspecified injury of other specified muscles, fascia and tendons at wrist and hand level**

√7ᵗʰ **S66.801 Unspecified injury of other specified muscles, fascia and tendons at wrist and hand level, right hand** PE

√7ᵗʰ **S66.802 Unspecified injury of other specified muscles, fascia and tendons at wrist and hand level, left hand** PE

√7ᵗʰ **S66.809 Unspecified injury of other specified muscles, fascia and tendons at wrist and hand level, unspecified hand** PE

√6ᵗʰ **S66.81 Strain of other specified muscles, fascia and tendons at wrist and hand level**

√7ᵗʰ **S66.811 Strain of other specified muscles, fascia and tendons at wrist and hand level, right hand**

√7ᵗʰ **S66.812 Strain of other specified muscles, fascia and tendons at wrist and hand level, left hand**

√7ᵗʰ **S66.819 Strain of other specified muscles, fascia and tendons at wrist and hand level, unspecified hand** PE

√6ᵗʰ **S66.82 Laceration of other specified muscles, fascia and tendons at wrist and hand level**

√7ᵗʰ **S66.821 Laceration of other specified muscles, fascia and tendons at wrist and hand level, right hand** CC PE

√7ᵗʰ **S66.822 Laceration of other specified muscles, fascia and tendons at wrist and hand level, left hand** CC PE

√7ᵗʰ **S66.829 Laceration of other specified muscles, fascia and tendons at wrist and hand level, unspecified hand** CC UNS PE

√6ᵗʰ **S66.89 Other injury of other specified muscles, fascia and tendons at wrist and hand level**

√7ᵗʰ **S66.891 Other injury of other specified muscles, fascia and tendons at wrist and hand level, right hand** PE

√7ᵗʰ **S66.892 Other injury of other specified muscles, fascia and tendons at wrist and hand level, left hand** PE

√7ᵗʰ **S66.899 Other injury of other specified muscles, fascia and tendons at wrist and hand level, unspecified hand** PE

√5ᵗʰ **S66.9 Injury of unspecified muscle, fascia and tendon at wrist and hand level**

√6ᵗʰ **S66.90 Unspecified injury of unspecified muscle, fascia and tendon at wrist and hand level**

√7ᵗʰ **S66.901 Unspecified injury of unspecified muscle, fascia and tendon at wrist and hand level, right hand** PE

√7ᵗʰ **S66.902 Unspecified injury of unspecified muscle, fascia and tendon at wrist and hand level, left hand** PE

√7ᵗʰ **S66.909 Unspecified injury of unspecified muscle, fascia and tendon at wrist and hand level, unspecified hand** PE

√6ᵗʰ **S66.91 Strain of unspecified muscle, fascia and tendon at wrist and hand level**

√7ᵗʰ **S66.911 Strain of unspecified muscle, fascia and tendon at wrist and hand level, right hand** PE

√7ᵗʰ **S66.912 Strain of unspecified muscle, fascia and tendon at wrist and hand level, left hand** PE

√7ᵗʰ **S66.919 Strain of unspecified muscle, fascia and tendon at wrist and hand level, unspecified hand** PE

√6ᵗʰ **S66.92 Laceration of unspecified muscle, fascia and tendon at wrist and hand level**

√7ᵗʰ **S66.921 Laceration of unspecified muscle, fascia and tendon at wrist and hand level, right hand** CC PE

√7ᵗʰ **S66.922 Laceration of unspecified muscle, fascia and tendon at wrist and hand level, left hand** CC PE

√7ᵗʰ **S66.929 Laceration of unspecified muscle, fascia and tendon at wrist and hand level, unspecified hand** CC UNS PE

√6ᵗʰ **S66.99 Other injury of unspecified muscle, fascia and tendon at wrist and hand level**

√7ᵗʰ **S66.991 Other injury of unspecified muscle, fascia and tendon at wrist and hand level, right hand** PE

√7ᵗʰ **S66.992 Other injury of unspecified muscle, fascia and tendon at wrist and hand level, left hand** PE

√7ᵗʰ **S66.999 Other injury of unspecified muscle, fascia and tendon at wrist and hand level, unspecified hand** PE

✓4th S67 Crushing injury of wrist, hand and fingers

Use additional code for all associated injuries, such as:
fracture of wrist and hand (S62.-)
open wound of wrist and hand (S61.-)

The appropriate 7th character is to be added to each code from category S67.
A   initial encounter
D   subsequent encounter
S   sequela

✓5th S67.0 Crushing injury of thumb
- **✓x7th S67.00** Crushing injury of unspecified thumb   PE
- **✓x7th S67.01** Crushing injury of right thumb   PE
- **✓x7th S67.02** Crushing injury of left thumb   PE

✓5th S67.1 Crushing injury of other and unspecified finger(s)
> EXCLUDES 2   crushing injury of thumb (S67.0-)
- **✓x7th S67.10** Crushing injury of unspecified finger(s)   PE
- **✓6th S67.19** Crushing injury of other finger(s)
  - **✓7th S67.190** Crushing injury of right index finger   PE
  - **✓7th S67.191** Crushing injury of left index finger   PE
  - **✓7th S67.192** Crushing injury of right middle finger   PE
  - **✓7th S67.193** Crushing injury of left middle finger   PE
  - **✓7th S67.194** Crushing injury of right ring finger   PE
  - **✓7th S67.195** Crushing injury of left ring finger   PE
  - **✓7th S67.196** Crushing injury of right little finger   PE
  - **✓7th S67.197** Crushing injury of left little finger   PE
  - **✓7th S67.198** Crushing injury of other finger   PE
    Crushing injury of specified finger with unspecified laterality

✓5th S67.2 Crushing injury of hand
> EXCLUDES 2   crushing injury of fingers (S67.1-)
> crushing injury of thumb (S67.0-)
- **✓x7th S67.20** Crushing injury of unspecified hand   PE
- **✓x7th S67.21** Crushing injury of right hand   PE
- **✓x7th S67.22** Crushing injury of left hand   PE

✓5th S67.3 Crushing injury of wrist
- **✓x7th S67.30** Crushing injury of unspecified wrist   PE
- **✓x7th S67.31** Crushing injury of right wrist   PE
- **✓x7th S67.32** Crushing injury of left wrist   PE

✓5th S67.4 Crushing injury of wrist and hand
> EXCLUDES 1   crushing injury of hand alone (S67.2-)
> crushing injury of wrist alone (S67.3-)
> EXCLUDES 2   crushing injury of fingers (S67.1-)
> crushing injury of thumb (S67.0-)
- **✓x7th S67.40** Crushing injury of unspecified wrist and hand   PE
- **✓x7th S67.41** Crushing injury of right wrist and hand   PE
- **✓x7th S67.42** Crushing injury of left wrist and hand   PE

✓5th S67.9 Crushing injury of unspecified part(s) of wrist, hand and fingers
- **✓x7th S67.90** Crushing injury of unspecified part(s) of unspecified wrist, hand and fingers   PE
- **✓x7th S67.91** Crushing injury of unspecified part(s) of right wrist, hand and fingers   PE
- **✓x7th S67.92** Crushing injury of unspecified part(s) of left wrist, hand and fingers   PE

✓4th S68 Traumatic amputation of wrist, hand and fingers

An amputation not identified as partial or complete should be coded to complete.

The appropriate 7th character is to be added to each code from category S68.
A   initial encounter
D   subsequent encounter
S   sequela

✓5th S68.0 Traumatic metacarpophalangeal amputation of thumb
Traumatic amputation of thumb NOS
- **✓6th S68.01** Complete traumatic metacarpophalangeal amputation of thumb
  - **✓7th S68.011** Complete traumatic metacarpophalangeal amputation of right thumb   PE
  - **✓7th S68.012** Complete traumatic metacarpophalangeal amputation of left thumb   PE

- **✓7th S68.019** Complete traumatic metacarpophalangeal amputation of unspecified thumb   PE
- **✓6th S68.02** Partial traumatic metacarpophalangeal amputation of thumb
  - **✓7th S68.021** Partial traumatic metacarpophalangeal amputation of right thumb   PE
  - **✓7th S68.022** Partial traumatic metacarpophalangeal amputation of left thumb   PE
  - **✓7th S68.029** Partial traumatic metacarpophalangeal amputation of unspecified thumb   PE

✓5th S68.1 Traumatic metacarpophalangeal amputation of other and unspecified finger
Traumatic amputation of finger NOS
> EXCLUDES 2   traumatic metacarpophalangeal amputation of thumb (S68.0-)
- **✓6th S68.11** Complete traumatic metacarpophalangeal amputation of other and unspecified finger
  - **✓7th S68.110** Complete traumatic metacarpophalangeal amputation of right index finger   PE
  - **✓7th S68.111** Complete traumatic metacarpophalangeal amputation of left index finger   PE
  - **✓7th S68.112** Complete traumatic metacarpophalangeal amputation of right middle finger   PE
  - **✓7th S68.113** Complete traumatic metacarpophalangeal amputation of left middle finger   PE
  - **✓7th S68.114** Complete traumatic metacarpophalangeal amputation of right ring finger   PE
  - **✓7th S68.115** Complete traumatic metacarpophalangeal amputation of left ring finger   PE
  - **✓7th S68.116** Complete traumatic metacarpophalangeal amputation of right little finger   PE
  - **✓7th S68.117** Complete traumatic metacarpophalangeal amputation of left little finger   PE
  - **✓7th S68.118** Complete traumatic metacarpophalangeal amputation of other finger   PE
    Complete traumatic metacarpophalangeal amputation of specified finger with unspecified laterality
  - **✓7th S68.119** Complete traumatic metacarpophalangeal amputation of unspecified finger   PE
- **✓6th S68.12** Partial traumatic metacarpophalangeal amputation of other and unspecified finger
  - **✓7th S68.120** Partial traumatic metacarpophalangeal amputation of right index finger   PE
  - **✓7th S68.121** Partial traumatic metacarpophalangeal amputation of left index finger   PE
  - **✓7th S68.122** Partial traumatic metacarpophalangeal amputation of right middle finger   PE
  - **✓7th S68.123** Partial traumatic metacarpophalangeal amputation of left middle finger   PE
  - **✓7th S68.124** Partial traumatic metacarpophalangeal amputation of right ring finger   PE
  - **✓7th S68.125** Partial traumatic metacarpophalangeal amputation of left ring finger   PE
  - **✓7th S68.126** Partial traumatic metacarpophalangeal amputation of right little finger   PE
  - **✓7th S68.127** Partial traumatic metacarpophalangeal amputation of left little finger   PE
  - **✓7th S68.128** Partial traumatic metacarpophalangeal amputation of other finger   PE
    Partial traumatic metacarpophalangeal amputation of specified finger with unspecified laterality
  - **✓7th S68.129** Partial traumatic metacarpophalangeal amputation of unspecified finger   PE

✓5th S68.4 Traumatic amputation of hand at wrist level
Traumatic amputation of hand NOS
Traumatic amputation of wrist
- **✓6th S68.41** Complete traumatic amputation of hand at wrist level
  - **✓7th S68.411** Complete traumatic amputation of right hand at wrist level   CC HCC PE
  - **✓7th S68.412** Complete traumatic amputation of left hand at wrist level   CC HCC PE
  - **✓7th S68.419** Complete traumatic amputation of unspecified hand at wrist level   CC UNS HCC PE
- **✓6th S68.42** Partial traumatic amputation of hand at wrist level
  - **✓7th S68.421** Partial traumatic amputation of right hand at wrist level   CC HCC PE

✓ Additional Character Required   ✓x7th Placeholder   Questionable PDx   Manifestation   Unspecified   UPD Unacceptable PDx   H1–H14 HAC   HCC CMS-HCC Dx   HIV HIV Dx

√7ᵗʰ **S68.422** **Partial traumatic amputation of** left **hand at wrist level** `CC` `HCC` `PE`

√7ᵗʰ **S68.429** **Partial traumatic amputation of unspecified hand at wrist level** `CC` `UNS` `HCC` `PE`

√5ᵗʰ **S68.5** **Traumatic** transphalangeal **amputation of** thumb
Traumatic interphalangeal joint amputation of thumb

√6ᵗʰ **S68.51** Complete **traumatic transphalangeal amputation of thumb**

√7ᵗʰ **S68.511** **Complete traumatic transphalangeal amputation of** right **thumb** `PE`

√7ᵗʰ **S68.512** **Complete traumatic transphalangeal amputation of** left **thumb** `PE`

√7ᵗʰ **S68.519** **Complete traumatic transphalangeal amputation of unspecified thumb** `PE`

√6ᵗʰ **S68.52** Partial **traumatic transphalangeal amputation of thumb**

√7ᵗʰ **S68.521** **Partial traumatic transphalangeal amputation of** right **thumb** `PE`

√7ᵗʰ **S68.522** **Partial traumatic transphalangeal amputation of** left **thumb** `PE`

√7ᵗʰ **S68.529** **Partial traumatic transphalangeal amputation of unspecified thumb** `PE`

√5ᵗʰ **S68.6** **Traumatic** transphalangeal **amputation of other and unspecified** finger

√6ᵗʰ **S68.61** Complete **traumatic transphalangeal amputation of other and unspecified finger(s)**

√7ᵗʰ **S68.610** **Complete traumatic transphalangeal amputation of** right index **finger** `PE`

√7ᵗʰ **S68.611** **Complete traumatic transphalangeal amputation of** left index **finger** `PE`

√7ᵗʰ **S68.612** **Complete traumatic transphalangeal amputation of** right middle **finger** `PE`

√7ᵗʰ **S68.613** **Complete traumatic transphalangeal amputation of** left middle **finger** `PE`

√7ᵗʰ **S68.614** **Complete traumatic transphalangeal amputation of** right ring **finger** `PE`

√7ᵗʰ **S68.615** **Complete traumatic transphalangeal amputation of** left ring **finger** `PE`

√7ᵗʰ **S68.616** **Complete traumatic transphalangeal amputation of** right little **finger** `PE`

√7ᵗʰ **S68.617** **Complete traumatic transphalangeal amputation of** left little **finger** `PE`

√7ᵗʰ **S68.618** **Complete traumatic transphalangeal amputation of other finger** `PE`
Complete traumatic transphalangeal amputation of specified finger with unspecified laterality

√7ᵗʰ **S68.619** **Complete traumatic transphalangeal amputation of unspecified finger** `PE`

√6ᵗʰ **S68.62** Partial **traumatic transphalangeal amputation of other and unspecified finger**

√7ᵗʰ **S68.620** **Partial traumatic transphalangeal amputation of** right index **finger** `PE`

√7ᵗʰ **S68.621** **Partial traumatic transphalangeal amputation of** left index **finger** `PE`

√7ᵗʰ **S68.622** **Partial traumatic transphalangeal amputation of** right middle **finger** `PE`

√7ᵗʰ **S68.623** **Partial traumatic transphalangeal amputation of** left middle **finger** `PE`

√7ᵗʰ **S68.624** **Partial traumatic transphalangeal amputation of** right ring **finger** `PE`

√7ᵗʰ **S68.625** **Partial traumatic transphalangeal amputation of** left ring **finger** `PE`

√7ᵗʰ **S68.626** **Partial traumatic transphalangeal amputation of** right little **finger** `PE`

√7ᵗʰ **S68.627** **Partial traumatic transphalangeal amputation of** left little **finger** `PE`

√7ᵗʰ **S68.628** **Partial traumatic transphalangeal amputation of other finger** `PE`
Partial traumatic transphalangeal amputation of specified finger with unspecified laterality

√7ᵗʰ **S68.629** **Partial traumatic transphalangeal amputation of unspecified finger** `PE`

√5ᵗʰ **S68.7** **Traumatic** transmetacarpal **amputation of** hand

√6ᵗʰ **S68.71** Complete **traumatic transmetacarpal amputation of hand**

√7ᵗʰ **S68.711** **Complete traumatic transmetacarpal amputation of** right **hand** `CC` `HCC` `PE`

√7ᵗʰ **S68.712** **Complete traumatic transmetacarpal amputation of** left **hand** `CC` `HCC` `PE`

√7ᵗʰ **S68.719** **Complete traumatic transmetacarpal amputation of unspecified hand** `CC` `UNS` `HCC` `PE`

√6ᵗʰ **S68.72** Partial **traumatic transmetacarpal amputation of hand**

√7ᵗʰ **S68.721** **Partial traumatic transmetacarpal amputation of** right **hand** `CC` `HCC` `PE`

√7ᵗʰ **S68.722** **Partial traumatic transmetacarpal amputation of** left **hand** `CC` `HCC` `PE`

√7ᵗʰ **S68.729** **Partial traumatic transmetacarpal amputation of unspecified hand** `CC` `UNS` `HCC` `PE`

√4ᵗʰ **S69** **Other and unspecified injuries of wrist, hand and finger(s)**

> The appropriate 7th character is to be added to each code from category S69.
> A   initial encounter
> D   subsequent encounter
> S   sequela

√5ᵗʰ **S69.8** **Other specified injuries of wrist, hand and finger(s)**

√x7ᵗʰ **S69.80** **Other specified injuries of unspecified wrist, hand and finger(s)** `PE`

√x7ᵗʰ **S69.81** **Other specified injuries of** right **wrist, hand and finger(s)** `PE`

√x7ᵗʰ **S69.82** **Other specified injuries of** left **wrist, hand and finger(s)** `PE`

√5ᵗʰ **S69.9** **Unspecified injury of wrist, hand and finger(s)**

√x7ᵗʰ **S69.90** **Unspecified injury of unspecified wrist, hand and finger(s)** `PE`

√x7ᵗʰ **S69.91** **Unspecified injury of** right **wrist, hand and finger(s)** `PE`

√x7ᵗʰ **S69.92** **Unspecified injury of** left **wrist, hand and finger(s)** `PE`

Injuries to the hip and thigh (S70-S79)

`EXCLUDES 2`   *burns and corrosions (T20-T32)*
frostbite (T33-T34)
snake bite (T63.0-)
venomous insect bite or sting (T63.4-)

√4ᵗʰ **S70** **Superficial injury of hip and thigh**

> The appropriate 7th character is to be added to each code from category S70.
> A   initial encounter
> D   subsequent encounter
> S   sequela

√5ᵗʰ **S70.0** **Contusion of** hip

√x7ᵗʰ **S70.00** **Contusion of unspecified hip** `PE`

√x7ᵗʰ **S70.01** **Contusion of** right **hip** `PE`

√x7ᵗʰ **S70.02** **Contusion of** left **hip** `PE`

√5ᵗʰ **S70.1** **Contusion of** thigh

√x7ᵗʰ **S70.10** **Contusion of unspecified thigh** `PE`

√x7ᵗʰ **S70.11** **Contusion of** right **thigh** `PE`

√x7ᵗʰ **S70.12** **Contusion of** left **thigh** `PE`

√5ᵗʰ **S70.2** **Other superficial injuries of** hip

√6ᵗʰ **S70.21** Abrasion **of hip**

√7ᵗʰ **S70.211** **Abrasion,** right **hip** `PE`

√7ᵗʰ **S70.212** **Abrasion,** left **hip** `PE`

√7ᵗʰ **S70.219** **Abrasion, unspecified hip** `PE`

√6ᵗʰ **S70.22** Blister **(nonthermal) of hip**

√7ᵗʰ **S70.221** **Blister (nonthermal),** right **hip** `PE`

√7ᵗʰ **S70.222** **Blister (nonthermal),** left **hip** `PE`

√7ᵗʰ **S70.229** **Blister (nonthermal), unspecified hip** `PE`

√6ᵗʰ **S70.24** External constriction **of hip**

√7ᵗʰ **S70.241** **External constriction,** right **hip** `PE`

√7ᵗʰ **S70.242** **External constriction,** left **hip** `PE`

√7ᵗʰ **S70.249** **External constriction, unspecified hip** `PE`

√6ᵗʰ **S70.25** **Superficial** foreign body **of hip**
Splinter in the hip

√7ᵗʰ **S70.251** **Superficial foreign body,** right **hip** `PE`

√7th **S70.252** Superficial foreign body, left hip   PE

√7th **S70.259** Superficial foreign body, unspecified hip   PE

√6th **S70.26** Insect bite (nonvenomous) of hip

√7th **S70.261** Insect bite (nonvenomous), right hip   PE

√7th **S70.262** Insect bite (nonvenomous), left hip   PE

√7th **S70.269** Insect bite (nonvenomous), unspecified hip   PE

√6th **S70.27** Other superficial bite of hip

EXCLUDES 1   *open bite of hip (S71.05-)*

√7th **S70.271** Other superficial bite of hip, right hip   PE

√7th **S70.272** Other superficial bite of hip, left hip   PE

√7th **S70.279** Other superficial bite of hip, unspecified hip   PE

√5th **S70.3** Other superficial injuries of thigh

√6th **S70.31** Abrasion of thigh

√7th **S70.311** Abrasion, right thigh   PE

√7th **S70.312** Abrasion, left thigh   PE

√7th **S70.319** Abrasion, unspecified thigh   PE

√6th **S70.32** Blister (nonthermal) of thigh

√7th **S70.321** Blister (nonthermal), right thigh   PE

√7th **S70.322** Blister (nonthermal), left thigh   PE

√7th **S70.329** Blister (nonthermal), unspecified thigh   PE

√6th **S70.34** External constriction of thigh

√7th **S70.341** External constriction, right thigh   PE

√7th **S70.342** External constriction, left thigh   PE

√7th **S70.349** External constriction, unspecified thigh   PE

√6th **S70.35** Superficial foreign body of thigh

Splinter in the thigh

√7th **S70.351** Superficial foreign body, right thigh   PE

√7th **S70.352** Superficial foreign body, left thigh   PE

√7th **S70.359** Superficial foreign body, unspecified thigh   PE

√6th **S70.36** Insect bite (nonvenomous) of thigh

√7th **S70.361** Insect bite (nonvenomous), right thigh   PE

√7th **S70.362** Insect bite (nonvenomous), left thigh   PE

√7th **S70.369** Insect bite (nonvenomous), unspecified thigh   PE

√6th **S70.37** Other superficial bite of thigh

EXCLUDES 1   *open bite of thigh (S71.15)*

√7th **S70.371** Other superficial bite of right thigh   PE

√7th **S70.372** Other superficial bite of left thigh   PE

√7th **S70.379** Other superficial bite of unspecified thigh   PE

√5th **S70.9** Unspecified superficial injury of hip and thigh

√6th **S70.91** Unspecified superficial injury of hip

√7th **S70.911** Unspecified superficial injury of right hip   PE

√7th **S70.912** Unspecified superficial injury of left hip   PE

√7th **S70.919** Unspecified superficial injury of unspecified hip   PE

√6th **S70.92** Unspecified superficial injury of thigh

√7th **S70.921** Unspecified superficial injury of right thigh   PE

√7th **S70.922** Unspecified superficial injury of left thigh   PE

√7th **S70.929** Unspecified superficial injury of unspecified thigh   PE

√4th **S71** Open wound of hip and thigh

Code also any associated wound infection

EXCLUDES 1   *open fracture of hip and thigh (S72.-)*
     traumatic amputation of hip and thigh (S78.-)

EXCLUDES 2   *bite of venomous animal (T63.-)*
     open wound of ankle, foot and toes (S91.-)
     open wound of knee and lower leg (S81.-)

> The appropriate 7th character is to be added to each code from category S71.
> A   initial encounter
> D   subsequent encounter
> S   sequela

√5th **S71.0** Open wound of hip

√6th **S71.00** Unspecified open wound of hip

√7th **S71.001** Unspecified open wound, right hip   PE

√7th **S71.002** Unspecified open wound, left hip   PE

√7th **S71.009** Unspecified open wound, unspecified hip   PE

√6th **S71.01** Laceration without foreign body of hip

√7th **S71.011** Laceration without foreign body, right hip   PE

√7th **S71.012** Laceration without foreign body, left hip   PE

√7th **S71.019** Laceration without foreign body, unspecified hip   PE

√6th **S71.02** Laceration with foreign body of hip

√7th **S71.021** Laceration with foreign body, right hip   PE

√7th **S71.022** Laceration with foreign body, left hip   PE

√7th **S71.029** Laceration with foreign body, unspecified hip   PE

√6th **S71.03** Puncture wound without foreign body of hip

√7th **S71.031** Puncture wound without foreign body, right hip   PE

√7th **S71.032** Puncture wound without foreign body, left hip   PE

√7th **S71.039** Puncture wound without foreign body, unspecified hip   PE

√6th **S71.04** Puncture wound with foreign body of hip

√7th **S71.041** Puncture wound with foreign body, right hip   PE

√7th **S71.042** Puncture wound with foreign body, left hip   PE

√7th **S71.049** Puncture wound with foreign body, unspecified hip   PE

√6th **S71.05** Open bite of hip

Bite of hip NOS

EXCLUDES 1   *superficial bite of hip (S70.26, S70.27)*

√7th **S71.051** Open bite, right hip   PE

√7th **S71.052** Open bite, left hip   PE

√7th **S71.059** Open bite, unspecified hip   PE

√5th **S71.1** Open wound of thigh

√6th **S71.10** Unspecified open wound of thigh

AHA: 2016,3Q,24

√7th **S71.101** Unspecified open wound, right thigh   PE

√7th **S71.102** Unspecified open wound, left thigh   PE

√7th **S71.109** Unspecified open wound, unspecified thigh   PE

√6th **S71.11** Laceration without foreign body of thigh

√7th **S71.111** Laceration without foreign body, right thigh   PE

√7th **S71.112** Laceration without foreign body, left thigh   PE

√7th **S71.119** Laceration without foreign body, unspecified thigh   PE

√6th **S71.12** Laceration with foreign body of thigh

√7th **S71.121** Laceration with foreign body, right thigh   PE

√7th **S71.122** Laceration with foreign body, left thigh   PE

√7th **S71.129** Laceration with foreign body, unspecified thigh   PE

✔ Additional Character Required   √x7th Placeholder   Questionable PDx   Manifestation   Unspecified   UPD Unacceptable PDx   H1 - H14 HAC   HCC CMS-HCC Dx   HIV Dx

ICD-10-CM 2025   **1077**

√6th **S71.13 Puncture wound without foreign body** of thigh

AHA: 2023,3Q,12; 2016,3Q,24

√7th **S71.131 Puncture wound without foreign body, right** thigh **PE**

√7th **S71.132 Puncture wound without foreign body, left** thigh **PE**

√7th **S71.139 Puncture wound without foreign body, unspecified thigh** **PE**

√6th **S71.14 Puncture wound with foreign body** of thigh

AHA: 2016,3Q,24

√7th **S71.141 Puncture wound with foreign body, right** thigh **PE**

√7th **S71.142 Puncture wound with foreign body, left** thigh **PE**

√7th **S71.149 Puncture wound with foreign body, unspecified thigh** **PE**

√6th **S71.15 Open bite** of thigh

Bite of thigh NOS

EXCLUDES 1 superficial bite of thigh (S70.37-)

√7th **S71.151 Open bite, right** thigh **PE**

√7th **S71.152 Open bite, left** thigh **PE**

√7th **S71.159 Open bite, unspecified thigh** **PE**

√4th **S72 Fracture of femur**

NOTE A fracture not indicated as displaced or nondisplaced should be coded to displaced.

A fracture not indicated as open or closed should be coded to closed.

The open fracture designations are based on the Gustilo open fracture classification.

EXCLUDES 1 traumatic amputation of hip and thigh (S78.-)

EXCLUDES 2 fracture of foot (S92.-)

fracture of lower leg and ankle (S82.-)

periprosthetic fracture of prosthetic implant of hip (M97.0-)

AHA: 2023,3Q,12; 2018,2Q,12; 2016,1Q,33; 2015,3Q,37-39; 2015,1Q,17; 2013,4Q,128

DEF: Diaphysis: Central shaft of a long bone.

DEF: Epiphysis: Proximal and distal rounded ends of a long bone communicates with the joint.

DEF: Metaphysis: Section of a long bone located between the epiphysis and diaphysis at the proximal and distal ends.

DEF: Physis (growth plate): Narrow zone of cartilaginous tissue between the epiphysis and metaphysis at each end of a long bone. In childhood, proliferation of cells in this zone lengthens the bone. As the bone matures, this area thins, ossification eventually fusing into solid bone and growth stops. *Synonym(s): Epiphyseal plate.*

The appropriate 7th character is to be added to all codes from category S72 [unless otherwise indicated].

A initial encounter for closed fracture

B initial encounter for open fracture type I or II

    initial encounter for open fracture NOS

C initial encounter for open fracture type IIIA, IIIB, or IIIC

D subsequent encounter for closed fracture with routine healing

E subsequent encounter for open fracture type I or II with routine healing

F subsequent encounter for open fracture type IIIA, IIIB, or IIIC with routine healing

G subsequent encounter for closed fracture with delayed healing

H subsequent encounter for open fracture type I or II with delayed healing

J subsequent encounter for open fracture type IIIA, IIIB, or IIIC with delayed healing

K subsequent encounter for closed fracture with nonunion

M subsequent encounter for open fracture type I or II with nonunion

N subsequent encounter for open fracture type IIIA, IIIB, or IIIC with nonunion

P subsequent encounter for closed fracture with malunion

Q subsequent encounter for open fracture type I or II with malunion

R subsequent encounter for open fracture type IIIA, IIIB, or IIIC with malunion

S sequela

√5th **S72.0 Fracture of head and neck** of femur

EXCLUDES 2 physeal fracture of lower end of femur (S79.1-)

physeal fracture of upper end of femur (S79.0-)

AHA: 2016,3Q,16

√6th **S72.00 Fracture of unspecified part of neck of femur**

Fracture of hip NOS

Fracture of neck of femur NOS

√7th **S72.001 Fracture of unspecified part of neck of right femur** **MCC** **CC** **H5** **HCC** **PE**

√7th **S72.002 Fracture of unspecified part of neck of left femur** **MCC** **CC** **H5** **HCC** **PE**

√7th **S72.009 Fracture of unspecified part of neck of unspecified femur** **MCC** **CC** **H5** **UNS** **HCC** **PE**

√6th **S72.01 Unspecified intracapsular fracture of femur**

Subcapital fracture of femur

√7th **S72.011 Unspecified intracapsular fracture of right femur** **MCC** **CC** **H5** **HCC** **PE**

√7th **S72.012 Unspecified intracapsular fracture of left femur** **MCC** **CC** **H5** **HCC** **PE**

√7th **S72.019 Unspecified intracapsular fracture of unspecified femur** **MCC** **CC** **H5** **UNS** **HCC** **PE**

N Newborn: 0 **P** Pediatric: 0-17 **M** Maternity: 9-64 **A** Adult: 15-124 **UNS** Unspecified Site **MCC** Major Complication/Comorbidity **CC** Complication/Comorbidity **PE** POA Exempt

1078

ICD-10-CM 2025

✓6ᵗʰ **S72.02** **Fracture of epiphysis (separation) (upper) of femur**

Transepiphyseal fracture of femur

EXCLUDES 1   capital femoral epiphyseal fracture (pediatric) of femur (S79.01-)

Salter-Harris Type I physeal fracture of upper end of femur (S79.01-)

✓7ᵗʰ **S72.021** **Displaced** fracture of epiphysis (separation) (upper) of **right** femur   `MCC` `CC` `H5` `HCC` `PE`

✓7ᵗʰ **S72.022** **Displaced** fracture of epiphysis (separation) (upper) of **left** femur   `MCC` `CC` `H5` `HCC` `PE`

✓7ᵗʰ **S72.023** **Displaced** fracture of epiphysis (separation) (upper) of unspecified femur   `MCC` `CC` `H5` `UNS` `HCC` `PE`

✓7ᵗʰ **S72.024** **Nondisplaced** fracture of epiphysis (separation) (upper) of **right** femur   `MCC` `CC` `H5` `HCC` `PE`

✓7ᵗʰ **S72.025** **Nondisplaced** fracture of epiphysis (separation) (upper) of **left** femur   `MCC` `CC` `H5` `HCC` `PE`

✓7ᵗʰ **S72.026** **Nondisplaced** fracture of epiphysis (separation) (upper) of unspecified femur   `MCC` `CC` `H5` `UNS` `HCC` `PE`

✓6ᵗʰ **S72.03** **Midcervical fracture of femur**

Transcervical fracture of femur NOS

✓7ᵗʰ **S72.031** **Displaced** midcervical fracture of **right** femur   `MCC` `CC` `H5` `HCC` `PE`

✓7ᵗʰ **S72.032** **Displaced** midcervical fracture of **left** femur   `MCC` `CC` `H5` `HCC` `PE`

✓7ᵗʰ **S72.033** **Displaced** midcervical fracture of unspecified femur   `MCC` `CC` `H5` `UNS` `HCC` `PE`

✓7ᵗʰ **S72.034** **Nondisplaced** midcervical fracture of **right** femur   `MCC` `CC` `H5` `HCC` `PE`

✓7ᵗʰ **S72.035** **Nondisplaced** midcervical fracture of **left** femur   `MCC` `CC` `H5` `HCC` `PE`

✓7ᵗʰ **S72.036** **Nondisplaced** midcervical fracture of unspecified femur   `MCC` `CC` `H5` `UNS` `HCC` `PE`

✓6ᵗʰ **S72.04** **Fracture of base of neck of femur**

Cervicotrochanteric fracture of femur

✓7ᵗʰ **S72.041** **Displaced** fracture of base of neck of **right** femur   `MCC` `CC` `H5` `HCC` `PE`

✓7ᵗʰ **S72.042** **Displaced** fracture of base of neck of **left** femur   `MCC` `CC` `H5` `HCC` `PE`

✓7ᵗʰ **S72.043** **Displaced** fracture of base of neck of unspecified femur   `MCC` `CC` `H5` `UNS` `HCC` `PE`

✓7ᵗʰ **S72.044** **Nondisplaced** fracture of base of neck of **right** femur   `MCC` `CC` `H5` `HCC` `PE`

✓7ᵗʰ **S72.045** **Nondisplaced** fracture of base of neck of **left** femur   `MCC` `CC` `H5` `HCC` `PE`

✓7ᵗʰ **S72.046** **Nondisplaced** fracture of base of neck of unspecified femur   `MCC` `CC` `H5` `UNS` `HCC` `PE`

✓6ᵗʰ **S72.05** **Unspecified fracture of head of femur**

Fracture of head of femur NOS

✓7ᵗʰ **S72.051** **Unspecified fracture of head of right** femur   `MCC` `CC` `H5` `HCC` `PE`

✓7ᵗʰ **S72.052** **Unspecified fracture of head of left** femur   `MCC` `CC` `H5` `HCC` `PE`

✓7ᵗʰ **S72.059** **Unspecified fracture of head of unspecified** femur   `MCC` `CC` `H5` `UNS` `HCC` `PE`

✓6ᵗʰ **S72.06** **Articular fracture of head of femur**

✓7ᵗʰ **S72.061** **Displaced articular fracture of head of right** femur   `MCC` `CC` `H5` `HCC` `PE`

✓7ᵗʰ **S72.062** **Displaced articular fracture of head of left** femur   `MCC` `CC` `H5` `HCC` `PE`

✓7ᵗʰ **S72.063** **Displaced articular fracture of head of unspecified** femur   `MCC` `CC` `H5` `UNS` `HCC` `PE`

✓7ᵗʰ **S72.064** **Nondisplaced articular fracture of head of right** femur   `MCC` `CC` `H5` `HCC` `PE`

✓7ᵗʰ **S72.065** **Nondisplaced articular fracture of head of left** femur   `MCC` `CC` `H5` `HCC` `PE`

✓7ᵗʰ **S72.066** **Nondisplaced articular fracture of head of unspecified** femur   `MCC` `CC` `H5` `UNS` `HCC` `PE`

✓6ᵗʰ **S72.09** **Other fracture of head and neck of femur**

✓7ᵗʰ **S72.091** **Other fracture of head and neck of right** femur   `MCC` `CC` `H5` `HCC` `PE`

✓7ᵗʰ **S72.092** **Other fracture of head and neck of left** femur   `MCC` `CC` `H5` `HCC` `PE`

✓7ᵗʰ **S72.099** **Other fracture of head and neck of unspecified** femur   `MCC` `CC` `H5` `UNS` `HCC` `PE`

✓5ᵗʰ **S72.1** **Pertrochanteric fracture**

AHA: 2016,3Q,16

✓6ᵗʰ **S72.10** **Unspecified trochanteric fracture of femur**

Fracture of trochanter NOS

✓7ᵗʰ **S72.101** **Unspecified trochanteric fracture of right** femur   `MCC` `CC` `H5` `HCC` `PE`

✓7ᵗʰ **S72.102** **Unspecified trochanteric fracture of left** femur   `MCC` `CC` `H5` `HCC` `PE`

✓7ᵗʰ **S72.109** **Unspecified trochanteric fracture of unspecified** femur   `MCC` `CC` `H5` `UNS` `HCC` `PE`

✓6ᵗʰ **S72.11** **Fracture of greater trochanter of femur**

✓7ᵗʰ **S72.111** **Displaced fracture of greater trochanter of right** femur   `MCC` `CC` `H5` `HCC` `PE`

✓7ᵗʰ **S72.112** **Displaced fracture of greater trochanter of left** femur   `MCC` `CC` `H5` `HCC` `PE`

✓7ᵗʰ **S72.113** **Displaced fracture of greater trochanter of unspecified** femur   `MCC` `CC` `H5` `UNS` `HCC` `PE`

✓7ᵗʰ **S72.114** **Nondisplaced fracture of greater trochanter of right** femur   `MCC` `CC` `H5` `HCC` `PE`

✓7ᵗʰ **S72.115** **Nondisplaced fracture of greater trochanter of left** femur   `MCC` `CC` `H5` `HCC` `PE`

✓7ᵗʰ **S72.116** **Nondisplaced fracture of greater trochanter of unspecified** femur   `MCC` `CC` `H5` `UNS` `HCC` `PE`

✓6ᵗʰ **S72.12** **Fracture of lesser trochanter of femur**

✓7ᵗʰ **S72.121** **Displaced fracture of lesser trochanter of right** femur   `MCC` `CC` `H5` `HCC` `PE`

✓7ᵗʰ **S72.122** **Displaced fracture of lesser trochanter of left** femur   `MCC` `CC` `H5` `HCC` `PE`

✓7ᵗʰ **S72.123** **Displaced fracture of lesser trochanter of unspecified** femur   `MCC` `CC` `H5` `UNS` `HCC` `PE`

✓7ᵗʰ **S72.124** **Nondisplaced fracture of lesser trochanter of right** femur   `MCC` `CC` `H5` `HCC` `PE`

✓7ᵗʰ **S72.125** **Nondisplaced fracture of lesser trochanter of left** femur   `MCC` `CC` `H5` `HCC` `PE`

✓7ᵗʰ **S72.126** **Nondisplaced fracture of lesser trochanter of unspecified** femur   `MCC` `CC` `H5` `UNS` `HCC` `PE`

✓6ᵗʰ **S72.13** **Apophyseal fracture of femur**

EXCLUDES 1   chronic (nontraumatic) slipped upper femoral epiphysis (M93.0-)

✓7ᵗʰ **S72.131** **Displaced apophyseal fracture of right** femur   `MCC` `CC` `H5` `HCC` `PE`

✓7ᵗʰ **S72.132** **Displaced apophyseal fracture of left** femur   `MCC` `CC` `H5` `HCC` `PE`

✓7ᵗʰ **S72.133** **Displaced apophyseal fracture of unspecified** femur   `MCC` `CC` `H5` `UNS` `HCC` `PE`

✓7ᵗʰ **S72.134** **Nondisplaced apophyseal fracture of right** femur   `MCC` `CC` `H5` `HCC` `PE`

✓7ᵗʰ **S72.135** **Nondisplaced apophyseal fracture of left** femur   `MCC` `CC` `H5` `HCC` `PE`

✓7ᵗʰ **S72.136** **Nondisplaced apophyseal fracture of unspecified** femur   `MCC` `CC` `H5` `UNS` `HCC` `PE`

✓6ᵗʰ **S72.14** **Intertrochanteric fracture of femur**

✓7ᵗʰ **S72.141** **Displaced intertrochanteric fracture of right** femur   `MCC` `CC` `H5` `HCC` `PE`

✓7ᵗʰ **S72.142** **Displaced intertrochanteric fracture of left** femur   `MCC` `CC` `H5` `HCC` `PE`

✓7ᵗʰ **S72.143** **Displaced intertrochanteric fracture of unspecified** femur   `MCC` `CC` `H5` `UNS` `HCC` `PE`

✓7ᵗʰ **S72.144** **Nondisplaced intertrochanteric fracture of right** femur   `MCC` `CC` `H5` `HCC` `PE`

✓ Additional Character Required   ✓x7ᵗʰ Placeholder   Questionable PDx   Manifestation   Unspecified   `UPD` Unacceptable PDx   `H1`-`H14` HAC   `HCC` CMS-HCC Dx   `HIV` HIV Dx

ICD-10-CM 2025   1079

√7ᵗʰ **S72.145** **Nondisplaced** intertrochanteric fracture of **left** femur   `MCC` `CC` `H5` `HCC` `PE`

√7ᵗʰ **S72.146** **Nondisplaced** intertrochanteric fracture of unspecified femur   `MCC` `CC` `H5` `UNS` `HCC` `PE`

√5ᵗʰ **S72.2** **Subtrochanteric** fracture of femur

√x 7ᵗʰ **S72.21** **Displaced** subtrochanteric fracture of **right** femur   `MCC` `CC` `H5` `HCC` `PE`

√x 7ᵗʰ **S72.22** **Displaced** subtrochanteric fracture of **left** femur   `MCC` `CC` `H5` `HCC` `PE`

√x 7ᵗʰ **S72.23** **Displaced** subtrochanteric fracture of unspecified femur   `MCC` `CC` `H5` `UNS` `HCC` `PE`

√x 7ᵗʰ **S72.24** **Nondisplaced** subtrochanteric fracture of **right** femur   `MCC` `CC` `H5` `HCC` `PE`

√x 7ᵗʰ **S72.25** **Nondisplaced** subtrochanteric fracture of **left** femur   `MCC` `CC` `H5` `HCC` `PE`

√x 7ᵗʰ **S72.26** **Nondisplaced** subtrochanteric fracture of unspecified femur   `MCC` `CC` `H5` `UNS` `HCC` `PE`

√5ᵗʰ **S72.3** Fracture of **shaft** of femur

√6ᵗʰ **S72.30** Unspecified fracture of shaft of femur

√7ᵗʰ **S72.301** Unspecified fracture of shaft of **right** femur   `MCC` `CC` `H5` `HCC` `PE`

√7ᵗʰ **S72.302** Unspecified fracture of shaft of **left** femur   `MCC` `CC` `H5` `HCC` `PE`

√7ᵗʰ **S72.309** Unspecified fracture of shaft of unspecified femur   `MCC` `CC` `H5` `UNS` `HCC` `PE`

√6ᵗʰ **S72.32** **Transverse** fracture of shaft of femur

√7ᵗʰ **S72.321** **Displaced** transverse fracture of shaft of **right** femur   `MCC` `CC` `H5` `HCC` `PE`

√7ᵗʰ **S72.322** **Displaced** transverse fracture of shaft of **left** femur   `MCC` `CC` `H5` `HCC` `PE`

√7ᵗʰ **S72.323** **Displaced** transverse fracture of shaft of unspecified femur   `MCC` `CC` `H5` `UNS` `HCC` `PE`

√7ᵗʰ **S72.324** **Nondisplaced** transverse fracture of shaft of **right** femur   `MCC` `CC` `H5` `HCC` `PE`

√7ᵗʰ **S72.325** **Nondisplaced** transverse fracture of shaft of **left** femur   `MCC` `CC` `H5` `HCC` `PE`

√7ᵗʰ **S72.326** **Nondisplaced** transverse fracture of shaft of unspecified femur   `MCC` `CC` `H5` `UNS` `HCC` `PE`

√6ᵗʰ **S72.33** **Oblique** fracture of shaft of femur

√7ᵗʰ **S72.331** **Displaced** oblique fracture of shaft of **right** femur   `MCC` `CC` `H5` `HCC` `PE`

√7ᵗʰ **S72.332** **Displaced** oblique fracture of shaft of **left** femur   `MCC` `CC` `H5` `HCC` `PE`

√7ᵗʰ **S72.333** **Displaced** oblique fracture of shaft of unspecified femur   `MCC` `CC` `H5` `UNS` `HCC` `PE`

√7ᵗʰ **S72.334** **Nondisplaced** oblique fracture of shaft of **right** femur   `MCC` `CC` `H5` `HCC` `PE`

√7ᵗʰ **S72.335** **Nondisplaced** oblique fracture of shaft of **left** femur   `MCC` `CC` `H5` `HCC` `PE`

√7ᵗʰ **S72.336** **Nondisplaced** oblique fracture of shaft of unspecified femur   `MCC` `CC` `H5` `UNS` `HCC` `PE`

√6ᵗʰ **S72.34** **Spiral** fracture of shaft of femur

√7ᵗʰ **S72.341** **Displaced** spiral fracture of shaft of **right** femur   `MCC` `CC` `H5` `HCC` `PE`

√7ᵗʰ **S72.342** **Displaced** spiral fracture of shaft of **left** femur   `MCC` `CC` `H5` `HCC` `PE`

√7ᵗʰ **S72.343** **Displaced** spiral fracture of shaft of unspecified femur   `MCC` `CC` `H5` `UNS` `HCC` `PE`

√7ᵗʰ **S72.344** **Nondisplaced** spiral fracture of shaft of **right** femur   `MCC` `CC` `H5` `HCC` `PE`

√7ᵗʰ **S72.345** **Nondisplaced** spiral fracture of shaft of **left** femur   `MCC` `CC` `H5` `HCC` `PE`

√7ᵗʰ **S72.346** **Nondisplaced** spiral fracture of shaft of unspecified femur   `MCC` `CC` `H5` `UNS` `HCC` `PE`

√6ᵗʰ **S72.35** **Comminuted** fracture of shaft of femur

√7ᵗʰ **S72.351** **Displaced** comminuted fracture of shaft of **right** femur   `MCC` `CC` `H5` `HCC` `PE`

√7ᵗʰ **S72.352** **Displaced** comminuted fracture of shaft of **left** femur   `MCC` `CC` `H5` `HCC` `PE`

√7ᵗʰ **S72.353** **Displaced** comminuted fracture of shaft of unspecified femur   `MCC` `CC` `H5` `UNS` `HCC` `PE`

√7ᵗʰ **S72.354** **Nondisplaced** comminuted fracture of shaft of **right** femur   `MCC` `CC` `H5` `HCC` `PE`

√7ᵗʰ **S72.355** **Nondisplaced** comminuted fracture of shaft of **left** femur   `MCC` `CC` `H5` `HCC` `PE`

√7ᵗʰ **S72.356** **Nondisplaced** comminuted fracture of shaft of unspecified femur   `MCC` `CC` `H5` `UNS` `HCC` `PE`

√6ᵗʰ **S72.36** **Segmental** fracture of shaft of femur

√7ᵗʰ **S72.361** **Displaced** segmental fracture of shaft of **right** femur   `MCC` `CC` `H5` `HCC` `PE`

√7ᵗʰ **S72.362** **Displaced** segmental fracture of shaft of **left** femur   `MCC` `CC` `H5` `HCC` `PE`

√7ᵗʰ **S72.363** **Displaced** segmental fracture of shaft of unspecified femur   `MCC` `CC` `H5` `UNS` `HCC` `PE`

√7ᵗʰ **S72.364** **Nondisplaced** segmental fracture of shaft of **right** femur   `MCC` `CC` `H5` `HCC` `PE`

√7ᵗʰ **S72.365** **Nondisplaced** segmental fracture of shaft of **left** femur   `MCC` `CC` `H5` `HCC` `PE`

√7ᵗʰ **S72.366** **Nondisplaced** segmental fracture of shaft of unspecified femur   `MCC` `CC` `H5` `UNS` `HCC` `PE`

√6ᵗʰ **S72.39** Other fracture of shaft of femur

√7ᵗʰ **S72.391** Other fracture of shaft of **right** femur   `MCC` `CC` `H5` `HCC` `PE`

√7ᵗʰ **S72.392** Other fracture of shaft of **left** femur   `MCC` `CC` `H5` `HCC` `PE`

√7ᵗʰ **S72.399** Other fracture of shaft of unspecified femur   `MCC` `CC` `H5` `UNS` `HCC` `PE`

√5ᵗʰ **S72.4** Fracture of **lower end** of femur

Fracture of distal end of femur

EXCLUDES 2   fracture of shaft of femur (S72.3-)

physeal fracture of lower end of femur (S79.1-)

AHA: 2016,4Q,42

√6ᵗʰ **S72.40** Unspecified fracture of lower end of femur

AHA: 2018,1Q,21; 2016,4Q,42

√7ᵗʰ **S72.401** Unspecified fracture of lower end of **right** femur   `MCC` `CC` `H5` `HCC` `PE`

√7ᵗʰ **S72.402** Unspecified fracture of lower end of **left** femur   `MCC` `CC` `H5` `HCC` `PE`

√7ᵗʰ **S72.409** Unspecified fracture of lower end of unspecified femur   `MCC` `CC` `H5` `UNS` `HCC` `PE`

√6ᵗʰ **S72.41** Unspecified **condyle** fracture of lower end of femur

Condyle fracture of femur NOS

√7ᵗʰ **S72.411** **Displaced** unspecified condyle fracture of lower end of **right** femur   `MCC` `CC` `H5` `HCC` `PE`

√7ᵗʰ **S72.412** **Displaced** unspecified condyle fracture of lower end of **left** femur   `MCC` `CC` `H5` `HCC` `PE`

√7ᵗʰ **S72.413** **Displaced** unspecified condyle fracture of lower end of unspecified femur   `MCC` `CC` `H5` `UNS` `HCC` `PE`

√7ᵗʰ **S72.414** **Nondisplaced** unspecified condyle fracture of lower end of **right** femur   `MCC` `CC` `H5` `HCC` `PE`

√7ᵗʰ **S72.415** **Nondisplaced** unspecified condyle fracture of lower end of **left** femur   `MCC` `CC` `H5` `HCC` `PE`

√7ᵗʰ **S72.416** **Nondisplaced** unspecified condyle fracture of lower end of unspecified femur   `MCC` `CC` `H5` `UNS` `HCC` `PE`

√6ᵗʰ **S72.42** Fracture of **lateral condyle** of femur

√7ᵗʰ **S72.421** **Displaced** fracture of lateral condyle of **right** femur   `MCC` `CC` `H5` `HCC` `PE`

√7ᵗʰ **S72.422** **Displaced** fracture of lateral condyle of **left** femur   `MCC` `CC` `H5` `HCC` `PE`

√7ᵗʰ **S72.423** **Displaced** fracture of lateral condyle of unspecified femur   `MCC` `CC` `H5` `UNS` `HCC` `PE`

√7ᵗʰ **S72.424** **Nondisplaced** fracture of lateral condyle of **right** femur   `MCC` `CC` `H5` `HCC` `PE`

√7ᵗʰ **S72.425** **Nondisplaced** fracture of lateral condyle of **left** femur   `MCC` `CC` `H5` `HCC` `PE`

`N` Newborn: 0   `P` Pediatric: 0-17   `M` Maternity: 9-64   `A` Adult: 15-124   `UNS` Unspecified Site   `MCC` Major Complication/Comorbidity   `CC` Complication/Comorbidity   `PE` POA Exempt

1080

ICD-10-CM 2025

√7th **S72.426** Nondisplaced fracture of lateral condyle of unspecified femur `MCC` `CC` `H5` `UNS` `HCC` `PE`

√6th **S72.43** Fracture of medial condyle of femur

√7th **S72.431** Displaced fracture of medial condyle of right femur `MCC` `CC` `H5` `HCC` `PE`

√7th **S72.432** Displaced fracture of medial condyle of left femur `MCC` `CC` `H5` `HCC` `PE`

√7th **S72.433** Displaced fracture of medial condyle of unspecified femur `MCC` `CC` `H5` `UNS` `HCC` `PE`

√7th **S72.434** Nondisplaced fracture of medial condyle of right femur `MCC` `CC` `H5` `HCC` `PE`

√7th **S72.435** Nondisplaced fracture of medial condyle of left femur `MCC` `CC` `H5` `HCC` `PE`

√7th **S72.436** Nondisplaced fracture of medial condyle of unspecified femur `MCC` `CC` `H5` `UNS` `HCC` `PE`

√6th **S72.44** Fracture of lower epiphysis (separation) of femur

    `EXCLUDES 1`   Salter-Harris Type I physeal fracture of lower end of femur (S79.11-)

√7th **S72.441** Displaced fracture of lower epiphysis (separation) of right femur `MCC` `CC` `H5` `HCC` `PE`

√7th **S72.442** Displaced fracture of lower epiphysis (separation) of left femur `MCC` `CC` `H5` `HCC` `PE`

√7th **S72.443** Displaced fracture of lower epiphysis (separation) of unspecified femur `MCC` `CC` `H5` `UNS` `HCC` `PE`

√7th **S72.444** Nondisplaced fracture of lower epiphysis (separation) of right femur `MCC` `CC` `H5` `HCC` `PE`

√7th **S72.445** Nondisplaced fracture of lower epiphysis (separation) of left femur `MCC` `CC` `H5` `HCC` `PE`

√7th **S72.446** Nondisplaced fracture of lower epiphysis (separation) of unspecified femur `MCC` `CC` `H5` `UNS` `HCC` `PE`

√6th **S72.45** Supracondylar fracture without intracondylar extension of lower end of femur

    Supracondylar fracture of lower end of femur NOS

    `EXCLUDES 1`   supracondylar fracture with intracondylar extension of lower end of femur (S72.46-)

√7th **S72.451** Displaced supracondylar fracture without intracondylar extension of lower end of right femur `MCC` `CC` `H5` `HCC` `PE`

√7th **S72.452** Displaced supracondylar fracture without intracondylar extension of lower end of left femur `MCC` `CC` `H5` `HCC` `PE`

√7th **S72.453** Displaced supracondylar fracture without intracondylar extension of lower end of unspecified femur `MCC` `CC` `H5` `UNS` `HCC` `PE`

√7th **S72.454** Nondisplaced supracondylar fracture without intracondylar extension of lower end of right femur `MCC` `CC` `H5` `HCC` `PE`

√7th **S72.455** Nondisplaced supracondylar fracture without intracondylar extension of lower end of left femur `MCC` `CC` `H5` `HCC` `PE`

√7th **S72.456** Nondisplaced supracondylar fracture without intracondylar extension of lower end of unspecified femur `MCC` `CC` `H5` `UNS` `HCC` `PE`

√6th **S72.46** Supracondylar fracture with intracondylar extension of lower end of femur

    `EXCLUDES 1`   supracondylar fracture without intracondylar extension of lower end of femur (S72.45-)

√7th **S72.461** Displaced supracondylar fracture with intracondylar extension of lower end of right femur `MCC` `CC` `H5` `HCC` `PE`

√7th **S72.462** Displaced supracondylar fracture with intracondylar extension of lower end of left femur `MCC` `CC` `H5` `HCC` `PE`

√7th **S72.463** Displaced supracondylar fracture with intracondylar extension of lower end of unspecified femur `MCC` `CC` `H5` `UNS` `HCC` `PE`

√7th **S72.464** Nondisplaced supracondylar fracture with intracondylar extension of lower end of right femur `MCC` `CC` `H5` `HCC` `PE`

√7th **S72.465** Nondisplaced supracondylar fracture with intracondylar extension of lower end of left femur `MCC` `CC` `H5` `HCC` `PE`

√7th **S72.466** Nondisplaced supracondylar fracture with intracondylar extension of lower end of unspecified femur `MCC` `CC` `H5` `UNS` `HCC` `PE`

√6th **S72.47** Torus fracture of lower end of femur

The appropriate 7th character is to be added to all codes in subcategory S72.47.

A   initial encounter for closed fracture

D   subsequent encounter for fracture with routine healing

G   subsequent encounter for fracture with delayed healing

K   subsequent encounter for fracture with nonunion

P   subsequent encounter for fracture with malunion

S   sequela

√7th **S72.471** Torus fracture of lower end of right femur `CC` `H5` `HCC` `PE`

√7th **S72.472** Torus fracture of lower end of left femur `CC` `H5` `HCC` `PE`

√7th **S72.479** Torus fracture of lower end of unspecified femur `CC` `H5` `UNS` `HCC` `PE`

√6th **S72.49** Other fracture of lower end of femur

√7th **S72.491** Other fracture of lower end of right femur `MCC` `CC` `H5` `HCC` `PE`

√7th **S72.492** Other fracture of lower end of left femur `MCC` `CC` `H5` `HCC` `PE`

√7th **S72.499** Other fracture of lower end of unspecified femur `MCC` `CC` `H5` `UNS` `HCC` `PE`

√5th **S72.8** Other fracture of femur

√6th **S72.8X** Other fracture of femur

√7th **S72.8X1** Other fracture of right femur `MCC` `CC` `H5` `HCC` `PE`

√7th **S72.8X2** Other fracture of left femur `MCC` `CC` `H5` `HCC` `PE`

√7th **S72.8X9** Other fracture of unspecified femur `MCC` `CC` `H5` `UNS` `HCC` `PE`

√5th **S72.9** Unspecified fracture of femur

    Fracture of thigh NOS

    Fracture of upper leg NOS

    `EXCLUDES 1`   fracture of hip NOS (S72.00-, S72.01-)

√x7th **S72.90** Unspecified fracture of unspecified femur `MCC` `CC` `H5` `UNS` `HCC` `PE`

    AHA: 2012,4Q,93

√x7th **S72.91** Unspecified fracture of right femur `MCC` `CC` `H5` `HCC` `PE`

√x7th **S72.92** Unspecified fracture of left femur `MCC` `CC` `H5` `HCC` `PE`

√4th **S73** Dislocation and sprain of joint and ligaments of hip

    `INCLUDES`   avulsion of joint or ligament of hip

              laceration of cartilage, joint or ligament of hip

              sprain of cartilage, joint or ligament of hip

              traumatic hemarthrosis of joint or ligament of hip

              traumatic rupture of joint or ligament of hip

              traumatic subluxation of joint or ligament of hip

              traumatic tear of joint or ligament of hip

Code also any associated open wound

    `EXCLUDES 2`   strain of muscle, fascia and tendon of hip and thigh (S76.-)

The appropriate 7th character is to be added to each code from category S73.

A   initial encounter

D   subsequent encounter

S   sequela

√5th **S73.0** Subluxation and dislocation of hip

    `EXCLUDES 2`   dislocation and subluxation of hip prosthesis (T84.020, T84.021)

√6th **S73.00** Unspecified subluxation and dislocation of hip

    Dislocation of hip NOS

    Subluxation of hip NOS

√7th **S73.001** Unspecified subluxation of right hip `CC` `H5` `HCC` `PE`

☑ Additional Character Required   √x7th Placeholder   Questionable PDx   Manifestation   Unspecified   `UPD` Unacceptable PDx   `H1`-`H14` HAC   `HCC` CMS-HCC Dx   `HIV` HIV Dx

ICD-10-CM 2025   1081

√7ᵗʰ **S73.002** Unspecified subluxation of left hip   CC H5 HCC PE

√7ᵗʰ **S73.003** Unspecified subluxation of unspecified hip   CC H5 UNS HCC PE

√7ᵗʰ **S73.004** Unspecified dislocation of right hip   CC H5 HCC PE

√7ᵗʰ **S73.005** Unspecified dislocation of left hip   CC H5 HCC PE

√7ᵗʰ **S73.006** Unspecified dislocation of unspecified hip   CC H5 UNS HCC PE

√6ᵗʰ **S73.01** Posterior subluxation and dislocation of hip

√7ᵗʰ **S73.011** Posterior subluxation of right hip   CC H5 HCC PE

√7ᵗʰ **S73.012** Posterior subluxation of left hip   CC H5 HCC PE

√7ᵗʰ **S73.013** Posterior subluxation of unspecified hip   CC H5 UNS HCC PE

√7ᵗʰ **S73.014** Posterior dislocation of right hip   CC H5 HCC PE

√7ᵗʰ **S73.015** Posterior dislocation of left hip   CC H5 HCC PE

√7ᵗʰ **S73.016** Posterior dislocation of unspecified hip   CC H5 UNS HCC PE

√6ᵗʰ **S73.02** Obturator subluxation and dislocation of hip

√7ᵗʰ **S73.021** Obturator subluxation of right hip   CC H5 HCC PE

√7ᵗʰ **S73.022** Obturator subluxation of left hip   CC H5 HCC PE

√7ᵗʰ **S73.023** Obturator subluxation of unspecified hip   CC H5 UNS HCC PE

√7ᵗʰ **S73.024** Obturator dislocation of right hip   CC H5 HCC PE

√7ᵗʰ **S73.025** Obturator dislocation of left hip   CC H5 HCC PE

√7ᵗʰ **S73.026** Obturator dislocation of unspecified hip   CC H5 UNS HCC PE

√6ᵗʰ **S73.03** Other anterior subluxation and dislocation of hip

√7ᵗʰ **S73.031** Other anterior subluxation of right hip   CC H5 HCC PE

√7ᵗʰ **S73.032** Other anterior subluxation of left hip   CC H5 HCC PE

√7ᵗʰ **S73.033** Other anterior subluxation of unspecified hip   CC H5 UNS HCC PE

√7ᵗʰ **S73.034** Other anterior dislocation of right hip   CC H5 HCC PE

√7ᵗʰ **S73.035** Other anterior dislocation of left hip   CC H5 HCC PE

√7ᵗʰ **S73.036** Other anterior dislocation of unspecified hip   CC H5 UNS HCC PE

√6ᵗʰ **S73.04** Central subluxation and dislocation of hip

√7ᵗʰ **S73.041** Central subluxation of right hip   CC H5 HCC PE

√7ᵗʰ **S73.042** Central subluxation of left hip   CC H5 HCC PE

√7ᵗʰ **S73.043** Central subluxation of unspecified hip   CC H5 UNS HCC PE

√7ᵗʰ **S73.044** Central dislocation of right hip   CC H5 HCC PE

√7ᵗʰ **S73.045** Central dislocation of left hip   CC H5 HCC PE

√7ᵗʰ **S73.046** Central dislocation of unspecified hip   CC H5 UNS HCC PE

√5ᵗʰ **S73.1** Sprain of hip

    AHA: 2014,4Q,25

√6ᵗʰ **S73.10** Unspecified sprain of hip

√7ᵗʰ **S73.101** Unspecified sprain of right hip   PE

√7ᵗʰ **S73.102** Unspecified sprain of left hip   PE

√7ᵗʰ **S73.109** Unspecified sprain of unspecified hip   PE

√6ᵗʰ **S73.11** Iliofemoral ligament sprain of hip

√7ᵗʰ **S73.111** Iliofemoral ligament sprain of right hip   PE

√7ᵗʰ **S73.112** Iliofemoral ligament sprain of left hip   PE

√7ᵗʰ **S73.119** Iliofemoral ligament sprain of unspecified hip   PE

√6ᵗʰ **S73.12** Ischiocapsular (ligament) sprain of hip

√7ᵗʰ **S73.121** Ischiocapsular ligament sprain of right hip   PE

√7ᵗʰ **S73.122** Ischiocapsular ligament sprain of left hip   PE

√7ᵗʰ **S73.129** Ischiocapsular ligament sprain of unspecified hip   PE

√6ᵗʰ **S73.19** Other sprain of hip

√7ᵗʰ **S73.191** Other sprain of right hip   PE

√7ᵗʰ **S73.192** Other sprain of left hip   PE

√7ᵗʰ **S73.199** Other sprain of unspecified hip   PE

√4ᵗʰ **S74** Injury of nerves at hip and thigh level

    Code also any associated open wound (S71.-)

     EXCLUDES 2   injury of nerves at ankle and foot level (S94.-)

                injury of nerves at lower leg level (S84.-)

> The appropriate 7th character is to be added to each code from category S74.
> A   initial encounter
> D   subsequent encounter
> S   sequela

√5ᵗʰ **S74.0** Injury of sciatic nerve at hip and thigh level

√x7ᵗʰ **S74.00** Injury of sciatic nerve at hip and thigh level, unspecified leg   PE

√x7ᵗʰ **S74.01** Injury of sciatic nerve at hip and thigh level, right leg   PE

√x7ᵗʰ **S74.02** Injury of sciatic nerve at hip and thigh level, left leg   PE

√5ᵗʰ **S74.1** Injury of femoral nerve at hip and thigh level

√x7ᵗʰ **S74.10** Injury of femoral nerve at hip and thigh level, unspecified leg   PE

√x7ᵗʰ **S74.11** Injury of femoral nerve at hip and thigh level, right leg   PE

√x7ᵗʰ **S74.12** Injury of femoral nerve at hip and thigh level, left leg   PE

√5ᵗʰ **S74.2** Injury of cutaneous sensory nerve at hip and thigh level

√x7ᵗʰ **S74.20** Injury of cutaneous sensory nerve at hip and thigh level, unspecified leg   PE

√x7ᵗʰ **S74.21** Injury of cutaneous sensory nerve at hip and high level, right leg   PE

√x7ᵗʰ **S74.22** Injury of cutaneous sensory nerve at hip and thigh level, left leg   PE

√5ᵗʰ **S74.8** Injury of other nerves at hip and thigh level

√6ᵗʰ **S74.8X** Injury of other nerves at hip and thigh level

√7ᵗʰ **S74.8X1** Injury of other nerves at hip and thigh level, right leg   PE

√7ᵗʰ **S74.8X2** Injury of other nerves at hip and thigh level, left leg   PE

√7ᵗʰ **S74.8X9** Injury of other nerves at hip and thigh level, unspecified leg   PE

√5ᵗʰ **S74.9** Injury of unspecified nerve at hip and thigh level

√x7ᵗʰ **S74.90** Injury of unspecified nerve at hip and thigh level, unspecified leg   PE

√x7ᵗʰ **S74.91** Injury of unspecified nerve at hip and thigh level, right leg   PE

√x7ᵗʰ **S74.92** Injury of unspecified nerve at hip and thigh level, left leg   PE

√4ᵗʰ **S75** Injury of blood vessels at hip and thigh level

    Code also any associated open wound (S71.-)

     EXCLUDES 2   injury of blood vessels at lower leg level (S85.-)

                injury of popliteal artery (S85.0)

> The appropriate 7th character is to be added to each code from category S75.
> A   initial encounter
> D   subsequent encounter
> S   sequela

√5ᵗʰ **S75.0** Injury of femoral artery

√6ᵗʰ **S75.00** Unspecified injury of femoral artery

√7ᵗʰ **S75.001** Unspecified injury of femoral artery, right leg   MCC PE

√7ᵗʰ **S75.002** Unspecified injury of femoral artery, left leg   MCC PE

√7ᵗʰ **S75.009** Unspecified injury of femoral artery, unspecified leg   MCC UNS PE

N Newborn: 0   P Pediatric: 0-17   M Maternity: 9-64   A Adult: 15-124   UNS Unspecified Site   MCC Major Complication/Comorbidity   CC Complication/Comorbidity   PE POA Exempt

1082   ICD-10-CM 2025

√6th **S75.01** Minor laceration of femoral artery
Incomplete transection of femoral artery
Laceration of femoral artery NOS
Superficial laceration of femoral artery

√7th **S75.011** Minor laceration of femoral artery, right leg `MCC` `PE`

√7th **S75.012** Minor laceration of femoral artery, left leg `MCC` `PE`

√7th **S75.019** Minor laceration of femoral artery, unspecified leg `MCC` `UNS` `PE`

√6th **S75.02** Major laceration of femoral artery
Complete transection of femoral artery
Traumatic rupture of femoral artery
AHA: 2023,3Q,12

√7th **S75.021** Major laceration of femoral artery, right leg `MCC` `PE`

√7th **S75.022** Major laceration of femoral artery, left leg `MCC` `PE`

√7th **S75.029** Major laceration of femoral artery, unspecified leg `MCC` `UNS` `PE`

√6th **S75.09** Other specified injury of femoral artery

√7th **S75.091** Other specified injury of femoral artery, right leg `MCC` `PE`

√7th **S75.092** Other specified injury of femoral artery, left leg `MCC` `PE`

√7th **S75.099** Other specified injury of femoral artery, unspecified leg `MCC` `UNS` `PE`

√5th **S75.1** Injury of femoral vein at hip and thigh level

√6th **S75.10** Unspecified injury of femoral vein at hip and thigh level

√7th **S75.101** Unspecified injury of femoral vein at hip and thigh level, right leg `MCC` `PE`

√7th **S75.102** Unspecified injury of femoral vein at hip and thigh level, left leg `MCC` `PE`

√7th **S75.109** Unspecified injury of femoral vein at hip and thigh level, unspecified leg `MCC` `UNS` `PE`

√6th **S75.11** Minor laceration of femoral vein at hip and thigh level
Incomplete transection of femoral vein at hip and thigh level
Laceration of femoral vein at hip and thigh level NOS
Superficial laceration of femoral vein at hip and thigh level

√7th **S75.111** Minor laceration of femoral vein at hip and thigh level, right leg `MCC` `PE`

√7th **S75.112** Minor laceration of femoral vein at hip and thigh level, left leg `MCC` `PE`

√7th **S75.119** Minor laceration of femoral vein at hip and thigh level, unspecified leg `MCC` `UNS` `PE`

√6th **S75.12** Major laceration of femoral vein at hip and thigh level
Complete transection of femoral vein at hip and thigh level
Traumatic rupture of femoral vein at hip and thigh level
AHA: 2023,3Q,12

√7th **S75.121** Major laceration of femoral vein at hip and thigh level, right leg `MCC` `PE`

√7th **S75.122** Major laceration of femoral vein at hip and thigh level, left leg `MCC` `PE`

√7th **S75.129** Major laceration of femoral vein at hip and thigh level, unspecified leg `MCC` `UNS` `PE`

√6th **S75.19** Other specified injury of femoral vein at hip and thigh level

√7th **S75.191** Other specified injury of femoral vein at hip and thigh level, right leg `MCC` `PE`

√7th **S75.192** Other specified injury of femoral vein at hip and thigh level, left leg `MCC` `PE`

√7th **S75.199** Other specified injury of femoral vein at hip and thigh level, unspecified leg `MCC` `UNS` `PE`

√5th **S75.2** Injury of greater saphenous vein at hip and thigh level
EXCLUDES 1 greater saphenous vein NOS (S85.3)

√6th **S75.20** Unspecified injury of greater saphenous vein at hip and thigh level

√7th **S75.201** Unspecified injury of greater saphenous vein at hip and thigh level, right leg `CC` `PE`

√7th **S75.202** Unspecified injury of greater saphenous vein at hip and thigh level, left leg `CC` `PE`

√7th **S75.209** Unspecified injury of greater saphenous vein at hip and thigh level, unspecified leg `CC` `UNS` `PE`

√6th **S75.21** Minor laceration of greater saphenous vein at hip and thigh level
Incomplete transection of greater saphenous vein at hip and thigh level
Laceration of greater saphenous vein at hip and thigh level NOS
Superficial laceration of greater saphenous vein at hip and thigh level

√7th **S75.211** Minor laceration of greater saphenous vein at hip and thigh level, right leg `CC` `PE`

√7th **S75.212** Minor laceration of greater saphenous vein at hip and thigh level, left leg `CC` `PE`

√7th **S75.219** Minor laceration of greater saphenous vein at hip and thigh level, unspecified leg `CC` `UNS` `PE`

√6th **S75.22** Major laceration of greater saphenous vein at hip and thigh level
Complete transection of greater saphenous vein at hip and thigh level
Traumatic rupture of greater saphenous vein at hip and thigh level

√7th **S75.221** Major laceration of greater saphenous vein at hip and thigh level, right leg `CC` `PE`

√7th **S75.222** Major laceration of greater saphenous vein at hip and thigh level, left leg `CC` `PE`

√7th **S75.229** Major laceration of greater saphenous vein at hip and thigh level, unspecified leg `CC` `UNS` `PE`

√6th **S75.29** Other specified injury of greater saphenous vein at hip and thigh level

√7th **S75.291** Other specified injury of greater saphenous vein at hip and thigh level, right leg `CC` `PE`

√7th **S75.292** Other specified injury of greater saphenous vein at hip and thigh level, left leg `CC` `PE`

√7th **S75.299** Other specified injury of greater saphenous vein at hip and thigh level, unspecified leg `CC` `UNS` `PE`

√5th **S75.8** Injury of other blood vessels at hip and thigh level

√6th **S75.80** Unspecified injury of other blood vessels at hip and thigh level

√7th **S75.801** Unspecified injury of other blood vessels at hip and thigh level, right leg `CC` `PE`

√7th **S75.802** Unspecified injury of other blood vessels at hip and thigh level, left leg `CC` `PE`

√7th **S75.809** Unspecified injury of other blood vessels at hip and thigh level, unspecified leg `CC` `UNS` `PE`

√6th **S75.81** Laceration of other blood vessels at hip and thigh level

√7th **S75.811** Laceration of other blood vessels at hip and thigh level, right leg `CC` `PE`

√7th **S75.812** Laceration of other blood vessels at hip and thigh level, left leg `CC` `PE`

√7th **S75.819** Laceration of other blood vessels at hip and thigh level, unspecified leg `CC` `UNS` `PE`

√6th **S75.89** Other specified injury of other blood vessels at hip and thigh level

√7th **S75.891** Other specified injury of other blood vessels at hip and thigh level, right leg `CC` `PE`

√7th **S75.892** Other specified injury of other blood vessels at hip and thigh level, left leg `CC` `PE`

√7th **S75.899** Other specified injury of other blood vessels at hip and thigh level, unspecified leg `CC` `UNS` `PE`

√5th **S75.9** Injury of unspecified blood vessel at hip and thigh level

√6th **S75.90** Unspecified injury of unspecified blood vessel at hip and thigh level

√7th **S75.901** Unspecified injury of unspecified blood vessel at hip and thigh level, right leg `CC` `PE`

√7th **S75.902** Unspecified injury of unspecified blood vessel at hip and thigh level, left leg `CC` `PE`

√7ᵗʰ **S75.909** Unspecified injury of unspecified blood vessel at hip and thigh level, unspecified leg `CC` `UNS` `PE`

√6ᵗʰ **S75.91** Laceration of unspecified blood vessel at hip and thigh level

√7ᵗʰ **S75.911** Laceration of unspecified blood vessel at hip and thigh level, right leg `CC` `PE`

√7ᵗʰ **S75.912** Laceration of unspecified blood vessel at hip and thigh level, left leg `CC` `PE`

√7ᵗʰ **S75.919** Laceration of unspecified blood vessel at hip and thigh level, unspecified leg `CC` `UNS` `PE`

√6ᵗʰ **S75.99** Other specified injury of unspecified blood vessel at hip and thigh level

√7ᵗʰ **S75.991** Other specified injury of unspecified blood vessel at hip and thigh level, right leg `CC` `PE`

√7ᵗʰ **S75.992** Other specified injury of unspecified blood vessel at hip and thigh level, left leg `CC` `PE`

√7ᵗʰ **S75.999** Other specified injury of unspecified blood vessel at hip and thigh level, unspecified leg `CC` `UNS` `PE`

√4ᵗʰ **S76 Injury of muscle, fascia and tendon at hip and thigh level**

Code also any associated open wound (S71.-)

EXCLUDES 2   injury of muscle, fascia and tendon at lower leg level (S86)
sprain of joint and ligament of hip (S73.1)

TIP: Refer to the Muscle/Tendon table at the beginning of this chapter.

The appropriate 7th character is to be added to each code from category S76.
A   initial encounter
D   subsequent encounter
S   sequela

√5ᵗʰ **S76.0** Injury of muscle, fascia and tendon of hip

√6ᵗʰ **S76.00** Unspecified injury of muscle, fascia and tendon of hip

√7ᵗʰ **S76.001** Unspecified injury of muscle, fascia and tendon of right hip `PE`

√7ᵗʰ **S76.002** Unspecified injury of muscle, fascia and tendon of left hip `PE`

√7ᵗʰ **S76.009** Unspecified injury of muscle, fascia and tendon of unspecified hip `PE`

√6ᵗʰ **S76.01** Strain of muscle, fascia and tendon of hip

√7ᵗʰ **S76.011** Strain of muscle, fascia and tendon of right hip `PE`

√7ᵗʰ **S76.012** Strain of muscle, fascia and tendon of left hip `PE`

√7ᵗʰ **S76.019** Strain of muscle, fascia and tendon of unspecified hip `PE`

√6ᵗʰ **S76.02** Laceration of muscle, fascia and tendon of hip

√7ᵗʰ **S76.021** Laceration of muscle, fascia and tendon of right hip `CC` `PE`

√7ᵗʰ **S76.022** Laceration of muscle, fascia and tendon of left hip `CC` `PE`

√7ᵗʰ **S76.029** Laceration of muscle, fascia and tendon of unspecified hip `CC` `UNS` `PE`

√6ᵗʰ **S76.09** Other specified injury of muscle, fascia and tendon of hip

√7ᵗʰ **S76.091** Other specified injury of muscle, fascia and tendon of right hip `PE`

√7ᵗʰ **S76.092** Other specified injury of muscle, fascia and tendon of left hip `PE`

√7ᵗʰ **S76.099** Other specified injury of muscle, fascia and tendon of unspecified hip `PE`

√5ᵗʰ **S76.1** Injury of quadriceps muscle, fascia and tendon

Injury of patellar ligament (tendon)

√6ᵗʰ **S76.10** Unspecified injury of quadriceps muscle, fascia and tendon

√7ᵗʰ **S76.101** Unspecified injury of right quadriceps muscle, fascia and tendon `PE`

√7ᵗʰ **S76.102** Unspecified injury of left quadriceps muscle, fascia and tendon `PE`

√7ᵗʰ **S76.109** Unspecified injury of unspecified quadriceps muscle, fascia and tendon `PE`

√6ᵗʰ **S76.11** Strain of quadriceps muscle, fascia and tendon

√7ᵗʰ **S76.111** Strain of right quadriceps muscle, fascia and tendon `PE`

√7ᵗʰ **S76.112** Strain of left quadriceps muscle, fascia and tendon `PE`

√7ᵗʰ **S76.119** Strain of unspecified quadriceps muscle, fascia and tendon `PE`

√6ᵗʰ **S76.12** Laceration of quadriceps muscle, fascia and tendon

√7ᵗʰ **S76.121** Laceration of right quadriceps muscle, fascia and tendon `CC` `PE`

√7ᵗʰ **S76.122** Laceration of left quadriceps muscle, fascia and tendon `CC` `PE`

√7ᵗʰ **S76.129** Laceration of unspecified quadriceps muscle, fascia and tendon `CC` `UNS` `PE`

√6ᵗʰ **S76.19** Other specified injury of quadriceps muscle, fascia and tendon

√7ᵗʰ **S76.191** Other specified injury of right quadriceps muscle, fascia and tendon `PE`

√7ᵗʰ **S76.192** Other specified injury of left quadriceps muscle, fascia and tendon `PE`

√7ᵗʰ **S76.199** Other specified injury of unspecified quadriceps muscle, fascia and tendon `PE`

√5ᵗʰ **S76.2** Injury of adductor muscle, fascia and tendon of thigh

√6ᵗʰ **S76.20** Unspecified injury of adductor muscle, fascia and tendon of thigh

√7ᵗʰ **S76.201** Unspecified injury of adductor muscle, fascia and tendon of right thigh `PE`

√7ᵗʰ **S76.202** Unspecified injury of adductor muscle, fascia and tendon of left thigh `PE`

√7ᵗʰ **S76.209** Unspecified injury of adductor muscle, fascia and tendon of unspecified thigh `PE`

√6ᵗʰ **S76.21** Strain of adductor muscle, fascia and tendon of thigh

√7ᵗʰ **S76.211** Strain of adductor muscle, fascia and tendon of right thigh `PE`

√7ᵗʰ **S76.212** Strain of adductor muscle, fascia and tendon of left thigh `PE`

√7ᵗʰ **S76.219** Strain of adductor muscle, fascia and tendon of unspecified thigh `PE`

√6ᵗʰ **S76.22** Laceration of adductor muscle, fascia and tendon of thigh

√7ᵗʰ **S76.221** Laceration of adductor muscle, fascia and tendon of right thigh `CC` `PE`

√7ᵗʰ **S76.222** Laceration of adductor muscle, fascia and tendon of left thigh `CC` `PE`

√7ᵗʰ **S76.229** Laceration of adductor muscle, fascia and tendon of unspecified thigh `CC` `UNS` `PE`

√6ᵗʰ **S76.29** Other injury of adductor muscle, fascia and tendon of thigh

√7ᵗʰ **S76.291** Other injury of adductor muscle, fascia and tendon of right thigh `PE`

√7ᵗʰ **S76.292** Other injury of adductor muscle, fascia and tendon of left thigh `PE`

√7ᵗʰ **S76.299** Other injury of adductor muscle, fascia and tendon of unspecified thigh `PE`

√5ᵗʰ **S76.3** Injury of muscle, fascia and tendon of the posterior muscle group at thigh level

√6ᵗʰ **S76.30** Unspecified injury of muscle, fascia and tendon of the posterior muscle group at thigh level

√7ᵗʰ **S76.301** Unspecified injury of muscle, fascia and tendon of the posterior muscle group at thigh level, right thigh `PE`

√7ᵗʰ **S76.302** Unspecified injury of muscle, fascia and tendon of the posterior muscle group at thigh level, left thigh `PE`

√7ᵗʰ **S76.309** Unspecified injury of muscle, fascia and tendon of the posterior muscle group at thigh level, unspecified thigh `PE`

√6ᵗʰ **S76.31** Strain of muscle, fascia and tendon of the posterior muscle group at thigh level

√7ᵗʰ **S76.311** Strain of muscle, fascia and tendon of the posterior muscle group at thigh level, right thigh `PE`

√7ᵗʰ **S76.312** Strain of muscle, fascia and tendon of the posterior muscle group at thigh level, left thigh `PE`

√7ᵗʰ **S76.319** Strain of muscle, fascia and tendon of the posterior muscle group at thigh level, unspecified thigh `PE`

`N` Newborn: 0   `P` Pediatric: 0-17   `M` Maternity: 9-64   `A` Adult: 15-124   `UNS` Unspecified Site   `MCC` Major Complication/Comorbidity   `CC` Complication/Comorbidity   `PE` POA Exempt

1084

ICD-10-CM 2025

✓6th **S76.32** **Laceration** of muscle, fascia and tendon of the posterior muscle group at thigh level

     ✓7th **S76.321** Laceration of muscle, fascia and tendon of the posterior muscle group at thigh level, **right** thigh `CC` `PE`

     ✓7th **S76.322** Laceration of muscle, fascia and tendon of the posterior muscle group at thigh level, **left** thigh `CC` `PE`

     ✓7th **S76.329** Laceration of muscle, fascia and tendon of the posterior muscle group at thigh level, unspecified thigh `CC` `UNS` `PE`

✓6th **S76.39** Other specified injury of muscle, fascia and tendon of the posterior muscle group at thigh level

     ✓7th **S76.391** Other specified injury of muscle, fascia and tendon of the posterior muscle group at thigh level, **right** thigh `PE`

     ✓7th **S76.392** Other specified injury of muscle, fascia and tendon of the posterior muscle group at thigh level, **left** thigh `PE`

     ✓7th **S76.399** Other specified injury of muscle, fascia and tendon of the posterior muscle group at thigh level, unspecified thigh `PE`

✓5th **S76.8** Injury of other specified muscles, fascia and tendons at **thigh level**

     ✓6th **S76.80** Unspecified injury of other specified muscles, fascia and tendons at thigh level

       ✓7th **S76.801** Unspecified injury of other specified muscles, fascia and tendons at thigh level, **right** thigh `PE`

       ✓7th **S76.802** Unspecified injury of other specified muscles, fascia and tendons at thigh level, **left** thigh `PE`

       ✓7th **S76.809** Unspecified injury of other specified muscles, fascia and tendons at thigh level, unspecified thigh `PE`

     ✓6th **S76.81** **Strain** of other specified muscles, fascia and tendons at thigh level

       ✓7th **S76.811** Strain of other specified muscles, fascia and tendons at thigh level, **right** thigh `PE`

       ✓7th **S76.812** Strain of other specified muscles, fascia and tendons at thigh level, **left** thigh `PE`

       ✓7th **S76.819** Strain of other specified muscles, fascia and tendons at thigh level, unspecified thigh `PE`

     ✓6th **S76.82** **Laceration** of other specified muscles, fascia and tendons at thigh level

       ✓7th **S76.821** Laceration of other specified muscles, fascia and tendons at thigh level, **right** thigh `CC` `PE`

       ✓7th **S76.822** Laceration of other specified muscles, fascia and tendons at thigh level, **left** thigh `CC` `PE`

       ✓7th **S76.829** Laceration of other specified muscles, fascia and tendons at thigh level, unspecified thigh `CC` `UNS` `PE`

     ✓6th **S76.89** Other injury of other specified muscles, fascia and tendons at thigh level

       ✓7th **S76.891** Other injury of other specified muscles, fascia and tendons at thigh level, **right** thigh `PE`

       ✓7th **S76.892** Other injury of other specified muscles, fascia and tendons at thigh level, **left** thigh `PE`

       ✓7th **S76.899** Other injury of other specified muscles, fascia and tendons at thigh level, unspecified thigh `PE`

✓5th **S76.9** Injury of unspecified muscles, fascia and tendons at **thigh level**

     ✓6th **S76.90** Unspecified injury of unspecified muscles, fascia and tendons at thigh level

       ✓7th **S76.901** Unspecified injury of unspecified muscles, fascia and tendons at thigh level, **right** thigh `PE`

       ✓7th **S76.902** Unspecified injury of unspecified muscles, fascia and tendons at thigh level, **left** thigh `PE`

       ✓7th **S76.909** Unspecified injury of unspecified muscles, fascia and tendons at thigh level, unspecified thigh `PE`

✓6th **S76.91** **Strain** of unspecified muscles, fascia and tendons at thigh level

     ✓7th **S76.911** Strain of unspecified muscles, fascia and tendons at thigh level, **right** thigh `PE`

     ✓7th **S76.912** Strain of unspecified muscles, fascia and tendons at thigh level, **left** thigh `PE`

     ✓7th **S76.919** Strain of unspecified muscles, fascia and tendons at thigh level, unspecified thigh `PE`

✓6th **S76.92** **Laceration** of unspecified muscles, fascia and tendons at thigh level

     ✓7th **S76.921** Laceration of unspecified muscles, fascia and tendons at thigh level, **right** thigh `CC` `PE`

     ✓7th **S76.922** Laceration of unspecified muscles, fascia and tendons at thigh level, **left** thigh `CC` `PE`

     ✓7th **S76.929** Laceration of unspecified muscles, fascia and tendons at thigh level, unspecified thigh `CC` `UNS` `PE`

✓6th **S76.99** Other specified injury of unspecified muscles, fascia and tendons at thigh level

     ✓7th **S76.991** Other specified injury of unspecified muscles, fascia and tendons at thigh level, **right** thigh `PE`

     ✓7th **S76.992** Other specified injury of unspecified muscles, fascia and tendons at thigh level, **left** thigh `PE`

     ✓7th **S76.999** Other specified injury of unspecified muscles, fascia and tendons at thigh level, unspecified thigh `PE`

✓4th **S77** **Crushing injury** of hip and thigh

Use additional code(s) for all associated injuries

EXCLUDES 2   crushing injury of ankle and foot (S97.-)

            crushing injury of lower leg (S87.-)

> The appropriate 7th character is to be added to each code from category S77.
> A   initial encounter
> D   subsequent encounter
> S   sequela

✓5th **S77.0** Crushing injury of **hip**

     ✓x7th **S77.00** Crushing injury of unspecified hip `CC` `H5` `UNS` `PE`

     ✓x7th **S77.01** Crushing injury of **right** hip `CC` `H5` `PE`

     ✓x7th **S77.02** Crushing injury of **left** hip `CC` `H5` `PE`

✓5th **S77.1** Crushing injury of **thigh**

     ✓x7th **S77.10** Crushing injury of unspecified thigh `CC` `H5` `UNS` `PE`

     ✓x7th **S77.11** Crushing injury of **right** thigh `CC` `H5` `PE`

     ✓x7th **S77.12** Crushing injury of **left** thigh `CC` `H5` `PE`

✓5th **S77.2** Crushing injury of **hip with thigh**

     ✓x7th **S77.20** Crushing injury of unspecified hip with thigh `PE`

     ✓x7th **S77.21** Crushing injury of **right** hip with thigh `PE`

     ✓x7th **S77.22** Crushing injury of **left** hip with thigh `PE`

✓4th **S78** **Traumatic amputation** of hip and thigh

An amputation not identified as partial or complete should be coded to complete

EXCLUDES 1   traumatic amputation of knee (S88.0-)

> The appropriate 7th character is to be added to each code from category S78.
> A   initial encounter
> D   subsequent encounter
> S   sequela

✓5th **S78.0** **Traumatic amputation** at **hip joint**

     ✓6th **S78.01** **Complete** traumatic amputation at hip joint

       ✓7th **S78.011** Complete traumatic amputation at **right** hip joint `CC` `HCC`

       ✓7th **S78.012** Complete traumatic amputation at **left** hip joint `CC` `HCC`

       ✓7th **S78.019** Complete traumatic amputation at unspecified hip joint `CC` `UNS` `HCC` `PE`

     ✓6th **S78.02** **Partial** traumatic amputation at hip joint

       ✓7th **S78.021** Partial traumatic amputation at **right** hip joint `CC` `HCC` `PE`

       ✓7th **S78.022** Partial traumatic amputation at **left** hip joint `CC` `HCC` `PE`

✓ Additional Character Required   ✓x7th Placeholder   Questionable PDx   Manifestation   Unspecified   `UPD` Unacceptable PDx   `H1`-`H14` HAC   `HCC` CMS-HCC Dx   `HIV` HIV Dx

ICD-10-CM 2025   1085

√7th **S78.029** Partial traumatic amputation at unspecified hip joint `CC` `UNS` `HCC` `PE`

√5th **S78.1** Traumatic amputation at level **between hip and knee**

> EXCLUDES 1   *traumatic amputation of knee (S88.0-)*

√6th **S78.11** **Complete** traumatic amputation at level between hip and knee

√7th **S78.111** Complete traumatic amputation at level between **right** hip and knee `CC` `HCC` `PE`

√7th **S78.112** Complete traumatic amputation at level between **left** hip and knee `CC` `HCC` `PE`

√7th **S78.119** Complete traumatic amputation at level between unspecified hip and knee `CC` `UNS` `HCC` `PE`

√6th **S78.12** **Partial** traumatic amputation at level between hip and knee

√7th **S78.121** Partial traumatic amputation at level between **right** hip and knee `CC` `HCC` `PE`

√7th **S78.122** Partial traumatic amputation at level between **left** hip and knee `CC` `HCC` `PE`

√7th **S78.129** Partial traumatic amputation at level between unspecified hip and knee `CC` `UNS` `HCC` `PE`

√5th **S78.9** Traumatic amputation of hip and thigh, level unspecified

√6th **S78.91** **Complete** traumatic amputation of hip and thigh, level unspecified

√7th **S78.911** Complete traumatic amputation of **right** hip and thigh, level unspecified `CC` `HCC` `PE`

√7th **S78.912** Complete traumatic amputation of **left** hip and thigh, level unspecified `CC` `HCC` `PE`

√7th **S78.919** Complete traumatic amputation of unspecified hip and thigh, level unspecified `CC` `UNS` `HCC` `PE`

√6th **S78.92** **Partial** traumatic amputation of hip and thigh, level unspecified

√7th **S78.921** Partial traumatic amputation of **right** hip and thigh, level unspecified `CC` `HCC` `PE`

√7th **S78.922** Partial traumatic amputation of **left** hip and thigh, level unspecified `CC` `HCC` `PE`

√7th **S78.929** Partial traumatic amputation of unspecified hip and thigh, level unspecified `CC` `UNS` `HCC` `PE`

√4th **S79** **Other and unspecified injuries of hip and thigh**

> NOTE   A fracture not indicated as open or closed should be coded to closed

AHA: 2018,2Q,12; 2018,1Q,3; 2015,3Q,37-39

> The appropriate 7th character is to be added to each code from subcategories S79.0 and S79.1.
> A   initial encounter for closed fracture
> D   subsequent encounter for fracture with routine healing
> G   subsequent encounter for fracture with delayed healing
> K   subsequent encounter for fracture with nonunion
> P   subsequent encounter for fracture with malunion
> S   sequela

√5th **S79.0** **Physeal** fracture of **upper end of femur**

> EXCLUDES 1   *apophyseal fracture of upper end of femur (S72.13-)*
> *nontraumatic slipped upper femoral epiphysis (M93.0-)*

AHA: 2019,4Q,56

√6th **S79.00** Unspecified physeal fracture of upper end of femur

√7th **S79.001** Unspecified physeal fracture of upper end of **right** femur `MCC` `CC` `H5` `HCC` `PE`

√7th **S79.002** Unspecified physeal fracture of upper end of **left** femur `MCC` `CC` `H5` `HCC` `PE`

√7th **S79.009** Unspecified physeal fracture of upper end of unspecified femur `MCC` `CC` `H5` `UNS` `HCC` `PE`

√6th **S79.01** **Salter-Harris Type I** physeal fracture of upper end of femur

Acute on chronic slipped capital femoral epiphysis (traumatic)
Acute slipped capital femoral epiphysis (traumatic)
Capital femoral epiphyseal fracture

> EXCLUDES 1   *chronic slipped upper femoral epiphysis (nontraumatic) (M93.02-)*

√7th **S79.011** Salter-Harris Type I physeal fracture of upper end of **right** femur `MCC` `CC` `H5` `HCC` `PE`

√7th **S79.012** Salter-Harris Type I physeal fracture of upper end of **left** femur `MCC` `CC` `H5` `HCC` `PE`

√7th **S79.019** Salter-Harris Type I physeal fracture of upper end of unspecified femur `MCC` `CC` `H5` `UNS` `HCC` `PE`

√6th **S79.09** Other physeal fracture of upper end of femur

√7th **S79.091** Other physeal fracture of upper end of **right** femur `MCC` `CC` `H5` `HCC` `PE`

√7th **S79.092** Other physeal fracture of upper end of **left** femur `MCC` `CC` `H5` `HCC` `PE`

√7th **S79.099** Other physeal fracture of upper end of unspecified femur `MCC` `CC` `H5` `UNS` `HCC` `PE`

√5th **S79.1** **Physeal** fracture of **lower end of femur**

AHA: 2019,4Q,56

√6th **S79.10** Unspecified physeal fracture of lower end of femur

√7th **S79.101** Unspecified physeal fracture of lower end of **right** femur `CC` `H5` `HCC` `PE`

√7th **S79.102** Unspecified physeal fracture of lower end of **left** femur `CC` `H5` `HCC` `PE`

√7th **S79.109** Unspecified physeal fracture of lower end of unspecified femur `CC` `H5` `UNS` `HCC` `PE`

√6th **S79.11** **Salter-Harris Type I** physeal fracture of lower end of femur

√7th **S79.111** Salter-Harris Type I physeal fracture of lower end of **right** femur `CC` `H5` `HCC` `PE`

√7th **S79.112** Salter-Harris Type I physeal fracture of lower end of **left** femur `CC` `H5` `HCC` `PE`

√7th **S79.119** Salter-Harris Type I physeal fracture of lower end of unspecified femur `CC` `H5` `UNS` `HCC` `PE`

√6th **S79.12** **Salter-Harris Type II** physeal fracture of lower end of femur

√7th **S79.121** Salter-Harris Type II physeal fracture of lower end of **right** femur `CC` `H5` `HCC` `PE`

√7th **S79.122** Salter-Harris Type II physeal fracture of lower end of **left** femur `CC` `H5` `HCC` `PE`

√7th **S79.129** Salter-Harris Type II physeal fracture of lower end of unspecified femur `CC` `H5` `UNS` `HCC` `PE`

√6th **S79.13** **Salter-Harris Type III** physeal fracture of lower end of femur

√7th **S79.131** Salter-Harris Type III physeal fracture of lower end of **right** femur `CC` `H5` `HCC` `PE`

√7th **S79.132** Salter-Harris Type III physeal fracture of lower end of **left** femur `CC` `H5` `HCC` `PE`

√7th **S79.139** Salter-Harris Type III physeal fracture of lower end of unspecified femur `CC` `H5` `UNS` `HCC` `PE`

√6th **S79.14** **Salter-Harris Type IV** physeal fracture of lower end of femur

√7th **S79.141** Salter-Harris Type IV physeal fracture of lower end of **right** femur `CC` `H5` `HCC` `PE`

√7th **S79.142** Salter-Harris Type IV physeal fracture of lower end of **left** femur `CC` `H5` `HCC` `PE`

√7th **S79.149** Salter-Harris Type IV physeal fracture of lower end of unspecified femur `CC` `H5` `UNS` `HCC` `PE`

√6th **S79.19** Other physeal fracture of lower end of femur

√7th **S79.191** Other physeal fracture of lower end of **right** femur `CC` `H5` `HCC` `PE`

√7th **S79.192** Other physeal fracture of lower end of **left** femur `CC` `H5` `HCC` `PE`

√7th **S79.199** Other physeal fracture of lower end of unspecified femur `CC` `H5` `UNS` `HCC` `PE`

√5th **S79.8** Other specified injuries of hip and thigh

> The appropriate 7th character is to be added to each code in subcategory S79.8.
> A   initial encounter
> D   subsequent encounter
> S   sequela

√6th **S79.81** Other specified injuries of **hip**

√7th **S79.811** Other specified injuries of **right** hip `PE`

√7th **S79.812** Other specified injuries of **left** hip `PE`

√7th **S79.819** Other specified injuries of unspecified hip `PE`

`N` Newborn: 0   `P` Pediatric: 0-17   `M` Maternity: 9-64   `A` Adult: 15-124   `UNS` Unspecified Site   `MCC` Major Complication/Comorbidity   `CC` Complication/Comorbidity   `PE` POA Exempt

1086
ICD-10-CM 2025

√6ᵗʰ **S79.82** Other specified injuries of **thigh**

     √7ᵗʰ **S79.821** Other specified injuries of **right** thigh   PE

     √7ᵗʰ **S79.822** Other specified injuries of **left** thigh   PE

     √7ᵗʰ **S79.829** Other specified injuries of unspecified thigh   PE

√5ᵗʰ **S79.9** Unspecified injury of hip and thigh

> The appropriate 7th character is to be added to each code in subcategory S79.9.
> A   initial encounter
> D   subsequent encounter
> S   sequela

√6ᵗʰ **S79.91** Unspecified injury of **hip**

     √7ᵗʰ **S79.911** Unspecified injury of **right** hip   PE

     √7ᵗʰ **S79.912** Unspecified injury of **left** hip   PE

     √7ᵗʰ **S79.919** Unspecified injury of unspecified hip   PE

√6ᵗʰ **S79.92** Unspecified injury of **thigh**

     √7ᵗʰ **S79.921** Unspecified injury of **right** thigh   PE

     √7ᵗʰ **S79.922** Unspecified injury of **left** thigh   PE

     √7ᵗʰ **S79.929** Unspecified injury of unspecified thigh   PE

Injuries to the knee and lower leg (S80-S89)

EXCLUDES 2   *burns and corrosions (T20-T32)*
            frostbite (T33-T34)
            injuries of ankle and foot, except fracture of ankle and malleolus (S90-S99)
            insect bite or sting, venomous (T63.4)

√4ᵗʰ **S80** Superficial injury of knee and lower leg

     EXCLUDES 2   *superficial injury of ankle and foot (S90.-)*

> The appropriate 7th character is to be added to each code from category S80.
> A   initial encounter
> D   subsequent encounter
> S   sequela

√5ᵗʰ **S80.0** Contusion of **knee**

     √x7ᵗʰ **S80.00** Contusion of unspecified knee   PE

     √x7ᵗʰ **S80.01** Contusion of **right** knee   PE

     √x7ᵗʰ **S80.02** Contusion of **left** knee   PE

√5ᵗʰ **S80.1** Contusion of **lower leg**

     √x7ᵗʰ **S80.10** Contusion of unspecified lower leg   PE

     √x7ᵗʰ **S80.11** Contusion of **right** lower leg   PE

     √x7ᵗʰ **S80.12** Contusion of **left** lower leg   PE

√5ᵗʰ **S80.2** Other superficial injuries of **knee**

     √6ᵗʰ **S80.21** **Abrasion** of knee

         √7ᵗʰ **S80.211** Abrasion, **right** knee   PE

         √7ᵗʰ **S80.212** Abrasion, **left** knee   PE

         √7ᵗʰ **S80.219** Abrasion, unspecified knee   PE

     √6ᵗʰ **S80.22** **Blister** (nonthermal) of knee

         √7ᵗʰ **S80.221** Blister (nonthermal), **right** knee   PE

         √7ᵗʰ **S80.222** Blister (nonthermal), **left** knee   PE

         √7ᵗʰ **S80.229** Blister (nonthermal), unspecified knee   PE

     √6ᵗʰ **S80.24** **External constriction** of knee

         √7ᵗʰ **S80.241** External constriction, **right** knee   PE

         √7ᵗʰ **S80.242** External constriction, **left** knee   PE

         √7ᵗʰ **S80.249** External constriction, unspecified knee   PE

     √6ᵗʰ **S80.25** Superficial **foreign body** of knee

         Splinter in the knee

         √7ᵗʰ **S80.251** Superficial foreign body, **right** knee   PE

         √7ᵗʰ **S80.252** Superficial foreign body, **left** knee   PE

         √7ᵗʰ **S80.259** Superficial foreign body, unspecified knee   PE

     √6ᵗʰ **S80.26** **Insect bite** (nonvenomous) of knee

         √7ᵗʰ **S80.261** Insect bite (nonvenomous), **right** knee   PE

         √7ᵗʰ **S80.262** Insect bite (nonvenomous), **left** knee   PE

         √7ᵗʰ **S80.269** Insect bite (nonvenomous), unspecified knee   PE

     √6ᵗʰ **S80.27** Other superficial **bite** of knee

         EXCLUDES 1   *open bite of knee (S81.05-)*

         √7ᵗʰ **S80.271** Other superficial bite of **right** knee   PE

         √7ᵗʰ **S80.272** Other superficial bite of **left** knee   PE

         √7ᵗʰ **S80.279** Other superficial bite of unspecified knee   PE

√5ᵗʰ **S80.8** Other superficial injuries of **lower leg**

     √6ᵗʰ **S80.81** **Abrasion** of lower leg

         √7ᵗʰ **S80.811** Abrasion, **right** lower leg   PE

         √7ᵗʰ **S80.812** Abrasion, **left** lower leg   PE

         √7ᵗʰ **S80.819** Abrasion, unspecified lower leg   PE

     √6ᵗʰ **S80.82** **Blister** (nonthermal) of lower leg

         √7ᵗʰ **S80.821** Blister (nonthermal), **right** lower leg   PE

         √7ᵗʰ **S80.822** Blister (nonthermal), **left** lower leg   PE

         √7ᵗʰ **S80.829** Blister (nonthermal), unspecified lower leg   PE

     √6ᵗʰ **S80.84** **External constriction** of lower leg

         √7ᵗʰ **S80.841** External constriction, **right** lower leg   PE

         √7ᵗʰ **S80.842** External constriction, **left** lower leg   PE

         √7ᵗʰ **S80.849** External constriction, unspecified lower leg   PE

     √6ᵗʰ **S80.85** Superficial **foreign body** of lower leg

         Splinter in the lower leg

         √7ᵗʰ **S80.851** Superficial foreign body, **right** lower leg   PE

         √7ᵗʰ **S80.852** Superficial foreign body, **left** lower leg   PE

         √7ᵗʰ **S80.859** Superficial foreign body, unspecified lower leg   PE

     √6ᵗʰ **S80.86** **Insect bite** (nonvenomous) of lower leg

         √7ᵗʰ **S80.861** Insect bite (nonvenomous), **right** lower leg   PE

         √7ᵗʰ **S80.862** Insect bite (nonvenomous), **left** lower leg   PE

         √7ᵗʰ **S80.869** Insect bite (nonvenomous), unspecified lower leg   PE

     √6ᵗʰ **S80.87** Other superficial **bite** of lower leg

         EXCLUDES 1   *open bite of lower leg (S81.85-)*

         √7ᵗʰ **S80.871** Other superficial bite, **right** lower leg   PE

         √7ᵗʰ **S80.872** Other superficial bite, **left** lower leg   PE

         √7ᵗʰ **S80.879** Other superficial bite, unspecified lower leg   PE

√5ᵗʰ **S80.9** Unspecified superficial injury of knee and lower leg

     √6ᵗʰ **S80.91** Unspecified superficial injury of **knee**

         √7ᵗʰ **S80.911** Unspecified superficial injury of **right** knee   PE

         √7ᵗʰ **S80.912** Unspecified superficial injury of **left** knee   PE

         √7ᵗʰ **S80.919** Unspecified superficial injury of unspecified knee   PE

     √6ᵗʰ **S80.92** Unspecified superficial injury of **lower leg**

         √7ᵗʰ **S80.921** Unspecified superficial injury of **right** lower leg   PE

         √7ᵗʰ **S80.922** Unspecified superficial injury of **left** lower leg   PE

         √7ᵗʰ **S80.929** Unspecified superficial injury of unspecified lower leg   PE

✓ Additional Character Required   √x7ᵗʰ Placeholder   Questionable PDx   Manifestation   Unspecified   UPD Unacceptable PDx   H1-H14 HAC   HCC CMS-HCC Dx   HIV HIV Dx

ICD-10-CM 2025   **1087**

✓4ᵗʰ **S81 Open wound of knee and lower leg**

Code also any associated wound infection

EXCLUDES 1   *open fracture of knee and lower leg (S82.-)*
             traumatic amputation of lower leg (S88.-)

EXCLUDES 2   *open wound of ankle and foot (S91.-)*

The appropriate 7th character is to be added to each code from category S81.
A   initial encounter
D   subsequent encounter
S   sequela

✓5ᵗʰ **S81.0 Open wound of knee**

  ✓6ᵗʰ **S81.00 Unspecified open wound of knee**

    ✓7ᵗʰ **S81.001 Unspecified open wound, right knee**   PE

    ✓7ᵗʰ **S81.002 Unspecified open wound, left knee**   PE

    ✓7ᵗʰ **S81.009 Unspecified open wound, unspecified knee**   PE

  ✓6ᵗʰ **S81.01 Laceration without foreign body of knee**

    ✓7ᵗʰ **S81.011 Laceration without foreign body, right knee**   PE

    ✓7ᵗʰ **S81.012 Laceration without foreign body, left knee**   PE

    ✓7ᵗʰ **S81.019 Laceration without foreign body, unspecified knee**   PE

  ✓6ᵗʰ **S81.02 Laceration with foreign body of knee**

    ✓7ᵗʰ **S81.021 Laceration with foreign body, right knee**   PE

    ✓7ᵗʰ **S81.022 Laceration with foreign body, left knee**   PE

    ✓7ᵗʰ **S81.029 Laceration with foreign body, unspecified knee**   PE

  ✓6ᵗʰ **S81.03 Puncture wound without foreign body of knee**

    ✓7ᵗʰ **S81.031 Puncture wound without foreign body, right knee**   PE

    ✓7ᵗʰ **S81.032 Puncture wound without foreign body, left knee**   PE

    ✓7ᵗʰ **S81.039 Puncture wound without foreign body, unspecified knee**   PE

  ✓6ᵗʰ **S81.04 Puncture wound with foreign body of knee**

    ✓7ᵗʰ **S81.041 Puncture wound with foreign body, right knee**   PE

    ✓7ᵗʰ **S81.042 Puncture wound with foreign body, left knee**   PE

    ✓7ᵗʰ **S81.049 Puncture wound with foreign body, unspecified knee**   PE

  ✓6ᵗʰ **S81.05 Open bite of knee**

    Bite of knee NOS

    EXCLUDES 1   *superficial bite of knee (S80.27-)*

    ✓7ᵗʰ **S81.051 Open bite, right knee**   PE

    ✓7ᵗʰ **S81.052 Open bite, left knee**   PE

    ✓7ᵗʰ **S81.059 Open bite, unspecified knee**   PE

✓5ᵗʰ **S81.8 Open wound of lower leg**

  ✓6ᵗʰ **S81.80 Unspecified open wound of lower leg**

    AHA: 2016,3Q,24

    ✓7ᵗʰ **S81.801 Unspecified open wound, right lower leg**   PE

    ✓7ᵗʰ **S81.802 Unspecified open wound, left lower leg**   PE

    ✓7ᵗʰ **S81.809 Unspecified open wound, unspecified lower leg**   PE

  ✓6ᵗʰ **S81.81 Laceration without foreign body of lower leg**

    ✓7ᵗʰ **S81.811 Laceration without foreign body, right lower leg**   PE

    ✓7ᵗʰ **S81.812 Laceration without foreign body, left lower leg**   PE

    ✓7ᵗʰ **S81.819 Laceration without foreign body, unspecified lower leg**   PE

  ✓6ᵗʰ **S81.82 Laceration with foreign body of lower leg**

    ✓7ᵗʰ **S81.821 Laceration with foreign body, right lower leg**   PE

    ✓7ᵗʰ **S81.822 Laceration with foreign body, left lower leg**   PE

    ✓7ᵗʰ **S81.829 Laceration with foreign body, unspecified lower leg**   PE

  ✓6ᵗʰ **S81.83 Puncture wound without foreign body of lower leg**

    AHA: 2016,3Q,24

    ✓7ᵗʰ **S81.831 Puncture wound without foreign body, right lower leg**   PE

    ✓7ᵗʰ **S81.832 Puncture wound without foreign body, left lower leg**   PE

    ✓7ᵗʰ **S81.839 Puncture wound without foreign body, unspecified lower leg**   PE

  ✓6ᵗʰ **S81.84 Puncture wound with foreign body of lower leg**

    AHA: 2016,3Q,24

    ✓7ᵗʰ **S81.841 Puncture wound with foreign body, right lower leg**   PE

    ✓7ᵗʰ **S81.842 Puncture wound with foreign body, left lower leg**   PE

    ✓7ᵗʰ **S81.849 Puncture wound with foreign body, unspecified lower leg**   PE

  ✓6ᵗʰ **S81.85 Open bite of lower leg**

    Bite of lower leg NOS

    EXCLUDES 1   *superficial bite of lower leg (S80.86-, S80.87-)*

    ✓7ᵗʰ **S81.851 Open bite, right lower leg**   PE

    ✓7ᵗʰ **S81.852 Open bite, left lower leg**   PE

    ✓7ᵗʰ **S81.859 Open bite, unspecified lower leg**   PE

✓4th S82 Fracture of lower leg, including ankle

NOTE A fracture not indicated as displaced or nondisplaced should be coded to displaced

A fracture not indicated as open or closed should be coded to closed

The open fracture designations are based on the Gustilo open fracture classification.

INCLUDES fracture of malleolus
EXCLUDES 1 *traumatic amputation of lower leg (S88.-)*
EXCLUDES 2 *fracture of foot, except ankle (S92.-)*
periprosthetic fracture around internal prosthetic ankle joint (M97.2)
periprosthetic fracture around internal prosthetic implant of knee joint (M97.1-)

AHA: 2018,2Q,12; 2016,1Q,33; 2015,3Q,37-39
DEF: Diaphysis: Central shaft of a long bone.
DEF: Epiphysis: Proximal and distal rounded ends of a long bone, communicates with the joint.
DEF: Metaphysis: Section of a long bone located between the epiphysis and diaphysis at the proximal and distal ends.
DEF: Physis (growth plate): Narrow zone of cartilaginous tissue between the epiphysis and metaphysis at each end of a long bone. In childhood, proliferation of cells in this zone lengthens the bone. As the bone matures, this area thins, ossification eventually fusing into solid bone and growth stops. *Synonym(s): Epiphyseal plate.*

The appropriate 7th character is to be added to all codes from category S82 [unless otherwise indicated].
A   initial encounter for closed fracture
B   initial encounter for open fracture type I or II
    initial encounter for open fracture NOS
C   initial encounter for open fracture type IIIA, IIIB, or IIIC
D   subsequent encounter for closed fracture with routine healing
E   subsequent encounter for open fracture type I or II with routine healing
F   subsequent encounter for open fracture type IIIA, IIIB, or IIIC with routine healing
G   subsequent encounter for closed fracture with delayed healing
H   subsequent encounter for open fracture type I or II with delayed healing
J   subsequent encounter for open fracture type IIIA, IIIB, or IIIC with delayed healing
K   subsequent encounter for closed fracture with nonunion
M   subsequent encounter for open fracture type I or II with nonunion
N   subsequent encounter for open fracture type IIIA, IIIB, or IIIC with nonunion
P   subsequent encounter for closed fracture with malunion
Q   subsequent encounter for open fracture type I or II with malunion
R   subsequent encounter for open fracture type IIIA, IIIB, or IIIC with malunion
S   sequela

✓5th S82.0 Fracture of patella
Knee cap

✓6th S82.00 Unspecified fracture of patella
- ✓7th **S82.001** Unspecified fracture of **right** patella   CC H5 PE
- ✓7th **S82.002** Unspecified fracture of **left** patella   CC H5 PE
- ✓7th **S82.009** Unspecified fracture of unspecified patella   CC H5 UNS PE

✓6th S82.01 Osteochondral fracture of patella
- ✓7th **S82.011** Displaced osteochondral fracture of **right** patella   CC H5 PE
- ✓7th **S82.012** Displaced osteochondral fracture of **left** patella   CC H5 PE
- ✓7th **S82.013** Displaced osteochondral fracture of unspecified patella   CC H5 UNS PE
- ✓7th **S82.014** Nondisplaced osteochondral fracture of **right** patella   CC H5 PE
- ✓7th **S82.015** Nondisplaced osteochondral fracture of **left** patella   CC H5 PE
- ✓7th **S82.016** Nondisplaced osteochondral fracture of unspecified patella   CC H5 UNS PE

✓6th S82.02 Longitudinal fracture of patella
- ✓7th **S82.021** Displaced longitudinal fracture of **right** patella   CC H5 PE
- ✓7th **S82.022** Displaced longitudinal fracture of **left** patella   CC H5 PE
- ✓7th **S82.023** Displaced longitudinal fracture of unspecified patella   CC H5 UNS PE
- ✓7th **S82.024** Nondisplaced longitudinal fracture of **right** patella   CC H5 PE
- ✓7th **S82.025** Nondisplaced longitudinal fracture of **left** patella   CC H5 PE
- ✓7th **S82.026** Nondisplaced longitudinal fracture of unspecified patella   CC H5 UNS PE

✓6th S82.03 Transverse fracture of patella
- ✓7th **S82.031** Displaced transverse fracture of **right** patella   CC H5 PE
- ✓7th **S82.032** Displaced transverse fracture of **left** patella   CC H5 PE
- ✓7th **S82.033** Displaced transverse fracture of unspecified patella   CC H5 UNS PE
- ✓7th **S82.034** Nondisplaced transverse fracture of **right** patella   CC H5 PE
- ✓7th **S82.035** Nondisplaced transverse fracture of **left** patella   CC H5 PE
- ✓7th **S82.036** Nondisplaced transverse fracture of unspecified patella   CC H5 UNS PE

✓6th S82.04 Comminuted fracture of patella
- ✓7th **S82.041** Displaced comminuted fracture of **right** patella   CC H5 PE
- ✓7th **S82.042** Displaced comminuted fracture of **left** patella   CC H5 PE
- ✓7th **S82.043** Displaced comminuted fracture of unspecified patella   CC H5 UNS PE
- ✓7th **S82.044** Nondisplaced comminuted fracture of **right** patella   CC H5 PE
- ✓7th **S82.045** Nondisplaced comminuted fracture of **left** patella   CC H5 PE
- ✓7th **S82.046** Nondisplaced comminuted fracture of unspecified patella   CC H5 UNS PE

✓6th S82.09 Other fracture of patella
- ✓7th **S82.091** Other fracture of **right** patella   CC H5 PE
- ✓7th **S82.092** Other fracture of **left** patella   CC H5 PE
- ✓7th **S82.099** Other fracture of unspecified patella   CC H5 UNS PE

✓5th S82.1 Fracture of upper end of tibia
Fracture of proximal end of tibia
EXCLUDES 2 *fracture of shaft of tibia (S82.2-)*
physeal fracture of upper end of tibia (S89.0-)

✓6th S82.10 Unspecified fracture of upper end of tibia
- ✓7th **S82.101** Unspecified fracture of upper end of **right** tibia   MCC CC H5 PE
- ✓7th **S82.102** Unspecified fracture of upper end of **left** tibia   MCC CC H5 PE
- ✓7th **S82.109** Unspecified fracture of upper end of unspecified tibia   MCC CC H5 UNS PE

✓6th S82.11 Fracture of tibial spine
- ✓7th **S82.111** Displaced fracture of **right** tibial spine   MCC CC H5 PE
- ✓7th **S82.112** Displaced fracture of **left** tibial spine   MCC CC H5 PE
- ✓7th **S82.113** Displaced fracture of unspecified tibial spine   MCC CC H5 UNS PE
- ✓7th **S82.114** Nondisplaced fracture of **right** tibial spine   MCC CC H5 PE
- ✓7th **S82.115** Nondisplaced fracture of **left** tibial spine   MCC CC H5 PE
- ✓7th **S82.116** Nondisplaced fracture of unspecified tibial spine   MCC CC H5 UNS PE

✓6th S82.12 Fracture of lateral condyle of tibia
- ✓7th **S82.121** Displaced fracture of lateral condyle of **right** tibia   MCC CC H5 PE
- ✓7th **S82.122** Displaced fracture of lateral condyle of **left** tibia   MCC CC H5 PE
- ✓7th **S82.123** Displaced fracture of lateral condyle of unspecified tibia   MCC CC H5 UNS PE
- ✓7th **S82.124** Nondisplaced fracture of lateral condyle of **right** tibia   MCC CC H5 PE
- ✓7th **S82.125** Nondisplaced fracture of lateral condyle of **left** tibia   MCC CC H5 PE

√7ᵗʰ **S82.126** **Nondisplaced** fracture of lateral condyle of unspecified tibia `MCC` `CC` `H5` `UNS` `PE`

√6ᵗʰ **S82.13** Fracture of **medial condyle** of tibia

√7ᵗʰ **S82.131** **Displaced** fracture of medial condyle of **right** tibia `MCC` `CC` `H5` `PE`

√7ᵗʰ **S82.132** **Displaced** fracture of medial condyle of **left** tibia `MCC` `CC` `H5` `PE`

√7ᵗʰ **S82.133** **Displaced** fracture of medial condyle of **unspecified** tibia `MCC` `CC` `H5` `UNS` `PE`

√7ᵗʰ **S82.134** **Nondisplaced** fracture of medial condyle of **right** tibia `MCC` `CC` `H5` `PE`

√7ᵗʰ **S82.135** **Nondisplaced** fracture of medial condyle of **left** tibia `MCC` `CC` `H5` `PE`

√7ᵗʰ **S82.136** **Nondisplaced** fracture of medial condyle of **unspecified** tibia `MCC` `CC` `H5` `UNS` `PE`

√6ᵗʰ **S82.14** **Bicondylar** fracture of tibia

Fracture of tibial plateau NOS

√7ᵗʰ **S82.141** **Displaced** bicondylar fracture of **right** tibia `MCC` `CC` `H5` `PE`

√7ᵗʰ **S82.142** **Displaced** bicondylar fracture of **left** tibia `MCC` `CC` `H5` `PE`

√7ᵗʰ **S82.143** **Displaced** bicondylar fracture of **unspecified** tibia `MCC` `CC` `H5` `UNS` `PE`

√7ᵗʰ **S82.144** **Nondisplaced** bicondylar fracture of **right** tibia `MCC` `CC` `H5` `PE`

√7ᵗʰ **S82.145** **Nondisplaced** bicondylar fracture of **left** tibia `MCC` `CC` `H5` `PE`

√7ᵗʰ **S82.146** **Nondisplaced** bicondylar fracture of **unspecified** tibia `MCC` `CC` `H5` `UNS` `PE`

√6ᵗʰ **S82.15** Fracture of **tibial tuberosity**

√7ᵗʰ **S82.151** **Displaced** fracture of **right** tibial tuberosity `MCC` `CC` `H5` `PE`

√7ᵗʰ **S82.152** **Displaced** fracture of **left** tibial tuberosity `MCC` `CC` `H5` `PE`

√7ᵗʰ **S82.153** **Displaced** fracture of unspecified tibial tuberosity `MCC` `CC` `H5` `UNS` `PE`

√7ᵗʰ **S82.154** **Nondisplaced** fracture of **right** tibial tuberosity `MCC` `CC` `H5` `PE`

√7ᵗʰ **S82.155** **Nondisplaced** fracture of **left** tibial tuberosity `MCC` `CC` `H5` `PE`

√7ᵗʰ **S82.156** **Nondisplaced** fracture of unspecified tibial tuberosity `MCC` `CC` `H5` `UNS` `PE`

√6ᵗʰ **S82.16** **Torus** fracture of upper end of tibia

> The appropriate 7th character is to be added to all codes in subcategory S82.16.
> A   initial encounter for closed fracture
> D   subsequent encounter for fracture with routine healing
> G   subsequent encounter for fracture with delayed healing
> K   subsequent encounter for fracture with nonunion
> P   subsequent encounter for fracture with malunion
> S   sequela

√7ᵗʰ **S82.161** **Torus** fracture of upper end of **right** tibia `CC` `H5` `PE`

√7ᵗʰ **S82.162** **Torus** fracture of upper end of **left** tibia `CC` `H5` `PE`

√7ᵗʰ **S82.169** **Torus** fracture of upper end of unspecified tibia `CC` `H5` `UNS` `PE`

√6ᵗʰ **S82.19** Other fracture of upper end of tibia

√7ᵗʰ **S82.191** Other fracture of upper end of **right** tibia `MCC` `CC` `H5` `PE`

√7ᵗʰ **S82.192** Other fracture of upper end of **left** tibia `MCC` `CC` `H5` `PE`

√7ᵗʰ **S82.199** Other fracture of upper end of unspecified tibia `MCC` `CC` `H5` `UNS` `PE`

√5ᵗʰ **S82.2** Fracture of **shaft of tibia**

√6ᵗʰ **S82.20** Unspecified fracture of shaft of tibia

Fracture of tibia NOS

√7ᵗʰ **S82.201** Unspecified fracture of shaft of **right** tibia `MCC` `CC` `H5` `PE`

√7ᵗʰ **S82.202** Unspecified fracture of shaft of **left** tibia `MCC` `CC` `H5` `PE`

√7ᵗʰ **S82.209** Unspecified fracture of shaft of unspecified tibia `MCC` `CC` `H5` `UNS` `PE`

√6ᵗʰ **S82.22** **Transverse** fracture of shaft of tibia

√7ᵗʰ **S82.221** **Displaced** transverse fracture of shaft of **right** tibia `MCC` `CC` `H5` `PE`

√7ᵗʰ **S82.222** **Displaced** transverse fracture of shaft of **left** tibia `MCC` `CC` `H5` `PE`

√7ᵗʰ **S82.223** **Displaced** transverse fracture of shaft of unspecified tibia `MCC` `CC` `H5` `UNS` `PE`

√7ᵗʰ **S82.224** **Nondisplaced** transverse fracture of shaft of **right** tibia `MCC` `CC` `H5` `PE`

√7ᵗʰ **S82.225** **Nondisplaced** transverse fracture of shaft of **left** tibia `MCC` `CC` `H5` `PE`

√7ᵗʰ **S82.226** **Nondisplaced** transverse fracture of shaft of unspecified tibia `MCC` `CC` `H5` `UNS` `PE`

√6ᵗʰ **S82.23** **Oblique** fracture of shaft of tibia

√7ᵗʰ **S82.231** **Displaced** oblique fracture of shaft of **right** tibia `MCC` `CC` `H5` `PE`

√7ᵗʰ **S82.232** **Displaced** oblique fracture of shaft of **left** tibia `MCC` `CC` `H5` `PE`

√7ᵗʰ **S82.233** **Displaced** oblique fracture of shaft of unspecified tibia `MCC` `CC` `H5` `UNS` `PE`

√7ᵗʰ **S82.234** **Nondisplaced** oblique fracture of shaft of **right** tibia `MCC` `CC` `H5` `PE`

√7ᵗʰ **S82.235** **Nondisplaced** oblique fracture of shaft of **left** tibia `MCC` `CC` `H5` `PE`

√7ᵗʰ **S82.236** **Nondisplaced** oblique fracture of shaft of unspecified tibia `MCC` `CC` `H5` `UNS` `PE`

√6ᵗʰ **S82.24** **Spiral** fracture of shaft of tibia

Toddler fracture

√7ᵗʰ **S82.241** **Displaced** spiral fracture of shaft of **right** tibia `MCC` `CC` `H5` `PE`

√7ᵗʰ **S82.242** **Displaced** spiral fracture of shaft of **left** tibia `MCC` `CC` `H5` `PE`

√7ᵗʰ **S82.243** **Displaced** spiral fracture of shaft of unspecified tibia `MCC` `CC` `H5` `UNS` `PE`

√7ᵗʰ **S82.244** **Nondisplaced** spiral fracture of shaft of **right** tibia `MCC` `CC` `H5` `PE`

√7ᵗʰ **S82.245** **Nondisplaced** spiral fracture of shaft of **left** tibia `MCC` `CC` `H5` `PE`

√7ᵗʰ **S82.246** **Nondisplaced** spiral fracture of shaft of unspecified tibia `MCC` `CC` `H5` `UNS` `PE`

√6ᵗʰ **S82.25** **Comminuted** fracture of shaft of tibia

√7ᵗʰ **S82.251** **Displaced** comminuted fracture of shaft of **right** tibia `MCC` `CC` `H5` `PE`

√7ᵗʰ **S82.252** **Displaced** comminuted fracture of shaft of **left** tibia `MCC` `CC` `H5` `PE`

√7ᵗʰ **S82.253** **Displaced** comminuted fracture of shaft of unspecified tibia `MCC` `CC` `H5` `UNS` `PE`

√7ᵗʰ **S82.254** **Nondisplaced** comminuted fracture of shaft of **right** tibia `MCC` `CC` `H5` `PE`

√7ᵗʰ **S82.255** **Nondisplaced** comminuted fracture of shaft of **left** tibia `MCC` `CC` `H5` `PE`

√7ᵗʰ **S82.256** **Nondisplaced** comminuted fracture of shaft of unspecified tibia `MCC` `CC` `H5` `UNS` `PE`

√6ᵗʰ **S82.26** **Segmental** fracture of shaft of tibia

√7ᵗʰ **S82.261** **Displaced** segmental fracture of shaft of **right** tibia `MCC` `CC` `H5` `PE`

√7ᵗʰ **S82.262** **Displaced** segmental fracture of shaft of **left** tibia `MCC` `CC` `H5` `PE`

√7ᵗʰ **S82.263** **Displaced** segmental fracture of shaft of unspecified tibia `MCC` `CC` `H5` `UNS` `PE`

√7ᵗʰ **S82.264** **Nondisplaced** segmental fracture of shaft of **right** tibia `MCC` `CC` `H5` `PE`

√7ᵗʰ **S82.265** **Nondisplaced** segmental fracture of shaft of **left** tibia `MCC` `CC` `H5` `PE`

√7ᵗʰ **S82.266** **Nondisplaced** segmental fracture of shaft of unspecified tibia `MCC` `CC` `H5` `UNS` `PE`

√6ᵗʰ **S82.29** Other fracture of shaft of tibia

√7ᵗʰ **S82.291** Other fracture of shaft of **right** tibia `MCC` `CC` `H5` `PE`

√7ᵗʰ **S82.292** Other fracture of shaft of **left** tibia `MCC` `CC` `H5` `PE`

√7ᵗʰ **S82.299** Other fracture of shaft of unspecified tibia `MCC` `CC` `H5` `UNS` `PE`

`N` Newborn: 0   `P` Pediatric: 0-17   `M` Maternity: 9-64   `A` Adult: 15-124   `UNS` Unspecified Site   `MCC` Major Complication/Comorbidity   `CC` Complication/Comorbidity   `PE` POA Exempt

1090

ICD-10-CM 2025

✓5ᵗʰ S82.3 Fracture of lower end of tibia

> EXCLUDES 1   bimalleolar fracture of lower leg (S82.84-)
> fracture of medial malleolus alone (S82.5-)
> Maisonneuve's fracture (S82.86-)
> pilon fracture of distal tibia (S82.87-)
> trimalleolar fractures of lower leg (S82.85-)

    ✓6ᵗʰ S82.30 Unspecified fracture of lower end of tibia

        ✓7ᵗʰ S82.301 Unspecified fracture of lower end of **right** tibia `CC` `H5` `PE`

        ✓7ᵗʰ S82.302 Unspecified fracture of lower end of **left** tibia `CC` `H5` `PE`

        ✓7ᵗʰ S82.309 Unspecified fracture of lower end of unspecified tibia `CC` `H5` `UNS` `PE`

    ✓6ᵗʰ S82.31 Torus fracture of lower end of tibia

> The appropriate 7th character is to be added to all codes in subcategory S82.31.
> A   initial encounter for closed fracture
> D   subsequent encounter for fracture with routine healing
> G   subsequent encounter for fracture with delayed healing
> K   subsequent encounter for fracture with nonunion
> P   subsequent encounter for fracture with malunion
> S   sequela

        ✓7ᵗʰ S82.311 Torus fracture of lower end of **right** tibia `CC` `H5` `PE`

        ✓7ᵗʰ S82.312 Torus fracture of lower end of **left** tibia `CC` `H5` `PE`

        ✓7ᵗʰ S82.319 Torus fracture of lower end of unspecified tibia `CC` `H5` `UNS` `PE`

    ✓6ᵗʰ S82.39 Other fracture of lower end of tibia

        AHA: 2015,1Q,25

        ✓7ᵗʰ S82.391 Other fracture of lower end of **right** tibia `CC` `H5` `PE`

        ✓7ᵗʰ S82.392 Other fracture of lower end of **left** tibia `CC` `H5` `PE`

        ✓7ᵗʰ S82.399 Other fracture of lower end of unspecified tibia `CC` `H5` `UNS` `PE`

✓5ᵗʰ S82.4 Fracture of shaft of fibula

> EXCLUDES 2   fracture of lateral malleolus alone (S82.6-)

    ✓6ᵗʰ S82.40 Unspecified fracture of shaft of fibula

        ✓7ᵗʰ S82.401 Unspecified fracture of shaft of **right** fibula `MCC` `CC` `H5` `PE`

        ✓7ᵗʰ S82.402 Unspecified fracture of shaft of **left** fibula `MCC` `CC` `H5` `PE`

        ✓7ᵗʰ S82.409 Unspecified fracture of shaft of unspecified fibula `MCC` `CC` `H5` `UNS` `PE`

    ✓6ᵗʰ S82.42 Transverse fracture of shaft of fibula

        ✓7ᵗʰ S82.421 Displaced transverse fracture of shaft of **right** fibula `MCC` `CC` `H5` `PE`

        ✓7ᵗʰ S82.422 Displaced transverse fracture of shaft of **left** fibula `MCC` `CC` `H5` `PE`

        ✓7ᵗʰ S82.423 Displaced transverse fracture of shaft of unspecified fibula `MCC` `CC` `H5` `UNS` `PE`

        ✓7ᵗʰ S82.424 Nondisplaced transverse fracture of shaft of **right** fibula `MCC` `CC` `H5` `PE`

        ✓7ᵗʰ S82.425 Nondisplaced transverse fracture of shaft of **left** fibula `MCC` `CC` `H5` `PE`

        ✓7ᵗʰ S82.426 Nondisplaced transverse fracture of shaft of unspecified fibula `MCC` `CC` `H5` `UNS` `PE`

    ✓6ᵗʰ S82.43 Oblique fracture of shaft of fibula

        ✓7ᵗʰ S82.431 Displaced oblique fracture of shaft of **right** fibula `MCC` `CC` `H5` `PE`

        ✓7ᵗʰ S82.432 Displaced oblique fracture of shaft of **left** fibula `MCC` `CC` `H5` `PE`

        ✓7ᵗʰ S82.433 Displaced oblique fracture of shaft of unspecified fibula `MCC` `CC` `H5` `UNS` `PE`

        ✓7ᵗʰ S82.434 Nondisplaced oblique fracture of shaft of **right** fibula `MCC` `CC` `H5` `PE`

        ✓7ᵗʰ S82.435 Nondisplaced oblique fracture of shaft of **left** fibula `MCC` `CC` `H5` `PE`

        ✓7ᵗʰ S82.436 Nondisplaced oblique fracture of shaft of unspecified fibula `MCC` `CC` `H5` `UNS` `PE`

    ✓6ᵗʰ S82.44 Spiral fracture of shaft of fibula

        ✓7ᵗʰ S82.441 Displaced spiral fracture of shaft of **right** fibula `MCC` `CC` `H5` `PE`

        ✓7ᵗʰ S82.442 Displaced spiral fracture of shaft of **left** fibula `MCC` `CC` `H5` `PE`

        ✓7ᵗʰ S82.443 Displaced spiral fracture of shaft of unspecified fibula `MCC` `CC` `H5` `UNS` `PE`

        ✓7ᵗʰ S82.444 Nondisplaced spiral fracture of shaft of **right** fibula `MCC` `CC` `H5` `PE`

        ✓7ᵗʰ S82.445 Nondisplaced spiral fracture of shaft of **left** fibula `MCC` `CC` `H5` `PE`

        ✓7ᵗʰ S82.446 Nondisplaced spiral fracture of shaft of unspecified fibula `MCC` `CC` `H5` `UNS` `PE`

    ✓6ᵗʰ S82.45 Comminuted fracture of shaft of fibula

        ✓7ᵗʰ S82.451 Displaced comminuted fracture of shaft of **right** fibula `MCC` `CC` `H5` `PE`

        ✓7ᵗʰ S82.452 Displaced comminuted fracture of shaft of **left** fibula `MCC` `CC` `H5` `PE`

        ✓7ᵗʰ S82.453 Displaced comminuted fracture of shaft of unspecified fibula `MCC` `CC` `H5` `UNS` `PE`

        ✓7ᵗʰ S82.454 Nondisplaced comminuted fracture of shaft of **right** fibula `MCC` `CC` `H5` `PE`

        ✓7ᵗʰ S82.455 Nondisplaced comminuted fracture of shaft of **left** fibula `MCC` `CC` `H5` `PE`

        ✓7ᵗʰ S82.456 Nondisplaced comminuted fracture of shaft of unspecified fibula `MCC` `CC` `H5` `UNS` `PE`

    ✓6ᵗʰ S82.46 Segmental fracture of shaft of fibula

        ✓7ᵗʰ S82.461 Displaced segmental fracture of shaft of **right** fibula `MCC` `CC` `H5` `PE`

        ✓7ᵗʰ S82.462 Displaced segmental fracture of shaft of **left** fibula `MCC` `CC` `H5` `PE`

        ✓7ᵗʰ S82.463 Displaced segmental fracture of shaft of unspecified fibula `MCC` `CC` `H5` `UNS` `PE`

        ✓7ᵗʰ S82.464 Nondisplaced segmental fracture of shaft of **right** fibula `MCC` `CC` `H5` `PE`

        ✓7ᵗʰ S82.465 Nondisplaced segmental fracture of shaft of **left** fibula `MCC` `CC` `H5` `PE`

        ✓7ᵗʰ S82.466 Nondisplaced segmental fracture of shaft of unspecified fibula `MCC` `CC` `H5` `UNS` `PE`

    ✓6ᵗʰ S82.49 Other fracture of shaft of fibula

        ✓7ᵗʰ S82.491 Other fracture of shaft of **right** fibula `MCC` `CC` `H5` `PE`

        ✓7ᵗʰ S82.492 Other fracture of shaft of **left** fibula `MCC` `CC` `H5` `PE`

        ✓7ᵗʰ S82.499 Other fracture of shaft of unspecified fibula `MCC` `CC` `H5` `UNS` `PE`

✓5ᵗʰ S82.5 Fracture of medial malleolus

> EXCLUDES 1   pilon fracture of distal tibia (S82.87-)
> Salter-Harris type III of lower end of tibia (S89.13-)
> Salter-Harris type IV of lower end of tibia (S89.14-)

    ✓x7ᵗʰ S82.51 Displaced fracture of medial malleolus of **right** tibia `CC` `H5` `PE`

    ✓x7ᵗʰ S82.52 Displaced fracture of medial malleolus of **left** tibia `CC` `H5` `PE`

    ✓x7ᵗʰ S82.53 Displaced fracture of medial malleolus of unspecified tibia `CC` `H5` `UNS` `PE`

    ✓x7ᵗʰ S82.54 Nondisplaced fracture of medial malleolus of **right** tibia `CC` `H5` `PE`

    ✓x7ᵗʰ S82.55 Nondisplaced fracture of medial malleolus of **left** tibia `CC` `H5` `PE`

    ✓x7ᵗʰ S82.56 Nondisplaced fracture of medial malleolus of unspecified tibia `CC` `H5` `UNS` `PE`

✓5ᵗʰ S82.6 Fracture of lateral malleolus

> EXCLUDES 1   pilon fracture of distal tibia (S82.87-)

    ✓x7ᵗʰ S82.61 Displaced fracture of lateral malleolus of **right** fibula `CC` `H5` `PE`

    ✓x7ᵗʰ S82.62 Displaced fracture of lateral malleolus of **left** fibula `CC` `H5` `PE`

    ✓x7ᵗʰ S82.63 Displaced fracture of lateral malleolus of unspecified fibula `CC` `H5` `UNS` `PE`

    ✓x7ᵗʰ S82.64 Nondisplaced fracture of lateral malleolus of **right** fibula `CC` `H5` `PE`

    ✓x7ᵗʰ S82.65 Nondisplaced fracture of lateral malleolus of **left** fibula `CC` `H5` `PE`

    ✓x7ᵗʰ S82.66 Nondisplaced fracture of lateral malleolus of unspecified fibula `CC` `H5` `UNS` `PE`

✓ Additional Character Required   ✓x7ᵗʰ Placeholder   Questionable PDx   Manifestation   Unspecified   `UPD` Unacceptable PDx   `H1`-`H14` HAC   `HCC` CMS-HCC Dx   `HIV` HIV Dx

ICD-10-CM 2025   1091

√5ᵗʰ S82.8 Other fractures of lower leg

√6ᵗʰ S82.81 Torus fracture of upper end of fibula

> The appropriate 7th character is to be added to all codes in subcategory S82.81
> A   initial encounter for closed fracture
> D   subsequent encounter for fracture with routine healing
> G   subsequent encounter for fracture with delayed healing
> K   subsequent encounter for fracture with nonunion
> P   subsequent encounter for fracture with malunion
> S   sequela

√7ᵗʰ **S82.811** Torus fracture of upper end of **right** fibula   CC PE

√7ᵗʰ **S82.812** Torus fracture of upper end of **left** fibula   CC PE

√7ᵗʰ **S82.819** Torus fracture of upper end of unspecified fibula   CC UNS PE

√6ᵗʰ S82.82 Torus fracture of lower end of fibula

> The appropriate 7th character is to be added to all codes in subcategory S82.82.
> A   initial encounter for closed fracture
> D   subsequent encounter for fracture with routine healing
> G   subsequent encounter for fracture with delayed healing
> K   subsequent encounter for fracture with nonunion
> P   subsequent encounter for fracture with malunion
> S   sequela

√7ᵗʰ **S82.821** Torus fracture of lower end of **right** fibula   CC PE

√7ᵗʰ **S82.822** Torus fracture of lower end of **left** fibula   CC PE

√7ᵗʰ **S82.829** Torus fracture of lower end of unspecified fibula   CC UNS PE

√6ᵗʰ S82.83 Other fracture of upper and lower end of fibula

     AHA: 2015,1Q,25

√7ᵗʰ **S82.831** Other fracture of upper and lower end of **right** fibula   MCC CC H5 PE

√7ᵗʰ **S82.832** Other fracture of upper and lower end of **left** fibula   MCC CC H5 PE

√7ᵗʰ **S82.839** Other fracture of upper and lower end of unspecified fibula   MCC CC H5 UNS PE

√6ᵗʰ S82.84 Bimalleolar fracture of lower leg

Right Bimalleolar Fracture

√7ᵗʰ **S82.841** Displaced bimalleolar fracture of **right** lower leg   CC H5 PE

√7ᵗʰ **S82.842** Displaced bimalleolar fracture of **left** lower leg   CC H5 PE

√7ᵗʰ **S82.843** Displaced bimalleolar fracture of unspecified lower leg   CC H5 UNS PE

√7ᵗʰ **S82.844** Nondisplaced bimalleolar fracture of **right** lower leg   CC H5 PE

√7ᵗʰ **S82.845** Nondisplaced bimalleolar fracture of **left** lower leg   CC H5 PE

√7ᵗʰ **S82.846** Nondisplaced bimalleolar fracture of unspecified lower leg   CC H5 UNS PE

√6ᵗʰ S82.85 Trimalleolar fracture of lower leg

√7ᵗʰ **S82.851** Displaced trimalleolar fracture of **right** lower leg   CC H5 PE

√7ᵗʰ **S82.852** Displaced trimalleolar fracture of **left** lower leg   CC H5 PE

√7ᵗʰ **S82.853** Displaced trimalleolar fracture of unspecified lower leg   CC H5 UNS PE

√7ᵗʰ **S82.854** Nondisplaced trimalleolar fracture of **right** lower leg   CC H5 PE

√7ᵗʰ **S82.855** Nondisplaced trimalleolar fracture of **left** lower leg   CC H5 PE

√7ᵗʰ **S82.856** Nondisplaced trimalleolar fracture of unspecified lower leg   CC H5 UNS PE

√6ᵗʰ S82.86 Maisonneuve's fracture

√7ᵗʰ **S82.861** Displaced Maisonneuve's fracture of **right** leg   MCC CC H5 PE

√7ᵗʰ **S82.862** Displaced Maisonneuve's fracture of **left** leg   MCC CC H5 PE

√7ᵗʰ **S82.863** Displaced Maisonneuve's fracture of unspecified leg   MCC CC H5 UNS PE

√7ᵗʰ **S82.864** Nondisplaced Maisonneuve's fracture of **right** leg   MCC CC H5 PE

√7ᵗʰ **S82.865** Nondisplaced Maisonneuve's fracture of **left** leg   MCC CC H5 PE

√7ᵗʰ **S82.866** Nondisplaced Maisonneuve's fracture of unspecified leg   MCC CC H5 UNS PE

√6ᵗʰ S82.87 Pilon fracture of tibia

√7ᵗʰ **S82.871** Displaced pilon fracture of **right** tibia   CC H5 PE

√7ᵗʰ **S82.872** Displaced pilon fracture of **left** tibia   CC H5 PE

√7ᵗʰ **S82.873** Displaced pilon fracture of unspecified tibia   CC H5 UNS PE

√7ᵗʰ **S82.874** Nondisplaced pilon fracture of **right** tibia   CC H5 PE

√7ᵗʰ **S82.875** Nondisplaced pilon fracture of **left** tibia   CC H5 PE

√7ᵗʰ **S82.876** Nondisplaced pilon fracture of unspecified tibia   CC H5 UNS PE

√6ᵗʰ S82.89 Other fractures of lower leg

     Fracture of ankle NOS

√7ᵗʰ **S82.891** Other fracture of **right** lower leg   CC H5 PE

√7ᵗʰ **S82.892** Other fracture of **left** lower leg   CC H5 PE

√7ᵗʰ **S82.899** Other fracture of unspecified lower leg   CC H5 UNS PE

√5ᵗʰ S82.9 Unspecified fracture of lower leg

√x7ᵗʰ **S82.90** Unspecified fracture of unspecified lower leg   CC H5 UNS PE

√x7ᵗʰ **S82.91** Unspecified fracture of **right** lower leg   CC H5 PE

√x7ᵗʰ **S82.92** Unspecified fracture of **left** lower leg   CC H5 PE

N Newborn: 0   P Pediatric: 0-17   M Maternity: 9-64   A Adult: 15-124   UNS Unspecified Site   MCC Major Complication/Comorbidity   CC Complication/Comorbidity   PE POA Exempt

1092   ICD-10-CM 2025

✓4th S83 Dislocation and sprain of joints and ligaments of knee

INCLUDES
avulsion of joint or ligament of knee
laceration of cartilage, joint or ligament of knee
sprain of cartilage, joint or ligament of knee
traumatic hemarthrosis of joint or ligament of knee
traumatic rupture of joint or ligament of knee
traumatic subluxation of joint or ligament of knee
traumatic tear of joint or ligament of knee

Code also any associated open wound

EXCLUDES 2
derangement of patella (M22.0-M22.3)
injury of patellar ligament (tendon) (S76.1-)
internal derangement of knee (M23.-)
old dislocation of knee (M24.36)
pathological dislocation of knee (M24.36)
recurrent dislocation of knee (M22.0)
strain of muscle, fascia and tendon of lower leg (S86.-)

The appropriate 7th character is to be added to each code from category S83.
A   initial encounter
D   subsequent encounter
S   sequela

✓5th S83.0 Subluxation and dislocation of patella

✓6th S83.00 Unspecified subluxation and dislocation of patella
- ✓7th S83.001 Unspecified subluxation of right patella PE
- ✓7th S83.002 Unspecified subluxation of left patella PE
- ✓7th S83.003 Unspecified subluxation of unspecified patella PE
- ✓7th S83.004 Unspecified dislocation of right patella PE
- ✓7th S83.005 Unspecified dislocation of left patella PE
- ✓7th S83.006 Unspecified dislocation of unspecified patella PE

✓6th S83.01 Lateral subluxation and dislocation of patella
- ✓7th S83.011 Lateral subluxation of right patella PE
- ✓7th S83.012 Lateral subluxation of left patella PE
- ✓7th S83.013 Lateral subluxation of unspecified patella PE
- ✓7th S83.014 Lateral dislocation of right patella PE
- ✓7th S83.015 Lateral dislocation of left patella PE
- ✓7th S83.016 Lateral dislocation of unspecified patella PE

✓6th S83.09 Other subluxation and dislocation of patella
- ✓7th S83.091 Other subluxation of right patella PE
- ✓7th S83.092 Other subluxation of left patella PE
- ✓7th S83.093 Other subluxation of unspecified patella PE
- ✓7th S83.094 Other dislocation of right patella PE
- ✓7th S83.095 Other dislocation of left patella PE
- ✓7th S83.096 Other dislocation of unspecified patella PE

✓5th S83.1 Subluxation and dislocation of knee

EXCLUDES 2   instability of knee prosthesis (T84.022, T84.023)

✓6th S83.10 Unspecified subluxation and dislocation of knee
- ✓7th S83.101 Unspecified subluxation of right knee PE
- ✓7th S83.102 Unspecified subluxation of left knee PE
- ✓7th S83.103 Unspecified subluxation of unspecified knee PE
- ✓7th S83.104 Unspecified dislocation of right knee PE
- ✓7th S83.105 Unspecified dislocation of left knee PE
- ✓7th S83.106 Unspecified dislocation of unspecified knee PE

✓6th S83.11 Anterior subluxation and dislocation of proximal end of tibia
Posterior subluxation and dislocation of distal end of femur
- ✓7th S83.111 Anterior subluxation of proximal end of tibia, right knee PE
- ✓7th S83.112 Anterior subluxation of proximal end of tibia, left knee PE
- ✓7th S83.113 Anterior subluxation of proximal end of tibia, unspecified knee PE
- ✓7th S83.114 Anterior dislocation of proximal end of tibia, right knee PE
- ✓7th S83.115 Anterior dislocation of proximal end of tibia, left knee PE
- ✓7th S83.116 Anterior dislocation of proximal end of tibia, unspecified knee PE

✓6th S83.12 Posterior subluxation and dislocation of proximal end of tibia
Anterior dislocation of distal end of femur
- ✓7th S83.121 Posterior subluxation of proximal end of tibia, right knee PE
- ✓7th S83.122 Posterior subluxation of proximal end of tibia, left knee PE
- ✓7th S83.123 Posterior subluxation of proximal end of tibia, unspecified knee PE
- ✓7th S83.124 Posterior dislocation of proximal end of tibia, right knee PE
- ✓7th S83.125 Posterior dislocation of proximal end of tibia, left knee PE
- ✓7th S83.126 Posterior dislocation of proximal end of tibia, unspecified knee PE

✓6th S83.13 Medial subluxation and dislocation of proximal end of tibia
- ✓7th S83.131 Medial subluxation of proximal end of tibia, right knee PE
- ✓7th S83.132 Medial subluxation of proximal end of tibia, left knee PE
- ✓7th S83.133 Medial subluxation of proximal end of tibia, unspecified knee PE
- ✓7th S83.134 Medial dislocation of proximal end of tibia, right knee PE
- ✓7th S83.135 Medial dislocation of proximal end of tibia, left knee PE
- ✓7th S83.136 Medial dislocation of proximal end of tibia, unspecified knee PE

✓6th S83.14 Lateral subluxation and dislocation of proximal end of tibia
- ✓7th S83.141 Lateral subluxation of proximal end of tibia, right knee PE
- ✓7th S83.142 Lateral subluxation of proximal end of tibia, left knee PE
- ✓7th S83.143 Lateral subluxation of proximal end of tibia, unspecified knee PE
- ✓7th S83.144 Lateral dislocation of proximal end of tibia, right knee PE
- ✓7th S83.145 Lateral dislocation of proximal end of tibia, left knee PE
- ✓7th S83.146 Lateral dislocation of proximal end of tibia, unspecified knee PE

✓6th S83.19 Other subluxation and dislocation of knee
- ✓7th S83.191 Other subluxation of right knee PE
- ✓7th S83.192 Other subluxation of left knee PE
- ✓7th S83.193 Other subluxation of unspecified knee PE
- ✓7th S83.194 Other dislocation of right knee PE
- ✓7th S83.195 Other dislocation of left knee PE
- ✓7th S83.196 Other dislocation of unspecified knee PE

✓5th S83.2 Tear of meniscus, current injury

EXCLUDES 1   old bucket-handle tear (M23.2)

AHA: 2019,2Q,26

✓6th S83.20 Tear of unspecified meniscus, current injury
Tear of meniscus of knee NOS
- ✓7th S83.200 Bucket-handle tear of unspecified meniscus, current injury, right knee PE
- ✓7th S83.201 Bucket-handle tear of unspecified meniscus, current injury, left knee PE
- ✓7th S83.202 Bucket-handle tear of unspecified meniscus, current injury, unspecified knee PE
- ✓7th S83.203 Other tear of unspecified meniscus, current injury, right knee PE
- ✓7th S83.204 Other tear of unspecified meniscus, current injury, left knee PE
- ✓7th S83.205 Other tear of unspecified meniscus, current injury, unspecified knee PE

✔ Additional Character Required   ✓x7th Placeholder   Questionable PDx   Manifestation   Unspecified   UPD Unacceptable PDx   H1-H14 HAC   HCC CMS-HCC Dx   HIV HIV Dx

√7th **S83.206** Unspecified tear of unspecified meniscus, current injury, **right** knee   PE

√7th **S83.207** Unspecified tear of unspecified meniscus, current injury, **left** knee   PE

√7th **S83.209** Unspecified tear of unspecified meniscus, current injury, unspecified knee   PE

√6th **S83.21** **Bucket-handle** tear of **medial** meniscus, current injury

√7th **S83.211** Bucket-handle tear of medial meniscus, current injury, **right** knee   PE

√7th **S83.212** Bucket-handle tear of medial meniscus, current injury, **left** knee   PE

√7th **S83.219** Bucket-handle tear of medial meniscus, current injury, unspecified knee   PE

√6th **S83.22** **Peripheral** tear of **medial** meniscus, current injury

√7th **S83.221** Peripheral tear of medial meniscus, current injury, **right** knee   PE

√7th **S83.222** Peripheral tear of medial meniscus, current injury, **left** knee   PE

√7th **S83.229** Peripheral tear of medial meniscus, current injury, unspecified knee   PE

√6th **S83.23** **Complex** tear of **medial** meniscus, current injury

√7th **S83.231** Complex tear of medial meniscus, current injury, **right** knee   PE

√7th **S83.232** Complex tear of medial meniscus, current injury, **left** knee   PE

√7th **S83.239** Complex tear of medial meniscus, current injury, unspecified knee   PE

√6th **S83.24** Other tear of **medial** meniscus, current injury

√7th **S83.241** Other tear of medial meniscus, current injury, **right** knee   PE

√7th **S83.242** Other tear of medial meniscus, current injury, **left** knee   PE

√7th **S83.249** Other tear of medial meniscus, current injury, unspecified knee   PE

√6th **S83.25** **Bucket-handle** tear of **lateral** meniscus, current injury

√7th **S83.251** Bucket-handle tear of lateral meniscus, current injury, **right** knee   PE

√7th **S83.252** Bucket-handle tear of lateral meniscus, current injury, **left** knee   PE

√7th **S83.259** Bucket-handle tear of lateral meniscus, current injury, unspecified knee   PE

√6th **S83.26** **Peripheral** tear of **lateral** meniscus, current injury

√7th **S83.261** Peripheral tear of lateral meniscus, current injury, **right** knee   PE

√7th **S83.262** Peripheral tear of lateral meniscus, current injury, **left** knee   PE

√7th **S83.269** Peripheral tear of lateral meniscus, current injury, unspecified knee   PE

√6th **S83.27** **Complex** tear of **lateral** meniscus, current injury

√7th **S83.271** Complex tear of lateral meniscus, current injury, **right** knee   PE

√7th **S83.272** Complex tear of lateral meniscus, current injury, **left** knee   PE

√7th **S83.279** Complex tear of lateral meniscus, current injury, unspecified knee   PE

√6th **S83.28** Other tear of **lateral** meniscus, current injury

√7th **S83.281** Other tear of lateral meniscus, current injury, **right** knee   PE

√7th **S83.282** Other tear of lateral meniscus, current injury, **left** knee   PE

√7th **S83.289** Other tear of lateral meniscus, current injury, unspecified knee   PE

√5th **S83.3** **Tear of articular cartilage** of knee, current

√x7th **S83.30** Tear of articular cartilage of unspecified knee, current   PE

√x7th **S83.31** Tear of articular cartilage of **right** knee, current   PE

√x7th **S83.32** Tear of articular cartilage of **left** knee, current   PE

√5th **S83.4** Sprain of **collateral ligament** of knee

√6th **S83.40** Sprain of unspecified collateral ligament of knee

√7th **S83.401** Sprain of unspecified collateral ligament of **right** knee   PE

√7th **S83.402** Sprain of unspecified collateral ligament of **left** knee   PE

√7th **S83.409** Sprain of unspecified collateral ligament of unspecified knee   PE

√6th **S83.41** Sprain of **medial** collateral ligament of knee

Sprain of tibial collateral ligament

√7th **S83.411** Sprain of medial collateral ligament of **right** knee   PE

√7th **S83.412** Sprain of medial collateral ligament of **left** knee   PE

√7th **S83.419** Sprain of medial collateral ligament of unspecified knee   PE

√6th **S83.42** Sprain of **lateral** collateral ligament of knee

Sprain of fibular collateral ligament

√7th **S83.421** Sprain of lateral collateral ligament of **right** knee   PE

√7th **S83.422** Sprain of lateral collateral ligament of **left** knee   PE

√7th **S83.429** Sprain of lateral collateral ligament of unspecified knee   PE

√5th **S83.5** Sprain of **cruciate ligament** of knee

AHA: 2016,2Q,3

√6th **S83.50** Sprain of unspecified cruciate ligament of knee

√7th **S83.501** Sprain of unspecified cruciate ligament of **right** knee   PE

√7th **S83.502** Sprain of unspecified cruciate ligament of **left** knee   PE

√7th **S83.509** Sprain of unspecified cruciate ligament of unspecified knee   PE

√6th **S83.51** Sprain of **anterior** cruciate ligament of knee

√7th **S83.511** Sprain of anterior cruciate ligament of **right** knee   PE

√7th **S83.512** Sprain of anterior cruciate ligament of **left** knee   PE

√7th **S83.519** Sprain of anterior cruciate ligament of unspecified knee   PE

√6th **S83.52** Sprain of **posterior** cruciate ligament of knee

√7th **S83.521** Sprain of posterior cruciate ligament of **right** knee   PE

√7th **S83.522** Sprain of posterior cruciate ligament of **left** knee   PE

√7th **S83.529** Sprain of posterior cruciate ligament of unspecified knee   PE

√5th **S83.6** Sprain of the **superior tibiofibular** joint and ligament

√x7th **S83.60** Sprain of the superior tibiofibular joint and ligament, unspecified knee   PE

√x7th **S83.61** Sprain of the superior tibiofibular joint and ligament, **right** knee   PE

√x7th **S83.62** Sprain of the superior tibiofibular joint and ligament, **left** knee   PE

√5th **S83.8** Sprain of other specified parts of knee

√6th **S83.8X** Sprain of other specified parts of knee

√7th **S83.8X1** Sprain of other specified parts of **right** knee   PE

√7th **S83.8X2** Sprain of other specified parts of **left** knee   PE

√7th **S83.8X9** Sprain of other specified parts of unspecified knee   PE

√5th **S83.9** Sprain of unspecified site of knee

√x7th **S83.90** Sprain of unspecified site of unspecified knee   PE

√x7th **S83.91** Sprain of unspecified site of **right** knee   PE

√x7th **S83.92** Sprain of unspecified site of **left** knee   PE

√4th **S84** **Injury of nerves at lower leg level**

Code also any associated open wound (S81.-)

EXCLUDES 2   injury of nerves at ankle and foot level (S94.-)

The appropriate 7th character is to be added to each code from category S84.
A   initial encounter
D   subsequent encounter
S   sequela

√5th **S84.0** Injury of **tibial nerve** at lower leg level

√x7th **S84.00** Injury of tibial nerve at lower leg level, unspecified leg   PE

√x7th **S84.01** Injury of tibial nerve at lower leg level, **right** leg   PE

√x7th **S84.02** Injury of tibial nerve at lower leg level, **left** leg   PE

√5th **S84.1** Injury of **peroneal nerve** at lower leg level

√x7th **S84.10** Injury of peroneal nerve at lower leg level, unspecified leg   PE

N Newborn: 0   **P** Pediatric: 0-17   **M** Maternity: 9-64   **A** Adult: 15-124   **UNS** Unspecified Site   **MCC** Major Complication/Comorbidity   **CC** Complication/Comorbidity   **PE** POA Exempt

1094   ICD-10-CM 2025

✓x 7th **S84.11**   **Injury of peroneal nerve at lower leg level, right leg** `PE`

✓x 7th **S84.12**   **Injury of peroneal nerve at lower leg level, left** `PE`

✓ 5th **S84.2**   **Injury of cutaneous sensory nerve at lower leg level**

✓x 7th **S84.20**   **Injury of cutaneous sensory nerve at lower leg level, unspecified leg** `PE`

✓x 7th **S84.21**   **Injury of cutaneous sensory nerve at lower leg level, right leg** `PE`

✓x 7th **S84.22**   **Injury of cutaneous sensory nerve at lower leg level, left leg** `PE`

✓ 5th **S84.8**   **Injury of other nerves at lower leg level**

✓ 6th **S84.80**   **Injury of other nerves at lower leg level**

✓ 7th **S84.801**   **Injury of other nerves at lower leg level, right leg** `PE`

✓ 7th **S84.802**   **Injury of other nerves at lower leg level, left leg** `PE`

✓ 7th **S84.809**   **Injury of other nerves at lower leg level, unspecified leg** `PE`

✓ 5th **S84.9**   **Injury of unspecified nerve at lower leg level**

✓x 7th **S84.90**   **Injury of unspecified nerve at lower leg level, unspecified leg** `PE`

✓x 7th **S84.91**   **Injury of unspecified nerve at lower leg level, right leg** `PE`

✓x 7th **S84.92**   **Injury of unspecified nerve at lower leg level, left leg** `PE`

✓ 4th **S85**   **Injury of blood vessels at lower leg level**

Code also any associated open wound (S81.-)

EXCLUDES 2   *injury of blood vessels at ankle and foot level (S95.-)*

The appropriate 7th character is to be added to each code from category S85.
A   initial encounter
D   subsequent encounter
S   sequela

✓ 5th **S85.0**   **Injury of popliteal artery**

✓ 6th **S85.00**   **Unspecified injury of popliteal artery**

✓ 7th **S85.001**   **Unspecified injury of popliteal artery, right leg** `MCC` `PE`

✓ 7th **S85.002**   **Unspecified injury of popliteal artery, left leg** `MCC` `PE`

✓ 7th **S85.009**   **Unspecified injury of popliteal artery, unspecified leg** `MCC` `UNS` `PE`

✓ 6th **S85.01**   **Laceration of popliteal artery**

✓ 7th **S85.011**   **Laceration of popliteal artery, right leg** `MCC` `PE`

✓ 7th **S85.012**   **Laceration of popliteal artery, left leg** `MCC` `PE`

✓ 7th **S85.019**   **Laceration of popliteal artery, unspecified leg** `MCC` `UNS` `PE`

✓ 6th **S85.09**   **Other specified injury of popliteal artery**

✓ 7th **S85.091**   **Other specified injury of popliteal artery, right leg** `MCC` `PE`

✓ 7th **S85.092**   **Other specified injury of popliteal artery, left leg** `MCC` `PE`

✓ 7th **S85.099**   **Other specified injury of popliteal artery, unspecified leg** `MCC` `UNS` `PE`

✓ 5th **S85.1**   **Injury of tibial artery**

✓ 6th **S85.10**   **Unspecified injury of unspecified tibial artery**

Injury of tibial artery NOS

✓ 7th **S85.101**   **Unspecified injury of unspecified tibial artery, right leg** `CC` `PE`

✓ 7th **S85.102**   **Unspecified injury of unspecified tibial artery, left leg** `CC` `PE`

✓ 7th **S85.109**   **Unspecified injury of unspecified tibial artery, unspecified leg** `CC` `UNS` `PE`

✓ 6th **S85.11**   **Laceration of unspecified tibial artery**

✓ 7th **S85.111**   **Laceration of unspecified tibial artery, right leg** `CC` `PE`

✓ 7th **S85.112**   **Laceration of unspecified tibial artery, left leg** `CC` `PE`

✓ 7th **S85.119**   **Laceration of unspecified tibial artery, unspecified leg** `CC` `UNS` `PE`

✓ 6th **S85.12**   **Other specified injury of unspecified tibial artery**

✓ 7th **S85.121**   **Other specified injury of unspecified tibial artery, right leg** `CC` `PE`

✓ 7th **S85.122**   **Other specified injury of unspecified tibial artery, left leg** `CC` `PE`

✓ 7th **S85.129**   **Other specified injury of unspecified tibial artery, unspecified leg** `CC` `UNS` `PE`

✓ 6th **S85.13**   **Unspecified injury of anterior tibial artery**

✓ 7th **S85.131**   **Unspecified injury of anterior tibial artery, right leg** `CC` `PE`

✓ 7th **S85.132**   **Unspecified injury of anterior tibial artery, left leg** `CC` `PE`

✓ 7th **S85.139**   **Unspecified injury of anterior tibial artery, unspecified leg** `CC` `UNS` `PE`

✓ 6th **S85.14**   **Laceration of anterior tibial artery**

✓ 7th **S85.141**   **Laceration of anterior tibial artery, right leg** `CC` `PE`

✓ 7th **S85.142**   **Laceration of anterior tibial artery, left leg** `CC` `PE`

✓ 7th **S85.149**   **Laceration of anterior tibial artery, unspecified leg** `CC` `UNS` `PE`

✓ 6th **S85.15**   **Other specified injury of anterior tibial artery**

✓ 7th **S85.151**   **Other specified injury of anterior tibial artery, right leg** `CC` `PE`

✓ 7th **S85.152**   **Other specified injury of anterior tibial artery, left leg** `CC` `PE`

✓ 7th **S85.159**   **Other specified injury of anterior tibial artery, unspecified leg** `CC` `UNS` `PE`

✓ 6th **S85.16**   **Unspecified injury of posterior tibial artery**

✓ 7th **S85.161**   **Unspecified injury of posterior tibial artery, right leg** `CC` `PE`

✓ 7th **S85.162**   **Unspecified injury of posterior tibial artery, left leg** `CC` `PE`

✓ 7th **S85.169**   **Unspecified injury of posterior tibial artery, unspecified leg** `CC` `UNS` `PE`

✓ 6th **S85.17**   **Laceration of posterior tibial artery**

✓ 7th **S85.171**   **Laceration of posterior tibial artery, right leg** `CC` `PE`

✓ 7th **S85.172**   **Laceration of posterior tibial artery, left leg** `CC` `PE`

✓ 7th **S85.179**   **Laceration of posterior tibial artery, unspecified leg** `CC` `UNS` `PE`

✓ 6th **S85.18**   **Other specified injury of posterior tibial artery**

✓ 7th **S85.181**   **Other specified injury of posterior tibial artery, right leg** `CC` `PE`

✓ 7th **S85.182**   **Other specified injury of posterior tibial artery, left leg** `CC` `PE`

✓ 7th **S85.189**   **Other specified injury of posterior tibial artery, unspecified leg** `CC` `UNS` `PE`

✓ 5th **S85.2**   **Injury of peroneal artery**

✓ 6th **S85.20**   **Unspecified injury of peroneal artery**

✓ 7th **S85.201**   **Unspecified injury of peroneal artery, right leg** `CC` `PE`

✓ 7th **S85.202**   **Unspecified injury of peroneal artery, left leg** `CC` `PE`

✓ 7th **S85.209**   **Unspecified injury of peroneal artery, unspecified leg** `CC` `UNS` `PE`

✓ 6th **S85.21**   **Laceration of peroneal artery**

✓ 7th **S85.211**   **Laceration of peroneal artery, right leg** `CC` `PE`

✓ 7th **S85.212**   **Laceration of peroneal artery, left leg** `CC` `PE`

✓ 7th **S85.219**   **Laceration of peroneal artery, unspecified leg** `CC` `UNS` `PE`

✓ 6th **S85.29**   **Other specified injury of peroneal artery**

✓ 7th **S85.291**   **Other specified injury of peroneal artery, right leg** `CC` `PE`

✓ 7th **S85.292**   **Other specified injury of peroneal artery, left leg** `CC` `PE`

✓ 7th **S85.299**   **Other specified injury of peroneal artery, unspecified leg** `CC` `UNS` `PE`

✓ 5th **S85.3**   **Injury of greater saphenous vein at lower leg level**

Injury of greater saphenous vein NOS
Injury of saphenous vein NOS

✓ 6th **S85.30**   **Unspecified injury of greater saphenous vein at lower leg level**

✓ 7th **S85.301**   **Unspecified injury of greater saphenous vein at lower leg level, right leg** `CC` `PE`

✓ 7th **S85.302**   **Unspecified injury of greater saphenous vein at lower leg level, left leg** `CC` `PE`

✔ Additional Character Required   ✓x 7th Placeholder   Questionable PDx   Manifestation   Unspecified   `UPD` Unacceptable PDx   `H1`-`H14` HAC   `HCC` CMS-HCC Dx   `HIV` HIV Dx

ICD-10-CM 2025   1095

√7th **S85.309** Unspecified injury of greater saphenous vein at lower leg level, unspecified leg `CC` `UNS` `PE`

√6th **S85.31** Laceration of greater saphenous vein at lower leg level

  √7th **S85.311** Laceration of greater saphenous vein at lower leg level, right leg `CC` `PE`

  √7th **S85.312** Laceration of greater saphenous vein at lower leg level, left leg `CC` `PE`

  √7th **S85.319** Laceration of greater saphenous vein at lower leg level, unspecified leg `CC` `UNS` `PE`

√6th **S85.39** Other specified injury of greater saphenous vein at lower leg level

  √7th **S85.391** Other specified injury of greater saphenous vein at lower leg level, right leg `CC` `PE`

  √7th **S85.392** Other specified injury of greater saphenous vein at lower leg level, left leg `CC` `PE`

  √7th **S85.399** Other specified injury of greater saphenous vein at lower leg level, unspecified leg `CC` `UNS` `PE`

√5th **S85.4** Injury of lesser saphenous vein at lower leg level

√6th **S85.40** Unspecified injury of lesser saphenous vein at lower leg level

  √7th **S85.401** Unspecified injury of lesser saphenous vein at lower leg level, right leg `CC` `PE`

  √7th **S85.402** Unspecified injury of lesser saphenous vein at lower leg level, left leg `CC` `PE`

  √7th **S85.409** Unspecified injury of lesser saphenous vein at lower leg level, unspecified leg `CC` `UNS` `PE`

√6th **S85.41** Laceration of lesser saphenous vein at lower leg level

  √7th **S85.411** Laceration of lesser saphenous vein at lower leg level, right leg `CC` `PE`

  √7th **S85.412** Laceration of lesser saphenous vein at lower leg level, left leg `CC` `PE`

  √7th **S85.419** Laceration of lesser saphenous vein at lower leg level, unspecified leg `CC` `UNS` `PE`

√6th **S85.49** Other specified injury of lesser saphenous vein at lower leg level

  √7th **S85.491** Other specified injury of lesser saphenous vein at lower leg level, right leg `CC` `PE`

  √7th **S85.492** Other specified injury of lesser saphenous vein at lower leg level, left leg `CC` `PE`

  √7th **S85.499** Other specified injury of lesser saphenous vein at lower leg level, unspecified leg `CC` `UNS` `PE`

√5th **S85.5** Injury of popliteal vein

√6th **S85.50** Unspecified injury of popliteal vein

  √7th **S85.501** Unspecified injury of popliteal vein, right leg `MCC` `PE`

  √7th **S85.502** Unspecified injury of popliteal vein, left leg `MCC` `PE`

  √7th **S85.509** Unspecified injury of popliteal vein, unspecified leg `MCC` `UNS` `PE`

√6th **S85.51** Laceration of popliteal vein

  √7th **S85.511** Laceration of popliteal vein, right leg `MCC` `PE`

  √7th **S85.512** Laceration of popliteal vein, left leg `MCC` `PE`

  √7th **S85.519** Laceration of popliteal vein, unspecified leg `MCC` `UNS` `PE`

√6th **S85.59** Other specified injury of popliteal vein

  √7th **S85.591** Other specified injury of popliteal vein, right leg `MCC` `PE`

  √7th **S85.592** Other specified injury of popliteal vein, left leg `MCC` `PE`

  √7th **S85.599** Other specified injury of popliteal vein, unspecified leg `MCC` `UNS` `PE`

√5th **S85.8** Injury of other blood vessels at lower leg level

√6th **S85.80** Unspecified injury of other blood vessels at lower leg level

  √7th **S85.801** Unspecified injury of other blood vessels at lower leg level, right leg `CC` `PE`

  √7th **S85.802** Unspecified injury of other blood vessels at lower leg level, left leg `CC` `PE`

√7th **S85.809** Unspecified injury of other blood vessels at lower leg level, unspecified leg `CC` `UNS` `PE`

√6th **S85.81** Laceration of other blood vessels at lower leg level

  √7th **S85.811** Laceration of other blood vessels at lower leg level, right leg `CC` `PE`

  √7th **S85.812** Laceration of other blood vessels at lower leg level, left leg `CC` `PE`

  √7th **S85.819** Laceration of other blood vessels at lower leg level, unspecified leg `CC` `UNS` `PE`

√6th **S85.89** Other specified injury of other blood vessels at lower leg level

  √7th **S85.891** Other specified injury of other blood vessels at lower leg level, right leg `CC` `PE`

  √7th **S85.892** Other specified injury of other blood vessels at lower leg level, left leg `CC` `PE`

  √7th **S85.899** Other specified injury of other blood vessels at lower leg level, unspecified leg `CC` `UNS` `PE`

√5th **S85.9** Injury of unspecified blood vessel at lower leg level

√6th **S85.90** Unspecified injury of unspecified blood vessel at lower leg level

  √7th **S85.901** Unspecified injury of unspecified blood vessel at lower leg level, right leg `CC` `PE`

  √7th **S85.902** Unspecified injury of unspecified blood vessel at lower leg level, left leg `CC` `PE`

  √7th **S85.909** Unspecified injury of unspecified blood vessel at lower leg level, unspecified leg `CC` `UNS` `PE`

√6th **S85.91** Laceration of unspecified blood vessel at lower leg level

  √7th **S85.911** Laceration of unspecified blood vessel at lower leg level, right leg `CC` `PE`

  √7th **S85.912** Laceration of unspecified blood vessel at lower leg level, left leg `CC` `PE`

  √7th **S85.919** Laceration of unspecified blood vessel at lower leg level, unspecified leg `CC` `UNS` `PE`

√6th **S85.99** Other specified injury of unspecified blood vessel at lower leg level

  √7th **S85.991** Other specified injury of unspecified blood vessel at lower leg level, right leg `CC` `PE`

  √7th **S85.992** Other specified injury of unspecified blood vessel at lower leg level, left leg `CC` `PE`

  √7th **S85.999** Other specified injury of unspecified blood vessel at lower leg level, unspecified leg `CC` `UNS` `PE`

√4th **S86** Injury of muscle, fascia and tendon at lower leg level

Code also any associated open wound (S81.-)

EXCLUDES 2   injury of muscle, fascia and tendon at ankle (S96.-)
     injury of patellar ligament (tendon) (S76.1-)
     sprain of joints and ligaments of knee (S83.-)

TIP: Refer to the Muscle/Tendon table at the beginning of this chapter.

> The appropriate 7th character is to be added to each code from category S86.
> A   initial encounter
> D   subsequent encounter
> S   sequela

√5th **S86.0** Injury of Achilles tendon

√6th **S86.00** Unspecified injury of Achilles tendon

  √7th **S86.001** Unspecified injury of right Achilles tendon `PE`

  √7th **S86.002** Unspecified injury of left Achilles tendon `PE`

  √7th **S86.009** Unspecified injury of unspecified Achilles tendon `PE`

√6th **S86.01** Strain of Achilles tendon

  √7th **S86.011** Strain of right Achilles tendon `PE`

  √7th **S86.012** Strain of left Achilles tendon `PE`

  √7th **S86.019** Strain of unspecified Achilles tendon `PE`

√6th **S86.02** Laceration of Achilles tendon

  √7th **S86.021** Laceration of right Achilles tendon `CC` `PE`

`N` Newborn: 0   `P` Pediatric: 0-17   `M` Maternity: 9-64   `A` Adult: 15-124   `UNS` Unspecified Site   `MCC` Major Complication/Comorbidity   `CC` Complication/Comorbidity   `PE` POA Exempt

1096

ICD-10-CM 2025

√7ᵗʰ **S86.022** Laceration of left Achilles tendon `CC` `PE`

√7ᵗʰ **S86.029** Laceration of unspecified Achilles tendon `CC` `UNS` `PE`

√6ᵗʰ **S86.09** Other specified injury of Achilles tendon

√7ᵗʰ **S86.091** Other specified injury of right Achilles tendon `PE`

√7ᵗʰ **S86.092** Other specified injury of left Achilles tendon `PE`

√7ᵗʰ **S86.099** Other specified injury of unspecified Achilles tendon `PE`

√5ᵗʰ **S86.1** Injury of other muscle(s) and tendon(s) of posterior muscle group at lower leg level

√6ᵗʰ **S86.10** Unspecified injury of other muscle(s) and tendon(s) of posterior muscle group at lower leg level

√7ᵗʰ **S86.101** Unspecified injury of other muscle(s) and tendon(s) of posterior muscle group at lower leg level, right leg `PE`

√7ᵗʰ **S86.102** Unspecified injury of other muscle(s) and tendon(s) of posterior muscle group at lower leg level, left leg `PE`

√7ᵗʰ **S86.109** Unspecified injury of other muscle(s) and tendon(s) of posterior muscle group at lower leg level, unspecified leg `PE`

√6ᵗʰ **S86.11** Strain of other muscle(s) and tendon(s) of posterior muscle group at lower leg level

√7ᵗʰ **S86.111** Strain of other muscle(s) and tendon(s) of posterior muscle group at lower leg level, right leg `PE`

√7ᵗʰ **S86.112** Strain of other muscle(s) and tendon(s) of posterior muscle group at lower leg level, left leg `PE`

√7ᵗʰ **S86.119** Strain of other muscle(s) and tendon(s) of posterior muscle group at lower leg level, unspecified leg `PE`

√6ᵗʰ **S86.12** Laceration of other muscle(s) and tendon(s) of posterior muscle group at lower leg level

√7ᵗʰ **S86.121** Laceration of other muscle(s) and tendon(s) of posterior muscle group at lower leg level, right leg `CC` `PE`

√7ᵗʰ **S86.122** Laceration of other muscle(s) and tendon(s) of posterior muscle group at lower leg level, left leg `CC` `PE`

√7ᵗʰ **S86.129** Laceration of other muscle(s) and tendon(s) of posterior muscle group at lower leg level, unspecified leg `CC` `UNS` `PE`

√6ᵗʰ **S86.19** Other injury of other muscle(s) and tendon(s) of posterior muscle group at lower leg level

√7ᵗʰ **S86.191** Other injury of other muscle(s) and tendon(s) of posterior muscle group at lower leg level, right leg `PE`

√7ᵗʰ **S86.192** Other injury of other muscle(s) and tendon(s) of posterior muscle group at lower leg level, left leg `PE`

√7ᵗʰ **S86.199** Other injury of other muscle(s) and tendon(s) of posterior muscle group at lower leg level, unspecified leg `PE`

√5ᵗʰ **S86.2** Injury of muscle(s) and tendon(s) of anterior muscle group at lower leg level

√6ᵗʰ **S86.20** Unspecified injury of muscle(s) and tendon(s) of anterior muscle group at lower leg level

√7ᵗʰ **S86.201** Unspecified injury of muscle(s) and tendon(s) of anterior muscle group at lower leg level, right leg `PE`

√7ᵗʰ **S86.202** Unspecified injury of muscle(s) and tendon(s) of anterior muscle group at lower leg level, left leg `PE`

√7ᵗʰ **S86.209** Unspecified injury of muscle(s) and tendon(s) of anterior muscle group at lower leg level, unspecified leg `PE`

√6ᵗʰ **S86.21** Strain of muscle(s) and tendon(s) of anterior muscle group at lower leg level

√7ᵗʰ **S86.211** Strain of muscle(s) and tendon(s) of anterior muscle group at lower leg level, right leg `PE`

√7ᵗʰ **S86.212** Strain of muscle(s) and tendon(s) of anterior muscle group at lower leg level, left leg `PE`

√7ᵗʰ **S86.219** Strain of muscle(s) and tendon(s) of anterior muscle group at lower leg level, unspecified leg `PE`

√6ᵗʰ **S86.22** Laceration of muscle(s) and tendon(s) of anterior muscle group at lower leg level

√7ᵗʰ **S86.221** Laceration of muscle(s) and tendon(s) of anterior muscle group at lower leg level, right leg `CC` `PE`

√7ᵗʰ **S86.222** Laceration of muscle(s) and tendon(s) of anterior muscle group at lower leg level, left leg `CC` `PE`

√7ᵗʰ **S86.229** Laceration of muscle(s) and tendon(s) of anterior muscle group at lower leg level, unspecified leg `CC` `UNS` `PE`

√6ᵗʰ **S86.29** Other injury of muscle(s) and tendon(s) of anterior muscle group at lower leg level

√7ᵗʰ **S86.291** Other injury of muscle(s) and tendon(s) of anterior muscle group at lower leg level, right leg `PE`

√7ᵗʰ **S86.292** Other injury of muscle(s) and tendon(s) of anterior muscle group at lower leg level, left leg `PE`

√7ᵗʰ **S86.299** Other injury of muscle(s) and tendon(s) of anterior muscle group at lower leg level, unspecified leg `PE`

√5ᵗʰ **S86.3** Injury of muscle(s) and tendon(s) of peroneal muscle group at lower leg level

√6ᵗʰ **S86.30** Unspecified injury of muscle(s) and tendon(s) of peroneal muscle group at lower leg level

√7ᵗʰ **S86.301** Unspecified injury of muscle(s) and tendon(s) of peroneal muscle group at lower leg level, right leg `PE`

√7ᵗʰ **S86.302** Unspecified injury of muscle(s) and tendon(s) of peroneal muscle group at lower leg level, left leg `PE`

√7ᵗʰ **S86.309** Unspecified injury of muscle(s) and tendon(s) of peroneal muscle group at lower leg level, unspecified leg `PE`

√6ᵗʰ **S86.31** Strain of muscle(s) and tendon(s) of peroneal muscle group at lower leg level

√7ᵗʰ **S86.311** Strain of muscle(s) and tendon(s) of peroneal muscle group at lower leg level, right leg `PE`

√7ᵗʰ **S86.312** Strain of muscle(s) and tendon(s) of peroneal muscle group at lower leg level, left leg `PE`

√7ᵗʰ **S86.319** Strain of muscle(s) and tendon(s) of peroneal muscle group at lower leg level, unspecified leg `PE`

√6ᵗʰ **S86.32** Laceration of muscle(s) and tendon(s) of peroneal muscle group at lower leg level

√7ᵗʰ **S86.321** Laceration of muscle(s) and tendon(s) of peroneal muscle group at lower leg level, right leg `CC` `PE`

√7ᵗʰ **S86.322** Laceration of muscle(s) and tendon(s) of peroneal muscle group at lower leg level, left leg `CC` `PE`

√7ᵗʰ **S86.329** Laceration of muscle(s) and tendon(s) of peroneal muscle group at lower leg level, unspecified leg `CC` `UNS` `PE`

√6ᵗʰ **S86.39** Other injury of muscle(s) and tendon(s) of peroneal muscle group at lower leg level

√7ᵗʰ **S86.391** Other injury of muscle(s) and tendon(s) of peroneal muscle group at lower leg level, right leg `PE`

√7ᵗʰ **S86.392** Other injury of muscle(s) and tendon(s) of peroneal muscle group at lower leg level, left leg `PE`

√7ᵗʰ **S86.399** Other injury of muscle(s) and tendon(s) of peroneal muscle group at lower leg level, unspecified leg `PE`

√5ᵗʰ **S86.8** Injury of other muscles and tendons at lower leg level

√6ᵗʰ **S86.80** Unspecified injury of other muscles and tendons at lower leg level

√7ᵗʰ **S86.801** Unspecified injury of other muscle(s) and tendon(s) at lower leg level, right leg `PE`

√7ᵗʰ **S86.802** Unspecified injury of other muscle(s) and tendon(s) at lower leg level, left leg `PE`

√7ᵗʰ **S86.809** Unspecified injury of other muscle(s) and tendon(s) at lower leg level, unspecified leg `PE`

√6ᵗʰ **S86.81** Strain of other muscles and tendons at lower leg level

√7ᵗʰ **S86.811** Strain of other muscle(s) and tendon(s) at lower leg level, right leg `PE`

✔ Additional Character Required   √x7ᵗʰ Placeholder   `Questionable PDx`   `Manifestation`   `Unspecified`   `UPD` Unacceptable PDx   `H1`-`H1C` HAC   `HCC` CMS-HCC Dx   `HIV` HIV Dx

√7th **S86.812** Strain of other muscle(s) and tendon(s) at lower leg level, **left** leg `PE`

√7th **S86.819** Strain of other muscle(s) and tendon(s) at lower leg level, unspecified leg `PE`

√6th **S86.82** **Laceration** of other muscles and tendons at lower leg level

√7th **S86.821** Laceration of other muscle(s) and tendon(s) at lower leg level, **right** leg `CC` `PE`

√7th **S86.822** Laceration of other muscle(s) and tendon(s) at lower leg level, **left** leg `CC` `PE`

√7th **S86.829** Laceration of other muscle(s) and tendon(s) at lower leg level, unspecified leg `CC` `UNS` `PE`

√6th **S86.89** Other injury of other muscles and tendons at lower leg level

√7th **S86.891** Other injury of other muscle(s) and tendon(s) at lower leg level, **right** leg `PE`

√7th **S86.892** Other injury of other muscle(s) and tendon(s) at lower leg level, **left** leg `PE`

√7th **S86.899** Other injury of other muscle(s) and tendon(s) at lower leg level, unspecified leg `PE`

√5th **S86.9** Injury of unspecified muscle and tendon at lower leg level

√6th **S86.90** Unspecified injury of unspecified muscle and tendon at lower leg level

√7th **S86.901** Unspecified injury of unspecified muscle(s) and tendon(s) at lower leg level, **right** leg

√7th **S86.902** Unspecified injury of unspecified muscle(s) and tendon(s) at lower leg level, **left** leg `PE`

√7th **S86.909** Unspecified injury of unspecified muscle(s) and tendon(s) at lower leg level, unspecified leg `PE`

√6th **S86.91** **Strain** of unspecified muscle and tendon at lower leg level

√7th **S86.911** Strain of unspecified muscle(s) and tendon(s) at lower leg level, **right** leg `PE`

√7th **S86.912** Strain of unspecified muscle(s) and tendon(s) at lower leg level, **left** leg `PE`

√7th **S86.919** Strain of unspecified muscle(s) and tendon(s) at lower leg level, unspecified leg `PE`

√6th **S86.92** **Laceration** of unspecified muscle and tendon at lower leg level

√7th **S86.921** Laceration of unspecified muscle(s) and tendon(s) at lower leg level, **right** leg `CC` `PE`

√7th **S86.922** Laceration of unspecified muscle(s) and tendon(s) at lower leg level, **left** leg `CC` `PE`

√7th **S86.929** Laceration of unspecified muscle(s) and tendon(s) at lower leg level, unspecified leg `CC` `UNS` `PE`

√6th **S86.99** Other injury of unspecified muscle and tendon at lower leg level

√7th **S86.991** Other injury of unspecified muscle(s) and tendon(s) at lower leg level, **right** leg `PE`

√7th **S86.992** Other injury of unspecified muscle(s) and tendon(s) at lower leg level, **left** leg `PE`

√7th **S86.999** Other injury of unspecified muscle(s) and tendon(s) at lower leg level, unspecified leg `PE`

√4th **S87** **Crushing injury** of lower leg

Use additional code(s) for all associated injuries

EXCLUDES 2   crushing injury of ankle and foot (S97.-)

The appropriate 7th character is to be added to each code from category S87.
A   initial encounter
D   subsequent encounter
S   sequela

√5th **S87.0** Crushing injury of **knee**

√x7th **S87.00** Crushing injury of unspecified knee `PE`

√x7th **S87.01** Crushing injury of **right** knee `PE`

√x7th **S87.02** Crushing injury of **left** knee `PE`

√5th **S87.8** Crushing injury of **lower leg**

√x7th **S87.80** Crushing injury of unspecified lower leg `PE`

√x7th **S87.81** Crushing injury of **right** lower leg `PE`

√x7th **S87.82** Crushing injury of **left** lower leg `PE`

√4th **S88** **Traumatic amputation of lower leg**

An amputation not identified as partial or complete should be coded to complete

EXCLUDES 1   traumatic amputation of ankle and foot (S98.-)

The appropriate 7th character is to be added to each code from category S88.
A   initial encounter
D   subsequent encounter
S   sequela

√5th **S88.0** Traumatic amputation at **knee level**

√6th **S88.01** **Complete** traumatic amputation at knee level

AHA: 2023,1Q,27,29

√7th **S88.011** Complete traumatic amputation at knee level, **right** lower leg `CC` `HCC` `PE`

√7th **S88.012** Complete traumatic amputation at knee level, **left** lower leg `CC` `HCC` `PE`

√7th **S88.019** Complete traumatic amputation at knee level, unspecified lower leg `CC` `UNS` `HCC` `PE`

√6th **S88.02** **Partial** traumatic amputation at knee level

√7th **S88.021** Partial traumatic amputation at knee level, **right** lower leg `CC` `HCC` `PE`

√7th **S88.022** Partial traumatic amputation at knee level, **left** lower leg `CC` `HCC` `PE`

√7th **S88.029** Partial traumatic amputation at knee level, unspecified lower leg `CC` `UNS` `HCC` `PE`

√5th **S88.1** Traumatic amputation at level **between knee and ankle**

√6th **S88.11** **Complete** traumatic amputation at level between knee and ankle

√7th **S88.111** Complete traumatic amputation at level between knee and ankle, **right** lower leg `CC` `HCC` `PE`

√7th **S88.112** Complete traumatic amputation at level between knee and ankle, **left** lower leg `CC` `HCC` `PE`

√7th **S88.119** Complete traumatic amputation at level between knee and ankle, unspecified lower leg `CC` `UNS` `HCC` `PE`

√6th **S88.12** **Partial** traumatic amputation at level between knee and ankle

√7th **S88.121** Partial traumatic amputation at level between knee and ankle, **right** lower leg `CC` `HCC` `PE`

√7th **S88.122** Partial traumatic amputation at level between knee and ankle, **left** lower leg `CC` `HCC` `PE`

√7th **S88.129** Partial traumatic amputation at level between knee and ankle, unspecified lower leg `CC` `UNS` `HCC` `PE`

√5th **S88.9** Traumatic amputation of lower leg, level unspecified

√6th **S88.91** **Complete** traumatic amputation of lower leg, level unspecified

√7th **S88.911** Complete traumatic amputation of **right** lower leg, level unspecified `CC` `HCC` `PE`

√7th **S88.912** Complete traumatic amputation of **left** lower leg, level unspecified `CC` `HCC` `PE`

√7th **S88.919** Complete traumatic amputation of unspecified lower leg, level unspecified `CC` `HCC` `PE`

√6th **S88.92** **Partial** traumatic amputation of lower leg, level unspecified

√7th **S88.921** Partial traumatic amputation of **right** lower leg, level unspecified `CC` `HCC` `PE`

√7th **S88.922** Partial traumatic amputation of **left** lower leg, level unspecified `CC` `HCC` `PE`

√7th **S88.929** Partial traumatic amputation of unspecified lower leg, level unspecified `CC` `UNS` `HCC` `PE`

`N` Newborn: 0   `P` Pediatric: 0-17   `M` Maternity: 9-64   `A` Adult: 15-124   `UNS` Unspecified Site   `MCC` Major Complication/Comorbidity   `CC` Complication/Comorbidity   `PE` POA Exempt

1098   ICD-10-CM 2025

☑4ᵗʰ **S89** **Other and unspecified injuries of lower leg**

> **NOTE**   A fracture not indicated as open or closed should be coded to closed.

EXCLUDES 2   *other and unspecified injuries of ankle and foot (S99.-)*

AHA: 2018,2Q,12; 2018,1Q,3; 2015,3Q,37-39

> The appropriate 7th character is to be added to each code from subcategories S89.0, S89.1, S89.2, and S89.3.
> A   initial encounter for closed fracture
> D   subsequent encounter for fracture with routine healing
> G   subsequent encounter for fracture with delayed healing
> K   subsequent encounter for fracture with nonunion
> P   subsequent encounter for fracture with malunion
> S   sequela

☑5ᵗʰ **S89.0** **Physeal fracture of upper end of tibia**

AHA: 2019,4Q,56

☑6ᵗʰ **S89.00** **Unspecified physeal fracture of upper end of tibia**

☑7ᵗʰ **S89.001** Unspecified physeal fracture of upper end of **right** tibia CC H5 PE

☑7ᵗʰ **S89.002** Unspecified physeal fracture of upper end of **left** tibia CC H5 PE

☑7ᵗʰ **S89.009** Unspecified physeal fracture of upper end of unspecified tibia CC H5 UNS PE

☑6ᵗʰ **S89.01** **Salter-Harris Type I physeal fracture of upper end of tibia**

☑7ᵗʰ **S89.011** Salter-Harris Type I physeal fracture of upper end of **right** tibia CC H5 PE

☑7ᵗʰ **S89.012** Salter-Harris Type I physeal fracture of upper end of **left** tibia CC H5 PE

☑7ᵗʰ **S89.019** Salter-Harris Type I physeal fracture of upper end of unspecified tibia CC H5 UNS PE

☑6ᵗʰ **S89.02** **Salter-Harris Type II physeal fracture of upper end of tibia**

☑7ᵗʰ **S89.021** Salter-Harris Type II physeal fracture of upper end of **right** tibia CC H5 PE

☑7ᵗʰ **S89.022** Salter-Harris Type II physeal fracture of upper end of **left** tibia CC H5 PE

☑7ᵗʰ **S89.029** Salter-Harris Type II physeal fracture of upper end of unspecified tibia CC H5 UNS PE

☑6ᵗʰ **S89.03** **Salter-Harris Type III physeal fracture of upper end of tibia**

☑7ᵗʰ **S89.031** Salter-Harris Type III physeal fracture of upper end of **right** tibia CC H5 PE

☑7ᵗʰ **S89.032** Salter-Harris Type III physeal fracture of upper end of **left** tibia CC H5 PE

☑7ᵗʰ **S89.039** Salter-Harris Type III physeal fracture of upper end of unspecified tibia CC H5 UNS PE

☑6ᵗʰ **S89.04** **Salter-Harris Type IV physeal fracture of upper end of tibia**

☑7ᵗʰ **S89.041** Salter-Harris Type IV physeal fracture of upper end of **right** tibia CC H5 PE

☑7ᵗʰ **S89.042** Salter-Harris Type IV physeal fracture of upper end of **left** tibia CC H5 PE

☑7ᵗʰ **S89.049** Salter-Harris Type IV physeal fracture of upper end of unspecified tibia CC H5 UNS PE

☑6ᵗʰ **S89.09** **Other physeal fracture of upper end of tibia**

☑7ᵗʰ **S89.091** Other physeal fracture of upper end of **right** tibia CC H5 PE

☑7ᵗʰ **S89.092** Other physeal fracture of upper end of **left** tibia CC H5 PE

☑7ᵗʰ **S89.099** Other physeal fracture of upper end of unspecified tibia CC H5 UNS PE

☑5ᵗʰ **S89.1** **Physeal fracture of lower end of tibia**

AHA: 2019,4Q,56

☑6ᵗʰ **S89.10** **Unspecified physeal fracture of lower end of tibia**

☑7ᵗʰ **S89.101** Unspecified physeal fracture of lower end of **right** tibia CC PE

☑7ᵗʰ **S89.102** Unspecified physeal fracture of lower end of **left** tibia CC PE

☑7ᵗʰ **S89.109** Unspecified physeal fracture of lower end of unspecified tibia CC UNS PE

☑6ᵗʰ **S89.11** **Salter-Harris Type I physeal fracture of lower end of tibia**

☑7ᵗʰ **S89.111** Salter-Harris Type I physeal fracture of lower end of **right** tibia CC PE

☑7ᵗʰ **S89.112** Salter-Harris Type I physeal fracture of lower end of **left** tibia CC PE

☑7ᵗʰ **S89.119** Salter-Harris Type I physeal fracture of lower end of unspecified tibia CC UNS PE

☑6ᵗʰ **S89.12** **Salter-Harris Type II physeal fracture of lower end of tibia**

☑7ᵗʰ **S89.121** Salter-Harris Type II physeal fracture of lower end of **right** tibia CC PE

☑7ᵗʰ **S89.122** Salter-Harris Type II physeal fracture of lower end of **left** tibia CC PE

☑7ᵗʰ **S89.129** Salter-Harris Type II physeal fracture of lower end of unspecified tibia CC UNS PE

☑6ᵗʰ **S89.13** **Salter-Harris Type III physeal fracture of lower end of tibia**

EXCLUDES 1   *fracture of medial malleolus (adult) (S82.5-)*

☑7ᵗʰ **S89.131** Salter-Harris Type III physeal fracture of lower end of **right** tibia CC PE

☑7ᵗʰ **S89.132** Salter-Harris Type III physeal fracture of lower end of **left** tibia CC PE

☑7ᵗʰ **S89.139** Salter-Harris Type III physeal fracture of lower end of unspecified tibia CC UNS PE

☑6ᵗʰ **S89.14** **Salter-Harris Type IV physeal fracture of lower end of tibia**

EXCLUDES 1   *fracture of medial malleolus (adult) (S82.5-)*

☑7ᵗʰ **S89.141** Salter-Harris Type IV physeal fracture of lower end of **right** tibia CC PE

☑7ᵗʰ **S89.142** Salter-Harris Type IV physeal fracture of lower end of **left** tibia CC PE

☑7ᵗʰ **S89.149** Salter-Harris Type IV physeal fracture of lower end of unspecified tibia CC UNS PE

☑6ᵗʰ **S89.19** **Other physeal fracture of lower end of tibia**

☑7ᵗʰ **S89.191** Other physeal fracture of lower end of **right** tibia CC PE

☑7ᵗʰ **S89.192** Other physeal fracture of lower end of **left** tibia CC PE

☑7ᵗʰ **S89.199** Other physeal fracture of lower end of unspecified tibia CC UNS PE

☑5ᵗʰ **S89.2** **Physeal fracture of upper end of fibula**

AHA: 2019,4Q,56

☑6ᵗʰ **S89.20** **Unspecified physeal fracture of upper end of fibula**

☑7ᵗʰ **S89.201** Unspecified physeal fracture of upper end of **right** fibula CC PE

☑7ᵗʰ **S89.202** Unspecified physeal fracture of upper end of **left** fibula CC PE

☑7ᵗʰ **S89.209** Unspecified physeal fracture of upper end of unspecified fibula CC UNS PE

☑6ᵗʰ **S89.21** **Salter-Harris Type I physeal fracture of upper end of fibula**

☑7ᵗʰ **S89.211** Salter-Harris Type I physeal fracture of upper end of **right** fibula CC PE

☑7ᵗʰ **S89.212** Salter-Harris Type I physeal fracture of upper end of **left** fibula CC PE

☑7ᵗʰ **S89.219** Salter-Harris Type I physeal fracture of upper end of unspecified fibula CC UNS PE

☑6ᵗʰ **S89.22** **Salter-Harris Type II physeal fracture of upper end of fibula**

☑7ᵗʰ **S89.221** Salter-Harris Type II physeal fracture of upper end of **right** fibula CC PE

☑7ᵗʰ **S89.222** Salter-Harris Type II physeal fracture of upper end of **left** fibula CC PE

☑7ᵗʰ **S89.229** Salter-Harris Type II physeal fracture of upper end of unspecified fibula CC UNS PE

☑6ᵗʰ **S89.29** **Other physeal fracture of upper end of fibula**

☑7ᵗʰ **S89.291** Other physeal fracture of upper end of **right** fibula CC PE

☑7ᵗʰ **S89.292** Other physeal fracture of upper end of **left** fibula CC PE

☑7ᵗʰ **S89.299** Other physeal fracture of upper end of unspecified fibula CC UNS PE

☑ Additional Character Required   ✓ₓ7ᵗʰ Placeholder   **Questionable PDx**   Manifestation   Unspecified   UPD Unacceptable PDx   H1-H14 HAC   HCC CMS-HCC Dx   HIV HIV Dx

ICD-10-CM 2025   1099

Chapter 19. Injury, Poisoning and Certain Other Consequences of External Causes

S89.3–S90.454

√5ᵗʰ **S89.3** **Physeal fracture of lower end of fibula**
AHA: 2019,4Q,56

√6ᵗʰ **S89.30** **Unspecified physeal fracture of lower end of fibula**

√7ᵗʰ **S89.301** Unspecified physeal fracture of lower end of **right** fibula   CC PE

√7ᵗʰ **S89.302** Unspecified physeal fracture of lower end of **left** fibula   CC PE

√7ᵗʰ **S89.309** Unspecified physeal fracture of lower end of unspecified fibula   CC UNS PE

√6ᵗʰ **S89.31** **Salter-Harris Type I physeal fracture of lower end of fibula**

√7ᵗʰ **S89.311** Salter-Harris Type I physeal fracture of lower end of **right** fibula   CC PE

√7ᵗʰ **S89.312** Salter-Harris Type I physeal fracture of lower end of **left** fibula   CC PE

√7ᵗʰ **S89.319** Salter-Harris Type I physeal fracture of lower end of unspecified fibula   CC UNS PE

√6ᵗʰ **S89.32** **Salter-Harris Type II physeal fracture of lower end of fibula**

√7ᵗʰ **S89.321** Salter-Harris Type II physeal fracture of lower end of **right** fibula   CC PE

√7ᵗʰ **S89.322** Salter-Harris Type II physeal fracture of lower end of **left** fibula   CC PE

√7ᵗʰ **S89.329** Salter-Harris Type II physeal fracture of lower end of unspecified fibula   CC UNS PE

√6ᵗʰ **S89.39** **Other physeal fracture of lower end of fibula**

√7ᵗʰ **S89.391** Other physeal fracture of lower end of right fibula   CC PE

√7ᵗʰ **S89.392** Other physeal fracture of lower end of left fibula   CC PE

√7ᵗʰ **S89.399** Other physeal fracture of lower end of unspecified fibula   CC UNS PE

√5ᵗʰ **S89.8** **Other specified injuries of lower leg**

The appropriate 7th character is to be added to each code in subcategory S89.8.
A   initial encounter
D   subsequent encounter
S   sequela

√x7ᵗʰ **S89.80** Other specified injuries of unspecified lower leg   PE

√x7ᵗʰ **S89.81** Other specified injuries of **right** lower leg   PE

√x7ᵗʰ **S89.82** Other specified injuries of **left** lower leg   PE

√5ᵗʰ **S89.9** **Unspecified injury of lower leg**

The appropriate 7th character is to be added to each code in subcategory S89.9.
A   initial encounter
D   subsequent encounter
S   sequela

√x7ᵗʰ **S89.90** Unspecified injury of unspecified lower leg   PE

√x7ᵗʰ **S89.91** Unspecified injury of **right** lower leg   PE

√x7ᵗʰ **S89.92** Unspecified injury of **left** lower leg   PE

Injuries to the ankle and foot (S90-S99)

EXCLUDES 2   burns and corrosions (T20-T32)
      fracture of ankle and malleolus (S82.-)
      frostbite (T33-T34)
      insect bite or sting, venomous (T63.4)

√4ᵗʰ **S90** **Superficial injury of ankle, foot and toes**

The appropriate 7th character is to be added to each code from category S90.
A   initial encounter
D   subsequent encounter
S   sequela

√5ᵗʰ **S90.0** **Contusion of ankle**

√x7ᵗʰ **S90.00** Contusion of unspecified ankle   PE

√x7ᵗʰ **S90.01** Contusion of **right** ankle   PE

√x7ᵗʰ **S90.02** Contusion of **left** ankle   PE

√5ᵗʰ **S90.1** **Contusion of toe without damage to nail**

√6ᵗʰ **S90.11** **Contusion of great toe without damage to nail**

√7ᵗʰ **S90.111** Contusion of **right** great toe without damage to nail   PE

√7ᵗʰ **S90.112** Contusion of **left** great toe without damage to nail   PE

√7ᵗʰ **S90.119** Contusion of unspecified great toe without damage to nail   PE

√6ᵗʰ **S90.12** **Contusion of lesser toe without damage to nail**

√7ᵗʰ **S90.121** Contusion of **right** lesser toe(s) without damage to nail   PE

√7ᵗʰ **S90.122** Contusion of **left** lesser toe(s) without damage to nail   PE

√7ᵗʰ **S90.129** Contusion of unspecified lesser toe(s) without damage to nail   PE
Contusion of toe NOS

√5ᵗʰ **S90.2** **Contusion of toe with damage to nail**

√6ᵗʰ **S90.21** **Contusion of great toe with damage to nail**

√7ᵗʰ **S90.211** Contusion of **right** great toe with damage to nail   PE

√7ᵗʰ **S90.212** Contusion of **left** great toe with damage to nail   PE

√7ᵗʰ **S90.219** Contusion of unspecified great toe with damage to nail   PE

√6ᵗʰ **S90.22** **Contusion of lesser toe with damage to nail**

√7ᵗʰ **S90.221** Contusion of **right** lesser toe(s) with damage to nail   PE

√7ᵗʰ **S90.222** Contusion of **left** lesser toe(s) with damage to nail   PE

√7ᵗʰ **S90.229** Contusion of unspecified lesser toe(s) with damage to nail   PE

√5ᵗʰ **S90.3** **Contusion of foot**
EXCLUDES 2   contusion of toes (S90.1-, S90.2-)

√x7ᵗʰ **S90.30** Contusion of unspecified foot   PE
Contusion of foot NOS

√x7ᵗʰ **S90.31** Contusion of **right** foot   PE

√x7ᵗʰ **S90.32** Contusion of **left** foot   PE

√5ᵗʰ **S90.4** **Other superficial injuries of toe**

√6ᵗʰ **S90.41** **Abrasion of toe**

√7ᵗʰ **S90.411** Abrasion, **right great** toe   PE

√7ᵗʰ **S90.412** Abrasion, **left great** toe   PE

√7ᵗʰ **S90.413** Abrasion, unspecified great toe   PE

√7ᵗʰ **S90.414** Abrasion, **right lesser** toe(s)   PE

√7ᵗʰ **S90.415** Abrasion, **left lesser** toe(s)   PE

√7ᵗʰ **S90.416** Abrasion, unspecified lesser toe(s)   PE

√6ᵗʰ **S90.42** **Blister (nonthermal) of toe**

√7ᵗʰ **S90.421** Blister (nonthermal), **right great** toe   PE

√7ᵗʰ **S90.422** Blister (nonthermal), **left great** toe   PE

√7ᵗʰ **S90.423** Blister (nonthermal), unspecified great toe   PE

√7ᵗʰ **S90.424** Blister (nonthermal), **right lesser** toe(s)   PE

√7ᵗʰ **S90.425** Blister (nonthermal), **left lesser** toe(s)   PE

√7ᵗʰ **S90.426** Blister (nonthermal), unspecified lesser toe(s)   PE

√6ᵗʰ **S90.44** **External constriction of toe**
Hair tourniquet syndrome of toe

√7ᵗʰ **S90.441** External constriction, **right great** toe   PE

√7ᵗʰ **S90.442** External constriction, **left great** toe   PE

√7ᵗʰ **S90.443** External constriction, unspecified great toe   PE

√7ᵗʰ **S90.444** External constriction, **right lesser** toe(s)   PE

√7ᵗʰ **S90.445** External constriction, **left lesser** toe(s)   PE

√7ᵗʰ **S90.446** External constriction, unspecified lesser toe(s)   PE

√6ᵗʰ **S90.45** **Superficial foreign body of toe**
Splinter in the toe

√7ᵗʰ **S90.451** Superficial foreign body, **right great** toe   PE

√7ᵗʰ **S90.452** Superficial foreign body, **left great** toe   PE

√7ᵗʰ **S90.453** Superficial foreign body, unspecified great toe   PE

√7ᵗʰ **S90.454** Superficial foreign body, **right lesser** toe(s)   PE

N Newborn: 0   P Pediatric: 0-17   M Maternity: 9-64   A Adult: 15-124   UNS Unspecified Site   MCC Major Complication/Comorbidity   CC Complication/Comorbidity   PE POA Exempt

√7ᵗʰ **S90.455** Superficial foreign body, **left lesser** toe(s) `PE`

√7ᵗʰ **S90.456** Superficial foreign body, unspecified lesser toe(s) `PE`

√6ᵗʰ **S90.46** Insect bite (nonvenomous) of toe

    √7ᵗʰ **S90.461** Insect bite (nonvenomous), **right great** toe `PE`

    √7ᵗʰ **S90.462** Insect bite (nonvenomous), **left great** toe `PE`

    √7ᵗʰ **S90.463** Insect bite (nonvenomous), unspecified great toe `PE`

    √7ᵗʰ **S90.464** Insect bite (nonvenomous), **right lesser** toe(s) `PE`

    √7ᵗʰ **S90.465** Insect bite (nonvenomous), **left lesser** toe(s) `PE`

    √7ᵗʰ **S90.466** Insect bite (nonvenomous), unspecified lesser toe(s) `PE`

√6ᵗʰ **S90.47** Other superficial bite of toe

    `EXCLUDES 1` *open bite of toe (S91.15-, S91.25-)*

    √7ᵗʰ **S90.471** Other superficial bite of **right great** toe `PE`

    √7ᵗʰ **S90.472** Other superficial bite of **left great** toe `PE`

    √7ᵗʰ **S90.473** Other superficial bite of unspecified great toe `PE`

    √7ᵗʰ **S90.474** Other superficial bite of **right lesser** toe(s) `PE`

    √7ᵗʰ **S90.475** Other superficial bite of **left lesser** toe(s) `PE`

    √7ᵗʰ **S90.476** Other superficial bite of unspecified lesser toe(s) `PE`

√5ᵗʰ **S90.5** Other superficial injuries of **ankle**

√6ᵗʰ **S90.51** **Abrasion** of ankle

    √7ᵗʰ **S90.511** Abrasion, **right** ankle `PE`

    √7ᵗʰ **S90.512** Abrasion, **left** ankle `PE`

    √7ᵗʰ **S90.519** Abrasion, unspecified ankle `PE`

√6ᵗʰ **S90.52** **Blister** (nonthermal) of ankle

    √7ᵗʰ **S90.521** Blister (nonthermal), **right** ankle `PE`

    √7ᵗʰ **S90.522** Blister (nonthermal), **left** ankle `PE`

    √7ᵗʰ **S90.529** Blister (nonthermal), unspecified ankle `PE`

√6ᵗʰ **S90.54** **External constriction** of ankle

    √7ᵗʰ **S90.541** External constriction, **right** ankle `PE`

    √7ᵗʰ **S90.542** External constriction, **left** ankle `PE`

    √7ᵗʰ **S90.549** External constriction, unspecified ankle `PE`

√6ᵗʰ **S90.55** Superficial **foreign body** of ankle

    Splinter in the ankle

    √7ᵗʰ **S90.551** Superficial foreign body, **right** ankle `PE`

    √7ᵗʰ **S90.552** Superficial foreign body, **left** ankle `PE`

    √7ᵗʰ **S90.559** Superficial foreign body, unspecified ankle `PE`

√6ᵗʰ **S90.56** **Insect bite** (nonvenomous) of ankle

    √7ᵗʰ **S90.561** Insect bite (nonvenomous), **right** ankle `PE`

    √7ᵗʰ **S90.562** Insect bite (nonvenomous), **left** ankle `PE`

    √7ᵗʰ **S90.569** Insect bite (nonvenomous), unspecified ankle `PE`

√6ᵗʰ **S90.57** Other superficial **bite** of ankle

    `EXCLUDES 1` *open bite of ankle (S91.05-)*

    √7ᵗʰ **S90.571** Other superficial bite of ankle, **right** ankle `PE`

    √7ᵗʰ **S90.572** Other superficial bite of ankle, **left** ankle `PE`

    √7ᵗʰ **S90.579** Other superficial bite of ankle, unspecified ankle `PE`

√5ᵗʰ **S90.8** Other superficial injuries of **foot**

√6ᵗʰ **S90.81** **Abrasion** of foot

    √7ᵗʰ **S90.811** Abrasion, **right** foot `PE`

    √7ᵗʰ **S90.812** Abrasion, **left** foot `PE`

    √7ᵗʰ **S90.819** Abrasion, unspecified foot `PE`

√6ᵗʰ **S90.82** **Blister** (nonthermal) of foot

    √7ᵗʰ **S90.821** Blister (nonthermal), **right** foot `PE`

    √7ᵗʰ **S90.822** Blister (nonthermal), **left** foot `PE`

    √7ᵗʰ **S90.829** Blister (nonthermal), unspecified foot `PE`

√6ᵗʰ **S90.84** **External constriction** of foot

    √7ᵗʰ **S90.841** External constriction, **right** foot `PE`

    √7ᵗʰ **S90.842** External constriction, **left** foot `PE`

    √7ᵗʰ **S90.849** External constriction, unspecified foot `PE`

√6ᵗʰ **S90.85** Superficial **foreign body** of foot

    Splinter in the foot

    √7ᵗʰ **S90.851** Superficial foreign body, **right** foot `PE`

    √7ᵗʰ **S90.852** Superficial foreign body, **left** foot `PE`

    √7ᵗʰ **S90.859** Superficial foreign body, unspecified foot `PE`

√6ᵗʰ **S90.86** **Insect bite** (nonvenomous) of foot

    √7ᵗʰ **S90.861** Insect bite (nonvenomous), **right** foot `PE`

    √7ᵗʰ **S90.862** Insect bite (nonvenomous), **left** foot `PE`

    √7ᵗʰ **S90.869** Insect bite (nonvenomous), unspecified foot `PE`

√6ᵗʰ **S90.87** Other superficial **bite** of foot

    `EXCLUDES 1` *open bite of foot (S91.35-)*

    √7ᵗʰ **S90.871** Other superficial bite of **right** foot `PE`

    √7ᵗʰ **S90.872** Other superficial bite of **left** foot `PE`

    √7ᵗʰ **S90.879** Other superficial bite of unspecified foot `PE`

√5ᵗʰ **S90.9** Unspecified superficial injury of ankle, foot and toe

√6ᵗʰ **S90.91** Unspecified superficial injury of **ankle**

    √7ᵗʰ **S90.911** Unspecified superficial injury of **right** ankle `PE`

    √7ᵗʰ **S90.912** Unspecified superficial injury of **left** ankle `PE`

    √7ᵗʰ **S90.919** Unspecified superficial injury of unspecified ankle `PE`

√6ᵗʰ **S90.92** Unspecified superficial injury of **foot**

    √7ᵗʰ **S90.921** Unspecified superficial injury of **right** foot `PE`

    √7ᵗʰ **S90.922** Unspecified superficial injury of **left** foot `PE`

    √7ᵗʰ **S90.929** Unspecified superficial injury of unspecified foot `PE`

√6ᵗʰ **S90.93** Unspecified superficial injury of **toes**

    √7ᵗʰ **S90.931** Unspecified superficial injury of **right great** toe `PE`

    √7ᵗʰ **S90.932** Unspecified superficial injury of **left great** toe `PE`

    √7ᵗʰ **S90.933** Unspecified superficial injury of unspecified great toe `PE`

    √7ᵗʰ **S90.934** Unspecified superficial injury of **right lesser** toe(s) `PE`

    √7ᵗʰ **S90.935** Unspecified superficial injury of **left lesser** toe(s) `PE`

    √7ᵗʰ **S90.936** Unspecified superficial injury of unspecified lesser toe(s) `PE`

√4ᵗʰ **S91** **Open wound of ankle, foot and toes**

Code also any associated wound infection

    `EXCLUDES 1` *open fracture of ankle, foot and toes (S92.- with 7th character B)*

          traumatic amputation of ankle and foot (S98.-)

AHA: 2021,1Q,7

The appropriate 7th character is to be added to each code from category S91.

A   initial encounter

D   subsequent encounter

S   sequela

√5ᵗʰ **S91.0** Open wound of **ankle**

√6ᵗʰ **S91.00** Unspecified open wound of ankle

    √7ᵗʰ **S91.001** Unspecified open wound, **right** ankle `PE`

    √7ᵗʰ **S91.002** Unspecified open wound, **left** ankle `PE`

    √7ᵗʰ **S91.009** Unspecified open wound, unspecified ankle `PE`

✔ Additional Character Required   ✓7ᵗʰ Placeholder   `Questionable PDx`   Manifestation   Unspecified   `UPD` Unacceptable PDx   `H1`-`H14` HAC   `HCC` CMS-HCC Dx   `HIV` HIV Dx

ICD-10-CM 2025   **1101**

√6th **S91.Ø1** **Laceration without foreign body** of ankle
- √7th **S91.Ø11** Laceration without foreign body, **right** ankle   PE
- √7th **S91.Ø12** Laceration without foreign body, **left** ankle   PE
- √7th **S91.Ø19** Laceration without foreign body, unspecified ankle   PE

√6th **S91.Ø2** **Laceration with foreign body** of ankle
- √7th **S91.Ø21** Laceration with foreign body, **right** ankle   PE
- √7th **S91.Ø22** Laceration with foreign body, **left** ankle   PE
- √7th **S91.Ø29** Laceration with foreign body, unspecified ankle   PE

√6th **S91.Ø3** **Puncture wound without foreign body** of ankle
- √7th **S91.Ø31** Puncture wound without foreign body, **right** ankle   PE
- √7th **S91.Ø32** Puncture wound without foreign body, **left** ankle   PE
- √7th **S91.Ø39** Puncture wound without foreign body, unspecified ankle   PE

√6th **S91.Ø4** **Puncture wound with foreign body** of ankle
- √7th **S91.Ø41** Puncture wound with foreign body, **right** ankle   PE
- √7th **S91.Ø42** Puncture wound with foreign body, **left** ankle   PE
- √7th **S91.Ø49** Puncture wound with foreign body, unspecified ankle   PE

√6th **S91.Ø5** **Open bite** of ankle
- **EXCLUDES 1**   superficial bite of ankle (S9Ø.56-, S9Ø.57-)
- √7th **S91.Ø51** Open bite, **right** ankle   PE
- √7th **S91.Ø52** Open bite, **left** ankle   PE
- √7th **S91.Ø59** Open bite, unspecified ankle   PE

√5th **S91.1** **Open wound** of **toe without damage to nail**

√6th **S91.1Ø** Unspecified open wound of toe without damage to nail
- √7th **S91.1Ø1** Unspecified open wound of **right great** toe without damage to nail   PE
- √7th **S91.1Ø2** Unspecified open wound of **left great** toe without damage to nail   PE
- √7th **S91.1Ø3** Unspecified open wound of unspecified great toe without damage to nail   PE
- √7th **S91.1Ø4** Unspecified open wound of **right lesser** toe(s) without damage to nail   PE
- √7th **S91.1Ø5** Unspecified open wound of **left lesser** toe(s) without damage to nail   PE
- √7th **S91.1Ø6** Unspecified open wound of unspecified lesser toe(s) without damage to nail   PE
- √7th **S91.1Ø9** Unspecified open wound of unspecified toe(s) without damage to nail   PE

√6th **S91.11** **Laceration without foreign body** of toe without damage to nail
- √7th **S91.111** Laceration without foreign body of **right great** toe without damage to nail   PE
- √7th **S91.112** Laceration without foreign body of **left great** toe without damage to nail   PE
- √7th **S91.113** Laceration without foreign body of unspecified great toe without damage to nail   PE
- √7th **S91.114** Laceration without foreign body of **right lesser** toe(s) without damage to nail   PE
- √7th **S91.115** Laceration without foreign body of **left lesser** toe(s) without damage to nail   PE
- √7th **S91.116** Laceration without foreign body of unspecified lesser toe(s) without damage to nail   PE
- √7th **S91.119** Laceration without foreign body of unspecified toe without damage to nail   PE

√6th **S91.12** **Laceration with foreign body** of toe without damage to nail
- √7th **S91.121** Laceration with foreign body of **right great** toe without damage to nail   PE
- √7th **S91.122** Laceration with foreign body of **left great** toe without damage to nail   PE
- √7th **S91.123** Laceration with foreign body of unspecified great toe without damage to nail   PE

- √7th **S91.124** Laceration with foreign body of **right lesser** toe(s) without damage to nail   PE
- √7th **S91.125** Laceration with foreign body of **left lesser** toe(s) without damage to nail   PE
- √7th **S91.126** Laceration with foreign body of unspecified lesser toe(s) without damage to nail   PE
- √7th **S91.129** Laceration with foreign body of unspecified toe(s) without damage to nail   PE

√6th **S91.13** **Puncture wound without foreign body** of toe without damage to nail
- √7th **S91.131** Puncture wound without foreign body of **right great** toe without damage to nail   PE
- √7th **S91.132** Puncture wound without foreign body of **left great** toe without damage to nail   PE
- √7th **S91.133** Puncture wound without foreign body of unspecified great toe without damage to nail   PE
- √7th **S91.134** Puncture wound without foreign body of **right lesser** toe(s) without damage to nail   PE
- √7th **S91.135** Puncture wound without foreign body of **left lesser** toe(s) without damage to nail   PE
- √7th **S91.136** Puncture wound without foreign body of unspecified lesser toe(s) without damage to nail   PE
- √7th **S91.139** Puncture wound without foreign body of unspecified toe(s) without damage to nail   PE

√6th **S91.14** **Puncture wound with foreign body** of toe without damage to nail
- √7th **S91.141** Puncture wound with foreign body of **right great** toe without damage to nail   PE
- √7th **S91.142** Puncture wound with foreign body of **left great** toe without damage to nail   PE
- √7th **S91.143** Puncture wound with foreign body of unspecified great toe without damage to nail   PE
- √7th **S91.144** Puncture wound with foreign body of **right lesser** toe(s) without damage to nail   PE
- √7th **S91.145** Puncture wound with foreign body of **left lesser** toe(s) without damage to nail   PE
- √7th **S91.146** Puncture wound with foreign body of unspecified lesser toe(s) without damage to nail   PE
- √7th **S91.149** Puncture wound with foreign body of unspecified toe(s) without damage to nail   PE

√6th **S91.15** **Open bite** of toe without damage to nail
- Bite of toe NOS
- **EXCLUDES 1**   superficial bite of toe (S9Ø.46-, S9Ø.47-)
- √7th **S91.151** Open bite of **right great** toe without damage to nail   PE
- √7th **S91.152** Open bite of **left great** toe without damage to nail   PE
- √7th **S91.153** Open bite of unspecified great toe without damage to nail   PE
- √7th **S91.154** Open bite of **right lesser** toe(s) without damage to nail   PE
- √7th **S91.155** Open bite of **left lesser** toe(s) without damage to nail   PE
- √7th **S91.156** Open bite of unspecified lesser toe(s) without damage to nail   PE
- √7th **S91.159** Open bite of unspecified toe(s) without damage to nail   PE

√5th **S91.2** **Open wound** of toe **with damage to nail**

√6th **S91.2Ø** Unspecified open wound of toe with damage to nail
- √7th **S91.2Ø1** Unspecified open wound of **right great** toe with damage to nail   PE
- √7th **S91.2Ø2** Unspecified open wound of **left great** toe with damage to nail   PE
- √7th **S91.2Ø3** Unspecified open wound of unspecified great toe with damage to nail   PE
- √7th **S91.2Ø4** Unspecified open wound of **right lesser** toe(s) with damage to nail   PE
- √7th **S91.2Ø5** Unspecified open wound of **left lesser** toe(s) with damage to nail   PE

N Newborn: 0   **P** Pediatric: 0-17   **M** Maternity: 9-64   **A** Adult: 15-124   **UNS** Unspecified Site   **MCC** Major Complication/Comorbidity   **CC** Complication/Comorbidity   **PE** POA Exempt

1102

ICD-10-CM 2025

√7ᵗʰ **S91.206** Unspecified open wound of unspecified lesser toe(s) with damage to nail   PE

√7ᵗʰ **S91.209** Unspecified open wound of unspecified toe(s) with damage to nail   PE

√6ᵗʰ **S91.21** Laceration without foreign body of toe with damage to nail

    √7ᵗʰ **S91.211** Laceration without foreign body of right great toe with damage to nail   PE

    √7ᵗʰ **S91.212** Laceration without foreign body of left great toe with damage to nail   PE

    √7ᵗʰ **S91.213** Laceration without foreign body of unspecified great toe with damage to nail   PE

    √7ᵗʰ **S91.214** Laceration without foreign body of right lesser toe(s) with damage to nail   PE

    √7ᵗʰ **S91.215** Laceration without foreign body of left lesser toe(s) with damage to nail   PE

    √7ᵗʰ **S91.216** Laceration without foreign body of unspecified lesser toe(s) with damage to nail   PE

    √7ᵗʰ **S91.219** Laceration without foreign body of unspecified toe(s) with damage to nail   PE

√6ᵗʰ **S91.22** Laceration with foreign body of toe with damage to nail

    √6ᵗʰ **S91.221** Laceration with foreign body of right great toe with damage to nail   PE

    √6ᵗʰ **S91.222** Laceration with foreign body of left great toe with damage to nail   PE

    √6ᵗʰ **S91.223** Laceration with foreign body of unspecified great toe with damage to nail   PE

    √6ᵗʰ **S91.224** Laceration with foreign body of right lesser toe(s) with damage to nail   PE

    √6ᵗʰ **S91.225** Laceration with foreign body of left lesser toe(s) with damage to nail   PE

    √6ᵗʰ **S91.226** Laceration with foreign body of unspecified lesser toe(s) with damage to nail   PE

    √6ᵗʰ **S91.229** Laceration with foreign body of unspecified toe(s) with damage to nail   PE

√6ᵗʰ **S91.23** Puncture wound without foreign body of toe with damage to nail

    √7ᵗʰ **S91.231** Puncture wound without foreign body of right great toe with damage to nail   PE

    √7ᵗʰ **S91.232** Puncture wound without foreign body of left great toe with damage to nail   PE

    √7ᵗʰ **S91.233** Puncture wound without foreign body of unspecified great toe with damage to nail   PE

    √7ᵗʰ **S91.234** Puncture wound without foreign body of right lesser toe(s) with damage to nail   PE

    √7ᵗʰ **S91.235** Puncture wound without foreign body of left lesser toe(s) with damage to nail   PE

    √7ᵗʰ **S91.236** Puncture wound without foreign body of unspecified lesser toe(s) with damage to nail   PE

    √7ᵗʰ **S91.239** Puncture wound without foreign body of unspecified toe(s) with damage to nail   PE

√6ᵗʰ **S91.24** Puncture wound with foreign body of toe with damage to nail

    √7ᵗʰ **S91.241** Puncture wound with foreign body of right great toe with damage to nail   PE

    √7ᵗʰ **S91.242** Puncture wound with foreign body of left great toe with damage to nail   PE

    √7ᵗʰ **S91.243** Puncture wound with foreign body of unspecified great toe with damage to nail   PE

    √7ᵗʰ **S91.244** Puncture wound with foreign body of right lesser toe(s) with damage to nail   PE

    √7ᵗʰ **S91.245** Puncture wound with foreign body of left lesser toe(s) with damage to nail   PE

    √7ᵗʰ **S91.246** Puncture wound with foreign body of unspecified lesser toe(s) with damage to nail   PE

    √7ᵗʰ **S91.249** Puncture wound with foreign body of unspecified toe(s) with damage to nail   PE

√6ᵗʰ **S91.25** Open bite of toe with damage to nail

    Bite of toe with damage to nail NOS

    EXCLUDES 1   superficial bite of toe (S90.46-, S90.47-)

    √7ᵗʰ **S91.251** Open bite of right great toe with damage to nail   PE

    √7ᵗʰ **S91.252** Open bite of left great toe with damage to nail   PE

    √7ᵗʰ **S91.253** Open bite of unspecified great toe with damage to nail   PE

    √7ᵗʰ **S91.254** Open bite of right lesser toe(s) with damage to nail   PE

    √7ᵗʰ **S91.255** Open bite of left lesser toe(s) with damage to nail   PE

    √7ᵗʰ **S91.256** Open bite of unspecified lesser toe(s) with damage to nail   PE

    √7ᵗʰ **S91.259** Open bite of unspecified toe(s) with damage to nail   PE

√5ᵗʰ **S91.3** Open wound of foot

  √6ᵗʰ **S91.30** Unspecified open wound of foot

    √7ᵗʰ **S91.301** Unspecified open wound, right foot   PE

    √7ᵗʰ **S91.302** Unspecified open wound, left foot   PE

    √7ᵗʰ **S91.309** Unspecified open wound, unspecified foot   PE

  √6ᵗʰ **S91.31** Laceration without foreign body of foot

    √7ᵗʰ **S91.311** Laceration without foreign body, right foot   PE

    √7ᵗʰ **S91.312** Laceration without foreign body, left foot   PE

    √7ᵗʰ **S91.319** Laceration without foreign body, unspecified foot   PE

  √6ᵗʰ **S91.32** Laceration with foreign body of foot

    √7ᵗʰ **S91.321** Laceration with foreign body, right foot   PE

    √7ᵗʰ **S91.322** Laceration with foreign body, left foot   PE

    √7ᵗʰ **S91.329** Laceration with foreign body, unspecified foot   PE

  √6ᵗʰ **S91.33** Puncture wound without foreign body of foot

    √7ᵗʰ **S91.331** Puncture wound without foreign body, right foot   PE

    √7ᵗʰ **S91.332** Puncture wound without foreign body, left foot   PE

    √7ᵗʰ **S91.339** Puncture wound without foreign body, unspecified foot   PE

  √6ᵗʰ **S91.34** Puncture wound with foreign body of foot

    √7ᵗʰ **S91.341** Puncture wound with foreign body, right foot   PE

    √7ᵗʰ **S91.342** Puncture wound with foreign body, left foot   PE

    √7ᵗʰ **S91.349** Puncture wound with foreign body, unspecified foot   PE

  √6ᵗʰ **S91.35** Open bite of foot

    EXCLUDES 1   superficial bite of foot (S90.86-, S90.87-)

    √7ᵗʰ **S91.351** Open bite, right foot   PE

    √7ᵗʰ **S91.352** Open bite, left foot   PE

    √7ᵗʰ **S91.359** Open bite, unspecified foot   PE

✔ Additional Character Required   √x7ᵗʰ Placeholder   Questionable PDx   Manifestation   Unspecified   UPD Unacceptable PDx   H1 - H14 HAC   HCC CMS-HCC Dx   HIV HIV Dx

ICD-10-CM 2025   1103

Chapter 19. Injury, Poisoning and Certain Other Consequences of External Causes

S92–S92.134

✓4ᵗʰ **S92 Fracture of foot and toe, except ankle**

> **NOTE**   A fracture not indicated as displaced or nondisplaced should be coded to displaced
>
> A fracture not indicated as open or closed should be coded to closed.

> **EXCLUDES 2**   fracture of ankle (S82.-)
> fracture of malleolus (S82.-)
> traumatic amputation of ankle and foot (S98.-)

AHA: 2018,2Q,12; 2015,3Q,37-39

> The appropriate 7th character is to be added to each code from category S92.
> A   initial encounter for closed fracture
> B   initial encounter for open fracture
> D   subsequent encounter for fracture with routine healing
> G   subsequent encounter for fracture with delayed healing
> K   subsequent encounter for fracture with nonunion
> P   subsequent encounter for fracture with malunion
> S   sequela

✓5ᵗʰ **S92.0 Fracture of calcaneus**
Heel bone
Os calcis
> **EXCLUDES 2**   physeal fracture of calcaneus (S99.0-)

✓6ᵗʰ **S92.00 Unspecified fracture of calcaneus**

✓7ᵗʰ **S92.001 Unspecified fracture of right calcaneus** CC H5 PE

✓7ᵗʰ **S92.002 Unspecified fracture of left calcaneus** CC H5 PE

✓7ᵗʰ **S92.009 Unspecified fracture of unspecified calcaneus** CC H5 UNS PE

✓6ᵗʰ **S92.01 Fracture of body of calcaneus**

✓7ᵗʰ **S92.011 Displaced fracture of body of right calcaneus** CC H5 PE

✓7ᵗʰ **S92.012 Displaced fracture of body of left calcaneus** CC H5 PE

✓7ᵗʰ **S92.013 Displaced fracture of body of unspecified calcaneus** CC H5 UNS PE

✓7ᵗʰ **S92.014 Nondisplaced fracture of body of right calcaneus** CC H5 PE

✓7ᵗʰ **S92.015 Nondisplaced fracture of body of left calcaneus** CC H5 PE

✓7ᵗʰ **S92.016 Nondisplaced fracture of body of unspecified calcaneus** CC H5 UNS PE

✓6ᵗʰ **S92.02 Fracture of anterior process of calcaneus**

✓7ᵗʰ **S92.021 Displaced fracture of anterior process of right calcaneus** CC H5 PE

✓7ᵗʰ **S92.022 Displaced fracture of anterior process of left calcaneus** CC H5 PE

✓7ᵗʰ **S92.023 Displaced fracture of anterior process of unspecified calcaneus** CC H5 UNS PE

✓7ᵗʰ **S92.024 Nondisplaced fracture of anterior process of right calcaneus** CC H5 PE

✓7ᵗʰ **S92.025 Nondisplaced fracture of anterior process of left calcaneus** CC H5 PE

✓7ᵗʰ **S92.026 Nondisplaced fracture of anterior process of unspecified calcaneus** CC H5 UNS PE

✓6ᵗʰ **S92.03 Avulsion fracture of tuberosity of calcaneus**

✓7ᵗʰ **S92.031 Displaced avulsion fracture of tuberosity of right calcaneus** CC H5 PE

✓7ᵗʰ **S92.032 Displaced avulsion fracture of tuberosity of left calcaneus** CC H5 PE

✓7ᵗʰ **S92.033 Displaced avulsion fracture of tuberosity of unspecified calcaneus** CC H5 UNS PE

✓7ᵗʰ **S92.034 Nondisplaced avulsion fracture of tuberosity of right calcaneus** CC H5 PE

✓7ᵗʰ **S92.035 Nondisplaced avulsion fracture of tuberosity of left calcaneus** CC H5 PE

✓7ᵗʰ **S92.036 Nondisplaced avulsion fracture of tuberosity of unspecified calcaneus** CC H5 UNS PE

✓6ᵗʰ **S92.04 Other fracture of tuberosity of calcaneus**

✓7ᵗʰ **S92.041 Displaced other fracture of tuberosity of right calcaneus** CC H5 PE

✓7ᵗʰ **S92.042 Displaced other fracture of tuberosity of left calcaneus** CC H5 PE

✓7ᵗʰ **S92.043 Displaced other fracture of tuberosity of unspecified calcaneus** CC H5 UNS PE

✓7ᵗʰ **S92.044 Nondisplaced other fracture of tuberosity of right calcaneus** CC H5 PE

✓7ᵗʰ **S92.045 Nondisplaced other fracture of tuberosity of left calcaneus** CC H5 PE

✓7ᵗʰ **S92.046 Nondisplaced other fracture of tuberosity of unspecified calcaneus** CC H5 UNS PE

✓6ᵗʰ **S92.05 Other extraarticular fracture of calcaneus**

✓7ᵗʰ **S92.051 Displaced other extraarticular fracture of right calcaneus** CC H5 PE

✓7ᵗʰ **S92.052 Displaced other extraarticular fracture of left calcaneus** CC H5 PE

✓7ᵗʰ **S92.053 Displaced other extraarticular fracture of unspecified calcaneus** CC H5 UNS PE

✓7ᵗʰ **S92.054 Nondisplaced other extraarticular fracture of right calcaneus** CC H5 PE

✓7ᵗʰ **S92.055 Nondisplaced other extraarticular fracture of left calcaneus** CC H5 PE

✓7ᵗʰ **S92.056 Nondisplaced other extraarticular fracture of unspecified calcaneus** CC H5 UNS PE

✓6ᵗʰ **S92.06 Intraarticular fracture of calcaneus**

✓7ᵗʰ **S92.061 Displaced intraarticular fracture of right calcaneus** CC H5 PE

✓7ᵗʰ **S92.062 Displaced intraarticular fracture of left calcaneus** CC H5 PE

✓7ᵗʰ **S92.063 Displaced intraarticular fracture of unspecified calcaneus** CC H5 UNS PE

✓7ᵗʰ **S92.064 Nondisplaced intraarticular fracture of right calcaneus** CC H5 PE

✓7ᵗʰ **S92.065 Nondisplaced intraarticular fracture of left calcaneus** CC H5 PE

✓7ᵗʰ **S92.066 Nondisplaced intraarticular fracture of unspecified calcaneus** CC H5 UNS PE

✓5ᵗʰ **S92.1 Fracture of talus**
Astragalus

✓6ᵗʰ **S92.10 Unspecified fracture of talus**

✓7ᵗʰ **S92.101 Unspecified fracture of right talus** CC H5 PE

✓7ᵗʰ **S92.102 Unspecified fracture of left talus** CC H5 PE

✓7ᵗʰ **S92.109 Unspecified fracture of unspecified talus** CC H5 UNS PE

✓6ᵗʰ **S92.11 Fracture of neck of talus**

✓7ᵗʰ **S92.111 Displaced fracture of neck of right talus** CC H5 PE

✓7ᵗʰ **S92.112 Displaced fracture of neck of left talus** CC H5 PE

✓7ᵗʰ **S92.113 Displaced fracture of neck of unspecified talus** CC H5 UNS PE

✓7ᵗʰ **S92.114 Nondisplaced fracture of neck of right talus** CC H5 PE

✓7ᵗʰ **S92.115 Nondisplaced fracture of neck of left talus** CC H5 PE

✓7ᵗʰ **S92.116 Nondisplaced fracture of neck of unspecified talus** CC H5 UNS PE

✓6ᵗʰ **S92.12 Fracture of body of talus**

✓7ᵗʰ **S92.121 Displaced fracture of body of right talus** CC H5 PE

✓7ᵗʰ **S92.122 Displaced fracture of body of left talus** CC H5 PE

✓7ᵗʰ **S92.123 Displaced fracture of body of unspecified talus** CC H5 UNS PE

✓7ᵗʰ **S92.124 Nondisplaced fracture of body of right talus** CC H5 PE

✓7ᵗʰ **S92.125 Nondisplaced fracture of body of left talus** CC H5 PE

✓7ᵗʰ **S92.126 Nondisplaced fracture of body of unspecified talus** CC H5 UNS PE

✓6ᵗʰ **S92.13 Fracture of posterior process of talus**

✓7ᵗʰ **S92.131 Displaced fracture of posterior process of right talus** CC H5 PE

✓7ᵗʰ **S92.132 Displaced fracture of posterior process of left talus** CC H5 PE

✓7ᵗʰ **S92.133 Displaced fracture of posterior process of unspecified talus** CC H5 UNS PE

✓7ᵗʰ **S92.134 Nondisplaced fracture of posterior process of right talus** CC H5 PE

N Newborn: 0   P Pediatric: 0-17   M Maternity: 9-64   A Adult: 15-124   UNS Unspecified Site   MCC Major Complication/Comorbidity   CC Complication/Comorbidity   PE POA Exempt

1104   ICD-10-CM 2025

√7th **S92.135** Nondisplaced fracture of posterior process of left talus `CC` `H5` `PE`

√7th **S92.136** Nondisplaced fracture of posterior process of unspecified talus `CC` `H5` `UNS` `PE`

√6th **S92.14** Dome fracture of talus

> EXCLUDES 1   osteochondritis dissecans (M93.2)

√7th **S92.141** Displaced dome fracture of right talus `CC` `H5` `PE`

√7th **S92.142** Displaced dome fracture of left talus `CC` `H5` `PE`

√7th **S92.143** Displaced dome fracture of unspecified talus `CC` `H5` `UNS` `PE`

√7th **S92.144** Nondisplaced dome fracture of right talus `CC` `H5` `PE`

√7th **S92.145** Nondisplaced dome fracture of left talus `CC` `H5` `PE`

√7th **S92.146** Nondisplaced dome fracture of unspecified talus `CC` `H5` `UNS` `PE`

√6th **S92.15** Avulsion fracture (chip fracture) of talus

√7th **S92.151** Displaced avulsion fracture (chip fracture) of right talus `CC` `H5` `PE`

√7th **S92.152** Displaced avulsion fracture (chip fracture) of left talus `CC` `H5` `PE`

√7th **S92.153** Displaced avulsion fracture (chip fracture) of unspecified talus `CC` `H5` `UNS` `PE`

√7th **S92.154** Nondisplaced avulsion fracture (chip fracture) of right talus `CC` `H5` `PE`

√7th **S92.155** Nondisplaced avulsion fracture (chip fracture) of left talus `CC` `H5` `PE`

√7th **S92.156** Nondisplaced avulsion fracture (chip fracture) of unspecified talus `CC` `H5` `UNS` `PE`

√6th **S92.19** Other fracture of talus

√7th **S92.191** Other fracture of right talus `CC` `H5` `PE`

√7th **S92.192** Other fracture of left talus `CC` `H5` `PE`

√7th **S92.199** Other fracture of unspecified talus `CC` `H5` `UNS` `PE`

√5th **S92.2** Fracture of other and unspecified tarsal bone(s)

√6th **S92.20** Fracture of unspecified tarsal bone(s)

√7th **S92.201** Fracture of unspecified tarsal bone(s) of right foot `CC` `H5` `PE`

√7th **S92.202** Fracture of unspecified tarsal bone(s) of left foot `CC` `H5` `PE`

√7th **S92.209** Fracture of unspecified tarsal bone(s) of unspecified foot `CC` `H5` `UNS` `PE`

√6th **S92.21** Fracture of cuboid bone

√7th **S92.211** Displaced fracture of cuboid bone of right foot `CC` `H5` `PE`

√7th **S92.212** Displaced fracture of cuboid bone of left foot `CC` `H5` `PE`

√7th **S92.213** Displaced fracture of cuboid bone of unspecified foot `CC` `H5` `UNS` `PE`

√7th **S92.214** Nondisplaced fracture of cuboid bone of right foot `CC` `H5` `PE`

√7th **S92.215** Nondisplaced fracture of cuboid bone of left foot `CC` `H5` `PE`

√7th **S92.216** Nondisplaced fracture of cuboid bone of unspecified foot `CC` `H5` `UNS` `PE`

√6th **S92.22** Fracture of lateral cuneiform

√7th **S92.221** Displaced fracture of lateral cuneiform of right foot `CC` `H5` `PE`

√7th **S92.222** Displaced fracture of lateral cuneiform of left foot `CC` `H5` `PE`

√7th **S92.223** Displaced fracture of lateral cuneiform of unspecified foot `CC` `H5` `UNS` `PE`

√7th **S92.224** Nondisplaced fracture of lateral cuneiform of right foot `CC` `H5` `PE`

√7th **S92.225** Nondisplaced fracture of lateral cuneiform of left foot `CC` `H5` `PE`

√7th **S92.226** Nondisplaced fracture of lateral cuneiform of unspecified foot `CC` `H5` `UNS` `PE`

√6th **S92.23** Fracture of intermediate cuneiform

√7th **S92.231** Displaced fracture of intermediate cuneiform of right foot `CC` `H5` `PE`

√7th **S92.232** Displaced fracture of intermediate cuneiform of left foot `CC` `H5` `PE`

√7th **S92.233** Displaced fracture of intermediate cuneiform of unspecified foot `CC` `H5` `UNS` `PE`

√7th **S92.234** Nondisplaced fracture of intermediate cuneiform of right foot `CC` `H5` `PE`

√7th **S92.235** Nondisplaced fracture of intermediate cuneiform of left foot `CC` `H5` `PE`

√7th **S92.236** Nondisplaced fracture of intermediate cuneiform of unspecified foot `CC` `H5` `UNS` `PE`

√6th **S92.24** Fracture of medial cuneiform

√7th **S92.241** Displaced fracture of medial cuneiform of right foot `CC` `H5` `PE`

√7th **S92.242** Displaced fracture of medial cuneiform of left foot `CC` `H5` `PE`

√7th **S92.243** Displaced fracture of medial cuneiform of unspecified foot `CC` `H5` `UNS` `PE`

√7th **S92.244** Nondisplaced fracture of medial cuneiform of right foot `CC` `H5` `PE`

√7th **S92.245** Nondisplaced fracture of medial cuneiform of left foot `CC` `H5` `PE`

√7th **S92.246** Nondisplaced fracture of medial cuneiform of unspecified foot `CC` `H5` `UNS` `PE`

√6th **S92.25** Fracture of navicular [scaphoid] of foot

√7th **S92.251** Displaced fracture of navicular [scaphoid] of right foot `CC` `H5` `PE`

√7th **S92.252** Displaced fracture of navicular [scaphoid] of left foot `CC` `H5` `PE`

√7th **S92.253** Displaced fracture of navicular [scaphoid] of unspecified foot `CC` `H5` `UNS` `PE`

√7th **S92.254** Nondisplaced fracture of navicular [scaphoid] of right foot `CC` `H5` `PE`

√7th **S92.255** Nondisplaced fracture of navicular [scaphoid] of left foot `CC` `H5` `PE`

√7th **S92.256** Nondisplaced fracture of navicular [scaphoid] of unspecified foot `CC` `H5` `UNS` `PE`

√5th **S92.3** Fracture of metatarsal bone(s)

> EXCLUDES 2   physeal fracture of metatarsal (S99.1-)

AHA: 2018,1Q,3

√6th **S92.30** Fracture of unspecified metatarsal bone(s)

√7th **S92.301** Fracture of unspecified metatarsal bone(s), right foot `CC` `H5` `PE`

√7th **S92.302** Fracture of unspecified metatarsal bone(s), left foot `CC` `H5` `PE`

√7th **S92.309** Fracture of unspecified metatarsal bone(s), unspecified foot `CC` `H5` `UNS` `PE`

√6th **S92.31** Fracture of first metatarsal bone

√7th **S92.311** Displaced fracture of first metatarsal bone, right foot `CC` `H5` `PE`

√7th **S92.312** Displaced fracture of first metatarsal bone, left foot `CC` `H5` `PE`

√7th **S92.313** Displaced fracture of first metatarsal bone, unspecified foot `CC` `H5` `UNS` `PE`

√7th **S92.314** Nondisplaced fracture of first metatarsal bone, right foot `CC` `H5` `PE`

√7th **S92.315** Nondisplaced fracture of first metatarsal bone, left foot `CC` `H5` `PE`

√7th **S92.316** Nondisplaced fracture of first metatarsal bone, unspecified foot `CC` `H5` `UNS` `PE`

√6th **S92.32** Fracture of second metatarsal bone

√7th **S92.321** Displaced fracture of second metatarsal bone, right foot `CC` `H5` `PE`

√7th **S92.322** Displaced fracture of second metatarsal bone, left foot `CC` `H5` `PE`

√7th **S92.323** Displaced fracture of second metatarsal bone, unspecified foot `CC` `H5` `UNS` `PE`

√7th **S92.324** Nondisplaced fracture of second metatarsal bone, right foot `CC` `H5` `PE`

√7th **S92.325** Nondisplaced fracture of second metatarsal bone, left foot `CC` `H5` `PE`

√7th **S92.326** Nondisplaced fracture of second metatarsal bone, unspecified foot `CC` `H5` `UNS` `PE`

√6th **S92.33** Fracture of third metatarsal bone

√7th **S92.331** Displaced fracture of third metatarsal bone, right foot `CC` `H5` `PE`

☑ Additional Character Required   √x7th Placeholder   Questionable PDx   Manifestation   Unspecified   `UPD` Unacceptable PDx   `H1`-`H14` HAC   `HCC` CMS-HCC Dx   `HIV` HIV Dx

ICD-10-CM 2025   1105

√7ᵗʰ **S92.332** **Displaced** fracture of third metatarsal bone, **left** foot `CC` `H5` `PE`

√7ᵗʰ **S92.333** **Displaced** fracture of third metatarsal bone, unspecified foot `CC` `H5` `UNS` `PE`

√7ᵗʰ **S92.334** **Nondisplaced** fracture of third metatarsal bone, **right** foot `CC` `H5` `PE`

√7ᵗʰ **S92.335** **Nondisplaced** fracture of third metatarsal bone, **left** foot `CC` `H5` `PE`

√7ᵗʰ **S92.336** **Nondisplaced** fracture of third metatarsal bone, unspecified foot `CC` `H5` `UNS` `PE`

√6ᵗʰ **S92.34** Fracture of **fourth** metatarsal bone

√7ᵗʰ **S92.341** **Displaced** fracture of fourth metatarsal bone, **right** foot `CC` `H5` `PE`

√7ᵗʰ **S92.342** **Displaced** fracture of fourth metatarsal bone, **left** foot `CC` `H5` `PE`

√7ᵗʰ **S92.343** **Displaced** fracture of fourth metatarsal bone, unspecified foot `CC` `H5` `UNS` `PE`

√7ᵗʰ **S92.344** **Nondisplaced** fracture of fourth metatarsal bone, **right** foot `CC` `H5` `PE`

√7ᵗʰ **S92.345** **Nondisplaced** fracture of fourth metatarsal bone, **left** foot `CC` `H5` `PE`

√7ᵗʰ **S92.346** **Nondisplaced** fracture of fourth metatarsal bone, unspecified foot `CC` `H5` `UNS` `PE`

√6ᵗʰ **S92.35** Fracture of **fifth** metatarsal bone

√7ᵗʰ **S92.351** **Displaced** fracture of fifth metatarsal bone, **right** foot `CC` `H5` `PE`

√7ᵗʰ **S92.352** **Displaced** fracture of fifth metatarsal bone, **left** foot `CC` `H5` `PE`

√7ᵗʰ **S92.353** **Displaced** fracture of fifth metatarsal bone, unspecified foot `CC` `H5` `UNS` `PE`

√7ᵗʰ **S92.354** **Nondisplaced** fracture of fifth metatarsal bone, **right** foot `CC` `H5` `PE`

√7ᵗʰ **S92.355** **Nondisplaced** fracture of fifth metatarsal bone, **left** foot `CC` `H5` `PE`

√7ᵗʰ **S92.356** **Nondisplaced** fracture of fifth metatarsal bone, unspecified foot `CC` `H5` `UNS` `PE`

√5ᵗʰ **S92.4** Fracture of **great toe**

> **EXCLUDES 2** physeal fracture of phalanx of toe (S99.2-)

√6ᵗʰ **S92.40** Unspecified fracture of great toe

√7ᵗʰ **S92.401** **Displaced** unspecified fracture of **right** great toe `CC` `PE`

√7ᵗʰ **S92.402** **Displaced** unspecified fracture of **left** great toe `CC` `PE`

√7ᵗʰ **S92.403** **Displaced** unspecified fracture of unspecified great toe `CC` `UNS` `PE`

√7ᵗʰ **S92.404** **Nondisplaced** unspecified fracture of **right** great toe `CC` `PE`

√7ᵗʰ **S92.405** **Nondisplaced** unspecified fracture of **left** great toe `CC` `PE`

√7ᵗʰ **S92.406** **Nondisplaced** unspecified fracture of unspecified great toe `CC` `UNS` `PE`

√6ᵗʰ **S92.41** Fracture of **proximal phalanx** of great toe

√7ᵗʰ **S92.411** **Displaced** fracture of proximal phalanx of **right** great toe `CC` `PE`

√7ᵗʰ **S92.412** **Displaced** fracture of proximal phalanx of **left** great toe `CC` `PE`

√7ᵗʰ **S92.413** **Displaced** fracture of proximal phalanx of unspecified great toe `CC` `UNS` `PE`

√7ᵗʰ **S92.414** **Nondisplaced** fracture of proximal phalanx of **right** great toe `CC` `PE`

√7ᵗʰ **S92.415** **Nondisplaced** fracture of proximal phalanx of **left** great toe `CC` `PE`

√7ᵗʰ **S92.416** **Nondisplaced** fracture of proximal phalanx of unspecified great toe `CC` `UNS` `PE`

√6ᵗʰ **S92.42** Fracture of **distal phalanx** of great toe

√7ᵗʰ **S92.421** **Displaced** fracture of distal phalanx of **right** great toe `CC` `PE`

√7ᵗʰ **S92.422** **Displaced** fracture of distal phalanx of **left** great toe `CC` `PE`

√7ᵗʰ **S92.423** **Displaced** fracture of distal phalanx of unspecified great toe `CC` `UNS` `PE`

√7ᵗʰ **S92.424** **Nondisplaced** fracture of distal phalanx of **right** great toe `CC` `PE`

√7ᵗʰ **S92.425** **Nondisplaced** fracture of distal phalanx of **left** great toe `CC` `PE`

√7ᵗʰ **S92.426** **Nondisplaced** fracture of distal phalanx of unspecified great toe `CC` `UNS` `PE`

√6ᵗʰ **S92.49** Other fracture of great toe

√7ᵗʰ **S92.491** Other fracture of **right** great toe `CC` `PE`

√7ᵗʰ **S92.492** Other fracture of **left** great toe `CC` `PE`

√7ᵗʰ **S92.499** Other fracture of unspecified great toe `CC` `UNS` `PE`

√5ᵗʰ **S92.5** Fracture of **lesser** toe(s)

> **EXCLUDES 2** physeal fracture of phalanx of toe (S99.2-)

√6ᵗʰ **S92.50** Unspecified fracture of lesser toe(s)

√7ᵗʰ **S92.501** **Displaced** unspecified fracture of **right** lesser toe(s) `CC` `PE`

√7ᵗʰ **S92.502** **Displaced** unspecified fracture of **left** lesser toe(s) `CC` `PE`

√7ᵗʰ **S92.503** **Displaced** unspecified fracture of unspecified lesser toe(s) `CC` `UNS` `PE`

√7ᵗʰ **S92.504** **Nondisplaced** unspecified fracture of **right** lesser toe(s) `CC` `PE`

√7ᵗʰ **S92.505** **Nondisplaced** unspecified fracture of **left** lesser toe(s) `CC` `PE`

√7ᵗʰ **S92.506** **Nondisplaced** unspecified fracture of unspecified lesser toe(s) `CC` `UNS` `PE`

√6ᵗʰ **S92.51** Fracture of **proximal phalanx** of lesser toe(s)

√7ᵗʰ **S92.511** **Displaced** fracture of proximal phalanx of **right** lesser toe(s) `CC` `PE`

√7ᵗʰ **S92.512** **Displaced** fracture of proximal phalanx of **left** lesser toe(s) `CC` `PE`

√7ᵗʰ **S92.513** **Displaced** fracture of proximal phalanx of unspecified lesser toe(s) `CC` `UNS` `PE`

√7ᵗʰ **S92.514** **Nondisplaced** fracture of proximal phalanx of **right** lesser toe(s) `CC` `PE`

√7ᵗʰ **S92.515** **Nondisplaced** fracture of proximal phalanx of **left** lesser toe(s) `CC` `PE`

√7ᵗʰ **S92.516** **Nondisplaced** fracture of proximal phalanx of unspecified lesser toe(s) `CC` `UNS` `PE`

√6ᵗʰ **S92.52** Fracture of **middle phalanx** of lesser toe(s)

√7ᵗʰ **S92.521** **Displaced** fracture of middle phalanx of **right** lesser toe(s) `CC` `PE`

√7ᵗʰ **S92.522** **Displaced** fracture of middle phalanx of **left** lesser toe(s) `CC` `PE`

√7ᵗʰ **S92.523** **Displaced** fracture of middle phalanx of unspecified lesser toe(s) `CC` `UNS` `PE`

√7ᵗʰ **S92.524** **Nondisplaced** fracture of middle phalanx of **right** lesser toe(s) `CC` `PE`

√7ᵗʰ **S92.525** **Nondisplaced** fracture of middle phalanx of **left** lesser toe(s) `CC` `PE`

√7ᵗʰ **S92.526** **Nondisplaced** fracture of middle phalanx of unspecified lesser toe(s) `CC` `UNS` `PE`

√6ᵗʰ **S92.53** Fracture of **distal phalanx** of lesser toe(s)

√7ᵗʰ **S92.531** **Displaced** fracture of distal phalanx of **right** lesser toe(s) `CC` `PE`

√7ᵗʰ **S92.532** **Displaced** fracture of distal phalanx of **left** lesser toe(s) `CC` `PE`

√7ᵗʰ **S92.533** **Displaced** fracture of distal phalanx of unspecified lesser toe(s) `CC` `UNS` `PE`

√7ᵗʰ **S92.534** **Nondisplaced** fracture of distal phalanx of **right** lesser toe(s) `CC` `PE`

√7ᵗʰ **S92.535** **Nondisplaced** fracture of distal phalanx of **left** lesser toe(s) `CC` `PE`

√7ᵗʰ **S92.536** **Nondisplaced** fracture of distal phalanx of unspecified lesser toe(s) `CC` `UNS` `PE`

√6ᵗʰ **S92.59** Other fracture of lesser toe(s)

√7ᵗʰ **S92.591** Other fracture of **right** lesser toe(s) `CC` `PE`

√7ᵗʰ **S92.592** Other fracture of **left** lesser toe(s) `CC` `PE`

√7ᵗʰ **S92.599** Other fracture of unspecified lesser toe(s) `CC` `UNS` `PE`

√5ᵗʰ **S92.8** Other fracture of foot, except ankle

√6ᵗʰ **S92.81** Other fracture of foot

> Sesamoid fracture of foot
> **AHA:** 2016,4Q,68

√7ᵗʰ **S92.811** Other fracture of **right** foot `CC` `H5` `PE`

√7ᵗʰ **S92.812** Other fracture of **left** foot `CC` `H5` `PE`

√7ᵗʰ **S92.819** Other fracture of unspecified foot `CC` `H5` `UNS` `PE`

✓5ᵗʰ S92.9 Unspecified fracture of foot and toe

  ✓6ᵗʰ S92.90 Unspecified fracture of foot

    ✓7ᵗʰ S92.901 Unspecified fracture of right foot `CC` `H5` `PE`

    ✓7ᵗʰ S92.902 Unspecified fracture of left foot `CC` `H5` `PE`

    ✓7ᵗʰ S92.909 Unspecified fracture of unspecified foot `CC` `H5` `UNS` `PE`

  ✓6ᵗʰ S92.91 Unspecified fracture of toe

    ✓7ᵗʰ S92.911 Unspecified fracture of right toe(s) `CC` `PE`

    ✓7ᵗʰ S92.912 Unspecified fracture of left toe(s) `CC` `PE`

    ✓7ᵗʰ S92.919 Unspecified fracture of unspecified toe(s) `CC` `UNS` `PE`

✓4ᵗʰ S93 Dislocation and sprain of joints and ligaments at ankle, foot and toe level

  INCLUDES avulsion of joint or ligament of ankle, foot and toe

        laceration of cartilage, joint or ligament of ankle, foot and toe

        sprain of cartilage, joint or ligament of ankle, foot and toe

        traumatic hemarthrosis of joint or ligament of ankle, foot and toe

        traumatic rupture of joint or ligament of ankle, foot and toe

        traumatic subluxation of joint or ligament of ankle, foot and toe

        traumatic tear of joint or ligament of ankle, foot and toe

  Code also any associated open wound

  EXCLUDES 2 *strain of muscle and tendon of ankle and foot (S96.-)*

  The appropriate 7th character is to be added to each code from category S93.

  A initial encounter

  D subsequent encounter

  S sequela

  ✓5ᵗʰ S93.0 Subluxation and dislocation of ankle joint

    Subluxation and dislocation of astragalus

    Subluxation and dislocation of fibula, lower end

    Subluxation and dislocation of talus

    Subluxation and dislocation of tibia, lower end

    ✓x7ᵗʰ S93.01 Subluxation of right ankle joint `PE`

    ✓x7ᵗʰ S93.02 Subluxation of left ankle joint `PE`

    ✓x7ᵗʰ S93.03 Subluxation of unspecified ankle joint `PE`

    ✓x7ᵗʰ S93.04 Dislocation of right ankle joint `PE`

    ✓x7ᵗʰ S93.05 Dislocation of left ankle joint `PE`

    ✓x7ᵗʰ S93.06 Dislocation of unspecified ankle joint `PE`

  ✓5ᵗʰ S93.1 Subluxation and dislocation of toe

    ✓6ᵗʰ S93.10 Unspecified subluxation and dislocation of toe

      Dislocation of toe NOS

      Subluxation of toe NOS

      ✓7ᵗʰ S93.101 Unspecified subluxation of right toe(s) `PE`

      ✓7ᵗʰ S93.102 Unspecified subluxation of left toe(s) `PE`

      ✓7ᵗʰ S93.103 Unspecified subluxation of unspecified toe(s) `PE`

      ✓7ᵗʰ S93.104 Unspecified dislocation of right toe(s) `PE`

      ✓7ᵗʰ S93.105 Unspecified dislocation of left toe(s) `PE`

      ✓7ᵗʰ S93.106 Unspecified dislocation of unspecified toe(s) `PE`

    ✓6ᵗʰ S93.11 Dislocation of interphalangeal joint

      ✓7ᵗʰ S93.111 Dislocation of interphalangeal joint of right great toe `PE`

      ✓7ᵗʰ S93.112 Dislocation of interphalangeal joint of left great toe `PE`

      ✓7ᵗʰ S93.113 Dislocation of interphalangeal joint of unspecified great toe `PE`

      ✓7ᵗʰ S93.114 Dislocation of interphalangeal joint of right lesser toe(s) `PE`

      ✓7ᵗʰ S93.115 Dislocation of interphalangeal joint of left lesser toe(s) `PE`

      ✓7ᵗʰ S93.116 Dislocation of interphalangeal joint of unspecified lesser toe(s) `PE`

      ✓7ᵗʰ S93.119 Dislocation of interphalangeal joint of unspecified toe(s) `PE`

✓6ᵗʰ S93.12 Dislocation of metatarsophalangeal joint

  ✓7ᵗʰ S93.121 Dislocation of metatarsophalangeal joint of right great toe `PE`

  ✓7ᵗʰ S93.122 Dislocation of metatarsophalangeal joint of left great toe `PE`

  ✓7ᵗʰ S93.123 Dislocation of metatarsophalangeal joint of unspecified great toe `PE`

  ✓7ᵗʰ S93.124 Dislocation of metatarsophalangeal joint of right lesser toe(s) `PE`

  ✓7ᵗʰ S93.125 Dislocation of metatarsophalangeal joint of left lesser toe(s) `PE`

  ✓7ᵗʰ S93.126 Dislocation of metatarsophalangeal joint of unspecified lesser toe(s) `PE`

  ✓7ᵗʰ S93.129 Dislocation of metatarsophalangeal joint of unspecified toe(s) `PE`

✓6ᵗʰ S93.13 Subluxation of interphalangeal joint

  ✓7ᵗʰ S93.131 Subluxation of interphalangeal joint of right great toe `PE`

  ✓7ᵗʰ S93.132 Subluxation of interphalangeal joint of left great toe `PE`

  ✓7ᵗʰ S93.133 Subluxation of interphalangeal joint of unspecified great toe `PE`

  ✓7ᵗʰ S93.134 Subluxation of interphalangeal joint of right lesser toe(s) `PE`

  ✓7ᵗʰ S93.135 Subluxation of interphalangeal joint of left lesser toe(s) `PE`

  ✓7ᵗʰ S93.136 Subluxation of interphalangeal joint of unspecified lesser toe(s) `PE`

  ✓7ᵗʰ S93.139 Subluxation of interphalangeal joint of unspecified toe(s) `PE`

✓6ᵗʰ S93.14 Subluxation of metatarsophalangeal joint

  ✓7ᵗʰ S93.141 Subluxation of metatarsophalangeal joint of right great toe `PE`

  ✓7ᵗʰ S93.142 Subluxation of metatarsophalangeal joint of left great toe `PE`

  ✓7ᵗʰ S93.143 Subluxation of metatarsophalangeal joint of unspecified great toe `PE`

  ✓7ᵗʰ S93.144 Subluxation of metatarsophalangeal joint of right lesser toe(s) `PE`

  ✓7ᵗʰ S93.145 Subluxation of metatarsophalangeal joint of left lesser toe(s) `PE`

  ✓7ᵗʰ S93.146 Subluxation of metatarsophalangeal joint of unspecified lesser toe(s) `PE`

  ✓7ᵗʰ S93.149 Subluxation of metatarsophalangeal joint of unspecified toe(s) `PE`

✓5ᵗʰ S93.3 Subluxation and dislocation of foot

  EXCLUDES 2 *dislocation of toe (S93.1-)*

  ✓6ᵗʰ S93.30 Unspecified subluxation and dislocation of foot

    Dislocation of foot NOS

    Subluxation of foot NOS

    ✓7ᵗʰ S93.301 Unspecified subluxation of right foot `PE`

    ✓7ᵗʰ S93.302 Unspecified subluxation of left foot `PE`

    ✓7ᵗʰ S93.303 Unspecified subluxation of unspecified foot `PE`

    ✓7ᵗʰ S93.304 Unspecified dislocation of right foot `PE`

    ✓7ᵗʰ S93.305 Unspecified dislocation of left foot `PE`

    ✓7ᵗʰ S93.306 Unspecified dislocation of unspecified foot `PE`

  ✓6ᵗʰ S93.31 Subluxation and dislocation of tarsal joint

    ✓7ᵗʰ S93.311 Subluxation of tarsal joint of right foot `PE`

    ✓7ᵗʰ S93.312 Subluxation of tarsal joint of left foot `PE`

    ✓7ᵗʰ S93.313 Subluxation of tarsal joint of unspecified foot `PE`

    ✓7ᵗʰ S93.314 Dislocation of tarsal joint of right foot `PE`

    ✓7ᵗʰ S93.315 Dislocation of tarsal joint of left foot `PE`

    ✓7ᵗʰ S93.316 Dislocation of tarsal joint of unspecified foot `PE`

  ✓6ᵗʰ S93.32 Subluxation and dislocation of tarsometatarsal joint

    ✓7ᵗʰ S93.321 Subluxation of tarsometatarsal joint of right foot `PE`

    ✓7ᵗʰ S93.322 Subluxation of tarsometatarsal joint of left foot `PE`

✔ Additional Character Required   ✓x7ᵗʰ Placeholder   Questionable PDx   Manifestation   Unspecified   UPD Unacceptable PDx   H1-H14 HAC   HCC CMS-HCC Dx   HIV HIV Dx

ICD-10-CM 2025

1107

√7ᵗʰ **S93.323** **Subluxation** of tarsometatarsal joint of unspecified foot **PE**

√7ᵗʰ **S93.324** **Dislocation** of tarsometatarsal joint of **right** foot **PE**

√7ᵗʰ **S93.325** **Dislocation** of tarsometatarsal joint of **left** foot **PE**

√7ᵗʰ **S93.326** **Dislocation** of tarsometatarsal joint of unspecified foot **PE**

√6ᵗʰ **S93.33** Other subluxation and dislocation of foot

√7ᵗʰ **S93.331** Other **subluxation** of **right** foot **PE**

√7ᵗʰ **S93.332** Other **subluxation** of **left** foot **PE**

√7ᵗʰ **S93.333** Other **subluxation** of unspecified foot **PE**

√7ᵗʰ **S93.334** Other **dislocation** of **right** foot **PE**

√7ᵗʰ **S93.335** Other **dislocation** of **left** foot **PE**

√7ᵗʰ **S93.336** Other **dislocation** of unspecified foot **PE**

√5ᵗʰ **S93.4** Sprain of **ankle**

EXCLUDES 2   injury of Achilles tendon (S86.0-)

√6ᵗʰ **S93.40** Sprain of unspecified ligament of ankle

Sprain of ankle NOS
Sprained ankle NOS

√7ᵗʰ **S93.401** Sprain of unspecified ligament of **right** ankle **PE**

√7ᵗʰ **S93.402** Sprain of unspecified ligament of **left** ankle **PE**

√7ᵗʰ **S93.409** Sprain of unspecified ligament of unspecified ankle **PE**

√6ᵗʰ **S93.41** Sprain of **calcaneofibular** ligament

√7ᵗʰ **S93.411** Sprain of calcaneofibular ligament of **right** ankle **PE**

√7ᵗʰ **S93.412** Sprain of calcaneofibular ligament of **left** ankle **PE**

√7ᵗʰ **S93.419** Sprain of calcaneofibular ligament of unspecified ankle **PE**

√6ᵗʰ **S93.42** Sprain of **deltoid** ligament

√7ᵗʰ **S93.421** Sprain of deltoid ligament of **right** ankle **PE**

√7ᵗʰ **S93.422** Sprain of deltoid ligament of **left** ankle **PE**

√7ᵗʰ **S93.429** Sprain of deltoid ligament of unspecified ankle **PE**

√6ᵗʰ **S93.43** Sprain of **tibiofibular** ligament

√7ᵗʰ **S93.431** Sprain of tibiofibular ligament of **right** ankle **PE**

√7ᵗʰ **S93.432** Sprain of tibiofibular ligament of **left** ankle **PE**

√7ᵗʰ **S93.439** Sprain of tibiofibular ligament of unspecified ankle **PE**

√6ᵗʰ **S93.49** Sprain of other ligament of ankle

Sprain of internal collateral ligament
Sprain of talofibular ligament

√7ᵗʰ **S93.491** Sprain of other ligament of **right** ankle **PE**

√7ᵗʰ **S93.492** Sprain of other ligament of **left** ankle **PE**

√7ᵗʰ **S93.499** Sprain of other ligament of unspecified ankle **PE**

√5ᵗʰ **S93.5** Sprain of **toe**

√6ᵗʰ **S93.50** Unspecified sprain of toe

√7ᵗʰ **S93.501** Unspecified sprain of **right great** toe **PE**

√7ᵗʰ **S93.502** Unspecified sprain of **left great** toe **PE**

√7ᵗʰ **S93.503** Unspecified sprain of unspecified great toe **PE**

√7ᵗʰ **S93.504** Unspecified sprain of **right lesser** toe(s) **PE**

√7ᵗʰ **S93.505** Unspecified sprain of **left lesser** toe(s) **PE**

√7ᵗʰ **S93.506** Unspecified sprain of unspecified lesser toe(s) **PE**

√7ᵗʰ **S93.509** Unspecified sprain of unspecified toe(s) **PE**

√6ᵗʰ **S93.51** Sprain of **interphalangeal joint** of toe

√7ᵗʰ **S93.511** Sprain of interphalangeal joint of **right great** toe **PE**

√7ᵗʰ **S93.512** Sprain of interphalangeal joint of **left great** toe **PE**

√7ᵗʰ **S93.513** Sprain of interphalangeal joint of unspecified great toe **PE**

√7ᵗʰ **S93.514** Sprain of interphalangeal joint of **right lesser** toe(s) **PE**

√7ᵗʰ **S93.515** Sprain of interphalangeal joint of **left lesser** toe(s) **PE**

√7ᵗʰ **S93.516** Sprain of interphalangeal joint of unspecified lesser toe(s) **PE**

√7ᵗʰ **S93.519** Sprain of interphalangeal joint of unspecified toe(s) **PE**

√6ᵗʰ **S93.52** Sprain of **metatarsophalangeal joint** of toe

√7ᵗʰ **S93.521** Sprain of metatarsophalangeal joint of **right great** toe **PE**

√7ᵗʰ **S93.522** Sprain of metatarsophalangeal joint of **left great** toe **PE**

√7ᵗʰ **S93.523** Sprain of metatarsophalangeal joint of unspecified great toe **PE**

√7ᵗʰ **S93.524** Sprain of metatarsophalangeal joint of **right lesser** toe(s) **PE**

√7ᵗʰ **S93.525** Sprain of metatarsophalangeal joint of **left lesser** toe(s) **PE**

√7ᵗʰ **S93.526** Sprain of metatarsophalangeal joint of unspecified lesser toe(s) **PE**

√7ᵗʰ **S93.529** Sprain of metatarsophalangeal joint of unspecified toe(s) **PE**

√5ᵗʰ **S93.6** Sprain of **foot**

EXCLUDES 2   sprain of metatarsophalangeal joint of toe (S93.52-)
sprain of toe (S93.5-)

√6ᵗʰ **S93.60** Unspecified sprain of foot

√7ᵗʰ **S93.601** Unspecified sprain of **right** foot **PE**

√7ᵗʰ **S93.602** Unspecified sprain of **left** foot **PE**

√7ᵗʰ **S93.609** Unspecified sprain of unspecified foot **PE**

√6ᵗʰ **S93.61** Sprain of **tarsal ligament** of foot

√7ᵗʰ **S93.611** Sprain of tarsal ligament of **right** foot **PE**

√7ᵗʰ **S93.612** Sprain of tarsal ligament of **left** foot **PE**

√7ᵗʰ **S93.619** Sprain of tarsal ligament of unspecified foot **PE**

√6ᵗʰ **S93.62** Sprain of **tarsometatarsal ligament** of foot

√7ᵗʰ **S93.621** Sprain of tarsometatarsal ligament of **right** foot **PE**

√7ᵗʰ **S93.622** Sprain of tarsometatarsal ligament of **left** foot **PE**

√7ᵗʰ **S93.629** Sprain of tarsometatarsal ligament of unspecified foot **PE**

√6ᵗʰ **S93.69** Other sprain of foot

√7ᵗʰ **S93.691** Other sprain of **right** foot **PE**

√7ᵗʰ **S93.692** Other sprain of **left** foot **PE**

√7ᵗʰ **S93.699** Other sprain of unspecified foot **PE**

√4ᵗʰ **S94** **Injury of nerves at ankle and foot level**

Code also any associated open wound (S91.-)

The appropriate 7th character is to be added to each code from category S94.
A   initial encounter
D   subsequent encounter
S   sequela

√5ᵗʰ **S94.0** Injury of **lateral plantar** nerve

√x7ᵗʰ **S94.00** Injury of lateral plantar nerve, unspecified leg **PE**

√x7ᵗʰ **S94.01** Injury of lateral plantar nerve, **right** leg **PE**

√x7ᵗʰ **S94.02** Injury of lateral plantar nerve, **left** leg **PE**

√5ᵗʰ **S94.1** Injury of **medial plantar** nerve

√x7ᵗʰ **S94.10** Injury of medial plantar nerve, unspecified leg **PE**

√x7ᵗʰ **S94.11** Injury of medial plantar nerve, **right** leg **PE**

√x7ᵗʰ **S94.12** Injury of medial plantar nerve, **left** leg **PE**

√5ᵗʰ **S94.2** Injury of **deep peroneal** nerve at ankle and foot level

Injury of terminal, lateral branch of deep peroneal nerve

√x7ᵗʰ **S94.20** Injury of deep peroneal nerve at ankle and foot level, unspecified leg **PE**

√x7ᵗʰ **S94.21** Injury of deep peroneal nerve at ankle and foot level, **right** leg **PE**

N Newborn: 0   **P** Pediatric: 0-17   **M** Maternity: 9-64   **A** Adult: 15-124   **UNS** Unspecified Site   **MCC** Major Complication/Comorbidity   **CC** Complication/Comorbidity   **PE** POA Exempt

1108   ICD-10-CM 2025

✓×7th **S94.22** Injury of deep peroneal nerve at ankle and foot level, **left** leg   PE

✓5th **S94.3** Injury of cutaneous sensory nerve at ankle and foot level

  ✓×7th **S94.30** Injury of cutaneous sensory nerve at ankle and foot level, unspecified leg   PE

  ✓×7th **S94.31** Injury of cutaneous sensory nerve at ankle and foot level, **right** leg   PE

  ✓×7th **S94.32** Injury of cutaneous sensory nerve at ankle and foot level, **left** leg   PE

✓5th **S94.8** Injury of other nerves at ankle and foot level

  ✓6th **S94.8X** Injury of other nerves at ankle and foot level

    ✓7th **S94.8X1** Injury of other nerves at ankle and foot level, **right** leg   PE

    ✓7th **S94.8X2** Injury of other nerves at ankle and foot level, **left** leg   PE

    ✓7th **S94.8X9** Injury of other nerves at ankle and foot level, unspecified leg   PE

✓5th **S94.9** Injury of unspecified nerve at ankle and foot level

  ✓×7th **S94.90** Injury of unspecified nerve at ankle and foot level, unspecified leg   PE

  ✓×7th **S94.91** Injury of unspecified nerve at ankle and foot level, **right** leg   PE

  ✓×7th **S94.92** Injury of unspecified nerve at ankle and foot level, **left** leg   PE

✓4th **S95 Injury of blood vessels at ankle and foot level**

Code also any associated open wound (S91.-)

EXCLUDES 2   injury of posterior tibial artery and vein (S85.1-, S85.8-)

The appropriate 7th character is to be added to each code from category S95.
A   initial encounter
D   subsequent encounter
S   sequela

✓5th **S95.0** Injury of dorsal artery of foot

  ✓6th **S95.00** Unspecified injury of dorsal artery of foot

    ✓7th **S95.001** Unspecified injury of dorsal artery of **right** foot   CC PE

    ✓7th **S95.002** Unspecified injury of dorsal artery of **left** foot   CC PE

    ✓7th **S95.009** Unspecified injury of dorsal artery of unspecified foot   CC UNS PE

  ✓6th **S95.01** Laceration of dorsal artery of foot

    ✓7th **S95.011** Laceration of dorsal artery of **right** foot   CC PE

    ✓7th **S95.012** Laceration of dorsal artery of **left** foot   CC PE

    ✓7th **S95.019** Laceration of dorsal artery of unspecified foot   CC UNS PE

  ✓6th **S95.09** Other specified injury of dorsal artery of foot

    ✓7th **S95.091** Other specified injury of dorsal artery of **right** foot   CC PE

    ✓7th **S95.092** Other specified injury of dorsal artery of **left** foot   CC PE

    ✓7th **S95.099** Other specified injury of dorsal artery of unspecified foot   CC UNS PE

✓5th **S95.1** Injury of plantar artery of foot

  ✓6th **S95.10** Unspecified injury of plantar artery of foot

    ✓7th **S95.101** Unspecified injury of plantar artery of **right** foot   CC PE

    ✓7th **S95.102** Unspecified injury of plantar artery of **left** foot   CC PE

    ✓7th **S95.109** Unspecified injury of plantar artery of unspecified foot   CC UNS PE

  ✓6th **S95.11** Laceration of plantar artery of foot

    ✓7th **S95.111** Laceration of plantar artery of **right** foot   CC PE

    ✓7th **S95.112** Laceration of plantar artery of **left** foot   CC PE

    ✓7th **S95.119** Laceration of plantar artery of unspecified foot   CC UNS PE

  ✓6th **S95.19** Other specified injury of plantar artery of foot

    ✓7th **S95.191** Other specified injury of plantar artery of **right** foot   CC PE

    ✓7th **S95.192** Other specified injury of plantar artery of **left** foot   CC PE

    ✓7th **S95.199** Other specified injury of plantar artery of unspecified foot   CC UNS PE

✓5th **S95.2** Injury of dorsal vein of foot

  ✓6th **S95.20** Unspecified injury of dorsal vein of foot

    ✓7th **S95.201** Unspecified injury of dorsal vein of **right** foot   CC PE

    ✓7th **S95.202** Unspecified injury of dorsal vein of **left** foot   CC PE

    ✓7th **S95.209** Unspecified injury of dorsal vein of unspecified foot   CC UNS PE

  ✓6th **S95.21** Laceration of dorsal vein of foot

    ✓7th **S95.211** Laceration of dorsal vein of **right** foot   CC PE

    ✓7th **S95.212** Laceration of dorsal vein of **left** foot   CC PE

    ✓7th **S95.219** Laceration of dorsal vein of unspecified foot   CC UNS PE

  ✓6th **S95.29** Other specified injury of dorsal vein of foot

    ✓7th **S95.291** Other specified injury of dorsal vein of **right** foot   CC PE

    ✓7th **S95.292** Other specified injury of dorsal vein of **left** foot   CC PE

    ✓7th **S95.299** Other specified injury of dorsal vein of unspecified foot   CC UNS PE

✓5th **S95.8** Injury of other blood vessels at ankle and foot level

  ✓6th **S95.80** Unspecified injury of other blood vessels at ankle and foot level

    ✓7th **S95.801** Unspecified injury of other blood vessels at ankle and foot level, **right** leg   CC PE

    ✓7th **S95.802** Unspecified injury of other blood vessels at ankle and foot level, **left** leg   CC PE

    ✓7th **S95.809** Unspecified injury of other blood vessels at ankle and foot level, unspecified leg   CC UNS PE

  ✓6th **S95.81** Laceration of other blood vessels at ankle and foot level

    ✓7th **S95.811** Laceration of other blood vessels at ankle and foot level, **right** leg   CC PE

    ✓7th **S95.812** Laceration of other blood vessels at ankle and foot level, **left** leg   CC PE

    ✓7th **S95.819** Laceration of other blood vessels at ankle and foot level, unspecified leg   CC UNS PE

  ✓6th **S95.89** Other specified injury of other blood vessels at ankle and foot level

    ✓7th **S95.891** Other specified injury of other blood vessels at ankle and foot level, **right** leg   CC PE

    ✓7th **S95.892** Other specified injury of other blood vessels at ankle and foot level, **left** leg   CC PE

    ✓7th **S95.899** Other specified injury of other blood vessels at ankle and foot level, unspecified leg   CC UNS PE

✓5th **S95.9** Injury of unspecified blood vessel at ankle and foot level

  ✓6th **S95.90** Unspecified injury of unspecified blood vessel at ankle and foot level

    ✓7th **S95.901** Unspecified injury of unspecified blood vessel at ankle and foot level, **right** leg   CC PE

    ✓7th **S95.902** Unspecified injury of unspecified blood vessel at ankle and foot level, **left** leg   CC PE

    ✓7th **S95.909** Unspecified injury of unspecified blood vessel at ankle and foot level, unspecified leg   CC UNS PE

  ✓6th **S95.91** Laceration of unspecified blood vessel at ankle and foot level

    ✓7th **S95.911** Laceration of unspecified blood vessel at ankle and foot level, **right** leg   CC PE

    ✓7th **S95.912** Laceration of unspecified blood vessel at ankle and foot level, **left** leg   CC PE

    ✓7th **S95.919** Laceration of unspecified blood vessel at ankle and foot level, unspecified leg   CC UNS PE

  ✓6th **S95.99** Other specified injury of unspecified blood vessel at ankle and foot level

    ✓7th **S95.991** Other specified injury of unspecified blood vessel at ankle and foot level, **right** leg   CC PE

✓ Additional Character Required   ✓×7th Placeholder   Questionable PDx   Manifestation   Unspecified   UPD Unacceptable PDx   H1-H14 HAC   HCC CMS-HCC Dx   HIV HIV Dx

ICD-10-CM 2025   1109

√7th **S95.992** Other specified injury of unspecified blood vessel at ankle and foot level, **left** leg `CC` `PE`

√7th **S95.999** Other specified injury of unspecified blood vessel at ankle and foot level, unspecified leg `CC` `UNS` `PE`

√4th **S96** **Injury of muscle and tendon at ankle and foot level**

Code also any associated open wound (S91.-)

EXCLUDES 2   injury of Achilles tendon (S86.Ø-)

sprain of joints and ligaments of ankle and foot (S93.-)

TIP: Refer to the Muscle/Tendon table at the beginning of this chapter.

The appropriate 7th character is to be added to each code from category S96.

A   initial encounter
D   subsequent encounter
S   sequela

√5th **S96.Ø** Injury of muscle and tendon of **long flexor muscle of toe** at ankle and foot level

√6th **S96.ØØ** Unspecified injury of muscle and tendon of long flexor muscle of toe at ankle and foot level

√7th **S96.ØØ1** Unspecified injury of muscle and tendon of long flexor muscle of toe at ankle and foot level, **right** foot `PE`

√7th **S96.ØØ2** Unspecified injury of muscle and tendon of long flexor muscle of toe at ankle and foot level, **left** foot `PE`

√7th **S96.ØØ9** Unspecified injury of muscle and tendon of long flexor muscle of toe at ankle and foot level, unspecified foot `PE`

√6th **S96.Ø1** **Strain** of muscle and tendon of long flexor muscle of toe at ankle and foot level

√7th **S96.Ø11** Strain of muscle and tendon of long flexor muscle of toe at ankle and foot level, **right** foot `PE`

√7th **S96.Ø12** Strain of muscle and tendon of long flexor muscle of toe at ankle and foot level, **left** foot `PE`

√7th **S96.Ø19** Strain of muscle and tendon of long flexor muscle of toe at ankle and foot level, unspecified foot `PE`

√6th **S96.Ø2** **Laceration** of muscle and tendon of long flexor muscle of toe at ankle and foot level

√7th **S96.Ø21** Laceration of muscle and tendon of long flexor muscle of toe at ankle and foot level, **right** foot `CC` `PE`

√7th **S96.Ø22** Laceration of muscle and tendon of long flexor muscle of toe at ankle and foot level, **left** foot `CC` `PE`

√7th **S96.Ø29** Laceration of muscle and tendon of long flexor muscle of toe at ankle and foot level, unspecified foot `CC` `UNS` `PE`

√6th **S96.Ø9** Other injury of muscle and tendon of long flexor muscle of toe at ankle and foot level

√7th **S96.Ø91** Other injury of muscle and tendon of long flexor muscle of toe at ankle and foot level, **right** foot `PE`

√7th **S96.Ø92** Other injury of muscle and tendon of long flexor muscle of toe at ankle and foot level, **left** foot `PE`

√7th **S96.Ø99** Other injury of muscle and tendon of long flexor muscle of toe at ankle and foot level, unspecified foot `PE`

√5th **S96.1** Injury of muscle and tendon of **long extensor muscle of toe** at ankle and foot level

√6th **S96.1Ø** Unspecified injury of muscle and tendon of long extensor muscle of toe at ankle and foot level

√7th **S96.1Ø1** Unspecified injury of muscle and tendon of long extensor muscle of toe at ankle and foot level, **right** foot `PE`

√7th **S96.1Ø2** Unspecified injury of muscle and tendon of long extensor muscle of toe at ankle and foot level, **left** foot `PE`

√7th **S96.1Ø9** Unspecified injury of muscle and tendon of long extensor muscle of toe at ankle and foot level, unspecified foot `PE`

√6th **S96.11** **Strain** of muscle and tendon of long extensor muscle of toe at ankle and foot level

√7th **S96.111** Strain of muscle and tendon of long extensor muscle of toe at ankle and foot level, **right** foot `PE`

√7th **S96.112** Strain of muscle and tendon of long extensor muscle of toe at ankle and foot level, **left** foot `PE`

√7th **S96.119** Strain of muscle and tendon of long extensor muscle of toe at ankle and foot level, unspecified foot `PE`

√6th **S96.12** **Laceration** of muscle and tendon of long extensor muscle of toe at ankle and foot level

√7th **S96.121** Laceration of muscle and tendon of long extensor muscle of toe at ankle and foot level, **right** foot `CC` `PE`

√7th **S96.122** Laceration of muscle and tendon of long extensor muscle of toe at ankle and foot level, **left** foot `CC` `PE`

√7th **S96.129** Laceration of muscle and tendon of long extensor muscle of toe at ankle and foot level, unspecified foot `CC` `UNS` `PE`

√6th **S96.19** Other specified injury of muscle and tendon of long extensor muscle of toe at ankle and foot level

√7th **S96.191** Other specified injury of muscle and tendon of long extensor muscle of toe at ankle and foot level, **right** foot

√7th **S96.192** Other specified injury of muscle and tendon of long extensor muscle of toe at ankle and foot level, **left** foot `PE`

√7th **S96.199** Other specified injury of muscle and tendon of long extensor muscle of toe at ankle and foot level, unspecified foot `PE`

√5th **S96.2** Injury of **intrinsic muscle and tendon** at ankle and foot level

√6th **S96.2Ø** Unspecified injury of intrinsic muscle and tendon at ankle and foot level

√7th **S96.2Ø1** Unspecified injury of intrinsic muscle and tendon at ankle and foot level, **right** foot `PE`

√7th **S96.2Ø2** Unspecified injury of intrinsic muscle and tendon at ankle and foot level, **left** foot `PE`

√7th **S96.2Ø9** Unspecified injury of intrinsic muscle and tendon at ankle and foot level, unspecified foot `PE`

√6th **S96.21** **Strain** of intrinsic muscle and tendon at ankle and foot level

√7th **S96.211** Strain of intrinsic muscle and tendon at ankle and foot level, **right** foot `PE`

√7th **S96.212** Strain of intrinsic muscle and tendon at ankle and foot level, **left** foot `PE`

√7th **S96.219** Strain of intrinsic muscle and tendon at ankle and foot level, unspecified foot `PE`

√6th **S96.22** **Laceration** of intrinsic muscle and tendon at ankle and foot level

√7th **S96.221** Laceration of intrinsic muscle and tendon at ankle and foot level, **right** foot `CC` `PE`

√7th **S96.222** Laceration of intrinsic muscle and tendon at ankle and foot level, **left** foot `CC` `PE`

√7th **S96.229** Laceration of intrinsic muscle and tendon at ankle and foot level, unspecified foot `CC` `UNS` `PE`

√6th **S96.29** Other specified injury of intrinsic muscle and tendon at ankle and foot level

√7th **S96.291** Other specified injury of intrinsic muscle and tendon at ankle and foot level, **right** foot `PE`

√7th **S96.292** Other specified injury of intrinsic muscle and tendon at ankle and foot level, **left** foot `PE`

√7th **S96.299** Other specified injury of intrinsic muscle and tendon at ankle and foot level, unspecified foot `PE`

√5th **S96.8** Injury of other specified muscles and tendons at ankle and foot level

√6th **S96.8Ø** Unspecified injury of other specified muscles and tendons at ankle and foot level

√7th **S96.8Ø1** Unspecified injury of other specified muscles and tendons at ankle and foot level, **right** foot `PE`

√7th **S96.8Ø2** Unspecified injury of other specified muscles and tendons at ankle and foot level, **left** foot `PE`

√7ᵗʰ **S96.809** Unspecified injury of other specified muscles and tendons at ankle and foot level, unspecified foot   PE

√6ᵗʰ **S96.81** **Strain** of other specified muscles and tendons at ankle and foot level

  √7ᵗʰ **S96.811** Strain of other specified muscles and tendons at ankle and foot level, **right** foot   PE

  √7ᵗʰ **S96.812** Strain of other specified muscles and tendons at ankle and foot level, **left** foot   PE

  √7ᵗʰ **S96.819** Strain of other specified muscles and tendons at ankle and foot level, unspecified foot   PE

√6ᵗʰ **S96.82** **Laceration** of other specified muscles and tendons at ankle and foot level

  √7ᵗʰ **S96.821** Laceration of other specified muscles and tendons at ankle and foot level, **right** foot   CC PE

  √7ᵗʰ **S96.822** Laceration of other specified muscles and tendons at ankle and foot level, **left** foot   CC PE

  √7ᵗʰ **S96.829** Laceration of other specified muscles and tendons at ankle and foot level, unspecified foot   CC UNS PE

√6ᵗʰ **S96.89** Other specified injury of other specified muscles and tendons at ankle and foot level

  √7ᵗʰ **S96.891** Other specified injury of other specified muscles and tendons at ankle and foot level, **right** foot   PE

  √7ᵗʰ **S96.892** Other specified injury of other specified muscles and tendons at ankle and foot level, **left** foot   PE

  √7ᵗʰ **S96.899** Other specified injury of other specified muscles and tendons at ankle and foot level, unspecified foot   PE

√5ᵗʰ **S96.9** Injury of unspecified muscle and tendon at ankle and foot level

√6ᵗʰ **S96.90** Unspecified injury of unspecified muscle and tendon at ankle and foot level

  √7ᵗʰ **S96.901** Unspecified injury of unspecified muscle and tendon at ankle and foot level, **right** foot   PE

  √7ᵗʰ **S96.902** Unspecified injury of unspecified muscle and tendon at ankle and foot level, **left** foot   PE

  √7ᵗʰ **S96.909** Unspecified injury of unspecified muscle and tendon at ankle and foot level, unspecified foot   PE

√6ᵗʰ **S96.91** **Strain** of unspecified muscle and tendon at ankle and foot level

  √7ᵗʰ **S96.911** Strain of unspecified muscle and tendon at ankle and foot level, **right** foot   PE

  √7ᵗʰ **S96.912** Strain of unspecified muscle and tendon at ankle and foot level, **left** foot   PE

  √7ᵗʰ **S96.919** Strain of unspecified muscle and tendon at ankle and foot level, unspecified foot   PE

√6ᵗʰ **S96.92** **Laceration** of unspecified muscle and tendon at ankle and foot level

  √7ᵗʰ **S96.921** Laceration of unspecified muscle and tendon at ankle and foot level, **right** foot   CC PE

  √7ᵗʰ **S96.922** Laceration of unspecified muscle and tendon at ankle and foot level, **left** foot   CC PE

  √7ᵗʰ **S96.929** Laceration of unspecified muscle and tendon at ankle and foot level, unspecified foot   CC UNS PE

√6ᵗʰ **S96.99** Other specified injury of unspecified muscle and tendon at ankle and foot level

  √7ᵗʰ **S96.991** Other specified injury of unspecified muscle and tendon at ankle and foot level, **right** foot   PE

  √7ᵗʰ **S96.992** Other specified injury of unspecified muscle and tendon at ankle and foot level, **left** foot   PE

  √7ᵗʰ **S96.999** Other specified injury of unspecified muscle and tendon at ankle and foot level, unspecified foot   PE

√4ᵗʰ **S97** **Crushing injury** of ankle and foot

Use additional code(s) for all associated injuries

The appropriate 7th character is to be added to each code from category S97.
A   initial encounter
D   subsequent encounter
S   sequela

√5ᵗʰ **S97.0** Crushing injury of **ankle**

  √x7ᵗʰ **S97.00** Crushing injury of unspecified ankle   PE

  √x7ᵗʰ **S97.01** Crushing injury of **right** ankle   PE

  √x7ᵗʰ **S97.02** Crushing injury of **left** ankle   PE

√5ᵗʰ **S97.1** Crushing injury of **toe**

√6ᵗʰ **S97.10** Crushing injury of unspecified toe(s)

  √7ᵗʰ **S97.101** Crushing injury of unspecified **right** toe(s)   PE

  √7ᵗʰ **S97.102** Crushing injury of unspecified **left** toe(s)   PE

  √7ᵗʰ **S97.109** Crushing injury of unspecified toe(s)   PE
     Crushing injury of toe NOS

√6ᵗʰ **S97.11** Crushing injury of **great toe**

  √7ᵗʰ **S97.111** Crushing injury of **right** great toe   PE

  √7ᵗʰ **S97.112** Crushing injury of **left** great toe   PE

  √7ᵗʰ **S97.119** Crushing injury of unspecified great toe   PE

√6ᵗʰ **S97.12** Crushing injury of **lesser toe**(s)

  √7ᵗʰ **S97.121** Crushing injury of **right** lesser toe(s)   PE

  √7ᵗʰ **S97.122** Crushing injury of **left** lesser toe(s)   PE

  √7ᵗʰ **S97.129** Crushing injury of unspecified lesser toe(s)   PE

√5ᵗʰ **S97.8** Crushing injury of **foot**

  √x7ᵗʰ **S97.80** Crushing injury of unspecified foot   PE
     Crushing injury of foot NOS

  √x7ᵗʰ **S97.81** Crushing injury of **right** foot   PE

  √x7ᵗʰ **S97.82** Crushing injury of **left** foot   PE

√4ᵗʰ **S98** **Traumatic amputation of ankle and foot**

An amputation not identified as partial or complete should be coded to complete

The appropriate 7th character is to be added to each code from category S98.
A   initial encounter
D   subsequent encounter
S   sequela

√5ᵗʰ **S98.0** Traumatic amputation of **foot at ankle level**

√6ᵗʰ **S98.01** **Complete** traumatic amputation of foot at ankle level

  √7ᵗʰ **S98.011** Complete traumatic amputation of **right** foot at ankle level   CC HCC PE

  √7ᵗʰ **S98.012** Complete traumatic amputation of **left** foot at ankle level   CC HCC PE

  √7ᵗʰ **S98.019** Complete traumatic amputation of unspecified foot at ankle level   CC UNS HCC PE

√6ᵗʰ **S98.02** **Partial** traumatic amputation of foot at ankle level

  √7ᵗʰ **S98.021** Partial traumatic amputation of **right** foot at ankle level   CC HCC PE

  √7ᵗʰ **S98.022** Partial traumatic amputation of **left** foot at ankle level   CC HCC PE

  √7ᵗʰ **S98.029** Partial traumatic amputation of unspecified foot at ankle level   CC UNS HCC PE

√5ᵗʰ **S98.1** Traumatic amputation of **one toe**

√6ᵗʰ **S98.11** **Complete** traumatic amputation of **great toe**

  √7ᵗʰ **S98.111** Complete traumatic amputation of **right** great toe   PE

  √7ᵗʰ **S98.112** Complete traumatic amputation of **left** great toe   PE

  √7ᵗʰ **S98.119** Complete traumatic amputation of unspecified great toe   PE

√6ᵗʰ **S98.12** **Partial** traumatic amputation of **great toe**

  √7ᵗʰ **S98.121** Partial traumatic amputation of **right** great toe   PE

  √7ᵗʰ **S98.122** Partial traumatic amputation of **left** great toe   PE

√7th **S98.129** Partial traumatic amputation of unspecified great toe PE

√6th **S98.13** **Complete** traumatic amputation of **one lesser toe**
Traumatic amputation of toe NOS

√7th **S98.131** Complete traumatic amputation of one **right** lesser toe PE

√7th **S98.132** Complete traumatic amputation of one **left** lesser toe PE

√7th **S98.139** Complete traumatic amputation of one unspecified lesser toe PE

√6th **S98.14** **Partial** traumatic amputation of **one lesser toe**

√7th **S98.141** Partial traumatic amputation of one **right** lesser toe PE

√7th **S98.142** Partial traumatic amputation of one **left** lesser toe PE

√7th **S98.149** Partial traumatic amputation of one unspecified lesser toe PE

√5th **S98.2** Traumatic amputation of **two or more lesser toes**

√6th **S98.21** **Complete** traumatic amputation of two or more lesser toes

√7th **S98.211** Complete traumatic amputation of two or more **right** lesser toes PE

√7th **S98.212** Complete traumatic amputation of two or more **left** lesser toes PE

√7th **S98.219** Complete traumatic amputation of two or more unspecified lesser toes PE

√6th **S98.22** **Partial** traumatic amputation of two or more lesser toes

√7th **S98.221** Partial traumatic amputation of two or more **right** lesser toes PE

√7th **S98.222** Partial traumatic amputation of two or more **left** lesser toes PE

√7th **S98.229** Partial traumatic amputation of two or more unspecified lesser toes PE

√5th **S98.3** Traumatic amputation of **midfoot**

√6th **S98.31** **Complete** traumatic amputation of midfoot

√7th **S98.311** Complete traumatic amputation of **right** midfoot CC HCC PE

√7th **S98.312** Complete traumatic amputation of **left** midfoot CC HCC PE

√7th **S98.319** Complete traumatic amputation of unspecified midfoot CC UNS HCC PE

√6th **S98.32** **Partial** traumatic amputation of midfoot

√7th **S98.321** Partial traumatic amputation of **right** midfoot CC HCC PE

√7th **S98.322** Partial traumatic amputation of **left** midfoot CC HCC PE

√7th **S98.329** Partial traumatic amputation of unspecified midfoot CC UNS HCC PE

√5th **S98.9** Traumatic amputation of foot, level unspecified

√6th **S98.91** **Complete** traumatic amputation of foot, level unspecified

√7th **S98.911** Complete traumatic amputation of **right** foot, level unspecified CC HCC PE

√7th **S98.912** Complete traumatic amputation of **left** foot, level unspecified CC HCC PE

√7th **S98.919** Complete traumatic amputation of unspecified foot, level unspecified CC UNS HCC PE

√6th **S98.92** **Partial** traumatic amputation of foot, level unspecified

√7th **S98.921** Partial traumatic amputation of **right** foot, level unspecified CC HCC PE

√7th **S98.922** Partial traumatic amputation of **left** foot, level unspecified CC HCC PE

√7th **S98.929** Partial traumatic amputation of unspecified foot, level unspecified CC UNS HCC PE

√4th **S99** **Other and unspecified injuries of ankle and foot**
AHA: 2018,2Q,12; 2018,1Q,3; 2016,4Q,68-69

√5th **S99.0** **Physeal fracture of calcaneus**
AHA: 2019,4Q,56

The appropriate 7th character is to be added to each code from subcategory S99.0.
A   initial encounter for closed fracture
B   initial encounter for open fracture
D   subsequent encounter for fracture with routine healing
G   subsequent encounter for fracture with delayed healing
K   subsequent encounter for fracture with nonunion
P   subsequent encounter for fracture with malunion
S   sequela

√6th **S99.00** **Unspecified physeal fracture of calcaneus**

√7th **S99.001** Unspecified physeal fracture of **right** calcaneus

√7th **S99.002** Unspecified physeal fracture of **left** calcaneus PE

√7th **S99.009** Unspecified physeal fracture of unspecified calcaneus PE

√6th **S99.01** **Salter-Harris Type I** physeal fracture of calcaneus

√7th **S99.011** Salter-Harris Type I physeal fracture of **right** calcaneus

√7th **S99.012** Salter-Harris Type I physeal fracture of **left** calcaneus PE

√7th **S99.019** Salter-Harris Type I physeal fracture of unspecified calcaneus PE

√6th **S99.02** **Salter-Harris Type II** physeal fracture of calcaneus

√7th **S99.021** Salter-Harris Type II physeal fracture of **right** calcaneus

√7th **S99.022** Salter-Harris Type II physeal fracture of **left** calcaneus PE

√7th **S99.029** Salter-Harris Type II physeal fracture of unspecified calcaneus

√6th **S99.03** **Salter-Harris Type III** physeal fracture of calcaneus

√7th **S99.031** Salter-Harris Type III physeal fracture of **right** calcaneus

√7th **S99.032** Salter-Harris Type III physeal fracture of **left** calcaneus PE

√7th **S99.039** Salter-Harris Type III physeal fracture of unspecified calcaneus PE

√6th **S99.04** **Salter-Harris Type IV** physeal fracture of calcaneus

√7th **S99.041** Salter-Harris Type IV physeal fracture of **right** calcaneus

√7th **S99.042** Salter-Harris Type IV physeal fracture of **left** calcaneus PE

√7th **S99.049** Salter-Harris Type IV physeal fracture of unspecified calcaneus PE

√6th **S99.09** **Other** physeal fracture of calcaneus

√7th **S99.091** Other physeal fracture of **right** calcaneus PE

√7th **S99.092** Other physeal fracture of **left** calcaneus PE

√7th **S99.099** Other physeal fracture of unspecified calcaneus PE

√5th **S99.1** **Physeal fracture of metatarsal**
AHA: 2019,4Q,56

The appropriate 7th character is to be added to each code from subcategory S99.1
A   initial encounter for closed fracture
B   initial encounter for open fracture
D   subsequent encounter for fracture with routine healing
G   subsequent encounter for fracture with delayed healing
K   subsequent encounter for fracture with nonunion
P   subsequent encounter for fracture with malunion
S   sequela

√6th **S99.10** **Unspecified physeal fracture of metatarsal**

√7th **S99.101** Unspecified physeal fracture of **right** metatarsal PE

√7th **S99.102** Unspecified physeal fracture of **left** metatarsal PE

√7th **S99.109** Unspecified physeal fracture of unspecified metatarsal PE

√6ᵗʰ **S99.11** Salter-Harris Type I physeal fracture of metatarsal

  √7ᵗʰ **S99.111** Salter-Harris Type I physeal fracture of right metatarsal PE

  √7ᵗʰ **S99.112** Salter-Harris Type I physeal fracture of left metatarsal PE

  √7ᵗʰ **S99.119** Salter-Harris Type I physeal fracture of unspecified metatarsal PE

√6ᵗʰ **S99.12** Salter-Harris Type II physeal fracture of metatarsal

  √7ᵗʰ **S99.121** Salter-Harris Type II physeal fracture of right metatarsal PE

  √7ᵗʰ **S99.122** Salter-Harris Type II physeal fracture of left metatarsal PE

  √7ᵗʰ **S99.129** Salter-Harris Type II physeal fracture of unspecified metatarsal PE

√6ᵗʰ **S99.13** Salter-Harris Type III physeal fracture of metatarsal

  √7ᵗʰ **S99.131** Salter-Harris Type III physeal fracture of right metatarsal PE

  √7ᵗʰ **S99.132** Salter-Harris Type III physeal fracture of left metatarsal PE

  √7ᵗʰ **S99.139** Salter-Harris Type III physeal fracture of unspecified metatarsal PE

√6ᵗʰ **S99.14** Salter-Harris Type IV physeal fracture of metatarsal

  √7ᵗʰ **S99.141** Salter-Harris Type IV physeal fracture of right metatarsal PE

  √7ᵗʰ **S99.142** Salter-Harris Type IV physeal fracture of left metatarsal PE

  √7ᵗʰ **S99.149** Salter-Harris Type IV physeal fracture of unspecified metatarsal PE

√6ᵗʰ **S99.19** Other physeal fracture of metatarsal

  √7ᵗʰ **S99.191** Other physeal fracture of right metatarsal PE

  √7ᵗʰ **S99.192** Other physeal fracture of left metatarsal PE

  √7ᵗʰ **S99.199** Other physeal fracture of unspecified metatarsal PE

√5ᵗʰ **S99.2** Physeal fracture of phalanx of toe

AHA: 2019,4Q,56

> The appropriate 7th character is to be added to each code from subcategories S99.2.
> A   initial encounter for closed fracture
> B   initial encounter for open fracture
> D   subsequent encounter for fracture with routine healing
> G   subsequent encounter for fracture with delayed healing
> K   subsequent encounter for fracture with nonunion
> P   subsequent encounter for fracture with malunion
> S   sequela

√6ᵗʰ **S99.20** Unspecified physeal fracture of phalanx of toe

  √7ᵗʰ **S99.201** Unspecified physeal fracture of phalanx of right toe PE

  √7ᵗʰ **S99.202** Unspecified physeal fracture of phalanx of left toe PE

  √7ᵗʰ **S99.209** Unspecified physeal fracture of phalanx of unspecified toe PE

√6ᵗʰ **S99.21** Salter-Harris Type I physeal fracture of phalanx of toe

  √7ᵗʰ **S99.211** Salter-Harris Type I physeal fracture of phalanx of right toe PE

  √7ᵗʰ **S99.212** Salter-Harris Type I physeal fracture of phalanx of left toe PE

  √7ᵗʰ **S99.219** Salter-Harris Type I physeal fracture of phalanx of unspecified toe PE

√6ᵗʰ **S99.22** Salter-Harris Type II physeal fracture of phalanx of toe

  √7ᵗʰ **S99.221** Salter-Harris Type II physeal fracture of phalanx of right toe PE

  √7ᵗʰ **S99.222** Salter-Harris Type II physeal fracture of phalanx of left toe PE

  √7ᵗʰ **S99.229** Salter-Harris Type II physeal fracture of phalanx of unspecified toe PE

√6ᵗʰ **S99.23** Salter-Harris Type III physeal fracture of phalanx of toe

  √7ᵗʰ **S99.231** Salter-Harris Type III physeal fracture of phalanx of right toe PE

  √7ᵗʰ **S99.232** Salter-Harris Type III physeal fracture of phalanx of left toe PE

  √7ᵗʰ **S99.239** Salter-Harris Type III physeal fracture of phalanx of unspecified toe PE

√6ᵗʰ **S99.24** Salter-Harris Type IV physeal fracture of phalanx of toe

  √7ᵗʰ **S99.241** Salter-Harris Type IV physeal fracture of phalanx of right toe PE

  √7ᵗʰ **S99.242** Salter-Harris Type IV physeal fracture of phalanx of left toe PE

  √7ᵗʰ **S99.249** Salter-Harris Type IV physeal fracture of phalanx of unspecified toe PE

√6ᵗʰ **S99.29** Other physeal fracture of phalanx of toe

  √7ᵗʰ **S99.291** Other physeal fracture of phalanx of right toe PE

  √7ᵗʰ **S99.292** Other physeal fracture of phalanx of left toe PE

  √7ᵗʰ **S99.299** Other physeal fracture of phalanx of unspecified toe PE

√5ᵗʰ **S99.8** Other specified injuries of ankle and foot

> The appropriate 7th character is to be added to each code from subcategory S99.8.
> A   initial encounter
> D   subsequent encounter
> S   sequela

√6ᵗʰ **S99.81** Other specified injuries of ankle

  √7ᵗʰ **S99.811** Other specified injuries of right ankle PE

  √7ᵗʰ **S99.812** Other specified injuries of left ankle PE

  √7ᵗʰ **S99.819** Other specified injuries of unspecified ankle PE

√6ᵗʰ **S99.82** Other specified injuries of foot

  √7ᵗʰ **S99.821** Other specified injuries of right foot PE

  √7ᵗʰ **S99.822** Other specified injuries of left foot PE

  √7ᵗʰ **S99.829** Other specified injuries of unspecified foot PE

√5ᵗʰ **S99.9** Unspecified injury of ankle and foot

> The appropriate 7th character is to be added to each code from subcategory S99.9.
> A   initial encounter
> D   subsequent encounter
> S   sequela

√6ᵗʰ **S99.91** Unspecified injury of ankle

  √7ᵗʰ **S99.911** Unspecified injury of right ankle PE

  √7ᵗʰ **S99.912** Unspecified injury of left ankle PE

  √7ᵗʰ **S99.919** Unspecified injury of unspecified ankle PE

√6ᵗʰ **S99.92** Unspecified injury of foot

  √7ᵗʰ **S99.921** Unspecified injury of right foot PE

  √7ᵗʰ **S99.922** Unspecified injury of left foot PE

  √7ᵗʰ **S99.929** Unspecified injury of unspecified foot PE

INJURY, POISONING AND CERTAIN OTHER CONSEQUENCES OF EXTERNAL CAUSES (T07-T88)

Injuries involving multiple body regions (T07)

> EXCLUDES 1   burns and corrosions (T20-T32)
> frostbite (T33-T34)
> insect bite or sting, venomous (T63.4)
> sunburn (L55.-)

√x7ᵗʰ **T07** Unspecified multiple injuries PE

> EXCLUDES 1   injury NOS (T14.90)

AHA: 2017,4Q,26

> The appropriate 7th character is to be added to code T07.
> A   initial encounter
> D   subsequent encounter
> S   sequela

✔ Additional Character Required   √x7ᵗʰ Placeholder   Questionable PDx   Manifestation   Unspecified   UPD Unacceptable PDx   H1-H14 HAC   HCC CMS-HCC Dx   HIV HIV Dx

ICD-10-CM 2025   1113

Injury of unspecified body region (T14)

✓4ᵗʰ T14 Injury of unspecified body region

> EXCLUDES 1   multiple unspecified injuries (T07)
>
> **AHA:** 2017,4Q,26
>
> The appropriate 7th character is to be added to each code from category T14.
> A   initial encounter
> D   subsequent encounter
> S   sequela

✓x7ᵗʰ T14.8 Other injury of unspecified body region   PE
> Abrasion NOS
> Contusion NOS
> Crush injury NOS
> Fracture NOS
> Skin injury NOS
> Vascular injury NOS
> Wound NOS

✓5ᵗʰ T14.9 Unspecified injury

    ✓x7ᵗʰ T14.90 Injury, unspecified   PE
> Injury NOS

    ✓x7ᵗʰ T14.91 Suicide attempt   HCC   PE
> Attempted suicide NOS

Effects of foreign body entering through natural orifice (T15-T19)

Use additional code, if known, for foreign body entering into or through a natural orifice (W44.-)

> EXCLUDES 2   foreign body accidentally left in operation wound (T81.5-)
> foreign body in penetrating wound - see open wound by body region
> residual foreign body in soft tissue (M79.5)
> splinter, without open wound - see superficial injury by body region

✓4ᵗʰ T15 Foreign body on external eye

> EXCLUDES 2   foreign body in penetrating wound of orbit and eye ball (S05.4-, S05.5-)
> open wound of eyelid and periocular area (S01.1-)
> retained foreign body in eyelid (H02.8-)
> retained (old) foreign body in penetrating wound of orbit and eye ball (H05.5-, H44.6-, H44.7-)
> superficial foreign body of eyelid and periocular area (S00.25-)
>
> The appropriate 7th character is to be added to each code from category T15.
> A   initial encounter
> D   subsequent encounter
> S   sequela

✓5ᵗʰ T15.0 Foreign body in cornea

    ✓x7ᵗʰ T15.00 Foreign body in cornea, unspecified eye   PE
    ✓x7ᵗʰ T15.01 Foreign body in cornea, right eye   PE
    ✓x7ᵗʰ T15.02 Foreign body in cornea, left eye   PE

✓5ᵗʰ T15.1 Foreign body in conjunctival sac

    ✓x7ᵗʰ T15.10 Foreign body in conjunctival sac, unspecified eye   PE
    ✓x7ᵗʰ T15.11 Foreign body in conjunctival sac, right eye   PE
    ✓x7ᵗʰ T15.12 Foreign body in conjunctival sac, left eye   PE

✓5ᵗʰ T15.8 Foreign body in other and multiple parts of external eye
> Foreign body in lacrimal punctum

    ✓x7ᵗʰ T15.80 Foreign body in other and multiple parts of external eye, unspecified eye   PE
    ✓x7ᵗʰ T15.81 Foreign body in other and multiple parts of external eye, right eye   PE
    ✓x7ᵗʰ T15.82 Foreign body in other and multiple parts of external eye, left eye   PE

✓5ᵗʰ T15.9 Foreign body on external eye, part unspecified

    ✓x7ᵗʰ T15.90 Foreign body on external eye, part unspecified, unspecified eye   PE
    ✓x7ᵗʰ T15.91 Foreign body on external eye, part unspecified, right eye   PE
    ✓x7ᵗʰ T15.92 Foreign body on external eye, part unspecified, left eye   PE

✓4ᵗʰ T16 Foreign body in ear

> INCLUDES   foreign body in auditory canal
>
> The appropriate 7th character is to be added to each code from category T16.
> A   initial encounter
> D   subsequent encounter
> S   sequela

✓x7ᵗʰ T16.1 Foreign body in right ear   PE
✓x7ᵗʰ T16.2 Foreign body in left ear   PE
✓x7ᵗʰ T16.9 Foreign body in ear, unspecified ear   PE

✓4ᵗʰ T17 Foreign body in respiratory tract

> The appropriate 7th character is to be added to each code from category T17.
> A   initial encounter
> D   subsequent encounter
> S   sequela

✓x7ᵗʰ T17.0 Foreign body in nasal sinus   PE

✓x7ᵗʰ T17.1 Foreign body in nostril   PE
> Foreign body in nose NOS

✓5ᵗʰ T17.2 Foreign body in pharynx
> Foreign body in nasopharynx
> Foreign body in throat NOS

    ✓6ᵗʰ T17.20 Unspecified foreign body in pharynx

      ✓7ᵗʰ T17.200 Unspecified foreign body in pharynx causing asphyxiation   PE
      ✓7ᵗʰ T17.208 Unspecified foreign body in pharynx causing other injury   PE

    ✓6ᵗʰ T17.21 Gastric contents in pharynx
> Aspiration of gastric contents into pharynx
> Vomitus in pharynx

      ✓7ᵗʰ T17.210 Gastric contents in pharynx causing asphyxiation   PE
      ✓7ᵗʰ T17.218 Gastric contents in pharynx causing other injury   PE

    ✓6ᵗʰ T17.22 Food in pharynx
> Bones in pharynx
> Seeds in pharynx

      ✓7ᵗʰ T17.220 Food in pharynx causing asphyxiation   PE
      ✓7ᵗʰ T17.228 Food in pharynx causing other injury   PE

    ✓6ᵗʰ T17.29 Other foreign object in pharynx

      ✓7ᵗʰ T17.290 Other foreign object in pharynx causing asphyxiation   PE
      ✓7ᵗʰ T17.298 Other foreign object in pharynx causing other injury   PE

✓5ᵗʰ T17.3 Foreign body in larynx

    ✓6ᵗʰ T17.30 Unspecified foreign body in larynx

      ✓7ᵗʰ T17.300 Unspecified foreign body in larynx causing asphyxiation   PE
      ✓7ᵗʰ T17.308 Unspecified foreign body in larynx causing other injury   PE

    ✓6ᵗʰ T17.31 Gastric contents in larynx
> Aspiration of gastric contents into larynx
> Vomitus in larynx

      ✓7ᵗʰ T17.310 Gastric contents in larynx causing asphyxiation   PE
      ✓7ᵗʰ T17.318 Gastric contents in larynx causing other injury   PE

    ✓6ᵗʰ T17.32 Food in larynx
> Bones in larynx
> Seeds in larynx

      ✓7ᵗʰ T17.320 Food in larynx causing asphyxiation   PE
      ✓7ᵗʰ T17.328 Food in larynx causing other injury   PE

    ✓6ᵗʰ T17.39 Other foreign object in larynx

      ✓7ᵗʰ T17.390 Other foreign object in larynx causing asphyxiation   PE
      ✓7ᵗʰ T17.398 Other foreign object in larynx causing other injury   PE

✓5ᵗʰ T17.4 Foreign body in trachea

    ✓6ᵗʰ T17.40 Unspecified foreign body in trachea

      ✓7ᵗʰ T17.400 Unspecified foreign body in trachea causing asphyxiation   CC   PE

✓7th **T17.408** Unspecified foreign body in trachea causing other injury   CC PE

✓6th **T17.41** Gastric contents in trachea
Aspiration of gastric contents into trachea
Vomitus in trachea

    ✓7th **T17.410** Gastric contents in trachea causing asphyxiation   CC PE

    ✓7th **T17.418** Gastric contents in trachea causing other injury   CC PE

✓6th **T17.42** Food in trachea
Bones in trachea
Seeds in trachea

    ✓7th **T17.420** Food in trachea causing asphyxiation   CC PE

    ✓7th **T17.428** Food in trachea causing other injury   CC PE

✓6th **T17.49** Other foreign object in trachea

    ✓7th **T17.490** Other foreign object in trachea causing asphyxiation   CC PE

    ✓7th **T17.498** Other foreign object in trachea causing other injury   CC PE

✓5th **T17.5** Foreign body in bronchus

✓6th **T17.50** Unspecified foreign body in bronchus

    ✓7th **T17.500** Unspecified foreign body in bronchus causing asphyxiation   CC PE

    ✓7th **T17.508** Unspecified foreign body in bronchus causing other injury   CC PE

✓6th **T17.51** Gastric contents in bronchus
Aspiration of gastric contents into bronchus
Vomitus in bronchus

    ✓7th **T17.510** Gastric contents in bronchus causing asphyxiation   CC PE

    ✓7th **T17.518** Gastric contents in bronchus causing other injury   CC PE

✓6th **T17.52** Food in bronchus
Bones in bronchus
Seeds in bronchus

    ✓7th **T17.520** Food in bronchus causing asphyxiation   CC PE

    ✓7th **T17.528** Food in bronchus causing other injury   CC PE

✓6th **T17.59** Other foreign object in bronchus

    ✓7th **T17.590** Other foreign object in bronchus causing asphyxiation   CC PE

    ✓7th **T17.598** Other foreign object in bronchus causing other injury   CC PE

✓5th **T17.8** Foreign body in other parts of respiratory tract
Foreign body in bronchioles
Foreign body in lung

✓6th **T17.80** Unspecified foreign body in other parts of respiratory tract

    ✓7th **T17.800** Unspecified foreign body in other parts of respiratory tract causing asphyxiation   CC PE

    ✓7th **T17.808** Unspecified foreign body in other parts of respiratory tract causing other injury   CC PE

✓6th **T17.81** Gastric contents in other parts of respiratory tract
Aspiration of gastric contents into other parts of respiratory tract
Vomitus in other parts of respiratory tract

    ✓7th **T17.810** Gastric contents in other parts of respiratory tract causing asphyxiation   CC PE

    ✓7th **T17.818** Gastric contents in other parts of respiratory tract causing other injury   CC PE

✓6th **T17.82** Food in other parts of respiratory tract
Bones in other parts of respiratory tract
Seeds in other parts of respiratory tract

    ✓7th **T17.820** Food in other parts of respiratory tract causing asphyxiation   CC PE

    ✓7th **T17.828** Food in other parts of respiratory tract causing other injury   CC PE

✓6th **T17.89** Other foreign object in other parts of respiratory tract

    ✓7th **T17.890** Other foreign object in other parts of respiratory tract causing asphyxiation   CC PE

✓7th **T17.898** Other foreign object in other parts of respiratory tract causing other injury   CC PE

✓5th **T17.9** Foreign body in respiratory tract, part unspecified

✓6th **T17.90** Unspecified foreign body in respiratory tract, part unspecified

    ✓7th **T17.900** Unspecified foreign body in respiratory tract, part unspecified causing asphyxiation   PE

    ✓7th **T17.908** Unspecified foreign body in respiratory tract, part unspecified causing other injury   PE

✓6th **T17.91** Gastric contents in respiratory tract, part unspecified
Aspiration of gastric contents into respiratory tract, part unspecified
Vomitus in trachea respiratory tract, part unspecified

    ✓7th **T17.910** Gastric contents in respiratory tract, part unspecified causing asphyxiation   PE

    ✓7th **T17.918** Gastric contents in respiratory tract, part unspecified causing other injury   PE

✓6th **T17.92** Food in respiratory tract, part unspecified
Bones in respiratory tract, part unspecified
Seeds in respiratory tract, part unspecified

    ✓7th **T17.920** Food in respiratory tract, part unspecified causing asphyxiation   PE

    ✓7th **T17.928** Food in respiratory tract, part unspecified causing other injury   PE

✓6th **T17.99** Other foreign object in respiratory tract, part unspecified

    ✓7th **T17.990** Other foreign object in respiratory tract, part unspecified in causing asphyxiation   PE
      AHA: 2019,3Q,15

    ✓7th **T17.998** Other foreign object in respiratory tract, part unspecified causing other injury   PE

✓4th **T18** Foreign body in alimentary tract

    EXCLUDES 2   *foreign body in pharynx (T17.2-)*

    The appropriate 7th character is to be added to each code from category T18.
    A   initial encounter
    D   subsequent encounter
    S   sequela

✓x7th **T18.0** Foreign body in mouth   PE

✓5th **T18.1** Foreign body in esophagus

    EXCLUDES 2   *foreign body in respiratory tract (T17.-)*

✓6th **T18.10** Unspecified foreign body in esophagus

    ✓7th **T18.100** Unspecified foreign body in esophagus causing compression of trachea   PE
      Unspecified foreign body in esophagus causing obstruction of respiration

    ✓7th **T18.108** Unspecified foreign body in esophagus causing other injury   PE

✓6th **T18.11** Gastric contents in esophagus
Vomitus in esophagus

    ✓7th **T18.110** Gastric contents in esophagus causing compression of trachea   PE
      Gastric contents in esophagus causing obstruction of respiration

    ✓7th **T18.118** Gastric contents in esophagus causing other injury   PE

✓6th **T18.12** Food in esophagus
Bones in esophagus
Seeds in esophagus

    ✓7th **T18.120** Food in esophagus causing compression of trachea   PE
      Food in esophagus causing obstruction of respiration

    ✓7th **T18.128** Food in esophagus causing other injury   PE

√6ᵗʰ **T18.19** **Other foreign object in esophagus**

    AHA: 2022,1Q,27; 2015,1Q,23

    √7ᵗʰ **T18.190** **Other foreign object in esophagus causing compression of trachea** PE

        Other foreign body in esophagus causing obstruction of respiration

        TIP: Any foreign object lodged in the esophagus requires immediate treatment and is considered an injury. Assign this code when there is respiratory compromise or compression. If no respiratory compromise or compression is documented, assign code T18.198-.

    √7ᵗʰ **T18.198** **Other foreign object in esophagus causing other injury** PE

        TIP: Any foreign object lodged in the esophagus requires immediate treatment and is considered an injury. Assign this code when there is no respiratory compromise or compression. If respiratory compromise or compression is documented, assign code T18.190-.

√x7ᵗʰ **T18.2** **Foreign body in stomach** PE

√x7ᵗʰ **T18.3** **Foreign body in small intestine** PE

√x7ᵗʰ **T18.4** **Foreign body in colon** PE

√x7ᵗʰ **T18.5** **Foreign body in anus and rectum** PE

    Foreign body in rectosigmoid (junction)

√x7ᵗʰ **T18.8** **Foreign body in other parts of alimentary tract** PE

√x7ᵗʰ **T18.9** **Foreign body of alimentary tract, part unspecified** PE

    Foreign body in digestive system NOS

    Swallowed foreign body NOS

√4ᵗʰ **T19** **Foreign body in genitourinary tract**

    EXCLUDES 2   *complications due to implanted mesh (T83.7-)*

        mechanical complications of contraceptive device (intrauterine) (vaginal) (T83.3-)

        presence of contraceptive device (intrauterine) (vaginal) (Z97.5)

    The appropriate 7th character is to be added to each code from category T19.

    A   initial encounter

    D   subsequent encounter

    S   sequela

√x7ᵗʰ **T19.0** **Foreign body in urethra** PE

√x7ᵗʰ **T19.1** **Foreign body in bladder** PE

√x7ᵗʰ **T19.2** **Foreign body in vulva and vagina** PE

√x7ᵗʰ **T19.3** **Foreign body in uterus** PE

√x7ᵗʰ **T19.4** **Foreign body in penis** PE

√x7ᵗʰ **T19.8** **Foreign body in other parts of genitourinary tract** PE

√x7ᵗʰ **T19.9** **Foreign body in genitourinary tract, part unspecified** PE

BURNS AND CORROSIONS (T20-T32)

INCLUDES   burns (thermal) from electrical heating appliances
     burns (thermal) from electricity
     burns (thermal) from flame
     burns (thermal) from friction
     burns (thermal) from hot air and hot gases
     burns (thermal) from hot objects
     burns (thermal) from lightning
     burns (thermal) from radiation
     chemical burn [corrosion] (external) (internal)
     scalds

EXCLUDES 2   *erythema [dermatitis] ab igne (L59.0)*
     radiation-related disorders of the skin and subcutaneous tissue (L55-L59)
     sunburn (L55.-)

AHA: 2016,2Q,4

Burns and corrosions of external body surface, specified by site (T20-T25)

INCLUDES   burns and corrosions of first degree [erythema]
     burns and corrosions of second degree [blisters] [epidermal loss]
     burns and corrosions of third degree [deep necrosis of underlying tissue] [full-thickness skin loss]

Use additional code from category T31 or T32 to identify extent of body surface involved

√4ᵗʰ **T20** **Burn and corrosion of head, face, and neck**

    EXCLUDES 2   *burn and corrosion of ear drum (T28.41, T28.91)*

        burn and corrosion of eye and adnexa (T26.-)

        burn and corrosion of mouth and pharynx (T28.0)

    AHA: 2015,1Q,18-19

    The appropriate 7th character is to be added to each code from category T20.

    A   initial encounter

    D   subsequent encounter

    S   sequela

√5ᵗʰ **T20.0** **Burn of unspecified degree of head, face, and neck**

    Use additional external cause code to identify the source, place and intent of the burn (X00-X19, X75-X77, X96-X98, Y92)

    √7ᵗʰ **T20.00** **Burn of unspecified degree of head, face, and neck, unspecified site** PE

    √6ᵗʰ **T20.01** **Burn of unspecified degree of ear [any part, except ear drum]**

        EXCLUDES 2   *burn of ear drum (T28.41-)*

        √7ᵗʰ **T20.011** **Burn of unspecified degree of right ear [any part, except ear drum]** PE

        √7ᵗʰ **T20.012** **Burn of unspecified degree of left ear [any part, except ear drum]** PE

        √7ᵗʰ **T20.019** **Burn of unspecified degree of unspecified ear [any part, except ear drum]** PE

    √7ᵗʰ **T20.02** **Burn of unspecified degree of lip(s)** PE

    √7ᵗʰ **T20.03** **Burn of unspecified degree of chin** PE

    √7ᵗʰ **T20.04** **Burn of unspecified degree of nose (septum)** PE

    √7ᵗʰ **T20.05** **Burn of unspecified degree of scalp [any part]** PE

    √7ᵗʰ **T20.06** **Burn of unspecified degree of forehead and cheek** PE

    √7ᵗʰ **T20.07** **Burn of unspecified degree of neck** PE

    √7ᵗʰ **T20.09** **Burn of unspecified degree of multiple sites of head, face, and neck** PE

√5ᵗʰ **T20.1** **Burn of first degree of head, face, and neck**

    Use additional external cause code to identify the source, place and intent of the burn (X00-X19, X75-X77, X96-X98, Y92)

    √7ᵗʰ **T20.10** **Burn of first degree of head, face, and neck, unspecified site** PE

    √6ᵗʰ **T20.11** **Burn of first degree of ear [any part, except ear drum]**

        EXCLUDES 2   *burn of ear drum (T28.41-)*

        √7ᵗʰ **T20.111** **Burn of first degree of right ear [any part, except ear drum]** PE

        √7ᵗʰ **T20.112** **Burn of first degree of left ear [any part, except ear drum]** PE

        √7ᵗʰ **T20.119** **Burn of first degree of unspecified ear [any part, except ear drum]** PE

    √7ᵗʰ **T20.12** **Burn of first degree of lip(s)** PE

    √7ᵗʰ **T20.13** **Burn of first degree of chin** PE

    √7ᵗʰ **T20.14** **Burn of first degree of nose (septum)** PE

    √7ᵗʰ **T20.15** **Burn of first degree of scalp [any part]** PE

    √7ᵗʰ **T20.16** **Burn of first degree of forehead and cheek** PE

    √7ᵗʰ **T20.17** **Burn of first degree of neck** PE

✓x 7th **T20.19** Burn of first degree of **multiple sites** of head, face, and neck   `PE`

Degree of Burns

Epidermis
Dermis
Subcutaneous

Normal   First Degree Burn

Epidermis
Dermis
Subcutaneous

Second Degree Burn   Third Degree Burn

✓5th **T20.2** Burn of **second degree** of head, face, and neck

Use additional external cause code to identify the source, place and intent of the burn (X00-X19, X75-X77, X96-X98, Y92)

✓x 7th **T20.20** Burn of second degree of head, face, and neck, unspecified site   `PE`

✓6th **T20.21** Burn of second degree of **ear** [any part, except ear drum]

     EXCLUDES 2   burn of ear drum (T28.41-)

   ✓7th **T20.211** Burn of second degree of **right** ear [any part, except ear drum]   `PE`

   ✓7th **T20.212** Burn of second degree of **left** ear [any part, except ear drum]   `PE`

   ✓7th **T20.219** Burn of second degree of unspecified ear [any part, except ear drum]   `PE`

✓x 7th **T20.22** Burn of second degree of **lip(s)**   `PE`

✓x 7th **T20.23** Burn of second degree of **chin**   `PE`

✓x 7th **T20.24** Burn of second degree of **nose** (septum)   `PE`

✓x 7th **T20.25** Burn of second degree of **scalp** [any part]   `PE`

✓x 7th **T20.26** Burn of second degree of **forehead and cheek**   `PE`

✓x 7th **T20.27** Burn of second degree of **neck**   `PE`

✓x 7th **T20.29** Burn of second degree of **multiple sites** of head, face, and neck   `PE`

✓5th **T20.3** Burn of **third degree** of head, face, and neck

Use additional external cause code to identify the source, place and intent of the burn (X00-X19, X75-X77, X96-X98, Y92)

✓x 7th **T20.30** Burn of third degree of head, face, and neck, unspecified site   `CC` `H5` `PE`

✓6th **T20.31** Burn of third degree of **ear** [any part, except ear drum]

     EXCLUDES 2   burn of ear drum (T28.41-)

     AHA: 2015,1Q,18

   ✓7th **T20.311** Burn of third degree of **right** ear [any part, except ear drum]   `CC` `H5` `PE`

   ✓7th **T20.312** Burn of third degree of **left** ear [any part, except ear drum]   `CC` `H5` `PE`

   ✓7th **T20.319** Burn of third degree of unspecified ear [any part, except ear drum]   `CC` `H5` `UNS` `PE`

✓x 7th **T20.32** Burn of third degree of **lip(s)**   `CC` `H5` `PE`

✓x 7th **T20.33** Burn of third degree of **chin**   `CC` `H5` `PE`

✓x 7th **T20.34** Burn of third degree of **nose** (septum)   `CC` `H5` `PE`

✓x 7th **T20.35** Burn of third degree of **scalp** [any part]   `CC` `H5` `PE`

✓x 7th **T20.36** Burn of third degree of **forehead and cheek**   `CC` `H5` `PE`

✓x 7th **T20.37** Burn of third degree of **neck**   `CC` `H5` `PE`

✓x 7th **T20.39** Burn of third degree of **multiple sites** of head, face, and neck   `CC` `H5` `PE`

✓5th **T20.4** Corrosion of unspecified degree of head, face, and neck

Code first (T51-T65) to identify chemical and intent
Use additional external cause code to identify place (Y92)

✓x 7th **T20.40** Corrosion of unspecified degree of head, face, and neck, unspecified site   `PE`

✓6th **T20.41** Corrosion of unspecified degree of **ear** [any part, except ear drum]

     EXCLUDES 2   corrosion of ear drum (T28.91-)

   ✓7th **T20.411** Corrosion of unspecified degree of **right** ear [any part, except ear drum]   `PE`

   ✓7th **T20.412** Corrosion of unspecified degree of **left** ear [any part, except ear drum]   `PE`

   ✓7th **T20.419** Corrosion of unspecified degree of unspecified ear [any part, except ear drum]   `PE`

✓x 7th **T20.42** Corrosion of unspecified degree of **lip(s)**   `PE`

✓x 7th **T20.43** Corrosion of unspecified degree of **chin**   `PE`

✓x 7th **T20.44** Corrosion of unspecified degree of **nose** (septum)   `PE`

✓x 7th **T20.45** Corrosion of unspecified degree of **scalp** [any part]   `PE`

✓x 7th **T20.46** Corrosion of unspecified degree of **forehead and cheek**   `PE`

✓x 7th **T20.47** Corrosion of unspecified degree of **neck**   `PE`

✓x 7th **T20.49** Corrosion of unspecified degree of **multiple sites** of head, face, and neck   `PE`

✓5th **T20.5** Corrosion of **first degree** of head, face, and neck

Code first (T51-T65) to identify chemical and intent
Use additional external cause code to identify place (Y92)

✓x 7th **T20.50** Corrosion of first degree of head, face, and neck, unspecified site   `PE`

✓6th **T20.51** Corrosion of first degree of **ear** [any part, except ear drum]

     EXCLUDES 2   corrosion of ear drum (T28.91-)

   ✓7th **T20.511** Corrosion of first degree of **right** ear [any part, except ear drum]   `PE`

   ✓7th **T20.512** Corrosion of first degree of **left** ear [any part, except ear drum]   `PE`

   ✓7th **T20.519** Corrosion of first degree of unspecified ear [any part, except ear drum]   `PE`

✓x 7th **T20.52** Corrosion of first degree of **lip(s)**   `PE`

✓x 7th **T20.53** Corrosion of first degree of **chin**   `PE`

✓x 7th **T20.54** Corrosion of first degree of **nose** (septum)   `PE`

✓x 7th **T20.55** Corrosion of first degree of **scalp** [any part]   `PE`

✓x 7th **T20.56** Corrosion of first degree of **forehead and cheek**   `PE`

✓x 7th **T20.57** Corrosion of first degree of **neck**   `PE`

✓x 7th **T20.59** Corrosion of first degree of **multiple sites** of head, face, and neck   `PE`

✓5th **T20.6** Corrosion of **second degree** of head, face, and neck

Code first (T51-T65) to identify chemical and intent
Use additional external cause code to identify place (Y92)

✓x 7th **T20.60** Corrosion of second degree of head, face, and neck, unspecified site   `PE`

✓6th **T20.61** Corrosion of second degree of **ear** [any part, except ear drum]

     EXCLUDES 2   corrosion of ear drum (T28.91-)

   ✓7th **T20.611** Corrosion of second degree of **right** ear [any part, except ear drum]   `PE`

   ✓7th **T20.612** Corrosion of second degree of **left** ear [any part, except ear drum]   `PE`

   ✓7th **T20.619** Corrosion of second degree of unspecified ear [any part, except ear drum]   `PE`

✓x 7th **T20.62** Corrosion of second degree of **lip(s)**   `PE`

✓x 7th **T20.63** Corrosion of second degree of **chin**   `PE`

✓x 7th **T20.64** Corrosion of second degree of **nose** (septum)   `PE`

✓x 7th **T20.65** Corrosion of second degree of **scalp** [any part]   `PE`

✓x 7th **T20.66** Corrosion of second degree of **forehead and cheek**   `PE`

✓x 7th **T20.67** Corrosion of second degree of **neck**   `PE`

✓x 7th **T20.69** Corrosion of second degree of **multiple sites** of head, face, and neck   `PE`

☑ Additional Character Required   ✓x 7th Placeholder   Questionable PDx   Manifestation   Unspecified   `UPD` Unacceptable PDx   `H1`-`H14` HAC   `HCC` CMS-HCC Dx   `HIV` HIV Dx

ICD-10-CM 2025   1117

√5ᵗʰ **T20.7 Corrosion of third degree of head, face, and neck**
Code first (T51-T65) to identify chemical and intent
Use additional external cause code to identify place (Y92)

√x7ᵗʰ **T20.70 Corrosion of third degree of head, face, and neck, unspecified site** `CC` `H5` `PE`

√6ᵗʰ **T20.71 Corrosion of third degree of ear [any part, except ear drum]**
EXCLUDES 2   corrosion of ear drum (T28.91-)

√7ᵗʰ **T20.711 Corrosion of third degree of right ear [any part, except ear drum]** `CC` `H5` `PE`

√7ᵗʰ **T20.712 Corrosion of third degree of left ear [any part, except ear drum]** `CC` `H5` `PE`

√7ᵗʰ **T20.719 Corrosion of third degree of unspecified ear [any part, except ear drum]** `CC` `H5` `UNS` `PE`

√x7ᵗʰ **T20.72 Corrosion of third degree of lip(s)** `CC` `H5` `PE`

√x7ᵗʰ **T20.73 Corrosion of third degree of chin** `CC` `H5` `PE`

√x7ᵗʰ **T20.74 Corrosion of third degree of nose (septum)** `CC` `H5` `PE`

√x7ᵗʰ **T20.75 Corrosion of third degree of scalp [any part]** `CC` `H5` `PE`

√x7ᵗʰ **T20.76 Corrosion of third degree of forehead and cheek** `CC` `H5` `PE`

√x7ᵗʰ **T20.77 Corrosion of third degree of neck** `CC` `H5` `PE`

√x7ᵗʰ **T20.79 Corrosion of third degree of multiple sites of head, face, and neck** `CC` `H5` `PE`

√4ᵗʰ **T21 Burn and corrosion of trunk**

INCLUDES   burns and corrosion of hip region
EXCLUDES 2   burns and corrosion of axilla (T22.- with fifth character 4)
burns and corrosion of scapular region (T22.- with fifth character 6)
burns and corrosion of shoulder (T22.- with fifth character 5)

The appropriate 7th character is to be added to each code from category T21.
A   initial encounter
D   subsequent encounter
S   sequela

√5ᵗʰ **T21.0 Burn of unspecified degree of trunk**
Use additional external cause code to identify the source, place and intent of the burn (X00-X19, X75-X77, X96-X98, Y92)

√x7ᵗʰ **T21.00 Burn of unspecified degree of trunk, unspecified site** `PE`

√x7ᵗʰ **T21.01 Burn of unspecified degree of chest wall** `PE`
Burn of unspecified degree of breast

√x7ᵗʰ **T21.02 Burn of unspecified degree of abdominal wall** `PE`
Burn of unspecified degree of flank
Burn of unspecified degree of groin

√x7ᵗʰ **T21.03 Burn of unspecified degree of upper back** `PE`
Burn of unspecified degree of interscapular region

√x7ᵗʰ **T21.04 Burn of unspecified degree of lower back** `PE`

√x7ᵗʰ **T21.05 Burn of unspecified degree of buttock** `PE`
Burn of unspecified degree of anus

√x7ᵗʰ **T21.06 Burn of unspecified degree of male genital region** `PE`
Burn of unspecified degree of penis
Burn of unspecified degree of scrotum
Burn of unspecified degree of testis

√x7ᵗʰ **T21.07 Burn of unspecified degree of female genital region** `PE`
Burn of unspecified degree of labium (majus) (minus)
Burn of unspecified degree of perineum
Burn of unspecified degree of vulva
EXCLUDES 2   burn of vagina (T28.3)

√x7ᵗʰ **T21.09 Burn of unspecified degree of other site of trunk** `PE`

√5ᵗʰ **T21.1 Burn of first degree of trunk**
Use additional external cause code to identify the source, place and intent of the burn (X00-X19, X75-X77, X96-X98, Y92)

√x7ᵗʰ **T21.10 Burn of first degree of trunk, unspecified site** `PE`

√x7ᵗʰ **T21.11 Burn of first degree of chest wall** `PE`
Burn of first degree of breast

√x7ᵗʰ **T21.12 Burn of first degree of abdominal wall** `PE`
Burn of first degree of flank
Burn of first degree of groin

√x7ᵗʰ **T21.13 Burn of first degree of upper back** `PE`
Burn of first degree of interscapular region

√x7ᵗʰ **T21.14 Burn of first degree of lower back** `PE`

√x7ᵗʰ **T21.15 Burn of first degree of buttock** `PE`
Burn of first degree of anus

√x7ᵗʰ **T21.16 Burn of first degree of male genital region** `PE`
Burn of first degree of penis
Burn of first degree of scrotum
Burn of first degree of testis

√x7ᵗʰ **T21.17 Burn of first degree of female genital region** `PE`
Burn of first degree of labium (majus) (minus)
Burn of first degree of perineum
Burn of first degree of vulva
EXCLUDES 2   burn of vagina (T28.3)

√x7ᵗʰ **T21.19 Burn of first degree of other site of trunk** `PE`

√5ᵗʰ **T21.2 Burn of second degree of trunk**
Use additional external cause code to identify the source, place and intent of the burn (X00-X19, X75-X77, X96-X98, Y92)

√x7ᵗʰ **T21.20 Burn of second degree of trunk, unspecified site** `PE`

√x7ᵗʰ **T21.21 Burn of second degree of chest wall** `PE`
Burn of second degree of breast

√x7ᵗʰ **T21.22 Burn of second degree of abdominal wall** `PE`
Burn of second degree of flank
Burn of second degree of groin

√x7ᵗʰ **T21.23 Burn of second degree of upper back** `PE`
Burn of second degree of interscapular region

√x7ᵗʰ **T21.24 Burn of second degree of lower back** `PE`

√x7ᵗʰ **T21.25 Burn of second degree of buttock** `PE`
Burn of second degree of anus

√x7ᵗʰ **T21.26 Burn of second degree of male genital region** `PE`
Burn of second degree of penis
Burn of second degree of scrotum
Burn of second degree of testis

√x7ᵗʰ **T21.27 Burn of second degree of female genital region** `PE`
Burn of second degree of labium (majus) (minus)
Burn of second degree of perineum
Burn of second degree of vulva
EXCLUDES 2   burn of vagina (T28.3)

√x7ᵗʰ **T21.29 Burn of second degree of other site of trunk** `PE`

√5ᵗʰ **T21.3 Burn of third degree of trunk**
Use additional external cause code to identify the source, place and intent of the burn (X00-X19, X75-X77, X96-X98, Y92)

√x7ᵗʰ **T21.30 Burn of third degree of trunk, unspecified site** `CC` `H5` `PE`

√x7ᵗʰ **T21.31 Burn of third degree of chest wall** `CC` `H5` `PE`
Burn of third degree of breast
AHA: 2016,2Q,5

√x7ᵗʰ **T21.32 Burn of third degree of abdominal wall** `CC` `H5` `PE`
Burn of third degree of flank
Burn of third degree of groin

√x7ᵗʰ **T21.33 Burn of third degree of upper back** `CC` `H5` `PE`
Burn of third degree of interscapular region

√x7ᵗʰ **T21.34 Burn of third degree of lower back** `CC` `H5` `PE`

√x7ᵗʰ **T21.35 Burn of third degree of buttock** `CC` `H5` `PE`
Burn of third degree of anus

√x7ᵗʰ **T21.36 Burn of third degree of male genital region** `CC` `H5` `PE`
Burn of third degree of penis
Burn of third degree of scrotum
Burn of third degree of testis

√x7ᵗʰ **T21.37 Burn of third degree of female genital region** `CC` `H5` `PE`
Burn of third degree of labium (majus) (minus)
Burn of third degree of perineum
Burn of third degree of vulva
EXCLUDES 2   burn of vagina (T28.3)

√x7ᵗʰ **T21.39 Burn of third degree of other site of trunk** `CC` `H5` `PE`

√5ᵗʰ **T21.4 Corrosion of unspecified degree of trunk**
Code first (T51-T65) to identify chemical and intent
Use additional external cause code to identify place (Y92)

√x7ᵗʰ **T21.40 Corrosion of unspecified degree of trunk, unspecified site** `PE`

√x 7ᵗʰ **T21.41** **Corrosion of unspecified degree of chest wall** PE
    Corrosion of unspecified degree of breast

√x 7ᵗʰ **T21.42** **Corrosion of unspecified degree of abdominal wall** PE
    Corrosion of unspecified degree of flank
    Corrosion of unspecified degree of groin

√x 7ᵗʰ **T21.43** **Corrosion of unspecified degree of upper back** PE
    Corrosion of unspecified degree of interscapular region

√x 7ᵗʰ **T21.44** **Corrosion of unspecified degree of lower back** PE

√x 7ᵗʰ **T21.45** **Corrosion of unspecified degree of buttock** PE
    Corrosion of unspecified degree of anus

√x 7ᵗʰ **T21.46** **Corrosion of unspecified degree of male genital region** PE
    Corrosion of unspecified degree of penis
    Corrosion of unspecified degree of scrotum
    Corrosion of unspecified degree of testis

√x 7ᵗʰ **T21.47** **Corrosion of unspecified degree of female genital region** PE
    Corrosion of unspecified degree of labium (majus) (minus)
    Corrosion of unspecified degree of perineum
    Corrosion of unspecified degree of vulva
    EXCLUDES 2   corrosion of vagina (T28.8)

√x 7ᵗʰ **T21.49** **Corrosion of unspecified degree of other site of trunk** PE

√5ᵗʰ **T21.5** **Corrosion of first degree of trunk**
    Code first (T51-T65) to identify chemical and intent
    Use additional external cause code to identify place (Y92)

√x 7ᵗʰ **T21.50** **Corrosion of first degree of trunk, unspecified site** PE

√x 7ᵗʰ **T21.51** **Corrosion of first degree of chest wall** PE
    Corrosion of first degree of breast

√x 7ᵗʰ **T21.52** **Corrosion of first degree of abdominal wall** PE
    Corrosion of first degree of flank
    Corrosion of first degree of groin

√x 7ᵗʰ **T21.53** **Corrosion of first degree of upper back** PE
    Corrosion of first degree of interscapular region

√x 7ᵗʰ **T21.54** **Corrosion of first degree of lower back** PE

√x 7ᵗʰ **T21.55** **Corrosion of first degree of buttock** PE
    Corrosion of first degree of anus

√x 7ᵗʰ **T21.56** **Corrosion of first degree of male genital region** PE
    Corrosion of first degree of penis
    Corrosion of first degree of scrotum
    Corrosion of first degree of testis

√x 7ᵗʰ **T21.57** **Corrosion of first degree of female genital region** PE
    Corrosion of first degree of labium (majus) (minus)
    Corrosion of first degree of perineum
    Corrosion of first degree of vulva
    EXCLUDES 2   corrosion of vagina (T28.8)

√x 7ᵗʰ **T21.59** **Corrosion of first degree of other site of trunk** PE

√5ᵗʰ **T21.6** **Corrosion of second degree of trunk**
    Code first (T51-T65) to identify chemical and intent
    Use additional external cause code to identify place (Y92)

√x 7ᵗʰ **T21.60** **Corrosion of second degree of trunk, unspecified site** PE

√x 7ᵗʰ **T21.61** **Corrosion of second degree of chest wall** PE
    Corrosion of second degree of breast

√x 7ᵗʰ **T21.62** **Corrosion of second degree of abdominal wall** PE
    Corrosion of second degree of flank
    Corrosion of second degree of groin

√x 7ᵗʰ **T21.63** **Corrosion of second degree of upper back** PE
    Corrosion of second degree of interscapular region

√x 7ᵗʰ **T21.64** **Corrosion of second degree of lower back** PE

√x 7ᵗʰ **T21.65** **Corrosion of second degree of buttock** PE
    Corrosion of second degree of anus

√x 7ᵗʰ **T21.66** **Corrosion of second degree of male genital region** PE
    Corrosion of second degree of penis
    Corrosion of second degree of scrotum
    Corrosion of second degree of testis

√x 7ᵗʰ **T21.67** **Corrosion of second degree of female genital region** PE
    Corrosion of second degree of labium (majus) (minus)
    Corrosion of second degree of perineum
    Corrosion of second degree of vulva
    EXCLUDES 2   corrosion of vagina (T28.8)

√x 7ᵗʰ **T21.69** **Corrosion of second degree of other site of trunk** PE

√5ᵗʰ **T21.7** **Corrosion of third degree of trunk**
    Code first (T51-T65) to identify chemical and intent
    Use additional external cause code to identify place (Y92)

√x 7ᵗʰ **T21.70** **Corrosion of third degree of trunk, unspecified site** CC H5 PE

√x 7ᵗʰ **T21.71** **Corrosion of third degree of chest wall** CC H5 PE
    Corrosion of third degree of breast

√x 7ᵗʰ **T21.72** **Corrosion of third degree of abdominal wall** CC H5 PE
    Corrosion of third degree of flank
    Corrosion of third degree of groin

√x 7ᵗʰ **T21.73** **Corrosion of third degree of upper back** CC H5 PE
    Corrosion of third degree of interscapular region

√x 7ᵗʰ **T21.74** **Corrosion of third degree of lower back** CC H5 PE

√x 7ᵗʰ **T21.75** **Corrosion of third degree of buttock** CC H5 PE
    Corrosion of third degree of anus

√x 7ᵗʰ **T21.76** **Corrosion of third degree of male genital region** CC H5 PE
    Corrosion of third degree of penis
    Corrosion of third degree of scrotum
    Corrosion of third degree of testis

√x 7ᵗʰ **T21.77** **Corrosion of third degree of female genital region** CC H5 PE
    Corrosion of third degree of labium (majus) (minus)
    Corrosion of third degree of perineum
    Corrosion of third degree of vulva
    EXCLUDES 2   corrosion of vagina (T28.8)

√x 7ᵗʰ **T21.79** **Corrosion of third degree of other site of trunk** CC H5 PE

√4ᵗʰ **T22** **Burn and corrosion of shoulder and upper limb, except wrist and hand**
    EXCLUDES 2   burn and corrosion of interscapular region (T21.-)
            burn and corrosion of wrist and hand (T23.-)

> The appropriate 7th character is to be added to each code from category T22.
> A   initial encounter
> D   subsequent encounter
> S   sequela

√5ᵗʰ **T22.0** **Burn of unspecified degree of shoulder and upper limb, except wrist and hand**
    Use additional external cause code to identify the source, place and intent of the burn (X00-X19, X75-X77, X96-X98, Y92)

√x 7ᵗʰ **T22.00** **Burn of unspecified degree of shoulder and upper limb, except wrist and hand, unspecified site** PE

√6ᵗʰ **T22.01** **Burn of unspecified degree of forearm**

    √7ᵗʰ **T22.011** **Burn of unspecified degree of right forearm** PE

    √7ᵗʰ **T22.012** **Burn of unspecified degree of left forearm** PE

    √7ᵗʰ **T22.019** **Burn of unspecified degree of unspecified forearm** PE

√6ᵗʰ **T22.02** **Burn of unspecified degree of elbow**

    √7ᵗʰ **T22.021** **Burn of unspecified degree of right elbow** PE

    √7ᵗʰ **T22.022** **Burn of unspecified degree of left elbow** PE

    √7ᵗʰ **T22.029** **Burn of unspecified degree of unspecified elbow** PE

√6ᵗʰ **T22.03** **Burn of unspecified degree of upper arm**

    √7ᵗʰ **T22.031** **Burn of unspecified degree of right upper arm** PE

    √7ᵗʰ **T22.032** **Burn of unspecified degree of left upper arm** PE

    √7ᵗʰ **T22.039** **Burn of unspecified degree of unspecified upper arm** PE

√6ᵗʰ **T22.04** **Burn of unspecified degree of axilla**

    √7ᵗʰ **T22.041** **Burn of unspecified degree of right axilla** PE

☑ Additional Character Required   √x 7ᵗʰ Placeholder   Questionable PDx   Manifestation   Unspecified   UPD Unacceptable PDx   H1 - H14 HAC   HCC CMS-HCC Dx   HIV HIV Dx

ICD-10-CM 2025   1119

Chapter 19. Injury, Poisoning and Certain Other Consequences of External Causes

√7ᵗʰ **T22.042** Burn of unspecified degree of left axilla `PE`

√7ᵗʰ **T22.049** Burn of unspecified degree of unspecified axilla `PE`

√6ᵗʰ **T22.05** Burn of unspecified degree of shoulder

√7ᵗʰ **T22.051** Burn of unspecified degree of right shoulder `PE`

√7ᵗʰ **T22.052** Burn of unspecified degree of left shoulder `PE`

√7ᵗʰ **T22.059** Burn of unspecified degree of unspecified shoulder `PE`

√6ᵗʰ **T22.06** Burn of unspecified degree of scapular region

√7ᵗʰ **T22.061** Burn of unspecified degree of right scapular region `PE`

√7ᵗʰ **T22.062** Burn of unspecified degree of left scapular region `PE`

√7ᵗʰ **T22.069** Burn of unspecified degree of unspecified scapular region `PE`

√6ᵗʰ **T22.09** Burn of unspecified degree of multiple sites of shoulder and upper limb, except wrist and hand

√7ᵗʰ **T22.091** Burn of unspecified degree of multiple sites of right shoulder and upper limb, except wrist and hand `PE`

√7ᵗʰ **T22.092** Burn of unspecified degree of multiple sites of left shoulder and upper limb, except wrist and hand `PE`

√7ᵗʰ **T22.099** Burn of unspecified degree of multiple sites of unspecified shoulder and upper limb, except wrist and hand `PE`

√5ᵗʰ **T22.1** Burn of first degree of shoulder and upper limb, except wrist and hand

Use additional external cause code to identify the source, place and intent of the burn (X00-X19, X75-X77, X96-X98, Y92)

√x 7ᵗʰ **T22.10** Burn of first degree of shoulder and upper limb, except wrist and hand, unspecified site `PE`

√6ᵗʰ **T22.11** Burn of first degree of forearm

√7ᵗʰ **T22.111** Burn of first degree of right forearm `PE`

√7ᵗʰ **T22.112** Burn of first degree of left forearm `PE`

√7ᵗʰ **T22.119** Burn of first degree of unspecified forearm `PE`

√6ᵗʰ **T22.12** Burn of first degree of elbow

√7ᵗʰ **T22.121** Burn of first degree of right elbow `PE`

√7ᵗʰ **T22.122** Burn of first degree of left elbow `PE`

√7ᵗʰ **T22.129** Burn of first degree of unspecified elbow `PE`

√6ᵗʰ **T22.13** Burn of first degree of upper arm

√7ᵗʰ **T22.131** Burn of first degree of right upper arm `PE`

√7ᵗʰ **T22.132** Burn of first degree of left upper arm `PE`

√7ᵗʰ **T22.139** Burn of first degree of unspecified upper arm `PE`

√6ᵗʰ **T22.14** Burn of first degree of axilla

√7ᵗʰ **T22.141** Burn of first degree of right axilla `PE`

√7ᵗʰ **T22.142** Burn of first degree of left axilla `PE`

√7ᵗʰ **T22.149** Burn of first degree of unspecified axilla `PE`

√6ᵗʰ **T22.15** Burn of first degree of shoulder

√7ᵗʰ **T22.151** Burn of first degree of right shoulder `PE`

√7ᵗʰ **T22.152** Burn of first degree of left shoulder `PE`

√7ᵗʰ **T22.159** Burn of first degree of unspecified shoulder `PE`

√6ᵗʰ **T22.16** Burn of first degree of scapular region

√7ᵗʰ **T22.161** Burn of first degree of right scapular region `PE`

√7ᵗʰ **T22.162** Burn of first degree of left scapular region `PE`

√7ᵗʰ **T22.169** Burn of first degree of unspecified scapular region `PE`

√6ᵗʰ **T22.19** Burn of first degree of multiple sites of shoulder and upper limb, except wrist and hand

√7ᵗʰ **T22.191** Burn of first degree of multiple sites of right shoulder and upper limb, except wrist and hand `PE`

√7ᵗʰ **T22.192** Burn of first degree of multiple sites of left shoulder and upper limb, except wrist and hand `PE`

√7ᵗʰ **T22.199** Burn of first degree of multiple sites of unspecified shoulder and upper limb, except wrist and hand `PE`

√5ᵗʰ **T22.2** Burn of second degree of shoulder and upper limb, except wrist and hand

Use additional external cause code to identify the source, place and intent of the burn (X00-X19, X75-X77, X96-X98, Y92)

√x 7ᵗʰ **T22.20** Burn of second degree of shoulder and upper limb, except wrist and hand, unspecified site `PE`

√6ᵗʰ **T22.21** Burn of second degree of forearm

√7ᵗʰ **T22.211** Burn of second degree of right forearm `PE`

√7ᵗʰ **T22.212** Burn of second degree of left forearm `PE`

√7ᵗʰ **T22.219** Burn of second degree of unspecified forearm `PE`

√6ᵗʰ **T22.22** Burn of second degree of elbow

√7ᵗʰ **T22.221** Burn of second degree of right elbow `PE`

√7ᵗʰ **T22.222** Burn of second degree of left elbow `PE`

√7ᵗʰ **T22.229** Burn of second degree of unspecified elbow `PE`

√6ᵗʰ **T22.23** Burn of second degree of upper arm

√7ᵗʰ **T22.231** Burn of second degree of right upper arm `PE`

√7ᵗʰ **T22.232** Burn of second degree of left upper arm `PE`

√7ᵗʰ **T22.239** Burn of second degree of unspecified upper arm `PE`

√6ᵗʰ **T22.24** Burn of second degree of axilla

√7ᵗʰ **T22.241** Burn of second degree of right axilla `PE`

√7ᵗʰ **T22.242** Burn of second degree of left axilla `PE`

√7ᵗʰ **T22.249** Burn of second degree of unspecified axilla `PE`

√6ᵗʰ **T22.25** Burn of second degree of shoulder

√7ᵗʰ **T22.251** Burn of second degree of right shoulder `PE`

√7ᵗʰ **T22.252** Burn of second degree of left shoulder `PE`

√7ᵗʰ **T22.259** Burn of second degree of unspecified shoulder `PE`

√6ᵗʰ **T22.26** Burn of second degree of scapular region

√7ᵗʰ **T22.261** Burn of second degree of right scapular region `PE`

√7ᵗʰ **T22.262** Burn of second degree of left scapular region `PE`

√7ᵗʰ **T22.269** Burn of second degree of unspecified scapular region `PE`

√6ᵗʰ **T22.29** Burn of second degree of multiple sites of shoulder and upper limb, except wrist and hand

√7ᵗʰ **T22.291** Burn of second degree of multiple sites of right shoulder and upper limb, except wrist and hand `PE`

√7ᵗʰ **T22.292** Burn of second degree of multiple sites of left shoulder and upper limb, except wrist and hand `PE`

√7ᵗʰ **T22.299** Burn of second degree of multiple sites of unspecified shoulder and upper limb, except wrist and hand `PE`

√5ᵗʰ **T22.3** Burn of third degree of shoulder and upper limb, except wrist and hand

Use additional external cause code to identify the source, place and intent of the burn (X00-X19, X75-X77, X96-X98, Y92)

√x 7ᵗʰ **T22.30** Burn of third degree of shoulder and upper limb, except wrist and hand, unspecified site `CC` `H5` `UNS` `PE`

√6ᵗʰ **T22.31** Burn of third degree of forearm

√7ᵗʰ **T22.311** Burn of third degree of right forearm `CC` `H5` `PE`

√7ᵗʰ **T22.312** Burn of third degree of left forearm `CC` `H5` `PE`

√7ᵗʰ **T22.319** Burn of third degree of unspecified forearm `CC` `H5` `UNS` `PE`

N Newborn: 0   **P** Pediatric: 0-17   **M** Maternity: 9-64   **A** Adult: 15-124   **UNS** Unspecified Site   **MCC** Major Complication/Comorbidity   **CC** Complication/Comorbidity   **PE** POA Exempt

1120

ICD-10-CM 2025

√6ᵗʰ **T22.32** Burn of third degree of **elbow**
- √7ᵗʰ **T22.321** Burn of third degree of **right** elbow `CC` `H5` `PE`
- √7ᵗʰ **T22.322** Burn of third degree of **left** elbow `CC` `H5` `PE`
- √7ᵗʰ **T22.329** Burn of third degree of unspecified elbow `CC` `H5` `UNS` `PE`

√6ᵗʰ **T22.33** Burn of third degree of **upper arm**
- √7ᵗʰ **T22.331** Burn of third degree of **right** upper arm `CC` `H5` `PE`
- √7ᵗʰ **T22.332** Burn of third degree of **left** upper arm `CC` `H5` `PE`
- √7ᵗʰ **T22.339** Burn of third degree of unspecified upper arm `CC` `H5` `UNS` `PE`

√6ᵗʰ **T22.34** Burn of third degree of **axilla**
- √7ᵗʰ **T22.341** Burn of third degree of **right** axilla `CC` `H5` `PE`
- √7ᵗʰ **T22.342** Burn of third degree of **left** axilla `CC` `H5` `PE`
- √7ᵗʰ **T22.349** Burn of third degree of unspecified axilla `CC` `H5` `UNS` `PE`

√6ᵗʰ **T22.35** Burn of third degree of **shoulder**
- √7ᵗʰ **T22.351** Burn of third degree of **right** shoulder `CC` `H5` `PE`
- √7ᵗʰ **T22.352** Burn of third degree of **left** shoulder `CC` `H5` `PE`
- √7ᵗʰ **T22.359** Burn of third degree of unspecified shoulder `CC` `H5` `UNS` `PE`

√6ᵗʰ **T22.36** Burn of third degree of **scapular region**
- √7ᵗʰ **T22.361** Burn of third degree of **right** scapular region `CC` `H5` `PE`
- √7ᵗʰ **T22.362** Burn of third degree of **left** scapular region `CC` `H5` `PE`
- √7ᵗʰ **T22.369** Burn of third degree of unspecified scapular region `CC` `H5` `UNS` `PE`

√6ᵗʰ **T22.39** Burn of third degree of **multiple sites** of shoulder and upper limb, except wrist and hand
- √7ᵗʰ **T22.391** Burn of third degree of multiple sites of **right** shoulder and upper limb, except wrist and hand `CC` `H5` `PE`
- √7ᵗʰ **T22.392** Burn of third degree of multiple sites of **left** shoulder and upper limb, except wrist and hand `CC` `H5` `PE`
- √7ᵗʰ **T22.399** Burn of third degree of multiple sites of unspecified shoulder and upper limb, except wrist and hand `CC` `H5` `PE`

√5ᵗʰ **T22.4** Corrosion of unspecified degree of shoulder and upper limb, except wrist and hand
> Code first (T51-T65) to identify chemical and intent
> Use additional external cause code to identify place (Y92)

√x 7ᵗʰ **T22.40** Corrosion of unspecified degree of shoulder and upper limb, except wrist and hand, unspecified site `PE`

√6ᵗʰ **T22.41** Corrosion of unspecified degree of **forearm**
- √7ᵗʰ **T22.411** Corrosion of unspecified degree of **right** forearm `PE`
- √7ᵗʰ **T22.412** Corrosion of unspecified degree of **left** forearm `PE`
- √7ᵗʰ **T22.419** Corrosion of unspecified degree of unspecified forearm `PE`

√6ᵗʰ **T22.42** Corrosion of unspecified degree of **elbow**
- √7ᵗʰ **T22.421** Corrosion of unspecified degree of **right** elbow `PE`
- √7ᵗʰ **T22.422** Corrosion of unspecified degree of **left** elbow `PE`
- √7ᵗʰ **T22.429** Corrosion of unspecified degree of unspecified elbow `PE`

√6ᵗʰ **T22.43** Corrosion of unspecified degree of **upper arm**
- √7ᵗʰ **T22.431** Corrosion of unspecified degree of **right** upper arm `PE`
- √7ᵗʰ **T22.432** Corrosion of unspecified degree of **left** upper arm `PE`
- √7ᵗʰ **T22.439** Corrosion of unspecified degree of unspecified upper arm `PE`

√6ᵗʰ **T22.44** Corrosion of unspecified degree of **axilla**
- √7ᵗʰ **T22.441** Corrosion of unspecified degree of **right** axilla `PE`

√7ᵗʰ **T22.442** Corrosion of unspecified degree of **left** axilla `PE`
- √7ᵗʰ **T22.449** Corrosion of unspecified degree of unspecified axilla `PE`

√6ᵗʰ **T22.45** Corrosion of unspecified degree of **shoulder**
- √7ᵗʰ **T22.451** Corrosion of unspecified degree of **right** shoulder `PE`
- √7ᵗʰ **T22.452** Corrosion of unspecified degree of **left** shoulder `PE`
- √7ᵗʰ **T22.459** Corrosion of unspecified degree of unspecified shoulder `PE`

√6ᵗʰ **T22.46** Corrosion of unspecified degree of **scapular region**
- √7ᵗʰ **T22.461** Corrosion of unspecified degree of **right** scapular region `PE`
- √7ᵗʰ **T22.462** Corrosion of unspecified degree of **left** scapular region `PE`
- √7ᵗʰ **T22.469** Corrosion of unspecified degree of unspecified scapular region `PE`

√6ᵗʰ **T22.49** Corrosion of unspecified degree of **multiple sites** of shoulder and upper limb, except wrist and hand
- √7ᵗʰ **T22.491** Corrosion of unspecified degree of multiple sites of **right** shoulder and upper limb, except wrist and hand `PE`
- √7ᵗʰ **T22.492** Corrosion of unspecified degree of multiple sites of **left** shoulder and upper limb, except wrist and hand `PE`
- √7ᵗʰ **T22.499** Corrosion of unspecified degree of multiple sites of unspecified shoulder and upper limb, except wrist and hand `PE`

√5ᵗʰ **T22.5** Corrosion of **first degree** of shoulder and upper limb, except wrist and hand
> Code first (T51-T65) to identify chemical and intent
> Use additional external cause code to identify place (Y92)

√x 7ᵗʰ **T22.50** Corrosion of first degree of shoulder and upper limb, except wrist and hand unspecified site `PE`

√6ᵗʰ **T22.51** Corrosion of first degree of **forearm**
- √7ᵗʰ **T22.511** Corrosion of first degree of **right** forearm `PE`
- √7ᵗʰ **T22.512** Corrosion of first degree of **left** forearm `PE`
- √7ᵗʰ **T22.519** Corrosion of first degree of unspecified forearm `PE`

√6ᵗʰ **T22.52** Corrosion of first degree of **elbow**
- √7ᵗʰ **T22.521** Corrosion of first degree of **right** elbow `PE`
- √7ᵗʰ **T22.522** Corrosion of first degree of **left** elbow `PE`
- √7ᵗʰ **T22.529** Corrosion of first degree of unspecified elbow `PE`

√6ᵗʰ **T22.53** Corrosion of first degree of **upper arm**
- √7ᵗʰ **T22.531** Corrosion of first degree of **right** upper arm `PE`
- √7ᵗʰ **T22.532** Corrosion of first degree of **left** upper arm `PE`
- √7ᵗʰ **T22.539** Corrosion of first degree of unspecified upper arm `PE`

√6ᵗʰ **T22.54** Corrosion of first degree of **axilla**
- √7ᵗʰ **T22.541** Corrosion of first degree of **right** axilla `PE`
- √7ᵗʰ **T22.542** Corrosion of first degree of **left** axilla `PE`
- √7ᵗʰ **T22.549** Corrosion of first degree of unspecified axilla `PE`

√6ᵗʰ **T22.55** Corrosion of first degree of **shoulder**
- √7ᵗʰ **T22.551** Corrosion of first degree of **right** shoulder `PE`
- √7ᵗʰ **T22.552** Corrosion of first degree of **left** shoulder `PE`
- √7ᵗʰ **T22.559** Corrosion of first degree of unspecified shoulder `PE`

√6ᵗʰ **T22.56** Corrosion of first degree of **scapular region**
- √7ᵗʰ **T22.561** Corrosion of first degree of **right** scapular region `PE`
- √7ᵗʰ **T22.562** Corrosion of first degree of **left** scapular region `PE`
- √7ᵗʰ **T22.569** Corrosion of first degree of unspecified scapular region `PE`

☑ Additional Character Required | √x 7ᵗʰ Placeholder | Questionable PDx | Manifestation | Unspecified | UPD Unacceptable PDx | H1 - H14 HAC | HCC CMS-HCC Dx | HIV HIV Dx

ICD-10-CM 2025   1121

Chapter 19. Injury, Poisoning and Certain Other Consequences of External Causes

T22.32–T22.569

√6th **T22.59** Corrosion of first degree of multiple sites of shoulder and upper limb, except wrist and hand

     √7th **T22.591** Corrosion of first degree of multiple sites of right shoulder and upper limb, except wrist and hand   PE

     √7th **T22.592** Corrosion of first degree of multiple sites of left shoulder and upper limb, except wrist and hand   PE

     √7th **T22.599** Corrosion of first degree of multiple sites of unspecified shoulder and upper limb, except wrist and hand   PE

√5th **T22.6** Corrosion of second degree of shoulder and upper limb, except wrist and hand

     Code first (T51-T65) to identify chemical and intent
     Use additional external cause code to identify place (Y92)

√x7th **T22.60** Corrosion of second degree of shoulder and upper limb, except wrist and hand, unspecified site   PE

√6th **T22.61** Corrosion of second degree of forearm

     √7th **T22.611** Corrosion of second degree of right forearm   PE

     √7th **T22.612** Corrosion of second degree of left forearm   PE

     √7th **T22.619** Corrosion of second degree of unspecified forearm   PE

√6th **T22.62** Corrosion of second degree of elbow

     √7th **T22.621** Corrosion of second degree of right elbow   PE

     √7th **T22.622** Corrosion of second degree of left elbow   PE

     √7th **T22.629** Corrosion of second degree of unspecified elbow   PE

√6th **T22.63** Corrosion of second degree of upper arm

     √7th **T22.631** Corrosion of second degree of right upper arm   PE

     √7th **T22.632** Corrosion of second degree of left upper arm   PE

     √7th **T22.639** Corrosion of second degree of unspecified upper arm   PE

√6th **T22.64** Corrosion of second degree of axilla

     √7th **T22.641** Corrosion of second degree of right axilla   PE

     √7th **T22.642** Corrosion of second degree of left axilla   PE

     √7th **T22.649** Corrosion of second degree of unspecified axilla   PE

√6th **T22.65** Corrosion of second degree of shoulder

     √7th **T22.651** Corrosion of second degree of right shoulder   PE

     √7th **T22.652** Corrosion of second degree of left shoulder   PE

     √7th **T22.659** Corrosion of second degree of unspecified shoulder   PE

√6th **T22.66** Corrosion of second degree of scapular region

     √7th **T22.661** Corrosion of second degree of right scapular region   PE

     √7th **T22.662** Corrosion of second degree of left scapular region   PE

     √7th **T22.669** Corrosion of second degree of unspecified scapular region   PE

√6th **T22.69** Corrosion of second degree of multiple sites of shoulder and upper limb, except wrist and hand

     √7th **T22.691** Corrosion of second degree of multiple sites of right shoulder and upper limb, except wrist and hand   PE

     √7th **T22.692** Corrosion of second degree of multiple sites of left shoulder and upper limb, except wrist and hand   PE

     √7th **T22.699** Corrosion of second degree of multiple sites of unspecified shoulder and upper limb, except wrist and hand   PE

√5th **T22.7** Corrosion of third degree of shoulder and upper limb, except wrist and hand

     Code first (T51-T65) to identify chemical and intent
     Use additional external cause code to identify place (Y92)

√x7th **T22.70** Corrosion of third degree of shoulder and upper limb, except wrist and hand, unspecified site   CC H5 UNS PE

√6th **T22.71** Corrosion of third degree of forearm

     √7th **T22.711** Corrosion of third degree of right forearm   CC H5 PE

     √7th **T22.712** Corrosion of third degree of left forearm   CC H5 PE

     √7th **T22.719** Corrosion of third degree of unspecified forearm   CC H5 UNS PE

√6th **T22.72** Corrosion of third degree of elbow

     √7th **T22.721** Corrosion of third degree of right elbow   CC H5 PE

     √7th **T22.722** Corrosion of third degree of left elbow   CC H5 PE

     √7th **T22.729** Corrosion of third degree of unspecified elbow   CC H5 UNS PE

√6th **T22.73** Corrosion of third degree of upper arm

     √7th **T22.731** Corrosion of third degree of right upper arm   CC H5 PE

     √7th **T22.732** Corrosion of third degree of left upper arm   CC H5 PE

     √7th **T22.739** Corrosion of third degree of unspecified upper arm   CC H5 UNS PE

√6th **T22.74** Corrosion of third degree of axilla

     √7th **T22.741** Corrosion of third degree of right axilla   CC H5 PE

     √7th **T22.742** Corrosion of third degree of left axilla   CC H5 PE

     √7th **T22.749** Corrosion of third degree of unspecified axilla   CC H5 UNS PE

√6th **T22.75** Corrosion of third degree of shoulder

     √7th **T22.751** Corrosion of third degree of right shoulder   CC H5 PE

     √7th **T22.752** Corrosion of third degree of left shoulder   CC H5 PE

     √7th **T22.759** Corrosion of third degree of unspecified shoulder   CC H5 UNS PE

√6th **T22.76** Corrosion of third degree of scapular region

     √7th **T22.761** Corrosion of third degree of right scapular region   CC H5 PE

     √7th **T22.762** Corrosion of third degree of left scapular region   CC H5 PE

     √7th **T22.769** Corrosion of third degree of unspecified scapular region   CC H5 UNS PE

√6th **T22.79** Corrosion of third degree of multiple sites of shoulder and upper limb, except wrist and hand

     √7th **T22.791** Corrosion of third degree of multiple sites of right shoulder and upper limb, except wrist and hand   CC H5 PE

     √7th **T22.792** Corrosion of third degree of multiple sites of left shoulder and upper limb, except wrist and hand   CC H5 PE

     √7th **T22.799** Corrosion of third degree of multiple sites of unspecified shoulder and upper limb, except wrist and hand   CC H5 PE

√4th **T23** Burn and corrosion of wrist and hand

     AHA: 2015,1Q,19

     The appropriate 7th character is to be added to each code from category T23.
     A   initial encounter
     D   subsequent encounter
     S   sequela

√5th **T23.0** Burn of unspecified degree of wrist and hand

     Use additional external cause code to identify the source, place and intent of the burn (X00-X19, X75-X77, X96-X98, Y92)

√6th **T23.00** Burn of unspecified degree of hand, unspecified site

     √7th **T23.001** Burn of unspecified degree of right hand, unspecified site   PE

     √7th **T23.002** Burn of unspecified degree of left hand, unspecified site   PE

     √7th **T23.009** Burn of unspecified degree of unspecified hand, unspecified site   PE

√6th **T23.01** Burn of unspecified degree of thumb (nail)

     √7th **T23.011** Burn of unspecified degree of right thumb (nail)   PE

     √7th **T23.012** Burn of unspecified degree of left thumb (nail)   PE

√7ᵗʰ **T23.019** Burn of unspecified degree of unspecified thumb (nail)   **PE**

√6ᵗʰ **T23.02** Burn of unspecified degree of single finger (nail) except thumb

√7ᵗʰ **T23.021** Burn of unspecified degree of single right finger (nail) except thumb   **PE**

√7ᵗʰ **T23.022** Burn of unspecified degree of single left finger (nail) except thumb   **PE**

√7ᵗʰ **T23.029** Burn of unspecified degree of unspecified single finger (nail) except thumb   **PE**

√6ᵗʰ **T23.03** Burn of unspecified degree of multiple fingers (nail), not including thumb

√7ᵗʰ **T23.031** Burn of unspecified degree of multiple right fingers (nail), not including thumb   **PE**

√7ᵗʰ **T23.032** Burn of unspecified degree of multiple left fingers (nail), not including thumb   **PE**

√7ᵗʰ **T23.039** Burn of unspecified degree of unspecified multiple fingers (nail), not including thumb   **PE**

√6ᵗʰ **T23.04** Burn of unspecified degree of multiple fingers (nail), including thumb

√7ᵗʰ **T23.041** Burn of unspecified degree of multiple right fingers (nail), including thumb   **PE**

√7ᵗʰ **T23.042** Burn of unspecified degree of multiple left fingers (nail), including thumb   **PE**

√7ᵗʰ **T23.049** Burn of unspecified degree of unspecified multiple fingers (nail), including thumb   **PE**

√6ᵗʰ **T23.05** Burn of unspecified degree of palm

√7ᵗʰ **T23.051** Burn of unspecified degree of right palm   **PE**

√7ᵗʰ **T23.052** Burn of unspecified degree of left palm   **PE**

√7ᵗʰ **T23.059** Burn of unspecified degree of unspecified palm   **PE**

√6ᵗʰ **T23.06** Burn of unspecified degree of back of hand

√7ᵗʰ **T23.061** Burn of unspecified degree of back of right hand   **PE**

√7ᵗʰ **T23.062** Burn of unspecified degree of back of left hand   **PE**

√7ᵗʰ **T23.069** Burn of unspecified degree of back of unspecified hand   **PE**

√6ᵗʰ **T23.07** Burn of unspecified degree of wrist

√7ᵗʰ **T23.071** Burn of unspecified degree of right wrist   **PE**

√7ᵗʰ **T23.072** Burn of unspecified degree of left wrist   **PE**

√7ᵗʰ **T23.079** Burn of unspecified degree of unspecified wrist   **PE**

√6ᵗʰ **T23.09** Burn of unspecified degree of multiple sites of wrist and hand

√7ᵗʰ **T23.091** Burn of unspecified degree of multiple sites of right wrist and hand   **PE**

√7ᵗʰ **T23.092** Burn of unspecified degree of multiple sites of left wrist and hand   **PE**

√7ᵗʰ **T23.099** Burn of unspecified degree of multiple sites of unspecified wrist and hand   **PE**

√5ᵗʰ **T23.1** Burn of first degree of wrist and hand

Use additional external cause code to identify the source, place and intent of the burn (X00-X19, X75-X77, X96-X98, Y92)

√6ᵗʰ **T23.10** Burn of first degree of hand, unspecified site

√7ᵗʰ **T23.101** Burn of first degree of right hand, unspecified site   **PE**

√7ᵗʰ **T23.102** Burn of first degree of left hand, unspecified site   **PE**

√7ᵗʰ **T23.109** Burn of first degree of unspecified hand, unspecified site   **PE**

√6ᵗʰ **T23.11** Burn of first degree of thumb (nail)

√7ᵗʰ **T23.111** Burn of first degree of right thumb (nail)   **PE**

√7ᵗʰ **T23.112** Burn of first degree of left thumb (nail)   **PE**

√7ᵗʰ **T23.119** Burn of first degree of unspecified thumb (nail)   **PE**

√6ᵗʰ **T23.12** Burn of first degree of single finger (nail) except thumb

√7ᵗʰ **T23.121** Burn of first degree of single right finger (nail) except thumb   **PE**

√7ᵗʰ **T23.122** Burn of first degree of single left finger (nail) except thumb   **PE**

√7ᵗʰ **T23.129** Burn of first degree of unspecified single finger (nail) except thumb   **PE**

√6ᵗʰ **T23.13** Burn of first degree of multiple fingers (nail), not including thumb

√7ᵗʰ **T23.131** Burn of first degree of multiple right fingers (nail), not including thumb   **PE**

√7ᵗʰ **T23.132** Burn of first degree of multiple left fingers (nail), not including thumb   **PE**

√7ᵗʰ **T23.139** Burn of first degree of unspecified multiple fingers (nail), not including thumb   **PE**

√6ᵗʰ **T23.14** Burn of first degree of multiple fingers (nail), including thumb

√7ᵗʰ **T23.141** Burn of first degree of multiple right fingers (nail), including thumb   **PE**

√7ᵗʰ **T23.142** Burn of first degree of multiple left fingers (nail), including thumb   **PE**

√7ᵗʰ **T23.149** Burn of first degree of unspecified multiple fingers (nail), including thumb   **PE**

√6ᵗʰ **T23.15** Burn of first degree of palm

√7ᵗʰ **T23.151** Burn of first degree of right palm   **PE**

√7ᵗʰ **T23.152** Burn of first degree of left palm   **PE**

√7ᵗʰ **T23.159** Burn of first degree of unspecified palm   **PE**

√6ᵗʰ **T23.16** Burn of first degree of back of hand

√7ᵗʰ **T23.161** Burn of first degree of back of right hand   **PE**

√7ᵗʰ **T23.162** Burn of first degree of back of left hand   **PE**

√7ᵗʰ **T23.169** Burn of first degree of back of unspecified hand   **PE**

√6ᵗʰ **T23.17** Burn of first degree of wrist

√7ᵗʰ **T23.171** Burn of first degree of right wrist   **PE**

√7ᵗʰ **T23.172** Burn of first degree of left wrist   **PE**

√7ᵗʰ **T23.179** Burn of first degree of unspecified wrist   **PE**

√6ᵗʰ **T23.19** Burn of first degree of multiple sites of wrist and hand

√7ᵗʰ **T23.191** Burn of first degree of multiple sites of right wrist and hand   **PE**

√7ᵗʰ **T23.192** Burn of first degree of multiple sites of left wrist and hand   **PE**

√7ᵗʰ **T23.199** Burn of first degree of multiple sites of unspecified wrist and hand   **PE**

√5ᵗʰ **T23.2** Burn of second degree of wrist and hand

Use additional external cause code to identify the source, place and intent of the burn (X00-X19, X75-X77, X96-X98, Y92)

√6ᵗʰ **T23.20** Burn of second degree of hand, unspecified site

√7ᵗʰ **T23.201** Burn of second degree of right hand, unspecified site   **PE**

√7ᵗʰ **T23.202** Burn of second degree of left hand, unspecified site   **PE**

√7ᵗʰ **T23.209** Burn of second degree of unspecified hand, unspecified site   **PE**

√6ᵗʰ **T23.21** Burn of second degree of thumb (nail)

√7ᵗʰ **T23.211** Burn of second degree of right thumb (nail)   **PE**

√7ᵗʰ **T23.212** Burn of second degree of left thumb (nail)   **PE**

√7ᵗʰ **T23.219** Burn of second degree of unspecified thumb (nail)   **PE**

√6ᵗʰ **T23.22** Burn of second degree of single finger (nail) except thumb

√7ᵗʰ **T23.221** Burn of second degree of single right finger (nail) except thumb   **PE**

√7ᵗʰ **T23.222** Burn of second degree of single left finger (nail) except thumb   **PE**

√7ᵗʰ **T23.229** Burn of second degree of unspecified single finger (nail) except thumb   **PE**

√6ᵗʰ **T23.23** Burn of second degree of multiple fingers (nail), not including thumb

√7ᵗʰ **T23.231** Burn of second degree of multiple right fingers (nail), not including thumb   **PE**

√7ᵗʰ **T23.232** Burn of second degree of multiple left fingers (nail), not including thumb   **PE**

√7ᵗʰ **T23.239** Burn of second degree of unspecified multiple fingers (nail), not including thumb   **PE**

√6ᵗʰ **T23.24** Burn of second degree of multiple fingers (nail), including thumb

√7ᵗʰ **T23.241** Burn of second degree of multiple right fingers (nail), including thumb **PE**

√7ᵗʰ **T23.242** Burn of second degree of multiple left fingers (nail), including thumb **PE**

√7ᵗʰ **T23.249** Burn of second degree of unspecified multiple fingers (nail), including thumb **PE**

√6ᵗʰ **T23.25** Burn of second degree of palm

√7ᵗʰ **T23.251** Burn of second degree of right palm **PE**

√7ᵗʰ **T23.252** Burn of second degree of left palm **PE**

√7ᵗʰ **T23.259** Burn of second degree of unspecified palm **PE**

√6ᵗʰ **T23.26** Burn of second degree of back of hand

√7ᵗʰ **T23.261** Burn of second degree of back of right hand **PE**

√7ᵗʰ **T23.262** Burn of second degree of back of left hand **PE**

√7ᵗʰ **T23.269** Burn of second degree of back of unspecified hand **PE**

√6ᵗʰ **T23.27** Burn of second degree of wrist

√7ᵗʰ **T23.271** Burn of second degree of right wrist **PE**

√7ᵗʰ **T23.272** Burn of second degree of left wrist **PE**

√7ᵗʰ **T23.279** Burn of second degree of unspecified wrist **PE**

√6ᵗʰ **T23.29** Burn of second degree of multiple sites of wrist and hand

√7ᵗʰ **T23.291** Burn of second degree of multiple sites of right wrist and hand **PE**

√7ᵗʰ **T23.292** Burn of second degree of multiple sites of left wrist and hand **PE**

√7ᵗʰ **T23.299** Burn of second degree of multiple sites of unspecified wrist and hand **PE**

√5ᵗʰ **T23.3** Burn of third degree of wrist and hand

Use additional external cause code to identify the source, place and intent of the burn (X00-X19, X75-X77, X96-X98, Y92)

√6ᵗʰ **T23.30** Burn of third degree of hand, unspecified site

AHA: 2016,2Q,5

√7ᵗʰ **T23.301** Burn of third degree of right hand, unspecified site **CC** **H5** **PE**

√7ᵗʰ **T23.302** Burn of third degree of left hand, unspecified site **CC** **H5** **PE**

√7ᵗʰ **T23.309** Burn of third degree of unspecified hand, unspecified site **CC** **H5** **UNS** **PE**

√6ᵗʰ **T23.31** Burn of third degree of thumb (nail)

√7ᵗʰ **T23.311** Burn of third degree of right thumb (nail) **CC** **H5** **PE**

√7ᵗʰ **T23.312** Burn of third degree of left thumb (nail) **CC** **H5** **PE**

√7ᵗʰ **T23.319** Burn of third degree of unspecified thumb (nail) **CC** **H5** **UNS** **PE**

√6ᵗʰ **T23.32** Burn of third degree of single finger (nail) except thumb

√7ᵗʰ **T23.321** Burn of third degree of single right finger (nail) except thumb **CC** **H5** **PE**

√7ᵗʰ **T23.322** Burn of third degree of single left finger (nail) except thumb **CC** **H5** **PE**

√7ᵗʰ **T23.329** Burn of third degree of unspecified single finger (nail) except thumb **CC** **H5** **UNS** **PE**

√6ᵗʰ **T23.33** Burn of third degree of multiple fingers (nail), not including thumb

√7ᵗʰ **T23.331** Burn of third degree of multiple right fingers (nail), not including thumb **CC** **H5** **PE**

√7ᵗʰ **T23.332** Burn of third degree of multiple left fingers (nail), not including thumb **CC** **H5** **PE**

√7ᵗʰ **T23.339** Burn of third degree of unspecified multiple fingers (nail), not including thumb **CC** **H5** **UNS** **PE**

√6ᵗʰ **T23.34** Burn of third degree of multiple fingers (nail), including thumb

√7ᵗʰ **T23.341** Burn of third degree of multiple right fingers (nail), including thumb **CC** **H5** **PE**

√7ᵗʰ **T23.342** Burn of third degree of multiple left fingers (nail), including thumb **CC** **H5** **PE**

√7ᵗʰ **T23.349** Burn of third degree of unspecified multiple fingers (nail), including thumb **CC** **H5** **UNS** **PE**

√6ᵗʰ **T23.35** Burn of third degree of palm

√7ᵗʰ **T23.351** Burn of third degree of right palm **CC** **H5** **PE**

√7ᵗʰ **T23.352** Burn of third degree of left palm **CC** **H5** **PE**

√7ᵗʰ **T23.359** Burn of third degree of unspecified palm **CC** **H5** **UNS** **PE**

√6ᵗʰ **T23.36** Burn of third degree of back of hand

√7ᵗʰ **T23.361** Burn of third degree of back of right hand **CC** **H5** **PE**

√7ᵗʰ **T23.362** Burn of third degree of back of left hand **CC** **H5** **PE**

√7ᵗʰ **T23.369** Burn of third degree of back of unspecified hand

√6ᵗʰ **T23.37** Burn of third degree of wrist

√7ᵗʰ **T23.371** Burn of third degree of right wrist **CC** **H5** **PE**

√7ᵗʰ **T23.372** Burn of third degree of left wrist **CC** **H5** **PE**

√7ᵗʰ **T23.379** Burn of third degree of unspecified wrist **CC** **H5** **UNS** **PE**

√6ᵗʰ **T23.39** Burn of third degree of multiple sites of wrist and hand

√7ᵗʰ **T23.391** Burn of third degree of multiple sites of right wrist and hand **CC** **H5** **PE**

√7ᵗʰ **T23.392** Burn of third degree of multiple sites of left wrist and hand **CC** **H5** **PE**

√7ᵗʰ **T23.399** Burn of third degree of multiple sites of unspecified wrist and hand **CC** **H5** **UNS** **PE**

√5ᵗʰ **T23.4** Corrosion of unspecified degree of wrist and hand

Code first (T51-T65) to identify chemical and intent

Use additional external cause code to identify place (Y92)

√6ᵗʰ **T23.40** Corrosion of unspecified degree of hand, unspecified site

√7ᵗʰ **T23.401** Corrosion of unspecified degree of right hand, unspecified site **PE**

√7ᵗʰ **T23.402** Corrosion of unspecified degree of left hand, unspecified site **PE**

√7ᵗʰ **T23.409** Corrosion of unspecified degree of unspecified hand, unspecified site **PE**

√6ᵗʰ **T23.41** Corrosion of unspecified degree of thumb (nail)

√7ᵗʰ **T23.411** Corrosion of unspecified degree of right thumb (nail) **PE**

√7ᵗʰ **T23.412** Corrosion of unspecified degree of left thumb (nail) **PE**

√7ᵗʰ **T23.419** Corrosion of unspecified degree of unspecified thumb (nail) **PE**

√6ᵗʰ **T23.42** Corrosion of unspecified degree of single finger (nail) except thumb

√7ᵗʰ **T23.421** Corrosion of unspecified degree of single right finger (nail) except thumb **PE**

√7ᵗʰ **T23.422** Corrosion of unspecified degree of single left finger (nail) except thumb **PE**

√7ᵗʰ **T23.429** Corrosion of unspecified degree of unspecified single finger (nail) except thumb **PE**

√6ᵗʰ **T23.43** Corrosion of unspecified degree of multiple fingers (nail), not including thumb

√7ᵗʰ **T23.431** Corrosion of unspecified degree of multiple right fingers (nail), not including thumb **PE**

√7ᵗʰ **T23.432** Corrosion of unspecified degree of multiple left fingers (nail), not including thumb **PE**

√7ᵗʰ **T23.439** Corrosion of unspecified degree of unspecified multiple fingers (nail), not including thumb **PE**

√6ᵗʰ **T23.44** Corrosion of unspecified degree of multiple fingers (nail), including thumb

√7ᵗʰ **T23.441** Corrosion of unspecified degree of multiple right fingers (nail), including thumb **PE**

√7ᵗʰ **T23.442** Corrosion of unspecified degree of multiple left fingers (nail), including thumb **PE**

N Newborn: 0 **P** Pediatric: 0-17 **M** Maternity: 9-64 **A** Adult: 15-124 **UNS** Unspecified Site **MCC** Major Complication/Comorbidity **CC** Complication/Comorbidity **PE** POA Exempt

1124

ICD-10-CM 2025

√7ᵗʰ **T23.449** Corrosion of unspecified degree of unspecified multiple fingers (nail), including thumb **PE**

√6ᵗʰ **T23.45** Corrosion of unspecified degree of **palm**

√7ᵗʰ **T23.451** Corrosion of unspecified degree of **right** palm **PE**

√7ᵗʰ **T23.452** Corrosion of unspecified degree of **left** palm **PE**

√7ᵗʰ **T23.459** Corrosion of unspecified degree of unspecified palm **PE**

√6ᵗʰ **T23.46** Corrosion of unspecified degree of **back of hand**

√7ᵗʰ **T23.461** Corrosion of unspecified degree of back of **right** hand **PE**

√7ᵗʰ **T23.462** Corrosion of unspecified degree of back of **left** hand **PE**

√7ᵗʰ **T23.469** Corrosion of unspecified degree of back of unspecified hand **PE**

√6ᵗʰ **T23.47** Corrosion of unspecified degree of **wrist**

√7ᵗʰ **T23.471** Corrosion of unspecified degree of **right** wrist **PE**

√7ᵗʰ **T23.472** Corrosion of unspecified degree of **left** wrist **PE**

√7ᵗʰ **T23.479** Corrosion of unspecified degree of unspecified wrist **PE**

√6ᵗʰ **T23.49** Corrosion of unspecified degree of **multiple sites** of wrist and hand

√7ᵗʰ **T23.491** Corrosion of unspecified degree of multiple sites of **right** wrist and hand **PE**

√7ᵗʰ **T23.492** Corrosion of unspecified degree of multiple sites of **left** wrist and hand **PE**

√7ᵗʰ **T23.499** Corrosion of unspecified degree of multiple sites of unspecified wrist and hand **PE**

√5ᵗʰ **T23.5** Corrosion of **first degree** of wrist and hand

Code first (T51-T65) to identify chemical and intent
Use additional external cause code to identify place (Y92)

√6ᵗʰ **T23.50** Corrosion of first degree of hand, unspecified site

√7ᵗʰ **T23.501** Corrosion of first degree of **right** hand, unspecified site **PE**

√7ᵗʰ **T23.502** Corrosion of first degree of **left** hand, unspecified site **PE**

√7ᵗʰ **T23.509** Corrosion of first degree of unspecified hand, unspecified site **PE**

√6ᵗʰ **T23.51** Corrosion of first degree of **thumb** (nail)

√7ᵗʰ **T23.511** Corrosion of first degree of **right** thumb (nail) **PE**

√7ᵗʰ **T23.512** Corrosion of first degree of **left** thumb (nail) **PE**

√7ᵗʰ **T23.519** Corrosion of first degree of unspecified thumb (nail) **PE**

√6ᵗʰ **T23.52** Corrosion of first degree of **single finger** (nail) except thumb

√7ᵗʰ **T23.521** Corrosion of first degree of single **right** finger (nail) except thumb **PE**

√7ᵗʰ **T23.522** Corrosion of first degree of single **left** finger (nail) except thumb **PE**

√7ᵗʰ **T23.529** Corrosion of first degree of unspecified single finger (nail) except thumb **PE**

√6ᵗʰ **T23.53** Corrosion of first degree of **multiple fingers** (nail), **not including thumb**

√7ᵗʰ **T23.531** Corrosion of first degree of multiple **right** fingers (nail), not including thumb **PE**

√7ᵗʰ **T23.532** Corrosion of first degree of multiple **left** fingers (nail), not including thumb **PE**

√7ᵗʰ **T23.539** Corrosion of first degree of unspecified multiple fingers (nail), not including thumb

√6ᵗʰ **T23.54** Corrosion of first degree of **multiple fingers** (nail), **including thumb**

√7ᵗʰ **T23.541** Corrosion of first degree of multiple **right** fingers (nail), including thumb **PE**

√7ᵗʰ **T23.542** Corrosion of first degree of multiple **left** fingers (nail), including thumb **PE**

√7ᵗʰ **T23.549** Corrosion of first degree of unspecified multiple fingers (nail), including thumb **PE**

√6ᵗʰ **T23.55** Corrosion of first degree of **palm**

√7ᵗʰ **T23.551** Corrosion of first degree of **right** palm **PE**

√7ᵗʰ **T23.552** Corrosion of first degree of **left** palm **PE**

√7ᵗʰ **T23.559** Corrosion of first degree of unspecified palm **PE**

√6ᵗʰ **T23.56** Corrosion of first degree of **back of hand**

√7ᵗʰ **T23.561** Corrosion of first degree of back of **right** hand **PE**

√7ᵗʰ **T23.562** Corrosion of first degree of back of **left** hand **PE**

√7ᵗʰ **T23.569** Corrosion of first degree of back of unspecified hand **PE**

√6ᵗʰ **T23.57** Corrosion of first degree of **wrist**

√7ᵗʰ **T23.571** Corrosion of first degree of **right** wrist **PE**

√7ᵗʰ **T23.572** Corrosion of first degree of **left** wrist **PE**

√7ᵗʰ **T23.579** Corrosion of first degree of unspecified wrist **PE**

√6ᵗʰ **T23.59** Corrosion of first degree of **multiple sites** of wrist and hand

√7ᵗʰ **T23.591** Corrosion of first degree of multiple sites of **right** wrist and hand **PE**

√7ᵗʰ **T23.592** Corrosion of first degree of multiple sites of **left** wrist and hand **PE**

√7ᵗʰ **T23.599** Corrosion of first degree of multiple sites of unspecified wrist and hand **PE**

√5ᵗʰ **T23.6** Corrosion of **second degree** of wrist and hand

Code first (T51-T65) to identify chemical and intent
Use additional external cause code to identify place (Y92)

√6ᵗʰ **T23.60** Corrosion of second degree of hand, unspecified site

√7ᵗʰ **T23.601** Corrosion of second degree of **right** hand, unspecified site **PE**

√7ᵗʰ **T23.602** Corrosion of second degree of **left** hand, unspecified site **PE**

√7ᵗʰ **T23.609** Corrosion of second degree of unspecified hand, unspecified site **PE**

√6ᵗʰ **T23.61** Corrosion of second degree of **thumb** (nail)

√7ᵗʰ **T23.611** Corrosion of second degree of **right** thumb (nail) **PE**

√7ᵗʰ **T23.612** Corrosion of second degree of **left** thumb (nail) **PE**

√7ᵗʰ **T23.619** Corrosion of second degree of unspecified thumb (nail) **PE**

√6ᵗʰ **T23.62** Corrosion of second degree of **single finger** (nail) except thumb

√7ᵗʰ **T23.621** Corrosion of second degree of single **right** finger (nail) except thumb **PE**

√7ᵗʰ **T23.622** Corrosion of second degree of single **left** finger (nail) except thumb **PE**

√7ᵗʰ **T23.629** Corrosion of second degree of unspecified single finger (nail) except thumb **PE**

√6ᵗʰ **T23.63** Corrosion of second degree of **multiple fingers** (nail), **not including thumb**

√7ᵗʰ **T23.631** Corrosion of second degree of multiple **right** fingers (nail), not including thumb **PE**

√7ᵗʰ **T23.632** Corrosion of second degree of multiple **left** fingers (nail), not including thumb **PE**

√7ᵗʰ **T23.639** Corrosion of second degree of unspecified multiple fingers (nail), not including thumb **PE**

√6ᵗʰ **T23.64** Corrosion of second degree of **multiple fingers** (nail), **including thumb**

√7ᵗʰ **T23.641** Corrosion of second degree of multiple **right** fingers (nail), including thumb **PE**

√7ᵗʰ **T23.642** Corrosion of second degree of multiple **left** fingers (nail), including thumb **PE**

√7ᵗʰ **T23.649** Corrosion of second degree of unspecified multiple fingers (nail), including thumb **PE**

√6ᵗʰ **T23.65** Corrosion of second degree of **palm**

√7ᵗʰ **T23.651** Corrosion of second degree of **right** palm **PE**

√7ᵗʰ **T23.652** Corrosion of second degree of **left** palm **PE**

☑ Additional Character Required   √x7ᵗʰ Placeholder   Questionable PDx   Manifestation   Unspecified   **UPD** Unacceptable PDx   **H1**-**H14** HAC   **HCC** CMS-HCC Dx   **HIV** HIV Dx

ICD-10-CM 2025   1125

√7ᵗʰ **T23.659** Corrosion of second degree of unspecified palm `PE`

√6ᵗʰ **T23.66** Corrosion of second degree of **back of hand**

√7ᵗʰ **T23.661** Corrosion of second degree back of **right** hand `PE`

√7ᵗʰ **T23.662** Corrosion of second degree back of **left** hand `PE`

√7ᵗʰ **T23.669** Corrosion of second degree back of unspecified hand `PE`

√6ᵗʰ **T23.67** Corrosion of second degree of **wrist**

√7ᵗʰ **T23.671** Corrosion of second degree of **right** wrist `PE`

√7ᵗʰ **T23.672** Corrosion of second degree of **left** wrist `PE`

√7ᵗʰ **T23.679** Corrosion of second degree of unspecified wrist `PE`

√6ᵗʰ **T23.69** Corrosion of second degree of **multiple sites** of wrist and hand

√7ᵗʰ **T23.691** Corrosion of second degree of multiple sites of **right** wrist and hand `PE`

√7ᵗʰ **T23.692** Corrosion of second degree of multiple sites of **left** wrist and hand `PE`

√7ᵗʰ **T23.699** Corrosion of second degree of multiple sites of unspecified wrist and hand `PE`

√5ᵗʰ **T23.7** Corrosion of **third degree** of wrist and hand

Code first (T51-T65) to identify chemical and intent

Use additional external cause code to identify place (Y92)

√6ᵗʰ **T23.70** Corrosion of third degree of hand, unspecified site

√7ᵗʰ **T23.701** Corrosion of third degree of **right** hand, unspecified site `CC` `H5` `PE`

√7ᵗʰ **T23.702** Corrosion of third degree of **left** hand, unspecified site `CC` `H5` `PE`

√7ᵗʰ **T23.709** Corrosion of third degree of unspecified hand, unspecified site `CC` `H5` `UNS` `PE`

√6ᵗʰ **T23.71** Corrosion of third degree of **thumb** (nail)

√7ᵗʰ **T23.711** Corrosion of third degree of **right** thumb (nail) `CC` `H5` `PE`

√7ᵗʰ **T23.712** Corrosion of third degree of **left** thumb (nail) `CC` `H5` `PE`

√7ᵗʰ **T23.719** Corrosion of third degree of unspecified thumb (nail) `CC` `H5` `UNS` `PE`

√6ᵗʰ **T23.72** Corrosion of third degree of **single finger** (nail) except thumb

√7ᵗʰ **T23.721** Corrosion of third degree of single **right** finger (nail) except thumb `CC` `H5` `PE`

√7ᵗʰ **T23.722** Corrosion of third degree of single **left** finger (nail) except thumb `CC` `H5` `PE`

√7ᵗʰ **T23.729** Corrosion of third degree of unspecified single finger (nail) except thumb `CC` `H5` `UNS` `PE`

√6ᵗʰ **T23.73** Corrosion of third degree of **multiple fingers** (nail), **not including thumb**

√7ᵗʰ **T23.731** Corrosion of third degree of multiple **right** fingers (nail), not including thumb `CC` `H5` `PE`

√7ᵗʰ **T23.732** Corrosion of third degree of multiple **left** fingers (nail), not including thumb `CC` `H5` `PE`

√7ᵗʰ **T23.739** Corrosion of third degree of unspecified multiple fingers (nail), not including thumb `CC` `H5` `UNS` `PE`

√6ᵗʰ **T23.74** Corrosion of third degree of **multiple fingers** (nail), **including thumb**

√7ᵗʰ **T23.741** Corrosion of third degree of multiple **right** fingers (nail), including thumb `CC` `H5` `PE`

√7ᵗʰ **T23.742** Corrosion of third degree of multiple **left** fingers (nail), including thumb `CC` `H5` `PE`

√7ᵗʰ **T23.749** Corrosion of third degree of unspecified multiple fingers (nail), including thumb `CC` `H5` `UNS` `PE`

√6ᵗʰ **T23.75** Corrosion of third degree of **palm**

√7ᵗʰ **T23.751** Corrosion of third degree of **right** palm `CC` `H5` `PE`

√7ᵗʰ **T23.752** Corrosion of third degree of **left** palm `CC` `H5` `PE`

√7ᵗʰ **T23.759** Corrosion of third degree of unspecified palm `CC` `H5` `UNS` `PE`

√6ᵗʰ **T23.76** Corrosion of third degree of **back of hand**

√7ᵗʰ **T23.761** Corrosion of third degree of back of **right** hand `CC` `H5` `PE`

√7ᵗʰ **T23.762** Corrosion of third degree of back of **left** hand `CC` `H5` `PE`

√7ᵗʰ **T23.769** Corrosion of third degree back of unspecified hand `CC` `H5` `UNS` `PE`

√6ᵗʰ **T23.77** Corrosion of third degree of **wrist**

√7ᵗʰ **T23.771** Corrosion of third degree of **right** wrist `CC` `H5` `PE`

√7ᵗʰ **T23.772** Corrosion of third degree of **left** wrist `CC` `H5` `PE`

√7ᵗʰ **T23.779** Corrosion of third degree of unspecified wrist `CC` `H5` `UNS` `PE`

√6ᵗʰ **T23.79** Corrosion of third degree of **multiple sites** of wrist and hand

√7ᵗʰ **T23.791** Corrosion of third degree of multiple sites of **right** wrist and hand `CC` `H5` `PE`

√7ᵗʰ **T23.792** Corrosion of third degree of multiple sites of **left** wrist and hand `CC` `H5` `PE`

√7ᵗʰ **T23.799** Corrosion of third degree of multiple sites of unspecified wrist and hand `CC` `H5` `UNS` `PE`

√4ᵗʰ **T24** Burn and corrosion of lower limb, except ankle and foot

EXCLUDES 2 | burn and corrosion of ankle and foot (T25.-)
burn and corrosion of hip region (T21.-)

The appropriate 7th character is to be added to each code from category T24.
A   initial encounter
D   subsequent encounter
S   sequela

√5ᵗʰ **T24.0** Burn of unspecified degree of lower limb, except ankle and foot

Use additional external cause code to identify the source, place and intent of the burn (X00-X19, X75-X77, X96-X98, Y92)

√6ᵗʰ **T24.00** Burn of unspecified degree of unspecified site of lower limb, except ankle and foot

√7ᵗʰ **T24.001** Burn of unspecified degree of unspecified site of **right** lower limb, except ankle and foot `PE`

√7ᵗʰ **T24.002** Burn of unspecified degree of unspecified site of **left** lower limb, except ankle and foot `PE`

√7ᵗʰ **T24.009** Burn of unspecified degree of unspecified site of unspecified lower limb, except ankle and foot `PE`

√6ᵗʰ **T24.01** Burn of unspecified degree of **thigh**

√7ᵗʰ **T24.011** Burn of unspecified degree of **right** thigh `PE`

√7ᵗʰ **T24.012** Burn of unspecified degree of **left** thigh `PE`

√7ᵗʰ **T24.019** Burn of unspecified degree of unspecified thigh `PE`

√6ᵗʰ **T24.02** Burn of unspecified degree of **knee**

√7ᵗʰ **T24.021** Burn of unspecified degree of **right** knee `PE`

√7ᵗʰ **T24.022** Burn of unspecified degree of **left** knee `PE`

√7ᵗʰ **T24.029** Burn of unspecified degree of unspecified knee `PE`

√6ᵗʰ **T24.03** Burn of unspecified degree of **lower leg**

√7ᵗʰ **T24.031** Burn of unspecified degree of **right** lower leg `PE`

√7ᵗʰ **T24.032** Burn of unspecified degree of **left** lower leg `PE`

√7ᵗʰ **T24.039** Burn of unspecified degree of unspecified lower leg `PE`

√6ᵗʰ **T24.09** Burn of unspecified degree of **multiple sites** of lower limb, except ankle and foot

√7ᵗʰ **T24.091** Burn of unspecified degree of multiple sites of **right** lower limb, except ankle and foot `PE`

√7ᵗʰ **T24.092** Burn of unspecified degree of multiple sites of **left** lower limb, except ankle and foot `PE`

√7ᵗʰ **T24.099** Burn of unspecified degree of multiple sites of unspecified lower limb, except ankle and foot `PE`

Chapter 19. Injury, Poisoning and Certain Other Consequences of External Causes

√5th **T24.1 Burn of first degree of lower limb, except ankle and foot**

Use additional external cause code to identify the source, place and intent of the burn (X00-X19, X75-X77, X96-X98, Y92)

√6th **T24.10** Burn of first degree of unspecified site of lower limb, except ankle and foot

√7th **T24.101** Burn of first degree of unspecified site of **right** lower limb, except ankle and foot `PE`

√7th **T24.102** Burn of first degree of unspecified site of **left** lower limb, except ankle and foot `PE`

√7th **T24.109** Burn of first degree of unspecified site of unspecified lower limb, except ankle and foot `PE`

√6th **T24.11** Burn of first degree of **thigh**

√7th **T24.111** Burn of first degree of **right** thigh `PE`

√7th **T24.112** Burn of first degree of **left** thigh `PE`

√7th **T24.119** Burn of first degree of unspecified thigh `PE`

√6th **T24.12** Burn of first degree of **knee**

√7th **T24.121** Burn of first degree of **right** knee `PE`

√7th **T24.122** Burn of first degree of **left** knee `PE`

√7th **T24.129** Burn of first degree of unspecified knee `PE`

√6th **T24.13** Burn of first degree of **lower leg**

√7th **T24.131** Burn of first degree of **right** lower leg `PE`

√7th **T24.132** Burn of first degree of **left** lower leg `PE`

√7th **T24.139** Burn of first degree of unspecified lower leg `PE`

√6th **T24.19** Burn of first degree of **multiple sites** of lower limb, except ankle and foot

√7th **T24.191** Burn of first degree of multiple sites of **right** lower limb, except ankle and foot `PE`

√7th **T24.192** Burn of first degree of multiple sites of **left** lower limb, except ankle and foot `PE`

√7th **T24.199** Burn of first degree of multiple sites of unspecified lower limb, except ankle and foot `PE`

√5th **T24.2 Burn of second degree of lower limb, except ankle and foot**

Use additional external cause code to identify the source, place and intent of the burn (X00-X19, X75-X77, X96-X98, Y92)

√6th **T24.20** Burn of second degree of unspecified site of lower limb, except ankle and foot

√7th **T24.201** Burn of second degree of unspecified site of **right** lower limb, except ankle and foot `PE`

√7th **T24.202** Burn of second degree of unspecified site of **left** lower limb, except ankle and foot `PE`

√7th **T24.209** Burn of second degree of unspecified site of unspecified lower limb, except ankle and foot `PE`

√6th **T24.21** Burn of second degree of **thigh**

√7th **T24.211** Burn of second degree of **right** thigh `PE`

√7th **T24.212** Burn of second degree of **left** thigh `PE`

√7th **T24.219** Burn of second degree of unspecified thigh `PE`

√6th **T24.22** Burn of second degree of **knee**

√7th **T24.221** Burn of second degree of **right** knee `PE`

√7th **T24.222** Burn of second degree of **left** knee `PE`

√7th **T24.229** Burn of second degree of unspecified knee `PE`

√6th **T24.23** Burn of second degree of **lower leg**

√7th **T24.231** Burn of second degree of **right** lower leg `PE`

√7th **T24.232** Burn of second degree of **left** lower leg `PE`

√7th **T24.239** Burn of second degree of unspecified lower leg `PE`

√6th **T24.29** Burn of second degree of **multiple sites** of lower limb, except ankle and foot

√7th **T24.291** Burn of second degree of multiple sites of **right** lower limb, except ankle and foot `PE`

√7th **T24.292** Burn of second degree of multiple sites of **left** lower limb, except ankle and foot `PE`

√7th **T24.299** Burn of second degree of multiple sites of unspecified lower limb, except ankle and foot `PE`

√5th **T24.3 Burn of third degree of lower limb, except ankle and foot**

Use additional external cause code to identify the source, place and intent of the burn (X00-X19, X75-X77, X96-X98, Y92)

√6th **T24.30** Burn of third degree of unspecified site of lower limb, except ankle and foot

√7th **T24.301** Burn of third degree of unspecified site of **right** lower limb, except ankle and foot `CC` `H5` `PE`

√7th **T24.302** Burn of third degree of unspecified site of **left** lower limb, except ankle and foot `CC` `H5` `PE`

√7th **T24.309** Burn of third degree of unspecified site of unspecified lower limb, except ankle and foot `CC` `H5` `UNS` `PE`

√6th **T24.31** Burn of third degree of **thigh**

√7th **T24.311** Burn of third degree of **right** thigh `CC` `H5` `PE`

√7th **T24.312** Burn of third degree of **left** thigh `CC` `H5` `PE`

√7th **T24.319** Burn of third degree of unspecified thigh `CC` `H5` `UNS` `PE`

√6th **T24.32** Burn of third degree of **knee**

√7th **T24.321** Burn of third degree of **right** knee `CC` `H5` `PE`

√7th **T24.322** Burn of third degree of **left** knee `CC` `H5` `PE`

√7th **T24.329** Burn of third degree of unspecified knee `CC` `H5` `UNS` `PE`

√6th **T24.33** Burn of third degree of **lower leg**

√7th **T24.331** Burn of third degree of **right** lower leg `CC` `H5` `PE`

√7th **T24.332** Burn of third degree of **left** lower leg `CC` `H5` `PE`

√7th **T24.339** Burn of third degree of unspecified lower leg `CC` `H5` `UNS` `PE`

√6th **T24.39** Burn of third degree of **multiple sites** of lower limb, except ankle and foot

AHA: 2016,2Q,4

√7th **T24.391** Burn of third degree of multiple sites of **right** lower limb, except ankle and foot `CC` `H5` `PE`

√7th **T24.392** Burn of third degree of multiple sites of **left** lower limb, except ankle and foot `CC` `H5` `PE`

√7th **T24.399** Burn of third degree of multiple sites of unspecified lower limb, except ankle and foot `CC` `H5` `UNS` `PE`

√5th **T24.4 Corrosion of unspecified degree of lower limb, except ankle and foot**

Code first (T51-T65) to identify chemical and intent
Use additional external cause code to identify place (Y92)

√6th **T24.40** Corrosion of unspecified degree of unspecified site of lower limb, except ankle and foot

√7th **T24.401** Corrosion of unspecified degree of unspecified site of **right** lower limb, except ankle and foot `PE`

√7th **T24.402** Corrosion of unspecified degree of unspecified site of **left** lower limb, except ankle and foot `PE`

√7th **T24.409** Corrosion of unspecified degree of unspecified site of unspecified lower limb, except ankle and foot `PE`

√6th **T24.41** Corrosion of unspecified degree of **thigh**

√7th **T24.411** Corrosion of unspecified degree of **right** thigh `PE`

√7th **T24.412** Corrosion of unspecified degree of **left** thigh `PE`

√7th **T24.419** Corrosion of unspecified degree of unspecified thigh `PE`

√6th **T24.42** Corrosion of unspecified degree of **knee**

√7th **T24.421** Corrosion of unspecified degree of **right** knee `PE`

✔ Additional Character Required   √x7th Placeholder   Questionable PDx   Manifestation   Unspecified   `UPD` Unacceptable PDx   `H1`-`H14` HAC   `HCC` CMS-HCC Dx   `HIV` HIV Dx

√7ᵗʰ **T24.422** Corrosion of unspecified degree of **left** knee   PE

√7ᵗʰ **T24.429** Corrosion of unspecified degree of unspecified knee   PE

√6ᵗʰ **T24.43** Corrosion of unspecified degree of **lower leg**

√7ᵗʰ **T24.431** Corrosion of unspecified degree of **right** lower leg   PE

√7ᵗʰ **T24.432** Corrosion of unspecified degree of **left** lower leg   PE

√7ᵗʰ **T24.439** Corrosion of unspecified degree of unspecified lower leg   PE

√6ᵗʰ **T24.49** Corrosion of unspecified degree of **multiple sites** of lower limb, except ankle and foot

√7ᵗʰ **T24.491** Corrosion of unspecified degree of **multiple sites** of **right** lower limb, except ankle and foot   PE

√7ᵗʰ **T24.492** Corrosion of unspecified degree of **multiple sites** of **left** lower limb, except ankle and foot   PE

√7ᵗʰ **T24.499** Corrosion of unspecified degree of multiple sites of unspecified lower limb, except ankle and foot   PE

√5ᵗʰ **T24.5** Corrosion of **first degree** of lower limb, except ankle and foot

Code first (T51-T65) to identify chemical and intent
Use additional external cause code to identify place (Y92)

√6ᵗʰ **T24.50** Corrosion of first degree of unspecified site of lower limb, except ankle and foot

√7ᵗʰ **T24.501** Corrosion of first degree of unspecified site of **right** lower limb, except ankle and foot   PE

√7ᵗʰ **T24.502** Corrosion of first degree of unspecified site of **left** lower limb, except ankle and foot   PE

√7ᵗʰ **T24.509** Corrosion of first degree of unspecified site of unspecified lower limb, except ankle and foot   PE

√6ᵗʰ **T24.51** Corrosion of first degree of **thigh**

√7ᵗʰ **T24.511** Corrosion of first degree of **right** thigh   PE

√7ᵗʰ **T24.512** Corrosion of first degree of **left** thigh   PE

√7ᵗʰ **T24.519** Corrosion of first degree of unspecified thigh   PE

√6ᵗʰ **T24.52** Corrosion of first degree of **knee**

√7ᵗʰ **T24.521** Corrosion of first degree of **right** knee   PE

√7ᵗʰ **T24.522** Corrosion of first degree of **left** knee   PE

√7ᵗʰ **T24.529** Corrosion of first degree of unspecified knee   PE

√6ᵗʰ **T24.53** Corrosion of first degree of **lower leg**

√7ᵗʰ **T24.531** Corrosion of first degree of **right** lower leg   PE

√7ᵗʰ **T24.532** Corrosion of first degree of **left** lower leg   PE

√7ᵗʰ **T24.539** Corrosion of first degree of unspecified lower leg   PE

√6ᵗʰ **T24.59** Corrosion of first degree of **multiple sites** of lower limb, except ankle and foot

√7ᵗʰ **T24.591** Corrosion of first degree of multiple sites of **right** lower limb, except ankle and foot   PE

√7ᵗʰ **T24.592** Corrosion of first degree of multiple sites of **left** lower limb, except ankle and foot   PE

√7ᵗʰ **T24.599** Corrosion of first degree of multiple sites of unspecified lower limb, except ankle and foot   PE

√5ᵗʰ **T24.6** Corrosion of **second degree** of lower limb, except ankle and foot

Code first (T51-T65) to identify chemical and intent
Use additional external cause code to identify place (Y92)

√6ᵗʰ **T24.60** Corrosion of second degree of unspecified site of lower limb, except ankle and foot

√7ᵗʰ **T24.601** Corrosion of second degree of unspecified site of **right** lower limb, except ankle and foot   PE

√7ᵗʰ **T24.602** Corrosion of second degree of unspecified site of **left** lower limb, except ankle and foot   PE

√7ᵗʰ **T24.609** Corrosion of second degree of unspecified site of unspecified lower limb, except ankle and foot   PE

√6ᵗʰ **T24.61** Corrosion of second degree of **thigh**

√7ᵗʰ **T24.611** Corrosion of second degree of **right** thigh   PE

√7ᵗʰ **T24.612** Corrosion of second degree of **left** thigh   PE

√7ᵗʰ **T24.619** Corrosion of second degree of unspecified thigh   PE

√6ᵗʰ **T24.62** Corrosion of second degree of **knee**

√7ᵗʰ **T24.621** Corrosion of second degree of **right** knee   PE

√7ᵗʰ **T24.622** Corrosion of second degree of **left** knee   PE

√7ᵗʰ **T24.629** Corrosion of second degree of unspecified knee   PE

√6ᵗʰ **T24.63** Corrosion of second degree of **lower leg**

√7ᵗʰ **T24.631** Corrosion of second degree of **right** lower leg   PE

√7ᵗʰ **T24.632** Corrosion of second degree of **left** lower leg   PE

√7ᵗʰ **T24.639** Corrosion of second degree of unspecified lower leg   PE

√6ᵗʰ **T24.69** Corrosion of second degree of **multiple sites** of lower limb, except ankle and foot

√7ᵗʰ **T24.691** Corrosion of second degree of multiple sites of **right** lower limb, except ankle and foot   PE

√7ᵗʰ **T24.692** Corrosion of second degree of multiple sites of **left** lower limb, except ankle and foot   PE

√7ᵗʰ **T24.699** Corrosion of second degree of multiple sites of unspecified lower limb, except ankle and foot   PE

√5ᵗʰ **T24.7** Corrosion of **third degree** of lower limb, except ankle and foot

Code first (T51-T65) to identify chemical and intent
Use additional external cause code to identify place (Y92)

√6ᵗʰ **T24.70** Corrosion of third degree of unspecified site of lower limb, except ankle and foot

√7ᵗʰ **T24.701** Corrosion of third degree of unspecified site of **right** lower limb, except ankle and foot   CC   H5

√7ᵗʰ **T24.702** Corrosion of third degree of unspecified site of **left** lower limb, except ankle and foot   CC   H5

√7ᵗʰ **T24.709** Corrosion of third degree of unspecified site of unspecified lower limb, except ankle and foot   CC   H5   UNS   PE

√6ᵗʰ **T24.71** Corrosion of third degree of **thigh**

√7ᵗʰ **T24.711** Corrosion of third degree of **right** thigh   CC   H5   PE

√7ᵗʰ **T24.712** Corrosion of third degree of **left** thigh   CC   H5   PE

√7ᵗʰ **T24.719** Corrosion of third degree of unspecified thigh   CC   H5   PE

√6ᵗʰ **T24.72** Corrosion of third degree of **knee**

√7ᵗʰ **T24.721** Corrosion of third degree of **right** knee   CC   H5   PE

√7ᵗʰ **T24.722** Corrosion of third degree of **left** knee   CC   H5   PE

√7ᵗʰ **T24.729** Corrosion of third degree of unspecified knee   CC   H5   UNS   PE

√6ᵗʰ **T24.73** Corrosion of third degree of **lower leg**

√7ᵗʰ **T24.731** Corrosion of third degree of **right** lower leg   CC   H5   PE

√7ᵗʰ **T24.732** Corrosion of third degree of **left** lower leg   CC   H5   PE

√7ᵗʰ **T24.739** Corrosion of third degree of unspecified lower leg   CC   H5   UNS   PE

√6ᵗʰ **T24.79** Corrosion of third degree of **multiple sites** of lower limb, except ankle and foot

√7ᵗʰ **T24.791** Corrosion of third degree of multiple sites of **right** lower limb, except ankle and foot   CC   H5   PE

√7ᵗʰ **T24.792** Corrosion of third degree of multiple sites of **left** lower limb, except ankle and foot   CC   H5   PE

N Newborn: 0   **P** Pediatric: 0-17   **M** Maternity: 9-64   **A** Adult: 15-124   **UNS** Unspecified Site   **MCC** Major Complication/Comorbidity   **CC** Complication/Comorbidity   **PE** POA Exempt

1128   ICD-10-CM 2025

√7ᵗʰ **T24.799** Corrosion of third degree of multiple sites of unspecified lower limb, except ankle and foot   CC H5 UNS PE

√4ᵗʰ **T25** **Burn and corrosion of ankle and foot**

> The appropriate 7th character is to be added to each code from category T25.
> A   initial encounter
> D   subsequent encounter
> S   sequela

√5ᵗʰ **T25.0** **Burn of unspecified degree of ankle and foot**

Use additional external cause code to identify the source, place and intent of the burn (X00-X19, X75-X77, X96-X98, Y92)

√6ᵗʰ **T25.01** Burn of unspecified degree of **ankle**

√7ᵗʰ **T25.011** Burn of unspecified degree of **right** ankle   PE

√7ᵗʰ **T25.012** Burn of unspecified degree of **left** ankle   PE

√7ᵗʰ **T25.019** Burn of unspecified degree of unspecified ankle   PE

√6ᵗʰ **T25.02** Burn of unspecified degree of **foot**

> EXCLUDES 2   burn of unspecified degree of toe(s) (nail) (T25.03-)

√7ᵗʰ **T25.021** Burn of unspecified degree of **right** foot   PE

√7ᵗʰ **T25.022** Burn of unspecified degree of **left** foot   PE

√7ᵗʰ **T25.029** Burn of unspecified degree of unspecified foot   PE

√6ᵗʰ **T25.03** Burn of unspecified degree of **toe**(s) (nail)

√7ᵗʰ **T25.031** Burn of unspecified degree of **right** toe(s) (nail)   PE

√7ᵗʰ **T25.032** Burn of unspecified degree of **left** toe(s) (nail)   PE

√7ᵗʰ **T25.039** Burn of unspecified degree of unspecified toe(s) (nail)   PE

√6ᵗʰ **T25.09** Burn of unspecified degree of **multiple sites** of ankle and foot

√7ᵗʰ **T25.091** Burn of unspecified degree of multiple sites of **right** ankle and foot   PE

√7ᵗʰ **T25.092** Burn of unspecified degree of multiple sites of **left** ankle and foot   PE

√7ᵗʰ **T25.099** Burn of unspecified degree of multiple sites of unspecified ankle and foot   PE

√5ᵗʰ **T25.1** **Burn of first degree of ankle and foot**

Use additional external cause code to identify the source, place and intent of the burn (X00-X19, X75-X77, X96-X98, Y92)

√6ᵗʰ **T25.11** Burn of first degree of **ankle**

√7ᵗʰ **T25.111** Burn of first degree of **right** ankle   PE

√7ᵗʰ **T25.112** Burn of first degree of **left** ankle   PE

√7ᵗʰ **T25.119** Burn of first degree of unspecified ankle   PE

√6ᵗʰ **T25.12** Burn of first degree of **foot**

> EXCLUDES 2   burn of first degree of toe(s) (nail) (T25.13-)

√7ᵗʰ **T25.121** Burn of first degree of **right** foot   PE

√7ᵗʰ **T25.122** Burn of first degree of **left** foot   PE

√7ᵗʰ **T25.129** Burn of first degree of unspecified foot   PE

√6ᵗʰ **T25.13** Burn of first degree of **toe**(s) (nail)

√7ᵗʰ **T25.131** Burn of first degree of **right** toe(s) (nail)   PE

√7ᵗʰ **T25.132** Burn of first degree of **left** toe(s) (nail)   PE

√7ᵗʰ **T25.139** Burn of first degree of unspecified toe(s) (nail)   PE

√6ᵗʰ **T25.19** Burn of first degree of **multiple sites** of ankle and foot

√7ᵗʰ **T25.191** Burn of first degree of multiple sites of **right** ankle and foot   PE

√7ᵗʰ **T25.192** Burn of first degree of multiple sites of **left** ankle and foot   PE

√7ᵗʰ **T25.199** Burn of first degree of multiple sites of unspecified ankle and foot   PE

√5ᵗʰ **T25.2** **Burn of second degree of ankle and foot**

Use additional external cause code to identify the source, place and intent of the burn (X00-X19, X75-X77, X96-X98, Y92)

√6ᵗʰ **T25.21** Burn of second degree of **ankle**

√7ᵗʰ **T25.211** Burn of second degree of **right** ankle   PE

√7ᵗʰ **T25.212** Burn of second degree of **left** ankle   PE

√7ᵗʰ **T25.219** Burn of second degree of unspecified ankle   PE

√6ᵗʰ **T25.22** Burn of second degree of **foot**

> EXCLUDES 2   burn of second degree of toe(s) (nail) (T25.23-)

√7ᵗʰ **T25.221** Burn of second degree of **right** foot   PE

√7ᵗʰ **T25.222** Burn of second degree of **left** foot   PE

√7ᵗʰ **T25.229** Burn of second degree of unspecified foot   PE

√6ᵗʰ **T25.23** Burn of second degree of **toe**(s) (nail)

√7ᵗʰ **T25.231** Burn of second degree of **right** toe(s) (nail)   PE

√7ᵗʰ **T25.232** Burn of second degree of **left** toe(s) (nail)   PE

√7ᵗʰ **T25.239** Burn of second degree of unspecified toe(s) (nail)   PE

√6ᵗʰ **T25.29** Burn of second degree of **multiple sites** of ankle and foot

√7ᵗʰ **T25.291** Burn of second degree of multiple sites of **right** ankle and foot   PE

√7ᵗʰ **T25.292** Burn of second degree of multiple sites of **left** ankle and foot   PE

√7ᵗʰ **T25.299** Burn of second degree of multiple sites of unspecified ankle and foot   PE

√5ᵗʰ **T25.3** **Burn of third degree of ankle and foot**

Use additional external cause code to identify the source, place and intent of the burn (X00-X19, X75-X77, X96-X98, Y92)

√6ᵗʰ **T25.31** Burn of third degree of **ankle**

√7ᵗʰ **T25.311** Burn of third degree of **right** ankle   CC H5 PE

√7ᵗʰ **T25.312** Burn of third degree of **left** ankle   CC H5 PE

√7ᵗʰ **T25.319** Burn of third degree of unspecified ankle   CC H5 UNS PE

√6ᵗʰ **T25.32** Burn of third degree of **foot**

> EXCLUDES 2   burn of third degree of toe(s) (nail) (T25.33-)

√7ᵗʰ **T25.321** Burn of third degree of **right** foot   CC H5 PE

√7ᵗʰ **T25.322** Burn of third degree of **left** foot   CC H5 PE

√7ᵗʰ **T25.329** Burn of third degree of unspecified foot   CC H5 UNS PE

√6ᵗʰ **T25.33** Burn of third degree of **toe**(s) (nail)

√7ᵗʰ **T25.331** Burn of third degree of **right** toe(s) (nail)   CC H5 PE

√7ᵗʰ **T25.332** Burn of third degree of **left** toe(s) (nail)   CC H5 PE

√7ᵗʰ **T25.339** Burn of third degree of unspecified toe(s) (nail)   CC H5 UNS PE

√6ᵗʰ **T25.39** Burn of third degree of **multiple sites** of ankle and foot

√7ᵗʰ **T25.391** Burn of third degree of multiple sites of **right** ankle and foot   CC H5 PE

√7ᵗʰ **T25.392** Burn of third degree of multiple sites of **left** ankle and foot   CC H5 PE

√7ᵗʰ **T25.399** Burn of third degree of multiple sites of unspecified ankle and foot   CC H5 UNS PE

√5ᵗʰ **T25.4** **Corrosion of unspecified degree of ankle and foot**

Code first (T51-T65) to identify chemical and intent
Use additional external cause code to identify place (Y92)

√6ᵗʰ **T25.41** Corrosion of unspecified degree of **ankle**

√7ᵗʰ **T25.411** Corrosion of unspecified degree of **right** ankle   PE

√7ᵗʰ **T25.412** Corrosion of unspecified degree of **left** ankle   PE

√7ᵗʰ **T25.419** Corrosion of unspecified degree of unspecified ankle   PE

✔ Additional Character Required   √x7ᵗʰ Placeholder   Questionable PDx   Manifestation   Unspecified   UPD Unacceptable PDx   H1-H14 HAC   HCC CMS-HCC Dx   HIV HIV Dx

ICD-10-CM 2025   1129

√6ᵗʰ **T25.42** **Corrosion of unspecified degree of foot**

     EXCLUDES 2   *corrosion of unspecified degree of toe(s) (nail) (T25.43-)*

     √7ᵗʰ **T25.421** **Corrosion of unspecified degree of right foot** **PE**

     √7ᵗʰ **T25.422** **Corrosion of unspecified degree of left foot** **PE**

     √7ᵗʰ **T25.429** **Corrosion of unspecified degree of unspecified foot** **PE**

√6ᵗʰ **T25.43** **Corrosion of unspecified degree of toe(s) (nail)**

     √7ᵗʰ **T25.431** **Corrosion of unspecified degree of right toe(s) (nail)** **PE**

     √7ᵗʰ **T25.432** **Corrosion of unspecified degree of left toe(s) (nail)** **PE**

     √7ᵗʰ **T25.439** **Corrosion of unspecified degree of unspecified toe(s) (nail)** **PE**

√6ᵗʰ **T25.49** **Corrosion of unspecified degree of multiple sites of ankle and foot**

     √7ᵗʰ **T25.491** **Corrosion of unspecified degree of multiple sites of right ankle and foot** **PE**

     √7ᵗʰ **T25.492** **Corrosion of unspecified degree of multiple sites of left ankle and foot** **PE**

     √7ᵗʰ **T25.499** **Corrosion of unspecified degree of multiple sites of unspecified ankle and foot** **PE**

√5ᵗʰ **T25.5** **Corrosion of first degree of ankle and foot**

     Code first (T51-T65) to identify chemical and intent
     Use additional external cause code to identify place (Y92)

√6ᵗʰ **T25.51** **Corrosion of first degree of ankle**

     √7ᵗʰ **T25.511** **Corrosion of first degree of right ankle** **PE**

     √7ᵗʰ **T25.512** **Corrosion of first degree of left ankle** **PE**

     √7ᵗʰ **T25.519** **Corrosion of first degree of unspecified ankle** **PE**

√6ᵗʰ **T25.52** **Corrosion of first degree of foot**

     EXCLUDES 2   *corrosion of first degree of toe(s) (nail) (T25.53-)*

     √7ᵗʰ **T25.521** **Corrosion of first degree of right foot** **PE**

     √7ᵗʰ **T25.522** **Corrosion of first degree of left foot** **PE**

     √7ᵗʰ **T25.529** **Corrosion of first degree of unspecified foot** **PE**

√6ᵗʰ **T25.53** **Corrosion of first degree of toe(s) (nail)**

     √7ᵗʰ **T25.531** **Corrosion of first degree of right toe(s) (nail)** **PE**

     √7ᵗʰ **T25.532** **Corrosion of first degree of left toe(s) (nail)** **PE**

     √7ᵗʰ **T25.539** **Corrosion of first degree of unspecified toe(s) (nail)** **PE**

√6ᵗʰ **T25.59** **Corrosion of first degree of multiple sites of ankle and foot**

     √7ᵗʰ **T25.591** **Corrosion of first degree of multiple sites of right ankle and foot** **PE**

     √7ᵗʰ **T25.592** **Corrosion of first degree of multiple sites of left ankle and foot** **PE**

     √7ᵗʰ **T25.599** **Corrosion of first degree of multiple sites of unspecified ankle and foot** **PE**

√5ᵗʰ **T25.6** **Corrosion of second degree of ankle and foot**

     Code first (T51-T65) to identify chemical and intent
     Use additional external cause code to identify place (Y92)

√6ᵗʰ **T25.61** **Corrosion of second degree of ankle**

     √7ᵗʰ **T25.611** **Corrosion of second degree of right ankle** **PE**

     √7ᵗʰ **T25.612** **Corrosion of second degree of left ankle** **PE**

     √7ᵗʰ **T25.619** **Corrosion of second degree of unspecified ankle** **PE**

√6ᵗʰ **T25.62** **Corrosion of second degree of foot**

     EXCLUDES 2   *corrosion of second degree of toe(s) (nail) (T25.63-)*

     √7ᵗʰ **T25.621** **Corrosion of second degree of right foot** **PE**

     √7ᵗʰ **T25.622** **Corrosion of second degree of left foot** **PE**

     √7ᵗʰ **T25.629** **Corrosion of second degree of unspecified foot** **PE**

√6ᵗʰ **T25.63** **Corrosion of second degree of toe(s) (nail)**

     √7ᵗʰ **T25.631** **Corrosion of second degree of right toe(s) (nail)** **PE**

     √7ᵗʰ **T25.632** **Corrosion of second degree of left toe(s) (nail)** **PE**

     √7ᵗʰ **T25.639** **Corrosion of second degree of unspecified toe(s) (nail)** **PE**

√6ᵗʰ **T25.69** **Corrosion of second degree of multiple sites of ankle and foot**

     √7ᵗʰ **T25.691** **Corrosion of second degree of right ankle and foot** **PE**

     √7ᵗʰ **T25.692** **Corrosion of second degree of left ankle and foot** **PE**

     √7ᵗʰ **T25.699** **Corrosion of second degree of unspecified ankle and foot** **PE**

√5ᵗʰ **T25.7** **Corrosion of third degree of ankle and foot**

     Code first (T51-T65) to identify chemical and intent
     Use additional external cause code to identify place (Y92)

√6ᵗʰ **T25.71** **Corrosion of third degree of ankle**

     √7ᵗʰ **T25.711** **Corrosion of third degree of right ankle** **CC** **H5** **PE**

     √7ᵗʰ **T25.712** **Corrosion of third degree of left ankle** **CC** **H5** **PE**

     √7ᵗʰ **T25.719** **Corrosion of third degree of unspecified ankle** **CC** **H5** **UNS** **PE**

√6ᵗʰ **T25.72** **Corrosion of third degree of foot**

     EXCLUDES 2   *corrosion of third degree of toe(s) (nail) (T25.73-)*

     √7ᵗʰ **T25.721** **Corrosion of third degree of right foot** **CC** **H5** **PE**

     √7ᵗʰ **T25.722** **Corrosion of third degree of left foot** **CC** **H5** **PE**

     √7ᵗʰ **T25.729** **Corrosion of third degree of unspecified foot** **CC** **H5** **UNS** **PE**

√6ᵗʰ **T25.73** **Corrosion of third degree of toe(s) (nail)**

     √7ᵗʰ **T25.731** **Corrosion of third degree of right toe(s) (nail)** **CC** **H5** **PE**

     √7ᵗʰ **T25.732** **Corrosion of third degree of left toe(s) (nail)** **CC** **H5** **PE**

     √7ᵗʰ **T25.739** **Corrosion of third degree of unspecified toe(s) (nail)** **CC** **H5** **UNS** **PE**

√6ᵗʰ **T25.79** **Corrosion of third degree of multiple sites of ankle and foot**

     √7ᵗʰ **T25.791** **Corrosion of third degree of multiple sites of right ankle and foot** **CC** **H5** **PE**

     √7ᵗʰ **T25.792** **Corrosion of third degree of multiple sites of left ankle and foot** **CC** **H5** **PE**

     √7ᵗʰ **T25.799** **Corrosion of third degree of multiple sites of unspecified ankle and foot** **CC** **H5** **UNS** **PE**

Burns and corrosions confined to eye and internal organs (T26-T28)

√4ᵗʰ **T26** **Burn and corrosion confined to eye and adnexa**

> The appropriate 7th character is to be added to each code from category T26.
> A   initial encounter
> D   subsequent encounter
> S   sequela

√5ᵗʰ **T26.0** **Burn of eyelid and periocular area**

     Use additional external cause code to identify the source, place and intent of the burn (X00-X19, X75-X77, X96-X98, Y92)

     √x7ᵗʰ **T26.00** **Burn of unspecified eyelid and periocular area** **PE**

     √x7ᵗʰ **T26.01** **Burn of right eyelid and periocular area** **PE**

     √x7ᵗʰ **T26.02** **Burn of left eyelid and periocular area** **PE**

√5ᵗʰ **T26.1** **Burn of cornea and conjunctival sac**

     Use additional external cause code to identify the source, place and intent of the burn (X00-X19, X75-X77, X96-X98, Y92)

     √x7ᵗʰ **T26.10** **Burn of cornea and conjunctival sac, unspecified eye** **PE**

     √x7ᵗʰ **T26.11** **Burn of cornea and conjunctival sac, right eye** **PE**

     √x7ᵗʰ **T26.12** **Burn of cornea and conjunctival sac, left eye** **PE**

N Newborn: 0   **P** Pediatric: 0-17   **M** Maternity: 9-64   **A** Adult: 15-124   **UNS** Unspecified Site   **MCC** Major Complication/Comorbidity   **CC** Complication/Comorbidity   **PE** POA Exempt

1130

ICD-10-CM 2025

√5th **T26.2** Burn with resulting **rupture and destruction of eyeball**

Use additional external cause code to identify the source, place and intent of the burn (X00-X19, X75-X77, X96-X98, Y92)

√x7th **T26.20** Burn with resulting rupture and destruction of unspecified eyeball   CC HE UNS PE

√x7th **T26.21** Burn with resulting rupture and destruction of **right** eyeball   CC H5 PE

√x7th **T26.22** Burn with resulting rupture and destruction of **left** eyeball   CC H5 PE

√5th **T26.3** Burns of other specified parts of eye and adnexa

Use additional external cause code to identify the source, place and intent of the burn (X00-X19, X75-X77, X96-X98, Y92)

√x7th **T26.30** Burns of other specified parts of unspecified eye and adnexa   PE

√x7th **T26.31** Burns of other specified parts of **right** eye and adnexa

√x7th **T26.32** Burns of other specified parts of **left** eye and adnexa   PE

√5th **T26.4** Burn of eye and adnexa, part unspecified

Use additional external cause code to identify the source, place and intent of the burn (X00-X19, X75-X77, X96-X98, Y92)

√x7th **T26.40** Burn of unspecified eye and adnexa, part unspecified   PE

√x7th **T26.41** Burn of **right** eye and adnexa, part unspecified   PE

√x7th **T26.42** Burn of **left** eye and adnexa, part unspecified   PE

√5th **T26.5** Corrosion of **eyelid and periocular area**

Code first (T51-T65) to identify chemical and intent
Use additional external cause code to identify place (Y92)

√x7th **T26.50** Corrosion of unspecified eyelid and periocular area   PE

√x7th **T26.51** Corrosion of **right** eyelid and periocular area   PE

√x7th **T26.52** Corrosion of **left** eyelid and periocular area   PE

√5th **T26.6** Corrosion of **cornea and conjunctival sac**

Code first (T51-T65) to identify chemical and intent
Use additional external cause code to identify place (Y92)

√x7th **T26.60** Corrosion of cornea and conjunctival sac, unspecified eye   PE

√x7th **T26.61** Corrosion of cornea and conjunctival sac, **right** eye   PE

√x7th **T26.62** Corrosion of cornea and conjunctival sac, **left** eye   PE

√5th **T26.7** Corrosion with resulting **rupture and destruction of eyeball**

Code first (T51-T65) to identify chemical and intent
Use additional external cause code to identify place (Y92)

√x7th **T26.70** Corrosion with resulting rupture and destruction of unspecified eyeball   CC H5 UNS PE

√x7th **T26.71** Corrosion with resulting rupture and destruction of **right** eyeball   CC H5 PE

√x7th **T26.72** Corrosion with resulting rupture and destruction of **left** eyeball   CC H5 PE

√5th **T26.8** Corrosions of other specified parts of eye and adnexa

Code first (T51-T65) to identify chemical and intent
Use additional external cause code to identify place (Y92)

√x7th **T26.80** Corrosions of other specified parts of unspecified eye and adnexa   PE

√x7th **T26.81** Corrosions of other specified parts of **right** eye and adnexa   PE

√x7th **T26.82** Corrosions of other specified parts of **left** eye and adnexa   PE

√5th **T26.9** Corrosion of eye and adnexa, part unspecified

Code first (T51-T65) to identify chemical and intent
Use additional external cause code to identify place (Y92)

√x7th **T26.90** Corrosion of unspecified eye and adnexa, part unspecified   PE

√x7th **T26.91** Corrosion of **right** eye and adnexa, part unspecified   PE

√x7th **T26.92** Corrosion of **left** eye and adnexa, part unspecified   PE

√4th **T27** Burn and corrosion of respiratory tract

Use additional external cause code to identify the source and intent of the burn (X00-X19, X75-X77, X96-X98)
Use additional external cause code to identify place (Y92)

The appropriate 7th character is to be added to each code from category T27.
A   initial encounter
D   subsequent encounter
S   sequela

√7th **T27.0** Burn of **larynx and trachea**   CC H5 PE

√7th **T27.1** Burn involving **larynx and trachea with lung**   CC H5 PE

√7th **T27.2** Burn of other parts of respiratory tract   CC H5 PE
Burn of thoracic cavity

√7th **T27.3** Burn of respiratory tract, part unspecified   CC H5 PE

√7th **T27.4** Corrosion of **larynx and trachea**   CC H5 PE
Code first (T51-T65) to identify chemical and intent

√7th **T27.5** Corrosion involving **larynx and trachea with lung**   CC H5 PE
Code first (T51-T65) to identify chemical and intent

√7th **T27.6** Corrosion of other parts of respiratory tract   CC H5 PE
Code first (T51-T65) to identify chemical and intent

√7th **T27.7** Corrosion of respiratory tract, part unspecified   CC H5 PE
Code first (T51-T65) to identify chemical and intent

√4th **T28** Burn and corrosion of other internal organs

Use additional external cause code to identify the source and intent of the burn (X00-X19, X75-X77, X96-X98)
Use additional external cause code to identify place (Y92)

The appropriate 7th character is to be added to each code from category T28.
A   initial encounter
D   subsequent encounter
S   sequela

√7th **T28.0** Burn of **mouth and pharynx**   PE

√7th **T28.1** Burn of **esophagus**   CC H5 PE

√7th **T28.2** Burn of other parts of alimentary tract   CC H5 PE

√7th **T28.3** Burn of **internal genitourinary organs**   PE

√5th **T28.4** Burns of other and unspecified internal organs

√7th **T28.40** Burn of unspecified internal organ   PE

√6th **T28.41** Burn of **ear drum**

√7th **T28.411** Burn of **right** ear drum   PE

√7th **T28.412** Burn of **left** ear drum   PE

√7th **T28.419** Burn of unspecified ear drum   PE

√7th **T28.49** Burn of other internal organ   PE

√7th **T28.5** Corrosion of **mouth and pharynx**
Code first (T51-T65) to identify chemical and intent

√7th **T28.6** Corrosion of **esophagus**   CC H5 PE
Code first (T51-T65) to identify chemical and intent

√7th **T28.7** Corrosion of other parts of alimentary tract   CC H5 PE
Code first (T51-T65) to identify chemical and intent

√7th **T28.8** Corrosion of internal **genitourinary organs**   PE
Code first (T51-T65) to identify chemical and intent

√5th **T28.9** Corrosions of other and unspecified internal organs
Code first (T51-T65) to identify chemical and intent

√7th **T28.90** Corrosions of unspecified internal organs   PE

√6th **T28.91** Corrosions of **ear drum**

√7th **T28.911** Corrosions of **right** ear drum   PE

√7th **T28.912** Corrosions of **left** ear drum   PE

√7th **T28.919** Corrosions of unspecified ear drum   PE

√7th **T28.99** Corrosions of other internal organs   PE

Burns and corrosions of multiple and unspecified body regions (T30-T32)

√4th **T30** Burn and corrosion, body region unspecified

T30.0 Burn of unspecified body region, unspecified degree
This code is not for inpatient use. Code to specified site and degree of burns
Burn NOS
Multiple burns NOS

✔ Additional Character Required   √x7th Placeholder   Questionable PDx   Manifestation   Unspecified   UPD Unacceptable PDx   H1 - H14 HAC   HCC CMS-HCC Dx   HIV HIV Dx

ICD-10-CM 2025   1131

Chapter 19. Injury, Poisoning and Certain Other Consequences of External Causes

T30.4   **Corrosion** of unspecified body region, unspecified degree
This code is not for inpatient use. Code to specified site and degree of corrosion
Corrosion NOS
Multiple corrosion NOS

✓4th   **T31**   **Burns** classified according to **extent of body surface involved**

NOTE   This category is to be used as the primary code only when the site of the burn is unspecified. It should be used as a supplementary code with categories T20-T25 when the site is specified.

T31.0   Burns involving **less than 10%** of body surface

✓5th   **T31.1**   Burns involving **10-19%** of body surface

     T31.10   Burns involving 10-19% of body surface with **0% to 9% third degree** burns   `CC` `H5`
       Burns involving 10-19% of body surface NOS

     T31.11   Burns involving 10-19% of body surface with **10-19% third degree** burns   `CC` `H5` `HCC`

✓5th   **T31.2**   Burns involving **20-29%** of body surface

     T31.20   Burns involving 20-29% of body surface with **0% to 9% third degree** burns   `CC` `H5`
       Burns involving 20-29% of body surface NOS

     T31.21   Burns involving 20-29% of body surface with **10-19% third degree** burns   `MCC` `H5` `HCC`

     T31.22   Burns involving 20-29% of body surface with **20-29% third degree** burns   `MCC` `H5` `HCC`

✓5th   **T31.3**   Burns involving **30-39%** of body surface

     T31.30   Burns involving 30-39% of body surface with **0% to 9% third degree** burns   `CC` `H5`
       Burns involving 30-39% of body surface NOS

     T31.31   Burns involving 30-39% of body surface with **10-19% third degree** burns   `MCC` `H5` `HCC`

     T31.32   Burns involving 30-39% of body surface with **20-29% third degree** burns   `MCC` `H5` `HCC`

     T31.33   Burns involving 30-39% of body surface with **30-39% third degree** burns   `MCC` `H5` `HCC`

✓5th   **T31.4**   Burns involving **40-49%** of body surface

     T31.40   Burns involving 40-49% of body surface with **0% to 9% third degree** burns   `CC` `H5`
       Burns involving 40-49% of body surface NOS

     T31.41   Burns involving 40-49% of body surface with **10-19% third degree** burns   `MCC` `H5` `HCC`

     T31.42   Burns involving 40-49% of body surface with **20-29% third degree** burns   `MCC` `H5` `HCC`

     T31.43   Burns involving 40-49% of body surface with **30-39% third degree** burns   `MCC` `H5` `HCC`

     T31.44   Burns involving 40-49% of body surface with **40-49% third degree** burns   `MCC` `H5` `HCC`

✓5th   **T31.5**   Burns involving **50-59%** of body surface

     T31.50   Burns involving 50-59% of body surface with **0% to 9% third degree** burns   `CC` `H5`
       Burns involving 50-59% of body surface NOS

     T31.51   Burns involving 50-59% of body surface with **10-19% third degree** burns   `MCC` `H5` `HCC`

     T31.52   Burns involving 50-59% of body surface with **20-29% third degree** burns   `MCC` `H5` `HCC`

     T31.53   Burns involving 50-59% of body surface with **30-39% third degree** burns   `MCC` `H5` `HCC`

     T31.54   Burns involving 50-59% of body surface with **40-49% third degree** burns   `MCC` `H5` `HCC`

     T31.55   Burns involving 50-59% of body surface with **50-59% third degree** burns   `MCC` `H5` `HCC`

✓5th   **T31.6**   Burns involving **60-69%** of body surface

     T31.60   Burns involving 60-69% of body surface with **0% to 9% third degree** burns   `CC` `H5`
       Burns involving 60-69% of body surface NOS

     T31.61   Burns involving 60-69% of body surface with **10-19% third degree** burns   `MCC` `H5` `HCC`

     T31.62   Burns involving 60-69% of body surface with **20-29% third degree** burns   `MCC` `H5` `HCC`

     T31.63   Burns involving 60-69% of body surface with **30-39% third degree** burns   `MCC` `H5` `HCC`

     T31.64   Burns involving 60-69% of body surface with **40-49% third degree** burns   `MCC` `H5` `HCC`

     T31.65   Burns involving 60-69% of body surface with **50-59% third degree** burns   `MCC` `H5` `HCC`

T31.66   Burns involving 60-69% of body surface with **60-69% third degree** burns   `MCC` `H5` `HCC`

✓5th   **T31.7**   Burns involving **70-79%** of body surface

     T31.70   Burns involving 70-79% of body surface with **0% to 9% third degree** burns   `CC` `H5`
       Burns involving 70-79% of body surface NOS

     T31.71   Burns involving 70-79% of body surface with **10-19% third degree** burns   `MCC` `H5` `HCC`

     T31.72   Burns involving 70-79% of body surface with **20-29% third degree** burns   `MCC` `H5` `HCC`

     T31.73   Burns involving 70-79% of body surface with **30-39% third degree** burns   `MCC` `H5` `HCC`

     T31.74   Burns involving 70-79% of body surface with **40-49% third degree** burns   `MCC` `H5` `HCC`

     T31.75   Burns involving 70-79% of body surface with **50-59% third degree** burns   `MCC` `H5` `HCC`

     T31.76   Burns involving 70-79% of body surface with **60-69% third degree** burns   `MCC` `H5` `HCC`

     T31.77   Burns involving 70-79% of body surface with **70-79% third degree** burns   `MCC` `H5` `HCC`

✓5th   **T31.8**   Burns involving **80-89%** of body surface

     T31.80   Burns involving 80-89% of body surface with **0% to 9% third degree** burns   `CC` `H5`
       Burns involving 80-89% of body surface NOS

     T31.81   Burns involving 80-89% of body surface with **10-19% third degree** burns   `MCC` `H5` `HCC`

     T31.82   Burns involving 80-89% of body surface with **20-29% third degree** burns   `MCC` `H5` `HCC`

     T31.83   Burns involving 80-89% of body surface with **30-39% third degree** burns   `MCC` `H5` `HCC`

     T31.84   Burns involving 80-89% of body surface with **40-49% third degree** burns   `MCC` `H5` `HCC`

     T31.85   Burns involving 80-89% of body surface with **50-59% third degree** burns   `MCC` `H5` `HCC`

     T31.86   Burns involving 80-89% of body surface with **60-69% third degree** burns   `MCC` `H5` `HCC`

     T31.87   Burns involving 80-89% of body surface with **70-79% third degree** burns   `MCC` `H5` `HCC`

     T31.88   Burns involving 80-89% of body surface with **80-89% third degree** burns   `MCC` `H5` `HCC`

✓5th   **T31.9**   Burns involving **90% or more** of body surface

     T31.90   Burns involving 90% or more of body surface with **0% to 9% third degree** burns   `CC` `H5`
       Burns involving 90% or more of body surface NOS

     T31.91   Burns involving 90% or more of body surface with **10-19% third degree** burns   `MCC` `H5` `HCC`

     T31.92   Burns involving 90% or more of body surface with **20-29% third degree** burns   `MCC` `H5` `HCC`

     T31.93   Burns involving 90% or more of body surface with **30-39% third degree** burns   `MCC` `H5` `HCC`

     T31.94   Burns involving 90% or more of body surface with **40-49% third degree** burns   `MCC` `H5` `HCC`

     T31.95   Burns involving 90% or more of body surface with **50-59% third degree** burns   `MCC` `H5` `HCC`

     T31.96   Burns involving 90% or more of body surface with **60-69% third degree** burns   `MCC` `H5` `HCC`

     T31.97   Burns involving 90% or more of body surface with **70-79% third degree** burns   `MCC` `H5` `HCC`

     T31.98   Burns involving 90% or more of body surface with **80-89% third degree** burns   `MCC` `H5` `HCC`

`N` Newborn: 0   `P` Pediatric: 0-17   `M` Maternity: 9-64   `A` Adult: 15-124   `UNS` Unspecified Site   `MCC` Major Complication/Comorbidity   `CC` Complication/Comorbidity   `PE` POA Exempt

1132   ICD-10-CM 2025

T31.99   Burns involving 90% or more of body surface with 90% or more third degree burns   `MCC` `H5` `HCC`

Rule of Nines Estimation of Total Body Surface Burned

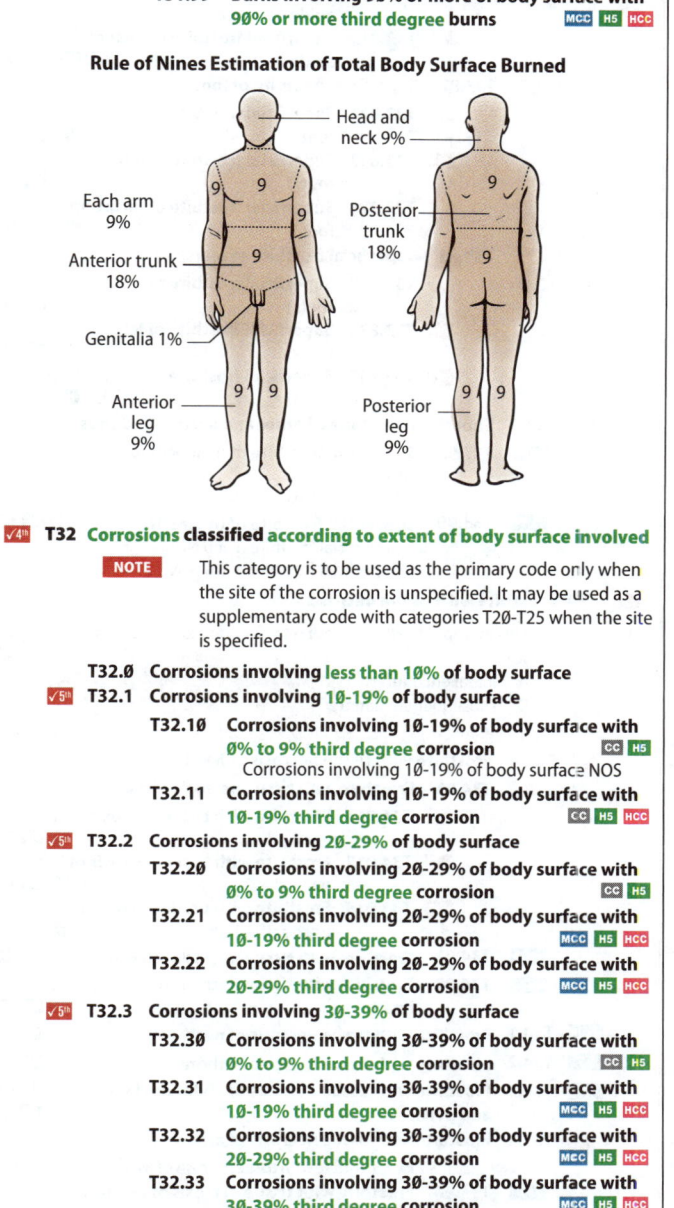

- Head and neck 9%
- Each arm 9%
- Posterior trunk 18%
- Anterior trunk 18%
- Genitalia 1%
- Anterior leg 9%
- Posterior leg 9%

✓4ᵗʰ T32   **Corrosions classified according to extent of body surface involved**

> **NOTE**   This category is to be used as the primary code only when the site of the corrosion is unspecified. It may be used as a supplementary code with categories T20-T25 when the site is specified.

T32.0   Corrosions involving less than 10% of body surface

✓5ᵗʰ T32.1   Corrosions involving 10-19% of body surface
- **T32.10**   Corrosions involving 10-19% of body surface with 0% to 9% third degree corrosion `CC` `H5`
  Corrosions involving 10-19% of body surface NOS
- **T32.11**   Corrosions involving 10-19% of body surface with 10-19% third degree corrosion `CC` `H5` `HCC`

✓5ᵗʰ T32.2   Corrosions involving 20-29% of body surface
- **T32.20**   Corrosions involving 20-29% of body surface with 0% to 9% third degree corrosion `CC` `H5`
- **T32.21**   Corrosions involving 20-29% of body surface with 10-19% third degree corrosion `MCC` `H5` `HCC`
- **T32.22**   Corrosions involving 20-29% of body surface with 20-29% third degree corrosion `MCC` `H5` `HCC`

✓5ᵗʰ T32.3   Corrosions involving 30-39% of body surface
- **T32.30**   Corrosions involving 30-39% of body surface with 0% to 9% third degree corrosion `CC` `H5`
- **T32.31**   Corrosions involving 30-39% of body surface with 10-19% third degree corrosion `MCC` `H5` `HCC`
- **T32.32**   Corrosions involving 30-39% of body surface with 20-29% third degree corrosion `MCC` `H5` `HCC`
- **T32.33**   Corrosions involving 30-39% of body surface with 30-39% third degree corrosion `MCC` `H5` `HCC`

✓5ᵗʰ T32.4   Corrosions involving 40-49% of body surface
- **T32.40**   Corrosions involving 40-49% of body surface with 0% to 9% third degree corrosion `CC` `H5`
- **T32.41**   Corrosions involving 40-49% of body surface with 10-19% third degree corrosion `MCC` `H5` `HCC`
- **T32.42**   Corrosions involving 40-49% of body surface with 20-29% third degree corrosion `MCC` `H5` `HCC`
- **T32.43**   Corrosions involving 40-49% of body surface with 30-39% third degree corrosion `MCC` `H5` `HCC`
- **T32.44**   Corrosions involving 40-49% of body surface with 40-49% third degree corrosion `MCC` `H5` `HCC`

✓5ᵗʰ T32.5   Corrosions involving 50-59% of body surface
- **T32.50**   Corrosions involving 50-59% of body surface with 0% to 9% third degree corrosion `CC` `H5`
- **T32.51**   Corrosions involving 50-59% of body surface with 10-19% third degree corrosion `MCC` `H5` `HCC`
- **T32.52**   Corrosions involving 50-59% of body surface with 20-29% third degree corrosion `MCC` `H5` `HCC`
- **T32.53**   Corrosions involving 50-59% of body surface with 30-39% third degree corrosion `MCC` `H5` `HCC`
- **T32.54**   Corrosions involving 50-59% of body surface with 40-49% third degree corrosion `MCC` `H5` `HCC`
- **T32.55**   Corrosions involving 50-59% of body surface with 50-59% third degree corrosion `MCC` `H5` `HCC`

✓5ᵗʰ T32.6   Corrosions involving 60-69% of body surface
- **T32.60**   Corrosions involving 60-69% of body surface with 0% to 9% third degree corrosion `CC` `H5`
- **T32.61**   Corrosions involving 60-69% of body surface with 10-19% third degree corrosion `MCC` `H5` `HCC`
- **T32.62**   Corrosions involving 60-69% of body surface with 20-29% third degree corrosion `MCC` `H5` `HCC`
- **T32.63**   Corrosions involving 60-69% of body surface with 30-39% third degree corrosion `MCC` `H5` `HCC`
- **T32.64**   Corrosions involving 60-69% of body surface with 40-49% third degree corrosion `MCC` `H5` `HCC`
- **T32.65**   Corrosions involving 60-69% of body surface with 50-59% third degree corrosion `MCC` `H5` `HCC`
- **T32.66**   Corrosions involving 60-69% of body surface with 60-69% third degree corrosion `MCC` `H5` `HCC`

✓5ᵗʰ T32.7   Corrosions involving 70-79% of body surface
- **T32.70**   Corrosions involving 70-79% of body surface with 0% to 9% third degree corrosion `CC` `H5`
- **T32.71**   Corrosions involving 70-79% of body surface with 10-19% third degree corrosion `MCC` `H5` `HCC`
- **T32.72**   Corrosions involving 70-79% of body surface with 20-29% third degree corrosion `MCC` `H5` `HCC`
- **T32.73**   Corrosions involving 70-79% of body surface with 30-39% third degree corrosion `MCC` `H5` `HCC`
- **T32.74**   Corrosions involving 70-79% of body surface with 40-49% third degree corrosion `MCC` `H5` `HCC`
- **T32.75**   Corrosions involving 70-79% of body surface with 50-59% third degree corrosion `MCC` `H5` `HCC`
- **T32.76**   Corrosions involving 70-79% of body surface with 60-69% third degree corrosion `MCC` `H5` `HCC`
- **T32.77**   Corrosions involving 70-79% of body surface with 70-79% third degree corrosion `MCC` `H5` `HCC`

✓5ᵗʰ T32.8   Corrosions involving 80-89% of body surface
- **T32.80**   Corrosions involving 80-89% of body surface with 0% to 9% third degree corrosion `CC` `H5`
- **T32.81**   Corrosions involving 80-89% of body surface with 10-19% third degree corrosion `MCC` `H5` `HCC`
- **T32.82**   Corrosions involving 80-89% of body surface with 20-29% third degree corrosion `MCC` `H5` `HCC`
- **T32.83**   Corrosions involving 80-89% of body surface with 30-39% third degree corrosion `MCC` `H5` `HCC`
- **T32.84**   Corrosions involving 80-89% of body surface with 40-49% third degree corrosion `MCC` `H5` `HCC`
- **T32.85**   Corrosions involving 80-89% of body surface with 50-59% third degree corrosion `MCC` `H5` `HCC`
- **T32.86**   Corrosions involving 80-89% of body surface with 60-69% third degree corrosion `MCC` `H5` `HCC`
- **T32.87**   Corrosions involving 80-89% of body surface with 70-79% third degree corrosion `MCC` `H5` `HCC`
- **T32.88**   Corrosions involving 80-89% of body surface with 80-89% third degree corrosion `MCC` `H5` `HCC`

✓5ᵗʰ T32.9   Corrosions involving 90% or more of body surface
- **T32.90**   Corrosions involving 90% or more of body surface with 0% to 9% third degree corrosion `CC` `H5`
- **T32.91**   Corrosions involving 90% or more of body surface with 10-19% third degree corrosion `MCC` `H5` `HCC`
- **T32.92**   Corrosions involving 90% or more of body surface with 20-29% third degree corrosion `MCC` `H5` `HCC`
- **T32.93**   Corrosions involving 90% or more of body surface with 30-39% third degree corrosion `MCC` `H5` `HCC`
- **T32.94**   Corrosions involving 90% or more of body surface with 40-49% third degree corrosion `MCC` `H5` `HCC`
- **T32.95**   Corrosions involving 90% or more of body surface with 50-59% third degree corrosion `MCC` `H5` `HCC`
- **T32.96**   Corrosions involving 90% or more of body surface with 60-69% third degree corrosion `MCC` `H5` `HCC`
- **T32.97**   Corrosions involving 90% or more of body surface with 70-79% third degree corrosion `MCC` `H5` `HCC`
- **T32.98**   Corrosions involving 90% or more of body surface with 80-89% third degree corrosion `MCC` `H5` `HCC`
- **T32.99**   Corrosions involving 90% or more of body surface with 90% or more third degree corrosion `MCC` `H5` `HCC`

✔ Additional Character Required   ✓x7ᵗʰ Placeholder   Questionable PDx   Manifestation   Unspecified   UPD Unacceptable PDx   H1-H14 HAC   HCC CMS-HCC Dx   HIV HIV Dx

ICD-10-CM 2025   1133

Chapter 19. Injury, Poisoning and Certain Other Consequences of External Causes

Frostbite (T33-T34)

EXCLUDES 2   hypothermia and other effects of reduced temperature (T68, T69.-)

√4th **T33 Superficial frostbite**

INCLUDES   frostbite with partial thickness skin loss

The appropriate 7th character is to be added to each code from category T33.
A   initial encounter
D   subsequent encounter
S   sequela

√5th **T33.0 Superficial frostbite of head**
- √6th **T33.01 Superficial frostbite of ear**
  - √7th **T33.011 Superficial frostbite of right ear** CC H5 PE
  - √7th **T33.012 Superficial frostbite of left ear** CC H5 PE
  - √7th **T33.019 Superficial frostbite of unspecified ear** CC H5 UNS PE
- √x7th **T33.02 Superficial frostbite of nose** CC H5 PE
- √x7th **T33.09 Superficial frostbite of other part of head** CC H5 PE

√x7th **T33.1 Superficial frostbite of neck** CC H5 PE

√x7th **T33.2 Superficial frostbite of thorax** CC H5 PE

√x7th **T33.3 Superficial frostbite of abdominal wall, lower back and pelvis** CC H5 PE

√5th **T33.4 Superficial frostbite of arm**
EXCLUDES 2   superficial frostbite of wrist and hand (T33.5-)
- √x7th **T33.40 Superficial frostbite of unspecified arm** CC H5 UNS PE
- √x7th **T33.41 Superficial frostbite of right arm** CC H5 PE
- √x7th **T33.42 Superficial frostbite of left arm** CC H5 PE

√5th **T33.5 Superficial frostbite of wrist, hand, and fingers**
- √6th **T33.51 Superficial frostbite of wrist**
  - √7th **T33.511 Superficial frostbite of right wrist** CC H5 PE
  - √7th **T33.512 Superficial frostbite of left wrist** CC H5 PE
  - √7th **T33.519 Superficial frostbite of unspecified wrist** CC H5 UNS PE
- √6th **T33.52 Superficial frostbite of hand**
  EXCLUDES 2   superficial frostbite of fingers (T33.53-)
  - √7th **T33.521 Superficial frostbite of right hand** CC H5 PE
  - √7th **T33.522 Superficial frostbite of left hand** CC H5 PE
  - √7th **T33.529 Superficial frostbite of unspecified hand** CC H5 UNS PE
- √6th **T33.53 Superficial frostbite of finger(s)**
  - √7th **T33.531 Superficial frostbite of right finger(s)** CC H5 PE
  - √7th **T33.532 Superficial frostbite of left finger(s)** CC H5 PE
  - √7th **T33.539 Superficial frostbite of unspecified finger(s)** CC H5 UNS PE

√5th **T33.6 Superficial frostbite of hip and thigh**
- √x7th **T33.60 Superficial frostbite of unspecified hip and thigh** CC H5 UNS PE
- √x7th **T33.61 Superficial frostbite of right hip and thigh** CC H5 PE
- √x7th **T33.62 Superficial frostbite of left hip and thigh** CC H5 PE

√5th **T33.7 Superficial frostbite of knee and lower leg**
EXCLUDES 2   superficial frostbite of ankle and foot (T33.8-)
- √x7th **T33.70 Superficial frostbite of unspecified knee and lower leg** CC H5 UNS PE
- √x7th **T33.71 Superficial frostbite of right knee and lower leg** CC H5 PE
- √x7th **T33.72 Superficial frostbite of left knee and lower leg** CC H5 PE

√5th **T33.8 Superficial frostbite of ankle, foot, and toe(s)**
- √6th **T33.81 Superficial frostbite of ankle**
  - √7th **T33.811 Superficial frostbite of right ankle** CC H5 PE

√7th **T33.812 Superficial frostbite of left ankle** CC H5 PE
√7th **T33.819 Superficial frostbite of unspecified ankle** CC H5 UNS PE
- √6th **T33.82 Superficial frostbite of foot**
  - √7th **T33.821 Superficial frostbite of right foot** CC H5 PE
  - √7th **T33.822 Superficial frostbite of left foot** CC H5 PE
  - √7th **T33.829 Superficial frostbite of unspecified foot** CC H5 UNS PE
- √6th **T33.83 Superficial frostbite of toe(s)**
  - √7th **T33.831 Superficial frostbite of right toe(s)** CC H5 PE
  - √7th **T33.832 Superficial frostbite of left toe(s)** CC H5 PE
  - √7th **T33.839 Superficial frostbite of unspecified toe(s)** CC H5 UNS PE

√5th **T33.9 Superficial frostbite of other and unspecified sites**
- √x7th **T33.90 Superficial frostbite of unspecified sites** CC H5 UNS PE
  Superficial frostbite NOS
- √x7th **T33.99 Superficial frostbite of other sites** CC H5 PE
  Superficial frostbite of leg NOS
  Superficial frostbite of trunk NOS

√4th **T34 Frostbite with tissue necrosis**

The appropriate 7th character is to be added to each code from category T34.
A   initial encounter
D   subsequent encounter
S   sequela

√5th **T34.0 Frostbite with tissue necrosis of head**
- √6th **T34.01 Frostbite with tissue necrosis of ear**
  - √7th **T34.011 Frostbite with tissue necrosis of right ear** CC H5 PE
  - √7th **T34.012 Frostbite with tissue necrosis of left ear** CC H5 PE
  - √7th **T34.019 Frostbite with tissue necrosis of unspecified ear** CC H5 UNS PE
- √x7th **T34.02 Frostbite with tissue necrosis of nose** CC H5 PE
- √x7th **T34.09 Frostbite with tissue necrosis of other part of head** CC H5 PE

√x7th **T34.1 Frostbite with tissue necrosis of neck** CC H5 PE

√x7th **T34.2 Frostbite with tissue necrosis of thorax** CC H5 PE

√x7th **T34.3 Frostbite with tissue necrosis of abdominal wall, lower back and pelvis** CC H5 PE

√5th **T34.4 Frostbite with tissue necrosis of arm**
EXCLUDES 2   frostbite with tissue necrosis of wrist and hand (T34.5-)
- √x7th **T34.40 Frostbite with tissue necrosis of unspecified arm** CC H5 UNS PE
- √x7th **T34.41 Frostbite with tissue necrosis of right arm** CC H5 PE
- √x7th **T34.42 Frostbite with tissue necrosis of left arm** CC H5 PE

√5th **T34.5 Frostbite with tissue necrosis of wrist, hand, and finger(s)**
- √6th **T34.51 Frostbite with tissue necrosis of wrist**
  - √7th **T34.511 Frostbite with tissue necrosis of right wrist** CC H5 PE
  - √7th **T34.512 Frostbite with tissue necrosis of left wrist** CC H5 PE
  - √7th **T34.519 Frostbite with tissue necrosis of unspecified wrist** CC H5 UNS PE
- √6th **T34.52 Frostbite with tissue necrosis of hand**
  EXCLUDES 2   frostbite with tissue necrosis of finger(s) (T34.53-)
  - √7th **T34.521 Frostbite with tissue necrosis of right hand** CC H5 PE
  - √7th **T34.522 Frostbite with tissue necrosis of left hand** CC H5 PE
  - √7th **T34.529 Frostbite with tissue necrosis of unspecified hand** CC H5 UNS PE
- √6th **T34.53 Frostbite with tissue necrosis of finger(s)**
  - √7th **T34.531 Frostbite with tissue necrosis of right finger(s)** CC H5 PE

N Newborn: 0   P Pediatric: 0-17   M Maternity: 9-64   A Adult: 15-124   UNS Unspecified Site   MCC Major Complication/Comorbidity   CC Complication/Comorbidity   PE POA Exempt

√7ᵗʰ　T34.532　Frostbite with tissue necrosis of left finger(s)　CC H5 PE

√7ᵗʰ　**T34.539**　Frostbite with tissue necrosis of unspecified finger(s)　CC HE UNS PE

√5ᵗʰ　**T34.6**　**Frostbite with tissue necrosis of hip and thigh**

√x7ᵗʰ　**T34.60**　Frostbite with tissue necrosis of unspecified hip and thigh　CC HE UNS PE

√x7ᵗʰ　T34.61　Frostbite with tissue necrosis of right hip and thigh　CC H5 PE

√x7ᵗʰ　T34.62　Frostbite with tissue necrosis of left hip and thigh　CC H5 PE

√5ᵗʰ　**T34.7**　**Frostbite with tissue necrosis of knee and lower leg**

　　EXCLUDES 2　*frostbite with tissue necrosis of ankle and foot (T34.8-)*

√x7ᵗʰ　**T34.70**　Frostbite with tissue necrosis of unspecified knee and lower leg　CC H5 UNS PE

√x7ᵗʰ　T34.71　Frostbite with tissue necrosis of right knee and lower leg　CC H5 PE

√x7ᵗʰ　T34.72　Frostbite with tissue necrosis of left knee and lower leg　CC H5 PE

√5ᵗʰ　**T34.8**　**Frostbite with tissue necrosis of ankle, foot, and toe(s)**

√6ᵗʰ　**T34.81**　Frostbite with tissue necrosis of ankle

√7ᵗʰ　T34.811　Frostbite with tissue necrosis of right ankle　CC H5 PE

√7ᵗʰ　T34.812　Frostbite with tissue necrosis of left ankle　CC H5 PE

√7ᵗʰ　**T34.819**　Frostbite with tissue necrosis of unspecified ankle　CC H5 UNS PE

√6ᵗʰ　**T34.82**　Frostbite with tissue necrosis of foot

√7ᵗʰ　T34.821　Frostbite with tissue necrosis of right foot　CC H5 PE

√7ᵗʰ　T34.822　Frostbite with tissue necrosis of left foot　CC H5 PE

√7ᵗʰ　**T34.829**　Frostbite with tissue necrosis of unspecified foot　CC H5 UNS PE

√6ᵗʰ　**T34.83**　Frostbite with tissue necrosis of toe(s)

√7ᵗʰ　T34.831　Frostbite with tissue necrosis of right toe(s)　CC H5 PE

√7ᵗʰ　T34.832　Frostbite with tissue necrosis of left toe(s)　CC H5 PE

√7ᵗʰ　**T34.839**　Frostbite with tissue necrosis of unspecified toe(s)　CC H5 UNS PE

√5ᵗʰ　**T34.9**　**Frostbite with tissue necrosis of other and unspecified sites**

√x7ᵗʰ　**T34.90**　Frostbite with tissue necrosis of unspecified sites　CC H5 UNS PE
　　　　Frostbite with tissue necrosis NOS

√x7ᵗʰ　**T34.99**　Frostbite with tissue necrosis of other sites　CC H5 PE
　　　　Frostbite with tissue necrosis of leg NOS
　　　　Frostbite with tissue necrosis of trunk NOS

Poisoning by, adverse effects of and underdosing of drugs, medicaments and biological substances (T36-T50)

INCLUDES　adverse effect of correct substance properly administered
poisoning by overdose of substance
poisoning by wrong substance given or taken in error
underdosing by (inadvertently) (deliberately) taking less substance than prescribed or instructed

Code first, for adverse effects, the nature of the adverse effect, such as:
adverse effect NOS (T88.7)
aspirin gastritis (K29.-)
blood disorders (D56-D76)
contact dermatitis (L23-L25)
dermatitis due to substances taken internally (L27.-)
nephropathy (N14.0-N14.2)

NOTE　The drug giving rise to the adverse effect should be identified by use of codes from categories T36-T50 with fifth or sixth character 5.

Use additional code(s) to specify:
manifestations of poisoning
underdosing or failure in dosage during medical and surgical care (Y63.6, Y63.8-Y63.9)
underdosing of medication regimen (Z91.12-, Z91.13-)
EXCLUDES 1　*toxic reaction to local anesthesia in pregnancy (O29.3-)*
EXCLUDES 2　*abuse and dependence of psychoactive substances (F10-F19)*
abuse of non-dependence-producing substances (F55.-)
drug reaction and poisoning affecting newborn (P00-P96)
immunodeficiency due to drugs (D84.821)
pathological drug intoxication (inebriation) (F10-F19)
AHA: 2018,4Q,71; 2016,2Q,8; 2015,3Q,22

√4ᵗʰ　**T36**　**Poisoning by, adverse effect of and underdosing of systemic antibiotics**

　　EXCLUDES 1　*antineoplastic antibiotics (T45.1-)*
　　　　locally applied antibiotic NEC (T49.0)
　　　　topically used antibiotic for ear, nose and throat (T49.6)
　　　　topically used antibiotic for eye (T49.5)

The appropriate 7th character is to be added to each code from category T36.
A　initial encounter
D　subsequent encounter
S　sequela

√5ᵗʰ　**T36.0**　**Poisoning by, adverse effect of and underdosing of penicillins**

√6ᵗʰ　**T36.0X**　Poisoning by, adverse effect of and underdosing of penicillins

√7ᵗʰ　T36.0X1　Poisoning by penicillins, accidental (unintentional)　PE
　　　　Poisoning by penicillins NOS

√7ᵗʰ　T36.0X2　Poisoning by penicillins, intentional self-harm　HCC PE

√7ᵗʰ　T36.0X3　Poisoning by penicillins, assault　PE

√7ᵗʰ　T36.0X4　Poisoning by penicillins, undetermined　PE

√7ᵗʰ　T36.0X5　Adverse effect of penicillins　UPD PE

√7ᵗʰ　T36.0X6　Underdosing of penicillins　UPD PE

√5ᵗʰ　**T36.1**　**Poisoning by, adverse effect of and underdosing of cephalosporins and other beta-lactam antibiotics**

√6ᵗʰ　**T36.1X**　Poisoning by, adverse effect of and underdosing of cephalosporins and other beta-lactam antibiotics

√7ᵗʰ　T36.1X1　Poisoning by cephalosporins and other beta-lactam antibiotics, accidental (unintentional)　PE
　　　　Poisoning by cephalosporins and other beta-lactam antibiotics NOS

√7ᵗʰ　T36.1X2　Poisoning by cephalosporins and other beta-lactam antibiotics, intentional self-harm　HCC PE

√7ᵗʰ　T36.1X3　Poisoning by cephalosporins and other beta-lactam antibiotics, assault　PE

√7ᵗʰ　T36.1X4　Poisoning by cephalosporins and other beta-lactam antibiotics, undetermined　PE

√7ᵗʰ　T36.1X5　Adverse effect of cephalosporins and other beta-lactam antibiotics　UPD PE

√7ᵗʰ　T36.1X6　Underdosing of cephalosporins and other beta-lactam antibiotics　UPD PE

Chapter 19. Injury, Poisoning and Certain Other Consequences of External Causes

√5th **T36.2** Poisoning by, adverse effect of and underdosing of chloramphenicol group

   √6th **T36.2X** Poisoning by, adverse effect of and underdosing of chloramphenicol group

      √7th **T36.2X1** Poisoning by chloramphenicol group, accidental (unintentional) **PE**
         Poisoning by chloramphenicol group NOS

      √7th **T36.2X2** Poisoning by chloramphenicol group, intentional self-harm **HCC** **PE**

      √7th **T36.2X3** Poisoning by chloramphenicol group, assault **PE**

      √7th **T36.2X4** Poisoning by chloramphenicol group, undetermined **PE**

      √7th **T36.2X5** Adverse effect of chloramphenicol group **UPD** **PE**

      √7th **T36.2X6** Underdosing of chloramphenicol group **UPD** **PE**

√5th **T36.3** Poisoning by, adverse effect of and underdosing of macrolides

   √6th **T36.3X** Poisoning by, adverse effect of and underdosing of macrolides

      √7th **T36.3X1** Poisoning by macrolides, accidental (unintentional) **PE**
         Poisoning by macrolides NOS

      √7th **T36.3X2** Poisoning by macrolides, intentional self-harm **HCC** **PE**

      √7th **T36.3X3** Poisoning by macrolides, assault **PE**

      √7th **T36.3X4** Poisoning by macrolides, undetermined **PE**

      √7th **T36.3X5** Adverse effect of macrolides **UPD** **PE**

      √7th **T36.3X6** Underdosing of macrolides **UPD** **PE**

√5th **T36.4** Poisoning by, adverse effect of and underdosing of tetracyclines

   √6th **T36.4X** Poisoning by, adverse effect of and underdosing of tetracyclines

      √7th **T36.4X1** Poisoning by tetracyclines, accidental (unintentional) **PE**
         Poisoning by tetracyclines NOS

      √7th **T36.4X2** Poisoning by tetracyclines, intentional self-harm **HCC** **PE**

      √7th **T36.4X3** Poisoning by tetracyclines, assault **PE**

      √7th **T36.4X4** Poisoning by tetracyclines, undetermined **PE**

      √7th **T36.4X5** Adverse effect of tetracyclines **UPD** **PE**

      √7th **T36.4X6** Underdosing of tetracyclines **UPD** **PE**

√5th **T36.5** Poisoning by, adverse effect of and underdosing of aminoglycosides
   Poisoning by, adverse effect of and underdosing of streptomycin

   √6th **T36.5X** Poisoning by, adverse effect of and underdosing of aminoglycosides

      √7th **T36.5X1** Poisoning by aminoglycosides, accidental (unintentional) **PE**
         Poisoning by aminoglycosides NOS

      √7th **T36.5X2** Poisoning by aminoglycosides, intentional self-harm **HCC** **PE**

      √7th **T36.5X3** Poisoning by aminoglycosides, assault **PE**

      √7th **T36.5X4** Poisoning by aminoglycosides, undetermined **PE**

      √7th **T36.5X5** Adverse effect of aminoglycosides **UPD** **PE**

      √7th **T36.5X6** Underdosing of aminoglycosides **UPD** **PE**

√5th **T36.6** Poisoning by, adverse effect of and underdosing of rifampicins

   √6th **T36.6X** Poisoning by, adverse effect of and underdosing of rifampicins

      √7th **T36.6X1** Poisoning by rifampicins, accidental (unintentional) **PE**
         Poisoning by rifampicins NOS

      √7th **T36.6X2** Poisoning by rifampicins, intentional self-harm **HCC** **PE**

      √7th **T36.6X3** Poisoning by rifampicins, assault **PE**

      √7th **T36.6X4** Poisoning by rifampicins, undetermined **PE**

      √7th **T36.6X5** Adverse effect of rifampicins **UPD** **PE**

      √7th **T36.6X6** Underdosing of rifampicins **UPD** **PE**

√5th **T36.7** Poisoning by, adverse effect of and underdosing of antifungal antibiotics, systemically used

   √6th **T36.7X** Poisoning by, adverse effect of and underdosing of antifungal antibiotics, systemically used

      √7th **T36.7X1** Poisoning by antifungal antibiotics, systemically used, accidental (unintentional) **PE**
         Poisoning by antifungal antibiotics, systemically used NOS

      √7th **T36.7X2** Poisoning by antifungal antibiotics, systemically used, intentional self-harm **HCC** **PE**

      √7th **T36.7X3** Poisoning by antifungal antibiotics, systemically used, assault **PE**

      √7th **T36.7X4** Poisoning by antifungal antibiotics, systemically used, undetermined **PE**

      √7th **T36.7X5** Adverse effect of antifungal antibiotics, systemically used **UPD** **PE**

      √7th **T36.7X6** Underdosing of antifungal antibiotics, systemically used **UPD** **PE**

√5th **T36.8** Poisoning by, adverse effect of and underdosing of other systemic antibiotics

   √6th **T36.8X** Poisoning by, adverse effect of and underdosing of other systemic antibiotics
     AHA: 2017,1Q,39

      √7th **T36.8X1** Poisoning by other systemic antibiotics, accidental (unintentional) **PE**
         Poisoning by other systemic antibiotics NOS

      √7th **T36.8X2** Poisoning by other systemic antibiotics, intentional self-harm **HCC** **PE**

      √7th **T36.8X3** Poisoning by other systemic antibiotics, assault **PE**

      √7th **T36.8X4** Poisoning by other systemic antibiotics, undetermined **PE**

      √7th **T36.8X5** Adverse effect of other systemic antibiotics **UPD** **PE**

      √7th **T36.8X6** Underdosing of other systemic antibiotics **UPD** **PE**

√5th **T36.9** Poisoning by, adverse effect of and underdosing of unspecified systemic antibiotic

   √x7th **T36.91** Poisoning by unspecified systemic antibiotic, accidental (unintentional) **PE**
         Poisoning by systemic antibiotic NOS

   √x7th **T36.92** Poisoning by unspecified systemic antibiotic, intentional self-harm **HCC** **PE**

   √x7th **T36.93** Poisoning by unspecified systemic antibiotic, assault **PE**

   √x7th **T36.94** Poisoning by unspecified systemic antibiotic, undetermined **PE**

   √x7th **T36.95** Adverse effect of unspecified systemic antibiotic **UPD** **PE**

   √x7th **T36.96** Underdosing of unspecified systemic antibiotic **UPD** **PE**

√4th **T37** Poisoning by, adverse effect of and underdosing of other systemic anti-infectives and antiparasitics

   EXCLUDES 1 anti-infectives topically used for ear, nose and throat (T49.6-)
     anti-infectives topically used for eye (T49.5-)
     locally applied anti-infectives NEC (T49.0-)

   The appropriate 7th character is to be added to each code from category T37.
   A   initial encounter
   D   subsequent encounter
   S   sequela

√5th **T37.0** Poisoning by, adverse effect of and underdosing of sulfonamides

   √6th **T37.0X** Poisoning by, adverse effect of and underdosing of sulfonamides

      √7th **T37.0X1** Poisoning by sulfonamides, accidental (unintentional) **PE**
         Poisoning by sulfonamides NOS

      √7th **T37.0X2** Poisoning by sulfonamides, intentional self-harm **HCC** **PE**

      √7th **T37.0X3** Poisoning by sulfonamides, assault **PE**

      √7th **T37.0X4** Poisoning by sulfonamides, undetermined **PE**

      √7th **T37.0X5** Adverse effect of sulfonamides **UPD** **PE**

      √7th **T37.0X6** Underdosing of sulfonamides **UPD** **PE**

N Newborn: 0   **P** Pediatric: 0-17   **M** Maternity: 9-64   **A** Adult: 15-124   **UNS** Unspecified Site   **MCC** Major Complication/Comorbidity   **CC** Complication/Comorbidity   **PE** POA Exempt

1136   ICD-10-CM 2025

√5th T37.1 Poisoning by, adverse effect of and underdosing of antimycobacterial drugs

EXCLUDES 1   *rifampicins (T36.6-)*
           streptomycin (T36.5-)

    √6th T37.1X Poisoning by, adverse effect of and underdosing of antimycobacterial drugs

       √7th T37.1X1 Poisoning by antimycobacterial drugs, accidental (unintentional) PE
               Poisoning by antimycobacterial drugs NOS

       √7th T37.1X2 Poisoning by antimycobacterial drugs, intentional self-harm HCC PE

       √7th T37.1X3 Poisoning by antimycobacterial drugs, assault PE

       √7th T37.1X4 Poisoning by antimycobacterial drugs, undetermined PE

       √7th T37.1X5 Adverse effect of antimycobacterial drugs UPD PE

       √7th T37.1X6 Underdosing of antimycobacterial drugs UPD PE

√5th T37.2 Poisoning by, adverse effect of and underdosing of antimalarials and drugs acting on other blood protozoa

EXCLUDES 1   *hydroxyquinoline derivatives (T37.8-)*

    √6th T37.2X Poisoning by, adverse effect of and underdosing of antimalarials and drugs acting on other blood protozoa

       √7th T37.2X1 Poisoning by antimalarials and drugs acting on other blood protozoa, accidental (unintentional) PE
               Poisoning by antimalarials and drugs acting on other blood protozoa NOS

       √7th T37.2X2 Poisoning by antimalarials and drugs acting on other blood protozoa, intentional self-harm HCC PE

       √7th T37.2X3 Poisoning by antimalarials and drugs acting on other blood protozoa, assault PE

       √7th T37.2X4 Poisoning by antimalarials and drugs acting on other blood protozoa, undetermined PE

       √7th T37.2X5 Adverse effect of antimalarials and drugs acting on other blood protozoa UPD PE

       √7th T37.2X6 Underdosing of antimalarials and drugs acting on other blood protozoa UPD PE

√5th T37.3 Poisoning by, adverse effect of and underdosing of other antiprotozoal drugs

    √6th T37.3X Poisoning by, adverse effect of and underdosing of other antiprotozoal drugs

       √7th T37.3X1 Poisoning by other antiprotozoal drugs, accidental (unintentional) PE
               Poisoning by other antiprotozoal drugs NOS

       √7th T37.3X2 Poisoning by other antiprotozoal drugs, intentional self-harm HCC PE

       √7th T37.3X3 Poisoning by other antiprotozoal drugs, assault PE

       √7th T37.3X4 Poisoning by other antiprotozoal drugs, undetermined PE

       √7th T37.3X5 Adverse effect of other antiprotozoal drugs UPD PE

       √7th T37.3X6 Underdosing of other antiprotozoal drugs UPD PE

√5th T37.4 Poisoning by, adverse effect of and underdosing of anthelminthics

    √6th T37.4X Poisoning by, adverse effect of and underdosing of anthelminthics

       √7th T37.4X1 Poisoning by anthelminthics, accidental (unintentional) PE
               Poisoning by anthelminthics NOS

       √7th T37.4X2 Poisoning by anthelminthics, intentional self-harm HCC PE

       √7th T37.4X3 Poisoning by anthelminthics, assault PE

       √7th T37.4X4 Poisoning by anthelminthics, undetermined PE

       √7th T37.4X5 Adverse effect of anthelminthics UPD PE

       √7th T37.4X6 Underdosing of anthelminthics UPD PE

√5th T37.5 Poisoning by, adverse effect of and underdosing of antiviral drugs

EXCLUDES 1   *amantadine (T42.8-)*
           cytarabine (T45.1-)

    √6th T37.5X Poisoning by, adverse effect of and underdosing of antiviral drugs

       √7th T37.5X1 Poisoning by antiviral drugs, accidental (unintentional) PE
               Poisoning by antiviral drugs NOS

       √7th T37.5X2 Poisoning by antiviral drugs, intentional self-harm HCC PE

       √7th T37.5X3 Poisoning by antiviral drugs, assault PE

       √7th T37.5X4 Poisoning by antiviral drugs, undetermined PE

       √7th T37.5X5 Adverse effect of antiviral drugs UPD PE

       √7th T37.5X6 Underdosing of antiviral drugs UPD PE

√5th T37.8 Poisoning by, adverse effect of and underdosing of other specified systemic anti-infectives and antiparasitics

Poisoning by, adverse effect of and underdosing of hydroxyquinoline derivatives

EXCLUDES 1   *antimalarial drugs (T37.2-)*

    √6th T37.8X Poisoning by, adverse effect of and underdosing of other specified systemic anti-infectives and antiparasitics

       √7th T37.8X1 Poisoning by other specified systemic anti-infectives and antiparasitics, accidental (unintentional) PE
               Poisoning by other specified systemic anti-infectives and antiparasitics NOS

       √7th T37.8X2 Poisoning by other specified systemic anti-infectives and antiparasitics, intentional self-harm HCC PE

       √7th T37.8X3 Poisoning by other specified systemic anti-infectives and antiparasitics, assault PE

       √7th T37.8X4 Poisoning by other specified systemic anti-infectives and antiparasitics, undetermined PE

       √7th T37.8X5 Adverse effect of other specified systemic anti-infectives and antiparasitics UPD PE

       √7th T37.8X6 Underdosing of other specified systemic anti-infectives and antiparasitics UPD PE

√5th T37.9 Poisoning by, adverse effect of and underdosing of unspecified systemic anti-infective and antiparasitics

    √x7th T37.91 Poisoning by unspecified systemic anti-infective and antiparasitics, accidental (unintentional) PE
               Poisoning by, adverse effect of and underdosing of systemic anti-infective and antiparasitics NOS

    √x7th T37.92 Poisoning by unspecified systemic anti-infective and antiparasitics, intentional self-harm HCC PE

    √x7th T37.93 Poisoning by unspecified systemic anti-infective and antiparasitics, assault PE

    √x7th T37.94 Poisoning by unspecified systemic anti-infective and antiparasitics, undetermined PE

    √x7th T37.95 Adverse effect of unspecified systemic anti-infective and antiparasitic UPD PE

    √x7th T37.96 Underdosing of unspecified systemic anti-infectives and antiparasitics UPD PE

✔ Additional Character Required   √x7th Placeholder   Questionable PDx   Manifestation   Unspecified   UPD Unacceptable PDx   H1 - H14 HAC   HCC CMS-HCC Dx   HIV HIV Dx

✓4ᵗʰ T38 Poisoning by, adverse effect of and underdosing of hormones and their synthetic substitutes and antagonists, not elsewhere classified

> EXCLUDES 1   mineralocorticoids and their antagonists (T50.0-)
> oxytocic hormones (T48.0-)
> parathyroid hormones and derivatives (T50.9-)

> The appropriate 7th character is to be added to each code from category T38.
> A   initial encounter
> D   subsequent encounter
> S   sequela

✓5ᵗʰ T38.0 Poisoning by, adverse effect of and underdosing of glucocorticoids and synthetic analogues

> EXCLUDES 1   glucocorticoids, topically used (T49.-)

✓6ᵗʰ T38.0X Poisoning by, adverse effect of and underdosing of glucocorticoids and synthetic analogues

     ✓7ᵗʰ **T38.0X1 Poisoning by glucocorticoids and synthetic analogues, accidental (unintentional)**   PE
         Poisoning by glucocorticoids and synthetic analogues NOS

     ✓7ᵗʰ **T38.0X2 Poisoning by glucocorticoids and synthetic analogues, intentional self-harm**   HCC PE

     ✓7ᵗʰ **T38.0X3 Poisoning by glucocorticoids and synthetic analogues, assault**   PE

     ✓7ᵗʰ **T38.0X4 Poisoning by glucocorticoids and synthetic analogues, undetermined**   PE

     ✓7ᵗʰ **T38.0X5 Adverse effect of glucocorticoids and synthetic analogues**   UPD PE

     ✓7ᵗʰ **T38.0X6 Underdosing of glucocorticoids and synthetic analogues**   UPD PE

✓5ᵗʰ T38.1 Poisoning by, adverse effect of and underdosing of thyroid hormones and substitutes

✓6ᵗʰ T38.1X Poisoning by, adverse effect of and underdosing of thyroid hormones and substitutes

     ✓7ᵗʰ **T38.1X1 Poisoning by thyroid hormones and substitutes, accidental (unintentional)**   PE
         Poisoning by thyroid hormones and substitutes NOS

     ✓7ᵗʰ **T38.1X2 Poisoning by thyroid hormones and substitutes, intentional self-harm**   HCC PE

     ✓7ᵗʰ **T38.1X3 Poisoning by thyroid hormones and substitutes, assault**   PE

     ✓7ᵗʰ **T38.1X4 Poisoning by thyroid hormones and substitutes, undetermined**   PE

     ✓7ᵗʰ **T38.1X5 Adverse effect of thyroid hormones and substitutes**   UPD PE

     ✓7ᵗʰ **T38.1X6 Underdosing of thyroid hormones and substitutes**   UPD PE

✓5ᵗʰ T38.2 Poisoning by, adverse effect of and underdosing of antithyroid drugs

✓6ᵗʰ T38.2X Poisoning by, adverse effect of and underdosing of antithyroid drugs

     ✓7ᵗʰ **T38.2X1 Poisoning by antithyroid drugs, accidental (unintentional)**   PE
         Poisoning by antithyroid drugs NOS

     ✓7ᵗʰ **T38.2X2 Poisoning by antithyroid drugs, intentional self-harm**   HCC PE

     ✓7ᵗʰ **T38.2X3 Poisoning by antithyroid drugs, assault**   PE

     ✓7ᵗʰ **T38.2X4 Poisoning by antithyroid drugs, undetermined**   PE

     ✓7ᵗʰ **T38.2X5 Adverse effect of antithyroid drugs**   UPD PE

     ✓7ᵗʰ **T38.2X6 Underdosing of antithyroid drugs**   UPD PE

✓5ᵗʰ T38.3 Poisoning by, adverse effect of and underdosing of insulin and oral hypoglycemic [antidiabetic] drugs

✓6ᵗʰ T38.3X Poisoning by, adverse effect of and underdosing of insulin and oral hypoglycemic [antidiabetic] drugs

     ✓7ᵗʰ **T38.3X1 Poisoning by insulin and oral hypoglycemic [antidiabetic] drugs, accidental (unintentional)**   PE
         Poisoning by insulin and oral hypoglycemic [antidiabetic] drugs NOS

     ✓7ᵗʰ **T38.3X2 Poisoning by insulin and oral hypoglycemic [antidiabetic] drugs, intentional self-harm**   HCC PE

     ✓7ᵗʰ **T38.3X3 Poisoning by insulin and oral hypoglycemic [antidiabetic] drugs, assault**   PE

     ✓7ᵗʰ **T38.3X4 Poisoning by insulin and oral hypoglycemic [antidiabetic] drugs, undetermined**   PE

     ✓7ᵗʰ **T38.3X5 Adverse effect of insulin and oral hypoglycemic [antidiabetic] drugs**   UPD PE

     ✓7ᵗʰ **T38.3X6 Underdosing of insulin and oral hypoglycemic [antidiabetic] drugs**   UPD PE

✓5ᵗʰ T38.4 Poisoning by, adverse effect of and underdosing of oral contraceptives

> Poisoning by, adverse effect of and underdosing of multiple- and single-ingredient oral contraceptive preparations

✓6ᵗʰ T38.4X Poisoning by, adverse effect of and underdosing of oral contraceptives

     ✓7ᵗʰ **T38.4X1 Poisoning by oral contraceptives, accidental (unintentional)**   PE
         Poisoning by oral contraceptives NOS

     ✓7ᵗʰ **T38.4X2 Poisoning by oral contraceptives, intentional self-harm**   HCC PE

     ✓7ᵗʰ **T38.4X3 Poisoning by oral contraceptives, assault**   PE

     ✓7ᵗʰ **T38.4X4 Poisoning by oral contraceptives, undetermined**   PE

     ✓7ᵗʰ **T38.4X5 Adverse effect of oral contraceptives**   UPD PE

     ✓7ᵗʰ **T38.4X6 Underdosing of oral contraceptives**   UPD PE

✓5ᵗʰ T38.5 Poisoning by, adverse effect of and underdosing of other estrogens and progestogens

> Poisoning by, adverse effect of and underdosing of estrogens and progestogens mixtures and substitutes

✓6ᵗʰ T38.5X Poisoning by, adverse effect of and underdosing of other estrogens and progestogens

     ✓7ᵗʰ **T38.5X1 Poisoning by other estrogens and progestogens, accidental (unintentional)**   PE
         Poisoning by other estrogens and progestogens NOS

     ✓7ᵗʰ **T38.5X2 Poisoning by other estrogens and progestogens, intentional self-harm**   HCC PE

     ✓7ᵗʰ **T38.5X3 Poisoning by other estrogens and progestogens, assault**   PE

     ✓7ᵗʰ **T38.5X4 Poisoning by other estrogens and progestogens, undetermined**   PE

     ✓7ᵗʰ **T38.5X5 Adverse effect of other estrogens and progestogens**   UPD PE

     ✓7ᵗʰ **T38.5X6 Underdosing of other estrogens and progestogens**   UPD PE

✓5ᵗʰ T38.6 Poisoning by, adverse effect of and underdosing of antigonadotrophins, antiestrogens, antiandrogens, not elsewhere classified

> Poisoning by, adverse effect of and underdosing of tamoxifen

✓6ᵗʰ T38.6X Poisoning by, adverse effect of and underdosing of antigonadotrophins, antiestrogens, antiandrogens, not elsewhere classified

     ✓7ᵗʰ **T38.6X1 Poisoning by antigonadotrophins, antiestrogens, antiandrogens, not elsewhere classified, accidental (unintentional)**   PE
         Poisoning by antigonadotrophins, antiestrogens, antiandrogens, not elsewhere classified NOS

     ✓7ᵗʰ **T38.6X2 Poisoning by antigonadotrophins, antiestrogens, antiandrogens, not elsewhere classified, intentional self-harm**   HCC PE

     ✓7ᵗʰ **T38.6X3 Poisoning by antigonadotrophins, antiestrogens, antiandrogens, not elsewhere classified, assault**   PE

     ✓7ᵗʰ **T38.6X4 Poisoning by antigonadotrophins, antiestrogens, antiandrogens, not elsewhere classified, undetermined**   PE

     ✓7ᵗʰ **T38.6X5 Adverse effect of antigonadotrophins, antiestrogens, antiandrogens, not elsewhere classified**   UPD PE

     ✓7ᵗʰ **T38.6X6 Underdosing of antigonadotrophins, antiestrogens, antiandrogens, not elsewhere classified**   UPD PE

N Newborn: 0   P Pediatric: 0-17   M Maternity: 9-64   A Adult: 15-124   UNS Unspecified Site   MCC Major Complication/Comorbidity   CC Complication/Comorbidity   PE POA Exempt

1138   ICD-10-CM 2025

☑5ᵗʰ **T38.7** **Poisoning by, adverse effect of and underdosing of androgens and anabolic congeners**

  ☑6ᵗʰ **T38.7X** **Poisoning by, adverse effect of and underdosing of androgens and anabolic congeners**

    ☑7ᵗʰ **T38.7X1** **Poisoning by androgens and anabolic congeners, accidental (unintentional)** PE
       Poisoning by androgens and anabolic congeners NOS

    ☑7ᵗʰ **T38.7X2** **Poisoning by androgens and anabolic congeners, intentional self-harm** HCC PE

    ☑7ᵗʰ **T38.7X3** **Poisoning by androgens and anabolic congeners, assault** PE

    ☑7ᵗʰ **T38.7X4** **Poisoning by androgens and anabolic congeners, undetermined** PE

    ☑7ᵗʰ **T38.7X5** **Adverse effect of androgens and anabolic congeners** UPD PE

    ☑7ᵗʰ **T38.7X6** **Underdosing of androgens and anabolic congeners** UPD PE

☑5ᵗʰ **T38.8** **Poisoning by, adverse effect of and underdosing of other and unspecified hormones and synthetic substitutes**

  ☑6ᵗʰ **T38.80** **Poisoning by, adverse effect of and underdosing of unspecified hormones and synthetic substitutes**

    ☑7ᵗʰ **T38.801** **Poisoning by unspecified hormones and synthetic substitutes, accidental (unintentional)** PE
       Poisoning by unspecified hormones and synthetic substitutes NOS

    ☑7ᵗʰ **T38.802** **Poisoning by unspecified hormones and synthetic substitutes, intentional self-harm** HCC PE

    ☑7ᵗʰ **T38.803** **Poisoning by unspecified hormones and synthetic substitutes, assault** PE

    ☑7ᵗʰ **T38.804** **Poisoning by unspecified hormones and synthetic substitutes, undetermined** PE

    ☑7ᵗʰ **T38.805** **Adverse effect of unspecified hormones and synthetic substitutes** UPD PE

    ☑7ᵗʰ **T38.806** **Underdosing of unspecified hormones and synthetic substitutes** UPD PE

  ☑6ᵗʰ **T38.81** **Poisoning by, adverse effect of and underdosing of anterior pituitary [adenohypophyseal] hormones**

    ☑7ᵗʰ **T38.811** **Poisoning by anterior pituitary [adenohypophyseal] hormones, accidental (unintentional)** PE
       Poisoning by anterior pituitary [adenohypophyseal] hormones NOS

    ☑7ᵗʰ **T38.812** **Poisoning by anterior pituitary [adenohypophyseal] hormones, intentional self-harm** HCC PE

    ☑7ᵗʰ **T38.813** **Poisoning by anterior pituitary [adenohypophyseal] hormones, assault** PE

    ☑7ᵗʰ **T38.814** **Poisoning by anterior pituitary [adenohypophyseal] hormones, undetermined** PE

    ☑7ᵗʰ **T38.815** **Adverse effect of anterior pituitary [adenohypophyseal] hormones** UPD PE

    ☑7ᵗʰ **T38.816** **Underdosing of anterior pituitary [adenohypophyseal] hormones** UPD PE

  ☑6ᵗʰ **T38.89** **Poisoning by, adverse effect of and underdosing of other hormones and synthetic substitutes**

    ☑7ᵗʰ **T38.891** **Poisoning by other hormones and synthetic substitutes, accidental (unintentional)** PE
       Poisoning by other hormones and synthetic substitutes NOS

    ☑7ᵗʰ **T38.892** **Poisoning by other hormones and synthetic substitutes, intentional self-harm** HCC PE

    ☑7ᵗʰ **T38.893** **Poisoning by other hormones and synthetic substitutes, assault** PE

    ☑7ᵗʰ **T38.894** **Poisoning by other hormones and synthetic substitutes, undetermined** PE

    ☑7ᵗʰ **T38.895** **Adverse effect of other hormones and synthetic substitutes** UPD PE

    ☑7ᵗʰ **T38.896** **Underdosing of other hormones and synthetic substitutes** UPD PE

☑5ᵗʰ **T38.9** **Poisoning by, adverse effect of and underdosing of other and unspecified hormone antagonists**

  ☑6ᵗʰ **T38.90** **Poisoning by, adverse effect of and underdosing of unspecified hormone antagonists**

    ☑7ᵗʰ **T38.901** **Poisoning by unspecified hormone antagonists, accidental (unintentional)** PE
       Poisoning by unspecified hormone antagonists NOS

    ☑7ᵗʰ **T38.902** **Poisoning by unspecified hormone antagonists, intentional self-harm** HCC PE

    ☑7ᵗʰ **T38.903** **Poisoning by unspecified hormone antagonists, assault** PE

    ☑7ᵗʰ **T38.904** **Poisoning by unspecified hormone antagonists, undetermined** PE

    ☑7ᵗʰ **T38.905** **Adverse effect of unspecified hormone antagonists** UPD PE

    ☑7ᵗʰ **T38.906** **Underdosing of unspecified hormone antagonists** UPD PE

  ☑6ᵗʰ **T38.99** **Poisoning by, adverse effect of and underdosing of other hormone antagonists**

    ☑7ᵗʰ **T38.991** **Poisoning by other hormone antagonists, accidental (unintentional)** PE
       Poisoning by other hormone antagonists NOS

    ☑7ᵗʰ **T38.992** **Poisoning by other hormone antagonists, intentional self-harm** HCC PE

    ☑7ᵗʰ **T38.993** **Poisoning by other hormone antagonists, assault** PE

    ☑7ᵗʰ **T38.994** **Poisoning by other hormone antagonists, undetermined** PE

    ☑7ᵗʰ **T38.995** **Adverse effect of other hormone antagonists** UPD PE

    ☑7ᵗʰ **T38.996** **Underdosing of other hormone antagonists** UPD PE

☑4ᵗʰ **T39** **Poisoning by, adverse effect of and underdosing of nonopioid analgesics, antipyretics and antirheumatics**

> The appropriate 7th character is to be added to each code from category T39.
> A   initial encounter
> D   subsequent encounter
> S   sequela

☑5ᵗʰ **T39.0** **Poisoning by, adverse effect of and underdosing of salicylates**

  ☑6ᵗʰ **T39.01** **Poisoning by, adverse effect of and underdosing of aspirin**
     Poisoning by, adverse effect of and underdosing of acetylsalicylic acid

    ☑7ᵗʰ **T39.011** **Poisoning by aspirin, accidental (unintentional)** PE

    ☑7ᵗʰ **T39.012** **Poisoning by aspirin, intentional self-harm** HCC PE

    ☑7ᵗʰ **T39.013** **Poisoning by aspirin, assault** PE

    ☑7ᵗʰ **T39.014** **Poisoning by aspirin, undetermined** PE

    ☑7ᵗʰ **T39.015** **Adverse effect of aspirin** UPD PE
       AHA: 2016,1Q,15

    ☑7ᵗʰ **T39.016** **Underdosing of aspirin** UPD PE

  ☑6ᵗʰ **T39.09** **Poisoning by, adverse effect of and underdosing of other salicylates**

    ☑7ᵗʰ **T39.091** **Poisoning by salicylates, accidental (unintentional)** PE
       Poisoning by salicylates NOS

    ☑7ᵗʰ **T39.092** **Poisoning by salicylates, intentional self-harm** HCC PE

    ☑7ᵗʰ **T39.093** **Poisoning by salicylates, assault** PE

    ☑7ᵗʰ **T39.094** **Poisoning by salicylates, undetermined** PE

    ☑7ᵗʰ **T39.095** **Adverse effect of salicylates** UPD PE

    ☑7ᵗʰ **T39.096** **Underdosing of salicylates** UPD PE

☑5ᵗʰ **T39.1** **Poisoning by, adverse effect of and underdosing of 4-Aminophenol derivatives**

  ☑6ᵗʰ **T39.1X** **Poisoning by, adverse effect of and underdosing of 4-Aminophenol derivatives**

    ☑7ᵗʰ **T39.1X1** **Poisoning by 4-Aminophenol derivatives, accidental (unintentional)** PE
       Poisoning by 4-Aminophenol derivatives NOS

☑ Additional Character Required   ✓x7ᵗʰ Placeholder   Questionable PDx   Manifestation   Unspecified   UPD Unacceptable PDx   H1-H14 HAC   HCC CMS-HCC Dx   HIV HIV Dx

ICD-10-CM 2025   1139

Chapter 19. Injury, Poisoning and Certain Other Consequences of External Causes

    ☑7th **T39.1X2** **Poisoning by 4-Aminophenol derivatives, intentional self-harm** `HCC` `PE`

    ☑7th **T39.1X3** **Poisoning by 4-Aminophenol derivatives, assault** `PE`

    ☑7th **T39.1X4** **Poisoning by 4-Aminophenol derivatives, undetermined** `PE`

    ☑7th **T39.1X5** **Adverse effect of 4-Aminophenol derivatives** `UPD` `PE`

    ☑7th **T39.1X6** **Underdosing of 4-Aminophenol derivatives** `UPD` `PE`

☑5th **T39.2** **Poisoning by, adverse effect of and underdosing of pyrazolone derivatives**

  ☑6th **T39.2X** **Poisoning by, adverse effect of and underdosing of pyrazolone derivatives**

    ☑7th **T39.2X1** **Poisoning by pyrazolone derivatives, accidental (unintentional)** `PE`
        Poisoning by pyrazolone derivatives NOS

    ☑7th **T39.2X2** **Poisoning by pyrazolone derivatives, intentional self-harm** `HCC` `PE`

    ☑7th **T39.2X3** **Poisoning by pyrazolone derivatives, assault** `PE`

    ☑7th **T39.2X4** **Poisoning by pyrazolone derivatives, undetermined** `PE`

    ☑7th **T39.2X5** **Adverse effect of pyrazolone derivatives** `UPD` `PE`

    ☑7th **T39.2X6** **Underdosing of pyrazolone derivatives** `UPD` `PE`

☑5th **T39.3** **Poisoning by, adverse effect of and underdosing of other nonsteroidal anti-inflammatory drugs [NSAID]**

  ☑6th **T39.31** **Poisoning by, adverse effect of and underdosing of propionic acid derivatives**
    Poisoning by, adverse effect of and underdosing of fenoprofen
    Poisoning by, adverse effect of and underdosing of flurbiprofen
    Poisoning by, adverse effect of and underdosing of ibuprofen
    Poisoning by, adverse effect of and underdosing of ketoprofen
    Poisoning by, adverse effect of and underdosing of naproxen
    Poisoning by, adverse effect of and underdosing of oxaprozin

    ☑7th **T39.311** **Poisoning by propionic acid derivatives, accidental (unintentional)** `PE`

    ☑7th **T39.312** **Poisoning by propionic acid derivatives, intentional self-harm** `HCC` `PE`

    ☑7th **T39.313** **Poisoning by propionic acid derivatives, assault** `PE`

    ☑7th **T39.314** **Poisoning by propionic acid derivatives, undetermined** `PE`

    ☑7th **T39.315** **Adverse effect of propionic acid derivatives** `UPD` `PE`

    ☑7th **T39.316** **Underdosing of propionic acid derivatives** `UPD` `PE`

  ☑6th **T39.39** **Poisoning by, adverse effect of and underdosing of other nonsteroidal anti-inflammatory drugs [NSAID]**

    ☑7th **T39.391** **Poisoning by other nonsteroidal anti-inflammatory drugs [NSAID], accidental (unintentional)** `PE`
        Poisoning by other nonsteroidal anti-inflammatory drugs NOS

    ☑7th **T39.392** **Poisoning by other nonsteroidal anti-inflammatory drugs [NSAID], intentional self-harm** `HCC` `PE`

    ☑7th **T39.393** **Poisoning by other nonsteroidal anti-inflammatory drugs [NSAID], assault** `PE`

    ☑7th **T39.394** **Poisoning by other nonsteroidal anti-inflammatory drugs [NSAID], undetermined** `PE`

    ☑7th **T39.395** **Adverse effect of other nonsteroidal anti-inflammatory drugs [NSAID]** `UPD` `PE`

    ☑7th **T39.396** **Underdosing of other nonsteroidal anti-inflammatory drugs [NSAID]** `UPD` `PE`

☑5th **T39.4** **Poisoning by, adverse effect of and underdosing of antirheumatics, not elsewhere classified**
    EXCLUDES 1   *poisoning by, adverse effect of and underdosing of glucocorticoids (T38.0-)*
        poisoning by, adverse effect of and underdosing of salicylates (T39.0-)

  ☑6th **T39.4X** **Poisoning by, adverse effect of and underdosing of antirheumatics, not elsewhere classified**

    ☑7th **T39.4X1** **Poisoning by antirheumatics, not elsewhere classified, accidental (unintentional)** `PE`
        Poisoning by antirheumatics, not elsewhere classified NOS

    ☑7th **T39.4X2** **Poisoning by antirheumatics, not elsewhere classified, intentional self-harm** `HCC` `PE`

    ☑7th **T39.4X3** **Poisoning by antirheumatics, not elsewhere classified, assault** `PE`

    ☑7th **T39.4X4** **Poisoning by antirheumatics, not elsewhere classified, undetermined** `PE`

    ☑7th **T39.4X5** **Adverse effect of antirheumatics, not elsewhere classified** `UPD` `PE`

    ☑7th **T39.4X6** **Underdosing of antirheumatics, not elsewhere classified** `UPD` `PE`

☑5th **T39.8** **Poisoning by, adverse effect of and underdosing of other nonopioid analgesics and antipyretics, not elsewhere classified**

  ☑6th **T39.8X** **Poisoning by, adverse effect of and underdosing of other nonopioid analgesics and antipyretics, not elsewhere classified**

    ☑7th **T39.8X1** **Poisoning by other nonopioid analgesics and antipyretics, not elsewhere classified, accidental (unintentional)** `PE`
        Poisoning by other nonopioid analgesics and antipyretics, not elsewhere classified NOS

    ☑7th **T39.8X2** **Poisoning by other nonopioid analgesics and antipyretics, not elsewhere classified, intentional self-harm** `HCC` `PE`

    ☑7th **T39.8X3** **Poisoning by other nonopioid analgesics and antipyretics, not elsewhere classified, assault** `PE`

    ☑7th **T39.8X4** **Poisoning by other nonopioid analgesics and antipyretics, not elsewhere classified, undetermined** `PE`

    ☑7th **T39.8X5** **Adverse effect of other nonopioid analgesics and antipyretics, not elsewhere classified** `UPD` `PE`

    ☑7th **T39.8X6** **Underdosing of other nonopioid analgesics and antipyretics, not elsewhere classified** `UPD` `PE`

☑5th **T39.9** **Poisoning by, adverse effect of and underdosing of unspecified nonopioid analgesic, antipyretic and antirheumatic**

  ☑x 7th **T39.91** **Poisoning by unspecified nonopioid analgesic, antipyretic and antirheumatic, accidental (unintentional)** `PE`
    Poisoning by nonopioid analgesic, antipyretic and antirheumatic NOS

  ☑x 7th **T39.92** **Poisoning by unspecified nonopioid analgesic, antipyretic and antirheumatic, intentional self-harm** `HCC` `PE`

  ☑x 7th **T39.93** **Poisoning by unspecified nonopioid analgesic, antipyretic and antirheumatic, assault** `PE`

  ☑x 7th **T39.94** **Poisoning by unspecified nonopioid analgesic, antipyretic and antirheumatic, undetermined** `PE`

  ☑x 7th **T39.95** **Adverse effect of unspecified nonopioid analgesic, antipyretic and antirheumatic** `UPD` `PE`

  ☑x 7th **T39.96** **Underdosing of unspecified nonopioid analgesic, antipyretic and antirheumatic** `UPD` `PE`

Chapter 19. Injury, Poisoning and Certain Other Consequences of External Causes

T39.1X2–T39.96

`N` Newborn: 0   `P` Pediatric: 0-17   `M` Maternity: 9-64   `A` Adult: 15-124   `UNS` Unspecified Site   `MCC` Major Complication/Comorbidity   `CC` Complication/Comorbidity   `PE` POA Exempt

1140   ICD-10-CM 2025

√4th T40 Poisoning by, adverse effect of and underdosing of narcotics and psychodysleptics [hallucinogens]

EXCLUDES 2   drug dependence and related mental and behavioral disorders due to psychoactive substance use (F10.-F19.-)

The appropriate 7th character is to be added to each code from category T40.
A   initial encounter
D   subsequent encounter
S   sequela

√5th T40.0 Poisoning by, adverse effect of and underdosing of opium

√6th T40.0X Poisoning by, adverse effect of and underdosing of opium

√7th T40.0X1   Poisoning by opium, accidental (unintentional)   HCC PE
Poisoning by opium NOS

√7th T40.0X2   Poisoning by opium, intentional self-harm   HCC PE

√7th T40.0X3   Poisoning by opium, assault   PE

√7th T40.0X4   Poisoning by opium, undetermined   HCC PE

√7th T40.0X5   Adverse effect of opium   UPD PE

√7th T40.0X6   Underdosing of opium   UPD PE

√5th T40.1 Poisoning by and adverse effect of heroin

√6th T40.1X Poisoning by and adverse effect of heroin

√7th T40.1X1   Poisoning by heroin, accidental (unintentional)   HCC PE
Poisoning by heroin NOS

√7th T40.1X2   Poisoning by heroin, intentional self-harm   HCC PE

√7th T40.1X3   Poisoning by heroin, assault   PE

√7th T40.1X4   Poisoning by heroin, undetermined   HCC PE

√5th T40.2 Poisoning by, adverse effect of and underdosing of other opioids

√6th T40.2X Poisoning by, adverse effect of and underdosing of other opioids

√7th T40.2X1   Poisoning by other opioids, accidental (unintentional)   HCC PE
Poisoning by other opioids NOS

√7th T40.2X2   Poisoning by other opioids, intentional self-harm   HCC PE

√7th T40.2X3   Poisoning by other opioids, assault   PE

√7th T40.2X4   Poisoning by other opioids, undetermined   HCC PE

√7th T40.2X5   Adverse effect of other opioids   UPD PE
AHA: 2020,2Q,24

√7th T40.2X6   Underdosing of other opioids   UPD PE

√5th T40.3 Poisoning by, adverse effect of and underdosing of methadone

√6th T40.3X Poisoning by, adverse effect of and underdosing of methadone

√7th T40.3X1   Poisoning by methadone, accidental (unintentional)   HCC PE
Poisoning by methadone NOS

√7th T40.3X2   Poisoning by methadone, intentional self-harm   HCC PE

√7th T40.3X3   Poisoning by methadone, assault   PE

√7th T40.3X4   Poisoning by methadone, undetermined   HCC PE

√7th T40.3X5   Adverse effect of methadone   UPD PE

√7th T40.3X6   Underdosing of methadone   UPD PE

√5th T40.4 Poisoning by, adverse effect of and underdosing of other synthetic narcotics
AHA: 2020,4Q,40

√6th T40.41 Poisoning by, adverse effect of and underdosing of fentanyl or fentanyl analogs

√7th T40.411   Poisoning by fentanyl or fentanyl analogs, accidental (unintentional)   HCC PE

√7th T40.412   Poisoning by fentanyl or fentanyl analogs, intentional self-harm   HCC PE

√7th T40.413   Poisoning by fentanyl or fentanyl analogs, assault   PE

√7th T40.414   Poisoning by fentanyl or fentanyl analogs, undetermined   HCC PE

√7th T40.415   Adverse effect of fentanyl or fentanyl analogs   UPD PE

√7th T40.416   Underdosing of fentanyl or fentanyl analogs   UPD PE

√6th T40.42 Poisoning by, adverse effect of and underdosing of tramadol

√7th T40.421   Poisoning by tramadol, accidental (unintentional)   HCC PE

√7th T40.422   Poisoning by tramadol, intentional self-harm   HCC PE

√7th T40.423   Poisoning by tramadol, assault   PE

√7th T40.424   Poisoning by tramadol, undetermined   HCC PE

√7th T40.425   Adverse effect of tramadol   UPD PE

√7th T40.426   Underdosing of tramadol   UPD PE

√6th T40.49 Poisoning by, adverse effect of and underdosing of other synthetic narcotics

√7th T40.491   Poisoning by other synthetic narcotics, accidental (unintentional)   HCC PE

√7th T40.492   Poisoning by other synthetic narcotics, intentional self-harm   HCC PE

√7th T40.493   Poisoning by other synthetic narcotics, assault   PE

√7th T40.494   Poisoning by other synthetic narcotics, undetermined   HCC PE

√7th T40.495   Adverse effect of other synthetic narcotics   UPD PE

√7th T40.496   Underdosing of other synthetic narcotics   UPD PE

√5th T40.5 Poisoning by, adverse effect of and underdosing of cocaine

√6th T40.5X Poisoning by, adverse effect of and underdosing of cocaine

√7th T40.5X1   Poisoning by cocaine, accidental (unintentional)   HCC PE
Poisoning by cocaine NOS
AHA: 2016,2Q,8

√7th T40.5X2   Poisoning by cocaine, intentional self-harm   HCC PE

√7th T40.5X3   Poisoning by cocaine, assault   PE

√7th T40.5X4   Poisoning by cocaine, undetermined   HCC PE

√7th T40.5X5   Adverse effect of cocaine   UPD PE

√7th T40.5X6   Underdosing of cocaine   UPD PE

√5th T40.6 Poisoning by, adverse effect of and underdosing of other and unspecified narcotics

√6th T40.60 Poisoning by, adverse effect of and underdosing of unspecified narcotics

√7th T40.601   Poisoning by unspecified narcotics, accidental (unintentional)   HCC PE
Poisoning by narcotics NOS

√7th T40.602   Poisoning by unspecified narcotics, intentional self-harm   HCC PE

√7th T40.603   Poisoning by unspecified narcotics, assault   PE

√7th T40.604   Poisoning by unspecified narcotics, undetermined   HCC PE

√7th T40.605   Adverse effect of unspecified narcotics   UPD PE

√7th T40.606   Underdosing of unspecified narcotics   UPD PE

√6th T40.69 Poisoning by, adverse effect of and underdosing of other narcotics

√7th T40.691   Poisoning by other narcotics, accidental (unintentional)   HCC PE
Poisoning by other narcotics NOS

√7th T40.692   Poisoning by other narcotics, intentional self-harm   HCC PE

√7th T40.693   Poisoning by other narcotics, assault   PE

√7th T40.694   Poisoning by other narcotics, undetermined   HCC PE

√7th T40.695   Adverse effect of other narcotics   UPD PE

√7th T40.696   Underdosing of other narcotics   UPD PE

√5th T40.7 Poisoning by, adverse effect of and underdosing of cannabis (derivatives)

√6th T40.71 Poisoning by, adverse effect of and underdosing of cannabis (derivatives)
AHA: 2021,4Q,30

√7th T40.711   Poisoning by cannabis, accidental (unintentional)   PE

√7th T40.712   Poisoning by cannabis, intentional self-harm   HCC PE

| ✓ Additional Character Required | √x7th Placeholder | Questionable PDx | Manifestation | Unspecified | UPD Unacceptable PDx | H1-H14 HAC | HCC CMS-HCC Dx | HIV HIV Dx |

ICD-10-CM 2025   1141

Chapter 19. Injury, Poisoning and Certain Other Consequences of External Causes

√7th **T40.713** Poisoning by cannabis, assault   PE

√7th **T40.714** Poisoning by cannabis, undetermined   PE

√7th **T40.715** Adverse effect of cannabis   UPD PE

√7th **T40.716** Underdosing of cannabis   UPD PE

√6th **T40.72** Poisoning by, adverse effect of and underdosing of synthetic cannabinoids

     AHA: 2021,4Q,30

√7th **T40.721** Poisoning by synthetic cannabinoids, accidental (unintentional)   PE

√7th **T40.722** Poisoning by synthetic cannabinoids, intentional self-harm   HCC PE

√7th **T40.723** Poisoning by synthetic cannabinoids, assault   PE

√7th **T40.724** Poisoning by synthetic cannabinoids, undetermined   PE

√7th **T40.725** Adverse effect of synthetic cannabinoids   UPD PE

√7th **T40.726** Underdosing of synthetic cannabinoids   UPD PE

√5th **T40.8** Poisoning by and adverse effect of lysergide [LSD]

√6th **T40.8X** Poisoning by and adverse effect of lysergide [LSD]

√7th **T40.8X1** Poisoning by lysergide [LSD], accidental (unintentional)   HCC PE
     Poisoning by lysergide [LSD] NOS

√7th **T40.8X2** Poisoning by lysergide [LSD], intentional self-harm   HCC PE

√7th **T40.8X3** Poisoning by lysergide [LSD], assault   PE

√7th **T40.8X4** Poisoning by lysergide [LSD], undetermined   HCC PE

√5th **T40.9** Poisoning by, adverse effect of and underdosing of other and unspecified psychodysleptics [hallucinogens]

√6th **T40.90** Poisoning by, adverse effect of and underdosing of unspecified psychodysleptics [hallucinogens]

√7th **T40.901** Poisoning by unspecified psychodysleptics [hallucinogens], accidental (unintentional)   HCC PE

√7th **T40.902** Poisoning by unspecified psychodysleptics [hallucinogens], intentional self-harm   HCC PE

√7th **T40.903** Poisoning by unspecified psychodysleptics [hallucinogens], assault   PE

√7th **T40.904** Poisoning by unspecified psychodysleptics [hallucinogens], undetermined   HCC PE

√7th **T40.905** Adverse effect of unspecified psychodysleptics [hallucinogens]   UPD PE

√7th **T40.906** Underdosing of unspecified psychodysleptics [hallucinogens]   UPD PE

√6th **T40.99** Poisoning by, adverse effect of and underdosing of other psychodysleptics [hallucinogens]

√7th **T40.991** Poisoning by other psychodysleptics [hallucinogens], accidental (unintentional)   HCC PE
     Poisoning by other psychodysleptics [hallucinogens] NOS

√7th **T40.992** Poisoning by other psychodysleptics [hallucinogens], intentional self-harm   HCC PE

√7th **T40.993** Poisoning by other psychodysleptics [hallucinogens], assault   PE

√7th **T40.994** Poisoning by other psychodysleptics [hallucinogens], undetermined   HCC PE

√7th **T40.995** Adverse effect of other psychodysleptics [hallucinogens]   UPD PE

√7th **T40.996** Underdosing of other psychodysleptics [hallucinogens]   UPD PE

√4th **T41** Poisoning by, adverse effect of and underdosing of anesthetics and therapeutic gases

     EXCLUDES 1   benzodiazepines (T42.4-)
         cocaine (T40.5-)
         complications of anesthesia during labor and delivery (O74.-)
         complications of anesthesia during pregnancy (O29.-)
         complications of anesthesia during the puerperium (O89.-)
         opioids (T40.0-T40.2-)

     The appropriate 7th character is to be added to each code from category T41.
     A   initial encounter
     D   subsequent encounter
     S   sequela

√5th **T41.0** Poisoning by, adverse effect of and underdosing of inhaled anesthetics

     EXCLUDES 1   oxygen (T41.5-)

√6th **T41.0X** Poisoning by, adverse effect of and underdosing of inhaled anesthetics

√7th **T41.0X1** Poisoning by inhaled anesthetics, accidental (unintentional)   PE
     Poisoning by inhaled anesthetics NOS

√7th **T41.0X2** Poisoning by inhaled anesthetics, intentional self-harm   HCC PE

√7th **T41.0X3** Poisoning by inhaled anesthetics, assault   PE

√7th **T41.0X4** Poisoning by inhaled anesthetics, undetermined   PE

√7th **T41.0X5** Adverse effect of inhaled anesthetics   UPD PE

√7th **T41.0X6** Underdosing of inhaled anesthetics   UPD PE

√5th **T41.1** Poisoning by, adverse effect of and underdosing of intravenous anesthetics

     Poisoning by, adverse effect of and underdosing of thiobarbiturates

√6th **T41.1X** Poisoning by, adverse effect of and underdosing of intravenous anesthetics

√7th **T41.1X1** Poisoning by intravenous anesthetics, accidental (unintentional)   PE
     Poisoning by intravenous anesthetics NOS

√7th **T41.1X2** Poisoning by intravenous anesthetics, intentional self-harm   HCC PE

√7th **T41.1X3** Poisoning by intravenous anesthetics, assault   PE

√7th **T41.1X4** Poisoning by intravenous anesthetics, undetermined   PE

√7th **T41.1X5** Adverse effect of intravenous anesthetics   UPD PE

√7th **T41.1X6** Underdosing of intravenous anesthetics   UPD PE

√5th **T41.2** Poisoning by, adverse effect of and underdosing of other and unspecified general anesthetics

√6th **T41.20** Poisoning by, adverse effect of and underdosing of unspecified general anesthetics

√7th **T41.201** Poisoning by unspecified general anesthetics, accidental (unintentional)   PE
     Poisoning by general anesthetics NOS

√7th **T41.202** Poisoning by unspecified general anesthetics, intentional self-harm   HCC PE

√7th **T41.203** Poisoning by unspecified general anesthetics, assault   PE

√7th **T41.204** Poisoning by unspecified general anesthetics, undetermined   PE

√7th **T41.205** Adverse effect of unspecified general anesthetics   UPD PE

     AHA: 2016,4Q,73

√7th **T41.206** Underdosing of unspecified general anesthetics   UPD PE

√6th **T41.29** Poisoning by, adverse effect of and underdosing of other general anesthetics

√7th **T41.291** Poisoning by other general anesthetics, accidental (unintentional)   PE
     Poisoning by other general anesthetics NOS

√7th **T41.292** Poisoning by other general anesthetics, intentional self-harm   HCC PE

√7th **T41.293** Poisoning by other general anesthetics, assault   PE

N Newborn: 0   P Pediatric: 0-17   M Maternity: 9-64   A Adult: 15-124   UNS Unspecified Site   MCC Major Complication/Comorbidity   CC Complication/Comorbidity   PE POA Exempt

1142   ICD-10-CM 2025

√7th **T41.294** Poisoning by other general anesthetics, undetermined PE

√7th **T41.295** Adverse effect of other general anesthetics UPD PE

√7th **T41.296** Underdosing of other general anesthetics UPD PE

√5th **T41.3** Poisoning by, adverse effect of and underdosing of local anesthetics
Cocaine (topical)
EXCLUDES 2 poisoning by cocaine used as a central nervous system stimulant (T40.5X1-T40.5X4)

√6th **T41.3X** Poisoning by, adverse effect of and underdosing of local anesthetics

√7th **T41.3X1** Poisoning by local anesthetics, accidental (unintentional) PE
Poisoning by local anesthetics NCS

√7th **T41.3X2** Poisoning by local anesthetics, intentional self-harm HCC PE

√7th **T41.3X3** Poisoning by local anesthetics, assault PE

√7th **T41.3X4** Poisoning by local anesthetics, undetermined PE

√7th **T41.3X5** Adverse effect of local anesthetics UPD PE

√7th **T41.3X6** Underdosing of local anesthetics UPD PE

√5th **T41.4** Poisoning by, adverse effect of and underdosing of unspecified anesthetic

√x7th **T41.41** Poisoning by unspecified anesthetic, accidental (unintentional) PE
Poisoning by anesthetic NOS

√x7th **T41.42** Poisoning by unspecified anesthetic, intentional self-harm HCC PE

√x7th **T41.43** Poisoning by unspecified anesthetic, assault PE

√x7th **T41.44** Poisoning by unspecified anesthetic, undetermined PE

√x7th **T41.45** Adverse effect of unspecified anesthetic UPD PE

√x7th **T41.46** Underdosing of unspecified anesthetics UPD PE

√5th **T41.5** Poisoning by, adverse effect of and underdosing of therapeutic gases

√6th **T41.5X** Poisoning by, adverse effect of and underdosing of therapeutic gases

√7th **T41.5X1** Poisoning by therapeutic gases, accidental (unintentional) PE
Poisoning by therapeutic gases NOS

√7th **T41.5X2** Poisoning by therapeutic gases, intentional self-harm HCC PE

√7th **T41.5X3** Poisoning by therapeutic gases, assault PE

√7th **T41.5X4** Poisoning by therapeutic gases, undetermined PE

√7th **T41.5X5** Adverse effect of therapeutic gases UPD PE

√7th **T41.5X6** Underdosing of therapeutic gases UPD PE

√4th **T42** Poisoning by, adverse effect of and underdosing of antiepileptic, sedative- hypnotic and antiparkinsonism drugs
EXCLUDES 2 drug dependence and related mental and behavioral disorders due to psychoactive substance use (F10.- - F19.-)

The appropriate 7th character is to be added to each code from category T42.
A initial encounter
D subsequent encounter
S sequela

√5th **T42.0** Poisoning by, adverse effect of and underdosing of hydantoin derivatives

√6th **T42.0X** Poisoning by, adverse effect of and underdosing of hydantoin derivatives

√7th **T42.0X1** Poisoning by hydantoin derivatives, accidental (unintentional) PE
Poisoning by hydantoin derivatives NOS

√7th **T42.0X2** Poisoning by hydantoin derivatives, intentional self-harm HCC PE

√7th **T42.0X3** Poisoning by hydantoin derivatives, assault PE

√7th **T42.0X4** Poisoning by hydantoin derivatives, undetermined PE

√7th **T42.0X5** Adverse effect of hydantoin derivatives UPD PE

√7th **T42.0X6** Underdosing of hydantoin derivatives UPD PE

√5th **T42.1** Poisoning by, adverse effect of and underdosing of iminostilbenes
Poisoning by, adverse effect of and underdosing of carbamazepine

√6th **T42.1X** Poisoning by, adverse effect of and underdosing of iminostilbenes

√7th **T42.1X1** Poisoning by iminostilbenes, accidental (unintentional) PE
Poisoning by iminostilbenes NOS

√7th **T42.1X2** Poisoning by iminostilbenes, intentional self-harm HCC PE

√7th **T42.1X3** Poisoning by iminostilbenes, assault PE

√7th **T42.1X4** Poisoning by iminostilbenes, undetermined PE

√7th **T42.1X5** Adverse effect of iminostilbenes UPD PE

√7th **T42.1X6** Underdosing of iminostilbenes UPD PE

√5th **T42.2** Poisoning by, adverse effect of and underdosing of succinimides and oxazolidinediones

√6th **T42.2X** Poisoning by, adverse effect of and underdosing of succinimides and oxazolidinediones

√7th **T42.2X1** Poisoning by succinimides and oxazolidinediones, accidental (unintentional) PE
Poisoning by succinimides and oxazolidinediones NOS

√7th **T42.2X2** Poisoning by succinimides and oxazolidinediones, intentional self-harm HCC PE

√7th **T42.2X3** Poisoning by succinimides and oxazolidinediones, assault PE

√7th **T42.2X4** Poisoning by succinimides and oxazolidinediones, undetermined PE

√7th **T42.2X5** Adverse effect of succinimides and oxazolidinediones UPD PE

√7th **T42.2X6** Underdosing of succinimides and oxazolidinediones UPD PE

√5th **T42.3** Poisoning by, adverse effect of and underdosing of barbiturates
EXCLUDES 1 poisoning by, adverse effect of and underdosing of thiobarbiturates (T41.1-)

√6th **T42.3X** Poisoning by, adverse effect of and underdosing of barbiturates

√7th **T42.3X1** Poisoning by barbiturates, accidental (unintentional) PE
Poisoning by barbiturates NOS

√7th **T42.3X2** Poisoning by barbiturates, intentional self-harm HCC PE

√7th **T42.3X3** Poisoning by barbiturates, assault PE

√7th **T42.3X4** Poisoning by barbiturates, undetermined PE

√7th **T42.3X5** Adverse effect of barbiturates UPD PE

√7th **T42.3X6** Underdosing of barbiturates UPD PE

√5th **T42.4** Poisoning by, adverse effect of and underdosing of benzodiazepines

√6th **T42.4X** Poisoning by, adverse effect of and underdosing of benzodiazepines

√7th **T42.4X1** Poisoning by benzodiazepines, accidental (unintentional) PE
Poisoning by benzodiazepines NOS

√7th **T42.4X2** Poisoning by benzodiazepines, intentional self-harm HCC PE

√7th **T42.4X3** Poisoning by benzodiazepines, assault PE

√7th **T42.4X4** Poisoning by benzodiazepines, undetermined PE

√7th **T42.4X5** Adverse effect of benzodiazepines UPD PE

√7th **T42.4X6** Underdosing of benzodiazepines UPD PE

√5th **T42.5** Poisoning by, adverse effect of and underdosing of mixed antiepileptics

√6th **T42.5X** Poisoning by, adverse effect of and underdosing of antiepileptics

√7th **T42.5X1** Poisoning by mixed antiepileptics, accidental (unintentional) PE
Poisoning by mixed antiepileptics NOS

✓7ᵗʰ **T42.5X2** **Poisoning by mixed antiepileptics, intentional self-harm** `HCC` `PE`

✓7ᵗʰ **T42.5X3** **Poisoning by mixed antiepileptics, assault** `PE`

✓7ᵗʰ **T42.5X4** **Poisoning by mixed antiepileptics, undetermined** `PE`

✓7ᵗʰ **T42.5X5** **Adverse effect of mixed antiepileptics** `UPD` `PE`

✓7ᵗʰ **T42.5X6** **Underdosing of mixed antiepileptics** `UPD` `PE`

✓5ᵗʰ **T42.6** **Poisoning by, adverse effect of and underdosing of other antiepileptic and sedative-hypnotic drugs**
Poisoning by, adverse effect of and underdosing of methaqualone
Poisoning by, adverse effect of and underdosing of valproic acid
EXCLUDES 1 *poisoning by, adverse effect of and underdosing of carbamazepine (T42.1-)*

✓6ᵗʰ **T42.6X** **Poisoning by, adverse effect of and underdosing of other antiepileptic and sedative-hypnotic drugs**

✓7ᵗʰ **T42.6X1** **Poisoning by other antiepileptic and sedative-hypnotic drugs, accidental (unintentional)** `PE`
Poisoning by other antiepileptic and sedative-hypnotic drugs NOS

✓7ᵗʰ **T42.6X2** **Poisoning by other antiepileptic and sedative-hypnotic drugs, intentional self-harm** `HCC` `PE`

✓7ᵗʰ **T42.6X3** **Poisoning by other antiepileptic and sedative-hypnotic drugs, assault** `PE`

✓7ᵗʰ **T42.6X4** **Poisoning by other antiepileptic and sedative-hypnotic drugs, undetermined** `PE`

✓7ᵗʰ **T42.6X5** **Adverse effect of other antiepileptic and sedative-hypnotic drugs** `UPD` `PE`

✓7ᵗʰ **T42.6X6** **Underdosing of other antiepileptic and sedative-hypnotic drugs** `UPD` `PE`

✓5ᵗʰ **T42.7** **Poisoning by, adverse effect of and underdosing of unspecified antiepileptic and sedative-hypnotic drugs**

✓x7ᵗʰ **T42.71** **Poisoning by unspecified antiepileptic and sedative-hypnotic drugs, accidental (unintentional)** `PE`
Poisoning by antiepileptic and sedative-hypnotic drugs NOS

✓x7ᵗʰ **T42.72** **Poisoning by unspecified antiepileptic and sedative-hypnotic drugs, intentional self-harm** `HCC` `PE`

✓x7ᵗʰ **T42.73** **Poisoning by unspecified antiepileptic and sedative-hypnotic drugs, assault** `PE`

✓x7ᵗʰ **T42.74** **Poisoning by unspecified antiepileptic and sedative-hypnotic drugs, undetermined** `PE`

✓x7ᵗʰ **T42.75** **Adverse effect of unspecified antiepileptic and sedative-hypnotic drugs** `UPD` `PE`

✓x7ᵗʰ **T42.76** **Underdosing of unspecified antiepileptic and sedative-hypnotic drugs** `UPD` `PE`

✓5ᵗʰ **T42.8** **Poisoning by, adverse effect of and underdosing of antiparkinsonism drugs and other central muscle-tone depressants**
Poisoning by, adverse effect of and underdosing of amantadine

✓6ᵗʰ **T42.8X** **Poisoning by, adverse effect of and underdosing of antiparkinsonism drugs and other central muscle-tone depressants**

✓7ᵗʰ **T42.8X1** **Poisoning by antiparkinsonism drugs and other central muscle-tone depressants, accidental (unintentional)** `PE`
Poisoning by antiparkinsonism drugs and other central muscle-tone depressants NOS

✓7ᵗʰ **T42.8X2** **Poisoning by antiparkinsonism drugs and other central muscle-tone depressants, intentional self-harm** `HCC` `PE`

✓7ᵗʰ **T42.8X3** **Poisoning by antiparkinsonism drugs and other central muscle-tone depressants, assault** `PE`

✓7ᵗʰ **T42.8X4** **Poisoning by antiparkinsonism drugs and other central muscle-tone depressants, undetermined** `PE`

✓7ᵗʰ **T42.8X5** **Adverse effect of antiparkinsonism drugs and other central muscle-tone depressants** `UPD` `PE`

✓7ᵗʰ **T42.8X6** **Underdosing of antiparkinsonism drugs and other central muscle-tone depressants** `UPD` `PE`

✓4ᵗʰ **T43** **Poisoning by, adverse effect of and underdosing of psychotropic drugs, not elsewhere classified**
EXCLUDES 1 *appetite depressants (T50.5-)*
barbiturates (T42.3-)
benzodiazepines (T42.4-)
methaqualone (T42.6-)
psychodysleptics [hallucinogens] (T40.7-T40.9-)
EXCLUDES 2 *drug dependence and related mental and behavioral disorders due to psychoactive substance use (F10.- – F19.-)*

The appropriate 7th character is to be added to each code from category T43.
A initial encounter
D subsequent encounter
S sequela

✓5ᵗʰ **T43.0** **Poisoning by, adverse effect of and underdosing of tricyclic and tetracyclic antidepressants**

✓6ᵗʰ **T43.01** **Poisoning by, adverse effect of and underdosing of tricyclic antidepressants**

✓7ᵗʰ **T43.011** **Poisoning by tricyclic antidepressants, accidental (unintentional)** `PE`
Poisoning by tricyclic antidepressants NOS

✓7ᵗʰ **T43.012** **Poisoning by tricyclic antidepressants, intentional self-harm** `HCC` `PE`

✓7ᵗʰ **T43.013** **Poisoning by tricyclic antidepressants, assault** `PE`

✓7ᵗʰ **T43.014** **Poisoning by tricyclic antidepressants, undetermined** `PE`

✓7ᵗʰ **T43.015** **Adverse effect of tricyclic antidepressants** `UPD` `PE`

✓7ᵗʰ **T43.016** **Underdosing of tricyclic antidepressants** `UPD` `PE`

✓6ᵗʰ **T43.02** **Poisoning by, adverse effect of and underdosing of tetracyclic antidepressants**

✓7ᵗʰ **T43.021** **Poisoning by tetracyclic antidepressants, accidental (unintentional)** `PE`
Poisoning by tetracyclic antidepressants NOS

✓7ᵗʰ **T43.022** **Poisoning by tetracyclic antidepressants, intentional self-harm** `HCC` `PE`

✓7ᵗʰ **T43.023** **Poisoning by tetracyclic antidepressants, assault** `PE`

✓7ᵗʰ **T43.024** **Poisoning by tetracyclic antidepressants, undetermined** `PE`

✓7ᵗʰ **T43.025** **Adverse effect of tetracyclic antidepressants** `UPD` `PE`

✓7ᵗʰ **T43.026** **Underdosing of tetracyclic antidepressants** `UPD` `PE`

✓5ᵗʰ **T43.1** **Poisoning by, adverse effect of and underdosing of monoamine-oxidase-inhibitor antidepressants**

✓6ᵗʰ **T43.1X** **Poisoning by, adverse effect of and underdosing of monoamine-oxidase-inhibitor antidepressants**

✓7ᵗʰ **T43.1X1** **Poisoning by monoamine-oxidase-inhibitor antidepressants, accidental (unintentional)** `PE`
Poisoning by monoamine-oxidase-inhibitor antidepressants NOS

✓7ᵗʰ **T43.1X2** **Poisoning by monoamine-oxidase-inhibitor antidepressants, intentional self-harm** `HCC` `PE`

✓7ᵗʰ **T43.1X3** **Poisoning by monoamine-oxidase-inhibitor antidepressants, assault** `PE`

✓7ᵗʰ **T43.1X4** **Poisoning by monoamine-oxidase-inhibitor antidepressants, undetermined** `PE`

✓7ᵗʰ **T43.1X5** **Adverse effect of monoamine-oxidase-inhibitor antidepressants** `UPD` `PE`

✓7ᵗʰ **T43.1X6** **Underdosing of monoamine-oxidase-inhibitor antidepressants** `UPD` `PE`

✓5th **T43.2** **Poisoning by, adverse effect of and underdosing of other and unspecified antidepressants**

  ✓6th **T43.20** **Poisoning by, adverse effect of and underdosing of unspecified antidepressants**

    ✓7th **T43.201** **Poisoning by unspecified antidepressants, accidental (unintentional)** PE
      Poisoning by antidepressants NOS

    ✓7th **T43.202** **Poisoning by unspecified antidepressants, intentional self-harm** HCC PE

    ✓7th **T43.203** **Poisoning by unspecified antidepressants, assault** PE

    ✓7th **T43.204** **Poisoning by unspecified antidepressants, undetermined** PE

    ✓7th **T43.205** **Adverse effect of unspecified antidepressants** UPD PE
      Antidepressant discontinuation syndrome

    ✓7th **T43.206** **Underdosing of unspecified antidepressants** UPD PE

  ✓6th **T43.21** **Poisoning by, adverse effect of and underdosing of selective serotonin and norepinephrine reuptake inhibitors**
    Poisoning by, adverse effect of and underdosing of SSNRI antidepressants

    ✓7th **T43.211** **Poisoning by selective serotonin and norepinephrine reuptake inhibitors, accidental (unintentional)** PE

    ✓7th **T43.212** **Poisoning by selective serotonin and norepinephrine reuptake inhibitors, intentional self-harm** HCC PE

    ✓7th **T43.213** **Poisoning by selective serotonin and norepinephrine reuptake inhibitors, assault** PE

    ✓7th **T43.214** **Poisoning by selective serotonin and norepinephrine reuptake inhibitors, undetermined** PE

    ✓7th **T43.215** **Adverse effect of selective serotonin and norepinephrine reuptake inhibitors** UPD PE

    ✓7th **T43.216** **Underdosing of selective serotonin and norepinephrine reuptake inhibitors** UPD PE

  ✓6th **T43.22** **Poisoning by, adverse effect of and underdosing of selective serotonin reuptake inhibitors**
    Poisoning by, adverse effect of and underdosing of SSRI antidepressants

    ✓7th **T43.221** **Poisoning by selective serotonin reuptake inhibitors, accidental (unintentional)** PE

    ✓7th **T43.222** **Poisoning by selective serotonin reuptake inhibitors, intentional self-harm** HCC PE

    ✓7th **T43.223** **Poisoning by selective serotonin reuptake inhibitors, assault** PE

    ✓7th **T43.224** **Poisoning by selective serotonin reuptake inhibitors, undetermined** PE

    ✓7th **T43.225** **Adverse effect of selective serotonin reuptake inhibitors** UPD PE
      AHA: 2022,2Q,11

    ✓7th **T43.226** **Underdosing of selective serotonin reuptake inhibitors** UPD PE

  ✓6th **T43.29** **Poisoning by, adverse effect of and underdosing of other antidepressants**

    ✓7th **T43.291** **Poisoning by other antidepressants, accidental (unintentional)** PE
      Poisoning by other antidepressants NOS

    ✓7th **T43.292** **Poisoning by other antidepressants, intentional self-harm** HCC PE

    ✓7th **T43.293** **Poisoning by other antidepressants, assault** PE

    ✓7th **T43.294** **Poisoning by other antidepressants, undetermined** PE

    ✓7th **T43.295** **Adverse effect of other antidepressants** UPD PE

    ✓7th **T43.296** **Underdosing of other antidepressants** UPD PE

✓5th **T43.3** **Poisoning by, adverse effect of and underdosing of phenothiazine antipsychotics and neuroleptics**

  ✓6th **T43.3X** **Poisoning by, adverse effect of and underdosing of phenothiazine antipsychotics and neuroleptics**

    ✓7th **T43.3X1** **Poisoning by phenothiazine antipsychotics and neuroleptics, accidental (unintentional)** PE
      Poisoning by phenothiazine antipsychotics and neuroleptics NOS

    ✓7th **T43.3X2** **Poisoning by phenothiazine antipsychotics and neuroleptics, intentional self-harm** HCC PE

    ✓7th **T43.3X3** **Poisoning by phenothiazine antipsychotics and neuroleptics, assault** PE

    ✓7th **T43.3X4** **Poisoning by phenothiazine antipsychotics and neuroleptics, undetermined** PE

    ✓7th **T43.3X5** **Adverse effect of phenothiazine antipsychotics and neuroleptics** UPD PE

    ✓7th **T43.3X6** **Underdosing of phenothiazine antipsychotics and neuroleptics** UPD PE

✓5th **T43.4** **Poisoning by, adverse effect of and underdosing of butyrophenone and thiothixene neuroleptics**

  ✓6th **T43.4X** **Poisoning by, adverse effect of and underdosing of butyrophenone and thiothixene neuroleptics**

    ✓7th **T43.4X1** **Poisoning by butyrophenone and thiothixene neuroleptics, accidental (unintentional)** PE
      Poisoning by butyrophenone and thiothixene neuroleptics NOS

    ✓7th **T43.4X2** **Poisoning by butyrophenone and thiothixene neuroleptics, intentional self-harm** HCC PE

    ✓7th **T43.4X3** **Poisoning by butyrophenone and thiothixene neuroleptics, assault** PE

    ✓7th **T43.4X4** **Poisoning by butyrophenone and thiothixene neuroleptics, undetermined** PE

    ✓7th **T43.4X5** **Adverse effect of butyrophenone and thiothixene neuroleptics** UPD PE

    ✓7th **T43.4X6** **Underdosing of butyrophenone and thiothixene neuroleptics** UPD PE

✓5th **T43.5** **Poisoning by, adverse effect of and underdosing of other and unspecified antipsychotics and neuroleptics**

    EXCLUDES 1   poisoning by, adverse effect of and underdosing of rauwolfia (T46.5-)

  ✓6th **T43.50** **Poisoning by, adverse effect of and underdosing of unspecified antipsychotics and neuroleptics**

    ✓7th **T43.501** **Poisoning by unspecified antipsychotics and neuroleptics, accidental (unintentional)** PE
      Poisoning by antipsychotics and neuroleptics NOS

    ✓7th **T43.502** **Poisoning by unspecified antipsychotics and neuroleptics, intentional self-harm** HCC PE

    ✓7th **T43.503** **Poisoning by unspecified antipsychotics and neuroleptics, assault** PE

    ✓7th **T43.504** **Poisoning by unspecified antipsychotics and neuroleptics, undetermined** PE

    ✓7th **T43.505** **Adverse effect of unspecified antipsychotics and neuroleptics** UPD PE
      AHA: 2022,4Q,24

    ✓7th **T43.506** **Underdosing of unspecified antipsychotics and neuroleptics** UPD PE

  ✓6th **T43.59** **Poisoning by, adverse effect of and underdosing of other antipsychotics and neuroleptics**
    AHA: 2017,1Q,40

    ✓7th **T43.591** **Poisoning by other antipsychotics and neuroleptics, accidental (unintentional)** PE
      Poisoning by other antipsychotics and neuroleptics NOS

    ✓7th **T43.592** **Poisoning by other antipsychotics and neuroleptics, intentional self-harm** HCC PE

    ✓7th **T43.593** **Poisoning by other antipsychotics and neuroleptics, assault** PE

    ✓7th **T43.594** **Poisoning by other antipsychotics and neuroleptics, undetermined** PE

✓ Additional Character Required   ✓x7th Placeholder   Questionable PDx   Manifestation   Unspecified   UPD Unacceptable PDx   H1 - H14 HAC   HCC CMS-HCC Dx   HIV HIV Dx

ICD-10-CM 2025   1145

√7ᵗʰ **T43.595** **Adverse effect** of other antipsychotics and neuroleptics `UPD` `PE`
AHA: 2022,2Q,11

√7ᵗʰ **T43.596** **Underdosing** of other antipsychotics and neuroleptics `UPD` `PE`

√5ᵗʰ **T43.6** **Poisoning by, adverse effect of and underdosing of psychostimulants**
EXCLUDES 1 *poisoning by, adverse effect of and underdosing of cocaine (T40.5-)*

√6ᵗʰ **T43.60** **Poisoning by, adverse effect of and underdosing of unspecified psychostimulant**

√7ᵗʰ **T43.601** **Poisoning by unspecified psychostimulants, accidental (unintentional)** `HCC` `PE`
Poisoning by psychostimulants NOS

√7ᵗʰ **T43.602** **Poisoning by unspecified psychostimulants, intentional self-harm** `HCC` `PE`

√7ᵗʰ **T43.603** **Poisoning by unspecified psychostimulants, assault** `PE`

√7ᵗʰ **T43.604** **Poisoning by unspecified psychostimulants, undetermined** `HCC` `PE`

√7ᵗʰ **T43.605** **Adverse effect** of unspecified psychostimulants `UPD` `PE`

√7ᵗʰ **T43.606** **Underdosing** of unspecified psychostimulants `UPD` `PE`

√6ᵗʰ **T43.61** **Poisoning by, adverse effect of and underdosing of caffeine**

√7ᵗʰ **T43.611** **Poisoning by caffeine, accidental (unintentional)** `HCC` `PE`
Poisoning by caffeine NOS

√7ᵗʰ **T43.612** **Poisoning by caffeine, intentional self-harm** `HCC` `PE`

√7ᵗʰ **T43.613** **Poisoning by caffeine, assault** `PE`

√7ᵗʰ **T43.614** **Poisoning by caffeine, undetermined** `HCC` `PE`

√7ᵗʰ **T43.615** **Adverse effect** of caffeine `UPD` `PE`

√7ᵗʰ **T43.616** **Underdosing** of caffeine `UPD` `PE`

√6ᵗʰ **T43.62** **Poisoning by, adverse effect of and underdosing of amphetamines**

√7ᵗʰ **T43.621** **Poisoning by amphetamines, accidental (unintentional)** `HCC` `PE`
Poisoning by amphetamines NOS
AHA: 2021,3Q,8

√7ᵗʰ **T43.622** **Poisoning by amphetamines, intentional self-harm** `HCC` `PE`

√7ᵗʰ **T43.623** **Poisoning by amphetamines, assault** `PE`

√7ᵗʰ **T43.624** **Poisoning by amphetamines, undetermined** `HCC` `PE`

√7ᵗʰ **T43.625** **Adverse effect** of amphetamines `UPD` `PE`

√7ᵗʰ **T43.626** **Underdosing** of amphetamines `UPD` `PE`

√6ᵗʰ **T43.63** **Poisoning by, adverse effect of and underdosing of methylphenidate**

√7ᵗʰ **T43.631** **Poisoning by methylphenidate, accidental (unintentional)** `HCC` `PE`
Poisoning by methylphenidate NOS

√7ᵗʰ **T43.632** **Poisoning by methylphenidate, intentional self-harm** `HCC` `PE`

√7ᵗʰ **T43.633** **Poisoning by methylphenidate, assault** `PE`

√7ᵗʰ **T43.634** **Poisoning by methylphenidate, undetermined** `HCC` `PE`

√7ᵗʰ **T43.635** **Adverse effect** of methylphenidate `UPD` `PE`

√7ᵗʰ **T43.636** **Underdosing** of methylphenidate `UPD` `PE`

√6ᵗʰ **T43.64** **Poisoning by ecstasy**
Poisoning by MDMA
Poisoning by 3,4-methylenedioxymethamphetamine
AHA: 2018,4Q,30-31

√7ᵗʰ **T43.641** **Poisoning by ecstasy, accidental (unintentional)** `HCC` `PE`
Poisoning by ecstasy NOS

√7ᵗʰ **T43.642** **Poisoning by ecstasy, intentional self-harm** `HCC` `PE`

√7ᵗʰ **T43.643** **Poisoning by ecstasy, assault** `PE`

√7ᵗʰ **T43.644** **Poisoning by ecstasy, undetermined** `HCC` `PE`

√6ᵗʰ **T43.65** **Poisoning by, adverse effect of and underdosing of methamphetamines**
AHA: 2022,4Q,45-47

√7ᵗʰ **T43.651** **Poisoning by methamphetamines accidental (unintentional)** `HCC` `PE`
Poisoning by methamphetamines NOS
AHA: 2022,4Q,46

√7ᵗʰ **T43.652** **Poisoning by methamphetamines intentional self-harm** `HCC` `PE`

√7ᵗʰ **T43.653** **Poisoning by methamphetamines, assault** `PE`

√7ᵗʰ **T43.654** **Poisoning by methamphetamines, undetermined** `HCC` `PE`

√7ᵗʰ **T43.655** **Adverse effect** of methamphetamines `UPD` `PE`
AHA: 2022,4Q,46

√7ᵗʰ **T43.656** **Underdosing** of methamphetamines `UPD` `PE`

√6ᵗʰ **T43.69** **Poisoning by, adverse effect of and underdosing of other psychostimulants**

√7ᵗʰ **T43.691** **Poisoning by other psychostimulants, accidental (unintentional)** `HCC` `PE`
Poisoning by other psychostimulants NOS

√7ᵗʰ **T43.692** **Poisoning by other psychostimulants, intentional self-harm** `HCC` `PE`

√7ᵗʰ **T43.693** **Poisoning by other psychostimulants, assault** `PE`

√7ᵗʰ **T43.694** **Poisoning by other psychostimulants, undetermined** `HCC` `PE`

√7ᵗʰ **T43.695** **Adverse effect** of other psychostimulants `UPD` `PE`

√7ᵗʰ **T43.696** **Underdosing** of other psychostimulants `UPD` `PE`

√5ᵗʰ **T43.8** **Poisoning by, adverse effect of and underdosing of other psychotropic drugs**

√6ᵗʰ **T43.8X** **Poisoning by, adverse effect of and underdosing of other psychotropic drugs**

√7ᵗʰ **T43.8X1** **Poisoning by other psychotropic drugs, accidental (unintentional)** `PE`
Poisoning by other psychotropic drugs NOS

√7ᵗʰ **T43.8X2** **Poisoning by other psychotropic drugs, intentional self-harm** `HCC` `PE`

√7ᵗʰ **T43.8X3** **Poisoning by other psychotropic drugs, assault** `PE`

√7ᵗʰ **T43.8X4** **Poisoning by other psychotropic drugs, undetermined** `PE`

√7ᵗʰ **T43.8X5** **Adverse effect** of other psychotropic drugs `UPD` `PE`

√7ᵗʰ **T43.8X6** **Underdosing** of other psychotropic drugs `UPD` `PE`

√5ᵗʰ **T43.9** **Poisoning by, adverse effect of and underdosing of unspecified psychotropic drug**

√x 7ᵗʰ **T43.91** **Poisoning by unspecified psychotropic drug, accidental (unintentional)** `PE`
Poisoning by psychotropic drug NOS

√x 7ᵗʰ **T43.92** **Poisoning by unspecified psychotropic drug, intentional self-harm** `HCC` `PE`

√x 7ᵗʰ **T43.93** **Poisoning by unspecified psychotropic drug, assault** `PE`

√x 7ᵗʰ **T43.94** **Poisoning by unspecified psychotropic drug, undetermined** `PE`

√x 7ᵗʰ **T43.95** **Adverse effect** of unspecified psychotropic drug `UPD` `PE`

√x 7ᵗʰ **T43.96** **Underdosing** of unspecified psychotropic drug `UPD` `PE`

✓4th **T44** **Poisoning by, adverse effect of and underdosing of drugs primarily affecting the autonomic nervous system**

> The appropriate 7th character is to be added to each code from category T44.
> A   initial encounter
> D   subsequent encounter
> S   sequela

✓5th **T44.0** **Poisoning by, adverse effect of and underdosing of anticholinesterase agents**

✓6th **T44.0X** **Poisoning by, adverse effect of and underdosing of anticholinesterase agents**

✓7th **T44.0X1** **Poisoning by anticholinesterase agents, accidental (unintentional)** `PE`
Poisoning by anticholinesterase agents NOS

✓7th **T44.0X2** **Poisoning by anticholinesterase agents, intentional self-harm** `HCC` `PE`

✓7th **T44.0X3** **Poisoning by anticholinesterase agents, assault** `PE`

✓7th **T44.0X4** **Poisoning by anticholinesterase agents, undetermined** `PE`

✓7th **T44.0X5** **Adverse effect of anticholinesterase agents** `UPD` `PE`

✓7th **T44.0X6** **Underdosing of anticholinesterase agents** `UPD` `PE`

✓5th **T44.1** **Poisoning by, adverse effect of and underdosing of other parasympathomimetics [cholinergics]**

✓6th **T44.1X** **Poisoning by, adverse effect of and underdosing of other parasympathomimetics [cholinergics]**

✓7th **T44.1X1** **Poisoning by other parasympathomimetics [cholinergics], accidental (unintentional)** `PE`
Poisoning by other parasympathomimetics [cholinergics] NOS

✓7th **T44.1X2** **Poisoning by other parasympathomimetics [cholinergics], intentional self-harm** `HCC` `PE`

✓7th **T44.1X3** **Poisoning by other parasympathomimetics [cholinergics], assault** `PE`

✓7th **T44.1X4** **Poisoning by other parasympathomimetics [cholinergics], undetermined** `PE`

✓7th **T44.1X5** **Adverse effect of other parasympathomimetics [cholinergics]** `UPD` `PE`

✓7th **T44.1X6** **Underdosing of other parasympathomimetics [cholinergics]** `UPD` `PE`

✓5th **T44.2** **Poisoning by, adverse effect of and underdosing of ganglionic blocking drugs**

✓6th **T44.2X** **Poisoning by, adverse effect of and underdosing of ganglionic blocking drugs**

✓7th **T44.2X1** **Poisoning by ganglionic blocking drugs, accidental (unintentional)** `PE`
Poisoning by ganglionic blocking drugs NCS

✓7th **T44.2X2** **Poisoning by ganglionic blocking drugs, intentional self-harm** `HCC` `PE`

✓7th **T44.2X3** **Poisoning by ganglionic blocking drugs, assault** `PE`

✓7th **T44.2X4** **Poisoning by ganglionic blocking drugs, undetermined** `PE`

✓7th **T44.2X5** **Adverse effect of ganglionic blocking drugs** `UPD` `PE`

✓7th **T44.2X6** **Underdosing of ganglionic blocking drugs** `UPD` `PE`

✓5th **T44.3** **Poisoning by, adverse effect of and underdosing of other parasympatholytics [anticholinergics and antimuscarinics] and spasmolytics**
Poisoning by, adverse effect of and underdosing of papaverine

✓6th **T44.3X** **Poisoning by, adverse effect of and underdosing of other parasympatholytics [anticholinergics and antimuscarinics] and spasmolytics**

✓7th **T44.3X1** **Poisoning by other parasympatholytics [anticholinergics and antimuscarinics] and spasmolytics, accidental (unintentional)** `PE`
Poisoning by other parasympatholytics [anticholinergics and antimuscarinics] and spasmolytics NOS

✓7th **T44.3X2** **Poisoning by other parasympatholytics [anticholinergics and antimuscarinics] and spasmolytics, intentional self-harm** `HCC` `PE`

✓7th **T44.3X3** **Poisoning by other parasympatholytics [anticholinergics and antimuscarinics] and spasmolytics, assault** `PE`

✓7th **T44.3X4** **Poisoning by other parasympatholytics [anticholinergics and antimuscarinics] and spasmolytics, undetermined** `PE`

✓7th **T44.3X5** **Adverse effect of other parasympatholytics [anticholinergics and antimuscarinics] and spasmolytics** `UPD` `PE`

✓7th **T44.3X6** **Underdosing of other parasympatholytics [anticholinergics and antimuscarinics] and spasmolytics** `UPD` `PE`

✓5th **T44.4** **Poisoning by, adverse effect of and underdosing of predominantly alpha-adrenoreceptor agonists**
Poisoning by, adverse effect of and underdosing of metaraminol

✓6th **T44.4X** **Poisoning by, adverse effect of and underdosing of predominantly alpha-adrenoreceptor agonists**

✓7th **T44.4X1** **Poisoning by predominantly alpha-adrenoreceptor agonists, accidental (unintentional)** `PE`
Poisoning by predominantly alpha-adrenoreceptor agonists NOS

✓7th **T44.4X2** **Poisoning by predominantly alpha-adrenoreceptor agonists, intentional self-harm** `HCC` `PE`

✓7th **T44.4X3** **Poisoning by predominantly alpha-adrenoreceptor agonists, assault** `PE`

✓7th **T44.4X4** **Poisoning by predominantly alpha-adrenoreceptor agonists, undetermined** `PE`

✓7th **T44.4X5** **Adverse effect of predominantly alpha-adrenoreceptor agonists** `UPD` `PE`

✓7th **T44.4X6** **Underdosing of predominantly alpha-adrenoreceptor agonists** `UPD` `PE`

✓5th **T44.5** **Poisoning by, adverse effect of and underdosing of predominantly beta-adrenoreceptor agonists**

> **EXCLUDES 1**   *poisoning by, adverse effect of and underdosing of beta-adrenoreceptor agonists used in asthma therapy (T48.6-)*

✓6th **T44.5X** **Poisoning by, adverse effect of and underdosing of predominantly beta-adrenoreceptor agonists**

✓7th **T44.5X1** **Poisoning by predominantly beta-adrenoreceptor agonists, accidental (unintentional)** `PE`
Poisoning by predominantly beta-adrenoreceptor agonists NOS

✓7th **T44.5X2** **Poisoning by predominantly beta-adrenoreceptor agonists, intentional self-harm** `HCC` `PE`

✓7th **T44.5X3** **Poisoning by predominantly beta-adrenoreceptor agonists, assault** `PE`

✓7th **T44.5X4** **Poisoning by predominantly beta-adrenoreceptor agonists, undetermined** `PE`

✓7th **T44.5X5** **Adverse effect of predominantly beta-adrenoreceptor agonists** `UPD` `PE`

✓7th **T44.5X6** **Underdosing of predominantly beta-adrenoreceptor agonists** `UPD` `PE`

✓5th **T44.6** **Poisoning by, adverse effect of and underdosing of alpha-adrenoreceptor antagonists**

> **EXCLUDES 1**   *poisoning by, adverse effect of and underdosing of ergot alkaloids (T48.0)*

✓6th **T44.6X** **Poisoning by, adverse effect of and underdosing of alpha-adrenoreceptor antagonists**

✓7th **T44.6X1** **Poisoning by alpha-adrenoreceptor antagonists, accidental (unintentional)** `PE`
Poisoning by alpha-adrenoreceptor antagonists NOS

✓7th **T44.6X2** **Poisoning by alpha-adrenoreceptor antagonists, intentional self-harm** `HCC` `PE`

✓7th **T44.6X3** **Poisoning by alpha-adrenoreceptor antagonists, assault** `PE`

✓7th **T44.6X4** **Poisoning by alpha-adrenoreceptor antagonists, undetermined** `PE`

✓7th **T44.6X5** **Adverse effect of alpha-adrenoreceptor antagonists** `UPD` `PE`

✓7th **T44.6X6** **Underdosing of alpha-adrenoreceptor antagonists** `UPD` `PE`

✔ Additional Character Required   ✓x7th Placeholder   `Questionable PDx`   Manifestation   Unspecified   `UPD` Unacceptable PDx   `H1`-`H14` HAC   `HCC` CMS-HCC Dx   `HIV` HIV Dx

Chapter 19. Injury, Poisoning and Certain Other Consequences of External Causes

T44.7–T45.1X6

√5th **T44.7** **Poisoning by, adverse effect of and underdosing of beta-adrenoreceptor antagonists**

√6th   **T44.7X**   **Poisoning by, adverse effect of and underdosing of beta-adrenoreceptor antagonists**

√7th   **T44.7X1**   **Poisoning by beta-adrenoreceptor antagonists, accidental (unintentional)** PE
Poisoning by beta-adrenoreceptor antagonists NOS

√7th   **T44.7X2**   **Poisoning by beta-adrenoreceptor antagonists, intentional self-harm** HCC PE

√7th   **T44.7X3**   **Poisoning by beta-adrenoreceptor antagonists, assault** PE

√7th   **T44.7X4**   **Poisoning by beta-adrenoreceptor antagonists, undetermined** PE

√7th   **T44.7X5**   **Adverse effect of beta-adrenoreceptor antagonists** UPD PE

√7th   **T44.7X6**   **Underdosing of beta-adrenoreceptor antagonists** UPD PE

√5th **T44.8** **Poisoning by, adverse effect of and underdosing of centrally-acting and adrenergic-neuron- blocking agents**
EXCLUDES 2   *poisoning by, adverse effect of and underdosing of clonidine (T46.5)*
poisoning by, adverse effect of and underdosing of guanethidine (T46.5)

√6th   **T44.8X**   **Poisoning by, adverse effect of and underdosing of centrally-acting and adrenergic- neuron-blocking agents**

√7th   **T44.8X1**   **Poisoning by centrally-acting and adrenergic-neuron-blocking agents, accidental (unintentional)** PE
Poisoning by centrally-acting and adrenergic-neuron-blocking agents NOS

√7th   **T44.8X2**   **Poisoning by centrally-acting and adrenergic-neuron-blocking agents, intentional self-harm** HCC PE

√7th   **T44.8X3**   **Poisoning by centrally-acting and adrenergic-neuron-blocking agents, assault** PE

√7th   **T44.8X4**   **Poisoning by centrally-acting and adrenergic-neuron-blocking agents, undetermined** PE

√7th   **T44.8X5**   **Adverse effect of centrally-acting and adrenergic-neuron-blocking agents** UPD PE

√7th   **T44.8X6**   **Underdosing of centrally-acting and adrenergic-neuron-blocking agents** UPD PE

√5th **T44.9** **Poisoning by, adverse effect of and underdosing of other and unspecified drugs primarily affecting the autonomic nervous system**
Poisoning by, adverse effect of and underdosing of drug stimulating both alpha and beta-adrenoreceptors

√6th   **T44.90**   **Poisoning by, adverse effect of and underdosing of unspecified drugs primarily affecting the autonomic nervous system**

√7th   **T44.901**   **Poisoning by unspecified drugs primarily affecting the autonomic nervous system, accidental (unintentional)** PE
Poisoning by unspecified drugs primarily affecting the autonomic nervous system NOS

√7th   **T44.902**   **Poisoning by unspecified drugs primarily affecting the autonomic nervous system, intentional self-harm** HCC PE

√7th   **T44.903**   **Poisoning by unspecified drugs primarily affecting the autonomic nervous system, assault** PE

√7th   **T44.904**   **Poisoning by unspecified drugs primarily affecting the autonomic nervous system, undetermined** PE

√7th   **T44.905**   **Adverse effect of unspecified drugs primarily affecting the autonomic nervous system** UPD PE

√7th   **T44.906**   **Underdosing of unspecified drugs primarily affecting the autonomic nervous system** UPD PE

√6th   **T44.99**   **Poisoning by, adverse effect of and underdosing of other drugs primarily affecting the autonomic nervous system**

√7th   **T44.991**   **Poisoning by other drug primarily affecting the autonomic nervous system, accidental (unintentional)** PE
Poisoning by other drugs primarily affecting the autonomic nervous system NOS

√7th   **T44.992**   **Poisoning by other drug primarily affecting the autonomic nervous system, intentional self-harm** HCC PE

√7th   **T44.993**   **Poisoning by other drug primarily affecting the autonomic nervous system, assault** PE

√7th   **T44.994**   **Poisoning by other drug primarily affecting the autonomic nervous system, undetermined** PE

√7th   **T44.995**   **Adverse effect of other drug primarily affecting the autonomic nervous system** UPD PE

√7th   **T44.996**   **Underdosing of other drug primarily affecting the autonomic nervous system** UPD PE

√4th **T45** **Poisoning by, adverse effect of and underdosing of primarily systemic and hematological agents, not elsewhere classified**

The appropriate 7th character is to be added to each code from category T45.
A   initial encounter
D   subsequent encounter
S   sequela

√5th **T45.0** **Poisoning by, adverse effect of and underdosing of antiallergic and antiemetic drugs**
EXCLUDES 1   *poisoning by, adverse effect of and underdosing of phenothiazine-based neuroleptics (T43.3)*

√6th   **T45.0X**   **Poisoning by, adverse effect of and underdosing of antiallergic and antiemetic drugs**

√7th   **T45.0X1**   **Poisoning by antiallergic and antiemetic drugs, accidental (unintentional)** PE
Poisoning by antiallergic and antiemetic drugs NOS

√7th   **T45.0X2**   **Poisoning by antiallergic and antiemetic drugs, intentional self-harm** HCC PE

√7th   **T45.0X3**   **Poisoning by antiallergic and antiemetic drugs, assault** PE

√7th   **T45.0X4**   **Poisoning by antiallergic and antiemetic drugs, undetermined** PE

√7th   **T45.0X5**   **Adverse effect of antiallergic and antiemetic drugs** UPD PE

√7th   **T45.0X6**   **Underdosing of antiallergic and antiemetic drugs** UPD PE

√5th **T45.1** **Poisoning by, adverse effect of and underdosing of antineoplastic and immunosuppressive drugs**
EXCLUDES 1   ▶*poisoning by, adverse effect of and underdosing of immune checkpoint inhibitors and immunostimulant drugs (T45.A)*◄
poisoning by, adverse effect of and underdosing of tamoxifen (T38.6)
AHA: 2019,1Q,17,20; 2014,4Q,22

√6th   **T45.1X**   **Poisoning by, adverse effect of and underdosing of antineoplastic and immunosuppressive drugs**

√7th   **T45.1X1**   **Poisoning by antineoplastic and immunosuppressive drugs, accidental (unintentional)** PE
Poisoning by antineoplastic and immunosuppressive drugs NOS

√7th   **T45.1X2**   **Poisoning by antineoplastic and immunosuppressive drugs, intentional self-harm** HCC PE

√7th   **T45.1X3**   **Poisoning by antineoplastic and immunosuppressive drugs, assault** PE

√7th   **T45.1X4**   **Poisoning by antineoplastic and immunosuppressive drugs, undetermined** PE

√7th   **T45.1X5**   **Adverse effect of antineoplastic and immunosuppressive drugs** UPD PE
AHA: 2024,1Q,25; 2023,2Q,10; 2021,3Q,4; 2020,4Q,11; 2020,3Q,22; 2019,2Q,24,28

√7th   **T45.1X6**   **Underdosing of antineoplastic and immunosuppressive drugs** UPD PE

√5th **T45.2 Poisoning by, adverse effect of and underdosing of vitamins**

> EXCLUDES 2   *poisoning by, adverse effect of and underdosing of iron (T45.4)*
>
> *poisoning by, adverse effect of and underdosing of nicotinic acid (derivatives) (T46.7)*
>
> *poisoning by, adverse effect of and underdosing of vitamin K (T45.7)*

√6th **T45.2X Poisoning by, adverse effect of and underdosing of vitamins**

√7th **T45.2X1 Poisoning by vitamins, accidental (unintentional)** PE
Poisoning by vitamins NOS

√7th **T45.2X2 Poisoning by vitamins, intentional self-harm** HCC PE

√7th **T45.2X3 Poisoning by vitamins, assault** PE

√7th **T45.2X4 Poisoning by vitamins, undetermined** PE

√7th **T45.2X5 Adverse effect of vitamins** UPD PE

√7th **T45.2X6 Underdosing of vitamins** UPD PE

> EXCLUDES 1   vitamin deficiencies (E50-E56)

√5th **T45.3 Poisoning by, adverse effect of and underdosing of enzymes**

√6th **T45.3X Poisoning by, adverse effect of and underdosing of enzymes**

√7th **T45.3X1 Poisoning by enzymes, accidental (unintentional)** PE
Poisoning by enzymes NOS

√7th **T45.3X2 Poisoning by enzymes, intentional self-harm** HCC PE

√7th **T45.3X3 Poisoning by enzymes, assault** PE

√7th **T45.3X4 Poisoning by enzymes, undetermined** PE

√7th **T45.3X5 Adverse effect of enzymes** UPD PE

√7th **T45.3X6 Underdosing of enzymes** UPD PE

√5th **T45.4 Poisoning by, adverse effect of and underdosing of iron and its compounds**

√6th **T45.4X Poisoning by, adverse effect of and underdosing of iron and its compounds**

√7th **T45.4X1 Poisoning by iron and its compounds, accidental (unintentional)** PE
Poisoning by iron and its compounds NOS

√7th **T45.4X2 Poisoning by iron and its compounds, intentional self-harm** HCC PE

√7th **T45.4X3 Poisoning by iron and its compounds, assault** PE

√7th **T45.4X4 Poisoning by iron and its compounds, undetermined** PE

√7th **T45.4X5 Adverse effect of iron and its compounds** UPD PE

√7th **T45.4X6 Underdosing of iron and its compounds** UPD PE

> EXCLUDES 1   iron deficiency (E61.1)

√5th **T45.5 Poisoning by, adverse effect of and underdosing of anticoagulants and antithrombotic drugs**

√6th **T45.51 Poisoning by, adverse effect of and underdosing of anticoagulants**

√7th **T45.511 Poisoning by anticoagulants, accidental (unintentional)** PE
Poisoning by anticoagulants NOS

√7th **T45.512 Poisoning by anticoagulants, intentional self-harm** HCC PE

√7th **T45.513 Poisoning by anticoagulants, assault** PE

√7th **T45.514 Poisoning by anticoagulants, undetermined** PE

√7th **T45.515 Adverse effect of anticoagulants** UPD PE
AHA: 2021,1Q,4; 2016,1Q,14; 2013,2Q,34

√7th **T45.516 Underdosing of anticoagulants** UPD PE

√6th **T45.52 Poisoning by, adverse effect of and underdosing of antithrombotic drugs**
Poisoning by, adverse effect of and underdosing of antiplatelet drugs

> EXCLUDES 2   *poisoning by, adverse effect of and underdosing of acetylsalicylic acid (T39.01-)*
>
> *poisoning by, adverse effect of and underdosing of aspirin (T39.01-)*

√7th **T45.521 Poisoning by antithrombotic drugs, accidental (unintentional)** PE
Poisoning by antithrombotic drug NOS

√7th **T45.522 Poisoning by antithrombotic drugs, intentional self-harm** HCC PE

√7th **T45.523 Poisoning by antithrombotic drugs, assault** PE

√7th **T45.524 Poisoning by antithrombotic drugs, undetermined** PE

√7th **T45.525 Adverse effect of antithrombotic drugs** UPD PE
AHA: 2016,1Q,15

√7th **T45.526 Underdosing of antithrombotic drugs** UPD PE

√5th **T45.6 Poisoning by, adverse effect of and underdosing of fibrinolysis-affecting drugs**

√6th **T45.60 Poisoning by, adverse effect of and underdosing of unspecified fibrinolysis-affecting drugs**

√7th **T45.601 Poisoning by unspecified fibrinolysis-affecting drugs, accidental (unintentional)** PE
Poisoning by fibrinolysis-affecting drug NOS

√7th **T45.602 Poisoning by unspecified fibrinolysis-affecting drugs, intentional self-harm** HCC PE

√7th **T45.603 Poisoning by unspecified fibrinolysis-affecting drugs, assault** PE

√7th **T45.604 Poisoning by unspecified fibrinolysis-affecting drugs, undetermined** PE

√7th **T45.605 Adverse effect of unspecified fibrinolysis-affecting drugs** UPD PE

√7th **T45.606 Underdosing of unspecified fibrinolysis-affecting drugs** UPD PE

√6th **T45.61 Poisoning by, adverse effect of and underdosing of thrombolytic drugs**

√7th **T45.611 Poisoning by thrombolytic drug, accidental (unintentional)** PE
Poisoning by thrombolytic drug NOS

√7th **T45.612 Poisoning by thrombolytic drug, intentional self-harm** HCC PE

√7th **T45.613 Poisoning by thrombolytic drug, assault** PE

√7th **T45.614 Poisoning by thrombolytic drug, undetermined** PE

√7th **T45.615 Adverse effect of thrombolytic drugs** UPD PE
AHA: 2017,2Q,9

√7th **T45.616 Underdosing of thrombolytic drugs** UPD PE

√6th **T45.62 Poisoning by, adverse effect of and underdosing of hemostatic drugs**

√7th **T45.621 Poisoning by hemostatic drug, accidental (unintentional)** PE
Poisoning by hemostatic drug NOS

√7th **T45.622 Poisoning by hemostatic drug, intentional self-harm** HCC PE

√7th **T45.623 Poisoning by hemostatic drug, assault** PE

√7th **T45.624 Poisoning by hemostatic drug, undetermined** PE

√7th **T45.625 Adverse effect of hemostatic drug** UPD PE

√7th **T45.626 Underdosing of hemostatic drugs** UPD PE

√6th **T45.69 Poisoning by, adverse effect of and underdosing of other fibrinolysis-affecting drugs**

√7th **T45.691 Poisoning by other fibrinolysis-affecting drugs, accidental (unintentional)** PE
Poisoning by other fibrinolysis-affecting drug NOS

✔ Additional Character Required   √x7th Placeholder   Questionable PDx   Manifestation   Unspecified   UPD Unacceptable PDx   H1-H14 HAC   HCC CMS-HCC Dx   HIV HIV Dx

ICD-10-CM 2025   1149

√7ᵗʰ **T45.692** Poisoning by other fibrinolysis-affecting drugs, intentional self-harm `HCC` `PE`

√7ᵗʰ **T45.693** Poisoning by other fibrinolysis-affecting drugs, assault `PE`

√7ᵗʰ **T45.694** Poisoning by other fibrinolysis-affecting drugs, undetermined `PE`

√7ᵗʰ **T45.695** Adverse effect of other fibrinolysis-affecting drugs `UPD` `PE`

√7ᵗʰ **T45.696** Underdosing of other fibrinolysis-affecting drugs `UPD` `PE`

√5ᵗʰ **T45.7** Poisoning by, adverse effect of and underdosing of anticoagulant antagonists, vitamin K and other coagulants

√6ᵗʰ **T45.7X** Poisoning by, adverse effect of and underdosing of anticoagulant antagonists, vitamin K and other coagulants

√7ᵗʰ **T45.7X1** Poisoning by anticoagulant antagonists, vitamin K and other coagulants, accidental (unintentional)
Poisoning by anticoagulant antagonists, vitamin K and other coagulants NOS

√7ᵗʰ **T45.7X2** Poisoning by anticoagulant antagonists, vitamin K and other coagulants, intentional self-harm `HCC` `PE`

√7ᵗʰ **T45.7X3** Poisoning by anticoagulant antagonists, vitamin K and other coagulants, assault `PE`

√7ᵗʰ **T45.7X4** Poisoning by anticoagulant antagonists, vitamin K and other coagulants, undetermined `PE`

√7ᵗʰ **T45.7X5** Adverse effect of anticoagulant antagonists, vitamin K and other coagulants `UPD` `PE`

√7ᵗʰ **T45.7X6** Underdosing of anticoagulant antagonist, vitamin K and other coagulants `UPD` `PE`
EXCLUDES 1   *vitamin K deficiency (E56.1)*

√5ᵗʰ **T45.8** Poisoning by, adverse effect of and underdosing of other primarily systemic and hematological agents
Poisoning by, adverse effect of and underdosing of liver preparations and other antianemic agents
Poisoning by, adverse effect of and underdosing of natural blood and blood products
Poisoning by, adverse effect of and underdosing of plasma substitute
EXCLUDES 2   *poisoning by, adverse effect of and underdosing of immunoglobulin (T50.Z1)*
poisoning by, adverse effect of and underdosing of iron (T45.4)
transfusion reactions (T80.-)

√6ᵗʰ **T45.8X** Poisoning by, adverse effect of and underdosing of other primarily systemic and hematological agents

√7ᵗʰ **T45.8X1** Poisoning by other primarily systemic and hematological agents, accidental (unintentional) `PE`
Poisoning by other primarily systemic and hematological agents NOS

√7ᵗʰ **T45.8X2** Poisoning by other primarily systemic and hematological agents, intentional self-harm `HCC` `PE`

√7ᵗʰ **T45.8X3** Poisoning by other primarily systemic and hematological agents, assault `PE`

√7ᵗʰ **T45.8X4** Poisoning by other primarily systemic and hematological agents, undetermined `PE`

√7ᵗʰ **T45.8X5** Adverse effect of other primarily systemic and hematological agents `UPD` `PE`
AHA: 2016,4Q,42

√7ᵗʰ **T45.8X6** Underdosing of other primarily systemic and hematological agents `UPD` `PE`

√5ᵗʰ **T45.9** Poisoning by, adverse effect of and underdosing of unspecified primarily systemic and hematological agent

√x7ᵗʰ **T45.91** Poisoning by unspecified primarily systemic and hematological agent, accidental (unintentional) `PE`
Poisoning by primarily systemic and hematological agent NOS

√x7ᵗʰ **T45.92** Poisoning by unspecified primarily systemic and hematological agent, intentional self-harm `HCC` `PE`

√x7ᵗʰ **T45.93** Poisoning by unspecified primarily systemic and hematological agent, assault `PE`

√x7ᵗʰ **T45.94** Poisoning by unspecified primarily systemic and hematological agent, undetermined `PE`

√x7ᵗʰ **T45.95** Adverse effect of unspecified primarily systemic and hematological agent `UPD` `PE`

√x7ᵗʰ **T45.96** Underdosing of unspecified primarily systemic and hematological agent `UPD` `PE`

● √5ᵗʰ **T45.A** Poisoning by, adverse effect of and underdosing of immune checkpoint inhibitors and immunostimulant drugs
EXCLUDES 1   *poisoning by, adverse effect of and underdosing of antineoplastic and immunosuppressive drug (T45.1)*

● √6ᵗʰ **T45.AX** Poisoning by, adverse effect of and underdosing of immune checkpoint inhibitors and immunostimulant drugs

√7ᵗʰ **T45.AX1** Poisoning by immune checkpoint inhibitors and immunostimulant drugs, accidental (unintentional) `PE`
Poisoning by immune checkpoint inhibitors and immunosuppressive drugs NOS

√7ᵗʰ **T45.AX2** Poisoning by immune checkpoint inhibitors and immunostimulant drugs, intentional self-harm `PE`

√7ᵗʰ **T45.AX3** Poisoning by immune checkpoint inhibitors and immunostimulant drugs, assault `PE`

√7ᵗʰ **T45.AX4** Poisoning by immune checkpoint inhibitors and immunostimulant drugs, undetermined `PE`

√7ᵗʰ **T45.AX5** Adverse effect of immune checkpoint inhibitors and immunostimulant drugs `PE`

√7ᵗʰ **T45.AX6** Underdosing of immune checkpoint inhibitors and immunostimulant drugs `PE`

√4ᵗʰ **T46** Poisoning by, adverse effect of and underdosing of agents primarily affecting the cardiovascular system
EXCLUDES 1   *poisoning by, adverse effect of and underdosing of metaraminol (T44.4)*

The appropriate 7th character is to be added to each code from category T46.
A   initial encounter
D   subsequent encounter
S   sequela

√5ᵗʰ **T46.0** Poisoning by, adverse effect of and underdosing of cardiac-stimulant glycosides and drugs of similar action

√6ᵗʰ **T46.0X** Poisoning by, adverse effect of and underdosing of cardiac-stimulant glycosides and drugs of similar action

√7ᵗʰ **T46.0X1** Poisoning by cardiac-stimulant glycosides and drugs of similar action, accidental (unintentional) `PE`
Poisoning by cardiac-stimulant glycosides and drugs of similar action NOS

√7ᵗʰ **T46.0X2** Poisoning by cardiac-stimulant glycosides and drugs of similar action, intentional self-harm `HCC` `PE`

√7ᵗʰ **T46.0X3** Poisoning by cardiac-stimulant glycosides and drugs of similar action, assault `PE`

√7ᵗʰ **T46.0X4** Poisoning by cardiac-stimulant glycosides and drugs of similar action, undetermined `PE`

√7ᵗʰ **T46.0X5** Adverse effect of cardiac-stimulant glycosides and drugs of similar action `UPD` `PE`

√7ᵗʰ **T46.0X6** Underdosing of cardiac-stimulant glycosides and drugs of similar action `UPD` `PE`

√5ᵗʰ **T46.1** Poisoning by, adverse effect of and underdosing of calcium-channel blockers

√6ᵗʰ **T46.1X** Poisoning by, adverse effect of and underdosing of calcium-channel blockers

√7ᵗʰ **T46.1X1** Poisoning by calcium-channel blockers, accidental (unintentional) `PE`
Poisoning by calcium-channel blockers NOS

√7ᵗʰ **T46.1X2** Poisoning by calcium-channel blockers, intentional self-harm `HCC` `PE`

√7ᵗʰ **T46.1X3** Poisoning by calcium-channel blockers, assault `PE`

√7ᵗʰ **T46.1X4** Poisoning by calcium-channel blockers, undetermined `PE`

√7ᵗʰ **T46.1X5** Adverse effect of calcium-channel blockers `UPD` `PE`

√7th **T46.1X6** Underdosing of calcium-channel blockers `UPD` `PE`
  AHA: 2023,1Q,39

√5th **T46.2** Poisoning by, adverse effect of and underdosing of other antidysrhythmic drugs, not elsewhere classified
  EXCLUDES 1 *poisoning by, adverse effect of and underdosing of beta-adrenoreceptor antagonists (T44.7-)*

√6th **T46.2X** Poisoning by, adverse effect of and underdosing of other antidysrhythmic drugs

√7th **T46.2X1** Poisoning by other antidysrhythmic drugs, accidental (unintentional) `PE`
  Poisoning by other antidysrhythmic drugs NOS

√7th **T46.2X2** Poisoning by other antidysrhythmic drugs, intentional self-harm `HCC` `PE`

√7th **T46.2X3** Poisoning by other antidysrhythmic drugs, assault `PE`

√7th **T46.2X4** Poisoning by other antidysrhythmic drugs, undetermined `PE`

√7th **T46.2X5** Adverse effect of other antidysrhythmic drugs `UPD` `PE`

√7th **T46.2X6** Underdosing of other antidysrhythmic drugs `UPD` `PE`

√5th **T46.3** Poisoning by, adverse effect of and underdosing of coronary vasodilators
  Poisoning by, adverse effect of and underdosing of dipyridamole
  EXCLUDES 1 *poisoning by, adverse effect of and underdosing of calcium-channel blockers (T46.1)*

√6th **T46.3X** Poisoning by, adverse effect of and underdosing of coronary vasodilators

√7th **T46.3X1** Poisoning by coronary vasodilators, accidental (unintentional) `PE`
  Poisoning by coronary vasodilators NOS

√7th **T46.3X2** Poisoning by coronary vasodilators, intentional self-harm `HCC` `PE`

√7th **T46.3X3** Poisoning by coronary vasodilators, assault `PE`

√7th **T46.3X4** Poisoning by coronary vasodilators, undetermined `PE`

√7th **T46.3X5** Adverse effect of coronary vasodilators `UPD` `PE`

√7th **T46.3X6** Underdosing of coronary vasodilators `UPD` `PE`

√5th **T46.4** Poisoning by, adverse effect of and underdosing of angiotensin-converting-enzyme inhibitors

√6th **T46.4X** Poisoning by, adverse effect of and underdosing of angiotensin-converting-enzyme inhibitors

√7th **T46.4X1** Poisoning by angiotensin-converting-enzyme inhibitors, accidental (unintentional) `PE`
  Poisoning by angiotensin-converting-enzyme inhibitors NOS

√7th **T46.4X2** Poisoning by angiotensin-converting-enzyme inhibitors, intentional self-harm `HCC` `PE`

√7th **T46.4X3** Poisoning by angiotensin-converting-enzyme inhibitors, assault `PE`

√7th **T46.4X4** Poisoning by angiotensin-converting-enzyme inhibitors, undetermined `PE`

√7th **T46.4X5** Adverse effect of angiotensin-converting-enzyme inhibitors `UPD` `PE`

√7th **T46.4X6** Underdosing of angiotensin-converting-enzyme inhibitors `UPD` `PE`

√5th **T46.5** Poisoning by, adverse effect of and underdosing of other antihypertensive drugs
  EXCLUDES 2 *poisoning by, adverse effect of and underdosing of beta-adrenoreceptor antagonists (T44.7)*
  poisoning by, adverse effect of and underdosing of calcium-channel blockers (T46.1)
  poisoning by, adverse effect of and underdosing of diuretics (T50.0-T50.2)

√6th **T46.5X** Poisoning by, adverse effect of and underdosing of other antihypertensive drugs

√7th **T46.5X1** Poisoning by other antihypertensive drugs, accidental (unintentional) `PE`
  Poisoning by other antihypertensive drugs NOS

√7th **T46.5X2** Poisoning by other antihypertensive drugs, intentional self-harm `HCC` `PE`

√7th **T46.5X3** Poisoning by other antihypertensive drugs, assault `PE`

√7th **T46.5X4** Poisoning by other antihypertensive drugs, undetermined `PE`

√7th **T46.5X5** Adverse effect of other antihypertensive drugs `UPD` `PE`

√7th **T46.5X6** Underdosing of other antihypertensive drugs `UPD` `PE`
  AHA: 2023,1Q,39; 2022,1Q,36

√5th **T46.6** Poisoning by, adverse effect of and underdosing of antihyperlipidemic and antiarteriosclerotic drugs

√6th **T46.6X** Poisoning by, adverse effect of and underdosing of antihyperlipidemic and antiarteriosclerotic drugs

√7th **T46.6X1** Poisoning by antihyperlipidemic and antiarteriosclerotic drugs, accidental (unintentional) `PE`
  Poisoning by antihyperlipidemic and antiarteriosclerotic drugs NOS

√7th **T46.6X2** Poisoning by antihyperlipidemic and antiarteriosclerotic drugs, intentional self-harm `HCC` `PE`

√7th **T46.6X3** Poisoning by antihyperlipidemic and antiarteriosclerotic drugs, assault `PE`

√7th **T46.6X4** Poisoning by antihyperlipidemic and antiarteriosclerotic drugs, undetermined `PE`

√7th **T46.6X5** Adverse effect of antihyperlipidemic and antiarteriosclerotic drugs `UPD` `PE`

√7th **T46.6X6** Underdosing of antihyperlipidemic and antiarteriosclerotic drugs `UPD` `PE`

√5th **T46.7** Poisoning by, adverse effect of and underdosing of peripheral vasodilators
  Poisoning by, adverse effect of and underdosing of nicotinic acid (derivatives)
  EXCLUDES 1 *poisoning by, adverse effect of and underdosing of papaverine (T44.3)*

√6th **T46.7X** Poisoning by, adverse effect of and underdosing of peripheral vasodilators

√7th **T46.7X1** Poisoning by peripheral vasodilators, accidental (unintentional) `PE`
  Poisoning by peripheral vasodilators NOS

√7th **T46.7X2** Poisoning by peripheral vasodilators, intentional self-harm `HCC` `PE`

√7th **T46.7X3** Poisoning by peripheral vasodilators, assault `PE`

√7th **T46.7X4** Poisoning by peripheral vasodilators, undetermined `PE`

√7th **T46.7X5** Adverse effect of peripheral vasodilators `UPD` `PE`

√7th **T46.7X6** Underdosing of peripheral vasodilators `UPD` `PE`

√5th **T46.8** Poisoning by, adverse effect of and underdosing of antivaricose drugs, including sclerosing agents

√6th **T46.8X** Poisoning by, adverse effect of and underdosing of antivaricose drugs, including sclerosing agents

√7th **T46.8X1** Poisoning by antivaricose drugs, including sclerosing agents, accidental (unintentional) `PE`
  Poisoning by antivaricose drugs, including sclerosing agents NOS

√7th **T46.8X2** Poisoning by antivaricose drugs, including sclerosing agents, intentional self-harm `HCC` `PE`

√7th **T46.8X3** Poisoning by antivaricose drugs, including sclerosing agents, assault `PE`

☑ Additional Character Required √x 7th Placeholder Questionable PDx Manifestation Unspecified `UPD` Unacceptable PDx `H1`-`H14` HAC `HCC` CMS-HCC Dx `HIV` HIV Dx

Chapter 19. Injury, Poisoning and Certain Other Consequences of External Causes

T46.8X4–T47.5X3

√7ᵗʰ **T46.8X4** Poisoning by antivaricose drugs, including sclerosing agents, undetermined PE

√7ᵗʰ **T46.8X5** Adverse effect of antivaricose drugs, including sclerosing agents UPD PE

√7ᵗʰ **T46.8X6** Underdosing of antivaricose drugs, including sclerosing agents UPD PE

√5ᵗʰ **T46.9** Poisoning by, adverse effect of and underdosing of other and unspecified agents primarily affecting the cardiovascular system

√6ᵗʰ **T46.90** Poisoning by, adverse effect of and underdosing of unspecified agents primarily affecting the cardiovascular system

√7ᵗʰ **T46.901** Poisoning by unspecified agents primarily affecting the cardiovascular system, accidental (unintentional) PE

√7ᵗʰ **T46.902** Poisoning by unspecified agents primarily affecting the cardiovascular system, intentional self-harm HCC PE

√7ᵗʰ **T46.903** Poisoning by unspecified agents primarily affecting the cardiovascular system, assault PE

√7ᵗʰ **T46.904** Poisoning by unspecified agents primarily affecting the cardiovascular system, undetermined PE

√7ᵗʰ **T46.905** Adverse effect of unspecified agents primarily affecting the cardiovascular system UPD PE

√7ᵗʰ **T46.906** Underdosing of unspecified agents primarily affecting the cardiovascular system UPD PE

√6ᵗʰ **T46.99** Poisoning by, adverse effect of and underdosing of other agents primarily affecting the cardiovascular system

√7ᵗʰ **T46.991** Poisoning by other agents primarily affecting the cardiovascular system, accidental (unintentional) PE

√7ᵗʰ **T46.992** Poisoning by other agents primarily affecting the cardiovascular system, intentional self-harm HCC PE

√7ᵗʰ **T46.993** Poisoning by other agents primarily affecting the cardiovascular system, assault PE

√7ᵗʰ **T46.994** Poisoning by other agents primarily affecting the cardiovascular system, undetermined PE

√7ᵗʰ **T46.995** Adverse effect of other agents primarily affecting the cardiovascular system UPD PE

√7ᵗʰ **T46.996** Underdosing of other agents primarily affecting the cardiovascular system UPD PE

√4ᵗʰ **T47** Poisoning by, adverse effect of and underdosing of agents primarily affecting the gastrointestinal system

The appropriate 7th character is to be added to each code from category T47.
A   initial encounter
D   subsequent encounter
S   sequela

√5ᵗʰ **T47.0** Poisoning by, adverse effect of and underdosing of histamine H2-receptor blockers

√6ᵗʰ **T47.0X** Poisoning by, adverse effect of and underdosing of histamine H2-receptor blockers

√7ᵗʰ **T47.0X1** Poisoning by histamine H2-receptor blockers, accidental (unintentional) PE
Poisoning by histamine H2-receptor blockers NOS

√7ᵗʰ **T47.0X2** Poisoning by histamine H2-receptor blockers, intentional self-harm HCC PE

√7ᵗʰ **T47.0X3** Poisoning by histamine H2-receptor blockers, assault PE

√7ᵗʰ **T47.0X4** Poisoning by histamine H2-receptor blockers, undetermined PE

√7ᵗʰ **T47.0X5** Adverse effect of histamine H2-receptor blockers UPD PE

√7ᵗʰ **T47.0X6** Underdosing of histamine H2-receptor blockers UPD PE

√5ᵗʰ **T47.1** Poisoning by, adverse effect of and underdosing of other antacids and anti-gastric-secretion drugs

√6ᵗʰ **T47.1X** Poisoning by, adverse effect of and underdosing of other antacids and anti-gastric-secretion drugs

√7ᵗʰ **T47.1X1** Poisoning by other antacids and anti-gastric-secretion drugs, accidental (unintentional) PE
Poisoning by other antacids and anti-gastric-secretion drugs NOS

√7ᵗʰ **T47.1X2** Poisoning by other antacids and anti-gastric-secretion drugs, intentional self-harm HCC PE

√7ᵗʰ **T47.1X3** Poisoning by other antacids and anti-gastric-secretion drugs, assault PE

√7ᵗʰ **T47.1X4** Poisoning by other antacids and anti-gastric-secretion drugs, undetermined PE

√7ᵗʰ **T47.1X5** Adverse effect of other antacids and anti-gastric-secretion drugs UPD PE

√7ᵗʰ **T47.1X6** Underdosing of other antacids and anti-gastric-secretion drugs UPD PE

√5ᵗʰ **T47.2** Poisoning by, adverse effect of and underdosing of stimulant laxatives

√6ᵗʰ **T47.2X** Poisoning by, adverse effect of and underdosing of stimulant laxatives

√7ᵗʰ **T47.2X1** Poisoning by stimulant laxatives, accidental (unintentional) PE
Poisoning by stimulant laxatives NOS

√7ᵗʰ **T47.2X2** Poisoning by stimulant laxatives, intentional self-harm HCC PE

√7ᵗʰ **T47.2X3** Poisoning by stimulant laxatives, assault PE

√7ᵗʰ **T47.2X4** Poisoning by stimulant laxatives, undetermined PE

√7ᵗʰ **T47.2X5** Adverse effect of stimulant laxatives UPD PE

√7ᵗʰ **T47.2X6** Underdosing of stimulant laxatives UPD PE

√5ᵗʰ **T47.3** Poisoning by, adverse effect of and underdosing of saline and osmotic laxatives

√6ᵗʰ **T47.3X** Poisoning by and adverse effect of saline and osmotic laxatives

√7ᵗʰ **T47.3X1** Poisoning by saline and osmotic laxatives, accidental (unintentional) PE
Poisoning by saline and osmotic laxatives NOS

√7ᵗʰ **T47.3X2** Poisoning by saline and osmotic laxatives, intentional self-harm HCC PE

√7ᵗʰ **T47.3X3** Poisoning by saline and osmotic laxatives, assault PE

√7ᵗʰ **T47.3X4** Poisoning by saline and osmotic laxatives, undetermined PE

√7ᵗʰ **T47.3X5** Adverse effect of saline and osmotic laxatives UPD PE

√7ᵗʰ **T47.3X6** Underdosing of saline and osmotic laxatives UPD PE

√5ᵗʰ **T47.4** Poisoning by, adverse effect of and underdosing of other laxatives

√6ᵗʰ **T47.4X** Poisoning by, adverse effect of and underdosing of other laxatives

√7ᵗʰ **T47.4X1** Poisoning by other laxatives, accidental (unintentional) PE
Poisoning by other laxatives NOS

√7ᵗʰ **T47.4X2** Poisoning by other laxatives, intentional self-harm HCC PE

√7ᵗʰ **T47.4X3** Poisoning by other laxatives, assault PE

√7ᵗʰ **T47.4X4** Poisoning by other laxatives, undetermined PE

√7ᵗʰ **T47.4X5** Adverse effect of other laxatives UPD PE

√7ᵗʰ **T47.4X6** Underdosing of other laxatives UPD PE

√5ᵗʰ **T47.5** Poisoning by, adverse effect of and underdosing of digestants

√6ᵗʰ **T47.5X** Poisoning by, adverse effect of and underdosing of digestants

√7ᵗʰ **T47.5X1** Poisoning by digestants, accidental (unintentional) PE
Poisoning by digestants NOS

√7ᵗʰ **T47.5X2** Poisoning by digestants, intentional self-harm HCC PE

√7ᵗʰ **T47.5X3** Poisoning by digestants, assault PE

√7ᵗʰ **T47.5X4** **Poisoning by digestants, undetermined** PE

√7ᵗʰ **T47.5X5** **Adverse effect of digestants** UPD PE

√7ᵗʰ **T47.5X6** **Underdosing of digestants** UPD PE

√5ᵗʰ **T47.6** **Poisoning by, adverse effect of and underdosing of antidiarrheal drugs**

EXCLUDES 2   poisoning by, adverse effect of and underdosing of systemic antibiotics and other anti-infectives (T36-T37)

√6ᵗʰ **T47.6X** **Poisoning by, adverse effect of and underdosing of antidiarrheal drugs**

√7ᵗʰ **T47.6X1** **Poisoning by antidiarrheal drugs, accidental (unintentional)** PE
Poisoning by antidiarrheal drugs NOS

√7ᵗʰ **T47.6X2** **Poisoning by antidiarrheal drugs, intentional self-harm** HCC PE

√7ᵗʰ **T47.6X3** **Poisoning by antidiarrheal drugs, assault** PE

√7ᵗʰ **T47.6X4** **Poisoning by antidiarrheal drugs, undetermined** PE

√7ᵗʰ **T47.6X5** **Adverse effect of antidiarrheal drugs** UPD PE

√7ᵗʰ **T47.6X6** **Underdosing of antidiarrheal drugs** UPD PE

√5ᵗʰ **T47.7** **Poisoning by, adverse effect of and underdosing of emetics**

√6ᵗʰ **T47.7X** **Poisoning by, adverse effect of and underdosing of emetics**

√7ᵗʰ **T47.7X1** **Poisoning by emetics, accidental (unintentional)** PE
Poisoning by emetics NOS

√7ᵗʰ **T47.7X2** **Poisoning by emetics, intentional self-harm** HCC PE

√7ᵗʰ **T47.7X3** **Poisoning by emetics, assault** PE

√7ᵗʰ **T47.7X4** **Poisoning by emetics, undetermined** PE

√7ᵗʰ **T47.7X5** **Adverse effect of emetics** UPD PE

√7ᵗʰ **T47.7X6** **Underdosing of emetics** UPD PE

√5ᵗʰ **T47.8** **Poisoning by, adverse effect of and underdosing of other agents primarily affecting gastrointestinal system**

√6ᵗʰ **T47.8X** **Poisoning by, adverse effect of and underdosing of other agents primarily affecting gastrointestinal system**

√7ᵗʰ **T47.8X1** **Poisoning by other agents primarily affecting gastrointestinal system, accidental (unintentional)** PE
Poisoning by other agents primarily affecting gastrointestinal system NOS

√7ᵗʰ **T47.8X2** **Poisoning by other agents primarily affecting gastrointestinal system, intentional self-harm** HCC PE

√7ᵗʰ **T47.8X3** **Poisoning by other agents primarily affecting gastrointestinal system, assault** PE

√7ᵗʰ **T47.8X4** **Poisoning by other agents primarily affecting gastrointestinal system, undetermined** PE

√7ᵗʰ **T47.8X5** **Adverse effect of other agents primarily affecting gastrointestinal system** UPD PE

√7ᵗʰ **T47.8X6** **Underdosing of other agents primarily affecting gastrointestinal system** UPD PE

√5ᵗʰ **T47.9** **Poisoning by, adverse effect of and underdosing of unspecified agents primarily affecting the gastrointestinal system**

√x7ᵗʰ **T47.91** **Poisoning by unspecified agents primarily affecting the gastrointestinal system, accidental (unintentional)** PE
Poisoning by agents primarily affecting the gastrointestinal system NOS

√x7ᵗʰ **T47.92** **Poisoning by unspecified agents primarily affecting the gastrointestinal system, intentional self-harm** HCC PE

√x7ᵗʰ **T47.93** **Poisoning by unspecified agents primarily affecting the gastrointestinal system, assault** PE

√x7ᵗʰ **T47.94** **Poisoning by unspecified agents primarily affecting the gastrointestinal system, undetermined** PE

√x7ᵗʰ **T47.95** **Adverse effect of unspecified agents primarily affecting the gastrointestinal system** UPD PE

√x7ᵗʰ **T47.96** **Underdosing of unspecified agents primarily affecting the gastrointestinal system** UPD PE

√4ᵗʰ **T48** **Poisoning by, adverse effect of and underdosing of agents primarily acting on smooth and skeletal muscles and the respiratory system**

The appropriate 7th character is to be added to each code from category T48.
A   initial encounter
D   subsequent encounter
S   sequela

√5ᵗʰ **T48.0** **Poisoning by, adverse effect of and underdosing of oxytocic drugs**

EXCLUDES 1   poisoning by, adverse effect of and underdosing of estrogens, progestogens and antagonists (T38.4-T38.6)

√6ᵗʰ **T48.0X** **Poisoning by, adverse effect of and underdosing of oxytocic drugs**

√7ᵗʰ **T48.0X1** **Poisoning by oxytocic drugs, accidental (unintentional)** PE
Poisoning by oxytocic drugs NOS

√7ᵗʰ **T48.0X2** **Poisoning by oxytocic drugs, intentional self-harm** HCC PE

√7ᵗʰ **T48.0X3** **Poisoning by oxytocic drugs, assault** PE

√7ᵗʰ **T48.0X4** **Poisoning by oxytocic drugs, undetermined** PE

√7ᵗʰ **T48.0X5** **Adverse effect of oxytocic drugs** UPD PE

√7ᵗʰ **T48.0X6** **Underdosing of oxytocic drugs** UPD PE

√5ᵗʰ **T48.1** **Poisoning by, adverse effect of and underdosing of skeletal muscle relaxants [neuromuscular blocking agents]**

√6ᵗʰ **T48.1X** **Poisoning by, adverse effect of and underdosing of skeletal muscle relaxants [neuromuscular blocking agents]**

√7ᵗʰ **T48.1X1** **Poisoning by skeletal muscle relaxants [neuromuscular blocking agents], accidental (unintentional)**
Poisoning by skeletal muscle relaxants [neuromuscular blocking agents] NOS

√7ᵗʰ **T48.1X2** **Poisoning by skeletal muscle relaxants [neuromuscular blocking agents], intentional self-harm** HCC PE

√7ᵗʰ **T48.1X3** **Poisoning by skeletal muscle relaxants [neuromuscular blocking agents], assault** PE

√7ᵗʰ **T48.1X4** **Poisoning by skeletal muscle relaxants [neuromuscular blocking agents], undetermined** PE

√7ᵗʰ **T48.1X5** **Adverse effect of skeletal muscle relaxants [neuromuscular blocking agents]** UPD PE

√7ᵗʰ **T48.1X6** **Underdosing of skeletal muscle relaxants [neuromuscular blocking agents]** UPD PE

√5ᵗʰ **T48.2** **Poisoning by, adverse effect of and underdosing of other and unspecified drugs acting on muscles**

√6ᵗʰ **T48.20** **Poisoning by, adverse effect of and underdosing of unspecified drugs acting on muscles**

√7ᵗʰ **T48.201** **Poisoning by unspecified drugs acting on muscles, accidental (unintentional)** PE
Poisoning by unspecified drugs acting on muscles NOS

√7ᵗʰ **T48.202** **Poisoning by unspecified drugs acting on muscles, intentional self-harm** HCC PE

√7ᵗʰ **T48.203** **Poisoning by unspecified drugs acting on muscles, assault** PE

√7ᵗʰ **T48.204** **Poisoning by unspecified drugs acting on muscles, undetermined** PE

√7ᵗʰ **T48.205** **Adverse effect of unspecified drugs acting on muscles** UPD PE

√7ᵗʰ **T48.206** **Underdosing of unspecified drugs acting on muscles** UPD PE

√6ᵗʰ **T48.29** **Poisoning by, adverse effect of and underdosing of other drugs acting on muscles**

√7ᵗʰ **T48.291** **Poisoning by other drugs acting on muscles, accidental (unintentional)** PE
Poisoning by other drugs acting on muscles NOS

√7ᵗʰ **T48.292** **Poisoning by other drugs acting on muscles, intentional self-harm** HCC PE

√7ᵗʰ **T48.293** **Poisoning by other drugs acting on muscles, assault** PE

√7ᵗʰ **T48.294** **Poisoning by other drugs acting on muscles, undetermined** PE

☑ Additional Character Required   √x7ᵗʰ Placeholder   Questionable PDx   Manifestation   Unspecified   UPD Unacceptable PDx   H1 - H14 HAC   HCC CMS-HCC Dx   HIV HIV Dx

ICD-10-CM 2025   1153

√7th **T48.295** Adverse effect of other drugs acting on muscles UPD PE

√7th **T48.296** Underdosing of other drugs acting on muscles UPD PE

√5th **T48.3** Poisoning by, adverse effect of and underdosing of antitussives

√6th **T48.3X** Poisoning by, adverse effect of and underdosing of antitussives

√7th **T48.3X1** Poisoning by antitussives, accidental (unintentional) PE
Poisoning by antitussives NOS

√7th **T48.3X2** Poisoning by antitussives, intentional self-harm HCC PE

√7th **T48.3X3** Poisoning by antitussives, assault PE

√7th **T48.3X4** Poisoning by antitussives, undetermined PE

√7th **T48.3X5** Adverse effect of antitussives UPD PE

√7th **T48.3X6** Underdosing of antitussives UPD PE

√5th **T48.4** Poisoning by, adverse effect of and underdosing of expectorants

√6th **T48.4X** Poisoning by, adverse effect of and underdosing of expectorants

√7th **T48.4X1** Poisoning by expectorants, accidental (unintentional) PE
Poisoning by expectorants NOS

√7th **T48.4X2** Poisoning by expectorants, intentional self-harm HCC PE

√7th **T48.4X3** Poisoning by expectorants, assault PE

√7th **T48.4X4** Poisoning by expectorants, undetermined PE

√7th **T48.4X5** Adverse effect of expectorants UPD PE

√7th **T48.4X6** Underdosing of expectorants UPD PE

√5th **T48.5** Poisoning by, adverse effect of and underdosing of other anti-common-cold drugs
Poisoning by, adverse effect of and underdosing of decongestants
EXCLUDES 2   poisoning by, adverse effect of and underdosing of antipyretics, NEC (T39.9-)
poisoning by, adverse effect of and underdosing of non-steroidal antiinflammatory drugs (T39.3-)
poisoning by, adverse effect of and underdosing of salicylates (T39.0-)

√6th **T48.5X** Poisoning by, adverse effect of and underdosing of other anti-common-cold drugs

√7th **T48.5X1** Poisoning by other anti-common-cold drugs, accidental (unintentional) PE
Poisoning by other anti-common-cold drugs NOS

√7th **T48.5X2** Poisoning by other anti-common-cold drugs, intentional self-harm HCC PE

√7th **T48.5X3** Poisoning by other anti-common-cold drugs, assault PE

√7th **T48.5X4** Poisoning by other anti-common-cold drugs, undetermined PE

√7th **T48.5X5** Adverse effect of other anti-common-cold drugs UPD PE

√7th **T48.5X6** Underdosing of other anti-common-cold drugs UPD PE

√5th **T48.6** Poisoning by, adverse effect of and underdosing of antiasthmatics, not elsewhere classified
Poisoning by, adverse effect of and underdosing of beta-adrenoreceptor agonists used in asthma therapy
EXCLUDES 1   poisoning by, adverse effect of and underdosing of anterior pituitary [adenohypophyseal] hormones (T38.8)
poisoning by, adverse effect of and underdosing of beta-adrenoreceptor agonists not used in asthma therapy (T44.5)

√6th **T48.6X** Poisoning by, adverse effect of and underdosing of antiasthmatics

√7th **T48.6X1** Poisoning by antiasthmatics, accidental (unintentional) PE
Poisoning by antiasthmatics NOS

√7th **T48.6X2** Poisoning by antiasthmatics, intentional self-harm HCC PE

√7th **T48.6X3** Poisoning by antiasthmatics, assault PE

√7th **T48.6X4** Poisoning by antiasthmatics, undetermined PE

√7th **T48.6X5** Adverse effect of antiasthmatics UPD PE

√7th **T48.6X6** Underdosing of antiasthmatics UPD PE
AHA: 2024,1Q,23

√5th **T48.9** Poisoning by, adverse effect of and underdosing of other and unspecified agents primarily acting on the respiratory system

√6th **T48.90** Poisoning by, adverse effect of and underdosing of unspecified agents primarily acting on the respiratory system

√7th **T48.901** Poisoning by unspecified agents primarily acting on the respiratory system, accidental (unintentional) PE

√7th **T48.902** Poisoning by unspecified agents primarily acting on the respiratory system, intentional self-harm HCC PE

√7th **T48.903** Poisoning by unspecified agents primarily acting on the respiratory system, assault PE

√7th **T48.904** Poisoning by unspecified agents primarily acting on the respiratory system, undetermined PE

√7th **T48.905** Adverse effect of unspecified agents primarily acting on the respiratory system UPD PE

√7th **T48.906** Underdosing of unspecified agents primarily acting on the respiratory system UPD PE

√6th **T48.99** Poisoning by, adverse effect of and underdosing of other agents primarily acting on the respiratory system

√7th **T48.991** Poisoning by other agents primarily acting on the respiratory system, accidental (unintentional) PE

√7th **T48.992** Poisoning by other agents primarily acting on the respiratory system, intentional self-harm HCC PE

√7th **T48.993** Poisoning by other agents primarily acting on the respiratory system, assault PE

√7th **T48.994** Poisoning by other agents primarily acting on the respiratory system, undetermined PE

√7th **T48.995** Adverse effect of other agents primarily acting on the respiratory system UPD PE

√7th **T48.996** Underdosing of other agents primarily acting on the respiratory system UPD PE

√4th **T49** Poisoning by, adverse effect of and underdosing of topical agents primarily affecting skin and mucous membrane and by ophthalmological, otorhinolaryngological and dental drugs
INCLUDES   poisoning by, adverse effect of and underdosing of glucocorticoids, topically used

> The appropriate 7th character is to be added to each code from category T49.
> A   initial encounter
> D   subsequent encounter
> S   sequela

√5th **T49.0** Poisoning by, adverse effect of and underdosing of local antifungal, anti-infective and anti-inflammatory drugs

√6th **T49.0X** Poisoning by, adverse effect of and underdosing of local antifungal, anti-infective and anti-inflammatory drugs

√7th **T49.0X1** Poisoning by local antifungal, anti-infective and anti-inflammatory drugs, accidental (unintentional) PE
Poisoning by local antifungal, anti-infective and anti-inflammatory drugs NOS

√7th **T49.0X2** Poisoning by local antifungal, anti-infective and anti-inflammatory drugs, intentional self-harm HCC PE

√7th **T49.0X3** Poisoning by local antifungal, anti-infective and anti-inflammatory drugs, assault PE

√7th **T49.0X4** Poisoning by local antifungal, anti-infective and anti-inflammatory drugs, undetermined PE

√7th **T49.0X5** Adverse effect of local antifungal, anti-infective and anti-inflammatory drugs UPD PE

√7th **T49.0X6** Underdosing of local antifungal, anti-infective and anti-inflammatory drugs UPD PE

N Newborn: 0   P Pediatric: 0-17   M Maternity: 9-64   A Adult: 15-124   UNS Unspecified Site   MCC Major Complication/Comorbidity   CC Complication/Comorbidity   PE POA Exempt

1154   ICD-10-CM 2025

✓5ᵗʰ **T49.1** Poisoning by, adverse effect of and underdosing of antipruritics

  ✓6ᵗʰ **T49.1X** Poisoning by, adverse effect of and underdosing of antipruritics

    ✓7ᵗʰ **T49.1X1** Poisoning by antipruritics, accidental (unintentional) PE
      Poisoning by antipruritics NOS

    ✓7ᵗʰ **T49.1X2** Poisoning by antipruritics, intentional self-harm HCC PE

    ✓7ᵗʰ **T49.1X3** Poisoning by antipruritics, assault PE

    ✓7ᵗʰ **T49.1X4** Poisoning by antipruritics, undetermined PE

    ✓7ᵗʰ **T49.1X5** Adverse effect of antipruritics UPD PE

    ✓7ᵗʰ **T49.1X6** Underdosing of antipruritics UPD PE

✓5ᵗʰ **T49.2** Poisoning by, adverse effect of and underdosing of local astringents and local detergents

  ✓6ᵗʰ **T49.2X** Poisoning by, adverse effect of and underdosing of local astringents and local detergents

    ✓7ᵗʰ **T49.2X1** Poisoning by local astringents and local detergents, accidental (unintentional) PE
      Poisoning by local astringents and local detergents NOS

    ✓7ᵗʰ **T49.2X2** Poisoning by local astringents and local detergents, intentional self-harm HCC PE

    ✓7ᵗʰ **T49.2X3** Poisoning by local astringents and local detergents, assault PE

    ✓7ᵗʰ **T49.2X4** Poisoning by local astringents and local detergents, undetermined PE

    ✓7ᵗʰ **T49.2X5** Adverse effect of local astringents and local detergents UPD PE

    ✓7ᵗʰ **T49.2X6** Underdosing of local astringents and local detergents UPD PE

✓5ᵗʰ **T49.3** Poisoning by, adverse effect of and underdosing of emollients, demulcents and protectants

  ✓6ᵗʰ **T49.3X** Poisoning by, adverse effect of and underdosing of emollients, demulcents and protectants

    ✓7ᵗʰ **T49.3X1** Poisoning by emollients, demulcents and protectants, accidental (unintentional) PE
      Poisoning by emollients, demulcents and protectants NOS

    ✓7ᵗʰ **T49.3X2** Poisoning by emollients, demulcents and protectants, intentional self-harm HCC PE

    ✓7ᵗʰ **T49.3X3** Poisoning by emollients, demulcents and protectants, assault PE

    ✓7ᵗʰ **T49.3X4** Poisoning by emollients, demulcents and protectants, undetermined PE

    ✓7ᵗʰ **T49.3X5** Adverse effect of emollients, demulcents and protectants UPD PE

    ✓7ᵗʰ **T49.3X6** Underdosing of emollients, demulcents and protectants UPD PE

✓5ᵗʰ **T49.4** Poisoning by, adverse effect of and underdosing of keratolytics, keratoplastics, and other hair treatment drugs and preparations

  ✓6ᵗʰ **T49.4X** Poisoning by, adverse effect of and underdosing of keratolytics, keratoplastics, and other hair treatment drugs and preparations

    ✓7ᵗʰ **T49.4X1** Poisoning by keratolytics, keratoplastics, and other hair treatment drugs and preparations, accidental (unintentional) PE
      Poisoning by keratolytics, keratoplastics, and other hair treatment drugs and preparations NOS

    ✓7ᵗʰ **T49.4X2** Poisoning by keratolytics, keratoplastics, and other hair treatment drugs and preparations, intentional self-harm HCC PE

    ✓7ᵗʰ **T49.4X3** Poisoning by keratolytics, keratoplastics, and other hair treatment drugs and preparations, assault PE

    ✓7ᵗʰ **T49.4X4** Poisoning by keratolytics, keratoplastics, and other hair treatment drugs and preparations, undetermined PE

    ✓7ᵗʰ **T49.4X5** Adverse effect of keratolytics, keratoplastics, and other hair treatment drugs and preparations UPD PE

    ✓7ᵗʰ **T49.4X6** Underdosing of keratolytics, keratoplastics, and other hair treatment drugs and preparations UPD PE

✓5ᵗʰ **T49.5** Poisoning by, adverse effect of and underdosing of ophthalmological drugs and preparations

  ✓6ᵗʰ **T49.5X** Poisoning by, adverse effect of and underdosing of ophthalmological drugs and preparations

    ✓7ᵗʰ **T49.5X1** Poisoning by ophthalmological drugs and preparations, accidental (unintentional) PE
      Poisoning by ophthalmological drugs and preparations NOS

    ✓7ᵗʰ **T49.5X2** Poisoning by ophthalmological drugs and preparations, intentional self-harm HCC PE

    ✓7ᵗʰ **T49.5X3** Poisoning by ophthalmological drugs and preparations, assault PE

    ✓7ᵗʰ **T49.5X4** Poisoning by ophthalmological drugs and preparations, undetermined PE

    ✓7ᵗʰ **T49.5X5** Adverse effect of ophthalmological drugs and preparations UPD PE

    ✓7ᵗʰ **T49.5X6** Underdosing of ophthalmological drugs and preparations UPD PE

✓5ᵗʰ **T49.6** Poisoning by, adverse effect of and underdosing of otorhinolaryngological drugs and preparations

  ✓6ᵗʰ **T49.6X** Poisoning by, adverse effect of and underdosing of otorhinolaryngological drugs and preparations

    ✓7ᵗʰ **T49.6X1** Poisoning by otorhinolaryngological drugs and preparations, accidental (unintentional) PE
      Poisoning by otorhinolaryngological drugs and preparations NOS

    ✓7ᵗʰ **T49.6X2** Poisoning by otorhinolaryngological drugs and preparations, intentional self-harm HCC PE

    ✓7ᵗʰ **T49.6X3** Poisoning by otorhinolaryngological drugs and preparations, assault PE

    ✓7ᵗʰ **T49.6X4** Poisoning by otorhinolaryngological drugs and preparations, undetermined PE

    ✓7ᵗʰ **T49.6X5** Adverse effect of otorhinolaryngological drugs and preparations UPD PE

    ✓7ᵗʰ **T49.6X6** Underdosing of otorhinolaryngological drugs and preparations UPD PE

✓5ᵗʰ **T49.7** Poisoning by, adverse effect of and underdosing of dental drugs, topically applied

  ✓6ᵗʰ **T49.7X** Poisoning by, adverse effect of and underdosing of dental drugs, topically applied

    ✓7ᵗʰ **T49.7X1** Poisoning by dental drugs, topically applied, accidental (unintentional) PE
      Poisoning by dental drugs, topically applied NOS

    ✓7ᵗʰ **T49.7X2** Poisoning by dental drugs, topically applied, intentional self-harm HCC PE

    ✓7ᵗʰ **T49.7X3** Poisoning by dental drugs, topically applied, assault PE

    ✓7ᵗʰ **T49.7X4** Poisoning by dental drugs, topically applied, undetermined PE

    ✓7ᵗʰ **T49.7X5** Adverse effect of dental drugs, topically applied UPD PE

    ✓7ᵗʰ **T49.7X6** Underdosing of dental drugs, topically applied UPD PE

✓5ᵗʰ **T49.8** Poisoning by, adverse effect of and underdosing of other topical agents
  Poisoning by, adverse effect of and underdosing of spermicides

  ✓6ᵗʰ **T49.8X** Poisoning by, adverse effect of and underdosing of other topical agents

    ✓7ᵗʰ **T49.8X1** Poisoning by other topical agents, accidental (unintentional) PE
      Poisoning by other topical agents NOS

    ✓7ᵗʰ **T49.8X2** Poisoning by other topical agents, intentional self-harm HCC PE

    ✓7ᵗʰ **T49.8X3** Poisoning by other topical agents, assault PE

    ✓7ᵗʰ **T49.8X4** Poisoning by other topical agents, undetermined PE

    ✓7ᵗʰ **T49.8X5** Adverse effect of other topical agents UPD PE

    ✓7ᵗʰ **T49.8X6** Underdosing of other topical agents UPD PE

Chapter 19. Injury, Poisoning and Certain Other Consequences of External Causes

T49.1–T49.8X6

✔ Additional Character Required   ✓x7ᵗʰ Placeholder   Questionable PDx   Manifestation   Unspecified   UPD Unacceptable PDx   H1-H14 HAC   HCC CMS-HCC Dx   HIV HIV Dx

ICD-10-CM 2025   **1155**

√5ᵗʰ **T49.9** Poisoning by, adverse effect of and underdosing of unspecified topical agent

  √x7ᵗʰ **T49.91** Poisoning by unspecified topical agent, accidental (unintentional)   PE

  √x7ᵗʰ **T49.92** Poisoning by unspecified topical agent, intentional self-harm   HCC PE

  √x7ᵗʰ **T49.93** Poisoning by unspecified topical agent, assault   PE

  √x7ᵗʰ **T49.94** Poisoning by unspecified topical agent, undetermined   PE

  √x7ᵗʰ **T49.95** Adverse effect of unspecified topical agent   UPD PE

  √x7ᵗʰ **T49.96** Underdosing of unspecified topical agent   UPD PE

√4ᵗʰ **T50** Poisoning by, adverse effect of and underdosing of diuretics and other and unspecified drugs, medicaments and biological substances

> The appropriate 7th character is to be added to each code from category T50.
> A   initial encounter
> D   subsequent encounter
> S   sequela

√5ᵗʰ **T50.0** Poisoning by, adverse effect of and underdosing of mineralocorticoids and their antagonists

  √6ᵗʰ **T50.0X** Poisoning by, adverse effect of and underdosing of mineralocorticoids and their antagonists

    √7ᵗʰ **T50.0X1** Poisoning by mineralocorticoids and their antagonists, accidental (unintentional)   PE
         Poisoning by mineralocorticoids and their antagonists NOS

    √7ᵗʰ **T50.0X2** Poisoning by mineralocorticoids and their antagonists, intentional self-harm   HCC PE

    √7ᵗʰ **T50.0X3** Poisoning by mineralocorticoids and their antagonists, assault   PE

    √7ᵗʰ **T50.0X4** Poisoning by mineralocorticoids and their antagonists, undetermined   PE

    √7ᵗʰ **T50.0X5** Adverse effect of mineralocorticoids and their antagonists   UPD PE

    √7ᵗʰ **T50.0X6** Underdosing of mineralocorticoids and their antagonists   UPD PE

√5ᵗʰ **T50.1** Poisoning by, adverse effect of and underdosing of loop [high-ceiling] diuretics

  √6ᵗʰ **T50.1X** Poisoning by, adverse effect of and underdosing of loop [high-ceiling] diuretics

    √7ᵗʰ **T50.1X1** Poisoning by loop [high-ceiling] diuretics, accidental (unintentional)   PE
         Poisoning by loop [high-ceiling] diuretics NOS

    √7ᵗʰ **T50.1X2** Poisoning by loop [high-ceiling] diuretics, intentional self-harm   HCC PE

    √7ᵗʰ **T50.1X3** Poisoning by loop [high-ceiling] diuretics, assault   PE

    √7ᵗʰ **T50.1X4** Poisoning by loop [high-ceiling] diuretics, undetermined   PE

    √7ᵗʰ **T50.1X5** Adverse effect of loop [high-ceiling] diuretics   UPD PE

    √7ᵗʰ **T50.1X6** Underdosing of loop [high-ceiling] diuretics   UPD PE

√5ᵗʰ **T50.2** Poisoning by, adverse effect of and underdosing of carbonic-anhydrase inhibitors, benzothiadiazides and other diuretics
   Poisoning by, adverse effect of and underdosing of acetazolamide

  √6ᵗʰ **T50.2X** Poisoning by, adverse effect of and underdosing of carbonic-anhydrase inhibitors, benzothiadiazides and other diuretics

    √7ᵗʰ **T50.2X1** Poisoning by carbonic-anhydrase inhibitors, benzothiadiazides and other diuretics, accidental (unintentional)   PE
         Poisoning by carbonic-anhydrase inhibitors, benzothiadiazides and other diuretics NOS

    √7ᵗʰ **T50.2X2** Poisoning by carbonic-anhydrase inhibitors, benzothiadiazides and other diuretics, intentional self-harm   HCC PE

    √7ᵗʰ **T50.2X3** Poisoning by carbonic-anhydrase inhibitors, benzothiadiazides and other diuretics, assault   PE

    √7ᵗʰ **T50.2X4** Poisoning by carbonic-anhydrase inhibitors, benzothiadiazides and other diuretics, undetermined   PE

    √7ᵗʰ **T50.2X5** Adverse effect of carbonic-anhydrase inhibitors, benzothiadiazides and other diuretics   UPD PE

    √7ᵗʰ **T50.2X6** Underdosing of carbonic-anhydrase inhibitors, benzothiadiazides and other diuretics

√5ᵗʰ **T50.3** Poisoning by, adverse effect of and underdosing of electrolytic, caloric and water-balance agents
   Poisoning by, adverse effect of and underdosing of oral rehydration salts

  √6ᵗʰ **T50.3X** Poisoning by, adverse effect of and underdosing of electrolytic, caloric and water-balance agents

    √7ᵗʰ **T50.3X1** Poisoning by electrolytic, caloric and water-balance agents, accidental (unintentional)   PE
         Poisoning by electrolytic, caloric and water-balance agents NOS

    √7ᵗʰ **T50.3X2** Poisoning by electrolytic, caloric and water-balance agents, intentional self-harm   HCC PE

    √7ᵗʰ **T50.3X3** Poisoning by electrolytic, caloric and water-balance agents, assault   PE

    √7ᵗʰ **T50.3X4** Poisoning by electrolytic, caloric and water-balance agents, undetermined   PE

    √7ᵗʰ **T50.3X5** Adverse effect of electrolytic, caloric and water-balance agents   UPD PE
         AHA: 2022,2Q,10

    √7ᵗʰ **T50.3X6** Underdosing of electrolytic, caloric and water-balance agents   UPD PE

√5ᵗʰ **T50.4** Poisoning by, adverse effect of and underdosing of drugs affecting uric acid metabolism

  √6ᵗʰ **T50.4X** Poisoning by, adverse effect of and underdosing of drugs affecting uric acid metabolism

    √7ᵗʰ **T50.4X1** Poisoning by drugs affecting uric acid metabolism, accidental (unintentional)   PE
         Poisoning by drugs affecting uric acid metabolism NOS

    √7ᵗʰ **T50.4X2** Poisoning by drugs affecting uric acid metabolism, intentional self-harm   HCC PE

    √7ᵗʰ **T50.4X3** Poisoning by drugs affecting uric acid metabolism, assault   PE

    √7ᵗʰ **T50.4X4** Poisoning by drugs affecting uric acid metabolism, undetermined   PE

    √7ᵗʰ **T50.4X5** Adverse effect of drugs affecting uric acid metabolism   UPD PE

    √7ᵗʰ **T50.4X6** Underdosing of drugs affecting uric acid metabolism   UPD PE

√5ᵗʰ **T50.5** Poisoning by, adverse effect of and underdosing of appetite depressants

  √6ᵗʰ **T50.5X** Poisoning by, adverse effect of and underdosing of appetite depressants

    √7ᵗʰ **T50.5X1** Poisoning by appetite depressants, accidental (unintentional)   PE
         Poisoning by appetite depressants NOS

    √7ᵗʰ **T50.5X2** Poisoning by appetite depressants, intentional self-harm   HCC PE

    √7ᵗʰ **T50.5X3** Poisoning by appetite depressants, assault   PE

    √7ᵗʰ **T50.5X4** Poisoning by appetite depressants, undetermined   PE

    √7ᵗʰ **T50.5X5** Adverse effect of appetite depressants   UPD PE

    √7ᵗʰ **T50.5X6** Underdosing of appetite depressants   UPD PE

√5ᵗʰ **T50.6** Poisoning by, adverse effect of and underdosing of antidotes and chelating agents
   Poisoning by, adverse effect of and underdosing of alcohol deterrents

  √6ᵗʰ **T50.6X** Poisoning by, adverse effect of and underdosing of antidotes and chelating agents

    √7ᵗʰ **T50.6X1** Poisoning by antidotes and chelating agents, accidental (unintentional)   PE
         Poisoning by antidotes and chelating agents NOS

    √7ᵗʰ **T50.6X2** Poisoning by antidotes and chelating agents, intentional self-harm   HCC PE

    √7ᵗʰ **T50.6X3** Poisoning by antidotes and chelating agents, assault   PE

N Newborn: 0   P Pediatric: 0-17   M Maternity: 9-64   A Adult: 15-124   UNS Unspecified Site   MCC Major Complication/Comorbidity   CC Complication/Comorbidity   PE POA Exempt

1156   ICD-10-CM 2025

√7th **T50.6X4** Poisoning by antidotes and chelating agents, **undetermined** `PE`

√7th **T50.6X5** **Adverse effect** of antidotes and chelating agents `UPD` `PE`

√7th **T50.6X6** **Underdosing** of antidotes and chelating agents `UPD` `PE`

√5th **T50.7** Poisoning by, adverse effect of and underdosing of analeptics and opioid receptor antagonists

√6th **T50.7X** Poisoning by, adverse effect of and underdosing of **analeptics and opioid receptor antagonists**

√7th **T50.7X1** Poisoning by analeptics and opioid receptor antagonists, **accidental (unintentional)** `PE`

Poisoning by analeptics and opioid receptor antagonists NOS

√7th **T50.7X2** Poisoning by analeptics and opioid receptor antagonists, **intentional self-harm** `HCC` `PE`

√7th **T50.7X3** Poisoning by analeptics and opioid receptor antagonists, **assault** `PE`

√7th **T50.7X4** Poisoning by analeptics and opioid receptor antagonists, **undetermined** `PE`

√7th **T50.7X5** **Adverse effect** of analeptics and opioid receptor antagonists `UPD` `PE`

√7th **T50.7X6** **Underdosing** of analeptics and opioid receptor antagonists `UPD` `PE`

√5th **T50.8** Poisoning by, adverse effect of and underdosing of diagnostic agents

√6th **T50.8X** Poisoning by, adverse effect of and underdosing of **diagnostic agents**

√7th **T50.8X1** Poisoning by diagnostic agents, **accidental (unintentional)** `FE`

Poisoning by diagnostic agents NOS

√7th **T50.8X2** Poisoning by diagnostic agents, **intentional self-harm** `HCC` `FE`

√7th **T50.8X3** Poisoning by diagnostic agents, **assault** `FE`

√7th **T50.8X4** Poisoning by diagnostic agents, **undetermined** `FE`

√7th **T50.8X5** **Adverse effect** of diagnostic agents `UPD` `FE`

AHA: 2023,3Q,4; 2022,4Q,33; 2021,3Q,9-10

√7th **T50.8X6** **Underdosing** of diagnostic agents `UPD` `PE`

√5th **T50.A** Poisoning by, adverse effect of and underdosing of bacterial vaccines

√6th **T50.A1** Poisoning by, adverse effect of and underdosing of **pertussis vaccine, including combinations with a pertussis component**

√7th **T50.A11** Poisoning by pertussis vaccine, including combinations with a pertussis component, **accidental (unintentional)** `PE`

√7th **T50.A12** Poisoning by pertussis vaccine, including combinations with a pertussis component, **intentional self-harm** `HCC` `PE`

√7th **T50.A13** Poisoning by pertussis vaccine, including combinations with a pertussis component, **assault** `PE`

√7th **T50.A14** Poisoning by pertussis vaccine, including combinations with a pertussis component, **undetermined** `PE`

√7th **T50.A15** **Adverse effect** of pertussis vaccine, including combinations with a pertussis component `UPD` `PE`

√7th **T50.A16** **Underdosing** of pertussis vaccine, including combinations with a pertussis component `UPD` `PE`

√6th **T50.A2** Poisoning by, adverse effect of and underdosing of **mixed bacterial vaccines without a pertussis component**

√7th **T50.A21** Poisoning by mixed bacterial vaccines without a pertussis component, **accidental (unintentional)** `PE`

√7th **T50.A22** Poisoning by mixed bacterial vaccines without a pertussis component, **intentional self-harm** `HCC` `PE`

√7th **T50.A23** Poisoning by mixed bacterial vaccines without a pertussis component, **assault** `PE`

√7th **T50.A24** Poisoning by mixed bacterial vaccines without a pertussis component, **undetermined** `PE`

√7th **T50.A25** **Adverse effect** of mixed bacterial vaccines without a pertussis component `UPD` `PE`

√7th **T50.A26** **Underdosing** of mixed bacterial vaccines without a pertussis component `UPD` `PE`

√6th **T50.A9** Poisoning by, adverse effect of and underdosing of **other bacterial vaccines**

√7th **T50.A91** Poisoning by other bacterial vaccines, **accidental (unintentional)** `PE`

√7th **T50.A92** Poisoning by other bacterial vaccines, **intentional self-harm** `HCC` `PE`

√7th **T50.A93** Poisoning by other bacterial vaccines, **assault** `PE`

√7th **T50.A94** Poisoning by other bacterial vaccines, **undetermined** `PE`

√7th **T50.A95** **Adverse effect** of other bacterial vaccines `UPD` `PE`

√7th **T50.A96** **Underdosing** of other bacterial vaccines `UPD` `PE`

√5th **T50.B** Poisoning by, adverse effect of and underdosing of viral vaccines

√6th **T50.B1** Poisoning by, adverse effect of and underdosing of **smallpox vaccines**

√7th **T50.B11** Poisoning by smallpox vaccines, **accidental (unintentional)** `PE`

√7th **T50.B12** Poisoning by smallpox vaccines, **intentional self-harm** `HCC` `PE`

√7th **T50.B13** Poisoning by smallpox vaccines, **assault** `PE`

√7th **T50.B14** Poisoning by smallpox vaccines, **undetermined** `PE`

√7th **T50.B15** **Adverse effect** of smallpox vaccines `UPD` `PE`

√7th **T50.B16** **Underdosing** of smallpox vaccines `UPD` `PE`

√6th **T50.B9** Poisoning by, adverse effect of and underdosing of **other viral vaccines**

√7th **T50.B91** Poisoning by other viral vaccines, **accidental (unintentional)** `PE`

√7th **T50.B92** Poisoning by other viral vaccines, **intentional self-harm** `HCC` `PE`

√7th **T50.B93** Poisoning by other viral vaccines, **assault** `PE`

√7th **T50.B94** Poisoning by other viral vaccines, **undetermined** `PE`

√7th **T50.B95** **Adverse effect** of other viral vaccines `UPD` `PE`

AHA: 2021,1Q,43

√7th **T50.B96** **Underdosing** of other viral vaccines `UPD` `PE`

√5th **T50.Z** Poisoning by, adverse effect of and underdosing of other vaccines and biological substances

√6th **T50.Z1** Poisoning by, adverse effect of and underdosing of **immunoglobulin**

√7th **T50.Z11** Poisoning by immunoglobulin, **accidental (unintentional)** `PE`

√7th **T50.Z12** Poisoning by immunoglobulin, **intentional self-harm** `HCC` `PE`

√7th **T50.Z13** Poisoning by immunoglobulin, **assault** `PE`

√7th **T50.Z14** Poisoning by immunoglobulin, **undetermined** `PE`

√7th **T50.Z15** **Adverse effect** of immunoglobulin `UPD` `PE`

√7th **T50.Z16** **Underdosing** of immunoglobulin `UPD` `PE`

√6th **T50.Z9** Poisoning by, adverse effect of and underdosing of **other vaccines and biological substances**

√7th **T50.Z91** Poisoning by other vaccines and biological substances, **accidental (unintentional)** `PE`

√7th **T50.Z92** Poisoning by other vaccines and biological substances, **intentional self-harm** `HCC` `PE`

√7th **T50.Z93** Poisoning by other vaccines and biological substances, **assault** `PE`

√7th **T50.Z94** Poisoning by other vaccines and biological substances, **undetermined** `PE`

√7th **T50.Z95** **Adverse effect** of other vaccines and biological substances   UPD PE
     AHA: 2020,1Q,18

√7th **T50.Z96** **Underdosing** of other vaccines and biological substances   UPD PE

√5th **T50.9** Poisoning by, adverse effect of and underdosing of other and unspecified drugs, medicaments and biological substances

√6th **T50.90** Poisoning by, adverse effect of and underdosing of unspecified drugs, medicaments and biological substances

√7th **T50.901** Poisoning by unspecified drugs, medicaments and biological substances, **accidental** (unintentional)   PE

√7th **T50.902** Poisoning by unspecified drugs, medicaments and biological substances, **intentional self-harm**   HCC PE

√7th **T50.903** Poisoning by unspecified drugs, medicaments and biological substances, **assault**   PE

√7th **T50.904** Poisoning by unspecified drugs, medicaments and biological substances, **undetermined**   PE

√7th **T50.905** **Adverse effect** of unspecified drugs, medicaments and biological substances   PE

√7th **T50.906** **Underdosing** of unspecified drugs, medicaments and biological substances   PE

√6th **T50.91** Poisoning by, adverse effect of and underdosing of multiple unspecified drugs, medicaments and biological substances
     Multiple drug ingestion NOS
     Code also any specific drugs, medicaments and biological substances

√7th **T50.911** Poisoning by multiple unspecified drugs, medicaments and biological substances, **accidental** (unintentional)   PE

√7th **T50.912** Poisoning by multiple unspecified drugs, medicaments and biological substances, **intentional self-harm**   HCC PE

√7th **T50.913** Poisoning by multiple unspecified drugs, medicaments and biological substances, **assault**   PE

√7th **T50.914** Poisoning by multiple unspecified drugs, medicaments and biological substances, **undetermined**   PE

√7th **T50.915** **Adverse effect** of multiple unspecified drugs, medicaments and biological substances   UPD PE

√7th **T50.916** **Underdosing** of multiple unspecified drugs, medicaments and biological substances   UPD PE

√6th **T50.99** Poisoning by, adverse effect of and underdosing of other drugs, medicaments and biological substances

√7th **T50.991** Poisoning by other drugs, medicaments and biological substances, **accidental** (unintentional)   PE

√7th **T50.992** Poisoning by other drugs, medicaments and biological substances, **intentional self-harm**   HCC PE

√7th **T50.993** Poisoning by other drugs, medicaments and biological substances, **assault**   PE

√7th **T50.994** Poisoning by other drugs, medicaments and biological substances, **undetermined**   PE

√7th **T50.995** **Adverse effect** of other drugs, medicaments and biological substances   PE
     AHA: 2023,3Q,4

√7th **T50.996** **Underdosing** of other drugs, medicaments and biological substances   PE

Toxic effects of substances chiefly nonmedicinal as to source (T51-T65)

NOTE   When no intent is indicated code to accidental. Undetermined intent is only for use when there is specific documentation in the record that the intent of the toxic effect cannot be determined.

Use additional code(s) for all associated manifestations of toxic effect, such as:
personal history of foreign body fully removed (Z87.821)
respiratory conditions due to external agents (J60-J70)
to identify any retained foreign body, if applicable (Z18.-)
EXCLUDES 1   contact with and (suspected) exposure to toxic substances (Z77.-)
AHA: 2017,1Q,39-40

√4th **T51** **Toxic effect of alcohol**

The appropriate 7th character is to be added to each code from category T51.
A   initial encounter
D   subsequent encounter
S   sequela

√5th **T51.0** **Toxic effect of ethanol**
     Toxic effect of ethyl alcohol
     EXCLUDES 2   acute alcohol intoxication or "hangover" effects (F10.129, F10.229, F10.929)
         drunkenness (F10.129, F10.229, F10.929)
         pathological alcohol intoxication (F10.129, F10.229, F10.929)

√6th **T51.0X** **Toxic effect of ethanol**

√7th **T51.0X1** Toxic effect of ethanol, **accidental** (unintentional)   PE
     Toxic effect of ethanol NOS

√7th **T51.0X2** Toxic effect of ethanol, **intentional self-harm**   HCC PE

√7th **T51.0X3** Toxic effect of ethanol, **assault**   PE

√7th **T51.0X4** Toxic effect of ethanol, **undetermined**   PE

√5th **T51.1** **Toxic effect of methanol**
     Toxic effect of methyl alcohol

√6th **T51.1X** **Toxic effect of methanol**

√7th **T51.1X1** Toxic effect of methanol, **accidental** (unintentional)   PE
     Toxic effect of methanol NOS

√7th **T51.1X2** Toxic effect of methanol, **intentional self-harm**   HCC PE

√7th **T51.1X3** Toxic effect of methanol, **assault**   PE

√7th **T51.1X4** Toxic effect of methanol, **undetermined**   PE

√5th **T51.2** **Toxic effect of 2-Propanol**
     Toxic effect of isopropyl alcohol

√6th **T51.2X** **Toxic effect of 2-Propanol**

√7th **T51.2X1** Toxic effect of 2-Propanol, **accidental** (unintentional)   PE
     Toxic effect of 2-Propanol NOS

√7th **T51.2X2** Toxic effect of 2-Propanol, **intentional self-harm**   HCC PE

√7th **T51.2X3** Toxic effect of 2-Propanol, **assault**   PE

√7th **T51.2X4** Toxic effect of 2-Propanol, **undetermined**   PE

√5th **T51.3** **Toxic effect of fusel oil**
     Toxic effect of amyl alcohol
     Toxic effect of butyl [1-butanol] alcohol
     Toxic effect of propyl [1-propanol] alcohol

√6th **T51.3X** **Toxic effect of fusel oil**

√7th **T51.3X1** Toxic effect of fusel oil, **accidental** (unintentional)   PE
     Toxic effect of fusel oil NOS

√7th **T51.3X2** Toxic effect of fusel oil, **intentional self-harm**   HCC PE

√7th **T51.3X3** Toxic effect of fusel oil, **assault**   PE

√7th **T51.3X4** Toxic effect of fusel oil, **undetermined**   PE

√5th **T51.8** **Toxic effect of other alcohols**

√6th **T51.8X** **Toxic effect of other alcohols**

√7th **T51.8X1** Toxic effect of other alcohols, **accidental** (unintentional)   PE
     Toxic effect of other alcohols NOS

√7th **T51.8X2** Toxic effect of other alcohols, **intentional self-harm**   HCC PE

✓7th **T51.8X3** **Toxic effect of other alcohols, assault** `PE`

✓7th **T51.8X4** **Toxic effect of other alcohols, undetermined** `PE`

✓5th **T51.9 Toxic effect of unspecified alcohol**

  ✓x7th **T51.91** **Toxic effect of unspecified alcohol, accidental (unintentional)** `PE`

  ✓x7th **T51.92** **Toxic effect of unspecified alcohol, intentional self-harm** `HCC` `PE`

  ✓x7th **T51.93** **Toxic effect of unspecified alcohol, assault** `PE`

  ✓x7th **T51.94** **Toxic effect of unspecified alcohol, undetermined** `PE`

✓4th **T52 Toxic effect of organic solvents**

  EXCLUDES 1   *halogen derivatives of aliphatic and aromatic hydrocarbons (T53.-)*

The appropriate 7th character is to be added to each code from category T52.
A   initial encounter
D   subsequent encounter
S   sequela

✓5th **T52.0 Toxic effects of petroleum products**
  Toxic effects of ether petroleum
  Toxic effects of gasoline [petrol]
  Toxic effects of kerosene [paraffin oil]
  Toxic effects of naphtha petroleum
  Toxic effects of paraffin wax
  Toxic effects of spirit petroleum

  ✓6th **T52.0X** **Toxic effects of petroleum products**

    ✓7th **T52.0X1** **Toxic effect of petroleum products, accidental (unintentional)** `PE`
      Toxic effects of petroleum products NOS

    ✓7th **T52.0X2** **Toxic effect of petroleum products, intentional self-harm** `HCC` `PE`

    ✓7th **T52.0X3** **Toxic effect of petroleum products, assault** `PE`

    ✓7th **T52.0X4** **Toxic effect of petroleum products, undetermined** `PE`

✓5th **T52.1 Toxic effects of benzene**

  EXCLUDES 1   *homologues of benzene (T52.2)*
                 nitroderivatives and aminoderivatives of benzene and its homologues (T65.3)

  ✓6th **T52.1X** **Toxic effects of benzene**

    ✓7th **T52.1X1** **Toxic effect of benzene, accidental (unintentional)** `PE`
      Toxic effects of benzene NOS

    ✓7th **T52.1X2** **Toxic effect of benzene, intentional self-harm** `HCC` `PE`

    ✓7th **T52.1X3** **Toxic effect of benzene, assault** `PE`

    ✓7th **T52.1X4** **Toxic effect of benzene, undetermined** `PE`

✓5th **T52.2 Toxic effects of homologues of benzene**
  Toxic effects of toluene [methylbenzene]
  Toxic effects of xylene [dimethylbenzene]

  ✓6th **T52.2X** **Toxic effects of homologues of benzene**

    ✓7th **T52.2X1** **Toxic effect of homologues of benzene, accidental (unintentional)** `PE`
      Toxic effects of homologues of benzene NOS

    ✓7th **T52.2X2** **Toxic effect of homologues of benzene, intentional self-harm** `HCC` `PE`

    ✓7th **T52.2X3** **Toxic effect of homologues of benzene, assault** `PE`

    ✓7th **T52.2X4** **Toxic effect of homologues of benzene, undetermined** `PE`

✓5th **T52.3 Toxic effects of glycols**

  ✓6th **T52.3X** **Toxic effects of glycols**

    ✓7th **T52.3X1** **Toxic effect of glycols, accidental (unintentional)** `PE`
      Toxic effects of glycols NOS

    ✓7th **T52.3X2** **Toxic effect of glycols, intentional self-harm** `HCC` `PE`

    ✓7th **T52.3X3** **Toxic effect of glycols, assault** `PE`

    ✓7th **T52.3X4** **Toxic effect of glycols, undetermined** `PE`

✓5th **T52.4 Toxic effects of ketones**

  ✓6th **T52.4X** **Toxic effects of ketones**

    ✓7th **T52.4X1** **Toxic effect of ketones, accidental (unintentional)** `PE`
      Toxic effects of ketones NOS

    ✓7th **T52.4X2** **Toxic effect of ketones, intentional self-harm** `HCC`

    ✓7th **T52.4X3** **Toxic effect of ketones, assault** `PE`

    ✓7th **T52.4X4** **Toxic effect of ketones, undetermined** `PE`

✓5th **T52.8 Toxic effects of other organic solvents**

  ✓6th **T52.8X** **Toxic effects of other organic solvents**

    ✓7th **T52.8X1** **Toxic effect of other organic solvents, accidental (unintentional)** `PE`
      Toxic effects of other organic solvents NOS

    ✓7th **T52.8X2** **Toxic effect of other organic solvents, intentional self-harm** `HCC`

    ✓7th **T52.8X3** **Toxic effect of other organic solvents, assault** `PE`

    ✓7th **T52.8X4** **Toxic effect of other organic solvents, undetermined** `PE`

✓5th **T52.9 Toxic effects of unspecified organic solvent**

  ✓x7th **T52.91** **Toxic effect of unspecified organic solvent, accidental (unintentional)** `PE`

  ✓x7th **T52.92** **Toxic effect of unspecified organic solvent, intentional self-harm** `HCC` `PE`

  ✓x7th **T52.93** **Toxic effect of unspecified organic solvent, assault** `PE`

  ✓x7th **T52.94** **Toxic effect of unspecified organic solvent, undetermined** `PE`

✓4th **T53 Toxic effect of halogen derivatives of aliphatic and aromatic hydrocarbons**

The appropriate 7th character is to be added to each code from category T53.
A   initial encounter
D   subsequent encounter
S   sequela

✓5th **T53.0 Toxic effects of carbon tetrachloride**
  Toxic effects of tetrachloromethane

  ✓6th **T53.0X** **Toxic effects of carbon tetrachloride**

    ✓7th **T53.0X1** **Toxic effect of carbon tetrachloride, accidental (unintentional)** `PE`
      Toxic effects of carbon tetrachloride NOS

    ✓7th **T53.0X2** **Toxic effect of carbon tetrachloride, intentional self-harm** `HCC` `PE`

    ✓7th **T53.0X3** **Toxic effect of carbon tetrachloride, assault** `PE`

    ✓7th **T53.0X4** **Toxic effect of carbon tetrachloride, undetermined** `PE`

✓5th **T53.1 Toxic effects of chloroform**
  Toxic effects of trichloromethane

  ✓6th **T53.1X** **Toxic effects of chloroform**

    ✓7th **T53.1X1** **Toxic effect of chloroform, accidental (unintentional)** `PE`
      Toxic effects of chloroform NOS

    ✓7th **T53.1X2** **Toxic effect of chloroform, intentional self-harm** `HCC` `PE`

    ✓7th **T53.1X3** **Toxic effect of chloroform, assault** `PE`

    ✓7th **T53.1X4** **Toxic effect of chloroform, undetermined** `PE`

✓5th **T53.2 Toxic effects of trichloroethylene**
  Toxic effects of trichloroethene

  ✓6th **T53.2X** **Toxic effects of trichloroethylene**

    ✓7th **T53.2X1** **Toxic effect of trichloroethylene, accidental (unintentional)** `PE`
      Toxic effects of trichloroethylene NOS

    ✓7th **T53.2X2** **Toxic effect of trichloroethylene, intentional self-harm** `HCC`

    ✓7th **T53.2X3** **Toxic effect of trichloroethylene, assault** `PE`

    ✓7th **T53.2X4** **Toxic effect of trichloroethylene, undetermined** `PE`

☑ Additional Character Required   ✓x7th Placeholder   Questionable PDx   Manifestation   Unspecified   `UPD` Unacceptable PDx   `H1`-`H14` HAC   `HCC` CMS-HCC Dx   `HIV` HIV Dx

√5ᵗʰ **T53.3 Toxic effects of tetrachloroethylene**
Toxic effects of perchloroethylene
Toxic effect of tetrachloroethene

   √6ᵗʰ **T53.3X Toxic effects of tetrachloroethylene**

     √7ᵗʰ **T53.3X1 Toxic effect of tetrachloroethylene, accidental (unintentional)** PE
Toxic effects of tetrachloroethylene NOS

     √7ᵗʰ **T53.3X2 Toxic effect of tetrachloroethylene, intentional self-harm** HCC PE

     √7ᵗʰ **T53.3X3 Toxic effect of tetrachloroethylene, assault** PE

     √7ᵗʰ **T53.3X4 Toxic effect of tetrachloroethylene, undetermined** PE

√5ᵗʰ **T53.4 Toxic effects of dichloromethane**
Toxic effects of methylene chloride

   √6ᵗʰ **T53.4X Toxic effects of dichloromethane**

     √7ᵗʰ **T53.4X1 Toxic effect of dichloromethane, accidental (unintentional)** PE
Toxic effects of dichloromethane NOS

     √7ᵗʰ **T53.4X2 Toxic effect of dichloromethane, intentional self-harm** HCC PE

     √7ᵗʰ **T53.4X3 Toxic effect of dichloromethane, assault** PE

     √7ᵗʰ **T53.4X4 Toxic effect of dichloromethane, undetermined** PE

√5ᵗʰ **T53.5 Toxic effects of chlorofluorocarbons**

   √6ᵗʰ **T53.5X Toxic effects of chlorofluorocarbons**

     √7ᵗʰ **T53.5X1 Toxic effect of chlorofluorocarbons, accidental (unintentional)** PE
Toxic effects of chlorofluorocarbons NOS

     √7ᵗʰ **T53.5X2 Toxic effect of chlorofluorocarbons, intentional self-harm** HCC PE

     √7ᵗʰ **T53.5X3 Toxic effect of chlorofluorocarbons, assault** PE

     √7ᵗʰ **T53.5X4 Toxic effect of chlorofluorocarbons, undetermined** PE

√5ᵗʰ **T53.6 Toxic effects of other halogen derivatives of aliphatic hydrocarbons**

   √6ᵗʰ **T53.6X Toxic effects of other halogen derivatives of aliphatic hydrocarbons**

     √7ᵗʰ **T53.6X1 Toxic effect of other halogen derivatives of aliphatic hydrocarbons, accidental (unintentional)** PE
Toxic effects of other halogen derivatives of aliphatic hydrocarbons NOS

     √7ᵗʰ **T53.6X2 Toxic effect of other halogen derivatives of aliphatic hydrocarbons, intentional self-harm** HCC PE

     √7ᵗʰ **T53.6X3 Toxic effect of other halogen derivatives of aliphatic hydrocarbons, assault** PE

     √7ᵗʰ **T53.6X4 Toxic effect of other halogen derivatives of aliphatic hydrocarbons, undetermined** PE

√5ᵗʰ **T53.7 Toxic effects of other halogen derivatives of aromatic hydrocarbons**

   √6ᵗʰ **T53.7X Toxic effects of other halogen derivatives of aromatic hydrocarbons**

     √7ᵗʰ **T53.7X1 Toxic effect of other halogen derivatives of aromatic hydrocarbons, accidental (unintentional)** PE
Toxic effects of other halogen derivatives of aromatic hydrocarbons NOS

     √7ᵗʰ **T53.7X2 Toxic effect of other halogen derivatives of aromatic hydrocarbons, intentional self-harm** HCC PE

     √7ᵗʰ **T53.7X3 Toxic effect of other halogen derivatives of aromatic hydrocarbons, assault** PE

     √7ᵗʰ **T53.7X4 Toxic effect of other halogen derivatives of aromatic hydrocarbons, undetermined** PE

√5ᵗʰ **T53.9 Toxic effects of unspecified halogen derivatives of aliphatic and aromatic hydrocarbons**

   √x 7ᵗʰ **T53.91 Toxic effect of unspecified halogen derivatives of aliphatic and aromatic hydrocarbons, accidental (unintentional)** PE

   √x 7ᵗʰ **T53.92 Toxic effect of unspecified halogen derivatives of aliphatic and aromatic hydrocarbons, intentional self-harm** HCC PE

   √x 7ᵗʰ **T53.93 Toxic effect of unspecified halogen derivatives of aliphatic and aromatic hydrocarbons, assault** PE

   √x 7ᵗʰ **T53.94 Toxic effect of unspecified halogen derivatives of aliphatic and aromatic hydrocarbons, undetermined** PE

√4ᵗʰ **T54 Toxic effect of corrosive substances**

> The appropriate 7th character is to be added to each code from category T54.
> A   initial encounter
> D   subsequent encounter
> S   sequela

√5ᵗʰ **T54.0 Toxic effects of phenol and phenol homologues**

   √6ᵗʰ **T54.0X Toxic effects of phenol and phenol homologues**

     √7ᵗʰ **T54.0X1 Toxic effect of phenol and phenol homologues, accidental (unintentional)** PE
Toxic effects of phenol and phenol homologues NOS

     √7ᵗʰ **T54.0X2 Toxic effect of phenol and phenol homologues, intentional self-harm** HCC PE

     √7ᵗʰ **T54.0X3 Toxic effect of phenol and phenol homologues, assault** PE

     √7ᵗʰ **T54.0X4 Toxic effect of phenol and phenol homologues, undetermined** PE

√5ᵗʰ **T54.1 Toxic effects of other corrosive organic compounds**

   √6ᵗʰ **T54.1X Toxic effects of other corrosive organic compounds**

     √7ᵗʰ **T54.1X1 Toxic effect of other corrosive organic compounds, accidental (unintentional)** PE
Toxic effects of other corrosive organic compounds NOS

     √7ᵗʰ **T54.1X2 Toxic effect of other corrosive organic compounds, intentional self-harm** HCC PE

     √7ᵗʰ **T54.1X3 Toxic effect of other corrosive organic compounds, assault** PE

     √7ᵗʰ **T54.1X4 Toxic effect of other corrosive organic compounds, undetermined** PE

√5ᵗʰ **T54.2 Toxic effects of corrosive acids and acid-like substances**
Toxic effects of hydrochloric acid
Toxic effects of sulfuric acid

   √6ᵗʰ **T54.2X Toxic effects of corrosive acids and acid-like substances**

     √7ᵗʰ **T54.2X1 Toxic effect of corrosive acids and acid-like substances, accidental (unintentional)** PE
Toxic effects of corrosive acids and acid-like substances NOS

     √7ᵗʰ **T54.2X2 Toxic effect of corrosive acids and acid-like substances, intentional self-harm** HCC PE

     √7ᵗʰ **T54.2X3 Toxic effect of corrosive acids and acid-like substances, assault** PE

     √7ᵗʰ **T54.2X4 Toxic effect of corrosive acids and acid-like substances, undetermined** PE

√5ᵗʰ **T54.3 Toxic effects of corrosive alkalis and alkali-like substances**
Toxic effects of potassium hydroxide
Toxic effects of sodium hydroxide

   √6ᵗʰ **T54.3X Toxic effects of corrosive alkalis and alkali-like substances**

     √7ᵗʰ **T54.3X1 Toxic effect of corrosive alkalis and alkali-like substances, accidental (unintentional)** PE
Toxic effects of corrosive alkalis and alkali-like substances NOS

     √7ᵗʰ **T54.3X2 Toxic effect of corrosive alkalis and alkali-like substances, intentional self-harm** HCC PE

     √7ᵗʰ **T54.3X3 Toxic effect of corrosive alkalis and alkali-like substances, assault** PE

     √7ᵗʰ **T54.3X4 Toxic effect of corrosive alkalis and alkali-like substances, undetermined** PE

√5ᵗʰ **T54.9 Toxic effects of unspecified corrosive substance**

   √x 7ᵗʰ **T54.91 Toxic effect of unspecified corrosive substance, accidental (unintentional)** PE

   √x 7ᵗʰ **T54.92 Toxic effect of unspecified corrosive substance, intentional self-harm** HCC PE

   √x 7ᵗʰ **T54.93 Toxic effect of unspecified corrosive substance, assault** PE

N Newborn: 0   **P** Pediatric: 0-17   **M** Maternity: 9-64   **A** Adult: 15-124   **UNS** Unspecified Site   **MCC** Major Complication/Comorbidity   **CC** Complication/Comorbidity   **PE** POA Exempt

1160   ICD-10-CM 2025

✓x7th **T54.94**   **Toxic effect of unspecified corrosive substance, undetermined**   PE

✓4th **T55**   **Toxic effect of soaps and detergents**

> The appropriate 7th character is to be added to each code from category T55.
> A   initial encounter
> D   subsequent encounter
> S   sequela

✓5th **T55.0**   **Toxic effect of soaps**

  ✓6th **T55.0X**   **Toxic effect of soaps**

    ✓7th **T55.0X1**   **Toxic effect of soaps, accidental (unintentional)**   PE
       Toxic effect of soaps NOS

    ✓7th **T55.0X2**   **Toxic effect of soaps, intentional self-harm**   HCC PE

    ✓7th **T55.0X3**   **Toxic effect of soaps, assault**   PE

    ✓7th **T55.0X4**   **Toxic effect of soaps, undetermined**   PE

✓5th **T55.1**   **Toxic effect of detergents**

  ✓6th **T55.1X**   **Toxic effect of detergents**

    ✓7th **T55.1X1**   **Toxic effect of detergents, accidental (unintentional)**   PE
       Toxic effect of detergents NOS

    ✓7th **T55.1X2**   **Toxic effect of detergents, intentional self-harm**   HCC PE

    ✓7th **T55.1X3**   **Toxic effect of detergents, assault**   PE

    ✓7th **T55.1X4**   **Toxic effect of detergents, undetermined**   PE

✓4th **T56**   **Toxic effect of metals**

> INCLUDES   toxic effects of fumes and vapors of metals
> toxic effects of metals from all sources, except medicinal substances
>
> Use additional code to identify any retained metal foreign body, if applicable (Z18.0-, T18.1-)
>
> EXCLUDES 1   arsenic and its compounds (T57.0)
> manganese and its compounds (T57.2)

> The appropriate 7th character is to be added to each code from category T56.
> A   initial encounter
> D   subsequent encounter
> S   sequela

✓5th **T56.0**   **Toxic effects of lead and its compounds**

  ✓6th **T56.0X**   **Toxic effects of lead and its compounds**

    ✓7th **T56.0X1**   **Toxic effect of lead and its compounds, accidental (unintentional)**   PE
       Toxic effects of lead and its compounds NOS

    ✓7th **T56.0X2**   **Toxic effect of lead and its compounds, intentional self-harm**   HCC PE

    ✓7th **T56.0X3**   **Toxic effect of lead and its compounds, assault**   PE

    ✓7th **T56.0X4**   **Toxic effect of lead and its compounds, undetermined**   PE

✓5th **T56.1**   **Toxic effects of mercury and its compounds**

  ✓6th **T56.1X**   **Toxic effects of mercury and its compounds**

    ✓7th **T56.1X1**   **Toxic effect of mercury and its compounds, accidental (unintentional)**   PE
       Toxic effect of mercury and its compounds NOS

    ✓7th **T56.1X2**   **Toxic effect of mercury and its compounds, intentional self-harm**   HCC PE

    ✓7th **T56.1X3**   **Toxic effect of mercury and its compounds, assault**   PE

    ✓7th **T56.1X4**   **Toxic effect of mercury and its compounds, undetermined**   PE

✓5th **T56.2**   **Toxic effects of chromium and its compounds**

  ✓6th **T56.2X**   **Toxic effects of chromium and its compounds**

    ✓7th **T56.2X1**   **Toxic effect of chromium and its compounds, accidental (unintentional)**   PE
       Toxic effects of chromium and its compounds NOS

    ✓7th **T56.2X2**   **Toxic effect of chromium and its compounds, intentional self-harm**   HCC PE

    ✓7th **T56.2X3**   **Toxic effect of chromium and its compounds, assault**   PE

    ✓7th **T56.2X4**   **Toxic effect of chromium and its compounds, undetermined**   PE

✓5th **T56.3**   **Toxic effects of cadmium and its compounds**

  ✓6th **T56.3X**   **Toxic effects of cadmium and its compounds**

    ✓7th **T56.3X1**   **Toxic effect of cadmium and its compounds, accidental (unintentional)**   PE
       Toxic effects of cadmium and its compounds NOS

    ✓7th **T56.3X2**   **Toxic effect of cadmium and its compounds, intentional self-harm**   HCC PE

    ✓7th **T56.3X3**   **Toxic effect of cadmium and its compounds, assault**   PE

    ✓7th **T56.3X4**   **Toxic effect of cadmium and its compounds, undetermined**   PE

✓5th **T56.4**   **Toxic effects of copper and its compounds**

  ✓6th **T56.4X**   **Toxic effects of copper and its compounds**

    ✓7th **T56.4X1**   **Toxic effect of copper and its compounds, accidental (unintentional)**   PE
       Toxic effects of copper and its compounds NOS

    ✓7th **T56.4X2**   **Toxic effect of copper and its compounds, intentional self-harm**   HCC PE

    ✓7th **T56.4X3**   **Toxic effect of copper and its compounds, assault**   PE

    ✓7th **T56.4X4**   **Toxic effect of copper and its compounds, undetermined**   PE

✓5th **T56.5**   **Toxic effects of zinc and its compounds**

  ✓6th **T56.5X**   **Toxic effects of zinc and its compounds**

    ✓7th **T56.5X1**   **Toxic effect of zinc and its compounds, accidental (unintentional)**   PE
       Toxic effects of zinc and its compounds NOS

    ✓7th **T56.5X2**   **Toxic effect of zinc and its compounds, intentional self-harm**   HCC PE

    ✓7th **T56.5X3**   **Toxic effect of zinc and its compounds, assault**   PE

    ✓7th **T56.5X4**   **Toxic effect of zinc and its compounds, undetermined**   PE

✓5th **T56.6**   **Toxic effects of tin and its compounds**

  ✓6th **T56.6X**   **Toxic effects of tin and its compounds**

    ✓7th **T56.6X1**   **Toxic effect of tin and its compounds, accidental (unintentional)**   PE
       Toxic effects of tin and its compounds NOS

    ✓7th **T56.6X2**   **Toxic effect of tin and its compounds, intentional self-harm**   HCC PE

    ✓7th **T56.6X3**   **Toxic effect of tin and its compounds, assault**   PE

    ✓7th **T56.6X4**   **Toxic effect of tin and its compounds, undetermined**   PE

✓5th **T56.7**   **Toxic effects of beryllium and its compounds**

  ✓6th **T56.7X**   **Toxic effects of beryllium and its compounds**

    ✓7th **T56.7X1**   **Toxic effect of beryllium and its compounds, accidental (unintentional)**   PE
       Toxic effects of beryllium and its compounds NOS

    ✓7th **T56.7X2**   **Toxic effect of beryllium and its compounds, intentional self-harm**   HCC PE

    ✓7th **T56.7X3**   **Toxic effect of beryllium and its compounds, assault**   PE

    ✓7th **T56.7X4**   **Toxic effect of beryllium and its compounds, undetermined**   PE

✓5th **T56.8**   **Toxic effects of other metals**

  ✓6th **T56.81**   **Toxic effect of thallium**

    ✓7th **T56.811**   **Toxic effect of thallium, accidental (unintentional)**   PE
       Toxic effect of thallium NOS

    ✓7th **T56.812**   **Toxic effect of thallium, intentional self-harm**   HCC PE

    ✓7th **T56.813**   **Toxic effect of thallium, assault**   PE

    ✓7th **T56.814**   **Toxic effect of thallium, undetermined**   PE

✔ Additional Character Required   ✓x7th Placeholder   Questionable PDx   Manifestation   Unspecified   UPD Unacceptable PDx   H1-H14 HAC   HCC CMS-HCC Dx   HIV HIV Dx

ICD-10-CM 2025   1161

☑6th **T56.82** **Toxic effect of gadolinium**

> EXCLUDES 1   adverse effect of diagnostic agents (T50.8X5-)
>
> **AHA:** 2023,4Q,44-45

  ☑7th **T56.821** **Toxic effect of gadolinium, accidental (unintentional)** PE
> Toxic effect of gadolinium NOS

  ☑7th **T56.822** **Toxic effect of gadolinium, intentional self-harm** HCC PE

  ☑7th **T56.823** **Toxic effect of gadolinium, assault** PE

  ☑7th **T56.824** **Toxic effect of gadolinium, undetermined** PE

☑6th **T56.89** **Toxic effects of other metals**

  ☑7th **T56.891** **Toxic effect of other metals, accidental (unintentional)** PE
> Toxic effects of other metals NOS

  ☑7th **T56.892** **Toxic effect of other metals, intentional self-harm** HCC PE

  ☑7th **T56.893** **Toxic effect of other metals, assault** PE

  ☑7th **T56.894** **Toxic effect of other metals, undetermined** PE

☑5th **T56.9** **Toxic effects of unspecified metal**

  ☑✗7th **T56.91** **Toxic effect of unspecified metal, accidental (unintentional)** PE

  ☑✗7th **T56.92** **Toxic effect of unspecified metal, intentional self-harm** HCC PE

  ☑✗7th **T56.93** **Toxic effect of unspecified metal, assault** PE

  ☑✗7th **T56.94** **Toxic effect of unspecified metal, undetermined** PE

☑4th **T57** **Toxic effect of other inorganic substances**

> The appropriate 7th character is to be added to each code from category T57.
> A   initial encounter
> D   subsequent encounter
> S   sequela

☑5th **T57.0** **Toxic effect of arsenic and its compounds**

  ☑6th **T57.0X** **Toxic effect of arsenic and its compounds**

    ☑7th **T57.0X1** **Toxic effect of arsenic and its compounds, accidental (unintentional)** PE
> Toxic effect of arsenic and its compounds NOS

    ☑7th **T57.0X2** **Toxic effect of arsenic and its compounds, intentional self-harm** HCC PE

    ☑7th **T57.0X3** **Toxic effect of arsenic and its compounds, assault** PE

    ☑7th **T57.0X4** **Toxic effect of arsenic and its compounds, undetermined** PE

☑5th **T57.1** **Toxic effect of phosphorus and its compounds**

> EXCLUDES 1   organophosphate insecticides (T60.0)

  ☑6th **T57.1X** **Toxic effect of phosphorus and its compounds**

    ☑7th **T57.1X1** **Toxic effect of phosphorus and its compounds, accidental (unintentional)** PE
> Toxic effect of phosphorus and its compounds NOS

    ☑7th **T57.1X2** **Toxic effect of phosphorus and its compounds, intentional self-harm** HCC PE

    ☑7th **T57.1X3** **Toxic effect of phosphorus and its compounds, assault** PE

    ☑7th **T57.1X4** **Toxic effect of phosphorus and its compounds, undetermined** PE

☑5th **T57.2** **Toxic effect of manganese and its compounds**

  ☑6th **T57.2X** **Toxic effect of manganese and its compounds**

    ☑7th **T57.2X1** **Toxic effect of manganese and its compounds, accidental (unintentional)** PE
> Toxic effect of manganese and its compounds NOS

    ☑7th **T57.2X2** **Toxic effect of manganese and its compounds, intentional self-harm** HCC PE

    ☑7th **T57.2X3** **Toxic effect of manganese and its compounds, assault** PE

    ☑7th **T57.2X4** **Toxic effect of manganese and its compounds, undetermined** PE

☑5th **T57.3** **Toxic effect of hydrogen cyanide**

  ☑6th **T57.3X** **Toxic effect of hydrogen cyanide**

    ☑7th **T57.3X1** **Toxic effect of hydrogen cyanide, accidental (unintentional)**
> Toxic effect of hydrogen cyanide NOS

    ☑7th **T57.3X2** **Toxic effect of hydrogen cyanide, intentional self-harm** HCC PE

    ☑7th **T57.3X3** **Toxic effect of hydrogen cyanide, assault**

    ☑7th **T57.3X4** **Toxic effect of hydrogen cyanide, undetermined** PE

☑5th **T57.8** **Toxic effect of other specified inorganic substances**

  ☑6th **T57.8X** **Toxic effect of other specified inorganic substances**

    ☑7th **T57.8X1** **Toxic effect of other specified inorganic substances, accidental (unintentional)**
> Toxic effect of other specified inorganic substances NOS

    ☑7th **T57.8X2** **Toxic effect of other specified inorganic substances, intentional self-harm** HCC PE

    ☑7th **T57.8X3** **Toxic effect of other specified inorganic substances, assault** PE

    ☑7th **T57.8X4** **Toxic effect of other specified inorganic substances, undetermined** PE

☑5th **T57.9** **Toxic effect of unspecified inorganic substance**

  ☑✗7th **T57.91** **Toxic effect of unspecified inorganic substance, accidental (unintentional)** PE

  ☑✗7th **T57.92** **Toxic effect of unspecified inorganic substance, intentional self-harm** HCC PE

  ☑✗7th **T57.93** **Toxic effect of unspecified inorganic substance, assault** PE

  ☑✗7th **T57.94** **Toxic effect of unspecified inorganic substance, undetermined** PE

☑4th **T58** **Toxic effect of carbon monoxide**

> INCLUDES   asphyxiation from carbon monoxide
> toxic effect of carbon monoxide from all sources

> The appropriate 7th character is to be added to each code from category T58.
> A   initial encounter
> D   subsequent encounter
> S   sequela

☑5th **T58.0** **Toxic effect of carbon monoxide from motor vehicle exhaust**
> Toxic effect of exhaust gas from gas engine
> Toxic effect of exhaust gas from motor pump

  ☑✗7th **T58.01** **Toxic effect of carbon monoxide from motor vehicle exhaust, accidental (unintentional)** PE

  ☑✗7th **T58.02** **Toxic effect of carbon monoxide from motor vehicle exhaust, intentional self-harm** HCC PE

  ☑✗7th **T58.03** **Toxic effect of carbon monoxide from motor vehicle exhaust, assault** PE

  ☑✗7th **T58.04** **Toxic effect of carbon monoxide from motor vehicle exhaust, undetermined** PE

☑5th **T58.1** **Toxic effect of carbon monoxide from utility gas**
> Toxic effect of acetylene
> Toxic effect of gas NOS used for lighting, heating, cooking
> Toxic effect of water gas

  ☑✗7th **T58.11** **Toxic effect of carbon monoxide from utility gas, accidental (unintentional)** PE

  ☑✗7th **T58.12** **Toxic effect of carbon monoxide from utility gas, intentional self-harm** HCC PE

  ☑✗7th **T58.13** **Toxic effect of carbon monoxide from utility gas, assault** PE

  ☑✗7th **T58.14** **Toxic effect of carbon monoxide from utility gas, undetermined** PE

☑5th **T58.2** **Toxic effect of carbon monoxide from incomplete combustion of other domestic fuels**
> Toxic effect of carbon monoxide from incomplete combustion of coal, coke, kerosene, wood

  ☑6th **T58.2X** **Toxic effect of carbon monoxide from incomplete combustion of other domestic fuels**

    ☑7th **T58.2X1** **Toxic effect of carbon monoxide from incomplete combustion of other domestic fuels, accidental (unintentional)** PE

    ☑7th **T58.2X2** **Toxic effect of carbon monoxide from incomplete combustion of other domestic fuels, intentional self-harm** HCC PE

N Newborn: 0   **P** Pediatric: 0-17   **M** Maternity: 9-64   **A** Adult: 15-124   **UNS** Unspecified Site   **MCC** Major Complication/Comorbidity   **CC** Complication/Comorbidity   **PE** POA Exempt

1162   ICD-10-CM 2025

✓7th **T58.2X3** Toxic effect of carbon monoxide from incomplete combustion of other domestic fuels, **assault** PE

✓7th **T58.2X4** Toxic effect of carbon monoxide from incomplete combustion of other domestic fuels, **undetermined** PE

✓5th **T58.8** Toxic effect of carbon monoxide from other source
     Toxic effect of carbon monoxide from blast furnace gas
     Toxic effect of carbon monoxide from fuels in industrial use
     Toxic effect of carbon monoxide from kiln vapor

✓6th **T58.8X** Toxic effect of carbon monoxide from other source

✓7th **T58.8X1** Toxic effect of carbon monoxide from other source, **accidental** (unintentional) PE

✓7th **T58.8X2** Toxic effect of carbon monoxide from other source, **intentional self-harm** HCC PE

✓7th **T58.8X3** Toxic effect of carbon monoxide from other source, **assault** PE

✓7th **T58.8X4** Toxic effect of carbon monoxide from other source, **undetermined** PE

✓5th **T58.9** Toxic effect of carbon monoxide from unspecified source

✓x7th **T58.91** Toxic effect of carbon monoxide from unspecified source, **accidental** (unintentional) PE

✓x7th **T58.92** Toxic effect of carbon monoxide from unspecified source, **intentional self-harm** HCC PE

✓x7th **T58.93** Toxic effect of carbon monoxide from unspecified source, **assault** PE

✓x7th **T58.94** Toxic effect of carbon monoxide from unspecified source, **undetermined** PE

✓4th **T59 Toxic effect of other gases, fumes and vapors**

INCLUDES   aerosol propellants
EXCLUDES 1   *chlorofluorocarbons (T53.5)*

The appropriate 7th character is to be added to each code from category T59.
A   initial encounter
D   subsequent encounter
S   sequela

✓5th **T59.0** Toxic effect of nitrogen oxides

✓6th **T59.0X** Toxic effect of nitrogen oxides

✓7th **T59.0X1** Toxic effect of nitrogen oxides, **accidental** (unintentional) PE
     Toxic effect of nitrogen oxides NOS

✓7th **T59.0X2** Toxic effect of nitrogen oxides, **intentional self-harm** HCC PE

✓7th **T59.0X3** Toxic effect of nitrogen oxides, **assault** PE

✓7th **T59.0X4** Toxic effect of nitrogen oxides, **undetermined** PE

✓5th **T59.1** Toxic effect of sulfur dioxide

✓6th **T59.1X** Toxic effect of sulfur dioxide

✓7th **T59.1X1** Toxic effect of sulfur dioxide, **accidental** (unintentional) PE
     Toxic effect of sulfur dioxide NOS

✓7th **T59.1X2** Toxic effect of sulfur dioxide, **intentional self-harm** HCC PE

✓7th **T59.1X3** Toxic effect of sulfur dioxide, **assault** PE

✓7th **T59.1X4** Toxic effect of sulfur dioxide, **undetermined** PE

✓5th **T59.2** Toxic effect of formaldehyde

✓6th **T59.2X** Toxic effect of formaldehyde

✓7th **T59.2X1** Toxic effect of formaldehyde, **accidental** (unintentional) PE
     Toxic effect of formaldehyde NOS

✓7th **T59.2X2** Toxic effect of formaldehyde, **intentional self-harm** HCC PE

✓7th **T59.2X3** Toxic effect of formaldehyde, **assault** PE

✓7th **T59.2X4** Toxic effect of formaldehyde, **undetermined** PE

✓5th **T59.3** Toxic effect of lacrimogenic gas
     Toxic effect of tear gas

✓6th **T59.3X** Toxic effect of lacrimogenic gas

✓7th **T59.3X1** Toxic effect of lacrimogenic gas, **accidental** (unintentional) PE
     Toxic effect of lacrimogenic gas NOS

✓7th **T59.3X2** Toxic effect of lacrimogenic gas, **intentional self-harm** HCC PE

✓7th **T59.3X3** Toxic effect of lacrimogenic gas, **assault** PE

✓7th **T59.3X4** Toxic effect of lacrimogenic gas, **undetermined** PE

✓5th **T59.4** Toxic effect of chlorine gas

✓6th **T59.4X** Toxic effect of chlorine gas

✓7th **T59.4X1** Toxic effect of chlorine gas, **accidental** (unintentional) PE
     Toxic effect of chlorine gas NOS

✓7th **T59.4X2** Toxic effect of chlorine gas, **intentional self-harm** HCC PE

✓7th **T59.4X3** Toxic effect of chlorine gas, **assault** PE

✓7th **T59.4X4** Toxic effect of chlorine gas, **undetermined** PE

✓5th **T59.5** Toxic effect of fluorine gas and hydrogen fluoride

✓6th **T59.5X** Toxic effect of fluorine gas and hydrogen fluoride

✓7th **T59.5X1** Toxic effect of fluorine gas and hydrogen fluoride, **accidental** (unintentional) PE
     Toxic effect of fluorine gas and hydrogen fluoride NOS

✓7th **T59.5X2** Toxic effect of fluorine gas and hydrogen fluoride, **intentional self-harm** HCC PE

✓7th **T59.5X3** Toxic effect of fluorine gas and hydrogen fluoride, **assault** PE

✓7th **T59.5X4** Toxic effect of fluorine gas and hydrogen fluoride, **undetermined** PE

✓5th **T59.6** Toxic effect of hydrogen sulfide

✓6th **T59.6X** Toxic effect of hydrogen sulfide

✓7th **T59.6X1** Toxic effect of hydrogen sulfide, **accidental** (unintentional) PE
     Toxic effect of hydrogen sulfide NOS

✓7th **T59.6X2** Toxic effect of hydrogen sulfide, **intentional self-harm** HCC PE

✓7th **T59.6X3** Toxic effect of hydrogen sulfide, **assault** PE

✓7th **T59.6X4** Toxic effect of hydrogen sulfide, **undetermined** PE

✓5th **T59.7** Toxic effect of carbon dioxide

✓6th **T59.7X** Toxic effect of carbon dioxide

✓7th **T59.7X1** Toxic effect of carbon dioxide, **accidental** (unintentional) PE
     Toxic effect of carbon dioxide NOS

✓7th **T59.7X2** Toxic effect of carbon dioxide, **intentional self-harm** HCC PE

✓7th **T59.7X3** Toxic effect of carbon dioxide, **assault** PE

✓7th **T59.7X4** Toxic effect of carbon dioxide, **undetermined** PE

✓5th **T59.8** Toxic effect of other specified gases, fumes and vapors

✓6th **T59.81** Toxic effect of smoke
     Smoke inhalation
     EXCLUDES 2   *toxic effect of cigarette (tobacco) smoke (T65.22-)*

✓7th **T59.811** Toxic effect of smoke, **accidental** (unintentional) PE
     Toxic effect of smoke NOS
     AHA: 2013,4Q,121

✓7th **T59.812** Toxic effect of smoke, **intentional self-harm** HCC PE

✓7th **T59.813** Toxic effect of smoke, **assault** PE

✓7th **T59.814** Toxic effect of smoke, **undetermined** PE

✓6th **T59.89** Toxic effect of other specified gases, fumes and vapors

✓7th **T59.891** Toxic effect of other specified gases, fumes and vapors, **accidental** (unintentional) PE

✓7th **T59.892** Toxic effect of other specified gases, fumes and vapors, **intentional self-harm** HCC PE

✓7th **T59.893** Toxic effect of other specified gases, fumes and vapors, **assault** PE

✓7th **T59.894** Toxic effect of other specified gases, fumes and vapors, **undetermined** PE

Chapter 19. Injury, Poisoning and Certain Other Consequences of External Causes

T59.9–T61.784

√5th **T59.9** **Toxic effect of unspecified gases, fumes and vapors**

√x7th **T59.91** **Toxic effect of unspecified gases, fumes and vapors, accidental (unintentional)** PE

√x7th **T59.92** **Toxic effect of unspecified gases, fumes and vapors, intentional self-harm** HCC PE

√x7th **T59.93** **Toxic effect of unspecified gases, fumes and vapors, assault** PE

√x7th **T59.94** **Toxic effect of unspecified gases, fumes and vapors, undetermined** PE

√4th **T60** **Toxic effect of pesticides**

INCLUDES   toxic effect of wood preservatives

The appropriate 7th character is to be added to each code from category T60.
A   initial encounter
D   subsequent encounter
S   sequela

√5th **T60.0** **Toxic effect of organophosphate and carbamate insecticides**

√6th **T60.0X** **Toxic effect of organophosphate and carbamate insecticides**

√7th **T60.0X1** **Toxic effect of organophosphate and carbamate insecticides, accidental (unintentional)** PE
Toxic effect of organophosphate and carbamate insecticides NOS

√7th **T60.0X2** **Toxic effect of organophosphate and carbamate insecticides, intentional self-harm** HCC PE

√7th **T60.0X3** **Toxic effect of organophosphate and carbamate insecticides, assault** PE

√7th **T60.0X4** **Toxic effect of organophosphate and carbamate insecticides, undetermined** PE

√5th **T60.1** **Toxic effect of halogenated insecticides**

EXCLUDES 1   chlorinated hydrocarbon (T53.-)

√6th **T60.1X** **Toxic effect of halogenated insecticides**

√7th **T60.1X1** **Toxic effect of halogenated insecticides, accidental (unintentional)** PE
Toxic effect of halogenated insecticides NOS

√7th **T60.1X2** **Toxic effect of halogenated insecticides, intentional self-harm** HCC PE

√7th **T60.1X3** **Toxic effect of halogenated insecticides, assault** PE

√7th **T60.1X4** **Toxic effect of halogenated insecticides, undetermined** PE

√5th **T60.2** **Toxic effect of other insecticides**

√6th **T60.2X** **Toxic effect of other insecticides**

√7th **T60.2X1** **Toxic effect of other insecticides, accidental (unintentional)** PE
Toxic effect of other insecticides NOS

√7th **T60.2X2** **Toxic effect of other insecticides, intentional self-harm** HCC PE

√7th **T60.2X3** **Toxic effect of other insecticides, assault** PE

√7th **T60.2X4** **Toxic effect of other insecticides, undetermined** PE

√5th **T60.3** **Toxic effect of herbicides and fungicides**

√6th **T60.3X** **Toxic effect of herbicides and fungicides**

√7th **T60.3X1** **Toxic effect of herbicides and fungicides, accidental (unintentional)** PE
Toxic effect of herbicides and fungicides NOS

√7th **T60.3X2** **Toxic effect of herbicides and fungicides, intentional self-harm** HCC PE

√7th **T60.3X3** **Toxic effect of herbicides and fungicides, assault** PE

√7th **T60.3X4** **Toxic effect of herbicides and fungicides, undetermined** PE

√5th **T60.4** **Toxic effect of rodenticides**

EXCLUDES 1   strychnine and its salts (T65.1)
thallium (T56.81-)

√6th **T60.4X** **Toxic effect of rodenticides**

√7th **T60.4X1** **Toxic effect of rodenticides, accidental (unintentional)** PE
Toxic effect of rodenticides NOS

√7th **T60.4X2** **Toxic effect of rodenticides, intentional self-harm** HCC PE

√7th **T60.4X3** **Toxic effect of rodenticides, assault** PE

√7th **T60.4X4** **Toxic effect of rodenticides, undetermined** PE

√5th **T60.8** **Toxic effect of other pesticides**

√6th **T60.8X** **Toxic effect of other pesticides**

√7th **T60.8X1** **Toxic effect of other pesticides, accidental (unintentional)** PE
Toxic effect of other pesticides NOS

√7th **T60.8X2** **Toxic effect of other pesticides, intentional self-harm** HCC PE

√7th **T60.8X3** **Toxic effect of other pesticides, assault** PE

√7th **T60.8X4** **Toxic effect of other pesticides, undetermined** PE

√5th **T60.9** **Toxic effect of unspecified pesticide**

√x7th **T60.91** **Toxic effect of unspecified pesticide, accidental (unintentional)** PE

√x7th **T60.92** **Toxic effect of unspecified pesticide, intentional self-harm** HCC PE

√x7th **T60.93** **Toxic effect of unspecified pesticide, assault** PE

√x7th **T60.94** **Toxic effect of unspecified pesticide, undetermined** PE

√4th **T61** **Toxic effect of noxious substances eaten as seafood**

EXCLUDES 1   allergic reaction to food, such as:
anaphylactic reaction or shock due to adverse food reaction (T78.0-)
bacterial foodborne intoxications (A05.-)
dermatitis (L23.6, L25.4, L27.2)
food protein-induced enterocolitis syndrome (K52.21)
food protein-induced enteropathy (K52.22)
gastroenteritis (noninfective) (K52.29)
toxic effect of aflatoxin and other mycotoxins (T64)
toxic effect of cyanides (T65.0-)
toxic effect of harmful algae bloom (T65.82-)
toxic effect of hydrogen cyanide (T57.3-)
toxic effect of mercury (T56.1-)
toxic effect of red tide (T65.82-)

The appropriate 7th character is to be added to each code from category T61.
A   initial encounter
D   subsequent encounter
S   sequela

√5th **T61.0** **Ciguatera fish poisoning**

√x7th **T61.01** **Ciguatera fish poisoning, accidental (unintentional)** PE

√x7th **T61.02** **Ciguatera fish poisoning, intentional self-harm** HCC PE

√x7th **T61.03** **Ciguatera fish poisoning, assault** PE

√x7th **T61.04** **Ciguatera fish poisoning, undetermined** PE

√5th **T61.1** **Scombroid fish poisoning**

Histamine-like syndrome

√x7th **T61.11** **Scombroid fish poisoning, accidental (unintentional)** PE

√x7th **T61.12** **Scombroid fish poisoning, intentional self-harm** HCC PE

√x7th **T61.13** **Scombroid fish poisoning, assault** PE

√x7th **T61.14** **Scombroid fish poisoning, undetermined** PE

√5th **T61.7** **Other fish and shellfish poisoning**

√6th **T61.77** **Other fish poisoning**

√7th **T61.771** **Other fish poisoning, accidental (unintentional)** PE

√7th **T61.772** **Other fish poisoning, intentional self-harm** HCC PE

√7th **T61.773** **Other fish poisoning, assault** PE

√7th **T61.774** **Other fish poisoning, undetermined** PE

√6th **T61.78** **Other shellfish poisoning**

√7th **T61.781** **Other shellfish poisoning, accidental (unintentional)** PE

√7th **T61.782** **Other shellfish poisoning, intentional self-harm** HCC PE

√7th **T61.783** **Other shellfish poisoning, assault** PE

√7th **T61.784** **Other shellfish poisoning, undetermined** PE

N Newborn: 0   P Pediatric: 0-17   M Maternity: 9-64   A Adult: 15-124   UNS Unspecified Site   MCC Major Complication/Comorbidity   CC Complication/Comorbidity   PE POA Exempt

1164   ICD-10-CM 2025

√5ᵗʰ **T61.8**   **Toxic effect of other seafood**

   √6ᵗʰ **T61.8X**   **Toxic effect of other seafood**

     √7ᵗʰ **T61.8X1**   **Toxic effect of other seafood, accidental (unintentional)**   PE

     √7ᵗʰ **T61.8X2**   **Toxic effect of other seafood, intentional self-harm**   HCC PE

     √7ᵗʰ **T61.8X3**   **Toxic effect of other seafood, assault**   PE

     √7ᵗʰ **T61.8X4**   **Toxic effect of other seafood, undetermined**   PE

√5ᵗʰ **T61.9**   **Toxic effect of unspecified seafood**

   √x7ᵗʰ **T61.91**   **Toxic effect of unspecified seafood, accidental (unintentional)**   PE

   √x7ᵗʰ **T61.92**   **Toxic effect of unspecified seafood, intentional self-harm**   HCC PE

   √x7ᵗʰ **T61.93**   **Toxic effect of unspecified seafood, assault**   PE

   √x7ᵗʰ **T61.94**   **Toxic effect of unspecified seafood, undetermined**   PE

√4ᵗʰ **T62**   **Toxic effect of other noxious substances eaten as food**

   EXCLUDES 1   allergic reaction to food, such as:

     anaphylactic shock (reaction) due to adverse food reaction (T78.0-)

     bacterial food borne intoxications (A05.-)

     dermatitis (L23.6, L25.4, L27.2)

     food protein-induced enterocolitis syndrome (K52.21)

     food protein-induced enteropathy (K52.22)

     gastroenteritis (noninfective) (K52.29)

     toxic effect of aflatoxin and other mycotoxins (T64)

     toxic effect of cyanides (T65.0-)

     toxic effect of hydrogen cyanide (T57.3-)

     toxic effect of mercury (T56.1-)

> The appropriate 7th character is to be added to each code from category T62.
> A   initial encounter
> D   subsequent encounter
> S   sequela

√5ᵗʰ **T62.0**   **Toxic effect of ingested mushrooms**

   √6ᵗʰ **T62.0X**   **Toxic effect of ingested mushrooms**

     √7ᵗʰ **T62.0X1**   **Toxic effect of ingested mushrooms, accidental (unintentional)**   PE
       Toxic effect of ingested mushrooms NOS

     √7ᵗʰ **T62.0X2**   **Toxic effect of ingested mushrooms, intentional self-harm**   HCC PE

     √7ᵗʰ **T62.0X3**   **Toxic effect of ingested mushrooms, assault**   PE

     √7ᵗʰ **T62.0X4**   **Toxic effect of ingested mushrooms, undetermined**   PE

√5ᵗʰ **T62.1**   **Toxic effect of ingested berries**

   √6ᵗʰ **T62.1X**   **Toxic effect of ingested berries**

     √7ᵗʰ **T62.1X1**   **Toxic effect of ingested berries, accidental (unintentional)**   PE
       Toxic effect of ingested berries NOS

     √7ᵗʰ **T62.1X2**   **Toxic effect of ingested berries, intentional self-harm**   HCC PE

     √7ᵗʰ **T62.1X3**   **Toxic effect of ingested berries, assault**   PE

     √7ᵗʰ **T62.1X4**   **Toxic effect of ingested berries, undetermined**   PE

√5ᵗʰ **T62.2**   **Toxic effect of other ingested (parts of) plant(s)**

   √6ᵗʰ **T62.2X**   **Toxic effect of other ingested (parts of) plant(s)**

     √7ᵗʰ **T62.2X1**   **Toxic effect of other ingested (parts of) plant(s), accidental (unintentional)**   PE
       Toxic effect of other ingested (parts of) plant(s) NOS

     √7ᵗʰ **T62.2X2**   **Toxic effect of other ingested (parts of) plant(s), intentional self-harm**   HCC PE

     √7ᵗʰ **T62.2X3**   **Toxic effect of other ingested (parts of) plant(s), assault**   PE

     √7ᵗʰ **T62.2X4**   **Toxic effect of other ingested (parts of) plant(s), undetermined**   PE

√5ᵗʰ **T62.8**   **Toxic effect of other specified noxious substances eaten as food**

   √6ᵗʰ **T62.8X**   **Toxic effect of other specified noxious substances eaten as food**

     √7ᵗʰ **T62.8X1**   **Toxic effect of other specified noxious substances eaten as food, accidental (unintentional)**   PE
       Toxic effect of other specified noxious substances eaten as food NOS

     √7ᵗʰ **T62.8X2**   **Toxic effect of other specified noxious substances eaten as food, intentional self-harm**   HCC PE

     √7ᵗʰ **T62.8X3**   **Toxic effect of other specified noxious substances eaten as food, assault**   PE

     √7ᵗʰ **T62.8X4**   **Toxic effect of other specified noxious substances eaten as food, undetermined**   PE

√5ᵗʰ **T62.9**   **Toxic effect of unspecified noxious substance eaten as food**

   √x7ᵗʰ **T62.91**   **Toxic effect of unspecified noxious substance eaten as food, accidental (unintentional)**   PE
     Toxic effect of unspecified noxious substance eaten as food NOS

   √x7ᵗʰ **T62.92**   **Toxic effect of unspecified noxious substance eaten as food, intentional self-harm**   HCC PE

   √x7ᵗʰ **T62.93**   **Toxic effect of unspecified noxious substance eaten as food, assault**   PE

   √x7ᵗʰ **T62.94**   **Toxic effect of unspecified noxious substance eaten as food, undetermined**   PE

√4ᵗʰ **T63**   **Toxic effect of contact with venomous animals and plants**

   INCLUDES   bite or touch of venomous animal
       pricked or stuck by thorn or leaf

   EXCLUDES 2   ingestion of toxic animal or plant (T61.-, T62.-)

> The appropriate 7th character is to be added to each code from category T63.
> A   initial encounter
> D   subsequent encounter
> S   sequela

√5ᵗʰ **T63.0**   **Toxic effect of snake venom**

   √6ᵗʰ **T63.00**   **Toxic effect of unspecified snake venom**

     √7ᵗʰ **T63.001**   **Toxic effect of unspecified snake venom, accidental (unintentional)**   PE
       Toxic effect of unspecified snake venom NOS

     √7ᵗʰ **T63.002**   **Toxic effect of unspecified snake venom, intentional self-harm**   HCC PE

     √7ᵗʰ **T63.003**   **Toxic effect of unspecified snake venom, assault**   PE

     √7ᵗʰ **T63.004**   **Toxic effect of unspecified snake venom, undetermined**   PE

   √6ᵗʰ **T63.01**   **Toxic effect of rattlesnake venom**

     √7ᵗʰ **T63.011**   **Toxic effect of rattlesnake venom, accidental (unintentional)**   PE
       Toxic effect of rattlesnake venom NOS

     √7ᵗʰ **T63.012**   **Toxic effect of rattlesnake venom, intentional self-harm**   HCC PE

     √7ᵗʰ **T63.013**   **Toxic effect of rattlesnake venom, assault**   PE

     √7ᵗʰ **T63.014**   **Toxic effect of rattlesnake venom, undetermined**   PE

   √6ᵗʰ **T63.02**   **Toxic effect of coral snake venom**

     √7ᵗʰ **T63.021**   **Toxic effect of coral snake venom, accidental (unintentional)**   PE
       Toxic effect of coral snake venom NOS

     √7ᵗʰ **T63.022**   **Toxic effect of coral snake venom, intentional self-harm**   HCC PE

     √7ᵗʰ **T63.023**   **Toxic effect of coral snake venom, assault**   PE

     √7ᵗʰ **T63.024**   **Toxic effect of coral snake venom, undetermined**   PE

   √6ᵗʰ **T63.03**   **Toxic effect of taipan venom**

     √7ᵗʰ **T63.031**   **Toxic effect of taipan venom, accidental (unintentional)**   PE
       Toxic effect of taipan venom NOS

     √7ᵗʰ **T63.032**   **Toxic effect of taipan venom, intentional self-harm**   HCC PE

     √7ᵗʰ **T63.033**   **Toxic effect of taipan venom, assault**   PE

     √7ᵗʰ **T63.034**   **Toxic effect of taipan venom, undetermined**   PE

✔ Additional Character Required   √x7ᵗʰ Placeholder   Questionable PDx   Manifestation   Unspecified   UPD Unacceptable PDx   H1 - H14 HAC   HCC CMS-HCC Dx   HIV HIV Dx

✓6ᵗʰ **T63.04**   **Toxic effect of cobra venom**
- ✓7ᵗʰ **T63.041**   Toxic effect of cobra venom, **accidental (unintentional)**   PE
  - Toxic effect of cobra venom NOS
- ✓7ᵗʰ **T63.042**   Toxic effect of cobra venom, **intentional self-harm**   HCC PE
- ✓7ᵗʰ **T63.043**   Toxic effect of cobra venom, **assault**   PE
- ✓7ᵗʰ **T63.044**   Toxic effect of cobra venom, **undetermined**   PE

✓6ᵗʰ **T63.06**   **Toxic effect of venom of other North and South American snake**
- ✓7ᵗʰ **T63.061**   Toxic effect of venom of other North and South American snake, **accidental (unintentional)**   PE
  - Toxic effect of venom of other North and South American snake NOS
- ✓7ᵗʰ **T63.062**   Toxic effect of venom of other North and South American snake, **intentional self-harm**   HCC PE
- ✓7ᵗʰ **T63.063**   Toxic effect of venom of other North and South American snake, **assault**   PE
- ✓7ᵗʰ **T63.064**   Toxic effect of venom of other North and South American snake, **undetermined**   PE

✓6ᵗʰ **T63.07**   **Toxic effect of venom of other Australian snake**
- ✓7ᵗʰ **T63.071**   Toxic effect of venom of other Australian snake, **accidental (unintentional)**   PE
  - Toxic effect of venom of other Australian snake NOS
- ✓7ᵗʰ **T63.072**   Toxic effect of venom of other Australian snake, **intentional self-harm**   HCC PE
- ✓7ᵗʰ **T63.073**   Toxic effect of venom of other Australian snake, **assault**   PE
- ✓7ᵗʰ **T63.074**   Toxic effect of venom of other Australian snake, **undetermined**   PE

✓6ᵗʰ **T63.08**   **Toxic effect of venom of other African and Asian snake**
- ✓7ᵗʰ **T63.081**   Toxic effect of venom of other African and Asian snake, **accidental (unintentional)**   PE
  - Toxic effect of venom of other African and Asian snake NOS
- ✓7ᵗʰ **T63.082**   Toxic effect of venom of other African and Asian snake, **intentional self-harm**   HCC PE
- ✓7ᵗʰ **T63.083**   Toxic effect of venom of other African and Asian snake, **assault**   PE
- ✓7ᵗʰ **T63.084**   Toxic effect of venom of other African and Asian snake, **undetermined**   PE

✓6ᵗʰ **T63.09**   **Toxic effect of venom of other snake**
- ✓7ᵗʰ **T63.091**   Toxic effect of venom of other snake, **accidental (unintentional)**   PE
  - Toxic effect of venom of other snake NOS
- ✓7ᵗʰ **T63.092**   Toxic effect of venom of other snake, **intentional self-harm**   HCC PE
- ✓7ᵗʰ **T63.093**   Toxic effect of venom of other snake, **assault**   PE
- ✓7ᵗʰ **T63.094**   Toxic effect of venom of other snake, **undetermined**   PE

✓5ᵗʰ **T63.1**   **Toxic effect of venom of other reptiles**
- ✓6ᵗʰ **T63.11**   **Toxic effect of venom of gila monster**
  - ✓7ᵗʰ **T63.111**   Toxic effect of venom of gila monster, **accidental (unintentional)**   PE
    - Toxic effect of venom of gila monster NOS
  - ✓7ᵗʰ **T63.112**   Toxic effect of venom of gila monster, **intentional self-harm**   HCC PE
  - ✓7ᵗʰ **T63.113**   Toxic effect of venom of gila monster, **assault**   PE
  - ✓7ᵗʰ **T63.114**   Toxic effect of venom of gila monster, **undetermined**   PE
- ✓6ᵗʰ **T63.12**   **Toxic effect of venom of other venomous lizard**
  - ✓7ᵗʰ **T63.121**   Toxic effect of venom of other venomous lizard, **accidental (unintentional)**   PE
    - Toxic effect of venom of other venomous lizard NOS
  - ✓7ᵗʰ **T63.122**   Toxic effect of venom of other venomous lizard, **intentional self-harm**   HCC PE
  - ✓7ᵗʰ **T63.123**   Toxic effect of venom of other venomous lizard, **assault**   PE

- ✓7ᵗʰ **T63.124**   Toxic effect of venom of other venomous lizard, **undetermined**   PE
- ✓6ᵗʰ **T63.19**   **Toxic effect of venom of other reptiles**
  - ✓7ᵗʰ **T63.191**   Toxic effect of venom of other reptiles, **accidental (unintentional)**   PE
    - Toxic effect of venom of other reptiles NOS
  - ✓7ᵗʰ **T63.192**   Toxic effect of venom of other reptiles, **intentional self-harm**   HCC PE
  - ✓7ᵗʰ **T63.193**   Toxic effect of venom of other reptiles, **assault**   PE
  - ✓7ᵗʰ **T63.194**   Toxic effect of venom of other reptiles, **undetermined**   PE

✓5ᵗʰ **T63.2**   **Toxic effect of venom of scorpion**
- ✓6ᵗʰ **T63.2X**   **Toxic effect of venom of scorpion**
  - ✓7ᵗʰ **T63.2X1**   Toxic effect of venom of scorpion, **accidental (unintentional)**   PE
    - Toxic effect of venom of scorpion NOS
  - ✓7ᵗʰ **T63.2X2**   Toxic effect of venom of scorpion, **intentional self-harm**   HCC PE
  - ✓7ᵗʰ **T63.2X3**   Toxic effect of venom of scorpion, **assault**   PE
  - ✓7ᵗʰ **T63.2X4**   Toxic effect of venom of scorpion, **undetermined**   PE

✓5ᵗʰ **T63.3**   **Toxic effect of venom of spider**
- ✓6ᵗʰ **T63.30**   **Toxic effect of unspecified spider venom**
  - ✓7ᵗʰ **T63.301**   Toxic effect of unspecified spider venom, **accidental (unintentional)**   PE
  - ✓7ᵗʰ **T63.302**   Toxic effect of unspecified spider venom, **intentional self-harm**   HCC PE
  - ✓7ᵗʰ **T63.303**   Toxic effect of unspecified spider venom, **assault**   PE
  - ✓7ᵗʰ **T63.304**   Toxic effect of unspecified spider venom, **undetermined**   PE
- ✓6ᵗʰ **T63.31**   **Toxic effect of venom of black widow spider**
  - ✓7ᵗʰ **T63.311**   Toxic effect of venom of black widow spider, **accidental (unintentional)**   PE
  - ✓7ᵗʰ **T63.312**   Toxic effect of venom of black widow spider, **intentional self-harm**   HCC PE
  - ✓7ᵗʰ **T63.313**   Toxic effect of venom of black widow spider, **assault**   PE
  - ✓7ᵗʰ **T63.314**   Toxic effect of venom of black widow spider, **undetermined**   PE
- ✓6ᵗʰ **T63.32**   **Toxic effect of venom of tarantula**
  - ✓7ᵗʰ **T63.321**   Toxic effect of venom of tarantula, **accidental (unintentional)**   PE
  - ✓7ᵗʰ **T63.322**   Toxic effect of venom of tarantula, **intentional self-harm**   HCC PE
  - ✓7ᵗʰ **T63.323**   Toxic effect of venom of tarantula, **assault**   PE
  - ✓7ᵗʰ **T63.324**   Toxic effect of venom of tarantula, **undetermined**   PE
- ✓6ᵗʰ **T63.33**   **Toxic effect of venom of brown recluse spider**
  - ✓7ᵗʰ **T63.331**   Toxic effect of venom of brown recluse spider, **accidental (unintentional)**   PE
  - ✓7ᵗʰ **T63.332**   Toxic effect of venom of brown recluse spider, **intentional self-harm**   HCC PE
  - ✓7ᵗʰ **T63.333**   Toxic effect of venom of brown recluse spider, **assault**   PE
  - ✓7ᵗʰ **T63.334**   Toxic effect of venom of brown recluse spider, **undetermined**   PE
- ✓6ᵗʰ **T63.39**   **Toxic effect of venom of other spider**
  - ✓7ᵗʰ **T63.391**   Toxic effect of venom of other spider, **accidental (unintentional)**   PE
  - ✓7ᵗʰ **T63.392**   Toxic effect of venom of other spider, **intentional self-harm**   HCC PE
  - ✓7ᵗʰ **T63.393**   Toxic effect of venom of other spider, **assault**   PE
  - ✓7ᵗʰ **T63.394**   Toxic effect of venom of other spider, **undetermined**   PE

✓5ᵗʰ **T63.4**   **Toxic effect of venom of other arthropods**
   ▶Use additional code, if applicable, for anaphylactic shock (T78.2)◀
- ✓6ᵗʰ **T63.41**   **Toxic effect of venom of centipedes and venomous millipedes**
  - ✓7ᵗʰ **T63.411**   Toxic effect of venom of centipedes and venomous millipedes, **accidental (unintentional)**   PE

N Newborn: 0   P Pediatric: 0-17   M Maternity: 9-64   A Adult: 15-124   UNS Unspecified Site   MCC Major Complication/Comorbidity   CC Complication/Comorbidity   PE POA Exempt

1166

ICD-10-CM 2025

√7ᵗʰ **T63.412** Toxic effect of venom of centipedes and venomous millipedes, intentional self-harm   HCC PE

√7ᵗʰ **T63.413** Toxic effect of venom of centipedes and venomous millipedes, assault   PE

√7ᵗʰ **T63.414** Toxic effect of venom of centipedes and venomous millipedes, undetermined   PE

√6ᵗʰ **T63.42** Toxic effect of venom of ants

√7ᵗʰ **T63.421** Toxic effect of venom of ants, accidental (unintentional)   PE

√7ᵗʰ **T63.422** Toxic effect of venom of ants, intentional self-harm   HCC PE

√7ᵗʰ **T63.423** Toxic effect of venom of ants, assault   PE

√7ᵗʰ **T63.424** Toxic effect of venom of ants, undetermined   PE

√6ᵗʰ **T63.43** Toxic effect of venom of caterpillars

√7ᵗʰ **T63.431** Toxic effect of venom of caterpillars, accidental (unintentional)   PE

√7ᵗʰ **T63.432** Toxic effect of venom of caterpillars, intentional self-harm   HCC PE

√7ᵗʰ **T63.433** Toxic effect of venom of caterpillars, assault   PE

√7ᵗʰ **T63.434** Toxic effect of venom of caterpillars, undetermined   PE

√6ᵗʰ **T63.44** Toxic effect of venom of bees

√7ᵗʰ **T63.441** Toxic effect of venom of bees, accidental (unintentional)   PE

√7ᵗʰ **T63.442** Toxic effect of venom of bees, intentional self-harm   HCC PE

√7ᵗʰ **T63.443** Toxic effect of venom of bees, assault   PE

√7ᵗʰ **T63.444** Toxic effect of venom of bees, undetermined   PE

√6ᵗʰ **T63.45** Toxic effect of venom of hornets

√7ᵗʰ **T63.451** Toxic effect of venom of hornets, accidental (unintentional)   PE

√7ᵗʰ **T63.452** Toxic effect of venom of hornets, intentional self-harm   HCC PE

√7ᵗʰ **T63.453** Toxic effect of venom of hornets, assault   PE

√7ᵗʰ **T63.454** Toxic effect of venom of hornets, undetermined   PE

√6ᵗʰ **T63.46** Toxic effect of venom of wasps

Toxic effect of yellow jacket

√7ᵗʰ **T63.461** Toxic effect of venom of wasps, accidental (unintentional)   PE

√7ᵗʰ **T63.462** Toxic effect of venom of wasps, intentional self-harm   HCC PE

√7ᵗʰ **T63.463** Toxic effect of venom of wasps, assault   PE

√7ᵗʰ **T63.464** Toxic effect of venom of wasps, undetermined   PE

√6ᵗʰ **T63.48** Toxic effect of venom of other arthropod

√7ᵗʰ **T63.481** Toxic effect of venom of other arthropod, accidental (unintentional)   PE

√7ᵗʰ **T63.482** Toxic effect of venom of other arthropod, intentional self-harm   HCC PE

√7ᵗʰ **T63.483** Toxic effect of venom of other arthropod, assault   PE

√7ᵗʰ **T63.484** Toxic effect of venom of other arthropod, undetermined   PE

√5ᵗʰ **T63.5** Toxic effect of contact with venomous fish

EXCLUDES 2   poisoning by ingestion of fish (T61.-)

√6ᵗʰ **T63.51** Toxic effect of contact with stingray

√7ᵗʰ **T63.511** Toxic effect of contact with stingray, accidental (unintentional)   PE

√7ᵗʰ **T63.512** Toxic effect of contact with stingray, intentional self-harm   HCC PE

√7ᵗʰ **T63.513** Toxic effect of contact with stingray, assault   PE

√7ᵗʰ **T63.514** Toxic effect of contact with stingray, undetermined   PE

√6ᵗʰ **T63.59** Toxic effect of contact with other venomous fish

√7ᵗʰ **T63.591** Toxic effect of contact with other venomous fish, accidental (unintentional)   PE

√7ᵗʰ **T63.592** Toxic effect of contact with other venomous fish, intentional self-harm   HCC PE

√7ᵗʰ **T63.593** Toxic effect of contact with other venomous fish, assault   PE

√7ᵗʰ **T63.594** Toxic effect of contact with other venomous fish, undetermined   PE

√5ᵗʰ **T63.6** Toxic effect of contact with other venomous marine animals

EXCLUDES 1   sea-snake venom (T63.09)

EXCLUDES 2   poisoning by ingestion of shellfish (T61.78-)

√6ᵗʰ **T63.61** Toxic effect of contact with Portuguese Man-o-war

Toxic effect of contact with bluebottle

√7ᵗʰ **T63.611** Toxic effect of contact with Portuguese Man-o-war, accidental (unintentional)   PE

√7ᵗʰ **T63.612** Toxic effect of contact with Portuguese Man-o-war, intentional self-harm   HCC PE

√7ᵗʰ **T63.613** Toxic effect of contact with Portuguese Man-o-war, assault   PE

√7ᵗʰ **T63.614** Toxic effect of contact with Portuguese Man-o-war, undetermined   PE

√6ᵗʰ **T63.62** Toxic effect of contact with other jellyfish

√7ᵗʰ **T63.621** Toxic effect of contact with other jellyfish, accidental (unintentional)   PE

√7ᵗʰ **T63.622** Toxic effect of contact with other jellyfish, intentional self-harm   HCC PE

√7ᵗʰ **T63.623** Toxic effect of contact with other jellyfish, assault   PE

√7ᵗʰ **T63.624** Toxic effect of contact with other jellyfish, undetermined   PE

√6ᵗʰ **T63.63** Toxic effect of contact with sea anemone

√7ᵗʰ **T63.631** Toxic effect of contact with sea anemone, accidental (unintentional)   PE

√7ᵗʰ **T63.632** Toxic effect of contact with sea anemone, intentional self-harm   HCC PE

√7ᵗʰ **T63.633** Toxic effect of contact with sea anemone, assault   PE

√7ᵗʰ **T63.634** Toxic effect of contact with sea anemone, undetermined   PE

√6ᵗʰ **T63.69** Toxic effect of contact with other venomous marine animals

√7ᵗʰ **T63.691** Toxic effect of contact with other venomous marine animals, accidental (unintentional)   PE

√7ᵗʰ **T63.692** Toxic effect of contact with other venomous marine animals, intentional self-harm   HCC PE

√7ᵗʰ **T63.693** Toxic effect of contact with other venomous marine animals, assault   PE

√7ᵗʰ **T63.694** Toxic effect of contact with other venomous marine animals, undetermined   PE

√5ᵗʰ **T63.7** Toxic effect of contact with venomous plant

√6ᵗʰ **T63.71** Toxic effect of contact with venomous marine plant

√7ᵗʰ **T63.711** Toxic effect of contact with venomous marine plant, accidental (unintentional)   PE

√7ᵗʰ **T63.712** Toxic effect of contact with venomous marine plant, intentional self-harm   HCC PE

√7ᵗʰ **T63.713** Toxic effect of contact with venomous marine plant, assault   PE

√7ᵗʰ **T63.714** Toxic effect of contact with venomous marine plant, undetermined   PE

√6ᵗʰ **T63.79** Toxic effect of contact with other venomous plant

√7ᵗʰ **T63.791** Toxic effect of contact with other venomous plant, accidental (unintentional)   PE

√7ᵗʰ **T63.792** Toxic effect of contact with other venomous plant, intentional self-harm   HCC PE

√7ᵗʰ **T63.793** Toxic effect of contact with other venomous plant, assault   PE

√7ᵗʰ **T63.794** Toxic effect of contact with other venomous plant, undetermined   PE

√5ᵗʰ **T63.8　Toxic effect of contact with other venomous animals**

√6ᵗʰ **T63.81　Toxic effect of contact with venomous frog**

EXCLUDES 1　*contact with nonvenomous frog (W62.0)*

√7ᵗʰ **T63.811　Toxic effect of contact with venomous frog, accidental (unintentional)**　PE

√7ᵗʰ **T63.812　Toxic effect of contact with venomous frog, intentional self-harm**　HCC PE

√7ᵗʰ **T63.813　Toxic effect of contact with venomous frog, assault**　PE

√7ᵗʰ **T63.814　Toxic effect of contact with venomous frog, undetermined**　PE

√6ᵗʰ **T63.82　Toxic effect of contact with venomous toad**

EXCLUDES 1　*contact with nonvenomous toad (W62.1)*

√7ᵗʰ **T63.821　Toxic effect of contact with venomous toad, accidental (unintentional)**　PE

√7ᵗʰ **T63.822　Toxic effect of contact with venomous toad, intentional self-harm**　HCC PE

√7ᵗʰ **T63.823　Toxic effect of contact with venomous toad, assault**　PE

√7ᵗʰ **T63.824　Toxic effect of contact with venomous toad, undetermined**　PE

√6ᵗʰ **T63.83　Toxic effect of contact with other venomous amphibian**

EXCLUDES 1　*contact with nonvenomous amphibian (W62.9)*

√7ᵗʰ **T63.831　Toxic effect of contact with other venomous amphibian, accidental (unintentional)**　PE

√7ᵗʰ **T63.832　Toxic effect of contact with other venomous amphibian, intentional self-harm**　HCC PE

√7ᵗʰ **T63.833　Toxic effect of contact with other venomous amphibian, assault**　PE

√7ᵗʰ **T63.834　Toxic effect of contact with other venomous amphibian, undetermined**　PE

√6ᵗʰ **T63.89　Toxic effect of contact with other venomous animals**

√7ᵗʰ **T63.891　Toxic effect of contact with other venomous animals, accidental (unintentional)**　PE

√7ᵗʰ **T63.892　Toxic effect of contact with other venomous animals, intentional self-harm**　HCC PE

√7ᵗʰ **T63.893　Toxic effect of contact with other venomous animals, assault**　PE

√7ᵗʰ **T63.894　Toxic effect of contact with other venomous animals, undetermined**　PE

√5ᵗʰ **T63.9　Toxic effect of contact with unspecified venomous animal**

√x7ᵗʰ **T63.91　Toxic effect of contact with unspecified venomous animal, accidental (unintentional)**　PE

√x7ᵗʰ **T63.92　Toxic effect of contact with unspecified venomous animal, intentional self-harm**　HCC PE

√x7ᵗʰ **T63.93　Toxic effect of contact with unspecified venomous animal, assault**　PE

√x7ᵗʰ **T63.94　Toxic effect of contact with unspecified venomous animal, undetermined**　PE

√4ᵗʰ **T64　Toxic effect of aflatoxin and other mycotoxin food contaminants**

The appropriate 7th character is to be added to each code from category T64.
A　initial encounter
D　subsequent encounter
S　sequela

√5ᵗʰ **T64.0　Toxic effect of aflatoxin**

√x7ᵗʰ **T64.01　Toxic effect of aflatoxin, accidental (unintentional)**　PE

√x7ᵗʰ **T64.02　Toxic effect of aflatoxin, intentional self-harm**　HCC PE

√x7ᵗʰ **T64.03　Toxic effect of aflatoxin, assault**　PE

√x7ᵗʰ **T64.04　Toxic effect of aflatoxin, undetermined**　PE

√5ᵗʰ **T64.8　Toxic effect of other mycotoxin food contaminants**

√x7ᵗʰ **T64.81　Toxic effect of other mycotoxin food contaminants, accidental (unintentional)**　PE

√x7ᵗʰ **T64.82　Toxic effect of other mycotoxin food contaminants, intentional self-harm**　HCC PE

√x7ᵗʰ **T64.83　Toxic effect of other mycotoxin food contaminants, assault**　PE

√x7ᵗʰ **T64.84　Toxic effect of other mycotoxin food contaminants, undetermined**　PE

√4ᵗʰ **T65　Toxic effect of other and unspecified substances**

The appropriate 7th character is to be added to each code from category T65.
A　initial encounter
D　subsequent encounter
S　sequela

√5ᵗʰ **T65.0　Toxic effect of cyanides**

EXCLUDES 1　*hydrogen cyanide (T57.3-)*

√6ᵗʰ **T65.0X　Toxic effect of cyanides**

√7ᵗʰ **T65.0X1　Toxic effect of cyanides, accidental (unintentional)**　PE
Toxic effect of cyanides NOS

√7ᵗʰ **T65.0X2　Toxic effect of cyanides, intentional self-harm**　HCC PE

√7ᵗʰ **T65.0X3　Toxic effect of cyanides, assault**　PE

√7ᵗʰ **T65.0X4　Toxic effect of cyanides, undetermined**　PE

√5ᵗʰ **T65.1　Toxic effect of strychnine and its salts**

√6ᵗʰ **T65.1X　Toxic effect of strychnine and its salts**

√7ᵗʰ **T65.1X1　Toxic effect of strychnine and its salts, accidental (unintentional)**　PE
Toxic effect of strychnine and its salts NOS

√7ᵗʰ **T65.1X2　Toxic effect of strychnine and its salts, intentional self-harm**　HCC PE

√7ᵗʰ **T65.1X3　Toxic effect of strychnine and its salts, assault**　PE

√7ᵗʰ **T65.1X4　Toxic effect of strychnine and its salts, undetermined**　PE

√5ᵗʰ **T65.2　Toxic effect of tobacco and nicotine**

EXCLUDES 2　*nicotine dependence (F17.-)*

√6ᵗʰ **T65.21　Toxic effect of chewing tobacco**

√7ᵗʰ **T65.211　Toxic effect of chewing tobacco, accidental (unintentional)**　PE
Toxic effect of chewing tobacco NOS

√7ᵗʰ **T65.212　Toxic effect of chewing tobacco, intentional self-harm**　HCC PE

√7ᵗʰ **T65.213　Toxic effect of chewing tobacco, assault**　PE

√7ᵗʰ **T65.214　Toxic effect of chewing tobacco, undetermined**　PE

√6ᵗʰ **T65.22　Toxic effect of tobacco cigarettes**
Toxic effect of tobacco smoke
Use additional code for exposure to second hand tobacco smoke (Z57.31, Z77.22)

√7ᵗʰ **T65.221　Toxic effect of tobacco cigarettes, accidental (unintentional)**　PE
Toxic effect of tobacco cigarettes NOS

√7ᵗʰ **T65.222　Toxic effect of tobacco cigarettes, intentional self-harm**　HCC PE

√7ᵗʰ **T65.223　Toxic effect of tobacco cigarettes, assault**　PE

√7ᵗʰ **T65.224　Toxic effect of tobacco cigarettes, undetermined**　PE

√6ᵗʰ **T65.29　Toxic effect of other tobacco and nicotine**

√7ᵗʰ **T65.291　Toxic effect of other tobacco and nicotine, accidental (unintentional)**　PE
Toxic effect of other tobacco and nicotine NOS

√7ᵗʰ **T65.292　Toxic effect of other tobacco and nicotine, intentional self-harm**　HCC PE

√7ᵗʰ **T65.293　Toxic effect of other tobacco and nicotine, assault**　PE

√7ᵗʰ **T65.294　Toxic effect of other tobacco and nicotine, undetermined**　PE

N Newborn: 0　**P** Pediatric: 0-17　**M** Maternity: 9-64　**A** Adult: 15-124　**UNS** Unspecified Site　**MCC** Major Complication/Comorbidity　**CC** Complication/Comorbidity　**PE** POA Exempt

1168

ICD-10-CM 2025

√5th **T65.3** **Toxic effect of nitroderivatives and aminoderivatives of benzene and its homologues**
► Toxic effect of aniline [benzenamine] ◄
Toxic effect of nitrobenzene
Toxic effect of trinitrotoluene

  √6th **T65.3X** **Toxic effect of nitroderivatives and aminoderivatives of benzene and its homologues**

    √7th **T65.3X1** **Toxic effect of nitroderivatives and aminoderivatives of benzene and its homologues, accidental (unintentional)** PE
Toxic effect of nitroderivatives and aminoderivatives of benzene and its homologues NOS

    √7th **T65.3X2** **Toxic effect of nitroderivatives and aminoderivatives of benzene and its homologues, intentional self-harm** HCC PE

    √7th **T65.3X3** **Toxic effect of nitroderivatives and aminoderivatives of benzene and its homologues, assault** PE

    √7th **T65.3X4** **Toxic effect of nitroderivatives and aminoderivatives of benzene and its homologues, undetermined** PE

√5th **T65.4** **Toxic effect of carbon disulfide**

  √6th **T65.4X** **Toxic effect of carbon disulfide**

    √7th **T65.4X1** **Toxic effect of carbon disulfide, accidental (unintentional)** PE
Toxic effect of carbon disulfide NOS

    √7th **T65.4X2** **Toxic effect of carbon disulfide, intentional self-harm** HCC PE

    √7th **T65.4X3** **Toxic effect of carbon disulfide, assault** PE

    √7th **T65.4X4** **Toxic effect of carbon disulfide, undetermined** PE

√5th **T65.5** **Toxic effect of nitroglycerin and other nitric acids and esters**
Toxic effect of 1,2,3-Propanetriol trinitrate

  √6th **T65.5X** **Toxic effect of nitroglycerin and other nitric acids and esters**

    √7th **T65.5X1** **Toxic effect of nitroglycerin and other nitric acids and esters, accidental (unintentional)** PE
Toxic effect of nitroglycerin and other nitric acids and esters NOS

    √7th **T65.5X2** **Toxic effect of nitroglycerin and other nitric acids and esters, intentional self-harm** HCC PE

    √7th **T65.5X3** **Toxic effect of nitroglycerin and other nitric acids and esters, assault** PE

    √7th **T65.5X4** **Toxic effect of nitroglycerin and other nitric acids and esters, undetermined** PE

√5th **T65.6** **Toxic effect of paints and dyes, not elsewhere classified**

  √6th **T65.6X** **Toxic effect of paints and dyes, not elsewhere classified**

    √7th **T65.6X1** **Toxic effect of paints and dyes, not elsewhere classified, accidental (unintentional)** PE
Toxic effect of paints and dyes NOS

    √7th **T65.6X2** **Toxic effect of paints and dyes, not elsewhere classified, intentional self-harm** HCC PE

    √7th **T65.6X3** **Toxic effect of paints and dyes, not elsewhere classified, assault** PE

    √7th **T65.6X4** **Toxic effect of paints and dyes, not elsewhere classified, undetermined** PE

√5th **T65.8** **Toxic effect of other specified substances**

  √6th **T65.81** **Toxic effect of latex**

    √7th **T65.811** **Toxic effect of latex, accidental (unintentional)** PE
Toxic effect of latex NOS

    √7th **T65.812** **Toxic effect of latex, intentional self-harm** HCC PE

    √7th **T65.813** **Toxic effect of latex, assault** PE

    √7th **T65.814** **Toxic effect of latex, undetermined** PE

  √6th **T65.82** **Toxic effect of harmful algae and algae toxins**
Toxic effect of (harmful) algae bloom NOS
Toxic effect of blue-green algae bloom
Toxic effect of brown tide
Toxic effect of cyanobacteria bloom
Toxic effect of Florida red tide
Toxic effect of pfiesteria piscicida
Toxic effect of red tide

    √7th **T65.821** **Toxic effect of harmful algae and algae toxins, accidental (unintentional)** PE
Toxic effect of harmful algae and algae toxins NOS

    √7th **T65.822** **Toxic effect of harmful algae and algae toxins, intentional self-harm** HCC PE

    √7th **T65.823** **Toxic effect of harmful algae and algae toxins, assault** PE

    √7th **T65.824** **Toxic effect of harmful algae and algae toxins, undetermined** PE

  √6th **T65.83** **Toxic effect of fiberglass**

    √7th **T65.831** **Toxic effect of fiberglass, accidental (unintentional)** PE
Toxic effect of fiberglass NOS

    √7th **T65.832** **Toxic effect of fiberglass, intentional self-harm** HCC PE

    √7th **T65.833** **Toxic effect of fiberglass, assault** PE

    √7th **T65.834** **Toxic effect of fiberglass, undetermined** PE

  √6th **T65.89** **Toxic effect of other specified substances**

    √7th **T65.891** **Toxic effect of other specified substances, accidental (unintentional)** PE
Toxic effect of other specified substances NOS
AHA: 2018,1Q,5

    √7th **T65.892** **Toxic effect of other specified substances, intentional self-harm** HCC PE

    √7th **T65.893** **Toxic effect of other specified substances, assault** PE

    √7th **T65.894** **Toxic effect of other specified substances, undetermined** PE

√5th **T65.9** **Toxic effect of unspecified substance**

  √x7th **T65.91** **Toxic effect of unspecified substance, accidental (unintentional)** PE
Poisoning NOS

  √x7th **T65.92** **Toxic effect of unspecified substance, intentional self-harm** HCC PE

  √x7th **T65.93** **Toxic effect of unspecified substance, assault** PE

  √x7th **T65.94** **Toxic effect of unspecified substance, undetermined** PE

Other and unspecified effects of external causes (T66-T78)

√x7th **T66** **Radiation sickness, unspecified** PE

  EXCLUDES 1   specified adverse effects of radiation, such as:
    burns (T20-T31)
    leukemia (C91-C95)
    radiation gastroenteritis and colitis (K52.0)
    radiation pneumonitis (J70.0)
    radiation related disorders of the skin and subcutaneous tissue (L55-L59)
    radiation sunburn (L55.-)

The appropriate 7th character is to be added to code T66.
A   initial encounter
D   subsequent encounter
S   sequela

☑ Additional Character Required   √x7th Placeholder   Questionable PDx   Manifestation   Unspecified   UPD Unacceptable PDx   H1-H14 HAC   HCC CMS-HCC Dx   HIV HIV Dx

ICD-10-CM 2025   1169

Chapter 19. Injury, Poisoning and Certain Other Consequences of External Causes

T67–T71.112

√4th **T67 Effects of heat and light**

> EXCLUDES 1   erythema [dermatitis] ab igne (L59.0)
> malignant hyperpyrexia due to anesthesia (T88.3)
> radiation-related disorders of the skin and subcutaneous tissue (L55-L59)
>
> EXCLUDES 2   burns (T20-T31)
> sunburn (L55.-)
> sweat disorder due to heat (L74-L75)

> The appropriate 7th character is to be added to each code from category T67.
> A   initial encounter
> D   subsequent encounter
> S   sequela

√5th **T67.0 Heatstroke and sunstroke**

> Use additional code(s) to identify any associated complications of heatstroke, such as:
> coma and stupor (R40.-)
> rhabdomyolysis (M62.82)
> systemic inflammatory response syndrome (R65.1-)
> **AHA:** 2019,4Q,17-18
> **DEF:** Headache, vertigo, cramps, and elevated body temperature due to prolonged exposure to high environmental temperatures that requires emergency intervention.

    √x 7th **T67.01 Heatstroke and sunstroke** `CC` `H5` `PE`
> Heat apoplexy
> Heat pyrexia
> Siriasis
> Thermoplegia

    √x 7th **T67.02 Exertional heatstroke** `CC` `H5` `PE`

    √x 7th **T67.09 Other heatstroke and sunstroke** `CC` `H5` `PE`

√x 7th **T67.1 Heat syncope** `PE`
> Heat collapse

√x 7th **T67.2 Heat cramp** `PE`

√x 7th **T67.3 Heat exhaustion, anhydrotic** `PE`
> Heat prostration due to water depletion
> EXCLUDES 1   heat exhaustion due to salt depletion (T67.4)

√x 7th **T67.4 Heat exhaustion due to salt depletion** `PE`
> Heat prostration due to salt (and water) depletion

√x 7th **T67.5 Heat exhaustion, unspecified** `PE`
> Heat prostration NOS

√x 7th **T67.6 Heat fatigue, transient** `PE`

√x 7th **T67.7 Heat edema** `PE`

√x 7th **T67.8 Other effects of heat and light** `PE`

√x 7th **T67.9 Effect of heat and light, unspecified** `PE`

√x 7th **T68 Hypothermia** `PE`
> Accidental hypothermia
> Hypothermia NOS
> Use additional code to identify source of exposure:
> exposure to excessive cold of man-made origin (W93)
> exposure to excessive cold of natural origin (X31)
> EXCLUDES 1   hypothermia following anesthesia (T88.51)
> hypothermia not associated with low environmental temperature (R68.0)
> hypothermia of newborn (P80.-)
> EXCLUDES 2   frostbite (T33-T34)

> The appropriate 7th character is to be added to code T68.
> A   initial encounter
> D   subsequent encounter
> S   sequela

√4th **T69 Other effects of reduced temperature**

> Use additional code to identify source of exposure:
> exposure to excessive cold of man-made origin (W93)
> exposure to excessive cold of natural origin (X31)
> EXCLUDES 2   frostbite (T33-T34)

> The appropriate 7th character is to be added to each code from category T69.
> A   initial encounter
> D   subsequent encounter
> S   sequela

√5th **T69.0 Immersion hand and foot**

    √6th **T69.01 Immersion hand**

       √7th **T69.011 Immersion hand, right hand** `PE`

       √7th **T69.012 Immersion hand, left hand** `PE`

       √7th **T69.019 Immersion hand, unspecified hand** `PE`

    √6th **T69.02 Immersion foot**
> Trench foot

       √7th **T69.021 Immersion foot, right foot** `CC` `H5` `PE`

       √7th **T69.022 Immersion foot, left foot** `CC` `H5` `PE`

       √7th **T69.029 Immersion foot, unspecified foot** `CC` `H5` `UNS` `PE`

√x 7th **T69.1 Chilblains** `PE`
> **DEF:** Red, swollen, itchy skin primarily affecting the fingers and toes, nose and ears, and legs. Chilblains follows damp-cold exposure, and can also be associated with pruritus and a burning feeling.

√x 7th **T69.8 Other specified effects of reduced temperature** `PE`

√x 7th **T69.9 Effect of reduced temperature, unspecified** `PE`

√4th **T70 Effects of air pressure and water pressure**

> The appropriate 7th character is to be added to each code from category T70.
> A   initial encounter
> D   subsequent encounter
> S   sequela

√x 7th **T70.0 Otitic barotrauma** `PE`
> Aero-otitis media
> Effects of change in ambient atmospheric pressure or water pressure on ears

√x 7th **T70.1 Sinus barotrauma** `PE`
> Aerosinusitis
> Effects of change in ambient atmospheric pressure on sinuses

√5th **T70.2 Other and unspecified effects of high altitude**
> EXCLUDES 2   polycythemia due to high altitude (D75.1)

    √x 7th **T70.20 Unspecified effects of high altitude** `PE`

    √x 7th **T70.29 Other effects of high altitude** `PE`
> Alpine sickness
> Anoxia due to high altitude
> Barotrauma NOS
> Hypobaropathy
> Mountain sickness

√x 7th **T70.3 Caisson disease [decompression sickness]** `CC` `H5` `PE`
> Compressed-air disease
> Diver's palsy or paralysis
> **DEF:** Rapid reduction in air pressure while breathing compressed air. Symptoms include skin lesions, joint pains, and respiratory and neurological problems.

√x 7th **T70.4 Effects of high-pressure fluids** `PE`
> Hydraulic jet injection (industrial)
> Pneumatic jet injection (industrial)
> Traumatic jet injection (industrial)

√x 7th **T70.8 Other effects of air pressure and water pressure** `PE`

√x 7th **T70.9 Effect of air pressure and water pressure, unspecified** `PE`

√4th **T71 Asphyxiation**
> Mechanical suffocation
> Traumatic suffocation
> EXCLUDES 1   acute respiratory distress (syndrome) (J80)
> anoxia due to high altitude (T70.2)
> asphyxia NOS (R09.01)
> asphyxia from carbon monoxide (T58.-)
> asphyxia from inhalation of food or foreign body (T17.-)
> asphyxia from other gases, fumes and vapors (T59.-)
> respiratory distress (syndrome) in newborn (P22.-)

> The appropriate 7th character is to be added to each code from category T71.
> A   initial encounter
> D   subsequent encounter
> S   sequela

√5th **T71.1 Asphyxiation due to mechanical threat to breathing**
> Suffocation due to mechanical threat to breathing

    √6th **T71.11 Asphyxiation due to smothering under pillow**

       √7th **T71.111 Asphyxiation due to smothering under pillow, accidental** `CC` `H5` `PE`
> Asphyxiation due to smothering under pillow NOS

       √7th **T71.112 Asphyxiation due to smothering under pillow, intentional self-harm** `CC` `H5` `HCC` `PE`

`N` Newborn: 0   `P` Pediatric: 0-17   `M` Maternity: 9-64   `A` Adult: 15-124   `UNS` Unspecified Site   `MCC` Major Complication/Comorbidity   `CC` Complication/Comorbidity   `PE` POA Exempt

1170   ICD-10-CM 2025

√7ᵗʰ   **T71.113**   **Asphyxiation due to smothering under pillow, assault**   CC H5 PE

√7ᵗʰ   **T71.114**   **Asphyxiation due to smothering under pillow, undetermined**   CC H5 PE

√6ᵗʰ   **T71.12**   **Asphyxiation due to plastic bag**

    √7ᵗʰ   **T71.121**   **Asphyxiation due to plastic bag, accidental**   CC H5 PE
       Asphyxiation due to plastic bag NOS

    √7ᵗʰ   **T71.122**   **Asphyxiation due to plastic bag, intentional self-harm**   CC H5 HCC PE

    √7ᵗʰ   **T71.123**   **Asphyxiation due to plastic bag, assault**   CC H5 PE

    √7ᵗʰ   **T71.124**   **Asphyxiation due to plastic bag, undetermined**   CC H5 PE

√6ᵗʰ   **T71.13**   **Asphyxiation due to being trapped in bed linens**

    √7ᵗʰ   **T71.131**   **Asphyxiation due to being trapped in bed linens, accidental**   CC H5 PE
       Asphyxiation due to being trapped in bed linens NOS

    √7ᵗʰ   **T71.132**   **Asphyxiation due to being trapped in bed linens, intentional self-harm**   CC H5 HCC PE

    √7ᵗʰ   **T71.133**   **Asphyxiation due to being trapped in bed linens, assault**   CC H5 PE

    √7ᵗʰ   **T71.134**   **Asphyxiation due to being trapped in bed linens, undetermined**   CC H5 PE

√6ᵗʰ   **T71.14**   **Asphyxiation due to smothering under another person's body (in bed)**

    √7ᵗʰ   **T71.141**   **Asphyxiation due to smothering under another person's body (in bed), accidental**   CC H5 PE
       Asphyxiation due to smothering under another person's body (in bed) NOS

    √7ᵗʰ   **T71.143**   **Asphyxiation due to smothering under another person's body (in bed), assault**   CC H5 PE

    √7ᵗʰ   **T71.144**   **Asphyxiation due to smothering under another person's body (in bed), undetermined**   CC H5 PE

√6ᵗʰ   **T71.15**   **Asphyxiation due to smothering in furniture**

    √7ᵗʰ   **T71.151**   **Asphyxiation due to smothering in furniture, accidental**   CC H5 PE
       Asphyxiation due to smothering in furniture NOS

    √7ᵗʰ   **T71.152**   **Asphyxiation due to smothering in furniture, intentional self-harm**   CC H5 HCC PE

    √7ᵗʰ   **T71.153**   **Asphyxiation due to smothering in furniture, assault**   CC H5 PE

    √7ᵗʰ   **T71.154**   **Asphyxiation due to smothering in furniture, undetermined**   CC H5 PE

√6ᵗʰ   **T71.16**   **Asphyxiation due to hanging**
    Hanging by window shade cord
    Use additional code for any associated injuries, such as:
       crushing injury of neck (S17.-)
       fracture of cervical vertebrae (S12.0-S12.2-)
       open wound of neck (S11.-)

    √7ᵗʰ   **T71.161**   **Asphyxiation due to hanging, accidental**   CC H5 PE
       Asphyxiation due to hanging NOS
       Hanging NOS

    √7ᵗʰ   **T71.162**   **Asphyxiation due to hanging, intentional self-harm**   CC H5 HCC PE

    √7ᵗʰ   **T71.163**   **Asphyxiation due to hanging, assault**   CC H5 PE

    √7ᵗʰ   **T71.164**   **Asphyxiation due to hanging, undetermined**   CC H5 PE

√6ᵗʰ   **T71.19**   **Asphyxiation due to mechanical threat to breathing due to other causes**

    √7ᵗʰ   **T71.191**   **Asphyxiation due to mechanical threat to breathing due to other causes, accidental**   CC H5 PE
       Asphyxiation due to other causes NOS

    √7ᵗʰ   **T71.192**   **Asphyxiation due to mechanical threat to breathing due to other causes, intentional self-harm**   CC H5 HCC PE

    √7ᵗʰ   **T71.193**   **Asphyxiation due to mechanical threat to breathing due to other causes, assault**   CC H5 PE

    √7ᵗʰ   **T71.194**   **Asphyxiation due to mechanical threat to breathing due to other causes, undetermined**   CC H5 PE

√5ᵗʰ   **T71.2**   **Asphyxiation due to systemic oxygen deficiency due to low oxygen content in ambient air**
    Suffocation due to systemic oxygen deficiency due to low oxygen content in ambient air

    √x7ᵗʰ   **T71.20**   **Asphyxiation due to systemic oxygen deficiency due to low oxygen content in ambient air due to unspecified cause**   CC H5 PE

    √x7ᵗʰ   **T71.21**   **Asphyxiation due to cave-in or falling earth**   CC H5 PE
       Use additional code for any associated cataclysm (X34-X38)

    √6ᵗʰ   **T71.22**   **Asphyxiation due to being trapped in a car trunk**

       √7ᵗʰ   **T71.221**   **Asphyxiation due to being trapped in a car trunk, accidental**   CC PE

       √7ᵗʰ   **T71.222**   **Asphyxiation due to being trapped in a car trunk, intentional self-harm**   CC HCC PE

       √7ᵗʰ   **T71.223**   **Asphyxiation due to being trapped in a car trunk, assault**   CC PE

       √7ᵗʰ   **T71.224**   **Asphyxiation due to being trapped in a car trunk, undetermined**   CC PE

    √6ᵗʰ   **T71.23**   **Asphyxiation due to being trapped in a (discarded) refrigerator**

       √7ᵗʰ   **T71.231**   **Asphyxiation due to being trapped in a (discarded) refrigerator, accidental**   CC PE

       √7ᵗʰ   **T71.232**   **Asphyxiation due to being trapped in a (discarded) refrigerator, intentional self-harm**   CC HCC PE

       √7ᵗʰ   **T71.233**   **Asphyxiation due to being trapped in a (discarded) refrigerator, assault**   CC PE

       √7ᵗʰ   **T71.234**   **Asphyxiation due to being trapped in a (discarded) refrigerator, undetermined**   CC PE

    √x7ᵗʰ   **T71.29**   **Asphyxiation due to being trapped in other low oxygen environment**   CC H5 PE

√x7ᵗʰ   **T71.9**   **Asphyxiation due to unspecified cause**   CC H5 PE
    Suffocation (by strangulation) due to unspecified cause
    Suffocation NOS
    Systemic oxygen deficiency due to low oxygen content in ambient air due to unspecified cause
    Systemic oxygen deficiency due to mechanical threat to breathing due to unspecified cause
    Traumatic asphyxia NOS

√4ᵗʰ   **T73**   **Effects of other deprivation**

> The appropriate 7th character is to be added to each code from category T73.
> A   initial encounter
> D   subsequent encounter
> S   sequela

√x7ᵗʰ   **T73.0**   **Starvation**   PE
    Deprivation of food

√x7ᵗʰ   **T73.1**   **Deprivation of water**   PE

√x7ᵗʰ   **T73.2**   **Exhaustion due to exposure**   PE

√x7ᵗʰ   **T73.3**   **Exhaustion due to excessive exertion**   PE
    Exhaustion due to overexertion

√x7ᵗʰ   **T73.8**   **Other effects of deprivation**   PE

√x7ᵗʰ   **T73.9**   **Effect of deprivation, unspecified**   PE

√4ᵗʰ   **T74**   **Adult and child abuse, neglect and other maltreatment, confirmed**
    Use additional code, if applicable, to identify any associated current injury
    Use additional external cause code to identify perpetrator, if known (Y07.-)
    EXCLUDES 1   abuse and maltreatment in pregnancy (O9A.3-, O9A.4-, O9A.5-)
       adult and child maltreatment, suspected (T76.-)

> The appropriate 7th character is to be added to each code from category T74.
> A   initial encounter
> D   subsequent encounter
> S   sequela

√5ᵗʰ   **T74.0**   **Neglect or abandonment, confirmed**

    √x7ᵗʰ   **T74.01**   **Adult neglect or abandonment, confirmed**   CC A PE

    √x7ᵗʰ   **T74.02**   **Child neglect or abandonment, confirmed**   CC P PE

☑ Additional Character Required   √x7ᵗʰ Placeholder   Questionable PDx   Manifestation   Unspecified   UPD Unacceptable PDx   H1-H14 HAC   HCC CMS-HCC Dx   HIV HIV Dx

ICD-10-CM 2025   1171

Chapter 19. Injury, Poisoning and Certain Other Consequences of External Causes

√5ᵗʰ **T74.1** **Physical abuse, confirmed**
     EXCLUDES 2   sexual abuse (T74.2-)
     √x7ᵗʰ **T74.11**   **Adult** physical abuse, confirmed   CC A PE
     √x7ᵗʰ **T74.12**   **Child** physical abuse, confirmed   CC P PE
         EXCLUDES 2   shaken infant syndrome (T74.4)

√5ᵗʰ **T74.2** **Sexual abuse, confirmed**
     Rape, confirmed
     Sexual assault, confirmed
     √x7ᵗʰ **T74.21**   **Adult** sexual abuse, confirmed   CC A PE
     √x7ᵗʰ **T74.22**   **Child** sexual abuse, confirmed   CC P PE

√5ᵗʰ **T74.3** **Psychological abuse, confirmed**
     Bullying and intimidation, confirmed
     Intimidation through social media, confirmed
     Target of threatened harm, confirmed
     Target of threatened physical violence, confirmed
     Target of threatened sexual abuse, confirmed
     √x7ᵗʰ **T74.31**   **Adult** psychological abuse, confirmed   A PE
     √x7ᵗʰ **T74.32**   **Child** psychological abuse, confirmed   CC P PE

√x7ᵗʰ **T74.4** **Shaken infant syndrome**   CC P PE

√5ᵗʰ **T74.5** **Forced sexual exploitation, confirmed**
     AHA: 2018,4Q,32-33,65
     √x7ᵗʰ **T74.51**   **Adult** forced sexual exploitation, confirmed   CC A PE
     √x7ᵗʰ **T74.52**   **Child** sexual exploitation, confirmed   CC P PE

√5ᵗʰ **T74.6** **Forced labor exploitation, confirmed**
     AHA: 2018,4Q,32-33,65
     √x7ᵗʰ **T74.61**   **Adult** forced labor exploitation, confirmed   CC A PE
     √x7ᵗʰ **T74.62**   **Child** forced labor exploitation, confirmed   CC P PE

√5ᵗʰ **T74.9** **Unspecified maltreatment, confirmed**
     √x7ᵗʰ **T74.91**   Unspecified **adult** maltreatment, confirmed   CC A PE
     √x7ᵗʰ **T74.92**   Unspecified **child** maltreatment, confirmed   CC P PE

√5ᵗʰ **T74.A** **Financial abuse, confirmed**
     AHA: 2023,1Q,4
     √x7ᵗʰ **T74.A1**   **Adult** financial abuse, confirmed   A PE
     √x7ᵗʰ **T74.A2**   **Child** financial abuse, confirmed   P PE

√4ᵗʰ **T75** **Other and unspecified effects of other external causes**
     EXCLUDES 1   adverse effects NEC (T78.-)
     EXCLUDES 2   burns (electric) (T20-T31)

> The appropriate 7th character is to be added to each code from category T75.
> A   initial encounter
> D   subsequent encounter
> S   sequela

√5ᵗʰ **T75.0** **Effects of lightning**
     Struck by lightning
     √x7ᵗʰ **T75.00**   Unspecified effects of lightning   PE
         Struck by lightning NOS
     √x7ᵗʰ **T75.01**   Shock due to being struck by lightning   PE
     √x7ᵗʰ **T75.09**   Other effects of lightning   PE
         Use additional code for other effects of lightning

√x7ᵗʰ **T75.1** **Unspecified effects of drowning and nonfatal submersion**   CC H5 PE
     Immersion
         EXCLUDES 1   specified effects of drowning - code to effects
     AHA: 2023,1Q,25

√5ᵗʰ **T75.2** **Effects of vibration**
     √x7ᵗʰ **T75.20**   Unspecified effects of vibration   PE
     √x7ᵗʰ **T75.21**   Pneumatic hammer syndrome   PE
     √x7ᵗʰ **T75.22**   Traumatic vasospastic syndrome   PE
     √x7ᵗʰ **T75.23**   Vertigo from infrasound   PE
         EXCLUDES 1   vertigo NOS (R42)
     √x7ᵗʰ **T75.29**   Other effects of vibration   PE

√x7ᵗʰ **T75.3** **Motion sickness**   PE
     Airsickness
     Seasickness
     Travel sickness
     Use additional external cause code to identify vehicle or type of motion (Y92.81-)

√x7ᵗʰ **T75.4** **Electrocution**   PE
     Shock from electric current
     Shock from electroshock gun (taser)

√5ᵗʰ **T75.8** **Other specified effects of external causes**
     √x7ᵗʰ **T75.81**   Effects of abnormal gravitation [G] forces   PE
     √x7ᵗʰ **T75.82**   Effects of weightlessness   PE
     √x7ᵗʰ **T75.89**   Other specified effects of external causes   PE

√4ᵗʰ **T76** **Adult and child abuse, neglect and other maltreatment, suspected**
     Use additional code, if applicable, to identify any associated current injury
     EXCLUDES 1   adult and child maltreatment, confirmed (T74.-)
         suspected abuse and maltreatment in pregnancy (O9A.3-, O9A.4-, O9A.5-)
         suspected adult physical abuse, ruled out (Z04.71)
         suspected adult sexual abuse, ruled out (Z04.41)
         suspected child physical abuse, ruled out (Z04.72)
         suspected child sexual abuse, ruled out (Z04.42)
     AHA: 2018,4Q,72

> The appropriate 7th character is to be added to each code from category T76.
> A   initial encounter
> D   subsequent encounter
> S   sequela

√5ᵗʰ **T76.0** **Neglect or abandonment, suspected**
     √x7ᵗʰ **T76.01**   **Adult** neglect or abandonment, suspected   CC A PE
     √x7ᵗʰ **T76.02**   **Child** neglect or abandonment, suspected   CC P PE

√5ᵗʰ **T76.1** **Physical abuse, suspected**
     √x7ᵗʰ **T76.11**   **Adult** physical abuse, suspected   CC A PE
     √x7ᵗʰ **T76.12**   **Child** physical abuse, suspected   CC P PE
         AHA: 2019,2Q,12

√5ᵗʰ **T76.2** **Sexual abuse, suspected**
     Rape, suspected
         EXCLUDES 1   alleged abuse, ruled out (Z04.7)
     √x7ᵗʰ **T76.21**   **Adult** sexual abuse, suspected   CC A PE
     √x7ᵗʰ **T76.22**   **Child** sexual abuse, suspected   CC P PE

√5ᵗʰ **T76.3** **Psychological abuse, suspected**
     Bullying and intimidation, suspected
     Intimidation through social media, suspected
     Target of threatened harm, suspected
     Target of threatened physical violence, suspected
     Target of threatened sexual abuse, suspected
     √x7ᵗʰ **T76.31**   **Adult** psychological abuse, suspected   A PE
     √x7ᵗʰ **T76.32**   **Child** psychological abuse, suspected   CC P PE

√5ᵗʰ **T76.5** **Forced sexual exploitation, suspected**
     AHA: 2018,4Q,32-33,65
     √x7ᵗʰ **T76.51**   **Adult** forced sexual exploitation, suspected   CC A PE
     √x7ᵗʰ **T76.52**   **Child** sexual exploitation, suspected   CC P PE

√5ᵗʰ **T76.6** **Forced labor exploitation, suspected**
     AHA: 2018,4Q,32-33,65
     √x7ᵗʰ **T76.61**   **Adult** forced labor exploitation, suspected   CC A PE
     √x7ᵗʰ **T76.62**   **Child** forced labor exploitation, suspected   CC P PE

√5ᵗʰ **T76.9** **Unspecified maltreatment, suspected**
     √x7ᵗʰ **T76.91**   Unspecified **adult** maltreatment, suspected   CC A PE
     √x7ᵗʰ **T76.92**   Unspecified **child** maltreatment, suspected   CC P PE

√5ᵗʰ **T76.A** **Financial abuse, suspected**
     AHA: 2023,1Q,4
     √x7ᵗʰ **T76.A1**   **Adult** financial abuse, suspected   A PE
     √x7ᵗʰ **T76.A2**   **Child** financial abuse, suspected   P PE

√4th **T78** **Adverse effects, not elsewhere classified**

    EXCLUDES 2 *complications of surgical and medical care NEC (T80–T88)*

> The appropriate 7th character is to be added to each code from category T78.
> A   initial encounter
> D   subsequent encounter
> S   sequela

√5th **T78.0** **Anaphylactic reaction due to food**

    Anaphylactic reaction due to adverse food reaction
    Anaphylactic shock or reaction due to nonpoisonous foods
    Anaphylactoid reaction due to food

    √x7th **T78.00** **Anaphylactic reaction due to unspecified food** CC PE

    √x7th **T78.01** **Anaphylactic reaction due to peanuts** CC PE

    √x7th **T78.02** **Anaphylactic reaction due to shellfish (crustaceans)** CC PE

    √x7th **T78.03** **Anaphylactic reaction due to other fish** CC PE

    √x7th **T78.04** **Anaphylactic reaction due to fruits and vegetables** CC PE

    √x7th **T78.05** **Anaphylactic reaction due to tree nuts and seeds** CC PE

        EXCLUDES 2 *anaphylactic reaction due to peanuts (T78.01)*

    √x7th **T78.06** **Anaphylactic reaction due to food additives** CC PE

    √x7th **T78.07** **Anaphylactic reaction due to milk and dairy products** CC PE

    √x7th **T78.08** **Anaphylactic reaction due to eggs** CC PE

    √x7th **T78.09** **Anaphylactic reaction due to other food products** CC PE

√x7th **T78.1** **Other adverse food reactions, not elsewhere classified** PE

    Use additional code to identify the type of reaction, if applicable

    EXCLUDES 1 *anaphylactic reaction or shock due to adverse food reaction (T78.0-)*
                anaphylactic reaction due to food (T78.0-)
                bacterial food borne intoxications (A05.-)

    EXCLUDES 2 *allergic and dietetic gastroenteritis and colitis (K52.29)*
                allergic rhinitis due to food (J30.5)
                dermatitis due to food in contact with skin (L23.6, L24.6, L25.4)
                dermatitis due to ingested food (L27.2)
                food protein-induced enterocolitis syndrome (K52.21)
                food protein-induced enteropathy (K52.22)

√x7th **T78.2** **Anaphylactic shock, unspecified** CC PE

    Allergic shock
    Anaphylactic reaction
    Anaphylaxis

    EXCLUDES 1 *anaphylactic reaction or shock due to adverse effect of correct medicinal substance properly administered (T88.6)*
                anaphylactic reaction or shock due to adverse food reaction (T78.0-)
                anaphylactic reaction or shock due to serum (T80.5-)

√x7th **T78.3** **Angioneurotic edema** PE

    Allergic angioedema
    Giant urticaria
    Quincke's edema

    EXCLUDES 1 *serum urticaria (T80.6-)*
                urticaria (L50.-)

√5th **T78.4** **Other and unspecified allergy**

    EXCLUDES 1 *specified types of allergic reaction such as:*
                allergic diarrhea (K52.29)
                allergic gastroenteritis and colitis (K52.29)
                dermatitis (L23-L25, L27.-)
                food protein-induced enterocolitis syndrome (K52.21)
                food protein-induced enteropathy (K52.22)
                hay fever (J30.1)

    √x7th **T78.40** **Allergy, unspecified** PE

        Allergic reaction NOS
        Hypersensitivity NOS

    √x7th **T78.41** **Arthus phenomenon** PE

        Arthus reaction

    √x7th **T78.49** **Other allergy** PE

        AHA: 2021,1Q,42

√x7th **T78.8** **Other adverse effects, not elsewhere classified** PE

Certain early complications of trauma (T79)

√4th **T79** **Certain early complications of trauma, not elsewhere classified**

    EXCLUDES 2 *acute respiratory distress syndrome (J80)*
                complications occurring during or following medical procedures (T80-T88)
                complications of surgical and medical care NEC (T80-T88)
                newborn respiratory distress syndrome (P22.0)

> The appropriate 7th character is to be added to each code from category T79.
> A   initial encounter
> D   subsequent encounter
> S   sequela

√x7th **T79.0** **Air embolism (traumatic)** MCC HCC PE

    EXCLUDES 1 *air embolism complicating abortion or ectopic or molar pregnancy (O00-O07, O08.2)*
                air embolism complicating pregnancy, childbirth and the puerperium (O88.0)
                air embolism following infusion, transfusion, and therapeutic injection (T80.0)
                air embolism following procedure NEC (T81.7-)

    DEF: Arterial or venous obstruction due to the introduction of air bubbles into the blood vessels following surgery or trauma.

√x7th **T79.1** **Fat embolism (traumatic)** MCC HCC PE

    EXCLUDES 1 *fat embolism complicating:*
                abortion or ectopic or molar pregnancy (O00-O07, O08.2)
                pregnancy, childbirth and the puerperium (O88.8)

    DEF: Arterial blockage due to the entrance of fat into the circulatory system after a fracture of the large bones or administration of corticosteroids.

√x7th **T79.2** **Traumatic secondary and recurrent hemorrhage and seroma** CC PE

√x7th **T79.4** **Traumatic shock** MCC HCC PE

    Shock (immediate) (delayed) following injury

    EXCLUDES 1 *anaphylactic shock due to adverse food reaction (T78.0-)*
                anaphylactic shock due to correct medicinal substance properly administered (T88.6)
                anaphylactic shock due to serum (T80.5-)
                anaphylactic shock NOS (T78.2)
                electric shock (T75.4)
                nontraumatic shock NEC (R57.-)
                obstetric shock (O75.1)
                postprocedural shock (T81.1-)
                septic shock (R65.21)
                shock complicating abortion or ectopic or molar pregnancy (O00-O07, O08.3)
                shock due to anesthesia (T88.2)
                shock due to lightning (T75.01)
                shock NOS (R57.9)

√x7th **T79.5** **Traumatic anuria** MCC PE

    Crush syndrome
    Renal failure following crushing

√x7th **T79.6** **Traumatic ischemia of muscle** PE

    Traumatic rhabdomyolysis
    Volkmann's ischemic contracture

    EXCLUDES 2 *anterior tibial syndrome (M76.8)*
                compartment syndrome (traumatic) (T79.A-)
                nontraumatic ischemia of muscle (M62.2-)

    AHA: 2019,2Q,12

√x7th **T79.7** **Traumatic subcutaneous emphysema** CC PE

    EXCLUDES 2 *emphysema NOS (J43)*
                emphysema (subcutaneous) resulting from a procedure (T81.82)

☑ Additional Character Required   √x7th Placeholder   Questionable PDx   Manifestation   Unspecified   UPD Unacceptable PDx   H1-H14 HAC   HCC CMS-HCC Dx   HIV HIV Dx

ICD-10-CM 2025   1173

Chapter 19. Injury, Poisoning and Certain Other Consequences of External Causes

✓5ᵗʰ **T79.A Traumatic compartment syndrome**

EXCLUDES 1 fibromyalgia (M79.7)
nontraumatic compartment syndrome (M79.A-)

EXCLUDES 2 traumatic ischemic infarction of muscle (T79.6)

DEF: Compression of nerves and blood vessels within an enclosed muscle space due to previous trauma, which leads to impaired blood flow and muscle and nerve damage.

✓x7ᵗʰ **T79.A0 Compartment syndrome, unspecified** CC PE
Compartment syndrome NOS

✓6ᵗʰ **T79.A1 Traumatic compartment syndrome of upper extremity**
Traumatic compartment syndrome of shoulder, arm, forearm, wrist, hand, and fingers

✓7ᵗʰ **T79.A11 Traumatic compartment syndrome of right upper extremity** CC PE

✓7ᵗʰ **T79.A12 Traumatic compartment syndrome of left upper extremity** CC PE

✓7ᵗʰ **T79.A19 Traumatic compartment syndrome of unspecified upper extremity** CC UNS PE

✓6ᵗʰ **T79.A2 Traumatic compartment syndrome of lower extremity**
Traumatic compartment syndrome of hip, buttock, thigh, leg, foot, and toes

✓7ᵗʰ **T79.A21 Traumatic compartment syndrome of right lower extremity** CC PE

✓7ᵗʰ **T79.A22 Traumatic compartment syndrome of left lower extremity** CC PE

✓7ᵗʰ **T79.A29 Traumatic compartment syndrome of unspecified lower extremity** CC UNS PE

✓x7ᵗʰ **T79.A3 Traumatic compartment syndrome of abdomen** CC PE

✓x7ᵗʰ **T79.A9 Traumatic compartment syndrome of other sites** CC PE

✓x7ᵗʰ **T79.8 Other early complications of trauma** PE

✓x7ᵗʰ **T79.9 Unspecified early complication of trauma** PE

Complications of surgical and medical care, not elsewhere classified (T80-T88)

Use additional code for adverse effect, if applicable, to identify drug (T36-T50 with fifth or sixth character 5)
Use additional code(s) to identify the specified condition resulting from the complication
Use additional code to identify devices involved and details of circumstances (Y62-Y82)

EXCLUDES 2 any encounters with medical care for postprocedural conditions in which no complications are present, such as:
artificial opening status (Z93.-)
closure of external stoma (Z43.-)
fitting and adjustment of external prosthetic device (Z44.-)
burns and corrosions from local applications and irradiation (T20-T32)
complications of surgical procedures during pregnancy, childbirth and the puerperium (O00-O9A)
mechanical complication of respirator [ventilator] (J95.850)
poisoning and toxic effects of drugs and chemicals (T36-T65 with fifth or sixth character 1-4 or 6)
postprocedural fever (R50.82)
specified complications classified elsewhere, such as:
cerebrospinal fluid leak from spinal puncture (G97.0)
colostomy malfunction (K94.0-)
disorders of fluid and electrolyte imbalance (E86-E87)
functional disturbances following cardiac surgery (I97.0-I97.1)
intraoperative and postprocedural complications of specified body systems (D78.-, E36.-, E89.-, G97.3-, G97.4, H59.3-, H59.-, H95.2-, H95.3, I97.4-, I97.5, J95.6-, J95.7, K91.6-, L76.-, M96.-, N99.-)
ostomy complications (J95.0-, K94.-, N99.5-)
postgastric surgery syndromes (K91.1)
postlaminectomy syndrome NEC (M96.1)
postmastectomy lymphedema syndrome (I97.2)
postsurgical blind-loop syndrome (K91.2)
ventilator associated pneumonia (J95.851)

AHA: 2015,1Q,15

✓4ᵗʰ **T80 Complications following infusion, transfusion and therapeutic injection**

INCLUDES complications following perfusion

EXCLUDES 2 bone marrow transplant rejection (T86.01)
febrile nonhemolytic transfusion reaction (R50.84)
fluid overload due to transfusion (E87.71)
posttransfusion purpura (D69.51)
transfusion associated circulatory overload (TACO) (E87.71)
transfusion (red blood cell) associated hemochromatosis (E83.111)
transfusion related acute lung injury (TRALI) (J95.84)

The appropriate 7th character is to be added to each code from category T80.
A initial encounter
D subsequent encounter
S sequela

✓x7ᵗʰ **T80.0 Air embolism following infusion, transfusion and therapeutic injection** MCC H2 PE

✓x7ᵗʰ **T80.1 Vascular complications following infusion, transfusion and therapeutic injection** CC PE
Use additional code to identify the vascular complication

EXCLUDES 2 extravasation of vesicant agent (T80.81-)
infiltration of vesicant agent (T80.81-)
postprocedural vascular complications (T81.7-)
vascular complications specified as due to prosthetic devices, implants and grafts (T82.8-, T83.8-, T84.8-, T85.8-)

√5th T80.2 Infections following infusion, transfusion and therapeutic injection

Use additional code to identify the specific infection, such as: sepsis (A41.9)

Use additional code (R65.2-) to identify severe sepsis, if applicable

EXCLUDES 2   infections specified as due to prosthetic devices, implants and grafts (T82.6-T82.7, T83.5-T83.6, T84.5-T84.7, T85.7)
postprocedural infections (T81.4-)

AHA: 2018,4Q,62

√6th T80.21 Infection due to central venous catheter

Infection due to pulmonary artery catheter (Swan-Ganz catheter)

AHA: 2019,1Q,13-14

DEF: Central venous catheter: Catheter positioned in the superior vena cava or right atrium and introduced through a large vein, such as the jugular or subclavian, and used to measure venous pressure or administer fluids or medication.

TIP: Code assignment is based on the location of the catheter and not how the catheter is being used; for example, for hemodialysis. Infections resulting from catheters that are not central lines should be coded to T82.7-.

√7th T80.211 Bloodstream infection due to central venous catheter CC H7 PE

Catheter-related bloodstream infection (CRBSI) NOS

Central line-associated bloodstream infection (CLABSI)

Bloodstream infection due to Hickman catheter

Bloodstream infection due to peripherally inserted central catheter (PICC)

Bloodstream infection due to portacath (port-a-cath)

Bloodstream infection due to pulmonary artery catheter

Bloodstream infection due to triple lumen catheter

Bloodstream infection due to umbilical venous catheter

AHA: 2019,1Q,13,14; 2018,4Q,89

√7th T80.212 Local infection due to central venous catheter CC H7 PE

Exit or insertion site infection

Local infection due to Hickman catheter

Local infection due to peripherally inserted central catheter (PICC)

Local infection due to portacath (port-a-cath)

Local infection due to pulmonary artery catheter

Local infection due to triple lumen catheter

Local infection due to umbilical venous catheter

Port or reservoir infection

Tunnel infection

√7th T80.218 Other infection due to central venous catheter CC H7 PE

Other central line-associated infection

Other infection due to Hickman catheter

Other infection due to peripherally inserted central catheter (PICC)

Other infection due to portacath (port-a-cath)

Other infection due to pulmonary artery catheter

Other infection due to triple lumen catheter

Other infection due to umbilical venous catheter

√7th T80.219 Unspecified infection due to central venous catheter CC H7 PE

Central line-associated infection NOS

Unspecified infection due to Hickman catheter

Unspecified infection due to peripherally inserted central catheter (PICC)

Unspecified infection due to portacath (port-a-cath)

Unspecified infection due to pulmonary artery catheter

Unspecified infection due to triple lumen catheter

Unspecified infection due to umbilical venous catheter

√x7th T80.22 Acute infection following transfusion, infusion, or injection of blood and blood products CC PE

√x7th T80.29 Infection following other infusion, transfusion and therapeutic injection CC PE

√5th T80.3 ABO incompatibility reaction due to transfusion of blood or blood products

EXCLUDES 1   minor blood group antigens reactions (Duffy) (E) (K) (Kell) (Kidd) (Lewis) (M) (N) (P) (S) (T80.A-)

√x7th T80.30 ABO incompatibility reaction due to transfusion of blood or blood products, unspecified CC H3 PE

ABO incompatibility blood transfusion NOS

Reaction to ABO incompatibility from transfusion NOS

√6th T80.31 ABO incompatibility with hemolytic transfusion reaction

√7th T80.310 ABO incompatibility with acute hemolytic transfusion reaction CC H3 PE

ABO incompatibility with hemolytic transfusion reaction less than 24 hours after transfusion

Acute hemolytic transfusion reaction (AHTR) due to ABO incompatibility

√7th T80.311 ABO incompatibility with delayed hemolytic transfusion reaction CC H3 PE

ABO incompatibility with hemolytic transfusion reaction 24 hours or more after transfusion

Delayed hemolytic transfusion reaction (DHTR) due to ABO incompatibility

√7th T80.319 ABO incompatibility with hemolytic transfusion reaction, unspecified CC H3 PE

ABO incompatibility with hemolytic transfusion reaction at unspecified time after transfusion

Hemolytic transfusion reaction (HTR) due to ABO incompatibility NOS

√x7th T80.39 Other ABO incompatibility reaction due to transfusion of blood or blood products CC H3 PE

Delayed serologic transfusion reaction (DSTR) from ABO incompatibility

Other ABO incompatible blood transfusion

Other reaction to ABO incompatible blood transfusion

√5th T80.4 Rh incompatibility reaction due to transfusion of blood or blood products

Reaction due to incompatibility of Rh antigens (C) (c) (D) (E) (e)

√x7th T80.40 Rh incompatibility reaction due to transfusion of blood or blood products, unspecified CC PE

Reaction due to Rh factor in transfusion NOS

Rh incompatible blood transfusion NOS

√6th T80.41 Rh incompatibility with hemolytic transfusion reaction

√7th T80.410 Rh incompatibility with acute hemolytic transfusion reaction CC PE

Acute hemolytic transfusion reaction (AHTR) due to Rh incompatibility

Rh incompatibility with hemolytic transfusion reaction less than 24 hours after transfusion

√7th T80.411 Rh incompatibility with delayed hemolytic transfusion reaction CC PE

Delayed hemolytic transfusion reaction (DHTR) due to Rh incompatibility

Rh incompatibility with hemolytic transfusion reaction 24 hours or more after transfusion

Chapter 19. Injury, Poisoning and Certain Other Consequences of External Causes

T80.2–T80.411

✓7th **T80.419 Rh incompatibility with hemolytic transfusion reaction, unspecified** CC PE

Rh incompatibility with hemolytic transfusion reaction at unspecified time after transfusion

Hemolytic transfusion reaction (HTR) due to Rh incompatibility NOS

✓x7th **T80.49 Other Rh incompatibility reaction due to transfusion of blood or blood products** CC PE

Delayed serologic transfusion reaction (DSTR) from Rh incompatibility

Other reaction to Rh incompatible blood transfusion

✓5th **T80.A Non-ABO incompatibility reaction due to transfusion of blood or blood products**

Reaction due to incompatibility of minor antigens (Duffy) (Kell) (Kidd) (Lewis) (M) (N) (P) (S)

✓x7th **T80.A0 Non-ABO incompatibility reaction due to transfusion of blood or blood products, unspecified** CC PE

Non-ABO antigen incompatibility reaction from transfusion NOS

✓6th **T80.A1 Non-ABO incompatibility with hemolytic transfusion reaction**

✓7th **T80.A10 Non-ABO incompatibility with acute hemolytic transfusion reaction** CC PE

Acute hemolytic transfusion reaction (AHTR) due to non-ABO incompatibility

Non-ABO incompatibility with hemolytic transfusion reaction less than 24 hours after transfusion

✓7th **T80.A11 Non-ABO incompatibility with delayed hemolytic transfusion reaction** CC PE

Delayed hemolytic transfusion reaction (DHTR) due to non-ABO incompatibility

Non-ABO incompatibility with hemolytic transfusion reaction 24 or more hours after transfusion

✓7th **T80.A19 Non-ABO incompatibility with hemolytic transfusion reaction, unspecified** CC PE

Hemolytic transfusion reaction (HTR) due to non-ABO incompatibility NOS

Non-ABO incompatibility with hemolytic transfusion reaction at unspecified time after transfusion

✓x7th **T80.A9 Other non-ABO incompatibility reaction due to transfusion of blood or blood products** CC PE

Delayed serologic transfusion reaction (DSTR) from non-ABO incompatibility

Other reaction to non-ABO incompatible blood transfusion

✓5th **T80.5 Anaphylactic reaction due to serum**

Allergic shock due to serum
Anaphylactic shock due to serum
Anaphylactoid reaction due to serum
Anaphylaxis due to serum

EXCLUDES 1   ABO incompatibility reaction due to transfusion of blood or blood products (T80.3-)

allergic reaction or shock NOS (T78.2)

anaphylactic reaction or shock NOS (T78.2)

anaphylactic reaction or shock due to adverse effect of correct medicinal substance properly administered (T88.6)

other serum reaction (T80.6-)

DEF: Life-threatening hypersensitivity to a foreign serum causing respiratory distress, vascular collapse, and shock.

✓x7th **T80.51 Anaphylactic reaction due to administration of blood and blood products** CC PE

✓x7th **T80.52 Anaphylactic reaction due to vaccination** CC PE

AHA: 2021,1Q,43

✓x7th **T80.59 Anaphylactic reaction due to other serum** CC PE

✓5th **T80.6 Other serum reactions**

Intoxication by serum
Protein sickness
Serum rash
Serum sickness
Serum urticaria

EXCLUDES 2   serum hepatitis (B16-B19)

DEF: Serum sickness: Hypersensitivity to a foreign serum that causes fever, hives, swelling, and lymphadenopathy.

✓x7th **T80.61 Other serum reaction due to administration of blood and blood products** CC PE

✓x7th **T80.62 Other serum reaction due to vaccination** CC PE

AHA: 2021,1Q,42

✓x7th **T80.69 Other serum reaction due to other serum** CC PE

Code also, if applicable, arthropathy in hypersensitivity reactions classified elsewhere (M36.4)

✓5th **T80.8 Other complications following infusion, transfusion and therapeutic injection**

✓6th **T80.81 Extravasation of vesicant agent**

Infiltration of vesicant agent

✓7th **T80.810 Extravasation of vesicant antineoplastic chemotherapy** CC PE

Infiltration of vesicant antineoplastic chemotherapy

✓7th **T80.818 Extravasation of other vesicant agent** CC PE

Infiltration of other vesicant agent

✓x7th **T80.82 Complication of immune effector cellular therapy** PE

Complication of chimeric antigen receptor (CAR-T) cell therapy

Complication of IEC therapy

Use additional code to identify the specific complication, such as:

cytokine release syndrome (D89.83-)

immune effector cell-associated neurotoxicity syndrome (G92.0-)

EXCLUDES 2   ▶adverse effect of immune checkpoint inhibitors and immunostimulant drugs (T45.AX5)◀

complication of bone marrow transplant (T86.0)

complication of stem cell transplant (T86.5)

AHA: 2021,4Q,31

✓x7th **T80.89 Other complications following infusion, transfusion and therapeutic injection** PE

Delayed serologic transfusion reaction (DSTR), unspecified incompatibility

Use additional code to identify graft-versus-host reaction, if applicable, (D89.81-)

AHA: 2020,4Q,14

✓5th **T80.9 Unspecified complication following infusion, transfusion and therapeutic injection**

✓x7th **T80.90 Unspecified complication following infusion and therapeutic injection** PE

✓6th **T80.91 Hemolytic transfusion reaction, unspecified incompatibility**

EXCLUDES 1   ABO incompatibility with hemolytic transfusion reaction (T80.31-)

non-ABO incompatibility with hemolytic transfusion reaction (T80.A1-)

Rh incompatibility with hemolytic transfusion reaction (T80.41-)

✓7th **T80.910 Acute hemolytic transfusion reaction, unspecified incompatibility** CC PE

✓7th **T80.911 Delayed hemolytic transfusion reaction, unspecified incompatibility** CC PE

✓7th **T80.919 Hemolytic transfusion reaction, unspecified incompatibility, unspecified as acute or delayed** CC PE

Hemolytic transfusion reaction NOS

✓x7th **T80.92 Unspecified transfusion reaction** PE

Transfusion reaction NOS

N Newborn: 0   P Pediatric: 0-17   M Maternity: 9-64   A Adult: 15-124   UNS Unspecified Site   MCC Major Complication/Comorbidity   CC Complication/Comorbidity   PE POA Exempt

1176   ICD-10-CM 2025

✓4ᵗʰ T81 Complications of procedures, not elsewhere classified

Use additional code for adverse effect, if applicable, to identify drug (T36-T50 with fifth or sixth character 5)

EXCLUDES 2   *complications following immunization (T88.0-T88.1)*
complications following infusion, transfusion and therapeutic injection (T80.-)
complications of transplanted organs and tissue (T86.-)
specified complications classified elsewhere, such as:
   complication of prosthetic devices, implants and grafts (T82-T85)
   dermatitis due to drugs and medicaments (L23.3, L24.4, L25.1, L27.0-L27.1)
   endosseous dental implant failure (M27.6-)
   floppy iris syndrome (IFIS) (intraoperative) (H21.81)
   intraoperative and postprocedural complications of specific body system (D78.-, E36.-, E89.-, G97.3-, G97.4, H59.3-, H59.-, H95.2-, H95.3, I97.4-, I97.5, J95, K91.-, L76.-, M96.-, N99.-)
   ostomy complications (J95.0-, K94.-, N99.5-)
   plateau iris syndrome (post-iridectomy) (postprocedural) H21.82
   poisoning and toxic effects of drugs and chemicals (T36-T65 with fifth or sixth character 1-4)

AHA: 2019,2Q,21

The appropriate 7th character is to be added to each code from category T81.
- A   initial encounter
- D   subsequent encounter
- S   sequela

✓5ᵗʰ T81.1 Postprocedural shock

Shock during or resulting from a procedure, not elsewhere classified

EXCLUDES 1   *anaphylactic shock NOS (T78.2)*
anaphylactic shock due to correct substance properly administered (T88.6)
anaphylactic shock due to serum (T80.5-)
electric shock (T75.4)
obstetric shock (O75.1)
shock due to anesthesia (T88.2)
shock following abortion or ectopic or molar pregnancy (O00-O07, O08.3)
traumatic shock (T79.4)

AHA: 2021,1Q,13

✓x7ᵗʰ T81.10 Postprocedural shock unspecified   CC PE

Collapse NOS during or resulting from a procedure, not elsewhere classified
Postprocedural failure of peripheral circulation
Postprocedural shock NOS

✓x7ᵗʰ T81.11 Postprocedural cardiogenic shock   MCC PE

✓x7ᵗʰ T81.12 Postprocedural septic shock   MCC UPD PE

Postprocedural endotoxic shock resulting from a procedure, not elsewhere classified
Postprocedural gram-negative shock resulting from a procedure, not elsewhere classified

Code first underlying infection
Use additional code, to identify any associated acute organ dysfunction, if applicable

AHA: 2018,4Q,63

✓x7ᵗʰ T81.19 Other postprocedural shock   MCC PE

Postprocedural hypovolemic shock

✓5ᵗʰ T81.3 Disruption of wound, not elsewhere classified

Disruption of any suture materials or other closure methods

EXCLUDES 1   *breakdown (mechanical) of permanent sutures (T85.612)*
displacement of permanent sutures (T85.622)
disruption of cesarean delivery wound (O90.0)
disruption of perineal obstetric wound (O90.1)
mechanical complication of permanent sutures NEC (T85.692)

AHA: 2014,1Q,23

✓x7ᵗʰ T81.30 Disruption of wound, unspecified   CC PE

Disruption of wound NOS

✓x7ᵗʰ T81.31 Disruption of external operation (surgical) wound, not elsewhere classified   CC PE

Dehiscence of operation wound NOS
Disruption of operation wound NOS
Disruption or dehiscence of closure of cornea
Disruption or dehiscence of closure of mucosa
Disruption or dehiscence of closure of skin and subcutaneous tissue
Full-thickness skin disruption or dehiscence
Superficial disruption or dehiscence of operation wound

EXCLUDES 1   *dehiscence of amputation stump (T87.81)*

✓6ᵗʰ T81.32 Disruption of internal operation (surgical) wound, not elsewhere classified

~~Deep disruption or dehiscence of operation wound NOS~~
~~Disruption or dehiscence of closure of internal organ or other internal tissue~~
~~Disruption or dehiscence of closure of muscle or muscle flap~~
~~Disruption or dehiscence of closure of ribs or rib cage~~
~~Disruption or dehiscence of closure of skull or craniotomy~~
~~Disruption or dehiscence of closure of sternum or sternotomy~~
~~Disruption or dehiscence of closure of tendon or ligament~~
~~Disruption or dehiscence of closure of superficial or muscular fascia~~

AHA: 2020,2Q,22; 2017,3Q,4

✓7ᵗʰ T81.320 Disruption or dehiscence of gastrointestinal tract anastomosis, repair, or closure   CC PE

✓7ᵗʰ T81.321 Disruption or dehiscence of closure of internal operation (surgical) wound of abdominal wall muscle or fascia   CC PE

✓7ᵗʰ T81.328 Disruption or dehiscence of closure of other specified internal operation (surgical) wound   CC PE

Disruption or dehiscence of closure of muscle or muscle flap (other than abdominal wall muscle)
Disruption or dehiscence of closure of ribs or rib cage
Disruption or dehiscence of closure of skull or craniotomy
Disruption or dehiscence of closure of sternum or sternotomy
Disruption or dehiscence of closure of tendon or ligament
Disruption or dehiscence of closure of superficial or muscular fascia (other than abdominal wall fascia)

✓7ᵗʰ T81.329 Deep disruption or dehiscence of operation wound, unspecified   CC PE

Deep disruption or dehiscence of operation wound NOS

✓x7ᵗʰ T81.33 Disruption of traumatic injury wound repair   CC PE

Disruption or dehiscence of closure of traumatic laceration (external) (internal)

✓5ᵗʰ T81.4 Infection following a procedure

Wound abscess following a procedure
▶Code also, if applicable, disruption of internal operation (surgical) wound (T81.32-)◀
Use additional code to identify infection
Use additional code (R65.2-) to identify severe sepsis, if applicable

EXCLUDES 2   *bleb associated endophthalmitis (H59.4-)*
infection due to infusion, transfusion and therapeutic injection (T80.2-)
infection due to prosthetic devices, implants and grafts (T82.6-T82.7, T83.5-T83.6, T84.5-T84.7, T85.7)
obstetric surgical wound infection (O86.0-)
postprocedural fever NOS (R50.82)
postprocedural retroperitoneal abscess (K68.11)

AHA: 2024,1Q,19; 2018,4Q,33-34,62; 2014,1Q,23

✓x7ᵗʰ T81.40 Infection following a procedure, unspecified   CC H11 H12 H13 PE

✓x7ᵗʰ T81.41 Infection following a procedure, superficial incisional surgical site   CC H11 H12 H13 PE

Subcutaneous abscess following a procedure
Stitch abscess following a procedure

✓ Additional Character Required   ✓x7ᵗʰ Placeholder   Questionable PDx   Manifestation   Unspecified   **UPD** Unacceptable PDx   H1-H14 HAC   HCC CMS-HCC Dx   HIV HIV Dx

✓x 7ᵗʰ T81.42 Infection following a procedure, deep incisional surgical site `CC` `H11` `H12` `H13` `PE`

Intra-muscular abscess following a procedure

✓x 7ᵗʰ T81.43 Infection following a procedure, organ and space surgical site `CC` `H11` `H12` `H13` `PE`

Intra-abdominal abscess following a procedure

Subphrenic abscess following a procedure

✓x 7ᵗʰ T81.44 Sepsis following a procedure `CC` `H11` `H12` `H13` `PE`

Use additional code to identify the sepsis

✓x 7ᵗʰ T81.49 Infection following a procedure, other surgical site `CC` `H11` `H12` `H13` `PE`

✓5ᵗʰ T81.5 Complications of foreign body accidentally left in body following procedure

AHA: 2014,4Q,24

  ✓6ᵗʰ T81.50 Unspecified complication of foreign body accidentally left in body following procedure

    ✓7ᵗʰ T81.500 Unspecified complication of foreign body accidentally left in body following surgical operation `CC` `H1` `PE`

    ✓7ᵗʰ T81.501 Unspecified complication of foreign body accidentally left in body following infusion or transfusion `CC` `H1` `PE`

    ✓7ᵗʰ T81.502 Unspecified complication of foreign body accidentally left in body following kidney dialysis `CC` `H1` `PE`

    ✓7ᵗʰ T81.503 Unspecified complication of foreign body accidentally left in body following injection or immunization `CC` `H1` `PE`

    ✓7ᵗʰ T81.504 Unspecified complication of foreign body accidentally left in body following endoscopic examination `CC` `H1` `PE`

    ✓7ᵗʰ T81.505 Unspecified complication of foreign body accidentally left in body following heart catheterization `CC` `H1` `PE`

    ✓7ᵗʰ T81.506 Unspecified complication of foreign body accidentally left in body following aspiration, puncture or other catheterization `CC` `H1` `PE`

    ✓7ᵗʰ T81.507 Unspecified complication of foreign body accidentally left in body following removal of catheter or packing `H1` `PE`

    ✓7ᵗʰ T81.508 Unspecified complication of foreign body accidentally left in body following other procedure `CC` `H1` `PE`

    ✓7ᵗʰ T81.509 Unspecified complication of foreign body accidentally left in body following unspecified procedure `CC` `H1` `PE`

  ✓6ᵗʰ T81.51 Adhesions due to foreign body accidentally left in body following procedure

    ✓7ᵗʰ T81.510 Adhesions due to foreign body accidentally left in body following surgical operation `CC` `H1` `PE`

    ✓7ᵗʰ T81.511 Adhesions due to foreign body accidentally left in body following infusion or transfusion `H1` `PE`

    ✓7ᵗʰ T81.512 Adhesions due to foreign body accidentally left in body following kidney dialysis `CC` `H1` `PE`

    ✓7ᵗʰ T81.513 Adhesions due to foreign body accidentally left in body following injection or immunization `CC` `H1` `PE`

    ✓7ᵗʰ T81.514 Adhesions due to foreign body accidentally left in body following endoscopic examination `CC` `H1` `PE`

    ✓7ᵗʰ T81.515 Adhesions due to foreign body accidentally left in body following heart catheterization `CC` `H1` `PE`

    ✓7ᵗʰ T81.516 Adhesions due to foreign body accidentally left in body following aspiration, puncture or other catheterization `CC` `H1` `PE`

    ✓7ᵗʰ T81.517 Adhesions due to foreign body accidentally left in body following removal of catheter or packing `CC` `H1` `PE`

    ✓7ᵗʰ T81.518 Adhesions due to foreign body accidentally left in body following other procedure `CC` `H1` `PE`

    ✓7ᵗʰ T81.519 Adhesions due to foreign body accidentally left in body following unspecified procedure `CC` `H1` `PE`

✓6ᵗʰ T81.52 Obstruction due to foreign body accidentally left in body following procedure

  ✓7ᵗʰ T81.520 Obstruction due to foreign body accidentally left in body following surgical operation `CC` `H1` `PE`

  ✓7ᵗʰ T81.521 Obstruction due to foreign body accidentally left in body following infusion or transfusion `CC` `H1` `PE`

  ✓7ᵗʰ T81.522 Obstruction due to foreign body accidentally left in body following kidney dialysis `CC` `H1` `PE`

  ✓7ᵗʰ T81.523 Obstruction due to foreign body accidentally left in body following injection or immunization `CC` `H1` `PE`

  ✓7ᵗʰ T81.524 Obstruction due to foreign body accidentally left in body following endoscopic examination `CC` `H1` `PE`

  ✓7ᵗʰ T81.525 Obstruction due to foreign body accidentally left in body following heart catheterization `CC` `H1` `PE`

  ✓7ᵗʰ T81.526 Obstruction due to foreign body accidentally left in body following aspiration, puncture or other catheterization `CC` `H1` `PE`

  ✓7ᵗʰ T81.527 Obstruction due to foreign body accidentally left in body following removal of catheter or packing `CC` `H1` `PE`

  ✓7ᵗʰ T81.528 Obstruction due to foreign body accidentally left in body following other procedure `CC` `H1` `PE`

  ✓7ᵗʰ T81.529 Obstruction due to foreign body accidentally left in body following unspecified procedure `CC` `H1` `PE`

✓6ᵗʰ T81.53 Perforation due to foreign body accidentally left in body following procedure

  ✓7ᵗʰ T81.530 Perforation due to foreign body accidentally left in body following surgical operation `CC` `H1` `PE`

  ✓7ᵗʰ T81.531 Perforation due to foreign body accidentally left in body following infusion or transfusion `CC` `H1` `PE`

  ✓7ᵗʰ T81.532 Perforation due to foreign body accidentally left in body following kidney dialysis `CC` `H1` `PE`

  ✓7ᵗʰ T81.533 Perforation due to foreign body accidentally left in body following injection or immunization `CC` `H1` `PE`

  ✓7ᵗʰ T81.534 Perforation due to foreign body accidentally left in body following endoscopic examination `CC` `H1` `PE`

  ✓7ᵗʰ T81.535 Perforation due to foreign body accidentally left in body following heart catheterization `CC` `H1` `PE`

  ✓7ᵗʰ T81.536 Perforation due to foreign body accidentally left in body following aspiration, puncture or other catheterization `CC` `H1` `PE`

  ✓7ᵗʰ T81.537 Perforation due to foreign body accidentally left in body following removal of catheter or packing `CC` `H1` `PE`

  ✓7ᵗʰ T81.538 Perforation due to foreign body accidentally left in body following other procedure `CC` `H1` `PE`

  ✓7ᵗʰ T81.539 Perforation due to foreign body accidentally left in body following unspecified procedure `CC` `H1` `PE`

✓6ᵗʰ T81.59 Other complications of foreign body accidentally left in body following procedure

EXCLUDES 2   obstruction or perforation due to prosthetic devices and implants intentionally left in body (T82.0-T82.5, T83.0-T83.4, T83.7, T84.0-T84.4, T85.0-T85.6)

  ✓7ᵗʰ T81.590 Other complications of foreign body accidentally left in body following surgical operation `CC` `H1` `PE`

  ✓7ᵗʰ T81.591 Other complications of foreign body accidentally left in body following infusion or transfusion `CC` `H1` `PE`

  ✓7ᵗʰ T81.592 Other complications of foreign body accidentally left in body following kidney dialysis `CC` `H1` `PE`

`N` Newborn: 0   `P` Pediatric: 0-17   `M` Maternity: 9-64   `A` Adult: 15-124   `UNS` Unspecified Site   `MCC` Major Complication/Comorbidity   `CC` Complication/Comorbidity   `PE` POA Exempt

1178

ICD-10-CM 2025

√7ᵗʰ **T81.593** **Other complications of foreign body accidentally left in body following injection or immunization** `CC` `H1` `PE`

√7ᵗʰ **T81.594** **Other complications of foreign body accidentally left in body following endoscopic examination** `CC` `H1` `PE`

√7ᵗʰ **T81.595** **Other complications of foreign body accidentally left in body following heart catheterization** `CC` `H1` `PE`

√7ᵗʰ **T81.596** **Other complications of foreign body accidentally left in body following aspiration, puncture or other catheterization** `CC` `H1` `PE`

√7ᵗʰ **T81.597** **Other complications of foreign body accidentally left in body following removal of catheter or packing** `CC` `H1` `PE`

√7ᵗʰ **T81.598** **Other complications of foreign body accidentally left in body following other procedure** `CC` `H1` `PE`

√7ᵗʰ **T81.599** **Other complications of foreign body accidentally left in body following unspecified procedure** `CC` `H1` `PE`

√5ᵗʰ **T81.6** **Acute reaction to foreign substance accidentally left during a procedure**

> **EXCLUDES 2**   *complications of foreign body accidentally left in body cavity or operation wound following procedure (T81.5-)*

√7ᵗʰ **T81.60** **Unspecified acute reaction to foreign substance accidentally left during a procedure** `CC` `H1` `PE`

√7ᵗʰ **T81.61** **Aseptic peritonitis due to foreign substance accidentally left during a procedure** `CC` `H1` `PE`
Chemical peritonitis

√7ᵗʰ **T81.69** **Other acute reaction to foreign substance accidentally left during a procedure** `CC` `H1` `PE`

√5ᵗʰ **T81.7** **Vascular complications following a procedure, not elsewhere classified**
Air embolism following procedure NEC
Phlebitis or thrombophlebitis resulting from a procedure

> **EXCLUDES 1**   *embolism complicating abortion or ectopic or molar pregnancy (O00-O07, O08.2)*
> *embolism complicating pregnancy, childbirth and the puerperium (O88.-)*
> *traumatic embolism (T79.0)*

> **EXCLUDES 2**   *embolism due to prosthetic devices, implants and grafts (T82.8-, T83.81, T84.8-, T85.81-)*
> *embolism following infusion, transfusion and therapeutic injection (T80.0)*

AHA: 2019,2Q,22

√6ᵗʰ **T81.71** **Complication of artery following a procedure, not elsewhere classified**

√7ᵗʰ **T81.710** **Complication of mesenteric artery following a procedure, not elsewhere classified** `CC` `PE`

√7ᵗʰ **T81.711** **Complication of renal artery following a procedure, not elsewhere classified** `CC` `PE`

√7ᵗʰ **T81.718** **Complication of other artery following a procedure, not elsewhere classified** `CC` `PE`
AHA: 2019,2Q,21-22

√7ᵗʰ **T81.719** **Complication of unspecified artery following a procedure, not elsewhere classified** `CC` `PE`

√7ᵗʰ **T81.72** **Complication of vein following a procedure, not elsewhere classified** `CC` `PE`

√5ᵗʰ **T81.8** **Other complications of procedures, not elsewhere classified**

> **EXCLUDES 2**   *hypothermia following anesthesia (T88.51)*
> *malignant hyperpyrexia due to anesthesia (T88.3)*

√7ᵗʰ **T81.81** **Complication of inhalation therapy** `PE`

√7ᵗʰ **T81.82** **Emphysema (subcutaneous) resulting from a procedure** `PE`

√7ᵗʰ **T81.83** **Persistent postprocedural fistula** `CC` `PE`
> ▶Code also, if applicable, disruption of internal operation (surgical) wound (T81.32-)◀
> Use additional code, if known, for site of fistula such as:
> anal fistula ▶(K60.3-)◀
> anorectal fistula ▶(K60.5-)◀
> bladder fistula (N32.2)
> other female intestinal-genital tract fistulae (N82.4)

AHA: 2023,1Q,30; 2017,3Q,3-4

√7ᵗʰ **T81.89** **Other complications of procedures, not elsewhere classified** `PE`
> Use additional code to specify complication, such as:
> postprocedural delirium (F05)

AHA: 2014,1Q,23

√7ᵗʰ **T81.9** **Unspecified complication of procedure** `PE`

√4ᵗʰ **T82** **Complications of cardiac and vascular prosthetic devices, implants and grafts**

> **EXCLUDES 2**   *failure and rejection of transplanted organs and tissue (T86.-)*

AHA: 2020,3Q,36-37

> The appropriate 7th character is to be added to each code from category T82.
> A   initial encounter
> D   subsequent encounter
> S   sequela

√5ᵗʰ **T82.0** **Mechanical complication of heart valve prosthesis**
Mechanical complication of artificial heart valve

> **EXCLUDES 1**   *mechanical complication of biological heart valve graft (T82.22-)*

√7ᵗʰ **T82.01** **Breakdown (mechanical) of heart valve prosthesis** `CC` `PE`

√7ᵗʰ **T82.02** **Displacement of heart valve prosthesis** `CC` `PE`
Malposition of heart valve prosthesis

√7ᵗʰ **T82.03** **Leakage of heart valve prosthesis** `CC` `PE`

√7ᵗʰ **T82.09** **Other mechanical complication of heart valve prosthesis**
Obstruction (mechanical) of heart valve prosthesis
Perforation of heart valve prosthesis
Protrusion of heart valve prosthesis

√5ᵗʰ **T82.1** **Mechanical complication of cardiac electronic device**

√6ᵗʰ **T82.11** **Breakdown (mechanical) of cardiac electronic device**

√7ᵗʰ **T82.110** **Breakdown (mechanical) of cardiac electrode** `CC` `PE`

√7ᵗʰ **T82.111** **Breakdown (mechanical) of cardiac pulse generator (battery)** `CC` `PE`

√7ᵗʰ **T82.118** **Breakdown (mechanical) of other cardiac electronic device** `CC` `PE`

√7ᵗʰ **T82.119** **Breakdown (mechanical) of unspecified cardiac electronic device** `CC` `PE`

√6ᵗʰ **T82.12** **Displacement of cardiac electronic device**
Malposition of cardiac electronic device

√7ᵗʰ **T82.120** **Displacement of cardiac electrode** `CC` `PE`

√7ᵗʰ **T82.121** **Displacement of cardiac pulse generator (battery)** `CC` `PE`

√7ᵗʰ **T82.128** **Displacement of other cardiac electronic device** `CC` `PE`

√7ᵗʰ **T82.129** **Displacement of unspecified cardiac electronic device** `CC` `PE`

√6ᵗʰ **T82.19** **Other mechanical complication of cardiac electronic device**
Leakage of cardiac electronic device
Obstruction of cardiac electronic device
Perforation of cardiac electronic device
Protrusion of cardiac electronic device

√7ᵗʰ **T82.190** **Other mechanical complication of cardiac electrode** `CC` `PE`

√7ᵗʰ **T82.191** **Other mechanical complication of cardiac pulse generator (battery)** `CC` `PE`

√7ᵗʰ **T82.198** **Other mechanical complication of other cardiac electronic device** `CC` `PE`

√7ᵗʰ **T82.199** **Other mechanical complication of unspecified cardiac device** `CC` `PE`

✔ Additional Character Required   √7ᵗʰ Placeholder   Questionable PDx   Manifestation   Unspecified   `UPD` Unacceptable PDx   `H1`-`H14` HAC   `HCC` CMS-HCC Dx   `HIV` HIV Dx

ICD-10-CM 2025   **1179**

√5ᵗʰ **T82.2 Mechanical complication of coronary artery bypass graft and biological heart valve graft**

> EXCLUDES 1 *mechanical complication of artificial heart valve prosthesis (T82.0-)*

√6ᵗʰ **T82.21 Mechanical complication of coronary artery bypass graft**

√7ᵗʰ **T82.211 Breakdown (mechanical) of coronary artery bypass graft** CC PE

√7ᵗʰ **T82.212 Displacement of coronary artery bypass graft** CC PE
Malposition of coronary artery bypass graft

√7ᵗʰ **T82.213 Leakage of coronary artery bypass graft** CC PE

√7ᵗʰ **T82.218 Other mechanical complication of coronary artery bypass graft** CC PE
Obstruction, mechanical of coronary artery bypass graft
Perforation of coronary artery bypass graft
Protrusion of coronary artery bypass graft

√6ᵗʰ **T82.22 Mechanical complication of biological heart valve graft**

√7ᵗʰ **T82.221 Breakdown (mechanical) of biological heart valve graft** CC PE

√7ᵗʰ **T82.222 Displacement of biological heart valve graft** CC PE
Malposition of biological heart valve graft

√7ᵗʰ **T82.223 Leakage of biological heart valve graft** CC PE

√7ᵗʰ **T82.228 Other mechanical complication of biological heart valve graft** CC PE
Obstruction of biological heart valve graft
Perforation of biological heart valve graft
Protrusion of biological heart valve graft

√5ᵗʰ **T82.3 Mechanical complication of other vascular grafts**

√6ᵗʰ **T82.31 Breakdown (mechanical) of other vascular grafts**

√7ᵗʰ **T82.310 Breakdown (mechanical) of aortic (bifurcation) graft (replacement)** CC PE
AHA: 2020,3Q,3-8

√7ᵗʰ **T82.311 Breakdown (mechanical) of carotid arterial graft (bypass)** CC PE

√7ᵗʰ **T82.312 Breakdown (mechanical) of femoral arterial graft (bypass)** CC PE

√7ᵗʰ **T82.318 Breakdown (mechanical) of other vascular grafts** CC PE

√7ᵗʰ **T82.319 Breakdown (mechanical) of unspecified vascular grafts** CC PE

√6ᵗʰ **T82.32 Displacement of other vascular grafts**
Malposition of other vascular grafts

√7ᵗʰ **T82.320 Displacement of aortic (bifurcation) graft (replacement)** CC PE

√7ᵗʰ **T82.321 Displacement of carotid arterial graft (bypass)** CC PE

√7ᵗʰ **T82.322 Displacement of femoral arterial graft (bypass)** CC PE

√7ᵗʰ **T82.328 Displacement of other vascular grafts** CC PE

√7ᵗʰ **T82.329 Displacement of unspecified vascular grafts** CC PE

√6ᵗʰ **T82.33 Leakage of other vascular grafts**

√7ᵗʰ **T82.330 Leakage of aortic (bifurcation) graft (replacement)** CC PE
AHA: 2020,3Q,3-8

√7ᵗʰ **T82.331 Leakage of carotid arterial graft (bypass)** CC PE

√7ᵗʰ **T82.332 Leakage of femoral arterial graft (bypass)** CC PE

√7ᵗʰ **T82.338 Leakage of other vascular grafts** CC PE

√7ᵗʰ **T82.339 Leakage of unspecified vascular graft** CC PE

√6ᵗʰ **T82.39 Other mechanical complication of other vascular grafts**
Obstruction (mechanical) of other vascular grafts
Perforation of other vascular grafts
Protrusion of other vascular grafts

√7ᵗʰ **T82.390 Other mechanical complication of aortic (bifurcation) graft (replacement)** CC PE
AHA: 2020,3Q,3-5

√7ᵗʰ **T82.391 Other mechanical complication of carotid arterial graft (bypass)** CC PE

√7ᵗʰ **T82.392 Other mechanical complication of femoral arterial graft (bypass)** CC PE

√7ᵗʰ **T82.398 Other mechanical complication of other vascular grafts** CC PE

√7ᵗʰ **T82.399 Other mechanical complication of unspecified vascular grafts** CC PE

√5ᵗʰ **T82.4 Mechanical complication of vascular dialysis catheter**
Mechanical complication of hemodialysis catheter

> EXCLUDES 1 *mechanical complication of intraperitoneal dialysis catheter (T85.62)*

√x7ᵗʰ **T82.41 Breakdown (mechanical) of vascular dialysis catheter** CC PE

√x7ᵗʰ **T82.42 Displacement of vascular dialysis catheter** CC PE
Malposition of vascular dialysis catheter

√x7ᵗʰ **T82.43 Leakage of vascular dialysis catheter** CC PE

√x7ᵗʰ **T82.49 Other complication of vascular dialysis catheter** CC PE
Obstruction (mechanical) of vascular dialysis catheter
Perforation of vascular dialysis catheter
Protrusion of vascular dialysis catheter

√5ᵗʰ **T82.5 Mechanical complication of other cardiac and vascular devices and implants**

> EXCLUDES 2 *mechanical complication of epidural and subdural infusion catheter (T85.61)*

√6ᵗʰ **T82.51 Breakdown (mechanical) of other cardiac and vascular devices and implants**

√7ᵗʰ **T82.510 Breakdown (mechanical) of surgically created arteriovenous fistula** CC PE
AHA: 2020,3Q,36

√7ᵗʰ **T82.511 Breakdown (mechanical) of surgically created arteriovenous shunt** CC PE
AHA: 2020,3Q,37

√7ᵗʰ **T82.512 Breakdown (mechanical) of artificial heart** CC HCC

√7ᵗʰ **T82.513 Breakdown (mechanical) of balloon (counterpulsation) device** CC PE

√7ᵗʰ **T82.514 Breakdown (mechanical) of infusion catheter** CC PE

√7ᵗʰ **T82.515 Breakdown (mechanical) of umbrella device** CC PE

√7ᵗʰ **T82.518 Breakdown (mechanical) of other cardiac and vascular devices and implants** CC PE

√7ᵗʰ **T82.519 Breakdown (mechanical) of unspecified cardiac and vascular devices and implants** CC PE

√6ᵗʰ **T82.52 Displacement of other cardiac and vascular devices and implants**
Malposition of other cardiac and vascular devices and implants

√7ᵗʰ **T82.520 Displacement of surgically created arteriovenous fistula** CC PE
AHA: 2020,3Q,36

√7ᵗʰ **T82.521 Displacement of surgically created arteriovenous shunt** CC PE

√7ᵗʰ **T82.522 Displacement of artificial heart** CC HCC PE

√7ᵗʰ **T82.523 Displacement of balloon (counterpulsation) device** CC PE

√7ᵗʰ **T82.524 Displacement of infusion catheter** CC PE
AHA: 2020,2Q,21; 2019,3Q,15

√7ᵗʰ **T82.525 Displacement of umbrella device** CC PE

√7ᵗʰ **T82.528 Displacement of other cardiac and vascular devices and implants** CC PE

√7ᵗʰ **T82.529 Displacement of unspecified cardiac and vascular devices and implants** CC PE

√6ᵗʰ **T82.53 Leakage of other cardiac and vascular devices and implants**

√7ᵗʰ **T82.530 Leakage of surgically created arteriovenous fistula** CC PE
AHA: 2020,3Q,36

√7ᵗʰ **T82.531 Leakage of surgically created arteriovenous shunt** CC PE

√7ᵗʰ **T82.532 Leakage of artificial heart** CC HCC

√7ᵗʰ **T82.533 Leakage of balloon (counterpulsation) device** CC PE

√7ᵗʰ **T82.534 Leakage of infusion catheter** CC PE

√7th **T82.535** Leakage of umbrella device   CC PE

√7th **T82.538** Leakage of other cardiac and vascular devices and implants

√7th **T82.539** Leakage of unspecified cardiac and vascular devices and implants   CC PE

√6th **T82.59** Other mechanical complication of other cardiac and vascular devices and implants

Obstruction (mechanical) of other cardiac and vascular devices and implants

Perforation of other cardiac and vascular devices and implants

Protrusion of other cardiac and vascular devices and implants

√7th **T82.590** Other mechanical complication of surgically created arteriovenous fistula   PE

AHA: 2020,3Q,36

√7th **T82.591** Other mechanical complication of surgically created arteriovenous shunt   CC PE

√7th **T82.592** Other mechanical complication of artificial heart   CC HCC PE

√7th **T82.593** Other mechanical complication of balloon (counterpulsation) device   CC PE

√7th **T82.594** Other mechanical complication of infusion catheter   CC PE

√7th **T82.595** Other mechanical complication of umbrella device   CC PE

√7th **T82.598** Other mechanical complication of other cardiac and vascular devices and implants   CC PE

√7th **T82.599** Other mechanical complication of unspecified cardiac and vascular devices and implants   CC PE

√x7th **T82.6** Infection and inflammatory reaction due to cardiac valve prosthesis   CC PE

Use additional code to identify infection

√x7th **T82.7** Infection and inflammatory reaction due to other cardiac and vascular devices, implants and grafts   CC H13 PE

Use additional code to identify infection

AHA: 2019,1Q,13-14

DEF: Midline catheter: Long peripheral catheter introduced via the cephalic, basilic, brachial, or median cubital veins in the upper arm and positioned so that the tip is level or near the level of the axilla and distal to the shoulder. Midline catheters are typically used for IV access, fluid replacement, and medication administration.

TIP: Assign this code for infections and/or cellulitis resulting from catheters that are not centrally placed (e.g., midline catheters).

√5th **T82.8** Other specified complications of cardiac and vascular prosthetic devices, implants and grafts

AHA: 2016,4Q,70

√6th **T82.81** Embolism due to cardiac and vascular prosthetic devices, implants and grafts

√7th **T82.817** Embolism due to cardiac prosthetic devices, implants and grafts   CC PE

√7th **T82.818** Embolism due to vascular prosthetic devices, implants and grafts   CC PE

√6th **T82.82** Fibrosis due to cardiac and vascular prosthetic devices, implants and grafts

√7th **T82.827** Fibrosis due to cardiac prosthetic devices, implants and grafts   CC PE

√7th **T82.828** Fibrosis due vascular prosthetic devices, implants and grafts   CC PE

√6th **T82.83** Hemorrhage due to cardiac and vascular prosthetic devices, implants and grafts

√7th **T82.837** Hemorrhage due to cardiac prosthetic devices, implants and grafts   CC PE

√7th **T82.838** Hemorrhage due to vascular prosthetic devices, implants and grafts   CC PE

AHA: 2020,3Q,36-37

√6th **T82.84** Pain due to cardiac and vascular prosthetic devices, implants and grafts

√7th **T82.847** Pain due to cardiac prosthetic devices, implants and grafts   CC PE

√7th **T82.848** Pain due to vascular prosthetic devices, implants and grafts   CC PE

√6th **T82.85** Stenosis due to cardiac and vascular prosthetic devices, implants and grafts

√7th **T82.855** Stenosis of coronary artery stent   CC PE

In-stent stenosis (restenosis) of coronary artery stent

Restenosis of coronary artery stent

AHA: 2021,3Q,6-7

√7th **T82.856** Stenosis of peripheral vascular stent   CC PE

In-stent stenosis (restenosis) of peripheral vascular stent

Restenosis of peripheral vascular stent

√7th **T82.857** Stenosis of other cardiac prosthetic devices, implants and grafts   CC PE

√7th **T82.858** Stenosis of other vascular prosthetic devices, implants and grafts   CC PE

√6th **T82.86** Thrombosis of cardiac and vascular prosthetic devices, implants and grafts

AHA: 2023,2Q,7

√7th **T82.867** Thrombosis due to cardiac prosthetic devices, implants and grafts   CC PE

√7th **T82.868** Thrombosis due to vascular prosthetic devices, implants and grafts   CC PE

√6th **T82.89** Other specified complication of cardiac and vascular prosthetic devices, implants and grafts

√7th **T82.897** Other specified complication of cardiac prosthetic devices, implants and grafts   CC PE

AHA: 2019,2Q,33

√7th **T82.898** Other specified complication of vascular prosthetic devices, implants and grafts   CC PE

AHA: 2020,3Q,3-5

√x7th **T82.9** Unspecified complication of cardiac and vascular prosthetic device, implant and graft   CC PE

√4th **T83** Complications of genitourinary prosthetic devices, implants and grafts

EXCLUDES 2   failure and rejection of transplanted organs and tissue (T86.-)

AHA: 2016,4Q,70-71

The appropriate 7th character is to be added to each code from category T83.

A   initial encounter
D   subsequent encounter
S   sequela

√5th **T83.0** Mechanical complication of urinary catheter

EXCLUDES 2   complications of stoma of urinary tract (N99.5-)

√6th **T83.01** Breakdown (mechanical) of urinary catheter

√7th **T83.010** Breakdown (mechanical) of cystostomy catheter   CC PE

√7th **T83.011** Breakdown (mechanical) of indwelling urethral catheter   PE

√7th **T83.012** Breakdown (mechanical) of nephrostomy catheter   PE

√7th **T83.018** Breakdown (mechanical) of other urinary catheter   PE

Breakdown (mechanical) of Hopkins catheter

Breakdown (mechanical) of ileostomy catheter

Breakdown (mechanical) urostomy catheter

√6th **T83.02** Displacement of urinary catheter

Malposition of urinary catheter

√7th **T83.020** Displacement of cystostomy catheter   CC PE

√7th **T83.021** Displacement of indwelling urethral catheter   PE

√7th **T83.022** Displacement of nephrostomy catheter   PE

√7th **T83.028** Displacement of other urinary catheter   PE

Displacement of Hopkins catheter
Displacement of ileostomy catheter
Displacement of urostomy catheter

√6th **T83.03** Leakage of urinary catheter

√7th **T83.030** Leakage of cystostomy catheter   CC PE

AHA: 2021,4Q,18

√7th **T83.031** Leakage of indwelling urethral catheter   PE

✓ Additional Character Required   √x7th Placeholder   Questionable PDx   Manifestation   Unspecified   UPD Unacceptable PDx   H1-H14 HAC   HCC CMS-HCC Dx   HIV HIV Dx

ICD-10-CM 2025   1181

Chapter 19. Injury, Poisoning and Certain Other Consequences of External Causes

    √7th   **T83.032**   Leakage of nephrostomy catheter   PE

    √7th   **T83.038**   Leakage of other urinary catheter   PE

       Leakage of Hopkins catheter

       Leakage of ileostomy catheter

       Leakage of urostomy catheter

√6th   **T83.09**   **Other mechanical complication of urinary catheter**

       Obstruction (mechanical) of urinary catheter

       Perforation of urinary catheter

       Protrusion of urinary catheter

    √7th   **T83.090**   **Other mechanical complication of cystostomy catheter**   CC   PE

    √7th   **T83.091**   **Other mechanical complication of indwelling urethral catheter**   PE

    √7th   **T83.092**   **Other mechanical complication of nephrostomy catheter**   PE

    √7th   **T83.098**   **Other mechanical complication of other urinary catheter**   PE

       Other mechanical complication of Hopkins catheter

       Other mechanical complication of ileostomy catheter

       Other mechanical complication of urostomy catheter

√5th   **T83.1**   **Mechanical complication of other urinary devices and implants**

  √6th   **T83.11**   **Breakdown (mechanical) of other urinary devices and implants**

    √7th   **T83.110**   **Breakdown (mechanical) of urinary electronic stimulator device**   CC   PE

       EXCLUDES 2   *breakdown (mechanical) of electrode (lead) for sacral nerve neurostimulator (T85.111)*

       breakdown (mechanical) of implanted electronic sacral neurostimulator, pulse generator or receiver (T85.113)

    √7th   **T83.111**   **Breakdown (mechanical) of implanted urinary sphincter**   CC   PE

    √7th   **T83.112**   **Breakdown (mechanical) of indwelling ureteral stent**   CC   PE

    √7th   **T83.113**   **Breakdown (mechanical) of other urinary stents**   CC

       Breakdown (mechanical) of ileal conduit stent

       Breakdown (mechanical) of nephroureteral stent

    √7th   **T83.118**   **Breakdown (mechanical) of other urinary devices and implants**   CC   PE

  √6th   **T83.12**   **Displacement of other urinary devices and implants**

       Malposition of other urinary devices and implants

    √7th   **T83.120**   **Displacement of urinary electronic stimulator device**   CC   PE

       EXCLUDES 2   *displacement of electrode (lead) for sacral nerve neurostimulator (T85.121)*

       displacement of implanted electronic sacral neurostimulator, pulse generator or receiver (T85.123)

    √7th   **T83.121**   **Displacement of implanted urinary sphincter**   CC   PE

    √7th   **T83.122**   **Displacement of indwelling ureteral stent**   CC   PE

    √7th   **T83.123**   **Displacement of other urinary stents**   CC

       Displacement of ileal conduit stent

       Displacement of nephroureteral stent

    √7th   **T83.128**   **Displacement of other urinary devices and implants**   CC   PE

√6th   **T83.19**   **Other mechanical complication of other urinary devices and implants**

       Leakage of other urinary devices and implants

       Obstruction (mechanical) of other urinary devices and implants

       Perforation of other urinary devices and implants

       Protrusion of other urinary devices and implants

    √7th   **T83.190**   **Other mechanical complication of urinary electronic stimulator device**   CC   PE

       EXCLUDES 2   *other mechanical complication of electrode (lead) for sacral nerve neurostimulator (T85.191)*

       other mechanical complication of implanted electronic sacral neurostimulator, pulse generator or receiver (T85.193)

    √7th   **T83.191**   **Other mechanical complication of implanted urinary sphincter**   CC   PE

    √7th   **T83.192**   **Other mechanical complication of indwelling ureteral stent**   CC   PE

    √7th   **T83.193**   **Other mechanical complication of other urinary stent**   CC   PE

       Other mechanical complication of ileal conduit stent

       Other mechanical complication of nephroureteral stent

    √7th   **T83.198**   **Other mechanical complication of other urinary devices and implants**   CC   PE

√5th   **T83.2**   **Mechanical complication of graft of urinary organ**

  √x7th   **T83.21**   **Breakdown (mechanical) of graft of urinary organ**   CC   PE

  √x7th   **T83.22**   **Displacement of graft of urinary organ**   CC   PE

       Malposition of graft of urinary organ

  √x7th   **T83.23**   **Leakage of graft of urinary organ**   CC   PE

  √x7th   **T83.24**   **Erosion of graft of urinary organ**   CC   PE

  √x7th   **T83.25**   **Exposure of graft of urinary organ**   CC   PE

  √x7th   **T83.29**   **Other mechanical complication of graft of urinary organ**   CC   PE

       Obstruction (mechanical) of graft of urinary organ

       Perforation of graft of urinary organ

       Protrusion of graft of urinary organ

√5th   **T83.3**   **Mechanical complication of intrauterine contraceptive device**

  √x7th   **T83.31**   **Breakdown (mechanical) of intrauterine contraceptive device**   PE

  √x7th   **T83.32**   **Displacement of intrauterine contraceptive device**   PE

       Malposition of intrauterine contraceptive device

       Missing string of intrauterine contraceptive device

       AHA: 2018,1Q,5

  √x7th   **T83.39**   **Other mechanical complication of intrauterine contraceptive device**   PE

       Leakage of intrauterine contraceptive device

       Obstruction (mechanical) of intrauterine contraceptive device

       Perforation of intrauterine contraceptive device

       Protrusion of intrauterine contraceptive device

√5th   **T83.4**   **Mechanical complication of other prosthetic devices, implants and grafts of genital tract**

  √6th   **T83.41**   **Breakdown (mechanical) of other prosthetic devices, implants and grafts of genital tract**

    √7th   **T83.410**   **Breakdown (mechanical) of implanted penile prosthesis**   CC   PE

       Breakdown (mechanical) of penile prosthesis cylinder

       Breakdown (mechanical) of penile prosthesis pump

       Breakdown (mechanical) of penile prosthesis reservoir

    √7th   **T83.411**   **Breakdown (mechanical) of implanted testicular prosthesis**   CC   PE

    √7th   **T83.418**   **Breakdown (mechanical) of other prosthetic devices, implants and grafts of genital tract**   CC   PE

N Newborn: 0   P Pediatric: 0-17   M Maternity: 9-64   A Adult: 15-124   UNS Unspecified Site   MCC Major Complication/Comorbidity   CC Complication/Comorbidity   PE POA Exempt

1182   ICD-10-CM 2025

√6th **T83.42** **Displacement** of other prosthetic devices, implants and grafts of genital tract
Malposition of other prosthetic devices, implants and grafts of genital tract

√7th **T83.420** **Displacement of implanted penile prosthesis** CC PE
Displacement of penile prosthesis cylinder
Displacement of penile prosthesis pump
Displacement of penile prosthesis reservoir

√7th **T83.421** **Displacement of implanted testicular prosthesis** CC PE

√7th **T83.428** **Displacement of other prosthetic devices, implants and grafts of genital tract** CC PE
AHA: 2018,1Q,5

√6th **T83.49** **Other mechanical complication of other prosthetic devices, implants and grafts of genital tract**
Leakage of other prosthetic devices, implants and grafts of genital tract
Obstruction, mechanical of other prosthetic devices, implants and grafts of genital tract
Perforation of other prosthetic devices, implants and grafts of genital tract
Protrusion of other prosthetic devices, implants and grafts of genital tract

√7th **T83.490** **Other mechanical complication of implanted penile prosthesis** CC PE
Other mechanical complication of penile prosthesis cylinder
Other mechanical complication of penile prosthesis pump
Other mechanical complication of penile prosthesis reservoir

√7th **T83.491** **Other mechanical complication of implanted testicular prosthesis** CC PE

√7th **T83.498** **Other mechanical complication of other prosthetic devices, implants and grafts of genital tract** CC PE

√5th **T83.5** **Infection and inflammatory reaction due to prosthetic device, implant and graft in urinary system**
Use additional code to identify infection

√6th **T83.51** **Infection and inflammatory reaction due to urinary catheter**
EXCLUDES 2   *complications of stoma of urinary tract (N99.5-)*
AHA: 2019,3Q,17

√7th **T83.510** **Infection and inflammatory reaction due to cystostomy catheter** CC PE

√7th **T83.511** **Infection and inflammatory reaction due to indwelling urethral catheter** CC H6 PE
AHA: 2022,2Q,7

√7th **T83.512** **Infection and inflammatory reaction due to nephrostomy catheter** CC PE

√7th **T83.518** **Infection and inflammatory reaction due to other urinary catheter** CC H6 PE
Infection and inflammatory reaction due to Hopkins catheter
Infection and inflammatory reaction due to ileostomy catheter
Infection and inflammatory reaction due to urostomy catheter

√6th **T83.59** **Infection and inflammatory reaction due to prosthetic device, implant and graft in urinary system**

√7th **T83.590** **Infection and inflammatory reaction due to implanted urinary neurostimulation device** CC PE
EXCLUDES 2   *infection and inflammatory reaction due to electrode lead of sacral nerve neurostimulator (T85.732)*
infection and inflammatory reaction due to pulse generator or receiver of sacral nerve neurostimulator (T85.734)

√7th **T83.591** **Infection and inflammatory reaction due to implanted urinary sphincter** CC PE

√7th **T83.592** **Infection and inflammatory reaction due to indwelling ureteral stent** CC PE

√7th **T83.593** **Infection and inflammatory reaction due to other urinary stents** CC PE
Infection and inflammatory reaction due to ileal conduit stents
Infection and inflammatory reaction due to nephroureteral stent

√7th **T83.598** **Infection and inflammatory reaction due to other prosthetic device, implant and graft in urinary system** CC PE
AHA: 2020,3Q,25

√5th **T83.6** **Infection and inflammatory reaction due to prosthetic device, implant and graft in genital tract**
Use additional code to identify infection

√x7th **T83.61** **Infection and inflammatory reaction due to implanted penile prosthesis** CC PE
Infection and inflammatory reaction due to penile prosthesis cylinder
Infection and inflammatory reaction due to penile prosthesis pump
Infection and inflammatory reaction due to penile prosthesis reservoir

√x7th **T83.62** **Infection and inflammatory reaction due to implanted testicular prosthesis** CC PE

√x7th **T83.69** **Infection and inflammatory reaction due to other prosthetic device, implant and graft in genital tract** CC PE

√5th **T83.7** **Complications due to implanted mesh and other prosthetic materials**

√6th **T83.71** **Erosion of implanted mesh and other prosthetic materials**

√7th **T83.711** **Erosion of implanted vaginal mesh to surrounding organ or tissue** PE
Erosion of implanted vaginal mesh into pelvic floor muscles

√7th **T83.712** **Erosion of implanted urethral mesh to surrounding organ or tissue** CC PE
Erosion of implanted female urethral sling
Erosion of implanted male urethral sling
Erosion of implanted urethral mesh into pelvic floor muscles

√7th **T83.713** **Erosion of implanted urethral bulking agent to surrounding organ or tissue** CC PE

√7th **T83.714** **Erosion of implanted ureteral bulking agent to surrounding organ or tissue** CC PE

√7th **T83.718** **Erosion of other implanted mesh to organ or tissue** CC PE

√7th **T83.719** **Erosion of other prosthetic materials to surrounding organ or tissue** CC PE

√6th **T83.72** **Exposure of implanted mesh and other prosthetic materials into surrounding organ or tissue**
Extrusion of implanted mesh

√7th **T83.721** **Exposure of implanted vaginal mesh into vagina** PE
Exposure of implanted vaginal mesh through vaginal wall

√7th **T83.722** **Exposure of implanted urethral mesh into urethra** CC PE
Exposure of implanted female urethral sling
Exposure of implanted male urethral sling
Exposure of implanted urethral mesh through urethral wall

√7th **T83.723** **Exposure of implanted urethral bulking agent into urethra** CC PE

√7th **T83.724** **Exposure of implanted ureteral bulking agent into ureter** CC PE

√7th **T83.728** **Exposure of other implanted mesh into organ or tissue** CC PE

√7th **T83.729** **Exposure of other prosthetic materials into organ or tissue** CC PE

√x7th **T83.79** **Other specified complications due to other genitourinary prosthetic materials** CC PE

√5th **T83.8** **Other specified complications of genitourinary prosthetic devices, implants and grafts**

√x7th **T83.81** **Embolism due to genitourinary prosthetic devices, implants and grafts** CC PE

√x7th **T83.82** **Fibrosis due to genitourinary prosthetic devices, implants and grafts** CC PE

√x7th **T83.83** **Hemorrhage due to genitourinary prosthetic devices, implants and grafts** CC PE

Chapter 19. Injury, Poisoning and Certain Other Consequences of External Causes

✓x 7ᵗʰ **T83.84** **Pain** due to genitourinary prosthetic devices, implants and grafts `CC` `PE`

✓x 7ᵗʰ **T83.85** **Stenosis** due to genitourinary prosthetic devices, implants and grafts `CC` `PE`

✓x 7ᵗʰ **T83.86** **Thrombosis** due to genitourinary prosthetic devices, implants and grafts `CC` `PE`

✓x 7ᵗʰ **T83.89** **Other specified complication** of genitourinary prosthetic devices, implants and grafts `CC` `PE`
AHA: 2022,3Q,13; 2016,1Q,19

✓x 7ᵗʰ **T83.9** **Unspecified complication** of genitourinary prosthetic device, implant and graft `CC` `PE`

✓4ᵗʰ **T84** **Complications of internal orthopedic prosthetic devices, implants and grafts**

> EXCLUDES 2   failure and rejection of transplanted organs and tissues (T86.-)
> fracture of bone following insertion of orthopedic implant, joint prosthesis or bone plate (M96.6)

> The appropriate 7th character is to be added to each code from category T84.
> A   initial encounter
> D   subsequent encounter
> S   sequela

✓5ᵗʰ **T84.0** **Mechanical complication** of **internal joint prosthesis**

✓6ᵗʰ **T84.01** **Broken** internal joint prosthesis
Breakage (fracture) of prosthetic joint
Broken prosthetic joint implant
EXCLUDES 1   periprosthetic joint implant fracture (M97.-)
AHA: 2016,4Q,42

✓7ᵗʰ **T84.010** **Broken internal right hip** prosthesis `CC` `PE`

✓7ᵗʰ **T84.011** **Broken internal left hip** prosthesis `CC` `PE`

✓7ᵗʰ **T84.012** **Broken internal right knee** prosthesis `CC` `PE`

✓7ᵗʰ **T84.013** **Broken internal left knee** prosthesis `CC` `PE`

✓7ᵗʰ **T84.018** **Broken internal joint prosthesis, other site** `CC` `PE`
Use additional code to identify the joint (Z96.6-)

✓7ᵗʰ **T84.019** **Broken internal joint prosthesis, unspecified site** `CC` `UNS` `PE`

✓6ᵗʰ **T84.02** **Dislocation** of internal joint prosthesis
Instability of internal joint prosthesis
Subluxation of internal joint prosthesis
AHA: 2019,2Q,27

✓7ᵗʰ **T84.020** **Dislocation of internal right hip** prosthesis `CC` `PE`

✓7ᵗʰ **T84.021** **Dislocation of internal left hip** prosthesis `CC` `PE`

✓7ᵗʰ **T84.022** **Instability of internal right knee** prosthesis `CC` `PE`

✓7ᵗʰ **T84.023** **Instability of internal left knee** prosthesis `CC` `PE`

✓7ᵗʰ **T84.028** **Dislocation of other internal joint** prosthesis `CC` `PE`
Use additional code to identify the joint (Z96.6-)

✓7ᵗʰ **T84.029** **Dislocation of unspecified internal joint** prosthesis `CC` `UNS` `PE`

✓6ᵗʰ **T84.03** **Mechanical loosening** of internal prosthetic joint
Aseptic loosening of prosthetic joint

✓7ᵗʰ **T84.030** **Mechanical loosening of internal right hip** prosthetic joint `CC` `PE`

✓7ᵗʰ **T84.031** **Mechanical loosening of internal left hip** prosthetic joint `CC` `PE`

✓7ᵗʰ **T84.032** **Mechanical loosening of internal right knee** prosthetic joint `CC` `PE`

✓7ᵗʰ **T84.033** **Mechanical loosening of internal left knee** prosthetic joint `CC` `PE`

✓7ᵗʰ **T84.038** **Mechanical loosening of other internal** prosthetic joint `CC` `PE`
Use additional code to identify the joint (Z96.6-)

✓7ᵗʰ **T84.039** **Mechanical loosening of unspecified internal prosthetic joint** `CC` `UNS` `PE`

✓6ᵗʰ **T84.05** **Periprosthetic osteolysis** of internal prosthetic joint
Use additional code to identify major osseous defect, if applicable (M89.7-)

✓7ᵗʰ **T84.050** **Periprosthetic osteolysis of internal prosthetic right hip joint** `CC` `PE`

✓7ᵗʰ **T84.051** **Periprosthetic osteolysis of internal prosthetic left hip joint** `CC` `PE`

✓7ᵗʰ **T84.052** **Periprosthetic osteolysis of internal prosthetic right knee joint** `CC` `PE`

✓7ᵗʰ **T84.053** **Periprosthetic osteolysis of internal prosthetic left knee joint** `CC` `PE`

✓7ᵗʰ **T84.058** **Periprosthetic osteolysis of other internal prosthetic joint** `CC` `PE`
Use additional code to identify the joint (Z96.6-)

✓7ᵗʰ **T84.059** **Periprosthetic osteolysis of unspecified internal prosthetic joint** `CC` `UNS` `PE`

✓6ᵗʰ **T84.06** **Wear of articular bearing surface** of internal prosthetic joint

✓7ᵗʰ **T84.060** **Wear of articular bearing surface of internal prosthetic right hip joint** `CC` `PE`

✓7ᵗʰ **T84.061** **Wear of articular bearing surface of internal prosthetic left hip joint** `CC` `PE`

✓7ᵗʰ **T84.062** **Wear of articular bearing surface of internal prosthetic right knee joint** `CC` `PE`

✓7ᵗʰ **T84.063** **Wear of articular bearing surface of internal prosthetic left knee joint** `CC` `PE`

✓7ᵗʰ **T84.068** **Wear of articular bearing surface of other internal prosthetic joint** `CC` `PE`
Use additional code to identify the joint (Z96.6-)

✓7ᵗʰ **T84.069** **Wear of articular bearing surface of unspecified internal prosthetic joint** `CC` `UNS` `PE`

✓6ᵗʰ **T84.09** **Other mechanical complication of internal joint prosthesis**
Prosthetic joint implant failure NOS
AHA: 2019,1Q,20

✓7ᵗʰ **T84.090** **Other mechanical complication of internal right hip prosthesis** `CC` `PE`

✓7ᵗʰ **T84.091** **Other mechanical complication of internal left hip prosthesis** `CC` `PE`

✓7ᵗʰ **T84.092** **Other mechanical complication of internal right knee prosthesis** `CC` `PE`

✓7ᵗʰ **T84.093** **Other mechanical complication of internal left knee prosthesis** `CC` `PE`

✓7ᵗʰ **T84.098** **Other mechanical complication of other internal joint prosthesis** `CC` `PE`
Use additional code to identify the joint (Z96.6-)

✓7ᵗʰ **T84.099** **Other mechanical complication of unspecified internal joint prosthesis** `CC` `UNS` `PE`

✓5ᵗʰ **T84.1** **Mechanical complication** of **internal fixation device** of **bones of limb**

> EXCLUDES 2   mechanical complication of internal fixation device of bones of feet (T84.2-)
> mechanical complication of internal fixation device of bones of fingers (T84.2-)
> mechanical complication of internal fixation device of bones of hands (T84.2-)
> mechanical complication of internal fixation device of bones of toes (T84.2-)

✓6ᵗʰ **T84.11** **Breakdown** (mechanical) of internal fixation device of bones of limb

✓7ᵗʰ **T84.110** **Breakdown (mechanical) of internal fixation device of right humerus** `CC` `PE`

✓7ᵗʰ **T84.111** **Breakdown (mechanical) of internal fixation device of left humerus** `CC` `PE`

✓7ᵗʰ **T84.112** **Breakdown (mechanical) of internal fixation device of bone of right forearm** `CC` `PE`

✓7ᵗʰ **T84.113** **Breakdown (mechanical) of internal fixation device of bone of left forearm** `CC` `PE`

✓7ᵗʰ **T84.114** **Breakdown (mechanical) of internal fixation device of right femur** `CC` `PE`

√7ᵗʰ **T84.115** Breakdown (mechanical) of internal fixation device of **left femur** `CC` `PE`

√7ᵗʰ **T84.116** Breakdown (mechanical) of internal fixation device of bone of **right lower leg** `CC` `PE`

√7ᵗʰ **T84.117** Breakdown (mechanical) of internal fixation device of bone of **left lower leg** `CC` `PE`

√7ᵗʰ **T84.119** Breakdown (mechanical) of internal fixation device of unspecified bone of limb `CC` `UNS` `PE`

√6ᵗʰ **T84.12** **Displacement** of internal fixation device of bones of limb
Malposition of internal fixation device of bones of limb

√7ᵗʰ **T84.120** Displacement of internal fixation device of **right humerus** `CC` `PE`

√7ᵗʰ **T84.121** Displacement of internal fixation device of **left humerus** `CC` `PE`

√7ᵗʰ **T84.122** Displacement of internal fixation device of bone of **right forearm** `CC` `PE`

√7ᵗʰ **T84.123** Displacement of internal fixation device of bone of **left forearm** `CC` `PE`

√7ᵗʰ **T84.124** Displacement of internal fixation device of **right femur** `CC` `PE`

√7ᵗʰ **T84.125** Displacement of internal fixation device of **left femur** `CC` `PE`

√7ᵗʰ **T84.126** Displacement of internal fixation device of bone of **right lower leg** `CC` `PE`

√7ᵗʰ **T84.127** Displacement of internal fixation device of bone of **left lower leg** `CC` `PE`

√7ᵗʰ **T84.129** Displacement of internal fixation device of unspecified bone of limb `CC` `UNS` `PE`

√6ᵗʰ **T84.19** Other mechanical complication of internal fixation device of bones of limb
Obstruction (mechanical) of internal fixation device of bones of limb
Perforation of internal fixation device of bones of limb
Protrusion of internal fixation device of bones of limb

√7ᵗʰ **T84.190** Other mechanical complication of internal fixation device of **right humerus** `CC` `PE`

√7ᵗʰ **T84.191** Other mechanical complication of internal fixation device of **left humerus** `CC` `PE`

√7ᵗʰ **T84.192** Other mechanical complication of internal fixation device of bone of **right forearm** `CC` `PE`

√7ᵗʰ **T84.193** Other mechanical complication of internal fixation device of bone of **left forearm** `CC` `PE`

√7ᵗʰ **T84.194** Other mechanical complication of internal fixation device of **right femur** `CC` `PE`

√7ᵗʰ **T84.195** Other mechanical complication of internal fixation device of **left femur** `CC` `PE`

√7ᵗʰ **T84.196** Other mechanical complication of internal fixation device of bone of **right lower leg** `CC` `PE`

√7ᵗʰ **T84.197** Other mechanical complication of internal fixation device of bone of **left lower leg** `CC` `PE`

√7ᵗʰ **T84.199** Other mechanical complication of internal fixation device of unspecified bone of limb `CC` `UNS` `PE`

√5ᵗʰ **T84.2** Mechanical complication of **internal fixation device** of **other bones**

√6ᵗʰ **T84.21** **Breakdown** (mechanical) of internal fixation device of other bones

√7ᵗʰ **T84.210** Breakdown (mechanical) of internal fixation device of bones of **hand and fingers** `CC` `PE`

√7ᵗʰ **T84.213** Breakdown (mechanical) of internal fixation device of bones of **foot and toes** `CC` `PE`

√7ᵗʰ **T84.216** Breakdown (mechanical) of internal fixation device of **vertebrae** `CC` `PE`

√7ᵗʰ **T84.218** Breakdown (mechanical) of internal fixation device of other bones `CC` `PE`

√6ᵗʰ **T84.22** **Displacement** of internal fixation device of other bones
Malposition of internal fixation device of other bones

√7ᵗʰ **T84.220** Displacement of internal fixation device of bones of **hand and fingers** `CC` `PE`

√7ᵗʰ **T84.223** Displacement of internal fixation device of bones of **foot and toes** `CC` `PE`

√7ᵗʰ **T84.226** Displacement of internal fixation device of **vertebrae** `CC` `PE`

√7ᵗʰ **T84.228** Displacement of internal fixation device of other bones `CC` `PE`

√6ᵗʰ **T84.29** Other mechanical complication of internal fixation device of other bones
Obstruction (mechanical) of internal fixation device of other bones
Perforation of internal fixation device of other bones
Protrusion of internal fixation device of other bones

√7ᵗʰ **T84.290** Other mechanical complication of internal fixation device of bones of **hand and fingers** `CC` `PE`

√7ᵗʰ **T84.293** Other mechanical complication of internal fixation device of bones of **foot and toes** `CC` `PE`

√7ᵗʰ **T84.296** Other mechanical complication of internal fixation device of **vertebrae**
AHA: AHA:2024,2Q,12

√7ᵗʰ **T84.298** Other mechanical complication of internal fixation device of other bones `CC` `PE`

√5ᵗʰ **T84.3** Mechanical complication of other bone devices, implants and grafts
`EXCLUDES 2`   other complications of bone graft (T86.83-)

√6ᵗʰ **T84.31** **Breakdown** (mechanical) of other bone devices, implants and grafts

√7ᵗʰ **T84.310** Breakdown (mechanical) of **electronic bone stimulator** `CC` `PE`

√7ᵗʰ **T84.318** Breakdown (mechanical) of other bone devices, implants and grafts `CC` `PE`

√6ᵗʰ **T84.32** **Displacement** of other bone devices, implants and grafts
Malposition of other bone devices, implants and grafts

√7ᵗʰ **T84.320** Displacement of **electronic bone stimulator** `CC` `PE`

√7ᵗʰ **T84.328** Displacement of other bone devices, implants and grafts `CC` `PE`
AHA: 2014,4Q,28

√6ᵗʰ **T84.39** Other mechanical complication of other bone devices, implants and grafts
Obstruction (mechanical) of other bone devices, implants and grafts
Perforation of other bone devices, implants and grafts
Protrusion of other bone devices, implants and grafts

√7ᵗʰ **T84.390** Other mechanical complication of **electronic bone stimulator** `CC` `PE`

√7ᵗʰ **T84.398** Other mechanical complication of other bone devices, implants and grafts `CC` `PE`

√5ᵗʰ **T84.4** Mechanical complication of other internal orthopedic devices, implants and grafts

√6ᵗʰ **T84.41** **Breakdown** (mechanical) of other internal orthopedic devices, implants and grafts

√7ᵗʰ **T84.410** Breakdown (mechanical) of **muscle and tendon graft** `CC` `PE`

√7ᵗʰ **T84.418** Breakdown (mechanical) of other internal orthopedic devices, implants and grafts `CC` `PE`

√6ᵗʰ **T84.42** **Displacement** of other internal orthopedic devices, implants and grafts
Malposition of other internal orthopedic devices, implants and grafts

√7ᵗʰ **T84.420** Displacement of **muscle and tendon graft** `CC` `PE`

√7ᵗʰ **T84.428** Displacement of other internal orthopedic devices, implants and grafts `CC` `PE`

√6ᵗʰ **T84.49** Other mechanical complication of other internal orthopedic devices, implants and grafts
Mechanical complication of other internal orthopedic devices, implants and grafts NOS
Obstruction (mechanical) of other internal orthopedic devices, implants and grafts
Perforation of other internal orthopedic devices, implants and grafts
Protrusion of other internal orthopedic devices, implants and grafts

√7ᵗʰ **T84.490** Other mechanical complication of **muscle and tendon graft** `CC` `PE`

√7ᵗʰ **T84.498** Other mechanical complication of other internal orthopedic devices, implants and grafts `CC` `PE`

✔ Additional Character Required   √x7ᵗʰ Placeholder   Questionable PDx   Manifestation   Unspecified   `UPD` Unacceptable PDx   `H1`-`H14` HAC   `HCC` CMS-HCC Dx   `HIV` HIV Dx

√5th **T84.5 Infection and inflammatory reaction due to internal joint prosthesis**
  Use additional code to identify infection
  AHA: 2019,3Q,16; 2015,1Q,16

√x7th **T84.50** Infection and inflammatory reaction due to unspecified internal joint prosthesis `CC` `UNS` `PE`

√x7th **T84.51** Infection and inflammatory reaction due to internal right hip prosthesis `CC` `PE`

√x7th **T84.52** Infection and inflammatory reaction due to internal left hip prosthesis `CC` `PE`

√x7th **T84.53** Infection and inflammatory reaction due to internal right knee prosthesis `CC` `PE`

√x7th **T84.54** Infection and inflammatory reaction due to internal left knee prosthesis `CC` `PE`

√x7th **T84.59** Infection and inflammatory reaction due to other internal joint prosthesis `CC` `PE`

√5th **T84.6 Infection and inflammatory reaction due to internal fixation device**
  Use additional code to identify infection

√x7th **T84.60** Infection and inflammatory reaction due to internal fixation device of unspecified site `CC` `H12` `UNS` `PE`

√6th **T84.61** Infection and inflammatory reaction due to internal fixation device of arm

√7th **T84.610** Infection and inflammatory reaction due to internal fixation device of right humerus `CC` `H12` `PE`

√7th **T84.611** Infection and inflammatory reaction due to internal fixation device of left humerus `CC` `H12` `PE`

√7th **T84.612** Infection and inflammatory reaction due to internal fixation device of right radius `CC` `H12` `PE`

√7th **T84.613** Infection and inflammatory reaction due to internal fixation device of left radius `CC` `H12` `PE`

√7th **T84.614** Infection and inflammatory reaction due to internal fixation device of right ulna `CC` `H12` `PE`

√7th **T84.615** Infection and inflammatory reaction due to internal fixation device of left ulna `CC` `H12` `PE`

√7th **T84.619** Infection and inflammatory reaction due to internal fixation device of unspecified bone of arm `CC` `H12` `UNS` `PE`

√6th **T84.62** Infection and inflammatory reaction due to internal fixation device of leg

√7th **T84.620** Infection and inflammatory reaction due to internal fixation device of right femur `CC` `PE`

√7th **T84.621** Infection and inflammatory reaction due to internal fixation device of left femur `CC` `PE`

√7th **T84.622** Infection and inflammatory reaction due to internal fixation device of right tibia `CC` `PE`

√7th **T84.623** Infection and inflammatory reaction due to internal fixation device of left tibia `CC` `PE`

√7th **T84.624** Infection and inflammatory reaction due to internal fixation device of right fibula `CC` `PE`

√7th **T84.625** Infection and inflammatory reaction due to internal fixation device of left fibula `CC` `PE`

√7th **T84.629** Infection and inflammatory reaction due to internal fixation device of unspecified bone of leg `CC` `UNS` `PE`

√x7th **T84.63** Infection and inflammatory reaction due to internal fixation device of spine `CC` `H12` `PE`

√x7th **T84.69** Infection and inflammatory reaction due to internal fixation device of other site `CC` `H12` `PE`

√x7th **T84.7 Infection and inflammatory reaction due to other internal orthopedic prosthetic devices, implants and grafts** `CC` `H12` `PE`
  Use additional code to identify infection

√5th **T84.8 Other specified complications of internal orthopedic prosthetic devices, implants and grafts**

√x7th **T84.81** Embolism due to internal orthopedic prosthetic devices, implants and grafts `CC` `PE`

√x7th **T84.82** Fibrosis due to internal orthopedic prosthetic devices, implants and grafts `CC` `PE`

√x7th **T84.83** Hemorrhage due to internal orthopedic prosthetic devices, implants and grafts `CC` `PE`

√x7th **T84.84** Pain due to internal orthopedic prosthetic devices, implants and grafts `CC` `PE`
  AHA: AHA:2024,2Q,12

√x7th **T84.85** Stenosis due to internal orthopedic prosthetic devices, implants and grafts `CC` `PE`

√x7th **T84.86** Thrombosis due to internal orthopedic prosthetic devices, implants and grafts `CC` `PE`

√x7th **T84.89** Other specified complication of internal orthopedic prosthetic devices, implants and grafts `CC` `PE`

√x7th **T84.9 Unspecified complication of internal orthopedic prosthetic device, implant and graft** `CC` `PE`

√4th **T85 Complications of other internal prosthetic devices, implants and grafts**
  EXCLUDES 2 failure and rejection of transplanted organs and tissue (T86.-)
  AHA: 2023,2Q,7; 2016,4Q,71-72

  The appropriate 7th character is to be added to each code from category T85.
  A   initial encounter
  D   subsequent encounter
  S   sequela

√5th **T85.0 Mechanical complication of ventricular intracranial (communicating) shunt**

√x7th **T85.01** Breakdown (mechanical) of ventricular intracranial (communicating) shunt `CC` `PE`

√x7th **T85.02** Displacement of ventricular intracranial (communicating) shunt `CC` `PE`
  Malposition of ventricular intracranial (communicating) shunt

√x7th **T85.03** Leakage of ventricular intracranial (communicating) shunt `CC` `PE`

√x7th **T85.09** Other mechanical complication of ventricular intracranial (communicating) shunt `CC` `PE`
  Obstruction (mechanical) of ventricular intracranial (communicating) shunt
  Perforation of ventricular intracranial (communicating) shunt
  Protrusion of ventricular intracranial (communicating) shunt

√5th **T85.1 Mechanical complication of implanted electronic stimulator of nervous system**

√6th **T85.11** Breakdown (mechanical) of implanted electronic stimulator of nervous system

√7th **T85.110** Breakdown (mechanical) of implanted electronic neurostimulator of brain electrode (lead) `CC` `PE`

√7th **T85.111** Breakdown (mechanical) of implanted electronic neurostimulator of peripheral nerve electrode (lead) `CC` `PE`
  Breakdown of electrode (lead) for cranial nerve neurostimulators
  Breakdown of electrode (lead) for gastric neurostimulator
  Breakdown of electrode (lead) for sacral nerve neurostimulator
  Breakdown of electrode (lead) for vagal nerve neurostimulators

√7th **T85.112** Breakdown (mechanical) of implanted electronic neurostimulator of spinal cord electrode (lead) `CC` `PE`

√7th **T85.113** Breakdown (mechanical) of implanted electronic neurostimulator, generator `CC` `PE`
  Breakdown (mechanical) of implanted electronic neurostimulator generator, brain, peripheral, gastric, spinal
  Breakdown (mechanical) of implanted electronic sacral neurostimulator, pulse generator or receiver

√7th **T85.118** Breakdown (mechanical) of other implanted electronic stimulator of nervous system `CC` `PE`

√6th **T85.12** Displacement of implanted electronic stimulator of nervous system
  Malposition of implanted electronic stimulator of nervous system

√7th **T85.120** Displacement of implanted electronic neurostimulator of brain electrode (lead) `CC` `PE`

√7ᵗʰ **T85.121 Displacement of implanted electronic neurostimulator of peripheral nerve electrode (lead)** CC PE
Displacement of electrode (lead) for cranial nerve neurostimulators
Displacement of electrode (lead) for gastric neurostimulator
Displacement of electrode (lead) for sacral nerve neurostimulator
Displacement of electrode (lead) for vagal nerve neurostimulators

√7ᵗʰ **T85.122 Displacement of implanted electronic neurostimulator of spinal cord electrode (lead)** CC PE

√7ᵗʰ **T85.123 Displacement of implanted electronic neurostimulator, generator** CC PE
Displacement of implanted electronic neurostimulator generator, brain, peripheral, gastric, spinal
Displacement of implanted electronic sacral neurostimulator, pulse generator or receiver

√7ᵗʰ **T85.128 Displacement of other implanted electronic stimulator of nervous system** CC PE

√6ᵗʰ **T85.19 Other mechanical complication of implanted electronic stimulator of nervous system**
Leakage of implanted electronic stimulator of nervous system
Obstruction (mechanical) of implanted electronic stimulator of nervous system
Perforation of implanted electronic stimulator of nervous system
Protrusion of implanted electronic stimulator of nervous system

√7ᵗʰ **T85.190 Other mechanical complication of implanted electronic neurostimulator of brain electrode (lead)** CC PE

√7ᵗʰ **T85.191 Other mechanical complication of implanted electronic neurostimulator of peripheral nerve electrode (lead)** CC PE
Other mechanical complication of electrode (lead) for cranial nerve neurostimulators
Other mechanical complication of electrode (lead) for gastric neurostimulator
Other mechanical complication of electrode (lead) for sacral nerve neurostimulator
Other mechanical complication of electrode (lead) for vagal nerve neurostimulators

√7ᵗʰ **T85.192 Other mechanical complication of implanted electronic neurostimulator of spinal cord electrode (lead)** CC PE

√7ᵗʰ **T85.193 Other mechanical complication of implanted electronic neurostimulator, generator** CC PE
Other mechanical complication of implanted electronic neurostimulator generator, brain, peripheral, gastric, spinal
Other mechanical complication of implanted electronic sacral neurostimulator, pulse generator or receiver

√7ᵗʰ **T85.199 Other mechanical complication of other implanted electronic stimulator of nervous system** CC PE

√5ᵗʰ **T85.2 Mechanical complication of intraocular lens**

√x7ᵗʰ **T85.21 Breakdown (mechanical) of intraocular lens** CC PE

√x7ᵗʰ **T85.22 Displacement of intraocular lens** CC PE
Malposition of intraocular lens

√x7ᵗʰ **T85.29 Other mechanical complication of intraocular lens**
Obstruction (mechanical) of intraocular lens
Perforation of intraocular lens
Protrusion of intraocular lens

√5ᵗʰ **T85.3 Mechanical complication of other ocular prosthetic devices, implants and grafts**
EXCLUDES 2   other complications of corneal graft (T86.84-)

√6ᵗʰ **T85.31 Breakdown (mechanical) of other ocular prosthetic devices, implants and grafts**

√7ᵗʰ **T85.310 Breakdown (mechanical) of prosthetic orbit of right eye**

√7ᵗʰ **T85.311 Breakdown (mechanical) of prosthetic orbit of left eye** CC PE

√7ᵗʰ **T85.318 Breakdown (mechanical) of other ocular prosthetic devices, implants and grafts** PE

√6ᵗʰ **T85.32 Displacement of other ocular prosthetic devices, implants and grafts**
Malposition of other ocular prosthetic devices, implants and grafts

√7ᵗʰ **T85.320 Displacement of prosthetic orbit of right eye** CC PE

√7ᵗʰ **T85.321 Displacement of prosthetic orbit of left eye** CC PE

√7ᵗʰ **T85.328 Displacement of other ocular prosthetic devices, implants and grafts** PE

√6ᵗʰ **T85.39 Other mechanical complication of other ocular prosthetic devices, implants and grafts**
Obstruction (mechanical) of other ocular prosthetic devices, implants and grafts
Perforation of other ocular prosthetic devices, implants and grafts
Protrusion of other ocular prosthetic devices, implants and grafts

√7ᵗʰ **T85.390 Other mechanical complication of prosthetic orbit of right eye** CC PE

√7ᵗʰ **T85.391 Other mechanical complication of prosthetic orbit of left eye** CC PE

√7ᵗʰ **T85.398 Other mechanical complication of other ocular prosthetic devices, implants and grafts** PE

√5ᵗʰ **T85.4 Mechanical complication of breast prosthesis and implant**

√x7ᵗʰ **T85.41 Breakdown (mechanical) of breast prosthesis and implant** CC PE

√x7ᵗʰ **T85.42 Displacement of breast prosthesis and implant** CC PE
Malposition of breast prosthesis and implant

√x7ᵗʰ **T85.43 Leakage of breast prosthesis and implant** CC PE

√x7ᵗʰ **T85.44 Capsular contracture of breast implant** CC PE

√x7ᵗʰ **T85.49 Other mechanical complication of breast prosthesis and implant** CC PE
Obstruction (mechanical) of breast prosthesis and implant
Perforation of breast prosthesis and implant
Protrusion of breast prosthesis and implant

√5ᵗʰ **T85.5 Mechanical complication of gastrointestinal prosthetic devices, implants and grafts**

√6ᵗʰ **T85.51 Breakdown (mechanical) of gastrointestinal prosthetic devices, implants and grafts**

√7ᵗʰ **T85.510 Breakdown (mechanical) of bile duct prosthesis**

√7ᵗʰ **T85.511 Breakdown (mechanical) of esophageal anti-reflux device** CC PE

√7ᵗʰ **T85.518 Breakdown (mechanical) of other gastrointestinal prosthetic devices, implants and grafts** CC PE

√6ᵗʰ **T85.52 Displacement of gastrointestinal prosthetic devices, implants and grafts**
Malposition of gastrointestinal prosthetic devices, implants and grafts

√7ᵗʰ **T85.520 Displacement of bile duct prosthesis** CC PE

√7ᵗʰ **T85.521 Displacement of esophageal anti-reflux device** CC PE

√7ᵗʰ **T85.528 Displacement of other gastrointestinal prosthetic devices, implants and grafts** CC PE

√6ᵗʰ **T85.59 Other mechanical complication of gastrointestinal prosthetic devices, implants and**
Obstruction, mechanical of gastrointestinal prosthetic devices, implants and grafts
Perforation of gastrointestinal prosthetic devices, implants and grafts
Protrusion of gastrointestinal prosthetic devices, implants and grafts

√7ᵗʰ **T85.590 Other mechanical complication of bile duct prosthesis** CC PE

√7ᵗʰ **T85.591 Other mechanical complication of esophageal anti-reflux device** CC PE

√7ᵗʰ **T85.598 Other mechanical complication of other gastrointestinal prosthetic devices, implants and grafts** CC PE

☑ Additional Character Required   √x7ᵗʰ Placeholder   Questionable PDx   Manifestation   Unspecified   UPD Unacceptable PDx   H1 - H14 HAC   HCC CMS-HCC Dx   HIV HIV Dx

ICD-10-CM 2025   1187

Chapter 19. Injury, Poisoning and Certain Other Consequences of External Causes

T85.6–T85.731

√5ᵗʰ **T85.6** **Mechanical complication of other specified internal and external prosthetic devices, implants and grafts**

√6ᵗʰ   **T85.61** **Breakdown (mechanical) of other specified internal prosthetic devices, implants and grafts**

√7ᵗʰ   **T85.610** **Breakdown (mechanical) of cranial or spinal infusion catheter** CC PE
       Breakdown (mechanical) of epidural infusion catheter
       Breakdown (mechanical) of intrathecal infusion catheter
       Breakdown (mechanical) of subarachnoid infusion catheter
       Breakdown (mechanical) of subdural infusion catheter

√7ᵗʰ   **T85.611** **Breakdown (mechanical) of intraperitoneal dialysis catheter** CC PE
       EXCLUDES 1   *mechanical complication of vascular dialysis catheter (T82.4-)*

√7ᵗʰ   **T85.612** **Breakdown (mechanical) of permanent sutures** CC PE
       EXCLUDES 1   *mechanical complication of permanent (wire) suture used in bone repair (T84.1-T84.2)*

√7ᵗʰ   **T85.613** **Breakdown (mechanical) of artificial skin graft and decellularized allodermis** CC PE
       Failure of artificial skin graft and decellularized allodermis
       Non-adherence of artificial skin graft and decellularized allodermis
       Poor incorporation of artificial skin graft and decellularized allodermis
       Shearing of artificial skin graft and decellularized allodermis

√7ᵗʰ   **T85.614** **Breakdown (mechanical) of insulin pump** CC PE

√7ᵗʰ   **T85.615** **Breakdown (mechanical) of other nervous system device, implant or graft** CC PE
       Breakdown (mechanical) of intrathecal infusion pump

√7ᵗʰ   **T85.618** **Breakdown (mechanical) of other specified internal prosthetic devices, implants and grafts** CC PE

√6ᵗʰ   **T85.62** **Displacement of other specified internal prosthetic devices, implants and grafts**
     Malposition of other specified internal prosthetic devices, implants and grafts

√7ᵗʰ   **T85.620** **Displacement of cranial or spinal infusion catheter** CC PE
       Displacement of epidural infusion catheter
       Displacement of intrathecal infusion catheter
       Displacement of subarachnoid infusion catheter
       Displacement of subdural infusion catheter

√7ᵗʰ   **T85.621** **Displacement of intraperitoneal dialysis catheter** CC PE
       EXCLUDES 1   *mechanical complication of vascular dialysis catheter (T82.4-)*

√7ᵗʰ   **T85.622** **Displacement of permanent sutures** CC PE
       EXCLUDES 1   *mechanical complication of permanent (wire) suture used in bone repair (T84.1-T84.2)*

√7ᵗʰ   **T85.623** **Displacement of artificial skin graft and decellularized allodermis** CC PE
       Dislodgement of artificial skin graft and decellularized allodermis

√7ᵗʰ   **T85.624** **Displacement of insulin pump** PE

√7ᵗʰ   **T85.625** **Displacement of other nervous system device, implant or graft** CC PE
       Displacement of intrathecal infusion pump

√7ᵗʰ   **T85.628** **Displacement of other specified internal prosthetic devices, implants and grafts** CC PE

√6ᵗʰ   **T85.63** **Leakage of other specified internal prosthetic devices, implants and grafts**

√7ᵗʰ   **T85.630** **Leakage of cranial or spinal infusion catheter**
       Leakage of epidural infusion catheter
       Leakage of intrathecal infusion catheter infusion catheter
       Leakage of subarachnoid infusion catheter
       Leakage of subdural infusion catheter
       AHA: 2022,3Q,24

√7ᵗʰ   **T85.631** **Leakage of intraperitoneal dialysis catheter** CC PE
       EXCLUDES 1   *mechanical complication of vascular dialysis catheter (T82.4)*

√7ᵗʰ   **T85.633** **Leakage of insulin pump** CC PE

√7ᵗʰ   **T85.635** **Leakage of other nervous system device, implant or graft** CC PE
       Leakage of intrathecal infusion pump

√7ᵗʰ   **T85.638** **Leakage of other specified internal prosthetic devices, implants and grafts** CC PE

√6ᵗʰ   **T85.69** **Other mechanical complication of other specified internal prosthetic devices, implants and grafts**
     Obstruction, mechanical of other specified internal prosthetic devices, implants and grafts
     Perforation of other specified internal prosthetic devices, implants and grafts
     Protrusion of other specified internal prosthetic devices, implants and grafts

√7ᵗʰ   **T85.690** **Other mechanical complication of cranial or spinal infusion catheter** CC PE
       Other mechanical complication of epidural infusion catheter
       Other mechanical complication of intrathecal infusion catheter
       Other mechanical complication of subarachnoid infusion catheter
       Other mechanical complication of subdural infusion catheter

√7ᵗʰ   **T85.691** **Other mechanical complication of intraperitoneal dialysis catheter** CC PE
       EXCLUDES 1   *mechanical complication of vascular dialysis catheter (T82.4)*

√7ᵗʰ   **T85.692** **Other mechanical complication of permanent sutures** CC PE
       EXCLUDES 1   *mechanical complication of permanent (wire) suture used in bone repair (T84.1-T84.2)*

√7ᵗʰ   **T85.693** **Other mechanical complication of artificial skin graft and decellularized allodermis** CC PE

√7ᵗʰ   **T85.694** **Other mechanical complication of insulin pump** CC PE

√7ᵗʰ   **T85.695** **Other mechanical complication of other nervous system device, implant or graft** CC PE
       Other mechanical complication of intrathecal infusion pump

√7ᵗʰ   **T85.698** **Other mechanical complication of other specified internal prosthetic devices, implants and grafts** CC PE
       Mechanical complication of nonabsorbable surgical material NOS

√5ᵗʰ **T85.7** **Infection and inflammatory reaction due to other internal prosthetic devices, implants and grafts**
     Use additional code to identify infection

√x7ᵗʰ   **T85.71** **Infection and inflammatory reaction due to peritoneal dialysis catheter** CC PE

√x7ᵗʰ   **T85.72** **Infection and inflammatory reaction due to insulin pump** CC PE

√6ᵗʰ   **T85.73** **Infection and inflammatory reaction due to nervous system devices, implants and graft**

√7ᵗʰ   **T85.730** **Infection and inflammatory reaction due to ventricular intracranial (communicating) shunt** CC PE

√7ᵗʰ   **T85.731** **Infection and inflammatory reaction due to implanted electronic neurostimulator of brain, electrode (lead)** CC PE

N Newborn: 0   P Pediatric: 0-17   M Maternity: 9-64   A Adult: 15-124   UNS Unspecified Site   MCC Major Complication/Comorbidity   CC Complication/Comorbidity   PE POA Exempt

1188   ICD-10-CM 2025

√7ᵗʰ **T85.732** **Infection and inflammatory reaction due to implanted electronic neurostimulator of peripheral nerve, electrode (lead)** `CC` `PE`

Infection and inflammatory reaction due to electrode (lead) for cranial nerve neurostimulators

Infection and inflammatory reaction due to electrode (lead) for gastric neurostimulator

Infection and inflammatory reaction due to electrode (lead) for sacral nerve neurostimulator

Infection and inflammatory reaction due to electrode (lead) for vagal nerve neurostimulators

√7ᵗʰ **T85.733** **Infection and inflammatory reaction due to implanted electronic neurostimulator of spinal cord, electrode (lead)** `CC` `PE`

√7ᵗʰ **T85.734** **Infection and inflammatory reaction due to implanted electronic neurostimulator, generator** `CC` `PE`

Generator pocket infection

√7ᵗʰ **T85.735** **Infection and inflammatory reaction due to cranial or spinal infusion catheter** `CC` `PE`

Infection and inflammatory reaction due to epidural catheter

Infection and inflammatory reaction due to intrathecal infusion catheter

Infection and inflammatory reaction due to subarachnoid catheter

Infection and inflammatory reaction due to subdural catheter

√7ᵗʰ **T85.738** **Infection and inflammatory reaction due to other nervous system device, implant or graft** `CC` `PE`

Infection and inflammatory reaction due to intrathecal infusion pump

√x7ᵗʰ **T85.79** **Infection and inflammatory reaction due to other internal prosthetic devices, implants and grafts** `CC` `PE`
AHA: 2023,2Q,27; 2022,2Q,7

√5ᵗʰ **T85.8** **Other specified complications of internal prosthetic devices, implants and grafts, not elsewhere classified**

√6ᵗʰ **T85.81** **Embolism due to internal prosthetic devices, implants and grafts, not elsewhere classified**

√7ᵗʰ **T85.810** **Embolism due to nervous system prosthetic devices, implants and grafts** `CC` `PE`

√7ᵗʰ **T85.818** **Embolism due to other internal prosthetic devices, implants and grafts** `PE`

√6ᵗʰ **T85.82** **Fibrosis due to internal prosthetic devices, implants and grafts, not elsewhere classified**

√7ᵗʰ **T85.820** **Fibrosis due to nervous system prosthetic devices, implants and grafts** `CC` `PE`

√7ᵗʰ **T85.828** **Fibrosis due to other internal prosthetic devices, implants and grafts** `PE`

√6ᵗʰ **T85.83** **Hemorrhage due to internal prosthetic devices, implants and grafts, not elsewhere classified**

√7ᵗʰ **T85.830** **Hemorrhage due to nervous system prosthetic devices, implants and grafts** `CC` `PE`

√7ᵗʰ **T85.838** **Hemorrhage due to other internal prosthetic devices, implants and grafts** `PE`

√6ᵗʰ **T85.84** **Pain due to internal prosthetic devices, implants and grafts, not elsewhere classified**

√7ᵗʰ **T85.840** **Pain due to nervous system prosthetic devices, implants and grafts** `CC` `PE`

√7ᵗʰ **T85.848** **Pain due to other internal prosthetic devices, implants and grafts** `PE`

√6ᵗʰ **T85.85** **Stenosis due to internal prosthetic devices, implants and grafts, not elsewhere classified**

√7ᵗʰ **T85.850** **Stenosis due to nervous system prosthetic devices, implants and grafts** `CC` `PE`

√7ᵗʰ **T85.858** **Stenosis due to other internal prosthetic devices, implants and grafts** `PE`

√6ᵗʰ **T85.86** **Thrombosis due to internal prosthetic devices, implants and grafts, not elsewhere classified**
AHA: AHA:2024,2Q,7

√7ᵗʰ **T85.860** **Thrombosis due to nervous system prosthetic devices, implants and grafts** `CC` `PE`

√7ᵗʰ **T85.868** **Thrombosis due to other internal prosthetic devices, implants and grafts** `PE`

√6ᵗʰ **T85.89** **Other specified complication of internal prosthetic devices, implants and grafts, not elsewhere classified**
Erosion or breakdown of subcutaneous device pocket
AHA: AHA:2024,2Q,8

√7ᵗʰ **T85.890** **Other specified complication of nervous system prosthetic devices, implants and grafts** `CC` `PE`

√7ᵗʰ **T85.898** **Other specified complication of other internal prosthetic devices, implants and grafts** `PE`

√x7ᵗʰ **T85.9** **Unspecified complication of internal prosthetic device, implant and graft** `PE`
Complication of internal prosthetic device, implant and graft NOS

√4ᵗʰ **T86** **Complications of transplanted organs and tissue**
Use additional code to identify other transplant complications, such as:
graft-versus-host disease (D89.81-)
malignancy associated with organ transplant (C80.2)
post-transplant lymphoproliferative disorders (PTLD) (D47.Z1)
AHA: 2020,1Q,18

√5ᵗʰ **T86.0** **Complications of bone marrow transplant**

T86.00 **Unspecified complication of bone marrow transplant** `CC` `HCC`

T86.01 **Bone marrow transplant rejection** `CC` `HCC`

T86.02 **Bone marrow transplant failure** `CC` `HCC`

T86.03 **Bone marrow transplant infection** `CC` `HCC`

T86.09 **Other complications of bone marrow transplant** `CC` `HCC`
AHA: 2023,3Q,19

√5ᵗʰ **T86.1** **Complications of kidney transplant**

T86.10 **Unspecified complication of kidney transplant** `CC`

T86.11 **Kidney transplant rejection** `CC`

T86.12 **Kidney transplant failure** `CC`
AHA: 2013,1Q,24

T86.13 **Kidney transplant infection** `CC`
Use additional code to specify infection

T86.19 **Other complication of kidney transplant** `CC`
AHA: 2019,2Q,7

√5ᵗʰ **T86.2** **Complications of heart transplant**

EXCLUDES 1   complication of:
artificial heart device (T82.5-)
heart-lung transplant (T86.3-)

T86.20 **Unspecified complication of heart transplant** `CC` `HCC`

T86.21 **Heart transplant rejection** `CC` `HCC`

T86.22 **Heart transplant failure** `CC` `HCC`

T86.23 **Heart transplant infection** `CC` `HCC`
Use additional code to specify infection

√6ᵗʰ **T86.29** **Other complications of heart transplant**

T86.290 **Cardiac allograft vasculopathy** `CC` `HCC`
EXCLUDES 1   atherosclerosis of coronary arteries (I25.75-, I25.76-, I25.81-)

T86.298 **Other complications of heart transplant** `CC` `HCC`

√5ᵗʰ **T86.3** **Complications of heart-lung transplant**

T86.30 **Unspecified complication of heart-lung transplant** `CC` `HCC`

T86.31 **Heart-lung transplant rejection** `CC` `HCC`

T86.32 **Heart-lung transplant failure** `CC` `HCC`

T86.33 **Heart-lung transplant infection** `CC` `HCC`
Use additional code to specify infection

T86.39 **Other complications of heart-lung transplant** `CC` `HCC`

√5ᵗʰ **T86.4** **Complications of liver transplant**

T86.40 **Unspecified complication of liver transplant** `CC` `HCC`

T86.41   **Liver transplant rejection** `CC` `HCC`

T86.42   **Liver transplant failure** `CC` `HCC`

T86.43   **Liver transplant infection** `CC` `HCC`

Use additional code to identify infection, such as: cytomegalovirus (CMV) infection (B25.-)

T86.49   **Other complications of liver transplant** `CC` `HCC`

T86.5   **Complications of stem cell transplant** `CC` `HCC`

Complications from stem cells from peripheral blood

Complications from stem cells from umbilical cord

AHA: 2020,4Q,14

✓5th **T86.8**   **Complications of other transplanted organs and tissues**

    ✓6th **T86.81**   **Complications of lung transplant**

      `EXCLUDES 1`   *complication of heart-lung transplant (T86.3-)*

      T86.810   **Lung transplant rejection** `CC` `HCC`

      T86.811   **Lung transplant failure** `CC` `HCC`

      T86.812   **Lung transplant infection** `CC` `HCC`

       Use additional code to specify infection

      T86.818   **Other complications of lung transplant** `CC` `HCC`

       AHA: 2019,2Q,6

      T86.819   **Unspecified complication of lung transplant** `CC` `HCC`

    ✓6th **T86.82**   **Complications of skin graft (allograft) (autograft)**

      `EXCLUDES 2`   *complication of artificial skin graft (T85.693)*

      T86.820   **Skin graft (allograft) rejection** `CC`

      T86.821   **Skin graft (allograft) (autograft) failure** `CC`

      T86.822   **Skin graft (allograft) (autograft) infection** `CC`

       Use additional code to specify infection

      T86.828   **Other complications of skin graft (allograft) (autograft)** `CC`

      T86.829   **Unspecified complication of skin graft (allograft) (autograft)** `CC`

    ✓6th **T86.83**   **Complications of bone graft**

      `EXCLUDES 2`   *mechanical complications of bone graft (T84.3-)*

      T86.830   **Bone graft rejection** `CC`

      T86.831   **Bone graft failure** `CC`

      T86.832   **Bone graft infection** `CC`

       Use additional code to specify infection

      T86.838   **Other complications of bone graft** `CC`

       AHA: 2023,1Q,30

      T86.839   **Unspecified complication of bone graft** `CC`

    ✓6th **T86.84**   **Complications of corneal transplant**

      `EXCLUDES 2`   *mechanical complications of corneal graft (T85.3-)*

      AHA: 2020,4Q,40

     ✓7th **T86.840**   **Corneal transplant rejection**

       T86.8401   **Corneal transplant rejection, right eye** `CC`

       T86.8402   **Corneal transplant rejection, left eye** `CC`

       T86.8403   **Corneal transplant rejection, bilateral** `CC`

       T86.8409   **Corneal transplant rejection, unspecified eye** `CC` `UNS`

     ✓7th **T86.841**   **Corneal transplant failure**

       T86.8411   **Corneal transplant failure, right eye** `CC`

       T86.8412   **Corneal transplant failure, left eye** `CC`

       T86.8413   **Corneal transplant failure, bilateral** `CC`

       T86.8419   **Corneal transplant failure, unspecified eye** `CC` `UNS`

     ✓7th **T86.842**   **Corneal transplant infection**

       Use additional code to specify infection

       T86.8421   **Corneal transplant infection, right eye** `CC`

       T86.8422   **Corneal transplant infection, left eye** `CC`

       T86.8423   **Corneal transplant infection, bilateral** `CC`

       T86.8429   **Corneal transplant infection, unspecified eye** `CC` `UNS`

     ✓7th **T86.848**   **Other complications of corneal transplant**

       T86.8481   **Other complications of corneal transplant, right eye** `CC`

       T86.8482   **Other complications of corneal transplant, left eye** `CC`

       T86.8483   **Other complications of corneal transplant, bilateral** `CC`

       T86.8489   **Other complications of corneal transplant, unspecified eye** `CC` `UNS`

     ✓7th **T86.849**   **Unspecified complication of corneal transplant**

       T86.8491   **Unspecified complication of corneal transplant, right eye** `CC`

       T86.8492   **Unspecified complication of corneal transplant, left eye** `CC`

       T86.8493   **Unspecified complication of corneal transplant, bilateral** `CC`

       T86.8499   **Unspecified complication of corneal transplant, unspecified eye** `CC` `UNS`

    ✓6th **T86.85**   **Complication of intestine transplant**

      T86.850   **Intestine transplant rejection** `CC` `HCC`

      T86.851   **Intestine transplant failure** `CC` `HCC`

      T86.852   **Intestine transplant infection** `CC` `HCC`

       Use additional code to specify infection

      T86.858   **Other complications of intestine transplant** `CC` `HCC`

      T86.859   **Unspecified complication of intestine transplant** `CC` `HCC`

    ✓6th **T86.89**   **Complications of other transplanted tissue**

      Transplant failure or rejection of pancreas

      AHA: 2020,1Q,18

      T86.890   **Other transplanted tissue rejection** `CC`

      T86.891   **Other transplanted tissue failure** `CC`

      T86.892   **Other transplanted tissue infection** `CC`

       Use additional code to specify infection

      T86.898   **Other complications of other transplanted tissue** `CC`

      T86.899   **Unspecified complication of other transplanted tissue** `CC`

   ✓5th **T86.9**   **Complication of unspecified transplanted organ and tissue**

      T86.90   **Unspecified complication of unspecified transplanted organ and tissue** `CC`

      T86.91   **Unspecified transplanted organ and tissue rejection** `CC`

      T86.92   **Unspecified transplanted organ and tissue failure** `CC`

      T86.93   **Unspecified transplanted organ and tissue infection** `CC`

       Use additional code to specify infection

      T86.99   **Other complications of unspecified transplanted organ and tissue** `CC`

✓4th **T87**   **Complications peculiar to reattachment and amputation**

   ✓5th **T87.0**   **Complications of reattached (part of) upper extremity**

    ✓6th **T87.0X**   **Complications of reattached (part of) upper extremity**

      T87.0X1   **Complications of reattached (part of) right upper extremity** `CC` `HCC`

      T87.0X2   **Complications of reattached (part of) left upper extremity** `CC` `HCC`

      T87.0X9   **Complications of reattached (part of) unspecified upper extremity** `CC` `UNS` `HCC`

   ✓5th **T87.1**   **Complications of reattached (part of) lower extremity**

    ✓6th **T87.1X**   **Complications of reattached (part of) lower extremity**

      T87.1X1   **Complications of reattached (part of) right lower extremity** `CC` `HCC`

      T87.1X2   **Complications of reattached (part of) left lower extremity** `CC` `HCC`

      T87.1X9   **Complications of reattached (part of) unspecified lower extremity** `CC` `UNS` `HCC`

   T87.2   **Complications of other reattached body part** `CC`

`N` Newborn: 0   `P` Pediatric: 0-17   `M` Maternity: 9-64   `A` Adult: 15-124   `UNS` Unspecified Site   `MCC` Major Complication/Comorbidity   `CC` Complication/Comorbidity   `PE` POA Exempt

1190

ICD-10-CM 2025

✓5ᵗʰ T87.3 Neuroma of amputation stump

DEF: Non-neoplastic tumor generated at the proximal end of severed, partially transected, or injured nerve following amputation.

    T87.30 Neuroma of amputation stump, unspecified extremity   `HCC`

    T87.31 Neuroma of amputation stump, **right upper** extremity   `HCC`

    T87.32 Neuroma of amputation stump, **left upper** extremity   `HCC`

    T87.33 Neuroma of amputation stump, **right lower** extremity   `HCC`

    T87.34 Neuroma of amputation stump, **left lower** extremity   `HCC`

✓5ᵗʰ T87.4 Infection of amputation stump

    T87.40 Infection of amputation stump, unspecified extremity   `CC` `UNS` `HCC`

    T87.41 Infection of amputation stump, **right upper** extremity   `CC` `HCC`

    T87.42 Infection of amputation stump, **left upper** extremity   `CC` `HCC`

    T87.43 Infection of amputation stump, **right lower** extremity   `CC` `HCC`

    T87.44 Infection of amputation stump, **left lower** extremity   `CC` `HCC`

✓5ᵗʰ T87.5 Necrosis of amputation stump

    T87.50 Necrosis of amputation stump, unspecified extremity   `HCC`

    T87.51 Necrosis of amputation stump, **right upper** extremity   `HCC`

    T87.52 Necrosis of amputation stump, **left upper** extremity   `HCC`

    T87.53 Necrosis of amputation stump, **right lower** extremity   `HCC`

    T87.54 Necrosis of amputation stump, **left lower** extremity   `HCC`

✓5ᵗʰ T87.8 Other complications of amputation stump

    T87.81 **Dehiscence** of amputation stump   `HCC`

    T87.89 Other complications of amputation stump   `HCC`

        Amputation stump contracture
        Amputation stump contracture of next proximal joint
        Amputation stump edema
        Amputation stump flexion
        Amputation stump hematoma

        EXCLUDES 2 *phantom limb syndrome (G54.6-G54.7)*

        AHA: 2022,3Q,11

    T87.9 **Unspecified complications of amputation stump**   `HCC`

✓4ᵗʰ T88 Other complications of surgical and medical care, not elsewhere classified

    EXCLUDES 2 *complication following infusion, transfusion and therapeutic injection (T80.-)*

        complication following procedure NEC (T81.-)
        complications of anesthesia in labor and delivery (O74.-)
        complications of anesthesia in pregnancy (O29.-)
        complications of anesthesia in puerperium (O89.-)
        complications of devices, implants and grafts (T82-T85)
        complications of obstetric surgery and procedure (O75.4)
        dermatitis due to drugs and medicaments (L23.3, L24.4, L25.1, L27.0-L27.1)
        poisoning and toxic effects of drugs and chemicals (T36-T65 with fifth or sixth character 1-4)
        specified complications classified elsewhere

> The appropriate 7th character is to be added to each code from category T88.
> A initial encounter
> D subsequent encounter
> S sequela

✓x7ᵗʰ T88.0 **Infection following immunization**   `CC` `PE`

    Sepsis following immunization

    AHA: 2018,4Q,62-63

✓x7ᵗʰ T88.1 **Other complications following immunization, not elsewhere classified**   `CC` `PE`

    Generalized vaccinia
    Rash following immunization

    EXCLUDES 1 *vaccinia not from vaccine (B08.011)*

    EXCLUDES 2 *anaphylactic shock due to serum (T80.5-)*
        other serum reactions (T80.6-)
        postimmunization arthropathy (M02.2)
        postimmunization encephalitis (G04.02)
        postimmunization fever (R50.83)

✓x7ᵗʰ T88.2 **Shock due to anesthesia**   `CC` `PE`

    Use additional code for adverse effect, if applicable, to identify drug (T41.- with fifth or sixth character 5)

    EXCLUDES 1 *complications of anesthesia (in):*
        labor and delivery (O74.-)
        postprocedural shock NOS (T81.1-)
        pregnancy (O29.-)
        puerperium (O89.-)

✓x7ᵗʰ T88.3 **Malignant hyperthermia due to anesthesia**   `CC` `PE`

    Use additional code for adverse effect, if applicable, to identify drug (T41.- with fifth or sixth character 5)

✓x7ᵗʰ T88.4 **Failed or difficult intubation**   `PE`

✓5ᵗʰ T88.5 **Other complications of anesthesia**

    Use additional code for adverse effect, if applicable, to identify drug (T41.- with fifth or sixth character 5)

    ✓x7ᵗʰ T88.51 **Hypothermia following anesthesia**   `PE`

    ✓x7ᵗʰ T88.52 **Failed moderate sedation during procedure**   `PE`

        Failed conscious sedation during procedure

        EXCLUDES 2 *personal history of failed moderate sedation (Z92.83)*

    ✓x7ᵗʰ T88.53 **Unintended awareness under general anesthesia during procedure**   `PE`

        EXCLUDES 2 *personal history of unintended awareness under general anesthesia (Z92.84)*

        AHA: 2016,4Q,72-73

    ✓x7ᵗʰ T88.59 **Other complications of anesthesia**   `PE`

✓x7ᵗʰ T88.6 **Anaphylactic reaction due to adverse effect of correct drug or medicament properly administered**   `CC` `PE`

    Anaphylactic shock due to adverse effect of correct drug or medicament properly administered
    Anaphylactoid reaction NOS

    Use additional code for adverse effect, if applicable, to identify drug (T36-T50 with fifth or sixth character 5)

    EXCLUDES 1 *anaphylactic reaction due to serum (T80.5-)*
        anaphylactic shock or reaction due to adverse food reaction (T78.0-)

    AHA: 2020,1Q,18

✓x7ᵗʰ T88.7 **Unspecified adverse effect of drug or medicament**   `PE`

    Drug hypersensitivity NOS
    Drug reaction NOS

    Use additional code for adverse effect, if applicable, to identify drug (T36-T50 with fifth or sixth character 5)

    EXCLUDES 1 *specified adverse effects of drugs and medicaments (A00-R94 and T80-T88.6, T88.8)*

✓x7ᵗʰ T88.8 **Other specified complications of surgical and medical care, not elsewhere classified**   `PE`

    Use additional code to identify the complication

    AHA: 2022,2Q,7

✓x7ᵗʰ T88.9 **Complication of surgical and medical care, unspecified**   `PE`

Chapter 20. External Causes of Morbidity (V00–Y99)

Chapter-specific Guidelines with Coding Examples

The chapter-specific guidelines from the ICD-10-CM Official Guidelines for Coding and Reporting have been provided below. Along with these guidelines are coding examples, contained in the shaded boxes, that have been developed to help illustrate the coding and/or sequencing guidance found in these guidelines.

The external causes of morbidity codes should never be sequenced as the first-listed or principal diagnosis.

External cause codes are intended to provide data for injury research and evaluation of injury prevention strategies. These codes capture how the injury or health condition happened (cause), the intent (unintentional or accidental; or intentional, such as suicide or assault), the place where the event occurred the activity of the patient at the time of the event, and the person's status (e.g., civilian, military).

There is no national requirement for mandatory ICD-10-CM external cause code reporting. Unless a provider is subject to a state-based external cause code reporting mandate or these codes are required by a particular payer, reporting of ICD-10-CM codes in Chapter 20, External Causes of Morbidity, is not required. In the absence of a mandatory reporting requirement, providers are encouraged to voluntarily report external cause codes, as they provide valuable data for injury research and evaluation of injury prevention strategies.

a. General external cause coding guidelines

1) Used with any code in the range of A00.0–T88.9, Z00–Z99

An external cause code may be used with any code in the range of A00.0–T88.9, Z00–Z99, classification that represents a health condition due to an external cause. Though they are most applicable to injuries, they are also valid for use with such things as infections or diseases due to an external source, and other health conditions, such as a heart attack that occurs during strenuous physical activity.

> Actinic reticuloid due to tanning bed use
>
> **L57.1**   **Actinic reticuloid**
>
> **W89.1XXA**   **Exposure to tanning bed, initial encounter**
>
> *Explanation:* An external cause code may be used with any code in the range of A00.0–T88.9, Z00–Z99, classifications that describe health conditions due to an external cause. Code W89.1 Exposure to tanning bed requires a seventh character of A to report this initial encounter, with a placeholder X for the fifth and sixth characters.

2) External cause code used for length of treatment

Assign the external cause code, with the appropriate 7th character (initial encounter, subsequent encounter or sequela) for each encounter for which the injury or condition is being treated.

Most categories in chapter 20 have a 7th character requirement for each applicable code. Most categories in this chapter have three 7th character values: A, initial encounter, D, subsequent encounter and S, sequela. While the patient may be seen by a new or different provider over the course of treatment for an injury or condition, assignment of the 7th character for external cause should match the 7th character of the code assigned for the associated injury or condition for the encounter.

3) Use the full range of external cause codes

Use the full range of external cause codes to completely describe the cause, the intent, the place of occurrence, and if applicable, the activity of the patient at the time of the event, and the patient's status, for all injuries, and other health conditions due to an external cause.

4) Assign as many external cause codes as necessary

Assign as many external cause codes as necessary to fully explain each cause. If only one external code can be recorded, assign the code most related to the principal diagnosis.

5) The selection of the appropriate external cause code

The selection of the appropriate external cause code is guided by the Alphabetic Index of External Causes and by Inclusion and Exclusion notes in the Tabular List.

6) External cause code can never be a principal diagnosis

An external cause code can never be a principal (first-listed) diagnosis.

7) Combination external cause codes

Certain of the external cause codes are combination codes that identify sequential events that result in an injury, such as a fall which results in striking against an object. The injury may be due to either event or both.

The combination external cause code used should correspond to the sequence of events regardless of which caused the most serious injury.

> Toddler tripped and fell while walking and struck his head on an end table, sustaining a scalp contusion
>
> **S00.03XA**   **Contusion of scalp, initial encounter**
>
> **W01.190A**   **Fall on same level from slipping, tripping and stumbling with subsequent striking against furniture, initial encounter**
>
> *Explanation:* Combination external cause codes identify sequential events that result in an injury, such as a fall resulting in striking against an object. The injury may be due to either or both events.

8) No external cause code needed in certain circumstances

No external cause code from Chapter 20 is needed if the external cause and intent are included in a code from another chapter (e.g., T36.0X1-, Poisoning by penicillins, accidental (unintentional)).

b. Place of occurrence guideline

Codes from category Y92, Place of occurrence of the external cause, are secondary codes for use after other external cause codes to identify the location of the patient at the time of injury or other condition.

Generally, a place of occurrence code is assigned only once, at the initial encounter for treatment. However, in the rare instance that a new injury occurs during hospitalization, an additional place of occurrence code may be assigned. No 7th characters are used for Y92.

Do not use place of occurrence code Y92.9 if the place is not stated or is not applicable.

> A farmer was working in his barn and sustained a foot contusion when the horse stepped on his left foot
>
> **S90.32XA**   **Contusion of left foot, initial encounter**
>
> **W55.19XA**   **Other contact with horse, initial encounter**
>
> **Y92.71**   **Barn as the place of occurrence of the external cause**
>
> *Explanation:* A place-of-occurrence code from category Y92 is assigned at the initial encounter to identify the location of the patient at the time the injury occurred.

c. Activity code

Assign a code from category Y93, Activity code, to describe the activity of the patient at the time the injury or other health condition occurred.

An activity code is used only once, at the initial encounter for treatment. Only one code from Y93 should be recorded on a medical record.

The activity codes are not applicable to poisonings, adverse effects, misadventures or sequela.

Do not assign Y93.9, Unspecified activity, if the activity is not stated.

A code from category Y93 is appropriate for use with external cause and intent codes if identifying the activity provides additional information about the event.

> Ranch hand who was grooming a horse sustained a foot contusion when the horse stepped on his left foot
>
> **S90.32XA**   **Contusion of left foot, initial encounter**
>
> **W55.19XA**   **Other contact with horse, initial encounter**
>
> **Y93.K3**   **Activity, grooming and shearing an animal**
>
> *Explanation:* One activity code from category Y93 is assigned at the initial encounter only to describe the activity of the patient at the time the injury occurred.

d. Place of occurrence, activity, and status codes used with other external cause code

When applicable, place of occurrence, activity, and external cause status codes are sequenced after the main external cause code(s). Regardless of the number of external cause codes assigned, generally there should be only one place of occurrence code, one activity code, and one external cause status code assigned to an encounter. However, in the rare instance that a new injury occurs during hospitalization, an additional place of occurrence code may be assigned.

e. If the reporting format limits the number of external cause codes

If the reporting format limits the number of external cause codes that can be used in reporting clinical data, report the code for the cause/intent most related to the principal diagnosis. If the format permits capture of additional external cause codes, the cause/intent, including medical misadventures, of the additional events should be reported rather than the codes for place, activity, or external status.

f. Multiple external cause coding guidelines

More than one external cause code is required to fully describe the external cause of an illness or injury. The assignment of external cause codes should be sequenced in the following priority:

If two or more events cause separate injuries, an external cause code should be assigned for each cause. The first-listed external cause code will be selected in the following order:

External codes for child and adult abuse take priority over all other external cause codes.

See Section I.C.19., Child and Adult abuse guidelines.

External cause codes for terrorism events take priority over all other external cause codes except child and adult abuse.

External cause codes for cataclysmic events take priority over all other external cause codes except child and adult abuse and terrorism.

External cause codes for transport accidents take priority over all other external cause codes except cataclysmic events, child and adult abuse and terrorism.

Activity and external cause status codes are assigned following all causal (intent) external cause codes.

The first-listed external cause code should correspond to the cause of the most serious diagnosis due to an assault, accident, or self-harm, following the order of hierarchy listed above..

30-year-old man accidentally discharged his hunting rifle, sustaining an open gunshot wound to the right thigh, which caused him to fall down the stairs, resulting in closed displaced comminuted fracture of his left radial shaft

S71.131A	Puncture wound without foreign body, right thigh, initial encounter
W33.02XA	Accidental discharge of hunting rifle, initial encounter
S52.352A	Displaced comminuted fracture of shaft of radius, left arm, initial encounter for closed fracture
W10.9XXA	Fall (on) (from) unspecified stairs and steps, initial encounter

Explanation: If two or more events cause separate injuries, an external cause code should be assigned for each cause.

---

g. Child and adult abuse guideline

Adult and child abuse, neglect and maltreatment are classified as assault. Any of the assault codes may be used to indicate the external cause of any injury resulting from the confirmed abuse.

For confirmed cases of abuse, neglect and maltreatment, when the perpetrator is known, a code from Y07, Perpetrator of maltreatment and neglect, should accompany any other assault codes.

See Section I.C.19. Adult and child abuse, neglect and other maltreatment

h. Unknown or undetermined intent guideline

If the intent (accident, self-harm, assault) of the cause of an injury or other condition is unknown or unspecified, code the intent as accidental intent. All transport accident categories assume accidental intent.

1) Use of undetermined intent

External cause codes for events of undetermined intent are only for use if the documentation in the record specifies that the intent cannot be determined.

i. Sequelae (late effects) of external cause guidelines

1) Sequelae external cause codes

Sequela are reported using the external cause code with the 7th character "S" for sequela. These codes should be used with any report of a late effect or sequela resulting from a previous injury.

See Section I.B.10. Sequela (Late Effects)

2) Sequela external cause code with a related current injury

A sequela external cause code should never be used with a related current nature of injury code.

3) Use of sequela external cause codes for subsequent visits

Use a late effect external cause code for subsequent visits when a late effect of the initial injury is being treated. Do not use a late effect external cause code for subsequent visits for follow-up care (e.g., to assess healing, to receive rehabilitative therapy) of the injury when no late effect of the injury has been documented.

j. Terrorism guidelines

1) Cause of injury identified by the Federal Government (FBI) as terrorism

When the cause of an injury is identified by the Federal Government (FBI) as terrorism, the first-listed external cause code should be a code from category Y38, Terrorism. The definition of terrorism employed by the FBI is found at the inclusion note at the beginning of category Y38. Use additional code for place of occurrence (Y92.-). More than one Y38 code may be assigned if the injury is the result of more than one mechanism of terrorism.

2) Cause of an injury is suspected to be the result of terrorism

When the cause of an injury is suspected to be the result of terrorism a code from category Y38 should not be assigned. Suspected cases should be classified as assault.

3) Code Y38.9, Terrorism, secondary effects

Assign code Y38.9, Terrorism, secondary effects, for conditions occurring subsequent to the terrorist event. This code should not be assigned for conditions that are due to the initial terrorist act.

It is acceptable to assign code Y38.9 with another code from Y38 if there is an injury due to the initial terrorist event and an injury that is a subsequent result of the terrorist event.

k. External cause status

A code from category Y99, External cause status, should be assigned whenever any other external cause code is assigned for an encounter, including an Activity code, except for the events noted below. Assign a code from category Y99, External cause status, to indicate the work status of the person at the time the event occurred. The status code indicates whether the event occurred during military activity, whether a non-military person was at work, whether an individual including a student or volunteer was involved in a non-work activity at the time of the causal event.

A code from Y99, External cause status, should be assigned, when applicable, with other external cause codes, such as transport accidents and falls. The external cause status codes are not applicable to poisonings, adverse effects, misadventures or late effects.

Do not assign a code from category Y99 if no other external cause codes (cause, activity) are applicable for the encounter.

An external cause status code is used only once, at the initial encounter for treatment. Only one code from Y99 should be recorded on a medical record.

Do not assign code Y99.9, Unspecified external cause status, if the status is not stated.

Chapter 20. External Causes of Morbidity (V00-Y99)

NOTE This chapter permits the classification of environmental events and circumstances as the cause of injury, and other adverse effects. Where a code from this section is applicable, it is intended that it shall be used secondary to a code from another chapter of the Classification indicating the nature of the condition. Most often, the condition will be classifiable to Chapter 19, Injury, poisoning and certain other consequences of external causes (S00-T88). Other conditions that may be stated to be due to external causes are classified in Chapters I to XVIII. For these conditions, codes from Chapter 20 should be used to provide additional information as to the cause of the condition.

AHA: 2018,4Q,58-60

This chapter contains the following blocks:

V00-X58	Accidents
V00-V99	Transport accidents
V00-V09	Pedestrian injured in transport accident
V10-V19	Pedal cycle rider injured in transport accident
V20-V29	Motorcycle rider injured in transport accident
V30-V39	Occupant of three-wheeled motor vehicle injured in transport accident
V40-V49	Car occupant injured in transport accident
V50-V59	Occupant of pick-up truck or van injured in transport accident
V60-V69	Occupant of heavy transport vehicle injured in transport accident
V70-V79	Bus occupant injured in transport accident
V80-V89	Other land transport accidents
V90-V94	Water transport accidents
V95-V97	Air and space transport accidents
V98-V99	Other and unspecified transport accidents
W00-X58	Other external causes of accidental injury
W00-W19	Slipping, tripping, stumbling and falls
W20-W49	Exposure to inanimate mechanical forces
W50-W64	Exposure to animate mechanical forces
W65-W74	Accidental non-transport drowning and submersion
W85-W99	Exposure to electric current, radiation and extreme ambient air temperature and pressure
X00-X08	Exposure to smoke, fire and flames
X10-X19	Contact with heat and hot substances
X30-X39	Exposure to forces of nature
X50	Overexertion and strenuous or repetitive movements
X52-X58	Accidental exposure to other specified factors
X71-X83	Intentional self-harm
X92-Y09	Assault
Y21-Y33	Event of undetermined intent
Y35-Y38	Legal intervention, operations of war, military operations, and terrorism
Y62-Y84	Complications of medical and surgical care
Y62-Y69	Misadventures to patients during surgical and medical care
Y70-Y82	Medical devices associated with adverse incidents in diagnostic and therapeutic use
Y83-Y84	Surgical and other medical procedures as the cause of abnormal reaction of the patient, or of later complication, without mention of misadventure at the time of the procedure
Y90-Y99	Supplementary factors related to causes of morbidity classified elsewhere

ACCIDENTS (V00-X58)

AHA: 2018,2Q,7-8

Transport accidents (V00-V99)

NOTE This section is structured in 12 groups. Those relating to land transport accidents (V00-V89) reflect the victim's mode of transport and are subdivided to identify the victim's 'counterpart' or the type of event. The vehicle of which the injured person is an occupant is identified in the first two characters since it is seen as the most important factor to identify for prevention purposes. A transport accident is one in which the vehicle involved must be moving or running or in use for transport purposes at the time of the accident.

Use additional code to identify:
   airbag injury (W22.1)
   type of street or road (Y92.4-)
   use of cellular telephone and other electronic equipment at the time of the transport accident (Y93.C-)

EXCLUDES 1　*agricultural vehicles in stationary use or maintenance (W31.-)*
assault by crashing of motor vehicle (Y03.-)
automobile or motor cycle in stationary use or maintenance - code to type of accident
crashing of motor vehicle, undetermined intent (Y32)
intentional self-harm by crashing of motor vehicle (X82)

EXCLUDES 2　*transport accidents due to cataclysm (X34-X38)*

NOTE Definitions related to transport accidents:

(a) A transport accident (V00-V99) is any accident involving a device designed primarily for, or used at the time primarily for, conveying persons or good from one place to another.

(b) A public highway [trafficway] or street is the entire width between property lines (or other boundary lines) of land open to the public as a matter of right or custom for purposes of moving persons or property from one place to another. A roadway is that part of the public highway designed, improved and customarily used for vehicular traffic.

(c) A traffic accident is any vehicle accident occurring on the public highway [i.e. originating on, terminating on, or involving a vehicle partially on the highway]. A vehicle accident is assumed to have occurred on the public highway unless another place is specified, except in the case of accidents involving only off-road motor vehicles, which are classified as nontraffic accidents unless the contrary is stated.

(d) A nontraffic accident is any vehicle accident that occurs entirely in any place other than a public highway.

(e) A pedestrian is any person involved in an accident who was not at the time of the accident riding in or on a motor vehicle, railway train, streetcar or animal-drawn or other vehicle, or on a pedal cycle or animal. This includes, a person changing a tire, working on a parked car, or a person on foot. It also includes the user of a pedestrian conveyance such as a baby stroller, ice-skates, skis, sled, roller skates, a skateboard, nonmotorized or motorized wheelchair, motorized mobility scooter, or nonmotorized scooter.

(f) A driver is an occupant of a transport vehicle who is operating or intending to operate it.

(g) A passenger is any occupant of a transport vehicle other than the driver, except a person traveling on the outside of the vehicle.

(h) A person on the outside of a vehicle is any person being transported by a vehicle but not occupying the space normally reserved for the driver or passengers, or the space intended for the transport of property. This includes a person travelling on the bodywork, bumper, fender, roof, running board or step of a vehicle, as well as, hanging on the outside of the vehicle.

(i) A pedal cycle is any land transport vehicle operated solely by nonmotorized pedals including a bicycle or tricycle.

(j) A pedal cyclist is any person riding a pedal cycle or in a sidecar or trailer attached to a pedal cycle.

(k) A motorcycle is a two-wheeled motor vehicle with one or two riding saddles and sometimes with a third wheel for the support of a sidecar. The sidecar is considered part of the motorcycle. This includes a moped, motor scooter, or motorized bicycle.

(l) A motorcycle rider is any person riding a motorcycle or in a sidecar or trailer attached to the motorcycle.

(m) A three-wheeled motor vehicle is a motorized tricycle designed primarily for on-road use. This includes a motor-driven tricycle, a motorized rickshaw, or a three-wheeled motor car.

(n) A car [automobile] is a four-wheeled motor vehicle designed primarily for carrying up to 7 persons. A trailer being towed by the car is considered part of the car. It does not include a van or minivan — see definition (o).

(o) A pick-up truck or van is a four or six-wheeled motor vehicle designed for carrying passengers as well as property or cargo weighing less than the local limit for classification as a heavy goods vehicle, and not requiring a special driver's license. This includes a minivan and a sport-utility vehicle (SUV).

(p) A heavy transport vehicle is a motor vehicle designed primarily for carrying property, meeting local criteria for classification as a heavy goods vehicle in terms of weight and requiring a special driver's license.

(q) A bus (coach) is a motor vehicle designed or adapted primarily for carrying more than 10 passengers, and requiring a special driver's license.

(r) A railway train or railway vehicle is any device, with or without freight or passenger cars couple to it, designed for traffic on a railway track. This includes subterranean (subways) or elevated trains.

(s) A streetcar, is a device designed and used primarily for transporting passengers within a municipality, running on rails, usually subject to normal traffic control signals, and operated principally on a right-of-way that forms part of the roadway. This includes a tram or trolley that runs on rails. A trailer being towed by a streetcar is considered part of the streetcar.

(t) A special vehicle mainly used on industrial premises is a motor vehicle designed primarily for use within the buildings and premises of industrial or commercial establishments. This includes battery-powered airport passenger vehicles or baggage/mail trucks, forklifts, coal-cars in a coal mine, logging cars and trucks used in mines or quarries.

(u) A special vehicle mainly used in agriculture is a motor vehicle designed specifically for use in farming and agriculture (horticulture), to work the land, tend and harvest crops and transport materials on the farm. This includes harvesters, farm machinery and tractor and trailers.

(v) A special construction vehicle is a motor vehicle designed specifically for use on construction and demolition sites. This includes bulldozers, diggers, earth levellers, dump trucks. backhoes, front-end loaders, pavers, and mechanical shovels.

☑ Additional Char Req　✓x7ᵗʰ Placeholder　Unacceptable PDx　Questionable PDx　Wrong Procedure　Manifestation　Unspecified　H1-H14 HAC　HCC CMS-HCC Dx　HIV HIV Dx

ICD-10-CM 2025　　　　　　　　　　　　　　　　　　　　　　　　　　　　　　　1195

Chapter 20. External Causes of Morbidity

(w) A special all-terrain vehicle is a motor vehicle of special design to enable it to negotiate over rough or soft ground, snow or sand. Examples of special design are high construction, special wheels and tires, tracks, and support on a cushion of air. This includes snow mobiles, All-terrain vehicles (ATV), and dune buggies. It does not include passenger vehicle designated as Sport Utility Vehicles. (SUV)

(x) A watercraft is any device designed for transporting passengers or goods on water. This includes motor or sailboats, ships, and hovercraft.

(y) An aircraft is any device for transporting passengers or goods in the air. This includes hot-air balloons, gliders, helicopters and airplanes.

(z) A military vehicle is any motorized vehicle operating on a public roadway owned by the military and being operated by a member of the military.

Pedestrian injured in transport accident (V00-V09)

INCLUDES   person changing tire on transport vehicle
person examining engine of vehicle broken down in (on side of) road
EXCLUDES 1   *fall due to non-transport collision with other person (W03)*
pedestrian on foot falling (slipping) on ice and snow (W00.-)
struck or bumped by another person (W51)

The appropriate 7th character is to be added to each code from categories V00-V09.
A   initial encounter
D   subsequent encounter
S   sequela

√4ᵗʰ **V00   Pedestrian conveyance accident**

Use additional place of occurrence and activity external cause codes, if known (Y92.-, Y93.-)

EXCLUDES 1   *collision with another person without fall (W51)*
fall due to person on foot colliding with another person on foot (W03)
fall from non-moving wheelchair, nonmotorized scooter and motorized mobility scooter without collision (W05.-)
pedestrian (conveyance) collision with other land transport vehicle (V01-V09)
pedestrian on foot falling (slipping) on ice and snow (W00.-)

√5ᵗʰ **V00.0   Pedestrian on foot injured in collision with pedestrian conveyance**

√x7ᵗʰ **V00.01   Pedestrian on foot injured in collision with roller-skater**

√x7ᵗʰ **V00.02   Pedestrian on foot injured in collision with skateboarder**

√6ᵗʰ **V00.03   Pedestrian on foot injured in collision with standing micro-mobility pedestrian conveyance**

√7ᵗʰ **V00.031   Pedestrian on foot injured in collision with rider of standing electric scooter**

√7ᵗʰ **V00.038   Pedestrian on foot injured in collision with rider of other standing micro-mobility pedestrian conveyance**

Pedestrian on foot injured in collision with rider of hoverboard
Pedestrian on foot injured in collision with rider of segway

√x7ᵗʰ **V00.09   Pedestrian on foot injured in collision with other pedestrian conveyance**

√5ᵗʰ **V00.1   Rolling-type pedestrian conveyance accident**

EXCLUDES 1   *accident with baby stroller (V00.82-)*
accident with motorized mobility scooter (V00.83-)
accident with wheelchair (powered) (V00.81-)

√6ᵗʰ **V00.11   In-line roller-skate accident**

√7ᵗʰ **V00.111   Fall from in-line roller-skates**

√7ᵗʰ **V00.112   In-line roller-skater colliding with stationary object**

√7ᵗʰ **V00.118   Other in-line roller-skate accident**

EXCLUDES 1   *roller-skater collision with other land transport vehicle (V01-V09 with 5th character 1)*

√6ᵗʰ **V00.12   Non-in-line roller-skate accident**

√7ᵗʰ **V00.121   Fall from non-in-line roller-skates**

√7ᵗʰ **V00.122   Non-in-line roller-skater colliding with stationary object**

√7ᵗʰ **V00.128   Other non-in-line roller-skating accident**

EXCLUDES 1   *roller-skater collision with other land transport vehicle (V01-V09 with 5th character 1)*

√6ᵗʰ **V00.13   Skateboard accident**

√7ᵗʰ **V00.131   Fall from skateboard**

√7ᵗʰ **V00.132   Skateboarder colliding with stationary object**

√7ᵗʰ **V00.138   Other skateboard accident**

EXCLUDES 1   *skateboarder collision with other land transport vehicle (V01-V09 with 5th character 2)*

√6ᵗʰ **V00.14   Scooter (nonmotorized) accident**

EXCLUDES 1   *motor scooter accident (V20-V29)*

√7ᵗʰ **V00.141   Fall from scooter (nonmotorized)**

√7ᵗʰ **V00.142   Scooter (nonmotorized) colliding with stationary object**

√7ᵗʰ **V00.148   Other scooter (nonmotorized) accident**

EXCLUDES 1   *scooter (nonmotorized) collision with other land transport vehicle (V01-V09 with fifth character 9)*

√6ᵗʰ **V00.15   Heelies accident**

Rolling shoe
Wheeled shoe
Wheelies accident

√7ᵗʰ **V00.151   Fall from heelies**

√7ᵗʰ **V00.152   Heelies colliding with stationary object**

√7ᵗʰ **V00.158   Other heelies accident**

√6ᵗʰ **V00.18   Accident on other rolling-type pedestrian conveyance**

√7ᵗʰ **V00.181   Fall from other rolling-type pedestrian conveyance**

√7ᵗʰ **V00.182   Pedestrian on other rolling-type pedestrian conveyance colliding with stationary object**

√7ᵗʰ **V00.188   Other accident on other rolling-type pedestrian conveyance**

√5ᵗʰ **V00.2   Gliding-type pedestrian conveyance accident**

√6ᵗʰ **V00.21   Ice-skates accident**

√7ᵗʰ **V00.211   Fall from ice-skates**

√7ᵗʰ **V00.212   Ice-skater colliding with stationary object**

√7ᵗʰ **V00.218   Other ice-skates accident**

EXCLUDES 1   *ice-skater collision with other land transport vehicle (V01-V09 with 5th character 9)*

√6ᵗʰ **V00.22   Sled accident**

√7ᵗʰ **V00.221   Fall from sled**

√7ᵗʰ **V00.222   Sledder colliding with stationary object**

√7ᵗʰ **V00.228   Other sled accident**

EXCLUDES 1   *sled collision with other land transport vehicle (V01-V09 with 5th character 9)*

√6ᵗʰ **V00.28   Other gliding-type pedestrian conveyance accident**

√7ᵗʰ **V00.281   Fall from other gliding-type pedestrian conveyance**

√7ᵗʰ **V00.282   Pedestrian on other gliding-type pedestrian conveyance colliding with stationary object**

√7ᵗʰ **V00.288   Other accident on other gliding-type pedestrian conveyance**

EXCLUDES 1   *gliding-type pedestrian conveyance collision with other land transport vehicle (V01-V09 with 5th character 9)*

√5ᵗʰ **V00.3   Flat-bottomed pedestrian conveyance accident**

√6ᵗʰ **V00.31   Snowboard accident**

√7ᵗʰ **V00.311   Fall from snowboard**

√7ᵗʰ **V00.312   Snowboarder colliding with stationary object**

N Newborn: 0   P Pediatric: 0-17   M Maternity: 9-64   A Adult: 15-124   UNS Unspecified Site   MCC Major Complication/Comorbidity   CC Complication/Comorbidity   PE POA Exempt

1196

V00–V00.312

ICD-10-CM 2025

    ☑7ᵗʰ **V00.318** Other snowboard accident

        EXCLUDES 1 *snowboarder collision with other land transport vehicle (V01-V09 with 5th character 9)*

  ✓6ᵗʰ **V00.32** Snow-ski accident

    ✓7ᵗʰ **V00.321** **Fall from** snow-skis

    ✓7ᵗʰ **V00.322** Snow-skier **colliding with stationary object**

    ✓7ᵗʰ **V00.328** Other snow-ski accident

        EXCLUDES 1 *snow-skier collision with other land transport vehicle (V01-V09 with 5th character 9)*

  ✓6ᵗʰ **V00.38** Other flat-bottomed pedestrian conveyance accident

    ✓7ᵗʰ **V00.381** **Fall from** other flat-bottomed pedestrian conveyance

    ✓7ᵗʰ **V00.382** Pedestrian on other flat-bottomed pedestrian conveyance **colliding with stationary object**

    ✓7ᵗʰ **V00.388** Other accident on other flat-bottomed pedestrian conveyance

✓5ᵗʰ **V00.8** Accident on other pedestrian conveyance

  ✓6ᵗʰ **V00.81** Accident with **wheelchair** (powered)

    ✓7ᵗʰ **V00.811** **Fall from** moving wheelchair (powered)

        EXCLUDES 1 *fall from non-moving wheelchair (W05.0)*

    ✓7ᵗʰ **V00.812** Wheelchair (powered) **colliding with stationary object**

    ✓7ᵗʰ **V00.818** Other accident with wheelchair (powered)

  ✓6ᵗʰ **V00.82** Accident with **baby stroller**

    ✓7ᵗʰ **V00.821** **Fall from** baby stroller

    ✓7ᵗʰ **V00.822** Baby stroller **colliding with stationary object**

    ✓7ᵗʰ **V00.828** Other accident with baby stroller

  ✓6ᵗʰ **V00.83** Accident with **motorized mobility scooter**

    ✓7ᵗʰ **V00.831** **Fall from** motorized mobility scooter

        EXCLUDES 1 *fall from non-moving motorized mobility scooter (W05.2)*

    ✓7ᵗʰ **V00.832** Motorized mobility scooter **colliding with stationary object**

    ✓7ᵗʰ **V00.838** Other accident with motorized mobility scooter

  ✓6ᵗʰ **V00.84** Accident with **standing micro-mobility pedestrian conveyance**

    ✓7ᵗʰ **V00.841** **Fall from** standing electric scooter

    ✓7ᵗʰ **V00.842** Pedestrian on standing electric scooter **colliding with stationary object**

    ✓7ᵗʰ **V00.848** Other accident with standing micro-mobility pedestrian conveyance

        Accident with hoverboard

        Accident with segway

  ✓6ᵗʰ **V00.89** Accident on other pedestrian conveyance

    ✓7ᵗʰ **V00.891** **Fall from** other pedestrian conveyance

    ✓7ᵗʰ **V00.892** Pedestrian on other pedestrian conveyance **colliding with stationary object**

    ✓7ᵗʰ **V00.898** Other accident on other pedestrian conveyance

        EXCLUDES 1 *other pedestrian (conveyance) collision with other land transport vehicle (V01-V09 with 5th character 9)*

✓4ᵗʰ **V01** Pedestrian injured in collision with pedal cycle

  ✓5ᵗʰ **V01.0** Pedestrian injured in collision with pedal cycle **in nontraffic accident**

    ✓x7ᵗʰ **V01.00** Pedestrian **on foot** injured in collision with pedal cycle in nontraffic accident

        Pedestrian NOS injured in collision with pedal cycle in nontraffic accident

    ✓x7ᵗʰ **V01.01** Pedestrian **on roller-skates** injured in collision with pedal cycle in nontraffic accident

    ✓x7ᵗʰ **V01.02** Pedestrian **on skateboard** injured in collision with pedal cycle in nontraffic accident

    ✓6ᵗʰ **V01.03** Pedestrian on standing micro-mobility pedestrian conveyance injured in collision with pedal cycle in nontraffic accident

      ✓7ᵗʰ **V01.031** Pedestrian **on standing electric scooter** injured in collision with pedal cycle in nontraffic accident

      ✓7ᵗʰ **V01.038** Pedestrian on other standing micro-mobility pedestrian conveyance injured in collision with pedal cycle in nontraffic accident

        Pedestrian on hoverboard injured in collision with pedal cycle in nontraffic accident

        Pedestrian on segway injured in collision with pedal cycle in nontraffic accident

    ✓x7ᵗʰ **V01.09** Pedestrian with other conveyance injured in collision with pedal cycle in nontraffic accident

        Pedestrian with baby stroller injured in collision with pedal cycle in nontraffic accident

        Pedestrian on ice-skates injured in collision with pedal cycle in nontraffic accident

        Pedestrian in motorized mobility scooter injured in collision with pedal cycle in nontraffic accident

        Pedestrian on nonmotorized scooter injured in collision with pedal cycle in nontraffic accident

        Pedestrian on sled injured in collision with pedal cycle in nontraffic accident

        Pedestrian on snowboard injured in collision with pedal cycle in nontraffic accident

        Pedestrian on snow-skis injured in collision with pedal cycle in nontraffic accident

        Pedestrian in wheelchair (powered) injured in collision with pedal cycle in nontraffic accident

  ✓5ᵗʰ **V01.1** Pedestrian injured in collision with pedal cycle **in traffic accident**

    ✓x7ᵗʰ **V01.10** Pedestrian **on foot** injured in collision with pedal cycle in traffic accident

        Pedestrian NOS injured in collision with pedal cycle in traffic accident

    ✓x7ᵗʰ **V01.11** Pedestrian **on roller-skates** injured in collision with pedal cycle in traffic accident

    ✓x7ᵗʰ **V01.12** Pedestrian **on skateboard** injured in collision with pedal cycle in traffic accident

    ✓6ᵗʰ **V01.13** Pedestrian on standing micro-mobility pedestrian conveyance injured in collision with pedal cycle in traffic accident

      ✓7ᵗʰ **V01.131** Pedestrian **on standing electric scooter** injured in collision with pedal cycle in traffic accident

      ✓7ᵗʰ **V01.138** Pedestrian on other standing micro-mobility pedestrian conveyance injured in collision with pedal cycle in traffic accident

        Pedestrian on hoverboard injured in collision with pedal cycle in traffic accident

        Pedestrian on segway injured in collision with pedal cycle in traffic accident

    ✓x7ᵗʰ **V01.19** Pedestrian with other conveyance injured in collision with pedal cycle in traffic accident

        Pedestrian with baby stroller injured in collision with pedal cycle in traffic accident

        Pedestrian on ice-skates injured in collision with pedal cycle in traffic accident

        Pedestrian in motorized mobility scooter injured in collision with pedal cycle in traffic accident

        Pedestrian on nonmotorized scooter injured in collision with pedal cycle in traffic accident

        Pedestrian on sled injured in collision with pedal cycle in traffic accident

        Pedestrian on snowboard injured in collision with pedal cycle in traffic accident

        Pedestrian on snow-skis injured in collision with pedal cycle in traffic accident

        Pedestrian in wheelchair (powered) injured in collision with pedal cycle in traffic accident

  ✓5ᵗʰ **V01.9** Pedestrian injured in collision with pedal cycle, unspecified whether traffic or nontraffic accident

    ✓x7ᵗʰ **V01.90** Pedestrian **on foot** injured in collision with pedal cycle, unspecified whether traffic or nontraffic accident

        Pedestrian NOS injured in collision with pedal cycle, unspecified whether traffic or nontraffic accident

☑ Additional Char Req   ✓x7ᵗʰ Placeholder   Unacceptable PDx   Questionable PDx   Wrong Procedure   Manifestation   Unspecified   H1-H14 HAC   HCC CMS-HCC Dx   HIV HIV Dx

ICD-10-CM 2025   1197

√x 7th **V01.91** Pedestrian **on roller-skates** injured in collision with pedal cycle, unspecified whether traffic or nontraffic accident

√x 7th **V01.92** Pedestrian **on skateboard** injured in collision with pedal cycle, unspecified whether traffic or nontraffic accident

√ 6th **V01.93** Pedestrian on standing micro-mobility pedestrian conveyance injured in collision with pedal cycle, unspecified whether traffic or nontraffic accident

√ 7th **V01.931** Pedestrian **on standing electric scooter** injured in collision with pedal cycle, unspecified whether traffic or nontraffic accident

√ 7th **V01.938** Pedestrian on other standing micro-mobility pedestrian conveyance injured in collision with pedal cycle, unspecified whether traffic or nontraffic accident

> Pedestrian on hoverboard injured in collision with pedal cycle, unspecified whether traffic or nontraffic accident
> Pedestrian on segway injured in collision with pedal cycle, unspecified whether traffic or nontraffic accident

√x 7th **V01.99** Pedestrian with other conveyance injured in collision with pedal cycle, unspecified whether traffic or nontraffic accident

> Pedestrian with baby stroller injured in collision with pedal cycle, unspecified whether traffic or nontraffic accident
> Pedestrian on ice-skates injured in collision with pedal cycle unspecified, whether traffic or nontraffic accident
> Pedestrian in motorized mobility scooter injured in collision with pedal cycle, unspecified whether traffic or nontraffic accident
> Pedestrian on nonmotorized scooter injured in collision with pedal cycle, unspecified whether traffic or nontraffic accident
> Pedestrian on sled injured in collision with pedal cycle unspecified, whether traffic or nontraffic accident
> Pedestrian on snowboard injured in collision with pedal cycle, unspecified whether traffic or nontraffic accident
> Pedestrian on snow-skis injured in collision with pedal cycle, unspecified whether traffic or nontraffic accident
> Pedestrian in wheelchair (powered) injured in collision with pedal cycle, unspecified whether traffic or nontraffic accident

√ 4th **V02** Pedestrian injured in collision with two- or three-wheeled motor vehicle

√ 5th **V02.0** Pedestrian injured in collision with two- or three-wheeled motor vehicle **in nontraffic accident**

√x 7th **V02.00** Pedestrian **on foot** injured in collision with two- or three-wheeled motor vehicle in nontraffic accident

> Pedestrian NOS injured in collision with two- or three-wheeled motor vehicle in nontraffic accident

√x 6th **V02.01** Pedestrian **on roller-skates** injured in collision with two- or three-wheeled motor vehicle in nontraffic accident

√x 7th **V02.02** Pedestrian **on skateboard** injured in collision with two- or three-wheeled motor vehicle in nontraffic accident

√ 6th **V02.03** Pedestrian on standing micro-mobility pedestrian conveyance injured in collision with two- or three-wheeled motor vehicle in nontraffic accident

√ 7th **V02.031** Pedestrian **on standing electric scooter** injured in collision with two- or three-wheeled motor vehicle in nontraffic accident

√ 7th **V02.038** Pedestrian on other standing micro-mobility pedestrian conveyance injured in collision with two- or three-wheeled motor vehicle in nontraffic accident

> Pedestrian on hoverboard injured in collision with two-or three wheeled motor vehicle in nontraffic accident
> Pedestrian on segway injured in collision with two- or three-wheeled motor vehicle in nontraffic accident

√x 7th **V02.09** Pedestrian with other conveyance injured in collision with two- or three-wheeled motor vehicle in nontraffic accident

> Pedestrian with baby stroller injured in collision with two- or three-wheeled motor vehicle in nontraffic accident
> Pedestrian on ice-skates injured in collision with two- or three-wheeled motor vehicle in nontraffic accident
> Pedestrian in motorized mobility scooter injured in collision with two- or three-wheeled motor vehicle in nontraffic accident
> Pedestrian on nonmotorized scooter injured in collision with two- or three-wheeled motor vehicle in nontraffic accident
> Pedestrian on sled injured in collision with two- or three-wheeled motor vehicle in nontraffic accident
> Pedestrian on snowboard injured in collision with two- or three-wheeled motor vehicle in nontraffic accident
> Pedestrian on snow-skis injured in collision with two- or three-wheeled motor vehicle in nontraffic accident
> Pedestrian in wheelchair (powered) injured in collision with two- or three-wheeled motor vehicle in nontraffic accident

√ 5th **V02.1** Pedestrian injured in collision with two- or three-wheeled motor vehicle **in traffic accident**

√x 7th **V02.10** Pedestrian **on foot** injured in collision with two- or three-wheeled motor vehicle in traffic accident

> Pedestrian NOS injured in collision with two- or three-wheeled motor vehicle in traffic accident

√x 7th **V02.11** Pedestrian **on roller-skates** injured in collision with two- or three-wheeled motor vehicle in traffic accident

√x 7th **V02.12** Pedestrian **on skateboard** injured in collision with two- or three-wheeled motor vehicle in traffic accident

√ 6th **V02.13** Pedestrian on standing micro-mobility pedestrian conveyance injured in collision with two- or three-wheeled motor vehicle in traffic accident

√ 7th **V02.131** Pedestrian **on standing electric scooter** injured in collision with two- or three-wheeled motor vehicle in traffic accident

√ 7th **V02.138** Pedestrian on other standing micro-mobility pedestrian conveyance injured in collision with two- or three-wheeled motor vehicle in traffic accident

> Pedestrian on hoverboard injured in collision with two-or three wheeled motor vehicle in traffic accident
> Pedestrian on segway injured in collision with two- or three-wheeled motor vehicle in traffic accident

√x 7th **V02.19** Pedestrian with other conveyance injured in collision with two- or three-wheeled motor vehicle in traffic accident

> Pedestrian with baby stroller injured in collision with two- or three-wheeled motor vehicle in traffic accident
> Pedestrian on ice-skates injured in collision with two- or three-wheeled motor vehicle in traffic accident
> Pedestrian in motorized mobility scooter injured in collision with two- or three-wheeled motor vehicle in traffic accident
> Pedestrian on nonmotorized scooter injured in collision with two- or three-wheeled motor vehicle in traffic accident
> Pedestrian on sled injured in collision with two- or three-wheeled motor vehicle in traffic accident
> Pedestrian on snowboard injured in collision with two- or three-wheeled motor vehicle in traffic accident
> Pedestrian on snow-skis injured in collision with two- or three-wheeled motor vehicle in traffic accident
> Pedestrian in wheelchair (powered) injured in collision with two- or three-wheeled motor vehicle in traffic accident

N Newborn: 0   P Pediatric: 0-17   M Maternity: 9-64   A Adult: 15-124   UNS Unspecified Site   MCC Major Complication/Comorbidity   CC Complication/Comorbidity   PE POA Exempt

1198   ICD-10-CM 2025

✓5ᵗʰ **V02.9 Pedestrian injured in collision with two- or three-wheeled motor vehicle, unspecified whether traffic or nontraffic accident**

✓x7ᵗʰ **V02.90 Pedestrian on foot injured in collision with two- or three-wheeled motor vehicle, unspecified whether traffic or nontraffic accident**
  Pedestrian NOS injured in collision with two- or three-wheeled motor vehicle, unspecified whether traffic or nontraffic accident

✓x7ᵗʰ **V02.91 Pedestrian on roller-skates injured in collision with two- or three-wheeled motor vehicle, unspecified whether traffic or nontraffic accident**

✓x7ᵗʰ **V02.92 Pedestrian on skateboard injured in collision with two- or three-wheeled motor vehicle, unspecified whether traffic or nontraffic accident**

✓6ᵗʰ **V02.93 Pedestrian on standing micro-mobility pedestrian conveyance injured in collision with two- or three-wheeled motor vehicle, unspecified whether traffic or nontraffic accident**

✓7ᵗʰ **V02.931 Pedestrian on standing electric scooter injured in collision with two- or three wheeled motor vehicle, unspecified whether traffic or nontraffic accident**

✓7ᵗʰ **V02.938 Pedestrian on other standing micro-mobility pedestrian conveyance injured in collision with two- or three wheeled motor vehicle, unspecified whether traffic or nontraffic accident**
  Pedestrian on hoverboard injured in collision with two-three-wheeled motor vehicle, unspecified whether traffic or nontraffic accident
  Pedestrian on segway injured in collision with two- or three wheeled motor vehicle, unspecified whether traffic or nontraffic accident

✓x7ᵗʰ **V02.99 Pedestrian with other conveyance injured in collision with two- or three-wheeled motor vehicle, unspecified whether traffic or nontraffic accident**
  Pedestrian with baby stroller injured in collision with two- or three-wheeled motor vehicle, unspecified whether traffic or nontraffic accident
  Pedestrian on ice-skates injured in collision with two- or three-wheeled motor vehicle, unspecified whether traffic or nontraffic accident
  Pedestrian on nonmotorized scooter injured in collision with two- or three-wheeled motor vehicle, unspecified whether traffic or nontraffic accident
  Pedestrian on sled injured in collision with two- or three-wheeled motor vehicle, unspecified whether traffic or nontraffic accident
  Pedestrian on snowboard injured in collision with two- or three-wheeled motor vehicle, unspecified whether traffic or nontraffic accident
  Pedestrian on snow-skis injured in collision with two- or three-wheeled motor vehicle, unspecified whether traffic or nontraffic accident
  Pedestrian in wheelchair (powered) injured in collision with two- or three-wheeled motor vehicle, unspecified whether traffic or nontraffic accident
  Pedestrian in motorized mobility scooter injured in collision with two- or three wheeled motor vehicle, unspecified whether traffic or nontraffic accident

✓4ᵗʰ **V03 Pedestrian injured in collision with car, pick-up truck or van**

✓5ᵗʰ **V03.0 Pedestrian injured in collision with car, pick-up truck or van in nontraffic accident**

✓x7ᵗʰ **V03.00 Pedestrian on foot injured in collision with car, pick-up truck or van in nontraffic accident**
  Pedestrian NOS injured in collision with car, pick-up truck or van in nontraffic accident

✓x7ᵗʰ **V03.01 Pedestrian on roller-skates injured in collision with car, pick-up truck or van in nontraffic accident**

✓x7ᵗʰ **V03.02 Pedestrian on skateboard injured in collision with car, pick-up truck or van in nontraffic accident**

✓6ᵗʰ **V03.03 Pedestrian on standing micro-mobility pedestrian conveyance injured in collision with car, pick-up or van in nontraffic accident**

✓7ᵗʰ **V03.031 Pedestrian on standing electric scooter injured in collision with car, pick-up or van in nontraffic accident**

✓7ᵗʰ **V03.038 Pedestrian on other standing micro-mobility pedestrian conveyance injured in collision with car, pick-up or van in nontraffic accident**
  Pedestrian on hoverboard injured in collision with car, pick-up or van in nontraffic accident
  Pedestrian on segway injured in collision with car, pick-up or van in nontraffic accident

✓x7ᵗʰ **V03.09 Pedestrian with other conveyance injured in collision with car, pick-up truck or van in nontraffic accident**
  Pedestrian with baby stroller injured in collision with car, pick-up truck or van in nontraffic accident
  Pedestrian on ice-skates injured in collision with car, pick-up truck or van in nontraffic accident
  Pedestrian in motorized mobility scooter injured in collision with car, pick-up truck or van in nontraffic accident
  Pedestrian on nonmotorized scooter injured in collision with car, pick-up truck or van in nontraffic accident
  Pedestrian on sled injured in collision with car, pick-up truck or van in nontraffic accident
  Pedestrian on snowboard injured in collision with car, pick-up truck or van in nontraffic accident
  Pedestrian on snow-skis injured in collision with car, pick-up truck or van in nontraffic accident
  Pedestrian in wheelchair (powered) injured in collision with car, pick-up truck or van in nontraffic accident

✓5ᵗʰ **V03.1 Pedestrian injured in collision with car, pick-up truck or van in traffic accident**

✓x7ᵗʰ **V03.10 Pedestrian on foot injured in collision with car, pick-up truck or van in traffic accident**
  Pedestrian NOS injured in collision with car, pick-up truck or van in traffic accident

✓x7ᵗʰ **V03.11 Pedestrian on roller-skates injured in collision with car, pick-up truck or van in traffic accident**

✓x7ᵗʰ **V03.12 Pedestrian on skateboard injured in collision with car, pick-up truck or van in traffic accident**

✓6ᵗʰ **V03.13 Pedestrian on standing micro-mobility pedestrian conveyance injured in collision with car, pick-up or van in traffic accident**

✓7ᵗʰ **V03.131 Pedestrian on standing electric scooter injured in collision with car, pick-up or van in traffic accident**

✓7ᵗʰ **V03.138 Pedestrian on other standing micro-mobility pedestrian conveyance injured in collision with car, pick-up or van in traffic accident**
  Pedestrian on hoverboard injured in collision with car, pick-up or van in traffic accident
  Pedestrian on segway injured in collision with car, pick-up or van in traffic accident

✓x7ᵗʰ **V03.19 Pedestrian with other conveyance injured in collision with car, pick-up truck or van in traffic accident**
  Pedestrian with baby stroller injured in collision with car, pick-up truck or van in traffic accident
  Pedestrian on ice-skates injured in collision with car, pick-up truck or van in traffic accident
  Pedestrian in motorized mobility scooter injured in collision with car, pick-up truck or van in nontraffic accident
  Pedestrian on nonmotorized scooter injured in collision with car, pick-up truck or van in nontraffic accident
  Pedestrian on sled injured in collision with car, pick-up truck or van in traffic accident
  Pedestrian on snowboard injured in collision with car, pick-up truck or van in traffic accident
  Pedestrian on snow-skis injured in collision with car, pick-up truck or van in traffic accident
  Pedestrian in wheelchair (powered) injured in collision with car, pick-up truck or van in traffic accident

✓5ᵗʰ **V03.9 Pedestrian injured in collision with car, pick-up truck or van, unspecified whether traffic or nontraffic accident**

✓x7ᵗʰ **V03.90 Pedestrian on foot injured in collision with car, pick-up truck or van, unspecified whether traffic or nontraffic accident**
  Pedestrian NOS injured in collision with car, pick-up truck or van, unspecified whether traffic or nontraffic accident

✓x7ᵗʰ **V03.91 Pedestrian on roller-skates injured in collision with car, pick-up truck or van, unspecified whether traffic or nontraffic accident**

✓x 7th **V03.92** Pedestrian **on skateboard** injured in collision with car, pick-up truck or van, unspecified whether traffic or nontraffic accident

✓ 6th **V03.93** Pedestrian on standing micro-mobility pedestrian conveyance injured in collision with car, pick-up or van, unspecified whether traffic or nontraffic accident

     ✓ 7th **V03.931** Pedestrian **on standing electric scooter** injured in collision with car, pick-up or van, unspecified whether traffic or nontraffic accident

     ✓ 7th **V03.938** Pedestrian on other standing micro-mobility pedestrian conveyance injured in collision with car, pick-up or van, unspecified whether traffic or nontraffic accident

         Pedestrian on hoverboard injured in collision with car, pick-up or van, unspecified whether traffic or nontraffic accident

         Pedestrian on segway injured in collision with car, pick-up or van, unspecified whether traffic or nontraffic accident

✓x 7th **V03.99** Pedestrian with other conveyance injured in collision with car, pick-up truck or van, unspecified whether traffic or nontraffic accident

     Pedestrian with baby stroller injured in collision with car, pick-up truck or van, unspecified whether traffic or nontraffic accident

     Pedestrian on ice-skates injured in collision with car, pick-up truck or van, unspecified whether traffic or nontraffic accident

     Pedestrian in motorized mobility scooter injured in collision with car, pick-up truck or van, unspecified whether traffic or nontraffic accident

     Pedestrian on nonmotorized scooter injured in collision with car, pick-up truck or van, unspecified whether traffic or nontraffic accident

     Pedestrian on sled injured in collision with car, pick-up truck or van in nontraffic accident

     Pedestrian on snowboard injured in collision with car, pick-up truck or van, unspecified whether traffic or nontraffic accident

     Pedestrian on snow-skis injured in collision with car, pick-up truck or van, unspecified whether traffic or nontraffic accident

     Pedestrian in wheelchair (powered) injured in collision with car, pick-up truck or van, unspecified whether traffic or nontraffic accident

✓ 4th **V04** **Pedestrian injured in collision with heavy transport vehicle or bus**

     EXCLUDES 1   *pedestrian injured in collision with military vehicle (V09.01, V09.21)*

✓ 5th **V04.0** Pedestrian injured in collision with heavy transport vehicle or bus **in nontraffic accident**

     ✓x 7th **V04.00** Pedestrian **on foot** injured in collision with heavy transport vehicle or bus in nontraffic accident

         Pedestrian NOS injured in collision with heavy transport vehicle or bus in nontraffic accident

     ✓x 7th **V04.01** Pedestrian **on roller-skates** injured in collision with heavy transport vehicle or bus in nontraffic accident

     ✓x 7th **V04.02** Pedestrian **on skateboard** injured in collision with heavy transport vehicle or bus in nontraffic accident

     ✓ 6th **V04.03** Pedestrian on standing micro-mobility pedestrian conveyance injured in collision with heavy transport vehicle or bus in nontraffic accident

         ✓ 7th **V04.031** Pedestrian **on standing electric scooter** injured in collision with heavy transport vehicle or bus in nontraffic accident

         ✓ 7th **V04.038** Pedestrian on other standing micro-mobility pedestrian conveyance injured in collision with heavy transport vehicle or bus in nontraffic accident

            Pedestrian on hoverboard injured in collision with heavy transport vehicle or bus in nontraffic accident

            Pedestrian on segway injured in collision with heavy transport vehicle or bus in nontraffic accident

✓x 7th **V04.09** Pedestrian with other conveyance injured in collision with heavy transport vehicle or bus in nontraffic accident

     Pedestrian with baby stroller injured in collision with heavy transport vehicle or bus in nontraffic accident

     Pedestrian on ice-skates injured in collision with heavy transport vehicle or bus in nontraffic accident

     Pedestrian in motorized mobility scooter injured in collision with heavy transport vehicle or bus in nontraffic accident

     Pedestrian on nonmotorized scooter injured in collision with heavy transport vehicle or bus in nontraffic accident

     Pedestrian on sled injured in collision with heavy transport vehicle or bus in nontraffic accident

     Pedestrian on snowboard injured in collision with heavy transport vehicle or bus in nontraffic accident

     Pedestrian on snow-skis injured in collision with heavy transport vehicle or bus in nontraffic accident

     Pedestrian in wheelchair (powered) injured in collision with heavy transport vehicle or bus in nontraffic accident

✓ 5th **V04.1** Pedestrian injured in collision with heavy transport vehicle or bus **in traffic accident**

     ✓x 7th **V04.10** Pedestrian **on foot** injured in collision with heavy transport vehicle or bus in traffic accident

         Pedestrian NOS injured in collision with heavy transport vehicle or bus in traffic accident

     ✓x 7th **V04.11** Pedestrian **on roller-skates** injured in collision with heavy transport vehicle or bus in traffic accident

     ✓x 7th **V04.12** Pedestrian **on skateboard** injured in collision with heavy transport vehicle or bus in traffic accident

     ✓ 6th **V04.13** Pedestrian on standing micro-mobility pedestrian conveyance injured in collision with heavy transport vehicle or bus in traffic accident

         ✓ 7th **V04.131** Pedestrian **on standing electric scooter** injured in collision with heavy transport vehicle or bus in traffic accident

         ✓ 7th **V04.138** Pedestrian on other standing micro-mobility pedestrian conveyance injured in collision with heavy transport vehicle or bus in traffic accident

            Pedestrian on hoverboard injured in collision with heavy transport vehicle or bus in traffic accident

            Pedestrian on segway injured in collision with heavy transport vehicle or bus in traffic accident

     ✓x 7th **V04.19** Pedestrian with other conveyance injured in collision with heavy transport vehicle or bus in traffic accident

         Pedestrian with baby stroller injured in collision with heavy transport vehicle or bus in traffic accident

         Pedestrian on ice-skates injured in collision with heavy transport vehicle or bus in traffic accident

         Pedestrian in motorized mobility scooter injured in collision with heavy transport vehicle or bus in traffic accident

         Pedestrian on nonmotorized scooter injured in collision with heavy transport vehicle or bus in traffic accident

         Pedestrian on sled injured in collision with heavy transport vehicle or bus in traffic accident

         Pedestrian on snowboard injured in collision with heavy transport vehicle or bus in traffic accident

         Pedestrian on snow-skis injured in collision with heavy transport vehicle or bus in traffic accident

         Pedestrian in wheelchair (powered) injured in collision with heavy transport vehicle or bus in traffic accident

✓ 5th **V04.9** Pedestrian injured in collision with heavy transport vehicle or bus, unspecified whether traffic or nontraffic accident

     ✓x 7th **V04.90** Pedestrian **on foot** injured in collision with heavy transport vehicle or bus, unspecified whether traffic or nontraffic accident

         Pedestrian NOS injured in collision with heavy transport vehicle or bus, unspecified whether traffic or nontraffic accident

     ✓x 7th **V04.91** Pedestrian **on roller-skates** injured in collision with heavy transport vehicle or bus, unspecified whether traffic or nontraffic accident

     ✓x 7th **V04.92** Pedestrian **on skateboard** injured in collision with heavy transport vehicle or bus, unspecified whether traffic or nontraffic accident

N Newborn: 0   **P** Pediatric: 0-17   **M** Maternity: 9-64   **A** Adult: 15-124   **UNS** Unspecified Site   **MCC** Major Complication/Comorbidity   **CC** Complication/Comorbidity   **PE** POA Exempt

1200   ICD-10-CM 2025

☑6th V04.93 Pedestrian on standing micro-mobility pedestrian conveyance injured in collision with heavy transport vehicle or bus, unspecified whether traffic or nontraffic accident

    ☑7th V04.931 Pedestrian on standing electric scooter injured in collision with heavy transport vehicle or bus, unspecified whether traffic or nontraffic accident

    ☑7th V04.938 Pedestrian on other standing micro-mobility pedestrian conveyance injured in collision with heavy transport vehicle or bus, unspecified whether traffic or nontraffic accident

         Pedestrian on hoverboard injured in collision with heavy transport vehicle or bus, unspecified whether traffic or nontraffic accident

         Pedestrian on segway injured in collision with heavy transport vehicle or bus, unspecified whether traffic or nontraffic accident

☑x7th V04.99 Pedestrian with other conveyance injured in collision with heavy transport vehicle or bus, unspecified whether traffic or nontraffic accident

     Pedestrian with baby stroller injured in collision with heavy transport vehicle or bus, unspecified whether traffic or nontraffic accident

     Pedestrian on ice-skates injured in collision with heavy transport vehicle or bus, unspecified whether traffic or nontraffic accident

     Pedestrian in motorized mobility scooter injured in collision with heavy transport vehicle or bus, unspecified whether traffic or nontraffic accident

     Pedestrian on nonmotorized scooter injured in collision with heavy transport vehicle or bus, unspecified whether traffic or nontraffic accident

     Pedestrian on sled injured in collision with heavy transport vehicle or bus, unspecified whether traffic or nontraffic accident

     Pedestrian on snowboard injured in collision with heavy transport vehicle or bus, unspecified whether traffic or nontraffic accident

     Pedestrian on snow-skis injured in collision with heavy transport vehicle or bus, unspecified whether traffic or nontraffic accident

     Pedestrian in wheelchair (powered) injured in collision with heavy transport vehicle or bus, unspecified whether traffic or nontraffic accident

☑4th V05 Pedestrian injured in collision with railway train or railway vehicle

    ☑5th V05.0 Pedestrian injured in collision with railway train or railway vehicle in nontraffic accident

        ☑x7th V05.00 Pedestrian on foot injured in collision with railway train or railway vehicle in nontraffic accident

             Pedestrian NOS injured in collision with railway train or railway vehicle in nontraffic accident

        ☑x7th V05.01 Pedestrian on roller-skates injured in collision with railway train or railway vehicle in nontraffic accident

        ☑x7th V05.02 Pedestrian on skateboard injured in collision with railway train or railway vehicle in nontraffic accident

        ☑6th V05.03 Pedestrian on standing micro-mobility pedestrian conveyance injured in collision with railway train or railway vehicle in nontraffic accident

            ☑7th V05.031 Pedestrian on standing electric scooter injured in collision with railway train or railway vehicle in nontraffic accident

            ☑7th V05.038 Pedestrian on other standing micro-mobility pedestrian conveyance injured in collision with railway train or railway vehicle in nontraffic accident

                 Pedestrian on hoverboard injured in collision with railway train or railway vehicle in nontraffic accident

                 Pedestrian on segway injured in collision with railway train or railway vehicle in nontraffic accident

☑x7th V05.09 Pedestrian with other conveyance injured in collision with railway train or railway vehicle in nontraffic accident

     Pedestrian with baby stroller injured in collision with railway train or railway vehicle in nontraffic accident

     Pedestrian on ice-skates injured in collision with railway train or railway vehicle in nontraffic accident

     Pedestrian in motorized mobility scooter injured in collision with railway train or railway vehicle in nontraffic accident

     Pedestrian on nonmotorized scooter injured in collision with railway train or railway vehicle in nontraffic accident

     Pedestrian on sled injured in collision with railway train or railway vehicle in nontraffic accident

     Pedestrian on snowboard injured in collision with railway train or railway vehicle in nontraffic accident

     Pedestrian on snow-skis injured in collision with railway train or railway vehicle in nontraffic accident

     Pedestrian in wheelchair (powered) injured in collision with railway train or railway vehicle in nontraffic accident

☑5th V05.1 Pedestrian injured in collision with railway train or railway vehicle in traffic accident

    ☑x7th V05.10 Pedestrian on foot injured in collision with railway train or railway vehicle in traffic accident

         Pedestrian NOS injured in collision with railway train or railway vehicle in traffic accident

    ☑x7th V05.11 Pedestrian on roller-skates injured in collision with railway train or railway vehicle in traffic accident

    ☑x7th V05.12 Pedestrian on skateboard injured in collision with railway train or railway vehicle in traffic accident

    ☑6th V05.13 Pedestrian on standing micro-mobility pedestrian conveyance injured in collision with railway train or railway vehicle in traffic accident

        ☑7th V05.131 Pedestrian on standing electric scooter injured in collision with railway train or railway vehicle in traffic accident

        ☑7th V05.138 Pedestrian on other standing micro-mobility pedestrian conveyance injured in collision with railway train or railway vehicle in traffic accident

             Pedestrian on hoverboard injured in collision with railway train or railway vehicle in traffic accident

             Pedestrian on segway injured in collision with railway train or railway vehicle in traffic accident

    ☑x7th V05.19 Pedestrian with other conveyance injured in collision with railway train or railway vehicle in traffic accident

         Pedestrian with baby stroller injured in collision with railway train or railway vehicle in traffic accident

         Pedestrian on ice-skates injured in collision with railway train or railway vehicle in traffic accident

         Pedestrian in motorized mobility scooter injured in collision with railway train or railway vehicle in traffic accident

         Pedestrian on nonmotorized scooter injured in collision with railway train or railway vehicle in traffic accident

         Pedestrian on sled injured in collision with railway train or railway vehicle in traffic accident

         Pedestrian on snowboard injured in collision with railway train or railway vehicle in traffic accident

         Pedestrian on snow-skis injured in collision with railway train or railway vehicle in traffic accident

         Pedestrian in wheelchair (powered) injured in collision with railway train or railway vehicle in traffic accident

☑5th V05.9 Pedestrian injured in collision with railway train or railway vehicle, unspecified whether traffic or nontraffic accident

    ☑x7th V05.90 Pedestrian on foot injured in collision with railway train or railway vehicle, unspecified whether traffic or nontraffic accident

         Pedestrian NOS injured in collision with railway train or railway vehicle, unspecified whether traffic or nontraffic accident

    ☑x7th V05.91 Pedestrian on roller-skates injured in collision with railway train or railway vehicle, unspecified whether traffic or nontraffic accident

    ☑x7th V05.92 Pedestrian on skateboard injured in collision with railway train or railway vehicle, unspecified whether traffic or nontraffic accident

☑ Additional Char Req   ☑x7th Placeholder   Unacceptable PDx   Questionable PDx   Wrong Procedure   Manifestation   Unspecified   H1-H14 HAC   HCC CMS-HCC Dx   HIV HIV Dx

ICD-10-CM 2025   1201

V04.93–V05.92

√6ᵗʰ **V05.93 Pedestrian on standing micro-mobility pedestrian conveyance injured in collision with railway train or railway vehicle, unspecified whether traffic or nontraffic accident**

√7ᵗʰ **V05.931 Pedestrian on standing electric scooter injured in collision with railway train or railway vehicle, unspecified whether traffic or nontraffic accident**

√7ᵗʰ **V05.938 Pedestrian on other standing micro-mobility pedestrian conveyance injured in collision with railway train or railway vehicle, unspecified whether traffic or nontraffic accident**

Pedestrian on hoverboard injured in collision with railway train or railway vehicle, unspecified whether traffic or nontraffic accident

Pedestrian on segway injured in collision with railway train or railway vehicle, unspecified whether traffic or nontraffic accident

√x7ᵗʰ **V05.99 Pedestrian with other conveyance injured in collision with railway train or railway vehicle, unspecified whether traffic or nontraffic accident**

Pedestrian with baby stroller injured in collision with railway train or railway vehicle, unspecified whether traffic or nontraffic

Pedestrian on ice-skates injured in collision with railway train or railway vehicle, unspecified whether traffic or nontraffic

Pedestrian on nonmotorized scooter injured in collision with railway train or railway vehicle, unspecified whether traffic or nontraffic

Pedestrian on sled injured in collision with railway train or railway vehicle, unspecified whether traffic or nontraffic

Pedestrian on snowboard injured in collision with railway train or railway vehicle, unspecified whether traffic or nontraffic

Pedestrian on snow-skis injured in collision with railway train or railway vehicle, unspecified whether traffic or nontraffic

Pedestrian in wheelchair (powered) injured in collision with railway train or railway vehicle, unspecified whether traffic or nontraffic

Pedestrian in motorized mobility scooter injured in collision with railway train or railway vehicle, unspecified whether traffic or nontraffic

√4ᵗʰ **V06 Pedestrian injured in collision with other nonmotor vehicle**

INCLUDES collision with animal-drawn vehicle, animal being ridden, nonpowered streetcar

EXCLUDES 1 pedestrian injured in collision with pedestrian conveyance (V00.0-)

√5ᵗʰ **V06.0 Pedestrian injured in collision with other nonmotor vehicle in nontraffic accident**

√x7ᵗʰ **V06.00 Pedestrian on foot injured in collision with other nonmotor vehicle in nontraffic accident**

Pedestrian NOS injured in collision with other nonmotor vehicle in nontraffic accident

√x7ᵗʰ **V06.01 Pedestrian on roller-skates injured in collision with other nonmotor vehicle in nontraffic accident**

√x7ᵗʰ **V06.02 Pedestrian on skateboard injured in collision with other nonmotor vehicle in nontraffic accident**

√6ᵗʰ **V06.03 Pedestrian on standing micro-mobility pedestrian conveyance injured in collision with other nonmotor vehicle in nontraffic accident**

√7ᵗʰ **V06.031 Pedestrian on standing electric scooter injured in collision with other nonmotor vehicle in nontraffic accident**

√7ᵗʰ **V06.038 Pedestrian on other standing micro-mobility pedestrian conveyance injured in collision with other nonmotor vehicle in nontraffic accident**

Pedestrian on hoverboard injured in collision with other nonmotor vehicle in nontraffic accident

Pedestrian on segway injured in collision with other nonmotor vehicle in nontraffic accident

√x7ᵗʰ **V06.09 Pedestrian with other conveyance injured in collision with other nonmotor vehicle in nontraffic accident**

Pedestrian with baby stroller injured in collision with other nonmotor vehicle in nontraffic accident

Pedestrian on ice-skates injured in collision with other nonmotor vehicle in nontraffic accident

Pedestrian in motorized mobility scooter injured in collision with other nonmotor vehicle in nontraffic accident

Pedestrian on nonmotorized scooter injured in collision with other nonmotor vehicle in nontraffic accident

Pedestrian on sled injured in collision with other nonmotor vehicle in nontraffic accident

Pedestrian on snowboard injured in collision with other nonmotor vehicle in nontraffic accident

Pedestrian on snow-skis injured in collision with other nonmotor vehicle in nontraffic accident

Pedestrian in wheelchair (powered) injured in collision with other nonmotor vehicle in nontraffic accident

√5ᵗʰ **V06.1 Pedestrian injured in collision with other nonmotor vehicle in traffic accident**

√x7ᵗʰ **V06.10 Pedestrian on foot injured in collision with other nonmotor vehicle in traffic accident**

Pedestrian NOS injured in collision with other nonmotor vehicle in traffic accident

√x7ᵗʰ **V06.11 Pedestrian on roller-skates injured in collision with other nonmotor vehicle in traffic accident**

√x7ᵗʰ **V06.12 Pedestrian on skateboard injured in collision with other nonmotor vehicle in traffic accident**

√6ᵗʰ **V06.13 Pedestrian on standing micro-mobility pedestrian conveyance injured in collision with other nonmotor vehicle in traffic accident**

√7ᵗʰ **V06.131 Pedestrian on standing electric scooter injured in collision with other nonmotor vehicle in traffic accident**

√7ᵗʰ **V06.138 Pedestrian on other standing micro-mobility pedestrian conveyance injured in collision with other nonmotor vehicle in traffic accident**

Pedestrian on hoverboard injured in collision with other nonmotor vehicle in traffic accident

Pedestrian on segway injured in collision with other nonmotor vehicle in traffic accident

√x7ᵗʰ **V06.19 Pedestrian with other conveyance injured in collision with other nonmotor vehicle in traffic accident**

Pedestrian with baby stroller injured in collision with other nonmotor vehicle in nontraffic accident

Pedestrian on ice-skates injured in collision with other nonmotor vehicle in traffic accident

Pedestrian in motorized mobility scooter injured in collision with other nonmotor vehicle in traffic accident

Pedestrian on nonmotorized scooter injured in collision with other nonmotor vehicle in traffic accident

Pedestrian on sled injured in collision with other nonmotor vehicle in traffic accident

Pedestrian on snowboard injured in collision with other nonmotor vehicle in traffic accident

Pedestrian on snow-skis injured in collision with other nonmotor vehicle in traffic accident

Pedestrian in wheelchair (powered) injured in collision with other nonmotor vehicle in traffic accident

√5ᵗʰ **V06.9 Pedestrian injured in collision with other nonmotor vehicle, unspecified whether traffic or nontraffic accident**

√x7ᵗʰ **V06.90 Pedestrian on foot injured in collision with other nonmotor vehicle, unspecified whether traffic or nontraffic accident**

Pedestrian NOS injured in collision with other nonmotor vehicle, unspecified whether traffic or nontraffic accident

√x7ᵗʰ **V06.91 Pedestrian on roller-skates injured in collision with other nonmotor vehicle, unspecified whether traffic or nontraffic accident**

√x7ᵗʰ **V06.92 Pedestrian on skateboard injured in collision with other nonmotor vehicle, unspecified whether traffic or nontraffic accident**

N Newborn: 0   **P** Pediatric: 0-17   **M** Maternity: 9-64   **A** Adult: 15-124   **UNS** Unspecified Site   **MCC** Major Complication/Comorbidity   **CC** Complication/Comorbidity   **PE** POA Exempt

1202   ICD-10-CM 2025

☑6ᵗʰ **V06.93**   **Pedestrian on standing micro-mobility pedestrian conveyance injured in collision with other nonmotor vehicle, unspecified whether traffic or nontraffic accident**

     ☑7ᵗʰ **V06.931**   **Pedestrian on standing electric scooter injured in collision with other nonmotor vehicle, unspecified whether traffic or nontraffic accident**

     ☑7ᵗʰ **V06.938**   **Pedestrian on other standing micro-mobility pedestrian conveyance injured in collision with other nonmotor vehicle, unspecified whether traffic or nontraffic accident**

         Pedestrian on hoverboard injured in collision with other nonmotor, unspecified whether traffic or nontraffic accident

         Pedestrian on segway injured in collision with other nonmotor vehicle, unspecified whether traffic or nontraffic accident

☑x7ᵗʰ **V06.99**   **Pedestrian with other conveyance injured in collision with other nonmotor vehicle, unspecified whether traffic or nontraffic accident**

     Pedestrian with baby stroller injured in collision with other nonmotor vehicle, unspecified whether traffic or nontraffic accident

     Pedestrian on ice-skates injured in collision with other nonmotor vehicle, unspecified whether traffic or nontraffic accident

     Pedestrian in motorized mobility scooter injured in collision with other nonmotorized vehicle, unspecified whether traffic or nontraffic accident

     Pedestrian on nonmotorized scooter injured in collision with other nonmotor vehicle, unspecified whether traffic or nontraffic accident

     Pedestrian on sled injured in collision with other nonmotor vehicle, unspecified whether traffic or nontraffic accident

     Pedestrian on snowboard injured in collision with other nonmotor vehicle, unspecified whether traffic or nontraffic accident

     Pedestrian on snow-skis injured in collision with other nonmotor vehicle, unspecified whether traffic or nontraffic accident

     Pedestrian in wheelchair (powered) injured in collision with other nonmotor vehicle, unspecified whether traffic or nontraffic accident

☑4ᵗʰ **V09**   **Pedestrian injured in other and unspecified transport accidents**

     ☑5ᵗʰ **V09.0**   **Pedestrian injured in nontraffic accident involving other and unspecified motor vehicles**

         ☑x7ᵗʰ **V09.00**   **Pedestrian injured in nontraffic accident involving unspecified motor vehicles**

         ☑x7ᵗʰ **V09.01**   **Pedestrian injured in nontraffic accident involving military vehicle**

         ☑x7ᵗʰ **V09.09**   **Pedestrian injured in nontraffic accident involving other motor vehicles**

             Pedestrian injured in nontraffic accident by special vehicle

     ☑x7ᵗʰ **V09.1**   **Pedestrian injured in unspecified nontraffic accident**

     ☑5ᵗʰ **V09.2**   **Pedestrian injured in traffic accident involving other and unspecified motor vehicles**

         ☑x7ᵗʰ **V09.20**   **Pedestrian injured in traffic accident involving unspecified motor vehicles**

         ☑x7ᵗʰ **V09.21**   **Pedestrian injured in traffic accident involving military vehicle**

         ☑x7ᵗʰ **V09.29**   **Pedestrian injured in traffic accident involving other motor vehicles**

     ☑x7ᵗʰ **V09.3**   **Pedestrian injured in unspecified traffic accident**

     ☑x7ᵗʰ **V09.9**   **Pedestrian injured in unspecified transport accident**

Pedal cycle rider injured in transport accident (V10-V19)

INCLUDES   any non-motorized vehicle, excluding an animal-drawn vehicle, or a sidecar or trailer attached to the pedal cycle

EXCLUDES 2   *rupture of pedal cycle tire (W37.0)*

The appropriate 7th character is to be added to each code from categories V10-V19.

A   initial encounter
D   subsequent encounter
S   sequela

☑4ᵗʰ **V10**   **Pedal cycle rider injured in collision with pedestrian or animal**

     EXCLUDES 1   *pedal cycle rider collision with animal-drawn vehicle or animal being ridden (V16.-)*

     ☑x7ᵗʰ **V10.0**   **Pedal cycle driver injured in collision with pedestrian or animal in nontraffic accident**

     ☑x7ᵗʰ **V10.1**   **Pedal cycle passenger injured in collision with pedestrian or animal in nontraffic accident**

     ☑x7ᵗʰ **V10.2**   **Unspecified pedal cyclist injured in collision with pedestrian or animal in nontraffic accident**

     ☑x7ᵗʰ **V10.3**   **Person boarding or alighting a pedal cycle injured in collision with pedestrian or animal**

     ☑x7ᵗʰ **V10.4**   **Pedal cycle driver injured in collision with pedestrian or animal in traffic accident**

     ☑x7ᵗʰ **V10.5**   **Pedal cycle passenger injured in collision with pedestrian or animal in traffic accident**

     ☑x7ᵗʰ **V10.9**   **Unspecified pedal cyclist injured in collision with pedestrian or animal in traffic accident**

☑4ᵗʰ **V11**   **Pedal cycle rider injured in collision with other pedal cycle**

     ☑x7ᵗʰ **V11.0**   **Pedal cycle driver injured in collision with other pedal cycle in nontraffic accident**

     ☑x7ᵗʰ **V11.1**   **Pedal cycle passenger injured in collision with other pedal cycle in nontraffic accident**

     ☑x7ᵗʰ **V11.2**   **Unspecified pedal cyclist injured in collision with other pedal cycle in nontraffic accident**

     ☑x7ᵗʰ **V11.3**   **Person boarding or alighting a pedal cycle injured in collision with other pedal cycle**

     ☑x7ᵗʰ **V11.4**   **Pedal cycle driver injured in collision with other pedal cycle in traffic accident**

     ☑x7ᵗʰ **V11.5**   **Pedal cycle passenger injured in collision with other pedal cycle in traffic accident**

     ☑x7ᵗʰ **V11.9**   **Unspecified pedal cyclist injured in collision with other pedal cycle in traffic accident**

☑4ᵗʰ **V12**   **Pedal cycle rider injured in collision with two- or three-wheeled motor vehicle**

     ☑x7ᵗʰ **V12.0**   **Pedal cycle driver injured in collision with two- or three-wheeled motor vehicle in nontraffic accident**

     ☑x7ᵗʰ **V12.1**   **Pedal cycle passenger injured in collision with two- or three-wheeled motor vehicle in nontraffic accident**

     ☑x7ᵗʰ **V12.2**   **Unspecified pedal cyclist injured in collision with two- or three-wheeled motor vehicle in nontraffic accident**

     ☑x7ᵗʰ **V12.3**   **Person boarding or alighting a pedal cycle injured in collision with two- or three-wheeled motor vehicle**

     ☑x7ᵗʰ **V12.4**   **Pedal cycle driver injured in collision with two- or three-wheeled motor vehicle in traffic accident**

     ☑x7ᵗʰ **V12.5**   **Pedal cycle passenger injured in collision with two- or three-wheeled motor vehicle in traffic accident**

     ☑x7ᵗʰ **V12.9**   **Unspecified pedal cyclist injured in collision with two- or three-wheeled motor vehicle in traffic accident**

☑4ᵗʰ **V13**   **Pedal cycle rider injured in collision with car, pick-up truck or van**

     ☑x7ᵗʰ **V13.0**   **Pedal cycle driver injured in collision with car, pick-up truck or van in nontraffic accident**

     ☑x7ᵗʰ **V13.1**   **Pedal cycle passenger injured in collision with car, pick-up truck or van in nontraffic accident**

     ☑x7ᵗʰ **V13.2**   **Unspecified pedal cyclist injured in collision with car, pick-up truck or van in nontraffic accident**

     ☑x7ᵗʰ **V13.3**   **Person boarding or alighting a pedal cycle injured in collision with car, pick-up truck or van**

     ☑x7ᵗʰ **V13.4**   **Pedal cycle driver injured in collision with car, pick-up truck or van in traffic accident**

     ☑x7ᵗʰ **V13.5**   **Pedal cycle passenger injured in collision with car, pick-up truck or van in traffic accident**

     ☑x7ᵗʰ **V13.9**   **Unspecified pedal cyclist injured in collision with car, pick-up truck or van in traffic accident**

☑4ᵗʰ **V14**   **Pedal cycle rider injured in collision with heavy transport vehicle or bus**

     EXCLUDES 1   *pedal cycle rider injured in collision with military vehicle (V19.81)*

     ☑x7ᵗʰ **V14.0**   **Pedal cycle driver injured in collision with heavy transport vehicle or bus in nontraffic accident**

☑ Additional Char Req   ☑x7ᵗʰ Placeholder   Unacceptable PDx   Questionable PDx   Wrong Procedure   Manifestation   Unspecified   H1 - H14 HAC   HCC CMS-HCC Dx   HIV HIV Dx

ICD-10-CM 2025   V06.93–V14.0   1203

Chapter 20. External Causes of Morbidity

Chapter 20. External Causes of Morbidity

V14.1–V20.11

√x7th **V14.1** Pedal cycle passenger injured in collision with heavy transport vehicle or bus in nontraffic accident

√x7th **V14.2** Unspecified pedal cyclist injured in collision with heavy transport vehicle or bus in nontraffic accident

√x7th **V14.3** Person boarding or alighting a pedal cycle injured in collision with heavy transport vehicle or bus

√x7th **V14.4** Pedal cycle driver injured in collision with heavy transport vehicle or bus in traffic accident

√x7th **V14.5** Pedal cycle passenger injured in collision with heavy transport vehicle or bus in traffic accident

√x7th **V14.9** Unspecified pedal cyclist injured in collision with heavy transport vehicle or bus in traffic accident

√4th **V15** Pedal cycle rider injured in collision with railway train or railway vehicle

√x7th **V15.0** Pedal cycle driver injured in collision with railway train or railway vehicle in nontraffic accident

√x7th **V15.1** Pedal cycle passenger injured in collision with railway train or railway vehicle in nontraffic accident

√x7th **V15.2** Unspecified pedal cyclist injured in collision with railway train or railway vehicle in nontraffic accident

√x7th **V15.3** Person boarding or alighting a pedal cycle injured in collision with railway train or railway vehicle

√x7th **V15.4** Pedal cycle driver injured in collision with railway train or railway vehicle in traffic accident

√x7th **V15.5** Pedal cycle passenger injured in collision with railway train or railway vehicle in traffic accident

√x7th **V15.9** Unspecified pedal cyclist injured in collision with railway train or railway vehicle in traffic accident

√4th **V16** Pedal cycle rider injured in collision with other nonmotor vehicle

INCLUDES   collision with animal-drawn vehicle, animal being ridden, streetcar

√x7th **V16.0** Pedal cycle driver injured in collision with other nonmotor vehicle in nontraffic accident

√x7th **V16.1** Pedal cycle passenger injured in collision with other nonmotor vehicle in nontraffic accident

√x7th **V16.2** Unspecified pedal cyclist injured in collision with other nonmotor vehicle in nontraffic accident

√x7th **V16.3** Person boarding or alighting a pedal cycle injured in collision with other nonmotor vehicle in nontraffic accident

√x7th **V16.4** Pedal cycle driver injured in collision with other nonmotor vehicle in traffic accident

√x7th **V16.5** Pedal cycle passenger injured in collision with other nonmotor vehicle in traffic accident

√x7th **V16.9** Unspecified pedal cyclist injured in collision with other nonmotor vehicle in traffic accident

√4th **V17** Pedal cycle rider injured in collision with fixed or stationary object

√x7th **V17.0** Pedal cycle driver injured in collision with fixed or stationary object in nontraffic accident

√x7th **V17.1** Pedal cycle passenger injured in collision with fixed or stationary object in nontraffic accident

√x7th **V17.2** Unspecified pedal cyclist injured in collision with fixed or stationary object in nontraffic accident

√x7th **V17.3** Person boarding or alighting a pedal cycle injured in collision with fixed or stationary object

√x7th **V17.4** Pedal cycle driver injured in collision with fixed or stationary object in traffic accident

√x7th **V17.5** Pedal cycle passenger injured in collision with fixed or stationary object in traffic accident

√x7th **V17.9** Unspecified pedal cyclist injured in collision with fixed or stationary object in traffic accident

√4th **V18** Pedal cycle rider injured in noncollision transport accident

INCLUDES   fall or thrown from pedal cycle (without antecedent collision)
overturning pedal cycle NOS
overturning pedal cycle without collision

√x7th **V18.0** Pedal cycle driver injured in noncollision transport accident in nontraffic accident

√x7th **V18.1** Pedal cycle passenger injured in noncollision transport accident in nontraffic accident

√x7th **V18.2** Unspecified pedal cyclist injured in noncollision transport accident in nontraffic accident

√x7th **V18.3** Person boarding or alighting a pedal cycle injured in noncollision transport accident

√x7th **V18.4** Pedal cycle driver injured in noncollision transport accident in traffic accident

√x7th **V18.5** Pedal cycle passenger injured in noncollision transport accident in traffic accident

√x7th **V18.9** Unspecified pedal cyclist injured in noncollision transport accident in traffic accident

√4th **V19** Pedal cycle rider injured in other and unspecified transport accidents

√5th **V19.0** Pedal cycle driver injured in collision with other and unspecified motor vehicles in nontraffic accident

√x7th **V19.00** Pedal cycle driver injured in collision with unspecified motor vehicles in nontraffic accident

√x7th **V19.09** Pedal cycle driver injured in collision with other motor vehicles in nontraffic accident

√5th **V19.1** Pedal cycle passenger injured in collision with other and unspecified motor vehicles in nontraffic accident

√x7th **V19.10** Pedal cycle passenger injured in collision with unspecified motor vehicles in nontraffic accident

√x7th **V19.19** Pedal cycle passenger injured in collision with other motor vehicles in nontraffic accident

√5th **V19.2** Unspecified pedal cyclist injured in collision with other and unspecified motor vehicles in nontraffic accident

√x7th **V19.20** Unspecified pedal cyclist injured in collision with unspecified motor vehicles in nontraffic accident
Pedal cycle collision NOS, nontraffic

√x7th **V19.29** Unspecified pedal cyclist injured in collision with other motor vehicles in nontraffic accident

√x7th **V19.3** Pedal cyclist (driver) (passenger) injured in unspecified nontraffic accident
Pedal cycle accident NOS, nontraffic
Pedal cyclist injured in nontraffic accident NOS

√5th **V19.4** Pedal cycle driver injured in collision with other and unspecified motor vehicles in traffic accident

√x7th **V19.40** Pedal cycle driver injured in collision with unspecified motor vehicles in traffic accident

√x7th **V19.49** Pedal cycle driver injured in collision with other motor vehicles in traffic accident

√5th **V19.5** Pedal cycle passenger injured in collision with other and unspecified motor vehicles in traffic accident

√x7th **V19.50** Pedal cycle passenger injured in collision with unspecified motor vehicles in traffic accident

√x7th **V19.59** Pedal cycle passenger injured in collision with other motor vehicles in traffic accident

√5th **V19.6** Unspecified pedal cyclist injured in collision with other and unspecified motor vehicles in traffic accident

√x7th **V19.60** Unspecified pedal cyclist injured in collision with unspecified motor vehicles in traffic accident
Pedal cycle collision NOS (traffic)

√x7th **V19.69** Unspecified pedal cyclist injured in collision with other motor vehicles in traffic accident

√5th **V19.8** Pedal cyclist (driver) (passenger) injured in other specified transport accidents

√x7th **V19.81** Pedal cyclist (driver) (passenger) injured in transport accident with military vehicle

√x7th **V19.88** Pedal cyclist (driver) (passenger) injured in other specified transport accidents

√x7th **V19.9** Pedal cyclist (driver) (passenger) injured in unspecified traffic accident
Pedal cycle accident NOS

Motorcycle rider injured in transport accident (V20-V29)

INCLUDES   electric bicycle
e-bike
e-bicycle
moped
motorcycle with sidecar
motorized bicycle
motor scooter

EXCLUDES 1   three-wheeled motor vehicle (V30-V39)

AHA: 2022,4Q,47

The appropriate 7th character is to be added to each code from categories V20-V29.
A   initial encounter
D   subsequent encounter
S   sequela

√4th **V20** Motorcycle rider injured in collision with pedestrian or animal

EXCLUDES 1   motorcycle rider collision with animal-drawn vehicle or animal being ridden (V26.-)

√5th **V20.0** Motorcycle driver injured in collision with pedestrian or animal in nontraffic accident

√x7th **V20.01** Electric (assisted) bicycle driver injured in collision with pedestrian or animal in nontraffic accident

√x7th **V20.09** Other motorcycle driver injured in collision with pedestrian or animal in nontraffic accident

√5th **V20.1** Motorcycle passenger injured in collision with pedestrian or animal in nontraffic accident

√x7th **V20.11** Electric (assisted) bicycle passenger injured in collision with pedestrian or animal in nontraffic accident

---

N Newborn: 0   P Pediatric: 0-17   M Maternity: 9-64   A Adult: 15-124   UNS Unspecified Site   MCC Major Complication/Comorbidity   CC Complication/Comorbidity   PE POA Exempt

1204   ICD-10-CM 2025

√7th **V20.19** Other motorcycle passenger injured in collision with pedestrian or animal in nontraffic accident

√5th **V20.2** Unspecified motorcycle rider injured in collision with pedestrian or animal **in nontraffic accident**

√7th **V20.21** Unspecified **electric (assisted) bicycle** rider injured in collision with pedestrian or animal in nontraffic accident

√7th **V20.29** Unspecified rider of other motorcycle injured in collision with pedestrian or animal in nontraffic accident

√5th **V20.3** **Person boarding or alighting** a motorcycle injured in collision with pedestrian or animal

√7th **V20.31** Person boarding or alighting an **electric (assisted) bicycle** injured in collision with pedestrian or animal

√7th **V20.39** Person boarding or alighting other motorcycle injured in collision with pedestrian or animal

√5th **V20.4** Motorcycle **driver** injured in collision with pedestrian or animal **in traffic accident**

√7th **V20.41** **Electric (assisted) bicycle** driver injured in collision with pedestrian or animal in traffic accident

√7th **V20.49** Other motorcycle driver injured in collision with pedestrian or animal in traffic accident

√5th **V20.5** Motorcycle **passenger** injured in collision with pedestrian or animal **in traffic accident**

√7th **V20.51** **Electric (assisted) bicycle** passenger injured in collision with pedestrian or animal in traffic accident

√7th **V20.59** Other motorcycle passenger injured in collision with pedestrian or animal in traffic accident

√5th **V20.9** Unspecified motorcycle rider injured in collision with pedestrian or animal **in traffic accident**

√7th **V20.91** Unspecified **electric (assisted) bicycle** rider injured in collision with pedestrian or animal in traffic accident

√7th **V20.99** Unspecified rider of other motorcycle injured in collision with pedestrian or animal in traffic accident

√4th **V21** Motorcycle rider injured in collision with pedal cycle

√5th **V21.0** Motorcycle **driver** injured in collision with pedal cycle **in nontraffic accident**

√7th **V21.01** **Electric (assisted) bicycle** driver injured in collision with pedal cycle in nontraffic accident

√7th **V21.09** Other motorcycle driver injured in collision with pedal cycle in nontraffic accident

√5th **V21.1** Motorcycle **passenger** injured in collision with pedal cycle **in nontraffic accident**

√7th **V21.11** **Electric (assisted) bicycle** passenger injured in collision with pedal cycle in nontraffic accident

√7th **V21.19** Other motorcycle passenger injured in collision with pedal cycle in nontraffic accident

√5th **V21.2** Unspecified motorcycle rider injured in collision with pedal cycle **in nontraffic accident**

√7th **V21.21** Unspecified **electric (assisted) bicycle** rider injured in collision with pedal cycle in nontraffic accident

√7th **V21.29** Unspecified rider of other motorcycle injured in collision with pedal cycle in nontraffic accident

√5th **V21.3** **Person boarding or alighting** a motorcycle injured in collision with pedal cycle

√7th **V21.31** Person boarding or alighting an **electric (assisted) bicycle** injured in collision with pedal cycle

√7th **V21.39** Person boarding or alighting other motorcycle injured in collision with pedal cycle

√5th **V21.4** Motorcycle **driver** injured in collision with pedal cycle **in traffic accident**

√7th **V21.41** **Electric (assisted) bicycle** driver injured in collision with pedal cycle in traffic accident

√7th **V21.49** Other motorcycle driver injured in collision with pedal cycle in traffic accident

√5th **V21.5** Motorcycle **passenger** injured in collision with pedal cycle **in traffic accident**

√7th **V21.51** **Electric (assisted) bicycle** passenger injured in collision with pedal cycle in traffic accident

√7th **V21.59** Other motorcycle passenger injured in collision with pedal cycle in traffic accident

√5th **V21.9** Unspecified motorcycle rider injured in collision with pedal cycle **in traffic accident**

√7th **V21.91** Unspecified **electric (assisted) bicycle** rider injured in collision with pedal cycle in traffic accident

√7th **V21.99** Unspecified rider of other motorcycle injured in collision with pedal cycle in traffic accident

√4th **V22** Motorcycle rider injured in collision with two- or three-wheeled motor vehicle

√5th **V22.0** Motorcycle **driver** injured in collision with two- three-wheeled motor vehicle **in nontraffic accident**

√7th **V22.01** **Electric (assisted) bicycle** driver injured in collision with two- or three-wheeled motor vehicle in nontraffic accident

√7th **V22.09** Other motorcycle driver injured in collision with two- or three-wheeled motor vehicle in nontraffic accident

√5th **V22.1** Motorcycle **passenger** injured in collision with two- three-wheeled motor vehicle **in nontraffic accident**

√7th **V22.11** **Electric (assisted) bicycle** passenger injured in collision with two- or three-wheeled motor vehicle in nontraffic accident

√7th **V22.19** Other motorcycle passenger injured in collision with two- or three-wheeled motor vehicle in nontraffic accident

√5th **V22.2** Unspecified motorcycle rider injured in collision with two- or three-wheeled motor vehicle **in nontraffic accident**

√7th **V22.21** Unspecified **electric (assisted) bicycle** rider injured in collision with two- or three-wheeled motor vehicle in nontraffic accident

√7th **V22.29** Unspecified rider of other motorcycle injured in collision with two- or three-wheeled motor vehicle in nontraffic accident

√5th **V22.3** **Person boarding or alighting** a motorcycle injured in collision with two- or three-wheeled motor vehicle

√7th **V22.31** Person boarding or alighting an **electric (assisted) bicycle** injured in collision with two- or three-wheeled motor vehicle

√7th **V22.39** Person boarding or alighting other motorcycle injured in collision with two- or three-wheeled motor vehicle

√5th **V22.4** Motorcycle **driver** injured in collision with two- or three-wheeled motor vehicle **in traffic accident**

√7th **V22.41** **Electric (assisted) bicycle** driver injured in collision with two- or three-wheeled motor vehicle in traffic accident

√7th **V22.49** Other motorcycle driver injured in collision with two- or three-wheeled motor vehicle in traffic accident

√5th **V22.5** Motorcycle **passenger** injured in collision with two- or three-wheeled motor vehicle **in traffic accident**

√7th **V22.51** **Electric (assisted) bicycle** passenger injured in collision with two- or three-wheeled motor vehicle in traffic accident

√7th **V22.59** Other motorcycle passenger injured in collision with two- or three-wheeled motor vehicle in traffic accident

√5th **V22.9** Unspecified motorcycle rider injured in collision with two- or three-wheeled motor vehicle **in traffic accident**

√7th **V22.91** Unspecified **electric (assisted) bicycle** rider injured in collision with two- or three-wheeled motor vehicle in traffic accident

√7th **V22.99** Unspecified rider of other motorcycle injured in collision with two- or three-wheeled motor vehicle in traffic accident

√4th **V23** Motorcycle rider injured in collision with car, pick-up truck or van

√5th **V23.0** Motorcycle **driver** injured in collision with car, pick-up truck or van **in nontraffic accident**

√7th **V23.01** **Electric (assisted) bicycle** driver injured in collision with car, pick-up truck or van in nontraffic accident

√7th **V23.09** Other motorcycle driver injured in collision with car, pick-up truck or van in nontraffic accident

√5th **V23.1** Motorcycle **passenger** injured in collision with car, pick-up truck or van **in nontraffic accident**

√7th **V23.11** **Electric (assisted) bicycle** passenger injured in collision with car, pick-up truck or van in nontraffic accident

√7th **V23.19** Other motorcycle passenger injured in collision with car, pick-up truck or van in nontraffic accident

√5th **V23.2** Unspecified motorcycle rider injured in collision with car, pick-up truck or van **in nontraffic accident**

√7th **V23.21** Unspecified **electric (assisted) bicycle** rider injured in collision with car, pick-up truck or van in nontraffic accident

√7th **V23.29** Unspecified rider of other motorcycle injured in collision with car, pick-up truck or van in nontraffic accident

√5th **V23.3** **Person boarding or alighting** a motorcycle injured in collision with car, pick-up truck or van

√7th **V23.31** Person boarding or alighting an **electric (assisted) bicycle** injured in collision with car, pick-up truck or van

✔ Additional Char Req   √7th Placeholder   Unacceptable PDx   Questionable PDx   Wrong Procedure   Manifestation   Unspecified   H1–H14 HAC   HCC CMS-HCC Dx   HIV HIV Dx

ICD-10-CM 2025   1205

☑x7ᵗʰ   **V23.39**   Person boarding or alighting other motorcycle injured in collision with car, pick-up truck or van

☑5ᵗʰ   **V23.4**   Motorcycle **driver** injured in collision with car, pick-up truck or van **in traffic accident**

     ☑x7ᵗʰ   **V23.41**   **Electric (assisted) bicycle** driver injured in collision with car, pick-up truck or van in traffic accident

     ☑x7ᵗʰ   **V23.49**   Other motorcycle driver injured in collision with car, pick-up truck or van in traffic accident

☑5ᵗʰ   **V23.5**   Motorcycle **passenger** injured in collision with car, pick-up truck or van **in traffic accident**

     ☑x7ᵗʰ   **V23.51**   **Electric (assisted) bicycle** passenger injured in collision with car, pick-up truck or van in traffic accident

     ☑x7ᵗʰ   **V23.59**   Other motorcycle passenger injured in collision with car, pick-up truck or van in traffic accident

☑5ᵗʰ   **V23.9**   Unspecified motorcycle rider injured in collision with car, pick-up truck or van **in traffic accident**

     ☑x7ᵗʰ   **V23.91**   Unspecified **electric (assisted) bicycle** rider injured in collision with car, pick-up truck or van in traffic accident

     ☑x7ᵗʰ   **V23.99**   Unspecified rider of other motorcycle injured in collision with car, pick-up truck or van in traffic accident

☑4ᵗʰ   **V24**   **Motorcycle rider injured in collision with heavy transport vehicle or bus**

     EXCLUDES 1   motorcycle rider injured in collision with military vehicle (V29.818)

☑5ᵗʰ   **V24.0**   Motorcycle **driver** injured in collision with heavy transport vehicle or bus **in nontraffic accident**

     ☑x7ᵗʰ   **V24.01**   **Electric (assisted) bicycle** driver injured in collision with heavy transport vehicle or bus in nontraffic accident

     ☑x7ᵗʰ   **V24.09**   Other motorcycle driver injured in collision with heavy transport vehicle or bus in nontraffic accident

☑5ᵗʰ   **V24.1**   Motorcycle **passenger** injured in collision with heavy transport vehicle or bus **in nontraffic accident**

     ☑x7ᵗʰ   **V24.11**   **Electric (assisted) bicycle** passenger injured in collision with heavy transport vehicle or bus in nontraffic accident

     ☑x7ᵗʰ   **V24.19**   Other motorcycle passenger injured in collision with heavy transport vehicle or bus in nontraffic accident

☑5ᵗʰ   **V24.2**   Unspecified motorcycle rider injured in collision with heavy transport vehicle or bus **in nontraffic accident**

     ☑x7ᵗʰ   **V24.21**   Unspecified **electric (assisted) bicycle** rider injured in collision with heavy transport vehicle or bus in nontraffic accident

     ☑x7ᵗʰ   **V24.29**   Unspecified rider of other motorcycle injured in collision with heavy transport vehicle or bus in nontraffic accident

☑5ᵗʰ   **V24.3**   **Person boarding or alighting** a motorcycle injured in collision with heavy transport vehicle or bus

     ☑x7ᵗʰ   **V24.31**   Person boarding or alighting an **electric (assisted) bicycle** injured in collision with heavy transport vehicle or bus

     ☑x7ᵗʰ   **V24.39**   Person boarding or alighting other injured in collision with heavy transport vehicle or bus

☑5ᵗʰ   **V24.4**   Motorcycle **driver** injured in collision with heavy transport vehicle or bus **in traffic accident**

     ☑x7ᵗʰ   **V24.41**   **Electric (assisted) bicycle** driver injured in collision with heavy transport vehicle or bus in traffic accident

     ☑x7ᵗʰ   **V24.49**   Other motorcycle driver injured in collision with heavy transport vehicle or bus in traffic accident

☑5ᵗʰ   **V24.5**   Motorcycle **passenger** injured in collision with heavy transport vehicle or bus **in traffic accident**

     ☑x7ᵗʰ   **V24.51**   **Electric (assisted) bicycle** passenger injured in collision with heavy transport vehicle or bus in traffic accident

     ☑x7ᵗʰ   **V24.59**   Other motorcycle passenger injured in collision with heavy transport vehicle or bus in traffic accident

☑5ᵗʰ   **V24.9**   Unspecified motorcycle rider injured in collision with heavy transport vehicle or bus **in traffic accident**

     ☑x7ᵗʰ   **V24.91**   Unspecified **electric (assisted) bicycle** rider injured in collision with heavy transport vehicle or bus in traffic accident

     ☑x7ᵗʰ   **V24.99**   Unspecified rider of other motorcycle injured in collision with heavy transport vehicle or bus in traffic accident

☑4ᵗʰ   **V25**   **Motorcycle rider injured in collision with railway train or railway vehicle**

☑5ᵗʰ   **V25.0**   Motorcycle **driver** injured in collision with railway train or railway vehicle **in nontraffic accident**

     ☑x7ᵗʰ   **V25.01**   **Electric (assisted) bicycle** driver injured in collision with railway train or railway vehicle in nontraffic accident

     ☑x7ᵗʰ   **V25.09**   Other motorcycle driver injured in collision with railway train or railway vehicle in nontraffic accident

☑5ᵗʰ   **V25.1**   Motorcycle **passenger** injured in collision with railway train or railway vehicle **in nontraffic accident**

     ☑x7ᵗʰ   **V25.11**   **Electric (assisted) bicycle** passenger injured in collision with railway train or railway vehicle in nontraffic accident

     ☑x7ᵗʰ   **V25.19**   Other motorcycle passenger injured in collision with railway train or railway vehicle in nontraffic accident

☑5ᵗʰ   **V25.2**   Unspecified motorcycle rider injured in collision with railway train or railway vehicle **in nontraffic accident**

     ☑x7ᵗʰ   **V25.21**   Unspecified **electric (assisted) bicycle** rider injured in collision with railway train or railway vehicle in nontraffic accident

     ☑x7ᵗʰ   **V25.29**   Unspecified rider of other motorcycle injured in collision with railway train or railway vehicle in nontraffic accident

☑5ᵗʰ   **V25.3**   **Person boarding or alighting** a motorcycle injured in collision with railway train or railway vehicle

     ☑x7ᵗʰ   **V25.31**   Person boarding or alighting an **electric (assisted) bicycle** injured in collision with railway train or railway vehicle

     ☑x7ᵗʰ   **V25.39**   Person boarding or alighting other motorcycle injured in collision with railway train or railway vehicle

☑5ᵗʰ   **V25.4**   Motorcycle **driver** injured in collision with railway train or railway vehicle **in traffic accident**

     ☑x7ᵗʰ   **V25.41**   **Electric (assisted) bicycle** driver injured in collision with railway train or railway vehicle in traffic accident

     ☑x7ᵗʰ   **V25.49**   Other motorcycle driver injured in collision with railway train or railway vehicle in traffic accident

☑5ᵗʰ   **V25.5**   Motorcycle **passenger** injured in collision with railway train or railway vehicle **in traffic accident**

     ☑x7ᵗʰ   **V25.51**   **Electric (assisted) bicycle** passenger injured in collision with railway train or railway vehicle in traffic accident

     ☑x7ᵗʰ   **V25.59**   Other motorcycle passenger injured in collision with railway train or railway vehicle in traffic accident

☑5ᵗʰ   **V25.9**   Unspecified motorcycle rider injured in collision with railway train or railway vehicle **in traffic accident**

     ☑x7ᵗʰ   **V25.91**   Unspecified **electric (assisted) bicycle** rider injured in collision with railway train or railway vehicle in traffic accident

     ☑x7ᵗʰ   **V25.99**   Unspecified rider of other motorcycle injured in collision with railway train or railway vehicle in traffic accident

☑4ᵗʰ   **V26**   **Motorcycle rider injured in collision with other nonmotor vehicle**

     INCLUDES   collision with animal-drawn vehicle, animal being ridden, streetcar

☑5ᵗʰ   **V26.0**   Motorcycle **driver** injured in collision with other nonmotor vehicle **in nontraffic accident**

     ☑x7ᵗʰ   **V26.01**   **Electric (assisted) bicycle** driver injured in collision with other nonmotor vehicle in nontraffic accident

     ☑x7ᵗʰ   **V26.09**   Other motorcycle driver injured in collision with other nonmotor vehicle in nontraffic accident

☑5ᵗʰ   **V26.1**   Motorcycle **passenger** injured in collision with other nonmotor vehicle **in nontraffic accident**

     ☑x7ᵗʰ   **V26.11**   **Electric (assisted) bicycle** passenger injured in collision with other nonmotor vehicle in nontraffic accident

     ☑x7ᵗʰ   **V26.19**   Other motorcycle passenger injured in collision with other nonmotor vehicle in nontraffic accident

☑5ᵗʰ   **V26.2**   Unspecified motorcycle rider injured in collision with other nonmotor vehicle **in nontraffic accident**

     ☑x7ᵗʰ   **V26.21**   Unspecified **electric (assisted) bicycle** rider injured in collision with other nonmotor vehicle in nontraffic accident

     ☑x7ᵗʰ   **V26.29**   Unspecified rider of other motorcycle injured in collision with other nonmotor vehicle in nontraffic accident

☑5ᵗʰ   **V26.3**   **Person boarding or alighting** a motorcycle injured in collision with other nonmotor vehicle

     ☑x7ᵗʰ   **V26.31**   Person boarding or alighting an **electric (assisted) bicycle** injured in collision with other nonmotor vehicle

N Newborn: 0   **P** Pediatric: 0-17   **M** Maternity: 9-64   **A** Adult: 15-124   **UNS** Unspecified Site   **MCC** Major Complication/Comorbidity   **CC** Complication/Comorbidity   **PE** POA Exempt

1206   ICD-10-CM 2025

☑x 7th **V26.39** Person boarding or alighting other motorcycle injured in collision with other nonmotor vehicle

☑5th **V26.4** Motorcycle **driver** injured in collision with other nonmotor vehicle **in traffic accident**

    ☑x 7th **V26.41** **Electric (assisted) bicycle** driver injured in collision with other nonmotor vehicle in traffic accident

    ☑x 7th **V26.49** Other motorcycle driver injured in collision with other nonmotor vehicle in traffic accident

☑5th **V26.5** Motorcycle **passenger** injured in collision with other nonmotor vehicle **in traffic accident**

    ☑x 7th **V26.51** **Electric (assisted) bicycle** passenger injured in collision with other nonmotor vehicle in traffic accident

    ☑x 7th **V26.59** Other motorcycle passenger injured in collision with other nonmotor vehicle in traffic accident

☑5th **V26.9** Unspecified motorcycle rider injured in collision with other nonmotor vehicle **in traffic accident**

    ☑x 7th **V26.91** Unspecified **electric (assisted) bicycle** rider injured in collision with other nonmotor vehicle in traffic accident

    ☑x 7th **V26.99** Unspecified rider of other motorcycle injured in collision with other nonmotor vehicle in traffic accident

☑4th **V27** Motorcycle rider injured in collision with fixed or stationary object

☑5th **V27.0** Motorcycle **driver** injured in collision with fixed or stationary object **in nontraffic accident**

    ☑x 7th **V27.01** **Electric (assisted) bicycle** driver injured in collision with fixed or stationary object in nontraffic accident

    ☑x 7th **V27.09** Other motorcycle driver injured in collision with fixed or stationary object in nontraffic accident

☑5th **V27.1** Motorcycle **passenger** injured in collision with fixed or stationary object **in nontraffic accident**

    ☑x 7th **V27.11** **Electric (assisted) bicycle** passenger injured in collision with fixed or stationary object in nontraffic accident

    ☑x 7th **V27.19** Other motorcycle passenger injured in collision with fixed or stationary object in nontraffic accident

☑5th **V27.2** Unspecified motorcycle rider injured in collision with fixed or stationary object **in nontraffic accident**

    ☑x 7th **V27.21** Unspecified **electric (assisted) bicycle** rider injured in collision with fixed or stationary object in nontraffic accident

    ☑x 7th **V27.29** Unspecified rider of other motorcycle injured in collision with fixed or stationary object in nontraffic accident

☑5th **V27.3** **Person boarding or alighting** a motorcycle injured in collision with fixed or stationary object

    ☑x 7th **V27.31** Person boarding or alighting an **electric (assisted) bicycle** injured in collision with fixed or stationary object

    ☑x 7th **V27.39** Person boarding or alighting other motorcycle injured in collision with fixed or stationary object

☑5th **V27.4** Motorcycle **driver** injured in collision with fixed or stationary object **in traffic accident**

    ☑x 7th **V27.41** **Electric (assisted) bicycle** driver injured in collision with fixed or stationary object in traffic accident

    ☑x 7th **V27.49** Other motorcycle driver injured in collision with fixed or stationary object in traffic accident

☑5th **V27.5** Motorcycle **passenger** injured in collision with fixed or stationary object **in traffic accident**

    ☑x 7th **V27.51** **Electric (assisted) bicycle** passenger injured in collision with fixed or stationary object in traffic accident

    ☑x 7th **V27.59** Other motorcycle passenger injured in collision with fixed or stationary object in traffic accident

☑5th **V27.9** Unspecified motorcycle rider injured in collision with fixed or stationary object **in traffic accident**

    ☑x 7th **V27.91** Unspecified **electric (assisted) bicycle** rider injured in collision with fixed or stationary object in traffic accident

    ☑x 7th **V27.99** Unspecified rider of other motorcycle injured in collision with fixed or stationary object in traffic accident

☑4th **V28** Motorcycle rider injured in noncollision transport accident

    INCLUDES   fall or thrown from motorcycle (without antecedent collision)
                  overturning motorcycle NOS
                  overturning motorcycle without collision

☑5th **V28.0** Motorcycle **driver** injured in noncollision transport accident **in nontraffic accident**

    ☑x 7th **V28.01** **Electric (assisted) bicycle** driver injured in noncollision transport accident in nontraffic accident

---

☑x 7th **V28.09** Other motorcycle driver injured in noncollision transport accident in nontraffic accident

☑5th **V28.1** Motorcycle **passenger** injured in noncollision transport accident **in nontraffic accident**

    ☑x 7th **V28.11** **Electric (assisted) bicycle** passenger injured in noncollision transport accident in nontraffic accident

    ☑x 7th **V28.19** Other motorcycle passenger injured in noncollision transport accident in nontraffic accident

☑5th **V28.2** Unspecified motorcycle rider injured in noncollision transport accident **in nontraffic accident**

    ☑x 7th **V28.21** Unspecified **electric (assisted) bicycle** rider injured in noncollision transport accident in nontraffic accident

    ☑x 7th **V28.29** Unspecified rider of other motorcycle injured in noncollision transport accident in nontraffic accident

☑5th **V28.3** **Person boarding or alighting** a motorcycle injured in noncollision transport accident

    ☑x 7th **V28.31** Person boarding or alighting an **electric (assisted) bicycle** injured in noncollision transport accident

    ☑x 7th **V28.39** Person boarding or alighting other motorcycle injured in noncollision transport accident

☑5th **V28.4** Motorcycle **driver** injured in noncollision transport accident **in traffic accident**

    ☑x 7th **V28.41** **Electric (assisted) bicycle** driver injured in noncollision transport accident in traffic accident

    ☑x 7th **V28.49** Other motorcycle driver injured in noncollision transport accident in traffic accident

☑5th **V28.5** Motorcycle **passenger** injured in noncollision transport accident **in traffic accident**

    ☑x 7th **V28.51** **Electric (assisted) bicycle** passenger injured in noncollision transport accident in traffic accident

    ☑x 7th **V28.59** Other motorcycle passenger injured in noncollision transport accident in traffic accident

☑5th **V28.9** Unspecified motorcycle rider injured in noncollision transport accident **in traffic accident**

    ☑x 7th **V28.91** Unspecified **electric (assisted) bicycle** rider injured in noncollision transport accident in traffic accident

    ☑x 7th **V28.99** Unspecified rider of other motorcycle injured in noncollision transport accident in traffic accident

☑4th **V29** Motorcycle rider injured in other and unspecified transport accidents

☑5th **V29.0** Motorcycle **driver** injured in collision with other and unspecified motor vehicles **in nontraffic accident**

    ☑6th **V29.00** Motorcycle driver injured in collision with unspecified motor vehicles in nontraffic accident

        ☑7th **V29.001** **Electric (assisted) bicycle** driver injured in collision with unspecified motor vehicles in nontraffic accident

        ☑7th **V29.008** Other motorcycle driver injured in collision with unspecified motor vehicles in nontraffic accident

    ☑6th **V29.09** Motorcycle driver injured in collision with other motor vehicles in nontraffic accident

        ☑7th **V29.091** **Electric (assisted) bicycle** driver injured in collision with other motor vehicles in nontraffic accident

        ☑7th **V29.098** Other motorcycle driver injured in collision with other motor vehicles in nontraffic accident

☑5th **V29.1** Motorcycle **passenger** injured in collision with other and unspecified motor vehicles **in nontraffic accident**

    ☑6th **V29.10** Motorcycle passenger injured in collision with unspecified motor vehicles in nontraffic accident

        ☑7th **V29.101** **Electric (assisted) bicycle** passenger injured in collision with unspecified motor vehicles in nontraffic accident

        ☑7th **V29.108** Other motorcycle passenger injured in collision with unspecified motor vehicles in nontraffic accident

    ☑6th **V29.19** Motorcycle passenger injured in collision with other motor vehicles in nontraffic accident

        ☑7th **V29.191** **Electric (assisted) bicycle** passenger injured in collision with other motor vehicles in nontraffic accident

        ☑7th **V29.198** Other motorcycle passenger injured in collision with other motor vehicles in nontraffic accident

☑5th **V29.2** Unspecified motorcycle rider injured in collision with other and unspecified motor vehicles **in nontraffic accident**

    ☑6th **V29.20** Unspecified motorcycle rider injured in collision with unspecified motor vehicles in nontraffic accident

        ☑7th **V29.201** Unspecified **electric (assisted) bicycle** rider injured in collision with unspecified motor vehicles in nontraffic accident

☑ Additional Char Req   ☑x 7th Placeholder   Unacceptable PDx   Questionable PDx   Wrong Procedure   Manifestation   Unspecified   H1-H14 HAC   HCC CMS-HCC Dx   HIV HIV Dx

ICD-10-CM 2025   1207

Chapter 20. External Causes of Morbidity

V29.2Ø8–V32.1

√7ᵗʰ **V29.2Ø8** Unspecified rider of other motorcycle injured in collision with unspecified motor vehicles in nontraffic accident
> Motorcycle collision NOS, nontraffic

√6ᵗʰ **V29.29** Unspecified motorcycle rider injured in collision with other motor vehicles in nontraffic accident

√7ᵗʰ **V29.291** Unspecified electric (assisted) bicycle rider injured in collision with other motor vehicles in nontraffic accident

√7ᵗʰ **V29.298** Unspecified rider of other motorcycle injured in collision with other motor vehicles in nontraffic accident

√5ᵗʰ **V29.3** Motorcycle rider (driver) (passenger) injured in unspecified nontraffic accident

√x7ᵗʰ **V29.31** Electric (assisted) bicycle (driver) (passenger) injured in unspecified nontraffic accident

√x7ᵗʰ **V29.39** Other motorcycle (driver) (passenger) injured in unspecified nontraffic accident
> Motorcycle accident NOS, nontraffic
> Motorcycle rider injured in nontraffic accident NOS

√5ᵗʰ **V29.4** Motorcycle driver injured in collision with other and unspecified motor vehicles in traffic accident

√6ᵗʰ **V29.4Ø** Motorcycle driver injured in collision with unspecified motor vehicles in traffic accident

√7ᵗʰ **V29.4Ø1** Electric (assisted) bicycle driver injured in collision with unspecified motor vehicles in traffic accident

√7ᵗʰ **V29.4Ø8** Other motorcycle driver injured in collision with unspecified motor vehicles in traffic accident

√6ᵗʰ **V29.49** Motorcycle driver injured in collision with other motor vehicles in traffic accident

√7ᵗʰ **V29.491** Electric (assisted) bicycle driver injured in collision with other motor vehicles in traffic accident

√7ᵗʰ **V29.498** Other motorcycle driver injured in collision with other motor vehicles in traffic accident

√5ᵗʰ **V29.5** Motorcycle passenger injured in collision with other and unspecified motor vehicles in traffic accident

√6ᵗʰ **V29.5Ø** Motorcycle passenger injured in collision with unspecified motor vehicles in traffic accident

√7ᵗʰ **V29.5Ø1** Electric (assisted) bicycle passenger injured in collision with unspecified motor vehicles in traffic accident

√7ᵗʰ **V29.5Ø8** Other motorcycle passenger injured in collision with unspecified motor vehicles in traffic accident

√6ᵗʰ **V29.59** Motorcycle passenger injured in collision with other motor vehicles in traffic accident

√7ᵗʰ **V29.591** Electric (assisted) bicycle passenger injured in collision with other motor vehicles in traffic accident

√7ᵗʰ **V29.598** Other motorcycle passenger injured in collision with other motor vehicles in traffic accident

√5ᵗʰ **V29.6** Unspecified motorcycle rider injured in collision with other and unspecified motor vehicles in traffic accident

√6ᵗʰ **V29.6Ø** Unspecified motorcycle rider injured in collision with unspecified motor vehicles in traffic accident

√7ᵗʰ **V29.6Ø1** Unspecified electric (assisted) bicycle rider injured in collision with unspecified motor vehicles in traffic accident

√7ᵗʰ **V29.6Ø8** Unspecified rider of other motorcycle injured in collision with unspecified motor vehicles in traffic accident
> Motorcycle collision NOS (traffic)

√6ᵗʰ **V29.69** Unspecified motorcycle rider injured in collision with other motor vehicles in traffic accident

√7ᵗʰ **V29.691** Unspecified electric (assisted) bicycle rider injured in collision with other motor vehicles in traffic accident

√7ᵗʰ **V29.698** Unspecified rider of other motorcycle injured in collision with other motor vehicles in traffic accident

√5ᵗʰ **V29.8** Motorcycle rider (driver) (passenger) injured in other specified transport accidents

√6ᵗʰ **V29.81** Motorcycle rider (driver) (passenger) injured in transport accident with military vehicle

√7ᵗʰ **V29.811** Electric (assisted) bicycle rider (driver) (passenger) injured in transport accident with military vehicle

√7ᵗʰ **V29.818** Rider (driver) (passenger) of other motorcycle injured in transport accident with military vehicle

√6ᵗʰ **V29.88** Motorcycle rider (driver) (passenger) injured in other specified transport accidents

√7ᵗʰ **V29.881** Electric (assisted) bicycle rider (driver) (passenger) injured in other specified transport accidents

√7ᵗʰ **V29.888** Rider (driver) (passenger) of other motorcycle injured in other specified transport accidents

√5ᵗʰ **V29.9** Motorcycle rider (driver) (passenger) injured in unspecified traffic accident

√x7ᵗʰ **V29.91** Electric (assisted) bicycle rider (driver) (passenger) injured in unspecified traffic accident

√x7ᵗʰ **V29.99** Rider (driver) (passenger) of other motorcycle injured in unspecified traffic accident
> Motorcycle accident NOS

Occupant of three-wheeled motor vehicle injured in transport accident (V3Ø-V39)

INCLUDES   motorized tricycle
> motorized rickshaw
> three-wheeled motor car

EXCLUDES 1   *all-terrain vehicles (V86.-)*
> *motorcycle with sidecar (V2Ø-V29)*
> *vehicle designed primarily for off-road use (V86.-)*

The appropriate 7th character is to be added to each code from categories V3Ø-V39.
A   initial encounter
D   subsequent encounter
S   sequela

√4ᵗʰ **V3Ø** Occupant of three-wheeled motor vehicle injured in collision with pedestrian or animal
> **EXCLUDES 1**   *three-wheeled motor vehicle collision with animal-drawn vehicle or animal being ridden (V36.-)*

√x7ᵗʰ **V3Ø.Ø** Driver of three-wheeled motor vehicle injured in collision with pedestrian or animal in nontraffic accident

√x7ᵗʰ **V3Ø.1** Passenger in three-wheeled motor vehicle injured in collision with pedestrian or animal in nontraffic accident

√x7ᵗʰ **V3Ø.2** Person on outside of three-wheeled motor vehicle injured in collision with pedestrian or animal in nontraffic accident

√x7ᵗʰ **V3Ø.3** Unspecified occupant of three-wheeled motor vehicle injured in collision with pedestrian or animal in nontraffic accident

√x7ᵗʰ **V3Ø.4** Person boarding or alighting a three-wheeled motor vehicle injured in collision with pedestrian or animal

√x7ᵗʰ **V3Ø.5** Driver of three-wheeled motor vehicle injured in collision with pedestrian or animal in traffic accident

√x7ᵗʰ **V3Ø.6** Passenger in three-wheeled motor vehicle injured in collision with pedestrian or animal in traffic accident

√x7ᵗʰ **V3Ø.7** Person on outside of three-wheeled motor vehicle injured in collision with pedestrian or animal in traffic accident

√x7ᵗʰ **V3Ø.9** Unspecified occupant of three-wheeled motor vehicle injured in collision with pedestrian or animal in traffic accident

√4ᵗʰ **V31** Occupant of three-wheeled motor vehicle injured in collision with pedal cycle

√x7ᵗʰ **V31.Ø** Driver of three-wheeled motor vehicle injured in collision with pedal cycle in nontraffic accident

√x7ᵗʰ **V31.1** Passenger in three-wheeled motor vehicle injured in collision with pedal cycle in nontraffic accident

√x7ᵗʰ **V31.2** Person on outside of three-wheeled motor vehicle injured in collision with pedal cycle in nontraffic accident

√x7ᵗʰ **V31.3** Unspecified occupant of three-wheeled motor vehicle injured in collision with pedal cycle in nontraffic accident

√x7ᵗʰ **V31.4** Person boarding or alighting a three-wheeled motor vehicle injured in collision with pedal cycle

√x7ᵗʰ **V31.5** Driver of three-wheeled motor vehicle injured in collision with pedal cycle in traffic accident

√x7ᵗʰ **V31.6** Passenger in three-wheeled motor vehicle injured in collision with pedal cycle in traffic accident

√x7ᵗʰ **V31.7** Person on outside of three-wheeled motor vehicle injured in collision with pedal cycle in traffic accident

√x7ᵗʰ **V31.9** Unspecified occupant of three-wheeled motor vehicle injured in collision with pedal cycle in traffic accident

√4ᵗʰ **V32** Occupant of three-wheeled motor vehicle injured in collision with two- or three-wheeled motor vehicle

√x7ᵗʰ **V32.Ø** Driver of three-wheeled motor vehicle injured in collision with two- or three-wheeled motor vehicle in nontraffic accident

√x7ᵗʰ **V32.1** Passenger in three-wheeled motor vehicle injured in collision with two- or three-wheeled motor vehicle in nontraffic accident

N Newborn: 0   **P** Pediatric: 0-17   **M** Maternity: 9-64   **A** Adult: 15-124   **UNS** Unspecified Site   **MCC** Major Complication/Comorbidity   **CC** Complication/Comorbidity   **PE** POA Exempt

1208   ICD-10-CM 2025

√x7th **V32.2** **Person on outside** of three-wheeled motor vehicle injured in collision with two- or three-wheeled motor vehicle **in nontraffic accident**

√x7th **V32.3** Unspecified occupant of three-wheeled motor vehicle injured in collision with two- or three-wheeled motor vehicle **in nontraffic accident**

√x7th **V32.4** **Person boarding or alighting** a three-wheeled motor vehicle injured in collision with two- or three-wheeled motor vehicle

√x7th **V32.5** **Driver** of three-wheeled motor vehicle injured in collision with two- or three-wheeled motor vehicle **in traffic accident**

√x7th **V32.6** **Passenger** in three-wheeled motor vehicle injured in collision with two- or three-wheeled motor vehicle **in traffic accident**

√x7th **V32.7** **Person on outside** of three-wheeled motor vehicle injured in collision with two- or three-wheeled motor vehicle **in traffic accident**

√x7th **V32.9** Unspecified occupant of three-wheeled motor vehicle injured in collision with two- or three-wheeled motor vehicle **in traffic accident**

√4th **V33** **Occupant of three-wheeled motor vehicle injured in collision with car, pick-up truck or van**

√x7th **V33.0** **Driver** of three-wheeled motor vehicle injured in collision with car, pick-up truck or van **in nontraffic accident**

√x7th **V33.1** **Passenger** in three-wheeled motor vehicle injured in collision with car, pick-up truck or van **in nontraffic accident**

√x7th **V33.2** **Person on outside** of three-wheeled motor vehicle injured in collision with car, pick-up truck or van **in nontraffic accident**

√x7th **V33.3** Unspecified occupant of three-wheeled motor vehicle injured in collision with car, pick-up truck or van **in nontraffic accident**

√x7th **V33.4** **Person boarding or alighting** a three-wheeled motor vehicle injured in collision with car, pick-up truck or van

√x7th **V33.5** **Driver** of three-wheeled motor vehicle injured in collision with car, pick-up truck or van **in traffic accident**

√x7th **V33.6** **Passenger** in three-wheeled motor vehicle injured in collision with car, pick-up truck or van **in traffic accident**

√x7th **V33.7** **Person on outside** of three-wheeled motor vehicle injured in collision with car, pick-up truck or van **in traffic accident**

√x7th **V33.9** Unspecified occupant of three-wheeled motor vehicle injured in collision with car, pick-up truck or van **in traffic accident**

√4th **V34** **Occupant of three-wheeled motor vehicle injured in collision with heavy transport vehicle or bus**

    EXCLUDES 1   *occupant of three-wheeled motor vehicle injured in collision with military vehicle (V39.81)*

√x7th **V34.0** **Driver** of three-wheeled motor vehicle injured in collision with heavy transport vehicle or bus **in nontraffic accident**

√x7th **V34.1** **Passenger** in three-wheeled motor vehicle injured in collision with heavy transport vehicle or bus **in nontraffic accident**

√x7th **V34.2** **Person on outside** of three-wheeled motor vehicle injured in collision with heavy transport vehicle or bus **in nontraffic accident**

√x7th **V34.3** Unspecified occupant of three-wheeled motor vehicle injured in collision with heavy transport vehicle or bus **in nontraffic accident**

√x7th **V34.4** **Person boarding or alighting** a three-wheeled motor vehicle injured in collision with heavy transport vehicle or bus

√x7th **V34.5** **Driver** of three-wheeled motor vehicle injured in collision with heavy transport vehicle or bus **in traffic accident**

√x7th **V34.6** **Passenger** in three-wheeled motor vehicle injured in collision with heavy transport vehicle or bus **in traffic accident**

√x7th **V34.7** **Person on outside** of three-wheeled motor vehicle injured in collision with heavy transport vehicle or bus **in traffic accident**

√x7th **V34.9** Unspecified occupant of three-wheeled motor vehicle injured in collision with heavy transport vehicle or bus **in traffic accident**

√4th **V35** **Occupant of three-wheeled motor vehicle injured in collision with railway train or railway vehicle**

√x7th **V35.0** **Driver** of three-wheeled motor vehicle injured in collision with railway train or railway vehicle **in nontraffic accident**

√x7th **V35.1** **Passenger** in three-wheeled motor vehicle injured in collision with railway train or railway vehicle **in nontraffic accident**

√x7th **V35.2** **Person on outside** of three-wheeled motor vehicle injured in collision with railway train or railway vehicle **in nontraffic accident**

√x7th **V35.3** Unspecified occupant of three-wheeled motor vehicle injured in collision with railway train or railway vehicle **in nontraffic accident**

√x7th **V35.4** **Person boarding or alighting** a three-wheeled motor vehicle injured in collision with railway train or railway vehicle

√x7th **V35.5** **Driver** of three-wheeled motor vehicle injured in collision with railway train or railway vehicle **in traffic accident**

√x7th **V35.6** **Passenger** in three-wheeled motor vehicle injured in collision with railway train or railway vehicle **in traffic accident**

√x7th **V35.7** **Person on outside** of three-wheeled motor vehicle injured in collision with railway train or railway vehicle **in traffic accident**

√x7th **V35.9** Unspecified occupant of three-wheeled motor vehicle injured in collision with railway train or railway vehicle **in traffic accident**

√4th **V36** **Occupant of three-wheeled motor vehicle injured in collision with other nonmotor vehicle**

    INCLUDES   collision with animal-drawn vehicle, animal being ridden, streetcar

√x7th **V36.0** **Driver** of three-wheeled motor vehicle injured in collision with other nonmotor vehicle **in nontraffic accident**

√x7th **V36.1** **Passenger** in three-wheeled motor vehicle injured in collision with other nonmotor vehicle **in nontraffic accident**

√x7th **V36.2** **Person on outside** of three-wheeled motor vehicle injured in collision with other nonmotor vehicle **in nontraffic accident**

√x7th **V36.3** Unspecified occupant of three-wheeled motor vehicle injured in collision with other nonmotor vehicle **in nontraffic accident**

√x7th **V36.4** **Person boarding or alighting** a three-wheeled motor vehicle injured in collision with other nonmotor vehicle

√x7th **V36.5** **Driver** of three-wheeled motor vehicle injured in collision with other nonmotor vehicle **in traffic accident**

√x7th **V36.6** **Passenger** in three-wheeled motor vehicle injured in collision with other nonmotor vehicle **in traffic accident**

√x7th **V36.7** **Person on outside** of three-wheeled motor vehicle injured in collision with other nonmotor vehicle **in traffic accident**

√x7th **V36.9** Unspecified occupant of three-wheeled motor vehicle injured in collision with other nonmotor vehicle **in traffic accident**

√4th **V37** **Occupant of three-wheeled motor vehicle injured in collision with fixed or stationary object**

√x7th **V37.0** **Driver** of three-wheeled motor vehicle injured in collision with fixed or stationary object **in nontraffic accident**

√x7th **V37.1** **Passenger** in three-wheeled motor vehicle injured in collision with fixed or stationary object **in nontraffic accident**

√x7th **V37.2** **Person on outside** of three-wheeled motor vehicle injured in collision with fixed or stationary object **in nontraffic accident**

√x7th **V37.3** Unspecified occupant of three-wheeled motor vehicle injured in collision with fixed or stationary object **in nontraffic accident**

√x7th **V37.4** **Person boarding or alighting** a three-wheeled motor vehicle injured in collision with fixed or stationary object

√x7th **V37.5** **Driver** of three-wheeled motor vehicle injured in collision with fixed or stationary object **in traffic accident**

√x7th **V37.6** **Passenger** in three-wheeled motor vehicle injured in collision with fixed or stationary object **in traffic accident**

√x7th **V37.7** **Person on outside** of three-wheeled motor vehicle injured in collision with fixed or stationary object **in traffic accident**

√x7th **V37.9** Unspecified occupant of three-wheeled motor vehicle injured in collision with fixed or stationary object **in traffic accident**

√4th **V38** **Occupant of three-wheeled motor vehicle injured in noncollision transport accident**

    INCLUDES   fall or thrown from three-wheeled motor vehicle
                    overturning of three-wheeled motor vehicle NOS
                    overturning of three-wheeled motor vehicle without collision

√x7th **V38.0** **Driver** of three-wheeled motor vehicle injured in noncollision transport accident **in nontraffic accident**

√x7th **V38.1** **Passenger** in three-wheeled motor vehicle injured in noncollision transport accident **in nontraffic accident**

√x7th **V38.2** **Person on outside** of three-wheeled motor vehicle injured in noncollision transport accident **in nontraffic accident**

√x7th **V38.3** Unspecified occupant of three-wheeled motor vehicle injured in noncollision transport accident **in nontraffic accident**

√x7th **V38.4** **Person boarding or alighting** a three-wheeled motor vehicle injured in noncollision transport accident

√x7th **V38.5** **Driver** of three-wheeled motor vehicle injured in noncollision transport accident **in traffic accident**

√x7th **V38.6** **Passenger** in three-wheeled motor vehicle injured in noncollision transport accident **in traffic accident**

√x7th **V38.7** **Person on outside** of three-wheeled motor vehicle injured in noncollision transport accident **in traffic accident**

√x7th **V38.9** Unspecified occupant of three-wheeled motor vehicle injured in noncollision transport accident **in traffic accident**

√4th **V39** **Occupant of three-wheeled motor vehicle injured in other and unspecified transport accidents**

√5th **V39.0** **Driver** of three-wheeled motor vehicle injured in collision with other and unspecified motor vehicles **in nontraffic accident**

√x7th **V39.00** Driver of three-wheeled motor vehicle injured in collision with unspecified motor vehicles in nontraffic accident

√x7th **V39.09** Driver of three-wheeled motor vehicle injured in collision with other motor vehicles in nontraffic accident

---

✔ Additional Char Req   √x7th Placeholder   Unacceptable PDx   Questionable PDx   Wrong Procedure   Manifestation   Unspecified   H1 - H14 HAC   HCC CMS-HCC Dx   HIV HIV Dx

√5ᵗʰ **V39.1** **Passenger** in three-wheeled motor vehicle injured in collision with other and unspecified motor vehicles **in nontraffic accident**

√x7ᵗʰ **V39.10** Passenger in three-wheeled motor vehicle injured in collision with unspecified motor vehicles in nontraffic accident

√x7ᵗʰ **V39.19** Passenger in three-wheeled motor vehicle injured in collision with other motor vehicles in nontraffic accident

√5ᵗʰ **V39.2** Unspecified occupant of three-wheeled motor vehicle injured in collision with other and unspecified motor vehicles **in nontraffic accident**

√x7ᵗʰ **V39.20** Unspecified occupant of three-wheeled motor vehicle injured in collision with unspecified motor vehicles in nontraffic accident

Collision NOS involving three-wheeled motor vehicle, nontraffic

√x7ᵗʰ **V39.29** Unspecified occupant of three-wheeled motor vehicle injured in collision with other motor vehicles in nontraffic accident

√x7ᵗʰ **V39.3** Occupant (driver) (passenger) of three-wheeled motor vehicle injured in unspecified nontraffic accident

Accident NOS involving three-wheeled motor vehicle, nontraffic
Occupant of three-wheeled motor vehicle injured in nontraffic accident NOS

√5ᵗʰ **V39.4** **Driver** of three-wheeled motor vehicle injured in collision with other and unspecified motor vehicles **in traffic accident**

√x7ᵗʰ **V39.40** Driver of three-wheeled motor vehicle injured in collision with unspecified motor vehicles in traffic accident

√x7ᵗʰ **V39.49** Driver of three-wheeled motor vehicle injured in collision with other motor vehicles in traffic accident

√5ᵗʰ **V39.5** **Passenger** in three-wheeled motor vehicle injured in collision with other and unspecified motor vehicles **in traffic accident**

√x7ᵗʰ **V39.50** Passenger in three-wheeled motor vehicle injured in collision with unspecified motor vehicles in traffic accident

√x7ᵗʰ **V39.59** Passenger in three-wheeled motor vehicle injured in collision with other motor vehicles in traffic accident

√5ᵗʰ **V39.6** Unspecified occupant of three-wheeled motor vehicle injured in collision with other and unspecified motor vehicles **in traffic accident**

√x7ᵗʰ **V39.60** Unspecified occupant of three-wheeled motor vehicle injured in collision with unspecified motor vehicles in traffic accident

Collision NOS involving three-wheeled motor vehicle (traffic)

√x7ᵗʰ **V39.69** Unspecified occupant of three-wheeled motor vehicle injured in collision with other motor vehicles in traffic accident

√5ᵗʰ **V39.8** Occupant (driver) (passenger) of three-wheeled motor vehicle injured in other specified transport accidents

√x7ᵗʰ **V39.81** Occupant (driver) (passenger) of three-wheeled motor vehicle injured in transport accident with **military vehicle**

√x7ᵗʰ **V39.89** Occupant (driver) (passenger) of three-wheeled motor vehicle injured in other specified transport accidents

√x7ᵗʰ **V39.9** Occupant (driver) (passenger) of three-wheeled motor vehicle injured in unspecified traffic accident

Accident NOS involving three-wheeled motor vehicle

Car occupant injured in transport accident (V40-V49)

INCLUDES a four-wheeled motor vehicle designed primarily for carrying passengers
automobile (pulling a trailer or camper)

EXCLUDES 1 bus (V50-V59)
minibus (V50-V59)
minivan (V50-V59)
motorcoach (V70-V79)
pick-up truck (V50-V59)
sport utility vehicle (SUV) (V50-V59)

The appropriate 7th character is to be added to each code from categories V40-V49.
A   initial encounter
D   subsequent encounter
S   sequela

√4ᵗʰ **V40** **Car occupant injured in collision with pedestrian or animal**

EXCLUDES 1 car collision with animal-drawn vehicle or animal being ridden (V46.-)

√x7ᵗʰ **V40.0** Car **driver** injured in collision with pedestrian or animal **in nontraffic accident**

√x7ᵗʰ **V40.1** Car **passenger** injured in collision with pedestrian or animal **in nontraffic accident**

√x7ᵗʰ **V40.2** **Person on outside** of car injured in collision with pedestrian or animal **in nontraffic accident**

√x7ᵗʰ **V40.3** Unspecified car occupant injured in collision with pedestrian or animal **in nontraffic accident**

√x7ᵗʰ **V40.4** **Person boarding or alighting** a car injured in collision with pedestrian or animal

√x7ᵗʰ **V40.5** Car **driver** injured in collision with pedestrian or animal **in traffic accident**

√x7ᵗʰ **V40.6** Car **passenger** injured in collision with pedestrian or animal **in traffic accident**

√x7ᵗʰ **V40.7** **Person on outside** of car injured in collision with pedestrian or animal **in traffic accident**

√x7ᵗʰ **V40.9** Unspecified car occupant injured in collision with pedestrian or animal **in traffic accident**

√4ᵗʰ **V41** **Car occupant injured in collision with pedal cycle**

√x7ᵗʰ **V41.0** Car **driver** injured in collision with pedal cycle **in nontraffic accident**

√x7ᵗʰ **V41.1** Car **passenger** injured in collision with pedal cycle **in nontraffic accident**

√x7ᵗʰ **V41.2** **Person on outside** of car injured in collision with pedal cycle **in nontraffic accident**

√x7ᵗʰ **V41.3** Unspecified car occupant injured in collision with pedal cycle **in nontraffic accident**

√x7ᵗʰ **V41.4** **Person boarding or alighting** a car injured in collision with pedal cycle

√x7ᵗʰ **V41.5** Car **driver** injured in collision with pedal cycle **in traffic accident**

√x7ᵗʰ **V41.6** Car **passenger** injured in collision with pedal cycle **in traffic accident**

√x7ᵗʰ **V41.7** **Person on outside** of car injured in collision with pedal cycle **in traffic accident**

√x7ᵗʰ **V41.9** Unspecified car occupant injured in collision with pedal cycle **in traffic accident**

√4ᵗʰ **V42** **Car occupant injured in collision with two- or three-wheeled motor vehicle**

√x7ᵗʰ **V42.0** Car **driver** injured in collision with two- or three-wheeled motor vehicle **in nontraffic accident**

√x7ᵗʰ **V42.1** Car **passenger** injured in collision with two- or three-wheeled motor vehicle **in nontraffic accident**

√x7ᵗʰ **V42.2** **Person on outside** of car injured in collision with two- or three-wheeled motor vehicle **in nontraffic accident**

√x7ᵗʰ **V42.3** Unspecified car occupant injured in collision with two- or three-wheeled motor vehicle **in nontraffic accident**

√x7ᵗʰ **V42.4** **Person boarding or alighting** a car injured in collision with two- or three-wheeled motor vehicle

√x7ᵗʰ **V42.5** Car **driver** injured in collision with two- or three-wheeled motor vehicle **in traffic accident**

√x7ᵗʰ **V42.6** Car **passenger** injured in collision with two- or three-wheeled motor vehicle **in traffic accident**

√x7ᵗʰ **V42.7** **Person on outside** of car injured in collision with two- or three-wheeled motor vehicle **in traffic accident**

√x7ᵗʰ **V42.9** Unspecified car occupant injured in collision with two- or three-wheeled motor vehicle **in traffic accident**

√4ᵗʰ **V43** **Car occupant injured in collision with car, pick-up truck or van**

√5ᵗʰ **V43.0** Car **driver** injured in collision with car, pick-up truck or van **in nontraffic accident**

√x7ᵗʰ **V43.01** Car driver injured in collision with **sport utility vehicle** in nontraffic accident

√x7ᵗʰ **V43.02** Car driver injured in collision with other type car in nontraffic accident

√x7ᵗʰ **V43.03** Car driver injured in collision with **pick-up truck** in nontraffic accident

√x7ᵗʰ **V43.04** Car driver injured in collision with **van** in nontraffic accident

√5ᵗʰ **V43.1** Car **passenger** injured in collision with car, pick-up truck or van **in nontraffic accident**

√x7ᵗʰ **V43.11** Car passenger injured in collision with **sport utility vehicle** in nontraffic accident

√x7ᵗʰ **V43.12** Car passenger injured in collision with other type car in nontraffic accident

√x7ᵗʰ **V43.13** Car passenger injured in collision with **pick-up truck** in nontraffic accident

√x7ᵗʰ **V43.14** Car passenger injured in collision with **van** in nontraffic accident

√5ᵗʰ **V43.2** **Person on outside** of car injured in collision with car, pick-up truck or van **in nontraffic accident**

√x7ᵗʰ **V43.21** Person on outside of car injured in collision with **sport utility vehicle** in nontraffic accident

N Newborn: 0   P Pediatric: 0-17   M Maternity: 9-64   A Adult: 15-124   UNS Unspecified Site   MCC Major Complication/Comorbidity   CC Complication/Comorbidity   PE POA Exempt

1210

ICD-10-CM 2025

V43.22 Person on outside of car injured in collision with other type car in nontraffic accident `✓x7th`

V43.23 Person on outside of car injured in collision with pick-up truck in nontraffic accident `✓x7th`

V43.24 Person on outside of car injured in collision with van in nontraffic accident `✓x7th`

`✓5th` **V43.3** Unspecified car occupant injured in collision with car, pick-up truck or van in nontraffic accident

V43.31 Unspecified car occupant injured in collision with sport utility vehicle in nontraffic accident `✓x7th`

V43.32 Unspecified car occupant injured in collision with other type car in nontraffic accident `✓x7th`

V43.33 Unspecified car occupant injured in collision with pick-up truck in nontraffic accident `✓x7th`

V43.34 Unspecified car occupant injured in collision with van in nontraffic accident `✓x7th`

`✓5th` **V43.4** Person boarding or alighting a car injured in collision with car, pick-up truck or van

V43.41 Person boarding or alighting a car injured in collision with sport utility vehicle `✓x7th`

V43.42 Person boarding or alighting a car injured in collision with other type car `✓x7th`

V43.43 Person boarding or alighting a car injured in collision with pick-up truck `✓x7th`

V43.44 Person boarding or alighting a car injured in collision with van `✓x7th`

`✓5th` **V43.5** Car driver injured in collision with car, pick-up truck or van in traffic accident

V43.51 Car driver injured in collision with sport utility vehicle in traffic accident `✓x7th`

V43.52 Car driver injured in collision with other type car in traffic accident `✓x7th`

V43.53 Car driver injured in collision with pick-up truck in traffic accident `✓x7th`

V43.54 Car driver injured in collision with van in traffic accident `✓x7th`

`✓5th` **V43.6** Car passenger injured in collision with car, pick-up truck or van in traffic accident

V43.61 Car passenger injured in collision with sport utility vehicle in traffic accident `✓x7th`

V43.62 Car passenger injured in collision with other type car in traffic accident `✓x7th`

V43.63 Car passenger injured in collision with pick-up truck in traffic accident `✓x7th`

V43.64 Car passenger injured in collision with van in traffic accident `✓x7th`

`✓5th` **V43.7** Person on outside of car injured in collision with car, pick-up truck or van in traffic accident

V43.71 Person on outside of car injured in collision with sport utility vehicle in traffic accident `✓x7th`

V43.72 Person on outside of car injured in collision with other type car in traffic accident `✓x7th`

V43.73 Person on outside of car injured in collision with pick-up truck in traffic accident `✓x7th`

V43.74 Person on outside of car injured in collision with van in traffic accident `✓x7th`

`✓5th` **V43.9** Unspecified car occupant injured in collision with car, pick-up truck or van in traffic accident

V43.91 Unspecified car occupant injured in collision with sport utility vehicle in traffic accident `✓x7th`

V43.92 Unspecified car occupant injured in collision with other type car in traffic accident `✓x7th`

V43.93 Unspecified car occupant injured in collision with pick-up truck in traffic accident `✓x7th`

V43.94 Unspecified car occupant injured in collision with van in traffic accident `✓x7th`

`✓4th` **V44** Car occupant injured in collision with heavy transport vehicle or bus

> **EXCLUDES 1**   car occupant injured in collision with military vehicle (V49.81)

V44.0 Car driver injured in collision with heavy transport vehicle or bus in nontraffic accident `✓x7th`

V44.1 Car passenger injured in collision with heavy transport vehicle or bus in nontraffic accident `✓x7th`

V44.2 Person on outside of car injured in collision with heavy transport vehicle or bus in nontraffic accident `✓x7th`

V44.3 Unspecified car occupant injured in collision with heavy transport vehicle or bus in nontraffic accident `✓x7th`

V44.4 Person boarding or alighting a car injured in collision with heavy transport vehicle or bus `✓x7th`

V44.5 Car driver injured in collision with heavy transport vehicle or bus in traffic accident `✓x7th`

V44.6 Car passenger injured in collision with heavy transport vehicle or bus in traffic accident `✓x7th`

V44.7 Person on outside of car injured in collision with heavy transport vehicle or bus in traffic accident `✓x7th`

V44.9 Unspecified car occupant injured in collision with heavy transport vehicle or bus in traffic accident `✓x7th`

`✓4th` **V45** Car occupant injured in collision with railway train or railway vehicle

V45.0 Car driver injured in collision with railway train or railway vehicle in nontraffic accident `✓x7th`

V45.1 Car passenger injured in collision with railway train or railway vehicle in nontraffic accident `✓x7th`

V45.2 Person on outside of car injured in collision with railway train or railway vehicle in nontraffic accident `✓x7th`

V45.3 Unspecified car occupant injured in collision with railway train or railway vehicle in nontraffic accident `✓x7th`

V45.4 Person boarding or alighting a car injured in collision with railway train or railway vehicle `✓x7th`

V45.5 Car driver injured in collision with railway train or railway vehicle in traffic accident `✓x7th`

V45.6 Car passenger injured in collision with railway train or railway vehicle in traffic accident `✓x7th`

V45.7 Person on outside of car injured in collision with railway train or railway vehicle in traffic accident `✓x7th`

V45.9 Unspecified car occupant injured in collision with railway train or railway vehicle in traffic accident `✓x7th`

`✓4th` **V46** Car occupant injured in collision with other nonmotor vehicle

> **INCLUDES**   collision with animal-drawn vehicle, animal being ridden, streetcar

V46.0 Car driver injured in collision with other nonmotor vehicle in nontraffic accident `✓x7th`

V46.1 Car passenger injured in collision with other nonmotor vehicle in nontraffic accident `✓x7th`

V46.2 Person on outside of car injured in collision with other nonmotor vehicle in nontraffic accident `✓x7th`

V46.3 Unspecified car occupant injured in collision with other nonmotor vehicle in nontraffic accident `✓x7th`

V46.4 Person boarding or alighting a car injured in collision with other nonmotor vehicle `✓x7th`

V46.5 Car driver injured in collision with other nonmotor vehicle in traffic accident `✓x7th`

V46.6 Car passenger injured in collision with other nonmotor vehicle in traffic accident `✓x7th`

V46.7 Person on outside of car injured in collision with other nonmotor vehicle in traffic accident `✓x7th`

V46.9 Unspecified car occupant injured in collision with other nonmotor vehicle in traffic accident `✓x7th`

`✓4th` **V47** Car occupant injured in collision with fixed or stationary object

> **AHA:** 2016,4Q,73

V47.0 Car driver injured in collision with fixed or stationary object in nontraffic accident `✓x7th`

V47.1 Car passenger injured in collision with fixed or stationary object in nontraffic accident `✓x7th`

V47.2 Person on outside of car injured in collision with fixed or stationary object in nontraffic accident `✓x7th`

V47.3 Unspecified car occupant injured in collision with fixed or stationary object in nontraffic accident `✓x7th`

V47.4 Person boarding or alighting a car injured in collision with fixed or stationary object `✓x7th`

V47.5 Car driver injured in collision with fixed or stationary object in traffic accident `✓x7th`

V47.6 Car passenger injured in collision with fixed or stationary object in traffic accident `✓x7th`

V47.7 Person on outside of car injured in collision with fixed or stationary object in traffic accident `✓x7th`

V47.9 Unspecified car occupant injured in collision with fixed or stationary object in traffic accident `✓x7th`

`✓4th` **V48** Car occupant injured in noncollision transport accident

> **INCLUDES**   overturning car NOS
> overturning car without collision

V48.0 Car driver injured in noncollision transport accident in nontraffic accident `✓x7th`

V48.1 Car passenger injured in noncollision transport accident in nontraffic accident `✓x7th`

V48.2 Person on outside of car injured in noncollision transport accident in nontraffic accident `✓x7th`

V48.3 Unspecified car occupant injured in noncollision transport accident in nontraffic accident `✓x7th`

V48.4 Person boarding or alighting a car injured in noncollision transport accident `✓x7th`

✔ Additional Char Req   `✓x7th` Placeholder   Unacceptable PDx   Questionable PDx   Wrong Procedure   Manifestation   Unspecified   H1-H14 HAC   HCC CMS-HCC Dx   HIV HIV Dx

√x 7th **V48.5** Car driver injured in noncollision transport accident in traffic accident

√x 7th **V48.6** Car passenger injured in noncollision transport accident in traffic accident

√x 7th **V48.7** Person on outside of car injured in noncollision transport accident in traffic accident

√x 7th **V48.9** Unspecified car occupant injured in noncollision transport accident in traffic accident

√4th **V49** Car occupant injured in other and unspecified transport accidents

  √5th **V49.0** Driver injured in collision with other and unspecified motor vehicles in nontraffic accident

    √x 7th **V49.00** Driver injured in collision with unspecified motor vehicles in nontraffic accident

    √x 7th **V49.09** Driver injured in collision with other motor vehicles in nontraffic accident

  √5th **V49.1** Passenger injured in collision with other and unspecified motor vehicles in nontraffic accident

    √x 7th **V49.10** Passenger injured in collision with unspecified motor vehicles in nontraffic accident

    √x 7th **V49.19** Passenger injured in collision with other motor vehicles in nontraffic accident

  √5th **V49.2** Unspecified car occupant injured in collision with other and unspecified motor vehicles in nontraffic accident

    √x 7th **V49.20** Unspecified car occupant injured in collision with unspecified motor vehicles in nontraffic accident
        Car collision NOS, nontraffic

    √x 7th **V49.29** Unspecified car occupant injured in collision with other motor vehicles in nontraffic accident

  √x 7th **V49.3** Car occupant (driver) (passenger) injured in unspecified nontraffic accident
      Car accident NOS, nontraffic
      Car occupant injured in nontraffic accident NOS

  √5th **V49.4** Driver injured in collision with other and unspecified motor vehicles in traffic accident

    √x 7th **V49.40** Driver injured in collision with unspecified motor vehicles in traffic accident

    √x 7th **V49.49** Driver injured in collision with other motor vehicles in traffic accident

  √5th **V49.5** Passenger injured in collision with other and unspecified motor vehicles in traffic accident

    √x 7th **V49.50** Passenger injured in collision with unspecified motor vehicles in traffic accident

    √x 7th **V49.59** Passenger injured in collision with other motor vehicles in traffic accident

  √5th **V49.6** Unspecified car occupant injured in collision with other and unspecified motor vehicles in traffic accident

    √x 7th **V49.60** Unspecified car occupant injured in collision with unspecified motor vehicles in traffic accident
        Car collision NOS (traffic)

    √x 7th **V49.69** Unspecified car occupant injured in collision with other motor vehicles in traffic accident

  √5th **V49.8** Car occupant (driver) (passenger) injured in other specified transport accidents

    √x 7th **V49.81** Car occupant (driver) (passenger) injured in transport accident with military vehicle

    √x 7th **V49.88** Car occupant (driver) (passenger) injured in other specified transport accidents

  √x 7th **V49.9** Car occupant (driver) (passenger) injured in unspecified traffic accident
      Car accident NOS

Occupant of pick-up truck or van injured in transport accident (V50-V59)

INCLUDES   a four or six wheel motor vehicle designed primarily for carrying passengers and property but weighing less than the local limit for classification as a heavy goods vehicle
    minibus
    minivan
    sport utility vehicle (SUV)
    truck
    van

EXCLUDES 1   *heavy transport vehicle (V60-V69)*

The appropriate 7th character is to be added to each code from categories V50-V59.
A   initial encounter
D   subsequent encounter
S   sequela

√4th **V50** Occupant of pick-up truck or van injured in collision with pedestrian or animal
    EXCLUDES 1   *pick-up truck or van collision with animal-drawn vehicle or animal being ridden (V56.-)*

  √x 7th **V50.0** Driver of pick-up truck or van injured in collision with pedestrian or animal in nontraffic accident

  √x 7th **V50.1** Passenger in pick-up truck or van injured in collision with pedestrian or animal in nontraffic accident

  √x 7th **V50.2** Person on outside of pick-up truck or van injured in collision with pedestrian or animal in nontraffic accident

  √x 7th **V50.3** Unspecified occupant of pick-up truck or van injured in collision with pedestrian or animal in nontraffic accident

  √x 7th **V50.4** Person boarding or alighting a pick-up truck or van injured in collision with pedestrian or animal

  √x 7th **V50.5** Driver of pick-up truck or van injured in collision with pedestrian or animal in traffic accident

  √x 7th **V50.6** Passenger in pick-up truck or van injured in collision with pedestrian or animal in traffic accident

  √x 7th **V50.7** Person on outside of pick-up truck or van injured in collision with pedestrian or animal in traffic accident

  √x 7th **V50.9** Unspecified occupant of pick-up truck or van injured in collision with pedestrian or animal in traffic accident

√4th **V51** Occupant of pick-up truck or van injured in collision with pedal cycle

  √x 7th **V51.0** Driver of pick-up truck or van injured in collision with pedal cycle in nontraffic accident

  √x 7th **V51.1** Passenger in pick-up truck or van injured in collision with pedal cycle in nontraffic accident

  √x 7th **V51.2** Person on outside of pick-up truck or van injured in collision with pedal cycle in nontraffic accident

  √x 7th **V51.3** Unspecified occupant of pick-up truck or van injured in collision with pedal cycle in nontraffic accident

  √x 7th **V51.4** Person boarding or alighting a pick-up truck or van injured in collision with pedal cycle

  √x 7th **V51.5** Driver of pick-up truck or van injured in collision with pedal cycle in traffic accident

  √x 7th **V51.6** Passenger in pick-up truck or van injured in collision with pedal cycle in traffic accident

  √x 7th **V51.7** Person on outside of pick-up truck or van injured in collision with pedal cycle in traffic accident

  √x 7th **V51.9** Unspecified occupant of pick-up truck or van injured in collision with pedal cycle in traffic accident

√4th **V52** Occupant of pick-up truck or van injured in collision with two- or three-wheeled motor vehicle

  √x 7th **V52.0** Driver of pick-up truck or van injured in collision with two- or three-wheeled motor vehicle in nontraffic accident

  √x 7th **V52.1** Passenger in pick-up truck or van injured in collision with two- or three-wheeled motor vehicle in nontraffic accident

  √x 7th **V52.2** Person on outside of pick-up truck or van injured in collision with two- or three-wheeled motor vehicle in nontraffic accident

  √x 7th **V52.3** Unspecified occupant of pick-up truck or van injured in collision with two- or three-wheeled motor vehicle in nontraffic accident

  √x 7th **V52.4** Person boarding or alighting a pick-up truck or van injured in collision with two- or three-wheeled motor vehicle

  √x 7th **V52.5** Driver of pick-up truck or van injured in collision with two- or three-wheeled motor vehicle in traffic accident

  √x 7th **V52.6** Passenger in pick-up truck or van injured in collision with two- or three-wheeled motor vehicle in traffic accident

  √x 7th **V52.7** Person on outside of pick-up truck or van injured in collision with two- or three-wheeled motor vehicle in traffic accident

  √x 7th **V52.9** Unspecified occupant of pick-up truck or van injured in collision with two- or three-wheeled motor vehicle in traffic accident

N Newborn: 0   **P** Pediatric: 0-17   **M** Maternity: 9-64   **A** Adult: 15-124   **UNS** Unspecified Site   **MCC** Major Complication/Comorbidity   **CC** Complication/Comorbidity   **PE** POA Exempt

1212   ICD-10-CM 2025

V53 Occupant of pick-up truck or van injured in collision with car, pick-up truck or van

- **V53.0** Driver of pick-up truck or van injured in collision with car, pick-up truck or van in nontraffic accident
- **V53.1** Passenger in pick-up truck or van injured in collision with car, pick-up truck or van in nontraffic accident
- **V53.2** Person on outside of pick-up truck or van injured in collision with car, pick-up truck or van in nontraffic accident
- **V53.3** Unspecified occupant of pick-up truck or van injured in collision with car, pick-up truck or van in nontraffic accident
- **V53.4** Person boarding or alighting a pick-up truck or van injured in collision with car, pick-up truck or van
- **V53.5** Driver of pick-up truck or van injured in collision with car, pick-up truck or van in traffic accident
- **V53.6** Passenger in pick-up truck or van injured in collision with car, pick-up truck or van in traffic accident
- **V53.7** Person on outside of pick-up truck or van injured in collision with car, pick-up truck or van in traffic accident
- **V53.9** Unspecified occupant of pick-up truck or van injured in collision with car, pick-up truck or van in traffic accident

V54 Occupant of pick-up truck or van injured in collision with heavy transport vehicle or bus

    EXCLUDES 1   occupant of pick-up truck or van injured in collision with military vehicle (V59.81)

- **V54.0** Driver of pick-up truck or van injured in collision with heavy transport vehicle or bus in nontraffic accident
- **V54.1** Passenger in pick-up truck or van injured in collision with heavy transport vehicle or bus in nontraffic accident
- **V54.2** Person on outside of pick-up truck or van injured in collision with heavy transport vehicle or bus in nontraffic accident
- **V54.3** Unspecified occupant of pick-up truck or van injured in collision with heavy transport vehicle or bus in nontraffic accident
- **V54.4** Person boarding or alighting a pick-up truck or van injured in collision with heavy transport vehicle or bus
- **V54.5** Driver of pick-up truck or van injured in collision with heavy transport vehicle or bus in traffic accident
- **V54.6** Passenger in pick-up truck or van injured in collision with heavy transport vehicle or bus in traffic accident
- **V54.7** Person on outside of pick-up truck or van injured in collision with heavy transport vehicle or bus in traffic accident
- **V54.9** Unspecified occupant of pick-up truck or van injured in collision with heavy transport vehicle or bus in traffic accident

V55 Occupant of pick-up truck or van injured in collision with railway train or railway vehicle

- **V55.0** Driver of pick-up truck or van injured in collision with railway train or railway vehicle in nontraffic accident
- **V55.1** Passenger in pick-up truck or van injured in collision with railway train or railway vehicle in nontraffic accident
- **V55.2** Person on outside of pick-up truck or van injured in collision with railway train or railway vehicle in nontraffic accident
- **V55.3** Unspecified occupant of pick-up truck or van injured in collision with railway train or railway vehicle in nontraffic accident
- **V55.4** Person boarding or alighting a pick-up truck or van injured in collision with railway train or railway vehicle
- **V55.5** Driver of pick-up truck or van injured in collision with railway train or railway vehicle in traffic accident
- **V55.6** Passenger in pick-up truck or van injured in collision with railway train or railway vehicle in traffic accident
- **V55.7** Person on outside of pick-up truck or van injured in collision with railway train or railway vehicle in traffic accident
- **V55.9** Unspecified occupant of pick-up truck or van injured in collision with railway train or railway vehicle in traffic accident

V56 Occupant of pick-up truck or van injured in collision with other nonmotor vehicle

    INCLUDES   collision with animal-drawn vehicle, animal being ridden, streetcar

- **V56.0** Driver of pick-up truck or van injured in collision with other nonmotor vehicle in nontraffic accident
- **V56.1** Passenger in pick-up truck or van injured in collision with other nonmotor vehicle in nontraffic accident
- **V56.2** Person on outside of pick-up truck or van injured in collision with other nonmotor vehicle in nontraffic accident
- **V56.3** Unspecified occupant of pick-up truck or van injured in collision with other nonmotor vehicle in nontraffic accident
- **V56.4** Person boarding or alighting a pick-up truck or van injured in collision with other nonmotor vehicle
- **V56.5** Driver of pick-up truck or van injured in collision with other nonmotor vehicle in traffic accident
- **V56.6** Passenger in pick-up truck or van injured in collision with other nonmotor vehicle in traffic accident
- **V56.7** Person on outside of pick-up truck or van injured in collision with other nonmotor vehicle in traffic accident
- **V56.9** Unspecified occupant of pick-up truck or van injured in collision with other nonmotor vehicle in traffic accident

V57 Occupant of pick-up truck or van injured in collision with fixed or stationary object

- **V57.0** Driver of pick-up truck or van injured in collision with fixed or stationary object in nontraffic accident
- **V57.1** Passenger in pick-up truck or van injured in collision with fixed or stationary object in nontraffic accident
- **V57.2** Person on outside of pick-up truck or van injured in collision with fixed or stationary object in nontraffic accident
- **V57.3** Unspecified occupant of pick-up truck or van injured in collision with fixed or stationary object in nontraffic accident
- **V57.4** Person boarding or alighting a pick-up truck or van injured in collision with fixed or stationary object
- **V57.5** Driver of pick-up truck or van injured in collision with fixed or stationary object in traffic accident
- **V57.6** Passenger in pick-up truck or van injured in collision with fixed or stationary object in traffic accident
- **V57.7** Person on outside of pick-up truck or van injured in collision with fixed or stationary object in traffic accident
- **V57.9** Unspecified occupant of pick-up truck or van injured in collision with fixed or stationary object in traffic accident

V58 Occupant of pick-up truck or van injured in noncollision transport accident

    INCLUDES   overturning pick-up truck or van NOS
            overturning pick-up truck or van without collision

- **V58.0** Driver of pick-up truck or van injured in noncollision transport accident in nontraffic accident
- **V58.1** Passenger in pick-up truck or van injured in noncollision transport accident in nontraffic accident
- **V58.2** Person on outside of pick-up truck or van injured in noncollision transport accident in nontraffic accident
- **V58.3** Unspecified occupant of pick-up truck or van injured in noncollision transport accident in nontraffic accident
- **V58.4** Person boarding or alighting a pick-up truck or van injured in noncollision transport accident
- **V58.5** Driver of pick-up truck or van injured in noncollision transport accident in traffic accident
- **V58.6** Passenger in pick-up truck or van injured in noncollision transport accident in traffic accident
- **V58.7** Person on outside of pick-up truck or van injured in noncollision transport accident in traffic accident
- **V58.9** Unspecified occupant of pick-up truck or van injured in noncollision transport accident in traffic accident

V59 Occupant of pick-up truck or van injured in other and unspecified transport accidents

- **V59.0** Driver of pick-up truck or van injured in collision with other and unspecified motor vehicles in nontraffic accident
  - **V59.00** Driver of pick-up truck or van injured in collision with unspecified motor vehicles in nontraffic accident
  - **V59.09** Driver of pick-up truck or van injured in collision with other motor vehicles in nontraffic accident
- **V59.1** Passenger in pick-up truck or van injured in collision with other and unspecified motor vehicles in nontraffic accident
  - **V59.10** Passenger in pick-up truck or van injured in collision with unspecified motor vehicles in nontraffic accident
  - **V59.19** Passenger in pick-up truck or van injured in collision with other motor vehicles in nontraffic accident
- **V59.2** Unspecified occupant of pick-up truck or van injured in collision with other and unspecified motor vehicles in nontraffic accident
  - **V59.20** Unspecified occupant of pick-up truck or van injured in collision with unspecified motor vehicles in nontraffic accident
    Collision NOS involving pick-up truck or van, nontraffic
  - **V59.29** Unspecified occupant of pick-up truck or van injured in collision with other motor vehicles in nontraffic accident
- **V59.3** Occupant (driver) (passenger) of pick-up truck or van injured in unspecified nontraffic accident
    Accident NOS involving pick-up truck or van, nontraffic
    Occupant of pick-up truck or van injured in nontraffic accident NOS
- **V59.4** Driver of pick-up truck or van injured in collision with other and unspecified motor vehicles in traffic accident
  - **V59.40** Driver of pick-up truck or van injured in collision with unspecified motor vehicles in traffic accident
  - **V59.49** Driver of pick-up truck or van injured in collision with other motor vehicles in traffic accident

✔ Additional Char Req   √x7ᵗʰ Placeholder   Unacceptable PDx   Questionable PDx   Wrong Procedure   Manifestation   Unspecified   H1-H14 HAC   HCC CMS-HCC Dx   HIV HIV Dx

ICD-10-CM 2025   1213

✓5ᵗʰ **V59.5** **Passenger** in pick-up truck or van injured in collision with other and unspecified motor vehicles **in traffic accident**

✓x7ᵗʰ **V59.50** Passenger in pick-up truck or van injured in collision with unspecified motor vehicles in traffic accident

✓x7ᵗʰ **V59.59** Passenger in pick-up truck or van injured in collision with other motor vehicles in traffic accident

✓5ᵗʰ **V59.6** Unspecified occupant of pick-up truck or van injured in collision with other and unspecified motor vehicles **in traffic accident**

✓x7ᵗʰ **V59.60** Unspecified occupant of pick-up truck or van injured in collision with unspecified motor vehicles in traffic accident
     Collision NOS involving pick-up truck or van (traffic)

✓x7ᵗʰ **V59.69** Unspecified occupant of pick-up truck or van injured in collision with other motor vehicles in traffic accident

✓5ᵗʰ **V59.8** Occupant (driver) (passenger) of pick-up truck or van injured in other specified transport accidents

✓x7ᵗʰ **V59.81** Occupant (driver) (passenger) of pick-up truck or van injured in transport accident with **military vehicle**

✓x7ᵗʰ **V59.88** Occupant (driver) (passenger) of pick-up truck or van injured in other specified transport accidents

✓x7ᵗʰ **V59.9** Occupant (driver) (passenger) of pick-up truck or van injured in unspecified traffic accident
     Accident NOS involving pick-up truck or van

Occupant of heavy transport vehicle injured in transport accident (V60-V69)

INCLUDES 18 wheeler
armored car
panel truck

EXCLUDES 1 *bus*
motorcoach

The appropriate 7th character is to be added to each code from categories V60-V69.
A   initial encounter
D   subsequent encounter
S   sequela

✓4ᵗʰ **V60** **Occupant of heavy transport vehicle injured in collision with pedestrian or animal**

EXCLUDES 1 *heavy transport vehicle collision with animal-drawn vehicle or animal being ridden (V66.-)*

✓x7ᵗʰ **V60.0** **Driver** of heavy transport vehicle injured in collision with pedestrian or animal **in nontraffic accident**

✓x7ᵗʰ **V60.1** **Passenger** in heavy transport vehicle injured in collision with pedestrian or animal **in nontraffic accident**

✓x7ᵗʰ **V60.2** **Person on outside** of heavy transport vehicle injured in collision with pedestrian or animal **in nontraffic accident**

✓x7ᵗʰ **V60.3** Unspecified occupant of heavy transport vehicle injured in collision with pedestrian or animal **in nontraffic accident**

✓x7ᵗʰ **V60.4** **Person boarding or alighting** a heavy transport vehicle injured in collision with pedestrian or animal

✓x7ᵗʰ **V60.5** **Driver** of heavy transport vehicle injured in collision with pedestrian or animal **in traffic accident**

✓x7ᵗʰ **V60.6** **Passenger** in heavy transport vehicle injured in collision with pedestrian or animal **in traffic accident**

✓x7ᵗʰ **V60.7** **Person on outside** of heavy transport vehicle injured in collision with pedestrian or animal **in traffic accident**

✓x7ᵗʰ **V60.9** Unspecified occupant of heavy transport vehicle injured in collision with pedestrian or animal **in traffic accident**

✓4ᵗʰ **V61** **Occupant of heavy transport vehicle injured in collision with pedal cycle**

✓x7ᵗʰ **V61.0** **Driver** of heavy transport vehicle injured in collision with pedal cycle **in nontraffic accident**

✓x7ᵗʰ **V61.1** **Passenger** in heavy transport vehicle injured in collision with pedal cycle **in nontraffic accident**

✓x7ᵗʰ **V61.2** **Person on outside** of heavy transport vehicle injured in collision with pedal cycle **in nontraffic accident**

✓x7ᵗʰ **V61.3** Unspecified occupant of heavy transport vehicle injured in collision with pedal cycle **in nontraffic accident**

✓x7ᵗʰ **V61.4** **Person boarding or alighting** a heavy transport vehicle injured in collision with pedal cycle while boarding or alighting

✓x7ᵗʰ **V61.5** **Driver** of heavy transport vehicle injured in collision with pedal cycle **in traffic accident**

✓x7ᵗʰ **V61.6** **Passenger** in heavy transport vehicle injured in collision with pedal cycle **in traffic accident**

✓x7ᵗʰ **V61.7** **Person on outside** of heavy transport vehicle injured in collision with pedal cycle **in traffic accident**

✓x7ᵗʰ **V61.9** Unspecified occupant of heavy transport vehicle injured in collision with pedal cycle **in traffic accident**

✓4ᵗʰ **V62** **Occupant of heavy transport vehicle injured in collision with two- or three-wheeled motor vehicle**

✓x7ᵗʰ **V62.0** **Driver** of heavy transport vehicle injured in collision with two- or three-wheeled motor vehicle **in nontraffic accident**

✓x7ᵗʰ **V62.1** **Passenger** in heavy transport vehicle injured in collision with two- or three-wheeled motor vehicle **in nontraffic accident**

✓x7ᵗʰ **V62.2** **Person on outside** of heavy transport vehicle injured in collision with two- or three-wheeled motor vehicle **in nontraffic accident**

✓x7ᵗʰ **V62.3** Unspecified occupant of heavy transport vehicle injured in collision with two- or three-wheeled motor vehicle **in nontraffic accident**

✓x7ᵗʰ **V62.4** **Person boarding or alighting** a heavy transport vehicle injured in collision with two- or three-wheeled motor vehicle

✓x7ᵗʰ **V62.5** **Driver** of heavy transport vehicle injured in collision with two- or three-wheeled motor vehicle **in traffic accident**

✓x7ᵗʰ **V62.6** **Passenger** in heavy transport vehicle injured in collision with two- or three-wheeled motor vehicle **in traffic accident**

✓x7ᵗʰ **V62.7** **Person on outside** of heavy transport vehicle injured in collision with two- or three-wheeled motor vehicle **in traffic accident**

✓x7ᵗʰ **V62.9** Unspecified occupant of heavy transport vehicle injured in collision with two- or three-wheeled motor vehicle **in traffic accident**

✓4ᵗʰ **V63** **Occupant of heavy transport vehicle injured in collision with car, pick-up truck or van**

✓x7ᵗʰ **V63.0** **Driver** of heavy transport vehicle injured in collision with car, pick-up truck or van **in nontraffic accident**

✓x7ᵗʰ **V63.1** **Passenger** in heavy transport vehicle injured in collision with car, pick-up truck or van **in nontraffic accident**

✓x7ᵗʰ **V63.2** **Person on outside** of heavy transport vehicle injured in collision with car, pick-up truck or van **in nontraffic accident**

✓x7ᵗʰ **V63.3** Unspecified occupant of heavy transport vehicle injured in collision with car, pick-up truck or van **in nontraffic accident**

✓x7ᵗʰ **V63.4** **Person boarding or alighting** a heavy transport vehicle injured in collision with car, pick-up truck or van

✓x7ᵗʰ **V63.5** **Driver** of heavy transport vehicle injured in collision with car, pick-up truck or van **in traffic accident**

✓x7ᵗʰ **V63.6** **Passenger** in heavy transport vehicle injured in collision with car, pick-up truck or van **in traffic accident**

✓x7ᵗʰ **V63.7** **Person on outside** of heavy transport vehicle injured in collision with car, pick-up truck or van **in traffic accident**

✓x7ᵗʰ **V63.9** Unspecified occupant of heavy transport vehicle injured in collision with car, pick-up truck or van **in traffic accident**

✓4ᵗʰ **V64** **Occupant of heavy transport vehicle injured in collision with heavy transport vehicle or bus**

EXCLUDES 1 *occupant of heavy transport vehicle injured in collision with military vehicle (V69.81)*

✓x7ᵗʰ **V64.0** **Driver** of heavy transport vehicle injured in collision with heavy transport vehicle or bus **in nontraffic accident**

✓x7ᵗʰ **V64.1** **Passenger** in heavy transport vehicle injured in collision with heavy transport vehicle or bus **in nontraffic accident**

✓x7ᵗʰ **V64.2** **Person on outside** of heavy transport vehicle injured in collision with heavy transport vehicle or bus **in nontraffic accident**

✓x7ᵗʰ **V64.3** Unspecified occupant of heavy transport vehicle injured in collision with heavy transport vehicle or bus **in nontraffic accident**

✓x7ᵗʰ **V64.4** **Person boarding or alighting** a heavy transport vehicle injured in collision with heavy transport vehicle or bus while boarding or alighting

✓x7ᵗʰ **V64.5** **Driver** of heavy transport vehicle injured in collision with heavy transport vehicle or bus **in traffic accident**

✓x7ᵗʰ **V64.6** **Passenger** in heavy transport vehicle injured in collision with heavy transport vehicle or bus **in traffic accident**

✓x7ᵗʰ **V64.7** **Person on outside** of heavy transport vehicle injured in collision with heavy transport vehicle or bus **in traffic accident**

✓x7ᵗʰ **V64.9** Unspecified occupant of heavy transport vehicle injured in collision with heavy transport vehicle or bus **in traffic accident**

✓4ᵗʰ **V65** **Occupant of heavy transport vehicle injured in collision with railway train or railway vehicle**

✓x7ᵗʰ **V65.0** **Driver** of heavy transport vehicle injured in collision with railway train or railway vehicle **in nontraffic accident**

✓x7ᵗʰ **V65.1** **Passenger** in heavy transport vehicle injured in collision with railway train or railway vehicle **in nontraffic accident**

✓x7ᵗʰ **V65.2** **Person on outside** of heavy transport vehicle injured in collision with railway train or railway vehicle **in nontraffic accident**

✓x7ᵗʰ **V65.3** Unspecified occupant of heavy transport vehicle injured in collision with railway train or railway vehicle **in nontraffic accident**

✓x7ᵗʰ **V65.4** **Person boarding or alighting** a heavy transport vehicle injured in collision with railway train or railway vehicle

✓x7ᵗʰ **V65.5** **Driver** of heavy transport vehicle injured in collision with railway train or railway vehicle **in traffic accident**

√x 7th **V65.6** **Passenger** in heavy transport vehicle injured in collision with railway train or railway vehicle **in traffic accident**

√x 7th **V65.7** **Person on outside** of heavy transport vehicle injured in collision with railway train or railway vehicle **in traffic accident**

√x 7th **V65.9** Unspecified occupant of heavy transport vehicle injured in collision with railway train or railway vehicle **in traffic accident**

✓4th **V66** **Occupant of heavy transport vehicle injured in collision with other nonmotor vehicle**

     INCLUDES   collision with animal-drawn vehicle, animal being ridden, streetcar

√x 7th **V66.0** **Driver** of heavy transport vehicle injured in collision with other nonmotor vehicle **in nontraffic accident**

√x 7th **V66.1** **Passenger** in heavy transport vehicle injured in collision with other nonmotor vehicle **in nontraffic accident**

√x 7th **V66.2** **Person on outside** of heavy transport vehicle injured in collision with other nonmotor vehicle **in nontraffic accident**

√x 7th **V66.3** Unspecified occupant of heavy transport vehicle injured in collision with other nonmotor vehicle **in nontraffic accident**

√x 7th **V66.4** **Person boarding or alighting** a heavy transport vehicle injured in collision with other nonmotor vehicle

√x 7th **V66.5** **Driver** of heavy transport vehicle injured in collision with other nonmotor vehicle **in traffic accident**

√x 7th **V66.6** **Passenger** in heavy transport vehicle injured in collision with other nonmotor vehicle **in traffic accident**

√x 7th **V66.7** **Person on outside** of heavy transport vehicle injured in collision with other nonmotor vehicle **in traffic accident**

√x 7th **V66.9** Unspecified occupant of heavy transport vehicle injured in collision with other nonmotor vehicle **in traffic accident**

✓4th **V67** **Occupant of heavy transport vehicle injured in collision with fixed or stationary object**

√x 7th **V67.0** **Driver** of heavy transport vehicle injured in collision with fixed or stationary object **in nontraffic accident**

√x 7th **V67.1** **Passenger** in heavy transport vehicle injured in collision with fixed or stationary object **in nontraffic accident**

√x 7th **V67.2** **Person on outside** of heavy transport vehicle injured in collision with fixed or stationary object **in nontraffic accident**

√x 7th **V67.3** Unspecified occupant of heavy transport vehicle injured in collision with fixed or stationary object **in nontraffic accident**

√x 7th **V67.4** **Person boarding or alighting** a heavy transport vehicle injured in collision with fixed or stationary object

√x 7th **V67.5** **Driver** of heavy transport vehicle injured in collision with fixed or stationary object **in traffic accident**

√x 7th **V67.6** **Passenger** in heavy transport vehicle injured in collision with fixed or stationary object **in traffic accident**

√x 7th **V67.7** **Person on outside** of heavy transport vehicle injured in collision with fixed or stationary object **in traffic accident**

√x 7th **V67.9** Unspecified occupant of heavy transport vehicle injured in collision with fixed or stationary object **in traffic accident**

✓4th **V68** **Occupant of heavy transport vehicle injured in noncollision transport accident**

     INCLUDES   overturning heavy transport vehicle NOS
                  overturning heavy transport vehicle without collision

√x 7th **V68.0** **Driver** of heavy transport vehicle injured in noncollision transport accident **in nontraffic accident**

√x 7th **V68.1** **Passenger** in heavy transport vehicle injured in noncollision transport accident **in nontraffic accident**

√x 7th **V68.2** **Person on outside** of heavy transport vehicle injured in noncollision transport accident **in nontraffic accident**

√x 7th **V68.3** Unspecified occupant of heavy transport vehicle injured in noncollision transport accident **in nontraffic accident**

√x 7th **V68.4** **Person boarding or alighting** a heavy transport vehicle injured in noncollision transport accident

√x 7th **V68.5** **Driver** of heavy transport vehicle injured in noncollision transport accident **in traffic accident**

√x 7th **V68.6** **Passenger** in heavy transport vehicle injured in noncollision transport accident **in traffic accident**

√x 7th **V68.7** **Person on outside** of heavy transport vehicle injured in noncollision transport accident **in traffic accident**

√x 7th **V68.9** Unspecified occupant of heavy transport vehicle injured in noncollision transport accident **in traffic accident**

✓4th **V69** **Occupant of heavy transport vehicle injured in other and unspecified transport accidents**

✓5th **V69.0** **Driver** of heavy transport vehicle injured in collision with other and unspecified motor vehicles **in nontraffic accident**

√x 7th **V69.00** Driver of heavy transport vehicle injured in collision with unspecified motor vehicles in nontraffic accident

√x 7th **V69.09** Driver of heavy transport vehicle injured in collision with other motor vehicles in nontraffic accident

√5th **V69.1** **Passenger** in heavy transport vehicle injured in collision with other and unspecified motor vehicles **in nontraffic accident**

√x 7th **V69.10** Passenger in heavy transport vehicle injured in collision with unspecified motor vehicles in nontraffic accident

√x 7th **V69.19** Passenger in heavy transport vehicle injured in collision with other motor vehicles in nontraffic accident

✓5th **V69.2** Unspecified occupant of heavy transport vehicle injured in collision with other and unspecified motor vehicles **in nontraffic accident**

√x 7th **V69.20** Unspecified occupant of heavy transport vehicle injured in collision with unspecified motor vehicles in nontraffic accident

         Collision NOS involving heavy transport vehicle, nontraffic

√x 7th **V69.29** Unspecified occupant of heavy transport vehicle injured in collision with other motor vehicles in nontraffic accident

√x 7th **V69.3** Occupant (driver) (passenger) of heavy transport vehicle injured in unspecified nontraffic accident

     Accident NOS involving heavy transport vehicle, nontraffic
     Occupant of heavy transport vehicle injured in nontraffic accident NOS

√5th **V69.4** **Driver** of heavy transport vehicle injured in collision with other and unspecified motor vehicles **in traffic accident**

√x 7th **V69.40** Driver of heavy transport vehicle injured in collision with unspecified motor vehicles in traffic accident

√x 7th **V69.49** Driver of heavy transport vehicle injured in collision with other motor vehicles in traffic accident

√5th **V69.5** **Passenger** in heavy transport vehicle injured in collision with other and unspecified motor vehicles **in traffic accident**

√x 7th **V69.50** Passenger in heavy transport vehicle injured in collision with unspecified motor vehicles in traffic accident

√x 7th **V69.59** Passenger in heavy transport vehicle injured in collision with other motor vehicles in traffic accident

√5th **V69.6** Unspecified occupant of heavy transport vehicle injured in collision with other and unspecified motor vehicles **in traffic accident**

√x 7th **V69.60** Unspecified occupant of heavy transport vehicle injured in collision with unspecified motor vehicles in traffic accident

         Collision NOS involving heavy transport vehicle (traffic)

√x 7th **V69.69** Unspecified occupant of heavy transport vehicle injured in collision with other motor vehicles in traffic accident

√5th **V69.8** Occupant (driver) (passenger) of heavy transport vehicle injured in other specified transport accidents

√x 7th **V69.81** Occupant (driver) (passenger) of heavy transport vehicle injured in transport accidents with **military vehicle**

√x 7th **V69.88** Occupant (driver) (passenger) of heavy transport vehicle injured in other specified transport accidents

√x 7th **V69.9** Occupant (driver) (passenger) of heavy transport vehicle injured in unspecified traffic accident

     Accident NOS involving heavy transport vehicle

Bus occupant injured in transport accident (V70-V79)

   INCLUDES   motorcoach
   EXCLUDES 1   minibus (V50-V59)

The appropriate 7th character is to be added to each code from categories V70-V79.
A   initial encounter
D   subsequent encounter
S   sequela

✓4th **V70** **Bus occupant injured in collision with pedestrian or animal**

     EXCLUDES 1   bus collision with animal-drawn vehicle or animal being ridden (V76.-)

√x 7th **V70.0** **Driver** of bus injured in collision with pedestrian or animal **in nontraffic accident**

√x 7th **V70.1** **Passenger** on bus injured in collision with pedestrian or animal **in nontraffic accident**

√x 7th **V70.2** **Person on outside** of bus injured in collision with pedestrian or animal **in nontraffic accident**

√x 7th **V70.3** Unspecified occupant of bus injured in collision with pedestrian or animal **in nontraffic accident**

√x 7th **V70.4** **Person boarding or alighting** from bus injured in collision with pedestrian or animal

√x 7th **V70.5** **Driver** of bus injured in collision with pedestrian or animal **in traffic accident**

√x7ᵗʰ **V70.6** Passenger on bus injured in collision with pedestrian or animal in traffic accident

√x7ᵗʰ **V70.7** Person on outside of bus injured in collision with pedestrian or animal in traffic accident

√x7ᵗʰ **V70.9** Unspecified occupant of bus injured in collision with pedestrian or animal in traffic accident

√4ᵗʰ **V71** Bus occupant injured in collision with pedal cycle

√x7ᵗʰ **V71.0** Driver of bus injured in collision with pedal cycle in nontraffic accident

√x7ᵗʰ **V71.1** Passenger on bus injured in collision with pedal cycle in nontraffic accident

√x7ᵗʰ **V71.2** Person on outside of bus injured in collision with pedal cycle in nontraffic accident

√x7ᵗʰ **V71.3** Unspecified occupant of bus injured in collision with pedal cycle in nontraffic accident

√x7ᵗʰ **V71.4** Person boarding or alighting from bus injured in collision with pedal cycle

√x7ᵗʰ **V71.5** Driver of bus injured in collision with pedal cycle in traffic accident

√x7ᵗʰ **V71.6** Passenger on bus injured in collision with pedal cycle in traffic accident

√x7ᵗʰ **V71.7** Person on outside of bus injured in collision with pedal cycle in traffic accident

√x7ᵗʰ **V71.9** Unspecified occupant of bus injured in collision with pedal cycle in traffic accident

√4ᵗʰ **V72** Bus occupant injured in collision with two- or three-wheeled motor vehicle

√x7ᵗʰ **V72.0** Driver of bus injured in collision with two- or three-wheeled motor vehicle in nontraffic accident

√x7ᵗʰ **V72.1** Passenger on bus injured in collision with two- or three-wheeled motor vehicle in nontraffic accident

√x7ᵗʰ **V72.2** Person on outside of bus injured in collision with two- or three-wheeled motor vehicle in nontraffic accident

√x7ᵗʰ **V72.3** Unspecified occupant of bus injured in collision with two- or three-wheeled motor vehicle in nontraffic accident

√x7ᵗʰ **V72.4** Person boarding or alighting from bus injured in collision with two- or three-wheeled motor vehicle

√x7ᵗʰ **V72.5** Driver of bus injured in collision with two- or three-wheeled motor vehicle in traffic accident

√x7ᵗʰ **V72.6** Passenger on bus injured in collision with two- or three-wheeled motor vehicle in traffic accident

√x7ᵗʰ **V72.7** Person on outside of bus injured in collision with two- or three-wheeled motor vehicle in traffic accident

√x7ᵗʰ **V72.9** Unspecified occupant of bus injured in collision with two- or three-wheeled motor vehicle in traffic accident

√4ᵗʰ **V73** Bus occupant injured in collision with car, pick-up truck or van

√x7ᵗʰ **V73.0** Driver of bus injured in collision with car, pick-up truck or van in nontraffic accident

√x7ᵗʰ **V73.1** Passenger on bus injured in collision with car, pick-up truck or van in nontraffic accident

√x7ᵗʰ **V73.2** Person on outside of bus injured in collision with car, pick-up truck or van in nontraffic accident

√x7ᵗʰ **V73.3** Unspecified occupant of bus injured in collision with car, pick-up truck or van in nontraffic accident

√x7ᵗʰ **V73.4** Person boarding or alighting from bus injured in collision with car, pick-up truck or van

√x7ᵗʰ **V73.5** Driver of bus injured in collision with car, pick-up truck or van in traffic accident

√x7ᵗʰ **V73.6** Passenger on bus injured in collision with car, pick-up truck or van in traffic accident

√x7ᵗʰ **V73.7** Person on outside of bus injured in collision with car, pick-up truck or van in traffic accident

√x7ᵗʰ **V73.9** Unspecified occupant of bus injured in collision with car, pick-up truck or van in traffic accident

√4ᵗʰ **V74** Bus occupant injured in collision with heavy transport vehicle or bus

EXCLUDES 1 *bus occupant injured in collision with military vehicle (V79.81)*

√x7ᵗʰ **V74.0** Driver of bus injured in collision with heavy transport vehicle or bus in nontraffic accident

√x7ᵗʰ **V74.1** Passenger on bus injured in collision with heavy transport vehicle or bus in nontraffic accident

√x7ᵗʰ **V74.2** Person on outside of bus injured in collision with heavy transport vehicle or bus in nontraffic accident

√x7ᵗʰ **V74.3** Unspecified occupant of bus injured in collision with heavy transport vehicle or bus in nontraffic accident

√x7ᵗʰ **V74.4** Person boarding or alighting from bus injured in collision with heavy transport vehicle or bus

√x7ᵗʰ **V74.5** Driver of bus injured in collision with heavy transport vehicle or bus in traffic accident

√x7ᵗʰ **V74.6** Passenger on bus injured in collision with heavy transport vehicle or bus in traffic accident

√x7ᵗʰ **V74.7** Person on outside of bus injured in collision with heavy transport vehicle or bus in traffic accident

√x7ᵗʰ **V74.9** Unspecified occupant of bus injured in collision with heavy transport vehicle or bus in traffic accident

√4ᵗʰ **V75** Bus occupant injured in collision with railway train or railway vehicle

√x7ᵗʰ **V75.0** Driver of bus injured in collision with railway train or railway vehicle in nontraffic accident

√x7ᵗʰ **V75.1** Passenger on bus injured in collision with railway train or railway vehicle in nontraffic accident

√x7ᵗʰ **V75.2** Person on outside of bus injured in collision with railway train or railway vehicle in nontraffic accident

√x7ᵗʰ **V75.3** Unspecified occupant of bus injured in collision with railway train or railway vehicle in nontraffic accident

√x7ᵗʰ **V75.4** Person boarding or alighting from bus injured in collision with railway train or railway vehicle

√x7ᵗʰ **V75.5** Driver of bus injured in collision with railway train or railway vehicle in traffic accident

√x7ᵗʰ **V75.6** Passenger on bus injured in collision with railway train or railway vehicle in traffic accident

√x7ᵗʰ **V75.7** Person on outside of bus injured in collision with railway train or railway vehicle in traffic accident

√x7ᵗʰ **V75.9** Unspecified occupant of bus injured in collision with railway train or railway vehicle in traffic accident

√4ᵗʰ **V76** Bus occupant injured in collision with other nonmotor vehicle

INCLUDES collision with animal-drawn vehicle, animal being ridden, streetcar

√x7ᵗʰ **V76.0** Driver of bus injured in collision with other nonmotor vehicle in nontraffic accident

√x7ᵗʰ **V76.1** Passenger on bus injured in collision with other nonmotor vehicle in nontraffic accident

√x7ᵗʰ **V76.2** Person on outside of bus injured in collision with other nonmotor vehicle in nontraffic accident

√x7ᵗʰ **V76.3** Unspecified occupant of bus injured in collision with other nonmotor vehicle in nontraffic accident

√x7ᵗʰ **V76.4** Person boarding or alighting from bus injured in collision with other nonmotor vehicle

√x7ᵗʰ **V76.5** Driver of bus injured in collision with other nonmotor vehicle in traffic accident

√x7ᵗʰ **V76.6** Passenger on bus injured in collision with other nonmotor vehicle in traffic accident

√x7ᵗʰ **V76.7** Person on outside of bus injured in collision with other nonmotor vehicle in traffic accident

√x7ᵗʰ **V76.9** Unspecified occupant of bus injured in collision with other nonmotor vehicle in traffic accident

√4ᵗʰ **V77** Bus occupant injured in collision with fixed or stationary object

√x7ᵗʰ **V77.0** Driver of bus injured in collision with fixed or stationary object in nontraffic accident

√x7ᵗʰ **V77.1** Passenger on bus injured in collision with fixed or stationary object in nontraffic accident

√x7ᵗʰ **V77.2** Person on outside of bus injured in collision with fixed or stationary object in nontraffic accident

√x7ᵗʰ **V77.3** Unspecified occupant of bus injured in collision with fixed or stationary object in nontraffic accident

√x7ᵗʰ **V77.4** Person boarding or alighting from bus injured in collision with fixed or stationary object

√x7ᵗʰ **V77.5** Driver of bus injured in collision with fixed or stationary object in traffic accident

√x7ᵗʰ **V77.6** Passenger on bus injured in collision with fixed or stationary object in traffic accident

√x7ᵗʰ **V77.7** Person on outside of bus injured in collision with fixed or stationary object in traffic accident

√x7ᵗʰ **V77.9** Unspecified occupant of bus injured in collision with fixed or stationary object in traffic accident

√4ᵗʰ **V78** Bus occupant injured in noncollision transport accident

INCLUDES overturning bus NOS
overturning bus without collision

√x7ᵗʰ **V78.0** Driver of bus injured in noncollision transport accident in nontraffic accident

√x7ᵗʰ **V78.1** Passenger on bus injured in noncollision transport accident in nontraffic accident

√x7ᵗʰ **V78.2** Person on outside of bus injured in noncollision transport accident in nontraffic accident

√x7ᵗʰ **V78.3** Unspecified occupant of bus injured in noncollision transport accident in nontraffic accident

√x7ᵗʰ **V78.4** Person boarding or alighting from bus injured in noncollision transport accident

N Newborn: 0 P Pediatric: 0-17 M Maternity: 9-64 A Adult: 15-124 UNS Unspecified Site MCC Major Complication/Comorbidity CC Complication/Comorbidity PE POA Exempt

√x 7ᵗʰ **V78.5** Driver of bus injured in noncollision transport accident in traffic accident

√x 7ᵗʰ **V78.6** Passenger on bus injured in noncollision transport accident in traffic accident

√x 7ᵗʰ **V78.7** Person on outside of bus injured in noncollision transport accident in traffic accident

√x 7ᵗʰ **V78.9** Unspecified occupant of bus injured in noncollision transport accident in traffic accident

√4ᵗʰ **V79 Bus occupant injured in other and unspecified transport accidents**

  √5ᵗʰ **V79.0** Driver of bus injured in collision with other and unspecified motor vehicles in nontraffic accident

    √x 7ᵗʰ **V79.00** Driver of bus injured in collision with unspecified motor vehicles in nontraffic accident

    √x 7ᵗʰ **V79.09** Driver of bus injured in collision with other motor vehicles in nontraffic accident

  √5ᵗʰ **V79.1** Passenger on bus injured in collision with other and unspecified motor vehicles in nontraffic accident

    √x 7ᵗʰ **V79.10** Passenger on bus injured in collision with unspecified motor vehicles in nontraffic accident

    √x 7ᵗʰ **V79.19** Passenger on bus injured in collision with other motor vehicles in nontraffic accident

  √5ᵗʰ **V79.2** Unspecified bus occupant injured in collision with other and unspecified motor vehicles in nontraffic accident

    √x 7ᵗʰ **V79.20** Unspecified bus occupant injured in collision with unspecified motor vehicles in nontraffic accident

      Bus collision NOS, nontraffic

    √x 7ᵗʰ **V79.29** Unspecified bus occupant injured in collision with other motor vehicles in nontraffic accident

  √x 7ᵗʰ **V79.3** Bus occupant (driver) (passenger) injured in unspecified nontraffic accident

    Bus accident NOS, nontraffic
    Bus occupant injured in nontraffic accident NOS

  √5ᵗʰ **V79.4** Driver of bus injured in collision with other and unspecified motor vehicles in traffic accident

    √x 7ᵗʰ **V79.40** Driver of bus injured in collision with unspecified motor vehicles in traffic accident

    √x 7ᵗʰ **V79.49** Driver of bus injured in collision with other motor vehicles in traffic accident

  √5ᵗʰ **V79.5** Passenger on bus injured in collision with other and unspecified motor vehicles in traffic accident

    √x 7ᵗʰ **V79.50** Passenger on bus injured in collision with unspecified motor vehicles in traffic accident

    √x 7ᵗʰ **V79.59** Passenger on bus injured in collision with other motor vehicles in traffic accident

  √5ᵗʰ **V79.6** Unspecified bus occupant injured in collision with other and unspecified motor vehicles in traffic accident

    √x 7ᵗʰ **V79.60** Unspecified bus occupant injured in collision with unspecified motor vehicles in traffic accident

      Bus collision NOS (traffic)

    √x 7ᵗʰ **V79.69** Unspecified bus occupant injured in collision with other motor vehicles in traffic accident

  √5ᵗʰ **V79.8** Bus occupant (driver) (passenger) injured in other specified transport accidents

    √x 7ᵗʰ **V79.81** Bus occupant (driver) (passenger) injured in transport accidents with military vehicle

    √x 7ᵗʰ **V79.88** Bus occupant (driver) (passenger) injured in other specified transport accidents

  √x 7ᵗʰ **V79.9** Bus occupant (driver) (passenger) injured in unspecified traffic accident

    Bus accident NOS

Other land transport accidents (V80-V89)

> The appropriate 7th character is to be added to each code from categories V80-V89.
> A   initial encounter
> D   subsequent encounter
> S   sequela

√4ᵗʰ **V80 Animal-rider or occupant of animal-drawn vehicle injured in transport accident**

  √5ᵗʰ **V80.0** Animal-rider or occupant of animal drawn vehicle injured by fall from or being thrown from animal or animal-drawn vehicle in noncollision accident

    √6ᵗʰ **V80.01** Animal-rider injured by fall from or being thrown from animal in noncollision accident

      √7ᵗʰ **V80.010** Animal-rider injured by fall from or being thrown from horse in noncollision accident

      √7ᵗʰ **V80.018** Animal-rider injured by fall from or being thrown from other animal in noncollision accident

    √x 7ᵗʰ **V80.02** Occupant of animal-drawn vehicle injured by fall from or being thrown from animal-drawn vehicle in noncollision accident

      Overturning animal-drawn vehicle NOS
      Overturning animal-drawn vehicle without collision

  √5ᵗʰ **V80.1** Animal-rider or occupant of animal-drawn vehicle injured in collision with pedestrian or animal

    EXCLUDES 1   animal-rider or animal-drawn vehicle collision with animal-drawn vehicle or animal being ridden (V80.7)

    √x 7ᵗʰ **V80.11** Animal-rider injured in collision with pedestrian or animal

    √x 7ᵗʰ **V80.12** Occupant of animal-drawn vehicle injured in collision with pedestrian or animal

  √5ᵗʰ **V80.2** Animal-rider or occupant of animal-drawn vehicle injured in collision with pedal cycle

    √x 7ᵗʰ **V80.21** Animal-rider injured in collision with pedal cycle

    √x 7ᵗʰ **V80.22** Occupant of animal-drawn vehicle injured in collision with pedal cycle

  √5ᵗʰ **V80.3** Animal-rider or occupant of animal-drawn vehicle injured in collision with two- or three-wheeled motor vehicle

    √x 7ᵗʰ **V80.31** Animal-rider injured in collision with two- or three-wheeled motor vehicle

    √x 7ᵗʰ **V80.32** Occupant of animal-drawn vehicle injured in collision with two- or three-wheeled motor vehicle

  √5ᵗʰ **V80.4** Animal-rider or occupant of animal-drawn vehicle injured in collision with car, pick-up truck, van, heavy transport vehicle or bus

    EXCLUDES 1   animal-rider injured in collision with military vehicle (V80.910)
      occupant of animal-drawn vehicle injured in collision with military vehicle (V80.920)

    √x 7ᵗʰ **V80.41** Animal-rider injured in collision with car, pick-up truck, van, heavy transport vehicle or bus

    √x 7ᵗʰ **V80.42** Occupant of animal-drawn vehicle injured in collision with car, pick-up truck, van, heavy transport vehicle or bus

  √5ᵗʰ **V80.5** Animal-rider or occupant of animal-drawn vehicle injured in collision with other specified motor vehicle

    √x 7ᵗʰ **V80.51** Animal-rider injured in collision with other specified motor vehicle

    √x 7ᵗʰ **V80.52** Occupant of animal-drawn vehicle injured in collision with other specified motor vehicle

  √5ᵗʰ **V80.6** Animal-rider or occupant of animal-drawn vehicle injured in collision with railway train or railway vehicle

    √x 7ᵗʰ **V80.61** Animal-rider injured in collision with railway train or railway vehicle

    √x 7ᵗʰ **V80.62** Occupant of animal-drawn vehicle injured in collision with railway train or railway vehicle

  √5ᵗʰ **V80.7** Animal-rider or occupant of animal-drawn vehicle injured in collision with other nonmotor vehicles

    √6ᵗʰ **V80.71** Animal-rider or occupant of animal-drawn vehicle injured in collision with animal being ridden

      √7ᵗʰ **V80.710** Animal-rider injured in collision with other animal being ridden

      √7ᵗʰ **V80.711** Occupant of animal-drawn vehicle injured in collision with animal being ridden

    √6ᵗʰ **V80.72** Animal-rider or occupant of animal-drawn vehicle injured in collision with other animal-drawn vehicle

      √7ᵗʰ **V80.720** Animal-rider injured in collision with animal-drawn vehicle

      √7ᵗʰ **V80.721** Occupant of animal-drawn vehicle injured in collision with other animal-drawn vehicle

    √6ᵗʰ **V80.73** Animal-rider or occupant of animal-drawn vehicle injured in collision with streetcar

      √7ᵗʰ **V80.730** Animal-rider injured in collision with streetcar

      √7ᵗʰ **V80.731** Occupant of animal-drawn vehicle injured in collision with streetcar

    √6ᵗʰ **V80.79** Animal-rider or occupant of animal-drawn vehicle injured in collision with other nonmotor vehicles

      √7ᵗʰ **V80.790** Animal-rider injured in collision with other nonmotor vehicles

      √7ᵗʰ **V80.791** Occupant of animal-drawn vehicle injured in collision with other nonmotor vehicles

  √5ᵗʰ **V80.8** Animal-rider or occupant of animal-drawn vehicle injured in collision with fixed or stationary object

    √x 7ᵗʰ **V80.81** Animal-rider injured in collision with fixed or stationary object

    √x 7ᵗʰ **V80.82** Occupant of animal-drawn vehicle injured in collision with fixed or stationary object

✔ Additional Char Req   √x 7ᵗʰ Placeholder   Unacceptable PDx   Questionable PDx   Wrong Procedure   Manifestation   Unspecified   H1 - H14 HAC   HCC CMS-HCC Dx   HIV HIV Dx

ICD-10-CM 2025   1217

☑5ᵗʰ **V80.9** Animal-rider or occupant of animal-drawn vehicle injured in other and unspecified transport accidents

    ☑6ᵗʰ **V80.91** Animal-rider injured in other and unspecified transport accidents

       ☑7ᵗʰ **V80.910** Animal-rider injured in transport accident with military vehicle

       ☑7ᵗʰ **V80.918** Animal-rider injured in other transport accident

       ☑7ᵗʰ **V80.919** Animal-rider injured in unspecified transport accident
          Animal rider accident NOS

    ☑6ᵗʰ **V80.92** Occupant of animal-drawn vehicle injured in other and unspecified transport accidents

       ☑7ᵗʰ **V80.920** Occupant of animal-drawn vehicle injured in transport accident with military vehicle

       ☑7ᵗʰ **V80.928** Occupant of animal-drawn vehicle injured in other transport accident

       ☑7ᵗʰ **V80.929** Occupant of animal-drawn vehicle injured in unspecified transport accident
          Animal-drawn vehicle accident NOS

☑4ᵗʰ **V81** Occupant of railway train or railway vehicle injured in transport accident

    INCLUDES   derailment of railway train or railway vehicle
             person on outside of train
    EXCLUDES 1   streetcar (V82.-)

    ✓x7ᵗʰ **V81.0** Occupant of railway train or railway vehicle injured in collision with motor vehicle in nontraffic accident
       EXCLUDES 1   occupant of railway train or railway vehicle injured due to collision with military vehicle (V81.83)

    ✓x7ᵗʰ **V81.1** Occupant of railway train or railway vehicle injured in collision with motor vehicle in traffic accident
       EXCLUDES 1   occupant of railway train or railway vehicle injured due to collision with military vehicle (V81.83)

    ✓x7ᵗʰ **V81.2** Occupant of railway train or railway vehicle injured in collision with or hit by rolling stock

    ✓x7ᵗʰ **V81.3** Occupant of railway train or railway vehicle injured in collision with other object
       Railway collision NOS

    ✓x7ᵗʰ **V81.4** Person injured while boarding or alighting from railway train or railway vehicle

    ✓x7ᵗʰ **V81.5** Occupant of railway train or railway vehicle injured by fall in railway train or railway vehicle

    ✓x7ᵗʰ **V81.6** Occupant of railway train or railway vehicle injured by fall from railway train or railway vehicle

    ✓x7ᵗʰ **V81.7** Occupant of railway train or railway vehicle injured in derailment without antecedent collision

    ☑5ᵗʰ **V81.8** Occupant of railway train or railway vehicle injured in other specified railway accidents

       ✓x7ᵗʰ **V81.81** Occupant of railway train or railway vehicle injured due to explosion or fire on train

       ✓x7ᵗʰ **V81.82** Occupant of railway train or railway vehicle injured due to object falling onto train
          Occupant of railway train or railway vehicle injured due to falling earth onto train
          Occupant of railway train or railway vehicle injured due to falling rocks onto train
          Occupant of railway train or railway vehicle injured due to falling snow onto train
          Occupant of railway train or railway vehicle injured due to falling trees onto train

       ✓x7ᵗʰ **V81.83** Occupant of railway train or railway vehicle injured due to collision with military vehicle

       ✓x7ᵗʰ **V81.89** Occupant of railway train or railway vehicle injured due to other specified railway accident

    ✓x7ᵗʰ **V81.9** Occupant of railway train or railway vehicle injured in unspecified railway accident
       Railway accident NOS

☑4ᵗʰ **V82** Occupant of powered streetcar injured in transport accident

    INCLUDES   interurban electric car
             person on outside of streetcar
             tram (car)
             trolley (car)
    EXCLUDES 1   bus (V70-V79)
             motorcoach (V70-V79)
             nonpowered streetcar (V76.-)
             train (V81.-)

    ✓x7ᵗʰ **V82.0** Occupant of streetcar injured in collision with motor vehicle in nontraffic accident

    ✓x7ᵗʰ **V82.1** Occupant of streetcar injured in collision with motor vehicle in traffic accident

    ✓x7ᵗʰ **V82.2** Occupant of streetcar injured in collision with or hit by rolling stock

    ✓x7ᵗʰ **V82.3** Occupant of streetcar injured in collision with other object
       EXCLUDES 1   collision with animal-drawn vehicle or animal being ridden (V82.8)

    ✓x7ᵗʰ **V82.4** Person injured while boarding or alighting from streetcar

    ✓x7ᵗʰ **V82.5** Occupant of streetcar injured by fall in streetcar
       EXCLUDES 1   fall in streetcar:
          while boarding or alighting (V82.4)
          with antecedent collision (V82.0-V82.3)

    ✓x7ᵗʰ **V82.6** Occupant of streetcar injured by fall from streetcar
       EXCLUDES 1   fall from streetcar:
          while boarding or alighting (V82.4)
          with antecedent collision (V82.0-V82.3)

    ✓x7ᵗʰ **V82.7** Occupant of streetcar injured in derailment without antecedent collision
       EXCLUDES 1   occupant of streetcar injured in derailment with antecedent collision (V82.0-V82.3)

    ✓x7ᵗʰ **V82.8** Occupant of streetcar injured in other specified transport accidents
       Streetcar collision with military vehicle
       Streetcar collision with train or nonmotor vehicles

    ✓x7ᵗʰ **V82.9** Occupant of streetcar injured in unspecified traffic accident
       Streetcar accident NOS

☑4ᵗʰ **V83** Occupant of special vehicle mainly used on industrial premises injured in transport accident

    INCLUDES   battery-powered airport passenger vehicle
             battery-powered truck (baggage) (mail)
             coal-car in mine
             forklift (truck)
             logging car
             self-propelled industrial truck
             station baggage truck (powered)
             tram, truck, or tub (powered) in mine or quarry
    EXCLUDES 1   special construction vehicles (V85.-)
             special industrial vehicle in stationary use or maintenance (W31.-)

    ✓x7ᵗʰ **V83.0** Driver of special industrial vehicle injured in traffic accident

    ✓x7ᵗʰ **V83.1** Passenger of special industrial vehicle injured in traffic accident

    ✓x7ᵗʰ **V83.2** Person on outside of special industrial vehicle injured in traffic accident

    ✓x7ᵗʰ **V83.3** Unspecified occupant of special industrial vehicle injured in traffic accident

    ✓x7ᵗʰ **V83.4** Person injured while boarding or alighting from special industrial vehicle

    ✓x7ᵗʰ **V83.5** Driver of special industrial vehicle injured in nontraffic accident

    ✓x7ᵗʰ **V83.6** Passenger of special industrial vehicle injured in nontraffic accident

    ✓x7ᵗʰ **V83.7** Person on outside of special industrial vehicle injured in nontraffic accident

    ✓x7ᵗʰ **V83.9** Unspecified occupant of special industrial vehicle injured in nontraffic accident
       Special-industrial-vehicle accident NOS

☑4ᵗʰ **V84** Occupant of special vehicle mainly used in agriculture injured in transport accident

    INCLUDES   self-propelled farm machinery
             tractor (and trailer)
    EXCLUDES 1   animal-powered farm machinery accident (W30.8-)
             contact with combine harvester (W30.0)
             special agricultural vehicle in stationary use or maintenance (W30.-)

    ✓x7ᵗʰ **V84.0** Driver of special agricultural vehicle injured in traffic accident

    ✓x7ᵗʰ **V84.1** Passenger of special agricultural vehicle injured in traffic accident

    ✓x7ᵗʰ **V84.2** Person on outside of special agricultural vehicle injured in traffic accident

    ✓x7ᵗʰ **V84.3** Unspecified occupant of special agricultural vehicle injured in traffic accident

    ✓x7ᵗʰ **V84.4** Person injured while boarding or alighting from special agricultural vehicle

    ✓x7ᵗʰ **V84.5** Driver of special agricultural vehicle injured in nontraffic accident

    ✓x7ᵗʰ **V84.6** Passenger of special agricultural vehicle injured in nontraffic accident

    ✓x7ᵗʰ **V84.7** Person on outside of special agricultural vehicle injured in nontraffic accident

N Newborn: 0   **P** Pediatric: 0-17   **M** Maternity: 9-64   **A** Adult: 15-124   **UNS** Unspecified Site   **MCC** Major Complication/Comorbidity   **CC** Complication/Comorbidity   **PE** POA Exempt

1218   ICD-10-CM 2025

✓x7ᵗʰ V84.9 Unspecified occupant of special agricultural vehicle injured in nontraffic accident
> Special-agricultural vehicle accident NOS

✓4ᵗʰ V85 Occupant of special construction vehicle injured in transport accident

> **INCLUDES** bulldozer
> digger
> dump truck
> earth-leveller
> mechanical shovel
> road-roller

> **EXCLUDES 1** special construction vehicle in stationary use or maintenance (W31.-)
> special industrial vehicle (V83.-)

✓x7ᵗʰ V85.0 Driver of special construction vehicle injured in traffic accident

✓x7ᵗʰ V85.1 Passenger of special construction vehicle injured in traffic accident

✓x7ᵗʰ V85.2 Person on outside of special construction vehicle injured in traffic accident

✓x7ᵗʰ V85.3 Unspecified occupant of special construction vehicle injured in traffic accident

✓x7ᵗʰ V85.4 Person injured while boarding or alighting from special construction vehicle

✓x7ᵗʰ V85.5 Driver of special construction vehicle injured in nontraffic accident

✓x7ᵗʰ V85.6 Passenger of special construction vehicle injured in nontraffic accident

✓x7ᵗʰ V85.7 Person on outside of special construction vehicle injured in nontraffic accident

✓x7ᵗʰ V85.9 Unspecified occupant of special construction vehicle injured in nontraffic accident
> Special-construction-vehicle accident NOS

✓4ᵗʰ V86 Occupant of special all-terrain or other off-road motor vehicle, injured in transport accident

> **EXCLUDES 1** special all-terrain vehicle in stationary use or maintenance (W31.-)
> sport-utility vehicle (V50-V59)
> three-wheeled motor vehicle designed for on-road use (V30-V39)

> **AHA:** 2017,4Q,26

✓5ᵗʰ V86.0 Driver of special all-terrain or other off-road motor vehicle injured in traffic accident

✓x7ᵗʰ V86.01 Driver of ambulance or fire engine injured in traffic accident

✓x7ᵗʰ V86.02 Driver of snowmobile injured in traffic accident

✓x7ᵗʰ V86.03 Driver of dune buggy injured in traffic accident

✓x7ᵗʰ V86.04 Driver of military vehicle injured in traffic accident

✓x7ᵗʰ V86.05 Driver of 3- or 4- wheeled all-terrain vehicle (ATV) injured in traffic accident

✓x7ᵗʰ V86.06 Driver of dirt bike or motor/cross bike injured in traffic accident

✓x7ᵗʰ V86.09 Driver of other special all-terrain or other off-road motor vehicle injured in traffic accident
> Driver of go cart injured in traffic accident
> Driver of golf cart injured in traffic accident

✓5ᵗʰ V86.1 Passenger of special all-terrain or other off-road motor vehicle injured in traffic accident

✓x7ᵗʰ V86.11 Passenger of ambulance or fire engine injured in traffic accident

✓x7ᵗʰ V86.12 Passenger of snowmobile injured in traffic accident

✓x7ᵗʰ V86.13 Passenger of dune buggy injured in traffic accident

✓x7ᵗʰ V86.14 Passenger of military vehicle injured in traffic accident

✓x7ᵗʰ V86.15 Passenger of 3- or 4- wheeled all-terrain vehicle (ATV) injured in traffic accident

✓x7ᵗʰ V86.16 Passenger of dirt bike or motor/cross bike injured in traffic accident

✓x7ᵗʰ V86.19 Passenger of other special all-terrain or other off-road motor vehicle injured in traffic accident
> Passenger of go cart injured in traffic accident
> Passenger of golf cart injured in traffic accident

✓5ᵗʰ V86.2 Person on outside of special all-terrain or other off-road motor vehicle injured in traffic accident

✓x7ᵗʰ V86.21 Person on outside of ambulance or fire engine injured in traffic accident

✓x7ᵗʰ V86.22 Person on outside of snowmobile injured in traffic accident

✓x7ᵗʰ V86.23 Person on outside of dune buggy injured in traffic accident

✓x7ᵗʰ V86.24 Person on outside of military vehicle injured in traffic accident

✓x7ᵗʰ V86.25 Person on outside of 3- or 4- wheeled all-terrain vehicle (ATV) injured in traffic accident

✓x7ᵗʰ V86.26 Person on outside of dirt bike or motor/cross bike injured in traffic accident

✓x7ᵗʰ V86.29 Person on outside of other special all-terrain or other off-road motor vehicle injured in traffic accident
> Person on outside of go cart in traffic accident
> Person on outside of golf cart injured in traffic accident

✓5ᵗʰ V86.3 Unspecified occupant of special all-terrain or other off-road motor vehicle injured in traffic accident

✓x7ᵗʰ V86.31 Unspecified occupant of ambulance or fire engine injured in traffic accident

✓x7ᵗʰ V86.32 Unspecified occupant of snowmobile injured in traffic accident

✓x7ᵗʰ V86.33 Unspecified occupant of dune buggy injured in traffic accident

✓x7ᵗʰ V86.34 Unspecified occupant of military vehicle injured in traffic accident

✓x7ᵗʰ V86.35 Unspecified occupant of 3- or 4- wheeled all-terrain vehicle (ATV) injured in traffic accident

✓x7ᵗʰ V86.36 Unspecified occupant of dirt bike or motor/cross bike injured in traffic accident

✓x7ᵗʰ V86.39 Unspecified occupant of other special all-terrain or other off-road motor vehicle injured in traffic accident
> Unspecified occupant of go cart injured in traffic accident
> Unspecified occupant of golf cart injured in traffic accident

✓5ᵗʰ V86.4 Person injured while boarding or alighting from special all-terrain or other off-road motor vehicle

✓x7ᵗʰ V86.41 Person injured while boarding or alighting from ambulance or fire engine

✓x7ᵗʰ V86.42 Person injured while boarding or alighting from snowmobile

✓x7ᵗʰ V86.43 Person injured while boarding or alighting from dune buggy

✓x7ᵗʰ V86.44 Person injured while boarding or alighting from military vehicle

✓x7ᵗʰ V86.45 Person injured while boarding or alighting from a 3- or 4- wheeled all-terrain vehicle (ATV)

✓x7ᵗʰ V86.46 Person injured while boarding or alighting from a dirt bike or motor/cross bike

✓x7ᵗʰ V86.49 Person injured while boarding or alighting from other special all-terrain or other off-road motor vehicle
> Person injured while boarding or alighting from go cart
> Person injured while boarding or alighting from golf cart

✓5ᵗʰ V86.5 Driver of special all-terrain or other off-road motor vehicle injured in nontraffic accident

✓x7ᵗʰ V86.51 Driver of ambulance or fire engine injured in nontraffic accident

✓x7ᵗʰ V86.52 Driver of snowmobile injured in nontraffic accident

✓x7ᵗʰ V86.53 Driver of dune buggy injured in nontraffic accident

✓x7ᵗʰ V86.54 Driver of military vehicle injured in nontraffic accident

✓x7ᵗʰ V86.55 Driver of 3- or 4- wheeled all-terrain vehicle (ATV) injured in nontraffic accident

✓x7ᵗʰ V86.56 Driver of dirt bike or motor/cross bike injured in nontraffic accident

✓x7ᵗʰ V86.59 Driver of other special all-terrain or other off-road motor vehicle injured in nontraffic accident
> Driver of go cart injured in nontraffic accident
> Driver of golf cart injured in nontraffic accident

✓5ᵗʰ V86.6 Passenger of special all-terrain or other off-road motor vehicle injured in nontraffic accident

✓x7ᵗʰ V86.61 Passenger of ambulance or fire engine injured in nontraffic accident

✓x7ᵗʰ V86.62 Passenger of snowmobile injured in nontraffic accident

✓x7ᵗʰ V86.63 Passenger of dune buggy injured in nontraffic accident

✓x7ᵗʰ V86.64 Passenger of military vehicle injured in nontraffic accident

✓x7ᵗʰ V86.65 Passenger of 3- or 4- wheeled all-terrain vehicle (ATV) injured in nontraffic accident

✓x7ᵗʰ V86.66 Passenger of dirt bike or motor/cross bike injured in nontraffic accident

✔ Additional Char Req   ✓x7ᵗʰ Placeholder   Unacceptable PDx   Questionable PDx   Wrong Procedure   Manifestation   Unspecified   H1-H14 HAC   HCC CMS-HCC Dx   HIV HIV Dx

ICD-10-CM 2025   1219

√x7th **V86.69** Passenger of other special all-terrain or other off-road motor vehicle injured in nontraffic accident
     Passenger of go cart injured in nontraffic accident
     Passenger of golf cart injured in nontraffic accident

√5th **V86.7** Person on outside of special all-terrain or other off-road motor vehicle injured in nontraffic accident

√x7th **V86.71** Person on outside of ambulance or fire engine injured in nontraffic accident

√x7th **V86.72** Person on outside of snowmobile injured in nontraffic accident

√x7th **V86.73** Person on outside of dune buggy injured in nontraffic accident

√x7th **V86.74** Person on outside of military vehicle injured in nontraffic accident

√x7th **V86.75** Person on outside of 3- or 4- wheeled all-terrain vehicle (ATV) injured in nontraffic accident

√x7th **V86.76** Person on outside of dirt bike or motor/cross bike injured in nontraffic accident

√x7th **V86.79** Person on outside of other special all-terrain or other off-road motor vehicles injured in nontraffic accident
     Person on outside of go cart injured in nontraffic accident
     Person on outside of golf cart injured in nontraffic accident

√5th **V86.9** Unspecified occupant of special all-terrain or other off-road motor vehicle injured in nontraffic accident

√x7th **V86.91** Unspecified occupant of ambulance or fire engine injured in nontraffic accident

√x7th **V86.92** Unspecified occupant of snowmobile injured in nontraffic accident

√x7th **V86.93** Unspecified occupant of dune buggy injured in nontraffic accident

√x7th **V86.94** Unspecified occupant of military vehicle injured in nontraffic accident

√x7th **V86.95** Unspecified occupant of 3- or 4- wheeled all-terrain vehicle (ATV) injured in nontraffic accident

√x7th **V86.96** Unspecified occupant of dirt bike or motor/cross bike injured in nontraffic accident

√x7th **V86.99** Unspecified occupant of other special all-terrain or other off-road motor vehicle injured in nontraffic accident
     Off-road motor-vehicle accident NOS
     Other motor-vehicle accident NOS
     Unspecified occupant of go cart injured in nontraffic accident
     Unspecified occupant of golf cart injured in nontraffic accident

√4th **V87** Traffic accident of specified type but victim's mode of transport unknown
     EXCLUDES 1   collision involving:
         pedal cycle (V10-V19)
         pedestrian (V01-V09)

√x7th **V87.0** Person injured in collision between car and two- or three-wheeled powered vehicle (traffic)

√x7th **V87.1** Person injured in collision between other motor vehicle and two- or three-wheeled motor vehicle (traffic)

√x7th **V87.2** Person injured in collision between car and pick-up truck or van (traffic)

√x7th **V87.3** Person injured in collision between car and bus (traffic)

√x7th **V87.4** Person injured in collision between car and heavy transport vehicle (traffic)

√x7th **V87.5** Person injured in collision between heavy transport vehicle and bus (traffic)

√x7th **V87.6** Person injured in collision between railway train or railway vehicle and car (traffic)

√x7th **V87.7** Person injured in collision between other specified motor vehicles (traffic)

√x7th **V87.8** Person injured in other specified noncollision transport accidents involving motor vehicle (traffic)

√x7th **V87.9** Person injured in other specified (collision)(noncollision) transport accidents involving nonmotor vehicle (traffic)

√4th **V88** Nontraffic accident of specified type but victim's mode of transport unknown
     EXCLUDES 1   collision involving:
         pedal cycle (V10-V19)
         pedestrian (V01-V09)

√x7th **V88.0** Person injured in collision between car and two- or three-wheeled motor vehicle, nontraffic

√x7th **V88.1** Person injured in collision between other motor vehicle and two- or three-wheeled motor vehicle, nontraffic

√x7th **V88.2** Person injured in collision between car and pick-up truck or van, nontraffic

√x7th **V88.3** Person injured in collision between car and bus, nontraffic

√x7th **V88.4** Person injured in collision between car and heavy transport vehicle, nontraffic

√x7th **V88.5** Person injured in collision between heavy transport vehicle and bus, nontraffic

√x7th **V88.6** Person injured in collision between railway train or railway vehicle and car, nontraffic

√x7th **V88.7** Person injured in collision between other specified motor vehicle, nontraffic

√x7th **V88.8** Person injured in other specified noncollision transport accidents involving motor vehicle, nontraffic

√x7th **V88.9** Person injured in other specified (collision)(noncollision) transport accidents involving nonmotor vehicle, nontraffic

√4th **V89** Motor- or nonmotor-vehicle accident, type of vehicle unspecified

√x7th **V89.0** Person injured in unspecified motor-vehicle accident, nontraffic
     Motor-vehicle accident NOS, nontraffic

√x7th **V89.1** Person injured in unspecified nonmotor-vehicle accident, nontraffic
     Nonmotor-vehicle accident NOS (nontraffic)

√x7th **V89.2** Person injured in unspecified motor-vehicle accident, traffic
     Motor-vehicle accident [MVA] NOS
     Road (traffic) accident [RTA] NOS

√x7th **V89.3** Person injured in unspecified nonmotor-vehicle accident, traffic
     Nonmotor-vehicle traffic accident NOS

√x7th **V89.9** Person injured in unspecified vehicle accident
     Collision NOS

Water transport accidents (V90-V94)

The appropriate 7th character is to be added to each code from categories V90-V94.
A   initial encounter
D   subsequent encounter
S   sequela

√4th **V90** Drowning and submersion due to accident to watercraft
     EXCLUDES 1   civilian water transport accident involving military watercraft (V94.81-)
         fall into water not from watercraft (W16.-)
         military watercraft accident in military or war operations (Y36.0-, Y37.0-)
         water-transport-related drowning or submersion without accident to watercraft (V92.-)

√5th **V90.0** Drowning and submersion due to watercraft overturning

√x7th **V90.00** Drowning and submersion due to merchant ship overturning

√x7th **V90.01** Drowning and submersion due to passenger ship overturning
     Drowning and submersion due to Ferry-boat overturning
     Drowning and submersion due to Liner overturning

√x7th **V90.02** Drowning and submersion due to fishing boat overturning

√x7th **V90.03** Drowning and submersion due to other powered watercraft overturning
     Drowning and submersion due to Hovercraft (on open water) overturning
     Drowning and submersion due to Jet ski overturning

√x7th **V90.04** Drowning and submersion due to sailboat overturning

√x7th **V90.05** Drowning and submersion due to canoe or kayak overturning

√x7th **V90.06** Drowning and submersion due to (nonpowered) inflatable craft overturning

√x7th **V90.08** Drowning and submersion due to other unpowered watercraft overturning
     Drowning and submersion due to windsurfer overturning

√x7th **V90.09** Drowning and submersion due to unspecified watercraft overturning
     Drowning and submersion due to boat NOS overturning
     Drowning and submersion due to ship NOS overturning
     Drowning and submersion due to watercraft NOS overturning

√5th **V90.1** Drowning and submersion due to watercraft sinking

√x7th **V90.10** Drowning and submersion due to merchant ship sinking

√x7th **V90.11** **Drowning and submersion due to passenger ship sinking**
    Drowning and submersion due to Ferry-boat sinking
    Drowning and submersion due to Liner sinking

√x7th **V90.12** **Drowning and submersion due to fishing boat sinking**

√x7th **V90.13** **Drowning and submersion due to other powered watercraft sinking**
    Drowning and submersion due to Hovercraft (on open water) sinking
    Drowning and submersion due to Jet ski sinking

√x7th **V90.14** **Drowning and submersion due to sailboat sinking**

√x7th **V90.15** **Drowning and submersion due to canoe or kayak sinking**

√x7th **V90.16** **Drowning and submersion due to (nonpowered) inflatable craft sinking**

√x7th **V90.18** **Drowning and submersion due to other unpowered watercraft sinking**

√x7th **V90.19** **Drowning and submersion due to unspecified watercraft sinking**
    Drowning and submersion due to boat NOS sinking
    Drowning and submersion due to ship NOS sinking
    Drowning and submersion due to watercraft NOS sinking

√5th **V90.2** **Drowning and submersion due to falling or jumping from burning watercraft**

√x7th **V90.20** **Drowning and submersion due to falling or jumping from burning merchant ship**

√x7th **V90.21** **Drowning and submersion due to falling or jumping from burning passenger ship**
    Drowning and submersion due to falling or jumping from burning Ferry-boat
    Drowning and submersion due to falling or jumping from burning Liner

√x7th **V90.22** **Drowning and submersion due to falling or jumping from burning fishing boat**

√x7th **V90.23** **Drowning and submersion due to falling or jumping from other burning powered watercraft**
    Drowning and submersion due to falling and jumping from burning Hovercraft (on open water)
    Drowning and submersion due to falling and jumping from burning Jet ski

√x7th **V90.24** **Drowning and submersion due to falling or jumping from burning sailboat**

√x7th **V90.25** **Drowning and submersion due to falling or jumping from burning canoe or kayak**

√x7th **V90.26** **Drowning and submersion due to falling or jumping from burning (nonpowered) inflatable craft**

√x7th **V90.27** **Drowning and submersion due to falling or jumping from burning water-skis**

√x7th **V90.28** **Drowning and submersion due to falling or jumping from other burning unpowered watercraft**
    Drowning and submersion due to falling and jumping from burning surf-board
    Drowning and submersion due to falling and jumping from burning windsurfer

√x7th **V90.29** **Drowning and submersion due to falling or jumping from unspecified burning watercraft**
    Drowning and submersion due to falling or jumping from burning boat NOS
    Drowning and submersion due to falling or jumping from burning ship NOS
    Drowning and submersion due to falling or jumping from burning watercraft NOS

√5th **V90.3** **Drowning and submersion due to falling or jumping from crushed watercraft**

√x7th **V90.30** **Drowning and submersion due to falling or jumping from crushed merchant ship**

√x7th **V90.31** **Drowning and submersion due to falling or jumping from crushed passenger ship**
    Drowning and submersion due to falling and jumping from crushed Ferry boat
    Drowning and submersion due to falling and jumping from crushed Liner

√x7th **V90.32** **Drowning and submersion due to falling or jumping from crushed fishing boat**

√x7th **V90.33** **Drowning and submersion due to falling or jumping from other crushed powered watercraft**
    Drowning and submersion due to falling and jumping from crushed Hovercraft
    Drowning and submersion due to falling and jumping from crushed Jet ski

√x7th **V90.34** **Drowning and submersion due to falling or jumping from crushed sailboat**

√x7th **V90.35** **Drowning and submersion due to falling or jumping from crushed canoe or kayak**

√x7th **V90.36** **Drowning and submersion due to falling or jumping from crushed (nonpowered) inflatable craft**

√x7th **V90.37** **Drowning and submersion due to falling or jumping from crushed water-skis**

√x7th **V90.38** **Drowning and submersion due to falling or jumping from other crushed unpowered watercraft**
    Drowning and submersion due to falling and jumping from crushed surf-board
    Drowning and submersion due to falling and jumping from crushed windsurfer

√x7th **V90.39** **Drowning and submersion due to falling or jumping from crushed unspecified watercraft**
    Drowning and submersion due to falling and jumping from crushed boat NOS
    Drowning and submersion due to falling and jumping from crushed ship NOS
    Drowning and submersion due to falling and jumping from crushed watercraft NOS

√5th **V90.8** **Drowning and submersion due to other accident to watercraft**

√x7th **V90.80** **Drowning and submersion due to other accident to merchant ship**

√x7th **V90.81** **Drowning and submersion due to other accident to passenger ship**
    Drowning and submersion due to other accident to Ferry-boat
    Drowning and submersion due to other accident to Liner

√x7th **V90.82** **Drowning and submersion due to other accident to fishing boat**

√x7th **V90.83** **Drowning and submersion due to other accident to other powered watercraft**
    Drowning and submersion due to other accident to Hovercraft (on open water)
    Drowning and submersion due to other accident to Jet ski

√x7th **V90.84** **Drowning and submersion due to other accident to sailboat**

√x7th **V90.85** **Drowning and submersion due to other accident to canoe or kayak**

√x7th **V90.86** **Drowning and submersion due to other accident to (nonpowered) inflatable craft**

√x7th **V90.87** **Drowning and submersion due to other accident to water-skis**

√x7th **V90.88** **Drowning and submersion due to other accident to other unpowered watercraft**
    Drowning and submersion due to other accident to surf-board
    Drowning and submersion due to other accident to windsurfer

√x7th **V90.89** **Drowning and submersion due to other accident to unspecified watercraft**
    Drowning and submersion due to other accident to boat NOS
    Drowning and submersion due to other accident to ship NOS
    Drowning and submersion due to other accident to watercraft NOS

√4th **V91** **Other injury due to accident to watercraft**

> **INCLUDES**   any injury except drowning and submersion as a result of an accident to watercraft
>
> **EXCLUDES 1**   *civilian water transport accident involving military watercraft (V94.81-)*
> *military watercraft accident in military or war operations (Y36, Y37.-)*
>
> **EXCLUDES 2**   *drowning and submersion due to accident to watercraft (V90.-)*

√5th **V91.0** **Burn due to watercraft on fire**

> **EXCLUDES 1**   *burn from localized fire or explosion on board ship without accident to watercraft (V93.-)*

√x7th **V91.00** **Burn due to merchant ship on fire**

√x7th **V91.01** **Burn due to passenger ship on fire**
    Burn due to Ferry-boat on fire
    Burn due to Liner on fire

√x7th **V91.02** **Burn due to fishing boat on fire**

√x7th **V91.03** **Burn due to other powered watercraft on fire**
    Burn due to Hovercraft (on open water) on fire
    Burn due to Jet ski on fire

√x7th **V91.04** **Burn due to sailboat on fire**

√x7th **V91.05** **Burn due to canoe or kayak on fire**

√x 7th **V91.06** **Burn due to (nonpowered) inflatable craft on fire**

√x 7th **V91.07** **Burn due to water-skis on fire**

√x 7th **V91.08** **Burn due to other unpowered watercraft on fire**

√x 7th **V91.09** **Burn due to unspecified watercraft on fire**
> Burn due to boat NOS on fire
> Burn due to ship NOS on fire
> Burn due to watercraft NOS on fire

√5th **V91.1** **Crushed between watercraft and other watercraft or other object due to collision**
> Crushed by lifeboat after abandoning ship in a collision

> **NOTE**   Select the specified type of watercraft that the victim was on at the time of the collision

√x 7th **V91.10** **Crushed between merchant ship and other watercraft or other object due to collision.**

√x 7th **V91.11** **Crushed between passenger ship and other watercraft or other object due to collision**
> Crushed between Ferry-boat and other watercraft or other object due to collision
> Crushed between Liner and other watercraft or other object due to collision

√x 7th **V91.12** **Crushed between fishing boat and other watercraft or other object due to collision**

√x 7th **V91.13** **Crushed between other powered watercraft and other watercraft or other object due to collision**
> Crushed between Hovercraft (on open water) and other watercraft or other object due to collision
> Crushed between Jet ski and other watercraft or other object due to collision

√x 7th **V91.14** **Crushed between sailboat and other watercraft or other object due to collision**

√x 7th **V91.15** **Crushed between canoe or kayak and other watercraft or other object due to collision**

√x 7th **V91.16** **Crushed between (nonpowered) inflatable craft and other watercraft or other object due to collision**

√x 7th **V91.18** **Crushed between other unpowered watercraft and other watercraft or other object due to collision**
> Crushed between surfboard and other watercraft or other object due to collision
> Crushed between windsurfer and other watercraft or other object due to collision

√x 7th **V91.19** **Crushed between unspecified watercraft and other watercraft or other object due to collision**
> Crushed between boat NOS and other watercraft or other object due to collision
> Crushed between ship NOS and other watercraft or other object due to collision
> Crushed between watercraft NOS and other watercraft or other object due to collision

√5th **V91.2** **Fall due to collision between watercraft and other watercraft or other object**
> Fall while remaining on watercraft after collision

> **NOTE**   Select the specified type of watercraft that the victim was on at the time of the collision

> **EXCLUDES 1**   crushed between watercraft and other watercraft and other object due to collision (V91.1-)
> drowning and submersion due to falling from crushed watercraft (V90.3-)

√x 7th **V91.20** **Fall due to collision between merchant ship and other watercraft or other object**

√x 7th **V91.21** **Fall due to collision between passenger ship and other watercraft or other object**
> Fall due to collision between Ferry-boat and other watercraft or other object
> Fall due to collision between Liner and other watercraft or other object

√x 7th **V91.22** **Fall due to collision between fishing boat and other watercraft or other object**

√x 7th **V91.23** **Fall due to collision between other powered watercraft and other watercraft or other object**
> Fall due to collision between Hovercraft (on open water) and other watercraft or other object
> Fall due to collision between Jet ski and other watercraft or other object

√x 7th **V91.24** **Fall due to collision between sailboat and other watercraft or other object**

√x 7th **V91.25** **Fall due to collision between canoe or kayak and other watercraft or other object**

√x 7th **V91.26** **Fall due to collision between (nonpowered) inflatable craft and other watercraft or other object**

√x 7th **V91.29** **Fall due to collision between unspecified watercraft and other watercraft or other object**
> Fall due to collision between boat NOS and other watercraft or other object
> Fall due to collision between ship NOS and other watercraft or other object
> Fall due to collision between watercraft NOS and other watercraft or other object

√5th **V91.3** **Hit or struck by falling object due to accident to watercraft**
> Hit or struck by falling object (part of damaged watercraft or other object) after falling or jumping from damaged watercraft

> **EXCLUDES 2**   drowning or submersion due to fall or jumping from damaged watercraft (V90.2-, V90.3-)

√x 7th **V91.30** **Hit or struck by falling object due to accident to merchant ship**

√x 7th **V91.31** **Hit or struck by falling object due to accident to passenger ship**
> Hit or struck by falling object due to accident to Ferry-boat
> Hit or struck by falling object due to accident to Liner

√x 7th **V91.32** **Hit or struck by falling object due to accident to fishing boat**

√x 7th **V91.33** **Hit or struck by falling object due to accident to other powered watercraft**
> Hit or struck by falling object due to accident to Hovercraft (on open water)
> Hit or struck by falling object due to accident to Jet ski

√x 7th **V91.34** **Hit or struck by falling object due to accident to sailboat**

√x 7th **V91.35** **Hit or struck by falling object due to accident to canoe or kayak**

√x 7th **V91.36** **Hit or struck by falling object due to accident to (nonpowered) inflatable craft**

√x 7th **V91.37** **Hit or struck by falling object due to accident to water-skis**
> Hit by water-skis after jumping off of waterskis

√x 7th **V91.38** **Hit or struck by falling object due to accident to other unpowered watercraft**
> Hit or struck by surf-board after falling off damaged surf-board
> Hit or struck by object after falling off damaged windsurfer

√x 7th **V91.39** **Hit or struck by falling object due to accident to unspecified watercraft**
> Hit or struck by falling object due to accident to boat NOS
> Hit or struck by falling object due to accident to ship NOS
> Hit or struck by falling object due to accident to watercraft NOS

√5th **V91.8** **Other injury due to other accident to watercraft**

√x 7th **V91.80** **Other injury due to other accident to merchant ship**

√x 7th **V91.81** **Other injury due to other accident to passenger ship**
> Other injury due to other accident to Ferry-boat
> Other injury due to other accident to Liner

√x 7th **V91.82** **Other injury due to other accident to fishing boat**

√x 7th **V91.83** **Other injury due to other accident to other powered watercraft**
> Other injury due to other accident to Hovercraft (on open water)
> Other injury due to other accident to Jet ski

√x 7th **V91.84** **Other injury due to other accident to sailboat**

√x 7th **V91.85** **Other injury due to other accident to canoe or kayak**

√x 7th **V91.86** **Other injury due to other accident to (nonpowered) inflatable craft**

√x 7th **V91.87** **Other injury due to other accident to water-skis**

√x 7th **V91.88** **Other injury due to other accident to other unpowered watercraft**
> Other injury due to other accident to surf-board
> Other injury due to other accident to windsurfer

√x 7th **V91.89** **Other injury due to other accident to unspecified watercraft**
> Other injury due to other accident to boat NOS
> Other injury due to other accident to ship NOS
> Other injury due to other accident to watercraft NOS

N Newborn: 0   **P** Pediatric: 0-17   **M** Maternity: 9-64   **A** Adult: 15-124   **UNS** Unspecified Site   **MCC** Major Complication/Comorbidity   **CC** Complication/Comorbidity   **PE** POA Exempt

1222   ICD-10-CM 2025

✓4ᵗʰ **V92** **Drowning and submersion due to accident on board watercraft, without accident to watercraft**

> EXCLUDES 1   *civilian water transport accident involving military watercraft (V94.81-)*
>
> *drowning or submersion due to accident to watercraft (V90-V91)*
>
> *drowning or submersion of diver who voluntarily jumps from boat not involved in an accident (W16.711, W16.721)*
>
> *fall into water without watercraft (W16.-)*
>
> *military watercraft accident in military or war operations (Y36, Y37)*

✓5ᵗʰ **V92.0** **Drowning and submersion due to fall off watercraft**

> Drowning and submersion due to fall from gangplank of watercraft
>
> Drowning and submersion due to fall overboard watercraft
>
> EXCLUDES 2   *hitting head on object or bottom of body of water due to fall from watercraft (V94.0-)*

✓x7ᵗʰ **V92.00** **Drowning and submersion due to fall off merchant ship**

✓x7ᵗʰ **V92.01** **Drowning and submersion due to fall off passenger ship**

> Drowning and submersion due to fall off Ferry-boat
> Drowning and submersion due to fall off Liner

✓x7ᵗʰ **V92.02** **Drowning and submersion due to fall off fishing boat**

✓x7ᵗʰ **V92.03** **Drowning and submersion due to fall off other powered watercraft**

> Drowning and submersion due to fall off Hovercraft (on open water)
> Drowning and submersion due to fall off Jet ski

✓x7ᵗʰ **V92.04** **Drowning and submersion due to fall off sailboat**

✓x7ᵗʰ **V92.05** **Drowning and submersion due to fall off canoe or kayak**

✓x7ᵗʰ **V92.06** **Drowning and submersion due to fall off (nonpowered) inflatable craft**

✓x7ᵗʰ **V92.07** **Drowning and submersion due to fall off water-skis**

> EXCLUDES 1   *drowning and submersion due to falling off burning water-skis (V90.27)*
>
> *drowning and submersion due to falling off crushed water-skis (V90.37)*
>
> *hit by boat while water-skiing NOS (V94.-)*

✓x7ᵗʰ **V92.08** **Drowning and submersion due to fall off other unpowered watercraft**

> Drowning and submersion due to fall off surf-board
> Drowning and submersion due to fall off windsurfer
>
> EXCLUDES 1   *drowning and submersion due to fall off burning unpowered watercraft (V90.28)*
>
> *drowning and submersion due to fall off crushed unpowered watercraft (V90.38)*
>
> *drowning and submersion due to fall off damaged unpowered watercraft (V90.88)*
>
> *drowning and submersion due to rider of nonpowered watercraft being hit by other watercraft (V94.-)*
>
> *other injury due to rider of nonpowered watercraft being hit by other watercraft (V94.-)*

✓x7ᵗʰ **V92.09** **Drowning and submersion due to fall off unspecified watercraft**

> Drowning and submersion due to fall off boat NOS
> Drowning and submersion due to fall off ship
> Drowning and submersion due to fall off watercraft NOS

✓5ᵗʰ **V92.1** **Drowning and submersion due to being thrown overboard by motion of watercraft**

> EXCLUDES 1   *drowning and submersion due to fall off surf-board (V92.08)*
>
> *drowning and submersion due to fall off water-skis (V92.07)*
>
> *drowning and submersion due to fall off windsurfer (V92.08)*

✓x7ᵗʰ **V92.10** **Drowning and submersion due to being thrown overboard by motion of merchant ship**

✓x7ᵗʰ **V92.11** **Drowning and submersion due to being thrown overboard by motion of passenger ship**

> Drowning and submersion due to being thrown overboard by motion of Ferry-boat
> Drowning and submersion due to being thrown overboard by motion of Liner

✓x7ᵗʰ **V92.12** **Drowning and submersion due to being thrown overboard by motion of fishing boat**

✓x7ᵗʰ **V92.13** **Drowning and submersion due to being thrown overboard by motion of other powered watercraft**

> Drowning and submersion due to being thrown overboard by motion of Hovercraft

✓x7ᵗʰ **V92.14** **Drowning and submersion due to being thrown overboard by motion of sailboat**

✓x7ᵗʰ **V92.15** **Drowning and submersion due to being thrown overboard by motion of canoe or kayak**

✓x7ᵗʰ **V92.16** **Drowning and submersion due to being thrown overboard by motion of (nonpowered) inflatable craft**

✓x7ᵗʰ **V92.19** **Drowning and submersion due to being thrown overboard by motion of unspecified watercraft**

> Drowning and submersion due to being thrown overboard by motion of boat NOS
> Drowning and submersion due to being thrown overboard by motion of ship NOS
> Drowning and submersion due to being thrown overboard by motion of watercraft NOS

✓5ᵗʰ **V92.2** **Drowning and submersion due to being washed overboard from watercraft**

> Code first any associated cataclysm (X37.0-)

✓x7ᵗʰ **V92.20** **Drowning and submersion due to being washed overboard from merchant ship**

✓x7ᵗʰ **V92.21** **Drowning and submersion due to being washed overboard from passenger ship**

> Drowning and submersion due to being washed overboard from Ferry-boat
> Drowning and submersion due to being washed overboard from Liner

✓x7ᵗʰ **V92.22** **Drowning and submersion due to being washed overboard from fishing boat**

✓x7ᵗʰ **V92.23** **Drowning and submersion due to being washed overboard from other powered watercraft**

> Drowning and submersion due to being washed overboard from Hovercraft (on open water)
> Drowning and submersion due to being washed overboard from Jet ski

✓x7ᵗʰ **V92.24** **Drowning and submersion due to being washed overboard from sailboat**

✓x7ᵗʰ **V92.25** **Drowning and submersion due to being washed overboard from canoe or kayak**

✓x7ᵗʰ **V92.26** **Drowning and submersion due to being washed overboard from (nonpowered) inflatable craft**

✓x7ᵗʰ **V92.27** **Drowning and submersion due to being washed overboard from water-skis**

> EXCLUDES 1   *drowning and submersion due to fall off water-skis (V92.07)*

✓x7ᵗʰ **V92.28** **Drowning and submersion due to being washed overboard from other unpowered watercraft**

> Drowning and submersion due to being washed overboard from surf-board
> Drowning and submersion due to being washed overboard from windsurfer

✓x7ᵗʰ **V92.29** **Drowning and submersion due to being washed overboard from unspecified watercraft**

> Drowning and submersion due to being washed overboard from boat NOS
> Drowning and submersion due to being washed overboard from ship NOS
> Drowning and submersion due to being washed overboard from watercraft NOS

✓4ᵗʰ **V93** **Other injury due to accident on board watercraft, without accident to watercraft**

> EXCLUDES 1   *civilian water transport accident involving military watercraft (V94.81-)*
>
> *military watercraft accident in military or war operations (Y36, Y37.-)*
>
> *other injury due to accident to watercraft (V91.-)*
>
> EXCLUDES 2   *drowning and submersion due to accident on board watercraft, without accident to watercraft (V92.-)*

✓5ᵗʰ **V93.0** **Burn due to localized fire on board watercraft**

> EXCLUDES 1   *burn due to watercraft on fire (V91.0-)*

✓x7ᵗʰ **V93.00** **Burn due to localized fire on board merchant vessel**

✅ Additional Char Req   ✓x7ᵗʰ Placeholder   Unacceptable PDx   Questionable PDx   Wrong Procedure   Manifestation   Unspecified   H1 - H14 HAC   HCC CMS-HCC Dx   HIV HIV Dx

ICD-10-CM 2025   1223

✓x7th **V93.Ø1** **Burn due to localized fire on board passenger vessel**
Burn due to localized fire on board Ferry-boat
Burn due to localized fire on board Liner

✓x7th **V93.Ø2** **Burn due to localized fire on board fishing boat**

✓x7th **V93.Ø3** **Burn due to localized fire on board other powered watercraft**
Burn due to localized fire on board Hovercraft
Burn due to localized fire on board Jet ski

✓x7th **V93.Ø4** **Burn due to localized fire on board sailboat**

✓x7th **V93.Ø9** **Burn due to localized fire on board unspecified watercraft**
Burn due to localized fire on board boat NOS
Burn due to localized fire on board ship NOS
Burn due to localized fire on board watercraft NOS

✓5th **V93.1** **Other burn on board watercraft**
Burn due to source other than fire on board watercraft
EXCLUDES 1   *burn due to watercraft on fire (V91.Ø-)*

✓x7th **V93.1Ø** **Other burn on board merchant vessel**

✓x7th **V93.11** **Other burn on board passenger vessel**
Other burn on board Ferry-boat
Other burn on board Liner

✓x7th **V93.12** **Other burn on board fishing boat**

✓x7th **V93.13** **Other burn on board other powered watercraft**
Other burn on board Hovercraft
Other burn on board Jet ski

✓x7th **V93.14** **Other burn on board sailboat**

✓x7th **V93.19** **Other burn on board unspecified watercraft**
Other burn on board boat NOS
Other burn on board ship NOS
Other burn on board watercraft NOS

✓5th **V93.2** **Heat exposure on board watercraft**
EXCLUDES 1   *exposure to man-made heat not aboard watercraft (W92)*
exposure to natural heat while on board watercraft (X3Ø)
exposure to sunlight while on board watercraft (X32)
EXCLUDES 2   *burn due to fire on board watercraft (V93.Ø-)*

✓x7th **V93.2Ø** **Heat exposure on board merchant ship**

✓x7th **V93.21** **Heat exposure on board passenger ship**
Heat exposure on board Ferry-boat
Heat exposure on board Liner

✓x7th **V93.22** **Heat exposure on board fishing boat**

✓x7th **V93.23** **Heat exposure on board other powered watercraft**
Heat exposure on board hovercraft

✓x7th **V93.24** **Heat exposure on board sailboat**

✓x7th **V93.29** **Heat exposure on board unspecified watercraft**
Heat exposure on board boat NOS
Heat exposure on board ship NOS
Heat exposure on board watercraft NOS

✓5th **V93.3** **Fall on board watercraft**
EXCLUDES 1   *fall due to collision of watercraft (V91.2-)*

✓x7th **V93.3Ø** **Fall on board merchant ship**

✓x7th **V93.31** **Fall on board passenger ship**
Fall on board Ferry-boat
Fall on board Liner

✓x7th **V93.32** **Fall on board fishing boat**

✓x7th **V93.33** **Fall on board other powered watercraft**
Fall on board Hovercraft (on open water)
Fall on board Jet ski

✓x7th **V93.34** **Fall on board sailboat**

✓x7th **V93.35** **Fall on board canoe or kayak**

✓x7th **V93.36** **Fall on board (nonpowered) inflatable craft**

✓x7th **V93.38** **Fall on board other unpowered watercraft**

✓x7th **V93.39** **Fall on board unspecified watercraft**
Fall on board boat NOS
Fall on board ship NOS
Fall on board watercraft NOS

✓5th **V93.4** **Struck by falling object on board watercraft**
Hit by falling object on board watercraft
EXCLUDES 1   *struck by falling object due to accident to watercraft (V91.3)*

✓x7th **V93.4Ø** **Struck by falling object on merchant ship**

✓x7th **V93.41** **Struck by falling object on passenger ship**
Struck by falling object on Ferry-boat
Struck by falling object on Liner

✓x7th **V93.42** **Struck by falling object on fishing boat**

✓x7th **V93.43** **Struck by falling object on other powered watercraft**
Struck by falling object on Hovercraft

✓x7th **V93.44** **Struck by falling object on sailboat**

✓x7th **V93.48** **Struck by falling object on other unpowered watercraft**

✓x7th **V93.49** **Struck by falling object on unspecified watercraft**

✓5th **V93.5** **Explosion on board watercraft**
Boiler explosion on steamship
EXCLUDES 2   *fire on board watercraft (V93.Ø-)*

✓x7th **V93.5Ø** **Explosion on board merchant ship**

✓x7th **V93.51** **Explosion on board passenger ship**
Explosion on board Ferry-boat
Explosion on board Liner

✓x7th **V93.52** **Explosion on board fishing boat**

✓x7th **V93.53** **Explosion on board other powered watercraft**
Explosion on board Hovercraft
Explosion on board Jet ski

✓x7th **V93.54** **Explosion on board sailboat**

✓x7th **V93.59** **Explosion on board unspecified watercraft**
Explosion on board boat NOS
Explosion on board ship NOS
Explosion on board watercraft NOS

✓5th **V93.6** **Machinery accident on board watercraft**
EXCLUDES 1   *machinery explosion on board watercraft (V93.4-)*
machinery fire on board watercraft (V93.Ø-)

✓x7th **V93.6Ø** **Machinery accident on board merchant ship**

✓x7th **V93.61** **Machinery accident on board passenger ship**
Machinery accident on board Ferry-boat
Machinery accident on board Liner

✓x7th **V93.62** **Machinery accident on board fishing boat**

✓x7th **V93.63** **Machinery accident on board other powered watercraft**
Machinery accident on board Hovercraft

✓x7th **V93.64** **Machinery accident on board sailboat**

✓x7th **V93.69** **Machinery accident on board unspecified watercraft**
Machinery accident on board boat NOS
Machinery accident on board ship NOS
Machinery accident on board watercraft NOS

✓5th **V93.8** **Other injury due to other accident on board watercraft**
Accidental poisoning by gases or fumes on watercraft

✓x7th **V93.8Ø** **Other injury due to other accident on board merchant ship**

✓x7th **V93.81** **Other injury due to other accident on board passenger ship**
Other injury due to other accident on board Ferry-boat
Other injury due to other accident on board Liner

✓x7th **V93.82** **Other injury due to other accident on board fishing boat**

✓x7th **V93.83** **Other injury due to other accident on board other powered watercraft**
Other injury due to other accident on board Hovercraft
Other injury due to other accident on board Jet ski

✓x7th **V93.84** **Other injury due to other accident on board sailboat**

✓x7th **V93.85** **Other injury due to other accident on board canoe or kayak**

✓x7th **V93.86** **Other injury due to other accident on board (nonpowered) inflatable craft**

✓x7th **V93.87** **Other injury due to other accident on board water-skis**
Hit or struck by object while waterskiing

✓x7th **V93.88** **Other injury due to other accident on board other unpowered watercraft**
Hit or struck by object while surfing
Hit or struck by object while on board windsurfer

✓x7th **V93.89** **Other injury due to other accident on board unspecified watercraft**
Other injury due to other accident on board boat NOS
Other injury due to other accident on board ship NOS
Other injury due to other accident on board watercraft NOS

✓4ᵗʰ V94 Other and unspecified water transport accidents

> EXCLUDES 1   *military watercraft accidents in military or war operations (Y36, Y37)*

✓x7ᵗʰ V94.0 Hitting object or bottom of body of water due to fall from watercraft

> EXCLUDES 2   *drowning and submersion due to fall from watercraft (V92.0-)*

✓5ᵗʰ V94.1 Bather struck by watercraft

> Swimmer hit by watercraft

✓x7ᵗʰ V94.11 Bather struck by powered watercraft

✓x7ᵗʰ V94.12 Bather struck by nonpowered watercraft

✓5ᵗʰ V94.2 Rider of nonpowered watercraft struck by other watercraft

✓x7ᵗʰ V94.21 Rider of nonpowered watercraft struck by other nonpowered watercraft

> Canoer hit by other nonpowered watercraft
> Surfer hit by other nonpowered watercraft
> Windsurfer hit by other nonpowered watercraft

✓x7ᵗʰ V94.22 Rider of nonpowered watercraft struck by powered watercraft

> Canoer hit by motorboat
> Surfer hit by motorboat
> Windsurfer hit by motorboat

✓5ᵗʰ V94.3 Injury to rider of (inflatable) watercraft being pulled behind other watercraft

✓x7ᵗʰ V94.31 Injury to rider of (inflatable) recreational watercraft being pulled behind other watercraft

> Injury to rider of inner-tube pulled behind motor boat

✓x7ᵗʰ V94.32 Injury to rider of non-recreational watercraft being pulled behind other watercraft

> Injury to occupant of dingy being pulled behind boat or ship
> Injury to occupant of life-raft being pulled behind boat or ship

✓x7ᵗʰ V94.4 Injury to barefoot water-skier

> Injury to person being pulled behind boat or ship

✓5ᵗʰ V94.8 Other water transport accident

✓6ᵗʰ V94.81 Water transport accident involving military watercraft

✓7ᵗʰ V94.810 Civilian watercraft involved in water transport accident with military watercraft

> Passenger on civilian watercraft injured due to accident with military watercraft

✓7ᵗʰ V94.811 Civilian in water injured by military watercraft

✓7ᵗʰ V94.818 Other water transport accident involving military watercraft

✓x7ᵗʰ V94.89 Other water transport accident

✓x7ᵗʰ V94.9 Unspecified water transport accident

> Water transport accident NOS

Air and space transport accidents (V95-V97)

> EXCLUDES 1   *military aircraft accidents in military or war operations (Y36, Y37)*

The appropriate 7th character is to be added to each code from categories V95-V97.
A   initial encounter
D   subsequent encounter
S   sequela

✓4ᵗʰ V95 Accident to powered aircraft causing injury to occupant

✓5ᵗʰ V95.0 Helicopter accident injuring occupant

✓x7ᵗʰ V95.00 Unspecified helicopter accident injuring occupant

✓x7ᵗʰ V95.01 Helicopter crash injuring occupant

✓x7ᵗʰ V95.02 Forced landing of helicopter injuring occupant

✓x7ᵗʰ V95.03 Helicopter collision injuring occupant

> Helicopter collision with any object, fixed, movable or moving

✓x7ᵗʰ V95.04 Helicopter fire injuring occupant

✓x7ᵗʰ V95.05 Helicopter explosion injuring occupant

✓x7ᵗʰ V95.09 Other helicopter accident injuring occupant

✓5ᵗʰ V95.1 Ultralight, microlight or powered-glider accident injuring occupant

✓x7ᵗʰ V95.10 Unspecified ultralight, microlight or powered-glider accident injuring occupant

✓x7ᵗʰ V95.11 Ultralight, microlight or powered-glider crash injuring occupant

✓x7ᵗʰ V95.12 Forced landing of ultralight, microlight or powered-glider injuring occupant

✓x7ᵗʰ V95.13 Ultralight, microlight or powered-glider collision injuring occupant

> Ultralight, microlight or powered-glider collision with any object, fixed, movable or moving

✓x7ᵗʰ V95.14 Ultralight, microlight or powered-glider fire injuring occupant

✓x7ᵗʰ V95.15 Ultralight, microlight or powered-glider explosion injuring occupant

✓x7ᵗʰ V95.19 Other ultralight, microlight or powered-glider accident injuring occupant

✓5ᵗʰ V95.2 Other private fixed-wing aircraft accident injuring occupant

✓x7ᵗʰ V95.20 Unspecified accident to other private fixed-wing aircraft, injuring occupant

✓x7ᵗʰ V95.21 Other private fixed-wing aircraft crash injuring occupant

✓x7ᵗʰ V95.22 Forced landing of other private fixed-wing aircraft injuring occupant

✓x7ᵗʰ V95.23 Other private fixed-wing aircraft collision injuring occupant

> Other private fixed-wing aircraft collision with any object, fixed, movable or moving

✓x7ᵗʰ V95.24 Other private fixed-wing aircraft fire injuring occupant

✓x7ᵗʰ V95.25 Other private fixed-wing aircraft explosion injuring occupant

✓x7ᵗʰ V95.29 Other accident to other private fixed-wing aircraft injuring occupant

✓5ᵗʰ V95.3 Commercial fixed-wing aircraft accident injuring occupant

✓x7ᵗʰ V95.30 Unspecified accident to commercial fixed-wing aircraft injuring occupant

✓x7ᵗʰ V95.31 Commercial fixed-wing aircraft crash injuring occupant

✓x7ᵗʰ V95.32 Forced landing of commercial fixed-wing aircraft injuring occupant

✓x7ᵗʰ V95.33 Commercial fixed-wing aircraft collision injuring occupant

> Commercial fixed-wing aircraft collision with any object, fixed, movable or moving

✓x7ᵗʰ V95.34 Commercial fixed-wing aircraft fire injuring occupant

✓x7ᵗʰ V95.35 Commercial fixed-wing aircraft explosion injuring occupant

✓x7ᵗʰ V95.39 Other accident to commercial fixed-wing aircraft injuring occupant

✓5ᵗʰ V95.4 Spacecraft accident injuring occupant

✓x7ᵗʰ V95.40 Unspecified spacecraft accident injuring occupant

✓x7ᵗʰ V95.41 Spacecraft crash injuring occupant

✓x7ᵗʰ V95.42 Forced landing of spacecraft injuring occupant

✓x7ᵗʰ V95.43 Spacecraft collision injuring occupant

> Spacecraft collision with any object, fixed, moveable or moving

✓x7ᵗʰ V95.44 Spacecraft fire injuring occupant

✓x7ᵗʰ V95.45 Spacecraft explosion injuring occupant

✓x7ᵗʰ V95.49 Other spacecraft accident injuring occupant

✓x7ᵗʰ V95.8 Other powered aircraft accidents injuring occupant

✓x7ᵗʰ V95.9 Unspecified aircraft accident injuring occupant

> Aircraft accident NOS
> Air transport accident NOS

✓4ᵗʰ V96 Accident to nonpowered aircraft causing injury to occupant

✓5ᵗʰ V96.0 Balloon accident injuring occupant

✓x7ᵗʰ V96.00 Unspecified balloon accident injuring occupant

✓x7ᵗʰ V96.01 Balloon crash injuring occupant

✓x7ᵗʰ V96.02 Forced landing of balloon injuring occupant

✓x7ᵗʰ V96.03 Balloon collision injuring occupant

> Balloon collision with any object, fixed, moveable or moving

✓x7ᵗʰ V96.04 Balloon fire injuring occupant

✓x7ᵗʰ V96.05 Balloon explosion injuring occupant

✓x7ᵗʰ V96.09 Other balloon accident injuring occupant

✓5ᵗʰ V96.1 Hang-glider accident injuring occupant

✓x7ᵗʰ V96.10 Unspecified hang-glider accident injuring occupant

✓x7ᵗʰ V96.11 Hang-glider crash injuring occupant

✓x7ᵗʰ V96.12 Forced landing of hang-glider injuring occupant

✔ Additional Char Req   ✓x7ᵗʰ Placeholder   Unacceptable PDx   Questionable PDx   Wrong Procedure   Manifestation   Unspecified   H1-H14 HAC   HCC CMS-HCC Dx   HIV HIV Dx

√x 7th **V96.13** **Hang-glider collision injuring occupant**
Hang-glider collision with any object, fixed, moveable or moving

√x 7th **V96.14** **Hang-glider fire injuring occupant**

√x 7th **V96.15** **Hang-glider explosion injuring occupant**

√x 7th **V96.19** **Other hang-glider accident injuring occupant**

✓5th **V96.2** **Glider (nonpowered) accident injuring occupant**

√x 7th **V96.20** **Unspecified glider (nonpowered) accident injuring occupant**

√x 7th **V96.21** **Glider (nonpowered) crash injuring occupant**

√x 7th **V96.22** **Forced landing of glider (nonpowered) injuring occupant**

√x 7th **V96.23** **Glider (nonpowered) collision injuring occupant**
Glider (nonpowered) collision with any object, fixed, moveable or moving

√x 7th **V96.24** **Glider (nonpowered) fire injuring occupant**

√x 7th **V96.25** **Glider (nonpowered) explosion injuring occupant**

√x 7th **V96.29** **Other glider (nonpowered) accident injuring occupant**

√x 7th **V96.8** **Other nonpowered-aircraft accidents injuring occupant**
Kite carrying a person accident injuring occupant

√x 7th **V96.9** **Unspecified nonpowered-aircraft accident injuring occupant**
Nonpowered-aircraft accident NOS

✓4th **V97** **Other specified air transport accidents**

√x 7th **V97.0** **Occupant of aircraft injured in other specified air transport accidents**
Fall in, on or from aircraft in air transport accident
EXCLUDES 1   accident while boarding or alighting aircraft (V97.1)

√x 7th **V97.1** **Person injured while boarding or alighting from aircraft**

✓5th **V97.2** **Parachutist accident**

√x 7th **V97.21** **Parachutist entangled in object**
Parachutist landing in tree

√x 7th **V97.22** **Parachutist injured on landing**

√x 7th **V97.29** **Other parachutist accident**

✓5th **V97.3** **Person on ground injured in air transport accident**

√x 7th **V97.31** **Hit by object falling from aircraft**
Hit by crashing aircraft
Injured by aircraft hitting house
Injured by aircraft hitting car

√x 7th **V97.32** **Injured by rotating propeller**

√x 7th **V97.33** **Sucked into jet engine**

√x 7th **V97.39** **Other injury to person on ground due to air transport accident**

✓5th **V97.8** **Other air transport accidents, not elsewhere classified**
EXCLUDES 1   aircraft accident NOS (V95.9)
exposure to changes in air pressure during ascent or descent (W94.-)

✓6th **V97.81** **Air transport accident involving military aircraft**

✓7th **V97.810** **Civilian aircraft involved in air transport accident with military aircraft**
Passenger in civilian aircraft injured due to accident with military aircraft

✓7th **V97.811** **Civilian injured by military aircraft**

✓7th **V97.818** **Other air transport accident involving military aircraft**

√x 7th **V97.89** **Other air transport accidents, not elsewhere classified**
Injury from machinery on aircraft

Other and unspecified transport accidents (V98-V99)

EXCLUDES 1   vehicle accident, type of vehicle unspecified (V89.-)

The appropriate 7th character is to be added to each code from categories V98-V99.
A   initial encounter
D   subsequent encounter
S   sequela

✓4th **V98** **Other specified transport accidents**

√x 7th **V98.0** **Accident to, on or involving cable-car, not on rails**
Caught or dragged by cable-car, not on rails
Fall or jump from cable-car, not on rails
Object thrown from or in cable-car, not on rails

√x 7th **V98.1** **Accident to, on or involving land-yacht**

√x 7th **V98.2** **Accident to, on or involving ice yacht**

√x 7th **V98.3** **Accident to, on or involving ski lift**
Accident to, on or involving ski chair-lift
Accident to, on or involving ski-lift with gondola

√x 7th **V98.8** **Other specified transport accidents**

√x 7th **V99** **Unspecified transport accident**

OTHER EXTERNAL CAUSES OF ACCIDENTAL INJURY (W00-X58)

Slipping, tripping, stumbling and falls (W00-W19)

EXCLUDES 1   assault involving a fall (Y01-Y02)
fall from animal (V80.-)
fall (in) (from) machinery (in operation) (W28-W31)
fall (in) (from) transport vehicle (V01-V99)
intentional self-harm involving a fall (X80-X81)

EXCLUDES 2   at risk for fall (history of fall) Z91.81
fall (in) (from) burning building (X00.-)
fall into fire (X00-X04, X08)

The appropriate 7th character is to be added to each code from categories W00-W19.
A   initial encounter
D   subsequent encounter
S   sequela

✓4th **W00** **Fall due to ice and snow**
INCLUDES   pedestrian on foot falling (slipping) on ice and snow
EXCLUDES 1   fall on (from) ice and snow involving pedestrian conveyance (V00.-)
fall from stairs and steps not due to ice and snow (W10.-)
AHA: 2016,2Q,4

√x 7th **W00.0** **Fall on same level due to ice and snow**

√x 7th **W00.1** **Fall from stairs and steps due to ice and snow**

√x 7th **W00.2** **Other fall from one level to another due to ice and snow**

√x 7th **W00.9** **Unspecified fall due to ice and snow**

✓4th **W01** **Fall on same level from slipping, tripping and stumbling**
INCLUDES   fall on moving sidewalk
EXCLUDES 1   fall due to bumping (striking) against object (W18.0-)
fall in shower or bathtub (W18.2-)
fall on same level NOS (W18.30)
fall on same level from slipping, tripping and stumbling due to ice or snow (W00.0)
fall off or from toilet (W18.1-)
slipping, tripping and stumbling NOS (W18.40)
slipping, tripping and stumbling without falling (W18.4-)

√x 7th **W01.0** **Fall on same level from slipping, tripping and stumbling without subsequent striking against object**
Falling over animal

✓5th **W01.1** **Fall on same level from slipping, tripping and stumbling with subsequent striking against object**

√x 7th **W01.10** **Fall on same level from slipping, tripping and stumbling with subsequent striking against unspecified object**

✓6th **W01.11** **Fall on same level from slipping, tripping and stumbling with subsequent striking against sharp object**

✓7th **W01.110** **Fall on same level from slipping, tripping and stumbling with subsequent striking against sharp glass**

✓7th **W01.111** **Fall on same level from slipping, tripping and stumbling with subsequent striking against power tool or machine**

✓7th **W01.118** **Fall on same level from slipping, tripping and stumbling with subsequent striking against other sharp object**

✓7th **W01.119** **Fall on same level from slipping, tripping and stumbling with subsequent striking against unspecified sharp object**

✓6th **W01.19** **Fall on same level from slipping, tripping and stumbling with subsequent striking against other object**

✓7th **W01.190** **Fall on same level from slipping, tripping and stumbling with subsequent striking against furniture**

✓7th **W01.198** **Fall on same level from slipping, tripping and stumbling with subsequent striking against other object**

✓x7ᵗʰ **W03** **Other fall on same level due to collision with another person**
> Fall due to non-transport collision with other person
> *EXCLUDES 1*   collision with another person without fall (W51)
> crushed or pushed by a crowd or human stampede (W52)
> fall due to ice or snow (W00)
> fall involving pedestrian conveyance (V00-V09)
> fall on same level NOS (W18.30)
> **AHA:** 2012,4Q,108

✓x7ᵗʰ **W04** **Fall while being carried or supported by other persons**
> Accidentally dropped while being carried

✓4ᵗʰ **W05** **Fall from non-moving wheelchair, nonmotorized scooter and motorized mobility scooter**
> *EXCLUDES 1*   fall from moving motorized mobility scooter (V00.831)
> fall from moving wheelchair (powered) (V00.811)
> fall from nonmotorized scooter (V00.141)

    ✓7ᵗʰ **W05.0** **Fall from non-moving wheelchair**
>   **AHA:** 2019,2Q,27

    ✓7ᵗʰ **W05.1** **Fall from non-moving nonmotorized scooter**

    ✓7ᵗʰ **W05.2** **Fall from non-moving motorized mobility scooter**

✓x7ᵗʰ **W06** **Fall from bed**

✓x7ᵗʰ **W07** **Fall from chair**

✓x7ᵗʰ **W08** **Fall from other furniture**
> Fall from stool

✓4ᵗʰ **W09** **Fall on and from playground equipment**
> *EXCLUDES 1*   fall involving recreational machinery (W31)

    ✓x7ᵗʰ **W09.0** **Fall on or from playground slide**

    ✓x7ᵗʰ **W09.1** **Fall from playground swing**

    ✓x7ᵗʰ **W09.2** **Fall on or from jungle gym**

    ✓x7ᵗʰ **W09.8** **Fall on or from other playground equipment**

✓4ᵗʰ **W10** **Fall on and from stairs and steps**
> *EXCLUDES 1*   Fall from stairs and steps due to ice and snow (W00.1)

    ✓x7ᵗʰ **W10.0** **Fall (on)(from) escalator**

    ✓x7ᵗʰ **W10.1** **Fall (on)(from) sidewalk curb**

    ✓x7ᵗʰ **W10.2** **Fall (on)(from) incline**
> Fall (on) (from) ramp

    ✓x7ᵗʰ **W10.8** **Fall (on) (from) other stairs and steps**

    ✓x7ᵗʰ **W10.9** **Fall (on) (from) unspecified stairs and steps**

✓x7ᵗʰ **W11** **Fall on and from ladder**

✓x7ᵗʰ **W12** **Fall on and from scaffolding**

✓4ᵗʰ **W13** **Fall from, out of or through building or structure**

    ✓x7ᵗʰ **W13.0** **Fall from, out of or through balcony**
> Fall from, out of or through railing

    ✓x7ᵗʰ **W13.1** **Fall from, out of or through bridge**

    ✓x7ᵗʰ **W13.2** **Fall from, out of or through roof**

    ✓x7ᵗʰ **W13.3** **Fall through floor**

    ✓x7ᵗʰ **W13.4** **Fall from, out of or through window**
> *EXCLUDES 2*   fall with subsequent striking against sharp glass (W01.110-)

    ✓x7ᵗʰ **W13.8** **Fall from, out of or through other building or structure**
> Fall from, out of or through viaduct
> Fall from, out of or through wall
> Fall from, out of or through flag-pole

    ✓x7ᵗʰ **W13.9** **Fall from, out of or through building, not otherwise specified**
> *EXCLUDES 1*   collapse of a building or structure (W20.-)
> fall or jump from burning building or structure (X00.-)

✓x7ᵗʰ **W14** **Fall from tree**

✓x7ᵗʰ **W15** **Fall from cliff**

✓4ᵗʰ **W16** **Fall, jump or diving into water**
> *EXCLUDES 1*   accidental non-watercraft drowning and submersion not involving fall (W65-W74)
> effects of air pressure from diving (W94.-)
> fall into water from watercraft (V90-V94)
> hitting an object or against bottom when falling from watercraft (V94.0)
> *EXCLUDES 2*   striking or hitting diving board (W21.4)

    ✓5ᵗʰ **W16.0** **Fall into swimming pool**
> Fall into swimming pool NOS
> *EXCLUDES 1*   fall into empty swimming pool (W17.3)

      ✓6ᵗʰ **W16.01** **Fall into swimming pool striking water surface**

        ✓7ᵗʰ **W16.011** **Fall into swimming pool striking water surface causing drowning and submersion**
> *EXCLUDES 1*   drowning and submersion while in swimming pool without fall (W67)

        ✓7ᵗʰ **W16.012** **Fall into swimming pool striking water surface causing other injury**

      ✓6ᵗʰ **W16.02** **Fall into swimming pool striking bottom**

        ✓7ᵗʰ **W16.021** **Fall into swimming pool striking bottom causing drowning and submersion**
> *EXCLUDES 1*   drowning and submersion while in swimming pool without fall (W67)

        ✓7ᵗʰ **W16.022** **Fall into swimming pool striking bottom causing other injury**

      ✓6ᵗʰ **W16.03** **Fall into swimming pool striking wall**

        ✓7ᵗʰ **W16.031** **Fall into swimming pool striking wall causing drowning and submersion**
> *EXCLUDES 1*   drowning and submersion while in swimming pool without fall (W67)

        ✓7ᵗʰ **W16.032** **Fall into swimming pool striking wall causing other injury**

    ✓5ᵗʰ **W16.1** **Fall into natural body of water**
> Fall into lake
> Fall into open sea
> Fall into river
> Fall into stream

      ✓6ᵗʰ **W16.11** **Fall into natural body of water striking water surface**

        ✓7ᵗʰ **W16.111** **Fall into natural body of water striking water surface causing drowning and submersion**
> *EXCLUDES 1*   drowning and submersion while in natural body of water without fall (W69)

        ✓7ᵗʰ **W16.112** **Fall into natural body of water striking water surface causing other injury**

      ✓6ᵗʰ **W16.12** **Fall into natural body of water striking bottom**

        ✓7ᵗʰ **W16.121** **Fall into natural body of water striking bottom causing drowning and submersion**
> *EXCLUDES 1*   drowning and submersion while in natural body of water without fall (W69)

        ✓7ᵗʰ **W16.122** **Fall into natural body of water striking bottom causing other injury**

      ✓6ᵗʰ **W16.13** **Fall into natural body of water striking side**

        ✓7ᵗʰ **W16.131** **Fall into natural body of water striking side causing drowning and submersion**
> *EXCLUDES 1*   drowning and submersion while in natural body of water without fall (W69)

        ✓7ᵗʰ **W16.132** **Fall into natural body of water striking side causing other injury**

    ✓5ᵗʰ **W16.2** **Fall in (into) filled bathtub or bucket of water**

      ✓6ᵗʰ **W16.21** **Fall in (into) filled bathtub**
> *EXCLUDES 1*   fall into empty bathtub (W18.2)

        ✓7ᵗʰ **W16.211** **Fall in (into) filled bathtub causing drowning and submersion**
> *EXCLUDES 1*   drowning and submersion while in filled bathtub without fall (W65)

        ✓7ᵗʰ **W16.212** **Fall in (into) filled bathtub causing other injury**

√6ᵗʰ **W16.22** **Fall in (into)** bucket of water

   √7ᵗʰ **W16.221** **Fall in (into) bucket of water causing** drowning and submersion

   √7ᵗʰ **W16.222** **Fall in (into) bucket of water causing other injury**

√5ᵗʰ **W16.3** **Fall into other water**

   Fall into fountain
   Fall into reservoir

  √6ᵗʰ **W16.31** **Fall into other water** striking water surface

    √7ᵗʰ **W16.311** **Fall into other water striking water surface causing** drowning and submersion

     EXCLUDES 1 *drowning and submersion while in other water without fall (W73)*

    √7ᵗʰ **W16.312** **Fall into other water striking water surface causing other injury**

  √6ᵗʰ **W16.32** **Fall into other water** striking bottom

    √7ᵗʰ **W16.321** **Fall into other water striking bottom causing** drowning and submersion

     EXCLUDES 1 *drowning and submersion while in other water without fall (W73)*

    √7ᵗʰ **W16.322** **Fall into other water striking bottom causing other injury**

  √6ᵗʰ **W16.33** **Fall into other water** striking wall

    √7ᵗʰ **W16.331** **Fall into other water striking wall causing** drowning and submersion

     EXCLUDES 1 *drowning and submersion while in other water without fall (W73)*

    √7ᵗʰ **W16.332** **Fall into other water striking wall causing other injury**

√5ᵗʰ **W16.4** **Fall into unspecified water**

  √x7ᵗʰ **W16.41** **Fall into unspecified water causing** drowning and submersion

  √x7ᵗʰ **W16.42** **Fall into unspecified water causing other injury**

√5ᵗʰ **W16.5** **Jumping or diving into** swimming pool

  √6ᵗʰ **W16.51** **Jumping or diving into swimming pool** striking water surface

    √7ᵗʰ **W16.511** **Jumping or diving into swimming pool striking water surface causing** drowning and submersion

     EXCLUDES 1 *drowning and submersion while in swimming pool without jumping or diving (W67)*

    √7ᵗʰ **W16.512** **Jumping or diving into swimming pool striking water surface causing other injury**

  √6ᵗʰ **W16.52** **Jumping or diving into swimming pool** striking bottom

    √7ᵗʰ **W16.521** **Jumping or diving into swimming pool striking bottom causing** drowning and submersion

     EXCLUDES 1 *drowning and submersion while in swimming pool without jumping or diving (W67)*

    √7ᵗʰ **W16.522** **Jumping or diving into swimming pool striking bottom causing other injury**

  √6ᵗʰ **W16.53** **Jumping or diving into swimming pool** striking wall

    √7ᵗʰ **W16.531** **Jumping or diving into swimming pool striking wall causing** drowning and submersion

     EXCLUDES 1 *drowning and submersion while in swimming pool without jumping or diving (W67)*

    √7ᵗʰ **W16.532** **Jumping or diving into swimming pool striking wall causing other injury**

√5ᵗʰ **W16.6** **Jumping or diving into** natural body of water

   Jumping or diving into lake
   Jumping or diving into open sea
   Jumping or diving into river
   Jumping or diving into stream

  √6ᵗʰ **W16.61** **Jumping or diving into natural body of water** striking water surface

    √7ᵗʰ **W16.611** **Jumping or diving into natural body of water striking water surface causing** drowning and submersion

     EXCLUDES 1 *drowning and submersion while in natural body of water without jumping or diving (W69)*

    √7ᵗʰ **W16.612** **Jumping or diving into natural body of water striking water surface causing other injury**

  √6ᵗʰ **W16.62** **Jumping or diving into natural body of water** striking bottom

    √7ᵗʰ **W16.621** **Jumping or diving into natural body of water striking bottom causing** drowning and submersion

     EXCLUDES 1 *drowning and submersion while in natural body of water without jumping or diving (W69)*

    √7ᵗʰ **W16.622** **Jumping or diving into natural body of water striking bottom causing other injury**

√5ᵗʰ **W16.7** **Jumping or diving** from boat

   EXCLUDES 1 *fall from boat into water - see watercraft accident (V90-V94)*

  √6ᵗʰ **W16.71** **Jumping or diving from boat** striking water surface

    √7ᵗʰ **W16.711** **Jumping or diving from boat striking water surface causing** drowning and submersion

    √7ᵗʰ **W16.712** **Jumping or diving from boat striking water surface causing other injury**

  √6ᵗʰ **W16.72** **Jumping or diving from boat** striking bottom

    √7ᵗʰ **W16.721** **Jumping or diving from boat striking bottom causing** drowning and submersion

    √7ᵗʰ **W16.722** **Jumping or diving from boat striking bottom causing other injury**

√5ᵗʰ **W16.8** **Jumping or diving into other water**

   Jumping or diving into fountain
   Jumping or diving into reservoir

  √6ᵗʰ **W16.81** **Jumping or diving into other water** striking water surface

    √7ᵗʰ **W16.811** **Jumping or diving into other water striking water surface causing** drowning and submersion

     EXCLUDES 1 *drowning and submersion while in other water without jumping or diving (W73)*

    √7ᵗʰ **W16.812** **Jumping or diving into other water striking water surface causing other injury**

  √6ᵗʰ **W16.82** **Jumping or diving into other water** striking bottom

    √7ᵗʰ **W16.821** **Jumping or diving into other water striking bottom causing** drowning and submersion

     EXCLUDES 1 *drowning and submersion while in other water without jumping or diving (W73)*

    √7ᵗʰ **W16.822** **Jumping or diving into other water striking bottom causing other injury**

  √6ᵗʰ **W16.83** **Jumping or diving into other water** striking wall

    √7ᵗʰ **W16.831** **Jumping or diving into other water striking wall causing** drowning and submersion

     EXCLUDES 1 *drowning and submersion while in other water without jumping or diving (W73)*

    √7ᵗʰ **W16.832** **Jumping or diving into other water striking wall causing other injury**

√5ᵗʰ **W16.9** **Jumping or diving into unspecified water**

  √x7ᵗʰ **W16.91** **Jumping or diving into unspecified water causing** drowning and submersion

  √x7ᵗʰ **W16.92** **Jumping or diving into unspecified water causing other injury**

√4ᵗʰ **W17** **Other fall from one level to another**

  √x7ᵗʰ **W17.0** **Fall into well**

  √x7ᵗʰ **W17.1** **Fall into storm drain or manhole**

N Newborn: 0   P Pediatric: 0-17   M Maternity: 9-64   A Adult: 15-124   UNS Unspecified Site   MCC Major Complication/Comorbidity   CC Complication/Comorbidity   PE POA Exempt

1228   ICD-10-CM 2025

Chapter 20. External Causes of Morbidity

√x7th **W17.2** **Fall into hole**
> Fall into pit

√x7th **W17.3** **Fall into empty swimming pool**
> > *EXCLUDES 1*   fall into filled swimming pool (W16.0-)

√x7th **W17.4** **Fall from dock**

√5th **W17.8** **Other fall from one level to another**

> √x7th **W17.81** **Fall down embankment (hill)**

> √x7th **W17.82** **Fall from (out of) grocery cart**
> > Fall due to grocery cart tipping over

> √x7th **W17.89** **Other fall from one level to another**
> > Fall from cherry picker
> > Fall from lifting device
> > Fall from mobile elevated work platform [MEWP]
> > Fall from sky lift
> > **AHA:** 2015,2Q,6

√4th **W18** **Other slipping, tripping and stumbling and falls**

> √5th **W18.0** **Fall due to bumping against object**
> > Striking against object with subsequent fall
> > > *EXCLUDES 1*   fall on same level due to slipping, tripping, or stumbling
> > > with subsequent striking against object (W01.1-)

> > √x7th **W18.00** **Striking against unspecified object with subsequent fall**

> > √x7th **W18.01** **Striking against sports equipment with subsequent fall**

> > √x7th **W18.02** **Striking against glass with subsequent fall**

> > √x7th **W18.09** **Striking against other object with subsequent fall**

> √5th **W18.1** **Fall from or off toilet**

> > √x7th **W18.11** **Fall from or off toilet without subsequent striking against object**
> > > Fall from (off) toilet NOS

> > √x7th **W18.12** **Fall from or off toilet with subsequent striking against object**

> √x7th **W18.2** **Fall in (into) shower or empty bathtub**
> > > *EXCLUDES 1*   fall in full bathtub causing drowning or submersion
> > > (W16.21-)

> √5th **W18.3** **Other and unspecified fall on same level**

> > √x7th **W18.30** **Fall on same level, unspecified**

> > √x7th **W18.31** **Fall on same level due to stepping on an object**
> > > Fall on same level due to stepping on an animal
> > > > *EXCLUDES 1*   slipping, tripping and stumbling without
> > > > fall due to stepping on animal
> > > > (W18.41)

> > √x7th **W18.39** **Other fall on same level**

> √5th **W18.4** **Slipping, tripping and stumbling without falling**
> > > *EXCLUDES 1*   collision with another person without fall (W51)

> > √x7th **W18.40** **Slipping, tripping and stumbling without falling, unspecified**

> > √x7th **W18.41** **Slipping, tripping and stumbling without falling due to stepping on object**
> > > Slipping, tripping and stumbling without falling due to stepping on animal
> > > > *EXCLUDES 1*   slipping, tripping and stumbling with fall
> > > > due to stepping on animal (W18.31)

> > √x7th **W18.42** **Slipping, tripping and stumbling without falling due to stepping into hole or opening**

> > √x7th **W18.43** **Slipping, tripping and stumbling without falling due to stepping from one level to another**

> > √x7th **W18.49** **Other slipping, tripping and stumbling without falling**

√x7th **W19** **Unspecified fall**
> Accidental fall NOS
> **AHA:** 2012,4Q,95

Exposure to inanimate mechanical forces (W20-W49)

> *EXCLUDES 1*   assault (X92-Y09)
> contact or collision with animals or persons (W50-W64)
> exposure to inanimate mechanical forces involving military or war
> operations (Y36.-, Y37.-)
> intentional self-harm (X71-X83)

The appropriate 7th character is to be added to each code from categories W20-W49.
A   initial encounter
D   subsequent encounter
S   sequela

√4th **W20** **Struck by thrown, projected or falling object**

> Code first any associated:
> cataclysm (X34-X39)
> lightning strike (T75.00)
> > *EXCLUDES 1*   falling object in machinery accident (W24, W28-W31)
> > falling object in transport accident (V01-V99)
> > object set in motion by explosion (W35-W40)
> > object set in motion by firearm (W32-W34)
> > struck by thrown sports equipment (W21.-)

> √x7th **W20.0** **Struck by falling object in cave-in**
> > > *EXCLUDES 2*   asphyxiation due to cave-in (T71.21)

> √x7th **W20.1** **Struck by object due to collapse of building**
> > > *EXCLUDES 1*   struck by object due to collapse of burning building
> > > (X00.2, X02.2)

> √x7th **W20.8** **Other cause of strike by thrown, projected or falling object**
> > > *EXCLUDES 1*   struck by thrown sports equipment (W21.-)

√4th **W21** **Striking against or struck by sports equipment**
> > *EXCLUDES 1*   assault with sports equipment (Y08.0-)
> > striking against or struck by sports equipment with subsequent
> > fall (W18.01)

> √5th **W21.0** **Struck by hit or thrown ball**

> > √x7th **W21.00** **Struck by hit or thrown ball, unspecified type**

> > √x7th **W21.01** **Struck by football**

> > √x7th **W21.02** **Struck by soccer ball**

> > √x7th **W21.03** **Struck by baseball**

> > √x7th **W21.04** **Struck by golf ball**

> > √x7th **W21.05** **Struck by basketball**

> > √x7th **W21.06** **Struck by volleyball**

> > √x7th **W21.07** **Struck by softball**

> > √x7th **W21.09** **Struck by other hit or thrown ball**

> √5th **W21.1** **Struck by bat, racquet or club**

> > √x7th **W21.11** **Struck by baseball bat**

> > √x7th **W21.12** **Struck by tennis racquet**

> > √x7th **W21.13** **Struck by golf club**

> > √x7th **W21.19** **Struck by other bat, racquet or club**

> √5th **W21.2** **Struck by hockey stick or puck**

> > √6th **W21.21** **Struck by hockey stick**

> > > √7th **W21.210** **Struck by ice hockey stick**

> > > √7th **W21.211** **Struck by field hockey stick**

> > √6th **W21.22** **Struck by hockey puck**

> > > √7th **W21.220** **Struck by ice hockey puck**

> > > √7th **W21.221** **Struck by field hockey puck**

> √5th **W21.3** **Struck by sports foot wear**

> > √x7th **W21.31** **Struck by shoe cleats**
> > > Stepped on by shoe cleats

> > √x7th **W21.32** **Struck by skate blades**
> > > Skated over by skate blades

> > √x7th **W21.39** **Struck by other sports foot wear**

> √x7th **W21.4** **Striking against diving board**
> > Use additional code for subsequent falling into water, if applicable (W16.-)

> √5th **W21.8** **Striking against or struck by other sports equipment**

> > √x7th **W21.81** **Striking against or struck by football helmet**

> > √x7th **W21.89** **Striking against or struck by other sports equipment**

> √x7th **W21.9** **Striking against or struck by unspecified sports equipment**

√4th **W22 Striking against or struck by other objects**

EXCLUDES 1 *striking against or struck by object with subsequent fall (W18.09)*

√5th **W22.0 Striking against stationary object**

EXCLUDES 1 *striking against stationary sports equipment (W21.8)*

√x7th **W22.01 Walked into wall**

√x7th **W22.02 Walked into lamppost**

√x7th **W22.03 Walked into furniture**

√6th **W22.04 Striking against wall of swimming pool**

√7th **W22.041 Striking against wall of swimming pool causing drowning and submersion**

EXCLUDES 1 *drowning and submersion while swimming without striking against wall (W67)*

√7th **W22.042 Striking against wall of swimming pool causing other injury**

√x7th **W22.09 Striking against other stationary object**

√5th **W22.1 Striking against or struck by automobile airbag**

√x7th **W22.10 Striking against or struck by unspecified automobile airbag**

√x7th **W22.11 Striking against or struck by driver side automobile airbag**

√x7th **W22.12 Striking against or struck by front passenger side automobile airbag**

√x7th **W22.19 Striking against or struck by other automobile airbag**

√x7th **W22.8 Striking against or struck by other objects**

Striking against or struck by object NOS

EXCLUDES 1 *struck by thrown, projected or falling object (W20.-)*

√4th **W23 Caught, crushed, jammed or pinched in or between objects**

EXCLUDES 1 *injury caused by cutting or piercing instruments (W25-W27)*

injury caused by firearms malfunction (W32.1, W33.1-, W34.1-)

injury caused by lifting and transmission devices (W24.-)

injury caused by machinery (W28-W31)

injury caused by nonpowered hand tools (W27.-)

injury caused by struck by thrown, projected or falling object (W20.-)

injury caused by transport vehicle being used as a means of transportation (V01-V99)

√x7th **W23.0 Caught, crushed, jammed, or pinched between moving objects**

√x7th **W23.1 Caught, crushed, jammed, or pinched between stationary objects**

√x7th **W23.2 Caught, crushed, jammed, or pinched between a moving and stationary object**

AHA: 2022,4Q,48

√4th **W24 Contact with lifting and transmission devices, not elsewhere classified**

EXCLUDES 1 *transport accidents (V01-V99)*

√x7th **W24.0 Contact with lifting devices, not elsewhere classified**

Contact with chain hoist

Contact with drive belt

Contact with pulley (block)

√x7th **W24.1 Contact with transmission devices, not elsewhere classified**

Contact with transmission belt or cable

√x7th **W25 Contact with sharp glass**

Code first any associated:

injury due to flying glass from explosion or firearm discharge (W32-W40)

transport accident (V00-V99)

EXCLUDES 1 *fall on same level due to slipping, tripping and stumbling with subsequent striking against sharp glass (W01.110-)*

striking against sharp glass with subsequent fall (W18.02-)

EXCLUDES 2 *glass embedded in skin (W45.-)*

√4th **W26 Contact with other sharp objects**

EXCLUDES 2 *sharp object(s) embedded in skin (W45.-)*

AHA: 2016,4Q,73

√x7th **W26.0 Contact with knife**

EXCLUDES 1 *contact with electric knife (W29.1)*

√x7th **W26.1 Contact with sword or dagger**

√x7th **W26.2 Contact with edge of stiff paper**

Paper cut

√x7th **W26.8 Contact with other sharp object(s), not elsewhere classified**

Contact with tin can lid

√x7th **W26.9 Contact with unspecified sharp object(s)**

√4th **W27 Contact with nonpowered hand tool**

√x7th **W27.0 Contact with workbench tool**

Contact with auger

Contact with axe

Contact with chisel

Contact with handsaw

Contact with screwdriver

√x7th **W27.1 Contact with garden tool**

Contact with hoe

Contact with nonpowered lawn mower

Contact with pitchfork

Contact with rake

√x7th **W27.2 Contact with scissors**

√x7th **W27.3 Contact with needle (sewing)**

EXCLUDES 1 *contact with hypodermic needle (W46.-)*

√x7th **W27.4 Contact with kitchen utensil**

Contact with fork

Contact with ice-pick

Contact with can-opener NOS

√x7th **W27.5 Contact with paper-cutter**

√x7th **W27.8 Contact with other nonpowered hand tool**

Contact with nonpowered sewing machine

Contact with shovel

√x7th **W28 Contact with powered lawn mower**

Powered lawn mower (commercial) (residential)

EXCLUDES 1 *contact with nonpowered lawn mower (W27.1)*

EXCLUDES 2 *exposure to electric current (W86.-)*

√4th **W29 Contact with other powered hand tools and household machinery**

EXCLUDES 1 *contact with commercial machinery (W31.82)*

contact with hot household appliance (X15)

contact with nonpowered hand tool (W27.-)

exposure to electric current (W86)

√x7th **W29.0 Contact with powered kitchen appliance**

Contact with blender

Contact with can-opener

Contact with garbage disposal

Contact with mixer

√x7th **W29.1 Contact with electric knife**

√x7th **W29.2 Contact with other powered household machinery**

Contact with electric fan

Contact with powered dryer (clothes) (powered) (spin)

Contact with sewing machine

Contact with washing-machine

√x7th **W29.3 Contact with powered garden and outdoor hand tools and machinery**

Contact with chainsaw

Contact with edger

Contact with garden cultivator (tiller)

Contact with hedge trimmer

Contact with other powered garden tool

EXCLUDES 1 *contact with powered lawn mower (W28)*

√x7th **W29.4 Contact with nail gun**

√x7th **W29.8 Contact with other powered hand tools and household machinery**

Contact with do-it-yourself tool NOS

√4th **W30 Contact with agricultural machinery**

INCLUDES animal-powered farm machine

EXCLUDES 1 *agricultural transport vehicle accident (V01-V99)*

explosion of grain store (W40.8)

exposure to electric current (W86.-)

√x7th **W30.0 Contact with combine harvester**

Contact with reaper

Contact with thresher

√x7th **W30.1 Contact with power take-off devices (PTO)**

√x7th **W30.2 Contact with hay derrick**

√x7th **W30.3 Contact with grain storage elevator**

EXCLUDES 1 *explosion of grain store (W40.8)*

√5th **W30.8 Contact with other specified agricultural machinery**

√x7th **W30.81 Contact with agricultural transport vehicle in stationary use**

Contact with agricultural transport vehicle under repair, not on public roadway

EXCLUDES 1 *agricultural transport vehicle accident (V01-V99)*

√x7th **W30.89 Contact with other specified agricultural machinery**

N Newborn: 0   P Pediatric: 0-17   M Maternity: 9-64   A Adult: 15-124   UNS Unspecified Site   MCC Major Complication/Comorbidity   CC Complication/Comorbidity   PE POA Exempt

1230

ICD-10-CM 2025

√x7ᵗʰ **W30.9**   **Contact with unspecified agricultural machinery**
     Contact with farm machinery NOS

4ᵗʰ **W31**   **Contact with other and unspecified machinery**
     EXCLUDES 1   *contact with agricultural machinery (W30.-)*
         contact with machinery in transport under own power or being towed by a vehicle (V01-V99)
         exposure to electric current (W86)

√x7ᵗʰ **W31.0**   **Contact with mining and earth-drilling machinery**
     Contact with bore or drill (land) (seabed)
     Contact with shaft hoist
     Contact with shaft lift
     Contact with undercutter

√x7ᵗʰ **W31.1**   **Contact with metalworking machines**
     Contact with abrasive wheel
     Contact with forging machine
     Contact with lathe
     Contact with mechanical shears
     Contact with metal drilling machine
     Contact with milling machine
     Contact with power press
     Contact with rolling-mill
     Contact with metal sawing machine

√x7ᵗʰ **W31.2**   **Contact with powered woodworking and forming machines**
     Contact with band saw
     Contact with bench saw
     Contact with circular saw
     Contact with molding machine
     Contact with overhead plane
     Contact with powered saw
     Contact with radial saw
     Contact with sander
     EXCLUDES 1   *nonpowered woodworking tools (W27.0)*

√x7ᵗʰ **W31.3**   **Contact with prime movers**
     Contact with gas turbine
     Contact with internal combustion engine
     Contact with steam engine
     Contact with water driven turbine

√5ᵗʰ **W31.8**   **Contact with other specified machinery**

√x7ᵗʰ **W31.81**   **Contact with recreational machinery**
     Contact with roller coaster

√x7ᵗʰ **W31.82**   **Contact with other commercial machinery**
     Contact with commercial electric fan
     Contact with commercial kitchen appliances
     Contact with commercial powered dryer (clothes) (powered) (spin)
     Contact with commercial sewing machine
     Contact with commercial washing-machine
     EXCLUDES 1   *contact with household machinery (W29.-)*
         contact with powered lawn mower (W28)

√x7ᵗʰ **W31.83**   **Contact with special construction vehicle in stationary use**
     Contact with special construction vehicle under repair, not on public roadway
     EXCLUDES 1   *special construction vehicle accident (V01-V99)*

√x7ᵗʰ **W31.89**   **Contact with other specified machinery**

√x7ᵗʰ **W31.9**   **Contact with unspecified machinery**
     Contact with machinery NOS

4ᵗʰ **W32**   **Accidental handgun discharge and malfunction**
     INCLUDES   accidental discharge and malfunction of gun for single hand use
         accidental discharge and malfunction of pistol
         accidental discharge and malfunction of revolver
         handgun discharge and malfunction NOS
     EXCLUDES 1   *accidental airgun discharge and malfunction (W34.010, W34.110)*
         accidental BB gun discharge and malfunction (W34.010, W34.110)
         accidental pellet gun discharge and malfunction (W34.010, W34.110)
         accidental shotgun discharge and malfunction (W33.01, W33.11)
         assault by handgun discharge (X93)
         handgun discharge involving legal intervention (Y35.0-)
         handgun discharge involving military or war operations (Y36.4-)
         intentional self-harm by handgun discharge (X72)
         Very pistol discharge and malfunction (W34.09, W34.19)

√x7ᵗʰ **W32.0**   **Accidental handgun discharge**

√x7ᵗʰ **W32.1**   **Accidental handgun malfunction**
     Injury due to explosion of handgun (parts)
     Injury due to malfunction of mechanism or component of handgun
     Injury due to recoil of handgun
     Powder burn from handgun

4ᵗʰ **W33**   **Accidental rifle, shotgun and larger firearm discharge and malfunction**
     INCLUDES   rifle, shotgun and larger firearm discharge and malfunction NOS
     EXCLUDES 1   *accidental airgun discharge and malfunction (W34.010, W34.110)*
         accidental BB gun discharge and malfunction (W34.010, W34.110)
         accidental handgun discharge and malfunction (W32.-)
         accidental pellet gun discharge and malfunction (W34.010, W34.110)
         assault by rifle, shotgun and larger firearm discharge (X94)
         firearm discharge involving legal intervention (Y35.0-)
         firearm discharge involving military or war operations (Y36.4-)
         intentional self-harm by rifle, shotgun and larger firearm discharge (X73)

√5ᵗʰ **W33.0**   **Accidental rifle, shotgun and larger firearm discharge**

√x7ᵗʰ **W33.00**   **Accidental discharge of unspecified larger firearm**
     Discharge of unspecified larger firearm NOS

√x7ᵗʰ **W33.01**   **Accidental discharge of shotgun**
     Discharge of shotgun NOS

√x7ᵗʰ **W33.02**   **Accidental discharge of hunting rifle**
     Discharge of hunting rifle NOS

√x7ᵗʰ **W33.03**   **Accidental discharge of machine gun**
     Discharge of machine gun NOS

√x7ᵗʰ **W33.09**   **Accidental discharge of other larger firearm**
     Discharge of other larger firearm NOS

√5ᵗʰ **W33.1**   **Accidental rifle, shotgun and larger firearm malfunction**
     Injury due to explosion of rifle, shotgun and larger firearm (parts)
     Injury due to malfunction of mechanism or component of rifle, shotgun and larger firearm
     Injury due to piercing, cutting, crushing or pinching due to (by) slide trigger mechanism, scope or other gun part
     Injury due to recoil of rifle, shotgun and larger firearm
     Powder burn from rifle, shotgun and larger firearm

√x7ᵗʰ **W33.10**   **Accidental malfunction of unspecified larger firearm**
     Malfunction of unspecified larger firearm NOS

√x7ᵗʰ **W33.11**   **Accidental malfunction of shotgun**
     Malfunction of shotgun NOS

√x7ᵗʰ **W33.12**   **Accidental malfunction of hunting rifle**
     Malfunction of hunting rifle NOS

√x7ᵗʰ **W33.13**   **Accidental malfunction of machine gun**
     Malfunction of machine gun NOS

√x7ᵗʰ **W33.19**   **Accidental malfunction of other larger firearm**
     Malfunction of other larger firearm NOS

✔ Additional Char Req   √x7ᵗʰ Placeholder   Unacceptable PDx   Questionable PDx   Wrong Procedure   Manifestation   Unspecified   H1-H14 HAC   HCC CMS-HCC Dx   HIV HIV Dx

ICD-10-CM 2025   **1231**

W34 Accidental discharge and malfunction from other and unspecified firearms and guns

W34.0 Accidental discharge from other and unspecified firearms and guns

W34.00 Accidental discharge from unspecified firearms or gun
Discharge from firearm NOS
Gunshot wound NOS
Shot NOS

W34.01 Accidental discharge of gas, air or spring-operated guns

W34.010 Accidental discharge of airgun
Accidental discharge of BB gun
Accidental discharge of pellet gun

W34.011 Accidental discharge of paintball gun
Accidental injury due to paintball discharge

W34.018 Accidental discharge of other gas, air or spring-operated gun

W34.09 Accidental discharge from other specified firearms
Accidental discharge from Very pistol [flare]

W34.1 Accidental malfunction from other and unspecified firearms and guns

W34.10 Accidental malfunction from unspecified firearms or gun
Firearm malfunction NOS

W34.11 Accidental malfunction of gas, air or spring-operated guns

W34.110 Accidental malfunction of airgun
Accidental malfunction of BB gun
Accidental malfunction of pellet gun

W34.111 Accidental malfunction of paintball gun
Accidental injury due to paintball gun malfunction

W34.118 Accidental malfunction of other gas, air or spring-operated gun

W34.19 Accidental malfunction from other specified firearms
Accidental malfunction from Very pistol [flare]

W35 Explosion and rupture of boiler
EXCLUDES 1 explosion and rupture of boiler on watercraft (V93.4)

W36 Explosion and rupture of gas cylinder

W36.1 Explosion and rupture of aerosol can

W36.2 Explosion and rupture of air tank

W36.3 Explosion and rupture of pressurized-gas tank

W36.8 Explosion and rupture of other gas cylinder

W36.9 Explosion and rupture of unspecified gas cylinder

W37 Explosion and rupture of pressurized tire, pipe or hose

W37.0 Explosion of bicycle tire

W37.8 Explosion and rupture of other pressurized tire, pipe or hose

W38 Explosion and rupture of other specified pressurized devices

W39 Discharge of firework

W40 Explosion of other materials
EXCLUDES 1 assault by explosive material (X96)
explosion involving legal intervention (Y35.1-)
explosion involving military or war operations (Y36.0-, Y36.2-)
intentional self-harm by explosive material (X75)

W40.0 Explosion of blasting material
Explosion of blasting cap
Explosion of detonator
Explosion of dynamite
Explosion of explosive (any) used in blasting operations

W40.1 Explosion of explosive gases
Explosion of acetylene
Explosion of butane
Explosion of coal gas
Explosion in mine NOS
Explosion of explosive gas
Explosion of fire damp
Explosion of gasoline fumes
Explosion of methane
Explosion of propane

W40.8 Explosion of other specified explosive materials
Explosion in dump NOS
Explosion in factory NOS
Explosion in grain store
Explosion in munitions
EXCLUDES 1 explosion involving legal intervention (Y35.1-)
explosion involving military or war operations (Y36.0-, Y36.2-)

W40.9 Explosion of unspecified explosive materials
Explosion NOS

W42 Exposure to noise

W42.0 Exposure to supersonic waves

W42.9 Exposure to other noise
Exposure to sound waves NOS

W44 Foreign body entering into or through a natural orifice
EXCLUDES 2 contact with other sharp objects (W26)
contact with sharp glass (W25)
foreign body or object entering through skin (W45)
AHA: 2023,4Q,45-46

W44.A Battery entering into or through a natural orifice

W44.A0 Battery unspecified, entering into or through a natural orifice

W44.A1 Button battery entering into or through a natural orifice

W44.A9 Other batteries entering into or through a natural orifice
Cylindrical battery

W44.B Plastic entering into or through a natural orifice

W44.B0 Plastic object unspecified, entering into or through a natural orifice

W44.B1 Plastic bead entering into or through a natural orifice
EXCLUDES 2 plastic jewelry entering into or through a natural orifice (W44.B4)

W44.B2 Plastic coin entering into or through a natural orifice

W44.B3 Plastic toy and toy part entering into or through a natural orifice

W44.B4 Plastic jewelry entering into or through a natural orifice
EXCLUDES 2 plastic bead entering into or through a natural orifice (W44.B1)

W44.B5 Plastic bottle entering into or through a natural orifice

W44.B9 Other plastic object entering into or through a natural orifice

W44.C Glass entering into or through a natural orifice

W44.C0 Glass unspecified, entering into or through a natural orifice

W44.C1 Sharp glass entering into or through a natural orifice
Glass shard entering into or through a natural orifice

W44.C2 Intact glass entering into or through a natural orifice
Intact glass bottle entering into or through a natural orifice

W44.D Magnetic metal entering into or through a natural orifice

W44.D0 Magnetic metal object unspecified, entering into or through a natural orifice

W44.D1 Magnetic metal bead entering into or through a natural orifice

W44.D2 Magnetic metal coin entering into or through a natural orifice

W44.D3 Magnetic metal toy entering into or through a natural orifice

W44.D4 Magnetic metal jewelry entering into or through a natural orifice

W44.D9 Other magnetic metal objects entering into or through a natural orifice

W44.E Non-magnetic metal entering into or through a natural orifice

W44.E0 Non-magnetic metal object unspecified, entering into or through a natural orifice

W44.E1 Non-magnetic metal bead entering into or through a natural orifice

W44.E2 Non-magnetic metal coin entering into or through a natural orifice

W44.E3 Non-magnetic metal toy entering into or through a natural orifice

W44.E4 Non-magnetic metal jewelry entering into or through a natural orifice

√x7th **W44.E9** **Other non-magnetic metal objects entering into or through a natural orifice**
    Bottle cap entering into or through a natural orifice
    Can lid entering into or through a natural orifice
    Pull tab entering into or through a natural orifice

√5th **W44.F** **Objects of natural or organic material entering into or through a natural orifice**

√x7th **W44.F0** **Objects of natural or organic material unspecified, entering into or through a natural orifice**

√x7th **W44.F1** **Bezoar entering into or through a natural orifice**

√x7th **W44.F2** **Rubber band entering into or through a natural orifice**

√x7th **W44.F3** **Food entering into or through a natural orifice**

√x7th **W44.F4** **Insect entering into or through a natural orifice**

√x7th **W44.F9** **Other object of natural or organic material, entering into or through a natural orifice**

√5th **W44.G** **Other non-organic objects entering into or through a natural orifice**

√x7th **W44.G0** **Other non-organic objects unspecified, entering into or through a natural orifice**

√x7th **W44.G1** **Audio device entering into or through a natural orifice**
    Ear buds
    Hearing aids

√x7th **W44.G2** **Combination metal and plastic toy and toy part entering into or through natural orifice**

√x7th **W44.G3** **Combination metal and plastic jewelry entering into or through a natural orifice**

√x7th **W44.G9** **Other non-organic objects entering into or through a natural orifice**

√5th **W44.H** **Other sharp object entering into or through a natural orifice**

√x7th **W44.H0** **Other sharp object unspecified, entering into or through a natural orifice**

√x7th **W44.H1** **Needle entering into or through a natural orifice**
    Dart entering into or through a natural orifice
    Hypodermic needle entering into or through a natural orifice
    Safety pin entering into or through a natural orifice
    Sewing needle entering into or through a natural orifice

√x7th **W44.H2** **Knife, sword or dagger entering into or through a natural orifice**

√x7th **W44.8** **Other foreign body entering into or through a natural orifice**

√x7th **W44.9** **Unspecified foreign body entering into or through a natural orifice**
    Foreign body NOS entering into or through a natural orifice

√4th **W45** **Foreign body or object entering through skin**

    INCLUDES   foreign body or object embedded in skin
                nail embedded in skin
    EXCLUDES 2   *contact with hand tools (nonpowered) (powered) (W27-W29)*
                contact with other sharp objects (W26.-)
                contact with sharp glass (W25.-)
                struck by objects (W20-W22)

√x7th **W45.0** **Nail entering through skin**

√x7th **W45.8** **Other foreign body or object entering through skin**
    Splinter in skin NOS

√4th **W46** **Contact with hypodermic needle**

√x7th **W46.0** **Contact with hypodermic needle**
    Hypodermic needle stick NOS

√x7th **W46.1** **Contact with contaminated hypodermic needle**

√4th **W49** **Exposure to other inanimate mechanical forces**

    INCLUDES   exposure to abnormal gravitational [G] forces
                exposure to inanimate mechanical forces NEC
    EXCLUDES 1   *exposure to inanimate mechanical forces involving military or war operations (Y36.-, Y37.-)*

√5th **W49.0** **Item causing external constriction**

√x7th **W49.01** **Hair causing external constriction**

√x7th **W49.02** **String or thread causing external constriction**

√x7th **W49.03** **Rubber band causing external constriction**

√x7th **W49.04** **Ring or other jewelry causing external constriction**

√x7th **W49.09** **Other specified item causing external constriction**

√x7th **W49.9** **Exposure to other inanimate mechanical forces**

Exposure to animate mechanical forces (W50-W64)

    EXCLUDES 1   *toxic effect of contact with venomous animals and plants (T63.-)*

The appropriate 7th character is to be added to each code from categories W50-W64.
A   initial encounter
D   subsequent encounter
S   sequela

√4th **W50** **Accidental hit, strike, kick, twist, bite or scratch by another person**

    INCLUDES   hit, strike, kick, twist, bite, or scratch by another person NOS
    EXCLUDES 1   *assault by bodily force (Y04)*
                struck by objects (W20-W22)

√x7th **W50.0** **Accidental hit or strike by another person**
    Hit or strike by another person NOS

√x7th **W50.1** **Accidental kick by another person**
    Kick by another person NOS

√x7th **W50.2** **Accidental twist by another person**
    Twist by another person NOS

√x7th **W50.3** **Accidental bite by another person**
    Human bite
    Bite by another person NOS

√x7th **W50.4** **Accidental scratch by another person**
    Scratch by another person NOS

√x7th **W51** **Accidental striking against or bumped into by another person**

    EXCLUDES 1   *assault by striking against or bumping into by another person (Y04.2)*
                fall due to collision with another person (W03)

√x7th **W52** **Crushed, pushed or stepped on by crowd or human stampede**
    Crushed, pushed or stepped on by crowd or human stampede with or without fall

√4th **W53** **Contact with rodent**

    INCLUDES   contact with saliva, feces or urine of rodent

√5th **W53.0** **Contact with mouse**

√x7th **W53.01** **Bitten by mouse**

√x7th **W53.09** **Other contact with mouse**

√5th **W53.1** **Contact with rat**

√x7th **W53.11** **Bitten by rat**

√x7th **W53.19** **Other contact with rat**

√5th **W53.2** **Contact with squirrel**

√x7th **W53.21** **Bitten by squirrel**

√x7th **W53.29** **Other contact with squirrel**

√5th **W53.8** **Contact with other rodent**

√x7th **W53.81** **Bitten by other rodent**

√x7th **W53.89** **Other contact with other rodent**

√4th **W54** **Contact with dog**

    INCLUDES   contact with saliva, feces or urine of dog

√x7th **W54.0** **Bitten by dog**

√x7th **W54.1** **Struck by dog**
    Knocked over by dog

√x7th **W54.8** **Other contact with dog**

√4th **W55** **Contact with other mammals**

    INCLUDES   contact with saliva, feces or urine of mammal
    EXCLUDES 1   *animal being ridden - see transport accidents*
                bitten or struck by dog (W54)
                bitten or struck by rodent (W53.-)
                contact with marine mammals (W56.-)

√5th **W55.0** **Contact with cat**

√x7th **W55.01** **Bitten by cat**

√x7th **W55.03** **Scratched by cat**

√x7th **W55.09** **Other contact with cat**

√5th **W55.1** **Contact with horse**

√x7th **W55.11** **Bitten by horse**

√x7th **W55.12** **Struck by horse**

√x7th **W55.19** **Other contact with horse**

√5th **W55.2** **Contact with cow**
    Contact with bull

√x7th **W55.21** **Bitten by cow**

Chapter 20. External Causes of Morbidity

W55.22–W61.69

- √x7ᵗʰ **W55.22** Struck by cow
  - Gored by bull
- √x7ᵗʰ **W55.29** Other contact with cow
- ✓5ᵗʰ **W55.3** Contact with other hoof stock
  - Contact with goats
  - Contact with sheep
  - √x7ᵗʰ **W55.31** Bitten by other hoof stock
  - √x7ᵗʰ **W55.32** Struck by other hoof stock
    - Gored by goat
    - Gored by ram
  - √x7ᵗʰ **W55.39** Other contact with other hoof stock
- ✓5ᵗʰ **W55.4** Contact with pig
  - √x7ᵗʰ **W55.41** Bitten by pig
  - √x7ᵗʰ **W55.42** Struck by pig
  - √x7ᵗʰ **W55.49** Other contact with pig
- ✓5ᵗʰ **W55.5** Contact with raccoon
  - √x7ᵗʰ **W55.51** Bitten by raccoon
  - √x7ᵗʰ **W55.52** Struck by raccoon
  - √x7ᵗʰ **W55.59** Other contact with raccoon
- ✓5ᵗʰ **W55.8** Contact with other mammals
  - √x7ᵗʰ **W55.81** Bitten by other mammals
  - √x7ᵗʰ **W55.82** Struck by other mammals
  - √x7ᵗʰ **W55.89** Other contact with other mammals
- ✓4ᵗʰ **W56** Contact with nonvenomous marine animal
  - EXCLUDES 1   contact with venomous marine animal (T63.-)
  - ✓5ᵗʰ **W56.0** Contact with dolphin
    - √x7ᵗʰ **W56.01** Bitten by dolphin
    - √x7ᵗʰ **W56.02** Struck by dolphin
    - √x7ᵗʰ **W56.09** Other contact with dolphin
  - ✓5ᵗʰ **W56.1** Contact with sea lion
    - √x7ᵗʰ **W56.11** Bitten by sea lion
    - √x7ᵗʰ **W56.12** Struck by sea lion
    - √x7ᵗʰ **W56.19** Other contact with sea lion
  - ✓5ᵗʰ **W56.2** Contact with orca
    - Contact with killer whale
    - √x7ᵗʰ **W56.21** Bitten by orca
    - √x7ᵗʰ **W56.22** Struck by orca
    - √x7ᵗʰ **W56.29** Other contact with orca
  - ✓5ᵗʰ **W56.3** Contact with other marine mammals
    - √x7ᵗʰ **W56.31** Bitten by other marine mammals
    - √x7ᵗʰ **W56.32** Struck by other marine mammals
    - √x7ᵗʰ **W56.39** Other contact with other marine mammals
  - ✓5ᵗʰ **W56.4** Contact with shark
    - √x7ᵗʰ **W56.41** Bitten by shark
    - √x7ᵗʰ **W56.42** Struck by shark
    - √x7ᵗʰ **W56.49** Other contact with shark
  - ✓5ᵗʰ **W56.5** Contact with other fish
    - √x7ᵗʰ **W56.51** Bitten by other fish
    - √x7ᵗʰ **W56.52** Struck by other fish
    - √x7ᵗʰ **W56.59** Other contact with other fish
  - ✓5ᵗʰ **W56.8** Contact with other nonvenomous marine animals
    - √x7ᵗʰ **W56.81** Bitten by other nonvenomous marine animals
    - √x7ᵗʰ **W56.82** Struck by other nonvenomous marine animals
    - √x7ᵗʰ **W56.89** Other contact with other nonvenomous marine animals
- √x7ᵗʰ **W57** Bitten or stung by nonvenomous insect and other nonvenomous arthropods
  - EXCLUDES 1   contact with venomous insects and arthropods (T63.2-, T63.3-, T63.4-)
- ✓4ᵗʰ **W58** Contact with crocodile or alligator
  - ✓5ᵗʰ **W58.0** Contact with alligator
    - √x7ᵗʰ **W58.01** Bitten by alligator
    - √x7ᵗʰ **W58.02** Struck by alligator
    - √x7ᵗʰ **W58.03** Crushed by alligator
    - √x7ᵗʰ **W58.09** Other contact with alligator

- ✓5ᵗʰ **W58.1** Contact with crocodile
  - √x7ᵗʰ **W58.11** Bitten by crocodile
  - √x7ᵗʰ **W58.12** Struck by crocodile
  - √x7ᵗʰ **W58.13** Crushed by crocodile
  - √x7ᵗʰ **W58.19** Other contact with crocodile
- ✓4ᵗʰ **W59** Contact with other nonvenomous reptiles
  - EXCLUDES 1   contact with venomous reptile (T63.0-, T63.1-)
  - ✓5ᵗʰ **W59.0** Contact with nonvenomous lizards
    - √x7ᵗʰ **W59.01** Bitten by nonvenomous lizards
    - √x7ᵗʰ **W59.02** Struck by nonvenomous lizards
    - √x7ᵗʰ **W59.09** Other contact with nonvenomous lizards
      - Exposure to nonvenomous lizards
  - ✓5ᵗʰ **W59.1** Contact with nonvenomous snakes
    - √x7ᵗʰ **W59.11** Bitten by nonvenomous snake
    - √x7ᵗʰ **W59.12** Struck by nonvenomous snake
    - √x7ᵗʰ **W59.13** Crushed by nonvenomous snake
    - √x7ᵗʰ **W59.19** Other contact with nonvenomous snake
  - ✓5ᵗʰ **W59.2** Contact with turtles
    - EXCLUDES 1   contact with tortoises (W59.8-)
    - √x7ᵗʰ **W59.21** Bitten by turtle
    - √x7ᵗʰ **W59.22** Struck by turtle
    - √x7ᵗʰ **W59.29** Other contact with turtle
      - Exposure to turtles
  - ✓5ᵗʰ **W59.8** Contact with other nonvenomous reptiles
    - √x7ᵗʰ **W59.81** Bitten by other nonvenomous reptiles
    - √x7ᵗʰ **W59.82** Struck by other nonvenomous reptiles
    - √x7ᵗʰ **W59.83** Crushed by other nonvenomous reptiles
    - √x7ᵗʰ **W59.89** Other contact with other nonvenomous reptiles
- √x7ᵗʰ **W60** Contact with nonvenomous plant thorns and spines and sharp leaves
  - EXCLUDES 1   contact with venomous plants (T63.7-)
- ✓4ᵗʰ **W61** Contact with birds (domestic) (wild)
  - INCLUDES   contact with excreta of birds
  - ✓5ᵗʰ **W61.0** Contact with parrot
    - √x7ᵗʰ **W61.01** Bitten by parrot
    - √x7ᵗʰ **W61.02** Struck by parrot
    - √x7ᵗʰ **W61.09** Other contact with parrot
      - Exposure to parrots
  - ✓5ᵗʰ **W61.1** Contact with macaw
    - √x7ᵗʰ **W61.11** Bitten by macaw
    - √x7ᵗʰ **W61.12** Struck by macaw
    - √x7ᵗʰ **W61.19** Other contact with macaw
      - Exposure to macaws
  - ✓5ᵗʰ **W61.2** Contact with other psittacines
    - √x7ᵗʰ **W61.21** Bitten by other psittacines
    - √x7ᵗʰ **W61.22** Struck by other psittacines
    - √x7ᵗʰ **W61.29** Other contact with other psittacines
      - Exposure to other psittacines
  - ✓5ᵗʰ **W61.3** Contact with chicken
    - √x7ᵗʰ **W61.32** Struck by chicken
    - √x7ᵗʰ **W61.33** Pecked by chicken
    - √x7ᵗʰ **W61.39** Other contact with chicken
      - Exposure to chickens
  - ✓5ᵗʰ **W61.4** Contact with turkey
    - √x7ᵗʰ **W61.42** Struck by turkey
    - √x7ᵗʰ **W61.43** Pecked by turkey
    - √x7ᵗʰ **W61.49** Other contact with turkey
  - ✓5ᵗʰ **W61.5** Contact with goose
    - √x7ᵗʰ **W61.51** Bitten by goose
    - √x7ᵗʰ **W61.52** Struck by goose
    - √x7ᵗʰ **W61.59** Other contact with goose
  - ✓5ᵗʰ **W61.6** Contact with duck
    - √x7ᵗʰ **W61.61** Bitten by duck
    - √x7ᵗʰ **W61.62** Struck by duck
    - √x7ᵗʰ **W61.69** Other contact with duck

N Newborn: 0   P Pediatric: 0-17   M Maternity: 9-64   A Adult: 15-124   UNS Unspecified Site   MCC Major Complication/Comorbidity   CC Complication/Comorbidity   PE POA Exempt

1234

ICD-10-CM 2025

✓5ᵗʰ **W61.9** **Contact with other birds**

  ✓x7ᵗʰ **W61.91** **Bitten** by other birds

  ✓x7ᵗʰ **W61.92** **Struck** by other birds

  ✓x7ᵗʰ **W61.99** **Other contact with other birds**
        Contact with bird NOS

✓4ᵗʰ **W62** **Contact with nonvenomous amphibians**

  EXCLUDES 1   contact with venomous amphibians (T63.81-T63.83)

  ✓x7ᵗʰ **W62.0** **Contact with nonvenomous frogs**

  ✓x7ᵗʰ **W62.1** **Contact with nonvenomous toads**

  ✓x7ᵗʰ **W62.9** **Contact with other nonvenomous amphibians**

✓x7ᵗʰ **W64** **Exposure to other animate mechanical forces**

  INCLUDES   exposure to nonvenomous animal NOS
  EXCLUDES 1   contact with venomous animal (T63.-)

Accidental non-transport drowning and submersion (W65-W74)

EXCLUDES 1   accidental drowning and submersion due to fall into water (W16.-)
        accidental drowning and submersion due to water transport accident (V90.-, V92.-)

EXCLUDES 2   accidental drowning and submersion due to cataclysm (X34-X39)

The appropriate 7th character is to be added to each code from categories W65-W74.
A   initial encounter
D   subsequent encounter
S   sequela

✓x7ᵗʰ **W65** **Accidental drowning and submersion while in bath-tub**

  EXCLUDES 1   accidental drowning and submersion due to fall in (into) bathtub (W16.211)

✓x7ᵗʰ **W67** **Accidental drowning and submersion while in swimming-pool**

  EXCLUDES 1   accidental drowning and submersion due to fall into swimming pool (W16.011, W16.021, W16.031)
        accidental drowning and submersion due to striking into wall of swimming pool (W22.041)

  AHA: 2023,1Q,25

✓x7ᵗʰ **W69** **Accidental drowning and submersion while in natural water**
    Accidental drowning and submersion while in lake
    Accidental drowning and submersion while in open sea
    Accidental drowning and submersion while in river
    Accidental drowning and submersion while in stream

  EXCLUDES 1   accidental drowning and submersion due to fall into natural body of water (W16.111, W16.121, W16.131)

✓x7ᵗʰ **W73** **Other specified cause of accidental non-transport drowning and submersion**
    Accidental drowning and submersion while in quenching tank
    Accidental drowning and submersion while in reservoir

  EXCLUDES 1   accidental drowning and submersion due to fall into other water (W16.311, W16.321, W16.331)

✓x7ᵗʰ **W74** **Unspecified cause of accidental drowning and submersion**
    Drowning NOS

Exposure to electric current, radiation and extreme ambient air temperature and pressure (W85-W99)

EXCLUDES 1   exposure to:
    failure in dosage of radiation or temperature during surgical and medical care (Y63.2-Y63.5)
    lightning (T75.0-)
    natural cold (X31)
    natural heat (X30)
    natural radiation NOS (X39)
    radiological procedure and radiotherapy (Y84.2)
    sunlight (X32)

AHA: 2018,2Q,7-8

The appropriate 7th character is to be added to each code from categories W85-W99.
A   initial encounter
D   subsequent encounter
S   sequela

✓x7ᵗʰ **W85** **Exposure to electric transmission lines**
    Broken power line

✓4ᵗʰ **W86** **Exposure to other specified electric current**

  ✓x7ᵗʰ **W86.0** **Exposure to domestic wiring and appliances**

  ✓x7ᵗʰ **W86.1** **Exposure to industrial wiring, appliances and electrical machinery**
    Exposure to conductors
    Exposure to control apparatus
    Exposure to electrical equipment and machinery
    Exposure to transformers

  ✓x7ᵗʰ **W86.8** **Exposure to other electric current**
    Exposure to wiring and appliances in or on farm (not farmhouse)
    Exposure to wiring and appliances outdoors
    Exposure to wiring and appliances in or on public building
    Exposure to wiring and appliances in or on residential institutions
    Exposure to wiring and appliances in or on schools

✓4ᵗʰ **W88** **Exposure to ionizing radiation**

  EXCLUDES 1   exposure to sunlight (X32)

  ✓x7ᵗʰ **W88.0** **Exposure to X-rays**

  ✓x7ᵗʰ **W88.1** **Exposure to radioactive isotopes**

  ✓x7ᵗʰ **W88.8** **Exposure to other ionizing radiation**

✓4ᵗʰ **W89** **Exposure to man-made visible and ultraviolet light**

  INCLUDES   exposure to welding light (arc)
  EXCLUDES 2   exposure to sunlight (X32)

  ✓x7ᵗʰ **W89.0** **Exposure to welding light (arc)**

  ✓x7ᵗʰ **W89.1** **Exposure to tanning bed**

  ✓x7ᵗʰ **W89.8** **Exposure to other man-made visible and ultraviolet light**

  ✓x7ᵗʰ **W89.9** **Exposure to unspecified man-made visible and ultraviolet light**

✓4ᵗʰ **W90** **Exposure to other nonionizing radiation**

  EXCLUDES 2   exposure to sunlight (X32)

  AHA: 2019,1Q,21

  ✓x7ᵗʰ **W90.0** **Exposure to radiofrequency**

  ✓x7ᵗʰ **W90.1** **Exposure to infrared radiation**

  ✓x7ᵗʰ **W90.2** **Exposure to laser radiation**

  ✓x7ᵗʰ **W90.8** **Exposure to other nonionizing radiation**

✓x7ᵗʰ **W92** **Exposure to excessive heat of man-made origin**

✓4ᵗʰ **W93** **Exposure to excessive cold of man-made origin**

  ✓5ᵗʰ **W93.0** **Contact with or inhalation of dry ice**

    ✓x7ᵗʰ **W93.01** **Contact with dry ice**

    ✓x7ᵗʰ **W93.02** **Inhalation of dry ice**

  ✓5ᵗʰ **W93.1** **Contact with or inhalation of liquid air**

    ✓x7ᵗʰ **W93.11** **Contact with liquid air**
        Contact with liquid hydrogen
        Contact with liquid nitrogen

    ✓x7ᵗʰ **W93.12** **Inhalation of liquid air**
        Inhalation of liquid hydrogen
        Inhalation of liquid nitrogen

  ✓x7ᵗʰ **W93.2** **Prolonged exposure in deep freeze unit or refrigerator**

  ✓x7ᵗʰ **W93.8** **Exposure to other excessive cold of man-made origin**

✓4ᵗʰ **W94** **Exposure to high and low air pressure and changes in air pressure**

  ✓x7ᵗʰ **W94.0** **Exposure to prolonged high air pressure**

  ✓5ᵗʰ **W94.1** **Exposure to prolonged low air pressure**

    ✓x7ᵗʰ **W94.11** **Exposure to residence or prolonged visit at high altitude**

    ✓x7ᵗʰ **W94.12** **Exposure to other prolonged low air pressure**

  ✓5ᵗʰ **W94.2** **Exposure to rapid changes in air pressure during ascent**

    ✓x7ᵗʰ **W94.21** **Exposure to reduction in atmospheric pressure while surfacing from deep-water diving**

    ✓x7ᵗʰ **W94.22** **Exposure to reduction in atmospheric pressure while surfacing from underground**

    ✓x7ᵗʰ **W94.23** **Exposure to sudden change in air pressure in aircraft during ascent**

    ✓x7ᵗʰ **W94.29** **Exposure to other rapid changes in air pressure during ascent**

  ✓5ᵗʰ **W94.3** **Exposure to rapid changes in air pressure during descent**

    ✓x7ᵗʰ **W94.31** **Exposure to sudden change in air pressure in aircraft during descent**

    ✓x7ᵗʰ **W94.32** **Exposure to high air pressure from rapid descent in water**

    ✓x7ᵗʰ **W94.39** **Exposure to other rapid changes in air pressure during descent**

✓x7ᵗʰ **W99** **Exposure to other man-made environmental factors**

Chapter 20. External Causes of Morbidity

Exposure to smoke, fire and flames (X00-X08)

EXCLUDES 1 arson (X97)
EXCLUDES 2 explosions (W35-W40)
          lightning (T75.0-)
          transport accident (V01-V99)

AHA: 2018,2Q,7-8

The appropriate 7th character is to be added to each code from categories X00-X08.
A   initial encounter
D   subsequent encounter
S   sequela

✓4th **X00 Exposure to uncontrolled fire in building or structure**
          INCLUDES conflagration in building or structure
          Code first any associated cataclysm
          EXCLUDES 2 exposure to ignition or melting of nightwear (X05)
                    exposure to ignition or melting of other clothing and apparel
                    (X06.-)
                    exposure to other specified smoke, fire and flames (X08.-)
          AHA: 2016,2Q,5

✓x7th X00.0 **Exposure to flames in uncontrolled fire in building or structure**
✓x7th X00.1 **Exposure to smoke in uncontrolled fire in building or structure**
✓x7th X00.2 **Injury due to collapse of burning building or structure in uncontrolled fire**
                    EXCLUDES 1 injury due to collapse of building not on fire (W20.1)
✓x7th X00.3 **Fall from burning building or structure in uncontrolled fire**
✓x7th X00.4 **Hit by object from burning building or structure in uncontrolled fire**
                    AHA: 2016,2Q,4
✓x7th X00.5 **Jump from burning building or structure in uncontrolled fire**
✓x7th X00.8 **Other exposure to uncontrolled fire in building or structure**

✓4th **X01 Exposure to uncontrolled fire, not in building or structure**
          INCLUDES exposure to forest fire
✓x7th X01.0 **Exposure to flames in uncontrolled fire, not in building or structure**
✓x7th X01.1 **Exposure to smoke in uncontrolled fire, not in building or structure**
✓x7th X01.3 **Fall due to uncontrolled fire, not in building or structure**
✓x7th X01.4 **Hit by object due to uncontrolled fire, not in building or structure**
✓x7th X01.8 **Other exposure to uncontrolled fire, not in building or structure**

✓4th **X02 Exposure to controlled fire in building or structure**
          INCLUDES exposure to fire in fireplace
                    exposure to fire in stove
✓x7th X02.0 **Exposure to flames in controlled fire in building or structure**
✓x7th X02.1 **Exposure to smoke in controlled fire in building or structure**
✓x7th X02.2 **Injury due to collapse of burning building or structure in controlled fire**
                    EXCLUDES 1 injury due to collapse of building not on fire (W20.1)
✓x7th X02.3 **Fall from burning building or structure in controlled fire**
✓x7th X02.4 **Hit by object from burning building or structure in controlled fire**
✓x7th X02.5 **Jump from burning building or structure in controlled fire**
✓x7th X02.8 **Other exposure to controlled fire in building or structure**

✓4th **X03 Exposure to controlled fire, not in building or structure**
          INCLUDES exposure to bon fire
                    exposure to camp-fire
                    exposure to trash fire
✓x7th X03.0 **Exposure to flames in controlled fire, not in building or structure**
✓x7th X03.1 **Exposure to smoke in controlled fire, not in building or structure**
✓x7th X03.3 **Fall due to controlled fire, not in building or structure**
✓x7th X03.4 **Hit by object due to controlled fire, not in building or structure**
✓x7th X03.8 **Other exposure to controlled fire, not in building or structure**

✓x7th **X04 Exposure to ignition of highly flammable material**
          Exposure to ignition of gasoline
          Exposure to ignition of kerosene
          Exposure to ignition of petrol
          EXCLUDES 2 exposure to ignition or melting of nightwear (X05)
                    exposure to ignition or melting of other clothing and apparel
                    (X06)
          AHA: 2016,2Q,4

✓x7th **X05 Exposure to ignition or melting of nightwear**
          EXCLUDES 2 exposure to uncontrolled fire in building or structure (X00.-)
                    exposure to uncontrolled fire, not in building or structure (X01.-)
                    exposure to controlled fire in building or structure (X02.-)
                    exposure to controlled fire, not in building or structure (X03.-)
                    exposure to ignition of highly flammable materials (X04.-)

✓4th **X06 Exposure to ignition or melting of other clothing and apparel**
          EXCLUDES 2 exposure to uncontrolled fire in building or structure (X00.-)
                    exposure to uncontrolled fire, not in building or structure (X01.-)
                    exposure to controlled fire in building or structure (X02.-)
                    exposure to controlled fire, not in building or structure (X03.-)
                    exposure to ignition of highly flammable materials (X04.-)

✓x7th X06.0 **Exposure to ignition of plastic jewelry**
✓x7th X06.1 **Exposure to melting of plastic jewelry**
✓x7th X06.2 **Exposure to ignition of other clothing and apparel**
✓x7th X06.3 **Exposure to melting of other clothing and apparel**

✓4th **X08 Exposure to other specified smoke, fire and flames**
✓5th X08.0 **Exposure to bed fire**
          Exposure to mattress fire
✓x7th   X08.00 **Exposure to bed fire due to unspecified burning material**
✓x7th   X08.01 **Exposure to bed fire due to burning cigarette**
✓x7th   X08.09 **Exposure to bed fire due to other burning material**
✓5th X08.1 **Exposure to sofa fire**
✓x7th   X08.10 **Exposure to sofa fire due to unspecified burning material**
✓x7th   X08.11 **Exposure to sofa fire due to burning cigarette**
✓x7th   X08.19 **Exposure to sofa fire due to other burning material**
✓5th X08.2 **Exposure to other furniture fire**
✓x7th   X08.20 **Exposure to other furniture fire due to unspecified burning material**
✓x7th   X08.21 **Exposure to other furniture fire due to burning cigarette**
✓x7th   X08.29 **Exposure to other furniture fire due to other burning material**
✓x7th X08.8 **Exposure to other specified smoke, fire and flames**

Contact with heat and hot substances (X10-X19)

EXCLUDES 1 exposure to excessive natural heat (X30)
          exposure to fire and flames (X00-X08)

AHA: 2018,2Q,7-8

The appropriate 7th character is to be added to each code from categories X10-X19.
A   initial encounter
D   subsequent encounter
S   sequela

✓4th **X10 Contact with hot drinks, food, fats and cooking oils**
✓x7th X10.0 **Contact with hot drinks**
✓x7th X10.1 **Contact with hot food**
✓x7th X10.2 **Contact with fats and cooking oils**

✓4th **X11 Contact with hot tap-water**
          INCLUDES contact with boiling tap-water
                    contact with boiling water NOS
          EXCLUDES 1 contact with water heated on stove (X12)
✓x7th X11.0 **Contact with hot water in bath or tub**
                    EXCLUDES 1 contact with running hot water in bath or tub (X11.1)
✓x7th X11.1 **Contact with running hot water**
          Contact with hot water running out of hose
          Contact with hot water running out of tap
✓x7th X11.8 **Contact with other hot tap-water**
          Contact with hot water in bucket
          Contact with hot tap-water NOS

✓x7th **X12 Contact with other hot fluids**
Contact with water heated on stove
EXCLUDES 1   *hot (liquid) metals (X18)*

✓4th **X13 Contact with steam and other hot vapors**
    ✓x7th **X13.0 Inhalation of steam and other hot vapors**
    ✓x7th **X13.1 Other contact with steam and other hot vapors**

✓4th **X14 Contact with hot air and other hot gases**
    ✓x7th **X14.0 Inhalation of hot air and gases**
    ✓x7th **X14.1 Other contact with hot air and other hot gases**

✓4th **X15 Contact with hot household appliances**
    EXCLUDES 1   *contact with heating appliances (X16)*
          contact with powered household appliances (W29.-)
          exposure to controlled fire in building or structure due to household appliance (X02.8)
          exposure to household appliances electrical current (W86.0)

    ✓x7th **X15.0 Contact with hot stove (kitchen)**
    ✓x7th **X15.1 Contact with hot toaster**
    ✓x7th **X15.2 Contact with hotplate**
    ✓x7th **X15.3 Contact with hot saucepan or skillet**
        Contact with hot cooking pan
        Contact with hot cooking pot
    ✓x7th **X15.8 Contact with other hot household appliances**
        Contact with cooker
        Contact with kettle
        Contact with light bulbs

✓x7th **X16 Contact with hot heating appliances, radiators and pipes**
    EXCLUDES 1   *contact with powered appliances (W29.-)*
          exposure to controlled fire in building or structure due to appliance (X02.8)
          exposure to industrial appliances electrical current (W86.1)

✓x7th **X17 Contact with hot engines, machinery and tools**
    EXCLUDES 1   *contact with hot heating appliances, radiators and pipes (X16)*
          contact with hot household appliances (X15)

✓x7th **X18 Contact with other hot metals**
        Contact with liquid metal

✓x7th **X19 Contact with other heat and hot substances**
    EXCLUDES 1   *objects that are not normally hot, e.g., an object made hot by a house fire (X00-X08)*

Exposure to forces of nature (X30-X39)

AHA: 2018,2Q,7-8

The appropriate 7th character is to be added to each code from categories X30-X39.
A   initial encounter
D   subsequent encounter
S   sequela

✓x7th **X30 Exposure to excessive natural heat**
        Exposure to excessive heat as the cause of sunstroke
        Exposure to heat NOS
    EXCLUDES 1   *excessive heat of man-made origin (W92)*
          exposure to man-made radiation (W89)
          exposure to sunlight (X32)
          exposure to tanning bed (W89)

✓x7th **X31 Exposure to excessive natural cold**
        Excessive cold as the cause of chilblains NOS
        Excessive cold as the cause of immersion foot or hand
        Exposure to cold NOS
        Exposure to weather conditions
    EXCLUDES 1   *cold of man-made origin (W93.-)*
          contact with or inhalation of dry ice (W93.-)
          contact with or inhalation of liquefied gas (W93.-)

✓x7th **X32 Exposure to sunlight**
    EXCLUDES 1   *man-made radiation (tanning bed) (W89)*
    EXCLUDES 2   *radiation-related disorders of the skin and subcutaneous tissue (L55-L59)*

✓x7th **X34 Earthquake**
    EXCLUDES 2   *tidal wave (tsunami) due to earthquake (X37.41)*

✓x7th **X35 Volcanic eruption**
    EXCLUDES 2   *tidal wave (tsunami) due to volcanic eruption (X37.41)*

✓4th **X36 Avalanche, landslide and other earth movements**
    INCLUDES   *victim of mudslide of cataclysmic nature*
    EXCLUDES 1   *earthquake (X34)*
    EXCLUDES 2   *transport accident involving collision with avalanche or landslide not in motion (V01-V99)*

    ✓x7th **X36.0 Collapse of dam or man-made structure causing earth movement**
    ✓x7th **X36.1 Avalanche, landslide, or mudslide**

✓4th **X37 Cataclysmic storm**
    ✓x7th **X37.0 Hurricane**
        Storm surge
        Typhoon
    ✓x7th **X37.1 Tornado**
        Cyclone
        Twister
    ✓x7th **X37.2 Blizzard (snow)(ice)**
    ✓x7th **X37.3 Dust storm**
    ✓5th **X37.4 Tidalwave**
       ✓x7th **X37.41 Tidal wave due to earthquake or volcanic eruption**
          Tidal wave NOS
          Tsunami
       ✓x7th **X37.42 Tidal wave due to storm**
       ✓x7th **X37.43 Tidal wave due to landslide**
    ✓x7th **X37.8 Other cataclysmic storms**
        Cloudburst
        Torrential rain
        EXCLUDES 2   *flood (X38)*
    ✓x7th **X37.9 Unspecified cataclysmic storm**
        Storm NOS
        EXCLUDES 1   *collapse of dam or man-made structure causing earth movement (X36.0)*

✓x7th **X38 Flood**
        Flood arising from remote storm
        Flood of cataclysmic nature arising from melting snow
        Flood resulting directly from storm
    EXCLUDES 1   *collapse of dam or man-made structure causing earth movement (X36.0)*
          tidal wave NOS (X37.41)
          tidal wave caused by storm (X37.42)

✓4th **X39 Exposure to other forces of nature**
    ✓5th **X39.0 Exposure to natural radiation**
        EXCLUDES 1   *contact with and (suspected) exposure to radon and other naturally occurring radiation (Z77.123)*
          exposure to man-made radiation (W88-W90)
          exposure to sunlight (X32)
       ✓x7th **X39.01 Exposure to radon**
       ✓x7th **X39.08 Exposure to other natural radiation**
    ✓x7th **X39.8 Other exposure to forces of nature**

Overexertion and strenuous or repetitive movements (X50)

✓4th **X50 Overexertion and strenuous or repetitive movements**
    AHA: 2018,2Q,7-8; 2016,4Q,73-74

The appropriate 7th character is to be added to each code from category X50.
A   initial encounter
D   subsequent encounter
S   sequela

    ✓x7th **X50.0 Overexertion from strenuous movement or load**
        Lifting heavy objects
        Lifting weights

Chapter 20. External Causes of Morbidity

✓x7ᵗʰ **X50.1 Overexertion from prolonged static or awkward postures**
- Prolonged bending
- Prolonged kneeling
- Prolonged reaching
- Prolonged sitting
- Prolonged standing
- Prolonged twisting
- Static bending
- Static kneeling
- Static reaching
- Static sitting
- Static standing
- Static twisting

✓x7ᵗʰ **X50.3 Overexertion from repetitive movements**
- Use of hand as hammer

  EXCLUDES 2   *overuse from prolonged static or awkward postures (X50.1)*

✓x7ᵗʰ **X50.9 Other and unspecified overexertion or strenuous movements or postures**
- Contact pressure
- Contact stress

Accidental exposure to other specified factors (X52-X58)

AHA: 2018,2Q,7-8

The appropriate 7th character is to be added to each code from categories X52-X58.
- A   initial encounter
- D   subsequent encounter
- S   sequela

✓x7ᵗʰ **X52 Prolonged stay in weightless environment**
- Weightlessness in spacecraft (simulator)

✓x7ᵗʰ **X58 Exposure to other specified factors**
- Accident NOS
- Exposure NOS

Intentional self-harm (X71-X83)

Purposely self-inflicted injury
Suicide (attempted)

The appropriate 7th character is to be added to each code from categories X71-X83.
- A   initial encounter
- D   subsequent encounter
- S   sequela

✓4ᵗʰ **X71 Intentional self-harm by drowning and submersion**

✓x7ᵗʰ **X71.0 Intentional self-harm by drowning and submersion while in bathtub** HCC

✓x7ᵗʰ **X71.1 Intentional self-harm by drowning and submersion while in swimming pool** HCC

✓x7ᵗʰ **X71.2 Intentional self-harm by drowning and submersion after jump into swimming pool** HCC

✓x7ᵗʰ **X71.3 Intentional self-harm by drowning and submersion in natural water** HCC

✓x7ᵗʰ **X71.8 Other intentional self-harm by drowning and submersion** HCC

✓x7ᵗʰ **X71.9 Intentional self-harm by drowning and submersion, unspecified** HCC

✓x7ᵗʰ **X72 Intentional self-harm by handgun discharge** HCC
- Intentional self-harm by gun for single hand use
- Intentional self-harm by pistol
- Intentional self-harm by revolver

  EXCLUDES 1   *Very pistol (X74.8)*

✓4ᵗʰ **X73 Intentional self-harm by rifle, shotgun and larger firearm discharge**

  EXCLUDES 1   *airgun (X74.01)*

✓x7ᵗʰ **X73.0 Intentional self-harm by shotgun discharge** HCC

✓x7ᵗʰ **X73.1 Intentional self-harm by hunting rifle discharge** HCC

✓x7ᵗʰ **X73.2 Intentional self-harm by machine gun discharge** HCC

✓x7ᵗʰ **X73.8 Intentional self-harm by other larger firearm discharge** HCC

✓x7ᵗʰ **X73.9 Intentional self-harm by unspecified larger firearm discharge** HCC

✓4ᵗʰ **X74 Intentional self-harm by other and unspecified firearm and gun discharge**

✓5ᵗʰ **X74.0 Intentional self-harm by gas, air or spring-operated guns**

✓x7ᵗʰ **X74.01 Intentional self-harm by airgun** HCC
- Intentional self-harm by BB gun discharge
- Intentional self-harm by pellet gun discharge

✓x7ᵗʰ **X74.02 Intentional self-harm by paintball gun** HCC

✓x7ᵗʰ **X74.09 Intentional self-harm by other gas, air or spring-operated gun** HCC

✓x7ᵗʰ **X74.8 Intentional self-harm by other firearm discharge** HCC
- Intentional self-harm by Very pistol [flare] discharge

✓x7ᵗʰ **X74.9 Intentional self-harm by unspecified firearm discharge** HCC

✓x7ᵗʰ **X75 Intentional self-harm by explosive material** HCC

✓x7ᵗʰ **X76 Intentional self-harm by smoke, fire and flames** HCC

✓4ᵗʰ **X77 Intentional self-harm by steam, hot vapors and hot objects**

✓x7ᵗʰ **X77.0 Intentional self-harm by steam or hot vapors** HCC

✓x7ᵗʰ **X77.1 Intentional self-harm by hot tap water** HCC

✓x7ᵗʰ **X77.2 Intentional self-harm by other hot fluids** HCC

✓x7ᵗʰ **X77.3 Intentional self-harm by hot household appliances** HCC

✓x7ᵗʰ **X77.8 Intentional self-harm by other hot objects** HCC

✓x7ᵗʰ **X77.9 Intentional self-harm by unspecified hot objects** HCC

✓4ᵗʰ **X78 Intentional self-harm by sharp object**

✓x7ᵗʰ **X78.0 Intentional self-harm by sharp glass** HCC

✓x7ᵗʰ **X78.1 Intentional self-harm by knife** HCC

✓x7ᵗʰ **X78.2 Intentional self-harm by sword or dagger** HCC

✓x7ᵗʰ **X78.8 Intentional self-harm by other sharp object** HCC

    AHA: 2022,1Q,27

✓x7ᵗʰ **X78.9 Intentional self-harm by unspecified sharp object** HCC

✓x7ᵗʰ **X79 Intentional self-harm by blunt object** HCC

✓x7ᵗʰ **X80 Intentional self-harm by jumping from a high place** HCC
- Intentional fall from one level to another

✓4ᵗʰ **X81 Intentional self-harm by jumping or lying in front of moving object**

✓x7ᵗʰ **X81.0 Intentional self-harm by jumping or lying in front of motor vehicle** HCC

✓x7ᵗʰ **X81.1 Intentional self-harm by jumping or lying in front of (subway) train** HCC

✓x7ᵗʰ **X81.8 Intentional self-harm by jumping or lying in front of other moving object** HCC

✓4ᵗʰ **X82 Intentional self-harm by crashing of motor vehicle**

✓x7ᵗʰ **X82.0 Intentional collision of motor vehicle with other motor vehicle** HCC

✓x7ᵗʰ **X82.1 Intentional collision of motor vehicle with train** HCC

✓x7ᵗʰ **X82.2 Intentional collision of motor vehicle with tree** HCC

✓x7ᵗʰ **X82.8 Other intentional self-harm by crashing of motor vehicle** HCC

✓4ᵗʰ **X83 Intentional self-harm by other specified means**

  EXCLUDES 1   *intentional self-harm by poisoning or contact with toxic substance - see Table of Drugs and Chemicals*

✓x7ᵗʰ **X83.0 Intentional self-harm by crashing of aircraft** HCC

✓x7ᵗʰ **X83.1 Intentional self-harm by electrocution** HCC

✓x7ᵗʰ **X83.2 Intentional self-harm by exposure to extremes of cold** HCC

✓x7ᵗʰ **X83.8 Intentional self-harm by other specified means** HCC

Assault (X92-Y09)

INCLUDES   homicide
    injuries inflicted by another person with intent to injure or kill, by any means

EXCLUDES 1   *injuries due to legal intervention (Y35.-)*
    injuries due to operations of war (Y36.-)
    injuries due to terrorism (Y38.-)

The appropriate 7th character is to be added to each code from categories X92-Y04 and Y08.
- A   initial encounter
- D   subsequent encounter
- S   sequela

✓4ᵗʰ **X92 Assault by drowning and submersion**

✓x7ᵗʰ **X92.0 Assault by drowning and submersion while in bathtub**

✓x7ᵗʰ **X92.1 Assault by drowning and submersion while in swimming pool**

✓x7ᵗʰ **X92.2 Assault by drowning and submersion after push into swimming pool**

✓x7ᵗʰ **X92.3 Assault by drowning and submersion in natural water**

✓x7ᵗʰ **X92.8 Other assault by drowning and submersion**

✓x7ᵗʰ **X92.9 Assault by drowning and submersion, unspecified**

N Newborn: 0   P Pediatric: 0-17   M Maternity: 9-64   A Adult: 15-124   UNS Unspecified Site   MCC Major Complication/Comorbidity   CC Complication/Comorbidity   PE POA Exempt

1238   ICD-10-CM 2025

X93 Assault by **handgun** discharge
Assault by discharge of gun for single hand use
Assault by discharge of pistol
Assault by discharge of revolver
EXCLUDES 1 Very pistol (X95.8)

X94 Assault by **rifle, shotgun and larger firearm** discharge
EXCLUDES 1 airgun (X95.01)
- X94.0 Assault by **shotgun**
- X94.1 Assault by **hunting rifle**
- X94.2 Assault by **machine gun**
- X94.8 Assault by other larger firearm discharge
- X94.9 Assault by unspecified larger firearm discharge

X95 Assault by other and unspecified firearm and gun discharge
- X95.0 Assault by **gas, air or spring-operated** guns
  - X95.01 Assault by **airgun** discharge
    Assault by BB gun discharge
    Assault by pellet gun discharge
  - X95.02 Assault by **paintball gun** discharge
  - X95.09 Assault by other gas, air or spring-operated gun
- X95.8 Assault by other firearm discharge
  Assault by Very pistol [flare] discharge
- X95.9 Assault by unspecified firearm discharge
  AHA: 2023,3Q,8,12

X96 Assault by explosive material
EXCLUDES 1 incendiary device (X97)
terrorism involving explosive material (Y38.2-)
- X96.0 Assault by **antipersonnel** bomb
  EXCLUDES 1 antipersonnel bomb use in military or war (Y36.2-)
- X96.1 Assault by **gasoline** bomb
- X96.2 Assault by **letter** bomb
- X96.3 Assault by **fertilizer** bomb
- X96.4 Assault by **pipe** bomb
- X96.8 Assault by other specified explosive
- X96.9 Assault by unspecified explosive

X97 Assault by smoke, fire and flames
Assault by arson
Assault by cigarettes
Assault by incendiary device

X98 Assault by steam, hot vapors and hot objects
- X98.0 Assault by **steam** or hot **vapors**
- X98.1 Assault by hot **tap water**
- X98.2 Assault by hot **fluids**
- X98.3 Assault by hot **household appliances**
- X98.8 Assault by other hot **objects**
- X98.9 Assault by unspecified hot objects

X99 Assault by sharp object
EXCLUDES 1 assault by strike by sports equipment (Y08.0-)
- X99.0 Assault by sharp **glass**
- X99.1 Assault by **knife**
- X99.2 Assault by **sword or dagger**
- X99.8 Assault by other sharp object
- X99.9 Assault by unspecified sharp object
  Assault by stabbing NOS

Y00 Assault by blunt object
EXCLUDES 1 assault by strike by sports equipment (Y08.0-)

Y01 Assault by pushing from high place

Y02 Assault by pushing or placing victim in front of moving object
- Y02.0 Assault by pushing or placing victim in front of **motor vehicle**
- Y02.1 Assault by pushing or placing victim in front of (subway) **train**
- Y02.8 Assault by pushing or placing victim in front of other moving object

Y03 Assault by crashing of motor vehicle
- Y03.0 Assault by being hit or run over by motor vehicle
- Y03.8 Other assault by crashing of motor vehicle

Y04 Assault by bodily force
EXCLUDES 1 assault by:
submersion (X92.-)
use of weapon (X93-X95, X99, Y00)
- Y04.0 Assault by **unarmed brawl or fight**
- Y04.1 Assault by **human bite**
- Y04.2 Assault by **strike** against or bumped into by another person
- Y04.8 Assault by other bodily force
  Assault by bodily force NOS

Y07 Perpetrator of assault, maltreatment and neglect
NOTE Codes from this category are for use only in cases of confirmed abuse (T74.-)
Selection of the correct perpetrator code is based on the relationship between the perpetrator and the victim
INCLUDES perpetrator of abandonment
perpetrator of emotional neglect
perpetrator of mental cruelty
perpetrator of physical abuse
perpetrator of physical neglect
perpetrator of sexual abuse
perpetrator of torture
perpetrator of verbal abuse
- Y07.0 **Spouse or partner,** perpetrator of maltreatment and neglect
  Spouse or partner, perpetrator of maltreatment and neglect against spouse or partner
  AHA: 2023,1Q,5
  - Y07.01 **Husband,** perpetrator of maltreatment and neglect
    - Y07.010 Husband, **current,** perpetrator of maltreatment and neglect PE
    - Y07.011 Husband, **former,** perpetrator of maltreatment and neglect PE
  - Y07.02 **Wife,** perpetrator of maltreatment and neglect
    - Y07.020 Wife, **current,** perpetrator of maltreatment and neglect PE
    - Y07.021 Wife, **former,** perpetrator of maltreatment and neglect PE
  - Y07.03 **Male partner,** perpetrator of maltreatment and neglect
    Male intimate or dating partner, perpetrator of maltreatment and neglect
    - Y07.030 Male partner, **current,** perpetrator of maltreatment and neglect PE
    - Y07.031 Male partner, **former,** perpetrator of maltreatment and neglect PE
  - Y07.04 **Female partner,** perpetrator of maltreatment and neglect
    Female intimate or dating partner, perpetrator of maltreatment and neglect
    - Y07.040 Female partner, **current,** perpetrator of maltreatment and neglect PE
    - Y07.041 Female partner, **former,** perpetrator of maltreatment and neglect PE
  - Y07.05 **Non-binary partner,** perpetrator of maltreatment and neglect
    Gender non-conforming partner, perpetrator of maltreatment and neglect
    - Y07.050 Non-binary partner, **current,** perpetrator of maltreatment and neglect PE
    - Y07.051 Non-binary partner, **former,** perpetrator of maltreatment and neglect PE
- Y07.1 **Parent** (adoptive) (biological), perpetrator of maltreatment and neglect
  - Y07.11 **Biological father,** perpetrator of maltreatment and neglect PE
  - Y07.12 **Biological mother,** perpetrator of maltreatment and neglect PE
  - Y07.13 **Adoptive father,** perpetrator of maltreatment and neglect PE
  - Y07.14 **Adoptive mother,** perpetrator of maltreatment and neglect PE

Chapter 20. External Causes of Morbidity

Y07.4–Y21.3

√5th **Y07.4** **Other family member, perpetrator of maltreatment and neglect**

    AHA: 2023,1Q,5

√6th **Y07.41** **Sibling, perpetrator of maltreatment and neglect**

       EXCLUDES 1   *stepsibling, perpetrator of maltreatment and neglect (Y07.435, Y07.436)*

     Y07.410 **Brother, perpetrator of maltreatment and neglect** PE

     Y07.411 **Sister, perpetrator of maltreatment and neglect** PE

√6th **Y07.42** **Foster parent, perpetrator of maltreatment and neglect**

     Y07.420 **Foster father, perpetrator of maltreatment and neglect** PE

     Y07.421 **Foster mother, perpetrator of maltreatment and neglect** PE

√6th **Y07.43** **Stepparent or stepsibling, perpetrator of maltreatment and neglect**

     Y07.430 **Stepfather, perpetrator of maltreatment and neglect** PE

     Y07.432 **Male friend of parent** (co-residing in household), **perpetrator of maltreatment and neglect** PE

     Y07.433 **Stepmother, perpetrator of maltreatment and neglect** PE

     Y07.434 **Female friend of parent** (co-residing in household), **perpetrator of maltreatment and neglect** PE

     Y07.435 **Stepbrother, perpetrator or maltreatment and neglect** PE

     Y07.436 **Stepsister, perpetrator of maltreatment and neglect** PE

   Y07.44 **Child, perpetrator of maltreatment and neglect** PE

     Adopted child, perpetrator of maltreatment and neglect

     Biological child, perpetrator of maltreatment and neglect

     Daughter, perpetrator of maltreatment and neglect

     Foster child, perpetrator of maltreatment and neglect

     In-law child, perpetrator of maltreatment and neglect

     Non-binary child, perpetrator of maltreatment and neglect

     Son, perpetrator of maltreatment and neglect

     Stepchild, perpetrator of maltreatment and neglect

   Y07.45 **Grandchild, perpetrator of maltreatment and neglect** PE

     Adopted grandchild, perpetrator of maltreatment and neglect

     Biological grandchild, perpetrator of maltreatment and neglect

     Foster grandchild, perpetrator of maltreatment and neglect

     Granddaughter, perpetrator of maltreatment and neglect

     Grandson, perpetrator of maltreatment and neglect

     In-law grandchild, perpetrator of maltreatment and neglect

     Non-binary grandchild, perpetrator of maltreatment and neglect

     Step grandchild, perpetrator of maltreatment and neglect

   Y07.46 **Grandparent, perpetrator of maltreatment and neglect** PE

     Grandfather, perpetrator of maltreatment and neglect

     Grandmother, perpetrator of maltreatment and neglect

     Non-binary grandparent, perpetrator of maltreatment and neglect

   Y07.47 **Parental sibling, perpetrator of maltreatment and neglect** PE

     Aunt, perpetrator of maltreatment and neglect

     Non-binary parental sibling, perpetrator of maltreatment and neglect

     Uncle, perpetrator of maltreatment and neglect

√6th **Y07.49** **Other family member, perpetrator of maltreatment and neglect**

     Y07.490 **Male cousin, perpetrator of maltreatment and neglect** PE

     Y07.491 **Female cousin, perpetrator of maltreatment and neglect** PE

     Y07.499 **Other family member, perpetrator of maltreatment and neglect** PE

√5th **Y07.5** **Non-family member, perpetrator of maltreatment and neglect**

    AHA: 2023,1Q,5

   Y07.50 **Unspecified non-family member, perpetrator of maltreatment and neglect** PE

√6th **Y07.51** **Daycare provider, perpetrator of maltreatment and neglect**

     Y07.510 **At-home childcare provider, perpetrator of maltreatment and neglect** PE

     Y07.511 **Daycare center childcare provider, perpetrator of maltreatment and neglect** PE

     Y07.512 **At-home adultcare provider, perpetrator of maltreatment and neglect** PE

     Y07.513 **Adultcare center provider, perpetrator of maltreatment and neglect** PE

     Y07.519 **Unspecified daycare provider, perpetrator of maltreatment and neglect** PE

√6th **Y07.52** **Healthcare provider, perpetrator of maltreatment and neglect**

     Y07.521 **Mental health provider, perpetrator of maltreatment and neglect** PE

     Y07.528 **Other therapist or healthcare provider, perpetrator of maltreatment and neglect** PE

       Nurse perpetrator of maltreatment and neglect

       Occupational therapist perpetrator of maltreatment and neglect

       Physical therapist perpetrator of maltreatment and neglect

       Speech therapist perpetrator of maltreatment and neglect

     Y07.529 **Unspecified healthcare provider, perpetrator of maltreatment and neglect** PE

   Y07.53 **Teacher or instructor, perpetrator of maltreatment and neglect**

     Coach, perpetrator of maltreatment and neglect

   Y07.54 **Acquaintance or friend, perpetrator of maltreatment and neglect** PE

   Y07.59 **Other non-family member, perpetrator of maltreatment and neglect** PE

   Y07.6 **Multiple perpetrators of maltreatment and neglect** PE

    AHA: 2018,4Q,32

   Y07.9 **Unspecified perpetrator of maltreatment and neglect** PE

√4th **Y08** **Assault by other specified means**

√5th **Y08.0** **Assault by strike by sport equipment**

   √x7th **Y08.01** **Assault by strike by hockey stick**

   √x7th **Y08.02** **Assault by strike by baseball bat**

   √x7th **Y08.09** **Assault by strike by other specified type of sport equipment**

√5th **Y08.8** **Assault by other specified means**

   √x7th **Y08.81** **Assault by crashing of aircraft**

   √x7th **Y08.89** **Assault by other specified means**

   Y09 **Assault by unspecified means**

     Assassination (attempted) NOS

     Homicide (attempted) NOS

     Manslaughter (attempted) NOS

     Murder (attempted) NOS

Event of undetermined intent (Y21-Y33)

Undetermined intent is only for use when there is specific documentation in the record that the intent of the injury cannot be determined. If no such documentation is present, code to accidental (unintentional).

The appropriate 7th character is to be added to each code from categories Y21-Y33.

A   initial encounter

D   subsequent encounter

S   sequela

√4th **Y21** **Drowning and submersion, undetermined intent**

   √x7th **Y21.0** **Drowning and submersion while in bathtub, undetermined intent**

   √x7th **Y21.1** **Drowning and submersion after fall into bathtub, undetermined intent**

   √x7th **Y21.2** **Drowning and submersion while in swimming pool, undetermined intent**

   √x7th **Y21.3** **Drowning and submersion after fall into swimming pool, undetermined intent**

N Newborn: 0   P Pediatric: 0-17   M Maternity: 9-64   A Adult: 15-124   UNS Unspecified Site   MCC Major Complication/Comorbidity   CC Complication/Comorbidity   PE POA Exempt

1240   ICD-10-CM 2025

✓x7ᵗʰ **Y21.4** Drowning and submersion in natural water, undetermined intent

✓x7ᵗʰ **Y21.8** Other drowning and submersion, undetermined intent

✓x7ᵗʰ **Y21.9** Unspecified drowning and submersion, undetermined intent

✓x7ᵗʰ **Y22** **Handgun** discharge, undetermined intent

> Discharge of gun for single hand use, undetermined intent
> Discharge of pistol, undetermined intent
> Discharge of revolver, undetermined intent
> EXCLUDES 2 *Very pistol (Y24.8)*

✓4ᵗʰ **Y23** **Rifle, shotgun and larger firearm** discharge, undetermined intent

> EXCLUDES 2 *airgun (Y24.0)*

✓x7ᵗʰ **Y23.0** **Shotgun** discharge, undetermined intent

✓x7ᵗʰ **Y23.1** **Hunting rifle** discharge, undetermined intent

✓x7ᵗʰ **Y23.2** **Military firearm** discharge, undetermined intent

✓x7ᵗʰ **Y23.3** **Machine gun** discharge, undetermined intent

✓x7ᵗʰ **Y23.8** Other larger firearm discharge, undetermined intent

✓x7ᵗʰ **Y23.9** Unspecified larger firearm discharge, undetermined intent

✓4ᵗʰ **Y24** Other and unspecified firearm discharge, undetermined intent

✓x7ᵗʰ **Y24.0** **Airgun** discharge, undetermined intent

> BB gun discharge, undetermined intent
> Pellet gun discharge, undetermined intent

✓x7ᵗʰ **Y24.8** Other firearm discharge, undetermined intent

> Paintball gun discharge, undetermined intent
> Very pistol [flare] discharge, undetermined intent

✓x7ᵗʰ **Y24.9** Unspecified firearm discharge, undetermined intent

✓x7ᵗʰ **Y25** Contact with explosive material, undetermined intent

✓x7ᵗʰ **Y26** Exposure to smoke, fire and flames, undetermined intent

✓4ᵗʰ **Y27** Contact with steam, hot vapors and hot objects, undetermined intent

✓x7ᵗʰ **Y27.0** Contact with **steam** and hot **vapors,** undetermined intent

✓x7ᵗʰ **Y27.1** Contact with hot **tap water,** undetermined intent

✓x7ᵗʰ **Y27.2** Contact with hot **fluids,** undetermined intent

✓x7ᵗʰ **Y27.3** Contact with hot **household appliance,** undetermined intent

✓x7ᵗʰ **Y27.8** Contact with other hot **objects,** undetermined intent

✓x7ᵗʰ **Y27.9** Contact with unspecified hot objects, undetermined intent

✓4ᵗʰ **Y28** Contact with sharp object, undetermined intent

✓x7ᵗʰ **Y28.0** Contact with sharp **glass,** undetermined intent

✓x7ᵗʰ **Y28.1** Contact with **knife,** undetermined intent

✓x7ᵗʰ **Y28.2** Contact with **sword or dagger,** undetermined intent

✓x7ᵗʰ **Y28.8** Contact with other sharp object, undetermined intent

✓x7ᵗʰ **Y28.9** Contact with unspecified sharp object, undetermined intent

✓x7ᵗʰ **Y29** Contact with blunt object, undetermined intent

✓x7ᵗʰ **Y30** Falling, jumping or pushed from a high place, undetermined intent

> Victim falling from one level to another, undetermined intent

✓x7ᵗʰ **Y31** Falling, lying or running before or into moving object, undetermined intent

✓x7ᵗʰ **Y32** Crashing of motor vehicle, undetermined intent

✓x7ᵗʰ **Y33** Other specified events, undetermined intent

Legal intervention, operations of war, military operations, and terrorism (Y35-Y38)

The appropriate 7th character is to be added to each code from categories Y35-Y38.
A   initial encounter
D   subsequent encounter
S   sequela

✓4ᵗʰ **Y35** **Legal intervention**

> INCLUDES   any injury sustained as a result of an encounter with any law enforcement official, serving in any capacity at the time of the encounter, whether on-duty or off-duty. Includes injury to law enforcement official, suspect and bystander
>
> **AHA:** 2019,4Q,18-19

✓5ᵗʰ **Y35.0** Legal intervention involving **firearm discharge**

✓6ᵗʰ **Y35.00** Legal intervention involving unspecified firearm discharge

> Legal intervention involving gunshot wound
> Legal intervention involving shot NOS

✓7ᵗʰ **Y35.001** **Legal intervention involving unspecified firearm discharge, law enforcement official injured**

✓7ᵗʰ **Y35.002** **Legal intervention involving unspecified firearm discharge, bystander injured**

✓7ᵗʰ **Y35.003** **Legal intervention involving unspecified firearm discharge, suspect injured**

✓7ᵗʰ **Y35.009** **Legal intervention involving unspecified firearm discharge, unspecified person injured**

✓6ᵗʰ **Y35.01** Legal intervention involving injury by **machine gun**

✓7ᵗʰ **Y35.011** **Legal intervention involving injury by machine gun, law enforcement official injured**

✓7ᵗʰ **Y35.012** **Legal intervention involving injury by machine gun, bystander injured**

✓7ᵗʰ **Y35.013** **Legal intervention involving injury by machine gun, suspect injured**

✓7ᵗʰ **Y35.019** **Legal intervention involving injury by machine gun, unspecified person injured**

✓6ᵗʰ **Y35.02** Legal intervention involving injury by **handgun**

✓7ᵗʰ **Y35.021** **Legal intervention involving injury by handgun, law enforcement official injured**

✓7ᵗʰ **Y35.022** **Legal intervention involving injury by handgun, bystander injured**

✓7ᵗʰ **Y35.023** **Legal intervention involving injury by handgun, suspect injured**

✓7ᵗʰ **Y35.029** **Legal intervention involving injury by handgun, unspecified person injured**

✓6ᵗʰ **Y35.03** Legal intervention involving injury by **rifle pellet**

✓7ᵗʰ **Y35.031** **Legal intervention involving injury by rifle pellet, law enforcement official injured**

✓7ᵗʰ **Y35.032** **Legal intervention involving injury by rifle pellet, bystander injured**

✓7ᵗʰ **Y35.033** **Legal intervention involving injury by rifle pellet, suspect injured**

✓7ᵗʰ **Y35.039** **Legal intervention involving injury by rifle pellet, unspecified person injured**

✓6ᵗʰ **Y35.04** Legal intervention involving injury by **rubber bullet**

✓7ᵗʰ **Y35.041** **Legal intervention involving injury by rubber bullet, law enforcement official injured**

✓7ᵗʰ **Y35.042** **Legal intervention involving injury by rubber bullet, bystander injured**

✓7ᵗʰ **Y35.043** **Legal intervention involving injury by rubber bullet, suspect injured**

✓7ᵗʰ **Y35.049** **Legal intervention involving injury by rubber bullet, unspecified person injured**

✓6ᵗʰ **Y35.09** Legal intervention involving other firearm discharge

✓7ᵗʰ **Y35.091** **Legal intervention involving other firearm discharge, law enforcement official injured**

✓7ᵗʰ **Y35.092** **Legal intervention involving other firearm discharge, bystander injured**

✓7ᵗʰ **Y35.093** **Legal intervention involving other firearm discharge, suspect injured**

✓7ᵗʰ **Y35.099** **Legal intervention involving other firearm discharge, unspecified person injured**

✓ Additional Char Req   ✓x7ᵗʰ Placeholder   Unacceptable PDx   Questionable PDx   Wrong Procedure   Manifestation   Unspecified   H1 - H14 HAC   HCC CMS-HCC Dx   HIV HIV Dx

ICD-10-CM 2025   **1241**

✓5th **Y35.1** **Legal intervention involving explosives**

  ✓6th **Y35.10** **Legal intervention involving unspecified explosives**

    ✓7th **Y35.101** Legal intervention involving unspecified explosives, **law enforcement official** injured

    ✓7th **Y35.102** Legal intervention involving unspecified explosives, **bystander** injured

    ✓7th **Y35.103** Legal intervention involving unspecified explosives, **suspect** injured

    ✓7th **Y35.109** Legal intervention involving unspecified explosives, unspecified person injured

  ✓6th **Y35.11** **Legal intervention involving injury by dynamite**

    ✓7th **Y35.111** Legal intervention involving injury by dynamite, **law enforcement official** injured

    ✓7th **Y35.112** Legal intervention involving injury by dynamite, **bystander** injured

    ✓7th **Y35.113** Legal intervention involving injury by dynamite, **suspect** injured

    ✓7th **Y35.119** Legal intervention involving injury by dynamite, unspecified person injured

  ✓6th **Y35.12** **Legal intervention involving injury by explosive shell**

    ✓7th **Y35.121** Legal intervention involving injury by explosive shell, **law enforcement official** injured

    ✓7th **Y35.122** Legal intervention involving injury by explosive shell, **bystander** injured

    ✓7th **Y35.123** Legal intervention involving injury by explosive shell, **suspect** injured

    ✓7th **Y35.129** Legal intervention involving injury by explosive shell, unspecified person injured

  ✓6th **Y35.19** **Legal intervention involving other explosives**

    Legal intervention involving injury by grenade
    Legal intervention involving injury by mortar bomb

    ✓7th **Y35.191** Legal intervention involving other explosives, **law enforcement official** injured

    ✓7th **Y35.192** Legal intervention involving other explosives, **bystander** injured

    ✓7th **Y35.193** Legal intervention involving other explosives, **suspect** injured

    ✓7th **Y35.199** Legal intervention involving other explosives, unspecified person injured

✓5th **Y35.2** **Legal intervention involving gas**

  Legal intervention involving asphyxiation by gas
  Legal intervention involving poisoning by gas

  ✓6th **Y35.20** **Legal intervention involving unspecified gas**

    ✓7th **Y35.201** Legal intervention involving unspecified gas, **law enforcement official** injured

    ✓7th **Y35.202** Legal intervention involving unspecified gas, **bystander** injured

    ✓7th **Y35.203** Legal intervention involving unspecified gas, **suspect** injured

    ✓7th **Y35.209** Legal intervention involving unspecified gas, unspecified person injured

  ✓6th **Y35.21** **Legal intervention involving injury by tear gas**

    ✓7th **Y35.211** Legal intervention involving injury by tear gas, **law enforcement official** injured

    ✓7th **Y35.212** Legal intervention involving injury by tear gas, **bystander** injured

    ✓7th **Y35.213** Legal intervention involving injury by tear gas, **suspect** injured

    ✓7th **Y35.219** Legal intervention involving injury by tear gas, unspecified person injured

  ✓6th **Y35.29** **Legal intervention involving other gas**

    ✓7th **Y35.291** Legal intervention involving other gas, **law enforcement official** injured

    ✓7th **Y35.292** Legal intervention involving other gas, **bystander** injured

    ✓7th **Y35.293** Legal intervention involving other gas, **suspect** injured

    ✓7th **Y35.299** Legal intervention involving other gas, unspecified person injured

✓5th **Y35.3** **Legal intervention involving blunt objects**

  Legal intervention involving being hit or struck by blunt object

  ✓6th **Y35.30** **Legal intervention involving unspecified blunt objects**

    ✓7th **Y35.301** Legal intervention involving unspecified blunt objects, **law enforcement official** injured

    ✓7th **Y35.302** Legal intervention involving unspecified blunt objects, **bystander** injured

    ✓7th **Y35.303** Legal intervention involving unspecified blunt objects, **suspect** injured

    ✓7th **Y35.309** Legal intervention involving unspecified blunt objects, unspecified person injured

  ✓6th **Y35.31** **Legal intervention involving baton**

    ✓7th **Y35.311** Legal intervention involving baton, **law enforcement official** injured

    ✓7th **Y35.312** Legal intervention involving baton, **bystander** injured

    ✓7th **Y35.313** Legal intervention involving baton, **suspect** injured

    ✓7th **Y35.319** Legal intervention involving baton, unspecified person injured

  ✓6th **Y35.39** **Legal intervention involving other blunt objects**

    ✓7th **Y35.391** Legal intervention involving other blunt objects, **law enforcement official** injured

    ✓7th **Y35.392** Legal intervention involving other blunt objects, **bystander** injured

    ✓7th **Y35.393** Legal intervention involving other blunt objects, **suspect** injured

    ✓7th **Y35.399** Legal intervention involving other blunt objects, unspecified person injured

✓5th **Y35.4** **Legal intervention involving sharp objects**

  Legal intervention involving being cut by sharp objects
  Legal intervention involving being stabbed by sharp objects

  ✓6th **Y35.40** **Legal intervention involving unspecified sharp objects**

    ✓7th **Y35.401** Legal intervention involving unspecified sharp objects, **law enforcement official** injured

    ✓7th **Y35.402** Legal intervention involving unspecified sharp objects, **bystander** injured

    ✓7th **Y35.403** Legal intervention involving unspecified sharp objects, **suspect** injured

    ✓7th **Y35.409** Legal intervention involving unspecified sharp objects, unspecified person injured

  ✓6th **Y35.41** **Legal intervention involving bayonet**

    ✓7th **Y35.411** Legal intervention involving bayonet, **law enforcement official** injured

    ✓7th **Y35.412** Legal intervention involving bayonet, **bystander** injured

    ✓7th **Y35.413** Legal intervention involving bayonet, **suspect** injured

    ✓7th **Y35.419** Legal intervention involving bayonet, unspecified person injured

  ✓6th **Y35.49** **Legal intervention involving other sharp objects**

    ✓7th **Y35.491** Legal intervention involving other sharp objects, **law enforcement official** injured

    ✓7th **Y35.492** Legal intervention involving other sharp objects, **bystander** injured

    ✓7th **Y35.493** Legal intervention involving other sharp objects, **suspect** injured

    ✓7th **Y35.499** Legal intervention involving other sharp objects, unspecified person injured

✓5th **Y35.8** **Legal intervention involving other specified means**

  AHA: 2019,4Q,19

  ✓6th **Y35.81** **Legal intervention involving manhandling**

    ✓7th **Y35.811** Legal intervention involving manhandling, **law enforcement official** injured

    ✓7th **Y35.812** Legal intervention involving manhandling, **bystander** injured

    ✓7th **Y35.813** Legal intervention involving manhandling, **suspect** injured

    ✓7th **Y35.819** Legal intervention involving manhandling, unspecified person injured

  ✓6th **Y35.83** **Legal intervention involving a conducted energy device**

    Electroshock device (taser)
    Stun gun

    ✓7th **Y35.831** Legal intervention involving a conducted energy device, **law enforcement official** injured

    ✓7th **Y35.832** Legal intervention involving a conducted energy device, **bystander** injured

    ✓7th **Y35.833** Legal intervention involving a conducted energy device, **suspect** injured

    ✓7th **Y35.839** Legal intervention involving a conducted energy device, unspecified person injured

N Newborn: 0   P Pediatric: 0-17   M Maternity: 9-64   A Adult: 15-124   UNS Unspecified Site   MCC Major Complication/Comorbidity   CC Complication/Comorbidity   PE POA Exempt

1242   ICD-10-CM 2025

√6ᵗʰ **Y35.89** Legal intervention involving other specified means

  √7ᵗʰ **Y35.891** Legal intervention involving other specified means, law enforcement official injured

  √7ᵗʰ **Y35.892** Legal intervention involving other specified means, bystander injured

  √7ᵗʰ **Y35.893** Legal intervention involving other specified means, suspect injured

    AHA: 2018,1Q,5

  √7ᵗʰ **Y35.899** Legal intervention involving other specified means, unspecified person injured

√5ᵗʰ **Y35.9** Legal intervention, means unspecified

  √x7ᵗʰ **Y35.91** Legal intervention, means unspecified, law enforcement official injured

  √x7ᵗʰ **Y35.92** Legal intervention, means unspecified, bystander injured

  √x7ᵗʰ **Y35.93** Legal intervention, means unspecified, suspect injured

  √x7ᵗʰ **Y35.99** Legal intervention, means unspecified, unspecified person injured

√4ᵗʰ **Y36 Operations of war**

  INCLUDES injuries to military personnel and civilians caused by war, civil insurrection, and peacekeeping missions

  EXCLUDES 1 *injury to military personnel occurring during peacetime military operations (Y37.-)*

    military vehicles involved in transport accidents with non-military vehicle during peacetime (V09.01, V09.21, V19.81, V29.818, V39.81, V49.81, V59.81, V69.81, V79.81)

  AHA: 2014,3Q,4

√5ᵗʰ **Y36.0** War operations involving explosion of marine weapons

  √6ᵗʰ **Y36.00** War operations involving explosion of unspecified marine weapon

    War operations involving underwater blast NOS

    √7ᵗʰ **Y36.000** War operations involving explosion of unspecified marine weapon, military personnel

    √7ᵗʰ **Y36.001** War operations involving explosion of unspecified marine weapon, civilian

  √6ᵗʰ **Y36.01** War operations involving explosion of depth-charge

    √7ᵗʰ **Y36.010** War operations involving explosion of depth-charge, military personnel

    √7ᵗʰ **Y36.011** War operations involving explosion of depth-charge, civilian

  √6ᵗʰ **Y36.02** War operations involving explosion of marine mine

    War operations involving explosion of marine mine, at sea or in harbor

    √7ᵗʰ **Y36.020** War operations involving explosion of marine mine, military personnel

    √7ᵗʰ **Y36.021** War operations involving explosion of marine mine, civilian

  √6ᵗʰ **Y36.03** War operations involving explosion of sea-based artillery shell

    √7ᵗʰ **Y36.030** War operations involving explosion of sea-based artillery shell, military personnel

    √7ᵗʰ **Y36.031** War operations involving explosion of sea-based artillery shell, civilian

  √6ᵗʰ **Y36.04** War operations involving explosion of torpedo

    √7ᵗʰ **Y36.040** War operations involving explosion of torpedo, military personnel

    √7ᵗʰ **Y36.041** War operations involving explosion of torpedo, civilian

  √6ᵗʰ **Y36.05** War operations involving accidental detonation of onboard marine weapons

    √7ᵗʰ **Y36.050** War operations involving accidental detonation of onboard marine weapons, military personnel

    √7ᵗʰ **Y36.051** War operations involving accidental detonation of onboard marine weapons, civilian

  √6ᵗʰ **Y36.09** War operations involving explosion of other marine weapons

    √7ᵗʰ **Y36.090** War operations involving explosion of other marine weapons, military personnel

    √7ᵗʰ **Y36.091** War operations involving explosion of other marine weapons, civilian

√5ᵗʰ **Y36.1** War operations involving destruction of aircraft

  √6ᵗʰ **Y36.10** War operations involving unspecified destruction of aircraft

    √7ᵗʰ **Y36.100** War operations involving unspecified destruction of aircraft, military personnel

    √7ᵗʰ **Y36.101** War operations involving unspecified destruction of aircraft, civilian

  √6ᵗʰ **Y36.11** War operations involving destruction of aircraft due to enemy fire or explosives

    War operations involving destruction of aircraft due to air to air missile

    War operations involving destruction of aircraft due to explosive placed on aircraft

    War operations involving destruction of aircraft due to rocket propelled grenade [RPG]

    War operations involving destruction of aircraft due to small arms fire

    War operations involving destruction of aircraft due to surface to air missile

    √7ᵗʰ **Y36.110** War operations involving destruction of aircraft due to enemy fire or explosives, military personnel

    √7ᵗʰ **Y36.111** War operations involving destruction of aircraft due to enemy fire or explosives, civilian

  √6ᵗʰ **Y36.12** War operations involving destruction of aircraft due to collision with other aircraft

    √7ᵗʰ **Y36.120** War operations involving destruction of aircraft due to collision with other aircraft, military personnel

    √7ᵗʰ **Y36.121** War operations involving destruction of aircraft due to collision with other aircraft, civilian

  √6ᵗʰ **Y36.13** War operations involving destruction of aircraft due to onboard fire

    √7ᵗʰ **Y36.130** War operations involving destruction of aircraft due to onboard fire, military personnel

    √7ᵗʰ **Y36.131** War operations involving destruction of aircraft due to onboard fire, civilian

  √6ᵗʰ **Y36.14** War operations involving destruction of aircraft due to accidental detonation of onboard munitions and explosives

    √7ᵗʰ **Y36.140** War operations involving destruction of aircraft due to accidental detonation of onboard munitions and explosives, military personnel

    √7ᵗʰ **Y36.141** War operations involving destruction of aircraft due to accidental detonation of onboard munitions and explosives, civilian

  √6ᵗʰ **Y36.19** War operations involving other destruction of aircraft

    √7ᵗʰ **Y36.190** War operations involving other destruction of aircraft, military personnel

    √7ᵗʰ **Y36.191** War operations involving other destruction of aircraft, civilian

√5ᵗʰ **Y36.2** War operations involving other explosions and fragments

  EXCLUDES 1 *war operations involving explosion of aircraft (Y36.1-)*

    war operations involving explosion of marine weapons (Y36.0-)

    war operations involving explosion of nuclear weapons (Y36.5-)

    war operations involving explosion occurring after cessation of hostilities (Y36.8-)

  √6ᵗʰ **Y36.20** War operations involving unspecified explosion and fragments

    War operations involving air blast NOS

    War operations involving blast NOS

    War operations involving blast fragments NOS

    War operations involving blast wave NOS

    War operations involving blast wind NOS

    War operations involving explosion NOS

    War operations involving explosion of bomb NOS

    √7ᵗʰ **Y36.200** War operations involving unspecified explosion and fragments, military personnel

    √7ᵗʰ **Y36.201** War operations involving unspecified explosion and fragments, civilian

  √6ᵗʰ **Y36.21** War operations involving explosion of aerial bomb

    √7ᵗʰ **Y36.210** War operations involving explosion of aerial bomb, military personnel

    √7ᵗʰ **Y36.211** War operations involving explosion of aerial bomb, civilian

✓6ᵗʰ **Y36.22** **War operations involving explosion of guided missile**

   ✓7ᵗʰ **Y36.220** **War operations involving explosion of guided missile, military personnel**

   ✓7ᵗʰ **Y36.221** **War operations involving explosion of guided missile, civilian**

✓6ᵗʰ **Y36.23** **War operations involving explosion of improvised explosive device [IED]**

   War operations involving explosion of person-borne improvised explosive device [IED]
   War operations involving explosion of vehicle-borne improvised explosive device [IED]
   War operations involving explosion of roadside improvised explosive device [IED]

   ✓7ᵗʰ **Y36.230** **War operations involving explosion of improvised explosive device [IED], military personnel**

   ✓7ᵗʰ **Y36.231** **War operations involving explosion of improvised explosive device [IED], civilian**

✓6ᵗʰ **Y36.24** **War operations involving explosion due to accidental detonation and discharge of own munitions or munitions launch device**

   ✓7ᵗʰ **Y36.240** **War operations involving explosion due to accidental detonation and discharge of own munitions or munitions launch device, military personnel**

   ✓7ᵗʰ **Y36.241** **War operations involving explosion due to accidental detonation and discharge of own munitions or munitions launch device, civilian**

✓6ᵗʰ **Y36.25** **War operations involving fragments from munitions**

   ✓7ᵗʰ **Y36.250** **War operations involving fragments from munitions, military personnel**

   ✓7ᵗʰ **Y36.251** **War operations involving fragments from munitions, civilian**

✓6ᵗʰ **Y36.26** **War operations involving fragments of improvised explosive device [IED]**

   War operations involving fragments of person-borne improvised explosive device [IED]
   War operations involving fragments of roadside improvised explosive device [IED]
   War operations involving fragments of vehicle-borne improvised explosive device [IED]

   ✓7ᵗʰ **Y36.260** **War operations involving fragments of improvised explosive device [IED], military personnel**

   ✓7ᵗʰ **Y36.261** **War operations involving fragments of improvised explosive device [IED], civilian**

✓6ᵗʰ **Y36.27** **War operations involving fragments from weapons**

   ✓7ᵗʰ **Y36.270** **War operations involving fragments from weapons, military personnel**

   ✓7ᵗʰ **Y36.271** **War operations involving fragments from weapons, civilian**

✓6ᵗʰ **Y36.29** **War operations involving other explosions and fragments**

   War operations involving explosion of grenade
   War operations involving explosions of land mine
   War operations involving shrapnel NOS

   ✓7ᵗʰ **Y36.290** **War operations involving other explosions and fragments, military personnel**

   ✓7ᵗʰ **Y36.291** **War operations involving other explosions and fragments, civilian**

✓5ᵗʰ **Y36.3** **War operations involving fires, conflagrations and hot substances**

   War operations involving smoke, fumes, and heat from fires, conflagrations and hot substances

   EXCLUDES 1 *war operations involving fires and conflagrations aboard military aircraft (Y36.1-)*
        war operations involving fires and conflagrations aboard military watercraft (Y36.0-)
        war operations involving fires and conflagrations caused indirectly by conventional weapons (Y36.2-)
        war operations involving fires and thermal effects of nuclear weapons (Y36.53-)

   ✓6ᵗʰ **Y36.30** **War operations involving unspecified fire, conflagration and hot substance**

      ✓7ᵗʰ **Y36.300** **War operations involving unspecified fire, conflagration and hot substance, military personnel**

      ✓7ᵗʰ **Y36.301** **War operations involving unspecified fire, conflagration and hot substance, civilian**

✓6ᵗʰ **Y36.31** **War operations involving gasoline bomb**

   War operations involving incendiary bomb
   War operations involving petrol bomb

   ✓7ᵗʰ **Y36.310** **War operations involving gasoline bomb, military personnel**

   ✓7ᵗʰ **Y36.311** **War operations involving gasoline bomb, civilian**

✓6ᵗʰ **Y36.32** **War operations involving incendiary bullet**

   ✓7ᵗʰ **Y36.320** **War operations involving incendiary bullet, military personnel**

   ✓7ᵗʰ **Y36.321** **War operations involving incendiary bullet, civilian**

✓6ᵗʰ **Y36.33** **War operations involving flamethrower**

   ✓7ᵗʰ **Y36.330** **War operations involving flamethrower, military personnel**

   ✓7ᵗʰ **Y36.331** **War operations involving flamethrower, civilian**

✓6ᵗʰ **Y36.39** **War operations involving other fires, conflagrations and hot substances**

   ✓7ᵗʰ **Y36.390** **War operations involving other fires, conflagrations and hot substances, military personnel**

   ✓7ᵗʰ **Y36.391** **War operations involving other fires, conflagrations and hot substances, civilian**

✓5ᵗʰ **Y36.4** **War operations involving firearm discharge and other forms of conventional warfare**

   ✓6ᵗʰ **Y36.41** **War operations involving rubber bullets**

      ✓7ᵗʰ **Y36.410** **War operations involving rubber bullets, military personnel**

      ✓7ᵗʰ **Y36.411** **War operations involving rubber bullets, civilian**

   ✓6ᵗʰ **Y36.42** **War operations involving firearms pellets**

      ✓7ᵗʰ **Y36.420** **War operations involving firearms pellets, military personnel**

      ✓7ᵗʰ **Y36.421** **War operations involving firearms pellets, civilian**

   ✓6ᵗʰ **Y36.43** **War operations involving other firearms discharge**

      War operations involving bullets NOS

      EXCLUDES 1 *war operations involving munitions fragments (Y36.25-)*
         war operations involving incendiary bullets (Y36.32-)

      ✓7ᵗʰ **Y36.430** **War operations involving other firearms discharge, military personnel**

      ✓7ᵗʰ **Y36.431** **War operations involving other firearms discharge, civilian**

   ✓6ᵗʰ **Y36.44** **War operations involving unarmed hand to hand combat**

      EXCLUDES 1 *war operations involving combat using blunt or piercing object (Y36.45-)*
         war operations involving intentional restriction of air and airway (Y36.46-)
         war operations involving unintentional restriction of air and airway (Y36.47-)

      ✓7ᵗʰ **Y36.440** **War operations involving unarmed hand to hand combat, military personnel**

      ✓7ᵗʰ **Y36.441** **War operations involving unarmed hand to hand combat, civilian**

   ✓6ᵗʰ **Y36.45** **War operations involving combat using blunt or piercing object**

      ✓7ᵗʰ **Y36.450** **War operations involving combat using blunt or piercing object, military personnel**

      ✓7ᵗʰ **Y36.451** **War operations involving combat using blunt or piercing object, civilian**

   ✓6ᵗʰ **Y36.46** **War operations involving intentional restriction of air and airway**

      ✓7ᵗʰ **Y36.460** **War operations involving intentional restriction of air and airway, military personnel**

      ✓7ᵗʰ **Y36.461** **War operations involving intentional restriction of air and airway, civilian**

   ✓6ᵗʰ **Y36.47** **War operations involving unintentional restriction of air and airway**

      ✓7ᵗʰ **Y36.470** **War operations involving unintentional restriction of air and airway, military personnel**

      ✓7ᵗʰ **Y36.471** **War operations involving unintentional restriction of air and airway, civilian**

☑6ᵗʰ **Y36.49** **War operations involving other forms of conventional warfare**

  ☑7ᵗʰ **Y36.490** War operations involving other forms of conventional warfare, **military personnel**

  ☑7ᵗʰ **Y36.491** War operations involving other forms of conventional warfare, **civilian**

☑5ᵗʰ **Y36.5** **War operations involving nuclear weapons**

  War operations involving dirty bomb NOS

☑6ᵗʰ **Y36.50** **War operations involving unspecified effect of nuclear weapon**

  ☑7ᵗʰ **Y36.500** War operations involving unspecified effect of nuclear weapon, **military personnel**

  ☑7ᵗʰ **Y36.501** War operations involving unspecified effect of nuclear weapon, **civilian**

☑6ᵗʰ **Y36.51** **War operations involving direct blast effect of nuclear weapon**

  War operations involving blast pressure of nuclear weapon

  ☑7ᵗʰ **Y36.510** War operations involving direct blast effect of nuclear weapon, **military personnel**

  ☑7ᵗʰ **Y36.511** War operations involving direct blast effect of nuclear weapon, **civilian**

☑6ᵗʰ **Y36.52** **War operations involving indirect blast effect of nuclear weapon**

  War operations involving being thrown by blast of nuclear weapon

  War operations involving being struck or crushed by blast debris of nuclear weapon

  ☑7ᵗʰ **Y36.520** War operations involving indirect blast effect of nuclear weapon, **military personnel**

  ☑7ᵗʰ **Y36.521** War operations involving indirect blast effect of nuclear weapon, **civilian**

☑6ᵗʰ **Y36.53** **War operations involving thermal radiation effect of nuclear weapon**

  War operations involving direct heat from nuclear weapon

  War operations involving fireball effects from nuclear weapon

  ☑7ᵗʰ **Y36.530** War operations involving thermal radiation effect of nuclear weapon, **military personnel**

  ☑7ᵗʰ **Y36.531** War operations involving thermal radiation effect of nuclear weapon, **civilian**

☑6ᵗʰ **Y36.54** **War operation involving nuclear radiation effects of nuclear weapon**

  War operation involving acute radiation exposure from nuclear weapon

  War operation involving exposure to immediate ionizing radiation from nuclear weapon

  War operation involving fallout exposure from nuclear weapon

  War operation involving secondary effects of nuclear weapons

  ☑7ᵗʰ **Y36.540** War operation involving nuclear radiation effects of nuclear weapon, **military personnel**

  ☑7ᵗʰ **Y36.541** War operation involving nuclear radiation effects of nuclear weapon, **civilian**

☑6ᵗʰ **Y36.59** **War operation involving other effects of nuclear weapons**

  ☑7ᵗʰ **Y36.590** War operation involving other effects of nuclear weapons, **military personnel**

  ☑7ᵗʰ **Y36.591** War operation involving other effects of nuclear weapons, **civilian**

☑5ᵗʰ **Y36.6** **War operations involving biological weapons**

☑6ᵗʰ **Y36.6X** **War operations involving biological weapons**

  ☑7ᵗʰ **Y36.6X0** War operations involving biological weapons, **military personnel**

  ☑7ᵗʰ **Y36.6X1** War operations involving biological weapons, **civilian**

☑5ᵗʰ **Y36.7** **War operations involving chemical weapons and other forms of unconventional warfare**

  EXCLUDES 1 *war operations involving incendiary devices (Y36.3-, Y36.5-)*

☑6ᵗʰ **Y36.7X** **War operations involving chemical weapons and other forms of unconventional warfare**

  ☑7ᵗʰ **Y36.7X0** War operations involving chemical weapons and other forms of unconventional warfare, **military personnel**

  ☑7ᵗʰ **Y36.7X1** War operations involving chemical weapons and other forms of unconventional warfare, **civilian**

☑5ᵗʰ **Y36.8** **War operations occurring after cessation of hostilities**

  War operations classifiable to categories Y36.0-Y36.8 but occurring after cessation of hostilities

☑6ᵗʰ **Y36.81** **Explosion of mine placed during war operations but exploding after cessation of hostilities**

  ☑7ᵗʰ **Y36.810** Explosion of mine placed during war operations but exploding after cessation of hostilities, **military personnel**

  ☑7ᵗʰ **Y36.811** Explosion of mine placed during war operations but exploding after cessation of hostilities, **civilian**

☑6ᵗʰ **Y36.82** **Explosion of bomb placed during war operations but exploding after cessation of hostilities**

  ☑7ᵗʰ **Y36.820** Explosion of bomb placed during war operations but exploding after cessation of hostilities, **military personnel**

  ☑7ᵗʰ **Y36.821** Explosion of bomb placed during war operations but exploding after cessation of hostilities, **civilian**

☑6ᵗʰ **Y36.88** **Other war operations occurring after cessation of hostilities**

  ☑7ᵗʰ **Y36.880** Other war operations occurring after cessation of hostilities, **military personnel**

  ☑7ᵗʰ **Y36.881** Other war operations occurring after cessation of hostilities, **civilian**

☑6ᵗʰ **Y36.89** **Unspecified war operations occurring after cessation of hostilities**

  ☑7ᵗʰ **Y36.890** Unspecified war operations occurring after cessation of hostilities, **military personnel**

  ☑7ᵗʰ **Y36.891** Unspecified war operations occurring after cessation of hostilities, **civilian**

☑5ᵗʰ **Y36.9** **Other and unspecified war operations**

  ☑x7ᵗʰ **Y36.90** **War operations, unspecified**

  ☑x7ᵗʰ **Y36.91** **War operations involving unspecified weapon of mass destruction [WMD]**

  ☑x7ᵗʰ **Y36.92** **War operations involving friendly fire**

☑4ᵗʰ **Y37** **Military operations**

  INCLUDES injuries to military personnel and civilians occurring during peacetime on military property and during routine military exercises and operations

  EXCLUDES 1 *military aircraft involved in aircraft accident with civilian aircraft (V97.81-)*

    military vehicles involved in transport accident with civilian vehicle (V09.01, V09.21, V19.81, V29.818, V39.81, V49.81, V59.81, V69.81, V79.81)

    military watercraft involved in water transport accident with civilian watercraft (V94.81-)

    war operations (Y36.-)

☑5ᵗʰ **Y37.0** **Military operations involving explosion of marine weapons**

☑6ᵗʰ **Y37.00** **Military operations involving explosion of unspecified marine weapon**

  Military operations involving underwater blast NOS

  ☑7ᵗʰ **Y37.000** Military operations involving explosion of unspecified marine weapon, **military personnel**

  ☑7ᵗʰ **Y37.001** Military operations involving explosion of unspecified marine weapon, **civilian**

☑6ᵗʰ **Y37.01** **Military operations involving explosion of depth-charge**

  ☑7ᵗʰ **Y37.010** Military operations involving explosion of depth-charge, **military personnel**

  ☑7ᵗʰ **Y37.011** Military operations involving explosion of depth-charge, **civilian**

☑6ᵗʰ **Y37.02** **Military operations involving explosion of marine mine**

  Military operations involving explosion of marine mine, at sea or in harbor

  ☑7ᵗʰ **Y37.020** Military operations involving explosion of marine mine, **military personnel**

  ☑7ᵗʰ **Y37.021** Military operations involving explosion of marine mine, **civilian**

☑6ᵗʰ **Y37.03** **Military operations involving explosion of sea-based artillery shell**

  ☑7ᵗʰ **Y37.030** Military operations involving explosion of sea-based artillery shell, **military personnel**

  ☑7ᵗʰ **Y37.031** Military operations involving explosion of sea-based artillery shell, **civilian**

☑ Additional Char Req   ☑x7ᵗʰ Placeholder   Unacceptable PDx   Questionable PDx   Wrong Procedure   Manifestation   Unspecified   H1-H14 HAC   HCC CMS-HCC Dx   HIV HIV Dx

ICD-10-CM 2025   1245

✓6ᵗʰ **Y37.04** Military operations involving explosion of torpedo

  ✓7ᵗʰ **Y37.040** Military operations involving explosion of torpedo, military personnel

  ✓7ᵗʰ **Y37.041** Military operations involving explosion of torpedo, civilian

✓6ᵗʰ **Y37.05** Military operations involving accidental detonation of onboard marine weapons

  ✓7ᵗʰ **Y37.050** Military operations involving accidental detonation of onboard marine weapons, military personnel

  ✓7ᵗʰ **Y37.051** Military operations involving accidental detonation of onboard marine weapons, civilian

✓6ᵗʰ **Y37.09** Military operations involving explosion of other marine weapons

  ✓7ᵗʰ **Y37.090** Military operations involving explosion of other marine weapons, military personnel

  ✓7ᵗʰ **Y37.091** Military operations involving explosion of other marine weapons, civilian

✓5ᵗʰ **Y37.1** Military operations involving destruction of aircraft

✓6ᵗʰ **Y37.10** Military operations involving unspecified destruction of aircraft

  ✓7ᵗʰ **Y37.100** Military operations involving unspecified destruction of aircraft, military personnel

  ✓7ᵗʰ **Y37.101** Military operations involving unspecified destruction of aircraft, civilian

✓6ᵗʰ **Y37.11** Military operations involving destruction of aircraft due to enemy fire or explosives

  Military operations involving destruction of aircraft due to air to air missile

  Military operations involving destruction of aircraft due to explosive placed on aircraft

  Military operations involving destruction of aircraft due to rocket propelled grenade [RPG]

  Military operations involving destruction of aircraft due to small arms fire

  Military operations involving destruction of aircraft due to surface to air missile

  ✓7ᵗʰ **Y37.110** Military operations involving destruction of aircraft due to enemy fire or explosives, military personnel

  ✓7ᵗʰ **Y37.111** Military operations involving destruction of aircraft due to enemy fire or explosives, civilian

✓6ᵗʰ **Y37.12** Military operations involving destruction of aircraft due to collision with other aircraft

  ✓7ᵗʰ **Y37.120** Military operations involving destruction of aircraft due to collision with other aircraft, military personnel

  ✓7ᵗʰ **Y37.121** Military operations involving destruction of aircraft due to collision with other aircraft, civilian

✓6ᵗʰ **Y37.13** Military operations involving destruction of aircraft due to onboard fire

  ✓7ᵗʰ **Y37.130** Military operations involving destruction of aircraft due to onboard fire, military personnel

  ✓7ᵗʰ **Y37.131** Military operations involving destruction of aircraft due to onboard fire, civilian

✓6ᵗʰ **Y37.14** Military operations involving destruction of aircraft due to accidental detonation of onboard munitions and explosives

  ✓7ᵗʰ **Y37.140** Military operations involving destruction of aircraft due to accidental detonation of onboard munitions and explosives, military personnel

  ✓7ᵗʰ **Y37.141** Military operations involving destruction of aircraft due to accidental detonation of onboard munitions and explosives, civilian

✓6ᵗʰ **Y37.19** Military operations involving other destruction of aircraft

  ✓7ᵗʰ **Y37.190** Military operations involving other destruction of aircraft, military personnel

  ✓7ᵗʰ **Y37.191** Military operations involving other destruction of aircraft, civilian

✓5ᵗʰ **Y37.2** Military operations involving other explosions and fragments

  EXCLUDES 1 *military operations involving explosion of aircraft (Y37.1-)*

  military operations involving explosion of marine weapons (Y37.0-)

  military operations involving explosion of nuclear weapons (Y37.5-)

✓6ᵗʰ **Y37.20** Military operations involving unspecified explosion and fragments

  Military operations involving air blast NOS

  Military operations involving blast NOS

  Military operations involving blast fragments NOS

  Military operations involving blast wave NOS

  Military operations involving blast wind NOS

  Military operations involving explosion NOS

  Military operations involving explosion of bomb NOS

  ✓7ᵗʰ **Y37.200** Military operations involving unspecified explosion and fragments, military personnel

  ✓7ᵗʰ **Y37.201** Military operations involving unspecified explosion and fragments, civilian

✓6ᵗʰ **Y37.21** Military operations involving explosion of aerial bomb

  ✓7ᵗʰ **Y37.210** Military operations involving explosion of aerial bomb, military personnel

  ✓7ᵗʰ **Y37.211** Military operations involving explosion of aerial bomb, civilian

✓6ᵗʰ **Y37.22** Military operations involving explosion of guided missile

  ✓7ᵗʰ **Y37.220** Military operations involving explosion of guided missile, military personnel

  ✓7ᵗʰ **Y37.221** Military operations involving explosion of guided missile, civilian

✓6ᵗʰ **Y37.23** Military operations involving explosion of improvised explosive device [IED]

  Military operations involving explosion of person-borne improvised explosive device [IED]

  Military operations involving explosion of vehicle-borne improvised explosive device [IED]

  Military operations involving explosion of roadside improvised explosive device [IED]

  ✓7ᵗʰ **Y37.230** Military operations involving explosion of improvised explosive device [IED], military personnel

  ✓7ᵗʰ **Y37.231** Military operations involving explosion of improvised explosive device [IED], civilian

✓6ᵗʰ **Y37.24** Military operations involving explosion due to accidental detonation and discharge of own munitions or munitions launch device

  ✓7ᵗʰ **Y37.240** Military operations involving explosion due to accidental detonation and discharge of own munitions or munitions launch device, military personnel

  ✓7ᵗʰ **Y37.241** Military operations involving explosion due to accidental detonation and discharge of own munitions or munitions launch device, civilian

✓6ᵗʰ **Y37.25** Military operations involving fragments from munitions

  ✓7ᵗʰ **Y37.250** Military operations involving fragments from munitions, military personnel

  ✓7ᵗʰ **Y37.251** Military operations involving fragments from munitions, civilian

✓6ᵗʰ **Y37.26** Military operations involving fragments of improvised explosive device [IED]

  Military operations involving fragments of person-borne improvised explosive device [IED]

  Military operations involving fragments of vehicle-borne improvised explosive device [IED]

  Military operations involving fragments of roadside improvised explosive device [IED]

  ✓7ᵗʰ **Y37.260** Military operations involving fragments of improvised explosive device [IED], military personnel

  ✓7ᵗʰ **Y37.261** Military operations involving fragments of improvised explosive device [IED], civilian

✓6ᵗʰ **Y37.27** Military operations involving fragments from weapons

  ✓7ᵗʰ **Y37.270** Military operations involving fragments from weapons, military personnel

  ✓7ᵗʰ **Y37.271** Military operations involving fragments from weapons, civilian

N Newborn: 0　**P** Pediatric: 0-17　**M** Maternity: 9-64　**A** Adult: 15-124　**UNS** Unspecified Site　**MCC** Major Complication/Comorbidity　**CC** Complication/Comorbidity　**PE** POA Exempt

1246　　ICD-10-CM 2025

Chapter 20. External Causes of Morbidity

√6ᵗʰ **Y37.29** **Military operations involving other explosions and fragments**
    Military operations involving explosion of grenade
    Military operations involving explosions of land mine
    Military operations involving shrapnel NOS

√7ᵗʰ **Y37.290** **Military operations involving other explosions and fragments, military personnel**

√7ᵗʰ **Y37.291** **Military operations involving other explosions and fragments, civilian**

√5ᵗʰ **Y37.3** **Military operations involving fires, conflagrations and hot substances**
    Military operations involving smoke, fumes, and heat from fires, conflagrations and hot substances
    EXCLUDES 1   *military operations involving fires and conflagrations aboard military aircraft (Y37.1-)*
        military operations involving fires and conflagrations aboard military watercraft (Y37.0-)
        military operations involving fires and conflagrations caused indirectly by conventional weapons (Y37.2-)
        military operations involving fires and thermal effects of nuclear weapons (Y36.53-)

√6ᵗʰ **Y37.30** **Military operations involving unspecified fire, conflagration and hot substance**

√7ᵗʰ **Y37.300** **Military operations involving unspecified fire, conflagration and hot substance, military personnel**

√7ᵗʰ **Y37.301** **Military operations involving unspecified fire, conflagration and hot substance, civilian**

√6ᵗʰ **Y37.31** **Military operations involving gasoline bomb**
    Military operations involving incendiary bomb
    Military operations involving petrol bomb

√7ᵗʰ **Y37.310** **Military operations involving gasoline bomb, military personnel**

√7ᵗʰ **Y37.311** **Military operations involving gasoline bomb, civilian**

√6ᵗʰ **Y37.32** **Military operations involving incendiary bullet**

√7ᵗʰ **Y37.320** **Military operations involving incendiary bullet, military personnel**

√7ᵗʰ **Y37.321** **Military operations involving incendiary bullet, civilian**

√6ᵗʰ **Y37.33** **Military operations involving flamethrower**

√7ᵗʰ **Y37.330** **Military operations involving flamethrower, military personnel**

√7ᵗʰ **Y37.331** **Military operations involving flamethrower, civilian**

√6ᵗʰ **Y37.39** **Military operations involving other fires, conflagrations and hot substances**

√7ᵗʰ **Y37.390** **Military operations involving other fires, conflagrations and hot substances, military personnel**

√7ᵗʰ **Y37.391** **Military operations involving other fires, conflagrations and hot substances, civilian**

√5ᵗʰ **Y37.4** **Military operations involving firearm discharge and other forms of conventional warfare**

√6ᵗʰ **Y37.41** **Military operations involving rubber bullets**

√7ᵗʰ **Y37.410** **Military operations involving rubber bullets, military personnel**

√7ᵗʰ **Y37.411** **Military operations involving rubber bullets, civilian**

√6ᵗʰ **Y37.42** **Military operations involving firearms pellets**

√7ᵗʰ **Y37.420** **Military operations involving firearms pellets, military personnel**

√7ᵗʰ **Y37.421** **Military operations involving firearms pellets, civilian**

√6ᵗʰ **Y37.43** **Military operations involving other firearms discharge**
    Military operations involving bullets NOS
    EXCLUDES 1   *military operations involving munitions fragments (Y37.25-)*
        military operations involving incendiary bullets (Y37.32-)

√7ᵗʰ **Y37.430** **Military operations involving other firearms discharge, military personnel**

√7ᵗʰ **Y37.431** **Military operations involving other firearms discharge, civilian**

√6ᵗʰ **Y37.44** **Military operations involving unarmed hand to hand combat**
    EXCLUDES 1   *military operations involving combat using blunt or piercing object (Y37.45-)*
        military operations involving intentional restriction of air and airway (Y37.46-)
        military operations involving unintentional restriction of air and airway (Y37.47-)

√7ᵗʰ **Y37.440** **Military operations involving unarmed hand to hand combat, military personnel**

√7ᵗʰ **Y37.441** **Military operations involving unarmed hand to hand combat, civilian**

√6ᵗʰ **Y37.45** **Military operations involving combat using blunt or piercing object**

√7ᵗʰ **Y37.450** **Military operations involving combat using blunt or piercing object, military personnel**

√7ᵗʰ **Y37.451** **Military operations involving combat using blunt or piercing object, civilian**

√6ᵗʰ **Y37.46** **Military operations involving intentional restriction of air and airway**

√7ᵗʰ **Y37.460** **Military operations involving intentional restriction of air and airway, military personnel**

√7ᵗʰ **Y37.461** **Military operations involving intentional restriction of air and airway, civilian**

√6ᵗʰ **Y37.47** **Military operations involving unintentional restriction of air and airway**

√7ᵗʰ **Y37.470** **Military operations involving unintentional restriction of air and airway, military personnel**

√7ᵗʰ **Y37.471** **Military operations involving unintentional restriction of air and airway, civilian**

√6ᵗʰ **Y37.49** **Military operations involving other forms of conventional warfare**

√7ᵗʰ **Y37.490** **Military operations involving other forms of conventional warfare, military personnel**

√7ᵗʰ **Y37.491** **Military operations involving other forms of conventional warfare, civilian**

√5ᵗʰ **Y37.5** **Military operations involving nuclear weapons**
    Military operation involving dirty bomb NOS

√6ᵗʰ **Y37.50** **Military operations involving unspecified effect of nuclear weapon**

√7ᵗʰ **Y37.500** **Military operations involving unspecified effect of nuclear weapon, military personnel**

√7ᵗʰ **Y37.501** **Military operations involving unspecified effect of nuclear weapon, civilian**

√6ᵗʰ **Y37.51** **Military operations involving direct blast effect of nuclear weapon**
    Military operations involving blast pressure of nuclear weapon

√7ᵗʰ **Y37.510** **Military operations involving direct blast effect of nuclear weapon, military personnel**

√7ᵗʰ **Y37.511** **Military operations involving direct blast effect of nuclear weapon, civilian**

√6ᵗʰ **Y37.52** **Military operations involving indirect blast effect of nuclear weapon**
    Military operations involving being thrown by blast of nuclear weapon
    Military operations involving being struck or crushed by blast debris of nuclear weapon

√7ᵗʰ **Y37.520** **Military operations involving indirect blast effect of nuclear weapon, military personnel**

√7ᵗʰ **Y37.521** **Military operations involving indirect blast effect of nuclear weapon, civilian**

√6ᵗʰ **Y37.53** **Military operations involving thermal radiation effect of nuclear weapon**
    Military operations involving direct heat from nuclear weapon
    Military operation involving fireball effects from nuclear weapon

√7ᵗʰ **Y37.530** **Military operations involving thermal radiation effect of nuclear weapon, military personnel**

√7ᵗʰ **Y37.531** **Military operations involving thermal radiation effect of nuclear weapon, civilian**

✔ Additional Char Req   √7ᵗʰ Placeholder   Unacceptable PDx   Questionable PDx   Wrong Procedure   Manifestation   Unspecified   H1 - H14 HAC   HCC CMS-HCC Dx   HIV HIV Dx

ICD-10-CM 2025   1247

☑6ᵗʰ **Y37.54 Military operation involving nuclear radiation effects of nuclear weapon**
Military operation involving acute radiation exposure from nuclear weapon
Military operation involving exposure to immediate ionizing radiation from nuclear weapon
Military operation involving fallout exposure from nuclear weapon
Military operation involving secondary effects of nuclear weapons

  ☑7ᵗʰ **Y37.540 Military operation involving nuclear radiation effects of nuclear weapon, military personnel**

  ☑7ᵗʰ **Y37.541 Military operation involving nuclear radiation effects of nuclear weapon, civilian**

☑6ᵗʰ **Y37.59 Military operation involving other effects of nuclear weapons**

  ☑7ᵗʰ **Y37.590 Military operation involving other effects of nuclear weapons, military personnel**

  ☑7ᵗʰ **Y37.591 Military operation involving other effects of nuclear weapons, civilian**

☑5ᵗʰ **Y37.6 Military operations involving biological weapons**

 ☑6ᵗʰ **Y37.6X Military operations involving biological weapons**

  ☑7ᵗʰ **Y37.6X0 Military operations involving biological weapons, military personnel**

  ☑7ᵗʰ **Y37.6X1 Military operations involving biological weapons, civilian**

☑5ᵗʰ **Y37.7 Military operations involving chemical weapons and other forms of unconventional warfare**

  EXCLUDES 1 *military operations involving incendiary devices (Y36.3-, Y36.5-)*

 ☑6ᵗʰ **Y37.7X Military operations involving chemical weapons and other forms of unconventional warfare**

  ☑7ᵗʰ **Y37.7X0 Military operations involving chemical weapons and other forms of unconventional warfare, military personnel**

  ☑7ᵗʰ **Y37.7X1 Military operations involving chemical weapons and other forms of unconventional warfare, civilian**

☑5ᵗʰ **Y37.9 Other and unspecified military operations**

 ☑x7ᵗʰ **Y37.90 Military operations, unspecified**

 ☑x7ᵗʰ **Y37.91 Military operations involving unspecified weapon of mass destruction [WMD]**

 ☑x7ᵗʰ **Y37.92 Military operations involving friendly fire**

☑4ᵗʰ **Y38 Terrorism**

NOTE These codes are for use to identify injuries resulting from the unlawful use of force or violence against persons or property to intimidate or coerce a Government, the civilian population, or any segment thereof, in furtherance of political or social objective

Use additional code for place of occurrence (Y92.-)

☑5ᵗʰ **Y38.0 Terrorism involving explosion of marine weapons**
Terrorism involving depth-charge
Terrorism involving marine mine
Terrorism involving mine NOS, at sea or in harbor
Terrorism involving sea-based artillery shell
Terrorism involving torpedo
Terrorism involving underwater blast

 ☑6ᵗʰ **Y38.0X Terrorism involving explosion of marine weapons**

  ☑7ᵗʰ **Y38.0X1 Terrorism involving explosion of marine weapons, public safety official injured**

  ☑7ᵗʰ **Y38.0X2 Terrorism involving explosion of marine weapons, civilian injured**

  ☑7ᵗʰ **Y38.0X3 Terrorism involving explosion of marine weapons, terrorist injured**

☑5ᵗʰ **Y38.1 Terrorism involving destruction of aircraft**
Terrorism involving aircraft burned
Terrorism involving aircraft exploded
Terrorism involving aircraft being shot down
Terrorism involving aircraft used as a weapon

 ☑6ᵗʰ **Y38.1X Terrorism involving destruction of aircraft**

  ☑7ᵗʰ **Y38.1X1 Terrorism involving destruction of aircraft, public safety official injured**

  ☑7ᵗʰ **Y38.1X2 Terrorism involving destruction of aircraft, civilian injured**

  ☑7ᵗʰ **Y38.1X3 Terrorism involving destruction of aircraft, terrorist injured**

☑5ᵗʰ **Y38.2 Terrorism involving other explosions and fragments**
Terrorism involving antipersonnel (fragments) bomb
Terrorism involving blast NOS
Terrorism involving explosion NOS
Terrorism involving explosion of breech block
Terrorism involving explosion of cannon block
Terrorism involving explosion (fragments) of artillery shell
Terrorism involving explosion (fragments) of bomb
Terrorism involving explosion (fragments) of grenade
Terrorism involving explosion (fragments) of guided missile
Terrorism involving explosion (fragments) of land mine
Terrorism involving explosion of mortar bomb
Terrorism involving explosion of munitions
Terrorism involving explosion (fragments) of rocket
Terrorism involving explosion (fragments) of shell
Terrorism involving shrapnel
Terrorism involving mine NOS, on land

  EXCLUDES 1 *terrorism involving explosion of nuclear weapon (Y38.5)*
    terrorism involving suicide bomber (Y38.81)

 ☑6ᵗʰ **Y38.2X Terrorism involving other explosions and fragments**

  ☑7ᵗʰ **Y38.2X1 Terrorism involving other explosions and fragments, public safety official injured**

  ☑7ᵗʰ **Y38.2X2 Terrorism involving other explosions and fragments, civilian injured**

  ☑7ᵗʰ **Y38.2X3 Terrorism involving other explosions and fragments, terrorist injured**

☑5ᵗʰ **Y38.3 Terrorism involving fires, conflagration and hot substances**
Terrorism involving conflagration NOS
Terrorism involving fire NOS
Terrorism involving petrol bomb

  EXCLUDES 1 *terrorism involving fire or heat of nuclear weapon (Y38.5)*

 ☑6ᵗʰ **Y38.3X Terrorism involving fires, conflagration and hot substances**

  ☑7ᵗʰ **Y38.3X1 Terrorism involving fires, conflagration and hot substances, public safety official injured**

  ☑7ᵗʰ **Y38.3X2 Terrorism involving fires, conflagration and hot substances, civilian injured**

  ☑7ᵗʰ **Y38.3X3 Terrorism involving fires, conflagration and hot substances, terrorist injured**

☑5ᵗʰ **Y38.4 Terrorism involving firearms**
Terrorism involving carbine bullet
Terrorism involving machine gun bullet
Terrorism involving pellets (shotgun)
Terrorism involving pistol bullet
Terrorism involving rifle bullet
Terrorism involving rubber (rifle) bullet

 ☑6ᵗʰ **Y38.4X Terrorism involving firearms**

  ☑7ᵗʰ **Y38.4X1 Terrorism involving firearms, public safety official injured**

  ☑7ᵗʰ **Y38.4X2 Terrorism involving firearms, civilian injured**

  ☑7ᵗʰ **Y38.4X3 Terrorism involving firearms, terrorist injured**

☑5ᵗʰ **Y38.5 Terrorism involving nuclear weapons**
Terrorism involving blast effects of nuclear weapon
Terrorism involving exposure to ionizing radiation from nuclear weapon
Terrorism involving fireball effect of nuclear weapon
Terrorism involving heat from nuclear weapon

 ☑6ᵗʰ **Y38.5X Terrorism involving nuclear weapons**

  ☑7ᵗʰ **Y38.5X1 Terrorism involving nuclear weapons, public safety official injured**

  ☑7ᵗʰ **Y38.5X2 Terrorism involving nuclear weapons, civilian injured**

  ☑7ᵗʰ **Y38.5X3 Terrorism involving nuclear weapons, terrorist injured**

☑5ᵗʰ **Y38.6 Terrorism involving biological weapons**
Terrorism involving anthrax
Terrorism involving cholera
Terrorism involving smallpox

 ☑6ᵗʰ **Y38.6X Terrorism involving biological weapons**

  ☑7ᵗʰ **Y38.6X1 Terrorism involving biological weapons, public safety official injured**

  ☑7ᵗʰ **Y38.6X2 Terrorism involving biological weapons, civilian injured**

  ☑7ᵗʰ **Y38.6X3 Terrorism involving biological weapons, terrorist injured**

N Newborn: 0   **P** Pediatric: 0-17   **M** Maternity: 9-64   **A** Adult: 15-124   **UNS** Unspecified Site   **MCC** Major Complication/Comorbidity   **CC** Complication/Comorbidity   **PE** POA Exempt

1248   ICD-10-CM 2025

✓5th **Y38.7** **Terrorism involving chemical weapons**
　　Terrorism involving gases, fumes, chemicals
　　Terrorism involving hydrogen cyanide
　　Terrorism involving phosgene
　　Terrorism involving sarin

　✓6th **Y38.7X** **Terrorism involving chemical weapons**

　　✓7th **Y38.7X1** **Terrorism involving chemical weapons, public safety official injured**

　　✓7th **Y38.7X2** **Terrorism involving chemical weapons, civilian injured**

　　✓7th **Y38.7X3** **Terrorism involving chemical weapons, terrorist injured**

✓5th **Y38.8** **Terrorism involving other and unspecified means**

　✓x7th **Y38.80** **Terrorism involving unspecified means**
　　Terrorism NOS

　✓6th **Y38.81** **Terrorism involving suicide bomber**

　　✓7th **Y38.811** **Terrorism involving suicide bomber, public safety official injured**

　　✓7th **Y38.812** **Terrorism involving suicide bomber, civilian injured**

　✓6th **Y38.89** **Terrorism involving other means**
　　Terrorism involving drowning and submersion
　　Terrorism involving lasers
　　Terrorism involving piercing or stabbing instruments

　　✓7th **Y38.891** **Terrorism involving other means, public safety official injured**

　　✓7th **Y38.892** **Terrorism involving other means, civilian injured**

　　✓7th **Y38.893** **Terrorism involving other means, terrorist injured**

✓5th **Y38.9** **Terrorism, secondary effects**

　　NOTE This code is for use to identify conditions occurring subsequent to a terrorist attack not those that are due to the initial terrorist attack

　✓6th **Y38.9X** **Terrorism, secondary effects**

　　✓7th **Y38.9X1** **Terrorism, secondary effects, public safety official injured**

　　✓7th **Y38.9X2** **Terrorism, secondary effects, civilian injured**

COMPLICATIONS OF MEDICAL AND SURGICAL CARE (Y62-Y84)

INCLUDES complications of medical devices
　surgical and medical procedures as the cause of abnormal reaction of the patient, or of later complication, without mention of misadventure at the time of the procedure

Misadventures to patients during surgical and medical care (Y62-Y69)

EXCLUDES 1 surgical and medical procedures as the cause of abnormal reaction of the patient, without mention of misadventure at the time of the procedure (Y83-Y84)

EXCLUDES 2 breakdown or malfunctioning of medical device (during procedure) (after implantation) (ongoing use) (Y70-Y82)

✓4th **Y62** **Failure of sterile precautions during surgical and medical care**

　Y62.0 **Failure of sterile precautions during surgical operation**

　Y62.1 **Failure of sterile precautions during infusion or transfusion**

　Y62.2 **Failure of sterile precautions during kidney dialysis and other perfusion**

　Y62.3 **Failure of sterile precautions during injection or immunization**

　Y62.4 **Failure of sterile precautions during endoscopic examination**

　Y62.5 **Failure of sterile precautions during heart catheterization**

　Y62.6 **Failure of sterile precautions during aspiration, puncture and other catheterization**

　Y62.8 **Failure of sterile precautions during other surgical and medical care**

　Y62.9 **Failure of sterile precautions during unspecified surgical and medical care**

✓4th **Y63** **Failure in dosage during surgical and medical care**

　EXCLUDES 2 accidental overdose of drug or wrong drug given in error (T36-T50)

　Y63.0 **Excessive amount of blood or other fluid given during transfusion or infusion**

　Y63.1 **Incorrect dilution of fluid used during infusion**

　Y63.2 **Overdose of radiation given during therapy**

　Y63.3 **Inadvertent exposure of patient to radiation during medical care**

　Y63.4 **Failure in dosage in electroshock or insulin-shock therapy**

　Y63.5 **Inappropriate temperature in local application and packing**

　Y63.6 **Underdosing and nonadministration of necessary drug, medicament or biological substance**
　　AHA: 2018,4Q,72

　Y63.8 **Failure in dosage during other surgical and medical care**
　　AHA: 2018,4Q,72

　Y63.9 **Failure in dosage during unspecified surgical and medical care**
　　AHA: 2018,4Q,72

✓4th **Y64** **Contaminated medical or biological substances**

　Y64.0 **Contaminated medical or biological substance, transfused or infused**

　Y64.1 **Contaminated medical or biological substance, injected or used for immunization**

　Y64.8 **Contaminated medical or biological substance administered by other means**

　Y64.9 **Contaminated medical or biological substance administered by unspecified means**
　　Administered contaminated medical or biological substance NOS

✓4th **Y65** **Other misadventures during surgical and medical care**

　Y65.0 **Mismatched blood in transfusion**

　Y65.1 **Wrong fluid used in infusion**

　Y65.2 **Failure in suture or ligature during surgical operation**

　Y65.3 **Endotracheal tube wrongly placed during anesthetic procedure**

　Y65.4 **Failure to introduce or to remove other tube or instrument**

　✓5th **Y65.5** **Performance of wrong procedure (operation)**

　　Y65.51 **Performance of wrong procedure (operation) on correct patient**
　　　Wrong device implanted into correct surgical site
　　　EXCLUDES 1 performance of correct procedure (operation) on wrong side or body part (Y65.53)

　　Y65.52 **Performance of procedure (operation) on patient not scheduled for surgery**
　　　Performance of procedure (operation) intended for another patient
　　　Performance of procedure (operation) on wrong patient

　　Y65.53 **Performance of correct procedure (operation) on wrong side or body part**
　　　Performance of correct procedure (operation) on wrong side
　　　Performance of correct procedure (operation) on wrong site

　Y65.8 **Other specified misadventures during surgical and medical care**
　　AHA: 2022,1Q,22; 2019,2Q,23-24

　Y66 **Nonadministration of surgical and medical care**
　　Premature cessation of surgical and medical care
　　EXCLUDES 1 DNR status (Z66)
　　　palliative care (Z51.5)

　Y69 **Unspecified misadventure during surgical and medical care**

Medical devices associated with adverse incidents in diagnostic and therapeutic use (Y70-Y82)

INCLUDES breakdown or malfunction of medical devices (during use) (after implantation) (ongoing use)

EXCLUDES 2 later complications following use of medical devices without breakdown or malfunctioning of device (Y83-Y84)
　misadventure to patients during surgical and medical care, classifiable to (Y62-Y69)
　surgical and other medical procedures as the cause of abnormal reaction of the patient, or of later complication, without mention of misadventure at the time of the procedure (Y83-Y84)

✓4th **Y70** **Anesthesiology devices associated with adverse incidents**

　Y70.0 **Diagnostic and monitoring anesthesiology devices associated with adverse incidents**

　Y70.1 **Therapeutic (nonsurgical) and rehabilitative anesthesiology devices associated with adverse incidents**

　Y70.2 **Prosthetic and other implants, materials and accessory anesthesiology devices associated with adverse incidents**

　Y70.3 **Surgical instruments, materials and anesthesiology devices (including sutures) associated with adverse incidents**

　Y70.8 **Miscellaneous anesthesiology devices associated with adverse incidents, not elsewhere classified**

✓4th **Y71** **Cardiovascular devices associated with adverse incidents**

　Y71.0 **Diagnostic and monitoring cardiovascular devices associated with adverse incidents**

　Y71.1 **Therapeutic (nonsurgical) and rehabilitative cardiovascular devices associated with adverse incidents**

Y71.2 **Prosthetic and other implants,** materials and accessory cardiovascular devices associated with adverse incidents

Y71.3 **Surgical instruments,** materials and cardiovascular devices (including sutures) associated with adverse incidents

Y71.8 Miscellaneous cardiovascular devices associated with adverse incidents, not elsewhere classified

☑4th **Y72** **Otorhinolaryngological** devices associated with adverse incidents

Y72.0 **Diagnostic and monitoring** otorhinolaryngological devices associated with adverse incidents

Y72.1 **Therapeutic** (nonsurgical) **and rehabilitative** otorhinolaryngological devices associated with adverse incidents

Y72.2 **Prosthetic and other implants,** materials and accessory otorhinolaryngological devices associated with adverse incidents

Y72.3 **Surgical instruments,** materials and otorhinolaryngological devices (including sutures) associated with adverse incidents

Y72.8 Miscellaneous otorhinolaryngological devices associated with adverse incidents, not elsewhere classified

☑4th **Y73** **Gastroenterology and urology** devices associated with adverse incidents

Y73.0 **Diagnostic and monitoring** gastroenterology and urology devices associated with adverse incidents

Y73.1 **Therapeutic** (nonsurgical) **and rehabilitative** gastroenterology and urology devices associated with adverse incidents

Y73.2 **Prosthetic and other implants,** materials and accessory gastroenterology and urology devices associated with adverse incidents

Y73.3 **Surgical instruments,** materials and gastroenterology and urology devices (including sutures) associated with adverse incidents

Y73.8 Miscellaneous gastroenterology and urology devices associated with adverse incidents, not elsewhere classified

☑4th **Y74** **General hospital** and personal-use devices associated with adverse incidents

Y74.0 **Diagnostic and monitoring** general hospital and personal-use devices associated with adverse incidents

Y74.1 **Therapeutic** (nonsurgical) **and rehabilitative** general hospital and personal-use devices associated with adverse incidents

Y74.2 **Prosthetic and other implants,** materials and accessory general hospital and personal-use devices associated with adverse incidents

Y74.3 **Surgical instruments,** materials and general hospital and personal-use devices (including sutures) associated with adverse incidents

Y74.8 Miscellaneous general hospital and personal-use devices associated with adverse incidents, not elsewhere classified

☑4th **Y75** **Neurological** devices associated with adverse incidents

Y75.0 **Diagnostic and monitoring** neurological devices associated with adverse incidents

Y75.1 **Therapeutic** (nonsurgical) **and rehabilitative** neurological devices associated with adverse incidents

Y75.2 **Prosthetic and other implants,** materials and neurological devices associated with adverse incidents

Y75.3 **Surgical instruments,** materials and neurological devices (including sutures) associated with adverse incidents

Y75.8 Miscellaneous neurological devices associated with adverse incidents, not elsewhere classified

☑4th **Y76** **Obstetric and gynecological** devices associated with adverse incidents

Y76.0 **Diagnostic and monitoring** obstetric and gynecological devices associated with adverse incidents

Y76.1 **Therapeutic** (nonsurgical) **and rehabilitative** obstetric and gynecological devices associated with adverse incidents

Y76.2 **Prosthetic and other implants,** materials and accessory obstetric and gynecological devices associated with adverse incidents

Y76.3 **Surgical instruments,** materials and obstetric and gynecological devices (including sutures) associated with adverse incidents

Y76.8 Miscellaneous obstetric and gynecological devices associated with adverse incidents, not elsewhere classified

☑4th **Y77** **Ophthalmic** devices associated with adverse incidents

Y77.0 **Diagnostic and monitoring** ophthalmic devices associated with adverse incidents

☑5th **Y77.1** **Therapeutic** (nonsurgical) **and rehabilitative** ophthalmic devices associated with adverse incidents
AHA: 2020,4Q,41

Y77.11 **Contact lens** associated with adverse incidents
Rigid gas permeable contact lens associated with adverse incidents
Soft (hydrophilic) contact lens associated with adverse incidents

Y77.19 Other therapeutic (nonsurgical) and rehabilitative ophthalmic devices associated with adverse incidents

Y77.2 **Prosthetic and other implants,** materials and accessory ophthalmic devices associated with adverse incidents

Y77.3 **Surgical instruments,** materials and ophthalmic devices (including sutures) associated with adverse incidents

Y77.8 Miscellaneous ophthalmic devices associated with adverse incidents, not elsewhere classified

☑4th **Y78** **Radiological** devices associated with adverse incidents

Y78.0 **Diagnostic and monitoring** radiological devices associated with adverse incidents

Y78.1 **Therapeutic** (nonsurgical) **and rehabilitative** radiological devices associated with adverse incidents

Y78.2 **Prosthetic and other implants,** materials and accessory radiological devices associated with adverse incidents

Y78.3 **Surgical instruments,** materials and radiological devices (including sutures) associated with adverse incidents

Y78.8 Miscellaneous radiological devices associated with adverse incidents, not elsewhere classified

☑4th **Y79** **Orthopedic** devices associated with adverse incidents

Y79.0 **Diagnostic and monitoring** orthopedic devices associated with adverse incidents

Y79.1 **Therapeutic** (nonsurgical) **and rehabilitative** orthopedic devices associated with adverse incidents

Y79.2 **Prosthetic and other implants,** materials and accessory orthopedic devices associated with adverse incidents

Y79.3 **Surgical instruments,** materials and orthopedic devices (including sutures) associated with adverse incidents

Y79.8 Miscellaneous orthopedic devices associated with adverse incidents, not elsewhere classified

☑4th **Y80** **Physical medicine** devices associated with adverse incidents

Y80.0 **Diagnostic and monitoring** physical medicine devices associated with adverse incidents

Y80.1 **Therapeutic** (nonsurgical) **and rehabilitative** physical medicine devices associated with adverse incidents

Y80.2 **Prosthetic and other implants,** materials and accessory physical medicine devices associated with adverse incidents

Y80.3 **Surgical instruments,** materials and physical medicine devices (including sutures) associated with adverse incidents

Y80.8 Miscellaneous physical medicine devices associated with adverse incidents, not elsewhere classified

☑4th **Y81** **General- and plastic-surgery** devices associated with adverse incidents

Y81.0 **Diagnostic and monitoring** general- and plastic-surgery devices associated with adverse incidents

Y81.1 **Therapeutic** (nonsurgical) **and rehabilitative** general- and plastic-surgery devices associated with adverse incidents

Y81.2 **Prosthetic and other implants,** materials and accessory general- and plastic-surgery devices associated with adverse incidents

Y81.3 **Surgical instruments,** materials and general- and plastic-surgery devices (including sutures) associated with adverse incidents

Y81.8 Miscellaneous general- and plastic-surgery devices associated with adverse incidents, not elsewhere classified

☑4th **Y82** **Other and unspecified** medical devices associated with adverse incidents

Y82.8 Other medical devices associated with adverse incidents

Y82.9 Unspecified medical devices associated with adverse incidents

Surgical and other medical procedures as the cause of abnormal reaction of the patient, or of later complication, without mention of misadventure at the time of the procedure (Y83-Y84)

EXCLUDES 1   *misadventures to patients during surgical and medical care, classifiable to (Y62-Y69)*

EXCLUDES 2   *breakdown or malfunctioning of medical device (during procedure) (after implantation) (ongoing use) (Y70-Y82)*

☑4ᵗʰ **Y83**   **Surgical operation** and other **surgical procedures** as the cause of abnormal reaction of the patient, or of later complication, without mention of misadventure at the time of the procedure

    Y83.0   Surgical operation **with transplant of whole organ** as the cause of abnormal reaction of the patient, or of later complication, without mention of misadventure at the time of the procedure

    Y83.1   Surgical operation **with implant of artificial internal device** as the cause of abnormal reaction of the patient, or of later complication, without mention of misadventure at the time of the procedure

    Y83.2   Surgical operation **with anastomosis, bypass or graft** as the cause of abnormal reaction of the patient, or of later complication, without mention of misadventure at the time of the procedure

    Y83.3   Surgical operation **with formation of external stoma** as the cause of abnormal reaction of the patient, or of later complication, without mention of misadventure at the time of the procedure

    Y83.4   Other reconstructive surgery as the cause of abnormal reaction of the patient, or of later complication, without mention of misadventure at the time of the procedure

    Y83.5   **Amputation of limb**(s) as the cause of abnormal reaction of the patient, or of later complication, without mention of misadventure at the time of the procedure

    Y83.6   **Removal of other organ** (partial) (total) as the cause of abnormal reaction of the patient, or of later complication, without mention of misadventure at the time of the procedure

    Y83.8   Other surgical procedures as the cause of abnormal reaction of the patient, or of later complication, without mention of misadventure at the time of the procedure

      AHA: 2023,2Q,14

    Y83.9   Surgical procedure, unspecified as the cause of abnormal reaction of the patient, or of later complication, without mention of misadventure at the time of the procedure

☑4ᵗʰ **Y84**   Other medical procedures as the cause of abnormal reaction of the patient, or of later complication, without mention of misadventure at the time of the procedure

    Y84.0   **Cardiac catheterization** as the cause of abnormal reaction of the patient, or of later complication, without mention of misadventure at the time of the procedure

    Y84.1   **Kidney dialysis** as the cause of abnormal reaction of the patient, or of later complication, without mention of misadventure at the time of the procedure

    Y84.2   **Radiological procedure and radiotherapy** as the cause of abnormal reaction of the patient, or of later complication, without mention of misadventure at the time of the procedure

      AHA: 2019,1Q,21; 2017,1Q,33

    Y84.3   **Shock therapy** as the cause of abnormal reaction of the patient, or of later complication, without mention of misadventure at the time of the procedure

    Y84.4   **Aspiration of fluid** as the cause of abnormal reaction of the patient, or of later complication, without mention of misadventure at the time of the procedure

    Y84.5   **Insertion of gastric or duodenal sound** as the cause of abnormal reaction of the patient, or of later complication, without mention of misadventure at the time of the procedure

    Y84.6   **Urinary catheterization** as the cause of abnormal reaction of the patient, or of later complication, without mention of misadventure at the time of the procedure

    Y84.7   **Blood-sampling** as the cause of abnormal reaction of the patient, or of later complication, without mention of misadventure at the time of the procedure

    Y84.8   Other medical procedures as the cause of abnormal reaction of the patient, or of later complication, without mention of misadventure at the time of the procedure

      AHA: 2024,1Q,26; 2023,2Q,28; 2021,1Q,5; 2014,4Q,24

    Y84.9   Medical procedure, unspecified as the cause of abnormal reaction of the patient, or of later complication, without mention of misadventure at the time of the procedure

Supplementary factors related to causes of morbidity classified elsewhere (Y90-Y99)

NOTE   These categories may be used to provide supplementary information concerning causes of morbidity. They are not to be used for single-condition coding.

☑4ᵗʰ **Y90**   **Evidence of alcohol involvement determined by blood alcohol level**

    Code first any associated alcohol related disorders (F10)

    Y90.0   Blood alcohol level of **less than 20 mg/100 ml**

    Y90.1   Blood alcohol level of **20-39 mg/100 ml**

    Y90.2   Blood alcohol level of **40-59 mg/100 ml**

    Y90.3   Blood alcohol level of **60-79 mg/100 ml**

    Y90.4   Blood alcohol level of **80-99 mg/100 ml**

    Y90.5   Blood alcohol level of **100-119 mg/100 ml**

    Y90.6   Blood alcohol level of **120-199 mg/100 ml**

    Y90.7   Blood alcohol level of **200-239 mg/100 ml**

    Y90.8   Blood alcohol level of **240 mg/100 ml or more**

    Y90.9   Presence of alcohol in blood, level not specified

☑4ᵗʰ **Y92**   **Place of occurrence of the external cause**

    The following category is for use, when relevant, to identify the place of occurrence of the external cause. Use in conjunction with an activity code.

    Place of occurrence should be recorded only at the initial encounter for treatment

☑5ᵗʰ **Y92.0**   **Non-institutional** (private) **residence** as the place of occurrence of the external cause

      EXCLUDES 1   *abandoned or derelict house (Y92.89)*

            home under construction but not yet occupied (Y92.6-)

            institutional place of residence (Y92.1-)

    ☑6ᵗʰ **Y92.00**   Unspecified non-institutional (private) residence as the place of occurrence of the external cause

      Y92.000   **Kitchen** of unspecified non-institutional (private) residence as the place of occurrence of the external cause   **PE**

      Y92.001   **Dining room** of unspecified non-institutional (private) residence as the place of occurrence of the external cause   **PE**

      Y92.002   **Bathroom** of unspecified non-institutional (private) residence as the place of occurrence of the external cause   **PE**

      Y92.003   **Bedroom** of unspecified non-institutional (private) residence as the place of occurrence of the external cause   **PE**

      Y92.007   **Garden or yard** of unspecified non-institutional (private) residence as the place of occurrence of the external cause   **PE**

      Y92.008   Other place in unspecified non-institutional (private) residence as the place of occurrence of the external cause   **PE**

      Y92.009   Unspecified place in unspecified non-institutional (private) residence as the place of occurrence of the external cause   **PE**

        Home (NOS) as the place of occurrence of the external cause

    ☑6ᵗʰ **Y92.01**   **Single-family** non-institutional (private) **house** as the place of occurrence of the external cause

       Farmhouse as the place of occurrence of the external cause

      EXCLUDES 1   *barn (Y92.71)*

            chicken coop or hen house (Y92.72)

            farm field (Y92.73)

            orchard (Y92.74)

            single family mobile home or trailer (Y92.02-)

            slaughter house (Y92.86)

      Y92.010   **Kitchen** of single-family (private) house as the place of occurrence of the external cause   **PE**

      Y92.011   **Dining room** of single-family (private) house as the place of occurrence of the external cause   **PE**

      Y92.012   **Bathroom** of single-family (private) house as the place of occurrence of the external cause   **PE**

☑ Additional Char Req   ☑x7ᵗʰ Placeholder   Unacceptable PDx   Questionable PDx   Wrong Procedure   Manifestation   Unspecified   H1 - H14 HAC   HCC CMS-HCC Dx   HIV HIV Dx

ICD-10-CM 2025   1251

Y92.013 **Bedroom** of single-family (private) house as the place of occurrence of the external cause PE

Y92.014 **Private driveway** to single-family (private) house as the place of occurrence of the external cause PE

Y92.015 **Private garage** of single-family (private) house as the place of occurrence of the external cause PE

Y92.016 **Swimming-pool** in single-family (private) house or garden as the place of occurrence of the external cause PE
AHA: 2023,1Q,25

Y92.017 **Garden or yard** in single-family (private) house as the place of occurrence of the external cause PE

Y92.018 Other place in single-family (private) house as the place of occurrence of the external cause PE

Y92.019 Unspecified place in single-family (private) house as the place of occurrence of the external cause PE

✓6th **Y92.02** **Mobile home** as the place of occurrence of the external cause

Y92.020 **Kitchen** in mobile home as the place of occurrence of the external cause PE

Y92.021 **Dining room** in mobile home as the place of occurrence of the external cause PE

Y92.022 **Bathroom** in mobile home as the place of occurrence of the external cause PE

Y92.023 **Bedroom** in mobile home as the place of occurrence of the external cause PE

Y92.024 **Driveway** of mobile home as the place of occurrence of the external cause PE

Y92.025 **Garage** of mobile home as the place of occurrence of the external cause PE

Y92.026 **Swimming-pool** of mobile home as the place of occurrence of the external cause PE

Y92.027 **Garden or yard** of mobile home as the place of occurrence of the external cause PE

Y92.028 Other place in mobile home as the place of occurrence of the external cause PE

Y92.029 Unspecified place in mobile home as the place of occurrence of the external cause PE

✓6th **Y92.03** **Apartment** as the place of occurrence of the external cause
Condominium as the place of occurrence of the external cause
Co-op apartment as the place of occurrence of the external cause

Y92.030 **Kitchen** in apartment as the place of occurrence of the external cause PE

Y92.031 · **Bathroom** in apartment as the place of occurrence of the external cause PE

Y92.032 **Bedroom** in apartment as the place of occurrence of the external cause PE

Y92.038 Other place in apartment as the place of occurrence of the external cause PE

Y92.039 Unspecified place in apartment as the place of occurrence of the external cause PE

✓6th **Y92.04** **Boarding-house** as the place of occurrence of the external cause

Y92.040 **Kitchen** in boarding-house as the place of occurrence of the external cause PE

Y92.041 **Bathroom** in boarding-house as the place of occurrence of the external cause PE

Y92.042 **Bedroom** in boarding-house as the place of occurrence of the external cause PE

Y92.043 **Driveway** of boarding-house as the place of occurrence of the external cause PE

Y92.044 **Garage** of boarding-house as the place of occurrence of the external cause PE

Y92.045 **Swimming-pool** of boarding-house as the place of occurrence of the external cause PE

Y92.046 **Garden or yard** of boarding-house as the place of occurrence of the external cause PE

Y92.048 Other place in boarding-house as the place of occurrence of the external cause PE

Y92.049 Unspecified place in boarding-house as the place of occurrence of the external cause PE

✓6th **Y92.09** Other non-institutional residence as the place of occurrence of the external cause
AHA: 2017,2Q,10

Y92.090 **Kitchen** in other non-institutional residence as the place of occurrence of the external cause PE

Y92.091 **Bathroom** in other non-institutional residence as the place of occurrence of the external cause PE

Y92.092 **Bedroom** in other non-institutional residence as the place of occurrence of the external cause PE

Y92.093 **Driveway** of other non-institutional residence as the place of occurrence of the external cause PE

Y92.094 **Garage** of other non-institutional residence as the place of occurrence of the external cause PE

Y92.095 **Swimming-pool** of other non-institutional residence as the place of occurrence of the external cause PE

Y92.096 **Garden or yard** of other non-institutional residence as the place of occurrence of the external cause PE

Y92.098 Other place in other non-institutional residence as the place of occurrence of the external cause PE

Y92.099 Unspecified place in other non-institutional residence as the place of occurrence of the external cause PE

✓5th **Y92.1** **Institutional** (nonprivate) **residence** as the place of occurrence of the external cause

Y92.10 Unspecified residential institution as the place of occurrence of the external cause PE

✓6th **Y92.11** **Children's home and orphanage** as the place of occurrence of the external cause

Y92.110 **Kitchen** in children's home and orphanage as the place of occurrence of the external cause PE

Y92.111 **Bathroom** in children's home and orphanage as the place of occurrence of the external cause PE

Y92.112 **Bedroom** in children's home and orphanage as the place of occurrence of the external cause PE

Y92.113 **Driveway** of children's home and orphanage as the place of occurrence of the external cause PE

Y92.114 **Garage** of children's home and orphanage as the place of occurrence of the external cause PE

Y92.115 **Swimming-pool** of children's home and orphanage as the place of occurrence of the external cause PE

Y92.116 **Garden or yard** of children's home and orphanage as the place of occurrence of the external cause PE

Y92.118 Other place in children's home and orphanage as the place of occurrence of the external cause PE

Y92.119 Unspecified place in children's home and orphanage as the place of occurrence of the external cause PE

✓6th **Y92.12** **Nursing home** as the place of occurrence of the external cause
Home for the sick as the place of occurrence of the external cause
Hospice as the place of occurrence of the external cause
AHA: 2017,2Q,10

Y92.120 **Kitchen** in nursing home as the place of occurrence of the external cause PE

Y92.121 **Bathroom** in nursing home as the place of occurrence of the external cause PE

Y92.122 **Bedroom** in nursing home as the place of occurrence of the external cause PE

Y92.123 **Driveway** of nursing home as the place of occurrence of the external cause PE

Y92.124 Garage of nursing home as the place of occurrence of the external cause **PE**

Y92.125 Swimming-pool of nursing home as the place of occurrence of the external cause **PE**

Y92.126 Garden or yard of nursing home as the place of occurrence of the external cause **PE**

Y92.128 Other place in nursing home as the place of occurrence of the external cause **PE**

Y92.129 Unspecified place in nursing home as the place of occurrence of the external cause **PE**

✓6ᵗʰ **Y92.13** Military base as the place of occurrence of the external cause

EXCLUDES 1   military training grounds (Y92.84)

Y92.130 Kitchen on military base as the place of occurrence of the external cause **PE**

Y92.131 Mess hall on military base as the place of occurrence of the external cause **PE**

Y92.133 Barracks on military base as the place of occurrence of the external cause **PE**

Y92.135 Garage on military base as the place of occurrence of the external cause **PE**

Y92.136 Swimming-pool on military base as the place of occurrence of the external cause **PE**

Y92.137 Garden or yard on military base as the place of occurrence of the external cause **PE**

Y92.138 Other place on military base as the place of occurrence of the external cause **PE**

Y92.139 Unspecified place military base as the place of occurrence of the external cause **PE**

✓6ᵗʰ **Y92.14** Prison as the place of occurrence of the external cause

Y92.140 Kitchen in prison as the place of occurrence of the external cause **PE**

Y92.141 Dining room in prison as the place of occurrence of the external cause **PE**

Y92.142 Bathroom in prison as the place of occurrence of the external cause **PE**

Y92.143 Cell of prison as the place of occurrence of the external cause **PE**

Y92.146 Swimming-pool of prison as the place of occurrence of the external cause **PE**

Y92.147 Courtyard of prison as the place of occurrence of the external cause **PE**

Y92.148 Other place in prison as the place of occurrence of the external cause **PE**

Y92.149 Unspecified place in prison as the place of occurrence of the external cause **PE**

✓6ᵗʰ **Y92.15** Reform school as the place of occurrence of the external cause

Y92.150 Kitchen in reform school as the place of occurrence of the external cause **PE**

Y92.151 Dining room in reform school as the place of occurrence of the external cause **PE**

Y92.152 Bathroom in reform school as the place of occurrence of the external cause **PE**

Y92.153 Bedroom in reform school as the place of occurrence of the external cause **PE**

Y92.154 Driveway of reform school as the place of occurrence of the external cause **PE**

Y92.155 Garage of reform school as the place of occurrence of the external cause **PE**

Y92.156 Swimming-pool of reform school as the place of occurrence of the external cause **PE**

Y92.157 Garden or yard of reform school as the place of occurrence of the external cause **PE**

Y92.158 Other place in reform school as the place of occurrence of the external cause **PE**

Y92.159 Unspecified place in reform school as the place of occurrence of the external cause **PE**

✓6ᵗʰ **Y92.16** School dormitory as the place of occurrence of the external cause

EXCLUDES 1   reform school as the place of occurrence of the external cause (Y92.15-)
school buildings and grounds as the place of occurrence of the external cause (Y92.2-)
school sports and athletic areas as the place of occurrence of the external cause (Y92.3-)

Y92.160 Kitchen in school dormitory as the place of occurrence of the external cause **PE**

Y92.161 Dining room in school dormitory as the place of occurrence of the external cause **PE**

Y92.162 Bathroom in school dormitory as the place of occurrence of the external cause **PE**

Y92.163 Bedroom in school dormitory as the place of occurrence of the external cause **PE**

Y92.168 Other place in school dormitory as the place of occurrence of the external cause **PE**

Y92.169 Unspecified place in school dormitory as the place of occurrence of the external cause **PE**

✓6ᵗʰ **Y92.19** Other specified residential institution as the place of occurrence of the external cause

AHA: 2017,2Q,10

Y92.190 Kitchen in other specified residential institution as the place of occurrence of the external cause **PE**

Y92.191 Dining room in other specified residential institution as the place of occurrence of the external cause **PE**

Y92.192 Bathroom in other specified residential institution as the place of occurrence of the external cause **PE**

Y92.193 Bedroom in other specified residential institution as the place of occurrence of the external cause **PE**

Y92.194 Driveway of other specified residential institution as the place of occurrence of the external cause **PE**

Y92.195 Garage of other specified residential institution as the place of occurrence of the external cause **PE**

Y92.196 Pool of other specified residential institution as the place of occurrence of the external cause **PE**

Y92.197 Garden or yard of other specified residential institution as the place of occurrence of the external cause **PE**

Y92.198 Other place in other specified residential institution as the place of occurrence of the external cause **PE**

Y92.199 Unspecified place in other specified residential institution as the place of occurrence of the external cause **PE**

✓5ᵗʰ **Y92.2** School, other institution and public administrative area as the place of occurrence of the external cause

Building and adjacent grounds used by the general public or by a particular group of the public

EXCLUDES 1   building under construction as the place of occurrence of the external cause (Y92.6)
residential institution as the place of occurrence of the external cause (Y92.1)
school dormitory as the place of occurrence of the external cause (Y92.16-)
sports and athletics area of schools as the place of occurrence of the external cause (Y92.3-)

✓6ᵗʰ **Y92.21** School (private) (public) (state) as the place of occurrence of the external cause

Y92.210 Daycare center as the place of occurrence of the external cause **PE**

Y92.211 Elementary school as the place of occurrence of the external cause **PE**
Kindergarten as the place of occurrence of the external cause

Y92.212 Middle school as the place of occurrence of the external cause **PE**

Y92.213 High school as the place of occurrence of the external cause `PE`
    AHA: 2012,4Q,108

Y92.214 College as the place of occurrence of the external cause `PE`
    University as the place of occurrence of the external cause

Y92.215 Trade school as the place of occurrence of the external cause `PE`

Y92.218 Other school as the place of occurrence of the external cause `PE`

Y92.219 Unspecified school as the place of occurrence of the external cause `PE`

Y92.22 Religious institution as the place of occurrence of the external cause `PE`
    Church as the place of occurrence of the external cause
    Mosque as the place of occurrence of the external cause
    Synagogue as the place of occurrence of the external cause

✓6ᵗʰ **Y92.23** Hospital as the place of occurrence of the external cause
    EXCLUDES 1   ambulatory (outpatient) health services establishments (Y92.53-)
        home for the sick as the place of occurrence of the external cause (Y92.12-)
        hospice as the place of occurrence of the external cause (Y92.12-)
        nursing home as the place of occurrence of the external cause (Y92.12-)

Y92.230 Patient room in hospital as the place of occurrence of the external cause

Y92.231 Patient bathroom in hospital as the place of occurrence of the external cause

Y92.232 Corridor of hospital as the place of occurrence of the external cause

Y92.233 Cafeteria of hospital as the place of occurrence of the external cause

Y92.234 Operating room of hospital as the place of occurrence of the external cause

Y92.238 Other place in hospital as the place of occurrence of the external cause

Y92.239 Unspecified place in hospital as the place of occurrence of the external cause

✓6ᵗʰ **Y92.24** Public administrative building as the place of occurrence of the external cause

Y92.240 Courthouse as the place of occurrence of the external cause `PE`

Y92.241 Library as the place of occurrence of the external cause `PE`

Y92.242 Post office as the place of occurrence of the external cause `PE`

Y92.243 City hall as the place of occurrence of the external cause `PE`

Y92.248 Other public administrative building as the place of occurrence of the external cause `PE`

✓6ᵗʰ **Y92.25** Cultural building as the place of occurrence of the external cause

Y92.250 Art Gallery as the place of occurrence of the external cause `PE`

Y92.251 Museum as the place of occurrence of the external cause `PE`

Y92.252 Music hall as the place of occurrence of the external cause `PE`

Y92.253 Opera house as the place of occurrence of the external cause `PE`

Y92.254 Theater (live) as the place of occurrence of the external cause `PE`

Y92.258 Other cultural public building as the place of occurrence of the external cause `PE`

Y92.26 Movie house or cinema as the place of occurrence of the external cause `PE`

Y92.29 Other specified public building as the place of occurrence of the external cause `PE`
    Assembly hall as the place of occurrence of the external cause
    Clubhouse as the place of occurrence of the external cause

✓5ᵗʰ **Y92.3** Sports and athletics area as the place of occurrence of the external cause

✓6ᵗʰ **Y92.31** Athletic court as the place of occurrence of the external cause
    EXCLUDES 1   tennis court in private home or garden (Y92.09)

Y92.310 Basketball court as the place of occurrence of the external cause `PE`

Y92.311 Squash court as the place of occurrence of the external cause `PE`

Y92.312 Tennis court as the place of occurrence of the external cause `PE`

Y92.318 Other athletic court as the place of occurrence of the external cause `PE`

✓6ᵗʰ **Y92.32** Athletic field as the place of occurrence of the external cause

Y92.320 Baseball field as the place of occurrence of the external cause `PE`

Y92.321 Football field as the place of occurrence of the external cause `PE`

Y92.322 Soccer field as the place of occurrence of the external cause `PE`

Y92.328 Other athletic field as the place of occurrence of the external cause `PE`
    Cricket field as the place of occurrence of the external cause
    Hockey field as the place of occurrence of the external cause

✓6ᵗʰ **Y92.33** Skating rink as the place of occurrence of the external cause

Y92.330 Ice skating rink (indoor) (outdoor) as the place of occurrence of the external cause `PE`

Y92.331 Roller skating rink as the place of occurrence of the external cause `PE`

Y92.34 Swimming pool (public) as the place of occurrence of the external cause `PE`
    EXCLUDES 1   swimming pool in private home or garden (Y92.016)

Y92.39 Other specified sports and athletic area as the place of occurrence of the external cause `PE`
    Golf-course as the place of occurrence of the external cause
    Gymnasium as the place of occurrence of the external cause
    Riding-school as the place of occurrence of the external cause
    Stadium as the place of occurrence of the external cause

✓5ᵗʰ **Y92.4** Street, highway and other paved roadways as the place of occurrence of the external cause
    EXCLUDES 1   private driveway of residence (Y92.014, Y92.024, Y92.043, Y92.093, Y92.113, Y92.123, Y92.154, Y92.194)

✓6ᵗʰ **Y92.41** Street and highway as the place of occurrence of the external cause

Y92.410 Unspecified street and highway as the place of occurrence of the external cause `PE`
    Road NOS as the place of occurrence of the external cause

Y92.411 Interstate highway as the place of occurrence of the external cause `PE`
    Freeway as the place of occurrence of the external cause
    Motorway as the place of occurrence of the external cause

Y92.412 Parkway as the place of occurrence of the external cause `PE`

Y92.413 State road as the place of occurrence of the external cause `PE`

Y92.414 Local residential or business street as the place of occurrence of the external cause `PE`

Y92.415 Exit ramp or entrance ramp of street or highway as the place of occurrence of the external cause `PE`

✓6ᵗʰ **Y92.48** Other paved roadways as the place of occurrence of the external cause

Y92.480 Sidewalk as the place of occurrence of the external cause `PE`

Y92.481 Parking lot as the place of occurrence of the external cause `PE`

Y92.482 Bike path as the place of occurrence of the external cause `PE`

Y92.488 Other paved roadways as the place of occurrence of the external cause `PE`

✓5ᵗʰ **Y92.5 Trade and service area** as the place of occurrence of the external cause

EXCLUDES 1   *garage in private home (Y92.015)*

schools and other public administration buildings (Y92.2-)

✓6ᵗʰ **Y92.51 Private commercial establishments** as the place of occurrence of the external cause

Y92.510 Bank as the place of occurrence of the external cause `PE`

Y92.511 Restaurant or cafe as the place of occurrence of the external cause `PE`

Y92.512 Supermarket, store or market as the place of occurrence of the external cause `PE`

Y92.513 Shop (commercial) as the place of occurrence of the external cause `PE`

✓6ᵗʰ **Y92.52 Service areas** as the place of occurrence of the external cause

Y92.520 Airport as the place of occurrence of the external cause `PE`

Y92.521 Bus station as the place of occurrence of the external cause `PE`

Y92.522 Railway station as the place of occurrence of the external cause `PE`

Y92.523 Highway rest stop as the place of occurrence of the external cause `PE`

Y92.524 Gas station as the place of occurrence of the external cause `PE`

Petroleum station as the place of occurrence of the external cause

Service station as the place of occurrence of the external cause

✓6ᵗʰ **Y92.53 Ambulatory health services establishments** as the place of occurrence of the external cause

Y92.530 Ambulatory surgery center as the place of occurrence of the external cause

Outpatient surgery center, including that connected with a hospital as the place of occurrence of the external cause

Same day surgery center, including that connected with a hospital as the place of occurrence of the external cause

Y92.531 Health care provider office as the place of occurrence of the external cause `PE`

Physician office as the place of occurrence of the external cause

Y92.532 Urgent care center as the place of occurrence of the external cause `PE`

Y92.538 Other ambulatory health services establishments as the place of occurrence of the external cause

AHA: 2019,1Q,21

Y92.59 Other trade areas as the place of occurrence of the external cause `PE`

Office building as the place of occurrence of the external cause

Casino as the place of occurrence of the external cause

Garage (commercial) as the place of occurrence of the external cause

Hotel as the place of occurrence of the external cause

Radio or television station as the place of occurrence of the external cause

Shopping mall as the place of occurrence of the external cause

Warehouse as the place of occurrence of the external cause

✓5ᵗʰ **Y92.6 Industrial and construction area** as the place of occurrence of the external cause

Y92.61 Building [any] **under construction** as the place of occurrence of the external cause `PE`

Y92.62 Dock or shipyard as the place of occurrence of the external cause `PE`

Dockyard as the place of occurrence of the external cause

Dry dock as the place of occurrence of the external cause

Shipyard as the place of occurrence of the external cause

Y92.63 Factory as the place of occurrence of the external cause `PE`

Factory building as the place of occurrence of the external cause

Factory premises as the place of occurrence of the external cause

Industrial yard as the place of occurrence of the external cause

Y92.64 Mine or pit as the place of occurrence of the external cause `PE`

Mine as the place of occurrence of the external cause

Y92.65 Oil rig as the place of occurrence of the external cause `PE`

Pit (coal) (gravel) (sand) as the place of occurrence of the external cause

Y92.69 Other specified industrial and construction area as the place of occurrence of the external cause `PE`

Gasworks as the place of occurrence of the external cause

Power-station (coal) (nuclear) (oil) as the place of occurrence of the external cause

Tunnel under construction as the place of occurrence of the external cause

Workshop as the place of occurrence of the external cause

✓5ᵗʰ **Y92.7 Farm** as the place of occurrence of the external cause

Ranch as the place of occurrence of the external cause

EXCLUDES 1   *farmhouse and home premises of farm (Y92.01-)*

Y92.71 Barn as the place of occurrence of the external cause `PE`

Y92.72 Chicken coop as the place of occurrence of the external cause `PE`

Hen house as the place of occurrence of the external cause

Y92.73 Farm field as the place of occurrence of the external cause `PE`

Y92.74 Orchard as the place of occurrence of the external cause `PE`

Y92.79 Other farm location as the place of occurrence of the external cause `PE`

✓5ᵗʰ **Y92.8 Other places** as the place of occurrence of the external cause

✓6ᵗʰ **Y92.81 Transport vehicle** as the place of occurrence of the external cause

EXCLUDES 1   *transport accidents (V00-V99)*

Y92.810 Car as the place of occurrence of the external cause `PE`

Y92.811 Bus as the place of occurrence of the external cause `PE`

Y92.812 Truck as the place of occurrence of the external cause `PE`

Y92.813 Airplane as the place of occurrence of the external cause `PE`

Y92.814 Boat as the place of occurrence of the external cause `PE`

Y92.815 Train as the place of occurrence of the external cause `PE`

Y92.816 Subway car as the place of occurrence of the external cause `PE`

Y92.818 Other transport vehicle as the place of occurrence of the external cause `PE`

✓6ᵗʰ **Y92.82 Wilderness area**

Y92.820 Desert as the place of occurrence of the external cause `PE`

Y92.821 Forest as the place of occurrence of the external cause `PE`

Y92.828 Other wilderness area as the place of occurrence of the external cause `PE`

Swamp as the place of occurrence of the external cause

Mountain as the place of occurrence of the external cause

Marsh as the place of occurrence of the external cause

Prairie as the place of occurrence of the external cause

✓6ᵗʰ **Y92.83 Recreation area** as the place of occurrence of the external cause

Y92.830 Public park as the place of occurrence of the external cause `PE`

Y92.831 Amusement park as the place of occurrence of the external cause `PE`

✅Additional Char Req   ✓x 7ᵗʰ Placeholder   Unacceptable PDx   Questionable PDx   Wrong Procedure   Manifestation   Unspecified   H1 -H14 HAC   HCC CMS-HCC Dx   HIV HIV Dx

ICD-10-CM 2025   1255

Y92.832   **Beach** as the place of occurrence of the external cause `PE`
Seashore as the place of occurrence of the external cause

Y92.833   **Campsite** as the place of occurrence of the external cause `PE`

Y92.834   **Zoological garden** (Zoo) as the place of occurrence of the external cause `PE`

Y92.838   **Other recreation area** as the place of occurrence of the external cause `PE`

Y92.84   **Military training ground** as the place of occurrence of the external cause `PE`

Y92.85   **Railroad track** as the place of occurrence of the external cause `PE`

Y92.86   **Slaughter house** as the place of occurrence of the external cause `PE`

Y92.89   **Other specified places** as the place of occurrence of the external cause `PE`
Derelict house as the place of occurrence of the external cause

Y92.9   **Unspecified place or not applicable** `PE`

✓4ᵗʰ Y93   Activity codes

> **NOTE**   Category Y93 is provided for use to indicate the activity of the person seeking healthcare for an injury or health condition, such as a heart attack while shoveling snow, which resulted from, or was contributed to, by the activity. These codes are appropriate for use for both acute injuries, such as those from chapter 19, and conditions that are due to the long-term, cumulative effects of an activity, such as those from chapter 13. They are also appropriate for use with external cause codes for cause and intent if identifying the activity provides additional information on the event. These codes should be used in conjunction with codes for external cause status (Y99) and place of occurrence (Y92).

This section contains the following broad activity categories:

Y93.0	Activities involving walking and running
Y93.1	Activities involving water and water craft
Y93.2	Activities involving ice and snow
Y93.3	Activities involving climbing, rappelling, and jumping off
Y93.4	Activities involving dancing and other rhythmic movement
Y93.5	Activities involving other sports and athletics played individually
Y93.6	Activities involving other sports and athletics played as a team or group
Y93.7	Activities involving other specified sports and athletics
Y93.A	Activities involving other cardiorespiratory exercise
Y93.B	Activities involving other muscle strengthening exercises
Y93.C	Activities involving computer technology and electronic devices
Y93.D	Activities involving arts and handcrafts
Y93.E	Activities involving personal hygiene and interior property and clothing maintenance
Y93.F	Activities involving caregiving
Y93.G	Activities involving food preparation, cooking and grilling
Y93.H	Activities involving exterior property and land maintenance, building and construction
Y93.I	Activities involving roller coasters and other types of external motion
Y93.J	Activities involving playing musical instrument
Y93.K	Activities involving animal care
Y93.8	Activities, other specified
Y93.9	Activity, unspecified

✓5ᵗʰ Y93.0   Activities involving walking and running

> `EXCLUDES 1`   activity, walking an animal (Y93.K1)
> activity, walking or running on a treadmill (Y93.A1)

Y93.01   **Activity, walking, marching and hiking**
Activity, walking, marching and hiking on level or elevated terrain
> `EXCLUDES 1`   activity, mountain climbing (Y93.31)

Y93.02   **Activity, running**

✓5ᵗʰ Y93.1   Activities involving water and water craft

> `EXCLUDES 1`   activities involving ice (Y93.2-)

Y93.11   **Activity, swimming**

Y93.12   **Activity, springboard and platform diving** `PE`

Y93.13   **Activity, water polo** `PE`

Y93.14   **Activity, water aerobics and water exercise** `PE`

Y93.15   **Activity, underwater diving and snorkeling** `PE`
Activity, SCUBA diving

Y93.16   **Activity, rowing, canoeing, kayaking, rafting and tubing** `PE`
Activity, canoeing, kayaking, rafting and tubing in calm and turbulent water

Y93.17   **Activity, water skiing and wake boarding** `PE`

Y93.18   **Activity, surfing, windsurfing and boogie boarding** `PE`
Activity, water sliding

Y93.19   **Activity, other involving water and watercraft** `PE`
Activity involving water NOS
Activity, parasailing
Activity, water survival training and testing

✓5ᵗʰ Y93.2   Activities involving ice and snow

> `EXCLUDES 1`   activity, shoveling ice and snow (Y93.H1)

Y93.21   **Activity, ice skating**
Activity, figure skating (singles) (pairs)
Activity, ice dancing
> `EXCLUDES 1`   activity, ice hockey (Y93.22)

Y93.22   **Activity, ice hockey** `PE`

Y93.23   **Activity, snow** (alpine) (downhill) **skiing, snowboarding, sledding, tobogganing and snow tubing** `PE`
> `EXCLUDES 1`   activity, cross country skiing (Y93.24)

Y93.24   **Activity, cross country skiing** `PE`
Activity, nordic skiing

Y93.29   **Activity, other involving ice and snow** `PE`
Activity involving ice and snow NOS

✓5ᵗʰ Y93.3   Activities involving climbing, rappelling and jumping off

> `EXCLUDES 1`   activity, hiking on level or elevated terrain (Y93.01)
> activity, jumping rope (Y93.56)
> activity, trampoline jumping (Y93.44)

Y93.31   **Activity, mountain climbing, rock climbing and wall climbing** `PE`

Y93.32   **Activity, rappelling** `PE`

Y93.33   **Activity, BASE jumping** `PE`
Activity, Building, Antenna, Span, Earth jumping

Y93.34   **Activity, bungee jumping** `PE`

Y93.35   **Activity, hang gliding** `PE`

Y93.39   **Activity, other involving climbing, rappelling and jumping off** `PE`

✓5ᵗʰ Y93.4   Activities involving dancing and other rhythmic movement

> `EXCLUDES 1`   activity, martial arts (Y93.75)

Y93.41   **Activity, dancing** `PE`
    AHA: 2012,4Q,108

Y93.42   **Activity, yoga** `PE`

Y93.43   **Activity, gymnastics** `PE`
Activity, rhythmic gymnastics
> `EXCLUDES 1`   activity, trampolining (Y93.44)

Y93.44   **Activity, trampolining** `PE`

Y93.45   **Activity, cheerleading** `PE`

Y93.49   **Activity, other involving dancing and other rhythmic movements** `PE`

✓5ᵗʰ Y93.5   Activities involving other sports and athletics played individually

> `EXCLUDES 1`   activity, dancing (Y93.41)
> activity, gymnastic (Y93.43)
> activity, trampolining (Y93.44)
> activity, yoga (Y93.42)

Y93.51   **Activity, roller skating** (inline) **and skateboarding** `PE`

Y93.52   **Activity, horseback riding** `PE`

Y93.53   **Activity, golf** `PE`

Y93.54   **Activity, bowling** `PE`

Y93.55   **Activity, bike riding** `PE`

Y93.56   **Activity, jumping rope** `PE`

Y93.57   **Activity, non-running track and field events** `PE`
> `EXCLUDES 1`   activity, running (any form) (Y93.02)

`N` Newborn: 0   `P` Pediatric: 0-17   `M` Maternity: 9-64   `A` Adult: 15-124   `UHS` Unspecified Site   `MCC` Major Complication/Comorbidity   `CC` Complication/Comorbidity   `PE` POA Exempt

1256   ICD-10-CM 2025

Y93.59   **Activity, other involving other sports and athletics played individually**   PE

> EXCLUDES 1   *activities involving climbing, rappelling, and jumping (Y93.3-)*
> *activities involving ice and snow (Y93.2-)*
> *activities involving walking and running (Y93.0-)*
> *activities involving water and watercraft (Y93.1-)*

✓5th **Y93.6**   **Activities involving other sports and athletics played as a team or group**

> EXCLUDES 1   *activity, ice hockey (Y93.22)*
> *activity, water polo (Y93.13)*

Y93.61   **Activity, American tackle football**   PE
    Activity, football NOS

Y93.62   **Activity, American flag or touch football**   PE

Y93.63   **Activity, rugby**   PE

Y93.64   **Activity, baseball**   PE
    Activity, softball

Y93.65   **Activity, lacrosse and field hockey**   PE

Y93.66   **Activity, soccer**   PE

Y93.67   **Activity, basketball**   PE

Y93.68   **Activity, volleyball** (beach) (court)   PE

Y93.6A   **Activity, physical games generally associated with school recess, summer camp and children**   PE
    Activity, capture the flag
    Activity, dodge ball
    Activity, four square
    Activity, kickball

Y93.69   **Activity, other involving other sports and athletics played as a team or group**   PE
    Activity, cricket

✓5th **Y93.7**   **Activities involving other specified sports and athletics**

Y93.71   **Activity, boxing**   PE

Y93.72   **Activity, wrestling**   PE

Y93.73   **Activity, racquet and hand sports**   PE
    Activity, handball
    Activity, racquetball
    Activity, squash
    Activity, tennis

Y93.74   **Activity, frisbee**   PE
    Activity, ultimate frisbee

Y93.75   **Activity, martial arts**   PE
    Activity, combatives

Y93.79   **Activity, other specified sports and athletics**   PE

> EXCLUDES 1   *sports and athletics activities specified in categories Y93.0-Y93.6*

✓5th **Y93.A**   **Activities involving other cardiorespiratory exercise**
    Activities involving physical training

Y93.A1   **Activity, exercise machines primarily for cardiorespiratory conditioning**   PE
    Activity, elliptical and stepper machines
    Activity, stationary bike
    Activity, treadmill

Y93.A2   **Activity, calisthenics**   PE
    Activity, jumping jacks
    Activity, warm up and cool down

Y93.A3   **Activity, aerobic and step exercise**   PE

Y93.A4   **Activity, circuit training**   PE

Y93.A5   **Activity, obstacle course**   PE
    Activity, challenge course
    Activity, confidence course

Y93.A6   **Activity, grass drills**   PE
    Activity, guerilla drills

Y93.A9   **Activity, other involving cardiorespiratory exercise**   PE

> EXCLUDES 1   *activities involving cardiorespiratory exercise specified in categories Y93.0-Y93.7*

✓5th **Y93.B**   **Activities involving other muscle strengthening exercises**

Y93.B1   **Activity, exercise machines primarily for muscle strengthening**   PE

Y93.B2   **Activity, push-ups, pull-ups, sit-ups**   PE

Y93.B3   **Activity, free weights**   PE
    Activity, barbells
    Activity, dumbbells

Y93.B4   **Activity, pilates**   PE

Y93.B9   **Activity, other involving muscle strengthening exercises**   PE

> EXCLUDES 1   *activities involving muscle strengthening specified in categories Y93.0-Y93.A*

✓5th **Y93.C**   **Activities involving computer technology and electronic devices**

> EXCLUDES 1   *activity, electronic musical keyboard or instruments (Y93.J-)*

Y93.C1   **Activity, computer keyboarding**   PE
    Activity, electronic game playing using keyboard or other stationary device

Y93.C2   **Activity, hand held interactive electronic device**   PE
    Activity, cellular telephone and communication device
    Activity, electronic game playing using interactive device

> EXCLUDES 1   *activity, electronic game playing using keyboard or other stationary device (Y93.C1)*

Y93.C9   **Activity, other involving computer technology and electronic devices**

✓5th **Y93.D**   **Activities involving arts and handcrafts**

> EXCLUDES 1   *activities involving playing musical instrument (Y93.J-)*

Y93.D1   **Activity, knitting and crocheting**   PE

Y93.D2   **Activity, sewing**   PE

Y93.D3   **Activity, furniture building and finishing**   PE
    Activity, furniture repair

Y93.D9   **Activity, other involving arts and handcrafts**   PE

✓5th **Y93.E**   **Activities involving personal hygiene and interior property and clothing maintenance**

> EXCLUDES 1   *activities involving cooking and grilling (Y93.G-)*
> *activities involving exterior property and land maintenance, building and construction (Y93.H-)*
> *activities involving caregiving (Y93.F-)*
> *activity, dishwashing (Y93.G1)*
> *activity, food preparation (Y93.G1)*
> *activity, gardening (Y93.H2)*

Y93.E1   **Activity, personal bathing and showering**   PE

Y93.E2   **Activity, laundry**   PE

Y93.E3   **Activity, vacuuming**   PE

Y93.E4   **Activity, ironing**   PE

Y93.E5   **Activity, floor mopping and cleaning**   PE

Y93.E6   **Activity, residential relocation**   PE
    Activity, packing up and unpacking involved in moving to a new residence

Y93.E8   **Activity, other personal hygiene**   PE

Y93.E9   **Activity, other interior property and clothing maintenance**   PE

✓5th **Y93.F**   **Activities involving caregiving**
    Activity involving the provider of caregiving

Y93.F1   **Activity, caregiving, bathing**   PE

Y93.F2   **Activity, caregiving, lifting**   PE

Y93.F9   **Activity, other caregiving**   PE

✓5th **Y93.G**   **Activities involving food preparation, cooking and grilling**

Y93.G1   **Activity, food preparation and clean up**   PE
    Activity, dishwashing

Y93.G2   **Activity, grilling and smoking food**   PE

Y93.G3   **Activity, cooking and baking**   PE
    Activity, use of stove, oven and microwave oven

Y93.G9   **Activity, other involving cooking and grilling**   PE

✓5th **Y93.H**   **Activities involving exterior property and land maintenance, building and construction**

Y93.H1   **Activity, digging, shoveling and raking**   PE
    Activity, dirt digging
    Activity, raking leaves
    Activity, snow shoveling

Y93.H2   **Activity, gardening and landscaping**   PE
    Activity, pruning, trimming shrubs, weeding

Y93.H3   **Activity, building and construction**   PE

Y93.H9   **Activity, other involving exterior property and land maintenance, building and construction**

✓5th **Y93.I**   **Activities involving roller coasters and other types of external motion**

Y93.I1   **Activity, rollercoaster riding**   PE

Y93.I9   **Activity, other involving external motion**   PE

✓ Additional Char Req   ✓7th Placeholder   Unacceptable PDx   Questionable PDx   Wrong Procedure   Manifestation   Unspecified   H1-H4 HAC   HCC CMS-HCC Dx   HIV HIV Dx

ICD-10-CM 2025   1257

Y93.59-Y93.I9

Chapter 20. External Causes of Morbidity

√5ᵗʰ **Y93.J** **Activities involving playing musical instrument**
Activity involving playing electric musical instrument

    Y93.J1 **Activity, piano playing** `PE`
        Activity, musical keyboard (electronic) playing

    Y93.J2 **Activity, drum and other percussion instrument playing** `PE`

    Y93.J3 **Activity, string instrument playing** `PE`

    Y93.J4 **Activity, winds and brass instrument playing** `PE`

√5ᵗʰ **Y93.K** **Activities involving animal care**
    EXCLUDES 1   activity, horseback riding (Y93.52)

    Y93.K1 **Activity, walking an animal** `PE`

    Y93.K2 **Activity, milking an animal** `PE`

    Y93.K3 **Activity, grooming and shearing an animal** `PE`

    Y93.K9 **Activity, other involving animal care** `PE`

√5ᵗʰ **Y93.8** **Activities, other specified**

    Y93.81 **Activity, refereeing a sports activity** `PE`

    Y93.82 **Activity, spectator at an event** `PE`

    Y93.83 **Activity, rough housing and horseplay** `PE`

    Y93.84 **Activity, sleeping** `PE`

    Y93.85 **Activity, choking game** `PE`
        Activity, blackout game
        Activity, fainting game
        Activity, pass out game
        AHA: 2016,4Q,74-76

    Y93.89 **Activity, other specified** `PE`

Y93.9 **Activity, unspecified** `PE`

Y95 **Nosocomial condition**
AHA: 2013,4Q,119

√4ᵗʰ **Y99** **External cause status**

    NOTE   A single code from category Y99 should be used in conjunction with the external cause code(s) assigned to a record to indicate the status of the person at the time the event occurred.

Y99.0 **Civilian activity done for income or pay** `PE`
    Civilian activity done for financial or other compensation
    EXCLUDES 1   military activity (Y99.1)
                volunteer activity (Y99.2)

Y99.1 **Military activity** `PE`
    EXCLUDES 1   activity of off duty military personnel (Y99.8)

Y99.2 **Volunteer activity** `PE`
    EXCLUDES 1   activity of child or other family member assisting in compensated work of other family member (Y99.8)

Y99.8 **Other external cause status** `PE`
    Activity NEC
    Activity of child or other family member assisting in compensated work of other family member
    Hobby not done for income
    Leisure activity
    Off-duty activity of military personnel
    Recreation or sport not for income or while a student
    Student activity
    EXCLUDES 1   civilian activity done for income or compensation (Y99.0)
                military activity (Y99.1)
    AHA: 2012,4Q,108

Y99.9 **Unspecified external cause status** `PE`

N Newborn: 0   P Pediatric: 0-17   M Maternity: 9-64   A Adult: 15-124   UNS Unspecified Site   MCC Major Complication/Comorbidity   CC Complication/Comorbidity   PE POA Exempt

1258

ICD-10-CM 2025

Chapter 21. Factors Influencing Health Status and Contact with Health Services (Z00–Z99)

Chapter-specific Guidelines with Coding Examples

The chapter-specific guidelines from the ICD-10-CM Official Guidelines for Coding and Reporting have been provided below. Along with these guidelines are coding examples, contained in the shaded boxes, that have been developed to help illustrate the coding and/or sequencing guidance found in these guidelines.

Note: The chapter-specific guidelines provide additional information about the use of Z codes for specified encounters.

a. Use of Z Codes in any healthcare setting

Z codes are for use in any healthcare setting. Z codes may be used as either a first-listed (principal diagnosis code in the inpatient setting) or secondary code, depending on the circumstances of the encounter. Certain Z codes may only be used as first-listed or principal diagnosis.

> Patient with middle lobe lung cancer admitted for initiation of chemotherapy
>
> **Z51.11**   **Encounter for antineoplastic chemotherapy**
>
> **C34.2**   **Malignant neoplasm of middle lobe, bronchus or lung**
>
> *Explanation:* A Z code can be used as first-listed in this situation based on guidelines in this chapter as well as chapter 2, "Neoplasms."

b. Z Codes indicate a reason for an encounter or provide additional information about a patient encounter

Z codes are not procedure codes. A corresponding procedure code must accompany a Z code to describe any procedure performed.

c. Categories of Z Codes

1) Contact/exposure

Category Z20 indicates contact with, and suspected exposure to, communicable diseases. These codes are for patients who are suspected to have been exposed to a disease by close personal contact with an infected individual or are in an area where a disease is epidemic.

Category Z77, Other contact with and (suspected) exposures hazardous to health, indicates contact with and suspected exposures hazardous to health. Contact/exposure codes may be used as a first-listed code to explain an encounter for testing, or, more commonly, as a secondary code to identify a potential risk.

2) Inoculations and vaccinations

Code Z23 is for encounters for inoculations and vaccinations. It indicates that a patient is being seen to receive a prophylactic inoculation against a disease. Procedure codes are required to identify the actual administration of the injection and the type(s) of immunizations given. Code Z23 may be used as a secondary code if the inoculation is given as a routine part of preventive health care, such as a well-baby visit.

3) Status

Status codes indicate that a patient is either a carrier of a disease or has the sequelae or residual of a past disease or condition. This includes such things as the presence of prosthetic or mechanical devices resulting from past treatment. A status code is informative, because the status may affect the course of treatment and its outcome. A status code is distinct from a history code. The history code indicates that the patient no longer has the condition.

A status code should not be used with a diagnosis code from one of the body system chapters, if the diagnosis code includes the information provided by the status code. For example, code Z94.1, Heart transplant status, should not be used with a code from subcategory T86.2, Complications of heart transplant. The status code does not provide additional information. The complication code indicates that the patient is a heart transplant patient.

For encounters for weaning from a mechanical ventilator, assign a code from subcategory J96.1, Chronic respiratory failure, followed by code Z99.11, Dependence on respirator [ventilator] status.

The status Z codes/categories are:

Z14   Genetic carrier
     Genetic carrier status indicates that a person carries a gene, associated with a particular disease, which may be passed to offspring who may develop that disease. The person does not have the disease and is not at risk of developing the disease.

Z15   Genetic susceptibility to disease
     Genetic susceptibility indicates that a person has a gene that increases the risk of that person developing the disease. Codes from category Z15 should not be used as principal or first-listed codes. If the patient has the condition to which he/she is susceptible, and that condition is the reason for the encounter, the code for the current condition should be sequenced first. If the patient is being seen for follow-up after completed treatment for this condition, and the condition no longer exists, a follow-up code should be sequenced first, followed by the appropriate personal history and genetic susceptibility codes. If the purpose of the encounter is genetic counseling associated with procreative

management, code Z31.5, Encounter for genetic counseling, should be assigned as the first-listed code, followed by a code from category Z15. Additional codes should be assigned for any applicable family or personal history.

Z16   Resistance to antimicrobial drugs
     This code indicates that a patient has a condition that is resistant to antimicrobial drug treatment. Sequence the infection code first.

> Penicillin resistant streptococcus pneumoniae meningitis
>
> **G00.1**   **Pneumococcal meningitis**
>
> **Z16.11**   **Resistance to penicillins**
>
> *Explanation:* The status Z code is used to describe the presence of a drug-resistant organism that most likely altered how the meningitis was treated.

Z17   Estrogen, **and other hormones and factors** receptor status

Z18   Retained foreign body fragments

Z19   Hormone sensitivity malignancy status

Z21   Asymptomatic HIV infection status
     This code indicates that a patient has tested positive for HIV but has manifested no signs or symptoms of the disease.

Z22   Carrier of infectious disease
     Carrier status indicates that a person harbors the specific organisms of a disease without manifest symptoms and is capable of transmitting the infection.

Z28.3   Underimmunization status
     See Section I.B.14. for underimmunization documentation by clinicians other than the patient's provider.

Z33.1   Pregnant state, incidental
     This code is a secondary code only for use when the pregnancy is in no way complicating the reason for visit. Otherwise, a code from the obstetric chapter is required.

Z66   Do not resuscitate
     This code may be used when it is documented by the provider that a patient is on do not resuscitate status at any time during the stay.

Z67   Blood type

Z68   Body mass index (BMI)
     BMI codes should only be assigned when there is an associated, reportable diagnosis (such as obesity). Do not assign BMI codes during pregnancy.
     See Section I.B.14. for BMI documentation by clinicians other than the patient's provider.

Z74.01   Bed confinement status

Z76.82   Awaiting organ transplant status

Z78   Other specified health status
     Code Z78.1, Physical restraint status, may be used when it is documented by the provider that a patient has been put in restraints during the current encounter. Please note that this code should not be reported when it is documented by the provider that a patient is temporarily restrained during a procedure.

Z79   Long-term (current) drug therapy
     Codes from this category indicate a patient's continuous use of a prescribed drug (including such things as aspirin therapy) for the long-term treatment of a condition or for prophylactic use. It is not for use for patients who have addictions to drugs. This subcategory is not for use of medications for detoxification or maintenance programs to prevent withdrawal symptoms (e.g., methadone maintenance for opiate dependence). Assign the appropriate code for the drug use, abuse, or dependence instead.
     Assign a code from Z79 if the patient is receiving a medication for an extended period as a prophylactic measure (such as for the prevention of deep vein thrombosis) or as treatment of a chronic condition (such as arthritis) or a disease requiring a lengthy course of treatment (such as cancer). Do not assign a code from category Z79 for medication being administered for a brief period of time to treat an acute illness or injury (such as a course of antibiotics to treat acute bronchitis).

Z88   Allergy status to drugs, medicaments and biological substances
     Except: Z88.9, Allergy status to unspecified drugs, medicaments and biological substances status

Z89   Acquired absence of limb

Z90   Acquired absence of organs, not elsewhere classified

Z91.0-   Allergy status, other than to drugs and biological substances

Z92.82   Status post administration of tPA (rtPA) in a different facility within the last 24 hours prior to admission to a current facility
     Assign code Z92.82, Status post administration of tPA (rtPA) in a different facility within the last 24 hours prior to admission to current facility, as a secondary diagnosis when a patient is received by transfer into a facility and documentation indicates they were administered tissue plasminogen activator (tPA) within the last 24 hours prior to admission to the current facility.

This guideline applies even if the patient is still receiving the tPA at the time they are received into the current facility.

The appropriate code for the condition for which the tPA was administered (such as cerebrovascular disease or myocardial infarction) should be assigned first.

Code Z92.82 is only applicable to the receiving facility record and not to the transferring facility record.

Z93   Artificial opening status
Z94   Transplanted organ and tissue status
Z95   Presence of cardiac and vascular implants and grafts
Z96   Presence of other functional implants
Z97   Presence of other devices
Z98   Other postprocedural states

Assign code Z98.85, Transplanted organ removal status, to indicate that a transplanted organ has been previously removed. This code should not be assigned for the encounter in which the transplanted organ is removed. The complication necessitating removal of the transplant organ should be assigned for that encounter.

See section I.C.19. for information on the coding of organ transplant complications.

Z99   Dependence on enabling machines and devices, not elsewhere classified

Note: Categories Z89–Z90 and Z93–Z99 are for use only if there are no complications or malfunctions of the organ or tissue replaced, the amputation site or the equipment on which the patient is dependent.

4) History (of)

There are two types of history Z codes, personal and family. Personal history codes explain a patient's past medical condition that no longer exists and is not receiving any treatment, but that has the potential for recurrence, and therefore may require continued monitoring.

Family history codes are for use when a patient has a family member(s) who has had a particular disease that causes the patient to be at higher risk of also contracting the disease.

Personal history codes may be used in conjunction with follow-up codes and family history codes may be used in conjunction with screening codes to explain the need for a test or procedure. History codes are also acceptable on any medical record regardless of the reason for visit. A history of an illness, even if no longer present, is important information that may alter the type of treatment ordered.

The reason for the encounter (for example, screening or counseling) should be sequenced first and the appropriate personal and/or family history code(s) should be assigned as additional diagnos(es).

The history Z code categories are:

Z80   Family history of primary malignant neoplasm
Z81   Family history of mental and behavioral disorders
Z82   Family history of certain disabilities and chronic diseases (leading to disablement)
Z83   Family history of other specific disorders
Z84   Family history of other conditions
Z85   Personal history of malignant neoplasm
Z86   Personal history of certain other diseases
Z87   Personal history of other diseases and conditions
Z91.4-   Personal history of psychological trauma, not elsewhere classified
Z91.5-   Personal history of self-harm
Z91.81   History of falling
Z91.82   Personal history of military deployment
Z91.85   Personal history of military service
Z92   Personal history of medical treatment

Except: Z92.0, Personal history of contraception
Except: Z92.82, Status post administration of tPA (rtPA) in a different facility within the last 24 hours prior to admission to a current facility

Patient has chronic lymphocytic leukemia for which the patient had previous chemotherapy and is now in remission

C91.11   **Chronic lymphocytic leukemia of B-cell type in remission**

Z92.21   **Personal history of antineoplastic chemotherapy**

Explanation: The personal history Z code is used to describe a secondary (supplementary) diagnosis to identify that this patient has had chemotherapy in the past.

5) Screening

Screening is the testing for disease or disease precursors in seemingly well individuals so that early detection and treatment can be provided for those who test positive for the disease (e.g., screening mammogram).

The testing of a person to rule out or confirm a suspected diagnosis because the patient has some sign or symptom is a diagnostic examination, not a screening. In these cases, the sign or symptom is used to explain the reason for the test.

A screening code may be a first-listed code if the reason for the visit is specifically the screening exam. It may also be used as an additional code if the screening is done during an office visit for other health problems. A screening code is not necessary if the screening is inherent to a routine examination, such as a pap smear done during a routine pelvic examination.

Should a condition be discovered during the screening then the code for the condition may be assigned as an additional diagnosis.

The Z code indicates that a screening exam is planned. A procedure code is required to confirm that the screening was performed.

The screening Z codes/categories:

Z11   Encounter for screening for infectious and parasitic diseases
Z12   Encounter for screening for malignant neoplasms
Z13   Encounter for screening for other diseases and disorders
      Except: Z13.9, Encounter for screening, unspecified
Z36   Encounter for antenatal screening for mother

6) Observation

There are three observation Z code categories. They are for use in very limited circumstances when a person is being observed for a suspected condition that is ruled out. The observation codes are not for use if an injury or illness or any signs or symptoms related to the suspected condition are present. In such cases the diagnosis/symptom code is used with the corresponding external cause code.

The observation codes are primarily to be used as a principal/first-listed diagnosis. An observation code may be assigned as a secondary diagnosis code when the patient is being observed for a condition that is ruled out and is unrelated to the principal/first-listed diagnosis Also, when the principal diagnosis is required to be a code from category Z38, Liveborn infants according to place of birth and type of delivery, then a code from category Z05, Encounter for observation and evaluation of newborn for suspected diseases and conditions ruled out, is sequenced after the Z38 code. Additional codes may be used in addition to the observation code, but only if they are unrelated to the suspected condition being observed.

Codes from subcategory Z03.7, Encounter for suspected maternal and fetal conditions ruled out, may either be used as a first-listed or as an additional code assignment depending on the case. They are for use in very limited circumstances on a maternal record when an encounter is for a suspected maternal or fetal condition that is ruled out during that encounter (for example, a maternal or fetal condition may be suspected due to an abnormal test result). These codes should not be used when the condition is confirmed. In those cases, the confirmed condition should be coded. In addition, these codes are not for use if an illness or any signs or symptoms related to the suspected condition or problem are present. In such cases the diagnosis/symptom code is used.

Additional codes may be used in addition to the code from subcategory Z03.7, but only if they are unrelated to the suspected condition being evaluated.

Codes from subcategory Z03.7 may not be used for encounters for antenatal screening of mother. *See Section I.C.21. Screening.*

For encounters for suspected fetal condition that are inconclusive following testing and evaluation, assign the appropriate code from category O35, O36, O40 or O41.

The observation Z code categories:

Z03   Encounter for medical observation for suspected diseases and conditions ruled out
Z04   Encounter for examination and observation for other reasons
      Except: Z04.9, Encounter for examination and observation for unspecified reason
Z05   Encounter for observation and evaluation of newborn for suspected diseases and conditions ruled out

Upon initial examination, a heart murmur was heard in a newborn infant delivered vaginally in the hospital; however, after further observation, any serious cardiac conditions were ruled out.

Z38.00   **Single liveborn infant, delivered vaginally**

Z05.0   **Observation and evaluation of newborn for suspected cardiac condition ruled out**

Explanation: Normally an observation code is used as the principal diagnosis except when the patient is a newborn. A code from category Z38 Liveborn infants according to place of birth and type of delivery code would be sequenced first, followed by the encounter for observation and evaluation of newborn for suspected diseases and conditions ruled out.

7) Aftercare

Aftercare visit codes cover situations when the initial treatment of a disease has been performed and the patient requires continued care during the healing or recovery phase, or for the long-term consequences of the disease. The aftercare Z code should not be used if treatment is directed at a current, acute disease. The diagnosis code is to be used in these cases. Exceptions to this rule are codes Z51.0, Encounter for antineoplastic radiation therapy, and codes from subcategory Z51.1, Encounter for antineoplastic chemotherapy and immunotherapy. These codes are to be first listed, followed by the diagnosis code when a patient's encounter is chiefly to receive radiation therapy, chemotherapy, or immunotherapy for the treatment of a neoplasm. If the reason for the encounter is more than one type of antineoplastic therapy, code Z51.0 and a code from subcategory Z51.1 may be assigned together, in which case one of these codes would be reported as a secondary diagnosis.

The aftercare Z codes should also not be used for aftercare for injuries. For aftercare of an injury, assign the acute injury code with the appropriate 7th character (for subsequent encounter).

The aftercare codes are generally first listed to explain the specific reason for the encounter. An aftercare code may be used as an additional code when some type of aftercare is provided in addition to the reason for admission and no diagnosis code is applicable. An example of this would be the closure of a colostomy during an encounter for treatment of another condition.

Aftercare codes should be used in conjunction with other aftercare codes or diagnosis codes to provide better detail on the specifics of an aftercare encounter visit, unless otherwise directed by the classification. The sequencing of multiple aftercare codes depends on the circumstances of the encounter.

Certain aftercare Z code categories need a secondary diagnosis code to describe the resolving condition or sequelae. For others, the condition is included in the code title.

Additional Z code aftercare category terms include fitting and adjustment, and attention to artificial openings.

Status Z codes may be used with aftercare Z codes to indicate the nature of the aftercare. For example code Z95.1, Presence of aortocoronary bypass graft, may be used with code Z48.812, Encounter for surgical aftercare following surgery on the circulatory system, to indicate the surgery for which the aftercare is being performed. A status code should not be used when the aftercare code indicates the type of status, such as using Z43.0, Encounter for attention to tracheostomy, with Z93.0, Tracheostomy status.

The aftercare Z category/codes:

Z42   Encounter for plastic and reconstructive surgery following medical procedure or healed injury
Z43   Encounter for attention to artificial openings
Z44   Encounter for fitting and adjustment of external prosthetic device
Z45   Encounter for adjustment and management of implanted device
Z46   Encounter for fitting and adjustment of other devices
Z47   Orthopedic aftercare
Z48   Encounter for other postprocedural aftercare
Z49   Encounter for care involving renal dialysis
Z51   Encounter for other aftercare and medical care

8) Follow-up

The follow-up codes are used to explain continuing surveillance following completed treatment of a disease, condition, or injury. They imply that the condition has been fully treated and no longer exists. They should not be confused with aftercare codes, or injury codes with a 7th character for subsequent encounter, that explain ongoing care of a healing condition or its sequelae. Follow-up codes may be used in conjunction with history codes to provide the full picture of the healed condition and its treatment. The follow-up code is sequenced first, followed by the history code.

A follow-up code may be used to explain multiple visits. Should a condition be found to have recurred on the follow-up visit, then the diagnosis code for the condition should be assigned in place of the follow-up code.

The follow-up Z codes/categories:

Z08   Encounter for follow-up examination after completed treatment for malignant neoplasm
Z09   Encounter for follow-up examination after completed treatment for conditions other than malignant neoplasm

Codes Z08, Encounter for follow-up examination after completed treatment for malignant neoplasm, and Z09, Encounter for follow up examination after completed treatment for conditions other than malignant neoplasm, may be assigned following any type of completed treatment modality (including both medical and surgical treatments).

Z39   Encounter for maternal postpartum care and examination

9) Donor

Codes in category Z52, Donors of organs and tissues, are used for living individuals who are donating blood or other body tissue. These codes are for individuals donating for others, as well as for self-donations. They are not used to identify cadaveric donations.

10) Counseling

Counseling Z codes are used when a patient or family member receives assistance in the aftermath of an illness or injury, or when support is required in coping with family or social problems.

The counseling Z codes/categories:

Z30.0-   Encounter for general counseling and advice on contraception
Z31.5   Encounter for procreative genetic counseling
Z31.6-   Encounter for general counseling and advice on procreation
Z32.2   Encounter for childbirth instruction
Z32.3   Encounter for childcare instruction
Z69   Encounter for mental health services for victim and perpetrator of abuse
Z70   Counseling related to sexual attitude, behavior and orientation
Z71   Persons encountering health services for other counseling and medical advice, not elsewhere classified
      Note: Code Z71.84, Encounter for health counseling related to travel, is to be used for health risk and safety counseling for future travel purposes.

Code Z71.85, Encounter for immunization safety counseling, is to be used for counseling of the patient or caregiver regarding the safety of a vaccine. This code should not be used for the provision of general information regarding risks and potential side effects during routine encounters for the administration of vaccines.

Code Z71.87, Encounter for pediatric-to-adult transition counseling, should be assigned when pediatric-to-adult transition counseling is the sole reason for the encounter or when this counseling is provided in addition to other services, such as treatment of a chronic condition. If both transition counseling and treatment of a medical condition are provided during the same encounter, the code(s) for the medical condition(s) treated and code Z71.87 should be assigned, with sequencing depending on the circumstances of the encounter.

Z76.81 Expectant mother prebirth pediatrician visit

11) Encounters for obstetrical and reproductive services

See Section I.C.15. Pregnancy, Childbirth, and the Puerperium, for further instruction on the use of these codes.

Z codes for pregnancy are for use in those circumstances when none of the problems or complications included in the codes from the Obstetrics chapter exist (a routine prenatal visit or postpartum care). Codes in category Z34, Encounter for supervision of normal pregnancy, are always first listed and are not to be used with any other code from the OB chapter.

Codes in category Z3A, Weeks of gestation, may be assigned to provide additional information about the pregnancy. Category Z3A codes should not be assigned for pregnancies with abortive outcomes (categories O00–O08), elective termination of pregnancy (code Z33.2), nor for postpartum conditions, as category Z3A is not applicable to these conditions. The date of the admission should be used to determine weeks of gestation for inpatient admissions that encompass more than one gestational week.

The outcome of delivery, category Z37, should be included on all maternal delivery records. It is always a secondary code.

Codes in category Z37 should not be used on the newborn record.

Z codes for family planning (contraceptive) or procreative management and counseling should be included on an obstetric record either during the pregnancy or the postpartum stage, if applicable.

Z codes/categories for obstetrical and reproductive services:

Z30   Encounter for contraceptive management
Z31   Encounter for procreative management
Z32.2   Encounter for childbirth instruction
Z32.3   Encounter for childcare instruction
Z33   Pregnant state
Z34   Encounter for supervision of normal pregnancy
Z36   Encounter for antenatal screening of mother
Z3A   Weeks of gestation
Z37   Outcome of delivery
Z39   Encounter for maternal postpartum care and examination
Z76.81 Expectant mother prebirth pediatrician visit

12) Newborns and infants

See Section I.C.16. Newborn (Perinatal) Guidelines, for further instruction on the use of these codes.

Newborn Z codes/categories:

Z76.1   Encounter for health supervision and care of foundling
Z00.1-   Encounter for routine child health examination
Z38   Liveborn infants according to place of birth and type of delivery

13) Routine and administrative examinations

The Z codes allow for the description of encounters for routine examinations, such as, a general check-up, or, examinations for administrative purposes, such as, a pre-employment physical. The codes are not to be used if the examination is for diagnosis of a suspected condition or for treatment purposes. In such cases the diagnosis code is used. During a routine exam, should a diagnosis or condition be discovered, it should be coded as an additional code. Pre-existing and chronic conditions and history codes may also be included as additional codes as long as the examination is for administrative purposes and not focused on any particular condition.

Some of the codes for routine health examinations distinguish between "with" and "without" abnormal findings. Code assignment depends on the information that is known at the time the encounter is being coded. For example, if no abnormal findings were found during the examination, but the encounter is being coded before test results are back, it is acceptable to assign the code for "without abnormal findings." When assigning a code for "with abnormal findings," additional code(s) should be assigned to identify the specific abnormal finding(s).

Pre-operative examination and pre-procedural laboratory examination Z codes are for use only in those situations when a patient is being cleared for a procedure or surgery and no treatment is given.

The Z codes/categories for routine and administrative examinations:

Z00   Encounter for general examination without complaint, suspected or reported diagnosis
Z01   Encounter for other special examination without complaint, suspected or reported diagnosis

Chapter 21. Factors Influencing Health Status and Contact with Health Services

Z02   Encounter for administrative examination
     Except: Z02.9, Encounter for administrative examinations, unspecified
Z32.0-   Encounter for pregnancy test

14) Miscellaneous Z codes

The miscellaneous Z codes capture a number of other health care encounters that do not fall into one of the other categories. Some of these codes identify the reason for the encounter; others are for use as additional codes that provide useful information on circumstances that may affect a patient's care and treatment.

Prophylactic organ removal

For encounters specifically for prophylactic removal of an organ (such as prophylactic removal of breasts due to a genetic susceptibility to cancer or a family history of cancer), the principal or first-listed code should be a code from category Z40, Encounter for prophylactic surgery, followed by the appropriate codes to identify the associated risk factor (such as genetic susceptibility or family history).

If the patient has a malignancy of one site and is having prophylactic removal at another site to prevent either a new primary malignancy or metastatic disease, a code for the malignancy should also be assigned in addition to a code from subcategory Z40.0, Encounter for prophylactic surgery for risk factors related to malignant neoplasms. A Z40.0 code should not be assigned if the patient is having organ removal for treatment of a malignancy, such as the removal of the testes for the treatment of prostate cancer.

Female patient with cancer in lower inner quadrant of right breast and positive BRCA 1 noted on testing is admitted for mastectomy of right breast and prophylactic removal of left breast

C50.311   **Malignant neoplasm of lower-inner quadrant of right female breast**

Z40.01   **Encounter for prophylactic removal of breast**

Z15.01   **Genetic susceptibility to malignant neoplasm of breast**

Explanation: Removal of the current neoplastic disease in the right breast was the focus of treatment for this admission and is sequenced first. The removal of the left breast was not required to treat a current disease process but as a means of prevention. The two Z codes are informational; they capture the reason behind the removal of what is currently a healthy left breast.

Miscellaneous Z codes/categories:

Z28   Immunization not carried out
     Except: Z28.3-, Underimmunization status
Z29   Encounter for other prophylactic measures
Z40   Encounter for prophylactic surgery
Z41   Encounter for procedures for purposes other than remedying health state
     Except: Z41.9, Encounter for procedure for purposes other than remedying health state, unspecified
Z53   Persons encountering health services for specific procedures and treatment, not carried out
Z72   Problems related to lifestyle
     Note: These codes should be assigned only when the documentation specifies that the patient has an associated problem
Z73   Problems related to life management difficulty
     Note: These codes should be assigned only when the documentation specifies that the patient has an associated problem.
Z74   Problems related to care provider dependency
     Except: Z74.01, Bed confinement status
Z75   Problems related to medical facilities and other health care
Z76.0   Encounter for issue of repeat prescription
Z76.3   Healthy person accompanying sick person
Z76.4   Other boarder to healthcare facility
Z76.5   Malingerer [conscious simulation]
Z91.1-   Patient's noncompliance with medical treatment and regimen
Z91.A-   Caregiver's noncompliance with patient's medical treatment and regimen
Z91.83   Wandering in diseases classified elsewhere
Z91.84- Oral health risk factors
Z91.89   Other specified personal risk factors, not elsewhere classified
See Section I.B.14. for Z55–Z65 Persons with potential health hazards related to socioeconomic and psychosocial circumstances, documentation by clinicians other than the patient's provider

15) Nonspecific Z codes

Certain Z codes are so non-specific, or potentially redundant with other codes in the classification, that there can be little justification for their use in the inpatient setting. Their use in the outpatient setting should be limited to those instances when there is no further documentation to permit more precise coding. Otherwise, any sign or symptom or any other reason for visit that is captured in another code should be used.
Nonspecific Z codes/categories:

Z02.9   Encounter for administrative examinations, unspecified
Z04.9   Encounter for examination and observation for unspecified reason

Z13.9   Encounter for screening, unspecified
Z41.9   Encounter for procedure for purposes other than remedying health state, unspecified
Z52.9   Donor of unspecified organ or tissue
Z86.59 Personal history of other mental and behavioral disorders
Z88.9   Allergy status to unspecified drugs, medicaments and biological substances status
Z92.0   Personal history of contraception

16) Z codes that may only be principal/first-listed diagnosis

The following Z codes/categories may only be reported as the principal/first-listed diagnosis, except when there are multiple encounters on the same day and the medical records for the encounters are combined:

Z00   Encounter for general examination without complaint, suspected or reported diagnosis
     Except: Z00.6
Z01   Encounter for other special examination without complaint, suspected or reported diagnosis
Z02   Encounter for administrative examination
Z04   Encounter for examination and observation for other reasons
Z33.2   Encounter for elective termination of pregnancy
Z31.81 Encounter for male factor infertility in female patient
Z31.83 Encounter for assisted reproductive fertility procedure cycle
Z31.84 Encounter for fertility preservation procedure
Z34   Encounter for supervision of normal pregnancy
Z39   Encounter for maternal postpartum care and examination
Z38   Liveborn infants according to place of birth and type of delivery
Z40   Encounter for prophylactic surgery
Z42   Encounter for plastic and reconstructive surgery following medical procedure or healed injury
Z51.0   Encounter for antineoplastic radiation therapy
Z51.1-   Encounter for antineoplastic chemotherapy and immunotherapy
Z52   Donors of organs and tissues
     Except: Z52.9, Donor of unspecified organ or tissue
Z76.1   Encounter for health supervision and care of foundling
Z76.2   Encounter for health supervision and care of other healthy infant and child
Z99.12 Encounter for respirator [ventilator] dependence during power failure

17) Social Determinants of Health

Social determinants of health (SDOH) codes describing social problems, conditions, or risk factors that influence a patient's health should be assigned when this information is documented in the patient's medical record. Assign as many SDOH codes as are necessary to describe all of the social problems, conditions, or risk factors documented during the current episode of care. For example, a patient who lives alone may suffer an acute injury temporarily impacting their ability to perform routine activities of daily living. When documented as such, this would support assignment of code Z60.2, Problems related to living alone. However, merely living alone, without documentation of a risk or unmet need for assistance at home, would not support assignment of code Z60.2. Documentation by a clinician (or patient-reported information that is signed off by a clinician) that the patient expressed concerns with access and availability of food would support assignment of code Z59.41, Food insecurity. Similarly, medical record documentation indicating the patient is homeless would support assignment of a code from subcategory Z59.0-, Homelessness.

For social determinants of health classified to chapter 21, such as information found in categories Z55-Z65, Persons with potential health hazards related to socioeconomic and psychosocial circumstances, code assignment may be based on medical record documentation from clinicians involved in the care of the patient who are not the patient's provider since this information represents social information, rather than medical diagnoses. For example, coding professionals may utilize documentation of social information from social workers, community health workers, case managers, or nurses, if their documentation is included in the official medical record.

Patient self-reported documentation may be used to assign codes for social determinants of health, as long as the patient self-reported information is signed-off by and incorporated into the medical record by either a clinician or provider.

Social determinants of health codes are located primarily in these Z code categories:

Z55   Problems related to education and literacy
Z56   Problems related to employment and unemployment
Z57   Occupational exposure to risk factors
Z58   Problems related to physical environment
Z59   Problems related to housing and economic circumstances
Z60   Problems related to social environment
Z62   Problems related to upbringing
Z63   Other problems related to primary support group, including family circumstances
Z64   Problems related to certain psychosocial circumstances
Z65   Problems related to other psychosocial circumstances

See Section I.B.14. Documentation by Clinicians Other than the Patient's Provider.

Chapter 21. Factors Influencing Health Status and Contact With Health Services (Z00-Z99)

NOTE Z codes represent reasons for encounters. A corresponding procedure code must accompany a Z code if a procedure is performed. Categories Z00-Z99 are provided for occasions when circumstances other than a disease, injury or external cause classifiable to categories A00-Y89 are recorded as "diagnoses" or "problems." This can arise in two main ways:

(a) When a person who may or may not be sick encounters the health services for some specific purpose, such as to receive limited care or service for a current condition, to donate an organ or tissue, to receive prophylactic vaccination (immunization), or to discuss a problem which is in itself not a disease or injury.

(b) When some circumstance or problem is present which influences the person's health status but is not in itself a current illness or injury.

AHA: 2018,4Q,60-61

This chapter contains the following blocks:

Z00-Z13	Persons encountering health services for examinations
Z14-Z15	Genetic carrier and genetic susceptibility to disease
Z16	Resistance to antimicrobial drugs
Z17	▶Estrogen, and other hormones and factors receptor status◀
Z18	Retained foreign body fragments
Z19	Hormone sensitivity malignancy status
Z20-Z29	Persons with potential health hazards related to communicable diseases
Z30-Z39	Persons encountering health services in circumstances related to reproduction
Z40-Z53	Encounters for other specific health care
Z55-Z65	Persons with potential health hazards related to socioeconomic and psychosocial circumstances
Z66	Do not resuscitate status
Z67	Blood type
Z68	Body mass index (BMI)
Z69-Z76	Persons encountering health services in other circumstances
Z77-Z99	Persons with potential health hazards related to family and personal history and certain conditions influencing health status

Persons encountering health services for examinations (Z00-Z13)

NOTE Nonspecific abnormal findings disclosed at the time of these examinations are classified to categories R70-R94.

EXCLUDES 1 examinations related to pregnancy and reproduction (Z30-Z36, Z39.-)

✓4ᵗʰ **Z00 Encounter for general examination without complaint, suspected or reported diagnosis**

EXCLUDES 1 encounter for examination for administrative purposes (Z02.-)

EXCLUDES 2 encounter for pre-procedural examinations (Z01.81-)
special screening examinations (Z11-Z13)

AHA: 2017,4Q,95

✓5ᵗʰ **Z00.0 Encounter for general adult medical examination**

Encounter for adult periodic examination (annual) (physical) and any associated laboratory and radiologic examinations

EXCLUDES 1 encounter for examination of sign or symptom - code to sign or symptom
general health check-up of infant or child (Z00.12.-)

Z00.00 Encounter for general adult medical examination without abnormal findings UPD A PE
Encounter for adult health check-up NOS
AHA: 2016,1Q,36

Z00.01 Encounter for general adult medical examination with abnormal findings UPD A PE
Use additional code to identify abnormal findings
AHA: 2016,1Q,35-36

✓5ᵗʰ **Z00.1 Encounter for newborn, infant and child health examinations**

✓6ᵗʰ **Z00.11 Newborn health examination**
Health check for child under 29 days old
Use additional code to identify any abnormal findings
EXCLUDES 1 health check for child over 28 days old (Z00.12-)

Z00.110 Health examination for newborn under 8 days old UPD N PE
Health check for newborn under 8 days old

Z00.111 Health examination for newborn 8 to 28 days old UPD N PE
Health check for newborn 8 to 28 days old
Newborn weight check

✓6ᵗʰ **Z00.12 Encounter for routine child health examination**
Health check (routine) for child over 28 days old
Immunizations appropriate for age
Routine developmental screening of infant or child
Routine vison and hearing testing
EXCLUDES 1 health check for child under 29 days old (Z00.11-)
health supervision of foundling or other healthy infant or child (Z76.1-Z76.2)
newborn health examination (Z00.11-)
AHA: 2018,4Q,36

Z00.121 Encounter for routine child health examination with abnormal findings UPD P PE
Use additional code to identify abnormal findings
AHA: 2016,1Q,34-35

Z00.129 Encounter for routine child health examination without abnormal findings UPD P PE
Encounter for routine child health examination NOS
AHA: 2016,1Q,34

Z00.2 Encounter for examination for period of rapid growth in childhood UPD P PE

Z00.3 Encounter for examination for adolescent development state UPD P PE
Encounter for puberty development state

Z00.5 Encounter for examination of potential donor of organ and tissue UPD PE

Z00.6 Encounter for examination for normal comparison and control in clinical research program PE
Examination of participant or control in clinical research program

✓5ᵗʰ **Z00.7 Encounter for examination for period of delayed growth in childhood**

Z00.70 Encounter for examination for period of delayed growth in childhood without abnormal findings UPD P PE

Z00.71 Encounter for examination for period of delayed growth in childhood with abnormal findings UPD P PE
Use additional code to identify abnormal findings

Z00.8 Encounter for other general examination UPD PE
Encounter for health examination in population surveys

✓4ᵗʰ **Z01 Encounter for other special examination without complaint, suspected or reported diagnosis**

INCLUDES routine examination of specific system

NOTE Codes from category Z01 represent the reason for the encounter. A separate procedure code is required to identify any examinations or procedures performed

EXCLUDES 1 encounter for examination for administrative purposes (Z02.-)
encounter for examination for suspected conditions, proven not to exist (Z03.-)
encounter for laboratory and radiologic examinations as a component of general medical examinations (Z00.0-)
encounter for laboratory, radiologic and imaging examinations for sign(s) and symptom(s) - code to the sign(s) or symptom(s)

EXCLUDES 2 screening examinations (Z11-Z13)

✓5ᵗʰ **Z01.0 Encounter for examination of eyes and vision**

EXCLUDES 1 examination for driving license (Z02.4)

Z01.00 Encounter for examination of eyes and vision without abnormal findings PE
Encounter for examination of eyes and vision NOS

Z01.01 Encounter for examination of eyes and vision with abnormal findings PE
Use additional code to identify abnormal findings
AHA: 2016,4Q,21

☑ Additional Character Required ✓x7ᵗʰ Placeholder Questionable PDx Manifestation Unspecified UPD Unacceptable PDx H1 -H14 HAC HCC CMS-HCC Dx HIV HIV Dx

ICD-10-CM 2025   **1263**

✓6ᵗʰ **Z01.02** **Encounter for examination of eyes and vision following failed vision screening**

     EXCLUDES 1   *encounter for examination of eyes and vision with abnormal findings (Z01.01)*

         encounter for examination of eyes and vision without abnormal findings (Z01.00)

     AHA: 2019,4Q,20

     Z01.020 **Encounter for examination of eyes and vision following failed vision screening without abnormal findings** PE

     Z01.021 **Encounter for examination of eyes and vision following failed vision screening with abnormal findings** PE

         Use additional code to identify abnormal findings

✓5ᵗʰ **Z01.1** **Encounter for examination of ears and hearing**

     Z01.10 **Encounter for examination of ears and hearing without abnormal findings** UPD PE

         Encounter for examination of ears and hearing NOS

         AHA: 2016,4Q,24

✓6ᵗʰ **Z01.11** **Encounter for examination of ears and hearing with abnormal findings**

         AHA: 2016,3Q,17-18

     Z01.110 **Encounter for hearing examination following failed hearing screening** UPD PE

     Z01.118 **Encounter for examination of ears and hearing with other abnormal findings** UPD PE

         Use additional code to identify abnormal findings

     Z01.12 **Encounter for hearing conservation and treatment** UPD PE

✓5ᵗʰ **Z01.2** **Encounter for dental examination and cleaning**

     Z01.20 **Encounter for dental examination and cleaning without abnormal findings** UPD PE

         Encounter for dental examination and cleaning NOS

     Z01.21 **Encounter for dental examination and cleaning with abnormal findings** UPD PE

         Use additional code to identify abnormal findings

✓5ᵗʰ **Z01.3** **Encounter for examination of blood pressure**

     Z01.30 **Encounter for examination of blood pressure without abnormal findings** UPD PE

         Encounter for examination of blood pressure NOS

     Z01.31 **Encounter for examination of blood pressure with abnormal findings** UPD PE

         Use additional code to identify abnormal findings

✓5ᵗʰ **Z01.4** **Encounter for gynecological examination**

     EXCLUDES 2   *pregnancy examination or test (Z32.0-)*

         routine examination for contraceptive maintenance (Z30.4-)

✓6ᵗʰ **Z01.41** **Encounter for routine gynecological examination**

     Encounter for general gynecological examination with or without cervical smear

     Encounter for gynecological examination (general) (routine) NOS

     Encounter for pelvic examination (annual) (periodic)

     Use additional code:

         for screening for human papillomavirus, if applicable, (Z11.51)

         for screening vaginal pap smear, if applicable (Z12.72)

         to identify acquired absence of uterus, if applicable (Z90.71-)

     EXCLUDES 1   *gynecologic examination status-post hysterectomy for malignant condition (Z08)*

         screening cervical pap smear not a part of a routine gynecological examination (Z12.4)

     Z01.411 **Encounter for gynecological examination (general) (routine) with abnormal findings** PE

         Use additional code to identify abnormal findings

     Z01.419 **Encounter for gynecological examination (general) (routine) without abnormal findings** PE

Z01.42 **Encounter for cervical smear to confirm findings of recent normal smear following initial abnormal smear** PE

✓5ᵗʰ **Z01.8** **Encounter for other specified special examinations**

✓6ᵗʰ **Z01.81** **Encounter for preprocedural examinations**

     Encounter for preoperative examinations

     Encounter for radiological and imaging examinations as part of preprocedural examination

     Z01.810 **Encounter for preprocedural cardiovascular examination** PE

     Z01.811 **Encounter for preprocedural respiratory examination** PE

     Z01.812 **Encounter for preprocedural laboratory examination**

         Blood and urine tests prior to treatment or procedure

         AHA: 2023,2Q,3; 2020,3Q,14

     Z01.818 **Encounter for other preprocedural examination** UPD PE

         Encounter for preprocedural examination NOS

         Encounter for examinations prior to antineoplastic chemotherapy

     Z01.82 **Encounter for allergy testing** UPD PE

     EXCLUDES 1   *encounter for antibody response examination (Z01.84)*

     Z01.83 **Encounter for blood typing** UPD PE

         Encounter for Rh typing

     Z01.84 **Encounter for antibody response examination** UPD PE

         Encounter for immunity status testing

     EXCLUDES 1   *encounter for allergy testing (Z01.82)*

         AHA: 2020,2Q,11

     Z01.89 **Encounter for other specified special examinations** UPD PE

✓4ᵗʰ **Z02** **Encounter for administrative examination**

     Z02.0 **Encounter for examination for admission to educational institution** UPD PE

         Encounter for examination for admission to preschool (education)

         Encounter for examination for re-admission to school following illness or medical treatment

     Z02.1 **Encounter for pre-employment examination** PE

     Z02.2 **Encounter for examination for admission to residential institution** UPD PE

     EXCLUDES 1   *examination for admission to prison (Z02.89)*

     Z02.3 **Encounter for examination for recruitment to armed forces** PE

     Z02.4 **Encounter for examination for driving license** UPD PE

     Z02.5 **Encounter for examination for participation in sport** UPD PE

     EXCLUDES 1   *blood-alcohol and blood-drug test (Z02.83)*

     Z02.6 **Encounter for examination for insurance purposes** UPD PE

✓5ᵗʰ **Z02.7** **Encounter for issue of medical certificate**

     EXCLUDES 1   *encounter for general medical examination (Z00-Z01, Z02.0-Z02.6, Z02.8-Z02.9)*

     Z02.71 **Encounter for disability determination** UPD PE

         Encounter for issue of medical certificate of incapacity

         Encounter for issue of medical certificate of invalidity

     Z02.79 **Encounter for issue of other medical certificate** UPD PE

✓5ᵗʰ **Z02.8** **Encounter for other administrative examinations**

     Z02.81 **Encounter for paternity testing** PE

     Z02.82 **Encounter for adoption services** UPD PE

     Z02.83 **Encounter for blood-alcohol and blood-drug test** PE

         Use additional code for findings of alcohol or drugs in blood (R78.-)

     Z02.84 **Encounter for child welfare exam** UPD P PE

         Encounter for child welfare screening exam

     EXCLUDES 2   *encounter for examination and observation for alleged child physical abuse (Z04.72)*

         encounter for examination and observation for alleged child rape (Z04.42)

         AHA: 2023,4Q,49

N Newborn: 0   P Pediatric: 0-17   M Maternity: 9-64   A Adult: 15-124   UNS Unspecified Site   MCC Major Complication/Comorbidity   CC Complication/Comorbidity   PE POA Exempt

1264   ICD-10-CM 2025

Z02.89 **Encounter for other administrative examinations**
Encounter for examination for admission to prison
Encounter for examination for admission to summer camp
Encounter for immigration examination
Encounter for naturalization examination
Encounter for premarital examination
EXCLUDES 1 *health supervision of foundling or other healthy infant or child (Z76.1-Z76.2)*

Z02.9 **Encounter for administrative examinations, unspecified** `UPD` `PE`

✓4ᵗʰ **Z03** **Encounter for medical observation for suspected diseases and conditions ruled out**
This category is to be used when a person without a diagnosis is suspected of having an abnormal condition, without signs or symptoms, which requires study, but after examination and observation, is ruled out. This category is also for use for administrative and legal observation status.
EXCLUDES 1 *contact with and (suspected) exposures hazardous to health (Z77.-)*
encounter for observation and evaluation of newborn for suspected diseases and conditions ruled out (Z05.-)
person with feared complaint in whom no diagnosis is made (Z71.1)
signs or symptoms under study - code to signs or symptoms
AHA: 2020,2Q,8; 2018,2Q,7-8; 2017,4Q,27

Z03.6 **Encounter for observation for suspected toxic effect from ingested substance ruled out** `PE`
Encounter for observation for suspected adverse effect from drug
Encounter for observation for suspected poisoning

✓5ᵗʰ **Z03.7** **Encounter for suspected maternal and fetal conditions ruled out**
Encounter for suspected maternal and fetal conditions not found
EXCLUDES 1 *known or suspected fetal anomalies affecting management of mother, not ruled out (O26.-, O35.-, O36.-, O40.-, O41.-)*

Z03.71 **Encounter for suspected problem with amniotic cavity and membrane ruled out** `UPD` `M` `PE`
Encounter for suspected oligohydramnios ruled out
Encounter for suspected polyhydramnios ruled out

Z03.72 **Encounter for suspected placental problem ruled out** `UPD` `M` `PE`

Z03.73 **Encounter for suspected fetal anomaly ruled out** `UPD` `M` `PE`

Z03.74 **Encounter for suspected problem with fetal growth ruled out** `UPD` `M` `PE`

Z03.75 **Encounter for suspected cervical shortening ruled out** `UPD` `M` `PE`

Z03.79 **Encounter for other suspected maternal and fetal conditions ruled out** `UPD` `M` `PE`

✓5ᵗʰ **Z03.8** **Encounter for observation for other suspected diseases and conditions ruled out**

✓6ᵗʰ **Z03.81** **Encounter for observation for suspected exposure to biological agents ruled out**

Z03.810 **Encounter for observation for suspected exposure to anthrax ruled out** `PE`

Z03.818 **Encounter for observation for suspected exposure to other biological agents ruled out** `PE`
AHA: 2020,2Q,8; 2020,1Q,34-36
TIP: Possible or actual exposure to COVID-19 should be coded using Z20.822 Contact with and (suspected) exposure to COVID-19, even when the COVID-19 infection has been ruled out.

✓6ᵗʰ **Z03.82** **Encounter for observation for suspected foreign body ruled out**
EXCLUDES 1 *retained foreign body (Z18.-)*
retained foreign body in eyelid (H02.81)
residual foreign body in soft tissue (M79.5)
EXCLUDES 2 *confirmed foreign body ingestion or aspiration including:*
foreign body in alimentary tract (T18)
foreign body in ear (T16)
foreign body on external eye (T15)
foreign body in respiratory tract (T17)
AHA: 2020,4Q,42

Z03.821 **Encounter for observation for suspected ingested foreign body ruled out** `UPD` `PE`

Z03.822 **Encounter for observation for suspected aspirated (inhaled) foreign body ruled out** `UPD` `PE`

Z03.823 **Encounter for observation for suspected inserted (injected) foreign body ruled out** `UPD` `PE`
Encounter for observation for suspected inserted (injected) foreign body in eye ruled out
Encounter for observation for suspected inserted (injected) foreign body in orifice ruled out
Encounter for observation for suspected inserted (injected) foreign body in skin ruled out

Z03.83 **Encounter for observation for suspected conditions related to home physiologic monitoring device ruled out** `UPD` `PE`
Encounter for observation for apnea alarm without findings
Encounter for observation for bradycardia alarm without findings
Encounter for observation for malfunction of home cardiorespiratory monitor
Encounter for observation for non-specific findings home physiologic monitoring device
Encounter for observation for pulse oximeter alarm without findings
EXCLUDES 1 *apnea NOS (R06.81)*
neonatal bradycardia (P29.12)
newborn apnea (P28.4-)
primary sleep apnea of newborn (P28.3-)
sleep apnea (G47.3-)
AHA: 2022,4Q,51

Z03.89 **Encounter for observation for other suspected diseases and conditions ruled out** `PE`

✓4ᵗʰ **Z04** **Encounter for examination and observation for other reasons**
INCLUDES encounter for examination for medicolegal reasons
This category is to be used when a person without a diagnosis is suspected of having an abnormal condition, without signs or symptoms, which requires study, but after examination and observation, is ruled-out. This category is also for use for administrative and legal observation status.
AHA: 2018,2Q,7-8

Z04.1 **Encounter for examination and observation following transport accident**
EXCLUDES 1 *encounter for examination and observation following work accident (Z04.2)*
AHA: 2019,2Q,11; 2018,2Q,8

Z04.2 **Encounter for examination and observation following work accident**

Z04.3 **Encounter for examination and observation following other accident**

✓5ᵗʰ **Z04.4** **Encounter for examination and observation following alleged rape**
Encounter for examination and observation of victim following alleged rape
Encounter for examination and observation of victim following alleged sexual abuse

Z04.41 **Encounter for examination and observation following alleged adult rape** `A`
Suspected adult rape, ruled out
Suspected adult sexual abuse, ruled out

Z04.42 **Encounter for examination and observation following alleged child rape** `P`
Suspected child rape, ruled out
Suspected child sexual abuse, ruled out

Z04.6 **Encounter for general psychiatric examination, requested by authority**

 Additional Character Required   ✓x7ᵗʰ Placeholder   Questionable PDx   Manifestation   Unspecified   `UPD` Unacceptable PDx   H1-H14 HAC   HCC CMS-HCC Dx   HIV HIV Dx

ICD-10-CM 2025   **1265**

✓5ᵗʰ **Z04.7** **Encounter for examination and observation following alleged physical abuse**

Z04.71 **Encounter for examination and observation following alleged adult physical abuse**   A

Suspected adult physical abuse, ruled out

EXCLUDES 1   *confirmed case of adult physical abuse (T74.-)*

encounter for examination and observation following alleged adult sexual abuse (Z04.41)

suspected case of adult physical abuse, not ruled out (T76.-)

Z04.72 **Encounter for examination and observation following alleged child physical abuse**   P

Suspected child physical abuse, ruled out

EXCLUDES 1   *confirmed case of child physical abuse (T74.-)*

encounter for examination and observation following alleged child sexual abuse (Z04.42)

suspected case of child physical abuse, not ruled out (T76.-)

✓5ᵗʰ **Z04.8** **Encounter for examination and observation for other specified reasons**

Encounter for examination and observation for request for expert evidence

AHA: 2018,4Q,32,35,72

Z04.81 **Encounter for examination and observation of victim following forced sexual exploitation**   PE

Z04.82 **Encounter for examination and observation of victim following forced labor exploitation**   PE

Z04.89 **Encounter for examination and observation for other specified reasons**   PE

Z04.9 **Encounter for examination and observation for unspecified reason**   UPD

Encounter for observation NOS

✓4ᵗʰ **Z05** **Encounter for observation and evaluation of newborn for suspected diseases and conditions ruled out**

This category is to be used for newborns, within the neonatal period (the first 28 days of life), who are suspected of having an abnormal condition, but without signs or symptoms, and which, after examination and observation, is ruled out.

AHA: 2022,1Q,17-18; 2017,4Q,27; 2016,4Q,77

Z05.0 **Observation and evaluation of newborn for suspected cardiac condition ruled out**   N PE

Z05.1 **Observation and evaluation of newborn for suspected infectious condition ruled out**   N PE

AHA: 2019,2Q,10

Z05.2 **Observation and evaluation of newborn for suspected neurological condition ruled out**   N PE

Z05.3 **Observation and evaluation of newborn for suspected respiratory condition ruled out**   N PE

✓5ᵗʰ **Z05.4** **Observation and evaluation of newborn for suspected genetic, metabolic or immunologic condition ruled out**

Z05.41 **Observation and evaluation of newborn for suspected genetic condition ruled out**   N PE

AHA: 2016,4Q,55

Z05.42 **Observation and evaluation of newborn for suspected metabolic condition ruled out**   N PE

Z05.43 **Observation and evaluation of newborn for suspected immunologic condition ruled out**   N PE

Z05.5 **Observation and evaluation of newborn for suspected gastrointestinal condition ruled out**   N PE

Z05.6 **Observation and evaluation of newborn for suspected genitourinary condition ruled out**   N PE

✓5ᵗʰ **Z05.7** **Observation and evaluation of newborn for suspected skin, subcutaneous, musculoskeletal and connective tissue condition ruled out**

Z05.71 **Observation and evaluation of newborn for suspected skin and subcutaneous tissue condition ruled out**   N PE

Z05.72 **Observation and evaluation of newborn for suspected musculoskeletal condition ruled out**   N PE

Z05.73 **Observation and evaluation of newborn for suspected connective tissue condition ruled out**   N PE

✓5ᵗʰ **Z05.8** **Observation and evaluation of newborn for other specified suspected condition ruled out**

AHA: 2023,4Q,48; 2022,1Q,17-18

Z05.81 **Observation and evaluation of newborn for suspected condition related to home physiologic monitoring device ruled out**   N PE

Encounter for observation of newborn for apnea alarm without findings

Encounter for observation of newborn for bradycardia alarm without findings

Encounter for observation of newborn for malfunction of home cardiorespiratory monitor

Encounter for observation of newborn for non-specific findings home physiologic monitoring device

Encounter for observation of newborn for pulse oximeter alarm without findings

EXCLUDES 1   *encounter for observation for suspected conditions related to home physiologic monitoring device ruled out (Z03.83)*

neonatal bradycardia (P29.12)

other newborn apnea (P28.4-)

primary sleep apnea of newborn (P28.3-)

Z05.89 **Observation and evaluation of newborn for other specified suspected condition ruled out**   N PE

Z05.9 **Observation and evaluation of newborn for unspecified suspected condition ruled out**   N PE

Z08 **Encounter for follow-up examination after completed treatment for malignant neoplasm**   UPD PE

Medical surveillance following completed treatment

Use additional code to identify any acquired absence of organs (Z90.-)

Use additional code to identify the personal history of malignant neoplasm (Z85.-)

EXCLUDES 1   *aftercare following medical care (Z43-Z49, Z51)*

AHA: 2020,3Q,30

Z09 **Encounter for follow-up examination after completed treatment for conditions other than malignant neoplasm**   UPD PE

Medical surveillance following completed treatment

Use additional code to identify any applicable history of disease code (Z86.-, Z87.-)

EXCLUDES 1   *aftercare following medical care (Z43-Z49, Z51)*

surveillance of contraception (Z30.4-)

surveillance of prosthetic and other medical devices (Z44-Z46)

AHA: 2022,3Q,4; 2021,1Q,33; 2020,2Q,10; 2017,1Q,9; 2015,1Q,8

✓4ᵗʰ **Z11** **Encounter for screening for infectious and parasitic diseases**

Screening is the testing for disease or disease precursors in asymptomatic individuals so that early detection and treatment can be provided for those who test positive for the disease.

EXCLUDES 1   *encounter for diagnostic examination - code to sign or symptom*

Z11.0 **Encounter for screening for intestinal infectious diseases**   UPD PE

Z11.1 **Encounter for screening for respiratory tuberculosis**   UPD PE

Encounter for screening for active tuberculosis disease

Z11.2 **Encounter for screening for other bacterial diseases**   UPD PE

Z11.3 **Encounter for screening for infections with a predominantly sexual mode of transmission**   UPD PE

EXCLUDES 2   *encounter for screening for human immunodeficiency virus [HIV] (Z11.4)*

encounter for screening for human papillomavirus (Z11.51)

Z11.4 **Encounter for screening for human immunodeficiency virus [HIV]**   UPD PE

✓5ᵗʰ **Z11.5** **Encounter for screening for other viral diseases**

EXCLUDES 2   *encounter for screening for viral intestinal disease (Z11.0)*

Z11.51 **Encounter for screening for human papillomavirus (HPV)**   UPD PE

Z11.52 **Encounter for screening for COVID-19**   UPD PE

AHA: 2023,2Q,3; 2021,1Q,27,37,41

Z11.59 **Encounter for screening for other viral diseases**   UPD PE

AHA: 2020,3Q,14

Z11.6 **Encounter for screening for other protozoal diseases and helminthiases**   UPD PE

EXCLUDES 2   *encounter for screening for protozoal intestinal disease (Z11.0)*

N Newborn: 0   P Pediatric: 0-17   M Maternity: 9-64   A Adult: 15-124   UNS Unspecified Site   MCC Major Complication/Comorbidity   CC Complication/Comorbidity   PE POA Exempt

1266   ICD-10-CM 2025

Z04.7–Z11.6

Z11.7 Encounter for testing for latent tuberculosis infection   `UPD` `PE`
> AHA: 2019,4Q,20

Z11.8 Encounter for screening for other infectious and parasitic diseases   `UPD` `PE`
> Encounter for screening for chlamydia
> Encounter for screening for rickettsial
> Encounter for screening for spirochetal
> Encounter for screening for mycoses

Z11.9 Encounter for screening for infectious and parasitic diseases, unspecified   `UPD` `PE`

√4ᵗʰ **Z12 Encounter for screening for malignant neoplasms**
> Screening is the testing for disease or disease precursors in asymptomatic individuals so that early detection and treatment can be provided for those who test positive for the disease.
>
> Use additional code to identify any family history of malignant neoplasm (Z80.-)
>
> EXCLUDES 1   encounter for diagnostic examination - code to sign or symptom

Z12.0 Encounter for screening for malignant neoplasm of stomach   `UPD` `PE`

√5ᵗʰ **Z12.1** Encounter for screening for malignant neoplasm of intestinal tract
> AHA: 2017,1Q,8,9

  Z12.10 Encounter for screening for malignant neoplasm of intestinal tract, unspecified   `UPD` `PE`

  Z12.11 Encounter for screening for malignant neoplasm of colon   `UPD` `PE`
> Encounter for screening colonoscopy NOS
> AHA: 2019,1Q,32-33; 2018,1Q,6

  Z12.12 Encounter for screening for malignant neoplasm of rectum   `UPD` `PE`
> AHA: 2018,1Q,6

  Z12.13 Encounter for screening for malignant neoplasm of small intestine   `UPD` `PE`

Z12.2 Encounter for screening for malignant neoplasm of respiratory organs   `UPD` `PE`

√5ᵗʰ **Z12.3** Encounter for screening for malignant neoplasm of breast

  Z12.31 Encounter for screening mammogram for malignant neoplasm of breast   `UPD` `PE`
> EXCLUDES 1   inconclusive mammogram (R92.2)
> AHA: 2023,4Q,44; 2015,1Q,24

  Z12.39 Encounter for other screening for malignant neoplasm of breast   `UPD` `PE`

Z12.4 Encounter for screening for malignant neoplasm of cervix   `UPD` `PE`
> Encounter for screening pap smear for malignant neoplasm of cervix
> EXCLUDES 1   when screening is part of general gynecological examination (Z01.4-)
> EXCLUDES 2   encounter for screening for human papillomavirus (Z11.51)

Z12.5 Encounter for screening for malignant neoplasm of prostate   `PE`

Z12.6 Encounter for screening for malignant neoplasm of bladder   `UPD` `PE`

√5ᵗʰ **Z12.7** Encounter for screening for malignant neoplasm of other genitourinary organs

  Z12.71 Encounter for screening for malignant neoplasm of testis   `UPD` `PE`

  Z12.72 Encounter for screening for malignant neoplasm of vagina   `UPD` `PE`
> Vaginal pap smear status-post hysterectomy for non-malignant condition
> Use additional code to identify acquired absence of uterus (Z90.71-)
> EXCLUDES 1   vaginal pap smear status-post hysterectomy for malignant conditions (Z08)

  Z12.73 Encounter for screening for malignant neoplasm of ovary   `UPD` `PE`

  Z12.79 Encounter for screening for malignant neoplasm of other genitourinary organs   `UPD` `PE`

√5ᵗʰ **Z12.8** Encounter for screening for malignant neoplasm of other sites

  Z12.81 Encounter for screening for malignant neoplasm of oral cavity   `UPD` `PE`

  Z12.82 Encounter for screening for malignant neoplasm of nervous system   `UPD` `PE`

  Z12.83 Encounter for screening for malignant neoplasm of skin   `UPD` `PE`

  Z12.89 Encounter for screening for malignant neoplasm of other sites   `UPD` `PE`
> AHA: 2021,1Q,14

Z12.9 Encounter for screening for malignant neoplasm, site unspecified   `UPD` `PE`

√4ᵗʰ **Z13 Encounter for screening for other diseases and disorders**
> Screening is the testing for disease or disease precursors in asymptomatic individuals so that early detection and treatment can be provided for those who test positive for the disease.
> EXCLUDES 1   encounter for diagnostic examination - code to sign or symptom

Z13.0 Encounter for screening for diseases of the blood and blood-forming organs and certain disorders involving the immune mechanism   `UPD` `PE`

Z13.1 Encounter for screening for diabetes mellitus   `UPD` `PE`

√5ᵗʰ **Z13.2** Encounter for screening for nutritional, metabolic and other endocrine disorders

  Z13.21 Encounter for screening for nutritional disorder   `UPD` `PE`

  √6ᵗʰ **Z13.22** Encounter for screening for metabolic disorder

    Z13.220 Encounter for screening for lipoid disorders   `UPD` `PE`
> Encounter for screening for cholesterol level
> Encounter for screening for hypercholesterolemia
> Encounter for screening for hyperlipidemia

    Z13.228 Encounter for screening for other metabolic disorders   `UPD` `PE`

  Z13.29 Encounter for screening for other suspected endocrine disorder   `UPD` `PE`
> EXCLUDES 2   encounter for screening for diabetes mellitus (Z13.1)

√5ᵗʰ **Z13.3** Encounter for screening examination for mental health and behavioral disorders
> AHA: 2018,4Q,35-36

  Z13.30 Encounter for screening examination for mental health and behavioral disorders, unspecified   `UPD` `PE`

  Z13.31 Encounter for screening for depression   `UPD` `PE`
> Encounter for screening for depression, adult
> Encounter for screening for depression for child or adolescent

  Z13.32 Encounter for screening for maternal depression   `UPD` `M` `PE`
> Encounter for screening for perinatal depression

  Z13.39 Encounter for screening examination for other mental health and behavioral disorders   `UPD` `PE`
> Encounter for screening for alcoholism
> Encounter for screening for intellectual disabilities

√5ᵗʰ **Z13.4** Encounter for screening for certain developmental disorders in childhood
> Encounter for development testing of infant or child
> Encounter for screening for developmental handicaps in early childhood
> EXCLUDES 2   encounter for routine child health examination (Z00.12-)
> AHA: 2018,4Q,36

  Z13.40 Encounter for screening for unspecified developmental delays   `UPD` `PE`

  Z13.41 Encounter for autism screening   `UPD` `PE`

  Z13.42 Encounter for screening for global developmental delays (milestones)   `UPD` `PE`
> Encounter for screening for developmental handicaps in early childhood

  Z13.49 Encounter for screening for other developmental delays   `UPD` `PE`

Z13.5 Encounter for screening for eye and ear disorders   `UPD` `PE`
> EXCLUDES 2   encounter for general hearing examination (Z01.1-)
>   encounter for general vision examination (Z01.0-)
> AHA: 2016,3Q,17

Z13.6 Encounter for screening for cardiovascular disorders   `UPD` `PE`

√5ᵗʰ **Z13.7** Encounter for screening for genetic and chromosomal anomalies
> EXCLUDES 1   genetic testing for procreative management (Z31.4-)

  Z13.71 Encounter for nonprocreative screening for genetic disease carrier status   `UPD` `PE`

  Z13.79 Encounter for other screening for genetic and chromosomal anomalies   `UPD` `PE`

| ✔ Additional Character Required | √×7ᵗʰ Placeholder | Questionable PDx | Manifestation | Unspecified | UPD Unacceptable PDx | H1 - H14 HAC | HCC CMS-HCC Dx | HIV HIV Dx |

ICD-10-CM 2025   **1267**

✓5ᵗʰ **Z13.8 Encounter for screening for other specified diseases and disorders**

> EXCLUDES 2   *screening for malignant neoplasms (Z12.-)*

✓6ᵗʰ **Z13.81 Encounter for screening for digestive system disorders**

Z13.810 Encounter for screening for upper gastrointestinal disorder UPD PE

Z13.811 Encounter for screening for lower gastrointestinal disorder UPD PE

> EXCLUDES 1   *encounter for screening for intestinal infectious disease (Z11.0)*

Z13.818 Encounter for screening for other digestive system disorders UPD PE

✓6ᵗʰ **Z13.82 Encounter for screening for musculoskeletal disorder**

Z13.820 Encounter for screening for osteoporosis UPD PE

Z13.828 Encounter for screening for other musculoskeletal disorder UPD PE

Z13.83 Encounter for screening for respiratory disorder NEC UPD PE

> EXCLUDES 1   *encounter for screening for respiratory tuberculosis (Z11.1)*

Z13.84 Encounter for screening for dental disorders UPD PE

✓6ᵗʰ **Z13.85 Encounter for screening for nervous system disorders**

Z13.850 Encounter for screening for traumatic brain injury UPD PE

Z13.858 Encounter for screening for other nervous system disorders

Z13.88 Encounter for screening for disorder due to exposure to contaminants UPD PE

> EXCLUDES 1   *those exposed to contaminants without suspected disorders (Z57.-, Z77.-)*

Z13.89 Encounter for screening for other disorder UPD PE
Encounter for screening for genitourinary disorders

Z13.9 Encounter for screening, unspecified UPD PE

Genetic carrier and genetic susceptibility to disease (Z14-Z15)

✓4ᵗʰ **Z14 Genetic carrier**

> **DEF:** Individuals carrying a gene mutation associated with a certain disease that typically do not develop the disease but are able to pass the mutated genes to offspring.

✓5ᵗʰ **Z14.0 Hemophilia A carrier**

Z14.01 Asymptomatic hemophilia A carrier UPD PE

Z14.02 Symptomatic hemophilia A carrier UPD PE

Z14.1 Cystic fibrosis carrier UPD PE

Z14.8 Genetic carrier of other disease UPD PE

✓4ᵗʰ **Z15 Genetic susceptibility to disease**

> INCLUDES   confirmed abnormal gene
>
> Use additional code, if applicable, for any associated family history of the disease (Z80-Z84)
>
> EXCLUDES 1   *chromosomal anomalies (Q90-Q99)*

✓5ᵗʰ **Z15.0 Genetic susceptibility to malignant neoplasm**

> Code first, if applicable, any current malignant neoplasm (C00-C75, C81-C96)
>
> Use additional code, if applicable, for any personal history of malignant neoplasm (Z85.-)

Z15.01 Genetic susceptibility to malignant neoplasm of breast UPD PE

Z15.02 Genetic susceptibility to malignant neoplasm of ovary UPD PE

Z15.03 Genetic susceptibility to malignant neoplasm of prostate UPD PE

Z15.04 Genetic susceptibility to malignant neoplasm of endometrium UPD PE

Z15.09 Genetic susceptibility to other malignant neoplasm UPD PE
AHA: 2021,1Q,14

Z15.1 Genetic susceptibility to epilepsy and neurodevelopmental disorders UPD PE

> Code also, if applicable, related disorders such as:
> developmental and epileptic encephalopathy (G93.45)
> developmental disorder of speech and language (F80.-)
> developmental disorders of scholastic skills (F81.-)
> epilepsy, by specific type (G40.-)
> intellectual disabilities (F70-F79)
> other neurodevelopmental disorder (F88)
> pervasive developmental disorders (F84.-)

Z15.2 Genetic susceptibility to obesity UPD PE

> Code also, if applicable, any associated manifestations, such as:
> other obesity (E66.8-)
> polyphagia (R63.2)
> Use additional code to identify body mass index (BMI), if known (Z68.-)

✓5ᵗʰ **Z15.8 Genetic susceptibility to other disease**

Z15.81 Genetic susceptibility to multiple endocrine neoplasia [MEN] UPD PE

> EXCLUDES 1   *multiple endocrine neoplasia [MEN] syndromes (E31.2-)*

> **DEF:** Group of conditions in which several endocrine glands grow excessively (such as in adenomatous hyperplasia) and/or develop benign or malignant tumors. Tumors and hyperplasia associated with MEN often produce excess hormones, which impede normal physiology. There is no comprehensive cure known for MEN syndrome. Treatment is directed at the hyperplasia or tumors in each individual gland. Tumors are usually surgically removed and oral medications or hormonal injections are used to correct hormone imbalances.

Z15.89 Genetic susceptibility to other disease UPD PE

Resistance to antimicrobial drugs (Z16)

✓4ᵗʰ **Z16 Resistance to antimicrobial drugs**

> NOTE   The codes in this category are provided for use as additional codes to identify the resistance and non-responsiveness of a condition to antimicrobial drugs.
>
> Code first the infection
>
> EXCLUDES 1   *Methicillin resistant Staphylococcus aureus infection (A49.02)*
> *Methicillin resistant Staphylococcus aureus pneumonia (J15.212)*
> *sepsis due to Methicillin resistant Staphylococcus aureus (A41.02)*

✓5ᵗʰ **Z16.1 Resistance to beta lactam antibiotics**

Z16.10 Resistance to unspecified beta lactam antibiotics CC UPD

Z16.11 Resistance to penicillins CC UPD
Resistance to amoxicillin
Resistance to ampicillin

Z16.12 Extended spectrum beta lactamase (ESBL) resistance CC UPD

> EXCLUDES 2   *Methicillin resistant Staphylococcus aureus infection in diseases classified elsewhere (B95.62)*

Z16.13 Resistance to carbapenem CC UPD
AHA: 2023,4Q,47

Z16.19 Resistance to other specified beta lactam antibiotics CC UPD
Resistance to cephalosporins

✓5ᵗʰ **Z16.2 Resistance to other antibiotics**

Z16.20 Resistance to unspecified antibiotic CC UPD
Resistance to antibiotics NOS

Z16.21 Resistance to vancomycin CC UPD

Z16.22 Resistance to vancomycin related antibiotics CC UPD

Z16.23 Resistance to quinolones and fluoroquinolones CC UPD

Z16.24 Resistance to multiple antibiotics CC UPD

Z16.29 Resistance to other single specified antibiotic CC UPD
Resistance to aminoglycosides
Resistance to macrolides
Resistance to sulfonamides
Resistance to tetracyclines

N Newborn: 0   P Pediatric: 0-17   M Maternity: 9-64   A Adult: 15-124   UNS Unspecified Site   MCC Major Complication/Comorbidity   CC Complication/Comorbidity   PE POA Exempt

1268   ICD-10-CM 2025

√5th **Z16.3 Resistance to other antimicrobial drugs**

    EXCLUDES 1   *resistance to antibiotics (Z16.1-, Z16.2-)*

Z16.30 Resistance to unspecified antimicrobial drugs CC UPD

    Drug resistance NOS

Z16.31 Resistance to antiparasitic drug(s) CC UPD

    Resistance to quinine and related compounds

Z16.32 Resistance to antifungal drug(s) CC UPD

Z16.33 Resistance to antiviral drug(s) CC UPD

√6th **Z16.34 Resistance to antimycobacterial drug(s)**

    Resistance to tuberculostatics

Z16.341 Resistance to single antimycobacterial drug CC UPD

    Resistance to antimycobacterial drug NOS

Z16.342 Resistance to multiple antimycobacterial drugs CC UPD

Z16.35 Resistance to multiple antimicrobial drugs CC UPD

    EXCLUDES 1   *resistance to multiple antibiotics only (Z16.24)*

Z16.39 Resistance to other specified antimicrobial drug CC UPD

▶ Estrogen, and other hormones and factors receptor status ◀ (Z17)

▲ √4th **Z17 Estrogen, and other hormones and factors receptor status**

    NOTE ▶Use one code, as available, for each receptor: Z17.0, Z17.1, Z17.2-, Z17.3-◀

    ▶ Code first malignant neoplasm, such as:◀

    malignant neoplasm of breast (C50.-)

    ▶malignant neoplasm of ovary (C56.-)◀

    AHA: 2022,3Q,14

    DEF: Receptor status of breast cancer cells for the hormone estrogen that is used to help determine treatment and evaluate prognosis. ER+ breast cancer responds to hormone therapies while ER- breast cancer does not.

Z17.0 Estrogen receptor positive status [ER+] UPD PE

Z17.1 Estrogen receptor negative status [ER-] UPD PE

● √5th **Z17.2 Progesterone receptor status**

●   **Z17.21 Progesterone receptor positive status** UPD PE

        PR+

●   **Z17.22 Progesterone receptor negative status** UPD PE

        PR-

● √5th **Z17.3 Human epidermal growth factor 2 receptor**

●   **Z17.31 Human epidermal growth factor receptor 2 positive status** UPD PE

        HER2+

●   **Z17.32 Human epidermal growth factor receptor 2 negative status** UPD PE

        HER2-

● √5th **Z17.4 Combined receptor status**

    NOTE   Assign a code from subcategory Z17.4- when only a combined receptor status is documented

● √6th **Z17.41 Hormone receptor positive**

        HR+

●   **Z17.410 Hormone receptor positive with human epidermal growth factor receptor 2 positive status** UPD PE

        HR+ with HER2+

●   **Z17.411 Hormone receptor positive with human epidermal growth factor receptor 2 negative status** UPD PE

        HR+ with HER2-

● √6th **Z17.42 Hormone receptor negative**

        HR-

●   **Z17.420 Hormone receptor negative with human epidermal growth factor receptor 2 positive status** UPD PE

        HR- with HER2+

●   **Z17.421 Hormone receptor negative with human epidermal growth factor receptor 2 negative status** UPD PE

        HR- with HER2-

        TNBC

        Triple negative breast cancer

Retained foreign body fragments (Z18)

√4th **Z18 Retained foreign body fragments**

    INCLUDES   embedded fragment (status)

        embedded splinter (status)

        retained foreign body status

    EXCLUDES 1   *artificial joint prosthesis status (Z96.6-)*

        foreign body accidentally left during a procedure (T81.5-)

        foreign body entering through orifice (T15-T19)

        in situ cardiac device (Z95.-)

        organ or tissue replaced by means other than transplant (Z96.-, Z97.-)

        organ or tissue replaced by transplant (Z94.-)

        personal history of retained foreign body fully removed Z87.821

        superficial foreign body (non-embedded splinter) - code to superficial foreign body, by site

    AHA: 2023,2Q,27

    DEF: Embedded or retained fragment, splinter, or foreign body, natural or synthetic that can cause infection.

√5th **Z18.0 Retained radioactive fragments**

    Z18.01 Retained depleted uranium fragments UPD PE

    Z18.09 Other retained radioactive fragments UPD PE

        Other retained depleted isotope fragments

        Retained nontherapeutic radioactive fragments

√5th **Z18.1 Retained metal fragments**

    EXCLUDES 1   *retained radioactive metal fragments (Z18.01-Z18.09)*

    Z18.10 Retained metal fragments, unspecified UPD PE

        Retained metal fragment NOS

    Z18.11 Retained magnetic metal fragments UPD PE

    Z18.12 Retained nonmagnetic metal fragments UPD PE

Z18.2 Retained plastic fragments UPD PE

    Acrylics fragments

    Diethylhexyl phthalates fragments

    Isocyanate fragments

√5th **Z18.3 Retained organic fragments**

    Z18.31 Retained animal quills or spines UPD PE

    Z18.32 Retained tooth UPD PE

    Z18.33 Retained wood fragments UPD PE

    Z18.39 Other retained organic fragments UPD PE

√5th **Z18.8 Other specified retained foreign body**

    Z18.81 Retained glass fragments UPD PE

    Z18.83 Retained stone or crystalline fragments UPD PE

        Retained concrete or cement fragments

    Z18.89 Other specified retained foreign body fragments UPD PE

Z18.9 Retained foreign body fragments, unspecified material UPD PE

Hormone sensitivity malignancy status (Z19)

√4th **Z19 Hormone sensitivity malignancy status**

    Code first malignant neoplasm — see Table of Neoplasms, by site, malignant

    AHA: 2016,4Q,76

Z19.1 Hormone sensitive malignancy status UPD PE

Z19.2 Hormone resistant malignancy status UPD PE

    Castrate resistant prostate malignancy status

Persons with potential health hazards related to communicable diseases (Z20-Z29)

√4th **Z20 Contact with and (suspected) exposure to communicable diseases**

    EXCLUDES 1   *carrier of infectious disease (Z22.-)*

        diagnosed current infectious or parasitic disease - see Alphabetic Index

    EXCLUDES 2   *personal history of infectious and parasitic diseases (Z86.1-)*

√5th **Z20.0 Contact with and (suspected) exposure to intestinal infectious diseases**

    Z20.01 Contact with and (suspected) exposure to intestinal infectious diseases due to Escherichia coli (E. coli)

    Z20.09 Contact with and (suspected) exposure to other intestinal infectious diseases UPD

Z20.1 Contact with and (suspected) exposure to tuberculosis UPD

Z20.2 Contact with and (suspected) exposure to infections with a predominantly sexual mode of transmission UPD

✓ Additional Character Required   √x7th Placeholder   Questionable PDx   ◆ Manifestation   Unspecified   UPD Unacceptable PDx   H1–H14 HAC   HCC CMS-HCC Dx   HIV HIV Dx

ICD-10-CM 2025   1269

Z20.3 Contact with and (suspected) exposure to rabies `UPD`

Z20.4 Contact with and (suspected) exposure to rubella `UPD`

Z20.5 Contact with and (suspected) exposure to viral hepatitis

Z20.6 Contact with and (suspected) exposure to human immunodeficiency virus [HIV]

EXCLUDES 1 asymptomatic human immunodeficiency virus [HIV] HIV infection status (Z21)

Z20.7 Contact with and (suspected) exposure to pediculosis, acariasis and other infestations `UPD`

✓5ᵗʰ **Z20.8** Contact with and (suspected) exposure to other communicable diseases

✓6ᵗʰ **Z20.81** Contact with and (suspected) exposure to other bacterial communicable diseases

Z20.810 Contact with and (suspected) exposure to anthrax `UPD`

Z20.811 Contact with and (suspected) exposure to meningococcus

Z20.818 Contact with and (suspected) exposure to other bacterial communicable diseases `UPD`

AHA: 2019,2Q,10

✓6ᵗʰ **Z20.82** Contact with and (suspected) exposure to other viral communicable diseases

Z20.820 Contact with and (suspected) exposure to varicella

Z20.821 Contact with and (suspected) exposure to Zika virus `UPD` `PE`

AHA: 2018,4Q,35,64

Z20.822 Contact with and (suspected) exposure to COVID-19 `UPD`

Contact with and (suspected) exposure to SARS-CoV-2

AHA: 2023,2Q,3; 2022,2Q,28-29; 2021,4Q,109; 2021,1Q,27-29,37-38;41

Z20.828 Contact with and (suspected) exposure to other viral communicable diseases

AHA: 2022,3Q,4; 2021,1Q,37-38; 2020,4Q,99; 2020,3Q,14-15; 2020,2Q,4,8; 2020,1Q,34-36

Z20.89 Contact with and (suspected) exposure to other communicable diseases `UPD`

Z20.9 Contact with and (suspected) exposure to unspecified communicable disease `UPD`

Z21 Asymptomatic human immunodeficiency virus [HIV] infection status `HCC`

HIV positive NOS

Code first human immunodeficiency virus [HIV] disease complicating pregnancy, childbirth and the puerperium, if applicable (O98.7-)

EXCLUDES 1 acquired immunodeficiency syndrome (B20)
contact with human immunodeficiency virus [HIV] (Z20.6)
exposure to human immunodeficiency virus [HIV] (Z20.6)
human immunodeficiency virus [HIV] disease (B20)
inconclusive laboratory evidence of human immunodeficiency virus [HIV] (R75)

AHA: 2022,1Q,36; 2019,1Q,8-11

DEF: Phase of human immunodeficiency virus (HIV) infection with no clinical symptoms. This phase may last for 10 years or more.

✓4ᵗʰ **Z22** Carrier of infectious disease

INCLUDES colonization status
suspected carrier

EXCLUDES 2 carrier of viral hepatitis (B18.-)

Z22.0 Carrier of typhoid `UPD` `PE`

Z22.1 Carrier of other intestinal infectious diseases `UPD` `PE`

Z22.2 Carrier of diphtheria `UPD` `PE`

✓5ᵗʰ **Z22.3** Carrier of other specified bacterial diseases

Z22.31 Carrier of bacterial disease due to meningococci `UPD` `PE`

✓6ᵗʰ **Z22.32** Carrier of bacterial disease due to staphylococci

Z22.321 Carrier or suspected carrier of Methicillin susceptible Staphylococcus aureus `UPD` `PE`

MSSA colonization

Z22.322 Carrier or suspected carrier of Methicillin resistant Staphylococcus aureus `UPD` `PE`

MRSA colonization

DEF: Carriers (colonization) of methicillin resistant *Staphylococcus aureus* (MRSA) have MRSA on their skin or in their body but do not exhibit signs of infection. These individuals are able to pass MRSA on to others who may develop an infection.

✓6ᵗʰ **Z22.33** Carrier of bacterial disease due to streptococci

Z22.330 Carrier of Group B streptococcus `UPD` `PE`

EXCLUDES 1 carrier of streptococcus group B (GBS) complicating pregnancy, childbirth and the puerperium (O99.82-)

Z22.338 Carrier of other streptococcus `UPD` `PE`

✓6ᵗʰ **Z22.34** Carrier of Acinetobacter baumannii

AHA: 2023,4Q,47

Z22.340 Carrier of carbapenem-resistant Acinetobacter baumannii `UPD` `PE`

Z22.341 Carrier of carbapenem-sensitive Acinetobacter baumannii `UPD` `PE`

Z22.349 Carrier of Acinetobacter baumannii, unspecified `UPD` `PE`

✓6ᵗʰ **Z22.35** Carrier of Enterobacterales

Carrier of E. coli
Carrier of K. pneumoniae

AHA: 2023,4Q,47

Z22.350 Carrier of carbapenem-resistant Enterobacterales `UPD` `PE`

Z22.358 Carrier of other Enterobacterales `UPD` `PE`

Carrier of carbapenem-sensitive Enterobacterales
Carrier of ESBL-producing Enterobacterales
Carrier of extended-spectrum beta-lactamase producing Enterobacterales

Z22.359 Carrier of Enterobacterales, unspecified

Z22.39 Carrier of other specified bacterial diseases `UPD` `PE`

Z22.4 Carrier of infections with a predominantly sexual mode of transmission `UPD` `PE`

Z22.6 Carrier of human T-lymphotropic virus type-1 [HTLV-1] infection `UPD` `PE`

Z22.7 Latent tuberculosis `UPD` `PE`

Latent tuberculosis infection (LTBI)

EXCLUDES 1 nonspecific reaction to cell mediated immunity measurement of gamma interferon antigen response without active tuberculosis (R76.12)
nonspecific reaction to tuberculin skin test without active tuberculosis (R76.11)

AHA: 2019,4Q,19

Z22.8 Carrier of other infectious diseases `UPD` `PE`

Z22.9 Carrier of infectious disease, unspecified `UPD` `PE`

Z23 Encounter for immunization `UPD` `PE`

`NOTE` Procedure codes are required to identify the types of immunizations given

Code first any routine childhood examination

Code also, if applicable, encounter for immunization safety counseling (Z71.85)

✓4ᵗʰ **Z28** Immunization not carried out and underimmunization status

INCLUDES vaccination not carried out

Code also, if applicable, encounter for immunization safety counseling (Z71.85)

✓5ᵗʰ **Z28.0** Immunization not carried out because of contraindication

DEF: Contraindication: Situation where a drug, surgery, or other procedure may negatively affect or cause harm to a patient.

Z28.01 Immunization not carried out because of acute illness of patient `UPD` `PE`

Z28.02 Immunization not carried out because of chronic illness or condition of patient `UPD` `PE`

Z28.03 Immunization not carried out because of immune compromised state of patient `UPD` `PE`

Z28.04 Immunization not carried out because of patient **allergy to vaccine or component** UPD PE

Z28.09 Immunization not carried out because of other contraindication UPD PE

Z28.1 Immunization not carried out because of patient decision for **reasons of belief or group pressure** UPD PE
   Immunization not carried out because of religious belief

✓5th **Z28.2** Immunization not carried out because of patient decision for **other and unspecified** reason

   Z28.20 Immunization not carried out because of patient decision for unspecified reason UPD PE

   Z28.21 Immunization not carried out because of patient **refusal** UPD PE

   Z28.29 Immunization not carried out because of patient decision for other reason UPD PE

✓5th **Z28.3** **Underimmunization status**

   Use additional code, if applicable, to identify:
   immunization not carried out because of contraindication (Z28.0-)
   immunization not carried out because of patient decision for other and unspecified reason (Z28.2-)
   immunization not carried out because of patient decision for reasons of belief or group pressure (Z28.1)
   immunization not carried out for other reason (Z28.8-)
   AHA: 2022,1Q,4-5

   ✓6th **Z28.31** **Underimmunization for COVID-19 status**

      NOTE These codes should not be used for individuals who are not eligible for the COVID-19 vaccines, as determined by the healthcare provider.

      Z28.310 **Unvaccinated** for COVID-19 UPD PE
      Z28.311 **Partially vaccinated** for COVID-19 UPD PE

   Z28.39 Other underimmunization status UPD PE
      Delinquent immunization status
      Lapsed immunization schedule status

✓5th **Z28.8** **Immunization not carried out for other reason**

   Z28.81 Immunization not carried out due to **patient having had the disease** UPD PE

   Z28.82 Immunization not carried out because of **caregiver refusal** UPD PE
      Immunization not carried out because of guardian refusal
      Immunization not carried out because of parent refusal
      EXCLUDES 1 *immunization not carried out because of caregiver refusal because of religious belief (Z28.1)*

   Z28.83 Immunization not carried out due to **unavailability of vaccine** UPD PE
      Delay in delivery of vaccine
      Lack of availability of vaccine
      Manufacturer delay of vaccine
      AHA: 2018,4Q,36

   Z28.89 Immunization not carried out for other reason UPD PE

Z28.9 Immunization not carried out for unspecified reason UPD PE

✓4th **Z29** **Encounter for other prophylactic measures**

   EXCLUDES 1 *desensitization to allergens (Z51.6)*
      prophylactic surgery (Z40.-)
   AHA: 2016,4Q,78-79

   ✓5th **Z29.1** **Encounter for prophylactic immunotherapy**
      Encounter for administration of immunoglobulin

      Z29.11 **Encounter for prophylactic immunotherapy for respiratory syncytial virus (RSV)** UPD PE

      Z29.12 Encounter for prophylactic **antivenin** UPD PE

      Z29.13 Encounter for prophylactic **Rho(D) immune globulin** UPD PE
         AHA: 2019,3Q,5

      Z29.14 Encounter for prophylactic **rabies immune globin** UPD PE

   Z29.3 Encounter for prophylactic **fluoride administration** UPD PE

✓5th **Z29.8** **Encounter for other specified prophylactic measures**
   AHA: 2023,4Q,49; 2022,2Q,27

   Z29.81 **Encounter for HIV pre-exposure prophylaxis** UPD PE
      Code also, if applicable, risk factors for HIV, such as:
      contact with and (suspected) exposure to human immunodeficiency virus [HIV] (Z20.6)
      high risk sexual behavior (Z72.5-)

   Z29.89 Encounter for other specified prophylactic measures UPD PE

Z29.9 Encounter for prophylactic measures, unspecified UPD PE

Persons encountering health services in circumstances related to reproduction (Z30-Z39)

✓4th **Z30** **Encounter for contraceptive management**
   AHA: 2016,4Q,78
   DEF: Contraceptive management to prevent pregnancy. Methods include oral medications, intrauterine devices, and surgical procedures for males and females (sterilization).

   ✓5th **Z30.0** **Encounter for general counseling and advice on contraception**

      ✓6th **Z30.01** **Encounter for initial prescription of contraceptives**
         EXCLUDES 1 *encounter for surveillance of contraceptives (Z30.4-)*

         Z30.011 **Encounter for initial prescription of contraceptive pills** UPD PE

         Z30.012 **Encounter for prescription of emergency contraception** UPD PE
            Encounter for postcoital contraception

         Z30.013 **Encounter for initial prescription of injectable contraceptive** UPD PE

         Z30.014 **Encounter for initial prescription of intrauterine contraceptive device** UPD PE
            EXCLUDES 1 *encounter for insertion of intrauterine contraceptive device (Z30.430, Z30.432)*

         Z30.015 Encounter for initial prescription of **vaginal ring hormonal** contraceptive UPD PE

         Z30.016 Encounter for initial prescription of **transdermal patch hormonal** contraceptive device UPD PE

         Z30.017 Encounter for initial prescription of **implantable subdermal** contraceptive UPD PE

         Z30.018 **Encounter for initial prescription of other contraceptives** UPD PE
            Encounter for initial prescription of barrier contraception
            Encounter for initial prescription of diaphragm

         Z30.019 **Encounter for initial prescription of contraceptives, unspecified** UPD PE

      Z30.02 Counseling and instruction in **natural family planning to avoid pregnancy** UPD PE

      Z30.09 Encounter for other general counseling and advice on contraception UPD PE
         Encounter for family planning advice NOS

   Z30.2 Encounter for **sterilization** PE
      AHA: 2021,3Q,13

   ✓5th **Z30.4** **Encounter for surveillance of contraceptives**

      Z30.40 **Encounter for surveillance of contraceptives, unspecified** UPD PE

      Z30.41 Encounter for surveillance of contraceptive **pills** UPD PE
         Encounter for repeat prescription for contraceptive pill

      Z30.42 **Encounter for surveillance of injectable contraceptive** UPD PE

      ✓6th **Z30.43** **Encounter for surveillance of intrauterine contraceptive device**

         Z30.430 **Encounter for insertion of intrauterine contraceptive device** UPD PE

         Z30.431 **Encounter for routine checking of intrauterine contraceptive device** UPD PE

         Z30.432 **Encounter for removal of intrauterine contraceptive device** UPD PE

✓ Additional Character Required   ✓x7th Placeholder   Questionable PDx   Manifestation   Unspecified   UPD Unacceptable PDx   H1-H14 HAC   HCC CMS-HCC Dx   HIV HIV Dx

ICD-10-CM 2025   1271

Z30.433   **Encounter for** removal and reinsertion **of intrauterine contraceptive device** `UPD` `PE`
Encounter for replacement of intrauterine contraceptive device

Z30.44   **Encounter for surveillance of** vaginal ring hormonal **contraceptive device** `UPD` `PE`

Z30.45   **Encounter for surveillance of** transdermal patch hormonal **contraceptive device** `UPD` `PE`

Z30.46   **Encounter for surveillance of** implantable subdermal **contraceptive** `UPD` `PE`
Encounter for checking, reinsertion or removal of implantable subdermal contraceptive

Z30.49   **Encounter for surveillance of other contraceptives** `UPD` `PE`
Encounter for surveillance of barrier contraception
Encounter for surveillance of diaphragm

Z30.8   **Encounter for other contraceptive management** `UPD` `PE`
Encounter for postvasectomy sperm count
Encounter for routine examination for contraceptive maintenance
EXCLUDES 1   *sperm count following sterilization reversal (Z31.42)*
sperm count for fertility testing (Z31.41)

Z30.9   **Encounter for contraceptive management, unspecified** `UPD` `PE`

√4ᵗʰ Z31   Encounter for procreative management
EXCLUDES 2   *complications associated with artificial fertilization (N98.-)*
female infertility (N97.-)
male infertility (N46.-)

Z31.0   **Encounter for** reversal of previous sterilization `PE`

√5ᵗʰ Z31.4   Encounter for procreative investigation and testing
EXCLUDES 1   *postvasectomy sperm count (Z30.8)*

Z31.41   **Encounter for** fertility testing `UPD` `PE`
Encounter for fallopian tube patency testing
Encounter for sperm count for fertility testing

Z31.42   **Aftercare following** sterilization reversal `UPD` `PE`
Sperm count following sterilization reversal

√6ᵗʰ Z31.43   Encounter for genetic testing of female **for procreative management**
Use additional code for recurrent pregnancy loss, if applicable (N96, O26.2-)
EXCLUDES 1   *nonprocreative genetic testing (Z13.7-)*

Z31.430   **Encounter of female for testing for genetic** disease carrier status **for procreative management** `UPD` `PE`

Z31.438   **Encounter for other genetic testing of female for procreative management** `UPD` `PE`

√6ᵗʰ Z31.44   Encounter for genetic testing of male **for procreative management**
EXCLUDES 1   *nonprocreative genetic testing (Z13.7-)*

Z31.440   **Encounter of male for testing for genetic** disease carrier status **for procreative management** `UPD` `PE`

Z31.441   **Encounter for testing of male partner of patient with** recurrent pregnancy loss `UPD` `A` `PE`

Z31.448   **Encounter for other genetic testing of male for procreative management** `UPD` `A` `PE`

Z31.49   **Encounter for other procreative investigation and testing** `UPD` `PE`

Z31.5   **Encounter for procreative genetic counseling** `UPD` `PE`
AHA: 2017,4Q,27

√5ᵗʰ Z31.6   Encounter for general counseling and advice on procreation

Z31.61   **Procreative counseling and advice using** natural family planning `UPD` `PE`

Z31.62   **Encounter for** fertility preservation **counseling** `UPD` `PE`
Encounter for fertility preservation counseling prior to cancer therapy
Encounter for fertility preservation counseling prior to surgical removal of gonads

Z31.69   **Encounter for other general counseling and advice on procreation** `UPD` `PE`

Z31.7   **Encounter for procreative management and counseling for gestational carrier** `UPD` `PE`
EXCLUDES 1   *pregnant state, gestational carrier (Z33.3)*
AHA: 2016,4Q,78

√5ᵗʰ Z31.8   Encounter for other procreative management

Z31.81   **Encounter for** male factor **infertility in female patient** `UPD` `PE`

Z31.82   **Encounter for** Rh incompatibility **status**
AHA: 2015,3Q,40; 2014,4Q,17

Z31.83   **Encounter for** assisted reproductive fertility procedure cycle `UPD` `PE`
Patient undergoing in vitro fertilization cycle
Use additional code to identify the type of infertility
EXCLUDES 1   *pre-cycle diagnosis and testing - code to reason for encounter*
AHA: 2022,2Q,15-16

Z31.84   **Encounter for** fertility preservation **procedure** `UPD` `PE`
Encounter for fertility preservation procedure prior to cancer therapy
Encounter for fertility preservation procedure prior to surgical removal of gonads

Z31.89   **Encounter for other procreative management** `UPD` `PE`

Z31.9   **Encounter for procreative management, unspecified** `UPD` `PE`

√4ᵗʰ Z32   Encounter for pregnancy test and childbirth and childcare instruction

√5ᵗʰ Z32.0   Encounter for pregnancy test

Z32.00   **Encounter for pregnancy test,** result unknown
Encounter for pregnancy test NOS

Z32.01   **Encounter for pregnancy test,** result positive `M`

Z32.02   **Encounter for pregnancy test,** result negative

Z32.2   **Encounter for** childbirth instruction `UPD`

Z32.3   **Encounter for** childcare instruction `UPD`
Encounter for prenatal or postpartum childcare instruction

√4ᵗʰ Z33   Pregnant state

Z33.1   **Pregnant state,** incidental `UPD` `M`
Pregnancy NOS
Pregnant state NOS
EXCLUDES 1   *complications of pregnancy (O00-O9A)*
pregnant state, gestational carrier (Z33.3)

Z33.2   **Encounter for** elective termination of pregnancy `M`
EXCLUDES 1   *early fetal death with retention of dead fetus (O02.1)*
late fetal death (O36.4)
spontaneous abortion (O03)
AHA: 2023,2Q,15; 2022,1Q,20
TIP: Do not assign a code from category Z3A with this code.

Z33.3   **Pregnant state,** gestational carrier `UPD` `M` `PE`
EXCLUDES 1   *encounter for procreative management and counseling for gestational carrier (Z31.7)*
AHA: 2016,4Q,78

√4ᵗʰ Z34   Encounter for supervision of normal pregnancy
EXCLUDES 1   *any complication of pregnancy (O00-O9A)*
encounter for pregnancy test (Z32.0-)
encounter for supervision of high risk pregnancy (O09.-)
AHA: 2019,3Q,5; 2014,4Q,17

√5ᵗʰ Z34.0   Encounter for supervision of normal first **pregnancy**

Z34.00   **Encounter for supervision of normal first pregnancy, unspecified trimester** `UPD` `M` `PE`

Z34.01   **Encounter for supervision of normal first pregnancy,** first trimester `UPD` `M` `PE`

Z34.02   **Encounter for supervision of normal first pregnancy,** second trimester `UPD` `M` `PE`

Z34.03   **Encounter for supervision of normal first pregnancy,** third trimester `UPD` `M` `PE`

√5ᵗʰ Z34.8   Encounter for supervision of other normal pregnancy

Z34.80   **Encounter for supervision of other normal pregnancy, unspecified trimester** `UPD` `M` `PE`

Z34.81   **Encounter for supervision of other normal pregnancy,** first trimester `UPD` `M` `PE`

Z34.82   **Encounter for supervision of other normal pregnancy,** second trimester `UPD` `M` `PE`

Z34.83   **Encounter for supervision of other normal pregnancy,** third trimester `UPD` `M` `PE`

√5ᵗʰ Z34.9   Encounter for supervision of normal pregnancy, unspecified

Z34.90   **Encounter for supervision of normal pregnancy, unspecified, unspecified trimester** `UPD` `M` `PE`

Z34.91   **Encounter for supervision of normal pregnancy, unspecified,** first trimester `UPD` `M` `PE`

`N` Newborn: 0   `P` Pediatric: 0-17   `M` Maternity: 9-64   `A` Adult: 15-124   `UHS` Unspecified Site   `MCC` Major Complication/Comorbidity   `CC` Complication/Comorbidity   `PE` POA Exempt

1272   ICD-10-CM 2025

Z34.92   Encounter for supervision of normal pregnancy, unspecified, **second trimester** `UPD` `M` `PE`

Z34.93   Encounter for supervision of normal pregnancy, unspecified, **third trimester** `UPD` `M` `PE`

✓4ᵗʰ **Z36** **Encounter for antenatal screening of mother**

`INCLUDES`   encounter for placental sample (taken vaginally)
screening is the testing for disease or disease precursors in asymptomatic individuals so that early detection and treatment can be provided for those who test positive for the disease.

`EXCLUDES 1`   diagnostic examination - code to sign or symptom
encounter for suspected maternal and fetal conditions ruled out (Z03.7-)
suspected fetal condition affecting management of pregnancy - code to condition in Chapter 15

`EXCLUDES 2`   abnormal findings on antenatal screening of mother (O28.-)
genetic counseling and testing (Z31.43-, Z31.5)
routine prenatal care (Z34)

AHA: 2017,4Q,28

Z36.0   Encounter for antenatal screening for **chromosomal anomalies** `M` `PE`

Z36.1   Encounter for antenatal screening for **raised alphafetoprotein level** `M` `PE`
Encounter for antenatal screening for elevated maternal serum alphafetoprotein level
DEF: High levels of alpha-fetoprotein (AFP) that may indicate a possibility of spina bifida and other neural tube defects, anencephaly, or omphalocele in the fetus.

Z36.2   Encounter for other antenatal screening follow-up `M` `PE`
Non-visualized anatomy on a previous scan

Z36.3   Encounter for antenatal screening for **malformations** `M` `PE`
Screening for a suspected anomaly

Z36.4   Encounter for antenatal screening for **fetal growth retardation** `M` `PE`
Intrauterine growth restriction (IUGR)/small-for-dates

Z36.5   Encounter for antenatal screening for **isoimmunization** `M` `PE`

✓5ᵗʰ **Z36.8**   **Encounter for other antenatal screening**

Z36.81   Encounter for antenatal screening for **hydrops fetalis** `M` `PE`
DEF: Hydrops fetalis: Abnormal accumulation of fluid in two or more parts of the fetus, such as ascites, effusion of the pleural or pericardial tissues, or edema.

Z36.82   Encounter for antenatal screening for **nuchal translucency** `M` `PE`

Z36.83   Encounter for fetal screening for **congenital cardiac abnormalities** `M` `PE`

Z36.84   Encounter for antenatal screening for **fetal lung maturity** `M` `PE`

Z36.85   Encounter for antenatal screening for **Streptococcus B** `M` `PE`

Z36.86   Encounter for antenatal screening for **cervical length** `M` `PE`
Screening for risk of pre-term labor

Z36.87   Encounter for antenatal screening for **uncertain dates** `M` `PE`

Z36.88   Encounter for antenatal screening for **fetal macrosomia** `M` `PE`
Screening for large-for-dates

Z36.89   Encounter for other specified antenatal screening `M` `PE`

Z36.8A   Encounter for antenatal screening for other genetic defects `M` `PE`

Z36.9   Encounter for antenatal screening, unspecified `M` `PE`

✓4ᵗʰ **Z3A** **Weeks of gestation**

`NOTE`   Codes from category Z3A are for use, only on the maternal record, to indicate the weeks of gestation of the pregnancy, if known.

Code first obstetric condition or encounter for delivery (O09-O60, O80-O82)
AHA: 2022,2Q,3; 2019,2Q,11; 2016,2Q,34; 2014,3Q,17; 2014,2Q,9; 2013,2Q,33
TIP: Do not assign a code from this category with codes from categories O00-O08 or code Z33.2.

✓5ᵗʰ **Z3A.0**   **Weeks of gestation of pregnancy, unspecified or less than 10 weeks**

Z3A.00   Weeks of gestation of pregnancy **not specified** `UPD` `M` `PE`

Z3A.01   **Less than 8 weeks** gestation of pregnancy `UPD` `M` `PE`

Z3A.08   **8 weeks** gestation of pregnancy `UPD` `M` `PE`

Z3A.09   **9 weeks** gestation of pregnancy `UPD` `M` `PE`

✓5ᵗʰ **Z3A.1**   Weeks of gestation of pregnancy, weeks **10-19**

Z3A.10   **10 weeks** gestation of pregnancy `UPD` `M` `PE`

Z3A.11   **11 weeks** gestation of pregnancy `UPD` `M` `PE`

Z3A.12   **12 weeks** gestation of pregnancy `UPD` `M` `PE`

Z3A.13   **13 weeks** gestation of pregnancy `UPD` `M` `PE`

Z3A.14   **14 weeks** gestation of pregnancy `UPD` `M` `PE`

Z3A.15   **15 weeks** gestation of pregnancy `UPD` `M` `PE`

Z3A.16   **16 weeks** gestation of pregnancy `UPD` `M` `PE`

Z3A.17   **17 weeks** gestation of pregnancy `UPD` `M` `PE`

Z3A.18   **18 weeks** gestation of pregnancy `UPD` `M` `PE`

Z3A.19   **19 weeks** gestation of pregnancy `UPD` `M` `PE`

✓5ᵗʰ **Z3A.2**   Weeks of gestation of pregnancy, weeks **20-29**

Z3A.20   **20 weeks** gestation of pregnancy `UPD` `M` `PE`

Z3A.21   **21 weeks** gestation of pregnancy `UPD` `M` `PE`

Z3A.22   **22 weeks** gestation of pregnancy `UPD` `M` `PE`

Z3A.23   **23 weeks** gestation of pregnancy `UPD` `M` `PE`

Z3A.24   **24 weeks** gestation of pregnancy `UPD` `M` `PE`

Z3A.25   **25 weeks** gestation of pregnancy `UPD` `M` `PE`

Z3A.26   **26 weeks** gestation of pregnancy `UPD` `M` `PE`

Z3A.27   **27 weeks** gestation of pregnancy `UPD` `M` `PE`

Z3A.28   **28 weeks** gestation of pregnancy `UPD` `M` `PE`

Z3A.29   **29 weeks** gestation of pregnancy `UPD` `M` `PE`

✓5ᵗʰ **Z3A.3**   Weeks of gestation of pregnancy, weeks **30-39**

Z3A.30   **30 weeks** gestation of pregnancy `UPD` `M` `PE`

Z3A.31   **31 weeks** gestation of pregnancy `UPD` `M` `PE`

Z3A.32   **32 weeks** gestation of pregnancy `UPD` `M` `PE`

Z3A.33   **33 weeks** gestation of pregnancy `UPD` `M` `PE`

Z3A.34   **34 weeks** gestation of pregnancy `UPD` `M` `PE`

Z3A.35   **35 weeks** gestation of pregnancy `UPD` `M` `PE`

Z3A.36   **36 weeks** gestation of pregnancy `UPD` `M` `PE`

Z3A.37   **37 weeks** gestation of pregnancy `UPD` `M` `PE`

Z3A.38   **38 weeks** gestation of pregnancy `UPD` `M` `PE`

Z3A.39   **39 weeks** gestation of pregnancy `UPD` `M` `PE`

✓5ᵗʰ **Z3A.4**   Weeks of gestation of pregnancy, weeks **40 or greater**
AHA: 2014,4Q,23

Z3A.40   **40 weeks** gestation of pregnancy `UPD` `M` `PE`

Z3A.41   **41 weeks** gestation of pregnancy `UPD` `M` `PE`

Z3A.42   **42 weeks** gestation of pregnancy `UPD` `M` `PE`

Z3A.49   **Greater than 42 weeks** gestation of pregnancy `UPD` `M` `PE`

✓4ᵗʰ **Z37** **Outcome of delivery**
This category is intended for use as an additional code to identify the outcome of delivery on the mother's record. It is not for use on the newborn record.

`EXCLUDES 1`   stillbirth (P95)

Z37.0   **Single live birth** `UPD` `M` `PE`
AHA: 2016,2Q,34; 2014,2Q,9

Z37.1   **Single stillbirth** `UPD` `M` `PE`

Z37.2   **Twins, both liveborn** `UPD` `M` `PE`

Z37.3   **Twins, one liveborn and one stillborn** `UPD` `M` `PE`

Z37.4   **Twins, both stillborn** `UPD` `M` `PE`

✓5ᵗʰ **Z37.5**   **Other multiple births, all liveborn**

Z37.50   Multiple births, unspecified, all liveborn `UPD` `M` `PE`

Z37.51   Triplets, all liveborn `UPD` `M` `PE`

Z37.52   Quadruplets, all liveborn `UPD` `M` `PE`

Z37.53   Quintuplets, all liveborn `UPD` `M` `PE`

Z37.54   Sextuplets, all liveborn `UPD` `M` `PE`

Z37.59   Other multiple births, all liveborn `UPD` `M` `PE`

✓5ᵗʰ **Z37.6**   **Other multiple births, some liveborn**

Z37.60   Multiple births, unspecified, some liveborn `UPD` `M` `PE`

Z37.61   Triplets, some liveborn `UPD` `M` `PE`

Z37.62   Quadruplets, some liveborn `UPD` `M` `PE`

Z37.63   Quintuplets, some liveborn `UPD` `M` `PE`

Z37.64   Sextuplets, some liveborn `UPD` `M` `PE`

Z37.69   Other multiple births, some liveborn `UPD` `M` `PE`

Z37.7   **Other multiple births, all stillborn** `UPD` `M` `PE`

Chapter 21. Factors Influencing Health Status and Contact With Health Services *(side margin)*

Z37.9   **Outcome of delivery, unspecified**   UPD M PE
Multiple birth NOS
Single birth NOS

✓4th **Z38**   **Liveborn infants according to place of birth and type of delivery**
This category is for use as the principal code on the initial record of a newborn baby. It is to be used for the initial birth record only. It is not to be used on the mother's record.
AHA: 2020,2Q,13; 2017,2Q,5-7; 2016,3Q,18; 2015,2Q,15

✓5th **Z38.0**   **Single liveborn infant, born in hospital**
Single liveborn infant, born in birthing center or other health care facility

    Z38.00   **Single liveborn infant, delivered vaginally**   N PE

    Z38.01   **Single liveborn infant, delivered by cesarean**   N PE

Z38.1   **Single liveborn infant, born outside hospital**   N PE

Z38.2   **Single liveborn infant, unspecified as to place of birth**   N PE
Single liveborn infant NOS

✓5th **Z38.3**   **Twin liveborn infant, born in hospital**

    Z38.30   **Twin liveborn infant, delivered vaginally**   N PE

    Z38.31   **Twin liveborn infant, delivered by cesarean**   N PE

Z38.4   **Twin liveborn infant, born outside hospital**   N PE

Z38.5   **Twin liveborn infant, unspecified as to place of birth**   N PE

✓5th **Z38.6**   **Other multiple liveborn infant, born in hospital**

    Z38.61   **Triplet liveborn infant, delivered vaginally**   N PE

    Z38.62   **Triplet liveborn infant, delivered by cesarean**   N PE

    Z38.63   **Quadruplet liveborn infant, delivered vaginally**   N PE

    Z38.64   **Quadruplet liveborn infant, delivered by cesarean**   N PE

    Z38.65   **Quintuplet liveborn infant, delivered vaginally**   N PE

    Z38.66   **Quintuplet liveborn infant, delivered by cesarean**   N PE

    Z38.68   **Other multiple liveborn infant, delivered vaginally**   N PE

    Z38.69   **Other multiple liveborn infant, delivered by cesarean**   N PE

Z38.7   **Other multiple liveborn infant, born outside hospital**   N PE

Z38.8   **Other multiple liveborn infant, unspecified as to place of birth**   N PE

✓4th **Z39**   **Encounter for maternal postpartum care and examination**

Z39.0   **Encounter for care and examination of mother immediately after delivery**   M PE
Care and observation in uncomplicated cases when the delivery occurs outside a healthcare facility
EXCLUDES 1   *care for postpartum complication - see Alphabetic Index*
AHA: 2021,3Q,13

Z39.1   **Encounter for care and examination of lactating mother**   UPD M PE
Encounter for supervision of lactation
EXCLUDES 1   *disorders of lactation (O92.-)*

Z39.2   **Encounter for routine postpartum follow-up**   UPD M PE

Encounters for other specific health care (Z40-Z53)

Categories Z40-Z53 are intended for use to indicate a reason for care. They may be used for patients who have already been treated for a disease or injury, but who are receiving aftercare or prophylactic care, or care to consolidate the treatment, or to deal with a residual state
EXCLUDES 2   *follow-up examination for medical surveillance after treatment (Z08-Z09)*

✓4th **Z40**   **Encounter for prophylactic surgery**
EXCLUDES 1   *organ donations (Z52.-)*
         therapeutic organ removal - code to condition
DEF: Treatment measure intended to prevent or ward off a disease or condition.

✓5th **Z40.0**   **Encounter for prophylactic surgery for risk factors related to malignant neoplasms**
Admission for prophylactic organ removal
Use additional code to identify risk factor
AHA: 2017,4Q,28-29

    Z40.00   **Encounter for prophylactic removal of unspecified organ**

    Z40.01   **Encounter for prophylactic removal of breast**

    Z40.02   **Encounter for prophylactic removal of ovary(s)**
Encounter for prophylactic removal of ovary(s) and fallopian tube(s)

    Z40.03   **Encounter for prophylactic removal of fallopian tube(s)**   PE

    Z40.09   **Encounter for prophylactic removal of other organ**

Z40.8   **Encounter for other prophylactic surgery**   UPD

Z40.9   **Encounter for prophylactic surgery, unspecified**   UPD

✓4th **Z41**   **Encounter for procedures for purposes other than remedying health state**

Z41.1   **Encounter for cosmetic surgery**   PE
Encounter for cosmetic breast implant
Encounter for cosmetic procedure
EXCLUDES 1   *encounter for plastic and reconstructive surgery following medical procedure or healed injury (Z42.-)*
         encounter for post-mastectomy breast implantation (Z42.1)

Z41.2   **Encounter for routine and ritual male circumcision**   PE
AHA: 2018,3Q,15
TIP: Do not report this code when circumcision is performed during the birth admission.

Z41.3   **Encounter for ear piercing**   UPD PE

Z41.8   **Encounter for other procedures for purposes other than remedying health state**   PE

Z41.9   **Encounter for procedure for purposes other than remedying health state, unspecified**   UPD PE

✓4th **Z42**   **Encounter for plastic and reconstructive surgery following medical procedure or healed injury**
EXCLUDES 1   *encounter for cosmetic plastic surgery (Z41.1)*
         encounter for plastic surgery for treatment of current injury - code to relevent injury

Z42.1   **Encounter for breast reconstruction following mastectomy**   A PE
EXCLUDES 1   *deformity and disproportion of reconstructed breast (N65.1-)*

Z42.8   **Encounter for other plastic and reconstructive surgery following medical procedure or healed injury**   PE
AHA: 2017,1Q,42

✓4th **Z43**   **Encounter for attention to artificial openings**
INCLUDES   closure of artificial openings
passage of sounds or bougies through artificial openings
reforming artificial openings
removal of catheter from artificial openings
toilet or cleansing of artificial openings
EXCLUDES 1   *complications of external stoma (J95.0-, K94.-, N99.5-)*
EXCLUDES 2   *fitting and adjustment of prosthetic and other devices (Z44-Z46)*
AHA: 2019,2Q,33

Z43.0   **Encounter for attention to tracheostomy**   HCC PE

Z43.1   **Encounter for attention to gastrostomy**   CC HCC PE
EXCLUDES 2   *artificial opening status only, without need for care (Z93.-)*

Z43.2   **Encounter for attention to ileostomy**   HCC PE

Z43.3   **Encounter for attention to colostomy**   HCC PE

Z43.4   **Encounter for attention to other artificial openings of digestive tract**   HCC PE

Z43.5   **Encounter for attention to cystostomy**   HCC PE

Z43.6   **Encounter for attention to other artificial openings of urinary tract**   HCC PE
Encounter for attention to nephrostomy
Encounter for attention to ureterostomy
Encounter for attention to urethrostomy

Z43.7   **Encounter for attention to artificial vagina**   PE

Z43.8   **Encounter for attention to other artificial openings**   HCC PE

Z43.9   **Encounter for attention to unspecified artificial opening**   UPD HCC PE

✓4th **Z44** **Encounter for fitting and adjustment of external prosthetic device**

INCLUDES removal or replacement of external prosthetic device

EXCLUDES 1 *malfunction or other complications of device - see Alphabetic Index*

presence of prosthetic device (Z97.-)

✓5th **Z44.0** **Encounter for fitting and adjustment of artificial arm**

✓6th **Z44.00** **Encounter for fitting and adjustment of unspecified artificial arm**

Z44.001 Encounter for fitting and adjustment of unspecified **right** artificial arm PE

Z44.002 Encounter for fitting and adjustment of unspecified **left** artificial arm PE

Z44.009 Encounter for fitting and adjustment of unspecified artificial arm, unspecified arm PE

✓6th **Z44.01** **Encounter for fitting and adjustment of complete artificial arm**

Z44.011 Encounter for fitting and adjustment of complete **right** artificial arm PE

Z44.012 Encounter for fitting and adjustment of complete **left** artificial arm PE

Z44.019 Encounter for fitting and adjustment of complete artificial arm, unspecified arm PE

✓6th **Z44.02** **Encounter for fitting and adjustment of partial artificial arm**

Z44.021 Encounter for fitting and adjustment of partial artificial **right** arm PE

Z44.022 Encounter for fitting and adjustment of partial artificial **left** arm PE

Z44.029 Encounter for fitting and adjustment of partial artificial arm, unspecified arm PE

✓5th **Z44.1** **Encounter for fitting and adjustment of artificial leg**

✓6th **Z44.10** **Encounter for fitting and adjustment of unspecified artificial leg**

Z44.101 Encounter for fitting and adjustment of unspecified **right** artificial leg HCC PE

Z44.102 Encounter for fitting and adjustment of unspecified **left** artificial leg HCC PE

Z44.109 Encounter for fitting and adjustment of unspecified artificial leg, unspecified leg HCC PE

✓6th **Z44.11** **Encounter for fitting and adjustment of complete artificial leg**

Z44.111 Encounter for fitting and adjustment of complete **right** artificial leg HCC PE

Z44.112 Encounter for fitting and adjustment of complete **left** artificial leg HCC PE

Z44.119 Encounter for fitting and adjustment of complete artificial leg, unspecified leg HCC PE

✓6th **Z44.12** **Encounter for fitting and adjustment of partial artificial leg**

Z44.121 Encounter for fitting and adjustment of partial artificial **right** leg HCC PE

Z44.122 Encounter for fitting and adjustment of partial artificial **left** leg HCC PE

Z44.129 Encounter for fitting and adjustment of partial artificial leg, unspecified leg HCC PE

✓5th **Z44.2** **Encounter for fitting and adjustment of artificial eye**

EXCLUDES 1 *mechanical complication of ocular prosthesis (T85.3)*

Z44.20 Encounter for fitting and adjustment of artificial eye, unspecified PE

Z44.21 Encounter for fitting and adjustment of artificial **right** eye PE

Z44.22 Encounter for fitting and adjustment of artificial **left** eye PE

✓5th **Z44.3** **Encounter for fitting and adjustment of external breast prosthesis**

EXCLUDES 1 *complications of breast implant (T85.4-)*

encounter for adjustment or removal of breast implant (Z45.81-)

encounter for initial breast implant insertion for cosmetic breast augmentation (Z41.1)

encounter for breast reconstruction following mastectomy (Z42.1)

Z44.30 Encounter for fitting and adjustment of external breast prosthesis, unspecified breast PE

Z44.31 Encounter for fitting and adjustment of external **right** breast prosthesis PE

Z44.32 Encounter for fitting and adjustment of external **left** breast prosthesis PE

Z44.8 **Encounter for fitting and adjustment of other external prosthetic devices** PE

Z44.9 **Encounter for fitting and adjustment of unspecified external prosthetic device** UPD PE

✓4th **Z45** **Encounter for adjustment and management of implanted device**

INCLUDES removal or replacement of implanted device

EXCLUDES 1 *malfunction or other complications of device - see Alphabetic Index*

EXCLUDES 2 *encounter for fitting and adjustment of non-implanted device (Z46.-)*

✓5th **Z45.0** **Encounter for adjustment and management of cardiac device**

TIP: Assign an additional code for the associated condition if that condition requires constant intervention from the device, as in cases of sick sinus syndrome. For conditions that do not require constant intervention from the device, as in cases of ventricular fibrillation, an additional code for the associated condition should be assigned only if the patient is experiencing the condition and the device is firing during the current admission.

✓6th **Z45.01** **Encounter for adjustment and management of cardiac pacemaker**

Encounter for adjustment and management of cardiac resynchronization therapy pacemaker (CRT-P)

EXCLUDES 1 *encounter for adjustment and management of automatic implantable cardiac defibrillator with synchronous cardiac pacemaker (Z45.02)*

Z45.010 **Encounter for checking and testing of cardiac pacemaker pulse generator [battery]** PE

Encounter for replacing cardiac pacemaker pulse generator [battery]

Z45.018 **Encounter for adjustment and management of other part of cardiac pacemaker** PE

EXCLUDES 1 *presence of other part of cardiac pacemaker (Z95.0)*

EXCLUDES 2 *presence of prosthetic and other devices (Z95.1-Z95.5, Z95.811-Z97)*

Z45.02 **Encounter for adjustment and management of automatic implantable cardiac defibrillator** PE

Encounter for adjustment and management of automatic implantable cardiac defibrillator with synchronous cardiac pacemaker

Encounter for adjustment and management of cardiac resynchronization therapy defibrillator (CRT-D)

AHA: 2024,1Q,21-22

Z45.09 **Encounter for adjustment and management of other cardiac device** PE

Z45.1 **Encounter for adjustment and management of infusion pump** PE

Z45.2 **Encounter for adjustment and management of vascular access device** PE

Encounter for adjustment and management of vascular catheters

EXCLUDES 1 *encounter for adjustment and management of renal dialysis catheter (Z49.01)*

AHA: 2020,2Q,21; 2018,3Q,20

✓5th **Z45.3** **Encounter for adjustment and management of implanted devices of the special senses**

Z45.31 **Encounter for adjustment and management of implanted visual substitution device** PE

✓ Additional Character Required ✓x7th Placeholder Questionable PDx Manifestation Unspecified UPD Unacceptable PDx H1 - H14 HAC HCC CMS-HCC Dx HIV HIV Dx

ICD-10-CM 2025 **1275**

√6th **Z45.32 Encounter for adjustment and management of implanted hearing device**
- EXCLUDES 1 ▶encounter for fitting and adjustment of hearing aid◀ (Z46.1)

     Z45.32Ø Encounter for adjustment and management of bone conduction device PE

     Z45.321 Encounter for adjustment and management of cochlear device PE

     Z45.328 Encounter for adjustment and management of other implanted hearing device PE

√5th **Z45.4 Encounter for adjustment and management of implanted nervous system device**

     Z45.41 Encounter for adjustment and management of cerebrospinal fluid drainage device PE
       Encounter for adjustment and management of cerebral ventricular (communicating) shunt

     Z45.42 Encounter for adjustment and management of neurostimulator PE
       Encounter for adjustment and management of brain neurostimulator
       Encounter for adjustment and management of gastric neurostimulator
       Encounter for adjustment and management of peripheral nerve neurostimulator
       Encounter for adjustment and management of sacral nerve neurostimulator
       Encounter for adjustment and management of spinal cord neurostimulator
       Encounter for adjustment and management of vagus nerve neurostimulator

     Z45.49 Encounter for adjustment and management of other implanted nervous system device PE
       AHA: 2014,3Q,19

√5th **Z45.8 Encounter for adjustment and management of other implanted devices**

√6th   **Z45.81 Encounter for adjustment or removal of breast implant**
       Encounter for elective implant exchange (different material) (different size)
       Encounter for removal of tissue expander with or without synchronous insertion of permanent implant
- EXCLUDES 1 complications of breast implant (T85.4-)
       encounter for initial breast implant insertion for cosmetic breast augmentation (Z41.1)
       encounter for breast reconstruction following mastectomy (Z42.1)

     Z45.811 Encounter for adjustment or removal of right breast implant PE

     Z45.812 Encounter for adjustment or removal of left breast implant PE

     Z45.819 Encounter for adjustment or removal of unspecified breast implant PE

     Z45.82 Encounter for adjustment or removal of myringotomy device (stent) (tube) UPD PE

     Z45.89 Encounter for adjustment and management of other implanted devices UPD PE
       AHA: 2014,4Q,26-28

   Z45.9 Encounter for adjustment and management of unspecified implanted device UPD PE

√4th **Z46 Encounter for fitting and adjustment of other devices**
- INCLUDES removal or replacement of other device
- EXCLUDES 1 malfunction or other complications of device - see Alphabetical Index
- EXCLUDES 2 encounter for fitting and management of implanted devices (Z45.-)
     issue of repeat prescription only (Z76.Ø)
     presence of prosthetic and other devices (Z95-Z97)

   Z46.Ø Encounter for fitting and adjustment of spectacles and contact lenses UPD PE

   Z46.1 Encounter for fitting and adjustment of hearing aid UPD PE
- EXCLUDES 1 encounter for adjustment and management of implanted hearing device (Z45.32-)

   Z46.2 Encounter for fitting and adjustment of other devices related to nervous system and special senses PE
- EXCLUDES 2 encounter for adjustment and management of implanted nervous system device (Z45.4-)
     encounter for adjustment and management of implanted visual substitution device (Z45.31)

   Z46.3 Encounter for fitting and adjustment of dental prosthetic device PE
     Encounter for fitting and adjustment of dentures

   Z46.4 Encounter for fitting and adjustment of orthodontic device UPD PE

√5th **Z46.5 Encounter for fitting and adjustment of other gastrointestinal appliance and device**
- EXCLUDES 1 encounter for attention to artificial openings of digestive tract (Z43.1-Z43.4)

     Z46.51 Encounter for fitting and adjustment of gastric lap band UPD PE

     Z46.59 Encounter for fitting and adjustment of other gastrointestinal appliance and device UPD PE

   Z46.6 Encounter for fitting and adjustment of urinary device UPD PE
- EXCLUDES 2 attention to artificial openings of urinary tract (Z43.5, Z43.6)

√5th **Z46.8 Encounter for fitting and adjustment of other specified devices**

     Z46.81 Encounter for fitting and adjustment of insulin pump UPD PE
       Encounter for insulin pump instruction and training
       Encounter for insulin pump titration

     Z46.82 Encounter for fitting and adjustment of non-vascular catheter PE

     Z46.89 Encounter for fitting and adjustment of other specified devices UPD PE
       Encounter for fitting and adjustment of wheelchair

   Z46.9 Encounter for fitting and adjustment of unspecified device UPD PE

√4th **Z47 Orthopedic aftercare**
- EXCLUDES 1 aftercare for healing fracture - code to fracture with 7th character D

   Z47.1 Aftercare following joint replacement surgery PE
     Use additional code to identify the joint (Z96.6-)
     AHA: 2020,1Q,23

   Z47.2 Encounter for removal of internal fixation device PE
- EXCLUDES 1 encounter for adjustment of internal fixation device for fracture treatment - code to fracture with appropriate 7th character
     encounter for removal of external fixation device - code to fracture with 7th character D
     infection or inflammatory reaction to internal fixation device (T84.6-)
     mechanical complication of internal fixation device (T84.1-)

√5th **Z47.3 Aftercare following explantation of joint prosthesis**
     Aftercare following explantation of joint prosthesis, staged procedure
     Encounter for joint prosthesis insertion following prior explantation of joint prosthesis
     AHA: 2020,1Q,23; 2015,1Q,16
     TIP: For staged removal of elbow joint prosthesis, assign code Z47.1.

     Z47.31 Aftercare following explantation of shoulder joint prosthesis PE
- EXCLUDES 1 acquired absence of shoulder joint following prior explantation of shoulder joint prosthesis (Z89.23-)
     shoulder joint prosthesis explantation status (Z89.23-)

     Z47.32 Aftercare following explantation of hip joint prosthesis PE
- EXCLUDES 1 acquired absence of hip joint following prior explantation of hip joint prosthesis (Z89.62-)
     hip joint prosthesis explantation status (Z89.62-)

N Newborn: 0   **P** Pediatric: 0-17   **M** Maternity: 9-64   **A** Adult: 15-124   **UNS** Unspecified Site   **MCC** Major Complication/Comorbidity   **CC** Complication/Comorbidity   **PE** POA Exempt

1276   ICD-10-CM 2025

Z47.33 **Aftercare following explantation of knee joint prosthesis** `PE`

> **EXCLUDES 1**   *acquired absence of knee joint following prior explantation of knee prosthesis (Z89.52-)*
> *knee joint prosthesis explantation status (Z89.52-)*

✓5ᵗʰ **Z47.8** **Encounter for other orthopedic aftercare**

Z47.81 **Encounter for orthopedic aftercare following surgical amputation** `PE`

> Use additional code to identify the limb amputated (Z89.-)

Z47.82 **Encounter for orthopedic aftercare following scoliosis surgery** `PE`

Z47.89 **Encounter for other orthopedic aftercare**
> **AHA:** 2015,1Q,8

✓4ᵗʰ **Z48** **Encounter for other postprocedural aftercare**

> **EXCLUDES 1**   *encounter for aftercare following injury - code to Injury, by site, with appropriate 7th character for subsequent encounter*
> *encounter for follow-up examination after completed treatment (Z08-Z09)*

> **EXCLUDES 2**   *encounter for attention to artificial openings (Z43.-)*
> *encounter for fitting and adjustment of prosthetic and other devices (Z44-Z46)*

> **AHA:** 2015,4Q,38; 2015,1Q,6-7

✓5ᵗʰ **Z48.0** **Encounter for attention to dressings, sutures and drains**

> **EXCLUDES 1**   *encounter for planned postprocedural wound closure (Z48.1)*

Z48.00 **Encounter for change or removal of nonsurgical wound dressing** `UPD` `PE`
> Encounter for change or removal of wound dressing NOS

Z48.01 **Encounter for change or removal of surgical wound dressing** `UPD` `PE`
> **AHA:** 2019,2Q,33

Z48.02 **Encounter for removal of sutures** `UPD` `PE`
> Encounter for removal of staples

Z48.03 **Encounter for change or removal of drains** `PE`
> **AHA:** 2019,2Q,33

Z48.1 **Encounter for planned postprocedural wound closure** `PE`

> **EXCLUDES 1**   *encounter for attention to dressings and sutures (Z48.0-)*

✓5ᵗʰ **Z48.2** **Encounter for aftercare following organ transplant**

Z48.21 **Encounter for aftercare following heart transplant** `CC` `HCC` `PE`

Z48.22 **Encounter for aftercare following kidney transplant** `CC` `PE`

Z48.23 **Encounter for aftercare following liver transplant** `CC` `HCC` `PE`

Z48.24 **Encounter for aftercare following lung transplant** `CC` `HCC` `PE`

✓6ᵗʰ **Z48.28** **Encounter for aftercare following multiple organ transplant**

Z48.280 **Encounter for aftercare following heart-lung transplant** `CC` `HCC` `PE`

Z48.288 **Encounter for aftercare following multiple organ transplant** `PE`

✓6ᵗʰ **Z48.29** **Encounter for aftercare following other organ transplant**

Z48.290 **Encounter for aftercare following bone marrow transplant** `CC` `HCC` `PE`

Z48.298 **Encounter for aftercare following other organ transplant** `PE`

Z48.3 **Aftercare following surgery for neoplasm** `PE`
> Use additional code to identify the neoplasm

✓5ᵗʰ **Z48.8** **Encounter for other specified postprocedural aftercare**

✓6ᵗʰ **Z48.81** **Encounter for surgical aftercare following surgery on specified body systems**
> These codes identify the body system requiring aftercare. They are for use in conjunction with other aftercare codes to fully explain the aftercare encounter. The condition treated should also be coded if still present.

> **EXCLUDES 1**   *aftercare for injury - code the injury with 7th character D*
> *aftercare following surgery for neoplasm (Z48.3)*

> **EXCLUDES 2**   *aftercare following organ transplant (Z48.2-)*
> *orthopedic aftercare (Z47.-)*

> **AHA:** 2015,4Q,38

Z48.810 **Encounter for surgical aftercare following surgery on the sense organs** `PE`

Z48.811 **Encounter for surgical aftercare following surgery on the nervous system** `PE`

> **EXCLUDES 2**   *encounter for surgical aftercare following surgery on the sense organs (Z48.810)*

Z48.812 **Encounter for surgical aftercare following surgery on the circulatory system** `PE`
> **AHA:** 2012,4Q,96

Z48.813 **Encounter for surgical aftercare following surgery on the respiratory system** `PE`
> **AHA:** 2019,2Q,33

Z48.814 **Encounter for surgical aftercare following surgery on the teeth or oral cavity** `PE`

Z48.815 **Encounter for surgical aftercare following surgery on the digestive system** `PE`

Z48.816 **Encounter for surgical aftercare following surgery on the genitourinary system** `PE`

> **EXCLUDES 1**   *encounter for aftercare following sterilization reversal (Z31.42)*

Z48.817 **Encounter for surgical aftercare following surgery on the skin and subcutaneous tissue** `PE`

Z48.89 **Encounter for other specified surgical aftercare** `PE`

✓4ᵗʰ **Z49** **Encounter for care involving renal dialysis**
> Code also associated end stage renal disease (N18.6)

✓5ᵗʰ **Z49.0** **Preparatory care for renal dialysis**
> Encounter for dialysis instruction and training

Z49.01 **Encounter for fitting and adjustment of extracorporeal dialysis catheter** `UPD` `PE`
> Removal or replacement of renal dialysis catheter
> Toilet or cleansing of renal dialysis catheter

Z49.02 **Encounter for fitting and adjustment of peritoneal dialysis catheter** `UPD` `PE`

✓5ᵗʰ **Z49.3** **Encounter for adequacy testing for dialysis**

Z49.31 **Encounter for adequacy testing for hemodialysis** `UPD` `PE`

Z49.32 **Encounter for adequacy testing for peritoneal dialysis** `UPD` `PE`
> Encounter for peritoneal equilibration test

✓4ᵗʰ **Z51** **Encounter for other aftercare and medical care**
> Code also condition requiring care

> **EXCLUDES 1**   *follow-up examination after treatment (Z08-Z09)*

Z51.0 **Encounter for antineoplastic radiation therapy** `PE`
> **AHA:** 2017,4Q,103
> **TIP:** Do not assign when admission is for insertion/implantation of radioactive elements. Assign a code for the malignancy instead. Any complications related to the radioactive elements should be assigned as secondary diagnoses.

✓5ᵗʰ **Z51.1** **Encounter for antineoplastic chemotherapy and immunotherapy**

> **EXCLUDES 2**   *encounter for chemotherapy and immunotherapy for nonneoplastic condition - code to condition*

Z51.11 **Encounter for antineoplastic chemotherapy** `PE`
> **AHA:** 2022,1Q,16; 2015,3Q,19

Z51.12 **Encounter for antineoplastic immunotherapy** `PE`
> **AHA:** 2024,1Q,24

✅ Additional Character Required   ✓x7ᵗʰ Placeholder   Questionable PDx   Manifestation   Unspecified   `UPD` Unacceptable PDx   `H1`-`H14` HAC   `HCC` CMS-HCC Dx   `HIV` HIV Dx

ICD-10-CM 2025   **1277**

Chapter 21. Factors Influencing Health Status and Contact With Health Services

Z51.5   Encounter for palliative care   PE
     AHA: 2022,1Q,18; 2020,4Q,98; 2017,1Q,48

Z51.6   Encounter for desensitization to allergens   UPD PE
     AHA: 2016,4Q,77

✓5ᵗʰ **Z51.8**   Encounter for other specified aftercare
      EXCLUDES 1   holiday relief care (Z75.5)

     Z51.81   Encounter for therapeutic drug level monitoring   PE
        Code also any long-term (current) drug therapy (Z79.-)
        EXCLUDES 1   encounter for blood-drug test for administrative or medicolegal reasons (Z02.83)
        DEF: Drug monitoring: Measurement of the level of a specific drug in the body or measurement of a specific function to assess effectiveness of a drug.

     Z51.89   Encounter for other specified aftercare   UPD PE
        AHA: 2012,4Q,95-97

● **Z51.A**   Encounter for sepsis aftercare   PE

✓4ᵗʰ **Z52**   Donors of organs and tissues
     INCLUDES   autologous and other living donors
     EXCLUDES 1   cadaveric donor - omit code
        examination of potential donor (Z00.5)
     AHA: 2012,4Q,99

   ✓5ᵗʰ **Z52.0**   Blood donor
     ✓6ᵗʰ **Z52.00**   Unspecified blood donor
        Z52.000   Unspecified donor, whole blood   UPD PE
        Z52.001   Unspecified donor, stem cells   UPD PE
        Z52.008   Unspecified donor, other blood   UPD PE

     ✓6ᵗʰ **Z52.01**   Autologous blood donor
        Z52.010   Autologous donor, whole blood   UPD PE
        Z52.011   Autologous donor, stem cells   UPD PE
        Z52.018   Autologous donor, other blood   UPD PE

     ✓6ᵗʰ **Z52.09**   Other blood donor
        Volunteer donor
        Z52.090   Other blood donor, whole blood   UPD PE
        Z52.091   Other blood donor, stem cells   UPD PE
        Z52.098   Other blood donor, other blood   UPD PE

   ✓5ᵗʰ **Z52.1**   Skin donor
     Z52.10   Skin donor, unspecified   PE
     Z52.11   Skin donor, autologous   PE
     Z52.19   Skin donor, other   PE

   ✓5ᵗʰ **Z52.2**   Bone donor
     Z52.20   Bone donor, unspecified   PE
     Z52.21   Bone donor, autologous   PE
     Z52.29   Bone donor, other   PE

   Z52.3   Bone marrow donor   PE
   Z52.4   Kidney donor   PE
   Z52.5   Cornea donor   PE
   Z52.6   Liver donor   PE

   ✓5ᵗʰ **Z52.8**   Donor of other specified organs or tissues
     ✓6ᵗʰ **Z52.81**   Egg (Oocyte) donor
        Z52.810   Egg (Oocyte) donor under age 35, anonymous recipient   UPD PE
          Egg donor under age 35 NOS
        Z52.811   Egg (Oocyte) donor under age 35, designated recipient   UPD PE
        Z52.812   Egg (Oocyte) donor age 35 and over, anonymous recipient   UPD PE
          Egg donor age 35 and over NOS
        Z52.813   Egg (Oocyte) donor age 35 and over, designated recipient   UPD PE
        Z52.819   Egg (Oocyte) donor, unspecified   UPD PE
     Z52.89   Donor of other specified organs or tissues   PE

   Z52.9   Donor of unspecified organ or tissue   PE
     Donor NOS

✓4ᵗʰ **Z53**   Persons encountering health services for specific procedures and treatment, not carried out
   ✓5ᵗʰ **Z53.0**   Procedure and treatment not carried out because of contraindication
     Z53.01   Procedure and treatment not carried out due to patient smoking   UPD

     Z53.09   Procedure and treatment not carried out because of other contraindication   UPD

   Z53.1   Procedure and treatment not carried out because of patient's decision for reasons of belief and group pressure   UPD

   ✓5ᵗʰ **Z53.2**   Procedure and treatment not carried out because of patient's decision for other and unspecified reasons
     Z53.20   Procedure and treatment not carried out because of patient's decision for unspecified reasons   UPD
     Z53.21   Procedure and treatment not carried out due to patient leaving prior to being seen by health care provider
     Z53.29   Procedure and treatment not carried out because of patient's decision for other reasons   UPD

   ✓5ᵗʰ **Z53.3**   Procedure converted to open procedure
     AHA: 2016,4Q,79
     Z53.31   Laparoscopic surgical procedure converted to open procedure   UPD PE
     Z53.32   Thoracoscopic surgical procedure converted to open procedure   UPD PE
     Z53.33   Arthroscopic surgical procedure converted to open procedure   UPD PE
     Z53.39   Other specified procedure converted to open procedure   UPD PE

   Z53.8   Procedure and treatment not carried out for other reasons   UPD
   Z53.9   Procedure and treatment not carried out, unspecified reason   UPD

Persons with potential health hazards related to socioeconomic and psychosocial circumstances (Z55-Z65)

AHA: 2021,4Q,34-37; 2019,4Q,66; 2018,4Q,58,73; 2018,1Q,18
DEF: Social determinants of health: Socioeconomic factors that can affect a person's health, including both environmental and societal conditions such as education and literacy, employment, health behaviors, housing, lack of adequate food or water, occupational exposure to risk factors, social support, transportation, and violence. Tracking social needs that impact patients allows providers to identify population health trends and to promote the personalized care that addresses the medical and social needs of individual patients. Synonym(s): SDOH.
TIP: Because codes in these categories represent social information rather than medical diagnoses, they can be assigned based on documentation by nonphysician clinicians involved in the care of these patients as well as self-reported documentation from the patient, as long as the information is approved and incorporated into the medical record by a clinician or provider.

✓4ᵗʰ **Z55**   Problems related to education and literacy
     EXCLUDES 1   disorders of psychological development (F80-F89)
   Z55.0   Illiteracy and low-level literacy   UPD PE
   Z55.1   Schooling unavailable and unattainable   UPD PE
   Z55.2   Failed school examinations   UPD PE
   Z55.3   Underachievement in school   UPD PE
   Z55.4   Educational maladjustment and discord with teachers and classmates   UPD PE
   Z55.5   Less than a high school diploma   UPD PE
     No general equivalence degree (GED)
   Z55.6   Problems related to health literacy   UPD PE
     Difficulty understanding health related information
     Difficulty understanding medication instructions
     Problem completing medical forms
     AHA: 2023,1Q,6
   Z55.8   Other problems related to education and literacy   UPD PE
     Problems related to inadequate teaching
   Z55.9   Problems related to education and literacy, unspecified   UPD PE
     Academic problems NOS

✓4ᵗʰ **Z56**   Problems related to employment and unemployment
     EXCLUDES 2   occupational exposure to risk factors (Z57.-)
        problems related to housing and economic circumstances (Z59.-)
   Z56.0   Unemployment, unspecified   UPD PE
   Z56.1   Change of job   UPD A PE
   Z56.2   Threat of job loss   UPD PE
   Z56.3   Stressful work schedule   UPD PE
   Z56.4   Discord with boss and workmates   UPD PE
   Z56.5   Uncongenial work environment   UPD PE
     Difficult conditions at work
   Z56.6   Other physical and mental strain related to work   UPD PE
   ✓5ᵗʰ **Z56.8**   Other problems related to employment
     Z56.81   Sexual harassment on the job   UPD PE

Z56.82   **Military deployment status**   UPD PE
Individual (civilian or military) currently deployed in theater or in support of military war, peacekeeping and humanitarian operations

Z56.89   **Other problems related to employment**   UPD PE

Z56.9   **Unspecified problems related to employment**   UPD PE
Occupational problems NOS

✓4ᵗʰ **Z57**   **Occupational exposure to risk factors**

Z57.0   **Occupational exposure to noise**   UPD PE

Z57.1   **Occupational exposure to radiation**   UPD PE

Z57.2   **Occupational exposure to dust**   UPD PE

✓5ᵗʰ **Z57.3**   **Occupational exposure to other air contaminants**

Z57.31   **Occupational exposure to environmental tobacco smoke**   UPD PE
EXCLUDES 2   *exposure to environmental tobacco smoke (Z77.22)*

Z57.39   **Occupational exposure to other air contaminants**   UPD PE

Z57.4   **Occupational exposure to toxic agents in agriculture**   UPD PE
Occupational exposure to solids, liquids, gases or vapors in agriculture

Z57.5   **Occupational exposure to toxic agents in other industries**   UPD PE
Occupational exposure to solids, liquids, gases or vapors in other industries

Z57.6   **Occupational exposure to extreme temperature**   UPD PE

Z57.7   **Occupational exposure to vibration**   UPD PE

Z57.8   **Occupational exposure to other risk factors**   UPD PE

Z57.9   **Occupational exposure to unspecified risk factor**   UPD PE

✓4ᵗʰ **Z58**   **Problems related to physical environment**   ▲
EXCLUDES 2   *occupational exposure (Z57.-)*

Z58.6   **Inadequate drinking-water supply**   UPD PE   ●
Lack of safe drinking water
EXCLUDES 2   *deprivation of water (T73.1)*

✓5ᵗʰ **Z58.8**   **Other problems related to physical environment**
AHA: 2023,1Q,6

Z58.81   **Basic services unavailable in physical environment**   UPD PE   ●
Unable to obtain internet service, due to unavailability in geographic area
Unable to obtain telephone service, due to unavailability in geographic area
Unable to obtain utilities, due to inadequate physical environment

Z58.89   **Other problems related to physical environment**   UPD PE

✓4ᵗʰ **Z59**   **Problems related to housing and economic circumstances**
EXCLUDES 2   *problems related to upbringing (Z62.-)*

✓5ᵗʰ **Z59.0**   **Homelessness**

Z59.00   **Homelessness unspecified**   CC UPD PE

Z59.01   **Sheltered homelessness**   CC UPD PE
Doubled up
Living in a shelter such as: motel, scattered site housing, temporary or transitional living situation

Z59.02   **Unsheltered homelessness**   CC UPD PE
Residing in place not meant for human habitation such as: abandoned buildings, cars, parks, sidewalk
Residing on the street

✓5ᵗʰ **Z59.1**   **Inadequate housing**
EXCLUDES 1   *problems related to the natural and physical environment (Z77.1-)*
EXCLUDES 2   ▶*problems related to the natural and physical environment (Z77.1-)*◀
AHA: 2023,1Q,6

Z59.10   **Inadequate housing, unspecified**   UPD PE
Inadequate housing NOS

Z59.11   **Inadequate housing environmental temperature**   UPD PE
Lack of air conditioning
Lack of heating

Z59.12   **Inadequate housing utilities**   UPD PE
Lack of electricity services
Lack of gas services
Lack of oil services
Lack of water services
EXCLUDES 2   *basic services unavailable in physical environment (Z58.81)*
lack of adequate food (Z59.4-)
other problems related to housing and economic circumstances (Z59.8-)

Z59.19   **Other inadequate housing**   UPD PE
Pest infestation
Restriction of space
Technical defects in home preventing adequate care
Unsatisfactory surroundings

Z59.2   **Discord with neighbors, lodgers and landlord**   UPD PE

Z59.3   **Problems related to living in residential institution**   UPD PE
Boarding-school resident
EXCLUDES 1   *institutional upbringing (Z62.22)*

✓5ᵗʰ **Z59.4**   **Lack of adequate food**
EXCLUDES 2   *deprivation of food (T73.0)*
effects of hunger (T73.0)
inappropriate diet or eating habits (Z72.4)
malnutrition (E40-E46)

Z59.41   **Food insecurity**   UPD PE

Z59.48   **Other specified lack of adequate food**   UPD PE
Inadequate food
Lack of food

Z59.5   **Extreme poverty**   UPD PE

Z59.6   **Low income**   UPD PE

✓5ᵗʰ **Z59.7**   **Insufficient social insurance and welfare support**
▶Insufficient social and welfare insurance◀

Z59.71   **Insufficient health insurance coverage**   UPD PE
Inadequate social insurance
Insufficient social insurance
No health insurance coverage

Z59.72   **Insufficient welfare support**   UPD PE
Inadequate welfare support

✓5ᵗʰ **Z59.8**   **Other problems related to housing and economic circumstances**
AHA: 2022,4Q,52

✓6ᵗʰ **Z59.81**   **Housing instability, housed**
Foreclosure on home loan
Past due on rent or mortgage
Unwanted multiple moves in the last 12 months

Z59.811   **Housing instability, housed, with risk of homelessness**   UPD PE
Imminent risk of homelessness

Z59.812   **Housing instability, housed, homelessness in past 12 months**   UPD PE

Z59.819   **Housing instability, housed unspecified**   UPD PE
EXCLUDES 2   *extreme poverty (Z59.5)*
financial insecurity (Z59.86)
low income (Z59.6)
material hardship due to limited financial resources, not elsewhere classified (Z59.87)

Z59.82   **Transportation insecurity**   UPD PE
Excessive transportation time
Inaccessible transportation
Inadequate transportation
Lack of transportation
Unaffordable transportation
Unreliable transportation
Unsafe transportation
EXCLUDES 2   *unavailability and inaccessibility of healthcare facilities (Z75.3)*

Z59.86–Z62.831   **Chapter 21. Factors Influencing Health Status and Contact With Health Services**   **ICD-10-CM 2025**

Chapter 21. Factors Influencing Health Status and Contact With Health Services

Z59.86–Z62.831

Z59.86   **Financial insecurity** `UPD` `PE`
- Bankruptcy
- Burdensome debt
- Economic strain
- Financial strain
- Money problems
- Running out of money
- Unable to make ends meet
  - **EXCLUDES 2**   *extreme poverty (Z59.5)*
    - *low income (Z59.6)*
    - *material hardship, not elsewhere classified (Z59.87)*

Z59.87   **Material hardship due to limited financial resources, not elsewhere classified** `UPD` `PE`
- Material deprivation due to limited financial resources
- Unable to obtain adequate childcare due to limited financial resources
- Unable to obtain adequate clothing due to limited financial resources
- Unable to obtain adequate utilities due to limited financial resources
- Unable to obtain basic needs due to limited financial resources
  - **EXCLUDES 2**   *extreme poverty (Z59.5)*
    - *financial insecurity, not elsewhere classified (Z59.86)*
    - *low income (Z59.6)*

Z59.89   **Other problems related to housing and economic circumstances** `UPD` `PE`
- Foreclosure on loan
- Isolated dwelling
- Problems with creditors

Z59.9   **Problem related to housing and economic circumstances, unspecified** `UPD` `PE`

√4ᵗʰ **Z60**   **Problems related to social environment**

Z60.0   **Problems of adjustment to life-cycle transitions** `UPD`
- Empty nest syndrome
- Phase of life problem
- Problem with adjustment to retirement [pension]

Z60.2   **Problems related to living alone** `UPD`

Z60.3   **Acculturation difficulty** `UPD`
- Problem with migration
- Problem with social transplantation
- **DEF:** Problem adapting to a different culture or environment not based on any coexisting mental disorder.

Z60.4   **Social exclusion and rejection** `UPD`
- Exclusion and rejection on the basis of personal characteristics, such as unusual physical appearance, illness or behavior.
- Social isolation
  - **EXCLUDES 1**   *target of adverse discrimination such as for racial or religious reasons (Z60.5)*

Z60.5   **Target of (perceived) adverse discrimination and persecution** `UPD`
- **EXCLUDES 1**   *social exclusion and rejection (Z60.4)*

Z60.8   **Other problems related to social environment** `UPD`
- Inadequate social support
- Lack of emotional support

Z60.9   **Problem related to social environment, unspecified** `UPD`

√4ᵗʰ **Z62**   **Problems related to upbringing**
- **INCLUDES**   current and past negative life events in childhood
  - current and past problems of a child related to upbringing
- **EXCLUDES 2**   *maltreatment syndrome (T74.-)*
  - *problems related to housing and economic circumstances (Z59.-)*

Z62.0   **Inadequate parental supervision and control** `UPD` `PE`

Z62.1   **Parental overprotection** `UPD` `PE`

√5ᵗʰ **Z62.2**   **Upbringing away from parents**
- **EXCLUDES 1**   *problems with boarding school (Z59.3)*
- **AHA:** 2023,4Q,49

Z62.21   **Child in welfare custody** `UPD` `P` `PE`
- Child in foster care
- Child in welfare guardianship

Z62.22   **Institutional upbringing** `UPD` `PE`
- Child living in group home
- Child living in orphanage
- Code also, if applicable, child in welfare custody (Z62.21)

Z62.23   **Child in custody of non-parental relative** `UPD` `P` `PE`
- Child in care of non-parental family member
- Child in custody of grandparent
- Child in kinship care
- Guardianship by non-parental relative
- Code also, if applicable, child in welfare custody (Z62.21)

Z62.24   **Child in custody of non-relative guardian** `UPD` `P` `PE`
- Code also, if applicable, child in welfare custody (Z62.21)

Z62.29   **Other upbringing away from parents** `UPD` `PE`

Z62.3   **Hostility towards and scapegoating of child** `UPD` `P` `PE`

Z62.6   **Inappropriate (excessive) parental pressure** `UPD` `PE`

√5ᵗʰ **Z62.8**   **Other specified problems related to upbringing**
- Code also, if applicable:
  - absence of family member (Z63.3-)
  - disappearance and death of family member (Z63.4)
  - disruption of family by separation and divorce (Z63.5)
  - other specified problems related to primary support group (Z63.8)
  - other stressful life events affecting family and household (Z63.7-)

√6ᵗʰ **Z62.81**   **Personal history of abuse in childhood**
- Personal history of abuse in adolescence
- **AHA:** 2023,1Q,6

Z62.810   **Personal history of physical and sexual abuse in childhood** `UPD` `PE`
- **EXCLUDES 1**   *current child physical abuse (T74.12, T76.12)*
  - *current child sexual abuse (T74.22, T76.22)*

Z62.811   **Personal history of psychological abuse in childhood** `UPD`
- **EXCLUDES 1**   *current child psychological abuse (T74.32, T76.32)*

Z62.812   **Personal history of neglect in childhood** `UPD` `PE`
- **EXCLUDES 1**   *current child neglect (T74.02, T76.02)*

Z62.813   **Personal history of forced labor or sexual exploitation in childhood** `UPD` `PE`
- **AHA:** 2018,4Q,32,35

Z62.814   **Personal history of child financial abuse** `UPD` `PE`
- **EXCLUDES 1**   *current child financial abuse (T74.A2)*

Z62.815   **Personal history of intimate partner abuse in childhood** `UPD` `PE`
- **EXCLUDES 2**   *adult and child abuse, neglect and other maltreatment, confirmed (T74.-)*

Z62.819   **Personal history of unspecified abuse in childhood** `UPD` `PE`
- **EXCLUDES 1**   *current child abuse NOS (T74.92, T76.92)*

√6ᵗʰ **Z62.82**   **Parent-child conflict**
- **AHA:** 2023,4Q,49

Z62.820   **Parent-biological child conflict** `UPD` `PE`
- Parent-child problem NOS

Z62.821   **Parent-adopted child conflict** `UPD` `PE`

Z62.822   **Parent-foster child conflict** `UPD` `PE`

Z62.823   **Parent-step child conflict** `UPD` `PE`

√6ᵗʰ **Z62.83**   **Non-parental relative or guardian-child conflict**
- **AHA:** 2023,4Q,50

Z62.831   **Non-parental relative-child conflict** `UPD` `PE`
- Grandparent-child conflict
- Kinship-care child conflict
- Non-parental relative legal guardian-child conflict
- Other relative-child conflict
  - **EXCLUDES 1**   *group home staff-child conflict (Z62.833)*

`N` Newborn: 0   `P` Pediatric: 0-17   `M` Maternity: 9-64   `A` Adult: 15-124   `UNS` Unspecified Site   `MCC` Major Complication/Comorbidity   `CC` Complication/Comorbidity   `PE` POA Exempt

1280   ICD-10-CM 2025

Z62.832 **Non-relative guardian-child conflict** `UPD` `PE`
  EXCLUDES 1   *group home staff-child conflict (Z62.833)*

Z62.833 **Group home staff-child conflict** `UPD` `PE`

✓⁶ᵗʰ Z62.89 **Other specified problems related to upbringing**

Z62.890 **Parent-child estrangement NEC** `UPD` `PE`
Z62.891 **Sibling rivalry** `UPD` `PE`
Z62.892 **Runaway [from current living environment]** `UPD` `PE`
  Child leaving living situation without permission
  AHA: 2023,4Q,50

Z62.898 **Other specified problems related to upbringing** `UPD` `PE`

Z62.9 **Problem related to upbringing, unspecified** `UPD` `PE`

✓⁴ᵗʰ Z63 **Other problems related to primary support group, including family circumstances**
  EXCLUDES 2   *maltreatment syndrome (T74.-, T76)*
  parent-child problems (Z62.-)
  problems related to negative life events in childhood (Z62.-)
  problems related to upbringing (Z62.-)

Z63.0 **Problems in relationship with spouse or partner** `UPD` `PE`
  Relationship distress with spouse or intimate partner
  EXCLUDES 1   *counseling for spousal or partner abuse problems (Z69.1)*
  counseling related to sexual attitude, behavior, and orientation (Z70.-)

Z63.1 **Problems in relationship with in-laws** `UPD` `PE`

✓⁵ᵗʰ Z63.3 **Absence of family member**
  EXCLUDES 1   *absence of family member due to disappearance and death (Z63.4)*
  absence of family member due to separation and divorce (Z63.5)

Z63.31 **Absence of family member due to military deployment** `UPD` `PE`
  Individual or family affected by other family member being on military deployment
  EXCLUDES 1   *family disruption due to return of family member from military deployment (Z63.71)*

Z63.32 **Other absence of family member** `UPD` `PE`

Z63.4 **Disappearance and death of family member** `UPD` `PE`
  Assumed death of family member
  Bereavement
  AHA: 2014,1Q,25

Z63.5 **Disruption of family by separation and divorce** `UPD` `PE`
  Marital estrangement

Z63.6 **Dependent relative needing care at home** `UPD` `PE`

✓⁵ᵗʰ Z63.7 **Other stressful life events affecting family and household**

Z63.71 **Stress on family due to return of family member from military deployment** `UPD` `PE`
  Individual or family affected by family member having returned from military deployment (current or past conflict)

Z63.72 **Alcoholism and drug addiction in family** `UPD` `PE`

Z63.79 **Other stressful life events affecting family and household** `UPD` `PE`
  Anxiety (normal) about sick person in family
  Health problems within family
  Ill or disturbed family member
  Isolated family

Z63.8 **Other specified problems related to primary support group** `UPD` `PE`
  Family discord NOS
  Family estrangement NOS
  High expressed emotional level within family
  Inadequate family support NOS
  Inadequate or distorted communication within family

Z63.9 **Problem related to primary support group, unspecified** `UPD` `PE`
  Relationship disorder NOS

✓⁴ᵗʰ Z64 **Problems related to certain psychosocial circumstances**

Z64.0 **Problems related to unwanted pregnancy** `UPD` `PE`
Z64.1 **Problems related to multiparity** `UPD` `PE`

Z64.4 **Discord with counselors** `UPD` `PE`
  Discord with probation officer
  Discord with social worker

✓⁴ᵗʰ Z65 **Problems related to other psychosocial circumstances**

Z65.0 **Conviction in civil and criminal proceedings without imprisonment** `UPD` `PE`

Z65.1 **Imprisonment and other incarceration** `UPD` `PE`

Z65.2 **Problems related to release from prison** `UPD` `PE`

Z65.3 **Problems related to other legal circumstances** `UPD` `PE`
  Arrest
  Child custody or support proceedings
  Litigation
  Prosecution

Z65.4 **Victim of crime and terrorism** `UPD` `PE`
  Victim of torture

Z65.5 **Exposure to disaster, war and other hostilities** `UPD` `PE`
  EXCLUDES 1   *target of perceived discrimination or persecution (Z60.5)*

Z65.8 **Other specified problems related to psychosocial circumstances** `UPD` `PE`
  At risk for feeling loneliness
  Religious or spiritual problem

Z65.9 **Problem related to unspecified psychosocial circumstances** `UPD` `PE`

Do not resuscitate status (Z66)

Z66 **Do not resuscitate** `UPD`
  DNR status
  DEF: Medical order written by a physician that instructs others not to perform cardiopulmonary resuscitation (CPR), intubation, or advanced cardiac life support (ACLS). It prevents unnecessary invasive treatment to prolong life should breathing stop or cardiac arrest occur.

Blood type (Z67)

✓⁴ᵗʰ Z67 **Blood type**
  AHA: 2015,3Q,40

✓⁵ᵗʰ Z67.1 **Type A blood**
Z67.10 **Type A blood, Rh positive** `UPD` `PE`
Z67.11 **Type A blood, Rh negative** `UPD` `PE`

✓⁵ᵗʰ Z67.2 **Type B blood**
Z67.20 **Type B blood, Rh positive** `UPD` `PE`
Z67.21 **Type B blood, Rh negative** `UPD` `PE`

✓⁵ᵗʰ Z67.3 **Type AB blood**
Z67.30 **Type AB blood, Rh positive** `UPD` `PE`
Z67.31 **Type AB blood, Rh negative** `UPD` `PE`

✓⁵ᵗʰ Z67.4 **Type O blood**
Z67.40 **Type O blood, Rh positive** `UPD` `PE`
Z67.41 **Type O blood, Rh negative** `UPD` `PE`

✓⁵ᵗʰ Z67.9 **Unspecified blood type**
Z67.90 **Unspecified blood type, Rh positive** `UPD` `PE`
Z67.91 **Unspecified blood type, Rh negative** `UPD` `PE`

✓⁵ᵗʰ Z67.A **Duffy phenotype**
Z67.A1 **Duffy null** `UPD` `PE`
  Duffy phenotype Fy(a-b-)
Z67.A2 **Duffy a positive** `UPD` `PE`
  Duffy phenotype Fy(a+b-)
Z67.A3 **Duffy b positive** `UPD` `PE`
  Duffy phenotype Fy(a-b+)
Z67.A4 **Duffy a and b positive** `UPD` `PE`
  Duffy phenotype Fy(a+b+)

☑ Additional Character Required   ✓ₓ⁷ᵗʰ Placeholder   Questionable PDx   Manifestation   Unspecified   `UPD` Unacceptable PDx   H1-H14 HAC   HCC CMS-HCC Dx   HIV HIV Dx

ICD-10-CM 2025   1281

Body mass index [BMI] (Z68)

√4th **Z68   Body mass index [BMI]**

Kilograms per meters squared

NOTE   BMI adult codes are for use for persons 20 years of age or older

BMI pediatric codes are for use for persons 2-19 years of age.

These percentiles are based on the growth charts published by the Centers for Disease Control and Prevention (CDC)

AHA: 2022,3Q,6; 2019,4Q,19,57; 2018,4Q,73,77-83; 2017,1Q,39
DEF: Index used to help determine whether an individual is underweight, a healthy weight, overweight, or obese.
TIP: Do not assign when used in association with fluctuations in body fluid during an encounter, such as fluid overload or fluid retention, or during pregnancy.
TIP: A BMI code may be assigned based on medical record documentation from clinicians who are not the patient's provider. However, the BMI must be associated with a condition that meets the definition of a reportable diagnosis, per the ICD-10-CM Official Guidelines for Coding and Reporting, and that condition can only be reported when documented by the patient's provider.

Z68.1   Body mass index [BMI] 19.9 or less, adult   CC UPD A PE

√5th **Z68.2   Body mass index [BMI] 20-29, adult**

Z68.20   Body mass index [BMI] 20.0-20.9, adult   UPD A PE
Z68.21   Body mass index [BMI] 21.0-21.9, adult   UPD A PE
Z68.22   Body mass index [BMI] 22.0-22.9, adult   UPD A PE
Z68.23   Body mass index [BMI] 23.0-23.9, adult   UPD A PE
Z68.24   Body mass index [BMI] 24.0-24.9, adult   UPD A PE
Z68.25   Body mass index [BMI] 25.0-25.9, adult   UPD A PE
Z68.26   Body mass index [BMI] 26.0-26.9, adult   UPD A PE
Z68.27   Body mass index [BMI] 27.0-27.9, adult   UPD A PE
Z68.28   Body mass index [BMI] 28.0-28.9, adult   UPD A PE
Z68.29   Body mass index [BMI] 29.0-29.9, adult   UPD A PE

√5th **Z68.3   Body mass index [BMI] 30-39, adult**

Z68.30   Body mass index [BMI] 30.0-30.9, adult   UPD A PE
Z68.31   Body mass index [BMI] 31.0-31.9, adult   UPD A PE
Z68.32   Body mass index [BMI] 32.0-32.9, adult   UPD A PE
Z68.33   Body mass index [BMI] 33.0-33.9, adult   UPD A PE
Z68.34   Body mass index [BMI] 34.0-34.9, adult   UPD A PE
Z68.35   Body mass index [BMI] 35.0-35.9, adult   UPD A PE
Z68.36   Body mass index [BMI] 36.0-36.9, adult   UPD A PE
Z68.37   Body mass index [BMI] 37.0-37.9, adult   UPD A PE
Z68.38   Body mass index [BMI] 38.0-38.9, adult   UPD A PE
Z68.39   Body mass index [BMI] 39.0-39.9, adult   UPD A PE

√5th **Z68.4   Body mass index [BMI] 40 or greater, adult**

Z68.41   Body mass index [BMI] 40.0-44.9, adult   CC UPD HCC A PE
Z68.42   Body mass index [BMI] 45.0-49.9, adult   CC UPD HCC A PE
Z68.43   Body mass index [BMI] 50.0-59.9, adult   CC UPD HCC A PE
Z68.44   Body mass index [BMI] 60.0-69.9, adult   CC UPD HCC A PE
Z68.45   Body mass index [BMI] 70 or greater, adult   CC UPD HCC A PE

√5th **Z68.5   Body mass index [BMI] pediatric**

AHA: 2018,4Q,81-82

Z68.51   Body mass index [BMI] pediatric, less than 5th percentile for age   UPD PE
Z68.52   Body mass index [BMI] pediatric, 5th percentile to less than 85th percentile for age   UPD PE
Z68.53   Body mass index [BMI] pediatric, 85th percentile to less than 95th percentile for age   UPD PE
▲ **Z68.54   Body mass index [BMI] pediatric, 95th percentile for age to less than 120% of the 95th percentile for age**   UPD PE
● **Z68.55   Body mass index [BMI] pediatric, 120% of the 95th percentile for age to less than 140% of the 95th percentile for age**   CC UPD PE
● **Z68.56   Body mass index [BMI] pediatric, greater than or equal to 140% of the 95th percentile for age**   CC UPD PE

Persons encountering health services in other circumstances (Z69-Z76)

√4th **Z69   Encounter for mental health services for victim and perpetrator of abuse**

INCLUDES   counseling for victims and perpetrators of abuse

√5th **Z69.0   Encounter for mental health services for child abuse problems**

√6th **Z69.01   Encounter for mental health services for parental child abuse**

Z69.010   Encounter for mental health services for victim of parental child abuse   P PE
Encounter for mental health services for victim of child abuse by parent
Encounter for mental health services for victim of child neglect by parent
Encounter for mental health services for victim of child psychological abuse by parent
Encounter for mental health services for victim of child sexual abuse by parent

Z69.011   Encounter for mental health services for perpetrator of parental child abuse   UPD PE
Encounter for mental health services for perpetrator of parental child neglect
Encounter for mental health services for perpetrator of parental child psychological abuse
Encounter for mental health services for perpetrator of parental child sexual abuse

EXCLUDES 1   encounter for mental health services for non-parental child abuse (Z69.02-)

√6th **Z69.02   Encounter for mental health services for non-parental child abuse**

Z69.020   Encounter for mental health services for victim of non-parental child abuse   P PE
Encounter for mental health services for victim of non-parental child neglect
Encounter for mental health services for victim of non-parental child psychological abuse
Encounter for mental health services for victim of non-parental child sexual abuse

Z69.021   Encounter for mental health services for perpetrator of non-parental child abuse   UPD PE
Encounter for mental health services for perpetrator of non-parental child neglect
Encounter for mental health services for perpetrator of non-parental child psychological abuse
Encounter for mental health services for perpetrator of non-parental child sexual abuse

√5th **Z69.1   Encounter for mental health services for spousal or partner abuse problems**

Z69.11   Encounter for mental health services for victim of spousal or partner abuse   UPD PE
Encounter for mental health services for victim of spouse or partner neglect
Encounter for mental health services for victim of spouse or partner psychological abuse
Encounter for mental health services for victim of spouse or partner violence, physical

Z69.12   Encounter for mental health services for perpetrator of spousal or partner abuse   UPD PE
Encounter for mental health services for perpetrator of spouse or partner neglect
Encounter for mental health services for perpetrator of spouse or partner psychological abuse
Encounter for mental health services for perpetrator of spouse or partner violence, physical
Encounter for mental health services for perpetrator of spouse or partner violence, sexual

√5ᵗʰ Z69.8 Encounter for mental health services for victim or perpetrator of other abuse

Z69.81 Encounter for mental health services for victim of other abuse `UPD` `PE`

Encounter for mental health services for victim of non-spousal adult abuse

Encounter for mental health services for victim of spouse or partner violence, sexual

Encounter for rape victim counseling

Z69.82 Encounter for mental health services for perpetrator of other abuse `UPD` `PE`

Encounter for mental health services for perpetrator of non-spousal adult abuse

√4ᵗʰ Z70 Counseling related to sexual attitude, behavior and orientation

INCLUDES encounter for mental health services for sexual attitude, behavior and orientation

EXCLUDES 2 contraceptive or procreative counseling (Z30-Z31)

Z70.0 Counseling related to sexual attitude `UPD` `PE`

Z70.1 Counseling related to patient's sexual behavior and orientation `UPD` `PE`

Patient concerned regarding impotence

Patient concerned regarding non-responsiveness

Patient concerned regarding promiscuity

Patient concerned regarding sexual orientation

Z70.2 Counseling related to sexual behavior and orientation of third party `UPD` `PE`

Advice sought regarding sexual behavior and orientation of child

Advice sought regarding sexual behavior and orientation of partner

Advice sought regarding sexual behavior and orientation of spouse

Z70.3 Counseling related to combined concerns regarding sexual attitude, behavior and orientation `UPD` `PE`

Z70.8 Other sex counseling `UPD` `PE`

Encounter for sex education

Z70.9 Sex counseling, unspecified `UPD` `PE`

√4ᵗʰ Z71 Persons encountering health services for other counseling and medical advice, not elsewhere classified

EXCLUDES 2 contraceptive or procreation counseling (Z30-Z31)

sex counseling (Z70.-)

Z71.0 Person encountering health services to consult on behalf of another person `UPD` `PE`

Person encountering health services to seek advice or treatment for non-attending third party

EXCLUDES 2 anxiety (normal) about sick person in family (Z63.7)

expectant (adoptive) parent(s) pre-birth pediatrician visit (Z76.81)

Z71.1 Person with feared health complaint in whom no diagnosis is made `UPD` `PE`

Person encountering health services with feared condition which was not demonstrated

Person encountering health services in which problem was normal state

"Worried well"

EXCLUDES 1 medical observation for suspected diseases and conditions proven not to exist (Z03.-)

Z71.2 Person consulting for explanation of examination or test findings `UPD` `PE`

Z71.3 Dietary counseling and surveillance `UPD` `PE`

Use additional code for any associated underlying medical condition

Use additional code to identify body mass index (BMI), if known (Z68.-)

√5ᵗʰ Z71.4 Alcohol abuse counseling and surveillance

Use additional code for alcohol abuse or dependence (F10.-)

Z71.41 Alcohol abuse counseling and surveillance of alcoholic `UPD` `PE`

Z71.42 Counseling for family member of alcoholic `UPD` `PE`

Counseling for significant other, partner, or friend of alcoholic

√5ᵗʰ Z71.5 Drug abuse counseling and surveillance

Use additional code for drug abuse or dependence (F11-F16, F18-F19)

Z71.51 Drug abuse counseling and surveillance of drug abuser `UPD` `PE`

Z71.52 Counseling for family member of drug abuser `UPD` `PE`

Counseling for significant other, partner, or friend of drug abuser

Z71.6 Tobacco abuse counseling `UPD` `PE`

Use additional code for nicotine dependence (F17.-)

Z71.7 Human immunodeficiency virus [HIV] counseling `UPD` `PE`

√5ᵗʰ Z71.8 Other specified counseling

EXCLUDES 2 counseling for contraception (Z30.0-)

AHA: 2017,4Q,27

Z71.81 Spiritual or religious counseling `UPD` `PE`

Z71.82 Exercise counseling `UPD` `PE`

Z71.83 Encounter for nonprocreative genetic counseling `PE`

EXCLUDES 1 counseling for procreative genetics (Z31.5)

counseling for procreative management (Z31.6)

Z71.84 Encounter for health counseling related to travel `UPD` `PE`

Encounter for health risk and safety counseling for (international) travel

Code also, if applicable, encounter for immunization (Z23)

EXCLUDES 2 encounter for administrative examination (Z02.-)

encounter for other special examination without complaint, suspected or reported diagnosis (Z01.-)

AHA: 2019,4Q,20,57

Z71.85 Encounter for immunization safety counseling `UPD` `PE`

Encounter for vaccine product safety counseling

Code also, if applicable, encounter for immunization (Z23)

Code also, if applicable, immunization not carried out (Z28.-)

EXCLUDES 1 encounter for health counseling related to travel (Z71.84)

AHA: 2021,4Q,34

Z71.87 Encounter for pediatric-to-adult transition counseling `UPD` `PE`

Code also chronic condition, if applicable, such as:

autism spectrum disorder (F84.0)

congenital malformations of the circulatory system (Q20-Q28)

cystic fibrosis (E84-)

sickle-cell disorder (D57-)

AHA: 2022,4Q,51

Z71.88 Encounter for counseling for socioeconomic factors `UPD` `PE`

AHA: 2022,4Q,51

Z71.89 Other specified counseling `UPD` `PE`

Z71.9 Counseling, unspecified `UPD` `PE`

Encounter for medical advice NOS

√4ᵗʰ Z72 Problems related to lifestyle

EXCLUDES 2 problems related to life-management difficulty (Z73.-)

problems related to socioeconomic and psychosocial circumstances (Z55-Z65)

Z72.0 Tobacco use `UPD` `PE`

Tobacco use NOS

EXCLUDES 1 history of tobacco dependence (Z87.891)

nicotine dependence (F17.2-)

tobacco dependence (F17.2-)

tobacco use during pregnancy (O99.33-)

Z72.3 Lack of physical exercise `UPD` `PE`

Z72.4 Inappropriate diet and eating habits `UPD` `PE`

EXCLUDES 1 behavioral eating disorders of infancy or childhood (F98.2-F98.3)

eating disorders (F50.-)

lack of adequate food (Z59.48)

malnutrition and other nutritional deficiencies (E40-E64)

✔ Additional Character Required   √x7ᵗʰ Placeholder   Questionable PDx   Manifestation   Unspecified   `UPD` Unacceptable PDx   H1-H14 HAC   HCC CMS-HCC Dx   HIV HIV Dx

Chapter 21. Factors Influencing Health Status and Contact With Health Services

Z72.5 **High risk sexual behavior** ✓5th
Promiscuity
EXCLUDES 1   *paraphilias (F65)*

   Z72.51   High risk **heterosexual** behavior   UPD PE
   Z72.52   High risk **homosexual** behavior   UPD PE
   Z72.53   High risk **bisexual** behavior   UPD PE

Z72.6 **Gambling and betting**   UPD PE
EXCLUDES 1   *compulsive or pathological gambling (F63.0)*

Z72.8 **Other problems related to lifestyle** ✓5th

   Z72.81 **Antisocial behavior** ✓6th
     EXCLUDES 1   *conduct disorders (F91.-)*

     Z72.810 **Child and adolescent** antisocial behavior   P PE
       Antisocial behavior (child) (adolescent) without manifest psychiatric disorder
       Delinquency NOS
       Group delinquency
       Offenses in the context of gang membership
       Stealing in company with others
       Truancy from school

     Z72.811 **Adult** antisocial behavior   A PE
       Adult antisocial behavior without manifest psychiatric disorder

   Z72.82 **Problems related to sleep** ✓6th

     Z72.820 **Sleep deprivation**   PE
       Lack of adequate sleep
       EXCLUDES 1   *insomnia (G47.0-)*

     Z72.821 **Inadequate** sleep hygiene   UPD PE
       Bad sleep habits
       Irregular sleep habits
       Unhealthy sleep wake schedule
       EXCLUDES 1   *insomnia (F51.0-, G47.0-)*

     Z72.823 **Risk of suffocation (smothering) under another while sleeping**   UPD
       Child-caregiver co-sleeping
       Infant bed-sharing
       AHA: 2022,4Q,51

   Z72.89 **Other problems related to lifestyle**   UPD PE
     Self-damaging behavior

Z72.9 **Problem related to lifestyle, unspecified**   UPD PE

Z73 **Problems related to life management difficulty** ✓4th
EXCLUDES 2   *problems related to socioeconomic and psychosocial circumstances (Z55-Z65)*
DEF: State of emotional, mental, and physical exhaustion causing difficulties in managing personal, school, or work circumstances. It is usually due to prolonged stress or poor interpersonal relationship skills or parenting skills.

Z73.0 **Burn-out**   UPD PE
Z73.1 **Type A behavior pattern**   UPD PE
Z73.2 **Lack of relaxation and leisure**   UPD PE
Z73.3 **Stress, not elsewhere classified**   UPD PE
   Physical and mental strain NOS
   EXCLUDES 1   *stress related to employment or unemployment (Z56.-)*
Z73.4 **Inadequate social skills, not elsewhere classified**   UPD PE
Z73.5 **Social role conflict, not elsewhere classified**   UPD PE
Z73.6 **Limitation of activities due to disability**   UPD PE
   EXCLUDES 1   *care-provider dependency (Z74.-)*
Z73.8 **Other problems related to life management difficulty** ✓5th

   Z73.81 **Behavioral insomnia of childhood** ✓6th
     DEF: Behaviors on the part of the child or caregivers that cause negative compliance with a child's sleep schedule resulting in lack of adequate sleep.

     Z73.810 **Behavioral insomnia of childhood, sleep-onset association** type   UPD P PE
     Z73.811 **Behavioral insomnia of childhood, limit setting** type   UPD P PE
     Z73.812 **Behavioral insomnia of childhood, combined** type   UPD P PE
     Z73.819 **Behavioral insomnia of childhood, unspecified** type   UPD P PE

   Z73.82 **Dual sensory impairment**   UPD PE
   Z73.89 **Other problems related to life management difficulty**   UPD PE

Z73.9 **Problem related to life management difficulty, unspecified**   UPD PE

Z74 **Problems related to care provider dependency** ✓4th
EXCLUDES 2   *dependence on enabling machines or devices NEC (Z99.-)*

Z74.0 **Reduced mobility** ✓5th

   Z74.01 **Bed confinement status**   UPD PE
     Bedridden

   Z74.09 **Other reduced mobility**   UPD
     Chair ridden
     Reduced mobility NOS
     EXCLUDES 2   *wheelchair dependence (Z99.3)*

Z74.1 **Need for assistance with personal care**   UPD
Z74.2 **Need for assistance at home and no other household member able to render care**   UPD
Z74.3 **Need for continuous supervision**   UPD
Z74.8 **Other problems related to care provider dependency**   UPD
Z74.9 **Problem related to care provider dependency, unspecified**   UPD

Z75 **Problems related to medical facilities and other health care** ✓4th

Z75.0 **Medical services not available in home**   UPD PE
   EXCLUDES 1   *no other household member able to render care (Z74.2)*
Z75.1 **Person awaiting admission to adequate facility elsewhere**
Z75.2 **Other waiting period for investigation and treatment**   UPD PE
Z75.3 **Unavailability and inaccessibility of health-care facilities**   UPD PE
   EXCLUDES 1   *bed unavailable (Z75.1)*
Z75.4 **Unavailability and inaccessibility of other helping agencies**   UPD PE
Z75.5 **Holiday relief care**
Z75.8 **Other problems related to medical facilities and other health care**   UPD PE
Z75.9 **Unspecified problem related to medical facilities and other health care**   UPD PE

Z76 **Persons encountering health services in other circumstances** ✓4th

Z76.0 **Encounter for issue of repeat prescription**   UPD PE
   Encounter for issue of repeat prescription for appliance
   Encounter for issue of repeat prescription for medicaments
   Encounter for issue of repeat prescription for spectacles
   EXCLUDES 2   *issue of medical certificate (Z02.7)*
     repeat prescription for contraceptive (Z30.4-)

Z76.1 **Encounter for health supervision and care of foundling**   PE
Z76.2 **Encounter for health supervision and care of other healthy infant and child**   UPD P PE
   Encounter for medical or nursing care or supervision of healthy infant under circumstances such as adverse socioeconomic conditions at home
   Encounter for medical or nursing care or supervision of healthy infant under circumstances such as awaiting foster or adoptive placement
   Encounter for medical or nursing care or supervision of healthy infant under circumstances such as maternal illness
   Encounter for medical or nursing care or supervision of healthy infant under circumstances such as number of children at home preventing or interfering with normal care

Z76.3 **Healthy person accompanying sick person**   PE
Z76.4 **Other boarder to healthcare facility**   PE
   EXCLUDES 1   *homelessness (Z59.0-)*
Z76.5 **Malingerer [conscious simulation]**   PE
   Person feigning illness (with obvious motivation)
   EXCLUDES 1   *factitious disorder (F68.1-, F68.A)*
     peregrinating patient (F68.1-)
   DEF: Act of intentionally exaggerating an illness or disability in order to receive personal gain or to avoid punishment or responsibility.

Z76.8 **Persons encountering health services in other specified circumstances** ✓5th

   Z76.81 **Expectant parent(s) prebirth pediatrician visit**   UPD PE
     Pre-adoption pediatrician visit for adoptive parent(s)
   Z76.82 **Awaiting organ transplant status**   UPD PE
     Patient waiting for organ availability
   Z76.89 **Persons encountering health services in other specified circumstances**   UPD PE
     Persons encountering health services NOS
     AHA: 2014,2Q,10

Persons with potential health hazards related to family and personal history and certain conditions influencing health status (Z77-Z99)

Code also any follow-up examination (Z08-Z09)

✓4ᵗʰ **Z77** **Other contact with and (suspected) exposures hazardous to health**

     [INCLUDES]   contact with and (suspected) exposures to potential hazards to health

     [EXCLUDES 2]   contact with and (suspected) exposure to communicable diseases (Z20.-)

       exposure to (parental) (environmental) tobacco smoke in the perinatal period (P96.81)

       newborn affected by noxious substances transmitted via placenta or breast milk (P04.-)

       occupational exposure to risk factors (Z57.-)

       retained foreign body (Z18.-)

       retained foreign body fully removed (Z87.821)

       toxic effects of substances chiefly nonmedicinal as to source (T51-T65)

✓5ᵗʰ **Z77.0** **Contact with and (suspected) exposure to hazardous, chiefly nonmedicinal, chemicals**

    ✓6ᵗʰ **Z77.01** **Contact with and (suspected) exposure to hazardous metals**

       Z77.010 **Contact with and (suspected) exposure to arsenic** [UPD]

       Z77.011 **Contact with and (suspected) exposure to lead** [UPD]

       Z77.012 **Contact with and (suspected) exposure to uranium** [UPD]

         [EXCLUDES 1]   retained depleted uranium fragments (Z18.01)

       Z77.018 **Contact with and (suspected) exposure to other hazardous metals** [UPD]

         Contact with and (suspected) exposure to chromium compounds

         Contact with and (suspected) exposure to nickel dust

    ✓6ᵗʰ **Z77.02** **Contact with and (suspected) exposure to hazardous aromatic compounds**

       Z77.020 **Contact with and (suspected) exposure to aromatic amines** [UPD]

       Z77.021 **Contact with and (suspected) exposure to benzene** [UPD]

       Z77.028 **Contact with and (suspected) exposure to other hazardous aromatic compounds** [UPD]

         Aromatic dyes NOS

         Polycyclic aromatic hydrocarbons

    ✓6ᵗʰ **Z77.09** **Contact with and (suspected) exposure to other hazardous, chiefly nonmedicinal, chemicals**

       Z77.090 **Contact with and (suspected) exposure to asbestos** [UPD]

       Z77.098 **Contact with and (suspected) exposure to other hazardous, chiefly nonmedicinal, chemicals** [UPD]

         Dyes NOS

✓5ᵗʰ **Z77.1** **Contact with and (suspected) exposure to environmental pollution and hazards in the physical environment**

    ✓6ᵗʰ **Z77.11** **Contact with and (suspected) exposure to environmental pollution**

       Z77.110 **Contact with and (suspected) exposure to air pollution** [UPD] [PE]

       Z77.111 **Contact with and (suspected) exposure to water pollution** [UPD] [PE]

       Z77.112 **Contact with and (suspected) exposure to soil pollution** [UPD] [PE]

       Z77.118 **Contact with and (suspected) exposure to other environmental pollution** [UPD] [PE]

    ✓6ᵗʰ **Z77.12** **Contact with and (suspected) exposure to hazards in the physical environment**

       Z77.120 **Contact with and (suspected) exposure to mold (toxic)** [UPD] [PE]

       Z77.121 **Contact with and (suspected) exposure to harmful algae and algae toxins** [UPD] [PE]

         Contact with and (suspected) exposure to (harmful) algae bloom NOS

         Contact with and (suspected) exposure to blue-green algae bloom

         Contact with and (suspected) exposure to brown tide

         Contact with and (suspected) exposure to cyanobacteria bloom

         Contact with and (suspected) exposure to Florida red tide

         Contact with and (suspected) exposure to pfiesteria piscicida

         Contact with and (suspected) exposure to red tide

       Z77.122 **Contact with and (suspected) exposure to noise** [UPD] [PE]

       Z77.123 **Contact with and (suspected) exposure to radon and other naturally occurring radiation** [UPD] [PE]

         [EXCLUDES 2]   radiation exposure as the cause of a confirmed condition (W88-W90, X39.0-)

           radiation sickness NOS (T66)

       Z77.128 **Contact with and (suspected) exposure to other hazards in the physical environment** [UPD] [PE]

✓5ᵗʰ **Z77.2** **Contact with and (suspected) exposure to other hazardous substances**

       Z77.21 **Contact with and (suspected) exposure to potentially hazardous body fluids** [UPD]

       Z77.22 **Contact with and (suspected) exposure to environmental tobacco smoke (acute) (chronic)** [UPD]

         Exposure to second hand tobacco smoke (acute) (chronic)

         Passive smoking (acute) (chronic)

         [EXCLUDES 1]   nicotine dependence (F17.-)

           tobacco use (Z72.0)

         [EXCLUDES 2]   occupational exposure to environmental tobacco smoke (Z57.31)

       Z77.29 **Contact with and (suspected) exposure to other hazardous substances** [UPD]

         AHA: 2016,2Q,33

   Z77.9 **Other contact with and (suspected) exposures hazardous to health** [UPD]

✓4ᵗʰ **Z78** **Other specified health status**

     [EXCLUDES 2]   asymptomatic human immunodeficiency virus [HIV] infection status (Z21)

       postprocedural status (Z93-Z99)

       sex reassignment status (Z87.890)

   Z78.0 **Asymptomatic menopausal state** [UPD] [A] [PE]

     Menopausal state NOS

     Postmenopausal status NOS

     [EXCLUDES 2]   symptomatic menopausal state (N95.1)

   Z78.1 **Physical restraint status** [UPD] [PE]

     [EXCLUDES 1]   physical restraint due to a procedure - omit code

     DEF: Application of mechanical restraining devices or manual restraints to limit physical mobility of a patient.

   Z78.9 **Other specified health status** [UPD] [PE]

✓4ᵗʰ **Z79** **Long term (current) drug therapy**

     [INCLUDES]   long term (current) drug use for prophylactic purposes

     Code also any therapeutic drug level monitoring (Z51.81)

     [EXCLUDES 2]   drug abuse and dependence (F11-F19)

       drug use complicating pregnancy, childbirth, and the puerperium (O99.32-)

   AHA: 2024,2Q,26; 2021,1Q,12

✓5ᵗʰ **Z79.0** **Long term (current) use of anticoagulants and antithrombotics/antiplatelets**

     [EXCLUDES 2]   long term (current) use of aspirin (Z79.82)

       Z79.01 **Long term (current) use of anticoagulants** [PE]

         AHA: 2023,2Q,28; 2022,2Q,17; 2021,1Q,4; 2020,2Q,20

       Z79.02 **Long term (current) use of antithrombotics/antiplatelets** [UPD] [PE]

✅ Additional Character Required   ✓x7ᵗʰ Placeholder   Questionable PDx   Manifestation   Unspecified   [UPD] Unacceptable PDx   H1-H14 HAC   HCC CMS-HCC Dx   HIV HIV Dx

ICD-10-CM 2025   **1285**

Chapter 21. Factors Influencing Health Status and Contact With Health Services

Z79.1 Long term (current) use of **non-steroidal anti-inflammatories (NSAID)** `UPD` `PE`
    EXCLUDES 2   *long term (current) use of aspirin (Z79.82)*

Z79.2 Long term (current) use of **antibiotics** `UPD` `PE`

Z79.3 Long term (current) use of **hormonal contraceptives** `PE`
    Long term (current) use of birth control pill or patch

Z79.4 Long term (current) use of **insulin** `HCC` `PE`
    EXCLUDES 2   *long-term (current) use of injectable non-insulin antidiabetic drugs (Z79.85)*
       long term (current) use of oral antidiabetic drugs (Z79.84)
       long term (current) use of oral hypoglycemic drugs (Z79.84)
    AHA: 2020,3Q,31

✓5ᵗʰ **Z79.5** Long term (current) use of steroids

    Z79.51 Long term (current) use of **inhaled steroids** `UPD` `PE`

    Z79.52 Long term (current) use of **systemic steroids** `UPD` `PE`

✓5ᵗʰ **Z79.6** Long term (current) use of immunomodulators and immunosuppressants
    EXCLUDES 2   *long term (current) use of steroids (Z79.5-)*
       long term (current) use of agents affecting estrogen receptors and estrogen levels (Z79.81-)
    AHA: 2022,4Q,50

    Z79.60 Long term (current) use of unspecified immunomodulators and immunosuppressants `UPD` `PE`

    Z79.61 Long term (current) use of **immunomodulator** `UPD` `PE`
       Long term (current) use of apremilast
       Long term (current) use of immunomodulatory imide drug
       Long term (current) use of lenalidomide
       Long term (current) use of pomalidomide

✓6ᵗʰ   **Z79.62** Long term (current) use of **immunosuppressant**

       Z79.620 Long term (current) use of **immunosuppressive biologic** `UPD` `PE`
          Long term (current) use of adalimumab
          Long term (current) use of etanercept
          Long term (current) use of infliximab
          Long term (current) use of monoclonal antibodies

       Z79.621 Long term (current) use of **calcineurin inhibitor** `UPD` `PE`
          Long term (current) use of cyclosporine
          Long term (current) use of tacrolimus

       Z79.622 Long term (current) use of **Janus kinase inhibitor** `UPD` `PE`
          Long term (current) use of tofacitinib

       Z79.623 Long term (current) use of **mammalian target of rapamycin (mTOR) inhibitor** `UPD` `PE`
          Long term (current) use of sirolimus

       Z79.624 Long term (current) use of **inhibitors of nucleotide synthesis** `UPD` `PE`
          Long term (current) use of azathioprine
          ►Long term (current) use of mycophenolate◄
          Long term (current) use of purine synthesis (IMDH) inhibitors

✓6ᵗʰ   **Z79.63** Long term (current) use of **chemotherapeutic agent**

       Z79.630 Long term (current) use of **alkylating agent** `UPD` `PE`
          Long term (current) use of chlorambucil
          Long term (current) use of cisplatin
          Long term (current) use of cyclophosphamide

       Z79.631 Long term (current) use of **antimetabolite agent** `UPD` `PE`
          Long term (current) use of 5-fluorouracil
          Long term (current) use of 6-mercaptopurine
          Long term (current) use of cytarabine
          Long term (current) use of methotrexate

       Z79.632 Long term (current) use of **antitumor antibiotic** `UPD` `PE`
          Long term (current) use of bleomycin
          Long term (current) use of doxorubicin
          Long term (current) use of mitomycin C

       Z79.633 Long term (current) use of **mitotic inhibitor** `UPD` `PE`
          Long term (current) use of paclitaxel
          Long term (current) use of plant alkaloids
          Long term (current) use of vinblastine
          Long term (current) use of vincristine

       Z79.634 Long term (current) use of **topoisomerase inhibitor** `UPD` `PE`
          Long term (current) use of etoposide
          Long term (current) use of irinotecan
          Long term (current) use of topotecan

    Z79.64 Long term (current) use of **myelosuppressive agent** `UPD` `PE`
       Long term (current) use of hydroxyurea

    Z79.69 Long term (current) use of other immunomodulators and immunosuppressants `UPD` `PE`

✓5ᵗʰ **Z79.8** Other long term (current) drug therapy

✓6ᵗʰ   **Z79.81** Long term (current) use of agents affecting estrogen receptors and estrogen levels
    Code first, if applicable:
       malignant neoplasm of breast (C50.-)
       malignant neoplasm of prostate (C61)
    Use additional code, if applicable, to identify:
       estrogen receptor positive status (Z17.0)
       family history of breast cancer (Z80.3)
       genetic susceptibility to malignant neoplasm (cancer) (Z15.0-)
       personal history of breast cancer (Z85.3)
       personal history of prostate cancer (Z85.46)
       postmenopausal status (Z78.0)
    EXCLUDES 1   *hormone replacement therapy (Z79.890)*
    AHA: 2022,3Q,14

       Z79.810 Long term (current) use of **selective estrogen receptor modulators (SERMs)** `UPD` `PE`
          Long term (current) use of raloxifene (Evista)
          Long term (current) use of tamoxifen (Nolvadex)
          Long term (current) use of toremifene (Fareston)

       Z79.811 Long term (current) use of **aromatase inhibitors** `UPD` `PE`
          Long term (current) use of anastrozole (Arimidex)
          Long term (current) use of exemestane (Aromasin)
          Long term (current) use of letrozole (Femara)

       Z79.818 Long term (current) use of **other agents affecting estrogen receptors and estrogen levels** `UPD` `PE`
          Long term (current) use of estrogen receptor downregulators
          Long term (current) use of fulvestrant (Faslodex)
          Long term (current) use of gonadotropin-releasing hormone (GnRH) agonist
          Long term (current) use of goserelin acetate (Zoladex)
          Long term (current) use of leuprolide acetate (leuprorelin) (Lupron)
          Long term (current) use of megestrol acetate (Megace)

    Z79.82 Long term (current) use of **aspirin** `PE`

    Z79.83 Long term (current) use of **bisphosphonates** `UPD` `PE`
       AHA: 2016,4Q,42

    Z79.84 Long term (current) use of **oral hypoglycemic drugs** `UPD` `PE`
       Long term (current) use of oral antidiabetic drugs
       EXCLUDES 2   *long-term (current) use of injectable non-insulin antidiabetic drugs (Z79.85)*
          long term (current) use of insulin (Z79.4)
       AHA: 2020,3Q,31; 2016,4Q,76

Z79.85   **Long-term (current) use of injectable non-insulin antidiabetic drugs**
EXCLUDES 2   *long term (current) use of insulin (Z79.4)*
long term (current) use of oral hypoglycemic drugs (Z79.84)
AHA: 2022,4Q,50

Z79.89   **Other long term (current) drug therapy**

Z79.890   **Hormone replacement therapy** UPD PE

Z79.891   **Long term (current) use of opiate analgesic** PE
Long term (current) use of methadone for pain management
EXCLUDES 1   *methadone use NOS (F11.9-)*
use of methadone for treatment of heroin addiction (F11.2-)

Z79.899   **Other long term (current) drug therapy** PE
AHA: 2023,3Q,17-18; 2020,4Q,11; 2020,3Q,31; 2020,2Q,14; 2015,4Q,34; 2015,3Q,21

Z80   **Family history of primary malignant neoplasm**

Z80.0   **Family history of malignant neoplasm of digestive organs** UPD PE
Conditions classifiable to C15-C26
AHA: 2018,1Q,6

Z80.1   **Family history of malignant neoplasm of trachea, bronchus and lung** UPD PE
Conditions classifiable to C33-C34

Z80.2   **Family history of malignant neoplasm of other respiratory and intrathoracic organs** UPD PE
Conditions classifiable to C30-C32, C37-C39

Z80.3   **Family history of malignant neoplasm of breast** UPD PE
Conditions classifiable to C50.-

Z80.4   **Family history of malignant neoplasm of genital organs**
Conditions classifiable to C51-C63

Z80.41   **Family history of malignant neoplasm of ovary** UPD PE

Z80.42   **Family history of malignant neoplasm of prostate** UPD PE

Z80.43   **Family history of malignant neoplasm of testis** UPD PE

Z80.49   **Family history of malignant neoplasm of other genital organs** UPD PE

Z80.5   **Family history of malignant neoplasm of urinary tract**
Conditions classifiable to C64-C68

Z80.51   **Family history of malignant neoplasm of kidney** UPD PE

Z80.52   **Family history of malignant neoplasm of bladder** UPD PE

Z80.59   **Family history of malignant neoplasm of other urinary tract organ** UPD PE

Z80.6   **Family history of leukemia** UPD PE
Conditions classifiable to C91-C95

Z80.7   **Family history of other malignant neoplasms of lymphoid, hematopoietic and related tissues** UPD PE
Conditions classifiable to C81-C90, C96.-

Z80.8   **Family history of malignant neoplasm of other organs or systems** UPD PE
Conditions classifiable to C00-C14, C40-C49, C69-C79

Z80.9   **Family history of malignant neoplasm, unspecified** UPD PE
Conditions classifiable to C80.1

Z81   **Family history of mental and behavioral disorders**

Z81.0   **Family history of intellectual disabilities** UPD PE
Conditions classifiable to F70-F79

Z81.1   **Family history of alcohol abuse and dependence** UPD PE
Conditions classifiable to F10.-

Z81.2   **Family history of tobacco abuse and dependence** UPD PE
Conditions classifiable to F17.-

Z81.3   **Family history of other psychoactive substance abuse and dependence** UPD PE
Conditions classifiable to F11-F16, F18-F19

Z81.4   **Family history of other substance abuse and dependence** UPD PE
Conditions classifiable to F55

Z81.8   **Family history of other mental and behavioral disorders** UPD PE
Conditions classifiable elsewhere in F01-F99

Z82   **Family history of certain disabilities and chronic diseases (leading to disablement)**

Z82.0   **Family history of epilepsy and other diseases of the nervous system** UPD PE
Conditions classifiable to G00-G99

Z82.1   **Family history of blindness and visual loss** UPD PE
Conditions classifiable to H54.-

Z82.2   **Family history of deafness and hearing loss** UPD PE
Conditions classifiable to H90-H91

Z82.3   **Family history of stroke** UPD PE
Conditions classifiable to I60-I64

Z82.4   **Family history of ischemic heart disease and other diseases of the circulatory system**
Conditions classifiable to I00-I5A, I65-I99

Z82.41   **Family history of sudden cardiac death** UPD PE

Z82.49   **Family history of ischemic heart disease and other diseases of the circulatory system** UPD PE

Z82.5   **Family history of asthma and other chronic lower respiratory diseases** UPD PE
Conditions classifiable to J40-J47
EXCLUDES 2   *family history of other diseases of the respiratory system (Z83.6)*

Z82.6   **Family history of arthritis and other diseases of the musculoskeletal system and connective tissue**
Conditions classifiable to M00-M99

Z82.61   **Family history of arthritis** UPD PE

Z82.62   **Family history of osteoporosis** UPD PE

Z82.69   **Family history of other diseases of the musculoskeletal system and connective tissue** UPD PE

Z82.7   **Family history of congenital malformations, deformations and chromosomal abnormalities**
Conditions classifiable to Q00-Q99

Z82.71   **Family history of polycystic kidney** UPD PE

Z82.79   **Family history of other congenital malformations, deformations and chromosomal abnormalities** UPD PE

Z82.8   **Family history of other disabilities and chronic diseases leading to disablement, not elsewhere classified** UPD PE

Z83   **Family history of other specific disorders**
EXCLUDES 2   *contact with and (suspected) exposure to communicable disease in the family (Z20.-)*

Z83.0   **Family history of human immunodeficiency virus [HIV] disease** UPD PE
Conditions classifiable to B20

Z83.1   **Family history of other infectious and parasitic diseases** UPD PE
Conditions classifiable to A00-B19, B25-B94, B99

Z83.2   **Family history of diseases of the blood and blood-forming organs and certain disorders involving the immune mechanism** UPD PE
Conditions classifiable to D50-D89

Z83.3   **Family history of diabetes mellitus** UPD PE
Conditions classifiable to E08-E13

Z83.4   **Family history of other endocrine, nutritional and metabolic diseases**
Conditions classifiable to E00-E07, E15-E88

Z83.41   **Family history of multiple endocrine neoplasia [MEN] syndrome** UPD PE

Z83.42   **Family history of familial hypercholesterolemia** UPD PE
AHA: 2016,4Q,77

Z83.43   **Family history of other disorder of lipoprotein metabolism and other lipidemias**
AHA: 2018,4Q,6,35

Z83.430   **Family history of elevated lipoprotein(a)** UPD PE
Family history of elevated Lp(a)

Z83.438   **Family history of other disorder of lipoprotein metabolism and other lipidemia** UPD PE
Family history of familial combined hyperlipidemia

Z83.49   **Family history of other endocrine, nutritional and metabolic diseases** UPD PE

Chapter 21. Factors Influencing Health Status and Contact With Health Services *(side margin)*

✓5ᵗʰ Z83.5 Family history of eye and ear disorders

    ✓6ᵗʰ Z83.51 Family history of eye disorders
        Conditions classifiable to H00-H53, H55-H59
        EXCLUDES 2   *family history of blindness and visual loss (Z82.1)*

        Z83.511 Family history of glaucoma UPD PE
        Z83.518 Family history of other specified eye disorder UPD PE

    Z83.52 Family history of ear disorders
        Conditions classifiable to H60-H83, H92-H95
        EXCLUDES 2   *family history of deafness and hearing loss (Z82.2)*

Z83.6 Family history of other diseases of the respiratory system UPD PE
    Conditions classifiable to J00-J39, J60-J99
    EXCLUDES 2   *family history of asthma and other chronic lower respiratory diseases (Z82.5)*

✓5ᵗʰ Z83.7 Family history of diseases of the digestive system
    Conditions classifiable to D12, K00-K93

    ✓6ᵗʰ Z83.71 Family history of colonic polyps
        EXCLUDES 2   *family history of malignant neoplasm of digestive organs (Z80.0)*
        AHA: 2023,4Q,47-48; 2021,1Q,14

        Z83.710 Family history of adenomatous and serrated polyps UPD PE
            Conditions classifiable to D12.-
            Family history of tubular adenoma polyps
            Family history of tubulovillous adenoma polyps
            Family history of villous adenoma polyps

        Z83.711 Family history of hyperplastic colon polyps UPD PE
        Z83.718 Other family history of colon polyps UPD PE
            Family history of inflammatory colon polyps
        Z83.719 Family history of colon polyps, unspecified UPD PE
            Family history of colon polyps NOS

    Z83.72 Family history of familial adenomatous polyposis UPD PE
    Z83.79 Family history of other diseases of the digestive system UPD PE

✓4ᵗʰ Z84 Family history of other conditions

    Z84.0 Family history of diseases of the skin and subcutaneous tissue UPD PE
        Conditions classifiable to L00-L99

    Z84.1 Family history of disorders of kidney and ureter UPD PE
        Conditions classifiable to N00-N29

    Z84.2 Family history of other diseases of the genitourinary system UPD PE
        Conditions classifiable to N30-N99

    Z84.3 Family history of consanguinity UPD PE

    ✓5ᵗʰ Z84.8 Family history of other specified conditions

        Z84.81 Family history of carrier of genetic disease UPD PE
            AHA: 2021,1Q,14

        Z84.82 Family history of sudden infant death syndrome UPD PE
            Family history of SIDS
            AHA: 2016,4Q,77

        Z84.89 Family history of other specified conditions UPD PE

✓4ᵗʰ Z85 Personal history of malignant neoplasm

    Code first any follow-up examination after treatment of malignant neoplasm (Z08)
    Use additional code to identify:
        alcohol use and dependence (F10.-)
        exposure to environmental tobacco smoke (Z77.22)
        history of tobacco dependence (Z87.891)
        occupational exposure to environmental tobacco smoke (Z57.31)
        tobacco dependence (F17.-)
        tobacco use (Z72.0)
    EXCLUDES 2   *personal history of benign neoplasm (Z86.01-)*
             personal history of carcinoma-in-situ (Z86.00-)
    AHA: 2022,3Q,28; 2020,3Q,30; 2018,4Q,64

    ✓5ᵗʰ Z85.0 Personal history of malignant neoplasm of digestive organs
        AHA: 2017,1Q,9

        Z85.00 Personal history of malignant neoplasm of unspecified digestive organ UPD PE
        Z85.01 Personal history of malignant neoplasm of esophagus UPD PE
            Conditions classifiable to C15

        ✓6ᵗʰ Z85.02 Personal history of malignant neoplasm of stomach
            Z85.020 Personal history of malignant carcinoid tumor of stomach UPD PE
                Conditions classifiable to C7A.092
            Z85.028 Personal history of other malignant neoplasm of stomach UPD PE
                Conditions classifiable to C16

        ✓6ᵗʰ Z85.03 Personal history of malignant neoplasm of large intestine
            Z85.030 Personal history of malignant carcinoid tumor of large intestine UPD PE
                Conditions classifiable to C7A.022-C7A.025, C7A.029
            Z85.038 Personal history of other malignant neoplasm of large intestine UPD PE
                Conditions classifiable to C18

        ✓6ᵗʰ Z85.04 Personal history of malignant neoplasm of rectum, rectosigmoid junction, and anus
            Z85.040 Personal history of malignant carcinoid tumor of rectum UPD PE
                Conditions classifiable to C7A.026
            Z85.048 Personal history of other malignant neoplasm of rectum, rectosigmoid junction, and anus UPD PE
                Conditions classifiable to C19-C21

        Z85.05 Personal history of malignant neoplasm of liver UPD PE
            Conditions classifiable to C22

        ✓6ᵗʰ Z85.06 Personal history of malignant neoplasm of small intestine
            Z85.060 Personal history of malignant carcinoid tumor of small intestine UPD PE
                Conditions classifiable to C7A.01-
            Z85.068 Personal history of other malignant neoplasm of small intestine UPD PE
                Conditions classifiable to C17

        Z85.07 Personal history of malignant neoplasm of pancreas UPD PE
            Conditions classifiable to C25

        Z85.09 Personal history of malignant neoplasm of other digestive organs UPD PE

    ✓5ᵗʰ Z85.1 Personal history of malignant neoplasm of trachea, bronchus and lung

        ✓6ᵗʰ Z85.11 Personal history of malignant neoplasm of bronchus and lung
            Z85.110 Personal history of malignant carcinoid tumor of bronchus and lung UPD PE
                Conditions classifiable to C7A.090
            Z85.118 Personal history of other malignant neoplasm of bronchus and lung UPD PE
                Conditions classifiable to C34

        Z85.12 Personal history of malignant neoplasm of trachea UPD PE
            Conditions classifiable to C33

    ✓5ᵗʰ Z85.2 Personal history of malignant neoplasm of other respiratory and intrathoracic organs

        Z85.20 Personal history of malignant neoplasm of unspecified respiratory organ UPD PE

N Newborn: 0   **P** Pediatric: 0-17   **M** Maternity: 9-64   **A** Adult: 15-124   **UNS** Unspecified Site   **MCC** Major Complication/Comorbidity   **CC** Complication/Comorbidity   **PE** POA Exempt

1288   ICD-10-CM 2025

Z85.21   **Personal history of malignant neoplasm of larynx**   UPD PE
    Conditions classifiable to C32

Z85.22   **Personal history of malignant neoplasm of nasal cavities, middle ear, and accessory sinuses**   UPD PE
    Conditions classifiable to C30-C31

✓6ᵗʰ Z85.23   **Personal history of malignant neoplasm of thymus**

    Z85.230   **Personal history of malignant carcinoid tumor of thymus**   UPD PE
       Conditions classifiable to C7A.091

    Z85.238   **Personal history of other malignant neoplasm of thymus**   UPD PE
       Conditions classifiable to C37

Z85.29   **Personal history of malignant neoplasm of other respiratory and intrathoracic organs**   UPD PE

Z85.3   **Personal history of malignant neoplasm of breast**   UPD PE
    Conditions classifiable to C50.-

✓5ᵗʰ Z85.4   **Personal history of malignant neoplasm of genital organs**
    Conditions classifiable to C51-C63

    Z85.40   **Personal history of malignant neoplasm of unspecified female genital organ**   UPD PE

    Z85.41   **Personal history of malignant neoplasm of cervix uteri**   UPD PE

    Z85.42   **Personal history of malignant neoplasm of other parts of uterus**   UPD PE

    Z85.43   **Personal history of malignant neoplasm of ovary**   UPD PE

    Z85.44   **Personal history of malignant neoplasm of other female genital organs**   UPD PE
       AHA: AHA:2024,2Q,11

    Z85.45   **Personal history of malignant neoplasm of unspecified male genital organ**   UPD PE

    Z85.46   **Personal history of malignant neoplasm of prostate**   UPD PE
       AHA: 2023,2Q,5

    Z85.47   **Personal history of malignant neoplasm of testis**   UPD PE

    Z85.48   **Personal history of malignant neoplasm of epididymis**   UPD PE

    Z85.49   **Personal history of malignant neoplasm of other male genital organs**   UPD PE

✓5ᵗʰ Z85.5   **Personal history of malignant neoplasm of urinary tract**
    Conditions classifiable to C64-C68

    Z85.50   **Personal history of malignant neoplasm of unspecified urinary tract organ**   UPD PE

    Z85.51   **Personal history of malignant neoplasm of bladder**   UPD PE

✓6ᵗʰ   Z85.52   **Personal history of malignant neoplasm of kidney**
       EXCLUDES 1   personal history of malignant neoplasm of renal pelvis (Z85.53)

    Z85.520   **Personal history of malignant carcinoid tumor of kidney**   UPD PE
       Conditions classifiable to C7A.093

    Z85.528   **Personal history of other malignant neoplasm of kidney**   UPD PE
       Conditions classifiable to C64

    Z85.53   **Personal history of malignant neoplasm of renal pelvis**   UPD PE

    Z85.54   **Personal history of malignant neoplasm of ureter**   UPD PE

    Z85.59   **Personal history of malignant neoplasm of other urinary tract organ**   UPD PE

Z85.6   **Personal history of leukemia**   UPD PE
    Conditions classifiable to C91-C95
       EXCLUDES 1   leukemia in remission C91.0-C95.9 with 5th character 1

✓5ᵗʰ Z85.7   **Personal history of other malignant neoplasms of lymphoid, hematopoietic and related tissues**

    Z85.71   **Personal history of Hodgkin lymphoma**   UPD PE
       Conditions classifiable to C81

    Z85.72   **Personal history of non-Hodgkin lymphomas**   UPD PE
       Conditions classifiable to C82-C85
       AHA: 2022,3Q,28

Z85.79   **Personal history of other malignant neoplasms of lymphoid, hematopoietic and related tissues**   UPD PE
    Conditions classifiable to C88-C90, C96
       EXCLUDES 1   multiple myeloma in remission (C90.01)
          plasma cell leukemia in remission (C90.11)
          plasmacytoma in remission (C90.21)

✓5ᵗʰ Z85.8   **Personal history of malignant neoplasms of other organs and systems**
    Conditions classifiable to C00-C14, C40-C49, C69-C75, C7A.098, C76-C79

✓6ᵗʰ Z85.81   **Personal history of malignant neoplasm of lip, oral cavity, and pharynx**
    Conditions classifiable to C00-C14

    Z85.810   **Personal history of malignant neoplasm of tongue**   UPD PE

    Z85.818   **Personal history of malignant neoplasm of other sites of lip, oral cavity, and pharynx**   UPD PE

    Z85.819   **Personal history of malignant neoplasm of unspecified site of lip, oral cavity, and pharynx**

✓6ᵗʰ Z85.82   **Personal history of malignant neoplasm of skin**

    Z85.820   **Personal history of malignant melanoma of skin**   UPD PE
       Conditions classifiable to C43
       AHA: 2022,3Q,9

    Z85.821   **Personal history of Merkel cell carcinoma**   UPD PE
       Conditions classifiable to C4A

    Z85.828   **Personal history of other malignant neoplasm of skin**   UPD PE
       Conditions classifiable to C44

✓6ᵗʰ Z85.83   **Personal history of malignant neoplasm of bone and soft tissue**
    Conditions classifiable to C40-C41; C45-C49

    Z85.830   **Personal history of malignant neoplasm of bone**   UPD PE

    Z85.831   **Personal history of malignant neoplasm of soft tissue**   UPD PE
       EXCLUDES 2   personal history of malignant neoplasm of skin (Z85.82-)

✓6ᵗʰ Z85.84   **Personal history of malignant neoplasm of eye and nervous tissue**
    Conditions classifiable to C69-C72

    Z85.840   **Personal history of malignant neoplasm of eye**   UPD PE

    Z85.841   **Personal history of malignant neoplasm of brain**   UPD PE

    Z85.848   **Personal history of malignant neoplasm of other parts of nervous tissue**   UPD PE

✓6ᵗʰ Z85.85   **Personal history of malignant neoplasm of endocrine glands**
    Conditions classifiable to C73-C75

    Z85.850   **Personal history of malignant neoplasm of thyroid**   UPD PE

    Z85.858   **Personal history of malignant neoplasm of other endocrine glands**   UPD PE
       AHA: AHA:2024,2Q,10

Z85.89   **Personal history of malignant neoplasm of other organs and systems**   UPD PE
    Conditions classifiable to C7A.098, C76, C77-C79

Z85.9   **Personal history of malignant neoplasm, unspecified**   UPD PE
    Conditions classifiable to C7A.00, C80.1

✓4ᵗʰ **Z86**   **Personal history of certain other diseases**
    Code first any follow-up examination after treatment (Z09)

✓5ᵗʰ Z86.0   **Personal history of in-situ and benign neoplasms and neoplasms of uncertain behavior**
       EXCLUDES 2   personal history of malignant neoplasms (Z85.-)
    AHA: 2017,1Q,9

✓6ᵗʰ Z86.00   **Personal history of in-situ neoplasm**
    Conditions classifiable to D00-D09
    AHA: 2019,4Q,20

    Z86.000   **Personal history of in-situ neoplasm of breast**   UPD PE
       Conditions classifiable to D05

✔ Additional Character Required   ✓x7ᵗʰ Placeholder   Questionable PDx   Manifestation   Unspecified   UPD Unacceptable PDx   H1-H14 HAC   HCC CMS-HCC Dx   HIV HIV Dx

Z86.001 Personal history of in-situ neoplasm of **cervix uteri** `UPD` `PE`
Conditions classifiable to D06
Personal history of cervical intraepithelial neoplasia III [CIN III]

Z86.002 Personal history of in-situ neoplasm of **other and unspecified genital organs** `UPD` `PE`
Conditions classifiable to D07
Personal history of high-grade prostatic intraepithelial neoplasia III [HGPIN III]
Personal history of vaginal intraepithelial neoplasia III [VAIN III]
Personal history of vulvar intraepithelial neoplasia III [VIN III]

Z86.003 Personal history of in-situ neoplasm of **oral cavity, esophagus and stomach** `UPD` `PE`
Conditions classifiable to D00

Z86.004 Personal history of in-situ neoplasm of **other and unspecified digestive organs** `UPD` `PE`
Conditions classifiable to D01
Personal history of anal intraepithelial neoplasia (AIN III)

Z86.005 Personal history of in-situ neoplasm of **middle ear and respiratory system** `UPD` `PE`
Conditions classifiable to D02

Z86.006 Personal history of **melanoma in-situ** `UPD` `PE`
Conditions classifiable to D03
EXCLUDES 2   sites other than skin - code to personal history of in-situ neoplasm of the site

Z86.007 Personal history of in-situ neoplasm of **skin** `UPD` `PE`
Conditions classifiable to D04
Personal history of carcinoma in situ of skin

Z86.008 Personal history of in-situ neoplasm of **other site** `UPD` `PE`
Conditions classifiable to D09

▲ √6ᵗʰ **Z86.01** Personal history of **benign neoplasm**

√7ᵗʰ **Z86.010** Personal history of **colon polyps**
▶Personal history of colorectal polyps◀
▶Personal history of rectal polyps◀
AHA: 2021,1Q,14; 2017,1Q,14

● **Z86.0100** Personal history of colon polyps, **unspecified** `UPD` `PE`
Personal history of colon polyps NOS

● **Z86.0101** Personal history of **adenomatous and serrated colon polyps** `UPD` `PE`
Personal history of tubular adenoma polyps
Personal history of sessile adenomatous colon polyp
Personal history of sessile serrated colon polyp
Personal history of tubulovillous adenoma polyps
Personal history of villous adenoma polyps
Personal history of traditional serrated adenoma polyps

● **Z86.0102** Personal history of **hyperplastic colon polyps** `UPD` `PE`

● **Z86.0109** Personal history of **other colon polyps** `UPD` `PE`

Z86.011 Personal history of benign neoplasm of the **brain** `UPD` `PE`

Z86.012 Personal history of benign **carcinoid tumor** `UPD` `PE`

Z86.018 Personal history of other benign **neoplasm** `UPD` `PE`
AHA: 2017,1Q,14

Z86.03 Personal history of **neoplasm of uncertain behavior** `UPD` `PE`

√5ᵗʰ **Z86.1** Personal history of **infectious and parasitic diseases**
Conditions classifiable to A00-B89, B99
EXCLUDES 1   personal history of infectious diseases specific to a body system
sequelae of infectious and parasitic diseases (B90-B94)

Z86.11 Personal history of **tuberculosis** `UPD` `PE`
Z86.12 Personal history of **poliomyelitis** `UPD` `PE`
Z86.13 Personal history of **malaria** `UPD` `PE`
Z86.14 Personal history of **Methicillin resistant Staphylococcus aureus** infection `UPD` `PE`
Personal history of MRSA infection

Z86.15 Personal history of **latent tuberculosis infection** `UPD` `PE`

Z86.16 Personal history of **COVID-19** `UPD` `PE`
EXCLUDES 1   post COVID-19 condition (U09.9)
AHA: 2021,4Q,107-108; 2021,1Q,28-29,33-35,40-41,44-45

Z86.19 Personal history of other infectious and parasitic **diseases** `UPD` `PE`
AHA: 2022,3Q,4; 2021,1Q,33-34,40; 2020,3Q,13; 2020,2Q,10,12

Z86.2 Personal history of diseases of the **blood and blood-forming organs** and certain disorders involving the **immune mechanism** `UPD` `PE`
Conditions classifiable to D50-D89

√5ᵗʰ **Z86.3** Personal history of **endocrine, nutritional and metabolic diseases**
Conditions classifiable to E00-E88

Z86.31 Personal history of **diabetic foot ulcer** `UPD` `PE`
EXCLUDES 2   current diabetic foot ulcer (E08.621, E09.621, E10.621, E11.621, E13.621)

Z86.32 Personal history of **gestational diabetes** `UPD` `PE`
Personal history of conditions classifiable to O24.4-
EXCLUDES 1   gestational diabetes mellitus in current pregnancy (O24.4-)

Z86.39 Personal history of other endocrine, nutritional and metabolic disease `UPD` `PE`
AHA: 2020,1Q,12

√5ᵗʰ **Z86.5** Personal history of **mental and behavioral disorders**
Conditions classifiable to F40-F59

Z86.51 Personal history of **combat and operational stress reaction** `UPD` `A` `PE`

Z86.59 Personal history of other mental and behavioral **disorders** `UPD` `PE`

√5ᵗʰ **Z86.6** Personal history of diseases of the **nervous system and sense organs**
Conditions classifiable to G00-G99, H00-H95

Z86.61 Personal history of **infections of the central nervous system** `UPD` `PE`
Personal history of encephalitis
Personal history of meningitis

Z86.69 Personal history of other diseases of the nervous system and sense organs `UPD` `PE`
AHA: 2016,4Q,24

√5ᵗʰ **Z86.7** Personal history of diseases of the **circulatory system**
Conditions classifiable to I00-I99
EXCLUDES 2   old myocardial infarction (I25.2)
personal history of anaphylactic shock (Z87.892)
postmyocardial infarction syndrome (I24.1)

√6ᵗʰ **Z86.71** Personal history of **venous thrombosis and embolism**

Z86.711 Personal history of **pulmonary embolism** `UPD` `PE`

Z86.718 Personal history of other venous thrombosis and embolism `UPD` `PE`
AHA: 2020,2Q,20

Z86.72 Personal history of **thrombophlebitis** `UPD` `PE`

Z86.73 Personal history of **transient ischemic attack** (TIA), and cerebral infarction without residual deficits `UPD` `PE`
Personal history of prolonged reversible ischemic neurological deficit (PRIND)
Personal history of stroke NOS without residual deficits
EXCLUDES 1   personal history of traumatic brain injury (Z87.820)
sequelae of cerebrovascular disease (I69.-)
AHA: 2023,1Q,37; 2012,4Q,92

`N` Newborn: 0   `P` Pediatric: 0-17   `M` Maternity: 9-64   `A` Adult: 15-124   `UNS` Unspecified Site   `MCC` Major Complication/Comorbidity   `CC` Complication/Comorbidity   `PE` POA Exempt

1290   ICD-10-CM 2025

Z86.74   **Personal history of sudden cardiac arrest** `UPD` `PE`
Personal history of sudden cardiac death successfully resuscitated
AHA: 2024,1Q,27

Z86.79   **Personal history of other diseases of the circulatory system** `UPD` `PE`
AHA: 2022,2Q,14; 2020,1Q,12

✓4ᵗʰ **Z87** **Personal history of other diseases and conditions**
Code first any follow-up examination after treatment (Z09)
AHA: 2022,4Q,50-51

✓5ᵗʰ **Z87.0**   **Personal history of diseases of the respiratory system**
Conditions classifiable to J00-J99

    Z87.01   **Personal history of pneumonia (recurrent)** `UPD` `PE`

    Z87.09   **Personal history of other diseases of the respiratory system** `UPD` `PE`

✓5ᵗʰ **Z87.1**   **Personal history of diseases of the digestive system**
Conditions classifiable to K00-K93

    Z87.11   **Personal history of peptic ulcer disease** `UPD` `PE`

    Z87.19   **Personal history of other diseases of the digestive system** `UPD` `PE`
AHA: 2017,1Q,14

Z87.2   **Personal history of diseases of the skin and subcutaneous tissue** `UPD` `PE`
Conditions classifiable to L00-L99
EXCLUDES 2   *personal history of diabetic foot ulcer (Z86.31)*

✓5ᵗʰ **Z87.3**   **Personal history of diseases of the musculoskeletal system and connective tissue**
Conditions classifiable to M00-M99
EXCLUDES 2   *personal history of (healed) traumatic fracture (Z87.81)*

✓6ᵗʰ **Z87.31**   **Personal history of (healed) nontraumatic fracture**

    Z87.310   **Personal history of (healed) osteoporosis fracture** `UPD` `PE`
Personal history of (healed) fragility fracture
Personal history of (healed) collapsed vertebra due to osteoporosis
TIP: Assign for history of osteoporosis fractures that have resolved, even when a code from category M80 indicating current osteoporosis fracture is also reported.

    Z87.311   **Personal history of (healed) other pathological fracture** `UPD` `PE`
Personal history of (healed) collapsed vertebra NOS
EXCLUDES 2   *personal history of osteoporosis fracture (Z87.310)*

    Z87.312   **Personal history of (healed) stress fracture** `UPD` `PE`
Personal history of (healed) fatigue fracture

    Z87.39   **Personal history of other diseases of the musculoskeletal system and connective tissue** `UPD` `PE`

✓5ᵗʰ **Z87.4**   **Personal history of diseases of the genitourinary system**
Conditions classifiable to N00-N99

✓6ᵗʰ **Z87.41**   **Personal history of dysplasia of the female genital tract**
EXCLUDES 1   *personal history of intraepithelial neoplasia III of female genital tract (Z86.001, Z86.008)*
personal history of malignant neoplasm of female genital tract (Z85.40-Z85.44)

    Z87.410   **Personal history of cervical dysplasia** `UPD` `PE`

    Z87.411   **Personal history of vaginal dysplasia** `UPD` `PE`

    Z87.412   **Personal history of vulvar dysplasia** `UPD` `PE`

    Z87.42   **Personal history of other diseases of the female genital tract** `UPD` `PE`

✓6ᵗʰ **Z87.43**   **Personal history of diseases of the male genital organs**

    Z87.430   **Personal history of prostatic dysplasia** `UPD` `PE`
EXCLUDES 1   *personal history of malignant neoplasm of prostate (Z85.46)*

    Z87.438   **Personal history of other diseases of male genital organs** `UPD` `PE`

✓6ᵗʰ **Z87.44**   **Personal history of diseases of the urinary system**
EXCLUDES 1   *personal history of malignant neoplasm of cervix uteri (Z85.41)*

    Z87.440   **Personal history of urinary (tract) infections** `UPD` `PE`

    Z87.441   **Personal history of nephrotic syndrome** `UPD` `PE`

    Z87.442   **Personal history of urinary calculi** `UPD` `PE`
Personal history of kidney stones

    Z87.448   **Personal history of other diseases of urinary system**

✓5ᵗʰ **Z87.5**   **Personal history of complications of pregnancy, childbirth and the puerperium**
Conditions classifiable to O00-O9A
EXCLUDES 2   *recurrent pregnancy loss (N96)*

    Z87.51   **Personal history of pre-term labor** `UPD` `PE`
EXCLUDES 1   *current pregnancy with history of pre-term labor (O09.21-)*

    Z87.59   **Personal history of other complications of pregnancy, childbirth and the puerperium** `UPD` `PE`
Personal history of trophoblastic disease

✓5ᵗʰ **Z87.6**   **Personal history of certain (corrected) conditions arising in the perinatal period**
Conditions classifiable to P00-P96
EXCLUDES 1   *personal history of (corrected) congenital malformations (Z87.7-)*

    Z87.61   **Personal history of (corrected) necrotizing enterocolitis of newborn** `UPD` `PE`

    Z87.68   **Personal history of other (corrected) conditions arising in the perinatal period** `UPD` `PE`

✓5ᵗʰ **Z87.7**   **Personal history of (corrected) congenital malformations**
Conditions classifiable to Q00-Q89 that have been repaired or corrected
EXCLUDES 2   *congenital malformations that have been partially corrected or repaired but which still require medical treatment - code to condition*
other postprocedural states (Z98.-)
personal history of medical treatment (Z92.-)
presence of cardiac and vascular implants and grafts (Z95.-)
presence of other devices (Z97.-)
presence of other functional implants (Z96.-)
transplanted organ and tissue status (Z94.-)

✓6ᵗʰ **Z87.71**   **Personal history of (corrected) congenital malformations of genitourinary system**

    Z87.710   **Personal history of (corrected) hypospadias** `UPD` `PE`

    Z87.718   **Personal history of other specified (corrected) congenital malformations of genitourinary system** `UPD` `PE`

✓6ᵗʰ **Z87.72**   **Personal history of (corrected) congenital malformations of nervous system and sense organs**

    Z87.720   **Personal history of (corrected) congenital malformations of eye** `UPD` `PE`

    Z87.721   **Personal history of (corrected) congenital malformations of ear** `UPD` `PE`

    Z87.728   **Personal history of other specified (corrected) congenital malformations of nervous system and sense organs** `UPD` `PE`

✓6ᵗʰ **Z87.73**   **Personal history of (corrected) congenital malformations of digestive system**

    Z87.730   **Personal history of (corrected) cleft lip and palate** `UPD` `PE`

    Z87.731   **Personal history of (corrected) tracheoesophageal fistula or atresia** `UPD` `PE`

    Z87.732   **Personal history of (corrected) persistent cloaca or cloacal malformations** `UPD` `PE`

    Z87.738   **Personal history of other specified (corrected) congenital malformations of digestive system** `UPD` `PE`

    Z87.74   **Personal history of (corrected) congenital malformations of heart and circulatory system** `UPD` `PE`

    Z87.75   **Personal history of (corrected) congenital malformations of respiratory system** `UPD` `PE`

✓ Additional Character Required   ✓x7ᵗʰ Placeholder   `Questionable PDx`   Manifestation   Unspecified   `UPD` Unacceptable PDx   `H1`-`H14` HAC   `HCC` CMS-HCC Dx   `HIV` HIV Dx

ICD-10-CM 2025   1291

✓6th **Z87.76** Personal history of (corrected) congenital malformations of integument, limbs and musculoskeletal system

   Z87.760 Personal history of (corrected) congenital diaphragmatic hernia or other congenital diaphragm malformations `UPD` `PE`

   Z87.761 Personal history of (corrected) gastroschisis `UPD` `PE`

   Z87.762 Personal history of (corrected) prune belly malformation

   Z87.763 Personal history of other (corrected) congenital abdominal wall malformations `UPD` `PE`

   Z87.768 Personal history of other specified (corrected) congenital malformations of integument, limbs and musculoskeletal system `UPD` `PE`

✓6th **Z87.79** Personal history of other (corrected) congenital malformations

   Z87.790 Personal history of (corrected) congenital malformations of face and neck `UPD` `PE`

   Z87.798 Personal history of other (corrected) congenital malformations `UPD` `PE`

✓5th **Z87.8** Personal history of other specified conditions

   EXCLUDES 2   personal history of self harm (Z91.5-)

   Z87.81 Personal history of (healed) traumatic fracture `UPD` `PE`

      EXCLUDES 2   personal history of (healed) nontraumatic fracture (Z87.31-)

✓6th **Z87.82** Personal history of other (healed) physical injury and trauma

   Conditions classifiable to S00-T88, except traumatic fractures

   Z87.820 Personal history of traumatic brain injury `UPD` `PE`

      EXCLUDES 1   personal history of transient ischemic attack (TIA), and cerebral infarction without residual deficits (Z86.73)

   Z87.821 Personal history of retained foreign body fully removed `UPD` `PE`

   Z87.828 Personal history of other (healed) physical injury and trauma `UPD` `PE`

✓6th **Z87.89** Personal history of other specified conditions

   Z87.890 Personal history of sex reassignment `PE`

   Z87.891 Personal history of nicotine dependence `UPD` `PE`

      EXCLUDES 1   current nicotine dependence (F17.2-)

      AHA: 2017,2Q,27

   Z87.892 Personal history of anaphylaxis `UPD` `PE`

      Code also allergy status such as:

         allergy status to drugs, medicaments and biological substances (Z88.-)

         allergy status, other than to drugs and biological substances (Z91.0-)

   Z87.898 Personal history of other specified conditions `UPD` `PE`

      AHA: 2013,1Q,21

✓4th **Z88** Allergy status to drugs, medicaments and biological substances

   EXCLUDES 2   allergy status, other than to drugs and biological substances (Z91.0-)

   AHA: 2015,3Q,23

Z88.0 Allergy status to penicillin `UPD` `PE`

Z88.1 Allergy status to other antibiotic agents `UPD` `PE`

Z88.2 Allergy status to sulfonamides `UPD` `PE`

Z88.3 Allergy status to other anti-infective agents `UPD` `PE`

Z88.4 Allergy status to anesthetic agent `UPD` `PE`

Z88.5 Allergy status to narcotic agent `UPD` `PE`

Z88.6 Allergy status to analgesic agent `UPD` `PE`

Z88.7 Allergy status to serum and vaccine `UPD` `PE`

Z88.8 Allergy status to other drugs, medicaments and biological substances `UPD` `PE`

Z88.9 Allergy status to unspecified drugs, medicaments and biological substances `UPD` `PE`

✓4th **Z89** Acquired absence of limb

   INCLUDES   amputation status

         postprocedural loss of limb

         post-traumatic loss of limb

   EXCLUDES 1   acquired deformities of limbs (M20-M21)

         congenital absence of limbs (Q71-Q73)

✓5th **Z89.0** Acquired absence of thumb and other finger(s)

   ✓6th **Z89.01** Acquired absence of thumb

      Z89.011 Acquired absence of right thumb `UPD` `PE`

      Z89.012 Acquired absence of left thumb `UPD` `PE`

      Z89.019 Acquired absence of unspecified thumb `UPD` `PE`

   ✓6th **Z89.02** Acquired absence of other finger(s)

      EXCLUDES 2   acquired absence of thumb (Z89.01-)

      Z89.021 Acquired absence of right finger(s) `UPD` `PE`

      Z89.022 Acquired absence of left finger(s) `UPD` `PE`

      Z89.029 Acquired absence of unspecified finger(s) `UPD` `PE`

✓5th **Z89.1** Acquired absence of hand and wrist

   ✓6th **Z89.11** Acquired absence of hand

      Z89.111 Acquired absence of right hand `UPD` `PE`

      Z89.112 Acquired absence of left hand `UPD` `PE`

      Z89.119 Acquired absence of unspecified hand `UPD` `PE`

   ✓6th **Z89.12** Acquired absence of wrist

      Disarticulation at wrist

      Z89.121 Acquired absence of right wrist `UPD` `PE`

      Z89.122 Acquired absence of left wrist `UPD` `PE`

      Z89.129 Acquired absence of unspecified wrist

✓5th **Z89.2** Acquired absence of upper limb above wrist

   ✓6th **Z89.20** Acquired absence of upper limb, unspecified level

      Z89.201 Acquired absence of right upper limb, unspecified level `UPD` `PE`

      Z89.202 Acquired absence of left upper limb, unspecified level `UPD` `PE`

      Z89.209 Acquired absence of unspecified upper limb, unspecified level `UPD` `PE`

      Acquired absence of arm NOS

   ✓6th **Z89.21** Acquired absence of upper limb below elbow

      Z89.211 Acquired absence of right upper limb below elbow `UPD` `PE`

      Z89.212 Acquired absence of left upper limb below elbow `UPD` `PE`

      Z89.219 Acquired absence of unspecified upper limb below elbow `UPD` `PE`

   ✓6th **Z89.22** Acquired absence of upper limb above elbow

      Disarticulation at elbow

      Z89.221 Acquired absence of right upper limb above elbow `UPD` `PE`

      Z89.222 Acquired absence of left upper limb above elbow `UPD` `PE`

      Z89.229 Acquired absence of unspecified upper limb above elbow `UPD` `PE`

   ✓6th **Z89.23** Acquired absence of shoulder

      Acquired absence of shoulder joint following explantation of shoulder joint prosthesis, with or without presence of antibiotic-impregnated cement spacer

      Z89.231 Acquired absence of right shoulder `UPD` `PE`

      Z89.232 Acquired absence of left shoulder `UPD` `PE`

      Z89.239 Acquired absence of unspecified shoulder `UPD` `PE`

✓5th **Z89.4** Acquired absence of toe(s), foot, and ankle

   ✓6th **Z89.41** Acquired absence of great toe

      Z89.411 Acquired absence of right great toe `UPD` `PE`

      Z89.412 Acquired absence of left great toe `UPD` `PE`

      Z89.419 Acquired absence of unspecified great toe `UPD` `PE`

N Newborn: 0   **P** Pediatric: 0-17   **M** Maternity: 9-64   **A** Adult: 15-124   **UNS** Unspecified Site   **MCC** Major Complication/Comorbidity   **CC** Complication/Comorbidity   **PE** POA Exempt

1292   ICD-10-CM 2025

√6th **Z89.42**   **Acquired absence of other toe(s)**
- EXCLUDES 2   *acquired absence of great toe (Z89.41-)*
- **Z89.421**   **Acquired absence of other right toe(s)**   UPD PE
- **Z89.422**   **Acquired absence of other left toe(s)**   UPD PE
- **Z89.429**   **Acquired absence of other toe(s), unspecified side**   UPD PE

√6th **Z89.43**   **Acquired absence of foot**
- **Z89.431**   **Acquired absence of right foot**   UPD HCC PE
- **Z89.432**   **Acquired absence of left foot**   UPD HCC PE
- **Z89.439**   **Acquired absence of unspecified foot**   UPD HCC PE

√6th **Z89.44**   **Acquired absence of ankle**
- Disarticulation of ankle
- **Z89.441**   **Acquired absence of right ankle**   UPD HCC PE
- **Z89.442**   **Acquired absence of left ankle**   UPD HCC PE
- **Z89.449**   **Acquired absence of unspecified ankle**   UPD HCC PE

√5th **Z89.5**   **Acquired absence of leg below knee**

√6th **Z89.51**   **Acquired absence of leg below knee**
- **Z89.511**   **Acquired absence of right leg below knee**   UPD HCC PE
- **Z89.512**   **Acquired absence of left leg below knee**   UPD HCC PE
- **Z89.519**   **Acquired absence of unspecified leg below knee**   UPD HCC PE

√6th **Z89.52**   **Acquired absence of knee**
- Acquired absence of knee joint following explantation of knee joint prosthesis, with or without presence of antibiotic-impregnated cement spacer
- **Z89.521**   **Acquired absence of right knee**   UPD PE
- **Z89.522**   **Acquired absence of left knee**   UPD PE
- **Z89.529**   **Acquired absence of unspecified knee**   UPD PE

√5th **Z89.6**   **Acquired absence of leg above knee**

√6th **Z89.61**   **Acquired absence of leg above knee**
- Acquired absence of leg NOS
- Disarticulation at knee
- **Z89.611**   **Acquired absence of right leg above knee**   UPD HCC PE
- **Z89.612**   **Acquired absence of left leg above knee**   UPD HCC PE
- **Z89.619**   **Acquired absence of unspecified leg above knee**   UPD HCC PE

√6th **Z89.62**   **Acquired absence of hip**
- Acquired absence of hip joint following explantation of hip joint prosthesis, with or without presence of antibiotic-impregnated cement spacer
- Disarticulation at hip
- **Z89.621**   **Acquired absence of right hip joint**   UPD PE
- **Z89.622**   **Acquired absence of left hip joint**   UPD PE
- **Z89.629**   **Acquired absence of unspecified hip joint**   UPD PE

Z89.9   **Acquired absence of limb, unspecified**   UPD PE

√4th **Z90**   **Acquired absence of organs, not elsewhere classified**
- INCLUDES   postprocedural or post-traumatic loss of body part NEC
- EXCLUDES 1   *congenital absence - see Alphabetical Index*
- EXCLUDES 2   *postprocedural absence of endocrine glands (E89.-)*

√5th **Z90.0**   **Acquired absence of part of head and neck**
- **Z90.01**   **Acquired absence of eye**   UPD PE
- **Z90.02**   **Acquired absence of larynx**   UPD PE
- **Z90.09**   **Acquired absence of other part of head and neck**   UPD PE
  - Acquired absence of nose
  - EXCLUDES 2   *teeth (K08.1)*

√5th **Z90.1**   **Acquired absence of breast and nipple**
- AHA: 2022,3Q,8
- **Z90.10**   **Acquired absence of unspecified breast and nipple**   PE

Z90.11   **Acquired absence of right breast and nipple**   PE

Z90.12   **Acquired absence of left breast and nipple**   PE

Z90.13   **Acquired absence of bilateral breasts and nipples**   PE

Z90.2   **Acquired absence of lung [part of]**   UPD PE

Z90.3   **Acquired absence of stomach [part of]**   UPD PE

√5th **Z90.4**   **Acquired absence of other specified parts of digestive tract**

√6th **Z90.41**   **Acquired absence of pancreas**
- Code also exocrine pancreatic insufficiency (K86.81)
- Use additional code to identify any associated: diabetes mellitus, postpancreatectomy (E13.-) insulin use (Z79.4)
- AHA: AHA:2024,2Q,10
- **Z90.410**   **Acquired total absence of pancreas**   UPD PE
  - Acquired absence of pancreas NOS
- **Z90.411**   **Acquired partial absence of pancreas**   UPD PE

Z90.49   **Acquired absence of other specified parts of digestive tract**   UPD PE

Z90.5   **Acquired absence of kidney**   UPD PE

Z90.6   **Acquired absence of other parts of urinary tract**   UPD PE
- Acquired absence of bladder

√5th **Z90.7**   **Acquired absence of genital organ(s)**
- EXCLUDES 1   *personal history of sex reassignment (Z87.890)*
- EXCLUDES 2   *female genital mutilation status (N90.81-)*

√6th **Z90.71**   **Acquired absence of cervix and uterus**
- **Z90.710**   **Acquired absence of both cervix and uterus**   UPD PE
  - Acquired absence of uterus NOS
  - Status post total hysterectomy
- **Z90.711**   **Acquired absence of uterus with remaining cervical stump**   UPD PE
  - Status post partial hysterectomy with remaining cervical stump
- **Z90.712**   **Acquired absence of cervix with remaining uterus**   UPD PE

√6th **Z90.72**   **Acquired absence of ovaries**
- **Z90.721**   **Acquired absence of ovaries, unilateral**   UPD PE
- **Z90.722**   **Acquired absence of ovaries, bilateral**   UPD PE

Z90.79   **Acquired absence of other genital organ(s)**   UPD PE
- AHA: 2023,2Q,5

√5th **Z90.8**   **Acquired absence of other organs**
- **Z90.81**   **Acquired absence of spleen**   UPD PE
- **Z90.89**   **Acquired absence of other organs**   UPD PE
  - AHA: 2023,3Q,13

√4th **Z91**   **Personal risk factors, not elsewhere classified**
- EXCLUDES 2   *contact with and (suspected) exposures hazardous to health (Z77.-)*
- *exposure to pollution and other problems related to physical environment (Z77.1-)*
- *female genital mutilation status (N90.81-)*
- *occupational exposure to risk factors (Z57.-)*
- *personal history of physical injury and trauma (Z87.81, Z87.82-)*

√5th **Z91.0**   **Allergy status, other than to drugs and biological substances**
- EXCLUDES 2   *allergy status to drugs, medicaments, and biological substances (Z88.-)*

√6th **Z91.01**   **Food allergy status**
- EXCLUDES 2   *food additives allergy status (Z91.02)*
- **Z91.010**   **Allergy to peanuts**   UPD PE
- **Z91.011**   **Allergy to milk products**   UPD PE
  - EXCLUDES 1   *lactose intolerance (E73.-)*
- **Z91.012**   **Allergy to eggs**   UPD PE
- **Z91.013**   **Allergy to seafood**   UPD PE
  - Allergy to octopus or squid ink
  - Allergy to shellfish

✓ Additional Character Required   √x7th Placeholder   Questionable PDx   Manifestation   Unspecified   UPD Unacceptable PDx   H1 - H14 HAC   HCC CMS-HCC Dx   HIV HIV Dx

Z91.Ø14 **Allergy to mammalian meats** `UPD` `PE`
    Allergy to beef
    Allergy to lamb
    Allergy to pork
    Allergy to red meats
    AHA: 2021,4Q,33

Z91.Ø18 **Allergy to other foods** `UPD` `PE`
    Allergy to nuts other than peanuts

Z91.Ø2 **Food additives allergy status** `UPD` `PE`

✓6ᵗʰ **Z91.Ø3** **Insect allergy status**

Z91.Ø3Ø **Bee allergy status** `UPD` `PE`

Z91.Ø38 **Other insect allergy status** `UPD` `PE`

✓6ᵗʰ **Z91.Ø4** **Nonmedicinal substance allergy status**

Z91.Ø4Ø **Latex allergy status** `UPD` `PE`
    Latex sensitivity status

Z91.Ø41 **Radiographic dye allergy status** `UPD` `PE`
    Allergy status to contrast media used for diagnostic X-ray procedure

Z91.Ø48 **Other nonmedicinal substance allergy status** `UPD` `PE`

Z91.Ø9 **Other allergy status, other than to drugs and biological substances** `UPD` `PE`

✓5ᵗʰ **Z91.1** **Patient's noncompliance with medical treatment and regimen**
    Code also, if applicable, to identify underdosing of specific drug (T36-T5Ø with final character 6)
    EXCLUDES 2 *caregiver noncompliance with patient's medical treatment and regimen (Z91.A-)*
    AHA: 2022,4Q,49

✓6ᵗʰ **Z91.11** **Patient's noncompliance with dietary regimen**
    Code also, if applicable, food insecurity (Z59.4-)

Z91.11Ø **Patient's noncompliance with dietary regimen due to financial hardship** `UPD` `PE`

Z91.118 **Patient's noncompliance with dietary regimen for other reason** `UPD` `PE`
    Inability to comply with dietary regimen

Z91.119 **Patient's noncompliance with dietary regimen due to unspecified reason** `UPD` `PE`

✓6ᵗʰ **Z91.12** **Patient's intentional underdosing of medication regimen**
    Code first underdosing of medication (T36-T5Ø) with fifth or sixth character 6
    EXCLUDES 1 *adverse effect of prescribed drug taken as directed - code to adverse effect*
    poisoning (overdose) - code to poisoning
    AHA: 2018,4Q,72

Z91.12Ø **Patient's intentional underdosing of medication regimen due to financial hardship** `UPD` `PE`

Z91.128 **Patient's intentional underdosing of medication regimen for other reason** `UPD` `PE`

✓6ᵗʰ **Z91.13** **Patient's unintentional underdosing of medication regimen**
    Code first underdosing of medication (T36-T5Ø) with fifth or sixth character 6
    EXCLUDES 1 *adverse effect of prescribed drug taken as directed - code to adverse effect*
    poisoning (overdose) - code to poisoning
    AHA: 2018,4Q,72

Z91.13Ø **Patient's unintentional underdosing of medication regimen due to age-related debility** `UPD` `PE`

Z91.138 **Patient's unintentional underdosing of medication regimen for other reason** `UPD` `PE`

✓6ᵗʰ **Z91.14** **Patient's other noncompliance with medication regimen**
    Patient's underdosing of medication NOS
    ▶Code first, if applicable, adverse effect of underdosing (T36-T5Ø)◀
    AHA: 2023,1Q,7; 2022,1Q,36; 2018,4Q,72

Z91.141 **Patient's other noncompliance with medication regimen due to financial hardship** `UPD` `PE`

Z91.148 **Patient's other noncompliance with medication regimen for other reason** `UPD` `PE`

✓6ᵗʰ **Z91.15** **Patient's noncompliance with renal dialysis**
    AHA: 2023,1Q,7

Z91.151 **Patient's noncompliance with renal dialysis due to financial hardship** `UPD` `PE`

Z91.158 **Patient's noncompliance with renal dialysis for other reason** `UPD` `PE`

✓6ᵗʰ **Z91.19** **Patient's noncompliance with other medical treatment and regimen**
    Patient's nonadherence to medical treatment

Z91.19Ø **Patient's noncompliance with other medical treatment and regimen due to financial hardship** `UPD` `PE`

Z91.198 **Patient's noncompliance with other medical treatment and regimen for other reason** `UPD` `PE`
    AHA: 2024,1Q,23

Z91.199 **Patient's noncompliance with other medical treatment and regimen due to unspecified reason** `UPD` `PE`

✓5ᵗʰ **Z91.A** **Caregiver's noncompliance with patient's medical treatment and regimen**
    AHA: 2023,4Q,48; 2022,4Q,49

✓6ᵗʰ **Z91.A1** **Caregiver's noncompliance with patient's dietary regimen**
    Caregiver's inability to comply with patient's dietary regimen
    Code also, if applicable, food insecurity (Z59.4-)

Z91.A1Ø **Caregiver's noncompliance with patient's dietary regimen due to financial hardship** `UPD` `PE`

Z91.A18 **Caregiver's noncompliance with patient's dietary regimen for other reason** `UPD` `PE`

✓6ᵗʰ **Z91.A2** **Caregiver's intentional underdosing of patient's medication regimen**
    Code first underdosing of medication (T36-T5Ø) with fifth or sixth character 6

Z91.A2Ø **Caregiver's intentional underdosing of patient's medication regimen due to financial hardship** `UPD` `PE`

Z91.A28 **Caregiver's intentional underdosing of medication regimen for other reason** `UPD` `PE`

Z91.A3 **Caregiver's unintentional underdosing of patient's medication regimen** `UPD` `PE`
    Code first underdosing of medication (T36-T5Ø) with fifth or sixth character 6

✓6ᵗʰ **Z91.A4** **Caregiver's other noncompliance with patient's medication regimen**
    Caregiver's underdosing of patient's medication NOS
    Caregiver's underdosing with patient's medication NOS

Z91.A41 **Caregiver's other noncompliance with patient's medication regimen due to financial hardship** `UPD` `PE`

Z91.A48 **Caregiver's other noncompliance with patient's medication regimen for other reason** `UPD` `PE`

✓6ᵗʰ **Z91.A5** **Caregiver's noncompliance with patient's renal dialysis**

Z91.A51 **Caregiver's noncompliance with patient's renal dialysis due to financial hardship** `UPD` `PE`

Z91.A58 **Caregiver's noncompliance with patient's renal dialysis for other reason** `UPD` `PE`

✓6ᵗʰ **Z91.A9** **Caregiver's noncompliance with patient's other medical treatment and regimen**
    Caregiver's nonadherence to patient's medical treatment

Z91.A91 **Caregiver's noncompliance with patient's other medical treatment and regimen due to financial hardship** `UPD` `PE`

Z91.A98 **Caregiver's noncompliance with patient's other medical treatment and regimen for other reason** `UPD` `PE`

✓5ᵗʰ **Z91.4** **Personal history of psychological trauma, not elsewhere classified**
AHA: 2023,1Q,7

✓6ᵗʰ **Z91.41** **Personal history of adult abuse**
EXCLUDES 2   personal history of abuse in childhood (Z62.81-)

Z91.410 **Personal history of adult physical and sexual abuse** UPD A PE
EXCLUDES 1   current adult physical abuse (T74.11, T76.11)
current adult sexual abuse (T74.21, T76.11)

Z91.411 **Personal history of adult psychological abuse** UPD A PE

Z91.412 **Personal history of adult neglect** UPD A PE
EXCLUDES 1   current adult neglect (T74.01, T76.01)

Z91.413 **Personal history of adult financial abuse** UPD PE

Z91.414 **Personal history of adult intimate partner abuse** UPD PE

Z91.419 **Personal history of unspecified adult abuse** UPD A PE

Z91.42 **Personal history of forced labor or sexual exploitation** UPD PE
AHA: 2018,4Q,32,35

Z91.49 **Other personal history of psychological trauma, not elsewhere classified** UPD PE

✓5ᵗʰ **Z91.5** **Personal history of self-harm**
Code also mental health disorder, if known
AHA: 2021,4Q,33

Z91.51 **Personal history of suicidal behavior** UPD PE
Personal history of parasuicide
Personal history of self-poisoning
Personal history of suicide attempt

Z91.52 **Personal history of nonsuicidal self-harm** UPD PE
Personal history of nonsuicidal self-injury
Personal history of self-inflicted injury without suicidal intent
Personal history of self-mutilation

✓5ᵗʰ **Z91.8** **Other specified personal risk factors, not elsewhere classified**

Z91.81 **History of falling** UPD PE
At risk for falling

Z91.82 **Personal history of military deployment** UPD A PE
Individual (civilian or military) with past history of military war, peacekeeping and humanitarian deployment (current or past conflict)
Returned from military deployment
EXCLUDES 2   personal history of military service (Z91.85)

Z91.83 ***Wandering in diseases classified elsewhere*** PE
Code first underlying disorder such as:
Alzheimer's disease (G30.-)
autism or pervasive developmental disorder (F84.-)
intellectual disabilities (F70-F79)
unspecified dementia with behavioral disturbance (F03.9-, F03.A-, F03.B-, F03.C-)

✓6ᵗʰ **Z91.84** **Oral health risk factors**
AHA: 2017,4Q,29

Z91.841 **Risk for dental caries, low** UPD PE

Z91.842 **Risk for dental caries, moderate** UPD PE

Z91.843 **Risk for dental caries, high** UPD PE

Z91.849 **Unspecified risk for dental caries** UPD PE

Z91.85 **Personal history of military service** UPD PE
Personal history of serving in the armed forces
Personal history of veteran
EXCLUDES 2   personal history of military deployment (Z91.82)
AHA: 2023,4Q,48

Z91.89 **Other specified personal risk factors, not elsewhere classified** UPD PE
Increased risk for social isolation
AHA: 2017,1Q,45

✓4ᵗʰ **Z92** **Personal history of medical treatment**
EXCLUDES 2   postprocedural states (Z98.-)

Z92.0 **Personal history of contraception** UPD PE
EXCLUDES 1   counseling or management of current contraceptive practices (Z30.-)
long term (current) use of contraception (Z79.3)
presence of (intrauterine) contraceptive device (Z97.5)

✓5ᵗʰ **Z92.2** **Personal history of drug therapy**
EXCLUDES 2   long term (current) drug therapy (Z79.-)

Z92.21 **Personal history of antineoplastic chemotherapy** UPD PE

Z92.22 **Personal history of monoclonal drug therapy** UPD PE
EXCLUDES 2   ▶personal history of immune checkpoint inhibitor therapy (Z92.26)◀

Z92.23 **Personal history of estrogen therapy** UPD PE

✓6ᵗʰ **Z92.24** **Personal history of steroid therapy**

Z92.240 **Personal history of inhaled steroid therapy** UPD PE

Z92.241 **Personal history of systemic steroid therapy** UPD PE
Personal history of steroid therapy NOS

Z92.25 **Personal history of immunosuppression therapy** UPD PE
EXCLUDES 2   personal history of steroid therapy (Z92.24)

Z92.26 **Personal history of immune checkpoint inhibitor therapy** UPD PE
Personal history of ICI drug therapy

Z92.29 **Personal history of other drug therapy** UPD PE

Z92.3 **Personal history of irradiation** UPD PE
Personal history of exposure to therapeutic radiation
EXCLUDES 1   exposure to radiation in the physical environment (Z77.12)
occupational exposure to radiation (Z57.1)

✓5ᵗʰ **Z92.8** **Personal history of other medical treatment**

Z92.81 **Personal history of extracorporeal membrane oxygenation (ECMO)** UPD PE

Z92.82 **Status post administration of tPA (rtPA) in a different facility within the last 24 hours prior to admission to current facility** UPD PE
Code first condition requiring tPA administration, such as:
acute cerebral infarction (I63.-)
acute myocardial infarction (I21.-, I22.-)
AHA: 2013,4Q,124

Z92.83 **Personal history of failed moderate sedation** UPD PE
Personal history of failed conscious sedation
EXCLUDES 2   failed moderate sedation during procedure (T88.52)

Z92.84 **Personal history of unintended awareness under general anesthesia** UPD PE
EXCLUDES 2   unintended awareness under general anesthesia during procedure (T88.53)
AHA: 2016,4Q,72-73,77

✓6ᵗʰ **Z92.85** **Personal history of cellular therapy**
EXCLUDES 2   ▶personal history of immune checkpoint inhibitor therapy (Z92.26)◀
AHA: 2021,4Q,33-34

Z92.850 **Personal history of Chimeric Antigen Receptor T-cell therapy** UPD PE
Personal history of CAR T-cell therapy

Z92.858 **Personal history of other cellular therapy** UPD PE

Z92.859 **Personal history of cellular therapy, unspecified** UPD PE

Z92.86 **Personal history of gene therapy** UPD PE
AHA: 2021,4Q,33-34

Z92.89 **Personal history of other medical treatment** UPD PE
AHA: 2020,1Q,18

✓ Additional Character Required   ✓x7ᵗʰ Placeholder   Questionable PDx   Manifestation   Unspecified   UPD Unacceptable PDx   H1-H14 HAC   HCC CMS-HCC Dx   HIV HIV Dx

Chapter 21. Factors Influencing Health Status and Contact With Health Services

Z93–Z96.619

√4th **Z93 Artificial opening status**

> EXCLUDES 1   *artificial openings requiring attention or management (Z43.-)*
> *complications of external stoma (J95.0-, K94.-, N99.5-)*

Z93.0 Tracheostomy status   UPD HCC PE
> **AHA:** 2013,4Q,129

Z93.1 Gastrostomy status   UPD HCC PE

Z93.2 Ileostomy status   UPD HCC PE
> ►Ileal pouch status◄
> ►Kock pouch status◄

Z93.3 Colostomy status   UPD HCC PE

Z93.4 Other artificial openings of gastrointestinal tract status   UPD HCC PE

√5th **Z93.5 Cystostomy status**

> **Z93.50 Unspecified cystostomy status**   UPD HCC PE
> **Z93.51 Cutaneous-vesicostomy status**   UPD HCC PE
> **Z93.52 Appendico-vesicostomy status**   UPD HCC PE
> **Z93.59 Other cystostomy status**   UPD HCC PE

Z93.6 Other artificial openings of urinary tract status   UPD HCC PE
> Nephrostomy status
> Ureterostomy status
> Urethrostomy status

Z93.8 Other artificial opening status   UPD HCC PE

Z93.9 Artificial opening status, unspecified   UPD HCC PE

√4th **Z94 Transplanted organ and tissue status**

> INCLUDES   organ or tissue replaced by heterogenous or homogenous transplant
> EXCLUDES 1   *complications of transplanted organ or tissue - see Alphabetical Index*
> EXCLUDES 2   *presence of vascular grafts (Z95.-)*

Z94.0 Kidney transplant status   CC UPD PE

Z94.1 Heart transplant status   CC UPD HCC PE
> EXCLUDES 1   *artificial heart status (Z95.812)*
> *heart-valve replacement status (Z95.2-Z95.4)*

Z94.2 Lung transplant status   CC UPD HCC PE

Z94.3 Heart and lungs transplant status   CC UPD HCC PE

Z94.4 Liver transplant status   CC UPD HCC PE

Z94.5 Skin transplant status   UPD PE
> Autogenous skin transplant status

Z94.6 Bone transplant status   UPD PE

Z94.7 Corneal transplant status   UPD PE

√5th **Z94.8 Other transplanted organ and tissue status**

> **Z94.81 Bone marrow transplant status**   CC UPD HCC PE
> **Z94.82 Intestine transplant status**   CC UPD HCC PE
> **Z94.83 Pancreas transplant status**   CC UPD HCC PE
> **Z94.84 Stem cells transplant status**   CC UPD HCC PE
> **Z94.89 Other transplanted organ and tissue status**   UPD PE

Z94.9 Transplanted organ and tissue status, unspecified   UPD PE

√4th **Z95 Presence of cardiac and vascular implants and grafts**

> EXCLUDES 2   *complications of cardiac and vascular devices, implants and grafts (T82.-)*

Z95.0 Presence of cardiac pacemaker   UPD PE
> Presence of cardiac resynchronization therapy (CRT-P) pacemaker
> EXCLUDES 1   *adjustment or management of cardiac device (Z45.0-)*
> *adjustment or management of cardiac pacemaker (Z45.0)*
> *presence of automatic (implantable) cardiac defibrillator with synchronous cardiac pacemaker (Z95.810)*
>
> **AHA:** 2022,2Q,14; 2019,1Q,33
> **TIP:** Assign an additional code for the associated condition if that condition requires constant intervention from the device, as in cases of sick sinus syndrome. For conditions that do not require constant intervention from the device, as in cases of ventricular fibrillation, an additional code for the associated condition should be assigned only if the patient is experiencing the condition and the device is firing during the current admission.

Z95.1 Presence of aortocoronary bypass graft   UPD PE
> Presence of coronary artery bypass graft

Z95.2 Presence of prosthetic heart valve   UPD PE
> Presence of heart valve NOS

Z95.3 Presence of xenogenic heart valve   UPD PE

Z95.4 Presence of other heart-valve replacement   UPD PE

Z95.5 Presence of coronary angioplasty implant and graft   UPD PE
> EXCLUDES 1   *coronary angioplasty status without implant and graft (Z98.61)*

√5th **Z95.8 Presence of other cardiac and vascular implants and grafts**

√6th **Z95.81 Presence of other cardiac implants and grafts**

> **Z95.810 Presence of automatic (implantable) cardiac defibrillator**   UPD PE
> Presence of automatic (implantable) cardiac defibrillator with synchronous cardiac pacemaker
> Presence of cardiac resynchronization therapy defibrillator (CRT-D)
> Presence of cardioverter-defibrillator (ICD)
> **AHA:** 2022,2Q,14; 2019,1Q,33
> **TIP:** Assign an additional code for the associated condition if that condition requires constant intervention from the device, as in cases of sick sinus syndrome. For conditions that do not require constant intervention from the device, as in cases of ventricular fibrillation, an additional code for the associated condition should be assigned only if the patient is experiencing the condition and the device is firing during the current admission.
>
> **Z95.811 Presence of heart assist device**   CC UPD HCC PE
> **Z95.812 Presence of fully implantable artificial heart**   CC UPD HCC PE
> **Z95.818 Presence of other cardiac implants and grafts**   UPD PE

√6th **Z95.82 Presence of other vascular implants and grafts**

> **Z95.820 Peripheral vascular angioplasty status with implants and grafts**   UPD PE
> EXCLUDES 1   *peripheral vascular angioplasty without implant and graft (Z98.62)*
>
> **Z95.828 Presence of other vascular implants and grafts**   UPD PE
> Presence of intravascular prosthesis NEC

Z95.9 Presence of cardiac and vascular implant and graft, unspecified   UPD PE

√4th **Z96 Presence of other functional implants**

> EXCLUDES 2   *complications of internal prosthetic devices, implants and grafts (T82-T85)*
> *fitting and adjustment of prosthetic and other devices (Z44-Z46)*

Z96.0 Presence of urogenital implants   UPD

Z96.1 Presence of intraocular lens   UPD
> Presence of pseudophakia

√5th **Z96.2 Presence of otological and audiological implants**

> **Z96.20 Presence of otological and audiological implant, unspecified**   UPD
> **Z96.21 Cochlear implant status**   UPD
> **Z96.22 Myringotomy tube(s) status**   UPD
> **Z96.29 Presence of other otological and audiological implants**   UPD
> Presence of bone-conduction hearing device
> Presence of eustachian tube stent
> Stapes replacement

Z96.3 Presence of artificial larynx   UPD

√5th **Z96.4 Presence of endocrine implants**

> **Z96.41 Presence of insulin pump (external) (internal)**   UPD
> **Z96.49 Presence of other endocrine implants**   UPD

Z96.5 Presence of tooth-root and mandibular implants   UPD

√5th **Z96.6 Presence of orthopedic joint implants**

> **AHA:** 2019,3Q,16
>
> **Z96.60 Presence of unspecified orthopedic joint implant**   UPD

√6th **Z96.61 Presence of artificial shoulder joint**

> **Z96.611 Presence of right artificial shoulder joint**   UPD
> **Z96.612 Presence of left artificial shoulder joint**   UPD
> **Z96.619 Presence of unspecified artificial shoulder joint**   UPD

✓6ᵗʰ **Z96.62** Presence of artificial elbow joint

    Z96.621 Presence of right artificial elbow joint `UPD`

    Z96.622 Presence of left artificial elbow joint `UPD`

    Z96.629 Presence of unspecified artificial elbow joint `UPD`

✓6ᵗʰ **Z96.63** Presence of artificial wrist joint

    Z96.631 Presence of right artificial wrist joint `UPD`

    Z96.632 Presence of left artificial wrist joint `UPD`

    Z96.639 Presence of unspecified artificial wrist joint `UPD`

✓6ᵗʰ **Z96.64** Presence of artificial hip joint

    Hip-joint replacement (partial) (total)

    Z96.641 Presence of right artificial hip joint `UPD`

    Z96.642 Presence of left artificial hip joint `UPD`

    Z96.643 Presence of artificial hip joint, bilateral `UPD`

    Z96.649 Presence of unspecified artificial hip joint `UPD`

✓6ᵗʰ **Z96.65** Presence of artificial knee joint

    Z96.651 Presence of right artificial knee joint `UPD`

    Z96.652 Presence of left artificial knee joint `UPD`

    Z96.653 Presence of artificial knee joint, bilateral `UPD`

    Z96.659 Presence of unspecified artificial knee joint `UPD`

✓6ᵗʰ **Z96.66** Presence of artificial ankle joint

    Z96.661 Presence of right artificial ankle joint `UPD`

    Z96.662 Presence of left artificial ankle joint `UPD`

    Z96.669 Presence of unspecified artificial ankle joint `UPD`

✓6ᵗʰ **Z96.69** Presence of other orthopedic joint implants

    Z96.691 Finger-joint replacement of right hand `UPD`

    Z96.692 Finger-joint replacement of left hand `UPD`

    Z96.693 Finger-joint replacement, bilateral `UPD`

    Z96.698 Presence of other orthopedic joint implants `UPD`

Z96.7 Presence of other bone and tendon implants `UPD`

    Presence of skull plate

✓5ᵗʰ **Z96.8** Presence of other specified functional implants

    Z96.81 Presence of artificial skin `UPD`

    Z96.82 Presence of neurostimulator `UPD` `PE`

      Presence of brain neurostimulator
      Presence of gastric neurostimulator
      Presence of peripheral nerve neurostimulator
      Presence of sacral nerve neurostimulator
      Presence of spinal cord neurostimulator
      Presence of vagus nerve neurostimulator
      AHA: 2019,4Q,19

    Z96.89 Presence of other specified functional implants `UPD`

Z96.9 Presence of functional implant, unspecified `UPD`

✓4ᵗʰ **Z97** Presence of other devices

    EXCLUDES 1 complications of internal prosthetic devices, implants and grafts (T82-T85)

    EXCLUDES 2 fitting and adjustment of prosthetic and other devices (Z44-Z46)
      presence of cerebrospinal fluid drainage device (Z98.2)

Z97.0 Presence of artificial eye `UPD` `PE`

✓5ᵗʰ **Z97.1** Presence of artificial limb (complete) (partial)

    Z97.10 Presence of artificial limb (complete) (partial), unspecified `UPD` `PE`

    Z97.11 Presence of artificial right arm (complete) (partial) `UPD` `PE`

    Z97.12 Presence of artificial left arm (complete) (partial) `UPD` `PE`

    Z97.13 Presence of artificial right leg (complete) (partial) `UPD` `HCC` `PE`

    Z97.14 Presence of artificial left leg (complete) (partial) `UPD` `HCC` `PE`

    Z97.15 Presence of artificial arms, bilateral (complete) (partial) `UPD` `PE`

    Z97.16 Presence of artificial legs, bilateral (complete) (partial) `UPD` `HCC` `PE`

Z97.2 Presence of dental prosthetic device (complete) (partial) `UPD` `PE`

    Presence of dentures (complete) (partial)

Z97.3 Presence of spectacles and contact lenses `UPD` `PE`

Z97.4 Presence of external hearing-aid `UPD` `PE`

Z97.5 Presence of (intrauterine) contraceptive device `UPD` `PE`

    EXCLUDES 1 checking, reinsertion or removal of implantable subdermal contraceptive (Z30.46)
      checking, reinsertion or removal of intrauterine contraceptive device (Z30.43-)

Z97.8 Presence of other specified devices `UPD` `PE`

✓4ᵗʰ **Z98** Other postprocedural states

    EXCLUDES 2 aftercare (Z43-Z49, Z51)
      follow-up medical care (Z08-Z09)
      postprocedural complication - see Alphabetical Index

Z98.0 Intestinal bypass and anastomosis status `UPD` `PE`

    EXCLUDES 2 bariatric surgery status (Z98.84)
      gastric bypass status (Z98.84)
      obesity surgery status (Z98.84)

Z98.1 Arthrodesis status `UPD` `PE`

    AHA: 2024,1Q,23

Z98.2 Presence of cerebrospinal fluid drainage device `UPD` `PE`

    Presence of CSF shunt

Z98.3 Post therapeutic collapse of lung status `UPD` `PE`

    Code first underlying disease

✓5ᵗʰ **Z98.4** Cataract extraction status

    Use additional code to identify intraocular lens implant status (Z96.1)

    EXCLUDES 1 aphakia (H27.0)

    Z98.41 Cataract extraction status, right eye `UPD` `PE`

    Z98.42 Cataract extraction status, left eye `UPD` `PE`

    Z98.49 Cataract extraction status, unspecified eye `UPD` `PE`

✓5ᵗʰ **Z98.5** Sterilization status

    EXCLUDES 1 female infertility (N97.-)
      male infertility (N46.-)

    Z98.51 Tubal ligation status `UPD` `PE`

    Z98.52 Vasectomy status `UPD` `A` `PE`

✓5ᵗʰ **Z98.6** Angioplasty status

    Z98.61 Coronary angioplasty status `UPD` `PE`

      EXCLUDES 1 coronary angioplasty status with implant and graft (Z95.5)

    Z98.62 Peripheral vascular angioplasty status `UPD` `PE`

      EXCLUDES 1 peripheral vascular angioplasty status with implant and graft (Z95.820)

✓5ᵗʰ **Z98.8** Other specified postprocedural states

    ✓6ᵗʰ **Z98.81** Dental procedure status

      Z98.810 Dental sealant status `UPD` `PE`

      Z98.811 Dental restoration status `UPD` `PE`

        Dental crown status
        Dental fillings status

      Z98.818 Other dental procedure status `UPD` `PE`

    Z98.82 Breast implant status `UPD` `PE`

      EXCLUDES 1 breast implant removal status (Z98.86)

      AHA: 2022,3Q,8

    Z98.83 Filtering (vitreous) bleb after glaucoma surgery status `UPD` `PE`

      EXCLUDES 1 inflammation (infection) of postprocedural bleb (H59.4-)

      AHA: 2020,3Q,29

    Z98.84 Bariatric surgery status `UPD` `PE`

      Gastric banding status
      Gastric bypass status for obesity
      Obesity surgery status

      EXCLUDES 1 bariatric surgery status complicating pregnancy, childbirth, or the puerperium (O99.84)

      EXCLUDES 2 intestinal bypass and anastomosis status (Z98.0)

      AHA: 2020,1Q,12

✓ Additional Character Required   ✓x7ᵗʰ Placeholder   Questionable PDx   Manifestation   Unspecified   `UPD` Unacceptable PDx   H1-H14 HAC   `HCC` CMS-HCC Dx   `HIV` HIV Dx

ICD-10-CM 2025   1297

Chapter 21. Factors Influencing Health Status and Contact With Health Services

Z98.85   **Transplanted organ removal status**   UPD PE
Transplanted organ previously removed due to complication, failure, rejection or infection
> EXCLUDES 1   *encounter for removal of transplanted organ - code to complication of transplanted organ (T86.-)*

Z98.86   **Personal history of breast implant removal**   UPD PE

√6th **Z98.87**   **Personal history of in utero procedure**

    Z98.870   **Personal history of in utero procedure during pregnancy**   UPD PE
> EXCLUDES 2   *complications from in utero procedure for current pregnancy (O35.7)*
> *supervision of current pregnancy with history of in utero procedure during previous pregnancy (O09.82-)*

    Z98.871   **Personal history of in utero procedure while a fetus**   UPD PE

√6th **Z98.89**   **Other specified postprocedural states**

    Z98.890   **Other specified postprocedural states**   UPD PE
Personal history of surgery, not elsewhere classified
AHA: 2023,3Q,13

    Z98.891   **History of uterine scar from previous surgery**   UPD PE
> EXCLUDES 1   *maternal care due to uterine scar from previous surgery (O34.2-)*
AHA: 2016,4Q,51-52,76

√4th **Z99**   **Dependence on enabling machines and devices, not elsewhere classified**
AHA: 2020,1Q,11

Z99.0   **Dependence on aspirator**   UPD PE

√5th **Z99.1**   **Dependence on respirator**
Dependence on ventilator

    Z99.11   **Dependence on respirator [ventilator] status**   CC HCC PE
AHA: 2015,1Q,21

    Z99.12   **Encounter for respirator [ventilator] dependence during power failure**   CC HCC PE
> EXCLUDES 1   *mechanical complication of respirator [ventilator] (J95.850)*

Z99.2   **Dependence on renal dialysis**   UPD PE
Hemodialysis status
Peritoneal dialysis status
Presence of arteriovenous shunt for dialysis
Renal dialysis status NOS
> EXCLUDES 1   *encounter for fitting and adjustment of dialysis catheter (Z49.0-)*
> EXCLUDES 2   *noncompliance with renal dialysis (Z91.15-)*
AHA: 2022,3Q,15; 2016,1Q,12; 2013,4Q,125

Z99.3   **Dependence on wheelchair**   UPD PE
Wheelchair confinement status
Code first cause of dependence, such as:
   muscular dystrophy (G71.0-)
   obesity (E66.-)

√5th **Z99.8**   **Dependence on other enabling machines and devices**

    Z99.81   **Dependence on supplemental oxygen**   UPD PE
Dependence on long-term oxygen
AHA: 2013,4Q,129

    Z99.89   **Dependence on other enabling machines and devices**   UPD PE
Dependence on machine or device NOS
AHA: 2020,1Q,11

Chapter 22. Codes for Special Purposes (UØØ–U85)

Chapter-specific Guidelines

UØ7.Ø	Vaping-related disorder (see Section I.C.10.e., Vaping-related disorders)
UØ7.1	COVID-19 (see Section I.C.1.g.1., COVID-19 infection)
UØ9.9	Post COVID-19 condition, unspecified (see Section I.C.1.g.1.m.)

Chapter 22. Codes for Special Purposes (U00-U85)

This chapter contains the following blocks:

U00-U49   Provisional assignment of new diseases of uncertain etiology or emergency use

Provisional assignment of new diseases of uncertain etiology or emergency use (U00-U49)

✓4ᵗʰ U07   Emergency use of U07

U07.0   Vaping-related disorder

Dabbing related lung damage
Dabbing related lung injury
E-cigarette, or vaping, product use associated lung injury [EVALI]
Electronic cigarette related lung damage
Electronic cigarette related lung injury

Use additional code, to identify manifestations, such as:
   abdominal pain (R10.84)
   acute respiratory distress syndrome (J80)
   diarrhea (R19.7)
   drug-induced interstitial lung disorder (J70.4)
   lipoid pneumonia (J69.1)
   weight loss (R63.4)

DEF: Respiratory illness or injury caused by harmful aerosolized substances and chemicals produced by electronic cigarettes, vapes, e-pipes, and other battery-powered vaping devices. Symptoms may include shortness of breath and fever, while some patients experience severe, sometimes fatal, lung damage.
Synonym(s): *e-cigarette and vaping product use-associated lung injury, EVALI.*

U07.1   COVID-19   HIV MCC

Use additional code to identify pneumonia or other manifestations, such as:
pneumonia due to COVID-19 (J12.82)
Use additional code, if applicable, for associated conditions such as:
   COVID-19 associated coagulopathy (D68.8)
   disseminated intravascular coagulation (D65)
   hypercoagulable states (D68.69)
   thrombophilia (D68.69)

EXCLUDES 2   *coronavirus as the cause of diseases classified elsewhere (B97.2-)*
     pneumonia due to SARS-associated coronavirus (J12.81)

AHA: 2022,2Q,28; 2021,4Q,101,107-108; 2021,1Q,25-30,31-49; 2020,4Q,14,99; 2020,3Q,9-16; 2020,2Q,3-13

DEF: First diagnosed in December 2019 in China, coronavirus disease 2019 (COVID-19) is a respiratory infection caused by a newly identified (novel) virus not previously seen in humans, known as severe acute respiratory syndrome coronavirus 2 (SARS-CoV-2). Symptoms of this lower respiratory illness include fever, dry cough, and tiredness that may progress to include difficulty breathing. Older patients and those with high blood pressure, heart problems, and diabetes are more likely to develop serious symptoms of the illness. **Synonym(s):** *SARS-CoV-2, coronavirus disease 2019.*

TIP: Only a confirmed diagnosis of COVID-19, either through a positive test result documented in the medical record or documentation by the provider, can be coded to U07.1.

TIP: Assign for asymptomatic individuals who test positive for COVID-19. Even though asymptomatic, the individual is considered to have the COVID-19 infection due to the positive test result.

TIP: Assign appropriate codes for presenting signs/symptoms associated with COVID-19 (cough, fever, shortness of breath) instead of U07.1, if a definitive diagnosis has not been established.

✓4ᵗʰ U09   Post COVID-19 condition

U09.9   Post COVID-19 condition, unspecified

NOTE   This code enables establishment of a link with COVID-19.

This code is not to be used in cases that are still presenting with active COVID-19. However, an exception is made in cases of re-infection with COVID-19, occurring with a condition related to prior COVID-19.

Post-acute sequela of COVID-19
Code first the specific condition related to COVID-19 if known, such as:
   chronic respiratory failure (J96.1-)
   loss of smell (R43.8)
   loss of taste (R43.8)
   multisystem inflammatory syndrome (M35.81)
   pulmonary embolism (I26.-)
   pulmonary fibrosis (J84.10)
AHA: 2021,4Q,31-32,102-106

Illustrations

Chapter 3. Diseases of the Blood and Blood-forming Organs and Certain Disorders Involving the Immune Mechanism (D5Ø–D89)

Red Blood Cells

White Blood Cell

Platelet

Coagulation

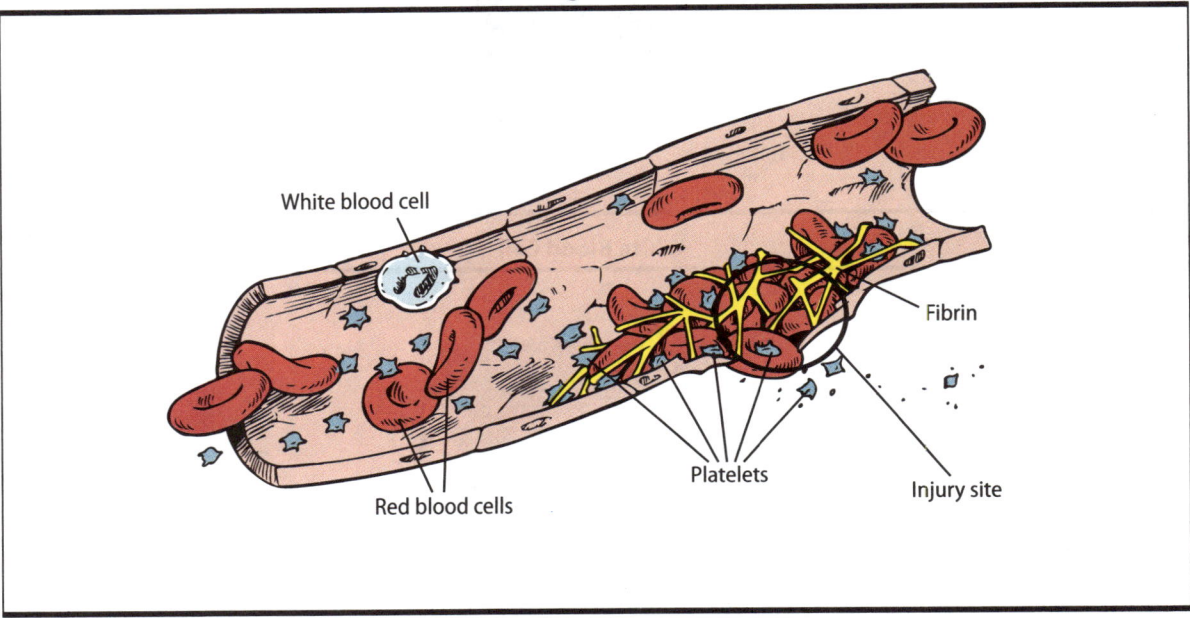

Spleen Anatomical Location and External Structures

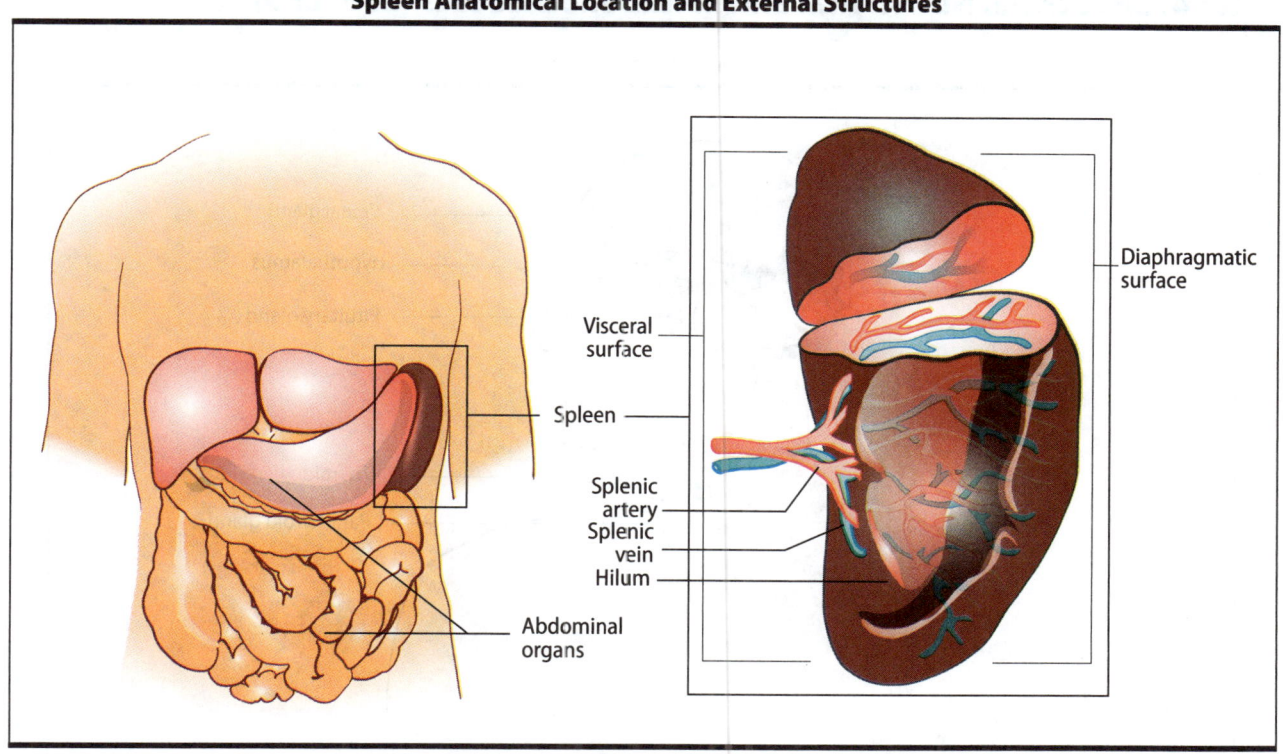

Spleen Interior Structures

Chapter 4. Endocrine, Nutritional and Metabolic Diseases (E00–E89)

Endocrine System

Thyroid

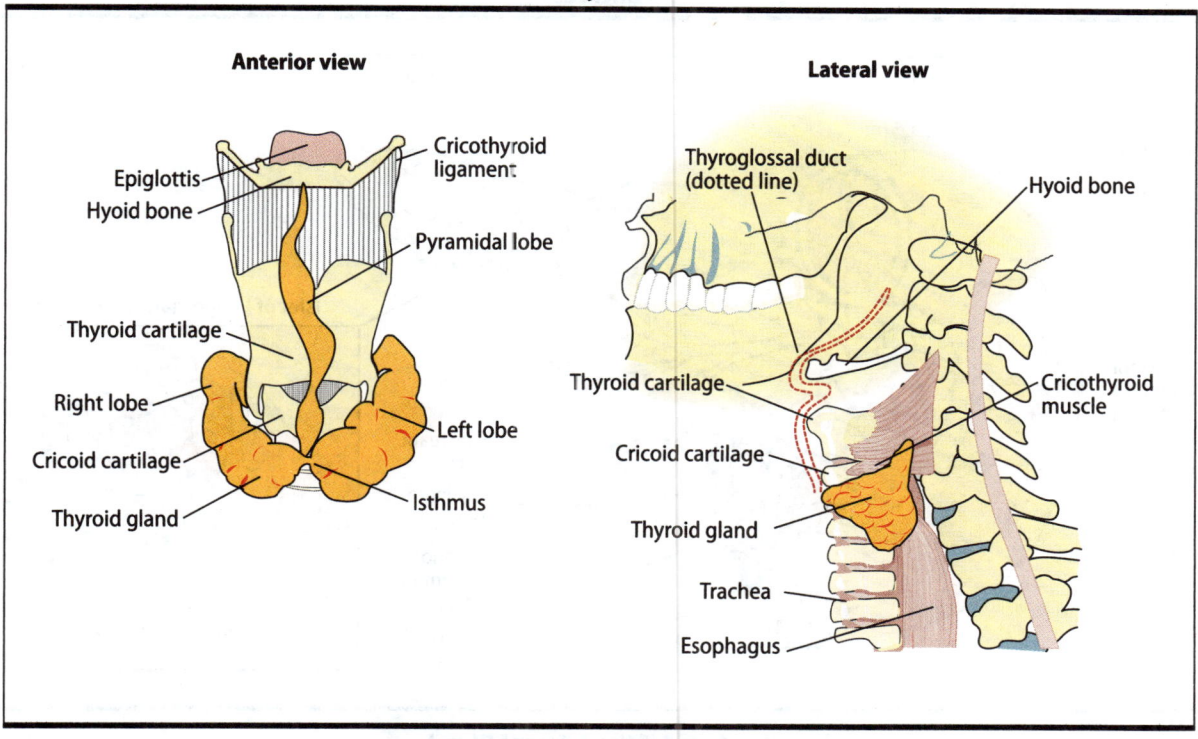

Thyroid and Parathyroid Glands

Pancreas

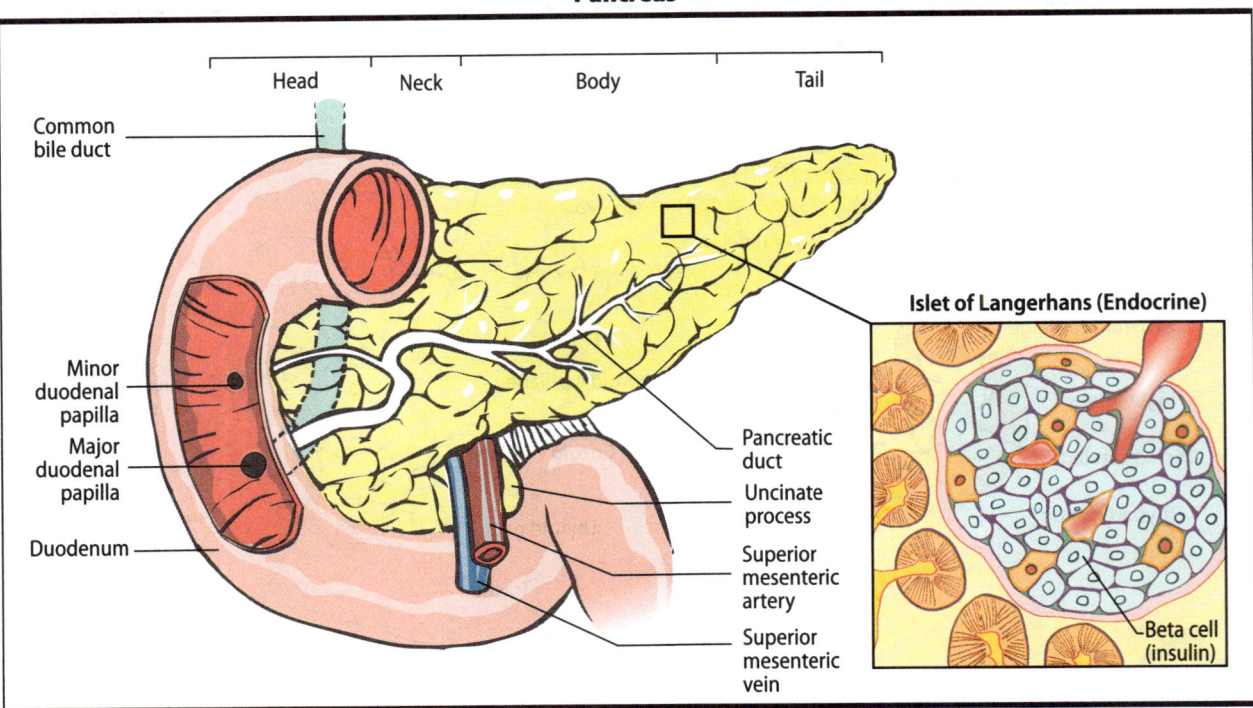

Head   Neck   Body   Tail

Common bile duct

Minor duodenal papilla

Major duodenal papilla

Duodenum

Pancreatic duct

Uncinate process

Superior mesenteric artery

Superior mesenteric vein

Islet of Langerhans (Endocrine)

Beta cell (insulin)

Anatomy of the Adrenal Gland

Adrenal glands

Kidney

Capsule

Cortex

Medulla

Structure of an Ovary

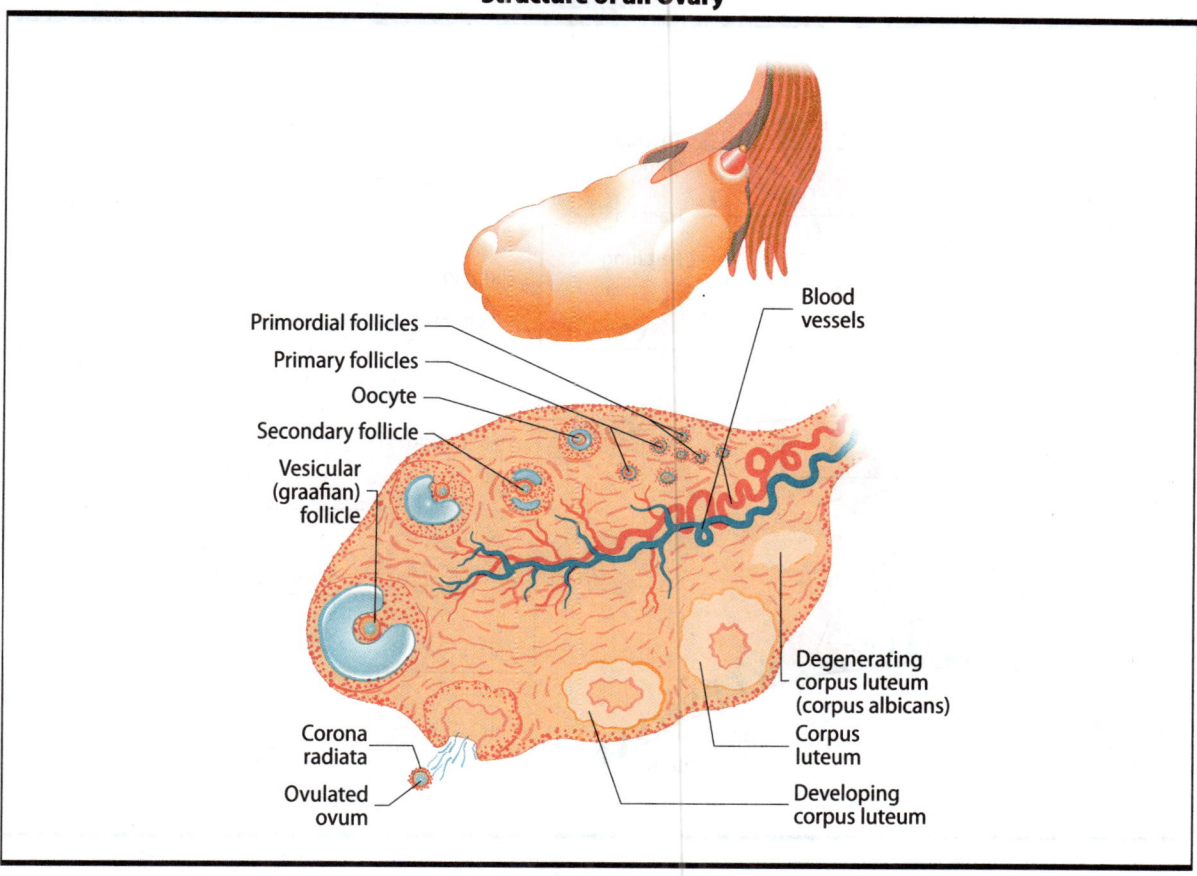

Testis and Associated Structures

Thymus

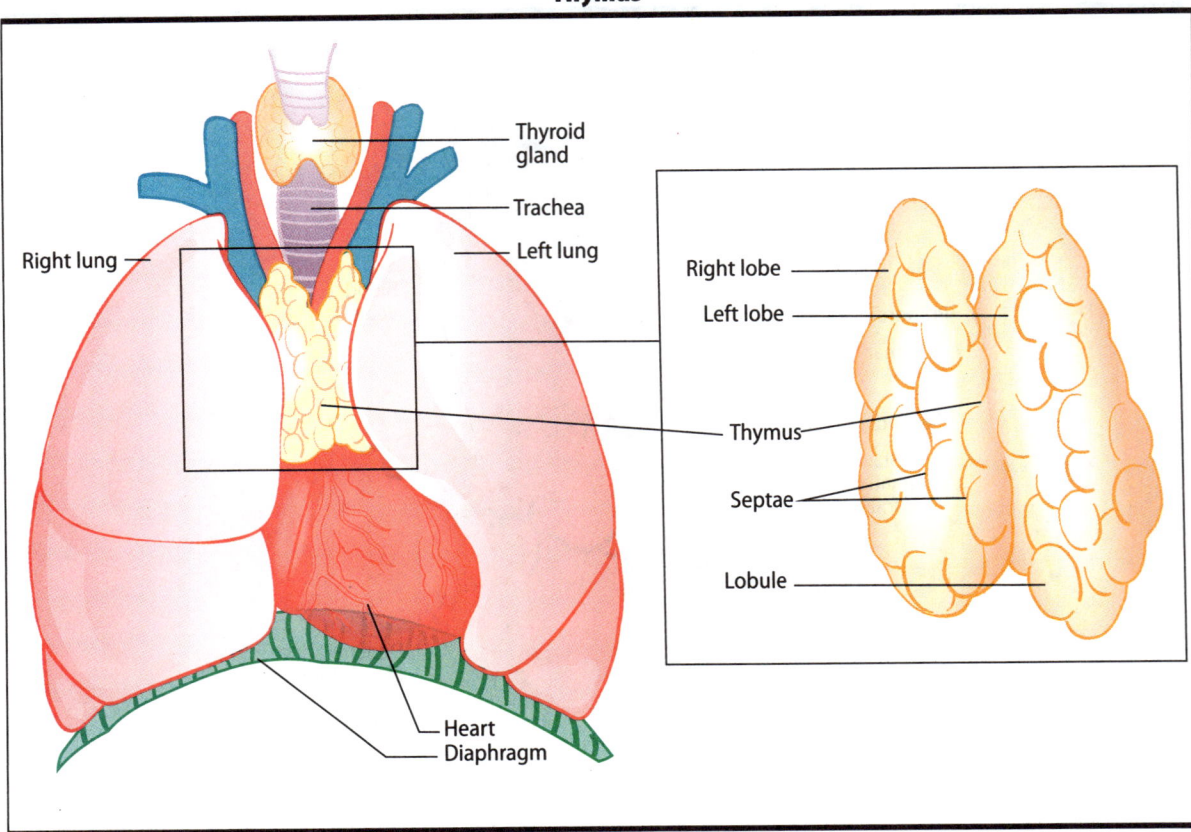

Chapter 6. Diseases of the Nervous System (G00–G99)

Brain

Cranial Nerves

Peripheral Nervous System

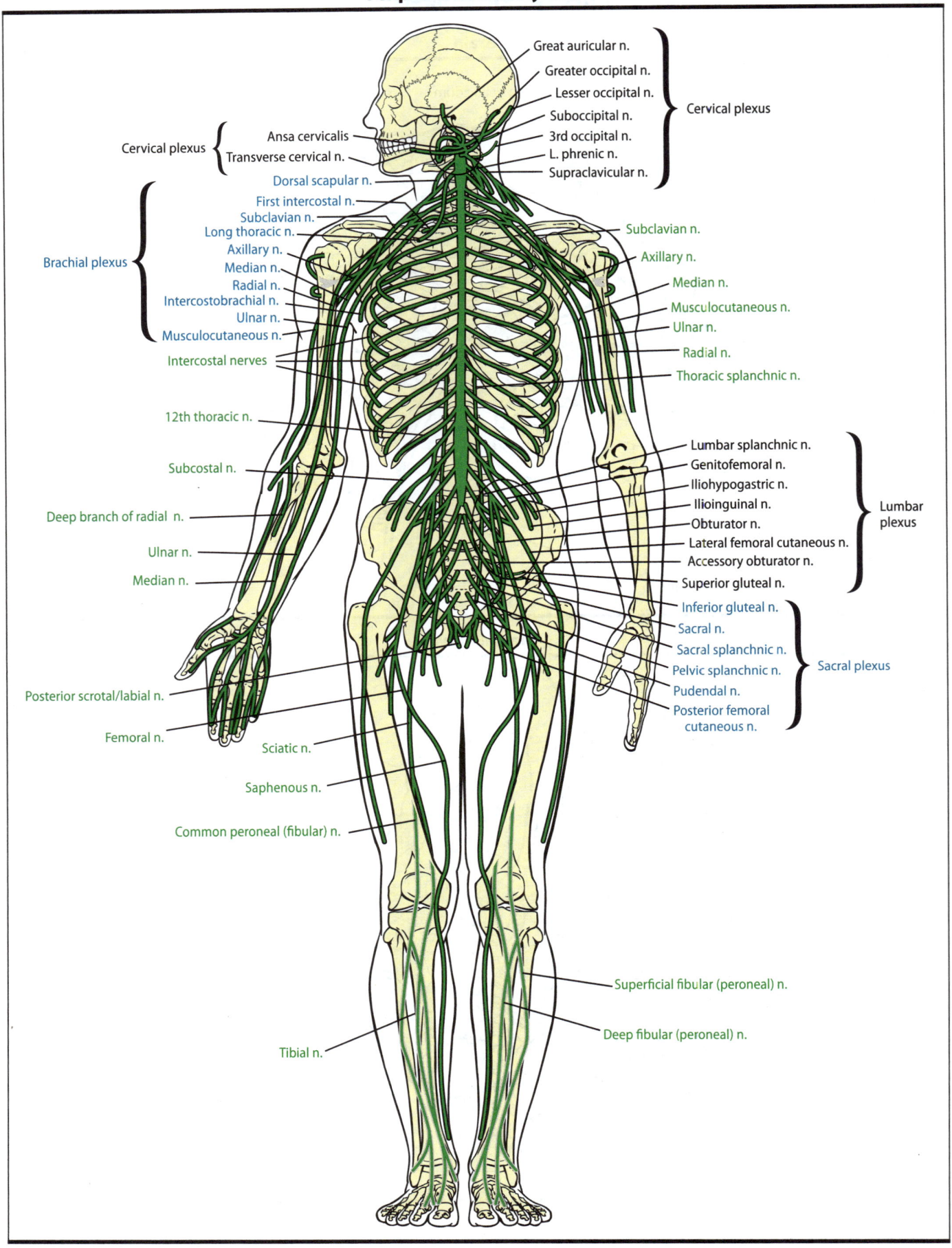

Spinal Cord and Spinal Nerves

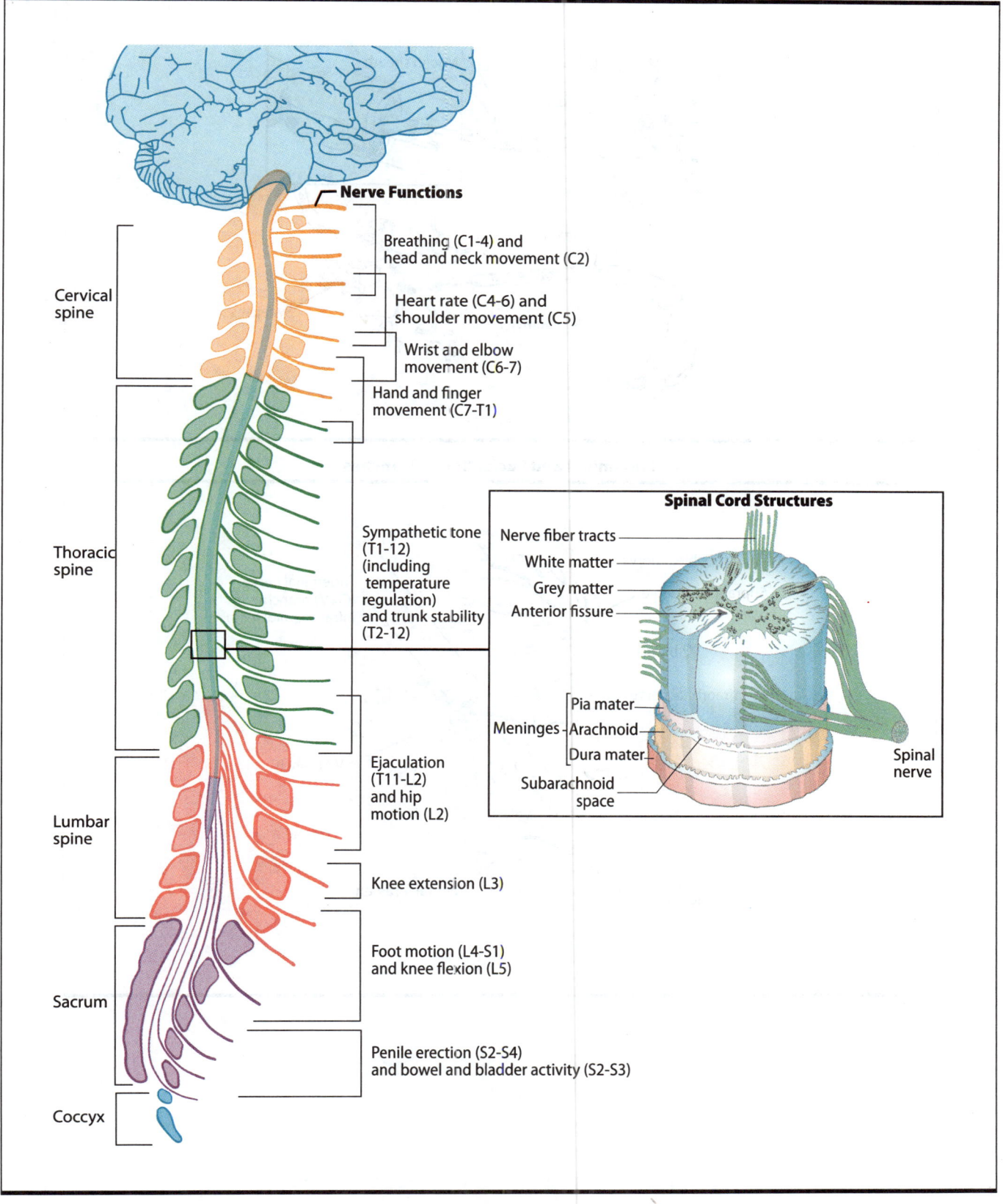

Nerve Functions

Breathing (C1-4) and
head and neck movement (C2)

Heart rate (C4-6) and
shoulder movement (C5)

Wrist and elbow
movement (C6-7)

Hand and finger
movement (C7-T1)

Sympathetic tone
(T1-12) (including
temperature
regulation)
and trunk stability
(T2-12)

Ejaculation
(T11-L2)
and hip
motion (L2)

Knee extension (L3)

Foot motion (L4-S1)
and knee flexion (L5)

Penile erection (S2-S4)
and bowel and bladder activity (S2-S3)

Cervical
spine

Thoracic
spine

Lumbar
spine

Sacrum

Coccyx

Spinal Cord Structures

Nerve fiber tracts

White matter

Grey matter

Anterior fissure

Meninges
- Pia mater
- Arachnoid
- Dura mater

Subarachnoid
space

Spinal
nerve

Nerve Cell

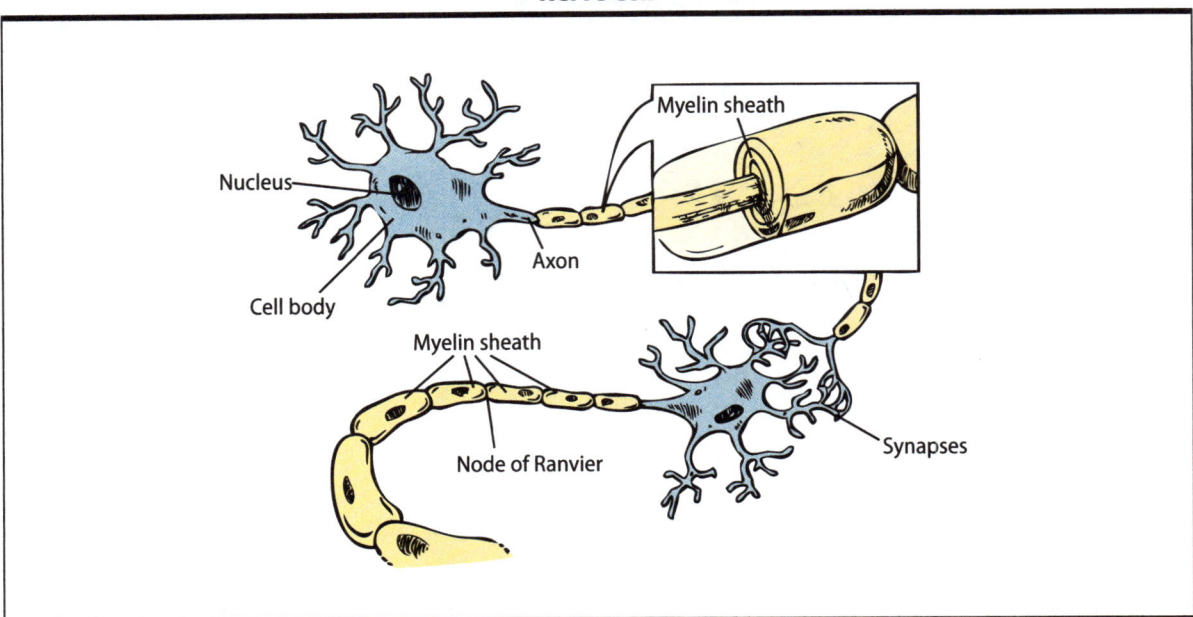

Trigeminal and Facial Nerve Branches

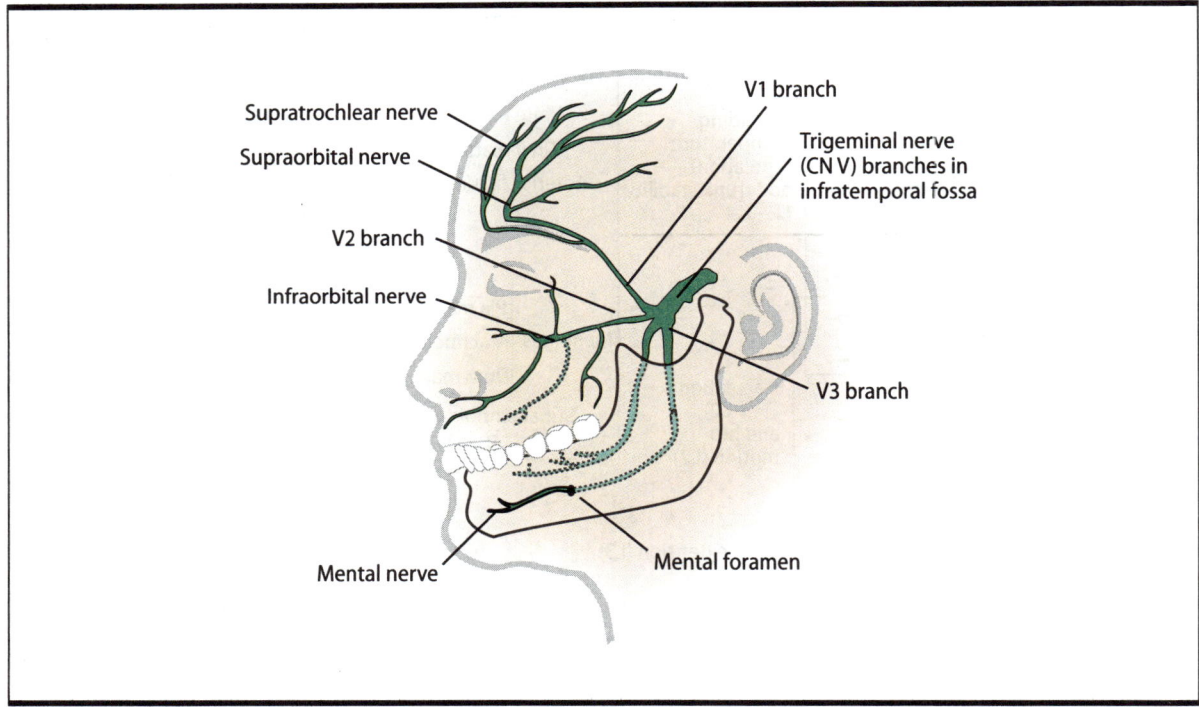

Chapter 7. Diseases of the Eye and Adnexa (H00–H59)

Eye

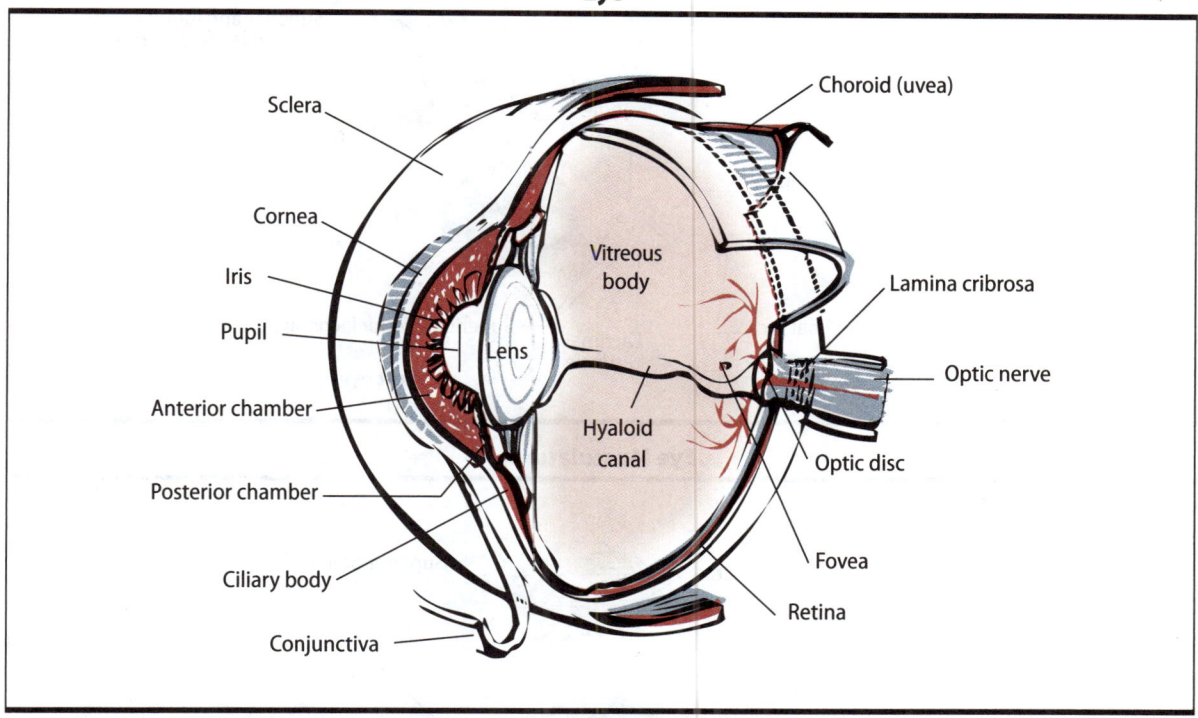

Posterior Pole of Globe/Flow of Aqueous Humor

Posterior Pole of Globe

Flow of Aqueous Humor

Lacrimal System

Eye Musculature

Eyelid Structures

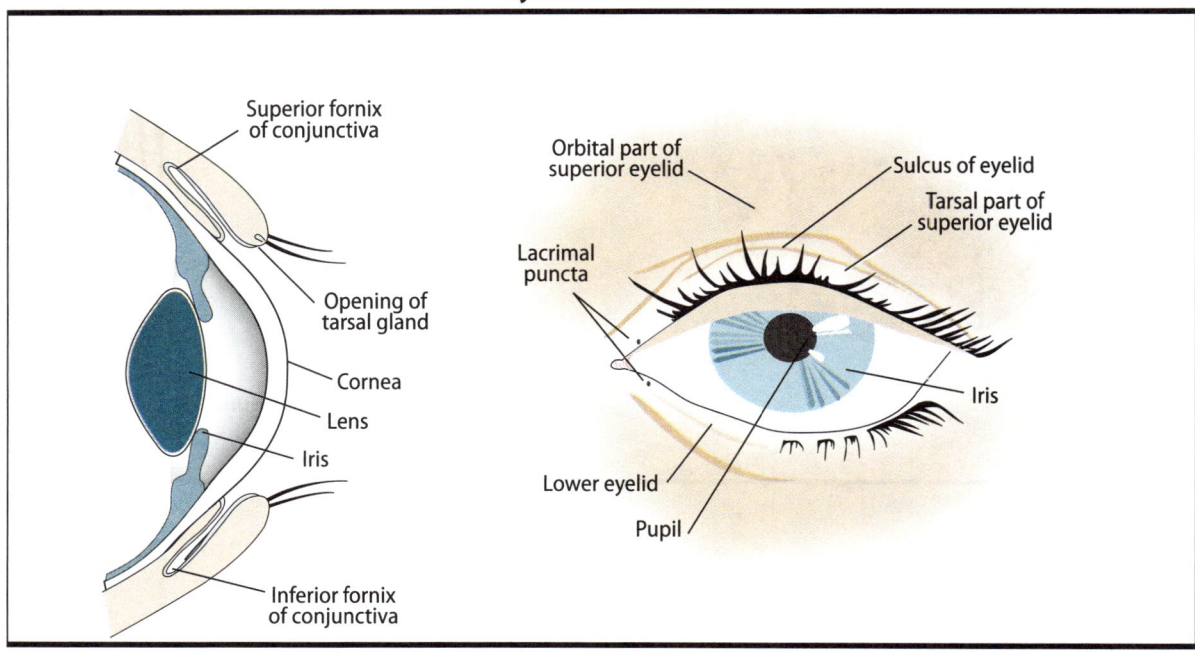

Chapter 8. Diseases of the Ear and Mastoid Process (H60–H95)

Ear Anatomy

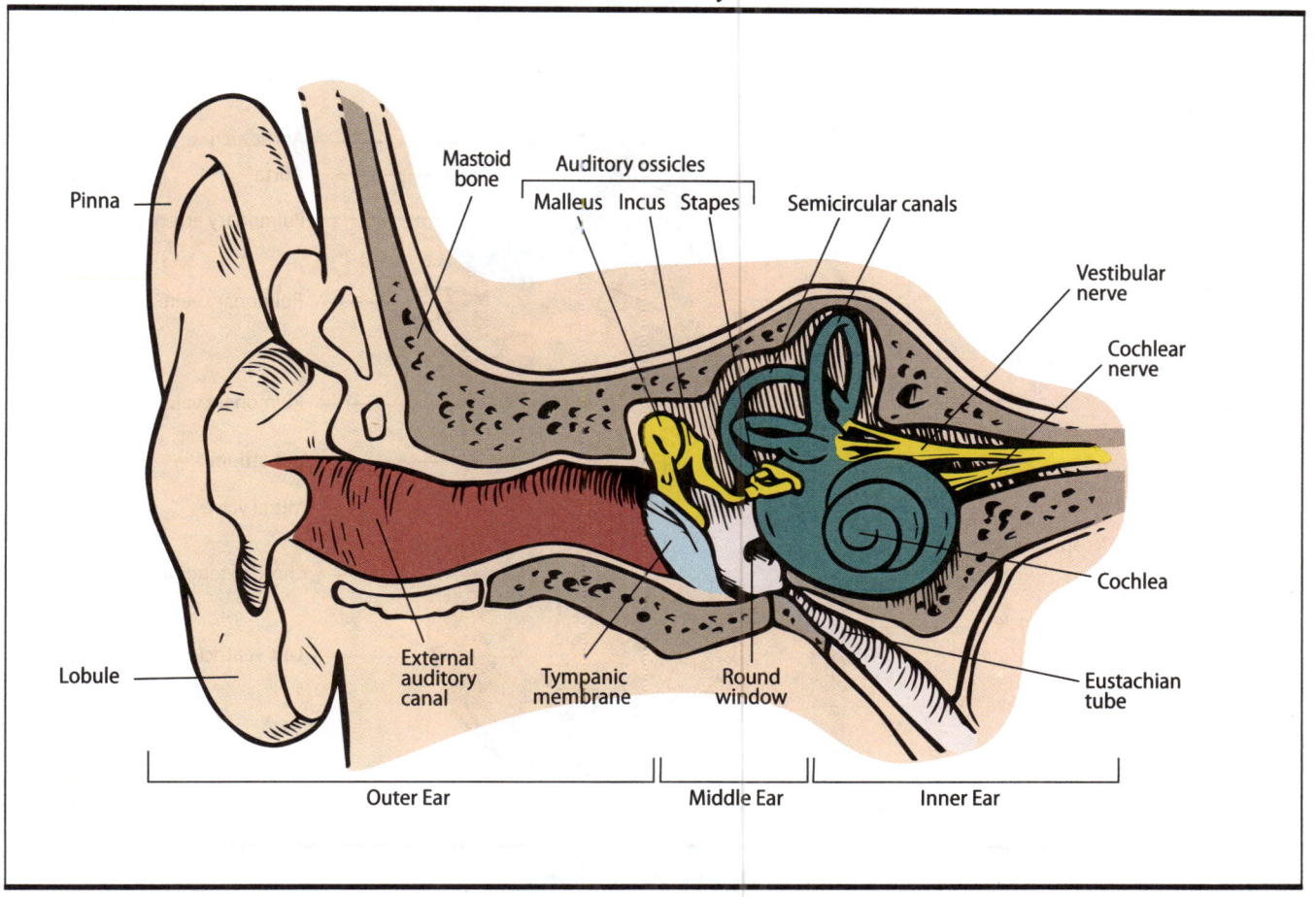

Chapter 9. Diseases of the Circulatory System (I00–I99)

Anatomy of the Heart

Heart Cross Section

Heart Valves

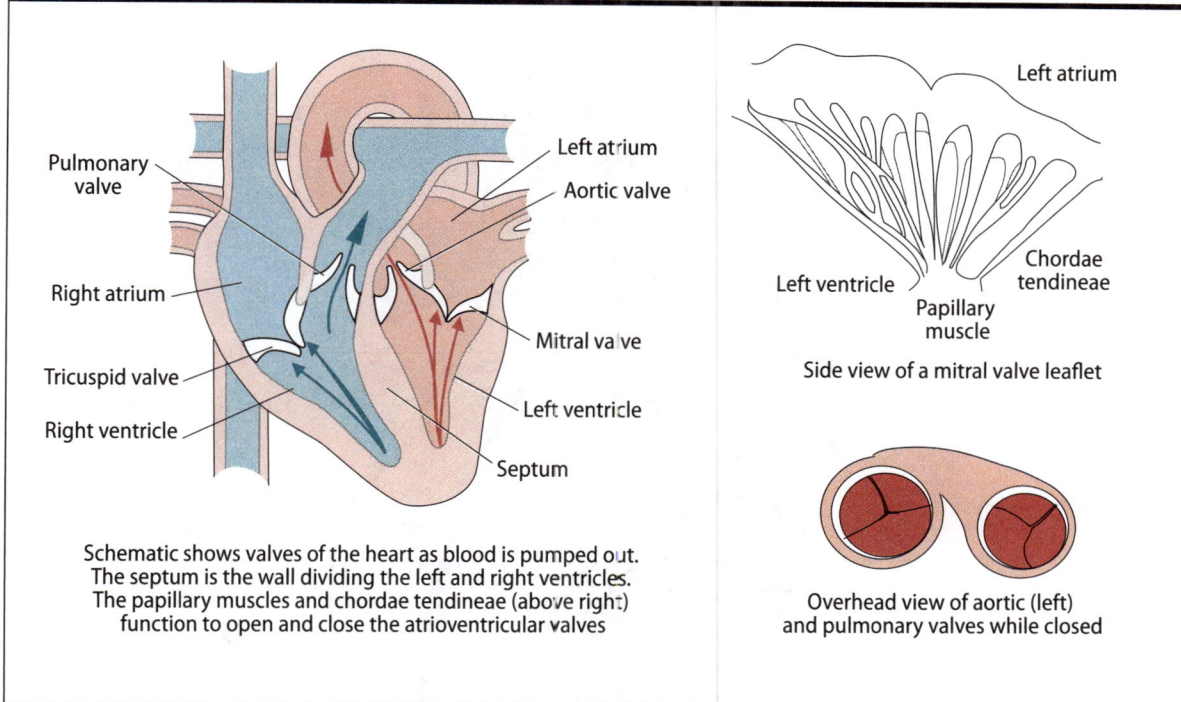

Pulmonary valve

Right atrium

Tricuspid valve

Right ventricle

Left atrium

Aortic valve

Mitral valve

Left ventricle

Septum

Left atrium

Chordae tendineae

Left ventricle

Papillary muscle

Side view of a mitral valve leaflet

Overhead view of aortic (left) and pulmonary valves while closed

Schematic shows valves of the heart as blood is pumped out. The septum is the wall dividing the left and right ventricles. The papillary muscles and chordae tendineae (above right) function to open and close the atrioventricular valves

Heart Conduction System

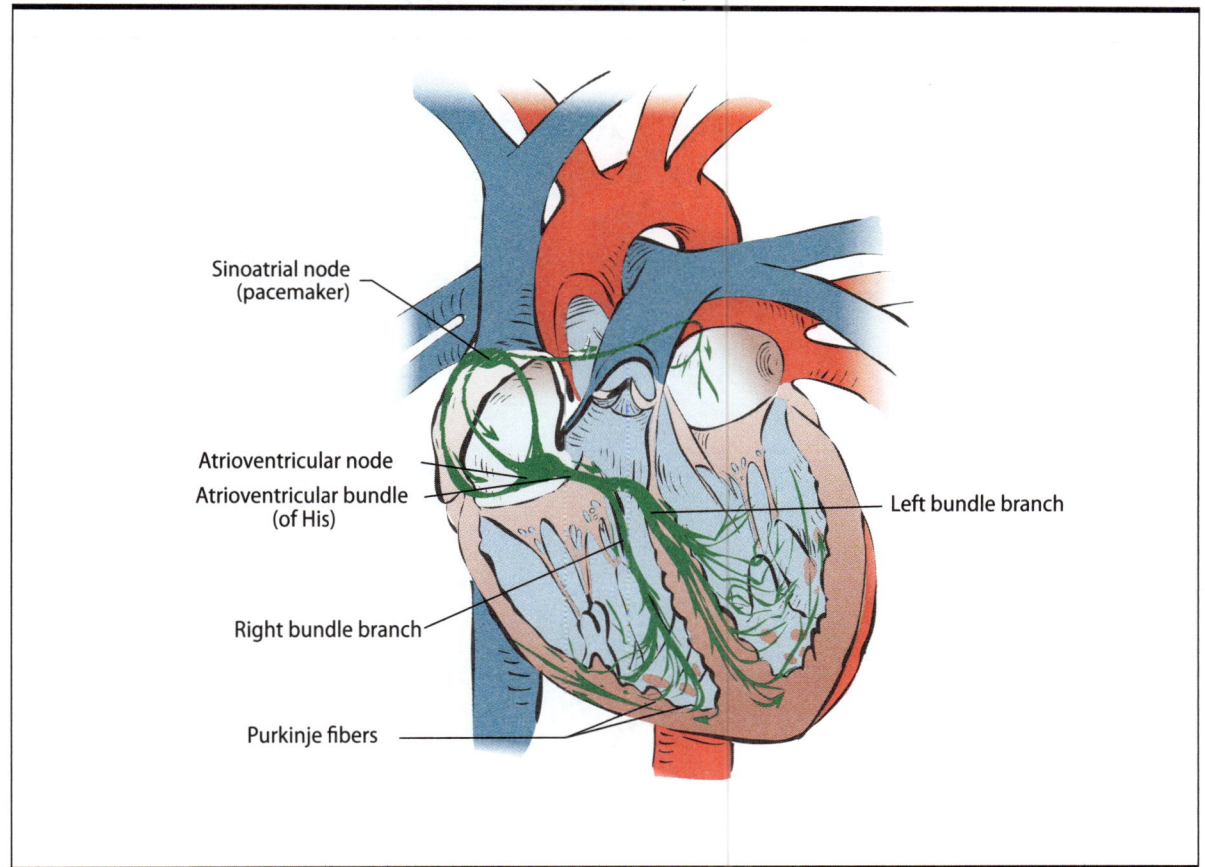

Sinoatrial node (pacemaker)

Atrioventricular node

Atrioventricular bundle (of His)

Right bundle branch

Purkinje fibers

Left bundle branch

Coronary Arteries

Arteries

Veins

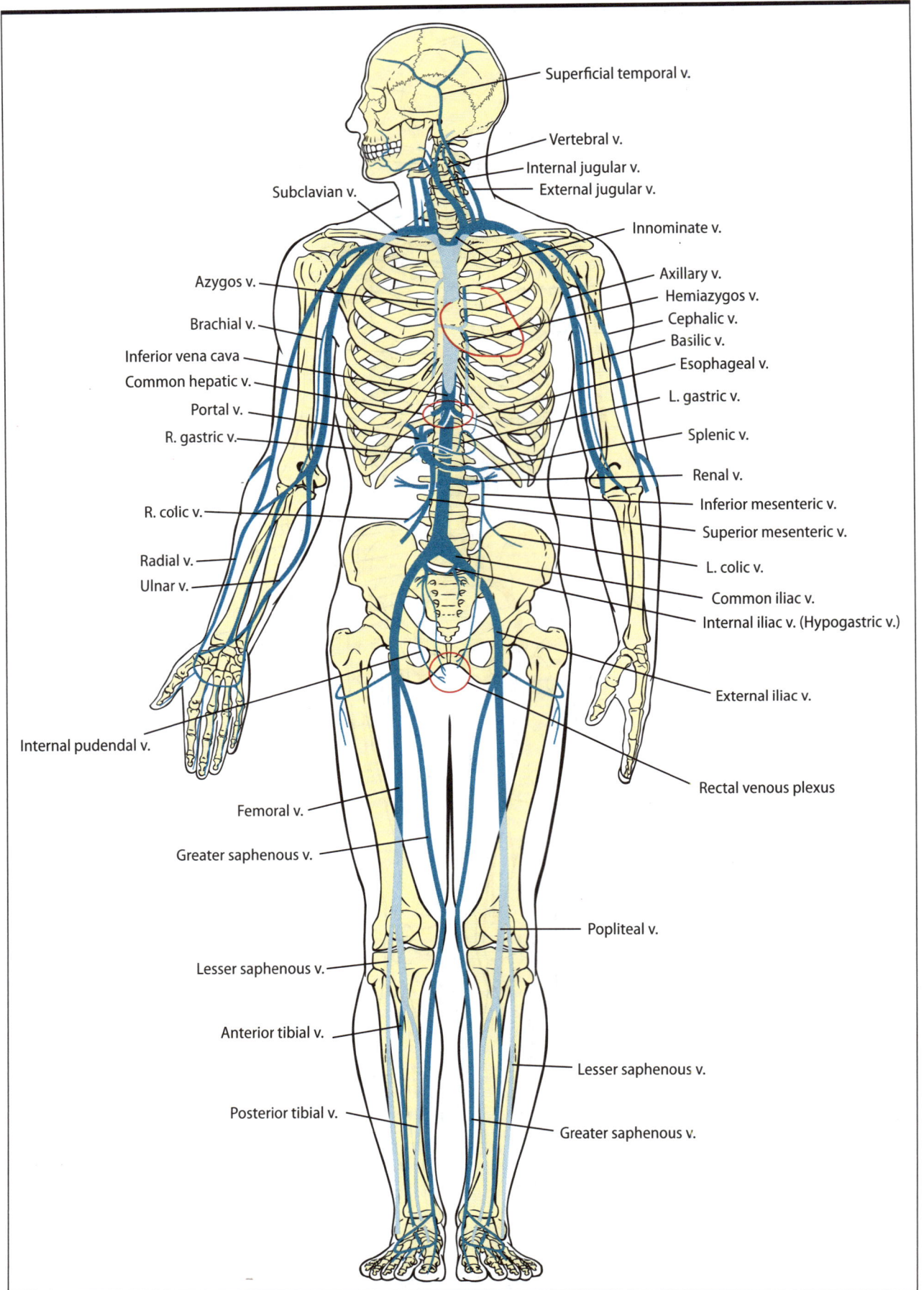

Internal Carotid and Vertebral Arteries and Branches

Side View

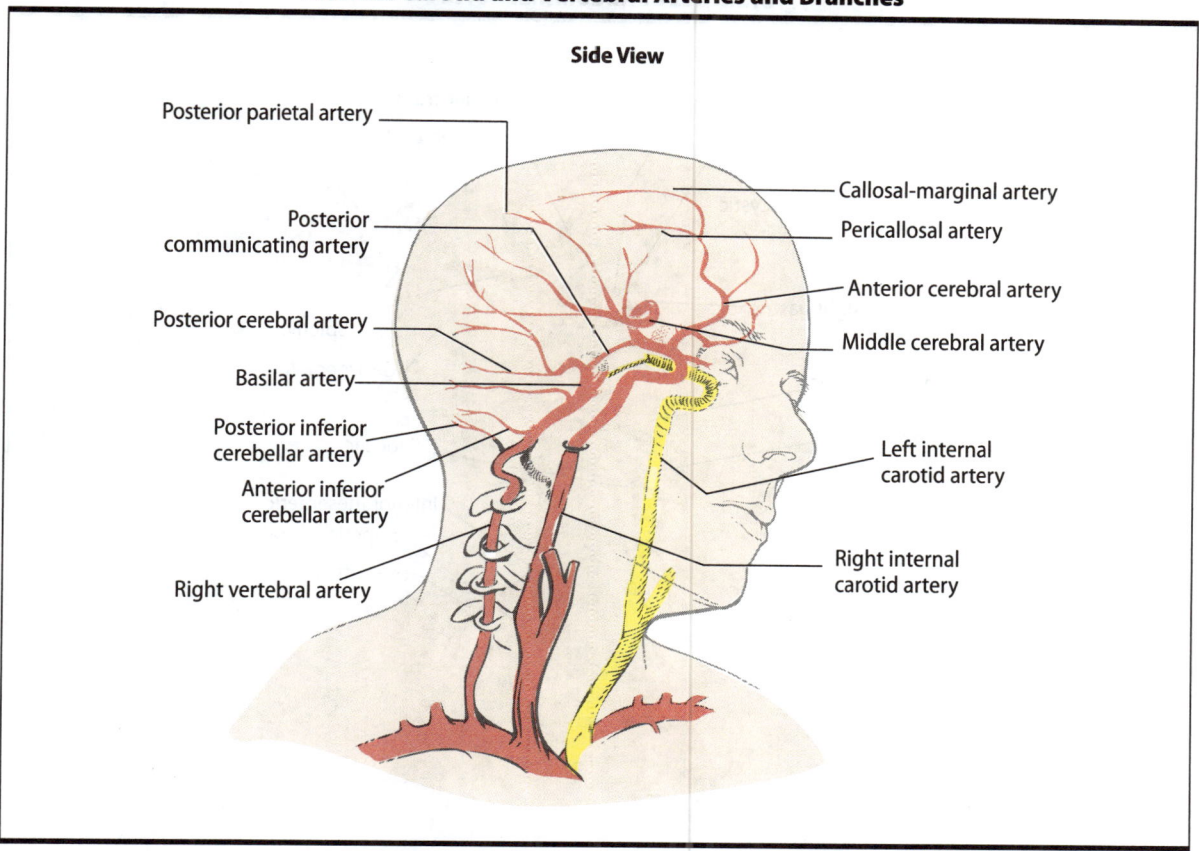

External Carotid Artery and Branches

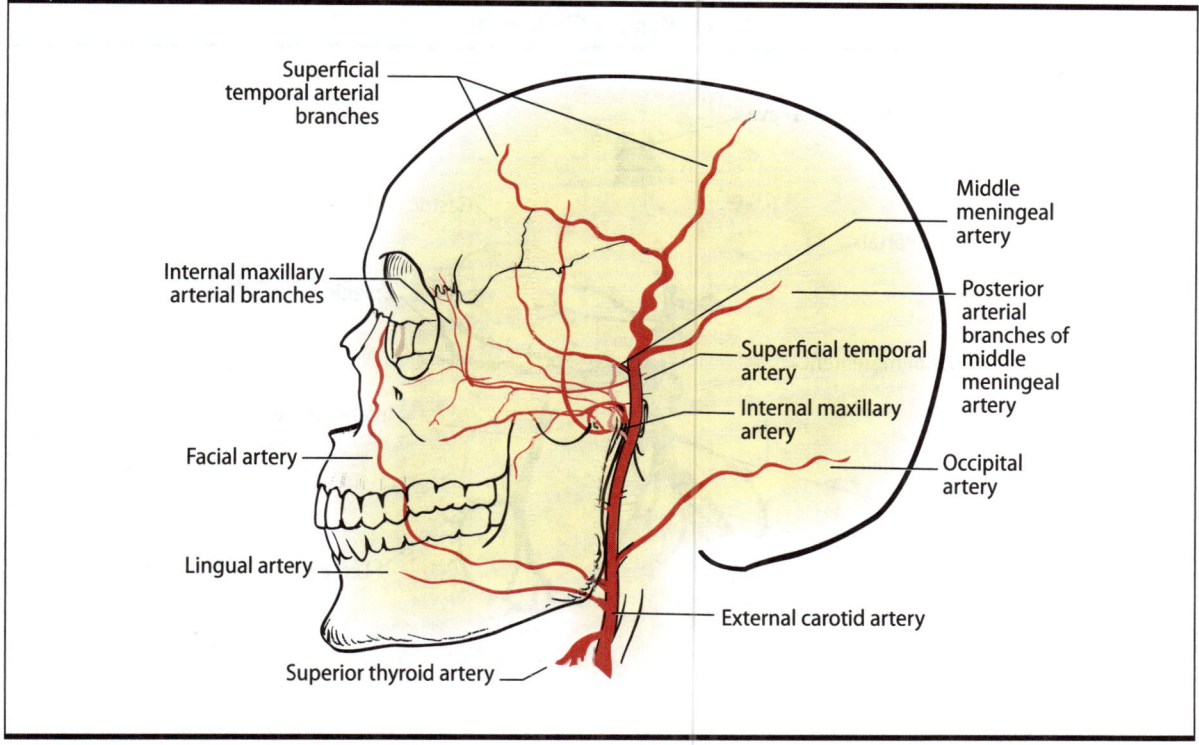

Branches of Abdominal Aorta

Portal Venous Circulation

Lymphatic System

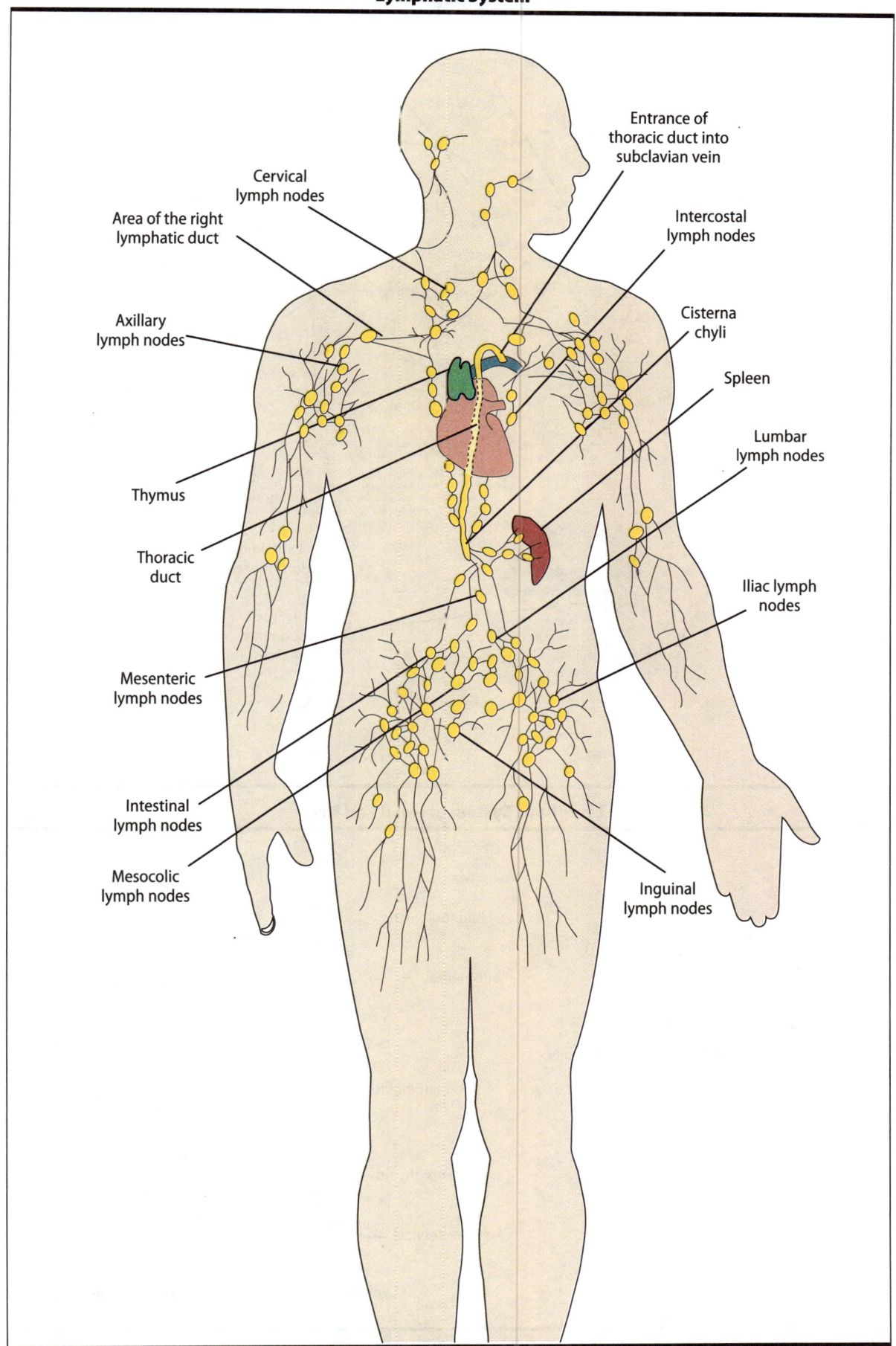

Axillary Lymph Nodes

Parasternal nodes

Sternum

Clavicle

Deltoid muscle

Brachialis muscle

Lateral nodes

Subscapular nodes

Pectoral nodes

Axillary lymph nodes

Central nodes

Latissimus dorsi muscle

Rectus abdominis muscle

Lymphatic System of Head and Neck

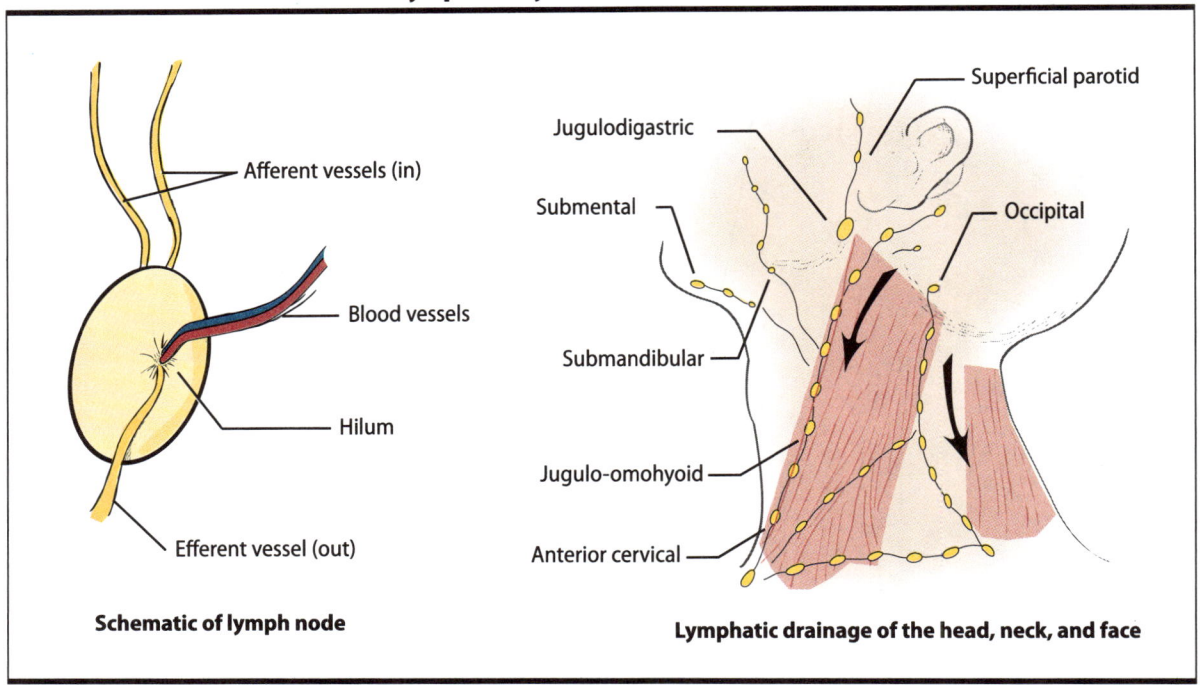

Afferent vessels (in)

Blood vessels

Hilum

Efferent vessel (out)

Schematic of lymph node

Jugulodigastric

Submental

Superficial parotid

Occipital

Submandibular

Jugulo-omohyoid

Anterior cervical

Lymphatic drainage of the head, neck, and face

Lymphatic Capillaries

Schematic of lymphatic capillaries

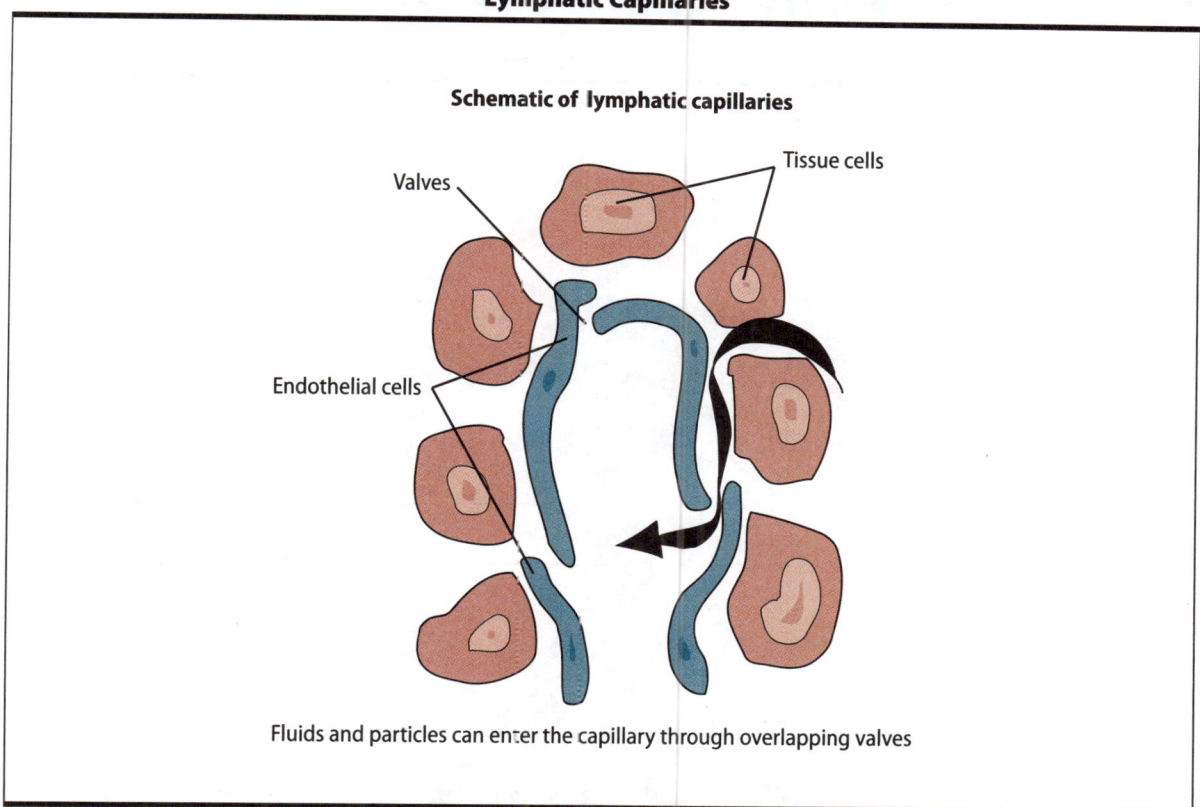

Fluids and particles can enter the capillary through overlapping valves

Lymphatic Drainage

Lymphatic drainage of the colon follows blood supply

Chapter 10. Diseases of the Respiratory System (J00–J99), U07.0

Respiratory System

Upper Respiratory System

Lower Respiratory System

Paranasal Sinuses

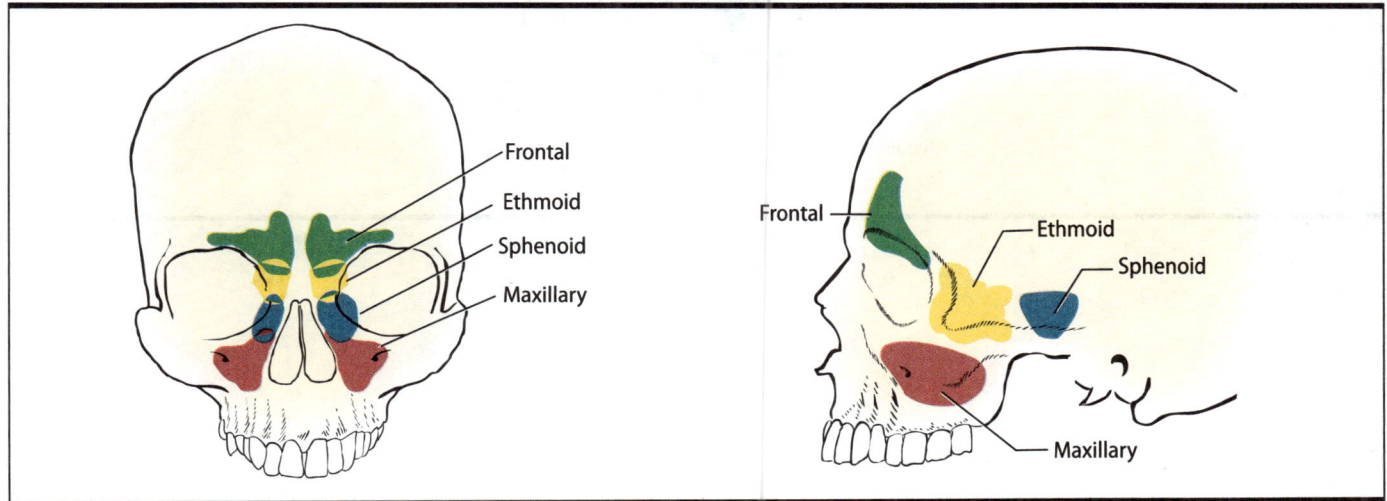

Lung Segments

Right lung

Left lung

Apical segment

Superior lobe

Posterior segment

Anterior segment

Apical-posterior segment

Anterior segment

Superior lingular segment

Inferior lingular segment

Superior lobe

Medial basal segment

Lateral segment

Superior segment

Middle lobe

Posterior basal segment

Inferior lobe

Anterior basal segment

Superior basal segment

Lateral basal segment

Anterior medial segment

Inferior lobe

Horizontal fissure

Oblique fissures

Alveoli

To trachea

Terminal bronchiole

Pulmonary arteriole

Elastic fibers

Capillary network over all alveoli

Alveoli

Alveolus

Chapter 11. Diseases of the Digestive System (K00–K95)

Digestive System

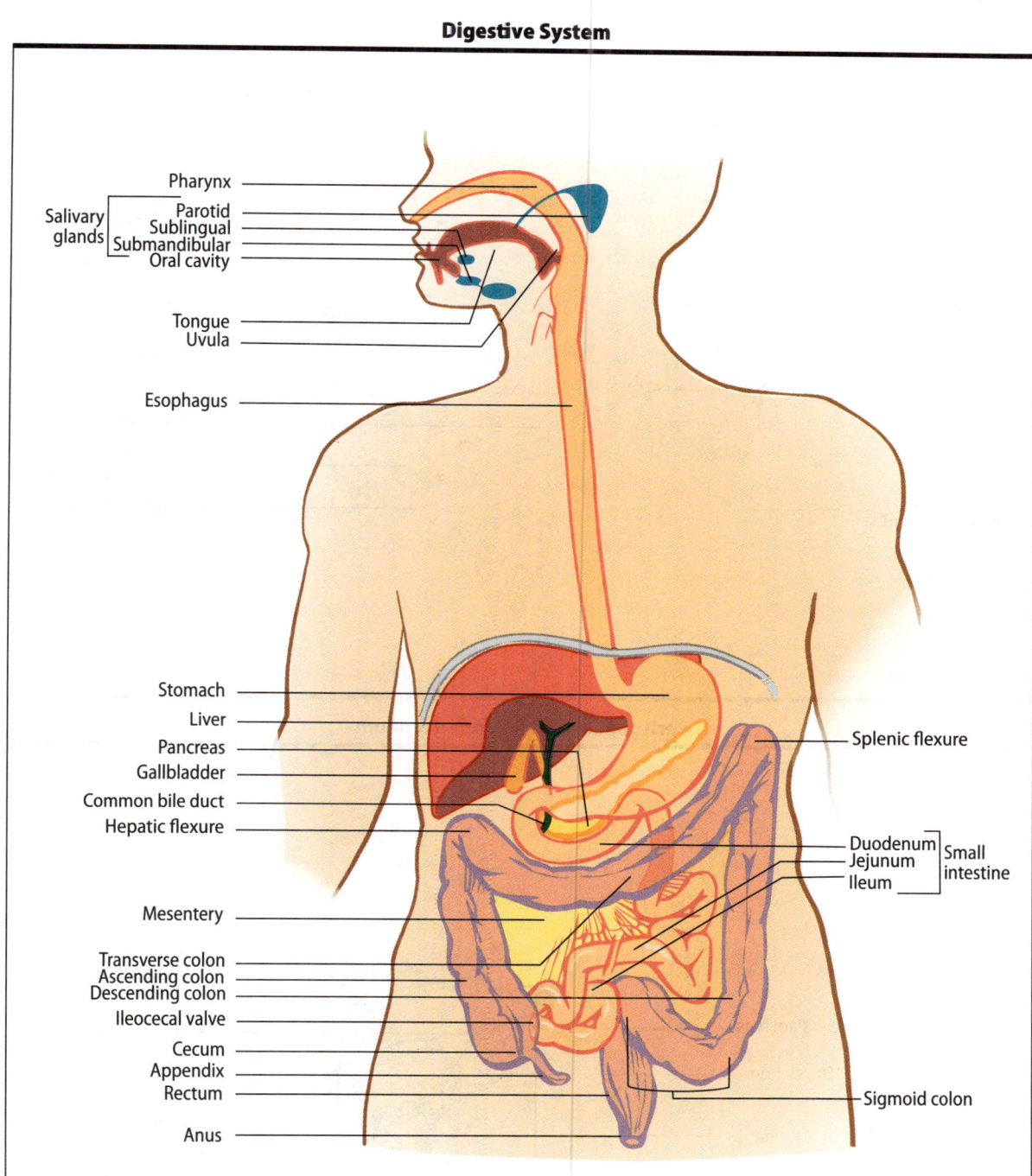

Omentum and Mesentery

Lesser omentum

Transverse colon

Ascending colon

Small intestine

Mesentery
(ascending mesocolon)

Greater omentum
(cut edge)

Descending
colon

Mesentery
(transverse mesocolon)

Mesentery proper

Mesentery
(descending mesocolon)

Sigmoid colon

Peritoneum and Retroperitoneum

Pancreas

Duodenum

Kidney

Ureter

Retroperitoneal space

Sigmoid colon

Bladder

Rectum

Diaphragm

Liver

Lesser omentum

Stomach

Transverse colon

Parietal peritoneum
(lines abdomen
and pelvis)

Peritoneal cavity

Visceral peritoneum
(covers organs)

Small intestine

Mesentery

Greater omentum

Chapter 12. Diseases of the Skin and Subcutaneous Tissue (L00–L99)

Nail Anatomy

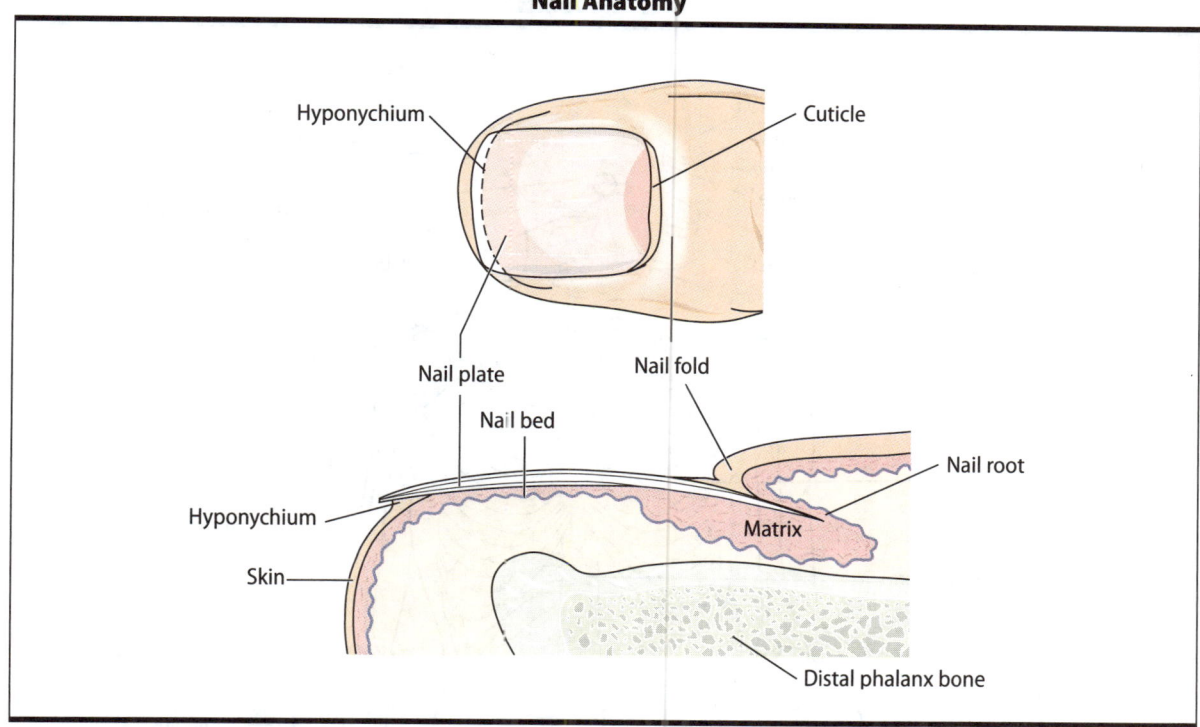

Skin and Subcutaneous Tissue

Chapter 13. Diseases of the Musculoskeletal System and Connective Tissue (MØØ–M99)

Bones and Joints

Shoulder Anterior View

Shoulder Posterior View

Elbow Anterior View

Elbow Posterior View

Hand

Hip Anterior View

Hip Posterior View

Knee Anterior View

Knee Posterior View

Foot

Muscles

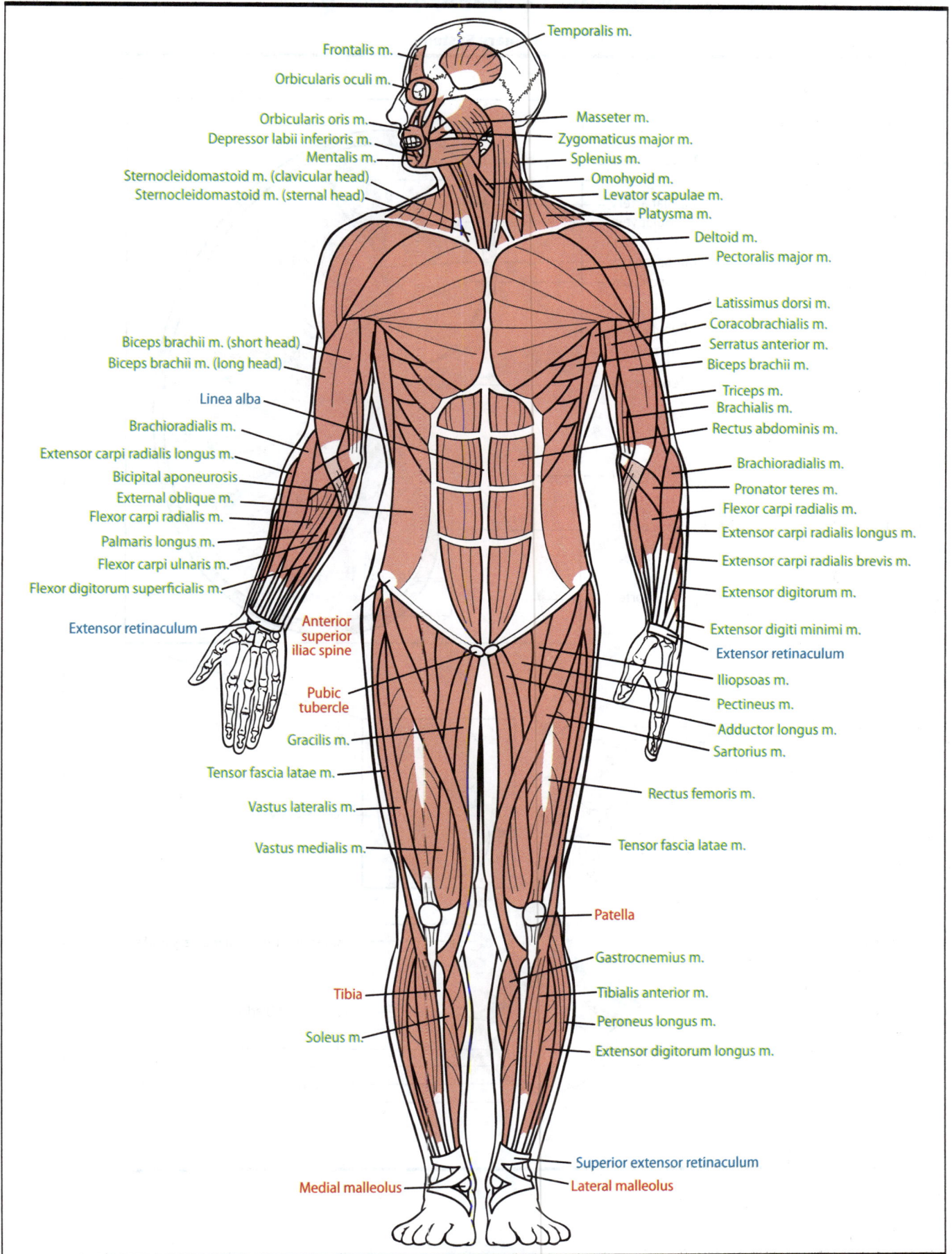

- Temporalis m.
- Frontalis m.
- Orbicularis oculi m.
- Orbicularis oris m.
- Masseter m.
- Depressor labii inferioris m.
- Zygomaticus major m.
- Mentalis m.
- Splenius m.
- Sternocleidomastoid m. (clavicular head)
- Omohyoid m.
- Sternocleidomastoid m. (sternal head)
- Levator scapulae m.
- Platysma m.
- Deltoid m.
- Pectoralis major m.
- Latissimus dorsi m.
- Coracobrachialis m.
- Biceps brachii m. (short head)
- Serratus anterior m.
- Biceps brachii m. (long head)
- Biceps brachii m.
- Triceps m.
- Linea alba
- Brachialis m.
- Brachioradialis m.
- Rectus abdominis m.
- Extensor carpi radialis longus m.
- Brachioradialis m.
- Bicipital aponeurosis
- Pronator teres m.
- External oblique m.
- Flexor carpi radialis m.
- Flexor carpi radialis m.
- Extensor carpi radialis longus m.
- Palmaris longus m.
- Extensor carpi radialis brevis m.
- Flexor carpi ulnaris m.
- Extensor digitorum m.
- Flexor digitorum superficialis m.
- Extensor digiti minimi m.
- Extensor retinaculum
- Extensor retinaculum
- Anterior superior iliac spine
- Iliopsoas m.
- Pectineus m.
- Pubic tubercle
- Adductor longus m.
- Sartorius m.
- Gracilis m.
- Tensor fascia latae m.
- Rectus femoris m.
- Vastus lateralis m.
- Tensor fascia latae m.
- Vastus medialis m.
- Patella
- Gastrocnemius m.
- Tibia
- Tibialis anterior m.
- Peroneus longus m.
- Soleus m.
- Extensor digitorum longus m.
- Superior extensor retinaculum
- Medial malleolus
- Lateral malleolus

Chapter 14. Diseases of the Genitourinary System (N00–N99)

Urinary System

Male Genitourinary System

Female Internal Genitalia

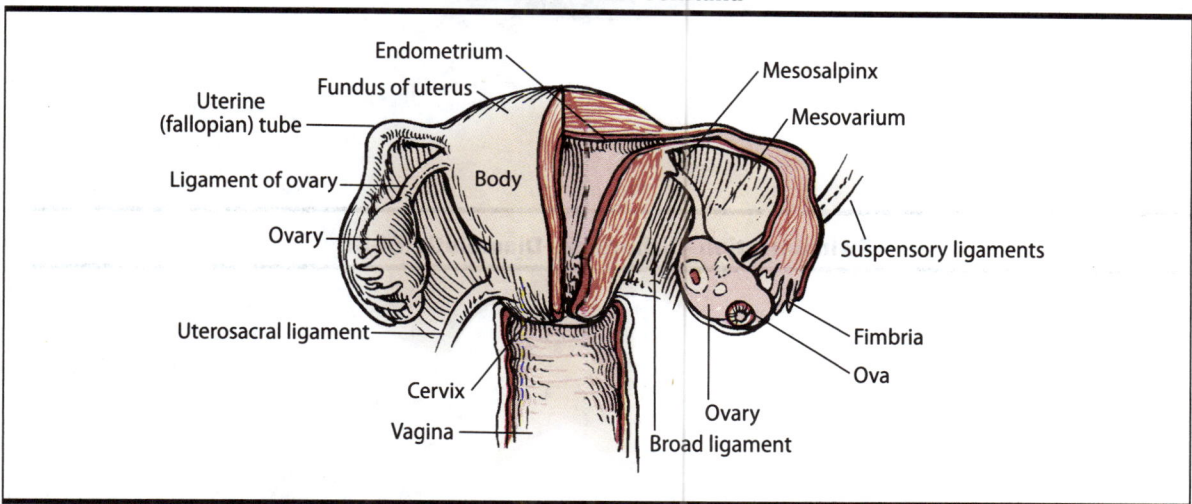

Female Genitourinary Tract Lateral View

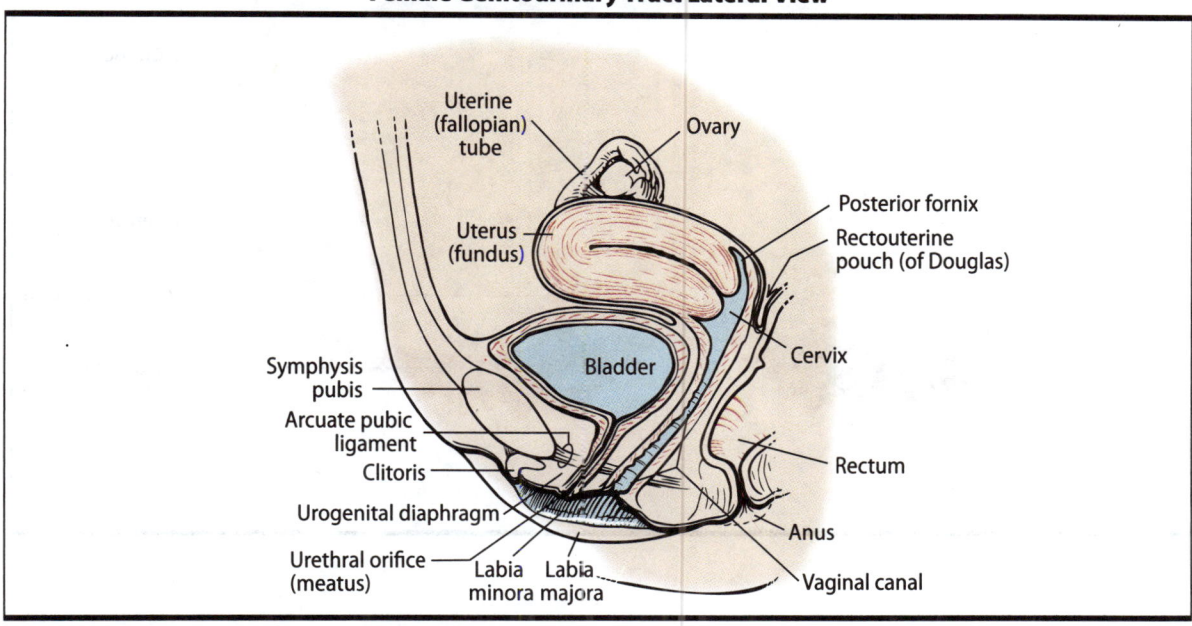

Chapter 15. Pregnancy, Childbirth and the Puerperium (O00–O9A)

Term Pregnancy – Single Gestation

Twin Gestation–Dichorionic–Diamniotic (DI-DI)

Twin Gestation–Monochorionic–Diamniotic (MO-DI)

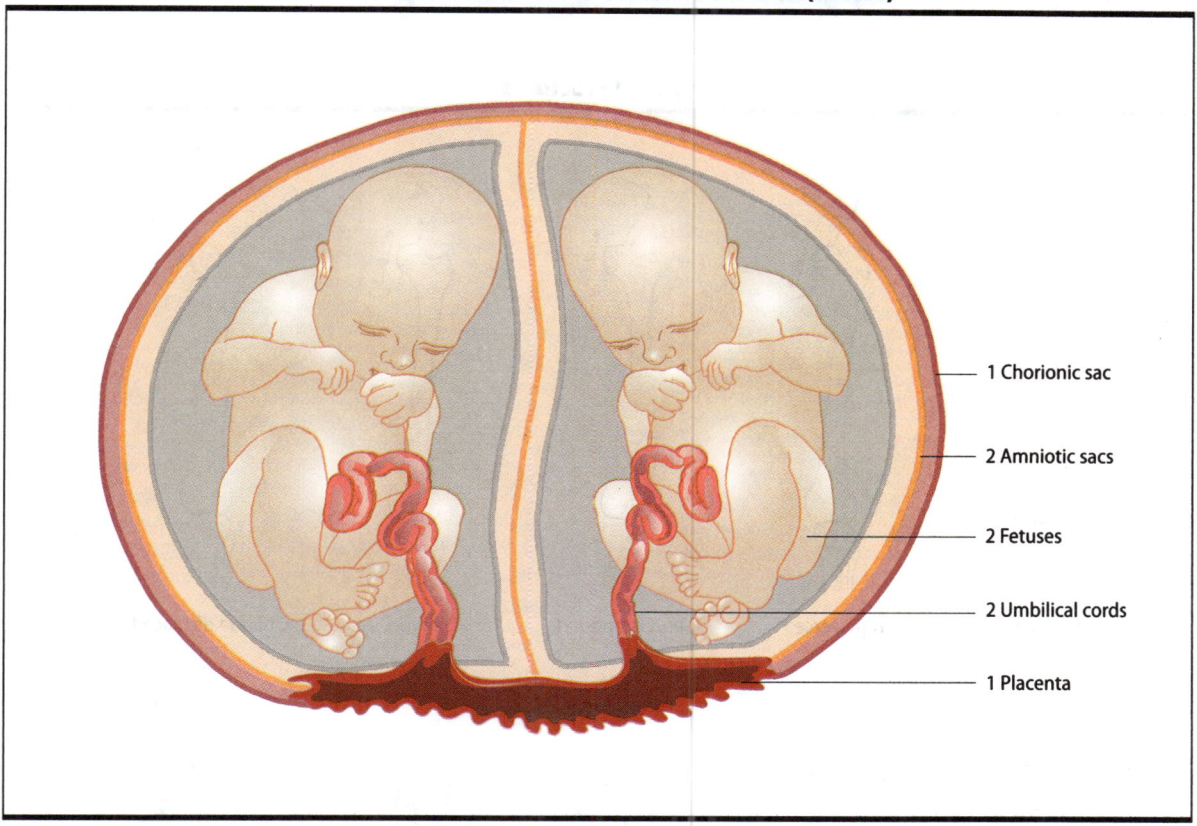

1 Chorionic sac

2 Amniotic sacs

2 Fetuses

2 Umbilical cords

1 Placenta

Twin Gestation–Monochorionic–Monoamniotic (MO-MO)

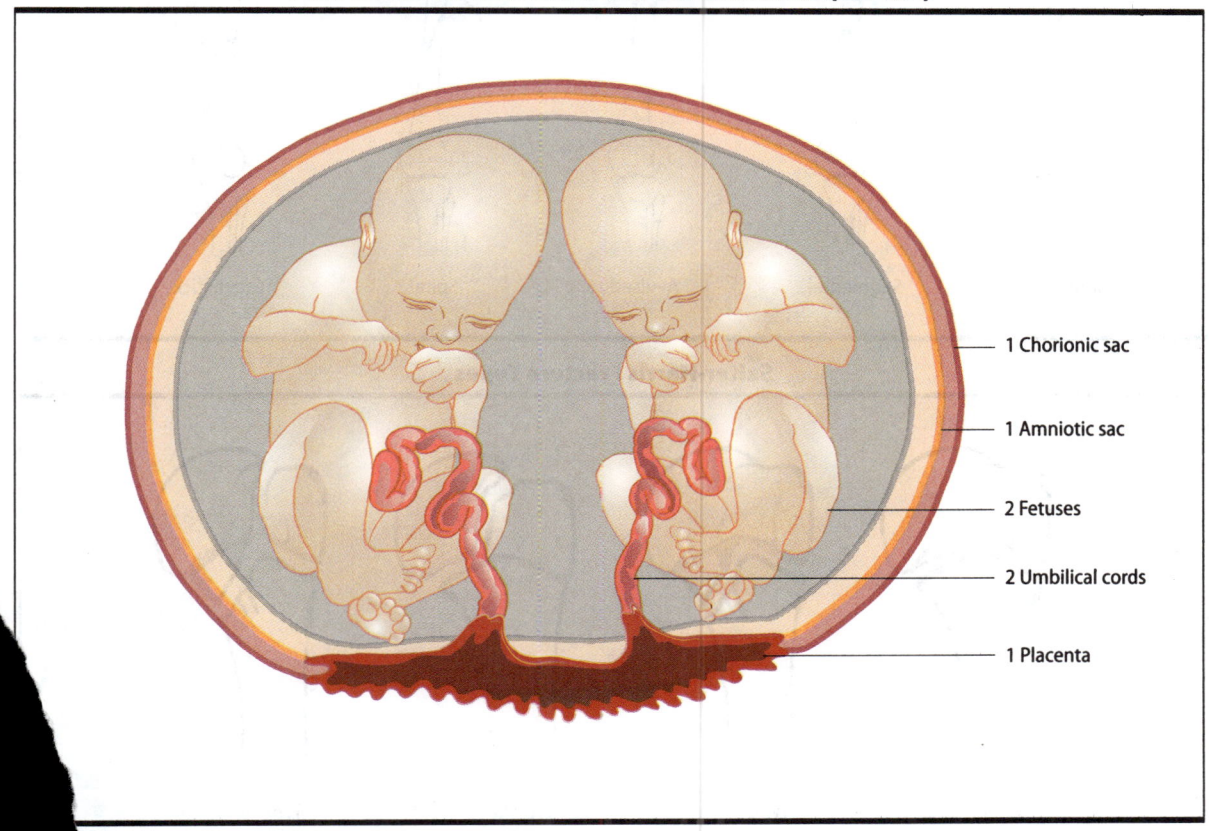

1 Chorionic sac

1 Amniotic sac

2 Fetuses

2 Umbilical cords

1 Placenta

Chapter 19. Injury, Poisoning and Certain Other Consequences of External Causes (SØØ–T88)

Types of Fractures

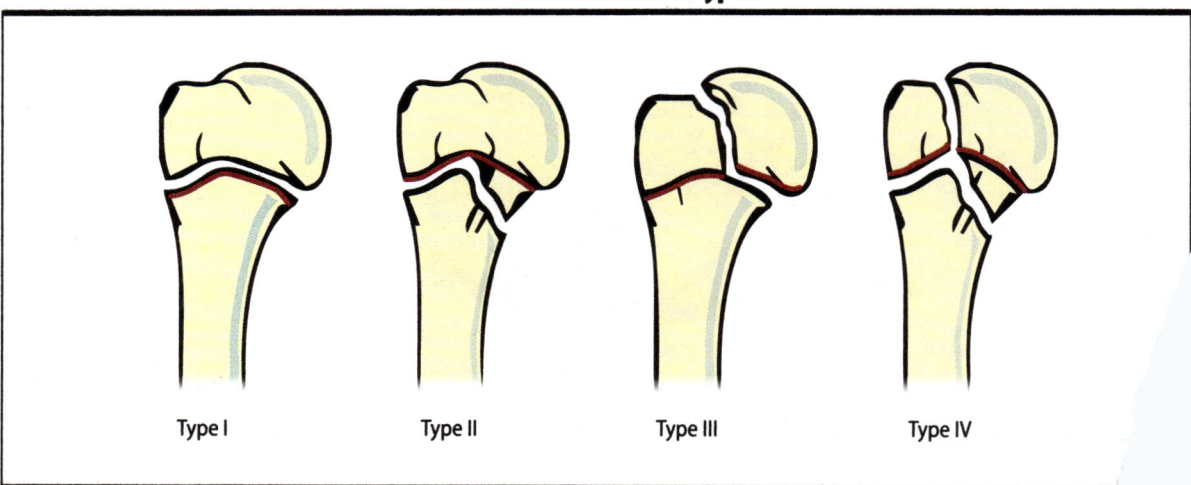

Normal   Transverse   Open/Compound   Oblique   Oblique displaced

Comminuted   Segmental   Avulsed   Spiral   Greenstick

Salter-Harris Fracture Types

Type I   Type II   Type III   Type IV